SEVENTH EDITION

Clinical Anesthesia

SEVENTH EDITION

Clinical Anesthesia

Edited By

Paul G. Barash, MD
Professor
Department of Anesthesiology
School of Medicine
Yale University School of Medicine
Attending Anesthesiologist
Yale-New Haven Hospital
New Haven, Connecticut

Bruce F. Cullen, MD
Emeritus Professor
Department of Anesthesiology
School of Medicine
University of Washington
Seattle, Washington

Robert K. Stoelting, MD
Emeritus Professor and Past Chair
Department of Anesthesia
School of Medicine
Indiana University
Indianapolis, Indiana

Michael K. Cahalan, MD
Professor and Chair
Department of Anesthesiology
School of Medicine
The University of Utah
Salt Lake City, Utah

M. Christine Stock, MD
Professor and Chair
Department of Anesthesiology
Feinberg School of Medicine
Northwestern University
Chicago, Illinois

Rafael Ortega, MD
Professor
Vice-Chairman of Academic Affairs
Department of Anesthesiology
School of Medicine
Boston University
Boston, Massachusetts

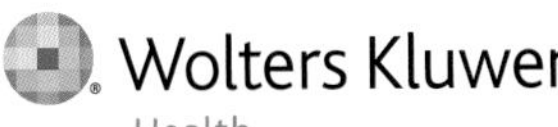

Lippincott Williams & Wilkins

Philadelphia • Baltimore • New York • London
Buenos Aires • Hong Kong • Sydney • Tokyo

Acquisitions Editor: Brian Brown
Managing Editor: Nicole T. Dernoski
Marketing Manager: Lisa Lawrence
Production Editor: Priscilla Crater
Senior Manufacturing Manager: Benjamin Rivera
Design Coordinator: Stephen Druding
Compositor: Aptara, Inc.

Two Commerce Square
2001 Market Street
Philadelphia, PA 19103 USA
LWW.com

Printed in China

Library of Congress Cataloging-in-Publication Data

Clinical anesthesia/edited by Paul G. Barash . . . [et al.]. – 7th ed.
p. ; cm.
Includes bibliographical references and index.
ISBN 978-1-4511-4419-2 (alk. paper)
I. Barash, Paul G.
[DNLM: 1. Anesthesia. 2. Anesthesiology. 3. Anesthetics. WO 200]

617.9′6–dc23 2012050848

Care has been taken to confirm the accuracy of the information presented and to describe generally accepted practices. However, the authors, editors, and publisher are not responsible for errors or omissions or for any consequences from application of the information in this book and make no warranty, expressed or implied, with respect to the currency, completeness, or accuracy of the contents of the publication. Application of this information in a particular situation remains the professional responsibility of the practitioner.

The authors, editors, and publisher have exerted every effort to ensure that drug selection and dosage set forth in this text are in accordance with current recommendations and practice at the time of publication. However, in view of ongoing research, changes in government regulations, and the constant flow of information relating to drug therapy and drug reactions, the reader is urged to check the package insert for each drug for any change in indications and dosage and for added warnings and precautions. This is particularly important when the recommended agent is a new or infrequently employed drug.

Some drugs and medical devices presented in this publication have Food and Drug Administration (FDA) clearance for limited use in restricted research settings. It is the responsibility of the health care provider to ascertain the FDA status of each drug or device planned for use in their clinical practice.

To purchase additional copies of this book, call our customer service department at (800) 638-3030 or fax orders to (301) 223-2320. International customers should call (301) 223-2300.

Visit Lippincott Williams & Wilkins on the Internet: at LWW.com. Lippincott Williams & Wilkins customer service representatives are available from 8:30 am to 6 pm, EST.

10 9 8 7 6 5 4 3 2 1

FOR ALL STUDENTS OF ANESTHESIOLOGY

CONTRIBUTING AUTHORS

Saint Adeogba, MD
Senior Research Fellow
Department of Anesthesiology and Pain Medicine
School of Medicine
University of Washington
Seattle, Washington

Shamsuddin Akhtar, MD
Associate Professor
Department of Anesthesiology
School of Medicine
Yale University
New Haven, Connecticut

Michael L. Ault, MD, FCCP, FCCM
Associate Professor
Departments of Anesthesiology, Neurological Surgery and Surgery
Feinberg School of Medicine
Northwestern University
Medical Director
Departments of Blood Gas Laboratory and Emergency Response Teams
Northwestern Memorial Hospital
Chicago, Illinois

Douglas R. Bacon, MD, MA
Professor and Chair
Department of Anesthesiology
School of Medicine
Wayne State University
Detroit, Michigan
Chair
Department of Anesthesiology
Saint Joseph Mercy Oakland
Pontiac, Michigan

Gina C. Badescu, MD
Assistant Professor
Department of Anesthesiology
School of Medicine
Division of Cardiothoracic Anesthesiology
Duke University Hospital
Durham, North Carolina

Dalia Banks, MD, FASE
Associate Professor
School of Medicine
University of California San Diego
Division of Cardiothoracic Anesthesiology Chief
Clinical Director for Sulpizio CVC and PTU
San Diego, California

Paul G. Barash, MD
Professor
Department of Anesthesiology
School of Medicine
Yale University
Attending Anesthesiologist
Yale-New Haven Hospital
New Haven, Connecticut

Honorio T. Benzon, MD
Professor of Anesthesiology
Department of Anesthesiology
Feinberg School of Medicine
Northwestern University
Attending Staff
Department of Anesthesiology
Northwestern Memorial Hospital
Chicago, Illinois

Christopher M. Bernards, MD*
Professor
Department of Anesthesiology
School of Medicine
Virginia Mason University
Seattle, Washington

Marcelle E. Blessing, MD
Assistant Professor
Department of Anesthesiology
School of Medicine
Yale University
New Haven, Connecticut

Michelle Y. Braunfeld, MD
Professor and Chair
Department of Anesthesiology
David Geffen School of Medicine
University of California Los Angeles
Greater Los Angeles VA Hospital
Los Angeles, California

Ferne R. Braveman, MD
Professor
Department of Anesthesiology
School of Medicine
Yale University
New Haven, Connecticut

Brenda A. Bucklin, MD
Professor
Department of Anesthesiology
School of Medicine
University of Colorado
Aurora, Colorado

Asokumar Buvanendran, MD
Professor
Department of Anesthesiology
Rush University Medical Center
Senior Attending Staff
Department of Anesthesiology
Rush University Medical Center
Chicago, Illinois

*Deceased

Michael K. Cahalan, MD
Professor and Chair
Department of Anesthesiology
School of Medicine
University of Utah
Salt Lake City, Utah

Levon M. Capan, MD
Professor
Department of Anesthesiology
School of Medicine
New York University
Associate Director
Department of Anesthesiology
Bellevue Hospital
New York, New York

Louanne M. Carabini, MD
Assistant Professor
Department of Anesthesiology
Feinberg School of Medicine
Northwestern University
Chicago, Illinois

C. Richard Chapman, PhD
Professor
Department of Anesthesiology
School of Medicine
University of Utah
Pain Research Center
Salt Lake City, Utah

Amalia Cochran, MD
Associate Professor
Department of Surgery
School of Medicine
University of Utah
Salt Lake City, Utah

Edmond Cohen, MD
Professor
Department of Anesthesiology
Director of Thoracic Anesthesia
Mount Sinai School of Medicine
New York, New York

Christopher W. Connor, MD, PhD
Assistant Professor
Departments of Anesthesiology, and Biomedical Engineering
School of Medicine
Boston University
Boston, Massachusetts

C. Michael Crowder, MD, PhD
Dr. Seymour and Rose T. Brown Professor
Department of Anesthesiology
School of Medicine
Washington University
St. Louis, Missouri

Marie Csete, MD, PhD
Division Director
Center for Cellular Therapies
AABB
Bethesda, Maryland
Adjunct Faculty
Department of Anesthesiology
USCD Medical Center
San Diego, California

Bruce F. Cullen, MD
Emeritus Professor
Department of Anesthesiology
School of Medicine
University of Washington
Seattle, Washington

Anthony Cunningham, MD
Professor
Foundation Dean
Pu-RCSI School of Medicine
Malaysia

Armagan Dagal, MD, FRCA
Assistant Professor
Department of Anesthesiology and Pain Medicine
School of Medicine
University of Washington
Chief of Spine and Orthopedic Anesthesia Services
Department of Anesthesiology and Pain Medicine
Harborview Medical Center
Seattle, Washington

Albert Dahan, MD
Professor
Department of Anesthesiology
Leiden University Medical Center
Leiden, The Netherlands

Steven Deem, MD
Professor
Department of Anesthesiology and Pain Medicine
School of Medicine
University of Washington
Director
Department of Neurocritical Care
Harborview Medical Center
Seattle, Washington

Timothy R. Deer, MD
Clinical Professor
Department of Anesthesiology
School of Medicine
West Virginia University
President and CEO
Center for Pain Relief, Inc.
Charleston, West Virginia

Stephen F. Dierdorf, MD
Professor and Vice Chair
Department of Anesthesia
School of Medicine
Indiana University
Indianapolis, Indiana

Karen B. Domino, MD, MPH
Professor
Department of Anesthesiology and Pain Medicine
School of Medicine
University of Washington
University of Washington Medical Center
Seattle, Washington

François Donati, MD, PhD, FRCPC
Professor
Department of Anesthesiology
Université de Montréal
Attending Anesthesiologist
Department of Anesthesiology
Hôpital Maisonneuve-Rosemont
Montréal, Québec, Canada

Michael B. Dorrough, MD
Staff Anesthesiologist
United Medical Center
Cheyenne, West Virginia

Randal O. Dull, MD, PhD
Vice Head for Research
Department of Anesthesiology
College of Medicine
University of Illinois at Chicago
Chicago, Illinois

Thomas J. Ebert, MD, PhD
Professor, Vice Chair for Education
Residency Program Director
Department of Anesthesiology
School of Medicine
Medical College of Wisconsin
Staff Anesthesiologist
Department of Anesthesiology
Zablocki VA Medical Center
Milwaukee, Wisconsin

Jan Ehrenwerth, MD
Professor
Department of Anesthesiology
School of Medicine
Yale University
Attending Staff
Department of Anesthesiology
Yale-New Haven Hospital
New Haven, Connecticut

John H. Eichhorn, MD
Professor
Department of Anesthesiology
College of Medicine
University of Kentucky
University of Kentucky Medical Center
Lexington, Kentucky

James B. Eisenkraft, MD
Professor
Department of Anesthesiology
Mount Sinai School of Medicine
New York, New York

Matthew R. Eng, MD
Resident
Department of Anesthesia
Cedars-Sinai Medical Center
Los Angeles, California

Alex S. Evers, MD
Henry Mallinckrodt Professor and Chair
Department of Anesthesiology
School of Medicine
Washington University
Anesthesiologist-in-Chief
Department of Anesthesiology
Barnes-Jewish Hospital
St. Louis, Missouri

Ana Fernandez-Bustamante, MD, PhD
Assistant Professor
Department of Anesthesiology
School of Medicine
University of Colorado, Denver
Aurora, Colorado

Lynne R. Ferrari, MD
Chief, Division of Perioperative Anesthesia
Department of Anesthesia
The Children's Hospital
Boston, Massachusetts

Scott M. Fishman, MD
Chief
Division of Pain Medicine
Professor of Clinical Anesthesiology
Department of Anesthesiology and Pain Medicine
School of Medicine
University of California, Davis
Sacramento, California

Lee A. Fleisher, MD
Robert Dunning Dripps Professor of Anesthesiology and Critical Care
Chair
Department of Anesthesiology and Critical Care
University of Pennsylvania Health System
Philadelphia, Pennsylvania

Michael A. Fowler, MD, MBA
Assistant Professor
Department of Anesthesiology
School of Medicine
Virginia Commonwealth University
Medical Director
Post Anesthesia Care Unit
Department of Anesthesia
VCU Health Systems
Richmond, Virginia

Kevin Friede, BA
Research Fellow
Perioperative Genomics Program
Division of Cardiothoracic Anesthesia and Critical Care
Department of Anesthesiology
Duke University Medical Center
Durham, North Carolina

J. Sean Funston, MD
Assistant Professor
Department of Anesthesiology
School of Medicine
University of Texas Medical Branch
Galveston, Texas

Tong J. Gan, MD
Professor
Department of Anesthesiology
Duke University Medical Center
Durham, North Carolina

Steven I. Gayer, MD, MBA
Professor
Department of Anesthesiology and Ophthalmology
Bascom Palmer Eye Institute
School of Medicine
University of Miami
Miami, Florida

Kevin J. Gingrich, MD
Professor
Department of Anesthesiology and Pain Management
College of Medicine
University of Texas Southwestern Medical Center
Dallas, Texas

Kathryn E. Glas, MD, MBA
Associate Professor
Department of Anesthesiology
School of Medicine
Emory University
Co-Director
Cardiothoracic Anesthesiology
Crawford Long Hospital
Atlanta, Georgia

Loreta Grecu, MD
Assistant Professor
Department of Anesthesiology
School of Medicine
Yale University
New Haven, Connecticut

Jay S. Grider, DO, PhD
Associate Professor
Department of Anesthesiology
School of Medicine
University of Kentucky
Division Chief
Regional Anesthesia and Pain Medicine
Department of Anesthesiology
University of Kentucky Chandler Medical Center
Lexington, Kentucky

Dhanesh K. Gupta, MD
Associate Professor
Departments of Anesthesiology and Neurological Surgery
Feinberg School of Medicine
Northwestern University
Director
Neuroanesthesia Research
Departments of Anesthesiology and Neurological Surgery
Northwestern Memorial Hospital
Chicago, Illinois

Steven C. Hall, MD
Professor
Department of Anesthesiology
Feinberg School of Medicine
Northwestern University
Anesthesiologist-in-Chief
Ann and Robert H. Lurie Children's Hospital
Chicago, Illinois

Matthew R. Hallman, MD
Assistant Professor
Department of Anesthesiology and Pain Medicine
School of Medicine
University of Washington
Harborview Medical Center
Seattle, Washington

J. Steven Hata, MD, FCCP, MSc
Director, Center for Critical Care
Departments of Cardiac Anesthesiology,
General Anesthesiology and Outcomes Research
Anesthesiology Institute
Cleveland Clinic
Cleveland, Ohio

Tara M. Hata, MD
Staff Anesthesiologist
Department of Pediatric Anesthesia
Anesthesia Institute
Cleveland Clinic
Cleveland, Ohio

Laurence M. Hausman, MD
Associate Professor
Director Ambulatory Anesthesia
Department of Anesthesia
Mount Sinai School of Medicine
New York, New York

Jeana E. Havidich, MD
Associate Professor
Department of Anesthesiology
School of Medicine
Dartmouth-Hitchcock
Lebanon, New Hampshire

Thomas K. Henthorn, MD
Professor and Chair
Department of Anesthesiology
School of Medicine
University of Colorado
Aurora, Colorado

Simon C. Hillier, MB, ChB
Professor
Departments of Anesthesia and Pediatrics
Dartmouth Hitchcock Medical Center
Lebanon, New Hampshire

Robert S. Holzman, MD
Professor of Anesthesia
School of Medicine
Harvard Medical School
Senior Associate in Perioperative Anesthesiology
Department of Anesthesiology, Perioperative and Pain Medicine
Boston Children's Hospital
Boston, Massachusetts

Harriet W. Hopf, MD
Professor and Vice Chair
Department of Anesthesiology
School of Medicine
University of Utah
Salt Lake City, Utah

Terese T. Horlocker, MD
Professor of Anesthesiology and Orthopaedics
Department of Anesthesiology
Mayo Clinic College of Medicine
Mayo Clinic
Rochester, Minnesota

Lucy S. Hostetter, MD
Staff Anesthesiologist
Physician's Anesthesia Service
Swedish Medical Center
Seattle, Washington

Robert W. Hurley, MD, PhD
Chief
Division of Pain Medicine
Departments of Anesthesiology, Neurology, Psychiatry, Orthopaedics and Rehabilitation
School of Medicine
University of Florida
Chest Pain Medicine
UF & Shands Hospital
Gainesville, Florida

Michael P. Hutchens, MD, MA
Assistant Professor
Department of Anesthesiology and Perioperative Medicine
School of Medicine
Oregon Health and Science University
Portland, Oregon

Adam K. Jacob, MD
Assistant Professor
Department of Anesthesiology
Mayo Clinic College of Medicine
Mayo Clinic
Rochester, Minnesota

Girish P. Joshi, MBBS, MD, FFARCSI
Professor
Department of Anesthesiology and Pain Management
University of Texas Southwestern Medical Center
Dallas, Texas

John P. Kampine, MD, PhD
Professor and Chair Emeritus
Department of Anesthesia
College of Medicine
Medical College of Wisconsin
Milwaukee, Wisconsin

Jonathan D. Katz, MD
Clinical Professor
Department of Anesthesiology
School of Medicine
Yale University
New Haven, Connecticut
Attending Anesthesiologist
Department of Anesthesia
St. Vincent Medical Center
Bridgeport, Connecticut

Sandra L. Kopp, MD
Associate Professor
Department of Anesthesiology
Mayo Clinic College of Medicine
Anesthesiologist
Mayo Clinic
Rochester, Minnesota

Catherine Kuhn, MD
Associate Professor
Department of Anesthesiology
School of Medicine
Duke University Medical Center
Durham, North Carolina

Arthur M. Lam, MD, FRCPC
Clinical Professor of Anesthesiology and Pain Medicine
School of Medicine
University of Washington
Medical Director of Neuroanesthesia and Neurocritical Care
Swedish Medical Center, Cherry Hill Campus
Seattle, Washington

Jerrold Lerman, MD, FRCPC, FANZCA
Clinical Professor
Department of Anesthesiology
School of Medicine
State University of New York
Women and Children's Hospital
Buffalo, New York
University of Rochester
Strong Hospital
Rochester, New York

Jerrold H. Levy, MD, FAHA, FCCM
Professor
Department of Anesthesiology
School of Medicine
Duke University
Durham, North Carolina

Adam D. Lichtman, MD
Assistant Professor of Anesthesiology
Department of Anesthesiology
Weill Cornell Medical Center
New York Presbyterian Hospital
New York, New York

J. Lance Lichtor, MD
Professor
Department of Anesthesiology
School of Medicine
Yale University
New Haven, Connecticut

Yi Lin, MD, PhD
Clinical Instructor of Anesthesiology
Department of Anesthesiology
Weill Medical College
Cornell University
Assistant Attending Anesthesiologist
Hospital for Special Surgery
New York, New York

Larry Lindenbaum, MD
Assistant Professor of Anesthesiology and Critical Care Medicine
Department of Anesthesiology
School of Medicine
Medical College of Wisconsin
Froedtert Memorial Lutheran Hospital
Milwaukee, Wisconsin

Spencer S. Liu, MD
Attending Anesthesiologist
Department of Anesthesiology
Hospital for Special Surgery
New York, New York

David A. Lubarsky, MD, MBA
CEO
UHealth Physician Practice
Emanuel M. Papper Professor and Chair
Department of Anesthesiology, Perioperative Medicine, and Pain Management
Miller School of Medicine
University of Miami
Department of Anesthesiology
Jackson Memorial Hospital
Miami, Florida

Stephen M. Macres, PharmD, MD
Clinical Professor of Anesthesiology
Department of Anesthesiology and Pain Medicine
School of Medicine
University of California, Davis
Director
Postoperative Pain and Regional Anesthesia Service
Sacramento, California

Gerard Manecke, MD
Clinical Professor and Chair
Department of Anesthesiology
UCSD Medical Center
San Diego, California

Joseph P. Mathew, MD
Professor
Department of Anesthesiology
Duke University Medical Center
Durham, North Carolina

Michael S. Mazurek, MD
Associate Professor of Clinical Anesthesia
Department of Anesthesia
School of Medicine
Indiana University
Division of Pediatric Anesthesia
Riley Hospital for Children
Indianapolis, Indiana

Kathryn E. McGoldrick, MD
Professor and Chair
Department of Anesthesiology
School of Medicine
New York Medical College
Director of Anesthesiology
Westchester Medical Center
Valhalla, New York

Sanford M. Miller, MD
Clinical Associate Professor
Department of Anesthesiology
School of Medicine
NYU School of Medicine
Assistant Director
Department of Anesthesiology
Bellevue Hospital Center
New York, New York

Timothy E. Miller, MBChB, FRCA
Assistant Professor
Department of Anesthesiology
School of Medicine
Duke University Medical Center
Durham, North Carolina

Peter G. Moore, MD, PhD
Professor and Chair
Department of Anesthesiology and Pain Medicine
School of Medicine
University of California, Davis
Sacramento, California

Michael J. Murray, MD, PhD, FCCM, FCCP
Colonel
US Army Medical Corp
Professor of Anesthesiology
Mayo Clinic College of Medicine
Mayo Clinic
Jacksonville, Florida

Charles D. Nargozian, MD
Assistant Professor
School of Medicine
Harvard Medical Center
Senior Associate in Anesthesia
Department of Anesthesiology, Perioperative and Pain Medicine
Boston Children's Hospital
Boston, Massachusetts

Steven M. Neustein, MD
Professor
Department of Anesthesiology
Mount Sinai School of Medicine
Attending Staff
Department of Anesthesiology
Mount Sinai Hospital
New York, New York

Marieke Niesters, MD
Department of Anesthesiology
Leiden University Medical Center
The Netherlands

Erik Olofsen, MSc
Research Associate
Department of Anesthesiology
Leiden University Medical Center
The Netherlands

Rafael Ortega, MD
Professor
Vice-Chairman of Academic Affairs
Department of Anesthesiology
School of Medicine
Boston University
Boston, Massachusetts

Charles W. Otto, MD, FCCM
Professor of Anesthesiology
Associate Professor of Medicine
College of Medicine
University of Arizona
Tucson, Arizona

Frank J. Overdyk, MSEE, MD
Professor
Department of Anesthesiology
School of Medicine
Hofstra North Shore-LIJ
Hempstead, New York

Nathan Leon Pace, MD, MStat
Professor
Department of Anesthesiology
School of Medicine
University of Utah
Salt Lake, Utah

Paul S. Pagel, MD, PhD
Professor and Director of Cardiac Anesthesia
Department of Anesthesiology
Clement J. Zablocki Veterans Affairs Medical Center
Milwaukee, Wisconsin

Ben Julian Palanca, MD, PhD
Assistant Professor
Department of Anesthesiology
School of Medicine
Washington University
St. Louis, Missouri

Albert C. Perrino, Jr., MD
Professor
Department of Anesthesiology
School of Medicine
Yale University
New Haven, Connecticut
Chief
Department of Anesthesiology
VA Connecticut
West Haven, Connecticut

Andrew J. Pittaway, FRCA
Assistant Professor
Department of Anesthesiology and Pain Medicine
School of Medicine
University of Washington
Attending Staff
Department of Anesthesiology and Pain Medicine
Seattle Children's Hospital
Seattle, Washington

Mihai V. Podgoreanu, MD
Associate Professor
Department of Anesthesiology
Director
Perioperative Genomics Program
School of Medicine
Duke University
Durham, North Carolina

Wanda M. Popescu, MD
Associate Professor
Department of Anesthesiology
School of Medicine
Yale University
Attending Physician
Yale New Haven Hospital
New Haven, Connecticut

Karen L. Posner, PhD
Research Professor
Department of Anesthesiology and Pain Medicine
School of Medicine
University of Washington
Seattle, Washington

Donald S. Prough, MD
Professor and Chair
Department of Anesthesiology
The University of Texas Medical Branch
Galveston, Texas

Glenn Ramsey, MD
Professor
Department of Pathology
Feinberg School of Medicine
Northwestern University
Medical Director
Blood Bank
Northwestern Memorial Hospital
Chicago, Illinois

Kevin T. Riutort, MD, MS
Anesthesiologist
South Denver Anesthesiologists, P.C.
Denver, Colorado

G. Alec Rooke, MD, PhD
Professor
Department of Anesthesiology and Pain Medicine
School of Medicine
University of Washington
Seattle, Washington

Stanley H. Rosenbaum, MA, MD
Professor
Departments of Anesthesiology, Internal Medicine, and Surgery
School of Medicine
Yale University
New Haven, Connecticut

Meg A. Rosenblatt, MD
Professor
Department of Anesthesiology and Orthopaedics
Mount Sinai School of Medicine
Mount Sinai Medical Center
New York, New York

William H. Rosenblatt, MD
Professor
Departments of Anesthesia and Surgery
Department of Anesthesiology
School of Medicine
Yale University
New Haven, Connecticut

Richard W. Rosenquist, MD
Chairman
Department of Pain Management
College of Medicine
Cleveland Clinic
Cleveland, Ohio

Aaron Sandler, MD, PhD
Associate Professor
Department of Anesthesiology
School of Medicine
Duke University Medical Center
Durham, North Carolina

Barbara M. Scavone, MD
Associate Professor
Departments of Anesthesia & Critical Care and Obstetrics & Gynecology
Pritzker School of Medicine
University of Chicago
Section Chief, Obstetric Anesthesia
Clinical Director, Labor and Delivery
The University of Chicago Medical Center
Chicago, Illinois

Katie Schenning, MD, MPH
Fellow
Departments of Anesthesiology and Perioperative Medicine
College of Medicine
Oregon Health and Science University
Portland, Oregon

Jeffrey J. Schwartz, MD
Associate Professor
Department of Anesthesiology
School of Medicine
Yale University
Attending Physician
Department of Anesthesiology
Yale New Haven Medical Center
New Haven, Connecticut

Harry A. Seifert, MD, MSCE
Adjunct Assistant Professor of Clinical Anesthesiology
Department of Anesthesiology and Critical Care
The Children's Hospital of Philadelphia
Philadelphia, Pennsylvania

Aarti Sharma, MD
Assistant Professor
Department of Anesthesiology
School of Medicine
Weill Cornell Medical Center
New York Presbyterian Hospital
New York, New York

Andrew Shaw, MB, FRCA, FCCM
Associate Professor
Department of Anesthesiology
School of Medicine
Duke University Medical Center
Durham, North Carolina

Benjamin M. Sherman, MD
Assistant Professor
School of Medicine
Yale University
VA Medical Center
Department of Cardiothoracic Anesthesiology
West Haven Connecticut

Nikolaos J. Skubas, MD, FASE
Director, Cardiac Anesthesia
Associate Professor of Anesthesiology
School of Medicine
Weill Cornell Medical College
Associate Attending of Anesthesiology
New York Hospital—Weill Cornell Medical Center
New York, New York

Todd J. Smaka, MD
Assistant Professor
Department of Anesthesiology, Perioperative Medicine and Pain Management
School of Medicine
University of Miami Miller
Jackson Memorial Hospital
Miami, Florida

Hugh M. Smith, MD
Assistant Professor
Department of Anesthesiology
Mayo Clinic College of Medicine
Mayo Clinic
Rochester, Minnesota

Terry Smith, PhD
Department of Anesthesiology
Leiden University Medical Center
The Netherlands

Karen J. Souter, MB, BS, MSc, FRCA
Associate Professor
Vice Chair for Education and Residency Program Director
Department of Anesthesiology and Pain Medicine
School of Medicine
University of Washington
University of Washington Medical Center
Seattle, Washington

Bruce D. Spiess, MD, FAHA
Professor
Departments of Anesthesiology and Emergency Medicine
Director of Virginia Commonwealth University Reanimation Engineering Shock Center
Virginia Commonwealth University Medical Center
Richmond, Virginia

Mark Stafford-Smith, MD, CM, FRCPC
Professor
Department of Anesthesiology
School of Medicine
Duke University Medical Center
Durham, North Carolina

Andrew F. Stasic, MD
Associate Professor
Department of Anesthesia
School of Medicine
Indiana University
Indianapolis, Indiana

Randolph H. Steadman, MD
Professor and Vice Chair
Department of Anesthesiology
Chief, Anesthesia of Liver Transplant
David Geffen School of Medicine
University of California, Los Angeles
Los Angeles, California

M. Christine Stock, MD
Professor and Chair
Department of Anesthesiology
Feinberg School of Medicine
Northwestern University
Chicago, Illinois

Robert K. Stoelting, MD
Emeritus Professor and Past Chair
Department of Anesthesia
School of Medicine
Indiana University
Indianapolis, Indiana

David F. Stowe, MD, PhD
Professor
Department of Anesthesiology
College of Medicine
Medical College of Wisconsin
Milwaukee, Wisconsin

Wariya Sukhupragarn, MD
Assistant Professor
Department of Anesthesiology
Chiang Mai University
Maharaj Nakorn Chiang Mai
Chiang Mai, Thailand

Santhanam Suresh, MD
Professor of Anesthesiology and Pediatrics
Chair, Department of Pediatric Anesthesiology
Feinberg School of Medicine
Northwestern University
Anesthesiologist-in-Chief
Ann and Robert H. Lurie Children's Hospital of Chicago
Chicago, Illinois

Christer H. Svensén, MD, PhD, DEAA, MSc
Professor of Anesthesiology, and Intensive Care
Department of Clinical Science and Education, Section of Anesthesiology and Intensive Care
Karolinska Institutet/Stockholm
South General, Stockholm, Sweden

Paul C. Tamul, DO
Assistant Professor
Department of Anesthesiology and Neurological Surgery
Feinberg School of Medicine
Northwestern University
Medical Director
Post-Anesthesia Care Unit
Northwestern Memorial Hospital
Chicago, Illinois

Stephen J. Thomas, MD
Topkin-Van Poznak Professor and Vice-Chairman
Department of Anesthesiology
Weill Medical College
Cornell University
Attending Anesthesiologist
New York Presbyterian Hospital
New York, New York

Miriam M. Treggiari, MD
Professor of Anesthesiology and Neurological Surgery
School of Medicine
University of Washington
Harborview Medical Center
Seattle, Washington

Ban C.H. Tsui, MSc, MD, FRCP(C)
Pediatric and Adult Anesthesiologist
Professor and Vice Chair (Research)
Department of Anesthesiology and Pain Management
Stollery Children's Hospital
University of Alberta Hospital
Edmonton, Alberta

J. Scott Walton, MD
Associate Professor
Department of Anesthesia and Perioperative Medicine
School of Medicine
Medical University of South Carolina
Charleston, South Carolina

Mary E. Warner, MD
Associate Professor
Department of Anesthesiology
Mayo Clinic College of Medicine
Mayo Clinic
Rochester, Minnesota

Denise J. Wedel, MD
Professor
Department of Anesthesiology
Mayo Clinic College of Medicine
Mayo Clinic
Rochester, Minnesota

Paul F. White, MD, PhD, FANZCA
Director of Research and Education
Department of Anesthesia
Cedars-Sinai Medical Center
Los Angeles, California
Visiting Scientist
Research Unit of Anesthesia and Intensive Care
Rizzoli Orthopedic Institute
University of Bologna
Italy

Scott W. Wolf, MD
Assistant Professor
Department of Anesthesiology
Feinberg School of Medicine
Northwestern University
Northwestern Memorial Hospital
Chicago, Illinois

Cynthia A. Wong, MD
Professor and Vice Chair
Section Chief, Obstetric Anesthesiology
Department of Anesthesiology
Feinberg School of Medicine
Northwestern University
Chicago, Illinois

James R. Zaidan, MD, MBA
Professor and Past Chair
Department of Anesthesiology
Emory University Hospital
Atlanta, Georgia

PREFACE

Seminal editions are an intrinsic part of the life cycle of textbooks. Certainly the first edition of *Clinical Anesthesia* in 1989 was decisive in shaping the goals and objectives that continue today. That goal was to create a single volume, comprehensive, yet clinically focused textbook that supports efficient and rapid acquisition of knowledge and meets the educational and clinical needs of all anesthesia providers including those with decades of experience and those just embarking on their careers.

The development of the *Clinical Anesthesia* series is designed to fulfill the more specific needs of our readers. First, the *Handbook of Clinical Anesthesia* meets the requests of the health care providers to have the essential information contained in the parent textbook in a more 'portable format'. Even with advent of personal computers, smart phones and tablets, the Handbook continues to have a vital role. Subsequently, a guided study book *Review of Clinical Anesthesia* edited by Drs. Neil Connelly and David Silverman facilitated integrated study of subject matter in the textbook. However, the hallmark of the series has been the continuous launching of electronic products to enhance the reader experience. As technology has evolved, so has *Clinical Anesthesia*. Clinical Anesthesia was one of the first textbooks in medicine to have an 'app' for a hand held electronic device, the Palm. This app was awarded the prestigious Folio Award for the Best Electronic Media in Science, Medicine and Technology. Using this as the electronic foundation, the *Lippincott-Raven Interactive Anesthesia Library* was developed and was highly successful as a study guide for Board examinations. Finally, in the previous edition, *Clinical Anesthesia* introduced Podcasts as enhancements to the educational process.

This brings us to *Clinical Anesthesia 7th Edition*, which has turned out to be a seminal edition and perhaps of even greater importance than the first. This is the first anesthesia textbook of the 21st Century to be designed from the 'ground up' as an electronic edition. In essence, we have created two distinct books, which share material. Previously, we and others have scanned the textbook pages to create an e-media version of a book. This not only results in a sub-optimal reader experience, but more importantly does not capture the strengths of e-publications, e.g. video clips, animation and updating etc. So for the book-lover, the printed textbook is still available with access to a completely enhanced and innovative digital experience powered by Inkling. Viewable through a browser or as a download to your smartphone or tablet, the electronic version has three hundred videos, animated tables, an enhanced search and navigation style and regular content updates. The readers will recognize that they are no longer reading an electronic version of the printed standard page, rather the presentation of information in a new and enhanced style.

This publication marks the addition of Dr. Rafael Ortega to the editorial board. Known internationally for the use of electronic media in education, Dr. Ortega incorporated electronic materials throughout the *7th Edition of Clinical Anesthesia*, a Herculean task. Drs. Michael Cahalan and Christine Stock continue to bring new and fresh ideas and have been instrumental in shaping its future.

In addition to being published in an electronic version, this edition of *Clinical Anesthesia* contains a new chapter on Laparoscopic and Robotic Surgery. Also, the Appendices on Electrocardiography and Pacemakers/Implantable Defibrillators are presented in a new graphic interface to improve reader comprehension of these important subjects. Finally, approximately twenty percent of the Chapters are written by new contributing authors who are leading authorities in their respective areas.

We wish to express our appreciation to all our contributors whose knowledge, hard work, dedication and timely submissions allowed us to maintain quality while working with a tight production schedule. Our readers also provided comments instrumental to the editors' continual improvement of *Clinical Anesthesia.* We are also grateful to our administrative assistants—Gail Norup, Ruby Wilson, Deanna Walker, and Mary Wynn. We would like to thank our editors at Lippincott Williams & Wilkins-Wolters Kluwer, Brian Brown and Lisa McAllister, for their commitment to excellence. Finally, we owe a debt of gratitude to Nicole Dernoski—Managing Editor at LWW, Chris Miller—Production Manager at Aptara, Lisa Lawrence—Marketing Manager at LWW whose day-to-day management of this endeavor resulted in a publication that exceeded the Editor's expectations.

The discovery and application of anesthesia is the single most important contribution of American medicine to mankind. The major achievements of modern surgery could not have taken place without the accompanying vision of the pioneers in Anesthesiology. This statement is echoed by surgeon-author Atul Gawande, who in the article *Two Hundred Years of Surgery* (*New England Journal of Medicine*) stated

> "The crucial spark of transformation—the moment that changed not just the future of surgery but of medicine as a whole—was the publication on November 18, 1846, of Henry Jacob Bigelow's groundbreaking report, 'Insensibility during Surgical Operations Produced by Inhalation'."

The Editors hope that every page of *Clinical Anesthesia* evokes the pride of being a part of the specialty of Anesthesiology and its achievements for the betterment of mankind.

Paul G. Barash, MD
Bruce F. Cullen, MD
Robert K. Stoelting, MD
Michael K. Cahalan, MD
M. Christine Stock, MD
Rafael Ortega, MD

CONTENTS

SECTION I
Introduction to Anesthesiology

SECTION II
Scientific Foundations of Anesthesia

SECTION III
Anatomy and Physiology

SECTION IV
Anesthetic Agents, Adjuvants, and Drug Interaction

SECTION V
Preanesthetic Evaluation and Preparation

SECTION VI
Anesthetic Management

SECTION VII
Anesthesia for Surgical Subspecialties

SECTION VIII
Perioperative and Consultative Services

SECTION I

Introduction to Anesthesiology

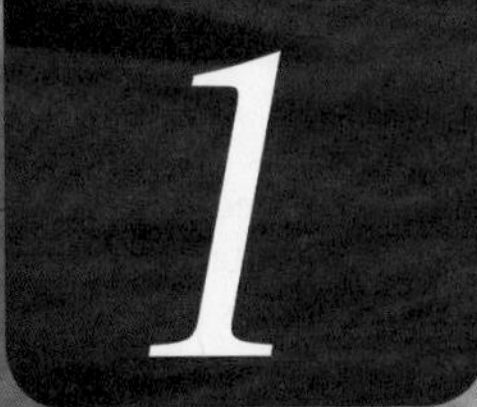

CHAPTER 1

The History of Anesthesia

ADAM K. JACOB • SANDRA L. KOPP • DOUGLAS R. BACON • HUGH M. SMITH

Key Points

1. Anesthesiology is a young specialty historically, especially when compared with surgery or internal medicine.
2. Discoveries in anesthesiology have taken decades to build upon the observations and experiments of many people, and in some instances we are still searching. For example, the ideal volatile anesthetic has yet to be discovered.
3. Much of our current anesthesia equipment is the direct result of anesthesiologists being unhappy with and needing better tools to properly anesthetize patients.
4. Many safety standards have been established through the work of anesthesiologists who were frustrated by the status quo.
5. Regional anesthesia is the direct outgrowth of a chance observation by an intern who would go on to become a successful ophthalmologist.
6. Pain medicine began as an outgrowth of regional anesthesia.
7. Organizations of anesthesia professionals have been critical in establishing high standards in education and proficiency, which in turn has defined the specialty.
8. Respiratory critical care medicine started as the need by anesthesiologists to use positive pressure ventilation to help polio victims.
9. Surgical anesthesia and physician specialization in its administration have allowed for increasingly complex operations to be performed on increasingly ill patients.

Multimedia

1. The Ether Monument
2. The Ether Controversy
3. ASA Seal

Surgery without adequate pain control may seem cruel to the modern reader, and in contemporary practice we are prone to forget the realities of preanesthesia surgery. Fanny Burney, a well-known literary artist from the early nineteenth century, described a mastectomy she endured after receiving a "wine cordial" as her sole anesthetic. As seven male assistants held her down, the surgery commenced: "When the dreadful steel was plunged into the breast-cutting through veins–arteries–flesh–nerves—I needed no injunction not to restrain my cries. I began a scream that lasted unintermittently during the whole time of the incision—& I almost marvel that it rings not in my Ears still! So excruciating was the agony. Oh Heaven!—I then felt the knife racking against the breast bone—scraping it! This performed while I yet remained in utterly speechless torture".[1] Burney's description illustrates the difficulty of overstating the impact of anesthesia on the human condition. An epitaph on a monument to William Thomas Green Morton, one of the founders of anesthesia, summarizes the contribution of anesthesia: "BEFORE WHOM in all time Surgery
1 was Agony".[2] Although most human civilizations evolved some method for diminishing patient discomfort, *anesthesia,* in its modern and effective meaning, is a comparatively recent discovery with traceable origins in the mid-nineteenth century. How we have changed perspectives from one in which surgical pain was terrible and expected to one in which patients reasonably assume they will be safe, pain-free, and unaware during extensive operations is a fascinating story and the subject of this chapter.

Anesthesiologists are like no other physicians: We are experts at controlling the airway and at emergency resuscitation; we are real-time cardiopulmonologists achieving hemodynamic and respiratory stability for the anesthetized patient; we are pharmacologists and physiologists, calculating appropriate doses and desired responses; we are gurus of postoperative care and patient safety; we are internists performing perianesthetic medical evaluations; we are the pain experts across all medical disciplines and apply specialized techniques in pain clinics and labor wards; we manage the severely sick and injured in critical care units; we are neurologists, selectively blocking sympathetic, sensory, or motor functions with our regional techniques; we are trained researchers exploring scientific mystery and clinical phenomenon.

Anesthesiology is an amalgam of specialized techniques, equipment, drugs, and knowledge that, like the growth rings of a tree, have built up over time. Current anesthesia practice is the summation of individual effort and fortuitous discovery of centuries. Every component of modern anesthesia was at some point a new discovery and reflects the experience, knowledge, and inventiveness of our predecessors. Historical examination enables understanding of how these individual components of anesthesia evolved. Knowledge of the history of anesthesia enhances our appreciation of current practice and intimates where our specialty might be headed.

ANESTHESIA BEFORE ETHER

Physical and Psychological Anesthesia

The Edwin Smith Surgical Papyrus, the oldest known written surgical document, describes 48 cases performed by an Egyptian surgeon from 3000 to 2500 BC. While this remarkable surgical treatise contains no direct mention of measures to lessen patient pain or suffering, Egyptian pictographs from the same era show a surgeon compressing a nerve in a patient's antecubital fossa while operating on the patient's hand. Another image displays a patient compressing his own brachial plexus while a procedure is performed on his palm.[3] In the sixteenth century, military surgeon Ambroise Paré became adept at nerve compression as a means of creating anesthesia.

Medical science has benefited from the natural refrigerating properties of ice and snow as well. For centuries anatomical dissections were performed only in winter because colder temperatures delayed deterioration of the cadaver, and in the Middle Ages the anesthetic effects of cold water and ice were recognized. In the seventeenth century, Marco Aurelio Severino described the technique of "refrigeration anesthesia" in which snow was placed in parallel lines across the incisional plane such that the surgical site became insensate within minutes. The technique never became widely used, likely because of the challenge of maintaining stores of snow year-round.[4] Severino is also known to have saved numerous lives during an epidemic of diphtheria by performing tracheostomies and inserting trocars to maintain patency of the airway.[5]

Formal manipulation of the psyche to relieve surgical pain was undertaken by French physicians Charles Dupotet and Jules Cloquet in the late 1820s with hypnosis, then called *mesmerism.* Although the work of Anton Mesmer was discredited by the French Academy of Science after formal inquiry several decades earlier, proponents like Dupotet and Cloquet continued with mesmeric experiments and pleaded to the Academie de Medicine to reconsider its utility.[6] In a well-attended demonstration in 1828, Cloquet removed the breast of a 64-year-old patient while she reportedly remained in a calm, mesmeric sleep. This demonstration made a lasting impression on British physician John Elliotson, who became a leading figure of the mesmeric movement in England in the 1830s and 1840s. Innovative and quick to adopt new advances, Elliotson performed mesmeric demonstrations and in 1843 published *Numerous Cases of Surgical Operations Without Pain in the Mesmeric State.* Support for mesmerism faded when in 1846 renowned surgeon Robert Liston performed the first operation using ether anesthesia in England and remarked, "This Yankee dodge beats mesmerism all hollow".[7]

Early Analgesics and Soporifics

Dioscorides, a Greek physician from the first century AD, commented on the analgesia of mandragora, a drug prepared from the bark and leaves of the mandrake plant. He observed that the plant substance could be boiled in wine, strained, and used "in the case of persons . . . about to be cut or cauterized, when they wish to produce anesthesia".[8] Mandragora was still being used to benefit patients as late as the seventeenth century. From the ninth to the thirteenth centuries, the *soporific sponge* was a dominant mode of providing pain relief during surgery. Mandrake leaves, along with black nightshade, poppies, and other herbs, were boiled together and cooked onto a sponge. The sponge was then reconstituted in hot water and placed under the patient's nose before surgery. Prior to the hypodermic syringe and routine venous access, ingestion and inhalation were the only known routes for administering medicines to gain systemic effects. Prepared as indicated by published reports of the time, the sponge generally contained morphine and scopolamine in varying amounts—drugs used in modern anesthesia.[9]

Alcohol was another element of the pre-ether armamentarium because it was thought to induce stupor and blunt the impact of pain. Although alcohol is a central nervous system depressant, in the amounts administered it produced little analgesia in the setting of true surgical pain. Fanny Burney's account underscores the ineffectiveness of alcohol as an anesthetic. Not only did alcohol provide minimal pain control, it did nothing to dull her recollection of events. Laudanum was an alcohol-based solution of opium first compounded by Paracelsus in the sixteenth century. It was wildly popular in the Victorian and Romantic periods and prescribed for a wide variety of ailments from the common cold to tuberculosis. Although appropriately used as an analgesic in some instances, it was frequently misused and abused. Laudanum was given by nursemaids to quiet wailing infants and abused by many upper-class women, poets, and artists who fell victim to its addictive potential.

Inhaled Anesthetics

Nitrous oxide was known for its ability to induce lightheadedness and was often inhaled by those seeking a thrill. It was not used for this purpose as frequently as ether because it was more difficult to synthesize and store. It was made by heating ammonium nitrate in the presence of iron filings. The evolved gas was passed through water to eliminate toxic oxides of nitrogen before being stored. Nitrous oxide was first prepared in 1773 by Joseph Priestley, an English clergyman and scientist, who ranks among the great pioneers of chemistry. Without formal scientific training, Priestley prepared and examined several gases, including nitrous oxide, ammonia, sulfur dioxide, oxygen, carbon monoxide, and carbon dioxide.

At the end of the eighteenth century in England, there was a strong interest in the supposed wholesome effects of mineral water and gases, particularly with regard to treatment of scurvy, tuberculosis, and other diseases. Thomas Beddoes opened his Pneumatic Institute close to the small spa of Hotwells, in the city of Bristol, to study the beneficial effects of inhaled gases. He hired Humphry Davy in 1798 to conduct research projects for the institute. Davy performed brilliant investigations of several gases but focused much of his attention on nitrous oxide. His human experimental results, combined with research on the physical properties of the gas, were published in *Nitrous Oxide,* a 580-page book published in 1800. This impressive treatise is now best remembered for a few incidental observations. Davy commented that nitrous oxide transiently relieved a severe headache, obliterated a minor headache, and briefly quenched an aggravating toothache. The most frequently quoted passage was a casual entry: "As nitrous oxide in its extensive operation appears capable of destroying physical pain, it may probably be used with advantage during surgical operations in which no great effusion of blood takes place".[10] This is perhaps the most famous of the "missed opportunities" to discover surgical anesthesia. Davy's lasting nitrous oxide legacy was coining the phrase "laughing gas" to describe its unique property.

Almost Discovery: Hickman, Clarke, Long, and Wells

2 As the nineteenth century progressed, societal attitudes toward pain changed, perhaps best exemplified in the writings of the Romantic poets.[11] Thus, efforts to relieve pain were undertaken and several more near-breakthroughs that occurred deserve mention. An English surgeon named Henry Hill Hickman searched intentionally for an inhaled anesthetic to relieve pain in his patients.[12] Hickman used high concentrations of carbon dioxide in his studies on mice and dogs. Carbon dioxide has some anesthetic properties, as shown by the absence of response to an incision in the animals of Hickman's study, but it was never determined if the animals were insensate because of hypoxia rather than anesthesia. Hickman's concept was magnificent; his choice of agent was regrettable.

The discovery of surgical anesthetics in the modern era remains linked to inhaled anesthetics. The compound now known as *diethyl ether* had been known for centuries; it may have been synthesized first by an eighth-century Arabian philosopher Jabir ibn Hayyan or possibly by Raymond Lully, a thirteenth century European alchemist. But diethyl ether was certainly known in the sixteenth century, to both Valerius Cordus and Paracelsus who prepared it by distilling sulfuric acid (oil of vitriol) with fortified wine to produce an *oleum vitrioli dulce* (sweet oil of vitriol). One of the first "missed" observations on the effects of inhaled agents, Paracelsus observed that ether caused chickens to fall asleep and awaken unharmed. He must have been aware of its analgesic qualities because he reported that it could be recommended for use in painful illnesses.

For three centuries thereafter, this simple compound remained a therapeutic agent with only occasional use. Some of its properties were examined but without sustained interest by distinguished British scientists Robert Boyle, Isaac Newton, and Michael Faraday, none of whom made the conceptual link to surgical anesthesia. Its only routine application came as an inexpensive recreational drug among the poor of Britain and Ireland, who sometimes drank an ounce or two of ether when taxes made gin prohibitively expensive.[13] An American variation of this practice was conducted by groups of students who held ether-soaked towels to their faces at nocturnal "ether frolics."

William E. Clarke, a medical student from Rochester, New York, may have given the first ether anesthetic in January 1842. From techniques learned as a chemistry student in 1839, Clarke entertained his companions with nitrous oxide and ether. Emboldened by these experiences, he administered ether, from a towel, to a young woman named Hobbie. One of her teeth was then extracted without pain by a dentist named Elijah Pope.[14] However, it was suggested that the woman's unconsciousness was due to hysteria and Clarke was advised to conduct no further anesthetic experiments.[15]

Two months later, on March 30, 1842, Crawford Williamson Long administered ether with a towel for surgical anesthesia in Jefferson, Georgia. His patient, James M. Venable, was a young man who was already familiar with ether's exhilarating effects, for he reported in a certificate that he had previously inhaled it and was fond of its use. Venable had two small tumors on his neck but refused to have them excised because he feared the pain that accompanied surgery. Knowing that Venable was familiar with ether's action, Dr. Long proposed that ether might alleviate pain and gained his patient's consent to proceed. After inhaling ether from the towel and having the procedure successfully completed, Venable reported that he was unaware of the removal of the tumors.[16] In determining the first fee for anesthesia and surgery, Long settled on a charge of $2.00.[17]

A common mid-nineteenth century problem facing dentists was that patients refused beneficial treatment of their teeth for fear of the pain of the procedure. From a dentist's perspective, pain was not so much life-threatening as it was livelihood-threatening. One of the first dentists to engender a solution was Horace Wells of Hartford, Connecticut, whose great moment of discovery came on December 10, 1844. He observed a lecture-exhibition on nitrous oxide by an itinerant "scientist," Gardner Quincy Colton, who encouraged members of the audience to inhale a sample of the gas. Wells observed a young man injure his leg without pain while under the influence of nitrous oxide. Sensing that it might provide pain relief during dental procedures, Wells contacted Colton and boldly proposed an experiment in which Wells was to be the subject. The following day, Colton gave Wells nitrous oxide before a fellow dentist, William Riggs, extracted a tooth.[18] Afterward Wells declared that he had not felt any pain and deemed the experiment a success. Colton taught Wells to prepare nitrous oxide, which the dentist administered with success to patients in his practice. His apparatus probably resembled that used by Colton: A wooden tube placed in the mouth through which nitrous oxide was breathed from a small bag filled with the gas.

Public Demonstration of Ether Anesthesia

Another New Englander, William Thomas Green Morton, briefly shared a dental practice with Wells in Hartford. Wells' daybook shows that he gave Morton a course of instruction in anesthesia, but Morton apparently moved to Boston without paying for the lessons.[19] In Boston, Morton continued his interest in anesthesia and sought instruction from chemist and physician Charles T. Jackson. After learning that ether dropped on the skin provided analgesia, he began experiments with inhaled ether, an agent that proved to be much more versatile than nitrous oxide. Bottles of liquid ether were easily transported, and the volatility of the drug permitted effective inhalation. The concentrations required for surgical anesthesia were so low that patients did not become hypoxic when breathing ether vaporized in air. It also possessed what would later be recognized as a unique property among all inhaled anesthetics: The quality of providing surgical anesthesia without causing respiratory depression. These properties, combined with a slow rate of induction, gave the patient a significant safety margin even in the hands of relatively unskilled anesthetists.[20]

After anesthetizing a pet dog, Morton became confident of his skills and anesthetized patients with ether in his dental office. Encouraged by his success, Morton sought an invitation to give a public demonstration in the Bullfinch amphitheater of the Massachusetts General Hospital, the same site as Wells' failed demonstration of the efficacy of nitrous oxide as a complete surgical anesthetic. Many details of the October 16, 1846, demonstration are well known. Morton secured permission to provide an anesthetic to Edward Gilbert Abbott, a patient of surgeon John Collins Warren. Warren planned to excise a vascular lesion from the left side of Abbott's neck and was about to proceed when Morton arrived late. He had been delayed because he was obliged to wait for an instrument maker to complete a new inhaler (Fig. 1-1). It consisted of a large glass bulb containing a sponge soaked with oil of orange mixed with ether and a spout that was placed in the patient's mouth. An opening on the opposite side of the bulb allowed air to enter and be drawn over the ether-soaked sponge with each breath.[21]

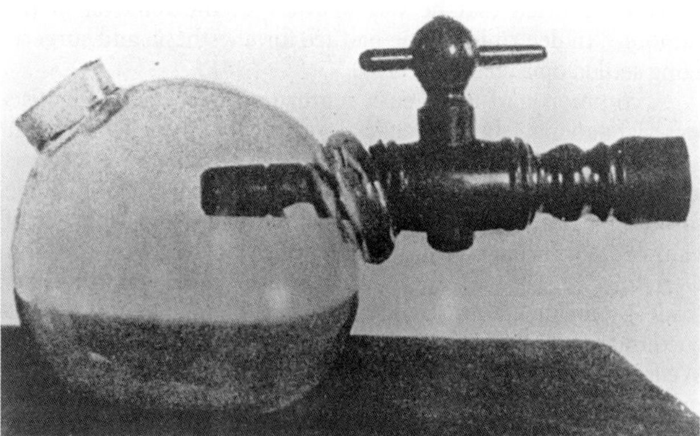

FIGURE 1-1. Morton's ether inhaler (1846).

The conversations of that morning were not accurately recorded; however, popular accounts state that the surgeon responded testily to Morton's apology for his tardy arrival by remarking, "Sir, your patient is ready." Morton directed his attention to his patient and first conducted a very abbreviated preoperative evaluation. He inquired, "Are you afraid?" Abbott responded that he was not and took the inhaler in his mouth. After a few minutes, Morton turned to the surgeon and said, "Sir, your patient is ready." Gilbert Abbott later reported that he was aware of the surgery but experienced no pain. When the procedure ended, Warren immediately turned to his audience and uttered the statement, "Gentlemen, this is no humbug".[22]

What would be recognized as America's greatest contribution to nineteenth century medicine had occurred. However, Morton, wishing to capitalize on his "discovery," refused to divulge what agent was in his inhaler. Some weeks passed before Morton admitted that the active component of the colored fluid, which he had called "Letheon," was simple diethyl ether. Morton, Wells, Jackson, and their supporters soon became drawn into a contentious, protracted, and fruitless debate over priority for the discovery. This debate has subsequently been termed *the ether controversy*. In short, Morton had applied for a patent for Letheon and, when it was granted, tried to receive royalties for the use of ether as an anesthetic.

When the details of Morton's anesthetic technique became public knowledge, the information was transmitted by train, stagecoach, and coastal vessels to other North American cities and by ship to the world. As ether was easy to prepare and administer, anesthetics were performed in Britain, France, Russia, South Africa, Australia, and other countries almost as soon as surgeons heard the welcome news of the extraordinary discovery. Even though surgery could now be performed with "pain put to sleep," the frequency of operations did not rise rapidly, and several years would pass before anesthesia was universally recommended.

Chloroform and Obstetrics

James Young Simpson was a successful obstetrician of Edinburgh, Scotland, and among the first to use ether for the relief of labor pain. Dissatisfied with ether, Simpson soon sought a more pleasant, rapid-acting anesthetic. He and his junior associates conducted a bold search by inhaling samples of several volatile chemicals collected for Simpson by British apothecaries. David Waldie suggested chloroform, which had first been prepared in 1831. Simpson and his friends inhaled it after dinner at a party in Simpson's home on the evening of November 4, 1847. They promptly fell unconscious and, when they awoke, were delighted with their success. Simpson quickly set about encouraging the use of chloroform. Within 2 weeks, he submitted his first account of its use for publication in *The Lancet.*

In the nineteenth century, the relief of obstetric pain had significant social ramifications and made anesthesia during childbirth a controversial subject. Simpson argued against the prevailing view, which held that relieving labor pain opposed God's will. The pain of the parturient was viewed as both a component of punishment and a means of atonement for Original Sin. Less than a year after administering the first anesthesia during childbirth, Simpson addressed these concerns in a pamphlet entitled *Answers to the Religious Objections Advanced Against the Employment of Anaesthetic Agents in Midwifery and Surgery and Obstetrics.* In it, Simpson recognized the Book of Genesis as being the root of this sentiment and noted that God promised to relieve the descendants of Adam and Eve of the curse. In addition, Simpson asserted that labor pain was a result of scientific and anatomic causes, and not the result of religious condemnation. He stated that the upright position of humans necessitated strong pelvic muscles to support the abdominal contents. As a result, he argued that the uterus necessarily developed strong musculature to overcome the resistance of the pelvic floor and that great contractile power caused great pain. Simpson's pamphlet probably did not have a significant impact on the prevailing attitudes, but he did articulate many concepts that his contemporaries were debating at the time.[23]

Chloroform gained considerable notoriety after John Snow used it to deliver the last two children of Queen Victoria. The Queen's consort, Prince Albert, interviewed John Snow before he was called to Buckingham Palace to administer chloroform at the request of the Queen's obstetrician. During the monarch's labor, Snow gave analgesic doses of chloroform on a folded handkerchief. This technique was soon termed *chloroform à la reine.* Victoria abhorred the pain of childbirth and enjoyed the relief that chloroform provided. She wrote in her journal, "Dr. Snow gave that blessed chloroform and the effect was soothing, quieting, and delightful beyond measure".[24] When the Queen, as head of the Church of England, endorsed obstetric anesthesia, religious debate over the management of labor pain terminated abruptly.

John Snow, already a respected physician, took an interest in anesthetic practice and was soon invited to work with many leading surgeons of the day. In 1848, Snow introduced a chloroform inhaler. He had recognized the versatility of the new agent and came to prefer it in his practice. At the same time, he initiated what was to become an extraordinary series of experiments that were remarkable in their scope and for anticipating sophisticated research performed a century later. Snow realized that successful anesthetics should abolish pain and unwanted movements. He anesthetized several species of animals with varying strengths of ether and chloroform to determine the concentration required to prevent reflex movement from sharp stimuli. This work approximated the modern concept of minimum alveolar concentration.[25] Snow assessed the anesthetic action of a large number of potential anesthetics but did not find any to rival chloroform or ether. His studies led him to recognize the relationship between solubility, vapor pressure, and anesthetic potency, which was not fully appreciated until after World War II. Snow published two remarkable books, *On the Inhalation of the Vapour of Ether* (1847) and *On Chloroform and Other Anaesthetics* (1858). The latter was almost completed when he died of a stroke at the age of 45 and was published posthumously.

ANESTHESIA PRINCIPLES, EQUIPMENT, AND STANDARDS

Control of the Airway

Definitive control of the airway, a skill anesthesiologists now consider paramount, developed only after many harrowing and apneic episodes spurred the development of safer airway management techniques. Preceding tracheal intubation, however, several important techniques were proposed toward the end of the nineteenth century that remain integral to anesthesiology education and practice. Joseph Clover was the first Englishman to urge the now universal practice of thrusting the patient's jaw forward to overcome obstruction of the upper airway by the tongue. Clover also published a landmark case report in 1877 in which he performed a surgical airway. Once his patient was asleep, Clover discovered that his patient had a tumor of the mouth that obstructed the airway completely, despite his trusted jaw-thrust maneuver. He averted disaster by inserting a small curved cannula of his design through the cricothyroid membrane. He continued anesthesia via the cannula until the tumor was excised. Clover, the model of the prepared anesthesiologist, remarked, "I have never used the cannula before although it has been my companion at some thousands of anaesthetic cases".[26]

Tracheal Intubation

The development of techniques and instruments for tracheal intubation ranks among the major advances in the history of anesthesiology. The first tracheal tubes were developed for the resuscitation of drowning victims, but were not used in anesthesia until 1878. The first use of elective oral intubation for an anesthetic was undertaken by Scottish surgeon William Macewan. He had practiced passing flexible metal tubes through the larynx of a cadaver before attempting the maneuver on an awake patient with an oral tumor at the Glasgow Royal Infirmary on July 5, 1878.[27] Since topical anesthesia was not yet known, the experience must have demanded fortitude on the part of Macewan's patient. Once the tube was correctly positioned, an assistant began a chloroform–air anesthetic via the tube. Once anesthetized, the patient soon stopped coughing. Unfortunately, Macewan abandoned the practice following a fatality in which a patient had been successfully intubated while awake but the tube became dislodged once the patient was asleep. After the tube was removed, an attempt to provide chloroform by mask anesthesia was unsuccessful and the patient died.

An American surgeon named Joseph O'Dwyer is remembered for his extraordinary dedication to the advancement of tracheal intubation. In 1885, O'Dwyer designed a series of metal laryngeal tubes, which he inserted blindly between the vocal cords of children suffering a diphtheritic crisis. Three years later, O'Dwyer designed a second rigid tube with a conical tip that occluded the larynx so effectively that it could be used for artificial ventilation when applied with the bellows and T-piece tube designed by George Fell. The Fell–O'Dwyer apparatus, as it came to be known, was used during thoracic surgery by Rudolph Matas of New Orleans. Matas was so pleased with it that he predicted, "The procedure that promises the most benefit in preventing pulmonary collapse in operations on the chest is . . . the rhythmical maintenance of artificial respiration by a tube in the glottis directly connected with a bellows."[22]

After O'Dwyer's death, the outstanding pioneer of tracheal intubation was Franz Kuhn, a surgeon of Kassel, Germany. From 1900 until 1912, Kuhn published several articles and a classic monograph, "*Die perorale Intubation,*" which were not well known in his lifetime but have since become widely appreciated.[25] His work might have had a more profound impact if it had been translated into English. Kuhn described techniques of oral and nasal intubation that he performed with flexible metal tubes composed of coiled tubing similar to those now used for the spout of metal gasoline cans. After applying cocaine to the airway, Kuhn introduced his tube over a curved metal stylet that he directed toward the larynx with his left index finger. While he was aware of the subglottic cuffs that had been used briefly by Victor Eisenmenger, Kuhn preferred to seal the larynx by positioning a supralaryngeal flange near the tube's tip before packing the pharynx with gauze. Kuhn even monitored the patient's breath sounds continuously through a monaural earpiece connected to an extension of the tracheal tube by a narrow tube.

Intubation of the trachea by palpation was an uncertain and sometimes traumatic act; surgeons even believed that it would be anatomically impossible to visualize the vocal cords directly. This misapprehension was overcome in 1895 by Alfred Kirstein in Berlin who devised the first direct-vision laryngoscope.[28] Kirstein was motivated by a friend's report that a patient's trachea had been accidentally intubated during esophagoscopy. Kirstein promptly fabricated a handheld instrument that at first resembled a shortened cylindrical esophagoscope. He soon substituted a semicircular blade that opened inferiorly. Kirstein could now examine the larynx while standing behind his seated patient, whose head had been placed in an attitude approximating the currently termed "sniffing position." Although Alfred Kirstein's "autoscope" was not used by anesthesiologists, it was the forerunner of all modern laryngoscopes. Endoscopy was refined by Chevalier Jackson in Philadelphia, who designed a U-shaped laryngoscope by adding a handgrip that was parallel to the blade. The Jackson blade has remained a standard instrument for endoscopists but was not favored by anesthesiologists. Two laryngoscopes that closely resembled modern L-shaped instruments were designed in 1910 and 1913 by two American surgeons, Henry Janeway and George Dorrance, but neither instrument achieved lasting use despite their excellent designs.[29]

Before the introduction of muscle relaxants in the 1940s, intubation of the trachea could be challenging. This challenge was made somewhat easier, however, with the advent of laryngoscope blades specifically designed to increase visualization of the vocal cords. Robert Miller of San Antonio, Texas, and Robert Macintosh of Oxford University created their respectively named blades within an interval of 2 years. In 1941, Miller brought forward the slender, straight blade with a slight curve near the tip to ease the passage of the tube through the larynx. Although Miller's blade was a refinement, the technique of its use was identical to that of earlier models as the epiglottis was lifted to expose the larynx.[30]

The Macintosh blade, which is placed in the vallecula rather than under the epiglottis, was invented as an incidental result of a tonsillectomy. Sir Robert Macintosh later described the circumstances of its discovery in an appreciation of the career of his technician, Mr. Richard Salt, who constructed the blade. As Sir Robert recalled, "A Boyle-Davis gag, a size larger than intended, was inserted for tonsillectomy, and when the mouth was fully opened the cords came into view. This was a surprise since conventional laryngoscopy, at that depth of anaesthesia, would have been impossible in those pre-relaxant days. Within a matter of hours, Salt had modified the blade of the Davis gag and attached a laryngoscope handle to it; and streamlined (after testing several models), the end result came into widespread use".[31] Macintosh underestimated the popularity of the blade, as more than 800,000 have been produced and many special-purpose versions have been marketed.

The most distinguished innovator in tracheal intubation was the self-trained British anesthetist Ivan (later, Sir Ivan) Magill.[32] In 1919, while serving in the Royal Army as a general medical officer, Magill was assigned to a military hospital near London. Although he had only rudimentary training in anesthesia, Magill was obliged to accept an assignment to the anesthesia service, where he worked with another neophyte, Stanley Rowbotham.[33] Together, Magill and Rowbotham attended casualties disfigured by severe facial injuries who underwent repeated restorative operations. These procedures required that the surgeon, Harold Gillies, have unrestricted access to the face and airway. These patients presented formidable challenges, but both Magill and Rowbotham became adept at tracheal intubation and quickly understood its current limitations. Because they learned from fortuitous observations, they soon extended the scope of tracheal anesthesia.

They gained expertise with blind nasal intubation after they learned to soften semirigid insufflation tubes for passage through the nostril. Even though their original intent was to position the tips of the nasal tubes in the posterior pharynx, the slender tubes frequently ended up in the trachea. Stimulated by this chance experience, they developed techniques of deliberate nasotracheal intubation. In 1920, Magill devised an aid to manipulating the catheter tip, the "Magill angulated forceps," which continues to be manufactured according to his original design over 90 years ago.

With the war over, Magill entered civilian practice and set out to develop a wide-bore tube that would resist kinking but be conformable to the contours of the upper airway. While in a hardware store, he found mineralized red rubber tubing that he cut, beveled, and smoothed to produce tubes that clinicians around the world would come to call "Magill tubes." His tubes remained the universal standard for more than 40 years until rubber products were supplanted by inert plastics. Magill also rediscovered the advantage of applying cocaine to the nasal mucosa, a technique that greatly facilitated awake blind nasal intubation.

In 1926, Arthur Guedel began a series of experiments that led to the introduction of the cuffed tube. Guedel transformed the basement of his Indianapolis home into a laboratory where he subjected each step of the preparation and application of his cuffs to a vigorous review.[34] He fashioned cuffs from the rubber of dental dams, condoms, and surgical gloves that were glued onto the outer wall of tubes. Using animal tracheas donated by the family butcher as his model, he considered whether the cuff should be positioned above, below, or at the level of the vocal cords. He recommended that the cuff be positioned just below the vocal cords to seal the airway. Ralph Waters later recommended that cuffs be constructed of two layers of soft rubber cemented together. These detachable cuffs were first manufactured by Waters' children, who sold them to the Foregger Company.

Guedel sought ways to show the safety and utility of the cuffed tube. He first filled the mouth of an anesthetized and intubated patient with water and showed that the cuff sealed the airway. Even though this exhibition was successful, he searched for a more dramatic technique to capture the attention of those unfamiliar with the advantages of intubation. He reasoned that if the cuff prevented water from entering the trachea of an intubated patient, it should also prevent an animal from drowning, even if it were submerged under water. To encourage physicians attending a medical convention to use his tracheal techniques, Guedel prepared the first of several "dunked dog" demonstrations (Fig. 1-2). An anesthetized and intubated dog, Guedel's own pet, "Airway," was immersed in an aquarium. After the demonstration was completed, the anesthetic

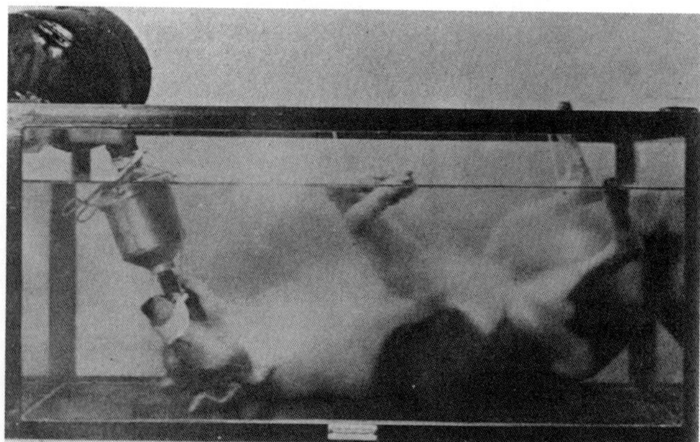

FIGURE 1-2. The "dunked dog."

was discontinued before the animal was removed from the water. According to legend, Airway awoke promptly, shook water over the onlookers, saluted a post, then trotted from the hall to the applause of the audience.

After a patient experienced an accidental endobronchial intubation, Ralph Waters reasoned that a very long cuffed tube could be used to isolate the lungs. The dependent lung could be ventilated while the upper lung was being resected.[35] On learning of his friend's success with intentional one-lung anesthesia, Arthur Guedel proposed an important modification for chest surgery, the double-cuffed single-lumen tube, which was introduced by Emery Rovenstine. These tubes were easily positioned, an advantage over bronchial blockers that had to be inserted by a skilled bronchoscopist. In 1953, single-lumen tubes were supplanted by double-lumen endobronchial tubes. The double-lumen tube currently most popular was designed by Frank Robertshaw of Manchester, England, and is prepared in both right- and left-sided versions. Robertshaw tubes were first manufactured from mineralized red rubber but are now made of extruded plastic, a technique refined by David Sheridan. Sheridan was also the first person to embed centimeter markings along the side of tracheal tubes, a safety feature that reduced the risk of the tube being incorrectly positioned.

Advanced Airway Devices

Conventional laryngoscopes proved inadequate for patients with "difficult airways." A few clinicians credit harrowing intubating experiences as the incentive for invention. In 1928, a rigid bronchoscope was specifically designed for examination of the large airways. Rigid bronchoscopes were refined and used by pulmonologists. Although it was known in 1870 that a thread of glass could transmit light along its length, technologic limitations were not overcome until 1964 when Shigeto Ikeda developed the first flexible fiberoptic bronchoscope. Fiberoptic-assisted tracheal intubation has become a common approach in the management of patients with difficult airways having surgery.

Roger Bullard desired a device to simultaneously examine the larynx and intubate the vocal cords. He had been frustrated by failed attempts to visualize the larynx of a patient with Pierre-Robin syndrome. In response, he developed the Bullard laryngoscope, whose fiberoptic bundles lie beside a curved blade. Similarly, the Wu-scope was designed by Tzu-Lang Wu in 1994 to combine and facilitate visualization and intubation of the trachea in patients with difficult airways.[36]

Dr. A. I. J. "Archie" Brain first recognized the principle of the laryngeal mask airway (LMA) in 1981 when, like many British clinicians, he provided dental anesthesia via a Goldman nasal mask. However, unlike any before him, he realized that just as the dental mask could be fitted closely about the nose, a comparable mask attached to a wide-bore tube might be positioned around the larynx. He not only conceived of this radical departure in airway management, which he first described in 1983,[37] but also spent years in single-handedly fabricating and testing several incremental modifications. Scores of Brain's prototypes are displayed in the Royal Berkshire Hospital, Reading, England, where they provide a detailed record of the evolution of the LMA. He fabricated his first models from Magill tubes and Goldman masks, then refined their shape by performing postmortem studies of the hypopharynx to determine the form of cuff that would be most functional. Before silicone rubber was selected, Brain had even mastered the technique of forming masks from liquid latex. Every detail of the LMA, the number and position of the aperture bars and the shape and the size of the masks, required repeated modification.

Early Anesthesia Delivery Systems

3 The transition from ether inhalers and chloroform-soaked handkerchiefs to more sophisticated anesthesia delivery equipment occurred gradually, with incremental advances supplanting older methods. One of the earliest anesthesia apparatus designs was that of John Snow, who had realized the inadequacies of ether inhalers through which patients rebreathed via a mouthpiece. After practicing anesthesia for only 2 weeks, Snow created the first of his series of ingenious ether inhalers.[38] His best-known apparatus featured unidirectional valves within a malleable, well-fitting mask of his own design, which closely resembles the form of a modern face mask. The face piece was connected to the vaporizer by a breathing tube, which Snow deliberately designed to be wider than the human trachea so that even rapid respirations would not be impeded. A metal coil within the vaporizer ensured that the patient's inspired breath was drawn over a large surface area to promote the uptake of ether. The device also incorporated a warm water bath to maintain the volatility of the agent (Fig. 1-3). Snow did not attempt to capitalize on his creativity, in contrast to William Morton; he closed his account of its preparation with

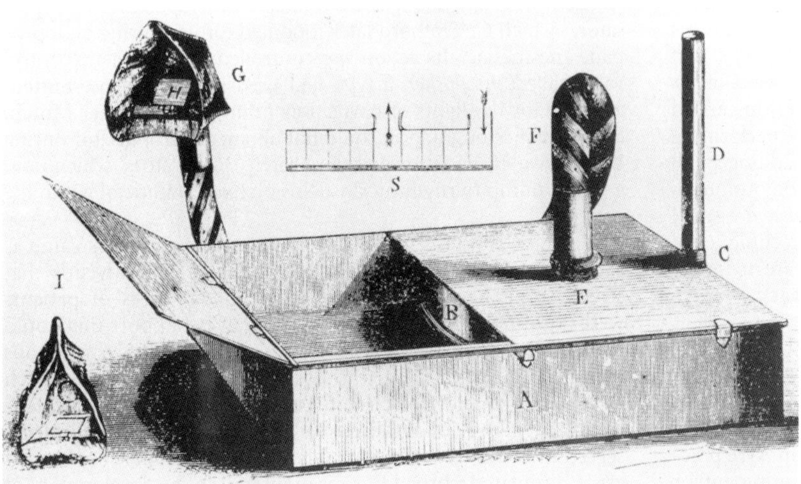

FIGURE 1-3. John Snow's inhaler (1847). The ether chamber (*B*) contained a spiral coil so that the air entering through the brass tube (*D*) was saturated by ether before ascending the flexible tube (*F*) to the face mask (*G*). The ether chamber rested in a bath of warm water (*A*).

the generous observation, "There is no restriction respecting the making of it".[39]

Joseph Clover, another British physician, was the first anesthetist to administer chloroform in known concentrations through the "Clover bag." He obtained a 4.5% concentration of chloroform in air by pumping a measured volume of air with a bellows through a warmed evaporating vessel containing a known volume of liquid chloroform.[40] Although it was realized that nitrous oxide diluted in air often gave a hypoxic mixture and that the oxygen–nitrous oxide mixture was safer, Chicago surgeon Edmund Andrews complained about the physical limitations of delivering anesthesia to patients in their homes. The large bag was conspicuous and awkward to carry along busy streets. He observed that "In city practice, among the higher classes, however, this is no obstacle as the bag can always be taken in a carriage, without attracting attention".[41] In 1872, Andrews was delighted to report the availability of liquefied nitrous oxide compressed under 750 pounds of pressure, which allowed a supply sufficient for three patients to be carried in a single cylinder.

Critical to increasing patient safety was the development of a machine capable of delivering a calibrated amount of gas and volatile anesthetic. In the late nineteenth century, demands in dentistry instigated development of the first freestanding anesthesia machines. Three American dentist-entrepreneurs, Samuel S. White, Charles Teter, and Jay Heidbrink, developed the original series of US instruments that used compressed cylinders of nitrous oxide and oxygen. Before 1900, the S. S. White Company modified Frederick Hewitt's apparatus and marketed its continuous-flow machine, which was refined by Teter in 1903. Heidbrink added reducing valves in 1912. In the same year, physicians initiated other important developments. Water–bubble flowmeters, introduced by Frederick Cotton and Walter Boothby of Harvard University, allowed the proportion of gases and their flow rate to be approximated. The Cotton and Boothby apparatus was transformed into a practical portable machine by James Tayloe Gwathmey of New York. The Gwathmey machine caught the attention of a London anesthetist Henry E. G. "Cockie" Boyle, who acknowledged his debt to the American when he incorporated Gwathmey's concepts in the first of the series of "Boyle" machines that were marketed by Coxeter and British Oxygen Corporation. During the same period in Lubeck, Germany, Heinrich Draeger and his son, Bernhaard, adapted compressed gas technology, which they had originally developed for mine rescue equipment, to manufacture ether and chloroform–oxygen machines.

In the years after World War I, several US manufacturers continued to bring forward widely admired anesthesia machines. Richard von Foregger was an engineer who was exceptionally receptive to clinicians' suggestions for additional features for his machines. Elmer McKesson became one of the country's first specialists in anesthesiology in 1910 and developed a series of gas machines. In an era of flammable anesthetics, McKesson carried nitrous oxide anesthesia to its therapeutic limit by performing inductions with 100% nitrous oxide and thereafter adding small volumes of oxygen. If the resultant cyanosis became too profound, McKesson depressed a valve on his machine that flushed a small volume of oxygen into the circuit. Even though his techniques of primary and secondary saturation with nitrous oxide are no longer used, the oxygen flush valve is part of McKesson's legacy.

Alternative Circuits

A valveless device, the Ayre's T-piece, has found wide application in the management of intubated patients. Phillip Ayre practiced anesthesia in England when the limitations of equipment for pediatric patients produced what he described as "a protracted and sanguine battle between surgeon and anaesthetist, with the poor unfortunate baby as the battlefield".[42] In 1937, Ayre introduced his valveless T-piece to reduce the effort of breathing in neurosurgical patients. The T-piece soon became particularly popular for cleft palate repairs, as the surgeon had free access to the mouth. Positive-pressure ventilation could be achieved when the anesthetist obstructed the expiratory limb. In time, this ingenious, lightweight, non-rebreathing device evolved through more than 100 modifications for a variety of special situations. A significant alteration was Gordon Jackson Rees' circuit, which permitted improved control of ventilation by substituting a breathing bag on the outflow limb.[43] An alternative method to reduce the amount of equipment near the patient is provided by the coaxial circuit of the Bain–Spoerel apparatus.[44] This lightweight tube-within-a-tube has served very well in many circumstances since its Canadian innovators described it in 1972.

Ventilators

Mechanical ventilators are now an integral part of the anesthesia machine. Patients are ventilated during general anesthesia by electrical or gas-powered devices that are simple to control yet sophisticated in their function. The history of mechanical positive-pressure ventilation began with attempts to resuscitate victims of drowning by a bellows attached to a mask or tracheal tube. These experiments found little role in anesthetic care for many years. At the beginning of the twentieth century, however, several modalities were explored before intermittent positive-pressure machines evolved.

A series of artificial environments were created in response to the frustration experienced by thoracic surgeons who found that the lung collapsed when they incised the pleura. Between 1900 and 1910, continuous positive- or negative-pressure devices were created to maintain inflation of the lungs of a spontaneously breathing patient once the chest was opened. Brauer (1904) and Murphy (1905) placed the patient's head and neck in a box in which positive pressure was continually maintained. Sauerbruch (1904) created a negative-pressure operating chamber encompassing both the surgical team and the patient's body and from which only the patient's head projected.[45]

In 1907, the first intermittent positive-pressure device, the Draeger "Pulmotor," was developed to rhythmically inflate the lungs. This instrument and later American models such as the E & J Resuscitator were used almost exclusively by firefighters and mine rescue workers. In 1934, a Swedish team developed the "Spiropulsator," which C. Crafoord later modified for use during cyclopropane anesthesia.[46] Its action was controlled by a magnetic control valve called *the flasher,* a type first used to provide intermittent gas flow for the lights of navigational buoys. When Trier Morch, a Danish anesthesiologist, could not obtain a Spiropulsator during World War II, he fabricated the Morch "Respirator," which used a piston pump to rhythmically deliver a fixed volume of gas to the patient.[45]

A major stimulus to the development of ventilators came as a consequence of a devastating epidemic of poliomyelitis that struck Copenhagen, Denmark, in 1952. As scores of patients were admitted, the only effective ventilatory support that could be provided to patients with bulbar paralysis was continuous manual ventilation via a tracheostomy employing devices such as Waters' "to-and-fro" circuit. This succeeded only through the dedicated efforts of hundreds of volunteers. Medical students served in relays to ventilate paralyzed patients. The Copenhagen crisis stimulated a broad European interest in the development of portable ventilators in anticipation of another epidemic of poliomyelitis. At this time, the common practice in North American hospitals was to place polio patients with respiratory involvement in "iron lungs," metal cylinders that encased the body below the neck. Inspiration was caused by intermittent negative pressure created by an electric motor acting on a piston-like device occupying the foot of the chamber.

Some early American ventilators were adaptations of respiratory-assist machines originally designed for the delivery of aerosolized drugs for respiratory therapy. Two types employed the Bennett or Bird "flow-sensitive" valves. The Bennett valve was designed during World War II when a team of physiologists at the University of Southern California encountered difficulties in separating inspiration from expiration in an experimental apparatus designed to provide positive-pressure breathing for aviators at high altitude. An engineer, Ray Bennett, visited their laboratory, observed their problem, and resolved it with a mechanical flow-sensitive automatic valve. A second valving mechanism was later designed by an aeronautical engineer, Forrest Bird.

The use of the Bird and Bennett valves gained anesthetic application when the gas flow from the valve was directed into a rigid plastic jar containing a breathing bag or bellows as part of an anesthesia circuit. These "bag-in-bottle" devices mimicked the action of the clinician's hand as the gas flow compressed the bag, thereby providing positive-pressure inspiration. Passive exhalation was promoted by the descent of a weight on the bag or bellows.

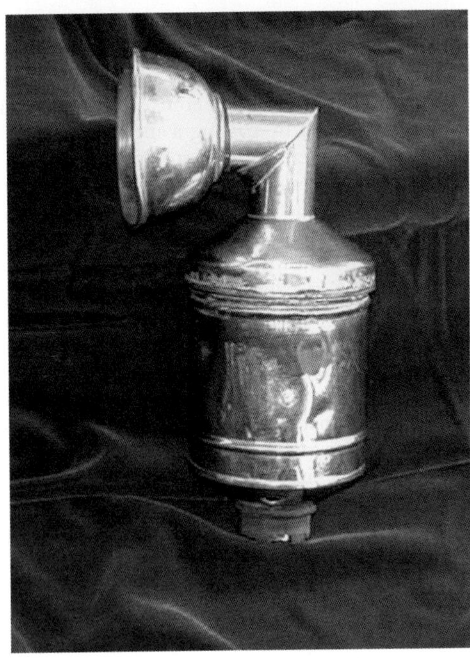

FIGURE 1-4. Waters' carbon dioxide absorbance canister.

Carbon Dioxide Absorption

Carbon dioxide (CO_2) absorbance is a basic element of modern anesthetic machines. It was initially developed to allow rebreathing of gas and minimize loss of flammable gases into the room, thereby reducing the risk of explosion. In current practice, it permits decreased utilization of oxygen and anesthetic, thus reducing cost. The first CO_2 absorber in anesthesia came in 1906 from the work of Franz Kuhn, a German surgeon. His use of canisters developed for mine rescues by Draeger was innovative, but his circuit had unfortunate limitations. The exceptionally narrow breathing tubes and a large dead space explain its very limited use, and Kuhn's device was ignored.

A few years later, the first American machine with a CO_2 absorber was independently fabricated by a pharmacologist named Dennis Jackson. In 1915, Jackson developed an early technique of CO_2 absorption that permitted the use of a closed anesthesia circuit. He used solutions of sodium and calcium hydroxide to absorb CO_2. As his laboratory was located in an area of St. Louis, Missouri, heavily laden with coal smoke, Jackson reported that the apparatus allowed him the first breaths of absolutely fresh air he had ever enjoyed in that city. The complexity of Jackson's apparatus limited its use in hospital practice, but his pioneering work in this field encouraged Ralph Waters to introduce a simpler device using soda lime granules 9 years later. Waters positioned a soda lime canister (Fig. 1-4) between a face mask and an adjacent breathing bag to which was attached the fresh gas flow. As long as the mask was held against the face, only small volumes of fresh gas flow were required and no valves were needed.[47]

Waters' device featured awkward positioning of the canister close to the patient's face. Brian Sword overcame this limitation in 1930 with a freestanding machine with unidirectional valves to create a circle system and an in-line CO_2 absorber.[48] James Elam and his coworkers at the Roswell Park Cancer Institute in Buffalo, New York, further refined the CO_2 absorber, increasing the efficiency of CO_2 removal with a minimum of resistance for breathing.[49] Consequently, the circle system introduced by Sword in the 1930s, with a few refinements, became the standard anesthesia circuit in North America.

Flowmeters

As closed and semiclosed circuits became practical, gas flow could be measured with greater accuracy. Bubble flowmeters were replaced with dry bobbins or ball-bearing flowmeters, which, although they did not leak fluids, could cause inaccurate measurements if they adhered to the glass column. In 1910, M. Neu had been the first to apply rotameters in anesthesia for the administration of nitrous oxide and oxygen, but his machine was not a commercial success, perhaps because of the great cost of nitrous oxide in Germany at that time. Rotameters designed for use in German industry were first employed in Britain in 1937 by Richard Salt; but as World War II approached, the English were denied access to these sophisticated flowmeters. After World War II rotameters became regularly employed in British anesthesia machines, although most American equipment still featured nonrotating floats. The now universal practice of displaying gas flow in liters per minute was not a customary part of all American machines until more than a decade after World War II.

Vaporizers

The art of a smooth induction with a potent anesthetic was a great challenge, particularly if the inspired concentration could not be determined with accuracy. Even the clinical introduction of halothane after 1956 might have been thwarted except for a fortunate coincidence: The prior development of calibrated vaporizers. Two types of calibrated vaporizers designed for other anesthetics had become available in the half decade before halothane was marketed. The prompt acceptance of halothane was in part because of an ability to provide it in carefully titrated concentrations.

The Copper Kettle was the first temperature-compensated, accurate vaporizer. It had been developed by Lucien Morris at the University of Wisconsin in response to Ralph Waters' plan to test chloroform by giving it in controlled concentrations.[50] Morris achieved this goal by passing a metered flow of oxygen through a vaporizer chamber that contained a sintered bronze disk to separate the oxygen into minute bubbles. The gas became fully saturated with anesthetic vapor as it percolated through the liquid. The concentration of the anesthetic inspired by the patient could be calculated by knowing the vapor pressure of the liquid anesthetic, the volume of oxygen flowing through the liquid, and the total volume of gases from all sources entering the anesthesia circuit. Although experimental models of Morris' vaporizer used a water bath to maintain stability, the excellent thermal conductivity of copper, especially when the device was attached to a metal anesthetic machine, was substituted in later models. When first marketed, the Copper Kettle did not feature a mechanism to indicate changes in the temperature (and vapor pressure) of the liquid. Shuh-Hsun Ngai proposed the incorporation of a thermometer, a suggestion that was later added to all vaporizers of that class.[51] The Copper Kettle (Foregger Company) and the Vernitrol (Ohio Medical Products) were universal vaporizers that could be charged with any anesthetic liquid, and, provided that its vapor pressure and temperature were known, the inspired concentration could be calculated quickly.

When halothane was first marketed in Britain, an effective temperature-compensated, agent-specific vaporizer had recently been placed in clinical use. The TECOTA (TEmperature COmpensated Trichloroethylene Air) vaporizer featured a bimetallic strip composed of brass and a nickel–steel alloy, two metals with different coefficients of expansion. As the anesthetic vapor cooled, the strip bent to move away from the orifice, thereby permitting more fresh gas to enter the vaporizing chamber. This maintained a constant inspired concentration despite changes in temperature and vapor pressure. After their TECOTA vaporizer was accepted into anesthetic practice, the technology was used to create the "Fluotec," the first of a series of agent-specific "tec" vaporizers for use in the operating room.

Patient Monitors

In many ways, the history of late-nineteenth and early-twentieth century anesthesiology is the quest for the safest anesthetic. The discovery and widespread use of electrocardiography, pulse oximetry, blood gas analysis, capnography, and neuromuscular blockade monitoring have reduced patient morbidity and mortality and revolutionized anesthesia practice. While safer machines assured clinicians that appropriate gas mixtures were delivered to the patient, monitors provided an early warning of acute physiologic deterioration before patients suffered irrevocable damage.

Joseph Clover was one of the first clinicians to routinely perform basic hemodynamic monitoring. Clover developed the habit of monitoring his patients' pulse but surprisingly, this was a contentious issue at the time. Prominent Scottish surgeons scorned Clover's emphasis on the action of chloroform on the heart. Baron Lister and others preferred that senior medical students give anesthetics and urged them to "strictly carry out certain simple instructions, among which is that of never touching the pulse, in order that their attention may not be distracted from the respiration".[52] Lister also counseled, "it appears that preliminary examination of the chest, often considered indispensable, is quite unnecessary, and more likely to induce the dreaded syncope, by alarming the patients, than to avert it".[53] Little progress in anesthesia could come from such reactionary statements. In contrast, Clover had observed the effect of chloroform on animals and urged other anesthetists to monitor the pulse at all times and to discontinue the anesthetic temporarily if any irregularity or weakness was observed in the strength of the pulse.

Two American surgeons, George W. Crile and Harvey Cushing, developed a strong interest in measuring blood pressure during anesthesia. Both men wrote thorough and detailed examinations of blood pressure monitoring; however, Cushing's contribution is better remembered because he was the first American to apply the Riva Rocci cuff, which he saw while visiting Italy. Cushing introduced the concept in 1902 and had blood pressure measurements recorded on anesthesia records.[54] In 1894, Cushing and a fellow student at Harvard Medical School, Charles Codman, initiated a system of recording patients' pulses to assess the course of the anesthetics they administered. In 1902, Cushing continued the practice of monitoring and recording patient blood pressures and pulses. The transition from manual to automated blood pressure devices, which first appeared in 1936 and operate on an oscillometric principle, has been gradual.

The first precordial stethoscope was believed to have been used by S. Griffith Davis at Johns Hopkins University.[38] He adapted a technique developed by Harvey Cushing in a laboratory in which dogs with surgically induced valvular lesions had stethoscopes attached to their chest wall so that medical students might listen to bruits characteristic of a specific malformation. Davis' technique was forgotten but was rehabilitated by Dr. Robert Smith, an energetic pioneer of pediatric anesthesiology in Boston in the 1940s. A Canadian contemporary, Albert Codesmith, of the Hospital for Sick Children, Toronto, became frustrated by the repeated dislodging of the chest piece under the surgical drapes and fabricated his first esophageal stethoscope from urethral catheters and Penrose drains. His brief report heralded its clinical role as a monitor of both normal and adventitious respiratory and cardiac sounds.[55]

Electrocardiography, Pulse Oximetry, and Capnography

Clinical electrocardiography began with Willem Einthoven's application of the string galvanometer in 1903. Within two decades, Thomas Lewis had described its role in the diagnosis of disturbances of cardiac rhythm, while James Herrick and Harold Pardee first drew attention to the changes produced by myocardial ischemia. After 1928, cathode ray oscilloscopes were available, but the risk of explosion owing to the presence of flammable anesthetics forestalled the introduction of the electrocardiogram into routine anesthetic practice until after World War II. At that time, the small screen of the heavily shielded "bullet" oscilloscope displayed only 3 seconds of data, but that information was highly prized.

Pulse oximetry, the optical measurement of oxygen saturation in tissues, is one of the more recent additions to the anesthesiologist's array of routine monitors. Although research in this area began in 1932, its first practical application came during World War II. An American physiologist, Glen Millikan, responded to a request from British colleagues in aviation research. Millikan set about preparing a series of devices to improve the supply of oxygen that was provided to pilots flying at high altitude in unpressurized aircraft. To monitor oxygen delivery and to prevent the pilot from succumbing to an unrecognized failure of his oxygen supply, Millikan created an oxygen-sensing monitor worn on the pilot's earlobe and coined the name *oximeter* to describe its action. Before his tragic death in a climbing accident in 1947, Millikan had begun to assess anesthetic applications of oximetry.

Refinements of oximetry by a Japanese engineer, Takuo Aoyagi, led to the development of pulse oximetry. As John Severinghaus recounted the episode, Aoyagi had attempted to eliminate the changes in a signal caused by pulsatile variations when he realized that this fluctuation could be used to measure both the pulse and oxygen saturation.[53]

Anesthesiologists have recognized a need for breath-by-breath measurement of respiratory and anesthetic gases. After 1954, infrared absorption techniques gave immediate displays of the exhaled concentration of CO_2. The ability to confirm endotracheal intubation and monitor ventilation, as reflected by concentrations of CO_2 in respired gas, began in 1943. At that time, K. Luft described the principle of infrared absorption by CO_2 and he developed an apparatus for measurement.[56] Routine application of capnography in anesthesia practice was pioneered by Dr. Bob Smalhout and Dr. Zden Kalenda in the Netherlands. Breath-to-breath continuous monitoring and a waveform display of CO_2 levels help anesthesiologists recognize abnormalities in metabolism, ventilation, and circulation. More recently, infrared analysis has been perfected to enable breath-by-breath measurement of anesthetic gases as well. This technology has largely replaced mass spectrometry, which initially had only industrial applications before Albert Faulconer of the Mayo Clinic first used it to monitor the concentration of an exhaled anesthetic in 1954.

Safety Standards

4 The introduction of safety features was coordinated by the American National Standards Institute (ANSI) Committee Z79, which was sponsored from 1956 until 1983 by the American Society of Anesthesiologists. Since 1983, representatives from industry, government, and health-care professions have met on Committee Z79 of the American Society for Testing and Materials. They establish voluntary goals that may become accepted national standards for the safety of anesthesia equipment.

Ralph Tovell voiced the first call for standards during World War II while he was the US Army Consultant in Anesthesiology for Europe. Tovell found that, as there were four different dimensions for connectors, tubes, masks, and breathing bags, supplies dispatched to field hospitals might not match their anesthesia machines. As Tovell observed, "When a sudden need for accessory equipment arose, nurses and corpsmen were likely to respond to it by bringing parts that would not fit".[57] Although Tovell's reports did not gain an immediate response, after the war Vincent Collins and Hamilton Davis took up his concern and formed the ANSI Committee Z79. One of the committee's most active members, Leslie Rendell-Baker, wrote an account of the committee's domestic and international achievements.[58] He reported that Tovell encouraged all manufacturers to select the now uniform orifice of 22 mm for all adult and pediatric face masks and to make every tracheal tube connector 15 mm in diameter. For the first time, a Z79-designed mask-tube elbow adapter would fit every mask and tracheal tube connector.

The Z79 Committee introduced other advances. Tracheal tubes of nontoxic plastic bear a Z79 or IT (*i*mplantation *t*ested) mark. The committee also mandated touch identification of oxygen flow control on the anesthesia machine at the suggestion of Roderick Calverley,[59] which reduced the risk that the wrong gas would be selected before internal mechanical controls prevented the selection of an hypoxic mixture. Pin indexing reduced the hazard of attaching a wrong cylinder in the place of oxygen. Diameter indexing of connectors prevented similar errors in high-pressure tubing. For many years, however, errors committed in reassembling hospital oxygen supply lines led to a series of tragedies before polarographic oxygen analyzers were added to the inspiratory limb of the anesthesia circuit.

THE HISTORY OF ANESTHETIC AGENTS AND ADJUVANTS

Inhaled Anesthetics

Throughout the second half of the nineteenth century, other compounds were examined for their anesthetic potential. The pattern of fortuitous discovery that brought nitrous oxide, diethyl ether, and chloroform forward between 1844 and 1847 continued. The next inhaled anesthetics to be used routinely, ethyl chloride and ethylene, were also discovered as a result of unexpected observations. Ethyl chloride and ethylene were first formulated in the eighteenth century. Ethyl chloride was used as a topical anesthetic and counterirritant; it was so volatile that the skin transiently "froze" after ethyl chloride was sprayed on it. Its rediscovery as an anesthetic came in 1894, when a Swedish dentist named Carlson sprayed ethyl chloride into a patient's mouth to "freeze" a dental abscess. Carlson was surprised to discover that his patient suddenly lost consciousness.

As the mechanisms to deliver drugs were refined, entirely new classes of medications were also developed, with the intention of providing safer, more pleasant pain control. Ethylene gas was the first alternative to ether and chloroform, but it had some major disadvantages. The rediscovery of ethylene in 1923 also came from a serendipitous observation. After it was learned that ethylene gas had been used to inhibit the opening of carnation buds in Chicago greenhouses, it was speculated that a gas that put flowers to sleep might also have an anesthetic action on humans. Arno Luckhardt was the first to publish a clinical study in February 1923. Within a month, Isabella Herb in Chicago and W. Easson Brown in Toronto presented two other independent studies. Ethylene was not a successful anesthetic because high concentrations were required and it was explosive. An additional significant shortcoming was a particularly unpleasant smell, which could only be partially disguised by the use of oil of orange or a cheap perfume. When cyclopropane was introduced, ethylene was abandoned.

The anesthetic action of cyclopropane was inadvertently discovered in 1929.[60] Brown and Henderson had previously shown that propylene had desirable properties as an anesthetic when freshly prepared, but after storage in a steel cylinder, it deteriorated to create a toxic material that produced nausea and cardiac irregularities in humans. Velyien Henderson, a professor of pharmacology at the University of Toronto, suggested that the toxic product be identified. After a chemist, George Lucas, identified cyclopropane among the chemicals in the tank, he prepared a sample in low concentration with oxygen and administered it to two kittens. The animals fell asleep quietly but quickly recovered unharmed. Rather than being a toxic contaminant, Lucas saw that cyclopropane was a potent anesthetic. After its effects in other animals were studied and cyclopropane proved to be stable after storage, human experimentation began.

Henderson was the first volunteer; Lucas followed. They then arranged a public demonstration in which Frederick Banting, a Nobel laureate for the discovery of insulin, was anesthetized before a group of physicians. Despite this promising beginning, further research was abruptly halted. Several anesthetic deaths in Toronto had been attributed to ethyl chloride, and concern about Canadian clinical trials of cyclopropane prevented human studies from proceeding. Rather than abandon the study, Henderson encouraged an American friend, Ralph Waters, to use cyclopropane at the University of Wisconsin. The Wisconsin group investigated the drug thoroughly and reported their clinical success in 1934.[61]

In 1930, Chauncey Leake and MeiYu Chen performed successful laboratory trials of vinethene (divinyl ether) but were thwarted in its further development by a professor of surgery in San Francisco. Ironically, Canadians, who had lost cyclopropane to Wisconsin, learned of vinethene from Leake and Chen in California and conducted the first human study in 1932 at the University of Alberta, Edmonton. International research collaboration enabled early anesthetic use of both cyclopropane and divinyl ether, advances that may not have occurred independently in either the United States or Canada.

All potent anesthetics of this period were explosive save for chloroform, whose hepatic and cardiac toxicity limited use in America. Anesthetic explosions remained a rare but devastating risk to both anesthesiologist and patient. To reduce the danger of explosion during the incendiary days of World War II, British anesthetists turned to trichloroethylene. This nonflammable anesthetic found limited application in America, as it decomposed to release phosgene when warmed in the presence of soda lime. By the end of World War II, however, another class of noninflammable anesthetics was prepared for laboratory trials. Ten years later, fluorinated hydrocarbons revolutionized inhalation anesthesia.

Fluorine, the lightest and most reactive halogen, forms exceptionally stable bonds. These bonds, although sometimes created with explosive force, resist separation by chemical or thermal means. For that reason, many early attempts to fluorinate hydrocarbons in a controlled manner were frustrated by the marked chemical activity of fluorine. In 1930, the first commercial application of fluorine chemistry came in the form of the refrigerant, Freon. This was followed by the first attempt to prepare a fluorinated anesthetic by Harold Booth and E. May Bixby in 1932. Although their drug, monochlorodifluoromethane, was devoid of anesthetic action, as were other drugs studied that decade, their report predicted future developments. "A survey of the properties of 166 known gases suggested that the best possibility of finding a new noncombustible anesthetic gas lay in the field of organic fluoride compounds. Fluorine substitution for other halogens lowers the boiling point, increases stability, and generally decreases toxicity".[62]

After the war, a team at the University of Maryland under professor of pharmacology John C. Krantz, Jr., investigated the anesthetic properties of dozens of hydrocarbons over a period of several years, but only one, ethyl vinyl ether, entered clinical use in 1947. Because it was flammable, Krantz requested that it be fluorinated. In response, Julius Shukys prepared several fluorinated analogs. One of these, trifluoroethyl vinyl ether, or fluroxene, became the first fluorinated anesthetic. Fluroxene, which was nonflammable in concentrations needed for anesthesia, was marketed from 1954 until 1974.

In 1951, Charles Suckling, a British chemist of Imperial Chemical Industries, was asked to create a new anesthetic. Suckling, who already had an expert understanding of fluorination, began by asking clinicians to describe the properties of an ideal anesthetic. He learned from this inquiry that his search must consider several limiting factors, including the volatility, inflammability, stability, and potency of the compounds. After 2 years of research and testing, Charles Suckling created halothane. He first determined that halothane possessed anesthetic action by anesthetizing mealworms and houseflies before he forwarded it to pharmacologist James Raventos. Suckling also made accurate predictions as to the concentrations required for anesthesia in higher animals. After Raventos completed a favorable review, halothane was offered to Michael Johnstone, a respected anesthetist of Manchester, England, who recognized its great advantages over other anesthetics available in 1956. After Johnstone's endorsement, halothane use spread quickly and widely within the practice of anesthesia.[63]

Halothane was followed in 1960 by methoxyflurane, an anesthetic that remained popular for a decade. By 1970, however, it was learned that dose-related nephrotoxicity following protracted methoxyflurane anesthesia was caused by inorganic fluoride. Similarly, because of persisting concern that rare cases of hepatitis following anesthesia might be a result of a metabolite of halothane, the search for newer inhaled anesthetics focused on the resistance to metabolic degradation.

Two fluorinated liquid anesthetics, enflurane and its isomer isoflurane, were results of the search for increased stability. They were synthesized by Ross Terrell in 1963 and 1965, respectively. Since enflurane was easier to create, it preceded isoflurane. Its application was restricted after it was shown to be a marked cardiovascular depressant and to have some convulsant properties. Isoflurane was nearly abandoned because of difficulties in its purification, but after Louise Speers overcame this problem, several successful trials were published in 1971. The release of isoflurane for clinical use was delayed again for more than half a decade by calls for repeated testing in lower animals, owing to an unfounded concern that the drug might be carcinogenic. As a consequence, isoflurane received more thorough testing than any other drug heretofore used in anesthesia. The era when an anesthetic could be introduced following a single fortuitous observation had given way to a cautious program of assessment and reassessment. Remarkably, no anesthetics were introduced into clinical use for another 20 years. Finally, desflurane was released in 1992 and sevoflurane was released in 1994. Xenon, a gas having many properties of the ideal anesthetic, was administered to a few patients in the early 1950s but it never gained popularity because of the extreme costs associated with its removal from air. However, interest in xenon has been renewed now that gas concentrations can be accurately measured when administered at low flows, and devices are available to scavenge and reuse the gas.

Intravenous Anesthetics

Prior to William Harvey's description of a complete and continuous intravascular circuit in *De Motu Cordis* (1628), it was widely held that blood emanated from the heart and was propelled to the periphery where it was consumed. The idea that substances could be injected intravascularly and travel systemically probably originated with Christopher Wren. In 1657, Wren injected aqueous opium into a dog through a goose quill attached to a pig's bladder, rendering the animal "stupefied".[64] Wren similarly injected intravenous *crocus metallorum,* an impure preparation of antimony, and observed the animals to vomit and then die. Knowledge of a circulatory system and intravascular access spurred investigations in other areas, and Wren's contemporary, Richard Lower, performed the first blood transfusions of lamb's blood into dogs and other animals.

In the mid-nineteenth century, equipment necessary for effective intravascular injections was conceived. Vaccination lancets were used in the 1830s to puncture the skin and force morphine paste subcutaneously for analgesia.[65] The hollow needle and hypodermic syringe were developed in the following decades but were not initially designed for intravenous use. In 1845, Dublin surgeon Francis Rynd created the hollow needle for injection of morphine into nerves in the treatment of "neuralgias." Similarly, Charles Gabriel Pravaz designed the first functional syringe in

1853 for perineural injections. Alexander Wood, however, is generally credited with perfecting the hypodermic glass syringe. In 1855, Wood published an article on the injection of opiates into painful spots by the use of hollow needle and his glass syringe.[66]

In 1872, Pierre Oré of Lyons performed what is perhaps the first successful intravenous surgical anesthetic by injecting chloral hydrate immediately prior to incision. His 1875 publication describes its use in 36 patients but several postoperative deaths lent little to recommend this method to other practitioners.[67] In 1909, Ludwig Burkhardt produced surgical anesthesia by intravenous injections of chloroform and ether in Germany. Seven years later, Elisabeth Bredenfeld of Switzerland reported the use of intravenous morphine and scopolamine. The trials failed to show an improvement over inhaled techniques. Intravenous anesthesia found little application or popularity, primarily because of a lack of suitable drugs. In the following decades, this would change.

The first barbiturate, barbital, was synthesized in 1903 by Fischer and von Mering. Phenobarbital and all other successors of barbital had very protracted action and found little use in anesthesia. After 1929, oral pentobarbital was used as a sedative before surgery, but when it was given in anesthetic concentrations, long periods of unconsciousness followed. The first short-acting oxybarbiturate was hexobarbital (Evipal), available clinically in 1932. Hexobarbital was enthusiastically received by the anesthesia communities in Europe and North America because its abbreviated induction time was unrivaled by any other technique. A London anesthetist, Ronald Jarman, found that it had a dramatic advantage over inhalation inductions for minor procedures. Jarman instructed his patients to raise one arm while he injected hexobarbital into a vein of the opposite forearm. When the upraised arm fell, indicating the onset of hypnosis, the surgeon could begin. Patients were also amazed in that many awoke unable to believe they had been anesthetized.[68]

Even though the prompt action of hexobarbital had a dramatic effect on the conduct of anesthesia, it was soon replaced by two thiobarbiturates. In 1932, Donalee Tabern and Ernest H. Volwiler of the Abbott Company synthesized thiopental (Pentothal®) and thiamylal (Surital®). The sulfated barbiturates proved to be more satisfactory, potent, and rapid acting than were their oxybarbiturate analogs. Thiopental was first administered to a patient at the University of Wisconsin in March 1934, but the successful introduction of thiopental into clinical practice followed a thorough investigation conducted by John Lundy and his colleagues at the Mayo Clinic in June 1934.

When first introduced, thiopental was often given in repeated increments as the primary anesthetic for protracted procedures. Its hazards were soon appreciated. At first, depression of respiration was monitored by the simple expedient of observing the motion of a wisp of cotton placed over the nose. Only a few skilled practitioners were prepared to pass a tracheal tube if the patient stopped breathing. Such practitioners realized that thiopental without supplementation did not suppress airway reflexes, and they therefore encouraged the prophylactic provision of topical anesthesia of the airway beforehand. The vasodilatory effects of thiobarbiturates were widely appreciated only when thiopental caused cardiovascular collapse in hypovolemic burned civilian and military patients in World War II. In response, fluid replacement was used more aggressively and thiopental administered with greater caution.

In 1962, ketamine was synthesized by Dr. Calvin Stevens at the Parke Davis Laboratories in Ann Arbor, Michigan. One of the cyclohexylamine compounds that includes phencyclidine, ketamine was the only drug of this group that gained clinical utility. The other compounds produced undesirable postanesthetic delirium and psychomimetic reactions. In 1966, the neologism "dissociative anesthesia" was created by Guenter Corrsen and Edward Domino to describe the trance-like state of profound analgesia produced by ketamine.[69] It was released for use in 1970, and although it remains primarily an agent for anesthetic induction, its analgesic properties are increasingly studied and used by pain specialists.

Etomidate was first described by Paul Janssen and his colleagues in 1964 and originally given the name hypnomidate. Its key advantages, minimal hemodynamic depression and lack of histamine release, account for its ongoing utility in clinical practice. It was released for use in 1974 and despite its drawbacks (pain on injection, myoclonus, postoperative nausea and vomiting [PONV], and inhibition of adrenal steroidogenesis), etomidate is often the drug of choice for anesthetizing hemodynamically unstable patients.

Propofol, or 2,6-diisopropylphenol, was first synthesized by Imperial Chemical Industries and tested clinically in 1977. Investigators found that it produced hypnosis quickly with minimal excitation and that patients awoke promptly once the drug was discontinued. In addition to its excellent induction characteristics, the antiemetic action of propofol made it an agent of choice in patient populations prone to nausea and emesis. Regrettably, Cremophor EL, the solvent with which it was formulated, produced several severe anaphylactic reactions and it was withdrawn from use. Once propofol was reformulated with egg lecithin, glycerol, and soybean oil, the drug reentered clinical practice and gained great success. Its popularity in Britain coincided with the introduction of the LMA, and it was soon noted that propofol suppressed pharyngeal reflexes to a degree that permitted the insertion of an LMA without a need for either muscle relaxants or potent inhaled anesthetics.

Local Anesthetics

Centuries after the conquest of Peru, Europeans became aware of the stimulating properties of a local, indigenous plant that the Peruvians called *khoka. Khoka,* which meant *the plant,* quickly became known as *coca* in Europe. In 1860, shortly after the Austrian Carl von Scherzer imported enough coca leaves to allow for analysis, German chemists Albert Niemann and Wilhelm Lossen isolated the main alkaloid and named it *cocaine.* Twenty-five years later, at the recommendation of his friend Sigmund Freud, Carl Koller became interested in the effects of cocaine. After several animal experiments, Koller successfully demonstrated the analgesic properties of cocaine applied to the eye in a patient with glaucoma.[70] Unfortunately, nearly simultaneous with the first reports of cocaine use, there were reports of central nervous system and cardiovascular toxicity.[71,72] As the popularity of cocaine grew, so did the frequency of toxic reactions and cocaine addictions.[73] Skepticism about the use of cocaine quickly grew within the medical community, forcing the pharmacologic industry to develop alternative local anesthetics.

In 1898, Alfred Eihorn synthesized nirvaquine, the first amino amide local anesthetic.[74] Nirvaquine proved to be an irritant to tissues and its use was immediately stopped. Returning his attention toward the development of amino ester local anesthetics, Eihorn synthesized benzocaine in 1900 and procaine (Novocaine) shortly after in 1905. Amino esters were commonly used for local infiltration and spinal anesthesia despite their low potency and high likelihood to cause allergic reactions. Tetracaine, the last (and probably safest) amino ester local anesthetic developed, proved to be quite useful for many years.

In 1944, Nils Löfgren and Bengt Lundquist developed lidocaine, an amino amide local anesthetic.[73] Lidocaine gained immediate popularity because of its potency, rapid onset, decreased incidence of allergic reactions, and overall effectiveness for all types of regional anesthetic blocks. Since the introduction of lidocaine, all local anesthetics developed and marketed have been of the amino amide variety.

Because of the increase in lengthy and sophisticated surgical procedures, the development of a long-acting local anesthetic took precedence. From that demand, bupivacaine was introduced in 1965. Synthesized by B. Ekenstam in 1957,[75] bupivacaine was initially discarded after it was found to be highly toxic. By 1980, several years after being introduced to the United States, there were several reports of almost simultaneous seizures *and* cardiovascular collapse following unintended intravascular injection.[76] Shortly after this, as a result of the cardiovascular toxicity associated with bupivacaine and the profound motor block associated with etidocaine, the pharmaceutical industry began searching for a new long-acting alternative. Introduced in 1996, ropivacaine is structurally similar to mepivacaine and bupivacaine, although it is prepared as a single levorotatory isomer rather than a racemic mixture. The levorotatory isomer has less potential for toxicity than the dextrorotatory isomer.[77] The potential safety of ropivacaine is controversial because ropivacaine is approximately 25% less potent than bupivacaine. Therefore, at equal-potent doses the margin of safety between ropivacaine and bupivacaine becomes less apparent, although systemic toxicity with ropivacaine may respond more quickly to conventional resuscitation.[78]

Each local anesthetic developed has had its own positive and negative attributes, which is why some are still used today and others have fallen out of favor. Currently, the pharmaceutical industry is in the process of developing extended-release local anesthetics using liposomes and microspheres.[79,80]

Opioids

Opioids (historically referred to as *narcotics,* although semantically incorrect—see Chapter 19) remain the analgesic workhorse in anesthesia practice. They are used routinely in the perioperative period, in the management of acute pain, and in a variety of terminal and chronic pain states. The availability of short-, medium-, and long-acting opioids, as well as the many routes of administration, gives physicians considerable flexibility in the use of these agents. The analgesic and sedating properties of opium have been known for more than two millennia. Certainly the Greeks and Chinese civilizations harnessed these properties in medical and cultural practices. Opium is derived from the seeds of the poppy (*Papaver somniferum*) and is an amalgam of more than 25 pharmacologic alkaloids. The first alkaloid isolated, morphine, was extracted by Prussian chemist Freidrich A. W. Sertürner in 1803. He named this alkaloid after the Greek god of dreams, Morpheus. Morphine became commonly used as a supplement to inhaled anesthesia and for postoperative pain control during the latter half of the nineteenth century. Codeine, another alkaloid of opium, was isolated in 1832 by Robiquet but its relatively weaker analgesic potency and nausea at higher doses limits its role in managing moderate-to-severe perioperative surgical pain.

Meperidine was the first synthetic opioid and was developed in 1939 by two German researchers at IG Farben, Otto Eisleb and O. Schaumann. Although many pharmacologists are remembered for the introduction of a single drug, one prolific researcher, Paul Janssen, has since 1953 brought forward more than 70 agents from among 70,000 chemicals created in his laboratory. His products have had profound effects on disciplines as disparate as parasitology and psychiatry. The pace of productive innovation in Janssen's research laboratory is astonishing. Chemical R4263 (fentanyl), synthesized in 1960, was followed only a year later by R4749 (droperidol), and then etomidate in 1964. Innovar, the fixed combination of fentanyl and droperidol, is less popular now but Janssen's phenylpiperidine derivatives, fentanyl, sufentanil, and alfentanil, are staples in the anesthesia pharmacopeia. Remifentanil, an ultra short-acting opioid introduced by Glaxo-Wellcome in 1996, is a departure from other opioids in that it has very rapid onset and equally rapid offset due to metabolism by nonspecific tissue esterases. Ketorolac, a nonsteroidal anti-inflammatory drug (NSAID) approved for use in 1990, was the first parenteral NSAID indicated for postoperative pain. With a 6 to 8 mg morphine equivalent analgesic potency, Ketorolac provides significant postoperative pain control and has particular use when an opioid-sparing approach is essential. Ketorolac use is limited by side effects and may be inappropriate in patients with underlying renal dysfunction, bleeding problems, or compromised bone healing.

Muscle Relaxants

Muscle relaxants entered anesthesia practice nearly a century after inhalational anesthetics (Table 1-1). Curare, the first known neuromuscular blocking agent, was originally used in hunting and tribal warfare by native peoples of South America. The curares are alkaloids prepared from plants native to equatorial rain forests. The refinement of the harmless sap of several species of vines into toxins that were lethal (through creation of total muscular paralysis and apnea) only when injected was an extraordinary triumph introduced by paleopharmacologists in loincloths. Their discovery was more remarkable because it was independently repeated on three separate continents—South America, Africa, and Asia. These jungle tribes also developed nearly identical methods of delivering the toxin by darts, which, after being dipped in curare, maintained their potency indefinitely until they were propelled through blowpipes to strike the flesh of monkeys and other animals of the treetops. Moreover, the American Indians knew of the juice of an herb that would counteract the effects of the poison if administered in time.[81]

The earliest clinical use of curare in humans was to ameliorate the tortuous muscle spasms of infectious tetanus. In 1858, New York physician Louis Albert Sayres reported two cases in which he attempted to treat severe tetanus with curare at the Bellevue Hospital. Both his patients died. Similar efforts were undertaken to use muscle relaxants to treat epilepsy, rabies, and choreiform disorders. Treatment of Parkinson-like rigidity and the prevention of trauma from seizure therapy also preceded the use of curare in anesthesia.[82]

Interestingly, curare antagonists were developed well before muscle relaxants were ever used in surgery. In 1900, Jacob Pal, a Viennese physician, recognized that curare could be antagonized by physostigmine. This substance had been isolated from the calabar bean some 36 years earlier by Scottish pharmacologist Sir T. R. Fraser. Neostigmine methylsulfate was synthesized in 1931 and was significantly more potent in antagonizing the effects of curare.[83]

In 1938, Richard and Ruth Gill returned to New York from South America, bringing with them 11.9 kg of crude curare collected near their Ecuadorian ranch. Their motivation was a mixture of personal and altruistic goals. Some months before, while on an earlier visit to the United States, Richard Gill learned that he had multiple sclerosis. His physician, Dr. Walter Freeman, mentioned the possibility that curare might have a therapeutic role in the management of spastic disorders. When the Gills returned to

TABLE 1-1. EVENTS IN THE DEVELOPMENT OF MUSCLE RELAXANTS

Year	Event
1516	Peter Martyr d'Anghera, *De orbe novo,* published account of South American Indian arrow poisons
1596	Sir Walter Raleigh provides detailed account of arrow poison effects and antidote
1745	Charles-Marie de la Condamine returns from Ecuador and conducts curare experiments with chickens and attempted to use sugar as an antidote
1780	Abbe Felix Fontana inserts curare directly into exposed sciatic nerve of rabbit without effect and concludes that mechanism is the destruction of the irritability of voluntary muscles. Publishes *On the American Poison Ticunas* (name of South American tribe)
1811	Benjamin Collins Brodie demonstrates that animals mechanically ventilated may survive significant doses of curare
1812	William Sewell suggests use of curare in "hydrophobia" (rabies) and tetanus
1844	Claude Bernard determines that death occurs by respiratory failure, motor nerves are unable to transmit stimuli from higher centers, differential effect on muscles with peripheral and thoracic muscles being affected before respiratory muscles. Bernard concludes that the site of action is the junction between muscles and nerves, neuromuscular junction
1858	Louis Albert Sayres, New York physician, uses curare to treat tetanus in two patients
1864	Physostigmine isolated from Calabar beans by Sir T. R. Fraser, a Scottish pharmacologist
1886–1897	R. Boehm, a German chemist, demonstrated three separate classes of alkaloids in each of three types of indigenous containers: Tube-curares, pot-curares, and calabash-curares
1900	Jacob Pal recognizes that physostigmine can antagonize the effects of curare
1906	Succinylcholine, prepared by Reid Hunt and R. Taveau, experimented on rabbits pretreated with curare to learn of cardiac effects and so paralysis went unrecognized
1912	Arthur Lawen uses curare in surgery but report published in German so it goes largely unrecognized
1938	Richard and Ruth Gill bring large quantity of curare to New York for further study by pharmaceutical company
1939	Abram E. Bennett uses curare in children with spastic disorders and to prevent trauma from metrazol therapy (precursor to electroconvulsive therapy [ECT])
1942	Harold Griffith and Enid Johnson use curare for abdominal relaxation in surgery
1942	H. A. Halody develops rabbit head-drop assay for standardization and large-scale production of curare and d-tubocurarine
1948	Decamethonium, a depolarizing relaxant, is synthesized
1949	Succinylcholine prepared by Daniel Bovet and the following year by J. C. Castillo and Edwin de Beer
1956	Distinction between depolarizing and non-depolarizing neuromuscular blockade is made by William D. M. Paton
1964	Pancuronium released for use in humans, synthesized by Savage and Hewett
1979	Vecuronium introduced, specifically designed to be more hepatically metabolized than pancuronium
1993	Mivacurium released for clinical use
1994	Rocuronium introduced to clinical practice

the United States with their supply of crude curare, they encouraged scientists at E. R. Squibb & Co. to take an interest in its unique properties. Squibb soon offered semirefined curare to two groups of American anesthesiologists, who assessed its action but quickly abandoned their studies when it caused total respiratory paralysis in two patients and the death of laboratory animals.

The earliest effective clinical application of curare in medicine occurred in physiatry. After A. R. McIntyre refined a portion of the raw curare in 1939, Abram E. Bennett of Omaha, Nebraska, injected it into children with spastic disorders. While no persistent benefit could be observed in these patients, he next administered it to patients about to receive metrazol, a precursor to electroconvulsive therapy. Because it eliminated seizure-induced fractures, they termed it a "shock absorber." By 1941, other psychiatrists followed this practice and, when they found that the action of curare was protracted, occasionally used neostigmine as an antidote.

Curare was used initially in surgery by Arthur Lawen in 1912, but the published report was written in German and was ignored for decades. Lawen, a physiologist and physician from Leipzig, used curare in his laboratory before boldly producing abdominal relaxation at a light level of anesthesia in a surgical patient. Lawen's efforts were not appreciated for decades, and while his pioneering work anticipated later clinical application, safe use would have to await the introduction of regular intubation of the trachea and controlled ventilation of the lungs.[84]

Thirty years after Lawen, Harold Griffith, the chief anesthetist of the Montreal Homeopathic Hospital, learned of A. E. Bennett's successful use of curare and resolved to apply it in anesthesia. As Griffith was already a master of tracheal intubation, he was much better prepared than were most of his contemporaries to attend to potential complications. On January 23, 1942, Griffith and his resident, Enid Johnson, anesthetized and intubated the trachea of a young man before injecting curare early in the course of his appendectomy. Satisfactory abdominal relaxation was obtained and the surgery proceeded without incident. Griffith and Johnson's report of the successful use of curare in the 25 patients of their series launched a revolution in anesthetic care.[85]

Anesthesiologists who practiced before muscle relaxants recall the anxiety they felt when a premature attempt to intubate the trachea under cyclopropane caused persisting laryngospasm. Before 1942, abdominal relaxation was possible only if the patient tolerated high concentrations of an inhaled anesthetic, which might bring profound respiratory depression and protracted recovery. Curare and the drugs that followed transformed anesthesia profoundly. Because intubation of the trachea could now be taught in a deliberate manner, a neophyte could fail on a first attempt

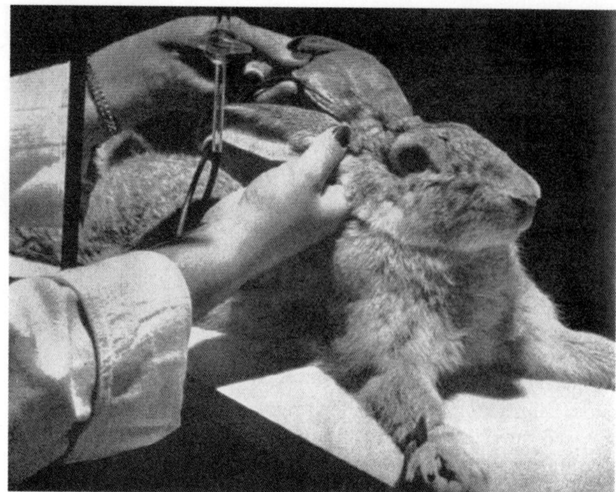

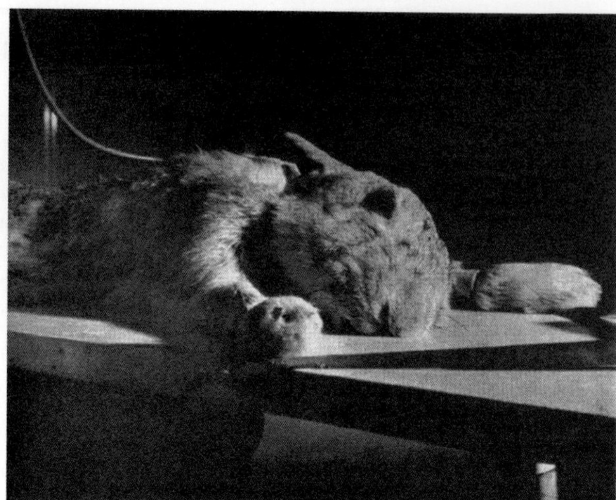

FIGURE 1-5. The rabbit head-drop assay. H. A. Halladay of Squibb pharmaceutical company developed a method of standardizing doses of curare and d-tubocurarine. A normal rabbit **(A)** had 0.1 mL of aqueous cecurane solution injected every 15 seconds until it could no longer raise its head **(B)**.

without compromising the safety of the patient. For the first time, abdominal relaxation could be attained when curare was supplemented by light planes of inhaled anesthetics or by a combination of intravenous agents providing "balanced anesthesia." New frontiers opened. Sedated and paralyzed patients could now successfully undergo the major physiologic trespasses of cardiopulmonary bypass, deliberate hypothermia, or long-term respiratory support after surgery.

Credit for successful and safe introduction of curare and d-tubocurarine into anesthesia must in part be given to a Squibb researcher named H. A. Holladay. Crude, unstandardized preparations of curare produced uncertain clinical effects and undesirable side effects related to various impurities. Isolation of d-tubocurarine in 1935 renewed clinical interest but a method for standardizing "Intocostrin" and its purer derivative, d-tubocurarine, had yet to be devised. In the early 1940s, in part as a result of Griffith and Johnson's successful trials, Squibb embarked on wide-scale production. Holaday developed a reliable, easily reproducible method for standardizing curare doses that became known as the rabbit head-drop assay (Fig. 1-5). The assay consisted of aqueous curare solution injected intravenously in 0.1 mL doses every 15 seconds until the end point, when the rabbit became unable to raise its head, was reached.[86]

Successful clinical use of curare led to the introduction of other muscle relaxants. By 1948, gallamine and decamethonium had been synthesized. Metubine, a curare "rediscovered" in the 1970s, was used clinically in the same year. Succinylcholine was prepared by the Nobel laureate Daniel Bovet in 1949 and was in wide international use before historians noted that the drug had been synthesized and tested long beforehand. In 1906, Reid Hunt and R. Taveaux prepared succinylcholine among a series of choline esters, which they had injected into rabbits to observe their cardiac effects. If their rabbits had not been previously paralyzed with curare, the depolarizing action of succinylcholine might have been recognized decades earlier.

The ability to monitor intraoperative neuromuscular blockade with nerve stimulators began in 1958. Working at St. Thomas' Hospital in London, T. H. Christie and H. Churchill-Davidson developed a method for monitoring peripheral neuromuscular blockade during anesthesia. It was not until 1970, however, that H. H. Ali and colleagues devised the technique of delivering four supramaximal impulses delivered at 2 Hz (0.5 seconds apart), or a "Train of Four," as a method of quantifying the degree of residual neuromuscular blockade.[87]

Research in relaxants was rekindled in 1960 when researchers became aware of the action of maloetine, a relaxant from the Congo basin. It was remarkable in that it had a steroidal nucleus. Investigations of maloetine led to pancuronium in 1968. In the 1970s and 1980s, research shifted toward identification of specific receptor biochemistry and development of receptor-specific drugs. From these isoquinolines, four related products emerged: Vecuronium, pipecuronium, rocuronium, and rapacuronium. Rapacuronium, released in the early 1990s, was withdrawn from clinical use after several cases of intractable bronchospasm led to brain damage or death. Four clinical products based on the steroid parent drug d-tubocurarine (atracurium, mivacurium, doxacurium, and *cis*-atracurium) also made it to clinical use. Recognition that atracurium and *cis*-atracurium undergo spontaneous degradation by Hoffmann elimination has defined a role for these muscle relaxants in patients with liver and renal insufficiency.

Antiemetics

Effective treatment for PONV evolved relatively recently and has been driven by incentives to limit hospitalization expenses and improve patient satisfaction. But PONV is an old problem for which late-nineteenth century practitioners recognized many causes including anxiety, severe pain, sudden changes in blood pressure, ileus, ingestion of blood, and the residual effects of opioids and inhalational anesthetics. Risk of pulmonary aspiration of gastric contents and subsequent death from asphyxia or aspiration pneumonia was a feared consequence of anesthetics, especially those preceding use of cuffed endotracheal tubes. Vomiting and aspiration during anesthesia led to the practice of maintaining an empty stomach preoperatively, a policy that continues today despite evidence that clear fluids up to 3 hours before surgery do not increase gastric volumes, change gastric pH, or increase the risk of aspiration.

A variety of treatments for nausea and vomiting were proposed by early anesthetists. James Gwathemy's 1914 publication, *Anesthesia,* commented that British surgeons customarily gave tincture of iodine in a teaspoonful of water every half hour for three or four doses. Inhalation of vinegar fumes and rectal injection of 30 to 40 drops of tincture of opium with 60 grains of sodium bromide were also thought to quiet the vomiting center.[88] Other practitioners attempted olfactory control by placing a piece of gauze moistened with essence of orange or an aromatic oil on the upper lip of the patient.[89] A 1937 anesthesia textbook encouraged treatment of PONV with lateral positioning, "iced soda water, strong black coffee, and chloretone".[90] Counterirritation, such as mustard leaf on the epigastrium, was also believed useful in limiting emesis.[91] As late as 1951, anesthesia texts recommended oxygen administration, whiffs of ammonia spirits, and control of blood pressure and positioning.[92] The complex central mechanisms of nausea and vomiting were largely unaffected by most of these treatments. Newer drugs capable of intervening at specific pathways were needed to have an impact on PONV. As more short-acting anesthetics were developed, the problem received sharper focus in awake postoperative patients in the recovery room. The nausea-attending use of newer chemotherapy agents provided additional impetus to the development of antiemetic medications.

In 1955, a nonrandomized study using the antihistamine cyclizine showed a reduction in PONV from 27% to 21% in a group of 3,000 patients. The following year, a more rigorous study by Knapp and Beecher reported a significant benefit from prophylaxis with the neuroleptic chlorpromazine. In 1957, promethazine (Phenergan) and chlorpromazine were both found to reduce PONV when used prophylactically. Thirteen years later, a double-blind study evaluating metoclopramide was published and that drug became a first-line drug in the management of PONV. Droperidol, released in the early 1960s, became widely used until 2001 when concerns regarding prolongation of QT intervals prompted a warning from the Food and Drug Administration about its continued use.

The antiemetic effects of corticosteroids were first recognized by oncologists treating intracranial edema from tumors.[93] Subsequent studies have borne out the antiemetic properties of this class of drugs in treating PONV. Recognition of the serotonin 5-HT3 pathway in PONV has led to a unique class of drugs devoted only to addressing this particular problem. Ondansetron, the first representative of this drug class, was approved by the Food and Drug Administration in 1991. Additional serotonin 5-HT3 antagonists have been approved and are available today.

ANESTHESIA SUBSPECIALTIES

Regional Anesthesia

5 Cocaine, an extract of the coca leaf, was the first effective local anesthetic. After Albert Niemann refined the active alkaloid and named it *cocaine,* it was used in experiments by a few investigators. It was noted that cocaine provided topical anesthesia and even produced local insensibility when injected, but Carl Koller, a Viennese surgical intern, first recognized the utility of cocaine in clinical practice.

In 1884, Carl Koller was completing his medical training at a time when many operations on the eye were performed without general anesthesia. Almost four decades after the discovery of ether, general anesthesia by mask still had limitations for ophthalmic surgery: Lack of patient cooperation, interference of the anesthesia apparatus with surgical access, and high incidence of PONV. At that time, since fine sutures were not available and surgical incisions of the eye were not closed, postoperative vomiting threatened the extrusion of the globe's contents, putting the patient at risk for irrevocable blindness.[94]

While a medical student, Koller had worked in a Viennese laboratory in a search of a topical ophthalmic anesthetic to overcome the limitations of general anesthesia. Unfortunately, the suspensions of morphine, chloral hydrate, and other drugs that he had used had been ineffectual. In 1884, Koller's friend, Sigmund Freud, became interested in the cerebral-stimulating effects of cocaine and gave him a small sample in an envelope, which he placed in his pocket. When the envelope leaked, a few grains of cocaine stuck to Koller's finger and he absentmindedly licked his tongue. When his tongue became numb, Koller instantly realized that he had found the object of his search. In his laboratory, he made a suspension of cocaine crystals that he and a laboratory associate tested in the eyes of a frog, a rabbit, and a dog. Satisfied with the anesthetic effects seen in the animal models, Koller dropped the solution onto his own cornea. To his amazement, his eyes were insensitive to the touch of a pin.[95] As an intern, Carl Koller could not afford to attend a Congress of German Ophthalmologists in Heidelberg on September 15, 1884. However, a friend presented his article at the meeting and a revolution in ophthalmic surgery and other surgical disciplines began. Within the next year, more than 100 articles supporting the use of cocaine appeared in European and American medical journals. In 1888, Koller immigrated to New York, where he practiced ophthalmology for the remainder of his career.

American surgeons quickly developed new applications for cocaine. Its efficacy in anesthetizing the nose, mouth, larynx, trachea, rectum, and urethra was described in October 1884. The next month, the first reports of its subcutaneous injection were published. In December 1884, two young surgeons, William Halsted and Richard Hall, described blocks of the sensory nerves of the face and arm. Halsted even performed a brachial plexus block but did so under direct vision while the patient received an inhaled anesthetic.[96] Unfortunately, self-experimentation with cocaine was hazardous, as both surgeons became addicted.[97] Addiction was an ill-understood but frequent problem in the late nineteenth century, especially when cocaine and morphine were present in many patent medicines and folk remedies.

Other regional anesthetic techniques were attempted before the end of the nineteenth century. The term *spinal anesthesia* was coined in 1885 by Leonard Corning, a neurologist who had observed Hall and Halsted. Corning wanted to assess the action of cocaine as a specific therapy for neurologic problems. After first assessing its action in a dog, producing a blockade of rapid onset that was confined to the animal's rear legs, he performed a neuraxial block using cocaine on a man "addicted to masturbation." Corning administered one dose without effect, then after a second dose, the patient's legs "felt sleepy." The man had impaired sensibility in his lower extremity after about 20 minutes and left Corning's office "none the worse for the experience".[98] Although Corning did not describe escape of cerebrospinal fluid (CSF) in either case, it is likely that the dog had a spinal anesthetic and that the man had an epidural anesthetic. No therapeutic benefit was described, but Corning closed his account and his attention to the subject by suggesting that cocainization might in time be "a substitute for etherization in genitourinary or other branches of surgery".[99]

Two other authors, August Bier and Theodor Tuffier, described authentic spinal anesthesia, with mention of CSF, injection of cocaine, and an appropriately short onset of action. In a comparative review of the original articles by Bier, Tuffier, and Corning, it was concluded that Corning's injection was extradural, and Bier merited the credit for introducing spinal anesthesia.[100]

Fourteen years passed before spinal anesthesia was performed for surgery. In the interval, Heinrich Quincke of Kiel, Germany, had described his technique of lumbar puncture. He offered the valuable observation that it was most safely performed at the level of the third or fourth lumbar interspace because entry at that level was below the termination of the spinal cord. Quincke's technique was used in Kiel for the first deliberate cocainization of the spinal cord in 1899 by his surgical colleague, August Bier. Six patients received small doses of cocaine intrathecally, but because some cried out during surgery while others vomited and experienced headaches, Bier considered it necessary to conduct further experiments before continuing this technique for surgery.

Professor Bier permitted his assistant, Dr. Hildebrandt, to perform a lumbar puncture, but after the needle penetrated the dura, Hildebrandt could not fit the syringe to the needle and a large volume of the professor's spinal fluid escaped. They were at the point of abandoning the study when Hildebrandt volunteered to be the subject of a second attempt. Their persistence was rewarded with an astonishing success. Twenty-three minutes after the spinal injection, Bier noted: "A strong blow with an iron hammer against the tibia was not felt as pain. After 25 minutes: Strong pressure and pulling on a testicle were not painful".[93] They celebrated their success with wine and cigars. That night, both developed violent headaches, which they attributed at first to their celebration. Bier's headache was relieved after 9 days of bed rest. Hildebrandt, as a house officer, did not have the luxury of continued rest. Bier postulated that their headaches were a result of the loss of large volumes of CSF and urged that this be avoided if possible. The high incidence of complications following lumbar puncture with wide-bore needles and the toxic reactions attributed to cocaine explain his later loss of interest in spinal anesthesia.[101]

Surgeons in several other countries soon practiced spinal anesthesia and progress occurred by many small contributions to the technique. Theodor Tuffier published the first series of 125 spinal anesthetics from France and he later counseled that the solution should not be injected before CSF was seen. The first American report was by Rudolph Matas of New Orleans, whose first patient developed postanesthetic meningismus, a frequent complication that was overcome in part by the use of hermetically sealed sterile solutions recommended by E. W. Lee of Philadelphia and sterile gloves as advocated by Halsted. During 1899, Dudley Tait and Guidlo Caglieri of San Francisco performed experimental studies in animals and therapeutic spinals for orthopedic patients. They encouraged the use of fine needles to lessen the escape of CSF and urged that the skin and deeper tissues be infiltrated beforehand with local anesthesia.[102] This had been suggested earlier by William Halsted and the foremost advocate of infiltration anesthesia, Carl Ludwig Schleich of Berlin. An early American specialist in anesthesia, Ormond Goldan, published an anesthesia record appropriate for recording the course of "intraspinal cocainization" in 1900. In the same year, Heinrich Braun learned of a newly described extract of the adrenal gland, epinephrine, which he used to prolong the action of local anesthetics with great success. Braun developed several new nerve blocks, coined the term *conduction anesthesia,* and is remembered by European writers as the "father of conduction anesthesia." Braun was the first person to use procaine, which, along with stovaine, was one of the first synthetic local anesthetics produced to reduce the toxicity of cocaine.

Before 1907, anesthesiologists were sometimes disappointed to observe that their spinal anesthetics were incomplete. Most believed that the drug spread solely by local diffusion before the property of baricity was investigated by Arthur Barker, a London surgeon.[103] Barker constructed a glass tube shaped to follow the curves of the human spine and used it to demonstrate the limited spread of colored solutions that he had injected through a T-piece in the lumbar region. Barker applied this observation to use solutions of stovaine made hyperbaric by the addition of 5% glucose, which worked in a more predictable fashion. After the injection was complete, Barker placed his patient's head on pillows to contain the anesthetic below the nipple line. Lincoln Sise acknowledged Barker's work in 1935 when he introduced the use of hyperbaric solutions of tetracaine (Pontocaine). John Adriani advanced the concept further in 1946 when he used a hyperbaric solution to produce "saddle block," or perineal anesthesia. Adriani's patients remained seated after injection as the drug descended to the sacral nerves.

Tait, Jonnesco, and other early masters of spinal anesthesia used a cervical approach for thyroidectomy and thoracic procedures, but this radical approach was supplanted in 1928 by the lumbar injection of hypobaric solutions of "light" nupercaine by G. P. Pitkin. Although the use of hypobaric solutions is now limited primarily to patients positioned in the jackknife position, their former use for thoracic procedures demanded skill and precise timing. The enthusiasts of hypobaric anesthesia devised formulas to attempt to predict the time in seconds needed for a warmed solution of hypobaric nupercaine to spread in patients of varying size from its site of injection in the lumbar area to the level of the fourth thoracic dermatome.

The recurring problem of inadequate duration of single-injection spinal anesthesia led a Philadelphia surgeon, William Lemmon, to devise an apparatus for continuous spinal anesthesia in 1940.[104] Lemmon began with the patient in the lateral position. The spinal tap was performed with a malleable silver needle, which was left in position. As the patient was turned supine, the needle was positioned through a hole in the mattress and table. Additional injections of local anesthetic could be performed as required. Malleable silver needles also found a less cumbersome and more common application in 1942 when Waldo Edwards and Robert Hingson encouraged the use of Lemmon's needles for continuous caudal anesthesia in obstetrics. In 1944, Edward Tuohy of the Mayo Clinic introduced two important modifications of the continuous spinal techniques. He developed the now familiar Tuohy needle[105] as a means of improving the ease of passage of lacquered silk ureteral catheters through which he injected incremental doses of local anesthetic.[106]

In 1949, Martinez Curbelo of Havana, Cuba, used Tuohy's needle and a ureteral catheter to perform the first continuous epidural anesthetic. Silk and gum elastic catheters were difficult to sterilize and sometimes caused dural infections before being superseded by disposable plastics. Yet, deliberate single-injection peridural anesthesia had been practiced occasionally for decades before continuous techniques brought it greater popularity. At the beginning of the twentieth century, two French clinicians experimented independently with caudal anesthesia. Neurologist Jean Athanase Sicard applied the technique for a nonsurgical purpose, the relief of back pain. Fernand Cathelin used caudal anesthesia as a less dangerous alternative to spinal anesthesia for hernia repairs. He also demonstrated that the epidural space terminated in the neck by injecting a solution of India ink into the caudal canal of a dog. The lumbar approach was first used solely for multiple paravertebral nerve blocks before the Pagés–Dogliotti single-injection technique became accepted. As they worked separately, the technique carries the names of both men. Captain Fidel Pagés prepared an elegant demonstration of segmental single-injection peridural anesthesia in 1921, but died soon after his article appeared in a Spanish military journal.[107] Ten years later, Achille M. Dogliotti of Turin,

Italy, wrote a classic study that made the epidural technique well known.[73] Whereas Pagés used a tactile approach to identify the epidural space, Dogliotti identified it by the loss-of-resistance technique.

Surgery on the extremities lent itself to other regional anesthesia techniques. In 1902, Harvey Cushing coined the phrase *regional anesthesia* for his technique of blocking either the brachial or sciatic plexus under direct vision during general anesthesia to reduce anesthesia requirements and provide postoperative pain relief.[54] Fifteen years before his publication, George Crile advanced a similar approach to reduce the stress and shock of surgery. Crile, a dedicated advocate of regional and infiltration techniques during general anesthesia, coined the term *anociassociation*.[108]

An intravenous regional technique with procaine was reported in 1908 by August Bier, the surgeon who had pioneered spinal anesthesia. Bier injected procaine into a vein of the upper limb between two tourniquets. Even though the technique is termed the *Bier block*, it was not used for many decades until it was reintroduced 55 years later by Mackinnon Holmes, who modified the technique by exsanguination before applying a single proximal cuff. Holmes used lidocaine, the very successful amide local anesthetic synthesized in 1943 by Lofgren and Lundquist of Sweden.

Several investigators achieved upper extremity anesthesia by percutaneous injections of the brachial plexus. In 1911, based on his intimate knowledge of the anatomy of the axillary area, Hirschel promoted a "blind" axillary injection. In the same year, Kulenkampff described a supraclavicular approach in which the operator sought out paresthesias of the plexus while keeping the needle at a point superficial to the first rib and the pleura. The risk of pneumothorax with Kulenkampff's approach led Mulley to attempt blocks more proximally by a lateral paravertebral approach, the precursor of what is now popularly known as the *Winnie block* (after Alon Winnie from Chicago).

Heinrich Braun wrote the earliest textbook of local anesthesia, which appeared in its first English translation in 1914. After 1922, Gaston Labat's *Regional Anesthesia* dominated the American market. Labat migrated from France to the Mayo Clinic in Minnesota, where he served briefly before taking a permanent position at the Bellevue Hospital in New York. He formed the first American Society for Regional Anesthesia.[109] After Labat's death, Emery A. Rovenstine was recruited to Bellevue to continue Labat's work, among other responsibilities. Rovenstein created the first American clinic for the treatment of chronic pain, where he and his associates refined techniques of lytic and therapeutic injections and used the American Society of Regional Anesthesia to further the knowledge of pain management across the United States.[110]

6 The development of the multidisciplinary pain clinic was one of the many contributions to anesthesiology made by John J. Bonica, a renowned teacher of regional techniques. During his periods of military, civilian, and university service at the University of Washington, Bonica formulated a series of improvements in the management of patients with chronic pain. His classic text *The Management of Pain*, now in its fourth edition, is regarded as a standard of the literature of anesthesia.

Cardiovascular Anesthesia

The earliest attempts to operate on the heart were limited to repairing cardiac wounds. These attempts generally failed until German surgeon Ludwig Rehn repaired a right ventricular stab wound in September 1896.[111] Despite this success, the field was not ready to advance. The taboo of cardiac surgery was summarized by Theodore Billroth when he supposedly said "any surgeon who would attempt an operation on the heart should lose the respect of his colleagues".[112] The resistance to such operations was partly because of fledgling anesthetic medications, lack of adequate monitors, and even a clear understanding of cardiovascular physiology that pervades modern anesthesia practice.

Fortunately, the turn of the twentieth century saw many advances in anesthesia practice, blood typing and transfusion, anticoagulation, antibiosis, as well as surgical instrumentation and technique. Some continued to attempt procedures like closed mitral valvotomy in the midst of these technologic advancements, but outcomes were still very poor with mortality rates exceeding 80%. Many believe that the successful ligation of a 7-year-old girl's patent ductus arteriosus by Robert Gross in 1938 served as the landmark case for modern cardiac surgery. Soon after Gross' achievement, a host of new procedures were developed for repairing congenital cardiac lesions, including the first Blalock–Taussig shunt performed on a 15-month-old "blue baby" in 1944.[65] Although the shunt had been successfully demonstrated in animal models, Austin Lamont, Chief of Anesthesia at Johns Hopkins, was not supportive of the procedure. He emphatically stated "I will not put that child to death" and left the open drop ether–oxygen anesthetic to resident anesthesiologist Merel Harmel.[113] Lamont attended on the second Blalock–Taussig shunt 2 months later. Together, Harmel and Lamont would publish the first article on anesthesia for cardiac surgery in 1946 based on 100 cases with Alfred Blalock and repair of congenital pulmonic stenosis.[114]

Closed cardiac surgery ensued and anesthesia pioneers like William McQuiston and Kenneth Keown worked side by side with surgeons during procedures like the first aortic–pulmonary anastomosis and the first transmyocardial mitral commissurotomy. Never before had anesthesia providers worked as intimately with surgeons for the patient's welfare. Anesthesiologist and World War II physician Max Samuel Sadove remarked, "the small-arms fire of the anesthesiologist joins the spy system of the lab to back up the surgeon's big artillery in a coordinated attack to conquer disease".[115]

Through the 1930s and 1940s, John Gibbon had been experimenting with several extracorporeal circuit designs and by 1947 was able to successfully place dogs on heart–lung bypass. The first successful use of Gibbon's cardiopulmonary bypass machine in humans in May 1953 was a monumental advance in the surgical treatment of complex cardiac pathology that stimulated international interest in open heart surgery and the specialty of cardiac anesthesia.

Over the next decade, rapid growth and expanded applications of cardiac surgery, including artificial valves and coronary artery bypass grafting, required many more anesthesiologists acquainted with these specialized techniques. In 1967, J. Earl Waynards published one of the first articles on anesthetic management of patients undergoing surgery for coronary artery disease.

As cardiac surgery evolved, so did the perioperative monitoring and care of patients undergoing cardiac surgery. Postoperative mechanical ventilation and surgical intensive care units appeared by the late 1960s. Devices like the left atrial pressure monitor and the intra-aortic balloon pump offered new methods of understanding cardiopulmonary physiology and treating postoperative ventricular failure. Cardiac anesthesiologists were quick to bring the pulmonary artery catheter (PAC) into the operating room, permitting more precise hemodynamic monitoring and intervention. Joel Kaplan, already known for using the V_5 lead to monitor for myocardial ischemia and nitroglycerin infusions to treat ischemia, popularized the use of the PAC to detect myocardial ischemia. At Texas Heart Institute, Stephen Slogoff and Arthur

Keats demonstrated the negative impact of myocardial ischemia on clinical outcome. By the end of the 1980s, the same duo would reveal that the choice of anesthetic agent had little impact on outcome, challenging the earlier paradigm of "isoflurane steal" proposed by Sebastian Reiz.

Developments like cold potassium cardioplegia, monitoring and reversal of heparin, and reduction of blood loss with aprotinin would change the practice of cardiac anesthesia. Transesophageal echocardiography, introduced into cardiac surgery by Roizen, Cahalan, and Kremer in the 1980s, helped to further define the subspecialty of cardiac anesthesia.

Neuroanesthesia

Brain surgery is considered by some to be the oldest of the practiced medical arts. Evidence of trepanation, a form of neurosurgery in which a hole is drilled or scraped into the skull to access the dura, was discovered in skulls dating back to 6500 BC at a French burial site. Prehistoric brain surgery was also practiced by civilizations in South America, Africa, and Asia.[116]

With the introduction of inhalational anesthesia in the mid-1800s, Scottish surgeon and neurosurgery pioneer Sir William Macewen used this novel practice while performing the first successful craniotomy for tumor removal in 1879. Macewen, well known for introducing the technique of orotracheal intubation, promoted the idea of teaching medical students at Glasgow Royal Infirmary the art of chloroform anesthesia.

Like Macewen, Sir Victor Horsely was a neurosurgeon with an interest in anesthesia. His experiments of how ether, chloroform, and morphine affected intracranial contents led him to conclude that "the agent of choice was chloroform and that morphine had some value because of its cerebral constriction effects".[117] He first published his anesthetic technique for brain surgery in the *British Medical Journal* in 1886.[118] Later, he omitted morphine from his regimen after discovering its tendency to produce respiratory depression.

Meanwhile, Harvard medical student and aspiring neurosurgeon Harvey Cushing developed the first charts to record heart rate, temperature, and respiration during anesthesia. Soon after, he would add blood pressure readings to the record. Cushing was one of the first surgeons to recognize the importance of dedicated, specially trained anesthesia personnel versed in neurosurgery. Charles Frazier, a neurosurgical contemporary of Cushing, also recognized this need, stating that "no [cranial] operation be undertaken unless the services of a skilled anesthetizer are available".[119]

Since ether and chloroform anesthesia had significant drawbacks, beginning in 1918 Cushing and his contemporaries explored the advantages of regional or local anesthesia for intracranial surgery. Part of the motivation driving this change was the increased duration in surgical time. Cushing and colleagues used a "slow" surgical technique for most surgical procedures, where the average duration for cranial operations was 5 hours.[120] In contrast, early neurosurgeons like Horseley and Sir Percy Sargeant could perform similar procedures in less than 90 minutes. Therefore, prolonged patient exposure to chloroform or ether anesthesia was likely to result in increased bleeding, postoperative headache, confusion, and/or vomiting. Cushing and his contemporaries thought the use of local or regional anesthesia lessened the risk of these complications.

After a decade, it was realized that the remote positioning of the anesthetist was troublesome when managing the airway of an awake or lightly sedated patient undergoing cranial surgery with regional anesthesia. Also, endotracheal tubes, although introduced at the beginning of the century, had become popular instruments for securing a patient's airway and providing inhalation anesthesia. Combined, these circumstances led to the rapid resurgence of popularity in general anesthesia for cranial surgery, a trend that would continue to the present day.

While the introduction of agents like thiopental, curare, and halothane advanced the practice of anesthesiology in general, the development of methods to measure brain electrical activity, cerebral blood flow, and metabolic rate by Kety and Schmidt and intracranial pressure by Lundburg "put neuroanesthesia practice on a scientific foundation and opened doors to neuroanesthesia research".[121] Clinician-scientists like John D. (Jack) Michenfelder, later known as the father of neuroanesthesia, conducted basic science and clinical research on cerebral blood flow and brain function and protection in response to various anesthetic agents and techniques. Many lessons learned during this period of groundbreaking research are still commonly used in modern neuroanesthesia practice.

Obstetric Anesthesia

Social attitudes about pain associated with childbirth began to change in the 1860s and women started demanding anesthesia for childbirth. Societal pressures were so great that physicians, although unconvinced of the benefits of analgesia, felt obligated to offer this service to their obstetric patients.[122] In 1907, an Austrian physician, Richard von Steinbüchel, used a combination of morphine and scopolamine to produce *Dämmerschlaff* or "Twilight Sleep".[123] Although these two drugs were well known, physicians remained skeptical that Twilight Sleep was essential to labor and delivery, which unfortunately contrasted with the opinion of most women. This method gained popularity after German obstetricians Carl Gauss and Bernhardt Krönig widely publicized the technique. Numerous advertisements touted the benefits of Twilight Sleep (analgesia, partial pain relief, and amnesia) as compared to ether and chloroform, which resulted in total unconsciousness.[124] Gauss recognized the narrow therapeutic margin of these medications and gave precise instructions on its use: The first injection (morphine 10 mg and scopolamine) was to be given shortly after active labor began—this was intended to blunt the pain of labor—and subsequent injections consisted of only scopolamine, which was dosed to obliterate the memory of labor. Because of the effects of scopolamine, many patients became disoriented and would scream and thrash about during labor and delivery. Gauss believed that he could minimize this reaction by decreasing the sensory input; therefore, he would put patients in a dark room, cover their eyes with gauze, and insert oil-soaked cotton into their ears. The patients were often confined to a padded bed and restrained with leather straps during the delivery.[125] Over time, the doses of morphine administered seemed to increase, although there were few, if any, reports of adverse neonatal effects. Virginia Apgar's system for evaluating newborns, developed in 1953, demonstrated that there actually was a difference in the neonates of mothers who had general versus regional anesthesia.[126]

The bulk of the interest in Twilight Sleep appears to have been popular rather than medical and, for a brief period, was intensely followed in the United States.[127] Public enthusiasm for Twilight Sleep quickly subsided after a prominent advocate of the method died during childbirth. Her physicians claimed her death was not related to complications from the method of Twilight Sleep that was used.[128]

The first articles describing the obstetric application of spinal, epidural, caudal, paravertebral, parasacral, and pudendal nerve blocks appeared between 1900 and 1930. However, their benefits were underappreciated for many years because the obstetricians seldom used these techniques.[128] Continuous caudal anesthesia was introduced in 1944 by Hingson and Edwards[129] and spinal anesthesia became popular shortly thereafter. Initially, spinal anesthesia could be administered by inexperienced personnel without monitoring. The combination of inexperienced providers and lack of patient monitoring led to higher rates of morbidity and mortality than those observed for general anesthesia.[130] Therefore, the use of spinal anesthesia was highly discouraged in the 1950s, leading to the "dark ages of obstetric anesthesia" when pain relief in obstetrics was essentially abandoned and women were forced to endure "natural childbirth" to avoid serious anesthesia-related complications.[131]

With an increased understanding of neuraxial anesthesia, involvement by well-trained anesthesiologists, and an appreciation for the physiologic changes during pregnancy, maternal and fetal safety greatly improved. In the past decade, anesthesia-related deaths during cesarean sections under general anesthesia have become more likely than neuraxial anesthesia-related deaths, making regional anesthesia the method of choice.[132,133] With the availability of safe and effective options for pain relief during labor and delivery, today's focus is on improving the quality of the birth experience for expectant parents.

Transfusion Medicine

Paleolithic cave drawings found in France depict a bear losing blood from multiple spear wounds, indicating that primitive man understood the simple relationship between blood and life.[134] More than 10,000 years later, modern anesthesiologists attempt to preserve this intimate relationship by replacing fluids and blood products when faced with intravascular volume depletion or diminished oxygen-carrying capacity from blood loss.

Blood transfusion was first attempted in 1667 by the physician to Louis XIV, Jean Baptiste Denis. Denis had learned of Richard Lower's transfusion of lamb's blood into a dog the previous year. Lamb's blood was most frequently used because the donating animal's essential qualities were thought to be transferred to the recipient. Despite this dangerous trans-species transfusion, Denis' first patient got better. His next two patients were not as fortunate, however, and Denis avoided further attempts. Given the poor outcomes of these early blood transfusions, and heated religious controversy regarding the implications of transferring animal-specific qualities across species, blood transfusion in humans was banned for more than a 100 years in both France and England beginning in 1670.[65]

In 1900, Karl Landsteiner and Samuel Shattock independently helped lay the scientific basis of all subsequent transfusions by recognizing that blood compatibility was based on different blood groups. Landsteiner, an Austrian physician, originally organized human blood into three groups based on substances present in the red blood cells. The fourth type, AB group, was identified in 1902 by two students, A. Decastrello and A. Sturli. On the basis of these findings, Reuben Ottenberg performed the first type-specific blood transfusion in 1907. Transfusion of physiologic solutions occurred in 1831, independently performed by O'Shaughnessy and Lewins in Great Britain. In his letter to *The Lancet,* Lewins described transfusing large volumes of saline solutions into patients with cholera. He reported that he would inject into adults 5 to 10 pounds of saline solution and repeat as needed.[135] Despite its publication in a prominent journal, Lewins' technique was apparently overlooked for decades, and balanced physiologic solution availability would have to await the coming of analytical chemistry.

PROFESSIONALISM AND ANESTHESIA PRACTICE

Organized Anesthesiology

7 Physician anesthetists sought to obtain respect among their surgical colleagues by organizing professional societies and improving the quality of training. The first American organization was founded by nine members on October 6, 1905, and called the Long Island Society of Anesthetists with annual dues of $1.00. In 1911, the annual assessment rose to $3.00 when the Long Island Society became the New York Society of Anesthetists. Although the new organization still carried a local title, it drew members from several states and had a membership of 70 physicians in 1915.[136]

One of the most noteworthy figures in the struggle to professionalize anesthesiology was Francis Hoffer McMechan. McMechan had been a practicing anesthesiologist in Cincinnati until 1911, when he suffered a severe first attack of rheumatoid arthritis, which eventually left him confined to a wheelchair and forced his retirement from the operating room in 1915. McMechan had been in practice for only 15 years, but he had written 18 clinical articles in this short time. A prolific researcher and writer, McMechan did not permit his crippling disease to sideline his career. Instead of pursuing goals in clinical medicine, he applied his talents to establishing anesthesiology societies.[137]

McMechan supported himself and his devoted wife through editing the *Quarterly Anesthesia Supplement* from 1914 until August 1926. He became editor of the first journal devoted to anesthesia, *Current Researches in Anesthesia and Analgesia,* the precursor of *Anesthesia and Analgesia,* the oldest journal of the specialty. As well as fostering the organization of the International Anesthesia Research Society (IARS) in 1925, McMechan and his wife, Laurette, became overseas ambassadors of American anesthesia. Since Laurette was French, it was understandable that McMechan combined his own ideas about anesthesiology with concepts from abroad.[121]

In 1926, McMechan held the Congress of Anesthetists in a joint conference with the Section on Anaesthetics of the British Medical Association. Subsequently, he traveled throughout Europe, giving lectures and networking physicians in the field. On his final return to America, he was gravely ill and was confined to bed for 2 years. His hard work and constant travel paid dividends, however: In 1929, the IARS, which McMechan founded in 1922, had members not only from North America but also from several European countries, Japan, India, Argentina, and Brazil.[120]

In the 1930s, McMechan expanded his mission from organizing anesthesiologists to promoting the academic aspects of the specialty. In 1931, work began on what would become the International College of Anesthetists. This body began to award fellowships in 1935. For the first time, physicians were recognized as specialists in anesthesiology. The certification qualifications were universal, and fellows were recognized as specialists in several countries. Although the criteria for certification were not strict, the college was a success in raising the standards of anesthesia practice in many nations.[138] In 1939, McMechan finally succumbed to illness, and the anesthesia world lost its tireless leader.

Other Americans promoted the growth of organized anesthesiology. Ralph Waters and John Lundy, among others, participated in evolving organized anesthesia. Waters' greatest contribution to the specialty was raising its academic standards. After completing his internship in 1913, he entered medical practice in Sioux City, Iowa, where he gradually limited his practice to anesthesia. His personal experience and extensive reading were supplemented by the only postgraduate training available, a 1-month course conducted in Ohio by E. I. McKesson. At that time, the custom of becoming a self-proclaimed specialist in medicine and surgery was not uncommon. Waters, who was frustrated by low standards and who would eventually have a great influence on establishing both anesthesia residency training and the formal examination process, recalled that, before 1920, "The requirements for specialization in many Midwestern hospitals consisted of the possession of sufficient audacity to attempt a procedure and persuasive power adequate to gain the consent of the patient or his family".[139]

Academic Anesthesia

In an effort to improve anesthetic care, Waters regularly corresponded with Dennis Jackson and other scientists. In 1925, he relocated to Kansas City with a goal of gaining an academic post at the University of Kansas, but the professor of surgery failed to support his proposal. The larger city did allow him to initiate his freestanding outpatient surgical facility, "The Downtown Surgical Clinic," which featured one of the first postanesthetic recovery rooms.[128] In 1927, Erwin Schmidt, professor of surgery at the University of Wisconsin's medical school, encouraged Dean 3
Charles Bardeen to recruit Waters.

In accepting the first American academic position in anesthesia, Waters described four objectives that have been since adopted by many other academic departments. His goals were as follows: "(1) to provide the best possible service to patients of the institution, (2) to teach what is known of the principles of Anesthesiology to all candidates for their medical degree, (3) to help long-term graduate students not only to gain a fundamental knowledge of the subject and to master the art of administration, but also to learn as much as possible of the effective methods of teaching, (4) to accompany these efforts with the encouragement of as much cooperative investigation as is consistent with achieving the first objectives".[127]

Waters' personal and professional qualities impressed talented young men and women who sought residency posts in his department. He encouraged residents to initiate research interests in which they collaborated with two pharmacologists whom Waters had known before arriving in Wisconsin, Arthur Loevenhart and Chauncey Leake, as well as others with whom he became associated in Madison. Clinical concerns were also investigated. As an example, anesthesia records were coded onto punch cards to form a database that was used to analyze departmental activities. Morbidity and mortality meetings, now a requirement of all training programs, also originated in Madison. Members of the department and distinguished visitors from other centers attended these meetings. As a consequence of their critical reviews of the conduct of anesthesia, responsibility for an operative tragedy gradually passed from the patient to the physician. In more casual times, a practitioner could complain, "The patient died because he did not take a good anesthetic." Alternatively, the death might be attributed to a mysterious force such as "status lymphaticus," of which Arthur Guedel, a master of sardonic humor, observed, "Certainly status lymphaticus is at times a great help to the anesthetist. When he has a fatality under anesthesia with no other cleansing explanation he is glad to recognize the condition as an entity".[127]

In 1929, John Lundy at the Mayo Clinic organized the Anaesthetists' Travel Club, whose members were leading American or Canadian teachers of anesthesia. Each year one member was the host for a group of 20 to 40 anesthesiologists who gathered for a program of informal discussions. There were demonstrations of promising innovations for the operating room and laboratory, which were all subjected to what is remembered as a "high-spirited, energetic, critical review".[125] The Travel Club would be critical in the upcoming battle to form the American Board of Anesthesiology.

Even during the lean years of the Depression, international guests also visited Waters' department. For Geoffrey Kaye of Australia, Torsten Gordh of Sweden, Robert Macintosh and Michael Nosworthy of England, and scores of others, Waters' department was their "mecca of anesthesia." Ralph Waters trained 60 residents during the 22 years he was the "Chief." From 1937 onward, the alumni, who declared themselves the "Aqualumni" in his honor, returned annually for a professional and social reunion. Thirty-four Aqualumni took academic positions and, of these, 14 became chairpersons of departments of anesthesia. They maintained Waters' professional principles and encouraged teaching careers for many of their own graduates.[140] His enduring legacy was once recognized by the dean who had recruited him in 1927, Charles Bardeen, who observed, "Ralph Waters was the first person the University hired to put people to sleep, but, instead, he awakened a world-wide interest in anesthesia".[141]

Establishing a Society

Waters and Lundy, along with Paul Wood of New York City, had an important role in establishing organized anesthesia and the definition of the specialty. In the heart of the Great Depression, these three physicians realized that anesthesiology needed to have a process to determine who was an anesthetic specialist with American Medical Association (AMA) backing. Using the New York Society of Anesthetists, of which Paul Wood was secretary-treasurer, a new class of members, "Fellows," was created. The Fellows criteria followed established AMA guidelines for specialty certification. However, the AMA wanted a national organization to sponsor a specialty board. The New York Society of Anesthetists changed its name to the American Society of Anesthetists (ASA) in 1936. Combined with the American Society of Regional Anesthesia, whose president was Emery Rovenstein, the American Board of Anesthesiology (ABA) was organized as a subordinate board to the American Board of Surgery in 1938. With McMechan's death in 1939, the AMA favored independence for the ABA, and in 1940, independence was granted.[124,129]

A few years later, the officers of the American Society of Anesthetists were challenged by Dr. M. J. Seifert, who wrote, "An Anesthetist is a technician and an Anesthesiologist is the specific authority on anesthesia and anesthetics. I cannot understand why you do not term yourselves the American Society of Anesthesiologists".[131] Ralph Waters was declared the first president of the newly named ASA in 1945. In that year, when World War II ended, 739 (37%) of 1,977 ASA members were in the armed forces. In the same year, the ASA's first Distinguished Service Award was presented to Paul M. Wood for his tireless service to the specialty, one element of which can be examined today in the extensive archives preserved in the Society's Wood Library-Museum at ASA headquarters, Park Ridge, Illinois.[141]

CONCLUSIONS

This overview of the development of anesthesiology is but a brief outline of our current roles in which anesthesiologists serve in hospitals, clinics, and laboratories. The operating room and obstetric delivery suite remain the central interest of most specialists. Aside from being the location where the techniques described in this chapter find regular application, service in these areas brings us into regular contact with new advances in pharmacology and bioengineering.

After surgery, patients are transported to the postanesthesia care unit or recovery room, an area that is now considered the anesthesiologist's "ward." Fifty years ago, patients were carried directly from the operating room to a surgical ward to be attended only by a junior nurse. That person lacked both the skills and equipment to intervene when complications occurred. After the experiences of World War II taught the value of centralized care, physicians and nurses created recovery rooms, which were soon mandated for all major hospitals. By 1960, the evolution of critical care progressed through the use of mechanical ventilators. Patients who required many days of intensive medical and nursing management were cared for in a curtained corner of the recovery room. In time, curtains drawn about one or two beds gave way to fixed partitions and the relocation of those areas to
8 form intensive care units. The principles of resuscitative and supportive care established by anesthesiologists transformed critical care medicine.

The future of anesthesiology is a bright one. The safer drugs that once revolutionized the care of patients undergoing surgery
9 are constantly being improved. The role of the anesthesiologist continues to broaden as physicians with backgrounds in the specialty have developed clinics for chronic pain control and centers for outpatient surgery and assumed a role as administrative heads of perioperative units in major medical centers. Anesthesia practice will continue to increase in scope, both inside and outside the operating suite, such that anesthesiologists will increasingly become an integral part of the entire perioperative experience.

References

1. Joyce H. *The Journals and Letters of Fanny Burney.* Oxford: Clarendon; 1975. As quoted in: Papper EM. *Romance, Poetry, and Surgical Sleep.* Westport, CT: Greenwood Press; 1995:12.
2. Epitaph to W.T.G. Morton on a memorial from the Mt. Auburn Cemetery, Cambridge, Massachusetts.
3. These Egyptian pictographs are dated approximately 2500 B.C. See Ellis ES: *Ancient Anodynes: Primitive Anaesthesia and Allied Conditions.* London: WM Heinemann Medical Books; 1946:80.
4. Bacon DR. Regional anesthesia and chronic pain therapy: A history. In: Brown DL, ed. *Regional Anesthesia and Analgesia.* Philadelphia, PA: WB Saunders; 1996:11.
5. Rutkow I. *Surgery, an Illustrated History.* St. Louis, MO: Mosby; 1993:215.
6. Winter A. *Mesmerized: Powers of Mind in Victorian Britain.* Chicago: University of Chicago Press; 1998:42.
7. Marmer MJ. *Hypnosis in Anesthesiology.* Springfield, IL: Charles C. Thomas; 1959:10.
8. Dioscorides: On mandragora. In: Dioscorides Opera Libra. Quoted in: Bergman N. *The Genesis of Surgical Anesthesia.* Park Ridge, IL: Wood Library-Museum of Anesthesiology; 1998:11.
9. Infusino M, O'Neill YV, Calmes S. Hog beans, poppies, and mandrake leaves—A test of the efficacy of the soporific sponge. In: Atkinson RS, Boulton TB, eds. *The History of Anaesthesia.* London: Parthenon Publishing Group; 1989:31.
10. Davy H. *Researches Chemical and Philosophical Chiefly Concerning Nitrous Oxide or Dephlogisticated Nitrous Air, and Its Respiration.* London: J Johnson; 1800:533.
11. Papper EM. *Romance, Poetry, and Surgical Sleep.* Westport, CT: Greenwood Press; 1995.
12. Hickman HH. A letter on suspended animation, containing experiments showing that it may be safely employed during operations on animals, with the view of ascertaining its probable utility in surgical operations on the human subject, addressed to T.A. Knight, Esq. Imprint Ironbridge, W. Smith, 1824.
13. Strickland RA. Ether drinking in Ireland. *Mayo Clin Proc.* 1996;71:1015.
14. Lyman HM. *Artificial Anaesthesia and Anaesthetics.* New York, NY: William Hood; 1881:6.
15. Stetson JB, William E. Clarke and the discovery of anesthesia. In: Fink BR, Morris L, Stephen ER, eds. *The History of Anesthesia: Third International Symposium Proceedings.* Park Ridge, IL: Wood Library-Museum of Anesthesiology; 1992:400.
16. Long CW. An account of the first use of sulphuric ether by inhalation as an anaesthetic in surgical operations. *South Med Surg J.* 1849;5:705.
17. Robinson V. *Victory Over Pain.* New York, NY: Henry Schuman; 1946:91.
18. Smith GB, Hirsch NP. Gardner Quincy Colton: Pioneer of nitrous oxide anesthesia. *Anesth Analg.* 1991;72:382.
19. Menczer LF. Horace Wells's "day book A": A transcription and analysis. In: Wolfe RJ, Menczer LF, eds. *I Awaken to Glory.* Boston, MA: Boston Medical Library; 1994:112.
20. Greene NM. A consideration of factors in the discovery of anesthesia and their effects on its development. *Anesthesiology.* 1971;35:515.
21. Fenster J. *Ether Day.* New York, NY: Harper Collins; 2001:76.
22. Duncum BM. *The Development of Inhalation Anaesthesia.* London: Oxford University Press; 1947:86.
23. Caton D. *What a Blessing She Had Chloroform.* New Haven: Yale University Press; 1999:103.
24. Journal of Queen Victoria, In: Strauss MB, ed. *Familiar Medical Quotations.* Boston, Little Brown; 1968:17.
25. Kuhn F. Nasotracheal intubation (trans). In: Faulconer A, Keys TE, eds. *Foundations of Anesthesiology.* Springfield, IL: Charles C Thomas; 1965:677.
26. Clover JT. Laryngotomy in chloroform anesthesia. *Br Med J.* 1877;1:132.
27. Macewan W. Clinical observations on the introduction of tracheal tubes by the mouth instead of performing tracheotomy or laryngotomy. *Br Med J.* 1880;2:122, 163.
28. Hirsch NP, Smith GB, Hirsch PO. Alfred Kirstein, pioneer of direct laryngoscopy. *Anaesthesia.* 1986;41:42.
29. Burkle CM, Zepeda FA, Bacon DR, et al. A historical perspective on use of the laryngoscope as a tool in anesthesiology. *Anesthesiology.* 2004;100:1003.
30. Miller RA. A new laryngoscope. *Anesthesiology.* 1941;2:317.
31. Macintosh RR. Richard Salt of Oxford, anaesthetic technician extraordinary. *Anaesthesia.* 1976;31:855.
32. Thomas KB. Sir Ivan Whiteside Magill, KCVO, DSc, MB, BCh, BAO, FRCS, FFARCS (Hon), FFARCSI (Hon), DA: A review of his publications and other references to his life and work. *Anaesthesia.* 1978;33:628.
33. Condon HA, Gilchrist E. Stanley Rowbotham: Twentieth century pioneer anaesthetist. *Anaesthesia.* 1986;41:46.
34. Calverley RK. Classical file. *Surv Anesth.* 1984;28:70.
35. Gale JW, Waters RM. Closed endobronchial anesthesia in thoracic surgery: Preliminary report. *Curr Res Anesth Analg.* 1932;11:283.
36. Wu TL, Chou HC. A new laryngoscope: The combination intubating device (letter). *Anesthesiology.* 1994;81:1085.
37. Brain AIJ. The laryngeal mask: A new concept in airway management. *Br J Anaesth.* 1983;55:801.
38. Calverley RK. An early ether vaporizer designed by John Snow, a Treasure of the Wood Library-Museum of Anesthesiology. In: Fink BR, Morris LE, Stephen CR, eds. *The History of Anesthesia.* Park Ridge, IL: Wood Library-Museum of Anesthesiology; 1992:91.
39. Snow J. *On the Inhalation of the Vapour of Ether (reprinted by the Wood Library-Museum of Anesthesiology).* London: J Churchill; 1847:23.
40. Calverley RK, Clover JT. A giant of Victorian anaesthesia. In: Rupreht J, van Lieburg MJ, Lee JA, Erdmann W, eds. *Anaesthesia: Essays on Its History.* Berlin: Springer-Verlag; 1985:21.
41. Andrews E. The oxygen mixture, a new anaesthetic combination. *Chicago Med Exam.* 1868;9:656.
42. Obituary of T. Philip Ayre. *Br Med J.* 1980;280:125.
43. Rees GJ. Anaesthesia in the newborn. *Br Med J.* 1950;2:1419.
44. Bain JA, Spoerel WE. A stream-lined anaesthetic system. *Can Anaesth Soc J.* 1972;19:426.
45. Mushin WW, Rendell-Baker L. *Thoracic Anaesthesia Past and Present (reprinted by the Wood Library-Museum of Anesthesiology 1991).* Springfield, IL: Charles C Thomas; 1953:44.
46. Shephard DAE. Harvey Cushing and anaesthesia. *Can Anaesth Soc J.* 1965;12:431.
47. Waters RM. Clinical scope and utility of carbon dioxide filtration in inhalation anesthesia. *Curr Res Anesth Analg.* 1923;3:20.
48. Sword BC. The closed circle method of administration of gas anesthesia. *Curr Res Anesth Analg.* 1930;9:198.
49. Sands RP, Bacon DR. An inventive mind: The career of James O. Elam, M.D. (1918–1995). *Anesthesiology.* 1998;88:1107.
50. Morris LE. A new vaporizer for liquid anesthetic agents. *Anesthesiology.* 1952;13:587.

51. Sands R, Bacon DR. The copper kettle: A historical perspective. *J Clin Anesthesiol.* 1996;8:528.
52. Duncum BM. *The Development of Inhalation Anaesthesia.* London: Oxford University Press; 1947:538.
53. Severinghaus JC, Honda Y. Pulse oximetry. *Int Anesthesiol Clin.* 1987;25:205.
54. Cushing H. On the avoidance of shock in major amputations by cocainization of large nerve trunks preliminary to their division: With observations on blood-pressure changes in surgical cases. *Ann Surg.* 1902;36:321.
55. Codesmith A. An endo-esophageal stethoscope. *Anesthesiology.* 1954;15:566.
56. Luft K. Methode der registrieren gas analyse mit hilfe der absorption ultraroten Strahlen ohne spectrale Zerlegung. *Z Tech Phys.* 1943;24:97.
57. Tovell RM. Problems in supply of anesthetic gases in the European theater of operations. *Anesthesiology.* 1947;8:303.
58. Rendell-Baker L. History of standards for anesthesia equipment. In: Rupreht J, van Lieburg MJ, Lee JA, Erdmann W, eds. *Anaesthesia: Essays on Its History.* Berlin: Springer-Verlag; 1985:161.
59. Calverley RK. A safety feature for anaesthesia machines: Touch identification of oxygen flow control. *Can Anaesth Soc J.* 1971;18:225.
60. Lucas GH. The discovery of cyclopropane. *Curr Res Anesth Analg.* 1961;40:15.
61. Seevers MH, Meek WJ, Rovenstine EA, et al. Cyclopropane study with espical reference to gas concentration, respiratory and electrocardiographic changes. *J Pharmacol Exp Ther.* 1934;51:1.
62. Calverley RK. Fluorinated anesthetics: I. The early years. *Surv Anesth.* 1986;29:170.
63. Suckling CW. Some chemical and physical factors in the development of fluothane. *Br J Anaesth.* 1957;29:466.
64. Wren PC. *Philosophical Transactions,* Vol I. London, Anno, 1665 and 1666.
65. Keys TE. *The History of Surgical Anesthesia.* New York, NY: Dover Publications; 1945:38.
66. Dundee J, Wyant G. *Intravenous Anesthesia.* Hong Kong: Churchill Livingstone; 1974:1.
67. Oré PC. *Etudes, cliniques sur l'anesthésie chirurgicale par la methode des injection de choral dans les veines.* Paris: JB Balliere et Fils; 1875. As quoted in: Hemelrijck JV, Kissin I: History of intravenous anesthesia. In: White PF, ed. *Textbook of Intravenous Anesthesia.* Baltimore: Williams & Wilkins; 1997:3.
68. Macintosh RR. Modern anaesthesia, with special reference to the chair of anaesthetics in Oxford. In: Rupreht J, van Lieburg MJ, Lee JA, Erdmann W, eds. *Anaesthesia: Essays on Its History.* Berlin: Springer-Verlag; 1985:352.
69. Hemelrijck JV, Kissin I. History of intravenous anesthesia. In: White PF, ed. *Textbook of Intravenous Anesthesia.* Baltimore: Williams & Wilkins; 1997:3.
70. Fink BR. Leaves and needles: The introduction of surgical local anesthesia. *Anesthesiology.* 1985;63:77–83.
71. Koller C. Über die Verwendung des Cocain zur Anästhesirung am Auge. *Wien Med Wochenschr.* 1884;34:1276.
72. Calatayud J, Gonzalez A. History of the development and evolution of local anesthesia since the coca leaf. *Anesthesiology.* 2003;98:1503.
73. Fink BR. History of local anesthesia. In: Cousins MJ, Bridenbaugh PO, eds. *Neural Blockade.* Philadelphia, PA: JB Lippincott; 1980:12.
74. Ruetsch YA, Boni T, Borgeat A. From cocaine to ropivacaine: The history of local anesthetic drugs. *Curr Top Med Chem.* 2001;1:175.
75. Ekenstam B, Egnev B, Pettersson G. Local anaesthetics: I. N-alkyl pyrrolidine and N-alkyl piperidine carboxylic acid amides. *Acta Chem Scand.* 1957;11:1183.
76. Albright GA. Cardiac arrest following regional anesthesia with etidocaine or bupivacaine. *Anesthesiology.* 1979;51:285.
77. Aberg G. Toxicological and local anaesthetic effects of optically active isomers of two local anaesthetic compounds. *Acta Pharmacol Toxicol (Copenh).* 1972;31:273.
78. Polley LS, Santos AC. Cardiac arrest following regional anesthesia with ropivacaine: Here we go again! *Anesthesiology.* 2003;99:1253.
79. Castillo J, Curley J, Hotz J, et al. Glucocorticoids prolong rat sciatic nerve blockade in vivo from bupivacaine microspheres. *Anesthesiology.* 1996;85:1157.
80. Mowat JJ, Mok MJ, MacLeod BA, et al. Liposomal bupivacaine. Extended duration nerve blockade using large unilamellar vesicles that exhibit a proton gradient. *Anesthesiology.* 1996;85:635.
81. McIntyre AR. *Curare, Its History, Nature, and Clinical Use.* Chicago: University of Chicago Press; 1947:6, 131.
82. Thomas BK. *Curare: Its History and Usage.* Philadelphia, PA: JB Lippincott Company; 1963:90.
83. Rushman GB, Davies NJH, Atkinson RS. *A Short History of Anaesthesia.* Oxford: Butterworth-Heinemann; 1996:78.
84. Knoefel PK. *Felice Fontana: Life and Works.* Trento: Societa de Studi Trentini; 1985:284.
85. Griffith HR, Johnson GE. The use of curare in general anesthesia. *Anesthesiology.* 1942;3:418.
86. McIntyre AR. Historical background, early use and development of muscle relaxants. *Anesthesiology.* 1959;20:412.
87. Ali HH, Utting JE, Gray C. Quantitative assessment of residual antidepolarizing block (part II). *Br J Anaesth.* 1971;43:478.
88. Gwathmey JT. *Anesthesia.* New York, NY: Appleton and Company; 1914:379.
89. Flagg PJ. *The Art of Anaesthesia.* Philadelphia, PA: JB Lippincott Company; 1918:80.
90. Chloretone (chlorobutanol) is prepared by mixing chloroform and acetone, and has a camphor-like odor that some find pleasant. Chloretone is now commonly used for euthanizing reptiles and amphibians.
91. Hewer CL. *Recent Advances in Anaesthesia and Analgesia.* Philadelphia, PA: P Blakiston's Son & Co. Inc..; 1937:237.
92. Collins VJ. *Principles and Practice of Anesthesiology.* Philadelphia, PA: Lea & Febiger; 1952:327.
93. Raeder J. History of postoperative nausea and vomiting. *Int Anesthesiol Clin.* 2003;41:1.
94. Koller C. Personal reminiscences of the first use of cocaine as local anesthetic in eye surgery. *Curr Res Anesth Analg.* 1928;7:9.
95. Becker HK. Carl Koller and cocaine. *Psychoanal Q.* 1963;32:309.
96. Halstead WS. Practical comments on the use and abuse of cocaine; suggested by its invariably successful employment in more than a thousand minor surgical operations. *N Y Med J.* 1885;42:294.
97. Olch PD, William S. Halstead and local anesthesia: Contributions and complications. *Anesthesiology.* 1975;42:479.
98. Marx G. The first spinal anesthesia: Who deserves the laurels? *Reg Anesth.* 1994;19:429.
99. Corning JL. Spinal anaesthesia and local medication of the cord. *N Y Med J.* 1885;42:483.
100. Bier AKG. Experiments in cocainization of the spinal cord, 1899. In: Faulconer A, Keys TE (trans), eds. *Foundations of Anesthesiology.* Springfield, IL: Charles C Thomas; 1965:854.
101. Goerig M, Agarwal K, Schulte am Esch J. The versatile August Bier (1861–1949), father of spinal anesthesia. *J Clin Anesth.* 2000;12:561.
102. Larson MD. Tait and Caglieri. The first spinal anesthetic in America. *Anesthesiology.* 1996;85:913.
103. Lee JA. Arthur Edward James Barker, 1850–1916: British pioneer of regional anaesthesia. *Anaesthesia.* 1979;34:885.
104. Lemmon WT. A method for continuous spinal anesthesia: A preliminary report. *Ann Surg.* 1940;111:141.
105. Martini JA, Bacon DR, Vasdev GM. Edward Tuohy: The man, his needle, and its place in obstetric anesthesia. *Reg Anesth Pain Med.* 2002;27:520.
106. Tuohy EB. Continuous spinal anesthesia: Its usefulness and technique involved. *Anesthesiology.* 1944;5:142.
107. Pagés F. Metameric anesthesia, 1921. In: Faulconer A, Keys TE (trans), eds. *Foundations of Anesthesiology.* Springfield, IL: Charles C Thomas; 1965:927.
108. Crile GW, Lower WE. *Anoci-Association.* Philadelphia, PA: WB Saunders Company; 1915.
109. Brown DL, Winnie AP. Biography of Louis Gaston Labat, M.D. *Reg Anesth.* 1992;17:248.
110. Bacon DR, Darwish H. Emery Rovenstine and regional anesthesia. *Reg Anesth.* 1997;22:273.
111. Rehn L. On penetrating cardiac injuries and cardiac suturing. *Arch Klin Chir.* 1897;55:315.
112. Naef AP. The mid-century revolution in thoracic and cardiovascular surgery: part 1. *Interact Cardiovasc Thorac Surg.* 2003;2:219.
113. Baum VC. Pediatric cardiac surgery: An historical appreciation. *Pediatr Anesth.* 2006;16:1213.
114. Harmel M, Lamont A. Anesthesia in the treatment of congenital pulmonary stenosis. *Anesthesiology.* 1948;7:477.
115. [Anon.] With Gas & Needle." Time. Monday, October 19, 1953.
116. Tracy PT, Hanigan WC. The history of neuroanesthesia. In: Greenblatt SH, ed. *The History of Neurosurgery.* New York, NY: Thieme; 1997:213.
117. Samuels SI. The history of neuroanesthesia: A contemporary review. *Int Anesthesiol Clin.* 1996;34:1.
118. Horsley V. Brain surgery. *Br Med J.* 1886;2:670.
119. Frazier C. Problems and procedures in cranial surgery. *JAMA.* 1909;52:1805.
120. Bacon DR. The World Federation of Societies of Anesthesiologists: McMechan's final legacy? *Anesth Analg.* 1997;84:1131.
121. Seldon TH. Francis Hoeffer McMechan. In: Volpitto PP, Vandam LD, eds. *Genesis of American Anesthesiology.* Springfield, IL: Charles C Thomas; 1982:5.
122. Canton D. The history of obstetric anesthesia. In: Chestnut DH, ed. *Obstetric Anesthesia: Principles and Practice.* Philadelphia, PA: Elsevier Mosby; 2004.
123. Barnett R. A horse named 'Twilight Sleep': The language of obstetric anaesthesia in 20th century Britain. *Int J Obstet Anesth.* 2005;14:310.
124. Canton D. *What a Blessing She Had Chloroform.* New Haven: Yale University Press; 1999.
125. MacKenzie RA, Bacon DR, Martin DP. Anaesthetists' Travel Club: A transformation of the Society of Clinical Surgery? *Bull Anesth Hist.* 2004;22:7.
126. Apgar V. A proposal for a new method of evaluation of the newborn infant. *Curr Res Anesth Analg.* 1953;32:260.
127. Guedel AE. *Inhalation Anesthesia: A Fundamental Guide.* New York, NY: MacMillan; 1937:129.
128. Waters RM. The down-town anesthesia clinic. *Am J Surg.* 1919;33:71.
129. Hingson RA. Continuous caudal analgesia in obstetrics, surgery, and therapeutics. *Br Med J.* 1949;2:777.
130. Gogarten W, Van Aken H. A century of regional analgesia in obstetrics. *Anesth Analg.* 2000;91:773.

131. Little DM Jr, Betcher AM. *The Diamond Jubilee 1905–1980.* Park Ridge, IL: American Society of Anesthesiologists; 1980:8.
132. Hawkins JL, Koonin LM, Palmer SK, et al. Anesthesia-related deaths during obstetric delivery in the United States, 1979–1990. *Anesthesiology.* 1997;86:277.
133. Hawkins JL. Anesthesia-related maternal mortality. *Clin Obstet Gynecol.* 2003;46:679.
134. Gottlieb AM. *A Pictorial History of Blood Practices and Transfusion.* Scottsdale, AZ: Arcane Publications; 1992:2.
135. Jenkins MT. *Epochs in Intravenous Fluid Therapy: From the Goose Quill and Pig Bladder to Balanced Salt Solutions.* Park Ridge, IL: The Lewis H. Wright Memorial Lecture, Wood Library-Museum Collection; 1993:4.
136. Betcher AM, Ciliberti BJ, Wood PM, et al. The jubilee year of organized anesthesia. *Anesthesiology.* 1956;17:226.
137. Bacon DR. The promise of one great anesthesia society. *Anesthesiology.* 1994; 80:929.
138. Bacon DR, Lema MJ. To define a specialty: A brief history of the American Board of Anesthesiology's first written examination. *J Clin Anesth.* 1992;4:489.
139. Waters RM. Pioneering in anesthesiology. *Postgrad Med.* 1948;4:265.
140. Bacon DR, Ament R. Ralph Waters and the beginnings of academic anesthesiology in the United States: The Wisconsin template. *J Clin Anesth.* 1995;7:534.
141. Bamforth BJ, Siebecker KL. Ralph M. Waters. In: Volpitto PP, Vandam LD, eds. *Genesis of American Anesthesiology.* Springfield, IL: Charles C Thomas; 1982.

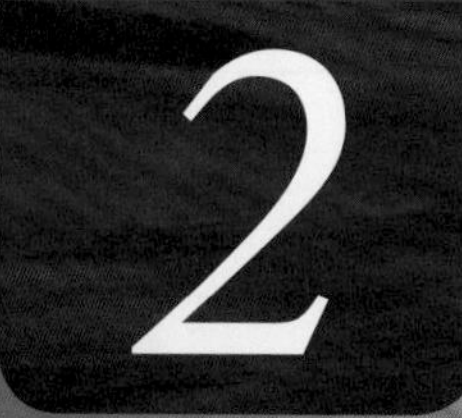

CHAPTER 2

Scope of Practice

JOHN H. EICHHORN • JAY S. GRIDER

Key Points

1. Anesthesia trainees, and many postgraduates also, tend to lack sufficient knowledge (with sometimes unfortunate results) about modes of practice or employment, financial matters of all types, and the forces that shape them, but contracting in particular. They must educate themselves and also seek expert advice and counsel to survive (and hopefully flourish) in today's exceedingly intricate medical practice milieu.
2. There are several very helpful detailed information resources concerning practice and OR management available from the American Society of Anesthesiologists and other sources. Factors influencing anesthesiology practice conditions are changing rapidly, and today's anesthesia professionals must be armed with detailed information about concepts (such as "pay for performance" and "accountable care organizations") that did not exist just a few years ago.
3. Securing hospital privileges is far more than a bureaucratic annoyance and must be taken seriously by anesthesiologists.
4. Anesthesiology is the leading medical specialty in establishing and promulgating standards of practice that have significantly influenced practice in a positive manner.
5. The immediate response to a major adverse anesthesia event is critical to the eventual result. An extremely valuable protocol is available at www.apsf.org, "Resource Center: Clinical Safety Tools."
6. Anesthesiologists must be involved, concerned, active participants and leaders in their institution and medical community in order to enhance their practice function and image.
7. The threatened negative impact of "managed care" largely failed to materialize regarding anesthesiology practice, but the impact of the "Great Recession" on all of the health-care system has been substantial and will resonate for the foreseeable future on budgets, availability of resources, and the economics of medical practice.
8. Anesthesiologists must participate in operating room (OR) management in their facilities and should play a central leadership role. OR scheduling, staffing, utilization, and patient flow issues are complex, and anesthesiologists should work hard to both thoroughly understand and positively influence them.
9. Anesthesiology personnel issues involve an elaborate balancing act that is subject to complex conflicting forces. Anesthesiology groups/departments should give these issues, as well as their constituent personnel, more attention and energy than has been done traditionally in the past.
10. Attention to the many often-underemphasized details of infrastructure, organization, and administration can transform a merely endurable anesthesia practice into one that is efficient, effective, productive, collegial, and even fun.

Multimedia

 AIMS

The structure and function of anesthesia practice, as well as of the entire health-care system, are evolving very rapidly in the United States. In the past, anesthesia professionals traditionally were little involved in the management of many components of their practice beyond the strictly medical elements of applied physiology and pharmacology, pathophysiology, and therapeutics. This was perhaps somewhat understandable because anesthesia professionals traditionally spent most of their usually very long work hours in a hospital operating room (OR). Business matters were often left to the one or two members of the traditional private practice group who were interested or willing to deal with an outside-contractor billing agency. In that era, very little formal teaching in practice management of any kind occurred. Today
1 the Anesthesiology Residency Review Committee of the Accreditation Council on Graduate Medical Education requires that the didactic curricula of anesthesiology residencies include material on practice management. Most training programs offer at least a cursory introduction to issues of practice management, but these can be insufficient to prepare satisfactorily the professional being graduated for the real infrastructure, administrative, business, and management challenges of the modern practice of anesthesiology.

This chapter presents a wide variety of topics that, until recently, were not included in anesthesiology textbooks or residency program curricula. Outlined are several basic components of the background, administrative, organizational (including both practice arrangements and daily functioning of the OR), and financial aspects of anesthesiology practice in the complex modern environment. Although many issues are undergoing almost constant change, it is important to understand the basic vocabulary and principles in this dynamic universe. Lack of understanding of these issues may put anesthesia professionals at a disadvantage when attempting to maximize the efficiency and impact of their daily activities, to create and execute practice arrangements, and to secure fair compensation in an increasingly complex health-care system featuring greater and greater competition for scarcer and scarcer resources.

ADMINISTRATIVE COMPONENTS OF ANESTHESIOLOGY PRACTICE

Operational and Information Resources

Outlined in this chapter is an overview summary intended as an introduction to organization, administration, and practice man-
2 agement in anesthesiology. Further, fortunately, the American Society of Anesthesiologists (ASA), the professional association for physician anesthesiologists in the United States, for many years has made available to its members extensive resource material regarding practice in general and specific arrangements for its execution. Citation and availability of this material can be found on the ASA web site, www.asahq.org. Elements are updated periodically by the ASA through its physician officers, committees, task forces, administrative and support staff, and its various offices. Although many of the documents and even the advice given in response to members' requests for help contain broad-brush generalities that must be interpreted in each individual practice situation, these nonetheless stand as a foundation on which many anesthesiology practices can be based. Prospective familiarity with the principles outlined in the ASA material likely could help avoid some of the problems leading to calls for help. Selected key documents have been compiled and bound into one volume (1). Also, each spring, the ASA offers a Practice Management Conference at which both reviews and current updates of a wide variety of relevant administrative and financial topics are covered.

Background

The ASA publishes the *Manual for Anesthesia Department Organization and Management*[1] that includes sections on physician responsibilities for medical care and on medical-administrative organization and responsibilities. Included are the ASA *Guidelines for the Ethical Practice of Anesthesiology,* which incorporate sections on the principles of medical ethics; the definition of medical direction of nonphysician personnel (including the specific statement that an anesthesiologist engaged in medical direction should not personally be administering another anesthetic); the anesthesiologist's relationship to patients and other physicians; the anesthesiologist's duties, responsibilities, and relationship to the hospital; and the anesthesiologist's relationship to nurse anesthetists and other nonphysician personnel. Further, beyond summaries such as this textbook chapter, reference to the great body of material created and presented by the ASA is an excellent starting point to help young anesthesia professionals during training prepare for the increasing rigors of starting and managing a career in practice. On the ASA web site, within the "For Members" area, the "Practice Management" section is functionally a gold mine that includes extensive information on the organization, administration, and business of anesthesia practice with reference to an extensive catalog of webinars and podcasts, as well as a compendium of chapters from the annual ASA Practice Management Conference.[2] Likewise, there is a great deal of information on the ASA web site concerning the most recent governmental regulations, rulings, and billing codes. Further, the *ASA Newsletter* contains the monthly columns "Washington Report" and "Practice Management," which disseminate related current administrative, organizational, and financial developments (and which are reprinted on the ASA web site).

In addition to the ASA and the American Association of Nurse Anesthetists, most anesthesiology subspecialty societies and interest groups have web locations, as do most journals. Particularly, the web site of the Anesthesia Patient Safety Foundation, www.apsf.org, has been cited as especially useful in promoting safe clinical practice. Electronic bulletin boards allow anesthesiology practitioners from around the world to exchange ideas in real time on diverse topics, both medical and administrative. One of the original sites that remains available is "GASnet," and a web search ("anesthesiology + bulletin board") reveals a great number of sites that contain a variety of discussions about all manner of anesthesiology-related topics, including practice organization, administration, finance, and management. In addition, references to the entirety of the medical literature are readily accessible to any practitioner (such as by starting with www.nlm.nih.gov to access Medline). A modern anesthesiology practice cannot reasonably exist without readily available high-speed Internet connections.

The Credentialing Process and Clinical Privileges

3 The system of credentialing a health-care professional and granting clinical privileges in a health-care facility is motivated by a fundamental assumption that appropriate education, training, and experience, along with the absence of excessive numbers of bad patient outcomes, increase the chances that the individual

will deliver acceptable-quality care. The process of credentialing health-care professionals has been the focus of considerable public attention (particularly in the mass media), in part the result of very rare incidents of untrained persons (impostors) infiltrating the health-care system and sometimes harming patients. The more common situation, however, involves health professionals who exaggerate past experience and credentials or fail to disclose adverse past experiences. In the past, there was justified publicity concerning physicians who lost their licenses sequentially in several states and simply moved on each time to start practice elsewhere (which should be much, much more difficult today).

Intense public and political pressure has been brought to bear on various lawmaking bodies, regulatory and licensing agencies, and health-care institution administrations to discover and purge both (1) fraudulent, criminal, and deviant health-care providers and (2) incompetent or simply poor-quality practitioners whose histories show sufficient poor patient outcomes to attract attention, usually through malpractice suits. Identifying and avoiding or correcting an incompetent practitioner is the goal. Verification of appropriate education, training, and experience on the part of a candidate for a clinical anesthesia position assumes special importance in light of the legal doctrine of *vicarious liability,* which can be described as follows: if an individual, group, or institution hires an anesthesia professional or even simply approves of that person (e.g., by granting clinical privileges through a hospital medical staff), those involved in the decision may later be held liable in the courts, along with the individual, for the individual's actions. This would be especially true if it were later discovered that the offending practitioner's past adverse outcomes had not been adequately investigated during the credentialing process.

Out of these various long-standing concerns has arisen the sometimes cumbersome process of obtaining state licenses to practice and of obtaining hospital privileges. The stringent credentialing process for health-care practice is intended both to protect patients and to safeguard the integrity of the profession. Central credentialing systems have been developed, including those affiliated with the American Medical Association, American Osteopathic Association, and, particularly, the Federation Credentials Verification Service of the Federation of State Medical Boards. These systems verify a physician's basic credentials (e.g., identity, citizenship or immigration status, medical education, postgraduate training, licensure examination history, prior licenses, and board actions) once, and then thereafter can certify the validity of these credentials to a state licensing board or medical facility. A few states do not yet accept this verification and most states seek specific supplemental information.

There are checklists of the requirements for the granting of medical staff privileges by hospitals (see the American Hospital Association Resource Center, www.aha.org/research/rc/index.shtml). In addition, the National Practitioner Data Bank and reporting system administered by the US government now contains many years' worth of information. This data bank is a central repository of licensing and credentials information about physicians. Many adverse situations involving a physician—particularly instances of substance abuse, malpractice litigation, or the revocation, suspension, or limitation of that physician's license to practice medicine or ability to hold hospital privileges—must be reported (via the particular state board of medical registration/licensure) to the National Practitioner Data Bank. It is a statutory requirement that all applications for hospital staff privileges be cross-checked against this national data bank. The potential medicolegal liability on the part of a facility's medical staff, and the anesthesiology group in particular, for failing to do so is significant. The data bank, however, is not a complete substitute for direct documentation and background checking. Often, practitioners reach private negotiated solutions following quality-driven medical staff problems, thereby avoiding the mandatory public reporting. In such cases, a practitioner in question may be given the option to resign medical staff privileges and avoid data bank reporting rather than undergo full involuntary privilege revocation (although most license and privilege applications contain a question specifically about this).

Documentation

The documentation for the credentialing process for each anesthesia practitioner must be complete. Privileges to administer anesthesia must be officially granted and delineated in writing. This can be straightforward or it can be more complex to accommodate institutional needs to identify practitioners specially qualified to practice in designated anesthesia subspecialty areas such as cardiac, infant/pediatric, obstetric, intensive care, or pain management. Specific documentation of the process of granting or renewing clinical privileges is required and, unlike some other administrative records, the documentation likely is protected as confidential peer review information. Any questions about complex sensitive issues such as this should be referred to an experienced attorney familiar with applicable federal and state law. Verification of an applicant's credentials and experience is mandatory. Because of another type of legal case, some examples of which have been highly publicized, medical practitioners may be hesitant to give an honest evaluation (or any evaluation at all) of individuals known to them who are seeking a professional position elsewhere. Obviously, someone writing a reference for a current or former coworker should be honest. Sticking to clearly documentable facts is advisable. Stating a fact that is in the public record (such as a malpractice case lost at trial) should not justify an objection from the subject of the reference. Whether such potentially "negative" facts can be omitted by a reference writer is complex. Including positive opinions and enthusiastic recommendations, of course, is no problem. Some fear that including facts that may be perceived as negative (e.g., the lost malpractice case or personal problems such as a history of treatment for substance abuse) and/or negative opinions will provoke a retaliatory lawsuit (such as for libel, defamation of character, or loss of livelihood) from the subject of the reference. Further, however, there have been cases of the facility doing the hiring suing reference writers for failing to mention (perceived as concealing) negative information about an applicant who later was charged with substandard practice. Because of the complexities and even apparent contradictions, many reference writers in these questionable situations confine their written material to brief, simple facts such as dates employed and position held. As always, questions about complex sensitive issues such as this should be referred to an experienced attorney familiar with applicable federal and state law.

Because there should be no hesitation for a reference writer to include positive facts and opinions, receipt of a reference that includes nothing more than dates worked and position held can be a suggestion that there may be more to the story (although some entities have adopted such a policy in all cases simply to eliminate any value judgments as to what is positive or negative information). Receipt of such a "dates/position only" reference about a person applying for a position should usually provoke a telephone call to the writer. A telephone call is likely advisable in all cases, independent of whatever the written reference contains. Frequently, pertinent questions over the telephone can elicit more candid information. In rare instances, there may be dishonesty through omission by the reference-giver even at this level. This may involve an applicant who an individual, a department or group, or an institution would like to see leave.

In all cases, new personnel in an anesthesia practice environment must be given a thorough and documented orientation and checkout. Policy, procedures, and equipment may be unfamiliar to even the most thoroughly trained, experienced, and safe practitioner. This may occasionally seem tedious, but it is a sound and critically important safety policy. Being in the midst of a crisis situation caused by unfamiliarity with a new setting is not the optimal orientation session.

After the initial granting of clinical privileges to practice anesthesia, anesthesia professionals must periodically renew their privileges within the institution or facility (e.g., annually or every other year). There are moral, ethical, and societal obligations on the part of the privilege-granting entity to take this process seriously. State licensing bodies often become aware of problems with health professionals very late in the evolution of any difficulties. An anesthesia professional's peers in the hospital or facility are much more likely to notice untoward developments as they first appear. However, privilege renewals are often essentially automatic and receive little of the necessary attention. Judicious checking of renewal applications and awareness of relevant peer review information are absolutely necessary. The anesthesia professionals or administrators responsible for evaluating staff members and reviewing their practices and privileges may be justifiably concerned about retaliatory legal action by a staff member who is censured or denied privilege renewal. Accordingly, such evaluating groups must be thoroughly objective (totally eliminating any hint of political or financial motives) and must have documentation that the staff person in question is in fact practicing below the standard of care. Court decisions have found liability by a hospital, its medical staff, or both, when the incompetence of a staff member was known or should have been known and was not acted upon.[3] Again, questions about complex sensitive issues such as this should be referred to an experienced attorney familiar with applicable federal and state law.

A major issue in the granting of clinical privileges, especially in procedure-oriented specialties such as anesthesiology, is whether it is reasonable to continue the common practice of "blanket" privileges. This process in effect authorizes the practitioner to attempt any treatment or procedure normally considered within the purview of the applicant's medical specialty. These considerations may have profound political and economic implications within medicine, such as which type of surgeon should be doing carotid endarterectomies or lumbar discectomies. More important, however, is whether the practitioner being evaluated is qualified to do everything traditionally associated with the specialty. Specifically, should the granting of privileges to practice anesthesia automatically approve the practitioner to handle pediatric cardiac cases, critically ill newborns (such as a day-old premature infant with a large diaphragmatic hernia), ablative pain therapy (such as an alcohol celiac plexus block under fluoroscopy), high-risk obstetric cases, and so forth? This question raises the issue of procedure-specific or limited privileges. The quality assurance (QA) and risk management considerations in this question are weighty if inexperienced or insufficiently qualified practitioners are allowed or even expected, because of peer or scheduling pressures, to undertake major challenges for which they are not prepared. The likelihood of complications and adverse outcome will be higher, and the difficulty of defending the practitioner against a malpractice claim in the event of catastrophe will be significantly increased.

There is no clear answer to the question of procedure-specific credentialing and granting of privileges. Ignoring issues regarding qualifications to undertake complex and challenging procedures has clear negative potential. On the other hand, stringent procedure-specific credentialing is impractical in smaller groups, and in larger groups encourages many small "fiefdoms," with a consequent further atrophy of the clinical skills outside the practitioner's specific area(s). Each anesthesia department or group needs to address these issues. At the very least, the common practice of every applicant for privileges (new or renewal) checking off every line on the printed list of anesthesia procedures should be reviewed. In addition, board certification for physicians is now essentially a standard of QA of the minimum skills required for the consultant practice of anesthesiology. Subspecialty boards, such as those in pain management, critical care, and transesophageal echocardiography, further objectify the credentialing process. This is now significant because initial board certification after the year 2000 by the American Board of Anesthesiology (ABA) is time-limited and subject to periodic testing and recertification (see Maintenance of Certification below). Many states, some institutions, and even some regulatory bodies have requirements for a minimum number of hours of continuing medical education (CME). Documentation of fulfilling such a standard again acts as one type of quality assurance mechanism for the individual practitioner, while providing another objective credentialing measurement for those granting licenses or privileges.

Maintenance of Certification in Anesthesiology

American anesthesiologists certified as diplomates by the ABA after January 1, 2000, are issued a "time-limited" board certification valid for 10 years. A formal process culminating in the recertification of an anesthesiologist for an additional and then subsequent 10-year intervals has evolved and now appropriately is called "Maintenance of Certification in Anesthesiology" (MOCA). Because certification by a medical specialty board is now often expected or actually required by medical staff bylaws in order to obtain and maintain medical facility privileges, even anesthesiologists who were certified (without a time limit) prior to the year 2000 likely will be engaging in the MOCA process.

In 1999, the American Board of Medical Specialties (ABMS) initiated a process to better insure continuing professional development of diplomates certified by the member boards. An enhancement of the traditional CME process, this initiative by the ABMS is designed to provide a transparent public system of accountability that physician skill and knowledge base do not wane while practicing after completion of formal training. Centered around the American Council for Graduate Medical Education core competencies of (1) patient-centered care, (2) medical knowledge, (3) interpersonal and communication skills, (4) professionalism, (5) system-based practice, and (6) practice-based learning improvement, each member board designs a curricular process to enhance and evaluate continued development of the competencies throughout the professional career of the certified clinician.

The MOCA program introduced in 2000 is subdivided into four components or modules: (1) professional standing, (2) lifelong learning and self-assessment, (3) cognitive examination, and (4) practice performance assessment and improvement.

Each module has specific requirements that must be completed within the 10-year cycle. For example, the professional standing component requires maintenance of an unrestricted medical license within the United States or Canada. The lifelong learning and self-assessment component includes up to 350 hours of category 1 CME from an accredited body with a recent requirement that 90 hours be from the ASA "Self Education and Evaluation" (SEE) or "Anesthesiology Continuing Education" (ACE) CME programs. Presently, the cognitive examination consists of 200 multiple-choice questions from the keyword content for

MOCA from the ABA. Practice performance assessment and improvement involves written evaluation of the practitioner's skill by a department chair or other anesthesiology colleagues in leadership positions within an institution highly familiar with that individual's clinical work. A newer component of the practice performance assessment and improvement module requires completion of a case scenario at one of the ASA-accredited simulation centers.

The ABA web site (www.theaba.org/home/MOCA *Tutorial*) provides a database for diplomates within the MOCA process which is referred to as a "portal account." This portal account is a password-protected repository in which collected MOCA material may be compiled during the 10-year cycle period. The site includes the ability to track the CME hours obtained in each year of the cycle. If the CME credits are not obtained through one of the ABA-approved sources, these CME hours are subject to audit by the ABA. Persons with time-limited certificates issued between 2000 and 2010 may have differing requirements for recertification as the process has been in continuous evolution since being instituted. As noted and importantly, American anesthesiologists certified before 2000 are increasingly finding that their institutions or medical staff bylaws require participation in the MOCA process, even if not mandated by the ABA. All practitioners should consult their individual medical staff bylaws and institutional regulations as well as the ABA web site to determine the best course of action to maintain primary certification in anesthesiology.

Clinicians with subspecialty training in Critical Care and Pain Medicine also have a MOCA process available. At present there are no CME hours or simulation case scenarios required to sit for these subspecialty examinations, though it seems reasonable to expect that these components will be forthcoming in the future as the ABMS strongly encourages that lifelong learning/self-assessment as well as evaluation through simulation are key components to the recertification process.

It is reasonable to project that the MOCA process will continue to evolve and likely will become more comprehensive over time as the overall emphasis on assuring both quality and efficiency of medical care in the United States increases further due to the expectations of accrediting bodies, government regulators, third-party payers, malpractice insurers, and, above all, the public.

Professional Staff Participation and Relationships

All medical care facilities and practice settings depend on their professional staffs, of course, for daily activities of the delivery of health care but, very importantly, they also depend on those staffs to provide administrative structure and support. Medical staff activities are increasingly important in achieving favorable accreditation status from the "Joint Commission" (formerly known as the Joint Commission for the Accreditation of Healthcare Organizations or JCAHO) and in meeting a wide variety of governmental regulations and reviews. Principal medical staff activities involve sometimes time-consuming efforts, such as duties as a staff officer or committee member. Anesthesiologists should be participants in—in fact, should play a significant role in—credentialing, peer review, tissue review, transfusion review, OR management, and medical direction of same-day surgery units, postanesthesia care units (PACUs), intensive care units (ICUs), and pain management units. Also, it is very important that anesthesiology personnel be involved in fund-raising activities, benefits, community outreach projects sponsored by the facility, and social events of the facility staff.

Anesthesia professionals as a group have a reputation for lack of involvement in medical staff and facility issues, allegedly because of lack of time due to long hours in the OR or simply lack of interest. In fact, anesthesiology professionals are all-too-often perceived in a facility as the ones who slip in and out of the building essentially anonymously (often dressed very casually or even in the pajama-like comfort of scrub suits) and virtually unnoticed. This is an unfortunate state of affairs, and it has frequently come back in various painful ways to haunt those who have not been involved, or even noticed, within their own facility. Anesthesia professionals sometimes respond that the demands for anesthesiology service are so great that they simply never have the time or the opportunity to become involved in their facility and with their peers. If this is really true, it is clear that more anesthesia professionals must be added at that facility, even if doing so slightly reduces the income of those already there.

If anesthesia professionals are not involved and not perceived as interested, dedicated "team players," they will be shut out of critical negotiations and decisions relevant to their practice. Although one obvious instance in which others could make decisions for uninvolved anesthesia professionals is the distribution of "bundled" practice fee income collected by a central "umbrella" medical practice organization, there are many such situations, and the excluded anesthesia professionals will be forced to comply with the resulting mandates.

Similarly, involvement with a facility, a professional staff, or a multispecialty group goes beyond formal organized governance and committee activity. Collegial relationships with professionals of other specialties and with administrators are central to maintenance of a recognized position and avoidance of the situation of exclusion just described. Being readily available for formal and informal consults, particularly regarding preoperative patient workup and the maximally efficient way to get surgeons' patients to the OR in a timely, expedient manner, is extremely important. No one individual can be everywhere all the time, but an anesthesiology group or department should strive to be always responsive to any request for help from physicians or administrators. It often appears that anesthesia professionals fail to appreciate just how great a positive impact a relatively simple involvement (starting an intravenous line for a pediatrician, helping an internist manage an ICU ventilator, or helping a facility administrator unclog a jammed recovery room) may have.

Establishing Standards of Practice and Understanding the Standard of Care

The increasing frequency and intensity of "production pressure",[4] with the tacit (or even explicit) directive to anesthesia professionals to "go fast" no matter what and to "do more with less," creates situations in which anesthesia professionals may conclude that they must cut corners and compromise safe patient care just to stay in business. This type of pressure has become even greater with the implementation of more and more protocols or parameters for practice, some from professional societies such as the ASA and some mandated by or developed in conjunction with purchasers of health care (government, insurance companies, or managed care organizations [MCOs]). Many of these protocols are devised to fast-track patients through the medical care system, especially when an elective procedure is involved, in as absolutely little time as possible, thus minimizing costs. Do these fast-track protocols constitute standards of care that health-care providers must implement? What are the implications of doing so? Of not doing so?

To better understand answers to such questions, it is important to have a basic background in the concept of the standard of care.

The *standard of care* is the conduct and skill of a prudent practitioner that can be expected by a reasonable patient. This is a very important medicolegal concept because a bad medical result due to failure to meet the standard of care is malpractice. Courts have traditionally relied on medical experts knowledgeable about the point in question to give opinions as to what is the standard of care and if it has been met in an individual case. This type of standard is somewhat different from the standards promulgated by various standard-setting bodies regarding, for example, the color of gas hoses connected to an anesthesia machine or the inability to open two vaporizers on that machine simultaneously. However, ignoring the equipment standards and tolerating an unsafe situation is a violation of the standard of care. Promulgated standards, such as the various safety codes and anesthesia machine specifications, rapidly become the standard of care because patients (through their attorneys, in the case of an untoward event) expect the published standards to be observed by the prudent practitioner.

Ultimately, the standard of care is what a jury says it is. However, it is possible to anticipate, at least in part, what knowledge and actions will be expected. There are two main sources of information as to exactly what is the expected standard of care. Traditionally, the beliefs offered by expert witnesses in medical liability lawsuits regarding what is actually being done in real life (de facto standards of care) were the main input juries had in deciding what was reasonable to expect from the defendant. The resulting problem is well known: except in the most egregious cases, it is usually possible for the lawyers to find experts who will support each of the two opposing sides, making the process more subjective than objective. (Because of this, there are even ASA *Guidelines for Expert Witness Qualifications and Testimony* and an equivalent document from the American Association of Nurse Anesthetists). Of course, there can be legitimate differences of opinion among thoughtful, insightful experts, but even in these cases the jury still must decide who is more believable, looks better, or sounds better. The second, much more objective, source for defining certain component parts of the standard of care is the published standards of care, guidelines, practice parameters, and protocols that have become more and more common since the idea was originally introduced.[5] These serve as more objective evidence of what can be reasonably expected of practitioners and can make it easier for a jury evaluating whether a malpractice defendant failed to meet the applicable standard of care. Several types of documents exist and have differing implications.

Leading the Way

4 Anesthesiology may be the medical specialty most involved with published standards of care. It has been suggested that the nature of anesthesia practice (having certain central critical functions relatively clearly defined and common to all situations and also having an emphasis on technology) makes it the most amenable of all the fields of medicine to the use of published standards. The original intraoperative monitoring standards[5] are a classic example. The ASA first adopted its own set of basic intraoperative monitoring standards in 1986 and has modified them several times. The text of all ASA standards, guidelines, statements, practice parameters, practice advisories, and other documents is readily available on the ASA web site home page under the "Practice Management" or "Patient Quality and Safety" tags.

The Standards for Basic Anesthetic Monitoring document includes clear specifications for the presence of personnel during an anesthetic episode and for continual evaluation of oxygenation, ventilation, circulation, and temperature. These ASA monitoring standards very quickly became part of the accepted standard of care in anesthesia practice. This means they are important to practice management because they have profound medicolegal implications: a catastrophic accident occurring while the standards are being actively ignored is very difficult to defend in the consequent malpractice suit, whereas an accident that occurs during well-documented full compliance with the standards will automatically have a strong defense because the standard of care was being met. Several states in the United States have made compliance with these ASA standards mandatory under state regulations or even statutes. Various malpractice insurance companies offer discounts on malpractice insurance policy premiums for compliance with these standards, something quite natural to insurers because they are familiar with the idea of managing known risks to help minimize financial loss to the company.

With many of the same elements of thinking, the ASA adopted "Basic Standards for Preanesthesia Care." This was supplemented significantly by another type of document, the ASA *Practice Advisory for Preanesthesia Evaluation.*[6] Also, the ASA adopted "Standards for Postanesthesia Care," in which there was consideration of and collaboration with the very detailed standards of practice for PACU care published by the American Society of Post Anesthesia Nurses (another good example of the sources of standards of care). This also was later supplemented by an extensive *Practice Guideline.*[7]

A slightly different situation exists with regard to the standards for conduct of anesthesia in obstetrics. These standards were originally passed by the ASA in 1988, in the same manner as the other ASA standards, but the ASA membership eventually questioned whether they reflected a realistic and desirable standard of care. Accordingly, the obstetric anesthesia standards were downgraded in 1990 to guidelines, specifically to remove the mandatory nature of the document. Because there was no agreement as to what should be prescribed as the standard of care, the medicolegal imperative of published standards in this instance has been temporarily set aside. From a management perspective, this makes the guidelines no less valuable because the intent of optimizing care through the avoidance of complications is no less operative. However, in the event of the need to defend against a malpractice claim in this area, it is clear from this sequence of events that the exact standard of care is debatable and not yet finally established (an extremely important medicolegal consideration). A different ASA document has since been generated, *Practice Guidelines for Obstetrical Anesthesia*, with more detail and specificity as well as an emphasis on the meta-analytic approach.[8]

Practice Guidelines

An important type of related ASA document is the *Practice Guideline* (formerly "Practice Parameter"). This has some of the same elements as a standard of practice but is more intended to guide judgment, largely through algorithms with some element of guidelines, in addition to directing the details of specific procedures as would a formal standard. Beyond the details of the minimum standards for carrying out the procedure, these practice parameters set forth algorithms and guidelines for helping to determine under what circumstances and with what timing to perform it. Understandably, purchasers of health care (government, insurance companies, and MCOs) with a strong desire to limit the costs of medical care have great interest in practice parameters as potential vehicles for helping to eliminate "unnecessary" procedures and limit even the necessary ones.

The ASA has been very active in creating and publishing practice guidelines. The first published parameter (since revised) concerned the use of pulmonary artery (PA) catheters.[9] It considered the clinical effectiveness of PA catheters, public policy issues (costs and concerns of patients and providers), and recommendations (indications and practice settings). Also, the ASA *Difficult Airway Algorithm* was published in an updated form in 2003.[10] This thoughtful document synthesizes a strategy summarized in a decision tree diagram for dealing acutely with airway problems. The difficult airway algorithm has been discussed extensively in the literature, including suggestions regarding the role of supraglottic airways and, more recently, adding the various airway video imaging technologies. This illustrates that all the ASA practice guidelines involve fluid concepts that are subject to reconsideration, reinterpretation, and revision as experience and technology evolve. Undoubtedly, the difficult airway algorithm has great clinical value and helps many patients. However, there is concern that, as with many modern things, that it starts to outdate as soon as it is published. Such considerations are important, both clinically and because all these documents are readily noticed by plaintiffs' lawyers as relevant to establishing the applicable standard of care.

An important and so-far undecided question is whether guidelines and practice parameters from recognized entities such as the ASA *define* the standard of care. There is no simple answer. This will be decided over time by practitioners' actions, debates in the literature, mandates from malpractice insurers, and, of course, court decisions. Some guidelines, such as the concepts in the US Food and Drug Administration (FDA) preanesthetic apparatus checkout, are accepted as the standard of care. There will be debate among experts, but the practitioner must make the decision as to how to apply practice parameters and guidelines such as those from the ASA. Practitioners have incorrectly assumed that they *must* do everything specified. This is clearly not true, yet there is a valid concern that these will someday be held up as defining the standard of care. Accordingly, prudent attention within the bounds of reason to the principles outlined in guidelines and parameters will put the practitioner in at least a reasonably defensible position, whereas radical deviation from them should be based only on obvious exigencies of the situation at that moment or clear, defensible alternative beliefs (with documentation).

The most recent type of document has been the "practice advisory," which can seem functionally similar to a guideline, but appears to have the implication of more consensus compromise than previous documents driven more by meta-analysis of the relevant literature. Examples of ASA Practice Advisories include "Intraoperative Awareness and Brain Function Monitoring," "Perioperative Management of Patients with Cardiac Rhythm Management Devices: Pacemakers and Implantable Cardioverter-Defibrillators," "Perioperative Visual Loss Associated with Spine Surgery," and "Practice Advisory on Anesthetic Care for Magnetic Resonance Imaging." At any given time, there are several additional topics under consideration and new advisories being prepared, indicating that anesthesia professionals would be wise to keep up to date on the documents published.

The potential QA and medicolegal implications of these documents are so important to anesthesia professionals and their practices that the ASA has what is essentially a guideline for the guidelines in its 2008 update of the "Policy Statement on Practice Parameters" in which the distinction is made between evidence-based documents and consensus-based documents with explanations of the background and formulation processes for each.

On the other hand, practice protocols, such as those for the fast-track management of coronary artery bypass graft patients, that are handed down by MCOs or health insurance companies are a different matter. Even though the desired implication is that practitioners must observe (or at least strongly consider) them, they do not have the same implications in defining the standard of care as the other documents. Practitioners must avoid getting trapped. It may well not be a valid legal defense to justify action or the lack of action because of a company or facility protocol. As difficult as it may be to reconcile with the payer, the practitioner still is subject to the classic definitions of standard of care.

The other types of standards associated with medical care are those of the Joint Commission, which is the best-known medical care quality regulatory agency. As noted, these standards were for many years concerned largely with structure (e.g., gas tanks chained down) and process (e.g., documentation complete), but in recent years they have been expanded to include reviews of the *outcome* of care. Joint Commission standards also focus on credentialing and privileges, verification that anesthesia services are of uniform quality throughout an institution, the qualifications of the director of the service, continuing education, and basic guidelines for anesthesia care (need for preoperative and postoperative evaluations, documentation, and so forth). Full Joint Commission accreditation of a health-care facility is usually for 3 years. Even the best hospitals and facilities receive some citations of problems or deficiencies that are expected to be corrected, and an interim report of efforts to do so is required. If there are enough problems, accreditation can be conditional for 1 year, with a complete reinspection at that time. Being ready for a Joint Commission inspection (which is unannounced and can come at any time) starts with verification that essential group/department structure is in place; an excellent outline/checklist exists.[1] The process of "constant preparation" ultimately involves a great deal of work, but because the standards usually do promote high-quality care, the majority of this work is highly constructive and of benefit to the institution and its medical staff.

Review Implications

"Peer review organizations"[11] were established in the 1980s and 1990s in every state, usually affiliated with state medical associations and/or state licensing agencies both to monitor quality of medical care and perform utilization reviews (URs), which were oriented to reducing health-care costs. These functions have migrated in recent years largely to the government insurers Medicare and Medicaid and have become fixated essentially exclusively on cost issues. Also, each private health insurance company has utilization review functions, whether internal or contracted out to a company that performs that function for the insurer.

The most likely interaction between a UR agency or office and anesthesia professionals will involve a request for perioperative admission of a patient whose care is mandated to be outpatient surgery (this could also occur in dealing with an MCO). If the anesthesiologist feels, for example, that either (1) preoperative admission for treatment to optimize cardiac, pulmonary, diabetic, or other medical status or (2) postoperative admission for monitoring of labile situations such as uncontrolled hypertension will reduce clear anesthetic risks for the patient, an application to UR for approval of admission must be made and vigorously supported. All too often, however, such issues surface a day or so before the scheduled procedure in a preanesthesia screening clinic or even in a preoperative holding area outside the OR on the day of surgery. This will continue to occur until anesthesia providers educate their constituent surgeon community as to what types of associated medical conditions may disqualify a proposed patient from the outpatient (ambulatory) surgical schedule. If adequate notice is given by the surgeon, the patient can be seen far enough in advance by an anesthesiologist to allow appropriate planning.

In the circumstance in which the first knowledge of a questionable patient comes 1 or 2 days before surgery, the anesthesiologist can try to have the procedure postponed, if possible, or can undertake the time-consuming task of multiple telephone calls to get the surgeon's agreement, get UR approval, and make the necessary arrangements. Because neither alternative is particularly attractive, especially from administrative and reimbursement perspectives, there may be a strong temptation to "let it slide" and try to deal with the patient as an outpatient even though this may be questionable. In almost all cases, it is likely that there would be no adverse result (the "get away with it" phenomenon). However, the patient might well be exposed to an avoidable risk. Both because of the workings of probability and because of the inevitable tendency to let sicker and sicker patients slip by as lax practitioners repeatedly "get away with it" and are lulled into a false sense of security, sooner or later there will be an unfortunate outcome or some preventable major morbidity or even mortality.

The situation is worsened when the first contact with a questionable ambulatory patient is preoperatively (or possibly even already in the OR) on the day of surgery. There may be intense pressure from the patient, the surgeon, or the OR administrator and staff to proceed with a case for which the anesthesia practitioner believes the patient is poorly prepared. The arguments made regarding patient inconvenience and anxiety are valid. However, they should not outweigh the best medical interests of the patient. Although this is a point in favor of screening all outpatients before the day of surgery, the anesthesia professional facing this situation on the day of operation should state clearly to all concerned the reasons for postponing the surgery, stressing the issue of avoidable risk and standards of care, and then help with alternative arrangements (including, if necessary, dealing with UR or an MCO).

Potential liability in this regard is the other side of the standard of care issue. Particularly concerning is the question of postoperative admission of ambulatory patients who have been unstable. It is an extremely poor defense against a malpractice claim to state that the patient was discharged home, only later to suffer a complication, because the UR process or an MCO deemed that operative procedure outpatient and not inpatient surgery. As bureaucratically annoying as it may be, it is a prudent management strategy to admit the patient if there is any legitimate question, thus minimizing the chance for complications, and later haggle with the UR bureaucracy.

Policy and Procedure

One important organizational point that is often overlooked in anesthesia practice is the need for a complete policy and procedure manual. Such a compilation of documents is necessary for all practices, from the largest departments covering multiple hospitals to a single-room outpatient facility with one anesthesia provider. Such a manual can be extraordinarily valuable, as, for example, when it provides crucial information during an emergency. Organizational and procedural elements should be included.

The organizational elements that should be present include a chart of organization and responsibilities that is not just a call schedule but a clear explanation of who is responsible for what functions of the department and when, with attendant details such as expectations for the practitioner's presence within the institution at designated hours, telephone availability, pager availability, the maximum permissible distance from the institution when on call, and so forth. Experience suggests it is especially important for there to be an absolutely clear specification of the availability of qualified anesthesiology personnel for emergency cesarean section, particularly in practice arrangements in which there are several people on call covering multiple locations. Sadly, these issues often are only considered after a disaster has occurred that involved miscommunication and the mistaken belief by one or more people that someone else would take care of an acute problem.

The organizational component of the policy and procedure manual should also include a clear explanation of the orientation and checkout procedure for new personnel, CME requirements and opportunities, the mechanisms for evaluating personnel and for communicating this evaluation to them, disaster plans (or reference to a separate disaster manual or protocol), QA activities of the department, and the format for statistical record keeping (number of procedures, types of anesthetics given, types of patients anesthetized, number and types of invasive monitoring procedures, number and type of responses to emergency calls, complications, or whatever the group/department decides).

The procedural component of the policy and procedure manual should give both handy practice tips and specific outlines of proposed courses of action for particular circumstances; it also should store little used but valuable information. Reference should be made to the statements, guidelines, practice parameters and advisories, and standards appearing on the ASA web site. Also included should be references to or specific protocols for the areas mentioned in the Joint Commission standards: preanesthetic evaluation, immediate preinduction reevaluation, safety of the patient during the anesthetic period, release of the patient from any PACU, recording of all pertinent events during anesthesia, recording of postanesthesia visits, guidelines defining the role of anesthesia services in hospital infection control, and guidelines for safe use of general anesthetic agents. Other appropriate topics include the following:

1. Recommendations for preanesthesia apparatus checkout, such as from the FDA[12] (see Chapter 24)
2. Guidelines for admission to, minimal monitoring and duration of stay of an infant, child, or adult in, and then discharge from the PACU
3. Procedures for transporting patients to/from the OR, PACU, or ICU
4. Policy on ambulatory surgical patients—for example, screening, use of regional anesthesia, discharge home criteria
5. Policy on evaluation and processing of same-day admissions
6. Policy on ICU admission and discharge
7. Policy on physicians responsible for writing orders in recovery room and ICU
8. Policy on informed consent for anesthesia and its documentation
9. Policy on the use of patients in clinical research (if applicable)
10. Guidelines for the support of cadaveric organ donors and its termination (plus organ donation after cardiac death if applicable)
11. Guidelines on environmental safety, including pollution with trace gases and electrical equipment inspection, maintenance, and hazard prevention
12. Procedure for change of personnel during an anesthetic and documentation (particularly if a printed hand-off protocol is used)
13. Procedure for the introduction of new equipment, drugs, or clinical practices
14. Procedure for epidural and spinal narcotic administration and subsequent patient monitoring (e.g., type, minimum time, nursing units)
15. Procedure for initial treatment of cardiac or respiratory arrest (updated Advanced Cardiac Life Support guidelines)
16. Policy for handling patient's refusal of blood or blood products, including the mechanism to obtain a court order to transfuse

17. Procedure for the management of malignant hyperthermia
18. Procedure for the induction and maintenance of barbiturate coma
19. Procedure for the evaluation of suspected pseudocholinesterase deficiency
20. Protocol for responding to an adverse anesthetic event (such as a copy of the update of the "Adverse Event Protocol"[13])
21. Policy on resuscitation of do-not-resuscitate patients in the OR

Individual departments will add to and modify these suggestions as dictated by their specific needs. A thorough, carefully conceived policy and procedure manual is a valuable tool. The manual should be reviewed and updated as needed but at least annually. Each member of a group or department should review the manual at least annually and sign off in a log indicating familiarity with current policies and procedures.

Meetings and Case Discussion

There must be regularly scheduled departmental or group meetings. Although didactic lectures and continuing education meetings are valuable and necessary, there also must be regular opportunities for open clinical discussion about interesting cases and problem cases. Also, the Joint Commission requires that there be at least monthly meetings at which risk management and QA activities are documented and reported. Whether these meetings are called case conferences, morbidity and mortality conferences, or deaths and complications conferences, the entire department or group should gather for an interchange of ideas. More recently, these gatherings have been called *QA meetings.* An open review of departmental statistics should be done, including all complications, even those that may appear trivial. Unusual patterns of small events may point toward a larger or systematic problem, especially if they are more frequently associated with one individual practitioner.

A problem case presented at the departmental meeting might be an overt accident, a near accident (critical incident), or an untoward outcome of unknown origin. Honest but constructive discussion, even of an anesthesia professional's technical deficiencies or lack of knowledge, should take place in the spirit of constructive peer review. The classic question, "What would you do differently next time?" is a good way to start the discussion. There may be situations in which inviting the surgeon or the internist involved in a specific case would be advantageous. The opportunity for each type of provider to hear the perspective of another discipline not only is inherently educational, but also can promote communication and cooperation in future potential problem cases.

Records of these meetings must be kept for accreditation purposes, but the enshrining of overly detailed minutes (potentially subject to discovery by a plaintiff's attorney at a later date) may inhibit true educational and corrective interchanges about untoward events. In the circumstance of discussion of a case that seems likely to provoke litigation, it is appropriate to be certain that the meeting is classified as official "peer review" and possibly even invite the hospital attorney or legal counsel from the relevant malpractice insurance carrier (to guarantee the privacy of the discussion and minutes).

Support Staff

There is a fundamental need for support staff in every anesthesia practice. Even independent practitioners rely in some measure on facilities, equipment, and services provided by the organization maintaining the anesthetizing location. In large, well-organized departments, reliance on support staff is often very great. What is often overlooked, however, is a process analogous to that of credentialing and privileges for anesthesia professionals, although at a somewhat different level. The people expected to provide clinical anesthesia practice support must be qualified and must at all times understand what they are expected to do and how to do it. It is singularly unfortunate to realize only after an anesthesia catastrophe has occurred that basic details of simple work assignments, such as the changing of carbon dioxide absorbent, were routinely ignored. This indicates the need for supervision and monitoring of the support staff by the involved practitioners. Further, such support personnel are favorite targets of cost-cutting administrators who do not understand the function of anesthesia technicians or their equivalent. In the modern era, many administrators seem driven almost exclusively by the "bottom line" and cannot appreciate the connection between valuable workers such as these and the "revenue stream." Even though it is obvious to all who work in an OR that the anesthesia support personnel make it possible for there to be patients flowing through the OR, it is their responsibility to convince the facility's fiscal administrator that elimination of such positions is genuinely false economy because of the attendant loss in efficiency, particularly in turning over the room between surgeries. Further, it is also false economy to reduce the number of personnel below that genuinely needed to retrieve, clean, sort, disassemble, sterilize, reassemble, store, and distribute the tools of daily anesthesia practice. Vigorous defense (or initiation of new positions if the staff is inadequate) by the anesthesia professionals should be undertaken, even sometimes with the realization that it may be necessary in some circumstances for them to supplement the budget from the facility with some of their practice income to guarantee an adequate complement of competent workers.

Business and organizational issues in the management of an anesthesia practice are also critically dependent on the existence of a sufficient number of appropriately trained support staff. One frequently overlooked issue that contributes to the negative impression generated by some anesthesiology practices centers on being certain there is someone available to answer the telephone *at all times* during the hours surgeons, other physicians, and OR scheduling desks are likely to call. This seemingly trivial component of practice management is very important to the success of an anesthesiology practice as a business whose principal customers are the surgeons. Certainly there is a commercial server–client relationship both with the patient and the purchaser of health care; however, the uniquely symbiotic nature of the relationship between surgeons and anesthesiologists is such that availability even for simple "just wanted to let you know" telephone calls is genuinely important. The person who answers the telephone is the representative of the practice to the world and must take that responsibility seriously. From a management standpoint, significant impact on the success of the practice as a business often hinges on such details. Further, anesthesia professionals should always have permanent personal electronic pagers (preferably with text and even more preferably two way) and reliable mobile telephones (or the radio equivalent) to facilitate communications from other members of the department or group and from support or facility personnel. This may sound intrusive, but the unusual position of anesthesia professionals in the spectrum of healthcare workers mandates this feature of managing an anesthesiology practice. Anesthesiology professionals should have no hesitation about spending their own practice income to do so. The symbolism alone is obvious.

Anesthesia Equipment and Equipment Maintenance

Problems with anesthesia equipment have been discussed extensively in the past.[14–16] However, compared with human error, overt equipment failure rarely causes intraoperative critical incidents[17] or deaths resulting from anesthesia care. Aside from the obvious human errors involving misuse of or unfamiliarity with the equipment, when the rare equipment failure does occur, it often appears that correct maintenance and servicing of the apparatus has not been done. These issues are part of anesthesia practice management efforts, which could have significant liability implications because there can often be confusion or even disputes about precisely who is responsible for arranging maintenance of the anesthesia equipment—the facility or the practitioners who use it and collect practice income from that activity. In many cases, the facility assumes the responsibility. In situations in which that is not true, however, it is necessary for the practitioners to recognize that responsibility and seek help securing a service arrangement, because this is likely an unfamiliar obligation for clinicians.

Programs for anesthesia equipment maintenance and service have been outlined.[1,18] A distinction is made between failure resulting from progressive deterioration of equipment, which should be preventable because it is observable and should provoke appropriate remedial action, and catastrophic failure, which, realistically, often cannot be predicted. Preventive maintenance for mechanical parts is critical and involves periodic performance checks every 4 to 6 months. Also, an annual safety inspection of each anesthetizing location and the equipment itself is necessary. For equipment service, an excellent mechanism is a relatively elaborate cross-reference system (possibly kept handwritten in a notebook but ideal for maintenance on an electronic spreadsheet program) to identify both the device needing service and also the mechanism to secure the needed maintenance or repair.

Equipment-handling principles are straightforward. Before purchase, it must be verified that a proposed piece of equipment meets all applicable standards, which will usually be true when dealing with new equipment from recognized major manufacturers. The renewed efforts of some facility administrators to save money by attempting to find "refurbished" anesthesia machines and monitoring systems (especially for "off-site," "satellite," or "office-based" locations) should provoke thorough review by the involved practitioners. On arrival, electrical equipment must be checked for absence of hazard (especially leakage of current) and compliance with applicable electrical standards. Complex equipment such as anesthesia machines and ventilators should be assembled and checked out by a representative from the manufacturer or manufacturer's agent. There are potential adverse medicolegal implications when relatively untrained personnel certify a particular piece of new equipment as functioning within specification, even if they do it perfectly. On arrival, a sheet or section in the departmental master equipment log must be created with the make, model, serial number, and in-house identification for each piece of capital equipment (anything with a serial number). This not only allows immediate identification of any equipment involved in a future recall or product alert, but also serves as the permanent repository of the record of every problem, problem resolution, maintenance, and servicing occurring until that particular equipment is scrapped. This log must be kept up-to-date at all times. There have been rare but frightening examples of potentially lethal problems with anesthesia machines leading to product alert notices requiring immediate identification of certain equipment and its service status. It is also very important to involve the manufacturer's representative in pre- and in-service training for those who will use the new equipment. Anesthesia systems with their ventilation and monitoring components have become significantly more integrated and more complex, particularly as they are increasingly electronic and less mechanical. Accordingly, it is critical that anesthesia professionals are properly trained to use their equipment safely. The perception that inadequate training is common and that this represents a threat to patient safety has led the Anesthesia Patient Safety Foundation to initiate a campaign urging anesthesia departments and groups to ensure organized verified complete training of all professionals who will use this new technology.[19]

Service

Beyond the administrative liability implications, precisely what type of support personnel should maintain and service major anesthesia equipment has been widely debated. Some groups or departments rely on factory service representatives from the equipment manufacturers for all attention to equipment, others engage independent service contractors, and still other (often larger) departments have access to personnel (either engineers and/or technicians) permanently within their facility. The single underlying principle is clear: The person(s) doing preventive maintenance and service on anesthesia equipment must be qualified. Anesthesia practitioners may wonder how they can assess these qualifications. The best way is to unhesitatingly ask pertinent questions about the education, training, and experience of those involved, including asking for references and speaking to supervisors and managers responsible for those doing the work. Whether an engineering technician who spent a week at a course at a factory can perform the most complex repairs depends on a variety of factors, which can be investigated by the practitioners ultimately using the equipment in the care of patients. Failure to be involved in this oversight function exposes the practice to increased liability in the event of an untoward outcome associated with improperly maintained or serviced equipment.

Replacement of obsolete anesthesia machines and monitoring equipment is a key element of a risk-modification program. Ten years is sometimes cited as an estimated useful life for an anesthesia machine, but although an ASA statement repeats that idea, it also notes that the ASA promulgated "Guidelines for Determining Anesthesia Machine Obsolescence" in 2004 that does not subscribe to any specific time interval. Very old anesthesia machines likely do not meet certain of the safety standards now in force (such as vaporizer lockout, fresh gas ratio protection, and automatic enabling of the oxygen analyzer). Further, it appears likely that this technology will continue to advance, particularly because of the adoption of anesthesia workstation standards by the European Economic Union that are affecting anesthesia machine design worldwide. Note that some anesthesia equipment manufacturers, anxious to minimize their own potential liability, have refused to support (with parts and service) some of the oldest of their pieces (particularly gas machines) still in use. This disowning of equipment by its own manufacturer is a very strong message to practitioners that such equipment must be replaced as soon as possible.

Should a piece of equipment fail, it must be removed from service and a replacement substituted. Groups, departments, and facilities are obligated to have sufficient backup equipment to cover any reasonable incidence of failure. The equipment removed from service must be clearly marked with a prominent label (so it is not returned into service by a well-meaning technician or practitioner) containing the date, time, person discovering, and the details of the problem. The responsible personnel must be notified so they can remove the equipment, make an entry in the log, and initiate the repair. As indicated in the protocol for response to an adverse event,[13] a piece of equipment involved or suspected in an anesthesia accident must be immediately sequestered and not touched by anybody—particularly not by any equipment service personnel. If a severe accident occurred, it may be necessary for the equipment in question to be inspected at a later time by a group consisting of qualified representatives of the manufacturer, the service personnel, the plaintiff's attorney, the insurance companies involved, and the practitioner's defense attorney. The equipment should thus be impounded following a catastrophic adverse event and treated similarly to any object in a forensic "chain of evidence," with careful documentation of parties in contact with and responsible for securing the equipment in question following such an event. Also, major equipment problems may, in some circumstances, reflect a pattern of failure due to a design or manufacturing fault. These problems should be reported to the FDA's Medical Device Problem Reporting system[20] via MedWatch on Form 3500 (found at www.fda.gov/medwatch/index.html, or telephone 800-FDA-1088). This system accepts voluntary reports from users and requires reports from manufacturers when there is knowledge of a medical device being involved in a serious incident. Whether or not filing such a report will have a positive impact in subsequent litigation is impossible to know, but it is a worthwhile practice management point that needs to be considered in the unlikely but important instance of a relevant event involving equipment failure.

Malpractice Insurance

All practitioners need liability insurance coverage specific for the specialty and role in which they are practicing. It is absolutely critical that applicants for medical liability insurance be completely honest in informing the insurer what duties and procedures they perform. Failure to do so, either from carelessness or from a foolishly misguided desire to reduce the resulting premium, may well result in retrospective denial of insurance coverage in the event of an untoward outcome from an activity the insurer did not know the insured engaged in.

Proof of adequate insurance coverage is usually required to secure or renew privileges to practice at a health-care facility. The facility may specify certain minimum policy limits in an attempt to limit its own liability exposure. It is difficult to suggest specific dollar amounts for policy limits because the details of practice vary so much among situations and locations. The malpractice crisis of the 1980s eased significantly in the early 1990s for anesthesia professionals, largely because of the decrease in number and severity of malpractice claims resulting from anesthesia catastrophes as anesthesia care in the United States became safer.[21–23] The exact analysis of this phenomenon can be debated,[24,25] but it is a simple fact that malpractice insurance risk ratings have been decreased and premiums for anesthesia professionals have not been increased at the same rate as for other specialties, in many cases, have actually decreased. Coverage limits of $1 million/$3 million were purchased by 72% of American anesthesiologists in 2010 (http://viewer.zmags.com/publication/68a45923#/68a45923/26). This policy specification usually means that the insurer will cover up to $1 million liability per claim and up to $3 million total per year, but this terminology is not necessarily universal. Therefore, anesthesia professionals must be absolutely certain what they are buying when they apply for malpractice insurance. Even though anesthesiologists have not recently suffered a great number of very large malpractice payments or jury verdicts,[26] in specific parts of the United States known for a pattern of exorbitant settlements and jury verdicts, liability coverage limits of $2 million/$5 million or even greater may be considered prudent. An additional feature in this regard is the potential to employ "umbrella" liability coverage above the limits of the base policy, as will be noted.

Background

The fundamental mechanism of medical malpractice insurance changed significantly some years ago because of the need for insurance companies to have better ways to predict their "losses" (amounts paid in settlements and judgments). Traditionally, medical liability insurance was sold on an "occurrence" basis, meaning that if the insurance policy was in force at the time of the occurrence of an incident resulting in a claim, whenever within the statute of limitations that claim might be filed, the practitioner would be covered. Occurrence insurance was somewhat more expensive than the alternative "claims-made" policies, but was seen as worth it by some (many) practitioners. These policies created some open-ended exposure for the insurer that sometimes led to unexpected large losses, even some large enough to threaten the existence of the insurance company. As a result, medical malpractice insurers have converted almost exclusively to "claims-made" insurance, which covers only claims that are filed while the insurance is in force. Premium rates for the first year a physician is in practice are relatively low because there is less likelihood of a claim coming in (a majority of malpractice suits are filed 1 to 3 years after the event in question). The premiums usually increase yearly for the first 5 years and then the policy is considered "mature." The issue comes when the physician later, for whatever reason, must change insurance companies (e.g., because of relocation to another state). If the physician simply discontinues the policy and a claim is filed the next year, there will be no insurance coverage. Therefore, the physician must secure "tail coverage," sometimes for a minimum number of years (e.g., 5) or, more often, indefinitely to guarantee liability insurance protection for claims filed after the physician is no longer primarily covered by that insurance policy. It may be possible in some circumstances to purchase tail coverage from a different insurer than was involved with the primary policy, but by far the most common thing done is to simply extend the existing insurance coverage for the period of the tail. This very often yields a bill for the entire tail coverage premium, which can be quite sizable, potentially staggering a physician who simply wants to move to another state where his or her existing insurance company is not licensed to or refuses to do business. Individual situations will vary widely, but it is reasonable for anesthesiologists organized into a fiscal entity to consider this issue at the time of the inception of the group and record their policy decisions in writing, rather than facing the potentially difficult question of how to treat one individual later. Other strategies have occasionally been employed when insuring the tail period, including converting the previous policy to part-time status for a period of years, and purchasing "nose" coverage from the new insurer—that is, paying an initial higher yearly premium with the new insurer, who then will cover claims that may occur during the tail period. Whatever strategy is adopted, it is critical that the individual practitioner is absolutely certain through personal verification that he or she is thoroughly covered at the time of any transition. The potential stakes are much too great to leave such important issues solely to an office clerk. Further, a practitioner arriving in a new location is often filling a need or void and is urged to begin clinical work as soon as possible by others who have been shouldering an increased load. It is essential that the new arrival verify with confirmation in writing (often called a "binder") that malpractice liability insurance coverage is in force before there is any patient contact.

Another component to the liability insurance situation is consideration of the advisability of purchasing yet another type of insurance called *umbrella coverage,* which is activated at the time of the need to pay a claim that exceeds the limits of coverage on the standard malpractice liability insurance policy. Because such an enormous claim is extremely unlikely, many practitioners are tempted to forgo the comparatively modest cost of such insurance coverage in the name of economy. As before, it is easy to see that this is potentially a very false economy—if there is a huge claim. Practitioners should consult with their financial managers and advisors, but it is likely that it would be considered wise management to purchase "umbrella" liability insurance coverage.

Medical malpractice insurers are becoming increasingly active in trying to prevent incidents that will lead to insurance claims. They often sponsor risk management seminars to teach practices and techniques to lessen the chances of liability claims and, in some cases, suggest (or even mandate) specific practices, such as strict documented compliance with the ASA "Standards for Basic Anesthetic Monitoring." In return for attendance at such events and/or the signing of contracts stating that the practitioner will follow certain guidelines or standards, the insurer often gives a discount on the liability insurance premium. Clearly, it is sound practice management strategy for practitioners to participate maximally in such programs. Likewise, some insurers make coverage conditional on the consistent implementation of certain strategies such as minimal monitoring, even stipulating that the practitioner will not be covered if it is found that the guidelines were being consciously ignored at the time of an untoward event. Again, it is obviously wise from a practice management standpoint to cooperate fully with such stipulations.

Response to an Adverse Event

5 In spite of the decreased incidence of anesthesia catastrophes, even with the very best of practice, it is statistically likely that each anesthesiologist at least once in his or her professional life will be involved in a major anesthesia accident (see Chapter 4). Precisely because such an event is rare, very few are prepared for it. It is probable that the involved personnel will have no relevant past experience regarding what to do. Although an obvious resource is another anesthetist who has had some exposure or experience, one of these may not be available either. Various authors have discussed what to do in that event.[27–29] Cooper et al.[30] thoughtfully presented the appropriate immediate response to an accident in a straightforward, logical, compact format (that has been updated[13] that should periodically be reviewed by all anesthesiology practitioners and should be included in all anesthesia policy and procedure manuals. This "adverse events protocol" is also always immediately available at www.apsf.org ("Resource Center," then "Clinical Safety Tools"). Unfortunately, however, the principal personnel involved in a significant untoward event may react with such surprise or shock as to temporarily lose sight of logic. At the moment of recognition that a major anesthetic complication has occurred or is occurring, help must be called. A sufficient number of people to deal with the situation must be assembled on site as quickly as possible. For example, in the unlikely but still possible event that an esophageal intubation goes unrecognized long enough to cause a cardiac arrest, the immediate need is for enough skilled personnel to conduct the resuscitative efforts, including making the correct diagnosis and replacing the tube into the trachea. Whether the anesthesiologist apparently responsible for the complication should direct the immediate remedial efforts will depend on the person and the situation. In such a circumstance, it would seem wise for a senior or supervising anesthesiologist quickly to evaluate the scenario and make a decision. This person becomes the "incident supervisor" and has responsibility for helping prevent continuation or recurrence of the incident, for investigating the incident, and for ensuring documentation while the original and helping anesthesiologists focus on caring for the patient. As noted, involved equipment must be sequestered and not touched until such time as it is certain that it was not involved in the incident.

If the accident is not fatal, continuing care of the patient is critical. Measures may be instituted to help limit damage from brain hypoxia. Consultants may be helpful and should be called without hesitation. If not already involved, the chief of anesthesiology must be notified as well as the facility administrator, risk manager, and the anesthesiologist's insurance company. These latter are critical to allow consideration of immediate efforts to limit later financial loss. (Likewise, there are often provisions in medical malpractice insurance policies that might limit or even deny insurance coverage if the company is not notified of any reportable event immediately.) If there is an involved surgeon of record, he or she probably will first notify the family, but the anesthesiologist and others (risk manager, insurance loss control officer, or even legal counsel) might appropriately be included at the outset. Full disclosure of facts as they are best known—with no confessions, opinions, speculation, or placing of blame—is currently still believed to be the best presentation. Any attempt to conceal or shade the truth will later only confound an already difficult situation. Obviously, comfort and support should be offered, including, if appropriate, the services of facility personnel such as clergy, social workers, and counselors. There is a relatively recent movement in medical risk management and insurance advocating immediate full disclosure to the victim or survivors, including "confessions" of medical judgment and performance errors with attendant sincere apologies. If indicated, early offers of reasonable compensation may be included. There have been instances when this overall strategy has prevented the filing of a malpractice lawsuit and has been applauded by all involved as an example of a shift from the "culture of blame" with punishment to a "just culture" with restitution. A widespread movement to implement immediate disclosure and apology has received support.[31,32]

Certain states have enacted or proposed the so-called "I'm sorry!" legislation intended to prevent any explanation or apology from being used as plaintiff's evidence in a subsequent malpractice suit. The importance of the patient's perspective on a serious adverse anesthesia event was highlighted in a riveting account of the stories of both survivors of anesthesia catastrophes and the families of patients who died.[33] In each case, one main message was the enormous negative impact of the perceived failure of the involved anesthesia professionals and their institutions to share detailed information about what exactly happened. A review summarized what patients want and expect following an adverse event.[34] Laudable as this policy of immediate full disclosure and apology may sound, it would be mandatory for an individual practitioner to check with the involved liability insurance carrier, the practice group, and the facility administration before attempting it.

The primary anesthesia provider and any others involved must document relevant information. Never, ever change any existing entries in the medical record. Write an amendment note if needed, with careful explanation of why amendment is necessary, particularly stressing explanations of professional judgments involved. State only facts as they are known. Make no judgments about causes or responsibility and do not "point fingers." The same guidelines hold true for the filing of the incident report in the facility, which should be done as soon as is practical. Further, all discussions with the patient or family should be carefully documented in the medical record. Recognizing that detailed memories of the events may fade in the 1 to 3 years before the practitioner may face deposition questions about exactly what happened, it is possible that it will be recommended, immediately after the incident, that the involved clinical personnel sit down as soon as practical and write out their own personal notes, which will include opinions and impressions as well as maximally detailed accounts of the events as they unfolded. These personal notes are not part of the medical record or the facility files. These notes should be written in the physical presence of an involved attorney representing the practitioner, even if this is not yet the specific defense attorney secured by the malpractice insurance company, and then that attorney should take possession of and keep those notes as case material. This strategy is intended to make the personal notes "attorney–client work product," and thus not subject to forced "discovery" (revelation) by other parties to the case.

Follow-up after the immediate handling of the incident will involve the primary anesthesiologist but should again be directed by a senior supervisor, who may or may not be the same person as the incident supervisor. The "follow-up supervisor" verifies the adequacy and coordination of ongoing care of the patient and facilitates communication among all involved, especially with the risk manager. Lastly, it is necessary to verify that adequate post-event documentation is taking place.

Of course, it is expected that such an adverse event will be discussed in the applicable morbidity and mortality meeting. It is necessary, however, to coordinate this activity with the involved risk manager and attorney so as to be completely certain that the contents and conclusions of the discussion are clearly considered peer review activity, and thus are shielded from discovery by the plaintiffs' attorney.

Unpleasant as this is to contemplate, it is better to have a clear plan and execute it in the event of an accident causing injury to a patient. Vigorous immediate intervention may improve the outcome for all concerned.

PRACTICE ESSENTIALS

The "Job Market" for Anesthesia Professionals

While it is true that in the mid-1990s, for the first time in the modern era, uncertainty faced residents finishing anesthesiology training because of a perception that there were not enough jobs for physician anesthesiologists available, that concept faded quickly. A tension between supply and demand developed, with a significant ongoing component of the idea that there was an overall shortage of anesthesia professionals. With the fading of the concept that managed care as envisioned in the 1990s would significantly reduce the demand for medical services and also the aging of the Baby Boom population, it appears that there may be a significant shortage of all medical professionals in the United States, and this also includes anesthesia professionals. To this end, several new medical schools have opened or will soon. Also, the total number of anesthesia residents and fellows in training increased 16% from academic year 2005–2006 to 2011–2012.[35] However, the dramatic economic downturn ("the Great Recession") late in the first decade of the 21st century complicated the issues of supply and demand. Some finishing residents (who would otherwise not have) sought fellowship training in order to be "more competitive" when seeking a practice position. Older practicing anesthesiologists who would have normally been expected to retire and thus open up practice spots may be postponing retirement due to financial uncertainties. Also, state and federal budget support for medical schools and residency training positions may be threatened by economic uncertainties while hospital budget pressures may influence subsidies for anesthesia practices. While there will always be a need for anesthesia professionals, probably increasing now and in the immediate future, there likely will be more factors to consider in seeking a practice position than ever before.

Types of Practice

Anesthesiology professionals finishing their training still need to choose among three fundamental possibilities: academic practice in a teaching hospital environment, a practice exclusively of patient care in the private practice marketplace, or a practice exclusively of patient care as an employee of a health-care system, organization, or facility.

Teaching hospitals with anesthesiology residency programs constitute only a very small fraction of the total number of facilities requiring anesthesia services. These academic departments tend to be among the largest groups of anesthesiologists, but the aggregate fraction of the entire anesthesiologist population is small. It is interesting, however, that by the nature of the system, most residents and fellows finishing their training have almost exclusively been exposed only to academic anesthesiology. Accordingly, finishing trainees in the past often were comparatively unprepared to evaluate and enter the anesthesiology job market.

Specialty certification by the ABA should be the goal of all anesthesia residency graduates. Some finishing trainees who know they are eventually headed for private practice have started their attending careers as full-time junior faculty in an academic department. This allows them to obtain some clinical practice and supervisory experience and offers them the opportunity to prepare for the ABA examinations in the nurturing, protected academic environment with which they are familiar. Most trainees, however, do not become junior faculty; they accept practice positions immediately. But they should take into account the need to become ABA-certified and build into their new practice arrangements the stipulation that there will be time and consideration given toward this goal.

Academic Practice

For those who choose to stay in academic practice, a number of specific characteristics of academic anesthesia departments can be used as screening questions.

How big is the department? Junior faculty sometimes can get lost in very big departments and be treated as little better than glorified senior residents. On the other hand, the availability of subspecialty service opportunities and significant research and educational resources can make large departments extremely attractive. In smaller academic departments, there may be fewer resources, but the likelihood of being quickly accepted as a valued and contributing member of the teaching faculty (and research team, if appropriate) may be higher. In very small departments, the number of expectations, projects, and involvements could potentially be overwhelming. In addition, a small department may lack a dedicated research infrastructure, so it may be necessary for the faculty in this situation to collaborate with other, larger departments to accomplish meaningful academic work.

What exactly is expected of junior faculty? If teaching one resident class every other week is standard, the candidate must enthusiastically accept that assignment and the attendant preparation work and time up front. Likewise, if it is expected that junior faculty will, by definition, be actively involved in publishable research, specific plans for projects to which the candidate is amenable must be made. In such situations, clear stipulations about start-up research funding and nonclinical time to carry out the projects should be obtained as much as possible (although clinical workload demands and revenue generation expectations may make this very difficult in some settings). Particularly important is determining what the expectation is concerning outside funding. For example, it can be a rude shock to realize that projects will suddenly halt after 2 years if extramural funding has not been secured.

What are the prospects for advancement? Many new junior faculty directly out of residency start with medical school appointments as instructors unless there is something else in their background that immediately qualifies them as assistant professors. It is wise to understand from the beginning what it takes in that department and medical school to facilitate academic advancement. There may be more than one academic "track"; the tenure track, for example, usually depends on published research whereas the clinical or teacher track relies more heavily on one's value in patient care and as a clinical educator. The criteria for promotion may be clearly spelled out by the institution—number of papers needed, involvement and recognition at various levels, grants submitted and funded, and so on—or the system may be less rigid and depend more heavily on the department chairman's and other faculty evaluations and recommendations. In either case, careful inquiry before accepting the position can avert later surprise and disappointment.

How much does it pay? Traditionally, academic anesthesiologists have not earned quite as much as those in private practice—in return for the advantage of more predictable schedules, continued intellectual stimulation, and the intangible rewards of academic success. There is now great activity and attention concerning reimbursement of anesthesiologists, and it is difficult to predict future income for any anesthesiology practice situation. However, all of the forces influencing payment for anesthesia care may significantly diminish the traditional income differential between academic and private practice. In some cases, a faculty member is exclusively an employee of the institution or a component financial entity, which bills and collects or negotiates group contracts for the patient care rendered by the faculty member, and then pays a negotiated amount (either an absolute dollar figure or a floating amount based on volume—or a combination of the two) that constitutes the faculty person's entire income. Under other much less common arrangements, faculty members themselves may be able to bill and collect or negotiate contracts for their clinical work. Some institutions have a (comparatively small) academic salary from the medical school for being on the faculty, but many do not; some channel variable amounts of money (from the so-called Part A clinical revenue) into the academic practice in recognition of teaching and administration or simply as a subsidy for needed service. Usually, the faculty will be members of some type of group or practice plan (either for the anesthesia department alone or the entire faculty as a whole) that bills and collects or negotiates contracts and then distributes the practice income to the faculty under an arrangement that must be examined by the candidate. In most academic institutions, practice expenses such as all overhead and malpractice insurance as well as reasonable benefits, including discretionary funds for meetings, subscriptions, books, dues, and so forth, are automatically part of the compensation package, which often may not be true in private practice and must be counted in making any comparison. An important corollary issue is that of the source of the salaries of the department's primary anesthesia providers—residents and, in some cases, nurse anesthetists. Although the hospital usually pays for at least some of these, arrangements vary, and it is important to ascertain whether the faculty practice income is also expected to cover the cost of the primary providers. Overall, it is appropriate for the candidate to ask probing questions about the commitment of the institution to the maintenance of reasonable compensation for faculty.

Private Practice in the Marketplace

Obviously, rotations to a private practice hospital in the final year of anesthesia residency could help greatly in this regard, but not all residency programs offer such opportunities. In that case, the finishing trainee who is certain about going into private practice must seek information on career development and mentors from the private sector.

Armed with as much information as possible, one fundamental initial choice is between independent individual practice and a position with a group (either a sole proprietorship, partnership, or corporation) that functions as a single financial entity. Independent practice may become increasingly less viable in many locations because of the need to be able to bid for contracts with either practice facilities or managed care entities. However, where independent practice is possible, it usually first involves attempting to secure clinical privileges at a number of hospitals or facilities in the area in which one chooses to live. This may not always be easy, and this issue has been the subject of many (frequently unsuccessful) antitrust suits over recent years (see Antitrust Considerations). Then the anesthesiologist makes it known to the respective surgeon communities that he or she is available to render anesthesia services and waits until there is a request for his or her services. The anesthesiologist obtains the requisite financial information from the patient and then either individually bills and collects for services rendered or employs a service to do billing and collection for a percentage fee (which will vary depending on the circumstances, especially the volume of business; for billing [without scheduling services] it would be unlikely to be more than 7% or, at the most, 8% of actual collections).

How much of the needed equipment and supplies will be provided by the hospital or facility and how much by the independent anesthesiologist varies widely. If an anesthesiologist spends considerable time in one operating suite, he or she may purchase an anesthesia machine exclusively for his or her own use and move it from room to room as needed. It is likely to be impractical to move a fully equipped anesthesia machine from hospital to hospital on a day-to-day basis. Among the features of this style of practice are the collegiality and relationships of a genuine private practice based on referrals and also the ability to decide independently how much time one wants to work. The downside is the potential unpredictability of the demand for service and the time needed to establish referral patterns and obtain bookings sufficient to generate a livable income.

When seeking a position with a private group, the applicant should search for potential practice opportunities through word of mouth, recruiting letters received by the training program, journal advertisements, and placement services (either commercial or professional, such as that provided at the ASA annual meeting). The growing availability and ease of access for online job searching has allowed prospective anesthesiologists and potential employers often to locate suitable candidates without the expense of commercial placement services. However, the most recent trend appears to be increasing reliance on placement services because these concerns vet an applicant for the practices, saving time and energy, and only present a qualified candidate who looks like a potential good fit for the practice. Traditional journal ads from private practices were rare in late 2012. Some of the screening questions by the applicant are the same as for an academic position, but there must be even more emphasis on the exact details of clinical expectations and financial arrangements.

Some trainees finish residency (or fellowship even more so) very highly skilled in complex, difficult anesthesia procedures. They can be surprised to find that in some private practice group situations, the junior-most anesthesiologist must wait some time, perhaps even years, before being eligible to do, for example, open heart anesthesia, and in the meantime will mostly be assigned more routine or less challenging anesthetics.

Financial arrangements in private group practices vary widely. Some groups are loose organizational alliances of independent practitioners who bill and collect separately and rotate clinical assignments and call for mutual convenience. Many groups act also as a fiscal entity, and there are many possible variations on this theme. In many circumstances in the past, new junior members started out as functional employees of the group for a probationary interval before being considered for full membership or partnership. This is not a classic employment situation because it is intended to be temporary as a prelude to full financial participation in the group. However, there have been enough instances of established groups abusing this arrangement that the ASA includes in its fundamental "Statement of Policy" the proviso: "Exploitation of anesthesiologists by other anesthesiologists is improper."[1] This goes on to say that after a reasonable trial period, income should reflect services rendered. These statements may have variable impact on groups in the marketplace. Some groups have a history of demanding excessively long trial periods during which the junior anesthesiologist's income is artificially low and then denying partnership and terminating the relationship to go on to employ a new probationer and start the cycle over again. Accordingly, new junior staff attempting to join groups should try to have such a "path to partnership" spelled out carefully in the agreement drafted by an expert representing the anesthesiologist. One key issue is the partnership "buy-in" once partnership is offered. This usually represents a percentage of the receivables (bills sent but not yet collected). As the cash outlay can be substantial, it is frequently "borrowed" from the group and paid back over time through a decrease in income, further delaying true equity participation in the group's profits. However, in times of great economic uncertainty and retrenchment, it could be theoretically possible that the equity partners in a group might take a cut in income while the employed junior associates continue to collect their full contracted compensation. At the very least, thorough investigation and understanding of the relationship is mandatory. Seeking assistance from an experienced medical practice contract attorney prior to any commitment is likely to be a very worthwhile investment.

Private Practice as an Employee

There has been what appears to be an increasing trend toward anesthesiologists becoming permanent employees of any one of various fiscal entities. The key difference is that there is no intention or hope of achieving an equity position (share of ownership, usually of a partnership, thus becoming a full partner). Hospitals, outpatient surgery centers, multidisciplinary clinics, other facilities tied to a specific location where surgery is performed, physician groups that have umbrella fiscal entities specifically created to serve as the employer of physicians, and even surgeons may seek to hire anesthesiologists as permanent employees. The common thread in this idea is that these fiscal entities want guaranteed anesthesia services they can control. Also, they likely see the anesthesiologists as additional ways of generating profits, or, worse yet, as a financial liability that must be mitigated. Again, in some cases it would appear that employees are not paid compensation that is commensurate with their production of receivables, at least considering traditional collection for anesthesia services in recent decades. That is, the fiscal entity will pay a salary plus appropriate overhead substantially below collections generated by the anesthesia professional's work. These arrangements are particularly favored by some large MCOs in certain geographic areas that view anesthesia professionals simply as expensive necessities that prevent facilities from realizing maximum profit (although sometimes there is a promise of a lighter or more manageable work schedule in these positions compared with marketplace private practice).

Negotiating for a position as a permanent full-time employee is somewhat simpler and more straightforward than it is in marketplace private practice. It parallels the usual understandings that apply to most regular employer–employee situations: job description, role expectations, working conditions, hours, pay, and benefits. The idea of anesthesiologists functionally becoming shift workers disturbs many in the profession because it contradicts the traditional professional model. Again, the complex nature and multiple levels of such considerations make it a personal issue that must be carefully evaluated by each individual with full awareness and consideration of the issues outlined here and commensurate research of ASA resources and available data about common regional circumstances and details of any specific medical community.

Practice as a Hospital Employee

While certified registered nurse anesthetists in some locations have traditionally practiced as hospital employees, until recently, it was less common outside full vertically integrated MCOs for physician anesthesiologists to be hospital (or facility) employees. In recent years, one of the responses of hospitals to requests for subsidies from exclusive-contract private practice groups of anesthesiologists has been to offer the anesthesiologists full-time employment status rather than subsidize an independent practice group that has its own significant administrative and overhead costs.[36] The hospital likely suggests that integrating the billing, collecting, and management functions as well as major overhead costs such as malpractice insurance into the existing larger hospital operation would be very cost-efficient, allowing more financial resources to go to physician salaries, and also with possibly a somewhat greater predictability in financially uncertain times. The hospital can also guarantee the availability of anesthesia care (a requirement to sustain the OR, one of the main hospital revenue sources) in an era when some anesthesiologist groups may simply walk away from a hospital in search of greater income elsewhere, leaving the hospital to seek a contract probably with one of the large and very expensive anesthesia management companies. Of course, in return for employee status, the anesthesiologists surrender some degree of independence and also, for the group's partners, their equity stake in sharing in any subsequent increased practice revenue. A hospital might counter that concern, particularly in the era of facilities subsidizing anesthesia practices, with the contention that traditional anesthesia fee-for-service private practice that has been so common for so long will *never again* yield enough revenue to maintain the compensation levels anesthesiologists have come to expect, so they will not be losing anything.

Practice for a Management Company

One prominent newer development is the growth and impact of large state, regional, or even national management companies that advertise the provision of comprehensive anesthesia services on a contract basis with hospitals, surgery centers, and clinics. These companies, some started and/or managed by anesthesia professionals, promise the facility availability of anesthesia care during the specified hours in return for a lucrative contract to do so. This relieves the facility from any concern about recruiting, hiring/contracting, and retaining anesthesia professionals, virtually eliminating concern about disruption of OR schedules due to limited availability of anesthesia care. The only requirement of the facility is approval of the already prepared credentialing information for each anesthesia professional. Unlike many locum tenens companies in which anesthesia professionals are considered independent contractors and paid fixed contract amounts per hour, per day, or per job for a limited interval with no benefits, some of the management companies may employ anesthesia professionals full time on a salary with benefits (paid vacation, health insurance, retirement contribution, and so forth). The employment agreement would stipulate whether travel for assignments in locations away from the employee's permanent home would be required as a condition of the full-time job or the position will always be in the practitioner's home community.

Practice in the Office-based Setting

Increasingly anesthesia professionals are being recruited into the office-based practice of sedation and general anesthesia for a growing number of procedures. While the governance and oversight of this practice is evolving there are several issues which are clear. A medical director must be appointed to determine the adequacy of facilities and to ensure that the procedures undertaken may be safely and effectively performed given the space, available equipment, and training of personnel involved. The anesthesia professional is a key component in determining patient selection. Practice situations should be avoided where the anesthesia professional does not have real input into the decision making about the patient and procedure. One danger in the office-based setting is that the hired anesthesia professional may feel intense production pressure if the owner/proceduralist (e.g., plastic surgeon, gastroenterologist, oral surgeon, etc.) is adamant about proceeding despite a discussion about the clinical concerns. Basic monitoring standards must be adhered to at all times and supervision of the patient until discharge from the facility must be factored into the time commitment on the part of the anesthesia professional. In addition, ensuring that all anesthesia equipment is up to date and in working order and that the protocols for cardiopulmonary emergencies and transfer of the patient to an outside facility are appropriate is required before accepting an office-based position. Some office-based centers allow the anesthesia professional to bill the patient directly for services rendered in a return to the older and more independent fee-for-service model. Those considering this avenue of practice should review the information and guidelines published by the ASA.[37]

Billing and Collecting

In practices in which anesthesiologists are directly involved with the financial management, they need to understand as much as possible about the complex world of health-care reimbursement. This significant task has been made easier by the ASA, which some time ago added a significant component to its Washington, DC, office (see www.asahq.org/government.htm) by adding a practice management coordinator to the staff. One of the associated assignments is helping ASA members understand and work with the sometimes confusing and convoluted issues of effective billing for anesthesiologists' services. There are often updates with the latest information and codes in the monthly ASA *Newsletter.*

There continue to be proposals for significant changes in billing for anesthesia care. However, the basics have changed only slightly in recent years. It is important to understand that many of the most contentious issues, such as the requirement for physician supervision of nurse anesthetists and the implications of that for reimbursement, apply in many circumstances mostly to Medicare and, in some states, Medicaid. Thus, the fraction of the patient population covered by these government payers is important in any consideration. Different practice situations have different arrangements regarding the financial relationships between anesthesiologists and nurse anesthetists, and this can affect the complex situation of who bills for what. The nurses may be employees of a hospital, of the anesthesiologists who medically direct them, or of no one in that they are independent contractors billing separately (even in cases in which physician supervision—not medical direction—is required but where those physicians do not bill for that component). In 1998, Medicare mandated that an anesthesia care team of a nurse anesthetist medically directed by an anesthesiologist could bill as a team no more than 100% of the fee that would apply if the anesthesiologist did the case alone. The implications of this change were complex and variable among anesthesiology practices. Also, complex related issues played out after that. In 2001, the federal government issued a new regulation allowing individual states to "opt out" of the requirement that nurse anesthetists be supervised by physicians and some states did so (17 states in one form or another as of this writing). This was opposed by the ASA. Because perioperative patient care, one component of which is administering anesthesia, is traditionally considered the practice of medicine, the implications of this change as far as the role of surgeons (or no one) supervising nurse anesthetists and the malpractice liability status of nurse anesthetists practicing independently were unclear. Further, the implications of all this for billing insurers other than Medicare and Medicaid are exceedingly complex.

Classic Methodology

Because there is still widespread application of the traditional method of billing for anesthesiology services, understanding it is important for anesthesia professionals starting practice. In this system, each anesthetic generates a value of so many "units," which represent effort and time. A conversion factor (dollars per unit) that can vary widely multiplied by the number of units generates an amount to be billed. Each anesthetic has a base value number of units (e.g., 8 for a cholecystectomy) and then the time taken for the anesthetic is divided into units, usually 15 minutes per unit. Thus, a cholecystectomy with anesthesia time of 1 hour and 50 minutes would have 8 base units and 7.33 time units for a total of 15.33 units. In some practice settings, it may be allowed to add modifiers, such as extra units for complex patients with multiple problems as reflected by an ASA physical status classification of 3–5 and/or E ("emergency") or for insertion of an arterial or PA catheter. The sum is the total billing unit value. Determining the base value for an anesthetic in units depends on full and correct understanding of what operation was done. Although this sounds easy, it is the most difficult component of traditional anesthesia billing. The process of determining the procedure done is known as *coding* because the procedure name listed on the anesthesia record is assigned an identifying code number from the universally used "current procedural terminology" (CPT)-4 coding book. This code is then translated through the ASA "Relative Value Guide," which assigns a base unit value to the type of procedure identified by the CPT-4 code. In the past, some anesthesiologists failed to understand the importance of correct coding to the success of the billing process. Placing this task in the hands of someone unfamiliar with the system and with surgical terminology can easily lead to incorrect coding. This can fail to capture charges and the resulting income to which the anesthesiologist is entitled or, worse, can systematically overcharge the payers, which will bring sanctions, penalties and, in certain cases, criminal prosecution. The international collection of diseases (ICD) terminology is the method by which providers and payers communicate concerning the type and classification of a given *diagnosis*. Usually, the diagnosis codes are entered by the facility billing for the time in the OR. The current system, ICD-9, has been in use since 1977 and was scheduled for replacement with ICD-10 in 1989. Due to the significant expansion of diagnosis codes, this implementation has been delayed by well over two decades, but is scheduled for October, 2013.

There has been a prevailing official attitude that there are no simple, innocent coding errors. All upcoding (charging for more expensive services than were actually delivered) is considered to be prima facie evidence of fraud and is subject to severe disciplinary and legal action. All practices should have detailed compliance programs in place to ensure correct coding for services rendered.[38] Outside expert help (such as from a health-care law firm that specializes in compliance programs) is highly desirable for the process of formulating and implementing a compliance plan regarding correct coding.

Assembly and transfer of the information necessary to generate bills must be efficient and complete. Traditionally, this involved depositing in a secure central location a paper extra copy of the anesthesia record and often a "billing sheet" with it, on which was inscribed the names of all the involved personnel and any additional information about other potentially billable services, such as invasive monitors. Any practice involved with a comprehensive electronic perioperative information management system in the facility should be using that to assemble this "front end" billing information. Short of that, some practices collect electronic information specifically generated by the anesthesia providers for that purpose. They have equipped each staff member with a handheld electronic device into which data are entered and then the device is synched with a departmental computer at the end of the day. If the OR suite has "Wi-Fi" (wireless electronic connection), the same function could be accomplished in real time with the providers entering the requisite information into a miniprogram on a laptop computer affixed to each anesthesia machine (or carried by each staff member) or a smartphone with the appropriate application installed. Once the information has been secured, a mechanism must be employed to generate the actual bill and communicate it to the payer (on paper, on disk, or, usually, directly computer to computer: "Electronic claims submission"). The possible exact arrangements for doing this vary widely.

Whether an anesthesia practice that will be billing and collecting for anesthesia services should employ its own in-house clerical and bookkeeping personnel to perform this function or should contract with an outside company whose sole function is medical billing and collecting (possibly, ideally, for anesthesiology only) can be debated endlessly. Whichever is chosen, knowledgeable oversight by the anesthesia professionals who ultimately will derive income from the revenue collected is required. Ultimately, the entity actually submitting the bill will verify that it has been paid (posting of receipts) and may or may not actually handle the incoming money. Very often, anesthesia practices or individuals who use a billing service (and even some who have in-house billing staffs) will arrange that the actual payments go directly to a bank lockbox, which is a post office box (better individual than shared, even if more expensive) to which the payments come and then go directly into a bank account. This system avoids the situation of having the people who generate the bill actually handle the incoming receipts, a practice that has led to theft and fraud in a few cases. Eventual decisions about how hard to try to collect from payers who deny coverage and then from patients directly will depend on the circumstances, including local customs.

Detailed summary statistics of the work done by an anesthesiology practice group are critical for logistic management of personnel, scheduling, and financial analysis. Spreadsheet and database computer programs customized for an individual practice's characteristics will be invaluable. A summary of the types of data an anesthesia practice should track is shown in Table 2-1. Once all the data are assembled and reviewed, at least monthly analysis by a business manager or equivalent as well as officers/leaders of the practice group can spot trends very early in their development and allow appropriate correction or planning. Often the responsible members of an anesthesiology group question how effective their financial services operation is, particularly regarding net collections. This is a complex issue[39] that, again, often requires outside help. Routine internal audits can be useful but could be self-serving. No billing office or company that is honest and completely above board should ever object to a client, in this case the anesthesiology practice group, engaging an independent outside auditor to come in and thoroughly examine both the efficiency of the operation and also "the books" concerning correctness and completeness of collections.

Anesthesia billing and collecting are among the most complex challenges in the medical reimbursement field. Traditional anesthesia reimbursement is unique in all of medicine. The experience of many people over the years has suggested that it often is well advised to deal with an entity that is not only very experienced in anesthesia billing, but also does anesthesia billing exclusively or as a large fraction of its efforts. It is very difficult for an anesthesiologist or a family member to do billing and collecting as a side activity to a normal life. This has led to inefficient and inadequate efforts in many cases, illustrating the value of paying a reasonable fee to a professional who will devote great time and energy to this challenging endeavor.

Antitrust Considerations

There can be antitrust implications of business arrangements involving anesthesiologists—particularly with all the realignments, consolidations, mergers, and contracts associated with the attempted implementation of managed care, the drive for cost efficiency and, most recently, the rise of accountable care organizations (ACOs). The applicable statutes and regulations are often poorly understood. Contrary to popular belief, the antitrust laws do not involve the rights of individuals to engage in business. Rather, the laws are concerned solely with the preservation of competition within a defined marketplace and the rights of the consumer, independent of whether any one vendor or provider of service is involved. When an anesthesiologist has been excluded from a particular hospital's staff or anesthesia group and then sues based on an alleged antitrust violation, the anesthesiologist loses virtually automatically. This is because there is still significant competition in the relevant medical care marketplace (community or region) and competition in that market is not threatened by the exclusion of one physician from one staff.

In essence, if there are *several* hospitals offering relatively similar services to an immediate community (the market), denial of privileges to one physician by one hospital is not anticompetitive. If, on the other hand, there is only *one* hospital in a smaller market, then the same act, the same set of circumstances, could be seen very differently. In that case, there would be a limitation of competition because the hospital dominates and, in fact, may control the market for hospital services. Exclusion of one physician, then, could limit access by the consumers to alternative competing services and hence would likely be judged an antitrust violation.

TABLE 2-1. TYPES OF DATA AN ANESTHESIOLOGY GROUP SHOULD TRACK AND MAINTAIN CONCERNING ITS OWN PRACTICE

Types of Data the Anesthesiology Group's Computer System Should Track	Type of Information to Generate from These Data

• Transaction-based system (track each case and charge as separate record)
  • Track individual charges by CPT-4 code
  • Track individual payments by payer
• Track all data elements on an interrelated basis
  • By place of service
  • By charge, broken down
    • by number of units (time and base)
    • by ASA modifiers
    • by number of lines
  • By CPT-4 code
  • By payer
  • By payment code (full payment, discount, write-off, or refund)
  • By diagnosis (ICD-9 code)
  • By surgeon
  • By anesthesiologist
  • By anesthesia care team provider
  • By start and stop times
  • By age
  • By gender
  • By employer
  • By ZIP code
	• Aggregate number of cases per year for the group
	• Total number of cases per year for each provider within the group
	  • Number of cases performed by anesthesiologists
	  • Number of cases performed by the anesthesia care team
	• Average number of units per case (as one measure of intensity per case)
	• Average number of units per CPT-4 code
	• Average time units per case and per CPT-4 code
	  • Group should be able to calculate time units per individual surgeon
	• Average line charge per case
	• Charges per case by CPT-4 code
	• Payments per case by payer
	• Patient mix
	  • Percent traditional indemnity
	  • Percent managed care (broken down by each MCO for which services are provided)
	  • Percent self-pay
	  • Percent Medicare
	  • Percent Medicaid
	• Collection rate for each population served
	• Overall collection rate
	• Costs per unit (total costs, excluding compensation ÷ total units) (costs include liability insurance, rent, collection costs, and legal and accounting fees)
	• Compensation costs per unit (total compensation ÷ total units) for MCO populations, utilization patterns by age, gender, and diagnosis

CPT, current procedural terminology; ASA, American Society of Anesthesiologists; ICD-9, International Classification of Diseases, ninth revision; MCO, managed care organization.

Reprinted from *Managed Care Reimbursement Mechanisms: A Guide for Anesthesiologists.* Park Ridge, IL: American Society of Anesthesiologists; 1994, with permission.

The Sherman Antitrust Act is a federal law more than 100 years old. Section 1 deals with contracts, combinations, conspiracy, and restraint of trade. By definition, two or more separate economic entities must be involved in an agreement that is challenged as illegal for this section to apply. Section 2 prohibits monopolies or conspiracy to create a monopoly, and it is possible that this could apply to a single economic entity that has illegally gained domination of a market. Consideration of possible monopolistic domination of a market involves a situation in which a single entity controls at least 50% of the business in that market. The stakes are high in that the antitrust legislation provides for triple damages if a lawsuit is successful. The US Department of Justice and the Federal Trade Commission are keenly interested in the current rapid evolution and consolidation in the health-care industry, and thus are actively involved in evaluating situations of possible antitrust violations.

There are two ways to judge violations. Under the *per se rule,* which is applied relatively rarely, conduct that is obviously limiting competition in a market is automatically illegal. The other type of violation is based on the *rule of reason,* which involves a careful analysis of the market and the state of competition. The majority of complaints against physicians are judged by this rule. The more competitors there are in a market, the less likely that any one act is anticompetitive. In a community with two hospitals, one smaller than the other, with an anesthesiology group practice exclusively at each, if the larger anesthesiology practice group buys out and absorbs the smaller, leaving only one group for the only two hospitals in the community, that may be anticompetitive, particularly if a new anesthesiologist seeks to practice solo at those hospitals and is refused privileges.

Legal Implications

In the current era of rapidly evolving practice arrangements, the antitrust laws are important. If physicians (individuals or groups) who normally would be competitors because they are separate economic entities meet and agree on the prices they will charge or the terms they will seek in a managed care or institutional contract, that can be anticompetitive, monopolistic, and hence possibly illegal. Note that sharing a common office and common billing service alone is not enough to constitute a true group. If, on the other hand, the same physicians join in a true economic partnership to form a new group (total integration) that is a single economic entity (and meets certain other criteria) that will set prices and negotiate contracts, that is perfectly legal. The other criteria are critical. There must be capital investment and also risk-sharing (if there is a profit or loss, it is distributed among the group members)—that is, total integration into a genuine partnership (that is usually incorporated, sometimes as a limited liability corporation). This issue is very important in considering the drive for new organizations to put together networks of physicians that then seek contracts with major employers to provide medical care. Sometimes, hospitals or clinics attempt to form a network comprising all the members of the medical staff so that the resulting entity can bid globally for total care contracts. Any network is a joint venture of independent practitioners. If the participating physicians of one specialty in a network are separate economic entities and the network advertises one price for their services, this would seem to suggest an antitrust violation (horizontal price fixing). In the past, if a network involved fewer than 20% of one type of medical specialist in a market, that was called a *safe harbor,* meaning that it was permissible for non-partners to get together and negotiate prices. The federal government has tried to encourage formation of such networks to help reduce health-care costs, and as a result made some relevant exceptions to the application of these rules. As long as the network is nonexclusive (other nonnetwork physicians of a given specialty are free to practice in the same facilities and compete for the same patients), the network can comprise up to 30% of the physicians of one specialty in a market. Note specifically that this does not allow a local specialty society in a big city to serve as a bargaining agent on fees for its members because it is very likely that >30% of the specialists in an area will be members of the society. The only real exception to this provision is in thinly populated rural areas where there may be just one physician network. In such cases (which are, so far, rare because the major managed care and network activity has occurred mainly in heavily populated urban areas), there is no limit on how many of one specialty can become network members and have the network negotiate fees, as long as the network is nonexclusive.

Relevant legislation, regulations, and court actions all happen rapidly and often. Mergers among anesthesiology groups in a market area for the purposes of both efficiency and strength in negotiating fees have been very popular as a response to the rapidly changing marketplace. A list of questions must be answered to determine if such a merger would have anticompetitive implications. Although compendia of relevant information are available to anesthesiologists,[40,41] they cannot substitute for expert advice and help. Obviously, anesthesiologists contemplating a merger or facing any one of a great number of other situations in the modern health-care arena must secure assistance from professional advisors, usually attorneys, whose job it is to be aware of the most recent developments, how they apply, and how best to forge agreements in formal contracts. Anesthesiologists hoping to find reputable advisors can start their search with word-of-mouth referrals from colleagues who have used such services. Local or state medical societies frequently know of attorneys who specialize in this area. Finally, the ASA Washington, DC, office has compiled a state-by-state list of advisors who have worked successfully with anesthesiologists in the past.

Exclusive Service Contracts

Often, one of the larger issues faced by anesthesiologists seeking to define practice arrangements concerns the desirability of considering an exclusive contract with a health-care facility to provide anesthesia services. An exclusive contract states that anesthesiologists practicing at a given facility must be members of the group holding the exclusive contract and, usually, that members of the group will practice nowhere else. A hospital may want to give an exclusive contract in return for a guarantee of coverage as part of the contract. Also, the hospital may believe that such a contract can help ensure the quality of practitioner because the contract can contain credentialing and performance criteria. It is important to understand that the hospital likely will exercise a degree of control over the anesthesiologists with such a contract in force, such as requiring them to participate as providers in any contracts the hospital makes with third-party payers and also tying hospital privileges to the existence of the contract (the so-called clean-sweep provision that bypasses any due process of the medical staff should the hospital terminate the contract). Certain of these types of provisions constitute *economic credentialing,* which is defined as the use of economic criteria unrelated to the quality of care or professional competency of physicians in granting or renewing hospital privileges (such as the acceptance of below-market fees associated with a hospital-negotiated care contract or even requiring financial contributions in some form to the hospital).

The ASA in the past has opposed economic credentialing. However, the anesthesiologists involved may accept such an exclusive services contract to guarantee that they alone will get the business from the surgeons on staff at that hospital, and hence the resulting income. There may be other considerations on both sides, and these have been outlined in extensive relevant ASA publications that also include a sample contract for information purposes only.[40] It is critical that anesthesiologists faced with important practice management decisions such as whether to enter into an exclusive contract must seek outside advice and counsel. There are a great many nuances to these issues,[40–43] and anesthesiologists are at risk attempting to negotiate such complex matters alone, just as patients would be at risk if a contract attorney attempted to induce general anesthesia.

Denial of hospital privileges as a result of the existence of an exclusive contract with the anesthesiologists in place at the facility has been the source of many lawsuits, including the well-known Louisiana case of *Hyde v Jefferson Parish.* In that case, the court found for the defendant anesthesiologists and the hospital, saying that there was no antitrust violation because there was no real adverse effect on competition as far as patients were concerned because there were several other hospitals within the market to which they could go, and therefore they could exercise their rights to take advantage of competition in the relevant market. Thus, existence of an exclusive contract only in the rare setting where anticompetitive effects on patients can be proved might lead to a legitimate antitrust claim by a physician denied privileges. This was proven true in the *Kessel v Monongahela County General Hospital* case in West Virginia in which an exclusive anesthesiology contract was held illegal. Therefore, again, these arrangements are by definition complex and fraught with hazard. Accordingly, outside advice and counsel are always necessary.

Hospital Subsidies

Modern economic realities have forced a great number of anesthesiology practice groups (in both private and academic settings) to recognize that their patient care revenue, after overhead is paid, does not provide sufficient compensation to attract and retain the number and quality of staff necessary to provide the expected clinical service (and fulfill any other group/department missions). Attempting to do the same (or more) work with fewer staff may temporarily provide increased financial compensation. Cutting benefits (discretionary personal professional expenses, retirement contributions, or even insurance coverage) may also be a component of a response to inadequate practice revenue. However, the resulting decrements in personal security, in convenience, and in quality of life as far as acute and chronic fatigue, decreased family and recreation time, and tension among colleagues fearful someone else is getting a "better deal" will quickly overcome any brief advantage of a somewhat higher income. Therefore, many practice groups in such situations are requesting their hospital (or other health-care facility where they practice) to pay them a direct cash subsidy that is used to augment practice revenue in order to maintain benefits and amenities while maintaining or even increasing the direct compensation to staff members, hopefully to a market-competitive level that will promote recruitment and retention of group members.

Obviously, requests by a practice group for a direct subsidy must be thoroughly justified to the facility administration receiving the petition. The group's business operation should already have been examined carefully for any possible defects or means to enhance revenue generation. Explanation of the general trend of declining reimbursements for anesthesia services should be carefully documented. Facts and figures on that and also the shortage of anesthesia providers can be obtained from journal articles and ASA publications, particularly the *Newsletter*. Demand for anesthesia coverage for the surgical schedule is a key component of this proposal. Scheduling and utilization, particularly if early-morning staffing is required for many ORs that are routinely unused later during the traditional work day, is a major issue to be understood and presented. Any other OR inefficiencies created by hospital support staff and previous efforts to deal with them should also be highlighted. Unfavorable payer mix, impact of contracts, and programs initiated by the hospital also often are major factors in situations of inadequate practice
6 revenue. Always, the group's good will with the surgeons and the community in general should be emphasized, as well as of the indirect or "behind the scenes" services and benefits the anesthesiology group provides to the hospital. Note that the necessity for such a subsidy request is precisely the time when the anesthesia professionals will benefit from being perceived as "good citizens" of the health-care facility. An overly aggressive effort beyond the bounds of logic could provoke the facility to consider alternative arrangements, even up to the point of putting out a request for proposal from other anesthesiology practice groups. Therefore, thoughtful calculations are required and a careful balance must be sought, seeking enough financial support to supplement practice revenues so that members' compensation is competitive but not so much as to be excessive. Supporting statements and documents about offers and potential earnings elsewhere must be completely honest and not exaggerated or credibility and good faith will be lost. Further, part of any agreement will be the full sharing of the group's detailed financial information with the facility administration, both at the time of the request and on an ongoing basis if the payment is more than a one-time "bail out." Plans for review and renewal should be made once a subsidy is paid.

Any subsidy will likely require a formal contract. There may be concern about malpractice liability implications for the hospital even though the practice group stays an independent entity as before. There may be "inurement" or "private benefit" concerns that could be perceived as a threat to the tax-exempt status of a nonprofit hospital. Lack of understanding of the applicable laws may lead to fears that a subsidy could be an illegal "kickback" or a violation of the Stark II self-referral prohibition. As is almost always the case, expert outside professional consultant advice, usually from an attorney who specializes exclusively in health-care finance contracting, is mandatory in such circumstances. The ASA Washington, DC, office maintains lists of consultants who have helped other anesthesiologists or groups in the past with various subjects, and the ASA has some basic information on subsidies to anesthesiology practice groups.[44–46]

Evolving Practice Arrangements

Even though managed care plans have not had the impact anticipated, various iterations still exist and have ongoing implications for anesthesiology practice. Further, concern about disproportionate increases in health-care spending as a percentage of US gross domestic product and the fear of the postulated bankruptcy of Medicare and Medicaid again raise the specter of new efforts to impose managed care or other new arrangements to control costs.

7 In the initial stages of the evolution of a managed care marketplace, the MCO usually seeks contracts with providers based on discounted fee-for-service arrangements. This preserves the basic traditional idea of production-based physician reimbursement (do more, bill more) but the price of each act of services is lower (the providers are induced to give deep discounts with the promise of significant volumes of patients); also, the MCO gatekeeper primary care physicians and the MCO reviewers are strongly encouraged to limit complex and costly services as much as possible. There are other features intermittently along the way, such as global fees and negotiated fee schedules (agreed-upon single prices for individual procedures, independent of length or complexity). In an application of the concept of risk-sharing (spend too much for patient care and lose income), this usually is initially manifest in the form of "withholds," the practice of the MCO holding back a fraction of the agreed-upon payment to the providers (e.g., 10% or 15%) and keeping this money until the end of the fiscal year. At that time, if there is any money left in the risk pool or withhold account after all the (partial) provider fees and MCO expenses are paid, it is distributed to the providers in proportion to their degree of participation during the year. This is a clever and powerful incentive to providers to reduce health-care expenses. It is not as powerful as the stage of full risk-sharing, however. As the managed care marketplace matures and MCOs grow and succeed, the existing organizations and, especially any new ones, intend to shift to prospective capitated payments for providers.

Prospective Payments

Prospective capitated payments constitute an entirely new world to health-care providers, involving prospective capitated payments for large populations of patients, in which each group of providers in the MCO receives a fixed amount per enrolled covered life (member) per month (PMPM) and agrees, except in the most unusual circumstances, to provide whatever care is needed by that population for that prospective payment. The most unusual circumstances involve "carve-out" arrangements in which specific very costly and unusual conditions or procedures (such as the birth of a child with disastrous multiple congenital anomalies) are covered separately on a discounted fee-for-service basis. If there were to ever be full capitation, the entire financial underpinning of American medical care would do a complete about-face from the traditional rewards for giving more care and doing more procedures to new rewards for giving and doing less. Some managed care contracts contain other features intended to protect the providers against unexpected overutilization by patients that would stretch the providers beyond the bounds of the original contract with the MCO. The provisions setting the boundaries are called *risk corridors,* and the "stop-loss clauses" add some discounted fee-for-service payment for the excess care beyond the risk corridor (capitated contract limit). Providers who were used to getting paid more for doing more can suddenly find themselves getting paid a fixed amount no matter how much or how little they do with regard to a specified population—hence, the perceived incentive to do, and consequently spend, less. If the providers render too much care within the defined boundary of the contract, they essentially will be working for free, the ultimate in risk-sharing.

There are clearly potential internal conflicts in such a system,[47] and how patients reacted initially to this radical change in attitude on the part of physicians where it was implemented demonstrated that this overall mechanism is unlikely to be readily embraced by the general public. Health-care providers (physicians, other health-care professionals, and facilities), in turn, allied themselves in a wide variety of organizations to create strength and desirable resources to present to the MCOs in contract negotiations. "Management service organizations" are joint-venture network arrangements that do not involve true economic integration among the practitioners, but merely offer common services to physicians who may, as a loosely organized informal group, elect to seek MCO contracts. "Preferred provider organizations" are network arrangements of otherwise economically independent physicians who form a new corporate entity to seek managed care contracts in which there are significant financial incentives to patients to use the network providers and financial penalties for going to out-of-network providers. This has proved a relatively popular model and appears to be gaining wide acceptance. Physician–hospital organizations are similar entities but involve understandings between groups of physicians and a hospital so that a large package or bundle of services can be constructed as essentially one-stop points of care. Independent practice associations are like preferred provider organizations but are specifically oriented toward capitated contracts for covered lives with significant risk-sharing by the providers. Groups (or clinics) "without walls" are collections of practitioners who fully integrate economically into a single fiscal entity (true partnership) and then compete for MCO contracts on the basis of risk-sharing incentives among the partners. Fully integrated groups or health maintenance organizations (such as Kaiser Permanente in California or Harvard Pilgrim Health in New England) house the group of partner provider physicians and associated support staff at a single location for the convenience of patients, a big selling point when they seek MCO or employer contracts.

Changing Paradigm

The era of solo independent practitioners may be ending in some locations where MCOs dominate because the organizations simply will not contract with one person. Independent hospital-based groups (likely still the most common private practice model) may face growing similar difficulties.[48] These smaller groups of anesthesiologists may find themselves at a competitive disadvantage unless they become part of a vertically integrated (multispecialty) or horizontally integrated (with other anesthesiologists) organization. Negotiations with MCOs require expert advice, probably even more so than the traditional exclusive contracts with hospitals as previously noted. Before any negotiation can even be considered, the MCO must provide significant amounts of information about the covered patient population. The projected health-care utilization pattern of a large group of white-collar workers (and their families) from major upscale employers in an urban area will be quite different from that of a relatively rural Medicaid population. Specific demographics and past utilization histories are absolutely mandatory for each proposed population to be covered, and this information should go directly to the advising experts for evaluation, whether the proposed negotiation is for discounted fee-for-service, a fee schedule, global bundled fees, or full capitation.

Significant questions were pointedly raised about the reimbursement implications for anesthesiologists of the putative managed care/practice reorganization revolution. Much of that discussion has been rendered moot by the failure of the pure prospective capitated payment model to gain widespread adoption. However, if an anesthesia practice or its parent financial entity is ever asked to enter negotiation for a "per member per month" payment for anesthesia services, immediate consultation with the Washington office of the ASA should occur.

Discounted fee-for-service arrangements are easier for anesthesiologists to understand because these are directly referable to existing fee structures. Reports of groups instituting 10% to 50% discounts off the starting point of 80% of usual and customary reimbursement in various practice circumstances were circulated at national meetings of anesthesiologists in years past. Were rigidly controlled fully mature managed care to dominate the practice community, it would be likely that the average income for anesthesiologists would decrease from past levels. However, it likely also would be true that anesthesia professionals would continue to have incomes still above average among all health-care professionals in that market.

Another common feature of this discussion has been the tendency of private (nongovernmental) contracting organizations to attempt to tie their payments for professional services to the government's Medicare rate for specific CPT-4 codes. It is common for both commercial indemnity insurance entities (e.g., Blue Shield, Aetna, Humana, United Health) and MCOs to offer primary care physicians, for example, 125% of the Medicare payment rate for specific services. Although groups of primary care physicians may view this as somewhat reasonable and, thus, they sign such contracts, anesthesiologists face unique challenges in this regard. Even with the hope of a Medicare reimbursement upgrade for anesthesia services, most anesthesia professionals still believe that the Medicare reimbursement rate is unfairly low for the work involved in providing anesthesia care. The Medicare rate likely would remain less than half the per unit "conversion factor" that the large indemnity carriers have been paying for anesthesia care in recent years. Therefore, 125% of what many anesthesia professionals consider woefully inadequate would still be inadequate. Thus, in spite of sometimes intense pressure, anesthesia professionals in many markets have been reluctant to accept indemnity insurance contract rates tied to Medicare rates. As always, anesthesia professionals faced with complex reimbursement situations and decisions should seek expert advice from the national offices of their professional practice organizations and from knowledgeable paid consultants and attorneys.

Pay for Performance

Commercial indemnity insurance entities, MCOs, and particularly, the federal Center for Medicare and Medicaid Services (CMS) are all fixated on the concept of "performance-based payments" as a significant new way to limit the growth of (and even reduce) health-care costs,[49] especially by reducing expensive complications of medical care. This "pay for performance" movement began with the federal Tax Relief and Healthcare Act of 2006 and continues with the Physician Quality Reporting Initiative in 2008. The potential implications for anesthesia practice have been summarized.[50]

In general, CMS made strenuous efforts to attempt to define and promulgate objective quality measures that could be documented as indicators of the "quality" of health care delivered. The main issue is the promotion of specific "best practices" care elements that help avoid expensive outcomes or complications that currently generate a disproportionate (preventable) fraction of health-care costs. The administration of aspirin and beta-blockers within a fixed brief interval after the arrival of an acute myocardial infarction patient is a good example, as are various parameters in the care of patients with community-acquired pneumonia or congestive heart failure. Defining and validating objective and easily quantifiable so-called quality measures that will prevent expensive complications of anesthesia care proved to be more difficult. The initial targeted parameter was somewhat indirect: the timing of the administration of prophylactic antibiotics prior to surgical incision. The anesthesia professional is judged to be in compliance when the antibiotic is administered within the 1 hour (2 hours for vancomycin and fluoroquinolones) prior to incision. This must be verifiably documented on the anesthesia record. Benchmark criteria such as 95% compliance for a specific financial entity billing Medicare and Medicaid must be met by members of the group or the reimbursement for anesthesia services by that financial entity will be reduced by a specific fraction (or a promised "bonus" will be withheld) as a compliance incentive, but also somewhat as an offset to the increased cost of the consequent complications associated with failure to comply. If performance is in compliance, CMS will pay the maximum allowable reimbursement (pay for performance).

The second target was catheter-related bloodstream infection, and the performance behavior expected of anesthesia professionals is observance of strict aseptic protocol during central vascular catheter placement (and avoiding the femoral route if at all possible). The third objective parameter of anesthesia care quality targeted temperature management of the surgical patient with the compliance behavior being met by achieving one of three possible goals: use of active warming intraoperatively or documented temperature ≥36°C either in the last 30 minutes of anesthesia or the first 30 minutes in the PACU. Future potential objective performance criteria intended to encourage avoidance of costly complications of anesthesia care may include glucose control in major surgery, use of pencil-point spinal needles in obstetric anesthesia, use of electronic medical records (EMRs), preoperative screening for sleep apnea, preoperative fasting instructions, meperidine administration for postoperative shivering, and several others. In all cases when a parameter is adopted, benchmark criteria for degree of compliance will be established and reimbursement will be reduced one way or another for failure to comply, as documented on the relevant records and self-reported by the billing financial entity (subject to audit, of course).

Hospitals will have even more at stake in the sense that the pay for performance movement is creating paradigms in which hospitals will not receive reimbursements for care associated with preventable complications such as catheter-related sepsis, ventilator-acquired pneumonia, and decubitus ulcers. This concept has several implications. One is that smaller hospitals often populated by less acute patients will be more likely and quicker to transfer sicker patients to larger referral facilities in order to avoid losing reimbursement associated with the development of patient complications. Concomitantly, documentation of the timing of the development of complications will become critical. If a hospital or department has documented the preexisting presence of a complication at the time of a patient's admission, it should not be penalized for the development of that condition. In this context, anesthesia professionals can have an important role documenting the existence of pneumonia or sacral decubitus ulcers in their records when they first see a newly admitted patient, usually for preoperative evaluation. This will be perceived as excellent institutional citizenship by the anesthesia professional because it may prevent significant reimbursement reduction to the hospital.

Accountable Care Organizations

The Patient Protection and Affordable Care Act (nicknamed "ObamaCare") was signed into law in 2010. While many of the details of implementation of this legislation are still being determined, one area of significance to anesthesiology professionals centers around the creation of ACOs. After review of the 698-page final rule it became clear to ASA that there was little consideration to the concept of preoperative care of the surgical patient in these provisions. To this end, ASA began advocacy for what is called a "surgical home" model of care, a concept that had been in early stages of formation over the prior decade and became very germane to the continued development of the professional practice of anesthesiology. In the surgical home model, anesthesiologists are identified (and ultimately compensated) for their roles in preoperative evaluation of increasingly complex patient populations, intraoperative management of the anesthetic, and postoperative management of pain and critical care issues of the surgical patient. Included in this is the idea that even routine postoperative care of the patient is within the domain of the anesthesiologist, as is follow-up care for those patients suffering from subacute pain following surgical procedures. The surgical home model represents a conceptual shift from the role of the anesthesiologist with a relatively limited scope of practice (as an intraoperative and immediately postoperative deliverer of care) to a more expanded role in perioperative medicine. Clearly, within the past decade a growing number of institutions have come to rely on anesthesiologist-directed preoperative assessment clinics to ensure adequate preparation of the surgical patient for their procedure. Likewise most institutions have physicians (usually anesthesiologists) practicing Pain Medicine/Management on staff. The surgical home model merely seeks to bring these elements along with critical care together to provide a vertical integration of care during the perioperative period. While most academic anesthesiology departments and some large community hospitals can assemble these teams into a "surgical home" model with relative ease, it remains to be seen how this concept could be executed in the medium to small community hospital setting or what partnerships would have to be developed to accomplish these goals. While the current language of the Affordable Care Act deals with the concept of primary care and does not comment on surgical care, the ACO format would in essence be similar to the prospective payment paradigm described previously with payment distributed to members of the care team based upon participation in care of the patient and any savings rendered from the efficient delivery of care distributed to the stakeholders in a given ACO.

Management Intricacies

The complexities of modern medical practice are significant and increasing rapidly. Management consultants, both large national firms that cross all industries and also boutique firms that specialize in only medical practices, are advertising their services to anesthesiology group practices. A recent analysis (that might seem more fitting as an MBA school case study) of business strategies relevant to anesthesiology group practices suggested there are key elements that detrimentally go unrecognized.[51] Whether a specific anesthesiology practice should consider bringing in an outside management consultant to help bolster the function, efficiency, and profitability of the practice obviously must be an individual carefully considered decision. However, even such a suggestion is a very recent phenomenon, reflecting the tensions of the modern medical marketplace. As in other related caveats, whenever considering engaging outside help, a rigorous vetting process is required, especially including reference checks and discussion with previous practices served by that consultant.

HIPAA

The 2003 implementation of the Privacy Rule of the Health Insurance Portability and Accountability Act (HIPAA) of 1996 required significant changes in how medical records and patient information are handled in the day-to-day delivery of health care. The impact on and requirements for anesthesiologists are summarized in a comprehensive publication from the ASA[52] that followed two educational summaries.[53,54]

Attention is focused on "protected health information" (identifiable as from a specific patient by name). Patients must be notified of their privacy rights. Usually this will be covered by the health-care facility in which anesthesia professionals work, but if separate private records are maintained, separate notification may be necessary. Privacy policies must be created, adopted, and promulgated to all practitioners, all of whom then must be trained in application of those policies. Often, anesthesiology groups can combine with the facilities in which they practice as an "organized health-care arrangement" so that the anesthesia practitioners can be covered in part by the HIPAA compliance activities of the facility. A "privacy officer" must be appointed for the practice group. Finally, and most importantly, medical records containing protected health information must be secured so they are not readily available to those who do not need them to render care.

One of the most obvious applications for many anesthesiologists is concern about the assembled preoperative information and charts for tomorrow's cases that frequently were placed prominently in the OR holding area at the end of one work day in readiness for the next day's cases. HIPAA provisions require that all that patient information be locked away overnight. Another classic example is what many ORs refer to as "the board." Often, a large white dry-marker board occupies a prominent wall near the front desk of an OR suite, and the rooms, cases, and personnel assignments are inscribed thereon at the beginning of the day and modified or crossed off as the day progresses. Under HIPAA, patients' names may not be used on such a board if there is any chance that anyone not directly involved in their care could see them. Alternatively, some facilities tape a copy of the day's OR schedule (including patients' names, ages, and operations) on the wall, which would also be a violation. The same is true for similar boards or posted schedules in OR holding areas and PACUs. Another issue often overlooked that is very problematic and probably the one that concerns patients the most is the obtaining of history information in a location, such as a "bed slot" behind just a curtain in the OR holding area, where sensitive medical and personal information is spoken out loud within earshot of other patients, other patients' families, and noninvolved caregivers. This concern is difficult to address and there is no one universally applicable suggestion. However, anesthesia professionals who interact with patients in such environments should be as sensitive as physically possible to being overheard and also should bring such concerns to the attention of the facility administrators.

Further, many anesthesiology practices also must apply HIPAA provisions to their billing operations; the details will vary depending on the mechanisms used and a great deal will depend on which type of electronic claims submission software is being used by the billing entity actually submitting the claims.[55] Telephone calls and faxes into offices must be handled specially if containing identifiable patient information. Presentation of patient information for QA or teaching purposes must be free of all identifiers unless specific individual permission has been obtained on prescribed printed forms. Requests for patient information from a wide variety of outside entities, including insurance companies and collection agencies, must be processed in HIPAA-compliant ways. HIPAA policy and actions, as well as enforcement activities, are being developed over time and as situations develop. This system depends in part on patient complaints for both enforcement and policy evolution. In many practices and practice locations, there have been few or even no formal complaints of violations of patient privacy, indicating that the initial implementation of HIPAA compliance may have largely had the desired effect.

Electronic Medical Records

Databases, spreadsheets, and electronic transfer of information are nonspecific features that have been applied to health care. Replacing the classic medical record, on the other hand, has required the creation of entirely new software in an attempt to duplicate the function of the handwritten or dictated traditional "chart." This has afforded opportunities to multiple competing commercial entities to attempt to fill this need. Usually, competing proprietary systems are incompatible and do not "talk to each other." This fact severely limits one of the highly touted benefits of medical practices "going electronic." Cost is another great barrier, as is the formidable task of entering the required information from the old paper records into the electronic system. There has been governmental and public pressure for health-care institutions, facilities, and practices to adopt electronic records because of the potential for increased legibility causing reduction in errors and confusion, greater speed of filing and retrieval, easy transmission of large amounts of information (such as from a surgeon's office to an anesthesia practice's booking office and also to a hospital's preoperative clinic or OR holding area), and QA monitoring of vast databases. Increased ease of transmission and filing of reimbursement claims and cost savings from clerical staff downsizing are claims intended to encourage physician practice groups to adopt EMRs. However, experience has suggested that the commercially available software systems (both for institutions and practice groups) are not as robust or reliable as advertised by their often aggressive manufacturers. Accordingly, the expected benefits have not materialized quite as predicted, particularly in that costs have been great, often far in excess of estimates, and cost savings have been minimal at best. Nonetheless, there is a federal mandate that health-care facilities and practices must implement "meaningful use" of EMR by the end of 2014 or face, starting in 2015, penalties in the form of reduced payments from Medicare and Medicaid. Practice groups of anesthesia professionals should consider all the noted points prior to investing in an EMR system. At minimum, careful study and evaluation of the same system already in place in another anesthesiology practice should be undertaken.

If basic EMR implementation has been problematic for practices, true electronic anesthesia information management systems have been even more difficult. These include preoperative, intraoperative, postoperative, billing, and QA components. For the actual OR anesthesia record, several commercial versions are available. Various anesthesia professionals have various opinions about ease of implementation and subsequent use. Unless one massive bolus of fully integrated new technology from a single manufacturer is installed all at one time, integration of a new EMR with the existing anesthesia machines and monitors to ensure full accurate capture of all data parameters can often be difficult and frustrating. The function and value of electronic anesthesia records can be debated endlessly. All of them today will require computers on or in the anesthesia machine. These computers should be Internet-enabled so that demographic and billing information can be automatically uploaded to the facility's and the practice's database. Any such system must also integrate with the billing systems of the facility and the practice or the touted benefits will be largely negated. Again, the best, and in some senses, the only way to evaluate seriously and thoroughly a proposed major investment of money, effort, and time is to visit a fully up-and-working installation of that electronic anesthesia information management system and talk directly in detail with the users. The costs, in all senses of the word, are so great that it remains a significant gamble to be the first to purchase and implement such a system.

Expansion into Perioperative Medicine, Hospital Care, and Hyperbaric Medicine

Some anesthesiologists now practice for at least some of their time in preoperative screening clinics because of the great fraction of OR patients who do not spend the night before surgery in the hospital or who do not come to a hospital at all. In such settings, these anesthesiologists frequently assume a role analogous to that of a primary care physician, planning and executing a workup of one or more significant medical or surgical problems before the patient can reasonably be expected to undergo surgery. Likewise, this concept would be excellent for the postoperative period. An anesthesiologist, on site in the hospital, immediately available and completely free of OR or other duties, could not only make at least twice-daily rounds on patients after surgery and provide exceedingly comprehensive pain management service, but also could follow the surgical progress and make reports (likely via an EMR or e-mail) to the surgeon's office or smartphone. A fundamental aspect of the practice of anesthesiology is the management of acute problems in the hospital setting. It is logical that anesthesiologists would be among the physicians best suited to provide primary care for hospitalized surgical patients. This concept is incorporated in the proposal noted above to create a recognized "surgical home" for patients as part of the structure of ACOs. It is clear that this would make the overall surgical episode more efficient. The involved anesthesiologists would need close working relationships with the participating surgeons so that the surgeons would remain involved in the technical and surgical details of the postoperative phase with which the anesthesiologists would be less familiar. Also, the financial aspects of such arrangements could be complex in that third-party payers are unlikely to agree to new costs for a new class of providers, and the surgeons may be reluctant to have their compensation proportionately reduced, even if the new arrangement would free up time for them to see more new patients and do more cases. An anesthesia group with great insight may well be willing to provide such labor-intense service without expecting additional compensation because doing so will help insure the security of their existing positions and traditionally relatively high incomes. In the Rovenstine Lecture at the 2005 ASA Annual Meeting,[56] there was an emphatic plea for significantly expanding the scope of practice for anesthesiologists in perioperative care, patient care in general, and in health systems (facilitated by increasing the number trained and increasing use of nonphysicians supervised by anesthesiologists to care for healthy patients) as a way to secure a role for anesthesiologists among the leaders of the future of American health care. To date, it appears that there has been little progress in this regard. The overall challenge persists for the young and upcoming generation of anesthesiologists.

An additional evolving opportunity within acute care hospitals is the creation and implementation of "rapid response teams." In essence, studies have revealed that patients on general care nursing floors sometimes begin to deteriorate and, for one reason or another (but often because of the responsible physician being unavailable or at a considerable distance at that moment), the patients are not evaluated or treated in a timely manner and often not until they have further deteriorated, sometimes to a critical status. Therefore, a national trend has developed in which hospitals create a team of knowledgeable professionals (who have other regular responsibilities) who usually have no prior knowledge of the deteriorating patient but who will respond within a very few minutes to the call from (usually) a floor nurse who detects a deteriorating patient (e.g., rapidly increasing fever, relative hypotension and tachycardia, absent urine output). Frequently, the rapid response team institutes immediate symptomatic treatment, arranges for a higher acuity level of care, and contacts the primary responsible physician. Importantly, in larger hospitals, it has been suggested that the in-house anesthesiologists are uniquely qualified to be key members of the rapid response team because the interventions almost always involve acute "bread-and-butter" resuscitative care. Although many anesthesiologists may believe they already have plenty of work in the OR, such participation when possible would be an outstanding and highly visible contribution to the hospital's mission of enhanced patient care. Also, such interventions potentially could be separately billable encounters as consultations or, alternatively, excellent support for the maintenance or even increase of the hospital's financial subsidy to its anesthesia professional group.

Finally, anesthesiologists in some locations have become involved in the practice of hyperbaric medicine and wound care. This is likely related to the familiarity of anesthesiologists with concepts of gas laws and physics, along with their constant presence in the hospital. The treatment of various medical conditions by the application of oxygen under increased pressure, usually 2 to 3 atmospheres absolute, at one time was one of the more rapidly growing hospital services. Anesthesiologists are among the leaders of this field, with unlimited opportunities for clinical care, teaching, and research. Even a brief discussion of this field is outside the scope of this chapter, and interested readers are referred to the Undersea and Hyperbaric Medical Society (www.umhs.org).

OPERATING ROOM MANAGEMENT

The role of anesthesiologists in OR management has changed dramatically. In a climate of a shortage of anesthesia professionals, hospitals subsidizing many anesthesiology group practices, and an increasing workload, participation in OR management is essentially mandatory. The current emphasis on cost containment and efficiency will force anesthesiologists to take an active role in eliminating many dysfunctional aspects of OR practice that were previously ignored. First-case morning start times have changed from a suggestion to a mandate. Delays of any sort are now often tracked electronically in real time and carefully scrutinized to eliminate waste and inefficiency. Together, anesthesiologists, surgeons, OR nurses and technicians, and increasingly, professional administrators/managers need to determine

who is best qualified to be a leader in the day-to-day management of the OR.[57] Clearly, different groups have different perspectives. However, anesthesiologists are in the best position to see the "big picture," both overall and on any given day. Surgeons are commonly elsewhere before and after their individual cases (and sometimes for the beginning and the end of their cases); nurses and administrators may lack the medical knowledge to make
8 appropriate, timely decisions, often "on the fly." It is the anesthesiologist with the insight, overview, and unique perspective who is best qualified to provide leadership in an OR community. The subsequent recognition and appreciation from the other groups (especially hospital administration) will clearly establish the anesthesiologists as concerned physicians genuinely interested in the welfare of the OR and the institution.

Organization

The symbiotic relationship between anesthesia professionals and surgeons remains unchanged. Both groups recognize this fact and also the common goal of having the OR function in a safe, expeditious manner. The age-old question, "Who is in charge of the operating room?" still confronts many hospitals/institutions. Because some anesthesiology groups are subsidized by the hospital, the OR organization in such cases has changed accordingly. Many hospital administrators want to have input regarding who is in charge of the OR with an eye to increasing efficiency and throughput while reducing cost. Their wishes have an even added significance when more of their dollars are involved through the anesthesiology group subsidy. Sometimes there can be no real answer to, "Who's in charge?" because of the complexity of the interpersonal relationships in the OR. Some institutions have a professional manager (often a former OR registered nurse) whose sole job is to organize and run the OR. This individual may be vested with enough authority to be recognized by all as the person in charge. Other institutions ostensibly have a "medical director of the OR." However, the implications to the surgeons that an anesthesiologist is in charge, or vice versa, have caused many institutions to abandon the title or retain the position but assign no authority to it. In such instances, institutions usually resolve disputes through some authority with a physician's perspective. If there is no medical director with authority to make decisions stick, central authority usually resides with the OR committee, most often populated by physicians, senior nurses, and administrators. Every OR has this forum for major policy and fiscal decisions. As part of committee function, the standard practices of negotiation, diplomacy, and lobbying for votes are regularly carried out. The impact of such an OR committee varies widely among institutions.

Despite the constantly changing dynamics of the OR management and the frequent major frustrations, anesthesiologists should pursue a greater role in day-to-day management in every possible applicable practice setting. An anesthesiologist who is capable of facilitating the start of cases with minimal delays and solving problems "on the fly" as they arise will be in an excellent position to serve his or her department. Succeeding in this role will have a dramatic positive impact on all the OR constituents. The surgeons will be less concerned about who is in charge because their cases are getting done. The hospital administration will welcome the effort because they want something extra in return for any money they are now giving to the anesthesiology groups as a subsidy. Furthermore, the OR committee (or whatever system for dispute resolution is in place) is still functional and has not been circumvented (and will be thankful for the absence of disputes needing resolution).

Some institutions use the term *Clinical Director of the OR*. The person awarded this designation should be a senior-level individual with firsthand knowledge of the OR environment and function. Anesthesiologists have a better understanding of the perioperative process. They possess the medical knowledge to make appropriate decisions. Their intimate association with surgeons and their patients allows them to best allocate resources. The American Association of Clinical Directors in 2002 reported that 71% of survey respondents stated that an anesthesiologist was designated as the Clinical Director of the OR.

Contact and Communication

An important issue for the anesthesia professionals in any OR setting is who among the group will be the contact person to interact with the OR and its related administrative functions. In situations in which everyone is an independent contractor, there may be a titular chief who by design is the contact person. The anesthesiologist in this role commonly changes yearly to spread the duties among all the members. Large groups or departments that function as the sole providing entity for that hospital/facility often identify an individual as the contact person to act as the voice for the department. Furthermore, these same groups delineate someone on a daily basis to be the operational clinical director, or the person "running the board." Frequently, this position is best filled by one from a small dedicated fraction of the group (e.g., three people) rather than rotating the responsibility among every member of the group. Experienced "board runners" have an instinctually derived better perspective on the nuances of managing the operating schedule in real time. Certain procedures may require specific training (e.g., transesophageal echocardiography skills) that not all members of the group possess. Clearly, changes sometimes have to be made in real time to match the ability of the anesthesia provider and the requirements of the procedure when urgent or emergent cases are posted.

Another benefit of a very small number of daily clinical directors is a relative consistency in the application of OR policies, particularly in relationship to the scheduling of cases, especially add-ons. One of the most frustrating aspects to both surgeons and OR personnel is unpredictability and inconsistency in the decisions made by the anesthesia group/department members. A patient deemed unacceptable for surgery by anesthesiologist X on Monday may be perfectly acceptable, in the same medical condition, for anesthesiologist Y on Tuesday. Differences of opinion are inevitable in any large group. However, day-to-day OR function may be hampered by a large number of these situations. Having one member of a very small group in charge will lead to more consistency in this process, especially if the board runner/clinical director has the authority to switch personnel to accommodate the situation. Without stifling individual practices, philosophies, and comfort levels, a certain amount of consistency applied to similar clinical scenarios will improve OR function immeasurably. These few dedicated directors should be able to accomplish both goals better than a large rotating group.

A newer potential component of intra-OR communications is the concept of checklists and team briefings. Analogous to the now-required "time-out" in each OR prior to surgical incision when the correct identity of the patient, the intended procedure, and any laterality involved are verified, some ORs are attempting to have a similar interprofessional communication involving all relevant OR personnel (the team) prior to the patient entering the actual OR, during which the involved surgeon, anesthesia professional, circulating nurse, scrub person, and support persons as indicated each acknowledge a summary of what is projected to take place in this case, any anticipated need for extra or unusual resources or equipment, any anticipated difficulties or increased risks, and specific plans to deal with any feature of any of these points that would require intervention. In many models, a printed single-page checklist with routine prompts and fill-in boxes is used to facilitate the process. One study reported a two-third reduction in "communication failures" that have otherwise likely caused problems, risks, or inefficiencies.[58]

The World Health Organization's recent "Surgery Safety Checklist" (http://whqlibdoc.who.int/publications/2009/9789241598590_eng_checklist.pdf) is primarily an accident-prevention tool, but also promotes communication among everyone in the OR, particularly regarding planning—before, during, and after the actual operation—which is directly related to maximally efficient and safe conduct of the procedure.

Materials Management

Usually, the institutional component of the anesthesia service staffs and maintains a location ("the workroom") containing the specific supplies unique to the practice of anesthesia. Objectives necessary for efficient materials management include the standardization of equipment, drugs, and supplies. Volume purchasing, inventory reduction, and avoidance of duplication are also worthwhile. There needs to be coordination with the OR staff as to who is responsible for acquisition of routine hospital supplies such as syringes, needles, IV tubing, and IV fluids. Decisions as to which brands of which supplies to purchase ideally should be made as a group. Often, when several companies compete against each other in an open market, lower prices are negotiable. In many cases, however, hospitals belong to large buying groups that determine what brands and models of equipment and supplies will be available, with no exceptions possible except at greatly increased cost. Sometimes, this is false economy if the provided items are inferior (cheap) or annoying and, for example, if it routinely takes opening three or four intravenous cannulae in the process of starting a preoperative intravenous line as opposed to the higher quality and reliable single one that may cost more per cannula but is less expensive overall because far fewer will be used. Dispassionate presentation of such logic by a respected team-player senior anesthesiologist to the OR committee or director of materials management may help resolve such conundrums.

Scheduling Cases

Anesthesiologists need to participate in the OR scheduling process at their facility or institution. In some facilities the scheduling office and the associated clerical personnel work under the anesthesia group. Commonly, scheduling falls under the OR staff's responsibility. Direct "control" of the schedule on a moment-to-moment basis often resides with the OR supervisor or charge person, frequently a nurse. Whatever the arrangements, the anesthesia group must have input and a direct line of communication to the scheduling system. The necessary number of anesthesia professionals that must be supplied often changes on a daily basis per the caseload and sometimes because of institutional policy decisions. After-hours call must be arranged, policy changes factored in, and additions/subtractions to the surgical load (day to day, week to week, and long term as surgical practices come and go in that OR) dealt with as well. These issues are important even when all the anesthesia professionals are independently contracted and are not affiliated with each other. In such situations, the titular chief of anesthesia should be the one to act as the link to the scheduling system. When the anesthesia group/department functions as a single entity, the chairman/chief, clinical director, or appointed spokesperson will be the individual who represents his or her group at meetings in which scheduling decisions are made in conjunction with the OR supervisors, surgeons, and hospital administrators.

There are as many different ways to create scheduling policies as there are OR suites. Most hospitals/facilities follow proprietary patterns established over the years. Despite all the efforts directed toward its creation, the OR schedule (both weekly time allotments and day-to-day scheduling of specific cases) remains one of the most contentious subjects for the OR. Recognizing the fact that it is impossible to satisfy everyone, the anesthesia group should endeavor to facilitate the process as much as possible. Initially, anesthesiologists need to be sympathetic toward all the surgeons' desires/demands (stated or implied) and attempt to coordinate these requests with the institution's ability to provide rooms, equipment, and staff. Secondly, the anesthesia group should make every possible effort to provide enough anesthesia services and personnel to realistically meet the goals of the institution. In light of the shortage of anesthesia professionals in this country, these efforts need to be made with a great deal of open communication among all contingencies of the OR committee as well as every member of the anesthesia group.

Regarding scheduling, surgeons essentially fall into one of three groups. One group wants to operate any time they can get their cases scheduled. This group wants the OR open 24/7. Another larger group wants "first case of the day" as often as possible so they can get to their offices. A smaller third group wants either the first time slot or an opening following that time slot, a several-hour hiatus, then to return to the OR after office hours to complete additional cases; usually starting after 5 PM. Clearly a compromise among these disparate constituencies must be reached. Anesthesiologists who approach the OR committee regarding this dilemma with a nonconfrontational attitude will greatly facilitate agreement on a compromise.

Types of Schedules

The majority of ORs use either block scheduling (preassigned guaranteed OR time for a surgeon or surgical service to schedule cases prior to an agreed-upon cut-off time; e.g., 24 or 48 hours before) or open scheduling (first come, first serve). Most large institutions have a combination of both. Block scheduling inherently contains several advantages for creating a schedule. Block scheduling allows for more predictability in the daily OR function as well as an easy review of utilization of allotted time. Historic utilization data should be reviewed with surgeons, OR staff, and the OR committee to determine its validity. Many operating suites have found it useful to assemble rather comprehensive statistics about what occurs in each OR. Some computerized scheduling systems (see later) are part of a larger computerized perioperative information management system that automatically generates statistics. Graphic examples are 13-month "statistical control charts" or "run charts" that show the number of cases, number of OR minutes used for those cases (and when: such as in block, exceeding block, evenings, nights, weekends, and so forth), number of cancellations (and multiple other related parameters if desired) by service, by individual surgeon, and total for the current month and the 12 prior months, always with "control limits" (usually 2 standard deviations from the 13-month moving average) clearly indicated. All these data are valuable in that they generate a clear picture of what is actually going on in the OR. It is also extremely valuable in that block time allocation should be reviewed periodically and adjusted based on changes, degree of utilization, and projected needs. Inflexible block time scheduling can create a major point of contention if the assigned blocks are not regularly reevaluated. The surgeon or surgical service with the early starting block that habitually runs beyond his or her block time will create problems for the following cases. If this surgeon were made to schedule into the later block on a rotating basis, delays in his or her start caused by others may provoke improved accuracy of his or her subsequent early case postings. Adjustments in availability of block time can also be made in the setting of the "release time," the time prior to the operative date that a given block is declared not filled and becomes available for open scheduling. Surgeons prefer as late a release time as possible in order to maintain their access to their OR block time. However, unused reserved block time wastes resources and prevents another service from scheduling. A single release time rarely fits all circumstances, but negotiating service-specific release times may lead to improved satisfaction for all. In the *ideal* system, enough OR time and equipment should exist to provide for each surgical service's genuine needs while retaining the ability to add to the schedule (via open scheduling) as needed. Such an environment does not exist. Invariably, in busy environments, surgical demand exceeds available block and open time, leading services to request additional block time. When this time is not granted, services may perversely then schedule procedures in open time before filling their block time. Surgeons who prefer open time would then be shut out of OR time. Open scheduling may reward those surgeons who run an efficient service, but it also may be a source of problems to those surgeons who have a significant portion of their service's cases arrive unscheduled, such as orthopedic surgeons. Some degree of flexibility will be necessary whichever system is used. The anesthesia group should adopt a neutral position in these discussions while being realistic about what can be accomplished given the number of ORs and the length of the normal operating day.

The handling of the urgent/emergent case posting precipitates a great deal of discussion in most OR environments. No studies allow determination of exactly what rate of OR utilization is the most cost-effective. However, many institutions subscribe to following parameters: adjusted utilization rates averaging below 70% are not associated with full use of available block time, wasting resources, while rates above 90% are frequently associated with the need for overtime hours.[59] Different OR constituencies have different comfort zones for degrees of utilization (Table 2-2). Most institutions cannot afford to have one or two ORs staffed, open, and waiting unless there is a reliable steady supply of late open-schedule additions, that is, urgent cases/emergencies, during the regular work day. A previously agreed-upon, clear algorithm for the acceptance and ordering of these cases will need to be adopted. In general, critical life-threatening emergencies and elective add-ons are fairly straightforward and at the two ends of the spectrum. The critical emergency goes in the next available room, whereas the elective case gets added to the end of the schedule. The so-called "urgent" patient requires the most judgment. Individual services should provide guidelines and limitations for their expected urgent cases. These "add-on case policy" guidelines[60] should be common knowledge to everyone involved in running the OR. Consequently, these cases, such as ectopic pregnancies, open fractures, the patient with obstructed bowel, and eye injuries, can then be triaged and inserted into the elective schedule as needed with minimal discussion from the delayed surgeon. The surgeons whose urgent case is presented as one that must immediately bump another service's patient, yet conversely could wait several hours if it is their own patient that will be delayed, will have to face their own previously agreed-upon standards in a future OR committee meeting. A simple way to express one logical policy for urgent cases (e.g., acute appendicitis, unruptured ectopic pregnancy, intestinal obstruction) is: (1) Bump the same surgeon's elective scheduled case; (2) if none, bump a scheduled case on the same service (gynecology, general A, and so forth); (3) if none, bump a scheduled case from an open-schedule surgical service; and (4) if none, bump a scheduled case from a block schedule service.[60] Some institutions require the attending surgeon of the posted urgent/emergent patient to speak personally with the surgeon of any bumped case.

Another area of burgeoning growth that must be accounted for in the daily work schedule is the non-OR "off-site" diagnostic test, or therapeutic intervention that requires anesthesia care. (In some locations, gastroenterologists expect anesthesia services for cases such as endoscopic retrograde cholangiopancreatography or other endoscopies on unusually sick patients, particularly after untoward emergencies beyond the capabilities of their sedation nurses have occurred and attracted attention in the facility.) In some instances the off-site procedures replace operations that, in the past, would have been posted on the OR schedule as urgent/emergency cases. For example, cerebral aneurysm coiling and computed tomography-guided abscess drainage, among other procedures, are done in imaging suites; some patients, adult as well as pediatric, require deep sedation or even general anesthesia for magnetic resonance imaging or computed tomography in radiology or for invasive procedures in catheterization laboratories. In addition, depending on distances involved and logistics, it may even be necessary to assign two people, a primary provider and an attending, exclusively to that one remote location when, had the case come to the OR, the attending may have been able to supervise one or more other cases also. Hospital administration or the OR committee may try to view these off-site cases as unrelated to OR function and, thus, purely

TABLE 2-2. OPERATING ROOM (OR) UTILIZATION: "COMFORT ZONES" OF THE OPERATING ROOM PERSONNEL CONSTITUENCIES

Block Time Utilization (%)	Facility Administration	Anesthesiology Group	OR Staff	Surgeons
>100	++	−−	−−−	−−−−
85–100	++++	++	−−	−−−
70–84	+++	++++	+	+/−
53–69	+	+++	+++	++
<55	−−	−	++	++++

"+"= favorable; "−"= unfavorable.

Reprinted from Mazzei WJ. OR management: State of the art. Proceedings of the 2003 Conference on Practice Management. Park Ridge, IL: American Society of Anesthesiologists; 2003:65, with permission.

a problem for the anesthesia group to solve. These cases must be treated the same as all the OR procedures.

In order to apportion hospital-based anesthesia resources reasonably, these off-site procedures should be subject to the same guidelines and processes for access and prioritization as any OR posting. Integration of the scheduling process with an institution-wide master program has been suggested as very helpful to maximize efficiency.[61] Most institutions have added at least one extra anesthetizing location ("line") to their formal operating schedule to designate these off-site procedures (occasionally with an imaginative classification such as "satellite," "road show," "outfield," or "safari"). For many of these off-site cases, there may be less or no reimbursement for anesthesia care. For example, government plans and also private insurance carriers may well not pay for the claustrophobic adult to receive monitored anesthesia care or even a general anesthetic for an obviously needed diagnostic magnetic resonance image, even though the patient, the surgeon, and the hospital benefit from the test results. The anesthesia group, the OR committee, and the hospital administration need to reach compromises for off-site procedures, regarding scheduling, allocation of anesthesia resources that would otherwise go to the OR, and even subsidization of the personnel costs in order to continue this obviously beneficial service that also does produce revenue for both the proceduralists and the facility.

Computerization

Computerized scheduling will likely benefit every OR regardless of size. Whether this scheduling function should be one component of a comprehensive EMR system is a complex question, as noted. In the OR, however, computerization allows for a faster, more efficient method of case posting than any handwritten system. Changes to the schedule can be made quickly without any loss of information. Rearranging the daily schedule is much simpler on a computer than erasing and rewriting on a ledger sheet. Furthermore, most hospitals have adopted a computer-determined average time for a given surgical procedure for a particular surgeon. Commonly, this time is the average of the last 10 (or 10 of the last 12, with the longest and shortest discarded) of the specific procedure (e.g., total knee replacement) with the potential to add a modifier (e.g., it is a repeat surgery) that shows a material difference in the projected time length (almost always longer) for one particular patient type. Suppose surgeon X has block time of 8 hours on a given day and wants to schedule four procedures in that allotted time. The computerized scheduling program looks at surgeon X's past performances and determines a projected length for each of the procedures that are identified to the computer usually by CPT-4 codes or possibly some other code developed locally for frequent procedures done by surgeon X. (Note that the recorded time length includes the turnover time, thus making the case time definition from the time the patient enters the OR until the time any following patient enters that OR [unless an "exception" is entered specifically for an unusual circumstance].) The use of agreed-upon codes instead of just text descriptions helps ensure accuracy because it eliminates any need for the scheduling clerk to guess what the surgeon intends to do. Bookings in most circumstances should not be taken without the accompanying codes (surgeons' offices objections not withstanding). The computer then decides whether surgeon X will finish the four procedures in the allotted block time. If the computer concludes that the fourth case would finish significantly (the definition of which can be determined and entered into the program) beyond the available block time, it will not accept the fourth case into that room's schedule on that particular day. The surgeon will accept the computer's assigned times and adjust accordingly, planning only three cases, or appeal for an "exception" based on some factor not in the booking that is claimed will materially decrease the time needed for at least one of the four cases, which the surgeon must explain to the "exception czar" (anesthesiology clinical director or OR charge nurse) of the day. An alternative method has the computer simply add (to each case except the last) a projected turnover time that is agreed upon by all involved at an (often contentious) OR committee meeting. Computerizing the scheduling process significantly reduces any personal biases and should smooth out the entire operating day. The long-standing ritual of mid-to-late-afternoon disputes between the surgeons and the anesthesia group and/or OR staff about whether or not to start the last scheduled case may be eliminated or at least reduced by this more realistic prospective OR scheduling method.

There are many variables to consider in any OR scheduling system. The patient population served and the nature of the institution dictate the overall structure of the OR schedule. Inner-city level 1 trauma centers must accommodate emergencies on a regular basis, 24 hours a day. These centers are unlikely to create a workable schedule more than a day in advance. An ambulatory surgery center serving plastic surgery patients may see only the rare emergency bring-back bleeding patient. Their schedule may be accurate many days in advance, with a high degree of expectation that the patient will arrive on time properly prepared for surgery. The anesthesia group at this ambulatory center may rarely have to make changes to the schedule, allowing them to proceed with a fairly predictable daily workload. At the inner-city trauma hospital, a great deal of flexibility and constant communication with the surgeons will be required in an attempt to get the cases done in a reasonable time frame with the inherent constraints placed on the OR staff's resources and the time available. These two extreme examples from opposite ends of the scheduling process spectrum can provide guidelines for the majority of the institutions that fall somewhere in between. Beyond open communication, how best to work toward this mutual understanding depends on the particulars of the people involved and the environment, but some ORs report benefits from team-building exercises, leadership retreats, and even OR-wide social events. ORs with a particularly malignant history of finger-pointing and bad feelings among the personnel groups may constitute one of the few instances an outside consultant may really be valuable in that there are workplace psychologists who specialize in analyzing dysfunctional work environments and implementing changes to improve the situation for all involved.

Preoperative Clinic

An anesthesia preoperative evaluation clinic (APEC) that provides a comprehensive perioperative medical evaluation usually results in a more efficient running of the OR schedule.[62–64] Unanticipated cancellations or delays are avoided when the anesthesia group evaluates complex patients prior to surgery. Even if the patient arrives to the OR on time the day of surgery, inadequate preoperative clearance mandating the ordering of additional tests will consume precious OR time during the delay waiting for results. Cancellations or delays adversely affect the efficiency of any OR. Subsequent cases in the delayed room, whether for the same or a different surgeon, may get significantly delayed or forced to be squeezed into an already busy schedule on another day. The financial impact of delays or cancellations on the institution is considerable. Revenue is lost with no offsetting absence of expenses. Worse, expenses may actually increase when overtime has to be paid, or the sterile equipment has to be discarded or repackaged after having been opened for the canceled procedure. Even worse, the inconvenienced patient and/or surgeon may go to another facility.

Optimal timing for preoperative evaluation should be related to the institution's scheduling preferences, patient convenience, and the overall health of the patient. Earlier completion of the preoperative evaluation may not reduce the overall cancellation rate when compared with a more proximate evaluation. However, an early evaluation and clearance may well provide a larger pool of patients available to place on the OR schedule (block or open) resulting in a more efficient use of OR time. In addition, a protocol-driven evaluation process can anticipate possible need for time-consuming investigations (such as a cardiology evaluation for the patient with likely angina). Early recognition of a failed preoperative test and need for postponement allows time for another patient to be moved into the now-vacant time slot. Also, early identification of certain problems requiring special care on the day of surgery (e.g., preoperative epidural, nerve block, or invasive monitoring placement) should lead to fewer unanticipated delays. Unfortunately, many issues precipitating delays are discovered on the day of surgery. Some of these preventable delays are unrelated to the patients' health status. Seemingly simple administrative issues such as verification of a ride home or incomplete financial information also contribute to unexpected delays. A properly functioning APEC may also be able to eliminate a majority of these annoying causes of preventable delays.

Regardless of the institutional specifics surrounding the service provided by the APEC, further cost savings can be obtained through its proper usage by the anesthesia group. The APEC frequently reduces dramatically the number of preoperative tests performed by focusing on which diagnostic tests and medical consults are really required for any specific patient (as opposed to the "shotgun approach" by some surgeons who order excessive testing simply with the intent of trying to avoid some last-minute request, whatever it might be, for more data). In some circumstances, the APEC may also function as an additional source of revenue for the anesthesia group when a formal preoperative consult on a complicated patient is ordered well in advance by the surgeon, in the same manner as would have otherwise been directed to a primary care physician for the often non-reassuring "clearance for surgery." The ability to centralize pertinent information including admission precertification/clearance, financial data, diagnostic and laboratory results, consult reports, and preoperative recommendations improves OR function by decreasing the time spent searching for all these items after changes have been made to the schedule. Patient and family education performed by the APEC frequently leads to an increase in patients' overall satisfaction of the perioperative experience. In addition, patient anxiety may be reduced secondary to the more in-depth contact possible inherent in the APEC process when compared with anesthesia practitioners meeting an ambulatory outpatient for the first time in an OR holding area immediately prior to surgery. The APEC model enables the anesthesia group to be more active and proactive in the perioperative process, improving their relations with the other OR constituents.

Anesthesiology Personnel Issues

In light of the putative shortage of anesthesia professionals, creating, managing, and maintaining an adequate supply of anesthesia practitioners promises to influence the OR landscape for years
9 to come.[65] Active recruiting for anesthesiologists appeared to be widespread and intense through approximately the end of 2010, sometimes involving creative marketing and incentives.[66] The lean resident recruiting years of the mid- to late-1990s continue to impact the profession. Even though applications to anesthesiology residencies from qualified applicants rebounded significantly,[65] it was projected many years of relatively large numbers of anesthesia graduates are needed to address the projected need for anesthesiologists, but the decreased number of CA-1 residents in 2009 portended in 2012 the first *decrease* in number of residency graduates in well over a decade.[67] The overall projected significant shortage of physicians in general has led to the opening and planning of several new medical schools in the United States. Regarding anesthesiology residency training programs, between 2005 and 2011, the number increased by two, from 129 to 131 and there was a 16% increase in the total number of anesthesia residents (while there was a 13% increase for all residents during the same interval).[35] Anesthesiology training programs continue to be challenged in maintaining support of their educational missions.[68] Furthermore, the relative supply of nonphysician anesthesia professionals is also dwindling. With the aging population of nurse anesthetists and the limited number of applications to schools in that profession, as well as the very limited number of training facilities for anesthesiology assistants, the overall supply of anesthesia professionals appeared potentially inadequate to meet current and, at least, short-term future demands. The need for anesthesia groups to create a flexible, attractive work environment in order to help retain professionals who might otherwise leave may increase. Note, however, that "the Great Recession" led to reduced turnover within practice groups because some anesthesia professionals, fearing economic uncertainty, chose to continue in practice positions that they likely would have vacated during normal economic conditions.

Another issue is consideration of what is a reasonable work load for an anesthesiologist and how best to measure, if possible, the clinical productivity of an anesthesia group/department. These questions have been the subject of considerable discussion.[69–72] Beyond the simple number of full-time equivalents, cases, and OR minutes, there must be consideration of factors such as the nature of the facility, types of surgical practice, patient acuity, and speed of the surgeons to allow fair comparisons. Thoughtful filtering of resulting data should take place before dissemination of the aggregate information to all members of a group because of the understandable extreme sensitivity among stressed and fatigued anesthesiologists to a suggestion that they are not working as hard as their group/department peers.

Except in highly unusual circumstances, flexible scheduling of anesthesia professionals and also fulfilling the demands placed on the group by the institution continues to be a constant balancing act. This demand assumes added significance because institutions now subsidize many anesthesia groups. Even when a majority of providers in a facility are independent contractors where it is required that a specific surgeon request their services, there are time conflicts ranging from no one at all being available to unwanted down time. When the anesthesia group/department accepts the responsibility of providing anesthesia services for an institution, they must schedule enough providers for that OR suite on each given day. Ideally, a sufficient number of professionals would be hired so that there would always be enough personnel to staff the minimum number of rooms scheduled on any given day, as well as after-hours call duty. This situation rarely exists because it would be financially disadvantageous to have an excess number of providers with no or minimal clinical activity. Having exactly the right number of anesthesia professionals in a group for the clinical load works well until one (or more) of them is out with an unplanned absence such as an extended illness or a family emergency. Many academic departments have a natural buffer with some clinicians assigned intervals of nonclinical time for research, teaching, or administrative duties. However, repeated loss of these nonclinical days because of inadequate clinical staffing in the OR leads to undermining the academic/research mission of the department. Continued loss of this time will eventually lead to faculty resignations (and possible migration to private practice), thus eliminating the original buffer. Consequently, anesthesia groups/departments need to anticipate available clinical personnel and match them to the OR demands. Ideally, this information should be accurate for several months into the future. Meeting this specification has become more difficult in the recent past. Hospital administrators must offer reasonable assurances to the anesthesia group providing service that a given OR utilization rate is likely, as well as accurate data regarding reimbursement (payer mix and any package contracts negotiated by the hospital). These data must be provided accurately and updated frequently if a health-care institution is to acquire and retain an anesthesia group staffed with the personnel to meet the expected demands.

Timing

Each operating environment has its own personnel scheduling system and expectations for the anesthesia group. Daily coordination between the anesthesia group's clinical director and the OR supervisor permits the construction of a reasonable schedule showing the number of ORs that day and when the schedule expects each of them to finish. Invariably, some cases take longer than anticipated or add-ons are posted, requiring the OR to run into the late afternoon or early evening. Many anesthesia professionals accept this occurrence as a matter of course. Few anesthesia professionals will tolerate this sequence of events as an essentially daily routine whether they are paid overtime or not. These practitioners become exhausted and resent the burdens continuously placed on them. If the OR schedule is such that add-ons frequently occur and elective cases run well into the evening, many anesthesia professionals will opt to protect their personal and family time and cut back their working hours or resign. Neither would be welcome in a tight market. Under these circumstances, hiring additional personnel who are scheduled to arrive at a later time, for example, 11:00 AM, and then providing lunch relief and staying late (e.g., 7:30 PM or later if needed) to finish the schedule may well be a very worthwhile investment.

Another possible solution to the demands of an extended OR schedule on an anesthesia group's personnel may revolve around employing part-time anesthesia professionals. Part-time opportunities could enhance a group's ability to attract additional staff. In the past, a disproportionately high percentage of women chose anesthesiology as a career. In 1970, women represented 7.6% of the physician population but were 14% of anesthesiologists; much more recently, they make up 45% of the physician population and only 20% of anesthesiologists, proportionately a significant reduction.[73] Beyond the basic demographic shift among all physicians, one likely partial explanation for the decreased number of women anesthesiologists may be the lack of part-time positions, which will hamper an anesthesia group's ability to attract and keep at least some of the female anesthesia professionals.

Scheduling after-hours coverage also adds to the personnel difficulties facing the anesthesia group. The variations of call schemes are endless. The nature of the institution and the workload determine the degree of late-night coverage. Major referral centers and level 1 trauma centers require in-house primary providers. If these providers include residents and/or nurse anesthetists, then the supervising attending staff likely will also be in-house 24 hours a day. A common solution employed at many institutions is to staff the evening/night call shifts for an average workload, recognizing that on some occasions there will be idle ORs, and on other nights, the surgical demand will exceed the call team's numbers.

There are also medicolegal issues surrounding the call team's availability. At a small community hospital with a limited number of independent attending practitioners, the practitioners may agree to cover call on a rotating basis. The individuals not on call are usually not obligated to the OR and may well be truly unreachable. What happens then when the on-call anesthesiologist is administering an anesthetic and another true emergency case arrives in the OR suite and the remaining staff anesthesiologists are legitimately unavailable? Does that anesthesiologist leave his or her current patient under the care of an OR nurse and go next door to tend to a more acutely (possibly critically) ill patient? Should the patient be transferred from the emergency department to another (hopefully nearby) hospital? These questions have no easy answers. Clearly, those practitioners on the scene have to assess in real time the relative risks and benefits and make the difficult decisions. If the call duty requires the practitioner(s) frequently to work much or all of the night, leaving the individual(s) stressed and fatigued, they should not be required to work the next day during normal working hours.

A more complicated answer involves what to do when the call assignment rarely requires a long night's work and the on-call anesthesia professionals routinely have rooms assigned to them the next day, but at least one person has just finished a difficult 24-hour shift being awake and working all night. Anesthesia groups need to decide how to handle the possible call shift scenarios, with permutations and combinations, and clearly communicate prospectively their decisions to the OR committee before any difficult decision has to be made one morning. As always, the medicolegal aspects of any decision such as this need to be taken into consideration. Whether or not fatigue was a factor, the practitioner who worked throughout the night before and appeared to contribute to an anesthetic catastrophe the next morning would have a very difficult defense in court. Further, the anesthesiology group may also be held liable in that their practice/policy was in place, allegedly authorizing the supposedly dangerous conduct.

COST AND QUALITY ISSUES

One of the more pervasive aspects of American medical care in today's environment is the drive to maintain and improve high-quality health care while reducing the cost of that care. Health-care costs account for a remarkable 17% of the gross domestic product, nearly triple the fraction a generation ago. Even more alarming, if costs continue to increase at the current rate, by 2019, it will be over 19% of the gross domestic product. Consequently, all physicians, including anesthesiologists, are urged constantly to include cost-consciousness in decisions balancing the natural desire to provide the highest possible quality of care with the overall priorities of both the health-care system and the individual patient, all while facing increasingly limited resources.[74] Anesthesiologists remain a target for limiting health-care expenditures. Anesthesia professionals (directly and indirectly) traditionally have represented 3% to 5% of the total health-care costs in the country.[75] Complicated decisions are required regarding which patients are suitable for ambulatory surgery, what preoperative studies to order, what anesthetic drugs or technique is best for the patient, what monitors or equipment are reasonably required to run an OR, and the list goes on and on. With this as background, anesthesiologists legitimately can include economic considerations in their practice management decision processes. When presented with multiple options to provide for therapeutic intervention or patient assessment, one should not automatically choose the more expensive approach (just to "cover all the bases") unless there is compelling evidence proving its value. Decisions that clearly materially increase cost should only be pursued when the benefit outweighs the risk. In anesthesia care as well as medicine in general, such decisions can be difficult regarding interventions that provide marginal benefit but contain significant cost increases.[76] Because cost containment initially requires accurate cost awareness, anesthesiologists need to find out the actual costs and benefits of their anesthesia care techniques. Details will be unique to each practice setting. Because they will be excited that the anesthesiologists actually care, usually it is possible to get the cooperation of the facility administration's financial department members in researching and calculating the actual cost of anesthesia care so that thoughtful evaluations of potential reductions can be initiated.

Anesthesia drug expenses represent a small portion of the total perioperative costs. However, the great number of doses actually administered contributes substantially to aggregate total cost to the institution in actual dollars. Prudent drug selection combined with appropriate anesthetic technique can result in substantial savings. Reducing fresh gas flow from 5 L/min to 2 L/min wherever possible has been estimated to potentially save approximately $100 million annually in the United States.[77] A majority of anesthesia professionals usually attempt a practical approach to cost savings, but they are more frequently faced with difficult choices regarding methods of anesthesia that likely produce similar outcomes but at substantially different cost. When comparing the total costs of more expensive anesthetic drugs and techniques to lesser expensive ones, many variables need to be added to the formula. The cost of anesthetic drugs needs to include the costs of additional equipment such as special vaporizers or extra infusion pumps and the associated maintenance. There are other indirect costs that may be difficult to quantitate and are commonly overlooked. Some of these indirect costs include increased setup time, possibly increasing room turnover time, extended PACU recovery time, and additional expensive drugs required to treat side effects. Sometimes, more expensive techniques reduce indirect costs. A propofol infusion, although more expensive than vapor, commonly results in a decreased PACU stay for a short noninvasive procedure. If fewer PACU staff are needed or patient throughput is increased, the more expensive drug can reduce overall cost. Conversely, using comparatively expensive propofol for a long procedure definitely requiring postoperative admission to an ICU is not cost justified. The impact of shorter-acting drugs and those with fewer side effects is context-specific. During long surgical procedures, such drugs may offer limited benefits over older, less expensive, longer-acting alternatives.[78] Under these conditions, advocating cost containment using educational efforts may decrease drug expenditures for several categories of drugs.[79] Drugs in the same therapeutic class have widely varying costs. The acquisition expenses may vary as much as 50-fold in some pharmacologic categories. It is estimated that the 10 highest expenditure drugs account for >80% of the anesthetic drug costs at some institutions.[80] Although newer, more expensive drugs may be easier to use, no data exist to support or refute the hypothesis that these drugs provide a "better" anesthetic experience when compared with carefully titrated older, less expensive, longer-acting drugs in the same class.

Evaluation of outcomes and their subsequent application to cost analysis can be derived from two principle sources: Data published in the literature and data collected from experience. As noted, computerized information management systems are useful tools to track outcomes and analyze the impact on the cost/benefit ledger. Using the collated data in the same manner as for OR utilization and case load, practitioners can readily apply a statistical process to evaluate outcomes in their practice, possibly including correlation with cost. This information may take on added importance in that published incidence studies may not exist for the specific outcome an anesthesia group is searching for. Cause-and-effect diagrams can track the parameters involved in the process and relate them to the various outcomes desired. Multiple pertinent examples could be constructed from the now-extensive body of literature on the factors contributing to postoperative nausea and vomiting and the various possible preventions and treatments, many of which involve expensive medications. Of course, this can be done locally within an institution. Information would be collected and stored in the database. Ideally, the database would identify and track as many variables as needed/possible to delineate sources for possible improvement and its ultimate cost analysis. Once these sources for improvement and the ensuing cost impact are known, the anesthesia group can determine whether or not to pursue changing their practice. Outcomes related to adverse effects can also be monitored. If analysis reveals a significant difference in an adverse outcome among practitioners, after all the other variables such as surgeon, patient mix, and so forth are eliminated, the outcome database can investigate the anesthetic technique used by that practitioner. If significant variations are identified, that practitioner would be able to learn of these variations in a nonthreatening manner because computer-derived data are used as opposed to a specific case analysis, which might lead that practitioner to feel singled out for public criticism. The database becomes a tool both for QA and professional education.

CONCLUSION

10 Practice and OR management in anesthesiology today is more complex and more important than ever before. Attention to details that previously either did not exist or were perceived as unimportant can likely make the difference between success and failure in anesthesiology practice.

Outlined here are basic descriptions and understandings of many different administrative, organizational, financial, and personnel components and factors in the practice of anesthesiology today. Ongoing significant changes in the health-care system will provide a continuing and expanding array of challenges. Application of the principles presented here will allow anesthesiologists to extrapolate creatively from these basics to their own individual circumstances and then forge ahead in anesthesiology practice that is efficient, effective, productive, collegial, and even fun.

References

1. American Society of Anesthesiologists: *2010 Manual for Anesthesia Department Organization and Management.* Park Ridge, IL: American Society of Anesthesiologists; 2010. See: https://www.asahq.org/For-Members/Practice-Management/ASA-Practice-Management-Resources.aspx; accessed 12/12/11.
2. American Society of Anesthesiologists: https://ecommerce.asahq.org/c-16-Practice-Management-Conference-Chapters.aspx; accessed 12/12/11.
3. Peters JD, Fineberg KS, Kroll DA, et al. *Anesthesiology and the Law.* Ann Arbor, MI: Health Administration Press; 1983.
4. Gaba DM, Howard SK, Jump B. Production pressure in the work environment. *Anesthesiology.* 1994;81:488.
5. Eichhorn JH, Cooper JB, Cullen DJ, et al. Anesthesia practice standards at Harvard: A review. *J Clin Anesth.* 1988;1:56.
6. American Society of Anesthesiologists Task Force on Preanesthesia Evaluation. Practice advisory for preanesthesia evaluation. *Anesthesiology.* 2002;96:485.
7. American Society of Anesthesiologists Task Force on Postanesthetic Care. Practice guidelines for postanesthetic care. *Anesthesiology.* 2002;96:742.
8. American Society of Anesthesiologists Task Force on Obstetric Anesthesia. Practice guidelines for obstetrical anesthesia. *Anesthesiology.* 2007;106:843.
9. American Society of Anesthesiologists Task Force on Pulmonary Artery Catheterization. Practice guidelines for pulmonary artery catheterization: An updated

report by the American Society of Anesthesiologists Task Force on Pulmonary Artery Catheterization. *Anesthesiology*. 2003;99:988.
10. American Society of Anesthesiologists Task Force on Management of the Difficult Airway. Practice guidelines for management of the difficult airway: An updated report by the American Society of Anesthesiologists Task Force on Management of the Difficult Airway. *Anesthesiology*. 2003;98:1269.
11. Dans PE, Weiner JP, Otter SE. Peer review organizations: Promises and potential pitfalls. *N Engl J Med*. 1985;313:1131.
12. Eichhorn JH. Anesthesia equipment: Checkout and quality assurance. In: Ehrenwerth J, Eisenkraft JB, eds. *Anesthesia Equipment: Principles and Applications*. St. Louis, MO: Mosby–Yearbook; 1992, p. 473.
13. Eichhorn JH. Organized response to major anesthesia accident will help limit damage: Update of "Adverse Event Protocol" provides valuable plan. *APSF Newsletter*. 2006;21:11.
14. Spooner RB, Kirby RR. Equipment-related anesthetic incidents. In: Pierce EC, Cooper JB, eds. *Analysis of Anesthetic Mishaps*. Boston, MA: International Anesthesiology Clinics; 1984;22:133.
15. Cooper JB, Newbower RS, Kitz RJ. An analysis of major errors and equipment failures in anesthesia management: Considerations for prevention and detection. *Anesthesiology*. 1984;60:34.
16. Caplan RA, Vistica M, Posner KL, et al. Adverse anesthetic outcomes arising from gas delivery equipment: A closed claims analysis. *Anesthesiology*. 1997;87:741.
17. Cooper JB, Newbower RS, Long CD, et al. Preventable anesthesia mishaps: A study of human factors. *Anesthesiology*. 1978;49:399.
18. Duberman S, Wald A. An integrated quality control program for anesthesia equipment. In: Chapman-Cliburn G, ed. *Risk Management and Quality Assurance, Issues and Interactions*. Chicago, IL: Joint Commission on the Accreditation of Hospitals; 1986, p. 105.
19. Olympio MA, Reinke B, Abramovich A. Challenges ahead in technology training: A report on the training initiative of the Committee on Technology. *APSF Newsletter*. 2006;21:43.
20. HHS Publication No. (FDA) 85–4196. Food and Drug Administration, Center for Devices and Radiologic Health, Rockville, MD 20857, p. 10.
21. Eichhorn JH. Influence of practice standards on anesthesia outcome. In: Desmonts JM, ed. *Outcome After Anesthesia and Surgery. Bailliere's Clinical Anaesthesiology—International Practice and Research*. 1992;6:663.
22. Eichhorn JH. Prevention of intraoperative anesthesia accidents and related severe injury through safety monitoring. *Anesthesiology*. 1989;70:572.
23. Keats AS. Anesthesia mortality in perspective. *Anesth Analg*. 1990;71:113.
24. Lagasse RS. Anesthesia safety: Model or myth? *Anesthesiology*. 2002;97:1609.
25. Cooper JB, Gaba DM. No myth: Anesthesia is a model for addressing patient safety. *Anesthesiology*. 2002;97:1335.
26. Peterson GN. Malpractice insurance: What are the limits? *ASA Newsletter*. 2007;71:14.
27. Bacon AK. Death on the table: Some thoughts on how to handle an anaesthetic-related death. *Anaesthesia*. 1989;44:245.
28. Runciman WB, Webb RK, Klepper ID, et al. Crisis management: Validation of an algorithm by analysis of 2000 incident reports. *Anaesth Intensive Care*. 1993;21:579.
29. Davies J, Webb RK. Adverse events in anaesthesia: The wrong drug. *Can J Anaesth*. 1994;41:83.
30. Cooper JB, Cullen DJ, Eichhorn JH, et al. Administrative guidelines for response to an adverse anesthesia event. *J Clin Anesth*. 1993;5:79.
31. Kraman SS, Hamm G. Risk management: Extreme honesty may be the best policy. *Ann Intern Med*. 1999;131:963.
32. Lazare A. Apology in medical practice: An emerging clinical skill. *JAMA*. 2006;296:1401.
33. Eichhorn JH. Patient perspective personalizes patient safety. *APSF Newsletter*. 2005;20:61.
34. Cox W. The five A's: What do patients want after an adverse event? *J Healthcare Risk Manag*. 2007;27:25.
35. Accreditation Council for Graduate Medical Education. *Data Resource Book, Academic Year 2010–2011*. Chicago, IL: ACGME; 2011.
36. Semo JJ. Our hospital wants to employ us: Now what? *Proceedings of the American Society of Anesthesiologists 2008 Conference on Practice Management*. Park Ridge, IL: American Society of Anesthesiologists; 2008:48.
37. American Society of Anesthesiologists. Office-Based Anesthesia: Considerations in Setting Up and Maintaining a Safe Office Anesthesia Environment. https://ecommerce.asahq.org/p-319-office-based-anesthesia-considerations-in-setting-up-and-maintaining-a-safe-office-anesthesia-environment.aspx; accessed 1/2/12.
38. Practice management: Compliance with Medicare and other payor billing requirements. Park Ridge, IL, American Society of Anesthesiologists, 1997; https://ecommerce.asahq.org/p-169-compliance-with-medicare-and-other-payor-billing-requirements-1997.aspx
39. Locke J. The net collections fallacy and other performance metric myths. *Proceedings of the American Society of Anesthesiologists 2003 Conference on Practice Management*. Park Ridge, IL: American Society of Anesthesiologists; 2003: 141.
40. Contracting Issues: A Primer for Anesthesiologists. Park Ridge, IL, American Society of Anesthesiologists, 1999; https://ecommerce.asahq.org/p-170-contracting-issues-a-primer-for-anesthesiologists-1999.aspx
41. Willett DE. Exclusive contracts: Update on legal issues. *Proceedings of the American Society of Anesthesiologists 2001 Conference on Practice Management*. Park Ridge, IL: American Society of Anesthesiologists; 2001:8.
42. Scott SJ, Blough GG. Exclusive contracts: Survey of hospital contracts. *Proceedings of the American Society of Anesthesiologists 2001 Conference on Practice Management*. Park Ridge, IL: American Society of Anesthesiologists; 2001:9.
43. Bierstein K. Pros and cons of exclusive contracts. *ASA Newsletter*. 2006;70(8):36.
44. Everett PC. Securing a hospital stipend: The business-like approach. *Proceedings of the American Society of Anesthesiologists 2003 Conference on Practice Management*. Park Ridge, IL: American Society of Anesthesiologists; 2003:189.
45. Semo JJ. Hospital stipend negotiations: Practical and legal issues. *Proceedings of the American Society of Anesthesiologists 2004 Conference on Practice Management*. Park Ridge, IL: American Society of Anesthesiologists; 2004:51.
46. Laden J, Monea M. Preparing the financial case for hospital support. *Proceedings of the American Society of Anesthesiologists 2008 Conference on Practice Management*. Park Ridge, IL: American Society of Anesthesiologists; 2008:258.
47. Rodin MA. Conflicts in managed care. *N Engl J Med*. 1995;332:604.
48. Adessa A. The vulnerability and potential extinction of independent, hospital-based practices. *Proceedings of the American Society of Anesthesiologists 2008 Conference on Practice Management*. Park Ridge, IL: American Society of Anesthesiologists; 2008:65.
49. Epstein AM, Lee TH, Hamel MB. Paying physicians for high-quality care. *N Engl J Med*. 2004;350:406.
50. Hannenberg AA. Progress report: Quality incentives in anesthesiology. *Proceedings of the American Society of Anesthesiologists 2008 Conference on Practice Management*. Park Ridge, IL: American Society of Anesthesiologists; 2008:57.
51. Scurlock C, Dexter F, Reich D, et al. Needs assessment for business strategies of anesthesiology groups' practices. *Anesth Analg*. 2011;113:170.
52. The HIPAA Privacy Rule in Anesthesia and Pain Medicine Practices. Park Ridge, IL, American Society of Anesthesiologists, 2003; https://ecommerce.asahq.org/p-254-practice-management-the-hipaa-privacy-rule-in-anesthesia-and-pain-medicine-practices-2003.aspx
53. Semo JJ. HIPAA privacy: What you need to know, what you need to do. *Proceedings of the American Society of Anesthesiologists 2003 Conference on Practice Management*. Park Ridge, IL: American Society of Anesthesiologists; 2003:96.
54. Semo JJ. HIPAA privacy update. *Proceedings of the American Society of Anesthesiologists 2004 Conference on Practice Management*. Park Ridge, IL: American Society of Anesthesiologists; 2004:123.
55. Johnson JF. Questions to ask your billing software vendor. *Proceedings of the American Society of Anesthesiologists 2003 Conference on Practice Management*. Park Ridge, IL: American Society of Anesthesiologists; 2003:130.
56. Warner M. Who better than anesthesiologists?: The 44th Rovenstine Lecture. *Anesthesiology*. 2006;104:1094.
57. Sexton J, Makary MA, Tersigni AR, et al. Teamwork in the operating room. *Anesthesiology*. 2006;105:877.
58. Lingard L, Regehr G, Orser B, et al. Evaluation of a preoperative checklist and team briefing among surgeons, nurses, and anesthesiologists to reduce failures in communication. *Arch Surg*. 2008;143:12.
59. Mazzei WJ. OR management. *Proceedings of the American Society of Anesthesiologists 2001 Conference on Practice Management*. Park Ridge, IL: American Society of Anesthesiologists ASA; 2001:12-1.
60. Malhotra V. Practical issues in OR management: The obvious and the not so obvious. *Proceedings of the American Society of Anesthesiologists 2004 Conference on Practice Management*. Park Ridge, IL: American Society of Anesthesiologists; 2004:43.
61. Dexter F, Xiao Y, Dow A, et al. Coordination of appointments for anesthesia care outside of operating rooms using an enterprise-wide scheduling system. *Anesth Analg*. 2007;105:1701.
62. Pollard JB, Zboray AL, Mazze RI. Economic benefits attributed to opening a preoperative evaluation clinic for outpatients. *Anesth Analg*. 1996;83:407.
63. Fischer SP. Development and effectiveness of an anesthesia preoperative evaluation clinic in a teaching hospital. *Anesthesiology*. 1996;85:196.
64. Yen C, Tsai M, Macario A. Preoperative evaluation clinics. *Curr Opin Anaesthesiol*. 2010;23:167.
65. Schubert A. Implications of a changing anesthesia workforce. *Proceedings of the American Society of Anesthesiologists 2008 Conference on Practice Management*. Park Ridge, IL: American Society of Anesthesiologists; 2008:297.
66. Blough GG, Scott SJ. Creative scheduling for anesthesiologists: Physician retention in a tight market. *Proceedings of the American Society of Anesthesiologists 2003 Conference on Practice Management*. Park Ridge, IL: American Society of Anesthesiologists; 2003:71.
67. Schubert A. 2009 Anesthesiology resident class sizes and graduates. *ASA Newsletter* 2009;74(2):324.
68. Kheterpal S, Tremper K, Shanks A, et al. Workforce and finances of the United States anesthesiology training programs: 2009–2010. *Anesth Analg*. 2011;112: 1480.
69. Abouleish AE, Prough DS, Zornow MH, et al. Designing meaningful industry metrics for clinical productivity for anesthesiology departments. *Anesth Analg*. 2001;93:309.
70. Abouleish AE, Prough DS, Whitten CW, et al. Comparing clinical productivity of anesthesiology departments. *Anesthesiology*. 2002;97:608.

71. Abouleish AE, Prough DS, Barker SJ, et al. Organizational factors affect comparisons of clinical productivity of academic anesthesiology departments. *Anesth Analg.* 2003;96:802.
72. Abouleish AE. Working hard: Hardly working; comparing clinical productivity of anesthesiology groups. *Proceedings of the American Society of Anesthesiologists 2004 Conference on Practice Management.* Park Ridge, IL: American Society of Anesthesiologists; 2004:195.
73. Calmes SH. Anesthesiology demographics: Women's changing specialty choices and implications for anesthesiology workforce shortage. *ASA Newsletter.* 2001;65 (8):22.
74. Tuman KJ, Ivankovich AD. High cost, high tech medicine—are we getting our money's worth? *J Clin Anesth.* 1993;5:168.
75. Johnstone RE, Martinec CL. Costs of anesthesia. *Anesth Analg.* 1993;76:840.
76. Eddy DM. Applying cost-effectiveness analysis: The inside story. *JAMA* 1992; 268:2575.
77. Baum JA. Low flow anaesthesia: The sensible and judicious use of inhalation anaesthetics. *Acta Anaesthesiol Scand Suppl.* 1997;111:264.
78. Szocik JF, Learned DW. Impact of a cost containment program on the use of volatile anesthetics and neuromuscular blocking drugs. *J Clin Anesth.* 1994;6: 378.
79. Barclay LP, Hatton RC, Doering PL, et al. Physicians' perceptions and knowledge of drug costs: Results of a survey. *Formulary.* 1995;30:268.
80. Johnstone R, Jozefczyk KG. Costs of anesthetic drugs: Experiences with a cost education trial. *Anesth Analg.* 1994;78:766.

CHAPTER

3 Occupational Health

JONATHAN D. KATZ • ROBERT S. HOLZMAN

Key Points

1. Exposure to waste anesthetic gases can be reduced to levels below those recommended by the National Institute for Occupational Safety and Health (NIOSH) by using waste gas scavenging equipment, routinely maintaining anesthesia machines, and following appropriate work practices.
2. Vigilance is one of the most critical tasks performed by anesthesiologists and may be adversely affected by several occupationally related issues including poor equipment engineering and design, excessive noise, interpersonal conflict-related interactions, production pressures, and fatigue.
3. Sleep deprivation and fatigue is common among anesthesiologists and can adversely affect patient safety. Sleep deprivation can have deleterious effects on the physician's cognition, mood, and health.
4. The risk of exposure to infectious pathogens can be reduced by the routine use of standard precautions, transmission-based precautions for infected patients, and safety devices designed to prevent needlestick injuries.
5. Hepatitis B vaccine is recommended for all anesthesia personnel because of the increased risk for occupational transmission of this blood-borne pathogen.
6. Many consider chemical dependency to be the primary occupational hazard among anesthesiologists. An incidence of controlled substance abuse of 1% to 2% has been repeatedly reported within anesthesia training programs.
7. Physician wellness is a topic integral to occupational health and patient safety. There is an evolving professional commitment to optimizing physician work style and lifestyle, as well as physical health (e.g., through better nutrition, fitness, and rest).
8. Mindfulness is an emerging and complementary concept to wellness that has specific relevance to vigilance. Functional imaging techniques as well as cognitive psychology are enhancing our understanding of this key component to anesthesia practice.

Multimedia

1 Fixation Errors

2 ASA Seal

3 Needle Stick

4 Chain of Communication

The health-care industry has the dubious distinction of being one of the most hazardous places to work in the United States. According to the U.S. Bureau of Labor, health care is second only to manufacturing in the number of occupational illnesses and injuries sustained by their workers.[1] Anesthesia personnel are at risk of acquiring a number of occupational illnesses and injuries that are specific to the high-intensity environment of the operating room. Workplace hazards include exposure to toxic chemicals and waste anesthetic gases, ionizing radiation, and infectious agents. They are vulnerable to injury from fires or explosions. In addition, anesthesia personnel are susceptible to emotional and psychological disorders, such as burnout and substance abuse, engendered at least in part by the high stress and other demands inherent in their work.

Only within the past few decades have comprehensive programs been developed to assess the health of anesthesia personnel and protect against and treat many of these occupational diseases. There are numerous potential health risks to anesthesia personnel, but with heightened awareness of the problems and the use of proper precautions, they are avoidable or manageable.

PHYSICAL HAZARDS

Anesthetic Gases

Concerns about possible toxic effects of occupational exposure to inhalation anesthetics have been expressed since their introduction into clinical practice. Investigations have included cellular research, in vitro and in vivo studies, and epidemiologic surveys. Specific focuses of the research have been whether or not occupational exposure to waste anesthetic gases is associated with cytotoxic and genotoxic changes, organ toxicity, adverse reproductive outcomes, impairment of psychomotor skills, or premature death.

Evidence exists to show that cellular damage can result from chronic exposure of cells to high concentrations of anesthetic gases in the laboratory.[2] However, it can be misleading to extrapolate data from studies in cellular cultures or experimental animals to the real-world experience of humans working in operating rooms. The reports regarding possible cellular injury from waste anesthetic gases are inconsistent. Several studies testing for chromosomal aberrations, sister chromatid exchanges, or changes in peripheral lymphocytes have found no evidence of cellular damage among clinicians exposed to the levels of anesthetic gases that are encountered in an adequately ventilated operating room.[3] On the other hand, individuals who are exposed to high ambient concentrations of waste gases, such as in anesthetizing locations where there is inadequate ventilation or scavenging, may be subject to a dose-dependent increase in cytotoxic changes.[4] Reports on cellular changes thought to result from waste anesthetic gas exposure are difficult to compare because of the inability to standardize other risk factors to which operating room personnel are exposed, such as radiation, long work hours, and stress. Most sources agree that occupational exposure to the low levels of anesthetics found in operating rooms with effective waste gas scavenging is not associated with significant cellular effects.[5]

Nitrous oxide exposure is a special situation.[6] Nitrous oxide can irreversibly oxidize the cobalt atom of vitamin B_{12} to an inactive state. This inhibits methionine synthetase and prevents the conversion of methyltetrahydrofolate to tetrahydrofolate, which is required for DNA synthesis, assembly of the myelin sheath, and methyl substitutions in neurotransmitters. At clinically utilized concentrations of nitrous oxide, this inhibition could result in anemia and polyneuropathy. As with the halogenated hydrocarbon anesthetics, these effects with nitrous oxide have not been demonstrated in operating rooms with effective waste gas scavenging.

Reproductive Outcomes

An adverse impact of waste anesthetic gases on reproductive outcomes has been a persistent concern. The earliest reports suggested an association between long-term exposure to waste anesthetic agents among health-care personnel and infertility, spontaneous abortions, and congenital abnormalities.[7] The American Society of Anesthesiologists (ASA) and the National Institute for Occupational Safety and Health (NIOSH) published a large retrospective study in 1974 in which 49,585 operating room personnel who had potential exposure to waste anesthetic gases were compared with a nonexposed group of 23,911 health-care professionals.[8] Among the findings in this study was an increased risk of spontaneous abortion and congenital abnormalities in children of women who worked in the operating room and an increased risk of congenital abnormalities in offspring of unexposed wives of male operating room personnel.

In response to criticism of the methodology and data analysis in this study, ASA commissioned a group of epidemiologists and biostatisticians to do a meta-analysis using data from this and 16 other published epidemiologic surveys.[9] They found only six studies on spontaneous abortion and congenital abnormalities in offspring of anesthesia personnel that they felt were free of errors in study design or statistical analysis. From these studies, they reported the relative risks of spontaneous abortion for female physicians and female nurses working in the operating room were 1.4 and 1.3, respectively (a relative risk of 1.3 represents a 30% increase in risk when compared with the risk of the control population). The increased relative risk for congenital abnormalities was of borderline statistical significance for exposed physicians only. Although they did find a statistically significant relative risk of spontaneous abortion and congenital abnormalities in women working in the operating room, the relative risk was small compared with other, better-documented maternal risk factors, such as cigarette smoking and long working hours. The reviewers also pointed out that duration and levels of anesthetic exposure were not measured in any of the studies and that other confounding factors were not adequately controlled.

Other medical specialties with occupational exposure to anesthetic gases have also conducted studies among their health-care professionals. Studies of female dental assistants have revealed a reduction in fecundability and an increased rate of spontaneous abortion among women who worked in offices not using scavenging equipment.[10,11] In offices where scavenging devices were used to vent waste nitrous oxide, there was no evidence of an increased risk for adverse reproductive outcomes. Findings from both of these studies of dental assistants must be viewed with caution because the estimates of nitrous oxide exposure were based solely on respondents' retrospective reports.

Veterinarians and others who work in animal hospitals are a third group of professionals who may have frequent exposure to waste anesthetic gases. In a study of 744 pregnant female veterinarians in Australia, there was a 2.5-fold increase in the risk of preterm delivery in those exposed to unscavenged anesthetic gases for one or more hours per week as compared with unexposed workers.[12] Data collected by the same group demonstrated no increased prevalence of birth defects as a result of maternal exposure to anesthetic gases.[13]

A meta-analysis in 1997, of 19 epidemiologic studies, which included hospital workers, dental assistants, veterinarians, and veterinary assistants, demonstrated an increased risk of spontaneous abortion in women with occupational exposure to anesthetic gases (RR—1.48).[14] Stratification by job category indicated that the relative risk was greatest for veterinarians (RR—2.45), followed by dental assistants (RR—1.89) and hospital workers (RR—1.30). When the meta-analysis was confined to five studies that controlled for several nonoccupational confounding variables, had appropriate control groups, and had a sufficient response rate, the relative risk for spontaneous abortion was 1.90. The author noted that the routine use of scavenging devices had been implemented since the time that most of the studies in this meta-analysis were performed and that there was no increased risk of spontaneous abortion in studies of personnel who worked in environments where waste gases were scavenged.

It is likely that other job-associated conditions besides exposure to trace anesthetic gases may account for many of the adverse reproductive outcomes reported among some health-care workers (HCWs). These include stress, infections, long work hours, shift work, and radiation exposure. A survey of 3,985 Swedish midwives demonstrated that night work was significantly associated with spontaneous abortions after the 12th week of pregnancy (odds ratio 3.33), while exposure to nitrous oxide appeared to have no effect.[15] Preterm birth in obstetric and neonatal nurses was associated with increased work hours, hours worked while standing, and occupational fatigue.[16] And in a study of female veterinarians, the risks of birth defects were highest among those exposed to radiation and to long working hours (>45 hours/week) but not to those exposed to waste anesthetic gases.[12]

Many of the epidemiologic studies suffer from important design
1 flaws. However, the evidence taken as a whole suggests that there is a slight increase in the relative risk of spontaneous abortion and congenital abnormalities in offspring of female health-care professionals working in the operating room. This risk is minimized when appropriate waste gas scavenging technology is applied.

Cancer

A 1968 report on the health of anesthesiologists concluded that male anesthesiologists had an increased risk of malignancies of the lymphoid and reticuloendothelial tissues but a lower death rate from lung cancer.[17] Data from a subsequent prospective study by the same group contradicted the original findings and found no evidence that lymphoid malignancies were an occupational hazard for anesthesiologists.[18]

The 1974 ASA-sponsored study (vide supra) found no differences in cancer rates between men exposed and those not exposed to trace concentrations of anesthetic gases.[8] There was a 1.3- to 2-fold increase in the occurrence of various forms of cancer among exposed women, predominantly from an increase in leukemia and lymphoma. The subsequent reanalysis of these data confirmed an increase in relative risk of cancer in exposed women (RR 1.4) but attributed the increase solely to cervical cancer (RR 2.8).[9] These authors also noted that the original study did not assess the effect of confounding variables, such as sexual or smoking history, that may have contributed to the findings. It is doubtful that these purported carcinogenic effects of anesthetics would be sex-related, and the conflicting results for men and women, especially in light of the low statistical significance of the data, cast doubt that anesthetics were the causative agents.

A subsequent ASA-sponsored study of anesthesiologists, covering the period from 1976 to 1995, used data on the cause of death from the National Death Index.[19] The mortality risks of a cohort of 40,242 anesthesiologists were compared with a matched cohort of internists. There was no difference between the two groups in overall mortality risk or mortality from cancer.

Behavioral Effects

One of the principal reasons identified by the NIOSH for limiting occupational exposure to waste anesthetic gases is to prevent "decrements in performance, cognition, audiovisual ability and dexterity".[20] The clearest evidence for behavioral effects from trace gas exposure comes from work with laboratory animals where concentration and duration of exposure can be precisely controlled. In a study of rats exposed for 30 days to 1/10 minimum alveolar concentration (MAC) of halothane, sevoflurane, or desflurane, there were significant alterations of exploratory activity, curiosity, anxiety, learning, and memory functions in the exposed animals.[21]

The effect on psychomotor performance among human volunteers varies considerably depending upon the concentration of anesthetic gas to which the subjects are exposed. Temporary lethargy and fatigue are the most common symptoms described after brief exposures to subanesthetic concentrations of anesthetic gases. Longer exposures and higher concentrations have been associated with changes such as headache, depression, anxiety, loss of appetite, loss of memory, decreased reaction time, and decrements in cognitive function. Most of the measurable psychomotor and cognitive impairments produced by brief exposures are short-lived and disappear within 5 minutes of cessation of exposure.[22]

One of the most dramatic demonstrations of psychomotor impairment resulting from chronic anesthetic gas exposure appeared as a case report in which two anesthesiologists in the same institution developed chronic toxic encephalopathy.[23] Each of them had spent many years doing pediatric cases requiring induction and maintenance of anesthesia by mask in two operating rooms that were subsequently shown to have insufficient fresh air supply resulting in high ambient concentrations of anesthetic gases. In both cases, symptoms gradually improved after the individuals were removed from the offending environment.

Levels of Trace Anesthetic Gases

The first report of occupational exposure to modern anesthetics was by Linde and Bruce[24] in 1969 who noted an average concentration of halothane of 10 ppm and of nitrous oxide of 130 ppm in the air surrounding an active anesthesia machine. End-expired air samples taken from anesthesiologists after work were as high as 12 ppm of halothane. It was later demonstrated that with appropriate scavenging equipment and with adequate air exchange in the operating room, levels of waste anesthetic gases could be significantly reduced.[25]

Elevated levels of volatile anesthetics have also been identified in the postanesthesia care unit (PACU). This typically occurs as a product of exhaled gases from recovering patients. In one study, the time-weighted average (TWA) concentrations for isoflurane, desflurane, and nitrous oxide were 1.1, 2.1, and 29 ppm, respectively, in the breathing zone of PACU nurses.[26] In this study, the tracheas of half of the patients were intubated on arrival in the PACU, suggesting that the patients were still partially anesthetized and were exhaling a greater concentration of anesthetic gases than if they had more completely recovered in the operating room. In contrast, in two institutions where nitrous oxide was discontinued at the end of surgery approximately 5 minutes before the patient left the operating room and adequate air exchanges were maintained in the PACU, the time-weighted nitrous oxide levels were less than 2.0 ppm.[27] Minimal levels of anesthetic gases can be obtained in the PACU by ensuring adequate room ventilation and fresh gas exchange and by discontinuing the anesthetic gases in sufficient time before leaving the operating room.

Recommendations of the National Institute of Occupational Safety and Health (NIOSH) and the Occupational Safety and Health Administration (OSHA)

In 1977, NIOSH issued a criteria document that included recommended exposure limits (RELs) for waste anesthetic gases of 2 ppm (1-hour ceiling) for halogenated anesthetic agents when used alone or 0.5 ppm for halogenated agent and 25 ppm of nitrous oxide when used together (TWA during the period of anesthetic administration).[20] In addition, it stated that operating room employees should be advised of the potential harmful effects of anesthetics. The guidelines proposed that annual medical and occupational histories be obtained from all personnel and that any abnormal outcomes of pregnancies should be documented. The publication also included information on scavenging procedures and equipment and methods for monitoring concentrations of waste anesthetic gases in the air.

In a subsequent publication, NIOSH issued an alert to warn health-care personnel that exposure to nitrous oxide may produce "harmful effects".[28] In this document, NIOSH recommends the following to reduce nitrous oxide exposure: Monitoring the air in operating rooms, implementation of appropriate engineering controls, work practices, and equipment maintenance procedures, and institution of a worker education program.

NIOSH has not yet developed RELs for the agents most commonly used in current practice (isoflurane, sevoflurane, and desflurane). These volatile agents have potencies, chemical characteristics, and rates and products of metabolism that differ significantly from older anesthetics.

Occupational Safety and Health Administration (OSHA), which is the federal agency that is responsible for enacting job health standards and investigating work site violations has never adopted the NIOSH criteria document and has not set a standard permissible exposure limit for waste anesthetic gases. However, most states have instituted regulations calling for routine measurement of ambient gases in operating rooms and have mandated that levels not exceed an arbitrary maximum. Other organizations, such as the American Conference of Governmental Industrial Hygienists (www.acgih.org), have established their own occupational exposure limits for waste anesthetic gases, in many cases greater than those recommended by NIOSH.

It is prudent to institute measures that reduce waste anesthetic levels in the operating room environment to as low as possible. To ensure reduced occupational exposure, facilities where anesthetics are administered should have procedures to monitor for detection of leaks in anesthesia machines and contamination as a result of faulty anesthetic techniques (e.g., poor mask fit, leaks around endotracheal tube cuffs and laryngeal mask airways, and scavenging system malfunctions) (Table 3-1). When there have been leaks of anesthetic gases, dispersion and removal of the pollutants depends upon adequate room ventilation, at least 15 to 21 air exchanges per hour with three bringing in outside air. Through the use of scavenging equipment, equipment maintenance procedures, appropriate anesthetic work practices, and efficient operating room ventilation systems, the environmental anesthetic concentration can be reduced to minimal levels.

TABLE 3-1. SOURCES OF OPERATING ROOM CONTAMINATION

Anesthetic Techniques
- Failure to turn off gas flow control valves at the end of an anesthetic
- Turning gas flow on before placing mask on patient
- Poorly fitting masks, especially with mask induction of anesthesia
- Flushing of the circuit
- Filling of anesthesia vaporizers
- Uncuffed or leaking tracheal tubes (e.g., pediatric) or poorly fitting laryngeal mask airways
- Pediatric circuits (e.g., Jackson-Rees version of the Mapleson D system)
- Sidestream sampling carbon dioxide and anesthetic gas analyzers

Anesthesia Machine Delivery System and Scavenging System
- Open/closed system
- Occlusion/malfunction of hospital disposal system
- Maladjustment of hospital disposal system vacuum
- Leaks
    - High-pressure hoses or connectors
    - Nitrous oxide tank mounting
    - O rings
    - CO_2 absorbent canisters
    - Low-pressure circuit

Other Sources
- Cryosurgery units
- Cardiopulmonary bypass circuits

Modified from: Task Force on Trace Anesthetic Gases of the Committee on Occupational Health of Operating Room Personnel. *Waste Anesthetic Gases: Information for Management in Anesthetizing Areas and the Postanesthesia Care Unit (PACU)*. Park Ridge, IL: American Society of Anesthesiologists; 1999, with permission from the American Society of Anesthesiologists. A copy of the full text can be obtained from the ASA, 520 N. Northwest Highway, Park Ridge, IL 60068-2573.

Chemicals

Methyl methacrylate is commonly used in various surgical procedures. Known cardiovascular complications of methyl methacrylate in surgical patients include hypotension, bradycardia, and cardiac arrest. Reported risks from repeated occupational exposure to methyl methacrylate include skin irritation and burns, allergic reactions and asthma, eye irritation including possible corneal ulceration, headache, and neurologic signs. Airborne concentrations greater than 170 ppm have been associated with chronic lung, liver, and kidney damage. In one report, a HCW suffered significant lower limb neuropathy after repeated occupational exposure to methyl methacrylate.[29] Concentrations as high as 280 ppm have been measured when methyl methacrylate is prepared for use in the operating room. OSHA recommends use of scavenging devices in order to maintain an 8-hour TWA exposure to methyl methacrylate of 100 ppm.

Allergic Reactions

Allergic reactions to volatile anesthetic agents and to some muscle relaxants have been associated with contact dermatitis, hepatitis, and anaphylaxis in individual anesthesiologists.[30,31] Analyses of sera from pediatric anesthesiologists exposed to halothane demonstrated an increased prevalence of autoantibodies to cytochrome P450 2E1 and hepatic endoplasmic reticulum protein (ERp58).[32]

TABLE 3-2. TYPES OF REACTIONS TO LATEX GLOVES

Reaction	Signs/Symptoms	Cause	Management
Irritant contact dermatitis	Scaling, drying, cracking of skin	Direct skin irritation by gloves, powder, soaps	Identify reaction, avoid irritant, possible use of glove liner, use of alternative product
Type IV—delayed hypersensitivity	Itching, blistering, crusting (delayed 6–72 h)	Chemical additives used in manufacturing (such as accelerators)	Identify offending chemical, possible use of alternative product without chemical additive, possible use of glove liner
Type I—immediate hypersensitivity	—	Proteins found in latex	Identify reaction; avoid latex-containing products; use of nonlatex or powder-free, low-protein gloves by coworkers
A. Localized contact urticaria	Itching, hives in area of contact with latex (immediate)		Antihistamines, topical/systemic steroids
B. Generalized reaction	Runny nose, swollen eyes, generalized rash or hives, bronchospasm, anaphylaxis		Anaphylaxis protocol

Reproduced from: American Society of Anesthesiologists Task Force on Latex Sensitivity of the Committee on Occupational Health of Operating Room Personnel. *Natural Rubber Latex Allergy: Considerations for Anesthesiologists.* Park Ridge, IL: American Society of Anesthesiologist; 2005 (http://www.asahq.org/puhlicationsAndServices/latexallergy.pdf), with permission from the American Society of Anesthesiologists. A copy of the full text can be obtained from the ASA, 520 N. Northwest Highway, Park Ridge, IL 60068-2573.

Despite the presence of these autoantibodies, only 1 of 105 anesthesiologists had findings of any hepatic injury. These data suggest that although autoantibodies may occur in anesthesiologists frequently exposed to volatile anesthetics, they do not appear to commonly cause anesthetic-induced hepatitis.

Latex in surgical and examination gloves has become a common source of allergic reactions among operating room personnel. In many cases, HCWs who are allergic to latex experience their first adverse reactions while they are patients undergoing surgery. The prevalence of latex sensitivity among anesthesiologists is approximately 12%.[33]

The latex found in medical products is actually a composite of many substances including proteins, polyisoprenes, lipids, and phospholipids combined with preservatives, accelerators, antioxidants, vulcanizing compounds, and lubricating agents (such as cornstarch or talc). The protein content is responsible for most of the generalized allergic reactions to latex-containing surgical gloves. These reactions are exacerbated by the presence of powder that enhances the potential of latex particles to aerosolize and to spread to the respiratory system of personnel and to environmental surfaces during the donning or removal of gloves.

Irritant or contact dermatitis accounts for the majority of reactions resulting from wearing latex-containing gloves (Table 3-2). True allergic reactions present as T-cell–mediated contact dermatitis (type IV) or as an immunoglobulin E–mediated anaphylactic reaction.

Anesthesiologists who believe that they are allergic to latex must avoid all direct contact with latex-containing products. It is also important that coworkers wear non-latex or powderless, low latex-allergen gloves to limit the levels of ambient allergens.

Radiation

Anesthesia personnel are at risk of exposure from both direct and indirect sources of ionizing radiation. Direct sources of radiation include exposure from the primary x-ray beam and leakage from other sites within the x-ray equipment. Indirect exposure results from scattered radiation reflected off surfaces such as tables, other equipment, and patient.

The biologic consequences of radiation exposure vary depending on age, gender, and specific organ site of exposure. The deterministic effects of radiation cause cell death and organ injury and are cumulative in a dose-related fashion. Common examples of deterministic injuries include skin damage, infertility, and certain types of cataracts. Stochastic effects of radiation are those that result in DNA injury and the development of cancer. There is no known threshold below which the risk of developing cancer completely disappears. And there can be a long latency period before the clinical presentation of an induced neoplasm.

OSHA has published occupational limits for workers exposed to ionizing radiation.[34] The annual limit is 5 rem with an allowable long-term limit of $(N - 18) \times 5$ rem where N is the age in years. The recommended maximum occupational exposure to a declared pregnant worker should not exceed a monthly limit of 0.5 mrem or a total exposure of 5 mrem (excluding medical and natural background radiation).

Early studies found the exposure to radiation among anesthesia personnel to be safely below the OSHA limits.[35] However, more recent studies, conducted subsequent to the increased utilization of ionizing radiation in operating rooms, cardiac catheterization, and other interventional radiology suites, have revealed a worrisome trend toward increased exposure among anesthesia personnel (although still well below OSHA limits).[36–38] In one study, there was a doubling of the aggregate radiation exposure to members of a department of anesthesiology in the year following the introduction of an electrophysiology laboratory[38] (Fig. 3-1). Anesthesia personnel in this study increased their average exposure to almost 500 mrem on an annualized basis. Preventative strategies for anesthesiologists to minimize their risk of radiation-induced injury include limiting the intensity and exposure time, distancing oneself from the source of the radiation, and using maximal shielding from both primary and scattered sources of radiation.

A second form of radiation with potential health hazards comes in the form of chronic exposure to low-frequency electromagnetic

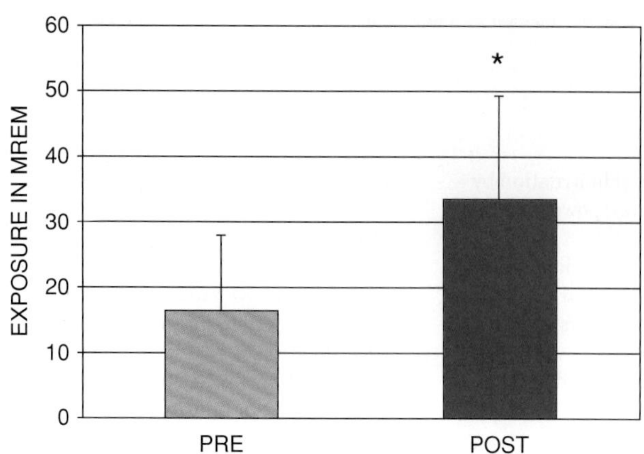

FIGURE 3-1. Radiation exposure in an electrophysiology lab. Aggregate radiation exposure to anesthesia personnel doubled after ("Post") as compared to before ("Pre") introduction of an electrophysiology service. *P=0.017, paired Student's t test.

TABLE 3-3. NOISE LEVELS IN A MODERN OPERATING ROOM FREQUENTLY EXCEED OSHA LIMITS

Operating Room	Noise
EPA recommendation	4.5 dB
Continuous suction	75–85 dB
Clang of instruments	75–85 dB
Surgical saw	80–105 dB
Music	75–105 dB
Average OR noise	77 dB
OSHA limit (8 h)	90 dB
Subway	100 dB
OSHA limit (0 h)	115 dB

fields such as those emitted by MRI equipment.[39] It is often necessary for the anesthesia care provider to remain in close proximity to the patient, and thus the magnet core, during MRI studies. Data are not yet available to determine the safety of long-term exposure to high-intensity magnetic fields. Therefore, until such time that safety thresholds have been determined for this type of exposure, anesthesiologists should obey the general admonition regarding all radiation exposure. That is, keep exposure as low as reasonably achievable.

Noise Pollution

Noise is quantified by determining both the intensity of the sound and the duration of the exposure. OSHA has determined that the maximum level for safe noise exposure is 90 dB for 8 hours.[40] Each increase in noise of 5 dB halves the permissible exposure time, so that 100 dB is acceptable for just 2 hours per day. The maximum allowable exposure in an industrial setting is 115 dB.

Noise levels in a modern operating room frequently exceed OSHA limits and are a potential health hazard. Ventilators, suction equipment, music, and conversation produce background noise at a level of 75 to 90 dB. Superimposed on these are sporadic noises caused by dropped equipment, surgical saws and drills, and alarms. Resultant noise levels can exceed 100 dB over 40% of the time with peak levels in excess of 120 dB, which is comparable to the clamor of a busy freeway or a rock and roll band[41] (Table 3-3).

Excessive levels of noise can adversely influence an anesthesiologist's capacity to perform common clinical tasks. Mental efficiency, short-term memory, and ability to multitask and perform complex psychomotor tasks are all diminished by exposure to excess noise.

Noise also interferes with the ability to hear alarms. This is especially apparent in the magnetic resonance imaging suite where noise from the scanner can mask many anesthesia alarms. Similarly, excessive noise can interfere with crucial verbal communication. Voice levels must be at least 20 dB above background noise to be heard and understood.

There are also chronic health ramifications of long-term exposure to excessive noise. Chronic exposure has been associated with elevated levels of endogenous catecholamines and heightened levels of stress, increased irritability, and elevated blood pressure.

Ultimately, exposure to excessive noise levels will result in hearing loss. Although no direct connection has been established with excess noise experienced in the operating room, it is interesting to note that more than 50% of anesthesiologists have a substantial hearing deficit and 7% have deficits that potentially interfere with their ability to hear operating room alarms.[42]

One form of background noise, music, can provide a number of beneficial effects. Music has proved advantageous as a supplement to sedation and analgesia for surgical patients.[43] Self-selected background music can contribute to reducing autonomic responses in surgeons and improving their performance.[44] The beneficial effects are less pronounced when a third party chooses the music. The selection of music, and the volume at which it is played, should be determined by mutual agreement of all parties present in the operating room.

Ergonomics/Human Factors

Human factor analysis, also called ergonomics, is the study of the interaction between humans and machines and the impact of equipment design on their use. It is a multidisciplinary science that applies diverse disciplines such as anthropometry, ethnography, biomechanics, industrial and social psychology, architecture, education, and information technology, toward developing user-friendly equipment and a safer workplace.

Human factor analysis has been most widely employed in industries such as aviation, nuclear power, and oil exploration where human error frequently has contributed significantly to catastrophic accidents. The work performed by an anesthesiologist shares many of the characteristics found in these industries, including the intricacy of the tasks, a narrow margin of error, and the vulnerability to human error.

A number of human factor difficulties exist in the anesthesiologist's workplace. For example, anesthesia equipment is often poorly designed or positioned. Anesthesia monitors are frequently placed so that the anesthesiologist's attention is directed away from the patient and surgical field. This was well demonstrated by observations that the insertion and monitoring of a transesophageal echocardiograph probe added significantly to the anesthesiologist's workload and diverted attention away from other patient-specific tasks.[45]

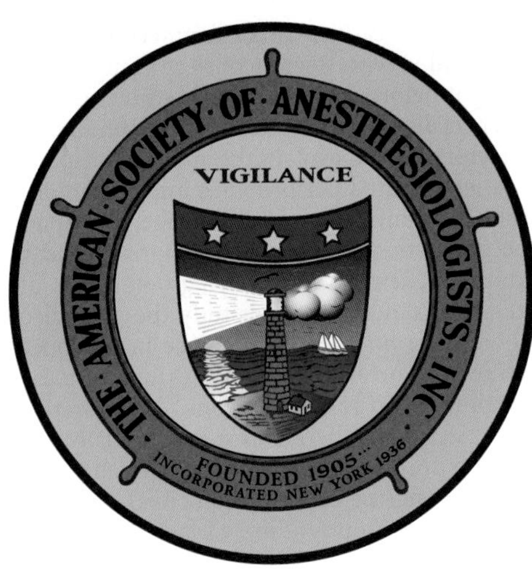

FIGURE 3-2. Official seal of the American Society of Anesthesiologists. The official seal of the ASA bears the inscription "Vigilance." Used with permission from the American Society of Anesthesiologists.

The ability to sustain complex monitoring tasks, such as maintaining vigilance,[a] and to respond to critical incidents are among those tasks that are most vulnerable to the distractions created by
2 poor equipment design or placement. The critical importance of the vigilance task to the practice of anesthesiology is evidenced by the fact that the seal of the ASA bears as its only motto "Vigilance"
2 (Fig. 3-2).

Vigilance tasks are generally performed at the level of 90% accuracy. In a setting where the stakes are high, such as during anesthesia and surgery, this leaves an unacceptable margin of
3 error. Human error, in part resulting from lapses in attention, accounts for a large proportion of the preventable deaths and serious injuries resulting from anesthetic mishaps in the United States annually.

A number of other work place factors conspire to interfere with anesthesiologists' ability to perform their complex tasks. Even seemingly trivial aspects of an anesthesiologist's work that require the expenditure of excessive energy produce a decrement in performance over the course of time. For example, if the anesthesiologist must make frequent rapid changes in observation from a dim, distant screen to a bright, nearby one, the continuous muscular activity required for pupil dilation and constriction and lens accommodation promotes fatigue and hinders performance.

The detrimental effects of unnecessary energy expenditure can be mental as well as physical. As a result of the ever-increasing number of monitors to be observed and amounts of data to be processed during the course of a surgical procedure, larger amounts of mental work must be expended. The cognitive burden varies directly with the difficulty encountered in extracting information from the monitors and displays that compete for the anesthesiologist's attention. Poor engineering of the monitor displays, so that mode of presentation, signal frequency, or strength is suboptimal, can adversely influence the operator's performance.

Even the alarms that have been developed with the specific goal of augmenting the task of vigilance can have considerable drawbacks. In general, alarms are nonspecific (the same alarm signaling as many as 12 different deviations from "normal") and can be a source of frustration and confusion. They are susceptible to many artifacts and false positives that can cause "alarm fatigue" and distract the observer from more clinically significant information. It is not unusual for distractive alarms to be ignored or inactivated.[46] A positive trend that is emerging in alarm technology is the development of "knowledge-based alarms" that can integrate information from more than one monitor and suggest a list of diagnostic and therapeutic possibilities.

4 Organizational issues, such as failed communication among team members, can adversely impact an anesthesiologist's performance. The potential for disaster as a result of poor communication has been well illustrated in a number of airline catastrophes. The possibility for miscommunication and resultant accident is heightened in the operating room where, in contrast to the structure inherent in an airline crew, there is absence of a well-defined hierarchical organization with overlaps in areas of expertise and responsibility. Poor communication can lead to conflict and compromised patient safety and has been identified as a root cause of many anesthesia-related sentinel events.

Effective conflict resolution is an important element of the teamwork necessary for successful surgical outcomes. Conflict and unpleasant interpersonal interactions among team members are among the most stressful aspects of the job of an anesthesiologist and can hinder safe anesthetic care. Some degree of conflict occurs during the management of as many as 78% of patients in high-intensity areas such as operating rooms or critical care units.[47]

Successful resolution of conflict is a skill that can be learned.[48] Mutual respect is required among team members along with a willingness to carefully listen and recognize differences of opinion. Intervention by a neutral third party is frequently helpful in finding an innovative solution. The airline industry has successfully implemented crew resource management programs to improve the performance of cockpit teams.[49]

"Production pressure" is an organizational concern that has the potential to create an environment in which issues of productivity supersede those of safety.[50] Production pressure has been associated with the commission of errors resulting from haste and/or deliberate deviations from known safe practices.

The application of simulation technology is gaining acceptance as a tool to study and teach human performance issues in anesthesiology. It appears to be particularly suited to training nontechnical skills such as resource management, teamwork, and communication.[51]

Work Hours, Night Call, and Fatigue

A circadian pattern of alertness and sleep is a fundamental element of healthy human physiology. Inadequate sleep caused by any number of factors, including obstructive sleep apnea or disruptive work schedules, can contribute to adverse health effects including cardiovascular disease and psychological illness such
3 as irritability, displaced anger, depression, and anxiety. Individuals who suffer from sleep deprivation also think and move more slowly and make more mistakes.

Sleep loss and fatigue can have deleterious effects upon work practices. In general, workers who are sleep deprived suffer a decrement in performance and are at greater risk of committing workplace errors. Fatigued individuals are more susceptible to "microsleeps" which are brief, uncontrolled, and spontaneous episodes of physiologic sleep that may last as little as a few seconds. Fatigued workers also incur more work-related accidents.[52] The susceptibility to accident is not limited to work hours and

[a]Vigilance is the ability to detect changes in a stimulus during prolonged monitoring tasks when the subject has no prior knowledge of whether or when any changes might occur.

extends to other activities of daily living, such as driving. The changes resulting from sleep deprivation bear a striking similarity to that seen with alcohol intoxication.[53] Significant individual variations in impairment due to fatigue have been identified.[54]

The contribution of sleep loss and fatigue to accidents has been well documented in many well-publicized industrial catastrophes. Sleep deprivation was a contributing factor to industrial accidents such as those that occurred at Chernobyl, Three Mile Island, Exxon-Valdez, and the Challenger space shuttle catastrophe.

A number of reports have also identified sleep deprivation as a causative factor in errors occurring in the health-care industry.[55] As early as 1971, Friedman et al. reported that interns made almost twice as many errors reading electrocardiograms after an extended work shift than after a night of sleep.[56] Intubation skills were reduced among emergency room physicians working night shifts when compared with other staff members working days.[57] Physicians in both groups were more likely to commit errors during a simulated triage test toward the end of their work shifts. And in a study that examined the management by medical interns of medical admissions, 35.9% more medical errors were committed while on a "traditional" schedule (24 hours plus work shifts) than when they worked a schedule that eliminated extended work shifts and reduced the number of hours worked per week.[58] Mistakes committed by these interns included 20.8% more medication errors and 5.6 times as many diagnostic errors.

Anesthesiologists who take night call commonly suffer from each of the three well-defined classes of sleep deprivation: Total, partial, and selective sleep deprivation. Interruption of sleep during call commonly occurs between the hours of 2 AM and 4 AM when humans are most vulnerable to fatigue-induced errors.

A number of specific consequences of sleep deprivation have the potential to adversely impact the conduct of a safe anesthetic, including impaired cognition, short-term memory and clinical decision making, prolonged reaction time, and reduced attention, vigilance, and performance. In a report by Howard et al.,[59] sleep-deprived residents managing a 4-hour simulated anesthetic demonstrated progressive impairment of alertness, mood, and performance and had longer response latency to vigilance probes.

Performance after sleep deprivation does not return to normal levels until 24 hours of rest and recovery has occurred after a period of sleep deprivation. Residents in their routine, non-post call state continue to suffer from chronic sleep deprivation and have the same degree of sleepiness as measured in residents finishing 24 hours of in-house call.[60]

An interesting phenomenon is the "end-spurt," in which previously deteriorated performance shows improvement when the subject expects that the task is nearly completed. However, if the procedure is unexpectedly prolonged, a "let-down" occurs with additional deterioration in performance.

Despite adequate evidence of performance impairment due to fatigue, the precise role of sleep deprivation on the specific end point of clinical outcomes remains unclear. A number of studies have reported a detrimental effect on patient outcomes of sleep deprivation among providers. In two studies of American anesthesia caregivers, more than 50% reported having committed an error in medical judgment that they attributed to fatigue.[50,61] And 58% of New Zealand anesthesiologists reported that they had exceeded their self-defined limit for safe continuous administration of anesthesia and 86% reported that they had committed a fatigue-related error.[62] Similar reports of fatigue-related complications appear in the surgical literature with as many as 16% of preventable adverse surgical events attributed to surgeon fatigue.[63,64] However, others have reported no evidence of suboptimal clinical management or poor outcomes from sleep-deprived clinicians. Chu et al. found no increase in mortality or major complications in 4,000 consecutive cardiac surgical procedures performed by surgeons who had varying degrees of sleep (ranging from 0 to >6 hours) the night before surgery.[65] Other studies of surgeons and critical care specialists have agreed with these findings.[66,67]

Several factors help to explain the apparent disparity between reports of fatigue-related performance impairment and the failure to conclusively link these with medical errors or adverse outcomes. The distinction between sleep deprived and well rested is often arbitrarily defined with varying definitions of the nonrested state. For example, in one study the general conclusion was that there were no overall difference in complication rates between surgeons who had operated during the previous night ("post-nighttime") and rested surgeons.[68] However, when sleep patterns were stratified, there was a substantially elevated rate of complication (6.2% vs. 3.4%) if the surgeon had less than 6 hours sleep during the on-call night. Also, there is great difficulty in eliminating confounding variables such as the impact of loss of continuity of care, errors that can occur during "handoffs" of critically ill patients, and the reallocation of many medical tasks from physicians to nonphysician providers. Finally, it can be difficult to extrapolate findings from simulation studies of volunteers in a laboratory to clinicians in real-life work conditions.

Medicine remains significantly behind other industries, most notably the transport and airline industries, in identifying and regulating work practices that permit excessively long shifts. It was not until the well-publicized Libby Zion case in 1984 (in which it was charged that fatal, avoidable mistakes were made by exhausted, unsupervised residents) that medical organizations and state legislatures took action to limit excessive work hours among residents. In 2000 the Accreditation Council for Graduate Medical Education (ACGME) established the first set of standards to limit resident duty hours. These standards were revised by the ACGME in 2011.[69] Policies established by the ACGME include the following:

1. Work hours must be limited to 80 hours per week, averaged over a 4-week period inclusive of all in-house call activities and all moonlighting.
2. Duty periods of PGY-1 residents must not exceed 16 hours in duration.
3. Duty hours of PGY-2 residents and above may be scheduled to a maximum of 24 hours of continuous duty in the hospital.
4. Strategic napping, especially after 16 hours of continuous duty and between the hours of 10:00 PM and 8:00 AM, is strongly suggested.
5. Residents *should* have 10 hours and *must* have 8 hours, free of duty between scheduled duty periods and at least 14 hours free of duty after 24 hours of in-house duty.

Somewhat ironically, at the end of a long list of duty hours restrictions, item VI.G.5.a-c states, "Residents in the final years of education (as defined by the Review Committee) must be prepared to enter the unsupervised practice of medicine and care for patients over irregular or extended periods." This statement recognizes that these restrictions on duty periods apply only to trainees and that work hours in medical practice remain unregulated.

Prolonged work hours and sleep deprivation are a ubiquitous component of many anesthesiologists' professional lives. Many academic faculty members now work longer hours than they did prior to house staff work hour limitations because of the shift of work from residents to faculty. Attending anesthesiologists and nurse anesthetists commonly work 10- to 12-hour workdays and 24-hour on-call shifts. Gravenstein et al. reported that the average anesthesiologist's work week was 56 hours and that 74% of the respondents had worked without a break for longer periods than they personally thought was safe.[61]

Several strategies have been devised to reduce fatigue and limit the adverse effects of sleep deprivation when long work periods are necessary. Recommendations include minimizing sleep debt by maximizing sleep before on-call shifts and utilizing maneuvers to overcome sleep inertia such as increasing ambient light levels and stretching, taking frequent breaks, and napping when possible. A number of pharmaceutical aids, such as caffeine and modafinil (a schedule IV drug), have been approved for military use and, if used under supervision and carefully monitored, arguably may be helpful for clinicians with shift-work sleep disorder.[70]

INFECTIOUS HAZARDS

Anesthesia personnel are at risk for acquiring infections from patients and from other personnel. This risk is likely to increase because as antimicrobial agents become more effective, the pathogens develop resistance and new survival strategies. In addition, increasingly immune-compromised patients become vectors for these resistant, opportunistic organisms. Furthermore, globalization brings with it increasing spread of organisms from less developed areas in the world, such as the 1999 outbreak in New York of West Nile Virus encephalitis and in 2003 of the epidemic of severe acute respiratory syndrome (SARS) in Hong Kong. Moreover, diseases that were once thought to be noninfectious, such as peptic ulcer disease (*Helicobacter pylori*), invasive cervical cancer (human papillomavirus), Kaposi's sarcoma (human herpesvirus type 8), and certain lymphomas (Epstein–Barr virus [EBV]) are now better understood as a long-term consequence of infection, making occupational health precautions even more important.

Viral infections are the most significant threat to HCWs. Most commonly, these are spread through the respiratory route. Other infections are spread by hand-to-hand transmission, and hand washing is the single most important protection strategy.[71] Immunity against some viral pathogens, such as hepatitis B, can be provided through vaccination.[72] Transmission of blood-borne pathogens such as hepatitis (HBV, HCV) and human immunodeficiency virus (HIV) can be prevented with mechanical barriers blocking portals of entry.[73] Current recommendations from the Centers for Disease Control and Prevention (CDC) for preemployment screening, infection control practices, vaccination, postexposure treatment, and work restrictions for infected personnel should be consulted for specific information related to each pathogen.[74–76]

OSHA Standards, Standard Precautions, and Transmission-Based Precautions

4 In the late 1980s the CDC formulated recommendations ("universal precautions") for preventing transmission of blood-borne infections to HCWs. The guidelines were based on the epidemiology of Hepatitis B Virus (HBV) as a worst-case model for transmission of blood-borne infections and available knowledge of the epidemiology of HIV and Hepatitis C Virus (HCV). Since asymptomatic carriers of many blood-borne viruses cannot be identified, universal precautions were recommended for use during all patient contact. Although exposure to blood carries the greatest risk of occupationally related transmission of pathogens, it was recognized that universal precautions should also be applied to semen, vaginal secretions, human tissues, and cerebrospinal, synovial, pleural, peritoneal, pericardial, and amniotic fluids. Subsequently, the CDC synthesized the major features of universal precautions into "standard precautions" that should be applied to all patients[77] (Table 3-4).

Standard precautions include the appropriate application and use of hand washing, personal protective equipment (PPE), and respiratory hygiene/cough etiquette. The selection of specific barriers or PPE should be commensurate with the task being performed. Gloves may be all that is necessary during many procedures that involve contact with mucous membranes or oral fluids, such as during routine endotracheal intubation or during insertion of a peripheral intravenous catheter. However, additional personal protection, such as gown, mask, and face shield, may be required during endotracheal intubation when the patient has hematemesis or during bronchoscopy or endotracheal suctioning. Respiratory hygiene/cough etiquette has been added to standard precautions to prevent droplet transmission of respiratory pathogens, especially during seasonal outbreaks.

OSHA has promulgated standards to protect employees from occupational exposure to blood-borne pathogens.[78] These standards require that there must be an exposure control plan specifically detailing the methods that the employer is providing to reduce employees' risk of exposure to blood-borne pathogens. Among other requirements, the employer must encourage strategies to reduce blood exposures, furnish appropriate PPE (e.g., gloves, gowns), offer the HBV vaccine at no charge to personnel, and provide an annual educational program to inform employees of their risk for blood-borne infection.

Implementation of standard precautions and OSHA regulations has been effective in decreasing the number of exposure incidents that result in HCW contact with patient blood and body fluids.

The institution's employee health service is required to obtain and record a contagious disease history from new employees and provide immunizations and annual purified protein derivative (PPD) skin testing. In addition, the employee health service must have protocols for dealing with workers exposed to contagious diseases and those percutaneously or mucosally exposed to the blood of patients infected with HIV or hepatitis B or C virus. Free consultation is available from the CDC Postexposure Prophylaxis Hotline (PEPline) at 1-888-HIV-4911. Protocols are also needed for dealing with caregivers who have common contagious diseases and for those who have less common but high-visibility public health problems.

Respiratory Viruses

Respiratory viruses account for half or more of all acute illnesses and are usually transmitted by one of two routes. First, small-particle aerosols from viruses such as influenza and measles are produced by coughing, sneezing, or talking and can be propelled over large distances. Second, large droplets that have been produced by coughing or sneezing can contaminate the donor's hands or an inanimate surface. The virus is then transferred to the oral, nasal, or conjunctival mucous membranes of a susceptible person by self-inoculation. Rhinovirus and human respiratory syncytial virus (HRSV) are spread by this process.

Influenza Viruses

Influenza viruses, members of the Orthomyxoviridae family, are designated as type A, B, or C based on characteristics of the nucleoprotein (NP) and matrix (M) protein antigens. Influenza A viruses are further subtyped on the basis of the surface hemagglutinin (H) and neuraminidase (N) antigens. Individual strains are designated according to the site of origin, isolate number, year of isolation, and subtype, for example, influenza A/California/07/2009 (the infamous H1N1). Influenza A has 16 H subtypes and 9 N subtypes, of which only H1, H2, H3, N1, and N2 have

TABLE 3-4. STANDARD PRECAUTIONS

Transmission-Based Precautions	
Modes of transmission	
Direct contact transmission	Transmission of an infectious agent directly from one person to another; may occur via contact of blood or secretions with mucous membranes, open cuts, or mites.
Indirect contact transmission	When an infectious agent is transmitted via an intermediate object (fomite) that has been previously contaminated. This may include (but is not limited to) patient-care devices, environmental surfaces, and clothing.
The particle size of emitted respiratory secretions is a continuum from aerosol size particles (≤5 μm) to droplets (>5 μm).	
Droplet transmission	(>5 μm) remain suspended for short periods of time and tend to be deposited within 3 feet of where they are generated. The distance that a droplet travels may be affected by such things as temperature, humidity, and air currents. Droplets are preferentially deposited in the upper airways, whereas aerosols penetrate deeper into the lower respiratory tract.
Airborne transmission	Organisms that can remain infectious when disseminated over distance and time as the droplet nuclei (<5 μm particles) are dispersed on air currents.
Standard precautions	Reduce the risk of transmission of infectious agents from patient to patient, patient to health-care worker (HCW), HCW to patient.
	Apply to all patients, as anyone may be infected or colonized with a transmissible disease.
	Wear gloves for all contact with blood, body fluids (except sweat), non-intact skin, and mucous membranes. Change gloves when they become soiled or when contact with a clean body part follows that with a contaminated part. Remove gloves after patient contact. Minimize environmental contamination.
	Perform hand hygiene before patient contact and upon removal of gloves. See section on hand hygiene.
	Gown, face, and eye protection should be worn if there is a risk of splash or spray.
	Environmental cleaning after contamination by body substances.
	Use a standard surgical mask when inserting a central line or performing neuraxial anesthesia.
	Needle and sharp safety—avoid recapping (when necessary, use one-handed technique), bending, or breaking used sharps. Dispose sharps in appropriate puncture-resistant container. See safe injection practices section.
	Practice and encourage respiratory hygiene/cough etiquette.
Contact precautions (in addition to standard precautions)	
	Private patient room or cohort patients. Spatial separation of 3 feet between patients recommended.
	Signage outside room to indicate level of precautions.
	Gown and glove upon entering room and with any patient or environmental contact.
	Face and eye protection if there is a risk of splash or spray.
	Remove gloves and gown before exiting room. Care must be used to avoid self-contamination when removing personal protective equipment (PPE).
	Perform hand hygiene after removal of PPE.
	Dedicated patient equipment whenever possible. Appropriately clean equipment prior to its use with other patients. See disinfection of equipment.
	Appropriate cleaning of room when vacated.
	Maintain contact precautions during transport and entire perioperative period.
	Communicate precaution level to those that will receive patient postoperatively.
Droplet precautions (in addition to standard precautions)	
	Single-patient room optimal. May cohort or keep patient with existing roommate when necessary.
	Spatial separation of patients 3 feet. If curtain present, keep drawn.
	Signage outside room to indicate level of precautions.
	HCWs should wear standard surgical mask, gloves, gown, and eye protection as required under standard precautions.
	Patient should wear standard mask (if tolerated) when transport outside room required.
	Respiratory hygiene/cough etiquette.
	Maintain precautions throughout perioperative period.
	Communicate precaution level to those that will receive patient postoperatively.

TABLE 3-4. STANDARD PRECAUTIONS (*continued*)

Transmission-Based Precautions	
Airborne precautions (in addition to standard precautions)	Place patient in an airborne isolation room (AIIR). See glossary. Signage outside room to indicate level of precautions. N95 respirator or greater protection should be used when in the same room as the patient. Patient should remain in AIIR with door closed at all times, except for medically necessary procedures. Elective procedures should be postponed until patient no longer requires respiratory isolation. Patients should wear a standard surgical mask when transported outside the AIIR. The purpose of the mask is to prevent respiratory droplets from being expelled into the environment where they can become droplet nuclei. Operating rooms (ORs) are designed to be positive pressure in relation to the environment. Therefore, it is important to choose the most appropriate OR to minimize the risk of contaminating the OR suite. Options include the OR that is most remote from others, one with an antechamber, install a portable negative pressure isolation chamber at the OR door. The surgical procedure should be scheduled at a time when it will minimize exposure of other patients and medical staff to the airborne infectious disease. Postanesthesia recovery must take place with the same level of respiratory precautions. Communicate precaution level to receiving personnel. Room should remain vacant after the patient leaves until adequate time has elapsed to result in a 99.9% air turnover (duration dependent on number of air exchanges per hour in room). http://www.cdc.gov/mmwr/preview/mmwrhtml/rr5417a1.htm?s_cid=rr5417a1_e

From Task Force on Infection Control of the Committee on Occupational Health of Operating Room Personnel. *Recommendations for Infection Control for the Practice of Anesthesiology,* 3rd ed. Park Ridge, IL: American Society of Anesthesiologists; 2011.

been associated with epidemics of disease in humans. Because influenza viruses are easily transmitted and are highly infectious, large outbreaks occur annually. Acutely ill patients shed virus for as long as 5 days after the onset of symptoms via small-particle aerosols. Because of their contact with nasopharyngeal secretions, anesthesiologists can easily become vectors in the spread of influenza virus in hospitals.

Anesthesia personnel who routinely care for patients in high-risk groups should be immunized annually (October or November) with the inactivated (killed virus) influenza virus vaccine.[76] There is evolving precedent to make this a condition of employment and medical staff credentialing.[79] Available inactivated vaccines have been highly purified and are associated with few reactions. Since the vaccine used in the United States and many other countries is produced in eggs, individuals with true hypersensitivity to egg products either should be desensitized or should not be vaccinated. A live attenuated influenza vaccine, approved for use in healthy nonpregnant persons 2 to 49 years of age and administered by intranasal spray, is now available.

Influenza Pandemics

Influenza outbreaks occur almost every year, although their extent and severity vary widely. In the past century, there have been three influenza pandemics (1918, 1957, and 1968) with the "Great Influenza" in 1918 killing between 40 and 50 million people worldwide. The most recent pandemic emerged in March 2009 and was caused by an influenza A/H1N1 virus that rapidly spread worldwide over several months. The large number of infected patients strained local and global resources, such as a large requirement for respirators for personnel and ventilators for patients. Containment to prevent spread requires early identification and isolation of infected individuals to limit disease transmission. For patients requiring hospitalization, specific wards should be established with dedicated staff. NIOSH-certified respirators (N95 or higher) should be used by personnel during activities or procedures likely to generate infectious respiratory aerosols.

Avian Influenza A

In 1997, human cases of influenza caused by avian influenza viruses (A/H5N1) were detected in Hong Kong during an extensive outbreak of influenza in poultry. Between that time and February 2010, 478 cases of avian influenza in humans were reported in Asia and the Middle East. Nearly all of these cases were associated with contact with infected poultry. Efficient person-to-person transmission was not observed. Mortality rates have been high (60%). Because of the absence of widespread immunity to the H5, H7, and H9 viruses, concern persists that avian-to-human transmission might also contribute to the emergence of a pandemic strain.[80] A vaccine for prophylaxis against avian influenza H5N1 was approved for use in the United States in 2007.

Human Respiratory Syncytial Virus

HRSV is the most common cause of serious bronchiolitis and lower respiratory tract disease in infants and young children worldwide. During periods when HRSV is prevalent in the community (usually late November through May in the United States), many hospitalized infants and children may carry the virus. Large amounts of virus are present in respiratory secretions of infected children, and although viable virus can be recovered for up to 6 hours on contaminated environmental surfaces, it is readily inactivated with soap and water and disinfectants. Infection of susceptible people occurs by self-inoculation when HRSV in secretions is transferred to the hands, which then contact the mucous membranes of the eyes or nose.[81] Although most children have been exposed to HRSV early in life, immunity is not permanent and reinfection is common.

HRSV may also be a significant cause of illness in healthy elderly patients and those with chronic cardiac or pulmonary disease.[82] HRSV is shed for approximately 7 days after infection. Hospitalized patients with the virus should be isolated, but during seasonal outbreaks large numbers of patients may make isolation impractical.[77] Careful hand washing and the use of standard precautions have been shown to reduce HRSV infection in hospital personnel.

Severe Acute Respiratory Syndrome (SARS)

SARS is a respiratory tract infection produced by SARS-associated coronavirus (SARS-CoV). SARS typically presents with a fever greater than 38.0°C followed by symptoms of headache, generalized aches, and cough. Severe pneumonia may lead to acute respiratory distress syndrome and death. The mechanisms of transmission of SARS are incompletely understood. Spread may occur by both large and small aerosols and perhaps by the fecal–oral route, as well as close person-to-person contact. Some ill individuals ("super-spreaders") appear to be hyperinfectious and are capable of transmitting infection to as many as 40 contacts.[83] The virus can also be spread when an individual touches a contaminated object and then inoculates the mouth, nose, or eyes. Aerosolization of respiratory secretions during coughing or endotracheal suctioning has been associated with transmission of the disease to HCWs, including anesthesiologists and critical care nurses.

After the first cases were reported from Asia in late 2002, the disease quickly spread globally in 2003 before being controlled. In most cases the infection was transmitted from human to human. The overall case fatality rate was 9.5%. Cases appeared to be somewhat milder in the United States with less severity among children. Since then, global surveillance for SARS-CoV has detected no confirmed cases.

Enteric Infections

Diarrheal disease is second only to lower respiratory infection as the most common infectious cause of death worldwide. Infectious agents include viruses, bacteria, and parasites, acting via noninflammatory (enterotoxin), inflammatory (cytotoxin), or penetrating mechanisms. Traveler's diarrhea is the most common travel-related infectious illness (20% to 50%), with *Escherichia coli* the most common organism. Rotavirus is most common among children less than 2 years of age, especially children in day care. Rotavirus can spread rapidly in day care centers and pediatric wards. *Giardia lamblia* is more common in older children, as is norovirus, and there is a high rate of secondary cases among family members.

Clostridium difficile is the main cause of nosocomial diarrhea among adult inpatients in the United States. One-third of elderly patients in nursing homes develop a significant diarrheal illness each year, and more than half of these are caused by *C. difficile*, especially following antibiotic therapy. Personal hygiene on the part of clinicians is directed to limiting secondary fecal–oral spread.

DNA Viruses

Herpes simplex viruses (HSV-1, HSV-2; *Herpesvirus hominis*) produce a variety of infections involving mucocutaneous surfaces, central nervous system (CNS), and sometimes visceral organs. Exposure to HSV at mucosal surfaces or abraded skin allows entry of the virus and initiation of viral replication. The primary infection with HSV type 1 is usually clinically unapparent but may involve severe oral lesions, fever, and adenopathy. After the primary infection subsides, the latent virus persists within the sensory nerve ganglion, awaiting reactivation. Gingivostomatitis and pharyngitis are the most common clinical manifestations of first-episode HSV-1 infection, while recurrent herpes labialis is the most common clinical manifestation of reactivation HSV-2. Herpetic whitlow—HSV infection of the finger—may occur as a complication of primary oral or genital herpes by inoculation of virus through a break in the epidermal surface or by direct introduction of virus into the hand, a particularly important point for HCWs. Additional organ systems affected include HSV infection of the eye, which is the most common cause of corneal blindness in the United States. Of all HSV-infected populations, infants younger than 6 weeks have the highest frequency of visceral and/or CNS infection. Without therapy, the overall rate of death from neonatal herpes is 65% in the United States. Of note especially for obstetrical anesthesia practice, antibody to HSV-2 has been detected in 32% of pregnant women with no history of genital herpes. Asymptomatic HSV shedding was detected in 0.43% of women in late pregnancy and during delivery, and a first episode of clinical genital herpes was recognized by 16% of women during their pregnancy.[84] HCWs may be inoculated by direct contact with body fluids laden with either HSV type 1 or 2.

Varicella-zoster virus (VZV) causes two distinct clinical diseases: Varicella (chickenpox) and zoster (shingles). Chickenpox, ubiquitous and extremely contagious, is usually a benign illness of childhood with transmission by the respiratory route. With reactivation of latent VZV, most common after the sixth decade of life, herpes zoster presents as a dermatomal vesicular rash, usually associated with severe pain. Infection during pregnancy may result in fetal death or (rarely) congenital defects. Patients and medical personnel with active VZV infection can transmit the virus to others. Anesthesiologists working in pain clinics may be exposed to VZV when caring for patients who have discomfort from herpes zoster.

Communicability begins 1 to 2 days before the onset of the rash and ends when all the lesions are crusted, usually 4 to 6 days after the rash appears.[85] Respiratory isolation should be used for patients with chickenpox or disseminated herpes zoster.[77] Use of gloves to avoid contact with vesicular fluid is adequate to prevent VZV spread from patients with localized herpes zoster.

Most adults in the United States have protective antibodies to VZV. Since there have been many reports of nosocomial transmission of VZV, it is recommended that all HCWs have immunity to the virus. Anesthesia personnel should be questioned about prior VZV infection, and those with a negative or unknown history of infection should be serologically tested.[85] All employees with negative titers should be restricted from caring for patients with active VZV infection and should be offered immunization with two doses of the live, attenuated varicella vaccine.

Susceptible personnel with a significant exposure to an individual with VZV infection are potentially infective from 10 to 21 days after exposure and should not contact patients during this period. They should be offered vaccination within 3 to 5 days of the exposure since it might modify the severity as well as the duration of the disease. Varicella-zoster immune globulin can also be considered but it is most effective when administered within 96 hours after exposure.[85] Personnel without VZV immunity should be reassigned to alternative locations so that they do not care for patients who have active VZV infections.

EBV, also a member of the family Herpesviridae, is the cause of heterophile-positive infectious mononucleosis, characterized by fever, sore throat, lymphadenopathy, and atypical lymphocytosis. About 15% of cases of Burkitt's lymphoma in the United States and 90% of those in Africa are associated with EBV. Anaplastic nasopharyngeal carcinoma is common in southern China and is uniformly associated with EBV. EBV has also been associated with Hodgkin's disease, especially the mixed-cellularity type.

EBV is spread by contact with oral secretions. The virus is frequently transmitted from asymptomatic adults to infants and among young adults by transfer of saliva during kissing. Transmission by less intimate contact is rare. EBV has been transmitted by blood transfusion and bone marrow transplantation. More than 90% of asymptomatic seropositive individuals shed the virus in oropharyngeal secretions. While B cells may become infected after contact with epithelial cells, studies suggest that lymphocytes in the tonsillar crypts can be infected directly.

Cytomegalovirus (CMV) infects between 50% and 85% of individuals in the United States before age 40, with most infections producing minimal symptoms. After the primary infection, the virus remains dormant, and recurrent disease only occurs with compromise of the individual's immune system. CMV is not readily spread by casual contact but rather by repeated or prolonged intimate exposure. It is unlikely that aerosols or small droplets play a role in CMV transmission.

Primary or recurrent CMV infection during pregnancy results in fetal infection in up to 2.5% of occurrences. Congenital CMV syndrome may be found in up to 10% of infected infants. Thus, although CMV infection usually does not result in morbidity in healthy adults, it may have significant sequelae in pregnant women, and therefore becomes an occupational health concern.

The two major populations with CMV infection in the hospital include infected infants and immunocompromised patients. Routine infection control procedures (standard precautions) are sufficient to prevent CMV infection in health-care personnel (Tables 3-4 and 3-5).[75] Pregnant personnel should be made aware of the risks associated with CMV infection during pregnancy and of appropriate infection control precautions to be used when caring for high-risk patients. There is no evidence to indicate that it is necessary to reassign pregnant women from patient-care areas in which they may have contact with CMV-positive patients.

Rubella

Outbreaks of rubella, or German measles, in hospital personnel have resulted in significant loss of employee working time, employee morbidity, and cost to the hospital. Although most adults in the United States are immune to rubella, up to 20% of women of childbearing age are still susceptible, allowing the potential for viral replication in the placenta and infection of fetal organs (congenital rubella syndrome [CRS]). The infection is persistent throughout fetal development and for up to 1 year after birth. Therefore, only individuals immune to rubella should have contact with infants who have CRS or who are congenitally infected with rubella virus but are not showing signs of CRS.

Rubella is transmitted by contact with nasopharyngeal droplets spread by infected individuals coughing or sneezing. Patients are most contagious while the rash is erupting but can transmit the virus from 1 week before to 5 to 7 days after the onset of the rash. Droplet precautions should be used to prevent transmission (Table 3-5).[77]

History is a poor indicator of immunity. Therefore, ensuring immunity at the time of employment (evidence of prior vaccination with live rubella vaccine or serologic confirmation) should prevent nosocomial transmission of rubella to personnel. A live, attenuated rubella virus vaccine (measles, mumps, rubella [MMR]) is available to produce immunity in susceptible personnel.[86,87] Many state or local health departments mandate rubella immunity for all HCWs, and local regulations should be consulted.

TABLE 3-5. PREVENTION OF OCCUPATIONALLY ACQUIRED INFECTIONS

Infection/Condition	Precautions	Comments
Abscess		
Draining/major	Contact	
Draining/minor	Standard	
Acquired immune deficiency virus (HIV)	Standard	Postexposure prophylaxis (PEP) for some exposures
Avian influenza	Droplet	Enhanced precautions (i.e., airborne may be recommended)
Bronchiolitis	Contact	
Clostridium		
Botulinum	Standard	Not transmitted person to person
Difficile	Contact	
Perfringens	Standard	Not transmitted person to person
Conjunctivitis		
Bacterial	Standard	
Viral	Contact	Most commonly: adenovirus, enterovirus, coxsackievirus A24
Creutzfeldt–Jakob disease	Standard	Single-use equipment preferred, special cleaning (NaOH, heat, and time requirements) for contaminated instruments and environment
Diphtheria pharyngeal	Droplet	Until two cultures >24 h apart are negative
Escherichia coli	Standard	Contact precautions if patient incontinent
Haemophilus influenza		
Seasonal	Droplet	Single-patient room or cohort, gown, and glove
Pandemic	Droplet	Enhanced precautions (airborne may be recommended)

(*continued*)

TABLE 3-5. PREVENTION OF OCCUPATIONALLY ACQUIRED INFECTIONS (*continued*)

Infection/Condition	Precautions	Comments
Hepatitis, viral		
A	Standard	Contact precautions for incontinent patients
B	Standard	
C	Standard	
E	Standard	Contact precautions for incontinent patients
Herpes, zoster (varicella-zoster)		
Disseminated	Airborne, contact	Health-care workers (HCW) without immunity should not care for patient if immune HCW available
Localized	Standard	
Impetigo	Contact	
Legionnaires' disease	Standard	Not transmitted person to person
Lice		
Head	Contact	
Body	Standard	
Pubic	Standard	
Lyme disease	Standard	
Malaria	Standard	
Measles	Airborne	Susceptible HCW should not care for patient if immune HCW available. Maintain precautions for 4 days after onset of rash. Nonimmune exposed individuals may be infectious from days 5 to 21 after exposure. PEP available (vaccine, immune globulin)
Meningitis		
Bacterial	Standard	
Fungal	Standard	
Neisseria	Droplet	
Streptococcus	Standard	PEP available
Multidrug-resistant organisms (MDROs: MRSA, VRE, VISA/VRSA, ESBLs, resistant *Streptococcus pneumoniae*)	Standard/contact	
Mumps	Droplet	Susceptible HCWs should not care for patient if immune HCW available
Mycoplasma	Droplet	
Mycobacterium tuberculosis	Airborne	
Parainfluenza	Contact	
Pertussis	Droplet	Single-patient room or cohort. PEP available. Tdap recommended
Poliomyelitis	Contact	
Rabies	Standard	
Respiratory syncytial virus	Contact	Standard mask should be worn
Rhinovirus	Droplet	
Rubella	Droplet	Susceptible HCW should not care for patient if immune HCW available. Vaccine available. Nonimmune exposed individuals may be contagious from days 5 to 21 after exposure
Salmonella	Standard	Contact precautions for incontinent patients
SARS-CoV	Airborne, droplet, contact	Maintain precautions until 10 days after resolution of fever
Shigella	Standard	Contact precautions for incontinent patients
Smallpox	Airborne, contact	Maintain precautions until all scabs have crusted and separated (3–4 weeks). Non-vaccinated HCW should not care for patient if immune HCW available
Staphylococcal		
Major, wound	Contact	
Streptococcal		
Major, wound	Contact, droplet	

MRSA, methicillin-resistant *Staphylococcus aureus;* VRE, vancomycin-resistant enterococci; VISA/VRSA, vancomycin-intermediate/resistant *Staphylococcus aureus;* ESBL, extended-spectrum beta-lactamase–producing organisms; SARS-CoV, severe acute respiratory syndrome-associated corona virus.
Adapted from CDC Guideline for Isolation Precautions: Preventing Transmission of Infectious Agents in Healthcare Settings, 2007.
For a complete list of organisms, see Appendix A. Type and duration of precautions recommended for selected infections and conditions. http://www.cdc.gov/ncidod/dhqp/pdf/guidelines/Isolation2007.pdf

Measles (Rubeola)

Measles virus is highly transmissible by large droplets and by the airborne route. The virus is found in the mucus of the nose and pharynx of the infected individual and is spread by coughing and sneezing. The disease can be transmitted from 4 days prior to the onset of the rash to 4 days after its onset. Airborne precautions should be used for infected patients (Table 3-5).[75,77] Secondary attack rates in susceptible household and institutional contacts generally exceed 90%. Introduction of the measles vaccine in the United States has successfully eliminated endemic cases of measles but importation of measles from other countries continues to occur.

Medical settings are well-recognized sites of measles virus transmission. Children may present to health-care facilities during the prodrome, when the diagnosis is not obvious although the child is infectious and is likely to infect susceptible contacts. Personnel are at increased risk for acquiring measles and transmitting the virus to susceptible coworkers and patients. The CDC recommends that medical personnel have adequate immunity to measles, as documented by one of the following: Evidence of two doses of live measles vaccine, a record of physician-diagnosed measles, or serologic evidence of measles immunity (Table 3-5).[86] Susceptible personnel born in or after 1957 should receive two doses of the live measles vaccine at the time of employment.

Viral Hepatitis

Many viruses produce hepatitis. The most common are type A (infectious hepatitis), type B (HBV, serum hepatitis), and type C (HCV and non-A, non-B hepatitis [NANBH]), which is responsible for most cases of parenterally transmitted hepatitis in the United States. Delta hepatitis (HDV), caused by an incomplete virus, occurs only in people infected with HBV. HEV, previously labeled *epidemic* or *enterically transmitted NANBH,* is an enterically transmitted virus that occurs primarily in India, Asia, Africa, and Central America. In these locations, HEV is the most common cause of acute hepatitis. All types of viral hepatitis produce clinically similar illnesses. These range from asymptomatic and inapparent to fulminant and fatal infections, as well as subclinical to chronic persistent liver disease with cirrhosis and hepatocellular carcinoma, common to the blood-borne types (HBV, HCV, and HDV). The greatest risks of occupational transmission to anesthesia personnel are associated with HBV and HCV (Table 3-6).

Hepatitis A virus is the cause of about 20% to 40% of viral hepatitis in adults in the United States. Hepatitis A is usually a self-limited illness, and no chronic carrier state exists. Spread is predominantly by the fecal–oral route, either by person-to-person contact or by ingestion of contaminated food or water. Outbreaks are usually found in institutions or other closed groups where there has been a breakdown in normal sanitary conditions. Inactivation of viral activity can be achieved by boiling water for 1 minute, by contact with formaldehyde and chlorine, or by ultraviolet irradiation. Hospital personnel do not appear to be at increased risk for hepatitis A and nosocomial transmission is rare. Personnel exposed to patients with hepatitis A should receive immune globulin intramuscularly as soon as possible but not more than 2 weeks after the exposure to reduce the likelihood of infection.[88] Immune globulin provides protection against hepatitis A through passive transfer of antibodies and is used for postexposure prophylaxis. Hepatitis A vaccine is not routinely recommended for health-care personnel except for those who may be working in countries where hepatitis A is endemic.[86,88]

Hepatitis B virus is a significant occupational hazard for nonimmune anesthesiologists and other medical personnel who have frequent contact with blood and blood products. The prevalence of hepatitis B in the United States during 1999 to 2006 (anti-HBc = 4.7% and hepatitis B surface antigen [HBsAg] = 0.27%) was not statistically different from what it was during 1988 to 1994 (5.4% and 0.38%, respectively). The prevalence of anti-HBc decreased among persons 6 to 19 years of age (from 1.9% to 0.6%; $P < 0.01$) and 20 to 49 years of age (from 5.9% to 4.6%; $P < 0.01$) but not among persons 50 years of age (7.2% vs. 7.7%).[89] The incidence of acute hepatitis B in the United States declined as much as 80% between 1987 and 2004, attributable to effective vaccination programs as well as universal precautions in needle use and in health care in general. Before the widespread administration of hepatitis B vaccine the prevalence of hepatitis B serologic markers in anesthesia personnel ranged from 19% to 49% and reflected the prevalence of HBV carriers in the referral population for the area.

TABLE 3-6. RISK OF OCCUPATIONAL INFECTION WITH BLOOD-BORNE PATHOGENS

1. The greatest risk of transmission of blood-borne infections with HIV, HBV, and HCV is from a blood-contaminated percutaneous injury.
2. The risk depends on the type of pathogen involved and increases when the source patient has higher viral titers (for HIV, HBV, HCV, respectively: Acute or terminal HIV illness; hepatitis B e antigen–positive source; increased HCV RNA titers) and with increased quantity of inoculum volume transferred from the patient source.

Average risk after an accidental parenteral exposure (needlestick or cut):		
Known HIV-infected patient	0.3%[a]	
	Clinical hepatitis risk	Seroconversion risk
Known hepatitis B surface antigen (HBsAg) positive/hepatitis B e antigen (HBeAg) negative	1–6%	23–37%
Known hepatitis B surface antigen (HBsAg) positive/hepatitis B e antigen (HBeAg) positive	22–31%	37–62%
Known hepatitis C positive		0.3–0.74%[b]

[a]Exceeds 0.3% for an exposure involving a greater infectious dose resulting from transfer of a larger blood volume, a higher HIV titer in the source patient's blood, or both. (Updated U.S. Public Health Service Guidelines for the Management of Occupational Exposures to HBV, HCV, and HIV and Recommendations for Postexposure Prophylaxis.)

[b]Jagger J, et al. Occupational transmission of hepatitis C virus. *JAMA.* 2002;288:1469.

Acute HBV infection may be asymptomatic and usually resolves without significant hepatic damage. Less than 1% of acutely infected patients develop fulminant hepatitis. Approximately 10% become chronic carriers of HBV (serologic evidence for >6 months). Within 2 years, half of the chronic carriers resolve their infection without significant hepatic impairment. Chronic active hepatitis, which may progress to cirrhosis and is linked to hepatocellular carcinoma, is found most commonly in individuals with chronic viral infection for >2 years.

The diagnosis and staging of HBV infection is made on the basis of serologic testing. The first marker detectable in serum within 1 to 12 weeks (usually between 8 and 12 weeks) is HBsAg. Circulating HBsAg precedes elevations of serum aminotransferase activity and clinical symptoms by 2 to 6 weeks and remains detectable during the entire icteric or symptomatic phase of acute hepatitis B and beyond. HBsAg becomes undetectable 1 to 2 months after the onset of jaundice and rarely persists beyond 6 months. After HBsAg disappears, antibody to HBsAg (anti-HBs) becomes detectable in serum and remains detectable indefinitely. Antibody to the surface antigen (anti-HBs) appears with resolution of the acute infection and confers lasting immunity against subsequent HBV infections. Chronic HBV carriers are likely to have HBsAg and antibody to the core antigen (anti-HBc) present in serum samples. The presence of hepatitis B e antigen (HBeAg) in serum is indicative of active viral replication in hepatocytes.

Anesthesia personnel are at risk for occupationally acquired HBV infection as a result of accidental percutaneous or mucosal contact with blood or body fluids from infected patients. Patient groups with a high prevalence of HBV include immigrants from endemic areas, users of illicit parenteral drugs, homosexual men, and patients on hemodialysis.[74] Carriers are frequently not identified during hospitalization because the clinical history and routine preoperative laboratory tests may be insufficient for diagnosis. The risk for infection after an HBV-contaminated percutaneous exposure, such as an accidental needlestick, is 37% to 62% if the source patient is HBeAg-positive and 23% to 37% if HBeAg-negative (Table 3-6). HBV can be found in saliva, but the rate of transmission is significantly less after mucosal contact with infected oral secretions than after percutaneous exposures to blood. HBV is a hardy virus that may be infectious for at least 1 week in dried blood on environmental surfaces.

Hepatitis B is now a preventable and treatable disease. The implementation of routine vaccination has dramatically reduced the incidence of new cases in the US population. In addition to vaccination, the use of standard precautions, safety devices, and postexposure prophylaxis have significantly reduced the risk of occupationally acquired HBV infection and its sequelae in health-care personnel.

Hepatitis B vaccine is the primary strategy to prevent occupational transmission of HBV to anesthesia personnel and other
5 health personnel at increased risk. Administration of three doses of vaccine into the deltoid muscle results in the production of protective antibodies (anti-HBs) in >90% of healthy personnel. Hospitals or anesthesia departments should have policies for educating, screening, and counseling personnel about their risk of acquiring HBV infection and should make vaccination available for susceptible personnel.

To ensure adequate postvaccination immunity, serologic testing for anti-HBs should take place within 1 to 2 months after the third dose of vaccine.[74] Protective antibodies develop in 30% to 50% of nonresponders (i.e., anti-HBs <10 mIU/mL) with a second three-dose vaccine series. Nonresponders to vaccination remain at risk for HBV infection and should be counseled on strategies to prevent infections and the need for postexposure prophylaxis.

Vaccine-induced antibodies decline over time, with maximum titers after vaccination correlating directly with duration of antibody persistence. The CDC states that for vaccinated adults with normal immune status, routine booster doses are not necessary and periodic monitoring of antibody concentration is not recommended.[74]

Hepatitis C virus causes most cases of parenterally transmitted NANBH and is a leading cause of chronic liver disease in the United States. Although antibody to HCV (anti-HCV) can be detected in most patients with hepatitis C, its presence does not correlate with resolution of the acute infection or progression of hepatitis, and it does not confer immunity against HCV infection.[90] Seropositivity for HCV RNA is a marker of chronic infection and continued viral presence (Table 3-6). After HCV seroconversion, only 15% to 25% will clear the virus spontaneously. Of those that develop chronic hepatitis, 20% will develop cirrhosis over the following 20 to 30 years and 1% to 2% of those will be diagnosed with hepatocellular carcinoma.[91] Six major genotypes of HCV have been identified with the specific genotype being predictive for the response to and the needed duration of antiviral therapy. Combination therapy with interferon alpha (standard or pegylated) and ribavirin has been effective in the treatment of some cases of acute and chronic hepatitis C.[92]

Like HBV, HCV is transmitted through blood, but the rate of occupational HCV infection is less than for HBV. Although HCV transmission has been documented in health-care settings, the prevalence of anti-HCV in HCW in the United States is not greater than that found in the general population (1.6%). The greatest risk of occupational HCV transmission is associated with exposure to blood from an HCV-positive source. HCV has been transmitted through blood splashes to the eye and with exposure via non-intact skin. HCV in dried blood on environmental surfaces may remain infectious for up to 16 hours, but environmental contamination does not appear to be a common route of transmission. HCV can be found in the saliva of infected individuals, but it is not believed to represent a great risk for occupational transmission.[74]

There is no vaccine or effective postexposure prophylaxis available to prevent HCV infection, and the use of immune globulin is no longer recommended after a known exposure.[74] Prevention of exposure remains the primary strategy for protection against HCV infection. Personnel who have had a percutaneous or mucosal exposure to HCV-positive blood should have serologic testing for anti-HCV and alanine aminotransferase and counseling at the time of the exposure and at 6 months. Absence of detectable HCV RNA 6 months after completion of treatment with combined interferon and ribavirin for 48 months shows some promise for the treatment of seroconversion.[74]

Pathogenic Human Retroviruses

The family Retroviridae includes seven subfamilies, two of which produce disease in humans—human T lymphotropic viruses (HTLV)-I and HTLV-II, which are transforming retroviruses, and the HIV-1 and HIV-2, which cause cytopathic effects either directly or indirectly. Tissue destruction may result directly from the viral infection or indirectly from malignant transformation of infected cells and an immune-deficient state in response to the virus, leading to neoplastic and infectious disease. HTLV-I infection is transmitted in at least three ways: From mother to child, especially via breast milk; through sexual activity; and through the blood via contaminated transfusions or contaminated needles. HIV infection/AIDS is a global pandemic, with cases reported from virtually every country. At the end of 2010, an estimated

33.3 million individuals were living with HIV infection according to the Joint United Nations Programme on HIV/AIDS (UNAIDS).[93] The global prevalence has increased approximately fourfold since 1990, reflecting the combined effects of continued high rates of new HIV infections and the beneficial (life-prolonging) impact of antiretroviral therapy. In 2009, there were an estimated 2.6 million new cases of HIV infection worldwide, including 370,000 in children <15 years. As of January 1, 2010, an estimated 1,108,611 cases of AIDS had been diagnosed in the United States. Approximately 1.1 million individuals in the United States were living with HIV infection, 21% of whom are unaware of their infection.

The initial infection with HIV begins as a mononucleosis-like syndrome with lymphadenopathy and rash. Although the patient then enters an asymptomatic period, monocyte-macrophage cells serve as a viral reservoir and CD4+ T cells harbor the virus in the blood. Within a few weeks, an antibody may be detected by an enzyme immunoassay or rapid HIV antibody test, but a positive result must be confirmed using Western blot or immunofluorescent assay. After a variable length period of asymptomatic HIV infection, there is an increase in viral titer and impaired host immunity, resulting in opportunistic infections and malignancies characteristic of AIDS.

HIV is spread by sexual contact (especially homosexual males), perinatally from infected mother to neonate, and through infected blood (transfusion or shared needles) and blood products. Transfusions of whole blood, packed red blood cells, platelets, leukocytes, and plasma are all capable of transmitting HIV infection. The risk of infection with HIV in the United States via transfused screened blood currently is approximately 1:1.5 million units. Although the virus can be found in saliva, tears, and urine, these body fluids have a low risk for viral transmission.

Risk of Occupational HIV Infection

There is a small but definite occupational risk of HIV transmission to HCWs, laboratory personnel, and others who work with HIV-containing materials. An estimated 600,000 to 800,000 HCWs are stuck with needles or other sharp medical instruments in the United States each year. Exposures that place personnel at potential risk of HIV infection are percutaneous injuries (a needlestick or cut with a sharp object) or contact of mucous membrane or non-intact skin with blood, tissue, or other potentially infectious body fluids. The risk of HIV transmission following skin puncture from a contaminated needle or a sharp object is 0.3% and after a mucous membrane exposure it is 0.09% if the injured and/or exposed person is not treated within 24 hours with antiretroviral drugs.[94,95] HIV transmission after non-intact skin exposure has been documented, but the average risk for transmission by this route has not been precisely determined. Transmission of HIV through intact skin has not been documented. Currently, virtually all puncture wounds and mucous membrane exposures in HCWs involving blood from a patient with documented HIV infection are treated prophylactically with combination antiretroviral therapy (cART). This practice has dramatically reduced the occurrence of puncture-related transmissions of HIV.

In the United States between 1981 and 2006, 57 HCWs for whom case investigations were completed had documented seroconversions to HIV following occupational exposures. The routes of exposure were 48 percutaneous (puncture/cut injury), 5 mucocutaneous (mucous membrane and/or skin), 2 both percutaneous and mucocutaneous, and 2 unknown route. Of the 57 people studied, 49 were exposed to HIV-infected blood, 3 to concentrated virus in a laboratory, 1 to visibly bloody fluid, and 4 to an unspecified fluid. The individuals with documented seroconversions included 19 laboratory workers (16 of whom were clinical laboratory workers), 24 nurses, 6 physicians, 2 surgical technicians, 1 dialysis technician, 1 respiratory therapist, 1 health aide, 1 embalmer/morgue technician, and 2 housekeeper/maintenance workers.

An increased risk for HIV infection following percutaneous exposures to HIV-infected blood is associated with exposures involving a relatively large quantity of blood, as in the case of a device visibly contaminated with the patient's blood, a procedure that involves a hollow-bore needle placed directly in a vein or artery, or a deep injury. Factors that might be associated with mucocutaneous transmission of HIV include exposure to an unusually large volume of blood, prolonged contact, and a potential portal of entry. The risk increases for exposures to blood from patients with advanced-stage disease or those patients in the acute stage of HIV infection because of higher levels of HIV in the blood.

Anesthesia personnel are frequently exposed to blood and body fluids during invasive procedures such as insertion of vascular catheters, arterial punctures, and endotracheal intubation.[96–98] Although many exposures are mucocutaneous and can be prevented by the use of gloves and protective clothing, these barriers do not prevent percutaneous exposures such as needlestick injuries, which carry a greater risk for pathogen transmission. Because of the tasks they perform, anesthesia personnel are likely to use and be injured by large-bore, hollow needles such as intravenous catheter stylets and needles on syringes.[93,98] Needleless or protected needle safety devices can be used to replace standard devices to reduce the risk of needlestick injuries. Safety devices usually are more expensive than a comparable non-safety item but may be more cost-effective when the cost of needlestick injury investigation and medical care for infected personnel is considered.

The occupational risk of HIV infection is a function of the annual number of blood exposures, the rate of HIV transmission with each exposure to infected blood, and the prevalence of HIV infection in the specific patient population. Greene et al. prospectively collected data on 138 contaminated percutaneous injuries to anesthesia personnel.[96] The rate of contaminated percutaneous injuries per year per full-time equivalent anesthesia worker was 0.42, and the average annual risk of HIV and HCV infection was estimated to be 0.0016% (0.16:10,000) and 0.015% (1.5:10,000), respectively.

Although HIV can be recovered in low titers from saliva in a small number of infected subjects, there is no convincing evidence that saliva can transmit HIV infection, either through kissing or through other exposures, such as those that occur occupationally. Saliva contains several antiviral factors including HIV-specific immunoglobulins (IgA, IgG, and IgM isotypes). Moreover, there is no evidence that HIV transmission can occur as a result of exposure to tears, sweat, or urine. However, there have been isolated cases of transmission of HIV infection by body fluids that may or may not have been contaminated with blood.

Since the beginning of the HIV epidemic, there have been rare instances where transmission of infection from a HCW to patients seemed highly probable. An HIV-infected dentist in Florida may have infected as many as six of his patients, putatively through contaminated instruments.[99,100] Nevertheless, the risk of HIV transmission from medical personnel to patient is extremely low. Several epidemiologic studies have been performed tracing thousands of patients of HIV-infected dentists, physicians, surgeons, obstetricians, and gynecologists, and no other cases of HIV transmission that could be linked to the health-care providers were identified.

Breaches in infection control and the reuse of contaminated syringes have also resulted in the transmission of HIV from patient to patient in hospitals, nursing homes, and outpatient settings. For example, in the only report of HIV transmission from patient to patient during a surgical procedure, several patients in Australia apparently were infected by an HIV-negative general surgeon during routine outpatient surgery.[101] Although the mechanism of transmission was not definitively identified, a failure on the part of the surgeon to sterilize instruments properly following prior surgery on an HIV-infected patient was considered a likely explanation for this outbreak.

Postexposure Treatment and Prophylactic Antiretroviral Therapy

When personnel have been exposed to patients' blood or body fluids, the incident should immediately be reported to the employee health service or the designated individual within the institution. Based on the nature of the injury, the exposed worker and the source individual should be tested for serologic evidence of HIV, HBV, and HCV infection.[102] Current local laws must be consulted to determine policies for testing the source patient, and confidentiality must be maintained. If the source patient is found to be HIV-positive, the employee should be retested for HIV antibodies at 6 and 12 weeks and at 6 months after exposure, although most infected people are expected to undergo seroconversion within the first 6 to 12 weeks. During this period, the exposed employee should follow CDC recommendations for preventing transmission of HIV to family members and patients.[102] If the source patient is found to be HIV-negative, no additional treatment is required.

Clinicians should consider potential occupational exposures to HIV as an urgent situation to ensure timely postexposure management and possible administration of postexposure antiretroviral prophylaxis (PEP). The wound should be immediately cleansed and antiseptic applied. Recommendations regarding PEP must take into account that a variety of circumstances determine the risk of transmission of HIV following occupational exposure. Increased risk for occupational transmission includes a deep injury, visible blood on the instrument causing the exposure, injury with a device that had been placed in the vein or artery of the source patient, terminal illness in the source patient, and lack of postexposure cART in the exposed HCW. Other important considerations when contemplating PEP in the HCW include known or suspected pregnancy or breast-feeding, the possibility of exposure to drug-resistant virus, and toxicities of PEP regimens.

If a decision is made to offer PEP, U.S. Public Health Service guidelines recommend either a combination of two nucleoside analogue reverse transcriptase inhibitors given for 4 weeks for less severe exposures or a combination of two nucleoside analogue reverse transcriptase inhibitors plus a third drug given for 4 weeks for more severe exposures. Most clinicians administer the latter regimen in all cases in which a decision is made to treat.[102] Failure of PEP has been attributed to a large viral inoculum, use of a single antiviral agent, drug resistance in the virus from the source patient, and delayed initiation or short duration of PEP therapy. For consultation on the treatment of occupational exposures to HIV and other blood-borne pathogens, the clinician managing the exposed patient can call the National Clinicians' Post-Exposure Prophylaxis Hotline (PEPline) at 1-888-448-4911.

Prion Diseases

Prions (from *pro*tein + infect*ion*) are composed of misfolded protein without nucleic acid. They are responsible for the transmissible spongiform encephalopathies: Bovine spongiform encephalopathy or "mad cow disease" in cattle and Creutzfeldt–Jakob disease (CJD) in humans. All are untreatable and fatal. When a prion enters a healthy organism, it provides a template to guide the misfolding of normal protein into the extremely stable prion form, highly resistant to denaturation by chemical and physical agents. This makes disinfection and sterilization of medical instruments a unique challenge in the health-care environment. Effective prion decontamination relies upon protein hydrolysis or reduction or destruction of protein tertiary structure.

Prions cause neurodegenerative disease by aggregating extracellularly within the CNS to form amyloid plaques resulting in the histologically characteristic spongy architecture. CJD, caused by an infectious protein or prion, may be unsuspected in patients presenting with dementia.[103] There are specific guidelines for the disinfection and sterilization of prion-contaminated medical instruments.[104]

Tuberculosis

Tuberculosis (TB), one of the oldest diseases known to man, is a major cause of death worldwide and, if properly treated, almost always curable. When untreated, TB can be fatal within 5 years in 50% to 65% of cases. More than 5.8 million new cases of TB were reported to the World Health Organization in 2009; 95% of cases were reported from developing countries, which represent about 63% (range 60% to 67%) of total estimated cases. In 2009, 11,545 cases of TB (0.38:10,000) were reported to the CDC.

Mycobacterium tuberculosis is most commonly transmitted from a person with infectious pulmonary TB to others by aerosolized droplet nuclei via coughing, sneezing, or speaking. As many as 3,000 infectious nuclei per cough can remain suspended in the air for several hours and can reach the terminal air passages when inhaled. The most infectious patients have cavitary pulmonary disease or, much less commonly, laryngeal TB and produce sputum containing as many as 10^5 to 10^7 acid-fast bacilli (AFB)/mL. Other routes of transmission are uncommon. Clinical illness directly following infection is classified as *primary TB* and is common among children in the first few years of life and among immune-compromised persons.

The best way to prevent TB is to diagnose and isolate infectious cases rapidly and to administer appropriate treatment until patients are noninfectious, usually 2 to 4 weeks after the start of proper treatment. Treatment also benefits the community by preventing spread of the infection.[105] In low-prevalence countries with adequate resources, screening of high-risk groups such as immigrants from high-prevalence countries, migratory workers, prisoners, homeless individuals, substance abusers, and HIV-seropositive persons is recommended.

Outbreaks of TB in health-care facilities have been attributed to delayed diagnosis of TB in the source patient, delayed initiation or inadequate deployment of airborne precautions, lapses in precautions during aerosol-generating procedures, and lack of adequate respiratory protection in health-care personnel.

Effective prevention of spread to medical personnel requires early identification of infected patients and immediate initiation of airborne infection isolation (Table 3-4).[106] Patients must remain in isolation until adequate treatment is documented. If patients with TB must leave their rooms, they should wear face masks to prevent spread of organisms into the air. Personnel should wear fit-tested respiratory protective devices when they enter an isolation room or when performing procedures that may induce coughing, such as endotracheal intubation or tracheal suctioning.[106] The CDC recommends that respiratory protective devices worn to protect against TB should be able to filter 95% of particles 1 mm in size at flow rates of 50 L/min and should fit the face with a leak rate of <10% around the seal, documented by fit testing.[106] High-efficiency particulate air (HEPA) respirators (classified as N95) are NIOSH-approved devices that meet the CDC criteria for respiratory protective devices against TB.[107] Elective surgery should be postponed until infected patients have had an adequate course of chemotherapy. If surgery is required, bacterial filters (HEPA filters) should be used on the anesthetic breathing circuit for patients with TB.[107] Patients must be recovered in a room that meets all the requirements for airborne precautions.

Routine periodic screening of employees for TB should be included as part of a hospital's employee health policy with the frequency of screening dependent on the prevalence of infected patients in the hospitalized population. When a new conversion is detected by skin testing, a history of exposure should be sought to determine the source patient. Treatment or preventive therapy is based on the drug-susceptibility pattern of the TB in the source patient, if known.

Viruses in Smoke Plumes

The use of lasers and electrosurgical devices is associated with several hazards to patients and to operating room personnel. Physical hazards include thermal burns, eye injuries, electrical hazards, fires, and explosions. Plume content consists of water and organic vapors, carbonized cell fragments, formaldehyde, acrolein, benzene, polyaromatic hydrocarbons, and carbon monoxide. While airborne cancer cells have not been detected in laser plumes, potentially harmful particles varying from 0.5 to 5.0 mm have been detected (for comparison, a red blood cell = 7.5 mm). Intact and infectious viral DNA can be detected with laser treatment of verrucae. Viable viruses can be found in plumes produced by both carbon dioxide and argon laser vaporization of a virus-loaded culture plate, but viable viruses are carried on larger particles that travel <100 mm from the site being vaporized.[108] A case report describes laryngeal papillomatosis in a surgeon who had used a laser to remove anogenital condylomas from several patients.[109] Although DNA analysis of the surgeon's papillomas revealed a viral type similar to that of the condylomas, proof of transmission was lacking.

Smoke does not qualify as blood or "other potentially infectious materials" according to OSHA (Bloodborne Pathogens) Standard 29 CFR 1910.1030. Smoke-vacuuming systems as well as PPE should be utilized when personnel are in proximity to surgical smoke.[110] The smoke-vacuuming systems should be held as close as 1 cm to within the target because at 2 cm there is a 50% loss of the evacuation ratio. HEPA or ultra-low penetration air filters should be used, and charcoal filters should be used for odor and gas absorption. Venting should be to the outdoors, if possible, and venting systems should have the ability to detect filter overloading (i.e., pressure drop). These filtration guidelines do not address fluid aspiration, which must be carried out independently. In addition, operating room personnel working in the vicinity of the laser plume should wear gloves, goggles, and high-efficiency filter masks (N95 respirators).[110]

EMOTIONAL CONSIDERATIONS

Stress

Occupational stress occurs when the demands of a job exceed the capabilities or resources of the worker. This can result in poor mental and physical health, industrial accidents, and injury. There are three identifiable components of the stress syndrome: The initiating stressors, the psychological filters that process and evaluate the stressors, and the coping mechanisms that are recruited in an attempt to control the stressful situation. The ultimate response to stress is very individualistic; what is unpleasant to one individual can be stimulating and pleasant to another, or even to the same individual under different circumstances.

Mild, brief, and controllable episodes of occupational stress are unavoidable and can serve as an impetus to personal achievement. As succinctly stated by Hans Selye, a pioneer in the modern study of stress, "The absence of stress is death".[111] On the other hand, extreme degrees of chronic stress are harmful and can result in a number of symptoms and diseases. Common stress-related illnesses include mood and sleep disturbances, disrupted relationships with family and friends, and various types of gastrointestinal, musculoskeletal, and cardiovascular diseases. Workplace stress-related outcomes include physical injuries at work, absenteeism, decreased productivity, and increased disability. Occupational stress costs organizations as much as $75 billion per year.

By any definition, anesthesiology is a stressful occupation.[112] The operating room imposes a background of chronic, low-level stress that is frequently interrupted by acute episodes of extreme stress. The demands are externally paced and usually out of the individual anesthesiologist's control. Random disturbances are intermittently and unpredictably inserted into the environment. Finally, failure to meet the demands imposed by the workplace can result in serious consequences.

Certain specific stressors are commonly reported by anesthesiologists. These include the unpredictability of the work, need for sustained vigilance during long intervals, production pressure, fear of litigation, difficult interpersonal relations, and economic uncertainties.

The process of inducing anesthesia can be among the most profound sources of acute stress for anesthesiologists. Tachycardia and dysrhythmia, elevation in blood pressure, and myocardial ischemia have all been observed among anesthesiologists during an anesthetic induction, especially those with the fewest years of experience.[113]

To many anesthesiologists, interpersonal relationships are the greatest source of workplace stress. Conflict and its constructive resolution have received less attention in the health-care industry than in many other industrial settings. Conflict can easily occur where the established hierarchy of command is blurred and overlapping areas of professional responsibility exist. The operating room, where surgeon and anesthesiologist simultaneously share responsibility but may have conflicting priorities, holds the potential of providing these conditions.[48] Recent work has focused upon applying the principles of crisis resource management, first developed in the aerospace industry, to improve communication and team work in the operating room.[114]

Exactly how an individual responds to stress is the product of a number of factors, including age, gender, experience, preexisting personality style, available defense and coping mechanisms, support systems, and concomitant events (such as sleep deprivation). Several personality traits can be predictive of maladaptive responses to stress, such as the obsessive-compulsive, dependent character structure. Individuals who have these personality characteristics typically manifest pessimism, passivity, self-doubt, and feelings of insecurity. They commonly respond to stress by internalization and becoming hypochondriacal and depressed. Undergraduate students who demonstrate these characteristics are more likely to have their medical careers disrupted by alcoholism or drug abuse, psychiatric illness, and marital disturbances.[115,116]

When appropriate defense mechanisms become overwhelmed, maladaptive behaviors begin to emerge such as personal and professional deterioration, burnout, drug addiction, and suicide.

Burnout

Burnout is a clinical syndrome that is characterized by physical and emotional exhaustion, poor judgment, cynicism, guilt, feelings of ineffectiveness, and a sense of depersonalization in relationships with coworkers or patients. Burnout primarily affects workers such as physicians and nurses whose job requires intense interactions with individuals who have great physical and emotional needs. Unfortunately, many of the characteristics that are found among the best health-care providers, such as idealism, perfectionism, and a heightened sense of responsibility, can also render these individuals at greater risk for feelings of inadequacy and burnout if their high standards are unmet.

Commonly cited causes of burnout among health-care providers are increased production requirements, excessive bureaucracy and regulation, long hours of work, lack of control of one's schedule, decreasing reimbursement, a rapidly expanding base of medical knowledge, and difficulty balancing personal and professional lives.

Physician burnout results in important personal and professional consequences. The quality of care provided by these physicians suffers and they are more prone to medical errors and malpractice lawsuits.[117,118] Their patients are more likely to be dissatisfied with their medical care and to be noncompliant with their medical treatment plans.[119] Burnout has also been shown to be a contributor to various illnesses, including cardiovascular disease[120] and substance abuse.[121]

Significant degrees of burnout have been identified in a number of medical specialties, including anesthesiology.[122,123] In one study approximately 40% of practicing anesthesiologists were reported to be at risk for burnout.[124] Although recovery from burnout is possible, prevention is the best strategy (see Wellness, vide infra).

Substance Use, Abuse, and Addiction

Illicit drug use remains one of our society's unresolved problems. It is estimated that 20 million Americans abuse substances and 5 million are addicted. *Substance abuse* is characterized by repeated use of a substance despite significant adverse consequences. The *addicted* individual continues to use the substance in spite of unsuccessful attempts to control its use, the need for larger amounts of the substance, symptoms of withdrawal, and the need to spend increasing amounts of time seeking the substance. The term *chemical dependence* is sometimes used interchangeably with addiction.

Approximately 10% to 12% of physicians will develop some form of substance abuse disorder during their careers.[125] The prevalence of alcoholism and overall substance abuse is approximately equal to that found in the general population.[126] However, physicians tend to abuse different substances than the general public and are less likely to abuse tobacco or illicit drugs and more likely to self-medicate with prescription drugs.

There is some debate whether there is an excess of substance abuse among anesthesiologists as compared to other physicians. Several older studies reported no increased prevalence of substance abuse among training[125,127] or attending anesthesiologists.[128] On the other hand, the majority of recent studies report a disproportionately high prevalence of substance abuse among both resident and practicing anesthesiologists.[129–131] These studies have reported an overrepresentation of anesthesiologists in substance abuse treatment centers that specialize in the treatment of addicted physicians and in state-run health programs that monitor physicians after treatment for substance abuse.[131,132]

Regardless of whether or not the specialty of anesthesiology has a disproportionate percentage of substance abusers, all agree that the disease is unacceptably high among anesthesiologists. In fact, substance abuse is considered by many authorities to be the number one occupational hazard of anesthesiology. For example, in a retrospective survey conducted among 260 graduates of one anesthesia training program, 32% had used illicit drugs to "get high" and 15.8% had been self-admitted problematic substance abusers.[133] Twenty percent of the respondents had observed their faculty members using alcohol and/or other drugs to the detriment of their teaching. A different survey found the incidence of known drug abuse to be 1.6% among anesthesiology residents and 1.0% among faculty members.[134]

One very troubling aspect of this problem is the persistently high incidence of substance abuse that is reported among anesthesiology residents. In a report from the Medical Association of Georgia Disabled Doctors' Program, anesthesiology residents constituted 33.7% of the resident population of the treatment group, despite representing only 4.6% of the resident population.[131] The incidence of controlled substance abuse within anesthesiology training programs continues to run close to 2% despite
6 increased residency requirements for educational programs and more stringent accounting of controlled substances.[134,135]

In addition to a high prevalence, the disease appears in a particularly virulent form among anesthesiologists because their drugs of choice tend toward the most addictive and harmful. Anesthesiologists are more likely than other physicians to develop an intravenous habit and to become addicted to potent drugs such as opioids or propofol that are potentially lethal.[130,136]

There is no single answer for the question of why there is a high prevalence of substance abuse and addiction among anesthesiologists. The disease occurs when a susceptible host is exposed to a "favorable" environment. Vulnerability in the host is an important factor and may account for a majority of the risk for addiction. What constitutes an instigating exposure to a drug in one person may have absolutely no effect on another. Other etiologic factors thought to be specific to certain anesthesiologists include a susceptible personality with low self-esteem, lack of external recognition, an orientation toward self-medication, and a stressful workplace. Unfortunately, there is no predictive tool to identify the susceptible individual until he or she gets the disease.

A prior history of recreational drug use and other high-risk behaviors may play a prominent role in the subsequent development of chemical dependency.[137] Self-prescription of drugs frequently precedes more extensive substance abuse and dependency. Of concern is the increasing recreational use among younger physicians and medical students of drugs, such as propofol, with enhanced potential for addiction.[138] It has been suggested that a drug-seeking individual may choose a career in anesthesiology motivated in part because of the known availability of powerful drugs.[135,139]

Other authors have focused upon the ease of access and chronic exposure to potent anesthetic drugs as a primary explanation for a high prevalence of substance abuse among anesthesiologists.[128] Anesthesiologists are unique among physicians because they frequently prescribe as well as personally administer these highly addictive psychoactive drugs. In contrast, physicians in most other specialties prescribe medications while other personnel administer them.

There is an apparent association between specific specialties and the preferred substance of abuse. The drugs of choice among most addicted anesthesiologists are anesthetic drugs. Early reports identified meperidine, diazepam, and barbiturates abuse among addicted anesthesiologists.[126] Subsequently, fentanyl and other synthetic narcotics and inhalation anesthetics became the most commonly abused substances.[134] Propofol is now emerging as the most commonly abused drug among anesthesia care providers. For example, in a survey of academic anesthesiology departments, 18% reported cases of abuse of propofol, as opposed to an incidence of about 10% for fentanyl addiction.[138]

Addiction is a chronic disease that produces a constellation of specific anatomic and physiologic changes and characteristic signs and symptoms. There is a predictable deterioration in professional, family, and social relationships (Table 3-7). The substance abuser becomes increasingly withdrawn and isolated in his or her personal as well as professional lives. Every attempt is made to maintain a facade of normality at work in order to preserve

TABLE 3-7. SIGNS OF SUBSTANCE ABUSE AND DEPENDENCE

What to Look for Outside the Hospital

1. Addiction is a disease of loneliness and isolation. Addicts quickly withdraw from family, friends, and leisure activities.
2. Addicts have unusual changes in behavior, including wide mood swings and periods of depression, anger, and irritability alternating with periods of euphoria.
3. Unexplained overspending, legal problems, gambling, extramarital affairs, and increased problems at work are commonly seen in addicts.
4. An obvious physical sign of alcoholism is the frequent smell of alcohol on the breath.
5. Domestic strife, fights, and arguments may increase in number and intensity.
6. Sexual drive may significantly decrease.
7. Children may develop behavioral problems.
8. Some addicts frequently change jobs over a period of several years in an attempt to find a "geographic cure" for their disease or to hide it from coworkers.
9. Addicts need to be near their drug source. For a health-care professional, this means long hours at the hospital, even when off duty. For alcoholics, it means calling in sick to work. Alcoholics may disappear without any explanation to bars or hiding places to drink secretly.
10. Addicts may suddenly develop the habit of locking themselves in the bathroom or other rooms while they are using drugs.
11. Addicts frequently hide pills, syringes, or alcohol bottles around the house.
12. Persons who inject drugs may leave bloody swabs and syringes containing blood-tinged liquid in conspicuous places.
13. Addicts may display evidence of withdrawal, especially diaphoresis (sweating) and tremors.
14. Narcotic addicts often have pinpoint pupils.
15. Weight loss and pale skin are also common signs of addiction.
16. Addicts may be seen injecting drugs.
17. Tragically, some addicts are found comatose or dead before any of these signs have been recognized by others.

What to Look for Inside the Hospital

1. Addicts sign out ever-increasing quantities of narcotics.
2. Addicts frequently have unusual changes in behavior, such as wide mood swings and periods of depression, anger, and irritability alternating with periods of euphoria.
3. Charting becomes increasingly sloppy and unreadable.
4. Addicts often sign out narcotics in inappropriately high doses for the operation being performed.
5. They refuse lunch and coffee relief.
6. Addicts like to work alone in order to use anesthetic techniques without narcotics, falsify records, and divert drugs for personal use.
7. They volunteer for extra cases, often where large amounts of narcotics are available (e.g., cardiac cases).
8. They frequently relieve others.
9. They are often at the hospital when off duty, staying close to their drug supply to prevent withdrawal.
10. They volunteer frequently for extra call.
11. They are often difficult to find between cases, taking short naps after using.
12. Addicted anesthesia personnel may insist on personally administering narcotics in the recovery room.
13. Addicts make frequent requests for bathroom relief. This is usually where they use drugs.
14. Addicts may wear long-sleeved gowns to hide needle tracks and also to combat the subjective feeling of cold they experience when using narcotics.
15. Narcotic addicts often have pinpoint pupils.
16. An addict's patients may come into the recovery room complaining of pain out of proportion to the amount of narcotic charted on the anesthesia records.
17. Weight loss and pale skin are also common signs of addiction.
18. Addicts may be seen injecting drugs.
19. Untreated addicts are found comatose.
20. Undetected addicts are found dead.

Adapted from: Farley WJ, Arnold WP. Videotape: Unmasking addiction: Chemical dependency in anesthesiology. Produced by Davids Production, Parsippany, NJ, funded by Janssen Pharmaceutica, Piscataway, NJ, 1991.
Reprinted with permission from: American Society of Anesthesiologists: Task Force on Chemical Dependence of the Committee on Occupational Health of Operating Room Personnel. *Chemical Dependence in Anesthesiologists: What You Need to Know When You Need to Know It.* Park Ridge, IL: American Society of Anesthesiologists; 1998.

access to the abused drugs. The disease is entering its end stage by the time that professional conduct is sufficiently impaired that it is apparent to the physician's colleagues.

If left untreated, addiction among physicians is frequently fatal. Alexander et al. calculated a relative risk of 2.79 for drug-related deaths among anesthesiologists compared to a matched cohort of internists.[19] Menk et al. found 14 drug-related deaths among the 79 drug abusers who had been reenrolled in anesthesiology residencies after treatment.[140] A more recent survey reported that there were 9 deaths in 100 residents who returned to and remained in anesthesiology training programs after treatment for chemical dependence.[135]

In addition to health hazards, addiction among physicians raises important legal considerations. State laws and regulations detail the necessary steps for handling the drug-abusing physician. In many states disciplinary action and criminal penalties can be imposed on physicians who knowingly fail to report an impaired colleague. Disciplinary action taken against an impaired physician must also be reported to the National Practitioner Data Bank to be in compliance with federal law. Most state medical societies have physicians' health programs. When chemically dependent physicians voluntarily seek treatment through this venue, the legal impact may be mitigated.

Physicians as a group are less likely than the general population to self-identify and seek professional assistance if a drug-related problem develops. Denial plays a major role in this reluctance to undergo counseling or therapy. Denial is learned early in a physician's professional life in order to endure the sleepless nights and the personal shortcomings that inevitably accompany the practice of medicine. A well-developed denial defense mechanism enables many physician-addicts to conclude that his or her problem is minor and that self-treatment is possible. Physicians typically enter programs for treatment only after they have reached the end stages of their illness.

Debate continues regarding the issue of compulsory random drug testing of anesthesiologists.[141] Preemployment and/or random drug screening is already well established in various industries, especially those with high public profiles (nuclear, aviation, military). Many chairs of academic anesthesiology programs have indicated a willingness to initiate a program of random drug screening of their staff.[133] Although random drug testing is an established element of most reentry contracts for recovering anesthesiologists, serious questions remain about the legality of this approach and its effectiveness in preventing substance abuse.

There is also controversy about the ultimate career path of the anesthesiologist in recovery.[142] The recidivism rate among the general population approaches 60% for patients who have been treated for addiction. Physicians are highly motivated and in general the prognosis for doctors' recovery exceeds that of the general public.[143] Reports have ranged from very optimistic to more pessimistic regarding predictions for successful rehabilitation and return to practice for addicted anesthesiologists. In one study, the rate of relapse among anesthesiologists was 40% and that of control physicians was 44%.[132] Sustained recovery for longer than 2 years occurred in 81% and 86%, respectively. A different study reported less favorable results, with a 66% failure rate for successful rehabilitation and return to practice among 79 opioid-dependent anesthesiology residents.[140] Even more alarming, there were 14 suicide or overdose deaths among the 79 returning trainees. A more recent study reported similar findings with only 46% of addicted anesthesia residents able to successfully complete their anesthesiology training.[135] Thirty-four percent entered a training program in another medical specialty, and 16% left medicine. There were 9 deaths among the 100 anesthesia residents that continued in anesthesia training programs after treatment.

Three factors have been closely associated with relapse among health-care professionals after completion of treatment for chemical dependency.[144] The risk of relapse is increased if there is a family history of substance abuse, when a major opioid is the abused drug, and when the individual has a coexisting psychiatric disorder (dual diagnosis). The risk of relapse is greatest when all three factors are present.

In order to reenter practice, the recovering physician must qualify for a valid license to practice medicine and must be re-credentialed at his/ her medical facility. This must be done in compliance with the state laws and regulations regarding return to practice for recovering physicians. Federal laws, such as the Americans with Disabilities Act, impose additional considerations. Finally, a carefully worded contract is an important step in the reentry process to define the obligations of the physician and the department.[145] The contract should include details on monitoring in a rehabilitation program and by a departmental supervisor and include an agreement to refrain from self-prescription of medication. It is frequently recommended that the returning anesthesiologist not take night or weekend call or handle opioids without direct supervision for at least the first 3 months. Despite all of these precautions, the potential for relapse must be anticipated.

Guidelines from physician treatment centers may be helpful to assist in the decisions surrounding reentry.[146] Individuals who, in most situations, can successfully return to the practice of anesthesiology immediately after treatment (category I) accept and understand their disease and have no evidence of accompanying psychiatric disorders. They have strong support from their family, demonstrate a balanced lifestyle, are committed to their recovery contract, and bond with Alcoholics Anonymous (AA; http://www.aa.org/) or Narcotics Anonymous (NA; http://www.na.org/). Their anesthesiology department and hospital must be supportive of their return, and the individual must have a sponsor that supports the return to anesthesiology. Category II includes those individuals who could possibly return to anesthesiology within a few years. They must have no or minimal denial regarding their disease and have no other psychiatric diagnoses. Their recovery skills are continually improving and they are involved, but not necessarily bonded, with AA/NA. Although their family situation may be characterized as dysfunctional, there should be tangible evidence of improvement. Individuals who should not return to anesthesiology and would best be redirected into another medical specialty are included in category III. These individuals may have had a history of prolonged intravenous substance use and have experienced relapses and prior treatment failures. Their disease remains active, and they have coexisting severe psychiatric diagnoses.

Because availability of drugs plays a role in the onset of this disease, attention has been directed toward programs to enforce increased accountability and regulation of controlled substances.[147] However, despite widespread application of protocols to enforce greater accountability, such as satellite pharmacies for operating suites, the frequency of substance abuse has changed little, if at all, in recent years.

Impairment and Disability

Impairment[b] and disability[c] can arise from physical, mental, emotional, sensory, or developmental causes. The onset can be

[b]Impairment is any loss of use of any body part, organ system, or organ function.

[c]Disability is an impairment that substantially limits one or more major life activities.

sudden, as occurs with injury or acute illness, or more gradual, as is the case with many chronic diseases.

Data regarding the number of impaired physicians[d] are difficult to obtain. Many cases of physician impairment are the result of substance-related disorders. Other factors that may result in physician impairment include physical or mental illness. Unwillingness or inability to keep up with current literature and techniques can be considered a form of impairment.

Depression is a prominent finding among impaired physicians. Unfortunately, many of the personality traits that ensure success as a physician, such as self-sacrifice, competitiveness, achievement orientation, denial of feelings, and intellectualization of emotions, may also serve as risk factors for depression. Observations of alcoholic physicians have provided some insight into the association of achievement orientation and emotional disturbance. In one study, more than half of the alcoholic physicians graduated in the upper one-third of their medical school class, 23% were in the upper one-tenth of their class, and only 5% were in the lower one-third of their class[148]. Similarly, a report on alcohol use in medical school demonstrated better first-year grades and higher scores on Part I National Board of Medical Examiners tests among those students identified as alcohol abusers.[149]

It can be very challenging to appropriately respond to all of the problems imposed by the impaired or unsafe anesthesiologist.[150] Management protocols for dealing with the impaired physician are covered in a series of articles by Canavan and Baxter.[151]

The Aging Anesthesiologist

Little attention has been given to the unique challenges faced by older anesthesiologists.[152] This is in contrast to the situation in many other industries where considerable attention is directed toward the well-being and competence of older workers. For example, older commercial airline pilots are required to take regular medical and competency examinations and adhere to strict policies on work hours.

Physiologic changes are routinely observed in many organ systems as a direct consequence of aging. Most notable for the safe practice of anesthesiology are the physical changes that appear in the CNS, such as decreases in neuronal density and brain weight, training-dependent plasticity, and ability of neurons to reorganize in response to training. Commonly observed physiologic changes include impairments in hearing, vision, short-term memory, creative thinking, and problem-solving abilities. Intellectual quickness, on-the-spot reasoning, learning, and reaction time all slow. These changes have the potential to limit the older anesthesiologist's ability to assimilate and apply new knowledge and to instantaneously process information, rapidly make complex decisions, and initiate the proper response.[153] These potential deficiencies are especially exposed in a stressful environment such as an operating room.

There are also important age-related changes in the cardiovascular and musculoskeletal systems. Older anesthesiologists often lack the stamina necessary to sustain the long, demanding work shifts common in anesthetic practice. Older individuals are particularly sensitive to disturbances of the sleep–wake cycle and are better suited to phase advances (morning work) than phase delays (nocturnal work). Demands associated with night call have been identified as the most stressful aspect of practice and most frequently cited impetus toward retirement.[152,154]

The physiologic changes that might impose a handicap on the older anesthesiologist are often compensated by advantages that accompany the normal aging process. These include wisdom, judgment, and the experience acquired by a lifelong practice of the specialty. There is a strong positive correlation between experience and performance.[155] However, this correlation does not necessarily exist between experience and complex cognitive skills. As pointed out by Weinger, experience is not synonymous with expertise.[156]

Aging among anesthesiologists raises complex legal and ethical issues. Neither state licensure nor hospital privileges are specifically limited by the chronologic age of the practitioner. In many cases, the decision to limit or retire from practice remains at the discretion of the individual anesthesiologist. A number of federal laws impact the aging anesthesiologist's rights and responsibilities regarding continuation of work. These include the Age Discrimination Act, Title VII of the Civil Rights Act, the Medical and Family Leave Act, the Fair Labor Standards Act, and the Employee Retirement Income Security Act.

Anesthesiology, similar to other high-stress professions, is often regarded as a young person's profession. This, in part, accounts for the observation that, on average, anesthesiologists retire at a younger age than many other physicians.[157] The decision to retire from anesthesiology is frequently precipitated by concerns about deteriorating clinical skills and the growing burdens of night call. In many cases, the retiring anesthesiologist just "felt it was time".[157]

As a result of a number of demographic factors, including the smaller residency class sizes observed during the mid-1990s, the mean age of the anesthesiology workforce is increasing. The greatest number (30%) of anesthesiologists are between 45 and 54 years of age, and 56% are 45 years of age and older (up from 49% 10 years ago).[158]

Mortality Among Anesthesiologists

There have been a number of conflicting reports regarding the average longevity of anesthesiologists. Employing different databases and methods, these studies have found a shortened[19,159] an average,[158,160] or a prolonged[161,162] life expectancy. A 2006 study reported a significant increase in life expectancy among anesthesiologists who had died in the period 1992 to 2001, such that the average age at death in the last year of the study was 78 years, the same as the national average for all Americans.[163]

The cause of death among anesthesiologists has also been extensively studied. Earlier work found an increased incidence of certain types of cancer, including leukemia and lymphoma.[8,17] More recent reports have failed to find any increase in cancer risk among anesthesiologists, but a consistent finding of increased numbers of drug-related deaths and suicide.[19]

Suicide

There is a disproportionately high incidence of suicide among both male[164] and female[165] physicians. Several reports have singled out anesthesiologists as being particularly vulnerable.[19,162,166] However, this conclusion has been questioned as a result of the methodologic difficulties in collecting accurate data on suicide and the frequent failure to adequately correct for confounding variables in the study populations.[167]

[d]An impaired physician is one whose performance as a professional person and as a practitioner of the healing arts is impaired because of alcoholism, drug abuse, mental illness, senility, or disabling disease.

A partial explanation for this alarming observation lies with the high degree of stress that is an integral part of the job. There is a close association in many individuals between stressful life events and major depressive disorders which can give way to despair and suicidal ideation.[168] Personality profiles collected from a number of suicide-susceptible individuals indicate common characteristics such as high anxiety, insecurity, low self-esteem, impulsiveness, and poor self-control. It is disturbing to note that in a study of personality traits of anesthesiologists, 20% manifested psychological profiles that reflected a predisposition to behavioral disintegration and attempted suicide when placed under extremes of stress.[169] This study raises the discomforting notion that "premorbid" personality characteristics exist before entering specialty training and are not being identified in the admission process.

One specific type of stress, that resulting from a malpractice lawsuit, may have a direct causative association with suicide. Newspaper reports have described the emotional deterioration and ultimate suicide of experienced physicians who have become involved in a malpractice suit. One study reported that 4 of 185 anesthesiologists being sued for medical malpractice attempted or committed suicide.[166]

Substance abuse among anesthesia personnel is another potential contributor to the increased suicide rate. Individuals with chemical dependence, who are not identified and are in the end stages of the disease, may die of drug overdose, a cause of death that can be difficult to distinguish from suicide. Drug abuse is among the highest causes of death and the most frequent method of suicide among anesthesiologists.[19] Drug overdose and death was the initial relapse symptom in 16% (13 of 79) of the parenteral opioid abusers who had reentered their residency in anesthesiology.[140] Physicians who are impaired from chemical dependence and whose privileges to practice medicine have been revoked are also at heightened risk for attempting suicide. Crawshaw et al. reported 8 successful and 2 near-miss suicide attempts among 43 physicians placed on probation for drug-related disability.[170]

WELLNESS

According to ethical guidelines of the ASA, anesthesiologists are obliged to maintain their "physical and mental health and special sensory capabilities."[171] Unfortunately, the emphasis on impairment labeling, intervention, and post-intervention monitoring of state medical boards' physician health committees provides little guidance and support for developing and sustaining a healthier lifestyle and no infrastructure for research and education. Hence, the formal incorporation of aspects of wellness as an integral
7 component of ASA's focus upon anesthesiologists' occupational health concerns is designed to address this emerging area.

The ability to balance normal occupational stress with the time necessary for maintenance of wellness occurs within the context of telescoped and overlapping life cycle events (Fig. 3-3). Compounded stresses at concurrent transition points can lead to maladaptive coping patterns and wellness choices. Stresses may occur when one or more cycles halt or move backward, when substantial overlap occurs, or when multiple stressful events occur, especially at transition points. External stressors such as disease, disability, divorce, death, malpractice actions or financial distress may have devastating short- or long-term effects.[112]

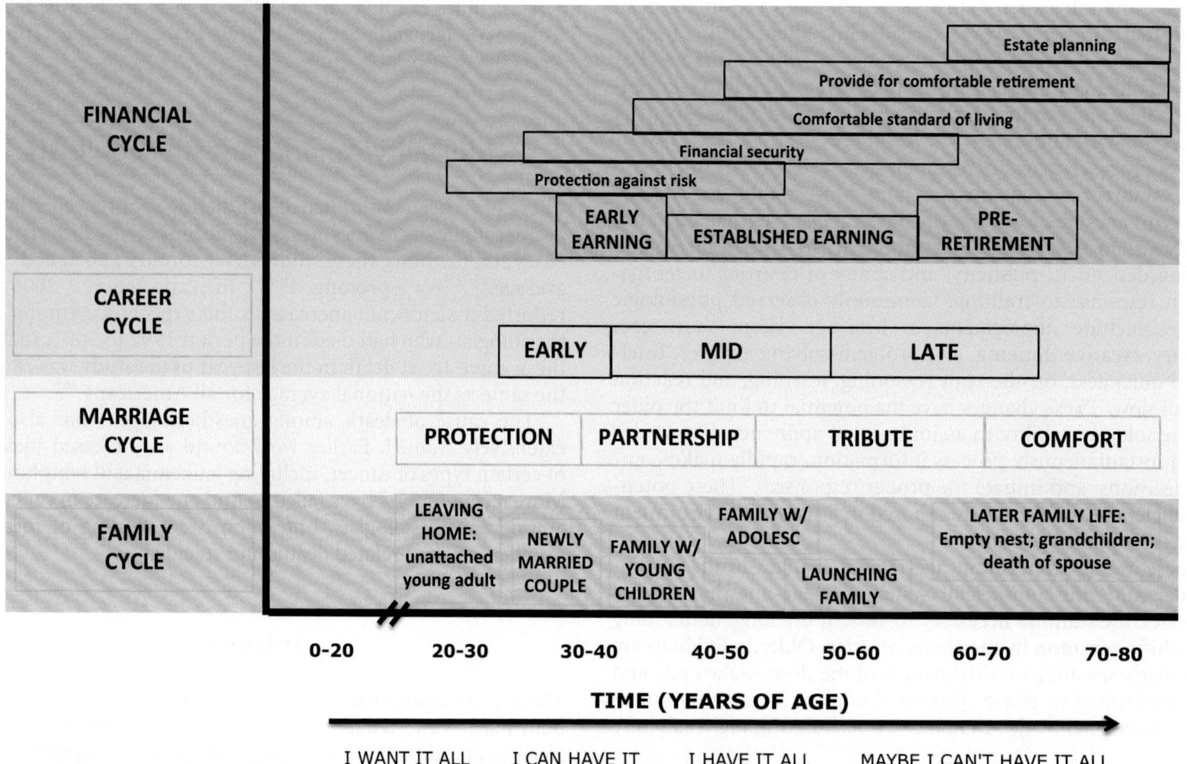

FIGURE 3-3. Life events. Life cycle events portrayed as multiple cycles moving through time. Because life plans are often deferred for long periods of education and training, many formative events are "shifted to the right," telescoping their concurrence and impact.

It has been estimated that half of the mortality in the United States is premature, and these deaths could be "deferred" with the modification of just 10 behaviors: Tobacco use, dietary pattern, physical activity level, alcohol consumption, exposure to microbial agents, exposure to toxic agents, use of firearms, sexual behavior, motor vehicle crashes, and illicit use of drugs. The first three accounted for nearly 800,000 deaths in 1990[172] and again in 2004.[173] It is a particular challenge for busy professionals to become informed about and adopt lifestyle changes related to diet and fitness.

Nutrition and Diet

Obesity is an evolving pandemic, with 380 million cases worldwide projected by 2025.[174] It is especially challenging for those with a more sedentary occupation coupled with a sedentary lifestyle. Adipose tissue is an endocrinologically active organ, releasing a large number of adipokines that affect food intake, peripheral insulin sensitivity, muscle glucose uptake, and hepatic glucose production.[175] Caloric restriction as an antiaging strategy has been recognized for a long time.[176] Putative mechanisms include increased DNA repair capacity, altered gene expression, decreased metabolic rate, and reduced oxidative stress.[177,178] Needless to say, anesthesiologists should not only have concern about obesity in their patients, but in themselves as well.

Fitness

Because skeletal muscle is the major site of whole-body fat and carbohydrate utilization, exercise, along with diet, plays a major role in wellness. Of 17,549 men who entered Harvard College between 1916 and 1950 and were reevaluated when aged 55 to 84 years (including a 16-year follow-up), a significant association was revealed between lower death rates and higher levels of walking, stair climbing, sports play, and various activity combinations. Compared to the one-third of men least active, the middle third experienced a 23% reduction in death rate during follow-up and the one-third of men most active, a 32% reduction. Light activities (<4 MET),[e] moderate activities (4 to 5 MET), and vigorous activities (>6 MET) each predicted lower death rates.[179]

At a molecular level, cell membrane substrate transporter genes GLUT4 (circulating glucose) and FAT/CD36 (fatty acid) are affected by various glycemic loads as well as exercise. After 60 minutes of cycling at 75% maximal oxygen consumption (VO_2max), subjects fed a high-glycemic index (HGI) or low-glycemic index (LGI) isocaloric meal demonstrated greater glucose and insulin responses following an HGI compared to an LGI diet.[180] Acute and chronic exercise also increases nitric oxide (NO) in sedentary and active men, but chronic exercise, especially in active men, results in a significantly greater level at baseline.[181] In addition, physical exercise has been shown in a rodent model to improve learning by modulating hippocampal mossy fiber sprouting and enhancing gamma-aminobutyric acid receptor A-alpha3 and cholescytokinin elaboration.[182]

[e]A *metabolic equivalent (MET)* expresses the energy cost of physical activities as multiples of resting metabolic rate (RMR) and is defined as the ratio of metabolic rate during a specific physical activity to a basal metabolic rate of 3.5 mL O_2/kg/min or 1 kcal/kg/h or 4.184 kJ/kg/h. One MET is considered as the RMR obtained during quiet sitting. MET values of physical activities range from 0.9 (sleeping) to 18 (running at 17.5 km/h).

Implementing Lifestyle Interventions for Lifestyle-Related Diseases

Weight loss requires a decrease in calories consumed and an increase in calories burned. A Cochrane review of 32 longitudinal analyses and 17 randomized controlled trials (RCTs) showed that intensive counseling strategies incorporating behavioral, dietary, and exercise components resulted in a weight loss of 3 to 4 kg over 1 to 3.3 years.[183] A meta-analysis of 32 RCTs involving obese patients showed that moderate and well-balanced calorie restriction is more effective than any other diet, resulting in an average weight loss of about 5 kg after 1 year.[184] A caloric deficit of about 500 kcals per day is the optimal goal for most.[185,186]

Strategies to reduce energy intake include consuming reduced portion sizes, a lower energy density diet, a Mediterranean diet, whole grains, fruits and vegetables, a low glycemic load, and decreased fat intake. These dietary changes can produce sustained weight loss and improvements in risk factors, as well as prevention of type 2 diabetes and improved control of hypertension.[187] Exercise is more important when trying to *maintain* weight loss than it is as an isolated weight loss strategy. Most RCTs show only modest weight loss with exercise alone, and slight increases in weight loss when exercise is added to dietary restriction.[188] A Cochrane review concluded that diet combined with exercise produced a 20% greater initial weight loss than diet alone and a greater likelihood that the weight loss would be sustained.[189] At least 10 MET of aerobic exercise (brisk walking, light jogging, or stationary cycling) is required for visceral fat reduction.

Mindfulness

Vigilance, referred to earlier as among the most important of an
8 anesthesiologist's tasks, is closely tied to concentration and attentiveness. An emerging area of interest is mindfulness,[f] especially in complex, dynamic environments like the operating room and ICU. The nuanced difference is that concentration is exclusive; mindfulness is inclusive and the opposite of multitasking,[190] which is often the perceived requirement of the data-laden critical care environment.

One reason multitasking (or task-switching) is so difficult is that it calls upon working memory (WM)—a brain resource that is extremely limited. High WM capacity is essential for the ability to differentiate between relevant and irrelevant information. In order to retain information during a delay, it is necessary to ignore interfering stimuli from the surroundings. Dual reaction time tasks engage additional cortical regions that are not activated by the component tasks, had they been performed as single tasks.[191] When attention needs to be divided between two concurrent processes there is a cost in performance. Most of the subjects during these studies reported using "chunking" of information as a strategy.[192,193] It is a point of professional pride that anesthesiologists can point to one of the best graphic displays of "chunked" information—the anesthesia record.

Mindful practice requires mentoring and guidance through progressive phases from denial to generalizations, insight, new behaviors, compassion, and presence[190] (Table 3-8).

[f]As used in cognitive psychology by Langer EJ. *Mindfulness.* Cambridge, MA: Da Capo Press; 1989.

TABLE 3-8. MINDFULNESS STAGES. CHARACTERISTICS OF MINDFUL PRACTICE, WITH A DESCRIPTIVE HIERARCHY

Mindful Practice	
Characteristics	
Active observation of oneself, the patient, and the problem	
Peripheral vision	
Preattentive processing	
Critical curiosity	
Courage to see the world as it is rather than as one would have it be	
Willingness to examine and set aside categories and prejudices	
Adoption of a beginner's mind	
Humility to tolerate awareness of one's areas of incompetence	
Connection between the knower and the known	
Compassion based on insight	
Presence	
Levels	**Description**
0	Denial and externalization
1	Imitation: Behavioral modeling
2	Curiosity: Cognitive understanding
3	Curiosity: Emotions and attitudes
4	Insight
5	Generalization, incorporation, and presence

Source: Epstein RM. Mindful practice. *JAMA.* 1999;282(9):833–839.

CONCLUSION

The perioperative and critical care environments challenge anesthesiologists in unique ways, from physical hazards such as exposure to toxic chemicals and waste anesthetic gases, to various forms of ionizing and nonionizing energies and numerous infectious agents, as well as risks of fire or explosion. In addition, the sustained cognitive, emotional, and psychological demands have significant bearing on performance and professional deportment. This chapter has reviewed some of the ongoing as well as emerging areas related to occupational illness and wellness of anesthesia personnel in these settings.

References

1. US Dept Labor Bureau of Labor Statistics. Fatal Occupational Injuries and Nonfatal Occupational Injuries and Illnesses, 2008 (http://www.bls.gov/iif/oshwc/osh/os/oshs2008_8.pdf). Accessed: 11/2011.
2. Matsuoka H, Kurosawa S, Horinouchi T, et al. Inhalation anesthetics induce apoptosis in normal peripheral lymphocytes in vitro. *Anesthesiology.* 2001;95:1467–1472.
3. Wiesner G, Hoerauf K, Schroegendorfer K, et al. High-level, but not low-level, occupational exposure to inhaled anesthetics is associated with genotoxicity in the micronucleus assay. *Anesth Analg.* 2001;92:118–122.
4. Chandrasekhar M, Rekhadevi PV, Sailaja N, et al. Evaluation of genetic damage in operating room personnel exposed to anaesthetic gases. *Mutagenesis.* 2006;21:249–254.
5. McGregor DG. Occupational exposure to trace concentrations of waste anesthetic gases. *Mayo Clin Proc.* 2000;75:273–277.
6. Sanders RD, Weimann J, Maze M. Biologic effects of nitrous oxide: A mechanistic and toxicologic review. *Anesthesiology.* 2008;109:707–722.
7. Cohen EN, Bellville JW, Brown BW Jr. Anesthesia, pregnancy, and miscarriage: A study of operating room nurses and anesthetists. *Anesthesiology.* 1971;35:343–347.
8. Occupational disease among operating room personnel: A national study. Report of an Ad Hoc Committee on the Effect of Trace Anesthetics on the Health of Operating Room Personnel, American Society of Anesthesiologists. *Anesthesiology.* 1974;41:321–340.
9. Buring JE, Hennekens CH, Mayrent SL, et al. Health experiences of operating room personnel. *Anesthesiology.* 1985;62:325–330.
10. Rowland AS, Baird DD, Shore DL, et al. Nitrous oxide and spontaneous abortion in female dental assistants. *Am J Epidemiol.* 1995;141:531–538.
11. Rowland AS, Baird DD, Weinberg CR, et al. Reduced fertility among women employed as dental assistants exposed to high levels of nitrous oxide. *N Engl J Med.* 1992;327:993–997.
12. Shirangi A, Fritschi L, Holman CD. Associations of unscavenged anesthetic gases and long working hours with preterm delivery in female veterinarians. *Obstet Gynecol.* 2009;113:1008–1017.
13. Shirangi A, Fritschi L, Holman CD, et al. Birth defects in offspring of female veterinarians. *J Occup Environ Med.* 2009;51:525–33.
14. Boivin JF. Risk of spontaneous abortion in women occupationally exposed to anaesthetic gases: A meta-analysis. *Occup Environ Med.* 1997;54:541–548.
15. Axelsson G, Ahlborg G Jr, Bodin L. Shift work, nitrous oxide exposure, and spontaneous abortion among Swedish midwives. *Occup Environ Med.* 1996;53:374–378.
16. Luke B, Mamelle N, Keith L, et al. The association between occupational factors and preterm birth: A United States nurses' study. Research Committee of the Association of Women's Health, Obstetric, and Neonatal Nurses. *Am J Obstet Gynecol.* 1995;173:849–862.
17. Bruce DL, Eide KA, Linde HW, et al. Causes of death among anesthesiologists: A 20-year survey. *Anesthesiology.* 1968;29:565–569.
18. Bruce DL, Eide KA, Smith NJ, et al. A prospective survey of anesthesiologist mortality, 1967–1971. *Anesthesiology.* 1974;41:71–74.
19. Alexander BH, Checkoway H, Nagahama SI, et al. Cause-specific mortality risks of anesthesiologists. *Anesthesiology.* 2000;93:922–930.
20. National Institute for Occupational Safety and Health (NIOSH): Criteria for a Recommended Standard: Occupational Exposure to Waste Anesthetic Gases and Vapors. Cincinnati, Ohio, Department of Health, Education, and Welfare (NIOSH), Publication No. 77-140. 1977.
21. Ozer M, Baris S, Karakaya D, et al. Behavioural effects of chronic exposure to subanesthetic concentrations of halothane, sevoflurane and desflurane in rats. *Can J Anaesth.* 2006;53:653–658.
22. Zacny JP, Yajnik S, Lichtor JL, et al. The acute and residual effects of subanesthetic concentrations of isoflurane/nitrous oxide combinations on cognitive and psychomotor performance in healthy volunteers. *Anesth Analg.* 1996;82:153–157.
23. Dreyfus E, Tramoni E, Lehucher-Michel MP. Persistent cognitive functioning deficits in operating rooms: Two cases. *Int Arch Occup Environ Health.* 2008;82:125–130.
24. Linde HW, Bruce DL. Occupational exposure of anesthetists to halothane, nitrous oxide and radiation. *Anesthesiology.* 1969;30:363–368.
25. Panni MK, Corn SB. Scavenging in the operating room. *Curr Opin Anesthesiol.* 2003;16:611–617.
26. Sessler DI, Badgwell JM. Exposure of postoperative nurses to exhaled anesthetic gases. *Anesth Analg.* 1998;87:1083–1088.
27. McGregor DG, Senjem DH, Mazze RI. Trace nitrous oxide levels in the postanesthesia care unit. *Anesth Analg.* 1999;89:472–475.
28. NIOSH Alert: Request for Assistance in Controlling Exposures to Nitrous Oxide During Anesthetic Administration. Cincinnati, Ohio, DHHS (NIOSH) Publication No. 94-100, 1994.
29. Sadoh DR, Sharief MK, Howard RS. Occupational exposure to methyl methacrylate monomer induces generalised neuropathy in a dental technician. *Br Dent J.* 1999;186:380–381.
30. Klatskin G, Kimberg DV. Recurrent hepatitis attributable to halothane sensitization in an anesthetist. *N Engl J Med.* 1969;280:515–522.
31. Vellore AD, Drought VJ, Sherwood-Jones D, et al. Occupational asthma and allergy to sevoflurane and isoflurane in anaesthetic staff. *Allergy.* 2006;61:1485–1486.
32. Njoku DB, Greenberg RS, Bourdi M, et al. Autoantibodies associated with volatile anesthetic hepatitis found in the sera of a large cohort of pediatric anesthesiologists. *Anesth Analg.* 2002;94:243–249.
33. Brown RH, Schauble JF, Hamilton RG. Prevalence of latex allergy among anesthesiologists: Identification of sensitized but asymptomatic individuals. *Anesthesiology.* 1998;89:292–299.
34. Occupational Safety and Health Administration, United States Department of Labor. Maximum Permissible Dose Equivalent for Occupational Exposure. http://www.osha.gov/SLTC/radiationionizing/introtoionizing/ionizingattachmentsix.html. Accessed 12/1/2011.
35. McGowan C, Heaton B, Stephenson RN. Occupational x-ray exposure of anaesthetists. *Br J Anaesth.* 1996;76:868–869.

36. Anastasian ZH, Strozyk D, Meyers PM, et al. Radiation exposure of the anesthesiologist in the neurointerventional suite. *Anesthesiology.* 2011;114:512–520.
37. Ismail S, Khan F, Sultan N, et al. Radiation exposure to anaesthetists during interventional radiology. *Anaesthesia.* 2010;65:54–60.
38. Katz JD. Radiation exposure to anesthesia personnel: The impact of an electrophysiology laboratory. *Anesth Analg.* 2005;101:1725–1726.
39. van Rongen E, Saunders RD, van Deventer ET, et al. Static fields: Biological effects and mechanisms relevant to exposure limits. *Health Phys.* 2007;92:584–590.
40. Occupational Safety and Health Administration. Occupational Noise Exposure. Standards 29CFR.1910.95(b)(2) 2008. June 3, 2010.
41. Kracht JM, Busch-Vishniac IJ, West JE. Noise in the operating rooms of Johns Hopkins Hospital. *J Acoust Soc Am.* 2007;121:2673–2680.
42. Wallace MS, Ashman MN, Matjasko MJ. Hearing acuity of anesthesiologists and alarm detection. *Anesthesiology.* 1994;81:13–28.
43. Nilsson U, Unosson M, Rawal N. Stress reduction and analgesia in patients exposed to calming music postoperatively: A randomized controlled trial. *Eur J Anaesthesiol.* 2005;22:96–102.
44. Allen K, Blascovich J. Effects of music on cardiovascular reactivity among surgeons. *JAMA.* 1994;272:882–884.
45. Weinger MB, Herndon OW, Gaba DM. The effect of electronic record keeping and transesophageal echocardiography on task distribution, workload, and vigilance during cardiac anesthesia. *Anesthesiology.* 1997;87:144–155.
46. Edworthy J, Hellier E. Alarms and human behaviour: Implications for medical alarms. *Br J Anaesth.* 2006;97:12–17.
47. Breen CM, Abernethy AP, Abbott KH, Tulsky JA. Conflict associated with decisions to limit life-sustaining treatment in intensive care units. *J Gen Intern Med.* 2001;16:283–289.
48. Katz JD. Conflict and its resolution in the operating room. *J Clin Anesth.* 2007;19:152–158.
49. Helmreich RL, Merritt AC, Wilhelm JA. The evolution of crew resource management training in commercial aviation. *Int J Aviat Psychol.* 1999;9:19–32.
50. Gaba DM, Howard SK, Jump B. Production pressure in the work environment: California anesthesiologists' attitudes and experiences. *Anesthesiology.* 1994;81:488–500.
51. Gaba DM, Howard SK, Fish KJ, et al. Simulation-based training in anesthesia crisis resource management (ARCM). A decade of experience. *Simul Gaming.* 2001;32:175–193.
52. Fisman DN, Harris AD, Rubin M, et al. Fatigue increases the risk of injury from sharp devices in medical trainees: Results from a case-crossover study. *Infect Control Hosp Epidemiol.* 2007;28:10–17.
53. Dawson D, Reid K. Fatigue, alcohol and performance impairment. *Nature.* 1997;388:235.
54. King AC, Belenky G, Van Dongen HP. Performance impairment consequent to sleep loss: Determinants of resistance and susceptibility. *Curr Opin Pulm Med.* 2009 15(6):559–564.
55. Barger LK, Ayas NT, Cade BE, et al. Impact of extended-duration shifts on medical errors, adverse events, and attentional failures. *PLoS Med.* 2006;3(12):e487. doi:10.1371/journal. pmed.0030487 (http://www.plosmedicine.org/article/info:doi/10.1371/journal.pmed.0030487).
56. Friedman RC, Bigger JT, Cornfield DS. The intern and sleep loss. *New Engl J Med.* 1971;285:201–203.
57. Smith-Coggins R, Rosekind MR, Hurd S, Buccino KR. Relationship of day versus night sleep to physician performance and mood. *Ann Emerg Med.* 1994;24: 928–934.
58. Landrigan CP, Rothschild JM, Cronin JW, et al. Effect of reducing interns' work hours on serious medical errors in intensive care units. *N Engl J Med.* 2004;351:1838–1848.
59. Howard SK, Gaba DM, Smith BE, et al. Simulation study of rested versus sleep-deprived anesthesiologists. *Anesthesiology.* 2003;98:1345–1355.
60. Howard SK, Gaba DM, Rosekind MR, Zarcone VP. The risks and implications of excessive daytime sleepiness in resident physicians. *Acad Med.* 2002;77:1019–1025.
61. Gravenstein JS, Cooper JB, Orkin FK. Work and rest cycles in anesthesia practice. *Anesthesiology.* 1990;72:737–742.
62. Gander PH, Merry A, Millar MM, et al. Hours of work and fatigue-related error: A survey of New Zealand anaesthetists. *Anaesth Intens Care.* 2000;28:178–183.
63. Gawande AA, Zinner MJ, Studdert DM, Brennan TA. Analysis of errors reported by surgeons at three teaching hospitals. *Surgery.* 2003;133:614–621.
64. Haynes DF, Schwedler M, Dyslin DC, et al. Are postoperative complications related to resident sleep deprivation? *South Med J.* 1995;88:283–289.
65. Chu MW, Stitt LW, Fox SA, et al. Prospective evaluation of consultant surgeon sleep deprivation and outcomes in more than 4000 consecutive cardiac surgical procedures. *Arch Surg.* 2011;146:1080–1085.
66. Ellman PI, Law MG, Tache-Leon C, et al. Sleep deprivation does not affect operative results in cardiac surgery. *Ann Thorac Surg.* 2004;78:906–911.
67. Schieman C, MacLean AR, Buie WD, et al. Does surgeon fatigue influence outcomes after anterior resection for rectal cancer? *Am J Surg.* 2008;195:684–687.
68. Rothschild JM, Keohane CA, Rogers S, et al. Risks of complications by attending physicians after performing nighttime procedures. *JAMA.* 2009;302:1565–1572.
69. The Accreditation Council for Graduate Medical Education (ACGME): Common Program Requirements, Effective: July 1, 2011 (approved: September 26, 2010). Accreditation Council for Graduate Medical Education. http://www.acgme-2010standards.org/approved-standards.html. Accessed: November 27/2011.
70. Caldwell JA, Caldwell JL. Fatigue in military aviation: An overview of US military-approved pharmacological countermeasures. *Aviat Space Envir Med.* 2005;76:C39–C51.
71. Katz JD. Hand washing and hand disinfection: More than your mother taught you. *Anesthesiol Clin North Am.* 2004;22:457–471.
72. Recommended adult immunization schedule: United States, 2011. *Ann Intern Med.* 2011;154:168–173.
73. What's new in the updated U.S. Public Health Service guidelines for the management of occupational exposures to HIV and recommendations for postexposure prophylaxis? *J Occup Environ Med.* 2006;48:750.
74. Updated U.S. Public Health Service Guidelines for the Management of Occupational Exposures to HBV, HCV, and HIV and Recommendations for Postexposure Prophylaxis. *MMWR Recomm Rep.* 2001;50:1.
75. Bolyard EA, Tablan OC, Williams WW, et al. Guideline for infection control in healthcare personnel, 1998. Hospital Infection Control Practices Advisory Committee. *Infect Control Hosp Epidemiol.* 1998;19:407–463.
76. Prevention and control of influenza with vaccines: Recommendations of the Advisory Committee on Immunization Practices (ACIP), 2011. *MMWR Morb Mortal Wkly Rep.* 2011;60:1128.
77. Siegel JD, Rhinehart E, Jackson M, et al. 2007 Guideline for Isolation Precautions: Preventing Transmission of Infectious Agents in Health Care Settings. *Am J Infect Control.* 2007;35:S65–S164.
78. Department of Labor, Occupational Safety and Health Administration: Occupational exposure to bloodborne pathogens: Needle-sticks and other sharp injuries: Final rule (29 CFR Part 1910.1030). *Fed Reg.* 2001;66:5318;.
79. Talbot T, Babcock H, Caplan A, et al. Revised SHEA position paper: Influenza vaccination of healthcare personnel. *Infect Control Hosp Epidemiol.* 2010;31: 987–995.
80. Abdel-Ghafar AN, Chotpitayasunondh T, Gao Z, et al. Update on avian influenza A (H5N1) virus infection in humans. *N Engl J Med.* 2008;358:261–273.
81. Tablan OC, Anderson LJ, Besser R, et al. Guidelines for preventing health-care–associated pneumonia, 2003: Recommendations of CDC and the Healthcare Infection Control Practices Advisory Committee. *MMWR Recomm Rep.* 2004;53: 1.
82. Falsey AR, Hennessey PA, Formica MA, et al. Respiratory syncytial virus infection in elderly and high-risk adults. *N Engl J Med.* 2005;352:1749–1759.
83. Severe acute respiratory syndrome—Singapore, 2003. *MMWR Morb Mortal Wkly Rep.* 2003;52:405.
84. Frenkel L, Garratty E, Shen J, et al. Clinical reactivation of herpes simplex virus type 2 infection in seropositive pregnant women with no history of genital herpes. *Ann Int Med.* 1993;118:414–418.
85. Marin M, Guris D, Chaves SS, et al. Prevention of varicella: Recommendations of the Advisory Committee on Immunization Practices (ACIP). *MMWR Recomm Rep.* 2007;56:1.
86. Recommended adult immunization schedule—United States, 2011. *MMWR Morb Mortal Wkly Rep.* 2011;60.
87. Watson JC, Hadler SC, Dykewicz CA, et al. Measles, mumps, and rubella–vaccine use and strategies for elimination of measles, rubella, and congenital rubella syndrome and control of mumps: Recommendations of the Advisory Committee on Immunization Practices (ACIP). *MMWR Recomm Rep.* 1998;47:1.
88. Fiore A, Wasley A, Bell B. Prevention of hepatitis A through active or passive immunization: Recommendations of the Advisory Committee on Immunization Practices (ACIP). *MMWR Morb Mortal Wkly Rep.* 2006;55:1.
89. Wasley A, Kruszon-Moran D, Kuhnert W, et al. The prevalence of hepatitis B virus infection in the United States in the era of vaccination. *J Infect Dis.* 2010;202:192–201.
90. Scott JD, Gretch DR. Molecular diagnostics of hepatitis C virus infection: A systematic review. *JAMA.* 2007;297:724–732.
91. Management of hepatitis C: 2002. *NIH Consens State Sci Statements.* 2002;19:1–46.
92. Hoofnagle JH, Seeff LB. Peginterferon and ribavirin for chronic hepatitis C. *N Engl J Med.* 2006;355:2444–2451.
93. Global Report: UNAIDS Report on the Global AIDS Epidemic 2010. Geneva: United Nations; 2010.
94. Bell DM. Occupational risk of human immunodeficiency virus infection in healthcare workers: An overview. *Am J Med.* 1997;102:9–15.
95. Ippolito G, Puro V, De Carli G. The risk of occupational human immunodeficiency virus infection in health care workers. Italian Multicenter Study. The Italian Study Group on Occupational Risk of HIV infection. *Arch Intern Med.* 1993;153:1451–1458.
96. Greene ES, Berry AJ, Jagger J, et al. Multicenter study of contaminated percutaneous injuries in anesthesia personnel. *Anesthesiology.* 1998;89:1362–1372.
97. Task Force on Infection Control of the Committee on Occupational Health of Operating Room Personnel. *Recommendations for Infection Control for the Practice of Anesthesiology,* 3rd ed. Park Ridge, IL: American Society of Anesthesiologists; 2011.
98. Greene ES, Berry AJ, Arnold WP 3rd, et al. Percutaneous injuries in anesthesia personnel. *Anesth Analg.* 1996;83:273–278.
99. Cicsiclski C, Marianos D, Ou C, et al. Transmission of human immunodeficiency virus in a dental practice. *Ann Intern Med.* 1992;116:798–805.

100. Barr S. The 1990 Florida Dental Investigation: Is the case really closed? *Ann Intern Med.* 1996;124:250–254.
101. Collignon P, Shields J, Chant K, et al. Patient-to-patient transmission of HIV. *Lancet.* 1994;343:415–416.
102. Panlilio AL, Cardo DM, Grohskopf LA, et al. Updated U.S. Public Health Service guidelines for the management of occupational exposures to HIV and recommendations for postexposure prophylaxis. *MMWR Recomm Rep.* 2005;54:1.
103. Johnson RT, Gibbs CJ, Jr. Creutzfeldt–Jakob disease and related transmissible spongiform encephalopathies. *N Engl J Med.* 1998;339:1994–2004.
104. Rutala W, Weber D. Guideline for disinfection and sterilization of prion-contaminated medical instruments. *Infect Control Hosp Epidemiol.* 2010;31:107–117.
105. Blumberg H, Burman W, Chaisson R, et al. American Thoracic Society/Centers for Disease Control and Prevention/Infectious Diseases Society of America: Treatment of tuberculosis. *Am J Respir Crit Care Med.* 2003;167:603–662.
106. Jensen P, Lambert L, Iademarco M, Ridzon R. Guidelines for preventing the transmission of Mycobacterium tuberculosis in health-care settings, 2005. *MMWR Recomm Rep.* 2005;54:1.
107. United States Department of Health and Human Services: 42 CRF Part 84: Respiratory protective devices; final rule and notice. *Fed Reg.* 1995;60:30336.
108. Matchette LS, Faaland RW, Royston DD, et al. In vitro production of viable bacteriophage in carbon dioxide and argon laser plumes. *Lasers Surg Med.* 1991;11:380–384.
109. Hallmo P, Naess O. Laryngeal papillomatosis with human papillomavirus DNA contracted by a laser surgeon. *Eur Arch Otorhinolaryngol.* 1991;248:425–427.
110. Sehulster L, Chinn RY. Guidelines for environmental infection control in health-care facilities. Recommendations of CDC and the Healthcare Infection Control Practices Advisory Committee (HICPAC). *MMWR Recomm Rep.* 2003;52:1.
111. Selye H. *The Stress of Life.* New York, NY: McGraw- Hill Book Co; 1984.
112. Jackson SH. The role of stress in anaesthetists' health and well-being. *Acta Anaesthesiol Scand.* 1999;43:583–602.
113. Kain ZN, Chan KM, Katz JD, et al. Anesthesiologists and acute perioperative stress: A cohort study. *Anesth Analg.* 2002;95:177–183.
114. Gaba DM. Crisis resource management and teamwork training in anaesthesia. *Br J Anaesth.* 2010;105:3–6.
115. McDonald JS, Lingam RP, Gupta B, et al. Psychologic testing as an aid to selection of residents in anesthesiology. *Anesth Analg.* 1994;78:542–547.
116. Vaillant GE, Brighton JR, McArthur C. Physicians' use of mood-altering drugs. A 20-year follow-up report. *N Engl J Med.* 1970;282:365–370.
117. Jones JW, Barge BN, Steffy BD, et al. Stress and medical malpractice: Organizational risk assessment and intervention. *J Appl Psychol.* 1988;73:727–735.
118. Shanafelt TD, Balch CM, Bechamps G, et al. Burnout and medical errors among American surgeons. *Ann Surg.* 2010;251:995–1000.
119. Haas JS, Cook EF, Puopolo AL, et al. Is the professional satisfaction of general internists associated with patient satisfaction? *J Gen Intern Med.* 2000;15:122–128.
120. Melamed S, Shirom A, Toker S, et al. Burnout and risk of cardiovascular disease: Evidence, possible causal paths, and promising research directions. *Psychol Bull.* 2006;132:327–353.
121. McCall SV. Chemically dependent health professionals. *West J Med.* 2001;174:50–54.
122. De Oliveira GS Jr, Ahmad S, Stock MC, et al. High incidence of burnout in academic chairpersons of *Anesthesiology:* Should we be taking better care of our leaders? *Anesthesiology.* 2011;114:181–193.
123. Hyman SA, Michaels DR, Berry JM, et al. Risk of burnout in perioperative clinicians: A survey study and literature review. *Anesthesiology.* 2011;114:194–204.
124. Nyssen AS, Hansez I, Baele P, et al. Occupational stress and burnout in anaesthesia. *Br J Anaesth.* 2003;90:333–337.
125. Hughes PH, Baldwin DC Jr, Sheehan DV, et al. Resident physician substance use, by specialty. *Am J Psychiatry.* 1992;149:1348–1354.
126. Hughes PH, Brandenburg N, Baldwin DC Jr, et al. Prevalence of substance use among US physicians. *JAMA.* 1992;267:2333–2339.
127. Lutsky I, Hopwood M, Abram SE, et al. Use of psychoactive substances in three medical specialties: Anaesthesia, medicine and surgery. *Can J Anaesth.* 1994;41:561–567.
128. Hughes PH, Storr CL, Brandenburg NA, et al. Physician substance use by medical specialty. *J Addict Dis.* 1999;18:23–37.
129. Gold MS, Melker RJ, Dennis DM, et al. Fentanyl abuse and dependence: Further evidence for second hand exposure hypothesis. *J Addict Dis.* 2006;25:15–21.
130. McLellan AT, Skipper GS, Campbell M, et al. Five year outcomes in a cohort study of physicians treated for substance use disorders in the United States. *Br Med J.* 2008;337:a2038.
131. Talbott GD, Gallegos KV, Wilson PO, et al. The Medical Association of Georgia's Impaired Physicians Program. Review of the first 1000 physicians: Analysis of specialty. *JAMA.* 1987;257:2927–2930.
132. Paris RT, Canavan DI. Physician substance abuse impairment: Anesthesiologists vs. other specialties. *J Addict Dis.* 1999;18:1–7.
133. Lutsky I, Abram SE, Jacobson GR, et al. Substance abuse by anesthesiology residents. *Acad Med.* 1991;66:164–166.
134. Booth JV, Grossman D, Moore J, et al. Substance abuse among physicians: A survey of academic *Anesthesiology* programs. *Anesth Analg.* 2002;95:1024–1030.
135. Collins GB, McAllister MS, Jensen M, et al. Chemical dependency treatment outcomes of residents in *Anesthesiology:* Results of a survey. *Anesth Analg.* 2005;101:1457–1462.
136. Skipper GE, Campbell MD, Dupont RL. Anesthesiologists with substance use disorders: A 5-year outcome study from 16 state physician health programs. *Anesth Analg.* 2009;109:891–896.
137. Moore RD, Mead L, Pearson TA. Youthful precursors of alcohol abuse in physicians. *Am J Med.* 1990;88:332–336.
138. Wischmeyer PE, Johnson BR, Wilson JE, et al. A survey of propofol abuse in academic anesthesia programs. *Anesth Analg.* 2007;105:1066–1071.
139. Yarborough WH. Substance use disorders in physician training programs. *J Okla State Med Assoc.* 1999;92:504–507.
140. Menk EJ, Baumgarten RK, Kingsley CP, et al. Success of reentry into anesthesiology training programs by residents with a history of substance abuse. *JAMA.* 1990;263:3060–3062.
141. Scott M, Fisher KS. The evolving legal context for drug testing programs. *Anesthesiology.* 1990;73:1022–1027.
142. Berge KH, Seppala MD, Lanier WL. The anesthesiology community's approach to opioid- and anesthetic-abusing personnel: Time to change course. *Anesthesiology.* 2008;109:762–764.
143. Marshall EJ. Doctors' health and fitness to practice: Treating addicted doctors. *Occup Med (Lond).* 2008;58:334–340.
144. Domino KB, Hornbein TF, Polissar NL, et al. Risk factors for relapse in health care professionals with substance use disorders. *JAMA.* 2005;293:1453–1460.
145. Task Force on Chemical Dependence of the Committee on Occupational Health of Operating Room Personnel. *Chemical Dependence in Anesthesiologists: What You Need to Know When You Need to Know It.* Park Ridge, IL: American Society of Anesthesiologists; 1998.
146. Angres DH, Talbott GD, Bettinardi-Angres K. Anesthesiologist's Return to Practice, in *Healing the Healer: The Addicted Physician.* Madison, CT: Psychosocial Press; 1998.
147. Epstein RH, Gratch DM, McNulty S, et al. Validation of a system to detect scheduled drug diversion by anesthesia care providers. *Anesth Analg.* 2011;113:160–164.
148. Bissell L, Jones RW. The alcoholic physician: A survey. *Am J Psychiatry.* 1976;133:1142–1146.
149. Clark DC, Eckenfels EJ, Daugherty SR, et al. Alcohol-use patterns through medical school. A longitudinal study of one class. *JAMA.* 1987;257:2921–2926.
150. Atkinson RS. The problem of the unsafe anaesthetist. *Br J Anaesth.* 1994;73:29–30.
151. Canavan DI, Baxter LE Sr. The twentieth anniversary of the Physicians' Health Program of the Medical Society of New Jersey. *N J Med.* 2003;100:27–29.
152. Katz JD. Issues of concern for the aging anesthesiologist. *Anesth Analg.* 2001;92:1487–1492.
153. Eva KW. The aging physician: Changes in cognitive processing and their impact on medical practice. *Acad Med.* 2002;77:S1–S6.
154. Travis KW, Mihevc NT, Orkin FK, et al. Age and anesthetic practice: A regional perspective. *J Clin Anesth.* 1999;11:175–186.
155. Dimick JB, Birkmeyer JD, Upchurch GR Jr. Measuring surgical quality: What's the role of provider volume? *World J Surg.* 2005;29:1217–1221.
156. Weinger M. Experience not equal expertise: Can simulation be used to tell the difference? *Anesthesiology.* 2007;107:691–694.
157. McNamee R, Keen RI, Corkill CM. Morbidity and early retirement among anaesthetists and other specialists. *Anaesthesia.* 1987;42:133–140.
158. Katz JD. Do anesthesiologists die at a younger age than other physicians? Age-adjusted death rates. *Anesth Analg.* 2004;98:1111–1113.
159. Svardsudd K, Wedel H, Gordh T. Mortality rates among Swedish physicians: A population-based nationwide study with special reference to anesthesiologists. *Acta Anaesthesiol Scand.* 2002;46:1187–1195.
160. Mostafa MS, Freeman RA. The specialty of physicians in relation to longevity and mortality, 1978-1979. *Ala Med.* 1985;54:13–8, 23.
161. Carpenter LM, Swerdlow AJ, Fear NT. Mortality of doctors in different 1: Findings from a cohort of 20000 NHS hospital consultants. *Occup Environ Med.* 1997;54:388–395.
162. Lew EA. Mortality experiences among anesthesiologists, 1954–1976. *Anesthesiology.* 1979;51:195–199.
163. Katz JD, Slade MD. Anesthesiologists are living longer: Mortality experience 1992 to 2001. *J Clin Anesth.* 2006;18:405–408.
164. Center C, Davis M, Detre T, et al. Confronting depression and suicide in physicians: A consensus statement. *JAMA.* 2003;289:3161–3166.
165. North CS, Ryall JE. Psychiatric illness in female physicians. Are high rates of depression an occupational hazard? *Postgrad Med.* 1997;101:233–236, 239–240, 242.
166. Birmingham PK, Ward RJ. A high-risk suicide group: The anesthesiologist involved in litigation. *Am J Psychiatry.* 1985;142:1225–1228.
167. Boxer PA, Burnett C, Swanson N. Suicide and occupation: A review of the literature. *J Occup Environ Med.* 1995;37:442–452.
168. Hammen C. Stress and depression. *Annu Rev Clin Psychol.* 2005;1:293–319.
169. Reeve PE. Personality characteristics of a sample of anaesthetists. *Anaesthesia.* 1980;35:559–568.

170. Crawshaw R, Bruce JA, Eraker PL, et al. An epidemic of suicide among physicians on probation. *JAMA.* 1980;243:1915–1917.
171. *Guidelines for the Ethical Practice of Anesthesiology.* Chicago: American Society of Anesthesiologists; 2008.
172. McGinnis J, Foege W. Actual causes of death in the United States. *JAMA.* 1993; 270:2207–2212.
173. Mokdad A, Marks J, Stroup D, et al. Actual causes of death in the United States, 2000. *JAMA.* 2004;291:1238–1245.
174. Hossain P, Kawar B, El Nahas M. Obesity and diabetes in the developing world—a growing challenge. *N Engl J Med.* 2007;356:213–215.
175. Rabe K, Lehrke M, Parhofer K, et al. Adipokines and insulin resistance. *Mol Med.* 2008;14:741–751.
176. Lee C, Klopp R, Weindruch R, et al. Gene expression profile of aging and its retardation by caloric restriction. *Science.* 1999;285:1390–1393.
177. Hansen B, ed. *Calorie Restriction: Effects on Body Composition, Insulin Signaling and Aging, Experimental Biology 2000.* San Diego, CA: American Society for Nutritional Sciences; 2000.
178. Park S, Prolla T. Gene expression profiling studies of aging in cardiac and skeletal muscles. *Cardiovasc Res.* 2005;66:205–212.
179. Paffenbarger R. Physical exercise to reduce cardiovascular disease risk. *Proc Nutr Soc.* 2000;59:421–422.
180. Cheng I, Liao S, Liu K, et al. Effect of dietary glycemic index on substrate transporter gene expression in human skeletal muscle after exercise. *Eur J Clin Nutr.* 2009;63:1404–1410.
181. Jenkins N, Witkowski S, Spangenburg E, et al. Effects of acute and chronic endurance exercise on intracellular nitric oxide in putative endothelial progenitor cells: Role of NAPDH oxidase. *Am J Physiol Heart Circ Physiol.* 2009;297:798–805.
182. Ni H, Li C, Tao L, et al. Physical exercise improves learning by modulating hippocampal mossy fiber sprouting and related gene expression in a developmental rat model of penicillin induced recurrent epilepticus. *Toxicol Lett.* 2009;191: 26–32.
183. McTigue K, Hess R, Ziouras J. Obesity in older adults: A systematic review of the evidence for diagnosis and treatment. *Obesity.* 2006;14:1485–1497.
184. Obesity: Weight loss without drugs: A balanced diet avoiding high-calorie foods, plus exercise. *Prescrire Int.* 2007;16:162–167.
185. Nonas C. A model for chronic care of obesity through dietary treatment. *J Am Diet Assoc.* 1998;98:S16–S22.
186. Rippe J, Crossley S, Ringer RJ. Obesity as a chronic disease: Modern medical and lifestyle management. *J Am Diet Assoc.* 1998;98:S9–S15.
187. Avenell A, Broom J, Brown T, et al. Systematic review of the long-term effects and economic consequences of treatments for obesity and implications for health improvement. *Health Technol Assess.* 2004;8:1–182.
188. Weiss E, Galuska D, Kettel Khan L, et al. Weight regain in U.S. adults who experienced substantial weight loss, 1999–2002. *Am J Prev Med.* 2007;33:34–40.
189. Curioni C, Lourenço P. Long-term weight loss after diet and exercise: A systematic review. *Int J Obes (Lond).* 2005;10:1168–1174.
190. Epstein R. Mindful practice. *JAMA.* 1999;282:833–839.
191. Herath P, Klingberg T, Young J, et al. Neural correlates of dual task interference can be dissociated from those of divided attention: An fMRI study. *Cereb Cortex.* 2001;11:796–805.
192. Olesen P, Macoveanu J, Tegnér J, et al. Brain activity related to working memory and distraction in children and adults. *Cereb Cortex.* 2007;17:1047–1054.
193. Olesen P, Westerberg H, Klingberg T. Increased prefrontal and parietal activity after training of working memory. *Nat Neurosci.* 2004;7:75–79.

CHAPTER

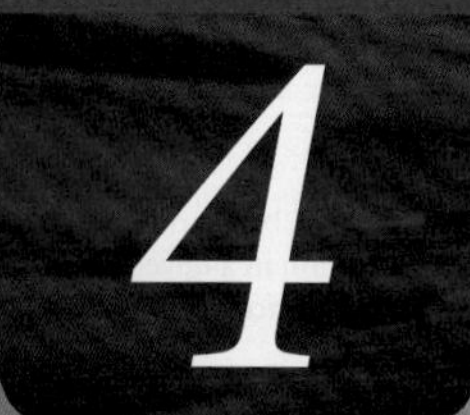

Anesthetic Risk, Quality Improvement, and Liability

KAREN L. POSNER • SAINT ADEOGBA • KAREN B. DOMINO

Key Points

1. Anesthetic mortality has decreased, but accidental deaths and disabling complications still occur.
2. Risk management programs are broadly oriented toward reducing the liability exposure of the organization. Risk management programs complement quality improvement programs in minimizing liability exposure while maximizing quality of patient care.
3. Quality improvement programs are generally guided by the requirements of the Joint Commission that accredits health-care organizations. Quality improvement programs focus on improving the structure, process, and outcome of care.
4. Continuous quality improvement (CQI) is a systems approach to identifying and improving quality of care.
5. Medical malpractice refers to the legal concept of professional negligence. The patient-plaintiff must prove that the anesthesiologist owed the patient a duty and failed to fulfill this duty, that the anesthesiologist's actions caused an injury, and that the injury resulted from a breach in the standard of anesthesia care.
6. The most common lawsuits against anesthesiologists (excluding dental injuries) are for death, brain damage, nerve damage, and airway injury. Chronic pain management is an increasing source of malpractice claims against anesthesiologists.

Multimedia

1 Rates of Selected Anesthetic Complications

2 Accident Causation

In anesthesia, as in other areas of life, everything does not always go as planned. Undesirable outcomes occur regardless of the quality of care provided. An anesthesia risk management program can work in conjunction with a program for quality improvement to minimize the liability risk of practice, while assuring the highest quality of care for patients. Payers such as Medicare are increasingly depending on accreditation through bodies such as the Joint Commission to ensure that mechanisms are in place to deliver quality and safe care to all patients. In addition, there has been a move toward performance measurement linked to reimbursement. The legal aspects of American medical practice have also become increasingly important as the public has turned to the courts for economic redress when their expectations of medical treatment are not met.

This chapter discusses anesthetic mortality and morbidity, risk management, continuous quality improvement (CQI), performance measurement, and medical liability. The chapter provides background for the practitioner concerning the role of risk management activity in minimizing and managing liability exposure. Also described are the medical legal system, the most frequent causes of lawsuits for anesthesiologists, and appropriate actions for physicians to take in the event of a malpractice suit.

ANESTHESIA RISK

Mortality and Major Morbidity Related to Anesthesia

1 Estimates of anesthesia-related morbidity and mortality are difficult to quantify. Not only are there difficulties obtaining data on complications, but different methods yield different estimates of anesthesia risk. Studies differ in their definitions of complications, in length of follow-up, and especially in approaches to evaluation of the contribution of anesthesia care to patient outcomes. A comprehensive review of anesthesia complications is beyond the scope of this chapter. A sampling of studies of anesthesia mortality and morbidity will be presented to provide historical perspective plus a limited overview of relatively recent findings.

Early studies estimated the anesthesia-related mortality rate as 1 per 1,560 anesthetics.[1] More recent studies using data from the 1990s and later estimate the anesthesia-related death rate in the United States to be <1 per 10,000 anesthetics.[2–6] Some examples of modern estimates of anesthesia-related death from throughout the world are provided in Table 4-1.[2–19] Differences in estimates may be influenced by different reporting methods, definitions, anesthesia practices, patient population, as well as actual differences in underlying complication rates. Nevertheless, it is generally accepted that anesthesia safety has improved over the past 50+ years.

1 Other complications related to anesthesia that have received relatively recent attention include postoperative nerve injury, awareness during general anesthesia, eye injuries and visual deficits, dental injury, and postoperative cognitive dysfunction in elderly patients (Table 4-2).[20–42] The incidence of ulnar neuropathy has been estimated to be 47 per 10,000 patients (Table 4-2).[21] Lower extremity neuropathy following surgery in the lithotomy position was observed in 151 per 10,000 patients (Table 4-2).[22] Permanent neurologic injury following neuraxial anesthesia was estimated at 0 to 4.2 per 10,000 spinal anesthetics and 0 to 7.6 per 10,000 epidural anesthetics.[20,24,25] Peripheral nerve injury following peripheral nerve blocks was estimated to occur at a rate of 1.7 to 4.2 per 10,000 anesthetics.[23,24,26] Awareness during general anesthesia has been estimated to occur in 15 to 100 per 10,000 patients.[27–31]

Eye injuries are a risk of anesthesia, including corneal abrasions as well as more rare complications such as blindness from ischemic optic neuropathy or central retinal artery occlusion (Table 4-2).[32–39] Corneal abrasion has occurred at a rate of 1.4 to 15.1 per 10,000 procedures.[32,34,39] Ischemic optic neuropathy has been observed at 0.57 to 2.8 per 10,000 spine surgeries.[32,35] Risk factors for ischemic optic neuropathy after spinal fusion have recently been identified and include a variety of patient, surgical, and anesthetic factors.[43] Among these include use of a Wilson surgical bed frame, obesity, and long anesthetic durations. All can contribute to increased venous congestion in the optic canal and potentially reduce optic nerve perfusion pressure. There was insufficient evidence to conclude that intraoperative anemia or transient periods of hypotension were causative factors.

Damage to teeth or dentures is perhaps the most common injury leading to anesthesia malpractice claims. Dental injury complaints are usually resolved by a hospital risk management department. Dental injuries after general endotracheal anesthesia were observed in 3.6 per 10,000 patients in the United States.[40]

Cognitive dysfunction is observed in many adult patients after major surgery, but only the elderly are at significant risk for long-term cognitive problems.[44] The cause for postoperative cognitive dysfunction is unknown.

Risk Management

Conceptual Introduction

2 Risk management and quality improvement programs work hand in hand to minimize liability exposure while maximizing quality of patient care. Although the functions of these programs vary from one institution to another, they overlap in their focus on patient safety. They can generally be distinguished by their basic
2 difference in orientation. A hospital risk management program is broadly oriented toward reducing the liability exposure of the organization. This includes not only professional liability (and therefore patient safety) but also contracts, employee safety, public safety, and any other liability exposure of the institution. Quality improvement programs have as their main goal the continuous maintenance and improvement of the quality of patient care. These programs may be broader in their patient safety focus than strictly risk management. Quality improvement (sometimes called *patient safety*) departments are responsible for providing the resources to provide safe, patient-centered, timely, efficient, effective, and equitable patient care.[45]

Risk Management in Anesthesia

Those aspects of risk management that are most directly relevant to the liability exposure of the anesthesiologist include prevention of patient injury, adherence to standards of care, documentation, and patient relations.

The key factors in the prevention of patient injury are vigilance, up-to-date knowledge, and adequate monitoring.[46] Physiologic monitoring of cardiopulmonary function, combined with monitoring of equipment function, might be expected to reduce anesthetic injury to a minimum. This was the rationale for the adoption by the American Society of Anesthesiologists (ASA) of *Standards for Basic Anesthetic Monitoring*.[a] Detailed information on anesthesia monitoring techniques can be found in Chapter 25.

The ASA web site should be reviewed yearly for any changes in these standards. It would also be reasonable to review the *Guidelines and Statements* published on the ASA web site. It should be noted that, although membership in the ASA is not required for the practice of anesthesiology, expert witnesses will, with virtual certainty, hold any practitioner to the ASA standards. It is also possible that, as a risk management strategy, a professional liability insurer or hospital may hold an individual anesthesiologist to standards higher than those promulgated by the ASA.

Another risk management tool is the use of checklists to prevent errors. Since the first pilot's checklists were developed for the military, checklists have been adopted by many industries wherein processes are too numerous and/or complex to rely on human memory. A checklist is a simple, yet powerful, tool that ensures no important detail is forgotten, and it removes variability, enhances consistency, and decreases likelihood of error. This patient safety tool helps to remind providers of key steps and thus works to facilitate a safe and effective health-care delivery.

Historically, checklists have been used in anesthesia for anesthesia machine checkout procedures. Information pertaining to anesthesia workstation pre-use procedures as well as safety considerations for workstations can be found in Chapter 24. Recently,

[a]http://www.asahq.org/For-Healthcare-Professionals/Standards-Guidelines-and-Statements.aspx

TABLE 4-1. ESTIMATES OF ANESTHESIA-RELATED DEATH

Reference	Country	Time	Data Sources/ Methods	Rate of Death
Flick et al.[4]	USA	1988–2005	Perioperative cardiac arrest in pediatric patients at a tertiary referral hospital (*n*—92,881 anesthetics)	Anesthesia-attributed deaths—0.22/10,000 anesthetics
Biboulet et al.[7]	France	1989–1995	ASA 1–4 patients undergoing anesthesia (*n*—101,769 anesthetics); cardiac arrest within 12 h postanesthesia (*n*—24)	Anesthesia-related death—0.6/10,000 anesthetics
Newland et al.[2]	USA	1989–1999	Cardiac arrests within 24 h of surgery (*n*—72,959 anesthetics) in a teaching hospital	Death related to anesthesia-attributable perioperative cardiac arrest—0.55/10,000 anesthetics
Eagle and Davis[8]	Western Australia	1990–1995	Deaths within 48 h or deaths in which anesthesia was considered a contributing factor (*n*—500 deaths)	Anesthesia-related death—0.025/10,000 anesthetics
Lagasse[3]	USA	(a) 1992–1994 (b) 1995–1999	(a) Suburban teaching hospital (*n*—115 deaths; *n*—37,924 anesthetics) (b) Urban teaching hospital (*n*—232 deaths; *n*—146,548 anesthetics)	Anesthesia-related death: (a) 0.79/10,000 anesthetics (b) 0.75/10,000 anesthetics
Khan and Khan[9]	Pakistan	1992–2003 (a) 1992–1998 (b) 1999–2003	University hospital. Deaths within 24 h of anesthesia (*n*—111,289 anesthetics)	3.14/10,000 anesthetics; deaths totally attributable to anesthesia 0.35/10,000; anesthesia partially responsible for death 0.7/10,000 (a) 0.68/10,000 anesthetics (b) 0.18/10,000 anesthetics
Ahmed et al.[10]	Pakistan	1992–2006	Perioperative cardiac arrest in pediatric patients at a university hospital (*n*—20,216 anesthetics)	Deaths primarily anesthesia-related 0.49/10,000 anesthetics
Davis[11]	Australia	1994–1996	Deaths reported to the committee (*n*—8,500,000 anesthetics)	Anesthesia-related death—0.16/10,000 anesthetics
Morray et al.[5]	USA	1994–1997	Pediatric patients from 63 hospitals (*n*—1,089,200 anesthetics)	Anesthesia-related death—0.36/10,000 anesthetics
Kawashima et al.[12]	Japan	1994–1998	Questionnaires to training hospitals (*n*—2,363,038 anesthetics)	Death totally attributable to anesthesia—0.21/10,000 anesthetics
Arbous et al.[13]	Holland	1995–1997	All deaths within 24 h or patients who remained unintentionally comatose 24 h postanesthesia (*n*—811 in 869,483 anesthetics)—64 hospitals	Anesthesia-related death—1.4/10,000 anesthetics
Braz et al.[14]	Brazil	1996–2005	Tertiary general teaching hospital (*n*—53,718 anesthetics)	Anesthesia-related death—1.12/10,000 anesthetics Totally attributed—0,56/10,000 Partially attributed—0.56/10,000
Lienhart et al.[15]	France	1999	Nationwide survey of anesthesia-related deaths	Death totally related to anesthesia—0.069/10,000 Death partially related to anesthesia—0.47/10,000
Kawashima et al.[16]	Japan	1999	Questionnaires to training hospitals (*n*—793,840 anesthetics)	Death totally attributable to anesthesia—0.13/10,000 anesthetics
Irita et al.[17]	Japan	1999–2002	Deaths as a result of life-threatening events in the operating room (*n*—3,855,384 anesthetics) in training hospitals	Death totally attributable to anesthetic management—0.1/10,000 anesthetics
Li et al.[6]	USA	1999–2005	Deaths with anesthesia-related complication codes from death certificate data (a) Population data from census records (b) National hospital discharge survey data (inpatients)	Anesthesia-related deaths (a) 1.1/million population/year (b) 8.2/million hospital surgical discharges
Charuluxananan et al.[18]	Thailand	2003–2004	Perioperative deaths within 24 h of surgery—20 hospitals (*n*—163,403 anesthetics)	Death directly related to anesthesia—1.7/10,000 Death partially related to anesthesia—4.0/10,000
Gibbs[19]	Australia	2003–2005	Deaths reported to Anesthesia Mortality Committees (n—5,983,704 anesthetics)	Anesthesia-related deaths 0.19/10,000

TABLE 4-2. RATES OF SELECTED ANESTHESIA COMPLICATIONS

Complication	Reference	Country	Time	Specific Complication	Results
Nerve injury	Brull et al.[20]	Various	1987–1999	Radiculopathy or peripheral neuropathy after spinal anesthesia	3.78/10,000 spinal anesthetics
				Radiculopathy or peripheral neuropathy after epidural anesthesia	2.19/10,000 epidural anesthetics
				Permanent neurologic injury after spinal anesthesia	0–4.2/10,000 spinal anesthetics
				Permanent neurologic injury after epidural anesthetic	0–7.6/10,000 epidural anesthetics
			Varies	Transient neurologic deficit after interscalene block	2.84/10,000 anesthetics
	Warner et al.[21]	USA	1995	Ulnar neuropathy in adults following noncardiac surgery (*n*—1,502)	47/10,000
	Warner et al.[22]	USA	1997–1998	Lower extremity neuropathy in adult patients ≥18 under general anesthesia (GA) while in lithotomy position (*n*—991)	151/10,000
	Welch et al.[23]	USA	1997–2007	Peripheral nerve injury within 48 h of sedation or anesthesia (*n*—380,680)	2.9/10,000
	Auroy et al.[24]	France	1998–1999	Serious peripheral neuropathy related to regional anesthesia	Non-obstetric spinal blocks (SBs) (*n*—35,439): 3.4/10,000 obstetric SBs (*n*—5,640): 3.5/10,000 Upper limb peripheral nerve blocks (PNBs) (*n*—23,784): 1.7/10,000 Lower limb PNBs (*n*—20,162): 4/10,000
	de Sèze et al.[25]	France	2000	Incapacitating neurologic complications lasting ≥3 months after central neuraxial blockade	Non-obstetric SBs (*n*—67,884): 0.15/10,000 Non-obstetric epidural blocks (EBs) (*n*—65,464): 0.015/10,000 obstetric EBs (*n*—116,639): 0.09/10,000
	Barrington et al.[26]	USA	2006–2008	Late neurologic complications after PNB or plexus block (*n*—7,156 blocks)	4.2/10,000 PNBs
Awareness	Errando et al.[27]	Spain	1995–1997 and 1998–2001	Awareness during GA (*n*—3,921)	99.5/10,000
	Sandin et al.[28]	Sweden	1997–1998	Awareness associated with GA (*n*—11,785)	15.3/10,000 procedures
	Sebel et al.[29]	USA	2001–2002	Awareness in patients ≥18 years old in seven academic medical centers (*n*—19,575)	12.8/10,000
	Avidan et al.[30]	USA	2005–2006	Single-center prospective study in patients ≥18 years old (*n*—1,941)	20.6/10,000
	Xu et al.[31]	China	NA	Multicenter cohort study of awareness after GA with muscle relaxants (*n*—11,101)	41.4/10,000

(continued)

TABLE 4-2. RATES OF SELECTED ANESTHESIA COMPLICATIONS (*continued*)

Complication	Reference	Country	Time	Specific Complication	Results
Vision loss and eye injuries	Chang and Miller[32]	USA	1983–2002	Vision loss due to perioperative ischemic optic neuropathy (ION) associated with spine surgery (*n*—14,102)	2.8/10,000
				Corneal abrasions	1.4/10,000
	Warner et al.[33]	USA	1986–1998	New-onset visual loss or visual changes lasting >30 days after noncardiac surgery (*n*—125,234)	0.08/10,000 patients
	Roth et al.[34]	USA	1988–1992	Eye injury after nonocular surgery (*n*—60,965)	5.6/10,000
				Corneal abrasions	3.4/10,000
				ION	0.16/10,000
	Patil et al.[35]	USA	1993–2002	Visual loss or disturbances after spine surgery (*n*—4,728,815)	Any visual disturbance: 9.4/10,000 ION: 0.57/10,000 Central retinal artery occlusion: 0.10/10,000
	Holy et al.[36]	USA	1998–2004	Retrospective chart review for ION (*n*—126,666)	ION: 1.3/10,000
	Shen et al.[37]	USA	1996–2005	Vision loss in surgery	Overall: 2.35/10,000 Cardiac surgery: 8.64/10,000 Spinal fusion: 3.09/10,000 Cholecystectomy 0.66/10,000 Appendectomy: 0.12/10,000
	Warner et al.[38]	USA	1999	New-onset blurred vision lasting ≥3 days (*n*—410,189 patients)	4.6/10,000
	Martin et al.[39]	USA	2005	Postoperative corneal injury (*n*—84,796) Baseline	15.1/10,000
			2006–2007	Performance initiative postoperative corneal injury	7.9/10,000
			2007–2008	Follow-up postoperative corneal injury	4.7/10,000
Dental injury	Warner et al.[40]	USA	1987–1997	Dental injuries within 7 days of anesthesia that required intervention (*n*—4,537)	2.2/10,000
				Dental injury under GA with tracheal intubation (*n*—2,805)	3.6/10,000
	Newland et al.[41]	USA	1989–2003	Dental injury with anesthesia (*n*—161,687 anesthetics)	4.8/10,000
	Gaudio et al.[42]	Italy	2000–2009	Dental injuries in surgical procedures under GA with tracheal intubation (*n*—62,898)	37.4/10,000

checklists for clinical care have been promoted to improve patient safety and medical management in various clinical settings, for example, central venous catheterization, intraoperative emergencies, and perioperative care. Catheter-related bloodstream infections were reduced significantly with the implementation of a standardized process that included a checklist for catheter placement and management.[47] The ASA has recently developed a checklist for central venous catheter access.[48] During simulated emergency scenarios, checklists have improved performance in the management of local anesthesia systemic toxicity[49] and

TABLE 4-3. WORLD HEALTH ORGANIZATION SURGICAL SAFETY CHECKLIST ELEMENTS

Pre-induction
- Patient confirms identity, site, procedure, and consent
- Site marked
- Anesthesia machine and medication check
- Pulse oximeter on and functioning
- Does the patient have
  - Known allergy?
  - Risk for difficult airway or aspiration?

Before incision
- Team members introduce themselves by name and role
- Confirm patient identity, procedure, and incision site
- Antibiotics within last 60 min
- Anticipated critical events:
  - Critical or nonroutine steps in procedure
  - Anticipated duration of surgery
  - Anticipated blood loss
  - Anesthesia concerns
  - Sterility confirmed
  - Equipment issues or concerns
- Essential imaging displayed

Before patient leaves operating room
- Confirm procedure
- Complete instrument, sponge, and needle counts
- Specimens labeled
- Address equipment problems
- What are the key concerns for recovery?

Based on the WHO Surgical Safety Checklist URL http://whqlibdoc.who.int/publications/2009/9789241598590_eng_Checklist.pdf

improved management of intraoperative crises such as malignant hyperthermia or massive hemorrhage.[50]

Perioperative use of the surgical safety checklist in a variety of global hospital settings reduced surgical complications and mortality.[51] In a staged fashion (prior to induction, prior to skin incision, prior to wound closure, and prior to patient leaving the OR), this checklist confirms patient information and presence of personnel, addresses potential case-specific concerns, and incorporates significant processes ranging from a surgical time-out to a post-procedural briefing (see Table 4-3). The surgical safety checklist has been widely incorporated into practice in the United States.

Although it may seem obvious, qualified anesthesia personnel should be in continuous attendance during the conduct of all anesthetics. The only exceptions should be those that lay people (i.e., judge and jury) can understand, such as radiation hazards or an unexpected life-threatening emergency elsewhere. Even then, provisions should be made for monitoring the patient adequately. Adequate supervision of nurse anesthetists and residents is also important, as is good communication with surgeons when adverse anesthetic outcomes occur.

Informed Consent

Informed consent regarding anesthesia should be documented with a general surgical consent, which should include a statement to the effect that "I understand that all anesthetics involve risks of complications, serious injury, or, rarely, death from both known and unknown causes." In addition, there should be a note in the patient's record that the risks of anesthesia and alternatives were discussed and that the patient accepted the proposed anesthetic plan. A brief documentation in the record that the common complications of the proposed technique were discussed is helpful. In some institutions, a separate written anesthesia consent form may be used, which may include more detail about risks. If it is necessary to change the agreed-on anesthesia plan significantly after the patient is premedicated or anesthetized, the reasons for the change should be documented in the record.

Shared decision-making is an enhanced form of informed consent applicable in elective situations when options for treatment are available to the patient. Shared decision-making is a strategy to empower the patient to actively make an evidenced-based choice in his/her treatment.[52] In shared decision-making, evidence-based information is shared with the patient using educational materials ("decision-aids"), and patient preferences and values are elicited during the decision-making process. When all parties are satisfied that they understand the options and expectations, an informed decision can be made regarding treatment.

There is an increasing body of evidence to suggest that sharing of information with patients, particularly when there may have been an adverse outcome, perhaps involving a medical error, can be beneficial. Effective disclosure can improve doctor–patient relations, facilitate better understanding of systems, and potentially decrease medical malpractice costs.[53]

Record Keeping

Good records can form a strong defense if they are adequate; however, records can be disastrous if inadequate. The anesthesia record itself should be as accurate, complete, and neat as possible. The use of automated anesthesia records may be helpful in the defense of malpractice cases, but they may also serve as damaging evidence for the lack of vigilance prior to an adverse event. In addition to documenting vital signs at least every 5 minutes, special attention should be paid to ensure that the patient's ASA classification, monitors used, fluids administered, and doses and times of all administered drugs are accurately charted. Because the principal causes of hypoxic brain damage and death during anesthesia are related to ventilation and/or oxygenation, all respiratory variables that are monitored should be documented accurately. It is important to note when there is a change of anesthesia personnel during the conduct of a case. Sloppy, inaccurate anesthesia records, with gaps during critical events, can be extremely damaging to the defense when enlarged and placed before a jury.

The use of electronic medical records (EMR) has been increasing in health care, and anesthesia information management systems (AIMS) have begun to supplant the traditional anesthesia paper record in the operating room. Basic AIMS are connected to the patient monitors and the anesthesia machine and capture perioperative data specific to anesthesia (e.g., vital signs, times of induction, intubation and emergence, medications and fluids). There is improved patient care and cost savings at institutions where EMR are fully incorporated.[54] When properly configured, AIMS can increase provider efficiency,[55] improve quality of care,[56] improve coding and billing accuracy[57,58] decrease paperwork, and be a legible, chronologic documentation of clinical care. Use of AIMS has substantial potential as a clinical-decision support.[59] AIMS can process information from multiple devices and the EMR, incorporate algorithms to remind physicians to perform critical clinical processes on time, and alert physicians to changes in patient status.

Some physicians are wary of EMRs and the possible increased risk of exposure to litigation. Concerns have been raised about the profuse amounts of data and the risk of electronic discovery being used in litigation.[60,61] Despite concerns, the digital data reviewed in court have not proven detrimental to the physician-defendant case. EMRs were associated with fewer paid malpractice claims in one study.[62] Although there is a growing cache of data accumulating, no definitive conclusions can yet be made regarding the risk of malpractice.[63]

What to Do After an Adverse Outcome

If a critical incident occurs during the conduct of an anesthetic, the anesthesiologist should document, in narrative form, what happened, which drugs were used, the time sequence, and who was present. This should be documented in the patient's progress notes, as a catastrophic intra-anesthetic event cannot be summarized adequately in a small amount of space on the usual anesthesia record. The critical incident note should be written as soon as possible. The report should be as consistent as possible with concurrent records, such as the anesthesia, operating room, recovery room, and cardiac arrest records. If significant inconsistencies exist, they should be explained. Records should never be altered after the fact. If an error is made in record keeping, a line should be drawn through the error, leaving it legible, and the correction should be initialed and timed. Litigation is a lengthy process, and a court appearance to explain the incident to a jury may be years away, when memories have faded.

Whenever an anesthetic complication becomes apparent, appropriate consultation should be obtained quickly, and the departmental or institutional risk management group should be notified. If the complication is apt to lead to prolonged hospitalization or permanent injury, the liability insurance carrier should be notified. The patient should be followed closely while in the hospital, with telephone follow-up, if indicated, after discharge. The anesthesiologist(s), surgeon(s), consulting physicians, and the institution should coordinate and be consistent in their explanations to the patient or the patient's family as to the cause of any complication.

If anesthetic complications occur, the anesthesiologist should be honest with both the patient and the family about the cause. The providers should provide the facts about the event, express regret to the patient and family about the outcome, and give a formal apology if the unanticipated outcome is the result of an error or system failure.[53,64] Some states have laws mandating disclosure of serious adverse events to patients, and disclosure has been incorporated into quality reporting. Some states prohibit use of disclosure discussions as evidence in malpractice litigation. Some institutions, health systems, and insurers have adopted "disclose and offer" approaches to adverse events.[65] These approaches vary in their details but share the underlying premise that early disclosure and an offer of compensation may provide satisfactory resolution to the patient and avoid formal litigation proceedings.

Special Circumstances: "Do Not Attempt Resuscitation" and Jehovah's Witnesses

It is important to recognize that patients have well-established rights, and that among these is the right to refuse specific treatments. Two situations most relevant to anesthesia care are "Do Not Attempt Resuscitation" (DNAR) orders and the special circumstance of blood transfusion for Jehovah's Witnesses.

Patients with severe medical conditions may elect to forgo resuscitation attempts in the event of cardiac arrest. Such DNAR orders may be specified at hospital admission or may be in place in the form of an advance directive prior to admission. DNAR orders or advance directives may be general or specific, such as refusal of tracheal intubation or mechanical ventilation. When a patient with DNAR status presents for anesthesia care, it is important to discuss this with the patient or patient's surrogate to clarify the patient's intentions. In many hospitals, the institutional policy is to suspend the DNAR order during the immediate perioperative period since the cause for a cardiac arrest may be easily identified and treated. In other institutions, the patient may choose to suspend the DNAR order during the entire perioperative period. It should be clarified when the DNAR order should be reinstated (e.g., discharge from recovery or possibly later, when the patient has recovered from the procedure) and documented in the patient's chart. The perioperative status of DNAR orders should also be clarified with the surgeon and other providers who will be involved in the patient's perioperative care. The ASA has published *Ethical Guidelines of the Anesthesia Care of Patients with Do-Not-Resuscitate Orders or Other Directives That Limit Treatment (2008)*.[b]

In the case of Jehovah's Witnesses, the treatment that may be refused is the administration of blood or blood products. A central religious belief of many Jehovah's Witnesses is that the faithful will be forbidden the pleasures of the afterlife if they receive blood or blood products. Thus, for them to receive a transfusion is a mortal sin, and many Jehovah's Witnesses would actually rather die in grace than live with no possibility of salvation. Anesthesiologists must recognize and respect these beliefs, but also be cognizant that these convictions may conflict with their own personal, religious, or ethical codes.

As a general rule, physicians are not obligated to treat all patients who apply for treatment in elective situations. It is well within the rights of a physician to decline to care for any patient who wishes to place burdensome constraints on the physician or to unacceptably limit the physician's ability to provide optimal care. When presented with the opportunity to provide elective care for a Jehovah's Witness, the physician may decline to provide any care or may limit, by mutual consent with the patient, his or her obligation to adhere to the patient's religious beliefs. If such an agreement is reached, it must be documented clearly in the medical record, and it is desirable to have the patient co-sign the note. Not all Jehovah's Witnesses have identical beliefs regarding blood transfusions or which methods of blood preservation or sequestration will be allowed. Some patients will not allow any blood that has left the body to be reinfused, yet others will accept autotransfusion if their blood remains in constant contact with the body (via tubing). Therefore, it is important to reach a clear understanding of which techniques for blood preservation are to be used and to document this plan in the record. Parents of a minor child may not legally prevent that child from receiving blood. It may be necessary to obtain a court order in this circumstance.

National Practitioner Data Bank

It is usually the obligation of the hospital risk management department to make reports and inquiries to the National Practitioner Data Bank (NPDB), a nationwide information system that theoretically allows licensing boards and hospitals a means of detecting adverse information about physicians.[66] Simply moving into another state does not provide safe haven for incompetent physicians.

[b]http://www.asahq.org/For-Healthcare-Professionals/Standards-Guidelines-and-Statements.aspx

The NPDB requires notification of the following actions: (1) medical malpractice payments, (2) license actions by medical boards, (3) license actions by states, and (4) negative actions or findings by a peer review organization or private accreditation entity.[67] In addition, any adverse actions on clinical privileges must be reported to the physician's state board of medical examiners (licensing board, or equivalent) which, in turn, must report to the NPDB. Revised reporting rules from 2010 consolidated reporting requirements from various agencies to reduce duplication of reporting. A major change in 2010 was the requirement to report any surrender of a medical license if formal license review proceedings had been initiated, even if those proceedings were closed without formal action.[67] There has been a great deal of effort to establish a minimum malpractice payment below which no report is necessary, but to date, any payment made on behalf of a physician in response to a written complaint or claim must be reported. Settlements made by cancellation of bills or settlements made on verbal complaints are not considered a reportable payment.

Once a report has been submitted, the physician is notified and may dispute the accuracy of the report. At this time, the reporting entity may correct the form or void it. Failing that, the physician has the option of putting a brief statement in the file or appealing to the US Secretary of Health and Human Services, who may also either correct or void the form. A practitioner may make a query about his or her file at any time. A physician may also add a statement to a report at any time. Such statements will be included in any reports that are sent in response to inquiries. The existence of the NPDB reporting requirements has made physicians reluctant to allow settlement of nuisance suits because it will cause their names to be added to the data bank.

QUALITY IMPROVEMENT AND PATIENT SAFETY IN ANESTHESIA

Quality is a concept that has continued to elude precise definition in medical practice. However, it is generally accepted that attention to quality will improve patient safety and satisfaction with anesthesia care. The field of quality improvement is continually evolving, as is the terminology used to describe such efforts. A more recent trend is emphasis on patient safety, the prevention of harm from medical care. At the time of this writing, patient safety initiatives are evolving and a movement toward "pay for performance" (direct linkage between care processes and outcomes and reimbursement) is on the horizon. These will be discussed in a separate section.

3 Anesthesia quality improvement programs at the service level are generally guided by requirements of the Joint Commission that accredits hospitals and health-care organizations. Quality improvement programs are basically oriented toward improvement of the structure, process, and outcome of health-care delivery. An understanding of the fundamental principles of quality improvement may clarify the relationship between the continually evolving Joint Commission requirements and mandated quality improvement and other reporting initiatives.

Structure, Process, and Outcome: The Building Blocks of Quality

Although quality of care is difficult to define, it is generally accepted that it is composed of three components: Structure, process, and outcome.[68] *Structure* refers to the setting in which care was provided, for example, personnel and facilities used to provide health-care services and the manner in which they are organized. This includes the qualifications and licensing of personnel, ratio of practitioners to patients, standards for the facilities and equipment used to provide care, and the organizational structure within which care is delivered. The *process* of care includes the sequence and coordination of patient care activities, that is, what was actually done. Was a preanesthetic evaluation performed and documented? Was the patient continuously attended and monitored throughout the anesthetic? *Outcome* of care refers to changes in health status of the patient following the delivery of medical care. A quality improvement program focuses on measuring and improving these basic components of care.

4 *Continuous quality improvement* takes a systems approach to identifying and improving quality of care.[69,70] The operator is just one part of a complex system. An important underlying premise is that poor results may be a result of either random or systematic error. Random errors are inherently difficult to prevent and programs focused in this direction are misguided. System errors, however, should be controllable and strategies to minimize them should be within reach. CQI is basically the process of continually evaluating anesthesia practice to identify systematic problems (opportunities for improvement) and implementing strategies to prevent their occurrence.

A CQI program may focus on undesirable outcomes as a way to identify opportunities for improvement in the structure and process of care. The focus is not on blame but rather on identification of the causes of undesirable outcomes. Instead of asking which practitioners have the highest patient mortality rates, a CQI program may focus on the relationship between the process of care and patient mortality. What proportion of deaths was related to the patient's disease process or debilitated condition? Are these patients being appropriately evaluated for anesthesia and surgery? Were there any controllable causes, such as lack of extra help during resuscitation? The latter may lead to a modification of personnel resources (structure) or assignments (process) to be sure that adequate personnel are available at all times.

Formally, the process of CQI involves the identification of opportunities for improvement through the continual assessment of important aspects of care. It is a process that is instituted from the bottom up, by those who are actually involved in the process to be improved, rather than from the top down by administrators. Identification of opportunities for improvement may be carried out by various means, from brainstorming sessions focusing on a systematic evaluation of care activities to the careful measurement of indicators of quality (such as morbidity and mortality). In any event, once areas are identified for improvement, their current status is measured and documented. This may involve measurement of outcomes, such as delayed recovery from anesthesia or peripheral nerve injury. The process of care leading to these problems is then analyzed. If a change is identified that should lead to improvement, it is implemented. After an appropriate time, the status is then measured again to determine whether improvement actually resulted. Attention may then be directed to continuing to improve this process or turning to a different process to target for improvement.

Difficulty of Outcome Measurement in Anesthesia

Improvement in quality of care is often measured by a reduction in the rate of adverse outcomes. However, adverse outcomes are relatively rare in anesthesia, making measurement of improvement difficult. For example, if an institution lowers its mortality rate of surgery patients from 1 in 1,000 to 0.5 in 1,000, this difference may not be statistically significant. In other words, it may be impossible to know if the change in outcome resulted from changes in care or is simply random fluctuation. Many adverse outcomes in anesthesia are sufficiently rare to render them problematic as quality improvement measures.

To complement outcome measurement, anesthesia CQI programs can focus on critical incidents, sentinel events, and human errors. *Critical incidents* are events that cause, or have the potential to cause, patient injury if not noticed and corrected in a timely manner. For example, a partial disconnect of the breathing circuit may be corrected before patient injury occurs, yet has the potential for causing hypoxic brain injury or death. Critical incidents are more common than adverse outcomes. Measurement of the occurrence rate of important critical incidents may serve as a proxy measure for rare outcomes in anesthesia in a CQI program designed to improve patient safety and prevent injury.

Sentinel events are single, isolated events that may indicate a systemic problem. The Joint Commission has a specific definition of sentinel events that will be discussed later. In general, a sentinel event may be a significant or alarming critical incident that did not result in patient injury, such as a syringe swap and administration of a potentially lethal dose of medication that was noted and treated promptly, avoiding catastrophe. Or a sentinel event may be an unexpected significant patient injury such as intraoperative death. In either case, a CQI program may investigate sentinel events in an attempt to uncover systemic problems in the delivery of care that can be corrected. For example, a syringe swap may be analyzed for confusing or unclear labeling of medications or unnecessary medications routinely stocked on the anesthesia cart, setting the scene for unintended mix-up. In the case of death, all aspects of the patient's hospital course from selection for surgery to anesthetic management may be analyzed to determine if similar deaths can be prevented by a change in the care delivery system.

Human error has garnered much attention since a government report that 98,000 Americans may die annually from medical errors in hospitals.[71] Human errors are inevitable yet potentially preventable by appropriate system safeguards. Errors of planning involve use of a wrong plan to achieve an aim.[72] Errors of execution are the failure of a planned action to be completed as intended.[72] Modern anesthesia equipment is designed with safeguards such as alarm systems to detect errors that could lead to patient injury. Other anesthesia care processes are also amenable to human factors design principles, such as color coding of drug labels. A quality improvement program may identify human errors and institute safety systems to aid in error prevention.

Joint Commission Requirements for Quality Improvement

Joint Commission requirements for quality improvement activities are updated on an annual basis. In general, a hospital must adopt a method for systematically assessing and improving important functions and processes of care and their outcomes in a cyclical fashion. The general outline for this CQI cycle is the design of a process or function, measurement of performance, assessment of performance measures through statistical analysis or comparison with other data sources, and improvement of the process or function. Then the cycle repeats. The Joint Commission provides specific standards that must be met, with examples of appropriate measures of performance. The goal of this cycle of design, measurement, assessment, and improvement of performance of important functions and processes is to improve patient safety and quality of care.

Anesthesia care is one important function of the care of patients monitored by the Joint Commission. It is important that policies and procedures for administration of anesthesia be consistent in all locations within the organization.

The Joint Commission has adopted and annually updates patient safety goals for accredited organizations. Recent patient safety goals include improved accuracy of patient identification, improved effectiveness of communication among caregivers, improved safety of medication usage including anticoagulation status and syringe labeling, reduction of health-care–associated infections, and prevention of mistakes in surgery. This latter goal includes adoption of a "time-out" prior to the procedure to assure that the entire team (anesthesiologist, surgeon, nursing staff) agrees that the procedure, patient, and procedural details are correct. The surgical check list, described earlier in this chapter, is often used for this purpose. Joint Commission accreditation visits are unannounced or conducted on short notice and involve the inspector watching patient care to see that safe and acceptable practices are routinely implemented. In the intraoperative environment, this may involve such processes as timely administration of antibiotics and proper labeling of all syringes on the anesthesia cart. Surveyors may also talk to any staff member about organizational policies and procedures.

The Joint Commission also requires all sentinel events (any unexpected occurrences involving death or serious physical or psychological injury or risk thereof) to undergo *root cause analysis*.[c] A root cause analysis is typically facilitated by the hospital and includes everyone involved in the care of the affected patient in reconstructing the events to identify system process flaws that facilitated medical error. Any surgery on the wrong patient or wrong body part is included in this policy. The Joint Commission publishes sentinel event alerts so health-care organizations can learn from the experiences of others and prevent future medical errors.

Pay for Performance

A relatively recent development related to quality improvement is P4P or "pay for performance." P4P programs provide monetary incentives for implementation of safe practices, measuring performance, and/or achieving performance goals. This is an evolving trend, so only a conceptual introduction will be provided here. Anesthesia providers and service groups will need to be cognizant of any P4P initiatives that are operative in their location and with their payers.

At the time of this writing, the Department of Health and Human Services (HHS) selected the National Quality Forum (NQF) to serve as the consensus-based entity to convene multistakeholder groups to identify performance measures for public reporting and performance-based payment programs under the Affordable Care Act. The basic concept involves payment for quality rather than simply payment for services. In some cases, quality incentive payments are provided for simply measuring processes. However, as measurement systems are implemented, it is expected that benchmarks for quality performance will be established and providers will need to show that they are meeting such performance benchmarks to receive incentive payments.

---

[c]The Joint Commission. Sentinel Event Policy and Procedures, Updated: January 4, 2011. http://www.jointcommission.org/Sentinel_Event_Policy_and_Procedures/

Eventually, providers falling short of benchmark performance may see their reimbursements reduced. P4P is being implemented at both the hospital and specific provider levels. Centers for Medicare & Medicaid Services (CMS) and other payers may eventually link reimbursement to individual provider profiles.

A multitude of performance measures are being developed to meet the benchmarking challenge. At present, individual institutions are not being held to particular benchmarks but are expected to adopt some of the major quality indicators for measurement and improvement. The NQF has a 2011 list of 29 serious reportable events (SREs).[d] Many, but not all of these events, are relevant to anesthesia care including surgery or invasive procedure on the wrong site or patient, wrong procedure, unintended retention of a foreign body, intraoperative or immediate postoperative death of an ASA 1 patient, patient death or injury associated with intravascular air embolism, death or serious injury associated with a medication error or unsafe administration of blood products, and patient burns. The list of SREs is reviewed and updated periodically by the NQF.

Medicare has adopted an incentive pay-for-performance program that includes quality measures relevant to anesthesiologists. Under the Physician Quality Reporting System,[e] physicians will receive incentive payments for satisfactory reporting of performance on these measures, with plans for future penalties for unsatisfactory reporting on these performance measures beginning in 2015. There are also incentive payments for maintenance of specialty board certification. The current CMS reporting measures relevant to anesthesiologists include timely administration of preoperative prophylactic antibiotics, adherence to the central venous catheter insertion protocol to prevent catheter-related bloodstream infections, and perioperative temperature management. Specific reporting requirements and incentive/disincentive payments may be revised annually.

The Anesthesia Quality Institute (AQI) is developing a National Anesthesia Clinical Outcomes Registry (NACOR) that may also serve as a benchmarking resource for anesthesiologists. The AQI is a resource chartered by ASA in 2009.[73] The AQI was developed to assist members in maintaining certification and meeting emerging standards and to collect digital case information. NACOR is the registry of accumulated digital data acquired through periodic transfer of case-specific data directly from one electronic system (electronic billing and health records, EMR, AIMS, etc.) to another. This registry is a rich bank of data for future outcomes analysis that may be used for personal benchmarking, comparing quality of care, maintaining licensure and certification, and research. Through NACOR, acquired data (practice demographics, case-specific data, outcome data, and risk adjustment data) can be analyzed, changes can be implemented, and health care can be improved.

PROFESSIONAL LIABILITY

This section addresses the basic concepts of medical liability. A more detailed discussion of liability issues and the steps of the lawsuit process and appropriate actions for physicians to take when sued is available from the ASA.[f]

The Tort System

5 Although physicians may become involved in the criminal law system in a professional capacity, they more commonly become involved in the legal system of civil laws. Civil law is broadly divided into *contract law* and *tort law.* A tort may be loosely defined as a civil wrongdoing; negligence is one type of tort. *Malpractice* actually refers to any professional misconduct, but its use in legal terms typically refers to professional negligence.

To be successful in a malpractice suit, the patient-plaintiff must prove four things:

1. Duty: That the anesthesiologist owed the patient a duty
2. Breach of duty: That the anesthesiologist failed to fulfill his or her duty
3. Causation: That a reasonably close causal relation exists between the anesthesiologist's acts and the resultant injury
4. Damages: That actual damage resulted because of a breach of the standard of care.

Failure to prove any one of these four elements will result in a decision for the defendant-anesthesiologist.

Duty

As a physician, the anesthesiologist establishes a duty to the patient when a doctor–patient relationship exists. When the patient is seen preoperatively and the anesthesiologist agrees to provide anesthesia care for the patient, a duty to the patient has been established. In the most general terms, the duty the anesthesiologist owes to the patient is to adhere to the *standard of care* for the treatment of the patient. Because it is virtually impossible to delineate specific standards for all aspects of medical practice and all eventualities, the courts have created the concept of the *reasonable and prudent* physician. For all specialties, there is a national standard that has displaced the local standard.

Breach of Duty

In a malpractice action, expert witnesses will review the medical records of the case and determine whether the anesthesiologist acted in a reasonable and prudent manner in the specific situation and fulfilled his or her duty to the patient. If they find that the anesthesiologist either did something that should not have been done or failed to do something that should have been done, then the duty to adhere to the standard of care has been breached. Therefore, the second requirement for a successful suit will have been met.

Causation

Judges and juries are interested in determining whether the breach of duty was the *proximate cause* of the injury. If the odds are better than even that the breach of duty led, however circuitously, to the injury, this requirement is met.

There are two common tests employed to establish causation. The first is the *but for* test and the second is the *substantial factor* test. If the injury would not have occurred but for the action of the defendant-anesthesiologist, or if the act of the anesthesiologist was a substantial factor in the injury despite other causes, then proximate cause is established.

Although the burden of proof of causation ordinarily falls on the patient-plaintiff, it may, under special circumstances, be shifted to the physician-defendant under the doctrine of *res ipsa*

[d]http://www.qualityforum.org/Topics/SREs/Serious_Reportable_Events.aspx
[e]https://www.cms.gov/PQRS
[f]ASA Committee on Professional Liability: Manual on Professional Liability. Park Ridge, IL: American Society of Anesthesiologists, 2010. https://ecommerce.asahq.org/p-136-manual-on-professional-liability.aspx

loquitur (literally, "the thing speaks for itself"). Applying this doctrine requires proving that

1. the injury is of a kind that typically would not occur in the absence of negligence,
2. the injury must be caused by something under the exclusive control of the anesthesiologist,
3. the injury must not be attributable to any contribution on the part of the patient, and
4. the evidence for the explanation of events must be more accessible to the anesthesiologist than to the patient.

Because anesthesiologists render patients insensible to their surroundings and unable to protect themselves from injury, the doctrine of *res ipsa loquitur* may be invoked in anesthesia malpractice cases. If the plaintiff can successfully argue that the injury would not have occurred in the absence of negligence, then the defendant-anesthesiologist must prove that he/she was not negligent in the case under consideration.

Damages

The law allows for three different types of damages. *General damages* are those such as pain and suffering that directly result from the injury. *Special damages* are those actual damages that are a consequence of the injury, such as medical expenses, lost income, and funeral expenses. *Punitive damages* are intended to punish the physician for negligence that was reckless, wanton, fraudulent, or willful. Punitive damages are exceedingly rare in medical malpractice cases. More likely in the case of gross negligence is a loss of the license to practice anesthesia. In extreme cases, criminal charges may be brought against the physician, although this is rare. Determination of the dollar amount is usually based on some assessment of the plaintiff's condition versus the condition he or she would have been in had there been no negligence. Plaintiffs' attorneys generally charge a percentage of the damages and will, therefore, seek to maximize the award given. Some states have legislated caps on damages. Such caps are more common for general damages, although some states cap total compensation for malpractice awards.

Standard of Care

Because medical malpractice usually involves issues beyond the comprehension of lay jurors and judges, the court establishes the standard of care in a particular case by the testimony of *expert witnesses.* These witnesses differ from factual witnesses mainly in that they may give opinions. The trial court judge has sole discretion in determining whether a witness may be qualified as an expert. Although any licensed physician may be an expert, information will be sought regarding the witness's education and training, the nature and scope of the person's practice, memberships and affiliations, and publications. The purpose in gathering this information is not only to establish the qualifications of the witness to provide expert testimony, but also to determine the weight to be given to that testimony by the jury. In many cases the success of a lawsuit depends primarily on the stature and believability of the expert witnesses.

Unfortunately, there is a tendency for experts to link severe injury with inappropriate care (i.e., a bias that "bad outcomes mean bad care"). To investigate the influence of the severity of the injury on the assessment of standard of care, a group of 112 practicing anesthesiologists judged appropriateness of care in 21 cases involving adverse anesthetic outcomes.[74] The original outcome in each case was either temporary or permanent. For each original case, a matching alternate case was created that was identical to the original in every respect, except that a plausible outcome of the opposite severity was substituted. Reviewers judged the standard of care in each case. Knowledge of the severity of injury produced a significant inverse effect on the judgment of appropriateness of care.[74] The proportion of ratings for appropriate care decreased when the outcome was changed from temporary to permanent and increased when the outcome was changed from permanent to temporary. These results suggest that outcome bias in the assessment of standard of care may contribute to the frequency and size of payments.

In certain circumstances, the standard of care may also be determined from published societal guidelines, written policies of a hospital or department, or textbooks and monographs. Some medical specialty societies have carefully avoided applying the term *standards* to their guidelines in the hope that no binding behavior or mandatory practices have been created. The essential difference between standards and guidelines is that guidelines *should* be adhered to and standards *must* be adhered to. The ASA publishes standards and guidelines for a variety of anesthesia-related activities.

Causes of Anesthesia-Related Lawsuits

Relatively few adverse outcomes end up in a malpractice suit. It has been estimated that less than 1 of 25 patient injuries result in malpractice litigation.[75] The ASA Committee on Professional Liability has conducted a nationwide analysis of malpractice claims against anesthesiologists, excluding dental damage, since
6 1985 (i.e., the *Closed Claims Project*).[76–78] The leading injuries in anesthesia-related malpractice claims in the 2000s were death (29%), nerve damage (21%), permanent brain damage (9%), and airway injury (6%; Fig. 4-1). Burns from cautery fires, especially during monitored anesthesia care, increased over previous decades.[79] The causes of death and permanent brain damage were predominantly problems in airway management (e.g., inadequate ventilation, difficult intubation, premature extubation) and other complications such as pulmonary embolism, inadequate fluid therapy, stroke, hemorrhage, and myocardial infarction.[80]

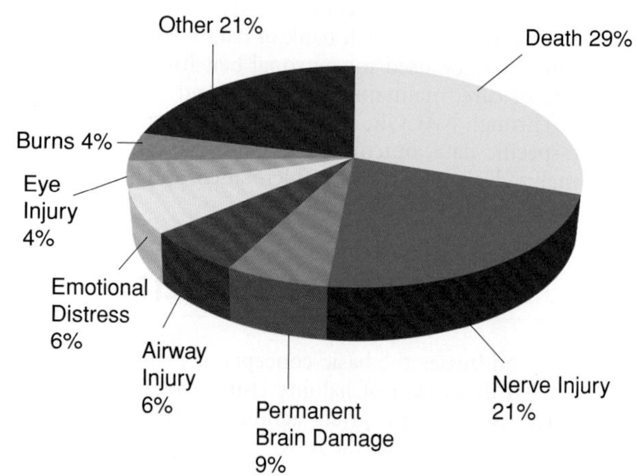

FIGURE 4-1. Most common injuries leading to anesthesia malpractice claims 2000 to 2009. Other category includes aspiration (4%), pneumothorax (3%), back pain (3%), myocardial infarction (3%), newborn injury (2%), headache (2%), and awareness/recall during general anesthesia (2%). Damage to teeth and dentures excluded. American Society of Anesthesiologists' Closed Claims Project (*n*—9,214).

Nerve damage, especially to the ulnar nerve, often occurs despite apparently adequate positioning.[81,82] Nerve injury was also the most common complication leading to claims after peripheral nerve blocks.[83] Spinal cord injury was the most common cause of nerve damage claims against anesthesiologists in the 1990s.[81] Chronic pain management is an increasing source of malpractice claims against anesthesiologists.[78,84] Medication management represented 17% of recent chronic pain management claims, with death as the most common outcome.[85] Cervical interventions for chronic pain management represented 22% of recent chronic pain management malpractice claims. Spinal cord damage was the outcome in 59% of these claims.[86]

The anesthesiologist is likely to be the target of a lawsuit if an untoward outcome occurs because the physician–patient relationship is usually tenuous at best. The patient rarely chooses the anesthesiologist, the preoperative visit is brief, and the anesthesiologist who sees the patient preoperatively may not actually anesthetize the patient. Communication between anesthesiologists and surgeons about complications is often lacking, and the tendency is for the surgeon to "blame anesthesia." In addition, anesthesiologists are often sued along with the surgeon in the case of an adverse outcome. This may occur even if the outcome was in no way related to the anesthetic care. However, as mentioned above, there is accumulating evidence that full disclosure of adverse events, probably best done by individuals properly trained in the process of disclosure, may significantly reduce the incidence of malpractice claims.[53,64]

What to Do When Sued

A lawsuit begins when the patient-plaintiff's attorney files a *complaint* and demands for jury trial with the court. The anesthesiologist is then served with the complaint and a summons requiring an answer to the complaint. Until this happens, no lawsuit has been filed. Insurance carriers must be notified immediately after the receipt of the complaint. The anesthesiologist will need assistance in answering the complaint, and there is a time limit placed on the response.

Specific actions at this point include the following:

1. Do not discuss the case with anyone, including colleagues who may have been involved, operating room personnel, or friends.
2. Never alter any records.
3. Gather together all pertinent records, including a copy of the anesthetic record, billing statements, and correspondence concerning the case.
4. Make notes recording all events recalled about the case.
5. Cooperate fully with the attorney provided by the insurer.

The first task the anesthesiologist must perform with an attorney is to prepare an answer to the complaint. The complaint contains certain facts and allegations with which the defense may either agree or disagree. Defense attorneys rely on the frank and totally candid observations of the physician in preparing an answer to the complaint. Physicians should be willing to educate their attorneys about the medical facts of the case, although most medical malpractice attorneys will be knowledgeable and medically sophisticated.

The next phase of the malpractice suit is called *discovery*. The purpose of discovery is the gathering of facts and clarification of issues in advance of the trial. In all likelihood the anesthesiologist will initially receive a written interrogatory, which will request factual information. In consultation with the defense attorney, the interrogatory should be answered in writing because carelessly or inadvertently misstated facts can become troublesome later.

Depositions are a second mechanism of discovery. The defendant-anesthesiologist will be deposed as a fact witness, and depositions will be obtained from other anesthesiologists who will act as expert witnesses. A nationally recognized expert in the area in question, recommended by the defendant but who is not a personal friend, and who agrees with the defense position, may be very valuable.

The plaintiff's attorney, not the defense attorney, will depose the anesthesiologist. Despite the apparent informality of the deposition, the anesthesiologist must be constantly aware that what is said during the deposition carries as much weight as what would be said in court. It is important to be factually prepared for the deposition by review of personal notes, the anesthetic record, and the medical record. The physician should dress conservatively and professionally because appearance and image are very important. The opposition is assessing the physician to see how he or she will appear to a jury. Answer only the question asked, and do not volunteer information. Rely on one's attorney for assistance when preparing for a deposition.

There will be depositions from expert witnesses, both for the plaintiff and for the defense. The anesthesiologist should work with his or her attorney to suggest questions and rebuttals. The better educated the attorney is about the medical facts, the reasons the anesthesiologist did what was done, and the alternative approaches, the better able the attorney will be to conduct these expert depositions.

If there is some merit in the case but the damages are minimal, or if proof of innocence will be difficult, there will probably be a settlement offer. There is a high cost incurred by both plaintiffs and defendants in pursuing a malpractice claim up through a jury trial. Unless there is a strong probability of a large dollar award, reputable plaintiffs' attorneys are not likely to pursue the claim. Thus, even if physicians believe that they are totally innocent of any wrongdoing, they should not be offended or angered about settling of the case: This is solely a matter of money, not medicine.

If a settlement is not reached during the discovery phase, a trial will occur. Only about 1 in 20 malpractice cases ever reach the point of a jury trial. Only those cases in which both sides think they can win, and which are likely to have significant financial impact, will proceed to trial.

The discussion of deposition testimony also applies to testimony in court, but there are a few additional points to consider during the trial. The members of the jury will not be as sophisticated medically as the attorneys who deposed the anesthesiologist during discovery. However, do not underestimate the intelligence of the jury. Talking down to them will create an unfavorable impression. If the answer to a question is not known, avoid guessing. If specific facts cannot be remembered, say so. Nobody expects total recall of events that may have occurred years before.

The defendant-physician should be present during the entire trial, even when not testifying, and should dress professionally. Displays of anger, remorse, relief, or hostility will hurt the physician in court. The physician should be able to give his or her testimony without using notes or documents. When it is necessary to refer to the medical record, it will be admitted into evidence. The anesthesiologist's goal is to convince the jury that he or she behaved in this case as any other competent and prudent anesthesiologist would have behaved.

It is important to keep in mind that *proof* in a malpractice case means only "more likely than not." The patient-plaintiff must "prove" the four elements of negligence, not to absolute certainty, but only to a probability greater than 50%. On the positive side, this means that the defendant-anesthesiologist must only show that his or her actions were, more likely than not, within an acceptable standard of care.

ACKNOWLEDGMENTS

The authors wish to thank F. W. Cheney, MD, and D. A. Kroll, MD, whose material from previous editions of this chapter has been retained in the current edition. They also thank Lynn Akerlund for her excellent secretarial assistance.

References

1. Beecher HK, Todd DP. A study of the deaths associated with anesthesia and surgery: Based on a study of 599,548 anesthesias in 10 institutions 1948–1952, inclusive. *Ann Surg.* 1954;140:2–35.
2. Newland MC, Ellis SJ, Lydiatt CA, et al. Anesthetic-related cardiac arrest and its mortality: A report covering 72,959 anesthetics over 10 years from a US teaching hospital. *Anesthesiology.* 2002;97:108–115.
3. Lagasse RS. Anesthesia safety: Model or myth? A review of the published literature and analysis of current original data. *Anesthesiology.* 2002;97:1609–1617.
4. Flick RP, Sprung J, Harrison TE, et al. Perioperative cardiac arrests in children between 1988 and 2005 at a tertiary referral center: A study of 92,881 patients. *Anesthesiology.* 2007;106:226–237.
5. Morray JP, Geiduschek JM, Ramamoorthy C, et al. Anesthesia-related cardiac arrest in children: Initial findings of the Pediatric Perioperative Cardiac Arrest (POCA) Registry. *Anesthesiology.* 2000;93:6–14.
6. Li G, Warner M, Lang BH, et al. Epidemiology of anesthesia-related mortality in the United States, 1999–2005. *Anesthesiology.* 2009;110(4):759–765.
7. Biboulet P, Aubas P, Dubourdieu J, et al. Fatal and non fatal cardiac arrests related to anesthesia. *Can J Anaesth.* 2001;48:326–328.
8. Eagle CC, Davis NJ. Report of the Anaesthetic Mortality Committee of Western Australia 1990–1995. *Anaesth Intensive Care.* 1997;25:51–59.
9. Khan M, Khan FA. Anesthetic deaths in a developing country. *Middle East J Anesthesiol.* 2007;19(1):159–172.
10. Ahmed A, Ali M, Khan M, et al. Perioperative cardiac arrests in children at a university teaching hospital of a developing country over 15 years. *Paediatr Anaesth.* 2009;19:581–586.
11. Davis NJ, ed. *Anaesthesia Related Mortality in Australia 1994.* Report of the Committee convened under the auspices of the Australian and New Zealand College of Anaesthetists. Melbourne: Capitol Press; 1999.
12. Kawashima Y, Takahashi S, Suzuki M, et al. Anesthesia-related mortality and morbidity over a 5-year period in 2,363,038 patients in Japan. *Acta Anaesthesiol Scand.* 2003;47:809–817.
13. Arbous MS, Grobbee DE, van Kleef JW, et al. Mortality associated with anaesthesia: A qualitative analysis to identify risk factors. *Anaesthesia.* 2001;56:1141–1153.
14. Braz LG, Modolo NSP, do Nascimento P, et al. Perioperative cardiac arrest: A study of 53,718 anaesthetics over 9 yr from a Brazilian teaching hospital. *Br J Anaesth.* 2006;96:569–575.
15. Lienhart A, Auroy Y, Pequignot F, et al. Survey of anesthesia-related mortality in France. *Anesthesiology.* 2006;105:1087–1097.
16. Kawashima Y, Seo N, Morita K, et al. Annual study of perioperative mortality and morbidity for the year of 1999 in Japan: The outlines report of the Japan Society of Anesthesiologists Committee on Operating Room Safety (in Japanese). *Masui.* 2001;50:1260–1274.
17. Irita K, Kawashima Y, Iwao Y, et al. Annual mortality and morbidity in operating rooms during 2002 and summary of morbidity and mortality between 1999 and 2002 in Japan: A brief review (in Japanese). *Masui.* 2004;53:320–335.
18. Charuluxananan S, Chinachoti T, Pulnitiporn A, et al. The Thai Anesthesia Incidents Study (THAI Study) of perioperative death: Analysis of risk factors. *J Med Assoc Thai.* 2005;88(7):S30–S40.
19. Gibbs N, ed. *Safety of Anaesthesia: A Review of Anaesthesia-Related Mortality Reporting in Australia and New Zealand 2003–2005.* Report of the mortality working group convened under the auspices of the Australian and New Zealand College of Anaesthetists. Melbourne: Australian and New Zealand College of Anaesthetists; 2009.
20. Brull R, McCartney CJ, Chan VW, et al. Neurological complications after regional anesthesia: Contemporary estimates of risk. *Anesth Analg.* 2007;104:965–974.
21. Warner MA, Warner DO, Matsumoto JY, et al. Ulnar neuropathy in surgical patients. *Anesthesiology.* 1999;90:54–59.
22. Warner MA, Warner DO, Harper CM, et al. Lower extremity neuropathies associated with lithotomy positions. *Anesthesiology.* 2000;93:938–942.
23. Welch MB, Brummett CM, Welch TD, et al. Perioperative peripheral nerve injuries: A retrospective study of 380,680 cases during a 10-year period at a single institution. *Anesthesiology.* 2009;111(3):490–497.
24. Auroy Y, Benhamou D, Bargues L, et al. Major complications of regional anesthesia in France: The SOS Regional Anesthesia Hotline Service. *Anesthesiology.* 2002;97:1274–1280.
25. de Sèze MP, Sztark F, Janvier G, et al. Severe and long-lasting complications of the nerve root and spinal cord after central neuraxial blockade. *Anesth Analg.* 2007;104:975–979.
26. Barrington MJ, Watts SA, Gledhill SR, et al. Preliminary results of the Australasian Regional Anaesthesia Collaboration: A prospective audit of more than 7000 peripheral nerve and plexus blocks for neurologic and other complications. *Reg Anesth Pain Med.* 2009;34:534–541.
27. Errando CL, Sigl JC, Robles M, et al. Awareness with recall during general anesthesia: A prospective observational evaluation of 4001 patients. *Br J Anaesth.* 2008;101:178–185.
28. Sandin RH, Enlund G, Samuelsson P, et al. Awareness during anaesthesia: A prospective case study. *Lancet.* 2000;355:707–711.
29. Sebel PS, Bowdle TA, Ghoneim MM, et al. The incidence of awareness during anesthesia: A multicenter United States study. *Anesth Analg.* 2004;99:833–839.
30. Avidan MS, Zhang L, Burnside BA, et al. Anesthesia awareness and the bispectral index. *N Engl J Med.* 2008;358:1097–1108.
31. Xu L, Wu AS, Yue Y. The incidence of intra-operative awareness during general anesthesia in China: A multi-center observational study. *Acta Anaesthesiol Scand.* 2009;53:873–882.
32. Chang SH, Miller NR. The incidence of vision loss due to perioperative ischemic optic neuropathy associated with spine surgery: The Johns Hopkins experience. *Spine.* 2005;30(11):1299–1302.
33. Warner ME, Warner MA, Garrity JA, et al. The frequency of perioperative vision loss. *Anesth Analg.* 2001;93:1417–1421.
34. Roth S, Thisted RA, Erickson JP, et al. Eye injuries after nonocular surgery. A study of 60,965 anesthetics from 1988 to 1992. *Anesthesiology.* 1996;85:1020–1027.
35. Patil CG, Lad EM, Lad SP, et al. Visual loss after spine surgery: A population-based study. *Spine.* 2008;33:1491–1496.
36. Holy SE, Tsai JH, McAllister RK, et al. Perioperative ischemic optic neuropathy: A case control analysis of 126,666 surgical procedures at a single institution. *Anesthesiology.* 2009;110:246–253.
37. Shen Y, Drum M, Roth S. The prevalence of perioperative visual loss in the United States: A 10-year study from 1996 to 2005 of spinal, orthopedic, cardiac, and general surgery. *Anesth Analg.* 2009;109:1534–1545.
38. Warner ME, Fronapfel PJ, Hebl JR, et al. Perioperative visual changes. *Anesthesiology.* 2002;96:855–859.
39. Martin DP, Weingarten TN, Gunn PW, et al. Performance improvement system and postoperative corneal injuries: Incidence and risk factors. *Anesthesiology.* 2009;111:320–326.
40. Warner ME, Benenfeld SM, Warner MA, et al. Perianesthetic dental injuries: Frequency, outcomes, and risk factors. *Anesthesiology.* 1999;90:1302–1305.
41. Newland MC, Ellis SJ, Peters KR, et al. Dental injury associated with anesthesia: A report of 161,687 anesthetics given over 14 years. *J Clin Anesth.* 2007;19:339–345.
42. Gaudio RM, Barbieri S, Feltracco P, et al. Traumatic dental injuries during anaesthesia. Part II: Medico-legal evaluation and liability. *Dent Traumatol.* 2011;27:40–45.
43. The Postoperative Visual Loss Study Group. Risk factors associated with ischemic optic neuropathy after spinal fusion surgery. *Anesthesiology.* 2012;116:15–24.
44. Monk TG, Weldon BC, Garvan CW, et al. Predictors of cognitive dysfunction after major noncardiac surgery. *Anesthesiology.* 2008;108:18–30.
45. Committee on Quality of Health Care in America, Institute of Medicine. *Crossing the Quality Chasm, A New Health System for the 21st Century.* Washington, DC: National Academy Press; 2001.
46. Gaba DM, Maxwell M, DeAnda A. Anesthetic mishaps: Breaking the chain of accident evolution. *Anesthesiology.* 1987;66:670–676.
47. Provonost P, Needham D, Berenholtz S, et al. An intervention to decrease catheter-related bloodstream infections in the ICU. *N Engl J Med.* 2006;355:2725–2732.
48. American Society of Anesthesiologists (ASA). Task Force on Central Venous Access. Practice guidelines for central venous access. *Anesthesiology.* 2012;116:539–573.
49. Neal JM, Hsiung RL, Mulroy MF, et al. ASRA checklist improves trainee performance during a simulated episode of local anesthetic systemic toxicity. *Reg Anesth Pain Med.* 2012;37:8–15.
50. Ziewacz JE, Arriaga AF, Bader AM, et al. Crisis checklists for the operating room: Development and pilot testing. *J Am Coll Surg.* 2011;213:212–219.
51. Haynes AB, Weiser TG, Berry WR, et al. A surgical safety checklist to reduce morbidity and mortality in a global population. *N Engl J Med.* 2009;360:491–499.
52. Charles C, Gafni A, Whelan T. Shared decision-making in the medical encounter: What does it mean? (Or it takes at least two to tango). *Soc Sci Med.* 1997;44:681–692.
53. Souter KJ, Gallagher TH. The disclosure of unanticipated outcomes of care and medical errors: What does this mean for anesthesiologists? *Anes Analg.* 2012;114:615–621.
54. Hillestad R, Bigelow J, Bower A, et al. Can electronic medical record systems transform health care? Potential health benefits, savings and costs. *Health Aff (Millwood).* 2005;24:1103–1117.

55. McLellan S, Galvin M, McMaugh D. Benefits measurement from the use of an automated anaesthetic record keeping system (AARK). *Electron J Health Inform.* 2011;6(1):e6. Available at http://www.ejhi.net
56. Chaudhry B, Wang J, Wu S, et al. Systematic review: Impact of health information technology on quality, efficiency, and costs of medical care. *Ann Intern Med.* 2006;144:742–752.
57. Reich DL, Kahn RA, Wax D, et al. Development of a module for point-of-care charge capture and submission using an anesthesia information management system. *Anesthesiology.* 2006;105:179–186.
58. Spring SF, Sandberg WS, Anupama S, et al. Automated documentation error detection and notification improves anesthesia billing performance. *Anesthesiology.* 2007;106:157–163.
59. Wanderer JP, Sandberg WS, Ehrenfeld JM. Real-time alerts and reminders using information systems. *Anesthesiol Clin.* 2011;29:389–396.
60. Vigoda MM, Lubarsky DA. Failure to recognize loss of incoming data in an anesthesia record-keeping system may have increased medical liability. *Anesth Analg.* 2006;102:1798–1802.
61. Miller AR, Tucker CE. Electronic discovery and electronic medical records: Does the threat of litigation affect firm decisions to adopt technology? Federal Trade Commission Bureau of Economics 2009-04-30. Available at: http://www.ftc.gov/be/seminardocs/090430amiller.pdf
62. Virapongse A, Bates DW, Shi P, et al. Electronic health records and malpractice claims in office practice. *Arch Intern Med.* 2008;168:2362–2367.
63. Mangalmurti SS, Murtagh L, Mello MM. Medical malpractice liability in the age of electronic health records. *N Engl J Med.* 2010;363:2060–2067.
64. Gallagher TH, Studdert D, Levinson W. Disclosing harmful medical errors to patients. *N Engl J Med.* 2007;356:2713–2719.
65. Mello MM, Gallagher TH. Malpractice reform – Opportunities for leadership by health care institutions and liability insurers. *N Engl J Med.* 2010;362:1353–1356.
66. Baldwin LM, Hart LG, Oshel RE, et al. Hospital peer review and the National Practitioner Data Bank: Clinical privileges action reports. *JAMA.* 1999;282:349–355.
67. Health Resources and Services Administration (HRSA), HHS. National Practitioner Data Bank for adverse information on physicians and other health care practitioners: Reporting on adverse and negative actions. Final rule. *Fed Regist.* 2010;75(18):4655–4682.
68. Donabedian A. The quality of care. How can it be assessed? *JAMA.* 1988;260:1743–1748.
69. Deming WE. *Out of the Crisis.* Cambridge: Massachusetts Institute of Technology; 1986.
70. Juran JM. *Juran on Planning for Quality.* New York, NY: Free Press; 1988.
71. Kohn LT, Corrigan JM, Donaldson MS, eds. *Committee on Quality of Health Care in America, Institute of Medicine. To Err Is Human: Building a Safer Health System.* Washington, DC: National Academy Press; 1999.
72. Reason JT. *Human Error.* Cambridge: Cambridge University Press; 1990.
73. Dutton RP, DuKatz A. Quality improvement using automated data sources: The Anesthesia Quality Institute. *Anesthesiology Clin.* 2011;29:439–454.
74. Caplan RA, Posner KL, Cheney FW. Effect of outcome on physician judgments of appropriateness of care. *JAMA.* 1991;265:1957–1960.
75. Localio AR, Lawthers AG, Brennan TA, et al. Relation between malpractice claims and adverse events due to negligence. Results of the Harvard Medical Practice Study III. *N Engl J Med.* 1991;325:245–251.
76. Cheney FW, Posner K, Caplan RA, et al. Standard of care and anesthesia liability. *JAMA.* 1989;261:1599–1603.
77. Cheney FW. The American Society of Anesthesiologists Closed Claims Project: What have we learned, how has it affected practice, and how will it affect practice in the future? *Anesthesiology.* 1999;91:552–556.
78. Metzner J, Posner KL, Lam MS, et al. Closed claims' analysis. *Best Pract Res Clin Anaesthesiol.* 2011;25:263–276.
79. Bhananker SM, Posner KL, Cheney FW, et al. Injury and liability associated with monitored anesthesia care. A closed claims analysis. *Anesthesiology.* 2006;104:228–234.
80. Cheney FW, Posner KL, Lee LA, et al. Trends in anesthesia-related death and brain damage: A closed claims analysis. *Anesthesiology.* 2006;105:1081–1086.
81. Cheney FW, Domino KB, Caplan RA, et al. Nerve injury associated with anesthesia: A closed claims analysis. *Anesthesiology.* 1999;90:1062–1069.
82. Warner MA, Warner ME, Martin JT. Ulnar neuropathy. Incidence, outcome, and risk factors in sedated or anesthetized patients. *Anesthesiology.* 1994;81:1332–1340.
83. Lee LA, Posner KL, Kent CD, et al. Complications associated with peripheral nerve blocks: Lessons from the ASA closed claims project. *Int Anesthesiol Clin.* 2011;49:56–67.
84. Fitzgibbon DR, Posner KL, Domino KB, et al. Chronic pain management: American Society of Anesthesiologists Closed Claims Project. *Anesthesiology.* 2004;100:98–105.
85. Fitzgibbon DR, Rathmell JP, Michna E, et al. Malpractice claims associated with medication management for chronic pain. *Anesthesiology.* 2010;112:948–956.
86. Rathmell JP, Michna E, Fitzgibbon DR, et al. Injury and liability associated with cervical procedures for chronic pain. *Anesthesiology.* 2011;114:918–926.

SECTION II

Scientific Foundations of Anesthesia

CHAPTER

5 Mechanisms of Anesthesia and Consciousness

C. MICHAEL CROWDER • BEN JULIAN PALANCA • ALEX S. EVERS

Key Points

1. The components of the anesthetic state include unconsciousness, amnesia, analgesia, immobility, and attenuation of autonomic responses to noxious stimulation.
2. Minimum alveolar concentration (MAC) remains the most robust measurement and the standard for determining the potency of volatile anesthetics.
3. Direct interactions of anesthetic molecules with proteins both satisfy the Meyer-Overton rule and provide the simplest explanation for compounds that deviate from this rule.
4. Current evidence strongly indicates protein rather than lipid as the molecular target for anesthetic action.
5. While current data still support the prevailing view that neuronal excitability is only slightly affected by general anesthetics, this small effect may nevertheless contribute significantly to the clinical actions of volatile anesthetics.
6. The synapse is generally thought to be the most likely relevant site of anesthetic action. Existing evidence indicates that even at this one site, anesthetics produce various effects, including presynaptic inhibition of neurotransmitter release, inhibition of excitatory neurotransmitter effect, and enhancement of inhibitory neurotransmitter effect. Furthermore, the effects of anesthetics on synaptic function differ among various anesthetic agents, neurotransmitters, and neuronal preparations.
7. Existing evidence suggests that most voltage-dependent calcium channels (VDCCs) are modestly sensitive or insensitive to anesthetics. However, some sodium channel subtypes are inhibited by volatile anesthetics and this effect may be responsible in part for a reduction in neurotransmitter release at some synapses.
8. Activation of background K^+ channels in mammalian vertebrates could be an important and general mechanism through which inhalational and gaseous anesthetics regulate neuronal resting membrane potential and thereby excitability.
9. Hyperpolarization-activated cyclic nucleotide-gated (HCN) channels are a recently discovered channel type inhibited by both volatile anesthetics and some intravenous anesthetics at clinical concentrations and could be a relevant anesthetic target.
10. A large body of evidence shows that clinical concentrations of many anesthetics potentiate γ-aminobutyric acid (GABA)-activated currents in the central nervous system (CNS). Other members of the ligand-activated ion channel family, including glycine receptors, neuronal nicotinic receptors, and 5-hydroxytryptamine (5-HT_3) receptors, are also affected by

clinical concentrations of anesthetics and remain plausible anesthetic targets.

11 Genetic experiments in mice provide definitive evidence for a role of specific $GABA_A$ receptor channels, two-pore potassium channels, and HCN1 channels in particular anesthetic behavioral effects. Genetically engineered mice also show that distinct anesthetic targets mediate different anesthetic end points and that not all anesthetics have the same targets.

12 While anesthetic action to produce immobility occurs largely at the spinal cord, specific molecular targets for amnesia lie in the hippocampus.

13 Anesthetic-induced unconsciousness can be viewed as impairment of both arousal and awareness. These actions are mediated by targets distributed across the brainstem, thalamus, and cerebral cortex.

14 Anesthetic ablation of arousal relies on disruption of redundant subcortical systems that regulate sleep and patterns of cortical activity.

15 Anesthetics alter the interaction of cortical networks responsible for cognitive functions and may thereby alter awareness by limiting the capacity to both represent and integrate information.

Multimedia

Meyer-Overton Rule

The introduction of general anesthetics into clinical practice over 150 years ago stands as one of the seminal innovations of medicine. This single discovery facilitated the development of modern surgery and spawned the specialty of anesthesiology. Despite the importance of general anesthetics and despite more than 100 years of active research, the molecular mechanisms responsible for anesthetic action remain one of the unsolved mysteries of science.

Why have mechanisms of anesthesia been so difficult to elucidate? Anesthetics, as a class of drugs, are challenging to study for three major reasons:

1. Anesthesia, by definition, is a change in the responses of an *intact animal* to external stimuli. Making a definitive link between anesthetic effects observed in vitro and the anesthetic state observed and defined in vivo has proven difficult.
2. No structure–activity relationships are apparent among anesthetics; a wide variety of structurally unrelated compounds, ranging from steroids to elemental xenon, are capable of producing clinical anesthesia. This suggests that there are multiple molecular mechanisms that can produce clinical anesthesia.
3. Anesthetics work at very high concentrations in comparison to drugs, neurotransmitters, and hormones that act at specific receptors. This implies that if anesthetics do act by binding to specific receptor sites, they must bind with very low affinity and probably stay bound to the receptor for very short periods of time. Low-affinity binding is much more difficult to observe and characterize than high-affinity binding.

Despite these difficulties, molecular and genetic tools are now available that should allow for major insights into anesthetic mechanisms in the next decade. The aim of this chapter is to provide a conceptual framework for the reader to catalog current knowledge and integrate future developments about mechanisms of anesthesia. Five specific questions will be addressed in this chapter:

1. What is anesthesia and how do we measure it?
2. What are the molecular targets of anesthetics?
3. What are the cellular neurophysiologic mechanisms of anesthesia (e.g., effects on synaptic function vs. effects on action potential generation) and what anesthetic effects on ion channels and other neuronal proteins underlie these mechanisms?
4. How are the molecular and cellular effects of anesthetics linked to the behavioral effects of anesthetics observed in vivo?
5. What are the major anatomic sites of anesthetic action in the CNS and how do anesthetics interfere with their interactions?

WHAT IS ANESTHESIA?

General anesthesia can be broadly defined as a drug-induced reversible depression of the CNS resulting in the loss of response to and perception of all external stimuli. Unfortunately, such a broad definition is inadequate for two reasons. First, the definition is not actually broad enough. Anesthesia is not simply a deafferented state; amnesia and unconsciousness are important aspects of the anesthetic state. Second, the definition is too broad, as all general anesthetics do not produce equal depression of all sensory modalities. For example, barbiturates are considered to be anesthetics, but they are not particularly effective analgesics. These conflicting problems with the definition can be bypassed by a more practical description of the anesthetic state as a collection
1 of "component" changes in behavior or perception. The components of the anesthetic state include unconsciousness, amnesia, analgesia, immobility, and attenuation of autonomic responses to noxious stimulation.

Regardless of which definition of anesthesia is used, rapid and reversible drug-induced changes in behavior or perception are essential to anesthesia. As such, anesthesia can only be defined and measured in the intact organism. Changes in behavior such as unconsciousness or amnesia can be intuitively understood in higher organisms such as mammals, but become increasingly difficult to define as one descends the phylogenetic tree. Thus, while anesthetics have effects on organisms ranging from worms to man, it is difficult to map with certainty the effects of anesthetics observed in lower organisms to any of our behavioral definitions of anesthesia. This contributes to the difficulty of using simple organisms as models in which to study the molecular mechanisms of anesthesia. Similarly, any cellular or molecular effects of anesthetics observed in higher organisms can be extremely difficult to link with the constellation of behaviors that constitute the anesthetic state. The absence of a simple and concise definition of anesthesia has clearly been one of the stumbling blocks to elucidating the mechanisms of anesthesia at a molecular and cellular level. Precise definitions for each of the component behaviors of the anesthetic state will be an important tool in dissecting the molecular and cellular mechanisms of each of the clinically important effects of anesthetic agents.

An additional difficulty in defining anesthesia is that our understanding of the mechanisms of consciousness is rather amorphous at present. One cannot easily define anesthesia when the neurobiologic phenomena ablated by anesthesia are not well understood. As discussed later in this chapter, the neural substrates for consciousness are beginning to be unraveled[1] and new theories[2] have incorporated this new anatomic knowledge leading to identification of surrogate physiologic markers of consciousness.[3] These new insights into mechanisms of consciousness are discussed in the section *Where in the Central Nervous System Do Anesthetics Work?*

Finally, it has long been assumed that anesthesia is a state that is achieved when an anesthetic agent reaches a specific concentration at its effect site in brain and that if tolerance to the anesthetic develops, increasing concentrations of anesthetic might be required to maintain a constant level of anesthesia during prolonged anesthetic administration. The recent finding that it takes a higher anesthetic brain concentration to induce anesthesia than to maintain anesthesia (i.e., emergence occurs at a significantly lower concentration than induction) contradicts these assumptions.[4] This phenomenon, referred to as neural inertia, adds a wrinkle to the definition of anesthesia and suggests that the mechanisms of anesthetic induction and emergence may be different.

HOW IS ANESTHESIA MEASURED?

In order to study the pharmacology of anesthetic action, quantitative measurements of anesthetic potency are absolutely essential. To this end, Quasha and colleagues[5] have defined the concept of MAC. MAC is defined as the alveolar partial pressure of a gas at which 50% of humans do not respond to a surgical incision. In animals, MAC is defined as the alveolar partial pressure of a gas at which 50% of animals do not respond to a noxious stimulus, such as tail clamp,[6] or at which they lose their righting reflex. The use of MAC as a measure of anesthetic potency has two major advantages. First, it is an extremely reproducible measurement that is remarkably constant over a wide range of species.[5] Second, the use of end-tidal gas concentration provides an index of the "free" concentration of drug required to produce anesthesia since the end-tidal gas concentration is in equilibrium with the free concentration in plasma. The MAC concept has several important limitations, particularly when trying to relate MAC values to anesthetic potency observed in vitro. First, the end point in a MAC determination is quantal: A subject is either anesthetized or unanesthetized; it cannot be partially anesthetized. Furthermore, MAC represents the average response of a whole population of subjects rather than the response of a single subject. The quantal nature of the MAC measurement makes it very difficult to compare MAC measurements to concentration–response curves obtained in vitro, where the graded response of a single preparation is measured as a function of anesthetic concentration. The second limitation of MAC measurements is that they can only be directly applied to anesthetic gases. Parenteral anesthetics (barbiturates, neurosteroids, propofol) cannot be assigned a MAC value, making it difficult to compare the potency of parenteral and volatile anesthetics. A MAC equivalent for parental anesthetics is the free concentration of the drug in plasma required to prevent response to a noxious stimulus in 50% of subjects; this value has been estimated for several parenteral anesthetics.[7] A third limitation of MAC is that it is highly dependent on the anesthetic end point used to define it. For example, if loss of response to a verbal command is used as an anesthetic end point, the MAC values obtained (MAC_{awake}) will be much lower than classic MAC values based on response to a noxious stimulus. Indeed, each behavioral component of the anesthetic state will likely have a different MAC value. Despite its limitations, MAC remains the most robust measurement and the standard for determining the potency of volatile anesthetics.

Because of the limitations of MAC, monitors that measure some correlate of anesthetic depth have been introduced into clinical practice.[8] The most popular of these monitors converts spontaneous electroencephalogram (EEG) waveforms into a single value that correlates with anesthetic depth for some general anesthetics. To date, these monitors have not been shown to be more effective at preventing awareness during anesthesia than simply maintaining an adequate end-tidal anesthetic concentration[9,10] or giving a standard dose of intravenous anesthetic. Nonetheless it is logical to think that different individuals may have different sensitivities to anesthetics and that measuring a surrogate end point such as a processed EEG value,[11] an evoked potential,[12] or a functional neuroimaging signal indicative of integrated cortical activity[1] might be a better indicator of anesthetic depth than merely measuring delivered concentration.

WHAT IS THE CHEMICAL NATURE OF THE ANESTHETIC TARGET SITES?

The Meyer–Overton Rule

More than 100 years ago, Meyer[13] and Overton[14] independently observed that the potency of gases as anesthetics was strongly correlated with their solubility in olive oil (Fig. 5-1). Since a wide variety of structurally unrelated compounds obey the Meyer–Overton rule, it has been reasoned that all anesthetics are likely to act at the same molecular site. This idea is referred to as the *unitary theory of anesthesia.* It has also been argued that since solubility in a specific solvent strongly correlates with anesthetic potency, the solvent showing the strongest correlation between anesthetic solubility and potency is likely to most closely mimic the chemical and physical properties of the anesthetic target site in the CNS. On the basis of this reasoning, the anesthetic target site was assumed to be hydrophobic in nature. Since olive oil/gas partition coefficients can be determined for gases and volatile liquids, but not for liquid anesthetics, attempts have been made to correlate anesthetic potency with solvent/water partition coefficients. To date, the octanol/water partition coefficient best correlates with anesthetic potency. This correlation holds for a variety of classes of anesthetics and spans a 10,000-fold range of anesthetic potencies.[15] The properties of the solvent octanol suggest that the anesthetic site is likely to be amphipathic, having both polar and nonpolar characteristics.

Exceptions to the Meyer–Overton Rule

Compounds exist that are structurally similar to halogenated anesthetics,[16] barbiturates,[17] and neurosteroids,[18] yet are convulsants rather than anesthetics. On the basis of olive oil/gas partition coefficients of the halogenated convulsant compounds,

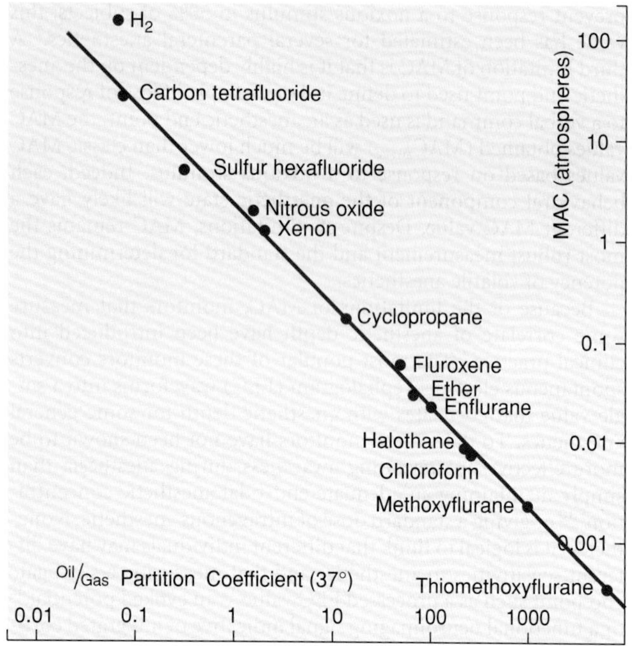

FIGURE 5-1. The Meyer–Overton rule. There is a linear relationship (on a log–log scale) between the oil/gas partition coefficient and the anesthetic potency (MAC) of a number of gases. The correlation between lipid solubility and MAC extends over a 70,000-fold difference in anesthetic potency. (Reproduced with permission from Tanfiuji Y, Eger EI, Terrell RC. Some characteristics of an exceptionally potent inhaled anesthetic: thiomethoxyflurane. *Anesth Analg.* 1977;56:387.)

anesthesia should have been achieved within the range of concentrations studied.[19] Halogenated compounds have also been identified that are neither anesthetic nor convulsant despite oil/gas partition coefficients that would predict they should be anesthetics.[19] Interestingly, some of these polyhalogenated compounds do produce amnesia in animals[20] and are thus referred to as *non-immobilizers* rather than as non-anesthetics. Finally, polyhalogenated alkanes, referred to as *transitional compounds,* have been identified that anesthetize mice, but only at concentrations 10 times those predicted by their oil/gas partition coefficients.[19]

In several homologous series of anesthetics, anesthetic potency increases with increasing chain length until a certain critical chain length is reached. Beyond this critical chain length, compounds are unable to produce anesthesia, even at the highest attainable concentrations. In the series of *n*-alkanols, for example, anesthetic potency increases from methanol through dodecanol; all longer alkanols are unable to produce anesthesia.[21] This phenomenon is referred to as the *cutoff effect.* Cutoff effects have been described for several homologous series of anesthetics including *n*-alkanes, *n*-alkanols, cycloalkanemethanols,[22] and perfluoroalkanes.[23] While the anesthetic potency in each of these homologous series of anesthetics shows a cutoff, a corresponding cutoff in octanol/water or oil/gas partition coefficients has not been demonstrated. Therefore, compounds above the cutoff represent a deviation from the Meyer–Overton rule.

A final deviation from the Meyer–Overton rule is the observation that enantiomers of anesthetics differ in their potency as anesthetics. Enantiomers (mirror-image compounds) are a class of stereoisomers that have identical physical properties, including identical solubility in solvents such as octanol or olive oil. Animal studies of barbiturate anesthetics,[24,25] ketamine,[26] neurosteroids,[27] etomidate,[28] and isoflurane[29] all show enantioselective differences in anesthetic potency. These differences in potency range in magnitude from a more than 10-fold difference between the enantiomers of etomidate or the neurosteroids to a 60% difference between the enantiomers of isoflurane. It is argued that a *major* difference in anesthetic potency between a pair of enantiomers can only be explained by a protein-binding site (see *Protein Theories of Anesthesia*); this appears to be the case for etomidate and the neurosteroids.

The exceptions to the Meyer–Overton rule do not obviate the importance of the rule. They do, however, indicate that the properties of a solvent such as octanol describe some, but not all, of the properties of an anesthetic-binding site. Compounds that deviate from the Meyer–Overton rule suggest that anesthetic target site(s) are also defined by other properties including size and shape.

In defining the molecular target(s) of anesthetic molecules, one must be able to account both for the Meyer–Overton rule and for the well-defined exceptions to this rule. It has sometimes been suggested that a correct molecular mechanism of anesthesia should also be able to account for pressure reversal. *Pressure reversal* is a phenomenon whereby the concentration of a given anesthetic needed to produce anesthesia is greatly increased if the anesthetic is administered to an animal under hyperbaric conditions. The idea that pressure reversal is a useful tool for elucidating mechanisms of anesthesia is based on the assumption that pressure reverses the specific physicochemical actions of the anesthetic that are responsible for producing anesthesia; that is to say, pressure and anesthetics act on the same molecular targets. However, evidence suggests that pressure reverses anesthesia by producing excitation that physiologically counteracts anesthetic depression, rather than by acting as an anesthetic antagonist at the anesthetic site of action.[30] Therefore, in the ensuing discussion of molecular targets of anesthesia, pressure reversal will not be further mentioned.

Lipid versus Protein Targets

Anesthetics might interact with several possible molecular targets to produce their effects on the *function* of ion channels and other proteins. Anesthetics might dissolve in the *lipid* bilayer, causing physicochemical changes in membrane structure that alter the ability of embedded membrane proteins to undergo conformational changes important for their function. Alternatively, anesthetics could bind directly to *proteins* (either ion channel proteins or modulatory proteins), thus either[1] interfering with binding of a ligand (e.g., a neurotransmitter, a substrate, a second messenger molecule) or[2] altering the ability of the protein to undergo conformational changes important for its function. The following section summarizes the arguments for and against lipid theories and protein theories of anesthesia.

Lipid Theories of Anesthesia

In its simplest incarnation, the lipid theory of anesthesia postulates that anesthetics dissolve in the lipid bilayers of biologic membranes and produce anesthesia when they reach a critical concentration in the membrane. Consistent with this hypothesis, the membrane/gas partition coefficients of anesthetic gases in pure lipid bilayers correlate strongly with anesthetic potency.[31] Also, consistent with the lipid theories, various membrane perturbations are produced by general anesthetics; however, the magnitude of these changes produced by clinical concentrations of anesthetics are quite small and are thought to be very unlikely to disrupt nervous system function.[32] While some of the more sophisticated lipid theories can account for the cutoff effect and for the ineffectiveness of nonimmobilizers, no lipid theory can plausibly explain all anesthetic pharmacology. Thus, most investigators do not consider lipids as the most likely target of general anesthetics.

Protein Theories of Anesthesia

The Meyer–Overton rule could also be explained by the direct interaction of anesthetics with hydrophobic sites on proteins. Three types of hydrophobic sites on proteins might interact with anesthetics:

1. Hydrophobic amino acids comprise the core of water-soluble proteins. Anesthetics could bind in hydrophobic pockets that are fortuitously present in the protein core.
2. Hydrophobic amino acids also form the lining of binding sites for hydrophobic ligands. For example, there are hydrophobic pockets in which fatty acids tightly bind on proteins such as albumin and the low-molecular-weight fatty acid–binding proteins. Anesthetics could compete with endogenous ligands for binding to such sites on either water-soluble or membrane proteins.
3. Hydrophobic amino acids are major constituents of the α-helices, which form the membrane-spanning regions of membrane proteins; hydrophobic amino acid side chains form the protein surface that faces the membrane lipid. Anesthetic molecules could interact with pockets formed between the α-helices or with the hydrophobic surface of these membrane proteins, disrupting normal lipid–protein interactions and possibly directly affecting protein conformation.

3 Direct interaction of anesthetic molecules with proteins not only satisfies the Meyer–Overton rule, but would also provide the simplest explanation for compounds that deviate from this rule. Any protein-binding site is likely to be defined by properties such as size and shape in addition to its solvent properties. Limitations in size and shape could reduce the binding affinity of compounds beyond the cutoff, thus explaining their lack of anesthetic effect. Enantioselectivity is also most easily explained by a direct binding of anesthetic molecules to defined sites on proteins; a protein-binding site of defined dimensions could readily distinguish between enantiomers on the basis of their different shapes. Protein-binding sites for anesthetics could also explain the convulsant effects of some polyhalogenated alkanes. Different compounds binding (in slightly different ways) to the same binding pocket can produce different effects on protein conformation and hence on protein function. For example, polyhalogenated alkanes (*non-immobilizers*) could be inverse agonists, binding at the same protein sites at which halogenated alkane anesthetics are agonists. The evidence for direct interactions between anesthetics and proteins is briefly reviewed in the following section.

Evidence for Anesthetic Binding to Proteins

A breakthrough in protein theories of anesthesia was the demonstration that a purified water-soluble protein, firefly luciferase, could be inhibited by general anesthetics. This provided the important proof of principle that anesthetics could bind to proteins in the absence of membranes. Numerous studies have extensively characterized the anesthetic inhibition of firefly luciferase activity and have shown that inhibition occurs at concentrations very similar to those required to produce clinical anesthesia, is consistent with the Meyer–Overton rule, is competitive with respect to the substrate D-luciferin, and exhibits a cutoff in anesthetic potency for both *n*-alkanes and *n*-alkanols.[33,34] These data suggest that the luciferin-binding pocket may have physical and chemical characteristics similar to those of a putative anesthetic-binding site in the CNS. To address proteins more relevant to anesthetic effects on the nervous system, numerous studies have employed site-directed mutagenesis of anesthetic-sensitive ion channels to identify amino acid residues that are crucial to anesthetic action. While the residues identified in these studies may contribute to anesthetic-binding sites, they may alternatively be sites that are essential for anesthetic-induced conformational changes in the protein. The literature on site-directed mutagenesis studies to identify putative anesthetic-binding sites on ion channels is extensively reviewed in the section *Anesthetic Actions on Ion Channels.*

More direct approaches to study anesthetic binding to proteins have included NMR spectroscopy and photoaffinity labeling. Early studies using ^{19}F-NMR spectroscopy demonstrated that isoflurane binds to the fatty acid–binding sites on bovine serum albumin (BSA) and that binding is competitively inhibited by halothane, methoxyflurane, sevoflurane, and octanol.[35,36] Using this BSA model, it was subsequently shown that anesthetic-binding sites could be identified and characterized using photoaffinity labeling with ^{14}C-labeled halothane.[37,38] Photoaffinity-labeling reagents have subsequently been developed for a variety of anesthetics including etomidate, propofol,[39,40] and neurosteroids and are a useful tool to validate results obtained using site-directed mutagenesis as well as to identify novel binding sites.

The most extensive photolabeling studies have used etomidate analogue photolabeling reagents to identify etomidate-binding sites on purified GABA$_A$ receptors. An initial study used azietomidate, a photolabeling reagent that preferentially labels nucleophilic amino acids, to photolabel-purified GABA$_A$ receptors from bovine brain.[41] This study identified two methionine residues that were sites of attachment for azi-etomidate: One site on the TM1 helix (Met-236) of the α_1 subunit and the other (Met-286) on the TM3 helix of the β_3 subunit. These data suggest an etomidate-binding pocket in the transmembrane domain at the interface between the α_1 and β_3 subunits. A subsequent study using TDBzl-etomidate, a photolabeling reagent with broader amino acid side chain reactivity, identified additional amino acids that confirmed and further defined this inter-subunit–binding site.[42] The combined results of site-directed mutagenesis studies and photoaffinity-labeling studies identified a specific, functionally relevant binding site for etomidate on GABA$_A$ receptors, definitively refuting lipid theories of anesthetic action. Photoaffinity-labeling studies with other anesthetic agents should provide similar levels of detail regarding anesthetic-binding sites on protein targets.

Although NMR and photoaffinity techniques can provide extensive information about anesthetic-binding sites on proteins, they cannot reveal the details of the three-dimensional structure of these sites. X-ray diffraction crystallography can provide this kind of three-dimensional detail and has been used to study anesthetic interactions with a small number of proteins. Firefly luciferase has been crystallized in the presence and absence of the anesthetic bromoform, confirming that anesthetics bind in the D-luciferin–binding pocket.[43] The firefly luciferase data demonstrate that anesthetics can bind to endogenous ligand–binding sites and that this binding strongly correlates with anesthetic inhibition of protein function. Human serum albumin has also been crystallized in the presence of either propofol or halothane, demonstrating binding of both anesthetics to preformed fatty acid–binding pockets. While these data provide insight into the structure of anesthetic-binding sites, x-ray crystallographic studies of anesthetic-binding sites on biologically relevant targets such as ion channels have been hampered by difficulties with crystallizing membrane proteins. Recently, a bacterial homolog of the ligand-gated ion channels, GLIC, has been crystallized and its crystal structure has been solved.[44] GLIC has been shown to be sensitive to clinical concentrations of anesthetics and the crystal structure of GLIC complexed with either desflurane or propofol has been solved.[45] These data reveal a preformed binding cavity in the interface between the transmembrane domains of each subunit of the ion channel. This landmark study opens the way to define the precise dimensions and location of anesthetic-binding pockets on their target proteins.

Summary

Evidence from studies using water-soluble proteins demonstrates that anesthetics can bind to hydrophobic pockets on proteins and that anesthetic–protein interactions can account for the Meyer–Overton rule and deviations from it. Photoaffinity-labeling studies demonstrate that etomidate binds to a pocket in the interface between the α_1 and β_3 subunits of the $GABA_A$ receptor. Mutagenesis of amino acids within this etomidate-binding pocket eliminates the anesthetic effect of etomidate, providing unequivocal evidence that anesthetic action can be mediated by binding to a specific protein site. Finally, recent x-ray crystallographic studies using the bacterial ion channel GLIC provide the first glimpse of
4 the three-dimensional structure of an anesthetic-binding site on a relevant protein model. While the long-standing controversy between lipid and protein theories of anesthesia may be behind us, numerous unanswered questions remain about the details of anesthetic–protein interactions, including:

1. What is the stoichiometry of anesthetic binding to a protein (i.e., do many anesthetic molecules interact with a single protein molecule or only a few)?
2. Do anesthetics compete with endogenous ligands for binding to hydrophobic pockets on protein targets or do they bind to fortuitous cavities in the protein?
3. Do all anesthetics bind to the same pocket on a protein or are there multiple hydrophobic pockets for different anesthetics?
4. How many proteins have hydrophobic pockets in which anesthetics can bind at clinically used concentrations?

HOW DO ANESTHETICS INTERFERE WITH THE ELECTROPHYSIOLOGIC FUNCTION OF THE NERVOUS SYSTEM?

The functional unit of the CNS is the neuron and ultimately general anesthetics must disrupt the function of neurons' mediating behavior, consciousness, and memory. In the simplest terms, anesthetics could accomplish this by altering the intrinsic firing rate of individual neurons, termed neuronal excitability, and/or by altering communication between neurons, generally occurring via synaptic transmission.

Neuronal Excitability

Neurons transmit information down their axons through action potentials. The propensity of a neuron to generate and propagate action potentials from the cell body to their nerve terminals is called its excitability. Intrinsic neuronal excitability is chiefly determined by three parameters: The resting membrane potential, the threshold potential for action potential generation, and the size/propagation of the action potential. Anesthetics can hyperpolarize (create a more negative resting membrane potential) both spinal motor neurons and cortical neurons,[46,47] and this ability to hyperpolarize neurons correlates with anesthetic potency. In general, the hyperpolarization produced by anesthetics is small in magnitude and is unlikely to alter *propagation* of an action potential down an axon. Small changes in resting potential may, however, inhibit the *initiation* of an action potential generated in response to synaptic excitation or in a spontaneously firing neuron. Indeed, isoflurane has been shown to hyperpolarize thalamic neurons, leading to an inhibition of tonic firing of action potentials.[48] Anesthetics have not been shown to alter reliably the threshold potential of a neuron for action potential generation. However, the data are conflicting on whether the size of the action potential, once initiated, is diminished by general anesthetics. A classic article by Larrabee and Posternak[49] demonstrated that concentrations of ether and chloroform that completely block synaptic transmission in mammalian sympathetic ganglia have no effect on the presynaptic action potential amplitude. Similar results have been obtained with fluorinated volatile anesthetics in mammalian brain preparations.[50,51] This dogma that the action potential is relatively resistant to general anesthetics has been challenged by more recent reports that volatile anesthetics at clinical concentrations produce a small but significant reduction in the size of the action potential in mammalian neurons.[52,53] At a large synapse, amenable to direct measurement of the action potential and transmitter release in the same neuron, the slightly smaller action potential was shown to produce a substantial reduction in transmitter release due to the
5 exponential relationship between the two.[53] Thus, while current data still support the prevailing view that neuronal excitability is only slightly affected by general anesthetics, this small effect may nevertheless contribute significantly to the clinical actions of volatile anesthetics.

Synaptic Transmission

Synaptic transmission is widely considered to be the most likely subcellular site of general anesthetic action. Neurotransmission across both excitatory and inhibitory synapses is markedly
6 altered by general anesthetics. General anesthetics inhibit excitatory synaptic transmission in a variety of preparations, including sympathetic ganglia,[49] olfactory cortex,[50] hippocampus,[51] and spinal cord.[54] However, not all excitatory synapses appear to be equally sensitive to anesthetics; indeed, transmission across some hippocampal excitatory synapses is enhanced by inhalational anesthetics.[30] In a similar fashion, general anesthetics both enhance and depress inhibitory synaptic transmission in various preparations. In a classic article in 1975, Nicoll et al.[55] showed that barbiturates enhanced inhibitory synaptic transmission by prolonging the decay of the GABAergic inhibitory postsynaptic current. Enhancement of inhibitory transmission has also been observed with many other general anesthetics including etomidate,[56] propofol,[57] inhalational anesthetics,[58] and neurosteroids.[59] Although anesthetic enhancement of inhibitory currents has received a great deal of attention as a potential mechanism of anesthesia,[32,60,61] it is important to note that there is also a large body of experimentation showing that clinical concentrations of general anesthetics can depress inhibitory postsynaptic potentials in hippocampus[62–64] and in spinal cord.[65] In summary, anesthetics do appear to have preferential effects on synapses, but there is

a great deal of heterogeneity in the manner in which anesthetic agents affect different synapses. This is not surprising given the large variation in synaptic structure, function (i.e., efficacy), and chemistry (neurotransmitters, modulators) extant in the nervous system.

Presynaptic Effects

Neurotransmitter release from glutamatergic synapses has consistently been found to be inhibited by clinical concentrations of volatile anesthetics. For example, a study by Perouansky and colleagues[66] conducted in mouse hippocampal slices showed that halothane inhibited excitatory postsynaptic potentials elicited by presynaptic electrical stimulation, but not those elicited by direct application of glutamate. This indicates that halothane must be acting to prevent the release of glutamate. MacIver and colleagues extended these observations by finding that the inhibition of glutamate release from hippocampal neurons is not due to effects at GABAergic synapses that could indirectly decrease transmitter release from glutamatergic neurons. Reduction of glutamate release by intravenous anesthetics has also been demonstrated, but the evidence is more limited and the effects potentially indirect.[67,68]

The data for anesthetic effects on inhibitory neurotransmitter release are mixed. Inhibition,[69] stimulation,[70,71] and no effect[72] on GABA release have been reported for both volatile and intravenous anesthetics. In a brain synaptosomal preparation where both GABA and glutamate release could be studied simultaneously, Westphalen and Hemmings[73] found that glutamate and, to a lesser degree, GABA release were inhibited by clinical concentrations of isoflurane. The mechanism underlying the anesthetic effects on transmitter release has not been established. The mechanism does not appear to involve reduced neurotransmitter synthesis or storage, but rather is a direct effect on neurosecretion. A variety of evidence argues that at some synapses a substantial portion of the anesthetic effect is upstream of the transmitter release machinery, perhaps on presynaptic sodium channels or potassium leak channels (see later discussion). However, genetic data in *Caenorhabditis elegans* show that mutations in the transmitter release machinery strongly influence volatile anesthetic sensitivity.[74,75] Recent evidence where the homologous rat mutant protein also reduced volatile anesthetic sensitivity against transmitter release suggests that this mechanism may be conserved in mammals.[76]

Postsynaptic Effects

Anesthetics alter the postsynaptic response to released neurotransmitter at a variety of synapses. Anesthetic modulation of excitatory neurotransmitter receptor function varies depending on the receptor type, anesthetic agent, and preparation. In a classic study, Richards and Smaje[77] examined the effects of several anesthetic agents on the response of olfactory cortical neurons to application of glutamate, the major excitatory neurotransmitter in the CNS. They found that while pentobarbital, diethyl ether, methoxyflurane, and alphaxalone depressed the electrical response to glutamate, halothane did not. In contrast, when acetylcholine was applied to the same olfactory cortical preparation, halothane and methoxyflurane stimulated the electrical response whereas pentobarbital had no effect; only alphaxalone depressed the electrical response to acetylcholine.[78] Anesthetic modulation of neuronal responses to inhibitory neurotransmitters is more consistent. A wide variety of anesthetics, including barbiturates, etomidate, neurosteroids, propofol, and fluorinated volatile anesthetics, have been shown to potentiate the electrical response to exogenously applied GABA [for reviews see (60,79)]. For example, Figure 5-2 illustrates the ability of enflurane to increase both the amplitude and the duration of the current elicited by application of GABA to hippocampal neurons.[80]

Summary

Anesthetics alter the two fundamental determinants of neuronal communication, neuronal excitability and synaptic transmission.

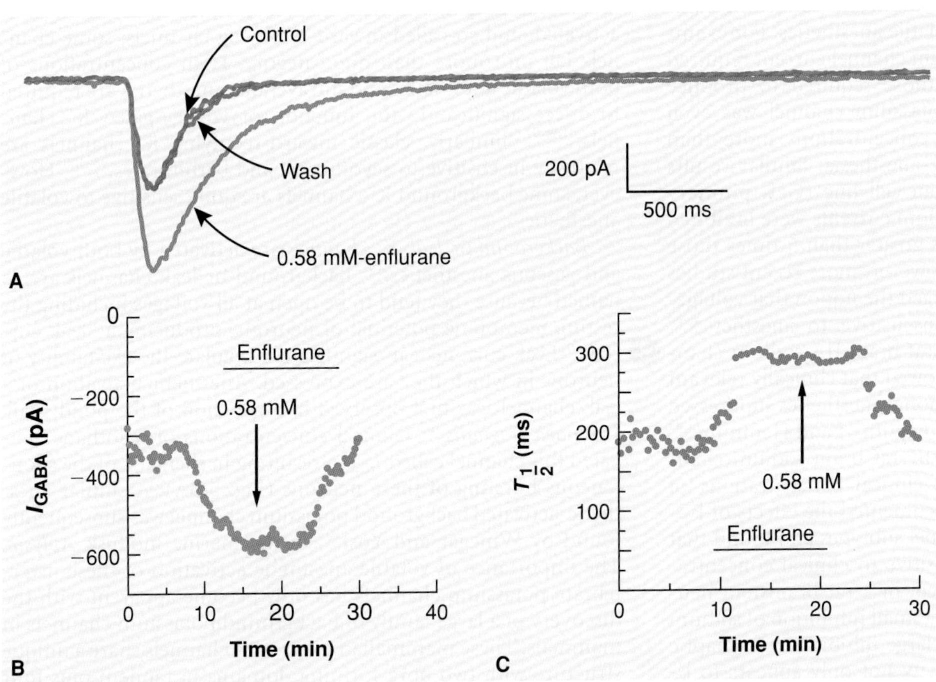

FIGURE 5-2. Enflurane potentiates the ability of GABA to activate a chloride current in cultured rat hippocampal cells. This potentiation is rapidly reversed by removal of enflurane (wash; **A**). Enflurane increases both the amplitude of the current **(B)** and the time ($T_{1/2}$) it takes for the current to decay **(C)**. (Reproduced with permission from Jones MV, Brooks PA, Harrison L: Enhancement of GABA-activated Cl^- currents in cultured rat hippocampal neurons by three volatile anaesthetics. *J Physiol.* 1992;449:289.)

Anesthetics have powerful and widespread effects on synaptic transmission that would logically contribute to general anesthesia. Thus, the synapse is generally thought to be the more relevant site of anesthetic action. Existing evidence indicates that even at the synapse, anesthetics have diverse actions, including presynaptic inhibition of neurotransmitter release, inhibition of excitatory neurotransmitter effect, and enhancement of inhibitory neurotransmitter effect. Furthermore, the synaptic effects of anesthetics differ among various anesthetic agents, neurotransmitters, and neuronal preparations.

ANESTHETIC ACTIONS ON ION CHANNELS

Ion channels are a likely target of anesthetic action. The advent of patch clamp techniques in the early 1980s made it possible to measure directly the currents from single ion channel proteins. Accordingly, during the 1980s and 1990s a major effort was directed at describing the effects of anesthetics on the various kinds of ion channels. The following section summarizes and distills this effort. For the purposes of this discussion, ion channels are cataloged according to the stimuli to which they respond by opening or closing (i.e., their mechanism of gating).

Anesthetic Effects on Voltage-Dependent Ion Channels

A variety of ion channels can sense a change in membrane potential and respond by either opening or closing their pore. These channels include voltage-dependent sodium, potassium, and calcium channels, all of which share significant structural
7 homologies. Voltage-dependent sodium and potassium channels are largely involved in generating and shaping action potentials. The effects of anesthetics on these channels have been extensively studied by Haydon and Urban[81] in the squid giant axon. These studies show that these invertebrate sodium and potassium channels are remarkably insensitive to volatile anesthetics. For example, 50% inhibition of the peak sodium channel current required halothane concentrations 8 times those required to produce anesthesia. The delayed rectifier potassium channel was even less sensitive, requiring halothane concentrations more than 20 times those required to produce anesthesia. Similar results have been obtained in a mammalian cell line (GH_3 pituitary cells) where both sodium and potassium currents were inhibited by halothane only at concentrations greater than 5 times those required to produce anesthesia.[82] However, more recent studies with volatile anesthetics have challenged the notion that voltage-dependent sodium channels are insensitive to anesthetics.[83] Rehberg and colleagues[84] expressed rat brain IIA sodium channels in a mammalian cell line and showed that clinically relevant concentrations of a variety of inhalational anesthetics suppressed voltage-elicited sodium currents. Ratnakumari and Hemmings[85] showed that sodium flux mediated by rat brain sodium channels was significantly inhibited by clinical concentrations of halothane. Shiraishi and Harris[86] documented the effects of isoflurane on a variety of sodium channel subtypes and found that several but not all subtypes are sensitive to clinical concentrations. Finally, as previously described, in a rat brainstem neuron, Wu and colleagues[53] found that a small inhibition of sodium currents by isoflurane resulted in a large inhibition of synaptic activity. Thus, sodium channel activity not only appears to be inhibited by volatile anesthetics, but this inhibition results in a significant reduction in synaptic function, at least at some mammalian synapses. Intravenous anesthetics have also been shown to inhibit sodium channels, but the concentrations for this effect are supra-clinical.[87,88]

VDCCs serve to couple electrical activity to specific cellular functions. In the nervous system, VDCCs located at presynaptic terminals respond to action potentials by opening. This allows calcium to enter the cell, activating calcium-dependent secretion of neurotransmitter into the synaptic cleft. At least six types of calcium channels (designated L, N, P, Q, R, and T) have been identified on the basis of electrophysiologic properties and a larger number based on amino acid sequence similarities. N-, P-, Q-, and R-type channels, as well as some of the untitled channels, are preferentially expressed in the nervous system and are thought to play a major role in synaptic transmission. L-type calcium channels, although expressed in brain, have been best studied in their role in excitation–contraction coupling in cardiac, skeletal, and smooth muscle and are thought to be less important in synaptic transmission. The anesthetic action on L- and T-type currents has been well characterized,[82,89,90] and some studies have reported the effects of anesthetics on N- and P-type currents.[91–93] As a general rule, these studies have shown that volatile anesthetics inhibit VDCCs (50% reduction in current) at concentrations 2 to 5 times those required to produce anesthesia in humans, with less than a 20% inhibition of calcium current at clinical concentrations of anesthetics. However, some studies have found VDCCs that are extremely sensitive to anesthetics. Takenoshita and Steinbach[94] reported a T-type calcium current in dorsal root ganglion neurons that was inhibited by subanesthetic concentrations of halothane. In addition, ffrench-Mullen and colleagues[95] have reported a VDCC of unspecified type in guinea pig hippocampus that is inhibited by pentobarbital at concentrations identical to those required to produce anesthesia. Thus, VDCCs could well mediate some actions of general anesthetics, but their general insensitivity makes them unlikely to be major targets.

Potassium channels are the most diverse of the ion channel types and include voltage-gated, background or leak channels that open over a wide range of voltages including at the resting membrane potential of neurons, second messenger and ligand-activated, and so-called inward-rectifying channels; some channels fall into more than one category. High concentrations of both volatile anesthetics and intravenous anesthetics are required to affect significantly the function of voltage-gated K^+ channels.[81,96,97] Similarly, classic inward-rectifying K^+ channels are relatively insensitive to sevoflurane and barbiturates.[98–100] However, some background K^+ channels are quite sensitive to volatile anesthetics.

Background or *leak K^+ channels* are activated by both volatile and gaseous anesthetics.[101] Background or leak channels are so named because they tend to be open at all voltages including the resting membrane potential of neurons, producing a "leak cur-
8 rent." Leak currents can significantly regulate the excitability of neurons in which they are expressed. Anesthetic activation of a leak channel was first observed in a ganglion of the pond snail, *Lymnaea stagnalis.*[102] Clinical concentrations of halothane activated this channel called $I_{K(AN)}$, resulting in silencing of the spontaneous bursting of these neurons (Fig. 5-3A). A similar anesthetic-activated background potassium channel was subsequently found by Winegar and Yost[103] in the marine mollusk *Aplysia.* The importance of volatile anesthetic activation of these invertebrate potassium channels has now become apparent with the discovery of a large family of background potassium channels in mammals. These mammalian potassium channels share a unique structure with two pore-forming domains in tandem plus four

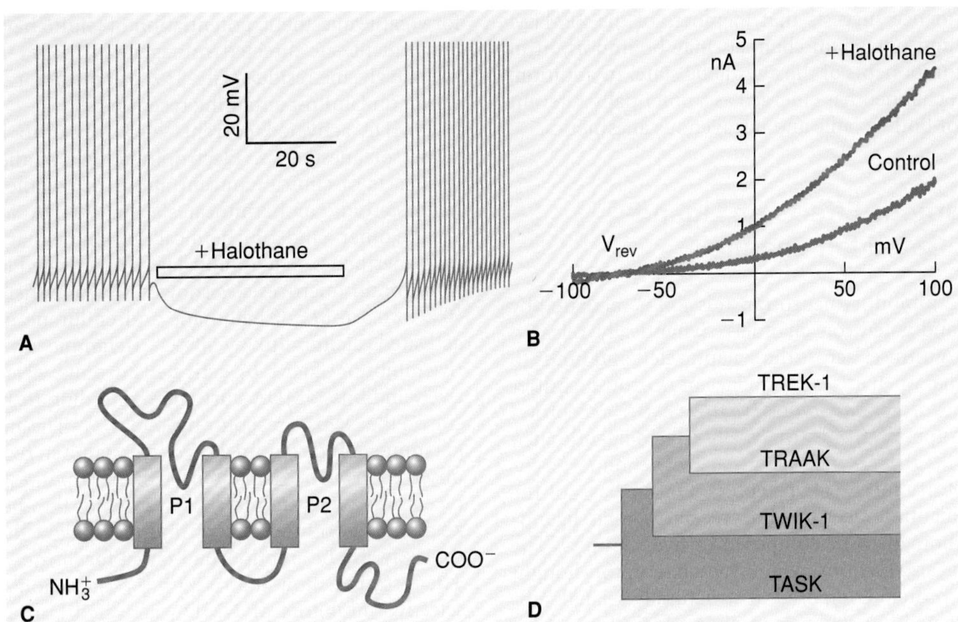

FIGURE 5-3. Volatile anesthetics activate background K⁺ channels. **A:** Halothane reversibly hyperpolarizes a pacemaker neuron from *L. stagnalis* (the pond snail) by activating $I_{K(AN)}$. **B:** Halothane (300 μM) activates human recombinant TREK-1 channels expressed in COS cells. The figure shows current–voltage relationships with reversal potential (V_{rev}) of –88 mV, indicative of a K⁺ channel. **C:** Predicted structure of a typical subunit of the mammalian background K⁺ channels. Note the four transmembrane-spanning segments (orange rectangles) and the two pore-forming domains (P1 and P2). Some but not all of these 2P/4TM K⁺ channels are activated by volatile anesthetics. **D:** Phylogenetic tree for the 2P/4TM family. (Reproduced with permission from Franks NP, Lieb WR: Background K⁺ channels: An important target for anesthetics? *Nat Neurosci.* 1999;2:395.)

transmembrane segments (2P/4TM; Fig. 5-3C, D).[104] Patel et al.[105] have studied the effects of volatile anesthetics on several members of the mammalian 2P/4TM family. They have shown that TREK-1 channels are activated by clinical concentrations of chloroform, diethyl ether, halothane, and isoflurane (Fig. 5-3B). In contrast, closely related TRAAK channels are insensitive to all the volatile anesthetics, and TASK channels are activated by halothane and isoflurane, inhibited by diethyl ether, and unaffected by chloroform. These authors further showed that the C-terminal regions of TASK and TREK-1 contain amino acids essential for anesthetic action. More recently, TREK-1 but not TASK was found to be activated by clinical concentrations of the gaseous anesthetics: Xenon, nitrous oxide, and cyclopropane.[106] Thus, activation of background K⁺ channels in mammalian vertebrates could be an important and general mechanism through which inhalational and gaseous anesthetics regulate neuronal resting membrane potential and thereby excitability. Indeed, genetic evidence argues for a role of these channels in producing anesthesia (see later discussion).

9 HCN channels are a relatively recently discovered channel type that is modulated by clinical concentrations of both volatile and some intravenous anesthetics. HCN channels pass a depolarizing current (termed I_h in the CNS) consisting of a mix of sodium and potassium ions and are activated by membrane hyperpolarization, the voltage dependence of which is shifted to a more depolarized range with the second messenger cyclic AMP.[107] Therefore, cyclic adenosine monophosphate (cAMP) activates HCN channels under most physiologic conditions. HCN channels are composed of homomeric and heteromeric combinations of four subunits—HCN1, 2, 3, 4—all of which are expressed in both brain and heart. HCN channels have been shown to regulate resting membrane potential and rhythmic firing of the sinoatrial node and spontaneously spiking neurons and thereby are important for synchronous oscillations of neuronal networks.[107]

Volatile anesthetics, propofol, and ketamine have been shown to inhibit HCN-mediated currents in both cell culture and native mouse neurons. The Bayliss group has shown that both halothane and isoflurane shifted activation of HCN1 channels expressed in cultured cells to a more negative membrane potential and reduced current amplitude.[108] In isolated spinal motor neurons, halothane reduced the I_h current, consistent with the inhibition of HCN channels. Similar inhibition of HCN1 channels was subsequently observed with clinical concentrations of propofol and ketamine.[109,110] The inhibition of HCN1 by ketamine was stereoselective in the same manner as its stereoselectivity for general anesthesia.[109] Notably, in this same study, etomidate was not found to inhibit HCN1 channel activation. Thus, HCN1 channels may be important for the actions of both volatile anesthetics and a subset of intravenous anesthetics. Genetic experiments described below argue that anesthetic inhibition of the HCN1 channel may contribute to ketamine and propofol anesthesia in vivo.

Summary

Existing evidence suggests that most voltage-dependent ion channels are modestly sensitive or insensitive to anesthetics. However, some sodium channel subtypes are inhibited by volatile anesthetics and this effect may be responsible in part for a reduction in neurotransmitter release at some synapses. Additional experimental data will be required to establish whether anesthetic-sensitive voltage-dependent ion channels are localized to specific synapses at which anesthetics have been shown to inhibit neurotransmitter release. Recent evidence suggests that members of the 2P/4TM family of background potassium channels may be important in producing some components of the anesthetic state. In addition, the HCN family of channels has emerged as a potentially relevant anesthetic target for both volatile and intravenous anesthetics.

Anesthetic Effects on Ligand-Gated Ion Channels

Fast excitatory and inhibitory neurotransmission is mediated by the actions of ligand-gated ion channels. Synaptically released glutamate or GABA diffuses across the synaptic cleft and binds to channel proteins that open as a consequence of neurotransmitter release. The channel proteins that bind GABA ($GABA_A$ receptors) are members of a superfamily of structurally related ligand-gated ion channel proteins that include nicotinic acetylcholine receptors, glycine receptors, and 5-HT_3 receptors. On the basis of the structure of the nicotinic acetylcholine receptor, each ligand-gated channel is thought to be composed of five subunits. The glutamate receptors also comprise a family, each receptor thought to be a tetrameric protein composed of structurally related subunits. The ligand-gated ion channels provide a logical target for anesthetic action because selective effects on these channels could inhibit fast excitatory synaptic transmission and/or facilitate fast inhibitory synaptic transmission. The effects of anesthetic agents on ligand-gated ion channels have been thoroughly cataloged in several reviews.[32,60,111,112] The following section provides a brief summary of this large body of work.

Glutamate-Activated Ion Channels

Glutamate-activated ion channels have been classified based on selective agonists, into three categories: AMPA receptors, kainate receptors, and NMDA receptors. 2-amino-3-(5-methyl-3-oxo-1,2- oxazol-4-yl)propanoic acid (AMPA) receptors, kainate receptors, and N-methyl-D-aspartic acid (NMDA)receptors are relatively nonselective monovalent cation channels involved in fast excitatory synaptic transmission, whereas NMDA channels conduct not only Na^+ and K^+ but also Ca^{2+} and are involved in long-term modulation of synaptic responses (long-term potentiation). Studies from the early 1980s in mouse and rat brain preparations showed that AMPA- and kainate-activated currents are insensitive to clinical concentrations of halothane,[113] enflurane,[114] and the neurosteroid allopregnanolone.[115] In contrast, kainate- and AMPA-activated currents were shown to be sensitive to barbiturates; in rat hippocampal neurons, 50 μM pentobarbital (pentobarbital produces anesthesia at approximately 50 μM) inhibited kainate and AMPA responses by 50%.[115] More recent studies using cloned and expressed glutamate receptor subunits show that submaximal agonist responses of GluR3 (AMPA-type) receptors are inhibited by fluorinated volatile anesthetics whereas agonist responses of GluR6 (kainate-type) receptors are enhanced.[116] In contrast, both GluR3 and GluR6 receptors are inhibited by pentobarbital. The directionally opposite effects of the volatile anesthetics on different glutamate receptor subtypes may explain the earlier inconclusive effects observed in tissue, where multiple subunit types are expressed. These opposite effects have also been used as a strategy to identify critical sites on the molecules involved in anesthetic effect. By producing GluR3/GluR6 receptor chimeras (receptors made up of various combinations of sections of the GluR3 and GluR6 receptors) and screening for volatile anesthetic effect, specific areas of the protein required for volatile anesthetic potentiation of GluR6 have been identified. Subsequent site-directed mutagenesis studies have identified a specific glycine residue (Gly-819) as critical for volatile anesthetic action on GluR6-containing receptors.[117]

NMDA-activated currents also appear to be sensitive to a subset of anesthetics. Electrophysiologic studies show virtually no effects of clinical concentrations of volatile anesthetics,[113,114] neurosteroids, or barbiturates[115] on NMDA-activated currents. On the other hand, biochemical flux studies have shown that volatile anesthetics may inhibit NMDA-activated channels. A study in rat brain microvesicles showed that anesthetic concentrations (0.2 to 0.3 mM) of halothane and enflurane inhibited NMDA-activated calcium flux by 50%.[118] Ketamine is a potent and selective inhibitor of NMDA-activated currents. Ketamine stereoselectively inhibits NMDA currents by binding to the phencyclidine site on the NMDA receptor protein.[119–121] The anesthetic effects of ketamine in intact animals show the same stereoselectivity as that observed in vitro,[26] consistent with the hypothesis that the NMDA receptor is a relevant molecular target for the anesthetic actions of ketamine. Two other recent findings suggest that NMDA receptors may also be an important target for nitrous oxide and xenon. These studies show that N_2O[122,123] and xenon[124] are potent and selective inhibitors of NMDA-activated currents. This is illustrated in Figure 5-4, showing that N_2O inhibits NMDA-elicited, but not GABA-elicited, currents in hippocampal neurons.

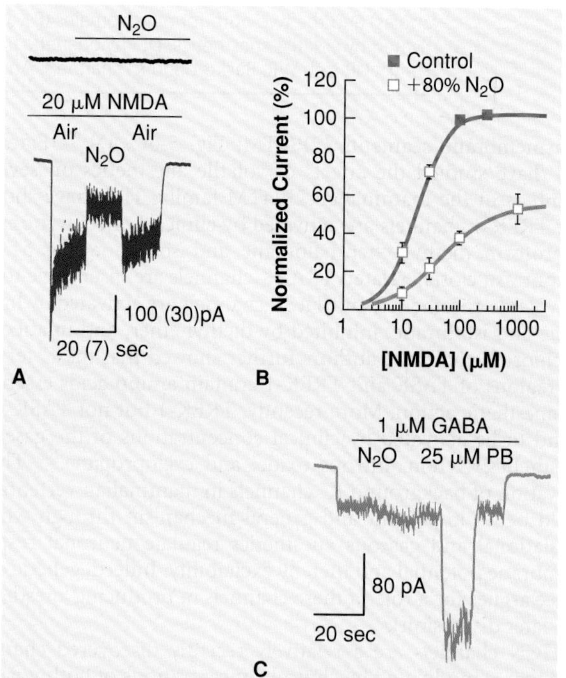

FIGURE 5-4. Nitrous oxide inhibits NMDA-elicited, but not GABA-elicited, currents in rat hippocampal neurons. **A:** Eighty percent N_2O has no effect on holding current (upper trace), but inhibits the current elicited by NMDA. **B:** N_2O causes a rightward and downward shift of the NMDA concentration–response curve, indicating a mixed competitive/noncompetitive antagonism. **C:** Eighty percent N_2O has little effect on GABA-elicited currents. In contrast, an equipotent anesthetic concentration of pentobarbital markedly enhances the GABA-elicited current. (Reproduced with permission from Jevtovic-Todorovic V, Todorovic SM, Mennerick S, et al.: Nitrous oxide (laughing gas) is an NMDA antagonist, neuroprotectant, and neurotoxin. *Nat Med.* 1998;4:460.)

GABA-Activated Ion Channels

GABA is the most important inhibitory neurotransmitter in the mammalian CNS. GABA-activated ion channels ($GABA_A$ receptors) mediate the postsynaptic response to synaptically released GABA by selectively allowing chloride ions to enter and thereby hyperpolarize neurons. $GABA_A$ receptors are multi-subunit proteins consisting of various combinations of α, β, δ, and ε subunits, and there are many subtypes of each of these subunits. The function of $GABA_A$ receptors is modulated by a wide variety of pharmacologic agents including convulsants, anticonvulsants, sedatives, anxiolytics, and anesthetics.[60] The effects of these various drugs on $GABA_A$ receptor function vary across brain regions and cell types. The following section briefly reviews the effects of anesthetics on $GABA_A$ receptor function.

Barbiturates, anesthetic steroids, benzodiazepines, propofol, etomidate, and volatile anesthetics all modulate $GABA_A$ receptor function.[80,125–128] These drugs produce three kinds of effects on the electrophysiologic behavior of the $GABA_A$ receptor channels: Potentiation, direct gating, and inhibition. *Potentiation* refers to the ability of anesthetics to increase markedly the current elicited by low concentrations of GABA, but to produce no increase in the current elicited by a maximally effective concentration of GABA. Potentiation is illustrated in Figure 5-5, showing the effects of halothane on currents elicited by a range of GABA concentrations in dissociated cortical neurons. Anesthetic potentiation of $GABA_A$ currents generally occurs at concentrations of anesthetics within the clinical range. *Direct gating* refers to the ability of anesthetics to activate $GABA_A$ channels in the absence of GABA. Generally, direct gating of $GABA_A$ currents occurs at anesthetic concentrations higher than those used clinically, but the concentration–response curves for potentiation and for direct gating can overlap. It is not known whether direct gating of $GABA_A$ channels is either required for or contributes to the effects of anesthetics on GABA-mediated inhibitory synaptic transmission in vivo. In the case of anesthetic steroids, strong evidence indicates that potentiation, rather than direct gating of $GABA_A$ currents, is required for producing anesthesia.[27] Anesthetics can also inhibit GABA-activated currents. *Inhibition* refers to the ability of anesthetics to prevent GABA from initiating current flow through $GABA_A$ channels and has generally been observed at high concentrations of both GABA and anesthetic.[129,130] Inhibition of $GABA_A$ channels may help to explain why volatile anesthetics have, in some cases, been observed to inhibit rather than facilitate inhibitory synaptic transmission.[62]

Effects of anesthetics have also been observed on the function of single $GABA_A$ channels. These studies show that barbiturates,[128] propofol,[126] and volatile anesthetics[131] do not alter the conductance (rate at which ions traverse the open channel) of the channel, but that they increase the frequency with which the channel opens and/or the average length of time that the channel remains open. Collectively, the whole cell and single channel data are most consistent with the idea that clinical concentrations of anesthetics produce a change in the conformation of $GABA_A$ receptors that increases the affinity of the receptor for GABA. This is consistent with the ability of anesthetics to increase the duration of inhibitory postsynaptic potentials since higher-affinity binding of GABA would slow the dissociation of GABA from postsynaptic $GABA_A$ channels. Anesthetics would not be expected to increase the peak amplitude of a GABAergic inhibitory postsynaptic potential since synaptically released GABA probably reaches very high concentrations in the synapse. Higher concentrations of anesthetics can produce additional effects, either directly activating or inhibiting $GABA_A$ channels. Consistent with these ideas, a study by Banks and Pearce[132] showed that isoflurane and enflurane simultaneously increased the duration and decreased the amplitude of GABAergic inhibitory postsynaptic currents in hippocampal slices.

Despite the similar effects of many anesthetics on $GABA_A$ receptor function, different anesthetics act on distinct subtypes of $GABA_A$ receptors. This is well illustrated for benzodiazepine sensitivity, which requires the presence of the γ_2 subunit subtype.[133] Similarly, sensitivity to etomidate has been shown to require the presence of a β_2 or β_3 subunit.[134]. The presence of a δ or ε subunit in a $GABA_A$ receptor has been shown to confer insensitivity to the potentiating effects of some anesthetics.[135,136] Interestingly, $GABA_A$ receptors composed of ρ-type subunits (referred to as

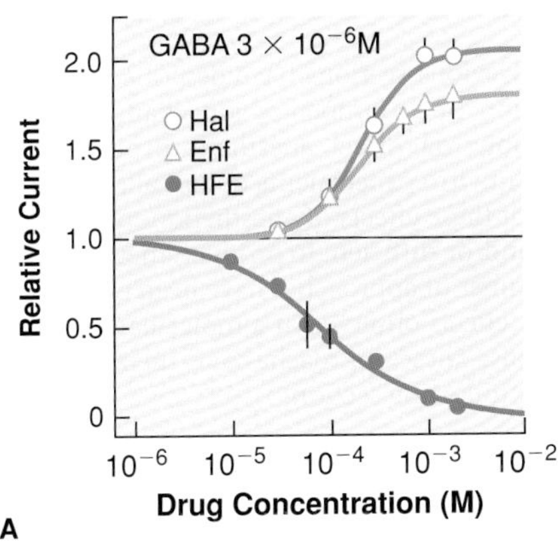

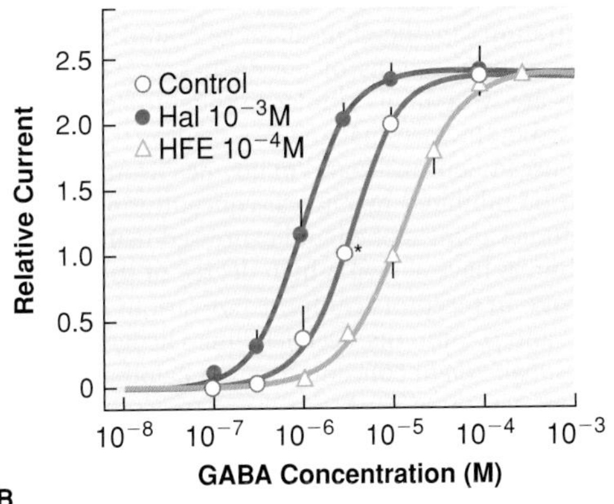

FIGURE 5-5. The effects of halothane (Hal), enflurane (Enf), and fluoroethyl (HFE) on GABA-activated chloride currents in dissociated rat CNS neurons. **A:** Clinical concentrations of halothane and enflurane potentiate the ability of GABA to elicit a chloride current. The convulsant fluoroethyl antagonizes the effects of GABA. **B:** GABA causes a concentration-dependent activation of a chloride current. Halothane shifts the GABA concentration–response curve to the left (increases the apparent affinity of the channel for GABA), whereas fluoroethyl shifts the curve to the right (decreases the apparent affinity of the channel for GABA). (Reproduced with permission from Wakamori M, Ikemoto Y, Akaike N: Effects of two volatile anesthetics and a volatile convulsant on the excitatory and inhibitory amino acid responses in dissociated CNS neurons of the rat. *J Neurophysiol.* 1991;66:2014.)

$GABA_C$ receptors) have been shown to be inhibited rather than potentiated by volatile anesthetics.[137] This property has been exploited to construct chimeric receptors composed of part of the ρ-receptor coupled to part of an α, β, or glycine receptor subunit. By screening these chimeras for anesthetic sensitivity, regions of the α, β, and glycine subunits responsible for anesthetic sensitivity have been identified. On the basis of the results of these chimeric studies, site-directed mutagenesis studies were performed to identify the specific amino acids responsible for conferring anesthetic sensitivity. These studies revealed two critical amino acids, near the extracellular regions of transmembrane domains 2 and 3 (TM2, TM3) of the glycine and $GABA_A$ receptors, that are required for the volatile anesthetic potentiation of agonist effect.[138] It is not yet clear whether these amino acids represent a volatile anesthetic-binding site or whether they are sites critical to transducing anesthetic-induced conformational changes in the receptor molecule. Interestingly, one of the amino acids shown to be critical to the volatile anesthetic effect (TM3 site) has also been shown to be required (in the β_2/β_3 subunit) for the potentiating effects of etomidate.[139] In contrast, the TM2 and TM3 sites do not appear to be required for potentiation by propofol, barbiturates, or neurosteroids.[140] A distinct amino acid in the TM3 region of the β_1 subunit of the $GABA_A$ receptor has been shown to selectively modulate the ability of propofol to potentiate GABA agonist effects. Neurosteroids actions on $GABA_A$ receptors occur via interactions with specific sites within the transmembrane-spanning regions of the α_1 and β_2 subunits that are distinct from those with which benzodiazepines and pentobarbital act.[141] Collectively, these data provide strong evidence that there are multiple unique sites for the action of anesthetics on the $GABA_A$ receptor protein.

Other Ligand-Activated Ion Channels

Ligand-gated receptors structurally similar to the $GABA_A$ receptor including the nicotinic acetylcholine receptors (muscle and neuronal types), glycine receptors, and 5-HT_3 receptors have been shown to be modulated by general anesthetics.[142] The muscle nicotinic receptor has served as a useful model because of its abundance and the wealth of knowledge about its structure. This nicotinic receptor subtype has been shown to be inhibited by anesthetic concentrations in the clinical range[143] and to be desensitized by higher concentrations of anesthetics.[144] Neuronal nicotinic receptors are structurally similar to the muscle type and are widely expressed in the mammalian CNS. Neuronal nicotinic receptors in molluscan neurons[145] and in bovine chromaffin cells[146] were found to be inhibited by clinical concentrations of volatile anesthetics. Studies using cloned and expressed neuronal nicotinic receptor subunits have shown a high degree of subunit and anesthetic selectivity. In receptors composed of various combinations of α_2, α_4, β_2, and β_4 subunits, acetylcholine-elicited currents are inhibited by *subanesthetic* concentrations of halothane[147] or isoflurane.[148] In contrast, these receptors are relatively insensitive to propofol, and receptors composed of only α_7 subunits are insensitive to both isoflurane and propofol.[148,149] Subsequent pharmacologic experiments using selective inhibitors of neuronal nicotinic receptors led to the conclusion that these receptors are unlikely to have a major role in immobilization by volatile anesthetics.[150,151] However, they might play a role in the amnestic or hypnotic effects of volatile anesthetics.[152]

Glycine is an important inhibitory neurotransmitter, particularly in the spinal cord and brainstem. The glycine receptor is a member of the ligand-activated channel superfamily that, like the $GABA_A$ receptor, is a chloride-selective ion channel. A large number of studies have shown that clinical concentrations of volatile anesthetics potentiate glycine-activated currents in intact neurons[113] and in cloned glycine receptors expressed in oocytes.[153,154] Volatile anesthetics appear to produce their potentiating effect by increasing the affinity of the receptor for glycine, much like for $GABA_A$ receptors.[152] Propofol,[126] alphaxalone, and pentobarbital also potentiate glycine-activated currents, whereas etomidate and ketamine do not.[154] Potentiation of glycine receptor function may contribute to the anesthetic action of volatile anesthetics and some parenteral anesthetics.

The 5-HT_3 receptors are also members of the genetically related superfamily of ligand-gated receptor channels. Clinical concentrations of volatile anesthetics potentiate currents activated by 5-HT_3 hydroxytryptamine in intact cells[155] and in cloned receptors expressed in oocytes.[156] In contrast, thiopental inhibits 5-HT_3 receptor currents[155] and propofol is without effect on these receptor channels.[156] The 5-HT_3 receptors may play some role in the anesthetic state produced by volatile anesthetics and may also contribute to some unpleasant anesthetic side effects such as nausea and vomiting.

Summary

Several ligand-gated ion channels are modulated by clinical concentrations of anesthetics. Ketamine, N_2O, and xenon inhibit NMDA-type glutamate receptors, and this effect may play a major role in their mechanism of action. A large body of evidence shows that clinical concentrations of many anesthetics potentiate GABA-activated currents in the CNS. This suggests that $GABA_A$ receptors
10 are a probable molecular target of anesthetics. Other members of the ligand-activated ion channel family, including glycine receptors, neuronal nicotinic receptors, and 5-HT_3 receptors, are also affected by clinical concentrations of anesthetics and remain plausible anesthetic targets.

HOW ARE THE MOLECULAR EFFECTS OF ANESTHETICS LINKED TO ANESTHESIA IN THE INTACT ORGANISM?

The previous sections have described how anesthetics affect the function of a number of ion channels and signaling proteins, probably via direct anesthetic–protein interactions. However, these in vitro experiments do not allow for determining which, if any, of these effects of anesthetics on protein function are necessary and/or sufficient to produce anesthesia in an intact organism. A number of approaches have been employed to try to link anesthetic effects observed at a molecular level to anesthesia in intact animals. These approaches and their pitfalls are briefly explored in the following section.

Pharmacologic Approaches

An experimental paradigm frequently used to study anesthetic mechanisms is to administer a drug thought to act specifically at a putative anesthetic target (e.g., a receptor agonist or antagonist, an ion channel activator or antagonist), then determine whether the drug has either increased or decreased the animal's sensitivity to a given anesthetic. The underlying assumption is that if a change in anesthetic sensitivity is observed, then the anesthetic is likely to act via an action on the specific target of the administered drug. However, conclusions from this approach must be tempered by a number of considerations. The drugs used to modulate anesthetic sensitivity usually have their own direct effects on CNS excitability and thus may *indirectly* affect anesthetic requirements. For example, while α_2-adrenergic agonists decrease halothane MAC,[157] they are profound CNS depressants in their own right and produce anesthesia by mechanisms distinct from those used by volatile anesthetics. Thus, the "MAC-sparing" effects of α_2-agonists provide little insight into how halothane works. A more useful pharmacologic strategy would be to identify drugs that have no effect on CNS excitability but prevent the effects of given anesthetics. Currently, however, there are no such anesthetic antagonists. Development of specific antagonists for anesthetic agents would provide a major tool for linking anesthetic effects at the molecular level to anesthesia in the intact organism and might also be of significant clinical utility.

An alternative pharmacologic approach is to develop "litmus tests" for the relevance of anesthetic effects observed in vitro. One such test takes advantage of compounds that are non-anesthetic despite the predictions of the Meyer–Overton rule.[19] Another test uses anesthetic stereoselectivity as the discriminator with the assumption that a target not affected with the same stereoselectivity as that observed for whole animal anesthesia is unlikely to be relevant to the production of anesthesia.[158] Although these tests may increase the plausibility of a particular target, they cannot be used to definitively rule out a potential target. For example, a non-anesthetic might depress CNS excitability via its actions on an important anesthetic target site while simultaneously producing counterbalancing excitatory effects at a second site. In this case the "litmus test" would incorrectly eliminate the anesthetic site as irrelevant to whole-animal anesthesia. This example is quite plausible given the convulsant effects of many of the non-anesthetic polyhalogenated hydrocarbons. Likewise, anesthetics may act stereoselectively on some relevant targets and non-stereoselectively on others. Another sort of litmus test is to antagonize the putative anesthetic target. If anesthetic effects are mediated through this target, inactivation of the target by the antagonist should result in anesthetic resistance. Using this logic, the modest MAC-sparing effects of $GABA_A$ and glycine receptor antagonists were used to argue that both $GABA_A$ and glycine receptors mediate some but not all of the immobilizing effects of volatile anesthetics in rodents.[159-161] This same group used the lack of effect of neuronal nicotinic antagonists on isoflurane MAC to conclude that these receptors had no role in volatile anesthetic immobilization.[150] Issues of specificity and efficacy of the antagonists prevent these experiments from being definitive. Nevertheless, these results are important and consistent with the conclusions that volatile anesthetics affect the function of a large number of important neuronal proteins and no one target is likely to mediate all of the effects of these drugs.

Genetic Approaches

An alternative approach to study the relationship between anesthetic effects observed in vitro and whole-animal anesthesia is to alter the structure or abundance of putative anesthetic targets and determine how this affects whole-animal anesthetic sensitivity. While they also have potential flaws, genetic techniques provide 11
the most specific and versatile methods for changing the structure or abundance of putative anesthetic targets. The first direct genetic screen for mutants with altered general anesthetic sensitivity was performed in the nematode C. elegans by Morgan and Cascorbi.[162] They screened for altered sensitivity to immobilization of *C. elegans* by halothane, which occurs at supra-clinical concentrations. The first mutant isolated had a 3-fold reduction in its EC_{50} for halothane and had an interesting locomotion defect in the absence of halothane called *fainting*. Normal *C. elegans* worms crawl almost continuously whereas "fainter" mutants spontaneously stop moving for extended periods of time. In testing other previously isolated fainter mutants, Sedensky found that, in general, fainters were hypersensitive to halothane.[163] Subsequent genetic screens and mapping of fainting mutants have led to a focus on a novel presumptive cation channel, NCA-1/NCA-2, that controls halothane sensitivity in both *C. elegans* and in the fruit fly *Drosophila.*[164] This remarkable conservation of the anesthetic hypersensitivity phenotype across such divergent species argues for a fundamental role of NCA-1/NCA-2 in the action of halothane.

Clinical concentrations of volatile anesthetics do not immobilize *C. elegans,* but they do produce behavioral effects including loss of coordinated movement.[165] Crowder and colleagues have screened for mutants that are resistant to anesthetic-induced uncoordination and found that mutations in a set of genes encoding proteins regulating neurotransmitter release control anesthetic sensitivity.[74,75] The gene with the largest effect encoded syntaxin 1A, a neuronal protein highly conserved from *C. elegans* to humans and essential for fusion of neurotransmitter vesicles with the presynaptic membrane.[75] Importantly, some syntaxin mutations produced hypersensitivity to volatile anesthetics while others conferred resistance. These allelic differences in anesthetic sensitivity could not be accounted for by effects on the process of transmitter release itself; rather, the genetic data argued that syntaxin interacts with a protein critical for volatile anesthetic action, perhaps an anesthetic target. Subsequent experiments by others in rat have shown that expression of the same mutant syntaxin in cultured rat neurons reduces the potency of isoflurane at inhibiting neurotransmitter release in mammals.[76] A highly evolutionarily conserved presynaptic protein called UNC-13 in *C. elegans* has been implicated in this syntaxin-regulated volatile anesthetic mechanism.[166] *C. elegans UNC-13* mutants are fully resistant to the effects of clinical concentration of isoflurane, and isoflurane prevents the normal synaptic localization of UNC-13 in *C. elegans.* Whether UNC-13 is a direct target of volatile anesthetics is unknown. This same laboratory has also shown by mutant analysis that an NMDA glutamate receptor subunit is essential for nitrous oxide sensitivity in *C. elegans*[167] and that another glutamate receptor subunit is required for the effects of xenon.[168]

In *Drosophila,* clinical concentrations of volatile anesthetics disrupt negative geotaxis behavior and response to a noxious light or heat stimulus.[169-171] Using one or more of these anesthetics effects, Krishnan and Nash[171] performed a forward genetic screen for halothane resistance. The results of this screen have led to a focus on the *Drosophila* homolog of *NCA-1/2.* As previously discussed, mutants in the *Drosophila* homolog of *NCA-1/2* are hypersensitive to halothane like the *C. elegans* mutants.[164] The synergy of both *Drosophila* and *C. elegans* genetics should lead to an understanding of how this channel controls volatile anesthetic sensitivity.

In mammals, the most powerful genetic model organism is mouse, where techniques have been developed to alter or delete any gene of interest. The $GABA_A$ receptor has been extensively studied using mouse genetic techniques.[172] Mice carrying mutations in α, β, and δ $GABA_A$ receptor subunits have been tested for their effects on anesthetic end points (Table 5-1). For α subunits, four knockout mutations (where the gene is fully inactivated) and one knockin mutation (where a functional but altered gene product is produced) have been examined. Knockout of the α_1 and α_4 subunits produced similar phenotypes with a large reduction of the efficacy of isoflurane at blocking learning and memory tasks in the mutant mice compared to

TABLE 5-1. MOUSE GENETICS OF ANESTHESIA

Gene Product	Mutation	Anesthetic Behavioral Effect				Reference
		Hypnosis	Immobility	Sedation	Amnesia	
GABA$_A$ α_1	Global and forebrain KO	**Hal**; *Iso, Pentobarb*	*Iso, Hal, Des*		Iso	Sonner Mol Pharm 2005, Blednov JPET 2003[173, 175]
GABA$_A$ α_1	S270H/L277A	**Iso, Enf, Etom**; *Hal*	*Iso, Hal, Des*	**Etom**; *Pentobarb*		Borghese JPET 2006, Sonner Anesth 2007, Werner 2006[178–180]
GABA$_A$ α_4	Global KO	**Hal**; *Iso*	*Iso, Hal*		**Iso**	Rau AA 2009[174]
GABA$_A$ α_5	Global KO	*Etom*		*Etom*	**Etom**; *Ket*	Cheng J Neurosci 2006, Martin Anesth 2009[176, 249]
GABA$_A$ α_6	Global KO	*Hal, Enf, Pentobarb*	*Enf*			Homanics Mol Pharm 1997[177]
GABA$_A$ β_2	Global KO	*Etom, Pentobarb*	*Etom*	**Etom**		Blednov JPET 2003, O'Meara Neuroreport 2004[173, 250]
GABA$_A$ β_2	N265S	**Etom**; *Prop, Pentobarb*	**Etom**; *Prop*	**Etom**; *Prop*		Reynolds J Neurosci 2003, Cirone Anesth 2004[189–190]
GABA$_A$ β_3	Global and forebrain KO	**Etom**; *Hal, Enf, Pentobarb*	**Hal, Enf**; *Iso*		**Iso**; *Etom*	Quinlan Anesth 1998, Rau AA 2011[251–252]
GABA$_A$ β_3	N265M	**Etom, Prop, Pentobarb**; *neurosteroids, Hal, Enf*	***Etom, Prop, Pentobarb***; **Hal, Iso, Enf, Cyclo**; *neurosteroids*	*Etom*	*Prop, Iso*	Zeller Mol Pharm 2007, Zeller BMC Pharm 2007, Jurd FASEB J 2003, Lambert Eur J Pharm 2005, Liao AA 2005[184–186,188,253]
GABA$_A$ δ	Global KO	**Neurosteroids**; *Etom, Prop, Ketam, Pentobarb, Hal, Enf*	*Hal, Enf*	*Neurosteroids*		Mihalek PNAS 1999[191]
TREK-1	Global KO	**Chloro, Des, Iso, Hal, Sevo**; *Pentobarb*	**Chloro, Des, Hal, Iso, Sevo**			Herteaux EMBO J 2004[192]
TASK-1	Global KO	**Iso**; *Hal*	**Hal**; *Iso*			Linden JPET 2006, Linden JPET 2008[194,254]
TASK-2	Global KO		*Hal, Iso, Des*			Gerstin AA 2003[98]
TASK-3	Global KO	**Hal**; *Cyclo, Prop*	**Hal**; *Iso*			Linden JPET 2007, Pang 2009[195,196]
HCN1	Global KO	**Ket, Prop**; *Etom*				Chen J Neurophys 2009[255]

Hal, halothane; Iso, Isoflurane; Pentobarb, pentobarbital; Des, desflurane; Enf, enflurane; Etom, etomidate; Prop, propofol; Cyclo, cyclopropane; Ketam, ketamine; Chloro, chloroform.

Bold indicates decreased sensitivity to that anesthetic; bold italics indicates lack of sensitivity; italics indicates normal sensitivity.

wild-type controls.[173–175] Similarly, an α_5 knockout mouse was strongly resistant to the amnestic effects of etomidate.[176] α_1 and α_4 knockouts also had small differences for halothane potency in assays of hypnosis. An α_6 knockout strain had normal sensitivities to halothane, enflurane, and pentobarbital in hypnosis and immobility assays.[177] A knockin α_1 mouse strain expressing a double-mutated α_1(S270H, L277A) subunit has also been tested for its anesthetic sensitivity.[178–180] The α_1(S270H) mutation had been shown to block GABA potentiation by volatile anesthetics,[181] but the mutation also increased native sensitivity to GABA, confounding interpretation of the data. Moreover, α_1(S270H) single-mutant mice are quite abnormal behaviorally and are prone to anesthetic-induced seizure activity.[182] Thus, a second mutation, L277A, was introduced into the α_1 subunit that compensated for the change in native gating properties.[178] The α_1(S270H, L277A) mice are viable and grossly behaviorally normal. These mice are mildly resistant to the hypnotic effects of isoflurane, enflurane, and etomidate as well as the ataxic effects of etomidate; however, the potency of the drugs in MAC and fear-conditioning assays (a measure of learning) are not altered by the double-mutant α_1 subunit.

While the anesthetic behavioral phenotypes of the α mutant mice were only incrementally different from wild-type mice, β subunit mutants have profound differences for the intravenous anesthetics etomidate and propofol. The electrophysiologic experiments that formed the foundation for generation of the mutant mice showed that etomidate potently inhibited β_2- and β_3-containing GABA$_A$ receptors and was much less potent against β_1-containing receptors.[134,139]. Mouse β_2 and β_3 both differ from β_1 at amino residue 265 in the second transmembrane domain where it is an asparagine (N) in β_2 and β_3 but is a serine (S) in β_1 and a methionine (M) in an etomidate-insensitive

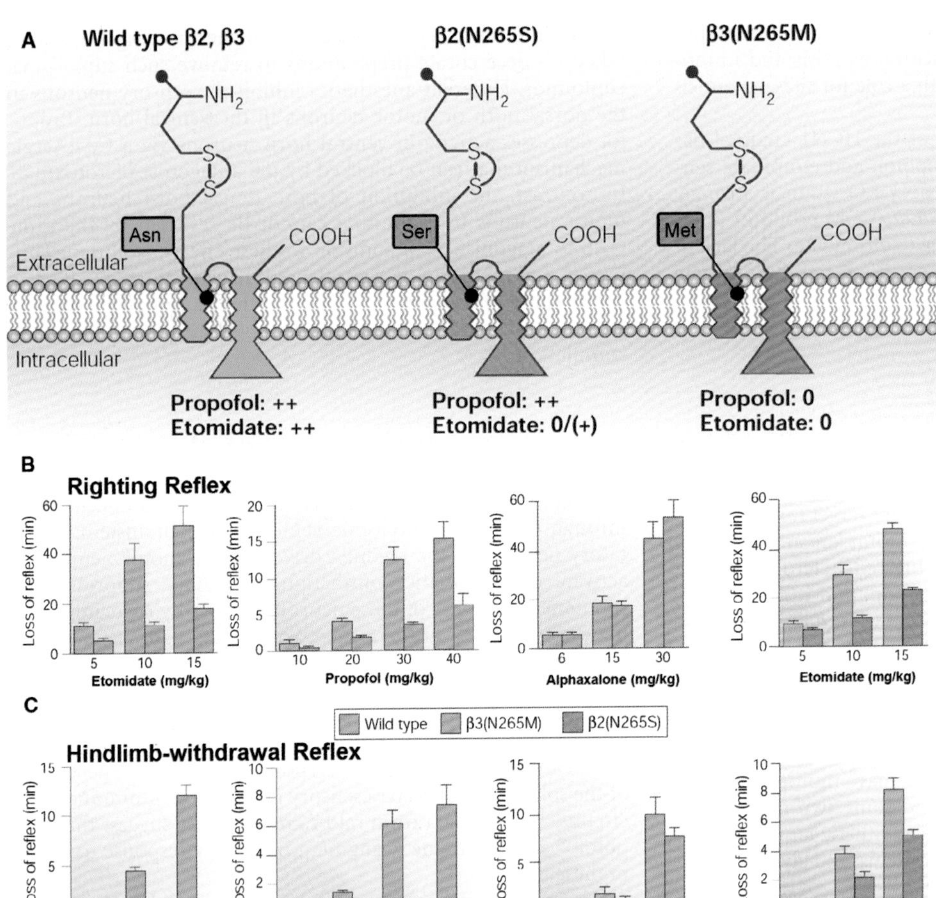

FIGURE 5-6. Mutations in the β_2 and β_3 subunits of the $GABA_A$ receptor reduce sensitivity to etomidate and propofol. **A:** Knockin transgenic mice were generated with mutation of a conserved asparagine (Asn) in the second transmembrane domain to a serine (Ser) in the β_2 subunit or a methionine (Met) in the β_3 subunit. **B:** The sensitivities of the wild type and the two knockin mice strains were measured in a LORR assay, which is thought to model hypnosis. Mutant sensitivities to etomidate and propofol are highly significantly different compared to wild type. The neurosteroid alphaxalone is equally potent in wild type and in the β_3(N265M) strain. **C:** The sensitivities of the wild type and the two knockin mice strains were measured in a hindlimb-withdrawal reflex to a painful stimulus assay, which is thought to model immobility. Note the lack of significant sensitivities to either etomidate or propofol in the β_3(N265M) strain. (Adapted from Rudolph U, Antkowiak B: Molecular and neuronal substrates for general anaesthetics. *Nat Rev Neurosci* 2004;5:709.)

insect GABA receptor. Electrophysiologic testing of recombinant β_3(N265M) receptors revealed that these mutations blocked potentiation of the receptor by etomidate and propofol.[139,183] An important confirmation of the relevance of these in vitro studies came from Rudolph and colleagues, who showed that a mouse β_3(N265M) knockin strain was fully resistant to the immobilizing effects of etomidate, propofol, and pentobarbital (Fig. 5-6).[184,185] These results provided the first definitive link between an anesthetic in vitro action and a mammalian behavioral end point. However, the β_3(N265M) mice were not completely resistant to the hypnotic action of these anesthetics, indicating that other targets mediate this behavioral effect (Table 5-1). Interestingly, the respiratory depressant effects of etomidate and propofol are also blocked by the β_3(N265M) mutation, but the cardiovascular and hypothermic actions of the drugs are not.[186,187] The β_3(N265M) mice also have a modest reduction in sensitivity to the immobilizing actions of volatile anesthetics, suggesting that the β_3 subunit may play a minor role in immobilization, but the mutant has unaltered sensitivity to the amnestic effects of isoflurane and propofol.[186,188] A similar approach for the β_2 subunit has shown that a β_2(N265S) mutant mouse has reduced sensitivity to etomidate although no anesthetic end point is fully blocked by this mutation (Fig. 5-6).[189,190] Finally, strains carrying a knockout mutation of the δ subunit of the $GABA_A$ receptor have a shorter duration of neurosteroid-induced loss of righting reflex (LORR) whereas their sensitivity to other intravenous and volatile anesthetics is unchanged.[191] Thus, the δ subunit may play a relatively specific role in neurosteroid action.

The roles in anesthetic sensitivity of two of the background potassium channels have been tested in limited mouse genetic studies. A TREK-1 knockout mouse was found to be significantly but not fully resistant to multiple volatile anesthetics for hypnotic and immobility end points.[192] The volatile anesthetic resistance of the TREK-1 knockout is substantial, particularly for halothane where MAC was increased by 48%. Importantly, the TREK-1 knockout mice have a normal sensitivity to pentobarbital, indicating specificity for volatile anesthetics consistent with previous electrophysiologic data. Recently, Westphalen et al. has used the TREK-1 knockout strain to test the hypothesis that TREK-1 mediates some of the presynaptic inhibitory effects of volatile anesthetics.[193] Indeed, glutamate release from synaptosomes prepared from the TREK-1 knockout strain is significantly resistant to inhibition by halothane compared to release from wild-type control synaptosomes. The role of TASK-2, another two-pore background potassium channel, has been similarly tested by measuring the MAC of a TASK-2 knockout mouse. However, unlike for TREK-1, the TASK-2 knockout has MAC values similar to wild-type controls for desflurane, halothane, and isoflurane.[98] This result is somewhat surprising given that TASK-2 is strongly activated by halothane and isoflurane and may be explained by an overall reduced expression in the nervous system compared to TREK-1.[101] Most recently, knockout strains for TASK-1 and TASK-3 have been tested. Both have modest but significant volatile anesthetic resistance to hypnosis and immobility[194–196] (Table 5-1), consistent with a role for these channels in anesthesia.

Finally, a knockout mouse strain of the HCN1 channel has been generated and its ketamine, propofol, and etomidate sensitivity for hypnosis tested.[109] The HCN1 KO strain is strongly resistant to ketamine (85% increased ED_{50}) and propofol (47% increased ED_{50}) and normally sensitive to etomidate. The lack of effect of etomidate indicates that the increase is not due to some nonspecific increase in sensitivities to all hypnotics.

Summary

Results from both invertebrate and vertebrate genetics indicate that multiple proteins control volatile anesthetic sensitivity. Some of these may be anesthetic targets and some not. The evidence for β_3-containing $GABA_A$ receptors as a relevant target for etomidate and propofol, however, is quite strong. Etomidate and propofol potentiate β_3-containing receptors expressed heterologously, a missense mutation blocks this potentiation, and mice expressing this mutant receptor are fully resistant to immobilization by etomidate, propofol, and pentobarbital but are normally sensitive to the neurosteroid anesthetic alphaxalone. Other anesthetic end points are not fully dependent on the β_3 subunit and other targets must be involved. For propofol, but not etomidate, both electrophysiologic and genetic data implicate the HCN1 channel as one such target. Volatile anesthetics appear to have multiple relevant targets, including $GABA_A$ receptors and some two-pore potassium channels. Other plausible volatile anesthetic targets such as certain sodium channels, presynaptic proteins, and glycine receptors remain to be examined genetically.

WHERE IN THE CENTRAL NERVOUS SYSTEM DO ANESTHETICS WORK?

Immobility

12 Several lines of evidence indicate that the spinal cord is the main site at which anesthetics act to inhibit movement in response to noxious stimulation. This is, of course, the end point used in most measurements of anesthetic potency. Rampil and colleagues[197,198] have shown that MAC values for fluorinated volatile anesthetics are unaffected in the rat by either decerebration[199] or cervical spinal cord transection.[198] Antognini and Schwartz[199] have used the strategy of isolating the cerebral circulation of goats to explore the contribution of brain and spinal cord to the determination of MAC. They found that when isoflurane is administered only to the brain, MAC is 2.9%, whereas when it is administered to the entire body, MAC is 1.2%. Surprisingly, when isoflurane was preferentially administered to the body and not to the brain, isoflurane MAC was reduced to 0.8%.[200] These provocative results suggest not only that anesthetic action at the spinal cord underlies MAC, but also that anesthetic action on the brain may actually sensitize the cord to noxious stimuli. Also, several in vitro electrophysiologic studies have demonstrated inhibition of excitatory synaptic transmission in the spinal cord by volatile anesthetics, arguing that they act, at least in part, directly on spinal neurons.[54,65,201,202] Recent work has revealed that neurons in the mesencephalic locomotor region may be responsible for supraspinal augmentation of locomotor circuits in the spinal cord at concentrations below 1 MAC.[203] Further investigations have relied on decerebrate preparations to remove such supraspinal confounds. Different anesthetics inhibit the sensory neurons in the dorsal horn or motor neurons in the ventral horn. Propofol depresses activity in ventral horn neurons via a GABAergic mechanism that can be blocked by the antagonist picrotoxin.[204] In contrast, the inhibition of both dorsal horn neurons and motor neurons by isoflurane cannot be reversed by the same GABA antagonist.[204] In addition to these effects, isoflurane suppresses interneurons of central pattern generators involved in coordinated movements.[205] Thus anesthetics can affect afferent, efferent, and modulation of reflex arcs in response to noxious stimulation.

Autonomic Control

Anesthetics exert profound effects on homeostatic mechanisms through effects on autonomic centers in the brainstem. Inspiratory neurons in the medulla drive phrenic motor neurons to activate diaphragmatic contraction. Halothane suppresses the spontaneous activity of these neurons in dogs by reducing glutamatergic input.[206] Cardiovascular perturbations are also mediated in part at autonomic centers. For example, the nucleus ambiguous contains cardiac vagal neurons whose efferents are critical in the regulation of heart rate by the parasympathetic nervous system. Both propofol and isoflurane augment the inhibitory potentials of rat cardiac vagal neurons in response to GABA.[207] The nucleus of the solitary tract receives sensory input from autonomic reflex circuits. In vitro data from rat brainstem slices suggest that propofol[208] and isoflurane[209] augment inhibitory response to GABA in these neurons.

Hypothalamic thermoregulation is also ablated by anesthetics. The preoptic area of the anterior hypothalamus contains neurons that are sensitive to either heat or cold and are also a point of convergence of input from peripheral sensors. Microinjection of norepinephrine into the preoptic area of rats anesthetized with isoflurane was sufficient in potentiating hypothermia whereas the antagonist prazosin reversed it.[210] The relationship between disruptions in temperature regulation and sleep homeostasis (also regulated by the preoptic area of the anterior hypothalamus) remains unclear.

Amnesia

While the neurobiologic mechanisms underlying learning, memory consolidation, and memory storage remain unclear, the hippocampus and the amygdala are plausible anesthetic targets for suppressing memory formation. Bilateral resection of these structures induces anterograde amnesia as demonstrated by the well-documented case of Henry Gustav Molaison, known as "Patient H.M." Similarly, anesthetics ablate the formation of new memories and substantially alter neural activity while leaving prior memories seemingly intact. Genetic and pharmacologic experiments support a crucial role of the hippocampus in the amnestic actions of anesthetics. The α_5 subtype of the $GABA_A$ receptor is primarily expressed in the hippocampus and has been implicated in learning and memory.[211] α_5 $GABA_A$ receptor knockout mice were fully resistant to etomidate in hippocampal-dependent memory tasks.[176] Furthermore, short-term memory deficits observed in wild-type mice after isoflurane or sevoflurane were absent in α_5 $GABA_A$ receptor knockout mice, and amnesia in wild-type mice was reversed by inhibitors of the α_5 $GABA_A$ receptors.[212]

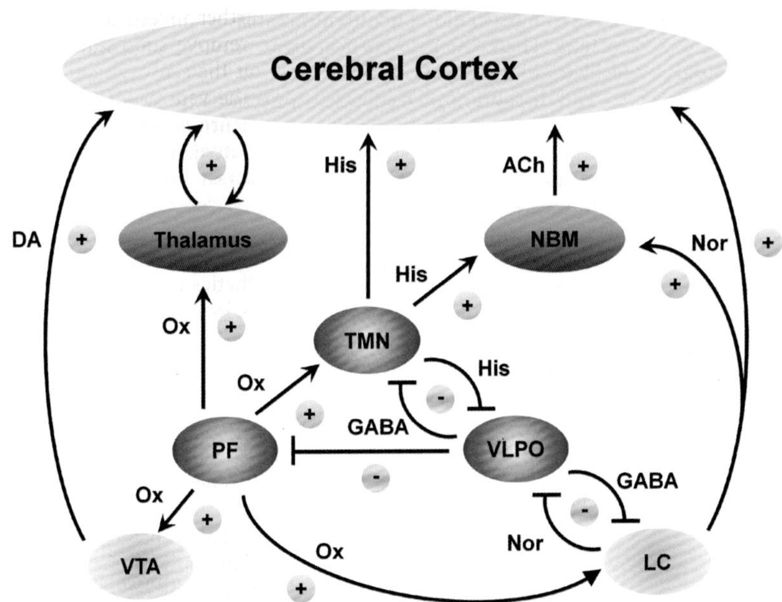

FIGURE 5-7. Diagram of subcortical arousal circuitry implicated in anesthetic-induced unconsciousness. The TMN and VLPO form a bistable sleep/wake switch. The TMN also provides critical histaminergic output to the cerebral cortex and enhances excitatory cholinergic release from the NBM. Orexin release from the perifornical area (PF) stabilizes the VLPO/TMN sleep switch and plays a key role in modulating outputs of the dopaminergic ventral tegmental area (VTA) and the noradrenergic locus coeruleus (LC), and thalamic outputs critical in maintaining recurrent thalamocortical excitability. Ox, orexin; Nor, norepinephrine; His, histamine; GABA, γ-aminobutyric acid; ACh, acetylcholine, DA, dopamine.

Unconsciousness

13 Consciousness is a complex state that can be operationally divided into the components of arousal and awareness, with both individually blocked by anesthetics.[213] *Awareness* is the ability to process and store information in order to interact with internal or external environment. In contrast, *arousal* or *wakefulness* is the state of receptivity to the external environment and is likely mediated through subcortical structures such as the reticular activating system (RAS) and other arousal centers (Fig. 5-7).

Reticular Activating System and Arousal Centers

The RAS is a diffuse collection of brainstem neurons that mediate arousal. Electrical stimulation of the RAS induces arousal in anesthetized animals.[214] The RAS includes the reticular formation, the tuberomammillary nucleus (TMN), the tegmentum, and the thalamic intralaminar nucleus.

The reticular formation (RF) is a heterogeneous collection of neurons in the midbrain and pons involved in the regulation of arousal and sleep. Lesions of the midbrain RF lead to coma. Moruzzi and Magoun have shown that electrical stimulation of the midbrain awakened sleeping animals. Electrical stimulation in the midbrain RF of anesthetized animals resulted in augmentation of EEG activity in rats rendered unresponsive by halothane or isoflurane.[215] GABA levels in the pontine RF are higher during wakefulness than during rapid eye movement (REM) sleep, suggesting that low GABAergic along with high cholinergic tone in the pontine RF leads to REM sleep.[216] Similarly, isoflurane reduces GABA levels in pontine RF.[217] GABA reuptake inhibitor injected into the pontine RF prolonged isoflurane induction while reductions in GABA production in the pontine RF shortened induction in rats.[217]

Multiple lines of evidence suggest that anesthetic inhibition of the TMN of the dorsal hypothalamus impairs arousal. The TMN is the sole source of excitatory histaminergic efferents in the CNS (Fig. 5-7). Rats with bilateral lesions of the TMN and rats with intraventricular injections of histamine receptor antagonists require less isoflurane to induce LORR and have impaired emergence.[218] The application of a GABAergic antagonist directly onto the TMN diminished the efficacy of the anesthetics propofol and pentobarbital.[219] GABAergic inhibitory postsynaptic potentials in TMN neurons taken from $GABA_A$ receptor β_3(N265M) mutant propofol-resistant mice show lack of potentiation by propofol, consistent with this nucleus being a relevant target for propofol.[220] The TMN forms a mutually inhibitory pair with the non-REM promoting ventrolateral posterior optic nucleus (VLPO). Inhibitory afferents of the VLPO suppress arousal pathways of the TMN, the locus coeruleus, and the perifornical area. Although anesthetics have been shown to activate VLPO neurons, VLPO ablation does not impair induction of general anesthesia.[221]

The perifornical area in the lateral hypothalamus appears to be critical in emergence from rather than induction of anesthetic-induced unconsciousness. It is the sole source of orexin, a neurotransmitter that stabilizes the flip-flopping of the VLPO/TMN sleep switch. Orexin knockout mice show frequent sleep/wake transitions akin to narcolepsy. Intraventricular injection of orexin A in isoflurane-anesthetized rats shifts EEG from burst suppression to patterns similar to arousal[222] and also expedites recovery of the righting reflex from propofol- or dexmedetomidine-induced unconsciousness.[220] While ablation of arousal by either isoflurane or sevoflurane is not affected in orexin knockout animals, recovery from anesthesia is delayed,[4] suggesting asymmetry in the neural mechanisms underlying induction and emergence.

Suppression of the nucleus basalis of Meynert (NBM) is also likely important in mediating anesthetic suppression of arousal and awareness. The NBM is the major source of excitatory cholinergic input to the thalamus, the RAS, and the cerebral cortex.

Histamine activation of the NBM during deep isoflurane anesthesia shifts surface EEG patterns from burst suppression to delta activity, consistent with diffuse cholinergic activation from this nucleus reversing anesthetic suppression of cortical activity.[218] Norepinephrine infused into NBM induces arousal at desflurane concentrations sufficient to ablate the righting reflex in rats, implying that ascending cholinergic stimulation can induce arousal and antagonize the effects of desflurane.[223] Similarly, histamine agonists injected into the NBM reversed EEG suppression and accelerated emergence from isoflurane anesthesia.[224]

The precise roles of dopaminergic and noradrenergic arousal centers in anesthetic-induced unconsciousness remain unclear. The locus coeruleus (LC) is a set of pontine noradrenergic neurons within the reticular formation. It is the primary adrenergic source to the cortex, thalamus, and hypothalamus. Dopaminergic inputs to the prefrontal cortical areas, hippocampus, and amygdala are produced by the ventral tegmental area. The dual norepinephrine/dopamine reuptake inhibitor, methylphenidate, restored righting reflex in rats anesthetized at the minimum isoflurane concentration required for unconsciousness.[225] In this study, restoration of behavioral and electrophysiologic patterns consistent with arousal and awareness was blocked by the receptor antagonist, droperidol. However, unlike in the TMN, LC neurons in $GABA_A$ receptor β_3(N265M) mutant mice were sensitive to propofol.[220] As discussed above these mutant mice are markedly resistant to the hypnotic effects of propofol; thus, the effects of propofol in the LC may not contribute significantly to loss of arousal.

Thalamus

The thalamus has been postulated as a likely target for anesthetic ablation of consciousness[226] but the precise mechanism remains unclear. Subgroups of neurons regulate widespread cortical excitability or relay information among neurons in cortical, striatal, limbic, and other subcortical structures. In this respect, the thalamus is likely critical for both arousal and awareness. Nuclei in the central thalamus have garnered particular attention as an extension of the RAS. Microinfusion to the central medial thalamus or the lateral thalamus of antibodies to the Kv1.2 potassium channel induced arousal in rats anesthetized with either desflurane or sevoflurane.[227] Nicotine injection into the central thalamus of rats reversed the LORR induced by sevoflurane.[228] However, the attenuation of information transfer through the thalamus does not appear necessary for anesthetic-induced unconsciousness. Anesthetized rats show reduced excitation in the somatosensory reticular thalamic nucleus but preserved activity in the ventroposterior lateral nucleus,[229] suggesting that while the reticular nucleus may contribute to ablating arousal, the nuclei involved in the transmission of sensory information to the thalamus remain intact. This is supported by data showing that flashed visual stimuli lead to excitation in primary visual cortex[230] of the anesthetized rats, even during burst suppression.[231] Thus, during deep anesthesia, the thalamus does not appear impermeable to the transmission of information from the external world to the cerebral cortex. As the thalamus forms recurrent feedback circuits with cortical neurons, altered patterns of excitability and oscillatory activity in the thalamus may substantially influence cortical processing. Simultaneous recordings from both structures in patients with Parkinson's disease have suggested that alterations in cortical activity during anesthetic induction precede those in the thalamus.[232] The intimate relationship of their connections will continue to impede an understanding of whether anesthetics induce unconsciousness primarily at the thalamus or the cerebral cortex.

Cerebral Cortex

The cerebral cortex is the major site for integration, storage, and retrieval of information for generating awareness of the external environment. Primary sensory areas provide focused feed-forward activity to association and attention areas in parietal and frontal cortices. These "higher" cortical areas provide reciprocal diffuse feedback to early cortical areas.

The disruption of feedback connections by anesthetics may contribute to impaired consciousness by attenuating the integration of information distributed among cortical regions. Analysis of rat visual neuron responses to flashed stimuli reveals that desflurane attenuates the late components of visual response.[233] These late components are products of feedback activity and mediate contextual modulation from higher cortical areas. Electrode recordings in rats have compared the direction of interactions between frontal and parietal cortical areas in both awake and anesthetized states. These interactions are balanced in the awake state but feedback interactions were reduced compared to feed-forward when rats were anesthetized by isoflurane.[234] Similarly, propofol preferentially reduces feedback activity from frontal to parietal areas in human EEG studies.[235–237] Recent fMRI data have also showed reductions in feedback connections between frontal and parietal areas.[238]

The effects of anesthetics on both cortical firing rates and timing of action potentials likely contribute to the ablation of awareness by limiting both the diversity of information that can be represented and the integration of neural information.[1] Anesthetics alter the topology of distinct networks of frontal, parietal, and temporal cortical areas subserving attention and higher cognitive processes based on patterns of correlated activity. Most notable are the alterations to the default mode network[239] associated with inwardly directed attention.[240,241] The weakening of correlated brain activity between cortical regions of different attention networks[239] is similar to that observed after induction of non-REM sleep.[242–244] Deep propofol sedation reduces the strength of correlated brain activity and integration between regions in these networks.[238] This blurring of boundaries between networks likely contributes to impaired consciousness by violating the generation and compartmentalization of neural representations.

Anesthetics weaken high-frequency synchronized oscillatory cortical activity that may normally be critical for integrating information across cortical areas into coherent representations.[245] In rats, isoflurane reduces high γ range (70 to 140 Hz) synchrony in the frontal cortex, visual cortex, and hippocampus.[246] Recordings from humans implanted with subdural electrocorticographic electrodes revealed a reduction in high γ band power (>75 Hz) on induction with propofol and recovery during emergence from propofol.[247] Analysis of EEG from humans rendered unresponsive by propofol revealed a reduction in information integration in the γ band[235] and multiple anesthetic agents cause widespread reduction in γ band power.[248]

Summary

Anesthetics suppress circuits in the spinal cord and brainstem to induce immobility and disruption of autonomic homeostasis. The hippocampus is the major site of anesthetic action for anterograde amnesia. As the neurobiologic underpinnings of arousal and awareness are distributed across brainstem, subcortical, and cortical structures, no single anatomic site is responsible for anes-
14 thetic-induced unconsciousness. Recent work has revealed that networks of subcortical and thalamic nuclei are altered in the ablation of arousal. Cortical networks critical for cognitive processing
15 of awareness are tentative substrates for eliminating subjective percepts, noxious and otherwise. Network perturbations in both frequency and temporal coding of information are putative mechanisms for altered integration and neural representation.

CONCLUSIONS

In this chapter, evidence has been reviewed concerning the anatomic, physiologic, and molecular loci of anesthetic action. It is clear that all anesthetic actions cannot be localized to a specific anatomic site in the CNS; indeed, considerable evidence supports the conclusion that different components of the anesthetic state are mediated by actions at disparate anatomic sites. The actions of anesthetics also cannot be localized to a single physiologic process. While there is consensus that anesthetics ultimately affect synaptic function as opposed to intrinsic neuronal excitability, the effects of anesthetics depend on the agent and synapse studied and can affect presynaptic and/or postsynaptic function. At a molecular level, volatile anesthetics show some selectivity, but still affect the function of multiple ion channels and synaptic proteins. The intravenous anesthetics, etomidate, propofol, and barbiturates, are more specific with the $GABA_A$ receptor as their major target. Although these effects are likely mediated via direct protein–anesthetic interactions, numerous proteins can directly interact with anesthetics. Genetic data plainly demonstrate that the unitary theory of anesthesia is not correct. No single mechanism is responsible for the effects of all general anesthetics, nor does a single mechanism account for all of the effects of a single anesthetic, at least where it has been examined. Figure 5-8 provides a simple model of the molecular and cellular effects of general anesthetics. This cartoon is not meant to include all potential targets of general anesthetics. Rather, only those molecules with strong evidence for importance in anesthetic action from multiple different approaches are shown.

Although the precise set of molecular interactions responsible for producing anesthesia has not been fully elucidated, anesthetics do act via selective effects on specific molecular targets. The technologic revolutions in molecular biology, genetics, neurophysiology, and neuroimaging make it likely that the next decade will provide additional answers to the anesthetic mechanism puzzle.

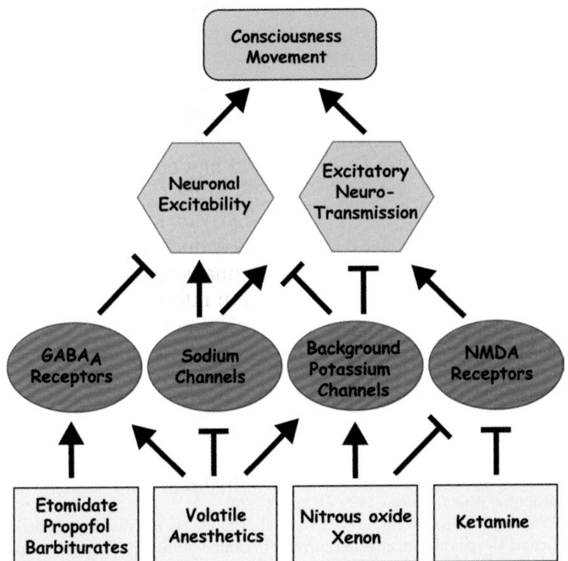

FIGURE 5-8. A multi-site model for anesthesia. Anesthetics are grouped according to similarity of mechanism. *Arrows* indicate activation or potentiation and "*T's*" indicate inhibition or antagonism. The neurophysiologic effects of general anesthetics are lumped into neuronal excitability (the probability of a neuron firing and propagating an axon potential) and excitatory neurotransmission (synaptic activity at excitatory synapses such as glutamatergic). Neuronal excitability in this context is the sum of both intrinsic and extrinsic factors (e.g., GABAergic inhibition).

ACKNOWLEDGMENTS

The authors acknowledge generous ongoing funding support from National Institute of General Medical Sciences, National Institute of Neurological Disorders and Stroke, National Center for Research Resources, and the Foundation for Anesthesia Education and Research, for ASE-P01 GM37846, CMC-R01 GM59781, RO1 NS045905, and BJP-FAER MRTG-CT, UL1 RR024992.

SCIENTIFIC FOUNDATIONS OF ANESTHESIA

References

1. Alkire MT, Hudetz AG, Tononi G. Consciousness and anesthesia. *Science.* 2008;322(5903):876–880.
2. Tononi G. Consciousness as integrated information: a provisional manifesto. *Biol Bull.* 2008;215(3):216–242.
3. Balduzzi D. Estimating integrated information with TMS pulses during wakefulness, sleep, and under anesthesia. *Conf Proc IEEE Eng Med Biol Soc.* 2011;2011:4717–4720.
4. Kelz MB, Sun Y, Chen J, et al. An essential role for orexins in emergence from general anesthesia. *Proc Natl Acad Sci USA.* 2008;105(4):1309–1314.
5. Quasha AL, Eger EI 2nd, Tinker JH. Determination and applications of MAC. *Anesthesiology.* 1980;53(4):315–334.
6. White PF, Johnston RR, Eger EI 2nd. Determination of anesthetic requirement in rats. *Anesthesiology.* 1974;40(1):52–57.
7. Franks NP, Lieb WR. Molecular and cellular mechanisms of general anaesthesia. *Nature.* 1994;367(6464):607–614.
8. Bowdle TA. Depth of anesthesia monitoring. *Anesthesiol Clin.* 2006;24(4):793–822.
9. Avidan MS, Jacobsohn E, Glick D, et al. Prevention of intraoperative awareness in a high-risk surgical population. *N Engl J Med.* 2011;365(7):591–600.
10. Avidan MS, Zhang L, Burnside BA, et al. Anesthesia awareness and the bispectral index. *N Engl J Med.* 2008;358(11):1097–1108.
11. Palanca BJ, Mashour GA, Avidan MS. Processed electroencephalogram in depth of anesthesia monitoring. *Curr Opin Anaesthesiol.* 2009;22(5):553–559.
12. Bruhn J, Myles PS, Sneyd R, et al. Depth of anaesthesia monitoring: what's available, what's validated and what's next? *Br J Anaesth.* 2006;97(1):85–94.
13. Meyer H. Theorie der alkoholnarkose. *Arch Exp Pathol Pharmakol.* 1899;42:109.
14. Overton CE. *Studies of Narcosis.* 1st ed. London: Chapman and Hall; 1891.
15. Franks NP, Lieb WR. Where do general anaesthetics act? *Nature.* 1978;274(5669):339–342.
16. Larson ER. Fluorine compounds in anesthesiology. In: Tarrant P, ed. *Fluorine Chemistry Reviews.* Vol. 3. New York, NY: Dekker; 1969.
17. Andrews PR, Jones GP, Poulton DB. Convulsant, anticonvulsant and anaesthetic barbiturates. In vivo activities of oxo- and thiobarbiturates related to pentobarbitone. *Eur J Pharmacol.* 1982;79(1-2):61–65.
18. Paul SM, Purdy RH. Neuroactive steroids. *FASEB J.* 1992;6(6):2311–2322.
19. Koblin DD, Chortkoff BS, Laster MJ, et al. Polyhalogenated and perfluorinated compounds that disobey the Meyer-Overton hypothesis. *Anesth Analg.* 1994;79(6):1043–1048.
20. Kandel L, Chortkoff BS, Sonner J, et al. Nonanesthetics can suppress learning. *Anesth Analg.* 1996;82(2):321–326.
21. Alifimoff JK, Firestone LL, Miller KW. Anaesthetic potencies of primary alkanols: implications for the molecular dimensions of the anaesthetic site. *Br J Pharmacol.* 1989;96(1):9–16.
22. Raines DE, Korten SE, Hill AG, et al. Anesthetic cutoff in cycloalkanemethanols. A test of current theories. *Anesthesiology.* 1993;78(5):918–927.
23. Liu J, Laster MJ, Koblin DD, et al. A cutoff in potency exists in the perfluoroalkanes. *Anesth Analg.* 1994;79(2):238–244.
24. Andrews PR, Mark LC. Structural specificity of barbiturates and related drugs. *Anesthesiology.* 1982;57(4):314–320.
25. Richter JA, Holtman JR Jr. Barbiturates: their in vivo effects and potential biochemical mechanisms. *Prog Neurobiol.* 1982;18(4):275–319.
26. Ryder S, Way WL, Trevor AJ. Comparative pharmacology of the optical isomers of ketamine in mice. *Eur J Pharmacol.* 1978;49(1):15–23.
27. Wittmer LL, Hu Y, Kalkbrenner M, et al. Enantioselectivity of steroid-induced gamma-aminobutyric acid A receptor modulation and anesthesia. *Mol Pharmacol.* 1996;50(6):1581–1586.
28. Tomlin SL, Jenkins A, Lieb WR, et al. Stereoselective effects of etomidate optical isomers on gamma-aminobutyric acid type A receptors and animals. *Anesthesiology.* 1998;88(3):708–717.

29. Lysko GS, Robinson JL, Casto R, et al. The stereospecific effects of isoflurane isomers in vivo. *Eur J Pharmacol.* 1994;263(1–2):25–29.
30. Kendig JJ, Grossman Y, MacIver MB. Pressure reversal of anaesthesia: a synaptic mechanism. *Br J Anaesth.* 1988;60(7):806–816.
31. Smith RA, Porter EG, Miller KW. The solubility of anesthetic gases in lipid bilayers. *Biochim Biophys Acta.* 1981;645(2):327–338.
32. Franks NP. Molecular targets underlying general anaesthesia. *Br J Pharmacol.* 2006;147(Suppl 1):S72–S81.
33. Franks NP, Lieb WR. Do general anaesthetics act by competitive binding to specific receptors? *Nature.* 1984;310(5978):599–601.
34. Franks NP, Lieb WR. Mapping of general anaesthetic target sites provides a molecular basis for cutoff effects. *Nature.* 1985;316(6026):349–351.
35. Dubois BW, Cherian SF, Evers AS. Volatile anesthetics compete for common binding sites on bovine serum albumin: a 19F-NMR study. *Proc Natl Acad Sci USA.* 1993;90(14):6478–6482.
36. Dubois BW, Evers AS. 19F-NMR spin-spin relaxation (T2) method for characterizing volatile anesthetic binding to proteins. Analysis of isoflurane binding to serum albumin. *Biochemistry.* 1992;31(31):7069–7076.
37. Eckenhoff RG. Amino acid resolution of halothane binding sites in serum albumin. *J Biol Chem.* 1996;271(26):15521–15526.
38. Eckenhoff RG, Shuman H. Halothane binding to soluble proteins determined by photoaffinity labeling. *Anesthesiology.* 1993;79(1):96–106.
39. Hall MA, Xi J, Lor C, et al. m-Aziproprofol (AziPm) a photoactive analogue of the intravenous general anesthetic propofol. *J Med Chem.* 2010;53(15):5667–5675.
40. Stewart DS, Savechenkov PY, Dostalova Z, et al. p-(4-Azipentyl)propofol: A potent photoreactive general anesthetic derivative of propofol. *J Med Chem.* 2011;54(23):8124–8135.
41. Li GD, Chiara DC, Sawyer GW, et al. Identification of a GABAA receptor anesthetic binding site at subunit interfaces by photolabeling with an etomidate analog. *J Neurosci.* 2006;26(45):11599–11605.
42. Chiara DC, Dostalova Z, Jayakar SS, et al. Mapping general anesthetic binding site(s) in human alpha1beta3 gamma-aminobutyric acid type A receptors with [(3) H]TDBzl-etomidate, a photoreactive etomidate analogue. *Biochemistry.* 2012;51 (4):836–847.
43. Franks NP, Jenkins A, Conti E, et al. Structural basis for the inhibition of firefly luciferase by a general anesthetic. *Biophys J.* 1998;75(5):2205–2211.
44. Bocquet N, Nury H, Baaden M, et al. X-ray structure of a pentameric ligand-gated ion channel in an apparently open conformation. *Nature.* 2009;457(7225): 111–114.
45. Nury H, Bocquet N, Le Poupon C, et al. Crystal structure of the extracellular domain of a bacterial ligand-gated ion channel. *J Mol Biol.* 2010;395(5):1114–1127.
46. MacIver MB, Kendig JJ. Anesthetic effects on resting membrane potential are voltage-dependent and agent-specific. *Anesthesiology.* 1991;74:83–88.
47. Madison DV, Nicoll RA. General anesthetics hyperpolarize neurons in the vertebrate central nervous system. *Science.* 1982;217:1055–1057.
48. Ries CR, Puil E. Mechanism of anesthesia revealed by shunting actions of isoflurane on thalamocortical neurons. *J Neurophysiol.* 1999;81(4):1795–1801.
49. Larrabee MG, Posternak JM. Selective action of anesthetics on synapses and axons in mammalian sympathetic ganglia. *J Neurophysiol.* 1952;15(2):91–114.
50. Richards CD, Russell WJ, Smaje JC. The action of ether and methoxyflurane on synaptic transmission in isolated preparations of the mammalian cortex. *J Physiol.* 1975;248(1):121–142.
51. Richards CD, White AE. The actions of volatile anaesthetics on synaptic transmission in the dentate gyrus. *J Physiol.* 1975;252(1):241–257.
52. Langmoen IA, Larsen M, Berg-Johnsen J. Volatile anaesthetics: Cellular mechanisms of action. *Eur J Anaesthesiol.* 1995;12(1):51–58.
53. Wu XS, Sun JY, Evers AS, et al. Isoflurane inhibits transmitter release and the presynaptic action potential. *Anesthesiology.* 2004;100(3):663–670.
54. Kullmann DM, Martin RL, Redman SJ. Reduction by general anaesthetics of group Ia excitatory postsynaptic potentials and currents in the cat spinal cord. *J Physiol.* 1989;412:277–296.
55. Nicoll RA, Eccles JC, Oshima T, et al. Prolongation of inhibitory postsynaptic potentials by barbiturates. *Nature.* 1975;258:625–627.
56. Proctor WR, Mynlieff M, Dunwiddie TV. Facilitatory action of etomidate and pentobarbital on recurrent inhibition in rat hippocampal pyramidal neurons. *J Neurosci.* 1986;6(11):3161–3168.
57. Collins GG. Effects of the anaesthetic 2,6-diisopropylphenol on synaptic transmission in the rat olfactory cortex slice. *Br J Pharmacol.* 1988;95(3):939–949.
58. Nicoll RA. The effects of anaesthetics on synaptic excitation and inhibition in the olfactory bulb. *J Physiol (Lond).* 1972;223:803–814.
59. Harrison NL, Vicini S, Barker JL. A steroid anesthetic prolongs inhibitory postsynaptic currents in cultured rat hippocampal neurons. *J Neurosci.* 1987;7(2):604–609.
60. Olsen R, Li G-D. $GABA_A$ receptors as molecular targets of general anesthetics: identification of binding sites provides clues to allosteric modulation. *Can J Anaesth.* 2011;58(2):206–215.
61. Solt K, Forman SA. Correlating the clinical actions and molecular mechanisms of general anesthetics. *Curr Opin Anaesthesiol.* 2007;20(4):300–306.
62. Fujiwara M, Higashi H, Nishi S, et al. Changes in spontaneous firing patterns of rat hippocampal neurones induced by volatile anaesthetics. *J Physiol (Lond).* 1988;402:155–175.
63. Mui P, Puil E. Isoflurane-induced impairment of synaptic transmission in hippocampal neurons. *Exp Brain Res.* 1989;75:354–360.
64. Yoshimura M, Higashi H, Fujita S, et al. Selective depression of hippocampal inhibitory postsynaptic potentials and spontaneous firing by volatile anesthetics. *Brain Res.* 1985;340:363–368.
65. Takenoshita M, Takahashi T. Mechanisms of halothane action on synaptic transmission in motoneurons of the newborn rat spinal cord in vitro. *Brain Res.* 1987;402:303–310.
66. Perouansky M, Baranov D, Salman M, et al. Effects of halothane on glutamate receptor-mediated excitatory post-synaptic currents: A patch-clamp study in adult mouse hippocampal slices. *Anesthesiology.* 1995;83(1):109–119.
67. Buggy DJ, Nicol B, Rowbotham DJ, et al. Effects of intravenous anesthetic agents on glutamate release: a role for GABAA receptor-mediated inhibition. *Br J Pharmacol.* 1988;95(3):939–949.
68. Kendall TJ, Minchin MC. The effects of anaesthetics on the uptake and release of amino acid neurotransmitters in thalamic slices. *Br J Pharmacol.* 1982;75: 219–227.
69. Larsen M, Haugstad TS, Berg-Johnsen J, et al. Effect of isoflurane on release and uptake of gamma-aminobutyric acid from rat cortical synaptosomes. *Br J Anaesth.* 1998;80(5):634–638.
70. Collins GGS. Release of endogenous amino acid neurotransmitter candidates from rat olfactory cortex slices: possible regulatory mechanisms and the effects of pentobarbitone. *Brain Res.* 1980;190:517–528.
71. Murugaiah KD, Hemmings HC Jr. Effects of intravenous general anesthetics on [3H]GABA release from rat cortical synaptosomes. *Anesthesiology.* 1998;89 (4):919–928.
72. Mantz J, Lecharny JB, Laudenbach V, et al. Anesthetics affect the uptake but not the depolarization-evoked release of GABA in rat striatal synaptosomes. *Anesthesiology.* 1995;82(2):502–511.
73. Westphalen RI, Hemmings HC Jr. Selective depression by general anesthetics of glutamate versus GABA release from isolated cortical nerve terminals. *J Pharmacol Exp Ther.* 2003;304(3):1188–1196.
74. Hawasli AH, Saifee O, Liu C, et al. Resistance to volatile anesthetics by mutations enhancing excitatory neurotransmitter release in Caenorhabditis elegans. *Genetics.* 2004;168(2):831–843.
75. van Swinderen B, Saifee O, Shebester L, et al. A neomorphic syntaxin mutation blocks volatile-anesthetic action in Caenorhabditis elegans. *Proc Natl Acad Sci USA.* 1999;96(5):2479–284.
76. Herring BE, Xie Z, Marks J, et al. Isoflurane inhibits the neurotransmitter release machinery. *J Neurophysiol.* 2009;102(2):1265–1273.
77. Richards CD, Smaje JC. Anaesthetics depress the sensitivity of cortical neurones to L-glutamate. *Br J Pharmacol.* 1976;58:347–357.
78. Smaje JC. General anaesthetics and the acetylcholine-sensitivity of cortical neurones. *Br J Pharmacol.* 1976;58:359–366.
79. Akk G, Steinbach JH. Structural studies of the actions of anesthetic drugs on the gamma-aminobutyric acid type A receptor. *Anesthesiology.* 2011;115(6):1338–1348.
80. Jones MV, Brooks PA, Harrison NL. Enhancements of gamma-aminobutyric acid-activated Cl^- currents in cultured rat hippocampal neurones by three volatile anesthetics. *J Physiol.* 1992;449:279–293.
81. Haydon DA, Urban BW. The actions of some general anaesthetics on the potassium current of the squid giant axon. *J Physiol.* 1986;373:311–327.
82. Herrington J, Stern RC, Evers AS, et al. Halothane inhibits two components of calcium current in clonal (GH_3) pituitary cells. *J Neurosci.* 1991;11(7):2226–2240.
83. Hemmings HC Jr. Sodium channels and the synaptic mechanisms of inhaled anaesthetics. *Br J Anaesth.* 2009;103(1):61–69.
84. Rehberg B, Xiao YH, Duch DS. Central nervous system sodium channels are significantly suppressed at clinical concentrations of volatile anesthetics. *Anesthesiology.* 1996;84(5):1223–1233.
85. Ratnakumari L, Hemmings HC Jr. Inhibition of presynaptic sodium channels by halothane. *Anesthesiology.* 1998;88(4):1043–1054.
86. Shiraishi M, Harris RA. Effects of alcohols and anesthetics on recombinant voltage-gated Na+ channels. *J Pharmacol Exp Ther.* 2004;309(3):987–994.
87. Frenkel C, Weckbecker K, Wartenberg HC, et al. Blocking effects of the anaesthetic etomidate on human brain sodium channels. *Neurosci Lett.* 1998;249(2–3):131–134.
88. Rehberg B, Duch DS. Suppression of central nervous system sodium channels by propofol. *Anesthesiology.* 1999;91(2):512–520.
89. Eskinder H, Rusch NJ, Supan FD, et al. The effects of volatile anesthetics on L- and T-type calcium channel currents in canine cardiac Purkinje cells. *Anesthesiology.* 1991;74(5):919–926.
90. Terrar DA. Structure and function of calcium channels and the actions of anaesthetics. *Br J Anaesth.* 1993;71(1):39–46.
91. Gundersen CB, Umbach JA, Swartz BE. Barbiturates depress currents through human brain calcium channels studied in Xenopus oocytes. *J Pharmacol Exp Ther.* 1988;247(3):824–829.
92. Hall AC, Lieb WR, Franks NP. Insensitivity of P-type calcium channels to inhalational and intravenous general anesthetics. *Anesthesiology.* 1994;81:117–123.
93. Study RE. Isoflurane inhibits multiple voltage-gated calcium currents in hippocampal pyramidal neurons. *Anesthesiology.* 1994;81:104–116.
94. Takenoshita M, Steinbach JH. Halothane blocks low-voltage-activated calcium current in rat sensory neurons. *J Neurosci.* 1991;11(5):1404–1412.

95. ffrench-Mullen JMH, Barker JL, Rogawski MA. Calcium current block by (-)-pentobarbital, phenobarbital, and CHEB but not (+)-pentobarbital in acutely isolated hippocampal CA1 neurons: Comparison with effects on GABA-activated Cl^- current. *J Neurosci.* 1993;13:3211–3221.
96. Correa AM. Gating kinetics of Shaker K+ channels are differentially modified by general anesthetics. *Am J Physiol.* 1998;275(4 Pt 1):C1009–C1021.
97. Friederich P, Urban BW. Interaction of intravenous anesthetics with human neuronal potassium currents in relation to clinical concentrations. *Anesthesiology.* 1999;91(6):1853–1860.
98. Gerstin KM, Gong DH, Abdallah M, et al. Mutation of KCNK5 or Kir3.2 potassium channels in mice does not change minimum alveolar anesthetic concentration. *Anesth Analg.* 2003;96(5):1345–1349.
99. Gibbons SJ, Núñez-Hernández R, Mazé G, et al. Inhibition of a fast inwardly rectifying potassium conductance by barbiturates. *Anesth Analg.* 1996;82(6): 1242–1246.
100. Stadnicka A, Bosnjak ZJ, Kampine JP, et al. Effects of sevoflurane on inward rectifier K+ current in guinea pig ventricular cardiomyocytes. *Am J Physiol.* 1997; 273(1 Pt 2):H324–H332.
101. Patel AJ, Honore E. Anesthetic-sensitive 2P domain K+ channels. *Anesthesiology.* 2001;95(4):1013–1021.
102. Franks NP, Lieb WR. Volatile general anaesthetics activate a novel neuronal K +current. *Nature.* 1988;333:662–664.
103. Winegar BD, Yost CS. Volatile anesthetics directly activate baseline S K^+ channels in aplysia neurons. *Brain Res.* 1998;807(1–2):255–262.
104. Honore E. The neuronal background K2P channels: Focus on TREK1. *Nat Rev Neurosci.* 2007;8(4):251–261.
105. Patel AJ, Honoré E, Lesage F, et al. Inhalational anesthetics activate two-pore-domain background K^+ channels. *Nat Neurosci.* 1999;2(5):422–426.
106. Gruss M, Bushell TJ, Bright DP, et al. Two-pore-domain K+ channels are a novel target for the anesthetic gases xenon, nitrous oxide, and cyclopropane. *Mol Pharmacol.* 2004;65(2):443–452.
107. Postea O, Biel M. Exploring HCN channels as novel drug targets. *Nat Rev Drug Discov.* 2011;10(12):903–914.
108. Chen X, Sirois JE, Lei Q, et al. HCN subunit-specific and cAMP-modulated effects of anesthetics on neuronal pacemaker currents. *J Neurosci.* 2005;25(24):5803–5814.
109. Chen X, Shu S, Bayliss DA. HCN1 channel subunits are a molecular substrate for hypnotic actions of ketamine. *J Neurosci.* 2009;29(3):600–609.
110. Cacheaux LP, Topf N, Tibbs GR, et al. Impairment of hyperpolarization-activated, cyclic nucleotide-gated channel function by the intravenous general anesthetic propofol. *J Pharmacol Exp Ther.* 2005;315(2):517–525.
111. Akk G, Mennerick S, Steinbach JH. Actions of anesthetics on excitatory transmitter-gated channels. *Handb Exp Pharmacol* 2008;(182):53–84.
112. Krasowski MD, Harrison NL. General anaesthetic actions on ligand-gated ion channels. *Cell Mol Life Sci.* 1999;55(10):1278–1303.
113. Wakamori M, Ikemoto Y, Akaike N. Effects of two volatile anesthetics and a volatile convulsant on the excitatory and inhibitory amino acid responses in dissociated CNS neurons of the rat. *J Neurophysiol.* 1991;66(6):2014–2021.
114. Lin L, Chen LL, Harris RA. Enflurane inhibits NMDA, AMPA and kainate-induced currents in Xenopus oocytes expressing mouse and human brain mRNA. *FASEB J.* 1992;7:479–485.
115. Weight FF, Lovinger DM, White G, et al. Alcohol and anesthetic actions on excitatory amino acid-activated ion channels. *Ann N Y Acad Sci.* 1991;625:97–107.
116. Dildy-Mayfield JE, Eger EI 2nd, Harris RA. Anesthetics produce subunit-selective actions on glutamate receptors. *J Pharmacol Exp Ther.* 1996;276(3):1058–1065.
117. Minami K, Wick MJ, Stern-Bach Y, et al. Sites of volatile anesthetic action on kainate (glutamate receptor 6) receptors. *J Biol Chem.* 1998;273(14):8248–8255.
118. Aronstam RS, Martin DC, Dennison RL. Volatile anesthetics inhibit NMDA-stimulated ^{45}Ca uptake by rat brain microvesicles. *Neurochem Res.* 1994;19(12): 1515–1520.
119. Anis NA, Berry SC, Burton NR, et al. The dissociative anaesthetics, ketamine and phencyclidine, selectively reduce excitation of central mammalian neurones by N-methyl-aspartate. *Br J Pharmacol.* 1983;79:565–575.
120. Lodge D, Anis NA, Burton NR. Effects of optical isomers of ketamine on excitation of cat and rat spinal neurons by amino acids and acetylcholine. *Neurosci Lett.* 1982;29:281–286.
121. Zeilhofer HU, Swandulla D, Geisslinger G, et al. Differential effects of ketamine enantiomers on NMDA receptor currents in cultured neurons. *Eur J Pharmacol.* 1992;213(1):155–158.
122. Jevtovi -Todorovi V, Todorovi SM, Mennerick S, et al. Nitrous oxide (laughing gas) is an NMDA antagonist, neuroprotectant and neurotoxin. *Nat Med.* 1998;4(4):460–463.
123. Mennerick S, Jevtovic-Todorovic V, Todorovic SM, et al. Effect of nitrous oxide on excitatory and inhibitory synaptic transmission in hippocampal cultures. *J Neurosci.* 1998;18(23):9716–9726.
124. Franks NP, Dickinson R, de Sousa SL, et al. How does xenon produce anaesthesia? [letter]. *Nature.* 1998;396:324.
125. Barker JL, Harrison NL, Lange GD, et al. Potentiation of gamma-aminobutyric-acid-activated chloride conductance by a steroid anesthetic in cultured rat spinal neurons. *J Physiol.* 1987;386:485–501.
126. Hales TH, Lambert JJ. Modulation of the $GABA_A$ receptor by propofol. *Br J Pharmacol.* 1988;93:84P.
127. Macdonald RL, Olsen RW. $GABA_A$ receptor channels. *Annu Rev Neurosci.* 1994;17:569–602.
128. Macdonald RL, Rogers CJ, Twyman RE. Barbiturate regulation of kinetic properties of the GABAA receptor channels of mouse spinal neurones in culture. *J Physiol.* 1989;417:483–500.
129. Hall AC, Lieb WR, Franks NP. Stereoselective and non-stereoselective actions of isoflurane on the $GABA_A$ receptor. *Br J Pharmacol.* 1994;112(3):906–910.
130. Nakahiro M, Yeh JZ, Brunner E, et al. General anesthetics modulate GABA receptor channel complex in rat dorsal root ganglion neurons. *FASEB J.* 1989;3: 1850–1854.
131. Yeh JZ, Quandt FN, Tanguy J, et al. General anesthetic action on gamma-aminobutyric acid-activated channels. *Ann N Y Acad Sci.* 1991;625:155–173.
132. Banks MI, Pearce RA. Dual actions of volatile anesthetics on GABA(A) IPSCs: Dissociation of blocking and prolonging effects. *Anesthesiology.* 1999;90(1):120–134.
133. Pritchett DB, Sontheimer H, Shivers BD. Importance of a novel $GABA_A$ receptor subunit for benzodiazepine pharmacology. *Nature.* 1989;338:582–585.
134. Hill-Venning C, Belelli D, Peters JA, et al. Subunit-dependent interaction of the general anaesthetic etomidate with the gamma-aminobutyric acid type A receptor. *Br J Pharmacol.* 1997;120(5):749–756.
135. Davies PA, Hanna MC, Hales TG, et al. Insensitivity to anaesthetic agents conferred by a class of $GABA_A$ receptor subunit. *Nature.* 1997;385:820–823.
136. Zhu WJ, Wang JF, Krueger KE, et al. Delta subunit inhibits neurosteroid modulation of GABAA receptors. *J Neurosci.* 1996;16:6648–6656.
137. Mihic SJ, Harris RA. Inhibition of rho1 receptor GABAergic currents by alcohols and volatile anesthetics. *J Pharmacol Exp Ther.* 1996;277:411–416.
138. Mihic SJ, Ye Q, Wick MJ, et al. Sites of alcohol and volatile anaesthetic action on GABA(A) and glycine receptors. *Nature.* 1997;389(6649):385–389.
139. Belelli D, Lambert JJ, Peters JA, et al. The interaction of the general anesthetic etomidate with the gamma-aminobutyric acid type A receptor is influenced by a single amino acid. *Proc Natl Acad Sci USA.* 1997;94(20):11031–11036.
140. Krasowski MD, Koltchine VV, Rick CE, et al. Propofol and other intravenous anesthetics have sites of action on the gamma-aminobutyric acid type A receptor distinct from that for isoflurane. *Mol Pharmacol.* 1998;53(3):530–538.
141. Hosie AM, Wilkins ME, da Silva HM, et al. Endogenous neurosteroids regulate GABAA receptors through two discrete transmembrane sites. *Nature.* 2006;444(7118):486–489.
142. Forman S, Miller K. Anesthetic sites and allosteric mechanisms of action on Cys-loop ligand-gated ion channels. *Can J Anaesth.* 2011;58(2):191–205.
143. Dilger JP, Vidal AM, Mody HI, et al. Evidence for direct actions of general anesthetics on an ion channel protein. An new look at a unified mode of action. *Anesthesiology.* 1994;81:431–442.
144. Firestone LL, Sauter JF, Braswell LM, et al. Actions of general anesthetics on acetylcholine receptor-rich membranes from Torpedo californica. *Anesthesiology.* 1986;64:694–702.
145. Franks NP, Lieb WR. Stereospecific effects of inhalational general anesthetic optical isomers on nerve ion channels. *Science.* 1991;254:427–430.
146. Charlesworth P, Richards CD. Anaesthetic modulation of nicotinic ion channel kinetics in bovine chromaffin cells. *Br J Pharmacol.* 1995;114(4):909–917.
147. Violet JM, Downie DL, Nakisa RC, et al. Differential sensitivities of mammalian neuronal and muscle nicotinic acetylcholine receptors to general anesthetics [see comments]. *Anesthesiology.* 1997;86(4):866–874.
148. Flood P, Ramirez-Latorre J, Role L. Alpha 4 beta 2 neuronal nicotinic acetylcholine receptors in the central nervous system are inhibited by isoflurane and propofol, but alpha 7-type nicotinic acetylcholine receptors are unaffected [see comments]. *Anesthesiology.* 1997;86(4):859–865.
149. Evers AS, Steinbach JH. Supersensitive sites in the central nervous system: Anesthetics block brain nicotinic receptors. *Anesthesiology.* 1997;86:760–762.
150. Eger EI 2nd, Zhang Y, Laster M, et al. Acetylcholine receptors do not mediate the immobilization produced by inhaled anesthetics. *Anesth Analg.* 2002;94(6): 1500–1504.
151. Wong SM, Sonner JM, Kendig JJ. Acetylcholine receptors do not mediate isoflurane's actions on spinal cord in vitro. *Anesth Analg.* 2002;94(6):1495–1499.
152. Raines DE, Claycomb RJ, Forman SA. Nonhalogenated anesthetic alkanes and perhalogenated nonimmobilizing alkanes inhibit alpha(4)beta(2) neuronal nicotinic acetylcholine receptors. *Anesth Analg.* 2002;95(3):573–577.
153. Downie DL, Hall AC, Lieb WR, et al. Effects of inhalational general anaesthetics on native glycine receptors in rat medullary neurons and recombinant glycine receptors in Xenopus oocytes. *Br J Pharmacol.* 1996;118:493–502.
154. Mascia MP, Machu TK, Harris RA. Enhancement of homomeric glycine receptor function by long-chain alcohols and anaesthetics. *Br J Pharmacol.* 1996;119(7):1331–1336.
155. Jenkins A, Franks NP, Lieb WR. Actions of general anaesthetics on 5-HT3 receptors in N1E-115 neuroblastoma cells. *Br J Pharmacol.* 1996;117:1507–1515.
156. Machu TK, Harris RA. Alcohols and anesthetics enhance the function of 5-hydroxytryptamine3 receptors expressed in Xenopus laevis oocytes. *J Pharmacol Exp Ther.* 1994;271:898–905.
157. Segal IS, Vickery RG, Walton JK, et al. Dexmedetomidine diminishes halothane anesthetic requirements in rats through a postsynaptic alpha 2 adrenergic receptor. *Anesthesiology.* 1988;69:818–823.
158. Moody EJ, Harris BD, Skolnick P. The potential for safer anaesthesia using stereoselective anaesthetics. *Trends Pharmacol Sci.* 1994;15(10):387–391.

159. Zhang Y, Laster MJ, Hara K, et al. Glycine receptors mediate part of the immobility produced by inhaled anesthetics. *Anesth Analg.* 2003;96(1):97–101.
160. Zhang Y, Sonner JM, Eger EI 2nd, et al. Gamma-aminobutyric acidA receptors do not mediate the immobility produced by isoflurane. *Anesth Analg.* 2004; 99(1):85–90.
161. Zhang Y, Wu S, Eger EI 2nd, et al. Neither GABA(A) nor strychnine-sensitive glycine receptors are the sole mediators of MAC for isoflurane. *Anesth Analg.* 2001;92(1):123–127.
162. Morgan PG, Cascorbi HF. Effect of anesthetics and a convulsant on normal and mutant Caenorhabditis elegans. *Anesthesiology.* 1985;62:738–744.
163. Sedensky MM, Meneely PM. Genetic analysis of halothane sensitivity in Caenorhabditis elegans. *Science.* 1987;236(4804):952–954.
164. Humphrey JA, Hamming KS, Thacker CM, et al. A putative cation channel and its novel regulator: Cross-species conservation of effects on general anesthesia. *Curr Biol.* 2007;17(7):624–629.
165. Crowder CM, Shebester LD, Schedl T. Behavioral effects of volatile anesthetics in Caenorhabditis elegans. *Anesthesiology.* 1996;85(4):901–912.
166. Metz LB, Dasgupta N, Liu C, et al. An evolutionarily conserved presynaptic protein is required for isoflurane sensitivity in Caenorhabditis elegans. *Anesthesiology.* 2007;107(6):971–982.
167. Nagele P, Metz LB, Crowder CM. Nitrous oxide (N2O) requires the N-methyl-D-aspartate receptor for its action in Caenorhabditis elegans. *Proc Natl Acad Sci USA.* 2004;101(23):8791–8796.
168. Nagele P, Metz LB, Crowder CM. Xenon acts by inhibition of non-N-methyl-D-aspartate receptor-mediated glutamatergic neurotransmission in Caenorhabditis elegans. *Anesthesiology.* 2005;103(3):508–513.
169. Campbell DB, Nash HA. Use of Drosophila mutants to distinguish among volatile general anesthetics. *Proc Natl Acad Sci USA.* 1994;91(6):2135–2139.
170. Campbell JL, Nash HA. The visually-induced jump response of Drosophila melanogaster is sensitive to volatile anesthetics. *J Neurogenet.* 1998;12(4):241–251.
171. Krishnan KS, Nash HA. A genetic study of the anesthetic response: mutants of Drosophila melanogaster altered in sensitivity to halothane. *Proc Natl Acad Sci USA.* 1990;87:8632–8636.
172. Drexler B, Antkowiak B, Engin E, et al. Identification and characterization of anesthetic targets by mouse molecular genetics approaches. *Can J Anaesth.* 2011; 58(2):178–190.
173. Blednov YA, Jung S, Alva H, et al. Deletion of the alpha1 or beta2 subunit of GABAA receptors reduces actions of alcohol and other drugs. *J Pharmacol Exp Ther.* 2003;304(1):30–36.
174. Rau V, Iyer SV, Oh I, et al. Gamma-aminobutyric acid type A receptor alpha 4 subunit knockout mice are resistant to the amnestic effect of isoflurane. *Anesth Analg.* 2009;109(6):1816–1822.
175. Sonner JM, Cascio M, Xing Y, et al. Alpha 1 subunit-containing GABA type A receptors in forebrain contribute to the effect of inhaled anesthetics on conditioned fear. *Mol Pharmacol.* 2005;68(1):61–68.
176. Cheng VY, Martin LJ, Elliott EM, et al. Alpha5GABAA receptors mediate the amnestic but not sedative-hypnotic effects of the general anesthetic etomidate. *J Neurosci.* 2006;26(14):3713–3720.
177. Homanics GE, Ferguson C, Quinlan JJ, et al. Gene knockout of the alpha6 subunit of the gamma-aminobutyric acid type A receptor: Lack of effect on responses to ethanol, pentobarbital, and general anesthetics. *Mol Pharmacol.* 1997;51(4):588–596.
178. Borghese CM, Werner DF, Topf N, et al. An isoflurane- and alcohol-insensitive mutant GABA(A) receptor alpha(1) subunit with near-normal apparent affinity for GABA: Characterization in heterologous systems and production of knockin mice. *J Pharmacol Exp Ther.* 2006;319(1):208–218.
179. Sonner JM, Werner DF, Elsen FP, et al. Effect of isoflurane and other potent inhaled anesthetics on minimum alveolar concentration, learning, and the righting reflex in mice engineered to express alpha1 gamma-aminobutyric acid type A receptors unresponsive to isoflurane. *Anesthesiology.* 2007;106(1):107–113.
180. Werner DF, Blednov YA, Ariwodola OJ, et al. Knockin mice with ethanol-insensitive alpha1-containing gamma-aminobutyric acid type A receptors display selective alterations in behavioral responses to ethanol. *J Pharmacol Exp Ther.* 2006; 319(1):219–227.
181. Nishikawa K, Jenkins A, Paraskevakis I, et al. Volatile anesthetic actions on the GABAA receptors: Contrasting effects of alpha 1(S270) and beta 2(N265) point mutations. *Neuropharmacology.* 2002;42(3):337–345.
182. Homanics GE, Elsen FP, Ying SW, et al. A gain-of-function mutation in the GABA receptor produces synaptic and behavioral abnormalities in the mouse. *Genes Brain Behav.* 2005;4(1):10–19.
183. Siegwart R, Jurd R, Rudolph U. Molecular determinants for the action of general anesthetics at recombinant alpha(2)beta(3)gamma(2)gamma-aminobutyric acid(A) receptors. *J Neurochem.* 2002;80(1):140–148.
184. Jurd R, Arras M, Lambert S, et al. General anesthetic actions in vivo strongly attenuated by a point mutation in the GABA(A) receptor beta3 subunit. *FASEB J.* 2003;17(2):250–252.
185. Zeller A, Arras M, Jurd R, et al. Identification of a molecular target mediating the general anesthetic actions of pentobarbital. *Mol Pharmacol.* 2007;71(3):852–859.
186. Zeller A, Arras M, Jurd R, et al. Mapping the contribution of beta3-containing GABAA receptors to volatile and intravenous general anesthetic actions. *BMC Pharmacol.* 2007;7:2.
187. Zeller A, Arras M, Lazaris A, et al. Distinct molecular targets for the central respiratory and cardiac actions of the general anesthetics etomidate and propofol. *FASEB J.* 2005;19(12):1677–1679.
188. Liao M, Sonner JM, Jurd R, et al. Beta3-containing gamma-aminobutyric acidA receptors are not major targets for the amnesic and immobilizing actions of isoflurane. *Anesth Analg.* 2005;101(2):412–418, table of contents.
189. Cirone J, Rosahl TW, Reynolds DS, et al. Gamma-aminobutyric acid type A receptor beta 2 subunit mediates the hypothermic effect of etomidate in mice. *Anesthesiology.* 2004;100(6):1438–1445.
190. Reynolds DS, Rosahl TW, Cirone J, et al. Sedation and anesthesia mediated by distinct GABA(A) receptor isoforms. *J Neurosci.* 2003;23(24):8608–8617.
191. Mihalek RM, Banerjee PK, Korpi ER, et al. Attenuated sensitivity to neuroactive steroids in gamma-aminobutyrate type A receptor delta subunit knockout mice. *Proc Natl Acad Sci USA.* 1999;96(22):12905–12910.
192. Heurteaux C, Guy N, Laigle C, et al. TREK-1, a K(+) channel involved in neuroprotection and general anesthesia. *EMBO J.* 2004;23(13):2684–2695.
193. Westphalen RI, Krivitski M, Amarosa A, et al. Reduced inhibition of cortical glutamate and GABA release by halothane in mice lacking the K+ channel, TREK-1. *Br J Pharmacol.* 2007;152(6):939–945.
194. Linden AM, Aller MI, Leppä E, et al. The in vivo contributions of TASK-1-containing channels to the actions of inhalation anesthetics, the alpha(2) adrenergic sedative dexmedetomidine, and cannabinoid agonists. *J Pharmacol Exp Ther.* 2006; 317(2):615–626.
195. Linden AM, Sandu C, Aller MI, et al. TASK-3 knockout mice exhibit exaggerated nocturnal activity, impairments in cognitive functions, and reduced sensitivity to inhalation anesthetics. *J Pharmacol Exp Ther.* 2007;323(3):924–934.
196. Pang DS, Robledo CJ, Carr DR, et al. An unexpected role for TASK-3 potassium channels in network oscillations with implications for sleep mechanisms and anesthetic action. *Proc Natl Acad Sci USA.* 2009;106(41):17546–17551.
197. Rampil IJ, Mason P, Singh H. Anesthetic potency (MAC) is independent of forebrain structures in the rat. *Anesthesiology.* 1993;78(4):707–712.
198. Rampil IJ. Anesthetic potency is not altered after hypothermic spinal cord transection in rats. *Anesthesiology.* 1994;80(3):606–610.
199. Antognini JF, Schwartz K. Exaggerated anesthetic requirements in the preferentially anesthetized brain. *Anesthesiology.* 1993;79(6):1244–1249.
200. Borges M, Antognini JF. Does the brain influence somatic responses to noxious stimuli during isoflurane anesthesia? *Anesthesiology.* 1994;81(6):1511–1515.
201. Zorychta E, Esplin DW, Capek R. Action of halothane on transmitter release in the spinal monosynaptic pathway. *Fed Proc Am Soc Exp Biol.* 1975;34:2999.
202. Takenoshita M, Takahashi T. Mechanisms of halothane action on synaptic transmission in motoneurons of the newborn rat spinal cord in vitro. *Brain Res* 1987;402:303–310.
203. Jinks SL, Bravo M, Satter O, et al. Brainstem regions affecting minimum alveolar concentration and movement pattern during isoflurane anesthesia. *Anesthesiology.* 2010;112(2):316–324.
204. Kungys G, Kim J, Jinks SL, et al. Propofol produces immobility via action in the ventral horn of the spinal cord by a GABAergic mechanism. *Anesth Analg.* 2009;108(5):1531–1537.
205. Jinks SL, Atherley RJ, Dominguez CL, et al. Isoflurane disrupts central pattern generator activity and coordination in the lamprey isolated spinal cord. *Anesthesiology.* 2005;103(3):567–575.
206. Stucke AG, Zuperku EJ, Tonkovic-Capin V, et al. Halothane depresses glutamatergic neurotransmission to brain stem inspiratory premotor neurons in a decerebrate dog model. *Anesthesiology.* 2003;98(4):897–905.
207. Wang X. Propofol and isoflurane enhancement of tonic gamma-aminobutyric acid type a current in cardiac vagal neurons in the nucleus ambiguus. *Anesth Analg.* 2009;108(1):142–148.
208. McDougall SJ, Bailey TW, Mendelowitz D, et al. Propofol enhances both tonic and phasic inhibitory currents in second-order neurons of the solitary tract nucleus (NTS). *Neuropharmacology.* 2008;54(3):552–563.
209. Peters JH, McDougall SJ, Mendelowitz D, et al. Isoflurane differentially modulates inhibitory and excitatory synaptic transmission to the solitary tract nucleus. *Anesthesiology.* 2008;108(4):675–683.
210. Kushikata T, Hirota K, Kotani N, et al. Isoflurane increases norepinephrine release in the rat preoptic area and the posterior hypothalamus in vivo and in vitro: Relevance to thermoregulation during anesthesia. *Neuroscience.* 2005;131(1): 79–86.
211. Collinson N, Kuenzi FM, Jarolimek W, et al. Enhanced learning and memory and altered GABAergic synaptic transmission in mice lacking the alpha 5 subunit of the GABAA receptor. *J Neurosci.* 2002;22(13):5572–5580.
212. Zurek AA, Bridgwater EM, Orser BA. Inhibition of alpha5 gamma-aminobutyric acid type A receptors restores recognition memory after general anesthesia. *Anesth Analg.* 2012;114(4):845–855.
213. Laureys S. The neural correlate of (un)awareness: lessons from the vegetative state. *Trends Cogn Sci.* 2005;9(12):556–559.
214. French JD, Verzeano M, Magoun HW. A neural basis of the anesthetic state. *AMA Arch Neurol Psychiatry.* 1953;69(4):519–529.
215. Orth M, Bravo E, Barter L, et al. The differential effects of halothane and isoflurane on electroencephalographic responses to electrical microstimulation of the reticular formation. *Anesth Analg.* 2006;102(6):1709–1714.

216. Vanini G, Wathen BL, Lydic R, et al. Endogenous GABA levels in the pontine reticular formation are greater during wakefulness than during rapid eye movement sleep. *J Neurosci.* 2011;31(7):2649–2656.
217. Vanini G, Watson CJ, Lydic R, et al. Gamma-aminobutyric acid-mediated neurotransmission in the pontine reticular formation modulates hypnosis, immobility, and breathing during isoflurane anesthesia. *Anesthesiology.* 2008;109(6):978–988.
218. Luo T, Leung LS. Involvement of tuberomamillary histaminergic neurons in isoflurane anesthesia. *Anesthesiology.* 2011;115(1):36–43.
219. Nelson LE, Guo TZ, Lu J, et al. The sedative component of anesthesia is mediated by GABA(A) receptors in an endogenous sleep pathway. *Nat Neurosci.* 2002;5(10):979–984.
220. Zecharia AY, Nelson LE, Gent TC, et al. The involvement of hypothalamic sleep pathways in general anesthesia: Testing the hypothesis using the GABAA receptor beta3N265M knock-in mouse. *J Neurosci.* 2009;29(7):2177–2187.
221. Eikermann M, Vetrivelan R, Grosse-Sundrup M, et al. The ventrolateral preoptic nucleus is not required for isoflurane general anesthesia. *Brain Res.* 2011;1426:30–37.
222. Yasuda Y, Takeda A, Fukuda S, et al. Orexin a elicits arousal electroencephalography without sympathetic cardiovascular activation in isoflurane-anesthetized rats. *Anesth Analg.* 2003;97(6):1663–1666.
223. Pillay S, Vizuete JA, McCallum JB, et al. Norepinephrine infusion into nucleus basalis elicits microarousal in desflurane-anesthetized rats. *Anesthesiology.* 2011;115(4):733–742.
224. Luo T, Leung LS. Basal forebrain histaminergic transmission modulates electroencephalographic activity and emergence from isoflurane anesthesia. *Anesthesiology.* 2009;111(4):725–733.
225. Solt K, Cotten JF, Cimenser A, et al. Methylphenidate actively induces emergence from general anesthesia. *Anesthesiology.* 2011;115(4):791–803.
226. Alkire MT, Haier RJ, Fallon JH. Toward a unified theory of narcosis: Brain imaging evidence for a thalamocortical switch as the neurophysiologic basis of anesthetic-induced unconsciousness. *Conscious Cogn.* 2000;9(3):370–386.
227. Alkire MT, Asher CD, Franciscus AM, et al. Thalamic microinfusion of antibody to a voltage-gated potassium channel restores consciousness during anesthesia. *Anesthesiology.* 2009;110(4):766–773.
228. Alkire MT, McReynolds JR, Hahn EL, et al. Thalamic microinjection of nicotine reverses sevoflurane-induced loss of righting reflex in the rat. *Anesthesiology.* 2007;107(2):264–272.
229. Yen CT, Shaw FZ. Reticular thalamic responses to nociceptive inputs in anesthetized rats. *Brain Res.* 2003;968(2):179–191.
230. Imas OA, Ropella KM, Wood JD, et al. Halothane augments event-related gamma oscillations in rat visual cortex. *Neuroscience.* 2004;123(1):269–278.
231. Hudetz AG, Imas OA. Burst activation of the cerebral cortex by flash stimuli during isoflurane anesthesia in rats. *Anesthesiology.* 2007;107(6):983–991.
232. Velly LJ, Rey MF, Bruder NJ, et al. Differential dynamic of action on cortical and subcortical structures of anesthetic agents during induction of anesthesia. *Anesthesiology.* 2007;107(2):202–212.
233. Hudetz AG, Vizuete JA, Imas OA. Desflurane selectively suppresses long-latency cortical neuronal response to flash in the rat. *Anesthesiology.* 2009;111(2):231–239.
234. Imas OA, Ropella KM, Ward BD, et al. Volatile anesthetics disrupt frontal-posterior recurrent information transfer at gamma frequencies in rat. *Neurosci Lett.* 2005;387(3):145–150.
235. Lee U, Mashour GA, Kim S, et al. Propofol induction reduces the capacity for neural information integration: Implications for the mechanism of consciousness and general anesthesia. *Conscious Cogn.* 2009;18(1):56–64.
236. Ku SW, Lee U, Noh GJ, et al. Preferential inhibition of frontal-to-parietal feedback connectivity is a neurophysiologic correlate of general anesthesia in surgical patients. *PLoS One.* 2011;6(10):e25155.
237. Lee U, Kim S, Noh GJ, et al. The directionality and functional organization of frontoparietal connectivity during consciousness and anesthesia in humans. *Conscious Cogn.* 2009;18(4):1069–1078.
238. Schrouff J, Perlbarg V, Boly M, et al. Brain functional integration decreases during propofol-induced loss of consciousness. *Neuroimage.* 2011;57(1):198–205.
239. Boveroux P, Vanhaudenhuyse A, Bruno MA, et al. Breakdown of within- and between-network resting state functional magnetic resonance imaging connectivity during propofol-induced loss of consciousness. *Anesthesiology.* 2010; 113(5):1038–1053.
240. Raichle ME, MacLeod AM, Snyder AZ, et al. A default mode of brain function. *Proc Natl Acad Sci USA.* 2001;98(2):676–682.
241. Greicius MD, Krasnow B, Reiss AL, et al. Functional connectivity in the resting brain: a network analysis of the default mode hypothesis. *Proc Natl Acad Sci USA.* 2003;100(1):253–258.
242. Samann PG, Wehrle R, Hoehn D, et al. Development of the brain's default mode network from wakefulness to slow wave sleep. *Cereb Cortex.* 2011;21(9):2082–2093.
243. Horovitz SG, Braun AR, Carr WS, et al. Decoupling of the brain's default mode network during deep sleep. *Proc Natl Acad Sci USA.* 2009;106(27):11376–11381.
244. Larson-Prior LJ, Power JD, Vincent JL, et al. Modulation of the brain's functional network architecture in the transition from wake to sleep. *Prog Brain Res.* 2011;193:277–294.
245. Mashour GA Consciousness unbound: toward a paradigm of general anesthesia. *Anesthesiology.* 2004;100(2):428–433.
246. Hudetz AG, Vizuete JA, Pillay S. Differential effects of isoflurane on high-frequency and low-frequency gamma oscillations in the cerebral cortex and hippocampus in freely moving rats. *Anesthesiology.* 2011;114(3):588–595.
247. Breshears JD, Roland JL, Sharma M, et al. Stable and dynamic cortical electrophysiology of induction and emergence with propofol anesthesia. *Proc Natl Acad Sci USA.* 2010;107(49):21170–21175.
248. John ER, Prichep LS, Kox W, et al. Invariant reversible QEEG effects of anesthetics. *Conscious Cogn.* 2001;10(2):165–183.
249. Martin LJ, Orser BA. Etomidate targets alpha5 gamma-aminobutyric acid subtype A receptors to regulate synaptic plasticity and memory blockade. *Anesthesiology.* 2009;111(5):1025–1035.
250. O'Meara GF, Newman RJ, Fradley RL, et al. The GABA-A beta3 subunit mediates anaesthesia induced by etomidate. *Neuroreport*;15(10):1653–1656.
251. Quinlan JJ, Homanics GE, Firestone LL. Anesthesia sensitivity in mice that lack the beta3 subunit of the gamma-aminobutyric acid receptor. *Anesthesiology*;88(3):775–780.
252. Rau V, Oh I, Liao M, et al. Gamma-aminobutyric acid type A receptor beta3 subunit forebrain-specific knockout mice are resistant to the amnestic effect of isoflurane. *Anesth Analg.* 2011;113(3):500–504.
253. Lambert S, Arras M, Vogt KE, et al. Isoflurane-induced surgical tolerance mediated only in part by beta3-containing GABA(A) receptors. *Eur J Pharmacol.* 2005; 516(1):23–27.
254. Linden AM, Aller MI, Leppa E, et al. K+ channel TASK-1 knockout mice show enhanced sensitivities to ataxic and hypnotic effects of GABA(A) receptor ligands. *J Pharmacol Exp Ther.* 2008;327(1):277–286.
255. Chen X, Shu S., Kennedy DP, et al. Subunit-specific effects of isoflurane on neuronal Ih in HCN1 knockout mice. *J Neurophysiol.* 2009;101(1):129–140.

CHAPTER

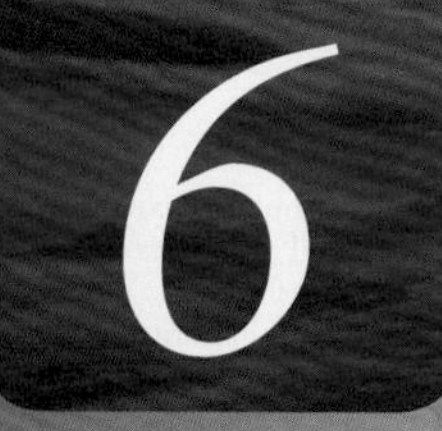

Genomic Basis of Perioperative Medicine

KEVIN FRIEDE • JOSEPH P. MATHEW • MIHAI V. PODGOREANU

Key Points

1. Despite the tremendous success of recent genome-wide association studies (GWAS) in identifying genetic variants associated with complex diseases, overall genetic variation has explained little of the high heritability of these traits, which limits their clinical utility.
2. Several candidate gene studies have suggested that susceptibility to adverse perioperative and long-term postoperative outcomes is genetically determined.
3. Potential applications of biomarkers in perioperative medicine include prognosis, diagnosis, and monitoring of adverse events, as well as informing therapeutic decisions. Very few have been rigorously evaluated to demonstrate incremental discriminatory accuracy when added to existing risk stratification models (clinical validity) or change therapy (clinical utility). Most promising among those are natriuretic peptides and C-reactive protein (CRP) for cardiovascular risk prediction.
4. Interindividual variability in response to anesthetic agents is as high as 24% and has underlying genetic mechanisms.
5. Individual variability in analgesic responsiveness is attributed to genetic control of peripheral nociceptive pathways and descending central pain modulatory pathways.
6. Pharmacogenomic variation in genes modulating drug actions explains part of the variability in drug response and has shown promising clinical utility for several classes of drugs used perioperatively.
7. Host responses to injury and the clinical trajectory of critically ill injured patients are genetically determined.
8. Genomic technology applications are beginning to fulfill the "5Ps" of perioperative medicine and pain management (personalized, preventive, predictive, participatory, and prospective).

Multimedia

1 Host Response to Injury

SCIENTIFIC RATIONALE FOR PERIOPERATIVE GENOMIC MEDICINE

Human biologic diversity involves interindividual variability in morphology, behavior, physiology, development, susceptibility to disease, and response to stressful stimuli and drug therapy (i.e., *phenotypes*). This phenotypic variation is determined, at least in part, by differences in the specific genetic makeup (i.e., *genotype*) of an individual. In 2003, the 50th anniversary of Watson and Crick's description of the DNA double-helix structure also marked the completion of the Human Genome Project.[1] This major accomplishment provides the discipline of genomics with basic resources to study the functions and interactions of all genes in a systematic fashion, including their interaction with environmental factors, and translate the findings into clinical and societal benefits. *Functional genomics* employs large-scale experimental methodologies and statistical analyses to investigate the regulation of gene expression in response to physiologic, pharmacologic, and pathologic changes. It also uses genetic information from clinical studies to examine the impact of genetic variability on disease characterization and outcome.[2] One of the major challenges and ongoing research efforts facing the post-genomic period is to connect the nearly 26,000 protein-coding genes of mammalian organisms to the genetic basis of complex polygenic diseases and the integrated function of complex biologic systems. The rapidly evolving field of *genomic medicine* proposes to use genomic information to assist medical decision-making and tailor health care to the individual patient.

A breathtaking acceleration on the path from the Human Genome Project to genomic medicine has been paved by landmark "big biology" efforts concentrated on the main themes of uncovering the function of human genes, identifying all human genomic variation, and elucidating the genetic basis for human diseases. Furthermore, dramatic improvements in sequencing technologies and cost reductions have fueled even more ambitious initiatives such as the ongoing Personal Genome Project,[3] which aims to publish the complete genomes and medical records of a number of volunteers in order to enable personalized medicine research. Nevertheless, it is fair to say a decade after its completion, although the Human Genome Project has revolutionized the pace and scope of biomedical science, it has failed so far to fulfill the promise and grand vision of "personalized medicine," leaving the scientific community somewhat sobered and divided.

Many common diseases such as atherosclerosis, coronary artery disease (CAD), hypertension, diabetes, cancer, and asthma and our responses to injury, drugs, and non-pharmacologic therapies are genetically complex. Characteristically they involve an interplay of many genetic variations in molecular and biochemical pathways (i.e., *polygenic*) and genetic–environmental interactions (i.e., *multifactorial*). In other words, complex phenotypes can be viewed as the integrated effect of many susceptibility genes and many environmental exposures. The proportion of phenotypic variance explained by genetic factors is referred to as *heritability* and can be estimated by examining the increased similarity of a phenotype in related as compared to unrelated individuals. According to the "common-disease/common-variants hypothesis",[4] individual susceptibility to common complex diseases and the manifestation, severity, and prognosis of the disease process is modulated by multiple common functional polymorphisms, each with only modest effect on disease risk. However, it is likely that
1 rare modest-risk alleles are important as well in polygenic disease, but their detection is more difficult due to sample size and sequencing constraints.

The perioperative period represents a unique and extreme example of such gene–environment interaction. As we appreciate in our daily practice in the operating rooms and intensive care units (ICUs), one hallmark of perioperative physiology is the striking variability in patient responses to the acute, robust, and generalized perioperative (environmental) perturbations induced by surgical injury, hemodynamic challenges, vascular cannulation, extracorporeal circulation, intra-aortic balloon counterpulsation, mechanical ventilation, partial/total organ resection, transient limb/organ ischemia, transfusions, anesthetic agents, and the pharmacopoeia used in the perioperative period. This translates into substantial interindividual variability in immediate perioperative adverse events (mortality or incidence/severity of organ dysfunction), as well as long-term outcomes (Table 6-1). For decades we have attributed this variability to many complexities such as age, nutritional state, and comorbidities—what we colloquially call "protoplasm"—or to the heterogeneity of the surgical insult. But given equivalent magnitudes of surgery or trauma, adequate antibiotic prophylaxis, and appropriate clinical and surgical skill, why is it that some patients never develop complications (e.g., infection, organ dysfunction) but others do? Moreover, why is it that when such complications do occur, some patients recover while others progress inexorably to multiple organ failure and death? It is becoming increasingly recognized that perioperative and posttraumatic morbidity arises as a direct result of exposure to the acute environmental stress of surgery or trauma occurring on a landscape of susceptibility determined by an individual's clinical and genetic characteristics (constitutive factors). It may even occur in otherwise healthy individuals. Thus, overall genetic predisposition to perioperative complications stems not only from genetic contributions to the development of comorbid risk factors (such as CAD and reduced preoperative cardiopulmonary reserve) during the patient's lifetime, but also from genetic variability in specific biologic pathways participating in the host response to surgical injury or trauma (Fig. 6-1). Such adverse outcomes will develop only in patients whose combined burden of genetic and environmental risk factors exceeds a certain threshold, which may vary with age. In fact, physiologic stress associated with life-threatening injury exposes genetic anomalies that might otherwise go unnoticed. Identification of such genetic contributions not only to disease causation and susceptibility, but that also influence the individual patient's *responses* to disease and drug therapy. Incorporation of genetic risk information in clinical decision-making, may lead to improved health outcomes and reduced costs.

With increasing evidence suggesting that genetic variation can significantly modulate risk of adverse perioperative events,[5–8] the emerging field of *perioperative genomics* aims to apply functional genomic approaches to discover underlying biologic mechanisms that explain why similar patients have such dramatically different outcomes after surgery and is justified by a unique combination of environmental insults and postoperative phenotypes that characterize surgical and critically ill patient populations. To integrate this new generation of genetic results into clinical practice, perioperative physicians need to understand the patterns of human genome variation, the methods of population-based genetic investigation, and the principles of gene and protein expression analysis. This chapter reviews general genetic/genomic concepts and highlights current and future applications of genomic technologies for perioperative risk stratification, outcome prediction, mechanistic understanding of surgical stress responses, as well as identification and validation of novel targets for perioperative organ protection.

TABLE 6-1. CATEGORIES OF PERIOPERATIVE PHENOTYPES

Immediate perioperative outcomes	• In-hospital mortality • Perioperative myocardial infarction • Perioperative low cardiac output syndrome/acute decompensated heart failure/ventricular dysfunction • Perioperative vasoplegic syndrome • Perioperative arrhythmias (atrial fibrillation, QTc prolongation) • Postoperative bleeding • Perioperative venous thrombosis • Acute postoperative stroke • Postoperative delirium • Perioperative acute kidney injury • Acute perioperative lung injury/prolonged postoperative mechanical ventilation • Acute allograft dysfunction/rejection • Postoperative sepsis • Multiple organ dysfunction syndrome • Postoperative nausea and vomiting • Acute postoperative pain • Variability in response to anesthetics, analgesics, and other perioperative drugs • Intermediate phenotypes (plasma biomarker levels)
Long-term postoperative outcomes	• Event-free survival/major adverse cardiac events • Progression of vein graft disease • Chronic allograft dysfunction/rejection • Postoperative cognitive dysfunction • Postoperative depression • Transition from acute to chronic pain • Cancer progression • Quality of life

Overview of Human Genomic Variation

Although the human DNA sequence is 99.9% identical between individuals, the variations may greatly affect a person's disease susceptibility. In elucidating the genetic basis of disease, much of what has been investigated in the pre-Human Genome Project era focused on identifying rare genetic variants (*mutations*) responsible for >1,500 monogenic disorders such as hypertrophic cardiomyopathy, long QT syndrome, sickle cell anemia, cystic fibrosis, or familial hypercholesterolemia, which are highly penetrant (carriers of the mutant gene will likely have the disease) and inherited in Mendelian fashion (hence termed Mendelian diseases). However, most of the genetic diversity in the population is attributable to more widespread DNA sequence variations (*polymorphisms*), typically single nucleotide base substitutions [*single nucleotide polymorphisms* (SNPs)], or to a broader category of previously overlooked *structural genetic variants* which include short sequence repeats (*microsatellites*), insertion/deletion (I/D) of one or more nucleotides (*indels*), inversions,

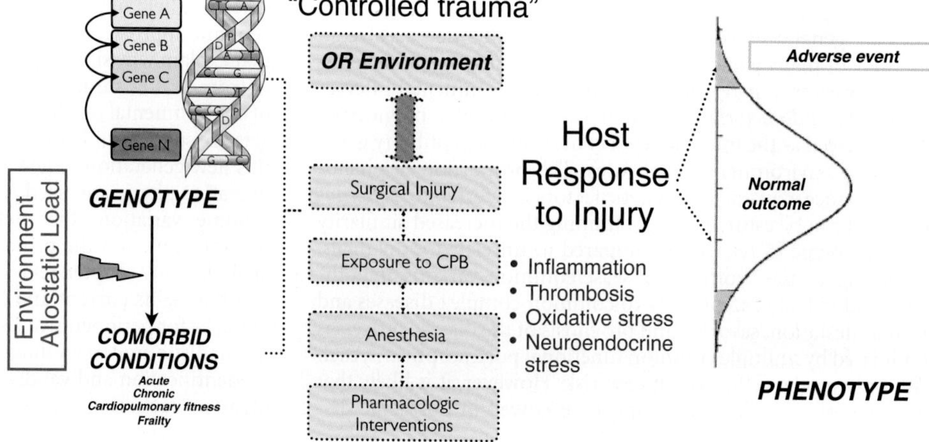

FIGURE 6-1. Perioperative adverse events are complex traits, characteristically involving an interaction between robust operative environmental perturbations (surgical trauma, hemodynamic challenges, exposure to extracorporeal circulation, drug administration) and multiple susceptibility genes. The observed variability in perioperative outcomes can in part be attributed to genetic variability modulating the host response to surgical injury. OR, operating room; CPB, cardiopulmonary bypass.

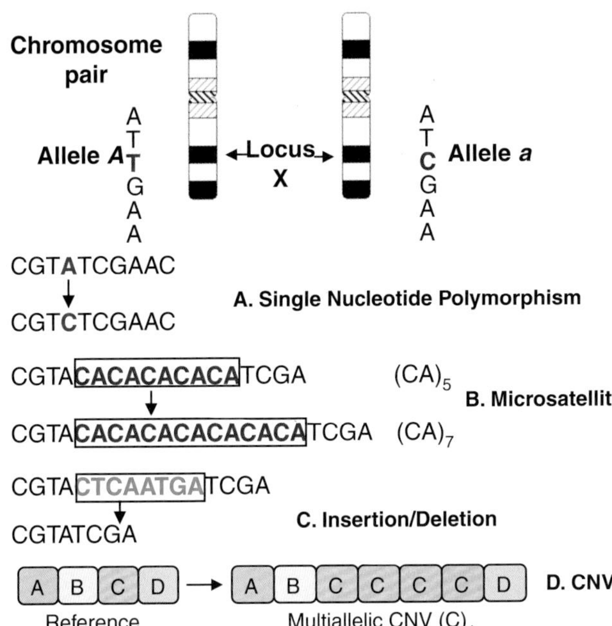

FIGURE 6-2. Categories of common human genetic variation. **A:** *Single nucleotide polymorphisms (SNPs)* can be silent or have functional consequences: Changes in amino acid sequence or premature termination of protein synthesis (if they occur in the coding regions of the gene) or alterations in the expression of the gene, resulting in more or less protein (if they occur in regulatory regions of the gene such as the promoter region or the intron/exon boundaries). Structural genetic variants include (**B**) *Microsatellites* with varying number of dinucleotide $(CA)_n$ repeats; (**C**) *insertions/deletions;* (**D**) copy number variation (CNV), (**A**)–(**D**) are long DNA segments, segment (**D**) shows variation in copy number. Glossary: *Locus,* the location of a gene/genetic marker in the genome; *alleles,* alternative forms of a gene/genetic marker; *genotype,* the observed alleles for an individual at a genetic locus; *heterozygous,* two different alleles are present at a locus; *homozygous,* two identical alleles are present at a locus. A SNP at position 1691 of a gene, with alleles G and A, would be written as 1691G > A.

and the recently discovered copy number variants (*CNVs,* large segments of DNA that vary in number of copies)[9] all of which may or may not be associated with a specific phenotype (Fig. 6-2). To be classified as a polymorphism, the DNA sequence alternatives (i.e., *alleles*) must exist with a frequency of at least 1% in the population. About 15 million SNPs are estimated to exist in the human genome, approximately once every 300 base pairs, located in genes as well as in the surrounding regions of the genome. Polymorphisms may directly alter the amino acid sequence and therefore potentially alter protein function or alter regulatory DNA sequences that modulate protein expression. Sets of nearby SNPs on a chromosome are inherited in blocks, referred to as *haplotypes.* As it will be shown later, haplotype analysis is a useful way of applying genotype information in disease gene discovery. On the other hand, CNVs involve approximately 12% of the human genome, often encompass genes (especially regulating inflammation and brain development), and may influence disease susceptibility through dosage imbalances. The year 2007 was marked by the realization that DNA differs from person to person much more than previously suspected; equipped with faster and cheaper DNA sequencing technologies, researchers have catalogued more than 3 million SNPs as part of the HapMap Project,[10] published the first diploid genome sequence of an individual human,[11] launched the 1000 Genomes Project (sequencing the genomes of 1,000 people from around the world), and begun charting CNVs and other structural variants, thus making understanding of human genetic variation the 2007 Science magazine "Breakthrough of the Year." Below, we review the common strategies used to incorporate genetic analysis into clinical studies.

Methodologic Approaches to Study the Genetic Architecture of Common Complex Diseases

Most ongoing research on complex disorders focuses on identifying genetic polymorphisms that enhance susceptibility to given conditions. Often the design of such studies is complicated by the presence of multiple risk factors, gene–environment interactions, and a lack of even rough estimates of the number of genes underlying such complex traits. Two broad strategies are being employed to identify complex trait loci. The *candidate gene* approach is motivated by what is known about the trait biologically and can be characterized as a hypothesis-testing approach, but is intrinsically biased. The second strategy is the *genome-wide scan,* in which thousands of markers uniformly distributed throughout the genome are used to locate regions that may harbor genes influencing the phenotypic variability. This is a hypothesis-free and unbiased approach, in the sense that no prior assumptions are being made about the biologic processes involved and no weight is given to known genes, thus allowing the detection of previously unknown trait loci. Both the candidate gene and the genome scan approaches can be implemented using one of two fundamental methods of identifying polymorphisms affecting common diseases: Linkage analysis or association studies in human populations.

Linkage Analysis. Used to identify the chromosomal location of gene variants related to a given disease by studying the distribution of disease alleles in affected individuals throughout a pedigree, linkage analysis has successfully mapped hundreds of genes for rare, monogenic disorders. However, common complex diseases are characterized by a multitude of genes with rare and/or common alleles, which create an apparently chaotic pattern of heterogeneity within and between families. The overall effect of this heterogeneity, together with the potentially weak influence of many loci, places a heavy burden on the statistical power needed to detect individual contributing genes and may be the reason why very few genome linkage scans so far have yielded disease loci that meet genome-wide significance criteria.[12] Furthermore, the nature of most complex diseases (especially for perioperative adverse events) precludes the study of extended multigenerational family pedigrees. Nevertheless, a few positive findings have emerged using this approach: A stroke susceptibility locus was mapped on chromosome 5q12,[13] risk of myocardial infarction was mapped to a single region on chromosome 14,[14] and a recent meta-analysis of several genome-wide scans for pulse pressure variation, an emerging risk factor for perioperative complications, has identified several linkage bins on chromosomes 22 and 10.[15]

Genetic Association Studies. Association studies examine the frequency of specific genetic polymorphisms in a population-based sample of unrelated diseased individuals and appropriately matched unaffected controls. The increased statistical power to uncover small clinical effects of multiple genes[16] and the fact that they do not require family-based sample collections are the main advantages of this approach over linkage analysis. Until very recently, most significant results in dissecting common complex diseases were gathered from candidate gene association studies, with genes selected because of a priori hypotheses about their potential etiologic role in disease based on current understanding of the disease pathophysiology.[17] For example, genetic variants within the renin–angiotensin system,[18] nitric oxide synthase (NOS),[19] and β_2-adrenergic receptors (AR),[20] known to modulate vascular tone, were tested and found to be associated with hypertension. Similarly, the possible effects of polymorphisms on genetic predisposition for CAD[21] or restenosis after angioplasty[22] have been extensively investigated; more recently, two large-scale association studies have identified gene variants that might affect susceptibility to myocardial infarction.[23] As it will be presented in more detail later, accumulating evidence from candidate gene association studies also suggests that specific genotypes are associated with a variety of organ-specific perioperative adverse outcomes, including myocardial infarction,[24,25] neurocognitive dysfunction,[26–28] renal compromise,[29–31] vein graft restenosis,[32,33] postoperative thrombosis,[34] vascular reactivity,[35] severe sepsis,[36,37] transplant rejection,[38] and death [for reviews, see (5,8)].

One of the main weaknesses of the candidate gene association approach is that, unless the marker of interest "travels" (i.e., is in *linkage disequilibrium*) with a functional variant, or the marker allele *is* the actual functional variant, the power to detect and map complex trait loci will be reduced. Other known limitations of genetic association studies include potential false-positive findings resulting from population stratification (i.e., admixture of different ethnic or genetic backgrounds in the case and control groups) and multiple comparison issues when large numbers of candidate genes are being assessed.[39] Replication of findings across different populations or related phenotypes remains the most reliable method of validating a true relationship between genetic polymorphisms and disease,[17] but poor reproducibility in subsequent studies has been one of the main criticisms of the candidate gene association approach.[40] However, a recent meta-analysis suggested that lack of statistical power may be the main contributor to this inconsistent replication and proposed more stringent statistical criteria to exclude false-positive results and the design of large collaborative association studies.[41]

At last, after several decades of frustrating limitations in the ability to find genetic variations responsible for common disease risk, with the completion of the second phase of the International HapMap Project (a high-resolution maps of human genetic variation and haplotypes)[10] and advances in high-throughput genotyping technologies, the year 2007 marked an explosion of adequately powered and successfully replicated *genome-wide association studies* (GWAS) that identified very significant genetic contributors to risk for common polygenic diseases like CAD,[42–44] myocardial infarction,[45] diabetes (types I and II),[46,47] atrial fibrillation,[48] obesity,[49] asthma, common cancers, rheumatoid arthritis, Crohn's disease, and others. GWAS make use of the known linkage disequilibrium pattern between SNPs from the human HapMap and the new high-density SNP chip technology to comprehensively interrogate between 65% and 80% of common variation across the genome, with even higher coverage being possible using statistical imputation techniques. The largest, most comprehensive GWAS to date was conducted by the Wellcome Trust Case-Control Consortium, investigating the association between 500,000 SNPs and 7 common diseases in 2,000 cases and 3,000 shared controls, which identified 25 independent association signals at stringent levels of significance ($P < 5 \times 10^{-7}$).[42] Interestingly, variants in or near *CDKN2A/B* (cyclin-dependent kinase inhibitor 2 A/B) conferred increased risk for both type II diabetes (odds ratio (OR) 1.2, $P = 7.8 \times 10^{-15}$) and myocardial infarction (OR 1.64, $P = 1.2 \times 10^{-20}$), which may lead to a mechanistic explanation for the link between the two disorders. This finding also highlights the power of GWAS to identify variants outside described genes: While one of the signals occurs in the *CDKN2A/B* region, the other much stronger association signal occurs >200 kb from these genes, in a gene desert, and thus would not have been picked up by a candidate gene approach. Identifying the mechanism by which this variant may affect *CDKN2A/B* expression will provide new insights into the regulation of these important genes.

Large-Scale Gene and Protein Expression Profiling: Static Versus Dynamic Genomic Markers of Perioperative Outcomes

Genomic approaches are anchored in the "central dogma" of molecular biology, the concept of transcription of messenger RNA (mRNA) from a DNA template, followed by translation of RNA into protein (Fig. 6-3). Since transcription is a key regulatory step that may eventually signal many other cascades of events, the study of RNA levels in a cell or organ (i.e., quantifying gene expression) can improve the understanding of a wide variety of biologic systems. Furthermore, while the human genome contains only about 25,000 genes, functional variability at the protein level is far more diverse, resulting from extensive posttranscriptional, translational, and posttranslational modifications. It is believed that there are approximately 200,000 distinct proteins in humans, which are further modified posttranslationally by phosphorylation, glycosylation, SUMOylation, oxidation, and disulfide structures. The "static" view of constitutive DNA sequence variants potentially involved in the pathophysiology of perioperative complications can be complemented by a "dynamic" view that integrates their functionality. There is increasing evidence that variability in gene expression levels underlies complex disease and is determined by regulatory DNA polymorphisms affecting transcription, splicing,

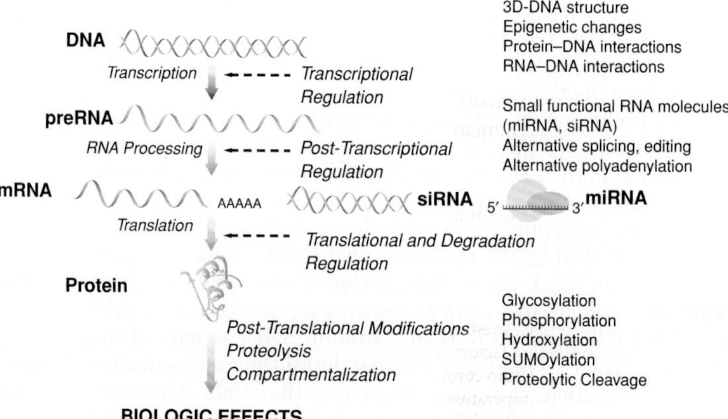

FIGURE 6-3. Increasing complexity of the central dogma of molecular biology. Protein expression involves two main processes, RNA synthesis (*transcription*) and protein synthesis (*translation*), with many intermediate regulatory steps. A single gene can give rise to multiple protein products (isoforms) via processing of preRNA molecules yielding multiple RNA products, including microRNA (miRNA) and small interfering RNA (siRNA) molecules, as well as alternative splicing and RNA editing. Thus functional variability at the protein level, ultimately responsible for biologic effects, is the cumulative result of genetic variability as well as extensive transcriptional, posttranscriptional, translational, and posttranslational modifications.

and translation efficiency in a tissue- and stimulus-specific manner.[50] Thus, analysis of large-scale variability in the pattern of RNA, microRNA (miRNA), and protein expression both at baseline and in response to the multidimensional perioperative stimuli (*dynamic genomics*) using microarray and proteomic approaches provides a much needed understanding of the overall regulatory networks involved in the pathophysiology of adverse postoperative outcomes. This information is complementary to the assessment of genetic variability at the DNA sequence level using various genotyping techniques as described in previous sections (*static genomics*). Such dynamic genomic markers can be incorporated in genomic classifiers and used clinically to improve perioperative risk stratification or monitor postoperative recovery.[51] This emergent concept of *molecular classification* involves the description of informational features in a training dataset using changes in relative RNA, miRNA, protein, or metabolite abundance in the context of genetic predisposition and applying to a test dataset to recognize a defined "fingerprint" characteristic of a particular perioperative phenotype (Table 6-2). For example, Feezor et al. used a combined genomic and proteomic approach to identify expression patterns of 138 genes from peripheral blood leukocytes and the concentrations of 7 circulating plasma proteins that discriminated patients who developed multiple organ dysfunction syndrome (MODS) after thoracoabdominal aortic aneurysm repair from those who did not. More importantly, these patterns of genome-wide gene expression and plasma protein concentration were observed before surgical trauma and visceral ischemia-reperfusion injury, suggesting that patients who developed MODS differed in either their genetic predisposition or their preexisting inflammatory state.[52]

Alternatively, dynamic genomic markers can be used to improve mechanistic understanding of perioperative stress, and to evaluate and catalogue organ-specific responses to surgical stress and severe systemic stimuli such as cardiopulmonary bypass (CPB)

SCIENTIFIC FOUNDATIONS OF ANESTHESIA

TABLE 6-2. SUMMARY OF GENE EXPRESSION STUDIES WITH IMPLICATIONS FOR PERIOPERATIVE CARDIOVASCULAR OUTCOMES

Tissue (Species)	Stimulus/Method	Genomic Signature: Number/Types of Genes	Reference
Myocardium (rat)	Ischemia/μA	14 (wound-healing, Ca-handling)	53
Myocardium (human)	CPB/circulatory arrest/μA	58 (inflammation, transcription activators, apoptosis, stress response)—adults	54
		50 (cardioprotective, antiproliferative, antihypertrophic)—neonates	55
Myocardium (rat)	IPC vs. APC/μA	566 differentially regulated/56 jointly regulated (cell defense)	56
Myocardium (rat)	APC vs. ApostC/μA	Opposing genomic profiles, 8 gene clusters, <2% jointly regulated genes	57
Myocardium (human)	APC, OPCAB, postoperative LV function/μA	319 upregulated and 281 downregulated gene sets in response to OPCAB; deregulation of fatty acid oxidation, DNA-damage signaling, and G-CSF survival (perioperative) and PGC-1α (constitutive) pathways predict improved LV function in sevoflurane-treated patients	58
PBMC (human)	APC, sevoflurane/μA	Deregulation of late preconditioning, PGC-1α, fatty acid oxidation, and L-selectin pathways	59
Atrial myocardium (pig)	Pacing-induced AF/μA + P	81 (MCL-2 ventricular/atrial isoform shift)	60
Atrial myocardium (human)	AF/μA	1,434 (ventricular-like genomic signature)	61
PBMC (human)	Cardiac surgery, PoAF/μA	1,302 genes uniquely deregulated in PoAF/401 upregulated (oxidative stress), 902 downregulated	62
PBMC (human)	Cardiac surgery, POCD/μA	1,201 genes uniquely deregulated in POCD/531 upregulated, 670 downregulated (inflammation, antigen presentation, cell adhesion, and apoptosis)	63
PBMC (human)	Heart transplant/μA	30 (profile correlated with biopsy-proven rejection; persistent immune activation in response to treatment)	64
PBMC (human)	Heart transplant/RT-PCR	11 (AlloMap, AlloMap score)	65
Myocardium (human)	Heart transplant/P	2 (increased αB-crystallin and tropomyosin serum levels)	66
PBMC, plasma (human)	TAAA/μA + P	138 genes and 7 plasma proteins predicted MODS	52
PBMC (human)	Obstructive CAD in nondiabetic patients/RT-PCR	23-gene expression signature	67
Ventricular myocardium (human)	End-stage cardiomyopathy on LVAD/μA	Combined signature of 28 microRNAs and 29 mRNAs had superior performance to classify status and predict recovery	68

AF, atrial fibrillation; APC, anesthetic preconditioning, ApostC, anesthetic postconditioning; CAD, coronary artery disease; CPB, cardiopulmonary bypass; G-CSF, granulocyte colony stimulating factor; IPC, ischemic preconditioning; LV, left ventricle; μA, microarray; MCL-2, myosin light chain 2; MODS, multiple organ dysfunction syndrome; OPCAB, off-pump coronary artery bypass; P, proteomics; PBMC, peripheral blood mononuclear cells; PGC-1α, peroxisome proliferators-activated receptor γ cofactor-1α; PoAF, postoperative atrial fibrillation; POCD, postoperative cognitive decline; RT-PCR, real-time polymerase chain reaction; TAAA, thoracoabdominal aortic aneurysm repair; LVAD, left ventricular assist device.

and endotoxemia, which can be subsequently used to identify and validate novel targets for organ-protective strategies.[69] Similarly, integrated transcriptomic and proteomic analyses have been used to characterize the peripheral blood molecular response signatures to cardiac surgery with and without CPB, a robust trigger of systemic inflammation.[70] The study demonstrated that, rather than being the primary source of serum cytokines, peripheral blood leukocytes only assume a "primed" phenotype upon contact with the extracorporeal circuit which facilitates their trapping and subsequent tissue-associated inflammatory response. Interestingly, many inflammatory mediators achieved similar systemic levels following off-pump surgery but with delayed kinetics, offering novel insights into the concepts of contact activation and compartmentalization of inflammatory responses to major surgery.

Several studies have profiled myocardial gene expression in the ischemic heart, demonstrating alterations in the expression of immediate-early genes (c-*fos*, *jun*B), as well as genes coding for calcium-handling proteins (calsequestrin, phospholamban), extracellular matrix, and cytoskeletal proteins.[53] Upregulation of transcripts mechanistically involved in cytoprotection (heat shock proteins), resistance to apoptosis, and cell growth has been found in stunned myocardium.[71] Moreover, cardiac gene expression profiling after CPB and cardioplegic arrest has identified the upregulation of inflammatory and transcription activators, apoptotic genes, and stress genes,[54] which appear to be age-related.[55] Microarray technology has also been utilized in the quest for novel cardioprotective genes, with the ultimate goal of designing strategies to activate these genes and prevent myocardial injury. Preconditioning is one of such well-studied models of cardioprotection, which can be induced by various triggers including intermittent ischemia, osmotic or redox stress, heat shock, toxins, and inhaled anesthetics. The main functional categories of genes identified as potentially involved in cardioprotective pathways include a host of transcription factors, heat shock proteins, antioxidant genes (heme-oxygenase, glutathione peroxidase), and growth factors, but different gene programs appear to be activated in ischemic versus anesthetic preconditioning, resulting in two distinct cardioprotective phenotypes.[56] More recently, a transcriptional response pattern consistent with late preconditioning has been reported in peripheral blood leukocytes following sevoflurane administration in healthy volunteers, characterized by reduced expression of L-selectin as well as downregulation of genes involved in fatty acid oxidation and the PCG1α (peroxisome-activated receptor γ coactivator 1α) pathway,[59] which mirrors changes observed in the myocardium from patients undergoing off-pump coronary artery bypass grafting (CABG) (OPCAB; Table 6-2).[58] Deregulation of these novel survival pathways thus appears to generalize across tissues, making them important targets for cardioprotection, but further studies are needed to correlate perioperative gene expression response patterns in end organs such as the myocardium to those in readily available potential surrogate tissues such as peripheral blood leukocytes.

The *transcriptome* (the complete collection of transcribed elements of the genome) is not fully representative of the *proteome* (the complete complement of proteins encoded by the genome), since many transcripts are not targeted for translation, as evidenced recently with the concept of gene silencing by RNA interference. Alternative splicing, a wide variety of posttranslational modifications, and protein–protein interactions responsible for biologic function would remain therefore undetected by gene expression profiling (Fig. 6-3). This has led to the emergence of a new field, *proteomics*, studying the sequence, modification, and function of many proteins in a biologic system at a given time. Rather than focusing on "static" DNA, proteomic studies examine dynamic protein products, with the goal of identifying proteins that undergo changes in abundance, modification, or localization in response to a particular disease state, trauma, stress, or therapeutic intervention [for a review, see (72)]. Thus, proteomics offers a more global and integrated view of biology, complementing other functional genomic approaches. Currently available methods for proteomic analysis include protein extraction, separation by two-dimensional gel electrophoresis or chromatography, followed by identification using mass spectrometry. Although rapidly improving, these methods are currently limited by sensitivity, specificity, and throughput. Several preclinical proteomic studies relevant to perioperative medicine have characterized the temporal changes in brain protein expression in response to various inhaled anesthetics[73,74] or following cardiac surgery with hypothermic circulatory arrest.[75] This may focus further studies aimed to identify new anesthetic binding sites and the development of neuroprotective strategies. Furthermore, detailed knowledge of the plasma proteome has profound implications in perioperative transfusion medicine,[76] in particular related to peptide and protein changes that occur during storage of blood products. The development of protein arrays and real-time proteomic analysis technologies has the potential to allow the use of these versatile and rigorous high-throughput methods for clinical applications and is the object of intense investigation.

GENOMICS AND PERIOPERATIVE RISK PROFILING

More than 40 million patients undergo surgery annually in the United States at a cost of $450 billion. Each year approximately 1 million patients sustain medical complications after surgery, resulting in costs of $25 billion annually. The proportion of the US population older than 65 is estimated to double in the next two decades, leading to a 25% increase in the number of surgeries, a 50% increase in surgery-related costs, and a 100% increase in complications from surgery. Recognizing the significant increase in surgical burden due to accelerated aging of the population and increased reliance on surgery for treatment of disease, the National Heart, Blood and Lung Institute has recently convened a working group on perioperative medicine. The group concluded that perioperative complications are significant, costly, variably reported, and often imprecisely detected, and identified a critical need for accurate comprehensive perioperative outcome databases. Furthermore, presurgical risk profiling is inconsistent and deserves further attention, especially for noncardiac, nonvascular surgery and older patients.[77]

Although many preoperative predictors have been identified and are constantly being refined, risk stratification based on clinical, procedural, and biologic markers explains only a small part of the variability in the incidence of perioperative complications. As mentioned above, it is becoming increasingly recognized that perioperative morbidity arises as a direct result of the environmental stress of surgery occurring on a landscape of susceptibility that is determined by an individual's clinical and genetic characteristics and may even occur in otherwise healthy individuals. Such adverse outcomes will develop only in patients whose combined burden of genetic and environmental risk factors exceeds a certain threshold, which may vary with age. Identification of such genetic contributions not only to disease causation and susceptibility, but also influencing the *response* to disease and drug therapy, and incorporation of genetic risk information in clinical decision-making, may lead to improved health outcomes and reduced costs. For instance, understanding the gene–environment interactions involved in

atherosclerotic cardiovascular disease and neurologic injury may facilitate preoperative patient optimization and resource utilization. Furthermore, understanding the role of allotypic variation in pro-inflammatory and pro-thrombotic pathways, the main pathophysiologic mechanisms responsible for perioperative complications, may contribute to the development of target-specific therapies, thereby limiting the incidence of adverse events in high-risk patients. Recently, rigorous methodologic frameworks for the design and analysis of studies aiming to evaluate the clinical validity and utility of genetic risk prediction have been developed,[78] together with detailed recommendations for reporting their
2 results.[79] To increase clinical relevance for the practicing perioperative and critical care physician, we summarize below existing evidence by specific outcome while highlighting candidate genes in relevant mechanistic pathways (Tables 6-3–6-5).

Predictive Biomarkers for Perioperative Adverse Cardiac Events

As part of the preoperative evaluation, anesthesiologists are involved in assessing the risks of perioperative complications. It is commonly accepted that patients who have underlying cardiovascular disease are at risk for adverse cardiac events after surgery, and several multifactorial risk indices have been developed and validated for patients undergoing noncardiac surgical procedures (such as the Goldman or the Lee Cardiac risk index), as well as cardiac surgery (such as the Hannan or Sergeant scores). However, identifying patients at the highest risk of perioperative infarction remains difficult, and risk scores, while potentially valuable for population studies, are not an ideal tool for directing care in an individual patient.[130] Genomic approaches have been used in the search for a better assessment of the individual coronary risk profile. Numerous reports from animal models, linkage analysis, family, twin, and population association studies have definitely proven the role of genetic influences in the incidence and progression of CAD, with a heritability of death from CAD as high as 58%; furthermore, hazardous patterns of angiographic CAD (left main and proximal disease), known major risk factors for perioperative cardiac complications, are also highly heritable. Similarly, genetic susceptibility to myocardial infarction (MI) has been established through multiple lines of evidence[14,23] including a recent well-powered and replicated GWAS.[45] While these studies do not directly address the heritability of adverse perioperative myocardial events, they do suggest a strong genetic contribution to the risk of adverse cardiovascular outcomes in general.

TABLE 6-3. **REPRESENTATIVE GENETIC POLYMORPHISMS ASSOCIATED WITH ALTERED SUSCEPTIBILITY TO ADVERSE PERIOPERATIVE CARDIOVASCULAR EVENTS**

Gene	Polymorphism	Type of Surgery	OR	Reference
Death, cardiovascular death				
AMPD1	−34C > T	Heart transplant	4.0	80
ANRIL (9p21 locus)	rs10116277	CABG	1.7[a]	81
THBD	A455V	CABG/CPB	2.4	82
Postoperative MACE and other composite adverse events (including late vein graft failure)				
ADRB1	R389G	Noncardiac with spinal block	1.87[a]	83
ADRB2	R16G	Cardiac surgery/CPB	1.96	84
	Q27E		2.82	
ACE	In/del	CABG/CPB	3.1[b]	85
ITGB3	L33P (Pl^{A2})	CABG/CPB	4.7	86
MTHFR	−677C > T	CABG	4.41	87
	A222V	PTCA and CABG/CBP	2.8	88
ADRB2	R16G	Cardiac surgery/CPB	1.96	84
	Q27E		2.82	
HP	Hp1/Hp2	CABG	n.r.	89
CR1, KDR, MICA, HLA-DPB1, VTN		CABG/CPB	n.r.	33
LPL	HindIII	CABG	n.r.	90
IL6	−174G > C	Noncardiac vascular surgery	2.14	91
	nt565G > A		1.84	
IL10	−1082G > A	Noncardiac vascular surgery	2.16	91
	−819C > T			
	−592C > A			
	ATA haplotype			
Perioperative myocardial infarction, ventricular dysfunction, early vein graft failure				
IL6	−572G > C	Cardiac/CPB	2.47	24
	−174G > C	Thoracic	1.8	92
ICAM-1	E469L	Cardiac/CPB	1.88	24
SELE	98G > T		0.16	24
MBL2	LYQA secretor haplotype	CABG/CPB	3.97	25
TNFA	−308G > A	Thoracic	2.5	92
TNFB (LTA)	TNFB2	Cardiac/CPB	3.84	93
IL10	−1082G > A	Cardiac/CPB	n.r.	94

(*continued*)

TABLE 6-3. REPRESENTATIVE GENETIC POLYMORPHISMS ASSOCIATED WITH ALTERED SUSCEPTIBILITY TO ADVERSE PERIOPERATIVE CARDIOVASCULAR EVENTS (*continued*)

Gene	Polymorphism	Type of Surgery	OR	Reference
F5	R506Q (FVL)	CABG/CPB	3.29	95
ITGB3	L33P (Pl^{A1}/Pl^{A2})	CABG/CPB	2.5[c]	96
		Major vascular	2.4	97
GP1BA	T145M	Major vascular	3.4	97
PAI-1	4G/5G	CABG	n.r.	98
CMA1	−1905A > G	CABG/CPB	n.r.	32
ANRIL	rs10116277G > T (9p21)	CABG	1.7	81
NPR3	rs700923A > G	CABG/CPB	4.28	99
	rs16890196A > G		4.09	
	rs765199C > T		4.27	
	rs700926A > C		3.89	
NPPA/NPPB	rs632793T > C	CABG/CPB	0.52	99
	rs6668352G > A		0.44	
	rs549596T > C		0.48	
	rs198388C > T		0.51	
	rs198389A > G		0.54	
ANRIL (chr 9p21 locus)	rs10116277G > T	CABG	1.79	100
	rs6475606C > T		1.79	
	rs2383207A > G		1.71	
Perioperative vasoplegia, vascular reactivity, coronary tone				
DDAH II	−449G > C	Cardiac/CPB	0.4	101
NOS3	E298D		n.r.	102,103
ACE	In/del		n.r.	35,104
ADRB2	Q27E	Tracheal intubation	11.7[d]	105
GNB3	825C > T	Response to α-AR agonists	n.r.	103
PON1	Q192R	Resting coronary tone	n.r.	103
TNFβ+250	−1082G > A	Hyperdynamic state		106
Postoperative arrhythmias: Atrial fibrillation, QTc prolongation				
IL6	−174G > C	CABG/CPB	3.25	107,108
		β-Blocker failure	n.r.	109
		Thoracic	1.8	92
RANTES	−403G > A	β-Blocker failure	n.r.	109
TNFA	−308G > A	Thoracic	2.5	92
ATFB5	rs2200733C > T	Cardiac/CPB	1.97	110
	rs2220427T > G		1.76	
IL1B	−511T > C	Cardiac/CPB	1.44	111
	5810G > A		0.66	
HSP70-Hom	−2437T > C	CABG	2.43	112
Cardiac allograft rejection				
TNFA	−308G > A	Cardiac transplant	n.r.	113
IL10	−1082G > A		n.r.	113
ICAM1	K469E		n.r.	114
IL1RN	86-bp VNTR	Thoracic transplant	2.02	115
IL1B	3953C > T		20.5[e]	115
TGF-β	915G > C	Cardiac transplant	n.r.	116

ACE, angiotensin converting enzyme; ADRB1, β_1-adrenergic receptor; ADRB2, β_2-adrenergic receptor; alpha-AR, alpha adrenergic receptors; AMPD1, adenosine monophosphate deaminase 1; ANRIL, antisense noncoding RNA in the INK4 locus; ATFB5, Atrial fibrillation, familial 5; CABG, coronary artery bypass grafting; CMA1, heart chymase; CPB, cardiopulmonary bypass; CR1, complement component 3b/4b; DDAH II, dimethylarginine dimethylaminohydrolase II; F5, factor V; FVL, factor V Leiden; GNB3, G-protein β_3 subunit; GP1BA, glycoprotein Ib*α*; HLA-DPB1, β-chain of class II major histocompatibility complex; HP, haptoglobin; HSP70, heat shock protein 70; ICAM1, intercellular adhesion molecule 1; IL1B, interleukin 1*β*; IL1RN, interleukin 1 receptor antagonist; IL6, interleukin 6; IL10, interleukin 10; ITGB3, glycoprotein IIIa; KDR, kinase inert domain receptor; LPL, lipoprotein lipase; MACE, major adverse cardiac events; MBL2, mannose-binding lectin 2; MICA, MHC I polypeptide; MTHFR, methylene-tetrahydrofolate reductase; n.r., not reported; NOS3, endothelial nitric oxide synthase; NPPA/NPPB, natriuretic peptide precursor A/B; NPR3, natriuretic peptide receptor 3 precursor; OR, odds ratio; PAI-1, plasminogen activator inhibitor-1; PON1, paraoxonase 1; PTCA, percutaneous transluminal coronary angioplasty; RANTES, regulated upon activation normally T-expressed and secreted; SELE, E-selectin; TGF-β, transforming growth factor-*β*; THBD, thrombomodulin; TNFA, tumor necrosis factor *α*; TNFB, tumor necrosis factor beta; VNTR, variable number tandem repeat; VTN, vitronectin.

[a] Hazard ratio.
[b] β-Coefficient.
[c] Relative risk
[d] *F*-value.
[e] In haplotype with IL1RN VNTR.

TABLE 6-4. REPRESENTATIVE GENETIC POLYMORPHISMS ASSOCIATED WITH ALTERED SUSCEPTIBILITY TO ADVERSE PERIOPERATIVE NEUROLOGIC EVENTS

Gene	Polymorphism	Type of Surgery	OR	Reference
Perioperative stroke, encephalopathy				
IL6	−174G > C	Cardiac/CPB	3.3	117
CRP	1846C > T			
SERPINE1 (PAI-1)	4G/4G	CPB	2.1	118
ITGB3	Pl^{A2}	PCI	4.1	119
Perioperative cognitive dysfunction, neuro-developmental dysfunction				
SELP	E298D	Cardiac/CPB	0.51	28
CRP	1059G > C	Cardiac/CPB	0.37	28
ITGB3	L33P (Pl^{A1}/Pl^{A2})	Cardiac/CPB	n.r.	27
APOE	ε4	CABG/CPB (adults)	n.r.	26
	ε2	Cardiac/CPB (children)	7; 11	120,121
Postoperative delirium				
APOE	ε4	Major noncardiac	3.64	122
		Critically ill	7.32	123

IL6, interleukin 6; CABG, coronary artery bypass grafting; CPB, cardiopulmonary bypass; CRP, C-reactive protein; PAI-1, plasminogen activator inhibitor-1; PCI, percutaneous coronary intervention; SELP, P-selectin; ITGB3, platelet glycoprotein IIIa; APOE, apolipoprotein E; OR, odds ratio; n.r., not reported.

TABLE 6-5. REPRESENTATIVE GENETIC POLYMORPHISMS ASSOCIATED WITH OTHER ADVERSE PERIOPERATIVE OUTCOMES

Gene	Polymorphism	Type of Surgery	OR	Reference
Perioperative thrombotic events				
F5	FVL	Noncardiac, cardiac	n.r.	34
Perioperative bleeding				
F5	R506Q (FVL)	Cardiac/CPB	−1.25[a]	124
PAI-1	4G/5G		10[b]	125
ITGA2	−52C > T, 807C > T	CABG/CPB	−0.15[a]	126
GP1BA	T145M		−0.22[a]	126
TF	−603A > G		−0.03[a]	126
TFPI	−399C > T		−0.05[a]	126
F2	20210G > A		0.38[a]	126
ACE	In/del		0.15[a]	126
ITGB3	L33P (Pl^{A1}/Pl^{A2})		n.r.	127
PAI-1	4G/5G	Cardiac/CPB	10[b]	125
TNFA	−238G > A	Brain AVM treatment	3.5[c]	128
APOE	ε2		10.9[c]	128
ELAM-1	98G/T 561A/C	CABG/CPB	n.r.	129
Perioperative acute kidney injury				
IL6	−572G > C	CABG/CPB	20.04[d]	29
AGT	M235T		32.19[d]	29
NOS3	E298D		4.29[d]	29
APOE	ε4		−0.13[a]	29,31
Perioperative severe sepsis				
APOE	ε3		0.28[e]	37

ACE, angiotensin converting enzyme; AGT, angiotensinogen; APOE, apolipoprotein E; AVM, arterio-venous malformation; CABG, coronary artery bypass grafting; CPB, cardiopulmonary bypass; ELAM-1, endothelial-leukocyte adhesion molecule-1; F2, prothrombin; F5, factor V; FVL, factor V Leiden; GP1BA, glycoprotein Ibα; IL6, interleukin 6; ITGA2, glycoprotein Ia/IIa; ITGB3, glycoprotein IIIa; NOS3, endothelial nitric oxide synthase; n.r., not reported; OR, odds ratio; PAI-1, plasminogen activator inhibitor-1; TF, tissue factor; TFPI, tissue factor pathway inhibitor; TNFA, tumor necrosis factor α.

[a] β-Coefficient.

[b] Odds ratio.

[c] Hazard ratio.

[d] *F*-value.

[e] Relative risk.

Despite advances in surgical, cardioprotective, and anesthetic techniques, the incidence of perioperative myocardial infarction (PMI) following cardiac and vascular surgery in several large randomized clinical trials has been reported at 7% to 19%[131,132] and is consistently associated with reduced short- and long-term survival. In the setting of cardiac surgery, PMI involves three major converging pathophysiologic processes, including systemic and local inflammation, "vulnerable" blood, and neuroendocrine stress.[5] In noncardiac surgery, pathophysiology of PMI is not so clearly understood, but a combination of two mechanisms appears predominant: (1) Plaque rupture and coronary thrombosis triggered by perioperative endothelial injury from catecholamine surges and pro-inflammatory and pro-thrombotic states; and (2) prolonged stress-induced ischemia and tachycardia in the setting of compromised perfusion. Extensive genetic variability exists in each of these mechanistic pathways, which may combine to modulate the magnitude of myocardial injury. However, only a paucity of studies exist relating genetic risk factors to adverse perioperative myocardial outcomes, mainly following CABG surgery (Table 6-3).[32,85,89]

Inflammation Biomarkers and Perioperative Adverse Cardiac Events

Although the role of inflammation in cardiovascular disease biology has long been established, we are just beginning to understand the relationship between genetically controlled variability in inflammatory responses to surgery and PMI pathogenesis. Consistent with the "inflammatory hypothesis" in the pathogenesis of perioperative organ injury, our group has recently identified three inflammatory gene polymorphisms that are independently predictive of PMI following cardiac surgery with CPB. These include the pro-inflammatory cytokine interleukin 6 (*IL6*)–572G > C (OR 2.47) and two adhesion molecules—intercellular adhesion molecule 1 (*ICAM1* Lys469Glu, OR 1.88) and E-selectin (SELE 98G > T, OR 0.16).[24] Importantly, inclusion of genotypic information from these SNPs improves prediction models for postcardiac surgery MI based on traditional risk factors alone. Using a similar definition of PMI, Collard et al. have reported that a combined haplotype in the mannose-binding lectin gene (*MBL2* LYQA secretor haplotype), an important recognition molecule in the lectin complement pathway, is independently associated with PMI in a cohort of Caucasian patients undergoing primary CABG with CPB.[25] Furthermore, genetic variants in *IL6* and *TNFA* are associated with increased incidence of postoperative cardiovascular complications (a composite outcome that included PMI) following lung resection for cancer.[92] Other genetic variants modulating the magnitude of postoperative inflammatory response have been identified. Polymorphisms in the promoter of the *IL6* gene (–572G > C and –174G > C) significantly increase the inflammatory response after heart surgery with CPB[133] and have been associated with length of hospitalization after CABG.[134] Furthermore, apolipoprotein E (APOE) genotype (the $\varepsilon 4$ allele),[135] several variants in the tumor necrosis factor (TNF) genes [tumor necrosis factor α (*TNFA*)–308G > A, lymphotoxin α (*LTA*) + 250G > A],[136] and a functional SNP in the macrophage migration inhibitory factor (MIF)[137] have been associated with pro-inflammatory effects in patients undergoing CPB and in some instances with postoperative ventricular dysfunction.[93] Conversely, a genetic variant modulating the release of the anti-inflammatory cytokine interleukin 10 (*IL10*) in response to CPB has been reported (*IL10*–1082G > A), with high levels of IL10 being associated with postoperative cardiovascular dysfunction.[94] In patients undergoing elective surgical revascularization for peripheral vascular disease, several SNPs in *IL6* and *IL10* were associated with endothelial dysfunction and increased risk of a composite endpoint of acute postoperative cardiovascular events.[91] Overall, while genetic factors may not be better predictors of outcomes than intermediate phenotypes (e.g., plasma cytokine levels), their greater ease of assessment, stability, and availability pre-procedure are significant advantages influencing potential future clinical utility.

C-reactive protein (CRP) is the prototypical acute-phase reactant and the most extensively studied inflammatory marker in clinical studies, and high-sensitivity CRP (hs-CRP) has emerged as a robust predictor of cardiovascular risk at all stages, from healthy subjects to patients with acute coronary syndromes and acute decompensated heart failure.[138] Whether CRP is merely a marker or is also a mediator of inflammatory processes is yet unclear, but several lines of evidence support the latter theory. In perioperative medicine, elevated preoperative CRP levels have been associated with increased short- and long-term morbidity and mortality in patients undergoing primary elective CABG (cutoff >3 mg/L)[139] as well as in higher-acuity CABG patients (cutoff >10 mg/L).[140] Interestingly, in a retrospective analysis of patients with elevated baseline hs-CRP levels undergoing OPCAB surgery, preoperative statin therapy was associated with reduced postoperative myocardial injury and need for dialysis.[141] In elective major noncardiac surgery patients, preoperative CRP levels (cutoff >3.4 mg/L) independently predicted perioperative major cardiovascular events (composite of MI, pulmonary edema, cardiovascular death) and significantly improved the predictive power of revised cardiac risk index (RCRI) in receiver operating characteristic analysis.[142] In addition to the already established heritability of elevated baseline plasma CRP levels, recent reports indicate that the acute-phase rise in postoperative plasma CRP levels is also genetically determined. The *CRP*1059G > C polymorphism was associated with lower peak postoperative serum CRP following both elective CABG with CPB[143] and esophagectomy for thoracic esophageal cancer.[144] Furthermore, *CRP*–717C > T polymorphism was associated with stress hyperglycemia in patients undergoing esophagectomy for cancer, leading to increased postoperative infectious complications and length of ICU stay.[145]

Thrombosis Biomarkers and Perioperative Adverse Cardiac Events

In addition to robust inflammatory activation, the host response to surgery is also characterized by an increase in fibrinogen concentration, platelet adhesiveness, and plasminogen activator inhibitor-1 (PAI-1) production. During cardiac surgery, alterations in the hemostatic system are even more complex and multifactorial, including the effects of hypothermia, hemodilution, and CPB-induced activation of coagulation, fibrinolytic, and inflammatory pathways. Perioperative thrombotic outcomes following cardiac surgery (e.g., coronary graft thrombosis, myocardial infarction, stroke, pulmonary embolism) represent one extreme on a continuum of coagulation dysfunction, with coagulopathy at the other end of the spectrum. Pathophysiologically, the balance between bleeding, normal hemostasis, and thrombosis is markedly influenced by the rate of thrombin formation and platelet activation. Recent evidence suggests genetic variability modulates the activation of each of these mechanistic pathways[146] suggesting significant heritability of the pro-thrombotic state (see Table 6-5 for an overview of genetic variants associated with postoperative bleeding). Several genotypes have been associated with increased risk of coronary graft thrombosis and myocardial injury following CABG. PAI-1 is an important negative regulator of fibrinolytic activity; a variant in the promoter of the *PAI-1* gene, consisting of an insertion (5G)/deletion (4G) polymorphism at position –675, has been consistently associated with changes in the plasma levels of PAI-1. The 4G allele is associated with increased risk of early graft thrombosis after CABG[98] and, in a recent meta-analysis, with increased incidence of MI.[147] Similarly, a polymorphism in the platelet glycoprotein IIIa gene (*ITGB3*), resulting in increased platelet aggregation (Pl^{A2} polymorphism), is associated with higher postoperative levels of troponin I following CABG[96] and increased risk for 1-year thrombotic coronary graft occlusion, myocardial infarction, and death following CABG.[86] On the other hand, in patients undergoing major vascular surgery, two SNPs in platelet glycoprotein receptors (*ITGB3* and *GP1BA*) are independent risk predictors of PMI and result in improved discrimination of an ischemia risk assessment tool when added to historic and procedural risk factors.[97] One of the most common inherited pro-thrombotic risk factors is a point mutation in coagulation factor V (1691G > A) resulting in resistance to activated protein C and referred to as factor V Leiden (FVL). FVL has been associated with various postoperative thrombotic complications following noncardiac surgery [for a review, see (34)], but interestingly, also associated with a significant reduction in postoperative blood loss and overall risk of transfusion in cardiac surgery patients.[124] In a prospective study of CABG patients with routine 3-month postoperative angiographic follow-up, a higher proportion of FVL carriers had graft occlusion compared to noncarriers.[95]

Natriuretic Peptides and Perioperative Adverse Cardiac Events

Circulating B-type natriuretic peptide (BNP) is a powerful biomarker of cardiovascular outcomes in many circumstances. Produced mainly in the ventricular myocardium, BNP is formed by cleavage of its prohormone by the enzyme corin into the biologically active C-terminal fragment (BNP) and an inactive N-terminal fragment (NT-proBNP). Known stimuli of BNP activation are myocardial mechanical stretch (from volume or pressure overload), acute ischemic injury, and a variety of other pro-inflammatory and neurohormonal stimuli inducing myocardial stress. Although secreted in 1:1 ratio, circulating levels of BNP and NT-proBNP differ considerably due to different clearance characteristics.

A large number of studies have reported consistent associations of baseline plasma BNP or NT-proBNP levels with a variety of postoperative short- and long-term morbidity and mortality endpoints, independent of the traditional risk factors. For noncardiac surgery, these have been summarized in two meta-analyses that overall indicate an approximately 20-fold increase in risk of adverse perioperative cardiovascular outcomes.[148,149] Similarly, for cardiac surgery patients, preoperative BNP was a strong independent predictor of in-hospital postoperative ventricular dysfunction, length of hospital stay, and 5-year mortality following primary CABG,[150] performing better than peak postoperative BNP.[151] The current guidelines for preoperative cardiac risk assessment in noncardiac surgery list BNP and NT-proBNP measurements as class IIa/level B indications.[152] However, despite the large number of studies conducted in both cardiac and noncardiac surgery, precise cutoff levels for BNP still need to be determined and adjusted for age, gender, and renal function. Similarly, no BNP-based goal-directed therapies have been reported in the
3 perioperative period. However, a role for BNP assays in monitoring aortic valve disease for optimal timing of surgery has been described.[153]

Furthermore, a recent study identified genetic variation in natriuretic peptide precursor genes (*NPPA/NPPB*) to be independently associated with decreased risk of postoperative ventricular dysfunction following primary CABG, whereas variants in natriuretic peptide receptor *NPR3* were associated with an increased risk (Table 6-3),[99] offering additional clues into the molecular mechanisms underlying postoperative ventricular dysfunction.

Genetic Variation in Vascular Reactivity and Perioperative Adverse Cardiac Events

Perioperative stress responses are also characterized by robust sympathetic nervous system activation, known to play a role in the pathophysiology of PMI; thus patients with CAD and specific AR genetic polymorphisms may be particularly susceptible to catecholamine toxicity and cardiac complications. Several functionally important SNPs modulating AR pathways have been characterized (for review, see Zaugg et al).[154] One such variant, the Arg389Gly polymorphism in β_1-AR gene (*ADRB1*), was recently associated with increased risk of a composite cardiovascular morbidity outcome at 1 year following noncardiac surgery under spinal anesthesia, while perioperative β-blockade had no significant effect.[83] The authors suggest that proper analysis of future perioperative β-blocker trials should be stratified by AR genotype, which may help identify patients likely to benefit from this therapy. Significantly increased vascular responsiveness to α-adrenergic stimulation (phenylephrine) was found in carriers of the endothelial *NOS3* 894G > T polymorphism,[102] and angiotensin converting enzyme (*ACE*) I/D polymorphism[35,104] undergoing cardiac surgery with CPB. Two studies have reported on the role of β_2-AR (*ADRB2*) genetic variants in perioperative vascular reactivity. Increased blood pressure responses to endotracheal intubation have been associated with a common functional *ADRB2* SNP (Glu27).[105] The second study, conducted in the obstetric population, showed that incidence and severity of maternal hypotension following spinal anesthesia for cesarean delivery, as well as the response to treatment, was affected by *ADRB2* genotype (Gly16 and/or Glu27 led to lower vasopressor use for the treatment of hypotension). In cardiac surgery patient, the development of vasoplegic syndrome is one manifestation of the perioperative systemic inflammatory response, but remains poorly predicted by clinical and procedural risk factors. Vasopressor requirement after surgery is associated with a common polymorphism in the dimethylarginine dimethylaminohydrolase II (*DDAH II*) gene, an important regulator of NOS activity.[101]

Emerging metabolomic tools have created the opportunity to establish metabolic signatures of myocardial injury. In a population of patients undergoing alcohol septal ablation for hypertrophic obstructive cardiomyopathy, a human model of planned (albeit chemical) myocardial infarction that recapitulates spontaneous myocardial infarction, targeted mass spectrometry–based metabolite profiling identified changes in circulating levels of metabolites participating in pyrimidine metabolism, the tricarboxylic acid (TCA) cycle, and the pentose phosphate pathway as early as 10 minutes after MI in an initial derivation group and were validated in a second, independent group. Coronary sinus sampling distinguished cardiac-derived peripheral metabolic changes. To assess generalizability, the planned MI-derived metabolic signature (consisting of aconitic acid, hypoxanthine, trimethylamine *N*-oxide, and threonine) differentiated with high accuracy patients with spontaneous MI.[155] We applied a similar approach to cardiac surgical patients undergoing planned global myocardial I/R and identified clear differences in metabolic fuel uptake based on the preexisting ventricular state (left ventricular dysfunction, CAD, or neither) as well as altered metabolic signatures predictive of postoperative hemodynamic course and PMI.[156] While simultaneous assessment of coronary sinus effluent in addition to the peripheral blood improves cardiac specificity of the observed signatures, direct measurement of metabolites in myocardial tissue allows marked enrichment and easier detection of potential biomarkers compared to plasma, as well as an assessment of how metabolic substrates are utilized in the tissue of interest. Such studies are possible in cardiac surgical patients where atrial tissues are routinely removed. Furthermore, rapid metabolic phenotyping approaches are emerging for both real-time intraoperative diagnostic (e.g., intelligent surgical knives for tissue/tumor diagnosis)[157] and perioperative prognostic stratification, monitoring, and optimization of surgical[158] and critically injured patients.[159]

Perioperative Atrial Fibrillation (PoAF)

New-onset PoAF remains a common complication of cardiac and major noncardiac thoracic surgical procedures (incidence 27% to 40%) and is associated with increased morbidity, hospital length of stay, rehospitalization, health-care costs, and reduced survival. Several large prospective multicenter trials have developed and validated comprehensive risk indices for occurrence of PoAF based on demographic, clinical, electrocardiographic, and procedural risk factors, but their predictive accuracy remains at best moderate,[160] suggesting an inherent genetic preoperative risk. Heritable forms of AF occur in the ambulatory nonsurgical population, and it appears that both monogenic forms like "lone" AF and polygenic predisposition to more common acquired forms like PoAF do exist.[161] A team led by researchers at deCODE genetics reported the results of a GWAS for AF; two polymorphisms on chromosome 4q25 demonstrated a highly significant association ($P = 3.3 \times 10^{-41}$) with AF,[48] with findings replicated in other populations from Sweden, the United States, and Hong Kong, and subsequently also associated with increased risk of ischemic strokes and AF recurrence after catheter ablation. Recently, this locus was also associated with new-onset PoAF after cardiac surgery with CPB (CABG with or without concurrent valve surgery).[110] The results were further validated in an independent study that also identified associations with increased risk of postoperative long-term AF and mortality, but not with long-term stroke, and, interestingly, suggested differential therapeutic responses in carriers of those SNPs (increased risk with β-blockers, reduced risk with statins).[162] The mechanism of action of the genetic locus identified by the two noncoding SNPs remains unknown, but it lies close to several genes involved in the development of the pulmonary myocardium or the sleeve of cardiomyocytes extending from the left atrium into the initial portion of the pulmonary veins. Clinical studies have demonstrated that ectopic foci of electric activity arising from within the pulmonary veins and posterior left atrium play a substantial role in initiating and maintaining AF.

Other candidate susceptibility genes for PoAF include those determining action potential duration (voltage-gated ion channels, ion transporters), responses to extracellular factors (adrenergic and other hormone receptors, heat shock proteins), remodeling processes, and magnitude of inflammatory and oxidative stress. It has been described that inflammation, reflected by elevated baseline CRP or IL6 levels and exaggerated postoperative leukocytosis, predicts the occurrence of PoAF. A link between inflammation and the development of PoAF is also supported by evidence that postoperative administration of nonsteroidal anti-inflammatory drugs may reduce the incidence of PoAF. Several recent studies have found that a functional SNP in the *IL6* promoter is associated with higher perioperative plasma IL6 levels and several adverse outcomes after CABG, including PoAF.[107,108,163] In noncardiac surgery, polymorphisms in *IL6* and *TNFA* genes have been shown to be associated with an increased risk of postoperative morbidity, including new-onset arrhythmias.[92] There is, however, a contradictory lack of association between CRP levels (strongly regulated by IL6) and PoAF in women undergoing cardiac surgery,[164] which may reflect gender-related differences. On the other hand, a recent study reported that both pre- and postoperative PAI-1 levels were independently associated with development of PoAF following cardiac surgery.[165]

Investigations of the transcriptional responses to AF in human atrial appendage myocardium collected at the time of cardiac surgery or in preclinical models (Table 6-2) have identified a ventricular-like genomic signature in fibrillating atria, with increased ratios of ventricular to atrial isoforms, suggesting dedifferentiation.[61] It remains unclear whether this "ventricularization" of atrial gene expression reflects a cause or an effect of AF, but it likely represents an adaptive energy-saving process to the high metabolic demand of fibrillating atrial myocardium, akin to chronic hibernation. Recently, a different mechanism has been proposed to be involved in PoAF. Patients who exhibit PoAF after cardiac surgery display a differential genomic response to CPB in their peripheral blood leukocytes, characterized by upregulation of oxidative stress genes, which correlates with a significantly larger increase in oxidant stress both systemically (as measured by total peroxide levels) and at the myocardial level (as measured in the right atrium).[62]

Finally, one study using high-resolution ^{1}H-NMR spectroscopy to conduct metabolomic analyses on atrial tissue samples obtained at the time of cardiac surgery identified alterations in myocardial ketone metabolism associated with persistent atrial fibrillation, and the ratio of glycolytic end products to end products of lipid metabolism correlated positively with time of onset of postoperative atrial fibrillation.[166]

Cardiac Allograft Rejection

Identification of peripheral blood gene- and protein-based biomarkers to noninvasively monitor, diagnose, and predict perioperative cardiac allograft rejection is an area of rapid scientific growth. While several polymorphisms in genes involved in alloimmune interactions, the renin–angiotensin–aldosterone system, and the transforming growth factor-β superfamily have been associated with cardiac transplant outcomes, their relevance as useful clinical monitoring tools remains uncertain. However, peripheral blood mononuclear cell–based molecular assays have shown much promise for monitoring the dynamic responses of the immune system to the transplanted heart, discriminating immunologic allograft quiescence and predicting future rejection.[167] A noninvasive molecular test to identify patients at risk for acute cellular rejection is commercially available (AlloMap, XDx), in which the expression levels of 20 genes are measured by quantitative real-time polymerase chain reaction (qRT-PCR) and translated using a mathematical algorithm into a clinically actionable AlloMap score that enhances the ability to deliver personalized monitoring and treatment to heart transplant patients. Furthermore, several clinically available protein-based biomarkers of alloimmune activation, microvascular injury (troponins), systemic inflammation (CRP), and wall stress and remodeling (BNP) correlate well with allograft failure and vasculopathy and have good negative predictive values, but require additional studies to guide their clinical use. Similarly, molecular signatures of functional recovery in end-stage heart failure following left ventricular assist device (LVAD) support using gene expression profiling have been reported[168] and could be used to monitor patients who received an LVAD as destination therapy or assess the timing of potential device explantation.

Several additional studies have identified genomic predictors of allograft dysfunction. Heart transplant patients carrying a polymorphism in the gene for adenosine monophosphate deaminase-1, which catalyzes deamination of adenosine monophosphate, require less inotropic support in the perioperative period but have higher all-cause and cardiac mortality at 1-year follow-up.[80] Levels of hypoxia-inducible factor-1α (a transcription factor for early growth response-1, vascular endothelial growth factor, and urokinase-type plasminogen activator pathways) in the donor heart predict primary graft dysfunction in the intraoperative and immediate postoperative period, which is in turn directly related to poor long-term outcomes of heart transplant.[169]

Predictive Biomarkers for Postoperative Event-Free Survival

Several large randomized clinical trials examining the benefits of CABG surgery and percutaneous coronary interventions relative to medical therapy and/or to one another have refined our knowledge of early and long-term survival after CABG. While these studies have helped define the subgroups of patients who benefit from surgical revascularization, they also demonstrated a substantial variability in long-term survival after CABG, altered by important demographic and environmental risk factors. Increasing evidence suggests that the *ACE* gene indel polymorphism may influence post-CABG complications, with carriers of the *D* allele having higher mortality and restenosis rates after CABG surgery compared with the *I* allele.[85] As discussed above, a prothrombotic amino acid alteration in the β_3-integrin chain of the glycoprotein IIb/IIIa platelet receptor (the Pl^{A2} polymorphism) is associated with an increased risk (OR 4.7) for major adverse cardiac events (MACE—a composite of myocardial infarction, coronary bypass graft occlusion, or death) following CABG surgery.[86] Subanalyses of two major trials, the Verona Heart Project study of CABG patients and the CABG arm of the MASS II trial of CAD patients, have linked the methylene-tetrahydrofolate reductase (*MTHFR*) C677T polymorphism with adverse perioperative outcomes. The polymorphism is linked to plasma homocysteinemia, which is in turn associated with a clear risk of MACE as well as all-cause mortality after CABG; however, univariate analyses linking the polymorphism directly to adverse outcomes did not consistently achieve statistical significance.[87,170] We found preliminary evidence for association of two functional polymorphisms modulating β_2-AR activity (Arg16Gly and Gln27Glu) with incidence of death or MACE following cardiac surgery[84] and recently identified in replicated analyses a functional polymorphism in thrombomodulin (*THBD* Ala455Val) to be independently associated with a 2.4-fold increased risk of 5-year mortality after CABG and to improve the predictive accuracy of the EuroSCORE[82] (Table 6-3).

To date, no true GWAS have been conducted specifically linking polymorphisms to periprocedural outcomes following cardiovascular interventions. However, several outcome studies have explored the chromosome 9p21 locus, previously associated in replicated GWAS to a multitude of cardiovascular diseases (including CAD, MI, and cerebral aneurysms among others) in ambulatory populations. In a prospective study of patients undergoing cardiac surgery, three different polymorphisms in the 9p21 region were associated with postoperative MI.[100] Muehlschlegel et al. further related the 9p21 variant with the strongest association to perioperative myocardial injury to all-cause mortality after primary CABG and found that it improved the prediction accuracy of the EuroSCORE model.[81]

A number of studies have begun to jointly examine polymorphisms in target sets of candidate genes. This can be accomplished either by calculating simple genetic risk scores (e.g., risk allele counts) or using regression analyses (e.g., weighted risk scores) or more complex analytic approaches such as support vector machines. With the rationale that single genetic variants individually explain little variability in multifactorial disease phenotypes, Eifert et al. profiled several genes known to be involved in the progression of CAD in patients undergoing CABG and incorporated genotypes into a risk profile to predict long-term MACE. The model, which included endothelial NOS, APOE, hepatic lipase, cholesterol ester transfer protein, PAI-1, and prothrombin genotypes, predicted long-term outcome better than traditional CAD risk prediction models.[171] Similarly, profiling a group of genes involved in atherosclerosis and inflammation identified seven polymorphisms associated with saphenous vein graft (SVG) patency at long-term follow-up after CABG.[33]

Predictive Biomarkers of Adverse Perioperative Neurologic Outcomes

Despite advances in surgical and anesthetic techniques, significant neurologic morbidity continues to occur following cardiac surgery, ranging in severity from coma and focal stroke (incidence 1% to 3%) to more subtle cognitive deficits (incidence up to 69%), with a substantial impact on the risk of perioperative death, quality of life, and resource utilization. Variability in the reported incidence of both early and late neurologic deficits remains poorly explained by procedural risk factors, suggesting that environmental (operative) and genetic factors may interact to determine disease onset, progression, and recovery. The pathophysiology of perioperative neurologic injury is thought to involve complex interactions between primary pathways associated with atherosclerosis and thrombosis and secondary response pathways like inflammation, vascular reactivity, and direct cellular injury. Many functional genetic variants have been reported in each of these mechanistic pathways involved in modulating the magnitude and the response to neurologic injury, which may have implications in chronic as well as acute perioperative neurocognitive outcomes. For example, Grocott et al. examined 26 SNPs in relationship to the incidence of acute postoperative ischemic stroke in 1,635 patients undergoing cardiac surgery and found that the interaction of minor alleles of the CRP (1846C > T) and IL6 promoter SNP −174G > C significantly increases the risk of acute stroke.[117] Similarly, a recent study suggests that P-selectin and CRP genes both contribute to modulating the susceptibility to postoperative cognitive decline (POCD) following cardiac surgery.[28] Specifically, the loss-of-function minor alleles of *CRP* 1059G > C and *SELP* 1087G > A are independently associated with a *reduction* in the observed incidence of POCD after adjustment for known clinical and demographic covariates (Table 6-4).

Our group has demonstrated a significant association between the *APOE* E4 genotype and adverse cerebral outcomes in cardiac surgery patients.[26,172] This is consistent with the role of the *APOE* genotype in recovery from acute brain injury, such as intracranial hemorrhage,[173] closed head injury,[174] and stroke,[175] as well as experimental models of cerebral ischemia–reperfusion injury[176]; two subsequent studies in CABG patients, however, have not replicated these initial findings. Furthermore, the incidence of postoperative delirium following major noncardiac surgery in the elderly[122] and critically ill patients[123] is increased in carriers of the *APOE* $\varepsilon 4$ allele. Unlike adult cardiac surgery patients, infants possessing the *APOE* $\varepsilon 2$ allele are at increased risk for developing adverse neuro-developmental sequelae following cardiac surgery.[120,121] The mechanisms by which the *APOE* genotypes might influence neurologic outcomes have yet to be determined. They do not seem to be related to alterations in global cerebral blood flow of oxygen metabolism during CPB[177]; however, genotypic effects in modulating the inflammatory response,[135] extent of aortic atheroma burden,[178] and risk for premature coronary atherosclerosis[179] may play a role.

Recent studies have suggested a role for platelet activation in the pathophysiology of adverse neurologic sequelae. Genetic variants in surface platelet membrane glycoproteins, important mediators of platelet adhesion and platelet–platelet interactions, have been shown to increase the susceptibility to pro-thrombotic events. Among these, the Pl^{A2} polymorphism in glycoprotein IIb/IIIa has been related to various adverse thrombotic outcomes, including acute coronary thrombosis[180] and atherothrombotic stroke.[181] We found the Pl^{A2} allele to be associated with more severe neurocognitive decline after CPB,[27] which could represent exacerbation of platelet-dependent thrombotic processes associated with plaque embolism.

Cardiac surgical patients who develop POCD demonstrate inherently different genetic responses to CPB from those without POCD, as evidenced by acute deregulation of gene expression pathways involving inflammation, antigen presentation, and cellular adhesion in peripheral blood leukocytes.[63] These findings corroborate with proteomic changes, in which patients with POCD similarly have significantly higher serologic inflammatory indices compared with those patients without POCD.[182,183] This adds to the increasing level of evidence that CPB does not cause an indiscriminate variation in gene expression but rather distinct patterns in specific pathways that are highly associated with the development of postoperative complications such as POCD. The implications for perioperative medicine include identifying populations at risk who might benefit not only from an improved informed consent, stratification, and resource allocation, but also from targeted anti-inflammatory strategies.

In noncardiac surgery, a study conducted in patients undergoing carotid endarterectomy has demonstrated that preoperative plasma levels of fibrinogen and hs-CRP were independently associated with new periprocedural cerebral ischemic lesions caused by microembolic events, as determined by MRI diffusion-weighted imaging.[184] However, we found no associations between APOE4 genotype, plasma levels of known biomarkers of brain injury, and POCD in patients undergoing major elective noncardiac surgery.[185]

Predictive Biomarkers of Perioperative Acute Kidney Injury

Acute kidney injury (AKI) is a common, serious complication of cardiac surgery; about 8% to 15% of patients develop moderate renal injury (>1.0 mg/dL peak creatinine rise), and up to 5% of them develop renal failure requiring dialysis.[186] Acute renal failure is independently associated with in-hospital mortality rates, exceeding 60% in patients requiring dialysis.[186] Several studies have demonstrated that inheritance of genetic polymorphisms in the APOE gene (ε4 allele, protective)[31,187] and in the promoter region of the *IL6* gene (–174C allele, deleterious)[163] is associated with AKI following CABG surgery (Table 6-5). We have reported that major differences in peak postoperative serum creatinine rise after CABG are predicted by possession of combinations of polymorphisms that interestingly differ by race: The angiotensinogen (*AGT*) 842T > C and *IL6*–572G > C variants in Caucasians and the endothelial *NOS3* 894G > T and *ACE* I/D in African Americans are associated with more than 50% reduction in postoperative glomerular filtration rate.[29] Another study of patients undergoing CABG reported the ACE I/D polymorphism, but not an angiotensin-II receptor polymorphism, to be associated with higher levels of AKI during the index hospitalization.[187] Recently, preoperative BNP levels have been shown to be associated with AKI following cardiac surgery (RR 1.87 and 3.17 for mild and severe AKI, respectively) and modestly improved risk prediction compared to clinical parameters alone.[188] Further identification of biomarkers predictive of adverse perioperative renal outcomes may facilitate individually tailored therapy, risk stratify the patients for interventional trials targeting the gene product itself, and aid in medical decision-making (e.g., selecting medical over surgical management).

Genetic Variants and Risk for Prolonged Postoperative Mechanical Ventilation

Prolonged mechanical ventilation (inability to extubate patient by 24 hours postoperatively) is a significant complication following cardiac surgery, occurring in 5.6% and 10.5% of patients undergoing first and repeat CABG surgery, respectively.[189] Several pulmonary and nonpulmonary causes have been identified, and scoring systems based on preoperative and procedural risk factors have been proposed and validated. Recently, genetic variants in the renin–angiotensin pathway and in pro-inflammatory cytokine genes have been associated with respiratory complications post-CPB. The *D* allele of a common functional I/D polymorphism in the *ACE* gene, accounting for 47% of variance in circulating ACE levels,[190] is associated with prolonged mechanical ventilation following CABG[191] and with susceptibility to and prognosis of adult respiratory distress syndrome (ARDS).[192] Furthermore, a hyposecretor haplotype in the neighboring genes *TNFA* and *LTA* on chromosome 6 (*TNFA*–308*G*/*LTA* + 250*G* haplotype)[193] and a functional polymorphism modulating postoperative IL6 levels (*IL6*–174G > C)[163] are independently associated with higher risk of prolonged mechanical ventilation post-CABG. The association is more dramatic in patients undergoing conventional CABG than in those undergoing OPCAB, suggesting that in high-risk patients identified by preoperative genetic screening OPCAB may be the optimal surgical procedure.

A next crucial step in understanding the complexity of adverse perioperative outcomes is to assess the contribution of variations in many genes simultaneously and their interaction with traditional risk factors to the longitudinal prediction of outcomes in individual patients. The use of such outcome predictive models incorporating genetic information may help stratify mortality and morbidity in surgical patients, improve prognostication, direct medical decision-making both intraoperatively and during postoperative follow-up, and even suggest novel targets for therapeutic intervention in the perioperative period.

PHARMACOGENOMICS AND ANESTHESIA

Interindividual variability in response to drug therapy, in terms of both efficacy and safety, is a rule by which anesthesiologists live. In fact, much of the art of anesthesiology is the astute clinician being prepared to deal with outliers. The term *pharmacogenomics* is used to describe how inherited variations in genes

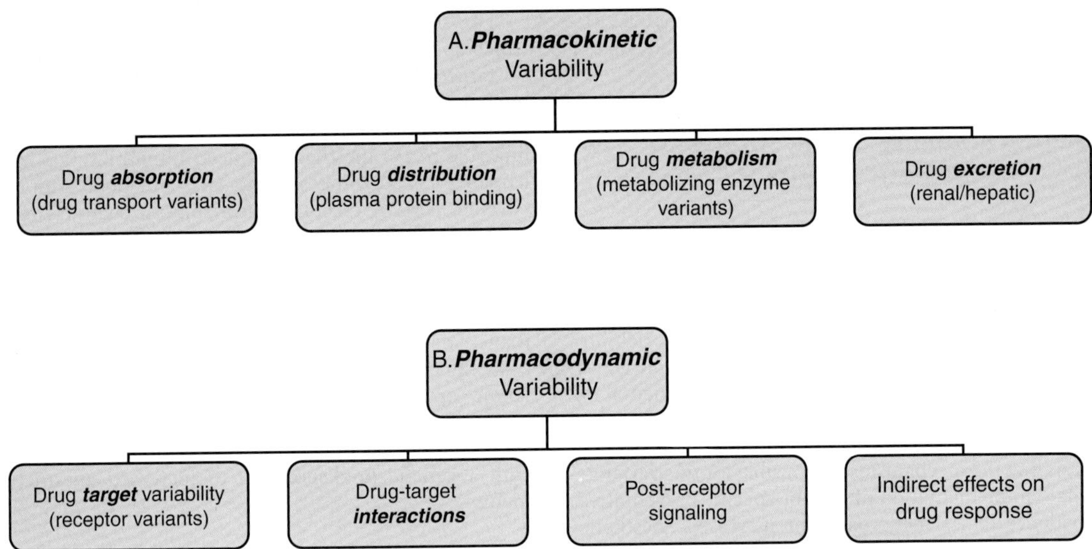

FIGURE 6-4. Pharmacogenomic determinants of individual drug response operated by pharmacokinetic and pharmacodynamic mechanisms. **A:** Genetic variants in *drug transporters* (e.g., ATP-binding cassette subfamily B member 1 or *ABCB1* gene) and *drug-metabolizing enzymes* (e.g., cytochrome P450 2D6 or *CYP2D6* gene, *CYP2C9* gene, *N*-acetyltransferase or *NAT2* gene, plasma cholinesterase or *BCHE* gene) are responsible for *pharmacokinetic* variability in drug response. **B:** Polymorphisms in *drug targets* (e.g., β_1 and β_2-adrenergic receptor *ADRB1, ADRB2* genes; angiotensin-I converting enzyme *ACE* gene), *post-receptor signaling molecules* (e.g., guanine nucleotide-binding protein $\beta 3$ or *GNB3* gene), or *molecules indirectly affecting drug response* (e.g., various ion channel genes involved in drug-induced arrhythmias) are sources of *pharmacodynamic* variability.

modulating drug actions are related to interindividual variability in drug response. Such variability in drug action may be *pharmacokinetic* or *pharmacodynamic* (Fig. 6-4). Pharmacokinetic variability refers to variability in a drug's absorption, distribution, metabolism, and excretion that mediates its efficacy and/or toxicity. The molecules involved in these processes include drug-metabolizing enzymes (such as members of the cytochrome P450, or CYP, superfamily) and drug transport molecules that mediate drug uptake into, and efflux from, intracellular sites. Pharmacodynamic variability refers to variable drug effects despite equivalent drug delivery to molecular sites of action. This may reflect variability in the function of the molecular target of the drug or in the pathophysiologic context in which the drug interacts with its receptor target (e.g., affinity, coupling, expression).[194] Thus, pharmacogenomics investigates complex, polygenically determined phenotypes of drug efficacy or toxicity, with the goal of identifying novel therapeutic targets and customizing drug therapy.

Pseudocholinesterase Deficiency

Historically, characterization of the genetic basis for plasma pseudocholinesterase deficiency in 1956 was of fundamental importance to anesthesia and the further development and understanding of genetically determined differences in drug response.[195] Individuals with an atypical form of pseudocholinesterase resulting in a markedly reduced rate of drug metabolism are at risk for excessive neuromuscular blockade and prolonged apnea. More than 20 variants have since been identified in the butyrylcholinesterase gene (*BCHE*), the most common of which are the A-variant (209A > G) and the K-variant (1615G > A), with various and somewhat poorly defined phenotypic consequences on prolonged neuromuscular blockade. Therefore, pharmacogenetic testing is currently not recommended in the population at large, but only as an explanation for an adverse event.[196]

Genetics of Malignant Hyperthermia

Malignant hyperthermia (MH) is a rare autosomal dominant genetic disease of skeletal muscle calcium metabolism, triggered by administration of general anesthesia with volatile anesthetic agents or succinylcholine in susceptible individuals. The clinical MH syndrome is characterized by skeletal muscle hypermetabolism and manifested as skeletal muscle rigidity, tachycardia, tachypnea, hemodynamic instability, increased oxygen consumption and CO_2 production, lactic acidosis, and fever, progressing to malignant ventricular arrhythmias, disseminated intravascular coagulation, and myoglobinuric renal failure. MH susceptibility has been initially linked to the ryonadine receptor (*RYRI*) gene locus on chromosome 19q.[197] However, subsequent studies have shown that MH may represent a common severe phenotype that originates not only from point mutations in the *RYRI* gene (Arg614Cys), but also within its functionally and/or structurally associated proteins regulating excitation–contraction coupling (such as *α1DHPR* and *FKBP12*). It is becoming increasingly apparent that MH susceptibility results from a complex interaction between multiple genes and environment (such as environmental toxins), suggested by the heterogeneity observed in the clinical MH syndrome and the variable penetrance of the MH phenotype.[198] Current diagnostic methods (the caffeine–halothane contracture test) are invasive and potentially nonspecific. Unfortunately, because of the polygenic determinism and variable penetrance, direct DNA testing in the general population for susceptibility to MH is currently not recommended; in contrast, testing in individuals from families with affected individuals had the potential to greatly reduce mortality and morbidity.[196] Furthermore, genomic approaches may help elucidate the molecular mechanisms involved in altered RYRI-mediated calcium signaling and identify novel, more specific therapeutic targets.

Genetic Variability and Response to Anesthetic Agents

Anesthetic potency, defined by the minimum alveolar concentration (MAC) of an inhaled anesthetic that abolishes purposeful movement in response to a noxious stimulus, varies among individuals, with a coefficient of variation (the ratio of standard deviation to mean) of approximately 10%.[199] This observed variability may be explained by interindividual differences in multiple genes that underlie responsiveness to anesthetics, by environmental or physiologic factors (brain temperature, age), or by measurement errors. With growing public concern over intraoperative awareness, understanding the mechanisms responsible for this variability may facilitate implementation of patient-specific preventative strategies. Evidence of a genetic basis for increased anesthetic requirements is beginning to emerge, suggested for instance by the observation that desflurane requirements are increased in subjects with red hair versus dark hair[200] and by recently reported variability in the immobilizing dose of sevoflurane (as much as 24%) in populations with different ethnic (and thus genetic) backgrounds.[201] Several studies evaluating the genetic control of anesthetic responses, coupled with molecular modeling, proteomic, neurophysiology, and pharmacologic approaches, have provided important developments in our understanding of general anesthetic mechanisms. Triggered by the seminal work of Franks and Lieb,[202] research shifted from the membrane lipid bilayer to protein receptors (specifically ligand- and voltage-gated ion channels) as potential anesthetic targets, ending a few decades of stagnation that was primarily due to an almost universal acceptance of the dogma of nonspecific anesthetic action (the so-called "lipid theory"). Some of the genes responsible for phenotypic differences in anesthetic effects have been mapped in various animal models and, following genomic manipulation of plausible candidate receptors to investigate their function in vitro, were evaluated in genetically engineered animals for their relationship to various anesthetic endpoints, such as immobility (i.e., MAC), hypnosis, amnesia, and analgesia (for reviews, see Sonner et al).[203] Several thousand different strains of knockout mice have been created and are used to investigate specific functions of particular genes and mechanisms of drug action, including the sensitivity to general anesthetic in animals lacking the β_3 subunit[204] or the α_6 subunit[205] of the $GABA_A$ receptor. On the other hand, *knockin* animals express a site-directed mutation in the targeted gene which remains under the control of endogenous regulatory elements, allowing the mutated gene to be expressed in the same amount, at the same time, and in the same tissues as the normal gene. This method has provided remarkable insight into the mechanisms of action of benzodiazepines[206] and IV anesthetics. In a seminal study by Jurd et al., a point mutation in the gene encoding the β_3 subunit of the $GABA_A$ receptor, previously known to render the receptor insensitive to etomidate and propofol in vitro,[207] was validated in vivo by creating a knockin mouse strain that also proved essentially insensitive to the immobilizing actions of etomidate and propofol.[208] A point mutation in the β_2 subunit of the $GABA_A$ receptor results in a knockin mouse with reduced sensitivity to the sedative[209] and hypothermic effects[210] of etomidate. Knockin mice harboring point mutations in the α_{2A}-AR have enabled the elucidation of the role of this receptor in anesthetic-sparing, analgesic, and sedative responses to dexmedetomidine.[211]

The situation is far more complex for inhaled anesthetics, which appear to mediate their effects by acting on several receptor targets. On the basis of combined pharmacologic and genetic in vivo studies to date, several receptors are unlikely to be direct mediators of MAC, including the $GABA_A$ (despite their compelling role in IV anesthetic-induced immobility), 5-HT_3, AMPA, kainate, acetylcholine and α_2-ARs, and potassium channels.[212] Glycine, NMDA receptors, and sodium channels remain likely candidates.[203] These conclusions, however, do not apply to other anesthetic endpoints, such as hypnosis, amnesia, and analgesia. Several preclinical proteomic analyses have identified in a more unbiased way a group of potential anesthetic targets for halothane,[72] desflurane,[73] and sevoflurane,[74] which should provide the
4 basis for more focused studies of anesthetic binding sites. Such "omic" approaches have the potential to evolve into preoperative screening profiles useful in guiding individualized therapeutic decisions, such as prevention of anesthetic awareness in patients with a genetic predisposition to increased anesthetic requirements.

Genetic Variability and Response to Pain

Similar to the observed variability in anesthetic potency, the response to painful stimuli and analgesic manipulations varies among individuals. The sources of variability in the report and experience of pain and analgesia (i.e., the "pain threshold") are multifactorial, including factors extrinsic to the organism (such as cultural factors, or circadian rhythms) and intrinsic factors (such as age, gender, hormonal status, or genetic makeup). Increasing evidence suggests that pain behavior in response to noxious stimuli and its modulation by the central nervous system in response to drug administration or environmental stress, as well as the development of persistent pain conditions through pain amplification, are strongly influenced by genetic factors.[213–215]

Results from studies in twins[216] and inbred mouse strains[217] indicate a moderate heritability for chronic pain syndromes and nociceptive sensitivity, which appears to be mediated by multiple genes. Various strains of knockout mice lacking target genes like neurotrophins and their receptors (e.g., nerve growth factor), peripheral mediators of nociception and hyperalgesia (e.g., substance P), opioid and non-opioid transmitters and their receptors, and intracellular signaling molecules have significantly contributed to the understanding of pain processing mechanisms.[218] A locus responsible for 28% of phenotypic variance in magnitude of systemic morphine analgesia in mouse has been mapped to chromosome 10, in or near the *OPRM* (μ-opioid receptor) gene. The μ-opioid receptor is also subject to pharmacodynamic variability; polymorphisms in the promoter region of the *OPRM* gene modulating interleukin 4–mediated gene expression have been correlated with morphine antinociception. The much quoted *OPRM*188A > G polymorphism is associated with decreased responses to morphine-6-glucuronide, resulting not only in altered analgesic requirements, but also in reduced incidence of postoperative nausea and vomiting and reduced risks of toxicity in renal failure patients. Conversely, variants of the melanocortin 1 receptor (*MC1R*) gene, which produce a red hair–fair skin phenotype, are associated with increased analgesic responses to κ-opioid agonists in women but not men, providing evidence for a gene-by-gender interaction in regulating analgesic response (for a review, see Somogyi et al.)[219] Very recent reports suggest that peripherally located β_2-ARs (*ADRB2*) also contribute to basal pain sensitivity, development of chronic pain states, as well as opioid-induced hyperalgesia.[215] Functionally important haplotypes in the

ADRB2[214] and catechol-*O*-methyltransferase (*COMT*)[220] genes are associated with enhanced pain sensitivity in humans.

In addition to the genetic control of peripheral nociceptive pathways, considerable evidence exists for genetic variability in the descending central pain modulatory pathways, further explaining the interindividual variability in analgesic responsiveness. One good example relevant to analgesic efficacy is cytochrome P450D6 (*CYP2D6*), a member of the superfamily of microsomal enzymes that catalyze phase I drug metabolism and responsible for the metabolism of a large number of therapeutic compounds. The relationship between the *CYP2D6* genotype and the enzyme metabolic rate has been extensively characterized, with at least 12 known mutations leading to a tetramodal distribution CYP2D6 activity: Ultrarapid metabolizers (5% to 7% of the population), extensive metabolizers (60%), intermediate metabolizers (25%), and poor metabolizers (10%). Currently, pharmacogenomic screening tests predict CYP2D6 phenotype with >95% reliabil-
5 ity. The consequences of inheriting an allele that compromises CYP2D6 function include the inability to metabolize codeine (a prodrug) to morphine by O-demethylation, leading to lack of analgesia but increased side effects from the parent drug (e.g., fatigue) in poor metabolizers.[196,213]

Genetic Variability in Response to Other Drugs Used Perioperatively

A wide variety of drugs used in the perioperative period display significant pharmacokinetic or pharmacodynamic variability that is genetically modulated (Table 6-6). Although such genetic variation in drug-metabolizing enzymes or drug targets usually result in unusually variable drug response, genetic markers associated with rare but life-threatening side effects have also been described. Of note, the most commonly cited categories of drugs involved in adverse drug reactions include cardiovascular, antibiotic, psychiatric, and analgesic medications, and interestingly, each category has a known genetic basis for increased risk of adverse reactions.

There are more than 30 families of drug-metabolizing enzymes in humans, most with genetic polymorphisms shown to influence enzymatic activity. Of special importance to the anesthesiologists is the *CYP2D6*, one of the most intensively studied and best understood examples of pharmacogenetic variation, involved in the metabolism of several drugs including analgesics (codeine, dextromethorphan), β-blockers, antiarrhythmics (flecainide, propafenone, quinidine), and diltiazem. Another important pharmacogenetic variation has been described in cytochrome P450C9 (*CYP2C9*), involved in metabolizing anticoagulants (warfarin), anticonvulsants (phenytoin), antidiabetic agents (glipizide, tolbutamide), and nonsteroidal anti-inflammatory drugs (celecoxib, ibuprofen), among others. Three known *CYP2C9* variant alleles result in different enzyme activities (extensive, intermediate, and slow metabolizer phenotypes) and have clinical implications in the increased risk of life-threatening bleeding complications in slow metabolizers during standard warfarin therapy. This illustrates the concept of "high-risk pharmacokinetics," which applies to drugs with low therapeutic ratios eliminated by a single pathway (in this case CYP2C9-mediated oxidation); genetic variation in that pathway may lead to large changes in drug clearance, concentrations, and effects.[194] Dose adjustments based on the pharmacogenetic phenotype have been proposed for drugs metabolized via both CYP2D6 and CYP2C9 pathways,[196] and a commercially available, FDA-approved test (CYP450 AmpliChip®, Roche Molecular Diagnostics) allows clinicians for the first time to test patients for a wide spectrum of genetic variation in drug-metabolizing enzymes. Using this technology, Candiotti et al. showed that patients carrying either three copies of the CYP2D6

TABLE 6-6. EXAMPLES OF GENETIC POLYMORPHISMS INVOLVED IN VARIABLE RESPONSES TO DRUGS USED IN THE PERIOPERATIVE PERIOD

Drug Class	Gene Name (Gene Symbol)	Effect of Polymorphism
Pharmacokinetic variability		
β-Blockers	Cytochrome P450 2D6 (*CYP2D6*)	Enhanced drug effect
Codeine, dextromethorphan	*CYP2D6*	Decreased drug effect
Ca-channel blockers	Cytochrome P450 3A4 (*CYP3A4*)	Uncertain
Alfentanil	*CYP3A4*	Enhanced drug response
Angiotensin-II receptor type 1 blockers	Cytochrome P450 2C9 (*CYP2C9*)	Enhanced blood pressure response
Warfarin	*CYP2C9*	Enhanced anticoagulant effect, risk of bleeding
Clopidogrel	*CYP2C19 (*2allele)*	Diminished response, risk of MACE
Phenytoin	*CYP2C9*	Enhanced drug effect
ACE inhibitors	Angiotensin-I converting enzyme (*ACE*)	Blood pressure response
Procainamide	*N*-acetyltransferase 2 (*NAT2*)	Enhanced drug effect
Succinylcholine	Butyrylcholinesterase (*BCHE*)	Enhanced drug effect
Digoxin	P-glycoprotein (*ABCB1, MDR1*)	Increased bioavailability
Pharmacodynamic variability		
β-Blockers	β_1- and β_2-adrenergic receptors (*ADRB1, ADRB2*)	Blood pressure and heart rate response, airway responsiveness to β_2-agonists
QT-prolonging drugs (antiarrhythmics, cisapride, erythromycin, etc.)	Sodium and potassium ion channels (*SCN5A, KCNH2, KCNE2, KCNQ1*)	Long QT syndrome, risk of torsade de pointes
Aspirin, glycoprotein IIb/IIIa inhibitors	Glycoprotein IIIa subunit of platelet glycoprotein IIb/IIIa (*ITGB3*)	Variability in antiplatelet effects
Phenylephrine	Endothelial nitric oxide synthase (*NOS3*)	Blood pressure response

gene, a genotype consistent with ultrarapid metabolism, or both have an increased risk of ondansetron failure for the prevention of postoperative vomiting but not nausea.[221] The strongest evidence to date for use of pharmacogenomic testing is to aid in the determination of warfarin dosage by using genotypes in the *CYP2C9* and vitamin K epoxide reductase complex 1 (*VKORC1*) genes, and at least four FDA-approved tests are now commercially available. Moreover, the genetic components of clopidogrel pharmacokinetics have been recently identified, with carriers of the *CYP2C19*2* allele being at increased risk of adverse long-term outcomes after PCI. The clinical utility of these pharmacogenomic markers is immediate. Other antiplatelet therapy options such as prasugrel and ticlopidine, believed not to be significantly affected by the above polymorphism, are available for patients who are poor metabolizers of clopidogrel. Importantly, a predictive model combining patients' clinical features and genetic testing is better than either genetic or clinical factors alone at gauging which patients treated with clopidogrel after PCI are at risk of experiencing stent thrombosis, with patients in the highest risk group using the combined model having seven times the risk of developing thrombosis than patients in the lowest risk group.[222] Although no randomized clinical trial has yet been conducted to assess whether genotyping CYP2C19 before prescribing clopidogrel can be implemented effectively in practice, efforts to further study the long-term outcomes of patients with different CYP2C19 genotypes and different antiplatelet regimens represent one of the most important potential successes of genomic and personalized medicine so far.[223]

Genetic variation in drug targets (receptors) can have profound effect on drug efficacy, and over 25 examples have already been identified. For example, functional polymorphisms in the β_2-AR (Arg16Gly, Gln27Glu) influence the bronchodilator and vascular responses to β-agonists, and β_1-AR variants (Arg389Gly) modulate responses to β-blockers and may impact postoperative
6 cardiovascular adverse events.[83,154] An excellent recent review by Nagele and Liggett[224] provides a strong rationale for using pharmacogenomic variation in β-blocker metabolism (*CYP2D6*) and receptor signaling pathway (both *ADRB1 ADRB2* and downstream genes) to determine the effectiveness and safety of perioperative β-blockade for prevention of PMI, particularly given the conflicting results raised by the POISE trial.[225]

Finally, clinically important genetic polymorphisms with indirect effects on drug response have been described. These include variants in candidate genes like sodium (*SCN5A*) and potassium ion channels (*KCNH2, KCNE2, KCNQ1*), which alter susceptibility to drug-induced long-QT syndrome and ventricular arrhythmias (torsade de pointes) associated with the use of drugs like erythromycin, terfenadine, disopyramide, sotalol, cisapride, or quinidine. Carriers of such susceptibility alleles have no manifest QT-interval prolongation or family history of sudden death until QT-prolonging drug challenge is superimposed.[194] Predisposition to QT-interval prolongation (considered a surrogate for risk of life-threatening ventricular arrhythmias) has been responsible for more drug withdrawals from the market than any other category of adverse event in recent times, so understanding genetic predisposing factors constitutes one of the highest priorities of current pharmacogenomic efforts.

Pharmacogenomics is emerging as an additional modifying component to anesthesia along with age, gender, comorbidities, and medication usage. Specific testing and treatment guidelines allowing clinicians to appropriately modify drug utilization (e.g., adjust dose or change drug) already exist for a few compounds[196] and will likely be expanded to all relevant therapeutic compounds, together with identification of novel therapeutic targets.

GENOMICS AND CRITICAL CARE

Genetic Variability in Response to Injury

Systemic injury (including trauma and surgical stress), shock, or infection triggers physiologic responses of fever, tachycardia, tachypnea, and leukocytosis that collectively define the systemic inflammatory response syndrome. This can progress to severe sepsis, septic shock, and MODS, the pathophysiology of which remains poorly understood. With the genomic revolution, a new paradigm has emerged in critical care medicine: Outcomes of critical illness are determined by the interplay between the *injury* and *repair* processes triggered by the initial insults.[226] Negative outcomes are thus the combined result of direct tissue injury, the side effects of resulting repair processes, and secondary injury mechanisms leading to suboptimal repair. This concept forms the basis of the new PIRO (*P*redisposition, *I*nfection/Insult, *R*esponse, *O*rgan dysfunction) staging system in critical illness.[227] Genomic factors play a role along this continuum, from inflammatory gene variants and modulators of pathogen–host interaction, to microbial genomics and rapid detection assays to identify pathogens, to biomarkers differentiating infection from inflammation, to dynamic measures of cellular responses to insult, apoptosis, cytopathic hypoxia, and cell stress. Regulation of these mechanisms is currently being extensively investigated at the genomic, proteomic, and pharmacogenomic level, aiming to model adaptive and maladaptive responses to injury, aid in development of diagnostic indices predictive of injury, monitor progress of repair, and eventually design novel therapeutic modalities that take into account the individual genetic makeup.

The large interindividual variability in the magnitude of response to injury, including activation of inflammatory and coagulation cascades, apoptosis, and fibrosis, suggests the involvement of genetic regulatory factors. Several functional genetic polymorphisms in molecules involved in various components of the inflammatory response have been associated with differences in susceptibility to and mortality from sepsis of different etiologies, including postoperative sepsis. These include polymorphisms in bacterial recognition molecules such as lipopolysaccharide-binding protein (*LBP*), bactericidal/permeability increasing protein (*BPI*), *CD14*, toll-like receptors (*TLR2, TLR4*), mannose-binding lectin (*MBL*); and pro-inflammatory cytokines such as *TNFA, LTA*, interleukin 1 (*IL1*) and IL1 receptor antagonist (*IL1RN*), *IL6* [for reviews, see (228,229)]. Similarly, functional genetic variants in the *PAI-1* and angiotensin-I converting enzyme (*ACE*) genes have been associated with poor outcomes in sepsis, reflecting the complex interaction between inflammation, coagulation, endothelial function, and vascular tone in the pathogenesis of sepsis-induced organ dysfunction.

This continuing effort to identify initial SNP–disease associations is followed by a process of selecting reliable predictive SNPs by validation in independent populations and determining which and how many markers will maximize the power to predict risk for sepsis or mortality following injury.

Functional Genomics of Injury

At a cellular level, injurious stimuli trigger adaptive stress responses determined by quantitative and qualitative changes in interdigitating cascades of biologic pathways interacting in complex, often redundant ways. As a result, numerous clinical trials attempting to block single inflammatory mediators, such as TNFα in sepsis, have been largely unsuccessful.[230] Given these complex interconnections, the standard "single gene" paradigm is insufficient to adequately describe the tissue response to severe systemic stimuli. Instead, organ injury might better be defined by patterns of altered gene and protein expression.[231] As previously discussed, DNA microarray technology has become a powerful high-throughput method of analyzing changes induced by various injuries on a genome-wide scale, by quantifying mRNA abundance and generating an expression profile for the cell or tissue of interest. Several studies have reported the gene expression profiles both in critically ill patients and in animal models of sepsis,[232,233] acute lung injury,[234] and burn injury.[235] Using gene expression profiling in peripheral blood neutrophils, Tang et al. have identified a set of 50 signature genes that correctly identified sepsis with a prediction accuracy of 91%. Importantly, this genomic classifier was a stronger predictor of sepsis than physiologic indices and cytokines, such as procalcitonin.[236] Once gene lists are identified, extracting biologic information has proven to be one of the most perplexing challenges. In human subjects administered endotoxin, the number of genes whose expression changed in blood leukocytes was greater than 4,000,[237] and in severely traumatized patients, the expression of over 6,000 genes changed in peripheral blood leukocytes.[238] It thus became evident that tools had to be developed that could categorize these genes and responses into "functional modules," "interactome maps," and signaling pathways.[237] Two large-scale national programs are using gene and protein expression profiles in circulating leukocytes to investigate the biologic reasons behind the extreme variability in patient outcomes after similar traumatic insults (the NIH-funded Trauma Glue Grant; www.gluegrant.org) and to elucidate regulatory mechanisms in response to septic challenge in high-risk patients (the German National Genome Research Network; http://www.ngfn.de/en/start.html).[231] Analytical and organizational approaches to a systematic evaluation of the variance associated with genome-wide expression analysis in human blood leukocytes in the "real world" have been reported by these groups and are very informative in the study of critical illness.[239]

Since only less than half of the changes at mRNA level are usually translated into changes in protein expression, transcriptional profiling has to be complemented by characterizing the injury proteome, for a more complete understanding of the host response to injury. Integrated analysis of neutrophils transcriptome and proteome in response to lipopolysaccharide stimulation has identified upregulation of a variety of genes including transcriptional regulators (NF-κB), cytokines (TNFα, IL6, IL1β), and chemokines (MCP-1, MIP-3α) and confirmed the poor concordance between transcriptional and translational responses.[240] A recent study has established an extensive reference protein database for trauma patients, providing a foundation for future high-throughput quantitative plasma proteomic investigations of the mechanisms underlying systemic inflam-
7 matory responses.[241] Changes in serum proteome associated with sepsis and septic shock have been reported[242] and may allow rapid subclassification of sepsis syndrome into variants that may better predict responsiveness to fluid resuscitation, IV steroids, activated protein C, anti-TNF drugs, or specific antibiotics.[72]

Modeling disease entities like sepsis and MODS, which are complex, nonlinear systems, require not only the ability to measure many diverse molecular events simultaneously, but also to integrate the data using novel analytical tools based on complex systems theory and nonlinear dynamics.[243] Such analysis might help identify the key signaling nodes against which therapeutics can be directed.

FUTURE DIRECTIONS

Systems Biology Approach to Perioperative Medicine: The "Perioptome"

Systems biology is a conceptual framework within which scientists attempt to correlate massive amounts of apparently unrelated data into a single unifying explanation of how biologic processes occur.[244] This evolving discipline that merges experimental and computational approaches to observe, record, and integrate information from the molecular, cellular, tissue, and whole organism level into testable models of a dynamic biologic process can be applied to understand the way patients respond to a multidimensional stimulus such as a surgical procedure and the mechanistic basis of perioperative morbidity Fig. 6-5). Such an approach involves multiple levels of data integration. First, delineating the composition of the *perioperative phenome* (the representation of all perioperative phenotypes expressed by a given patient) requires standardized definitions, controlled vocabularies, and data dictionaries (a perioperative phenotype ontology), new (molecular) imaging technologies, and the availability of comprehensive data warehousing capabilities which will allow cataloguing individual perioperative phenotypes as well as correlations between combinations of phenotypes (organ cross-talk, multiple organ failure). Second, orthogonal integration of whole-genome genotypic, transcriptomic, proteomic, and metabolomic data, augmented by more recent functional genomic and proteomic approaches including protein–protein, protein–DNA, or other "component–component" interaction mapping (*interactome*), transcript or protein three-dimensional localization mapping (*localizome*),[245] and literature data within individual biologic systems involved in perioperative morbidity. This highest level of data integration is the mapping of the integrated high-throughput static and dynamic genomic data into regulatory networks in order to model interactions of the different components of the system, identify modules of highly interconnected genes, and hub points that can be prioritized as therapeutic targets. Ultimately, mathematical models require experimental validation in animal models of disease or tissue culture, in an iterative process that is one of the core characteristics of systems biology.[246] Such integrative approaches to study not only cardiovascular function (the Cardiome Project) but also perioperative morbidity (the Perioptome)[247] have already been outlined and promise to increase the identification of key drivers of perioperative adverse events beyond what could be achieved by genetic associations alone.

Targeted Therapeutic Applications: The "5Ps" of Perioperative Medicine and Pain Management

Genomic and proteomic approaches are rapidly becoming platforms for all aspects of drug discovery and development, from target identification and validation to individualization of drug therapy. As mentioned above, the human genome contains about 25,000 genes encoding for approximately 200,000 proteins which represent potential drug targets. However, only about 120 drug targets are currently being marketed, thus making identification of novel therapeutic targets an area of intense research. Following gene identification, its therapeutic potential needs to be validated by defining the sequence function and its role in disease and demonstrating that the gene product can be manipulated with

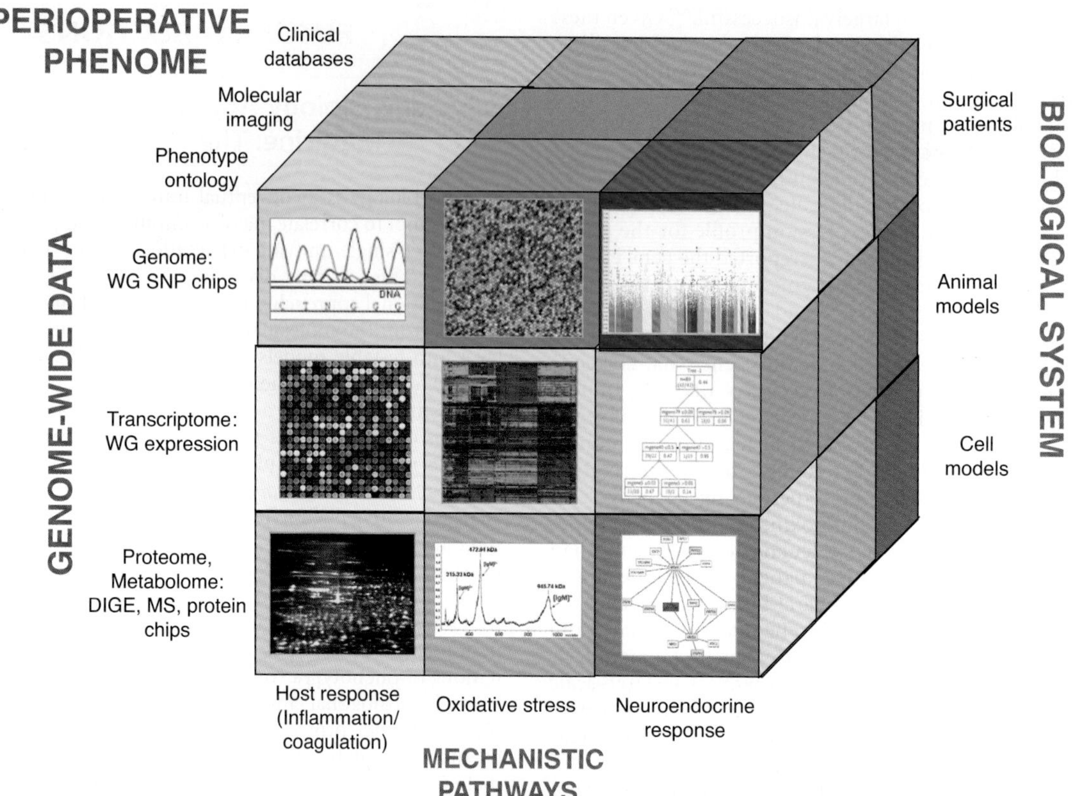

FIGURE 6-5. Levels of integration in perioperative systems biology—the "perioptome." Cellular function is organized as a multilayered set of interdependent processes controlled at the level of the *genome* (DNA), *transcriptome* (messenger RNA), *proteome* (the collection of all proteins encoded within the DNA of a genome), and *metabolome* (the complete set of small-molecule metabolites to be found in a biologic system), which can all be interrogated using high-throughput technologies. Accurate representation of the perioperative *phenome* (the set of all perioperative phenotypes expressed by an individual patient) requires integration of standardized phenotype definitions (phenotype ontology), state-of-the-art imaging technologies, and comprehensive clinical data warehousing. Relating genome variability to specific perioperative phenotypes through systems biology approaches involves the orthogonal integration of multiple levels of biologic organization provided by genome-wide datasets with clinical data and literature data, modeling the regulatory networks involved in adverse perioperative outcomes, and identifying critical regulatory nodes for therapeutic manipulation. WG, whole genome; DIGE, differential in-gel electrophoresis; MS, mass spectrometry; SNP, single nucleotide polymorphism.

beneficial effect and no toxic effects. A developing field, *toxicogenomics*, studies the influence of toxic or potentially toxic substances on different model organisms by evaluating the gene expression changes induced by novel drugs in a given tissue. Sponsored by the National Institutes of Health, a nationwide collaborative effort called the Pharmacogenetics Research Network (http://www.nigms.nih.gov/pharmacogenetics/) is aiming to establish a strong pharmacogenomics knowledge base (http://www.pharmgkb.org/) as well as create a shared computational and experimental infrastructure required to connect human sequence variation with drug responses and translate information into novel therapeutics.

The epidemiologic framework for assessing the applicability of previously identified biomarkers of perioperative morbidity and the successful implementation of molecular diagnostics in perioperative medicine is contingent upon demonstrating their *clinical validity, analytical validity,* and *clinical utility.*[248] Perioperative genomic investigators are currently conducting replication studies in different surgical patient populations to formally assess the clinical validity of the markers reported so far. For genomic classifiers the emphasis during external validation is placed on prospectively testing the accuracy of the entire molecular fingerprint in a new patient population rather than corroborating results in individual genes. In perioperative and critical care settings it is vital to have fast turnaround time (several hours) and easy-to-use testing capabilities, so that meaningful therapeutic interventions can take place. In this regard, new molecular diagnostic systems based on the random access technology such as the GeneXpert® (Cepheid), eSensor® (Osmetech), and Liat™ Analyzer (Iquum) are already becoming available. Clinical utility (targeted interventions to reduce perioperative morbidity among patients with a certain genomic profile) remains to be evaluated in future genomically stratified perioperative trials. Indeed, a landmark study on the effects of a 5-lipooxygenase-activating protein (FLAP) inhibitor on biomarkers associated with the risk of MI demonstrates that by defining at-risk patients for two genes in the leukotriene pathway, one can predict who will respond to targeted drug therapy. Specifically, in patients carrying the at-risk variants in the FLAP and in the leukotriene A4 hydrolase genes, use of a FLAP inhibitor in a randomized controlled trial resulted in significant and dose-dependent suppression of biomarkers associated with increased risk of MI.[249] It is expected that similar principles of targeted therapeutics could be operational in the perioperative period, thus beginning to fulfill the 5Ps of modern medicine (*P*ersonalized, *P*reventive, *P*redictive, *P*articipatory, and *P*rospective).

Ethical Considerations

Although one of the aims of the Human Genome Project is to improve therapy through genome-based prediction, the birth of personal genomics opens up a Pandora's Box of ethical issues, including privacy and the risk for discrimination against individuals who are genetically predisposed for a medical disorder. Such discrimination may include barriers to obtaining health, life, or long-term care insurance, or obtaining employment. Thus, extensive efforts are made to protect patients participating in genetic research from prejudice, discrimination, or uses of genetic information that will adversely affect them. To address the concerns of both biomedical research and health communities, the U.S. Senate has approved in 2003 the Genetic Information and Nondiscrimination Act, which provides the strong safeguards required to protect the public participating in human genome research.

Another ethical concern is the transferability of genetic tests across ethnic groups, particularly in the prediction of adverse drug responses. It is known that most polymorphisms associated with variability in drug response show significant differences in allele frequencies among populations and racial groups. Furthermore, the patterns of linkage disequilibrium are markedly different between ethnic groups, which may lead to spurious findings when markers, instead of causal variants, are used in diagnostic tests extrapolated across populations. In exploring racial disparities in health and disease outcomes, considerable debate has focused on whether race and ethnic identity are primarily social or biologic constructs and the contribution of genetic variability in explaining observed differences in the rates of disease between racial groups. With the goal of personalized medicine being the prediction of risk and treatment of disease on the basis of an individual's genetic profile, some have argued that biologic consideration of race will become obsolete. However, in this discovery phase of the post-genome era, continuing to incorporate racial information in genetic studies should improve our understanding of the architecture of the human genome and its implications for novel strategies aiming at identifying variants protecting against, or conferring susceptibility to, common diseases and modulating drug effects.[250]

CONCLUSIONS

The Human Genome Project has revolutionized all aspects of medicine, allowing us to assess the impact of genetic variability on disease taxonomy, characterization, and outcome and individual responses to various drugs and injuries. Mechanistically, information gleaned through genomic approaches is already unraveling long-standing mysteries behind general anesthetic action and adverse responses to drugs used perioperatively. Most studies published so far in the field of periprocedural genetic risk prediction are limited in size, mostly unreplicated, and not focused on the development of clinico-genomic predictive scores, and few report the predictive accuracy of their models. Rigorous future development and validation of clinico-genomic risk prediction models to identify patients who would benefit from increased or different interventions and monitoring, combined with high-quality methodology and reporting, is key to impacting the health of patients undergoing cardiovascular interventions. Therefore, a strong need remains for prospective, well-powered genetic studies in highly phenotyped surgical populations, which require the development of multidimensional perioperative databases.

For the anesthesiologist, this may soon translate into prospective risk assessment incorporating genetic profiling of markers important in thrombotic, inflammatory, vascular, and neurologic responses to perioperative stress, with implications ranging from individualized additional preoperative testing and physiologic optimization, to choice of perioperative monitoring strategies and critical care resource utilization. Furthermore, genetic profiling of drug-metabolizing enzymes, carrier proteins, and receptors, using currently available high-throughput molecular technologies, will enable personalized choice of drugs and dosage regimens tailored to suit a patient's pharmacogenetic profile. At that point, perioperative physicians will have far more robust information to use in designing the most appropriate and safest anesthetic plan for a given patient.

Future trends and challenges in perioperative genomics are still being defined, but mainly concern interdisciplinary studies designed to combine an analytical system approach, mathematical modeling, and engineering principles with the multiple molecular and genetic factors and stimuli and the macroscale interactions which determine the pathophysiologic response to surgery.

ACKNOWLEDGMENTS

Supported in part by NIH grants HL075273 and HL092071 (to MVP).

SCIENTIFIC FOUNDATIONS OF ANESTHESIA

References

1. Collins FS, Green ED, Guttmacher AE, et al. A vision for the future of genomics research. *Nature.* 2003;422:835–847.
2. Schwinn DA, Booth JV. Genetics infuses new life into human physiology: Implications of the human genome project for anesthesiology and perioperative medicine. *Anesthesiology.* 2002;96:261–263.
3. Lunshof JE, Bobe J, Aach J, et al. Personal genomes in progress: From the human genome project to the personal genome project. *Dialogues Clin Neurosci.* 2010;12:47–60.
4. Lander ES. The new genomics: Global views of biology. *Science.* 1996;274: 536–539.
5. Podgoreanu MV, Schwinn DA. New paradigms in cardiovascular medicine: Emerging technologies and practices: Perioperative genomics. *J Am Coll Cardiol.* 2005;46:1965–1977.
6. Fox AA, Shernan SK, Body SC. Predictive genomics of adverse events after cardiac surgery. *Semin Cardiothorac Vasc Anesth.* 2004;8:297–315.
7. Stuber F, Hoeft A. The influence of genomics on outcome after cardiovascular surgery. *Curr Opin Anaesthesiol.* 2002;15:3–8.
8. Ziegeler S, Tsusaki BE, Collard CD. Influence of genotype on perioperative risk and outcome. *Anesthesiology.* 2003;99:212–219.
9. Redon R, Ishikawa S, Fitch KR, et al. Global variation in copy number in the human genome. *Nature.* 2006;444:444–454.
10. Frazer KA, Ballinger DG, Cox DR, et al. A second generation human haplotype map of over 3.1 million SNPs. *Nature.* 2007;449:851–861.
11. Levy S, Sutton G, Ng PC, et al. The diploid genome sequence of an individual human. *PLoS Biol.* 2007;5:e254.
12. Podgoreanu MV, Schwinn DA. Genomics and the circulation. *Br J Anaesth.* 2004; 93:140–148.
13. Gretarsdottir S, Sveinbjornsdottir S, Jonsson HH, et al. Localization of a susceptibility gene for common forms of stroke to 5q12. *Am J Hum Genet.* 2002;70: 593–603.
14. Broeckel U, Hengstenberg C, Mayer B, et al. A comprehensive linkage analysis for myocardial infarction and its related risk factors. *Nat Genet.* 2002;30:210–214.
15. Zintzaras E, Kitsios G, Kent D, et al. Genome-wide scans meta-analysis for pulse pressure. *Hypertension.* 2007;50:557–564.
16. Risch N, Merikangas K. The future of genetic studies of complex human diseases. *Science.* 1996;273:1516–1517.
17. Tabor HK, Risch NJ, Myers RM. Opinion: Candidate-gene approaches for studying complex genetic traits: Practical considerations. *Nat Rev Genet.* 2002;3: 391–397.
18. Zhu X, Chang YP, Yan D, et al. Associations between hypertension and genes in the renin-angiotensin system. *Hypertension.* 2003;41:1027–1034.
19. Jachymova M, Horky K, Bultas J, et al. Association of the glu298asp polymorphism in the endothelial nitric oxide synthase gene with essential hypertension resistant to conventional therapy. *Biochem Biophys Res Commun.* 2001;284: 426–430.

20. Tomaszewski M, Brain NJ, Charchar FJ, et al. Essential hypertension and beta2-adrenergic receptor gene: Linkage and association analysis. *Hypertension.* 2002;40:286–291.
21. Winkelmann BR, Hager J. Genetic variation in coronary heart disease and myocardial infarction: Methodological overview and clinical evidence. *Pharmacogenomics.* 2000;1:73–94.
22. Agema WR, Jukema JW, Pimstone SN, et al. Genetic aspects of restenosis after percutaneous coronary interventions: Towards more tailored therapy. *Eur Heart J.* 2001;22:2058–2074.
23. Ozaki K, Ohnishi Y, Iida A, et al. Functional SNPs in the lymphotoxin-alpha gene that are associated with susceptibility to myocardial infarction. *Nat Genet.* 2002;32:650–654.
24. Podgoreanu MV, White WD, Morris RW, et al. Inflammatory gene polymorphisms and risk of postoperative myocardial infarction after cardiac surgery. *Circulation.* 2006;114:I275–I281.
25. Collard CD, Shernan SK, Fox AA, et al. The mbl2 'lyqa secretor' haplotype is an independent predictor of postoperative myocardial infarction in whites undergoing coronary artery bypass graft surgery. *Circulation.* 2007;116:I106–I112.
26. Tardiff BE, Newman MF, Saunders AM, et al. Preliminary report of a genetic basis for cognitive decline after cardiac operations. The Neurologic Outcome Research Group of the Duke Heart Center. *Ann Thorac Surg.* 1997;64:715–720.
27. Mathew JP, Rinder CS, Howe JG, et al. Platelet pla2 polymorphism enhances risk of neurocognitive decline after cardiopulmonary bypass. Multicenter study of perioperative ischemia (McSPI) research group. *Ann Thorac Surg.* 2001;71:663–666.
28. Mathew JP, Podgoreanu MV, Grocott HP, et al. Genetic variants in P-selectin and C-reactive protein influence susceptibility to cognitive decline after cardiac surgery. *J Am Coll Cardiol.* 2007;49:1934–1942.
29. Stafford-Smith M, Podgoreanu M, Swaminathan M, et al. Association of genetic polymorphisms with risk of renal injury after coronary bypass graft surgery. *Am J Kidney Dis.* 2005;45:519–530.
30. Chew ST, Newman MF, White WD, et al. Preliminary report on the association of apolipoprotein E polymorphisms, with postoperative peak serum creatinine concentrations in cardiac surgical patients. *Anesthesiology.* 2000;93:325–331.
31. MacKensen GB, Swaminathan M, Ti LK, et al. Preliminary report on the interaction of apolipoprotein E polymorphism with aortic atherosclerosis and acute nephropathy after CABG. *Ann Thorac Surg.* 2004;78:520–526.
32. Ortlepp JR, Janssens U, Bleckmann F, et al. A chymase gene variant is associated with atherosclerosis in venous coronary artery bypass grafts. *Coron Artery Dis.* 2001;12:493–497.
33. Ellis SG, Chen MS, Jia G, et al. Relation of polymorphisms in five genes to long-term aortocoronary saphenous vein graft patency. *Am J Cardiol.* 2007;99:1087–1089.
34. Donahue BS. Factor V Leiden and perioperative risk. *Anesth Analg.* 2004;98:1623–1634, table of contents.
35. Lasocki S, Iglarz M, Seince PF, et al. Involvement of renin-angiotensin system in pressure-flow relationship: Role of angiotensin-converting enzyme gene polymorphism. *Anesthesiology.* 2002;96:271–275.
36. Stuber F, Petersen M, Bokelmann F, et al. A genomic polymorphism within the tumor necrosis factor locus influences plasma tumor necrosis factor-alpha concentrations and outcome of patients with severe sepsis. *Crit Care Med.* 1996;24:381–384.
37. Moretti EW, Morris RW, Podgoreanu M, et al. APOE polymorphism is associated with risk of severe sepsis in surgical patients. *Crit Care Med.* 2005;33:2521–2526.
38. Slavcheva E, Albanis E, Jiao Q, et al. Cytotoxic T-lymphocyte antigen 4 gene polymorphisms and susceptibility to acute allograft rejection. *Transplantation.* 2001;72:935–940.
39. Cardon LR, Bell JI. Association study designs for complex diseases. *Nat Rev Genet.* 2001;2:91–99.
40. Hirschhorn JN, Lohmueller K, Byrne E, et al. A comprehensive review of genetic association studies. *Genet Med.* 2002;4:45–61.
41. Lohmueller KE, Pearce CL, Pike M, et al. Meta-analysis of genetic association studies supports a contribution of common variants to susceptibility to common disease. *Nat Genet.* 2003;33:177–182.
42. TWTC-C Consortium. Genome-wide association study of 14,000 cases of seven common diseases and 3,000 shared controls. *Nature.* 2007;447:661–678.
43. Samani NJ, Erdmann J, Hall AS, et al. Genomewide association analysis of coronary artery disease. *N Engl J Med.* 2007;357:443–453.
44. McPherson R, Pertsemlidis A, Kavaslar N, et al. A common allele on chromosome 9 associated with coronary heart disease. *Science.* 2007;316:1488–1491.
45. Helgadottir A, Thorleifsson G, Manolescu A, et al. A common variant on chromosome 9p21 affects the risk of myocardial infarction. *Science.* 2007;316:1491–1493.
46. Todd JA, Walker NM, Cooper JD, et al. Robust associations of four new chromosome regions from genome-wide analyses of type 1 diabetes. *Nat Genet.* 2007;39:857–864.
47. Saxena R, Voight BF, Lyssenko V, et al. Genome-wide association analysis identifies loci for type 2 diabetes and triglyceride levels. *Science.* 2007;316:1331–1336.
48. Gudbjartsson DF, Arnar DO, Helgadottir A, et al. Variants conferring risk of atrial fibrillation on chromosome 4q25. *Nature.* 2007;448:353–357.
49. Scuteri A, Sanna S, Chen WM, et al. Genome-wide association scan shows genetic variants in the FTO gene are associated with obesity-related traits. *PLoS Genet.* 2007;3:e115.
50. Stranger BE, Nica AC, Forrest MS, et al. Population genomics of human gene expression. *Nat Genet.* 2007;39:1217–1224.
51. Hopf HW. Molecular diagnostics of injury and repair responses in critical illness: What is the future of "monitoring" in the intensive care unit? *Crit Care Med.* 2003;31:S518–S523.
52. Feezor RJ, Baker HV, Xiao W, et al. Genomic and proteomic determinants of outcome in patients undergoing thoracoabdominal aortic aneurysm repair. *J Immunol.* 2004;172:7103–7109.
53. Sehl PD, Tai JT, Hillan KJ, et al. Application of cDNA microarrays in determining molecular phenotype in cardiac growth, development, and response to injury. *Circulation.* 2000;101:1990–1999.
54. Ruel M, Bianchi C, Khan TA, et al. Gene expression profile after cardiopulmonary bypass and cardioplegic arrest. *J Thorac Cardiovasc Surg.* 2003;126:1521–1530.
55. Konstantinov IE, Coles JG, Boscarino C, et al. Gene expression profiles in children undergoing cardiac surgery for right heart obstructive lesions. *J Thorac Cardiovasc Surg.* 2004;127:746–754.
56. Sergeev P, da Silva R, Lucchinetti E, et al. Trigger-dependent gene expression profiles in cardiac preconditioning: Evidence for distinct genetic programs in ischemic and anesthetic preconditioning. *Anesthesiology.* 2004;100:474–488.
57. Lucchinetti E, da Silva R, Pasch T, et al. Anaesthetic preconditioning but not postconditioning prevents early activation of the deleterious cardiac remodelling programme: Evidence of opposing genomic responses in cardioprotection by pre- and postconditioning. *Br J Anaesth.* 2005;95:140–152.
58. Lucchinetti E, Hofer C, Bestmann L, et al. Gene regulatory control of myocardial energy metabolism predicts postoperative cardiac function in patients undergoing off-pump coronary artery bypass graft surgery: Inhalational versus intravenous anesthetics. *Anesthesiology.* 2007;106:444–457.
59. Lucchinetti E, Aguirre J, Feng J, et al. Molecular evidence of late preconditioning after sevoflurane inhalation in healthy volunteers. *Anesth Analg.* 2007;105:629–640.
60. Lai LP, Lin JL, Lin CS, et al. Functional genomic study on atrial fibrillation using cDNA microarray and two-dimensional protein electrophoresis techniques and identification of the myosin regulatory light chain isoform reprogramming in atrial fibrillation. *J Cardiovasc Electrophysiol.* 2004;15:214–223.
61. Barth AS, Merk S, Arnoldi E, et al. Reprogramming of the human atrial transcriptome in permanent atrial fibrillation: Expression of a ventricular-like genomic signature. *Circ Res.* 2005;96:1022–1029.
62. Ramlawi B, Otu H, Mieno S, et al. Oxidative stress and atrial fibrillation after cardiac surgery: A case-control study. *Ann Thorac Surg.* 2007;84:1166–1172, discussion 1172–1163.
63. Ramlawi B, Otu H, Rudolph JL, et al. Genomic expression pathways associated with brain injury after cardiopulmonary bypass. *J Thorac Cardiovasc Surg.* 2007;134:996–1005.
64. Horwitz PA, Tsai EJ, Putt ME, et al. Detection of cardiac allograft rejection and response to immunosuppressive therapy with peripheral blood gene expression. *Circulation.* 2004;110:3815–3821.
65. Pham MX, Teuteberg JJ, Kfoury AG, et al. Gene-expression profiling for rejection surveillance after cardiac transplantation. *N Engl J Med.* 2010;362:1890–1900.
66. Borozdenkova S, Westbrook JA, Patel V, et al. Use of proteomics to discover novel markers of cardiac allograft rejection. *J Proteome Res.* 2004;3:282–288.
67. Rosenberg S, Elashoff MR, Beineke P, et al. Multicenter validation of the diagnostic accuracy of a blood-based gene expression test for assessing obstructive coronary artery disease in nondiabetic patients. *Ann Intern Med.* 2010;153:425–434.
68. Matkovich SJ, Van Booven DJ, Youker KA, et al. Reciprocal regulation of myocardial microRNAs and messenger RNA in human cardiomyopathy and reversal of the microRNA signature by biomechanical support. *Circulation.* 2009;119:1263–1271.
69. Hughes TR, Marton MJ, Jones AR, et al. Functional discovery via a compendium of expression profiles. *Cell.* 2000;102:109–126.
70. Tomic V, Russwurm S, Moller E, et al. Transcriptomic and proteomic patterns of systemic inflammation in on-pump and off-pump coronary artery bypass grafting. *Circulation.* 2005;112:2912–2920.
71. Depre C, Tomlinson JE, Kudej RK, et al. Gene program for cardiac cell survival induced by transient ischemia in conscious pigs. *Proc Natl Acad Sci U S A.* 2001;98:9336–9341.
72. Atkins JH, Johansson JS. Technologies to shape the future: Proteomics applications in anesthesiology and critical care medicine. *Anesth Analg.* 2006;102:1207–1216.
73. Futterer CD, Maurer MH, Schmitt A, et al. Alterations in rat brain proteins after desflurane anesthesia. *Anesthesiology.* 2004;100:302–308.
74. Kalenka A, Hinkelbein J, Feldmann RE Jr, et al. The effects of sevoflurane anesthesia on rat brain proteins: A proteomic time-course analysis. *Anesth Analg.* 2007;104:1129–1135, table of contents.
75. Sheikh AM, Barrett C, Villamizar N, et al. Proteomics of cerebral injury in a neonatal model of cardiopulmonary bypass with deep hypothermic circulatory arrest. *J Thorac Cardiovasc Surg.* 2006;132:820–828.
76. Queloz PA, Thadikkaran L, Crettaz D, et al. Proteomics and transfusion medicine: Future perspectives. *Proteomics.* 2006;6:5605–5614.
77. Mangano DT. Perioperative medicine: NHLBI working group deliberations and recommendations. *J Cardiothorac Vasc Anesth.* 2004;18:1–6.
78. Janssens AC, van Duijn CM. Genome-based prediction of common diseases: Methodological considerations for future research. *Genome Med.* 2009;1:20.

79. Janssens AC, Ioannidis JP, Bedrosian S, et al. Strengthening the reporting of genetic risk prediction studies (GRIPS): Explanation and elaboration. *Eur J Clin Invest.* 2011;41:1010–1035.
80. Taegtmeyer AB, Breen JB, Rogers P, et al. Effect of adenosine monophosphate deaminase-1 c34t allele on the requirement for donor inotropic support and on the incidence of early graft dysfunction after cardiac transplantation. *Am J Cardiol.* 2009;103:1457–1462.
81. Muehlschlegel JD, Liu KY, Perry TE, et al. Chromosome 9p21 variant predicts mortality after coronary artery bypass graft surgery. *Circulation.* 2010;122: S60–S65.
82. Lobato RL, White WD, Mathew JP, et al. Thrombomodulin gene variants are associated with increased mortality after coronary artery bypass surgery in replicated analyses. *Circulation.* 2011;124:S143–S148.
83. Zaugg M, Bestmann L, Wacker J, et al. Adrenergic receptor genotype but not perioperative bisoprolol therapy may determine cardiovascular outcome in at-risk patients undergoing surgery with spinal block: The Swiss Beta Blocker in Spinal Anesthesia (BBSA) study: A double-blinded, placebo-controlled, multicenter trial with 1-year follow-up. *Anesthesiology.* 2007;107:33–44.
84. Podgoreanu MV, Booth JV, White WD, et al. Beta adrenergic receptor polymorphisms and risk of adverse events following cardiac surgery. *Circulation.* 2003;108:IV-434.
85. Volzke H, Engel J, Kleine V, et al. Angiotensin I-converting enzyme insertion/deletion polymorphism and cardiac mortality and morbidity after coronary artery bypass graft surgery. *Chest.* 2002;122:31–36.
86. Zotz RB, Klein M, Dauben HP, et al. Prospective analysis after coronary-artery bypass grafting: Platelet GP IIIa polymorphism (HPA-1b/PIA2) is a risk factor for bypass occlusion, myocardial infarction, and death. *Thromb Haemost.* 2000; 83:404–407.
87. Pereira AC, Miyakawa AA, Lopes NH, et al. Dynamic regulation of MTHFR mRNA expression and C677T genotype modulate mortality in coronary artery disease patients after revascularization. *Thromb Res.* 2007;121:25–32.
88. Botto N, Andreassi MG, Rizza A, et al. C677t polymorphism of the methylenetetrahydrofolate reductase gene is a risk factor of adverse events after coronary revascularization. *Int J Cardiol.* 2004;96:341–345.
89. Delanghe J, Cambier B, Langlois M, et al. Haptoglobin polymorphism, a genetic risk factor in coronary artery bypass surgery. *Atherosclerosis.* 1997;132:215–219.
90. Taylor KD, Scheuner MT, Yang H, et al. Lipoprotein lipase locus and progression of atherosclerosis in coronary-artery bypass grafts. *Genet Med.* 2004;6:481–486.
91. Stoica AL, Stoica E, Constantinescu I, et al. Interleukin-6 and interleukin-10 gene polymorphism, endothelial dysfunction, and postoperative prognosis in patients with peripheral arterial disease. *J Vasc Surg.* 2010;52:103–109.
92. Shaw AD, Vaporciyan AA, Wu X, et al. Inflammatory gene polymorphisms influence risk of postoperative morbidity after lung resection. *Ann Thorac Surg.* 2005;79:1704–1710.
93. Tomasdottir H, Hjartarson H, Ricksten A, et al. Tumor necrosis factor gene polymorphism is associated with enhanced systemic inflammatory response and increased cardiopulmonary morbidity after cardiac surgery. *Anesth Analg.* 2003;97:944–949, table of contents.
94. Galley HF, Lowe PR, Carmichael RL, et al. Genotype and interleukin-10 responses after cardiopulmonary bypass. *Br J Anaesth.* 2003;91:424–426.
95. Moor E, Silveira A, van't Hooft F, et al. Coagulation factor V (Arg506–>Gln) mutation and early saphenous vein graft occlusion after coronary artery bypass grafting. *Thromb Haemost.* 1998;80:220–224.
96. Rinder CS, Mathew JP, Rinder HM, et al. Platelet PLA2 polymorphism and platelet activation are associated with increased troponin I release after cardiopulmonary bypass. *Anesthesiology.* 2002;97:1118–1122.
97. Faraday N, Martinez EA, Scharpf RB, et al. Platelet gene polymorphisms and cardiac risk assessment in vascular surgical patients. *Anesthesiology.* 2004;101: 1291–1297.
98. Rifon J, Paramo JA, Panizo C, et al. The increase of plasminogen activator inhibitor activity is associated with graft occlusion in patients undergoing aorto-coronary bypass surgery. *Br J Haematol.* 1997;99:262–267.
99. Fox AA, Collard CD, Shernan SK, et al. Natriuretic peptide system gene variants are associated with ventricular dysfunction after coronary artery bypass grafting. *Anesthesiology.* 2009;110:738–747.
100. Liu KY, Muehlschlegel JD, Perry TE, et al. Common genetic variants on chromosome 9p21 predict perioperative myocardial injury after coronary artery bypass graft surgery. *J Thorac Cardiovasc Surg.* 2010;139:483–488, 488.e1– e2.
101. Ryan R, Thornton J, Duggan E, et al. Gene polymorphism and requirement for vasopressor infusion after cardiac surgery. *Ann Thorac Surg.* 2006;82:895–901.
102. Philip I, Plantefeve G, Vuillaumier-Barrot S, et al. G894t polymorphism in the endothelial nitric oxide synthase gene is associated with an enhanced vascular responsiveness to phenylephrine. *Circulation.* 1999;99:3096–3098.
103. Heusch G, Erbel R, Siffert W. Genetic determinants of coronary vasomotor tone in humans. *Am J Physiol Heart Circ Physiol.* 2001;281:H1465–H1468.
104. Henrion D, Benessiano J, Philip I, et al. The deletion genotype of the angiotensin I-converting enzyme is associated with an increased vascular reactivity in vivo and in vitro. *J Am Coll Cardiol.* 1999;34:830–836.
105. Kim NS, Lee IO, Lee MK, et al. The effects of beta2 adrenoceptor gene polymorphisms on pressor response during laryngoscopy and tracheal intubation. *Anaesthesia.* 2002;57:227–232.
106. Iribarren JL, Sagasti FM, Jimenez JJ, et al. TNFbeta+250 polymorphism and hyperdynamic state in cardiac surgery with extracorporeal circulation. *Interact Cardiovasc Thorac Surg.* 2008;7:1071–1074.
107. Gaudino M, Andreotti F, Zamparelli R, et al. The -174 g/c interleukin-6 polymorphism influences postoperative interleukin-6 levels and postoperative atrial fibrillation. Is atrial fibrillation an inflammatory complication? *Circulation.* 2003;108(Suppl 1):II195–II199.
108. Motsinger AA, Donahue BS, Brown NJ, et al. Risk factor interactions and genetic effects associated with post-operative atrial fibrillation. *Pac Symp Biocomput.* 2006:584–595.
109. Donahue BS, Roden D. Inflammatory cytokine polymorphisms are associated with beta-blocker failure in preventing postoperative atrial fibrillation. *Anesth Analg.* 2005;100:SCA30 (abstract).
110. Body SC, Collard CD, Shernan SK, et al. Variation in the 4q25 chromosomal locus predicts atrial fibrillation after coronary artery bypass graft surgery. *Circ Cardiovasc Genet.* 2009;2:499–506.
111. Podgoreanu MV, Morris R, Zhang Q, et al. Gene variants in interleukin 1-beta are associated with early QTc prolongation after cardiac surgery. *Anesthesiology.* 2007;107:A1287 (abstract).
112. Afzal AR, Mandal K, Nyamweya S, et al. Association of Met439Thr substitution in heat shock protein 70 gene with postoperative atrial fibrillation and serum HSP70 protein levels. *Cardiology.* 2008;110:45–52.
113. Holweg CT, Weimar W, Uitterlinden AG, et al. Clinical impact of cytokine gene polymorphisms in heart and lung transplantation. *J Heart Lung Transplant.* 2004; 23:1017–1026.
114. Borozdenkova S, Smith J, Marshall S, et al. Identification of ICAM-1 polymorphism that is associated with protection from transplant associated vasculopathy after cardiac transplantation. *Hum Immunol.* 2001;62:247–255.
115. Vamvakopoulos JE, Taylor CJ, Green C, et al. Interleukin 1 and chronic rejection: Possible genetic links in human heart allografts. *Am J Transplant.* 2002;2:76–83.
116. Benza RL, Coffey CS, Pekarek DM, et al. Transforming growth factor-beta polymorphisms and cardiac allograft rejection. *J Heart Lung Transplant.* 2009;28: 1057–1062.
117. Grocott HP, White WD, Morris RW, et al. Genetic polymorphisms and the risk of stroke after cardiac surgery. *Stroke.* 2005;36:1854–1858.
118. Sirgo G, Perez-Vela JL, Morales P, et al. Association between 4g/5g polymorphism of the plasminogen activator inhibitor 1 gene with stroke or encephalopathy after cardiac surgery. *Intensive Care Med.* 2006;32:668–675.
119. Galasso G, Santulli G, Piscione F, et al. The GPIIIA PLA2 polymorphism is associated with an increased risk of cardiovascular adverse events. *BMC Cardiovasc Disord.* 2010;10:41.
120. Gaynor JW, Gerdes M, Zackai EH, et al. Apolipoprotein e genotype and neurodevelopmental sequelae of infant cardiac surgery. *J Thorac Cardiovasc Surg.* 2003; 126:1736–1745.
121. Zeltser I, Jarvik GP, Bernbaum J, et al. Genetic factors are important determinants of neurodevelopmental outcome after repair of tetralogy of fallot. *J Thorac Cardiovasc Surg.* 2008;135:91–97.
122. Leung JM, Sands LP, Wang Y, et al. Apolipoprotein E e4 allele increases the risk of early postoperative delirium in older patients undergoing noncardiac surgery. *Anesthesiology.* 2007;107:406–411.
123. Ely EW, Girard TD, Shintani AK, et al. Apolipoprotein e4 polymorphism as a genetic predisposition to delirium in critically ill patients. *Crit Care Med.* 2007; 35:112–117.
124. Donahue BS, Gailani D, Higgins MS, et al. Factor V Leiden protects against blood loss and transfusion after cardiac surgery. *Circulation.* 2003;107:1003–1008.
125. Duggan E, O'Dwyer MJ, Caraher E, et al. Coagulopathy after cardiac surgery may be influenced by a functional plasminogen activator inhibitor polymorphism. *Anesth Analg.* 2007;104:1343–1347, table of contents.
126. Welsby IJ, Podgoreanu MV, Phillips-Bute B, et al. Genetic factors contribute to bleeding after cardiac surgery. *J Thromb Haemost.* 2005;3:1206–1212.
127. Morawski W, Sanak M, Cisowski M, et al. Prediction of the excessive perioperative bleeding in patients undergoing coronary artery bypass grafting: Role of aspirin and platelet glycoprotein IIIa polymorphism. *J Thorac Cardiovasc Surg.* 2005;130:791–796.
128. Achrol AS, Kim H, Pawlikowska L, et al. Association of tumor necrosis factor-alpha-238G>A and apolipoprotein E2 polymorphisms with intracranial hemorrhage after brain arteriovenous malformation treatment. *Neurosurgery.* 2007;61: 731–739, discussion 740.
129. Welsby IJ, Podgoreanu MV, Phillips-Bute B, et al. Association of the 98T ELAM-1 polymorphism with increased bleeding after cardiac surgery. *J Cardiothorac Vasc Anesth.* 2010;24:427–433.
130. Howell SJ, Sear JW. Perioperative myocardial injury: Individual and population implications. *Br J Anaesth.* 2004;93:3–8.
131. Mangano DT. Effects of acadesine on myocardial infarction, stroke, and death following surgery. A meta-analysis of the 5 international randomized trials. The Multicenter Study of Perioperative Ischemia (McSPI) Research Group. *JAMA.* 1997;277:325–332.
132. Mahaffey KW, Roe MT, Kilaru R, et al. Creatine kinase-MB elevation after coronary artery bypass grafting surgery in patients with non-ST-segment elevation acute coronary syndromes predict worse outcomes: Results from four large clinical trials. *Eur Heart J.* 2007;28:425–432.

133. Brull DJ, Montgomery HE, Sanders J, et al. Interleukin-6 gene -174g>c and -572g>c promoter polymorphisms are strong predictors of plasma interleukin-6 levels after coronary artery bypass surgery. *Arterioscler Thromb Vasc Biol.* 2001; 21:1458–1463.
134. Burzotta F, Iacoviello L, Di Castelnuovo A, et al. Relation of the -174 g/c polymorphism of interleukin-6 to interleukin-6 plasma levels and to length of hospitalization after surgical coronary revascularization. *Am J Cardiol.* 2001;88:1125–1128.
135. Grocott HP, Newman MF, El-Moalem H, et al. Apolipoprotein e genotype differentially influences the proinflammatory and anti-inflammatory response to cardiopulmonary bypass. *J Thorac Cardiovasc Surg.* 2001;122:622–623.
136. Roth-Isigkeit A, Hasselbach L, Ocklitz E, et al. Inter-individual differences in cytokine release in patients undergoing cardiac surgery with cardiopulmonary bypass. *Clin Exp Immunol.* 2001;125:80–88.
137. Lehmann LE, Schroeder S, Hartmann W, et al. A single nucleotide polymorphism of macrophage migration inhibitory factor is related to inflammatory response in coronary bypass surgery using cardiopulmonary bypass. *Eur J Cardiothorac Surg.* 2006;30:59–63.
138. Willerson JT, Ridker PM. Inflammation as a cardiovascular risk factor. *Circulation.* 2004;109:II2–II10.
139. Perry TE, Muehlschlegel JD, Liu KY, et al. Preoperative C-reactive protein predicts long-term mortality and hospital length of stay after primary, nonemergent coronary artery bypass grafting. *Anesthesiology.* 2010;112:607–613.
140. Kangasniemi OP, Biancari F, Luukkonen J, et al. Preoperative C-reactive protein is predictive of long-term outcome after coronary artery bypass surgery. *Eur J Cardiothorac Surg.* 2006;29:983–985.
141. Song Y, Kwak YL, Choi YS, et al. Effect of preoperative statin therapy on myocardial protection and morbidity endpoints following off-pump coronary bypass surgery in patients with elevated C-reactive protein level. *Korean J Anesthesiol.* 2010;58:136–141.
142. Choi JH, Cho DK, Song YB, et al. Preoperative NT-proBNP and CRP predict perioperative major cardiovascular events in non-cardiac surgery. *Heart.* 2010; 96:56–62.
143. Perry TE, Muehlschlegel JD, Liu KY, et al. C-reactive protein gene variants are associated with postoperative C-reactive protein levels after coronary artery bypass surgery. *BMC Med Genet.* 2009;10:38.
144. Motoyama S, Miura M, Hinai Y, et al. C-reactive protein 1059G>C genetic polymorphism influences serum C-reactive protein levels after esophagectomy in patients with thoracic esophageal cancer. *J Am Coll Surg.* 2009;209:477–483.
145. Motoyama S, Miura M, Hinai Y, et al. C-reactive protein -717c>t genetic polymorphism associates with esophagectomy-induced stress hyperglycemia. *World J Surg.* 2010;34:1001–1007.
146. Voetsch B, Loscalzo J. Genetic determinants of arterial thrombosis. *Arterioscler Thromb Vasc Biol.* 2004;24:216–229.
147. Iacoviello L, Burzotta F, Di Castelnuovo A, et al. The 4G/5G polymorphism of PAI-1 promoter gene and the risk of myocardial infarction: A meta-analysis. *Thromb Haemost.* 1998;80:1029–1030.
148. Karthikeyan G, Moncur RA, Levine O, et al. Is a pre-operative brain natriuretic peptide or N-terminal pro-B-type natriuretic peptide measurement an independent predictor of adverse cardiovascular outcomes within 30 days of noncardiac surgery? A systematic review and meta-analysis of observational studies. *J Am Coll Cardiol.* 2009;54:1599–1606.
149. Ryding AD, Kumar S, Worthington AM, et al. Prognostic value of brain natriuretic peptide in noncardiac surgery: A meta-analysis. *Anesthesiology.* 2009;111: 311–319.
150. Fox AA, Shernan SK, Collard CD, et al. Preoperative B-type natriuretic peptide is an independent predictor of ventricular dysfunction and mortality after primary coronary artery bypass grafting. *J Thorac Cardiovasc Surg.* 2008;136:452–461.
151. Fox AA, Muehlschlegel JD, Body SC, et al. Comparison of the utility of preoperative versus postoperative B-type natriuretic peptide for predicting hospital length of stay and mortality after primary coronary artery bypass grafting. *Anesthesiology.* 2010;112:842–851.
152. Poldermans D, Bax JJ, Boersma E, et al. Guidelines for pre-operative cardiac risk assessment and perioperative cardiac management in non-cardiac surgery. *Eur Heart J.* 2009;30:2769–2812.
153. Shaw SM, Lewis NT, Williams SG, et al. A role for BNP assays in monitoring aortic valve disease for optimal timing of surgery. *Int J Cardiol.* 2008;127:328–330.
154. Zaugg M, Schaub MC. Genetic modulation of adrenergic activity in the heart and vasculature: Implications for perioperative medicine. *Anesthesiology.* 2005;102:429–446.
155. Lewis GD, Wei R, Liu E, et al. Metabolite profiling of blood from individuals undergoing planned myocardial infarction reveals early markers of myocardial injury. *J Clin Invest.* 2008;118:3503–3512.
156. Turer AT, Stevens RD, Bain JR, et al. Metabolomic profiling reveals distinct patterns of myocardial substrate use in humans with coronary artery disease or left ventricular dysfunction during surgical ischemia/reperfusion. *Circulation.* 2009; 119:1736–1746.
157. Balog J, Szaniszlo T, Schaefer KC, et al. Identification of biological tissues by rapid evaporative ionization mass spectrometry. *Anal Chem.* 2010;82:7343–7350.
158. Kinross JM, Holmes E, Darzi AW, et al. Metabolic phenotyping for monitoring surgical patients. *Lancet.* 2011;377:1817–1819.
159. Cohen MJ, Grossman AD, Morabito D, et al. Identification of complex metabolic states in critically injured patients using bioinformatic cluster analysis. *Crit Care.* 2010;14:R10.
160. Mathew JP, Fontes ML, Tudor IC, et al. A multicenter risk index for atrial fibrillation after cardiac surgery. *JAMA.* 2004;291:1720–1729.
161. Brugada R. Is atrial fibrillation a genetic disease? *J Cardiovasc Electrophysiol.* 2005;16:553–556.
162. Virani SS, Brautbar A, Lee VV, et al. Usefulness of single nucleotide polymorphism in chromosome 4q25 to predict in-hospital and long-term development of atrial fibrillation and survival in patients undergoing coronary artery bypass grafting. *Am J Cardiol.* 2011;107:1504–1509.
163. Gaudino M, Di Castelnuovo A, Zamparelli R, et al. Genetic control of postoperative systemic inflammatory reaction and pulmonary and renal complications after coronary artery surgery. *J Thorac Cardiovasc Surg.* 2003;126:1107–1112.
164. Hogue CW Jr, Palin CA, Kailasam R, et al. C-reactive protein levels and atrial fibrillation after cardiac surgery in women. *Ann Thorac Surg.* 2006;82:97–102.
165. Pretorius M, Donahue BS, Yu C, et al. Plasminogen activator inhibitor-1 as a predictor of postoperative atrial fibrillation after cardiopulmonary bypass. *Circulation.* 2007;116:I1–I7.
166. Mayr M, Yusuf S, Weir G, et al. Combined metabolomic and proteomic analysis of human atrial fibrillation. *J Am Coll Cardiol.* 2008;51:585–594.
167. Mehra MR, Feller E, Rosenberg S. The promise of protein-based and gene-based clinical markers in heart transplantation: From bench to bedside. *Nat Clin Pract Cardiovasc Med.* 2006;3:136–143.
168. Hall JL, Birks EJ, Grindle S, et al. Molecular signature of recovery following combination left ventricular assist device (LVAD) support and pharmacologic therapy. *Eur Heart J.* 2007;28:613–627.
169. Aharinejad S, Schafer R, Krenn K, et al. Donor myocardial HIF-1alpha is an independent predictor of cardiac allograft dysfunction: A 7-year prospective, exploratory study. *Am J Transplant.* 2007;7:2012–2019.
170. Girelli D, Martinelli N, Olivieri O, et al. Hyperhomocysteinemia and mortality after coronary artery bypass grafting. *PLoS One.* 2006;1:e83.
171. Eifert S, Rasch A, Beiras-Fernandez A, et al. Gene polymorphisms in APOE, NOS3, and LIPC genes may be risk factors for cardiac adverse events after primary CABG. *J Cardiothorac Surg.* 2009;4:46.
172. Newman MF, Booth JV, Laskowitz DT, et al. Genetic predictors of perioperative neurological and cognitive injury and recovery. *Best Pract Res Clin Anesthesiol.* 2001;15:247–276.
173. Alberts MJ, Graffagnino C, McClenny C, et al. ApoE genotype and survival from intracerebral haemorrhage. *Lancet.* 1995;346:575.
174. Teasdale GM, Nicoll JA, Murray G, et al. Association of apolipoprotein E polymorphism with outcome after head injury. *Lancet.* 1997;350:1069–1071.
175. Slooter AJ, Tang MX, van Duijn CM, et al. Apolipoprotein E epsilon4 and the risk of dementia with stroke. A population-based investigation. *JAMA.* 1997;277: 818–821.
176. Sheng H, Laskowitz DT, Bennett E, et al. Apolipoprotein E isoform-specific differences in outcome from focal ischemia in transgenic mice. *J Cereb Blood Flow Metab.* 1998;18:361–366.
177. Ti LK, Mathew JP, Mackensen GB, et al. Effect of apolipoprotein E genotype on cerebral autoregulation during cardiopulmonary bypass. *Stroke.* 2001;32: 1514–1519.
178. Ti LK, Mackensen GB, Grocott HP, et al. Apolipoprotein e4 increases aortic atheroma burden in cardiac surgical patients. *J Thorac Cardiovasc Surg.* 2003; 125:211–213.
179. Newman MF, Laskowitz DT, White WD, et al. Apolipoprotein E polymorphisms and age at first coronary artery bypass graft. *Anesth Analg.* 2001;92:824–829.
180. Weiss EJ, Bray PF, Tayback M, et al. A polymorphism of a platelet glycoprotein receptor as an inherited risk factor for coronary thrombosis. *N Engl J Med.* 1996;334:1090–1094.
181. Carter AM, Catto AJ, Bamford JM, et al. Platelet GP IIIa PLA and GP ib variable number tandem repeat polymorphisms and markers of platelet activation in acute stroke. *Arterioscler Thromb Vasc Biol.* 1998;18:1124–1131.
182. Ramlawi B, Rudolph JL, Mieno S, et al. C-reactive protein and inflammatory response associated to neurocognitive decline following cardiac surgery. *Surgery.* 2006;140:221–226.
183. Ramlawi B, Rudolph JL, Mieno S, et al. Serologic markers of brain injury and cognitive function after cardiopulmonary bypass. *Ann Surg.* 2006;244:593–601.
184. Heider P, Poppert H, Wolf O, et al. Fibrinogen and high-sensitive C-reactive protein as serologic predictors for perioperative cerebral microembolic lesions after carotid endarterectomy. *J Vasc Surg.* 2007;46:449–454.
185. McDonagh DL, Mathew JP, White WD, et al. Cognitive function after major noncardiac surgery, apolipoprotein e4 genotype, and biomarkers of brain injury. *Anesthesiology.* 2010;112:852–859.
186. Mangano CM, Diamondstone LS, Ramsay JG, et al. Renal dysfunction after myocardial revascularization: Risk factors, adverse outcomes, and hospital resource utilization. The multicenter study of Perioperative Ischemia Research Group. *Ann Intern Med.* 1998;128:194–203.
187. Isbir SC, Tekeli A, Ergen A, et al. Genetic polymorphisms contribute to acute kidney injury after coronary artery bypass grafting. *Heart Surg Forum.* 2007; 10:E439–E444.

188. Patel UD, Garg AX, Krumholz HM, et al. Pre-operative serum brain natriuretic peptide and risk of acute kidney injury after cardiac surgery. *Circulation.* 2012;125(11):1347–1355.
189. Yende S, Wunderink R. Causes of prolonged mechanical ventilation after coronary artery bypass surgery. *Chest.* 2002;122:245–252.
190. Rigat B, Hubert C, Alhenc-Gelas F, et al. An insertion/deletion polymorphism in the angiotensin I-converting enzyme gene accounting for half the variance of serum enzyme levels. *J Clin Invest.* 1990;86:1343–1346.
191. Yende S, Quasney MW, Tolley EA, et al. Clinical relevance of angiotensin-converting enzyme gene polymorphisms to predict risk of mechanical ventilation after coronary artery bypass graft surgery. *Crit Care Med.* 2004;32:922–927.
192. Marshall RP, Webb S, Bellingan GJ, et al. Angiotensin converting enzyme insertion/deletion polymorphism is associated with susceptibility and outcome in acute respiratory distress syndrome. *Am J Respir Crit Care Med.* 2002;166:646–650.
193. Yende S, Quasney MW, Tolley E, et al. Association of tumor necrosis factor gene polymorphisms and prolonged mechanical ventilation after coronary artery bypass surgery. *Crit Care Med.* 2003;31:133–140.
194. Roden DM. Cardiovascular pharmacogenomics. *Circulation.* 2003;108:3071–3074.
195. Lehmann H, Ryan E. The familial incidence of low pseudocholinesterase level. *Lancet.* 1956;271:124.
196. Bukaveckas BL, Valdes R Jr, Linder MW. Pharmacogenetics as related to the practice of cardiothoracic and vascular anesthesia. *J Cardiothorac Vasc Anesth.* 2004;18:353–365.
197. McCarthy TV, Healy JM, Heffron JJ, et al. Localization of the malignant hyperthermia susceptibility locus to human chromosome 19q12-13.2. *Nature.* 1990;343:562–564.
198. Pessah IN, Allen PD. Malignant hyperthermia. *Best Pract Res Clin Anesthesiol.* 2001;15:277–288.
199. Eger EI 2nd. *Anesthetic Uptake and Action.* Baltimore, MD: Williams and Wilkins; 1974.
200. Liem EB, Lin CM, Suleman MI, et al. Anesthetic requirement is increased in redheads. *Anesthesiology.* 2004;101:279–283.
201. Ezri T, Sessler D, Weisenberg M, et al. Association of ethnicity with the minimum alveolar concentration of sevoflurane. *Anesthesiology.* 2007;107:9–14.
202. Franks NP, Lieb WR. Molecular and cellular mechanisms of general anaesthesia. *Nature.* 1994;367:607–614.
203. Sonner JM, Antognini JF, Dutton RC, et al. Inhaled anesthetics and immobility: Mechanisms, mysteries, and minimum alveolar anesthetic concentration. *Anesth Analg.* 2003;97:718–740.
204. Wong SM, Cheng G, Homanics GE, et al. Enflurane actions on spinal cords from mice that lack the beta3 subunit of the GABA(A) receptor. *Anesthesiology.* 2001;95:154–164.
205. Homanics GE, Ferguson C, Quinlan JJ, et al. Gene knockout of the alpha6 subunit of the gamma-aminobutyric acid type a receptor: Lack of effect on responses to ethanol, pentobarbital, and general anesthetics. *Mol Pharmacol.* 1997;51:588–596.
206. Rudolph U, Crestani F, Benke D, et al. Benzodiazepine actions mediated by specific gamma-aminobutyric acid(a) receptor subtypes. *Nature.* 1999;401:796–800.
207. Belelli D, Lambert JJ, Peters JA, et al. The interaction of the general anesthetic etomidate with the gamma-aminobutyric acid type a receptor is influenced by a single amino acid. *Proc Natl Acad Sci U S A.* 1997;94:11031–11036.
208. Jurd R, Arras M, Lambert S, et al. General anesthetic actions in vivo strongly attenuated by a point mutation in the GABA(A) receptor beta3 subunit. *FASEB J.* 2003;17:250–252.
209. Reynolds DS, Rosahl TW, Cirone J, et al. Sedation and anesthesia mediated by distinct GABA(A) receptor isoforms. *J Neurosci.* 2003;23:8608–8617.
210. Cirone J, Rosahl TW, Reynolds DS, et al. Gamma-aminobutyric acid type a receptor beta 2 subunit mediates the hypothermic effect of etomidate in mice. *Anesthesiology.* 2004;100:1438–1445.
211. Lakhlani PP, MacMillan LB, Guo TZ, et al. Substitution of a mutant alpha2a-adrenergic receptor via "hit and run" gene targeting reveals the role of this subtype in sedative, analgesic, and anesthetic-sparing responses in vivo. *Proc Natl Acad Sci U S A.* 1997;94:9950–9955.
212. Gerstin KM, Gong DH, Abdallah M, et al. Mutation of KCNK5 or Kir3.2 potassium channels in mice does not change minimum alveolar anesthetic concentration. *Anesth Analg.* 2003;96:1345–1349, table of contents.
213. Sternberg WF, Mogil JF. Genetic and hormonal basis of pain states. *Best Pract Res Clin Anesthesiol.* 2001;15:229–245.
214. Diatchenko L, Anderson AD, Slade GD, et al. Three major haplotypes of the beta2 adrenergic receptor define psychological profile, blood pressure, and the risk for development of a common musculoskeletal pain disorder. *Am J Med Genet B Neuropsychiatr Genet.* 2006;141:449–462.
215. Diatchenko L, Nackley AG, Tchivileva IE, et al. Genetic architecture of human pain perception. *Trends Genet.* 2007;23:605–613.
216. Bengtsson B, Thorson J. Back pain: A study of twins. *Acta Genet Med Gemellol (Roma).* 1991;40:83–90.
217. Mogil JS, Wilson SG, Bon K, et al. Heritability of nociception I: Responses of 11 inbred mouse strains on 12 measures of nociception. *Pain.* 1999;80:67–82.
218. Lacroix-Fralish ML, Ledoux JB, Mogil JS. The pain genes database: An interactive web browser of pain-related transgenic knockout studies. *Pain.* 2007;131:3e1–3e4.
219. Somogyi AA, Barratt DT, Coller JK. Pharmacogenetics of opioids. *Clin Pharmacol Ther.* 2007;81:429–444.
220. Diatchenko L, Nackley AG, Slade GD, et al. Catechol-O-methyltransferase gene polymorphisms are associated with multiple pain-evoking stimuli. *Pain.* 2006;125:216–224.
221. Candiotti KA, Birnbach DJ, Lubarsky DA, et al. The impact of pharmacogenomics on postoperative nausea and vomiting: Do cyp2d6 allele copy number and polymorphisms affect the success or failure of ondansetron prophylaxis? *Anesthesiology.* 2005;102:543–549.
222. Cayla G, Hulot JS, O'Connor SA, et al. Clinical, angiographic, and genetic factors associated with early coronary stent thrombosis. *JAMA.* 2011;306:1765–1774.
223. Sorich MJ, Vitry A, Ward MB, et al. Prasugrel vs. clopidogrel for cytochrome P450 2C19-genotyped subgroups: Integration of the TRITON-TIMI 38 trial data. *J Thromb Haemost.* 2010;8:1678–1684.
224. Nagele P, Liggett SB. Genetic variation, beta-blockers, and perioperative myocardial infarction. *Anesthesiology.* 2011;115:1316–1327.
225. Devereaux PJ, Yang H, Yusuf S, et al. Effects of extended-release metoprolol succinate in patients undergoing non-cardiac surgery (POISE trial): A randomised controlled trial. *Lancet.* 2008;371:1839–1847.
226. Lin LH, Hopf HW. Paradigm of the injury-repair continuum during critical illness. *Crit Care Med.* 2003;31:S493–S495.
227. Angus DC, Burgner D, Wunderink R, et al. The piro concept: P is for predisposition. *Crit Care.* 2003;7:248–251.
228. Lin MT, Albertson TE. Genomic polymorphisms in sepsis. *Crit Care Med.* 2004; 32:569–579.
229. De Maio A, Torres MB, Reeves RH. Genetic determinants influencing the response to injury, inflammation, and sepsis. *Shock.* 2005;23:11–17.
230. Zeni F, Freeman B, Natanson C. Anti-inflammatory therapies to treat sepsis and septic shock: A reassessment. *Crit Care Med.* 1997;25:1095–1100.
231. Cobb JP, O'Keefe GE. Injury research in the genomic era. *Lancet.* 2004;363:2076–2083.
232. Prucha M, Ruryk A, Boriss H, et al. Expression profiling: Toward an application in sepsis diagnostics. *Shock.* 2004;22:29–33.
233. Cobb JP, Laramie JM, Stormo GD, et al. Sepsis gene expression profiling: Murine splenic compared with hepatic responses determined by using complementary DNA microarrays. *Crit Care Med.* 2002;30:2711–2721.
234. Leikauf GD, McDowell SA, Wesselkamper SC, et al. Acute lung injury: Functional genomics and genetic susceptibility. *Chest.* 2002;121:70S–75S.
235. Dasu MR, Cobb JP, Laramie JM, et al. Gene expression profiles of livers from thermally injured rats. *Gene.* 2004;327:51–60.
236. Tang BM, McLean AS, Dawes IW, et al. The use of gene-expression profiling to identify candidate genes in human sepsis. *Am J Respir Crit Care Med.* 2007; 176:676–684.
237. Calvano SE, Xiao W, Richards DR, et al. A network-based analysis of systemic inflammation in humans. *Nature.* 2005;437:1032–1037.
238. Laudanski K, Miller-Graziano C, Xiao W, et al. Cell-specific expression and pathway analyses reveal alterations in trauma-related human T cell and monocyte pathways. *Proc Natl Acad Sci U S A.* 2006;103:15564–15569.
239. Cobb JP, Mindrinos MN, Miller-Graziano C, et al. Application of genome-wide expression analysis to human health and disease. *Proc Natl Acad Sci U S A.* 2005;102:4801–4806.
240. Fessler MB, Malcolm KC, Duncan MW, et al. A genomic and proteomic analysis of activation of the human neutrophil by lipopolysaccharide and its mediation by p38 mitogen-activated protein kinase. *J Biol Chem.* 2002;277:31291–31302.
241. Liu T, Qian WJ, Gritsenko MA, et al. High dynamic range characterization of the trauma patient plasma proteome. *Mol Cell Proteomics.* 2006;5:1899–1913.
242. Kalenka A, Feldmann RE Jr, Otero K, et al. Changes in the serum proteome of patients with sepsis and septic shock. *Anesth Analg.* 2006;103:1522–1526.
243. Buchman TG, Cobb JP, Lapedes AS, et al. Complex systems analysis: A tool for shock research. *Shock.* 2001;16:248–251.
244. Strange K. The end of "naive reductionism": Rise of systems biology or renaissance of physiology? *Am J Physiol Cell Physiol.* 2005;288:C968–C974.
245. Ge H, Walhout AJ, Vidal M. Integrating 'omic' information: A bridge between genomics and systems biology. *Trends Genet.* 2003;19:551–560.
246. Lusis AJ. A thematic review series: Systems biology approaches to metabolic and cardiovascular disorders. *J Lipid Res.* 2006;47:1887–1890.
247. Shaw A. Exploring the perioptome: The role of genomics in thoracic surgery and anaesthesia. *Curr Opin Anaesthesiol.* 2007;20:32–36.
248. Khoury MJ, Yang Q, Gwinn M, et al. An epidemiologic assessment of genomic profiling for measuring susceptibility to common diseases and targeting interventions. *Genet Med.* 2004;6:38–47.
249. Hakonarson H, Thorvaldsson S, Helgadottir A, et al. Effects of a 5-lipoxygenase-activating protein inhibitor on biomarkers associated with risk of myocardial infarction: A randomized trial. *JAMA.* 2005;293:2245–2256.
250. Phimister EG. Medicine and the racial divide. *N Engl J Med.* 2003;348:1081–1082.

CHAPTER

7 Basic Principles of Clinical Pharmacology

DHANESH K. GUPTA • THOMAS K. HENTHORN

Key Points

1. Most drugs must pass through cell membranes to reach their sites of action. Consequently, drugs tend to be relatively lipophilic, rather than hydrophilic.
2. The highly lipophilic anesthetic drugs have a rapid onset of action because they rapidly diffuse into the highly perfused brain tissue. They have a very short duration of action because of redistribution of drug from the CNS to the blood.
3. The cytochrome P450 (CYP) superfamily is the most important group of enzymes involved in drug metabolism. The CYP family, along with other drug-metabolizing enzymes exhibit genetic polymorphisms.
4. The kidneys eliminate hydrophilic drugs and relatively hydrophilic metabolites of lipophilic drugs. Renal elimination of lipophilic compounds is negligible.
5. The liver is the most important organ for metabolism of drugs. Hepatic drug clearance depends on three factors: The intrinsic ability of the liver to metabolize a drug, hepatic blood flow, and the extent of binding of the drug to blood components.
6. The volume of distribution quantifies the extent of drug distribution. The greater the affinity of tissues for a drug relative to blood, the greater its volume of distribution (i.e., lipophilic drugs have greater volumes of distribution).
7. Elimination clearance is the parameter that characterizes the ability of drug-eliminating organs to irreversibly remove drugs from the body. The efficiency of the body to remove drug from the body is proportional to the elimination clearance.
8. All else being equal, an increase in the volume of distribution of a drug will increase its elimination half-life; while an increase in elimination clearance will decrease elimination half-life.
9. Most drugs bring about a pharmacologic effect by binding to a specific receptor that brings about a change in cellular function to produce the pharmacologic effect.
10. Although most pharmacologic effects can be characterized by both dose-response curves and concentration-response curves, the dose-response curves are unable to determine whether variations in pharmacologic response are caused by differences in pharmacokinetics, pharmacodynamics, or both.
11. Integrated pharmacokinetic–pharmacodynamic models allow temporal characterization of the relationship between dose, plasma concentration, and pharmacologic effect.
12. In vitro drug–drug interactions due to pharmacological (physiochemical) properties of drugs can significantly alter drug bioavailability and produce unintended toxic byproducts.
13. Novel approaches to antagonizing neuromuscular blockade have been developed that take advantage of in vivo physiochemical drug–drug interactions, thereby avoiding some of the systemic side effects associated with inhibition of plasma acetylcholinesterase.
14. Distribution clearance is influenced by changes in cardiac output and regional blood flow.
15. Inhibition of CYP isozyme activity can make it difficult to achieve adequate analgesia when using opioids, such as codeine and tramadol, that require CYP 2D6 activity for conversion to the biologically active opioid.
16. Serotonin syndrome can be precipitated by a wide array of drugs that are associated with serotonergic activity, including selective serotonin reuptake inhibitors (SSRIs), serotonin–norepinephrine reuptake inhibitors (SNRIs), and phenylpiperidine opioids.

17 Simulations of multicompartmental pharmacokinetic models that describe intravenous anesthetics demonstrate that for most anesthetic dosing regimens, the distribution of drug from the plasma to the inert peripheral tissues has a greater influence on the plasma concentration profile of the drug than the elimination of drug from the body.

18 Target-controlled infusions are achieved with computer-controlled infusion pumps worldwide (not yet FDA-approved in the United States), and permit clinicians to make use of the drug concentration–effect relationship, optimally accounting for pharmacokinetics, and predicting the offset of drug effect.

19 Classic pharmacokinetic models inaccurately describe the initial several minutes of drug distribution that occur during the time of drug onset, and therefore, overestimate the interindividual pharmacodynamic variability.

20 By understanding the interactions between the opioids and the sedative-hypnotics (e.g., response surface models), it is possible to select target concentration pairs of the two drugs that produce the desired clinical effect, while minimizing unwanted side effects associated with high concentrations of a single drug.

Multimedia

1 Dose Response Relationships

2 Drug Concentration and Effect

In 1943, Halford labeled thiopental as "an ideal method of euthanasia" for war surgical patients and pronounced that "open-drop ether still retains primacy!"[1] Based on this recount of the experience with thiopental at Pearl Harbor, it is impressive that cooler heads prevailed—Adams and Gray detailed a case of a civilian gunshot wound where they carefully titrated incremental doses of thiopental without any adverse respiratory or cardiovascular events.[2] To highlight the importance of the quiet case report versus the animated condemnation of intravenous anesthesia for patients with hemorrhagic shock, an anonymous editorial appeared in the same issue of *Anesthesiology* that attempted to give some scientific justification for the discrepancy in opinions.[3] As the editorial detailed, thiopental had a small therapeutic index and that the tolerance to normal doses was decreased in extreme physical conditions (e.g., blood loss, sepsis). Therefore, just like with open-drop ether, small doses of thiopental should be titrated to achieve the desired effects and avoid side effects associated with overdose. Fortunately, the anesthesia community did not simply abandon the use of thiopental, and in 1960, Price utilized mathematical models in order to describe the effects of hypovolemia on thiopental distribution.[4]

Anesthetic drugs are administered with the goal of rapidly establishing and maintaining a therapeutic effect while minimizing undesired side effects. Although open-drop ether and chloroform were administered using knowledge of a dose-effect relationship, the more potent volatile agents, along with the intravenous hypnotics, neuromuscular junction blocking agents, and intravenous opioids, all require a sound knowledge of pharmacokinetics and pharmacodynamics in order to accurately achieve the desired pharmacologic effect for the desired period of time without any drug toxicity.

This chapter attempts to guide the reader through the fundamental knowledge of what the body does to a drug (i.e., pharmacokinetics) and what a drug does to the body (i.e., pharmacodynamics). The initial section of this chapter discusses the biologic and pharmacologic factors that influence the absorption, distribution, and elimination of a drug from the body. Where necessary, quantitative analyses of these processes are discussed to give readers insight into the intricacies of pharmacokinetics that cannot be easily described by text alone. The second section concentrates on the factors that determine the relationship between drug concentration and pharmacologic effect. Once again, mathematical models are presented as needed in order to clarify pharmacodynamic concepts. The third section applies the knowledge from the first two sections in order to describe the clinically important drug–drug interactions that are encountered in the perioperative period. The final section builds on the reader's knowledge gained from the first two sections to apply the principles of pharmacokinetics and pharmacodynamics to determine the target concentration of intravenous anesthetics required and the dosing strategies necessary to produce an adequate anesthetic state. Understanding these concepts should allow the reader to integrate the anesthetic drugs of the future into a rational anesthetic regimen. Although specific drugs are utilized to illustrate pharmacokinetic and pharmacodynamic principles throughout this chapter, detailed pharmacologic information of anesthetic pharmacopeia are presented in subsequent chapters of this book.

PHARMACOKINETIC PRINCIPLES

Drug Absorption and Routes of Administration

Transfer of Drugs across Membranes

1 For even the simplest drug that is directly administered into the blood to exert its action, it must move across at least one cell membrane to its site of action. Because biologic membranes are lipid bilayers composed of a lipophilic core sandwiched between two hydrophilic layers, only small lipophilic drugs can passively diffuse across the membrane down its concentration gradient. For water-soluble drugs to passively diffuse across the membrane down its concentration gradient, transmembrane proteins that form a hydrophilic channel are required. Because of the abundance of these nonspecific hydrophilic channels in the capillary endothelium of all organs except for the central nervous system (CNS), where the blood–brain barrier capillary endothelial cells have very limited numbers of transmembrane hydrophilic channels, passive transport of drugs from the intravascular space into the interstitium of various organs is limited by blood flow, not by the lipid solubility of the drug.[5]

Hydrophilic drugs can only enter the CNS after binding to drug specific transmembrane proteins that actively transport the hydrophilic drug across the capillary endothelium into the CNS interstitium. When these transmembrane carrier proteins require energy to transport the drug across the membrane, they are able to shuttle proteins against their concentration gradients, a process called *active transport.* In contrast, when these carrier proteins do not require energy to shuttle drugs, they cannot overcome concentration gradients, a process called *facilitated diffusion.* Therefore, active transport is not limited to the CNS, but is also found in the organs related to drug elimination (e.g., hepatocytes, renal tubular cells, pulmonary capillary endothelium), where the ability to transport drugs against the concentration gradient has specific biologic advantages. Both active transport and facilitated diffusion of drugs are saturable processes that are only limited by the number of carrier proteins available to shuttle a specific drug.[5]

For lipophilic compounds transporters are not needed for the drug to diffuse across the capillary wall into tissues, but the presence of transporters does affect the concentration gradients that exist. For instance, some lipophilic drugs are transported out of tissues by ATP-dependent transporters such as p-glycoprotein (P-gp). The lipophilic potent μ-opioid agonist, loperamide, used for the treatment of diarrhea, has limited bioavailability because of P-gp transporters at the intestine-portal capillary interface and then what does reach the circulation has its CNS penetrance limited by P-gp at the blood–brain barrier.[6] Conversely, lipophilic compounds can be transported into tissues, increasing the tissue concentration of the drug beyond what would be accomplished by passive diffusion. The class of transporters called organic anion polypeptide transporters (OATPs), like P-gp, is located in the microvascular endothelium of the brain and transport endogenous opioids into the brain.[7,8] These OATPs also transport drugs. The degree to which transporter proteins may account for intra- and interindividual responses to anesthetic drugs has not been well studied to date.[9]

Intravenous Administration

For a drug to be delivered to its site of action, the drug must be absorbed into the systemic circulation. Therefore, intravenous administration results in rapid increases in drug concentration. Although this can lead to a very rapid onset of drug effect, for drugs that have a low *therapeutic index* (the ratio of the intravenous dose that produces a toxic effect in 50% of the population to the intravenous dose that produces a therapeutic effect in 50% of the population), rapid overshoot of the desired plasma concentration can potentially result in immediate and severe side effects. Except for intravenous (IV) administration, the absorption of a drug into the systemic circulation is an important determinant of the time course of drug action and the maximum drug effect produced. As the absorption of drug is slowed, the maximum plasma concentration and drug effect achieved is limited. However, as long as the plasma concentration is maintained at a level above the minimum effective plasma concentration, the drug will produce an effect.[10] Therefore, non-intravenous methods of administration can produce a sustained and significant effect that may be more advantageous than administering drugs by the intravenous route.[11]

Bioavailability is the *relative amount* of a drug dose that reaches the systemic circulation unchanged and the *rate* at which this occurs. For most intravenously administered drugs, the absolute bioavailability of the drug available is close to unity and the rate is nearly instantaneous. However, the pulmonary endothelium can slow the rate at which intravenously administered drugs reach the systemic circulation if distribution into the alveolar endothelium is extensive such as that occurs with the pulmonary uptake of fentanyl. The pulmonary endothelium also contains enzymes that may metabolize intravenously administered drugs (e.g., propofol) on first pass and reduce their absolute bioavailability.[12]

Oral Administration

For almost all therapeutic agents used across all fields of medicine, oral administration is perhaps the safest and most convenient method of administration. However, this route is not utilized significantly in anesthetic practice because of the limited and variable rate of bioavailability. The absorption rate in the gastrointestinal tract is highly variable because the main determinant of the timing of absorption is gastric emptying into the small intestines, where the surface area for absorption is several orders of magnitude greater than that of the stomach or large intestines. Additionally, the active metabolism of drug by the small intestine mucosal epithelium, and the obligatory path through the portal circulation before entering the systemic circulation, contribute to decreased bioavailability of orally administered drugs.[13] In fact, the metabolic capacity of the liver for drugs is so high that only a small fraction of most lipophilic drugs actually reach the systemic circulation. Because of this extensive *first-pass metabolism,* the oral dose of most drugs must be significantly higher to generate a therapeutic plasma concentration. Coupled with the prolonged and variable time until peak concentrations are usually achieved from oral administration (between tens of minutes to hours), it is nearly impractical to utilize this mode to administer perioperative anesthetic agents.

Highly lipophilic drugs that can maintain a high contact time with nasal or oral (sublingual) mucosa can be absorbed without needing to traverse the gastrointestinal tract. Sublingual administration of drug has the additional advantage over gastrointestinal absorption in that absorbed drug directly enters the systemic venous circulation and therefore is able to bypass the metabolically active intestinal mucosa and the hepatic first pass metabolism. Therefore, small amounts of drug can rapidly produce a significant plasma concentration and therapeutic effect.[14] However, because of formulation limitations and the small amount of surface area available for absorption, sublingual administration is limited to drugs that fortuitously meet these requirements and require a rapid onset of drug action (e.g., nitroglycerine, fentanyl).

Transcutaneous Administration

A few lipophilic drugs have been manufactured in formulations that are sufficient to allow penetration of intact skin. Although scopolamine, nitroglycerin, opioids, and clonidine all produce therapeutic systemic plasma concentrations when administered as "drug patches," the extended amount of time that it takes to achieve an effective therapeutic concentration limits practical application except for maintenance therapy. Attempts to speed the passive diffusion of these drugs utilizing an electric current has been described for fentanyl,[15] but it is still limited in its practicality.

Intramuscular and Subcutaneous Administration

Absorption of drugs from the depots in the subcutaneous tissue or in muscle tissue is directly dependent on the drug formulation and the blood flow to the depot. Because of the high blood flow to muscles in most physiologic states, intramuscular absorption of drugs in solution is relatively rapid and complete. Therefore, some aqueous drugs can be administered as intramuscular injection with rapid and predictable effects (e.g., neuromuscular junction blocking agents). The subcutaneous route of drug absorption is more variable in its onset because of the variability of subcutaneous blood flow during varying physiologic states—this is the primary reason that subcutaneous heparin and regular insulin administered perioperatively have a variable time of onset and maximum effect.

Intrathecal, Epidural, and Perineural Injection

Because the spinal cord is the primary site of action of many anesthetic agents, direct injection of local anesthetics and opioids directly into the intrathecal space bypasses the limitations of drug absorption and distribution compared to any other route of administration. However, this is not the case for epidural and perineural administration of local anesthetics, because not delivering the drug directly into the cerebrospinal fluid necessitates that the drug be absorbed through the dura or nerve sheath in order to reach the site of drug action. The major downside to all of these techniques is the relative expertise required to perform regional anesthetics relative to oral, intravenous, and inhalational administration of drug.

Inhalational Administration

The large surface area of the pulmonary alveoli available for exchange with the large volumetric flow of blood found in the pulmonary capillaries makes inhalational administration an extremely attractive method by which to administer drugs.[16] New technologies have been developed that can rapidly and predictably aerosolize a wide range of drugs and thus approximate intravenous administration.[17] These devices are currently in Phase II FDA trials.

Drug Distribution

Once drug has entered the systemic circulation, it is transported through bulk flow of blood to all of the organs throughout the body. The relative distribution of cardiac output among organ vascular beds determines the speed at which organs are exposed to the drug. The highly perfused core circulatory components—the brain, lungs, heart, and kidneys receive the highest relative distribution of cardiac output, and therefore, are the initial organs to reach equilibrium with plasma drug concentrations.[4] Drug concentrations then equilibrate with the less well-perfused muscles and liver and then, finally, with the relatively poorly perfused splanchnic vasculature, adipose tissue, and bone.

Whether by passive diffusion or transporter-mediation, drug transport at the capillaries is not usually saturable; hence the amount of drug uptake by tissues and organs is limited by the blood flow they receive (i.e., flow-limited drug uptake).

Although the rate of initial drug delivery may be dependent on the relative blood flow of the organ, the rate of drug equilibration by the tissue is dependent on the ratio of blood flow to tissue content. Therefore, drug uptake rapidly approaches equilibrium in the highly perfused, but low volume brain, kidneys, and lungs in a matter of minutes, whereas drug transfer to the less well perfused, intermediate volume muscle tissue, may take hours to approach equilibrium, and drug transfer to the poorly perfused, large cellular volumes of adipose tissue, does not equilibrate for days.[11]

Redistribution

2 Highly lipophilic drugs, such as thiopental and propofol, rapidly begin to diffuse into the highly perfused brain tissue usually less than a minute after intravenous injection. Because of the low tissue volume and high perfusion of the brain, the drug concentration in the cerebral arterial blood rapidly equilibrates, usually within 3 minutes, with the concentration in the brain tissue. As the drug continues to be taken up by other tissues with lower blood flows and higher tissue mass, the plasma concentration of the drug continues to rapidly decrease. Once the concentration of drug in the brain tissue is higher than the plasma concentration of the drug, there is a reversal of the drug concentration gradient so that the lipophilic drug readily diffuses back into the blood and is *redistributed* to the other tissues that are still taking up the drug.[4,18,19] This process continues for each of the organ beds until ultimately, the adipose tissue will contain the majority of the lipophilic drug that has not been removed from the body by metabolism or excretion. However, after a single bolus of a highly lipophilic drug, the brain's tissue concentration rapidly decreases below therapeutic levels due to redistribution of drug to muscle tissue, which has a larger perfusion than adipose tissue.[4,19] Although single, moderate doses of highly lipophilic drugs have a very short CNS duration of action because of redistribution of drug from the CNS to the blood and other, less well-perfused tissues, repeated injections of a drug allows the rapid establishment of significant peripheral tissue concentrations. When the tissue concentrations of a drug are high enough, the decrease in plasma drug concentration below therapeutic threshold becomes solely dependent on drug elimination from the body.[20]

Drug Elimination

Besides being excreted unchanged from the body, a drug can be biotransformed (metabolized) into one or more new compounds that are then eliminated from the body. Either mechanism of elimination will decrease the drug concentration in the body such that the concentration will eventually be negligible and therefore unable to produce drug effect. Elimination is the pharmacokinetic term that describes all the processes that remove a drug from the body. Although the liver and the kidneys are considered the major organs of drug elimination, drug metabolism can occur at many other locations that contain active drug metabolizing enzymes (e.g., pulmonary vasculature, red blood cells) and the drug can be excreted unchanged from other organs (e.g., lungs).

Elimination clearance (drug clearance) is the theoretical volume of blood from which drug is completely and irreversibly removed in a unit of time.[21] Elimination clearance has the units of flow—[volume per time]. *Total* drug clearance can be calculated with pharmacokinetic models of blood concentration versus time data.

Biotransformation Reactions

Most drugs that are excreted unchanged from the body are hydrophilic and therefore readily passed into urine or stool. Drugs that are not sufficiently hydrophilic to be able to be excreted unchanged, require modification into more hydrophilic, excretable compounds. Enzymatic reactions that metabolize drugs can be classified into Phase I and Phase II biotransformation reactions. Phase I reactions tend to transform a drug into one or more polar, and hence potentially excretable, compounds. Phase II reactions transform the original drug by conjugating a variety of endogenous compounds to a polar functional group of the drug, making the metabolite even more hydrophilic. Often drugs will undergo a Phase I reaction to produce a new compound with a polar functional group that will then undergo a Phase II reaction. However, it is possible for a drug to undergo either a Phase I or a Phase II reaction alone.

Phase I Reactions

Phase I reactions may hydrolyze, oxidize, or reduce the parent compound. *Hydrolysis* is the insertion of a molecule of water into another molecule, which forms an unstable intermediate compound that subsequently splits apart. Thus, hydrolysis cleaves the original substance into two separate molecules. Hydrolytic reactions are the primary way amides, such as lidocaine and other amide local anesthetics, and esters, such as succinylcholine, are metabolized.

Many drugs are biotransformed by oxidative reactions. *Oxidations* are defined as reactions that remove electrons from a molecule. The common element of most, if not all, oxidations is an enzymatically mediated reaction that inserts a hydroxyl group (OH) into the drug molecule. In some instances, this action produces a chemically stable, more polar hydroxylated metabolite. However, hydroxylation usually creates unstable compounds that spontaneously split into separate molecules. Many different biotransformations are effected by this basic mechanism. Dealkylation (removal of a carbon-containing group), deamination (removal of nitrogen-containing groups), oxidation of nitrogen-containing groups, desulfuration, dehalogenation, and dehydrogenation all follow an initial hydroxylation. Hydrolysis and hydroxylation are comparable processes. Both have an initial, enzymatically mediated step that produces an unstable compound that rapidly dissociates into separate molecules.

Some drugs are metabolized by *reductive reactions,* that is, reactions that add electrons to a molecule. In contrast to oxidations, where electrons are transferred from NADPH to an oxygen atom, the electrons are transferred to the drug molecule. Oxidation of xenobiotics requires oxygen, but reductive biotransformation is inhibited by oxygen, so it is facilitated when the intracellular oxygen tension is low.

Cytochrome P450 Enzymes

3 The cytochrome P450 (CYP) is the superfamily of constitutive and inducible enzymes that catalyze most Phase I biotransformations. CYP3A4 is the single most important enzyme, accounting for 40% to 45% of all CYP-mediated drug metabolism. CYP enzymes are incorporated into the smooth endoplasmic reticulum of hepatocytes and the membranes of the upper intestinal enterocytes in high concentrations. CYP are also found in the lungs, kidneys, and skin, but in much smaller amounts. CYP isoenzymes oxidize their substrates primarily by the insertion of an atom of oxygen in the form of a hydroxyl group, while another oxygen atom is reduced to water.

Several constitutive CYPs are involved in the production of various endogenous compounds, such as cholesterol, steroid hormones, prostaglandins, and eicosanoids. In addition to the constitutive forms, production of various CYPs can be induced by a wide variety of xenobiotics. CYP drug-metabolizing activity increases after exposure to various exogenous chemicals, including many drugs. The number and type of CYPs present at any time depends on exposure to different xenobiotics. The CYP system is able to protect the organism from the deleterious effects of accumulation of exogenous compounds because of its two fundamental characteristics—broad substrate specificity and the capability to adapt to exposure to different substances by induction of different CYP isoenzymes. Table 7-1 groups drugs encountered in anesthetic practice according to the CYP isoenzymes responsible for their biotransformation.

Biotransformations can be inhibited if different substrates compete for the drug-binding site on the same CYP member. The effect of two competing substrates on each other's metabolism depends on their relative affinities for the enzyme. Biotransformation of the compound with the lower affinity is inhibited to a greater degree. This is the mechanism by which the H_2 receptor antagonist cimetidine inhibits the metabolism of many drugs, including meperidine, propranolol, and diazepam. The newer H_2 antagonist ranitidine has a different structure and causes fewer clinically significant drug interactions. Other drugs, notably calcium channel blockers and antidepressants, also inhibit oxidative drug metabolism in humans. This information allows clinicians to predict which combinations of drugs are more likely to lead to clinically significant interactions because of altered drug metabolism by the cytochrome P450 system.

TABLE 7-1. SUBSTRATES FOR CYTOCHROME P450 (CYP) ISOENZYMES ENCOUNTERED IN ANESTHESIOLOGY

CYP3A4	CYP2D6	CYP2B6	CYP2C9	CYP2C19
Acetaminophen	Captopril	Methadone	Diclofenac	Diazepam
Alfentanil	Codeine	Propofol	Ibuprofen	Omeprazole
Alprazolam	Hydrocodone		Indomethacin	Propranolol
Bupivacaine	Metoprolol			Warfarin
Cisapride	Ondansetron			
Codeine	Oxycodone			
Diazepam	Propranolol			
Digitoxin	Timolol			
Diltiazem				
Fentanyl				
Lidocaine				
Midazolam				
Nicardipine				
Nifedipine				
Omeprazole				
Ropivacaine				
Statins				
Sufentanil				
Verapamil				
Warfarin				

Phase II Reactions

Phase II reactions are also known as *conjugation* or *synthetic reactions.* Many drugs do not have a polar chemical group suitable for conjugation, so it occurs only after a Phase I reaction. Other drugs, such as morphine, already have a polar group that serves as a "handle" for conjugation, and they undergo these reactions directly. Various endogenous compounds can be attached to parent drugs or their Phase I metabolites to form different conjugation products. These endogenous substrates include glucuronic acid, acetate, and amino acids. Mercapturic acid conjugates result from the binding of exogenous compounds to glutathione. Other conjugation reactions produce sulfated or methylated derivatives of drugs or their metabolites. Like the cytochrome P450 system, the enzymes that catalyze Phase II reactions are inducible. Phase II reactions produce conjugates that are polar, water-soluble compounds. This facilitates the ultimate excretion of the drug via the kidneys or hepatobiliary secretion. Like CYP, there are different families and superfamilies of the enzymes that catalyze Phase II biotransformations.

Genetic Variations in Drug Metabolism

For most enzymes involved in Phase I and Phase II reactions, there are several biologically available isoforms. Drug metabolism varies substantially among individuals because of variability in the genes controlling the numerous enzymes responsible for biotransformation. For most drugs, individual subjects' rates of metabolism have a unimodal distribution. However, distinct subpopulations with different rates of elimination of some drugs have been identified. The resulting multimodal distribution of individual rates of metabolism is known as *polymorphism.* For example, different genotypes result in either normal, low, or (rarely) absent plasma pseudocholinesterase activity, accounting for the well-known differences in individuals' responses to succinylcholine, which is hydrolyzed by this enzyme. Many drug-metabolizing enzymes exhibit genetic polymorphism, including CYP and various transferases that catalyze phase II reactions. However, none of these have a sex-related difference.

Chronologic Variations in Drug Metabolism

The activity and capacity of the CYP enzymes increase from subnormal levels in the fetal and neonatal period, to reach normal levels at about 1 year of age. Although age is a covariate in mathematical models of drug elimination, it is not clear if these changes are related to chronologic changes in organ function (age-related organ dysfunction) or a decrease in CYP levels with increasing age. In contrast, it is clear that the neonate has a limited ability to perform phase II conjugation reactions, but after normalizing phase II activity over the initial year of life, advanced age does not affect the capacity to perform phase II reactions.

Renal Drug Clearance

4 The primary role of the kidneys in drug elimination is to excrete into urine the unchanged, hydrophilic drugs, and the hepatic derived metabolites from Phase I and Phase II reactions of lipophilic drugs. The passive elimination of drugs by passive glomerular filtration is a very inefficient process—any significant degree of binding of the drug to plasma proteins or erythrocytes will decrease the renal clearance below the glomerular filtration rate of 20% of renal blood flow. In order to make renal elimination more efficient, discrete active transporters of organic acids and bases exist in the proximal renal tubular cells. Although these transporters are saturable, they allow for the renal clearance of drugs to approach the entire renal blood flow.

In reality, renal drug clearance of actively secreted drugs can be inhibited by both passive tubular reabsorption of lipophilic drugs and active, carrier-mediated tubular reabsorption of hydrophilic drugs. Therefore, the small amount of filtered and secreted lipophilic drug is easily reabsorbed in the distal tubules, making the net renal clearance negligible. In contrast, the large amount of filtered and secreted hydrophilic drug can be passively reabsorbed if renal tubular flow decreases substantially (e.g., oliguria) and/or the urine pH favors the unionized form of the hydrophilic drug. Because overall renal function is readily estimated by clearance of endogenous creatinine, renal drug clearance, even for drugs eliminated primarily by tubular secretion, is dependent on renal function. Therefore, in patients with acute and chronic causes of decreased renal function, including advanced age, low cardiac output states, and hepatorenal syndrome, drug dosing must be altered in order to avoid accumulation of parent compounds and potentially toxic metabolites (e.g., lidocaine, meperidine) (Table 7-2).

TABLE 7-2. DRUGS WITH SIGNIFICANT RENAL EXCRETION ENCOUNTERED IN ANESTHESIOLOGY

Aminoglycosides	Pancuronium
Atenolol	Penicillins
Cephalosporins	Procainamide
Digoxin	Pyridostigmine
Edrophonium	Quinolones
Nadolol	Rocuronium
Neostigmine	Sugammadex

Hepatic Drug Clearance

5 Drug elimination by the liver depends on the intrinsic ability of the liver to metabolize the drug (intrinsic clearance, Cl_I), and the amount of drug available to diffuse into the liver. Many types of mathematical models have been developed to attempt to accurately model the relationship between hepatic artery blood flow, portal artery blood flow, intrinsic clearance, and drug binding to plasma proteins.[22,23] According to these models, the unbound concentration of drug in the hepatic venous blood (C_v) is in equilibrium with the drug within the liver that is available for elimination. These models also make the assumption that the entire drug delivered to the liver is available for elimination and that the elimination is a first-order process—a constant *fraction* of the available drug is eliminated per unit time. The fraction of the drug removed from the blood passing through the liver is the hepatic extraction ratio, *E:*

$$E = \frac{C_a - C_v}{C_a} \qquad (7\text{-}1)$$

where C_a is the mixed hepatic arterial–portal venous drug concentration and C_v is the mixed hepatic venous drug concentration. The total hepatic drug clearance, Cl_H, is:

$$Cl_H = Q \cdot E \qquad (7\text{-}2)$$

where Q is the hepatic blood flow. Therefore, hepatic clearance is a function of hepatic blood flow and the ability of the liver to extract drug from the blood.

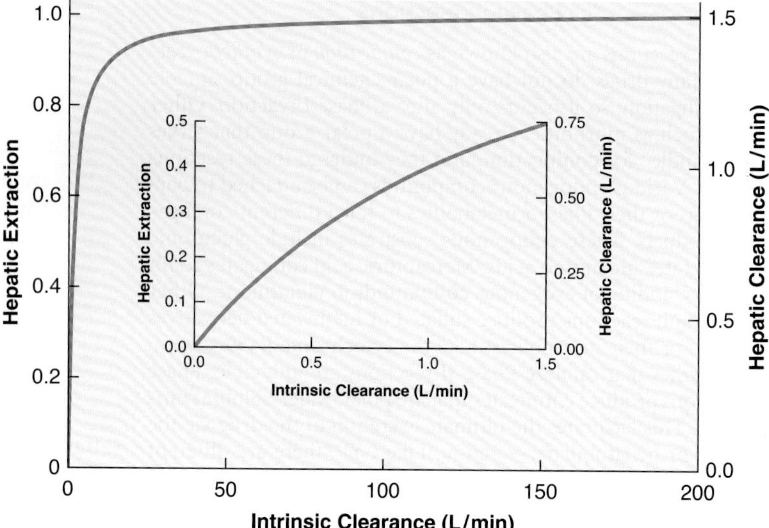

FIGURE 7-1. The relationship between hepatic extraction ratio (E, left y-axis), intrinsic clearance (Cl_I, x-axis), and hepatic clearance (Cl_H, right y-axis) at the normal hepatic blood flow (Q) of 1.5 L/min. For drugs with a high intrinsic clearance ($Cl_I >> Q$), increasing intrinsic clearance has little effect on hepatic extraction and total hepatic clearance and total hepatic clearance approaches hepatic blood flow. In contrast, if the intrinsic clearance is small ($Cl_I \leq Q$), the extraction ratio is similar to the intrinsic clearance (inset). (Adapted from: Wilkinson GR, Shand DG: A physiologic approach to hepatic drug clearance. *Clin Pharmacol Ther.* 1975;18:377.)

The ability to extract drug depends on the activity of drug-metabolizing enzymes and the capacity for hepatobiliary excretion—the intrinsic clearance of the liver (Cl_I).

Intrinsic clearance represents the ability of the liver to remove drug from the blood in the absence of any limitations imposed by blood flow or drug binding. The relationship of total hepatic drug clearance to the extraction ratio and intrinsic clearance, Cl_I, is:

$$Cl_H = Q \cdot E = Q\left(\frac{Cl_1}{Q + Cl_1}\right) \tag{7-3}$$

The right-hand side of Equation 7-3 indicates that if intrinsic clearance is very high (many times larger than hepatic blood flow, $Cl_I >> Q$), total hepatic clearance approaches hepatic blood flow. On the other hand, if intrinsic clearance is very small ($Q + Cl_I \approx Q$), hepatic clearance will be similar to intrinsic clearance. These relationships are shown in Figure 7-1.

Thus, hepatic drug clearance and extraction are determined by two independent variables, intrinsic clearance and hepatic blood flow. Changes in either will change hepatic clearance. However, the extent of the change depends on the initial relationship between intrinsic clearance and hepatic blood flow, according to the nonlinear relationship:

$$E = \frac{Cl_1}{Q + Cl_1} \tag{7-4}$$

If the initial intrinsic clearance is small relative to hepatic blood flow, then the extraction ratio is also small, and Equation 7-4 reduces to the following relationship:

$$E = \frac{Cl_I}{Q} \ll 1 \tag{7-4a}$$

Equation 7-4a indicates that doubling intrinsic clearance will produce an almost proportional increment as in the extraction ratio, and, consequently, hepatic elimination clearance (Fig. 7-1, inset). However, if intrinsic clearance is much greater than hepatic blood flow, Equation 7-4 reduces to the following relationship:

$$E = \frac{Cl_I}{Cl_I} \approx 1 \tag{7-4b}$$

Equation 7-4b demonstrates that the extraction ratio is independent of intrinsic clearance and therefore a change in intrinsic clearance has a negligible effect on the extraction ratio and hepatic drug clearance (Fig. 7-1). In nonmathematical terms, high intrinsic clearance indicates efficient hepatic elimination. It is hard to enhance an already efficient process, whereas it is relatively easy to improve on inefficient drug clearance because of low intrinsic clearance.

For drugs with a high extraction ratio and a high intrinsic clearance, hepatic elimination clearance is directly proportional to hepatic blood flow. Therefore, any manipulation of hepatic blood flow will be directly reflected by a proportional change in hepatic elimination clearance (Fig. 7-2). In contrast, when the intrinsic

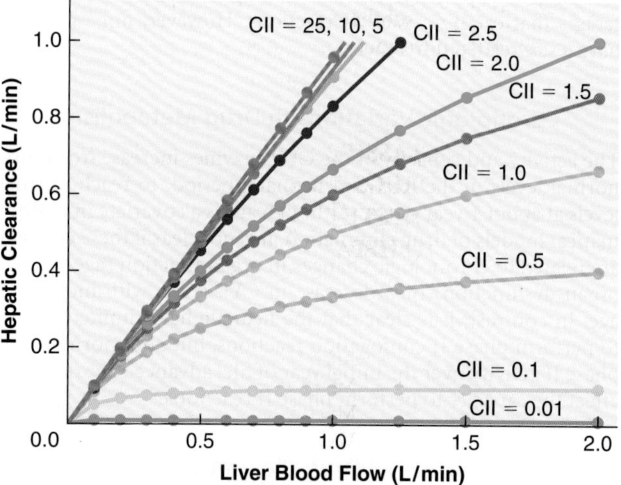

FIGURE 7-2. The relationship between liver blood flow (Q, x-axis) and hepatic clearance (Cl_H, y-axis) for different values of intrinsic clearance (Cl_I). When the intrinsic clearance is low, hepatic elimination clearance is independent of liver blood flow—the drug elimination is limited by the capacity of the liver to metabolize the drug (i.e., the intrinsic clearance). In contrast, as intrinsic clearance increases, the hepatic elimination becomes more dependent on hepatic blood flow—the liver is able to metabolize all of the drug that it is exposed to and therefore only limited by the amount of drug that is delivered to the liver (i.e., flow limited metabolism).

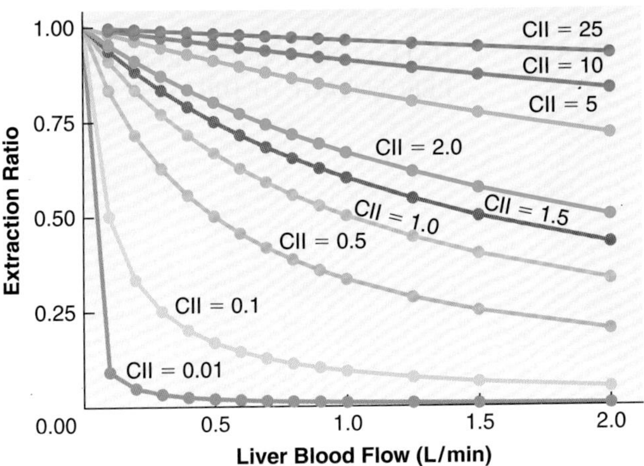

FIGURE 7-3. The relationship between liver blood flow (*Q*, x-axis) and hepatic extraction ratio (*E*, y-axis) for different values of intrinsic clearance (*Cl$_I$*). When the intrinsic clearance is low, increases in hepatic blood flows cause a decrease in the extraction ratio because the liver has limited metabolic capabilities. In contrast, when the intrinsic clearance is high, the extraction ratio is essentially independent of hepatic blood flow because the liver's ability to eliminate drug is well above the amount of drug provided by normal hepatic blood flow.

clearance is low, changes in hepatic blood flow produce inversely proportional changes in extraction ratio (Fig. 7-3), and therefore the hepatic elimination clearance is essentially independent of hepatic blood flow and exquisitely related to intrinsic clearance (Fig. 7-3). Therefore, classifying drugs as having either low, intermediate, or high extraction ratios (Table 7-3), allows predictions to be made on how intrinsic hepatic clearance and blood flow affect hepatic elimination clearance. This allows gross adjustments to be made in hepatically metabolized drug dosing to avoid excess accumulation of drugs (decreased hepatic elimination without dose adjustment) or subtherapeutic dosing strategies (increased hepatic elimination without dose adjustment).

TABLE 7-3. CLASSIFICATION OF DRUGS ENCOUNTERED IN ANESTHESIOLOGY ACCORDING TO HEPATIC EXTRACTION RATIOS

Low	Intermediate	High
Diazepam	Alfentanil	Alprenolol
Lorazepam	Methohexital	Bupivacaine
Methadone	Midazolam	Diltiazem
Phenytoin	Vecuronium	Fentanyl
Rocuronium		Ketamine
Theophylline		Lidocaine
Thiopental		Meperidine
		Metoprolol
		Morphine
		Naloxone
		Nifedipine
		Propofol
		Propranolol
		Sufentanil

Pharmacologic and pathologic manipulations of cardiac output with its consequences on hepatic/splanchnic blood flow and renal blood flow are important covariates when designing drug dosing strategies.[24] As detailed above, in states where cardiac output is decreased (e.g., heart failure, shock, spinal anesthesia), high extraction ratio drugs will have a decrease in hepatic elimination, whereas low extraction rate drugs will have minimal change in clearance.[25,26] In contrast, autoregulation of renal blood flow maintains a relatively constant renal elimination clearance until low urine output states eventually allow increased reabsorption of drugs from the distal tubules.[27]

Pharmacokinetic Models

The concentration of drug at its site or sites of action is the fundamental determinant of a drug's pharmacologic effects. Although the blood is rarely the site of action, the tissue drug concentration of an individual organ is a function of the blood flow to the organ, the concentration of drug in the arterial inflow of the organ, the capacity of the organ to take up drug, and the ability of the drug to diffuse between the blood and the organ.

Physiologic versus Compartment Models

Initial pharmacokinetic models of intravenous and inhalational anesthetics used physiologic or perfusion models.[4] In these models, body tissues were lumped into groups that had similar distribution of cardiac output and capacity for drug uptake. Highly perfused tissues with a large amount of blood flow per volume of tissue were classified as the vessel rich group, whereas tissues with a balanced amount of blood flow per volume of tissue were classified as the lean tissue group or fast tissue group. The vessel-poor group (slow tissue group) was comprised of tissues that had a large capacity for drug uptake but a limited tissue perfusion. Although identification of the exact organs that made up each tissue group was not possible from the mathematical model, it was apparent that the highly perfused tissues were comprised of the brain, lungs, kidneys, and a subset of muscle, the fast equilibrating tissue would be consistent with the majority of muscle and some of the splanchnic bed (e.g., liver), and the slowly equilibrating tissues contained the majority of the adipose tissue and the remainder of the splanchnic organs.

Based on the computationally and experimentally intense physiologic models, Price was able to demonstrate that awakening after a single dose of thiopental was primarily a result of redistribution of thiopental from the brain to the muscle with little contribution by distribution to less well-perfused tissues or drug metabolism.[4,18] This fundamental concept of redistribution applies to all lipophilic drugs and was not delineated until an accurate pharmacokinetic model had been constructed.

Perfusion-based physiologic pharmacokinetic models have provided significant insights into how physiologic, pharmacologic, and pathologic distribution of cardiac output can effect drug distribution and elimination.[28,29] However, verification of the predictions of these models requires measurement of drug concentrations in many different tissues, which is experimentally inefficient and destructive to the system. Therefore, simpler mathematical models have been developed. In these models, the body is comprised of one or more compartments. Drug concentrations in the blood are used to define the relationship between dose and the time course of changes in the drug concentration. The compartments of the compartmental pharmacokinetic models cannot be equated with the tissue groups that make up physiologic pharmacokinetic models because the compartments are theoretical entities that are used to mathematically characterize the blood concentration profile of a drug. These models allow the derivation of pharmacokinetic parameters that can be used to quantify drug distribution and elimination—volume of distribution, clearance, and half-lives.

Although the simplicity of compartmental models, compared to physiologic pharmacokinetic models, has its advantages, it also has some disadvantages. For example, cardiac output is not a parameter of compartmental models, and therefore cannot be used to predict directly the effect of cardiac failure on drug disposition.[30] However, compartmental pharmacokinetic models can still quantify the effects of reduced cardiac output on the disposition of a drug if a group of patients with cardiac failure is compared to a group of otherwise healthy subjects.

The discipline of pharmacokinetics is, to the despair of many, mathematically based. In the succeeding sections, formulas are used to illustrate the concepts needed to understand and interpret pharmacokinetic studies. Readers are encouraged to concentrate on the concepts, not the formulas.

Pharmacokinetic Concepts

Rate Constants and Half-lives

The disposition of most drugs follows *first-order* kinetics. A first-order kinetic process is one in which a constant fraction of the drug is removed during a finite period of time regardless of the drug amount or concentration. This fraction is equivalent to the rate constant of the process. Rate constants are usually denoted by the letter k and have units of "inverse time," such as min^{-1} or h^{-1}. If 10% of the drug is eliminated per minute, then the rate constant is $0.1\ \text{min}^{-1}$. Since a constant fraction is removed per unit of time in first-order kinetics, the absolute amount of drug removed is proportional to the concentration of the drug. It follows that, in first-order kinetics, the rate of change of the amount of drug at any given time is proportional to the concentration present at that time. When the concentration is high, more drug will be removed than when it is low. First-order kinetics apply not only to elimination, but also to absorption and distribution.

Rather than using rate constants, the rapidity of pharmacokinetic processes is often described with half-lives—the time required for the concentration to change by a factor of 2. Half-lives are calculated directly from the corresponding rate constants with this simple equation:

$$t_{1/2} = \frac{\ln 2}{k} = \frac{0.693}{k} \qquad (7\text{-}6)$$

Thus, a rate constant of $0.1\ \text{min}^{-1}$ translates into a half-life of 6.93 minutes. The half-life of any first-order kinetic process, including drug absorption, distribution, and elimination, can be calculated. First-order processes asymptotically approach completion, because a constant fraction of the drug, not an absolute amount, is removed per unit of time. However, after five half-lives, the process will be almost 97% complete (Table 7-4). For practical purposes, this is essentially 100% and therefore there is a negligible amount of drug remaining in the body.

Volume of Distribution

6 The volume of distribution quantifies the extent of drug distribution. The physiologic factor that governs the extent of drug distribution is the overall capacity of tissues versus the capacity of blood for that drug. Overall tissue capacity for uptake of a drug is in turn a function of the total mass of the tissues into which a drug distributes and their average affinity for the drug.

TABLE 7-4. HALF-LIVES AND CORRESPONDING PERCENTAGE OF DRUG REMOVED

Number of Half-Lives	Percentage of Drug Remaining	Percentage of Drug Removed
0	100	0
1	50	50
2	25	75
3	12.5	87.5
4	6.25	93.75
5	3.125	96.875

In compartmental pharmacokinetic models, drugs are envisaged as distributing into one or more "boxes," or compartments. These compartments cannot be equated directly with specific tissues. Rather, they are hypothetical entities that permit analysis of drug distribution and elimination and description of the drug concentration versus time profile.

The volume of distribution is an "apparent" volume because it represents the size of these hypothetical boxes, that are necessary to explain the concentration of drug in a reference compartment, usually called the *central* or *plasma compartment.* The volume of distribution, V_d, relates the total amount of drug present to the concentration observed in the central compartment:

$$V_d = \frac{\textit{amount of drug administered}}{\textit{initial drug plasma concentration}} \qquad (7\text{-}7)$$

If a drug is extensively distributed, then the concentration will be lower relative to the amount of drug present, which equates to a larger volume of distribution. For example, if a total of 10 mg of drug is present and the concentration is 2 mg/L, then the apparent volume of distribution is 5 L. On the other hand, if the concentration was 4 mg/L, then the volume of distribution would be 2.5 L.

Simply stated, the apparent volume of distribution is a numeric index of the extent of drug distribution that does not have any relationship to the actual volume of any tissue or group of tissues. It may be as small as plasma volume, or, if overall tissue uptake is extensive, the apparent volume of distribution may greatly exceed the actual total volume of the body. In general, lipophilic drugs have larger volumes of distribution than hydrophilic drugs. Since the volume of distribution is a mathematical construct to model the distribution of a drug in the body, it cannot provide any information regarding the actual tissue concentration in any specific real organ in the body. However, this simple mathematical construct provides a useful summary description of the behavior of the drug in the body. In fact, the loading dose of drug required to achieve a target plasma concentration can be easily calculated by rearranging Equation 7-7 as follows:

$$\textit{Loading Dose} = V_d \times \textit{Target Concentration} \qquad (7\text{-}7a)$$

On the basis of this equation, it is clear that an increase in the volume of distribution means that a larger loading dose will be required to "fill up the box" and achieve the same concentration. Therefore, any change in state because of changes in physiologic and pathologic conditions can alter the volume of distribution, necessitating therapeutic adjustments.

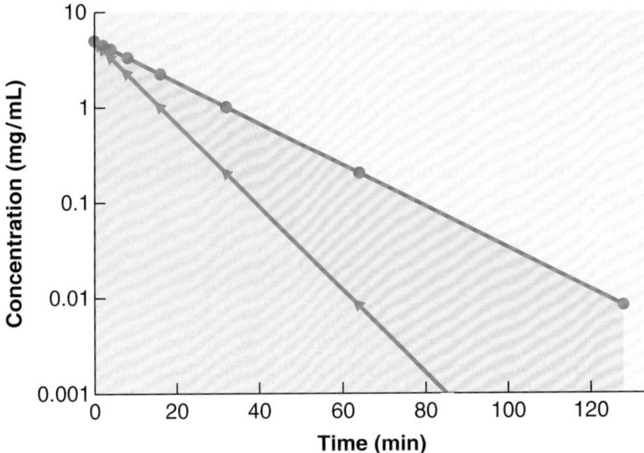

FIGURE 7-4. The plasma concentration (y-axis) versus time (x-axis) curve for two drugs that only differ in their elimination clearance. Notice that the areas under the curves are different, signifying that the drug that has the smaller area under the curve is more rapidly eliminated from the body than the drug that has the slower elimination clearance.

Total Drug (Elimination) Clearance

7 *Elimination clearance* (drug clearance) is the theoretical volume of blood from which the drug is completely and irreversibly removed in a unit of time. Elimination clearance has the units of flow (volume per time). *Total* drug clearance can be calculated with pharmacokinetic models of blood concentration versus time data. Drug clearance is often corrected for weight or body surface area, in which case the units are mL/min/kg or mL/min/m^2, respectively.

Elimination clearance, *Cl*, can be calculated from the declining blood levels observed after an IV injection, as follows:

$$Cl = \frac{dose\ of\ drug\ administered}{area\ under\ the\ concentration\ versus\ time\ curve} \quad (7\text{-}8)$$

If a drug is rapidly removed from the plasma, its concentration will fall more quickly than the concentration of a drug that is less readily eliminated. This results in a smaller area under the concentration versus time curve, which equates to greater clearance (Fig. 7-4).

Without additional organ-specific data (e.g., urine drug concentration measurements, drug arterial inflow concentration), calculating elimination clearance from compartmental pharmacokinetic models usually does not specify the relative contribution of different organs to drug elimination. Nonetheless, estimation of drug clearance with these models has made important contributions to clinical pharmacology. In particular, these models have provided a great deal of clinically useful information regarding altered drug elimination in various pathologic conditions.

Elimination Half-life

Although the elimination clearance is the pharmacokinetic parameter that best describes the physiologic process of drug elimination (i.e., drug delivery to organs of elimination coupled with the capacity of the organ to eliminate the drug), the variable most often reported in textbooks and literature is the *elimination half-life* of a drug ($t_{1/2\beta}$). The elimination half-life is the time during which the amount of drug in the body decreases by 50%. Although this parameter appears to be a simple summary of the physiology of drug elimination, it is actually a complex parameter, influenced by the distribution and the elimination of the drug as follows:

$$t_{1/2_\beta} = \frac{\ln 2}{k_\beta} = 0.693 \times \frac{V_d}{Cl_E} \quad (7\text{-}9)$$

Therefore, when a physiologic or pathologic perturbation changes the elimination half-life of a drug, it is not a simple reflection of the change in the body's ability to metabolize or eliminate the drug. For example, the elimination half-life of thiopental is prolonged in the elderly, however, the elimination clearance is unchanged and the volume of distribution is increased.[31] Therefore, elderly patients need dosing strategies that accommodate for the change in the distribution rather than a decreased metabolism of the drug. In contrast, in patients with renal insufficiency, the increase in the elimination half-life of pancuronium is due to a simple decrease in renal elimination of the drug while the volume of distribution is unchanged.[32]

Besides its inability to give insight into the mechanism by which a drug is retained in the body, the elimination half-life is unable to give insight into the time that it takes for a single or a series of repeated drug doses to terminate its effect. Although elimination of drug from the body begins the moment the drug is delivered to the organs of elimination, the rapid termination of effect of a bolus of an intravenous agent is due to redistribution of drug from the brain to the blood and subsequently other tissue (e.g., muscle). Therefore, the effects of most anesthetics have waned long before even one elimination half-life has been completed, making this measure of drug kinetics incapable of providing useful information regarding the duration of action following the administration of intravenous agents. Thus the elimination half-life has limited utility in anesthetic practice.[10]

Effect of Hepatic or Renal Disease on Pharmacokinetic Parameters

Diverse pathophysiologic changes preclude precise prediction of the pharmacokinetics of a given drug in individual patients with hepatic or renal disease. In addition, liver function tests (e.g., transaminases) are unreliable predictors of the degree of liver function and the remaining metabolic capacity for drug elimination. However, some generalizations can be made. In patients with hepatic disease, the elimination half-life of drugs metabolized or excreted by the liver is often increased because of decreased clearance, and possibly, increased volume of distribution caused by ascites and altered protein binding.[10,33] Drug concentration at steady state is inversely proportional to elimination clearance. Therefore, when hepatic drug clearance is reduced, repeated bolus dosing or continuous infusion of drugs such as benzodiazepines, opioids, and barbiturates may result in excessive accumulation of drug as well as excessive and prolonged pharmacologic effects. Since recovery from small doses of drugs such as thiopental and fentanyl is largely the result of redistribution, recovery from conservative doses will be minimally affected by reductions in elimination clearance. In patients with renal failure, similar concerns apply to the administration of drugs excreted by the kidneys. It is almost always better to underestimate a patient's dose requirement, observe the response, and give additional drug if necessary.

Nonlinear Pharmacokinetics

The physiologic and compartmental models thus far discussed are based on the assumption that drug distribution and elimination are first-order processes. Therefore, their parameters, such as clearance and elimination half-life, are independent of the dose or concentration of the drug. However, the rate of elimination of a few drugs is dose-dependent, or *nonlinear.*

Elimination of drugs involves interactions with either enzymes catalyzing biotransformation reactions or carrier proteins for transmembrane transport. If sufficient drug is present, the capacity of the drug-eliminating systems can be exceeded. When this occurs, it is no longer possible to excrete a constant fraction of the drug present to the eliminating system, and a constant amount of drug is excreted per unit time. Phenytoin is a well-known example of a drug that exhibits nonlinear elimination at therapeutic concentrations,[34] whereas in anesthetic practice, the extremely high doses of thiopental utilized for cerebral protection can demonstrate zero-order elimination.[35] In theory, all drugs are cleared in a nonlinear fashion. In practice, the capacity to eliminate most drugs is so great that this is usually not evident, even with toxic concentrations.

Compartmental Pharmacokinetic Models

One-compartment Model

Although for most drugs the one-compartment model is an oversimplification, it does serve to illustrate the basic relationship among clearance, volume of distribution, and the elimination half-life. In this model, the body is envisaged as a single homogeneous compartment. Drug distribution after injection is assumed to be instantaneous, so there are no concentration gradients within the compartment. The concentration can decrease only by elimination of drug from the system. The plasma concentration versus time curve for a hypothetical drug with one-compartment kinetics is shown in Figure 7-5. The decrease in plasma concentration (C) with time from the initial concentration (C_0) can be characterized by the simple monoexponential function:

$$C(t) = C_0 \times e^{-k_e \times t} \qquad (7\text{-}10)$$

With the concentration plotted on a logarithmic scale, the concentration versus time curve becomes a straight line. The slope of the logarithm of concentration versus time is equal to the first-order elimination rate constant (k_e).

In the one-compartment model, drug clearance, Cl, is equal to the product of the elimination rate constant, k_e, and the volume of distribution:

$$Cl = k_e \cdot V_d \qquad (7\text{-}11)$$

Combining Equations 7-6 and 7-10 yields Equation 7-9 (where $k_e = k_\beta$):

$$t_{1/2_\beta} = \frac{\ln 2}{k_e} = 0.693 \times \frac{V_d}{Cl_E} \qquad (7\text{-}9)$$

Therefore, when it is appropriate to make the simplifying assumption of instantaneous mixing of drug into a single compartment, the elimination half-life is inversely proportional to the slope of the concentration time curve. For drugs that require consideration of their multicompartmental pharmacokinetics, the relationship among clearance, volume of distribution, and the elimination half-life is not a simple linear one such as Equation 7-9. However,
8 the same principles apply. All else being equal, the greater the clearance, the shorter the elimination half-life; the larger the volume of distribution, the longer the elimination half-life. Thus, the elimination half-life depends on two other variables, clearance and volume of distribution that characterize, respectively, the extent of drug distribution and efficiency of drug elimination.

Two-compartment Model

For many drugs, a graph of the logarithm of the plasma concentration versus time after an IV injection is similar to the schematic graph shown in Figure 7-6. There are two discrete phases in the decline of the plasma concentration. The first phase after injection is characterized by a very rapid decrease in concentration. The rapid decrease in concentration during this "distribution phase" is largely caused by passage of drug from the plasma into tissues. The distribution phase is followed by a slower decline of the concentration owing to drug elimination. Elimination also begins immediately after injection, but its contribution to the drop in plasma concentration is initially much smaller than the fall in concentration because of drug distribution.

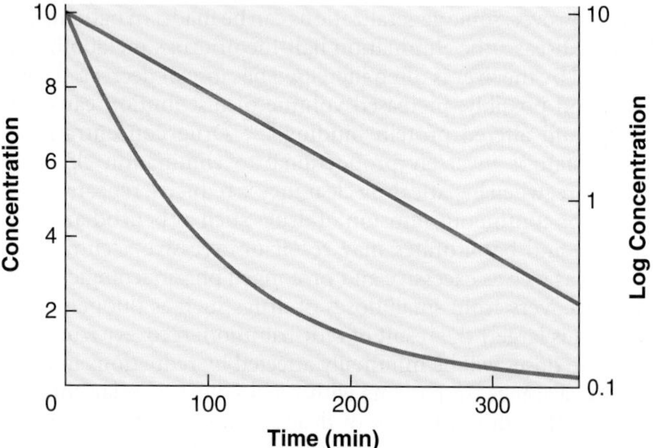

FIGURE 7-5. The plasma concentration versus time profile plotted on both linear (*blue line,* left y-axis) and logarithmic (*red line,* right y-axis) scales for a hypothetical drug exhibiting one-compartment, first-order pharmacokinetics. Note that the slope of the logarithmic concentration profile is equal to the elimination rate constant (k_e) and related to the elimination half-life ($t_{1/2\beta}$) as described in Equation 7-9.

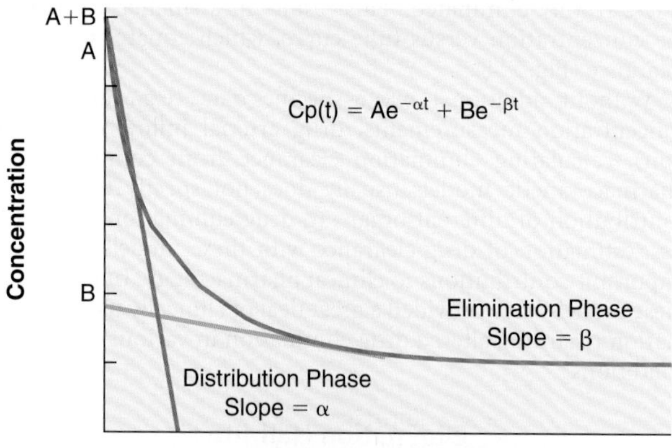

FIGURE 7-6. The logarithmic plasma concentration versus time profile for a hypothetical drug exhibiting two-compartment, first-order pharmacokinetics. Note that the distribution phase has a slope that is significantly larger than that of the elimination phase, indicating that the process of distribution is not only more rapid than elimination of the drug from the body, but also responsible for the majority of the decline in plasma concentration in the several minutes after drug administration.

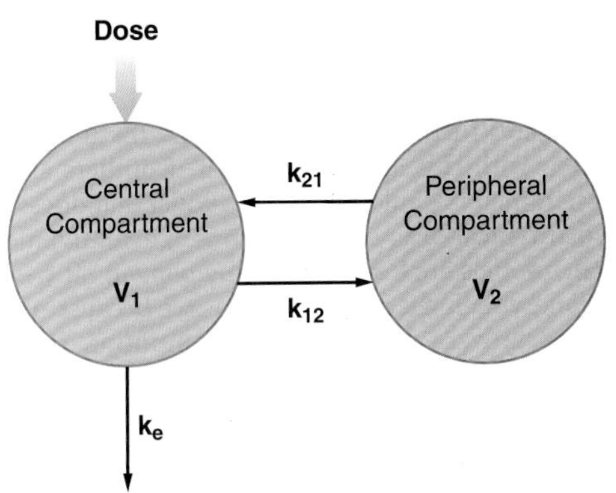

FIGURE 7-7. A schematic of a two-compartment pharmacokinetic model. See text for explanation.

To account for this biphasic behavior, one must consider the body to be made up of two compartments, a central compartment, which includes the plasma, and a peripheral compartment (Fig. 7-7). This two-compartment model assumes that it is the central compartment into which the drug is injected and from which the blood samples for measurement of concentration are obtained, and that drug is eliminated only from the central compartment. Drug distribution within the central compartment is considered to be instantaneous. In reality, this last assumption cannot be true. However, drug uptake into some of the highly perfused tissues is so rapid that it cannot be detected as a discrete phase on the plasma concentration versus time curve.

The distribution and elimination phases can be characterized by graphic analysis of the plasma concentration versus time curve, as shown in Figure 7-6. The elimination phase line is extrapolated back to time zero (the time of injection). In Figure 7-6, the zero time intercepts of the distribution and elimination lines are points A and B, respectively. The *hybrid rate constants,* α and β, are equal to the slopes of the two lines, and are used to calculate the distribution and elimination half-lives; α and β are called hybrid rate constants because they depend on both distribution and elimination processes.

At any time after an IV injection, the plasma concentration of drugs with two-compartment kinetics is equal to the sum of two exponential terms:

$$C_p(t) = Ae^{-\alpha t} + Be^{-\beta t} \quad (7\text{-}12)$$

where t = time, $C_p(t)$ = plasma concentration at time t, A = y-axis intercept of the distribution phase line, α = hybrid rate constant of the distribution phase, B = y-axis intercept of the elimination phase line, and β = hybrid rate constant of the elimination phase. The first term characterizes the distribution phase and the second term characterizes the elimination phase. Immediately after injection, the first term represents a much larger fraction of the total plasma concentration than the second term. After several distribution half-lives, the value of the first term approaches zero, and the plasma concentration is essentially equal to the value of the second term (see Fig. 7-6).

In multicompartmental models, the drug is initially distributed only within the central compartment. Therefore, the initial apparent volume of distribution is the volume of the central compartment. Immediately after injection, the amount of drug present is the dose, and the concentration is the extrapolated concentration at time $t = 0$, which is equal to the sum of the intercepts of the distribution and elimination lines. The volume of the central compartment, V_1, is calculated by modifying Equation 7-7:

$$V_1 = \frac{dose}{initial\ plasma\ concentration} = \frac{dose}{A + B} \quad (7\text{-}13)$$

The volume of the central compartment is important in clinical anesthesiology because it is the pharmacokinetic parameter that determines the peak plasma concentration after an IV bolus injection. Hypovolemia, for example, reduces the volume of the central compartment. If doses are not correspondingly reduced, the higher plasma concentrations will increase the incidence of adverse pharmacologic effects.

Immediately after IV injection, the entire drug is in the central compartment. Simultaneously, three processes begin. Drug moves from the central to the peripheral compartment, which also has a volume, V_2. This intercompartmental transfer is a first-order process, and its magnitude is quantified by the rate constant k_{12}. As soon as the drug appears in the peripheral compartment, some passes back to the central compartment, a process characterized by the rate constant k_{21}. The transfer of drug between the central and peripheral compartments is quantified by the *distributional* or *intercompartmental clearance:*

$$Intercompartmental\ Clearance = Cl_{12} = Cl_{21} = V_1 \times k_{12} = V_2 \times k_{21} \quad (7\text{-}14)$$

The third process that begins immediately after administration of the drug is the irreversible removal of drug from the system via the central compartment. As in the one-compartment model, the elimination rate constant is k_e, and *elimination clearance* is:

$$Elimination\ Clearance = Cl_E = V_1 \times k_e \quad (7\text{-}15)$$

The rapidity of the decrease in the central compartment concentration after IV injection depends on the magnitude of the compartmental volumes, the intercompartmental clearance, and the elimination clearance.

At equilibrium, the drug is distributed between the central and the peripheral compartments, and by definition, the drug concentrations in the compartments are equal. Therefore, the ultimate volume of distribution, termed the volume of distribution at steady state (V_{ss}), is the sum of V_1 and V_2. Extensive tissue uptake of a drug is reflected by a large volume of the peripheral compartment, which, in turn, results in a large V_{ss}. Consequently, V_{ss} can greatly exceed the actual volume of the body.

As in the single-compartment model, the elimination clearance in multicompartment models is equal to the dose divided by the area under the concentration versus time curve. This area, as well as the compartmental volumes and intercompartmental clearances, can be calculated from the intercepts and hybrid rate constants, without having to reach steady-state conditions.

Three-compartment Model

After IV injection of some drugs, the initial, rapid distribution phase is followed by a second, slower distribution phase before the elimination phase becomes evident. Therefore, the plasma concentration is the sum of three exponential terms:

$$C_p(t) = Ae^{-\alpha t} + Be^{-\beta t} + Ge^{-\gamma t} \quad (7\text{-}16)$$

where t = time, $C_p(t)$ = plasma concentration at time t, A = intercept of the rapid distribution phase line, α = hybrid rate constant of the rapid distribution phase, B = intercept of the slower

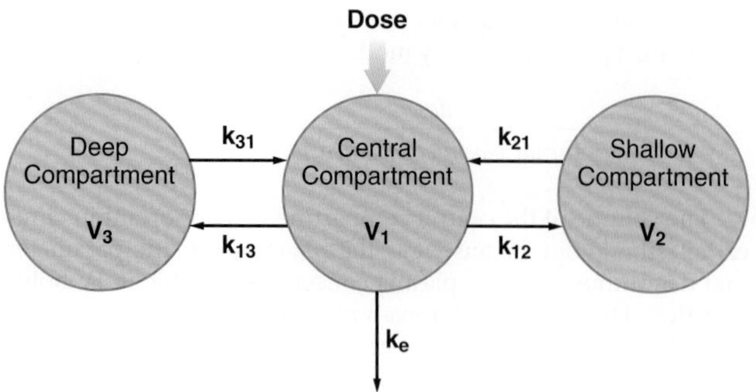

FIGURE 7-8. A schematic of a three-compartment pharmacokinetic model. See text for details.

distribution phase line, β = hybrid rate constant of the slower distribution phase, G = intercept of the elimination phase line, and γ = hybrid rate constant of the elimination phase. This triphasic behavior is explained by a three-compartment pharmacokinetic model (Fig. 7-8). As in the two-compartment model, the drug is injected into and eliminated from the central compartment. Drug is reversibly transferred between the central compartment and two peripheral compartments, which accounts for two distribution phases. Drug transfer between the central compartment and the more rapidly equilibrating, or "shallow," peripheral compartment is characterized by the first-order rate constants k_{12} and k_{21}. Transfer in and out of the more slowly equilibrating, "deep" compartment is characterized by the rate constants k_{13} and k_{31}. In this model, there are three compartmental volumes: V_1, V_2, and V_3, whose sum equals V_{ss}; and there are three clearances: The rapid intercompartmental clearance, the slow intercompartmental clearance, and elimination clearance.

The pharmacokinetic parameters of interest to clinicians, such as clearance, volumes of distribution, and distribution and elimination half-lives, are determined by calculations analogous to those used in the two-compartment model. Accurate estimates of these parameters depend on accurate characterization of the measured plasma concentration versus time data. A frequently encountered problem is that the duration of sampling is not long enough to define accurately the elimination phase. Similar problems arise if the assay cannot detect low concentrations of the drug. Conversely, samples are sometimes obtained too infrequently following drug administration to be able to characterize the distribution phases accurately.[36,37] Whether a drug exhibits two- or three-compartment kinetics is of no clinical consequence.[10] In fact, some drugs have two-compartment kinetics in some patients and three-compartment kinetics in others. In selecting a pharmacokinetic model, the most important factor is that it accurately characterizes the measured concentrations.

In general, the model with the smallest number of compartments or exponents that accurately reflects the data is used. However, it is good to consider that the data collected in a particular study may not be reflective of the clinical pharmacologic issues of concern in another situation, making published pharmacokinetic model parameters potentially irrelevant. For instance, new data indicates that hypotension following intravenous administration of drug X is related to peak arterial plasma drug X concentrations 1 minute after injection, but previous pharmacokinetic models are based on venous plasma drug X concentrations beginning 5 minutes after the dose. In this case, the pharmacokinetic models will not be of use in designing dosing regimens for drug X that avoid toxic drug concentrations at 1 minute.[10,38,39]

Almost all earlier pharmacokinetic studies used *two-stage modeling.* With this technique, pharmacokinetic parameters were estimated independently for each subject and then averaged to provide estimates of the typical parameters for the population. One problem with this approach is that if outliers are present, averaging parameters could result in a model that does not accurately predict typical drug concentrations. Currently, most pharmacokinetic models are developed using *population pharmacokinetic modeling,* which has been made feasible because of advances in modeling software and increased computing power. With these techniques, the pharmacokinetic parameters are estimated using all the concentration versus time data from the entire group of subjects in a single stage, using sophisticated nonlinear regression methods. This modeling technique provides single estimates of the typical parameter values for the population.

Non-compartmental (Stochastic) Pharmacokinetic Models

Often investigators performing pharmacokinetic analyses of drugs want to avoid the experimental requirements of a physiologic model—data or empirical estimations of individual organ inflow and outflow concentration profiles and organ tissue drug concentrations are required in order to identify the components of the model.[40] Although compartmental models do not assume any physiologic or anatomic basis for the model structure, investigators often attribute anatomic and physiologic functions to these empiric models.[41] Even if the disciplined clinical pharmacologist avoids overinterpretation of the meaning of compartment models, the simple fact that several competing models can provide equally good descriptions of the mathematical data or that some subjects in a dataset may be better fit with a three-compartment model rather than the two-compartment model, which provides the best fit for the other dataset subjects, leads many to question whether there is a true best model architecture for any given drug. Therefore, some investigators choose to employ mathematical techniques to characterize a pharmacokinetic dataset that attempt to avoid any preconceived notion of structure and yet yield the pharmacokinetic parameters that summarize drug distribution and elimination. These techniques are classified as non-compartmental techniques or stochastic techniques, and they are similar to the methods based on moment analysis utilized in process analysis of chemical engineering systems. Although these techniques are often called model-independent, like any mathematical construct, assumptions must be made to simplify the mathematics. The basic assumptions of non-compartmental analysis are that all of the elimination clearance occurs directly from the plasma, the distribution and elimination of drug is a linear and first-order process, and the pharmacokinetics of the system does not vary over the time of the data collection (time-invariant). All of these assumptions are also made in the basic compartmental and most physiologic models. Therefore, the main advantage of the non-compartmental pharmacokinetic methods is that a general description of drug absorption, distribution, and elimination can be made without resorting to more complex mathematical modeling techniques.[40]

Another appealing facet of non-compartmental analysis is that the parameters that describe drug distribution (volume of distribution at steady state, Vd_{ss}) and drug elimination (elimination clearance, Cl_E) are analogous to parameters found in other pharmacokinetic techniques. In fact, when properly defined, the estimates of these parameters from the non-compartmental approach and a well-defined compartmental model yield similar values. The main unique parameter of non-compartmental analysis is the mean residence time (MRT), which is the average time a drug molecule spends in the body before being eliminated.[42] The MRT unfortunately suffers from the main failings of the elimination half-life derived from compartmental models—not only does it fail to capture the contribution of extensive distribution versus limited elimination to allow a drug to linger in the body, but both parameters also fail to describe the situation where the drug effect can dissipate by redistribution of drug from the site of action back into blood and then into other, less well-perfused tissues.[43]

PHARMACODYNAMIC PRINCIPLES

Much of the clinical pharmacology efforts of the late 1980s through 1990s were devoted to applying new computational power of desktop personal computers to deciphering the pharmacokinetics of intravenous anesthetics. However, the premise behind developing models to better characterize and understand the effects of various physiologic and pathologic states on drug distribution and elimination was that the efforts of the previous 30 years had clearly characterized the relationship between a dose of drug and its effect(s). As computational power and drug assay technology grew, it became possible to characterize the relationship between a drug concentration and the associated pharmacologic effect. As a result, pharmacodynamic studies since the 1990s have focused on the quantitative analysis of the relationship between the drug concentration in the blood and the resultant effects of the drug on physiologic processes.

Drug–Receptor Interactions

9 Most pharmacologic agents produce their physiologic effects by binding to a drug-specific receptor, which brings about a change in cellular function. The majority of pharmacologic receptors are cell membrane–bound proteins, although some receptors are located in the cytoplasm or the nucleoplasm of the cell.

Binding of drugs to receptors, like the binding of drugs to plasma proteins, is usually reversible, and follows the law of mass action:

$$[drug] + [receptor] \leftrightarrow [drug - receptor\ complex] \quad (7\text{-}17)$$

This relationship demonstrates that the higher the concentration of free drug or unoccupied receptor, the greater the tendency to form the drug–receptor complex. Plotting the percentage of receptors occupied by a drug against the logarithm of the concentration of the drug yields a sigmoid curve, as shown in Figure 7-9.[44]

The percentage of receptors occupied by a drug is not equivalent to the percentage of maximal effect produced by the drug. In fact, most receptor systems have more receptors than required to obtain the maximum drug effect.[45] The presence of "extra" unoccupied receptors will promote the formation of the drug–receptor complex (law of mass action, Eq. 7-17), therefore, near-maximal drug effects can occur at very low drug concentrations. This process not only allows extremely efficient responses to drugs, but it provides a large margin of safety—an extremely large number of drugs receptors must be bound to an antagonist before the drug is unable to produce its pharmacologic effect. For example, at the neuromuscular junction, only 20% to 25% of the postjunctional nicotinic cholinergic receptors need to bind acetylcholine to produce contraction of all the fibers in the muscle, while 75% of the receptors must be blocked by a non-depolarizing neuromuscular antagonist to produce a significant drop in muscle strength. This accounts for the "margin of safety" of neuromuscular transmission.[45]

The binding of drugs to receptors and the resulting changes in cellular function are the last two steps in the complex series of events between administration of the drug and production of its pharmacologic effects. There are two primary schemes by which the binding of an agonist to a receptor changes cellular function: Receptor-linked membrane ion channels called *ionophores,* and guanine nucleotide binding proteins, referred to as *G-proteins.* The nicotinic cholinergic receptor in the neuromuscular postsynaptic membrane is one example of a receptor–ionophore complex. Binding of acetylcholine opens the cation ionophore, leading to an influx of Na^+ ions, propagation of an action potential, and, ultimately, muscle contraction. The β-amino butyric acid (GABA) receptor–chloride ionophore complex is another example of this type of effector mechanism. Binding of either endogenous neurotransmitters (GABA) or exogenous agonists (benzodiazepines and IV anesthetics) increases Cl^- conductance, which hyperpolarizes the neuron and decreases its excitability. Adrenergic receptors are the proto-typical G-protein coupled receptors. G-proteins change the intracellular concentrations of various *second messengers,* such as Ca^{2+} and cyclic AMP, in order to transduce their signal and modify cellular behavior.

Desensitization and Downregulation of Receptors

Receptors are not static entities. Rather, they are dynamic cellular components that adapt to their environment. Prolonged exposure of a receptor to its agonist leads to desensitization—subsequent doses of the agonist will produce lower maximal effects. With

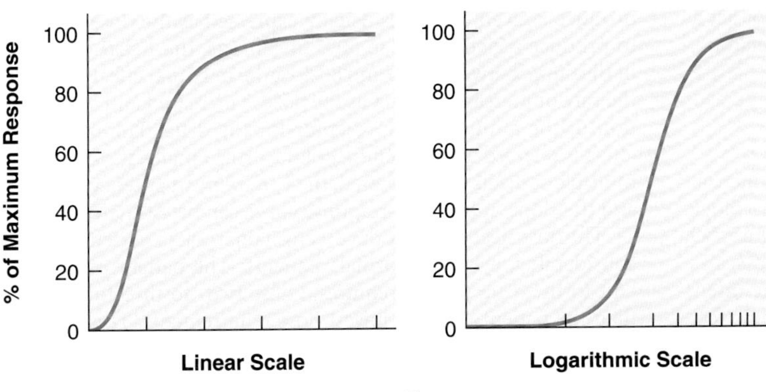

FIGURE 7-9. A schematic curve of the effect of a drug plotted against dose. In the left panel, the response data is plotted against the dose data on a linear scale. In the right panel, the same response data are plotted against the dose data on a logarithmic scale yielding a sigmoid dose-response curve that is linear between 20% and 80% of the maximal effect.

SCIENTIFIC FOUNDATIONS OF ANESTHESIA

sustained elevation of the cytosolic second messengers downstream of the G-proteins, pathways to prevent further G-protein signaling are activated. Phosphorylation by G-protein receptor kinases and arrestin-mediated blockage of the coupling site needed to form the active heterotrimeric G-protein complex prevents G-protein–coupled receptors from becoming active. Arrestins and other cell membrane proteins can tag receptors that have sustained activity so that these non-G-protein receptors are internalized and sequestered, making them no longer accessible to agonists. Similar mechanisms will prevent the trafficking of stored receptors to the cell membrane. The combined increased rate of internalization and decreased rate of replenishing of receptor results in *downregulation*—a decrease in the total number of receptors. Signals that produce downregulation with sustained receptor activation are essentially reversed in the face of constant receptor inactivity. Therefore, chronically denervated neuromuscular junctions just like cardiac tissue constantly bathed with adrenergic antagonists will both upregulate the specific receptors in an attempt to produce a signal in the face of lower concentrations of agonists.

Agonists, Partial Agonists, and Antagonists

Drugs that bind to receptors and produce an effect are called *agonists*. Different drugs may be capable of producing the same maximal effect (E_{MAX}), although they may differ in concentration that produces the effect (i.e., potency). Agonists that differ in potency but bind to the same receptors will have parallel concentration-response curves (curves *A* and *B* in Fig. 7-10). Differences in potency of agonists reflect differences in affinity for the receptor. *Partial agonists* are drugs that are not capable of producing the maximal effect, even at very high concentrations (curve *C* in Fig. 7-10).

Compounds that bind to receptors without producing any changes in cellular function are referred to as *antagonists*—from blocking the active binding site(s) inhibit agonist binding to the receptors. *Competitive antagonists* bind reversibly to receptors, and their blocking effect can be overcome by high concentrations of an agonist (i.e., competition). Therefore, competitive antagonists produce a parallel shift in the dose-response curve, but the maximum effect is not altered (see Fig. 7-10, curves *A* and *B*). *Noncompetitive antagonists* bind irreversibly to receptors. This has the same effect as reducing the number of receptors and shifts the dose-response curve downward and to the right, decreasing both the slope and the maximum effect (curves *A* and *C* in Fig. 7-10). The effect of noncompetitive antagonists is reversed only by synthesis of new receptor molecules.

Agonists produce a structural change in the receptor molecule that initiates changes in cellular function. Partial agonists may produce a qualitatively different change in the receptor, whereas antagonists bind without producing a change in the receptor that results in altered cellular function. The underlying mechanisms by which different compounds that bind to the same receptor act as agonists, partial agonists, or antagonists are not fully understood.

Dose-response Relationships

Dose-response studies determine the relationship between increasing doses of a drug and the ensuing changes in pharmacologic effects. Schematic dose-response curves are shown in Figure 7-9, with the dose plotted on both linear and logarithmic scales. There is a curvilinear relationship between dose and the intensity of response. Low doses produce little pharmacologic effect. Once effects become evident, a small increase in dose produces a relatively large change in effect. At near-maximal response, large increases in dose produce little change in effect. Usually the dose 10
is plotted on a logarithmic scale (see Fig. 7-9, right panel), which demonstrates the linear relationship between the logarithm of the dose and the intensity of the response between 20% and 80% of the maximum effect.

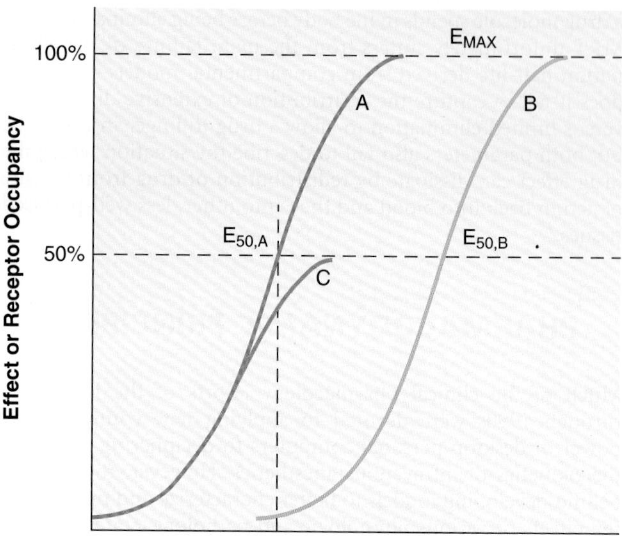

FIGURE 7-10. Schematic pharmacodynamic curves, with dose or concentration on the x-axis and effect or receptor occupancy on the y-axis, that illustrate agonism, partial agonism, and antagonism. Drug A produces a maximum effect, E_{MAX}, and a 50% of maximal effect at dose or concentration $E_{50,A}$. Drug B, a full agonist, can produce the maximum effect, E_{MAX}, however, it is less potent ($E_{50,B} > E_{50,A}$). Drug C, a partial agonist, can only produce a maximum effect of approximately 50% E_{MAX}. If a competitive antagonist is given to a patient, the dose response for the agonist would shift from curve A to curve B—although the receptors would have the same affinity for the agonist, the presence of the competitor would necessitate an increase in agonist in order to produce an effect. In fact, the agonist would still be able to produce a maximal effect, if a sufficient overdose was given to displace the competitive antagonist. However, the competitive antagonist would not change the binding characteristics of the receptor for the agonist and so curve B is simply shifted to the right but remains parallel to curve A. In contrast, if a noncompetitive antagonist binds to the receptor, the agonist would no longer be able to produce a maximal effect, no matter how much of an overdose is administered (curve C).

Acquiring the pharmacologic effect data from a population of subjects exposed to a variety of doses of a drug provides four key characteristics of the drug dose-response relationship—potency, drug–receptor affinity, efficacy, and population pharmacodynamic variability. The *potency* of the drug—the dose required to produce a given effect—is usually expressed as the dose required to produce a given effect in 50% of subjects, the *ED50*. The *slope* of the curve between 20% and 80% of the maximal effect indicates the rate of increase in effect as the dose is increased and is a reflection of the affinity of the receptor for the drug. The maximum effect is referred to as the *efficacy* of the drug. Finally, if curves from multiple subjects are generated, the *variability* in potency, efficacy, and the slope of the dose-response curve can be estimated.

The dose needed to produce a given pharmacologic effect varies considerably, even in "normal" patients. The patient most resistant to the drug usually requires a dose two- to threefold greater than the patient with the lowest dose requirements. This variability is caused by differences among individuals in the relationship between drug concentration and pharmacologic effect, superimposed on differences in pharmacokinetics. Dose-response studies have the disadvantage of not being able to determine whether variations in pharmacologic responses are caused by differences in pharmacokinetics, pharmacodynamics, or both.

Concentration-response Relationships

The onset and duration of pharmacologic effects depend not only on pharmacokinetic factors but also on the pharmacodynamic factors governing the degree of temporal disequilibrium between changes in concentration and changes in effect. The magnitude of the pharmacologic effect is a function of the amount of drug present at the site of action, hence increasing the dose increases the peak effect. Larger doses have a more rapid onset of action because pharmacologically active concentrations at the site of action occur sooner. Increasing the dose also increases the duration of action because pharmacologically effective concentrations are maintained for a longer time.

Ideally, the concentration of drug at its site of action should be used to define the concentration-response relationship. Unfortunately, these data are rarely available, so the relationship between the concentration of drug in the blood and pharmacologic effect is studied instead. This relationship is easiest to understand if the changes in pharmacologic effect that occur during and after an IV infusion of a hypothetical drug are considered. If a drug is infused
2 at a constant rate, the plasma concentration initially increases rapidly and asymptotically approaches a steady-state level after approximately five elimination half-lives have elapsed (Fig. 7-11). The effect of the drug initially increases very slowly, then more rapidly, and eventually also reaches a steady state. When the infusion is discontinued, indicated by point *C* in Figure 7-11, the plasma concentration immediately decreases because of drug distribution and elimination. However, the effect stays the same for a short period, and then also begins to decrease—there is always a time lag between changes in plasma concentration and changes in pharmacologic response. Figure 7-11 also demonstrates that the same plasma concentration is associated with different responses if the concentration is changing. At points *A* and *B* in Figure 7-11, the plasma concentrations are the same, but the effects at each time differ. When the concentration is increasing, there is a concentration gradient from blood to the site of action. When the infusion is discontinued, the concentration gradient is reversed. Therefore, at the same plasma concentration, the concentration at the site of action is higher after, compared to during, the infusion. This is associated with a correspondingly greater effect.

In theory, there must be some degree of temporal disequilibrium between plasma concentration and drug effect for all drugs with extravascular sites of action. However, for some drugs, the time lag may be so short that it cannot be demonstrated. The magnitude of this temporal disequilibrium depends on several factors:

1. The perfusion of the organ on which the drug acts
2. The tissue:blood partition coefficient of the drug
3. The rate of diffusion or transport of the drug from the blood to the cellular site of action
4. The rate and affinity of drug–receptor binding
5. The time required for processes initiated by the drug–receptor interaction to produce changes in cellular function

The consequence of this time lag between changes in concentration and changes in effects is that the plasma concentration will have an unvarying relationship with pharmacologic effect only under steady-state conditions. At steady state, the plasma concentration is in equilibrium with the concentrations throughout the body, and is thus directly proportional to the steady-state concentration at the site of action. Plotting the logarithm of the steady-state plasma concentration versus response generates a curve identical in appearance to the dose-response curve shown in the right panel of Figure 7-9. The $Cp_{ss}50$, the steady-state plasma concentration producing 50% of the maximal response, is determined from the concentration-response curve. Like the ED50, the $Cp_{ss}50$ is a measure of sensitivity to a drug, but the $Cp_{ss}50$ has the advantage of being unaffected by pharmacokinetic variability. Because it takes five elimination half-lives to approach steady-state conditions, it is not practical to determine the $Cp_{ss}50$ directly. For drugs with long elimination half-lives, the pseudoequilibrium during the elimination phase can be used to approximate steady-state conditions, because the concentrations in plasma and at the site of action are changing very slowly.

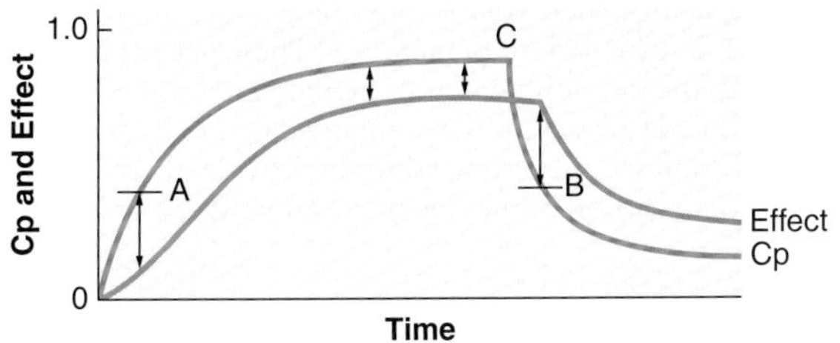

FIGURE 7-11. The changes in plasma drug concentration and pharmacologic effect during and after an intravenous infusion. See text for explanation. (Reprinted with permission from Stanski DR, Sheiner LB. Pharmacokinetics and pharmacodynamics of muscle relaxants. *Anesthesiology.* 1979;51:103.)

Combined Pharmacokinetic–Pharmacodynamic Models

11 Integrated pharmacokinetic–pharmacodynamic (PK–PD) models fully characterize the relationships among time, dose, plasma concentration, and pharmacologic effect. This is accomplished by adding a hypothetical "effect compartment" (biophase) to a standard compartmental pharmacokinetic model (Fig. 7-12).[46–48] Transfer of drug between central compartment and the effect compartment is assumed to be a first-order process, and the pharmacologic effect is assumed to be directly related to the concentration in the biophase. The biophase is a "virtual" compartment, although linked to the pharmacokinetic model, does not actually receive or return drug to the model and, therefore, ensures that the effect-site processes do not influence the pharmacokinetics of the rest of the body. By simultaneously characterizing the pharmacokinetics of the drug and the time course of drug effect, the combined—PK–PD model is able to quantify the temporal dissociation between the plasma (central compartment) concentration and effect with the rate constant for equilibration between the plasma and the biophase, k_{e0}. By quantifying the time lag between changes in plasma concentration and changes in pharmacologic effect, these models can also define the $Cp_{ss}50$, even without steady-state conditions. These models have contributed greatly to our understanding of factors influencing the response to intravenous anesthetics, opioids, and non-depolarizing muscle relaxants in humans.

The rate of equilibration between the plasma and the biophase, k_{e0}, can also be characterized by the half-life of effect-site equilibration ($T_{1/2k_{e0}}$) using the formula:

$$T_{1/2k_{e0}} = \frac{\ln 2}{k_{e0}} = \frac{0.693}{k_{e0}} \quad (7\text{-}18)$$

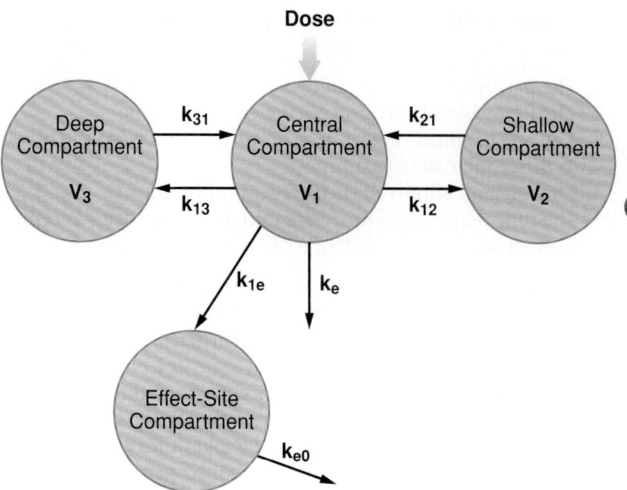

FIGURE 7-12. A schematic of a three-compartment pharmacokinetic model with the effect site linked to the central compartment. The rate constant for transfer between the plasma (central compartment) and the effect site, k_{1e}, and the volume of the effect site are both presumed to be negligible to ensure that the effect site does not influence the pharmacokinetic model. The rate constant for drug removal from the effect site, which relates the concentration in the central compartment to the pharmacologic effect is k_{e0}.

$T_{1/2ke0}$ is the time for the effect-site concentration to reach 50% of the plasma concentration when the plasma concentration is held constant. For anesthetics with a short $T_{1/2ke0}$ (high k_{e0}), equilibration between the plasma and the biophase is rapid, and therefore, there is little delay before an effect is reached when a bolus of drug is administered or an infusion of drug is initiated. However, because the decline in the effect-site concentration will also depend on the concentration gradient between the effect site and the plasma, drugs that rapidly equilibrate with the biophase may take longer to redistribute away.[49] Therefore, the offset of drug effect is more dependent on the pharmacokinetics of the body than on the rapidity of biophase-plasma equilibration.[20,49]

DRUG INTERACTIONS

Taking into account premedication, perioperative antibiotics, IV agents used for induction or maintenance, inhalational anesthetics, opioids, muscle relaxants, the drugs used to restore neuromuscular transmission, and postoperative analgesics, ten or more drugs may be given for a relatively "routine" anesthetic. Consequently, thorough understanding of the mechanisms of drug interactions and knowledge of specific interactions with drugs used in anesthesia are essential to the safe practice of anesthesiology. Indeed, anesthesiologists often deliberately take advantage of drug interactions. For example, moderate to high doses of opioid are often utilized to decrease the amount of volatile anesthetic required to provide immobility and hemodynamic stability to surgical incision (e.g., MAC^a and MAC_{BAR}), thereby avoiding the side effects of higher concentrations of inhaled anesthetics (e.g., vasodilation, prolonged awakening). In this section, we will examine the major classes of drug–drug interactions by detailing common examples encountered in the perioperative period.

Pharmaceutical (Physiochemical) Interactions: In Vitro

Anesthesiologists often overlook the drug interactions produced by pharmaceutical (physicochemical) properties because the majority of perioperative drugs are administered intravenously or
12 via inhalation, and therefore have a high bioavailability. However, in vitro drug–drug interactions due to physiochemical properties of drugs can significantly alter drug bioavailability and produce unintended toxic byproducts. Basic acid–base chemistry can predict many of the observed in vitro interactions. One classic example of a physiochemical drug–drug interaction that alters drug bioavailability is the formation of insoluble salts that precipitate when acidic drugs, such as thiopental, and basic drugs, such as opioids or muscle relaxants, are "mixed" when the two drugs are administered into intravenous tubing with an insufficient fluid flow rate.[50] Another example is the observation that commercial preparations of local anesthetic solutions that contain epinephrine would have a lower pH than local anesthetic solutions to which epinephrine is added shortly prior to administration because of the high acidity of the antioxidant stabilizers used in commercial preparations (i.e., sodium bisulfite or sodium pyrosulfite).[51] The unintended consequence of this commercial formulation is that the local anesthetic appears less effective due to the increased concentration of the less permeable, ionized form local anesthetic that exists in acidic environments.

Although physiochemical drug interactions that affect the bioavailability of drugs are relatively easy to avoid or, at least, overcome by increasing the drug dose, some physiochemical interactions can result in unintended toxic compounds. One chemical agent often overlooked by anesthesiologists is the soda lime or Baralyme that are used in modern anesthesia machines to remove carbon dioxide from the exhaled gases. Although patients are not directly administered this agent, the gas that they inhale from the anesthesia machine often contain the byproducts of the interaction between the constituents of the exhaled gas and the carbon dioxide absorbent. While this allows the patient to receive a "heated and humidified" inhaled gas mixture, if conditions are correct, the halogenated volatile anesthetics can undergo degradation by the strong base (i.e., sodium and/or potassium hydroxide) contained in the carbon dioxide absorber.[52] This chemical reaction led the FDA to recommend that sevoflurane exposure should not exceed 2 MAC-hours at using fresh gas flow rates of 1 to <2 L/min, in order to minimize exposure to the potentially nephrotoxic haloalkene ("compound A") formed by dehydrofluroniation of sevoflurane by soda lime or Baralyme.[53] Although the effects of compound A on human renal function are not of great clinical concern, the strong bases in some carbon dioxide absorbents can also degrade the difluoromethyl-containing halogenated volatile anesthetics (i.e., desflurane and isoflurane) to form carbon monoxide.[54] These patient safety concerns led to the development and the increased use of Amsorb®, a carbon dioxide adsorbent that contains calcium hydroxide lime in place of sodium and/or potassium hydroxide, therefore causes minimal to no carbon monoxide or compound A formation.[55]

Pharmaceutical (Physiochemical) Interactions: In Vivo

13 Whereas many of the in vitro physiochemical interactions can result in unintended toxicity due to exposure to either subtherapeutic drug concentrations or toxic degradation products,

physiochemical interactions have been exploited to develop two novel approaches to antagonize neuromuscular junction blocking agents. The first approach, which was approved for use in the European Union in 2008, is the selective relaxant binding agent, sugammadex. Sugammadex is a synthetic cyclodextrin that encapsulates and electrostatically binds rocuronium. By essentially irreversibly binding plasma rocuronium, sugammadex acts as a chelator that not only rapidly decreases the free plasma rocuronium concentration but also promotes redistribution of rocuronium from the neuromuscular junction (extracellular space) to the intravascular space.[56] Therefore, if there is an excess of sugammadex molecules relative to rocuronium molecules, the neuromuscular blockade is antagonized. An alternative approach to neuromuscular blockade antagonism is to design a molecule that can be inactivated via nonbiologic routes. This approach has led to Phase 1 studies of a new class of non-depolarizing neuromuscular blocking drugs called the asymmetric mixed-onium cholorofumerates. These molecules are rapidly inactivated by the nonenzymatic formation of cysteine adducts when combined with plasma cysteine.[57] Therefore, cysteine administration antagonizes the neuromuscular blockade. These two novel approaches to drug development could be used to develop designer drugs that can be readily antagonized via nonbiologic routes, if the important receptor targets for sedation and amnesia components of general anesthesia are identified.

Pharmacokinetic Interactions

Drugs can alter each other's absorption, distribution, and elimination. Understanding the basis for alterations in the pharmacokinetics allows anesthesiologists to not only avoid unintentional supratherapeutic or subtherapeutic concentrations of the perioperative medications, but also to strategically employ alterations in pharmacokinetics to achieve the desired concentration profile.

Absorption (Uptake)

Some drugs can alter the absorption of other drugs, by either altering the delivery of drug to the site of drug absorption (uptake) or by altering the local blood flow to the site of drug administration. Although this type of drug–drug interaction will alter bioavailability, it should not alter any other pharmacokinetic parameter. Drugs like ranitidine, which alters gastric pH, and metoclopramide, which speeds gastric emptying, alter absorption from the GI tract. Vasoconstrictors that decrease local blood flow and decrease systemic uptake of drug can be beneficial when added to local anesthetic solutions because they prolong the duration of action of the local anesthetic at the site of injection and can decrease the risk of systemic toxicity from rapid absorption. However, when systemically administered, vasoactive drugs can decrease blood flow to skin and muscle, and decrease the systemic uptake of drugs given by subcutaneous or intramuscular injection. In a similar manner, vasoactive agents can alter the ventilation–perfusion ratio, thereby altering pulmonary uptake of volatile anesthetics, despite a constant inspired concentration. Because of the variability produced by vasoactive agents in drug uptake, careful thought must be given when choosing to administer drugs via nonintravenous route in perioperative patients.

Distribution

Some drugs can alter the systemic distribution of other drugs. Alterations in drug distribution will change some or all of a pharmacokinetic model's volume parameters. It can also alter one or all of the *intercompartmental* clearance parameters of a multicompartmental pharmacokinetic model. There are two main mechanisms purported in textbooks and the clinical pharmacology literature by which drug–drug interactions alter drug distribution—(a) changing the volume of tissue available for drug uptake and (b) changing the amount of drug available for tissue uptake. Since the drug dose required to achieve a desired drug concentration is intimately linked to systemic drug distribution, understanding what common drug–drug interactions produce real alterations in drug distribution can avoid unintentional exposure to subtherapeutic and supratherapeutic drug concentrations.

Although a drug cannot alter the actual volume of tissue available for drug uptake, changing the exposure of blood to different tissue beds changes a drug's apparent tissue volume of
14 distribution. Therefore, drug induced alterations of cardiac output and the distribution of cardiac output to tissues can change the distribution clearance of other drugs. Once again, vasoactive agents can alter tissue distribution by altering regional blood flow even if the total cardiac output is unchanged. Since the change in the plasma drug concentration produced by a prescribed dosing regimen is inversely related to the distribution clearance, the drug dose must be decreased when vasoactive drugs decrease cardiac output or the distribution of cardiac output, otherwise the patient will be exposed to supratherapeutic drug concentrations.[58–60] In addition, the unintended cardiovascular effects of anesthetic drugs, such as the decrease in cardiac output with increasing doses of the direct myocardial depressant, halothane, or the direct arterial dilator, isoflurane, can lead to similar increases in the plasma drug concentration.[61,62]

There is an over abundance of clinical pharmacology literature that examines the ability of one drug to displace another drug from its protein-binding site(s), thereby increasing the concentration of unbound drug in the blood that could cause supratherapeutic concentrations and potential toxicity. When examining specific pharmacokinetic parameters, an increase in the fraction of unbound drug in the plasma could theoretically increase the total apparent volume of distribution (V_{ss}), as more molecules of drug are available for distribution into the tissue. Although most changes in protein binding will not influence clinical drug exposure, analysis of the equations governing the steady-state pharmacokinetics suggests that drugs that are extensively protein bound, have a high hepatic extraction ratio, and have a low therapeutic index may be the exception that require dose adjustment.[63] However, the clinical importance of protein binding in anesthetic drugs is based on several common misconceptions regarding drug distribution. First, the number of unoccupied binding sites is several orders of magnitude higher than the number of molecules of anesthetic drug administered in clinical practice. Therefore, it is hard to envision a scenario where a significant amount of displacement could occur. Even if a drug could displace a significant amount of another drug from its protein-binding site, the liver has the capacity available to metabolize this sudden influx of free drug, thereby returning the free drug concentration to the pre-displacement concentrations (i.e., flow-limited metabolism). Finally, the theoretical argument supporting the importance of protein binding on highly lipophilic drugs ignores the fact that lipophilic drugs not only have flow-limited elimination clearance, but also flow-limited tissue distribution. Therefore, the equations supporting the negligible role of protein binding on flow-limited elimination clearance also generalize to include flow-limited tissue distribution.[63] Indirect proof of this is provided by the fact that there are no examples in the literature that drug–drug interactions that produce changes in protein binding of opioids and hypnotics are clinically relevant.[64]

TABLE 7-5. INDUCERS AND INHIBITORS OF HEPATIC DRUG METABOLISM

Inducers	Inhibitors
Carbamazepine	Azole antifungal drugs (i.e., Ketoconazole, Itraconazole)
Ethanol	Cimetidine
Glucocorticoids	Disulfiram
Phenobarbital	Grapefruit Juice
Phenytoin	Macrolide antibiotics (i.e., Clarithromycin and Erythromycin)
Rifampin	Protease inhibitors (i.e., Ritonavir, Indinavir, Saquinavir)
St John's Wort	Quinidine
Tamoxifen	Selective serotonin reuptake inhibitors (i.e., Fluoxetine and Sertraline) CYP 3A4 and CYP2D6

Metabolism

Drugs that alter hepatic blood flow (i.e., vasoactive drugs, volatile anesthetics) can proportionally alter hepatic metabolism of drugs with flow-limited clearance.[58–62] In addition, drugs that inhibit or induce the enzymes that catalyze biotransformation reactions can affect clearance of other concomitantly administered drugs (Table 7-5). The concomitant use of CYP isozyme inducers can usually be overcome by increasing the administered dose, especially if an easy measure of biologic activity is available or the therapeutic concentration range is known. For example, the anticonvulsant phenytoin shortens the duration of action of the non-depolarizing neuromuscular junction blocking agents by inducing CYP3A4 and therefore increasing elimination clearance of the drug.[65] In contrast, when CYP isozyme inhibition is present, it is more difficult to adjust the drug dose without achieving supratherapeutic, and possibly toxic drug concentrations, unless a suitable rapidly responsive measure of biologic activity is available. While it may be possible to safely administer opioids in the presence of protease inhibitors such as ritonavir, because opioids can be titrated in small doses to clinical effect, it is more difficult to titrate warfarin or glyburide when instituting short-term antifungal therapy. Furthermore, pro-drugs that require CYP isozyme activity for conversion to active moieties may be difficult to titrate to adequate clinical effect if there are other
15 sources of interindividual variability in drug dose-response. The opioid pro-drugs codeine, oxycodone, hydrocodone, and tramadol all require CYP2D6 for conversion to the biologically active opioid.[64] Because of the high polymorphic character of the CYP2D6 enzyme, it is difficult to determine which patients who are taking selective serotonin reuptake inhibitors (SSRIs), which also inhibit CYP2D6 activity, would receive adequate analgesia from these opioids. Therefore, other opioids may have less variability in opioid dose-response and be better choices than these pro-drugs.

Pharmacodynamic Interactions

Pharmacodynamic interactions fall into two broad classifications. Drugs can interact, either directly or indirectly, at the same receptors. Opioid antagonists directly displace opioids from opiate receptors. Cholinesterase inhibitors indirectly antagonize the effects of neuromuscular blockers by increasing the amount of acetylcholine, which displaces the blocking drug from nicotinic receptors. Pharmacodynamic interactions can also occur if two drugs affect a physiologic system at different sites.[66,67] For example, μ-opioid receptor mediated ventilatory depression can be selectively antagonized by ampakines that potentiate AMPA receptor-mediated glutamatergic excitation without mitigating opioid induced analgesia.[68]

The most common example of pharmacodynamic interactions that are used to the advantage of anesthesiologists (and their patients) is the interaction between hypnotics and opioids. Hypnotics and opioids, each acting on their own specific receptors, appear to interact synergistically.[69] The pharmacodynamic interaction between two drugs can be characterized utilizing response surface models.[70–75] The three dimensional models are useful in delineating the concentration pairs of a hypnotic (e.g., volatile anesthetic, propofol, midazolam) and an opioid (e.g., remifentanil, alfentanil, fentanyl) that produce adequate anesthesia while minimizing undesired side effects.[76] (See Response Surface Models of Drug–Drug Interactions, below.)

Serotonin Syndrome

16 One pharmacodynamic interaction that has become more common with the widespread use of medications that modulate the serotonergic pathway is the potentially fatal serotonin syndrome (syndrome toxicity).[77,78] High CNS concentrations of serotonin can produce mental status changes (confusion, hyperactivity, memory problems), muscle twitching, excessive sweating, shivering, and fever. Classically, excessive CNS serotonin levels are associated with inhibition of monoamine oxidase, an enzyme responsible for breaking down serotonin in the brain. However, excessive intrasynaptic serotonin levels from decreased reuptake of serotonin have been associated with other antidepressant medications, including serotonin reuptake inhibitors and serotonin norepinephrine reuptake inhibitors (Table 7-6). The interaction of meperidine with MAOIs is the most classic drug–drug interactions associated with serotonin syndrome. It is important to know that other common perioperative medications, such as methylene blue, which is a potent reversible MAOI, and the phenylpiperidine series of opioids (i.e., fentanyl and its congeners, methadone, meperidine, tramadol), which act as weak serotonin reuptake inhibitors, have been reported to be associated with serotonin toxicity in small case reports.[78–81] Ideally, the serotonergic drug would be held until sufficient CNS drug washout can occur to mitigate any interaction. Because the SSRIs with long elimination half-lives require more than 4 weeks for adequate CNS washout, withholding these drugs can result in worsening depression or neuropathic pain, depending on the indication for the initial serotonergic medication. Therefore, when adequate washout cannot be obtained and methylene blue must be administered, the serotonergic drug should stopped and not reinstated for 24 hours after the last dose of methylene blue.[80] When methylene blue or phenylpiperidine opioids must be administered to patients taking serotonergic psychiatric medications, clinicians should have a high clinical suspicion for the development of serotonin toxicity. This is especially important in the perioperative period when other more common clinical states, such as postoperative delirium or perioperative fever, can be associated with the common symptoms of serotonin toxicity, thereby delaying diagnosis. Although cyproheptadine, a serotonin receptor antagonist, is the most common treatment of moderate to severe serotonin toxicity, it is only available as an oral formulation, thereby limiting its bioavailability in the critically ill perioperative patients. Intravenous chlorpromazine is an alternative serotonin receptor antagonist that has been used successfully with concomitant supportive care.

TABLE 7-6. SEROTONERGIC PSYCHIATRIC DRUGS IMPLICATED IN THE CASES OF SEROTONIN SYNDROME WITH METHYLENE BLUE[a]

Class	Generic	Brand Name(s)
Selective Serotonin Reuptake Inhibitors (SSRIs)	Paroxetine	Paxil, Paxil CR, Pexeva
	Fluvoxamine	Luvox, Luvox CR
	Fluoxetine	Prozac, Sarafem, Symbyax
	Sertraline	Zoloft
	Citalopram	Celexa
	Escitalopram	Lexapro
	Vilazodone	Viibryd
Serotonin-Norepinephrine Reuptake Inhibitors (SNRIs)	Venlafaxine	Effexor, Effexor XR
	Desvenlafaxine	Pristiq
	Duloxetine	Cymbalta
Tricyclic Antidepressants (TCAs)	Amitriptyline	Amitid, Amitril, Elavil, Endep, Etrafon, Limbitrol, Triavil
	Desipramine	Norpramin, Pertofrane
	Clomipramine	Anafranil
	Imipramine	Tofranil, Tofranil PM, Janimine, Pramine, Presamine
	Nortriptyline	Pamelor, Aventyl hydrochloride
	Protriptyline	Vivactil
	Doxepin	Sinequan, Zonalon, Silenor
	Trimipramine	Surmontil
Monoamine Oxidase Inhibitors (MAOIs)	Isocarboxazid	Marplan
	Phenelzine	Nardil
	Selegiline	Emsam, Eldepryl, Zelapar
	Tranylcypromine	Parnate
Others	Amoxapine	Asendin
	Maprotiline	Ludiomil
	Nefazodone	Serzone
	Trazodone	Desyrel, Oleptro, Trialodine
	Bupropion	Wellbutrin, Wellbutrin SR, Wellbutrin XL, Zyban, Aplenzin
	Buspirone	Buspar
	Mirtazapine	Remeron, Remeron Soltab

[a]Adapted from U.S. Food & Drug Administration website, updated 11/08/2011 (http://www.fda.gov/Drugs/DrugSafety/ucm276119.htm).

CLINICAL APPLICATIONS OF PHARMACOKINETICS AND PHARMACODYNAMICS TO THE ADMINISTRATION OF INTRAVENOUS ANESTHETICS

While no new inhaled anesthetics have been synthesized since the 1960s, intravenous drugs that act on the CNS continue to be developed. Anesthesiologists have become accustomed to the exquisite control of anesthetic blood (and effect site) concentrations afforded by modern volatile anesthetic agents and their vaporizers, coupled to end-tidal anesthetic gas monitoring. Although pharmacokinetic and pharmacodynamic principles and data have contributed greatly to our understanding of the behavior of intravenous anesthetics, their primary utility and ultimate purpose are to determine optimal dosing with as much mathematical precision and clinical accuracy as possible. In most pharmacotherapeutic scenarios outside of anesthesia care, the time scales for onset of drug effect, its maintenance, and its offset are measured in days, weeks, or even years. In such cases, global pharmacokinetic variables (and one-compartment models) such as total volume of distribution (V_{SS}), elimination clearance (Cl_e), and half-life ($t_{1/2}$) are sufficient and utilitarian parameters for calculating dose regimens. However, in the operating room and the intensive care unit, the temporal tolerances for onset and offset of desired drug effects are measured in minutes.[38,39] Consequently, these global variables are insufficient to describe the details of kinetic behavior of drugs in the minutes following intravenous administration. This is particularly true of lipid-soluble hypnotics and opioids that rapidly and extensively distribute throughout the various tissues of the body, because distribution processes dominate pharmacokinetic behavior during the time frame of most anesthetics. Additionally, the therapeutic indices of many intravenous anesthetic drugs are small and two-tailed (i.e., an underdose, resulting in awareness, which is a "toxic" effect). Optimal dosing in these situations requires use of all the variables of a multicompartmental pharmacokinetic model to account for drug distribution in blood and other tissues.

It is not easy to intuit the pharmacokinetic behavior of a multicompartmental system by simple examination of the kinetic variables.[10] Computer simulation is required to meaningfully interpret dosing or to accurately devise new dosing regimens. In addition, there are several pharmacokinetic concepts that are uniquely applicable to intravenous administration of drugs with multicompartmental kinetics and must be taken into account when administering intravenous infusions.

To achieve similar degrees of control of intravenously administered anesthetic drug concentrations in blood and in the CNS, new technologies aimed at improving intravenous infusion devices, as well as new software to manage the daunting pharmacokinetic principles involved, are needed. This section examines the current state of infusion devices and the pharmacokinetic and pharmacodynamic principles specifically required for precise delivery of anesthetic agents.

Rise to Steady-state Concentration

The drug concentration versus time profile for the rise to steady state is the mirror image of its elimination profile. In a one-compartment model with a decline in concentration versus time that is monoexponential following a single dose, the rise of drug concentration to the steady-state concentration (C_{SS}) is likewise monoexponential during a continuous infusion. That is, in one elimination half-life, an infusion is halfway to its eventual steady-state concentration, in another half-life it reaches half of what remains between halfway and steady state (i.e., 75% of the eventual steady state is reached in two elimination half-lives), and so on for each half-life increment. The equation describing this behavior is:

$$C_p(t) = C_{ss}[1 - e^{-kt}] \qquad (7\text{-}19)$$

where $C_p(t)$ = the concentration at time t, k is the rate constant related to the elimination half-life, and t is the time from the start of the infusion. This relationship can also be described by:

$$C_p(n) = C_{SS}[1 - (1/2)^n] \qquad (7\text{-}20)$$

in which $C_p(n)$ is the concentration at n half-lives. Equation 7-20 indicates that during a constant infusion, the concentration reaches 90% of C_{ss} after 3.3 half-lives, which is usually deemed close enough for clinical purposes.

However, for a drug such as propofol, which partitions extensively to pharmacologically inert body tissues (e.g., muscle, gut), a monoexponential equation, or single-compartment model, is insufficient to describe the time course of propofol concentrations in the first minutes and hours after beginning drug administration. Instead, a multicompartmental or multiexponential model must be used. With such a model, the picture changes drastically for the plasma drug concentration rise toward steady state. The rate of rise toward steady state is determined by the distribution rate constants to the degree that their respective exponential terms contribute to the total area under the concentration versus time curve. Thus, for the three-compartment model describing the pharmacokinetics of propofol, Equation 7-19 becomes:

$$C_p(t) = C_{SS}\left[\frac{A}{A+B+G}(1-e^{-\alpha t}) + \frac{B}{A+B+G}(1-e^{-\beta t}) + \frac{G}{A+B+G}(1-e^{-\gamma t})\right] \qquad (7\text{-}21)$$

in which t = time; $C_p(t)$ = plasma concentration at time; A = coefficient of the rapid distribution phase and α = hybrid rate constant of the rapid distribution phase; B = coefficient of the slower distribution phase and β = hybrid rate constant of the slower distribution; and G = coefficient of elimination phase and γ = hybrid rate constant of the elimination phase. A + B + G is the sum of the coefficients of all the exponential terms. For most lipophilic anesthetics and opioids, A is typically one order of magnitude greater than B, and B is in turn an order of magnitude greater than G. Therefore, distribution-phase kinetics for intravenous anesthetics have a much greater influence on the time to reach C_{SS} than do elimination-phase kinetics.[49]

For example, with propofol having an elimination half-life of approximately six hours, the simple one-compartment rule in Equation 7-20 tells us that it would take 6 hours from the start of a constant rate infusion to reach even 50% of the eventual steady-state propofol plasma concentration and 12 hours to reach 75%. In contrast, with a full three-compartment propofol kinetic model, Equation 7-21 accurately predicts that 50% of steady state is reached in less than 30 minutes and 75% will be reached in less than 4 hours. This example emphasizes the necessity of using multicompartment models to describe the clinical pharmacokinetics of intravenous anesthetics.

Manual Bolus and Infusion Dosing Schemes

Based on a one compartment pharmacokinetic model, a stable steady-state plasma concentration ($C_{p,ss}$) can be maintained by administering an infusion at a rate (I) that is proportional to the elimination of drug from the body (Cl_E)—

$$I = C_{p,SS} \times Cl_E \qquad (7\text{-}22)$$

However, if the drug was only administered by initiating and maintaining this infusion, it would take one-elimination half-time to reach 50% of the target plasma concentration and three times that long to reach 90% of the target plasma concentration. In order to decrease the time until the target plasma concentration is achieved, an initial bolus (loading dose) of drug can be administered that would produce the target plasma concentration:

$$Bolus = C_{p,SS} \times V_{d,SS} \qquad (7\text{-}23)$$

Although this method is very efficient in achieving and maintaining the target plasma concentration of a drug that instantaneously mixes and equilibrates throughout the tissues of the body (e.g., drugs modeled with a one-compartment pharmacokinetic model), utilizing the steady-state elimination clearance and volume of distribution to calculate the loading dose and maintenance infusion rate will result in plasma drug concentrations that are higher throughout the initial distribution phase (see Fig. 7-13).

Utilizing Equations 7-22 and 7-23 and $V_{d,SS}$ = 262 L and Cl_E = 1.7 L/min (for a 50-year-old male who is 178 cm tall and weighs 70 kg from Schnider, et al.), the loading dose and infusion rate of propofol that is needed to achieve a steady-state plasma concentration of 5 mcg/mL is 1300 mg (18 mg/kg) and 120 mcg/kg/min. Obviously, the loading dose of propofol is too high, compared with clinically utilized doses (1–2 mg/kg), while the infusion rate appears to be a clinically acceptable dose. The erroneous estimate of the loading dose is due to the fact that the initial bolus of drug is not instantaneously mixed and equilibrated with the entire volume of tissue that will eventually take up the drug. Therefore, manual dosing strategies for intravenous anesthetics need to be modified to account for the fact that when a bolus of drug

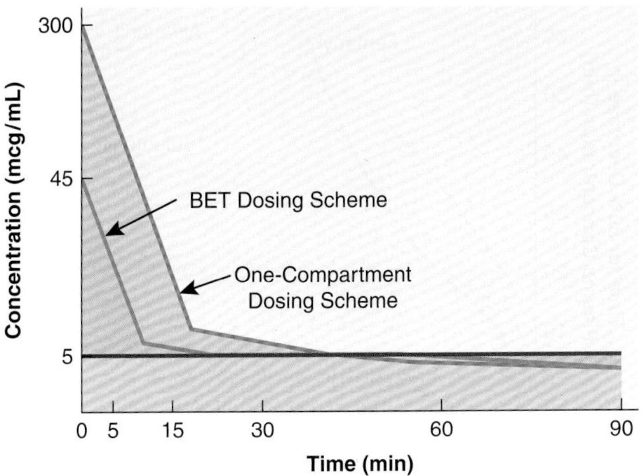

FIGURE 7-13. A computer simulation of the plasma propofol concentration profile during and after the administration of a single bolus and infusion scheme calculated using the steady state, one-compartment pharmacokinetic parameters (*red line*) and the BET scheme from Table 7-7 (*blue line*) to achieve a plasma concentration of 5 mcg/mL. $V_{d,SS}$ = 262 L and Cl_E = 1.7 L/min for a 50-year-old male who is 178 cm tall and weighs 70 kg.

is administered, it rapidly mixes and equilibrates with the blood and only a small volume of tissue (e.g., the central compartment), and then will distribute over time into other tissues.

To design a manual bolus that more precisely achieves the desired target plasma concentration, it is necessary to choose a bolus that is based on the small, initial volume of distribution (V_c). To maintain the target plasma concentration, a series of infusions of decreasing rate can be used that match the elimination clearance and compensates for drug loss from the central to the peripheral compartments during the initial period of extensive drug distribution and the second period of moderate drug distribution. This manual dosing scheme has been termed the BET scheme, where B is the loading bolus dose, E is the infusion to replace drug removed by elimination clearance, and T is a continuously decreasing infusion that compensates for transfer of drug to the peripheral tissues (i.e., distribution).[82] An example of a BET scheme for propofol to achieve a target plasma concentration of 5 mcg/mL is shown in Table 7-7.

TABLE 7-7. THE BOLUS-ELIMINATION-INFUSION (BET) SCHEME TO ACHIEVE A PROPOFOL PLASMA CONCENTRATION OF 5 mcg/mL FOR 120 MINUTES

Dose		Time (min)
Bolus Dose	2.8 mg/kg	
Infusion	238 mcg/kg/min	0–10
	187 mcg/kg/min	10–20
	136 mcg/kg/min	20–60
	112 mcg/kg/min	60–120

Isoconcentration Nomogram

To make the calculations of the various infusion rates required to maintain a target plasma concentration for a drug that follows multicompartment pharmacokinetics, a clinician would need access to a basic computer and the software to perform the appropriate simulations. With the appropriate formulas, this is quite feasible to do on any basic computer with any basic spreadsheet. However, even with more sophisticated pharmacokinetic software (e.g., SAAM II, WinNonLin, RugLoop, Stanpump), this is a time consuming process that diverts the clinician's attention from the patient. In 1994, Shafer introduced an isoconcentration nomogram for propofol that utilized the rise toward steady state described by a multicompartmental system (Fig. 7-14).[83] This graphical tool allows users to employ concentration-effect, rather than dose-effect relationships when determining optimal dosing of intravenous anesthetic agents. The nomogram is constructed by calculating the plasma drug concentration versus time curve for a constant-rate infusion from a set of pharmacokinetic variables for a particular drug. From this single simulation, one can readily visualize (and estimate) the rise toward steady-state plasma drug concentration described by the drug's pharmacokinetic model. By simulating a range of potential infusion rates, a series of curves of identical shape are then plotted on a single graph with drug concentrations at any time that are directly proportional to the infusion rate.

By placing a horizontal line at the desired plasma drug concentration (y-axis), the times (x-axis) at which the horizontal intersects

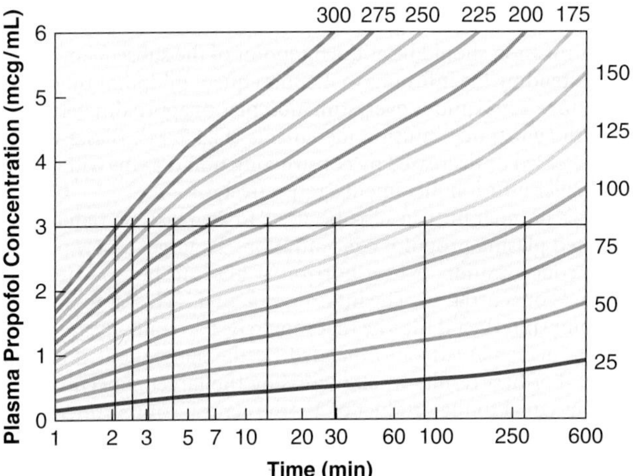

FIGURE 7-14. Isoconcentration nomogram for determining propofol infusion rates designed to maintain a desired plasma propofol concentration. This nomogram is based on the pharmacokinetics of Schnider et al., and plotted on a log–log scale to better delineate the early time points. Curved lines represent the plasma propofol concentration versus time plots, resulting from the various continuous infusion rates indicated along the right and upper borders (units in μg/kg/min). A horizontal line is placed at the desired target plasma propofol concentration (3 μg/mL in this case) and vertical lines are placed at each intersection of a curved concentration-time plot. The vertical lines indicate the times that the infusion rate should be set to the one represented by the next intersected curve as one moves from left to right along the horizontal line drawn at 3 μg/mL. In this example the infusion rate would be reduced from 300 μg/kg/min to 275 μg/kg/min at 2.5 minutes, to 250 μg/kg/min at 3 minutes, to 225 μg/kg/min at 4.5 minutes, and so on until it is turned to 100 μg/kg/min at 260 minutes.

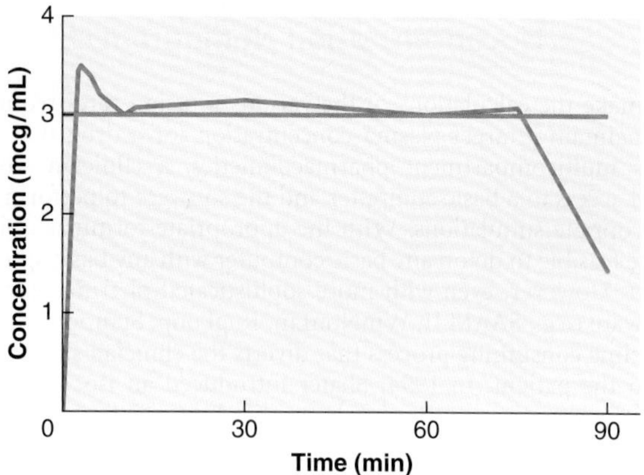

FIGURE 7-15. Simulated plasma propofol concentration history resulting from the information in the isoconcentration nomogram in Figure 7-14 and extending the times to switch the infusion to the next lower increment to the midpoint of the subsequent time segment (i.e., the switch from 250 to 225 μg/kg/min was at 5 minutes, rather than at 4.5 minutes). Note that for the first 30 minutes, this sequence predicts plasma propofol concentrations that are always slightly above 3 μg/mL (see text). The infusion is stopped at 90 minutes in this case.

the line for a particular infusion rate will represent the times at which the infusion rate should be set to the rate on the intercepting line. In the example shown (see Fig. 7-14) with 25 μg/kg/min increments, the predicted plasma propofol concentrations remain within 10% of the target from 2 minutes onward with a bias of underestimation. If never allowing the estimated concentration to fall below the target is desired, then the time to decrease to the next lower infusion should be at the midpoint of the subsequent interval. Extending the infusions to the subsequent midpoint times will introduce a maximum overestimation bias of approximately 17% with the illustrated infusion increments (Fig. 7-14). Biases would be increased or decreased by constructing nomograms with larger or smaller infusion increments, respectively.

The nomogram can also be used to increase or reduce the targeted plasma propofol concentration. To target a new plasma drug concentration, a new horizontal line can be drawn at the desired concentration. The infusion rate that is closest to the current time intersect is the one that should be used initially, followed by the decremented rates dictated by the subsequent intercept times. For best results when increasing the target concentration, a bolus equal to the product of V_c (the central compartment volume) and the incremental change in concentration should be administered. Likewise, when decreasing the concentration the best strategy is to turn off the infusion for the duration predicted by the applicable context-sensitive decrement time and resume the infusion rate predicted for the current time plus the context-sensitive decrement time. For instance, if after 30 minutes one wishes to decrease the target plasma propofol concentration from 3 μg/mL to 2 μg/mL (a 33% decrement at a time context of 30 minutes), one would shut off the infusion for 1 minute and 10 seconds to let the concentration fall by 33% and then restart at 75 μg/kg/min. The estimated plasma propofol concentrations from this nomogram-guided dosing scheme are shown in Figure 7-15.

Context-sensitive Decrement Times

During an infusion, the drug is taken up by the inert, peripheral tissues (18). Once drug delivery is terminated, recovery occurs

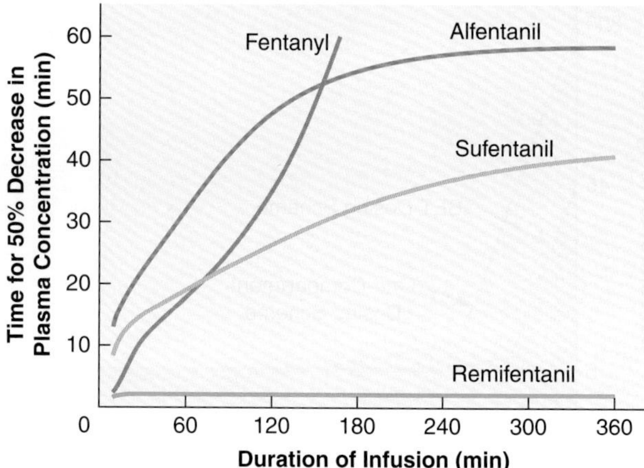

FIGURE 7-16. The context-sensitive plasma half-time for fentanyl, alfentanil, sufentanil, and remifentanil.

when the effect-site concentration decreases below a threshold concentration for producing a pharmacologic effect (e.g., MAC-AWAKE—the concentration where 50% of patients follow com-
17 mands).[49,75] Although the rate of elimination of the drug from the body can give some indication for the time required to reach a subtherapeutic effect-site drug concentration, distribution to and from the peripheral tissues also contributes to the time course of decreasing drug concentrations of the central compartment and the effected site. For drugs with multicompartmental kinetics, the elimination half-life will always overestimate the time to recovery from anesthetic drugs. The *context-sensitive half-time* is defined as the time required for the drug concentration of the plasma to decrease by 50%, where the context is the duration of the infusion[84]. The context-sensitive half-time for the common synthetic opioids fentanyl, alfentanil, sufentanil, and remifentanil are illustrated in Figure 7-16.

The context-sensitive half time is not a pharmacokinetic parameter per se. It is calculated by simulating a TCI of a particular length (the length is the context) and then observing the time required for the plasma concentration to reach one-half of the target concentration from the time the infusion is terminated. As the length of the infusion increases, the value of the half-time increases and will eventually asymptotically approach a maximum half-time at steady state. Generally, for multicompartmental pharmacokinetic models, the half-time will always be less than the elimination half-life.

When an infusion is terminated at steady state, input into the system's central compartment is lost and net transfer of the drug is no longer zero. Instead, net drug distribution immediately begins moving toward the central compartment from the peripheral compartments rather than away, as was the case during infusion, and the elimination from the central compartment continues unabated by the infusion's input. Plasma or central compartment concentrations will fall relatively rapidly, compared to the elimination half-life, until set concentration ratios of central:fast and central:slow are achieved. These ratios with higher peripheral compartment drug concentrations will achieve the net drug distribution flux into the central compartment that will balance the elimination flux to create a constant elimination rate.

During the elimination phase, the multicompartmental system behaves kinetically as a single compartment, but only does so because there are (fixed) drug concentration ratios among the compartments. With a short infusion, the peripheral compartment drug concentrations will have only achieved low drug concentrations and the plasma drug concentration will have to fall quite far to reach the central:peripheral drug concentration ratios needed to enter the constant elimination phase. Thus, the half-time is less with shorter infusion contexts. After a very long infusion with peripheral compartment drug concentrations reaching higher drug concentrations as they approach their steady state, plasma drug concentrations will not need to fall as much to reach the concentration ratios required for the elimination phase, and the rate of plasma drug decline will begin approaching the elimination half-life sooner, resulting in longer half-times.

One must be aware of the limitations of the context-sensitive half-time concept.[10,20] First, it is not a kinetic parameter; it only describes a specific simulation event. This means it cannot be extrapolated backward or, more importantly, forward to lesser or greater drug concentration decrements, as is possible with true kinetic parameters. Second, it cannot be directly calculated from other kinetic parameters. Rather, a model of the specific drug pharmacokinetics is programmed into a simulation with a set drug infusion regimen; tedious for pencil and paper or hand-held calculator, but a simple matter for even a modest computing device (e.g., TCA pumps and applications for smartphones). Third, the most relevant concentration decrease may not be one half. It could be less than one half or, as is likelier in practice, more than one half. Therefore, simulating both the specific infusion context, as well as the required percentage decrease from the target concentration, should be done to get the best estimate of when a drug's effect will reach the clinically desired endpoint.

Although a 50% decrease in plasma concentration is an appealing and comprehensible parameter, larger or smaller decreases in plasma concentrations may be required for recovery from the drug. Simulations show that the time for different percent decreases in plasma concentration are not linear.[10,20] Therefore, if a 25% or 75% decrease in plasma concentration is required, simulations must be performed to calculate the context-sensitive 25% decrement time or context-sensitive 75% decrement time (Fig. 7-17). In addition, if the concentration of interest is the effect-site concentration rather than the plasma concentration, simulations can be performed to calculate the context-sensitive effect-site decrement time. Finally, if a constant plasma or effect-site concentration is not maintained throughout the delivery of the drug (which is typically the case with manual bolus and infusion schemes and also with varying drug requirements depending on surgical stimulation, etc.), the context-sensitive decrement times are guidelines of recovery rather than an absolute prediction of the decay in drug concentration. If precise drug

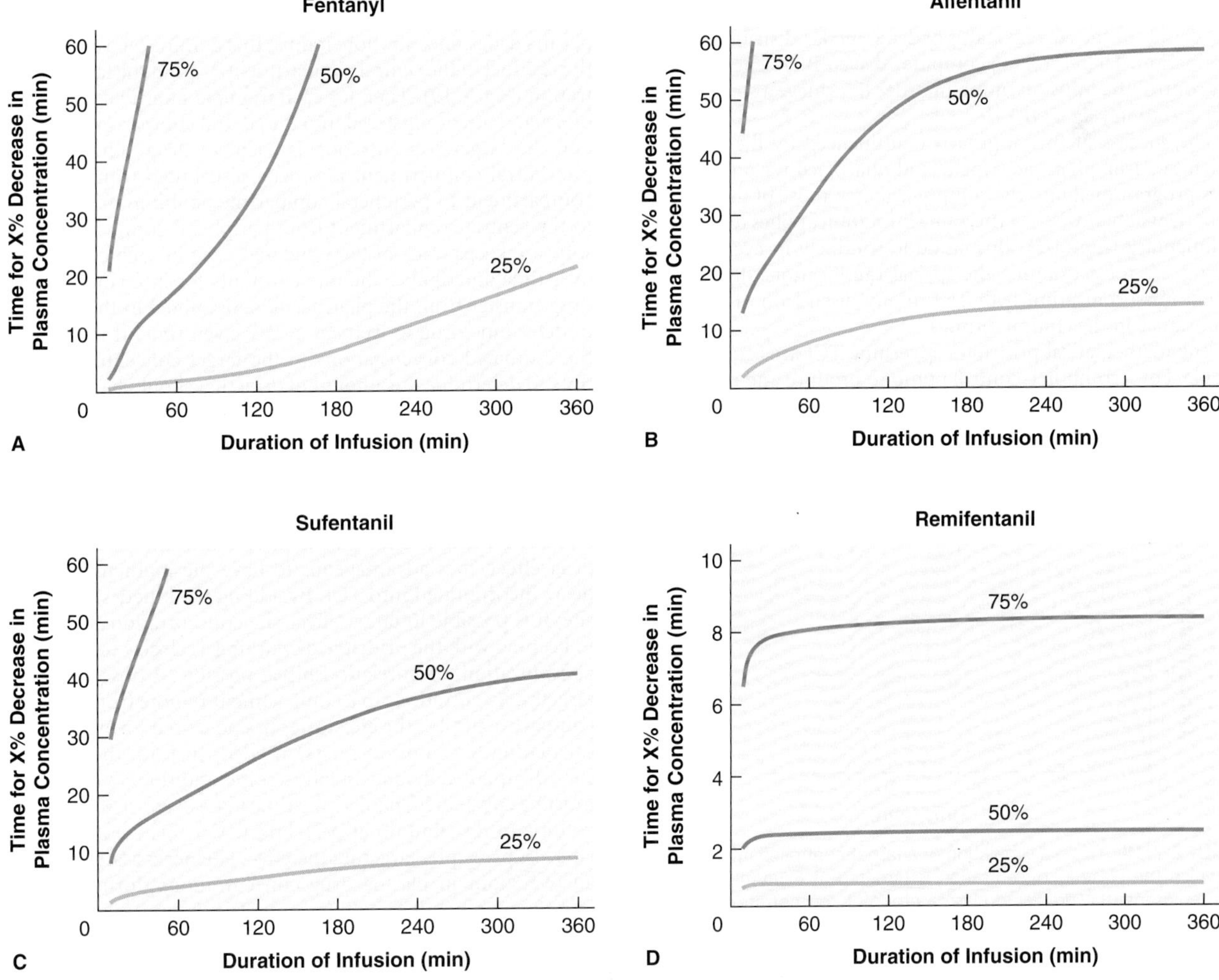

FIGURE 7-17. The context-sensitive 25%, 50%, and 75% plasma decrement times for fentanyl, alfentanil, sufentanil, and remifentanil.

administration data are known, it is possible to compute the context-sensitive decrement time for the individual situation or context. Even though the context-sensitive decrement times are limited, this concept has changed the way that intravenous anesthetics are described and has helped foster an increase in accurately and safely administering intravenous anesthetics.

Target-controlled Infusions

Prior to performing an anesthetic, it is possible to perform the calculations above and derive a BET scheme targeted to a predetermined plasma or effect-site concentration. However, in the operating room, once the anesthetic has commenced, without the help of a computer, software, and possibly an assistant, it is laborious and difficult to make any calculations to determine how to adjust the infusion or how to bolus (or stop the infusion) to increase or decrease the target plasma concentration.[85] By linking a computer with the appropriate pharmacokinetic model to an infusion pump, it is possible for the physician to enter the desired target plasma concentration of a drug and for the computer to nearly instantaneously calculate the appropriate infusion scheme to achieve this target in a matter of seconds.[86] Because drug accumulates at various rates among the various tissues and organs in the body, the computer continually calculates the current drug concentration and adjusts the infusion pump in order to account for the current status of drug uptake, distribution, and elimination. Therefore, the computer driven BET scheme can in fact control the infusion pump in order to achieve a steady target concentration (Fig. 7-18).

The success of this approach is influenced by the extent to which the drug pharmacokinetic and pharmacodynamic parameters programmed into the computer match those of the particular patient at hand. While this same limitation applies to the more rudimentary (non-TCI) dosing done routinely in every clinical setting, we must examine the special ramifications of—PK–PD model misspecification with TCI in any discussion of its future importance in the clinical setting.

The mathematical principles governing TCI are actually quite simple. For a computer-control pump to produce and maintain a

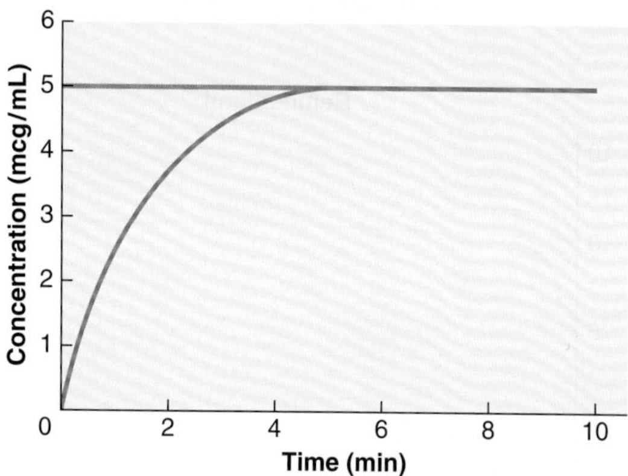

FIGURE 7-18. This is a simulation of a target-controlled infusion (TCI) in which the plasma concentration is targeted at 5 μg/mL. The *blue line* represents the predicted plasma propofol concentration of 5 μg/mL, which in theory is attained at time t = 0 and is then maintained by a variable rate infusion. The *red line* is the predicted effect-site concentration under the conditions of a constant pseudo–steady-state plasma concentration. Note that 95% of the target concentration is reached in the effect site at approximately 4 minutes.

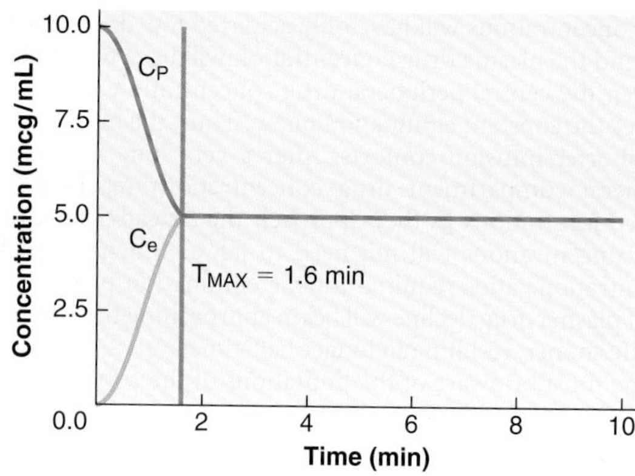

FIGURE 7-19. This is a simulation of a target-controlled infusion (TCI) in which the effect-site concentration is targeted at 5 μg/mL. The *solid line* represents the predicted plasma propofol concentration that results from a bolus dose, given at time t = 0 that is predicted to purposely overshoot the plasma propofol concentration target until time t = T_{MAX} (1.6 minutes). At T_{MAX}, pseudo-equilibration between the effect site and the plasma occurs and both concentrations are then predicted to be the same until the target is changed. Note that the effect site attains the target in less than half the time with effect site targeting compared to the plasma concentration targeting seen in Figure 7-18.

plasma drug concentration, it must first administer a dose equal to the product of the central compartment, V_1, and the target concentration (Fig. 7-19). Then for each moment after that, the amount of drug to be administered into the central compartment to maintain the target concentration is equal to drug eliminated from the central compartment *plus* drug distributed from the central compartment to peripheral compartments *minus* drug returning to the central compartment from peripheral compartments. The software keeps track of the estimated drug in each compartment over time and applies the rate constants for intercompartmental drug transfer from the pharmacokinetic model to these amounts to determine drug movement at any given time. It then matches the estimated concentrations to the target concentration at any time to determine the amount of drug that should be infused. The software can also predict future concentrations, usually with the assumption that the infusion will be stopped so that emergence from anesthesia or the dissipation of drug effect will occur optimally according to the context-sensitive decrement time.

Because there is a delay or hysteresis between the attainment of a drug concentration in the plasma and the production of a drug effect, it is advantageous to have the mathematics of this delay incorporated into TCI. By adding the kinetics of the effect site, it is possible to target effect-site concentrations as would be in keeping with the principle of working as closely to the relevant concentration-effect relationship as possible. A dose scheme that targets concentrations in a compartment remote from the central compartment (i.e., the effect site) has no closed form solution for calculating the infusion rate(s) needed. Instead, the solution is solved numerically and involves some additional concepts that must be considered, namely the time to peak effect, T_{MAX}, and the volume of distribution at peak effect, V_{DPE}. These are discussed later. In principle, targeting the effect site necessitates producing an overshoot in plasma drug concentrations during induction and for subsequent target increases. This is similar in concept to over-pressurizing inhaled anesthetic concentrations to achieve a targeted end-tidal concentration. However, unlike the inspiratory limb of an anesthesia circuit, the plasma compartment seems to be closely linked to cardiovascular effects, and large overshoots in plasma drug concentration may produce unwanted side effects.

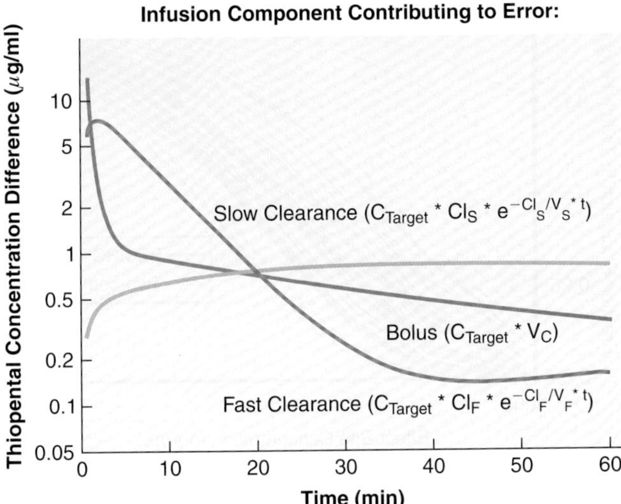

FIGURE 7-20. The influence of the misspecification of each of the components of the traditional three-compartment pharmacokinetic models on the prolonged discrepancy (overshoot) between predicted and targeted concentrations with target-controlled infusions (TCI). The error resulting from elimination clearance was negligible and therefore not illustrated. Notice that the loading dose (based on V_C) produces a large amount of error in the initial minutes, however, from 1 to 20 minutes, the deviation from the target concentration is largely due to the overestimation of Cl_F. The equations listed are for the respective BET infusions of the TCI system. (From: Avram MJ and Krejcie TC. Using front-end kinetics to optimize target-controlled drug infusions. *Anesthesiology.* 2003;99:1078–1086.)

The performance of TCI is influenced by the pharmacokinetic model chosen. Although most modern TCI models, whether they target the plasma or the effect site, seem to be similar in performance, they all produce overshoot for 10 to 20 minutes when increasing the target concentration.[36] This is because the dose adjustments made are based on calculations that utilize a central compartment that ignores the complexity of intravascular mixing, thereby overestimating the central compartment's true volume (V_C) and overestimating the rate of transfer to the fast peripheral tissue (Cl_F) and the size of the peripheral tissue compartment (V_F) (Fig. 7-20). The performance of TCI is also influenced by the variance between pharmacokinetic parameters determined from group or population studies and the individual patient. Median absolute performance errors for fentanyl,[87] alfentanil,[88] sufentanil,[89] midazolam,[90,91] and propofol[91,92] are in the range of ±30% when literature values for pharmacokinetic parameters are used to drive the TCI device and fall to approximately ±7% when the average kinetics of the test subjects themselves are used.[88] Divergence (the percentage change of the absolute performance error) is generally quite low (approximately 1%) when target concentrations remain relatively stable, but increase to nearly 20% when the frequency of concentration steps is as frequent as every 12 minutes.[36,92] These data suggest that while a considerable error may exist (±30%) between the targeted drug concentration and the one actually achieved in a patient, the concentration attained will not vary much over time. Thus, incremental adjustments in the target should result in incremental and stable new concentrations in the patient as long as the incremental adjustments are not too frequent.

18 The introduction of the concept of TCI was first described by Schwilden et al. in early 1980s. Other software systems were developed in North America by groups at Stanford University and Duke University. By the late 1990s a commercially available TCI system for propofol (Diprifusor®) was introduced. This greatly increased both anesthesiologists' interest in this mode of delivery and their understanding of the concentration-effect relationships for hypnotics and opioids. In most of the world, devices for delivering propofol by TCI are commercially available from at least three companies (Graseby, Alaris, and Fresenius) with similar performance parameters.[93] In the United States, there are still no FDA-approved devices. For investigational purposes, STANPUMP (developed by Steve Shafer at Stanford University) can be interfaced via an RS232 port to an infusion pump. STANPUMP currently provides pharmacokinetic parameters for 19 different drugs, but has the ability to accept any kinetic model for any drug provided by the user. (Information regarding STANPUMP is available at *http://opentci.org/doku.php?id=code:code&s[]=stanpump* Accessed December 10, 2012.). RUGLOOP© is the TCI software (developed by Michel Struys of Ghent University), which is similar to STANPUMP but operates in Windows® rather than DOS® and is capable of controlling multiple drug infusions simultaneously. (Information regarding RUGLOOP is available at *http://www.demed.be/index.html;* Accessed December 10, 2007.)

While the pharmacologic principle of relating a concentration rather than a dose is scientifically sound, few studies have actually attempted to determine whether TCI improves clinical performance or outcome. Only a few limited studies have actually compared manual infusion control versus TCI. Some have shown better control and a more predictable emergence with TCI,[93,94] whereas others have simply shown no advantage.[95,96]

TCI principles continue to be developed beyond the scope of intravenous anesthesia techniques. TCI has been used to provide postoperative analgesia with alfentanil.[97,98] In this system, a desired target plasma alfentanil concentration was set in the range of 40 to 100 ng/mL. A demand by the patient automatically increased the target level by 5 ng/mL. Lack of a demand caused the system to gradually reduce the targeted level. The quality of analgesia was judged to be superior to standard morphine patient controlled analgesia (PCA).

Similarly, TCI has been used to provide patient-controlled sedation with propofol.[99,100] The TCI was set to 1 μg/mL and a demand by the patient increased the level by 0.2 μg/mL. As with the TCI analgesia system, the lack of a demand caused the system to gradually reduce the targeted plasma propofol concentration. The timing and increment of the decrease were adjusted by the clinician. Over 90% of patients were satisfied with this method of sedation.

Time to Maximum Effect Compartment Concentration (T_{MAX})

Earlier in this chapter, the delay between attaining a plasma concentration and an effect-site concentration was described (Fig. 7-11). This delay, or hysteresis, is presumed to be a result of transfer of drug between the plasma compartment, V_C, and an effect compartment, V_e, as well as the time required for a cellular response. By simultaneously modeling the plasma drug concentration versus time data (pharmacokinetics) and the measured drug effect (pharmacodynamics), an estimate of the drug transfer rate constant, k_{e0}, between plasma and the putative effect site can be estimated.[47] However, estimates of k_{e0}, like all rate constants, are model specific.[101,102] That is, k_{e0} cannot be transported from one set of kinetic parameters determined in one specific—PK–PD study to any another set of pharmacokinetic parameters. Likewise, it is not valid to compare estimates of k_{e0} among studies of the same drug or across different drugs and, therefore, one should not be surprised that reported values for k_{e0} for the same drug vary markedly among studies. The model-independent parameter that characterizes the delay between the plasma and effect site is the time to maximal effect, or T_{MAX}.[102] Accordingly, if the T_{MAX} and the pharmacokinetics for a drug are known from independent studies, a k_{e0} can be estimated by numeric techniques for the independent kinetic set that would produce the known effect-site T_{MAX}.

The concept of a transportable, model-independent parameter that characterizes the kinetics of the effect site is important for robust effect site–targeted, computer-controlled infusions. This is because there are many more pharmacokinetic studies characterizing a wider variety of patient types and groups in the literature than there are complete—PK–PD studies. By making the generally valid assumption that interindividual differences are small in a drug's rate of effect-site equilibration, it is possible with a known T_{MAX} to estimate effect-site kinetics for a drug across a wide variety of patient groups where only the pharmacokinetics are known. This cannot be done in a valid manner using k_{E0} or $t½_{Ke0}$ alone.[101,102]

Volume of Distribution at Peak Effect (V_{DPE})

While the plasma concentration can be brought rapidly to the targeted drug concentration by administering a bolus dose to the central compartment ($C \times V_C$) and then held there by a computer-controlled infusion (Fig. 7-18), the time for the effect site to reach the target concentration will be much longer than T_{MAX} (4 minutes for propofol effect-site concentration to reach 95% of that targeted). It is possible to calculate a bolus dose that will attain the estimated effect-site concentration at T_{MAX} without overshoot in the effect site. However, plasma drug concentration will overshoot (Fig. 7-19). This is done by combining the concept of describing drug distribution as an expanding volume of distribution that starts at V_C and approaches V_β (the apparent volume of distribution during the elimination phase) over time with the concept of T_{MAX}.[103,104]

Volume of distribution over time is calculated by dividing the total amount of drug remaining in the body by the plasma drug concentration at each time, *t*. The time-dependent volume at the time of peak effect (or T_{MAX}) is V_{DPE}. The product of the targeted effect-site concentration and V_{DPE} plus the amount lost to elimination in the time to T_{MAX} becomes the proper bolus dose that will attain the target concentration at the effect site as rapidly as possible without overshoot. In practical terms, this bolus is given at time t = 0, after which the infusion stops until time $t = T_{MAX}$. It then resumes infusing drug in its normal "stop loss" manner.

Some software programs for controlling TCIs include this concept in their algorithms. In the case of the propofol kinetics used to construct the isoconcentration nomogram in Figure 7-14, the—PK–PD parameter set of Schnider et al.,[105] predicts a T_{MAX} of 1.6 minutes, a V_{DPE} of 16.62 L, and an elimination loss of 23.8% of the dose over 1.6 minutes in a 70 kg man. Thus the proper propofol bolus for a targeted effect-site propofol concentration of 5 μg/mL is 109 mg. The computer-controlled infusion pump will deliver this dose as rapidly as possible and then begin a targeted infusion for 5 μg/mL at t = 1.6 minutes (see Fig. 7-19).

Front-end Pharmacokinetics

Classic PK–PD models make the simplifying assumptions that there is instantaneous and complete mixing of drug in the intra-

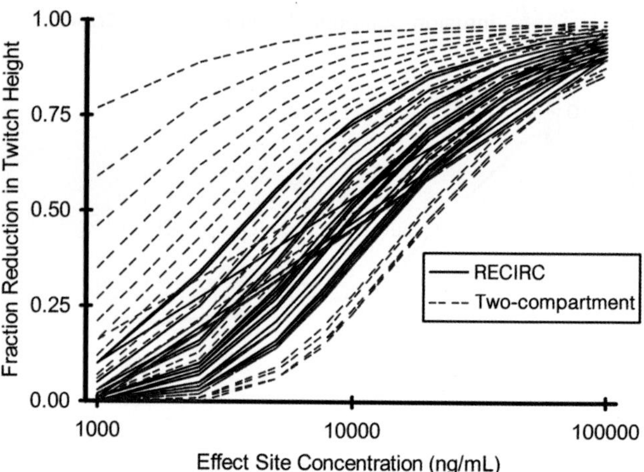

FIGURE 7-21. The misestimation of the central distribution volume (V_c) by a traditional compartmental PK–PD model results in more interindividual variability in pharmacodynamic estimates than pharmacodynamic estimates from a high-resolution, recirculatory PK–PD model. This figure uses Monte Carlo simulation of the effect-site concentration—pharmacologic-effect relationships to demonstrate the interindividual variability from a traditional compartmental PK–PD model (Two-compartment, blue dashed lines) and a high-resolution recirculatory PK–PD model (RECIRC, *black solid lines*). (Adapted from the rocuronium data of Kuipers JA, Boer F, Olofsen E, et al., Recirculatory pharmacokinetics and pharmacodynamics of rocuronium in patients: The influence of cardiac output. *Anesthesiology.* 2001;94:47–55.)

vascular space—a mathematical construct without regard for the physiology that drives drug disposition.[106–108] Therefore, the classic PK models inaccurately describe the initial/central distribution volume (V_C), as a result of which they misestimate intercompartmental clearances and are unable to characterize cardiac output and
19 its distribution.[36,39,58,106,108–111] Misspecification of V_C also results in misspecification of the effect-site kinetics and compensates by overestimating interindividual PD variability.[36,108,111] Physiologically based PK–PD models that can accurately estimate distribution volumes and clearances result in more realistic estimates of PD variability (Fig. 7-21).[111] Another source of PK and PD variability is cardiac output and its distribution.[58,108,109,111,112] Cardiac output and its distribution influences PK by modifying the distribution of drug to tissue compartments. In addition, cardiac output influences PD by changing the blood to effect-site equilibration rate (Fig. 7-22).[111] Because they cannot characterize cardiac output and its distribution, classic PK–PD models will be unable to identify the changes in cardiac output and its distribution that are the result of alterations in physiology related to sex, age, body composition or pathologic processes.[113,114] Therefore, classic PK–PD models will not identify factors that solely alter cardiac output and its distribution as a source of PK variability and will overestimate the true PD.[36,111,115,116]

The term "front-end pharmacokinetics" refers to the intravascular mixing, pulmonary uptake, and recirculation events that occur in the first few minutes during and after intravenous drug administration.[39] These kinetic events and the drug concentration versus time profile that results are important because the peak effect of rapidly acting drugs occurs during this temporal window.[38,111,117,118] Although it has been suggested that front-end pharmacokinetics be utilized to guide drug dosing,[36] current TCI does not incorporate front-end kinetics into the models from

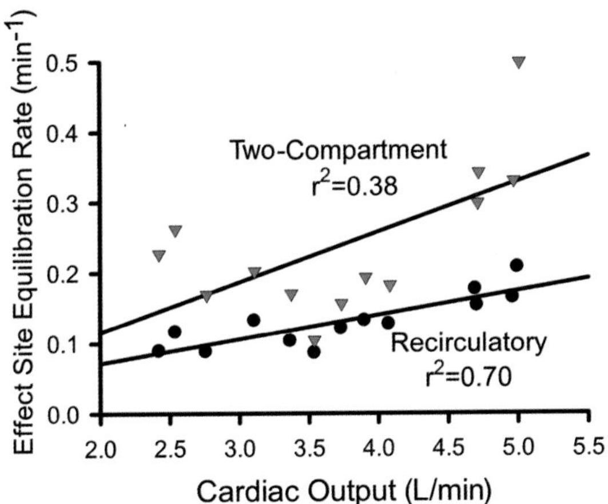

FIGURE 7-22. The effects of cardiac output on the blood—effect-site equilibration rate (k_{e0}) when the PK–PD model is a high-resolution "recirculatory" model (*black circles*) versus a traditional compartmental model (*triangles*). While the traditional model has a moderate correlation between measured cardiac output and k_{e0} and significant systematic error (*gray line*), the high-resolution recirculatory model has a very strong correlation between measured cardiac output and k_{e0} (*black line*). Therefore, for lipophilic drugs with flow limited tissue-distribution (i.e., opioids, hypnotics), a high-resolution PK–PD model provides a physiologic basis for transfer of drug from the blood to the effect site. In addition, these high-resolution PK–PD models can quantitate the effects of physiologic perturbations on the PK and PD of these drugs more accurately than the traditional compartmental models. (Adapted from the rocuronium data of Kuipers JA, Boer F, Olofsen E, et al., Recirculatory pharmacokinetics and pharmacodynamics of rocuronium in patients: The influence of cardiac output. *Anesthesiology.* 2001;94:47–55.)

which drug infusion rates are calculated. As described above, not doing so introduces further error.

TCI relies on pharmacokinetic models that are based on the simplifying assumption of instantaneous and complete mixing within V_C. However, the determination of V_C is routinely overestimated in most pharmacokinetic studies. Overestimation of V_C, when used to calculate TCI infusion rates, results in plasma drug concentrations that overshoot the desired target concentration, especially in the first few minutes after beginning TCI. Furthermore, correct description of drug distribution to tissues is dependent on an accurate V_C estimate, so inaccuracies caused by not taking front-end pharmacokinetics into account may be persistent and result in undershoot as well as overshoot. Simulation indicates that pharmacokinetic parameters derived from studies in which the drug is administered by a short (approximately 2 minutes) infusion better estimate V_C and tissue-distribution kinetics than those from a rapid intravenous bolus infusion.[36,37] When the latter drug administration method is used, full characterization of the front-end recirculatory pharmacokinetics is required to obtain valid estimates of V for use in TCI.[36,37]

Closed-loop Infusions

When a valid, and nearly continuous, measure of drug effect is available, drug delivery can be automatically titrated by feedback control. Such systems have been used experimentally for control of blood pressure,[119] oxygen delivery,[120] blood glucose,[121] neuromuscular blockade,[122] and depth of anesthesia.[123–129] A target value for the desired effect measure (the output of the system) is selected and the rate of drug delivery (the input into the system) is dependent on whether the effect measure is above, below, or at the target value. Thus the output feeds back and controls the input. Standard controllers (referred to as *proportional-integral-derivative* [or PID] *controllers*) adjust drug delivery based on either the integral, or magnitude, of the deviation from target and the rate of deviation, or the derivative.

Under a range of responses, standard PID controllers work quite well. However, they have been shown to develop unstable characteristics in situations where the output may vary rapidly and widely. Schwilden et al.[130] have proposed a controller in which the output (measured response) controls not only the input (drug infusion rate), but also the pharmacokinetic model driving the infusion rate. This is a so-called *model-driven* or *adaptive* closed-loop system. Such a system has performed well in clinical trials,[124] and in a simulation of extreme conditions it was demonstrated to outperform a standard PID controller.[127]

Closed-loop systems for anesthesia are the most difficult to design and implement because the precise definition of "anesthesia" remains elusive, as does a robust monitor for "anesthetic depth".[75] Because modification of consciousness must accompany anesthesia, processed electroencephalographic (EEG) parameters that correlate with level of consciousness, such as the bispectral index (BIS), electroencephalographic entropy, and auditory evoked potentials, make it possible to undertake closed-loop control of anesthesia. There is keen interest in further developing these tools to make them more reliable because, advances in pharmacokinetic modeling, including the effect compartment, the implementation of such models into drug delivery systems, and the creation of adaptive controllers based on these models, has made routine closed-loop delivery of anesthesia imaginable.[123] So far it has been difficult to bring a true closed-loop system to market in medical applications because of the regulatory agency hurdles. From a regulatory point of view, an open-loop TCI system is much easier to attain and offers many of the benefits of actual closed-loop systems. Unless there is a regulatory or a design "breakthrough," closed-loop systems for anesthesia will likely remain in the theoretical and experimental realms.

Response Surface Models of Drug–Drug Interactions

During the course of an operation, the level of anesthetic drug administered is adjusted to ensure amnesia to ongoing events, provide immobility to noxious stimulation, and blunt the sympathetic response to noxious stimulation. Although it is possible to achieve an adequate anesthetic state with a high dose of a sedative-hypnotic alone (i.e., a volatile anesthetic or propofol), the effect-site drug concentration necessary is often associated with excessive hemodynamic depression[67] and excessively deep plane of hypnosis that may be associated with long standing morbidity or mortality.[131,132] Therefore, to limit side effects, an opioid and a sedative-hypnotic are administered together. Although the administration of two volatile anesthetics or a volatile anesthetic and propofol produce a net-additive effect, the combination of an opioid and a sedative-hypnotic are synergistic for most pharmacologic effects. By understanding the interactions between the opioids and the sedative-hypnotics, it is possible to select target concentration pairs of the two drugs that produce the desired clinical effect while minimizing unwanted side effects associated with high concentrations of a single drug (e.g., hemodynamic instability, prolonged respiratory depression).

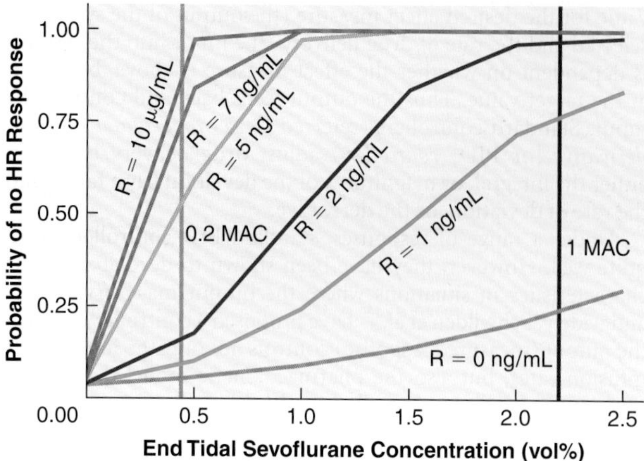

FIGURE 7-23. The effect of adding remifentanil on the concentration-effect curve for sevoflurane-induced analgesia (no hemodynamic response to a 5 second, 50 milliamp tetanic stimulation in volunteers). Each curve represents the concentration-effect relation for sevoflurane with a fixed effect-site concentration of remifentanil. The leftward shift in the curves indicates that remifentanil decreases the amount of sevoflurane needed to produce adequate analgesia. The changes in the slopes of the concentration-response curves indicate that there is significant pharmacodynamic synergy between sevoflurane–remifentanil. Also note that there is a ceiling effect to this pharmacodynamic interaction—the magnitude of the leftward shift decreases as the remifentanil concentration increases. HR, heart rate; MAC, minimum alveolar concentration. (Adapted from: Manyam SC, Gupta DK, Johnson KB, et al., Opioid-volatile anesthetic synergy: A response surface model with remifentanil and sevoflurane as prototypes. *Anesthesiology*. 2006;105:267–278.)

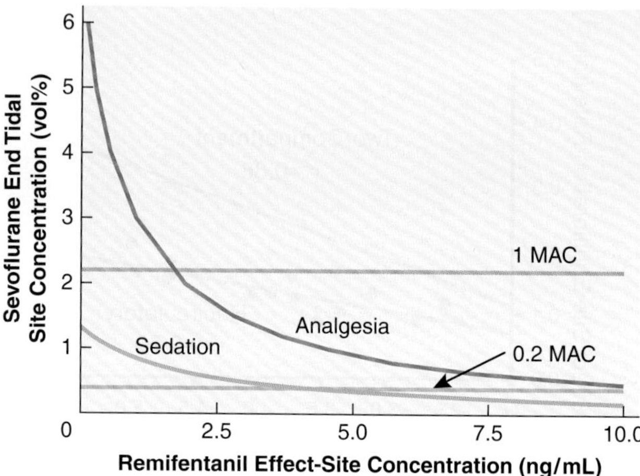

FIGURE 7-24. Remifentanil–sevoflurane interaction for sedation (*green line*) and analgesia to electrical tetanic stimulation (*red line*) for volunteers. The respective 95% isoboles demonstrate the myriad of target concentration pairs of remifentanil and sevoflurane that have a 95% probability of producing the desired pharmacodynamic endpoint. MAC, minimum alveolar concentration. (Adapted from: Manyam SC, Gupta DK, Johnson KB, et al., Opioid-volatile anesthetic synergy: A response surface model with remifentanil and sevoflurane as prototypes. *Anesthesiology.* 2006;105:267–278.)

Studies designed to evaluate the pharmacodynamic interactions between an opioid and a sedative-hypnotic have traditionally focused on the effects of adding one or two fixed doses or concentrations of the opioid to several defined concentrations or doses of the sedative-hypnotic.[66,67,133–140] Graphical demonstration of these interaction data are most commonly performed by demonstrating a shift of parallel dose-response curves (Fig. 7-23). An alternative mathematical model is the isobologram—isoeffect curves that show dose combinations that result in equal effect (Fig. 7-24). Isobolographic analysis has the additional benefit of characterizing the interaction between the two drugs as additive, antagonistic, or synergistic (Fig. 7-25), whereas shifts of dose-response curves requires more complex concentrations to determine if the interaction, demonstrated by a left-ward shift in the curve, is more than additive.

An alternative mathematical model that can fully characterize the complete spectrum of interaction between two drugs for all possible levels of concentration and effects is the response surface model.[71,74] The surface morphology of a response surface not only demonstrates whether the interaction is additive, synergistic, or antagonistic, but the model itself can quantitatively describe the degree of interaction between the two drugs. Furthermore, isobolograms can be derived from the projection of the response surface onto the appropriate horizontal effect plane (Fig. 7-26), and concentration-response curves can be derived from taking a vertical slice through a response surface in the plane perpendicular to the fixed-opioid concentration of interest (Fig. 7-26).[71,74,75] Therefore, response surface models can be viewed as generalizations of the traditional pharmacodynamic methods of analysis. The major limitation of response surface models is that they require a large number of pharmacodynamic measurements across all possible concentration pair combinations to accurately characterize the entire surface.[141] This is most efficiently done in the laboratory setting utilizing volunteers who can be exposed to subtherapeutic (e.g., below the level that guarantees amnesia) and supratherapeutic drug concentration pairs. However, because response surface models characterize the drug concentration pairs that provide adequate anesthesia and also adequate recoveries from anesthesia, these models provide information that are not normally available from studies that generate an isobologram from surgical patients.

Isobolograms and response surface models clearly demonstrate that there are multiple target concentration pairs of

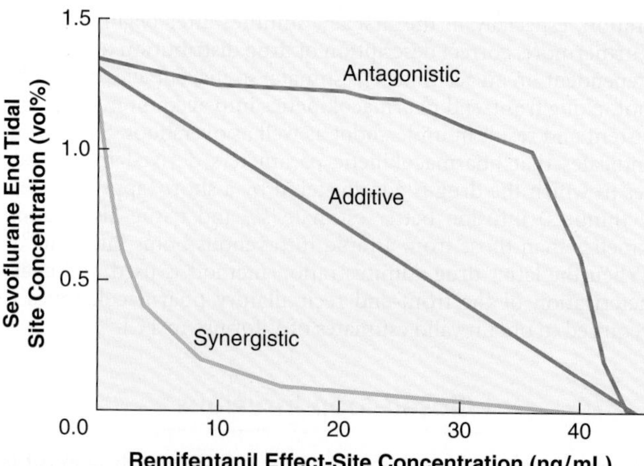

FIGURE 7-25. Isoboles to demonstrate additive (*blue line*), synergistic (*green line*), and antagonistic (*red line*) interactions between Drug A and Drug B.

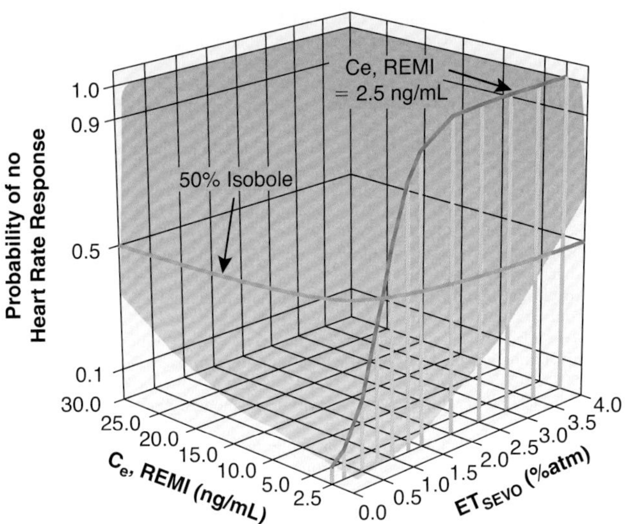

FIGURE 7-26. A response surface model characterizing the remifentanil–sevoflurane interaction for analgesia to electrical tetanic stimulation. The projection of the response surface onto the 50% probability horizontal plane results in the 50% effect isobole while the projection of the response surface onto the 2.5 ng/mL remifentanil effect–site concentration vertical plane results in the sevoflurane concentration-response curve under 2.5 ng/mL of remifentanil. (Adapted from: Manyam SC, Gupta DK, Johnson KB, et al. Opioid-volatile anesthetic synergy: A response surface model with remifentanil and sevoflurane as prototypes. *Anesthesiology.* 2006;105:267–278.)

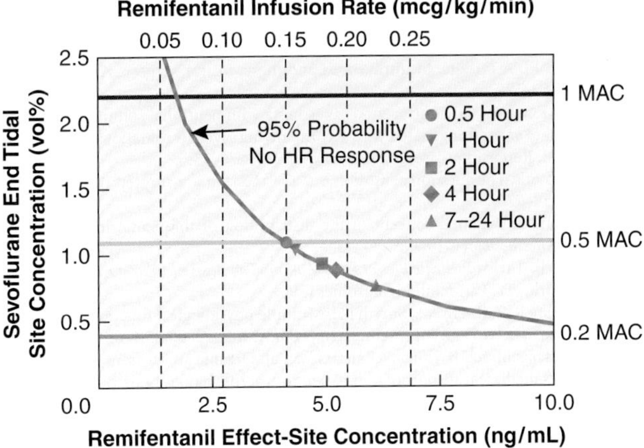

FIGURE 7-27. The optimal target concentration pairs of remifentanil and sevoflurane to maintain adequate analgesia (95% isobole for analgesia to electrical tetanic stimulation) result in the most rapid emergence for anesthetics of various durations. For example, for a 2-hour anesthetic, target concentrations of 0.93 vol% sevoflurane and 4.9 ng/mL remifentanil would result in a 5.8-minute time to awakening. As the duration of anesthesia increases, a minimum sevoflurane target concentration of 0.75 vol% is reached. HR, heart rate; MAC, minimum alveolar concentration. (Adapted from: Manyam SC, Gupta DK, Johnson KB, et al. Opioid-volatile anesthetic synergy: A response surface model with remifentanil and sevoflurane as prototypes. *Anesthesiology.* 2006;105:267–278.)

an opioid and a sedative-hypnotic that can provide adequate anesthesia—a 95% probability of no hemodynamic response to a noxious stimulus and 95% probability of clinically adequate seda-
20 tion.[72,73,76] Combining the response surface pharmacodynamic models with pharmacokinetic models allows computer simulations to be performed to identify the target concentration pair of the opioid and the sedative-hypnotic that produces an adequate anesthetic, and yet optimizes one or more pharmacodynamic endpoints, such as the speed of awakening from anesthesia, drug induced respiratory depression, or drug acquisition costs.[69,73] For sevoflurane-remifentanil anesthetics, these types of pharmacokinetic–pharmacodynamic simulations demonstrate the benefit of minimizing the administered dose of even the low solubility volatile anesthetic sevoflurane to near 0.5 MAC to take advantage of the pharmacokinetic efficiency of remifentanil, especially as the duration of anesthesia increases (Fig. 7-27 and Table 7-8).[73]

CONCLUSION

Since World War II, we have moved from characterizing all anesthetics by a dose-response relationship to developing sophisticated models to characterize the synergistic interaction between sedative-hypnotics and opioids and having the physical devices and the computer support to accurately administer drugs to achieve the desired concentrations at the effect site of drug action. The rational selection of drug target concentrations required to achieve adequate anesthesia and minimize side effects (e.g., prolonged awakening, hemodynamic depression) and the methods by which to efficiently achieve those concentration targets with minimal overshoot requires a solid understanding of the clinical pharmacology of anesthetics. As new drugs enter the anesthetic armaterium, careful characterization of their pharmacokinetic and pharmacodynamic properties will allow them to be safely and appropriately utilized as part of a balanced anesthetic.[75]

TABLE 7-8. THE OPTIMAL TARGET CONCENTRATION PAIRS OF SEVOFLURANE AND REMIFENTANIL FOR ANESTHETICS 30 TO 900 MINUTES IN DURATION

Duration of Anesthetic (h)	Shortest Recovery Time (min)	Effect-Site Remifentanil Concentration (ng/mL)	Remifentanil Infusion Rate (mcg/kg/min)	End Tidal Sevoflurane Concentration (vol%)
0.5	4.5	4.1	0.15	1.1
1	5.0	4.3	0.16	1.05
2	5.8	4.9	0.18	0.93
4	6.7	5.2	0.19	0.88
7–24	7.2–7.7	6.1	0.22	0.75

References

1. Halford FJ. A critique of intravenous anesthesia in war surgery. *Anesthesiology.* 1943;4:67–69.
2. Adams RC, Gray HK. Intravenous anesthesia with pentothal sodium in the case of gunshot wound associated with accompanying severe traumatic shock and loss of blood: Report of a case. *Anesthesiology.* 1943;4:70–73.
3. Anonymous. The question of intravenous anesthesia in war surgery. *Anesthesiology.* 1943;4:74–77.
4. Price HL. A dynamic concept of the distribution of thiopental in the human body. *Anesthesiology.* 1960;21:40–45.
5. Pratt WB, Taylor P. *Principles of Drug Action: The Basis of Pharmacology.* 3rd ed. New York, NY: Churchill Livingstone; 1990.
6. Johnstone RW, Ruefli AA, Smyth MJ. Multiple physiological functions for multidrug transporter P-glycoprotein? *Trends Biochem Sci.* 2000;25:1–6.
7. Gao B, Hagenbuch B, Kullak-Ublick GA, et al. Organic anion-transporting polypeptides mediate transport of opioid peptides across blood–brain barrier. *J Pharmacol Exp Ther.* 2000;294:73–79.
8. Hagenbuch B, Gao B, Meier PJ. Transport of xenobiotics across the blood–brain barrier. *News Physiol Sci.* 2002;17:231–234.
9. Upton RN. Cerebral uptake of drugs in humans. *Clin Exp Pharmacol Physiol.* 2007;34:695–701.
10. Shafer SL, Stanski DR. Improving the clinical utility of anesthetic drug pharmacokinetics. *Anesthesiology.* 1992;76:327–330.
11. Stanski DR, Greenblatt DJ, Lowenstein E. Kinetics of intravenous and intramuscular morphine. *Clin Pharmacol Ther.* 1978;24:52–59.
12. Kuipers JA, Boer F, Olieman W, et al. First-pass lung uptake and pulmonary clearance of propofol: Assessment with a recirculatory indocyanine green pharmacokinetic model. *Anesthesiology.* 1999;91:1780–1787.
13. Ding X, Kaminsky LS. Human extrahepatic cytochromes P450: Function in xenobiotic metabolism and tissue-selective chemical toxicity in the respiratory and gastrointestinal tracts. *Annu Rev Pharmacol Toxicol.* 2003;43:149–173.
14. Stanley TH, Hague B, Mock DL, et al. Oral transmucosal fentanyl citrate (lollipop) premedication in human volunteers. *Anesth Analg.* 1989;69:21–27.
15. Ashburn MA, Streisand J, Zhang J, et al. The iontophoresis of fentanyl citrate in humans. *Anesthesiology.* 1995;82:1146–1153.
16. Eger EI 2nd, Severinghaus JW. Effect of uneven pulmonary distribution of blood and gas on induction with inhalation anesthetics. *Anesthesiology.* 1964;25: 620–626.
17. Avram MJ, Henthorn TK, Spyker DA, et al. Recirculatory pharmacokinetic model of the uptake, distribution, and bioavailability of prochlorperazine administered as a thermally generated aerosol in a single breath to dogs. *Drug Metab Dispos.* 2007;35:262–267.
18. Price HL, Kovnat PJ, Safer JN, et al. The uptake of thiopental by body tissues and its relationship to the duration of narcosis. *Clin Pharmacol Ther.* 1960;1:16.
19. Saidman LJ, Eger EI 2nd. The effect of thiopental metabolism on duration of anesthesia. *Anesthesiology.* 1966;27:118–126.
20. Shafer SL, Varvel JR. Pharmacokinetics, pharmacodynamics, and rational opioid selection. *Anesthesiology.* 1991;74:53–63.
21. Wilkinson GR. Clearance approaches in pharmacology. *Pharmacol Rev.* 1987; 39:1–47.
22. Ahmad AB, Bennett PN, Rowland M. Models of hepatic drug clearance: Discrimination between the 'well stirred' and 'parallel-tube' models. *J Pharm Pharmacol.* 1983;35:219–224.
23. Wilkinson GR, Shand DG. Commentary: A physiological approach to hepatic drug clearance. *Clin Pharmacol Ther.* 1975;18:377–390.
24. Weiss M, Krejcie TC, Avram MJ. Transit time dispersion in pulmonary and systemic circulation: Effects of cardiac output and solute diffusivity. *Am J Physiol Heart Circ Physiol.* 2006;291:H861–H870.
25. Nies AS, Shand DG, Wilkinson GR. Altered hepatic blood flow and drug disposition. *Clin Pharmacokinet.* 1976;1:135–155.
26. Wilkinson GR. Pharmacokinetics of drug disposition: Hemodynamic considerations. *Annu Rev Pharmacol.* 1975;15:11–27.
27. Rane A, Villeneuve JP, Stone WJ, et al. Plasma binding and disposition of furosemide in the nephrotic syndrome and in uremia. *Clin Pharmacol Ther.* 1978;24: 199–207.
28. Ebling WF, Wada DR, Stanski DR. From piecewise to full physiologic pharmacokinetic modeling: applied to thiopental disposition in the rat. *J Pharmacokinet Biopharm.* 1994;22:259–292.
29. Wada DR, Björkman S, Ebling WF, et al. Computer simulation of the effects of alterations in blood flows and body composition on thiopental pharmacokinetics in humans. *Anesthesiology.* 1997;87:884–899.
30. Henthorn TK, Avram MJ, Krejcie TC. Intravascular mixing and drug distribution: The concurrent disposition of thiopental and indocyanine green. *Clin Pharmacol Ther.* 1989;45:56–65.
31. Homer TD, Stanski DR. The effect of increasing age on thiopental disposition and anesthetic requirement. *Anesthesiology.* 1985;62:714–724.
32. Miller RD, Stevens WC, Way WL. The effect of renal failure and hyperkalemia on the duration of pancuronium neuromuscular blockade in man. *Anesth Analg.* 1973;52:661–666.
33. Patwardhan RV, Johnson RF, Hoyumpa A Jr, et al. Normal metabolism of morphine in cirrhosis. *Gastroenterology.* 1981;81:1006–1011.
34. Lund L, Alvan G, Berlin A, et al. Pharmacokinetics of single and multiple doses of phenytoin in man. *Eur J Clin Pharmacol.* 1974;7:81–86.
35. Stanski DR, Mihm FG, Rosenthal MH, et al. Pharmacokinetics of high-dose thiopental used in cerebral resuscitation. *Anesthesiology.* 1980;53:169–171.
36. Avram MJ, Krejcie TC. Using front-end kinetics to optimize target-controlled drug infusions. *Anesthesiology.* 2003;99:1078–1086.
37. Chiou WL, Peng GW, Nation RL. Rapid estimation of volume of distribution after a short intravenous infusion and its application to dosing adjustments. *J Clin Pharmacol.* 1978;18:266–271.
38. Fisher DM. (Almost) everything you learned about pharmacokinetics was (somewhat) wrong! *Anesth Analg.* 1996;83:901–903.
39. Krejcie TC, Avram MJ. What determines anesthetic induction dose? It's the front-end kinetics, doctor! *Anesth Analg.* 1999;89:541–544.
40. Weiss M, Krejcie TC, Avram MJ. A minimal physiological model of thiopental distribution kinetics based on a multiple indicator approach. *Drug Metab Dispos.* 2007;35:1525–1532.
41. Hull CJ. How far can we go with compartmental models? *Anesthesiology.* 1990;72: 399–402.
42. Kong AN, Jusko WJ. Definitions and applications of mean transit and residence times in reference to the two-compartment mammillary plasma clearance model. *J Pharm Sci.* 1988;77:157–165.
43. Jacobs JR, Shafer SL, Larsen JL, et al. Two equally valid interpretations of the linear multicompartment mammillary pharmacokinetic model. *J Pharm Sci.* 1990; 79:331–333.
44. Norman J. Drug-receptor reactions. *Br J Anaesth.* 1979;51:595–601.
45. Waud BE, Waud DR. The margin of safety of neuromuscular transmission in the muscle of the diaphragm. *Anesthesiology.* 1972;37:417–422.
46. Segre G. Kinetics of interaction between drugs and biological systems. *Farmaco [Sci].* 1968;23:907–918.
47. Sheiner LB, Stanski DR, Vozeh S, et al. Simultaneous modeling of pharmacokinetics and pharmacodynamics: Application to d-tubocurarine. *Clin Pharmacol Ther.* 1979;25:358–371.
48. Kern SE, Stanski DR. Pharmacokinetics and pharmacodynamics of intravenously administered anesthetic drugs: Concepts and lessons for drug development. *Clin Pharmacol Ther.* 2008;84:153–157.
49. Jacobs JR, Reves JG. Effect site equilibration time is a determinant of induction dose requirement. *Anesth Analg.* 1993;76:1–6.
50. Morton WD, Lerman J. The effect of pancuronium on the solubility of aqueous thiopentone. *Can J Anaesth.* 1987;34:87–89.
51. Dejong RH, Cullen SC. Buffer-demand and pH of local anesthetic solutions containing epinephrine. *Anesthesiology.* 1963;24:801–807.
52. Anders MW. Formation and toxicity of anesthetic degradation products. *Annu Rev Pharmacol Toxicol.* 2005;45:147–176.
53. Kharasch ED. Adverse drug reactions with halogenated anesthetics. *Clin Pharmacol Ther.* 2008;84:158–162.
54. Baxter PJ, Garton K, Kharasch ED. Mechanistic aspects of carbon monoxide formation from volatile anesthetics. *Anesthesiology.* 1998;89:929–941.
55. Kharasch ED, Powers KM, Artru AA. Comparison of Amsorb, sodalime, and Baralyme degradation of volatile anesthetics and formation of carbon monoxide and compound a in swine in vivo. *Anesthesiology.* 2002;96:173–182.
56. Bom A, Bradley M, Cameron K, et al. A novel concept of reversing neuromuscular block: Chemical encapsulation of rocuronium bromide by a cyclodextrin-based synthetic host. *Angew Chem Int Ed Engl.* 2002;41:266–270.
57. Heerdt PM, Malhotra JK, Pan BY, et al. Pharmacodynamics and cardiopulmonary side effects of CW002, a cysteine-reversible neuromuscular blocking drug in dogs. *Anesthesiology.* 2010;112:910–916.
58. Avram MJ, Krejcie TC, Henthorn TK, et al. Beta-adrenergic blockade affects initial drug distribution due to decreased cardiac output and altered blood flow distribution. *J Pharmacol Exp Ther.* 2004;311:617–624.
59. Niemann CU, Henthorn TK, Krejcie TC, et al. Indocyanine green kinetics characterize blood volume and flow distribution and their alteration by propranolol. *Clin Pharmacol Ther.* 2000;67:342–350.
60. Krejcie TC, Wang Z, Avram MJ. Drug-induced hemodynamic perturbations alter the disposition of markers of blood volume, extracellular fluid, and total body water. *J Pharmacol Exp Ther.* 2001;296:922–930.
61. Avram MJ, Krejcie TC, Niemann CU, et al. Isoflurane alters the recirculatory pharmacokinetics of physiologic markers. *Anesthesiology.* 2000;92:1757–1768.
62. Avram MJ, Krejcie TC, Niemann CU, et al. The effect of halothane on the recirculatory pharmacokinetics of physiologic markers. *Anesthesiology.* 1997;87: 1381–1393.
63. Benet LZ, Hoener BA. Changes in plasma protein binding have little clinical relevance. *Clin Pharmacol Ther.* 2002;71:115–121.
64. Gupta DK, Krejcie TC, Avram MJ. Pharmacokinetics of opioids. In: Evers A, Maze M, Kharasch ED, eds. *Anesthetic Pharmacology: Physiologic Principles and Clinical Practice.* 2nd ed. Cambridge, UK: Cambridge University Press; 2011: 509–530.
65. Wright PM, McCarthy G, Szenohradszky J, et al. Influence of chronic phenytoin administration on the pharmacokinetics and pharmacodynamics of vecuronium. *Anesthesiology.* 2004;100:626–633.

66. Zbinden AM, Maggiorini M, Petersen-Felix S, et al. Anesthetic depth defined using multiple noxious stimuli during isoflurane/oxygen anesthesia. I. Motor reactions. *Anesthesiology.* 1994;80:253–260.
67. Zbinden AM, Petersen-Felix S, Thomson DA. Anesthetic depth defined using multiple noxious stimuli during isoflurane/oxygen anesthesia. II. Hemodynamic responses. *Anesthesiology.* 1994;80:261–267.
68. Oertel BG, Felden L, Tran PV, et al. Selective antagonism of opioid-induced ventilatory depression by an ampakine molecule in humans without loss of opioid analgesia. *Clin Pharmacol Ther.* 2010;87:204–211.
69. Vuyk J, Mertens MJ, Olofsen E, et al. Propofol anesthesia and rational opioid selection: Determination of optimal EC50-EC95 propofol-opioid concentrations that assure adequate anesthesia and a rapid return of consciousness. *Anesthesiology.* 1997;87:1549–1562.
70. Bouillon TW, Bruhn J, Radulescu L, et al. Pharmacodynamic interaction between propofol and remifentanil regarding hypnosis, tolerance of laryngoscopy, bispectral index, and electroencephalographic approximate entropy. *Anesthesiology.* 2004;100:1353–1372.
71. Greco WR, Bravo G, Parsons JC. The search for synergy: A critical review from a response surface perspective. *Pharmacol Rev.* 1995;47:331–385.
72. Kern SE, Xie G, White JL, et al. A response surface analysis of propofol-remifentanil pharmacodynamic interaction in volunteers. *Anesthesiology.* 2004; 100:1373–1381.
73. Manyam SC, Gupta DK, Johnson KB, et al. Opioid-volatile anesthetic synergy: A response surface model with remifentanil and sevoflurane as prototypes. *Anesthesiology.* 2006;105:267–278.
74. Minto CF, Schnider TW, Short TG, et al. Response surface model for anesthetic drug interactions. *Anesthesiology.* 2000;92:1603–1616.
75. Shafer SL, Stanski DR. Defining depth of anesthesia. *Handb Exp Pharmacol.* 2008:409–423.
76. Manyam SC, Gupta DK, Johnson KB, et al. When is a bispectral index of 60 too low?: Rational processed electroencephalographic targets are dependent on the sedative-opioid ratio. *Anesthesiology.* 2007;106:472–483.
77. Boyer EW, Shannon M. The serotonin syndrome. *N Engl J Med.* 2005;352: 1112–1120.
78. Rastogi R, Swarm RA, Patel TA. Case scenario: Opioid association with serotonin syndrome: Implications to the practitioners. *Anesthesiology.* 2011;115:1291–1298.
79. Gillman PK. Monoamine oxidase inhibitors, opioid analgesics and serotonin toxicity. *Br J Anaesth.* 2005;95:434–441.
80. Gillman PK. CNS toxicity involving methylene blue: The exemplar for understanding and predicting drug interactions that precipitate serotonin toxicity. *J Psychopharmacol.* 2011;25:429–436.
81. Schwiebert C, Irving C, Gillman PK. Small doses of methylene blue, previously considered safe, can precipitate serotonin toxicity. *Anaesthesia.* 2009;64:924.
82. Schüttler J, Schwilden H, Stoekel H. Pharmacokinetics as applied to total intravenous anaesthesia. Practical implications. *Anaesthesia.* 1983;38(Suppl):53–56.
83. Shafer SL. Towards optimal intravenous dosing strategies. *Semin Anesth.* 1994; 12:222.
84. Hughes MA, Glass PS, Jacobs JR. Context-sensitive half-time in multicompartment pharmacokinetic models for intravenous anesthetic drugs. *Anesthesiology.* 1992;76:334–341.
85. Maitre PO, Shafer SL. A simple pocket calculator approach to predict anesthetic drug concentrations from pharmacokinetic data. *Anesthesiology.* 1990;73: 332–336.
86. Egan TD. Target-controlled drug delivery: Progress toward an intravenous "vaporizer" and automated anesthetic administration. *Anesthesiology.* 2003;99: 1214–1219.
87. Shafer SL, Varvel JR, Aziz N, et al. Pharmacokinetics of fentanyl administered by computer-controlled infusion pump. *Anesthesiology.* 1990;73:1091–1102.
88. Barvais L, Cantraine F, D'Hollander A, et al. Predictive accuracy of continuous alfentanil infusion in volunteers: Variability of different pharmacokinetic sets. *Anesth Analg.* 1993;77:801–810.
89. Barvais L, Heitz D, Schmartz D, et al. Pharmacokinetic model-driven infusion of sufentanil and midazolam during cardiac surgery: Assessment of the prospective predictive accuracy and the quality of anesthesia. *J Cardiothorac Vasc Anesth.* 2000;14:402–408.
90. Barvais L, D'Hollander AA, Cantraine F, et al. Predictive accuracy of midazolam in adult patients scheduled for coronary surgery. *J Clin Anesth.* 1994;6:297–302.
91. Veselis RA, Glass P, Dnistrian A, et al. Performance of computer-assisted continuous infusion at low concentrations of intravenous sedatives. *Anesth Analg.* 1997;84:1049–1057.
92. Vuyk J, Engbers FH, Burm AG, et al. Performance of computer-controlled infusion of propofol: An evaluation of five pharmacokinetic parameter sets. *Anesth Analg.* 1995;81:1275–1282.
93. Schraag S, Flaschar J. Delivery performance of commercial target-controlled infusion devices with Diprifusor module. *Eur J Anaesthesiol.* 2002;19:357–360.
94. Passot S, Servin F, Allary R, et al. Target-controlled versus manually-controlled infusion of propofol for direct laryngoscopy and bronchoscopy. *Anesth Analg.* 2002;94:1212–1216.
95. Gale T, Leslie K, Kluger M. Propofol anaesthesia via target controlled infusion or manually controlled infusion: Effects on the bispectral index as a measure of anaesthetic depth. *Anaesth Intensive Care.* 2001;29:579–584.
96. Suttner S, Boldt J, Schmidt C, et al. Cost analysis of target-controlled infusion-based anesthesia compared with standard anesthesia regimens. *Anesth Analg.* 1999;88:77–82.
97. Checketts MR, Gilhooly CJ, Kenny GN. Patient-maintained analgesia with target-controlled alfentanil infusion after cardiac surgery: A comparison with morphine PCA. *Br J Anaesth.* 1998;80:748–751.
98. van den Nieuwenhuyzen MC, Engbers FH, Burm AG, et al. Target-controlled infusion of alfentanil for postoperative analgesia: Contribution of plasma protein binding to intra-patient and inter-patient variability. *Br J Anaesth.* 1999;82:580–585.
99. Campbell L, Imrie G, Doherty P, et al. Patient maintained sedation for colonoscopy using a target controlled infusion of propofol. *Anaesthesia.* 2004;59:127–132.
100. Irwin MG, Thompson N, Kenny GN. Patient-maintained propofol sedation. Assessment of a target-controlled infusion system. *Anaesthesia.* 1997;52:525–530.
101. Gentry WB, Krejcie TC, Henthorn TK, et al. Effect of infusion rate on thiopental dose-response relationships. Assessment of a pharmacokinetic-pharmacodynamic model. *Anesthesiology.* 1994;81:316–324.
102. Minto CF, Schnider TW, Gregg KM, et al. Using the time of maximum effect site concentration to combine pharmacokinetics and pharmacodynamics. *Anesthesiology.* 2003;99:324–333.
103. Henthorn TK, Krejcie TC, Shanks CA, et al. Time-dependent distribution volume and kinetics of the pharmacodynamic effector site. *J Pharm Sci.* 1992;81:1136–1138.
104. Shafer SL, Gregg KM. Algorithms to rapidly achieve and maintain stable drug concentrations at the site of drug effect with a computer-controlled infusion pump. *J Pharmacokinet Biopharm.* 1992;20:147–169.
105. Schnider TW, Minto CF, Gambus PL, et al. The influence of method of administration and covariates on the pharmacokinetics of propofol in adult volunteers. *Anesthesiology.* 1998;88:1170–1182.
106. Chiou WL. Potential pitfalls in the conventional pharmacokinetic studies: Effects of the initial mixing of drug in blood and the pulmonary first-pass elimination. *J Pharmacokinet Biopharm.* 1979;7:527–536.
107. Henthorn TK. The effect of altered physiological states on intravenous anesthetics. *Handb Exp Pharmacol.* 2008: (182): 363–377.
108. Henthorn TK, Krejcie TC, Avram MJ. Early drug distribution: a generally neglected aspect of pharmacokinetics of particular relevance to intravenously administered anesthetic agents. *Clin Pharmacol Ther.* 2008;84:18–22.
109. Krejcie TC, Henthorn TK, Gentry WB, et al. Modifications of blood volume alter the disposition of markers of blood volume, extracellular fluid, and total body water. *J Pharmacol Exp Ther.* 1999;291:1308–1316.
110. Krejcie TC, Henthorn TK, Niemann CU, et al. Recirculatory pharmacokinetic models of markers of blood, extracellular fluid and total body water administered concomitantly. *J Pharmacol Exp Ther.* 1996;278:1050–1057.
111. Kuipers JA, Boer F, Olofsen E, et al. Recirculatory pharmacokinetics and pharmacodynamics of rocuronium in patients: The influence of cardiac output. *Anesthesiology.* 2001;94:47–55.
112. Avram MJ, Sanghvi R, Henthorn TK, et al. Determinants of thiopental induction dose requirements. *Anesth Analg.* 1993;76:10–17.
113. Forbes GB, Hursh JB. Age and sex trends in lean body mass calculated from K40 measurements: With a note on the theoretical basis for the procedure. *Ann N Y Acad Sci.* 1963;110:255–263.
114. Sathyaprabha TN, Pradhan C, Rashmi G, et al. Noninvasive cardiac output measurement by transthoracic electrical bioimpedence: Influence of age and gender. *J Clin Monit Comput.* 2008;22:401–408.
115. Avram MJ, Henthorn TK, Spyker DA, et al. Recirculatory kinetic model of fentanyl administered as a thermally generated aerosol to volunteers. *Anesthesiology.* 2008;109:A815.
116. Avram MJ, Henthorn TK, Spyker DA, et al. Recirculatory pharmacokinetic model of fentanyl aerosol in volunteers. *Clin Pharmacol Ther.* 2008;83:PI-76.
117. Avram MJ, Krejcie TC, Henthorn TK. The concordance of early antipyrine and thiopental distribution kinetics. *J Pharmacol Exp Ther.* 2002;302:594–600.
118. Kuipers JA, Boer F, Olofsen E, et al. Recirculatory and compartmental pharmacokinetic modeling of alfentanil in pigs: The influence of cardiac output. *Anesthesiology.* 1999;90:1146–1157.
119. Woodruff EA, Martin JF, Omens M. A model for the design and evaluation of algorithms for closed-loop cardiovascular therapy. *IEEE Trans Biomed Eng.* 1997;44:694–705.
120. Tehrani F, Rogers M, Lo T, et al. Closed-loop control if the inspired fraction of oxygen in mechanical ventilation. *J Clin Monit Comput.* 2002;17:367–376.
121. Renard E. Implantable closed-loop glucose-sensing and insulin delivery: The future for insulin pump therapy. *Curr Opin Pharmacol.* 2002;2:708–716.
122. O'Hara DA, Hexem JG, Derbyshire GJ, et al. The use of a PID controller to model vecuronium pharmacokinetics and pharmacodynamics during liver transplantation. Proportional-integral-derivative. *IEEE Trans Biomed Eng.* 1997;44:610–619.
123. De Smet T, Struys MM, Greenwald S, et al. Estimation of optimal modeling weights for a Bayesian-based closed-loop system for propofol administration using the bispectral index as a controlled variable: A simulation study. *Anesth Analg.* 2007;105:1629–1638.
124. Mortier E, Struys M, De Smet T, et al. Closed-loop controlled administration of propofol using bispectral analysis. *Anaesthesia.* 1998;53:749–754.
125. Schwilden H, Schüttler J, Stoeckel H. Closed-loop feedback control of methohexital anesthesia by quantitative EEG analysis in humans. *Anesthesiology.* 1987; 67:341–347.

126. Schwilden H, Stoeckel H. Effective therapeutic infusions produced by closed-loop feedback control of methohexital administration during total intravenous anesthesia with fentanyl. *Anesthesiology.* 1990;73:225–229.
127. Struys MM, De Smet T, Greenwald S, et al. Performance evaluation of two published closed-loop control systems using bispectral index monitoring: A simulation study. *Anesthesiology.* 2004;100:640–647.
128. Struys MM, De Smet T, Mortier EP. Closed-loop control of anaesthesia. *Curr Opin Anaesthesiol.* 2002;15:421–425.
129. Struys MM, De Smet T, Versichelen LF, et al. Comparison of closed-loop controlled administration of propofol using Bispectral Index as the controlled variable versus "standard practice" controlled administration. *Anesthesiology.* 2001;95:6–17.
130. Tzabazis A, Ihmsen H, Schywalsky M, et al. EEG-controlled closed-loop dosing of propofol in rats. *Br J Anaesth.* 2004;92:564–569.
131. Monk TG, Saini V, Weldon BC, et al. Anesthetic management and one-year mortality after noncardiac surgery. *Anesth Analg.* 2005;100:4–10.
132. Monk TG, Weldon BC, Garvan CW, et al. Predictors of cognitive dysfunction after major noncardiac surgery. *Anesthesiology.* 2008;108:18–30.
133. Katoh T, Ikeda K. The effects of fentanyl on sevoflurane requirements for loss of consciousness and skin incision. *Anesthesiology.* 1998;88:18–24.
134. Katoh T, Kobayashi S, Suzuki A, et al. The effect of fentanyl on sevoflurane requirements for somatic and sympathetic responses to surgical incision. *Anesthesiology.* 1999;90:398–405.
135. Katoh T, Nakajima Y, Moriwaki G, et al. Sevoflurane requirements for tracheal intubation with and without fentanyl. *Br J Anaesth.* 1999;82:561–565.
136. Katoh T, Uchiyama T, Ikeda K. Effect of fentanyl on awakening concentration of sevoflurane. *Br J Anaesth.* 1994;73:322–325.
137. McEwan AI, Smith C, Dyar O, et al. Isoflurane minimum alveolar concentration reduction by fentanyl. *Anesthesiology.* 1993;78:864–869.
138. Sebel PS, Glass PS, Fletcher JE, et al. Reduction of the MAC of desflurane with fentanyl. *Anesthesiology.* 1992;76:52–59.
139. Vuyk J, Lim T, Engbers FH, et al. Pharmacodynamics of alfentanil as a supplement to propofol or nitrous oxide for lower abdominal surgery in female patients. *Anesthesiology.* 1993;78:1036–1045.
140. Vuyk J, Lim T, Engbers FH, et al. The pharmacodynamic interaction of propofol and alfentanil during lower abdominal surgery in women. *Anesthesiology.* 1995;83:8–22.
141. Short TG, Ho TY, Minto CF, et al. Efficient trial design for eliciting a pharmacokinetic-pharmacodynamic model-based response surface describing the interaction between two intravenous anesthetic drugs. *Anesthesiology.* 2002;96:400–408.

CHAPTER

8 Electrical and Fire Safety*

JAN EHRENWERTH • HARRY A. SEIFERT

Key Points

1. A basic principle of electricity is known as *Ohm's law* (Voltage = Current × Resistance).
2. To have the completed circuit necessary for current flow, a closed loop must exist and a voltage source must drive the current through the impedance.
3. To receive a shock, one must contact the electrical circuit at two points, and there must be a voltage source that causes the current to flow through an individual.
4. In electrical terminology, *grounding* is applied to two separate concepts: The grounding of electrical power and the grounding of electrical equipment.
5. To provide an extra measure of safety from gross electrical shock (macroshock), the power supplied to most operating rooms (ORs) is ungrounded.
6. The line isolation monitor (LIM) is a device that continuously monitors the integrity of an isolated power system.
7. The ground fault circuit interrupter is a popular device used to prevent individuals from receiving an electrical shock in a grounded power system.
8. An electrically susceptible patient (i.e., one who has a direct, external connection to the heart) may be at risk from very small currents; this is called *microshock*.
9. Problems can arise if the electrosurgical return plate is improperly applied to the patient or if the cord connecting the return plate to the electrosurgical unit (ESU) is damaged or broken.
10. Fires in the OR are just as much a danger today as they were 100 years ago when patients were anesthetized with flammable anesthetic agents.
11. The necessary components for a fire consist of the triad of heat or an ignition source, a fuel, and an oxidizer.
12. The two major ignition sources for OR fires are the ESU and the laser.
13. It is known that desiccated carbon dioxide absorbent can, in rare circumstances, react with sevoflurane to produce a fire.
14. All OR personnel should be familiar with the location and operation of fire extinguishers.

Multimedia

1 Grounded Electrical Power
2 Electric Plugs
3 Line Isolation
4 Line Isolation Monitor
5 Return Plate
6 Fire in the Operating Room

---

*This chapter and images were developed in whole for both Barash PG, Cullen BF, Stoelting RK, et al., eds. *Clinical Anesthesia* 7th ed. Philadelphia, PA: Wolters Kluwer Health/Lippincott Williams and Wilkins and Ehrenwerth J, Eisenkraft JB, Berry JM, eds. Anesthesia Equipment: Principals and Applications. 2nd ed. Philadelphia, PA: Elsevier, with permission of the editors and publishers.

The myriad of electrical and electronic devices in the modern operating room (OR) greatly improve patient care and safety. However, these devices also subject both the patient and OR personnel to increased risks. To reduce the risk of electrical shock, most ORs have electrical systems that incorporate special safety features. It is incumbent upon the anesthesiologist to have a thorough understanding of the basic principles of electricity and an appreciation of the concepts of electrical safety applicable to the OR environment.

PRINCIPLES OF ELECTRICITY

1 A basic principle of electricity is known as *Ohm's law*, which is represented by the equation:

$$E = I \times R$$

where E is electromotive force (in volts), I is current (in amperes), and R is resistance (in ohms). Ohm's law forms the basis for the physiologic equation BP = CO × SVR; that is, blood pressure (BP) is equal to the cardiac output (CO) times the systemic vascular resistance (SVR). In this case, the blood pressure of the vascular system is analogous to voltage, the cardiac output to current, and the systemic vascular resistance to the forces opposing the flow of electrons. Electrical power (P) is measured in watts (W). Power is the product of the voltage (E) and the current (I), as defined by the formula:

$$P = E \times I$$

The amount of electrical work done is measured in watts multiplied by a unit of time. The watt-second (a joule, J) is a common designation for electrical energy expended in doing work. The energy produced by a defibrillator is measured in watt-seconds (or joules). The kilowatt-hour is used by electrical utility companies to measure larger quantities of electrical energy.

Power can be thought of as a measure not only of work done but also of heat produced in any electrical circuit. Substituting Ohm's law in the formula:

$$P = E \times I$$
$$P = (I \times R) \times I$$
$$P = I^2 \times R$$

Thus, power is equal to the square of the current I^2 (amperage) times the resistance R. Using these formulas, it is possible to calculate the number of amperes and the resistance of a given device if the wattage and the voltage are known. For example, a 60-watt light bulb operating on a household 120-volt circuit would require 0.5 ampere of current for operation. Rearranging the formula so that:

$$I = P/E$$

We have:

$$I = (60 \text{ watts})/(120 \text{ volts})$$
$$I = 0.5 \text{ ampere}$$

Using this in Ohm's law:

$$R = E/I$$

The resistance can be calculated to be 240 ohms:

$$R = (120 \text{ volts})/(0.5 \text{ ampere})$$
$$R = 240 \text{ ohms}$$

It is obvious from the previous discussion that 1 volt of electromotive force (EMF) flowing through a 1-ohm resistance will generate 1 ampere of current. Similarly, 1 ampere of current induced by 1 volt of EMF will generate 1 watt of power.

Direct and Alternating Currents

Any substance that permits the flow of electrons is called a *conductor*. Current is characterized by electrons flowing through a conductor. If the electron flow is always in the same direction, it is referred to as *direct current* (DC). However, if the electron flow reverses direction at a regular interval, it is termed *alternating current* (AC). Either of these types of current can be pulsed or continuous in nature.

The previous discussion of Ohm's law is accurate when applied to DC circuits. However, when dealing with AC circuits, the situation is more complex because the flow of the current is opposed by a more complicated form of resistance, known as *impedance*.

Impedance

Impedance, designated by the letter Z, is defined as the sum of the forces that oppose electron movement in an AC circuit. Impedance consists of resistance (ohms) but also takes capacitance and inductance into account. In actuality, when referring to AC circuits, Ohm's law is defined as:

$$E = I \times Z$$

An *insulator* is a substance that opposes the flow of electrons. Therefore, an insulator has a high impedance to electron flow, whereas a conductor has a low impedance to electron flow.

In AC circuits, the capacitance and inductance can be important factors in determining the total impedance. Both capacitance and inductance are influenced by the frequency (cycles per second or hertz, Hz) at which the AC current reverses direction. The impedance is directly proportional to the frequency (f) times the inductance (IND):

$$Z \propto (f \times \text{IND})$$

and the impedance is inversely proportional to the product of the frequency (f) and the capacitance (CAP):

$$Z \propto 1/(f \times \text{CAP})$$

As the AC current increases in frequency, the net effect of both capacitance and inductance increases. However, because impedance and capacitance are inversely related, total impedance decreases as the product of the frequency and the capacitance increases. Thus, as frequency increases, impedance falls and more current is allowed to pass.

Capacitance

A *capacitor* consists of any two parallel conductors that are separated by an insulator (Fig. 8-1). A capacitor has the ability to store charge. *Capacitance* is the measure of that substance's ability to store charge. In a DC circuit the capacitor plates are charged by a voltage source (i.e., a battery) and there is only a momentary current flow. The circuit is not completed and no further current can flow unless a resistance is connected between the two plates and the capacitor is discharged.

In contrast to DC circuits, a capacitor in an AC circuit permits current flow even when the circuit is not completed by a resistance. This is because of the nature of AC circuits, in which the current flow is constantly being reversed. Because current flow

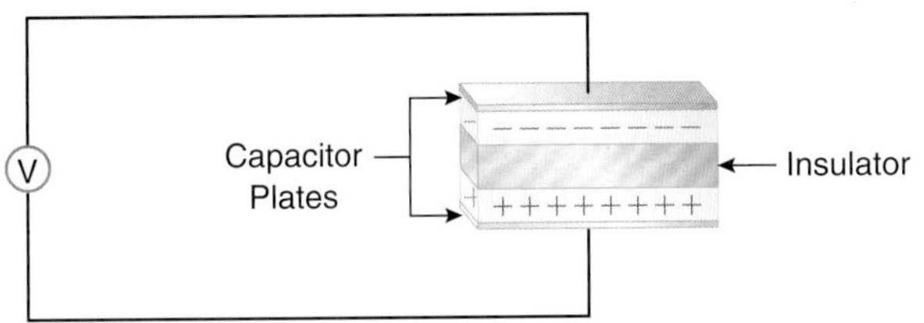

FIGURE 8-1. A capacitor consists of two parallel conductors separated by an insulator. The capacitor is capable of storing charge supplied by a voltage source.

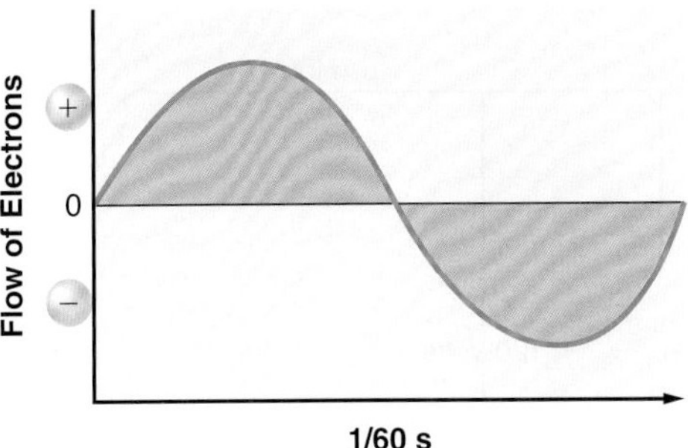

FIGURE 8-2. Sine wave flow of electrons in a 60 Hz AC.

results from the movement of electrons, the capacitor plates are alternately charged—first positive and then negative with every reversal of the AC current direction—resulting in an effective current flow as far as the remainder of the circuit is concerned, even though the circuit is not completed.

Since the effect of capacitance on impedance varies directly with the AC frequency in hertz, the greater the AC frequency, the lower the impedance. Therefore, high-frequency currents (0.5 to 2 million Hz), such as those used by electrosurgical units (ESUs), will cause a marked decrease in impedance.

Electrical devices use capacitors for various beneficial purposes. There is, however, a phenomenon known as *stray capacitance*—capacitance that was not designed into the system but is incidental to the construction of the equipment. All AC-operated equipment produces stray capacitance. An ordinary power cord, for example, consisting of two insulated wires running next to each other will generate significant capacitance simply by being plugged into a 120-volt circuit, even though the piece of equipment is not turned on. Another example of stray capacitance is found in electric motors. The circuit wiring in electric motors generates stray capacitance to the metal housing of the motor. The clinical importance of capacitance will be emphasized later in the chapter.

Inductance

Whenever electrons flow in a wire, a magnetic field is induced around the wire. If the wire is coiled repeatedly around an iron core, as in a transformer, the magnetic field can be very strong. *Inductance* is a property of AC circuits in which an opposing EMF can be electromagnetically generated in the circuit. The net effect of inductance is to increase impedance. Since the effect of inductance on impedance also depends on AC frequency, increases in frequency will increase the total impedance. Therefore, the total impedance of a coil will be much greater than its simple resistance.

ELECTRICAL SHOCK HAZARDS

Alternating and Direct Currents

Whenever an individual contacts an external source of electricity, an electrical shock is possible. An electrical current can stimulate skeletal muscle cells to contract, and thus can be used therapeutically in devices such as pacemakers or defibrillators. However, casual contact with an electrical current, whether AC or DC, can lead to injury or death. Although it takes approximately 3 times as much DC as AC to cause ventricular fibrillation, this by no means renders DC harmless. Devices such as an automobile battery or a DC defibrillator can be sources of DC shocks.

In the United States, utility companies supply electrical energy in the form of ACs of 120 volts at a frequency of 60 Hz. The 120 volts of EMF and 1 ampere of current are the effective voltage and amperage in an AC circuit. This is also referred to as *RMS* (root-mean-square). It takes 1.414 amperes of peak amperage in the sinusoidal curve to give an effective amperage of 1 ampere. Similarly, it takes 170 volts (120 × 1.414) at the peak of the AC curve to get an effective voltage of 120 volts. The 60 Hz refers to the number of times in 1 second that the current reverses its direction of flow. Both the voltage and current waveforms form a sinusoidal pattern (Fig. 8-2).

To have the completed circuit necessary for current flow, a
2 closed loop must exist and a voltage source must drive the current through the impedance. If current is to flow in the electrical circuit, there has to be a *voltage differential,* or a drop in the driving pressure across the impedance. According to Ohm's law, if the resistance is held constant, then the greater the current flow, the larger the voltage drop must be.

The power company attempts to maintain the line voltage constant at 120 volts. Therefore, by Ohm's law, the current flow is inversely proportional to the impedance. A typical power cord consists of two conductors. One, designated as *hot* carries the current to the impedance; the other is *neutral,* and it returns the current to the source. The potential difference between the two is effectively 120 volts (Fig. 8-3). The amount of current flowing through a given device is frequently referred to as the *load.* The load of the circuit depends on the impedance. A very high impedance circuit allows only a small current to flow and thus has a small load. A very low impedance circuit will draw a large

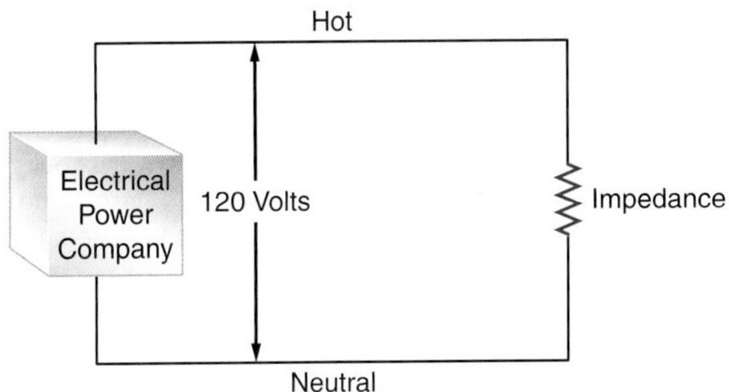

FIGURE 8-3. A typical AC circuit where there is a potential difference of 120 volts between the hot and neutral sides of the circuit. The current flows through a resistance, which in AC circuits is more accurately referred to as *impedance,* and then returns to the electrical power company.

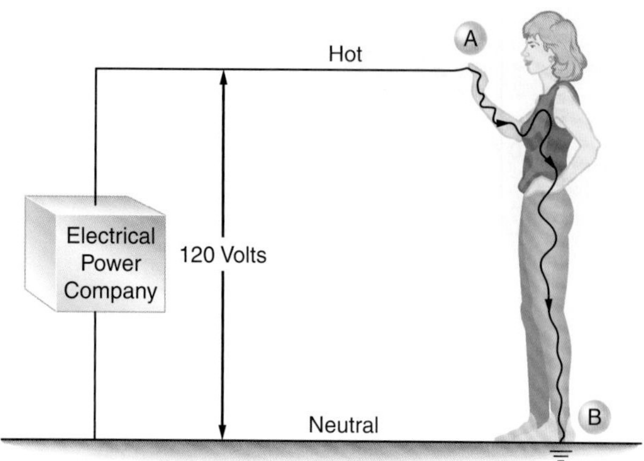

FIGURE 8-4. An individual can complete an electric circuit and receive a shock by coming in contact with the hot side of the circuit (point *A*). This is because he or she is standing on the ground (point *B*) and the contact point *A* and the ground point *B* provide the two contact points necessary for a completed circuit. The severity of the shock that the individual receives depends on his or her skin resistance.

TABLE 8-1. EFFECTS OF 60-HZ CURRENT ON AN AVERAGE HUMAN FOR A 1-SECOND CONTACT

Current	Effect
Macroshock	
1 mA (0.001 A)	Threshold of perception
5 mA (0.005 A)	Accepted as maximum harmless current intensity
10–20 mA (0.01–0.02 A)	"Let-go" current before sustained muscle contraction
50 mA (0.05 A)	Pain, possible fainting, mechanical injury; heart and respiratory functions continue
100–300 mA (0.1–0.3 A)	Ventricular fibrillation will start, but respiratory center remains intact
6,000 mA (6 A)	Sustained myocardial contraction, followed by normal heart rhythm; temporary respiratory paralysis; burns if current density is high
Microshock	
100 μA (0.1 mA)	Ventricular fibrillation
10 μA (0.01 mA)	Recommended maximum 60-Hz leakage current

A, amperes; mA, milliamperes; μA, microamperes.

current and is said to be a large load. A *short circuit* occurs when there is a zero impedance load with a very high current flow.[1]

Source of Shocks

Electrical accidents or shocks occur when a person becomes part
3 of, or completes, an electrical circuit. To receive a shock, one must contact the electrical circuit at two points, and there must be a voltage source that causes the current to flow through an individual (Fig. 8-4).

When an individual contacts a source of electricity, damage occurs in one of two ways. First, the electrical current can disrupt the normal electrical function of cells. Depending on its magnitude, the current can contract muscles, alter brain function, paralyze respiration, or disrupt normal heart function, leading to ventricular fibrillation. The second mechanism involves the dissipation of electrical energy throughout the body's tissues. An electrical current passing through any resistance raises the temperature of that substance. If enough thermal energy is released, the temperature will rise sufficiently to produce a burn. Accidents involving household currents usually do not result in severe burns. However, in accidents involving very high voltages (i.e., power transmission lines), severe burns are common.

The severity of an electrical shock is determined by the amount of current (number of amperes) and the duration of the current flow. For the purpose of this discussion, electrical shocks are divided into two categories. *Macroshock* refers to large amounts of current flowing through a person, which can cause harm or death. *Microshock* refers to very small amounts of current and applies only to the electrically susceptible patient. This is an individual who has an external conduit that is in direct contact with the heart. This can be a pacing wire or a saline-filled catheter such as a central venous or pulmonary artery catheter. In the case of the electrically susceptible patient, even minute amounts of current (microshock) may cause ventricular fibrillation.

Table 8-1 shows the effects typically produced by various currents following a 1-second contact with a 60 Hz current. When an individual contacts a 120-volt household current, the severity of the shock will depend on his or her skin resistance, the duration of the contact, and the current density. Skin resistance can vary from a few thousand to 1 million ohms. If a person with a skin resistance of 1,000 ohms contacts a 120-volt circuit, he or she would receive 120 milliamperes (mA) of current, which would probably be lethal. However, if that same person's skin resistance is 100,000 ohms, the current flow would be 1.2 mA, which would barely be perceptible.

$$I = E/R = (120 \text{ volts})/(1{,}000 \text{ ohms}) = 120 \text{ mA}$$

$$I = E/R = (120 \text{ volts})/(100{,}000 \text{ ohms}) = 1.2 \text{ mA}$$

The longer an individual is in contact with the electrical source, the more dire the consequences, because more energy will be released and more tissue damaged. Also, there will be a greater chance of ventricular fibrillation from excitation of the heart during the vulnerable period of the electrocardiogram (ECG) cycle.

Current density is a way of expressing the amount of current that is applied per unit area of tissue. The diffusion of current in the body tends to be in all directions. The greater the current or the smaller the area to which it is applied, the higher the current density. In relation to the heart, a current of 100 mA (100,000 μA) is generally required to produce ventricular fibrillation when applied to the surface of the body. However, only 100 μA (0.1 mA) is required to produce ventricular fibrillation when that minute current is applied directly to the myocardium through an instrument having a very small contact area, such as a pacing wire electrode. In this case, the current density is 1,000-fold greater when applied directly to the heart; therefore, only 1/1,000 of the energy is required to cause ventricular fibrillation. In this case, the electrically susceptible patient can be electrocuted with currents well below 1 mA, which is the threshold of perception for humans. The frequency at which the current reverses is also an important

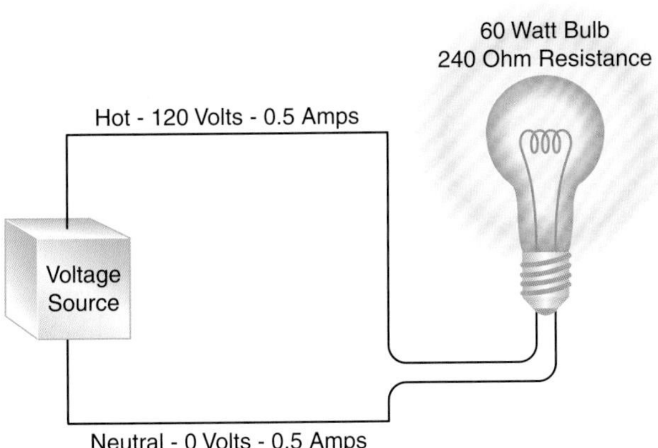

FIGURE 8-5. A 60-watt light bulb has an internal resistance of 240 ohms and draws 0.5 ampere of current. The voltage drop in the circuit is from 120 in the hot wire to 0 in the neutral wire, but the current is 0.5 ampere in both the hot and neutral wires.

factor in determining the amount of current an individual can safely contact. Utility companies in the United States produce electricity at a frequency of 60 Hz. They use 60 Hz because higher frequencies cause greater power loss through transmission lines and lower frequencies cause a detectable flicker from light sources.[2] The "let-go" current is defined as that current above which sustained muscular contraction occurs and at which an individual would be unable to let go of an energized wire. The let-go current for a 60 Hz AC power is 10 to 20 mA,[1,3,4] whereas at a frequency of 1 million Hz, up to 3 amperes (3,000 mA) is generally considered safe. It should be noted that very high frequency currents do not excite contractile tissue; consequently, they do not cause cardiac dysrhythmias.

It can be seen that Ohm's law governs the flow of electricity. For a completed circuit to exist, there must be a closed loop with a driving pressure to force a current through a resistance, just as in the cardiovascular system there must be a blood pressure to drive the cardiac output through the peripheral resistance. Figure 8-5 illustrates that a hot wire carrying a 120-volt pressure through the resistance of a 60-watt light bulb produces a current flow of 0.5 ampere. The voltage in the neutral wire is approximately 0 volts, while the current in the neutral wire remains at 0.5 ampere. This correlates with our cardiovascular analogy, where a mean blood pressure decrease of 80 mm Hg between the aortic root and the right atrium forces a cardiac output of 6 L/min through a systemic vascular resistance of 13.3 resistance units. However, the flow (in this case, the cardiac output, or in the case of the electrical model, the current) is still the same everywhere in the circuit. That is, the cardiac output on the arterial side is the same as the cardiac output on the venous side.

Grounding

To fully understand electrical shock hazards and their prevention, one must have a thorough knowledge of the concepts of grounding. These concepts of grounding probably constitute the most
4 confusing aspects of electrical safety because the same term is used to describe several different principles. In electrical terminology, grounding is applied to two separate concepts. The first is the grounding of electrical *power,* and the second is the grounding of electrical *equipment.* Thus, the concepts that (1) power can

TABLE 8-2. DIFFERENCES BETWEEN POWER AND EQUIPMENT GROUNDING IN THE HOME AND THE OPERATING ROOM

	Power	Equipment
Home	+	±
Operating room	–	+

+, grounded; –, ungrounded; ±, may or may not be grounded.

be grounded or ungrounded and that (2) power can supply electrical devices that are themselves grounded or ungrounded are not mutually exclusive. It is vital to understand this point as the basis of electrical safety (Table 8-2). Whereas electrical *power* is grounded in the home, it is usually ungrounded in the OR. In the home, electrical *equipment* may be grounded or ungrounded, but it should always be grounded in the OR.

ELECTRICAL POWER: GROUNDED

Electrical utilities universally provide power that is grounded (by convention, the earth-ground potential is zero, and all voltages represent a difference between potentials). That is, one of the wires supplying the power to a home is intentionally connected to the earth. The utility companies do this as a safety measure to prevent electrical charges from building up in their wiring during electrical storms. This also prevents the very high voltages used in transmitting power by the utility from entering the home in the event of an equipment failure in their high-voltage system.

The power enters the typical home via two wires. These two wires are attached to the main fuse or the circuit breaker box at the service entrance. The "hot" wire supplies power to the "hot" distribution strip. The neutral wire is connected to the neutral distribution strip and to a service entrance ground (i.e., a pipe buried in the earth; Fig. 8-6). From the fuse box, three wires leave to supply the electrical outlets in the house. In the United States, the hot wire is color-coded black and carries a voltage 120 volts above ground potential. The second wire is the neutral wire color-coded white; the third wire is the ground wire, which is either color-coded green or is uninsulated (bare wire). The ground and the neutral wires are attached at the same point in the circuit breaker box and then further connected to a cold-water pipe (Figs. 8-7 and 8-8). Thus, this grounded power system is also referred to as a *neutral grounded power system.* The black wire is not connected to the ground, as this would create a short circuit. The black wire is attached to the hot (i.e., 120 volts above ground) distribution strip on which the circuit breakers or fuses are located. From here, numerous branch circuits supply electrical power to the outlets in the house. Each branch circuit is protected by a circuit breaker or fuse that limits current to a specific maximum amperage. Most electrical circuits in the house are 15- or 20-ampere circuits. These typically supply power to the electrical outlets and lights in the house. Several higher amperage circuits are also provided for devices such as an electric stove or an electric clothes dryer. These devices are powered by 240-volt circuits, which can draw from 30 to 50 amperes of current. The circuit breaker or fuse will interrupt

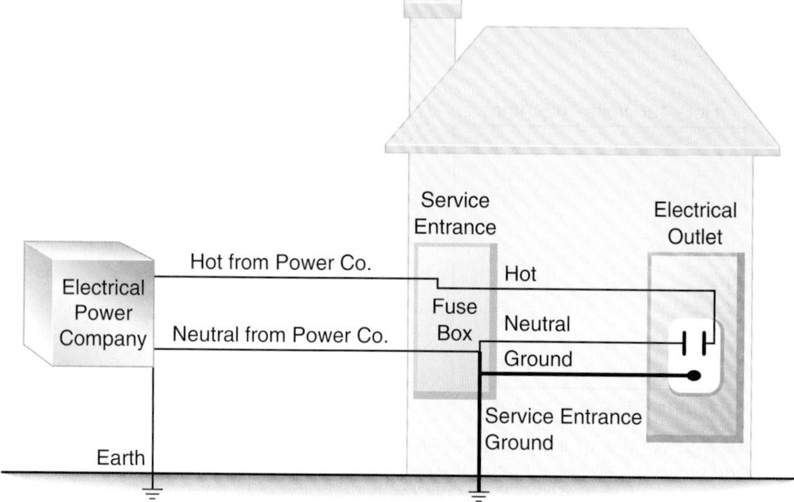

FIGURE 8-6. In a neutral grounded power system, the electric company supplies two lines to the typical home. The neutral wire is connected to ground by the power company and again connected to a service entrance ground when it enters the fuse box. Both the neutral and ground wires are connected together in the fuse box at the neutral bus bar, which is also attached to the service entrance ground.

the flow of current on the hot side of the line in the event of a short circuit or if the demand placed on that circuit is too high. For example, a 15-ampere branch circuit will be capable of supporting 1,800 watts of power.

$$P = E \times I$$

$$P = 120 \text{ volts} \times 15 \text{ amperes}$$

$$P = 1{,}800 \text{ watts}$$

Therefore, if two 1,500-watt hair dryers were simultaneously plugged into one outlet, the load would be too great for a 15-ampere circuit, and the circuit breaker would open (trip) or the fuse would melt. This is done to prevent the supply wires in the circuit from melting and starting a fire. The amperage of the circuit breaker on the branch circuit is determined by the thickness of the wire that it supplies. If a 20-ampere breaker is used with wire rated for only 15 amperes, the wire could melt and start a fire before the circuit breaker would trip. It is important to note that a 15-ampere circuit breaker does not protect an individual from lethal shocks. The 15 amperes of current that would trip the circuit breaker far exceeds the 100 to 200 mA that will produce ventricular fibrillation.

The wires that leave the circuit breaker supply the electrical outlets and lighting for the rest of the house. In older homes, the electrical cable consists of two wires, a hot and a neutral, which supply power to the electrical outlets (Fig. 8-9). In newer homes, a third wire has been added to the electrical cable (Fig. 8-10). This third wire is either green or uninsulated (bare) and serves as a ground wire for the power receptacle (Fig. 8-11). On one end, the ground wire is attached to the electrical outlet (Fig. 8-12); on the other, it is connected to the neutral distribution strip in the circuit breaker box along with the neutral (white) wires (Fig. 8-13).

It should be realized that in both the old and new situations, the power is grounded. That is, a 120-volt potential exists between the hot (black) and the neutral (white) wire and between the hot wire and ground. In this case, the ground is the earth (Fig. 8-14). In modern home construction, there is still a 120-volt potential difference between the hot (black) and the neutral (white) wire

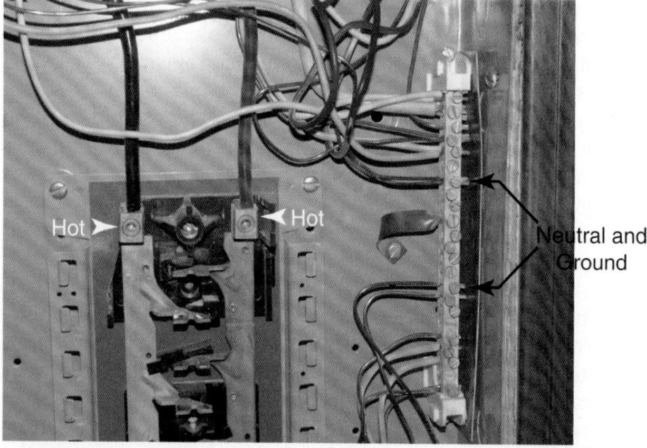

FIGURE 8-7. Inside a fuse box with the circuit breakers removed. The *arrowheads* indicate the hot wires energizing the strips where the circuit breakers are located. The *arrows* point to the neutral bus bar where the neutral and ground wires are connected.

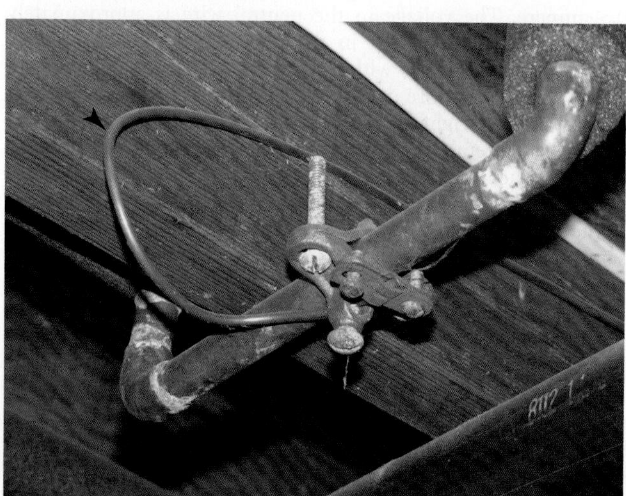

FIGURE 8-8. The *arrowhead* indicates the ground wire from the circuit breaker box attached to a cold-water pipe.

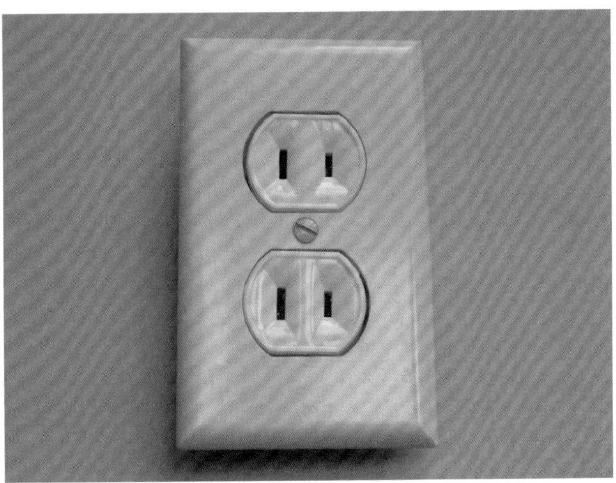

FIGURE 8-9. An older style electrical outlet consisting of just two wires (a hot and a neutral). There is no ground wire.

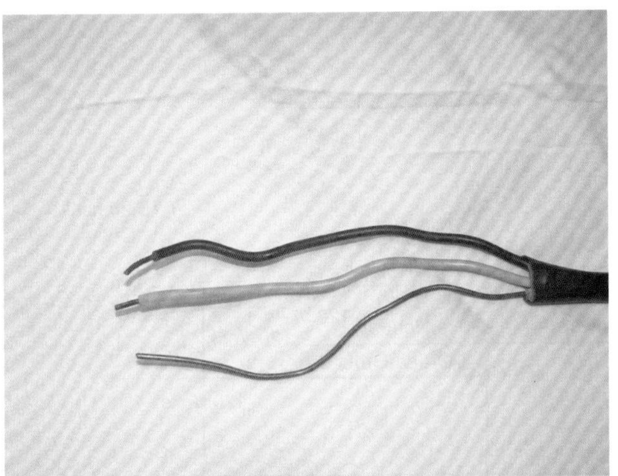

FIGURE 8-10. Modern electrical cable in which a third, or ground wire has been added.

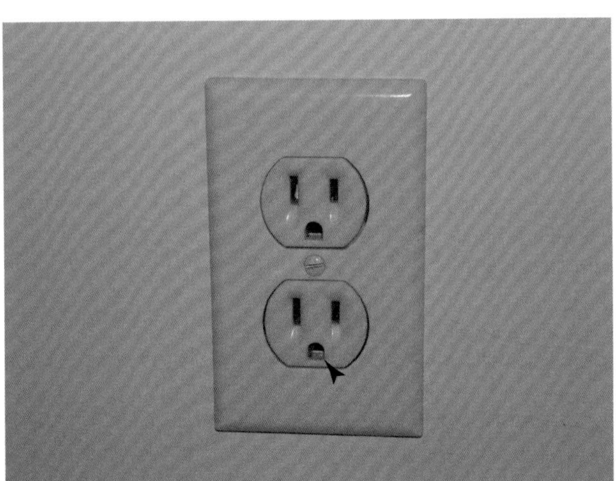

FIGURE 8-11. Modern electrical outlet in which the ground wire is present. The *arrowhead* points to the part of the receptacle where the ground wire connects.

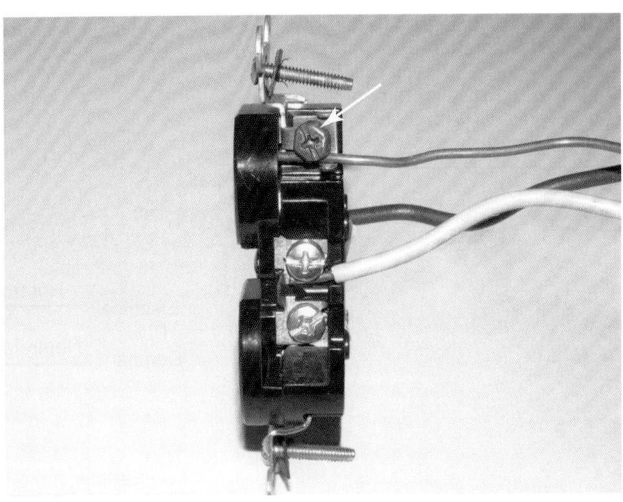

FIGURE 8-12. Detail of modern electrical power receptacle. The *arrow* points to the ground wire (bare wire), which is attached to the green grounding screw on the power receptacle.

as well as a 120-volt difference between the equipment ground wire (which is the third wire), and between the hot wire and earth (Fig. 8-15).

A 60-watt light bulb can be used as an example to further illustrate this point. Normally, the hot and neutral wires are connected to the two wires of the light bulb socket, and throwing the switch will illuminate the bulb (Fig. 8-16). Similarly, if the hot wire is connected to one side of the bulb socket and the other wire from the light bulb is connected to the equipment ground wire, the bulb will still illuminate. If there is no equipment ground wire, the bulb will still light if the second wire is connected to any grounded metallic object such as a water pipe or a faucet. This illustrates the fact that the 120-volt potential difference exists not only between the hot and the neutral wires but also between the hot wire and any grounded object. Thus, in a grounded power system, the current will flow between the hot wire and any conductor with an earth ground.

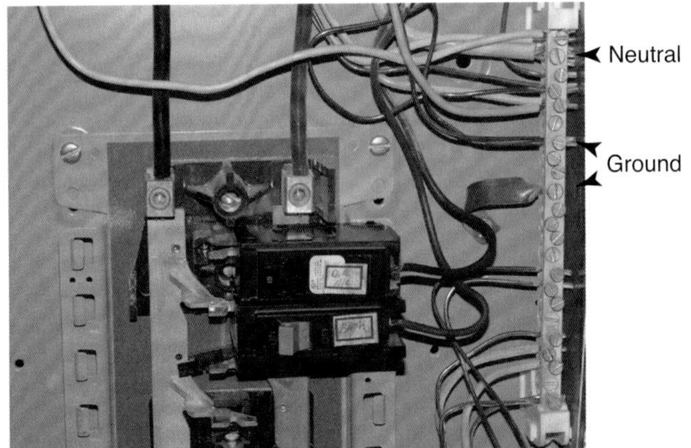

FIGURE 8-13. The ground wires (bare wires) from the power outlet are run to the neutral bus bar, where they are connected with the neutral wires (white wires) (*arrowheads*).

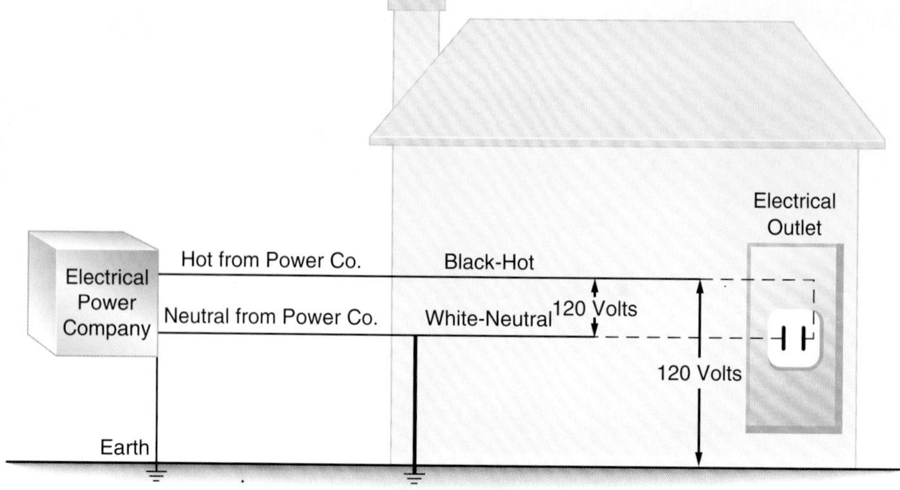

FIGURE 8-14. Diagram of a house with older style wiring that does not contain a ground wire. A 120-volt potential difference exists between the hot and the neutral wires, as well as between the hot wire and the earth.

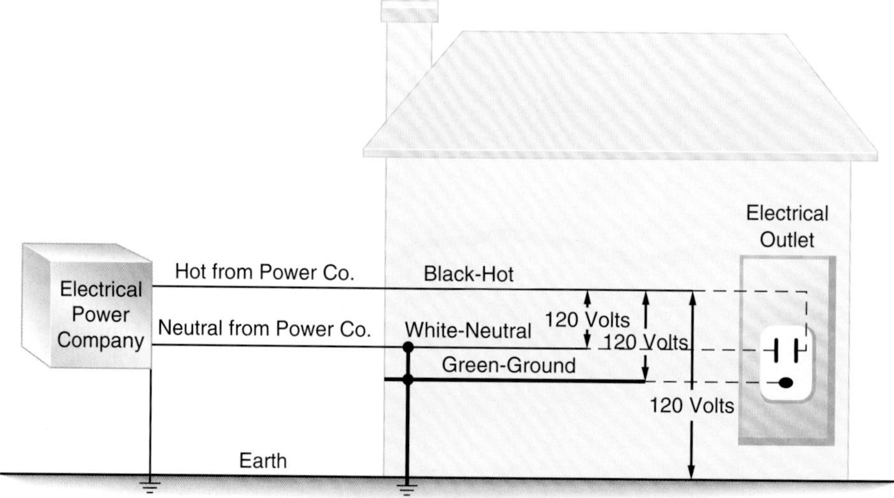

FIGURE 8-15. Diagram of a house with modern wiring in which the third, or ground, wire has been added. The 120-volt potential difference exists between the hot and neutral wires, the hot and the ground wires, and the hot wire and the earth.

As previously stated, current flow requires a closed loop with a source of voltage. For an individual to receive an electric shock, he or she must contact the loop at two points. Because we may be standing on the ground or be in contact with an object that is referenced to ground, only one additional contact point is necessary to complete the circuit and thus receive an electrical shock. This is an unfortunate and inherently dangerous consequence of grounded power systems. Modern wiring systems have added the third wire, the equipment ground wire, as a safety measure to reduce the severity of a potential electrical shock. This is accomplished by providing an alternate, low-resistance pathway through which the current can flow to ground.

Over time, the insulation covering wires may deteriorate. It is then possible for a bare, hot wire to contact the metal case or frame of an electrical device. The case would then become energized and constitute a shock hazard to someone coming in contact with it. Figure 8-17 illustrates a typical short circuit, where the individual has come in contact with the hot case of an instrument. This illustrates the type of wiring found in older homes. There is no ground wire in the electrical outlet, nor is the electrical apparatus equipped with a ground wire. Here, the individual completes the circuit and receives a severe shock. Figure 8-18 illustrates a similar

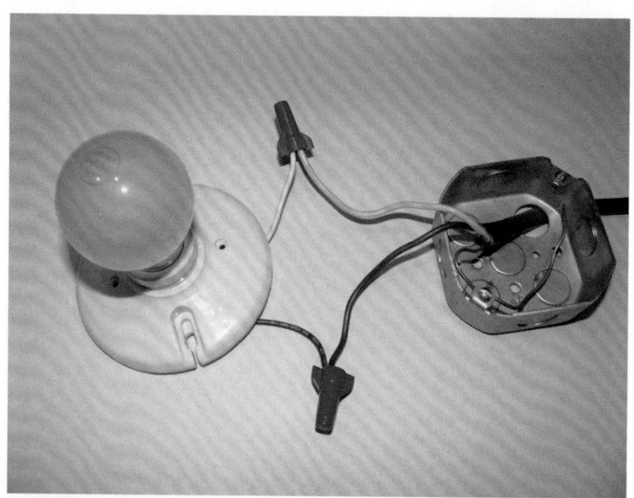

FIGURE 8-16. A simple light bulb circuit in which the hot (black) and neutral (white) wires are connected with the corresponding wires from the light bulb fixture.

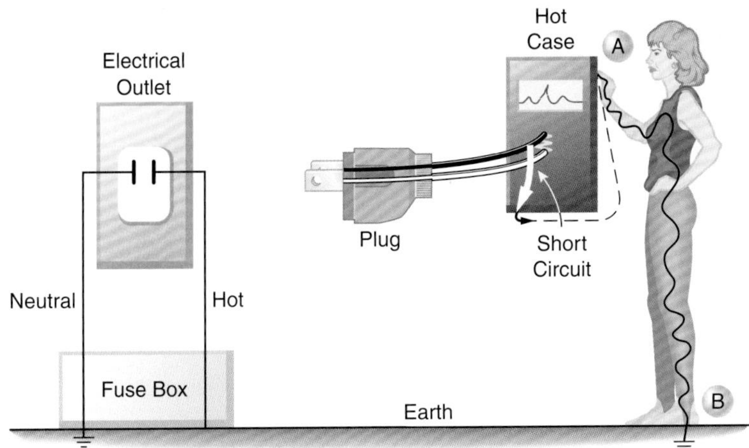

FIGURE 8-17. When a faulty piece of equipment without an equipment ground wire is plugged into an electrical outlet not containing a ground wire, the case of the instrument will become hot. An individual touching the hot case (point *A*) will receive a shock because he or she is standing on the earth (point *B*) and completes the circuit. The current (*dashed line*) will flow from the instrument through the individual touching the hot case.

example, except that now the equipment ground wire is part of the electrical distribution system. In this example, the equipment ground wire provides a pathway of low impedance through which the current can travel; therefore, most of the current would travel through the ground wire. In this case, the person may get a shock, but it is unlikely to be fatal.

The electrical power supplied to homes is always grounded. A 120-volt potential always exists between the hot conductor and the ground or earth. The third or equipment ground wire used in modern electrical wiring systems does not normally have current flowing through it. In the event of a short circuit, an electrical device with a three-prong plug (i.e., a ground wire connected to its case) will conduct the majority of the short-circuited or "fault" current through the ground wire and away from the individual. This provides a significant safety benefit to someone accidentally contacting the defective device. If a large enough fault current exists, the ground wire also will provide a means to complete the short circuit back to the circuit breaker or fuse, and this will either melt the fuse or trip the circuit breaker. Thus, in a grounded power system, it is possible to have either grounded or ungrounded equipment, depending on when the wiring was installed and whether the electrical device is equipped with a three-prong plug containing a ground wire. Obviously, attempts to bypass the safety system of the equipment ground should be avoided. Devices such as a "cheater plug" (Fig. 8-19) should never be used because they defeat the safety feature of the equipment ground wire.

ELECTRICAL POWER: UNGROUNDED

Numerous electronic devices, together with power cords and puddles of saline solutions on the floor, make the OR an electrically hazardous environment for both patients and personnel. Bruner et al.[5] found that 40% of electrical accidents in hospitals occurred in the OR. The complexity of electrical equipment in the modern OR demands that electrical safety be a factor of paramount importance.
5 To provide an extra measure of safety from macroshock, the power supplied to most ORs is ungrounded. In this ungrounded power system, the current is isolated from the ground potential. The 120-volt potential difference exists only between the two wires of the isolated power system (IPS), but no circuit exists between the ground and either of the isolated power lines.

Supplying ungrounded power to the OR requires the use of an *isolation transformer* (Fig. 8-20). This device uses electromagnetic induction to induce a current in the ungrounded or secondary winding of the transformer from energy supplied to the primary winding. There is no direct electrical connection between the power supplied by the utility company on the primary side and the power induced by the transformer on the ungrounded or secondary side. Thus, the power supplied to the OR is isolated from the ground (Fig. 8-21). Since the 120-volt potential exists only between the two wires of the isolated circuit, neither wire is hot nor neutral with reference to ground. In this case, they are simply

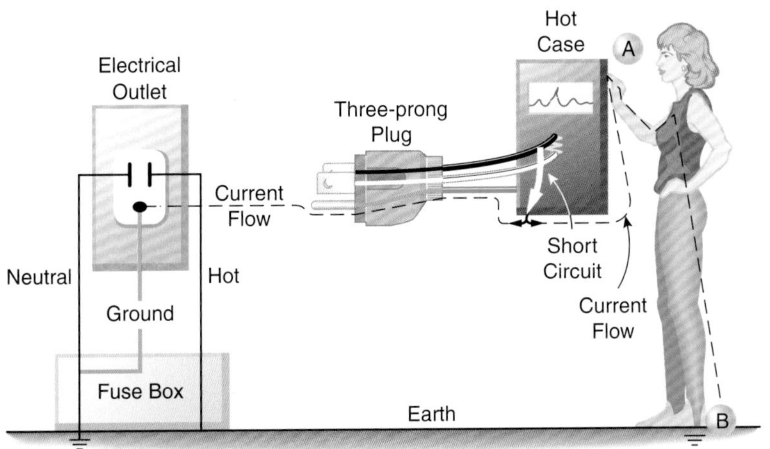

FIGURE 8-18. When a faulty piece of equipment containing an equipment ground wire is properly connected to an electrical outlet with a grounding connection, the current (*dashed line*) will preferentially flow down the low-resistance ground wire. An individual touching the case (point *A*) while standing on the ground (point *B*) will still complete the circuit; however, only a small part of the current will go through the individual.

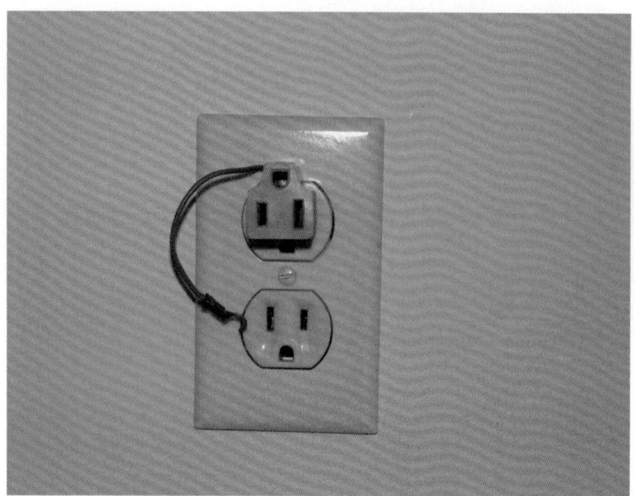

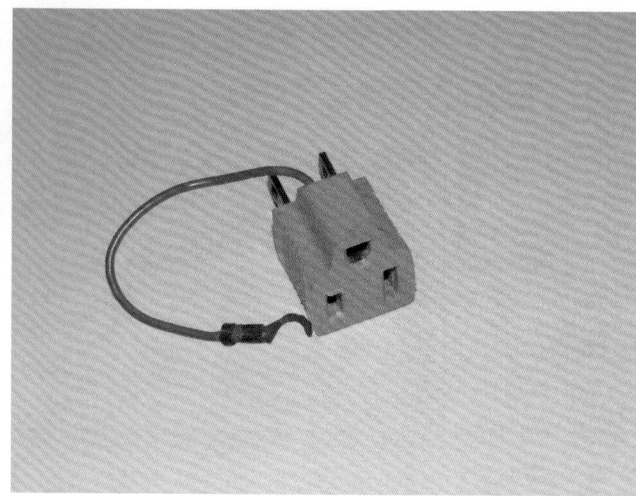

FIGURE 8-19. Right: A "cheater plug" that converts a three-prong power cord to a two-prong cord. **Left:** The wire attached to the cheater plug is rarely connected to the screw in the middle of the outlet. This totally defeats the purpose of the equipment ground wire.

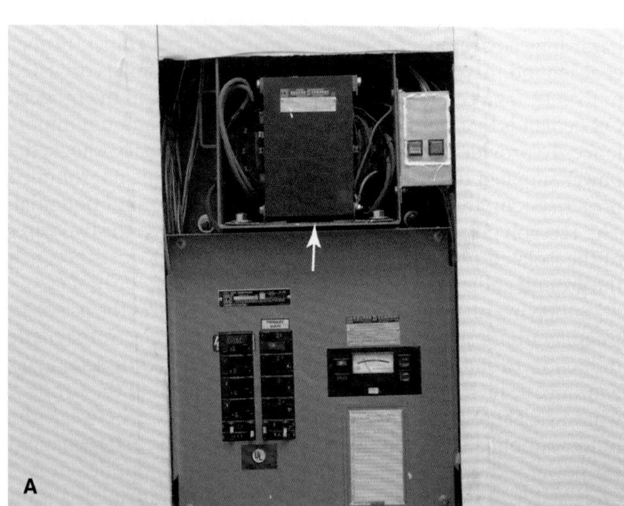

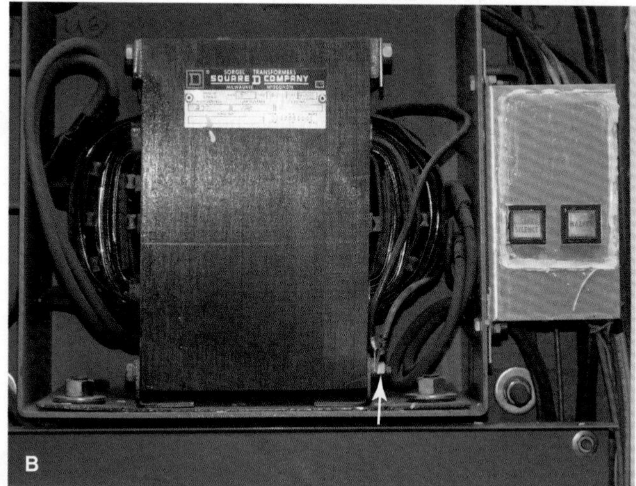

FIGURE 8-20. A: Isolated power panel showing circuit breakers, LIM, and isolation transformer (*arrow*). **B:** Detail of an isolation transformer with the attached warning lights. The arrow points to ground wire connection on the primary side of the transformer. Note that no similar connection exists on the secondary side of the transformer.

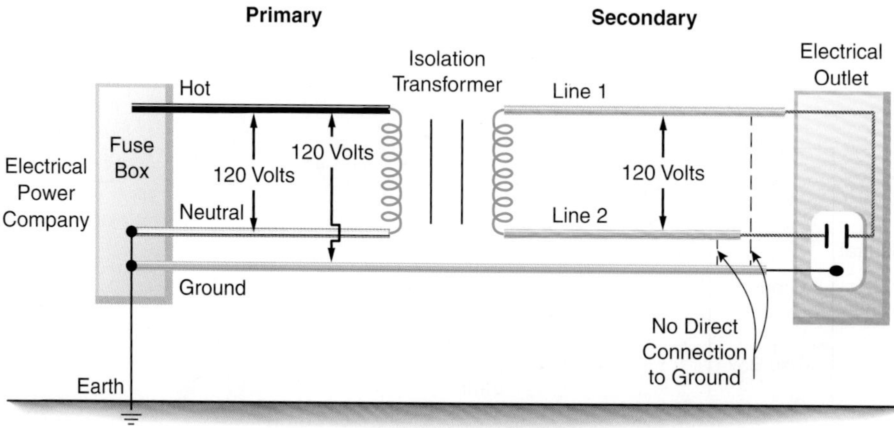

FIGURE 8-21. In the OR, the isolation transformer converts the grounded power on the primary side to an ungrounded power system on the secondary side of the transformer. A 120-volt potential difference exists between line 1 and line 2. There is no direct connection from the power on the secondary side to ground. The equipment ground wire, however, is still present.

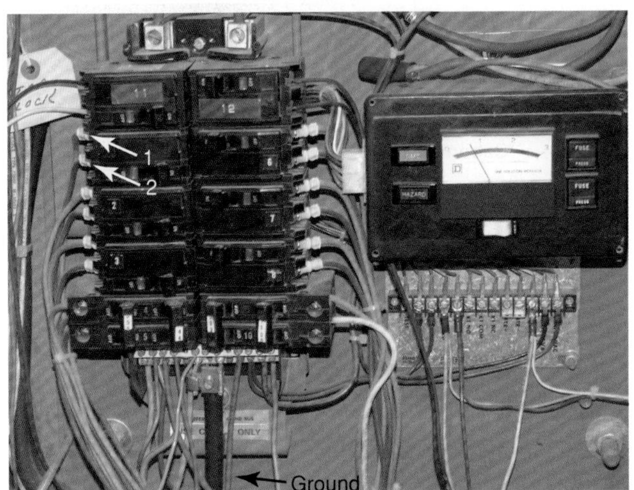

FIGURE 8-22. Detail of the inside of a circuit breaker box in an isolated power system. The *bottom arrow* points to ground (green) wires meeting at the common ground terminal. *Arrows 1* and *2* indicate lines 1 and 2 (orange and brown) from the isolated power circuit breaker. Neither line 1 nor line 2 is connected to the same terminals as the ground wires. This is in marked contrast to Figure 8-13, where the neutral and ground wires are attached at the same point.

referred to as line 1 and line 2 (Fig. 8-22). Using the example of the light bulb, if one connects the two wires of the bulb socket to the two wires of the IPS, the light will illuminate. However, if one connects one of the wires to one side of the isolated power and the other wire to the ground, the light will not illuminate. If the wires of the IPS are connected, the short circuit will trip the circuit breaker. In comparing the two systems, the standard grounded power has a direct connection to ground, whereas the isolated system imposes a very high impedance to any current flow to ground. The added safety of this system can be seen in Figure 8-23. In this case, a person has come in contact with one side of the IPS (point *A*). Since standing on the ground (point *B*) does not constitute a part of the isolated circuit, the individual does not complete the loop and will not receive a shock. This is because the ground is part of the primary circuit (*solid lines*), and the person is contacting only one side of the isolated secondary circuit (*cross-hatched lines*). The person does not complete either circuit (i.e., have two contact points); therefore, this situation does not pose an electric shock hazard. Of course, if the person contacts both lines of the IPS (an unlikely event), he or she would receive a shock.

If a faulty electrical appliance with an intact equipment ground wire is plugged into a standard household outlet, and the home wiring has a properly connected ground wire, then the amount of electrical current that will flow through the individual is considerably less than what will flow through the low-resistance ground wire. Here, an individual would be fairly well protected from a serious shock. However, if that ground wire were broken, the individual might receive a lethal shock. No shock would occur if the same faulty piece of equipment were plugged into the IPS, even if the equipment ground wire were broken. Thus, the IPS provides a significant amount of protection from macroshock. Another feature of the IPS is that the faulty piece of equipment, even though it may be partially short-circuited, will not usually trip the circuit breaker. This is an important feature because the faulty piece of equipment may be part of a life-support system for a patient. It is important to note that even though the power is isolated from ground, the case or frame of all electrical equipment is still connected to an equipment ground. The third wire (equipment ground wire) is necessary for a total electrical safety program.

Figure 8-24 illustrates a scenario involving a faulty piece of equipment connected to the IPS. This does not represent a hazard; it merely converts the isolated power back to a grounded power system as exists outside the OR. In fact, a *second* fault is necessary to create a hazard.

The previous discussion assumes that the IPS is perfectly isolated from ground. Actually, perfect isolation is impossible to achieve. All AC-operated power systems and electrical devices manifest some degree of capacitance. As previously discussed, electrical power cords, wires, and electrical motors exhibit capacitive coupling to the ground wire and metal conduits and "leak" small amounts of current to the ground (Fig. 8-25). This so-called *leakage current* partially ungrounds the IPS. This does not usually amount to more than a few milliamperes in an OR. So an individual coming in contact with one side of the IPS would receive only a very small shock (1 to 2 mA). Although this amount of current would be perceptible, it would not be dangerous.

THE LINE ISOLATION MONITOR

The *line isolation monitor* (LIM) is a device that continuously
6 monitors the integrity of an IPS. If a faulty piece of equipment is connected to the IPS, this will, in effect, change the system back to

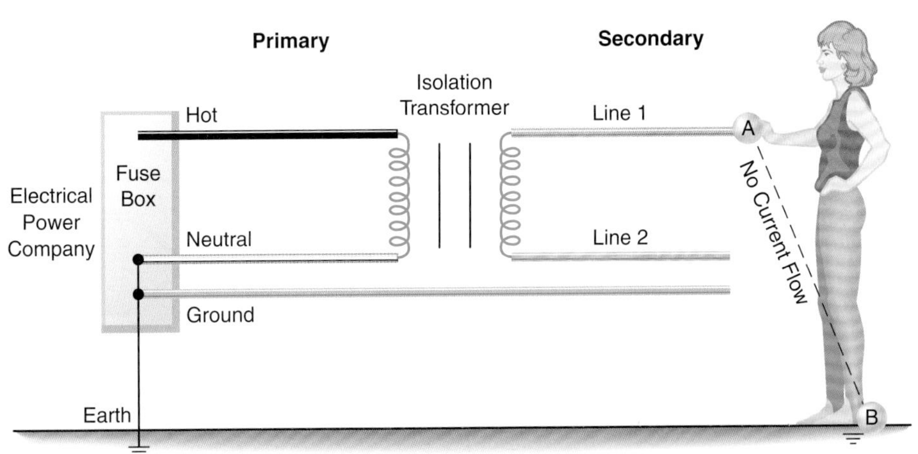

FIGURE 8-23. A safety feature of the isolated power system is illustrated. An individual contacting one side of the isolated power system (point *A*) and standing on the ground (point *B*) will not receive a shock. In this instance, the individual is not contacting the circuit at two points and thus is not completing the circuit. Point *A* is part of the isolated power system, and point *B* is part of the primary or grounded side of the circuit.

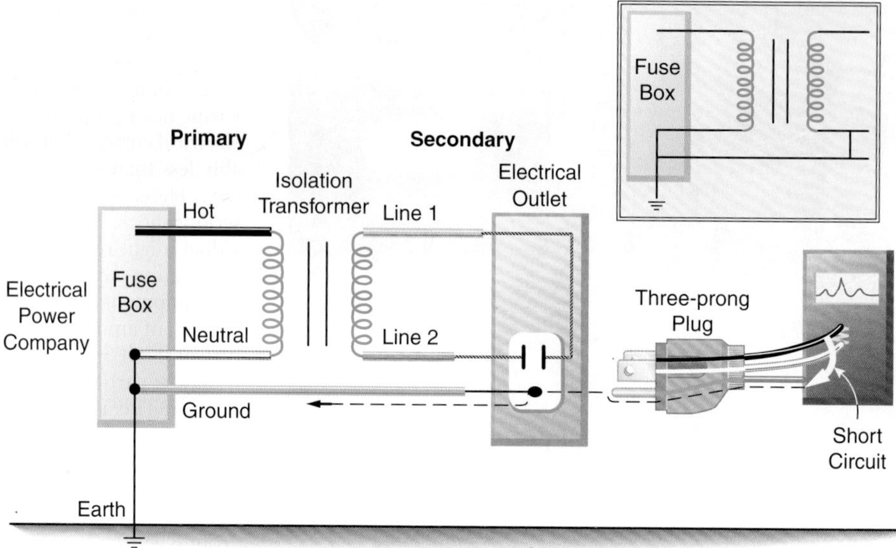

FIGURE 8-24. A faulty piece of equipment plugged into the isolated power system does not present a shock hazard. It merely converts the isolated power system into a grounded power system. The figure inset illustrates that the isolated power system is now identical to the grounded power system. The *dashed line* indicates current flow in the ground wire.

a conventional grounded system. Also, the faulty piece of equipment will continue to function normally. Therefore, it is essential that a warning system be in place to alert the personnel that the power is no longer ungrounded. The LIM continuously monitors the isolated power to ensure that it is indeed isolated from ground, and the device has a meter that displays a continuous indication of the integrity of the system (Fig. 8-26). The LIM is actually measuring the impedance to the ground of each side of the IPS. As previously discussed, with perfect isolation, impedance would be infinitely high and there would be no current flow in the event of a first fault situation ($Z = E/I$; if $I = 0$, then $Z = \infty$). Because all AC wiring and all AC-operated electrical devices have some capacitance, small leakage currents are present that partially degrade the isolation of the system. The meter of the LIM will indicate (in milliamperes) the total amount of leakage in the system resulting from capacitance, electrical wiring, and any devices plugged into the IPS.

The reading on the LIM meter does not mean that current is actually flowing; rather, it indicates how much current would flow in the event of a first fault. The LIM is set to alarm at 2 or 5 mA, depending on the age and brand of the system. Once this preset limit is exceeded, visual and audible alarms are triggered to indicate that the isolation from the ground has been degraded beyond a predetermined limit (Fig. 8-27). This does not necessarily mean that there is a hazardous situation, but rather that the system is no longer totally isolated from ground. It would require a second fault to create a dangerous situation.

For example, if the LIM were set to alarm at 2 mA, using Ohm's law, the impedance for either side of the IPS would be 60,000 ohms:

$$Z = E/I$$

$$Z = (120 \text{ volts})/(0.002 \text{ ampere})$$

$$Z = 60{,}000 \text{ ohms}$$

Therefore, if either side of the IPS had less than 60,000 ohms impedance to the ground, the LIM would trigger an alarm. This might occur in two situations. In the first situation, a faulty piece of equipment is plugged into the IPS. In this case, a true fault to ground exists from one line to ground. Now the system would be converted to the equivalent of a grounded power system. This faulty piece of equipment should be removed and serviced as soon as possible. However, this piece of equipment could still be used safely if it were essential for the care of the patient. It should

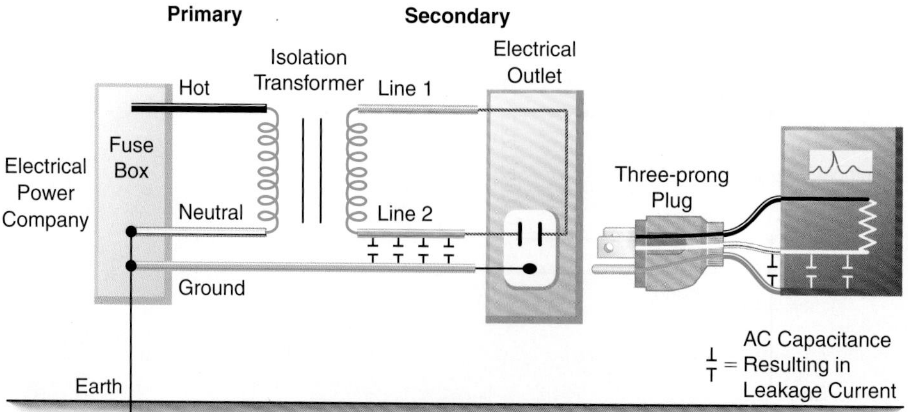

FIGURE 8-25. The capacitance that exists in alternating current (AC) power lines and AC-operated equipment results in small "leakage currents" that partially degrade the isolated power system.

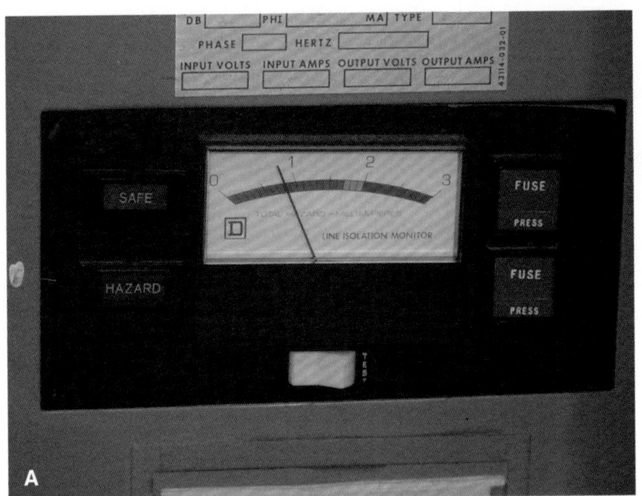

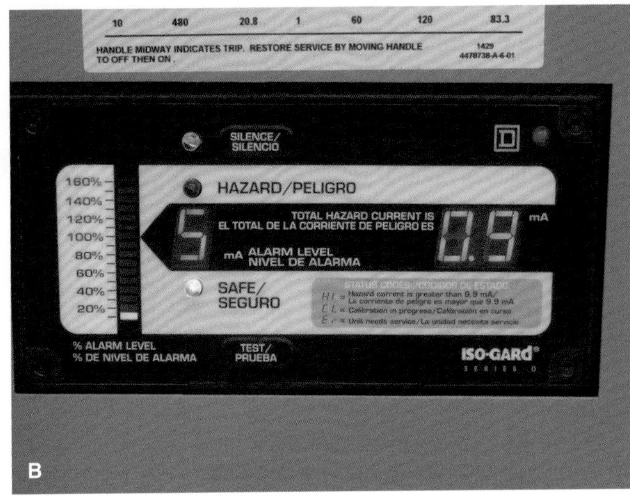

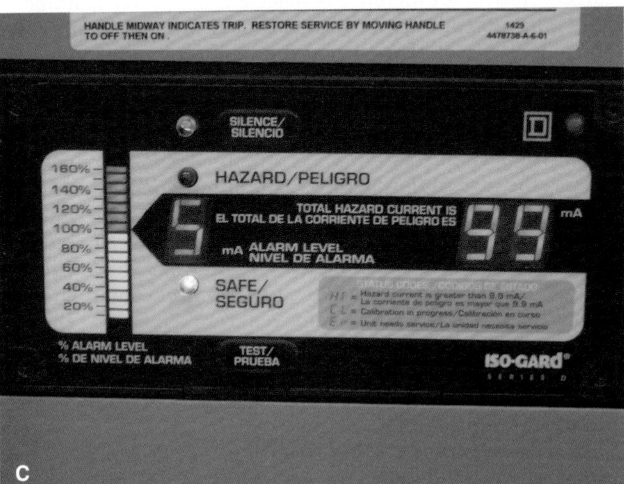

FIGURE 8-26. The meter of the LIM is calibrated in milliamperes. If the isolation of the power system is degraded such that >2 mA (5 mA in newer systems) of current could flow, the hazard light will illuminate and a warning buzzer will sound. Note the button for testing the hazard warning system. **(A)** Older LIM that will trigger an alarm at 2 mA. **(B)** Newer LIM that will trigger an alarm at 5 mA. **(C)** The LIM alarm is triggered, and the red hazard stripe is illuminated, while the number on the right shows 9.9 mA of potential current flow.

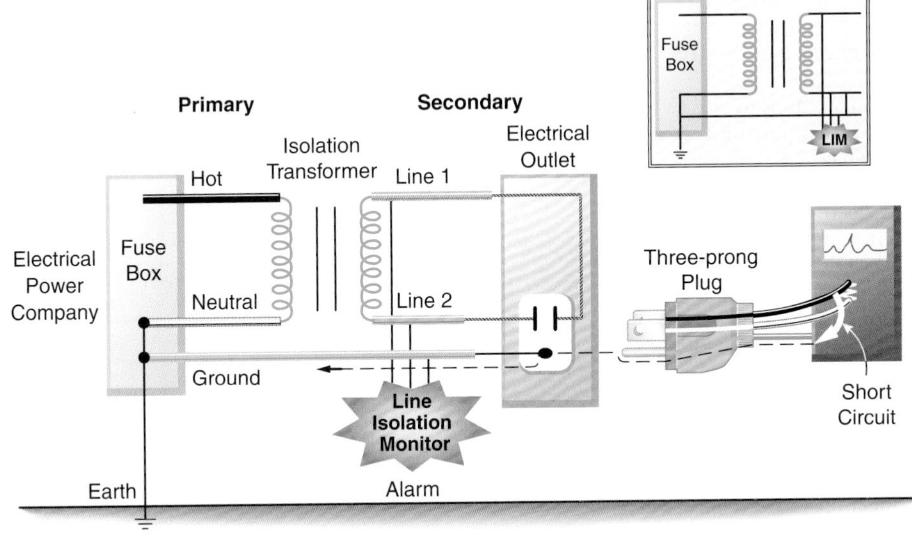

FIGURE 8-27. When a faulty piece of equipment is plugged into the isolated power system, it will markedly decrease the impedance from line 1 or line 2 to ground. This will be detected by the LIM, which will sound an alarm.

be remembered, however, that continuing to use this faulty piece of equipment would create the potential for a serious electrical shock. This would occur if a second faulty piece of equipment were simultaneously connected to the IPS.

The second situation involves connecting many perfectly normal pieces of equipment to the IPS. Although each piece of equipment has only a small amount of leakage current, if the total leakage exceeds 2 mA, the LIM will trigger an alarm. Assume that in the same OR there are 30 electrical devices, each having 100 μA of leakage current. The total leakage current (30 × 100 μA) would be 3 mA. The impedance to ground would still be 40,000 ohms (120/0.003). The LIM alarm would sound because the 2 mA set point was violated. However, the system is still safe and represents a state significantly different from that in the first situation. For this reason, the newer LIMs are set to alarm at 5 mA instead of 2 mA.

The newest LIMs are referred to as *third-generation monitors.* The first-generation monitor, or static LIM, was unable to detect balanced faults (i.e., a situation in which there are equal faults to ground from both line 1 and line 2). The second-generation, or dynamic, LIM did not have this problem but could interfere with physiologic monitoring. Both of these monitors would trigger an alarm at 2 mA, which led to annoying "false" alarms. The third-generation LIM corrects the problems of its predecessors and has the alarm threshold set at 5 mA.[6] Proper functioning of the LIM depends on having both intact equipment ground wires as well as its own connection to ground. First- and second-generation LIMs could not detect the loss of the LIM ground connection. The third-generation LIM can detect this loss of ground to the monitor. In this case the LIM alarm would sound and the red hazard light would illuminate, but the LIM meter would read zero. This condition will alert the staff that the LIM needs to be repaired. However, the LIM still cannot detect broken equipment ground wires. An example of the third-generation LIM is the *Iso-Gard* made by the Square D Company (Monroe, NC).

The equipment ground wire is again an important part of the safety system. If this wire is broken, a faulty piece of equipment that is plugged into an outlet would operate normally, but the LIM would not alarm. A second fault could therefore cause a shock, without any alarm from the LIM. Also, in the event of a second fault, the equipment ground wire provides a low-resistance path to ground for most of the fault current (see Fig. 8-24). The LIM will only be able to register leakage currents from pieces of equipment that are connected to the IPS and have intact ground wires.

If the LIM alarm is triggered, the first thing to do is to check the gauge to determine if it is a true fault. The other possibility is that too many pieces of electrical equipment have been plugged in and the 2 mA limit has been exceeded. If the gauge is between 2 and 5 mA, it is probable that too much electrical equipment has been plugged in. If the gauge reads >5 mA, most likely there is a faulty piece of equipment present in the OR. The next step is to identify the faulty equipment, which is done by unplugging each piece of equipment until the alarm ceases. If the faulty piece of equipment is not of a life-support nature, it should be removed from the OR. If it is a vital piece of life-support equipment, it can be safely used. (Note: If a critical piece of life support equipment—like the cardio-pulmonary bypass machine—is suspected as causing the alarm, do not disconnect it until it is no longer needed.) However, it must be remembered that the protection of the IPS and the LIM is no longer operative. Therefore, if possible, no other electrical equipment should be connected during the remainder of the case, or until the faulty piece of equipment can be safely removed.

GROUND FAULT CIRCUIT INTERRUPTER

7 The ground fault circuit interrupter (GFCI, or occasionally abbreviated as GFI) is another popular device used to prevent individuals from receiving an electrical shock in a grounded power system. Electrical codes for most new construction require that a GFCI circuit be present in potentially hazardous (e.g., wet) areas such as bathrooms, kitchens, or outdoor electrical outlets. The GFCI may be installed as an individual power outlet (Fig. 8-28) or may be a special circuit breaker to which all the individual protected outlets are connected at a single point. The special GFCI circuit breaker is located in the main fuse/circuit breaker box and can be distinguished by its red test button (Fig. 8-29). As Figure 8-5 demonstrates, the current flowing in both the hot and neutral wires is usually equal. The GFCI monitors both sides of the circuit for the equality of current flow; if a difference is detected, the power is immediately interrupted. If an individual should contact a faulty piece of equipment such that current flowed through the individual, an imbalance between the two sides of the circuit would be created, which would be detected by the GFCI. Since the GFCI can detect very small current differences (in the range of 5 mA), the GFCI will open the circuit in a few milliseconds, thereby interrupting the current flow before a significant shock occurs. Thus, the GFCI provides a high level of protection at a very modest cost. If the OR has a GFCI that tripped, then one should first attempt to reset it by pushing the reset button. This is because a surge may have caused the GFCI to trip. If it cannot be reset, then the equipment must be removed from service and checked by the biomedical engineering staff. It is essential that when GFCIs are used in an OR, only one outlet be protected by each GFCI. They should never be "daisy-chained," so that one GFCI protects multiple outlets.

The disadvantage of using a GFCI in the OR is that it interrupts the power without warning. A defective piece of equipment could no longer be used, which might be a problem if it were of a life-support nature, whereas if the same faulty piece of equipment were plugged into an IPS, the LIM would alarm but the equipment could still be used.

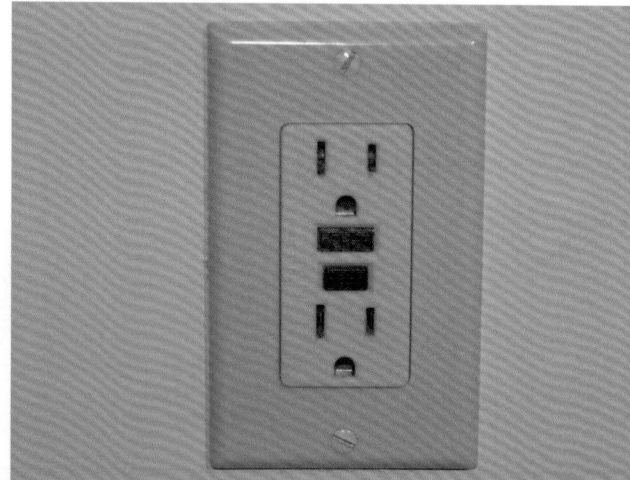

FIGURE 8-28. A GFCI electrical outlet with integrated test (black) and reset (red) buttons.

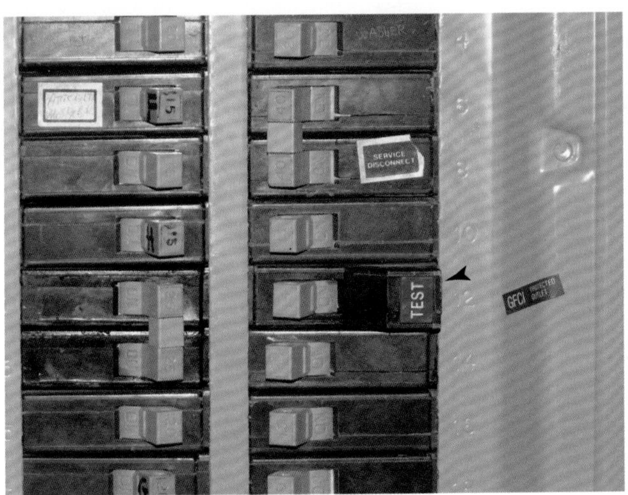

FIGURE 8-29. Special GFCI circuit breaker. The *arrowhead* points to the distinguishing red test button.

DOUBLE INSULATION

There is one instance in which it is acceptable for a piece of equipment to have only a two-prong and not a three-prong plug. This is permitted when the instrument has what is termed *double insulation.* These instruments have two layers of insulation and usually have a plastic exterior. Double insulation is found in many home power tools and is seen in hospital equipment such as infusion pumps. Double-insulated equipment is permissible in the OR with IPSs. However, if water or saline should get inside the unit, there could be a hazard because the double insulation is bypassed. This is even more serious if the OR has no isolated power or GFCIs.[7]

MICROSHOCK

As previously discussed, macroshock involves relatively large amounts of current applied to the surface of the body. The current is conducted through all the tissues in proportion to their conductivity and area in a plane perpendicular to the current. Consequently, the "density" of the current (amperes per meter squared) that reaches the heart is considerably less than what is applied to the body surface. However, an electrically suscep-
8 tible patient (i.e., one who has a direct, external connection to the heart, such as through a central venous pressure catheter or transvenous cardiac pacing wires) may be at risk from very small currents; this is called *microshock.*[8] The catheter orifice or electrical wire with a very small surface area in contact with the heart produces a relatively large current density at the heart.[9] Stated another way, even very small amounts of current applied directly to the myocardium will cause ventricular fibrillation. Microshock is a particularly difficult problem because of the insidious nature of the hazard.

In the electrically susceptible patient, ventricular fibrillation can be produced by a current that is below the threshold of human perception. The exact amount of current necessary to cause ventricular fibrillation in this type of patient is unknown. Whalen et al.[10] were able to produce fibrillation with 20 μA of current applied directly to the myocardium of dogs. Raftery et al.[11] produced fibrillation with 80 μA of current in some patients. Hull[12] used data obtained by Watson et al.[13] to show that 50% of patients would fibrillate at currents of 200 μA. Since 1,000 μA (1 mA) is generally regarded as the threshold of human perception with 60 Hz AC, the electrically susceptible patient can be electrocuted with one-tenth the normally perceptible currents. This is not only of academic interest but also of practical concern because many cases of ventricular fibrillation from microshock have been reported.[14–18]

The stray capacitance that is part of any AC-powered electrical instrument may result in significant amounts of charge buildup on the case of the instrument. If an individual simultaneously touches the case of an instrument where this has occurred and the electrically susceptible patient, he or she may unknowingly cause a discharge to the patient that results in ventricular fibrillation. Once again, the equipment ground wire constitutes the major source of protection against microshock for the electrically susceptible patient. In this case, the equipment ground wire provides a low-resistance path by which most of the leakage current is dissipated instead of stored as a charge.

Figure 8-30 illustrates a situation involving a patient with a saline-filled catheter in the heart with a resistance of ~500 ohms. The ground wire with a resistance of 1 ohm is connected to the instrument case. A leakage current of 100 μA will divide according to the relative resistances of the two paths. In this case, 99.8 μA will flow through the equipment ground wire and only 0.2 μA will flow through the fluid-filled catheter. This extremely small current does

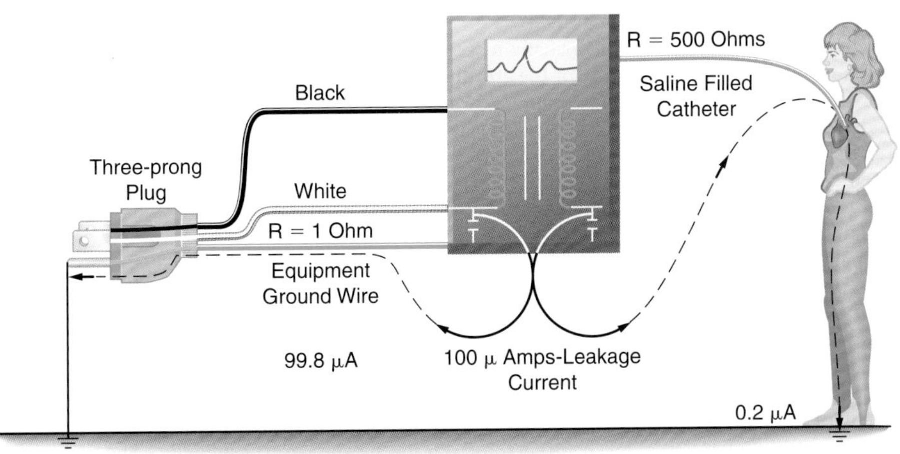

FIGURE 8-30. The electrically susceptible patient is protected from microshock by the presence of an intact equipment ground wire. The equipment ground wire provides a low-impedance path in which the majority of the leakage current (*dashed lines*) can flow. R, resistance.

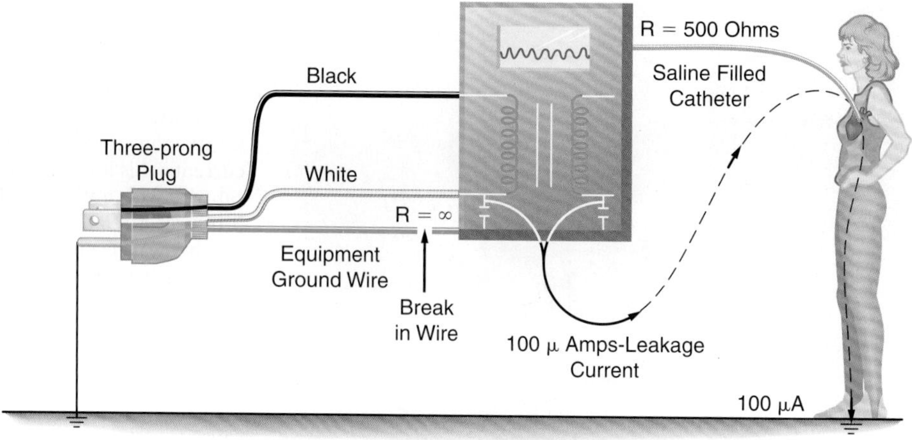

FIGURE 8-31. A broken equipment ground wire results in a significant hazard to the electrically susceptible patient. In this case, the entire leakage current can be conducted to the heart and may result in ventricular fibrillation. R, resistance.

not endanger the patient. However, if the equipment ground wire were broken, the electrically susceptible patient would be at great risk because all 100 μA of leakage current could flow through the catheter and cause ventricular fibrillation (Fig. 8-31). Currently, electronic equipment is permitted 100 μA of leakage current.

Modern patient monitors incorporate another mechanism to reduce the risk of microshock for electrically susceptible patients.[19] This mechanism involves electrically isolating all direct patient connections from the power supply of the monitor by placing a very high impedance between the patient and any device. This limits the amount of internal leakage through the patient connection to a very small value. The standard currently is <10 μA. For instance, the output of an ECG monitor's power supply is electrically isolated from the patient by placing a very high impedance between the monitor and the patient's ECG leads.[20] Isolation techniques are designed to inhibit hazardous electrical pathways between the patient and the monitor while allowing the passage of the physiologic signal.

An intact equipment ground wire is probably the most important factor in preventing microshock. There are, however, other things that the anesthesiologist can do to reduce the incidence of microshock. One should never simultaneously touch an electrical device and a saline-filled central catheter or external pacing wires. Whenever one is handling a central catheter or pacing wires, it is best to insulate oneself by wearing rubber gloves. Also, one should never let any external current source, such as a nerve stimulator, come into contact with the catheter or wires. Finally, one should be alert to potential sources of energy that can be transmitted to the patient. Even stray radiofrequency current from the ESU (cautery) can, with the right conditions, be a source of microshock.[21] It must be remembered that the LIM is not designed to provide protection from microshock. The microampere currents involved in microshock are far below the LIM threshold of protection. In addition, the LIM does not register the leakage of individual monitors, but rather indicates the status of the total system. The LIM reading indicates the total amount of leakage current resulting from the entire capacitance of the system. This is the amount of current that would flow to ground in the event of a first-fault situation.

The essence of electrical safety is a thorough understanding of all the principles of grounding. The objective of electrical safety is to make it difficult for electrical current to pass through people. For this reason, both the patient and the anesthesiologist should be isolated from ground as much as possible. That is, their resistance to current flow should be as high as is technologically feasible. In the inherently unsafe electrical environment of an OR, several measures can be taken to help protect against contacting hazardous current flows. First, the grounded power provided by the utility company can be converted to ungrounded power by means of an isolation transformer. The LIM will continuously monitor the status of this isolation from ground and warn that the isolation of the power (from ground) has been lost in the event that a defective piece of equipment is plugged into one of the isolated circuit outlets. In addition, the shock that an individual could receive from a faulty piece of equipment is determined by the capacitance of the system and is limited to a few milliamperes. Second, all equipment plugged into the IPS has an equipment ground wire that is attached to the case of the instrument. This equipment ground wire provides an alternative low-resistance pathway enabling potentially dangerous currents to flow to ground. Thus, the patient and the anesthesiologist should be as insulated from ground as possible and all electrical equipment should be grounded.

The equipment ground wire serves three functions. First, it provides a low-resistance path for fault currents to reduce the risk of macroshock. Second, it dissipates leakage currents that are potentially harmful to the electrically susceptible patient. Third, it provides information to the LIM on the status of the ungrounded power system. If the equipment ground wire is broken, a significant factor in the prevention of electrical shock is lost. Additionally, the IPS will appear safer than it actually is because the LIM is unable to detect broken equipment ground wires.

Because power cord plugs and receptacles are subjected to greater abuse in the hospital than in the home, the Underwriters Laboratories (Melville, NY) has issued a strict specification for special "hospital-grade" plugs and receptacles (Fig. 8-32). The plugs and receptacles that conform to this specification are marked by a green dot.[22] The hospital-grade plug is one that can be visually inspected or easily disassembled to ensure the integrity of the ground wire connection. Molded opaque plugs are not acceptable. Edwards[23] reported that of 3,000 non–hospital-grade receptacles installed in a new hospital building, 1,800 (60%) were defective after 3 years. When 2,000 of the non–hospital-grade receptacles were replaced with ones of hospital grade, no failures had occurred after 18 months of use.

ELECTROSURGERY

On that fateful October day in 1926 when Dr. Harvey W. Cushing first used an electrosurgical (ESU) machine invented by Professor William T. Bovie to resect a brain tumor, the course of modern surgery and anesthesia was forever altered.[24] The ubiquitous

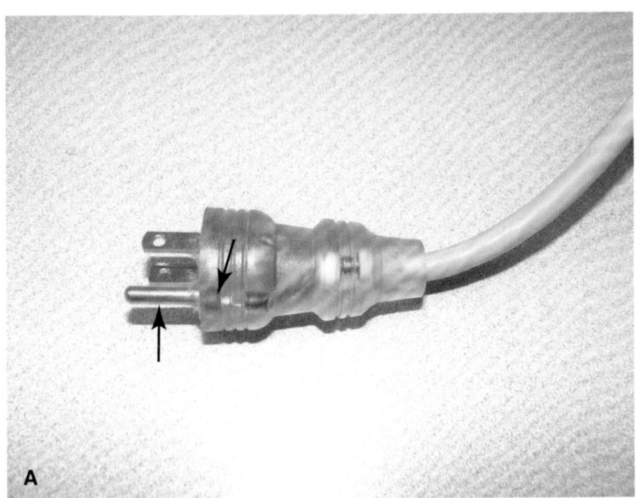

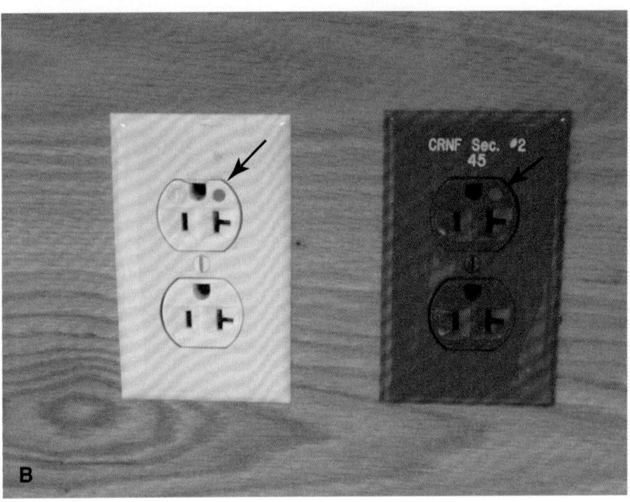

FIGURE 8-32. A: A hospital-grade plug that can be visually inspected. The *arrow* points to the equipment ground wire whose integrity can be readily verified Note that the prong for the ground wire (*arrow*) is longer than the hot or neutral prong, so that it is the first to enter the receptacle. **B:** The *arrows* point to the green dot denoting a hospital-grade power outlet. The red outlet on the right is connected to the emergency power (generator) system.

use of electrosurgery attests to the success of Professor Bovie's invention. However, this technology was not adopted without a cost. The widespread use of electrocautery has, at the very least, hastened the elimination of explosive anesthetic agents from the OR. In addition, as every anesthesiologist is aware, few things in the OR are immune to interference from the "Bovie." The high-frequency electrical energy generated by the ESU interferes with everything from the ECG signal to cardiac output computers, pulse oximeters, and even implanted cardiac pacemakers.[25]

The ESU operates by generating very-high-frequency currents (radiofrequency range) of anywhere from 500,000 to 1 million Hz. Heat is generated whenever a current passes through a resistance. The amount of heat (H) produced is proportional to the square of the current and inversely proportional to the area through which the current passes ($H = I^2/A$).[26] By concentrating the energy at the tip of the "Bovie pencil," the surgeon can produce either a cut or a coagulation at any given spot. This very-high-frequency current behaves differently from the standard 60 Hz AC current and can pass directly across the precordium without causing ventricular fibrillation.[26] This is because high-frequency currents have a low tissue penetration and do not excite contractile cells.

Although the ESU is used safely hundreds of thousands of times each year, there is evidence that under certain circumstances it has been the cause of ventricular fibrillation.[27–30] The mechanism is thought to be low frequency (50 to 60 Hz) "stray current" that is generated when the ESU is activated. Current in the 50 to 60 Hz range can cause ventricular fibrillation. These cases have been associated with the use of the coagulation mode, when the surgeon is using the device near the heart, and when the patient has a conductor in the heart such as a CVP or pulmonary artery catheter. However, the exact mechanism has not been elucidated.

The large amount of energy generated by the ESU can pose other problems to the operator and the patient. Dr. Cushing became aware of one such problem. He wrote, "Once the operator received a shock which passed through a metal retractor to his arm and out by a wire from his headlight, which was unpleasant to say the least".[31] The ESU cannot be safely operated unless the energy is properly routed from the ESU through the patient and back to the unit. Ideally, the current generated by the active electrode is concentrated at the ESU tip, constituting a very small surface area. This energy has a high current density and is able to generate enough heat to produce a therapeutic cut or coagulation. The energy then
5 passes through the patient to a dispersive electrode of large surface area that returns the energy safely to the ESU (Fig. 8-33).

One unfortunate quirk in terminology concerns the return (dispersive) plate of the ESU. This plate, often incorrectly referred to as a *ground plate,* is actually a dispersive electrode of large surface area that safely returns the generated energy to the ESU via a low current density pathway. When inquiring whether the dispersive electrode has been attached to the patient, OR personnel frequently ask, "Is the patient grounded?" Because the aim of electrical safety is to isolate the patient from the ground, this expression is worse than erroneous; it can lead to confusion. Because the area of the return plate is large, the current density is low; therefore, no harmful heat is generated and no tissue destruction occurs. In a properly functioning system, the only tissue effect is at the site of the active electrode that is held by the surgeon.

Problems can arise if the electrosurgical return plate is improperly applied to the patient or if the cord connecting the
9 return plate to the ESU is damaged or broken. In these instances, the high-frequency current generated by the ESU will seek an alternate return pathway. Anything attached to the patient, such as ECG leads or a temperature probe, can provide this alternate return pathway. The current density at the ECG pad will be considerably higher than normal because its surface area is much less than that of the ESU return plate. This may result in a serious burn at this alternate return site. Similarly, a burn may occur at the site of the ESU return plate if it is not properly applied to the patient or if it becomes partially dislodged during the operation (Fig. 8-34). This is not merely a theoretical possibility but is evidenced by the numerous case reports involving patients who have received ESU burns.[32–37]

The original ESUs were manufactured with the power supply connected directly to the ground by the equipment ground wire. These devices made it extremely easy for ESU current to return by alternate pathways. The ESU would continue to operate normally even without the return plate connected to the patient. In most modern ESUs, the power supply is isolated from ground to

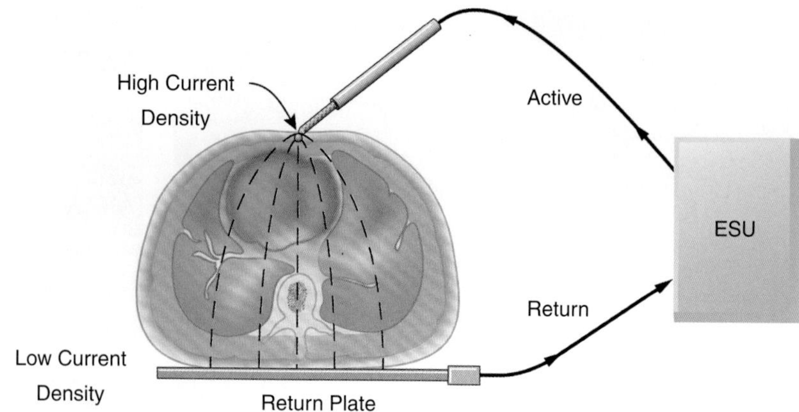

FIGURE 8-33. A properly applied electrosurgical unit (ESU) return plate. The current density at the return plate is low, resulting in no danger to the patient.

protect the patient from burns.[38] It was hoped that by isolating the return pathway from ground, the only route for current flow would be via the return electrode. Theoretically, this would eliminate alternate return pathways and greatly reduce the incidence of burns. However, Mitchell[39] found two situations in which the current could return via alternate pathways, even with the isolated ESU circuit. If the return plate were left either on top of an uninsulated ESU cabinet or in contact with the bottom of the OR table, then the ESU could operate fairly normally and the current would return via alternate pathways. It will be recalled that the impedance is inversely proportional to the capacitance times the current frequency. The ESU operates at 500,000 to >1,000,000 Hz, which greatly enhances the effect of capacitive coupling and causes a marked reduction in impedance. Therefore, even with isolated ESUs, the decrease in impedance allows the current to return to the ESU by alternate pathways. In addition, the isolated ESU does not protect the patient from burns if the return electrode does not make proper contact with the patient. Although the isolated ESU does provide additional patient safety, it is by no means foolproof protection against the patient receiving a burn.

Preventing patient burns from the ESU is the responsibility of all professional staff in the OR. Not only the circulating nurse, but also the surgeon and the anesthesiologist must be aware of proper techniques and be vigilant to potential problems. The most important factor is the proper application of the return plate. It is essential that the return plate has the appropriate amount of electrolyte gel and an intact return wire. Reusable return plates must be properly cleaned after each use, and disposable plates must be checked to ensure that the electrolyte has not dried out during storage. In addition, it is prudent to place the return plate as close as possible to the site of the operation. ECG pads should be placed as far from the site of the operation as is feasible. OR personnel must be alert to the possibility that pools of flammable "prep" solutions such as alcohol and acetone can ignite when the ESU is used. If the ESU must be used on a patient with a demand pacemaker, the return electrode should be located below the thorax, and preparations for treating potential dysrhythmias should be available, including a magnet to convert the pacemaker to a fixed rate, a defibrillator, and an external pacemaker. It is best to keep the pacemaker out of the path between the surgical site and the dispersal plate.

The ESU has also caused other problems in patients with pacemakers, including reprogramming and microshock.[40,41] If the surgeon requests higher than normal power settings on the ESU, this should alert both the circulating nurse and the anesthesiologist to a potential problem. The return plate and cable must be immediately inspected to ensure that it is functioning and properly positioned. If this does not correct the problem, the return plate should be replaced.[42,43] If the problem remains, the entire ESU should be taken out of service. Finally, an ESU that is dropped or damaged must be removed immediately from the OR and thoroughly tested by a qualified biomedical engineer. Following these simple safety steps will prevent most patient burns from the ESU.

The previous discussion concerned only *unipolar* ESUs. There is a second type of ESU, in which the current passes only between the two blades of a pair of forceps. This type of device is referred

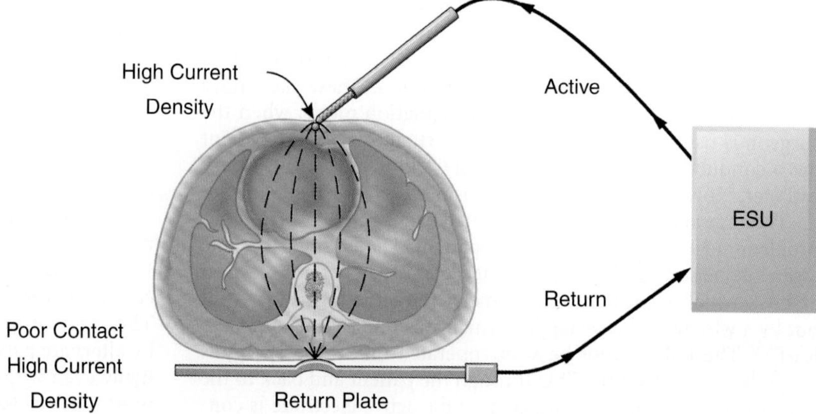

FIGURE 8-34. An improperly applied electrosurgical unit (ESU) return plate. Poor contact with the return plate results in a high current density and a possible burn to the patient.

to as a *bipolar* ESU. Because the active and return electrodes are the two blades of the forceps, it is not necessary to attach another dispersive electrode to the patient, unless a unipolar ESU is also being used. The bipolar ESU generates considerably less power than the unipolar and is mainly used for ophthalmic and neurologic surgery.

In 1980 Mirowski et al.[44] reported the first human implantation of a device to treat intractable ventricular tachydysrhythmias. This device, known as the *automatic implantable cardioverter-defibrillator* (AICD), is capable of sensing ventricular tachycardia and ventricular fibrillation and then automatically defibrillating the patient. Since 1980, thousands of patients have received AICD implants.[45,46] Because some of these patients may present for noncardiac surgery, it is important that the anesthesiologist be aware of potential problems.[47] The use of a unipolar ESU may cause electrical interference that could be interpreted by the AICD as a ventricular tachydysrhythmia. This would trigger a defibrillation pulse to be delivered to the patient and would likely cause an actual episode of ventricular tachycardia or ventricular fibrillation. The patient with an AICD is also at risk for ventricular fibrillation during electroconvulsive therapy.[47] In both cases, the AICD should be disabled by placing a magnet over the device or by use of a specific protocol to shut it off. Therefore, it is best to consult with someone experienced with the device before starting surgery. The device can be reactivated by reversing the process. Also, an external defibrillator and a noninvasive pacemaker should be in the OR whenever a patient with an AICD is anesthetized.

Electrical safety in the OR is a matter of combining common sense with some basic principles of electricity. Once OR personnel understand the importance of safe electrical practice, they are able to develop a heightened awareness to potential problems. All electrical equipment must undergo routine maintenance, service, and inspection to ensure that it conforms to designated electrical safety standards. Records of these test results must be kept for future inspection because human error can easily compound electrical hazards. Starmer et al.[48] cited one case concerning a newly constructed laboratory where the ground wire was not attached to a receptacle. In another study Albisser et al.[49] found a 14% (198/1,424) incidence of improperly or incorrectly wired outlets. Furthermore, potentially hazardous situations should be recognized and corrected before they become a problem. For instance, electrical power cords are frequently placed on the floor where they can be crushed by various carts or the anesthesia machine. These cords could be located overhead or placed in an area of low traffic flow. Multiple-plug extension boxes should not be left on the floor where they can come in contact with electrolyte solutions. These could easily be mounted on a cart or the anesthesia machine. Pieces of equipment that have been damaged or have obvious defects in the power cord must not be used until they have been properly repaired. If everyone is aware of what constitutes a potential hazard, dangerous situations can be prevented with minimal effort.

Sparks generated by the ESU may provide the ignition source for a fire with resulting burns to the patient and OR personnel. This is a particular risk when the ESU is used in an oxygen-enriched environment as may be present in the patient's airway or in close proximity to the patient's face. The administration of high-flow nasal oxygen to a sedated patient during procedures on the face and eye is particularly hazardous. Most plastics such as tracheal tubes and components of the anesthetic breathing system that would not burn in room air will ignite in the presence of oxygen and/or nitrous oxide. Tenting of the drapes to allow dispersion of any accumulated oxygen and/or its dilution by room air will decrease the risk of ignition from a spark generated by a nearby ESU. The risk of fire can also be reduced by use of a circle anesthesia breathing system with minimal to no leak of gases around the anesthesia mask.

Conductive Flooring

In past years, conductive flooring was mandated for ORs where flammable anesthetic agents were being administered. This would minimize the buildup of static charges that could cause a flammable anesthetic agent to ignite. The standards have now been changed to eliminate the necessity for conductive flooring in anesthetizing areas where flammable agents are no longer used.

ENVIRONMENTAL HAZARDS

There are a number of potential electrically related hazards in the OR that are of concern to the anesthesiologist. There is the potential for electrical shock not only to the patient but also to OR personnel. In addition, cables and power cords to electrical equipment and monitoring devices can become hazardous. Finally, all OR personnel should have a plan of what to do in the event of a power failure.

In today's OR, there are literally dozens of pieces of electrical equipment. It is not uncommon to have numerous power cords lying on the floor, where they are vulnerable to damage. If the insulation on the power cable becomes damaged, it is fairly easy for the hot wire to come in contact with a piece of metal equipment. If the OR does not have isolated power, that piece of equipment would become energized and be a potential electrical shock hazard.[50] Having isolated power minimizes the risk to the patient and OR personnel. Clearly, getting electrical power cords off the floor is desirable. This can be accomplished by having electrical outlets in the ceiling or by having ceiling-mounted articulated arms that contain electrical outlets. Also, the use of multi-outlet extension boxes that sit on the floor can be hazardous and should be avoided. These can be contaminated with fluids, which could easily trip the circuit breaker. In one case, it apparently tripped the main circuit breaker for the entire OR, resulting in a loss of all electrical power except for the overhead lights.[51]

Modern monitoring devices have many safety features incorporated into them. Virtually all of them have isolated the patient input from the power supply of the device. This is frequently done with optocoupler isolation circuits, which transfer electrical signals by utilizing light waves. This was an important feature that was lacking from the original ECG monitors. In the early days, patients could actually become part of the electrical circuit of the monitor. There have been relatively few problems with patients and monitoring devices since the advent of isolated inputs. However, between 1985 and 1994, the Food and Drug Administration (FDA) received approximately 24 reports in which infants and children had received an electrical shock, including five children who died by electrocution.[52,53] These electrical accidents occurred because the electrode lead wires from either an ECG monitor or an apnea monitor were plugged directly into a 120-volt electrical outlet instead of the appropriate patient cable. In 1997, the FDA issued a new performance standard for electrode lead wires and patient cables that requires that the exposed male connector pins from the electrode lead wires be eliminated. Therefore, the lead wires must have female connections and the connector pins must be housed in a protected patient cable (Fig. 8-35). This effectively eliminates the possibility of the patient being connected directly to an AC source since there are no exposed connector pins on the lead wires.

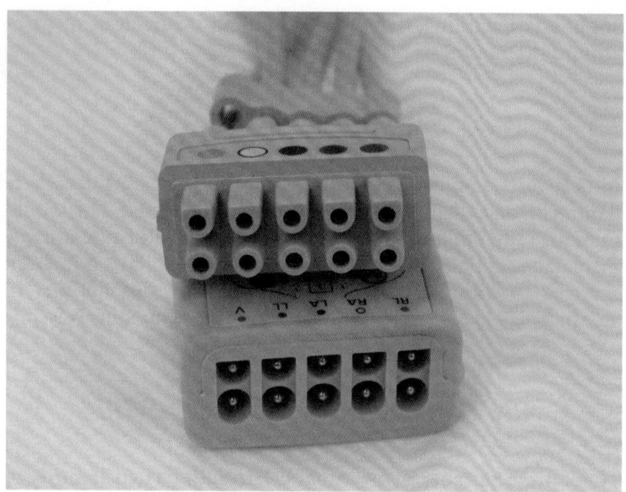

FIGURE 8-35. The current standard for patient lead wires **(top)** requires a female connector. The patient cable **(bottom)** has shielded connector pins that the lead wires plug into.

All health care facilities are required to have a source of emergency power. This generally consists of one or more electrical generators. These generators are configured to start up automatically and provide power to the facility within 10 seconds after detecting the loss of power from the utility company. The facility is required to test these generators on a regular basis. However, in the past, not all health care facilities tested them under actual load. There are numerous anecdotal reports of generators not functioning properly during an actual power failure. If the generators are not tested under actual load, it is possible that many years will pass before a real power outage puts a severe demand on the generator. If the facility has several generators and one of them fails, the increased demand on the others may be enough to cause them to fail in rapid succession. Hospitals (under the current National Fire Protection Association [NFPA] 99 standards) must test their emergency power supply systems (generators) under connected load once a month for at least 30 minutes. If the generator is oversized for the application and cannot be loaded to at least 30% of its rating, it must be load-banked and run for a total of 2 hours every year. A fairly recent requirement is for emergency power supply systems to be tested once every 3 years for 4 continuous hours, with a recommendation that this be performed during peak usage of the system.[54,55]

Although all hospitals are required to have emergency generators to power essential equipment in the event of a power failure, these generators do not function in every circumstance. If there is a loss of power from the electrical utility, then this is detected by a relay switch, which in turn causes a series of events to activate the transfer of the power generation to the backup system. This usually happens seamlessly. However, if the transfer switch or the generator fails, then there will be no backup electricity.

Another cause of partial or total power failure has to do with construction mishaps. As hospitals frequently remodel, add new wings, or upgrade existing facilities, there is always a chance that the power will be accidentally interrupted. This may be due to a worker tripping a GFI, or a relay failure that caused a power transfer to a nonworking generator.[56,57] Since the electrical utility is still supplying power, the generators may not be activated.

It is vitally important that each OR has a contingency plan for a power failure. There should be a supply of battery-operated light sources available in each OR. A laryngoscope can serve as a readily available source of light that allows one to find flashlights and other pieces of equipment. The overhead lights in the OR should also be connected to some sort of battery-operated lighting system. Most anesthesia machines have a backup battery that will last 30 to 60 minutes. If the power failure lasts longer than that, the anesthesiologist must make plans on how to continue the anesthetic. The newer electronic machines may be more problematic than older traditional machines, since they may have electronic gas or vaporization systems. The department should have a supply of battery-powered monitors, but it is unlikely that there will be enough for every OR. Syringe pumps typically have a battery, and blood pressures can be taken with a manual sphygmomanometer. Since many ORs employ automated drug dispensing systems, these devices will not work without power and a communication link to the hospital information system. In reality, the backup generators will usually supply power in the event of an emergency. However, there are many circumstances where the hospital can experience partial or total power loss. The cost of these contingencies is relatively small but the benefits can be incomparable in an emergency.

ELECTROMAGNETIC INTERFERENCE

Rapid advances in technology have led to an explosion in the number of wireless communication devices in the marketplace. These devices include cellular telephones, cordless telephones, walkie-talkies, and wireless Internet access devices. All of these devices have something in common: They emit electromagnetic interference (EMI). This most commonly manifests itself when traveling on airplanes. Most airlines require that these devices be turned off when the plane is taking off or landing or, in some cases, during the entire flight. There is concern that the EMI emitted by these devices may interfere with the plane's navigation and communication equipment.

In recent years, the number of people who own these devices has increased exponentially. Indeed, in some hospitals, they form a vital link in the regular or emergency communication system. It is not uncommon for physicians, nurses, paramedics, and other personnel to have their own cellular telephones. In addition, patients and visitors may also have cellular telephones and other types of communication devices. Hospital maintenance and security personnel frequently have walkie-talkie–type radios and some hospitals have even instituted an in-house cellular telephone network that augments or replaces the paging system. There has been concern that the EMI emitted by these devices may interfere with implanted pacemakers or various types of monitoring devices and ventilators in critical care areas.[58] One case of a patient death has been reported when a ventilator malfunctioned secondary to EMI.[59]

Several studies have been done to find out if cellular telephones cause problems with cardiac pacemakers. One report by Hayes et al.[60] studied 980 patients with five different types of cellular telephones. They conducted more than 5,000 tests and found that in more than 20% of the cases they could detect some interference from the cellular telephone. Patients were symptomatic in 7.2% of the cases, and clinically significant interference occurred in 6.6% of the cases. When the telephone was held in the normal position over the ear, clinically significant interference was not detected. In fact, the interference that caused clinical symptoms occurred only if the telephone was directly over the pacemaker. Other studies have demonstrated changes such as erroneous sensing and pacer inhibition.[61,62] Again, these occurred only when the telephone was close to the pacemaker. The changes were temporary, and the pacemaker reverted to normal when the cellular telephone was moved to a safe distance. Currently, the FDA guidelines are that the cellular telephones be kept at least 6 inches from the pacemaker. Therefore, a patient with a pacemaker should not carry a cellular telephone in the shirt pocket, which is adjacent to the pacemaker. There appears to be little risk if hospital personnel carry a cellular telephone and if they ensure that it is kept at a reasonable distance from patients with a pacemaker.

AICDs comprise another group of devices of concern to biomedical engineers. Fetter et al.[63] conducted a study of 41 patients who had AICDs. They concluded that the cellular telephones did not interfere with the AICDs. They did, however, recommend keeping the cellular telephone at least 6 inches from the device.

EMI extends well beyond that of cellular telephones. Walkie-talkies, which are frequently used by hospital maintenance and security personnel, paging systems, police radios, and even televisions all emit EMI, which could potentially interfere with medical devices of any nature. Although there are many anecdotal reports, the amount of available scientific information on this problem is scant. Reports of interference include ventilator and infusion pumps that have been shut down or reprogrammed, interference with ECG monitors, and even an electronic wheelchair that was accidentally started because of EMI. It is a difficult problem to study because there are many different types of devices that emit EMI and a vast array of medical equipment that has the potential to interact with these devices. Even though a device may seem "safe" in the medical environment, if two or three cellular telephones or walkie-talkies are brought together in the same area at the same time, there may be unanticipated problems or interference.

Any time a cellular telephone is turned on, it is actually communicating with the cellular network, even though a call is not in progress. Therefore, the potential to interfere with devices exists. The ECRI Institute reported in October 1999 that walkie-talkies were far more likely to cause problems with medical devices than cellular telephones.[64] This is because they operate on a lower frequency than cellular telephones and have a higher power output. The ECRI recommends that cellular telephones be maintained at a distance of 1 meter from medical devices, while walkie-talkies be kept at a distance of 6 to 8 meters.

Some hospitals have made restrictive policies on the use of cellular telephones, particularly in critical care areas.[65] These policies are supported by little scientific documentation and are nearly impossible to enforce. The ubiquitous presence of cellular telephones carried by hospital personnel and visitors makes enforcing a ban virtually impossible. Even when people try to comply with the ban, failure is nearly inevitable because the general public is usually unaware that a cellular telephone in the standby mode is still communicating with the tower and generating EMI.

The real solution is to "harden" devices against EMI. This is difficult to do because of the many different frequencies on which these devices operate. Education of medical personnel is essential. When working in an OR or critical care area, all personnel must be alert to the fact that electronic devices and pacemakers can be interfered by EMI. Creating a restrictive policy would certainly irritate personnel and visitors, and in some cases, may actually compromise emergency communications.[66]

CONSTRUCTION OF NEW OPERATING ROOMS

Frequently, an anesthesiologist is asked to consult with hospital administrators and architects in designing new, or remodeling older, ORs. In the past, a strict electrical code was enforced because of the use of flammable anesthetic agents. This code included a requirement for IPSs and LIMs. The NFPA revised its standard for health care facilities in 1984 (NFPA 99-1984). These standards did not require IPS or LIMs in areas designated for use of nonflammable anesthetic agents only.[67,68] Although not mandatory, NFPA standards are usually adopted by local authorities when revising their electrical codes.

This change in the standard created a dilemma. The NFPA 99-2012—*Health Care Facilities Code,* mandates that "wet procedure locations shall be provided with special protection against electrical shock." Section 6.3.2.2.8.2 further states that "this special protection shall be provided as follows: (1) Power distribution system that inherently limits the possible ground-fault current due to a first fault to a low value, without interrupting the power supply, (2) power distribution system in which the power supply is interrupted if the ground-fault current does, in fact, exceed the trip value of a Class A GFCI."[69]

The decision of whether to install isolated power hinged on two factors. The first was whether or not the OR was considered a wet location, and, if so, whether an interruptible power supply was tolerable. When power interruption was tolerable, a GFCI was permitted as the protective means. However, the standard also stated that "the use of an isolated power system (IPS) shall be permitted as a protective means capable of limiting ground fault current without power interruption."

Most people who have worked in an OR would attest to its being a wet procedure location. The presence of blood, body fluids, and saline solutions spilled on the floor all contribute to making this a wet environment. The cystoscopy suite serves as a good example.

Once the premise that the OR is a wet location is accepted, it must be determined whether a GFCI can provide the means of protection. The argument against using GFCIs in the OR is illustrated by the following example. Assume that during an open heart procedure, the cardiopulmonary bypass pump and the patient monitors are plugged into outlets on the same branch circuit. Also assume that during bypass, the circulating nurse plugs in a faulty headlight. If there is a GFCI protecting the circuit, the fault will be detected and the GFCI will interrupt all power to the pump and the monitors. This undoubtedly would cause a great deal of confusion and consternation among the OR personnel and may place the patient at risk for injury. The pump would have to be manually operated while the problem was being resolved. In addition, the GFCI could not be reset (and power restored) until the headlight is identified as the cause of the fault and unplugged from the outlet. However, if the OR were protected with an IPS and LIM, the same scenario would cause the LIM to alarm, but the pump and patient monitors would continue to operate normally. There would be no interruption of power and the problem could be resolved without risk to the patient.

It should be realized that a GFCI is an active system. That is, a potentially hazardous current is already flowing and must be actively interrupted, whereas the IPS (with LIM) is designed to be safe during a first-fault situation. Thus, it is a passive system because no mechanical action is required to activate the protection.[70]

Many hospital administrators and engineers wanted to eliminate IPSs in new OR construction by advocating that it was unnecessary and costly. They also grossly inflated the maintenance costs of the IPS. In fact, the maintenance costs of modern systems are minimal, and the installation costs are approximately 1% to 2% of the cost of constructing a new OR. The American Society of Anesthesiologists (ASA) and others, however, had advocated for the retention of IPSs.[70–73] In 2006, the ASA, through its representatives to NFPA-99 and its technical committee on Electrical Systems, launched a major campaign to have ORs default to being a wet procedure location. This was vigorously opposed by the American Hospital Association and the American Society of Healthcare engineers. The final version of the NFPA-99, 2012 edition, contains the following language: "Section 6.3.2.2.8.4 ORs shall be considered to be a wet procedure location, unless a risk assessment conducted by the health care governing body determines otherwise." In addition section 6.3.2.2.8.7 states: "Operating rooms defined as wet procedure locations shall be protected by either isolated power or ground fault circuit interrupters." Although, this code applies only to new or remodeled ORs, it is nonetheless a major victory for ASA, our patients, and OR personnel. In the event that the health care facility wants to classify an OR as a "dry" location, then they have to do a risk assessment, and the NFPA-99 annex (A.6.3.2.2.8.4) states that among others this should include clinicians.[69]

Although not perfect,[74] the IPS and LIM do provide both the patient and OR personnel with a significant amount of protection in an electrically hazardous environment. IPSs provide clean stable voltages, which is important for sensitive diagnostic equipment.[75] Also, modern LIMs, which are microprocessor-based, require only yearly instead of monthly testing.

The value of the IPS is illustrated in a report by Day[76] in 1994. He reported four instances of electrical shock to OR personnel in a 1-year period. The operating suite had been renovated and the IPS removed, and it was not until the OR personnel received a shock that a problem was discovered. Also, in 2010, Wills et al. reported an incident where an OR nurse received a severe electrical shock while plugging in a piece of equipment.[77] This case further illustrates the consequences of having a wet floor in an OR with no IPS or GFCIs.

Anesthesiologists need to be aware of these new regulations and strongly encourage that new ORs be constructed with IPSs. The relatively small cost savings that the alternative would represent do not justify the elimination of such a useful safety system. The use of GFCIs in the OR environment can be acceptable if carefully planned and engineered. In order to avoid the loss of power to multiple instruments and monitors at one time, each outlet must be an individual GFCI. If that is done, then a fault will result in only one piece of equipment losing power. Using GFCIs also precludes the use of multiple plug strips in the OR.

Finally, in 2011, August reported on the opening of 24 new ORs in his facility. To their dismay, they found that the electrical service panels outside each OR were locked, and that the ORs had been reclassified as "dry" locations, without the knowledge of the anesthesia department.[78] Barker also reported an incident where a PACU monitor overheated and was billowing smoke. An attempt to shut off the power, was met with a locked circuit breaker box.[79] He too, commented on the need to have ORs designated as wet procedure locations.

Hopefully, with the new NFPA-99 code, there will be far fewer incidents of new ORs being designated as "dry" locations, especially without the knowledge of the anesthesia department. Electrical safety should be the concern of everyone in the OR. Accidents can be prevented only if proper installation and maintenance of the appropriate safety equipment in the OR have occurred and the OR personnel understand the concepts of electrical safety and are vigilant in their efforts to detect new hazards.[80]

FIRE SAFETY

Fires in the OR are just as much a danger today as they were 100
10 years ago when patients were anesthetized with flammable anesthetic agents.[81,82] Because the potential consequences of a fire or explosion with ether or cyclopropane were well known and potentially devastating, OR fire safety practices were routinely followed.[83,84]

Today, the risk of an OR fire is probably as great or greater than the days when ether and cyclopropane were used, in part because of the routine use of potential sources of ignition (including electrosurgical cauteries) in an environment rich in fuel sources (i.e., flammable materials) and oxidizers (e.g., oxygen and nitrous oxide). Although the number of OR fires that occur annually in the United States is unknown, some estimates suggest that there are 550 to 650 fires each year, with as many as 5% to 10% associated with serious injury or death.[85] In contrast to the era of flammable anesthetics, there currently appears to be a lack of awareness of the potential for an OR fire. In response to the risks presented by this situation, in 2008 the ASA released a Practice Advisory on the Prevention and Management of Operating Room Fires[86] (Table 8-3).

For a fire to start, three components are necessary. The limbs
11 of the "fire triad" are a heat or ignition source, fuel, and an oxidizer[87] (Fig. 8-36). A fire occurs when there is a chemical reaction
6 of a fuel rapidly combining with an oxidizer to release energy in the form of heat and light. In the OR, there are many heat or igni-
12 tion sources, such as the ESU, lasers, and the ends of fiberoptic light cords. The main oxidizers in the OR are air, oxygen, and nitrous oxide. Oxygen and nitrous oxide function equally well as oxidizers, so a combination of 50% oxygen and 50% nitrous oxide would avidly support combustion, as would 100% oxygen. Fuel for a fire can be found everywhere in the OR. Paper drapes, which have largely replaced cloth drapes, are much easier to ignite and can burn with greater intensity.[88,89] Other sources of fuel include gauze dressings, endotracheal tubes, gel mattress pads, and even facial or body hair[90] (Table 8-4).

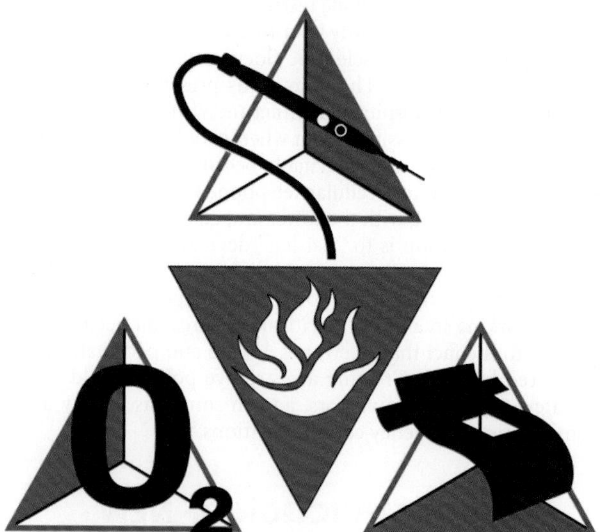

FIGURE 8-36. The fire triangle. ©ECRI Institute. Used with permission.

TABLE 8-3. RECOMMENDATIONS FOR THE PREVENTION AND MANAGEMENT OF OPERATING ROOM FIRES

Preparation
- Train personnel in OR fire management
- Practice responses to fires (fire drills)
- Assure that fire-management equipment is readily available
- Determine if a high-risk situation exists
- Team decides how to prevent/manage a fire
- Each person assigned a task (e.g., remove endotracheal tube or disconnect circuit)

Prevention
- Allow flammable skin preparations to dry before draping
- Configure surgical drapes to avoid buildup of oxidizer
- Anesthesiologist collaborates with team throughout the procedure to minimize oxidizer-enriched environment near ignition source
- Keep O_2 concentration as low as clinically possible
- Avoid N_2O
- Notify surgeon if oxidizer ↔ ignition source are in proximity to each other
- Moisten gauze and sponges that are near an ignition source

Management
- Look for early warning sign of a fire (e.g., pop, flash, or smoke)
- Stop procedure and each team member immediately carries out assigned task

Airway fire
- *Simultaneously* remove the endotracheal tube and stop gases/disconnect circuit
- Pour saline into airway
- Remove burning materials
- Mask ventilate patient, assess injury, consider bronchoscopy, reintubate

Fire on the patient
- Turn off gases
- Remove drapes and burning materials
- Extinguish flames with water, saline, or fire extinguisher
- Assess patient's status, devise care plan, assess for smoke inhalation

Failure to extinguish
- Use CO_2 fire extinguisher
- Activate fire alarm
- Consider evacuation of room: Close door and do not reopen
- Turn off medical gas supply to room

Risk management
- Preserve scene
- Notify hospital risk manager
- Follow local regulatory reporting requirements
- Treat fire as an adverse event
- FIRE DRILLS

Adapted from: Practice Advisory for the Prevention and Management of Operating Room Fires. Park Ridge, IL: American Society of Anesthesiologists. Approved by the ASA House of Delegates in October 2007; published in *Anesthesiology*, May 2008.

Fire prevention is accomplished by not allowing all three of the elements of the fire triad to come together at the same time.[91] The challenge in the OR is that frequently each of the limbs of the fire triad is controlled by a different individual. For instance, the surgeon is frequently in charge of the ignition source, the anesthesiologist is usually administering the oxidizer, and the OR nurse frequently controls the fuel sources. It is not always evident to any one individual that all of these elements may be coming together at the same time. This is especially true in any case in which there is the possibility of oxygen or an oxygen-nitrous oxide mixture being delivered around the surgical site. In these circumstances, the risk of an OR fire is markedly increased and the need for communication among the surgeon, the anesthesiologist, and the OR nurses throughout the procedure is essential.

There are several dangers that may result from an OR fire. The most obvious is that the patient and OR personnel can suffer severe burns. However, a less obvious but potentially more deadly risk can be posed by the products of combustion (called *toxicants*). When materials such as plastics burn, a variety of injurious compounds can be produced. These include carbon monoxide, ammonia, hydrogen chloride, an even cyanide. Toxicants can produce injury by damaging airways and lung tissue, and can cause asphyxia. OR fires can often produce significant amounts of smoke and toxicants, but may not cause enough heat to activate overhead sprinkler systems. If enough smoke is produced, the OR personnel may have to evacuate the area. Therefore, it is essential to have an evacuation plan for both the OR personnel and the patient, which was planned and carefully considered before a fire could occur.

OR fires can be divided into two different types. The more common type of fire occurs *in* or *on* the patient, especially during high-risk procedures in which an ignition source is used in an oxidizer-rich environment. These would include airway fires (including endotracheal tube fires, fires in the oropharynx, which may occur during a tonsillectomy, fires in the breathing circuit), and fires during laparoscopy. In 2005, Katz and Campbell reported on a fire during a thoracotomy.[92] A dry gauze lap pad was set on fire, because 100% oxygen was present in the thoracic cavity while the surgeon was using the electrocautery. Cases that involve stripping of the pleura or resection of pulmonary blebs, can easily result in high concentrations of oxygen in the thoracic cavity when the lung is reinflated due to gas leakage. Solutions to this problem include making sure that the lap pads are always wet, and if the surgeon needs the lung inflated, then doing CPAP with air instead of oxygen will greatly reduce the risk of a fire.

Fires occurring on the patient mainly involve head and neck surgery done under regional anesthesia or monitored anesthesia care (MAC) when the patient is receiving high flows of supplemental oxygen. Because these fires occur in an oxygen-enriched environment, items such as surgical towels, drapes, or even the body hair can be readily ignited and produce a severe burn. The ECRI Institute warns that "oxygen enriched atmospheres lower the temperature at which a fuel will ignite".[85] In addition, these fires will burn more vigorously, and spread faster. The other type of OR fire is one that is remote from the patient. This would include an electrical fire in a piece of equipment, or a carbon dioxide (CO_2) absorber fire.

All materials burn in the presence of an oxygen-enriched environment. Wolf et al. tested a number of surgical drape materials in 21%, 50%, and 95% oxygen.[93] They found that the higher the concentration of oxygen, the more readily the material could be set on fire. In 50% and 95% O_2, all the materials burned. In the case of the cotton huck towel, the time to ignition in 21% O_2 was a mean of 12 seconds. The same material ignited in 0.1 seconds in 95% O_2.

TABLE 8-4. **FUEL SOURCES COMMONLY FOUND IN THE OPERATING ROOM**

"Prep" agents
- Alcohol
- Degreasers (acetone, ether)
- Adhesives (tincture of benzoin, Aeroplast)™
- Chlorhexidine digluconate (Hibitane)™
- Iodophor (Dura-Prep)™

Drapes and covers
- Patient drapes (paper, plastic, cloth)
- Equipment drapes (paper, plastic, cloth)
- Blankets and sheets
- Pillows, mattresses, and padding
- Gowns
- Masks
- Shoe covers
- Gloves (latex, nonlatex)
- Clothing
- Compression (anti-embolism) stockings

Patient
- Hair
- Alimentary tract gases (methane, hydrogen)
- Desiccated tissue

Dressings
- Gauze and sponges
- Petrolatum-impregnated dressings
- Xeroform™
- Adhesive tape (cloth, plastic, paper)
- Elastic bandages
- Stockinettes
- Sutures
- Steri-strips
- Collodion

Ointments
- Petrolatum
- Antibiotics (bacitracin, neomycin, polymyxin B)
- Nitropaste (Nitro-Bid)™
- EMLA™
- Lip balms

Anesthesia equipment
- Breathing circuit hoses
- Masks
- Endotracheal tubes
- Oral and nasal airways
- Laryngeal mask airways
- Nasogastric tubes
- Suction catheters and tubing
- Scavenger hoses
- Volatile anesthetics
- CO_2 absorbers
- Intravenous tubing
- Pressure monitor tubing and plastic transducers

Other equipment
- Charts and records
- Cardboard, wooden, and particleboard boxes and cabinets
- Packing materials (cardboard, expanded polystyrene [Styrofoam])
- Fiberoptic cable covers
- Wire covers and insulation
- Fiberoptic endoscope coverings
- Sphygmomanometer cuffs and tubing
- Pneumatic tourniquet cuffs and tubing
- Stethoscope tubing™
- Vascular shunts (Gore-tex, Dacron)™
- Dialysis and extracorporeal circulation circuits
- Wound drains and collection systems
- Mops and brooms
- Textbooks and instruction manuals

The two major ignition sources for OR fires are the ESU and the laser. However, the ends of some fiberoptic light cords can also become hot enough to start a fire if they are placed on paper drapes. Although the ESU is responsible for igniting the majority of the fires,[94] it is the laser that has generated the most attention and research. Laser is the acronym for *l*ight *a*mplification by *s*timulated *e*mission of *r*adiation. A laser consists of an energy source and material that the energy excites to emit light.[95–97] The material that the energy excites is called the *lasing medium* and provides the name of the particular type of laser. The important property of laser light is that it is coherent radiation, meaning that is monochromatic (of a single wavelength), coherent (photons are in phase with each other), and collimated (the beam does not disperse as the distance from the source increases). This coherent light can be focused into very small spots that have very high power density.

There are many different types of medical lasers, and each has a specific application. The argon laser is used in eye and dermatologic procedures because it is absorbed by hemoglobin and has a modest tissue penetration of between 0.05 and 2.0 mm. The potassium titanyl phosphate (KTP) or frequency-doubled yttrium aluminum garnet (YAG) lasers are also absorbed by hemoglobin and have tissue penetrations similar to that of the argon laser. The tunable dye laser has a wavelength that is easily changed and can be used in different applications, particularly in dermatologic procedures. The neodymium-doped yttrium aluminum garnet (Nd:YAG) laser is the most powerful of the medical lasers. Since the tissue penetration is between 2 and 6 mm, it can be used for tumor debulking, particularly in the trachea and main stem bronchi, or in the upper airway. The energy can be transmitted through a fiberoptic cable that is placed down the suction port of a fiberoptic bronchoscope (FOB). The laser can then be used in a contact mode to treat a tumor mass. The CO_2 laser has very little tissue penetration and can be used where great precision is needed. It is also absorbed by water, so that minimal heat is dispersed to surrounding tissues. The CO_2 laser is used primarily for procedures in the oropharynx and in and around the vocal cords. The helium–neon laser (He–Ne) produces an intense red light and thus can be used for aiming the CO_2 and the Nd:YAG lasers. It has very low power and thus will present no significant danger to OR personnel.

One of the most devastating types of OR fires occurs when an endotracheal tube is ignited *in* the patient.[98–103] If the patient is being ventilated with oxygen and/or nitrous oxide, the endotracheal tube will essentially emit a blowtorch type of flame that can result in severe injury to the trachea, lungs, and surrounding tissues (Fig. 8-37). Red rubber, polyvinyl chloride, and silicone

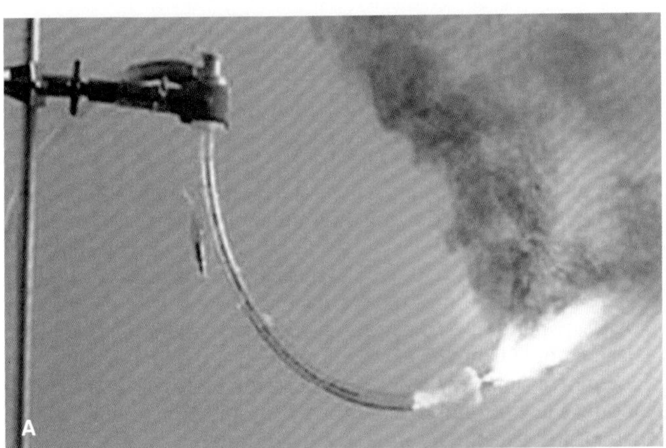

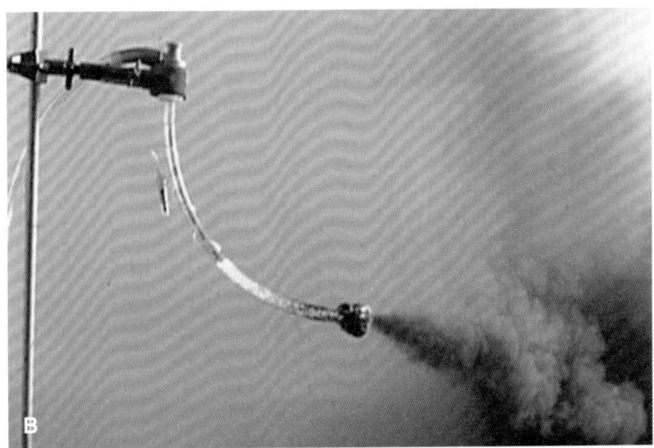

FIGURE 8-37. **A:** A burning ET tube with a high concentration of O_2 or O_2/N_2O will exhibit a "blowtorch" effect. © ECRI Institute. Used with permission. **B:** A burning ET tube will produce a large amount of debris. © ECRI Institute. Used with permission.

endotracheal tubes all have oxygen-flammability indices (defined as the minimum O_2 fraction in N_2 that will just support a candle-like flame for a given fuel source using a standard ignition source) [104] of <26%.[105] Historically, anesthesiologists attempted to improve the safety of these tubes by wrapping red rubber or polyvinyl chloride tubes with some sort of reflective tape. However, taped–wrapped tubes often became kinked, gaps in the tape exposed areas of the tube to the laser, and non–laser-resistant tape was sometimes unintentionally used. To prevent these problems during high-risk procedures, "laser-resistant" endotracheal tubes have been developed.[106–108] Anesthesiologists can now use an endotracheal tube that is designed to be resistant to ignition by the specific type of laser that will be used during surgery. For instance, when using the CO_2 laser, the LaserFlex (Mallinckrodt, Pleasanton, CA) (Fig. 8-38) is an excellent choice. This is a flexible metal tube that has two cuffs that can be inflated with saline colored with methylene blue. The methylene blue enables the surgeon to easily recognize if he or she has accidentally penetrated one of the cuffs. The LaserFlex™ tube is highly resistant to being struck by the laser. If the Nd:YAG laser is being used, then the Lasertubus™ (Rüsch Inc., Duluth, GA) can be used (Fig. 8-39). The Lasertubus™ has a soft rubber shaft that is covered by a corrugated silver foil that is in turn covered in a Merocel sponge jacket. In order to provide maximum protection, the Merocel must be kept moist with saline. It should be noted that only the portion of the tube covered with the Merocel is laser resistant.

Another potential source of ignition for an OR fire is the ESU.[109,110] A typical example of how an ESU could cause ignition would be during a tonsillectomy in a child in whom the anesthesiologist was using an uncuffed, flammable endotracheal tube. In this case, the oxygen or oxygen–nitrous oxide mixture could leak around the endotracheal tube and pool at the operative site, providing an oxidizer-enriched environment. When the surgeon uses the ESU (or laser) to cauterize the tonsil bed, the combination of a high concentration of oxidizer (oxygen or oxygen–nitrous oxide mixture), fuel (endotracheal tube), and ignition source (the ESU or laser) could easily start a fire.[111,112]

The best way to prevent this type of fire is to take steps to prevent the three legs of the fire triad from coming together. For example, mixing the oxygen with air will keep the inspired oxygen concentration as low as possible, thus reducing the available oxidizer. Another possibility would be to place wet pledgets around the endotracheal tube, which would prevent the escape of oxygen or oxygen–nitrous oxide mixture from the trachea into the operative

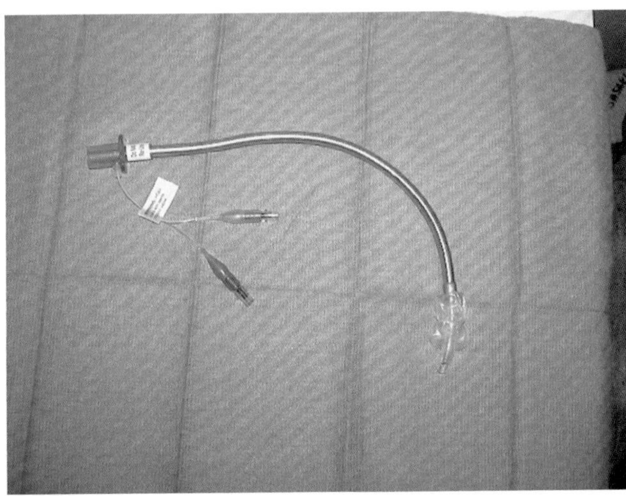

FIGURE 8-38. LaserFlex laser resistant ET tube.

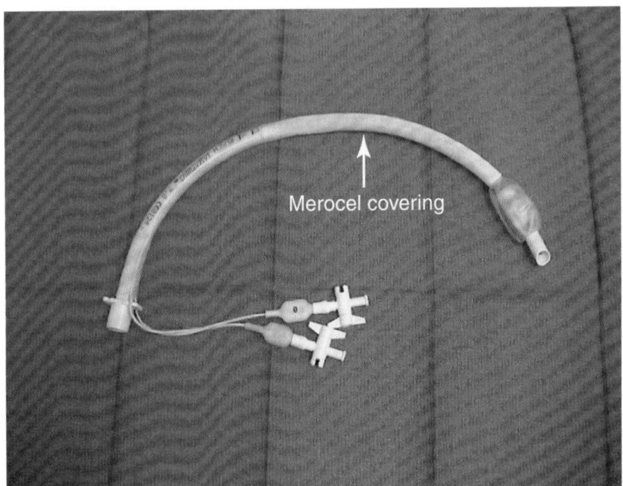

FIGURE 8-39. Lasertubus laser resistant ET tube.

field. This reduces the available oxidizer and would keep the endotracheal tube and tissues from becoming desiccated, thus reducing their suitability as fuel sources. However, the pledgets must be kept moist, lest they dry out and become an additional source of fuel for a fire.

A related situation that requires a different solution can arise when a critically ill patient requires a tracheostomy.[113,114] These patients may require very high concentrations of inspired oxygen to maintain tissue oxygenation so that any decrease in inspired oxygen concentration or interruption of ventilation would not be tolerated. In this circumstance, the best option for preventing a fire would be to avoid the use of electrocautery (ignition source) when the surgeon enters the trachea.

The Nd:YAG laser can be used to treat tumors of the lower trachea and main stem bronchi. Most commonly, the surgeon will use a FOB and pass the laser fiber through the suction port of the bronchoscope. The FOB can be used in conjunction with a rigid metal bronchoscope or passed through an 8.5 or 9.0 mm polyvinyl chloride endotracheal tube. A special laser-resistant tube would not be used in this circumstance because the FOB and laser fiber pass through the endotracheal tube and focus on tissue distal to the tube. Fire safety precautions available in this setting include titrating the concentration of inspired oxygen to as low a concentration as the patient can tolerate while maintaining a saturation of between 90% and 95% (ideally keeping the inspired oxygen below 30%), keeping the tip of the endotracheal tube and FOB away from the site of surgery and out of the "line of fire" of the laser, and removing charred and desiccated tissue from the surgical field.

The use of a rigid metal bronchoscope instead of an endotracheal tube will eliminate the possibility of setting the tube on fire but does not eliminate the possibility of setting the FOB on fire. This would also necessitate the use of a jet Venturi system to ventilate the patient, which would, in turn, deliver an inspired oxygen concentration of between 40% and 60%.

There are a number of basic safety precautions that should be taken whenever a laser is used in surgery. Since laser light can be reflected off any metal surface, it is important that all OR personnel wear protective goggles that are specific to the type of laser being used. The anesthesiologist needs to be aware that the laser goggles may make it difficult to read certain monitor displays. In addition, it is important that the patient's eyes be covered with wet gauze or eye packs. OR personnel should also wear high filtration masks because the laser "plume" may contain vaporized virus particles or chemical toxins. Finally, all doors to the OR should have warning signs that a laser is in use, and all windows should be covered with black window shades.

Laparoscopic surgery in the abdomen is another potential risk for a surgically related fire. Ordinarily, the abdomen is inflated with CO_2, which does not support combustion. It is important to verify that, indeed, only CO_2 is being used, as erroneous inclusion of oxygen can be disastrous.[115,116] Also, nitrous oxide administered to the patient as part of the anesthetic can, over 30 minutes, diffuse into the abdominal cavity and attain a concentration that could support combustion.[117] In fact, when sampling the abdominal gas contents after 30 minutes, the mean nitrous oxide concentration was 36%; however, in certain patients it reached a concentration of 47%. Both methane and hydrogen are flammable gases that are frequently present in bowel gas in significant concentrations. Methane concentration in bowel gas can be up to 56% and hydrogen has been reported as high as 69%. With the maximum abdominal concentration of 47% nitrous oxide mixed with CO_2, it would require the maximum of 56% of methane to be flammable. Therefore, this represents a relatively small hazard. In contrast, a concentration of 69% hydrogen is flammable if the nitrous oxide concentration is >29%. Therefore, a fire is possible if the surgeon, while using the ESU, enters the bowel with a high concentration of hydrogen and the intra-abdominal nitrous oxide content is >29%.

In recent years, fires *on* the patient seem to have become the most frequent type of OR fire. These cases occur most often during surgery in and around the head and neck, where the patient is receiving MAC and supplemental oxygen is being administered by either a face mask or nasal cannulae.[118–122] In these cases, the oxygen can collect under the drapes if not properly vented, and when the surgeon uses the ESU or the laser, a fire can easily start. There are many things that can act as fuel, such as the surgical towels, paper drapes, disinfecting preparation solutions, sponges, plastic tubing from the oxygen face mask, and even the body hair. These fires start very quickly and can turn into an intense blaze in only a few seconds. Even if the fire is quickly extinguished, the patient will usually sustain a significant burn.

Currently, the majority of OR fires occur with MAC during head and neck surgery. Invariably, this involves an oxygen-enriched atmosphere since 75% of surgical fires are oxygen enriched. Currently, the Anesthesia Patient Safety Foundation (APSF), and ECRI Institute recommend that there be no open delivery of oxygen during these cases.[85,123] If the patient needs increased levels of sedation during a time when the surgeon is using the ESU or laser, then the airway needs to be secured with an LMA or an endotracheal tube. Occasionally, there are cases during which the patient and the anesthesiologist need to communicate. An example of this might be an awake craniotomy or a carotid endarterectomy under regional anesthesia. In these cases it is prudent to use an FIO_2 of less than 30%. Preferably, the patient should receive only room air during these cases.

The most important principle that the anesthesiologist has to keep in mind to minimize the risk of fire is to titrate the inspired oxygen to the lowest concentration necessary to keep patient's oxygenation within safe levels. If the anesthesia machine has the ability to deliver air, then the nasal cannula or face mask can be attached to the anesthesia circuit by using a small no. 3 or no. 4, 15 mm endotracheal tube adapter.[124] This is attached to the right-angle elbow of the circuit. If the anesthesia machine is equipped with an auxiliary oxygen flowmeter that has a removable nipple adapter, then a humidifier can be installed in place of the nipple adapter. The humidifier has a Venturi mechanism through which room air is entrained and thus the oxygen concentration that is delivered to the face mask can be varied from 28% to 100%. Finally, if this machine has a common gas outlet that is easily accessible, a nasal cannula or face mask can be attached at this point using the same small 3 or 4 mm endotracheal tube adaptor (Fig. 8-40). If it is necessary to deliver >30% oxygen to the patient, then delivering 5 to 10 L/min of air under the drapes will dilute the oxygen. The oxygen should always be discontinued at least one minute before the surgeon uses the ESU. Also the bipolar ESU is preferable to the monopolar ESU. It is important that the drapes be arranged in such a manner that there is no oxygen buildup beneath them. Venting the drapes and having the surgeon use an adhesive sticky drape that seals the operative site from the oxygen flow are steps that will help reduce the risk of a fire.

It is potentially possible to discontinue the use of oxygen before the surgeon plans to use the electrocautery or laser. This would have to be done several minutes beforehand in order to allow any oxygen that has built up to dissipate. If the surgeon is planning to use the electrocautery or laser during the entire case, this may not be practical. Also the bipolar ESU is preferable to the monopolar ESU.

Some newer surgical preparation solutions can contribute to surgically related fires.[125,126] These solutions typically come prepackaged in a "paint stick" applicator with a sponge on the end

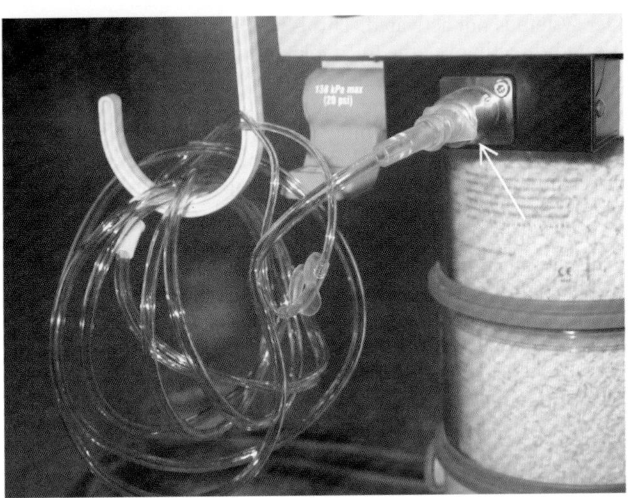

FIGURE 8-40. A nasal cannula connected to the alternate fresh gas outlet (*arrow*) on a GE-Datex-Ohmeda Aestiva anesthesia machine.

(e.g., DuraPrep™, St. Paul, MN). It consists of Iodophor mixed with 74% isopropyl alcohol. This is highly flammable and can easily be the fuel for an OR fire. In 2001, Barker and Polson[118] reported such a case. In a laboratory recreation, they found that if the DuraPrep™ had been allowed to dry completely (4 to 5 minutes), the fire did not occur (Fig. 8-41). The other problem with these types of preparation solutions is that small pools of the solution can accumulate if the person doing the preparation is not careful. The alcohol in these small puddles will continue to evaporate for a period of time, and the alcohol vapors are also extremely flammable. Flammable skin preparation solutions should be allowed to dry and puddles removed before the site is draped (Fig. 8-42).

It is important to bear in mind that halogenation of hydrocarbon anesthetics confers relative, but not absolute, resistance to combustion. Even the newer, "nonflammable" volatile anesthetics can, under certain circumstances, present fire hazards. For example, sevoflurane is nonflammable in air, but can serve as a fuel at concentrations as low as 11% in oxygen and 10% in nitrous
13 oxide.[127] In addition, sevoflurane and desiccated CO_2 absorbent (either soda lime or Baralyme™) can undergo exothermic chemical reactions that have been implicated in several fires that involved

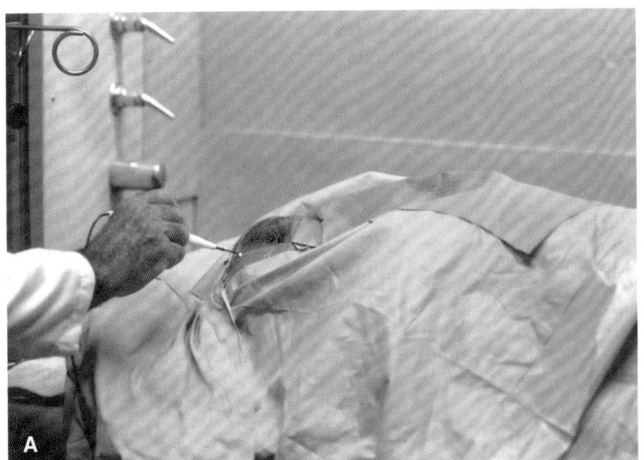

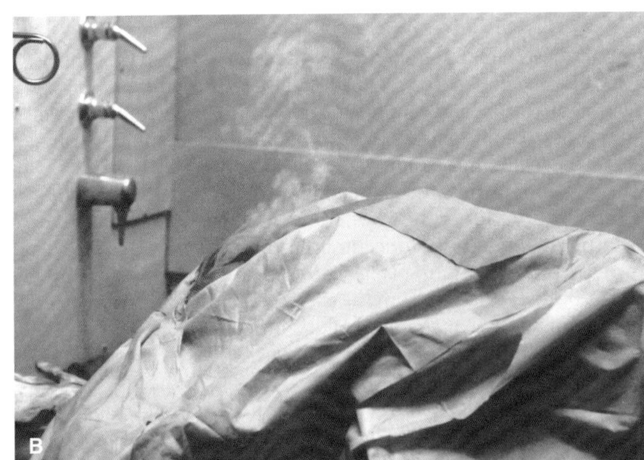

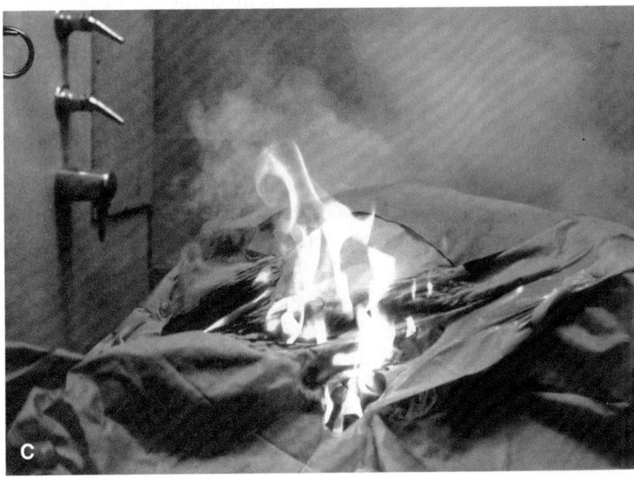

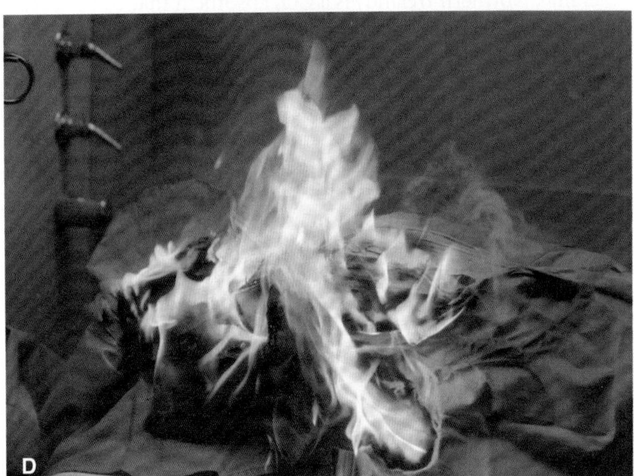

FIGURE 8-41. Simulation of fire caused by ESU electrode during surgery. **A:** Mannequin prepared and draped for surgery. Electrosurgical unit monopolar pencil electrode applied to operative site at start of surgery. **B:** Six seconds after electrosurgical unit application. Smoke appears from under the drapes. **C:** Fourteen seconds after electrosurgical unit application. Flames burst through the drapes. **D:** Twenty-four seconds after electrosurgical unit application. Entire patient head and drapes in flames. (Adapted from: Barker SJ, Polson JS. Fire in the operating room: A case report and laboratory study. *Anesth Analg.* 2001;93:960, with permission.)

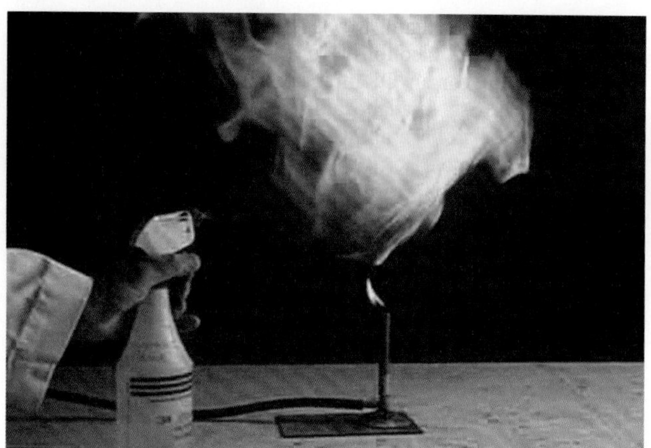

FIGURE 8-42. A demonstration of the intense heat and flame that is present in an alcohol fire. (Photograph courtesy of Marc Bruley of Emergency Care Research Institute. Reprinted with permission, Copyright 2009, ECRI Institute. www.ecri.org.)

the anesthesia breathing circuit.[128–131] In 2003, the manufacturer of sevoflurane published a "Dear Health Care Provider" letter and advisory alert.[132] To prevent future fires, the manufacturer of sevoflurane has recommended that anesthesiologists employ several measures, including avoiding the use of desiccated CO_2 absorbent and monitoring the temperature of the absorbers and the inspired concentration of sevoflurane; if elevated temperature or an inspired sevoflurane concentration that differed unexpectedly from the vaporizer setting is detected, it is recommended that the patient be disconnected from the anesthesia circuit and monitored for signs of thermal or chemical injury, and that the CO_2 absorbent be removed from the circuit and/or replaced.

Another way to prevent this type of fire is to use a CO_2 absorbent that does not contain a strong alkali, as do soda lime and Baralyme™ (Chemetron Medical Division, Allied Healthcare Products, St. Louis, Missouri). Amsorb™ (Amstrong Medical Limited, Coleraine, Northern Ireland) is a CO_2 absorbent that contains calcium hydroxide and calcium chloride, but no strong alkali.[133] In experimental studies, it was found that Amsorb is unreactive with currently used volatile anesthetics and does not produce carbon monoxide or Compound A with desiccated absorbent. Therefore, it would not interact with sevoflurane and undergo an exothermic chemical reaction.

If a fire does occur, it is important to extinguish it as soon as possible. The first step is to interrupt the fire triad by removing one component. This is usually best accomplished by removing the oxidizer from the fire. Therefore, if a tracheal tube is on fire, disconnecting the circuit from the tube or disconnecting the inspiratory limb of the circuit will usually result in the fire immediately going out. Simultaneously the surgeon should remove the burning endotracheal tube. Once the fire is extinguished, the airway is inspected via bronchoscopy, and the patient reintubated.

If the fire is on the patient, then extinguishing it with a basin of saline may be the most rapid and effective method to deal with this type of fire. There is also a method to use a sheet or towel to extinguish the fire. If the drapes are burning, particularly if they are paper drapes, then they must be removed and placed on the floor. Paper drapes are impervious to water; thus, throwing water or saline on them will do little to extinguish the fire. Once the burning drapes are removed from the patient, the fire can then be extinguished with a fire extinguisher. In most OR fires, the sprinkler system is not activated. This is because the sprinklers are not located directly over the OR table and because OR fires seldom get hot enough to activate the sprinklers.

All OR personnel should receive OR fire safety education,
14 which should include training in institutional fire safety protocols and learning the location and operation of the fire extinguishers. Fire safety education, including fire drills, allows each member of the OR team to learn and practice what his or her responsibilities and actions should be if a fire were to occur. Fire drills are an important part of the plan and can help personnel become familiar with the exits, evacuation routes, location of fire extinguishers, and how to shut off medical gas and electrical supplies. Although institutional fire safety protocols vary, the general principles of responding to an OR fire can be summarized by the mnemonic ERASE: *E*xtinguish, *r*escue, *a*ctivate, *s*hut, and *e*valuate. In sequence: First, the team should generally attempt to extinguish a fire on, in, or near the patient. Depending on the situation, this may include the use of saline or a CO_2 fire extinguisher (see later discussion). If the initial attempts at extinguishing the fire are unsuccessful, the patient and all other persons at risk should be *r*escued and the OR evacuated, if possible, and the fire *a*larm should be activated. Once the OR is emptied of personnel, the doors should be *s*hut and the medical gas supply to the room should be *s*hut off. The patient should then be *e*valuated and any injuries should be appropriately managed.

Fire extinguishers are divided into three classes, termed *A, B,* and *C,* based on the types of fires for which they are best suited. Class A extinguishers are used on paper, cloth, and plastic materials; Class B extinguishers are used for fires when liquids or grease are involved; Class C extinguishers are used for energized electrical equipment. A single fire extinguisher may be useful for any one, two, or all three types of fires. Probably the best fire extinguisher for the OR is the CO_2 extinguisher. This can be used on Class B and C fires and some Class A fires. Other extinguishers are water mist and new environmentally friendly fluorocarbons that replaced the Halon fire extinguisher. Finally, many ORs are equipped with a fire hose that supplies pressurized water at a rate of 50 gallons per minute. Such equipment is best left to the fire department to use, unless there is a need to rescue someone from a fire. In order to effectively use a fire extinguisher, the acronym "PASS" can be used. This stands for *p*ull the pin to activate the fire extinguisher, *a*im at the base of the fire, *s*queeze the trigger, and *s*weep the extinguisher back and forth across the base of the fire. When responding to a fire, the acronym RACE is useful. This stands for *r*escue; *a*larm; *c*onfine; *e*xtinguish. Clearly, having a plan that everyone is familiar with will greatly facilitate extinguishing the fire and minimizing the harm to the patient and equipment.

However, neither fire drills nor the presence and use of fire extinguishers should be relied on to provide a fire-safe operating environment. Only through heightened awareness, continuing education, and ongoing communication can the legs of the fire triad be kept apart and the risk of an OR fire minimized.

References

1. Harpell TR. Electrical shock hazards in the hospital environment: Their causes and cures. *Can Hosp.* 1970;47(11):48.
2. Buczko GB, McKay WP. Electrical safety in the operating room. *Can J Anaesth.* 1987;34(3 Pt 1):315.
3. Wald A. Electrical safety in medicine. In: Skalak R, Chien S, eds. *Handbook of Bioengineering.* New York, NY: McGraw-Hill; 1987:34.1.
4. Dalziel CF, Massoglia FP. Let-go currents and voltages. *AIEE Trans.* 1956;75:49.
5. Bruner JM, Aronow S, Cavicchi RV. Electrical incidents in a large hospital: A 42 month register. *J Assoc Adv Med Instrum.* 1972;6:222.
6. Bernstein MS. Isolated power and line isolation monitors. *Biomed Instrum Technol.* 1990;24:221.

7. Gibby GL. Shock and electrocution. In: Lobato EB, Gravenstein N, Kirby RR, eds. *Complications in Anesthesiology*. Philadelphia, PA: Wolters Kluwer/Lippincott Williams & Wilkins; 2008:780.
8. Weinberg DI, Artley JL, Whalen RE, et al. Electric shock hazards in cardiac catheterization. *Circ Res*. 1962;11:1004.
9. Starmer CF, Whalen RE. Current density and electrically induced ventricular fibrillation. *Med Instrum*. 1973;7:158.
10. Whalen RE, Starmer CF, McIntosh HD. Electrical hazards associated with cardiac pacemaking. *Ann N Y Acad Sci*. 1964;111:922.
11. Raftery EB, Green HL, Yacoub MH. Disturbances of heart rhythm produced by 50-Hz leakage currents in human subjects. *Cardiovasc Res*. 1975;9:263.
12. Hull CJ. Electrocution hazards in the operating theatre. *Br J Anaesth*. 1978;50:647.
13. Watson AB, Wright JS, Loughman J. Electrical thresholds for ventricular fibrillation in man. *Med J Aust*. 1973;1:1179.
14. Furman S, Schwedel JB, Robinson G, et al. Use of an intracardiac pacemaker in the control of heart block. *Surgery*. 1961;49:98.
15. Noordijk JA, Oey FJI, Tebra W. Myocardial electrodes and the danger of ventricular fibrillation. *Lancet*. 1961;1:975.
16. Pengelly LD, Klassen GA. Myocardial electrodes and the danger of ventricular fibrillation. *Lancet*. 1961;1:1234.
17. Rowe GG, Zarnstorff WC. Ventricular fibrillation during selective angiocardiography. *JAMA*. 1965;192:947.
18. Hopps JA, Roy OS. Electrical hazards in cardiac diagnosis and treatment. *Med Electr Biol Eng*. 1963;1:133.
19. Baas LS, Beery TA, Hickey CS. Care and safety of pacemaker electrodes in intensive care and telemetry nursing units. *Am J Crit Care*. 1997;6:302.
20. Leeming MN. Protection of the electrically susceptible patient: A discussion of systems and methods. *Anesthesiology*. 1973;38:370.
21. McNulty SE, Cooper M, Staudt S. Transmitted radiofrequency current through a flow directed pulmonary artery catheter. *Anesth Analg*. 1994;78:587.
22. Cromwell L, Weibell FJ, Pfeiffer EA. *Biomedical Instrumentation and Measurements*. 2nd ed. Englewood Cliffs, NJ: Prentice-Hall; 1980:430.
23. Edwards NK. Specialized electrical grounding needs. *Clin Perinatol*. 1976;3:367.
24. Goldwyn RM. Bovie: The man and the machine. *Ann Plast Surg*. 1979;2:135.
25. Lichter I, Borrie J, Miller WM. Radio-frequency hazards with cardiac pacemakers. *Br Med J*. 1965;1:1513.
26. Dornette WHL. An electrically safe surgical environment. *Arch Surg*. 1973;107:567.
27. Klop WM, Lohuis PJ, Strating RP, et al. Ventricular fibrillation caused by electrocoagulation during laparoscopic surgery. *Surg Endosc*. 2002;16:362.
28. Fu Q, Cao P, Mi WD, et al. Ventricular fibrillation caused by electrocoagulation during thoracic surgery. *Acta Anaesthesiol Scand*. 2010;54:256.
29. Yan CY, Cai XJ, Wang YF, et al. Ventricular fibrillation caused by electrocoagulation in monopolar mode during laparoscopic subphrenic mass resection. *Surg Endosc*. 2011;25:309–311.
30. Dalibon N, Pelle-Lancien E, Puyo P, et al. Recurrent asystole during electrocauterization: An uncommon hazard in common situations. *Eur J Anaesthesiol*. 2005;22:476–478.
31. Cushing H. Electro-surgery as an aid to the removal of intracranial tumors: With a preliminary note on a new surgical-current generator by W.T. Bovie. *Surg Gynecol Obstet*. 1928;47:751.
32. Meathe EA. Electrical safety for patients and anesthetists. In: Saidman LJ, Smith NT, eds. *Monitoring in Anesthesia*. 2nd ed. Boston, MA: Butterworth; 1984:497.
33. Rolly G. Two cases of burns caused by misuse of coagulation unit and monitoring. *Acta Anaesthesiol Belg*. 1978;29:313.
34. Parker EO 3rd. Electrosurgical burn at the site of an esophageal temperature probe. *Anesthesiology*. 1984;61:93.
35. Schneider AJL, Apple HP, Braun RT. Electrosurgical burns at skin temperature probes. *Anesthesiology*. 1977;47:72.
36. Bloch EC, Burton LW. Electrosurgical burn while using a battery-operated Doppler monitor. *Anesth Analg*. 1979;58:339.
37. Becker CM, Malhotra IV, Hedley-Whyte J. The distribution of radiofrequency current and burns. *Anesthesiology*. 1973;38:106.
38. Jones CM, Pierre KB, Nicoud IB, et al. Electrosurgery. *Current Surgery*. 2006;63:458–463.
39. Mitchell JP. The isolated circuit diathermy. *Ann R Coll Surg Engl*. 1979;61:287.
40. Titel JH, el Etr AA. Fibrillation resulting from pacemaker electrodes and electrocautery during surgery. *Anesthesiology*. 1968;29:845.
41. Domino KB, Smith TC. Electrocautery-induced reprogramming of a pacemaker using a precordial magnet. *Anesth Analg*. 1983;62:609.
42. Damaged reusable ESU return electrode cables. *Health Devices*. 1985;14:214.
43. Sparking from and ignition of damaged electrosurgical electrode cables. *Health Devices*. 1998;27:301.
44. Mirowski M, Reid PR, Mower MM, et al. Termination of malignant ventricular arrhythmias with an implanted automatic defibrillator in human beings. *N Engl J Med*. 1980;303:322.
45. Crozier IG, Ward DE. Automatic implantable defibrillators. *Br J Hosp Med*. 1988;40:136.
46. Elefteriades JA, Biblo LA, Batsford WP, et al. Evolving patterns in the surgical treatment of malignant ventricular tachyarrhythmias. *Ann Thorac Surg*. 1990; 49:94.
47. Carr CM, Whiteley SM. The automatic implantable cardioverter-defibrillator. *Anaesthesia*. 1991;46:737.
48. Starmer CF, McIntosh HD, Whalen RE. Electrical hazards and cardiovascular function. *N Engl J Med*. 1971;284:181.
49. Albisser AM, Parson ID, Pask BA. A survey of the grounding systems in several large hospitals. *Med Instrum*. 1973;7:297.
50. McLaughlin AJ, Campkin NT. Electrical safety: A reminder (letter). *Anaesthesia*. 1998;53:608.
51. Nixon MC, Ghurye M. Electrical failure in theatre—A consequence of complacency? *Anaesthesia*. 1997;52:88.
52. Medical Devices; Establishment of a Performance Standard for Electrode Lead Wires and Patient Cables, Federal Register 1997;62:25477.
53. Emergency Care Research Institute. FDA establishes performance standards for electrode lead wires. *Health Devices*. 1998;27:34.
54. National Fire Protection Association. *NFPA 99, Health Care Facilities Code, 2012 Edition, Article 6.4.4.1.1.2 Maintenance and Testing of Alternate Power Source and Transfer Switches*. Quincy, MA.
55. National Fire Protection Association. NFPA 110, Standard for Emergency and Standby Power Systems, Chapter 8, Quincy MA.
56. Carpenter T, Robinson ST. Response to a partial power failure in the operating room. *Anesth Analg*. 2010;110:1644–1646.
57. Eichhorn JH, Hessel EA. Electrical power failure in the operating room: A neglected topic in anesthesia safety. *Anesth Analg*. 2010;110:1519–1521.
58. Jones RP, Conway DH. The effect of electromagnetic interference from mobile communication on the performance of intensive care ventilators. *Eur J Anaesthesiol*. 2005;22:578.
59. Lawrentschuk N, Bolton DM. Mobile phone interference with medical equipment and its clinical relevance: A systematic review. *Med J Aust*. 2004;181:145.
60. Hayes DL, Wang PJ, Reynolds DW, et al. Interference with cardiac pacemakers by cellular telephones. *N Engl J Med*. 1997;336:1473.
61. Schlegel RE, Grant FH, Raman S, et al. Electromagnetic compatibility study of the *in vitro* interaction of wireless phones with cardiac pacemakers. *Biomed Instrum Technol*. 1998;32:645.
62. Chen WH, Lau CP, Leung SK, et al. Interference of cellular phones with implanted permanent pacemakers. *Clin Cardiol*. 1996;19:881.
63. Fetter JG, Ivans V, Benditt DG, et al. Digital cellular telephone interaction with implantable cardioverter-defibrillators. *J Am Coll Cardiol*. 1998;21:623.
64. Emergency Care Research Institute. Cell phones and walkie-talkies: Is it time to relax your restrictive policies? *Health Devices*. 1999;28:409.
65. Adler D, Margulies L, Mahler Y, et al. Measurements of electromagnetic fields radiated from communication equipment and of environmental electromagnetic noise: Impact on the use of communication equipment within the hospital. *Biomed Instrum Technol*. 1998;32:581.
66. Schwartz JJ, Ehrenwerth J. Electrical safety. In: Lake CL, Hines RH, Blitt C, eds. *Clinical Monitoring: Practical Applications for Anesthesia and Critical Care*. Philadelphia, PA: WB Saunders; 2000.
67. Kermit E, Staewen WS. Isolated power systems: Historical perspective and update on regulations. *Biomed Tech Today*. 1986;1:86.
68. National Fire Protection Association. National electric code (ANSI/NFPA 70-1984). Quincy, MA: National Fire Protection Association; 1984.
69. National Fire Protection Association. NFPA-99, Health Care Facilities Code. 2012 edition. Quincy, MA.
70. Bruner JMR, Leonard PF. *Electricity, Safety and the Patient*. Chicago, IL: Year Book Medical Publishers; 1989:300.
71. Matjasko MJ, Ashman MN. All you need to know about electrical safety in the operating room. In: Barash PG, Deutsch S, Tinker J, eds. *ASA Refresher Courses in Anesthesiology, vol 18*. Philadelphia, PA: JB Lippincott; 1990:251.
72. Lennon RL, Leonard PF. A hitherto unreported virtue of the isolated power system (letter). *Anesth Analg*. 1987;66:1056.
73. Barker SJ, Doyle DJ. Electrical safety in the operating room: dry versus wet. *Anesth Analg*. 2010;110:1517–1518.
74. Gilbert TB, Shaffer M, Matthews M. Electrical shock by dislodged spark gap in bipolar electrosurgical device. *Anesth Analg*. 1991;73:355.
75. Van Kerckhove K. Re-evaluating the isolated power equation. *Electrical Products and Solutions*. March 2008:25–27.
76. Day FJ. Electrical safety revisited: A new wrinkle. *Anesthesiology*. 1994;80:220.
77. Wills JH, Ehrenwerth J, Rogers D. Electrical injury to a nurse due to conductive fluid in an operating room designated as a dry location. *Anesth Analg*. 2010; 110:1647–1649.
78. August DA. Locked out of a box and a process. *Anesth Analg*. 2011;112:1248–1249.
79. Barker SJ. In response to August DA. *Anesth Analg*. 2011;112:1249.
80. Litt L, Ehrenwerth J. Electrical safety in the operating room: Important old wine, disguised in new bottles. *Anesth Analg*. 1994;78:417.
81. Seifert HA. Fire safety in the operating room. In: Eisenkraft JB, ed. *Progress in Anesthesiology*. Philadelphia, PA: WB Saunders; 1994.
82. Neufeld GR. Fires and explosions. In: Orkin K, Cooperman LH, eds. *Complications in Anesthesiology*. Philadelphia, PA: Lippincott; 1983:671.
83. Moxon MA. Fire in the operating room. *Anaesthesia*. 1986;41:543.
84. Vickers MD. Fire and explosion hazards in operating theatres. *Br J Anaesth*. 1978; 50:659.
85. ECRI Institute. New clinical guide to surgical fire prevention. *Health Devices*. 2009;38(10):314–332.

86. Caplan RA, Barker SJ, Connis RT, et al. Practice advisory for the prevention and management of operating room fires. *Anesthesiology.* 2008;108:786–801.
87. de Richemond AL. The patient is on fire! *Health Devices.* 1992;21:19.
88. Cameron BG, Ingram GS. Flammability of drape materials in nitrous oxide and oxygen. *Anesthesiology.* 1971;26:218.
89. Johnson RM, Smith CV, Leggett K. Flammability of disposable surgical drapes. *Arch Ophthalmol.* 1976;94:1327.
90. Simpson JI, Wolf GL. Flammability of esophageal stethoscopes, nasogastric tubes, feeding tubes, and nasopharyngeal airways in oxygen- and nitrous oxide-enriched atmospheres. *Anesth Analg.* 1988;67:1093.
91. Ponath RE. Preventing surgical fires. *JAMA.* 1984;252:1762.
92. Katz J, Campbell L. Fire during thoracotomy: A need to control the inspired oxygen concentration. *Anesth Analg.* 2005;101:612.
93. Wolf G, Sidebotham GW, Lazard JL. Laser ignition of surgical drape materials in air 50% oxygen, and 95% oxygen. *Anesthesiology.* 2004;100:1167–1171.
94. Food and Drug Administration. Surgical Fires Reported January 1995—June 1998. FDA Databases MDR/MAUDE, 1999.
95. Rampil IJ. Anesthetic considerations for laser surgery. *Anesth Analg.* 1992;74:424.
96. Pashayan AG, Ehrenwerth J. Lasers and electrical safety in the operating room. In: Ehrenwerth J, Eisenkraft JB, eds. *Anesthesia Equipment: Principles and Applications.* St. Louis, MO: Mosby; 1993.
97. Emergency Care Research Institute. Lasers in medicine—An introduction. *Health Devices.* 1984;13:151.
98. Casey KR, Fairfax WR, Smith SJ, et al. Intratracheal fire ignited by the Nd:YAG laser during treatment of tracheal stenosis. *Chest.* 1983;84:295.
99. Burgess GE, LeJeune FE. Endotracheal tube ignition during laser surgery of the larynx. *Arch Otolaryngol.* 1979;105:561.
100. Cozine K, Rosenbaum LM, Askanazi J, et al. Laser induced endotracheal tube fire. *Anesthesiology.* 1981;55:583.
101. Geffin B, Shapshay SM, Bellack GS, et al. Flammability of endotracheal tubes during Nd:YAG laser application in the airway. *Anesthesiology.* 1986;65:511.
102. Hirshman CA, Smith J. Indirect ignition of the endotracheal tube during carbon dioxide laser surgery. *Arch Otolaryngol.* 1980;106:639.
103. Krawtz S, Mehta AC, Weidemann HP, et al. Nd:YAG laser-induced endobronchial burn. *Chest.* 1989;95:916.
104. Goldblum KB. Oxygen index: Key to precise flammability ratings. *Soc Plast Eng J.* 1969;25:50–52.
105. Wolf GL, Simpson JI. Flammability of endotracheal tubes in oxygen and nitrous oxide enriched atmosphere. *Anesthesiology.* 1987;67:236.
106. de Richemond AL. Laser resistant endotracheal tubes—Protection against oxygen-enriched airway fires during surgery? In: Stoltzfus JM, McIlroy K, eds. *Flammability and Sensitivity of Material in Oxygen-Enriched Atmospheres, vol 5 (ASTM STP 1111).* Philadelphia, PA: American Society for Testing and Materials; 1991:157.
107. Emergency Care Research Institute. Airway fires: Reducing the risk during laser surgery. *Health Devices.* 1990;19:109.
108. Emergency Care Research Institute. Laser-resistant tracheal tubes (evaluation). *Health Devices.* 1992;21:4.
109. Aly A, McIlwain M, Ward M. Electrosurgery-induced endotracheal tube ignition during tracheotomy. *Ann Otol Rhinol Laryngol.* 1991;100:31.
110. Simpson JI, Wolf GL. Endotracheal tube fire ignited by pharyngeal electrocautery. *Anesthesiology.* 1986;65:76.
111. Gupte SR. Gauze fire in the oral cavity: A case report. *Anesth Analg.* 1972;51:645.
112. Snow JC, Norton ML, Saluja TS, et al. Fire hazard during CO_2 laser microsurgery on the larynx and trachea. *Anesth Analg.* 1975;55:146.
113. Lew EO, Mittleman RE, Murray D. Tube ignition by electrocautery during tracheostomy: Case report with autopsy findings. *J Forensic Sci.* 1991;36:1586.
114. Marsh B, Riley DH. Double-lumen tube fire during tracheostomy. *Anesthesiology.* 1992;76:480.
115. Neuman GG, Sidebotham G, Negoianu E, et al. Laparoscopy explosion hazards with nitrous oxide. *Anesthesiology.* 1993;78:875.
116. Di Pierro GB, Besmer I, Hefermehl LJ, et al. Intra-abdominal fire due to insufflating oxygen instead of carbon dioxide during robot-assisted radical prostatectomy: case report and literature review. *Eur Urol.* 2010;58:626–628.
117. Greilich PE, Greilich NB, Froelich EG. Intraabdominal fire during laparoscopic cholecystectomy. *Anesthesiology.* 1995;83:871.
118. Barker SJ, Polson JS. Fire in the operating room: A case report and laboratory study. *Anesth Analg.* 2001;93:960.
119. Bruley ME, Lavanchy C. *Oxygen-enriched fires during surgery of the head and neck, Symposium on Flammability and Sensitivity of Material in Oxygen-Enriched Atmospheres (ASTM STP 1040).* Philadelphia, PA: American Society for Testing and Materials; 1989:392.
120. de Richemond AL, Bruley ME. Head and neck surgical fires. In: Eisele DW, ed. *Complications in Head and Neck Surgery.* St. Louis, MO: Mosby; 1993.
121. Emergency Care Research Institute. Fires during surgery of the head and neck area (hazard). *Health Devices.* 1979;9:50.
122. Ramanathan S, Capan L, Chalon J, et al. Mini-environmental control under the drapes during operations on eyes of conscious patients. *Anesthesiology.* 1978;48:286.
123. Anesthesia Patient safety Foundation. Prevention and management of operating room fires (Video). *Apsf org.* 2010.
124. Lampotang S, Gravenstein N, Paulus DA, et al. Reducing the incidence of surgical fires: Supplying nasal cannulae with sub-100% O_2 gas mixtures from anesthesia machines. *Anesth Analg.* 2005;101:1407–1412.
125. Patel R, Chavda KD, Hukkeri S. Surgical field fire and skin burns caused by alcohol-based skin preparation. *J Emerg Trauma Shock.* 2010;3(3):305.
126. Prasad R, Quezado Z, St. Andre A, et al. Fires in the operating room and intensive care unit: Awareness is the key to prevention. *Anesth Analg.* 2006;102:172–174.
127. Wallin RF, Regan BM, Napoli MD, et al. Sevoflurane: A new inhalational anesthetic agent. *Anesth Analg.* 1975;54:758.
128. Fatheree RS, Leighton BL. Acute respiratory syndrome after an exothermic baralymeR-sevoflurane reaction. *Anesthesiology.* 2004;101:531.
129. Castro BA, Freedman LA, Craig WL, et al. Explosion within an anesthesia machine: BaralymeR, high fresh gas flows and sevoflurane concentration. *Anesthesiology.* 2004;101:537.
130. Wu J, Previte JP, Adler E, et al. Spontaneous ignition, explosion and fire with sevoflurane and barium hydroxide lime. *Anesthesiology.* 2004;101:534.
131. Abbott A. Dear healthcare provider (letter). November 17, 2003. [http://www.fda.gov/downloads/Safety/MedWatch/SafetyInformation/SafetyAlertsforHumanMedicalProducts/UCM169499.pdf].
132. Murray JM, Renfrew CW, Bedi A, et al. Amsorb: A new carbon dioxide absorbent for use in anesthetic breathing systems. *Anesthesiology.* 1999;91:1342.
133. Laster M, Roth P, Eger EI. Fires from the interaction of anesthetics with desiccated absorbent. *Anesth Analg.* 2004;99:769.

CHAPTER

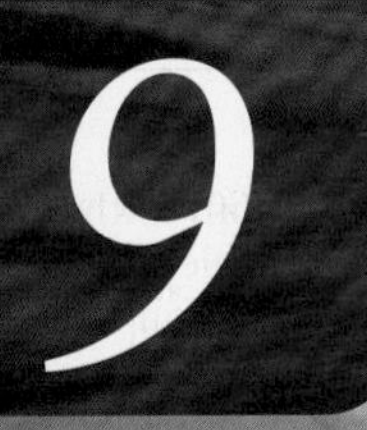

Experimental Design and Statistics

NATHAN LEON PACE

Key Points

1. Statistics and mathematics are the language of scientific medicine.
2. Good research planning includes a clear biologic hypothesis, the specification of outcome variables, the choice of anticipated statistical methods, and sample size planning.
3. To minimize the risk of bias in clinical research of interventions, the crucial elements of good research design include concurrent control groups; random allocation of subjects to treatment groups; concealment of random allocation; blinding of treatment assignment to patients, caregivers, and outcome assessors; and full reporting of outcomes for all study patients.
4. Visual presentation of data by graphs, descriptive statistics (e.g., mean, standard deviation), and inferential statistics (e.g., *t* test, confidence interval) are all essential methods for the presentation of research results.
5. Bayesian statistical methods report research results as a function of both observed data and historical (prior) knowledge; the more common Frequentist statistical methods report research results only as a function of observed data.
6. Multivariable logistic regression and propensity score matching are statistical techniques for identifying associations between risk factors and outcomes in nonrandomized studies.
7. Systematic review and meta-analysis summarize the results of individual studies and permit more powerful inferences for the comparison of interventions.
8. Resources and guidance for experimental design and statistical methods include policy statements, textbooks, journal articles, and public domain software.

Multimedia

 Graphing Data

INTRODUCTION

Medical journal reports are replete with numbers including weights, lengths, pressures, volumes, flows, concentrations, counts, temperatures, rates, currents, energies, forces, and so forth. The analysis and interpretation of these numbers require the use of
1 statistical techniques. The design of the experiment to acquire these numbers is also part of statistical competence. The methods of probability and statistics have been formulated to solve concrete problems, such as betting on cards, understanding biologic inheritance, and improving food processing. Studies in anesthesia have even inspired new statistics. The development of statistical techniques is manifest in the increasing use of more sophisticated research designs and statistical tests in anesthesia research.

If a physician is to be a practitioner of scientific medicine, he or she must read the language of science to be able to independently assess and interpret the scientific report. Without exception, the language of the medical report is increasingly statistical. Readers of the anesthesia literature, whether in a community hospital or a university environment, cannot and should not totally depend on the editors of journals to banish all errors of statistical analysis and interpretation. In addition, there are regularly questions about simple statistics in examinations required for anesthesiologists. Finally, certain statistical methods have everyday applications in clinical medicine. This chapter briefly scans some elements of experimental design and statistical analysis.

DESIGN OF RESEARCH STUDIES

The scientific investigator should view himself or herself as an
2 experimenter and not merely as a naturalist. The naturalist goes out into the field ready to capture and report the numbers that flit into view; this is a worthy activity, typified by the *case report.* Case reports engender interest, suspicion, doubt, wonder, and perhaps the desire to experiment; however, the case report is not sufficient evidence to advance scientific medicine. The experimenter attempts to constrain and control, as much as possible, the environment in which he or she collects numbers to test a hypothesis. The elements of experimental design are intended to prevent and minimize the possibility of bias, that is, a deviation of results or inferences from the truth.

Sampling

Two words of great importance to statisticians are *population* and *sample.* In statistical language, each has a specialized meaning. Instead of referring only to the count of individuals in a geographic or political region, population refers to any target group of things (animate or inanimate) in which there is interest. For anesthesia researchers, a typical target population might be mothers in the first stage of labor or head-trauma victims undergoing craniotomy. A target population could also be cell cultures, isolated organ preparations, or hospital bills. A sample is a subset of the target population. Samples are taken because of the impossibility of observing the entire population; it is generally not affordable, convenient, or practical to examine more than a relatively small fraction of the population. Nevertheless, the researcher wishes to generalize from the results of the small sample group to the entire population.

Although the subjects of a population are alike in at least one way, these population members are generally quite diverse in other ways. Because the researcher can work only with a subset of the population, he or she hopes that the sample of subjects in the experiment is representative of the population's diversity. Head-injury patients can have open or closed wounds, a variety of coexisting diseases, and normal or increased intracranial pressure. These subgroups within a population are called *strata.* Often the researcher wishes to increase the sameness or homogeneity of the target population by further restricting it to just a few strata; perhaps only closed and not open head injuries will be included. Restricting the target population to eliminate too much diversity must be balanced against the desire to have the results be applicable to the broadest possible population of patients.

The best hope for a representative sample of the population would be realized if every subject in the population had the same chance of being in the experiment; this is called *random sampling.* If there were several strata of importance, random sampling from each stratum would be appropriate. Unfortunately, in most clinical anesthesia studies researchers are limited to using those patients who happen to show up at their hospitals; this is called *convenience sampling.* Convenience sampling is also subject to the nuances of the surgical schedule, the goodwill of the referring physician and attending surgeon, and the willingness of the patient to cooperate. At best, the convenience sample is representative of patients at that institution, with no assurance that these patients are similar to those elsewhere. Convenience sampling is also the rule in studying new anesthetic drugs; such studies are typically performed on healthy, young volunteers.

Experimental Constraints

The researcher must define the conditions to which the sample members will be exposed. Particularly in clinical research, one must decide whether these conditions should be rigidly standardized or whether the experimental circumstances should be adjusted or individualized to the patient. In anesthetic drug research, should a fixed dose be given to all members of the sample or should the dose be adjusted to produce an effect or to achieve a specific end point? Standardizing the treatment groups by fixed doses simplifies the research work. There are risks to this standardization, however (1) a fixed dose may produce excessive numbers of side effects in some patients; (2) a fixed dose may be therapeutically insufficient in others; and (3) a treatment standardized for an experimental protocol may be so artificial that it has no broad clinical relevance, even if demonstrated to be superior. The researcher should carefully choose and report the adjustment/individualization of experimental treatments.

Control Groups

Even if a researcher is studying just one experimental group, the results of the experiment are usually not interpreted solely in terms of that one group but are also contrasted and compared
3 with other experimental groups. Examining the effects of a new drug on blood pressure during anesthetic induction is important, but what is more important is comparing those results with the effects of one or more standard drugs commonly used in the same situation. Where can the researcher obtain these comparative data? There are several possibilities: (1) each patient could receive the standard drug under identical experimental circumstances at another time, (2) another group of patients receiving the standard drug could be studied simultaneously, (3) a group of patients could have been studied previously with the standard drug under similar circumstances, and (4) literature reports of

the effects of the drug under related but not necessarily identical circumstances could be used. Under the first two possibilities, the control group is contemporaneous—either a *self-control* (crossover) or *parallel control* group. The second two possibilities are examples of the use of *historical controls.*

Since historical controls already exist, they are convenient and seemingly cheap to use. Unfortunately, the history of medicine is littered with the "debris" of therapies enthusiastically accepted on the basis of comparison with past experience. A classic example is operative ligation of the internal mammary artery for the treatment of angina pectoris—a procedure now known to be of no value. Proposed as a method to improve coronary artery blood flow, the lack of benefit was demonstrated in a trial where some patients had the procedure and some had a sham procedure; both groups showed benefit.[1] There is now firm empirical evidence that studies using historical controls usually show a favorable outcome for a new therapy, whereas studies with concurrent controls, that is, parallel control group or self-control, less often reveal a benefit.[2] Nothing seems to increase the enthusiasm for a new treatment as much as the omission of a concurrent control group. If the outcome with an old treatment is not studied simultaneously with the outcome of a new treatment, one cannot know if any differences in results are a consequence of the two treatments, or of unsuspected and unknowable differences between the patients, or of other changes over time in the general medical environment. One possible exception would be in studying a disease that is uniformly fatal (100% mortality) over a very short time.

Random Allocation of Treatment Groups

Having accepted the necessity of an experiment with a control group, the question arises as to the method by which each subject should be assigned to the predetermined experimental groups. Should it depend on the whim of the investigator, the day of the week, the preference of a referring physician, the wish of the patient, the assignment of the previous subject, the availability of a study drug, a hospital chart number, or some other arbitrary criterion? All such methods have been used and are still used, but all can ruin the purity and usefulness of the experiment. It is important to remember the purpose of sampling: By exposing a small number of subjects from the target population to the various experimental conditions, one hopes to make conclusions about the entire population. Thus, the experimental groups should be as similar as possible to each other in reflecting the target population; if the groups are different, selection bias is introduced into the experiment. Although randomly allocating subjects of a sample to one or another of the experimental groups requires additional work, this principle prevents selection bias by the researcher, minimizes (but cannot always prevent) the possibility that important differences exist among the experimental groups, and disarms the critics' complaints about research methods. Random allocation is most commonly accomplished by the use of computer-generated random numbers. Even with a random allocation process, selection bias can occur if research personnel are allowed knowledge of the group assignment of the next patient to be recruited for a study. Failure to conceal random allocation leads to biases in the results of clinical studies.[3,4]

Blinding

Blinding refers to the masking from the view of patient and experimenters the experimental group to which the subject has been or will be assigned. In clinical trials, the necessity for blinding starts even before a patient is enrolled in the research study; this is called the *concealment of random allocation.* There is good evidence that, if the process of random allocation is accessible to view, the referring physicians, the research team members, or both are tempted to manipulate the entrance of specific patients into the study to influence their assignment to a specific treatment group[5]; they do so having formed a personal opinion about the relative merits of the treatment groups and desiring to get the "best" for someone they favor. This creates bias in the experimental groups.

Each subject should remain, if possible, ignorant of the assigned treatment group after entrance into the research protocol. The patient's expectation of improvement, a placebo effect, is a real and useful part of clinical care. But when studying a new treatment, one must ensure that the fame or infamy of the treatments does not induce a bias in outcome by changing patient expectations. A researcher's knowledge of the treatment assignment can bias his or her ability to administer the research protocol and to observe and record data faithfully; this is true for clinical, animal, and in vitro research. If the treatment group is known, those who observe data cannot trust themselves to record the data impartially and dispassionately. The appellations *single-blind* and *double-blind* to describe blinding are commonly used in research reports, but often applied inconsistently; the researcher should carefully plan and report exactly who is blinded.

Types of Research Design

Ultimately, research design consists of choosing what subjects to study, what experimental conditions and constraints to enforce, and which observations to collect at what intervals. A few key features in this research design largely determine the strength of scientific inference on the collected data. These key features allow the classification of research reports (Table 9-1). This classification reveals the variety of experimental approaches and indicates strengths and weaknesses of the same design applied to many research problems.

The first distinction is between *longitudinal* and *cross-sectional* studies. The former is the study of changes over time, whereas the latter describes a phenomenon at a certain point in time. For example, reporting the frequency with which certain drugs are used during anesthesia is a cross-sectional study, whereas investigating the hemodynamic effects of different drugs during anesthesia is a longitudinal one.

Longitudinal studies are next classified by the method with which the research subjects are selected. These methods for choosing research subjects can be either *prospective* or *retrospective;* these two approaches are also known as *cohort* (prospective) or

TABLE 9-1. CLASSIFICATION OF CLINICAL RESEARCH REPORTS

I. Longitudinal studies
   A. Prospective (cohort) studies
      1. Studies of deliberate intervention
         a. Concurrent controls
         b. Historical controls
      2. Observational studies
   B. Retrospective (case-control) studies
II. Cross-sectional studies

case-control (retrospective). A prospective study assembles groups of subjects by some input characteristic that is thought to change an output characteristic; a typical input characteristic would be the opioid drug administered during anesthesia; for example, remifentanil or fentanyl. A retrospective study gathers subjects by an output characteristic; an output characteristic is the status of the subject after an event; for example, the occurrence of a myocardial infarction. A prospective (cohort) study would be one in which a group of patients undergoing neurologic surgery was divided in two groups, given two different opioids (remifentanil or fentanyl), and followed for the development of a perioperative myocardial infarction. In a retrospective (case-control) study, patients who suffered a perioperative myocardial infarction would be identified from hospital records; a group of subjects of similar age, gender, and disease who did not suffer a perioperative myocardial infarction would also be chosen, and the two groups would then be compared for the relative use of the two opioids (remifentanil or fentanyl). Retrospective studies are a primary tool of epidemiology. A case-control study can often identify an association between an input and an output characteristic, but the causal link or relationship between the two is more difficult to specify.

Prospective studies are further divided into those in which the investigator performs a deliberate intervention and those in which the investigator merely observes. In a study of *deliberate intervention,* the investigator would choose several anesthetic maintenance techniques and compare the incidence of postoperative nausea and vomiting. If it were performed as an *observational study,* the investigator would observe a group of patients receiving anesthetics chosen at the discretion of each patient's anesthesiologist and compare the incidence of postoperative nausea and vomiting (PONV) among the anesthetics used. Obviously, in this example of an observational study, there has been an intervention; an anesthetic has been given. The crucial distinction is whether the investigator controlled the intervention. An observational study may reveal differences among treatment groups, but whether such differences are the consequence of the treatments or of other differences among the patients receiving the treatments will remain obscure.

Studies of deliberate intervention are further subdivided into those with concurrent controls and those with historical controls. Concurrent controls are either a simultaneous parallel control group or a self-control study; historical controls include previous studies and literature reports. A *randomized controlled trial* (RCT) is thus a longitudinal, prospective study of deliberate intervention with concurrent controls.

Although most of this discussion about experimental design has focused on human experimentation, the same principles apply and should be followed in animal experimentation. The randomized, controlled clinical trial is the most potent scientific tool for evaluating medical treatment; randomization into treatment groups is relied on to equally weight the subjects of the treatment groups for baseline attributes that might predispose or protect the subjects from the outcome of interest.

DATA AND DESCRIPTIVE STATISTICS

Statistics is a method for working with *sets* of numbers, a set being a group of objects. Statistics involves the description of number sets, comparison of number sets with theoretical models, comparison between number sets, and comparison of recently acquired number sets with those from the past. A typical scientific hypothesis asks which of two methods (treatments), X and Y, is better. A statistical hypothesis is formulated concerning the sets of numbers collected under the conditions of treatments X and Y. Statistics provides methods for deciding if the set of values associated with X are different from the values associated with Y. Statistical methods are necessary because there are sources of variation in any data set, including random biologic variation and measurement error. These errors in the data cause difficulties in avoiding bias and in being precise. Bias keeps the true value from being known and fosters incorrect decisions; precision deals with the problem of the data scatter and with quantifying the uncertainty about the value in the population from which a sample is drawn. These statistical methods are relatively independent of the particular field of study. Regardless of whether the numbers in sets X and Y are systolic pressures, body weights, or serum chlorides, the approach for comparing sets X and Y is usually the same.

Data Structure

Data collected in an experiment include the defining characteristics of the experiment and the values of events or attributes that vary over time or conditions. The former are called *explanatory variables* and the latter are called *response variables.* The researcher records his or her observations on data sheets or case record forms, which may be one to many pages in length, and assembles them together for statistical analysis. Variables such as gender, age, and doses of accompanying drugs reflect the variability of the experimental subjects. Explanatory variables, it is hoped, explain the systematic variations in the response variables. In a sense, the response variables depend on the explanatory variables.

Response variables are also called *dependent variables.* Response variables reflect the primary properties of experimental interest in the subjects. Research in anesthesiology is particularly likely to have repeated measurement variables; that is, a particular measurement recorded more than once for each individual. Some variables can be both explanatory and response; these are called *intermediate response variables.* Suppose an experiment is conducted comparing electrocardiography and myocardial responses between five doses of an opioid. One might analyze how ST segments depended on the dose of opioids; here, maximum ST segment depression is a response variable. Maximum ST segment depression might also be used as an explanatory variable to address the subtler question of the extent to which the effect of an opioid dose on postoperative myocardial infarction can be accounted for by ST segment changes.

The mathematical characteristics of the possible values of a variable fit into five classifications (Table 9-2). Properly assigning a variable to the correct data type is essential for choosing the correct statistical technique. For *interval variables,* there is equal distance between successive intervals; the difference between 15 and 10 is the same as the difference between 25 and 20. *Discrete interval data* can have only integer values; for example, number of living children. *Continuous interval data* are measured on a continuum and can be a decimal fraction; for example, blood pressure can be described as accurately as desired (e.g., 136, 136.1, or 136.14 mm Hg). The same statistical techniques are used for discrete and continuous data.

Putting observations into two or more discrete categories derives *categorical variables;* for statistical analysis, numeric values are assigned as labels to the categories. *Dichotomous data* allow only two possible values; for example, male versus female. *Ordinal data* have three or more categories that can logically be ranked or ordered; however, the ranking or ordering of the variable indicates only relative and not absolute differences between values; there is not necessarily the same difference between American Society of Anesthesiologists Physical Status score I and II as there

TABLE 9-2. DATA TYPES

Data Type	Definition	Examples
Interval		
Discrete	Data measured with an integer-only scale	Parity Number of teeth
Continuous	Data measured with a constant scale interval	Blood pressure, temperature
Categorical		
Dichotomous	Binary data	Mortality, gender
Nominal	Qualitative data that cannot be ordered or ranked	Eye color, drug category
Ordinal	Data ordered, ranked, or measured without a constant scale interval	ASA physical status score, pain score

is between III and IV. Although ordinal data are often treated as interval data in choosing a statistical technique, such analysis may be suspect; alternative techniques for ordinal data are available. *Nominal variables* are placed into categories that have no logical ordering. The eye colors blue, hazel, and brown might be assigned the numbers 1, 2, and 3, but it is nonsense to say that blue < hazel < brown.

Descriptive Statistics

A typical hypothetical data set could be a sample of ages (the response or dependent variable) of 12 residents in an anesthe-
4 sia training program (the population). Although the results of a particular experiment might be presented by repeatedly showing the entire set of numbers, there are concise ways of summarizing the information content of the data set into a few numbers. These numbers are called *sample* or *summary statistics;* summary statistics are calculated using the numbers of the sample. By convention, the symbols of summary statistics are roman letters. The two summary statistics most frequently used for interval variables are the *central location* and the *variability,* but there are other summary statistics. Other data types have analogous summary statistics. Although the first purpose of descriptive statistics is to describe the sample of numbers obtained, there is also the desire to use the summary statistics from the sample to characterize the population from which the sample was obtained. For example, what can be said about the age of all anesthesia residents from the information in a sample? The population also has measures of central location and variability called the *parameters* of the population; Greek letters denote population parameters. Usually, the population parameters cannot be directly calculated because data from all population members cannot be obtained. The beauty of properly chosen summary statistics is that they are the best possible estimators of the population parameters.

These sampling statistics can be used in conjunction with a probability density function to provide additional descriptions of the sample and its population. Also commonly described as a probability distribution, a probability density function is an algebraic equation, $f(x)$, which gives a theoretical percentage distribution of x. Each value of x has a probability of occurrence given by $f(x)$. The most important probability distribution is the *normal* or *Gaussian function* $f(x) = \frac{1}{\sqrt{2\pi\sigma^2}}\exp\left[-\frac{1}{2}\left(\frac{x-\mu}{\sigma}\right)^2\right]$. There are two parameters (population mean and population variance) in the equation of the normal function that are denoted μ and σ^2. Often called the *normal equation,* it can be plotted and produces the familiar bell-shaped curve. Why are the mathematical properties of this curve so important to biostatistics? First, it has been empirically noted that when a biologic variable is sampled repeatedly, the pattern of the numbers plotted as a histogram resembles the normal curve; thus, most biologic data are said to follow or to obey a normal distribution. Second, if it is reasonable to assume that a sample is from a normal population, the mathematical properties of the normal equation can be used with the sampling statistic estimators of the population parameters to describe the sample and the population. Third, a mathematical theorem (the central limit theorem) allows the use of the assumption of normality for certain purposes, even if the population is not normally distributed.

Central Location

The three most common summary statistics of central location for interval variables are the arithmetic *mean,* the *median,* and the *mode.* The mean is merely the average of the numbers in the data set. Being a summary statistic of the sample, the arithmetic mean is denoted by the Roman letter x under a bar or $\bar{x} = \frac{1}{n}\sum_{i=1}^{n} x_i$, where i is the index of summation and n is the count of objects in the sample. If all values in the population could be obtained, then the population mean μ could be calculated similarly. Since all values of the population cannot be obtained, the sample mean is used. (Statisticians describe the sample mean as the unbiased, consistent, minimum variance, sufficient estimator of the population mean. Estimators are denoted by a hat over a greek letter; for example, $\hat{\mu}$. Thus, the sample mean $\bar{x}$ is the estimator $\hat{\mu}$ of the population mean μ.)

The median is the middlemost number or the number that divides the sample into two equal parts—first, ranking the sample values from lowest to highest and then counting up halfway to obtain the median. The concept of ranking is used in nonparametric statistics. A virtue of the median is that it is hardly affected by a few extremely high or low values. The mode is the most popular number of a sample; that is, the number that occurs most frequently. A sample may have ties for the most common value and be bi- or polymodal; these modes may be widely separated or adjacent. The raw data should be inspected for this unusual appearance. The mode is always mentioned in discussions of descriptive statistics, but it is rarely used in statistical practice.

Spread or Variability

Any set of interval data has variability unless all the numbers are identical. The range of ages from lowest to highest expresses the largest difference. This spread, diversity, and variability can also be expressed in a concise manner. Variability is specified by calculating the *deviation* or *deviate* of each individual x_i from the center (mean) of all the x_i's. The *sum of the squared deviates* is always positive unless all set values are identical. This sum is then divided by the number of individual measurements. The result is the *averaged squared deviation;* the average squared deviation is ubiquitous in statistics.

The concept of describing the spread of a set of numbers by calculating the average distance from each number to the center of the numbers applies to both a sample and a population; this average squared distance is called the *variance.* The population variance is a parameter and is represented by σ^2. As with the population mean, the population variance is not usually known and cannot be calculated. Just as the sample mean is used in place of the population mean, the sample variance is used in place of the population variance. The sample variance is

$$\text{VAR} = \text{SD}^2 = \frac{\sum_{i=1}^{n}(x_i - \bar{x})^2}{(n-1)}$$

Statistical theory demonstrates that if the divisor in the formula for SD^2 is $(n - 1)$ rather than n, the sample variance is an unbiased estimator of the population variance. While the variance is used extensively in statistical calculations, the units of variance are squared units of the original observations. The square root of the variance has the same units as the original observations; the square roots of the sample and population variances are called the *sample* (SD) and *population* (σ) *standard deviations.*

It was previously mentioned that most biologic observations appear to come from populations with normal distributions. By accepting this assumption of a normal distribution, further meaning can be given to the sample summary statistics (mean and SD) that have been calculated. This involves the use of the expression $\bar{x} \pm k \times \text{SD}$, where $k = 1, 2, 3$, and so forth. If the population from which the sample is taken is unimodal and roughly symmetric, then the bounds for 1, 2, and 3 encompasses roughly 68%, 95%, and 99% of the sample and population members.

HYPOTHESES AND PARAMETERS

Hypothesis Formulation

The researcher starts work with some intuitive feel for the phenomenon to be studied. Whether stated explicitly or not, this is the *biologic hypothesis;* it is a statement of experimental expectations to be accomplished by the use of experimental tools, instruments, or methods accessible to the research team. An example would be the hope that isoflurane would produce less myocardial ischemia than fentanyl; the experimental method might be the electrocardiography determination of ST segment changes. The biologic hypothesis of the researcher becomes a *statistical hypothesis* during research planning. The researcher measures quantities that can vary—variables such as heart rate or temperature or ST segment change—in samples from populations of interest. In a statistical hypothesis, statements are made about the relationship among parameters of one or more populations. (To restate, a *parameter* is a number describing a variable of a population; Greek letters are used to denote parameters.) The typical statistical hypothesis can be established in a somewhat rote fashion for every research project, regardless of the methods, materials, or goals. The most frequently used method of setting up the algebraic formulation of the statistical hypothesis is to create two mutually exclusive statements about some parameters of the study population (Table 9-3); estimates for the values for these parameters are acquired by sampling data. In the hypothetical example comparing isoflurane and fentanyl, ϕ_1 and ϕ_2 would represent the ST segment changes with isoflurane and with fentanyl. The *null hypothesis* is the hypothesis of no difference of ST segment changes between isoflurane and fentanyl. The *alternative hypothesis* is usually nondirectional, that is, either $\phi_1 < \phi_2$ or $\phi_1 > \phi_2$; this is known as a *two-tail alternative hypothesis.* This is a more conservative alternative hypothesis than assuming that the inequality can only be either less than or greater than.

TABLE 9-3. ALGEBRAIC STATEMENT OF STATISTICAL HYPOTHESES

H_0: $\phi_1 = \phi_2$ (null hypothesis)
H_a: $\phi_1 \neq \phi_2$ (alternative hypothesis)
ϕ_1 = Parameter estimated from sample of first population
ϕ_2 = Parameter estimated from sample of second population

Logic of Proof

One particular decision strategy is used most commonly to choose between the null and the alternative hypothesis. The decision strategy is similar to a method of indirect proof used in mathematics called *reductio ad absurdum* (proof by contradiction). If a theorem cannot be proved directly, assume that it is not true; show that the falsity of this theorem will lead to contradictions and absurdities; thus, reject the original assumption of the falseness of the theorem. For statistics, the approach is to assume that the null hypothesis is true even though the goal of the experiment is to show that there is a difference. One examines the consequences of this assumption by examining the actual sample values obtained for the variable(s) of interest. This is done by calculating what is called a *sample test statistic;* sample test statistics are calculated from the sample numbers. Associated with a sample test statistic is a *probability.* One also chooses the *level of significance;* the level of significance is the probability level considered too low to warrant support of the null hypothesis being tested. If sample values are sufficiently unlikely to have occurred by chance (i.e., the probability of the sample test statistic is less than the chosen level of significance), the null hypothesis is rejected; otherwise, the null hypothesis is not rejected.

Because the statistics deal with probabilities, not certainties, there is a chance that the decision concerning the null hypothesis is erroneous. These errors are best displayed in table form (Table 9-4); condition 1 and condition 2 could be different drugs, two doses of the same drug, or different patient groups. Of the four possible outcomes, two decisions are clearly undesirable. The error of wrongly rejecting the null hypothesis (false positive) is called the *type I* or *alpha error.* The experimenter should choose a probability value for alpha before collecting data; the experimenter decides how cautious to be against falsely claiming a difference. The most common choice for the value of alpha is 0.05. What are the consequences of choosing an alpha of 0.05? Assuming that there is, in fact, no difference between the two conditions and that the experiment is to be repeated 20 times, then during one of these experimental replications (5% of 20) a mistaken conclusion that there is a difference would be made. The probability of a type I error depends on the chosen level of significance and the existence or nonexistence of a difference between the two experimental conditions. The smaller the chosen alpha, the smaller will be the risk of a type I error.

The error of failing to reject a false null hypothesis (false negative) is called a *type II* or *beta error.* (The power of a test is 1 minus beta). The probability of a type II error depends on four factors.

TABLE 9-4. ERRORS IN HYPOTHESIS TESTING: THE TWO-WAY TRUTH TABLE

		Reality (Population Parameters)	
		Conditions 1 and 2 Equivalent	Conditions 1 and 2 Not Equivalent
Conclusion from sample (sample statistics)	**Conditions 1 and 2 equivalent**[a]	Correct conclusion	False-negative type II error (beta error)
	Conditions 1 and 2 not equivalent[b]	False-positive type I error (alpha error)	Correct conclusion

[a]Do not reject the null hypothesis: condition 1 = condition 2.
[b]Reject the null hypothesis: condition 1 ≠ condition 2.

Unfortunately, the smaller the alpha, the greater the chance of a false-negative conclusion; this fact keeps the experimenter from automatically choosing a very small alpha. Second, the more variability there is in the populations being compared, the greater the chance of a type II error. This is analogous to listening to a noisy radio broadcast; the more static there is, the harder it will be to discriminate between words. Next, increasing the number of subjects will lower the probability of a type II error. The fourth and most important factor is the magnitude of the difference between the two experimental conditions. The probability of a type II error goes from very high, when there is only a small difference, to extremely low, when the two conditions produce large differences in population parameters.

Inferential Statistics

The testing of hypotheses or *significance testing* has been the main focus of inferential statistics. Hypothesis testing allows the experimenter to use data from the sample to make inferences about the population. Statisticians have created formulas that use the values of the samples to calculate test statistics. Statisticians have also explored the properties of various theoretical probability distributions. Depending on the assumptions about how data are collected, the appropriate probability distribution is chosen as the source of critical values to accept or reject the null hypothesis. If the value of the test statistic calculated from the sample(s) is greater than the critical value, the null hypothesis is rejected. The critical value is chosen from the appropriate probability distribution after the magnitude of the type I error is specified.

There are parameters within the equation that generate any particular probability distribution; for the normal probability distribution, the parameters are μ and σ^2. For the normal distribution, each set of values for μ and σ^2 will generate a different shape for the bell-like normal curve. All probability distributions contain one or more parameters and can be plotted as curves; these parameters may be discrete (integer only) or continuous. Each value or combination of values for these parameters will create a different curve for the probability distribution being used. Thus, each probability distribution is actually a family of probability curves. Some additional parameters of theoretical probability distributions have been given the special name *degrees of freedom* and are represented by Latin letters such as *m*, *n*, and *s*.

Associated with the formula for computing a test statistic is a rule for assigning integer values to the one or more parameters called degrees of freedom. The number of degrees of freedom and the value for each degree of freedom depend on (1) the number of subjects, (2) the number of experimental groups, (3) the specifics of the statistical hypothesis, and (4) the type of statistical test. The correct curve of the probability distribution from which to obtain a critical value for comparison with the value of the test statistic is obtained with the values of one or more degrees of freedom.

To accept or reject the null hypothesis, the following steps are performed: (1) confirm that experimental data conform to the assumptions of the intended statistical test; (2) choose a significance level (alpha); (3) calculate the test statistic; (4) determine the degree(s) of freedom; (5) find the critical value for the chosen alpha and the degree(s) of freedom from the appropriate probability distribution; (6) if the test statistic exceeds the critical value, reject the null hypothesis; (7) if the test statistic does not exceed the critical value, do not reject the null hypothesis. There are general guidelines that relate the variable type and the experimental design to the choice of statistical test (Table 9-5).

Sample Size Calculations

Formerly, researchers typically ignored the latter error in experimental design. The practical importance of worrying about

TABLE 9-5. WHEN TO USE WHAT

Variable Type	One-sample Tests	Two-sample Tests	Multiple-sample Tests
Dichotomous or nominal	Binomial distribution	Chi-square test, Fisher's exact test	Chi-square test
Ordinal	Chi-square test	Chi-square test, nonparametric tests	Chi-square test, nonparametric tests
Continuous or discrete	*z* distribution or *t* distribution	Unpaired *t* test, paired *t* test, nonparametric tests	Analysis of variance, nonparametric analysis of variance

type II errors reached the consciousness of the medical research community several decades ago. Some controlled clinical trials that claimed to find no advantage of new therapies compared with standard therapies lacked sufficient statistical power to discriminate between the experimental groups and would have missed an important therapeutic improvement. As an example, the formula for calculating the size of each sample in a study comparing the means of two populations is $n = 2\left[\frac{(z_\alpha - z_\beta)\sigma}{\mu_1 - \mu_2}\right]^2$. The z values are taken from the normal probability distribution and represent assumptions about the prespecified alpha and beta; the sigma (σ) is the assumed common SD; the mu's (μ) are the assumed population values. There are four options for decreasing type II error (increasing statistical power): (1) raise alpha, (2) reduce population variability, (3) make the sample bigger, and (4) make the difference between the conditions greater. Under most circumstances, only the sample size can be varied. Sample size planning has become an important part of research design for controlled clinical trials. Some published research still fails the test of adequate sample size planning.

The Bayesian Alternative

In 1965, the statistician and epidemiologist A. B. Hill suggested guidelines for assessing evidence of causation when presented with an observed association between the environment and disease; on his list of features, the second criteria was Consistency. "Has it been repeatedly observed by different persons, in different places, circumstances and times?".[6] Be it an RCT or an observational study report, the results and claims of medical research are not and should not be considered in isolation from prior knowledge. Yet the most commonly used methods of statistical inference used in medical research (see supra) explicitly use only the newly obtained data. This is the Frequentist approach or inference, so called because the precise definition of probability values depends on assumptions about hypothetical repeated replication of data collection. The new information of a study is a function only of the data.

A competing approach is called Bayesian inference that explicitly reports the new information of a study as a function of both
5 observed data and historical (prior) knowledge. Both Frequentist and Bayesian inferences make statements about parameters. But Bayesian methods involve the multiplication of the prior knowledge represented as a probability distribution of the parameter(s) times the likelihood of the observed data; the product is the new (posterior) probability distribution of the parameters (Table 9-6).[7,8] Bayesian methods have been proposed to resolve the conundrum that some highly cited clinical research whose evidence is interpreted by a Frequentist p value is later contradicted or found to be excessively optimistic in the magnitude of effect.[9–12] Among reasons for the slower adoption of Bayesian methods are concerns about the subjectivity in defining the prior probability distribution and the considerably greater computational difficulty in performing an analysis.

TABLE 9-6. COMPARISON OF FREQUENTIST AND BAYESIAN APPROACHES TO STATISTICAL INFERENCE

Let us assume that we want to evaluate whether a new drug improves 1-year survival after myocardial infarction by using data from a placebo-controlled trial. We do this by estimating the risk ratio—the risk of death in patients treated with the new drug divided by the risk of death in the control group. If the risk ratio is 0.5, then the new drug reduces the risk of death by 50%. If the risk ratio is 1, then the drug has no effect.

Frequentist Statistics	Bayesian Statistics
We use the data to make inferences about the true (but unknown) population value of the risk ratio.	Bayesians take a subjective approach. We start with our prior opinion about the risk ratio, expressed as a probability distribution. We use the data to modify that opinion (we derive the posterior probability distribution for the risk ratio based on both the data and the prior distribution).
The 95% confidence interval gives us a plausible range of values for the population risk ratio; 95% of the times we derive such a range it will contain the true (but unknown) population value.	A 95% credible interval is one that has a 95% chance of containing the population risk ratio.
The P value is the probability of getting a risk ratio at least as far from the null value of 1 as the one found in our study.	The posterior distribution can be used to derive direct probability statements about the risk ratio, for example, the probability that the drug increases the risk of death.

If our prior opinion about the risk ratio is vague (we consider a wide range of values to be equally likely) then the results of a Frequentist analysis are similar to the results of a Bayesian analysis; both are based on what statisticians call the likelihood for the data:

- The 95% confidence interval is the same as the 95% credible interval, except that the latter has the meaning often incorrectly ascribed to a confidence interval.
- The (one-sided) P value is the same as the Bayesian posterior probability that the drug increases the risk of death (assuming that we found a protective effect of the drug).

The two approaches, however, will give different results if our prior opinion is not vague, relative to the amount of information contained in the data.

Adapted with permission from: BMJ Publishing Group Limited. Sterne JA, Davey Smith G. Sifting the evidence: What's wrong with significance tests? *BMJ.* 2001;322: 226–231.

STATISTICAL TESTS AND MODELS

Interval Data

Parametric statistics are the usual choice in the analysis of interval data, both discrete and continuous. The purpose of such analysis is to test the hypothesis of a difference between population means. The population means are unknown and are estimated by the sample means. A typical example would be the comparison of the mean heart rates of patients receiving and not receiving atropine. Parametric test statistics have been developed by using the properties of the normal probability distribution and two related probability distributions, the *t* and the *F* distributions. In using such parametric methods, the assumption is made that the sample or samples is/are drawn from population(s) with a normal distribution. The parametric test statistics that have been created for interval data all have the form of a ratio. In general terms, the numerator of this ratio is the variability of the means of the samples; the denominator of this ratio is the variability among all the members of the samples. These variabilities are similar to the variances developed for descriptive statistics. The test statistic is thus a ratio of variabilities or variances. All parametric test statistics are used in the same fashion; if the test statistic ratio becomes large, the null hypothesis of no difference is rejected. The critical values against which to compare the test statistic are taken from tables of the three relevant probability distributions (normal, *t*, or *F*). In hypothesis testing at least one of the population means is unknown, but the population variance(s) may or may not be known. Parametric statistics can be divided into two groups according to whether or not the population variances are known. If the population variance is known, the test statistic used is called the *z* score; critical values are obtained from the normal distribution. In most biomedical applications, the population variance is rarely known and the *z* score is little used.

Confidence Intervals

The other major areas of statistical inference are the estimation of parameters with associated *confidence intervals* (CIs). In statistics, a CI is an interval estimate of a population parameter. A CI describes how likely it is that the population parameter is estimated by any particular sample statistic such as the mean. (The technical definition of the CI of the mean is more rigorous. A 95% CI implies that if the experiment were done over and over again, 95 of each 100 CIs would be expected to contain the true value of the mean.) CIs are a range of the following form: Summary statistic ± (confidence factor) × (precision factor).

The *precision factor* is derived from the sample itself, whereas the *confidence factor* is taken from a probability distribution and also depends on the specified confidence level chosen. For a sample of interval data taken from a normally distributed population for which CIs are to be chosen for $\bar{x}$, the precision factor is called the *standard error of the mean* and is obtained by dividing SD by the square root of the sample size or $\mathrm{SE} = \frac{\mathrm{SD}}{\sqrt{n}} = \sqrt{\sum_{i=1}^{n}(x_i - \bar{x})^2/n(n-1)}$.

The confidence factors are the same as those used for the dispersion or spread of the sample and are obtained from the normal distribution. The CIs for confidence factors 1, 2, and 3 have roughly a 68%, 95%, and 99% chance of containing the population mean. Strictly speaking, when the SD must be estimated from sample values, the confidence factors should be taken from the *t distribution*, another probability distribution. These coefficients will be larger than those used previously. This is usually ignored if the sample size is reasonable; for example, $n > 25$. Even when the sample size is only 5 or greater, the use of the coefficients 1, 2, and 3 is simple and sufficiently accurate for quick mental calculations of CIs on parameter estimates.

Almost all research reports include the use of SE, regardless of the probability distribution of the populations sampled. This use is a consequence of the *central limit theorem*, one of the most remarkable theorems in all of mathematics. The central limit theorem states that the SE can always be used, if the sample size is sufficiently large, to specify CIs around the sample mean. These CIs are calculated as previously described. This is true even if the population distribution is so different from normal that SD cannot be used to characterize the dispersion of the population members. Only rough guidelines can be given for the necessary sample size; for interval data, 25 and above is large enough and 4 and below is too small.

Although the SE is often discussed along with other descriptive statistics, it is really an inferential statistic. SE and SD are usually mentioned together because of their similarities of computation, but there is often confusion about their use in research reports in the form "mean ± number." Some confusion results from the failure of the author to specify whether the number after the ± sign is the one or the other. More importantly, the choice between using SD and using SE has become controversial. Because SE is always less than SD, it has been argued that authors seek to deceive by using SE to make the data look better than they really are. The choice is actually simple. When describing the spread, scatter, or dispersion of the sample, use SD; when describing the precision with which the population mean is known, use SE.

t Test

An important advance in statistical inference came early in the twentieth century with the creation of *Student's t test statistic* and the *t distribution*, which allowed the testing of hypotheses when the population variance is not known. The most common use of Student's *t* test is to compare the mean values of two populations. There are two types of *t* test. If each subject has two measurements taken, for example, one before (x_i) and one after (y_i) a drug, then a one-sample or *paired t test* procedure is used; each control measurement taken before drug administration is paired with a measurement in the same patient after drug administration. Of course, this is a self-control experiment. This pairing of measurements in the same patient reduces variability and increases statistical power. The difference $d_i = x_i - y_i$ of each pair of values is calculated and the average $\bar{d}$ is calculated. In the formula for Student's *t* statistic, the numerator is $\bar{d}$, whereas the denominator is the SE of $\bar{d}$ denoted ($\mathrm{SE}_{\bar{d}}$) so the test statistic is $t = \frac{\bar{d}}{\mathrm{SE}_{\bar{d}}}$.

All *t* statistics are created in this way; the numerator is the difference of two means, whereas the denominator is the SE of the two means. If the difference between the two means is large compared with their variability, then the null hypothesis of no difference is rejected. The critical values for the *t* statistic are taken from the *t* probability distribution. The *t* distribution is symmetric and bell-shaped but more spread out than the normal distribution. The *t* distribution has a single integer parameter; for a paired *t* test, the value of this single degree of freedom is the sample size minus one. There can be some confusion about the use of the letter *t*. It refers both to the value of the test statistic calculated by the formula and to the critical value from the theoretical probability distribution. The critical *t* value is determined by looking in a *t* table after a significance level is chosen and the degree of freedom is computed.

More commonly, measurements are taken on two separate groups of subjects. For example, one group receives blood pressure treatment with sample values x_i, whereas no treatment is given to a control group with sample values y_i. The number of subjects in each group might or might not be identical; regardless of this, in no sense is an individual measurement in the first group matched or paired with a specific measurement in the second group. An *unpaired* or *two-sample t test* is used to compare the means of the two groups. The numerator of the *t* statistic is $\bar{x} - \bar{y}$. The denominator is a weighted average of the SDs of each sample so that the test statistic *t* is

$$t = \frac{\bar{x} - \bar{y}}{\sqrt{\left(\frac{1}{n_x} + \frac{1}{n_y}\right)\left(\frac{(n_x - 1)s_x^2 + (n_y - 1)s_y^2}{n_x + n_y - 2}\right)}}.$$

The degree of freedom for an unpaired *t* test is calculated as the sum of the subjects of the two groups minus two. As with the paired *t* test, if the *t* ratio becomes large, the null hypothesis is rejected.

Analysis of Variance

Experiments in anesthesia, whether they are with humans or with animals, may not be limited to one or two groups of data for each variable. It is very common to follow a variable longitudinally; heart rate, for example, might be measured five times before and during anesthetic induction. These are also called *repeated measurement experiments;* the experimenter will wish to compare changes between the initial heart rate measurement and those obtained during induction. The experimental design might also include several groups receiving different induction drugs; for example, comparing heart rate across groups immediately after laryngoscopy. Researchers have mistakenly handled these analysis problems with just the *t* test. If heart rate is collected five times, these collection times could be labeled *A, B, C, D,* and *E.* Then *A* could be compared with *B, C, D,* and *E; B* could be compared with *C, D,* and *E;* and so forth. The total of possible pairings is 10; thus, 10 paired *t* tests could be calculated for all the possible pairings of *A, B, C, D,* and *E.* A similar approach can be used for comparing more than two groups for unpaired data.

The use of *t* tests in this fashion is inappropriate. In testing a statistical hypothesis, the experimenter sets the level of type I error; this is usually chosen to be 0.05. When using many *t* tests, as in the example given earlier, the chosen error rate for performing all these *t* tests is much higher than 0.05, even though the type I error is set at 0.05 for each individual comparison. In fact, the type I error rate for all *t* tests simultaneously, that is, the chance of finding at least one of the multiple *t* test statistics significant merely by chance, is given by the formula $\alpha = 1 - 0.95^{\kappa}$. If 13 *t* tests are performed ($\kappa = 13$), the real error rate is 49%. Applying *t* tests over and over again to all the possible pairings of a variable will misleadingly identify statistical significance when in fact there is none.

The most versatile approach for handling comparisons of means between more than two groups or between several measurements in the same group is called *analysis of variance* and is frequently cited by the acronym ANOVA. Analysis of variance consists of rules for creating test statistics on means when there are more than two groups. These test statistics are called *F ratios,* after Ronald Fisher; the critical values for the *F* test statistic are taken from the *F* probability distribution that Fisher derived.

Suppose that data for three groups are obtained. What can be said about the mean values of the three target populations? The *F* test is actually asking several questions simultaneously: Is group 1 different from group 2; is group 2 different from group 3; and is group 1 different from group 3? As with the *t* test, the *F* test statistic is a ratio; in general terms, the numerator expresses the variability of the mean values of the three groups, whereas the denominator expresses the average variability or difference of each sample value from the mean of all sample values. The formulas to create the test statistic are computationally elegant but are rather hard to appreciate intuitively. The *F* statistic has two degrees of freedom, denoted *m* and *n;* the value of *m* is a function of the number of experimental groups; the value for *n* is a function of the number of subjects in all experimental groups. The analysis of multigroup data is not necessarily finished after the ANOVAs are calculated. If the null hypothesis is rejected and it is accepted that there are differences among the groups tested, how can it be decided where the differences are? A variety of techniques are available to make what are called *multiple comparisons* after the ANOVA test is performed.

Robustness and Nonparametric Tests

Most statistical tests depend on certain assumptions about the nature of the distribution of values in the underlying populations from which experimental samples are taken. For the parametric statistics, that is, *t* tests and ANOVA, it is assumed that the populations follow the normal distribution. However, for some data, experience or historical reasons suggests that these assumptions of a normal distribution do not hold; some examples include proportions, percentages, and response times. What should the experimenter do if he or she fears that the data are not normally distributed?

The experimenter might choose to ignore the problem of nonnormal data and inhomogeneity of variance, hoping that everything will work out. Such insouciance is actually a very practical and reasonable approach to the problem. Parametric statistics are called *robust* statistics; they stand up to much adversity. To a statistician, robustness implies that the magnitude of type I errors is not seriously affected by ill-conditioned data. Parametric statistics are sufficiently robust that the accuracy of decisions reached by means of *t* tests and ANOVA remains very credible, even for moderately severe departures from the assumptions.

Another possibility would be to use statistics that do not require any assumptions about probability distributions of the populations. Such statistics are known as *nonparametric tests;* they can be used whenever there is very serious concern about the shape of the data. Nonparametric statistics are also the tests of choice for ordinal data. The basic concept behind nonparametric statistics is the ability to rank or order the observations; nonparametric tests are also called *order statistics.*

Most nonparametric statistics still require the use of theoretical probability distributions; the critical values that must be exceeded by the test statistic are taken from the binomial, normal, and chi-square distributions, depending on the nonparametric test being used. The *nonparametric sign test, Mann–Whitney rank sum test,* and *Kruskal–Wallis one-way ANOVA* are analogous to the paired *t* test, unpaired *t* test, and one-way ANOVA, respectively. The currently available nonparametric tests are not used more commonly because they do not adapt well to complex statistical models and because they are less able than parametric tests to distinguish between the null and alternative hypotheses if the data are, in fact, normally distributed.

Binary Variables

Confidence Intervals on Proportions

Categorical binary data, also called *enumeration data,* provide counts of subject responses. Given a sample of subjects of whom some have a certain characteristic (e.g., death, female sex), a ratio of responders to the number of subjects can be easily calculated as $p = x/n$; this ratio or rate can be expressed as a decimal fraction or as a percentage. It should be clear that this is a measure of central location of binary data. In the population from which the sample is taken, the ratio of responders to total subjects is a population parameter, denoted π. (This is not related to the geometry constant $\pi = 3.14159....$) The sample proportion p is the estimator ($\hat{\pi}$) of the population proportion π. As with other data types, π is usually not known, but must be estimated from the sample. The sample ratio p is the best estimate of π.

Since the population is not generally known, the experimenter usually wishes to estimate π by the sample ratio p and to specify with what precision π is known. If the sample is sufficiently large ($n \times p \geq 5$; $n \times (1-p) \geq 5$), advantage is taken of the central limit theorem to derive an SE analogous to that derived for interval data: $\text{SE} = \sqrt{\frac{p \times (1-p)}{n}}$. This sample SE is exactly analogous to the sample SE of the mean for interval data, except that it is an SE of the proportion. Just as a 95% CI of the mean was calculated, so may a CI on the proportion may be obtained. Larger samples will make the CI more precise.

If nothing goes wrong, is everything all right? This question was proposed by Henley and Lippman-Hand to discuss the interpretations of zero numerators using the 3 over n rule.[13] Consider an observational study that reports no morbidity in 167 patients receiving a new intravenous anesthetic. Is there really no risk? While the best estimate of the population parameter π is 0/167 or 0%, an upper bound on the 95% CI is relevant to consider how high the rate of adverse events might be. As the probability of binary data is provided by the *binomial probability distribution function*, this upper bound may be derived from $1-(0.05)^{1/n}$ where n is the denominator; for $n > 30$, this is well approximated by $3/n = 3/167 \approx 1.8\%$.

The zero numerator example can be used to illustrate a difference between a Bayesian and a Frequentist approach. If there is no prior information (Bayes–Laplace *beta probability distribution function*), the upper bound is $3/(n+1) = 3/168 \approx 1.8\%$; the Bayesian equivalent of a CI is called a Credible Interval (CI).[14] As the sample size increases, $3/n$ and $3/(n+1)$ become closer and closer. By contrast, when there is prior information Bayesian inference will provide a more informative CI than a Frequentist approach. Suppose a prior study with the same new anesthetic had found 15 morbid events in 10,000 (0.15%) patients. Then with the new data the estimate of the population rate of morbidity is 0.12% (upper bound 95% CI = 0.36%).[14] Using prior information and the new data of 0 events in 167 patients, the population rate estimate has been reduced from 0.15% to 0.12% and the upper bound of the 95% CI is much lower (0.36% vs. 1.8%) than by Frequentist estimation.

Hypothesis Testing

In the experiment negating the value of mammary artery ligation, five of eight patients (62.5%) having ligation showed benefit while five of nine patients (55.6%) having sham surgery also had benefit.[1] Is this difference real? This experiment sampled patients from two populations—those having the real procedure and those having the sham procedure. A variety of statistical techniques allow a comparison of the success rate. These include *Fisher's exact test* and (*Pearson's*) *chi-square test*. The chi-square test offers the advantage of being computationally simpler; it can also analyze contingency tables with more than two rows and two columns; however, certain assumptions of sample size and response rate are not achieved by this experiment. Fisher's exact test fails to reject the null hypothesis for these data.

The results of such experiments are often presented as rate ratios. The rate of improvement for the experimental group (5/8 = 62.5%) is divided by the rate of improvement for the control group (5/9 = 55.6%). A rate ratio of 1.00 (100%) fails to show a difference of benefit or harm between the two groups. In this example the rate ratio is 1.125. Thus, the experimental group had a 12.5% greater chance of improvement compared with the control group. A CI can be calculated for the rate ratio; in this example it is (0.40, 3.13), thus widely spread to either side of the rate ratio of no difference. (If such experiment were performed now, the sample size would be much larger to have adequate statistical power.)

Linear and Logistic Regression

Simple Linear Regression

Often a goal of an experiment is to find relationships between two variables so that in new patients the prediction of the value of one characteristic may be made by knowledge of another characteristic. The most commonly used technique for this purpose is linear regression analysis. Experiments for this purpose collect data pairs (x_i, y_i); these data pairs may be captured in either clinical trials or observational studies. The y variable is called the dependent or response variable while the x variable is denoted the independent or explanatory variable. These data should be displayed in a scatter plot; in the simplest type, a straight line (linear relationship) is assumed between two variables; the y variable is considered a function of the x variable. This is expressed as the linear regression equation $y = a + bx$; the parameters of the regression equation are a and b. The parameter b is the slope of the straight line relating x and y; for each 1 unit change in x, there are b unit changes in y. The parameter a is the intercept (value of y when x equals 0). Estimates of the parameters are obtained from a least squares method that sets the slope b value to minimize the sum of the vertical distances from the data pairs to the regression line: $b = \frac{\sum_{i=1}^{n}(x_i - \bar{x})(y_i - \bar{y})}{\sum_{i=1}^{n}(x_i - \bar{x})^2}$; $a = \bar{y} + b\bar{x}$. The parameter of greatest interest in regression is usually the slope, especially whether the slope is nonzero; a zero-valued slope implies that x and y are not linearly related. A t test statistic is used to check the statistical significance of the slope.

While there is the additional assumption of bivariate normality (both x and y normally distributed), the same (x_i, y_i) data pairs are usually subjected to correlation analysis. The correlation coefficient r is a measure of the linear covariation of x and y; r ranges from –1 to 1. There is no linear correlation between x and y if r is zero valued. It is estimated by $r = \frac{\sum_{i=1}^{n}(x_i - \bar{x})(y_i - \bar{y})}{\sqrt{\sum_{i=1}^{n}(x_i - \bar{x})^2}\sqrt{\sum_{i=1}^{n}(y_i - \bar{y})^2}}$.

The test of the statistical significance of r is equivalent to the test for the significance of the regression slope b. The squared value of r known as the coefficient of determination (r^2) varies between 0 and 1 and is sometimes expressed as a percentage. The coefficient of determination has a very useful interpretation: The fraction of the variation of y explained by the variation of x.

As a hypothetical example, suppose that age and a plasma biomarker of physical maturity are collected in 11 children. The (x_i, y_i) values recorded are (10, 8.04), (8, 6.95), (13, 7.58), (9, 8.81), (11, 8.33), (14, 9.96), (6, 7.24), (4, 4.26), (12, 10.84), (7, 4.82), and

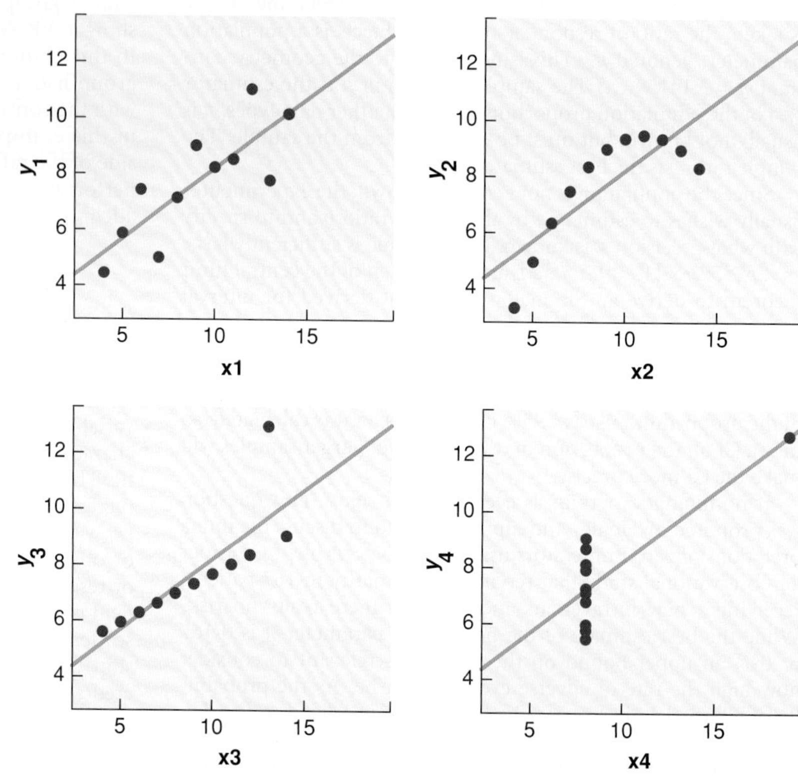

FIGURE 9-1. Four scatter plots from the Anscombe data sets. For each data set, $n = 11$, $\bar{x} = 9.00$, $SD_x = 3.31$, $\bar{y} = 7.50$, $SD_y = 2.03$, $y = 3.00 + 0.50x$, $SE_a = 1.12$, $SE_b = 0.12$, $r^2 = 0.67$, and so forth. All statistics are equal up to the fourth decimal place.

(5, 5.68). Neither an inspection of these values nor of the summary statistics ($\bar{x} = 9.00, \bar{y} = 7.50$) permit the reader to detect any relationship. The calculation of the coefficient of determination ($r^2 = 0.67$) does allow the inference that 67% of the variation in the biomarker is explained by the variation in age.

A researcher or reader should not be satisfied to see only the
1 statistical results of regression and correlation. The statistician Anscombe created four hypothetical data sets to illustrate the importance of visual inspection of data.[15] Each data set has 11 paired (x_i, y_i) observations (Fig. 9-1). The hypothetical example given above is displayed in the upper left quadrant; a linear relationship is displayed. For the data in the upper right quadrant, the relationship between x and y is curvilinear (quadratic). For the lower right quadrant, there is no relationship between x and y; with one exception all data pairs have the same x value. For the lower left quadrant, there is a near perfect correlation between x and y except for one data pair with a much higher y value. Nevertheless, all summary statistics, regression, and correlation values of the four data sets including means, SDs, slopes, intercepts, standard errors of regression parameters, statistical significance of regression parameters, and correlation coefficients are equal. There are clearly four different patterns that can only be detected by visual inspection. Even this simplest form of regression and correlation analysis is based on the strong assumption of an underlying linear relationship between x and y; failure of that assumption leads to erroneous statistical inference. Using just the summary, regression, and correlation statistics, the four data sets would have been thought to have very similar/identical underlying relationships.

Multivariable Linear Regression

Regression methods can be extended to data sets in which one response variable is thought to be linearly related to many explanatory variables. This regression includes methods for choosing which of the explanatory variables have a statistically significant (i.e., nonzero) regression slope. Multivariable linear regression is the creation of a model relating some continuous response such as heart rate to k explanatory variables; these are also called covari-
6 ates. This regression starts with data from n patients of the form (y_i, $x_{i,1}$, $x_{i,2}$, ..., $x_{i,k}$) where the subscript i denotes the ith patient, y_i is the response in the ith patient, x_i is the value of a covariate in the ith patient, and the second subscript of x_i denotes the 1 to k covariates. The linear model equation for the ith individual is

$$\mu_i = \beta_0 + \beta_1 x_{i,1} + \beta_2 x_{i,2} + \cdots + \beta_k x_{i,k} = \sum_{j=1}^{k} \beta_j x_{i,j}.$$

The β_js are the unknown coefficients (parameters) of the model that will be estimated from the observed data. For the ith individual, the expected value of the model, μ_i, is the linear sum of each covariate value multiplied by its coefficient. The difference between the observed (y_i) and expected values (μ_i) reflects biologic variability, measurement error, and so forth.

Univariable and Multivariable Logistic Regression

If the response variable is binary (alive/dead, complication/no complication), linear regression has been extended; thus, the typically sigmoidally shaped regression of a binary outcome (e.g., movement) versus anesthetic dose. There are multiple methods for regression of binary outcomes, the most common being logistic regression. The most commonly used format of the logistic method is the multivariable logistic regression model. The response variable y_i denotes the value of the binary outcome in the ith individual and is generally coded as 0 or 1 representing the absence or presence of an event (e.g., day-of-surgery mortality). Letting π represent the probability that the response variable has value 1, then the logit transformation, log of the odds ratio = $\ln\left(\frac{\pi}{1-\pi}\right)$, allows π to be expressed as the linear combination of the covariates:

$$\ln\left(\frac{\pi_i}{1-\pi_i}\right) = \beta_0 + \beta_1 x_{i,1} + \beta_2 x_{i,2} + \cdots + \beta_k x_{i,k} = \sum_{j=1}^{k} \beta_j x_{i,j}.$$

The logit transformation is the link function relating the the sum of the covariates to the probability of the binary outcome.

Multivariable regression is used to control for confounding. Confounding occurs when the apparent association between a covariate and an outcome is affected by the relationship of a third variable to the covariate and to the outcome; the third variable is a confounder. As contrasted to sequentially regressing each covariate against the response variable, this is done by fitting all explanatory variables simultaneously.[16] For example in exploring the relationship between tobacco and myocardial infarction, male sex, poverty, and sedentary lifestyle could be confounders because they are associated with both smoking and coronary heart disease.

Each year thousands of reports are published in the medical literature using stepwise, multivariable logistic regression on observational data to identify "independent" predictors for various clinical outcomes.[17] In the anesthesia literature PONV has been a very common topic for such statistical modeling.[18–21] Stepwise, multivariable logistic regression is an automatic procedure where there are a large number of potential explanatory variables and no underlying theory on which to base the selection of prediction model risk factors.[22] Once these prediction models have been created, there is a framework for assessing their performance.[23–25] Great skepticism should be shown for most of these prognostic models, especially those concerning mortality, as they usually have not been validated, have modest accuracy, and do not have documented clinical utility.[26,27]

Propensity Score Matching and Analysis

Another approach for providing estimation of treatment effect in nonrandomized studies (NRSs) is the methodology of propensity score matching. This use of NRS data is intended to investigate the effect of treatment X on a specified dichotomous outcome Y; the good outcome can be denoted Y^+, for example survival, with Y^- being the opposite. It is usually the case that one or more baseline prognostic covariates (confounders $C_1, C_2, \ldots, C_k$) may be imbalanced between the patients that did (X^+) and did not (X^-) receive the treatment of interest. The favorable outcome, conditional on receiving treatment X^+, is denoted $Y^+|X^+$ with $Y^+|X^-$ being a favorable outcome in those not receiving the treatment. Any difference between interventions on the outcome Y may be a consequence of the confounders influencing both the treatment and the outcome; a failure to observe a difference in outcome may also be a consequence of confounding. As an example, pulmonary artery catheterization (PAC) in the care of the critically ill was adopted about 40 years ago and widely disseminated without rigorous evaluation. The enthusiasm of intensivists for such monitoring even forced the cessation of an RCT comparing care with and without PACs because of the unwillingness of physicians to allow patient participation in the study.[28] Using data of 5,735 critically ill patients, Connors et al. reported lower 6-month survival in the 2,184 patients with PACs ($Y^+|X^+ = 46.3\%$ vs. $Y^+|X^- = 53.7\%$), but far more X^+ patients had multiorgan system failure (MOSF: 57% vs. 35%) at the time of PAC placement; there were other imbalances of initial covariates.[29] Was the higher mortality attributable to the use of PACs or to a greater severity of illness? Using propensity matching, Connors created a pair of subsets (1,008 patients vs. 1,008 patients) with similar proportions of prognostic factors in both groups (e.g., MOSF: 34%); 6-month survival was still lower ($Y^+|X^+ = 46.0\%$ vs. $Y^+|X^- = 51.2\%$).

Propensity score matching is a statistical technique within the general concept of matching. If only one prognostic factor was important, for example, sex, then a pair of matched subsets could be created easily by repeatedly and randomly placing one man and one woman into each subset—matching the groups just by sex. However, there is usually a great deal of baseline information about patients observed in an NRS; Connors had details for about 40+ baseline covariates.[29] In addition, it is often not evident which baseline characteristics are predictive of outcome. Creating matched groups by simple matching is not generally possible using more than a very few covariates.

The propensity score is defined as a subject's probability of receiving a specific treatment conditional on the many baseline covariates. The propensity score is usually estimated by multivariable logistic regression. In contrast to the attempt to create parsimonious model with a few independent predictors of outcome by logistic regression modeling of NRS data, all available covariates are left in the model for a propensity score whether or not they are statistically significant. These covariates must be restricted to those that are known prior to the intervention. In the study by Connors, the presence/absence of MOSF on hospital admission should be included in propensity score; MOSF developing a week later should not.

For each patient in the data set, the z score obtained from the sum of each covariate times its regression coefficient is calculated:

$$z = \beta_0 + \beta_1 C_{i,1} + \beta_2 C_{i,2} + \cdots + \beta_k C_{i,k} = \sum_{j=1}^{k} \beta_j C_{i,j}.$$

Taking the anti-logit of the z score $\left(p = \frac{1}{1+e^{-z}}\right)$ yields the probability that a patient with those covariate values received the intervention. Of course, it is in fact known whether or not a patient received the intervention. Propensity-matched subsets of patients are created by randomly choosing and matching one patient receiving the intervention to one patient not receiving the intervention with the same probability from the z score; usually the propensity probabilities (scores) are matched to the third or greater decimal place. The success of propensity score matching in balancing many covariates was well displayed in an observational comparison of epidural anesthesia for intermediate- to high-risk noncardiac surgery by Wijeysundera et al.[30] As graphed by Gayat et al. (Fig. 9-2), 45 baseline characteristics of two matched subsets of about 44,000 patients each became extremely well balanced.[31] In the original data set, an arterial line was used in 59% versus 33%; after balancing, an arterial line was used in 48% for both. The total patients in the two matched subsets will always be less than the total count of patients in the NRS data set; some patients cannot be matched. Simple paired statistics are used to compare the outcomes of the two subsets.

Propensity score methods are being used in NRSs to reduce the effect of selection bias in estimating causal treatment effects. Besides propensity score matching, the effect of selection bias can also be reduced by using propensity scores for stratification, regression adjustment, and weighting. It is now routine to see NRS using propensity analysis in the intensive care and anesthesia literature—most commonly using matching.[31] A propensity score matching analysis should include (1) details of propensity score building; (2) matching method; and (3) demonstration of covariate balancing by tabular or graphical display.[31] The

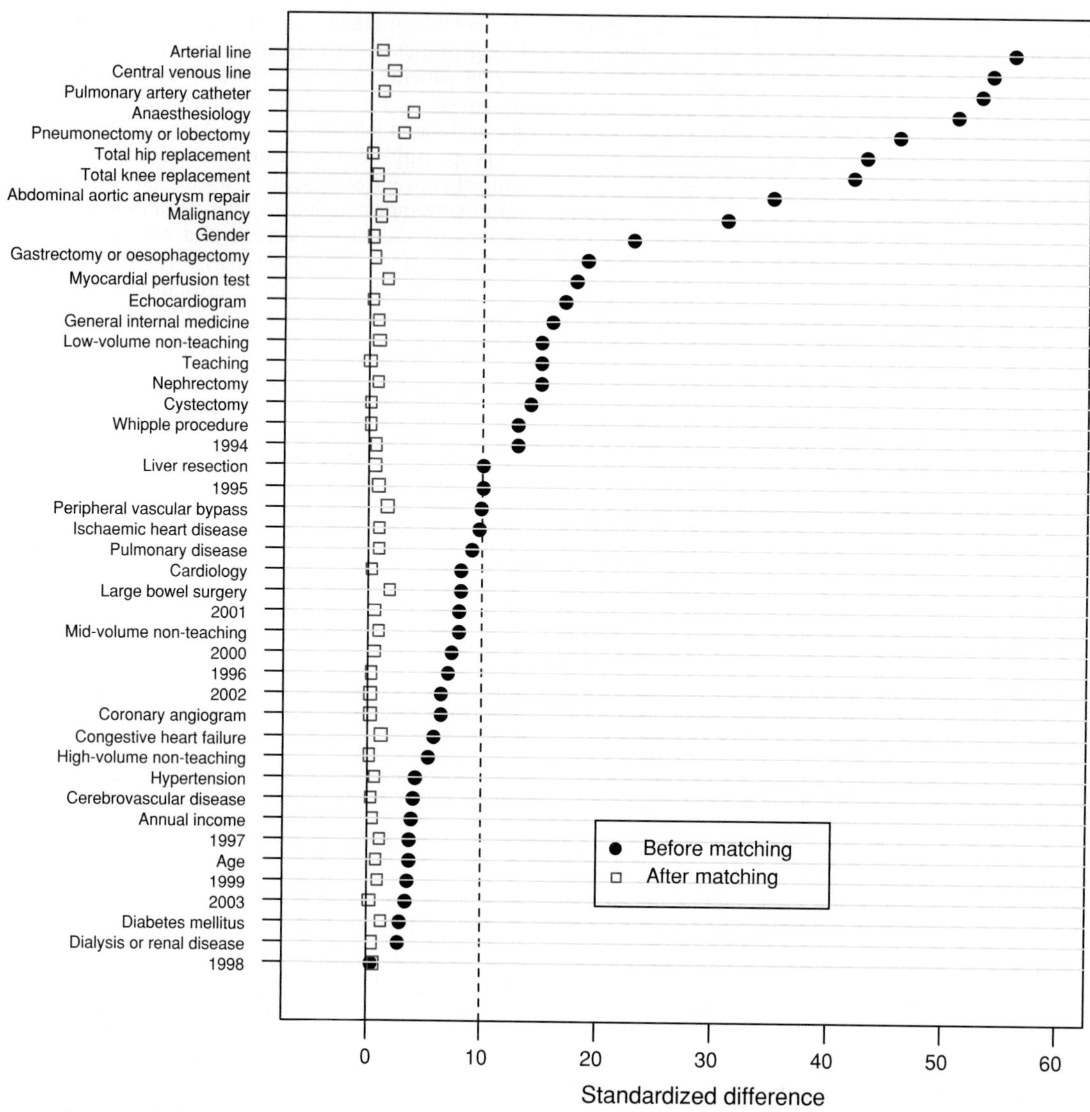

FIGURE 9-2. Graphical representation of 45 baseline covariates before and after propensity score matching using data from: Wijeysundera DN, Beattie WS, Austin PC, et al. Epidural anaesthesia and survival after intermediate-to-high risk non-cardiac surgery: A population-based cohort study. *Lancet.* 2008;372:562–569. The standardized difference for each covariate is the average difference between groups divided by the average standard deviation of the two groups. The standardized difference increases directly with increasing imbalance between groups. With propensity score matching, the standardized difference is close to zero for all covariates. With kind permission from Springer Science+Business Media: Gayat E, Pirracchio R, Resche-Rigon M, et al. Propensity scores in intensive care and anaesthesiology literature: A systematic review. *Intensive Care Med.* 2010;36:1997, figure 2.

propensity score can reduce bias due to observed covariates. But propensity score methods cannot replace the RCT since randomization minimizes covariate imbalance between treatment groups for observed, unobserved, and unobservable covariates.

Systematic Reviews and Meta-analyses

It is over 20 years since the first systematic review (SR) with an accompanying meta-analysis (MA) was published in an anesthesia journal[32] and reports using these research methods are now 7 commonplace in anesthesia journals.[33–37] The focused question of an SR of interventions can be subsumed by the acronym PICO: P = Population, I = Intervention, C = Comparison, and O = Outcome. As an example, in the Cochrane Library SR *Pulmonary Artery Catheters for Adult Patients in Intensive Care* the population of interest were adults receiving intensive care; the intervention was the use of pulmonary artery catheters; the comparison was the nonuse of pulmonary artery catheters; and the outcome was hospital mortality.[38] The structured title of an SR usually contains most of the PICO elements: *Transient Neurologic Symptoms (TNS)* [Outcome] *following Spinal Anaesthesia with Lidocaine* [Intervention] *versus Other Local Anaesthetics* [Comparison].[39]

Data are obtained from controlled trials (usually randomized) already in the medical literature rather than from newly conducted clinical trials; the basic unit of analysis of this observational research is the published study. A structured protocol is followed that includes in part (1) choice of study inclusion/exclusion criteria, (2) explicitly defined literature searching, (3) abstraction of data from included studies, (4) appraisal of risk bias within each study, (5) systematic pooling of data, and (6) discussion of inferences. This structured protocol is intended to minimize bias. Even RCTs may have sources of bias such as (1) selection bias: Systematic differences between the patients receiving each intervention; (2) performance bias: Systematic differences in care being given to study patients other than the preplanned interventions being evaluated; (3) attrition bias: Systematic differences in the withdrawal of patients from each of the two intervention groups; and (4) detection bias: Systematic differences in the ascertainment and recording of outcomes. The main focus of bias detection in the trials incorporated into an SR is (1) the randomization process, (2) the concealment of random allocation, (3) the use of blinding, and (4) the reporting/analysis of dropouts.

Binary outcomes (yes/no, alive/dead, presence/absence) within a study are usually compared by the relative risk (RR) or odds ratio (OR) statistic. The RR, OR, and mean difference of continuous variables are each an effect size of the intervention. If there is sufficient clinical similarity among the included studies, a summary value of the overall effect size of the intervention versus comparison treatments is estimated by MA. MA is a set of statistical techniques for combining results from different studies. The results of an MA are usually present in a figure called a *Forest plot* (Fig. 9-3). The far left column identifies the included studies; the center left columns display the observed data. The center right columns list the RRs with 95% CIs for the individual studies and the summary statistics. The horizontal lines and diamond shapes in the figures of the far right column are graphical representations of individual study RR and summary RR, respectively. There are also descriptive and inferential statistics concerning the statistical heterogeneity of the MA and the significance of the summary statistics.

An examination of Figure 9-3 shows that 11 of 15 individual comparisons had wide, nonsignificant CIs that touch or cross the RR of identity (RR = 1). However, the overall consistency of effect is easily seen with lidocaine being favored in only one study. The RR calculated from all studies was 7.31 with a 95% CI [4.16, 12.86]. The power of summary statistics to combine evidence is clear. About every seventh patient (92/637) who had a lidocaine spinal block had TNS; this risk of TNS was about seven times higher compared to other local anesthetics.[39]

The production of SRs comes from several sources. Many come from the individual initiative of researchers who publish their results as stand-alone reports in the journals of medicine and anesthesia. The American Society of Anesthesiologists has developed a process for the creation of practice parameters that includes among other things a variant form of SRs. The most prominent proponent of SRs is the Cochrane Collaboration, Oxford, United Kingdom. "The Cochrane Collaboration, established in 1993, is an international network of more than 28,000 dedicated people from over 100 countries. We work together to help health care providers, policy-makers, patients, their advocates and carers, make well-informed decisions about health care, based on the best available research evidence, by preparing, updating and promoting the accessibility of Cochrane Reviews—over 4,600 so far, published online in The Cochrane Library."[a] The Cochrane Collaboration has extensive documentation, tutorials, and software available electronically explaining the techniques of SRs and MA. There are more than 50 collaborative review groups with the Cochrane Collaboration that provide the editorial control and supervision of SRs; one of these, located in Copenhagen, is ".... responsible for producing and regularly updating reviews of interventions in the areas of anaesthesia, perioperative medicine, intensive care medicine, prehospital medicine, resuscitation, and emergency medicine"[b] [40].

There is a continuing expansion in the resources giving guidance in methodology.[41–44] Much of the improvement has been driven by epidemiologists and statisticians associated with the Cochrane Collaboration. Researchers publishing SRs have often adopted Cochrane methods and used Cochrane software. An important distinction between Cochrane and non-Cochrane SRs is an obligation by the authors to maintain and update Cochrane SRs periodically as new research reports become available; an SR is provisional, an update with new evidence always being possible. It has been noted that the initial estimates of benefit—the effect size—are generally inflated when compared to the effect size estimated when the SR is later updated.[45] Standards for the reporting of the clinical trials and observational studies and for the SR and MA techniques include (1) the 2010 CONSORT (Consolidated Standards of Reporting Trials) statement[46,47]; (2) the STROBE (Strengthening the Reporting of Observational Studies in Epidemiology) statement[48,49]; (3) the PRISMA (Preferred Reporting Items for Systematic reviews and Meta-Analyses) statement[50,51]; and (4) the MOOSE (Meta-analysis of Observational Studies in Epidemiology) statement.[52]

Interpretation of Results

Scientific studies do not end with the statistical test. The experimenter must submit an opinion as to the generalizability of his or her work to the rest of the world. Even if there is a statistically significant difference, the experimenter must decide if this difference is medically or physiologically important. Statistical significance does not always equate with biologic relevance. The questions an experimenter should ask about the interpretation of results are highly dependent on the specifics of the experiment. First, even small, clinically unimportant differences between groups can be detected if the sample size is sufficiently large. On the other hand, if the sample size is small, one must always worry that identified or unidentified confounding variables may explain any difference; as the sample size decreases, randomization is less successful in assuring homogenous groups. Second, if the experimental groups are given three or more doses of a drug, do the results suggest a steadily increasing or decreasing dose–response relationship? Suppose the observed effect for an intermediate dose is either much higher or much lower than that for both the highest and lowest doses; a dose–response relationship may exist, but some skepticism about the experimental methods is warranted. Third, for clinical studies comparing different drugs, devices, and operations on patient outcome, are the patients, clinical care, and studied therapies sufficiently similar to those provided at other locations to be of interest to a wide group of practitioners? This is the distinction between *efficacy* (does it work under the best (research) circumstances?) and *effectiveness* (does it work under the typical circumstances of routine clinical care?).

Finally, in comparing alternative therapies, the confidence that a claim for a superior therapy is true depends on the study design. The strength of the evidence concerning efficacy will be least for an anecdotal case report; next in importance will be a retrospective study, then a prospective series of patients compared with historical controls, and finally a randomized, controlled clinical trial. The greatest strength for a therapeutic claim is a series of randomized, controlled clinical trials confirming the same hypothesis.

[a]See http://www.cochrane.org/about-us

[b]See http://carg.cochrane.org/scope-our-work

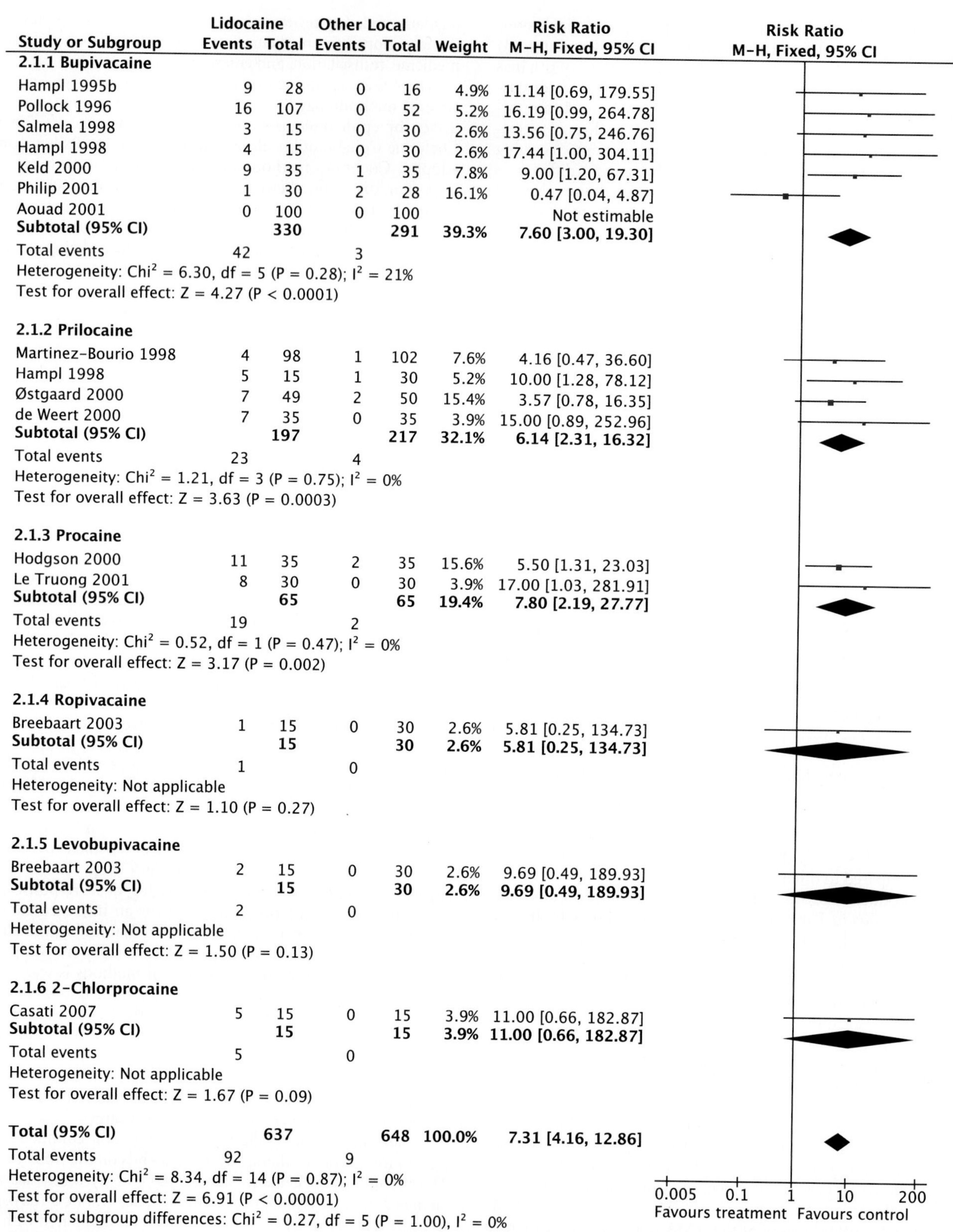

Study or Subgroup	Lidocaine Events	Lidocaine Total	Other Local Events	Other Local Total	Weight	Risk Ratio M-H, Fixed, 95% CI
2.1.1 Bupivacaine						
Hampl 1995b	9	28	0	16	4.9%	11.14 [0.69, 179.55]
Pollock 1996	16	107	0	52	5.2%	16.19 [0.99, 264.78]
Salmela 1998	3	15	0	30	2.6%	13.56 [0.75, 246.76]
Hampl 1998	4	15	0	30	2.6%	17.44 [1.00, 304.11]
Keld 2000	9	35	1	35	7.8%	9.00 [1.20, 67.31]
Philip 2001	1	30	2	28	16.1%	0.47 [0.04, 4.87]
Aouad 2001	0	100	0	100		Not estimable
Subtotal (95% CI)		**330**		**291**	**39.3%**	**7.60 [3.00, 19.30]**
Total events	42		3			
Heterogeneity: $Chi^2 = 6.30$, df = 5 (P = 0.28); $I^2 = 21\%$						
Test for overall effect: Z = 4.27 (P < 0.0001)						
2.1.2 Prilocaine						
Martinez-Bourio 1998	4	98	1	102	7.6%	4.16 [0.47, 36.60]
Hampl 1998	5	15	1	30	5.2%	10.00 [1.28, 78.12]
Østgaard 2000	7	49	2	50	15.4%	3.57 [0.78, 16.35]
de Weert 2000	7	35	0	35	3.9%	15.00 [0.89, 252.96]
Subtotal (95% CI)		**197**		**217**	**32.1%**	**6.14 [2.31, 16.32]**
Total events	23		4			
Heterogeneity: $Chi^2 = 1.21$, df = 3 (P = 0.75); $I^2 = 0\%$						
Test for overall effect: Z = 3.63 (P = 0.0003)						
2.1.3 Procaine						
Hodgson 2000	11	35	2	35	15.6%	5.50 [1.31, 23.03]
Le Truong 2001	8	30	0	30	3.9%	17.00 [1.03, 281.91]
Subtotal (95% CI)		**65**		**65**	**19.4%**	**7.80 [2.19, 27.77]**
Total events	19		2			
Heterogeneity: $Chi^2 = 0.52$, df = 1 (P = 0.47); $I^2 = 0\%$						
Test for overall effect: Z = 3.17 (P = 0.002)						
2.1.4 Ropivacaine						
Breebaart 2003	1	15	0	30	2.6%	5.81 [0.25, 134.73]
Subtotal (95% CI)		**15**		**30**	**2.6%**	**5.81 [0.25, 134.73]**
Total events	1		0			
Heterogeneity: Not applicable						
Test for overall effect: Z = 1.10 (P = 0.27)						
2.1.5 Levobupivacaine						
Breebaart 2003	2	15	0	30	2.6%	9.69 [0.49, 189.93]
Subtotal (95% CI)		**15**		**30**	**2.6%**	**9.69 [0.49, 189.93]**
Total events	2		0			
Heterogeneity: Not applicable						
Test for overall effect: Z = 1.50 (P = 0.13)						
2.1.6 2-Chlorprocaine						
Casati 2007	5	15	0	15	3.9%	11.00 [0.66, 182.87]
Subtotal (95% CI)		**15**		**15**	**3.9%**	**11.00 [0.66, 182.87]**
Total events	5		0			
Heterogeneity: Not applicable						
Test for overall effect: Z = 1.67 (P = 0.09)						
Total (95% CI)		**637**		**648**	**100.0%**	**7.31 [4.16, 12.86]**
Total events	92		9			
Heterogeneity: $Chi^2 = 8.34$, df = 14 (P = 0.87); $I^2 = 0\%$						
Test for overall effect: Z = 6.91 (P < 0.00001)						
Test for subgroup differences: $Chi^2 = 0.27$, df = 5 (P = 1.00), $I^2 = 0\%$						

FIGURE 9-3. A Forest plot illustrates the relative strength of treatment effect across multiple studies. The point estimate for each study is represented by a square with 95% CIs represented by horizontal lines. In a Forest plot of RRs or ORs, the *x*-axis of the graph is on a logarithmic scale so that CIs are symmetrical about the point estimate. The vertical line of no effect is at 1. The area of each square is proportional to the weight of that study in the summary RR. The summary RRs are diamonds whose lateral points indicate the 95% CI of the summary value. (This figure is reprinted with permission and is published within a Cochrane Review in the Cochrane Database of Systematic Reviews 2011, Issue 12. Cochrane Reviews are regularly updated as new evidence emerges and in response to comments and criticisms, and the Cochrane Database of Systematic Reviews should be consulted for the most recent version of the review. The source systematic review is: Zaric D, Pace NL. Transient neurologic symptoms (TNS) following spinal anaesthesia with lidocaine versus other local anaesthetics. *Cochrane Database Syst Rev.* 2009, Issue 2. Art.No.: CD003006. DOI: http://dx.doi.org/10.1002/14651858.CD003006.pub3.)

CONCLUSIONS

Statistical Resources

Accompanying the exponential growth of medical information since World War II has been the creation of a wealth of biostatistical knowledge. Textbooks oriented toward medical statistics and with expositions of basic, intermediate, and advanced statistics abound.[53–58] There are new journals of biomedical statistics, including *Trials, Statistics in Medicine,* and *Statistical Methods in Medical Research,* whose audiences are both statisticians and
8 biomedical researchers. Some medical journals, for example, the *British Medical Journal,* regularly publish expositions of both basic and newer advanced statistical methods. Extensive Internet resources including electronic textbooks of basic statistical methods, online statistical calculators, standard data sets, reviews of statistical software, and so on can be easily found. High-performance statistical software is freely available from the R Foundation for Statistical Computing, Vienna, Austria.[c]

Statistics and Anesthesia

One intent of this chapter is to present the basic scope of support that the discipline of statistics can provide to anesthesia research. Journals of anesthesia now include many newer methods that have not been described. To mention just four: (1) studies of the pharmacokinetics and pharmacokinetics of a drug or a combination of drugs typically use linear mixed effects or generalized linear mixed effects models; (2) techniques of survival analysis are applied to hospital discharge times or postoperative morbidity/mortality outcomes; (3) methods of interim analysis or sequential trial design are used in RCTs to stop futile or dangerous treatments; and (4) the description and implications of diagnostic tests.

Although an intuitive understanding of certain basic principles is emphasized, these basic principles are not necessarily simple and have been developed by statisticians with great mathematical rigor. Academic anesthesia needs more workers to immerse themselves in these statistical fundamentals. Having done so, these statistically knowledgeable academic anesthesiologists will be prepared to improve their own research projects, to assist their colleagues in research, to efficiently seek consultation from the professional statistician, to strengthen the editorial review of journal articles, and to expound to the clinical reader the whys and wherefores of statistics. The clinical reader also needs to expend his or her own effort to acquire some basic statistical skills. Journals are increasingly difficult to understand without some basic statistical understanding. Some clinical problems can be best understood with a perspective based on probability. Finally, understanding principles of experimental design can prevent premature acceptances of new therapies from faulty studies.

References

1. Cobb LA, Thomas GI, Dillard DH, et al. An evaluation of internal-mammary-artery ligation by a double-blind technic. *N Engl J Med.* 1959;260:1115–1118.
2. Sacks H, Chalmers TC, Smith HJ. Randomized versus historical controls for clinical trials. *Am J Med.* 1982;72:233–240.
3. Kunz R, Oxman AD. The unpredictability paradox: Review of empirical comparisons of randomised and non-randomised clinical trials. *BMJ.* 1998;317:1185–1190.

[c]See http://www.R-project.org

4. Herbison P, Hay-Smith J, Gillespie WJ. Different methods of allocation to groups in randomized trials are associated with different levels of bias. A meta-epidemiological study. *J Clin Epidemiol.* 2011;64:1070–1075.
5. Schulz KF, Chalmers I, Hayes RJ, et al. Empirical evidence of bias. Dimensions of methodological quality associated with estimates of treatment effects in controlled trials. *JAMA.* 1995;273:408–412.
6. Hill AB. The environment and disease: Association or causation? *Proc R Soc Med.* 1965;58:295–300.
7. Little RJ. Calibrated Bayes: A Bayes/Frequentist roadmap. *Am Stat.* 2006;60:213–223.
8. Sterne JA, Davey Smith G. Sifting the evidence: What's wrong with significance tests? *BMJ.* 2001;322:226–231.
9. Ioannidis JP. Why most published research findings are false. *PLoS Med.* 2005;2:e124.
10. Ioannidis JP. Contradicted and initially stronger effects in highly cited clinical research. *JAMA.* 2005;294:218–228.
11. Ioannidis JP. Effect of formal statistical significance on the credibility of observational associations. *Am J Epidemiol.* 2008;168:374–383, discussion 384–390.
12. Katki HA. Invited commentary: Evidence-based evaluation of p values and Bayes factors. *Am J Epidemiol.* 2008;168:384–388.
13. Hanley JA, Lippman-Hand A. If nothing goes wrong, is everything all right? Interpreting zero numerators. *JAMA.* 1983;249:1743–1745.
14. Tuyl F, Gerlach R, Mengersen K. A comparison of Bayes-Laplace, Jeffreys, and other priors: The case of zero events. *Am Stat.* 2008;62:40–44.
15. Anscombe FJ. Graphs in statistical analysis. *Am Stat.* 1973;27:17–21.
16. Katz MH. Multivariable analysis: A primer for readers of medical research. *Ann Intern Med.* 2003;138:644–650.
17. Brotman DJ, Walker E, Lauer MS, et al. In search of fewer independent risk factors. *Arch Intern Med.* 2005;165:138–145.
18. Eberhart LHJ, Morin AM. Risk scores for predicting postoperative nausea and vomiting are clinically useful tools and should be used in every patient: Con - 'life is really simple, but we insist on making it complicated'. *Eur J Anaesthesiol.* 2011;28:155–159.
19. Kranke P. Effective management of postoperative nausea and vomiting: Let us practise what we preach! *Eur J Anaesthesiol.* 2011;28:152–154.
20. Pierre S. Risk scores for predicting post-operative nausea and vomiting are clinically useful tools and should be used in every patient: 'Don't throw the baby out with the bathwater'. *Eur J Anaesthesiol.* 2011;28:160–163.
21. Pace NL, Eberhart LHJ, Kranke PR. Quantifying prognosis with risk predictions. *Eur J Anaesthesiol.* 2012;29:7–16.
22. Pace NL. Independent predictors from stepwise logistic regression may be nothing more than publishable p values. *Anesth Analg.* 2008;107:1775–1778.
23. Cook NR. Statistical evaluation of prognostic versus diagnostic models: Beyond the ROC curve. *Clin Chem.* 2008;54:17–23.
24. Cook NR, Ridker PM. Advances in measuring the effect of individual predictors of cardiovascular risk: The role of reclassification measures. *Ann Intern Med.* 2009;150:795–802.
25. Steyerberg EW, Vickers AJ, Cook NR, et al. Assessing the performance of prediction models: A framework for traditional and novel measures. *Epidemiology.* 2010;21:128–138.
26. Siontis GC, Tzoulaki I, Ioannidis JP. Predicting death: An empirical evaluation of predictive tools for mortality. *Arch Intern Med.* 2011;171:1721–1726.
27. Wyatt JC, Altman DG. Prognostic models: Clinically useful or quickly forgotten? *Br Med J.* 1995;311:1539–1541.
28. Guyatt G. A randomized control trial of right-heart catheterization in critically ill patients. Ontario Intensive Care Study Group. *J Intensive Care Med.* 1991;6:91–95.
29. Connors AF Jr, Speroff T, Dawson NV, et al. The effectiveness of right heart catheterization in the initial care of critically ill patients. SUPPORT Investigators. *JAMA.* 1996;276:889–897.
30. Wijeysundera DN, Beattie WS, Austin PC, et al. Epidural anaesthesia and survival after intermediate-to-high risk non-cardiac surgery: A population-based cohort study. *Lancet.* 2008;372:562–569.
31. Gayat E, Pirracchio R, Resche-Rigon M, et al. Propensity scores in intensive care and anaesthesiology literature: A systematic review. *Intensive Care Med.* 2010;36:1993–2003.
32. Pace NL. Prevention of succinylcholine myalgias: A meta-analysis. *Anesth Analg.* 1990;70:477–483.
33. Biondi-Zoccai G, Lotrionte M, Landoni G, et al. The rough guide to systematic reviews and meta-analyses. *HSR Proc Intensive Care Cardiovasc Anesth.* 2011;3:161–173.
34. Carlisle JB. Systematic reviews: How they work and how to use them. *Anaesthesia.* 2007;62:702–707.
35. Kranke P. Evidence-based practice: How to perform and use systematic reviews for clinical decision-making. *Eur J Anaesthesiol.* 2010;27:763–772.
36. Pace NL. Research methods for meta-analyses. *Best Pract Res Clin Anaesthesiol.* 2011;25:523–533.
37. Pace N. The meta-analysis of a systematic review. In: Møller A, Pedersen T, Cracknell J, eds. *Evidence-Based Anaesthesia and Intensive Care.* New York, NY: Cambridge University Press; 2006:46–60.

38. Harvey S, Young D, Brampton W, et al. Pulmonary artery catheters for adult patients in intensive care. *Cochrane Database Syst Rev.* 2006;3:CD003408.
39. Zaric D, Pace NL. Transient neurologic symptoms (TNS) following spinal anaesthesia with lidocaine versus other local anaesthetics. *Cochrane Database Syst Rev.* 2009;4:CD003006.
40. Pedersen T, Møller A. The Cochrane Collaboration and the Cochrane Anaesthesia Review Group. In: Møller A, Pedersen T, Cracknell J, eds. *Evidence-Based Anaesthesia and Intensive Care.* New York, NY: Cambridge University Press; 2006: 77–87.
41. Higgins JPT, Green S, eds. *Cochrane Handbook for Systematic Reviews of Interventions Version 5.1.0.* The Cochrane Collaboration; 2011.
42. Cooper H, Hedges LV, Valentine JC. *The Handbook of Research Synthesis and Meta-analysis.* 2nd ed. New York: Russell Sage Foundation; 2009.
43. Eden J, Levit L, Berg A, et al. Finding what works. In: *Health Care: Standards for Systematic Reviews.* Washington, DC: The National Academies Press; 2011.
44. Egger M, Smith GD, Altman DG. *Systematic Reviews in Health Care: Meta-analysis in Context.* 2nd ed. London: BMJ Books; 2001.
45. Pereira TV, Ioannidis JP. Statistically significant meta-analyses of clinical trials have modest credibility and inflated effects. *J Clin Epidemiol.* 2011;64:1060–1069.
46. Moher D, Hopewell S, Schulz KF, et al. CONSORT 2010 explanation and elaboration: Updated guidelines for reporting parallel group randomised trials. *BMJ.* 2010;340:c869.
47. Schulz KF, Altman DG, Moher D. CONSORT 2010 statement: Updated guidelines for reporting parallel group randomised trials. *BMJ.* 2010;340:c332.
48. Vandenbroucke JP, von Elm E, Altman DG, et al. Strengthening the Reporting of Observational Studies in Epidemiology (STROBE): Explanation and elaboration. *PLoS Med.* 2007;4:e297.
49. von Elm E, Altman DG, Egger M, et al. Strengthening the Reporting of Observational Studies in Epidemiology (STROBE) statement: Guidelines for reporting observational studies. *BMJ.* 2007;335:806–808.
50. Liberati A, Altman DG, Tetzlaff J, et al. The PRISMA statement for reporting systematic reviews and meta-analyses of studies that evaluate healthcare interventions: Explanation and elaboration. *BMJ.* 2009;339:b2700.
51. Moher D, Liberati A, Tetzlaff J, et al. Preferred reporting items for systematic reviews and meta-analyses: The PRISMA statement. *BMJ.* 2009;339:b2535.
52. Stroup DF, Berlin JA, Morton SC, et al. Meta-analysis of observational studies in epidemiology: A proposal for reporting. Meta-analysis of Observational Studies in Epidemiology (MOOSE) group. *JAMA.* 2000;283:2008–2012.
53. Campbell MJ, Machin D, Walters SJ. *Medical Statistics: A Textbook for the Health Sciences.* 4th ed. Chichester, England: John Wiley & Sons; 2007.
54. Dalgaard P. *Introductory Statistics with R.* 2nd ed. New York, NY: Springer; 2008.
55. Dawson B, Trapp R. *Basic & Clinical Biostatistics.* 4th ed. New York, NY: McGraw-Hill; 2004.
56. Glantz SA. *Primer of Biostatistics.* 7th ed. New York, NY: McGraw-Hill; 2012.
57. Guyatt G, Rennie D, Meade MO, et al. *Users Guides' Manual for Evidence-Based Clinical Practice.* 2nd ed. New York, NY: McGraw-Hill; 2008.
58. Riffenburgh RH. *Statistics in Medicine.* 2nd ed. San Diego, CA: Academic Press; 2006.

SECTION III

Anatomy and Physiology

CHAPTER

10 Cardiac Anatomy and Physiology

PAUL S. PAGEL • JOHN P. KAMPINE • DAVID F. STOWE

Key Points

1. The mechanical capabilities of the heart are determined by its cartilaginous skeleton, myocardial fiber orientation, valves, coronary blood supply, and conduction system.
2. The cardiac myocyte is engineered for contraction and relaxation, but not protein synthesis.
3. Alterations in sarcomere muscle tension and length as observed in isolated cardiac muscle are translated to changes in pressure and volume in the intact heart as applied by the Law of Laplace.
4. The pressure–volume diagram provides a useful framework for the analysis of systolic and diastolic function.
5. The end-systolic and end-diastolic pressure–volume relations determine the operating range of each cardiac chamber.
6. The determinants of pump performance are heart rate, preload, afterload, and myocardial contractility.
7. The quantity of blood that a chamber contains immediately before contraction is termed "preload."
8. The external resistance to the emptying of a chamber after the onset of contraction is known as "afterload."
9. Myocardial contractility is the force of contraction under controlled heart rate and loading conditions and may be quantified using the pressure–volume relation, isovolumic contraction, and ejection phase analysis.
10. The ability of a cardiac chamber to effectively collect blood at a normal filling pressure is defined by its diastolic function.
11. No single index completely describes diastolic function because this phase of the cardiac cycle is a complicated sequence of temporally related, but heterogeneous events.
12. Heart failure may be due to left ventricular diastolic dysfunction in as many as 50% of patients.
13. Invasive analysis of diastolic function may be conducted using the pressure–volume model.
14. Transmitral and pulmonary venous blood flow velocities are commonly used to noninvasively measure diastolic function.
15. The restraining forces of the pericardium are important determinants of chamber filling and ventricular interdependence.
16. The atria act as reservoirs, conduits, and contractile chambers.

Multimedia

Coronary Blood Flow

Laplace

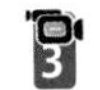
Pressure–Volume Loop

INTRODUCTION

The heart is a phasic, variable speed, muscular pump that is electrically self-sustaining and provides its own blood supply. The two pair of atria and ventricles of the heart are elastic chambers that are arranged to supply equal amounts of blood to the pulmonary and systemic vasculature. Atrial and ventricular myocardium responds to stimulation rate and muscle stretch before (preload) and after (afterload) contraction begins. Coronary arterial blood vessels supply oxygen and metabolic substrates to the heart. The mechanical characteristics of the myocardium and its response to changes in autonomic nervous system activity allow the heart to adapt to rapidly changing physiologic requirements. The contractile function of the atria and ventricles and the ability of these chambers to adequately fill without excessive pressure determine overall cardiac performance. Thus, abnormalities in systolic or diastolic function may lead to heart failure. Comprehensive knowledge of cardiac anatomy and physiology is crucial for modern anesthesia practice. This chapter describes the fundamentals of cardiac anatomy and physiology, and fluency in this subject is essential for modern anesthesia practice. The authors will focus on the left atria and ventricle (LA and LV, respectively) for the vast majority of the subsequent discussion.

GROSS ANATOMY

Architecture

1 A flexible, cartilaginous structure forms the heart's skeleton and is composed of the annuli of the cardiac valves, the aortic and pulmonary arterial (PA) roots, the central fibrous body, and the left and right fibrous trigones. This foundation of cartilage creates support for the valves and maintains the heart's structural integrity in the presence of developed internal pressures. Some superficial subepicardial muscles also insert into the cartilaginous skeleton, but most of the atrial and ventricular muscles directly arise from and insert within adjacent surrounding myocardium. The atrial and ventricular myocardia are continuously interwoven and cannot be separated into distinct "layers." The atria contain two, relatively thin, orthogonally oriented bands of myocardium, whereas the LV and, to a lesser extent the right ventricle (RV), consist of the interdigitating deep sinospiral, the superficial sinospiral, and the superficial bulbospiral muscles (Fig. 10-1). The angle of the myocardial fibers changes across the thickness of the ventricular myocardium from the endocardium to the epicardium. Subendocardial and subepicardial muscle fibers of the LV are oriented in perpendicular, oblique, and helical planes from the heart's base (superior in the mediastinum) to its apex. This arrangement reverses direction at approximately the LV's midpoint, creating an overall fiber architecture that appears as a flattened "figure of eight" or a "raked turban." This orientation allows both LV chamber shortening along the heart's longitudinal axis and a distinctive "twisting" motion. This latter effect substantially enhances LV systolic force, and loss of this helical–rotational action contributes to a decrease in ejection fraction during the development of congestive heart failure (CHF).[1] Elastic recoil of systolic twist during LV relaxation is also important for early diastolic filling, especially during hypovolemia and exercise.[2] In contrast to the subepicardial and subendocardial layers, midmyocardial fibers are arranged in a circumferential orientation and act to reduce chamber diameter during contraction.

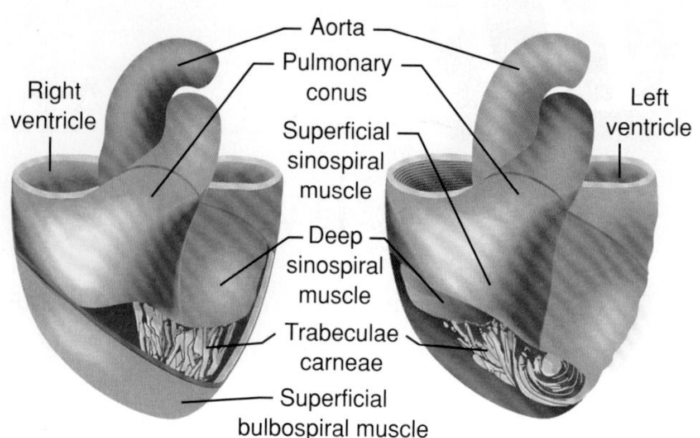

FIGURE 10-1. Illustration depicting the components of the myocardium. The outer muscle layers pull the apex of the heart toward the base. The inner circumferential layers constrict the lumen, particularly of the LV. (Reproduced with permission from: Barash PG, Cullen BF, Stoelting RK, et al. *Clinical Anesthesia*, 6th ed., Lippincott Williams & Wilkins, Figure 10-1, p. 210.)

The LV free walls taper in thickness from base to apex because the relative amount of midmyocardium gradually declines. LV and RV subendocardium and LV midmyocardium extend from the LV anterior wall to form the interventricular septum. As a result, the septum thickens toward the LV chamber during contraction under normal conditions. However, RV distention or chronic pressure-overload may produce paradoxical motion of the interventricular septum. Notably, regional differences in LV wall thickness and fiber orientation contribute to load-dependent alterations in LV mechanics.[3] The trabeculae carneae are irregular ridges of subendocardium of unknown significance that are present within the LV apex and, to a greater extent, within the RV chamber.

The LV apex and interventricular septum are relatively fixed in space within the mediastinum, whereas the lateral and posterior walls shift position to the anterior and the right during contraction. This motion effectively changes the LV longitudinal axis from a plane that favors LV filling to a position that facilitates ejection. The systolic movement of the lateral and posterior LV walls also produces the palpable point of maximum impulse. The LV base descends toward the apex during systole as a result of the combined effects of subendocardial and subepicardial contraction, papillary muscle shortening, and recoil caused by ejection of blood into the aortic root. Taken as a whole, synchronous activation of the LV causes its long axis to shorten, reduces its chamber diameter, and produces rotation of its apex in an anterior-right direction (Fig. 10-2). Differential changes in wall tension also create an apex-to-base intraventricular pressure gradient during LV ejection; this effect serves to enhance the transfer efficiency of stroke volume from the LV to the aortic root.

The crescent-shaped RV is anatomically anterior and to the right of the LV. This chamber propels deoxygenated venous blood into the relatively compliant, low-pressure PA tree. As a result, the RV wall is thinner and contains fewer cardiac myocytes compared with the LV, which is subjected to substantially greater wall stress during ejection of blood into the high-pressure systemic vasculature. Embryologically distinct inflow and outflow tracts exist in the RV, which causes RV contraction to be less temporally uniform than the LV. The RV relies on the interventricular septum against which the RV free wall contracts. The LV also contributes to RV contractility. The combination of these factors provides a mechanical advantage to the RV that compensates for its thinner

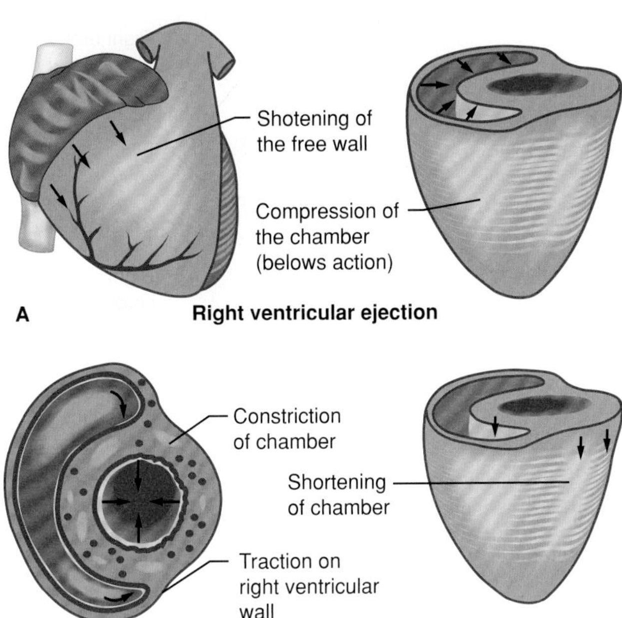

FIGURE 10-2. Illustration depicting the contraction characteristics and modes of emptying of the RV and LV. The volumes ejected by each ventricle are equal, but the LV requires a more circumferential muscular wall to eject its volume at a pressure that is approximately four to five times greater than that in the right ventricle. (Reproduced with permission from: Barash PG, Cullen BF, Stoelting RK, et al. *Clinical Anesthesia*, 6th ed., Lippincott Williams and Wilkins, Figure 10-2, p. 210.)

wall dimension, thereby allowing it to pump a stroke volume that is equal to the LV stroke volume during each beat. Nevertheless, the RV more easily decompensates with acute increases in afterload than the LV because the RV is able to produce less than 20% of the total pressure–volume (stroke) work than the thicker, more muscular LV. However, the RV is highly compliant and is able to accommodate to acute changes in intraventricular volume to a greater degree than the LV.

Valve Structure

Two pairs of translucent, macroscopically avascular valves guarantee unidirectional movement of blood through the heart. The pulmonic and aortic valves separate the RV and LV from the PA and aorta, respectively. These valves open and close and operate passively with changes in pressure resulting from RV and LV contraction and relaxation. The pulmonic valve leaflets are named for their anatomic locations (right, left, and anterior) within the mediastinum, whereas each aortic valve leaflet is identified on the basis of a corresponding coronary artery (e.g., the right coronary leaflet lies adjacent to the ostium of the right coronary artery). At the time of maximal blood flow during ejection, the orifice areas of the pulmonic and aortic valves are nearly equivalent to the corresponding annulus cross-sectional areas. The sinuses of Valsalva are dilated segments in the proximal aortic root that are located immediately superior to each aortic leaflet. Hydraulic flow vortices (eddy currents) occur within the sinuses of Valsalva that prevent adherence of the valve leaflets to the walls of the aortic root during systole and also aid closure of the valve by facilitating leaflet mobility during diastole.[4] These actions assure that the aortic valve leaflets do not inadvertently occlude the coronary ostia. Sinuses of Valsalva are absent in the proximal PA.

The mitral valve is located between the LA and the LV, contains two leaflets (the oval-shaped anterior and the crescent-shaped posterior), and resembles a saddle when viewed in three dimensions. Coaptation of the leaflets occurs along a central curve with the posterior leaflet creating its concave border. Despite the differences in their shapes, the anterior and posterior leaflets have similar cross-sectional areas because the posterior leaflet occupies a greater percentage of the annular circumference. Anterior–lateral and posterior–medial commissures connect the leaflets and are located above the corresponding papillary muscles. The mitral valve opens in response to a positive pressure gradient between the LA and LV that occurs during the late phase of relaxation. This process is facilitated by untwisting and elastic recoil of the LV as the chamber relaxes. Closure of the leaflets occurs as retrograde blood flow moves toward the valve during early systole. The chordae tendineae act as "cable stays" to prevent leaflet prolapse and inversion during LV contraction. Primary and secondary chordae tendineae are attached to the leaflet edges and bodies, respectively, whereas tertiary chordae insert into the distal posterior leaflet or the myocardium adjacent to the annulus. The papillary muscles are composed of subendocardial myocardium that contract with the LV. Each papillary muscle has chordal attachments to both mitral leaflets; contraction of the papillary muscles effectively tensions the chordae. As a result, motion of the leaflets beyond the coaptation zone is restricted. Closure of the mitral leaflets is also facilitated by tightening of the annulus because the surrounding subepicardium contracts in a sphincter-like manner. The mitral valve apparatus is critical for overall LV function. The valve apparatus guarantees that blood flow from the LA to the LV is unidirectional because blood is prevented from refluxing into the LA and pulmonary veins during LV contraction. Thus, ischemia or infarction of a papillary muscle may cause dysfunction of the mitral apparatus and is often accompanied by acute mitral regurgitation. In addition, the mitral apparatus plays an essential role in LV systolic function because papillary muscle shortening assists LV apical contraction. This latter action is particularly important during mitral valve replacement because severing attachments between the chordae tendineae and the papillary muscles is invariably associated with a reduction in LV ejection fraction.

The tricuspid valve is composed of anterior, posterior, and septal leaflets, and assures unidirectional movement of blood from the RA and RV. The posterior leaflet is usually smaller than the anterior and septal leaflets. The morphologic RV may be distinguished from the LV by the presence of a septal papillary muscle in patients with transposition of the great vessels and other forms of congenital heart disease. The moderator band is a lateral segment of myocardium stretching between the anterior and septal papillary muscles and separates the embryologic RV inflow and outflow tracts. The RV often has coarser trabeculae carnae than the LV, but the physiologic implications of these differences in subendocardial structure remain a mystery. In contrast to the mitral valve, the tricuspid valve does not have a collagenous annulus. Instead, the tricuspid leaflets originate from the atrioventricular groove that separates the RA from the RV. Notably, the atrioventricular groove also contains the proximal right coronary artery, and this vessel must be carefully avoided during tricuspid valve repair or replacement surgery.

Coronary Blood Supply

The left anterior descending, left circumflex, and right coronary arteries (LAD, LCCA, and RCA, respectively) supply blood to the

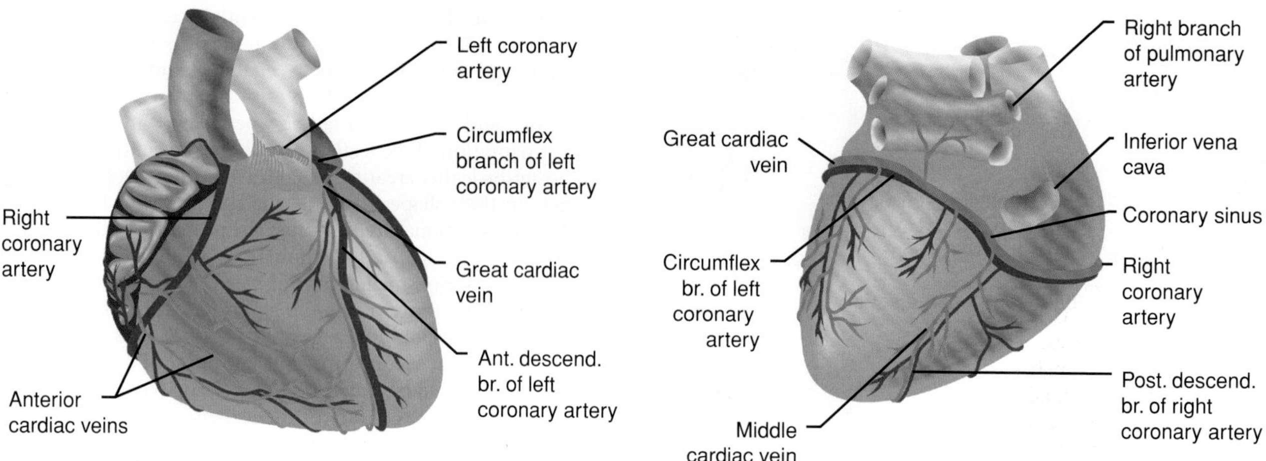

FIGURE 10-3. An anterior view of the heart **(left)** shows right coronary and left anterior descending coronary arteries. A posterior view **(right)** shows left circumflex and posterior descending coronary arteries. The anterior cardiac veins from the RV and the coronary sinus, which drain primarily the LV, empty into the RA. (Reproduced with permission from: Barash PG, Cullen BF, Stoelting RK, et al. *Clinical Anesthesia*, 6th ed., Lippincott Williams and Wilkins, Figure 10-16, p. 222.)

LV (Fig. 10-3). Most coronary blood flow to the LV myocardium occurs during diastole because aortic blood pressure is greater than LV pressure. A critical stenosis or acute occlusion of one of these three vessels may produce myocardial ischemia or infarction accompanied by abnormal regional contractile function based on the known distribution of each coronary artery's blood supply. The medial LV anterior wall, the anterior two-thirds of the interventricular septum, and the LV apex are supplied by the LCA and its branches; the anterior and posterior aspects of the lateral wall are perfused by the LCCA; and the medial portions of the posterior wall and the posterior one-third of the interventricular septum are supplied by the RCA. The "dominance" of the coronary circulation is determined on the basis of which major coronary artery feeds the posterior descending coronary artery (PDA). A "right dominant" circulation occurs when the RCA supplies blood to the PDA and is observed in approximately 80% of patients. A "left dominant" circulation in which the PDA is supplied by the LCCA is observed in the remaining 20% of patients. Distal connections or collateral blood vessels between the major coronary arteries may also provide perfusion to regions of myocardium that lie distal to a severe stenosis or occlusion. A single coronary artery (2:1 ratio of RCA to LCCA) provides blood flow to the posterior–medial papillary muscle in two-thirds of patients. Thus, RCA or LCCA occlusion may produce acute posterior–medial papillary muscle ischemia or infarction and, as a result, new mitral valve dysfunction. However, this is not always the case, as both vessels perfuse the posterior–medial papillary muscle in the remaining patients.[5] In contrast to the posterior–medial papillary muscle, the anterior–lateral papillary muscle has a dual blood supply (LAD and LCCA), rendering this papillary muscle less susceptible to ischemic dysfunction than its counterpart.

RA, LA, and RV coronary perfusion occurs during both systole and diastole because aortic blood pressure always exceeds the pressure within each of these chambers (Fig. 10-4). Most of the RV is supplied by the RCA and its branches; the RV anterior wall is also perfused by distal diagonal and septal branches of the LAD. These observations indicate that either RCA or LAD occlusion may lead to RV dysfunction. Branches of the LCCA are

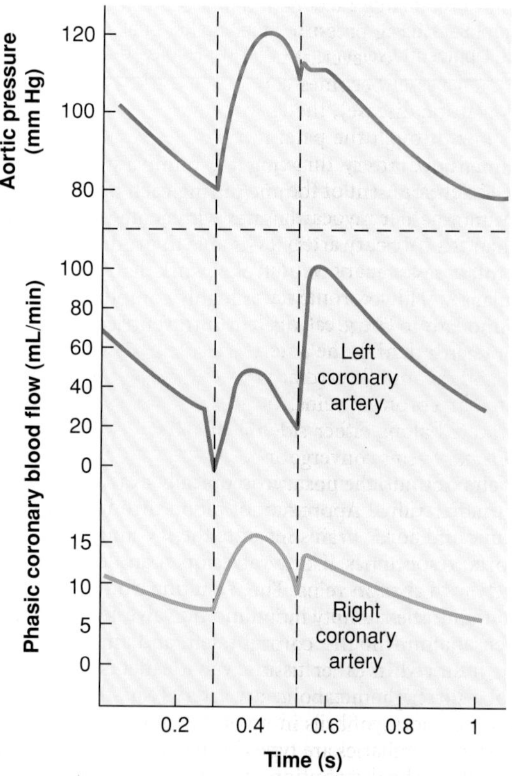

FIGURE 10-4. Schematic representation of blood flow in the left and right coronary arteries during phases of the cardiac cycle. Note that most left coronary flow occurs during diastole, while right coronary flow (and coronary sinus flow) occurs mostly during late systole and early diastole. (Reproduced with permission from: Barash PG, Cullen BF, Stoelting RK, et al. *Clinical Anesthesia*, 6th ed., Lippincott Williams and Wilkins, Figure 10-19, p. 224.)

the major sources of blood supply to the LA. As a result, LCCA occlusion often causes LA contractile dysfunction, whereas a compensatory increase in LA contractility may be observed if the LAD becomes acutely occluded.[6] The RA is supplied by branches of both the RCA and the LCCA. For example, the sinoatrial (SA) node may be perfused by either the RCA (55% of patients) or the LCCA (45%). The atrioventricular (AV) node is more commonly supplied by the RCA, but also may be perfused by the LCCA depending on the right or left dominance of the coronary circulation. The clinical implications of these anatomical relationships are clear: Critical stenosis or acute occlusion of either the RCA or LCCA may interrupt normal conduction and cause bradyarrhythmias.

The proximal branches of the RCA, LCCA, and LAD are located on the epicardial surface of the heart and give rise to multiple intramural vessels that penetrate perpendicularly or obliquely deep into the ventricular walls. Except for the thin tissue layer on the endocardial surface, the heart's blood supply is almost entirely derived from these three major coronary arteries. The penetrating branches divide into dense capillary networks located roughly along the courses of the myocardial bundles. Arterial branches with diameters between 50 and 500 μm form interconnecting anastomoses throughout the endocardium of the RV and LV walls (Fig. 10-5). Another network of subendocardial vessels between 100 and 200 μm in diameter forms a plexus of deep anastomoses. A coronary collateral circulation may also arise from different branches of the same coronary artery or from branches of two different coronary arteries. Flow through a coronary collateral is usually negligible because the driving pressure at the two ends of the connection is nearly equal. However, if the artery supplying one branch of a collateral vessel becomes severely stenotic or occluded (e.g., atherosclerotic disease), the large pressure reduction will divert blood flow through the patent artery and into the distribution of the occluded artery through the collateral vessel. Thus, the extent of development of the coronary collateral circulation may determine whether myocardial ischemia or infarction is likely in patients with coronary artery disease.

The main coronary venous drainage tends to retrace the course of the major coronary arteries along the AV and interventricular grooves. The great cardiac vein (that runs along the AV groove and the LAD), the anterior cardiac vein (located with the RCA), and the middle cardiac vein (associated with PDA) are the three major coronary veins. In general, there are two coronary veins located along either side of each coronary arterial branch. The coronary veins converge and terminate in the coronary sinus, which empties into the posterior aspect of the right atrium above the tricuspid valve. Approximately 85% of the total coronary blood flow to the LV drains into the coronary sinus. The remaining blood flow empties directly into the atrial and ventricular cavities via the Thebesian veins. The RV veins drain into the anterior cardiac veins; these empty individually into the right atrium.

The structure of the coronary capillary network is similar to that observed in other tissue beds. Because the heart has an exceptionally high metabolic demand, the density of capillary blood vessels to myofibrils in myocardium is approximately 1:1, and adjacent capillaries are typically separated by the diameter of one myocyte. The distribution of capillaries is quite uniform and ranges between 3,000 and 4,000/mm^2 of tissue. Notably, capillary density is reduced in the AV node and interventricular septum; this observation may explain why the conducting system is more susceptible to ischemia. As in other capillary beds, coronary capillaries are the sites for exchange of O_2 and CO_2, and for the movement of larger molecules across the endothelium without the impediment of vascular smooth muscle.

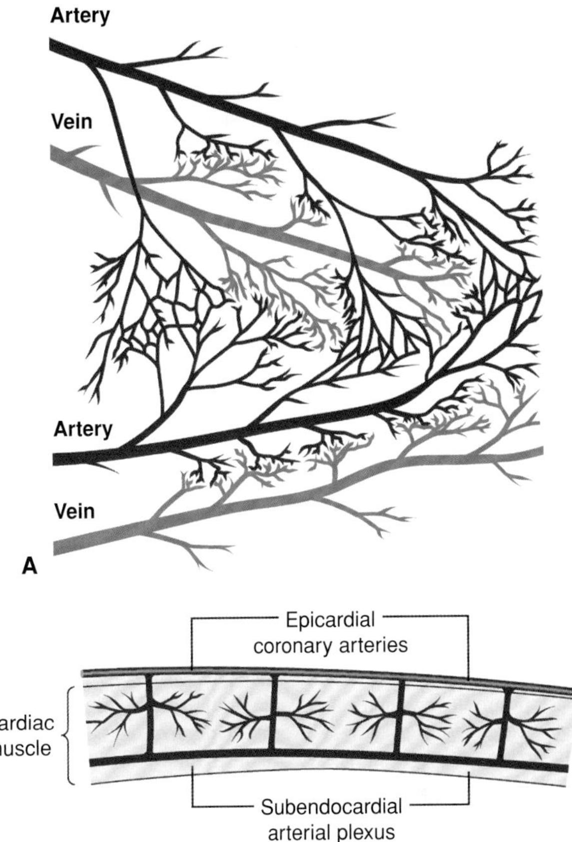

FIGURE 10-5. A: Diagram of the arterial-to-arterial and venous-to-venous anastomoses of the coronary arterial system, which allows diversion of flow if one distribution becomes blocked. **B:** Diagram of the epicardial coronary vessels lying on the cardiac muscle surface, the penetrating deep vessels, and the subendocardial arterial plexus connecting the deep vessels. (Reproduced with permission from: Barash PG, Cullen BF, Stoelting RK, et al. *Clinical Anesthesia*, 6th ed., *Lippincott Williams and Wilkins*, Figure 10-17, p. 223.)

Impulse Conduction

How the heart is electrically activated is essential to its mechanical performance. The primary cardiac pacemaker is the SA node, although declines in firing rate, delays or blockade of normal conduction, or the presence of secondary pacemakers (e.g., AV node, bundle of His) may supersede the dominance of SA automaticity. The initial SA node depolarization is rapidly transmitted across the RA to the AV node by the anterior, middle (Wenckebach), and posterior (Thorel) internodal pathways. The SA node depolarization is also transmitted to the LA through the atrial septum by Bachmann's bundle (a branch of the anterior internodal pathway). It is important to note that examination of myocyte histology rarely differentiates the internodal pathways, although these structures may be clearly identified in the electrophysiology laboratory. The atria are electrically isolated from the ventricles by the heart's cartilaginous skeleton. As a result, atrial depolarization is directed solely to the RV and the LV through the AV node. Because AV node conduction is relatively slow compared with the pathways proximal and distal to it, the AV node is responsible for the sequential contraction pattern of the atria and the ventricles. Clearly, accessory pathways that bypass the AV node and establish abnormal conduction between the atria and ventricles may produce supraventricular tachyarrhythmias. This is the putative mechanism by which the bundle of Kent produces Wolff–Parkinson–White syndrome. The AV node transmits its depolarization to the His bundle, which further transmits the signal to the RV and LV via the right and left bundle branches, respectively, through Purkinje fibers within the endocardium. The conduction velocity through the His bundle, the bundle branches, and the Purkinje network is very rapid, assuring coordinated RV and LV depolarization and contraction. In contrast, exogenous cardiac pacing does not rely on the normal conduction sequence and may cause dyssynchronous LV activation, which may be misinterpreted as a new ischemia-induced regional wall motion abnormality during cardiac surgery. Similarly, contractile dyssynchrony produced by chronic RV apical pacing may also lead to LV dysfunction.[7] Indeed, cardiac resynchronization therapy in patients with CHF is based on reestablishing the normal sequence of electrical activation because LV contractile synchrony is restored.[8]

CORONARY PHYSIOLOGY

Blood supply to the LV is directly dependent on the difference between the aortic pressure and LV end-diastolic pressure (coronary perfusion pressure) and inversely related to the vascular resistance to flow, which varies to the fourth power of the radius of the vessel (Poiseuille's law). Two other determinants of coronary flow are vessel length and viscosity of the blood, but these factors are relatively constant. Resting coronary blood flow in the adult is approximately 250 mL/min (1 mL/min/g) or 5% of total cardiac output. The changes in aortic pressure and the impedance to flow resulting from physical compression of the intramural coronary arteries during the cardiac cycle govern the pulsatile pattern of coronary flow in the LV. The LV subendocardium is exposed to a higher pressure than the subepicardial layer during systole. Indeed, the systolic intraventricular pressure may be higher than the peak LV systolic pressure. Because of these differences in tissue pressure, the subendocardial layer is more susceptible to ischemia in the presence of coronary artery stenoses, pressure-overload hypertrophy, or pronounced tachycardia. Coronary blood flow may also be compromised when aortic diastolic pressure is reduced (e.g., severe aortic insufficiency). Elevated LV end-diastolic pressure, as observed during CHF, also reduces coronary blood flow because of decreased coronary perfusion pressure. Coronary sinus (venous) blood flow is maximal during late systole because of the extravascular compression and the low RA pressure.

The two major determinants of coronary blood flow (perfusion pressure and vascular resistance) also vary substantially during the cardiac cycle. Coronary perfusion pressure certainly changes in response to aortic, intramyocardial, and coronary venous pressures, but the major factor that regulates coronary blood flow is the variable resistance produced by coronary vascular smooth muscle. Sympathetic nervous system activation increases coronary vascular smooth muscle tone. The degree of stretch of smooth muscle (termed the "myogenic factor") also affects coronary vascular tone. However, metabolic factors are the primary physiologic determinants of coronary vascular tone and, hence, myocardial perfusion. The ratio of epicardial to endocardial blood flow ratio remains near 1.0 throughout the cardiac cycle despite systolic compressive forces exerted on the subendocardium. The more pronounced resistance to flow in the subendocardium is offset by beta-adrenoceptor–mediated vasodilation and by local metabolic autocrine factors (e.g., release of the vasodilator adenosine during hypoxic conditions) produced by the myocardium itself. The relative maintenance of subendocardial blood flow may also be related to the extensive number of redundant arteriolar and capillary anastomoses within the subendocardium.

The heart normally extracts between 75% and 80% of arterial O_2 content, by far the greatest O_2 extraction of all the body's organs. The majority of O_2 consumption results from the rate and magnitude of LV pressure development during isovolumic contraction. Oxygen consumption is also affected by the diameter of the LV as dictated by the Law of Laplace (see below). Heart rate is the primary determinant of myocardial O_2 demand in the intact heart. Increases in myocardial contractility, preload, and afterload are also associated with elevations in myocardial O_2 demand. Cardiac O_2 extraction is near maximal under resting conditions and cannot be substantially increased during exercise. Thus, the primary mechanism by which myocardium meets its O_2 demand is through enhanced O_2 delivery, which is proportional to coronary blood flow when hemoglobin concentration is constant. Coronary blood flow and myocardial O_2 consumption increase fourfold to fivefold during strenuous physical exercise. The difference between maximal and resting coronary blood flow is termed "coronary reserve." Myocardial O_2 consumption is a major determinant of coronary blood flow. For example, coronary vascular resistance is greater in the rested, perfused heart than in the contracting heart, indicating that coronary blood flow increases in response to a higher rate of O_2 consumption. The mechanism(s) responsible for the correlation between myocardial work, O_2 consumption, and coronary vessel dilatation has yet to be precisely determined. In addition to metabolically induced vasodilation, the factors responsible for coronary autoregulation (maintenance of coronary blood flow with a change in perfusion pressure) and reactive hyperemia (the severalfold increase in blood flow above baseline after a brief period of ischemia) are also not well understood. Metabolic coronary vasodilation occurs, at least in part, as a result of activation of the sympathetic nerves to the heart and coronary vasculature during an increase in heart rate and myocardial contractility. This sympathetic nerve stimulation produces a feed-forward vasodilation of small coronary arterioles via activation of beta-adrenoceptors.[9] An alpha–adrenoceptor-induced vasoconstriction also occurs in larger coronary arteries during exercise. This vasoconstriction occurs upstream from coronary small coronary arterioles and serves two important functions: reduction of vascular compliance and attenuation of coronary blood flow oscillations during the cardiac cycle. These actions act to preserve coronary blood flow to the more vulnerable LV endocardium when heart rate, contractility, and myocardial O_2 consumption are elevated. Interestingly, cardiac parasympathetic nerves have a prominent role in regulating heart rate, but these nerves appear to have a negligible direct effect on the regulation of coronary blood flow.

The conclusions about sympathetic nervous system control of the coronary circulation are based on alterations in the slope of the O_2 consumption–coronary venous O_2 tension relation during graded exercise in the presence of exogenous alpha- or beta-adrenoceptor blockade. Current evidence implicating the beta-adrenoceptor in coronary vasodilation accounts for only about 25% of the total coronary vasodilation observed during exercise-induced hyperemia. These data suggest that the other 75% of coronary vasodilation during exercise may be produced by as yet undefined local metabolic factors that act on coronary vascular smooth muscle with or without the influence of endothelium. Recent evidence indicates that this process may be mediated, at least in part, by the release of adenine nucleotides released from red blood cells that subsequently activate endothelial purinergic receptors to produce vasodilation during exercise.[10] Many metabolic factors have been proposed to individually or collectively modulate coronary flow at the arteriolar or capillary level, including adenosine, nitric oxide, arterial oxygen or CO_2 tension, pH, osmolarity, K^+, Ca^{2+}, and prostaglandins. Many of these factors exert predictable direct effects. For example, hypoxia or ischemia decreases arterial oxygen tension and pH and increases CO_2 tension, adenosine, and K^+ and Ca^{2+} concentrations. These changes may augment coronary blood flow, but none individually appear to be the sole determinant of vasodilation during exercise. For example, adenosine receptor blockade does not alter coronary blood flow under resting conditions or during exercise. Similarly, inhibition of nitric oxide (NO) production or ATP-sensitive K^+ (K_{ATP}) channels does not alter the slope of the myocardial O_2 consumption–coronary venous O_2 relationship during graded exercise. Despite these data, it is abundantly clear that NO and K_{ATP} channels are important regulators of myocardial O_2 supply–demand relations under resting conditions. Adenosine released during hypoxia or ischemia causes coronary vasodilation; this effect is mediated by K_{ATP} channel activation. Adenosine and K_{ATP} channels have also shown to play a role in reactive hyperemia after ischemia, but these mediators do not appear to be required for coronary autoregulation. Moreover, the K_{ATP} channel may act to reduce coronary vascular smooth muscle tone, and thus, maintain a higher basal coronary blood flow, during resting conditions. While not acting as a local metabolic vasodilator, NO may react to increased downstream arterial dilation by dilating larger, upstream epicardial coronary arteries, thereby preventing excessive sheer stress on coronary endothelium.

CARDIAC MYOCYTE ANATOMY AND FUNCTION

Ultrastructure

The heart contracts and relaxes nearly 3 billion times during an average lifetime, based on a heart rate of 70 beats per minute and a life expectancy of 75 years. A review of cardiac myocyte ultrastructure provides important insights into how the heart accomplishes this astonishing performance. The sarcolemma is the external membrane of the cardiac muscle cell. The sarcolemma contains ion channels (e.g., Na^+, K^+, Ca^{2+}), ion pumps and exchangers (e.g., Na^+–K^+ ATPase, Ca^{2+}-ATPase, Na^+–Ca^{2+} or Na^+–H^+ exchangers), G-protein–coupled and other receptors (e.g., beta$_1$-adrenergic, adenosine, opioid), and transporter enzymes that regulate intracellular ion concentrations, facilitate signal transduction, and provide metabolic substrates required for energy production. Deep invaginations of the sarcolemma, known as transverse ("T") tubules, penetrate the internal structure of the myocyte at regular intervals, thereby assuring rapid, uniform transmission of the depolarizing impulses that initiate contraction to be simultaneously distributed throughout the cell. Unlike the skeletal muscle cell, the cardiac myocyte is densely packed with mitochondria, which are responsible for generation of the large quantities of high-energy phosphates (e.g., adenosine triphosphate [ATP]) required for the heart's phasic cycle of contraction and relaxation. The fundamental contractile unit of cardiac muscle is the sarcomere. The myofilaments within each sarcomere are arranged in parallel cross-striated bundles of thin (containing actin, tropomyosin, and the troponin complex) and thick (primarily composed of myosin and its supporting proteins) fibers. Sarcomeres are connected in series, thereby producing characteristic shortening and thickening of the long and short axes of each myocyte, respectively, during contraction.

The structure of each sarcomere is described based on observations from light and electron microscopy. The area of overlap of thick and thin fibers characterizes the "A" band. This band lengthens as the sarcomere shortens during contraction. The "I" band represents the region of the sarcomere that contains thin filaments alone, and this band is reduced in width as the cell contracts. Each "I" band is bisected by a "Z" (from the German *zuckung* [twitch]) line), which delineates the border between two adjacent sarcomeres. Thus, the length of each sarcomere contains a complete "A" band and two one-half "I" band units located between "Z" lines. A central "M" band is also present within the "A" band and is composed of thick filaments spatially constrained in a cross-sectional hexagonal matrix by myosin-binding protein C. An extensively intertwined network of sarcoplasmic reticulum (SR) invests each bundle of contractile proteins and functions as a Ca^{2+} reservoir, thereby assuring homogenous distribution and reuptake of activator Ca^{2+} throughout the myofilaments during contraction and relaxation, respectively. The subsarcolemmal cisternae of the SR are specialized structures located immediately adjacent to, but not continuous with, the sarcolemmal and transverse tubular membranes and contain large numbers of ryanodine receptors that function as the primary Ca^{2+} release channel for the SR. The contractile machinery and the mitochondria that power it occupy >80%, whereas the cytosol and nucleus fill <15%, of the
2 total volume of the cardiac myocyte. This observation emphasizes that contraction and relaxation, and not new protein synthesis, are the predominant functions of the cardiac myocyte. Intercalated discs mechanically connect adjacent myocytes through the fascia adherens and desmosomes, which link actin and other proteins between cells, respectively. The intercalated discs also provide a seamless electrical connection between myocytes via large, nonspecific ion channels known as gap junctions that facilitate intercellular cytosolic diffusion of ions and small molecules.

Contractile Apparatus

Myosin, actin, tropomyosin, and the three-protein troponin complex compose the six major components of the contractile apparatus. Myosin (molecular weight of approximately 500 kDa; length, 0.17 μm) contains two interwoven chain helices with two globular heads that bind to actin and two additional pairs of light chains. Enzymatic digestion of myosin divides the structure into light (containing the tail section of the complex) and heavy (composed of the globular heads and the light chains) meromyosin. The elongated tail section of the myosin complex functions as the architectural support of the molecule (Fig. 10-6). The globular heads of the myosin dimer contain two "hinges" located at the junction of the distal light chains and the tail helix that play a critical role in myofilament shortening during contraction. These globular structures bind to actin, thereby activating an ATPase that plays a central role in hinge rotation and release of actin during contraction and relaxation, respectively. The maximum velocity of sarcomere shortening has been shown to be dependent on the activity of this actin-activated myosin ATPase. Notably, adult and neonatal atrial and ventricular myocardia contain several different myosin ATPase isoforms that are distinguished by their relative ATPase activity. The myosin molecules are primarily arranged in series along the length of the thick filament, but are abutted "tail-to-tail" in the center of the thick filament. This orientation facilitates shortening of the distance between "Z" lines during contraction as the thin filaments are drawn progressively toward the center of the sarcomere.

The light chains contained within the myosin complex serve either "regulatory" or "essential" roles. Regulatory myosin light

FIGURE 10-6. Schematic illustration of the myosin molecule demonstrating double helix tail, globular heads that form cross-bridges with actin during contraction, two pairs of light chains, and "hinges" (cleavage sites of proteolytic enzymes) that divide the molecule into meromyosin fragments (see text). (Reproduced with permission from: Barash PG, Cullen BF, Stoelting RK, et al. *Clinical Anesthesia*, 6th ed., Lippincott Williams and Wilkins, Figure 10-6, p. 214.)

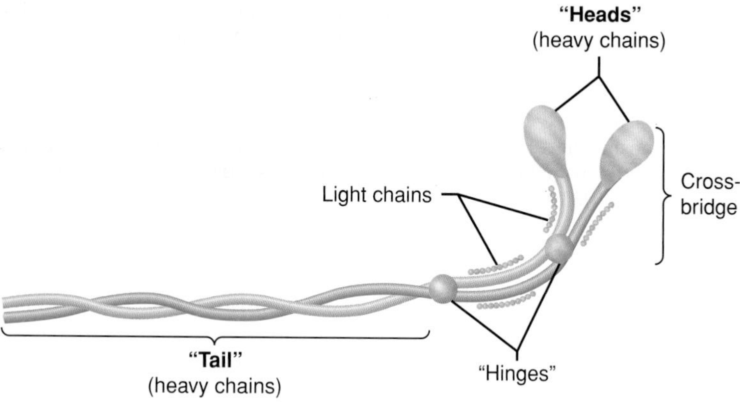

chains may favorably modulate myosin–actin interaction through Ca^{2+}-dependent protein kinase phosphorylation, whereas essential light chains serve an as yet undefined obligate function in myosin activity, as their removal denatures the myosin molecule. Discussion of myosin light chain isoforms is beyond the scope of the current chapter, but isoform switches from ventricular to atrial forms have been observed in left ventricular hypertrophy that may contribute to contractile dysfunction.[11] In addition to myosin and its binding protein, thick filaments contain titin, a long elastic protein that attaches myosin to the "Z" lines. Titin has been postulated to be a "length sensor" similar to a bidirectional spring that establishes progressively greater passive restoring forces as sarcomere length approaches its maximum or minimum.[12] Compression and stretching of titin occur during decreases and increases in muscle load, thereby resisting further sarcomere shortening and lengthening, respectively. Thus, titin is a third important elastic element (in addition to actin and myosin) that contributes to the stress-strain biomechanical properties of cardiac muscle.[13]

Actin is the major component of the thin filament. Actin is a 42 kDa, ovoid-shaped, globular protein ("G" form; 5.5 nm in diameter) that exists in a polymerized filamentous ("F") form in cardiac muscle. F-actin binds adenosine diphosphate (ADP) and a divalent cation (Ca^{2+} or Mg^{2+}), but unlike myosin, the molecule does not directly hydrolyze high-energy nucleotides such as ATP. F-actin is wound in double-stranded helical chains of G-actin monomers that resemble two intertwined strands of pearls. A single complete helical revolution of filamentous actin is approximately 77 nm in length and contains 14 G-actin monomers. Actin derives its name from its function as the "activator" of myosin ATPase through its reversible binding with myosin. The hydrolysis of ATP by this actin–myosin complex provides the chemical energy required to produce the conformational changes in the myosin heads that drive the cycle of contraction and relaxation within the sarcomere. Tropomyosin is one of two major inhibitors of actin–myosin interaction. Tropomyosin (length of 40 nm; weight between 68 and 72 kDa) is a rigid double-stranded alpha-helix protein linked by a single disulfide bond. Human tropomyosin contains both alpha and beta isoforms (34 and 36 kDa, respectively) and may be present as either a homo- or a heterodimer.[14] Tropomyosin stiffens the thin filament through its position within the longitudinal cleft between intertwined F-actin polymers (Fig. 10-7), but its Ca^{2+}-dependent interaction with troponin complex proteins is the mechanism that links sarcolemmal membrane depolarization to actin–myosin interaction in the cardiac myocyte (excitation–contraction coupling). The thin filaments are anchored to "Z" lines by cytoskeletal proteins including alpha- and beta-actinin and nebulette.[15]

The troponin proteins serve complementary but distinct roles as critical regulators of the contractile apparatus.[16] The troponin complexes are arranged at 40 nm intervals along the length of the thin filament. Troponin C (so named because this molecule binds Ca^{2+}) exists in a highly conserved, single isoform in cardiac muscle. Troponin C is composed of a central nine-turn alpha-helix separating two globular regions that contain four discrete amino acid sequences capable of binding divalent cations including Ca^{2+} and Mg^{2+}. Of this quartet of amino acid–cation binding sequences, two (termed sites I and II) are Ca^{2+}-specific, thereby allowing the troponin C molecule to respond to the acute changes in intracellular Ca^{2+} concentration that accompany contraction and relaxation. Troponin I ("inhibitor") is a 23 kDa protein that exists in a single isoform in cardiac muscle. Troponin I alone weakly prevents the interaction between actin and myosin, but when combined with tropomyosin, the troponin I–tropomyosin complex becomes the major inhibitor of actin–myosin binding. The troponin I molecule contains a serine residue that may be phosphorylated by protein kinase A (PKA) via the intracellular second messenger cAMP, thereby reducing troponin C–Ca^{2+} binding and enhancing relaxation during administration of $beta_1$-adrenoceptor agonists (e.g., dobutamine) or phosphodiesterase fraction III inhibitors (e.g., milrinone). Troponin T (so denoted because it binds other troponin molecules and tropomyosin) is the largest of the troponin proteins and exists in four major isoforms in human cardiac muscle. Troponin T anchors the other

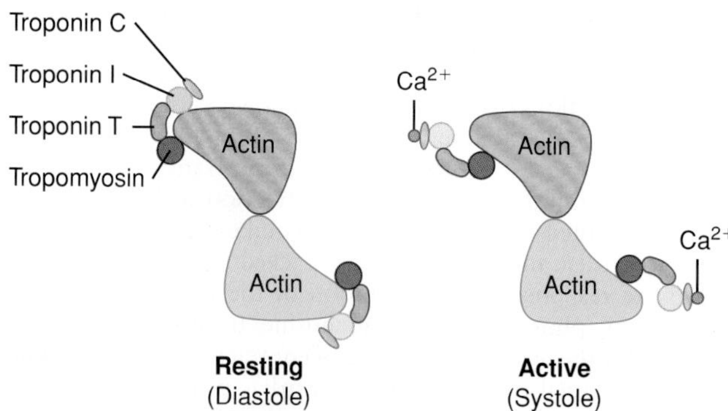

FIGURE 10-7. Cross-sectional schematic illustration demonstrating the structural relationship between the troponin–tropomyosin complex and actin under resting conditions **(left panel)** and after Ca^{2+} binding to troponin C (**right panel**, see text). (Reproduced with permission from: Barash PG, Cullen BF, Stoelting RK, et al. *Clinical Anesthesia*, 6th ed., Lippincott Williams and Wilkins, Figure 10-7, p. 215.)

troponin molecules and may also influence the relative Ca^{2+} sensitivity of the complex.[17]

Calcium–Myofilament Interaction

Binding of Ca^{2+} to troponin C precipitates a series of conformational changes in the troponin–tropomyosin complex that lead to the exposure of the myosin-binding site on the actin molecule. During conditions in which intracellular Ca^{2+} concentration is low (10^{-7} M; diastole), very little Ca^{2+} is bound to troponin C, and each tropomyosin molecule is constrained to the outer region of the groove between F-actin filaments by a troponin complex. This structural configuration prevents myosin–actin interaction by effectively blocking cross-bridge formation. Thus, an inhibitory state produced by the troponin–tropomyosin complex exists in cardiac muscle under resting conditions. A 100-fold increase in intracellular Ca^{2+} concentration (10^{-5} M; systole) occurs as a consequence of sarcolemmal depolarization, which opens L- and T-type sarcolemmal Ca^{2+} channels, thereby allowing Ca^{2+} influx into the myocyte from the extracellular compartment and stimulating Ca^{2+}-dependent Ca^{2+} release from the SR via its ryanodine receptors. When Ca^{2+} is bound to troponin C under these conditions, the shape of the troponin C protein becomes elongated and its interactions with troponin I and T are enhanced. These Ca^{2+}-induced allosteric rearrangements in troponin complex structure weaken the interaction between troponin I and actin, allow repositioning of the tropomyosin molecule along the F-actin filaments, and reverse the baseline inhibition of actin–myosin binding by tropomyosin.[18] In this way, Ca^{2+} binding to troponin C may be directly linked to a series of changes in regulatory protein chemical structure that block inhibition of the binding site for myosin on the actin molecule and allow cross-bridge formation and contraction to occur. This antagonism of inhibition is fully reversible, as relaxation is facilitated by dissociation of Ca^{2+} from troponin C concomitant with rapid restoration of the original conformation of the troponin–tropomyosin complex on F-actin.

Most Ca^{2+} ions are removed from the myofilaments and the cytosol after membrane repolarization by a Ca^{2+}-ATPase located in the SR membrane (sarcoendoplasmic reticulum Ca^{2+}-ATPase, SERCA). This Ca^{2+} is stored (concentration of approximately 10^{-3} M) in the SR bound to calsequestrin and calreticulin until the subsequent sarcolemmal depolarization is initiated. The Na^+/Ca^{2+} exchanger and a Ca^{2+}-ATPase located within the sarcolemmal membrane also remove a small quantity of Ca^{2+}, similar to that which originally entered the myocyte from the extracellular space during depolarization. Phospholamban is a small protein (6 kDa) located in the SR membrane that partially inhibits the activity of the dominant form (type 2a) of cardiac SERCA under baseline conditions. However, phosphorylation of this protein by PKA blocks this inhibition and enhances the rate of SERCA uptake of Ca^{2+} into the SR,[19] thereby increasing the rate and extent of relaxation (positive lusitropic effect) and augmenting the amount of Ca^{2+} stored for the next cycle of contraction (positive inotropic effect). Thus, SERCA activity is regulated by a cAMP-dependent PKA that is responsive to beta$_1$-adrenoceptor stimulation or phosphodiesterase fraction III inhibition. In addition to PKA-mediated phosphorylation of troponin I that facilitates Ca^{2+} release from troponin C, these observations explain why positive inotropic drugs such as dobutamine and milrinone also augment relaxation.

Myosin–Actin Interaction

The biochemistry of cardiac muscle contraction is most often described using a simplified four-component model (Fig. 10-8).[20] Binding of ATP with high affinity to the catalytic domain of myosin initiates the series of chemical and mechanical events that cause contraction of the sarcomere to occur. The myosin ATPase enzyme hydrolyzes the ATP molecule into ADP and inorganic phosphate, but these reaction products do not immediately dissociate from myosin. Instead, the ATP hydrolysis products and myosin form an "active" complex that retains the chemical energy released from the reaction as potential energy. In the absence of actin, subsequent dissociation of ADP and phosphate from myosin is the rate-limiting step of myosin ATPase and the muscle remains relaxed. However, the activity of myosin ATPase is markedly accelerated when the myosin–ADP–phosphate complex

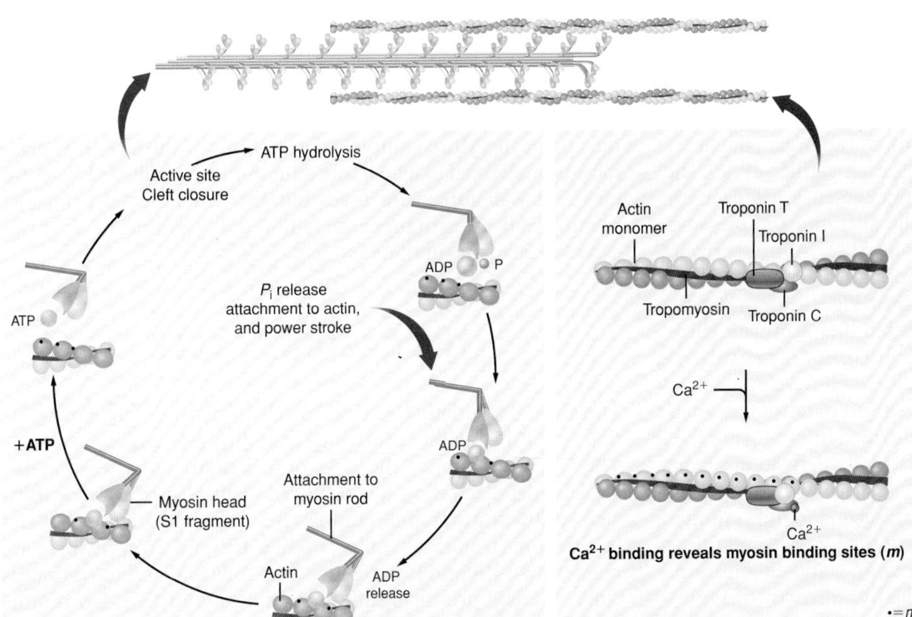

FIGURE 10-8. Schematic illustration of the actin filaments and its individual monomers and active myosin bindings sites (*m*; **left panel**). The myosin head is dissociated from actin by binding with adenosine triphosphate (ATP). Subsequent ATP hydrolysis and release of inorganic phosphate (P_i) "cocks" the head group into a tension-generating configuration. Attachment of the myosin head to actin allows the head to apply tension to the myosin rod and the actin filament. The right panel illustrates Ca^{2+} binding to troponin C, which causes troponin I to decrease its affinity for actin. As a result, in a conformational shift in tropomyosin position (see text), seven sites on actin monomers are revealed. (Reproduced with permission from: Barash PG, Cullen BF, Stoelting RK, et al. *Clinical Anesthesia*, 6th ed., Lippincott Williams and Wilkins, Figure 10-9, p. 216.)

is bound to actin, and under these circumstances, the chemical energy obtained from ATP hydrolysis becomes directly transferred into mechanical work. Attachment of myosin to its binding site on the actin molecule releases the phosphate anion from the myosin head, thereby producing a molecular conformation within this cross-bridge structure that generates tension in both myofilaments.[21] Release of ADP and the stored potential energy from this activated conformation produce rotation of the cross-bridge ("power stroke") at the hinge point separating the helix tail region from the globular myosin head and its associated light chain proteins. Each cross-bridge rotation generates 3 to 4×10^{-12} newtons of force and moves myosin approximately 11 nm along the actin molecule.[22] Completion of myosin head rotation and ADP release does not dissociate the myosin-active complex but leaves it in a low-energy bound ("rigor") state. Separation of myosin and actin occurs when a new ATP molecule binds to myosin, and the process is subsequently repeated, provided that energy supply is adequate and the myosin-binding site on actin remains unimpeded by troponin–tropomyosin inhibition.

Several factors may affect the efficiency of cross-bridge biochemistry and myocardial contractility independent of autonomic nervous system tone or administration of exogenous vasoactive drugs. There is a direct relationship between myosin ATPase activity and the maximal velocity of unloaded muscle shortening (V_{max}). The normal increase in intracellular Ca^{2+} concentration (from 10^{-7} to 10^{-5} M) that occurs after sarcolemmal depolarization enhances baseline myosin ATPase activity fivefold before it interacts with actin, thereby increasing V_{max}. Contractile force depends on sarcomere length immediately before sarcolemmal depolarization. This length-dependent activation (Frank–Starling effect) may be related to an increase in myofilament sensitivity to Ca^{2+}, favorable alterations in spacing between myofilaments, or titin-induced elastic recoil. Abrupt increases in load during contraction (Anrep effect) or those that occur after a prolonged pause between beats (Woodworth phenomenon) causes transient increases in contractile force through a length-dependent activation mechanism. An increase in cardiac muscle stimulation frequency also augments contractile force (treppe phenomenon) via enhanced myofilament Ca^{2+} sensitivity and greater SR Ca^{2+} release.

LAW OF LAPLACE

On a cellular level, each individual cardiac myocyte shortens and develops tension during contraction and subsequently, lengthens and releases this tension during relaxation. As an organ, the heart
3 produces pressure–volume work during each cardiac cycle. The Law of Laplace allows translation of changes in tension and length observed in the cardiac myocyte into the alterations in pressure
2 and volume that occur in the intact heart.[23] A pressurized, spherical shell is a simple model for relating cardiac myocyte tension and length to LV pressure and volume (Fig. 10-9). In reality, the geometry of the LV more closely resembles a prolate ellipsoid,[24] but for the purposes of the current discussion, a pressurized sphere model of the LV is quite useful. Tension development in each cardiac myocyte increases LV wall stress (σ; tension exerted over a cross-sectional area) that is transformed into pressure (p). Three assumptions are used in the most basic derivation of the Law of Laplace: First, the LV is spherical in shape with an internal radius (r) and uniform wall thickness (h); second, σ is presumed to be constant throughout the thickness of the LV wall; and third, the LV is not actively contracting, that is, in static equilibrium. Thus, "p" is the force acting to distend the LV, whereas "σ" represents the force resisting this distension. It can be easily shown that

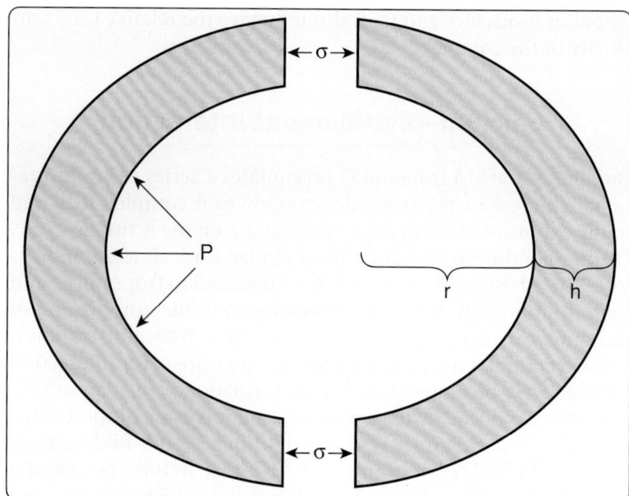

FIGURE 10-9. This schematic diagram depicts the opposing forces within a theoretical LV sphere that determine the Law of Laplace. LV pressure (P) pushes the sphere apart, whereas wall stress (σ) holds the sphere together. r, LV radius; h, LV thickness. (Reproduced with permission from: Kaplan JA, Reich DL, Savino JS. *Kaplan's Cardiac Anesthesia: The Echo Era*, 6th ed., St. Louis, Elsevier Saunders, 2011, Figure 5-6, p. 105.)

$\sigma = pr/2h$, indicating that wall stress varies directly with pressure and radius and inversely with wall thickness. Despite the model's broad assumptions and remarkable simplicity, this version of the Law of Laplace allows appreciation of the factors that alter LV wall stress and how they may be affected by cardiac pathology. For example, the chronically elevated LV pressure (p) that occurs in the presence of severe aortic stenosis or uncontrolled essential hypertension clearly increases wall stress because these variables are directly related. Similarly, LV dilation associated with chronic mitral insufficiency also increases LV wall stress because the internal diameter (r) of the LV is greater. Notably, increases in wall stress under either circumstance cause a greater myocardial oxygen demand because each myocyte requires more energy to develop enhanced tension.[25] Conversely, an increase in wall thickness (h) decreases wall stress. This observation emphasizes that hypertrophy is an essential compensatory response to elevated wall stress that reduces the tension developed in each cardiac myocyte. More complete descriptions of the Law of Laplace have been derived in which more anatomically realistic LV geometry and wall forces are used, but the fundamental principles relating wall stress to pressure, radius, and wall thickness remain essential elements in these models as well.[26]

THE CARDIAC CYCLE

The time-dependent electrical, mechanical, and valvular events that occur during the cardiac cycle are illustrated in Figure 10-10. The QRS complex of the electrocardiogram indicates that RV and LV depolarization has occurred. This electrical event initiates contraction (systole) and is associated with rapid increases in pressure in both chambers. When RV and LV pressures are greater than RA and LA pressures, the tricuspid and mitral valves close, thereby producing the first heart sound (S_1). Isovolumic contraction, rapid ejection, and slower ejection phases are the

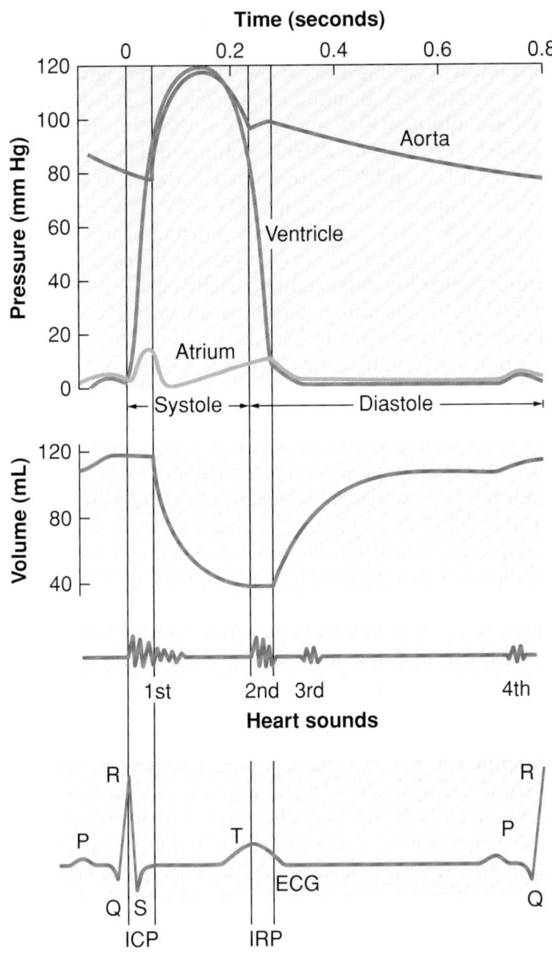

FIGURE 10-10. Mechanical and electrical events of the cardiac cycle showing also the LV volume curve and the heart sounds. Note the LV isovolumic contraction (ICP) and the relaxation period (IRP) during which there is no change in LV volume because aortic and mitral valves are closed. The LV decreases in volume as it ejects its contents into the aorta. During the first third of systolic ejection (the rapid ejection period), the curve of emptying is steep. ECG, electrocardiogram. (Reproduced with permission from: Barash PG, Cullen BF, Stoelting RK, et al. *Clinical Anesthesia*, 6th ed., Lippincott Williams and Wilkins, Figure 10-4, p. 212.)

three major phases of LV systole. During LV isovolumic contraction, LV volume is constant because both the aortic and mitral valves are closed. However, LV shape becomes more spherical because base-to-apex length decreases. The maximum rate of rise of LV pressure (+dP/dt), a commonly used index of myocardial contractility, also occurs during LV isovolumic contraction. In contrast to the synchronous LV, the peristaltic contractions of the RV inflow and outflow tracts preclude isovolumic contraction in the RV.[27] The pressures in the aortic and pulmonic roots reach their minima before the corresponding valves open. When LV and RV pressures are greater than aortic and PA pressures, respectively, rapid ejection of approximately two-thirds of the end-diastolic volume of each chamber occurs. The kinetic energy of LV and RV contraction is stored as potential energy in the aorta and PA, respectively, and is then released to the distal vascular beds during diastole. The magnitude of this potential energy is determined by the relative compliance of the proximal systemic and PA vasculature. As aortic and PA pressures reach their maximum values, LV and RV ejection falls dramatically and then stops entirely when the LV and RV begin to repolarize. Aortic and PA pressures briefly exceed LV and RV pressures as this slower ejection phase comes to an end, and the aortic and pulmonic valves close in response to these pressure gradient reversals. Closure of the aortic and pulmonic valves causes the second heart sound (S_2); this event denotes end-systole. S_2 is normally split because the aortic valve closes slightly before the pulmonic valve.

Isovolumic relaxation, early ventricular filling, diastasis, and atrial systole are the four phases of LV diastole. LV volume is constant during isovolumic relaxation because both the aortic and mitral valves are closed. LV pressure very rapidly declines as the myofilaments relax. The mitral valve opens when LA pressure exceeds LV pressure, and the pressure gradient between the chambers drives blood stored in the LA into the LV. Sarcomere relaxation is completed and recoil of compressed elastic components cause LV pressure to continue to decrease after the mitral valve has opened,[28] thereby establishing a time-dependent pressure gradient between the LA and LV.[29] The instantaneous LA pressure immediately before mitral valve opening combined with the rate and extent with which LV pressure decreases are the primary determinants of the pressure gradient between chambers.[30] Early LV filling is rapid; the peak velocities of mitral blood flow during early filling and aortic outflow during ejection are similar.[31] Vortex ring formation within the LV accompanies the mitral inflow jet and facilitates selective filling of the LV outflow tract.[32] Age and cardiac disease (e.g., myocardial ischemia, pressure-overload hypertrophy) often delay LV relaxation, which blunts early LV filling by reducing the LA-to-LV pressure gradient. It is important to note that LV pressure continues to fall to subatmospheric values if blood flow across the mitral valve is experimentally prevented.[33] This "diastolic suction" effect assures that the LV will continue to fill even if LA pressure is zero (e.g., during profound hypovolemia).[34] The early filling phase of diastole normally provides 70% to 75% of final stroke volume. During the third phase of diastole, the LA acts as a conduit to transfer pulmonary venous blood flow through the open mitral valve. Less than 5% of total stroke volume enters the LV during diastasis, which may be shortened or eliminated during pronounced tachycardia.[35] The final phase of ventricular diastole is atrial systole. A positive pressure gradient for renewed LA to LV flow is created by LA contraction. Retrograde blood flow into the pulmonary veins is largely prevented by the sphincter-like anatomy of the pulmonary venous–LA junction. Atrial systole generates 15% to 25% of final stroke volume, but its importance is accentuated when delayed LV relaxation or reduced LV compliance is present. Thus, it is common for patients with these abnormalities to develop cardiovascular instability or CHF when LA contraction is improperly timed (e.g., AV conduction blockade) or absent (e.g., atrial fibrillation).

Three major deflections are observed in the LA pressure waveform during sinus rhythm. The P wave of atrial depolarization is followed by LA contraction, which produces the "a" wave of atrial systole. An increase in LA preload or contractility augments the magnitude of the "a" wave. LA relaxation may be quantified using the rate of deceleration of the "a" wave.[36] A second small increase in LA pressure occurs with the onset of LV contraction because of mitral valve closure. This deflection is known as the "c" wave. The "v" wave results from LA filling during LV systole and early relaxation as pulmonary venous return enters the LA. Mitral regurgitation or reductions in LA compliance enhances the magnitude of the "v" wave.[37] Similar changes in the RA pressure waveform deflections also occur, and this RA "a-c-v" morphology may be easily seen in the jugular veins during the physical examination.

THE PRESSURE–VOLUME DIAGRAM

4 Continuous LV pressure and volume may be plotted against each other to obtain a time-dependent diagram that is useful for analysis of LV systolic and diastolic function (Fig. 10-11). The LV pressure–volume (P–V) diagram proceeds in a counterclockwise direction over time. End-diastole initiates the cardiac cycle (point A, Fig. 10-11). This is followed by isovolumic contraction, in which a rapid increase in LV pressure that occurs without change in LV volume. When LV pressure is greater than aorta pressure, the aortic valve opens (point B, Fig. 10-11). Ejection of blood from the LV into the proximal great vessels causes a precipitous decline in LV volume. The aortic valve closes when LV pressure drops below aortic pressure (point C, Fig. 10-11). When LV pressure falls below LA pressure during isovolumic relaxation, the mitral valve opens (point D, Fig. 10-11) and LV filling occurs, thereby increasing LV volume during the remainder of diastole
3 concomitant with small increases in LV pressure. This final stage completes the P–V diagram.

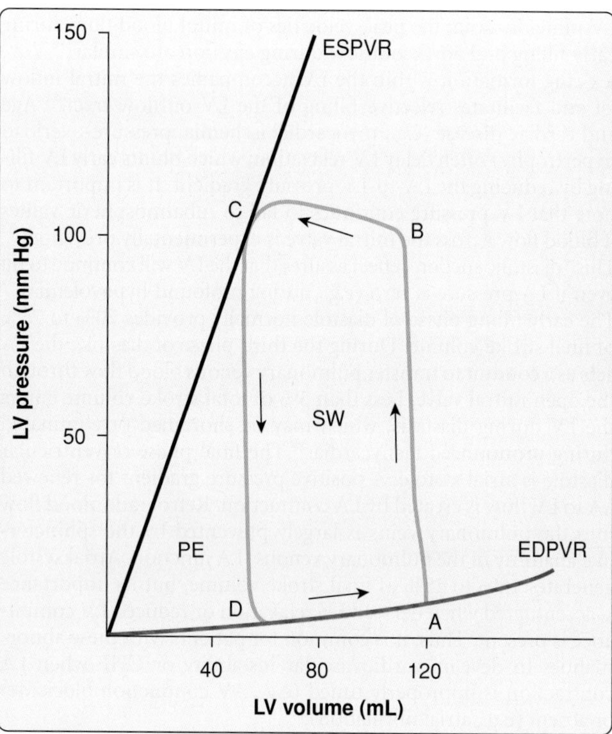

FIGURE 10-11. This illustration depicts the steady state LV pressure–volume diagram. The cardiac cycle proceeds in a time-dependent counterclockwise direction (*arrows*). Points A, B, C, and D correspond to LV end-diastole (closure of the mitral valve), opening of the aortic valve, LV end-systole (closure of the aortic valve), and opening of the mitral valve, respectively. Segments AB, BC, CD, and DA represent isovolumic contraction, ejection, isovolumic relaxation, and filling, respectively. The LV is constrained to operate within the boundaries of the end-systolic and end-diastolic pressure–volume relations (ESPVR and EDPVR, respectively). The area inscribed by the LV pressure–volume diagram is stroke work (SW) performed during the cardiac cycle. The area to the left of the LV pressure–volume diagram between ESPVR and EDPVR is the remaining potential energy (PE) of the system. (Reproduced with permission from: Kaplan JA, Reich DL, Savino JS. *Kaplan's Cardiac Anesthesia: The Echo Era*, 6th ed., St. Louis, Elsevier Saunders, 2011, Figure 5-9, p. 107.)

The LV P–V diagram allows simple recognition of major cardiac events without electrocardiographic correlation (e.g., aortic and mitral valve opening and closing). The lower right and upper left corners of the P–V diagram identify the LV end-diastolic and end-systolic volumes (EDV and ESV, respectively). This observation facilitates calculation of stroke volume and ejection fraction. The normal EDV and ESV are approximately 120 and 40 mL, respectively. Thus, stroke volume (EDV–ESV) is 80 mL and ejection fraction (SV/EDV) is 67% in the normal heart. The area of the LV P–V diagram defines stroke work for the cardiac cycle. An increase in preload is indicated by a rightward shift of the right side of the LV P–V diagram. In contrast, greater LV pressure associated with an increase in afterload causes the LV P–V diagram to increase in height and become narrower. A series of LV P–V diagrams may be acquired as a result of an acute change in LV loading conditions over several cardiac cycles and is useful for determining contractile state, chamber compliance, and mechanical efficiency. Changes in preload or afterload may be briefly induced mechanically (e.g., transient occlusion of the inferior vena cava) or pharmacologically (e.g., intravenous infusion of nitroglycerin) to generate a nested set of differentially loaded LV P–V diagrams. These loops may then be used to determine the end-systolic pressure–volume relation (ESPVR), the slope of which ("end-systolic elastance" [E_{es}]) is an index of myocardial contractility in vivo.[38] Similarly, LV compliance may be quantified using the same set of LV P–V diagrams to calculate the end-diastolic pressure–volume relationship (EDPVR).[23] The LV functions within the constraints of the boundaries established by ESPVR and EDPVR, which define the LV's mechanical characteristics during systole and diastole, respectively.[39] In addition, the triangular space that lies between ESPVR and EDPVR to the left of the steady state LV P–V diagram itself is the potential energy remaining in the system. This area may be used to quantify the energetics and
5 mechanical efficiency of the LV.[40] The principles of pressure–volume theory have also been successfully applied to the study of RV and LA function.[41,42]

CHF resulting from LV systolic or diastolic dysfunction may be clearly depicted using P–V analysis.[43] Pure LV systolic dysfunction is represented by a reduction in the ESPVR slope and often occurs in conjunction with LV dilation, as illustrated by a right shift of the P–V diagram without a change in the position of EDPVR (Fig. 10-12). Thus, a compensatory increase in preload serves to maintain stroke volume in the presence of reduced myocardial contractility, but LV filling pressures are greater as a result. A decrease in LV compliance is indicated by an increase in EDPVR; this defines LV diastolic dysfunction because LV pressure is greater for a given LV volume. In pure diastolic heart failure, myocardial contractility is preserved (ESPVR is unchanged), but clinical symptoms are present because LV filling pressures are elevated. The combination of LV systolic and diastolic dysfunction is indicated by simultaneously decreased ESPVR and elevated EDPVR. Under these circumstances, the LV operates with a very restricted range of preload and afterload conditions and stroke volume may be substantially compromised as a result.

FACTORS THAT DETERMINE SYSTOLIC FUNCTION

The pumping ability of the LV (and the other cardiac chambers) is determined by its ability to collect and eject blood. Cardiac output and ejection fraction are most often used to quantify LV systolic function. The amount of blood contained within the LV

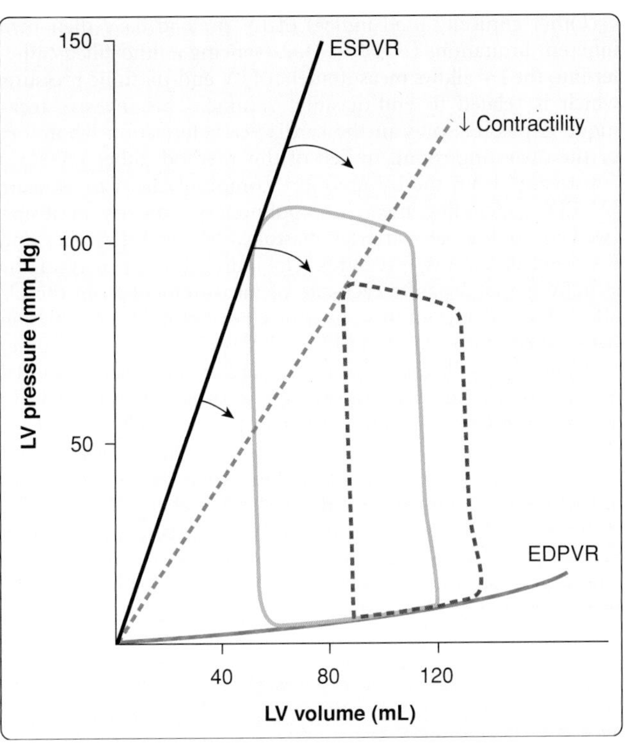

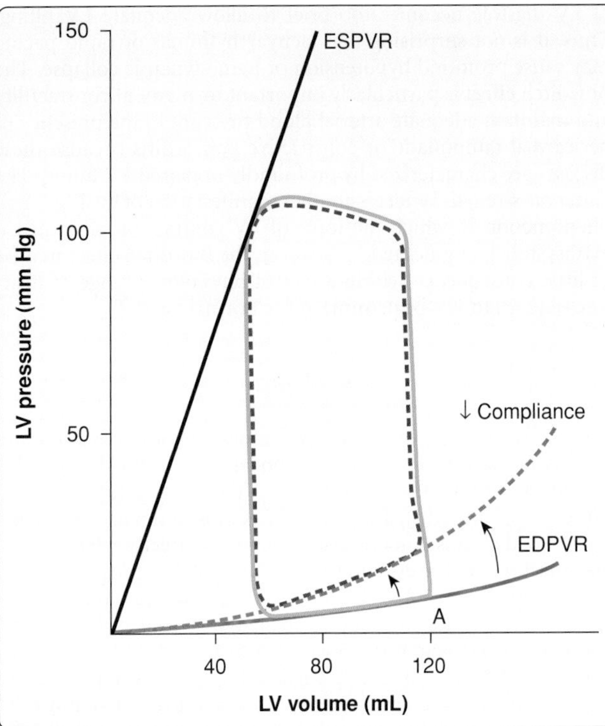

FIGURE 10-12. These schematic illustrations demonstrate alterations in the steady state LV pressure–volume diagram produced by a reduction in myocardial contractility as indicated by a decrease in the slope of the end-systolic pressure–volume relation (ESPVR; **left panel**) and a decrease in LV compliance as indicated by an increase in the position of the end-diastolic pressure–volume relation (EDPVR; **right panel**). These diagrams emphasize that heart failure may result from LV systolic or diastolic dysfunction independently. (Reproduced with permission from: Kaplan JA, Reich DL, Savino JS. *Kaplan's Cardiac Anesthesia: The Echo Era*, 6th ed., St. Louis, Elsevier Saunders, 2011, Figure 5-11, p. 109.)

before the onset of contraction, the arterial resistance to emptying that the LV must overcome, and the contractile properties of the LV itself determine the stroke volume for each cardiac cycle
6 (Fig. 10-13). These three factors combine with the heart rate and rhythm to determine cardiac output. Clearly, the LV's structural integrity is essential to its efficiency as a hydraulic pump. For example, an anomalous route of blood flow from the chamber

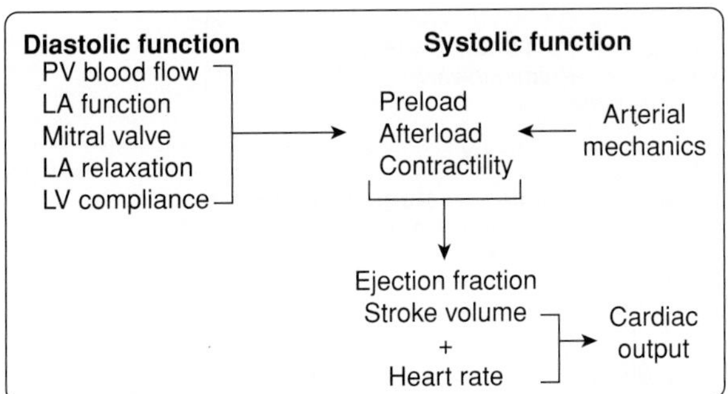

FIGURE 10-13. This illustration depicts the major factors that determine LV diastolic **(left)** and systolic **(right)** function. Note that pulmonary venous (PV) blood flow, LA function, mitral valve integrity, LA relaxation, and LV compliance combine to determine LV preload. (Reproduced with permission from: Kaplan JA, Reich DL, Savino JS. *Kaplan's Cardiac Anesthesia: The Echo Era*, 6th ed., St. Louis, Elsevier Saunders, 2011, Figure 5-15, p. 111.)

(e.g., a ventricular septal defect with right to left shunt) or valvular dysfunction (e.g., severe mitral regurgitation) may reduce forward flow and limit the utility of cardiac output and ejection fraction as indices of LV systolic function. The ability of the LV to fill properly at normal pressure (approximately 10 mm Hg) is determined by pulmonary venous blood flow, LA and mitral function, pericardial forces, and the active (relaxation) and passive (compliance) properties of the LV during diastole.[44] LV diastolic dysfunction caused by perturbations in any of these variables often precludes proper LV filling without elevated pressure and may independently contribute to clinical signs and symptoms of CHF without LV systolic dysfunction per se.

Heart Rate

The contractile state of isolated cardiac muscle is directly related to its stimulation frequency. This phenomenon is known as the Bowditch, "staircase," or "treppe" effect or the "force–frequency" relationship and has been attributed to improved Ca^{2+} cycling efficiency and increased myofilament Ca^{2+} sensitivity. Maximal contractile force is generated at 150 to 180 stimulations/min in isolated cardiac muscle; these experimental data support the clinical observation of optimal matching of cardiac output to venous return at heart rates approaching 175 beats/min during intense aerobic exercise. Nevertheless, contractility may subsequently decline at heart rates greater than 175 beats/min because LV relaxation abnormalities begin to develop as a result of insufficient Ca^{2+} uptake from the contractile apparatus and because the duration of LV diastole becomes too brief to allow adequate LV filling. Thus, it is not surprising that tachyarrhythmias or rapid pacing may cause profound hypotension or hemodynamic collapse. The Bowditch effect is particularly important to augment contractility and maintain adequate arterial blood pressure in the presence of pericardial tamponade or constrictive pericarditis because these diseases are characterized by profoundly impaired LV filling. The "interval-strength" effect is another manifestation of the Bowditch phenomenon in which the force of LV contraction after an LV extrasystole is augmented.[45] However, the Bowditch effect may be of little consequence within a typical physiologic range of heart rate (e.g., 50 to 150 beats/min) in the normal heart.[46]

Preload

7 Sarcomere length immediately before myocyte contraction is a useful way to envision the concept of "preload," but this definition is unrealistic considering the LV's complex three-dimensional structure. Instead, EDV is most often used to define LV preload because this volume of blood is directly related to LV end-diastolic wall stress and implicitly establishes the precontraction length of each LV sarcomere. Real-time quantification of LV EDV continues to be quite challenging from a clinical perspective. Experimental methods used to measure LV EDV (e.g., sonomicrometry, conductance technology) are very precise but impractical because they require invasive instrumentation.[47,48] Noninvasive methods including radionuclide angiography or dynamic magnetic resonance imaging may also be used to measure LV EDV, but these imaging techniques cannot be used in the operating room or intensive care unit. Three-dimensional transesophageal echocardiography (TEE) offers perhaps the best technique to quantify real-time LV EDV, but this technology is relatively new and has yet to be widely applied outside the setting of cardiac surgery. More often, anesthesiologists estimate LV EDV using two-dimensional TEE by examining transgastric LV midpapillary short axis imaging plane to measure LV end-diastolic area or diameter. Using this technique, a decrease in LV preload may be inferred when there is a reduction in end-diastolic area and diameter. Clearly, TEE assessment of LV preload cannot be practically performed in a conscious patient and requires that the anesthesiologist obtain specialized training to properly interpret the data.

Other clinically used indices of LV preload have their own inherent limitations (Fig. 10-14). Advancing a fluid-filled catheter into the LV allows measurement of LV end-diastolic pressure, which is related to end-diastolic volume. This invasive technique is possible only in the cardiac catheterization laboratory or the operating room. In lieu of this method, other pressures "upstream" from the LV are more commonly used to estimate LV EDV, including mean LA, pulmonary capillary occlusion (wedge), pulmonary arterial diastolic, RV end-diastolic, and RA (central venous) pressures. Obviously, the integrity of the structures that separate each site of measurement from the LV affects the accuracy of these methods. For example, a correlation between central venous and LV end-diastolic pressures assumes that pulmonary disease, airway pressure during respiration, RV or pulmonary vascular disease, LA dysfunction, mitral valve abnormalities, or LV compliance have not adversely affected the fluid column between the RA and the LV. This is certainly not the case in patients with significant pulmonary or cardiac disease, as there is a well-known lack of correlation between LV end-diastolic volume, pulmonary artery occlusion pressure, and central venous pressure in patients with LV systolic dysfunction[49] in whom accurate measurement of LV preload may be especially important to optimize cardiac output.

Afterload

8 The additional load to which cardiac muscle is exposed after contraction has begun is termed "afterload." This concept is intuitive when studying isolated cardiac muscle under experimental conditions, but it is more difficult to quantify when the heart's interaction with the arterial vasculature is considered in vivo. Four components combine to determine LV afterload in the intact cardiovascular system. These include the size and mechanical behavior of arterial blood vessels; terminal arteriolar vascular tone, which establishes total arterial resistance; LV end-systolic wall stress, which is defined by LV pressure development and the changes in LV geometry needed to generate it; and the physical properties and volume of blood as a hydraulic fluid. The methods used to estimate RV afterload are similar to those used to characterize LV afterload; this discussion will focus on LV afterload as a result. The reader should appreciate that two major differences

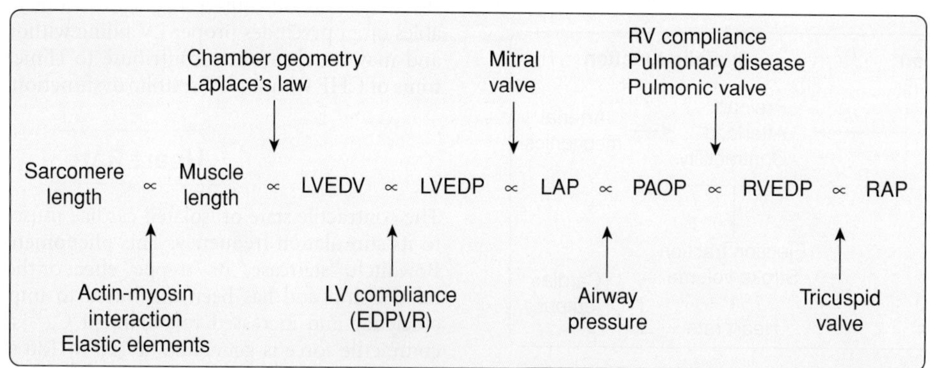

FIGURE 10-14. This schematic diagram depicts factors that influence experimental and clinical estimates of sarcomere length as a pure index of the preload of the contracting LV myocyte. LVEDV, LV end-diastolic volume; LVEDP, LV end-diastolic pressure; EDPVR, end-diastolic pressure–volume relation; LAP, left atrial pressure; PAOP, pulmonary artery occlusion pressure; RV, right ventricle; RVEDP, RV end-diastolic pressure; RAP, right atrial pressure. (Reproduced with permission from: Kaplan JA, Reich DL, Savino JS. *Kaplan's Cardiac Anesthesia: The Echo Era*, 6th ed., St. Louis, Elsevier Saunders, 2011, Figure 5-16, p. 112.)

exist between RV and LV afterload systems: The pulmonary arterial circulation is substantially more compliant than systemic vasculature and, as mentioned previously, the RV is more sensitive to changes in afterload than the LV.

The most comprehensive description of LV afterload is aortic input impedance [$Z_{in}(\omega)$] defined as the ratio of continuous aortic pressure (the forces acting on the blood) to blood flow (the motion that those forces creates). Power spectral or Fourier series analysis is used to calculate $Z_{in}(\omega)$ from high-fidelity measurements of pressure and flow. $Z_{in}(\omega)$ includes the frequency dependent characteristics of the arterial vasculature with its viscoelastic effects and its wave reflection properties. This methodology is quite useful from an experimental perspective, but has limited practical applicability. Another definition of LV afterload quantifies the mechanical forces to which the LV is exposed during ejection as LV end-systolic wall stress. A large decline in LV volume occurs after the aortic valve opens concomitant with elevated LV pressure and increased wall thickness. As indicated by the Law of Laplace, changes in these variables cause a profound increase in LV end-systolic wall stress, which reaches its maximum value during early LV ejection and subsequently declines.[50] The alterations in LV systolic wall stress during ejection are important. Maximal LV systolic wall stress has been shown to be a stimulus for LV concentric hypertrophy in the presence of chronic increases in afterload, such as may be observed in patients with essential hypertension or severe aortic valve stenosis.[51] The area under the LV systolic wall stress curve is directly related to myocardial oxygen demand.[52] At end-systole, the forces driving further ejection and those resisting it are equal. Thus, LV end-systolic wall stress is a determinant of stroke volume and ejection fraction.

Afterload may also be approached from a mechanical systems perspective because the LV and the arterial vascular tree must be appropriately coupled to assure optimal energy transfer between them. In this model, the LV and arterial circulation are considered elastic chambers in series, and LV-arterial coupling is described using the ratio of LV elastance (E_{es}) and effective arterial elastance (E_a) determined using P–V analysis (Fig. 10-15).[40,53] E_a may also be estimated as the ratio of end-systolic arterial pressure to LV end-systolic pressure, and has been clinically applied to approximate LV afterload using this definition. E_a has been shown to be affected by arteriolar resistance and the compliance of the proximal great vessels, and as such, is often used to estimate LV afterload that resembles LV end-systolic wall stress. However, E_a does not include arterial frequency dependence or arterial wave reflection properties and cannot be used as a quantitative index of LV afterload as a result.

The most commonly used clinical estimate of LV afterload is systemic vascular resistance calculated as ((MAP-RAP) • 80)/CO, where MAP and RAP are mean arterial and right atrial pressures, respectively, CO is cardiac output, and 80 is a constant that converts mm Hg•min^{-1}•L^{-1} to dynes•sec•cm^{-5}. Similar to LV end-systolic wall stress and E_a, systemic vascular resistance does not consider the mechanical properties of the blood and arterial walls, ignores the frequency-dependence of arterial pressure and blood flow, and does not account for arterial wave reflection. Notably, these components of LV afterload are of greater importance in elderly patients or in the presence of peripheral vascular disease,[54] clinical circumstances in which quantitative evaluation of afterload may be more important to optimize cardiac output. In general, systemic vascular resistance is best used as a nonparametric estimate,[55] but not as a quantitative index, of LV afterload produced by vasoactive medications or cardiovascular disease.

The failing LV is especially sensitive to increases in afterload.[56] Activation of the sympathetic nervous system serves to improve contractility in the presence of LV systolic dysfunction, but this response also causes unintentional but equally important increases in LV afterload that may negate any potential increase in cardiac output. LV hypertrophy is also an important adaptation response to chronic increases in LV afterload that reduces LV wall stress by increasing wall thickness (Fig. 10-16). However, this compensatory response also inadvertently increases myocardial oxygen demand and reduces LV compliance. These effects make the hypertrophied LV more susceptible to myocardial ischemia and diastolic dysfunction, respectively. Thus, decreasing LV afterload by reducing the inciting stress is a crucial objective in the clinical management of CHF.

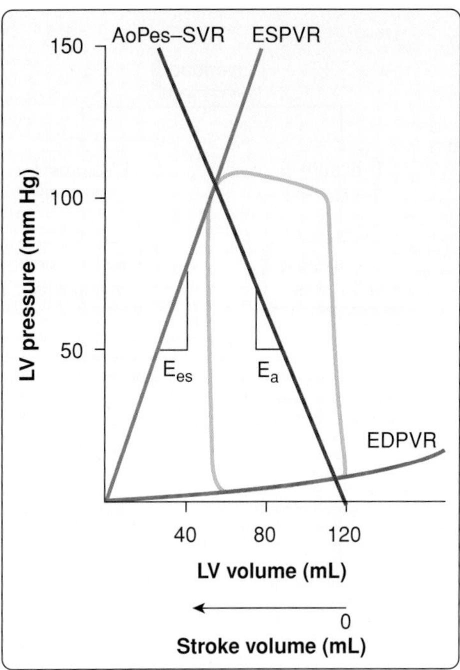

FIGURE 10-15. This schematic diagram illustrates the LV end-systolic pressure–volume and aortic end-systolic pressure–stroke volume relations (ESPVR and A_oP_{es}–SVR, respectively) used to determine LV-arterial coupling as the ratio of end-systolic elastance (E_{es}; the slope of ESPVR) and effective arterial elastance (E_a; the slope of A_oP_{es}–SVR). EDPVR, end-diastolic pressure–volume relation. (Reproduced with permission from: Kaplan JA, Reich DL, Savino JS. *Kaplan's Cardiac Anesthesia: The Echo Era*, 6th ed., St. Louis, Elsevier Saunders, 2011, Figure 5-19, p. 114.)

Myocardial Contractility

9 Myocardial contractility (also known as inotropic state) is the specific force that cardiac muscle is capable of producing during contraction under controlled loading conditions and stimulation rate. Such a measurement is certainly possible in isolated cardiac muscle, but determining contractility in the intact heart is remarkably difficult. This is clearly an important clinical objective because the ability to quantify inotropic state has substantial implications during the management of patients with LV or RV contractile dysfunction. Nevertheless, a "gold standard" of myocardial contractility that is truly independent of heart rate and loading conditions has not been developed. Indeed, it is essential to recognize that inotropic state and loading conditions are intimately interrelated in the sarcomere,[57] and hence, it may be impossible to measure contractility as a truly independent variable. To date, indices

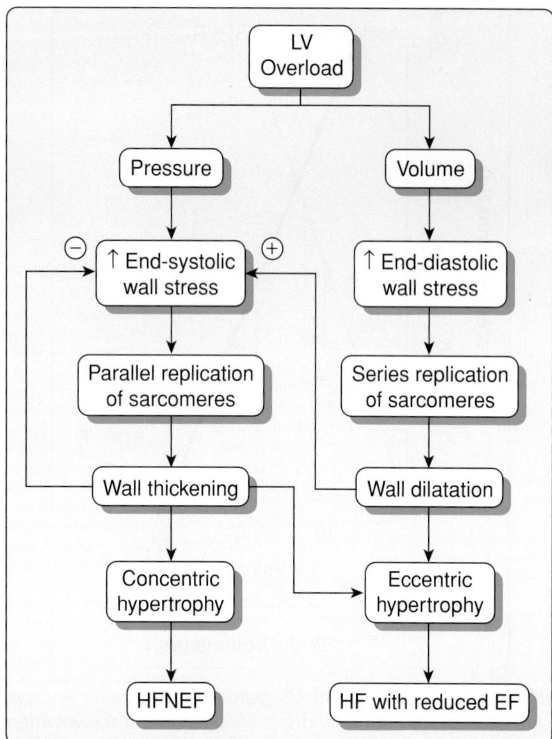

FIGURE 10-16. LV pressure- and volume-overload produce compensatory responses based on the nature of the inciting stress. Wall thickening reduces (–) whereas chamber dilation increases (+) end-systolic wall stress as predicted by the Law of Laplace. LV pressure-overload hypertrophy has been linked to heart failure with normal ejection fraction (HFNEF), but LV volume-overload most often causes heart failure (HF) with reduced ejection fraction (EF). (Reproduced with permission from: Kaplan JA, Reich DL, Savino JS. *Kaplan's Cardiac Anesthesia: The Echo Era*, 6th ed., St. Louis, Elsevier Saunders, 2011, Figure 5-21, p. 114.)

derived from LV P–V analysis, isovolumic contraction, and ejection are the major approaches to the measurement of contractility in vivo.

The ratio of continuous LV pressure-to-volume during the cardiac cycle has been characterized as "time-varying elastance," such that $E(t) = P(t)/[V(t) - V_0]$, where E(t) is the time-varying elastance, P(t) and V(t) are the time-dependent changes in LV pressure and volume, respectively, and V_0 is unstressed LV volume.[58] In this model, maximal LV elastance (E_{max}) typically occurs at or very close to the left upper corner of the steady state LV P–V diagram. As mentioned previously, a nested set of LV P–V diagrams may be generated by an acute change in loading conditions; each loop in this set has a distinct E_{max}. These E_{max} values are linearly related, and establish the ESPVR for the LV (Fig. 10-17). The slope of ESPVR is termed "end-systolic elastance" (E_{es}) and is an afterload-insensitive index of contractility because the analysis from which it is derived is performed at end-systole. Alterations in contractile state are reflected in changes in E_{es}. For example, intravenous administration of a positive inotropic medication such as dobutamine causes an increase in E_{es} to occur, the magnitude of which quantifies the change in contractility that has occurred. Another contractile index may be derived from the same series of LV P–V diagrams and is based on the Frank–Starling principle relating preload to cardiac output. There is linear relationship between the area of each LV P–V diagram (stroke work; SW) within this nested set of loops and its corresponding EDV, such that $SW = M_{sw} \cdot (EDV - V_{sw})$, where M_{sw} and V_{sw} are the slope and volume intercept of the relation. The slope of this "preload recruitable stroke work" relation has also been shown to quantify changes in contractility in a relatively load-independent manner.[59] E_{es} and M_{sw} are not used on a routine basis in clinical anesthesiology because invasive measurement of LV pressure and volume is required for its derivation and extensive off-line analysis must be performed. However, both indices of inotropic provide important conceptual tools with which to understand LV, RV, and atrial contractile function in the intact heart.

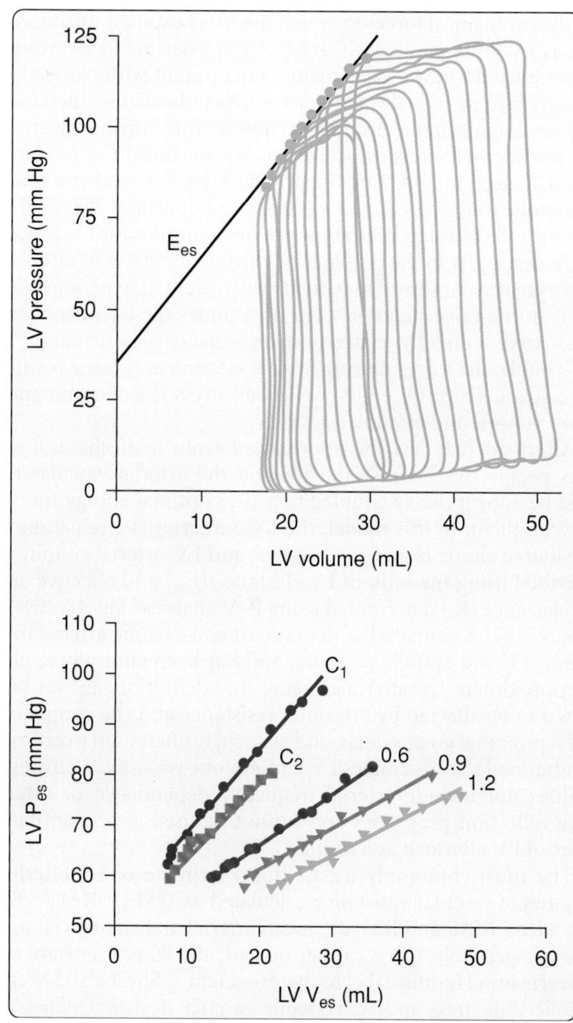

FIGURE 10-17. This illustration depicts the method used to derive the LV end-systolic pressure–volume relation (ESPVR) from a series of differentially loaded LV pressure–volume diagrams generated by abrupt occlusion of the inferior vena cava in a canine heart in vivo. The maximal elastance (E_{max}; pressure/volume ratio) for each pressure–volume diagram is identified as its left upper corner, and a linear regression analysis is used to define the slope (E_{es}; end-systolic elastance) and volume intercept of the ESPVR **(top panel)**. The effects of isoflurane (0.6, 0.9, and 1.2 minimum alveolar concentration) on the ESPVR are illustrated in the bottom panel. C_1, Control 1 (before isoflurane); C_2, Control 2 (after isoflurane). (Reproduced with permission from: Kaplan JA, Reich DL, Savino JS. *Kaplan's Cardiac Anesthesia: The Echo Era*, 6th ed., St. Louis, Elsevier Saunders, 2011, Figure 5-23, p. 116.)

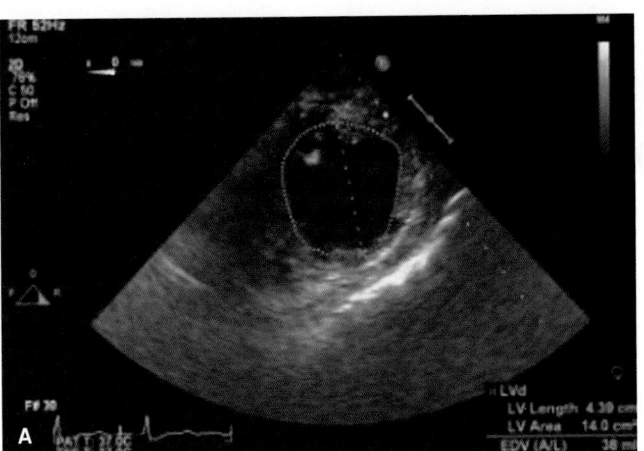

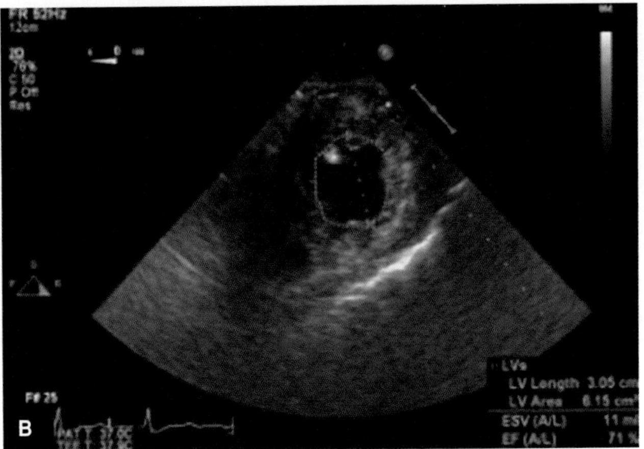

FIGURE 10-18. Calculation of fractional area change from LV midpapillary short axis images obtained at end-diastole **(left panel)** and end-systole **(right panel)**. The LV endocardial border is manually traced (excluding the papillary muscles). The software integrates the area inscribed of the LV chamber. (Reproduced with permission from: Kaplan JA, Reich DL, Savino JS. *Kaplan's Cardiac Anesthesia: The Echo Era*, 6th ed., St. Louis, Elsevier Saunders, 2011, Figure 5-27, p. 119.)

Indices of global myocardial contractility may also be derived using parameters obtained from the LV pressure waveform alone during isovolumic contraction. The most commonly used isovolumic index of contractility is the maximum rate of increase of LV pressure (+dP/dt). This index is typically obtained in the cardiac catheterization laboratory and usually requires invasive measurement of continuous LV pressure, but +dP/dt may also be estimated noninvasively using TEE.[60] LV +dP/dt sensitively indicates changes in contractile state, but its absolute value is less important than the magnitude of its change in response to an inotropic intervention (e.g., administration of epinephrine). LV +dP/dt is generally considered to be afterload-independent because the aortic valve opens after the maximal rate of rise of LV pressure occurs during isovolumic contraction. In contrast, +dP/dt is highly dependent on preload, although an index of contractility based on LV P–V analysis that compensates for this preload-dependence has been developed and validated.[61] LV +dP/dt is also affected by LV mass, chamber geometry, and valve disease. Declines in global LV inotropic state caused by regional myocardial ischemia may also not be accurately quantified with +dP/dt because compensatory increases in contractility may occur in the surrounding normal myocardium. Other isovolumic indices of contractility based on +dP/dt, including the rate of rise of LV pressure at a predetermined LV pressure (e.g., dP/dt measured at 40 mm Hg) or the ratio of dP/dt to maximum LV pressure (dP/dt/P) have also been used, but these measures do not provide unique additional information compared with +dP/dt.

Ejection fraction (EF; the ratio of stroke volume to EDV) is the most common clinical measure of LV contractility. Echocardiography is most often used to calculate EF, but other methods, including radionuclide angiography and dynamic magnetic resonance imaging, also provide very reliable estimates of this ejection phase index of inotropic state. In the operating room, two-dimensional TEE midesophageal four- or two-chamber windows are obtained at end-systole and end-diastole and are then analyzed using Simpson's rule of discs to determine EF. However, this technique is rather time consuming and may be impractical during rapidly changing hemodynamic conditions. Instead, regional approximations of EF such as fractional shortening and fractional area change (FAC) are often used by examining midpapillary short axis diameter and area, respectively, at end-systole and end-diastole. For example, FAC is determined as EDA–ESA/EDA, where EDA and ESA are end-diastolic and end-systolic areas, respectively, obtained by manually tracing the endocardial borders of the LV (Fig. 10-18). However, it is important to recognize that all ejection phase indices of contractility are dependent on both loading conditions and inotropic state. Thus, interpretation of EF, FAC, or fractional shortening must be considered within the clinical circumstances in which the value was obtained. The frequent observation of profoundly depressed EF in a patient with newly recognized CHF resulting may occur because afterload is markedly increased and not because of pure LV systolic dysfunction. Ejection phase indices may also be inaccurate when mitral or aortic valve disease is present. Hence, EF may be greater than normal during severe mitral regurgitation because a large percentage of blood flow from the LV is diverted into the low pressure LA during systole.

FACTORS THAT DETERMINE DIASTOLIC FUNCTION

10 Each chamber of the heart must fill adequately under normal pressures to facilitate optimal function during the subsequent contraction. We will emphasize LV diastolic function in the current section of this chapter, but the readers should be aware that the diastolic properties of the RV and atria are critically important
11 for the overall performance of the heart as well. Because diastole is an inherently complex sequence of temporally related events (Table 10-1), no single index of LV diastolic function completely characterizes this phase of the cardiac cycle or selectively predicts those patients who may be a greatest risk of developing CHF
12 related to abnormal diastolic function.[62] Notably, nearly one-half of patients with CHF do not have overt clinical evidence of LV contractile dysfunction (e.g., a reduction in LV EF).[63] Hypertensive elderly women who are obese or are affected by renal insufficiency, anemia, or atrial fibrillation appear to be at greatest risk of developing this "heart failure with normal ejection fraction" (HFNEF; also known as "diastolic heart failure").[64] Delayed LV relaxation, reduced compliance, and abnormal coupling

TABLE 10-1. DETERMINANTS OF LEFT VENTRICULAR DIASTOLIC FUNCTION

Heart rate and rhythm
LV systolic function
Wall thickness
Chamber geometry
Duration, rate, and extent of myocyte relaxation
LV untwisting and elastic recoil
Magnitude of diastolic suction
LA–LV pressure gradient
Passive elastic properties of LV myocardium
Viscoelastic effects (rapid LV filling and atrial systole)
LA structure and function
Mitral valve structure and function
Pulmonary venous blood flow
Pericardial restraint
RV loading conditions and function
Ventricular interdependence
Coronary blood flow and vascular engorgement
Compression by mediastinal masses

Abbreviation: LV, left ventricle; LA, left atrium; RV, right ventricle.
Reproduced with permission from: Kaplan JA, Reich DL, Savino JS. *Kaplan's Cardiac Anesthesia: The Echo Era*, 6th ed., St. Louis, Elsevier Saunders, 2011:121.

between the LV and the arterial circulation have been implicated in the pathophysiology of HFNEF (Table 10-1).[65,66] Thus, LV diastolic dysfunction is a primary cause of HFNEF, the severity and response to medical therapy of which are key factors that establish exercise tolerance[67] and may predict prognosis[68] in patients with heart failure independent of abnormal LV contractility. From the anesthesiologist's perspective, the LV response to changes in loading conditions (such as those observed in the operating room) is determined primarily by LV diastolic function. In addition, many commonly used volatile and intravenous anesthetics affect LV relaxation and filling in the normal and failing heart.[69] As a result, preoperative determination of the presence, cause (Table 10-2), and severity of LV diastolic dysfunction is important when caring for patients undergoing surgery in which large shifts in intravascular volume are anticipated.

Invasive Assessment of LV Relaxation

Removal of Ca^{2+} from the contractile apparatus and the sarcoplasm is an active, energy-dependent process that causes rapid dissociation of contractile proteins and recoil of compressed elastic elements. These events are essential for relaxation of cardiac muscle to occur. Clearly, failure of actin–myosin cross-bridges to properly dissociate or dysfunctional removal of intracellular Ca^{2+} may contribute to delays in relaxation in the intact LV.[70] Such abnormalities are important because early LV filling is dependent on the rate and extent of LV relaxation and hence, may be substantially attenuated if relaxation is delayed. Under these circumstances, the final EDV required for the next LV contraction becomes more dependent on the contribution of atrial systole. Thus, CHF is often precipitated by the acute onset of atrial fibrillation in patients with heart diseases characterized by delayed LV relaxation (e.g., pressure-overload hypertrophy, hypertrophic obstructive cardiomyopathy). Myocardial ischemia caused by acute occlusion of a major coronary artery is also a frequent cause of delayed LV relaxation and may be accompanied by reductions in LV compliance that further limit LV filling.[71]

13 Quantitative evaluation of LV relaxation is most often performed by assessing the rate of LV pressure decline during isovolumic relaxation. This type of analysis generally requires invasive measurement of continuous LV pressure and may be conducted in the cardiac catheterization laboratory. Several indices of LV relaxation may be derived using this method, among which the maximum rate at which LV pressure decreases (–dP/dt; analogous to +dP/dt during isovolumic contraction) and a time constant of LV relaxation (τ) are the most common. LV –dP/dt is not an ideal as an index of LV relaxation because this parameter is essentially a "snapshot" of relaxation at a single point in time that is primarily determined by the value of LV end-systolic pressure. LV pressure decay during relaxation is exponential between aortic valve closure and mitral valve opening; a time constant (τ) is often used to quantify LV relaxation using from the equation $P(t) = P_0e^{-t/\tau}$, where P(t) is time-dependent LV pressure, P_0 is LV pressure at end-systole, e is the natural exponent, and t is time after LV end-systole. Despite its inherent limitations,[33,72] an increase in τ indicates that a delay in LV relaxation has occurred. This technique has been used to quantify delays in LV relaxation during cardiac disease [e.g., myocardial ischemia,[73] pressure-overload hypertrophy][74] or as a result of administration of negative inotropic medications (e.g., volatile anesthetics).[75] In contrast, reductions in τ are observed during tachycardia, sympathetic nervous system activation, or administration of positive inotropic medications and indicate accelerated LV relaxation. From a clinical perspective, LV relaxation and its pharmacologic modulation are very important in CHF. LV relaxation is modestly dependent on afterload under normal conditions,[23] but this afterload-dependence of LV relaxation is especially pronounced in the failing heart.[76] Thus, medications that reduce afterload augment LV systolic function and simultaneously enhance LV relaxation (decrease τ) in patients with CHF.[56] This latter effect improves early LV filling dynamics, thereby decreasing congestive signs and symptoms.

TABLE 10-2. COMMON CAUSES OF LEFT VENTRICULAR DIASTOLIC DYSFUNCTION

Age >60 years
Acute myocardial ischemia (supply or demand)
Myocardial stunning, hibernation, or infarction
Ventricular remodeling after infarction
Pressure-overload hypertrophy (e.g., aortic stenosis, hypertension)
Volume-overload hypertrophy (e.g., aortic or mitral regurgitation)
Hypertrophic obstructive cardiomyopathy
Dilated cardiomyopathy
Restrictive cardiomyopathy (e.g., amyloidosis, hemochromatosis)
Pericardial diseases (e.g., tamponade, constrictive pericarditis)

Reproduced with permission from: Kaplan JA, Reich DL, Savino JS. *Kaplan's Cardiac Anesthesia: The Echo Era*, 6th ed., St. Louis, Elsevier Saunders, 2011:121.

Invasive Assessment of LV Filling and Compliance

Indices of LV filling may be calculated using invasive or noninvasive (e.g., echocardiography, radionuclide angiography, dynamic MRI) measurement of continuous LV volume. A biphasic waveform with peaks occurring during early LV filling ("E") and atrial systole ("A") is obtained when the LV volume waveform is differentiated with respect to time (dV/dt). This dV/dt waveform resembles the transmitral blood flow velocity signal acquired during LV filling using Doppler echocardiography (see later). Development of CHF has been shown to cause changes in the morphology of the dV/dt waveform that are very similar to the "delayed relaxation," "pseudonormal," and "restrictive" filling patterns measures using Doppler echocardiography (Fig. 10-19).[77] Invasive analysis of LV filling with continuous LV volume and its first derivative is limited almost exclusively to the laboratory and is of little practical value in clinical anesthesiology.

As mentioned previously, EDPVR is an index of LV compliance derived from a nested set of LV P–V diagrams. The relationship between EDP and EDV is exponential: $EDP = Ae^{K(EDV)} + B$, where K is the modulus of chamber stiffness and A and B are curve-fitting constants. Thus, an increase in K indicates that the LV is less compliant and therefore, requires higher LV pressure to distend the LV to a given volume. Parallel upward shifts in the EDPVR, such as those observed during pericardial tamponade, represent an exception, the value of K is not affected under these circumstances even though LV pressure is greater at each LV volume.[43] Thus, the relative position of the EDPVR may be more important than the actual value of K itself because a shift in EDPVR up or to the left indicates that a higher LV pressure is required to achieve a similar LV volume.[78] The diastolic stress–strain relation is another model frequently used to experimentally characterize LV compliance. Myocardium is an elastic material that follows Hooke's law, that is, cardiac muscle develops resisting forces (stress; σ) as muscle length (strain; ε) increases during LV filling. The relation is exponential: $\sigma = \alpha(e^{\beta\varepsilon} - 1)$, where α is the coefficient of gain and β is the modulus of myocardial stiffness.[79] Similar to the EDPVR, an increase in β occurs when the stress–strain relationship shifts up or to the left and may be observed in pathologic conditions characterized by fundamental structural abnormalities that adversely influence myocardial stiffness (e.g., hypertrophic cardiomyopathy, amyloidosis). EDPVR and myocardial stress–strain relations are generally not used clinically because analysis required to examine these relationships is complicated, time consuming, and not feasible during rapidly changing hemodynamic conditions.

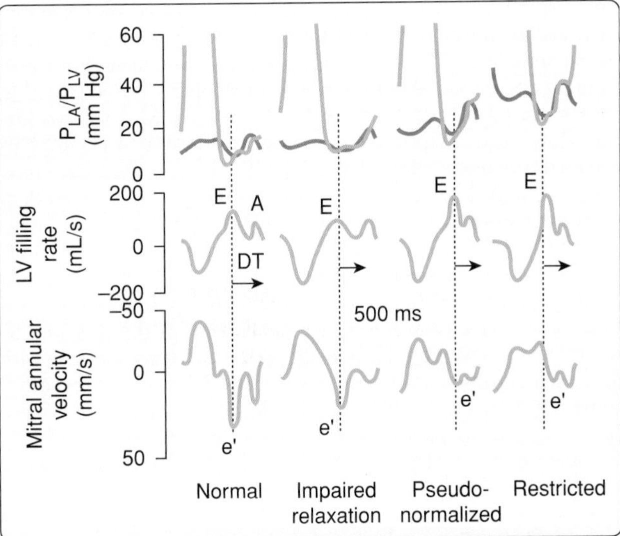

FIGURE 10-19. This illustration depicts the simultaneous relationships between LA and LV pressures (P_{LA} and P_{LV}, respectively; **top panel**), LV filling rate during early filling (E) and atrial systole (A; **middle panel**), and early mitral annular velocity (e′; **bottom panel**) under normal conditions and during evolving diastolic dysfunction (impaired relaxation, pseudonormal, and restrictive). Note the initial lengthening of E wave deceleration time (DT) during impaired relaxation and the subsequent shortening of DT as diastolic function worsens. (Reproduced with permission from: Kaplan JA, Reich DL, Savino JS. *Kaplan's Cardiac Anesthesia: The Echo Era*, 6th ed., St. Louis, Elsevier Saunders, 2011, Figure 5-29, p. 122.)

Noninvasive Evaluation of Diastolic Function

The duration between aortic valve closure and mitral valve opening defines isovolumic relaxation time (IVRT), which is often used as a noninvasive index of LV relaxation. IVRT is the time interval between the end of aortic blood flow (end-systole) and the opening of the mitral valve (beginning of transmitral blood flow) and is usually measured using M-mode or Doppler echocardiography. In the absence of aortic or mitral valve disease, IVRT is determined by the rate of LV relaxation and the difference between LV end-systolic pressure and LA pressure when the mitral valve opens.[80] Thus, IVRT is dependent on both LV relaxation and loading conditions. IVRT is seldom used alone, but is most often combined with the transmitral blood flow velocity pattern (see later) to define the rate and extent of LV relaxation.

Noninvasive analysis of LV diastolic function is based on Doppler echocardiographic evaluation of transmitral blood flow velocity.[81] A pulse-wave Doppler echocardiography sample volume is placed between the mitral leaflets to obtain a high-resolution transmitral blood flow velocity waveform. The normal pattern of transmitral blood flow velocity has two peaks: An early "E" peak associated with early LV filling and a late "A" peak corresponding to LA systole.[82] The ratio of these peak E and A wave velocities is commonly used to quantify the relative contributions of early LV filling and atrial systole to EDV. The time elapsed as the E wave velocity falls to zero is known as the deceleration time; this parameter may be used with or without IVRT to assess LV relaxation. For example, an increase in E wave deceleration time indicates that early LV filling is prolonged because LV relaxation is delayed. Age affects LV diastolic function because a gradual slowing of LV relaxation occurs. Under these circumstances IVRT, deceleration time, and A wave velocity increase, whereas E wave velocity and E/A ratio decrease.[83] These changes occur because the heart becomes less compliant with age, especially in the presence of coexisting essential hypertension and LV hypertrophy. These age-related changes in LV diastolic function predispose the elderly patients to develop CHF.[84]

The reversal of E/A secondary to age is an example of "delayed relaxation." This transmitral blood flow velocity pattern is the least severe of three abnormal LV filling patterns that describe the continuum of LV diastolic dysfunction. Clinical symptoms, exercise tolerance, New York Heart Association (NYHA) functional class, and mortality are closely correlated with the relative severity of LV diastolic dysfunction as indicated using this method.[85] The "delayed relaxation" pattern is characterized by a reduced peak E velocity and an increased peak A velocity (E/A < 1) and indicates that early LV filling is attenuated concomitant

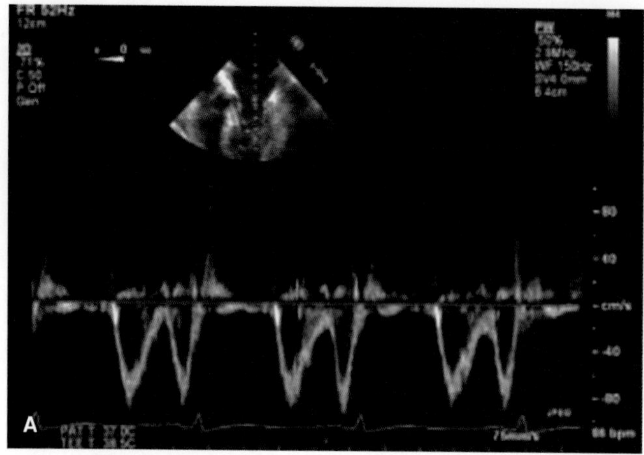

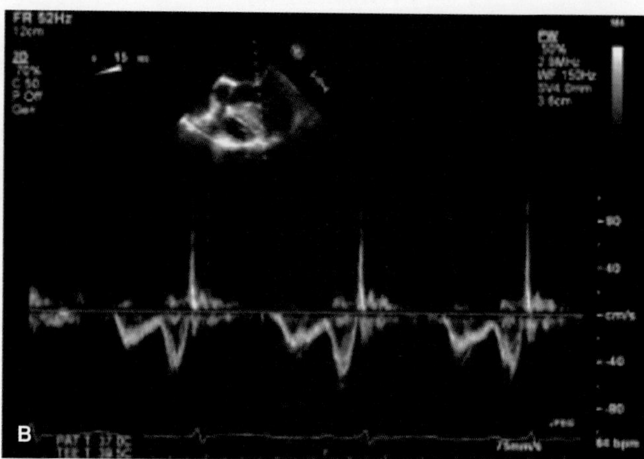

FIGURE 10-20. Transmitral blood flow velocity waveforms obtained using pulse wave Doppler echocardiography under normal conditions **(left)** and during delayed relaxation **(right)**. (Reproduced with permission from: Kaplan JA, Reich DL, Savino JS. *Kaplan's Cardiac Anesthesia: The Echo Era*, 6th ed., St. Louis, Elsevier Saunders, 2011, Figure 5-31, p. 123.)

with enhanced LA "kick.[77]" The "delayed relaxation" pattern is often observed in patients with essential hypertension, pressure-overload LV hypertrophy, and ischemic heart disease (Fig. 10-20).

As diastolic dysfunction worsens, a "pseudonormal" pattern replaces after the "delayed relaxation" profile. The pseudonormal pattern occurs because E/A becomes >1 as LA pressures progressively increase. As a result, E wave velocity "normalizes" because the LA–LV pressure gradient increases when the mitral valve opens. The "pseudonormal" pattern may be distinguished from a normal pattern by using other indices of diastolic function (e.g., pulmonary venous blood flow velocity, tissue Doppler imaging) or by administration of a vasodilator which may convert a pseudonormal profile to a delayed relaxation pattern.[86] A "restrictive pattern" of transmitral blood flow velocity indicates severe LV diastolic dysfunction in which LA pressure is markedly elevated and LV compliance is further reduced. The E/A becomes >2 as the LA–LV pressure gradient is further augmented by increased LA pressure (causing a larger peak E wave velocity) concomitant with progressive LA contractile dysfunction (decline in peak A wave velocity). Failure of a "restrictive" filling pattern to respond to administration of a vasodilator and revert to a pseudonormal or delayed relaxation pattern is associated with a poor prognosis in patients with heart failure[81].

Abnormal LV diastolic function may also be determined using analysis of the pulmonary venous blood flow velocity pattern
14 obtained with pulse-wave Doppler echocardiography.[87] Most often, the pulmonary venous blood flow velocity is used in conjunction with transmitral blood flow velocity when quantifying the severity of LV diastolic dysfunction.[88] Two large positive deflections (indicating forward flow from the pulmonary veins into the LA) and a single, small negative reflection (demonstrating retrograde flow from the LA to the pulmonary veins, termed "atrial reversal") make up the normal pulmonary venous blood flow velocity pattern. The first positive deflection is known as the "S" (systolic) wave, and occurs during LV systole and early isovolumic relaxation before the mitral valve opens.[89] This "S" wave results from LA relaxation, which facilitates movement of blood from the pulmonary veins into the LA. The mitral valve annulus also descends toward the LV apex during systole, drawing additional blood from the pulmonary veins into the LA.[90] Thus, it is not surprising that LA filling is adversely affected by depressed myocardial contractility. Additional LA filling occurs as a result of transmission of the RV systolic pressure pulse through the pulmonary circulation. After the mitral valve opens, blood stored in the LA during LV systole enters the LV, an event which allows further flow from the pulmonary veins into the LA to occur. This causes the second positive deflection ("D" wave) of the pulmonary venous blood flow velocity pattern. The "D" wave is dependent on the extent of early LV filling and LV compliance.[91] The "atrial reversal" ("Ar") wave is determined by LA preload, LA contractile state, and LV pressure during late diastole.[92]

Like transmitral blood flow velocity, the pulmonary venous blood flow velocity profile is age-dependent, as the ratio of "S" to "D" waves and the peak velocity of the "Ar" wave increase with age.[82] These observations emphasize that LA function becomes more important to LV filling in the elderly. As LV diastolic function worsens, LA pressures increase and the "S" wave gradually becomes blunted (Fig. 10-21); this allows distinction between

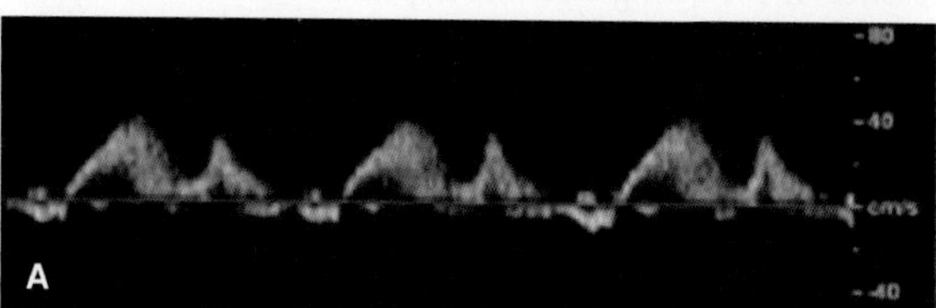

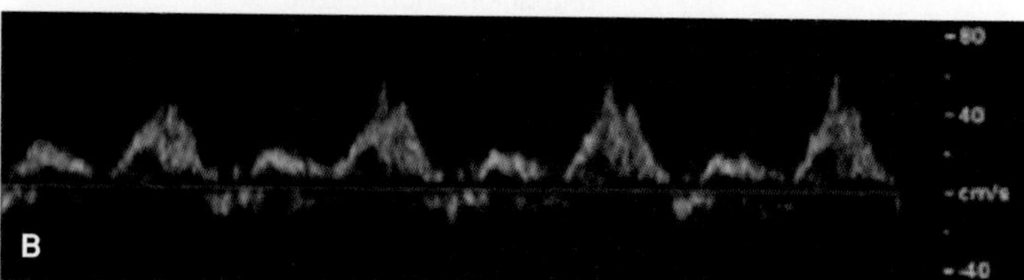

FIGURE 10-21. Pulmonary venous blood flow velocity waveforms obtained using pulse wave Doppler echocardiography under normal conditions **(left panel)** and in the presence of increased LA pressure **(right panel)**. (Reproduced with permission from: Kaplan JA, Reich DL, Savino JS. *Kaplan's Cardiac Anesthesia: The Echo Era,* 6th ed., St. Louis, Elsevier Saunders, 2011, Figure 5-33, p. 125.)

normal and pseudonormal transmitral blood flow velocity patterns because the "S" to "D" ratio falls below one in the latter condition.[87] These changes become even more exaggerated in the presence of a restrictive filling pattern because LV diastolic and LA pressures are further elevated. The "S" wave may be completely abolished or even reversed concomitant with an enhanced "D" wave under these circumstances. Thus, pulmonary venous blood flow velocity patterns also provide very useful information about the pathophysiologic changes associated with developing LV diastolic dysfunction. Other indices of diastolic function, including tissue Doppler imaging[93] and color M-mode propagation velocity,[94] may also be used to define the progression of LV diastolic dysfunction. They will be discussed in detail in Chapter 26.

Pericardium

The heart, proximal great vessels, venae cavae, and pulmonary veins are contained in the pericardium. The pericardium separates the heart from other structures in the mediastinum and limits the heart's displacement through its diaphragmatic and great vessel attachments. The fluid in the pericardium (plasma ultrafiltrate, lymph, and myocardial interstitial fluid; total volume of 15 to 35 mL) acts as a lubricant that facilitates cardiac movement. The pericardium is much less compliant than LV myocardium, and has very limited volume reserve (Fig. 10-22).[95] As a result, acute increases in pericardial volume (e.g., tamponade) cause pronounced elevations in pericardial pressure that restricts filling of the LV and other cardiac chambers.[96] Since the atria and RV have thinner walls than the LV, pericardial restraint is most apparent in these chambers. Indeed, the diastolic pressure and volume of the RA, LA, and RV is determined primarily by pericardial restraint and not by the relative compliance of these chambers alone. LV filling is also profoundly affected by the pericardium.[97] A parallel upward shift of the EDPVR occurs as a result of an acute increase in pericardial pressure.[98] This shift in the EDPVR indicates that LV pressure must be increased for each LV volume and explains why LV filling is impaired in the presence of pericardial tamponade. Whereas the pericardium is acutely noncompliant, a chronic, gradual increase in pericardial pressure (e.g., a slowly developing pericardial effusion or biventricular dilatation) causes the pericardium to stretch. This compensatory response increases the pericardium's compliance and reduces its restraining effects, allowing the heart to continue functioning without precipitous hemodynamic collapse.

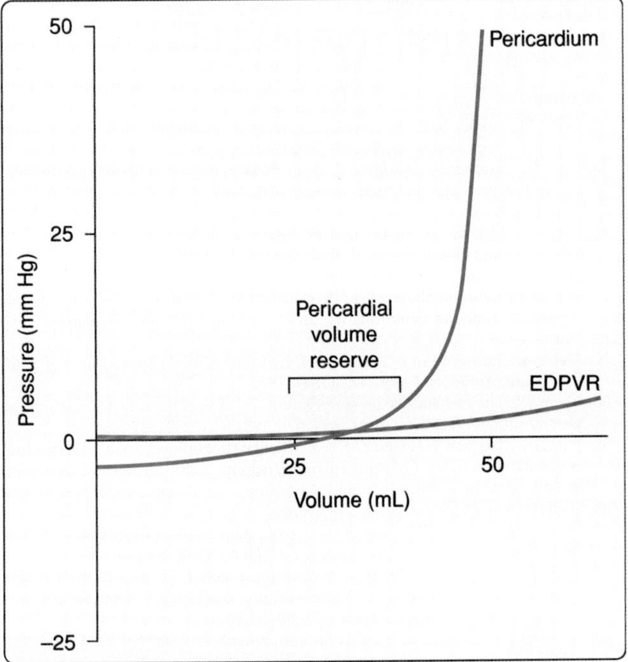

FIGURE 10-22. Pressure–volume relation of the pericardium (*blue*) compared with the LV end-diastolic pressure–volume relation (EDPVR; *orange*). Note that large increases in pericardial occur after reserve volume is exceeded. (Reproduced with permission from: Kaplan JA, Reich DL, Savino JS. *Kaplan's Cardiac Anesthesia: The Echo Era*, 6th ed., St. Louis, Elsevier Saunders, 2011, Figure 5-35, p. 127.)

The influence of the pressure and volume of one ventricle on the function of the other is known as ventricular interdepen-
15 dence. The pericardium plays a crucial role in ventricular interdependence because it equally restrains the RV and the LV. As a result, an acute increase in RV pressure and volume (e.g., volume overload) causes the pressure within the pericardium to increase as well. This action compresses the LV, reducing its effective compliance and impairing its filling.[99] Not surprisingly, LV distention has a similar effect on the RV and limits RV filling through an identical mechanism.[100] Ventricular interdependence may be readily appreciated by examining changes in RV and LV filling during spontaneous ventilation.[101] Since intrathoracic pressure declines during inspiration, venous return to the right side of the heart increases and produces modest dilation of the RV. The result of this RV distention is a corresponding increase in pericardial restraint of the LV, which limits LV filling and causes a small decrease in stroke volume and mean arterial pressure. This ventricular interaction effect between the RV and the LV is reversed during expiration. Notably, pericardial tamponade[102] or constrictive pericarditis[103] exaggerates the normal respiratory changes in RV and LV filling and produces the phenomenon known as pulsus paradoxus. It is important to realize that spontaneous ventilation is critical in these conditions because negative intrathoracic pressure assists venous return, whereas cardiovascular collapse may ensue with the initiation of positive pressure ventilation because venous return may be profoundly limited.

Atrial Function

The mechanical properties of the LA are often overlooked in dis-
16 cussions of cardiac physiology. This is unfortunate because the LA acts as a contractile chamber, a reservoir (storage of blood before mitral valve opening), and a conduit (analogous to an extension of the pulmonary veins) and its function is crucial to LV performance. The maximum velocity of shortening of LA myocardium is equal to or greater than LV myocardium under similar loading conditions.[104]. LA emptying fraction (similar to LV EF) is dependent on LA contractility and preload unless the LA is dilated to the point at which its myofilaments are stretched far beyond normal operating length,[105] such as may occur when LA pressures are chronically elevated as a result of severe LV diastolic dysfunction or mitral regurgitation. Under these conditions, the LA may no longer be capable of contributing to EDV as a contractile chamber. The LA response to changes in autonomic nervous system activity, inotropic medications, and anesthetics is very similar to that of the LV.[106,107] The afterload faced by the LA during contraction is determined by LV compliance and pressure during late diastole. This observation implies that the LA must perform greater work in the presence of LV diastolic dysfunction because its afterload is increased. Like the RV, the LA

is more susceptible to acute increases in afterload than the LV because the LA has thinner walls and less muscle mass. Thus, the LA emptying fraction may initially increase early during developing LV failure.[108] Subsequently, LA contractile dysfunction occurs as the chamber dilates in response to reduced LV compliance and increased pressure.[109] LV diastolic dysfunction also causes remodeling and reduced compliance of the LA, which further limit pulmonary venous return.

The LA also serves reservoir and conduit functions. The reservoir function of the LA is determined by LA relaxation, LV base descent during systole, transmission of RV stroke volume, and LA compliance. Thus, LA ischemia, hypertrophy, or dilation often attenuate reservoir function, as do LV or RV contractile dysfunction.[90,92] Diseases in which LA compliance is reduced are also associated with impaired LA filling and contribute to pulmonary venous congestion.[37,110] The LA appendage plays an important role in LA filling, as exclusion or excision of the LA appendage reduces the compliance of the LA as a whole.[111,112]

Exercise enhances both LA contractility and reservoir function.[113] The latter effect is important because greater reservoir capacity causes a larger LA–LV pressure gradient during early LV filling, thereby facilitating additional blood flow to the LV during conditions requiring greater LV stroke volume and cardiac output. Conduit function is also been augmented in endurance athletes.[114] Compensatory increases in LA emptying fraction and declines in passive LA emptying occur as the LA begins to dilate in healthy elderly subjects. [115] LA dilation initially augments the ratio of LA reservoir to LV stroke volume (termed "storage fraction"),[116] but comes at a cost because this dilation increases in LA wall stress and contributes to eventual LA contractile dysfunction and the onset of atrial arrhythmias in the elderly.[117]

References

1. Buckberg GD, Coghlan HC, Torrent-Guasp F. The structure and function of the helical heart and its buttress wrapping. VI. Geometric concepts of heart failure and use for structural correction. *Semin Thorac Cardiovasc Surg.* 2001;13: 386–401.
2. Cheng CP, Noda T, Nozawa T, et al. Effect of heart failure on the mechanism of exercise-induced augmentation of mitral valve flow. *Circ Res.* 1993;72:795–806.
3. Takayama Y, Costa KD, Covell JW. Contribution of laminar myofiber architecture to load-dependent changes in mechanics of LV myocardium. *Am J Physiol Heart Circ Physiol.* 2002;282:H1510–H1520.
4. Gharib M, Rambod E, Kheradvar A, et al. Optimal vortex formation as an index of cardiac health. *Proc Natl Acad Sci U S A.* 2006;103:6305–6308.
5. Voci P, Bilotta F, Caretta Q, et al. Papillary muscle perfusion pattern. A hypothesis for ischemic papillary muscle dysfunction. *Circulation.* 1995;91:1714–1718.
6. Stefanadis C, Dernellis J, Tsiamis E, et al. Effects of pacing-induced and balloon coronary occlusion ischemia on left atrial function in patients with coronary artery disease. *J Am Coll Cardiol* 1999;33:687–696.
7. Tops LF, Schalij MJ, Bax JJ. The effects of right ventricular apical pacing on ventricular function and dyssynchrony implications for therapy. *J Am Coll Cardiol.* 2009;54:764–776.
8. Epstein AE, DiMarco JP, Ellenbogen KA, et al. ACC/AHA/HRS 2008 Guidelines for Device-Based Therapy of Cardiac Rhythm Abnormalities: A report of the American College of Cardiology/American Heart Association Task Force on Practice Guidelines (Writing Committee to Revise the ACC/AHA/NASPE 2002 Guideline Update for Implantation of Cardiac Pacemakers and Antiarrhythmia Devices): Developed in collaboration with the American Association for Thoracic Surgery and Society of Thoracic Surgeons. *Circulation.* 2008;117:e350–e408.
9. Gorman MW, Tune JD, Richmond KN, et al. Feedforward sympathetic coronary vasodilation in exercising dogs. *J Appl Physiol.* 2000;89:1892–1902.
10. Gorman MW, Rooke GA, Savage MV, et al. Adenine nucleotide control of coronary blood flow during exercise. *Am J Physiol Heart Circ Physiol.* 2010;299: H1981–H1989.
11. Schaub MC, Hefti MA, Zuellig RA, et al. Modulation of contractility in human cardiac hypertrophy by myosin essential light chain isoforms. *Cardiovasc Res.* 1998;37:381–404.
12. Cazorla O, Vassort G, Garnier D, et al. Length modulation of active force in rat cardiac myocytes: Is titin the sensor? *J Mol Cell Cardiol.* 1999;31:1215–1227.
13. Helmes M, Trombitas K, Granzier H. Titin develops restoring force in rat cardiac myocytes. *Circ Res* 1996;79:619–626.
14. Schiaffino S, Reggiani C. Molecular diversity of myofibrillar proteins: Gene regulation and molecular significance. *Physiol Rev.* 1996;76:371–423.
15. Moncman CL, Wang K. Nebulette: A 107 kD nebulin-like protein in cardiac muscle. *Cell Motil Cytoskeleton.* 1995;32:205–225.
16. Solaro RJ, Rarick HM. Troponin and tropomyosin. Proteins that switch on and tune in the activity of cardiac myofilaments. *Circ Res.* 1998;83:471–480.
17. Tobacman LS. Thin filament-mediated regulation of cardiac contraction. *Annu Rev Physiol.* 1996;58:447–481.
18. Solaro RJ, Van Eyk J. Altered interactions among thin filaments proteins modulate cardiac function. *J Mol Cell Cardiol.* 1999;28:217–230.
19. Luo W, Grupp IL, Harrer J, et al. Targeted ablation of the phospholamban gene is associated with markedly enhanced myocardial contractility and loss of beta agonist stimulation. *Circ Res.* 1994;75:401–409.
20. Rayment I, Holden HM, Whittaker M, et al. Structure of the actin-myosin complex and its implications for muscle contraction. *Science.* 1993;261:58–65.
21. Dominguez R, Freyzon Y, Trybus KM, et al. Crystal structure of a vertebrate smooth muscle myosin motor domain and its complex with the essential light chain: Visualization of the pre-power stroke state. *Cell.* 1998;94:559–571.
22. Finer JT, Simmons RM, Spudich JA. Single myosin molecule mechanics: Piconewton forces and nanometer steps. *Nature.* 1994;368:113–119.
23. Gilbert JC, Glantz SA. Determinants of left ventricular filling and of the diastolic pressure-volume relation. *Circ Res.* 1989;64:827–852.
24. Stefanadis C, Dernellis J, Stratos C, et al. Assessment of left atrial pressure-area relation in humans by means of retrograde left atrial catheterization and echocardiographic automatic boundary detection: Effects of dobutamine. *J Am Coll Cardiol.* 1998;31:426–436.
25. Florenzano F, Glantz SA. Left ventricular mechanical adaptation to chronic aortic regurgitation in intact dogs. *Am J Physiol.* 1987;252:H969–H984.
26. Regen DM, Anversa P, Capasso JM. Segmental calculation of left ventricular wall stresses. *Am J Physiol.* 1993;264:H1411–H1421.
27. Haddad F, Couture P, Tousignant C, et al. The right ventricle in cardiac surgery, a perioperative perspective: I. Anatomy, physiology, and assessment. *Anesth Analg.* 2009;108:407–421.
28. Cheng CP, Freeman GL, Santamore WP, et al. Effect of loading conditions, contractile state, and heart rate on early diastolic left ventricular filling in conscious dogs. *Circ Res.* 1990;66:814–823.
29. Courtois M, Kovacs SJ Jr, Ludbrook PA. Transmitral pressure-flow velocity relation. Importance of regional pressure gradients in the left ventricle during diastole. *Circulation.* 1988;78:661–671.
30. Ishida Y, Meisner JS, Tsujioka K, et al. Left ventricular filling dynamics: Influence of left ventricular relaxation and left atrial pressure. *Circulation.* 1986;74:187–196.
31. Little WC, Oh JK. Echocardiographic evaluation of diastolic function can be used to guide clinical care. *Circulation.* 2009;120:802–809.
32. Kheradvar A, Gharib M. On mitral valve dynamics and its connection to early diastolic flow. *Ann Biomed Eng.* 2009;37:1–13.
33. Yellin EL, Nikolic S, Frater RWM. Left ventricular filling dynamics and diastolic function. *Prog Cardiovasc Dis.* 1990;32:247–271.
34. Suga H, Yasumura Y, Nozawa T, et al. Pressure-volume relation around zero transmural pressure in excised cross-circulated dog left ventricle. *Circ Res.* 1988; 63:361–372.
35. Keren G, Meisner JS, Sherez J, et al. Interrelationship of mid-diastolic mitral valve motion, pulmonary venous flow, and transmitral flow. *Circulation.* 1986;74: 36–44.
36. Barbier P, Solomon SB, Schiller NB, et al. Left atrial relaxation and left ventricular systolic function determine left atrial reservoir function. *Circulation.* 1999; 100:427–436.
37. Mehta S, Charbonneau F, Fitchett DH, et al. The clinical consequences of a stiff left atrium. *Am Heart J.* 1991;122:1184–1191.
38. Sagawa K. The end-systolic pressure-volume relation of the ventricle: Definition, modifications and clinical use. *Circulation.* 1981;63:1223–1227.
39. Kass DA, Maughan WL, Guo ZM, et al. Comparative influence of load versus inotropic states on indexes of ventricular contractility: Experimental and theoretical analysis based on pressure-volume relationships. *Circulation.* 1987;76:1422–1436.
40. Suga H. Ventricular energetics. *Physiol Rev.* 1990;70:247–277.
41. Brown KA, Ditchey RV. Human right ventricular end-systolic pressure-volume relation defined by maximal elastance. *Circulation.* 1988;78:81–91.
42. Pagel PS, Kehl F, Gare M, et al. Mechanical function of the left atrium: New insights based on analysis of pressure-volume relations and Doppler echocardiography. *Anesthesiology.* 2003;98:975–994.
43. Grossman W. Diastolic dysfunction and congestive heart failure. *Circulation.* 1990;81(2 Suppl):III1–III7.
44. Little WC, Downes TR. Clinical evaluation of left ventricular diastolic performance. *Prog Cardiovasc Dis.* 1990;32:273–290.
45. Wier W, Yue DT. Intracellular calcium transients underlying the short-term force-interval relationship in ferret ventricular myocardium. *J Physiol.* 1986; 376:507–530.
46. Vatner SF. Sympathetic mechanisms regulating myocardial contractility in conscious animals. In Fozzard HA, Haber E, Jennings RB, et al., eds. *The Heart and*

Cardiovascular System: Scientific Foundations, 2nd Ed. New York: Raven Press: 1991:1709–1728.
47. Little WC, Freeman GL, O'Rourke RA. Simultaneous determination of left ventricular end-systolic pressure-volume and pressure-dimension relationships in closed-chest dogs. *Circulation.* 1985;71:1301–1308.
48. Burkhoff D. The conductance method of left ventricular volume estimation. Methodologic limitations put into perspective. *Circulation.* 1990;81:703–706.
49. Hansen RM, Viquerat CE, Matthay MA, et al. Poor correlation between pulmonary arterial wedge pressure and left ventricular end-diastolic volume after coronary artery bypass graft surgery. *Anesthesiology.* 1986;64:764–770.
50. Grossman W, Jones D, McLaurin LP. Wall stress and patterns of hypertrophy in the human left ventricle. *J Clin Invest.* 1975;56:56–64.
51. Borow KM, Colan SD, Neumann A. Altered left ventricular mechanics in patients with valvular aortic stenosis and coarctation of the aorta: Effects on systolic performance and late outcome. *Circulation.* 1985;72:515–522.
52. Weber KT, Janicki JS. Myocardial oxygen consumption: The role of wall force and shortening. *Am J Physiol.* 1977;233:H421–H430.
53. Little WC, Cheng CP. Left ventricular-arterial coupling in conscious dogs. *Am J Physiol.* 1991;261:H70–H76.
54. Nichols WW, Nicolini FA, Pepine CJ. Determinants of isolated systolic hypertension in the elderly. *J Hypertens Suppl.* 1992;10:S73–S77.
55. Lang RM, Borow KM, Neumann A, et al. Systemic vascular resistance: An unreliable index of left ventricular afterload. *Circulation.* 1986;74:1114–1123.
56. Little WC. Enhanced load dependence of relaxation in heart failure. Clinical implications. *Circulation.* 1992;85:2326–2328.
57. De Tombe PP, Little WC. Inotropic effects of ejection are myocardial properties. *Am J Physiol.* 1994;266:H1202–H1213.
58. Suga H, Sagawa K, Shoukas AA. Load-independence of the instantaneous pressure-volume ratio of the canine left ventricle and effects of epinephrine and heart rate on the ratio. *Circ Res.* 1973;32:314–322.
59. Glower DD, Spratt JA, Snow ND, et al. Linearity of the Frank–Starling relationship in the intact heart: The concept of preload recruitable stroke work. *Circulation.* 1985;71:994–1009.
60. Chen C, Rodriguez L, Guerrero JL, et al. Noninvasive estimation of the instantaneous first derivative of left ventricular pressure using continuous-wave Doppler echocardiography. *Circulation.* 1991;83:2101–2110.
61. Little WC. The left ventricular dP/dt_{max}-end-diastolic volume relation in closed-chest dogs. *Circ Res.* 1985;56:808–815.
62. Yew WYW. Evaluation of left ventricular diastolic function. *Circulation.* 1989;79:1393–1397.
63. Gaasch WH, Zile MR. Left ventricular diastolic dysfunction and diastolic heart failure. *Annu Rev Med.* 2004;55:373–394.
64. Maeder MT, Kaye DM. Heart failure with normal left ventricular ejection fraction. *J Am Coll Cardiol.* 2009;53:905–918.
65. Zile MR, Baicu CF, Gaasch WH. Diastolic heart failure – abnormalities in active relaxation and passive stiffness of the left ventricle. *N Engl J Med.* 2004;350: 1953–1959.
66. Bench T, Burkhoff D, O'Connell JB, et al. Heart failure with normal ejection fraction: Consideration of mechanisms other than diastolic dysfunction. *Curr Heart Fail Rep.* 2009;6:57–64.
67. Grewal J, McCully RB, Kane GC, et al. Left ventricular function and exercise capacity. *JAMA.* 2009;301:286–294.
68. Traversi E, Pozzoli M, Cioffi G, et al. Mitral flow velocity changes after 6 months of optimized therapy provides important hemodynamic and prognostic information in patients with heart failure. *Am Heart J.* 1996;132:809–819.
69. Pagel PS, Farber NE, Pratt Jr PF, et al. Cardiovascular pharmacology, in Miller RD (ed), *Miller's Anesthesia*, 7th edition. Philadelphia: Elsevier Churchill Livingstone, 2009, pp. 595–632.
70. Morgan JP, Erny RE, Allen PD, et al. Abnormal intracellular calcium handling, a major cause of systolic and diastolic dysfunction in ventricular myocardium from patients with heart failure. *Circulation.* 1990;81(2 Suppl):III21–III32.
71. Carroll JD, Hess OM, Hirzel HO, et al. Left ventricular systolic and diastolic function in coronary artery disease: Effects of revascularization on exercise-induced ischemia. *Circulation.* 1985;72:119–129.
72. Raff GL, Glantz SA. Volume loading slows left ventricular isovolumic relaxation rate. Evidence of load-dependent relaxation in the intact dog heart. *Circ Res.* 1981; 48:813–824.
73. Serizawa T, Vogel WM, Apstein CS, et al. Comparison of acute alterations in left ventricular relaxation and diastolic chamber stiffness induced by hypoxia and ischemia. Role of myocardial oxygen supply-demand imbalance. *J Clin Invest.* 1981;68:91–102.
74. Eichhorn P, Grimm J, Koch R, et al. Left ventricular relaxation in patients with left ventricular hypertrophy secondary to aortic valve disease. *Circulation.* 1982;65:1395–1404.
75. Pagel PS, Kampine JP, Schmeling WT, et al. Alteration of left ventricular diastolic function by desflurane, isoflurane, and halothane in the chronically instrumented dog with autonomic nervous system blockade. *Anesthesiology.* 1991;74:1103–1114.
76. Eichhorn EJ, Willard JE, Alvarez L, et al. Are contraction and relaxation coupled in patients with and without congestive heart failure? *Circulation.* 1992;85:2132–2139.
77. Ohno M, Cheng CP, Little WC. Mechanism of altered patterns of left ventricular filling during the development of congestive heart failure. *Circulation.* 1994; 89:2241–2250.
78. Glantz SA. Computing indices of diastolic stiffness has been counterproductive. *Fed Proc.* 1980;39:162–168.
79. Mirsky I. Assessment of diastolic function: Suggested methods and future considerations. *Circulation.* 1984;69:836–841.
80. Myreng Y, Smiseth OA. Assessment of left ventricular relaxation by Doppler echocardiography. Comparison of isovolumic relaxation time and transmitral flow velocities with time constant of isovolumic relaxation. *Circulation.* 1990; 81:260–266.
81. Nishimura RA, Tajik AJ. Evaluation of diastolic filling of left ventricle in health and disease: Doppler echocardiography is the clinician's Rosetta stone. *J Am Coll Cardiol.* 1997;30:8–18.
82. Nagueh SF, Appleton CP, Gillebert TC, et al. Recommendations for the evaluation of left ventricular diastolic function by echocardiography. *J Am Soc Echocardiogr.* 2009;22:107–133.
83. Klein AL, Burstow DJ, Tajik AJ, et al. Effects of age on left ventricular dimensions and filling dynamics in 117 normal persons. *Mayo Clin Proc.* 1994;69:212–224.
84. Genovesi-Ebert A, Marabotti C, Palombo C, et al. Left ventricular filling: Relationship with arterial blood pressure, left ventricular mass, age, heart rate, and body build. *J Hypertens.* 1991;9:345–353.
85. Cohen GI, Pietrolungo JF, Thomas JD, et al. A practical guide to assessment of ventricular diastolic function using Doppler echocardiography. *J Am Coll Cardiol.* 1996;27:1753–1760.
86. Hurrell DG, Nishimura RA, Ilstrup DM, et al. Utility of preload alteration in assessment of left ventricular filling pressure by Doppler echocardiography: A simultaneous catheterization and Doppler echocardiographic study. *J Am Coll Cardiol.* 1997;30:459–467.
87. Rakowski H, Appleton C, Chan KL, et al. Canadian consensus recommendations for the measurement and reporting of diastolic dysfunction by echocardiography: From the Investigators of Consensus on Diastolic Dysfunction by Echocardiography. *J Am Soc Echocardiogr.* 1996;9:736–760.
88. Dini FL, Dell'Anna R, Micheli A, et al. Impact of blunted pulmonary venous flow on the outcome of patients with left ventricular systolic dysfunction secondary to either ischemic or idiopathic dilated cardiomyopathy. *Am J Cardiol.* 2000;85:1455–1460.
89. Smiseth OA, Thompson CR, Lohavanichbutr K, et al. The pulmonary venous systolic flow pulse. Its origin and relationship to left atrial pressure. *J Am Coll Cardiol.* 1999;34:802–809.
90. Fujii K, Ozaki M, Yamagishi T, et al. Effect of left ventricular contractile performance on passive left atrial filling– clinical study using radionuclide angiography. *Clin Cardiol.* 1994;17:258–262.
91. Appleton CP, Gonzalez MS, Basnight MA. Relationship of left atrial pressure and pulmonary venous flow velocities: Importance of baseline mitral and pulmonary venous flow velocity patterns in lightly sedated dogs. *J Am Soc Echocardiogr.* 1994;7:264–275.
92. Keren G, Bier A, Sherez J, et al. Atrial contraction is an important determinant of pulmonary venous flow. *J Am Coll Cardiol.* 1986;7:693–695.
93. Garcia MJ, Thomas JD, Klein AL. New Doppler echocardiographic applications for the study of diastolic function. *J Am Coll Cardiol.* 1998;32:865–875.
94. Takatsuji H, Mikami T, Urasawa K, et al. A new approach for evaluation of left ventricular diastolic function: Spatial and temporal analysis of left ventricular filling flow propagation by color M-mode Doppler echocardiography. *J Am Coll Cardiol.* 1996;27:365–371.
95. Watkins MW, LeWinter MM. Physiologic role of the normal pericardium. *Annu Rev Med.* 1993;44:171–180.
96. Maruyama Y, Ashikawa K, Isoyama S, et al. Mechanical interactions between four heart chambers with and without the pericardium in canine hearts. *Circ Res.* 1982;50:86–100.
97. Refsum H, Jünemann M, Lipton MJ, et al. Ventricular diastolic pressure-volume relations and the pericardium. Effects of changes in blood volume and pericardial effusion in dogs. *Circulation.* 1981;64:997–1004.
98. Jünemann M, Smiseth OA, Refsum H, et al. Quantification of effect of pericardium on LV diastolic PV relation in dogs. *Am J Physiol.* 1987;252:H963–H968.
99. Santamore WP, Dell'Italia LJ. Ventricular interdependence: Significant left ventricular contributions to right ventricular systolic function. *Prog Cardiovasc Dis.* 1998;40:289–308.
100. Weber KT, Janicki JS, Shroff S, et al. Contractile mechanics and interaction of the right and left ventricles. *Am J Cardiol.* 1981;47:686–695.
101. Gonzalez MS, Basnight MA, Appleton CP. Experimental cardiac tamponade: A hemodynamic and Doppler echocardiographic reexamination of the relation of right and left heart ejection dynamics to the phase of respiration. *J Am Coll Cardiol.* 1991;18:243–252.
102. Santamore WP, Heckman JL, Bove AA. Right and left ventricular pressure-volume response to elevated pericardial pressure. *Am Rev Respir Dis.* 1986;134:101–107.
103. Santamore WP, Bartlett R, Van Buren SJ, et al. Ventricular coupling in constrictive pericarditis. *Circulation.* 1986;74:597–602.
104. Goldman S, Olajos M, Morkin E. Comparison of left atrial and left ventricular performance in conscious dogs. *Cardiovasc Res.* 1984;18:604–612.

105. Payne RM, Stone HL, Engelken EJ. Atrial function during volume loading. *J Appl Physiol.* 1971;31:326–331.
106. Dernellis J, Tsiamis E, Stefanadis C, et al. Effects of postural changes on left atrial function in patients with hypertrophic cardiomyopathy. *Am Heart J.* 1998; 136:982–987.
107. Gare M, Schwabe DA, Hettrick DA, et al. Desflurane, sevoflurane, and isoflurane affect left atrial active and passive mechanical properties and impair left atrial-left ventricular coupling in vivo. Analysis using pressure-volume relations. *Anesthesiology.* 2001;95:689–698.
108. Prioli A, Marino P, Lanzoni L, et al. Increasing degrees of left ventricular filling impairment modulate left atrial function in humans. *Am J Cardiol.* 1998;82: 756–761.
109. Ito T, Suwa M, Kobashi A, et al. Reversible left atrial dysfunction possibly due to afterload mismatch in patients with left ventricular dysfunction. *J Am Soc Echocardiogr.* 1998;11:274–279.
110. Plehn JF, Southworth J, Cornwell GG 3rd. Brief report: Atrial systolic failure in primary amyloidosis. *N Engl J Med.* 1992;327:1570–1573.
111. Tabata T, Oki T, Yamada H, et al. Role of left atrial appendage in left atrial reservoir function as evaluated by left atrial appendage clamping during cardiac surgery. *Am J Cardiol.* 1998;81:327–332.
112. Hoit BD, Shao Y, Tsai LM, et al. Altered left atrial compliance after atrial appendectomy. Influence on left atrial and ventricular filling. *Circ Res.* 1993;72:167–175.
113. Nishikawa Y, Roberts JP, Tan P, et al. Effect of dynamic exercise on left atrial function in conscious dogs. *J Physiol.* 1994;481:457–468.
114. Toutouzas K, Trikas A, Pitsavos C, et al. Echocardiographic features of left atrium in elite male athletes. *Am J Cardiol.* 1996;78:1314–1317.
115. Triposkiadis F, Tentolouris K, Androulakis A, et al. Left atrial mechanical function in the healthy elderly: New insights from a combined assessment of changes in atrial volume and transmitral flow velocity. *J Am Soc Echocardiogr.* 1995;8:801–809.
116. Nishigaki K, Arakawa M, Miwa H, et al. A study of left atrial transport function. Effect of age or left ventricular ejection fraction on left atrial storage function. *Angiology.* 1994;45:953–962.
117. Zuccala G, Cocchi A, Lattanzio F, et al. Effect of age on left atrial function in patients with coronary artery disease. *Cardiology.* 1994;85:8–13.

CHAPTER

11 Respiratory Function in Anesthesia

PAUL C. TAMUL • MICHAEL L. AULT

Key Points

1. In a person with normal lungs, breathing can be performed exclusively by the diaphragm.
2. In the adult, the tip of an orotracheal tube moves an average of 3.8 cm with flexion and extension of the neck, but can travel up to 6.4 cm. In infants and children, displacement of even 1 cm can move the tube above the vocal cords or below the carina.
3. The following anatomy should be considered when contemplating the use of a double-lumen tube. The adult right mainstem bronchus is ~2.5 cm long before it branches into lobar bronchi. In 10% of adults, the right upper lobe bronchus departs from the right mainstem bronchus less than 2.5 cm below the carina. In 2% to 3% of adults, the right upper lobe bronchus opens directly into the trachea, above the carina.
4. When lung compliance is reduced, larger changes in pleural pressure are needed to create the same tidal volume (V_T). Patients with low lung compliance breathe with smaller V_T and more rapidly, making spontaneous respiratory rate the most sensitive clinical index of lung compliance.
5. Carotid and aortic bodies are stimulated by Pao_2 values less than 60 to 65 mm Hg. Thus, patients who depend on hypoxic ventilatory drive do not have Pao_2 values >65 mm Hg. The response of the peripheral receptors will not reliably increase ventilatory rate or minute ventilation to herald the onset of hypoxemia during general anesthesia or recovery.
6. There are three etiologies of hyperventilation: Arterial hypoxemia, metabolic acidemia, and central etiologies (e.g., intracranial hypertension, hepatic cirrhosis, anxiety, pharmacologic agents).
7. Increases in dead space ventilation primarily affect CO_2 elimination (with minimal influence on arterial oxygenation), and physiologic shunt increase primarily affects arterial oxygenation (with minimal influence on CO_2 elimination).
8. During spontaneous ventilation, the ratio of alveolar ventilation to dead space ventilation is 2:1. The alveolar-to-dead space ventilation ratio during positive-pressure ventilation is 1:1. Thus, minute ventilation during mechanical ventilatory support must be greater than that during spontaneous ventilation to achieve the same $Paco_2$.
9. $Paco_2 \geq P_{ETCO_2}$ unless the patient inspires or receives exogenous CO_2. The difference between $Paco_2$ and P_{ETCO_2} is due to dead space ventilation. The most common reason for an acute increase in dead space ventilation is decreased cardiac output.
10. Calculation of the shunt fraction is the best tool for evaluating the lungs' efficiency in oxygenating the arterial blood. It is the only index of oxygenation that takes into account the contribution of mixed venous blood to arterial oxygenation.
11. When functional residual capacity (FRC) is reduced, lung compliance falls and results in tachypnea, and venous admixture increases, creating arterial hypoxemia.

12 There is no compelling evidence that defines rules or parameters for ordering preoperative pulmonary function tests. Rather, they should be obtained to ascertain the presence of reversible pulmonary dysfunction (bronchospasm) or to define the severity of advanced pulmonary disease.

13 Patients who smoke should be advised to *stop* smoking at least 2 months prior to an elective operation to decrease the risk of postoperative pulmonary complications (PPCs).

14 The operative site is one of the most important determinants of the risk of PPC. The highest risk for PPC is associated with nonlaparoscopic upper abdominal operations, followed by lower abdominal and intrathoracic operations.

15 The single most important aspect of postoperative pulmonary care and prevention of PPC is early ambulation. Patients should be encouraged to get out of bed and walk.

Multimedia

1 Law of Laplace

2 Lung Volumes

3 Lung Blood Flow Distribution

4 Continuum of Ventilation and Perfusion

5 Flow Volume

Anesthesiologists directly manipulate pulmonary function. Thus, a sound and thorough working knowledge of applied pulmonary physiology is essential to the safe conduct of anesthesia. This chapter discusses pulmonary anatomy, the control of ventilation, oxygen and carbon dioxide transport, ventilation–perfusion relationships, lung volumes and pulmonary function testing, abnormal physiology and anesthesia, the effect of smoking on pulmonary function, and assessing risk for postoperative pulmonary complications (PPCs).

FUNCTIONAL ANATOMY OF THE LUNGS

This section emphasizes functional lung anatomy, with structure described as it applies to the mechanical and physiologic function of the lungs.

Thorax

The thoracic cage is shaped like a truncated cone, with a small superior aperture and a larger inferior opening to which the diaphragm is attached. The sternal angle is located in the horizontal plane that passes through the vertebral column at the T4 or T5 level. This plane separates the superior from the inferior mediastinum. During ventilation, the predominant changes in thoracic diameter occur in the anteroposterior direction in the upper thoracic region and in the lateral or transverse direction in the lower thorax.

Muscles of Ventilation

Work of breathing is the energy expenditure of ventilatory muscles. Similar to other skeletal muscles, the ventilatory muscles are endurance muscles subject to fatigue from inadequate oxygen delivery, poor nutrition, increased work secondary to chronic obstructive pulmonary disease (COPD) with gas trapping, or increased airway resistance. The ventilatory muscles include the diaphragm, intercostal muscles, abdominal muscles, cervical strap muscles, sternocleidomastoid muscles, and the large back and intervertebral muscles of the shoulder girdle. During non-strenuous breathing, the diaphragm performs most of the muscle work. Work contribution from the intercostal muscles in non-strenuous breathing is minor. Normally, at rest, inspiration requires work while exhalation is passive. As work of breathing increases, abdominal muscles assist with rib depression and increase intra-abdominal pressure to facilitate forced exhalation causing the "stitch," or rib pain that athletes experience when they actively exhale. With a further increase in work is required, the cervical strap muscles are recruited to help elevate the sternum and upper portions of the chest to optimize the dimensions of the thoracic cavity. Finally, during periods of maximal work, recruitment of large back and paravertebral muscles of the shoulder girdle contribute to ventilatory effort. The muscles of the abdomi-
1 nal wall, the most powerful muscles of expiration, are important for expulsive efforts such as coughing.[1] However, with normal lungs, breathing can be performed solely by the diaphragm.

Breathing is an endurance phenomenon involving fatigue-resistant muscle fibers, characterized by a slow-twitch response to electrical stimulation that must create sufficient force to lift the ribs and generate subatmospheric pressure in the intrapleural space. These fatigue-resistant fibers comprise approximately 50% of the total diaphragmatic muscle fibers. The high oxidative capacity of these fibers creates endurance units.[2] Fast-twitch muscle fibers, more susceptible to fatigue, have rapid responses to electrical stimulation imparting strength and allowing greater force over less time. The combination of fast-twitch fibers useful during brief periods of maximal ventilatory effort (coughing, sneezing) and slow-twitch fibers providing endurance (breathing without rest) underscore the unique dual function of the diaphragm as a muscle.[3]

A working muscle like the diaphragm must be firmly anchored at both its origin and insertion. However, its unique insertion is mobile—a central tendon originates from fibers attached to the vertebral bodies as well as the lower ribs and sternum. Diaphragmatic contraction results in descent of the diaphragmatic dome and expansion of the thoracic base creating decreases in intrathoracic and intrapleural pressure and an increase in intra-abdominal pressure.

The cervical strap muscles, active even during breathing at rest, are the most important inspiratory accessory muscles. When diaphragm function is impaired, as in patients with cervical spinal cord transection they can become the primary inspiratory muscles.

Lung Structures

In an intact respiratory system, the expandable lung tissue fills the pleural cavity. The visceral and parietal pleurae oppose each other,

TABLE 11-1. MAJOR DIVISIONS OF THE LUNG

Lung Side/Lobe	Bronchopulmonary Segment
Right	
Upper	Apical
	Anterior
	Posterior
Middle	Medial
	Lateral
Lower	Superior
	Medial basal
	Lateral basal
	Anterior basal
	Posterior basal
Left	
Upper	Apical posterior
	Anterior
Lingula	Superior
	Inferior
Lower	Superior
	Posterior basal
	Anteromedial basal
	Lateral basal

creating a potential intrapleural space where pressure decreases when the diaphragm descends and the rib cage expands. At the end of inspiration, the resultant subatmospheric intrapleural pressure is a reflection of the opposing and equal forces between the natural tendency of the lungs to collapse and the chest wall musculature to remain expanded. These equal and opposing forces at end inspiration result in the functional residual capacity (FRC), the volume of gas remaining in the lungs at passive end expiration. At FRC, the intrapleural space normally has a slightly sub-ambient pressure (–2 to –3 mm Hg). Major divisions of the right and left lung are listed in Table 11-1. Knowledge of the bronchopulmonary segments is important for localizing lung pathology, interpreting lung radiographs, identifying lung regions during bronchoscopy, and operating on the lung. Each bronchopulmonary segment is separated from its adjacent segments by well-defined connective tissue planes, which often anatomically confine initial primary lung pathologies.

The lung parenchyma can be subdivided into three airway categories based on functional lung anatomy (Table 11-2). The conductive airways allow or conduct basic gas transport without gas exchange. The next group of airways, which have smaller diameters, are transitional airways. Transitional airways are not only conduits for gas movement, but also allow limited gas diffusion and exchange. Finally, the smallest respiratory airways' primary function is gas exchange.

Conventionally, large airways with diameters of >2 mm create 90% of total airway resistance. The number of alveoli increases progressively with age, from approximately 24 million at birth and reaches its final adult count of 300 million by the age of 8 or 9 years. These alveoli are associated with about 250 million precapillaries and 280 billion capillary segments, resulting in a surface area of ~70 m^2 for gas exchange.

Conductive Airways

In the adult, the trachea is a fibromuscular tube ~10 to 12 cm long with an outer diameter of ~20 mm. Structural support is provided by 20 U-shaped structures composed of hyaline cartilage, with the opening of the U facing posteriorly. The cricoid membrane tethers the trachea to the cricoid cartilage at the level of the sixth cervical vertebral body. The trachea enters the superior mediastinum and bifurcates at the sternal angle (the lower border of the fourth thoracic vertebral body). Normally, half of the trachea is intrathoracic and half is extrathoracic. Since both ends of the trachea are attached to mobile structures, the adult carina can move superiorly as much as 5 cm from its normal resting position. Awareness of airway "motion" is essential to proper care of the intubated patient. In the adult, the tip of an orotracheal tube
2 moves an average of 3.8 cm with flexion and extension of the neck but can travel as far as 6.4 cm.[4] In infants and children, tracheal tube movement with respect to the trachea is even more critical: Displacement of even 1 cm can result in unintentional extubation or bronchial intubation.

The next airway generation below the carina is composed of the right and left mainstem bronchi. The diameter of the right bronchus is generally greater than that of the left. In the adult, the right bronchus leaves the trachea at ~25 degrees from the vertical tracheal axis, whereas the angle of the left bronchus is ~45 degrees. Thus, unintentional endobronchial intubation or aspiration of foreign material is more likely to occur on the right than the left. Furthermore, the right upper lobe bronchus dives almost directly posterior at ~90 degrees from the right main bronchus, facilitating aspiration of foreign bodies and fluid into the right upper lobe in the supine patient. In children younger than 3 years of age, the angles created by the right and left mainstem bronchi are approximately equal, with takeoff angles of about 55 degrees.

The adult right main bronchus is ~2.5 cm long before it initially branches into lobar bronchi. However, in 10% of adults,
3 the right upper lobe bronchus departs from the right mainstem bronchus less than 2.5 cm from the carina. Furthermore, in ~2% to 3% of adults, the right upper lobe bronchus opens into the trachea, superior to the carina. Patients with these anomalies require special consideration when placing double-lumen tracheal tubes, especially if one contemplates inserting a right-sided endobronchial tube. After the right upper and middle lobe bronchi divide from the right main bronchus, the main channel becomes the right lower lobe bronchus.

The left main bronchus is ~5 cm long before its initial branching point to the left upper lobe and the lingula; it then continues as the left lower lobe bronchus.

The bronchioles, typically 1 mm in diameter, are devoid of cartilaginous support and have the highest proportion of smooth muscle in their walls. Of the three to four bronchiolar generations, the final generation is the terminal bronchiole, which is the last airway component incapable of gas exchange.

TABLE 11-2. FUNCTIONAL AIRWAY DIVISIONS

Type	Function	Structure
Conductive	Bulk gas movement	Trachea to terminal bronchioles
Transitional	Bulk gas movement	Respiratory bronchioles
	Limited gas exchange	Alveolar ducts
Respiratory	Gas exchange	Alveoli
		Alveolar sacs

Transitional Airways

The respiratory bronchiole, which follows the terminal bronchiole, is the first site in the tracheobronchial tree where gas exchange occurs. In adults, two or three generations of respiratory bronchioles lead to alveolar ducts, of which there are four to five generations, each with multiple openings into alveolar sacs. The final divisions of alveolar ducts terminate in alveolar sacs that open into alveolar clusters.

Respiratory Airways and the Alveolar–Capillary Membrane

The alveolar–capillary membrane has two primary functions: Transport of respiratory gases (oxygen and carbon dioxide), and the production of a wide variety of local and humoral substances. Gas transport is facilitated by the pulmonary capillary beds, which logically are the densest capillary networks in the body. This extensive vascular branching system starts with pulmonary arterioles in the region of the respiratory bronchioles. Each alveolus is closely associated with ~1,000 short capillary segments.

The alveolar–capillary interface is complicated but well designed to facilitate gas exchange. Viewed with electron microscopy, the alveolar wall consists of a thin capillary epithelial cell, a basement membrane, a pulmonary capillary endothelial cell, and a surfactant lining layer. The flattened, squamous type I alveolar cells cover ~80% of the alveolar surface. Type I cells contain flattened nuclei and extremely thin cytoplasmic extensions that provide the surface suitable for gas exchange. Type I cells are highly differentiated and metabolically limited, which makes them highly susceptible to injury. When type I cells are damaged severely (during acute lung injury or adult respiratory distress syndrome), type II cells replicate and modify to form new type I cells.[5]

Type II alveolar cells are interspersed among type I cells, primarily at alveolar–septal junctions. These polygonal cells have vast metabolic and enzymatic activity, and manufacture surfactant. The enzymatic activity required to produce surfactant is only 50% of the total enzymatic activity present in type II alveolar cells.[6] The remaining enzymatic activity modulates local electrolyte balance, as well as endothelial and lymphatic cell functions. Both type I and type II alveolar cells have tight intracellular junctions, providing a relatively impermeable barrier to fluids.

Type III alveolar cells, alveolar macrophages, are an important element of immunologic lung defense. Their migratory and phagocytic activities permit ingestion of foreign materials within alveolar spaces.[7] Although functional pulmonary macrophages reduce the incidence of lung infection,[8] they also play an integral role in the organ-wide pulmonary inflammatory response. Thus, it is highly controversial whether the presence of these cells is beneficial (reducing the sequelae of infection) or harmful (contributing to the inflammatory response).[9]

Pulmonary Vascular Systems

Two major circulatory systems supply blood to the lungs: The pulmonary and bronchial vascular networks. The pulmonary vascular system delivers mixed venous blood from the right ventricle to the pulmonary capillary bed via two pulmonary arteries. After gas exchange occurs in the pulmonary capillary bed, blood is returned to the left atrium via four pulmonary veins. The pulmonary veins run independently along the intralobar connective tissue planes. The pulmonary capillary system adequately provides the metabolic and oxygen needs of the alveolar parenchyma. The bronchial arterial system provides oxygen to the conductive airways and pulmonary vessels. Anatomic connections between the bronchial and pulmonary venous circulations create an absolute shunt of ~2% to 5% of the total cardiac output, and represents "normal" shunt.

LUNG MECHANICS

Lung movement occurs secondary to forces external to the lungs. During spontaneous ventilation, the external forces are produced by ventilatory muscles. The response of the lungs to these external forces is governed by two main characteristics: (1) ease of elastic recoil of the chest wall and (2) resistance to gas flow within airways.

Elastic Work

The natural tendency of the lungs is to collapse because of elastic recoil; thus, expiration at rest is normally passive as gas flows out of the lungs. The thoracic cage exerts an outward-directed force, and the lungs exert an inward-directed force and because the outward force of the thoracic cage exceeds the inward force of the lung, the overall tendency of the lung within the thoracic cage is to remain inflated. FRC represents the gas volume in the lungs when the outward and inward forces on the lung are equal. Gravitational forces create a more subatmospheric pressure in nondependent areas of the lung than in dependent areas. In the upright adult, the difference in intrapleural pressure from the top to the bottom of the lung is ~7 cm H_2O.

Surface tension at an air–fluid interface produces forces that tend to further reduce the area of interface. For a bubble to remain inflated, the gas pressure within a bubble which is contained by surface tension must be higher than the surrounding gas pressure. Alveoli resemble bubbles in this respect, but unlike a bubble, alveolar gas communicates with the atmosphere via the airways. The Laplace equation describes this phenomenon: $P = 2T/R$, where P is the pressure within the bubble ($dyne \cdot cm^{-2}$), T is the surface tension of the liquid ($dyne \cdot cm^{-1}$), and R is the radius of the bubble (cm).

During inspiration, the surface tension of the liquid in the lung increases to 40 mN/m, a value close to that of plasma. During expiration, this surface tension falls to 19 mN/m, a value lower than that of most other fluids. This change in surface tension creates hysteresis of the alveoli, the phenomenon of different pressure–volume relationships of the alveoli during inspiration versus expiration. Unlike a bubble, the pressure within an alveolus decreases as the radius of curvature decreases, creating gas flow from larger to smaller alveoli which maintains structural stability and prevents lung collapse.

The alveolar transmural pressure gradient, or transpulmonary pressure, is the difference between intrapleural and alveolar pressure and is directly proportional to lung volume. Intrapleural pressure can be safely measured with a percutaneously inserted catheter[10]; however, clinicians rarely perform this technique. When measured with an esophageal balloon in the midesophagus, esophageal pressure can be used as a reflection of intrapleural pressure.[11] Commercially available esophageal pressure monitors increase the ease and accuracy of measuring esophageal pressure as a reflection of intrapleural pressure.[12] These monitors are useful for estimating the elastic work performed by the patient during spontaneous ventilation, mechanical ventilation, or a combination of spontaneous and mechanical ventilation. By estimating intrapleural pressure on a real-time basis, it is possible to quantitate the

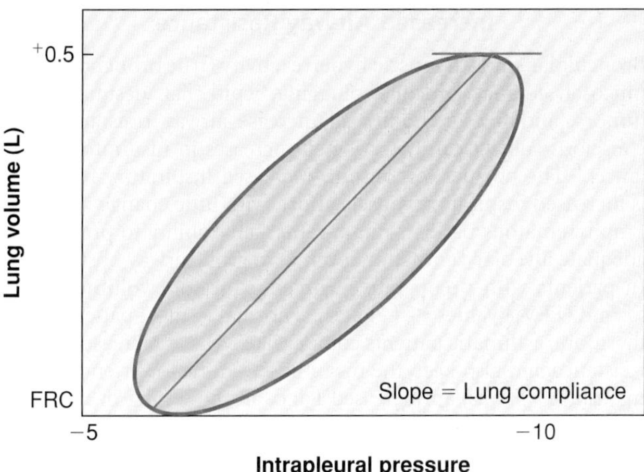

FIGURE 11-1. Dynamic pressure–volume loop of resting tidal volume. Quiet, normal breathing is characterized by hysteresis of the pressure–volume loop. The lung is more resistant to deformation than expected and returns to its original configuration less easily than expected. The slope of the line connecting the zenith and nadir lung volumes is lung compliance, ~500 mL/3 cm H_2O = 167 mL/cm H_2O. FRC, functional residual capacity.

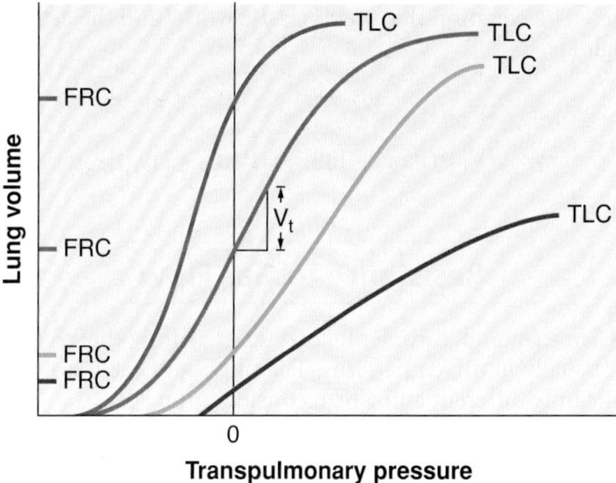

FIGURE 11-2. Pulmonary pressure–volume relationships at different values of total lung capacity (TLC), ignoring hysteresis. The *blue line* depicts the normal pulmonary pressure–volume relationships. Humans normally breathe on the linear, steep part of this sigmoidal curve, where the slope, which is equal to compliance, is greatest. The *black vertical line* at zero defines functional residual capacity (FRC), regardless of the position of the curve on the graph. Mild restrictive lung disease, indicated by the *green line,* shifts the curve to the right with little change in slope. However, with restrictive disease, the patient breathes on a lower FRC, at a point on the curve where the slope is less. Severe restrictive pulmonary disease profoundly depresses the FRC and diminishes the slope of the entire curve (*red line*). Obstructive disease (*orange line*) elevates both FRC and compliance.

patient's work of breathing and changes secondary to intervention. For example, low levels of inspiratory pressure support can compensate for the work of breathing imposed by the endotracheal tube.[13]

Physiologic work of breathing includes elastic work (inspiratory work required to overcome the elastic recoil of the pulmonary system) and resistive work (work to overcome resistance to gas flow in the airway). For a patient in whom breathing apparatus is employed, the concept of total work of breathing encompasses physiologic work plus equipment-imposed ventilatory work to overcome the resistance imposed by the breathing apparatus, for example, an endotracheal tube or a ventilator demand valve.

If the lungs are slowly inflated and deflated, the pressure–volume curve during inflation differs from that obtained during deflation. The two curves form a hysteresis loop that becomes progressively broader as the tidal volume is increased (Fig. 11-1). To inflate the lungs, pressure greater than the recoil pressure of deflation is needed, which means that the lung accepts deformation poorly and, once deformed, reforms to its original shape slowly. Elastic hysteresis is important for the maintenance of normal lung compliance but is not clinically significant.

2 The sum of the pressure–volume relationships of the thorax and lung results in a sigmoidal curve (Fig. 11-2). The vertical line drawn at end expiration coincides with FRC. Normally, humans breathe on the steepest part of the sigmoidal curve, where compliance ($\Delta V/\Delta P$) or slope is highest. In restrictive pulmonary diseases, the compliance curve shifts to the right, has decreased slope ($\Delta V/\Delta P$), or both. This decreased lung compliance results in smaller FRCs. When lung compliance is reduced, larger changes in intrapleural pressure are required to create the same tidal volume; that is, the thorax has to work harder to acquire the same volume of gas into the lungs. The body, being an energy conserving organism, prefers to move less gas with each breath rather than
4 working harder to achieve the same tidal volume. Thus, patients with restrictive lung disease typically breathe with smaller tidal volumes at more rapid rates, making spontaneous ventilatory rate one of the most sensitive indices of lung compliance. When lung compliance is decreased, the benefit of therapeutic continuous positive airway pressure (CPAP) is its ability to shift the vertical line (defined as FRC) to the right, allowing the patient to breathe on a steeper, more efficient portion of the volume–pressure curve. In other words, CPAP can increase the FRC, which allows for a slower ventilatory rate with a larger tidal volume.

At the other end of the spectrum, patients with diseases which increase lung compliance expend less elastic work to inspire but have decreased elastic recoil, resulting in larger than normal FRC (gas trapping). In such cases, their pressure–volume curves shift to the left and steepen. Chronic obstructive lung disease and acute asthma are the most common examples of diseases with high lung compliance. If lung compliance and FRC are sufficiently high that elastic recoil is minimal, the patient must use ventilatory muscles to actively exhale. The difficulty these patients experience in emptying the lungs is compounded by the increased airway resistance.

Both compliance and inspiratory elastic work can be measured for a single breath by measuring airway (Paw), intrapleural (Ppl) pressures, and tidal volume. If esophageal pressure is measured correctly, the esophageal pressure values can be substituted for Ppl values. Lung compliance, C_L, the slope of the volume–pressure curve, is given by the equation

$$C_L = \frac{\Delta V}{\Delta P_L} + \frac{V_T}{P_{L_i} - P_{L_e}} = \frac{V_T}{(Paw_i - Ppl_i) - (Paw_e - Ppl_e)} \quad (11\text{-}1)$$

where P_L is transpulmonary pressure, P_{L_i} and P_{L_e} are transpulmonary pressure at end-inspiratory and end-expiratory, V_T is tidal volume, Paw_e and Paw_i are expiratory and inspiratory airway pressures, and Ppl_e and Ppl_i are expiratory and inspiratory intrapleural pressures.

Elastic work (W_{el}) is performed during inspiration only because expiration is passive during normal breathing. The area within the triangle in Figure 11-2 describes the work required to inspire. The equation that yields elastic work (and the area of the triangle) is

$$W_{el} = \tfrac{1}{2}(V_T)(P_{L_i} - P_{L_e})$$
$$= \tfrac{1}{2}(V_T)[(Paw_i - Ppl_i) - (Paw_e - Ppl_e)] \quad (11\text{-}2)$$

Resistance to Gas Flow

Both laminar and turbulent flows exist within the respiratory tract, usually in mixed patterns. The physics of each, however, is significantly different and worth consideration.

Laminar Flow

Below critical flow rates that create turbulent flow, gas proceeds through a straight tube as a series of concentric cylinders that slide over one another. Fully developed flow has a parabolic profile with a velocity of zero at the cylinder wall and a maximum velocity at the center of the advancing "cone." This type of streamlined flow is usually inaudible. The advancing conical front means that some fresh gas reaches the end of the tube before the tube has been completely filled with fresh gas. Thus, laminar flow in the airways results in alveolar ventilation that can occur even when the tidal volume (V_T) is less than anatomic dead space. This phenomenon certainly has significant clinical implications, and as noted by Rohrer in 1915,[14] it allows high-frequency ventilation to achieve adequate alveolar ventilation.

Resistance to laminar gas flows in a straight, unbranched cylinder can be calculated by the following equation:

$$R = \frac{8 \times \text{length} \times \text{viscosity}}{\pi \times (\text{radius})^4} = \frac{P_B - P_A}{\text{flow}} \quad (11\text{-}3)$$

where P_B and P_A are barometric and alveolar pressures. It is essential to note that as radius decreases in narrowed airways, resistance will increase by a power of four. Viscosity is the only physical gas property that is relevant under conditions of laminar flow. Helium has a low density, but its viscosity is close to that of air. Therefore, helium will not improve gas flow if the flow is laminar. However, if flow is turbulent due to critical airway narrowing or abnormally high airway resistance, low-density helium is useful therapy (see next section).

Turbulent Flow

High flow rates, particularly through branched or irregularly shaped tubes, disrupt the orderly flow of laminar gas. When resistance to gas flow is significant, turbulent flow occurs and is usually audible. Turbulent flow usually presents with a square front so fresh gas will not reach the end of the tube until the amount of gas entering the tube is almost equal to the volume of the tube. Thus, turbulent flow effectively purges the contents of a tube. Four conditions that will change laminar flow to turbulent flow are high gas flows, sharp angles within the tube, branching in the tube, and a decrease in the diameter of the tube. During laminar flow, resistance is inversely proportional to gas flow rate. Conversely, during turbulent flow, resistance increases significantly in proportion to the flow rate. A detailed description of these phenomena is beyond the scope of this chapter, but the reader is referred to descriptions by Nunn.[15]

Increased Airway Resistance

Bronchiolar smooth muscle hyperreactivity (true bronchospasm), mucosal edema, mucous plugging, epithelial desquamation, tumors, and foreign bodies all increase airway resistance. The conscious subject can detect small increases in inspiratory resistance.[16] The normal response to increased inspiratory resistance is increased inspiratory muscle effort, with little change in FRC.[17] Emphysematous patients retain remarkable ability to preserve an adequate alveolar ventilation, even with gross airway obstruction. In patients with preoperative Forced expiratory volume in one second (FEV_1) values <1 L, $Paco_2$ is normal in most patients. Furthermore, asthmatic patients compensate well for increased airway resistance and also keep the mean $Paco_2$ in the lower end of normal range.[18] Thus, an increased $Paco_2$ in the setting of increased airway resistance warrants serious attention as it may signal that the patient's compensatory mechanisms are nearly exhausted. Mild expiratory resistance does not result in muscle use for active exhalation in conscious or anesthetized subjects. Instead, the initial work to overcome expiratory resistance is performed by augmenting inspiratory force until a sufficiently high lung volume is achieved, which allows elastic recoil to overcome expiratory resistance.[19] Only when expiratory resistance becomes excessive are accessory muscles recruited to expel gas from the lungs. During acute increases in expiratory resistance, this response can be well tolerated by most patients. However, chronic use of accessory muscles to exhale significantly increases the risk of ventilatory failure if work of breathing is further increased. When work of breathing exceeds physiologic reserves, work of breathing becomes detrimental to physiologic homeostasis and increases the risk of ventilatory failure. Acute ventilatory failure secondary to ventilatory muscle fatigue is evidenced by an acute increase in arterial carbon dioxide. Commonly, this is precipitated by pneumonia or heart failure.

Physiologic Changes in Respiratory Function Associated with Aging

Physiologic aging of the lung is associated with dilation of the alveoli, enlargement of the airspaces, decrease in exchange surface area, and loss of supporting tissue. Changes in the aging lung and chest wall result in decreased lung recoil (elastance), creating an increased residual volume and FRC. In addition, compliance of the chest wall diminishes, thereby increasing the work of breathing compared with younger subjects. Respiratory muscle strength decreases with aging and is strongly correlated with nutritional status and cardiac index. Expiratory flow rates decrease with a flow–volume curve suggestive of small airway resistance. Despite these changes, the respiratory system is normally able to maintain adequate gas exchange at rest and during exertion throughout life, with only modest decrements in Pao_2 and no change in $Paco_2$. With aging, respiratory centers in the nervous system demonstrate decreased sensitivity to hypoxemia and hypercapnia resulting in a blunted ventilatory response when challenged by heart failure, airway obstruction, or pneumonia.[20]

CONTROL OF VENTILATION

Mechanisms that control ventilation are extremely complex, requiring integration with many parts of the central and peripheral nervous systems (Fig. 11-3). LeGallois, who localized the respiratory centers in the brainstem in 1812, demonstrated that breathing does not depend on an intact cerebrum. Rather, breathing depends on a small region of the medulla near the origin of

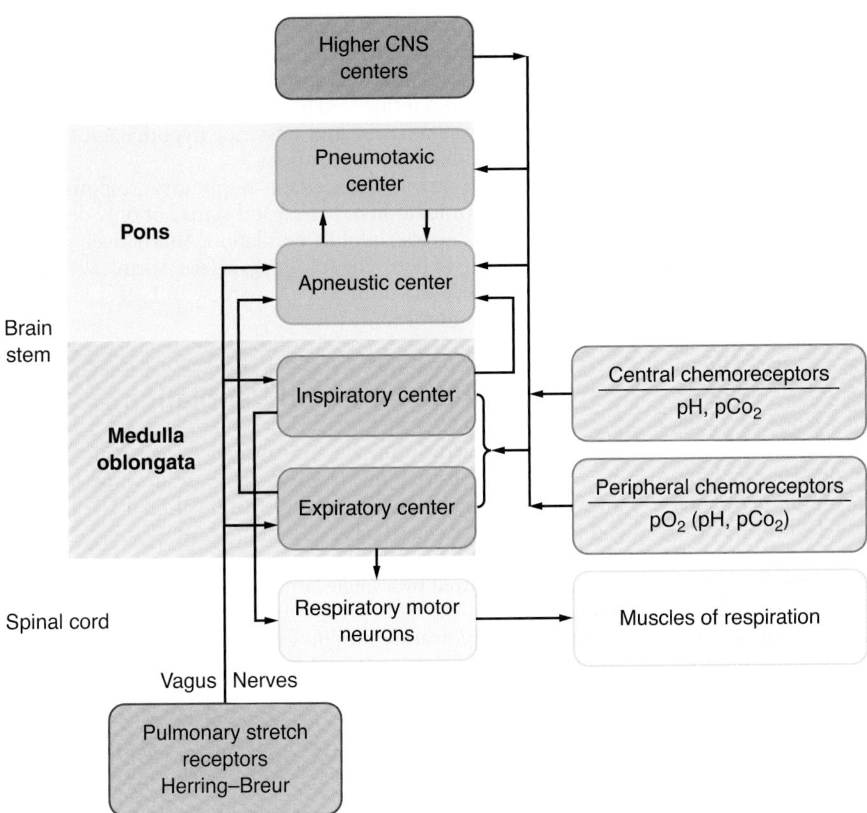

FIGURE 11-3. Classic central nervous system (CNS) respiratory centers. Diagram illustrates major respiratory centers, neurofeedback circuits, primary neurohumoral sensory inputs, and mechanical outputs.

the vagus nerves.[21] Countless studies in the past two centuries have greatly increased our knowledge and understanding of the anatomic components of ventilatory control. However, experimental work performed in animals is difficult to apply to humans because of interspecies variation.

Terminology

Breathing, ventilation, and respiration are often used interchangeably. However, it is important to realize that these terms have distinct meanings. The term *breathing* refers to the act of inspiring and exhaling that requires energy utilization for muscle work and thus, is limited by energy reserves. *Ventilation,* on the other hand, is the movement of gas in and out of the lungs. When spontaneous, ventilation requires energy for muscle work and is thus, breathing. *Respiration* occurs when energy is released from organic molecules. Such energy release is dependent on the movement of gas molecules such as carbon dioxide and oxygen across membranes whether alveolar or mitochondrial. Thus, humans breathe to ventilate and ventilate to respire. Despite what appears to be clear distinctions in terminology, vernacular use of these terms are often confused in daily dialog. For example, *respirators* are used to treat those who have succumbed to *respiratory* arrest and do not have a *respiratory* rate, and residents are sometimes advised to *breathe* down a patient using potent anesthetic agent.

Generation of Ventilatory Pattern

Refer to Table 11-3 for definitions of terms used in this section. A *respiratory center* is a specific area in the brain that integrates neural traffic resulting in spontaneous ventilation. Within the pontine and medullary reticular formations, there are several discrete respiratory centers that function as the control system (see Fig. 11-3).

Initial descriptions of brainstem respiratory functions are based on classic ablation and electrical stimulation studies. Another method for localizing respiratory centers entails recording action potentials from different areas of the brainstem with microelectrodes. This method is based on the assumption that

TABLE 11-3. DEFINITION OF RESPIRATORY PATTERN TERMINOLOGY

Word	Definition
Eupnea	"Good breathing": Continuous inspiratory and expiratory movement without interruption
Apnea	"No breathing": Cessation of ventilatory effort at passive end-expiration (lung volume = FRC)
Apneusis	Cessation of ventilatory effort with lungs filled at TLC
Apneustic ventilation	Apneusis with periodic expiratory spasms
Biot	Ventilatory gasps interposed between periods of ventilation apnea; *also* "agonal ventilation"

FRC, functional residual capacity; TLC, total lung capacity.

local brain activity that occurs in phase with respiratory activity is evidence that the area under study has "respiratory neurons".[22] These techniques are imperfect for precisely localizing discrete respiratory centers.

Medullary Centers

The medulla oblongata contains the most basic ventilatory control centers in the brain. Specific medullary areas are primarily active during inspiration or during expiration, with many neural inspiratory or expiratory interconnections. The inspiratory centers that reside in the dorsal respiratory group (DRG) are located in the dorsal medullary reticular formation. The DRG is the source of elementary ventilatory rhythmicity[23,24] and serves as the "pacemaker" for the respiratory system.[25] Whereas resting lung volume occurs at end expiration, the electrical activity of the ventilatory centers is at rest at end inspiration. The rhythmic activity of the DRG persists even when all incoming peripheral and interconnecting nerves are sectioned or blocked completely. Isolating the DRG in this manner results in ataxic, gasping ventilation with frequent maximum inspiratory efforts: Apneustic breathing.

The ventral respiratory group (VRG), which is located in the ventral medullary reticular formation, serves as the expiratory coordinating center. The inspiratory and expiratory neurons function by a system of reciprocal innervation, or negative feedback.[22] When the DRG creates an impulse to inspire, inspiration occurs and the DRG impulse is quenched by a reciprocating VRG impulse. This VRG transmission prohibits further use of the inspiratory muscles, thus allowing passive expiration to occur.

Pontine Centers

The pontine centers process information that originates in the medulla. The apneustic center is located in the middle or lower pons. With activation, this center sends impulses to inspiratory DRG neurons and is designed to sustain inspiration. Electrical stimulation of this area results in inspiratory spasm.[26] The middle and lower pons contain specific areas for phase-spanning neurons.[27] These neurons assist with the transition between inspiration and expiration, and do not exert direct control over ventilatory muscles.

The pneumotaxic respiratory center is in the rostral pons. A simple transection through the brainstem that isolates this portion of the pons from the upper brainstem reduces ventilatory rate and increases tidal volume. If both vagus nerves are additionally transected, apneusis results.[28] Thus, the primary function of the pneumotaxic center is to limit the depth of inspiration. When maximally activated, the pneumotaxic center secondarily increases ventilatory frequency. However, the pneumotaxic center performs no pacemaking function and has no intrinsic rhythmicity.

Higher Respiratory Centers

Many higher brain structures clearly affect ventilatory control processes. In the midbrain, stimulation of the reticular activating system increases the rate and amplitude of ventilation.[29] The cerebral cortex also affects breathing pattern, although precise neural pathways are not known. Occasionally, the ventilatory control process becomes subservient to other regulatory centers. For example, the respiratory system plays an important role in the control of body temperature because it supplies a large surface area for heat exchange. This is especially important in animals in which panting is a primary means of dissipating heat. Thus, the, ventilatory pattern is influenced by neural input from descending pathways from the anterior and posterior hypothalamus to the pneumotaxic center of the upper pons.

Vasomotor control and certain respiratory responses are closely linked. Stimulation of the carotid sinus not only decreases vasomotor tone, but also inhibits ventilation. Alternatively, stimulation of the carotid body chemoreceptors (see Chemical Control of Ventilation section) results in an increase in both ventilatory activity and vasomotor tone.

Reflex Control of Ventilation

Reflexes that directly influence ventilatory pattern usually do so to prevent airway obstruction. *Deglutition,* or swallowing, involves the glossopharyngeal and vagus nerves. Stimulation of the anterior and posterior pharyngeal pillars of the posterior pharynx induces swallowing. During swallowing, inspiration ceases momentarily, it is usually followed by a single large breath, and briefly increases ventilation.

Vomiting significantly modifies normal ventilatory activity.[30] Swallowing, salivation, gastrointestinal reflexes, rhythmic spasmodic ventilatory movements, and significant diaphragmatic and abdominal muscular activity must be coordinated over a very brief interval. Because of the obvious risk of aspirating gastric contents, it is advantageous to inhibit inspiration during vomiting. Input into the respiratory centers occurs from both cranial and spinal cord nerves.

Coughing results from stimulation of the tracheal subepithelium, especially along the posterior tracheal wall and carina.[31] Coughing also requires coordination of both airway and ventilatory muscle activity. An effective cough requires deep inspiration and then forced exhalation against a momentarily closed glottis to increase intrathoracic pressure, thus allowing an expulsive expiratory maneuver.

Proprioception in the pulmonary system, the qualitative knowledge of the gas volume within the lungs, probably arises from smooth muscle spindle receptors. These proprioceptors, which are located within the smooth muscle of all airways, are sensitive to pressure changes. Airway stretch reflexes can be demonstrated during distention of isolated airways so airway pressure, rather than volume distention, appears to be the primary stimulation.[32] Clinical conditions in which pulmonary airway stretch receptors are stimulated include pulmonary edema and atelectasis.

Golgi tendon organs (tendon spindles), which are arranged in series within ventilatory muscles, facilitate proprioception. The intercostal muscles are rich in tendon spindles, whereas the diaphragm has a limited number. Thus, the pulmonary stretch reflex primarily involves the intercostal muscles but not the diaphragm. When the lungs are full and the chest wall is stretched, these receptors send signals to the brainstem that inhibit further inspiration.

In 1868, Hering and Breuer reported that lightly anesthetized, spontaneously breathing animals would cease or decrease ventilatory effort during sustained lung distention.[33] This response was blocked by bilateral vagotomy. The *Hering–Breuer reflex* is prominent in lower-order mammals and is sufficiently active in lower mammals that even 5 cm H_2O CPAP will induce apnea. In humans, however, the reflex is only weakly present, as evidenced by the fact that humans will continue to breathe spontaneously with CPAP in excess of 40 cm H_2O.

Chemical Control of Ventilation

Peripheral Chemoreceptors

In a simplistic view of chemical ventilatory control, the peripheral chemoreceptors respond primarily to lack of oxygen, and the central nervous system (CNS) receptors respond primarily to changes in PCO_2, pH, and acid–base disturbances.

The peripheral chemoreceptors are composed of the carotid and aortic bodies. The carotid bodies, located at the bifurcation of the common carotid artery, have predominantly ventilatory effects. The aortic bodies, which are scattered about the aortic arch and its branches, have predominantly circulatory effects. The neural output from the carotid body reaches the central respiratory centers via the afferent glossopharyngeal nerves. Output from the aortic bodies travels to the medullary centers via the vagus nerve. Both carotid and aortic bodies are stimulated by decreased
5 PaO_2, but not by decreased SaO_2 or CaO_2. When PaO_2 falls to less than 100 mm Hg, neural activity from these receptors begins to increase. However, it is not until the PaO_2 reaches 60 to 65 mm Hg that neural activity increases sufficiently to substantially augment minute ventilation. Thus, patients who depend on hypoxic ventilatory drive have PaO_2 values in the mid-60s. Once the PaO_2 values of these patients exceed 60 to 65 mm Hg, ventilatory drive diminishes and PaO_2 falls until ventilation is again stimulated by arterial hypoxemia. Thus, during withdrawal of mechanical ventilatory support in the patient who depends on hypoxic ventilatory drive, the PaO_2 must fall to less than 65 mm Hg for spontaneous ventilation to resume.

The carotid bodies are also sensitive to decreased pH_a, but this response is minor. Similarly, changes in $PaCO_2$ do not stimulate these receptors sufficiently to alter minute ventilation. Increases in blood temperature, hypoperfusion of the carotid bodies themselves, and some chemicals will stimulate these receptors. Sympathetic ganglion stimulation by nicotine or acetylcholine will stimulate the carotid and aortic bodies; this effect is blocked by hexamethonium. Blockade of the cytochrome electron transport system by cyanide will prevent oxidative metabolism and will also stimulate these receptors.

Ventilatory effects resulting from stimulation of these receptors are increased ventilatory rate and tidal volume. Hemodynamic changes resulting from stimulation of these receptors include bradycardia, hypertension, increases in bronchiolar tone, and increases in adrenal secretion. The carotid body chemical receptors have been termed *ultimum moriens* ("last to die"). Although the response of peripheral receptors to hypoxemia was formerly believed to be resistant to the influences of anesthesia, potent inhaled anesthetics appear to depress hypoxic ventilatory response by depressing carotid body response to hypoxemia.[34] The response of the peripheral receptors is not sufficiently robust to reliably increase ventilatory rate or minute ventilation to herald the onset of arterial hypoxemia during general anesthesia or recovery from anesthesia. Furthermore, flumazenil, in a 1 mg intravenous dose, only partially reversed the diazepam-induced depression of hypoxic ventilatory drive.[35] Mora's data further suggest that humans may develop tolerance to respiratory depressant effects of diazepam.

Central Chemoreceptors

Approximately 80% of the ventilatory response to inhaled carbon dioxide originates in the central medullary centers. Acid–base regulation involving carbon dioxide, H^+, and bicarbonate is related primarily to chemosensitive receptors located in the medulla close to or in contact with the cerebrospinal fluid (CSF). The chemosensitive areas of the brainstem are in the inferolateral aspects of the medulla near the origin of cranial nerves IX and X. The area just beneath the surface of the ventral medulla is exquisitely sensitive to the extracellular fluid H^+ concentration.[36] Although the central response is the major factor in the regulation of breathing by carbon dioxide, carbon dioxide has little direct stimulating effect on these chemosensitive areas. These receptors are primarily sensitive to changes in H^+ concentration. Carbon dioxide has a potent but indirect effect by reacting with water to form carbonic acid, which dissociates into hydrogen and bicarbonate ions.[37]

An acute increase in $PaCO_2$ is a more potent ventilatory stimulus than an acute increase in arterial H^+ concentration from a metabolic source. Carbon dioxide, but not H^+, passes readily through the blood–brain and blood–CSF barriers. Local buffering systems immediately neutralize H^+ in arterial blood and body fluids. In contrast, the CSF has minimal buffering capacity. Thus, once carbon dioxide crosses into the CSF, H^+ are created and trapped in the CSF, resulting in a CSF H^+ concentration considerably greater than that found in the blood. Because carbon dioxide crosses the blood–brain barrier readily, the PCO_2 values in the CSF, cerebral tissue, and jugular venous blood rise quickly and to the same degree as the $PaCO_2$, although the central values are ~10 mm Hg higher than those measured in arterial blood.

The ventilatory response to changes in $PaCO_2$ (increased V_T, increased respiratory rate) is rapid and peaks within 1 to 2 minutes after an acute change in $PaCO_2$. With the same, persistent level of carbon dioxide stimulation, the resultant increase in ventilation declines over a period of several hours, probably as a result of bicarbonate ions that are actively transported from the blood into the CSF through the arachnoid villi, thereby increasing CSF pH toward the normal range.[38]

With chronic carbon dioxide retention, CSF pH is renormalized which determines ventilatory response to subsequent changes in arterial carbon dioxide tension. This phenomenon explains the differing effects of acute hypercapnia versus chronic hypercapnia on the CNS mediated ventilatory response. The goals of mechanical ventilatory support in a patient with chronic CO_2 retention are different from a normal patient. In this instance, providing mechanical support which allows a $PaCO_2$ range to generate a pH which is normal for that specific patient is referred to as "eucapnic ventilation." Attempting to achieve a normal $PaCO_2$, "normocarbia," in such a patient will iatrogenically result in alkalemia, further increasing CSF pH and raising the apneic threshold.[39] Finally, central medullary chemoreceptors also respond to temperature change. Cold CSF (with normal pH) or local anesthetic applied to the medullary surface will depress ventilation.

Ventilatory Response to Altitude

Ventilatory response and adaptation to high altitude are good examples of the integration of peripheral and central chemoreceptor control of ventilation. The following mechanism of acclimatization was proposed by Severinghaus and coworkers in 1963 and has since been confirmed.[40]

Following ascent from sea level to 4,000 m, acute exposure to high altitude and low PIO_2 results in arterial hypoxemia. This decrease in PaO_2 activates the peripheral hypoxemic ventilatory drive by stimulating the carotid and aortic bodies, and causes increased minute ventilation. As minute ventilation increases, $PaCO_2$ and CSF PCO_2 decrease, causing concomitant increases in pH_a and CSF pH. The alkaline shift of the CSF decreases ventilatory drive via medullary chemoreceptors, partially offsetting hypoxemic drive. A temporary equilibrium is attained within minutes, with $PaCO_2$ only 2 to 5 mm Hg less than normal and

Pa_{O_2} approximately 45 mm Hg. This initially profound hypoxemia probably causes the acute respiratory distress and other associated symptoms (headache, diarrhea) associated with rapid ascent. However, the CNS is able to restore CSF pH to normal (7.326) by pumping bicarbonate ions out of the CSF over 2 to 3 days. In 2 to 3 days, CSF bicarbonate concentration decreases approximately 5 mEq/L and restores CSF pH to within 0.01 pH unit of values at sea level. Then, centrally mediated ventilatory drive returns to normal, and hypoxic drive and stimulation of peripheral receptors can proceed unopposed. Thus, after 3 days' exposure to 4,000 m altitude, ventilatory adaptation would result in a new equilibrium, with Pa_{CO_2} approximately 30 mm Hg and Pa_{O_2} approximately 55 mm Hg. Following descent to sea level, the low CSF bicarbonate concentration persists for several days, and the climber "overbreathes" until CSF bicarbonate and pH values return to normal.

Breath-holding

Most adults with normal lungs and gas exchange can hold their breath for ~1 minute when breathing room air without previously hyperventilating. After 1 minute of breath-holding under these circumstances, Pa_{O_2} decreases to ~65 to 70 mm Hg and Pa_{CO_2} increases by ~12 mm Hg. In the absence of supplemental oxygen and hyperventilation, the "breakpoint" at which normal people are compelled to breathe is remarkably constant at a Pa_{CO_2} of 50 mm Hg.[41,42] However, if the individual breathes 100% oxygen before breath-holding, he or she should be able to hold his or her breath for 2 to 3 minutes, or until Pa_{CO_2} rises to 60 mm Hg. Hyperventilation before breath-holding reducing Pa_{CO_2} to 20 mm Hg can lengthen the period of breath-holding to 3 to 4 minutes.[43] Hyperventilation with 100% oxygen before breath-holding should extend the apneic period to 6 to 10 minutes. The rate of Pa_{CO_2} rise in awake, preoxygenated adults with normal lungs who hold their breath without previous hyperventilation is 7 mm Hg/min in the first 10 seconds, 2 mm Hg/min in the next 10 seconds, and 6 mm Hg/min thereafter.[42]

The duration of voluntary breath-holding is directly proportional to lung volume at onset, and is probably related both to oxygen stores in the alveoli and to the rate at which Pa_{CO_2} rises. With smaller lung volumes, the same amount of carbon dioxide is emptied into a smaller volume during the apneic period, thus increasing the carbon dioxide concentration more rapidly than occurs with larger lung volumes. Of note, apneic patients during general anesthesia actually "breath-hold" at FRC rather than at vital capacity (VC), which tends to accelerate the rate of Pa_{CO_2} rise. Despite this difference in lung volume, the rate of rise of Pa_{CO_2} in apneic anesthetized patients is 12 mm Hg during the first minute and 3.5 mm Hg/min thereafter, significantly lower than in the awake state.[43,44] During anesthesia, metabolic rate and carbon dioxide production are significantly less than during ambulatory wakefulness, which likely accounts for the lower rate of Pa_{CO_2} rise under anesthesia.

Hyperventilation with room air prior to prolonged breath-holding during exercise is inadvisable. During underwater swimming after poolside hyperventilation, the urge to breathe is first stimulated by a rising Pa_{CO_2}. Because an increased arterial carbon dioxide tension provides the stimulus to inspire, swimmers who hyperventilate with room air before swimming long distances frequently lose consciousness from arterial hypoxemia before the Pa_{CO_2} is sufficiently increased to stimulate the "need" to breathe.

Hyperventilation is rarely followed by an apneic period in awake humans, despite a markedly depressed Pa_{CO_2}. However, minute ventilation may decrease significantly. Aggressive intermittent positive-pressure breathing treatments for patients with COPD who continue to have a carbon dioxide based ventilatory drive can depress minute ventilation sufficiently to create arterial hypoxemia if they breathe room air after cessation of therapy.[45] In contrast, even mild hyperventilation during general anesthesia will produce prolonged apneic periods.[46]

Quantitative Aspects of Chemical Control of Breathing

The ventilatory responses to oxygen and carbon dioxide can be assessed quantitatively. Unfortunately, the quantitative indices of hypoxemic sensitivity are not clinically useful because the normal range is wide and confounded by many environmental factors. The reader is referred to a classical discussion of the quantitative indices of hypoxemic sensitivity.[47]

Ventilatory responses to Pa_{CO_2} changes are measured in several ways, provided that carbon dioxide production remains constant. When subjects voluntarily increase minute ventilation to a prescribed level, the Pa_{CO_2} decreases hyperbolically. The plot of minute ventilation (independent variable) and Pa_{CO_2} (dependent variable) is the metabolic hyperbola (Fig. 11-4). The metabolic hyperbola is cumbersome to evaluate and difficult to use clinically.

The curve more commonly used is the Pa_{CO_2} ventilatory response curve (see Fig. 11-4). It describes the effect of changing Pa_{CO_2} on the resultant minute ventilation. Usually, subjects inspire carbon dioxide to raise Pa_{CO_2}, and the effect on minute ventilation is measured. Creating these curves and observing how they change in various circumstances allows quantitative study of factors that affect the chemical carbon dioxide control of ventilation. The carbon dioxide response curve approaches linearity in

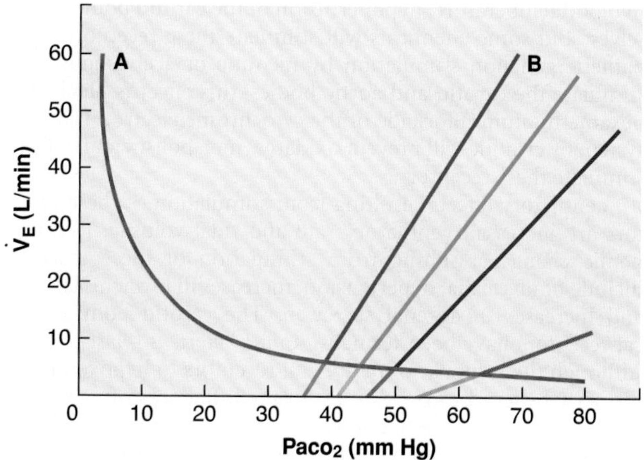

FIGURE 11-4. Carbon dioxide–ventilatory response curve. The metabolic hyperbola, curve A, is generated by varying $\dot{V}_A/\dot{Q}_E$ and measuring changes in carbon dioxide concentration. The hyperbolic configuration makes it cumbersome for clinical use. The carbon dioxide–ventilatory response curve, B, is linear between approximately 20 and 80 mm Hg. It is generated by varying Pa_{CO_2} (usually by controlling inspired carbon dioxide concentration) and measuring the resultant $\dot{V}_A/\dot{Q}_E$. This is the most commonly used test of ventilatory response. The slope defines "sensitivity"; the set point, or resting Pa_{CO_2}, occurs at the intersection of the metabolic hyperbola and the carbon dioxide–ventilatory response curve; and the apneic threshold can be obtained by extrapolating the carbon dioxide–ventilatory response curve to the *x*-intercept. In the absence of surgical stimulation, increasing doses of potent inhaled anesthesia or opioids will shift the curve to the right and eventually depress the slope (*green, red, and brown lines*). Painful stimulation will reverse these changes to varying and unpredictable degrees.

the range most often encountered in life: At $Paco_2$ values between 20 and 80 mm Hg. Once the $Paco_2$ exceeds 80 mm Hg, the curve becomes parabolic, with its peak ventilatory response at a $Paco_2$ between 100 and 120 mm Hg. Increasing the $Paco_2$ to higher than 100 mm Hg allows carbon dioxide to act as a ventilatory and CNS depressant, the origin of the term "carbon dioxide narcosis," with one minimum alveolar concentration (MAC) being approximately 200 mm Hg.

The slope of the carbon dioxide response curve is considered to represent carbon dioxide sensitivity. When $Paco_2$ reaches 100 mm Hg, carbon dioxide sensitivity is at its peak. The *set point*, the point of intersection of the carbon dioxide response curve and the metabolic hyperbola, defines normal resting $Paco_2$. Extrapolation of the carbon dioxide response curve to the *x*-intercept (where minute ventilation is 0) defines the apneic threshold. In awake, normal adults, the apneic threshold normally occurs at a $Paco_2$ of ~32 mm Hg, although awake adults usually continue to breathe when they achieve the apneic threshold because the sensation of apnea is disturbing. The slope of the curve is a measure of the response of the entire ventilatory mechanism to carbon dioxide stimulation.

Once Pao_2 exceeds 100 mm Hg, it no longer influences the carbon dioxide response curve. When the Pao_2 is between 65 and 100 mm Hg, its effect on the carbon dioxide response curve is small. However, when Pao_2 falls to less than 65 mm Hg, the carbon dioxide response curve shifts to the left and its slope increases, probably as a result of increased ventilatory drive stimulated by the peripheral chemoreceptors. Thus, during measurements of carbon dioxide ventilatory response, the subject should breathe supplemental oxygen to prevent hypoxic ventilatory drive interference.

The carbon dioxide response curve can be generated rapidly by increasing the fraction of inspired carbon dioxide ($FICO_2$) and requiring the subject to rebreathe exhaled gas. The results obtained with this technique are less pure because the $FICO_2$ is not controlled.

Three clinical states result in a left shift and/or a steepened slope of the carbon dioxide response curve. These same three situations are the only causes of true hyperventilation, that is, an increase in minute ventilation such that the decreased $Paco_2$ creates respiratory alkalosis (either primary or compensatory). The three causes of hyperventilation (enhanced carbon dioxide
6 response) are arterial hypoxemia, metabolic acidemia, and CNS etiologies. Examples of central etiologies that cause hyperventilation include drug administration, intracranial hypertension, hepatic cirrhosis, and nonspecific arousal states such as anxiety and fear. Aminophylline, doxapram, salicylates, and norepinephrine stimulate ventilation independent of peripheral chemoreceptors. Opioid antagonists, given in the absence of opioids do not stimulate ventilation. However, when given after opiate administration, they do reverse the effects of opioids on the carbon dioxide response curve.

Ventilatory depressants either displace the carbon dioxide response curve to the right, decrease its slope, or both. Changes in physiology that depress ventilation include metabolic alkalemia, denervation of peripheral chemoreceptors, normal sleep, and drugs. During normal sleep, the carbon dioxide response curve is displaced to the right, with the degree of displacement depending on the depth of sleep. Usually, $Paco_2$ increases up to 10 mm Hg during deep sleep. Hypoxemic responses are not impaired by sleep, which is convenient for continued survival at high altitude while sleeping.

Opioids displace the carbon dioxide response curve to the right with little change in slope at sedative doses. With higher, "anesthetic" doses, the curve shifts farther to the right and its slope is depressed, simulating the effect of potent inhalation agents on the carbon dioxide response curve (see Fig. 11-4). In the absence of other ventilatory depressant drugs, opioids induce pathognomonic changes in ventilatory patterns: A decreased ventilatory rate with an increased tidal volume. Not until opioids nearly induce apnea is tidal volume decreased. Large narcotic doses usually result in apnea responsive to verbal encouragement before consciousness is lost.

Barbiturates in sedative or light hypnotic doses have little effect on the carbon dioxide response curve. However, in doses adequate to allow skin incision, barbiturates shift the carbon dioxide response curve to the right. The ventilatory pattern resulting from barbiturate administration is characterized by decreased tidal volume and increased ventilatory rate. Potent inhaled anesthetics displace the carbon dioxide response curve to the right and decrease the slope, the degree of which depends on the anesthetic dose and the level of surgical stimulation. Like barbiturates, the ventilatory pattern following administration of potent inhaled anesthetics is initially represented by a decreased tidal volume and increased ventilatory rate. As more potent anesthetic agent is administered, however, ventilatory rate decreases toward an apneic endpoint. This clinical response occurs when the carbon dioxide response curve eventually becomes horizontal (slope = 0), resulting in essentially no ventilatory response to $Paco_2$ changes.

Potent inhaled anesthetics and opioids displace the set point to the right, implying that the resting, steady state $Paco_2$ is higher and minute ventilation lower. Furthermore, when the carbon dioxide response curve shifts to the right, the apneic threshold also increases (see Fig. 11-4). Surgical stimulation reverses the ventilatory response changes induced by inhaled anesthetics and opioids, but the degree of reversal is not predictable.

OXYGEN AND CARBON DIOXIDE TRANSPORT

This chapter discusses only external respiration, in which oxygen moves from the ambient environment into the pulmonary capillaries, and carbon dioxide leaves the pulmonary capillaries to enter the atmosphere. The movement of gas across the alveolar–capillary membrane depends on the integrity of the pulmonary and cardiac systems. Unless it is otherwise stated, the reader should assume that the ventilation and perfusion of alveolar–capillary units are normal. Abnormal distribution of ventilation or perfusion of the lungs is discussed later (see Ventilation–Perfusion Relationships section).

Bulk Flow of Gas (Convection)

Convection, in which all gas molecules move in the same direction, is the primary mechanism responsible for gas flow in large and most small airways, from the bronchi down to the bronchiolar airways of the 14th or 15th generation. Resistance can be defined with Poiseuille's law as $R = 8nl/\pi r^4$, where n = viscosity, l = length, r = radius. Therefore, resistance decreases rapidly as the diameter, radius, or cross-sectional area of a tube increases. Although a single isolated 14th generation bronchiolar airway may have greater resistance to air flow compared to the bronchi, the overall total resistance in a system is also dependent on the number of parallel pathways present. The overall total resistance of the system will be less than any individual tube's resistance, as illustrated by the equation: $1/R_{total} = 1/R_1 + 1/R_2 + 1/R_3 +$ etc. The anatomy of the tracheobronchial tree is organized in such a way that there is an increase in total parallel pathways and total cross-sectional area with each generation toward the periphery. Therefore, total airway resistance to gas flow is lower at the periphery compared to the bronchi.

The exponential increase in total cross-sectional area of parallel airways toward the lung periphery also affects airflow velocity. Similar to airflow resistance, velocity is inversely proportional to a system's overall total cross-sectional area. Therefore, airflow velocity at the lower generations of the tracheobronchial tree is lower than that of the bronchi. In other words, the velocity of airflow decreases from the trachea down to the peripheral distal airways. During normal quiet ventilation, gas flow within convective airways is mainly laminar.

Gas Diffusion

Diffusion within a gas-filled space is random molecular motion that results in complete mixing of all gases. In the distal airways of the lung beginning with the terminal bronchioles (16th airway generation), diffusion becomes the predominant mode of gas transport. Once gas reaches the small alveolar ducts, alveolar sacs, and alveoli, both diffusion and regional $\dot{V}/\dot{Q}$ relationships influence gas transport. Historically, clinicians assumed that defects in gas diffusion were responsible for arterial hypoxemia. However, the most frequent cause of arterial hypoxemia is shunt effect (see Ventilation–Perfusion Relationships section).[48]

The other usage of "diffusion" refers to the passive movement of molecules across a membrane that is governed primarily by concentration gradient. In this sense, carbon dioxide is 20 times more diffusible across human membranes than is oxygen; therefore, carbon dioxide crosses alveoli easily. As a result, hypercapnia is *never* the result of defective diffusion; rather, it is the result of inadequate alveolar ventilation with respect to carbon dioxide production.

True diffusion defects that create arterial hypoxemia are rare. The most common reason for a measured decrease in diffusing capacity (see Pulmonary Function Testing section) is mismatched ventilation and perfusion, which functionally results in a decreased surface area available for diffusion.

Distribution of Ventilation and Perfusion

The efficiency with which oxygen and carbon dioxide exchange at the alveolar–capillary level highly depends on the matching of capillary perfusion and alveolar ventilation. At this level, the marriage between the lung and the circulatory system must be well matched and intimate.

Distribution of Blood Flow

Blood flow within the lung is mainly gravity dependent. Because the alveolar–capillary beds are not composed of rigid vessels, the pressure of the surrounding tissues can influence the resistance to flow through the individual capillaries. Thus, blood flow depends on the relationship between pulmonary artery pressure (P_{pa}), alveolar pressure (P_A), and pulmonary venous pressure (P_{pv}) (Fig. 11-5). West created a lung model that divides the lung into three zones.[48,49] Zone 1 conditions occur in the most gravity-independent part of the lung (lung apex). In this region, alveolar pressure is approximately equal to atmospheric pressure. Pulmonary artery pressure always exceeds pulmonary venous pressure, which is subatmospheric in Zone 1. Therefore, Zone 1 can be described by the following relationship: $P_A > P_{pa} > P_{pv}$. In Zone 1, alveolar pressure transmitted to the pulmonary capillaries promotes their collapse, with a consequent theoretical blood flow of zero to this lung region. Thus, Zone 1 receives ventilation in the absence of perfusion. This relationship is referred to as alveolar dead space ventilation. Normally, Zone 1 areas exist only to a limited extent. However, in conditions of decreased pulmonary artery pressure, such as hypovolemic shock, Zone 1 enlarges, thus increasing alveolar dead space ventilation.

Zone 2 occurs from the lower limit of Zone 1 to the upper limit of Zone 3, where $P_{pa} > P_A > P_{pv}$. The pressure difference between pulmonary artery and alveolar pressure determines blood flow in Zone 2. Pulmonary venous pressure has little influence. Well-matched ventilation and perfusion occur in Zone 2, which contains the majority of alveoli.

Finally, Zone 3 occurs in the most gravity-dependent areas of the lung where $P_{pa} > P_{pv} > P_A$ and blood flow is primarily governed by the pulmonary arterial to venous pressure difference. Because gravity also increases pulmonary venous pressure, the pulmonary capillaries become distended. Thus, perfusion in Zone 3 is lush, resulting in capillary perfusion in excess of ventilation, or physiologic shunt.

Distribution of Ventilation

Alveolar pressure is the same throughout the lung; therefore, the more negative intrapleural pressure at the apex (or the least gravity-dependent area) results in larger, more distended apical alveoli than in other areas of the lung. The transpulmonary pressure (Paw − Ppl), or distending pressure of the lung, is greater

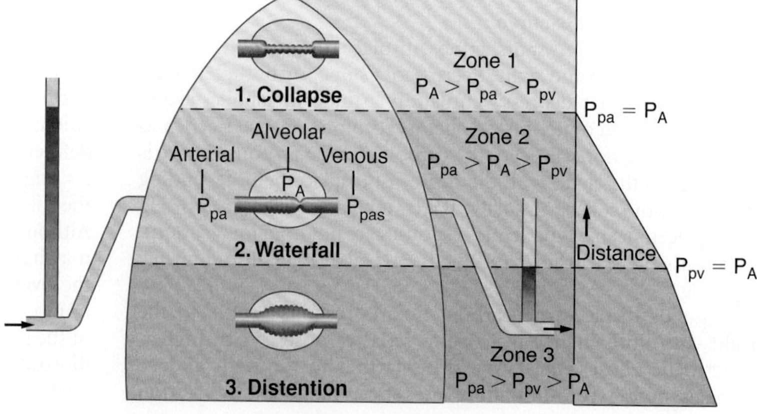

FIGURE 11-5. Distribution of blood flow in the isolated lung. In Zone 1, alveolar pressure (P_A) exceeds pulmonary artery pressure (P_{pa}), and no flow occurs because the vessels are collapsed. In Zone 2, arterial pressure exceeds alveolar pressure, but alveolar pressure exceeds pulmonary venous pressure (P_{pv}). Flow in Zone 2 is determined by the arterial–alveolar pressure difference ($P_{pa} - P_A$), which steadily increases down the zone. In Zone 3, pulmonary venous pressure exceeds alveolar pressure, and flow is determined by the arterial–venous pressure difference ($P_{pa} - P_{pv}$), which is constant down this pulmonary zone. However, the pressure across the vessel walls increases down the zone so their caliber increases, as does the flow. (With permission from: West JB, Dollery CT, Naimark A. Distribution of blood flow in isolated lung: Relation to vascular and alveolar pressures. *J Appl Physiol.* 1964;19:713.)

at the top and lower at the bottom, where intrapleural pressure is less negative. Despite the smaller alveolar size, more ventilation is delivered to dependent pulmonary areas. The decrease in intrapleural pressure at the base of the lungs during inspiration is greater than at the apex because of diaphragmatic proximity. Thus, because the dependent area of the lung generates the greatest change in transpulmonary pressure, more gas is sucked into dependent areas of the lung.

Ventilation–Perfusion Relationships

As discussed previously, the majority of blood flow is distributed to the gravity-dependent part of the lung. During a spontaneous breath, the largest portion of the tidal volume also reaches the gravity-dependent part of the lung. Thus, the nondependent area of the lung receives a lower proportion of both ventilation and perfusion, and dependent lung receives greater proportions of ventilation and perfusion. Nevertheless, ventilation and perfusion are not matched perfectly, and various $\dot{V}_A/\dot{Q}$ ratios result throughout the lung. The ideal $\dot{V}_A/\dot{Q}$ ratio of 1 is believed to occur at approximately the level of the third rib. Above this level, ventilation occurs slightly in excess of perfusion, whereas below the third rib the $\dot{V}_A/\dot{Q}$ ratio becomes less than 1 (Fig. 11-6).

In a simplified model, gas exchange units can be divided into normal ($\dot{V}_A/\dot{Q}$ = 1:1), dead space ($\dot{V}_A/\dot{Q}$ = 1:0), shunt ($\dot{V}_A/\dot{Q}$ = 0:1),
4 or a silent unit ($\dot{V}_A/\dot{Q}$ = 0:0) (Fig. 11-7). Although this model is helpful in understanding $\dot{V}_A/\dot{Q}$ relationships and their influences on gas exchange, $\dot{V}_A/\dot{Q}$ really occurs as a continuum. In the lungs of a healthy, upright, spontaneously breathing individual, the majority of alveolar–capillary units are normal gas exchange units. The $\dot{V}_A/\dot{Q}$ ratio varies between absolute shunt (in which $\dot{V}_A/\dot{Q} = 0$) to absolute dead space (in which $\dot{V}_A/\dot{Q} = \infty$). Rather than absolute shunt, most units with low $\dot{V}_A/\dot{Q}$ mismatch receive a small amount of ventilation relative to blood flow. Similarly, most dead space units are not absolute, but rather are characterized by low blood flow relative to ventilation. During acute lung injury and adult respiratory distress syndrome, areas of low $\dot{V}_A/\dot{Q}$ matching commonly lie adjacent to areas of high $\dot{V}_A/\dot{Q}$ matching.[50] Thus, the West lung zone model should be used to aid the understanding of pulmonary physiology and not be regarded as an incontrovertible anatomic truism.

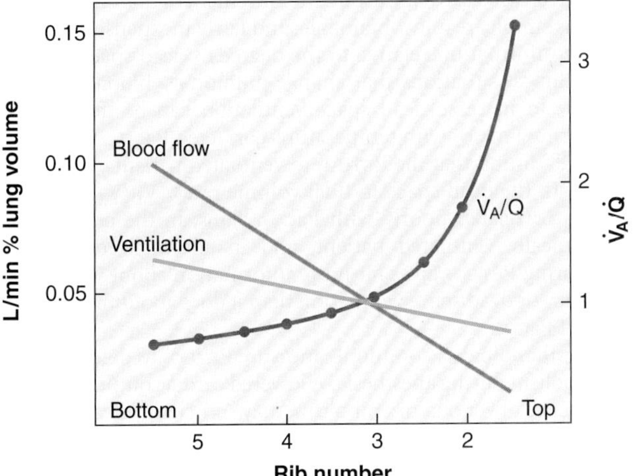

FIGURE 11-6. Distribution of ventilation, blood flow, and ventilation–perfusion ratio in the normal, upright lung. Straight lines have been drawn through the ventilation and blood flow data. Because blood flow falls more rapidly than ventilation with distance up the lung, ventilation–perfusion ratio rises, slowly at first, then rapidly. (With permission from: West JB. *Ventilation/blood flow and gas exchange*, 4th ed. Oxford, England, Blackwell Scientific, 1985.)

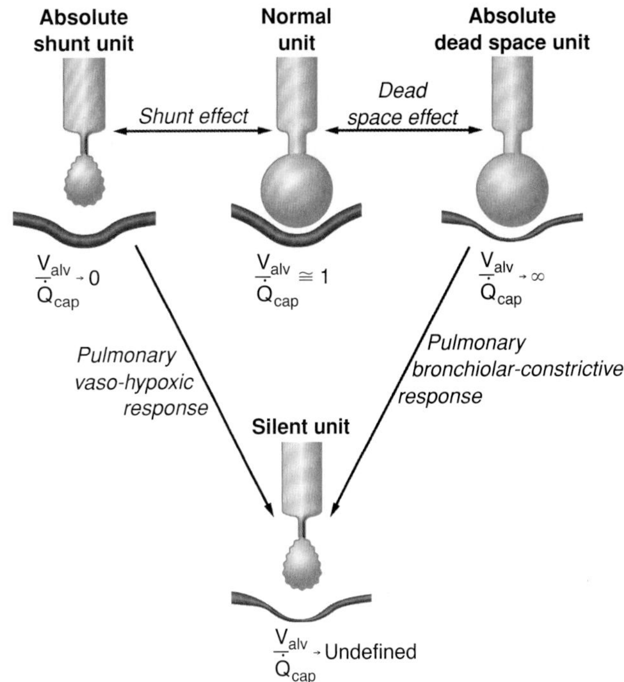

FIGURE 11-7. Continuum of ventilation–perfusion relationships. Gas exchange is maximally effective in normal lung units and only partially effective in shunt and dead space effect units. It is totally absent in silent units, absolute shunt, and dead space units.

Hypoxic pulmonary vasoconstriction and bronchoconstriction allow the lungs to maintain optimal $\dot{V}_A/\dot{Q}$ matching. Hypoxic pulmonary vasoconstriction, stimulated by alveolar hypoxia, severely decreases blood flow. Thus, poorly ventilated alveoli also receive minuscule blood flow. Furthermore, decreased regional pulmonary blood flow results in bronchiolar constriction and diminishes the degree of dead space ventilation.[51,52] When either phenomena occurs, the shunt or dead space units effectively become silent units in which little ventilation or perfusion occurs.

Many pulmonary diseases result in both physiologic shunt and dead space abnormalities. However, most disease processes can be characterized as producing either primarily shunt or dead space in their early stages. Increases in dead space ventilation primarily affect carbon dioxide elimination and have little influence on arterial oxygenation until dead space ventilation exceeds 80% to 90% of minute ventilation ($\dot{V}_E$). Similarly, physiologic shunt primar-
7 ily affects arterial oxygenation with little effect on carbon dioxide elimination until the physiologic shunt fraction exceeds 75% to 80% of the cardiac output. Defective to absent gas exchange can be the net effect of either abnormality in the extreme.

Physiologic Dead Space

Each inspired breath is composed of gas that contributes to alveolar ventilation (V_A) and gas that becomes dead space ventilation (V_D). Thus, tidal volume (V_T) = V_A + V_D. In the normal, spontaneously breathing person, the ratio of alveolar-to-dead space ventilation for each breath is 2:1. Conveniently, the rule of "1, 2, 3" applies to normal, spontaneously breathing persons. For each breath, 1 mL/lb (lean body weight) becomes V_D, 2 mL · lb^{-1} becomes Va, and 3 mL · lb^{-1} constitutes the V_T.

Physiologic dead space consists of anatomic and alveolar dead space. Anatomic dead space ventilation, approximately 2 mL/kg ideal body weight, accounts for the majority of physiologic dead space. It arises from ventilation of structures that do not exchange respiratory gases: The oronasopharynx to the terminal and respiratory bronchioles. Clinical conditions that modify anatomic dead space include tracheal intubation, tracheostomy, and large lengths of ventilator tubing between the tracheal tube and the ventilator Y-piece. It is important to note that ventilation occurs because gas flows into and out of the alveoli. In contrast, the inspiratory or expiratory limb of anesthesia circle system has unidirectional flow, and therefore, is not a component of anatomic dead space ventilation.

Alveolar dead space ventilation arises from ventilation of alveoli with inadequate or no perfusion. Since disease produces little change in anatomic dead space, physiologic dead space is primarily influenced by changes in alveolar dead space. Rapid changes in physiologic dead space ventilation most often arise from changes in pulmonary blood flow, resulting in decreased perfusion to ventilated alveoli. The most common etiology of acutely increased physiologic dead space is an abrupt decrease in cardiac output. Another pathologic condition that interferes with pulmonary blood flow, and thereby creates dead space, is pulmonary embolism, whether due to thrombus, fat, air, or amniotic fluid. Although there may be obstruction to blood flow with some types of pulmonary emboli, the greatest decrease in pulmonary blood flow is due to vasoconstriction induced by locally released vasoactive substances such as leukotrienes.

Chronic pulmonary diseases create dead space ventilation by irreversibly changing the relationship between alveolar ventilation and blood flow; this alteration is especially prominent in patients with COPD. In general, individuals with acute exacerbations of COPD will have a greater degree of ventilation defect than perfusion defect due to obstruction caused by inflammation, mucous plugging, or bronchospasm. However, individuals with chronic COPD may develop decreased perfusion in areas of poor ventilation from hypoxic vasoconstriction and collateral ventilation can occur, leading to a smaller than expected V/Q mismatch. Similar to acute exacerbations of COPD, acute diseases such as adult respiratory distress syndrome can cause an increase in dead space ventilation owing to intense pulmonary vasoconstriction. Finally, therapeutic or supportive manipulations such as positive-pressure ventilation or positive airway pressure therapy can increase alveolar dead space because depressed venous return to the right heart will decrease cardiac output and blood flow through the pulmonary vasculature, leading to decreased perfusion of the alveoli despite improved ventilation with positive pressure therapy. However, this can usually be overcome by intravenous fluid administration. Occasionally, therapeutics that create intrapulmonary positive pressure may increase physiologic shunt, when blood flow to a previously silent area of $\dot{V}_A/\dot{Q}$ matching now receives blood redistributed by positive pressure from more compliant areas of the lung.

Assessment of Physiologic Dead Space

As the lung receives nearly 100% of the cardiac output, assessment of physiologic dead space ventilation in the acute setting yields valuable information about pulmonary blood flow and, ultimately, about cardiac output. If pulmonary blood flow decreases, the most likely cause is a decreased cardiac output. Thus, it is clinically useful to be able to readily assess the degree of physiologic dead space ventilation.

There are two easy and several difficult ways to assess dead space ventilation. A comparison of minute ventilation and $Paco_2$ allows a gross qualitative assessment of physiologic dead space ventilation. The $Paco_2$ is determined only by alveolar ventilation and $\dot{V}co_2$. If $\dot{V}co_2$ remains constant, $Paco_2$ will also remain constant as long as minute ventilation supplies the same degree of alveolar ventilation. If the spontaneously breathing individual must increase minute ventilation to maintain the same $Paco_2$, he or she will experience an increase in dead space ventilation because less of the minute ventilation is contributing to alveolar ventilation. Alternatively, a mechanically ventilated patient with a fixed minute ventilation and no increase in $\dot{V}co_2$ also experiences an increased dead space ventilation if the $Paco_2$ rises. Hence, when $Paco_2$ in a mechanically ventilated patient increases, it is necessary to determine if the cause is increased dead space ventilation or an increased $\dot{V}co_2$.

Because positive pressure ventilation increases alveolar pressure, the mechanically ventilated patient with normal lungs has a dead space to alveolar ventilation ratio (V_D/V_A) of 1:1 (more West Zone 1) rather than 1:2, as during spontaneous ventilation. If mechanical V_T is 1,000 mL, 500 mL contributes to V_A, and 500 mL contributes to V_D. At rest, the required $\dot{V}_A$ with normal $\dot{V}co_2$ is approximately 60 mL/kg/min. A 70 kg man would then require a $\dot{V}_A$ of 4,200 mL/min. During spontaneous breathing, the required $\dot{V}_E$ would be 6,300 mL/min, but during mechanical ventilation $\dot{V}_E$ would have to be 8,400 mL/min. Using this cal-
8 culation, if a 70 kg resting patient requires $\dot{V}_E$ much in excess of 8,400 mL/min, either $\dot{V}_D$ or $\dot{V}co_2$ is increased. A rule of thumb for mechanically ventilated patients is that doubling baseline minute ventilation decreases $Paco_2$ from 40 to 30 mm Hg, and quadrupling minute ventilation decreases $Paco_2$ from 40 to 20 mm Hg.

The $Paco_2$ will be greater than or equal to end-tidal $Paco_2$ ($P_{ET}co_2$) unless the patient inspires or receives exogenous carbon dioxide (e.g., from peritoneal insufflation). The difference between $P_{ET}co_2$ and $Paco_2$ is due to dead space ventilation. The
9 most common reason for an acute increase in dead space ventilation is decreased cardiac output. Measurement of this difference—which is simple, readily obtainable, and fairly inexpensive—yields reliable information relative to the degree of dead space ventilation. Clinical situations that change pulmonary blood flow sufficiently to increase dead space ventilation can be detected by comparing $P_{ET}co_2$ with temperature-corrected $Paco_2$. Yamanaka and Sue[53] found that the $P_{ET}co_2$ in ventilated patients varied linearly with the dead space to tidal volume ratio (V_D/V_T) and that $P_{ET}co_2$ correlated poorly with $Paco_2$. Thus, in the critically ill, mechanically ventilated patient, and in anesthetized patients, monitoring $P_{ET}co_2$ gives far more information about ventilatory efficiency or dead space ventilation than it does about the absolute value of $Paco_2$.

Anesthesiologists commonly measure $P_{ET}co_2$ to detect venous air embolism during anesthesia. A lowered cardiac output alone, in the absence of venous air embolism, may sufficiently decrease pulmonary perfusion so dead space ventilation increases and $P_{ET}co_2$ falls. Thus, a depressed $P_{ET}co_2$ is sensitive for decreased cardiac output but not specific for pulmonary embolism. Air in the pulmonary arteries mechanically interferes with blood flow and also causes pulmonary arterial constriction, further decreasing pulmonary blood flow. A decreased $P_{ET}co_2$ suggests that a physiologically significant air embolism has occurred. The same physiologic considerations apply to detecting pulmonary thromboembolism.

Some clinicians use the divergence of $P_{ET}co_2$ from $Paco_2$ as a reflection of pulmonary blood flow for other applications. During intentional pharmacologic or surgical manipulation of pulmonary blood flow, the difference between $Paco_2$ and $PETco_2$ serves as a useful physiologic monitor for the effectiveness of these interventions. Furthermore, $PETco_2$ as a reflection of pulmonary perfusion is a useful tool for studying and monitoring the effectiveness of resuscitation efforts and may provide a marker for survival after resuscitation.[54]

The most quantitative technique used to measure physiologic dead space uses a modification of the Bohr equation:

$$\frac{V_D}{V_T} = \frac{PaCO_2 - P\bar{E}CO_2}{PaCO_2} \qquad (11\text{-}4)$$

where $P\bar{E}co_2$ is the Pco_2 from the mixture of all expired gases over the period of time during which measurements are made. This calculation estimates the fraction of each breath that does not contribute to gas exchange. In spontaneously breathing patients, normal V_D/V_T is between 0.2 and 0.4, or ~0.33. In patients receiving positive-pressure ventilation, V_D/V_T becomes ~0.5. The major limitation of performing this calculation is the difficulty in collecting exhaled gas for $P\bar{E}co_2$ measurement. Exhaled gases, collected in cumbersome Douglass bags, can be easily contaminated with inspired air or supplemental oxygen. The measurement will also be inaccurate if the patient does not maintain a steady ventilatory pattern. Therefore, extreme care must be taken to ensure all measurements are performed accurately. In practice, this measurement is rarely performed.

Physiologic Shunt

Whereas physiologic dead space ventilation applies to areas of the lung that are ventilated but poorly perfused, physiologic shunt occurs in the lung that is perfused but poorly ventilated. The physiologic shunt ($\dot{Q}_{SP}$) is that portion of the total cardiac output ($\dot{Q}_T$) that returns to the left heart and systemic circulation without receiving oxygen in the lung. When pulmonary blood is not exposed to alveoli or when those alveoli are devoid of ventilation, the result is *absolute or true shunt*, in which $\dot{V}_A/\dot{Q} = 0$. *Shunt effect*, or *venous admixture*, is the more common clinical phenomenon and occurs in areas where alveolar ventilation is deficient compared with the degree of perfusion: $0 < \dot{V}_A/\dot{Q} < 1$.

Because blood passing through areas of absolute shunt receives no oxygen, arterial hypoxemia resulting from absolute shunt is minimally reversed with supplemental oxygen. Alternatively, supplemental oxygen supplied to patients with arterial hypoxemia due to venous admixture will increase the Pao_2. Although ventilation to these alveoli is deficient, they do carry a small amount of oxygen to the capillary bed. Thus, assessment of arterial oxygen responsiveness to supplemental oxygen administration is a helpful diagnostic tool.

A small percentage of venous blood normally bypasses the right ventricle and empties directly into the left atrium. This anatomic, absolute, or true shunt arises from the venous return of the pleural, bronchiolar, and Thebesian veins. This venous admixture accounts for 2% to 5% of total cardiac output and represents the small shunt that normally occurs. Anatomic shunts of greatest magnitude are usually associated with congenital heart diseases that cause right-to-left shunt. Intrapulmonary anatomic shunts can also cause anatomic shunt. For example, the arterial hypoxemia associated with advanced hepatic failure (hepatopulmonary syndrome) is due, in part, to arteriovenous malformations.[55,56] Diseases that may cause absolute or true shunt include acute lobar atelectasis, extensive acute lung injury, advanced pulmonary edema, and consolidated pneumonia. Disease entities that tend to produce venous admixture include mild pulmonary edema, postoperative atelectasis, and COPD.

Assessment of Arterial Oxygenation and Physiologic Shunt

The simplest assessment of oxygenation is qualitative comparison of the patient's Fio_2 and Pao_2. The highest possible Pao_2 for any given Fio_2 (and $Paco_2$) can be calculated from the alveolar gas equation:

$$P_{AO_2} = F_{IO_2}(P_b - P_{H_2O}) - \frac{P_{ACO_2}}{R} \qquad (11\text{-}5)$$

where PAO_2 and $PACO_2$ are alveolar Po_2 and Pco_2, PH_2O is water vapor pressure at 100% saturation and 37°C, P_b is barometric pressure, and R is respiratory quotient. Assuming one makes the calculation for a well-perfused alveolus, the alveolar and arterial Pco_2 are equal. Therefore, $Paco_2$ can be substituted for $PACO_2$. Respiratory quotient (R) is the ratio of O_2 consumed ($\dot{V}o_2$) to CO_2 produced ($\dot{V}co_2$):

$$\frac{\dot{V}co_2}{\dot{V}o_2} = \frac{200\ \text{mL/min}}{250\ \text{mL/min}} = 0.8 \qquad (11\text{-}6)$$

Oxygen tension–based indices do not reflect mixed venous contribution to arterial oxygenation and can be misleading.[57] Even if venous admixture is small, mixed venous blood with very low oxygen content will magnify the effect of a small shunt. Oxygen tension–based indices, for example, Pao_2/Fio_2, alveolar to arterial Po_2 difference ($PA\text{-}ao_2$), and ratio Pao_2/PAO_2, do not take into account the influence of $C\bar{v}o_2$ on arterial oxygenation. Therefore, in critically ill patients who are hypoxemic, the insertion of a pulmonary artery catheter to assess shunt and to measure cardiac output may be essential to understanding the influence of cardiac function on arterial oxygenation.

The alveolar gas equation has important clinical utility in recognizing alveolar hypoventilation due to its effect on arterial oxygenation. Dalton's law refers to the fact that each gas in a mixture will exert its partial pressure and in sum will equal the total pressure of the mixture.[58] The first term in the equation describes the partial pressure of oxygen in the alveolus, while the second represents carbon dioxide. In the event of significant alveolar hypoventilation, carbon dioxide accumulates in arterial blood and subsequently the alveolus. While inspiring room air, this will reduce the concentration of oxygen and arterial hypoxemia will occur. Using a $PaCO_2$ value of 80 mm Hg, the alveolar gas equation will calculate the PAO_2 as approximately 50 mm Hg. Assuming a normal P_{50} for hemoglobin and normal A-a gradient, this arterial oxygen tension will correspond to an arterial saturation value in the 80% range, modestly above the value for mixed venous saturation.[39] In response to hypoxemia, alveolar hyperventilation produces a decrease in arterial carbon dioxide tension and $PACO_2$. While inspiring room air, if the $PaCO_2$ were to decrease, a concomitant increase in the partial pressure of oxygen must occur to preserve the total pressure in the alveolus. For example, if the $PaCO_2$ were to decrease to 20 mm Hg, the resulting PAO_2 would increase by approximately 25 mm Hg, thereby increasing arterial oxygen saturation, oxygen content, and oxygen delivery.

$P(A\text{-}a)o_2$ is a useful quantitative assessment of arterial oxygenation mainly when arterial hemoglobin is well saturated when normal $D(A\text{-}a)o_2$ is <5 mm Hg. When Pao_2 is less than 150 mm Hg (and certainly when it is less than 100 mm Hg), the relationship between oxygen content and oxygen tension is nonlinear, thus making $D(A\text{-}a)O_2$ more difficult to interpret.

The assessment of arterial oxygenation requires, at least, knowledge of FIO_2 and either PaO_2 or SaO_2. Oxygen tension–based indices of oxygenation are useful, but they do not take into account the contribution of mixed venous blood to arterial oxygenation. Mixed venous blood can become extremely desaturated in the critically ill patient owing to inadequate cardiac output, anemia, arterial hypoxemia, increased $\dot{V}O_2$, or abnormal hemoglobin moieties. The best knowledge of the efficiency with which the lungs oxygenate the arterial blood can be obtained only by calculating shunt fraction or ventilation–perfusion ratio (VQI).

Physiologic Shunt Calculation

The clinical reference standard for the calculation of physiologic shunt fraction is derived from a two-compartment pulmonary blood flow model. One compartment performs ideal gas exchange and contains perfectly married alveolar–capillary units, whereas the other is the shunt compartment and contains pulmonary capillaries that have no exposure to ventilated alveoli. Using the Fick relationship, the following equation can be derived:

$$\frac{\dot{Q}_{SP}}{\dot{Q}_T} = \frac{Cc'O_2 - CaO_2}{Cc'O_2 - C\bar{v}O_2} \qquad (11\text{-}7)$$

where $\dot{Q}_{SP}/\dot{Q}_T$ is the shunt fraction ($\dot{Q}_{SP}$ is blood flow through the physiologic shunt compartment, $\dot{Q}_T$ is total cardiac output), and $Cc'O_2$ and $C\bar{v}O_2$ are end-capillary and mixed venous oxygen contents, respectively. Normal intrapulmonary shunt is approximately 5%. Because this equation is based on an artificial two-compartment model, the absolute value is physically meaningless. A calculated $\dot{Q}_{SP}/\dot{Q}_T$ of 25% means that if the lung existed in two compartments, 25% of the cardiac output would travel through the shunt compartment. Since the lung does not truly exist in two compartments, this equation grossly estimates pulmonary oxygen exchange defects. Nevertheless, it remains our best tool for clinically evaluating the lungs' efficiency in oxygenating arterial blood. Observing changes in shunt fraction corresponding to therapeutic intervention or disease progression is more valuable than knowing the absolute value per se.

Since hemoglobin concentration is uniform throughout the vascular system, the oxygen contents in the shunt equation are determined primarily by oxyhemoglobin saturation. Thus, the shunt equation can be approximated by substituting saturation values for each term; the new value, called *ventilation–perfusion ratio* (VQI),[56] is determined as follows:

$$VQI = \frac{Sc'O_2 - SaO_2}{Sc'O_2 - S\bar{v}O_2} \cong \frac{1 - SaO_2}{1 - S\bar{v}O_2} \qquad (11\text{-}8)$$

If the patient is neither breathing a hypoxic gas mixture nor has a methemoglobin or carboxyhemoglobin value in excess of 5% to 6%, $Sc'O_2$ must equal 1 because the model requires a perfect alveolar–capillary interface. This substitution results in the final expression in the previous equation. The absolute values of VQI are meaningless, although "normal" should be 0 to 4%. Like $\dot{Q}_{SP}/\dot{Q}_T$, the importance of these values lies in their trend as disease and treatment progress.

SaO_2 and $S\bar{v}O_2$ can be estimated continuously with pulse oximetry and by using a pulmonary artery catheter with oximetry
10 capability. By interfacing the outputs of these two devices with a computer, VQI can be calculated continuously. The greatest advantage of calculating $\dot{Q}_{SP}/\dot{Q}_T$ or VQI to assess arterial oxygenation efficiency is that these values include the contribution of mixed venous blood.

PULMONARY FUNCTION TESTING

Anesthesiologists frequently care for patients with significant pulmonary dysfunction. It is important for the anesthesiologist to be able to interpret tests of pulmonary function intelligently and to know which tests will help define dysfunction if the patient's history and physical examinations are suggestive of disease. This section discusses lung volumes, tests of pulmonary mechanics, and diffusing capacity.

Lung Volumes and Capacities

Known, reproducible pulmonary gas volumes and capacities provide a reliable basis for comparison between normal and abnormal measurements.[59] Because normal measurements vary with size, height is most frequently used to define "normal." Lung capacities are composed of two or more lung volumes. Lung volumes and capacities are schematically illustrated in Figure 11-8.

Tidal volume is the volume of gas that moves in and out of the lungs during quiet breathing and is ~6 to 8 mL/kg. Tidal volume falls with decreased lung compliance or when the patient has reduced ventilatory muscle strength.

Vital capacity is usually ~60 mL/kg but may vary as much as 20% from normal in healthy individuals. VC correlates well with the capability for deep breathing and effective coughing. It is decreased by restrictive pulmonary disease such as pulmonary edema or atelectasis. VC may also be reduced by mechanically induced extrapulmonary restriction seen in pleural effusion,

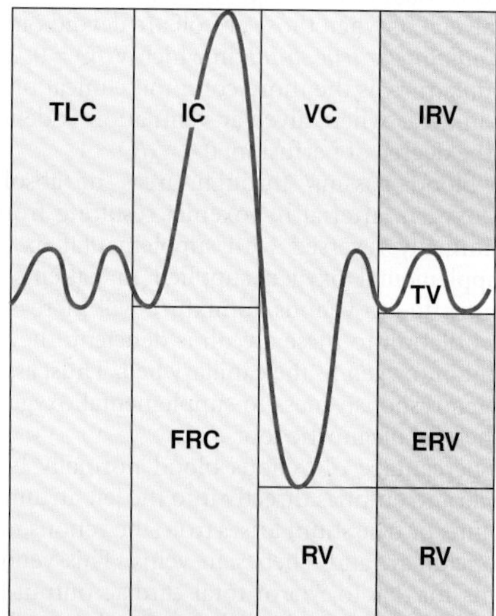

FIGURE 11-8. Lung volumes and capacities. The darkest shaded bar on the far right depicts the four basic lung volumes that sum to create TLC. Other lung capacities are composed of two or more lung volumes. The overlying spirographic tracing orients the reader to the relationship between the lung volumes and capacities and the spirogram. ERV, expiratory reserve volume; FRC, functional residual capacity; IC, inspiratory capacity; IRV, inspiratory reserve volume; RV, residual volume; TLC, total lung capacity; VC, vital capacity; VT, tidal volume.

pneumothorax, pregnancy, large ascites, or ventilatory muscle weakness.

The *inspiratory capacity* is the largest volume of gas that can be inspired from the resting expiratory level and is frequently decreased in the presence of significant extrathoracic airway obstruction. This measurement is one of the few simple tests that can detect extrathoracic airway obstruction. Most routine pulmonary function tests measure only exhaled flows and volumes, which may be relatively unaffected by extrathoracic obstruction until it is severe. Changes in the absolute volume of inspiratory capacity usually parallel changes in VC. *Expiratory reserve volume* is not of great diagnostic value.

Functional residual capacity (FRC) is the volume of gas remaining in the lungs at passive end expiration. *Residual volume* is the gas remaining within the lungs at the end of forced maximal expiration. The FRC serves two primary physiologic functions. First, it determines the point on the pulmonary volume–pressure curve for resting ventilation (see Fig. 11-2). The tangent defined by the midportion pulmonary volume–pressure curve at FRC defines lung compliance. Thus, FRC determines the elastic pressure–volume relationships within the lung. Furthermore, FRC is the resting expiratory volume of the lung and is the primary determinant of oxygen reserve in humans when apnea occurs. As such, it greatly influences ventilation–
11 perfusion relationships within the lung. When FRC is reduced, venous admixture (low $\dot{V}_A/\dot{Q}$) increases and results in arterial hypoxemia (see Oxygen and Carbon Dioxide Transport and Lung Mechanics sections).

Further, the FRC may be used to quantify the degree of pulmonary restriction. Disease processes that reduce FRC and lung compliance include acute lung injury, pulmonary edema, pulmonary fibrotic processes, and atelectasis. Mechanical factors also reduce FRC, for example, pregnancy, obesity, pleural effusion, and posture. The FRC decreases 10% when a healthy subject lies down. Ventilatory muscle weakness or paralysis will also decrease FRC. In contrast, patients with COPD have excessively compliant lungs that recoil less forcibly. Their lungs retain an abnormally large volume at the end of passive expiration, a phenomenon called *gas trapping*.

FRC Measurement

The FRC and residual volume must be measured indirectly because residual volume cannot be removed from the lung. The multiple-breath nitrogen washout test is performed by having the subject breathe 100% oxygen for several minutes so that alveolar nitrogen is gradually "washed out." With each breath, the volume of gas and the concentration of nitrogen in the exhaled gas are measured. A rapid nitrogen analyzer coupled to a spirometer or pneumotachometer provides a breath-by-breath analysis of nitrogen washout. Electronic signals proportional to nitrogen concentrations and exhaled volumes (or flow, if a pneumotachometer is used) are integrated to derive the exhaled volume of nitrogen for each breath. Then, the values for all breaths are summed to provide a total volume of nitrogen washed out of the lungs. The test proceeds until the alveolar nitrogen concentration is reduced to less than 7%, usually requiring 7 to 10 minutes. FRC is calculated using the equation:

$$\text{FRC} = \text{N}_2 \text{ volume} \times \frac{[\text{N}_2]_f}{[\text{N}_2]_i} \qquad (11\text{-}9)$$

where $[N_2]_i$ and $[N_2]_f$ are the fractional concentrations of alveolar nitrogen at the beginning and end of the test, respectively.

Pulmonary Function Tests

Forced Vital Capacity

The forced vital capacity (FVC) is the volume of gas that can be expired as forcefully and rapidly as possible after maximal inspiration. Normally, FVC is equal to VC. Although forced expiration significantly increases intrapleural pressures but changes airway pressure minimally, bronchiolar collapse, obstructive lesions, and gas trapping are exaggerated. Thus, FVC may be reduced in chronic obstructive diseases even when the VC appears near normal. FVC is nearly always decreased by restrictive diseases. FVC values <15 mL/kg are associated with an increased incidence of PPCs, probably because these patients cough ineffectively.[60] FVC reduced to this level represents a profound defect, most commonly seen in quadriplegics or severe neuromuscular disease. Finally, FVC is largely dependent on patient effort and cooperation.

Forced Expiratory Volume

FEV_T is the forced expiratory volume of gas over a given time interval during the FVC maneuver. The interval, described by the subscript T, is the time elapsed in seconds from the onset of expiration. Because FEV_T records a volume of gas expired over time, it is actually a measure of flow. By measuring expiratory flow at specific intervals, the severity of airway obstruction can be ascertained. Decreased FEV_T values are common in both obstructive and restrictive disease patterns. The most important application of FEV_T is its comparison with the patient's FVC. Normal subjects can expire at least three-fourths of FVC within the first second of the forced expiratory maneuver. The FEV_1, the most frequently employed value, is normally greater than or equal to 75% of the FVC, or $FEV_1/FVC \geq 0.75$.

Normally, an individual can expire 50% to 60% of FVC in 0.5 second, 75% to 85% in 1 second, 94% in 2 seconds, and 97% in 3 seconds. Cooperative patients with obstructive disease will exhibit a reduced FEV_1/FVC in most cases. However, patients with restrictive disease usually have normal FEV_1/FVC ratios. The validity of the evaluation of the FEV_1/FVC is highly dependent on patient cooperation and effort. It is possible to deliberately produce an artificially low FEV_1/FVC.

Forced Expiratory Flow

$FEF_{25-75\%}$ is the average forced expiratory flow during the middle half of the FEV maneuver. This test is also called maximum midexpiratory flow rate. The length of time required for a subject to expire the middle half of the FVC is divided into 50% of the FVC. The spirogram in Figure 11-9 marks the place from 25% to 75% of FVC, constituting the middle 50% of FVC. The straight line connecting the 25% and 75% volumes has a slope approximately equal to average flow. A normal value for a healthy 70 kg man is approximately 4.7 L/s (or 280 mL/min). Normally, both the absolute value and the percentage of predicted value for the individual being studied are recorded. A normal value is 100 ± 25% of that predicted. Decreased flow rates from this middle 50% of FVC anatomically represents flow in medium size airways, and when decreased, is indicative of obstructive disease of medium size airways. This value is typically normal in restrictive diseases. This test is fairly sensitive in the early stages of obstructive airway disease. Decreased $FEV_{25-75\%}$ frequently will be observed before other obstructive manifestations occur. Although somewhat effort-dependent, the test is much more reliable and reproducible than FEV_1/FVC.

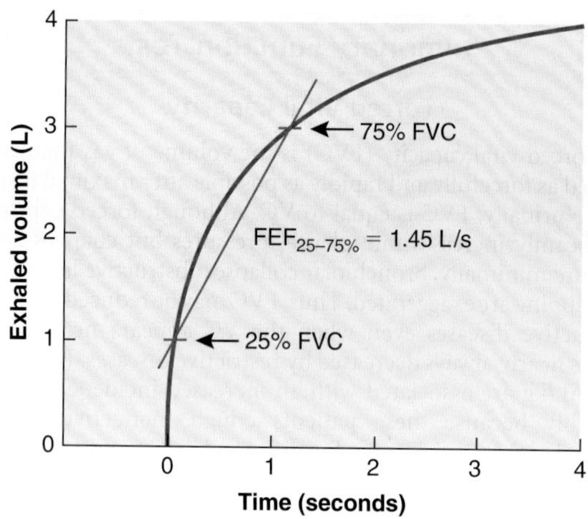

FIGURE 11-9. $FEF_{25-75\%}$. The spirogram depicts a 4 L FVC on which the points representing 25% and 75% FVC are marked. The slope of the line connecting these points is the $FEF_{25-75\%}$. FEF, forced expiratory flow; FVC, forced vital capacity.

Maximum Voluntary Ventilation

Maximum voluntary ventilation (MVV) is the largest volume of gas that can be breathed in 1 minute by voluntary effort. The MVV is measured by having the subject breathe as deeply and as rapidly as possible for 10, 12, or 15 seconds. The results are extrapolated to 1 minute. The subject is instructed to set his or her own ventilatory rate and move more than tidal volume but less than VC in each breath.

MVV measures the endurance of the ventilatory muscles and indirectly reflects lung–thorax compliance and airway resistance. MVV is the best ventilatory endurance test that can be performed in the laboratory. Values that vary by as much as 30% from predicted values may be normal so only large reductions in MVV are significant. Healthy, young adults average ~170 L/min. Values are lower in women and decrease with age in both sexes. Because this maneuver exaggerates air trapping and exerts the ventilatory muscles, MVV is decreased greatly in patients with moderate to severe obstructive disease. MVV is usually normal in patients with restrictive disease.

Flow–Volume Loops

The flow–volume loop graphically demonstrates the flow generated during a forced expiratory maneuver followed by a forced inspiratory maneuver, plotted against the volume of gas expired (Fig. 11-10). The subject forcefully exhales completely, then immediately forcefully inhales to VC. The expired and inspired volumes are plotted on the abscissa and flow is plotted on the ordinate. Although various numbers can be generated from the flow–volume loop, the configuration of the loop itself is probably the most informative part of the test.

Flow–volume loops were formerly useful in the diagnosis of large airway and extrathoracic airway obstruction prior to the availability of precise imaging techniques. Imaging techniques such as MRI give more precise and useful information in the diagnosis of upper airway and extrathoracic obstruction and superseded the use of flow–volume loops for diagnosis of these conditions. Therefore, it is rare that flow–volume loops are useful for preoperative pulmonary evaluation in the modern era of imaging.

Carbon Monoxide Diffusing Capacity

Since P_{O_2} in the pulmonary capillary blood varies with time as it moves through the pulmonary capillary bed, oxygen cannot be used to assess diffusing capacity. Instead, a gas mixture containing carbon monoxide is the traditional diagnostic gas used to measure diffusing capacity. The partial pressure of carbon monoxide in the blood is nearly zero, and its affinity for hemoglobin is 200 times that of oxygen.[61] Carbon monoxide diffusing capacity (D_{LCO}) collectively measures all the factors that affect the diffusion of gas across the alveolar–capillary membrane. The D_{LCO} is recorded in mL CO/min/mm Hg at STPD (standard temperature and pressure, dry). In persons with normal hemoglobin concentrations and normal $\dot{V}_A/\dot{Q}$ matching, the main factor limiting diffusion is the alveolar–capillary membrane. Small amounts of carbon dioxide and inspired gas can produce measurable changes in the concentration of inspired gas compared with expired gas. There are several methods for determining D_{LCO}, but all methods measure diffusing capacity according to the equation:

$$D_{LCO} = \frac{\text{mL CO transferred/min}}{\text{mean } P_{ACO_2} - \text{mean capillary } P_{CO_2}} \qquad (11\text{-}10)$$

The average value for resting subjects when the single-breath method is used is 25 mL CO/min/mm Hg. D_{LCO} values can increase to two or three times normal during exercise.

The D_{LO_2} may be estimated from the D_{LCO} by multiplying D_{LCO} by 1.23, although the D_{LCO} is usually the reported value. D_{LCO} can be divided by the lung volume at which the measurement was made to obtain an expression of diffusing capacity per unit lung volume.

Some of the other factors that can influence D_{LCO} are as follows:

1. Hemoglobin concentration: Decreased hemoglobin concentration decreases the D_{LCO}
2. Alveolar P_{CO_2}: An increased P_{ACO_2} raises D_{LCO}
3. Body position: The supine position increases D_{LCO}
4. Pulmonary capillary blood volume

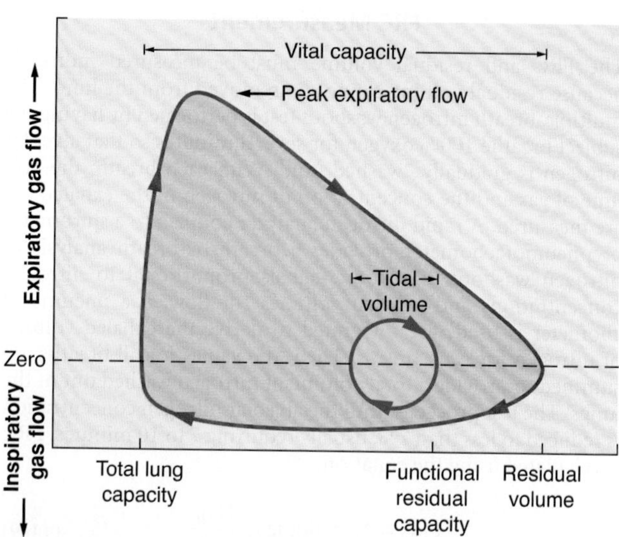

FIGURE 11-10. Flow–volume loop. The figure depicts a normally configured adult flow–volume loop. The slope of the loop after the subject reaches peak expiratory flow is nearly linear.

Diffusing capacity is decreased in alveolar fibrosis associated with sarcoidosis, asbestosis, berylliosis, oxygen toxicity, and pulmonary edema. These states are frequently categorized as diffusion defects, but low D_{LCO} is probably more closely related to loss of lung volume or capillary bed perfusion. D_{LCO} is decreased in obstructive disease because of the decreased alveolar surface area, loss of capillary bed, the increased distance from the terminal bronchiole to the alveolar–capillary membrane, and $\dot{V}_A/\dot{Q}$ mismatching. In short, few disease states truly inhibit oxygen diffusion across the alveolar–capillary membrane.

Practical Application of Pulmonary Function Tests

Although we have a host of pulmonary function tests from which to choose, spirometry is the most useful, cost-effective, and commonly used test.[62] Screening spirometry yields VC, FVC, and FEV_1. From these values, two basic types of pulmonary dysfunction can be identified and quantitated: Obstructive defects and restrictive defects. The primary criterion for airflow obstruction is decreased FEV_1/FVC ratio. Other measurements, such as $FEF_{25-75\%}$, can be used to support the diagnosis of an obstructive defect or to assist in making decisions (e.g., whether to institute bronchodilation). A restrictive defect is a proportional decrease in all lung volumes; thus, VC, FVC, and FEV_1 all are reduced, but FEV_1/FVC remains normal. When there is a question about whether a decreased VC is due to restriction, total lung capacity (TLC) should be measured. Reduced TLC defines a restrictive defect but is not necessary unless VC on screening spirometry is reduced. The American Thoracic Society published an experts' consensus concerning interpretation of lung function tests.[63] Table 11-4 summarizes the distinction between pulmonary function results obtained from those with restrictive and obstructive defects. Refer to the "Pulmonary Function Postoperatively" section for a discussion on the use of pulmonary testing.

TABLE 11-4. PULMONARY FUNCTION TESTS IN RESTRICTIVE AND OBSTRUCTIVE LUNG DISEASE

Value	Restrictive Disease	Obstructive Disease
Definition	Proportional decreases in all lung volumes	Small airway obstruction to expiratory flow
FVC	↓↓↓	Normal or slightly ↑
FEV_1	↓↓↓	Normal or slightly ↓
FEV_1/FVC	Normal	↓↓↓
$FEF_{25-75\%}$	Normal	↓↓↓
FRC	↓↓↓	Normal or ↑ if gas trapping
TLC	↓↓↓	Normal or ↑ if gas trapping

FEV, forced expiratory volume; FRC, functional residual capacity; FVC, forced vital capacity; TLC, total lung capacity; ↓↓↓, ↑↑↑ = large decrease or increase, respectively; ↓, ↑ = small/moderate decrease or increase, respectively.

Preoperative Pulmonary Assessment

Markedly impaired pulmonary function is likely in patients who have the following:

1. Any chronic disease that involves the lung
2. Smoking history, persistent cough, and/or wheezing
3. Chest wall and spinal deformities
4. Morbid obesity
5. Requirement for single-lung anesthesia or lung resection
6. Severe neuromuscular disease

Preoperative pulmonary evaluation must include history and physical examination, and may include chest radiograph, arterial blood gas analysis, and screening spirometry, depending on the patient's history. A history of sputum production, wheezing or dyspnea, exercise intolerance, or limited daily activities may yield more practical information than does formal testing. Arterial blood analysis, which should be sampled while the patient breathes room air, adds information regarding gas exchange and acid–base balance. Arterial blood gas sampling is primarily useful if the patient's history suggests that he or she may be chronically hypoxemic or may "retain" CO_2 (i.e., a patient with a chronic, compensated arterial acidemia) and can be used to guide ventilatory management goals. These values may be interpreted in the context of previously measured bicarbonate levels, as they are frequently elevated in those with chronic acidemia.

The goals one might hope to achieve through preoperative pulmonary function would be to predict the likelihood of pulmonary complications, obtain quantitative baseline information concerning pulmonary function which guides decision making, and identify patients who may benefit from therapy to improve pulmonary function preoperatively. For patients who will have lung resections, pulmonary function testing does provide some predictive benefit.[64] For all other patients, however, overwhelming evidence suggests that preoperative pulmonary function testing does not predict or assign risk for PPCs.[65,66]

In 2002, the American Society of Anesthesiologists' Taskforce on Preanesthetic Evaluation published an updated practice advisory[67] wherein they recommended that "there is insufficient evidence to identify explicit decision parameters or rules for ordering preoperative tests on the basis of specific clinical characteristics." Review of the literature[68] also reveals that specific measurements of lung function do not predict PPCs. Rather, they should be obtained to ascertain the presence of reversible
12 pulmonary disease (bronchospasm) or to define the severity of advanced pulmonary disease. Instead, the clinician obtains more information from the patient's history. In a series of 272 adults undergoing nonthoracic surgery, McAlister et al.[69] found that the following historical factors independently increased the risk of PPC: Age >65 years, smoking >40 pack-years, COPD, asthma, productive cough, and exercise tolerance of less than one flight of stairs.

The need to obtain baseline pulmonary function data should be reserved for those patients with severely impaired preoperative pulmonary function, such as quadriplegics or myasthenics, so assessment for liberation from mechanical ventilation and/or tracheal extubation might be based on the patient's baseline pulmonary function.

Arterial blood gases (ABG) are not indicated unless the patient's history suggests arterial hypoxemia or severe enough COPD that one suspects CO_2 retention. Then, the ABG should be used in essentially the same manner as one might use preoperative PFTs: To look for reversible disease, or to define the severity of the disease at its baseline. Defining baseline Pa_{O_2} and Pa_{CO_2} is

TABLE 11-5. RESPIRATORY FORMULAS

Formula	Normal Values (70 kg)
Alveolar oxygen tension	110 mm Hg
$P_{AO_2} = (P_B - 47)\ F_{IO_2} - (P_{ACO_2}/R)$	($F_{IO_2} = 0.21$)
Alveolar–arterial oxygen gradient	<10 mm Hg
$A\text{-}aO_2 = P_{AO_2} - PaO_2$	($F_{IO_2} = 0.21$)
Arterial-to-alveolar oxygen ratio, a/A ratio	>0.75
Arterial oxygen content	20 mL/10
$Cao_2 = (Sao_2)\ (Hb \times 1.34) + Pao_2\ (0.0031)$	0 mL blood
Mixed venous oxygen content	15 mL/100 mL blood
$C\bar{v}O_2 = (S\bar{v}o_2)\ (Hb \times 1.34) + P\bar{v}o_2\ (0.0031)$	
Arterial–venous oxygen content difference	4–6 mL/100 mL blood
$Ca\text{-}\bar{v}o_2 = Cao_2 - C\bar{v}o_2$	
Intrapulmonary shunt	<5%
$\dot{Q}_{SP}/\dot{Q}_T = (Cc'o_2 - Cao_2)/(Cc'O_2 - C\bar{v}o_2)$	
where $Cc'o_2 = (Hb \times 1.34) + (P_{AO_2} \times 0.0031)$	
Physiologic dead space	0.33
$V_D/V_T = (Paco_2 - P\bar{E}co_2)/Paco_2$	
Oxygen consumption	250 mL/min
$\dot{V}o_2 = CO\ (Cao_2 - C\bar{v}o_2)$	
Oxygen transport	1,000 mL/min
$O_2T = CO\ (Cao_2)$	
Respiratory quotient	0.8
$\dot{V}co_2/\dot{V}o_2 = R$	

Cao_2, arterial oxygen content; $C\bar{v}o_2$, mixed venous oxygen content; $Cc'o_2$, end-pulmonary capillary oxygen content; CO, cardiac output; F_{IO_2}, fraction inspired oxygen; Hb, hemoglobin concentration; O_2T, oxygen transport; PB, barometric pressure; $\dot{Q}_{SP}/\dot{Q}_T$, intrapulmonary shunt; P_{ACO_2}, alveolar carbon dioxide tension; $Paco_2$, arterial carbon dioxide tension; P_{AO_2}, alveolar oxygen tension; Pao_2, arterial oxygen tension; $P\bar{E}co_2$, mixed expired carbon dioxide tension; $P\bar{v}o_2$, mixed venous oxygen tension; Sao_2, arterial oxygen saturation; $S\bar{v}o_2$, mixed venous oxygen saturation; V_D, dead space gas volume; V_T, tidal volume; $\dot{V}co_2$, oxygen consumption (mL/min); $\dot{V}co_2$, carbon dioxide production (mL/min); R, respiratory quotient.

particularly important if one anticipates postoperatively ventilating a patient who has severe COPD. Table 11-5 summarizes the respiratory physiology formulas discussed in this chapter.

ANESTHESIA AND OBSTRUCTIVE PULMONARY DISEASE

Patients with marked obstructive pulmonary disease are at increased risk for both intraoperative and PPCs. For example, patients with reduced FEV_1/FVC or reduced midexpiratory flow not only suffer airway obstruction, but also usually exhibit increased airway reactivity. Because of the hazard of provoking reflex bronchoconstriction during laryngoscopy and tracheal intubation, patients with COPD or asthma should receive aggressive bronchodilator therapy preoperatively, prior to instrumentation of the airway. High alveolar concentrations of most potent inhalational anesthetics will blunt airway reflexes and reflex bronchoconstriction but require a fairly robust cardiovascular system. Adjunctive intravenous administration of opioids and lidocaine prior to airway instrumentation will decrease airway reactivity by deepening anesthesia. Furthermore, a single dose of corticosteroids may help prevent postoperative increases in airway resistance.

Spontaneous ventilation during general anesthesia in patients with severe obstructive disease is more likely to result in hypercapnia than in patients with normal pulmonary function.[70] Preoperative FEV_1 reduction correlates with the $Paco_2$ increase during anesthesia. Slower rates of mechanical ventilation (8–10 breaths · min^{-1}) should be used to allow time for exhalation. Low ventilatory rates necessitate larger tidal volume if one desires a normal $Paco_2$, but larger V_T and resultant higher peak airway pressure may predispose the patient to pulmonary barotrauma. Tidal volume and inspiratory flows should be adjusted to keep peak airway pressure less than 40 cm H_2O,[71,72] if possible. Higher inspiratory flows produce a shorter inspiratory time and, usually, a high peak airway pressure. Thus, a balance that avoids high peak airway pressure and excessively large V_T that allows the longest possible expiratory time should be sought.

Ideally, depending on the procedure and the duration of anesthesia, one would extubate the patient's trachea at the end of the operation. The irritating tracheal tube increases both airway resistance and reflex bronchoconstriction, limits the ability of the patient to clear secretions effectively, and increases the risk of iatrogenic infection. For some patients with obstructive disease (e.g., the young asthmatic), many advocate tracheal extubation during deep anesthesia at the conclusion of the operation.

ANESTHESIA AND RESTRICTIVE PULMONARY DISEASE

Restrictive disease is characterized by proportional decreases in all lung volumes. The decreased FRC produces low lung compliance and also results in arterial hypoxemia because of low $\dot{V}_A/\dot{Q}$ mismatching. These patients typically breathe rapidly and shallowly.

Positive-pressure ventilation of patients with restrictive disease is fraught with high peak airway pressures because more pressure is required to expand stiff lungs. Lower mechanical tidal volumes at more rapid rates reduce the risk of barotrauma but augment ventilation-induced cardiovascular depression and increase the chances of developing atelectasis. Larger tidal volumes should be avoided, because of the increased risk of both barotrauma[73] and volutrauma.[50] Various lung protective strategies have been developed to ventilate patients with profound restrictive lung disease (see Chapters 36 and 56).

Because the FRC is reduced, a lower oxygen store is available during apneic periods. Even preoxygenation with an F_{IO_2} of 1 can result in arterial hypoxemia seconds after the cessation of breathing or disconnection from a ventilator circuit. Patients with severe restrictive diseases tolerate apnea poorly. Because arterial hypoxemia develops so rapidly, transportation of these patients within the hospital should be performed with a pulse oximeter.

Even healthy individuals develop mild restrictive defects during anesthesia. FRC decreases 10% to 15% when healthy, spontaneously breathing individuals lie supine. Tracheal intubation also minimally reduces FRC. General anesthesia consistently decreases FRC by a further 5% to 10%,[74]) which usually results in decreased lung compliance.[75] The FRC reaches its nadir within the first 10 minutes of anesthesia[74,76,77] and is independent of whether ventilation is spontaneous or controlled. The diminished FRC persists in the postoperative period but may be restored postoperatively by the use of positive end-expiratory pressure or CPAP.[74,78,79]. However, once positive airway pressure is removed, FRC plummets to previously diminished levels, which reach a postoperative nadir 12 hours after operation.[80]

EFFECTS OF CIGARETTE SMOKING ON PULMONARY FUNCTION

Smoking affects pulmonary function in many ways. The irritant smoke decreases ciliary motility and increases sputum production. Thus, these patients have a high volume of sputum and decreased ability to clear it effectively. As smoking habits persist, airway reactivity and the development of obstructive disease become problematic. Studies of the pathogenesis of COPD suggest that smoking results in an excess of pulmonary proteolytic enzymes, which directly cause damage to the lung parenchyma.[81] Exposure to smoke increases synthesis and release of elastolytic enzymes from alveolar macrophages—cells instrumental in the genesis of COPD due to smoking. Further damage to the lung tissue is probably caused by reactive metabolites of oxygen, such as hydroxyl radicals and hydrogen peroxide, which are usually used by the macrophages to kill microorganisms. The immunoregulatory function of the macrophages is also changed by cigarette smoking, with changes occurring in the presentation of antigens and interaction with T lymphocytes.[82] Other direct effects on lung tissue caused by smoking include increased epithelial permeability[83] and changed pulmonary surfactant.[84] The airway irritation or small airway reactivity evoked by inhaling cigarette smoke is the result of activation of sensory endings located in the central airways, which is primarily caused by nicotine.[85]

Early in the disease, mild $\dot{V}_A/\dot{Q}$ mismatch, bronchitis, and airway hyperreactivity are primary problems. Later, these problems are accompanied by the hallmarks of COPD: Gas trapping, flattened diaphragmatic configuration (which decreases the diaphragm's efficiency), and barrel chest deformity. Lung compliance increases significantly so limited elastic recoil prevents complete passive emptying. As a result, many patients exhale forcibly to reduce gas trapping.

With gas trapping, ventilation and perfusion become increasingly mismatched. Large areas of dead space ventilation and venous admixture occur. Carbon dioxide elimination is inefficient because of dead space ventilation. The typical minute ventilation for patients with advanced obstructive lung disease can be 1.5 to 2 times normal. In addition, venous admixture produces arterial hypoxemia that is exquisitely sensitive to low concentrations of supplemental oxygen. Gas exchange is further impaired by the increased carboxyhemoglobin concentration that results from inspiring smoke. Normal carboxyhemoglobin concentration in nonsmokers is approximately 1%; in smokers, however, it can be as high as 8% to 10%. Cessation of smoking, even for 12 to 24 hours preoperatively, can decrease CO concentration to near normal.

Smoking is one of the main and most prevalent risk factors associated with postoperative morbidity.[86] COPD patients who smoke have a twofold to sixfold[87] risk of developing postoperative pneumonia compared with nonsmokers. Furthermore, smokers' relative risk of PPC is doubled, even if they do not have evidence of clinical pulmonary disease or abnormal pulmonary function.[88] The incidence of PPC in smokers can be reduced by abstinence from smoking, although there is no consensus on the minimal or optimal duration of preoperative smoking abstinence.[89–91] Warner et al.[86] studied 200 patients undergoing coronary artery bypass grafting and found that patients who continued to smoke or stopped less than 8 weeks before the operation had a complication rate nearly four times that of patients who had quit smoking more than 8 weeks preoperatively. The data further demonstrated that those who quit smoking less than 8 weeks preoperatively had a higher rate of complication than those who continued to smoke. Normalization of mucociliary function requires 2 to 3 weeks of abstinence from smoking, during which time sputum increases. Several months of smoking abstinence is required to return sputum clearance to normal.[92] In a study of bupropion-assisted smoking cessation, Hurt and coworkers demonstrated decreased risk of postoperative complications even after 4 weeks of abstinence from smoking.[93]

Nonetheless, Public Health Service guidelines published in 2,000 emphasize the responsibility of health care facilities to coordinate interventions aimed at tobacco dependence treatment. In addition to the guidelines noting that tobacco dependence often necessitates repeated interventions, "every patient who uses tobacco should be offered at least brief treatment" as brief tobacco dependence therapy has been shown to be effective. These guidelines recognize five first-line pharmacologic adjuncts that increase smoking cessation success: Bupropion SR, nicotine gum, nicotine inhaler, nicotine nasal spray, and nicotine patch. Additionally, clonidine and nortriptyline were identified as second-line pharmacologic adjuncts.[94]

Following publication of these 2,000 guidelines, a randomized controlled trial utilizing the partial nicotinic acetylcholine agonist, varenicline, showed improved smoking abstinence rates at all times evaluated during the study when compared to bupropion

SR treatment.[95] On the basis of this information, the utilization of varenicline in a smoking cessation program should be considered.

Smokers who decrease, but do not stop, cigarette consumption without the aid of nicotine replacement therapy, continue to acquire equal amounts of nicotine from fewer cigarettes by changing their technique of smoking to maximize nicotine intake.[96] Levels of serum nicotine and cotinine and urinary mutagenesis levels remain unchanged. Thus, *reduction* in the number of cigarettes smoked will likely have little effect on the risk of
13 developing PPCs.[87] Smoking patients should be advised to *stop* smoking 2 months prior to elective operations to maximize the effect of smoking cessation,[86] or for at least 4 weeks to benefit from improved mucociliary function and some reduction in PPC rate. If patients cannot stop smoking for 4 to 8 weeks preoperatively, it is controversial whether they should be advised to stop smoking 24 hours preoperatively. A 24-hour smoking abstinence would allow carboxyhemoglobin levels to fall to normal but may increase the risk of PPC.

PULMONARY FUNCTION POSTOPERATIVELY

Risk of Postoperative Pulmonary Complications

Postoperative Pulmonary Function

The changes in pulmonary function that occur postoperatively are primarily restrictive, with proportional decreases in all lung volumes and no change in airway resistance. The decrease in FRC, however, is the yardstick by which the severity of the restrictive defect is gauged. This defect is generated by abdominal contents that impinge on and prevent normal movement of the diaphragm, and by an abnormal respiratory pattern devoid of sighs and characterized by shallow, rapid respirations. The normal resting respiratory rate for adults is 12 breaths per minute, whereas the postoperative patient usually breathes approximately 20 breaths per minute. Furthermore, most (but not all) factors that tend to make the restrictive defect worse are also those associated with a higher risk of PPCs.

The operative site is one of the single most important determi-
14 nants of the degree of pulmonary restriction and the risk of PPCs. Nonlaparoscopic upper abdominal operations cause the most profound restrictive defect, precipitating a 40% to 50% decrease in FRC compared with preoperative levels, when conventional postoperative analgesia is employed. Lower abdominal and thoracic operations cause the next most severe change in pulmonary function, with decreases in FRC to 30% of preoperative levels. Most other operative sites—intracranial, peripheral vascular, otolaryngologic—have approximately the same effect on FRC, with reductions to 15% to 20% of preoperative levels.

Postoperative Pulmonary Complications

Two problems confound interpretation of the literature examining PPCs. First, there is no clear definition of what constitutes a PPC. For example, some clinical studies include only pneumonia, whereas others add atelectasis and/or ventilatory failure. Thus, to interpret data concerning rates of PPCs, it is important to discern what complications are specifically being addressed. Second, the criteria by which the diagnosis of postoperative pneumonia or atelectasis is made vary from study to study. For this discussion, PPCs include atelectasis and pneumonia only. Reasonable, well-accepted diagnostic criteria for these diagnoses include change in the color and quantity of sputum, oral temperature exceeding 38.5°C, and a new infiltrate on chest radiograph.

The operative site is an important risk factor for the development of PPCs. Nonlaparoscopic upper abdominal operations increase risk for PPC at least twofold,[90] with rates of occurrence varying from 20% to 70%.[96]) Lower abdominal and intrathoracic operations are associated with slightly less risk, but still higher risk than extremity, intracranial, and head/neck operations.

Patients with COPD are at risk for PPC. Their risks can be minimized by ensuring that they do not have an active pulmonary infection and any increased resistance associated with reactive airways disease is minimized by the use of bronchodilator therapy. Interestingly, those with asthma are not at increased risk for atelectasis or pneumonia. However, exacerbation of asthma in the postoperative period can be problematic. Careful attention must be given to ensuring the continuation of bronchodilating regimens and steroid administration (either inhaled or systemic) through the perioperative period.

There are several strategies by which it is possible to reduce risk of PPC: The use of lung-expanding therapies postoperatively, choice of analgesia,[97] and cessation of smoking. After upper abdominal operations, which are associated with the highest incidence of PPCs, FRC recovers over 3 to 7 days. With the use of intermittent CPAP by mask, FRC will recover within 72 hours.[98] Patients correctly use incentive spirometers only 10% of the time unless therapy is supervised.[99] Stir-up regimens are as effective as incentive spirometry at preventing PPCs,[100] and they are less expensive than supervised incentive spirometry; thus, they are preferred over incentive spirometry therapy.

After median sternotomy for cardiac operations, FRC does not return to normal for several weeks, regardless of postoperative pulmonary therapy.[101] The persistently low FRC in this population is probably due to mechanical factors such as a wid-
15 ened mediastinum, intrapleural fluid, and altered chest wall compliance. The single most important aspect of postoperative pulmonary care is getting the patient out of bed, preferably walking.

The choice of anesthetic technique for intraoperative anesthesia does not change the risk for PPC independent of the operative site or duration of the operation. Operations exceeding 3 hours are associated with a higher rate of PPC. Choice of postoperative analgesia strongly influences the risk of PPC.[90] The use of postoperative epidural analgesia, particularly for abdominal and thoracic operations, markedly decreases the risk of PPC and appears to decrease length of stay in the hospital.

Although obesity is associated with marked restrictive defects, some studies demonstrate that obesity does not independently increase the risk of PPC, whereas others do demonstrate increased independent risk for PPCs in the obese population.[102] However, there is data to support[102] advanced age as an independent risk factor for PPCs.

Several authors have attempted to assess the influence of overall health on PPC risk. The use of indices that weigh and score various aspects of physiology and health shows that patients who are in a poor state of health preoperatively tend to be at higher risk of PPC.[91]

Patients with obstructive airway disease and decreased expiratory flows may benefit from preoperative bronchodilator therapy and formal pulmonary toilet.[103] High-risk patients with COPD who receive bronchodilation, chest physical therapy, deep breathing, forced oral fluids (>3 L/day), and preoperative instruction in postoperative respiratory techniques, as well as those who stop smoking for more than 2 months preoperatively, experience a PPC rate approximately equal to that observed in normal patients.[104] Interestingly, although a regimen of this nature significantly reduces the incidence of PPCs,[105] airway obstruction and arterial hypoxemia are not measurably reversed during the 48 to 72 hours of preoperative therapy.[106] It is possible that the reduced complication rate results from the additional attention that these patients receive rather than from the specific regimen employed.

References

1. Lieberman DA, Faulkner JA, Craig AB Jr, et al. Performance and histochemical composition of guinea-pig and human diaphragm. *J Appl Physiol.* 1973;34(2): 233–237.
2. Roussos CS, Macklem PT. Diaphragmatic fatigue in man. *J Appl Physiol.* 1977; 43(2):189–197.
3. Campbell EJM, Green JH. The behavior of the abdominal muscles and the intra-abdominal pressure during quiet breathing and increased pulmonary ventilation; a study in man. *J Physiol.* 1955;127:423–426.
4. Conrady PA, Goodman LR, Lainge F, et al. Alteration of endotracheal tube position. Flexion and extension of the neck. *Crit Care Med.* 1976;4:8.
5. Bachofen M, Weibel ER. Basic pattern of tissue repair in human lungs following unspecific injury. *Chest.* 1974;65(4):14S–19S.
6. Fishman A. Nonrespiratory functions of the lungs. *Chest.* 1977;72(1): 84–89.
7. Hocking WG, Golde DW. The pulmonary-alveolar macrophage (first of two parts). *N Engl J Med.* 1979;301(11):580–587.
8. Whitehead TC, Zhang H, Mullen B, et al. Effect of mechanical ventilation on cytokine response to intratracheal lipopolysaccharide. *Anesthesiology.* 2004;101(1): 52–58.
9. Dreyfuss D, Rouby JJ. Mechanical ventilation-induced lung release of cytokines: A key for the future or pandora's box? *Anesthesiology.* 2004;101(1):1–3.
10. Downs JB. A technique for direct measurement of intrapleural pressure. *Crit Care Med.* 1976;4(4):207–210.
11. Baydur A, Behrakis PK, Zin WA, et al. A simple method for assessing the validity of the esophageal balloon technique. *Am Rev Respir Dis.* 1982;126(5):788–791.
12. Banner MJ, Kirby RR, Gabrielli A, et al. Partially and totally unloading respiratory muscles based on real-time measurements of work of breathing. A clinical approach. *Chest.* 1994;106(6):1835–1842.
13. Brochard L, Rua F, Lorino H, et al. Inspiratory pressure support compensates for the additional work of breathing caused by the endotracheal-tube. *Anesthesiology.* 1991;75(5):739–745.
14. Rohrer F. Der Strömungswiderstand in den menschlichen Atemwegen. *Pflugers Arch.* 1915;162:225.
15. Nunn J. Resistance to gas flow and airway closure. In: *Applied Respiratory Physiology.* Boston, Butterworths, 1987, pp 50.
16. Campbell EJ, Freedman S, Smith PS, et al. The ability of man to detect added elastic loads to breathing. *Clin Sci.* 1961;20:223–231.
17. Fink BR, Ngai SH, Holaday DA. Effect of air flow resistance on ventilation and respiratory muscle activity. *J Am Med Assoc.* 1958;168(17):2245–2249.
18. Palmer KN, Diament ML. Effect of aerosol isoprenaline on blood-gas tensions in severe bronchial asthma. *Lancet.* 1967;2(7528):1232–1233.
19. Campbell E. The effects of increased resistance to expiration on the respiratory behavior of the abdominal muscles and intra-abdominal pressure. *J Physiol.* 1957; 136:556–552.
20. Janssens JP, Pache JC, Nicod LP. Physiologic changes in respiratory function associated with ageing. *Eur Respir J.* 1999;13:197–205.
21. LeGallois CJJ. Expériences sur le Principe de la Vie. Paris, D'Hautel, 1812:325.
22. Salmoiraghi GB, Burns BD. Localization and patterns of discharge of respiratory neurons in the brainstem of a cat. *J Neurophysiol.* 1960;23:2–13.
23. Cohen MI. Neurogenesis of respiratory rhythm in the mammal. *Physiol Rev.* 1979;59(4):1105–1173.
24. Guz A. Regulation of respiration in man. *Annu Rev Physiol.* 1975;37:303–323.
25. Pitts RF, Magoun HW, Ranson SW. The origin of respiratory rhythmicity. *Am J Physiol.* 1939;127:654–670.
26. Lumsden T. Observations on the respiratory centers in the cat. *J Physiol.* 1923; 57:153–160.
27. Cohen MI, Wang SC. Respiratory neuronal activity in pons of the cat. *Am J Physiol.* 1956;187(3):592–592.
28. Stella G. On the mechanism of production and the physiologic significance of "apneusis." *J Physiol*. 1938;93:10–23.
29. Kabat H. Electrical stimulation of points in the forebrain and mid-brain: The resultant alterations in respiration. *J Comp Neurol.* 1936;64:187.
30. Wang SC, Borison HL. The vomiting center; a critical experimental analysis. *Arch Neurol Psychiatry.* 1950;63(6):928–941.
31. Gaylor J. The intrinsic nervous mechanisms of the human lung. *Brain.* 1934; 57:143.
32. Davis HL, Fowler WS, Lambert EH. Effect of volume and rate of inflation and deflation on transpulmonary pressure and response of pulmonary stretch receptors. *Am J Physiol.* 1956;187(3):558–566.
33. Hering E, Breuer J. Die selbsteuerung der athmung durch den nervus vagus sitzber. *Akad Wiss Wien.* 1868;57:672–676.
34. Ide T, Sakurai Y, Aono M, et al. Contribution of peripheral chemoreception to the depression of the hypoxic ventilatory response during halothane anesthesia in cats. *Anesthesiology.* 1999;90(4):1084–1091.
35. Mora CT, Torjman M, White PF. Effects of diazepam and flumazenil on sedation and hypoxic ventilatory response. *Anesth Analg.* 1989;68(4):473–478.
36. Leusen I. Regulation of cerebrospinal fluid composition with reference to breathing. *Physiol Rev.* 1972;52(1):1–56.
37. Cohen MI. Discharge patterns of brain-stem respiratory neurons in relation to carbon dioxide tension. *J Neurophysiol.* 1968;31:142–165.
38. Heinemann HO, Goldring RM. Bicarbonate and the regulation of ventilation. *Am J Med.* 1974;57(3):361–370.
39. Shapiro BA, Peruzzi WT, Kozlowski-Templin R, ed. *Clinical Application of Blood Gases, 5th Edition.* Mosby; 1993.
40. Severinghaus JM, Mitchell RA, Richardson BW, et al. Respiratory control at high altitude suggesting active transport regulation of CSF pH. *J Appl Physiol.* 1963;18:1155–1156.
41. Ferris EE, Engel GL, Stevens CD, et al. Voluntary breath holding. *J Clin Invest.* 1946;25:734.
42. Stock MD, Downs JB, McDonald JS, et al. The carbon dioxide rate of rise in awake apneic humans. *J Clin Anesth.* 1988;1:96.
43. Eger EI, Severinghaus JW. The rate of rise of PaCO2 in the apneic anesthetized patient. *Anesthesiology.* 1961;22:419–425.
44. Stock MC, Schisler JQ, McSweeney TD. The PaCO2 rate of rise in anesthetized patients with airway obstruction. *J Clin Anesth.* 1989;1(5):328–332.
45. Wright FG Jr, Foley MF, Downs JB, et al. Hypoxemia and hypocarbia following intermittent positive-pressure breathing. *Anesth Analg.* 1976;55(4):555–559.
46. Fink BR. The stimulant effect of wakefulness on respiration: Clinical aspects. *Br J Anaesth.* 1961;33:97–101.
47. Berger AJ, Mitchell RA, Severinghaus JW. Regulation of respiration (third of three parts). *N Engl J Med.* 1977;297(4):194–201.
48. West JB, Dollery CT, Naimark A. Distribution of blood flow in isolated lung; relation to vascular and alveolar pressures. *J Appl Physiol.* 1964;19:713–724.
49. West JB, Dollery CT. Distribution of blood flow and the pressure-flow relations of the whole lung. *J Appl Physiol.* 1965;20:175.
50. Gattinoni L, Pesenti A, Avalli L, et al. Pressure-volume curve of total respiratory system in acute respiratory-failure. Computed tomographic scan study. *Am Rev Respir Dis.* 1987;136(3):730–736.
51. Benumof JP, Pirlo AF, Johanson I, et al. Interaction of PVO2 with PAO2 on hypoxic pulmonary vasoconstriction. *J Appl Physiol.* 1981;51:871–874.
52. Swenson EW, Finley TN , Guzman SV . Unilateral hypoventilation in man during temporary occlusion of one pulmonary artery. *J Clin Invest.* 1961;40(5):828–835.
53. Yamanaka MK, Sue DY. Comparison of arterial-end-tidal PCO2 difference and dead space/tidal volume ratio in respiratory failure. *Chest.* 1987;92:832–835.
54. Tyburski JG, Collinge JD, Wilson RF, et al. End-tidal CO2-derived values during emergency trauma surgery correlated with outcome: A prospective study. *J Trauma.* 2002;53(4):738–743.
55. Huffmyer JL, Nemergut EC. Respiratory dysfunction and pulmonary disease in cirrhosis and other hepatic disorders. *Respir Care.* 2007;52(8):1030–1036.
56. Gaines DI, Fallon MB. Hepatopulmonary syndrome. *Liver Int.* 2004;24(5): 397–401.
57. Räsänen JD, Downs JB, Malec DJ, et al. Oxygen tensions and oxyhemoglobin saturations in the assessment of pulmonary gas exchange. *Crit Care Med.* 1987; 15:1058–1061.
58. Cruickshank S, Hirschauer N. The alveolar gas equation. *Contin Educ Anaesth Crit Care Pain.* 2004;4(1):24–27.
59. Christie RV. Lung volume and its subdivisions: I. Methods of measurement. *J Clin Invest.* 1932;11:1099–1118.
60. Tisi GM. Preoperative evaluation of pulmonary function. Validity, indications, and benefits. *Am Rev Respir Dis.* 1979;119(2):293–310.
61. Apthorp GH, Marshall R. Pulmonary diffusing capacity: A comparison of breath-holding and steady state methods using carbon monoxide. *J Clin Invest.* 1961;40:1775–1784.
62. Crapo RO. Pulmonary function testing—Reply. *N Engl J Med.* 1994;331(19): 1314–1314.
63. American Thoracic Society. Lung function testing: Selection of reference values and interpretive strategies. *Am Rev Respir Dis.* 1991;144:1202–1218.
64. Kearney DJ, Lee TH, Reilly JJ, et al. Assessment of operative risk in patients undergoing lung resection. Importance of predicted pulmonary function. *Chest.* 1994;105(3):753–759.
65. Ferguson MK. Preoperative assessment of pulmonary risk. *Chest.* 1999;115(5): 58S–63S.
66. Bapoje SR, Whitaker WJ, Schulz T, et al. Preoperative evaluation of the patient with pulmonary disease. *Chest.* 2007;132:1637–1645.
67. Practice advisory for preanesthesia evaluation: A report by the American Society of Anesthesiologists Task Force on Preanesthesia Evaluation. *Anesthesiology.* 2002;96:485–496.

68. Zollinger A, Hofer CK, Pasch T. Preoperative pulmonary evaluation: Facts and myths. *Curr Opin Anaesth.* 2002;14:59–63.
69. McAlister FA, Khan NA, Strauss SE, et al. Accuracy of the preoperative assessment in predicting pulmonary risk after nonthoracic surgery. *Am J Respir Crit Care Med.* 2003;167:741–744.
70. Pietak S, Weenig CS, Hickey R, et al. Anesthetic effects on ventilation in patients with chronic obstructive pulmonary disease. *Anesthesiology.* 1975;42(2):160–166.
71. Connors AF Jr, McCaffree DR, Gray BA. Effect of inspiratory flow rate on gas exchange during mechanical ventilation. *Am Rev Respir Dis.* 1981;124(5):537–543.
72. Tuxen DL, Lane S. The effects of ventilatory pattern on hyperinflation, airway pressures, and circulation in mechanical ventilation of patients with severe airflow obstruction. *Am Rev Respir Dis.* 1987;136:872–879.
73. Petersen GW, Baier H. Incidence of pulmonary barotrauma in a medical ICU. *Crit Care Med.* 1983;11(2):67–69.
74. Brisner BH, Hedenstierna G, Lundquist H, et al. Pulmonary densities during anesthesia with muscular relaxation: A proposal of atelectasis. *Anesthesiology.* 1985;62:422–428.
75. Don HF, Robson JG. The mechanics of the respiratory system during anesthesia. The effects of atropine and carbon dioxide. *Anesthesiology.* 1965;26:168–178.
76. Don HW, Wahba M, Cuadrado L, et al. The effects of anesthesia and 100 percent oxygen on the functional residual capacity of the lungs. *Anesthesiology.* 1970; 32:521–529.
77. Westbrook PR, Stubbs SE, Sessler AD, et al. Effects of anesthesia and muscle paralysis on respiratory mechanics in normal man. *J Appl Physiol.* 1973;34(1):81–86.
78. Wyche MQ Jr, Teichner RL, Kallos T, et al. Effects of continuous positive-pressure breathing on functional residual capacity and arterial oxygenation during intra-abdominal operation: Studies in man during nitrous oxide and d-tubocurarine anesthesia. *Anesthesiology.* 1973;38:68–74.
79. Rose DM, Downs JB, Heenan TJ. Temporal responses of functional residual capacity and oxygen tension to changes in positive end-expiratory pressure. *Crit Care Med.* 1981;9(2):79–82.
80. Craig DB. Postoperative recovery of pulmonary function. *Anesth Analg.* 1981;60 (1):46–52.
81. Diamond L, Lai YL. Augmentation of elastase-induced emphysema by cigarette smoke: Effects of reducing tar and nicotine content. *J Toxicol Environ Health.* 1987;20(3):287–301.
82. deShazo RD, Banks DE, Diem JE, et al. Bronchoalveolar lavage cell–lymphocyte interactions in normal nonsmokers and smokers. Analysis with a novel system. *Am Rev Respir Dis.* 1983;127:545–548.
83. Hogg JC. The effect of smoking on airway permeability. *Chest.* 1983;83(1):1–2.
84. Clements JA. Smoking and pulmonary surfactant. *N Engl J Med.* 1972;286(5): 261–262.
85. Lee L-Y, Gerhardstein DC, Wang AL, et al. Nicotine is responsible for airway irritation evoked by cigarette smoke inhalation in men. *J Appl Physiol.* 1993;75: 1955–1961.
86. Warner MA, Divertie MB, Tinker JH. Preoperative cessation of smoking and pulmonary complications in coronary artery bypass patients. *Anesthesiology.* 1984;60(4):380–383.
87. Bluman LG, Mosca L, Newman N, et al. Preoperative smoking habits and postoperative pulmonary complications. *Chest.* 1998;113(4):883–889.
88. Chalon J, Tayyab MA, Ramanathan S. Cytology of respiratory epithelium as a predictor of respiratory complications after operation. *Chest.* 1975;67(1):32–35.
89. Theadom A, Cropley M. Effects of preoperative smoking cessation on the incidence and risk of intraoperative and postoperative complications in adult smokers: A systematic review. *Tob control.* 2006;15:352–358.
90. Quraishi SA, Orkin OF, Roizen MF. The anesthesia preoperative assessment: An opportunity for smoking cessation intervention. *J Clin Anesth.* 2006;18:635–640.
91. Warner MA, Offord KP, Warner ME, et al. Role of preoperative cessation of smoking and other factors in postoperative pulmonary complications: A blinded prospective study of coronary artery bypass patients. *Mayo Clin Proc.* 1989;64(6):609–616.
92. Beckers S, Camu F. The anesthetic risk of tobacco smoking. *Acta Anaesthesiol Belg.* 1991;42(1):45–56.
93. Hurt RD, Sachs DP, Glover ED, et al. A comparison of sustained-release bupropion and placebo for smoking cessation. *N Engl J Med.* 1997;337(17):1195–1202.
94. Fiore MC. US public health service clinical practice guideline: Treating tobacco use and dependence. *Respir Care.* 2000;45(10):1200–1262.
95. Gonzales D, Rennard SI, Nides M, et al. Varenicline, an alpha4beta2 nicotinic acetylcholine receptor partial agonist, vs sustained-release bupropion and placebo for smoking cessation: A randomized controlled trial. *JAMA.* 2006;296(1):47–55.
96. Benowitz NL, Jacob P 3rd, Kozlowski LT, et al. Influence of smoking fewer cigarettes on exposure to tar, nicotine, and carbon monoxide. *N Engl J Med.* 1986;315(21):1310–1313.
97. Liu SS, Wu CL. Effect of postoperative analgesia on major postoperative complications: a systematic update of the evidence. *Anesth Analg.* 2007;104: 689–702.
98. Gust R, Pecher S, Gust A, et al. Effect of patient-controlled analgesia on pulmonary complications after coronary artery bypass grafting. *Crit Care Med.* 1999;27 (10):2218–2223.
99. Stock MC, Downs JB, Gauer PK, et al. Prevention of postoperative pulmonary complications with CPAP, incentive spirometry, and conservative therapy. *Chest.* 1985;87(2):151–157.
100. Lyager SW, Wernberg M, Rajani N, et al. Can postoperative pulmonary complications be improved by treatment with Bartlett-Edwards incentive spirometer after upper abdominal surgery?. *Acta Anaesthesiol Scand.* 1979;23:312–319.
101. Stock MC, Downs JB, Cooper RB, et al. Comparison of continuous positive airway pressure, incentive spirometry, and conservative therapy after cardiac operations. *Crit Care Med.* 1984;12(11):969–972.
102. Smentana GW, Lawrence VA, Cornell JE. Preoperative pulmonary risk stratification for noncardiothoracic surgery: Systematic review for the American College of Physicians. *Ann Intern Med.* 2006;144:581.
103. Chumillas S, Ponce JL, Delgado F, et al. Prevention of postoperative pulmonary complications through respiratory rehabilitation: A controlled clinical study. *Arch Phys Med Rehabil.* 1998;79(1):5–9.
104. Brooks-Brunn JA. Validation of a predictive model for postoperative pulmonary complications. *Heart Lung.* 1998;27(3):151–158.
105. Gracey DR, Divertie MB, Didier EP. Preoperative pulmonary preparation of patients with chronic obstructive pulmonary disease: A prospective study. *Chest.* 1979;76(2):123–129.
106. Petty TL, Brink GA, Miller MW, et al. Objective functional improvement in chronic airway obstruction. *Chest.* 1970;57(3):216–223.

CHAPTER

12 The Allergic Response

JERROLD H. LEVY

Key Points

1. Anesthesiologists routinely manage patients during their perioperative medical care where they are exposed to multiple agents that can produce an allergic response including drugs (antibiotics, anesthetic agents, neuromuscular blocking agents [NMBAs], sedative-hypnotics), polypeptides (i.e., protamine), blood products, and environmental antigens (i.e., latex).
2. Antibodies are specific proteins called immunoglobulins that can recognize and bind to a specific antigen, and usually IgE or IgG is implicated.
3. Cytokines are inflammatory cell activators that are synthesized to act as secondary messengers and activate endothelial cells and white cells.
4. Immune competence during surgery can be affected by direct and hormonal effects of anesthetic drugs, by immunologic effects of other drugs used, by the surgery, by coincident infection, and by transfused blood products.
5. Most of the allergic reactions evoked by intravenous drugs occur within 5 minutes of administration. In the anesthetized patient, the most common life-threatening manifestation of an allergic reaction is circulatory collapse, reflecting vasodilation with resulting decreased venous return.
6. Many diverse molecules administered during the perioperative period release histamine in a dose-dependent, nonimmunologic fashion.
7. A plan for treating anaphylactic reactions must be established before the event. Airway maintenance, 100% oxygen administration, intravascular volume expansion, and epinephrine are essential to treat the hypotension and hypoxia that result from vasodilation, increased capillary permeability, and bronchospasm. Vasopressin and additional diagnostic monitoring should be considered for refractory shock.
8. After an anaphylactic reaction, it is important to attempt to identify the causative agent to prevent readministration.
9. Health-care workers and children with spina bifida, urogenital abnormalities, or certain food allergies have been recognized as people at increased risk for anaphylaxis to latex.
10. NMBAs have several unique molecular features that make them potential antigens.

Multimedia

 Type 3 Immune Complex Reaction

 Anaphylaxis

ANATOMY AND PHYSIOLOGY

INTRODUCTION

1 Allergic reactions represent an important cause of perioperative complications. Anesthesiologists routinely administer multiple drugs and blood products and manage patients during their perioperative medical care where they are exposed to multiple agents including drugs (i.e., antibiotics, anesthetic agents, neuromuscular blocking agents [NMBAs], sedative-hypnotics), polypeptides (protamine, aprotinin), blood products, and environmental antigens (i.e., latex). Anesthesiologists must be able to rapidly recognize and treat anaphylaxis, the most life-threatening form of an allergic reaction.[1]

The allergic response represents just one aspect of the pathologic response that the immune system evolved to recognize foreign substances. As part of normal host surveillance mechanisms, a series of cellular and humoral elements oversees foreign surfaces of cell surfaces and molecular structures called *antigens* to provide host defense. These foreign substances (antigens) consist of molecular arrangements found on cells, bacteria, viruses, proteins, or complex macromolecules.[2,3] Immunologic mechanisms (1) involve antigen interaction with antibodies or specific effector cells; (2) are reproducible; and (3) are specific and adaptive, distinguishing foreign substances and amplifying reactivity through a series of inflammatory cells and proteins. The immune system serves to protect the body against external microorganisms and toxins, as well as internal threats from neoplastic cells; however, it can respond inappropriately to cause hypersensitive (allergic) reactions. Life-threatening allergic reactions to drugs and other foreign substances observed perioperatively may represent different expressions of the immune response.[2,3]

BASIC IMMUNOLOGIC PRINCIPLES

The immune system protects the body from invasion by organisms by recognizing and removing foreign substances called *antigens* that are molecular structures, usually proteins and/or carbohydrates. However, the body also has mechanisms to tolerate similar molecular configurations of the host (self-tolerance); however, problems arise when the immune system is dysfunctional as in cases of autoimmunity that can give rise to serious diseases including rheumatoid arthritis and lupus. The immune response includes both cell-mediated immunity and humoral immunity. Cell-mediated immunity involves immune cell directed at elimination or destruction of pathogens or cells. Humoral immunity comprises different antibodies and proteins such as complement that can directly or in concert with cellular immunity orchestrate cell injury and destruction. The purpose is to provide host defense mechanisms.

As part of humoral immune responses, protein mediators called cytokines and chemokines are released initially by inflammatory responses to bring other immune cells to the site of the injury or infection, and cause further inflammatory responses and fever, and to increase capillary permeability to allow other immune cells to migrate and translocate to the site of injury. This inflammatory response also causes hemostatic activation and produces pain, erythema, and edema locally and potentially systemically depending on the extent of the injury. Cytokines have an extensive spectrum of inflammatory effects, an issue studied more extensively in sepsis.[4] The immune response can be variable in onset from immediate in anaphylaxis, to days, and can remember antigens for many years, especially following immunization.

TABLE 12-1. AGENTS ADMINISTERED DURING ANESTHESIA THAT ACT AS ANTIGENS

Haptens	Macromolecules
Penicillin and its derivatives	Aprotinin Blood products
Anesthetic drugs	Chymopapain Colloid volume expanders Neuromuscular blocking agents Protamine Latex

Although this is a simplified review of the immune system, it is important to consider individual aspects of the immune response and their importance below.

Antigens

As mentioned, molecules stimulating an immune response (antibody production or lymphocyte stimulation) are called *antigens.*[5,6] Only a few drugs used by anesthesiologists, such as polypeptides (protamine) and other large macromolecules (dextrans), are complete antigens (Table 12-1). Most commonly used drugs are simple organic compounds of low molecular weight (around 1,000 Da). For such a small molecule to become immunogenic, it must form a stable bond with circulating proteins or tissue micromolecules to result in an antigen (hapten-macromolecular complex). Small molecular weight substances such as drugs or drug metabolites that bind to host proteins or cell membranes to sensitize patients are called *haptens.* Haptens are not antigenic by themselves. Often, a reactive drug metabolite (i.e., penicilloyl derivative of penicillin) is believed to bind with macromolecules to become antigens, but for most drugs this has not been proved. Some molecular structures in bacteria or fungi are immediately recognized as foreign.

Thymus-derived (T-cell) and Bursa-derived (B-cell) Lymphocytes

The thymus of the fetus differentiates immature lymphocytes into thymus-derived cells (T cells). T cells have receptors that are activated by binding with foreign antigens and secrete mediators that regulate the immune response. The subpopulations of T cells that exist in humans include helper, suppressor, cytotoxic, and killer cells.[5,6] The two types of regulatory T cells are helper cells (OKT4) and suppressor cells (OKT8). Helper cells are important for key effector cell responses, whereas suppressor cells inhibit immune function. Infection of helper T cells with a retrovirus, the human immunodeficiency virus, produces a specific increase in the number of suppressor cells. Cytotoxic T cells destroy mycobacteria, fungi, and viruses. Other lymphocytes, called natural killer cells, do not need specific antigen stimulation to set up their role. Both the cytotoxic T cells and natural killer cells take part in defense against tumor cells and in transplant rejection. T cells produce mediators that influence the response

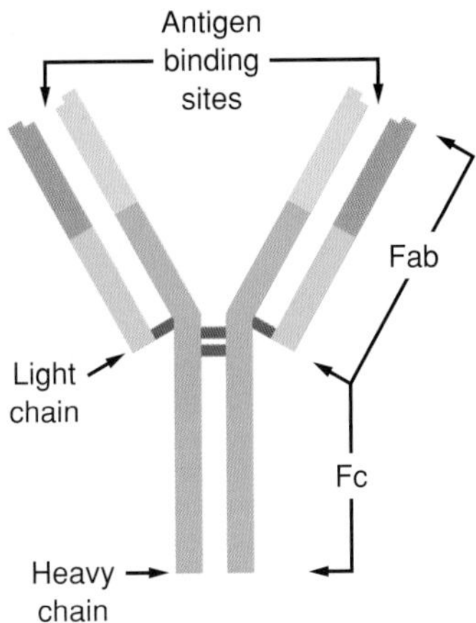

FIGURE 12-1. Basic structural configuration of the antibody molecule representing human immunoglobulin G (IgG). Immunoglobulins are composed of two heavy chains and two light chains bound by disulfide linkages (represented by *crossbars*). Papain cleaves the molecule into two Fab fragments and one Fc fragment. Antigen binding occurs on the Fab fragments, whereas the Fc segment is responsible for membrane binding or complement activation. (Reprinted with permission from: Levy JH. *Anaphylactic Reactions in Anesthesia and Intensive Care.* 2nd ed. Boston, MA: Butterworth-Heinemann; 1992.)

of other cell types involved in the recognition and destruction of foreign substances.[5,6]

B cells represent a specific lymphocyte cell line that can differentiate into specific plasma cells that synthesize antibodies, a step controlled by both helper and suppressor T-cell lymphocytes. B cells are also called bursa-derived cells because in birds, the bursa of Fabricius is important in producing cells responsible for antibody synthesis.

Antibodies

2 Antibodies are specific proteins called *immunoglobulins* (Igs) that can recognize and bind to a specific antigen. The basic structure of the antibody molecule is illustrated in Figure 12-1. Each antibody has at least two heavy chains and two light chains that are bound together by disulfide bonds. The Fab fragment has the ability to bind antigen, and the Fc, or crystallizable, fragment is responsible for the unique biologic properties of the different classes of Igs (cell binding and complement activation). Antibodies function as specific receptor molecules for immune cells and proteins. When antigen binds covalently to the Fab fragments, the antibody undergoes conformational changes to activate the Fc receptor. The results of antigen–antibody binding depend on the cell type, which causes a specific type of activation (i.e., lymphocyte proliferation and differentiation into antibody-secreting cells, mast cell degranulation, and complement activation).

Five major classes of antibodies occur in humans: IgG, IgA, IgM, IgD, and IgE. The heavy chain determines the structure and the function of each molecule. The basic properties of each antibody are listed in Table 12-2.

Effector Cells and Proteins of the Immune Response

Cells

Monocytes, neutrophils (polymorphonuclear leukocytes [PMNs]), and eosinophils represent important effector cells that migrate into areas of inflammation in response to specific chemotactic factors, including lymphokines, cytokines, and complement-derived mediators. The deposition of antibody or complement fragments on the surface of foreign cells is called *opsonization,* a process that promotes killing foreign cells by effector cells. In addition, lymphokines and cytokines produce chemotaxis of other inflammatory cells in a manner described in the following sections.[5,6] Activation of these cellular process is orchestrated by multiple mechanisms, as best recently reviewed.[7]

Monocytes and Macrophages

Macrophages regulate immune responses by processing and presenting antigens to effect inflammatory, tumoricidal, and microbicidal functions. Macrophages arise from circulating monocytes or may be confined to specific organs such as the lung. They are recruited and activated in response to microorganisms or tissue injury. Macrophages ingest antigens before they interact with receptors on the lymphocyte surface to regulate their action.

TABLE 12-2. BIOLOGIC CHARACTERISTICS OF IMMUNOGLOBULINS

	IgG	IgM	IgA	IgE	IgD
Heavy chain	γ	μ	α	ε	δ
Molecular weight	160,000	900,000	170,000	188,000	184,000
Subclasses	1, 2, 3, 4	1, 2	1, 2		
Serum concentration (mg/dL)	6–14	0.5–1.5	1–3	$<-0.5 \times 10^3$	<0.1
Complement activation	All but IgG_4	+	–	–	–
Placental transfer	+	–	–	–	–
Serum half-life (days)	23	5	6	1–5	2–8
Cell binding	Mast cells (IgG_4) Neutrophils Lymphocytes Mononuclear cells Platelets	Lymphocytes		Mast cells Basophils	Neutrophils Lymphocytes

Modified with permission from: Levy JH. *Anaphylactic Reactions in Anesthesia and Intensive Care.* 2nd ed. Boston, MA: Butterworth-Heinemann; 1992.

Macrophages synthesize mediators to facilitate both B-lymphocyte and T-lymphocyte responses.

Polymorphonuclear Leukocytes (Neutrophils)

The first cells to appear in acute inflammatory reaction are neutrophils that contain acid hydrolases, neutral proteases, and lysosomes. Once activated, they produce hydroxyl radicals, superoxide, and hydrogen peroxide, which aid in microbial killing.

Eosinophils

The exact function of the eosinophil in host defense is unclear; however, inflammatory cells recruit eosinophils to collect at sites of parasitic infections, tumors, and allergic reactions.

Basophils

Basophils comprise 0.5% to 1% of circulating granulocytes in the blood. On the surface of basophils are IgE receptors, which function similarly to those on mast cells.

Mast Cells

Mast cells are important cells for immediate hypersensitivity responses. They are tissue fixed and located in the perivascular spaces of the skin, lung, and intestine. On the surface of mast cells are IgE receptors, which bind to specific antigens. Once activated, these cells release physiologically active mediators important to immediate hypersensitivity responses (see IgE-mediated Pathophysiology section under Anaphylactic Reactions). Mast cells can be activated by a series of both immune and nonimmune stimuli.

Proteins

Cytokines/Interleukins

3 Cytokines are inflammatory cell activators that are synthesized by macrophages to act as secondary messengers and activate endothelial cells and white cells.[8] Interleukin-1 and tumor necrosis factor are examples of cytokines considered to be important mediators of the biologic responses to infection and other inflammatory reactions. Liberation of interleukin-1 and tumor necrosis factor produces fever, neuropeptide release, endothelial cell activation, increased adhesion molecule expression, neutrophil priming, hypotension, myocardial suppression, and a catabolic state.[8] The term *interleukin* was coined for a group of cytokines that promotes communication between and among ("inter") leukocytes ("leukin"). Interleukins are a group of different regulatory proteins that act to control many aspects of the immune and inflammatory responses. The interleukins are polypeptides synthesized in response to cellular activation; they produce their inflammatory effects by activating specific receptors on inflammatory cells and vasculature. T-cell lymphocytes influence the activity of other immunologic and nonimmunologic cells by producing an array of interleukins that they secrete. Different interleukins of this class have been isolated and characterized; they function as short-range or intracellular soluble mediators of the immune and inflammatory responses. The interleukin family of cytokines has been rapidly growing in number because of advances in gene cloning.

Complement

The primary humoral response to antigen and antibody binding is activation of the complement system.[9,10] The complement system consists of around 20 different proteins that bind to activated antibodies, other complement proteins, and cell membranes. The complement system is an important effector system of inflammation. Complement activation can be initiated by IgG or IgM binding to antigen, by plasmin through the classic pathway, by endotoxin, or by drugs through the alternate (properdin) pathway (Fig. 12-2). Specific fragments released during complement activation include C3a, C4a, and C5a, which have important humoral and chemotactic properties (see Non-IgE–mediated Reactions section). The major function of the complement system is to recognize bacteria both directly and indirectly by attracting phagocytes (chemotaxis), as well as the increased adhesion of phagocytes to antigens (opsonization), and cell lysis by activation of the complete cascade.[9,10]

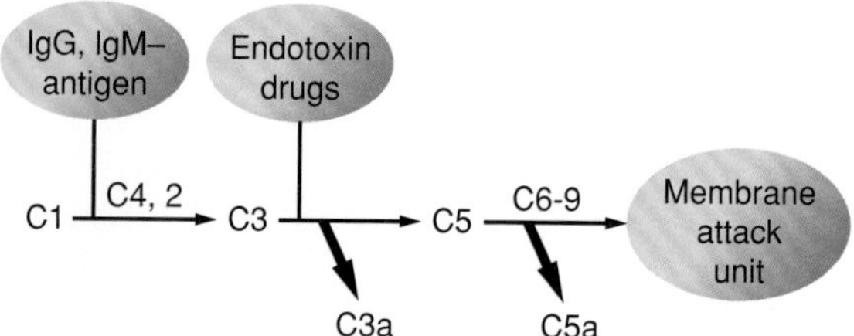

FIGURE 12-2. Diagram of complement activation. Complement system can be activated by either the classic pathway (IgG, IgM–antigen interaction) or the alternate pathway (endotoxin, drug interaction). Small peptide fragments of C3 and C5 called anaphylatoxins (C3a, C5a) that are released during activation are potent vasoactive mediators. Formation of the complete complement cascade produces a membrane attack unit that lyses cell walls and membranes. An inhibitor of the complement cascade, the C1 esterase inhibitor, ensures the complement system is turned off most of the time.

A series of inhibitors regulates activation to ensure regulation of the complement system. Hereditary (autosomal dominant) or acquired (associated with lymphoma, lymphosarcoma, chronic lymphatic leukemia, and macroglobulinemia) angioneurotic edema is an example of a deficiency in an inhibitor of the C1 complement system (C1 esterase deficiency). This syndrome is characterized by recurrent increased vascular permeability of specific subcutaneous and serosal tissues (angioedema), which produces laryngeal obstruction and respiratory and cardiovascular abnormalities after tissue trauma and surgery, or even without any obvious precipitating factor.[11] One of the important pathologic manifestations of complement activation is acute pulmonary vasoconstriction associated with protamine administration.[1]

Effects of Anesthesia on Immune Function

Anesthesia and surgery depress nonspecific host resistance mechanisms, including lymphocyte activation and phagocytosis.[12]
4 Immune competence during surgery can be affected by direct and hormonal effects of anesthetic drugs, by immunologic effects of other drugs used, by the surgery, by coincident infections, and by transfused blood products. Blood represents a complex of humoral and cellular elements that may alter immunomodulation to various antigens. Although multiple studies demonstrate in vitro changes of immune function, no studies have ever proved their importance.[12] Besides, such changes are likely of minor importance compared with the hormonal aspects of stress responses.

HYPERSENSITIVITY RESPONSES (ALLERGY)

Gell and Coombs first described a scheme for classifying immune responses to understand specific diseases mediated by immunologic processes. The immune pathway functions as a protective mechanism, but can also react inappropriately to produce a hypersensitivity or allergic response. They defined four basic types of hypersensitivity, types I to IV. It is useful first to review all four mechanisms to understand the different immune reactions that occur in humans.

Type I Reactions

Type I reactions are anaphylactic or immediate-type hypersensitivity reactions (Fig. 12-3). Physiologically active mediators are released from mast cells and basophils after antigen binding to IgE antibodies on the membranes of these cells. Type I hypersensitivity reactions include anaphylaxis, extrinsic asthma, and allergic rhinitis.

Type II Reactions

Type II reactions are also known as antibody-dependent cell-mediated cytotoxic hypersensitivity or cytotoxic reactions (antibody-dependent cell-mediated cytotoxic) (Fig. 12-4). These reactions are mediated by either IgG or IgM antibodies directed against antigens on the surface of foreign cells. These antigens may be either integral cell membrane components (A or B blood group antigens in ABO incompatibility reactions) or haptens that absorb to the surface of a cell, stimulating the production of antihapten antibodies (autoimmune hemolytic anemia). The cell damage in type II reactions is produced by (1) direct cell lysis after complete complement cascade activation, (2) increased phagocytosis by macrophages, or (3) killer T-cell lymphocytes producing antibody-dependent cell-mediated cytotoxic effects. Examples of type II reactions in humans are ABO-incompatible transfusion reactions, drug-induced immune hemolytic anemia, and heparin-induced thrombocytopenia.

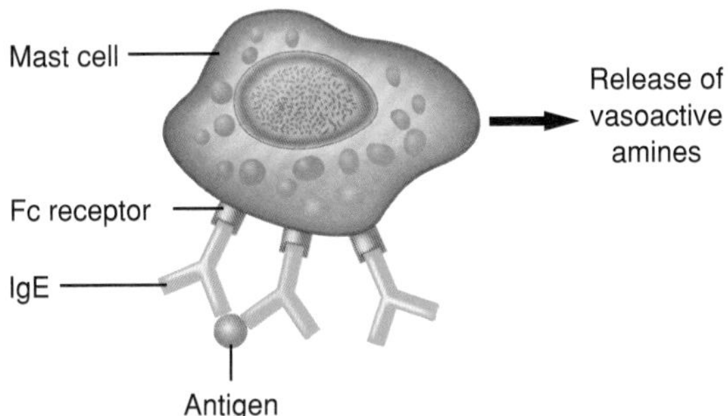

FIGURE 12-3. Type I immediate hypersensitivity reactions (anaphylaxis) involve IgE antibodies binding to mast cells or basophils by way of their Fc receptors. On encountering immunospecific antigens, the IgE becomes cross-linked, inducing degranulation, intracellular activation, and release of mediators. This reaction is independent of complement.

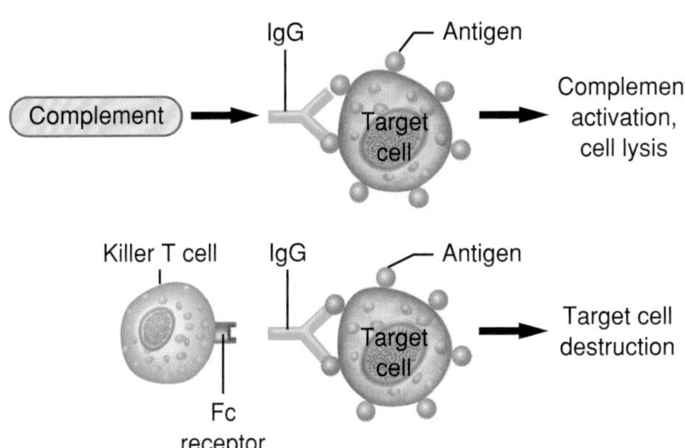

FIGURE 12-4. Type II or cytotoxic reactions. Antibody of an IgG or IgM class is directed against antigens on an individual's own cells (target cells). The antigens may be integral membrane components or foreign molecules that have been absorbed. This may lead to complement activation, including cell lysis (*upper figure*) or cytotoxic action by killer T-cell lymphocytes (*lower figure*).

Type III Reactions (Immune Complex Reactions)

Type III reactions result from circulating soluble antigens and antibodies that bind to form insoluble complexes that deposit in the microvasculature (Fig. 12-5). Complement is activated, and neutrophils are localized to the site of complement deposition to produce tissue damage. Type III reactions include classic serum sickness observed after snake antisera or antithymocyte globulin, and immune complex vascular injury, and may occur through mechanisms of protamine-mediated pulmonary vasoconstriction.[1]

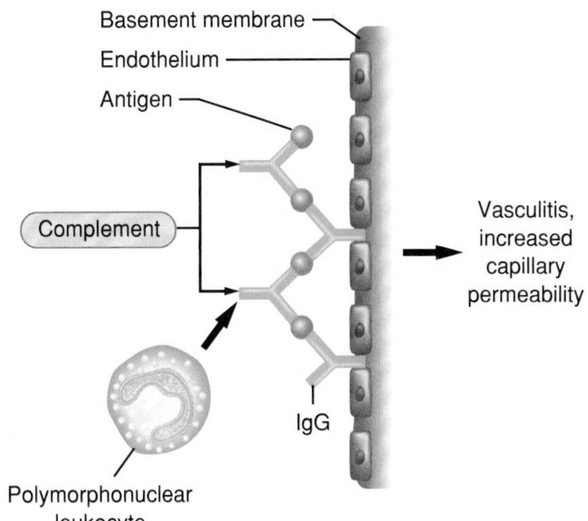

FIGURE 12-5. Type III immune complex reactions. Antibodies of an IgG or IgM type bind to the antigen in the soluble base and are subsequently deposited in the microvasculature. Complement is activated, resulting in chemotaxis and activation of polymorphonuclear leukocytes at the site of antigen–antibody complexes and subsequent tissue injury.

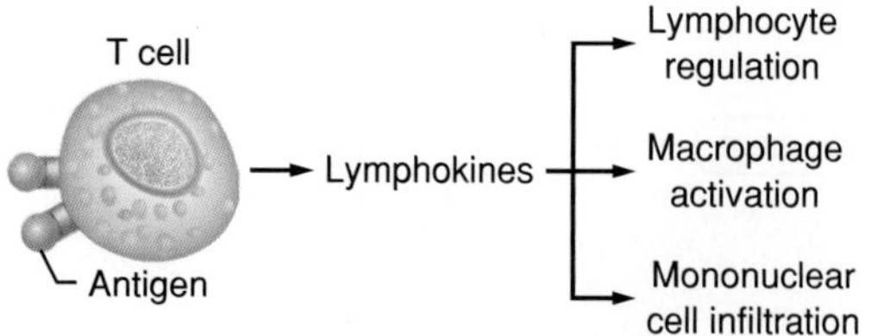

FIGURE 12-6. Type IV immune complex reactions (delayed hypersensitivity or cell-mediated immunity). Antigen binds to sensitized T-cell lymphocytes to release lymphokines after a second contact with the same antigen. This reaction is independent of circulating antibody or complement activation. Lymphokines induce inflammatory reactions and activate, as well as attract, macrophages and other mononuclear cells to produce delayed tissue injury.

Type IV Reactions (Delayed Hypersensitivity Reactions)

Type IV reactions result from the interactions of sensitized lymphocytes with specific antigens (Fig. 12-6). Delayed hypersensitivity reactions are mainly mononuclear, manifest in 18 to 24 hours, peak at 40 to 80 hours, and disappear in 72 to 96 hours. Antigen–lymphocyte binding produces lymphokine synthesis, lymphocyte proliferation, and generation of cytotoxic T cells, and attracting macrophages and other inflammatory cells. Cytotoxic T cells are produced specifically to kill target cells that bear antigens identical with those that triggered the reaction. This form of immunity is important in tissue rejection, graft-versus-host reactions, contact dermatitis (e.g., poison ivy), and tuberculin immunity.

Intraoperative Allergic Reactions

Understanding perioperative anaphylaxis is important because of the potential for morbidity and mortality.[13] However, most estimates of the incidence are based on retrospective data, which may account for variability in the incidence. The risk of perioperative anaphylaxis is reported as between 1:3,500 and 1:20,000, with a mortality rate of 4% and an additional 2% surviving with
5 severe brain damage.[13,14] More than 90% of the allergic reactions evoked by intravenous drugs occur within 5 minutes of administration. In the anesthetized patient, the most common life-threatening manifestation of an allergic reaction is circulatory collapse, reflecting vasodilation with resulting decreased venous return (Table 12-3). The only manifestation of an allergic reaction may be refractory hypotension. Portier and Richet first used the word *anaphylaxis* (from *ana,* "against," and *prophylaxis,* "protection") to describe the profound shock and resulting death that sometimes occurred in dogs immediately after a second challenge with a foreign antigen.[15] When life-threatening allergic reactions mediated by antibodies occur, they are defined as anaphylactic. Although the term *anaphylactoid* has been used in the past to describe nonimmunologic reactions, this term is now rarely used.

ANAPHYLACTIC REACTIONS

IgE-mediated Pathophysiology

Antigen binding to IgE antibodies initiates anaphylaxis (Fig. 12-7). Prior exposure to the antigen or to a substance of similar structure is needed to produce sensitization, although an allergic history

TABLE 12-3. RECOGNITION OF ANAPHYLAXIS DURING REGIONAL AND GENERAL ANESTHESIA

Systems	Symptoms	Signs
Respiratory	Dyspnea Chest discomfort	Coughing Wheezing Sneezing Laryngeal edema Decreased pulmonary compliance Fulminant pulmonary edema Acute respiratory failure
Cardiovascular	Dizziness Malaise Retrosternal oppression	Disorientation Diaphoresis Loss of consciousness Hypotension Tachycardia Dysrhythmias Decreased systemic vascular resistance Cardiac arrest Pulmonary hypertension
Cutaneous	Itching Burning Tingling	Urticaria (hives) Flushing Periorbital edema Perioral edema

Reprinted with permission from: Levy JH. *Anaphylactic Reactions in Anesthesia and Intensive Care.* 2nd ed. Boston, MA: Butterworth-Heinemann; 1992.

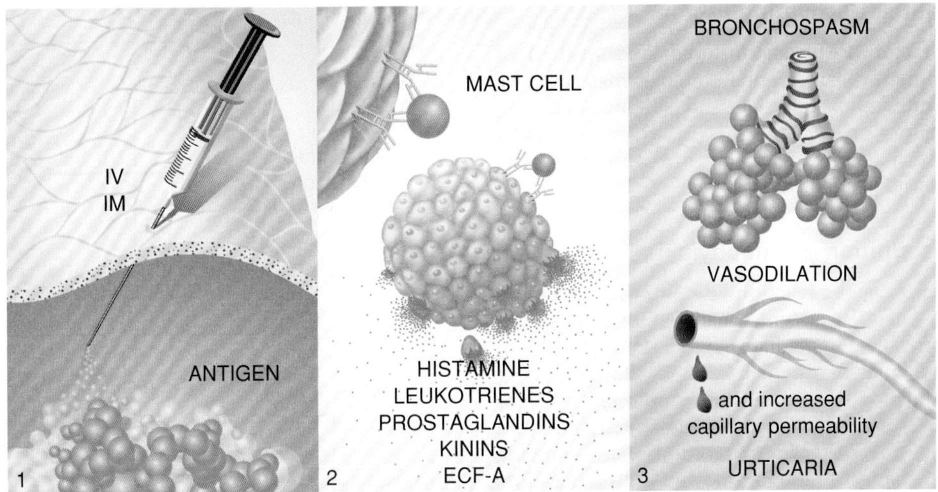

FIGURE 12-7. During anaphylaxis (type I immediate hypersensitivity reaction), (1) antigen enters a patient during anesthesia through a parenteral route. (2) It bridges two IgE antibodies on the surface of mast cells or basophils. In a calcium-dependent and energy-dependent process, cells release various substances—histamine, eosinophilic chemotactic factor of anaphylaxis, leukotrienes, prostaglandins, and kinins. (3) These released mediators produce the characteristic effects in the pulmonary, cardiovascular, and cutaneous systems. The most severe and life-threatening effects of the vasoactive mediators occur in the respiratory and cardiovascular systems. (Reprinted with permission from: Levy JH. *Identification and Treatment of Anaphylaxis: Mechanisms of Action and Strategies for Treatment Under General Anesthesia.* Chicago, IL: Smith Laboratories; 1983.)

may be unknown to the patient. On reexposure, binding of the antigen to bridge two immunospecific IgE antibodies found on the surfaces of mast cells and basophils releases stored mediators, including histamine, tryptase, and chemotactic factors.[13,16,17] Arachidonic acid metabolites (leukotrienes and prostaglandins), kinins, and cytokines are subsequently synthesized and released in response to cellular activation.[18] The released mediators produce a symptom complex of bronchospasm and upper airway edema in the respiratory system, vasodilation and increased capillary permeability in the cardiovascular system, and urticaria in the cutaneous system. Different mediators are released from mast cells and basophils after activation.

Chemical Mediators of Anaphylaxis

Histamine stimulates H_1, H_2, and H_3 receptors. H_1 receptor activation releases endothelium-derived relaxing factor (nitric oxide) from vascular endothelium, increases capillary permeability, and contracts airway and vascular smooth muscle.[16,19] H_2 receptor activation causes gastric secretion, inhibits mast cell activation, and contributes to vasodilation. When injected into skin, histamine produces the classic wheal (increased capillary permeability producing tissue edema) and flare (cutaneous vasodilation) response in humans.[20,21] Histamine undergoes rapid metabolism in humans by the enzymes histamine *N*-methyltransferase and diamine oxidase found in endothelial cells.

Peptide Mediators of Anaphylaxis

Factors are released from mast cells and basophils that cause granulocyte migration (chemotaxis) and collection at the site of the inflammatory stimulus.[17,18] Eosinophilic chemotactic factor of anaphylaxis (ECF-A) is a small molecular weight peptide chemotactic for eosinophils.[22] Although the exact role of ECF-A or the eosinophil in acute allergic response is unclear, eosinophils release enzymes that can inactivate histamine and leukotrienes.[18] In addition, a neutrophilic chemotactic factor is released that causes chemotaxis and activation.[18,23] Neutrophil activation may be responsible for recurrent manifestations of anaphylaxis.

Arachidonic Acid Metabolites

Leukotrienes and prostaglandins are both synthesized after mast cell activation from arachidonic acid metabolism of phospholipid cell membranes through either lipoxygenase or cyclooxygenase pathways.[22] The classic slow-reacting substance of anaphylaxis is a combination of leukotrienes C_4, D_4, and E_4. Leukotrienes produce bronchoconstriction (more intense than that produced by histamine), increased capillary permeability, vasodilation, coronary vasoconstriction, and myocardial depression.[24] Prostaglandins are potent mast cell mediators that produce vasodilation, bronchospasm, pulmonary hypertension, and increased capillary permeability. Prostaglandin D_2, the major metabolite of mast cells, produces bronchospasm and vasodilation. Elevated plasma levels of thromboxane B_2 (the metabolite of thromboxane A_2), also a prostaglandin synthesized by mast cells as well as by PMNs, have been demonstrated after protamine reactions associated with pulmonary hypertension.

Kinins

Small peptides called *kinins* are synthesized in mast cells and basophils to produce vasodilation, increased capillary permeability, and bronchoconstriction. Kinins can stimulate vascular endothelium to release vasoactive factors, including prostacyclin, and endothelial-derived relaxing factors such as nitric oxide.

Platelet-activating Factor

Platelet-activating factor (PAF), an unstored lipid synthesized in activated human mast cells, is a potent biologic material. PAF aggregates and activates human platelets, and perhaps leukocytes, to release inflammatory products. PAF levels were significantly higher in patients with anaphylaxis than controls and were correlated with the severity of anaphylaxis.[23]

Recognition of Anaphylaxis

The onset and severity of the reaction relate to the mediator's specific end-organ effects. Antigenic challenge in a sensitized individual usually produces immediate clinical manifestations of anaphylaxis, but the onset may be delayed 2 to 20 minutes.[24–27] The reaction may include some or all the symptoms and signs listed in Table 12-3. Individuals vary in their manifestations and course of anaphylaxis. A spectrum of reactions exists, ranging from minor clinical changes to the full-blown syndrome leading to death.[24,28] The enigma of anaphylaxis lies in the unpredictability of happening, the severity of the attack, and the lack of a prior allergic history.

Non-IgE–mediated Reactions

Other immunologic and nonimmunologic mechanisms release many of the mediators previously discussed independent of IgE, creating a clinical syndrome identical with anaphylaxis. Specific pathways important in producing the same clinical manifestations are considered later.

Complement Activation

Complement activation follows both immunologic (antibody mediated; i.e., classic pathway) or nonimmunologic (alternative) pathways to include a series of multimolecular, self-assembling proteins that release biologically active complement fragments of C3 and C5.[9,10] C3a and C5a are called *anaphylatoxins* because they release histamine from mast cells and basophils, contract smooth muscle, increase capillary permeability, and cause interleukin synthesis (Table 12-4). C5a interacts with specific high-affinity receptors on PMNs and platelets, causing leukocyte chemotaxis, aggregation, and activation.[9,10] Aggregated leukocytes embolize to various organs, producing microvascular occlusion and liberation of inflammatory products such as arachidonic acid metabolites, oxygen free radicals, and lysosomal enzymes (Fig. 12-8). Antibodies of the IgG class directed against antigenic determinants or granulocyte surfaces can also produce leukocyte aggregation.[29] These antibodies are called *leukoagglutinins.* Investigators have associated complement activation and PMN aggregation in producing the clinical expression of transfusion reactions, pulmonary vasoconstriction after protamine reactions, adult respiratory distress syndrome, and septic shock.[1]

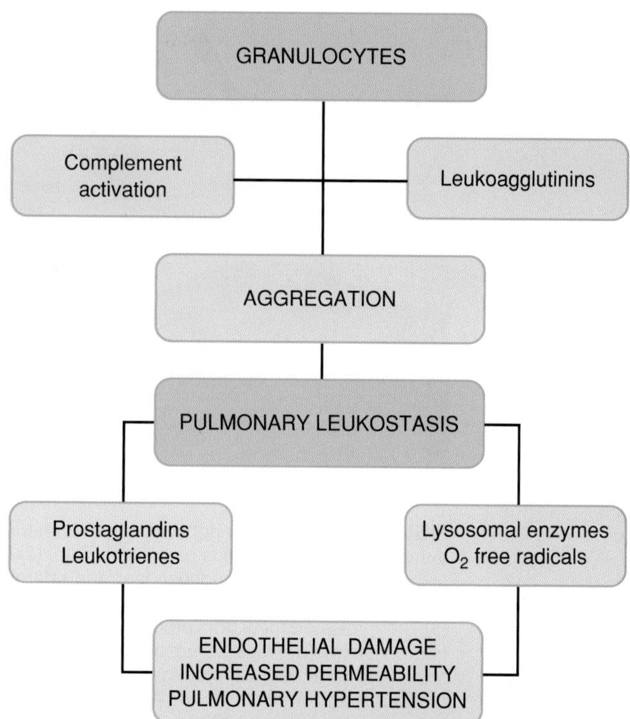

FIGURE 12-8. Sequence of events producing granulocyte aggregation, pulmonary leukostasis, and cardiopulmonary dysfunction. (Reprinted from: Levy JH. *Anaphylactic Reactions in Anesthesia and Intensive Care.* 2nd ed. Boston, MA: Butterworth-Heinemann; 1992.)

TABLE 12-4. BIOLOGIC EFFECTS OF ANAPHYLATOXINS

Biologic Effects	C3a	C5a
Histamine release	+	+
Smooth muscle contraction	+	+
Increased vascular permeability	+	+
Chemotaxis		+
Leukocyte and platelet aggregation		+
Interleukin release	+	+

Angioedema can also occur from complement deficiency states as well allergic reactions.[11] A syndrome called hereditary angioedema (HAE) can present with life-threatening episodes of edema of airway and gastrointestinal areas resulting in intensive care unit admission. Several variants of HAE exist that occur due to unopposed activation of multiple kinins and mediators including kallikrein and bradykinin causing increased vascular permeability and edema.[11] Older treatment was anabolic steroids and antifibrinolytics. In Europe, C1 esterase inhibitor (C1-INH) concentrates have been used since 1974 for both preventing and terminating attacks and are currently licensed in the United States for use in HAE patients, one for prophylaxis (Cinryze, ViroPharma, administered every 3 or 4 days for routine prophylaxis against angioedema attacks in HAE patients) and the other for treating acute abdominal and facial HAE attacks (Berinert P, CSL Behring).[11] The first kinin pathway modulator, ecallantide (Kalbitor, Dyax), has also been licensed recently in the United States for treating HAE attacks.[11]

Nonimmunologic Release of Histamine

6 Many diverse molecules administered during the perioperative period release histamine in a dose-dependent, nonimmunologic fashion (Table 12-5 and Fig. 12-9).[1] The mechanisms involved in nonimmunologic histamine release are not well understood, but represent selective mast cell and not basophil activation

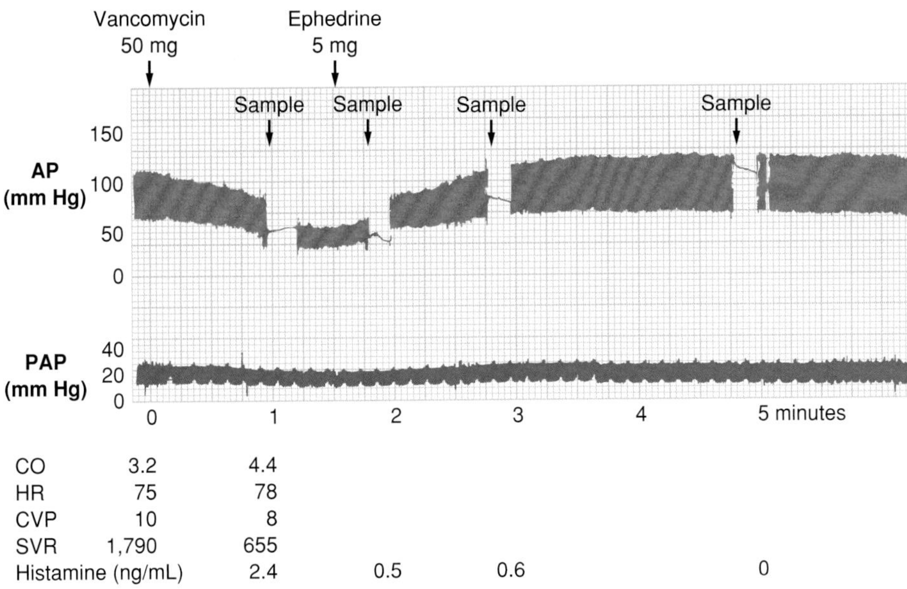

FIGURE 12-9. Example of an anaphylactic reaction after rapid vancomycin administration in a patient. Hypotension is associated with an increased cardiac output and decreased calculated systemic vascular resistance. Plasma histamine levels 1 minute after vancomycin administration were 2.4 ng/mL and subsequently decreased to zero. The patient was given ephedrine 5 mg, and blood pressure returned to baseline values. AP=arterial pressure, PAP=pulmonary artery pressure, CO=cardiac output, HR=heart rate, CVP=central venous pressure, SVR=systemic vascular resistance. (Reprinted from: Levy JH, Kettlekamp N, Goertz P, et al. Histamine release by vancomycin: A mechanism for hypotension in man. *Anesthesiology.* 1987;67:122.)

(Fig. 12-10).[30,31] Human cutaneous mast cells are the only cell population that releases histamine in response to both drugs and endogenous stimuli (neuropeptides). Nonimmunologic histamine release may involve mast cell activation through specific cell-signaling activation (Fig. 12-11). Different molecular structures release histamine in humans, which suggests that different mechanisms are involved. Histamine release is not dependent on the μ-receptor because fentanyl and sufentanil, the most potent μ-receptor agonists clinically available, do not release histamine in human skin.[32] Although the newer muscle relaxants may be more potent at the neuromuscular junction, drugs that are mast cell degranulators are equally capable of releasing histamine.[33] On an equimolar basis, atracurium is as potent as *d*-tubocurarine or metocurine in its ability to degranulate mast cells.[33] Newer aminosteroidal agents such as rocuronium and rapacuronium at clinically recommended doses have minimal effects on histamine release.[34,35]

Antihistamine pretreatment before administration of drugs that are known to release histamine in humans does not inhibit histamine release; rather, the antihistamines compete with histamine at the receptor and may attenuate decreases in systemic vascular resistance.[1] However, the effect of any drug on systemic vascular resistance may depend on other factors in addition to histamine release.

TABLE 12-5. DRUGS CAPABLE OF NONIMMUNOLOGIC HISTAMINE RELEASE

Antibiotics (vancomycin, pentamidine)
Basic compounds
Hyperosmotic agents
Muscle relaxants (*d*-tubocurarine, metocurine, atracurium, mivacurium, doxacurium)
Opioids (morphine, meperidine, codeine)
Thiobarbiturates

Treatment Plan

7 A plan for treating anaphylactic reactions must be established before the event. Airway maintenance, 100% oxygen administration, intravascular volume expansion, and epinephrine are essential to treat the hypotension and hypoxia that result from

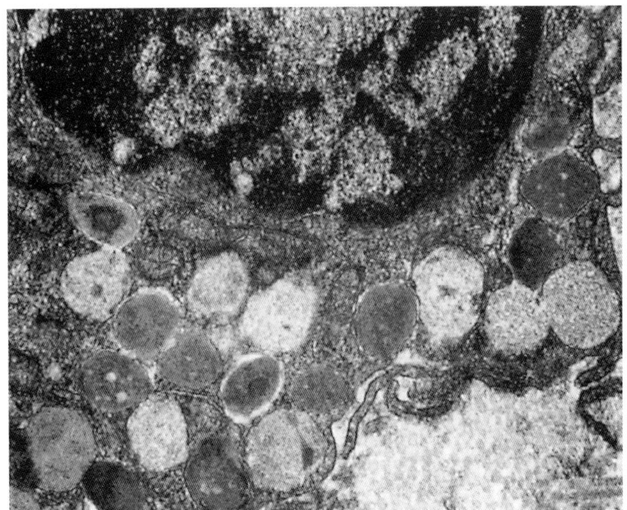

FIGURE 12-10. Electron micrograph of human cutaneous mast cell after injection of dynorphin, a κ-opioid agonist. The cell outline is rounded and most of the cytoplasmic granules are swollen, exhibiting varying degrees of decreased electron density and flocculence consistent with ongoing degranulation. The perigranular membranes of the adjacent granules at the periphery of the cell are fused to each other and to plasma membrane. Original magnification ×72,000. (Reprinted from: Casale TB, Bowman S, Kaliner M. Induction of human cutaneous mast cell degranulation by opiates and endogenous opioid peptides: Evidence for opiate and nonopiate receptor participation. *J Allergy Clin Immunol.* 1984;73:778.)

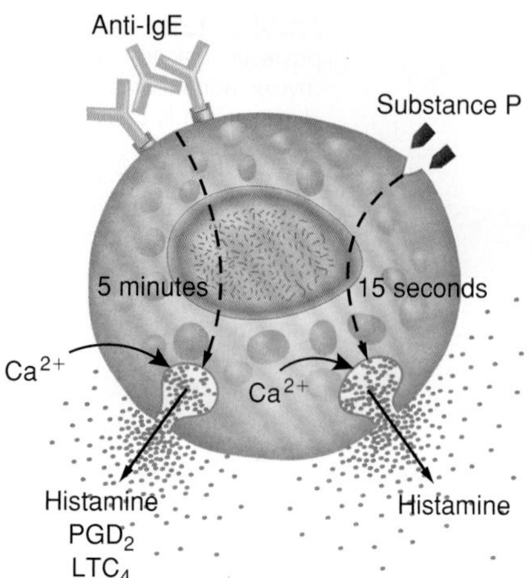

FIGURE 12-11. Different mechanisms of mediator release from human cutaneous mast cells stimulated immunologically by anti-IgE and by nonimmunologic stimuli with substance P. Anti-IgE stimulation, like antigen stimulation, initiates the release of histamine, prostaglandin D_2 (PGD_2), or leukotriene C_4 (LTC_4) by a mechanism that takes 5 minutes to reach completion and requires the influx of intracellular calcium. Nonimmunologic activation with drugs or substance P releases histamine but not PGD_2 or LTC_4 by a mechanism that is complete within 15 seconds and uses calcium mobilized from intracellular sources. (Reprinted from: Caulfield JP, El-Lati S, Thomas G, Church MK. Dissociated human foreskin mast cells degranulate in response to anti-IgE and substance P. *Lab Invest.* 1990;63:502.)

vasodilation, increased capillary permeability, and bronchospasm.[1] Table 12-6 lists a protocol for managing anaphylaxis during general anesthesia, with representative doses for a 70 kg adult. The treatment plan is the same for life-threatening anaphylactic or anaphylactoid reactions. Therapy must be titrated to needed effects with careful monitoring.[1] Severe reactions need aggressive therapy and may be protracted, with persistent hypotension, pulmonary hypertension, lower respiratory obstruction, or laryngeal obstruction that may persist 5 to 32 hours despite vigorous therapy. All patients who have experienced an anaphylactic reaction should be admitted to an intensive care unit for 24 hours of monitoring because manifestations may recur after successful treatment.

TABLE 12-6. MANAGEMENT OF ANAPHYLAXIS DURING GENERAL ANESTHESIA

Initial therapy
1. Stop administration of antigen
2. Maintain airway and administer 100% O_2
3. Discontinue all anesthetic agents
4. Start intravascular volume expansion (2–4 L of crystalloid/colloid with hypotension)
5. Give epinephrine (5–10 μg IV bolus with hypotension, titrate as needed; 0.1–1.0 mg IV with cardiovascular collapse)

Secondary treatment
1. Antihistamines (0.5–1 mg/kg diphenhydramine)
2. Catecholamine infusions (starting doses: Epinephrine 4–8 μg/min; norepinephrine 4–8 μg/min; or isoproterenol 0.5–1 μg/min as an infusion; titrated to desired effects)
3. Bronchodilators: Inhaled albuterol, terbutaline, and/or anticholinergic agents with persistent bronchospasm)
4. Corticosteroids (0.25–1 g hydrocortisone; alternatively, 1–2 g methylprednisolone)[a]
5. Sodium bicarbonate (0.5–1 mEq/kg with persistent hypotension or acidosis)
6. Airway evaluation (before extubation)
7. Vasopressin for refractory shock

[a]Methylprednisolone may be the drug of choice if the reaction is suspected to be mediated by complement.
IV, intravenous(ly).
Reprinted with permission from: Levy JH. *Anaphylactic Reactions in Anesthesia and Intensive Care.* 2nd ed. Boston, MA: Butterworth-Heinemann; 1992:162.

Initial Therapy

Although it may not be possible to stop the administration of antigen, limiting antigen administration may prevent further mast cell and basophil activation.

Maintain Airway and Administer 100% Oxygen

Profound ventilation–perfusion abnormalities producing hypoxemia can occur with anaphylactic reactions. Always administer 100% oxygen with ventilatory support as needed. Arterial blood gas values may be useful to follow during resuscitation.

Discontinue All Anesthetic Drugs

Inhalational anesthetic drugs are not the bronchodilators of choice in treating bronchospasm after anaphylaxis, especially during hypotension. These drugs interfere with the body's compensatory response to cardiovascular collapse, and halothane sensitizes the myocardium to epinephrine.

Provide Volume Expansion

Hypovolemia rapidly follows during anaphylactic shock with up to 40% loss of intravascular fluid into the interstitial space during reactions. Therefore, volume expansion is important with epinephrine in correcting the acute hypotension. Initially, 2 to 4 L of lactated Ringer's solution, or colloid or normal saline, should be administered, keeping in mind that an additional 25 to 50 mL/kg may be necessary if hypotension persists. Refractory hypotension after volume and epinephrine administration requires additional hemodynamic monitoring. The use of transesophageal echocardiography for rapid assessment of intraventricular volume and ventricular function, and to determine other occult causes of acute cardiovascular dysfunction, can be important for accurate assessment of intravascular volume and guidance of rational therapeutic interventions.[1] Fulminant noncardiogenic pulmonary edema with loss of intravascular volume can occur after anaphylaxis. This condition requires intravascular volume repletion with careful hemodynamic monitoring until the capillary defect improves. Colloid volume expansion has not proved to be more effective than crystalloid volume expansion for treating anaphylactic shock.

Administer Epinephrine

Epinephrine is the drug of choice when resuscitating patients during anaphylactic shock. α-adrenergic effects vasoconstrict to reverse hypotension; β_2-receptor stimulation bronchodilates and inhibits mediator release by increasing cyclic adenosine monophosphate (cAMP) in mast cells and basophils. The route of epinephrine administration and the dose depend on the patient's condition. Rapid and timely intervention is important when treating anaphylaxis. Furthermore, patients under general anesthesia may have altered sympathoadrenergic responses to acute anaphylactic shock, whereas the patient under spinal or epidural anesthesia may be partially sympathectomized and may need even larger doses of catecholamines.

In hypotensive patients, 5 to 10 μg boluses of epinephrine should be administered intravenously and incrementally titrated to restore blood pressure. (This dose of epinephrine can be obtained with 0.05 to 0.1 mL of a 1:10,000 dilution [100 μg/mL] or by mixing 2 mg epinephrine with 250 mL of fluid to yield an 8 μg/mL solution.) Additional volume and incrementally increased doses of epinephrine should be administered until hypotension is corrected. Although infusion is an ideal method of administering epinephrine, it is usually impossible to infuse the drug through peripheral intravenous access lines during acute volume resuscitation. With cardiovascular collapse, full intravenous cardiopulmonary resuscitative doses of epinephrine, 0.1 to 1.0 mg, should be administered and repeated until hemodynamic stability resumes. Patients with laryngeal edema without hypotension should receive subcutaneous epinephrine. Epinephrine should not be administered IV to patients with normal blood pressures.

Secondary Treatment

Antihistamines

Because H_1 receptors mediate many of the adverse effects of histamine, the intravenous administration of 0.5 to 1 mg/kg of an H_1 antagonist such as diphenhydramine may be useful in treating acute anaphylaxis. Antihistamines do not inhibit anaphylactic reactions or histamine release, but compete with histamine at receptor sites. H_1 antagonists are indicated in all forms of anaphylaxis. The H_1 antagonists available for parenteral administration may have antidopaminergic effects and should be given slowly to prevent precipitous hypotension in potentially hypovolemic patients.[1] The indications for administering an H_2 antagonist once anaphylaxis has occurred remain unclear.

Catecholamines

Epinephrine infusions may be useful in patients with persistent hypotension or bronchospasm after initial resuscitation.[1] Epinephrine infusions should be started at 0.05 to 0.1 μg/kg/min (5 to 10 μg/min) and titrated to correct hypotension. Norepinephrine infusions may be needed in patients with refractory hypotension due to decreased systemic vascular resistance. It may be started at 0.05 to 0.1 μg/kg/min (5 to 10 μg/min) and adjusted to correct hypotension.[1]

Bronchodilators

Inhaled β-adrenergic agents include inhaled albuterol or terbutaline if bronchospasm is a major feature.[36] Inhaled ipratropium may be especially useful for treatment of bronchospasm in patients receiving β-adrenergic blockers.[36] Special adaptors allow administration of bronchodilators through the endotracheal tube.

Corticosteroids

Corticosteroids have a series of anti-inflammatory effects mediated by multiple mechanisms, including altering the activation and migration of other inflammatory cells (i.e., PMNs) after an acute reaction. Consider infusing high-dose corticosteroids early in the course of therapy although beneficial effects are delayed at least 4 to 6 hours.[36] Despite their unproven usefulness in treating acute reactions, they are often administered as adjuncts to therapy when refractory bronchospasm or refractory shock occurs after resuscitative therapy. Although the exact corticosteroid dose and preparation are unclear, investigators have recommended 0.25 to 1 g intravenously of hydrocortisone in IgE-mediated reactions. Alternatively, 1 to 2 g of methylprednisolone (30 to 35 mg/kg) intravenously may be useful in reactions believed to be complement mediated, such as catastrophic pulmonary vasoconstriction after protamine transfusion reactions. Administering corticosteroids after an anaphylactic reaction may also be important in attenuating the late-phase reactions reported to occur 12 to 24 hours after anaphylaxis.

Bicarbonate

Acidosis develops rapidly in patients with persistent hypotension. This reduces the effect of epinephrine on the heart and systemic vasculature. Therefore, with refractory hypotension or acidemia, sodium bicarbonate, 0.5 to 1 mEq/kg, may be given and repeated every 5 minutes or as dictated by arterial blood gas values.

Airway Evaluation

Because profound laryngeal edema can occur, the airway should be evaluated before extubation of the trachea. Persistent facial edema suggests airway edema. The trachea of these patients should remain intubated until the edema subsides. Developing a significant air leak after endotracheal tube cuff deflation and before extubation of the trachea is useful in assessing airway patency. If there is any question of airway edema, direct laryngoscopy should be performed before the trachea is extubated.

Refractory Hypotension

Vasopressin is an important drug for refractory shock, including vasodilatory shock associated with anaphylaxis. Vasodilatory shock is characterized by hypotension association with a high cardiac output and is thought to be due to the multiple activation of vasodilator mechanisms and the inability of α-adrenergic mechanisms to compensate. Starting doses to consider are 0.01 units/minute as an infusion, although bolus administration is part of Advanced Cardiopulmonary Life Support (ACLS) guidelines.[36] Vasopressin may attenuate pathologic-induced vasodilation. Further, additional monitoring, including echocardiography and preferably transesophageal, should be considered in patients with refractory hypotension to better evaluate cardiac function or hypovolemia.

PERIOPERATIVE MANAGEMENT OF THE PATIENT WITH ALLERGIES

Allergic drug reactions account for 6% to 10% of all adverse reactions and the risk of an allergic drug reaction occurring is approximately 1% to 3% for most drugs, and around 5% of adults in the United States may be allergic to one or more drugs.[37–39] Unfortunately, patients often refer to adverse drug effects as being allergic in nature. For example, opioid administration can produce nausea, vomiting, or even local release of histamine along the vein of administration. Patients will say they are "allergic" to a specific drug when in fact their adverse reaction is independent of allergy. Nearly 15% of adults in the United States believe they are allergic to specific medication(s) and therefore may be denied treatment with an indicated drug. To understand allergic reactions, the spectrum of adverse reactions to drugs needs to be considered.

Predictable adverse drug reactions account for about 80% of adverse drug effects. They are often dose dependent, related to known pharmacologic actions of the drug, and typically occur in normal patients. Most serious, predictable adverse drug reactions are toxic and are directly related to the drug in the body (overdosage) or to an unintentional route of administration (e.g., lidocaine-induced seizures or cardiovascular collapse). Side effects are the most common adverse drug reactions and are undesirable pharmacologic actions of the drugs occurring at usual prescribed dosages. Most anesthetic drugs present multiple side effects that can produce precipitous hypotension. For example, morphine dilates the venous capacitance bed, thereby decreasing preload; releases histamine from cutaneous mast cells, thereby producing arterial and venous dilation; slows the heart rate; and decreases sympathetic tone. However, the net effects of morphine on blood pressure and myocardial function depend on the patient's blood volume, sympathetic tone, and ventricular function. Hypotension rapidly develops in a volume-depleted trauma patient in pain who is given morphine. Drug interactions also represent important predictable adverse drug reactions. Intravenous fentanyl administration to a patient who has just received intravenous benzodiazepines or other sedative-hypnotic drugs may produce precipitous hypotension that results from decreased sympathetic tone or direct vasodilation from propofol administration.[40] This represents a dose-dependent, predictable adverse drug reaction that is independent of allergy.

Unpredictable adverse drug reactions are usually dose independent and usually not related to the drug's pharmacologic actions, but are often related to the immunologic response (allergy) of the individual. On occasion, adverse reactions can be related to genetic differences (i.e., idiosyncratic) in a susceptible individual who has an isolated genetic enzyme deficiency. In most allergic drug reactions, an immunologic mechanism is present or, more often, presumed. Determining whether the causing event involves a reaction between the drug or drug metabolites with drug-specific antibodies or sensitized T lymphocytes is often impractical. Without direct immunologic evidence that may be helpful in distinguishing an allergic reaction from other adverse reactions include allergic reactions occur in only a small percentage of patients receiving the drug, and the clinical manifestations do not resemble known pharmacologic actions. In the absence of prior drug exposure, allergic symptoms rarely appear after less than 1 week of continuous treatment. After sensitization, the reaction develops rapidly on reexposure to the drug. In general, drugs that have been administered without complications for several months or longer are rarely responsible for producing drug allergy. The time span between exposure to the drug and noticed manifestations is often the most vital information in deciding which drugs administered were the cause of a suspected allergic reaction.

Although the reaction may produce a life-threatening response in the cardiopulmonary system (anaphylaxis), various cutaneous manifestations, fever, and pulmonary reactions have been attributed to drug hypersensitivity. Usually, the reaction may be reproduced by small doses of the suspected drug or other agents having similar or cross-reacting chemical structures. On occasion, drug-specific antibodies or lymphocytes have been identified that react with the suspected drug, although the relationship is seldom diagnostically useful in practice. Even when an immune response to a drug is demonstrated, it may not be associated with a clinical allergic reaction. As with adverse drug reactions in general, the reaction usually subsides within several days of discontinuation of the drug.

Immunologic Mechanisms of Drug Allergy

Different immunologic responses to any antigen can occur. Drugs have been associated with all the immunologic mechanisms proposed by Gell and Coombs. Although more than one mechanism may contribute to a particular reaction, any one can occur. Penicillin may produce different reactions in different patients or a spectrum of reactions in the same patient. In one patient, penicillin can produce anaphylaxis (type I reaction), hemolytic anemia (type II reaction), serum sickness (type III reaction), and contact dermatitis (type IV reaction).[5,6] Therefore, any one antigen has the ability to produce a diffuse spectrum of allergic responses in humans. Why some patients have localized rashes or angioneurotic edema in response to penicillin whereas others suffer complete cardiopulmonary collapse is unknown. Most anesthetic drugs and agents administered perioperatively have been reported to produce anaphylactic reactions (Table 12-7).[31,39] Muscle relaxants are the most common drugs responsible for evoking intraoperative allergic reactions. In this regard, there is cross-sensitivity between succinylcholine and the nondepolarizing muscle relaxants. Unexplained intraoperative cardiovascular collapse has been attributed to anaphylaxis triggered by latex (natural rubber), and certain patients, including those with a history of spina bifida, are at a greater risk for reactions.

Life-threatening allergic reactions are potentially thought to occur more likely in patients with a history of allergy, atopy, or asthma, although this concept is also controversial and in part based on older data.[41] Nevertheless, because the incidence is low, the history is not a reliable predictor that an allergic reaction will occur and does not mandate that such patients should be investigated or pretreated or that specific drugs be selected or avoided. Although different mechanisms have been proposed, no one theory has been proved. The drugs and foreign substances listed in Table 12-7 may have both immunologic and nonimmunologic mechanisms for adverse drug reactions in humans.

Evaluation of Patients with Allergic Reactions

Identifying the drug responsible for a suspected allergic reaction still depends on circumstantial evidence suggesting the temporal sequence of drug administration. Conventional in vivo and in vitro methods of diagnosing allergic reactions to most anesthetic drugs are unavailable or not applicable. The most important factor in diagnosis is the awareness of the physician that an untoward event may be related to a drug the patient received. The physician must always be aware of the capacity of any drug to produce an allergic reaction. The history is important when evaluating whether an adverse drug reaction is allergic and whether the drug can be readministered. Although a prior allergic reaction to the drug in question is important, this is rarely the case. Direct challenge of a patient with a test dose of drug is the only way to prove a reaction, but this is potentially

TABLE 12-7. AGENTS IMPLICATED IN ALLERGIC REACTIONS DURING ANESTHESIA

Anesthetic agents
Induction agents (cremophor-solubilized drugs, barbiturates, etomidate, propofol)
Local anesthetics (*para*-aminobenzoic ester agents)
Muscle relaxants (succinylcholine, gallamine, pancuronium, *d*-tubocurarine, metocurine, atracurium, vecuronium, mivacurium, doxacurium)
Opioids (meperidine, morphine, fentanyl)
Other agents
Antibiotics (cephalosporins, penicillin, sulfonamides, vancomycin)
Aprotinin
Blood products (whole blood, packed cells, fresh frozen plasma, platelets, cryoprecipitate, fibrinin glue, gamma globulin)
Bone cement
Chymopapain
Corticosteriods
Cyclosporin
Drug additives (preservatives)
Furosemide
Insulin
Mannitol
Methylmethacrylate
Nonsteroidal anti-inflammatory drugs
Protamine
Radiocontrast dye
Latex (natural rubber)
Streptokinase
Vascular graft material
Vitamin K
Colloid volume expanders (dextrans, protein fractions, albumin, hydroxyethyl starch)

Reprinted with permission from: Levy JH. *Anaphylactic Reactions in Anesthesia and Intensive Care.* 2nd ed. Boston, MA: Butterworth-Heinemann; 1992.

dangerous and not recommended. Although the anesthesiologist commonly gives small test doses of anesthetic drugs, these are pharmacologic test doses and have nothing to do with immunologic dosages. The demonstration of drug-specific IgE antibodies is accepted as evidence that the patient may be at risk for anaphylaxis if the drug is administered. Different clinical tests are of historical interest, and few of them are actually available to confirm or diagnose drug allergy but are considered in the following section.

Testing for Allergy

8 After an anaphylactic reaction, it is important to identify the causative agent to prevent readministration. When one particular drug has been administered and there is a clear correlation between the time of administration and the occurrence of a reaction, testing may be unnecessary, and general avoidance of the drug should be instituted. However, when patients have simultaneously received multiple drugs (e.g., an opioid, muscle relaxant, hypnotic, and antibiotic), it is often difficult to prove which particular drug caused the reaction. Further, the reaction might have been caused by the vehicle or by one of the preservatives. For patients who want to know which drug was responsible and for patients scheduled for subsequent procedures, some degree of allergy evaluation should be undertaken to evaluate the drug at risk. Unfortunately, few *laboratory* tests exist for anesthetic drugs; therefore, the available allergy tests are discussed.

Leukocyte Histamine Release

Leukocyte histamine is performed by incubating the patient's leukocytes with the offending drug and measuring histamine release as a marker for basophil activation, although false-positive results can occur. This test is not easy to perform, although variations allow the use of whole blood instead of isolated PMNs, and is generally not available nor used.

Radioallergosorbent Test

The radioallergosorbent test (RAST) allows *laboratory* detection of specific IgE directed toward particular antigens. In this test, antigens are linked to insoluble material to make an immunoabsorbent. When incubated with the serum in question, antibodies of different classes directed toward the antigen bind to it. After washing, the antigen–antibody complex on the immunoabsorbent is incubated with radiolabeled antibodies directed against human IgE and counted in a scintillation counter. The concentration of specific IgE in the patient's serum directed toward the allergen is measured. The RAST is more quantitative than skin tests and avoids the potential of reexposure. RAST testing has previously been used to detect the presence of antibodies to meperidine, succinylcholine, and thiopental. Two major limitations to this test include the commercial availability of the drug prepared as an antigen and false-positive test results in patients with high IgE levels; however, because of radioactivity involved, RAST testing is rarely performed.

Enzyme-linked Immunosorbent Assay

The enzyme-linked immunosorbent assay (ELISA) measures antigen-specific antibodies. The basis of the ELISA is similar to that of the RAST; however, immunospecific IgE directed against the antigen in question is determined by adding an anti-IgE coupled to an enzyme such as peroxidase that acts as a chromogen. A colorless substrate is acted on by peroxidase to produce a colored byproduct. The ELISA has been used to prove IgE antibodies to chymopapain and protamine and has been developed to screen for other antibodies to diverse agents and has become the mainstay of immunologic testing. Although antibodies can occur, patients may be asymptomatic.

Intradermal Testing (Skin Testing)

Skin testing is the method most often used in patients after anaphylactic reaction to anesthetic drugs after the history has suggested the relevant antigens for testing.[42] Within minutes after antigen introduction, histamine released from cutaneous mast cells causes vasodilation (flare) and localized edema from increased vascular permeability (wheal). Fisher suggested that this is a simple, safe, and useful method of establishing a diagnosis in most cases of anaphylactic reactions occurring in the perioperative period. If the strict protocols established by Fisher are used, intradermal reactions are helpful.[42] Intradermal testing is of no value in reactions to contrast media or colloid volume expanders. Cross-sensitivity between drugs of similar structures can often be evaluated based on skin testing.

Agents Implicated in Allergic Reactions

Any drug or biologic agent can cause anaphylaxis in a patient. However, the agents most often implicated in the perioperative period include antibiotics, blood products, chlorhexidine, neuromuscular blocking drugs (NMBDs), polypeptides (aprotinin, latex, and protamine), and intravascular volume expanders. Most of the information about perioperative anaphylaxis is from Australia, Europe, the United Kingdom, and New Zealand, where centers exist for many years to investigate perioperative anaphylaxis when it occurs.[43–48] In one of the largest reports, perioperative anaphylaxis was evaluated over an 8-year period from 1997 to 2004 in France. Among the 2,516 patients with anaphylaxis, IgE-mediated reactions occurred in 1,816 cases (72.2%). The most common causes for the IgE-mediated events were NMBDs in 58% (n = 1,067), latex in 19.6% (n = 316), and antibiotics in 12.8% (n = 236).[49] One of the concerns regarding NMBA allergy is that if patients are allergic to a muscle relaxant, there is a potential for cross-reactivity because of the similarity of the active site, a quaternary ammonium molecule, among the different types of relaxants, and alternatives cannot be chosen without some degree of immunologic testing.

From the United States/North American perspective, there are few reports describing the incidence or agents implicated for perioperative anaphylaxis. Two noteworthy reports include one in 1990 where barbiturates were the most likely causative agent for 38% of IgE-mediated anaphylaxis.[50] These findings are different from European reports where the most frequent agent reported for perioperative IgE-mediated anaphylaxis is NMBAs.[51] A recent report examined a skin test database of 38 patients with perioperative anaphylaxis who were tested to medications implicated in the reactions.[52] The history obtained by an allergist, skin test results, and tryptase measurements were reported.[52] Of note, 40% of the surgical procedures were aborted, and 58% of events resulted in intensive care unit admissions suggesting the severity of the responses.[52] Of the 38 patients, 18 were considered IgE-mediated reactions by skin testing, 6 were non-IgE–mediated anaphylactic reactions as determined by elevated tryptase levels and negative skin testing, and 14 were probable non-IgE–mediated anaphylactic reactions because tryptase levels were normal or not obtained and skin testing was negative. Of the IgE-mediated anaphylactic reactions, antibiotics were the causative agents in half of the patients while NMBAs were implicated solely as a likely causative agent in only one reaction. The authors noted causative agents could not be determined in the other half of the patients and suggested this placed them at risk of a subsequent reexposure to the same allergen or potentially unnecessary avoidance of needed medications.[52] Of note is that the authors identified only one true IgE-mediated reaction to an NMBA. Another patient had positive skin tests to three agents including vecuronium, propofol, and cefazolin making the diagnosis uncertain. A previous Danish study reported 68 patients, of which 36 underwent complete investigations with in vitro testing and skin testing, and found that only one patient tested positive for NMBAs (4.8%: 1/21), while chlorhexidine accounted for 19.1% of reactions and antibiotics 14.3%.[53] In the current study chlorhexidine was tested in only 4% of cases and may account for some of the undiagnosed reactions with elevated tryptase.[52] Because of this information, antibiotics, latex, and NMBAs will be considered in more detail, along with local anesthetic agents.

Antibiotics

Most surgical patients receive an antibiotic that includes a cephalosporin or vancomycin for prophylaxis. Despite their widespread use, the incidence of antibiotic allergy and its reported prevalence vary widely, as cutaneous manifestations are often the presenting reaction.[39] As reviewed in a recent article,[1] anaphylaxis to penicillins is low, occurring in an estimated 0.004% to 0.015%, but this widely quoted reference is old and penicillin is rarely used.[54] Further, data on anaphylaxis to cephalosporins is also uncommon, occurring from 0.0001% to 0.1%; however this number is not zero.[55] Anaphylactic reactions to vancomycin are rare, but as we have demonstrated, it is a potent histamine-releasing agent that can cause severe hypotension and flushing on administration especially with rapid infusion.[30,31]

As reviewed previously, managing the patient with a history of penicillin allergy when the surgeon requests cephalosporin administration is still not clear based on reported data.[1] Older data suggest cross-reactivity to cephalosporins among penicillin-allergic patients is high and suggest choosing another agent, a practice that developed from case reports[56] of anaphylaxis following first-generation cephalosporins together with in vitro and skin testing which showed extensive cross-reactivity between penicillins and first-generation cephalosporins.[1] The clinical relevance of this in vitro cross-reactivity was never demonstrated.[56] However, the risk of acute cephalosporin reactions among patients with positive penicillin skin tests is reported to be ~4.4%, compared with 0.6% among patients with negative penicillin skin tests.[56,57] Anaphylactic reactors were selectively omitted from these open studies. Further, an allergic reaction to a cephalosporin may occur independently of prior penicillin sensitization. One authority has concluded that most patients who have a history of penicillin allergy will tolerate cephalosporins, but that indiscriminate administration cannot be recommended, especially for patients who have had serious acute reactions to any β-lactam antibiotic.[39] Penicillin skin testing when available can be useful in identifying the 85% of patients with histories of penicillin allergy who no longer have (or never had) IgE antibodies to major and minor determinants and are therefore at negligible risk of cephalosporin reactions. For the remaining patients who are skin test positive, gradual escalation of the first dose of a cephalosporin under careful observation will further mitigate against uncommon but potentially serious acute reactions.

If a patient has a penicillin allergy history that is consistent with anaphylaxis and penicillin skin testing is unavailable, then cephalosporins should be used with caution, with graded dose escalation of the first dose. A patient who has experienced an allergic reaction to a specific cephalosporin should probably not receive that cephalosporin again. However, the risk of an acute reaction when a different cephalosporin is administered appears to be low, but systemic evaluations of reaction risks when administering other cephalosporins or β-lactam antibiotics to patients with IgE antibodies to a particular cephalosporin are not available. Unfortunately, patient histories are often unreliable in this circumstance.

Latex Allergy

For the anesthesiologist, latex represents an environmental agent often implicated as an important cause of perioperative anaphylaxis. Latex is the milky sap derived from the tree *Hevea brasiliensis* to which multiple agents, including preservatives, accelerators, and antioxidants are added to make the final rubber product. Latex is present in a variety of different products. Latex allergy is an IgE-dependent immediate hypersensitivity reaction to latex proteins. The first case of an allergic reaction because of latex was reported in 1979 and was manifested by contact urticaria. In 1989, the first reports of intraoperative anaphylaxis because of latex were reported.

9 Health-care workers and children with spina bifida, urogenital abnormalities, or certain food allergies have also been recognized as people at increased risk for anaphylaxis to latex. Brown et al. reported a 24% incidence of irritant or contact dermatitis and a 12.5% incidence of latex-specific IgE positivity in anesthesiologists. Of this group, 10% were clinically asymptomatic, although IgE positive.[58] A history of atopy was also a significant risk factor for latex sensitization. Brown et al. suggested that these people are in their early stages of sensitization and perhaps, by avoiding latex exposure, their progression to symptomatic disease can be prevented.[58] Patients allergic to bananas, avocados, and kiwis have also been reported to have antibodies that cross-react with latex.[59,60] Multiple attempts are being made to reduce latex exposure to both health-care workers and patients. If latex allergy occurs, then strict avoidance of latex from gloves and other sources needs to be considered, following recommendations as reported by Holzman.[61,62] Since latex is such a common environmental antigen, this ongoing effort by suppliers of hospital equipment has significantly reduced the latex exposure over recent years.

More importantly, anesthesiologists must be prepared to treat the life-threatening cardiopulmonary collapse that occurs after anaphylaxis, as previously discussed. The most important preventive therapy is to avoid antigen exposure; although clinicians have used pretreatment with antihistamine (diphenhydramine and cimetidine) and corticosteroids, there are no data in the literature to suggest that pretreatment prevents anaphylaxis or decreases its severity.[1] Patients in whom latex allergy is suspected should be referred to an allergist for proper evaluation and potential testing for definitive diagnosis. When this is not possible, patients should be treated as if they were latex allergic, and the antigen avoided. Patients with a documented history of latex allergy should wear Medic Alert bracelets.

Local Anesthetics

Skin testing to local anesthetics (LA) is considered a direct challenge or provocative dose testing. Local anesthetic drugs are injected in increasing quantities under controlled circumstances. This testing decides if the person can safely receive amide derivatives (e.g., lidocaine) and can also be used to decide if the person is sensitive to *para*-aminobenzoic ester agents (e.g., procaine, tetracaine). Because the immediate hypersensitivity reactions to local anesthetics is unknown, they are commonly regarded as "pseudoallergic" or "nonimmune type" anaphylaxis as immunologically mediated reactions have rarely been observed with positive skin-prick tests.[63] Other ingredients in LA preparations have to be considered as elicitors, for example, preservatives like benzoates or sulfites or latex contaminants in injection bottles. Practical management of patients with a history of LA reaction includes a careful allergy history and skin-prick and intradermal tests. Undiluted LA solutions may elicit false-positive intradermal test reactions. If prick and intradermal tests are negative, the procedure of subcutaneous provocation testing is applied in a placebo-controlled manner. When patients are constantly reacting to placebo, a regimen of "reverse placebo provocation" with injection of an LA (verum) is applied while the patient is informed about receiving placebo in order to "rule out psychosomatic involvement." With this regimen it is possible to eliminate anxiousness and fear, and the patient has proof that he has tolerated the respective LA substance.[63]

However, the diagnostic evaluation of patients with suspected allergy to local anesthetics who have experienced a reaction remains controversial. One of the largest reports of skin testing for local anesthetic allergy evaluation is a retrospective chart review of patients following local anesthetic skin testing who underwent prick and intradermal skin testing followed by incremental subcutaneous and open subcutaneous challenge.[64] A total of 178 patients underwent 227 local anesthetic skin tests of which 220 (97%) were negative, and 214 (97%) had negative challenge or probable non-IgE–mediated events during challenge while 3 patients with 6 negative skin tests had a local reaction during the challenge. Only seven skin tests per five patients met the criteria for a positive skin test, and one patient had a skin reaction without systemic effects, three patients had a negative subcutaneous challenge, and one patient did not undergo a challenge. Overall, 98% of patients receiving local anesthetics after open subcutaneous challenge tolerated the medications. The negative predictive value of the local anesthetic skin test was 97% with few positive skin tests. Positive local anesthetic skin tests are uncommon and the local anesthetic skin tests have an excellent negative predictive value.[64]

Neuromuscular Blocking Agents

10 NMBAs have several unique molecular features that make them potential allergens. All NMBAs are functionally divalent and are thus capable of cross-linking cell-surface IgE and causing mediator release from mast cells and basophils without binding or haptenating to larger carrier molecules. NMBAs have also been implicated in epidemiologic studies of anesthetic drug-induced anaphylaxis. Epidemiologic data from France suggest that NMBAs are responsible for 62% to 81% of reactions, depending on the time period evaluated.

In more recent years, NMBAs, especially steroid-derived agents, have been reported as potential causative agents of anaphylactic reactions during anesthesia. The data associating NMBAs in the most recent reports from France are mainly based on skin testing; however, studies have previously reported the steroidal-derived NMBAs and other molecules produce false-positive skin tests (i.e., weal and flare). One of the major problems is that anaphylaxis to NMBAs is rare in the United States, but has been reported more often in Europe. Although suggestions have been made that this is because of underreporting, the severity of anaphylaxis and its sequelae to produce adverse outcomes clearly make this unlikely based on the current medicolegal climate that exists in the United States. One of the only ways to explain this widely divergent perspective is to understand how the diagnosis is made because the recommended threshold test concentrations have not been defined, resulting in unreliable results.

We previously reported in several studies that steroid-derived agents could induce positive weal and flare responses independent of mast cell degranulation, even at low concentrations, following intradermal injection. This effect is likely because of a direct effect on the cutaneous vasculature that occurs for most NMBAs at concentrations as low as 10^{-5} M using intradermal skin tests in 30 volunteers. A positive cutaneous reaction without evidence of mast cell degranulation was noted at low concentrations (100 mcg/mL) of rocuronium in almost all the volunteers. We have used intradermal injections to compare cutaneous effects of anesthetic and other agents.

Other investigators have also reported similar results. Because prick tests are often used for authenticating NMBAs as causative drugs, Dhonneur et al. evaluated 30 volunteers, using prick testing. Each subject received 10 prick tests (50 μL) on both forearms.[65] The investigators studied the weal and flare responses to prick tests with rocuronium and vecuronium, using four dilutions (1/1,000,

1/100, 1/10, and 1) and two controls, and measured weal and flare immediately after and at 15 minutes. They noted 50% and 40% of the subjects had a positive skin reaction to undiluted rocuronium and vecuronium, respectively. To avoid false-positive results, they suggested that prick testing with rocuronium and vecuronium should be performed in subjects who have experienced a hypersensitivity reaction during anesthesia, with concentrations below that commonly inducing positive reactions in anesthesia-naive, healthy subjects (i.e., for men in a dilution of 1/10 and for women in a dilution of 1/100).[65] Guidelines for prick testing that are internationally agreed on need to be established. Many of these differences may explain the various incidences of allergy to NMBAs among countries. Concentration–skin response curves to rocuronium and vecuronium have showed that prick tests should be performed with dilution of the commercially available preparation. Female volunteers significantly ($P < 0.01$) reacted to lower vecuronium and rocuronium concentrations than males. In female subjects, positive skin reactions were reported with dilutions of 1/100 of both relaxants. In male subjects, positive skin reactions were noted with the undiluted concentration, except for one volunteer who reacted to rocuronium (1/10 dilution).[65]

SUMMARY

Although the immune system functions to provide host defense, it can respond inappropriately to produce hypersensitivity or allergic reactions. A spectrum of life-threatening allergic reactions to any drug or agent can occur in the perioperative period. The enigma of these reactions lies in their unpredictable nature. Certain patients undergoing high-risk procedures with multiple blood product exposures are also at higher risk. However, a high index of suspicion, prompt recognition, and appropriate and aggressive therapy can help avoid a disastrous outcome.

References

1. Levy JH, Adkinson NF Jr. Anaphylaxis during cardiac surgery: Implications for clinicians. *Anesth Analg.* 2008;106:392–403.
2. Kay AB. Allergy and allergic diseases. First of two parts. *N Engl J Med.* 2001; 344:30–37.
3. Kay AB. Allergy and allergic diseases. Second of two parts. *N Engl J Med.* 2001; 344:109–113.
4. Hotchkiss RS, Karl IE. The pathophysiology and treatment of sepsis. *N Engl J Med.* 2003;348:138–150.
5. Delves PJ, Roitt IM. The immune system. Second of two parts. *N Engl J Med.* 2000; 343:108–117.
6. Delves PJ, Roitt IM. The immune system. First of two parts. *N Engl J Med.* 2000;343:37–49.
7. Skrupky LP, Kerby PW, Hotchkiss RS. Advances in the management of sepsis and the understanding of key immunologic defects. *Anesthesiology.* 2011;115: 1349–1362.
8. Pober JS, Cotran RS. Cytokines and endothelial cell biology. *Physiol Rev.* 1990; 70:427–451.
9. Walport MJ. Complement. Second of two parts. *N Engl J Med.* 2001;344:1140–1144.
10. Walport MJ. Complement. First of two parts. *N Engl J Med.* 2001;344:1058–1066.
11. Levy JH, Freiberger DJ, Roback J. Hereditary angioedema: Current and emerging treatment options. *Anesth Analg.* 2010;110:1271–1280.
12. Stevenson GW, Hall SC, Rudnick S, et al. The effect of anesthetic agents on the human immune response. *Anesthesiology.* 1990;72:542–552.
13. Sampson HA, Munoz-Furlong A, Bock SA, et al. Symposium on the definition and management of anaphylaxis: Summary report. *J Allergy Clin Immunol.* 2005;115:584–591.
14. Mertes PM, Laxenaire MC, Alla F. Anaphylactic and anaphylactoid reactions occurring during anesthesia in France in 1999-2000. *Anesthesiology.* 2003;99: 536–545.
15. Portier P, Richet CR. De l'action anaphylactique de certains venins. *C R Soc Biol.* 1902;54:170–172.
16. MacGlashan D Jr. Histamine: A mediator of inflammation. *J Allergy Clin Immunol.* 2003;112:S53–S59.
17. Kalesnikoff J, Galli SJ. Anaphylaxis: Mechanisms of mast cell activation. *Chem Immunol Allergy.* 2011;95:45–66.
18. Wedemeyer J, Tsai M, Galli SJ. Roles of mast cells and basophils in innate and acquired immunity. *Curr Opin Immunol.* 2000;12:624–631.
19. Marone G, Bova M, Detoraki A, et al. The human heart as a shock organ in anaphylaxis. *Novartis Found Symp.* 2004;257:133–149, discussion 149–160, 276–285.
20. Majno G, Palade GE. Studies on inflammation. 1. The effect of histamine and serotonin on vascular permeability: An electron microscopic study. *J Biophys Biochem Cytol.* 1961;11:571–605.
21. Majno G, Palade GE, Schoefl GI. Studies on inflammation. II. The site of action of histamine and serotonin along the vascular tree: A topographic study. *J Biophys Biochem Cytol.* 1961;11:607–626.
22. Holgate ST, Peters-Golden M, Panettieri RA, et al. Roles of cysteinyl leukotrienes in airway inflammation, smooth muscle function, and remodeling. *J Allergy Clin Immunol.* 2003;111:S18–S34, discussion S34–S36.
23. Vadas P, Gold M, Perelman B, et al. Platelet-activating factor, PAF acetylhydrolase, and severe anaphylaxis. *N Engl J Med.* 2008;358:28–35.
24. Pumphrey RS. Lessons for management of anaphylaxis from a study of fatal reactions. *Clin Exp Allergy.* 2000;30:1144–1150.
25. Pumphrey R. Anaphylaxis: Can we tell who is at risk of a fatal reaction? *Curr Opin Allergy Clin Immunol.* 2004;4:285–290.
26. Pumphrey RS. Fatal anaphylaxis in the UK, 1992–2001. *Novartis Found Symp.* 2004;257:116–128, discussion 128–132, 157–160, 276–285.
27. Delage C, Irey NS. Anaphylactic deaths: A clinicopathologic study of 43 cases. *J Forensic Sci.* 1972;17:525–540.
28. Pumphrey RS, Roberts IS. Postmortem findings after fatal anaphylactic reactions. *J Clin Pathol.* 2000;53:273–276.
29. Sheppard CA, Logdberg LE, Zimring JC, et al. Transfusion-related acute lung injury. *Hematol Oncol Clin North Am.* 2007;21:163–176.
30. Veien M, Szlam F, Holden JT, et al. Mechanisms of nonimmunological histamine and tryptase release from human cutaneous mast cells. *Anesthesiology.* 2000;92:1074–1081.
31. Levy JH, Kettlekamp N, Goertz P, et al. Histamine release by vancomycin: A mechanism for hypotension in man. *Anesthesiology.* 1987;67:122–125.
32. Levy JH, Brister NW, Shearin A, et al. Wheal and flare responses to opioids in humans. *Anesthesiology.* 1989;70:756–760.
33. Levy JH, Adelson D, Walker B. Wheal and flare responses to muscle relaxants in humans. *Agents Actions.* 1991;34:302–308.
34. Levy JH, Davis GK, Duggan J, et al. Determination of the hemodynamics and histamine release of rocuronium (Org 9426) when administered in increased doses under N2O/O2-sufentanil anesthesia. *Anesth Analg.* 1994;78:318–321.
35. Levy JH, Pitts M, Thanopoulos A, et al. The effects of rapacuronium on histamine release and hemodynamics in adult patients undergoing general anesthesia. *Anesth Analg.* 1999;89:290–295.
36. 2005 CARE AHAGFCRAEC: Part 10.6: Anaphylaxis. *Circulation.* 2005;112: IV-143–IV-145.
37. DeSwarte RD. Drug allergy–problems and strategies. *J Allergy Clin Immunol.* 1984;74:209–224.
38. Gruchalla RS. Drug allergy. *J Allergy Clin Immunol.* 2003;111:S548–S559.
39. Gruchalla RS, Pirmohamed M. Clinical practice. Antibiotic allergy. *N Engl J Med.* 2006;354:601–609.
40. Reich DL, Hossain S, Krol M, et al. Predictors of hypotension after induction of general anesthesia. *Anesth Analg.* 2005;101:622–628.
41. Laforest M, More D, Fisher M. Predisposing factors in anaphylactoid reactions to anaesthetic drugs in an Australian population: The role of allergy, atopy and previous anaesthesia. *Anaesth Intensive Care.* 1980;8:454–459.
42. Fisher MM, Bowey CJ. Intradermal compared with prick testing in the diagnosis of anaesthetic allergy. *Br J Anaesth.* 1997;79:59–63.
43. Galletly DC, Treuren BC. Anaphylactoid reactions during anaesthesia. Seven years' experience of intradermal testing. *Anaesthesia.* 1985;40:329–333.
44. Laxenaire MC. Drugs and other agents involved in anaphylactic shock occurring during anaesthesia. A French multicenter epidemiological inquiry. *Ann Fr Anesth Reanim.* 1993;12:91–96.
45. Laxenaire MC, Mertes PM. Anaphylaxis during anaesthesia. Results of a two-year survey in France. *Br J Anaesth.* 2001;87:549–558.
46. Harboe T, Guttormsen AB, Irgens A, et al. Anaphylaxis during anesthesia in Norway: A 6-year single-center follow-up study. *Anesthesiology.* 2005;102:897–903.
47. Mertes PM. Anaphylactic reactions during anaesthesia–let us treat the problem rather than debating its existence. *Acta Anaesthesiol Scand.* 2005;49:431–433.
48. Fisher M, Baldo BA. Anaphylaxis during anaesthesia: Current aspects of diagnosis and prevention. *Eur J Anaesthesiol.* 1994;11:263–284.
49. Mertes PM, Alla F, Trechot P, et al. Anaphylaxis during anesthesia in France: An 8-year national survey. *J Allergy Clin Immunol.* 2011;128(2):366–367. Epub 2011 Apr 17.
50. Moscicki RA, Sockin SM, Corsello BF, et al. Anaphylaxis during induction of general anesthesia: Subsequent evaluation and management. *J Allergy Clin Immunol.* 1990;86:325–332.
51. Levy JH. Anaphylactic reactions to neuromuscular blocking drugs: Are we making the correct diagnosis? *Anesth Analg.* 2004;98:881–882.

52. Gurrieri C, Weingarten TN, Martin DP, et al. Allergic reactions during anesthesia at a large United States referral center. *Anesth Analg.* 2011;113(5):1202–1212.
53. Garvey LH, Roed-Petersen J, Menne T, et al. Danish anaesthesia allergy centre - preliminary results. *Acta Anaesthesiol Scand.* 2001;45:1204–1209.
54. Idsoe O, Guthe T, Willcox RR, et al. Nature and extent of penicillin side-reactions, with particular reference to fatalities from anaphylactic shock. *Bull World Health Organ.* 1968;38:159–188.
55. Kelkar PS, Li JT. Cephalosporin allergy. *N Engl J Med.* 2001;345:804–809.
56. Pichichero ME. A review of evidence supporting the American Academy of Pediatrics recommendation for prescribing cephalosporin antibiotics for penicillin-allergic patients. *Pediatrics.* 2005;115:1048–1057.
57. Pichichero ME. Cephalosporins can be prescribed safely for penicillin-allergic patients. *J Fam Pract.* 2006;55:106–112.
58. Brown RH, Schauble JF, Hamilton RG. Prevalence of latex allergy among anesthesiologists: Identification of sensitized but asymptomatic individuals. *Anesthesiology.* 1998;89:292–299.
59. Lavaud F, Prevost A, Cossart C, et al. Allergy to latex, avocado pear, and banana: Evidence for a 30 kd antigen in immunoblotting. *J Allergy Clin Immunol.* 1995; 95:557–564.
60. Blanco C, Carrillo T, Castillo R, et al. Latex allergy: Clinical features and cross-reactivity with fruits. *Ann Allergy.* 1994;73:309–314.
61. Holzman RS. Clinical management of latex-allergic children. *Anesth Analg.* 1997; 85:529–533.
62. Holzman RS, Katz JD. Occupational latex allergy: The end of the innocence. *Anesthesiology.* 1998;89:287–289.
63. Ring J, Franz R, Brockow K. Anaphylactic reactions to local anesthetics. *Chem Immunol Allergy.* 2011;95:190–200.
64. McClimon B, Rank M, Li J. The predictive value of skin testing in the diagnosis of local anesthetic allergy. *Allergy Asthma Proc.* 2011;32:95–98.
65. Dhonneur G, Combes X, Chassard D, et al. Skin sensitivity to rocuronium and vecuronium: A randomized controlled prick-testing study in healthy volunteers. *Anesth Analg.* 2004;98:986–989.

CHAPTER

13 Inflammation, Wound Healing, and Infection

HARRIET W. HOPF • C. RICHARD CHAPMAN • AMALIA COCHRAN • MICHAEL B. DORROUGH • RANDAL O. DULL

Key Points

1. The most crucial component of infection prevention is frequent and effective hand hygiene.
2. The ideal hand hygiene agent kills a broad spectrum of microbes, has antimicrobial activity that persists for at least 6 hours after application, is simple to use, and has few side effects.
3. Wearing gloves does not reduce the need for hand hygiene.
4. Antibiotic prophylaxis has become standard for surgeries in which there is more than a minimum risk of infection. The most commonly used antibiotic for surgical prophylaxis is cefazolin, a first-generation cephalosporin, as the potential pathogens for most surgeries are gram-positive cocci from the skin.
5. The exact timing for the administration of the antibiotic depends on the pharmacology and half-life of the drug, but should generally be 0 to 60 minutes before incision. Prophylactic antibiotics should be discontinued by 24 hours following surgery if postoperative dosing is selected at all. Prolonging the course of prophylactic antibiotics does not reduce the risk of infection but does increase the risk of adverse consequences of antibiotic administration, including resistance, *Clostridium difficile* infection, and sensitization.
6. Anesthesiologists should work in consultation with surgeons to use guidelines determined by the local infection control committee to take initiative for administering prophylactic antibiotics because they have access to the patient during the 60 minutes prior to incision and can optimize timing of administration.
7. The standard teaching that oxygen delivery depends more on hemoglobin-bound oxygen (oxygen content) than on arterial PO_2 may be true of working muscle, but it is not true of wound healing.
8. Although oxygen consumption is relatively low in wounds, it is consumed by processes that require oxygen at a high concentration.
9. High oxygen tensions (>100 mm Hg) can be reached in wounds but only if perfusion is rapid and arterial PO_2 is high.
10. Peripheral vasoconstriction, which results from central sympathetic control of subcutaneous vascular tone, is probably the most frequent and clinically the most important impediment to wound oxygenation.
11. Prevention or correction of hypothermia and blood volume deficits has been shown to decrease wound infections and increase collagen deposition in patients undergoing major abdominal surgery.
12. Modifiable risks include smoking, malnutrition, obesity, hyperglycemia, hypercholesterolemia, and hypertension. These should be assessed and corrected when possible prior to surgery.
13. Maintenance of a high room temperature or active warming before, during, and after the operation is significantly more effective than other methods of warming, such as circulating water blankets placed on the surface of the operating table and humidification of the breathing circuit.
14. Optimizing the volume of perioperative fluid administration to minimize morbidity and mortality remains a significant and controversial challenge.
15. Current best recommendations for volume management include replacing fluid losses based on standard recommendations for the type of surgery, replacement of blood loss, and replacement of other ongoing fluid losses (e.g., high urine output due to diuretic or dye administration, hyperglycemia, or thermoregulatory vasoconstriction).
16. Wounds are most vulnerable in the first few hours after surgery.
17. All vasoconstrictive stimuli must be corrected simultaneously to allow optimal healing.
18. Local perfusion is not assured until patients have a normal blood volume, are warm and pain-free, and are receiving no vasoconstrictive drugs; that is, until the sympathetic nervous system is inactivated.
19. Urine output is a poor, often misleading guide to peripheral perfusion.
20. Physical examination of the patient is a better guide to hypovolemia and vasoconstriction.

21 Administration of supplemental oxygen via face mask or nasal cannulae increases safety in patients receiving systemic opioids. As a side benefit, it may also improve wound healing. Pain control also appears important since it favorably influences both pulmonary function and vascular tone.

 22 In patients with moderate to high risk of surgical site infection, anesthesiologists have the opportunity to enhance wound healing and reduce the incidence of wound infections by simple, inexpensive, and readily available means.

Multimedia

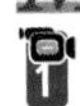 Oxygen Tension in Wound Module

Despite major advances in the management of patients undergoing surgery—including aseptic technique, prophylactic antibiotics, and advances in surgical approaches such as laparoscopic surgery—surgical wound infection and wound failure remain common complications of surgery (Fig. 13-1). Wound complications are associated with prolonged hospitalization, increased resource consumption, and even increased mortality. More than 300,000 surgical site infections (SSIs; Table 13-1) occur each year in the United States at an estimated cost of more than $1 billion.[2] A growing body of literature supports the concept that patient factors are a major determinant of wound outcome following surgery. Comorbidities such as diabetes and cardiac disease clearly contribute, but environmental stressors as well the individual response to stress may be equally important. In particular, wounds are exquisitely sensitive to hypoxia, which is both common and preventable. Perioperative management can be adapted to promote postoperative wound healing and resistance to infection. Along with aseptic technique and prophylactic antibiotics, maintaining perfusion and oxygenation of the wound is paramount. This chapter discusses how knowledge of the principles of infection control and the biology and physiology of wound repair and resistance to infection can improve outcomes.

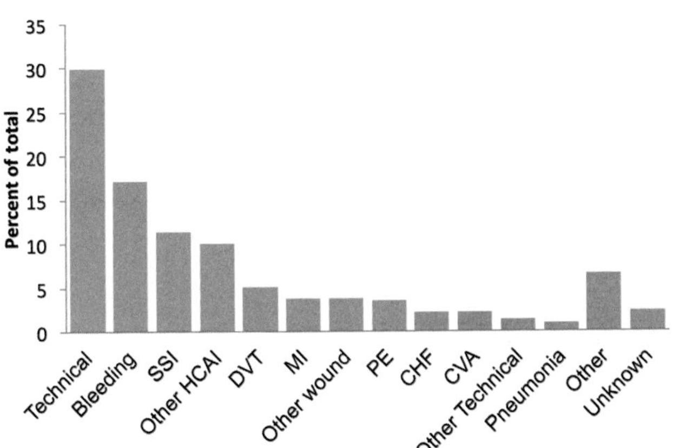

FIGURE 13-1. Thomas et al.[1] reviewed the records of 15,000 nonpsychiatric patients discharged from a representative sample of Utah and Colorado hospitals in 1992 for adverse events. There were 17,912 adverse events identified, or 2.9 ± 0.2% of hospitalizations. Of these, almost half (45%) were related to operative care. The graph shows the distribution of adverse events within the subcategory of operative care (7,716 operative adverse events). Note that about 20% were infection related and about 15% were wound related. SSI, surgical site infection; HCAI, health care–associated infection; DVT, deep venous thrombosis; MI, myocardial infarction; PE, pulmonary embolus; CHF, congestive heart failure; CVA, cerebrovascular accident. (Data from: Thomas EJ, Studdert DM, Burstin HR, et al. Incidence and types of adverse events and negligent care in Utah and Colorado. *Med Care* 2000;38:261–271.)

INFECTION CONTROL

Hand Hygiene

1 Perhaps the most crucial component of infection prevention is frequent and effective hand hygiene. In 1847 Ignaz Semmelweis made the observation that women who delivered their babies in the First Clinic at the General Hospital of Vienna, staffed by medical students and physicians, had a mortality rate of 5% to 15%, largely the result of puerperal infections; this was substantially higher than the 2% rate of women who delivered at Clinic 2, which was staffed by midwife students and midwives.[3] Students and physicians at Clinic 1 usually started the day performing autopsies (including on patients who died of puerperal fever) and then moved on to the clinic, where they performed examinations on women in labor. Semmelweis made the connection, and although germ theory was some years off, he insisted that physicians and medical students wash their hands in a chlorinated solution when leaving the pathology laboratory. This reduced the rate of puerperal fever to the same rate as at Clinic 2. Soon, Semmelweis identified cases of transmission from an infected to an uninfected patient, and instituted the use of chlorinated solution hand washing between cases as well. He also demonstrated that the chlorinated solution was more effective than soap and water. Unfortunately, his innovation was not widely adopted, resulting from a combination of his delay in publishing his results, the reluctance of his colleagues to accept that they might be responsible for transmitting disease, and his lack of tact in trying to convince health care workers to adopt his measures. Despite our current knowledge of germ theory, hand hygiene remains an inexplicably neglected component of infection control: Studies consistently demonstrate about a 40% rate of adherence (range, 5% to 81%) to hand hygiene guidelines.[4]

Bacteria are resident in the skin and can never be completely eliminated.[4] Resident flora are embedded in the deeper folds of the skin and are more resistant to removal, but are also infrequently pathogenic. Coagulase-negative staphylococci and diphtheroids

TABLE 13-1. CRITERIA FOR DEFINING A SURGICAL SITE INFECTION (SSI)

Superficial Incisional SSI

- Infection occurs within 30 days after the operation
  and
- Infection involves only skin or subcutaneous tissue of the incision
  and
- At least *one* of the following:
  1. Purulent drainage, with or without laboratory confirmation, from the superficial incision
  2. Organisms isolated from an aseptically obtained culture of fluid or tissue from the superficial incision
  3. At least one of the following signs or symptoms of infection: Pain or tenderness, localized swelling, redness, or heat *and* superficial incision is deliberately opened by the surgeon, *unless* the incision is culture-negative
  4. Diagnosis of superficial incisional SSI by the surgeon or attending physician
- Do *not* report the following conditions as superficial incisional SSI:
  1. Stitch abscess (minimal inflammation and discharge confined to the points of suture penetration)
  2. Infection of an episiotomy or newborn circumcision site
  3. Infected burn wound
  4. Incisional SSI that extends into the facial and muscle layers (see "Deep Incisional SSI")

Note: Specific criteria are used for identifying infected episiotomy and circumcision sites and burn wounds

Deep Incisional SSI

- Infection occurs within 30 days after the operation if no implant is left in place or within 1 year if implant is in place and the infection appears to be related to the operation
  and
- Infection involves deep soft tissues (e.g., fascial and muscle layers) of the incision
  and
- At least *one* of the following:
  1. Purulent drainage from the deep incision but not from the organ/space component of the surgical site
  2. A deep incision spontaneously dehisces or is deliberately opened by a surgeon when the patient has at least one of the following signs or symptoms: Fever (>38°C), localized pain, or tenderness, unless site is culture-negative
  3. An abscess or other evidence of infection involving the deep incision is found on direct examination, during reoperation, or by histopathologic or radiologic examination
  4. Diagnosis of a deep incisional SSI by a surgeon or attending physician

Notes:

1. Report infection that involves both superficial and deep incision sites as deep incisional SSI
2. Report an organ/space SSI that drains through the incision as a deep incisional SSI

Organ/Space SSI

- Infection occurs within 30 days after the operation if no implant is left in place or within 1 year if implant is in place and the infection appears to be related to the operation
  and
- Infection involves any part of the anatomy (e.g., organs or spaces), other than the incision, which was opened or manipulated during an operation
  and
- At least *one* of the following:
  1. Purulent drainage from a drain that is placed through a stab wound into the organ/space
  2. Organisms isolated from an aseptically obtained culture of fluid or tissue in the organ/space
  3. An abscess or other evidence of infection involving the organ/space that is found on direct examination, during reoperation, or by histopathologic or radiologic examination
  4. Diagnosis of an organ/space SSI by a surgeon or attending physician

From: Mangram AJ, Horan TC, Pearson ML, et al. Guideline for Prevention of Surgical Site Infection, 1999. Centers for Disease Control and Prevention (CDC) Hospital Infection Control Practices Advisory Committee. *Am J Infect Control.* 1999;27:97–132, with permission.

are the most common. Transient flora colonize the superficial layers of the skin and thus are easier to remove with hand hygiene. Transient flora are also the source of most health care–associated infections, as health care worker skin can become contaminated from patient contact or contact with contaminated surfaces. Contamination from surfaces is most commonly with organisms such as staphylococci and enterococci, which are resistant to drying. Even "clean" activities such as taking a patient's pulse or applying monitors can lead to hand contamination: 100 to 1,000 colony-forming units of *Klebsiella* species were measured on nurses' hands following such activities in one study.[5] No studies have related hand contamination to actual transmission of infection to patients; however, numerous studies, starting with those of Semmelweis, have demonstrated a reduction in health care–associated infections following institution of hand hygiene or improved adherence to hand hygiene.[4]

A number of products are available for hand hygiene. The
2 ideal agent kills a broad spectrum of microbes, has antimicrobial

activity that persists for at least 6 hours after application, is simple to use, and has few side effects. The most commonly used and efficacious agents are reviewed here.

Plain (not antiseptic) soap and water are generally the least effective at reducing hand contamination.[6] Although obvious dirt is removed by the detergent effect of soap and the mechanical action of washing, bacterial load is not greatly reduced. Further, soap and water hand hygiene is associated with high rates of skin irritation and drying, both of which are risk factors for an increased bacterial load. Soap and water are, however, the most effective at removing spores, and therefore should be used when contamination with *Clostridium difficile* or *Bacillus anthracis* is a concern.[4]

Alcohol-based rinses, gels, and foams denature proteins, and this confers their antimicrobial activity.[4] Ethanol is most commonly used because it has more antiviral activity than isopropanol. Antiseptics containing 60% to 95% ethanol with a water base are germicidal and effective against gram-positive and gram-negative bacteria, lipophilic viruses such as herpes simplex, human immunodeficiency, influenza, respiratory syncytial, and vaccinia viruses, and hepatitis B and C viruses. They have little persistent activity, although regrowth of bacteria does occur slowly after use of alcohol-based products. Combination with low doses of other agents such as chlorhexidine, quaternary ammonium compounds, or triclosan can confer persistent activity. Efficacy depends on volume applied (3 mL is superior to 1 mL) and duration of contact (ideally, 30 seconds).

Chlorhexidine is a cationic bisbiguanide that disrupts cytoplasmic membranes, resulting in precipitation of cellular contents.[4] It is germicidal against gram-positive bacteria and lipophilic viruses, with somewhat less activity against gram-negative bacteria and fungi, and minimal against tubercle bacilli. It has substantial persistence on the skin, and the Centers for Disease Control and Prevention (CDC) has identified it as the topical agent of choice for skin preparation in central venous catheter insertion. It may cause severe corneal damage after direct contact with the eye, ototoxicity after direct contact with the inner or middle ear, and neurotoxicity after direct contact with the brain or meninges. There are reports of bacteria that have acquired reduced susceptibility to chlorhexidine, but these are of questionable clinical pertinence since the concentrations at which resistance was found were substantially lower than that of commercially available products. Recent reports have identified immunoglobulin E–mediated allergic reactions to chlorhexidine.[7] Cases are likely underreported because of the difficulty identifying the source of anaphylactic reactions perioperatively. Chlorhexidine is present in a wide range of medical and community based products, including wipes, impregnated central venous catheters, toothpaste, mouthwash, contact lens cleanser, and food preservatives. Therefore, potentially sensitizing exposures are common.

Iodine and iodophors (iodine with a polymer carrier) penetrate the cell wall and impair protein synthesis and cell membrane function.[4] They are bactericidal against gram-positive, gram-negative, and some spore-forming bacteria including clostridia and *Bacillus* species, although inactive against spores. They also have activity against mycobacteria, viruses, and fungi. Their persistence is generally fairly poor. They cause more contact dermatitis than other commonly used agents, and allergies to this class of topical agent are common. Iodophors generally cause fewer side effects than iodine agents.

The choice of an antiseptic depends on the expected pathogens, acceptability by health care workers, and cost. In general, antiseptics cost about $1 per patient day, far less than the cost of health care–associated infections. In nine studies that examined the effect of improved hand hygiene adherence on health care–associated infections, the majority demonstrated that as hand hygiene practices improved, infection rates decreased.[4]

Barriers to hand hygiene include skin irritation and fear of skin irritation, inaccessibility, time, and health care worker acceptance (largely related to the other factors mentioned). Although alcohol-based agents have long been believed to cause more skin irritation, several recent trials have demonstrated less skin irritation and better acceptance with emollient-containing, alcohol-based hand rubs compared with either antimicrobial or nonantimicrobial soaps. The use of appropriate (glove-compatible) lotions twice a day also reduces skin irritation—as well as leading to a 50% increase in hand hygiene frequency in one study.[4] Alcohol-based gels and foams are also generally more accessible than antiseptic soap and water, as the dispenser may be pocket-sized or placed conveniently near sites of patient care. It has been estimated that alcohol-based gels and foams require only about 25% of the time of going to a sink to wash one's hands. However, soap and water should be used to remove particulate matter including blood and other body fluids or after five to ten applications of alcohol-based agent.

Adherence to hand hygiene guidelines (Tables 13-2 to 13-4) generally decreases as the frequency of indicated hand washing increases, as the workload increases, and as staffing decreases. CDC guidelines for health care providers traditionally focused on hand hygiene prior to entering and after leaving a patient room. More recently, the World Health Organization has developed a campaign highlighting the "5 Moments" of hand hygiene (Fig. 13-2). The campaign emphasizes the need to perform hand hygiene after each contact with a patient or their immediate environment.[8]

In an intensive care unit (ICU), hand hygiene for nurses is generally indicated about 20 times per hour, as compared with a normal ward where this number decreases to 8 times per hour.[4] In the operating room (OR), frequent patient contact by the anesthesiologist requires frequent hand hygiene, probably at about the level of nurses in the ICU, while accessibility is often quite limited. Sinks are available only outside the OR. Therefore, alcohol-based agents should be available within hand's reach of the anesthesia machine. Loftus et al.[9] studied bacterial contamination of the anesthesia work area (adjustable pressure limiting valve complex and agent flowmeter) and cross-contamination of the sterile anesthesia stopcock during 61 first cases in their OR. They found an average increase in bacterial contamination of the work area of 115 colonies per surface area sampled during cases (95% confidence interval: 62–169; $p < 0.001$). Transmission of bacteria from the work area to the sterile stopcock in the patients' intravenous tubing occurred in 32% of cases, including transmission of methicillin-resistant *Staphylococcus aureus* (MRSA) in two cases and vancomycin-resistant *Enterococcus* in one case. A high level of contamination of the work area (>100 colonies per surface area sampled) increased the risk of stopcock contamination 4.7 fold (95% confidence interval: 1.42–15.42; $p = 0.011$).

In a follow-up study, Koff et al.[10] demonstrated that increased hand hygiene episodes (7–9 per hour compared to <0.5 per hour during the control period) triggered by an alarm and encouraged by education decreased work area contamination, decreased stopcock contamination from 32% to 8%, and decreased health care–associated infections significantly. Opportunities were not measured and hand hygiene episodes were not necessarily coordinated with one of the 5 Moments. Thus, transmission of bacterial contamination by the anesthesia provider appears to be common, a potential source of nosocomial infections, and largely preventable.[9] Frequent hand hygiene by anesthesia providers has a direct and positive impact on patient outcomes.

3 Wearing gloves does not reduce the need for hand hygiene. Although gloves provide protection, bacterial flora from patients

TABLE 13-2. INDICATIONS FOR HAND HYGIENE

- When hands are visibly dirty or contaminated with proteinaceous material or are visibly soiled with blood or other body fluids, wash hands with either a nonantimicrobial soap and water or an antimicrobial soap and water.
- If hands are not visibly soiled, use an alcohol-based hand rub for routinely decontaminating hands. Alternatively, wash hands with an antimicrobial soap and water.
- Decontaminate hands before having direct contact with patients.
- Decontaminate hands before donning sterile gloves when inserting a central intravascular catheter.
- Decontaminate hands before inserting indwelling urinary catheters, peripheral vascular catheters, or other invasive devices that do not require a surgical procedure.
- Decontaminate hands after contact with a patient's intact skin (e.g., applying monitors, moving patient).
- Decontaminate hands after contact with body fluids or excretions, mucous membranes, nonintact skin, and wound dressings if hands are not visibly soiled.
- Decontaminate hands if moving from a contaminated-body site (e.g., mouth during tracheal intubation) to a clean-body site (e.g., adjusting gas flow, turning on ventilator, starting IV) during patient care.
- Decontaminate hands after contact with inanimate objects (including medical equipment) in the immediate vicinity of the patient. Take care to reduce contamination of the anesthesia machine (e.g., after tracheal intubation) as well!
- Decontaminate hands after removing gloves.
- Before eating and after using a restroom, wash hands with a nonantimicrobial soap and water or with an antimicrobial soap and water.
- Antimicrobial-impregnated wipes (i.e., towelettes) may be considered as an alternative to washing hands with nonantimicrobial soap and water. Because they are not as effective as alcohol-based hand rubs or washing hands with an antimicrobial soap and water for reducing bacterial counts on the hands of HCWs, they are not a substitute for using an alcohol-based hand rub or antimicrobial soap.

IV, intravenous (tube); HCW, health care worker.
Modified from: Boyce JM, Pittet D. Guideline for hand hygiene in health-care settings. Recommendations of the Healthcare Infection Control Practices Advisory Committee and the HIPAC/SHEA/APIC/IDSA Hand Hygiene Task Force. *Am J Infect Control.* 2002;30(8):S1.

may be cultured from up to 30% of health care workers who wear gloves during patient contact.[4] Therefore, hand hygiene should be practiced both before putting on gloves and immediately after removal. Moreover, gloves should be removed or changed immediately after each procedure, including vascular access, intubation, and neuraxial anesthesia, because gloves become contaminated by patient contact just as hands do. Balancing hand hygiene with close attention to the patient during critical portions of the case (e.g., securing the airway) can be challenging. Double gloving and providing a convenient location for contaminated equipment have been suggested as effective approaches.[11]

Artificial and long fingernails, as well as chipped fingernail polish, are associated with higher concentrations of bacteria on the hands of health care workers. Artificial nails have been identified as a source in several hospital-associated outbreaks of infection with gram-negative bacilli and yeast, and CDC guidelines discourage wearing of artificial nails by health care workers in high-risk settings; many hospitals have banned wearing of artificial nails by any employee who has direct patient contact.[4] It may also be appropriate to counsel patients scheduled for surgery that artificial nails may increase their risk of infection, although this has not been investigated. Large quantities of bacteria are

TABLE 13-3. HAND HYGIENE TECHNIQUE

- When decontaminating hands with an alcohol-based hand rub, apply the recommended volume of product to the palm of one hand and rub hands together, covering all surfaces of hands and fingers, until hands are dry.
- When washing hands with soap and water, wet hands first with water, apply an amount of the product recommended by the manufacturer to hands, and rub hands together vigorously for at least 15 seconds, covering all surfaces of the hands and fingers. Rinse hands with water and dry thoroughly with a disposable towel. Use towel to turn off the faucet. Avoid using hot water because repeated exposure to hot water may increase the risk of dermatitis.
- Liquid, bar, leaflet, or powdered forms of plain soap are acceptable when washing hands with a nonantimicrobial soap and water. When bar soap is used, soap racks that facilitate drainage and small bars of soap should be used.

Modified from: Boyce JM, Pittet D. Guideline for hand hygiene in health-care settings. Recommendations of the Healthcare Infection Control Practices Advisory Committee and the HIPAC/SHEA/APIC/IDSA Hand Hygiene Task Force. *Am J Infect Control.* 2002;30(8):S1.

TABLE 13-4. SKIN CARE

- Provide health care workers with hand lotions or creams to minimize the occurrence of irritant contact dermatitis associated with hand antisepsis or hand washing.
- Solicit information from manufacturers regarding any effects that hand lotions, creams, or alcohol-based hand antiseptics may have on the persistent effects of antimicrobial soaps being used in the institution, as well as on glove integrity. Select a combination of products that minimizes these effects.

Modified from: Boyce JM, Pittet D. Guideline for hand hygiene in health-care settings. Recommendations of the Healthcare Infection Control Practices Advisory Committee and the HIPAC/SHEA/APIC/IDSA Hand Hygiene Task Force. *Am J Infect Control.* 2002;30(8):S1.

Your 5 moments for HAND HYGIENE

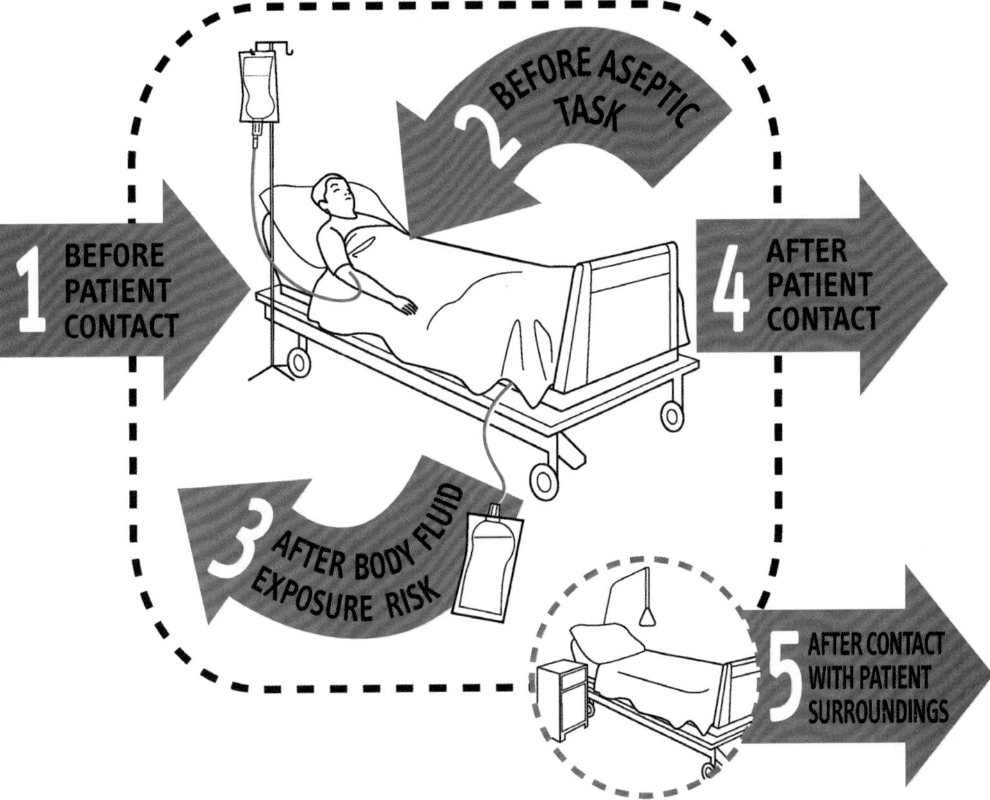

1 BEFORE PATIENT CONTACT	WHEN? Clean your hands before touching a patient when approaching him or her WHY? To protect the patient against harmful germs carried on your hands
2 BEFORE AN ASEPTIC TASK	WHEN? Clean your hands immediately before any aseptic task WHY? To protect the patient against harmful germs, including the patient's own germs, entering his or her body
3 AFTER BODY FLUID EXPOSURE RISK	WHEN? Clean your hands immediately after an exposure risk to body fluids (and after glove removal) WHY? To protect yourself and the health care environment from harmful patient germs
4 AFTER PATIENT CONTACT	WHEN? Clean your hands after touching a patient and his or her immediate surroundings when leaving WHY? To protect yourself and the health care environment from harmful patient germs
5 AFTER CONTACT WITH PATIENT SURROUNDINGS	WHEN? Clean your hands after touching any object or furniture in the patient's immediate surroundings, when leaving - even without touching the patient WHY? To protect yourself and the health care environment from harmful patient germs

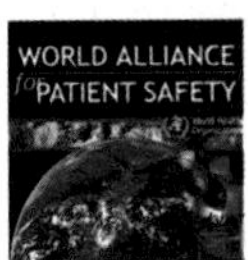

WHO acknowledges the Hôpitaux Universitaires de Genève (HUG), in particular the members of the Infection Control Programme, for their active participation in developing this material.

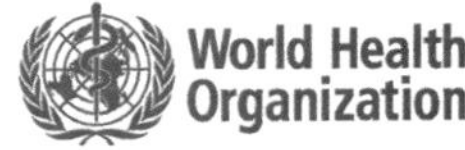

October 2006, version 1.

FIGURE 13-2. World Health Organization schematic of the "5 Moments" for hand hygiene.

typically trapped under the fingernails, and 2002 CDC guidelines recommend that health care workers keep their nail tips trimmed to less than ¼ inch.[4]

Bacteria may be cultured at higher concentrations from the skin beneath a ring. On the other hand, wearing a ring does not increase overall bacterial levels measured on the hands of health care workers. Therefore, it remains unclear whether transmission of infection could be reduced by prohibiting health care workers from wearing rings.[4]

Antisepsis

Masks have long been advocated as preventing SSI, and are used almost universally in the US operating rooms. Tunevall.[12] studied the rate of wound infections in 3,088 patients over 115 weeks. In alternating weeks, OR personnel either wore masks or did not (personnel with active respiratory infections continued to wear masks). There was no difference in the rate of surgical wound infections (4.7% vs. 3.5%, respectively) in the two groups, nor in bacterial species cultured from the wounds. Friberg et al.[13] demonstrated comparable air and surface contamination during sham surgery in a horizontal laminar airflow unit whether OR personnel wore a nonsterile hood and mask or a sterilized helmet aspirator system. When the head cover but not the mask was omitted, however, contamination increased three- to five-fold. These data suggest that wearing a head cover is useful for preventing SSI, while wearing a mask is not. Nonetheless, the study by Tunevall is a small one, and most hospital personnel continue to require a mask in the OR while surgical instruments are open. Moreover, the mask does serve the purpose of protecting the health care provider, particularly when combined with eye protection, and thus should most likely be used during tracheal intubation, emergence from anesthesia, and at other times when exposure to body fluids is likely.

Although the preponderance of postoperative surgical infections is caused by flora that are endogenous to the patient, environmental and airborne contaminants may also play a causative role. An important, but frequently overlooked, consideration is the role that traffic patterns into an OR can play in patient exposure to airborne organisms. A recent Israeli study of risk factors for surgical infection after total knee replacement demonstrated a trend toward increased infection rates within increased number of orthopedic surgeons or anesthetists present in the OR.[14] This study reconfirmed a prior study showing a trend toward increased incidence of SSI as the number of people in the operating suite increases.[15] However, it has been noted in one audit that physicians and nurses did little to limit the number of people through ORs during procedures.[16] Current recommended practices are that traffic patterns should limit the flow of people through an OR that is in use, and that no more people than necessary should be in an OR during a procedure.[17] The anesthesiologist is clearly in a position to play a leadership role in controlling human traffic through the OR.

Mermel et al.[18] in 1991 demonstrated that central venous lines placed by the anesthesiologist in the OR became infected more often (relative risk [RR], 2.1; $p = 0.03$) than those placed by surgeons or other providers, whether in or out of the OR. Contributing factors appeared to be site of placement and the stringency of aseptic technique. Internal jugular vein insertion has a greater risk of infection (RR, 4.3; $p < 0.01$) compared with subclavian vein, although its other benefits may outweigh this risk. Raad et al.[19] demonstrated that use of a maximal sterile barrier technique versus sterile gloves and small sterile drapes led to a significant reduction in central venous catheter-related infection from 7.2% to 2.2% ($p = 0.03$). Therefore, gowning and gloving, careful aseptic technique, and use of a wide sterile field should be routine.[20] In anesthetized patients, the central line is ideally placed before the surgical site is draped in order to avoid contamination of the wire on the underside of the surgical drape.

Epidural abscess formation is an extremely rare but potentially catastrophic complication of neuraxial anesthesia and epidural catheter placement. Therefore, careful attention to aseptic technique and infection control is required. The most important consideration is to prevent contamination of the needle and catheter. Thus, hand washing, skin preparation, draping, and maintenance of a sterile field should be carefully observed. Gowning and wearing a mask likely play a smaller role, but are reasonable given the devastating consequences of infection. Finally, epidurals should probably be avoided in patients known or suspected to have bacteremia or deferred until after appropriate antibiotics are administered.

Antibiotic Prophylaxis

After antibiotics came into widespread use in the 1940s and 1950s, there was much debate over the possibility that antibiotic prophylaxis might prevent SSI. In 1957 Miles et al.[21] used a guinea pig model for the proof of principle that administration of an antibiotic prior to contamination (incision) could reduce the risk of SSI. When appropriate antibiotics were given within 2 hours before or after intradermal injection of bacteria, they were effective in preventing invasive infection and necrosis. When given outside this window, they were not effective. This gave rise to the concept of a "decisive period" in which antibiotics will be effective, which remains a guiding principle of antibiotic prophylaxis. Miles et al. also demonstrated that injection of epinephrine intradermally prior to administration of antibiotics led to antibiotic failure, as demonstrated in an increased wound infection rate. This demonstrated the crucial role of local perfusion in delivering antibiotics to the site. Knighton et al.,[22] using the same model, demonstrated that increased inspired oxygen was equally as effective as antibiotics in preventing infection, and that the two effects were additive (Fig. 13-3). Knighton et al.[23] also delayed the administration of oxygen for up to 6 hours after inoculation and demonstrated no reduction in effect. Thus, the decisive period for oxygen is considerably longer than that of antibiotics.

Two surgeons at Washington University in St. Louis, Harvey Bernard and William Cole,[24] reported on the first controlled clinical trial of the efficacy of antibiotic prophylaxis in 1964 and demonstrated a benefit in abdominal operations. Thereafter, numerous clinical trials were performed with somewhat variable results. Eventually these served to define the timing and population in which prophylactic antibiotics work. By the 1970s antibiotic prophylaxis for high-risk surgery—meaning clean-contaminated and contaminated cases—was becoming well accepted and widely used, although some skeptics remained. In 1992, Classen et al.[25] published their prospective series including 2,847 patients undergoing clean or clean-contaminated surgical procedures at LDS Hospital in Salt Lake City, UT (Fig. 13-4). They demonstrated that the decisive period for SSI in humans undergoing surgery was essentially the same as for experimental infections in guinea pigs. That is, they found the lowest infection rate when antibiotics were given within 2 hours before or after incision and a rapid increase in SSI rate when they were given outside that range. The best results, though only by a small margin and not statistically significant, were within 0 to 60 minutes of surgery, and this subsequently became the clinical standard.

Antibiotic prophylaxis has now become standard for surger-
4 ies in which there is more than a minimum risk of infection.

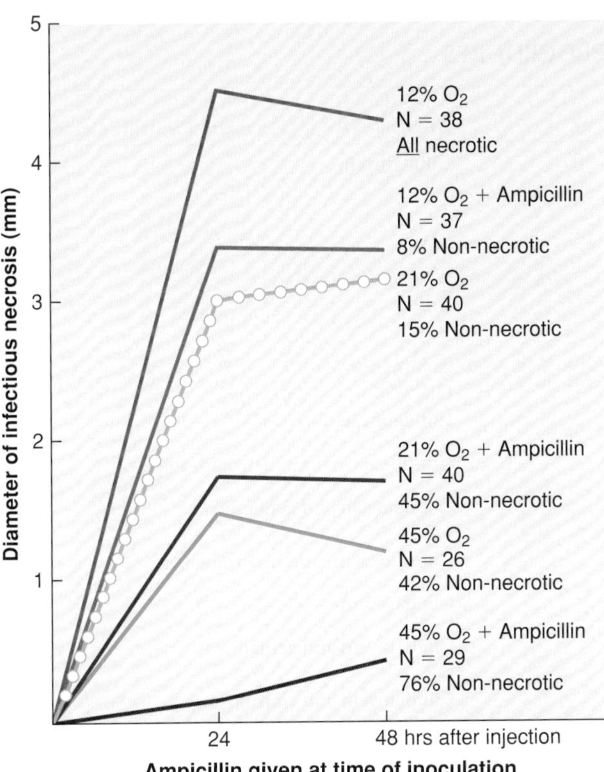

FIGURE 13-3. The effect of oxygen and/or antibiotics on lesion diameter after intradermal injection of bacteria into guinea pigs. Note that at every level, oxygen adds to the effect of antibiotics and that increasing oxygen in the breathing mixture from 12% to 20% or from 20% to 45% exerts an effect comparable to that of appropriately timed antibiotics. (From: Rabkin J, Hunt TK. *Infection and oxygen, Problem wounds: The Role of Oxygen*. Edited by Davis J, Hunt TK. New York, Elsevier, 1988, pp 1, with permission.)

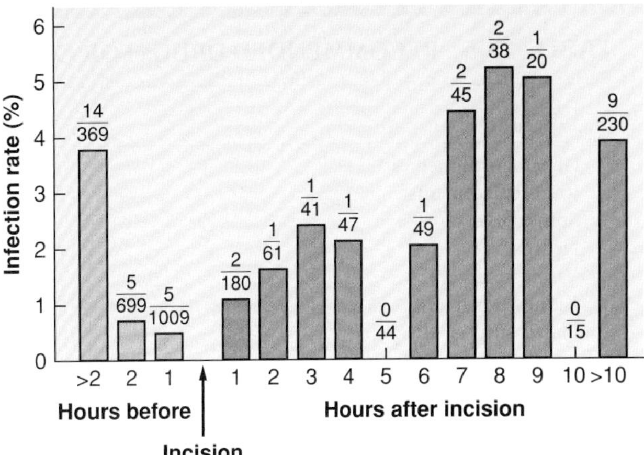

FIGURE 13-4. The figure demonstrates rates of surgical wound infection corresponding to the temporal relation between antibiotic administration and the start of surgery. The number of infections and the number of patients for each hourly interval appear as the numerator and denominator, respectively, of the fraction for that interval. The trend toward higher rates of infection for each hour that antibiotic administration was delayed after the surgical incision was significant (z score = 2.00; $p < 0.05$ by the Wilcoxon test). (From: Classen DC, Evans RS, Pestotnik KS, et al. The timing of prophylactic administration of antibiotics and the risk of surgical-wound infection. *N Engl J Med.* 1992:326;281, with permission.)

Although not every surgery and situation has been studied, a strong rationale for the approach to prophylactic antibiotics has emerged. Several groups separately developed guidelines for use, culminating in recommendations published in 2004 by the National Surgical Infection Prevention Project.[26] These guidelines emphasize timing and choice of appropriate agents. Guidelines generally do not specify antibiotic agents, although they give rationales for various choices.[26] The agent for antibiotic prophylaxis must cover the most likely spectrum of bacteria presented in the surgical field (see Tables 13-5 and 13-6). The most commonly used antibiotic for surgical prophylaxis is cefazolin, a first-generation cephalosporin, as the potential pathogens for most surgeries are gram-positive cocci from the skin.[26,27]

By definition, prophylactic antibiotics are given pre- or intraoperatively. The exact timing for the administration of the antibi-
5 otic depends on the pharmacology and half-life of the drug. It has been suggested that administration of prophylatic antibiotics is ideal within 30 minutes to 1 hour of incision.[27,28] Drugs given by bolus administration (e.g., cefazolin) achieve adequate tissue concentration rapidly, so that giving these drugs within 0 to 30 minutes of incisions appears equally efficacious. Giving the antibiotics too early (so that the incision is more than 60 minutes after the dose) is a recurrent issue at many hospitals, especially for cases that require complex patient positioning. Giving the antibiotics closer to the incision time prevents this problem. Providing timely prophylactic antibiotics is relatively uncomplicated for antibiotics that can be given as a bolus dose (e.g., cephalosporins) or as an infusion over a few minutes (e.g., clindamycin) and thus provide tissue levels within minutes. For drugs like vancomycin that require infusion over an hour, coordination of administration is more complex. In general, it is considered acceptable if the infusion is started prior to incision. When a tourniquet is used, the infusion must be complete prior to inflation of the tourniquet. An appropriate dose based on body weight and volume of distribution should be given. Depending on the half-life, antibiotics should be repeated during long operations or operations with large blood loss.[29] For example, cefazolin is normally dosed every 8 hours but the dose should be repeated every 4 hours intraoperatively.[29] Finally, prophylactic antibiotics should be discontinued by 24 hours following surgery if postoperative dosing is selected at all. Prolonging the course of prophylactic antibiotics does not reduce the risk of infection but does increase the risk of adverse consequences of antibiotic administration,[22] including resistance, *Clostridium difficile* infection, and sensitization.

Unfortunately, MRSA is becoming a more common pathogen. Although it varies by country, region, and hospital, about 60% of *S. aureus* are MRSA. Independent risk factors identified for MRSA infection include prolonged use of prophylaxis, use of drains for more than 24 hours, and increasing number of procedures performed on the patient. Hand hygiene is among the most effective means of preventing development of MRSA since alcohol-based gel or foam used properly kills over 99.9% of all transient pathogens including MRSA. There does not appear to be a justification for using antibiotics effective against MRSA for prophylaxis in most clinical settings.

Because they have access to the patient during the 60 minutes prior to incision and can optimize timing of administration, anesthesiologists should work in consultation with the surgeon to use
6 guidelines determined by the local infection control committee

TABLE 13-5. RECOMMENDED DRUGS FOR COMMON PROCEDURES

Procedure	Primary Drug	Alternate Drug (If Primary Contraindicated)
General orthopedics Joint replacements[a] Spine surgery Neurosurgery Vascular surgery Kidney transplant Plastic surgery	Cefazolin	Clindamycin
Cardiothoracic[a]	Cefazolin	Cefuroxime OR Clindamycin
Colorectal	Cefoxitin	Ciprofloxacin[b] and metronidazole
Gynecology Abdominal hysterectomy	Cefazolin	Clindamycin and gentamicin OR Ciprofloxacin[b] and metronidazole
Open gastric and biliary—low risk	Cefazolin	Clindamycin
Open gastric and biliary—high risk Biliary stent or other foreign body placement	Cefoxitin	Clindamycin and gentamicin OR Clindamycin and ciprofloxacin[b]
Head and neck—low risk	Cefazolin	Clindamycin and gentamicin
Head and neck— high risk Oral cavity involvement	Clindamycin	Clindamycin and gentamicin OR Ertapenem
Genitourinary—low risk	Cefazolin	Clindamycin
Genitourinary— high risk ESWL with nonsterile urine Implant or other foreign body placement	Ciprofloxacin[b]	
Low-risk elective procedures without implants • Laparoscopic cholecystectomy • Breast biopsy • Inguinal hernia repair • Anorectal surgery • ESWL with sterile urine • Thyroidectomy	Cefazolin OR No antibiotics	Clindamycin OR No antibiotics
Cases in which therapeutic antibiotics have already been given in ER (e.g., appendicitis, acute cholecystitis)	Continue antibiotics started in ER. Re-dose using guidelines for intraoperative re-dosing for the given antibiotic	

NOTE:
- Always confirm with surgeons at the time-out or earlier.
  - The surgeon may wish to delay antibiotics until after culture
  - Antibiotics may not be indicated (e.g., low risk, elective procedures such as laparoscopic cholecystectomy or breast biopsy where implants will not be used)
  - Make sure to record the reason for not giving antibiotics on the record
- Ideally an antibiotic infusion should be completed before incision, but CMS guidelines consider starting the infusion before incision adequate. When possible, for drugs requiring slow (>30 min) infusion, the infusion should be initiated preoperatively.
  - When a tourniquet is used, the dose must be completed at least 5 minutes before the tourniquet is inflated.
- Additional intraoperative doses should be given when there is significant blood loss (~half to one blood volume). Use the recommended second dose for this purpose.
- When *therapeutic* antibiotics are given for an infection or presumed infection (e.g., acute appendicitis), prophylactic antibiotics are not required. Each situation should be examined individually: When was the antibiotic given? Which antibiotic was used? In some cases, coverage of skin flora may be appropriate prior to skin incision, but often continuation of the therapeutic antibiotics is all that is required.

[a]Vancomycin is indicated only for patients undergoing cardiothoracic or joint replacement surgery who are at high risk for MRSA (e.g. transferred from a skilled nursing facility, jail, or long-term care facility). Recent studies [Lee BY, Wiringa AE, Bailey RR, Goyal V, Tsui B, Lewis GJ, Muder RR, Harrison LH. The economic effect of screening orthopedic surgery patients preoperatively for methicillin-resistant Staphylococcus aureus. *Infect Control Hosp Epidemiol.* 2010 Nov;31(11):1130–1138.] suggest screening for MRSA may be a useful approach to identifying patients at high risk.

[b]Note that ciprofloxacin is infused over an hour. Ideally the infusion should be completed before incision, but CMS guidelines consider starting the infusion before incision adequate.

Used with permission from the University of Utah Health Care.

TABLE 13-6. DRUGS AND DOSES AVAILABLE ROUTINELY FOR ANTIBIOTIC PROPHYLAXIS

Drug	Initial Dose (<80 kg)	Initial Dose (≥80 kg)	Timing	Repeat Dose[d] (Interval)	Interval for Serum Creatinine >3
Drugs to Be Given in the operating room (OR) by the Anesthesia Team					
Cefazolin	1 g	2 g	0–60 min before incision	1 g (4 hr)	12 hr
Cefoxitin	2 g	2 g	0–60 min before incision	1 g Q3h	12 hr
Cefuroxime	1.5 g	1.5 g	0–60 min before incision	1.5 g Q4h No repeat dose for serum creatinine >3	No re-dose
Clindamycin	600 mg	900 mg	Infuse over 10–15 min[a]	600 mg Q6h	12 hr
Gentamicin	1.5 mg/kg	1.5 mg/kg	Infuse over 10–15 min[a]	1 mg/kg Q6h	12 hr
Metronidazole	500 mg	500 mg	Infuse over 30 min[a]	500 mg Q6h	12 hr
Aztreonam[b]	2 g	2 g	Infuse over 30 min[a]	1 g Q4h	12 hr
Ertapenem[c]	1 g	1 g	Infuse over 30 min[a]	Q24h	Q24h
Re-dose for Therapeutic Antibiotics Started Preoperatively					
Piperacillin/Tazobactam (Zosyn)[c]	3.375 g	3.375 g	Infuse over 30 min[a]	Re-dose prior to incision if most recent dose >2 hr before incision; then re-dose Q4h	12 hr
Ampicillin/Sulbactam (Unasyn)	1.5 g	3 g	Infuse over 30 min[a]	Re-dose prior to incision if most recent dose >2 hr before incision; then re-dose Q4h	12 hr
Meropenem[c]	500 mg	500 mg	Infuse over 30 min[a]	Re-dose prior to incision if most recent dose >2 hr before incision; then re-dose Q4h	12 hr
Cefazolin[c]	1 g	2 g	0–60 min before incision	Re-dose prior to incision if most recent dose >2 hr before incision; then re-dose 1 g Q4h	12 hr

Drug	Initial Dose	Timing	Repeat Dose (Interval)
Drugs to be Given in the Preoperative Setting by a Ragistered Nurse			
Vancomycin[e] (<110 kg)	1.5 g	Infuse over 1.5 hr; Complete within 0–60 min prior to incision	Single re-dose at 8 hr No repeat dose for serum creatinine >2
Vancomycin[e] (≥ 110 kg)	2 g	Infuse over 2 hr; Complete within 0–60 min prior to incision	Single re-dose at 8 hr No repeat dose for serum creatinine >2
Levofloxacin	500 mg	Infuse over 60 min Complete within 0–60 min prior to incision	500 mg Q12h
Ciprofloxacin (IV)[f]	400 mg	Infuse over 60 min Complete within 0–60 min prior to incision	400 mg Q6h
Ciprofloxacin (Oral)[f]	500 mg	Take p.o. 60 min prior to OR	400 mg IV Q6h

[a]Infusion must begin prior to incision (CMS guidelines). Ideally, it should be completed before incision as well.
[b]Aztreonam is indicated only for ventricular assist device placement; it is given in addition to vancomycin in those patients.
[c]Protocol used when therapeutic antibiotics are started preoperatively (e.g., in the Emergency Department) to treat actual or presumed infections, e.g., appendicitis or acute cholecystitis. Either the same drug can be continued or the usual prophylactic antibiotic agent for that procedure may be used. Note that, procedurally, these cases are not counted in our compliance monitoring, because these are therapeutic rather than prophylactic guidelines. These cases were created to provide guidance to providers in determining when to re-dose the antibiotics from the perspective of patient benefit.
[d]Note that dosing schedule is more frequent than for therapeutic use to maintain wound tissue levels throughout surgery and ongoing contamination.
Used with permission from the University of Utah Healthcare.
[e]Vancomycin is indicated only for patients undergoing cardiac or joint replacement surgery who are at high risk of MRSA infection based on surveillance. These patients should be identified in the preoperative clinic. They should never be scheduled as first case, and should be asked to come in 3–4 hours before surgery so that vancomycin can be initiated in the preoperative setting.
[f]Oral administration is acceptable for urology cases.

to take initiative for administering prophylactic antibiotics. In this way, anesthesiologists can make a major contribution to preventing SSI. The Centers for Medicare and Medicaid Services has identified timely and appropriate antibiotic prophylaxis administration as a cornerstone of SSI prevention. Physician and hospital reimbursements are increasingly tied to such performance measures, meaning anesthesiologists also have an economic interest in ensuring adherence to guidelines.

MECHANISMS OF WOUND REPAIR

Wound healing is a complex process, requiring a coordinated repair response including inflammation, matrix production, angiogenesis, epithelization, and remodeling (Fig. 13-5). Many factors may impair wound healing. Systemic factors such as medical comorbidities, nutrition,[30] sympathetic nervous system activation,[31] and age[32–34] have a substantial effect on the repair process. Local environmental factors in and around the wound including bacterial load,[35] degree of inflammation, moisture content,[36] oxygen tension,[37] and vascular perfusion[38] also have a profound effect on healing. Although all of these factors are important, perhaps the most critical element is oxygen supply to the wound. Wound hypoxia impairs each of the components of healing.[39]

Although the role of oxygen is usually thought of in terms of aerobic respiration and energy production via oxidative phosphorylation, in wound healing oxygen is required as a cofactor for enzymatic processes and for cell-signaling mechanisms. Oxygen is a rate-limiting component in leukocyte-mediated bacterial killing and collagen formation because specific enzymes require oxygen at a partial pressure of at least 40 mm Hg.[40,41] The mechanisms by which the other processes are oxygen-dependent are less clear, but these processes also require oxygen at a concentration much above that required for cellular respiration.[42–45]

The Initial Response to Injury

A surgical incision disrupts the skin barrier, creating an acute wound, and an effective initial response to injury depends on the ability to clean foreign material and to resist infection. This response initiates a sequence of events that starts with any source of injury that disrupts homeostasis in the local environment and eventually leads to healing.

Wound healing has traditionally been described in four separate phases: Hemostasis, inflammation, proliferation, and remodeling.[46]

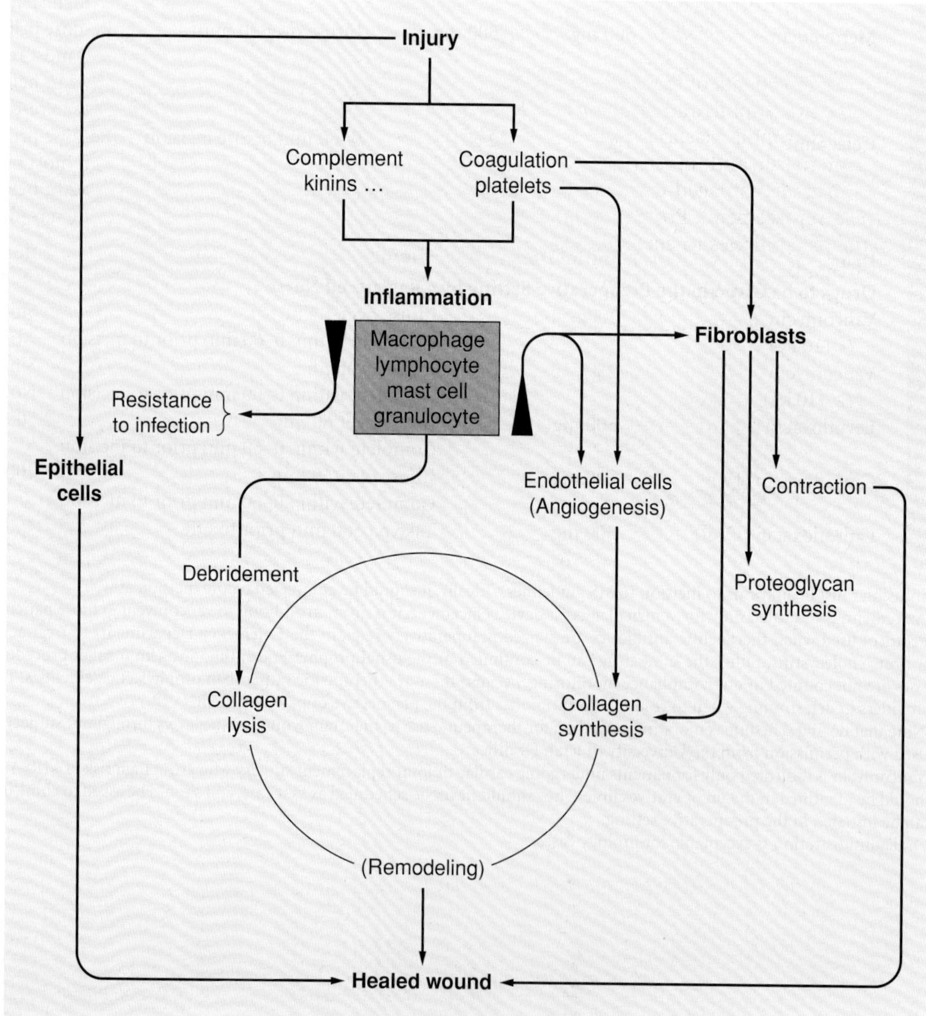

FIGURE 13-5. Schematic of the processes of wound healing. (From Hunt T. *Fundamentals of wound management in surgery, wound healing: Disorders of Repair.* South Plainfield, NJ, Chirugecom, Inc., 1976, with permission.)

Considerable overlap exists between each of these phases, and differentiating precisely when one phase ends and the next begins is virtually impossible. Each phase is composed of complex interactions between host cells, contaminants, cytokines, and other chemical mediators that, when functioning properly, lead to repair of injury. These processes are highly conserved across species,[47] indicating the critical importance of the inflammatory response that directs the process of cellular/tissue repair. When any component of healing is disturbed and interrupts the orderly progression of repair, wound failure may result.[48]

Injury damages the local circulation and causes platelets to aggregate and release a variety of substances, including chemoattractants and growth factors.[46] The initial result is coagulation, which prevents exsanguination but also widens the area that is no longer perfused. Platelet degranulation releases platelet-derived growth factor, transforming growth factor beta (TGF-β), epidermal growth factor, and insulin-like growth factor-1 (IGF-1), which conjointly initiate the inflammatory process.[46] Bradykinin, complement, and histamine released by mast cells cause vasodilation and increased vascular permeability. Polymorphonuclear leukocytes arrive at the wound almost immediately and are followed by macrophages at 24 to 48 hours. These inflammatory cells activate in response to endothelial integrins, selectins, cell adhesion molecules, cadherins, fibrin, lactate, hypoxia, foreign bodies, infectious agents, and growth factors.[46] In turn, macrophages and lymphocytes produce more lactate[49] and growth factors, including IGF-1, leukocyte growth factor, interleukins (ILs) 1 and 2, TGF-β, and vascular endothelial growth factor (VEGF).[50] This early inflammatory phase is characterized by erythema and edema of the wound edges.

Activated neutrophils and macrophages also release proteases, including neutrophil elastase, neutrophil collagenase, matrix metalloproteinase, and macrophage metalloelastase.[46] These proteases degrade damaged extracellular matrix components to allow their replacement. Proteases also degrade the basement membrane of capillaries to enable inflammatory cells to migrate into the wound.

In wounds, local blood supply is compromised at the same time that metabolic demand is increased. As a result, the wound environment becomes hypoxic and acidotic with high lactate levels.[51,52] This represents the sum of three effects: (1) decreased oxygen supply due to vascular damage and coagulation, (2) increased metabolic demand due to the heightened cellular response (anaerobic glycolysis), and (3) aerobic glycolysis by inflammatory cells.[53,54] Leukocytes contain few mitochondria and therefore acquire energy from glucose, primarily by production of lactate and even in the presence of adequate oxygen supply.[53] In activated neutrophils, the respiratory burst, in which oxygen and glucose are converted to superoxide, hydrogen ion, and lactate, accounts for up to 98% of oxygen consumption; in the setting of injury, this activity increases by up to 50-fold over baseline.[55,56]

Local hypoxia is a normal and inevitable result of tissue injury.[57,58] Hypoxia acts as a stimulus to repair,[59] but also leads to poor healing[37] and increased susceptibility to infection.[60,61] Numerous experimental models[21,60,62,63] as well as human clinical experience[61,64] have led to the conclusion that wound healing is delayed in hypoxic wounds. The partial pressure of oxygen in dermal wounds is heterogeneous, ranging from 0 to 10 mm Hg in the central ("dead space") portion of the wound, to 80 to 100 mm Hg (near arterial) adjacent to perfused arterioles and capillaries (Fig. 13-6).[58] The PO_2 of a given area depends on diffusion of oxygen from perfused capillaries, and thus wound PO_2 depends on capillary density, arterial PO_2, and the metabolic activity of the cells, with some contribution from shifts in the oxyhemoglobin dissociation curve associated with wound pH and temperature.

Resistance to Infection

After a disruption of the normal skin barrier, successful wound healing requires the ability to clear foreign material and resist infection. Neutrophils provide nonspecific immunity and prevent infection. Leukocytes migrate in tissue toward the site of injury via chemotaxis, defined as locomotion oriented along a chemical gradient.[46] Chemical gradients can be produced both exogenously and endogenously. Exogenous gradients result from bacterial

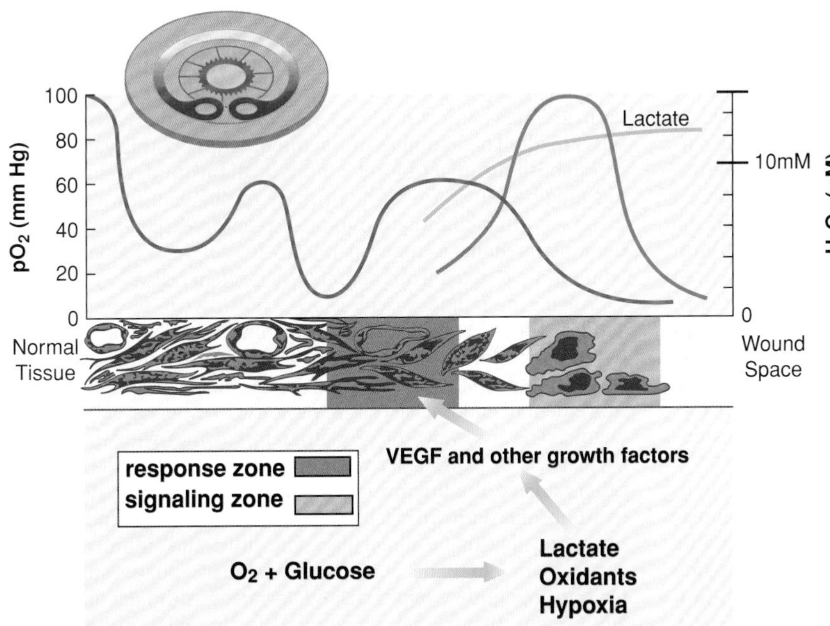

FIGURE 13-6. The varying oxygen tension in the wound module. Cross-section of the wound module in a rabbit ear chamber is in left upper corner of figure. Note that PO_2, depicted graphically above the cross-section (red line), is highest next to the vessels, with a gradient down to zero at the wound edge. Note also the lactate gradient (green line), high in the dead space and lower (but still above plasma) toward the vasculature. Hydrogen peroxide (H_2O_2) is present at fairly high concentrations (blue line) and is also a major stimulus to wound repair.[65] Growth factors such as VEGF are produced by inflammatory cells in the hypoxic, high lactate, high hydrogen peroxide "Signaling Zone" and then diffuse to the "Response Zone" where they act on fibroblasts and endothelial cells to promote healing. VEGF, vascular endothelial growth factor. (Modified version reprinted from: IA Silver. *The physiology of wound healing, Fundamentals of wound management.* Edited by TK Hunt, JE Dunphy. New York, Appleton-Century-Crofts, 1980, p 30, with permission.)

ANATOMY AND PHYSIOLOGY

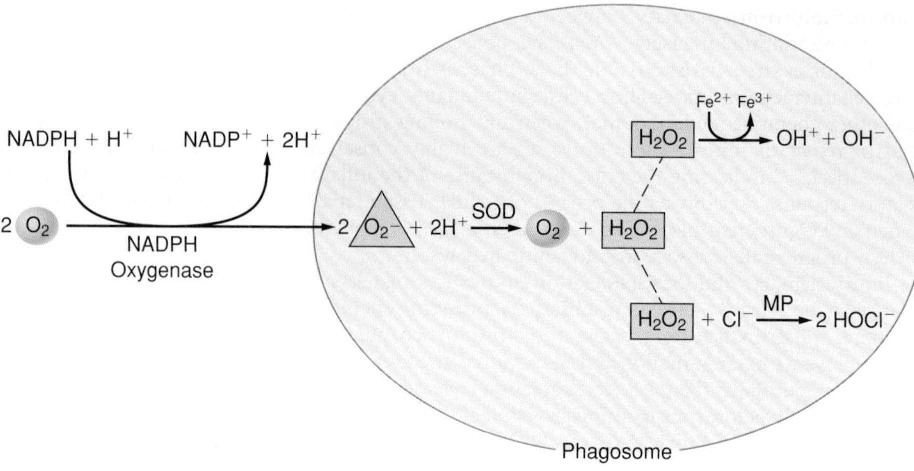

FIGURE 13-7. Schematic of superoxide and other oxidant production within the phagosome. NADPH, nicotinamide adenine dinucleotide phosphate-oxidase; NADP, nicotinamide adenine dinucleotide phosphate; SOD, superoxide dismutase; MP, myeloperoxidase. (From: Hunt TK, Hopf HW. Wound healing and wound infection. What surgeons and anesthesiologists can do. *Surg Clin North Am* 1997;77(3):587–606, with permission.)

products present in contaminated tissues. Endogenous mediators include components of the complement system (C5a), products of lipoxygenase pathway (leukotriene B4), and cytokines (IL-1, 8), along with lactate.[66] Together, these chemical mediators help to organize and control leukocyte invasion, bacterial killing, necrotic tissue removal, and the initiation of angiogenesis and matrix production. In the absence of infection, neutrophils disappear by about 48 hours. Nonspecific phagocytosis and intracellular killing are the major immune pathways activated in wounds.[67]

Neutrophils are the primary cells responsible for nonspecific immunity, and their function depends on a high partial pressure of oxygen.[41,68] This is because reactive oxygen species are the major component of the bactericidal defense against wound pathogens.[67] Phagocytosis of the pathogen activates the phagosomal oxidase (also known as the primary oxidase or nicotinamide adenine dinucleotide phosphate-oxidase [NADPH]-linked oxygenase), present in the phagocytic membrane, which uses oxygen as the substrate to catalyze the formation of superoxide. Superoxide itself is bactericidal, but more importantly it initiates a series of cascades that produce other oxidants within the phagosome that increase bacterial-killing capacity (Fig. 13-7). For example, in the presence of superoxide dismutase, superoxide is reduced to hydrogen peroxide (H_2O_2). H_2O_2 combines with chloride and in the presence of myeloperoxidase forms the bactericidal hypochlorous acid, more commonly recognized as the active ingredient in bleach.[68,69] Since intraphagosomal oxidant production depends on conversion of oxygen to superoxide, the process is exquisitely sensitive to the partial pressure of oxygen in the tissue. The K_m (half-maximal velocity) for the phagosomal oxidase using oxygen as a substrate is 40 to 80 mm Hg.[41] This means that resistance to infection is critically impaired by wound hypoxia and becomes more efficient as PO_2 increases even to very high levels (500 to 1,000 mm Hg).[41] Such levels do not occur naturally in tissue, but can be achieved by the administration of hyperbaric oxygen.[70–72] This is one mechanism for the proposed benefit of hyperbaric oxygen therapy as an adjunctive treatment for necrotizing infections and chronic refractory osteomyelitis.[73,74]

Oxidants produced by inflammatory cells have a dual role in wound repair. Not only are they central to resistance to infection, but they also play a major role in initiating and directing the healing process. Oxidants, and in particular hydrogen peroxide produced via the respiratory burst, increase neovascularization and collagen deposition in vitro and in vivo.[65]

Proliferation

The proliferative phase normally begins approximately 4 days after injury, concurrent with a waning of the inflammatory phase. It consists of granulation tissue formation and epithelization. Granulation involves neovascularization and synthesis of collagen and connective tissue proteins.

Neovascularization

New blood vessels must replace the injured microcirculation. Neovascularization in wounds proceeds both by angiogenesis and vasculogenesis. Angiogenesis is the phenomenon of new vessel growth via budding from existing vessels. In the setting of wounds, new vessels grow from mature vessels, usually intact, postcapillary venules in the undamaged tissue immediately adjacent to the site of injury. Normally, the oxygen tension in adjacent tissue is sufficient to support this process. The new vessel growth extends and enters into the damaged areas that are typically high in lactate and have a low partial pressure of oxygen. Mature extracellular matrix is required for ingrowth of mature vessels.[75]

In vasculogenesis, bone marrow–derived endothelial precursor cells (EPCs) populate the tissue and differentiate and grow into new vessel tubules. In wounds, these tubules appear in the damaged area before any direct anastomosis with preexisting vessels is made. These tubules must connect with existing vasculature to establish an intact blood supply in the wound. Angiogenesis has long been held to be the primary mechanism for new blood vessel growth in granulation tissue. Recent research, however, has demonstrated that as many as 15% to 20% of new blood vessels in wounds are derived from hematopoietic stem cells.[75–77]

Angiogenesis and vasculogenesis both occur in response to similar stimuli, consisting of some combination of redox stress, hypoxia, and lactate. However, the specific mechanisms by which they proceed appear to differ somewhat. Angiogenesis involves the movement of endothelial cells in response to three waves of growth factors. The first wave of growth factors comes with the release by platelets of platelet-derived growth factor, TGF-β, IGF-1, and others during the inflammatory phase. The second wave comes from fibroblast growth factor released from normal binding sites on connective tissue molecules. The third and dominant wave comes from VEGF, delivered largely by macrophages stimulated by fibrinopeptides, hypoxia, and lactate.[78] Although it is usually present, hypoxia is not required for granulation because of constitutive (aerobic) lactate production by inflammatory cells and fibroblasts. Too little lactate leads to inadequate granulation, while levels in excess of about 15 mM—usually associated with inflammation or infection—delay granulation.[79] The capillary endothelial response to angiogenic agents requires oxygen so that angiogenesis progresses in proportion to blood perfusion and arterial PO_2.[80]

Vasculogenesis occurs in response to similar stressors as angiogenesis. EPCs are mobilized from the bone marrow into the circulation via a nitric oxide–mediated mechanism. Tissue hypoxia induces release of VEGF-A, which activates bone marrow stromal nitric oxide synthase. Increased bone marrow nitric oxide leads to release of EPCs into the circulation. These circulating EPCs home to the wound via tissue-hypoxia–induced upregulation of stromal cell-derived factor 1-α. Within the wound, EPCs undergo differentiation and participate in the formation of new blood vessels.[76]

Collagen and Extracellular Matrix Deposition

New blood vessels grow into the matrix that is produced by fibroblasts. Although fibroblasts replicate and migrate mainly in response to growth factors and chemoattractants, production of mature collagen requires oxygen.[40,81,82] Lactate, hypoxia, and some growth factors induce collagen mRNA synthesis and procollagen production. Posttranslational modification by prolyl and lysyl hydroxylases is required to allow collagen peptides to aggregate into triple helices. Collagen can only be exported from the cell when it is in this triple helical structure. The helical configuration is also primarily responsible for tissue strength. The activity of the hydroxylases is critically dependent on vitamin C and tissue oxygen tension, with a K_m for oxygen of about 25 mm Hg.[40,81–83] Wound strength, which results from collagen deposition, is therefore highly vulnerable to wound hypoxia.[37]

Neovascularization and extracellular matrix (primarily collagen) production are closely linked. Fibroblasts cannot produce mature collagen in the absence of mature blood vessels that deliver oxygen to the site. New blood vessels cannot mature without a strong collagen matrix. Mice kept in a hypoxic environment of 13% inspired oxygen develop some new blood vessels in a test wound with the addition of exogenous VEGF or lactate, but these vessels are immature with little surrounding matrix and demonstrate frequent areas of hemorrhage.[42]

Epithelization

Epithelization is characterized by replication and migration of epithelial cells across the skin edges in response to growth factors. Cell migration may begin from any site that contains living keratinocytes, including remnants of hair follicles, sebaceous glands, islands of living epidermis, or the normal wound edge. In acute wounds that are primarily closed, epithelization is normally completed in 1 to 3 days. In open wounds healing by secondary intention, epithelization is the final phase of healing and cannot progress until the wound bed is fully granulated. Like immunity and granulation, epithelization depends on growth factors and oxygen. Silver[84] and Medawar[45] demonstrated in vivo that the rate of epithelization depends on local oxygen. Topical oxygen applied in a manner that does not dry out epithelial cells has been advocated as a method to increase the rate of epithelization.[85] Ngo et al.[86] demonstrated oxygen-dependent differentiation and cell growth in human keratinocyte culture. In contrast, O'Toole et al.[87] demonstrated that hypoxia increases epithelial migration in vitro. This may be explained, at least in part, by the dependence of epithelization on the presence of a bed of healthy granulation tissue, which is known to be oxygen-dependent.

Maturation and Remodeling

The final phase of wound repair is maturation, which involves ongoing remodeling of the granulation tissue and increasing wound tensile strength. As the matrix becomes denser with thicker, stronger collagen fibrils, it becomes stiffer and less compliant. Fibroblasts are capable of adapting to changing mechanical stress and loading. Fibroblasts migrate throughout the matrix to help mold the wound to new stresses. Matrix metalloproteinases and other proteases help with fibroblast migration and continued matrix remodeling in response to mechanical stress. Some fibroblasts differentiate into myofibroblasts under the influence of TGF-β, resulting in contractile cells. As the myofibroblasts contract, the collagenous matrix cross-links in the shortened position. This helps to strengthen the matrix and minimize scar size. Contraction is inhibited by the use of high doses of corticosteroids.[88] Even steroids given several days after injury have this effect. In those wounds where contraction is detrimental, this effect can be used for benefit. Although there is little definitive evidence, one dose of dexamethasone intraoperatively to prevent postoperative nausea and vomiting does not appear to impair healing.

Net collagen synthesis continues for at least 6 weeks and up to 6 months after wounding. Over time, the initial collagen threads are reabsorbed and deposited along stress lines, conferring greater tensile strength. Collagen found in granulation tissue is biochemically different from collagen of uninjured skin, and a scar never achieves the tensile strength of uninjured skin. Hydroxylation and glycosylation of lysine residues in granulation tissue collagen lead to thinner collagen fibers. At 1 week, a wound closed by primary intention has only reached 3% of the tensile strength of normal skin. By 3 weeks it is at 30%, and it only reaches 80% after 3 to 6 months.

Some wounds heal to excess. Hypertrophic scar and keloid are common forms of abnormal scar due to abnormal responses to healing. Hypertrophic scarring may be thought of as "exuberant" scarring in which the inflammatory process that allows wound healing remains excessively active, resulting in stiff, rubbery, nonmobile scar tissue. Hypertrophic scars are most commonly seen following burns and are thought to correlate with the length of time required to close the wound, although other factors are also believed to play a role and are being actively explored. Keloids are scars that outgrow the boundaries of the initial scar, and are most typically seen following surgical incisions. Keloid formation is most likely due to a genetic predisposition, although exogenous inflammatory factors may also play a role.

WOUND PERFUSION AND OXYGENATION

Complications of wounds include failure to heal, infection, and excessive scarring or contracture. Rapid repair has the least potential for infection and excess scarring. The perioperative physician's goals, therefore, are to avoid contamination, ensure rapid tissue synthesis, and optimize the immune response. All surgical procedures lead to some degree of contamination that must be controlled by local host defenses. The initial hours after contamination represent a decisive period during which inadequate local defenses may allow an infection to become established.

Normally, wounds on the extremities and trunk heal more slowly than those on the face. The major difference in these wounds is the degree of tissue perfusion and thus the wound tissue oxygen tension. As a rule, repair proceeds most rapidly and immunity is strongest when wound oxygen levels are high, and this is only achieved by maintaining perfusion of injured tissue.[89] Ischemic or hypoxic tissue, on the other hand, is highly susceptible to infection and heals poorly, if at all.[64] Wound tissue oxygenation is complex and depends on the interaction of blood perfusion, arterial oxygen tension, hemoglobin dissociation conditions, carrying capacity, mass transfer resistances, and local oxygen consumption. Wound oxygen delivery depends on vascular anatomy, the degree of vasoconstriction, and arterial PO_2.

The standard teaching that oxygen delivery depends more on
7 hemoglobin-bound oxygen (oxygen content) than on arterial PO_2 may be true of working muscle, but it is not true of wound healing. In muscle, intercapillary distances are small and oxygen consumption is high. In contrast, intercapillary distances are large and oxygen consumption is relatively low in subcutaneous tissue.[44] In wounds, where the microvasculature is damaged, diffusion distances are substantially increased. Peripheral vasoconstriction further increases diffusion distance.[58] The driving force of diffusion is partial pressure. Hence, a high PO_2 is needed to force oxygen into injured and healing tissues, particularly in subcutaneous tissue, fascia, tendon, and bone, the tissues most at risk for poor healing.

Although oxygen consumption is relatively low in wounds,
8 it is consumed by processes that require oxygen at a high concentration. Inflammatory cells use little oxygen for respiration, producing energy largely via the hexose monophosphate shunt.[41] Most of the oxygen consumed in wounds is used for oxidant production (bacterial killing), with a significant contribution as well for collagen synthesis, angiogenesis, and epithelization. The rate constants (K_m) for oxygen for these components of repair all fall within the physiologic range of 25 to 100 mm Hg.[40,41,45,68,81,90]

Because of the high rate constants for oxygen substrate for the components of repair, the rate at which repair proceeds varies according to tissue PO_2 from zero to at least 250 mm Hg. In vitro fibroblast replication is optimal at a PO_2 of about 40 to 60 mm Hg. Neutrophils lose their ability to kill bacteria in vitro below a PO_2 of about 40 mm Hg.[91,92] These in vitro observations are clinically relevant. "Normal" subcutaneous PO_2, measured in test wounds in uninjured, euthermic, euvolemic volunteers breathing room air, is 65 ± 7 mm Hg.[93] Thus, any reduction in wound PO_2 may impair immunity and repair. In surgical patients, the rate of wound infections is inversely proportional[61] and collagen deposition is directly proportional[37] to postoperative subcutaneous wound tissue oxygen tension.

High oxygen tensions (>100 mm Hg) can be reached in
9 wounds but only if perfusion is rapid and arterial PO_2 is high.[37,89] This is because subcutaneous tissue serves a reservoir function, so there is normally flow in excess of nutritional needs and wound cells consume relatively little oxygen, about 0.7/100 mL of blood flow at a normal perfusion rate.[43,44] When arterial oxygen tension (PaO_2) is high, this small volume can be carried by plasma alone. Contrary to popular belief, therefore, oxygen-carrying capacity, that is, hemoglobin concentration, is not particularly important to wound healing, provided that perfusion is normal.[94,95] Wound PO_2 and collagen synthesis remain normal in individuals who have hematocrit levels as low as 15% to 18% provided they can appropriately increase cardiac output, and vasoconstriction is prevented.[95,96]

Peripheral vasoconstriction, which results from central sym-
10 pathetic control of subcutaneous vascular tone, is probably the most frequent and clinically the most important impediment to wound oxygenation. Subcutaneous tissue is both a reservoir to maintain central volume and a major site of thermoregulation. There is little local regulation of blood flow, except by local heating.[97] Therefore, subcutaneous tissue is particularly vulnerable to vasoconstriction. Sympathetically induced peripheral vasoconstriction is stimulated by cold, pain, fear, and blood volume deficit,[98,99] and by various pharmacologic agents including nicotine,[93] β-adrenergic antagonists, and α_1-agonists, all commonly present in the perioperative environment. Perioperative hypothermia is common and results from anesthetic drugs, exposure to cold, and redistribution of body heat from the core to the periphery.[100] Blood loss and increases in insensible losses increase fluid requirements in the perioperative period, thereby leaving the patient vulnerable to inadequate fluid replacement. Thus, vasomotor tone is, to a large degree, under the perioperative physician's control.[98,99]

Prevention or correction of hypothermia[101] and blood vol-
11 ume deficits[102] have been shown to decrease wound infections and increase collagen deposition in patients undergoing major abdominal surgery. Preoperative systemic (forced air warmer) or local (warming bandage) warming have also been shown to decrease wound infections, even in clean, low-risk surgeries such as breast surgery and inguinal hernia repair.[103] Subcutaneous tissue oxygen tension is significantly higher in patients with good pain control than those with poor pain control after arthroscopic knee surgery.[104] Stress also causes wound hypoxia and significantly impairs wound healing and resistance to infection.[105,106] These effects are clearly mediated, in large part, by changes in the partial pressure of oxygen in the injured tissue.

A number of groups have evaluated whether increasing inspired oxygen during surgery can reduce SSI by increasing wound oxygen levels. Most found benefit. Greif et al.[107] demonstrated in a randomized, controlled, double-blind trial including 500 patients that in warm, volume-replete patients with good pain control undergoing major colon surgery, administration of 80% versus 30% oxygen intraoperatively and for the first 2 hours after surgery significantly reduced the wound infection rate by 50%. Wound oxygen levels were significantly higher (almost double) intraoperatively and in the PACU in the 80% oxygen group. Belda et al.[108] replicated these results (significant 40% reduction in SSI) in a randomized, controlled, double-blind trial in 300 colon surgery patients randomized to 80% versus 30% oxygen intraoperatively and during the first 6 hours after surgery. Surgical and anesthetic management were standardized and intended to support optimal perfusion. Myles et al.[109] demonstrated a significant reduction in major postoperative complications, as well as specifically wound infections in 2,050 major surgery patients randomized to 80% oxygen in 20% nitrogen versus 30% oxygen in 70% nitrous oxide intraoperatively. Bickel et al.[110] demonstrated a significant reduction in SSI (5.6% vs. 13.5%; $p = 0.04$) in patients undergoing open appendectomy ($n = 210$) who received 80% oxygen intraoperatively and high flow oxygen for 2 hours after surgery versus those who received 30% oxygen intraoperatively. Schietroma et al.[111] demonstrated in patients undergoing major rectal cancer surgery ($n = 72$) that the risk of anastomotic leak was 46% lower in the 80% inspired oxygen group (RR, 0.63; 95% confidence interval, 0.42–0.98) versus the 30% group. In a retrospective case control study of patient undergoing spine surgery,[112] intraoperative administered fraction of inspired oxygen of less than 50% was the strongest predictor of SSI (OR, 12; 94% CI, 4.5–33; $P < 0.001$).

Pryor et al.[113] demonstrated a doubling of SSI in patients randomized to 80% versus 35% oxygen intraoperatively ($n = 165$). There were a number of methodologic flaws in the study, but, more importantly, the two groups of patients were not equivalent, which likely explained the increase in infections seen in the 80% oxygen group. Meyhoff et al.[114] found no difference in SSI rate (20.1% vs. 19.1%, p = NS) as a function of oxygen administration in 1,400 patients undergoing colon and gynecologic surgery. A major difference in design from the studies that demonstrated benefit was the use of a highly restricted volume replacement regimen. The stated aim was that patients were to gain no more than 1 kg by the second day after operation. Without data on wound oxygen (which was not measured), it is difficult to determine the reason for the difference in outcome compared to the Greif, Belda, and Myles studies, but wound vasoconstriction and a resulting lack of increase in wound oxygen tension is a strong possibility.

Although the preponderance of evidence indicates that use of high-inspired oxygen intraoperatively and providing supplemental oxygen postoperatively in *well-perfused* patients undergoing major abdominal surgery will reduce the risk of wound infection, there remains controversy about the benefits of high-inspired oxygen. One factor in the hesitation to adopt high-inspired oxygen is concern about potential side effects or toxicity of 80% oxygen. Two of the above studies examined this question in detail and found no difference in pulmonary complications or atelectasis.[114,115] A recent study[116] in patients at low risk for SSI (n = 100) found no difference in postoperative oxygen requirement in patients randomized to 30% oxygen intraoperatively versus those randomized to >90%. Thus, high-inspired oxygen appears to be a low-risk approach to enhancing host defenses and reducing SSI.

Perfusion and oxygen also play a key role in the effectiveness of antibiotic prophylaxis. Delivery of antibiotics depends on perfusion. Parenteral antibiotics given so that high levels are present in the blood at the time of wounding clearly diminish but do not eliminate wound infections.[25] In about one-third of all wound infections, the bacteria cultured from the wound are sensitive to the prophylactic antibiotic given to the patient, even when the antibiotics were given according to standard procedure.[25] The vulnerable third of patients appear to be the hypoxic and vasoconstricted group. When antibiotics are present in the wound at the time of injury, they are trapped in the fibrin clot at the wound site where they may have efficacy against contaminating organisms. Antibiotics diffuse poorly into the fibrin clot; however, so that later administration, whether more than 2 hours after injury or in response to wound infection, will have little effect. On the other hand, oxygen diffuses easily through the fibrin clots and is effective even 6 hours after contamination.[23]

Bactericidal antibiotics currently in use employ oxygen to kill organisms in much the same way as phagocytes. Kohanski[117] has demonstrated that quinolones, β-lactams, and aminoglycosides kill *S. aureus* and *Escherichia coli* by stimulating hydroxyl radical production from oxygen, even though all have different mechanisms for entering bacteria. Suller and Lloyd[118] observed a logarithmic reduction in bacterial cell counts in 10–15 hours in aerobic conditions compared with more than 60 hours to achieve the same result in an anaerobic environment for four facultative anaerobic staphylococcal strains exposed to vancomycin in air-equilibrated versus hypoxic conditions. Thus, maintaining conditions that optimize wound oxygen will also optimize the effectiveness of many commonly used antibiotics.

Role of Dysregulation in Impaired Wound Healing

Human beings challenged by adverse physical or psychosocial events mount a coordinated, adaptive reaction characterized by physiologic arousal. This response is often associated psychologically with the experience of threat or other negative effect. The term for such an arousal reaction is *stress response*, and any event that triggers such a response is a stressor. The major mechanisms of the stress response are the hypothalamic–pituitary–adrenocortical (HPA) axis and the sympatho-adrenomedullary (SAM) axis.[119] Psychosocial stressors evoke cognitive responses such as appraisal, memory, expectation, and the attribution of meaning. These endogenous processes heavily involve the prefrontal and frontal cortices of the brain, and these cortices exert control over aspects of the hypothalamus, including the periventricular nucleus (PVN). The PVN initiates the HPA stress response and controls it through negative feedback mechanisms. The PVN triggers further stress response in the SAM axis by recruiting catecholaminergic cells in the rostral ventrolateral medulla. This structure is a cardiovascular regulatory area involved, together with the solitary nucleus, in the control of blood pressure. The rostral ventrolateral medulla activates the solitary nucleus and, together with it, provides tonic excitatory drive to sympathetic vasoconstrictor nerves that maintain resting blood pressure levels. A normal stress response involves a complex pattern of autonomic arousal that includes increased blood pressure followed by a period of recovery when blood pressure and other aspects of arousal return to normal.

Human life often involves repetitive stressors or a series of stressors. When the HPA axis must mount a new stress response before the previous stress response has fully recovered, it incurs risk of system dysregulation. That is, processes normally self-regulating through negative feedback become unregulated and dysfunctional, with maladaptive consequences. SAM dysregulation, which may involve altered medullary GABAergic neurotransmission,[120] can result in abnormal blood flow of indefinite duration. This, in turn, can compromise oxygenation of the healing wound.

PATIENT MANAGEMENT

Preoperative Preparation

Given knowledge of the physiology of wound healing, what are the best strategies to ensure optimal healing? Wound infection, healing failure, and dehiscence are dreaded complications of surgery. To the degree they are predictable, interventions can be targeted at those patients most at risk (Table 13-7).

The CDC, in the "Study of the Effect of Nosocomial Infection Control" (SENIC),[121] developed a remarkably useful and simple predictive tool based on a score of 0 or 1 for each of the following four patient factors: An abdominal operation, an operation that lasts 2 hours or more, a surgical site that is contaminated or infected, and a patient who will have three or more diagnoses at discharge, exclusive of wound infection. The risk of infection with a score of 0 is 1%, with a score of 1 is 3.6%, with a score of 2 is 9%, with a score of 3 is 17%, and with a score of 4 is 27%. These percentages may seem high, but this index was constructed on 3% of the American surgical patients in 1975–1976 and 1983, and the overall results are consistent with numerous other studies. More recent risk analyses by the same group, based on simpler predictors (e.g., American Society of Anesthesiologists Physical Status Classification) have yielded less sensitivity, but about the same overall infection rate.[122]

Modifiable risks include smoking, malnutrition, obesity,
12 hyperglycemia, hypercholesterolemia, and hypertension. These should be assessed and corrected when possible prior to surgery.

TABLE 13-7. PREOPERATIVE CHECKLIST

- Assess and optimize cardiopulmonary function. Correct hypertension.
- Treat vasoconstriction: Attend to blood volume, thermoregulatory vasoconstriction, pain, and anxiety.
- Assess recent nutrition and treat as appropriate.
- Treat existing infection. Among other actions, clean and treat skin infections.
- Assess wound risk by SENIC[a] score in order to decide on the extent to which prophylactic measures should be taken.
- Start vitamin A or anabolic steroids in patients taking prednisone.
- Improve or maintain blood sugar control.

[a]See text and reference.[114]
From: Hunt TK, Hopf HW. Wound healing and wound infection. What surgeons and anesthesiologists can do. *Surg Clin North Am,* 1997;77:587, with permission.

The decision to delay surgery must take into account both the urgency of the surgery and the severity of the risk.

Stress dysregulation also predisposes to poor wound healing. Human and murine studies are consistent in showing that exposing a subject to a stressor delays wound repair. Animal stress models typically involve restraint or social disruption, while human models usually employ a public speaking challenge.[123] Laboratory stress is short term and associated with increased cortisol and corticosterone levels that downregulate the early inflammatory response. This directly implicates the HPA axis, but the background processes are more extensive. Human studies can also take advantage of naturally occurring stressors such as academic examination or marital discord. Such studies compare stressed and nonstressed populations in rate of healing following a punch biopsy or induced blister. This approach allows investigators to study chronic conditions associated with dysregulation such as depression.

The mechanisms behind wound healing are more extensive than altered HPA axis function alone, and so negative clinical outcomes can take multiple forms. The nervous, endocrine, and immune systems operate interdependently through a common chemical language composed of neurotransmitters, hormones, cytokines, peptides, and endocannabinoids.[119] Simple stress can slow wound healing, but stress-induced dysregulation can lead to enduring dysfunction in autonomic nervous system, endocrine function, and/or immune function. Immune complications include impaired bacterial clearance at the wound,[105] the sickness responses associated with proinflammatory cytokines,[124] and systemic imbalance in the T-helper 1/T-helper 2 (Th1/Th2) cytokine profile. This profile represents balance in the contributions of helper T-cell subsets: Th1 is proinflammatory and Th2 anti-inflammatory. Th1-dominant imbalance indicates excessive inflammation with resultant fatigue, aching joints, and loss of appetite. Surgery sometimes creates a Th2 imbalance, which puts the patient at risk for sepsis, edema, and other complications such as poor sleep. Th1/Th2 balance normally recovers after surgery, but some patients come to surgery already chronically dysregulated in cytokine profile, which may predispose them to poor wound healing and other negative outcomes.

Adverse psychosocial circumstances at the time of surgery may put patients at risk for poor wound healing. Kiecolt-Glaser et al.[125] studied the impact of hostile marital interactions on the healing of experimental blister wounds. High-hostile couples produced more proinflammatory cytokines and healed more slowly than low-hostile couples. Using a tape-stripping model, Muizzuddin et al.[126] investigated the effect of marital dissolution on skin barrier recovery and found that high stress was associated with slower recovery. Bosch et al.[127] studied the healing of a circular wound on the oral hard palate in subjects who varied in depression and/or dysphoria. High-dysphoric individuals had higher wound sizes from day 2 onward and depressive symptoms predicted slower wound healing. Collectively, these studies point to links between psychosocial distress, dysregulation at the system level, and impaired capacity for wound healing. It seems likely that stress-reduction techniques will reduce wound complications, and well-designed clinical trials are needed in this area.

Intraoperative Management

Careful surgical technique is fundamental to optimal wound healing (Table 13-8). Delicate handling of the tissue, adequate hemostasis, and surgeon experience lead to healthier wounds. Incisions should be planned with regard to blood supply, particularly when operating near or in old incisions. Mechanical retractors should be released from time to time to allow perfusion to the wound edges. Judicious antibiotic irrigation of contaminated areas may be effective. Because dried wounds lose perfusion, wounds should be kept moist, especially during long operations. Not all wounds can be anatomically closed. Edema, obesity, the possibility of unacceptable respiratory compromise, or the need to debride grossly contaminated or necrotic soft tissues can all interfere with closure of the wound.

As the operation proceeds, new wounds are made and contamination continues. All anesthetic agents tend to cause hypothermia—first, by causing vasodilation, which redistributes heat from core to periphery in previously vasoconstricted patients, and second, by increasing heat loss and decreasing heat production.[100] Vasoconstriction is uncommon intraoperatively, as the threshold for thermoregulatory vasoconstriction is decreased, but is often severe in the immediate postoperative period when anesthesia is discontinued and the thermoregulatory threshold returns to normal in the face of core hypothermia. The onset of pain with emergence from anesthesia adds to this vasoconstriction because of the associated catecholamine release.[104] Rapid rewarming using a forced air warmer for hypothermic patients

TABLE 13-8. INTRAOPERATIVE MANAGEMENT

- Appropriate prophylactic antibiotics should be given at the start of any procedure in which infection is highly probable and/or has potentially disastrous consequences. Maintain antibiotic levels during long operations.
- Keep patients warm.
- Observe gentle surgical technique with minimal use of ties and cautery.
- Keep wounds moist.
- Antibiotic irrigation in contaminated cases.
- Elevate Pa_{O_2}.
- Delayed closure for heavily contaminated wounds.
- Use appropriate sutures (and skin tapes).
- Use appropriate dressings.

From: Hunt TK, Hopf HW. Wound healing and wound infection. What surgeons and anesthesiologists can do. *Surg Clin North Am.* 1997;77:587, with permission.

in the postanesthesia care unit (PACU) does appear to be effective,[128] although prevention of hypothermia is clearly the goal.[101] Maintenance of a high room temperature or active warming 13 before, during, and after the operation is significantly more effective than other methods of warming such as circulating water blankets placed on the operating table surface and humidification of the breathing circuit.[129]

Forced air warming was the first practical means of keeping patients warm intraoperatively. More recently, a number of other effective approaches have been introduced, including resistive warming, negative pressure warming, and thin, adhesive circulating water pads that are applied directly to the skin.[130]

Volume Management

Surgical stress results in increased intravenous fluid requirements. The increased fluid requirement may be partly due to substances like IL-6, TNF, substance-P, and bradykinin, which are released in response to, and in proportion to, surgical stress.[131] These inflammatory mediators cause both vasodilation and an increase in vascular permeability.[132] This loss of functional intravascular volume is in addition to other known causes of perioperative hypovolemia or fluid loss. These include preoperative mechanical bowel preparation, lack of oral intake, fever, preexisting medical conditions, and medications such as diuretics, as well surgical fluid losses, which include evaporation and blood loss.

There are known serious complications of both hypervolemia and hypovolemia, particularly in the perioperative period. The major complications associated with hypervolemia include pulmonary edema, congestive heart failure, edema of gut with prolonged ileus, and possibly an increase in cardiac arrhythmias.[133] The major complications of hypovolemia, aside from hemodynamic instability, include decreased oxygenation of surgical wounds (which predisposes to wound infection),[37,61,89,134–136] decreased collagen formation,[37,102] impaired wound healing, and increased wound breakdown.

Optimizing the volume of perioperative fluid administra-
14 tion to minimize morbidity and mortality remains a significant and controversial challenge. Estimates of blood loss, third-space fluid losses, and maintenance requirements are notoriously inaccurate and may lead to either over- or under-replacement if used as guides. Currently, most practitioners rely on clinical acumen, vital signs such as heart rate and blood pressure, and urine output to manage perioperative fluids. Surgical patients can be markedly hypovolemic without a change in any one of these variables because of the compensatory action of peripheral vasoconstriction.[37,89,136] Unfortunately, this shunts blood away from skin, increases wound hypoxemia, and increases the risk of surgical wound infection. Kabon et al.[137] performed a randomized, controlled trial to compare standard (8 mL/kg/hr) versus high (16 to 18 mL/kg/hr) volume administration in 253 patients undergoing elective colon resection. They found a trend toward reduced wound infections in the group that received high volume (8.5% vs. 11.3%), which would be a clinically significant reduction. Unfortunately, the study was terminated early, so it had inadequate power. Patients at high risk for heart failure or with end-stage renal disease were excluded, so the study also has limited generalizability.

A number of methods, both invasive and minimally invasive, have been investigated as more sensitive measures of volume status. Hartmann et al.[102] used subcutaneous PO_2 to guide perioperative volume management in a randomized controlled trial in abdominal surgery patients. Patients randomized to the intervention group (vs. usual management) received more fluid, had significantly higher wound oxygen tension, and deposited more collagen in a test wound.

Pulmonary arterial catheters have also been used in an attempt to optimize volume management, generally with little success. Most of these studies were performed in an ICU setting, rather than during surgery. In one study in 4,059 patients undergoing abdominal surgery,[132] those who received a pulmonary artery (PA) catheter had worse outcomes than those who did not. In fact, the rate of major postoperative cardiac events was 15.4% in the PA catheter group versus 3.6% in the control group. This could be partly due to the observation that many clinicians misinterpret PA data.[138] With recent studies demonstrating a lack of patient benefit with PA catheters and the increase in use and availability of less invasive monitors like echocardiography, the future of these catheters is uncertain.[139]

Esophageal Doppler has been advocated as a useful monitor of intraoperative volume status. Mythen and Webb[140] used esophageal Doppler to optimize intraoperative volume management in 60 cardiac patients and demonstrated that the patients with esophageal Doppler-guided fluid management received more IV fluid and had decreased gut hypoperfusion (7% vs. 56%) compared with traditional management. There were also fewer "major complications" (0 vs. 6), although the study was too small to achieve statistical significance. Sinclair et al.[141] randomized 40 patients undergoing surgical repair of proximal femoral fractures to esophageal Doppler-guided volume management or traditional management. The patients with the Doppler-guided fluid management had faster recoveries and more rapid hospital discharge. Esophageal Doppler can be difficult to use reliably. However, the same principles that are used in esophageal Doppler are available in much more advanced technologies like transesophageal echocardiography. Thus, TEE shows promise for guiding volume management in both cardiac and noncardiac surgeries. Identification of the appropriate markers and interventions, however, remains inadequately studied.

A final topic of debate is whether colloids or crystalloids are preferable for intraoperative fluid administration. Synthetic colloids have been associated with coagulopathy when large volumes are delivered, which appears to be in large part mediated by dilution of coagulation factors.[142] Crystalloids, on the other hand, may cause a hypercoagulable state.[143] The intravascular half-life of colloids, either albumin or synthetic colloids, is much longer than that of crystalloids, allowing the total volume of fluid administered to be reduced by including colloids in surgical fluid resuscitation.[144] Edema formation may also be decreased. A number of studies[133,144,145] purport to evaluate intraoperative or postoperative fluid administration in terms of restrictive versus traditional fluid management. Virtually all have compared colloid ("restrictive" group) with crystalloid ("traditional" group) administration. Thus, the "restricted" volume group likely received a larger amount of effective intravascular volume than the traditional or "liberal" group. In general, these studies have demonstrated improved outcomes (reduction in SSI, earlier return of bowel function) for the colloid group. The mechanism for the benefit is unclear, however, as on the basis of effective intravascular volume delivered, the crystalloid groups might actually have been less well volume replaced than the colloid groups.

Current best recommendations include replacing fluid losses
15 based on standard recommendations (Table 13-9) for the type of surgery, replacement of blood loss, and replacement of other ongoing fluid losses (e.g., high urine output due to diuretic or dye administration, hyperglycemia, or thermoregulatory vasoconstriction). Maintenance of normothermia is also critical to optimal volume management. Warm patients are unlikely to develop pulmonary edema with a high rate of fluid administration because they have excess capacitance due to vasodilation. Cold patients, on the other hand, are highly susceptible to pulmonary edema

TABLE 13-9. STANDARD VOLUME MANAGEMENT GUIDELINES FOR SURGICAL PATIENTS

Fluid Requirement = Deficit + Maintenance (baseline plus replacement) + estimated blood loss and other sensible fluid losses
Deficit = Maintenance (1.5 mL/kg/hr) × hours NPO
Adjust for fever, high NG output, bowel preparation, and other sources of ongoing preoperative increased fluid loss
Replace EBL 3:1 with crystalloid, 1:1 with colloid

Maintenance requirements for different surgeries:
Superficial surgical trauma: 1–2 mL/kg/hr
Peripheral surgery
Minimal surgical trauma: 3–4 mL/kg/hr
Head and neck, hernia, knee surgery
Moderate surgical trauma: 5–6 mL/kg/hr
Major surgery without exposed abdominal contents
Severe surgical trauma: 8–10 mL/kg/hr (or more)
Major abdominal, especially with exposed abdominal contents

NPO, nothing by mouth; NG, nasogastric; EBL, estimated blood loss.

even after relatively small fluid boluses. Thermoregulatory vasoconstriction increases afterload, causing increased cardiac work. Moreover, administered fluid cannot open up constricted vessels until the hypothermic stimulus is removed; thus, there is virtually no excess capacitance in the system.

Pain control should be addressed intraoperatively so that patients do not have severe pain on emergence. Achieving the goal is more important than the technique used to do so. Although regional anesthesia and analgesia may provide superior pain relief, the effects of specific analgesic regimens on wound outcome have not yet been adequately studied.

Postoperative Management

Wounds are most vulnerable in the first few hours after surgery
16 (Table 13-10). Although antibiotics lose their effectiveness after the first hours, oxygen-mediated natural wound immunity lasts longer.[22] Even a short period of vasoconstriction during the first day is sufficient to reduce oxygen supply and increase infection risk.[61] Correction and prevention of vasoconstriction in the first 24 to 48 hours after surgery will have significant beneficial effects.[61] Given the large number of diabetic patients who undergo surgery, along with the fact that the stress response frequently induces hyperglycemia intraoperatively even in nondiabetic patients, guidelines for controlling blood sugar in perioperative patients are critical to prevention of SSI. Unfortunately, balancing a narrow therapeutic window between hypoglycemia and hyperglycemia is a complex issue in blood sugar control. Clinical trials have provided conflicting results. A 2001 randomized controlled trial demonstrated a 25% reduction in risk of septicemia in critically ill surgical patients whose blood glucose levels were more tightly controlled than a comparison group.[146] On the other hand, in 2007 Gandhi et al.[147] found no difference in SSI in 400 cardiac surgery patients comparing a target blood sugar of 80–100 versus <200 mg/dL. The NICE-SUGAR study

TABLE 13-10. POSTOPERATIVE MANAGEMENT

- Keep patients warm.
- Provide analgesia to keep patients comfortable, if not pain free. Patient report and the ability to move freely are the best signs of adequate pain relief.
- Only one more dose of antibiotic unless an infection is present or contamination continues.
- Keep up with third-space losses. Remember that fever increases fluid losses.
- Assess perfusion and react to abnormalities.
- Avoid diuresis until pain is gone and patient is warm.
- Assess losses (including thermal losses) if wound is open.
- Assess need for parenteral or enteral nutrition and respond.
- Continue to control hypertension and hyperglycemia.

From: Hunt TK, Hopf HW. Wound healing and wound infection. What surgeons and anesthesiologists can do. *Surg Clin North Am.* 1997;77:587, with permission.

in 6,104 ICU patients demonstrated excess mortality in the tight control[81–111] versus standard (<180) group.[148] The current recommendation is to keep glucose close to normal (e.g., 100 to 180 or 200 mg/dL).[149]

All vasoconstrictive stimuli must be corrected simultaneously
17 to allow optimal healing. Volume is the last to be corrected because vasoconstriction for other reasons induces diuresis and renders the patient relatively hypovolemic (peripherally, not centrally). These measures are particularly important in any patients at high risk for wound complications for other reasons (e.g., malnutrition, steroid use, diabetes), or when vasoconstrictive drugs such as beta-blockers and α-agonists are required for other reasons.

Local perfusion is not assured until patients have a normal
18 blood volume, are warm and pain free, and are receiving no vasoconstrictive drugs; that is, until the sympathetic nervous system is inactivated. Warming should continue until patients are thoroughly awake and active and can maintain their own thermal balance. After major operations, warming may be useful for many hours or even days. The goal is to achieve warmth at the skin; wound vasoconstriction due to cold surroundings often coexists with core hyperthermia. Moderate hyperthermia is not, itself, a problem. When extensive wounds are left open, warmth should be continued, and heat losses due to evaporation should be prevented to avoid vasoconstriction and to minimize caloric losses.

Assessing perfusion, especially in the PACU, is critical. Unfortunately, urine output is a poor, often misleading guide to periph-
19 eral perfusion.[135] Markedly low output may indicate decreased renal perfusion, but normal or even high urine output has little correlation to wound or tissue PO_2. Many factors commonly present in the perioperative period, including hyperglycemia, dye administration, thermoregulatory vasoconstriction, adrenal insufficiency, and various drugs, may cause inappropriate diuresis in the face of mild hypovolemia.

Physical examination of the patient is a better guide to hypo-
20 volemia and vasoconstriction. Assess vasoconstriction by a capillary return time of >2 to 3 seconds at the forehead and >5 seconds over the patella. Eye turgor is another good measure of volume status. Finally, patients can usually distinguish thirst from a dry mouth. Skin should be warm and dry.

After major abdominal surgery, third-space losses continue for about 12 to 24 hours, so that increased fluid requirements continue. In general, for large abdominal cases, 2 to 3 mL/kg/hr of IV fluids is sufficient for the first 12 to 24 postoperative hours. After that period, the IV rate should be decreased below calculated maintenance levels because edema fluid begins to be mobilized, thus increasing circulating intravascular volume.

When excessive tissue fluids have accumulated, diuresis should be undertaken gently so that transcapillary refill can maintain blood volume. This applies to patients who need renal dialysis as well. The average dialysis patient vasoconstricts sufficiently to lower tissue PO_2 by 30% or more during dialysis and needs about 24 hours to return vasomotor tone and wound and tissue PO_2 to normal.[150] Fluid losses from the vascular system are not necessarily replaced from the tissues as rapidly as they are sustained. Tissue edema may be the price paid for adequate intravascular volume. Edema increases intracapillary distance, so that there may be a delicate balance between excessive edema and peripheral vasoconstriction (which worsens the hypoxia caused by edema).

Vasoconstrictive drugs should be avoided. The most common and most avoidable is nicotine in the form of cigarettes. Beta-blockers should be used only when clearly medically indicated. Both are known to reduce wound and tissue PO_2. Clonidine is an alternative drug for heart rate control[151,152] that also induces vasodilation and may increase wound PO_2.[153] High-dose α-adrenergic agonists or other vasopressors may cause harm by decreasing tissue PO_2, but in a limited experience we have found that lower doses have little or no effect on wound/tissue PO_2. It is important to remember that decreasing cardiac output may also reduce wound perfusion. Thus, a balance must be maintained between minimizing use of vasopressors and maintaining adequate cardiac output.

Maintenance of tissue PO_2 requires attention to pulmonary
21 function postoperatively. Administration of supplemental oxygen via face mask or nasal cannulae increases safety in patients receiving systemic opioids[154] and one study demonstrated a reduction in SSI after lower extremity revascularization.[155] Pain control also appears important since it favorably influences both pulmonary function and vascular tone. This is particularly true in patients at high risk for pulmonary complications postoperatively, such as morbidly obese patients and those with pulmonary disease.[156] Epidural analgesia may be the route of choice in these patients. It has several advantages over parenterally administered opioids in that it generally achieves lower pain scores with less sedation. Nonetheless, opioid-induced pruritus is more common with epidural administration, and in some patients may be severe enough to counteract the benefits of pain control.

Patient-controlled analgesia is also quite effective at achieving low pain scores. It also has the benefit of giving control to the patient, leading to patient satisfaction as high as with epidural analgesia in many cases.[157] Nurse-administered, as-needed doses of IV or intramuscular opioids should be avoided as inadequate pain control often exceeds 50% using this approach.[158] The key to pain control is recognition of the need for analgesia and attention to the patient's complaints of pain. Opioid requirements vary enormously and are not always predictable, but even tolerant patients (IV drug abusers or those with cancer pain) can be given adequate pain relief with sufficient attention. Multimodal analgesia appears to be a valuable approach, reducing pain while minimizing respiratory depression.

SUMMARY

In patients with moderate to high risk of SSI, anesthesiologists
22 have the opportunity to enhance wound healing and reduce the incidence of wound infections by simple, inexpensive, and readily available means. Intraoperatively, appropriate antibiotic use, prevention of vasoconstriction through volume and warming, and maintenance of a high PaO_2 (300 to 500 mm Hg) are key. Postoperatively, the focus should remain on prevention of vasoconstriction through pain relief, warming, and adequate volume administration in the PACU. The addition of measures to reduce and prevent the stress response is likely to be effective as well, although further study is required.

Areas for Future Research

- When and why should a mask be worn in the OR?
- Should IVs be placed using sterile technique? A-lines?
- Is delay of antibiotics for culture justified?
- Can you modulate more than the sympathetic nervous system?
- Psychological preparation and intervention can modulate both HPA axis and SAM axis aspects of the stress response. Will this reduce wound complications?
- Do nonsteroidal anti-inflammatory agents increase risk of wound complications?
- Does dexamethasone for postoperative nausea and vomiting prophylaxis increase the risk of wound complications?
- Do epidurals reduce the risk of SSI? Are they cost-effective (vs. time and risk)?
- Who should get a high FIO_2? Is there potential toxicity?
- Does postoperative oxygen reduce wound complications? How long should patients receive supplemental oxygen postoperatively?

References

1. Brennan TA, Leape LL, Laird NM, et al. Incidence of adverse events and negligence in hospitalized patients. Results of the Harvard Medical Practice Study I. *N Engl J Med*. 1991;324:370–376.
2. Kaye KS, Sands K, Donahue JG, et al. Preoperative drug dispensing as predictor of surgical site infection. *Emerg Infect Dis*. 2001;7:57–65.
3. Noakes TD, Borresen J, Hew-Butler T, et al. Semmelweis and the aetiology of puerperal sepsis 160 years on: An historical review. *Epidemiol Infect*. 2007; 136(1):1–9.
4. Boyce JM, Pittet D, Healthcare Infection Control Practices Advisory Committee; HICPAC/SHEA/APIC/IDSA Hand Hygiene Task Force. Guideline for Hand Hygiene in Health-Care Settings. Recommendations of the Healthcare Infection Control Practices Advisory Committee and the HIPAC/SHEA/APIC/IDSA Hand Hygiene Task Force. *Am J Infect Control*. 2002;30:S1–S46.
5. Casewell M, Phillips I. Hands as route of transmission for Klebsiella species. *Br Med J*. 1977;2:1315–1317.
6. Ehrenkranz NJ, Alfonso BC. Failure of bland soap handwash to prevent hand transfer of patient bacteria to urethral catheters. *Infect Control Hosp Epidemiol*. 1991;12:654–662.
7. Sivathasan N, Goodfellow PB. Skin cleansers: The risks of chlorhexidine. *J Clin Pharmacol*. 2011;51:785–786.
8. Sax H, Allegranzi B, Uçkay I, et al. 'My five moments for hand hygiene': A user-centered design approach to understand, train, monitor and report hand hygiene. *J Hosp Infect*. 2007;67:9–21.
9. Loftus RW, Koff MD, Burchman CC, et al. Transmission of pathogenic bacterial organisms in the anesthesia work area. *Anesthesiology*. 2008;109:399–407.
10. Koff MD, Loftus RW, Burchman CC, et al. Reduction in intraoperative bacterial contamination of peripheral intravenous tubing through the use of a novel device. *Anesthesiology*. 2009;110:978–985.
11. Mecham E, Hopf HW. A proposal to minimize work area contamination during induction. *Anesthesiology*. 2011;116:712.
12. Tunevall TG. Postoperative wound infections and surgical face masks: A controlled study. *World J Surg*. 1991;15:383–387.
13. Friberg B, Friberg S, Ostensson R, et al. Surgical area contamination–comparable bacterial counts using disposable head and mask and helmet aspirator system, but dramatic increase upon omission of head-gear: An experimental study in horizontal laminar air-flow. *J Hosp Infect*. 2001;47:110–115.
14. Babkin Y, Raveh D, Lifschitz M, et al. Incidence and risk factors for surgical infection after total knee replacement. *Scand J Infect Dis*. 2007;39:890–895.
15. Pryor F, Messmer PR. The effect of traffic patterns in the OR on surgical site infections. *AORN J*. 1998;68:649–660.

16. Moro ML. Health care-associated infections. *Surg Infect (Larchmt).* 2006;7: S21–S23.
17. Allo MD, Tedesco M. Operating room management: Operative suite considerations, infection control. *Surg Clin North Am.* 2005;85:1291–1297.
18. Mermel LA, McCormick RD, Springman SR, et al. The pathogenesis and epidemiology of catheter-related infection with pulmonary artery Swan-Ganz catheters: A prospective study utilizing molecular subtyping. *Am J Med.* 1991;91: 197S–205S.
19. Raad II, Hohn DC, Gilbreath BJ, et al. Prevention of central venous catheter-related infections by using maximal sterile barrier precautions during insertion. *Infect Control Hosp Epidemiol.* 1994;15:231–238.
20. O'Grady NP, Alexander M, Dellinger EP, et al. Guidelines for the prevention of intravascular catheter-related infections. *Infect Control Hosp Epidemiol.* 2002;23:759–769.
21. Miles AA, Miles EM, Burke J. The value and duration of defence reactions of the skin to the primary lodgement of bacteria. *Br J Exp Pathol.* 1957;38:79–96.
22. Knighton DR, Halliday B, Hunt TK. Oxygen as an antibiotic. The effect of inspired oxygen on infection. *Arch Surg.* 1984;119:199–204.
23. Knighton DR, Halliday B, Hunt TK. Oxygen as an antibiotic. A comparison of the effects of inspired oxygen concentration and antibiotic administration on in vivo bacterial clearance. *Arch Surg.* 1986;121:191–195.
24. Bernard HR, Cole WR. The prophylaxis of surgical infection: The effect of prophylactic antimicrobial drugs on the incidence of infection following potentially contaminated operations. *Surgery.* 1964;56:151–157.
25. Classen D, Evans R, Pestotnik S, et al. The timing of prophylactic administration of antibiotics and the risk of surgical-wound infection. *N Engl J Med.* 1992;326:281–286.
26. Bratzler DW, Houck PM. Antimicrobial prophylaxis for surgery: An advisory statement from the National Surgical Infection Prevention Project. *Clin Infect Dis.* 2004;38:1706–1715.
27. Nichols RL, Condon RE, Barie PS. Antibiotic prophylaxis in surgery–2005 and beyond. *Surg Infect (Larchmt).* 2005;6:349–361.
28. Burke JP. Maximizing appropriate antibiotic prophylaxis for surgical patients: An update from LDS Hospital, Salt Lake City. *Clin Infect Dis.* 2001;33(Suppl 2): S78–S83.
29. Scher KS. Studies on the duration of antibiotic administration for surgical prophylaxis. *Am Surg.* 1997;63:59–62.
30. Arnold M, Barbul A. Nutrition and wound healing. *Plast Reconstr Surg.* 2006; 117:42S–58S.
31. Jensen JA, Jonsson K, Goodson WH 3rd, et al. Epinephrine lowers subcutaneous wound oxygen tension. *Curr Surg.* 1985;42:472–474.
32. Mogford JE, Tawil N, Chen A, et al. Effect of age and hypoxia on TGFbeta1 receptor expression and signal transduction in human dermal fibroblasts: Impact on cell migration. *J Cell Physiol.* 2002;190:259–265.
33. Mogford JE, Sisco M, Bonomo SR, et al. Impact of aging on gene expression in a rat model of ischemic cutaneous wound healing. *J Surg Res.* 2004;118: 190–196.
34. Lenhardt R, Hopf HW, Marker E, et al. Perioperative collagen deposition in elderly and young men and women. *Arch Surg.* 2000;135:71–74.
35. Robson MC, Mannari RJ, Smith PD, et al. Maintenance of wound bacterial balance. *Am J Surg.* 1999;178:399–402.
36. Winter GD. Formation of the scab and the rate of epithelisation of superficial wounds in the skin of the young domestic pig. 1962. *J Wound Care.* 1995;4:366–367; discussion 368–371.
37. Jonsson K, Jensen J, Goodson W, et al. Tissue oxygenation, anemia, and perfusion in relation to wound healing in surgical patients. *Ann Surg.* 1991;214:605–613.
38. Hopf HW, Ueno C, Aslam R, et al. Guidelines for the treatment of arterial insufficiency ulcers. *Wound Repair Regen.* 2006;14:693–710.
39. Ueno C, Hunt TK, Hopf HW. Using physiology to improve surgical wound outcomes. *Plast Reconstr Surg.* 2006;117:59S–71S.
40. De Jong L, Kemp A. Stoichiometry and kinetics of the prolyl 4-hydroxylase partial reaction. *Biochim Biophys Acta.* 1984;787:105–111.
41. Allen DB, Maguire JJ, Mahdavian M, et al. Wound hypoxia and acidosis limit neutrophil bacterial killing mechanisms. *Arch Surg.* 1997;132:991–996.
42. Hopf HW, Gibson JJ, Angeles AP, et al. Hyperoxia and angiogenesis. *Wound Repair Regen.* 2005;13:558–564.
43. Hopf H, Hunt T, Jensen J. Calculation of subcutaneous tissue blood flow. *Surgical Forum.* 1988;39:33–36.
44. Evans NTS, Naylor PFD. Steady states of oxygen tension in human dermis. *Respir Physiol.* 1966;2:46–60.
45. Medawar PS. The behavior of mammalian skin epithelium under strictly anaerobic conditions. *Q J Microsc Sci.* 1947;88:27.
46. Schulz G. *Molecular Regulation of Wound Healing, Acute and Chronic Wounds: Current Management Concepts.* 3rd edn. In: Bryant R, Nix D, eds. St. Louis: Mosby Elsevier; 2006:82–99.
47. Adams JC. Functions of the conserved thrombospondin carboxy-terminal cassette in cell-extracellular matrix interactions and signaling. *Int J Biochem Cell Biol.* 2004;36:1102–1114.
48. Mast BA, Schultz GS. Interactions of cytokines, growth factors, and proteases in acute and chronic wounds. *Wound Repair Regen.* 1996;4:411–420.
49. Constant J, Suh D, Hussain M, et al. Wound healing angiogenesis: The metabolic basis of repair. In *Molecular, Cellular, and Clinical Aspects of Angiogenesis.* New York, NY: Plenum Press; 1996:151–159.
50. Dvonch VM, Murphey RJ, Matsuoka J, et al. Changes in growth factor levels in human wound fluid. *Surgery.* 1992;112:18–23.
51. Zabel DD, Feng JJ, Scheuenstuhl H, et al. Lactate stimulation of macrophage-derived angiogenic activity is associated with inhibition of poly(ADP-ribose) synthesis. *Lab Invest.* 1996;74:644–649.
52. Heppenstall RB, Littooy FN, Fuchs R, et al. Gas tensions in healing tissues of traumatized patients. *Surgery.* 1974;75:874–880.
53. Trabold O, Wagner S, Wicke C, et al. Lactate and oxygen constitute a fundamental regulatory mechanism in wound healing. *Wound Repair Regen.* 2003;11: 504–509.
54. Caldwell MD, Shearer J, Morris A, et al. Evidence for aerobic glycolysis in lambda-carrageenan-wounded skeletal muscle. *J Surg Res.* 1984;37:63–68.
55. Klebanoff SJ. Oxygen metabolism and the toxic properties of phagocytes. *Ann Intern Med.* 1980;93:480–489.
56. Remensnyder JP, Majno G. Oxygen gradients in healing wounds. *Am J Pathol.* 1968;52:301–323.
57. Niinikoski J, Hunt TK, Dunphy JE. Oxygen supply in healing tissue. *Am J Surg.* 1972;123:247–252.
58. Silver IA. Cellular microenvironment in healing and non-healing wounds. In: Hunt TK, Heppenstall RB, Pines E, eds. *Soft and Hard Tissue Repair.* New York, NY: Praeger; 1984:50–66.
59. Falcone PA, Caldwell MD. Wound metabolism. *Clin Plast Surg.* 1990;17:443–456.
60. Chang N, Mathes SJ. Comparison of the effect of bacterial inoculation in musculocutaneous and random-pattern flaps. *Plast Reconstr Surg.* 1982;70(1):1–10.
61. Hopf HW, Hunt TK, West JM, et al. Wound tissue oxygen tension predicts the risk of wound infection in surgical patients. *Arch Surg.* 1997;132:997–1004; discussion 1005.
62. Schwentker A, Evans SM, Partington M, et al. A model of wound healing in chronically radiation-damaged rat skin. *Cancer Lett.* 1998;128:71–78.
63. Bauer SM, Goldstein LJ, Bauer RJ, et al. The bone marrow-derived endothelial progenitor cell response is impaired in delayed wound healing from ischemia. *J Vasc Surg.* 2006;43:134–141.
64. Wütschert R, Bounameaux H. Determination of amputation level in ischemic limbs. Reappraisal of the measurement of TcPo2. *Diabetes Care.* 1997;20: 1315–1318.
65. Sen CK, Khanna S, Babior BM, et al. Oxidant-induced vascular endothelial growth factor expression in human keratinocytes and cutaneous wound healing. *J Biol Chem.* 2002;277:33284–33290.
66. Beckert S, Farrahi F, Aslam RS, et al. Lactate stimulates endothelial cell migration. *Wound Repair Regen.* 2006;14:321–324.
67. Babior BM. Oxygen-dependent microbial killing by phagocytes (first of two parts). *N Engl J Med.* 1978;298:659–668.
68. Edwards S, Hallett MB, Campbell AK. Oxygen-radical production during inflammation may be limited by oxygen concentration. *Biochem J.* 1984;217:851–854.
69. Gabig TG, Bearman SI, Babior BM. Effects of oxygen tension and pH on the respiratory burst of human neutrophils. *Blood.* 1979;53:1133–1139.
70. Smith BM, Desvigne LD, Slade JB, et al. Transcutaneous oxygen measurements predict healing of leg wounds with hyperbaric therapy. *Wound Repair Regen.* 1996;4:224–229.
71. Fife CE, Buyukcakir C, Otto GH, et al. The predictive value of transcutaneous oxygen tension measurement in diabetic lower extremity ulcers treated with hyperbaric oxygen therapy: A retrospective analysis of 1,144 patients. *Wound Repair Regen.* 2002;10:198–207.
72. Rollins MD, Gibson JJ, Hunt TK, et al. Wound oxygen levels during hyperbaric oxygen treatment in healing wounds. *Undersea Hyperb Med.* 2006;33:17–25.
73. Mader JT. Phagocytic killing and hyperbaric oxygen: Antibacterial mechanisms. *HBO Reviews.* 1981;2:37–49.
74. Mader JT, Brown GL, Guckian JC, et al. A mechanism for the amelioration by hyperbaric oxygen of experimental staphylococcal osteomyelitis in rabbits. *J Infect Dis.* 1980;142:915–922.
75. Hunt TK, Aslam RS, Beckert S, et al. Aerobically derived lactate stimulates revascularization and tissue repair via redox mechanisms. *Antioxid Redox Signal.* 2007;9:1115–1124.
76. Velazquez OC. Angiogenesis and vasculogenesis: Inducing the growth of new blood vessels and wound healing by stimulation of bone marrow-derived progenitor cell mobilization and homing. *J Vasc Surg.* 2007;45(Suppl A):A39–A47.
77. Capla JM, Ceradini DJ, Tepper OM, et al. Skin graft vascularization involves precisely regulated regression and replacement of endothelial cells through both angiogenesis and vasculogenesis. *Plast Reconstr Surg.* 2006;117:836–844.
78. Schultz GS, Grant MB. Neovascular growth factors. *Eye (Lond).* 1991;5:170–180.
79. Beckert S, Hierlemann H, Muschenborn N, et al. Experimental ischemic wounds: Correlation of cell proliferation and insulin-like growth factor I expression and its modification by different local IGF-I release systems. *Wound Repair Regen.* 2005;13:278–283.
80. Knighton DR, Silver IA, Hunt TK. Regulation of wound-healing angiogenesis-effect of oxygen gradients and inspired oxygen concentration. *Surgery.* 1981;90: 262–270.

81. Myllyla R, Tuderman L, Kivirikko KI. Mechanism of the prolyl hydroxylase reaction. 2. Kinetic analysis of the reaction sequence. *Eur J Biochem.* 1977;80:349–357.
82. Prockop DJ, Kivirikko KI, Tuderman L, et al. The biosynthesis of collagen and its disorders (first of two parts). *N Engl J Med.* 1979;301:13–23.
83. Uitto J, Prockop DJ. Synthesis and secretion of under-hydroxylated procollagen at various temperatures by cells subject to temporary anoxia. *Biochem Biophys Res Commun.* 1974;60:414.
84. Silver IA. Oxygen tension and epithelialization. In: Maibach HI, Rovee DT, eds. *Epidermal Wound Healing.* Chicago: Year Book Medical Publishers; 1972:291.
85. Feldmeier JJ, Hopf HW, Warriner RA 3rd, et al. UHMS position statement: Topical oxygen for chronic wounds. *Undersea Hyperb Med.* 2005;32:157–168.
86. Ngo MA, Sinitsyna NN, Qin Q, et al. Oxygen-dependent differentiation of human keratinocytes. *J Invest Dermatol.* 2007;127:354–361.
87. O'Toole EA, Marinkovich MP, Peavey CL, et al. Hypoxia increases human keratinocyte motility on connective tissue. *J Clin Invest.* 1997;100:2881–2891.
88. Doughty DB. Preventing and managing surgical wound dehiscence. *Adv Skin Wound Care.* 2005;18:319–322.
89. Gottrup F, Firmin R, Rabkin J, et al. Directly measured tissue oxygen tension and arterial oxygen tension assess tissue perfusion. *Crit Care Med.* 1987;15:1030–1036.
90. Hutton JJ, Tappel AL, Udenfriend S. Cofactor and substrate requirements of collagen proline hydroxylase. *Arch Biochem Biophys.* 1967;118:231–240.
91. Jönsson K, Hunt TK, Mathes SJ. Oxygen as an isolated variable influences resistance to infection. *Ann Surg.* 1988;208:783–787.
92. Hohn DC, MacKay RD, Halliday B, et al. Effect of O2 tension on microbicidal function of leukocytes in wounds and in vitro. *Surg Forum.* 1976;27:18–20.
93. Jensen JA, Goodson WH, Hopf HW, et al. Cigarette smoking decreases tissue oxygen. *Arch Surg.* 1991;126:1131–1134.
94. Hopf HW, Viele M, Watson JJ, et al. Subcutaneous perfusion and oxygen during acute severe isovolemic hemodilution in healthy volunteers. *Arch Surg.* 2000;135:1443–1449.
95. Hopf H, Hunt T. Does— and if so, to what extent— normovolemic dilutional anemia influence post-operative wound healing? *Chirugische Gastroenterologie.* 1992;8:148–150.
96. Jensen JA, Goodson WH 3rd, Vasconez LO, et al. Wound healing in anemia. *West J Med.* 1986;144:465–467.
97. Sheffield CW, Sessler DI, Hopf HW, et al. Centrally and locally mediated thermoregulatory responses alter subcutaneous oxygen tension. *Wound Repair Regen.* 1996;4:339–345.
98. Derbyshire DR, Smith G. Sympathoadrenal responses to anaesthesia and surgery. *Br J Anaesth.* 1984;56:725–739.
99. Halter JB, Pflug AE, Porte D Jr. Mechanism of plasma catecholamine increases during surgical stress in man. *J Clin Endocrinol Metab.* 1977;45:936–944.
100. Matsukawa T, Sessler DI, Sessler AM, et al. Heat flow and distribution during induction of general anesthesia. *Anesthesiology.* 1995;82:662–673.
101. Kurz A, Sessler DI, Lenhardt R. Perioperative normothermia to reduce the incidence of surgical-wound infection and shorten hospitalization. Study of Wound Infection and Temperature Group. *N Engl J Med.* 1996;334:1209–1215.
102. Hartmann M, Jönsson K, Zederfeldt B. Effect of tissue perfusion and oxygenation on accumulation of collagen in healing wounds. Randomized study in patients after major abdominal operations. *Eur J Surg.* 1992;158:521–526.
103. Melling AC, Ali B, Scott EM, et al. Effects of preoperative warming on the incidence of wound infection after clean surgery: A randomised controlled trial. *Lancet.* 2001;358:876–880.
104. Akça O, Melischek M, Scheck T, et al. Postoperative pain and subcutaneous oxygen tension [letter]. *Lancet.* 1999;354:41–42.
105. Rojas IG, Padgett DA, Sheridan JF, et al. Stress-induced susceptibility to bacterial infection during cutaneous wound healing. *Brain Behav Immun.* 2002;16: 74–84.
106. Horan MP, Quan N, Subramanian SV, et al. Impaired wound contraction and delayed myofibroblast differentiation in restraint-stressed mice. *Brain Behav Immun.* 2005;19:207–216.
107. Greif R, Akça O, Horn EP, et al. Supplemental perioperative oxygen to reduce the incidence of surgical-wound infection. Outcomes Research Group. *N Engl J Med.* 2000;342:161–167.
108. Belda FJ, Aguilera L, Garcia de la Asuncion J, et al. Supplemental perioperative oxygen and the risk of surgical wound infection: A randomized controlled trial. *JAMA.* 2005;294:2035–2042.
109. Myles PS, Leslie K, Chan MT, et al. Avoidance of nitrous oxide for patients undergoing major surgery: A randomized controlled trial. *Anesthesiology.* 2007;107: 221–231.
110. Bickel A, Gurevits M, Vamos R, et al. Perioperative hyperoxygenation and wound site infection following surgery for acute appendicitis: A randomized, prospective, controlled trial. *Arch Surg.* 2011;146:464–470.
111. Schietroma M, Carlei F, Cecilia E, et al. Colorectal infraperitoneal anastomosis: The effects of perioperative supplemental oxygen administration on the anastomotic dehiscence. *J Gastrointest Surg.* 2012;16:427–434.
112. Maragakis LL, Cosgrove SE, Martinez EA, et al. Intraoperative fraction of inspired oxygen is a modifiable risk factor for surgical site infection after spinal surgery. *Anesthesiology.* 2009;110:556–562.
113. Pryor KO, Fahey TJ 3rd, Lien CA, et al. Surgical site infection and the routine use of perioperative hyperoxia in a general surgical population: A randomized controlled trial. *JAMA.* 2004;291:79–87.
114. Meyhoff C, Wetterslev J, Jorgensen LN, et al. Effect of high perioperative oxygen fraction on surgical site infection and pulmonary complications after abdominal surgery: The PROXI Randomized Clinical Trial. *JAMA.* 2009;302: 1543–1550.
115. Akça O, Podolsky A, Eisenhuber E, et al. Comparable postoperative pulmonary atelectasis in patients given 30% or 80% oxygen during and 2 hours after colon resection. *Anesthesiology.* 1999;91:991–998.
116. Mackintosh N, Gertsch MC, Hopf HW, et al. High intraoperative inspired oxygen does not increase postoperative supplemental oxygen requirements. *Anesthesiology.* 2012;117:271–279.
117. Kohanski MA, Dwyer DJ, Hayete B, et al. A common mechanism of cellular death induced by bactericidal antibiotics. *Cell.* 2007;130:797–810.
118. Suller MT, Lloyd D. The antibacterial activity of vancomycin towards Staphylococcus aureus under aerobic and anaerobic conditions. *J Appl Microbiol.* 2002;92:866–872.
119. Chapman CR, Tuckett RP, Song CW. Pain and stress in a systems perspective: Reciprocal neural, endocrine and immune interactions. *J Pain.* 2008;9:122–145.
120. Buck BJ, Kerman IA, Burghardt PR, et al. Upregulation of GAD65 mRNA in the medulla of the rat model of metabolic syndrome. *Neurosci Lett.* 2007;419: 178–183.
121. Haley RW, Culver DH, Morgan WM, et al. Identifying patients at high risk of surgical wound infection. A simple multivariate index of patient susceptibility and wound contamination. *Am J Epidemiol.* 1985;121:206–215.
122. Culver DH, Horan TC, Gaynes RP, et al. Surgical wound infection rates by wound class, operative procedure, and patient risk index. National Nosocomial Infections Surveillance System. *Am J Med.* 1991;91:152S–157S.
123. Sheridan JF, Padgett DA, Avitsur R, et al. Experimental models of stress and wound healing. *World J Surg.* 2004;28:327–330.
124. Dantzer R, Kelley KW. Twenty years of research on cytokine-induced sickness behavior. *Brain Behav Immun.* 2007;21:153–160.
125. Kiecolt-Glaser JK, Loving TJ, Stowell JR, et al. Hostile marital interactions, proinflammatory cytokine production, and wound healing. *Arch Gen Psychiatry.* 2005;62:1377–1384.
126. Muizzuddin N, Matsui MS, Marenus KD, et al. Impact of stress of marital dissolution on skin barrier recovery: Tape stripping and measurement of trans-epidermal water loss (TEWL). *Skin Res Technol.* 2003;9:34–38.
127. Bosch JA, Engeland CG, Cacioppo JT, et al. Depressive symptoms predict mucosal wound healing. *Psychosom Med.* 2007;69:597–605.
128. West J, Hopf H, Sessler D, et al. The effect of rapid postoperative rewarming on tissue oxygen. *Wound Repair Regen.* 1993;1:93.
129. Kurz A, Kurz M, Poeschl G, et al. Forced-air warming maintains intraoperative normothermia better than circulating water mattresses. *Anesth Analg.* 1993; 77:89–95.
130. Galvão CM, Marck PB, Sawada NO, et al. A systematic review of the effectiveness of cutaneous warming systems to prevent hypothermia. *J Clin Nurs.* 2010;18: 627–636.
131. Kehlet H. Surgical stress response: Does endoscopic surgery confer an advantage? *World J Surg.* 1999;23:801–807.
132. Holte K, Sharrock NE, Kehlet H. Pathophysiology and clinical implications of perioperative fluid excess. *Br J Anaesth.* 2002;89:622–632.
133. Nisanevich V, Felsenstein I, Almogy G, et al. Effect of intraoperative fluid management on outcome after intraabdominal surgery. *Anesthesiology.* 2005;103: 25–32.
134. Arkiliç CF, Taguchi A, Sharma N, et al. Supplemental perioperative fluid administration increases tissue oxygen pressure. *Surgery.* 2003;133:49–55.
135. Jonsson K, Jensen JA, Goodson WH 3rd, et al. Assessment of perfusion in postoperative patients using tissue oxygen measurements. *Br J Surg.* 1987;74:263–267.
136. Gosain A, Rabkin J, Reymond JP, et al. Tissue oxygen tension and other indicators of blood loss or organ perfusion during graded hemorrhage. *Surgery.* 1991;109:523–532.
137. Kabon B, Akca O, Taguchi A, et al. Supplemental intravenous crystalloid administration does not reduce the risk of surgical wound infection. *Anesth Analg.* 2005;101:1546–1553.
138. Iberti TJ, Fischer EP, Leibowitz AB, et al. A multicenter study of physicians' knowledge of the pulmonary artery catheter. Pulmonary Artery Catheter Study Group. *JAMA.* 1990;264:2928–2932.
139. Rubenfeld GD, McNamara-Aslin E, Rubinson L. The pulmonary artery catheter, 1967–2007: Rest in peace? *JAMA.* 2007;298:458–461.
140. Mythen MG, Webb AR. Perioperative plasma volume expansion reduces the incidence of gut mucosal hypoperfusion during cardiac surgery. *Arch Surg.* 1995;130:423–429.
141. Sinclair S, James S, Singer M. Intraoperative intravascular volume optimisation and length of hospital stay after repair of proximal femoral fracture: Randomised controlled trial. *BMJ.* 1997;315:909–912.
142. Grocott MP, Mythen MG, Gan TJ. Perioperative fluid management and clinical outcomes in adults. *Anesth Analg.* 2005;100:1093–1106.

143. Ruttmann TG, James MF, Aronson I. In vivo investigation into the effects of haemodilution with hydroxyethyl starch (200/0.5) and normal saline on coagulation. *Br J Anaesth.* 1998;80:612–616.
144. Chappell D, Jacob M, Hofmann-Kiefer K, et al. A rational approach to perioperative fluid management. *Anesthesiology.* 2008;109:723–740.
145. Lobo DN, Bostock KA, Neal KR, et al. Effect of salt and water balance on recovery of gastrointestinal function after elective colonic resection: A randomised controlled trial. *Lancet.* 2002;359:1812–1818.
146. van den Berghe G, Wouters P, Weekers F, et al. Intensive insulin therapy in the critically ill patients. *N Engl J Med.* 2001;345:1359–1367.
147. Gandhi GY, Nuttall GA, Abel MD, et al. Intensive intraoperative insulin therapy versus conventional glucose management during cardiac surgery: a randomized trial. *Ann Intern Med.* 2007;146:233–243.
148. Finfer S, Chittock DR, Su SY, et al. Intensive versus conventional glucose control in critically ill patients. *N Engl J Med.* 2009;360:1283–1297.
149. Griesdale DE, de Souza RJ, van Dam RM, et al. Intensive insulin therapy and mortality among critically ill patients: A meta-analysis including NICE-SUGAR study data. *CMAJ.* 2009;180:821–827.
150. Jensen JA, Goodson WH 3rd, Omachi RS, et al. Subcutaneous tissue oxygen tension falls during hemodialysis. *Surgery.* 1987;101:416–421.
151. Stühmeier K, Mainzer B, Cierpka J, et al. Small, oral dose of clonidine reduces the incidence of intraoperative myocardial ischemia in patients having vascular surgery. *Anesthesiology.* 1996;85:706–712.
152. Wallace AW, Galindez D, Salahieh A, et al. Effect of clonidine on cardiovascular morbidity and mortality after noncardiac surgery. *Anesthesiology.* 2004;101:284–293.
153. Hopf H, West J, Hunt T. Clonidine increases tissue oxygen in patients with local tissue hypoxia in non-healing wounds. *Wound Repair Regen.* 1996;4:A129.
154. Stone JG, Cozine KA, Wald A. Nocturnal oxygenation during patient-controlled analgesia. *Anesth Analg.* 1999;89:104–110.
155. Turtiainen J, Saimanen E, Partio T, et al. Supplemental postoperative oxygen in the prevention of surgical wound infection after lower limb vascular surgery: A randomized controlled trial. *World J Surg.* 2011;35:1387–1395.
156. Wisner D. A stepwise logistic regression analysis of factors affecting morbidity and mortality after thoracic trauma: Effect of epidural analgesia. *J Trauma.* 1990;30:799–804.
157. Owen H, McMillan V, Rogowski D. Postoperative pain therapy: a survey of patients' expectations and their experiences. *Pain.* 1990;41:303–307.
158. Donovan M, Dillon P, McGuire L. Incidence and characteristics of pain in a sample of medical-surgical inpatients. *Pain.* 1987;30:69–78.

CHAPTER

14 Fluids, Electrolytes, and Acid–Base Physiology

DONALD S. PROUGH • J. SEAN FUNSTON • CHRISTER H. SVENSÉN • SCOTT W. WOLF

Key Points

1. The Henderson–Hasselbalch equation describes the relationship between pH, $Paco_2$, and serum bicarbonate. The Henderson equation defines the previous relationship but substitutes hydrogen concentration for pH.
2. The pathophysiology of metabolic alkalosis is divided into generating and maintenance factors. A particularly important maintenance factor is renal hypoperfusion, often due to hypovolemia.
3. The addition of iatrogenic respiratory alkalosis to metabolic alkalosis can produce severe alkalemia.
4. Metabolic acidosis occurs as a consequence of the use of bicarbonate to buffer endogenous organic acids or as a consequence of external bicarbonate loss. The former causes an increase in the anion gap ($Na^+ - [Cl^- + [HCO_3^-]]$).
5. When substituting mechanical ventilation for spontaneous ventilation in a patient with severe metabolic acidosis, it is important to maintain an appropriate level of ventilatory compensation, pending effective treatment of the primary cause for the metabolic acidosis.
6. Sodium bicarbonate, never proved to alter outcome in patients with lactic acidosis, should be reserved for those patients with severe acidemia.
7. Control of blood glucose in critically ill surgical patients has been associated with improvements in clinical outcomes. However, a blood glucose target of 180 mg/dL or less is associated with a lower mortality than a target of 81 to 108 mg/dL.
8. In patients undergoing moderate surgical procedures, generous administration of fluids is associated with fewer minor complications, such as nausea, vomiting, and drowsiness.
9. In patients undergoing colon surgery, careful perioperative fluid restriction has been associated with lower mortality and better wound healing.
10. Homeostatic mechanisms are usually adequate for the maintenance of electrolyte balance. However, critical illnesses and their treatment strategies can cause significant perturbations in electrolyte status, possibly leading to worsened patient outcome.
11. Disorders of the concentration of sodium, the principal extracellular cation, depend on the total body water (TBW) concentration and can lead to neurologic dysfunction. Disorders of potassium, the principal intracellular cation, are influenced primarily by insults that result in increased total body losses of potassium or changes in distribution.
12. Calcium, phosphorus, and magnesium are all essential for maintenance and function of the cardiovascular system. In addition, they also provide the milieu that ensures neuromuscular transmission. Disorders affecting any one of these electrolytes may lead to significant dysfunction and possibly result in cardiopulmonary arrest.

Multimedia

1 Renal Regulation of Water

2 Hyponatremia Rapid Correction

3 Hyperkalemia

As a consequence of underlying diseases and of therapeutic manipulations, surgical patients develop potentially harmful disorders of acid–base equilibrium, intravascular and extravascular volume, and serum electrolytes. Precise perioperative management of acid–base status, fluids, and electrolytes may limit perioperative morbidity and mortality.

ACID–BASE INTERPRETATION AND TREATMENT

Management of perioperative acid–base disturbances requires an understanding of the four simple acid–base disorders—metabolic alkalosis, metabolic acidosis, respiratory alkalosis, and respiratory acidosis—as well as more complex combinations of disturbances. This section will review the pathogenesis, major complications, physiologic compensatory mechanisms, and treatment of common perioperative acid–base abnormalities.

Overview of Acid–Base Equilibrium

Conventionally, acid–base equilibrium is described using the
1 Henderson–Hasselbalch equation:

$$\text{pH} = 6.1 + \log \frac{[\text{HCO}_3^-]}{0.03 \times \text{Paco}_2} \quad (14\text{-}1)$$

where 6.1 = the pK_a of carbonic acid and 0.03 is the solubility coefficient in blood of carbon dioxide (CO_2). Within this context, pH is the dependent variable while the bicarbonate concentration $[HCO_3^-]$ and $Paco_2$ are independent variables; therefore, metabolic alkalosis and acidosis are defined as disturbances in which $[HCO_3^-]$ is primarily increased or decreased and respiratory alkalosis and acidosis are defined as disturbances in which $Paco_2$ is primarily decreased or increased. pH, the negative logarithm of the hydrogen ion concentration ($[H^+]$), defines the acidity or alkalinity of solutions or blood. The simpler Henderson equation, after conversion of pH to $[H^+]$, also describes the relationship between the three major variables measured or calculated in blood gas samples:

$$[\text{H}^+] = \frac{24 \times \text{Paco}_2}{[\text{HCO}_3^-]} \quad (14\text{-}2)$$

To approximate the logarithmic relationship of pH to $[H^+]$, assume that $[H^+]$ is 40 mmol/L at a pH of 7.4; that an increase in pH of 0.10 pH units reduces $[H^+]$ to 0.8 × the starting $[H^+]$ concentration; that a decrease in pH of 0.10 pH units increases the $[H^+]$ by a factor of 1.25; and that small changes (i.e., <0.05 pH units) produce reciprocal increases or decreases of approximately 1 mmol/L in $[H^+]$ for each 0.01 decrease or increase in pH units.

The alternative "Stewart" approach to acid–base interpretation distinguishes between the independent variables and dependent variables that determine pH.[1,2] The independent variables are $Paco_2$, the strong (i.e., highly dissociated) ion difference, and the concentration of proteins, which usually are not strong ions. The strong ions include sodium (Na^+), potassium (K^+), chloride (Cl^-), and lactate. The strong ion difference, calculated as ($Na^+ + K^+ - Cl^-$), under normal circumstances is approximately 42 mEq/L. In general, the Stewart approach provides more insight into the mechanisms underlying acid–base disturbances, in contrast to the more descriptive Henderson–Hasselbalch approach. However, the clinical interpretation or treatment of common acid–base disturbances is rarely handicapped by the simpler constructs of the conventional Henderson–Hasselbalch or Henderson equations.

Metabolic Alkalosis

Metabolic alkalosis, characterized by hyperbicarbonatemia (>27 mEq/L) and usually by an alkalemic pH (>7.45), occurs frequently in postoperative patients and critically ill patients. Factors that generate metabolic alkalosis include vomiting and diuretic
2 administration (Table 14-1).[3] Maintenance of metabolic alkalosis depends on a continued stimulus, such as renal hypoperfusion, hypokalemia, hypochloremia, or hypovolemia, for distal tubular reabsorption of $[HCO_3^-]$ (Table 14-2).[3]

Metabolic alkalosis is associated with hypokalemia, ionized hypocalcemia, secondary ventricular arrhythmias, increased digoxin toxicity, and compensatory hypoventilation (hypercarbia), although compensation rarely results in $Paco_2$ >55 mm Hg (Table 14-3). Alkalemia may reduce tissue oxygen availability by
3 shifting the oxyhemoglobin dissociation curve to the left and by decreasing cardiac output. During anesthetic management, inadvertent addition of iatrogenic respiratory alkalosis to preexisting metabolic alkalosis may produce severe alkalemia and precipitate cardiovascular depression, dysrhythmias, and hypokalemia.

TABLE 14-1. GENERATION OF METABOLIC ALKALOSIS

Generation	Examples
I. Loss of acid from extracellular space	
A. Loss of gastric fluid (HCl)	Vomiting
B. Acid loss in the urine: Increased distal Na delivery in presence of hyperaldosteronism	Primary aldosteronism plus diuretic
C. Acid shifts into cells	Potassium deficiency
D. Loss of acid into stool	Congenital chloride-losing diarrhea
II. Excessive HCO_3^- loads	
A. Absolute	
1. Oral or parenteral HCO_3^-	Milk–alkali syndrome
2. Metabolic conversion of the salts of organic acids to HCO	Lactate, acetate, or citrate administration
B. Relative	$NaHCO_3$ dialysis
III. Posthypercapnic states	Correction (e.g., by mechanical ventilatory support) of chronic hypercapnia

Modified from: Khanna A, Kurtzman NA. Metabolic alkalosis. *J Nephrol.* 2006;19(suppl 9):S86–S96, with permission.

TABLE 14-2. FACTORS THAT MAINTAIN METABOLIC ALKALOSIS

Factor	Proposed Mechanism
Decreased GFR	Increases fractional HCO_3^- reabsorption and prevents the elevated plasma $[HCO_3^-]$ from exceeding Tm
Volume contraction	Stimulates proximal tubular HCO_3 reabsorption
Hypokalemia	Decreases GFR and increases proximal tubular HCO_3^- reabsorption; stimulates Na-independent/K-dependent (low) secretion in CCT
Hypochloremia[a]	Increases renin, decreases GFR, and decreases distal chloride delivery (↑ proton secretion in MCT)
Passive backflux of HCO_3^-	Creates a favorable concentration gradient for passive HCO_3^- movement from proximal tubular lumen to blood
Aldosterone	Increases Na-dependent proton secretion in CCT and Na-independent proton secretion in CCT and MCT

All factors decrease urinary HCO_3 excretion in vivo.
[a]Animal models are associated with hypokalemia; thus, the precise role of chloride in humans is not clearly understood.
GFR, glomerular filtration rate; CCT, cortical collecting tubule; MCT, medullary collecting tubule.
Modified from: Khanna A, Kurtzman NA. Metabolic alkalosis. *J Nephrol.* 2006;19(suppl 9):S86–S96, with permission.

In patients in whom arterial blood gasses have not yet been obtained, serum electrolytes and a history of major risk factors, such as vomiting, nasogastric suction, or chronic diuretic use, can suggest metabolic alkalosis. Total CO_2 (usually abbreviated on electrolyte reports as CO_2) should be about 1 mEq/L greater than $[HCO_3^-]$ on simultaneously obtained arterial blood gasses. If either calculated $[HCO_3^-]$ on the arterial blood gasses or "CO_2" on the serum electrolytes exceeds normal (24 and 25 mEq/L, respectively) by >4 mEq/L, either the patient has a primary metabolic alkalosis or has conserved bicarbonate in response to chronic hypercarbia. Recognition of hyperbicarbonatemia on the preoperative serum electrolytes justifies arterial blood gas analysis and should alert the anesthesiologist to the likelihood of factors that generate or maintain metabolic alkalosis (see Tables 14-1 and 14-2).

Treatment of metabolic alkalosis consists of etiologic and nonetiologic therapies. Etiologic therapy consists of measures such as expansion of intravascular volume or the administration of potassium. Infusion of 0.9% saline will dose-dependently increase serum $[Cl^-]$ and decrease serum $[HCO_3^-]$.[4] Nonetiologic therapy includes administration of acetazolamide (a carbonic anhydrase inhibitor that causes renal bicarbonate wasting), infusion of $[H^+]$ in the form of ammonium chloride, arginine hydrochloride, or 0.1 N hydrochloric acid (100 mmol/L), or dialysis against a high-chloride/low bicarbonate dialysate.[3] Of the previously mentioned factors, 0.1 N hydrochloric acid most rapidly corrects life-threatening metabolic alkalosis but must be infused into a central vein; peripheral infusion will cause severe tissue damage.

TABLE 14-3. RESPIRATORY COMPENSATION IN RESPONSE TO METABOLIC ALKALOSIS AND METABOLIC ACIDOSIS

Metabolic alkalosis

1. $Paco_2$ increases ~0.5–0.6 mm Hg per 1 mEq/L increase in $[HCO_3^-]$
2. The last two digits of the pH should approximate the $[HCO_3^-] + 15$

Metabolic acidosis

1. $Paco_2 \sim [HCO_3^-] \times 1.5 + 8$
2. $Paco_2$ decreases 1.2 mm Hg per 1 mEq/L in $[HCO_3^-]$ to a minimum of 10–15 mm Hg
3. The last two digits of the pH ~ $[HCO_3^-] + 15$

Metabolic Acidosis

Metabolic acidosis, characterized by hypobicarbonatemia (<21 mEq/L) and usually by an acidemic pH (<7.35), can be innocuous or reflect a life-threatening emergency. Metabolic acidosis occurs as a consequence of buffering by bicarbonate of endogenous or exogenous acid loads or as a consequence of abnormal external loss of bicarbonate.[5–7] Approximately, 70 mmol of acid metabolites are produced, buffered, and excreted daily; these
4 include about 25 mmol of sulfuric acid from amino acid metabolism, 40 mmol of organic acids, and phosphoric and other acids. Extracellular volume (ECV) in a 70 kg adult contains 336 mmol of bicarbonate buffer (24 mEq/L × 14 L of ECV). Glomerular filtration of plasma volume (PV) necessitates reabsorption of 4,500 mmol of bicarbonate daily, of which 85% is reabsorbed in the proximal tubule, 10% in the thick ascending limb, and the remainder is titrated by proton secretion in the collecting duct.

Calculation of the anion gap $[(Na^+ - ([Cl^-] + [HCO_3^-])]$ distinguishes between two types of metabolic acidosis (Table 14-4).[8] The anion gap is normal (<13 mEq/L) in situations such as diarrhea, biliary drainage, and renal tubular acidosis in which bicarbonate is lost externally. The anion gap is also normal or reduced in hyperchloremic acidosis associated with perioperative infusion of substantial quantities of 0.9% saline.[4,9] Metabolic acidosis associated with a high anion gap (>13 mEq/L) occurs because of excess production or decreased excretion of organic acids or ingestion of one of several toxic compounds (Table 14-4). In metabolic acidosis associated with a high anion gap, bicarbonate ions are consumed in buffering hydrogen ions, while the associated anion replaces bicarbonate in serum. Because three quarters of the normal anion gap consists of albumin, the calculated anion gap should be corrected for hypoalbuminemia by adding to the calculated anion gap, the difference between measured serum albumin and normal albumin concentration of 4 g/dL multiplied by 2 to 2.5.[10] In general, an increase in the albumin-corrected anion gap (ΔAG) should be approximately matched by a decrease in the serum $[HCO_3^-]$ (ΔHCO_3^-).[11] A ratio of $\Delta AG:\Delta HCO_3^-$ that

TABLE 14-4. DIFFERENTIAL DIAGNOSIS OF METABOLIC ACIDOSIS

Elevated Anion Gap[a]	Normal Anion Gap[b]
Three Diseases	1. Renal tubular acidosis
1. Uremia	2. Diarrhea
2. Ketoacidosis	3. Carbonic anhydrase inhibition
3. Lactic acidosis	4. Ureteral diversions
Toxins	5. Early renal failure
1. Methanol	6. Hydronephrosis
2. Ethylene glycol	7. HCl administration
3. Salicylates	8. Saline administration
4. Paraldehyde	

[a]Correction of the anion gap for hypoalbuminemia is essential for effective perioperative use.
[b]To correct the anion gap for hypoalbuminemia, add to the calculated anion gap twice the difference between normal serum albumin (4 g/L) and actual serum albumin.

is <0.8 or >1.2 should prompt consideration of a mixed acid–base disturbance.

Sufficient reductions in pH may reduce myocardial contractility, increase pulmonary vascular resistance, and decrease systemic vascular resistance. It is particularly important to note that failure
5 of a patient to appropriately hyperventilate in response to metabolic acidosis is physiologically equivalent to respiratory acidosis and suggests clinical deterioration. If a patient with metabolic acidosis requires mechanical ventilation, for example, during general anesthesia, every attempt should be made to maintain an appropriate level of ventilatory compensation (see Table 14-3) until the primary process can be corrected. Table 14-5 illustrates failure to maintain compensatory hyperventilation.

The anesthetic implications of metabolic acidosis are proportional to the severity of the underlying process. Although a patient with hyperchloremic metabolic acidosis may be relatively healthy, those with lactic acidosis, ketoacidosis, uremia, or toxic ingestions will be chronically or acutely ill. Preoperative assessment should emphasize volume status and renal function. If shock has caused metabolic acidosis, direct arterial pressure monitoring and preload may require assessment via echocardiography or pulmonary arterial catheterization. Intraoperatively, one should be concerned about the possibility of exaggerated hypotensive responses to drugs and positive pressure ventilation. In planning intravenous fluid therapy, consider that balanced salt solutions tend to increase [HCO_3^-] (e.g., by metabolism of lactate to bicarbonate) and pH and 0.9% saline tends to decrease [HCO_3^-] and pH.

The treatment of metabolic acidosis consists of the treatment of the primary pathophysiologic process, that is, hypoperfusion, hypoxia, and if pH is severely decreased, administration of $NaHCO_3^-$. Hyperventilation, although an important compensatory response to metabolic acidosis, is not a definitive therapy for metabolic acidosis. The initial dose of $NaHCO_3$ can be calculated as:

$$NaHCO_3\,(\text{mEq/L}) = \frac{\text{Wt(kg)} \times 0.3(24\ \text{mEq/L} - \text{Actual } HCO_3^-)}{2} \quad (14\text{-}3)$$

where 0.3 = the assumed distribution space for bicarbonate and 24 mEq/L is the normal value for [HCO_3^-] on arterial blood gas determination. The calculation markedly underestimates dosage in severe metabolic acidosis. In infants and children, a customary initial dose is 1 to 2 mEq/kg of body weight.

Both evidence and opinion suggest that $NaHCO_3$ should rarely be used to treat acidemia induced by metabolic acidosis.[5,6,12] In critically ill patients with lactic acidosis, there were no important differences between the physiologic effects (other than changes in pH) of 0.9 M $NaHCO_3$ and 0.9 M sodium chloride.[13] Importantly,
6 $NaHCO_3$ did not improve the cardiovascular response to catecholamines and actually reduced plasma ionized calcium.[13] Although many clinicians continue to administer $NaHCO_3$ to patients with persistent lactic acidosis and ongoing deterioration, neither $NaHCO_3$ nor dichloroacetate[14] has improved outcome. The buffer THAM (*tris*-hydroxymethyl aminomethane) effectively reduces [H^+], does not increase plasma [Na^+], does not generate CO_2 as a byproduct of buffering, and does not decrease plasma [K^+][15]; however, there is no generally accepted indication for THAM.

Respiratory Alkalosis

Respiratory alkalosis, always characterized by hypocarbia ($Paco_2 \leq$ 35 mm Hg) and usually characterized by an alkalemic pH (>7.45), results from an increase in minute ventilation that is greater than that required to excrete metabolic CO_2 production. Because respiratory alkalosis may be a sign of pain, anxiety, hypoxemia, central nervous system disease, or systemic sepsis, the development of spontaneous respiratory alkalosis in a previously normocarbic patient requires prompt evaluation. The hyperventilation syndrome, a diagnosis of exclusion, is most often encountered in the emergency department.[16]

Respiratory alkalosis, such as metabolic alkalosis, may produce hypokalemia, hypocalcemia, cardiac dysrhythmias, bronchoconstriction, and hypotension, and may potentiate the toxicity of digoxin. In addition, both brain pH and cerebral blood flow are tightly regulated and respond rapidly to changes in systemic pH.[17]

TABLE 14-5. FAILURE TO MAINTAIN APPROPRIATE VENTILATORY COMPENSATION FOR METABOLIC ACIDOSIS[a]

		Spontaneous Ventilation		Mechanical Hypoventilation
Arterial	pH	7.29		7.13
Blood gasses	$Paco_2$ (mm Hg)	29	→→→→→→→	49
	[HCO_3^-] (mEq/L)	14		16

[a]In the presence of metabolic acidosis, an otherwise modest increase in $Paco_2$ may create a life-threatening decrease in pH.

Doubling minute ventilation reduces $Paco_2$ to 20 mm Hg and halves cerebral blood flow; conversely, halving minute ventilation doubles $Paco_2$ and doubles cerebral blood flow. Therefore, acute hyperventilation may be useful in neurosurgical procedures to reduce brain bulk and to control intracranial pressure (ICP) during emergent surgery for noncranial injuries associated with acute closed head trauma. In those situations, intraoperative monitoring of arterial blood gasses, correlated with capnography, will document adequate reduction of $Paco_2$. Acute profound hypocapnia (<20 mm Hg) may produce electroencephalographic evidence of cerebral ischemia. If $Paco_2$ is maintained at abnormally high or low levels for 8 to 24 hours, cerebral blood flow will return toward previous levels, associated with a return of cerebrospinal fluid [HCO_3^-] toward normal.

Treatment of respiratory alkalosis per se is often not required. The most important steps are recognition and treatment of the underlying cause.[16] For instance, correction of hypoxemia or hypoperfusion-induced lactic acidosis should result in resolution of the associated increases in respiratory drive. Preoperative recognition of chronic hyperventilation necessitates intraoperative maintenance of a similar $Paco_2$.

Respiratory Acidosis

Respiratory acidosis, always characterized by hypercarbia ($Paco_2 \leq 45$ mm Hg) and usually characterized by a low pH (<7.35), occurs because of a decrease in minute alveolar ventilation (V_A), an increase in production of carbon dioxide (V_{CO_2}) or both, from the equation:

$$Pa_{CO_2} = K\frac{V_{CO_2}}{V_A} \qquad (14\text{-}4)$$

where K = constant (rebreathing of exhaled, carbon dioxide–containing gas may also increase $Paco_2$). Respiratory acidosis may be either acute, without compensation by renal [HCO_3^-] retention, or chronic, with [HCO_3^-] retention offsetting the decrease in pH (Table 14-6). A reduction in V_A may be due to an overall decrease in minute ventilation (V_E) or to an increase in the amount of wasted ventilation (V_D), according to the equation:

$$V_A = V_E - V_D \qquad (14\text{-}5)$$

Decreases in V_E may occur because of central ventilatory depression by drugs or central nervous system injury because of increased work of breathing, or because of airway obstruction or neuromuscular dysfunction. Increases in V_D occur with chronic obstructive pulmonary disease, pulmonary embolism, and most acute forms of respiratory failure. V_{CO_2} may be increased by sepsis, high-glucose parenteral feeding, or fever.

Patients with chronic hypercarbia due to intrinsic pulmonary disease require careful preoperative evaluation. The ventilatory restriction imposed by upper abdominal or thoracic surgery may aggravate ventilatory insufficiency after surgery. Administration of narcotics and sedatives, even in small doses, may cause hazardous ventilatory depression. Preoperative evaluation should consider direct arterial pressure monitoring and frequent intraoperative blood gas determinations, as well as strategies to manage postoperative pain with minimal doses of systemic opioids. Intraoperatively, a patient with chronically compensated hypercapnia should be ventilated to maintain a normal pH. Inadvertent restoration of normal V_A may result in profound alkalemia. Postoperatively, prophylactic ventilatory support may be required for selected patients with chronic hypercarbia.

The treatment of respiratory acidosis depends on whether the process is acute or chronic. Acute respiratory acidosis may require mechanical ventilation unless a simple etiologic factor (i.e., narcotic overdosage or residual muscular blockade) can be treated quickly. Bicarbonate administration is rarely indicated unless severe metabolic acidosis is also present or unless mechanical ventilation is ineffective in reducing acute hypercarbia. In contrast, chronic respiratory acidosis is rarely managed with ventilation but rather with efforts to improve pulmonary function. In patients requiring mechanical ventilation for acute respiratory failure, ventilation with a lung-protective strategy may result in hypercapnia, which occasionally may require administration of buffers to avoid excessive acidemia.[18]

TABLE 14-6. CHANGES OF [HCO_3^-] AND pH IN RESPONSE TO ACUTE AND CHRONIC CHANGES IN $Paco_2$

Decreased $Paco_2$
1. pH increases 0.10 per 10 mm Hg decrease in $Paco_2$
2. [HCO_3^-] decreases 2 mEq/L per 10 mm Hg decrease in $Paco_2$
3. pH will nearly normalize if hypocarbia is sustained
4. [HCO_3^-] will decrease 5–6 mEq/L per 10 mm Hg chronic ↓ in $Paco_2$[a]

Increased $Paco_2$
1. pH will decrease 0.05 per acute 10 mm Hg increase $Paco_2$
2. [HCO_3^-] will increase 1 mEq/L per 10 mm Hg increase $Paco_2$
3. pH will return toward normal if hypercarbia is sustained
4. [HCO_3^-] will increase 4–5 mEq/L per chronic 10 mm Hg increase in $Paco_2$

[a]Hospitalized patients rarely develop chronic compensation for hypocarbia because of stimuli that enhance distal tubular reabsorption of sodium.

PRACTICAL APPROACH TO ACID–BASE INTERPRETATION

Rapid interpretation of a patient's acid–base status involves the integration of three sets of data: Arterial blood gasses, electrolytes, and history. A systematic, sequential approach facilitates interpretation (Table 14-7). Acid–base assessment usually can be completed before initiating therapy; however, inspection of arterial blood gas data may disclose disturbances (e.g., respiratory acidosis or metabolic acidosis with pH < 7.1) that require immediate attention.

The second step is to determine whether a patient is acidemic (pH < 7.35) or alkalemic (pH > 7.45). The pH status will usually indicate the predominant primary process, that is, acidosis produces acidemia and alkalosis produces alkalemia. Note that the suffix "-osis" indicates a primary process that, if unopposed, will produce the corresponding pH change. The suffix "-emia" refers to the pH. A compensatory process is not considered an "-osis." Of course, a patient may have mixed "-oses," that is, more than one primary process.

The third step is to determine whether the entire arterial blood gas picture is consistent with a simple acute respiratory alkalosis or acidosis (see Table 14-6). For example, a patient with

TABLE 14-7. SEQUENTIAL APPROACH TO ACID–BASE INTERPRETATION

1. Is the pH life-threatening, requiring immediate intervention?
2. Is the pH acidemic or alkalemic?
3. Could the entire arterial blood gas picture represent only an acute increase or decrease in $Paco_2$?
4. If the answer to question 3 is "No," is there evidence of a chronic respiratory disturbance or of an acute metabolic disturbance?
5. If an acute metabolic disturbance is present, is it accompanied by appropriate respiratory compensatory changes?
6. Is an anion gap present?
7. Are the clinical data consistent with the proposed interpretation?

acute hypocapnia ($Paco_2$ 30 mm Hg) would have a pH increase of 0.10 units to a pH of 7.50 and a decrease of calculated $[HCO_3^-]$ to 22 mEq/L.

As the fourth step, if changes in $Paco_2$, pH, and $[HCO_3^-]$ are not consistent with a simple acute respiratory disturbance, chronic respiratory acidosis (≥24 hours) or metabolic acidosis or alkalosis should be considered. In chronic respiratory acidosis, pH returns to nearly normal as bicarbonate is retained by the kidneys (Table 14-6), usually at a ratio of 4 to 5 mEq/L per 10 mm Hg chronic increase in $Paco_2$.[19] For example, chronic hypoventilation at a $Paco_2$ of 60 mm Hg would be associated with an increase in $[HCO_3^-]$ of 8 to 10 mEq/L so that $[HCO_3^-]$ would be expected to range from 32 to 34 mEq/L and pH would be expected to be within the low normal range (7.35 to 7.38). If neither an acute nor chronic respiratory change appears to explain the arterial blood gas data, then a metabolic disturbance must also be present.

The fifth question addresses respiratory compensation for metabolic disturbances. Respiratory compensation for metabolic disturbances occurs more rapidly than renal compensation for respiratory disturbances (Table 14-3). Several general rules describe compensation. First, overcompensation is rare. Second, inadequate or excessive compensation suggests an additional primary disturbance. Third, hypobicarbonatemia associated with an increased anion gap is never compensatory.

The sixth question, whether an anion gap is present, should be assessed even if the arterial blood gasses appear straightforward. The simultaneous occurrence of metabolic alkalosis and metabolic acidosis may result in an unremarkable pH and $[HCO_3^-]$; therefore, the combined abnormality may only be appreciated by examining the anion gap (if the cause of the metabolic acidosis is associated with a high anion gap). As noted previously, correct assessment of the anion gap requires correction for hypoalbuminemia.[10] Metabolic acidoses associated with increased anion gaps require specific treatments, thus necessitating a correct diagnosis and differentiation from hyperchloremic metabolic acidosis. For instance, if metabolic acidosis results from administration of large volumes of 0.9% saline, no specific treatment of metabolic acidosis would usually be necessary.

The seventh and final question is whether the clinical data are consistent with the proposed acid–base interpretation. Failure to integrate clinical findings with arterial blood gas and plasma electrolyte data may lead to serious errors in interpretation and management.

TABLE 14-8. HYPERCHLOREMIC METABOLIC ACIDOSIS DURING PROLONGED SURGERY

Arterial blood gasses	pH	7.40
	$Paco_2$	32 mm Hg
	$[HCO_3^-]$	19 mEq/L
Electrolytes	$[Na^+]$	140 mEq/L
	$[Cl^-]$	114 mEq/L
	CO_2	20 mEq/L
	Anion gap	8 mEq/L
Serum albumin		3 g/dL

Examples

The following two hypothetical cases illustrate the use of the algorithm and rules of thumb previously discussed.

Example Number 1

A 65-year-old woman has undergone 12 hours of an expected 16-hour radical neck dissection and flap construction. Estimated blood loss is 1,000 mL. She has received three units of packed red blood cells and 6 L of 0.9% saline. Her blood pressure and heart rate have remained stable while anesthetized with 0.5% to 1% isoflurane in 70:30 nitrous oxide and oxygen. Urinary output is adequate. Arterial blood gas levels are shown in Table 14-8.

The step-by-step interpretation is as follows:

1. The pH requires no immediate treatment.
2. The pH is normal.
3. The arterial blood gasses cannot be adequately explained by acute hypocarbia. The predicted pH would be 7.48 and the predicted $[HCO_3^-]$ would be 22 mEq/L (see Table 14-6).
4. A metabolic acidosis appears to be present.
5. Patients under general anesthesia with controlled mechanical ventilation cannot compensate for metabolic acidosis. However, spontaneous hypocapnia of this magnitude would represent slight overcompensation for metabolic acidosis (see Table 14-3) and would suggest the presence of a primary respiratory alkalosis.
6. Metabolic acidosis occurring during prolonged anesthesia and surgery could suggest lactic acidosis and prompt additional fluid therapy or other attempts to improve perfusion. However, serum electrolytes reveal an anion gap that is slightly less than normal (Table 14-8), indicating that the metabolic acidosis is probably the result of dilution of the ECV with a high-chloride fluid. Correction of the anion gap for the serum albumin of 3 g/dL only increases the anion gap to 10 to 11 mEq/L, again consistent with hyperchloremic metabolic acidosis. After differentiation from high anion gap metabolic acidoses, hyperchloremic acidosis secondary to infusion of high-chloride fluid usually requires no treatment. The arterial blood gasses and serum electrolytes are compatible with the clinical picture.

Example Number 2

A 35-year-old man, 3 days after appendectomy, develops nausea with recurrent emesis persisting for 48 hours. An arterial

TABLE 14-9. METABOLIC ALKALOSIS SECONDARY TO NAUSEA AND VOMITING WITH SUBSEQUENT LACTIC ACIDOSIS SECONDARY TO HYPOVOLEMIA

		Normal	Metabolic Alkalosis	Metabolic Acidosis
Blood gasses	PH	7.40	7.50	7.40
	$Paco_2$ (mm Hg)	40	46	40
	$[HCO_3^-]$ (mEq/L)	24	35	24
Serum electrolytes	$[Na^+]$ (mEq/L)	140	140	140
	$[Cl^-]$ (mEq/L)	105	94	94
	CO_2 (mEq/L)	25	36	25
	Anion gap (mEq/L)	10	10	21

blood gas reveals the results shown in the middle column of Table 14-9.

1. The pH of 7.50 requires no immediate intervention.
2. The pH is alkalemic, suggesting a primary alkalosis.
3. An acute $Paco_2$ of 46 mm Hg would yield a pH of approximately 7.37; therefore, this is not simply an acute ventilatory disturbance.
4. The patient has a primary metabolic alkalosis as suggested by the $[HCO_3^-]$ of 35 mEq/L.
5. The limits of respiratory compensation for metabolic alkalosis are wide and difficult to predict for individual patients. The rules of thumb, summarized in Table 14-3, suggest that $[HCO_3^-]$ + 15 should equal the last two digits of the pH and that the $Paco_2$ should increase 5 to 6 mm Hg for every 10 mEq/L change in serum $[HCO_3^-]$; that is, a pH of 7.50 and a $Paco_2$ of 46 mm Hg are within the expected range.
6. The anion gap is 10 mEq/L.
7. The diagnosis of a primary metabolic alkalosis with compensatory hypoventilation is consistent with the history of recurrent vomiting. Consider how the arterial blood gasses could change if vomiting were sufficiently severe to produce hypovolemic shock and lactic acidosis (third column, Table 14-9).

This sequence illustrates the important concept that the final pH, $Paco_2$, and $[HCO_3^-]$ represent the result of all of the vectors operating on acid–base status. Complex or "triple disturbances" can only be interpreted using a thorough, stepwise approach.

FLUID MANAGEMENT

Physiology

Body Fluid Compartments

Accurate replacement of fluid deficits necessitates an understanding of the expected distribution spaces of water, sodium, and colloid. The sum of intracellular volume (ICV), which constitutes 40% of total body weight, and extracellular volume, which constitutes 20% of body weight, comprises total body water (TBW), which therefore approximates 60% of total body weight. PV, equals about one-fifth of ECV, the remainder of which is interstitial fluid volume (IFV). Red cell volume, approximately 2 L, is part of ICV.

The distribution volume of sodium-free water is TBW. The distribution volume of infused sodium is ECV, which contains equal sodium concentrations ($[Na^+]$) in the PV and IF. Plasma $[Na^+]$ is approximately 140 mEq/L. The predominant intracellular cation, potassium, has an intracellular concentration ($[K^+]$) approximating 150 mEq/L. Albumin, the most important oncotically active constituent of ECV, is unequally distributed in PV (~4 g/dL) and IFV (~1 g/dL). The IFV concentration of albumin varies greatly among tissues; however, ECV is the distribution volume for colloid solutions.

Distribution of Infused Fluids

Conventionally, clinical prediction of PV expansion after fluid infusion assumes that body fluid spaces are static. Kinetic analysis of PV expansion replaces the static assumption with a dynamic description. As an example of the static approach, assume that a 70 kg patient has suffered an acute blood loss of 2,000 mL, approximately 40% of the predicted 5 L blood volume. The formula describing the effects of replacement with 5% dextrose in water (D_5W), lactated Ringer solution, or 5% or 25% human serum albumin is as follows:

$$\text{Expected PV increment} = \text{volume infused} \times \text{normal PV/distribution volume} \quad (14\text{-}6)$$

Rearranging the equation yields the following:

$$\text{Volume infused} = \text{expected PV increment} \times \text{distribution volume/normal PV} \quad (14\text{-}7)$$

To restore blood volume using D_5W, assuming a distribution volume for sodium-free water of TBW, requires 28 L:

$$28\,\text{L} = 2\,\text{L} \times 42\,\text{L}/3\,\text{L} \quad (14\text{-}8)$$

where 2 L is the desired PV increment, 42 L = TBW in a 70 kg person, and 3 L is the normal estimated PV.

To restore blood volume using lactated Ringer solution requires 9.1 L:

$$9.1\,\text{L} = 2\,\text{L} \times 14\,\text{L}/3\,\text{L} \quad (14\text{-}9)$$

where 14 L = ECV in a 70 kg person.

If 5% albumin, which exerts colloid osmotic pressure similar to plasma, were infused, the infused volume initially would remain in the PV, perhaps attracting additional interstitial fluid intravascularly. Twenty-five percent human serum albumin, a concentrated colloid, expands PV by approximately 400 mL for each 100 mL infused.

However, these static analyses are simplistic. Infused fluid does not simply equilibrate throughout an assumed distribution volume but is added to a highly regulated system that attempts to maintain intravascular, interstitial, and intracellular volume. A more comprehensive kinetic model was proposed by Svensén and Hahn.[20] Kinetic models of intravenous fluid therapy allow clinicians to predict more accurately the time course of volume changes produced by infusions of fluids of various compositions. Kinetic analysis permits estimation of peak volume expansion and rates of clearance of infused fluid and complements analysis of "pharmacodynamic" effects, such as changes in cardiac output or cardiac filling pressures.[21]

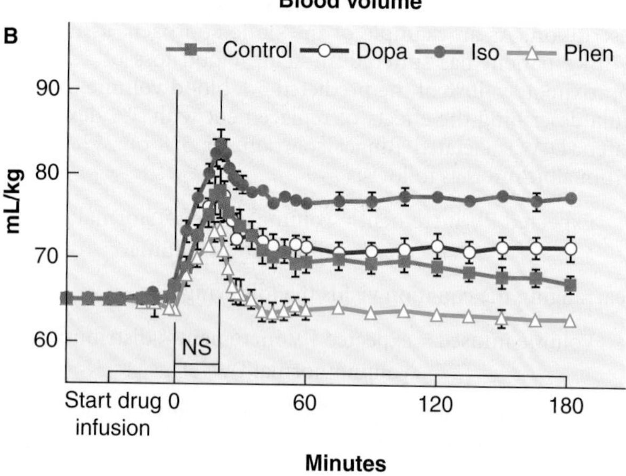

FIGURE 14-1. A: Blood hemoglobin (mean ± SEM) sampled at three baseline periods during a 30-minute catecholamine infusion and for 3 hours after starting a 20-minute 0.9% NaCl bolus of 24 mL/kg. Catecholamine protocols are dopamine (Dopa, *open diamonds*), isoproterenol (Iso, closed circles), phenylephrine (Phen, open triangles), and no-drug control (Control, closed squares). The 0.9% NaCl bolus decreased hemoglobin in all protocols at the end of the 20-minute 0.9% NaCl infusion and in all protocols except the Phen protocol thereafter. Post infusion protocol differences were Phen > Dopa = Control > Iso. **B:** Calculated blood volume (mean ± SEM) at three baseline periods during a catecholamine infusion and for 3 hours after starting a 20-minute 0.9% NaCl bolus of 24 mL/kg. The 0.9% NaCl bolus increased blood volume in all protocols at T_{20} and in all protocols except the Phen protocol thereafter. Post infusion protocol differences were Iso > Dopa = Control > Phen. NS, normal saline bolus. (From: Vane LA, Prough DS, Kinsky MA, et al. Effects of different catecholamines on the dynamics of volume expansion of crystalloid infusion. *Anesthesiology.* 2004;101:1136–1144, with permission.)

Using a kinetic approach to fluid therapy permits analysis of the effects of common physiologic and pharmacologic influences on fluid distribution in experimental animals or humans. For example, in chronically instrumented sheep, isoflurane anesthesia and the conscious state were associated with similar kinetics of PV expansion after fluid infusion, but reduced urinary output in anesthetized sheep demonstrated that expansion of extravascular volume was relatively greater during anesthesia; this effect was attributable to isoflurane and not to mechanical ventilation during anesthesia.[22] Also in chronically instrumented sheep, administration of catecholamine infusions before and during fluid infusions profoundly altered intravascular fluid retention, with phenylephrine diminishing and isoproterenol enhancing intravascular fluid retention (Fig. 14-1).[23]

Regulation of Extracellular Fluid Volume

TBW content is regulated by the intake and output of water. Water intake includes ingested liquids plus an average of 750 mL ingested in solid food and 350 mL that is generated metabolically. Insensible losses are normally 1 L/day and gastrointestinal losses are 100 to 150 mL/day. Thirst, the primary mechanism of controlling water intake, is triggered by an increase in body fluid tonicity or by a decrease in ECV.

Reabsorption of filtered water and sodium is enhanced by changes mediated by the hormonal factors antidiuretic hormone (ADH), atrial natriuretic peptide (ANP), and aldosterone. Renal water handling has three important components: (1) Delivery of tubular fluid to the diluting segments of the nephron, (2) separation of solute and water in the diluting segment, and (3) variable reabsorption of water in the collecting ducts. In the descending loop of Henle, water is reabsorbed while solute is retained to achieve a final osmolality of tubular fluid of approximately 1,200 mOsm/kg (Fig. 14-2). This concentrated fluid is then diluted by the active reabsorption of electrolytes in the ascending limb of the loop of Henle and in the distal tubule, both of which are relatively impermeable to water. As fluid exits the distal tubule and enters the collecting duct, osmolality is approximately 50 mOsm/kg. Within the collecting duct, water reabsorption is modulated by ADH (also called *vasopressin*). Vasopressin binds to V_2 receptors along the basolateral membrane of the collecting duct cells, then stimulates the synthesis and insertion of the aquaporin-2 water channel into the luminal membrane of collecting duct cells.[24]

Plasma hypotonicity suppresses ADH release, resulting in excretion of dilute urine. Hypertonicity stimulates ADH secretion, which increases the permeability of the collecting duct to water and enhances water reabsorption. In response to changing plasma [Na^+], changing secretion of ADH can vary urinary osmolality from 50 to 1,200 mOsm/kg and urinary volume from 0.4 to 20 L/day (Fig. 14-3).[25] Other factors that stimulate ADH secretion, although none as powerfully as plasma tonicity, include hypotension, hypovolemia, and nonosmotic stimuli such as nausea, pain, and medications, including opiates.

Two powerful hormonal systems regulate total body sodium. The natriuretic peptides, ANP, brain natriuretic peptide, and C-type natriuretic peptide, defend against sodium overload[26–28] and the renin–angiotensin–aldosterone axis defends against sodium depletion and hypovolemia. ANP, released from the cardiac atria in response to increased atrial stretch, exerts vasodilatory effects and increases the renal excretion of sodium and water. ANP secretion is decreased during hypovolemia. Even in patients with chronic (nonoliguric) renal insufficiency, infusion of ANP in low, nonhypotensive doses increased sodium excretion and augmented urinary losses of retained solutes.[29]

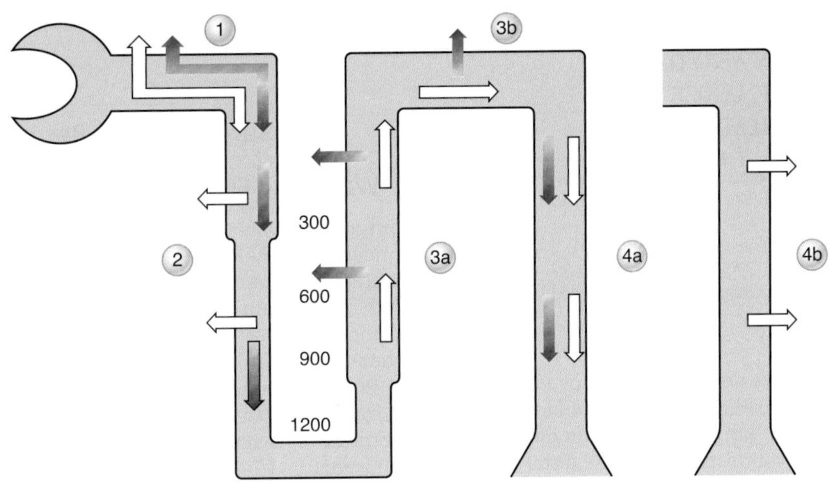

FIGURE 14-2. Renal filtration, reabsorption, and excretion of water. *Open arrows* represent water and *solid arrows* represent electrolytes. Water and electrolytes are filtered by the glomerulus. In the proximal tubule (1), water and electrolytes are absorbed isotonically. In the descending loop of Henle (2), water is absorbed to achieve osmotic equilibrium with the interstitium while electrolytes are retained. The numbers (300, 600, 900, and 1200) between the descending and ascending limbs represent the osmolality of the interstitium in milliosmoles per kilogram. The delivery of solute and fluid to the distal nephron is a function of proximal tubular reabsorption; as proximal tubular reabsorption increases, delivery of solute to the medullary (3a) and cortical (3b) diluting sites decreases. In the diluting sites, electrolyte-free water is generated through selective reabsorption of electrolytes while water is retained in the tubular lumen, generating a dilute tubular fluid. In the absence of vasopressin, the collecting duct (4a) remains relatively impermeable to water and diluted urine is excreted. When vasopressin acts on the collecting ducts (4b), water is reabsorbed from these vasopressin-responsive nephron segments, allowing the excretion of concentrated urine. (From: Fried LF, Palevsky PM. Hyponatremia and hypernatremia. In: Saklayen MG, ed. *The Medical Clinics of North America. Renal Disease.* Philadelphia, PA: WB Saunders Company; 1997:585–609, with permission.)

Aldosterone is the final common pathway in a complex response to decreased effective arterial volume, whether decreased effective arterial volume is true or relative, as in edematous states or hypoalbuminemia. In this pathway, decreased stretch in the baroreceptors of the aortic arch and carotid body and stretch receptors in the great veins, pulmonary vasculature, and atria result in increased sympathetic tone. Increased sympathetic tone, in combination with decreased renal perfusion, leads to renin release and formation of angiotensin I from angiotensinogen. Angiotensin-converting enzyme (ACE) converts angiotensin I to angiotensin II, which stimulates the adrenal cortex to synthesize and release aldosterone.[30] Acting primarily in the distal tubules, high concentrations of aldosterone cause sodium reabsorption and may reduce urinary excretion of sodium nearly to

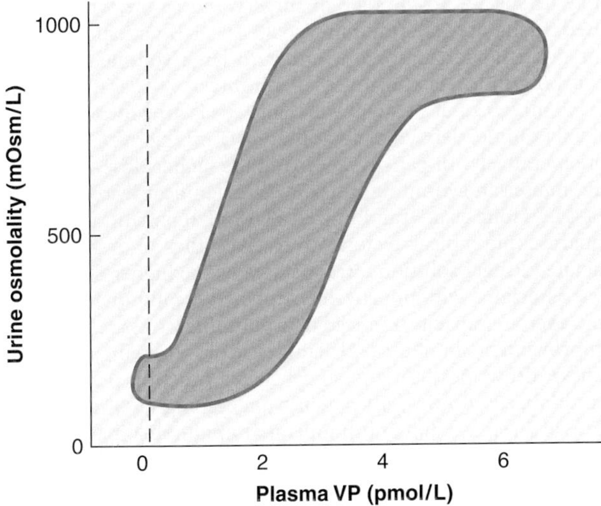

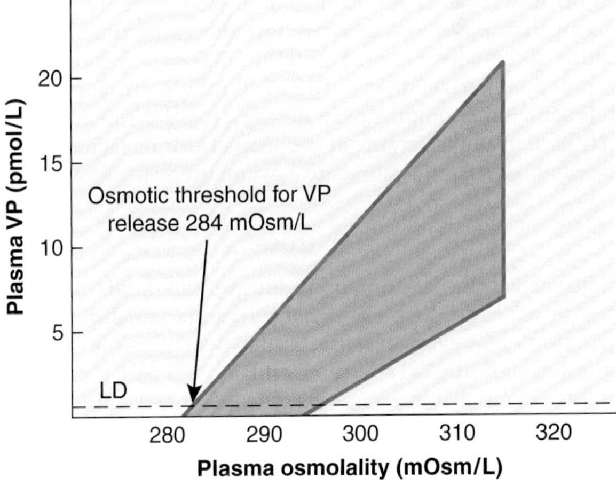

FIGURE 14-3. Left: The sigmoid relationship between plasma vasopressin (VP) and urinary osmolality. Data were obtained during water loading and fluid restriction in a group of healthy adults. Maximum urinary concentration is achieved by plasma VP values of 3 to 4 pmol/L. **Right:** The linear relationship between plasma osmolality and plasma VP. Increases in VP in response to hypertonicity induced by infusion of 855 mmol/L saline in a group of healthy adults. The shaded area represents the reference range response. LD represents the limit of detection of the VP assay, 0.3 pmol/L. (From: Ball SG. Vasopressin and disorders of water balance: the physiology and pathophysiology of vasopressin. *Ann Clin Biochem.* 2007;44:417–431, with permission.)

TABLE 14-10. HOURLY AND DAILY MAINTENANCE WATER REQUIREMENTS

Weight (kg)	Water (mL/kg/hr)	Water (mL/kg/day)
1–10	4	100
11–20	2	50
21–n+	1	20

zero. Intrarenal physical factors are also important in regulating sodium balance. Sodium loading decreases colloid osmotic pressure, thereby increasing the glomerular filtration rate (GFR), decreasing net sodium reabsorption and increasing distal sodium delivery, which, in turn, suppresses renin secretion.

Fluid Replacement Therapy

Maintenance Requirements for Water, Sodium, and Potassium

Calculation of maintenance fluid requirements is of limited value in determining intraoperative fluid requirements. However, calculation of maintenance fluid requirements (Table 14-10) is useful for estimating water and electrolyte deficits that result from preoperative restriction of oral food and fluids and for estimating the ongoing requirements for patients with prolonged postoperative bowel dysfunction. In healthy adults, sufficient water is required to balance gastrointestinal losses of 100 to 200 mL/day, insensible losses of 500 to 1,000 mL/day (half of which is respiratory and half is cutaneous), and urinary losses of 1,000 mL/day. Urinary losses exceeding 1,000 mL/day may represent an appropriate physiologic response to ECV expansion or pathophysiologic inability to conserve salt or water.

Daily adult requirements for sodium and potassium are approximately 75 and 40 mEq/kg respectively, although wider ranges of sodium intake than potassium intake are physiologically tolerated because renal sodium conservation and excretion are more efficient than potassium conservation and excretion. Therefore, healthy, 70 kg adults require 2,500 mL/day of water containing [Na^+] of 30 mEq/L and [K^+] of 15 to 20 mEq/L. Intraoperatively, fluids containing sodium-free water (i.e., [Na^+] < 130 mEq/L) are rarely used in adults because of the necessity for replacing isotonic losses and the risk of postoperative hyponatremia.

Dextrose

Traditionally, glucose-containing intravenous fluids have been given in an effort to prevent hypoglycemia and limit protein catabolism. However, because of the hyperglycemic response associated with surgical stress, only infants and patients receiving insulin or drugs that interfere with glucose synthesis are at risk for hypoglycemia. Iatrogenic hyperglycemia can limit the effectiveness of fluid resuscitation by inducing an osmotic diuresis and, in animals, may aggravate ischemic neurologic injury.[31] Although associated with worsened outcome after subarachnoid hemorrhage[32] and traumatic brain injury[33] in humans, hyperglycemia may also constitute a hormonally mediated response to more severe injury. In critically ill patients, some evidence suggests that
7 tight control of plasma glucose (maintenance of plasma glucose between 80 and 110 mg/dL) is associated with better outcomes, but other evidence does not, and in fact, suggests that tight control may increase mortality.[34–37]

Surgical Fluid Requirements

Water and Electrolyte Composition of Fluid Losses

Surgical patients require replacement of PV and ECV losses secondary to wound or burn edema, ascites, and gastrointestinal secretions. Wound and burn edema and ascitic fluid are protein-rich and contain electrolytes in concentrations similar to plasma. Although gastrointestinal secretions vary greatly in composition, the composition of replacement fluid need not be closely matched if ECV is adequate and renal and cardiovascular functions are normal. Substantial loss of gastrointestinal fluids requires more accurate replacement of electrolytes (i.e., potassium, magnesium, phosphate). Chronic gastric losses may produce hypochloremic metabolic alkalosis that can be corrected with 0.9% saline; chronic diarrhea may produce hyperchloremic metabolic acidosis that may be prevented or corrected by infusion of fluid containing bicarbonate or bicarbonate substrate (e.g., lactate). If cardiovascular or renal function is impaired, more precise replacement may require frequent assessment of serum electrolytes.

Influence of Perioperative Fluid Infusion Rates on Clinical Outcomes

Conventionally, intraoperative fluid management has included replacement of fluid that is assumed to accumulate extravascularly in surgically manipulated tissue.[38] Until recently, periopera-
8 tive clinical practice included, in addition to maintenance fluids and replacement of estimated blood loss, 4 to 6 mL/kg/hr for procedures involving minimal tissue trauma, 6 to 8 mL/kg/hr for those involving moderate trauma, and 8 to 12 mL/kg/hr for those involving extreme trauma.

However, recent clinical trials strongly link perioperative fluid management to potentially important alterations of both minor and major morbidities. Moreover, the influence of fluid volume may be specific to the type of surgery and to the types of fluid
9 used. Maharaj et al.[39] randomized 80 ASA I-II patients scheduled for gynecologic laparoscopy either to large volume, defined as 2 mL/kg/hr of fasting over 20 minutes preoperatively (e.g., 1,440 mL/60 kg in a patient who had been fasting for 12 hours) or small volume, defined as total fluid of 3 mL/kg over 20 minutes preoperatively. In patients receiving the higher dose, postoperative nausea and vomiting and pain were significantly reduced (Fig. 14-4).[39] Holte et al.[40] randomized 48 ASA I-II patients undergoing laparoscopic cholecystectomy to receive either 15 or 40 mL/kg of lactated Ringer solution intraoperatively; the higher dose of fluid was associated with improved postoperative pulmonary function and exercise capacity, reduced neurohumoral stress response, and improvements in nausea, general sense of well-being, thirst, dizziness, drowsiness, fatigue, and balance function. Holte et al.[41] randomized 48 ASA I-III patients undergoing fast-track elective knee arthroplasty under intraoperative epidural/spinal anesthesia and postoperative epidural analgesia to either liberal or restricted fluids. Median intravenous fluid administered intraoperatively and in the postanesthesia care unit in the restrictive group was 1,740 mL (range: 1,100 to 2,165 mL) of lactated Ringer solution and in the liberal group was 3,275 mL (range: 2,400 to 4,000 mL). Restrictive fluid administration was associated with a higher incidence of vomiting but less hypercoagulability and no difference in short-term postoperative mobility or ileus. Therefore, fluid restriction appears to be less well tolerated than more liberal fluid

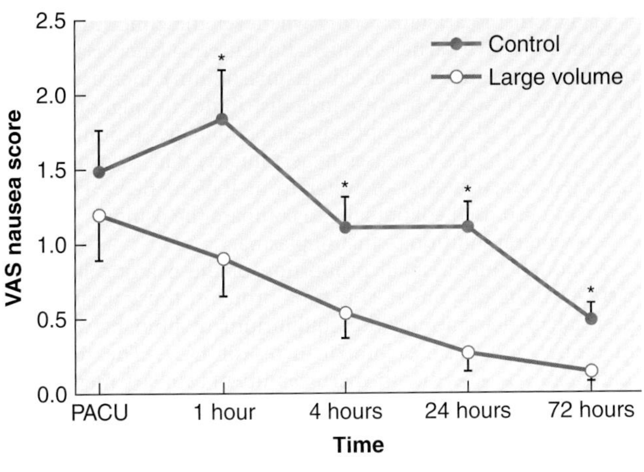

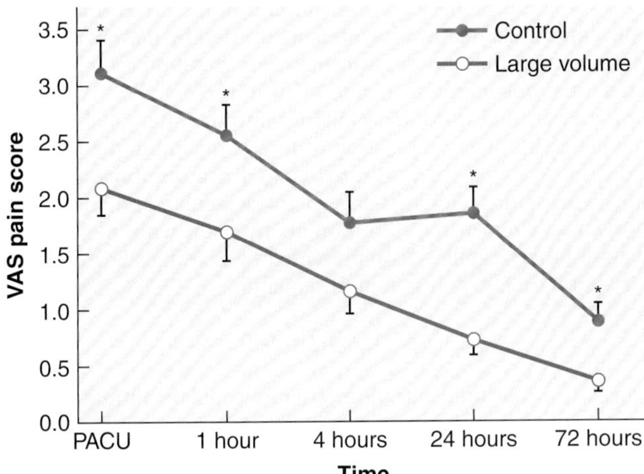

FIGURE 14-4. Top: Mean postoperative verbal analog scale (VAS) nausea scores in each group over the first 72 postoperative hours. Mean VAS nausea scores were significantly lower in the group that received the large-volume intravenous fluid infusion compared with the control group at 1, 4, 24, and 72 hours postoperatively. **Bottom:** Mean postoperative VAS pain scores in each group over the first 72 postoperative hours. Mean VAS pain scores were significantly lower in the group that received the large-volume intravenous fluid infusion compared with the control group at 0, 1, 24, and 72 hours postoperatively. *Significantly higher ($p < 0.05$, *t*-test postanalysis of variance) VAS score compared with the large volume group. PACU, postanesthesia care unit. (From: Maharaj CH, Kallam SR, Malik A, et al. Preoperative intravenous fluid therapy decreases postoperative nausea and pain in high risk patients. *Anesth Analg.* 2005;100:675–682, with permission.)

therapy in patients undergoing surgery of limited scope, but perhaps at the expense of hypercoagulability.

In patients undergoing major intra-abdominal surgery, recent randomized controlled trials also suggest that restrictive fluid administration is associated with a combination of positive and negative effects. Brandstrup et al.[42] randomized 172 elective colon surgery patients to either restrictive perioperative fluid management or standard perioperative fluid management, with the primary goal of maintaining preoperative body weight in the fluid-restricted group. By design, the fluid-restricted group received less perioperative fluid and acutely gained <1 kg in contrast to >3 kg in the standard therapy group. More importantly, cardiopulmonary complications, tissue-healing complications, and total postoperative complications were significantly fewer in the fluid-restricted group. In 152 patients undergoing intra-abdominal surgery, including colon surgery, Nisanevich et al.[43] reported less prompt return of gastrointestinal function and longer hospital stays in patients receiving conventional fluid therapy (10 mL/kg/hr of lactated Ringer solution) than in patients receiving restricted fluid therapy (4 mL/kg/hr). In a small clinical trial comparing gastric emptying in patients randomized to receive the postoperative fluids at a restricted (≤2 L/day of water; ≤77 mEq/day) or liberal regimen (≥3 L/day of water; ≥154 mEq/day), gastric emptying time for both liquids and solids was significantly reduced in patients receiving restricted fluids (Fig. 14-5).[44] Khoo et al.[45] randomized 70 ASA I-III patients undergoing elective colorectal surgery to conventional perioperative management, including intraoperative

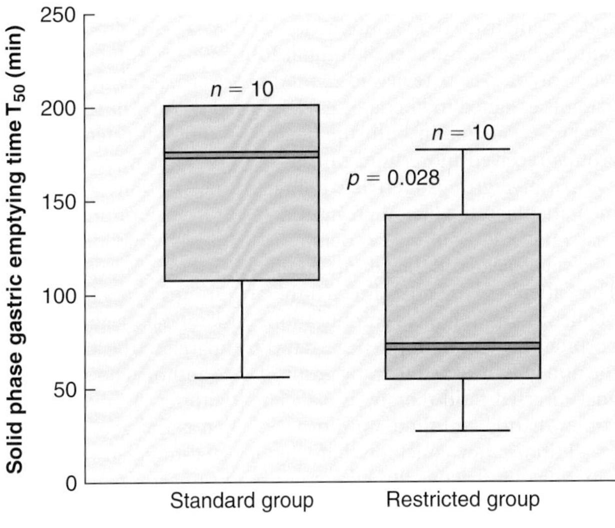

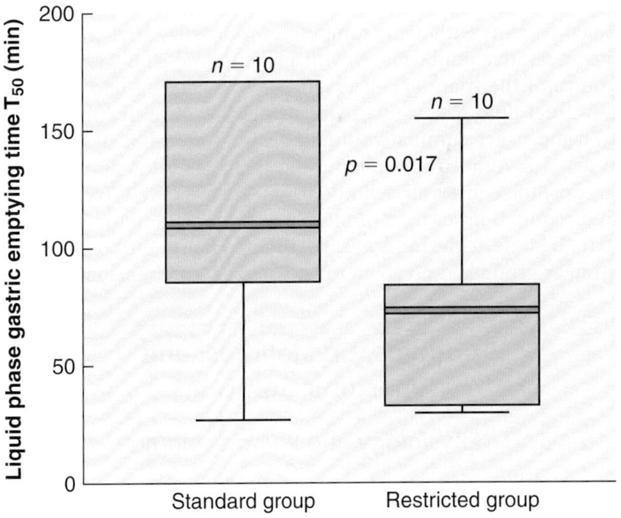

FIGURE 14-5. Solid and liquid phase gastric emptying times (T_{50}) after 4 days of standard or restricted intravenous postoperative fluid therapy. Solid lines are medians, shaded areas interquartile ranges, and whiskers represent extreme values. Differences between medians for solid and liquid phase T_{50} were 56 minutes (95% confidence interval: 12 to 132 minutes) and 52 minutes (9 to 95 minutes), respectively. (Reprinted with permission from: Lobo DN, Bostock KA, Neal KR, et al. Effect of salt and water balance on recovery of gastrointestinal function after elective colonic resection: A randomised controlled trial. *Lancet.* 2002;359:1812.)

fluid management at the discretion of the anesthesiologist, or to multimodal perioperative management, including intraoperative fluid restriction, unrestricted postoperative oral intake, prokinetic agents, early ambulation, and postoperative epidural analgesia. Multimodal perioperative management was associated with a reduced median stay (5 vs. 7 days) and fewer cardiorespiratory and anastomotic complications, but more hospital readmissions. Holte et al.[46] randomized 32 ASA I-III patients undergoing "fast-track" colon resection under combined epidural/general anesthesia to intraoperative fluid administration using either a restrictive (median: 1,640 mL; range: 935 to 2,250 mL) or liberal (median: 5,050 mL; range: 3,563 to 8,050 mL) regimen. Fluid-restricted patients had significantly improved postoperative forced vital capacity and fewer, less severe episodes of oxygen desaturation but at the expense of increased stress responses (aldosterone, ADH, and angiotensin II measurements) and a statistically insignificantly increased number of complications. In a recent meta-analysis, Corcoran et al. reviewed 23 randomized trials involving 3,861 patients assigned to liberal or goal-directed therapy during major surgery.[47] Patients in both the liberal and goal-directed therapy groups received more fluid during surgery than their respective comparative groups (restrictive fluid administration). However, the patients in the liberal groups had a higher risk of pneumonia (risk ratio 2.2), pulmonary edema (risk ratio 3.8), and longer hospital stay (mean difference 2 days) than their comparative groups. The patients in the goal-directed therapy groups had a lower risk of pneumonia and renal complications (risk ratio 0.7), and shorter hospital stay (mean difference 2 days) compared to the patients in the non goal-directed therapy group. These authors conclude that goal-directed fluid therapy is associated with fewer adverse outcomes than liberal fluid administration that is not goal directed. In addition, they conclude that whether goal-directed therapy is superior to restrictive fluid therapy remains uncertain.

Critically ill patients with acute lung injury represent an important group that may benefit from careful regulation of fluid intake. The ARDS Clinical Trials Network[48] randomized 1,000 patients with acute lung injury to a 7-day trial comparing a conservative fluid strategy with a liberal fluid strategy. Over the course of the trial the conservative strategy group had a cumulative net fluid balance that was slightly negative in comparison to a mean net cumulative fluid balance in the liberal group of nearly 7 L. Although overall mortality was no different in the two groups, the conservative fluid group had improved oxygenation and required fewer days of mechanical ventilation and intensive care. Despite achieving a negative fluid balance, the conservative strategy group had no greater incidence of acute renal failure.

Colloids, Crystalloids, and Hypertonic Solutions

Physiology and Pharmacology

Osmotically active particles attract water across semipermeable membranes until equilibrium is attained. The *osmolarity* of a solution refers to the number of osmotically active particles per *liter* of solvent; *osmolality*, a measurement of the number of osmotically active particles per *kilogram*, can be estimated as follows:

$$\text{Osmolality} = ([\text{Na}^+] \times 2) + (\text{Glucose}/18) + (\text{BUN}/2.3) \quad (14\text{-}10)$$

where osmolality is expressed in mmol/kg, $[\text{Na}^+]$ is expressed in mEq/L, serum glucose is expressed in mg/dL, and BUN is blood urea nitrogen expressed in mg/dL. Sugars, alcohols, and radiographic dyes increase measured osmolality, generating an increased "osmolal gap" between the measured and calculated values.

A hyperosmolar state occurs whenever the concentration of osmotically active particles is high. Both uremia (increased BUN) and hypernatremia (increased serum sodium) increase serum osmolality. However, because urea distributes throughout TBW, an increase in BUN does not cause *hypertonicity*. Sodium, largely restricted to the ECV, causes hypertonicity, that is, osmotically mediated redistribution of water from ICV to ECV. The term *tonicity* is also used colloquially to compare the osmotic pressure of a parenteral solution to that of plasma.

Although only a small proportion of the osmotically active particles in blood consist of plasma proteins, those particles are essential in determining the equilibrium of fluid between the interstitial and plasma compartments of ECV. The reflection coefficient (σ) describes the permeability of capillary membranes to individual solutes, with 0 representing free permeability and 1 representing complete impermeability. The reflection coefficient for albumin ranges from 0.6 to 0.9 in various capillary beds. Because capillary protein concentrations exceed interstitial concentrations, the osmotic pressure exerted by plasma proteins (termed *colloid osmotic pressure* or *oncotic pressure*) is higher than interstitial oncotic pressure and tends to preserve PV. The filtration rate of fluid from the capillaries into the interstitial space is the net result of a combination of forces, including the gradient from intravascular to interstitial colloid osmotic pressures and the hydrostatic gradient between intravascular and interstitial pressures. The net fluid filtration at any point within a systemic or pulmonary capillary is represented by Starling's law of capillary filtration, as expressed in the equation:

$$Q = \underline{k}\underline{A}\,[(P_c - P_i) + \sigma(\pi_i - \pi_c)] \quad (14\text{-}11)$$

where Q is the fluid filtration, $\underline{k}$ is the capillary filtration coefficient (conductivity of water), $\underline{A}$ is the area of the capillary membrane, P_c is the capillary hydrostatic pressure, P_i is the interstitial hydrostatic pressure, σ is the reflection coefficient for albumin, π_i is the interstitial colloid osmotic pressure, and π_c is the capillary colloid osmotic pressure.

The IFV is determined by the relative rates of capillary filtration and lymphatic drainage. P_c, the most powerful factor promoting fluid filtration, is determined by capillary flow, arterial resistance, venous resistance, and venous pressure. If capillary filtration increases, the rates of water and sodium filtration usually exceed protein filtration, resulting in preservation of π_c, dilution of π_i, and preservation of the oncotic pressure gradient, the most powerful factor opposing fluid filtration. When coupled with increased lymphatic drainage, preservation of the oncotic pressure gradient limits the accumulation of IF. If P_c increases at a time when lymphatic drainage is maximal, then IFV accumulates, forming edema.

Clinical Implications of Choices Between Alternative Fluids

If membrane permeability is intact, colloids such as albumin or hydroxyethyl starch preferentially expand PV rather than IFV. Concentrated colloid-containing solutions (e.g., 25% albumin) exert sufficient oncotic pressure to translocate substantial volumes of IFV into the PV, thereby increasing PV by a volume that exceeds the original infused volume. PV expansion unaccompanied by IFV expansion offers apparent advantages: Lower fluid requirements, less peripheral and pulmonary edema accumulation, and reduced concern about the cardiopulmonary consequences of later fluid mobilization (Table 14-11).

However, exhaustive research has failed to establish the superiority of either colloid-containing or crystalloid-containing fluids for either intraoperative or postoperative use. Moretti et al.[49] reported that patients who were randomized to receive

TABLE 14-11. CLAIMED ADVANTAGES AND DISADVANTAGES OF COLLOID VERSUS CRYSTALLOID INTRAVENOUS FLUIDS

Solution	Advantages	Disadvantages
Colloid	Smaller infused volume	Greater cost
	Prolonged increase in plasma volume	Coagulopathy (dextran > HES)
	Less peripheral edema	Pulmonary edema (capillary leak states)
		Decreased GFR
		Osmotic diuresis (low-molecular-weight dextran)
		Greater duration of excessive volume expansion
Crystalloid	Lower cost	Transient increase in intravascular volume
	Greater urinary flow	Transient hemodynamic improvement
	Interstitial fluid replacement	Peripheral edema (protein dilution)
		Pulmonary edema (protein dilution plus high PAOP)

HES, hydroxyethyl starch; GFR, glomerular filtration rate; PAOP, pulmonary arterial occlusion pressure.

6% hetastarch had less postoperative nausea and vomiting than those who received lactated Ringer solution without colloid. In addition, colloid administration appears to have been an essential component of perioperative management strategies that demonstrated improved morbidity after colon surgery[42] and after major surgery in conjunction with goal-directed fluid challenges.[50,51]

In critically ill patients and patients undergoing more extensive surgery, systematic reviews of available comparisons of colloid versus crystalloid and albumin versus crystalloid suggested that the choice of fluid did not influence mortality.[52] A recent randomized controlled trial comparing 4% albumin with 0.9% saline for fluid maintenance in 6,997 critically ill patients supports the conclusion that choice of colloid or crystalloid does not influence mortality.[53] Baseline serum albumin concentration did not alter the lack of effect of albumin management on outcome.[54] However, subgroup analyses suggested that crystalloid treatment could be superior in patients after trauma and that colloid could be superior in patients with severe sepsis.[53] Subsequent 2-year follow-up of a subset of 460 patients with traumatic brain injury (Glasgow Coma Scale score ≤13) demonstrated a nearly twofold increased risk of death in patients receiving colloid fluid management.[55]

Although hydroxyethyl starch, the most commonly used synthetic colloid, is less expensive than albumin, large doses (exceeding 20 mL/kg/day) produce laboratory evidence of coagulopathy.[56,57] While newer and potentially improved formulations continue to become available, the Cochrane Systematic Reviews published the results of a meta-analysis of 70 trials published between 1974 and 2007 involving 4,375 patients and concluded that "there is no evidence that one colloid is more effective or safer than any other". However, in patients with severe sepsis, the most recent data indicate that fluid resuscitation with hydroxyl ethyl starch 13/0.42 results in a significantly higher death rate (51% vs. 43%), higher need for renal replacement therapy (22% vs. 16%), and higher rate of severe bleeding (10% vs. 6%) compared with treatment with Ringer's lactate.[58]

Implications of Crystalloid and Colloid Infusions on Intracranial Pressure

Because the cerebral capillary membrane, the blood–brain barrier, is highly impermeable to sodium, abrupt changes in serum osmolality produced by changes in serum sodium, produce reciprocal changes in brain water. In anesthetized rabbits, reducing plasma osmolality from 295 to 282 mOsm/kg (which decreases plasma osmotic pressure by ~250 mm Hg) increased cortical water content and ICP; in contrast reducing colloid osmotic pressure from 20 to 7 mm Hg produced no significant change in either variable.[59] Similar independence of brain water and ICP from colloid osmotic pressure has been demonstrated with prolonged hypoalbuminemia[60] and in animals after forebrain ischemia[61] and focal cryogenic injury.[62] Although rats had reduced brain water after fluid percussion traumatic brain injury if colloid oncotic pressure was increased with hetastarch,[63] these observations must be balanced against the apparent increase in mortality in traumatic brain injury patients managed with albumin rather than 0.9% saline during intensive care.[55]

Clinical Implications of Hypertonic Fluid Administration

An ideal alternative to conventional crystalloid and colloid fluids would be inexpensive, would produce minimal peripheral or pulmonary edema, would generate sustained hemodynamic effects, and would be effective even if administered in small volumes. Hypertonic, hypernatremic solutions, with or without added colloid, appear to fulfill some of these criteria (Table 14-12).

Current enthusiasm for hypertonic resuscitation was stimulated by the work of Velasco et al.,[64] who successfully used small volumes (6 mL/kg) of 7.5% hypertonic saline as the sole resuscitative measure in dogs after severe hemorrhage. Hypertonic solutions exert favorable effects on cerebral hemodynamics, in part because of the reciprocal relationship between plasma osmolality and brain water.[59] ICP increased during resuscitation from hemorrhagic shock with lactated Ringer solution but remained unchanged if 7.5% saline was infused in a sufficient volume to comparably improve systemic hemodynamics.[65] However, improvements in ICP gradually are lost. Delayed increases in ICP were reported after hypertonic resuscitation from hypovolemic shock accompanied by an intracranial mass lesion.[66] In addition, systemic hemodynamic improvement produced by hypertonic resuscitation is short-lived.[65] Strategies to prolong the therapeutic effects beyond 30 to 60 minutes include continued infusion of hypertonic saline, subsequent infusion of blood or conventional fluids, or addition of colloid to hypertonic resuscitation.

Despite concerns about central nervous system dysfunction due to hypertonicity and hypernatremia associated with hypertonic saline, acute increases in serum sodium to 155 to 160 mEq/L

TABLE 14-12. HYPERTONIC RESUSCITATION FLUIDS: ADVANTAGES AND DISADVANTAGES

Solution	Advantages	Disadvantages
Hypertonic crystalloid	Inexpensive Promotes urinary flow Small initial volume Arteriolar dilation Reduced peripheral edema Lower intracranial pressure	Hypertonicity Subdural hemorrhage Transient effect Potential rebound intracranial hypertension
Hypertonic crystalloid plus colloid (in comparison to hypertonic crystalloid alone)	Sustained hemodynamic response Reduced subsequent volume requirements	Added expense Osmotic diuresis Hypertonicity

From: Prough DS, Johnston WE. Fluid resuscitation in septic shock: no solution yet. *Anesth Analg.* 1989;69:699–704, with permission.

produced no apparent harm in humans resuscitated with hypertonic saline.[67] Central pontine myelinolysis, which follows rapid correction of severe, chronic hyponatremia, has not been observed in clinical trials of hypertonic resuscitation. Despite theoretical considerations favoring the use of hypertonic saline in resuscitation of patients with traumatic brain injury, a recent randomized trial failed to demonstrate an improvement in outcome.[68]

Will clinicians routinely use hypertonic or combination hypertonic/hyperoncotic fluids for resuscitation in the future? Pending further preclinical work, the theoretical advantages of such fluids appear most attractive in the acute resuscitation of hypovolemic patients who have decreased intracranial compliance.[69]

Fluid Status: Assessment and Monitoring

For most surgical patients, conventional clinical assessment of the adequacy of intravascular volume is appropriate. For high-risk patients, goal-directed hemodynamic management may be superior.

Conventional Clinical Assessment

Clinical quantification of blood volume and ECV begins with recognition of deficit-generating settings such as bowel obstruction, preoperative bowel preparation, chronic diuretic use, sepsis, burns, and trauma. Physical signs that suggest hypovolemia include oliguria, supine hypotension, and a positive tilt test. Oliguria implies hypovolemia, although hypovolemic patients may be nonoliguric and normovolemic patients may be oliguric because of renal failure or stress-induced endocrine responses.[70] Supine hypotension implies a blood volume deficit exceeding 30%, although arterial blood pressure within the normal range could represent relative hypotension in an elderly or chronically hypertensive patient.

In the tilt test, a positive response is defined as an increase in heart rate ≥20 beats/ minute and a decrease in systolic blood pressure ≥20 mm Hg when the subject assumes the upright position. However, young, healthy subjects can withstand acute loss of 20% of blood volume while exhibiting only postural tachycardia and variable postural hypotension. In contrast, orthostasis may occur in 20% to 30% of elderly patients despite normal blood volume. In volunteers, withdrawal of 500 mL of blood[71] was associated with a greater increase in heart rate on standing than before blood withdrawal, but with no significant difference in the response of blood pressure or cardiac index.

Laboratory evidence that suggests hypovolemia or ECV depletion includes azotemia, low urinary sodium, metabolic alkalosis (if hypovolemia is mild), and metabolic acidosis (if hypovolemia is severe). Hematocrit is virtually unchanged by acute hemorrhage until fluids are administered or until fluid shifts from the interstitial to the intravascular space. BUN, normally 8 to 20 mg/dL, is increased by hypovolemia, high-protein intake, gastrointestinal bleeding, or accelerated catabolism and decreased by severe hepatic dysfunction. Serum creatinine (SCr), a product of muscle catabolism, may be misleadingly low in elderly adults, females, and debilitated or malnourished patients. In contrast, in muscular or acutely catabolic patients, SCr may exceed the normal range (0.5 to 1.5 mg/dL) because of greater muscle protein metabolism. A ratio of BUN to SCr exceeding the normal range (10 to 20) suggests dehydration. In prerenal oliguria, enhanced sodium reabsorption should reduce urinary [Na^+] to ≤20 mEq/L and enhanced water reabsorption should increase urinary concentration (i.e., urinary osmolality >400, urine/plasma creatinine ratio >40:1). However, the sensitivity and specificity of measurements of urinary variables may be misleading. Although hypovolemia does not generate metabolic alkalosis, ECV depletion is a potent stimulus for the maintenance of metabolic alkalosis. Severe hypovolemia may result in systemic hypoperfusion and lactic acidosis.

Intraoperative Clinical Assessment

Visual estimation, the simplest technique for quantifying intraoperative blood loss, assesses the amount of blood absorbed by gauze squares and laparotomy pads and adds an estimate of blood accumulation on the floor and surgical drapes and in suction containers. Both surgeons and anesthesia providers tend to underestimate losses.

Assessment of the adequacy of intraoperative fluid resuscitation integrates multiple clinical variables, including heart rate, blood pressure, urinary output, arterial oxygenation, and pH. Tachycardia is an insensitive, nonspecific indicator of hypovolemia. In patients receiving potent inhalational agents, maintenance of a satisfactory blood pressure implies adequate intravascular volume. Preservation of blood pressure, accompanied by a central venous pressure (CVP) of 6 to 12 mm Hg, more strongly suggests adequate replacement. During profound hypovolemia, indirect measurements of blood pressure may significantly underestimate true blood pressure. In patients undergoing extensive procedures, direct arterial pressure measurements are more accurate than indirect techniques and provide convenient access for obtaining arterial blood samples. An additional advantage of direct arterial pressure monitoring may be recognition of increased systolic blood pressure variation accompanying positive pressure ventilation in the presence of hypovolemia.[72,73] However, in a large multicenter prospective trial, pulse pressure variation (PPV) during mechanical ventilation was compared with CVP as a means to predict cardiac output increase in response to fluid challenge. Although PPV was superior to CVP, it was inconclusive in approximately 25% of patients.[74] Specifically, when PPV is between 9% and 13% in patients under general anesthesia, fluid responsiveness cannot be reliably predicted.

Urinary output usually declines precipitously during moderate to severe hypovolemia. Therefore, in the absence of glycosuria or diuretic administration, a urinary output of 0.5 to 1 mL/kg/hr during anesthesia suggests adequate renal perfusion. Arterial pH may decrease only when tissue hypoperfusion becomes severe. Cardiac output can be normal despite severely reduced regional blood flow. Mixed venous hemoglobin desaturation, a specific indicator of poor systemic perfusion, reflects average perfusion in multiple organs and cannot supplant regional monitors such as urinary output.

A technique for assessing the adequacy of cardiac preload during high-risk surgical procedures is the use of esophageal Doppler that measures blood flow in the descending thoracic aorta and that also measures the duration of aortic systole, which, if corrected for heart rate, correlates with left ventricular preload.[75] In general, a corrected flow time <0.35 second suggests that volume expansion should improve cardiac output, while a corrected flow time >0.40 second suggests that further volume expansion will be ineffective.

Oxygen Delivery as a Goal of Management

No intraoperative monitor is sufficiently sensitive or specific to detect hypoperfusion in all patients. One key variable that has been associated with improved outcome in high-risk surgical patients and critically ill patients is a systemic oxygen delivery (Do_2) ≥600 mL O_2/m^2 min (equivalent to a cardiac index [CI] of 3 L/m^2 min, a [Hgb] of 14 g/dL, and 98% oxyhemoglobin saturation). At present, available data are consistent with two inferences. First, there is no apparent benefit for patients other than surgical patients and patients undergoing initial resuscitation from septic shock in the emergency department.[76] In surgical patients, early initiation of goal-directed resuscitation is associated with better outcome than delayed initiation.[77] Second, outcome may be strongly influenced by the choice of methods to increase oxygen delivery, that is, the choice of fluid administration or various inotropic agents. Lobo et al.[78] randomized 50 high-risk patients, defined as elderly patients with coexistent pathologies who were undergoing major elective surgery, to goal-directed hemodynamic therapy either with fluids alone or with fluids plus dobutamine. Hemodynamic goals intraoperatively and for the first 24 hours postoperatively consisted of DO_2I >600 mL O_2/m^2 min. Postoperative cardiovascular complications occurred significantly more frequently in the group receiving fluids alone (13/25, 52% vs. 4/25, 16%; relative risk, 3.25; 95% CI, 1.22–8.60; $p < 0.05$) and mortality was greater, but not statistically significantly greater in this small series. Increased fluid given as part of goal-oriented resuscitation has been associated with an increased incidence of abdominal compartment syndrome in trauma patients.[79] Wilson et al.[80] randomized 138 patients undergoing major elective surgery into three groups. One group received routine perioperative care; one received fluid and dopexamine preoperatively, intraoperatively, and postoperatively to maintain oxygen delivery ≥600 mL O_2/m^2 min; and the third received fluid plus epinephrine preoperatively, intraoperatively, and postoperatively to achieve the same end points. In the two groups in which oxygen delivery was supported, only 3 of 92 died, compared with 8 of 46 control patients. However, the complication rate was significantly lower in the dopexamine group than in the epinephrine group.

Several studies have reported improved outcome based on adjustment of perioperative fluids through the use of an esophageal Doppler monitor.[81] Using the esophageal Doppler to guide administration of colloid boluses, Venn et al.[49] and Gan et al.[50] have reported shortened length of hospital stay after hip surgery and major surgery, respectively. Of note, Horowitz and Kumar[82] speculated that the infusion of colloid rather than the monitor-driven algorithm was responsible for the improved results.

ELECTROLYTES

Sodium

Physiologic Role

Sodium, the principal extracellular cation and solute, is essential
10 for generation of action potentials in neurologic and cardiac tissues. Disorders (pathologic increases or decreases) of *total body sodium* are associated with corresponding increases or decreases of ECV and PV. Disorders of sodium *concentration,* that is, hyponatremia and hypernatremia, usually result from relative excesses or deficits, respectively, of water. Regulation of total body sodium and [Na^+] is accomplished primarily by the endocrine and renal systems (Table 14-13). Secretion of aldosterone and ANP control *total body sodium.* ADH, which is secreted in response to increased osmolality or decreased blood pressure, primarily regulates [Na^+]. Therefore, primary hyperaldosteronism is associated with hypervolemia and with hypertension, but not with abnormal [Na^+].[83,84]

Hyponatremia

Hyponatremia, defined as [Na^+] < 130 mEq/L, is the most common electrolyte disturbance in hospitalized patients. In the

TABLE 14-13. REGULATION OF TOTAL BODY ELECTROLYTE MASS AND PLASMA CONCENTRATIONS

Electrolyte	Regulated by
Sodium	Total body sodium regulated by aldosterone, ANP, [Na^+] altered by ADH
Potassium	Total body potassium regulated by aldosterone, intrinsic renal mechanisms; [K^+] regulated by epinephrine, insulin
Calcium	Both total body calcium and [Ca^{++}] regulated by PTH, vitamin D
Phosphate	Both total body phosphate and [HPO_4^{--}] regulated primarily by renal mechanisms with a minor contribution from PTH
Magnesium	Both total body magnesium and [Mg^{++}] regulated primarily by renal mechanisms with a minor contribution from PTH and vitamin D

ANP, atrial natriuretic peptide; [Na^+], sodium concentration; ADH, antidiuretic hormone; PTH, parathyroid hormone.

majority of hyponatremic patients, total body sodium is normal or increased. The most common clinical scenarios associated with hyponatremia include the postoperative state, acute intracranial disease, malignant disease, medications, and acute pulmonary disease. Hyponatremia is associated with increased mortality, both as a direct effect of hyponatremia and because of the association between hyponatremia and severe systemic disease.

The signs and symptoms of hyponatremia depend on both the rate and severity of the decrease in plasma [Na^+]. Symptoms that can accompany severe hyponatremia ([Na^+] <120 mEq/L) include loss of appetite, nausea, vomiting, cramps, weakness, altered level of consciousness, coma, and seizures.

Acute central nervous system manifestations of hyponatremia result from brain overhydration. Because the blood–brain barrier is poorly permeable to sodium but freely permeable to water, a rapid decrease in plasma [Na^+] promptly increases both extracellular and intracellular brain water. Because the brain rapidly compensates for changes in osmolality, acute hyponatremia produces more severe symptoms than chronic hyponatremia. The symptoms of chronic hyponatremia probably relate to depletion of brain electrolytes. Once brain volume has compensated for hyponatremia, rapid increases in [Na^+] may lead to abrupt brain dehydration.

In hyponatremic patients, serum osmolality may be normal, high, or low (Fig. 14-6). Hyponatremia with a normal or high serum osmolality results from the presence of a nonsodium solute, such as glucose or mannitol, which holds water within the extracellular space and results in dilutional hyponatremia. The presence of a nonsodium solute may be inferred if measured osmolality exceeds calculated osmolality by >10 mOsm/kg. For example, plasma [Na^+] decreases approximately 2.4 mEq/L for each 100 mg/dL rise in glucose concentration with perhaps even greater decreases as glucose concentration >400 mg/dL.[85] In anesthesia practice, a common cause of hyponatremia associated with a normal osmolality is the absorption of large volumes of sodium-free irrigating solutions (containing mannitol, glycerin, or sorbitol as the solute) during transurethral resection of the prostate.[86] Neurologic symptoms are minimal if mannitol is used

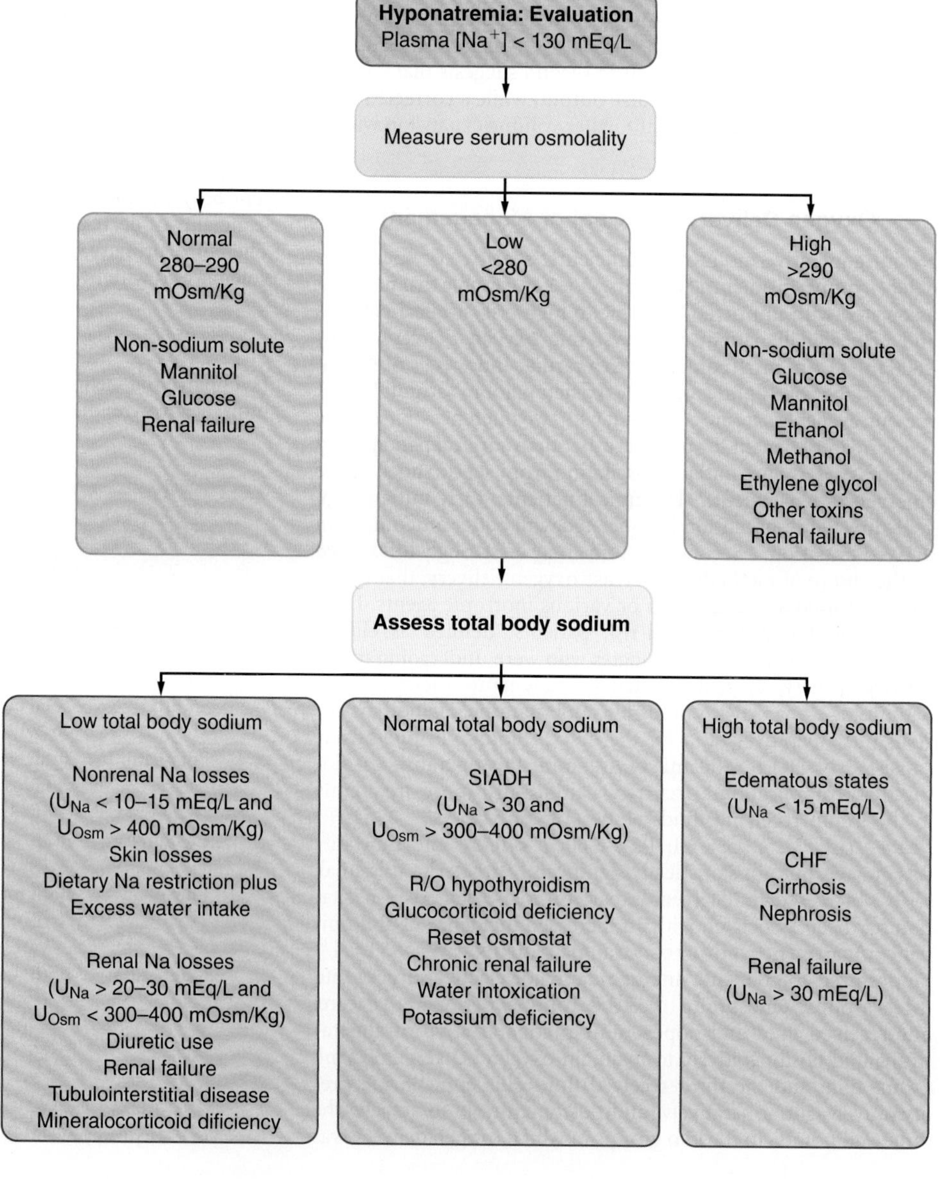

FIGURE 14-6. Algorithm by which hyponatremia can be evaluated. SIADH, syndrome of inappropriate antidiuretic hormone secretion; R/O, rule out; CHF, congestive heart failure.

because the agent does not cross the blood–brain barrier and is excreted with water in the urine. In contrast, as glycine or sorbitol is metabolized, hyposmolality will gradually develop and cerebral edema may appear as a late complication, that is, hypoosmolality is more important in generating symptoms than hyponatremia per se.[86] Hyponatremia with a normal or elevated serum osmolality also may accompany renal insufficiency. BUN, included in the calculation of total osmolality, distributes throughout both ECV and ICV. Calculation of *effective* osmolality (2[Na^+] + glucose/18) excludes the contribution of urea to tonicity and demonstrates true hypotonicity.

Hyponatremia with low serum osmolality may be associated with a high, low, or normal total body sodium and PV. Therefore, hyponatremia with hyposmolality (Fig. 14-6) is evaluated by assessing total body sodium content, BUN, SCr, urinary osmolality, and urinary [Na^+]. Hyponatremia with increased total body sodium is characteristic of edematous states, that is, congestive heart failure, cirrhosis, nephrosis, and renal failure. Aquaporin 2, the vasopressin-regulated water channel, is upregulated in experimental congestive heart failure[87] and cirrhosis[88] and decreased by chronic vasopressin stimulation.[89] In patients with renal insufficiency, reduced urinary diluting capacity can lead to hyponatremia if excess free water is given. In general, diseases that prompt hospitalization generate numerous stimuli for secretion of arginine vasopressin (AVP), which has prompted some experts to suggest that hyponatremic fluids rarely be given to hospitalized patients.[90]

The underlying mechanism of hypovolemic hyponatremia is secretion of AVP synonymous with ADH in response to volume contraction in association with ongoing oral or intravenous intake of hypotonic fluid.[91] Angiotensin II also decreases renal free water clearance. Thiazide diuretics, unlike loop diuretics, promote hypovolemic hyponatremia by interfering with urinary dilution in the distal tubule.[91] Hypovolemic hyponatremia associated with a urinary [Na^+] > 20 mmol/L suggests mineralocorticoid deficiency, especially if serum [K^+], BUN, and SCr are increased.[91]

The cerebral salt-wasting syndrome is an often severe, symptomatic salt-losing diathesis that appears to be mediated by brain natriuretic peptide and in which, in contrast to the syndrome of inappropriate antidiuretic hormone secretion (SIADH), secretion of AVP is *appropriate*[91]; patients at risk for the cerebral salt-wasting syndrome include those with cerebral lesions due to trauma, subarachnoid hemorrhage, tumors, and infection. In patients after subarachnoid hemorrhage, administration of hydrocortisone 1,200 mg/day prevented the cerebral salt-wasting syndrome.[92]

Euvolemic hyponatremia is most commonly associated with nonosmotic vasopressin secretion, for example, glucocorticoid deficiency, hypothyroidism, thiazide-induced hyponatremia, SIADH, and the reset osmostat syndrome. Total body sodium and ECV are relatively normal and edema is rarely evident. SIADH may be idiopathic but also is associated with diseases of the central nervous system and with pulmonary disease (Table 14-14). Euvolemic hyponatremia is usually associated with exogenous AVP administration, pharmacologic potentiation of AVP action, drugs that mimic the action of AVP in the renal tubules, or excessive ectopic AVP secretion. Tissues from some small cell lung cancers, duodenal cancers, and pancreatic cancers increase AVP production in response to osmotic stimulation.[91]

At least 4% of postoperative patients develop plasma [Na^+] <130 mEq/L. Although neurologic manifestations usually do not accompany postoperative hyponatremia, signs of hypervolemia are occasionally present. Much less frequently, postoperative hyponatremia is accompanied by mental status changes, seizures, and transtentorial herniation,[93] attributable in part to intravenous administration of hypotonic fluids, secretion of AVP, and other factors, including drugs and altered renal function that influence perioperative water balance. Women appear to be more vulnerable than men and premenopausal women appear to be more

ANATOMY AND PHYSIOLOGY

TABLE 14-14. COMMON ASSOCIATIONS WITH THE SYNDROME OF INAPPROPRIATE ANTIDIURETIC HORMONE SECRETION

Neoplastic Disease	**Chest Disorders**
Carcinoma (e.g., lung)	Pneumonia
Thymoma	Tuberculosis
Mesothelioma	Empyema
Lymphoma, leukemia	Cystic fibrosis
Ewing sarcoma	Pneumothorax
Carcinoid	Aspergillosis
Bronchial adenoma	**Drugs**
Neurologic Disorders	Sulfonylureas
Head injury, neurosurgery	Opiates
Brain abscess or tumor	Thiazides and loop diuretics
Meningitis, encephalitis	Dopamine antagonists
Cerebral hemorrhage	Anticonvulsants
Guillain–Barré syndrome	Tricyclic antidepressants
Hydrocephalus	SSRIs
Alcohol Withdrawal	**Miscellaneous**
Peripheral neuropathy	Idiopathic
Seizures	Psychosis
Subdural hematoma	Porphyria

SSRI, selective serotonin reuptake inhibitor.
Modified from: Ball SG. Vasopressin and disorders of water balance: The physiology and pathophysiology of vasopressin. *Ann Clin Biochem.* 2007;44:417–431, with permission.

vulnerable than postmenopausal women to brain damage secondary to postoperative hyponatremia.[94] Postoperative hyponatremia can develop even with infusion of isotonic fluids if AVP is persistently increased. Twenty-four hours after surgery, mean plasma [Na^+] in 22 women (mean age, 42 years) undergoing uncomplicated gynecologic surgery had decreased from 140 ± 1 to 136 ± 0.5 mEq/L.[95] Although the patients retained sodium perioperatively, they retained proportionately more water (an average of 1.1 L of electrolyte-free water). Careful postoperative attention to fluid and electrolyte balance may minimize the occurrence of symptomatic hyponatremia.

If both [Na^+] and measured osmolality are below the normal range, hyponatremia is further evaluated by first assessing volume status using physical findings and laboratory data. In hypovolemic patients or edematous patients, the ratio of BUN to SCr should be >20:1. Urinary [Na^+] is generally <15 mEq/L in edematous states and volume depletion and >20 mEq/L in hyponatremia secondary to renal salt wasting or renal failure with water retention.

The criteria for the diagnosis of SIADH are listed in Table 14-15. Urinary [Na^+] should be >20 mEq/L unless fluids have been restricted. Arieff[96] has argued that the diagnosis of SIADH may be inaccurately applied to functionally hypovolemic postoperative patients, in whom, by definition, AVP secretion would be "appropriate."

Treatment of hyponatremia associated with a normal or high serum osmolality requires reduction of the elevated concentrations of the responsible solute, for example, urea or mannitol. Uremic patients are treated by free water restriction or dialysis. Treatment of edematous (hypervolemic) patients necessitates restriction of both sodium and water, usually accompanied by efforts to improve cardiac output and renal perfusion and to use diuretics to inhibit sodium reabsorption (Fig. 14-7). In hypovolemic, hyponatremic patients, blood volume must be restored, usually by infusion of 0.9% saline, and excessive sodium losses must be curtailed. Correction of hypovolemia usually results in removal of the stimulus for AVP release, accompanied by a rapid water diuresis.

The cornerstone of SIADH management is free water restriction and elimination of precipitating causes. Water restriction, sufficient to decrease TBW by 0.5 to 1 L per day, decreases ECV even if excessive AVP secretion continues. The resultant reduction

TABLE 14-15. DIAGNOSTIC CRITERIA FOR SYNDROME OF INAPPROPRIATE ANTIDIURETIC HORMONE SECRETION

Hyponatremia with appropriately low plasma osmolality
Urinary osmolality greater than plasma osmolality
Renal sodium excretion >20 mmol/L
Absence of hypotension, hypovolemia, and edematous states
Normal renal and adrenal functions
Absence of drugs that directly influence renal water and sodium handling

Modified from: Ball SG. Vasopressin and disorders of water balance: The physiology and pathophysiology of vasopressin. *Ann Clin Biochem.* 2007;44:417–431, with permission.

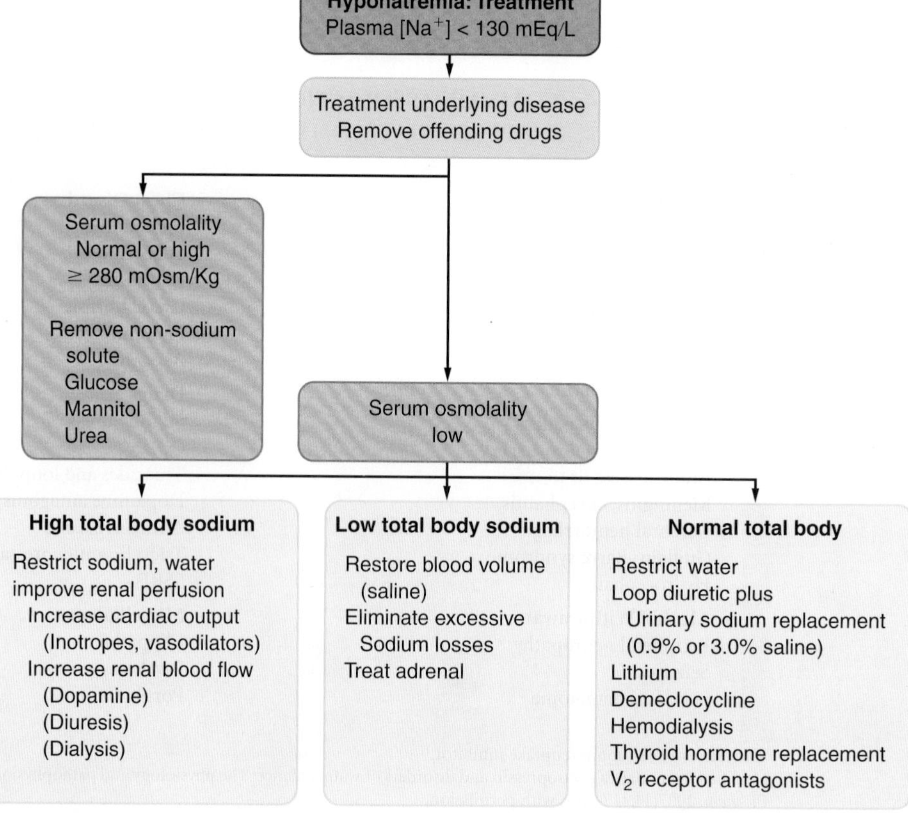

FIGURE 14-7. Hyponatremia is treated according to the etiology of the disturbance, the level of serum osmolality, and a clinical estimation of total body sodium.

in GFR enhances proximal tubular reabsorption of salt and water, thereby decreasing free water generation, and stimulates aldosterone secretion. As long as free water losses (i.e., renal, skin, gastrointestinal) exceed free water intake, plasma [Na$^+$] will increase. During treatment of hyponatremia, increases in plasma [Na$^+$] are determined both by the composition of the infused fluid and by the rate of renal free water excretion.[97] Free water excretion can be increased by administering furosemide.

Recently, vasopressin receptor blocking agents have been developed that inhibit the action of AVP on the renal collecting ducts.[98–101] These agents have proven to be safe and efficacious in hyponatremic patients, appearing to have particular value in patients with hypervolemic hyponatremia secondary to congestive heart failure.[98] Conivaptan, which inhibits both $V_{1\alpha}$ and V_2 receptors, has been approved for the treatment of normovolemic and hypervolemic, hyponatremic patients.[100] However, potential decreases in blood pressure associated with $V_{1\alpha}$ receptor blockade necessitate caution in patients with borderline low blood pressure.[101] Tolvaptan, a selective V_2 receptor antagonist, also has proven effective in clinical trials.[102] Within a few years, vaptans will likely become a mainstay of therapy for normovolemic and hypervolemic hypernatremia.[101]

Neurologic symptoms or profound hyponatremia ([Na$^+$] < 115 to 120 mEq/L) requires more aggressive therapy. Hypertonic (3%) saline is most clearly indicated in patients who have seizures or patients who acutely develop symptoms of water intoxication secondary to intravenous fluid administration. In such cases, 3% saline may be administered at a rate of 1 to 2 mL/kg/hr, to increase plasma [Na$^+$] by 1 to 2 mEq/L/hr; however, this treatment should not continue for more than a few hours. Three percent saline may only transiently increase plasma [Na$^+$] because ECV expansion results in increased urinary sodium excretion. Intravenous furosemide, combined with quantitative replacement of urinary sodium losses with 0.9% or 3% saline, can rapidly increase plasma [Na$^+$], in part by increasing free water clearance.

The rate of treatment of hyponatremia continues to generate controversy, extending from "too fast, too soon" to "too slow, too late." Although delayed correction may result in neurologic injury, inappropriately rapid correction may result in abrupt brain dehydration (Fig. 14-8) or permanent neurologic sequelae (i.e., osmotic demyelination syndrome),[103] cerebral hemorrhage, or congestive heart failure. The symptoms of the osmotic demyelination syndrome vary from mild (transient behavioral disturbances or seizures) to severe (including pseudobulbar palsy and quadriparesis). The principal determinants of neurologic injury appear to be the magnitude and chronicity of hyponatremia and the rate of correction. The osmotic demyelination syndrome is more likely when hyponatremia has persisted >48 hours. Most patients in whom the osmotic demyelination syndrome is fatal have undergone correction of plasma [Na$^+$] of more than 20 mEq/L/day. Other risk factors for the development of osmotic demyelination syndrome include alcoholism, poor nutritional status, liver disease, burns, and hypokalemia.

The clinician faces formidable difficulties in predicting the rate at which plasma [Na$^+$] will increase because increases in plasma [Na$^+$] are determined both by the composition of the infused fluid and by the rate of renal free water excretion. The expected change in plasma [Na$^+$] resulting from 1 L of selected infusate can be estimated using the following equation[104]:

$$\Delta[\mathrm{Na}^+]_S = \frac{[\mathrm{Na}^+]_{\mathrm{inf}} - [\mathrm{Na}^+]_s}{\mathrm{TBW} + 1} \qquad (14\text{-}12)$$

where $\Delta[\mathrm{Na}^+]_s$ is the change in the patient's serum [Na$^+$], $[\mathrm{Na}^+]_{\mathrm{inf}}$ is the [Na$^+$] of the infusate, $[\mathrm{Na}^+]_s$ is the patient's serum [Na$^+$], TBW is the patient's estimated total body water in liters, and 1 is a factor added to take into account the volume of infusate.

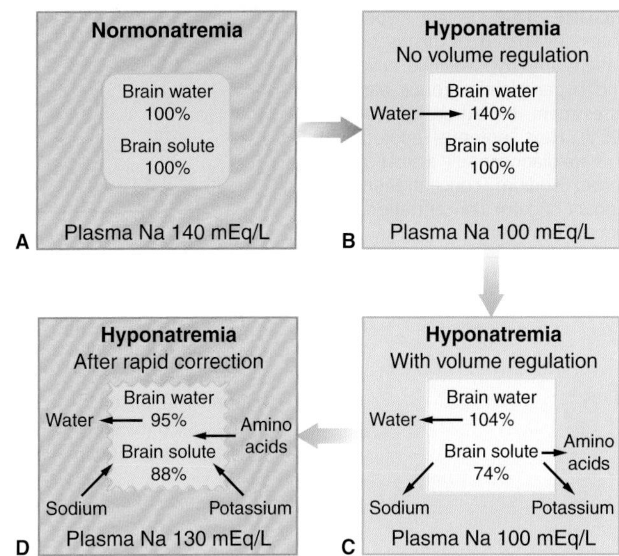

FIGURE 14-8. Brain water and solute in concentrations in hyponatremia. If normal plasma sodium (Na) **(A)** suddenly decreased, the increase in brain water theoretically would be proportional to the decrease in plasma Na **(B)**. However, because of adaptive loss of cerebral intracellular solute, cerebral edema is minimized in chronic hyponatremia **(C)**. Once adaptation has occurred, a rapid return of plasma Na concentration toward a normal level results in brain dehydration **(D)**. (From: Sterns RH. Vignettes in clinical pathophysiology. Neurological deterioration following treatment for hyponatremia. *Am J Kidney Dis.* 1989;XIII:434–437, with permission.)

Treatment should be interrupted or slowed when symptoms improve. Frequent determinations of [Na$^+$] are important to prevent correction at a rate >1 to 2 mEq/L in any 1 hour and >8 mEq/L in 24 hours.[105] Initially, plasma [Na$^+$] may be increased by 1 to 2 mEq/L/hr; however, the rate of correction should then be slowed to avoid excessively rapid correction. Hypernatremia should be avoided. Once plasma [Na$^+$] exceeds 120 to 125 mEq/L, water restriction alone is usually sufficient to normalize [Na$^+$]. As acute hyponatremia is corrected, central nervous system signs and symptoms usually improve within 24 hours, although 96 hours may be necessary for maximal recovery.

For patients who require long-term pharmacologic therapy of hyponatremia, vasopressin receptor antagonists are the current most promising therapies.[106] Hemodialysis is occasionally necessary in severely hyponatremic patients who cannot be adequately managed with drugs or hypertonic saline. Once hyponatremia has improved, careful fluid restriction is necessary to avoid recurrence of hyponatremia.

Hypernatremia

Hypernatremia ([Na$^+$] > 150 mEq/L) indicates an absolute or relative water deficit. Normally, slight increases in tonicity or [Na$^+$] stimulate thirst and AVP secretion. Therefore, severe, persistent hypernatremia occurs only in patients who cannot respond to thirst by voluntary ingestion of fluid, that is, obtunded patients, anesthetized patients, and infants.

Hypernatremia produces neurologic symptoms (including stupor, coma, and seizures), hypovolemia, renal insufficiency (occasionally progressing to renal failure), and decreased urinary

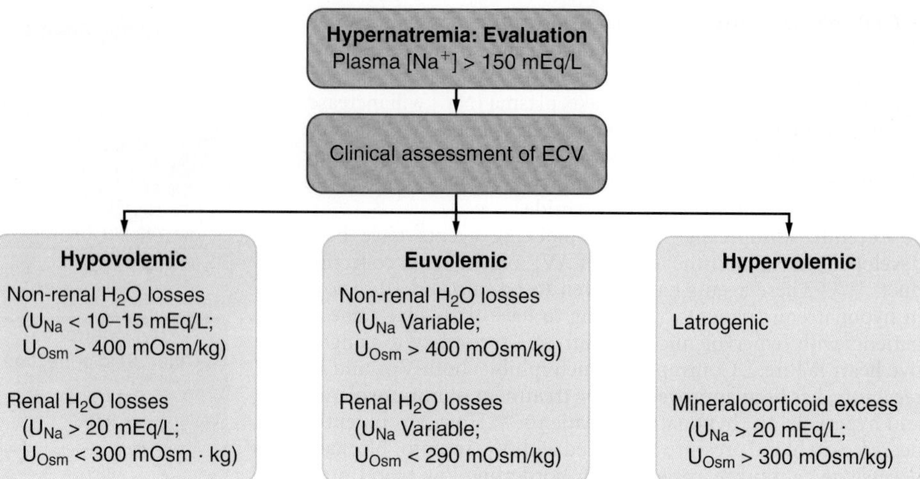

FIGURE 14-9. Severe hypernatremia is evaluated by first separating patients into hypovolemic, euvolemic, and hypervolemic groups based on assessment of extracellular volume (ECV). Next, potential etiologic factors are diagnostically assessed. [Na$^+$], serum sodium concentration; U_{Na}, urinary sodium concentration; U_{Osm}, urinary osmolality.

concentrating ability. Because hypernatremia frequently results from diabetes insipidus (DI) or osmotically induced losses of sodium and water, many patients are hypovolemic or bear the stigmata of renal disease. Postoperative neurosurgical patients who have undergone pituitary surgery are at particular risk of developing transient or prolonged DI. Polyuria may be present for only a few days within the first week of surgery, may be permanent, or may demonstrate a triphasic sequence: Early DI, return of urinary concentrating ability, then recurrent DI.[107]

The clinical consequences of hypernatremia are most serious at the extremes of age and when hypernatremia develops abruptly. Geriatric patients are at increased risk of hypernatremia because of decreased renal concentrating ability and decreased thirst. Brain shrinkage secondary to rapidly developing hypernatremia may damage delicate cerebral vessels, leading to subdural hematoma, subcortical parenchymal hemorrhage, subarachnoid hemorrhage, and venous thrombosis. Polyuria may cause bladder distention, hydronephrosis, and permanent renal damage. Although the mortality of hypernatremia is 40% to 55%, it is unclear whether hypernatremia contributes to mortality or is simply a marker of severe associated disease.

Surprisingly, if plasma [Na$^+$] is initially normal, moderate acute increases in plasma [Na$^+$] do not appear to precipitate central pontine myelinolysis. However, larger accidental increases in plasma [Na$^+$] have produced severe consequences in children. In experimental animals, acute severe hypernatremia (acute increase from 146 to 170 mEq/L) caused neuronal damage at 24 hours, suggestive of early central pontine myelinolysis.[108]

By definition, hypernatremia indicates an absolute or relative water deficit and is always associated with hypertonicity. Hypernatremia can be generated by hypotonic fluid loss, as in burns, gastrointestinal losses, diuretic therapy, osmotic diuresis, renal disease, mineralocorticoid excess or deficiency, and iatrogenic causes or can be generated by isolated water loss, as in central or nephrogenic DI. The acquired form of nephrogenic DI is more common and usually less severe than the congenital form. As chronic renal failure advances, most patients have defective concentrating ability, resulting in resistance to AVP associated with hypotonic urine. Because hypovolemia accompanies most pathologic water loss, signs of hypoperfusion also may be present. In many patients, before the development of hypernatremia, an increased volume of hypotonic urine suggests an abnormality in water balance. Although uncommon as a cause of hypernatremia, isolated sodium gain occasionally occurs in patients who receive large quantities of sodium, such as treatment of metabolic acidosis with 8.4% sodium bicarbonate, in which [Na$^+$] is approximately 1,000 mEq/L, or perioperative or prehospital treatment with hypertonic saline resuscitation solutions.

Hypernatremic patients can be separated into three groups, based on clinical assessment of ECV (Fig. 14-9). Note that plasma [Na$^+$] does not reflect total body sodium, which must be estimated separately based on signs of the adequacy of ECV. Polyuric, hypernatremic patients may be undergoing solute diuresis or may have DI. Measurement of urinary sodium and osmolality can help to differentiate the various causes. A urinary osmolality <150 mOsm/kg in the setting of hypertonicity and polyuria is diagnostic of DI.

Treatment of hypernatremia produced by water loss requires repletion of water as well of associated deficits in total body sodium and other electrolytes (Table 14-16). Common errors in treating hypernatremia include excessively rapid correction as well as failing to appreciate the magnitude of the water deficit and failing to account for ongoing maintenance requirements and continued fluid losses in planning therapy.

TABLE 14-16. HYPERNATREMIA: ACUTE TREATMENT

Sodium Depletion (Hypovolemia)
Hypovolemia correction (0.9% saline)
Hypernatremia correction (hypotonic fluids)
Sodium overload (hypervolemia)
Enhance sodium removal (loop diuretics, dialysis)
Replace water deficit (hypotonic fluids)
Normal total body sodium (euvolemia)
Replace water deficit (hypotonic fluids)
Control diabetes insipidus
Central diabetes insipidus:
DDAVP, 10–20 μg intranasally; 2–4 μg SC
Aqueous vasopressin, 5 U q2–4h IM or SC
Nephrogenic diabetes insipidus:
Restrict sodium, water intake
Thiazide diuretics

DDAVP, desmopressin.

The first step in treating hypernatremia is to estimate the TBW deficit, which can be accomplished by inserting the measured plasma [Na$^+$] into the equation:

$$\text{TBW deficit} = 0.6 \times \text{body weight (kg)} \times [(([\text{Na}^+] - 140)/140] \quad (14\text{-}13)$$

where 140 is the middle of the normal range for [Na$^+$]. Adrogué and Madias[109] proposed an equation (see Eq. 14-12) that can be used in hypernatremic patients as it can be in hyponatremic patients to predict the expected decrease in serum [Na$^+$] produced by infusion of 1 L of infusate.[104] The accuracy of this equation has recently been validated in a large clinical series of hypernatremic and hyponatremic patients.[110]

Hypernatremia must be corrected slowly because of the risk of neurologic sequelae such as seizures or cerebral edema (Fig. 14-10). At the cellular level, restoration of cell volume occurs remarkably quickly after tonicity is altered; as a consequence, acute treatment of hypertonicity may result in overshooting the original, normotonic cell volume. The water deficit should be replaced over 24 to 48 hours, and the plasma [Na$^+$] should not be reduced by more than 1 to 2 mEq/L/hr. Reversible underlying causes should be treated. Hypovolemia should be corrected promptly with 0.9% saline. Although the [Na$^+$] of 0.9% saline is 154 mEq/L, the solution is effective in treating volume deficits and will reduce [Na$^+$] that exceeds 154 mEq/L in hypovolemic, hypernatremic patients. Once hypovolemia is corrected, water can be replaced orally or with intravenous hypotonic fluids, depending on the ability of the patient to tolerate oral hydration. In the occasional sodium-overloaded patient, sodium excretion can be accelerated using loop diuretics or dialysis.

The management of hypernatremia secondary to DI varies according to whether the cause is central or nephrogenic (see Table 14-16). The two most suitable agents for correcting central DI (an AVP deficiency syndrome) are desmopressin (DDAVP) and aqueous vasopressin. DDAVP, given subcutaneously in a dose of 1 to 4 μg or intranasally in a dose of 5 to 20 μg every 12 to 24 hours, is effective in most patients. DDAVP is preferred because it has a longer duration of action than AVP and lacks vasoconstrictor effects.[111] Incomplete AVP deficits (partial DI) often are effectively managed with pharmacologic agents that stimulate AVP release or enhance the renal response to AVP. Chlorpropamide, which potentiates the renal effects of vasopressin, and carbamazepine, which enhances vasopressin secretion, have been used to treat partial central DI, but are associated with clinically important side effects. In nephrogenic DI, salt and water restriction or thiazide diuretics induce contraction of ECV, thereby enhancing fluid reabsorption in the proximal tubules. If less filtrate passes through into the collecting ducts, less water will be excreted.

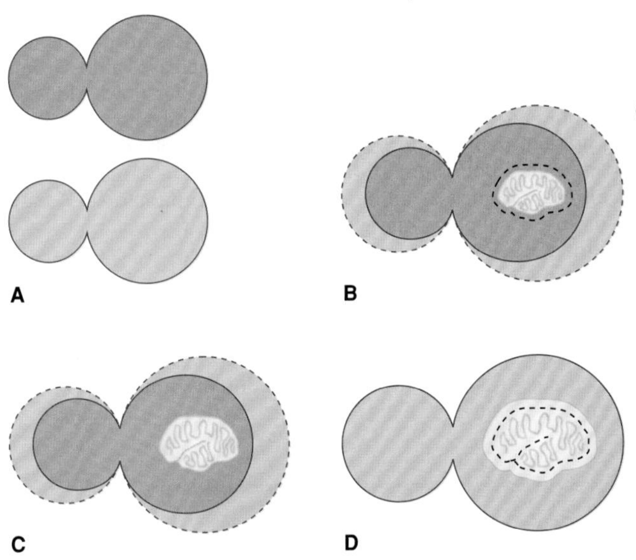

FIGURE 14-10. A: The concentration of sodium is reflected in the intensity of the stippling: the upper figure, representing extracellular volume (smaller circle) and intracellular volume (larger circle), is more heavily stippled, that is, serum sodium is higher. **B:** In response to an acute increase in serum sodium resulting from water loss, both the intracellular and the extracellular volume substantially decrease. The brain (schematically illustrated) shrinks in proportion to the reduction in intracellular volume in other tissues. **C:** However, owing to the production of idiogenic osmoles, the brain rapidly restores its intracellular volume, despite the persistent reduction in intracellular volume in other tissues and in extracellular volume. **D:** With excessively rapid correction of hypernatremia (the reduction in serum sodium is reflected in the decrease in the intensity of stippling), the brain expands to greater than its original size. The resulting increase in cerebral edema and intracranial pressure can cause severe neurologic damage. (Modified from: Feig PU. Hypernatremia and hypertonic syndromes. *Med Clin North Am.* 1981;65:271–290, with permission.)

Potassium

Physiologic Role

11 Potassium plays an important role in cell membrane physiology, especially in maintaining resting membrane potentials and in generating action potentials in the central nervous system and heart. Potassium is actively transported into cells by a Na/K adenosine triphosphatase (ATPase) pump, which maintains an intracellular [K$^+$] that is at least 30-fold greater than extracellular [K$^+$]. Intracellular potassium concentration ([K$^+$]) is normally 150 mEq/L while the extracellular concentration is only 3.5 to 5 mEq/L. Serum [K$^+$] measures about 0.5 mEq/L higher than plasma [K$^+$] because of cell lysis during clotting. Total body potassium in a 70 kg adult is approximately 4,256 mEq, of which 4,200 mEq is intracellular; of the 56 mEq in the ECV, only 12 mEq is located in the PV. The ratio of intracellular to extracellular potassium contributes to the resting potential difference across cell membranes and therefore to the integrity of cardiac and neuromuscular transmissions. The primary mechanism that maintains potassium inside cells is the negative voltage created by the transport of three sodium ions out of the cell for every two potassium ions transported in. Both insulin and β-agonists promote potassium entry into cells.[112,113] Metabolic and respiratory acidoses tend to shift potassium out of cells, while metabolic and respiratory alkaloses favor movement into cells.

Usual potassium intake varies between 50 and 150 mEq/day. Freely filtered at the glomerulus, most potassium excretion is urinary, with some fecal elimination. Most filtered potassium is reabsorbed; usually, excretion is approximately equal to daily intake. As long as GFR is >8 mL/min, dietary potassium intake, unless greater than normal, can be excreted. Assuming a plasma [K$^+$] of 4 mEq/L and a normal GFR of 180 L/day, 720 mEq of potassium is filtered daily, of which 85% to 90% is reabsorbed in the proximal convoluted tubule and loop of Henle. The remaining 10% to 15% reaches the distal convoluted tubule, which is the major site at which potassium excretion is regulated. Excretion of potassium ions is a function of open potassium channels and the electrical driving force in the cortical collecting duct.

The two most important regulators of potassium excretion are plasma [K$^+$] and aldosterone. Potassium secretion into the distal convoluted tubules and cortical collecting ducts is increased by hyperkalemia, aldosterone, alkalemia, increased delivery of Na$^+$ to the distal tubule and collecting duct, high urinary flow rates, and the presence in luminal fluid of nonreabsorbable anions such as carbenicillin, phosphates, and sulfates. As sodium reabsorption increases, the electrical driving force opposing reabsorption of potassium is increased. Aldosterone increases sodium reabsorption by inducing a more open configuration of the epithelial sodium channel; potassium-sparing diuretics (amiloride and triamterene) and trimethoprim block the epithelial sodium channel, thereby increasing potassium reabsorption. Magnesium depletion contributes to renal potassium wasting.

Hypokalemia

Uncommon among healthy persons, hypokalemia ([K$^+$] < 3.5 mEq/L) is a frequent complication of treatment with diuretic drugs and occasionally complicates other diseases and treatment regimens (Table 14-17). Plasma [K$^+$] poorly reflects total body potassium; hypokalemia may occur with normal, low, or high total body potassium. However, as a general rule, a chronic decrement of 1 mEq/L in the plasma [K$^+$] corresponds to a total body deficit of approximately 200 to 300 mEq. In uncomplicated hypokalemia, the total body potassium deficit exceeds 300 mEq if plasma [K$^+$] is <3 mEq/L and 700 mEq if plasma [K$^+$] is <2 mEq/L.

The symptoms and signs of hypokalemia primarily relate to neuromuscular and cardiovascular functions. Hypokalemia causes muscle weakness and, when severe, may even cause paralysis. With chronic potassium loss, the ratio of intracellular to extracellular [K$^+$] remains relatively stable; in contrast, acute redistribution of potassium from the extracellular to the intracellular space substantially changes resting membrane potentials. Cardiac rhythm disturbances are among the most dangerous complications of potassium deficiency. Acute hypokalemia causes hyperpolarization of the cardiac cell and may lead to ventricular escape activity, reentrant phenomena, ectopic tachycardias, and delayed conduction. In patients treated with digoxin, hypokalemia increases toxicity by increasing myocardial digoxin binding and pharmacologic effectiveness. Hypokalemia contributes to systemic hypertension, especially when combined with a high-sodium diet. In diabetic patients, hypokalemia impairs insulin secretion and end-organ sensitivity to insulin. Although no clear threshold has been defined for a level of hypokalemia below which safe conduct of anesthesia is compromised, [K$^+$] <3.5 mEq/L in cardiac surgical patients has been associated with an increased incidence of perioperative dysrhythmias, especially atrial fibrillation/flutter.[114]

Potassium depletion also induces defects in renal concentrating ability, resulting in polyuria and a reduction in GFR. Potassium replacement improves GFR, although the concentrating deficit may not improve for several months after treatment. If hypokalemia is sufficiently prolonged, chronic renal interstitial damage may occur. In experimental animals, hypokalemia was associated with intrarenal vasoconstriction and a pattern of renal injury similar to that produced by ischemia.[115]

Hypokalemia may result from chronic depletion of total body potassium or from acute redistribution of potassium from the ECV to the ICV. Redistribution of potassium into cells occurs when the activity of the sodium–potassium ATPase pump is acutely increased by extracellular hyperkalemia or increased intracellular concentrations of sodium, as well as by insulin, carbohydrate loading (which stimulates release of endogenous insulin), β_2-agonists, and aldosterone. Both metabolic and respiratory alkaloses lead to decreases in plasma [K$^+$].

Causes of chronic hypokalemia include those etiologies associated with renal potassium conservation (extrarenal potassium losses; low urinary [K$^+$]) and those with renal potassium wasting (Fig. 14-11).[116] A low urinary [K$^+$] suggests inadequate dietary intake or extrarenal depletion (in the absence of recent diuretic use). Diuretic-induced urinary potassium losses are frequently associated with hypokalemia, secondary to increased aldosterone secretion, alkalemia, and increased renal tubular flow. Aldosterone does not cause renal potassium wasting unless sodium ions are present; that is, aldosterone primarily controls sodium reabsorption, not potassium excretion. Renal tubular damage due to nephrotoxins such as aminoglycosides or amphotericin B may also cause renal potassium wasting.

Initial evaluation of hypokalemia includes a medical history (e.g., diarrhea, vomiting, diuretic, or laxative use), physical examination (e.g., hypertension, cushingoid features, edema), measurement of serum electrolytes (e.g., magnesium), arterial pH assessment, and evaluation of the electrocardiogram (ECG). Measurement of 24-hour urinary excretion of sodium and potassium may distinguish extrarenal from renal causes. Magnesium

TABLE 14-17. CAUSES OF RENAL POTASSIUM LOSS

Drugs	**Bicarbonaturia**
Diuretics	Distal renal tubular acidosis
Thiazide diuretics	Treatment of proximal renal tubular acidosis
Loop diuretics	Correction phase of metabolic alkalosis
Osmotic diuretics	**Magnesium Deficiency**
Antibiotics	**Other Less Common Causes**
Penicillin and penicillin analogs	Cisplatin
Amphotericin B	Carbonic anhydrase inhibitors
Aminoglycosides	Leukemia
Hormones	Diuretic phase of acute tubular necrosis
Aldosterone	**Intrinsic renal transport defects**
Glucocorticoids	Bartter syndrome
	Gitelman syndrome

Modified from: Weiner ID, Wingo CS. Hypokalemia – consequences, causes, and correction. *J Am Soc Nephrol.* 1997;8:1179–1188, with permission.

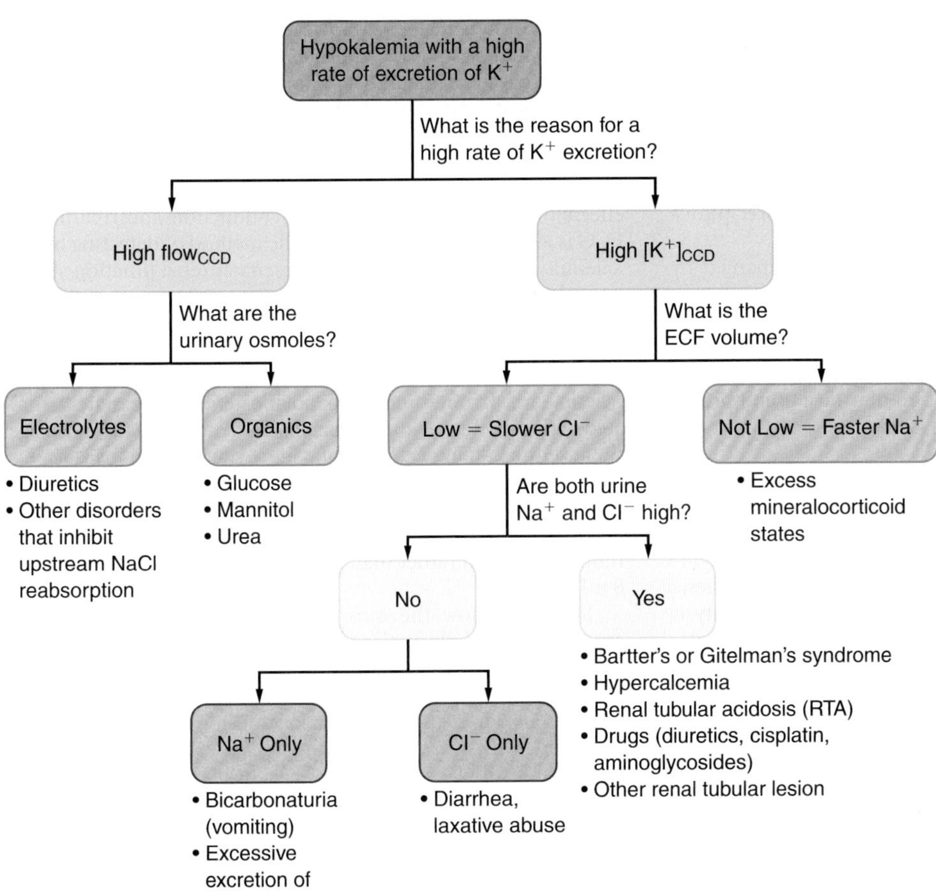

FIGURE 14-11. A diagnostic flow chart for hypokalemia with a high rate of K^+ excretion. ECF, extracellular fluid. (From: Lin SH, Halperin ML. Hypokalemia: a practical approach to diagnosis and its genetic basis. *Curr Med Chem.* 2007;14:1551–1565, with permission.)

deficiency, associated with aminoglycoside and cisplatin therapy, can generate hypokalemia that is resistant to replacement therapy. Plasma renin and aldosterone levels may be helpful in the differential diagnosis of hypokalemia of unclear origin, especially if primary hyperaldosteronism is suspected.[117] Characteristic electrocardiographic changes associated with hypokalemia include flat or inverted T waves, prominent U waves, and ST segment depression.

The treatment of hypokalemia consists of potassium repletion, correction of alkalemia, and removal of offending drugs (Table 14-18). Hypokalemia secondary only to acute redistribution (e.g., secondary to acute alkalemia) may not require treatment. There is no urgent need for potassium replacement therapy in mild-to-moderate hypokalemia (3 to 3.5 mEq/L) in patients who have no symptoms. If total body potassium is decreased, oral potassium supplementation is preferable to intravenous replacement. Potassium is usually replaced as the chloride salt because coexisting chloride deficiency may limit the ability of the kidney to conserve potassium.

Intravenous potassium repletion, when necessary, must be performed cautiously (i.e., usually at a rate ≤10 to 20 mEq/hr) because the magnitude of potassium deficits is unpredictable. The plasma $[K^+]$ and the ECG must be monitored during rapid repletion (10 to 20 mEq/hr) to avoid hyperkalemic complications. The plasma $[K^+]$ and ECG should be monitored to detect inadvertent hyperkalemia. Particular care should be taken in patients who have concurrent acidemia, type IV renal tubular acidosis, diabetes mellitus, or in those patients receiving nonsteroidal anti-inflammatory agents, ACE inhibitors, or β_2-blockers, all of which delay movement of extracellular potassium into cells. β_1-blockers do not delay movement of extracellular potassium into cells or predispose patients to hyperkalemia.[118]

However, in patients with life-threatening dysrhythmias secondary to hypokalemia, serum $[K^+]$ must be rapidly increased. Assuming that PV in a 70 kg adult is 3 L, administration of 6 mEq/L of potassium in 1 minute will acutely increase serum $[K^+]$ by no more than 2 mEq/L because redistribution into interstitial fluid and ICV will decrease the quantity remaining in the PV.

Hypokalemia associated with hyperaldosteronemia (e.g., primary aldosteronism, Cushing syndrome) usually responds favorably to reduced sodium intake and increased potassium intake.

TABLE 14-18. HYPOKALEMIA: TREATMENT

Correct Precipitating Factors
Increased pH
Decreased $[Mg^{2+}]$
Drugs
Mild Hypokalemia ($[K^+] > 2$ mEq/L)
Intravenous KCl infusion ≤10 mEq/hr
Severe Hypokalemia ($[K^+] \leq 2$ mEq/L, paralysis or ECG changes)
Intravenous KCl infusion ≤40 mEq/hr
Continuous ECG monitoring
If life-threatening, 5–6 mEq bolus

ECG, electrocardiogram.

Hypomagnesemia, if present, aggravates the effects of hypokalemia, impairs potassium conservation, and should be treated. Potassium supplements or potassium-sparing diuretics should be given cautiously to patients who have diabetes mellitus or renal insufficiency, which limit compensation for acute hyperkalemia. In patients such as those who have diabetic ketoacidosis, who are both hypokalemic and acidemic, potassium administration should precede correction of acidosis to avoid a precipitous decrease in plasma [K⁺] as pH increases.

In patients with normal serum potassium accompanied by symptoms of potassium depletion (e.g., muscle fatigue), history of potassium loss or insufficient intake, or in patients in whom potassium depletion may be of special threat (e.g., patients on diuretics, digitalis, or β_2-agonists), muscle biopsy with measurement of muscle potassium concentration may be a useful procedure to detect and quantify potassium depletion.

Hyperkalemia

The most lethal manifestations of hyperkalemia ([K⁺] >5 mEq/L) involve the cardiac conducting system and include dysrhythmias, conduction abnormalities, and cardiac arrest. In anesthesia practice, the classic example of hyperkalemic cardiac toxicity is associated with the administration of succinylcholine to paraplegic, quadriplegic, or severely burned[119] patients. If plasma [K⁺] is <6 mEq/L, cardiac effects are negligible. As the concentration increases further, the ECG shows tall, peaked T waves, especially in the precordial leads. With further increases, the PR interval becomes prolonged, followed by a decrease in the amplitude of the P wave. Finally, the QRS complex widens into a pattern resembling a sine wave, as a prelude to cardiac standstill (Fig. 14-12).[112] Hyperkalemic cardiotoxicity is enhanced by hyponatremia, hypocalcemia, or acidosis. Because progression to fatal cardiotoxicity is unpredictable and often swift, the presence of hyperkalemic ECG

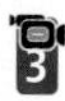

changes mandates immediate therapy. The life-threatening cardiac effects usually require more urgent treatment than other manifestations of hyperkalemia. However, ascending muscle weakness appears when plasma [K⁺] approaches 7 mEq/L, and may progress to flaccid paralysis, inability to phonate, and respiratory arrest.

The most important diagnostic issues are medical history, emphasizing recent drug therapy, and assessment of renal function. Although the ECG may provide the first suggestion of hyperkalemia in some patients, and despite the well-described effects of hyperkalemia on cardiac conduction and rhythm, the ECG is an insensitive and nonspecific method of detecting hyperkalemia. If hyponatremia is also present, adrenal function should be evaluated.

Hyperkalemia may occur with normal, high, or low total body potassium stores. A deficiency of aldosterone, a major regulator of potassium excretion, leads to hyperkalemia in adrenal insufficiency and hyporeninemic hypoaldosteronism, a state associated with diabetes mellitus, renal insufficiency, and advanced age. Because the kidneys excrete potassium, severe renal insufficiency commonly causes hyperkalemia. Patients with chronic renal insufficiency can maintain normal plasma [K⁺] despite markedly decreased GFR because urinary potassium excretion depends on tubular secretion rather than glomerular filtration if GFR exceeds 8 mL/min.

Drugs are now the most common cause of hyperkalemia, especially in elderly patients. Drugs that may limit potassium excretion include nonsteroidal anti-inflammatory drugs, ACE inhibitors, cyclosporin, and potassium-sparing diuretics such as triamterene. Drug-induced hyperkalemia most commonly occurs in patients with other predisposing factors, such as diabetes mellitus, renal insufficiency, advanced age, or hyporeninemic hypoaldosteronism. ACE inhibitors are particularly likely to produce hyperkalemia in patients who have congestive heart failure.[120]

In patients who have normal total body potassium, hyperkalemia may accompany a sudden shift of potassium from the ICV to the ECV because of acidemia, increased catabolism, or rhabdomyolysis. Metabolic acidosis and respiratory acidosis tend to cause an increase in plasma [K⁺]. However, organic acidoses (i.e., lactic

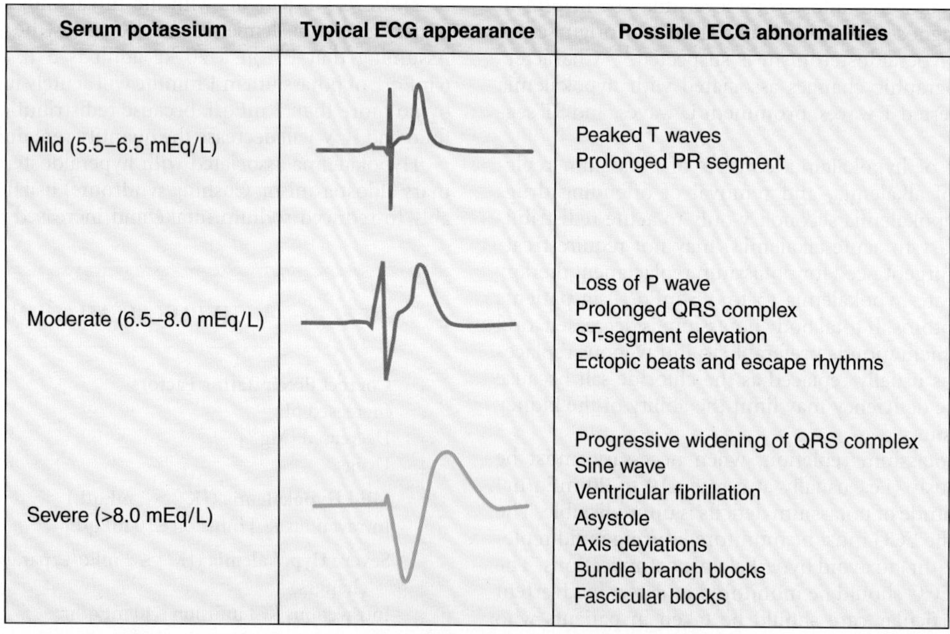

FIGURE 14-12. Electrocardiographic (ECG) manifestations of hyperkalemia. (From: Sood MM, Sood AR, Richardson R. Emergency management and commonly encountered outpatient scenarios in patients with hyperkalemia. *Mayo Clin Proc.* 2007;82:1553–1561, with permission.)

acidosis, ketoacidosis) have little effect on [K^+], whereas mineral acids cause significant cellular shifts. In response to increased hydrogen ion activity because of addition of acids, potassium will increase if the anion remains in the ECV. Neither lactate nor keto-acids remain in the extracellular fluid. Therefore, hyperkalemia in these circumstances reflects tissue injury or lack of insulin. Pseudohyperkalemia, which occurs when potassium is released from cells in blood collection tubes, can be diagnosed by comparing serum and plasma K^+ levels from the same blood sample. Hyperkalemia usually accompanies malignant hyperthermia.

The treatment of hyperkalemia is aimed at eliminating the cause, reversing membrane hyperexcitability, and removing potassium from the body (Fig. 14-13).[112,113,120,121] Mineralocorticoid deficiency can be treated with 9-α-fludrocortisone (0.025 to 0.10 mg/day). Hyperkalemia secondary to digitalis intoxication may be resistant to therapy because attempts to shift potassium from the ECV to

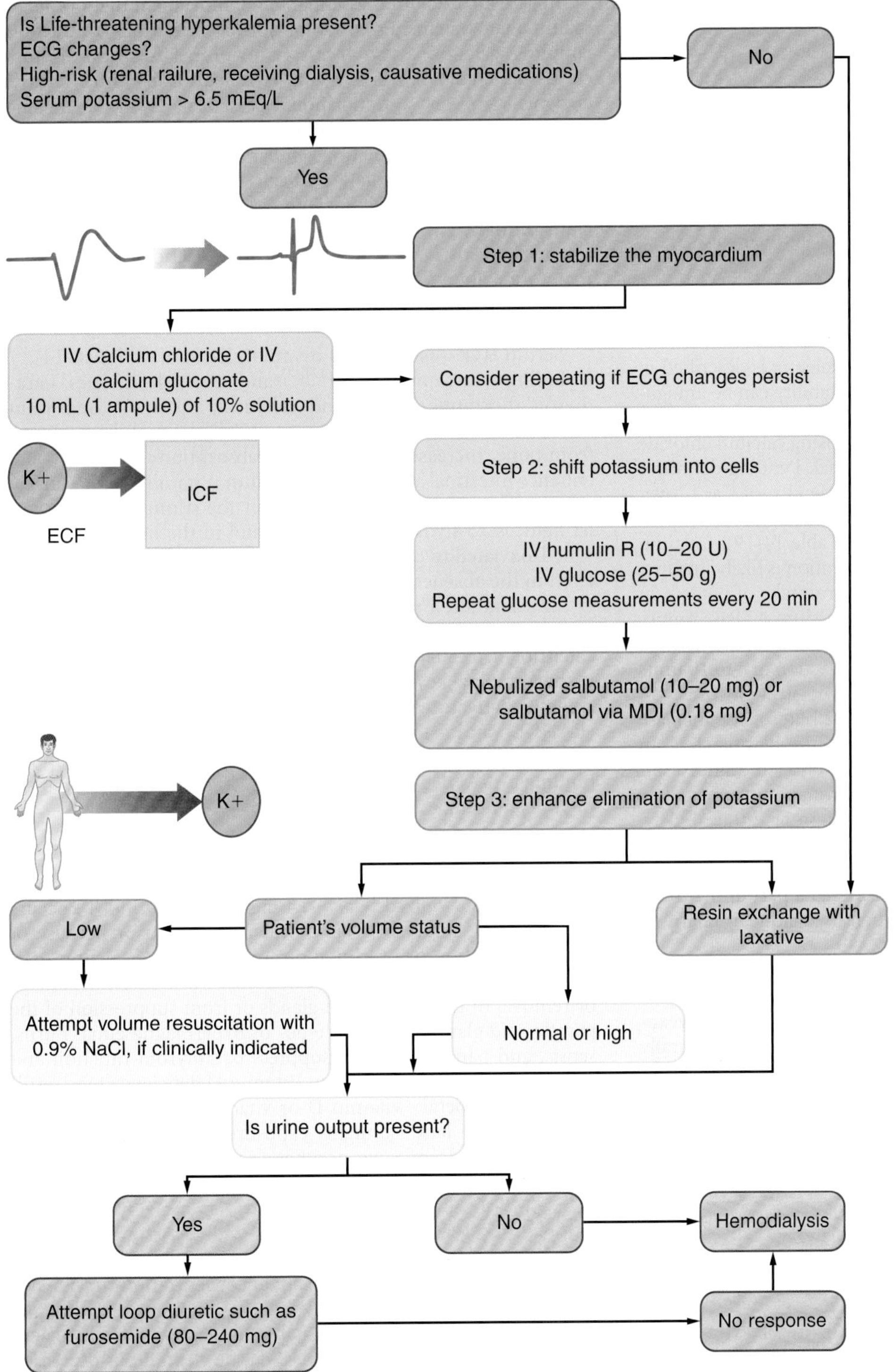

FIGURE 14-13. Algorithmic management of hyperkalemia. ECG, electrocardiographic; IV, intravenous; K, potassium; ECF, extracellular fluid; ICF, intracellular fluid; MDI, metered-dose inhaler; NaCl, sodium chloride. (From: Sood MM, Sood AR, Richardson R. Emergency management and commonly encountered outpatient scenarios in patients with hyperkalemia. *Mayo Clin Proc.* 2007;82:1553–1561, with permission.)

TABLE 14-19. SEVERE HYPERKALEMIA[a] TREATMENT

Reverse membrane effects
Calcium (10 mL of 10% calcium chloride IV over 10 min)
Transfer extracellular [K^+] into cells
Glucose and insulin ($D_{10}W$ + 5–10 U regular insulin per 25–50 g glucose)
Sodium bicarbonate (50–100 mEq over 5–10 min)
β_2-agonists
Remove potassium from body
Diuretics, proximal or loop
Potassium-exchange resins (sodium polystyrene sulfonate)
Hemodialysis
Monitor ECG and serum [K^+] level

[a]Potassium concentration ([K^+]) >7 mEq/L or electrocardiographic changes. IV, intravenous; $D_{10}W$, 10% dextrose in water; ECG, electrocardiogram.

the ICV are often ineffective. In this situation, use of digoxin-specific antibodies has been successful.

Emergent management of severe hyperkalemia is described in detail in Table 14-19. Membrane hyperexcitability can be antagonized by translocating potassium from the ECV to the ICV, removing excess potassium, or (transiently) by infusing calcium chloride to depress the membrane threshold potential. Pending definitive treatment, rapid infusion of calcium chloride (1 g of $CaCl_2$ over 3 minutes, or two to three ampules of 10% calcium gluconate over 5 minutes) may stabilize cardiac rhythm (Table 14-19). Calcium should be given cautiously if digitalis intoxication is likely. Insulin, in a dose-dependent fashion, causes cellular uptake of potassium by increasing the activity of the sodium/potassium ATPase pump. Insulin increases cellular uptake of potassium best when high insulin levels are achieved by intravenous injection of 5 to 10 units of regular insulin, accompanied by 50 mL of 50% glucose.[112,120] β_2-adrenergic drugs such as salbutamol and albuterol also increase potassium uptake by skeletal muscle and reduce plasma [K^+], an action that may explain hypokalemia with severe, acute illness. Salbutamol, a selective β_2-agonist, decreases serum potassium acutely by 1 mEq/L or more when given by inhalation or intravenously, although cardiac dysrhythmias may occasionally complicate treatment with selective β_2-agonists.[112] Although administration of sodium bicarbonate has long been considered a part of the treatment of hyperkalemia, bicarbonate, when used alone, is relatively ineffective and is no longer favored.[120]

Potassium may be removed from the body by the renal or gastrointestinal routes. Furosemide promotes kaliuresis in a dose-dependent fashion. Sodium polystyrene sulfonate resin (Kayexalate), which exchanges sodium for potassium, can be given orally (30 g) or as a retention enema (50 g in 200 mL of 20% sorbitol). However, sodium overload and hypervolemia are potential risks. Rarely, when temporizing measures are insufficient, emergency hemodialysis may remove 25 to 50 mEq/hr. Peritoneal dialysis is less efficient.

Calcium

Physiologic Role

Calcium is a divalent cation found primarily in the extracellular fluid. The free calcium concentration [Ca^{2+}] in ECV is approximately 1 mM, whereas the free [Ca^{2+}] in the ICV approximates 100 mM, a gradient of 10,000 to 1. Circulating calcium consists
12 of a protein-bound fraction (40% to 50%), a fraction bound to inorganic anions (10% to 15%), and an ionized fraction (45% to 50%), which is the physiologically active and homeostatically regulated component. Acute acidemia increases and acute alkalemia decreases ionized calcium.[122] Because mathematical formulae that "correct" total calcium measurements for albumin concentration are inaccurate in critically ill patients,[123] ionized calcium should be directly measured.

In general, calcium is essential for all movement that occurs in mammalian systems. Essential for normal excitation–contraction coupling, calcium is also necessary for proper function of muscle tissue, ciliary movement, mitosis, neurotransmitter release, enzyme secretion, and hormonal secretion. Cyclic adenosine monophosphate (cAMP) and phosphoinositides, which are major second messengers regulating cellular metabolism, function primarily through the regulation of calcium movement. Activation of numerous intracellular enzyme systems requires calcium. Calcium is important both for generation of the cardiac pacemaker activity and for generation of the cardiac action potential and therefore is the primary ion responsible for the plateau phase of the action potential. Calcium also plays vital functions in membrane and bone structure.

Serum [Ca^{2+}] is regulated by multiple factors (Fig. 14-14),[124] including a calcium receptor[124,125] and several hormones. Parathyroid hormone (PTH) and calcitriol, the most important neurohumoral mediators of serum [Ca^{2+}],[126] mobilize calcium from bone, increase renal tubular reabsorption of calcium, and enhance intestinal absorption of calcium. Vitamin D, after ingestion or cutaneous manufacture under the stimulus of ultraviolet light, is 25-hydroxylated to calcidiol in the liver and then is 1-hydroxylated to calcitriol, the active metabolite, in the kidney. Even in the absence of dietary calcium intake, PTH and vitamin D can maintain a normal circulating [Ca^{2+}] by mobilizing calcium from bone. In addition to the key roles played by PTH and calcitriol in regulating serum [Ca^{2+}], other recently described pathways play key molecular roles in bone resorption. The receptor activator of nuclear factor κB (RANK), RANK ligand (RANKL), and osteoprotegerin play key molecular roles; binding of RANKL to RANK stimulates osteoclast activity, whereas binding of RANKL to osteoprotegerin, a soluble decoy receptor, disrupts binding to RANK.[127]

Hypocalcemia

Hypocalcemia (ionized [Ca^{2+}] < 4 mg/dL or <1 mmol/L) occurs as a result of failure of PTH or calcitriol action or because of calcium chelation or precipitation, not because of calcium deficiency alone. PTH deficiency can result from surgical damage or removal of the parathyroid glands or from suppression of the parathyroid glands by severe hypo- or hypermagnesemia. Burns, sepsis, and pancreatitis may suppress parathyroid function and interfere with vitamin D action. Vitamin D deficiency may result from lack of dietary vitamin D or vitamin D malabsorption in patients who lack sunlight exposure. Hyperphosphatemia-induced hypocalcemia may occur as a consequence of overzealous phosphate therapy, from cell lysis secondary to chemotherapy, or as a result of cellular destruction from rhabdomyolysis. Precipitation of $CaHPO_4$ complexes occurs with hyperphosphatemia. However, ionized [Ca^{2+}] only decreases approximately 0.019 mM for each 1 mM increase in phosphate concentration. In massive transfusion, citrate may produce hypocalcemia by chelating calcium; however, decreases are usually transient and produce negligible cardiovascular effects, unless citrate clearance is decreased

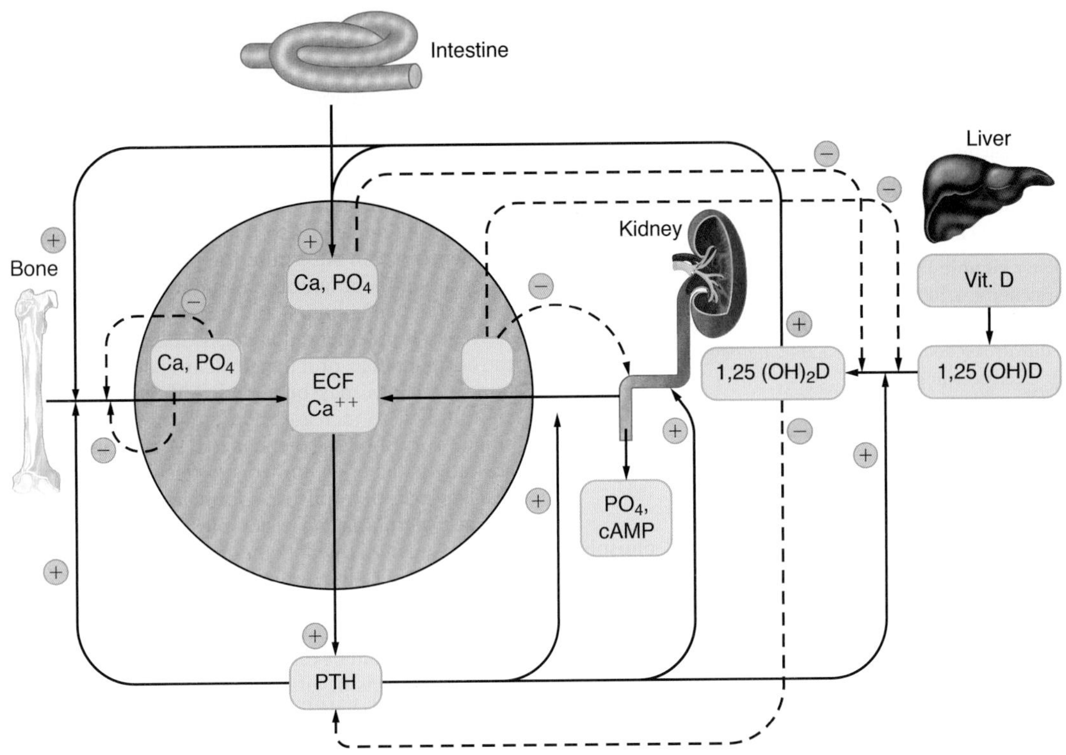

FIGURE 14-14. Schematic representation of the regulatory system maintaining Ca^{2+} homeostasis. The *solid arrows* and *lines* delineate effects of parathyroid hormone (PTH) and 1,25 $(OH)_2D_3$ (dihydroxyvitamin D) on their target tissues; *dashed arrows* and *lines* show examples of how extracellular Ca^{2+} or phosphate ions act directly on tissues regulating mineral ion metabolism. Ca, calcium; PO_4, phosphate; ECF, extracellular fluid; cAMP, cyclic adenosine monophosphate; 25(OH)D, 25-hydroxyvitamin D; negative signs indicate inhibitory actions and plus signs indicate stimulatory effects. (Reprinted with permission from: Brown EM, Pollak M, Hebert SC. The extracellular calcium-sensing receptor: Its role in health and disease. *Annu Rev Med.* 1998;49:15–29).

(e.g., by hepatic or renal disease or hypothermia) or blood transfusion exceeds 5 units of packed red blood cells.[128] Alkalemia resulting from hyperventilation or sodium bicarbonate injection can acutely decrease [Ca^{2+}].

The hallmark of hypocalcemia is increased neuronal membrane irritability and tetany (Table 14-20). Early symptoms include sensations of numbness and tingling involving fingers, toes, and the circumoral region. In frank tetany, tonic contraction of respiratory muscles may lead to laryngospasm, bronchospasm, or respiratory arrest. Smooth muscle spasm can result in abdominal cramping and urinary frequency. Mental status alterations include irritability, depression, psychosis, and dementia. Hypocalcemia may impair cardiovascular function and has been associated with heart failure, hypotension, dysrhythmias, insensitivity to digitalis, and impaired β-adrenergic action.

Reduced *ionized* serum calcium occurs in as many as 88% of critically ill patients, 66% of less severely ill intensive care unit patients and 26% of hospitalized non-intensive care unit patients.[129] Patients at particular risk include patients after multiple trauma and cardiopulmonary bypass. In most such patients, ionized hypocalcemia is clinically mild ([Ca^{2+}] 0.8 to 1 mmol/L).

Initial diagnostic evaluation should concentrate on history and physical examination, laboratory evaluation of renal function, and measurement of serum phosphate concentration. Latent hypocalcemia can be diagnosed by tapping on the facial nerve to elicit Chvostek sign or by inflating a sphygmomanometer to 20 mm Hg above systolic pressure, which produces radial and ulnar nerve ischemia and causes carpal spasm known as *Trousseau sign.* The differential diagnosis of hypocalcemia can be approached by addressing four issues: Age of the patient, serum phosphate concentration, general clinical status, and duration of hypocalcemia.[130] Low or normal phosphate concentrations imply vitamin D or magnesium deficiency. An otherwise healthy patient with chronic hypocalcemia probably is hypoparathyroid. High phosphate concentrations suggest renal failure or

TABLE 14-20. HYPOCALCEMIA: CLINICAL MANIFESTATIONS

Cardiovascular	**Respiratory**
Dysrhythmias	Apnea
Digitalis insensitivity	Laryngeal spasm
ECG changes	Bronchospasm
Heart failure	**Psychiatric**
Hypotension	Anxiety
Neuromuscular	Dementia
Tetany	Depression
Muscle spasm	Psychosis
Papilledema	
Seizures	
Weakness	
Fatigue	

ECG, electrocardiogram.

ANATOMY AND PHYSIOLOGY

TABLE 14-21. HYPOCALCEMIA: ACUTE TREATMENT

Administer calcium
- IV: 10 mL 10% calcium gluconate[a] over 10 min, followed by elemental calcium 0.3–2 mg/kg/hr
- Oral: 500–100 mg elemental calcium q6h

Administer vitamin D
- Ergocalciferol, 1,200 μg/day ($T_{1/2}$ = 30 days)
- Dihydrotachysterol, 200–400 μg/day ($T_{1/2}$ = 7 days)
- 1,25-dihydroxycholecalciferol, 0.25–1 μg/day ($T_{1/2}$ = 1 day)

Monitor electrocardiogram

[a]Calcium gluconate contains 93 mg elemental calcium per 10 mL vial.
IV, intravenous; $T_{1/2}$, half-life.

hypoparathyroidism. In renal insufficiency, reduced phosphorus excretion results in hyperphosphatemia, which downregulates the 1α-hydroxylase responsible for the renal conversion of calcidiol to calcitriol. This, in combination with decreased production of calcitriol secondary to reduced renal mass, causes reduced intestinal absorption of calcium and hypocalcemia.[126] Chronically ill adults with hypocalcemia often have disorders such as malabsorption, osteomalacia, or osteoblastic metastases.

The definitive treatment of hypocalcemia necessitates identification and treatment of the underlying cause (Table 14-21). Symptomatic hypocalcemia usually occurs when serum ionized [Ca^{2+}] is <0.7 mM.

Unnecessary offending drugs should be discontinued. Hypocalcemia resulting from hypomagnesemia or hyperphosphatemia is treated by repletion of magnesium or removal of phosphate. Treatment of a patient who has tetany and hyperphosphatemia requires coordination of therapy to avoid the consequences of metastatic soft-tissue calcification.[131] Potassium and other electrolytes should be measured and abnormalities should be corrected. Hyperkalemia and hypomagnesemia potentiate hypocalcemia-induced cardiac and neuromuscular irritability. In contrast, hypokalemia protects against hypocalcemic tetany; therefore, correction of hypokalemia without correction of hypocalcemia may provoke tetany.

Mild, ionized hypocalcemia should not be overtreated. For instance, in most patients after cardiac surgery, administration of calcium only increases blood pressure and actually attenuates the β-adrenergic effects of epinephrine. In normocalcemic dogs, calcium chloride primarily acts as a peripheral vasoconstrictor, with transient reduction of myocardial contractility; in hypocalcemic dogs, calcium infusion significantly improves contractile performance and blood pressure.[132] Therefore, calcium infusions should be of limited value in surgical patients unless there is demonstrable evidence of ionized hypocalcemia. Calcium salts appear to confer no benefit to patients already receiving inotropic or vasoactive agents.

The cornerstone of therapy for confirmed, symptomatic, ionized hypocalcemia ([Ca^{2+}] < 0.7 mM) is calcium administration. In patients who have severe hypocalcemia or hypocalcemic symptoms, calcium should be administered intravenously. In emergency situations, in an averaged-sized adult, the "rule of 10s" advises infusion of 10 mL of 10% calcium gluconate (93 mg elemental calcium) over 10 minutes, followed by a continuous infusion of elemental calcium, 0.3 to 2 mg/kg/hr (i.e., 3 to 16 mL/hr of 10% calcium gluconate for a 70 kg adult). Calcium salts should be diluted in 50 to 100 mL D_5W (to limit venous irritation and thrombosis), should not be mixed with bicarbonate (to prevent precipitation), and must be given cautiously to digitalized patients because calcium increases the toxicity of digoxin. Continuous ECG monitoring during initial therapy will detect cardiotoxicity (e.g., heart block, ventricular fibrillation). During calcium replacement, the clinician should monitor serum calcium, magnesium, phosphate, potassium, and creatinine. Once the ionized [Ca^{2+}] is stable in the range of 4 to 5 mg/dL (1 to 1.25 mM), oral calcium supplements can substitute for parenteral therapy. Urinary calcium should be monitored in an attempt to avoid hypercalciuria (>5 mg/kg per 24 hours) and urinary tract stone formation.

When supplementation fails to maintain serum calcium within the normal range, or if hypercalciuria develops, vitamin D or vitamin D analogs may be added. Although the principal effect of vitamin D is to increase enteric calcium absorption, osseous calcium resorption is also enhanced. When rapid changes in dosage are anticipated or an immediate effect is required (e.g., postoperative hypoparathyroidism), shorter-acting calciferols such as dihydrotachysterol may be preferable. Because the effect of vitamin D is not regulated, the dosages of calcium and vitamin D should be adjusted to raise the serum calcium into the low normal range.

Adverse reactions to calcium and vitamin D include hypercalcemia and hypercalciuria. If hypercalcemia develops, calcium and vitamin D should be discontinued and appropriate therapy given. The toxic effects of vitamin D metabolites persist in proportion to their biologic half-lives (ergocalciferol, 20 to 60 days; dihydrotachysterol, 5 to 15 days; calcitriol, 2 to 10 days). Glucocorticoids antagonize the toxic effects of vitamin D metabolites.

Hypercalcemia

Although ionized [Ca^{2+}] most accurately defines hypercalcemia (ionized [Ca^{2+}] > 1.5 mmol/L or total serum calcium > 10.5 mg/dL), hypercalcemia customarily is discussed in terms of total serum calcium. In hypoalbuminemic patients, total serum calcium can be estimated (albeit inaccurately) by assuming an increase of 0.8 mg/dL for every 1 g/dL of albumin concentration below 4 g/dL. Patients in whom total serum calcium is <11.5 mg/dL are usually asymptomatic. Patients with moderate hypercalcemia (total serum calcium 11.5 to 13 mg/dL) may show symptoms of lethargy, anorexia, nausea, and polyuria. Severe hypercalcemia (total serum calcium > 13 mg/dL) is associated with more severe neuromyopathic symptoms, including muscle weakness, depression, impaired memory, emotional lability, lethargy, stupor, and coma. The cardiovascular effects of hypercalcemia include hypertension, arrhythmias, heart block, cardiac arrest, and digitalis sensitivity. Skeletal disease may occur secondary to direct osteolysis or humoral bone resorption.

Hypercalcemia impairs urinary concentrating ability and renal excretory capacity for calcium by irreversibly precipitating calcium salts within the renal parenchyma and by reducing renal blood flow and GFR. In response to hypovolemia, renal tubular reabsorption of sodium enhances renal calcium reabsorption. Effective treatment of severe hypercalcemia is necessary to prevent progressive dehydration and renal failure leading to further increases in total serum calcium, because volume depletion exacerbates hypercalcemia.[133] Hypercalcemia occurs when calcium enters the ECV more rapidly than the kidneys can excrete the excess. Clinically, hypercalcemia most commonly results from an excess of bone resorption over bone formation, usually secondary to malignant disease, hyperparathyroidism, hypocalciuric hypercalcemia, thyrotoxicosis, immobilization, and granulomatous diseases. Granulomatous diseases produce hypercalciuria and hypercalcemia because of conversion by granulomatous tissue of calcidiol to calcitriol.[126]

Malignancy may produce hypercalcemia either through bone destruction or secretion by malignant tissue of hormones that promote hypercalcemia. Examples of malignancy-associated hormonal effects include secretion by solid tumors of parathormone-like peptides and derangement of the RANKL/osteoprotegerin system in multiple myeloma.[134] Primary hyperparathyroidism is associated with weakness, weight loss, and anemia, symptoms that suggest malignancy but may result simply from hyperparathyroidism. Hypercalcemia associated with granulomatous diseases (e.g., sarcoidosis) results from the production of calcitriol by granulomatous tissue. To compensate for increased gut absorption or bone resorption of calcium, renal excretion can readily increase from 100 to more than 400 mg/day. Factors that promote hypercalcemia may be offset by coexisting disorders such as pancreatitis, sepsis, or hyperphosphatemia that cause hypocalcemia.

Although definitive treatment of hypercalcemia requires correction of underlying causes, temporizing therapy may be necessary to avoid complications and to relieve symptoms. Total serum calcium exceeding 14 mg/dL represents a medical emergency. General supportive treatment includes hydration, correction of associated electrolyte abnormalities, removal of offending drugs, dietary calcium restriction, and increased physical activity. Because anorexia and antagonism by calcium of ADH action invariably lead to sodium and water depletion, infusion of 0.9% saline will dilute serum calcium, promote renal excretion, and can reduce total serum calcium by 1.5 to 3 mg/dL. Urinary output should be maintained at 200 to 300 mL/hr. As GFR increases, sodium ions increase calcium excretion by competing with calcium ions for reabsorption in the proximal renal tubules and the loop of Henle.

Furosemide further enhances calcium excretion by increasing tubular sodium. Patients who have renal impairment may require higher doses of furosemide. During saline infusion and forced diuresis, careful monitoring of cardiopulmonary status and electrolytes, especially magnesium and potassium, is required. Intensive diuresis and saline administration can achieve net calcium excretion rates of 2,000 to 4,000 mg per 24 hours, a rate eight times greater than saline alone, but still somewhat less than the 6,000 mg every 8 hours that can be removed by hemodialysis. Patients treated with phosphates for hypercalcemia should be well hydrated.

Bone resorption, the primary cause of hypercalcemia, can be minimized by increasing physical activity and initiating drug therapy with biphosphonates, calcitonin, glucocorticoids, or calcimetrics.[135] Bisphosphonates, currently the first-line therapy for acute hypercalcemia, inhibit osteoclast function and viability. Bisphosphonates are the principal drugs for the management of hypercalcemia mediated by osteoclastic bone resorption.[134] Pamidronate, unlike earlier biphosphonates, does not appear to worsen renal insufficiency. More recently released biphosphonates include alendronate, risedronate, and zoledronate. Risedronate has been associated with less gastrointestinal morbidity than alendronate.[136,137] Zoledronate has the most rapid onset of action among the biphosphonates and prolongs the duration before relapse of hypercalcemia; however, zoledronate has been associated with compromised renal function.[135] Biphosphonates also are used to control osteoporosis in both men and women.[138,139]

Calcitonin, usually reserved as a secondary treatment for life-threatening hypercalcemia, lowers serum calcium within 24 to 48 hours and is more effective when combined with glucocorticoids.[134,135] Usually calcitonin reduces total serum calcium by only 1 to 2 mg/dL. Although calcitonin is relatively nontoxic, more than 25% of patients may not respond. Thus, calcitonin is unsuitable as a first-line drug during life-threatening hypercalcemia. Hydrocortisone is effective in treating hypercalcemic patients with lymphatic malignancies, vitamin D or A intoxication, and diseases associated with production by tumor or granulomas of 1,25$(OH)_2$D or osteoclast-activating factor. Glucocorticoids rarely improve hypercalcemia secondary to malignancy or hyperparathyroidism.

In the near future, calcimimetics may become the treatment of choice for suppressing primary, secondary, and tertiary hyperparathyroidism. With the first agent, cinacalcet, recently released for clinical use in the United States and others undergoing clinical trials, calcimimetic agents also reduce inorganic phosphate concentration (Pi) and the calcium × phosphate product.[140–142] Although hyperparathyroidectomy remains the treatment of choice for primary hyperparathyroidism, calcimimetics represent an alternative for patients who are not acceptable candidates for surgery.[142] In hyperparathyroidism secondary to chronic renal failure, conventional treatment with calcium supplements, phosphate binders, and vitamin D analogs reduces the associated secondary hyperparathyroidism but also generate undesirable side effects, including hypercalcemia.[140] In effect, such patients develop a variation of the milk–alkali syndrome.[143] In chronic renal failure patients, calcimimetics reduce serum calcium, Pi and the calcium × phosphate product by sensitizing the parathyroid calcium receptor to calcium.[141] In addition, calcimimetics appear to be effective in tertiary hyperparathyroidism, which develops after renal transplantation in 25% to 50% of renal allograft recipients.[142]

Phosphates lower serum calcium by causing deposition of calcium in bone and soft tissue. Because the risk of extraskeletal calcification of organs such as the kidneys and myocardium is less if phosphates are given orally, the intravenous route should be reserved for patients with life-threatening hypercalcemia and those in whom other measures have failed.

Phosphate

Physiologic Role

Phosphorus, in the form of inorganic phosphate (Pi), is distributed in similar concentrations throughout the intracellular and the extracellular fluid. Of total body phosphorus, 90% exists in bone, 10% is intracellular, and the remainder, <1%, is found in the extracellular fluid. Phosphate circulates as the free ion (55%), complexed ion (33%), and in a protein-bound form (12%). Blood levels vary widely: The normal total Pi ranges from 2.7 to 4.5 mg/dL in adults.

Control of Pi is achieved by altered renal excretion and redistribution within the body compartments. Absorption occurs in the duodenum and jejunum and is largely unregulated. Phosphate reabsorption in the kidney is primarily regulated by PTH, dietary intake, and insulin-like growth factor. Phosphate is freely filtered at the glomerulus and its concentration in the glomerular ultrafiltrate is similar to that of plasma. The filtered phosphate is then reabsorbed in the proximal tubule where it is cotransported with sodium. Proximal tubular reabsorption of phosphorus occurs by passive cotransport with sodium. Cotransport is regulated by phosphorus intake and PTH. Phosphate excretion is increased by volume expansion and decreased by respiratory alkalosis.

Phosphates provide the primary energy bond in ATP and creatine phosphate. Therefore, severe phosphate depletion results in cellular energy depletion. Phosphorus is an essential element of second-messenger systems, including cAMP and phosphoinositides, and a major component of nucleic acids, phospholipids, and cell membranes. As part of 2,3-diphosphoglycerate, phosphate promotes release of oxygen from the hemoglobin molecule. Phosphorus also functions in protein phosphorylation and acts as a urinary buffer.

Hypophosphatemia

Hypophosphatemia is characterized by low levels of phosphate-containing cellular components, including ATP, 2,3-diphosphoglycerate, and membrane phospholipids. Serious life-threatening organ dysfunction may occur when the serum Pi falls below 1 mg/dL. Neurologic manifestations of hypophosphatemia include paresthesias, myopathy, encephalopathy, delirium, seizures, and coma.[144] Hematologic abnormalities include dysfunction of erythrocytes, platelets, and leukocytes. Because hypophosphatemia limits the chemotactic, phagocytic, and bactericidal activity of granulocytes, associated immune dysfunction may contribute to the susceptibility of hypophosphatemic patients to sepsis.[145] Muscle weakness and malaise are common. Respiratory muscle failure and myocardial dysfunction are potential problems of particular concern to anesthesiologists. Rhabdomyolysis is a complication of severe hypophosphatemia.

Common in postoperative and traumatized patients, hypophosphatemia (Pi < 2.5 mg/dL) is caused by three primary abnormalities in Pi homeostasis: An intracellular shift of Pi, an increase in renal Pi loss, and a decrease in gastrointestinal Pi absorption. Carbohydrate-induced hypophosphatemia (the "refeeding syndrome"),[146] mediated by insulin-induced cellular Pi uptake, is the type most commonly encountered in hospitalized patients. Hypophosphatemia may also occur as catabolic patients become anabolic and during medical management of diabetic ketoacidosis. Acute alkalemia, which may reduce serum Pi to 1 to 2 mg/dL, increases intracellular consumption of Pi by increasing the rate of glycolysis. Hyperventilation significantly reduces Pi and, importantly, the effect is progressive after cessation of hyperventilation.[147] Acute correction of respiratory acidemia may also result in severe hypophosphatemia. Respiratory alkalosis probably explains the hypophosphatemia associated with Gram-negative bacteremia and salicylate poisoning. Excessive renal loss of Pi explains the hypophosphatemia associated with hyperparathyroidism, hypomagnesemia, hypothermia, diuretic therapy, and renal tubular defects in Pi absorption. Excess gastrointestinal loss of Pi is most commonly secondary to the use of Pi-binding antacids or to malabsorption syndromes.

Measurement of urinary Pi aids in differentiation of hypophosphatemia due to renal losses from that are due to excessive gastrointestinal losses or redistribution of Pi into cells. Extrarenal causes of hypophosphatemia cause avid renal tubular Pi reabsorption, reducing urinary excretion to <100 mg/day.

Patients who have severe (<1 mg/dL) or symptomatic hypophosphatemia require intravenous phosphate administration (Table 14-22).[144,147] In chronically hypophosphatemic patients, 0.2 to 0.68 mmol/kg (5 to 16 mg/kg elemental phosphorus) should be infused over 12 hours. For moderately hypophosphatemic adult patients suffering from critical illness, the use of 15 mmol boluses (465 mg) mixed with 100 mL of 0.9% sodium chloride and given over a 2-hour period safely repletes phosphate.[148] The dosage is then adjusted as indicated by the serum Pi level because the cumulative deficit cannot be predicted accurately. Oral therapy can be substituted for parenteral Pi once the serum Pi level exceeds 2 mg/dL. Continued therapy with Pi supplements is required for 5 to 10 days in order to replenish body stores.

TABLE 14-22. HYPOPHOSPHATEMIA: ACUTE TREATMENT

Parenteral phosphate, 0.2 mM–0.68 mM/kg (5–16 mg/kg) over 12 h
Potassium phosphate (93 mg/mL of phosphate)
Sodium phosphate (93 mg/mL of phosphate)

Phosphate should be administered cautiously to hypocalcemic patients because of the risk of precipitating more severe hypocalcemia. In hypercalcemic patients, Pi may cause soft-tissue calcification. Phosphorus must be given cautiously to patients with renal insufficiency because of impaired excretory ability. During treatment, close monitoring of serum Pi, calcium, magnesium, and potassium is essential to avoid complications.

Hyperphosphatemia

The clinical features of hyperphosphatemia (Pi > 5 mg/dL) relate primarily to the development of hypocalcemia and ectopic calcification. Hyperphosphatemia is caused by three basic mechanisms: Inadequate renal excretion, increased movement of Pi out of cells, and increased Pi or vitamin D intake. Rapid cell lysis from chemotherapy, rhabdomyolysis, and sepsis can cause hyperphosphatemia, especially when renal function is impaired. Renal failure is the most common cause of hyperphosphatemia.

Renal excretion of Pi remains adequate until the GFR falls below 20 to 25 mL/min. Accumulation of Pi in patients with chronic renal failure merits the inclusion of Pi as a uremic toxin.[149]

Measurements of BUN, creatinine, GFR, and urinary Pi are helpful in the differential diagnosis of hyperphosphatemia. Normal renal function accompanied by high Pi excretion (>1,500 mg/day) indicates an oversupply of Pi. An elevated BUN, elevated creatinine, and low GFR suggest impaired renal excretion of Pi. Normal renal function and Pi excretion <1,500 mg/day suggest increased Pi reabsorption (i.e., hypoparathyroidism).

Hyperphosphatemia is corrected by eliminating the cause of the Pi elevation and correcting the associated hypocalcemia. Calcium supplementation of hypocalcemic patients should be delayed until serum phosphate has fallen below 2 mmol/L (6 mg/dL).[126] The serum concentration of Pi is reduced by restricting intake, increasing urinary excretion with saline and acetazolamide (500 mg every 6 hours), and increasing gastrointestinal losses by enteric administration of aluminum hydroxide (30 to 45 mL every 6 hours).

Although calcimimetics may replace Pi-binders for managing hyperphosphatemia in patients with chronic renal failure, several remain in common use. Calcium-based binders may contribute to hypercalcemia, sevelamer hydrochloride binds bile acids, and lanthanum carbonate offers the advantage of requiring patients to ingest fewer pills.[150] Hemodialysis and peritoneal dialysis are effective in removing Pi in patients who have renal failure.

Magnesium

Physiologic Role

Magnesium is an important, multifunctional, divalent cation located primarily in the intracellular space. Approximately 50% of the typical adult's 24 g of magnesium is located in bone, 12 g is located intracellularly (approximately one-half or 6 g in muscle), and <1% (<240 mg) of total body magnesium circulates in the serum.[151] Of the normal circulating total magnesium concentration (1.5 to 1.9 mEq/L or 0.75 to 0.95 mmol/L or 1.5 to 1.9 mg/dL), there are three components: Protein-bound (30%), anion-bound (15%), and ionized (55%), of which only ionized magnesium is active.

Magnesium is necessary for enzymatic reactions involving DNA and protein synthesis, energy metabolism, glucose utilization, and fatty acid synthesis and breakdown.[152] As a primary regulator or cofactor in many enzyme systems, magnesium is important for the regulation of the sodium–potassium pump, Ca-ATPase enzymes, adenyl cyclase, proton pumps, and slow calcium channels. Magnesium has been called an *endogenous calcium antagonist* because regulation of slow calcium channels contributes to maintenance of normal vascular tone, prevention of vasospasm, and perhaps the prevention of calcium overload in many tissues. Because magnesium partially regulates PTH secretion and is important for the maintenance of end-organ sensitivity to both PTH and vitamin D, abnormalities in ionized magnesium concentration ($[Mg^{2+}]$) may result in abnormal calcium metabolism. Magnesium functions in potassium metabolism primarily through regulating sodium–potassium ATPase, an enzyme that controls potassium entry into cells, especially in potassium-depleted states, and controls reabsorption of potassium by the renal tubules. In addition, magnesium functions as a regulator of membrane excitability and serves as a structural component in both cell membranes and the skeleton.

Because magnesium stabilizes axonal membranes, hypomagnesemia decreases the threshold of axonal stimulation and increases nerve conduction velocity. Magnesium also influences the release of neurotransmitters at the neuromuscular junction by competitively inhibiting the entry of calcium into the presynaptic nerve terminals. The concentration of calcium required to trigger calcium release and the rate at which calcium is released from the sarcoplasmic reticulum are inversely related to the ambient magnesium concentration. Thus, the net effect of hypomagnesemia is muscle that contracts more in response to stimuli and is tetany-prone.

Magnesium is widely available in foods and is absorbed through the gastrointestinal tract, although dietary consumption appears to have decreased over several decades.[152] Seventy percent of plasma magnesium is filtered through the glomerular membrane; of the filtered magnesium, 30% is absorbed in the proximal tubule, 60% in the thick ascending loop of Henle, and 10% to 15% in the distal tubule.[151] While both magnesium and Pi are primarily regulated by intrinsic renal mechanisms, PTH exerts a greater effect on renal loss of Pi.

Magnesium has been used to help manage an impressive array of clinical problems in patients who are not hypomagnesemic. Therapeutic hypermagnesemia is used to treat patients with premature labor, preeclampsia, and eclampsia. Because magnesium blocks the release of catecholamines from adrenergic nerve terminals and the adrenal glands, magnesium has been used to reduce the effects of catecholamine excess in patients with tetanus and pheochromocytoma.[153] In patients awaiting liver transplantation, one study showed that administration of magnesium significantly reversed hypocoagulability.[154] Although clinical data are inconsistent, magnesium also may exert an analgesic effect on postoperative pain,[153,155] perhaps in part due to magnesium's antagonism of the *N*-methyl-D-aspartate glutamate receptor.[153] Magnesium has been proposed as part of an antivasospasm regimen after subarachnoid hemorrhage, but its efficacy may be limited by induction of increasing magnesium levels of hypocalcemia, which in turn could aggravate cerebral vasospasm.[156] Surprisingly, redistribution of magnesium after subarachnoid hemorrhage has been correlated with ECG changes.[157]

Magnesium administration may influence dysrhythmias by direct effects on myocardial membranes, by altering cellular potassium and sodium concentrations, by inhibiting cellular calcium entry, by improving myocardial oxygen supply and demand, by prolonging the effective refractory period, by depressing conduction, by antagonizing catecholamine action on the conducting system, and by preventing vasospasm. Administration of magnesium reduces the incidence of dysrhythmias after myocardial infarction and in patients with congestive heart failure.[158] In humans with ischemic myocardium, magnesium prevented ischemic increases in action potential duration and membrane repolarization.[159] After acute myocardial infarction, intravenous magnesium administration decreased short-term mortality.[160] In addition, magnesium may be useful as treatment for torsades de pointes, even in normomagnesemic patients.[161] Treatment of hypomagnesemia during cardiopulmonary bypass decreased the incidence of postoperative ventricular tachycardia from 30% to 7% and increased the frequency of continuous sinus rhythm from 5% to 34%.[162]

Hypomagnesemia

The clinical features of hypomagnesemia ($[Mg^{2+}] < 1.8$ mg/dL), like those of hypocalcemia, are characterized by increased neuronal irritability and tetany (Table 14-23).[151] Symptoms are rare when the serum $[Mg^{2+}]$ is 1.5 to 1.7 mg/dL; in most symptomatic patients serum $[Mg^{2+}]$ is <1.2 mg/dL. Patients frequently complain of weakness, lethargy, muscle spasms, paresthesias, and depression. When severe, hypomagnesemia may induce seizures, confusion, and coma. Cardiovascular abnormalities include coronary artery spasm, cardiac failure, dysrhythmias, and hypotension. Severe hypomagnesemia may reduce the response of adenylate cyclase to stimulation of the PTH receptor.[163] Hypomagnesemia can aggravate digoxin toxicity and congestive heart failure.

Rarely resulting from inadequate dietary intake, hypomagnesemia most commonly is caused by inadequate gastrointestinal absorption, excessive magnesium losses, or failure of renal magnesium conservation. Hypomagnesemia is particularly frequent in alcoholic patients.[151] Of alcoholic patients admitted to the hospital, 30% are hypomagnesemic.[164] Excessive loss of magnesium is associated with prolonged nasogastric suctioning, gastrointestinal or biliary fistulas, and intestinal drains. Inability of the renal tubules to conserve magnesium complicates a variety of systemic and renal diseases, although advanced renal disease with a decreased GFR may lead to magnesium retention. Polyuria, whether secondary to ECV expansion or to pharmacologic or pathologic diuresis, may result in excessive urinary magnesium excretion. Various drugs, including aminoglycosides, *cis*-platinum, cardiac glycosides, and diuretics, enhance urinary magnesium excretion. Intracellular shifts of magnesium as a result of thyroid hormone or insulin administration may also decrease serum $[Mg^{2+}]$.

Because the sodium–potassium pump is magnesium-dependent, hypomagnesemia increases myocardial sensitivity to digitalis preparations and may cause hypokalemia as a result of renal potassium wasting. Attempts to correct potassium deficits with potassium-replacement therapy alone may not be successful without simultaneous magnesium therapy. Magnesium is important in the regulation of potassium channels. The interrelationships of magnesium and potassium in cardiac tissue have probably the greatest clinical relevance in terms of dysrhythmias, digoxin toxicity, and myocardial infarction. Both severe hypomagnesemia and hypermagnesemia suppress PTH secretion and can cause hypocalcemia. Severe hypomagnesemia may also impair end-organ response to PTH.

Hypomagnesemia is associated with hypokalemia, hyponatremia, hypophosphatemia, and hypocalcemia. The reported prevalence of hypomagnesemia in hospitalized and critically ill patients varies from 11% to 61%, with the variability attributable to differences in measurement technique.[165] Recent development of a specific electrode to measure ionized $[Mg^{2+}]$ has demonstrated an association between hypomagnesemia, use of diuretics, and

TABLE 14-23. MANIFESTATIONS OF ALTERED SERUM MAGNESIUM CONCENTRATIONS

Magnesium Level			
mg/dL	mEq/L	mmol/L	Manifestation
<1.2	<1	<0.5	Tetany Seizures Arrhythmias
1.2–1.8	1–1.5	0.5–0.75	Neuromuscular irritability Hypocalcemia Hypokalemia
1.8–2.5	1.5–2.1	0.75–1.05	Normal magnesium level
2.5–5	2.1–4.2	1.05–2.1	Typically asymptomatic
5–7	4.2–5.8	2.1–2.9	Lethargy Drowsiness Flushing Nausea and vomiting Diminished deep tendon reflex
7–12	5.8–10	2.9–5	Somnolence Loss of deep tendon reflexes Hypotension ECG changes
>12	>10	>5	Complete heart block Cardiac arrest Apnea Paralysis Coma

Anatomy and Physiology.
ECG, electrocardiogram.
Reprinted from: Topf JM, Murray PT. Hypomagnesemia and hypermagnesemia. *Rev Endocr Metab Disord.* 2003;4:195–206, with permission.

development of sepsis.[165] Patients who develop hypomagnesemia while in intensive care have an increased mortality.[165] Serum [Mg^{2+}] may not reflect intracellular magnesium content. Peripheral lymphocyte magnesium concentration correlates well with skeletal and cardiac magnesium content.

Measurement of 24-hour urinary magnesium excretion is useful in separating renal from nonrenal causes of hypomagnesemia. Normal kidneys can reduce magnesium excretion to <1 to 2 mEq/day in response to magnesium depletion. Hypomagnesemia accompanied by high urinary excretion of magnesium (>3 to 4 mEq/day) suggests a renal etiology. In the magnesium-loading test, urinary [Mg^{2+}] excretion is measured for 24 hours after an intravenous magnesium load.[166]

Magnesium deficiency is treated by the administration of magnesium supplements (Table 14-24). One gram of magnesium sulfate provides approximately 4 mmol (8 mEq or 98 mg) of elemental magnesium. Mild deficiencies can be treated with diet alone. Replacement must be added to daily magnesium requirements (0.3 to 0.4 mEq/kg/day). Symptomatic or severe hypomagnesemia ([Mg^{2+}] < 1 mg/dL) should be treated with parenteral magnesium: 1 to 2 g (8 to 16 mEq) of magnesium sulfate as an intravenous bolus over the first hour, followed by a continuous infusion of 2 to 4 mEq/hr. Therapy should be guided subsequently by the serum magnesium level. The rate of infusion should not exceed 1 mEq/min, even in emergency situations, and the patient should receive continuous cardiac monitoring to detect cardiotoxicity. Because magnesium antagonizes calcium, blood pressure and cardiac function should be monitored, although blood pressure and cardiac output usually change little during magnesium infusion.

During repletion, patellar reflexes should be monitored frequently and magnesium withheld if they become suppressed. Patients who have renal insufficiency have a diminished ability to excrete magnesium and require careful monitoring during therapy. Repletion of systemic magnesium stores usually requires 5 to 7 days of therapy, after which daily maintenance doses of magnesium should be provided. Magnesium can be given orally, usually in a dose of 60 to 90 mEq/day of magnesium oxide. Hypocalcemic, hypomagnesemic patients should receive magnesium as the chloride salt because the sulfate ion can chelate calcium and further reduce the serum [Ca^{2+}].

TABLE 14-24. HYPOMAGNESEMIA: ACUTE TREATMENT

Intravenous Mg^{a}: 8–16 mEq (1–2 g $MgSO_4$) bolus over 1 h, followed by 2–4 mEq/hr (250–500 mg/hr $MgSO_4$) as continuous infusion
Intramuscular Mg^{a}: 10 mEq q4–6h

[a] $MgSO_4$: 1 g = 8 mEq/mg; $MgCl_2$: 1 g = 10 mEq/mg.

Hypermagnesemia

Most cases of hypermagnesemia ($[Mg^{2+}] > 2.5$ mg/dL) are iatrogenic, resulting from the administration of magnesium in antacids, enemas, or parenteral nutrition, especially to patients with impaired renal function. Other rarer causes of mild hypermagnesemia are hypothyroidism, Addison disease, lithium intoxication, and familial hypocalciuric hypercalcemia. Hypermagnesemia is rarely detected in routine electrolyte determinations.[151] Hypermagnesemia antagonizes the release and effect of acetylcholine at the neuromuscular junction. The result is depressed skeletal muscle function and neuromuscular blockade. Magnesium potentiates the action of nondepolarizing muscle relaxants and decreases potassium release in response to succinylcholine. The clinical features of progressive hypermagnesemia are listed in Table 14-23.[151]

The neuromuscular and cardiac toxicity of hypermagnesemia can be acutely, but transiently, antagonized by giving intravenous calcium (5 to 10 mEq) to buy time while more definitive therapy is instituted.[151] All magnesium-containing preparations must be stopped. Urinary excretion of magnesium can be increased by expanding ECV and inducing diuresis with a combination of saline and furosemide. In emergency situations and in patients with renal failure, magnesium may be removed by dialysis.

References

1. Corey HE. Stewart and beyond: New models of acid-base balance. *Kidney Int.* 2004;64:777.
2. Moviat M, van Haren F, van der Hoeven H. Conventional or physicochemical approach in intensive care unit patients with metabolic acidosis. *Crit Care.* 2003;7:219.
3. Khanna A, Kurtzman NA. Metabolic alkalosis. *J Nephrol.* 2006;19(suppl 9):S86.
4. Prough DS, Bidani A. Hyperchloremic metabolic acidosis is a predictable consequence of intraoperative infusion of 0.9% saline. *Anesthesiology.* 1999;90:1247.
5. Adrogué HJ. Metabolic acidosis: Pathophysiology, diagnosis and management. *J Nephrol.* 2006;19(suppl 9):S62.
6. Morris CG, Low J. Metabolic acidosis in the critically ill: Part 2. Causes and treatment. *Anaesthesia.* 2008;63:396.
7. Morris CG, Low J. Metabolic acidosis in the critically ill: Part 1. Classification and pathophysiology. *Anaesthesia.* 2008;63:294.
8. Kraut JA, Madias NE. Serum anion gap: Its uses and limitations in clinical medicine. *Clin J Am Soc Nephrol.* 2007;2:162.
9. Scheingraber S, Rehm M, Sehmisch C, et al. Rapid saline infusion produces hyperchloremic acidosis in patients undergoing gynecologic surgery. *Anesthesiology.* 1999;90:1265.
10. Carvounis CP, Feinfeld DA. A simple estimate of the effect of the serum albumin level on the anion Gap. *Am J Nephrol.* 2000;20:369.
11. Rastegar A. Use of the DeltaAG/DeltaHCO3$^-$ ratio in the diagnosis of mixed acid-base disorders. *J Am Soc Nephrol.* 2007;18:2429.
12. Gehlbach BK, Schmidt GA. Bench-to-bedside review: Treating acid-base abnormalities in the intensive care unit—the role of buffers. *Crit Care.* 2004;8:259.
13. Cooper DJ, Walley KR, Wiggs BR, et al. Bicarbonate does not improve hemodynamics in critically ill patients who have lactic acidosis. A prospective, controlled clinical study. *Ann Intern Med.* 1990;112:492.
14. Stacpoole PW, Wright EC, Baumgartner TG, et al. Dichloroacetate-Lactic Acidosis Study Group: A controlled clinical trial of dichloroacetate for treatment of lactic acidosis in adults. *N Engl J Med.* 1992;327:1564.
15. Hoste EA, Colpaert K, Vanholder RC, et al. Sodium bicarbonate versus THAM in ICU patients with mild metabolic acidosis. *J Nephrol.* 2005;18:303.
16. Foster GT, Vaziri ND, Sassoon CSH. Respiratory alkalosis. *Respir Care.* 2001; 46:384.
17. Chesler M. Regulation and modulation of pH in the brain. *Physiol Rev.* 2003; 83:1183.
18. Kallet RH, Liu K, Tang J. Management of acidosis during lung-protective ventilation in acute respiratory distress syndrome. *Respir Care Clin N Am.* 2003;9:437.
19. Martinu T, Menzies D, Dial S. Re-evaluation of acid-base prediction rules in patients with chronic respiratory acidosis. *Can Respir J.* 2003;10:311.
20. Svensén C, Hahn RG. Volume kinetics of Ringer solution, dextran 70, and hypertonic saline in male volunteers. *Anesthesiology.* 1997;87:204.
21. Svensen CH, Rodhe PM, Prough DS. Pharmacokinetic aspects of fluid therapy. *Best Pract Res Clin Anaesthesiol.* 2009;23:213-224.
22. Connolly CM, Kramer GC, Hahn RG, et al. Isoflurane but not mechanical ventilation promotes extravascular fluid accumulation during crystalloid volume loading. *Anesthesiology.* 2003;98:670.
23. Vane LA, Prough DS, Kinsky MA, et al. Effects of different catecholamines on the dynamics of volume expansion of crystalloid infusion. *Anesthesiology.* 2004;101:1136.
24. Schrier RW. The sea within us: Disorders of body water homeostasis. *Curr Opin Investig Drugs.* 2007;8:304.
25. Ball SG. Vasopressin and disorders of water balance: The physiology and pathophysiology of vasopressin. *Ann Clin Biochem.* 2007;44:417.
26. Martinez-Rumayor A, Richards AM, Burnett JC, et al. Biology of the natriuretic peptides. *Am J Cardiol.* 2008;101:3.
27. Akashi YJ, Springer J, Lainscak M, et al. Atrial natriuretic peptide and related peptides. *Clin Chem Lab Med.* 2007;45:1259.
28. Silver MA. The natriuretic peptide system: Kidney and cardiovascular effects. *Curr Opin Nephrol Hypertens.* 2006;15:14.
29. Conte G, Bellizzi V, Cianciaruso B, et al. Physiologic role and diuretic efficacy of atrial natriuretic peptide in health and chronic renal disease. *Kidney Int.* 1997;51:S28.
30. Atlas SA. The renin-angiotensin aldosterone system: Pathophysiological role and pharmacologic inhibition. *J Manag Care Pharm.* 2007;13:9.
31. Baughman VL. Brain protection during neurosurgery. *Anesthesiol Clin North America.* 2002;20:315.
32. Lanzino G, Kassell NF, Germanson T, et al. Plasma glucose levels and outcome after aneurysmal subarachnoid hemorrhage. *J Neurosurg.* 1993;79:885.
33. Rovlias A, Kotsou S. The influence of hyperglycemia on neurological outcome in patients with severe head injury. *Neurosurgery.* 2000;46:335.
34. Weiner RS, Weiner DC, Larson RJ. Benefits and risks of tight glucose control in critically ill adults: A meta-analysis. *JAMA.* 2008;300:933.
35. Akhtar S, Barash PG, Inzucchi SE. Scientific principles and clinical implications of perioperative glucose regulation and control. *Anesth Analg.* 2010;110:478–497.
36. Finfer S, Chittock DR, Su SY, et al. Intensive versus conventional glucose control in critically ill patients. *N Engl J Med.* 2009;360:1283–1297.
37. Kansagara D, Fu R, Freeman M, et al. Intensive insulin therapy in hospitalized patients: A systematic review. *Ann Intern Med.* 2011;154:268–282.
38. Jacob M, Chappell D, Rehm M. The 'third space'–fact or fiction? *Best Pract Res Clin Anaesthesiol.* 2009;23:144.
39. Maharaj CH, Kallam SR, Malik A, et al. Preoperative intravenous fluid therapy decreases postoperative nausea and pain in high risk patients. *Anesth Analg.* 2005;100:675.
40. Holte K, Klarskov B, Christensen DS, et al. Liberal versus restrictive fluid administration to improve recovery after laparoscopic cholecystectomy: A randomized, double-blind study. *Ann Surg.* 2004;240:892.
41. Holte K, Kristensen BB, Valentiner L, et al. Liberal versus restrictive fluid management in knee arthroplasty: A randomized, double-blind study. *Anesth Analg.* 2007;105:465.
42. Brandstrup B, Tonnesen H, Beier-Holgersen R, et al. Effects of intravenous fluid restriction on postoperative complications: Comparison of two perioperative fluid regimens—a randomized assessor-blinded multicenter trial. *Ann Surg.* 2003; 238:641.
43. Nisanevich V, Felsenstein I, Almogy G, et al. Effect of intraoperative fluid management on outcome after intraabdominal surgery. *Anesthesiology.* 2005;103:25.
44. Lobo DN, Bostock KA, Neal KR, et al. Effect of salt and water balance on recovery of gastrointestinal function after elective colonic resection: A randomised controlled trial. *Lancet.* 2002;359:1812.
45. Khoo CK, Vickery CJ, Forsyth N, et al. A prospective randomized controlled trial of multimodal perioperative management protocol in patients undergoing elective colorectal resection for cancer. *Ann Surg.* 2007;245:867.
46. Holte K, Foss NB, Andersen J, et al. Liberal or restrictive fluid administration in fast-track colonic surgery: A randomized, double-blind study. *Br J Anaesth.* 2007;99:500.
47. Corcoran T, Rhodes JE, Clarke S, et al. Perioperative fluid management strategies in major surgery: A stratified meta-analysis. *Anesth Analg.* 2012;114:640.
48. Wiedemann HP, Wheeler AP, Bernard GR, et al. Comparison of two fluid-management strategies in acute lung injury. *N Engl J Med.* 2006;354:2564.
49. Moretti EW, Robertson KM, El Moalem H, et al. Intraoperative colloid administration reduces postoperative nausea and vomiting and improves postoperative outcomes compared with crystalloid administration. *Anesth Analg.* 2003;96:611.
50. Venn R, Steele A, Richardson P, et al. Randomized controlled trial to investigate influence of the fluid challenge on duration of hospital stay and perioperative morbidity in patients with hip fractures. *Br J Anaesth.* 2002;88:65.
51. Gan TJ, Soppitt A, Maroof M, et al. Goal-directed intraoperative fluid administration reduces length of hospital stay after major surgery. *Anesthesiology.* 2002; 97:820.
52. Roberts I, Blackhall K, Alderson P, et al. Colloids versus crystalloids for fluid resuscitation in critically ill patients. *Cochrane Database Syst Rev.* 2011;CD001208.
53. Finfer S, Bellomo R, Boyce N, et al. A comparison of albumin and saline for fluid resuscitation in the intensive care unit. *N Engl J Med.* 2004;350:2247.
54. Finfer S, Bellomo R, McEvoy S, et al. Effect of baseline serum albumin concentration on outcome of resuscitation with albumin or saline in patients in intensive care units: Analysis of data from the saline versus albumin fluid evaluation (SAFE) study. *BMJ.* 2006;333:1044.
55. Myburgh J, Cooper DJ, Finfer S, et al. Saline or albumin for fluid resuscitation in patients with traumatic brain injury. *N Engl J Med.* 2007;357:874.

56. Kozek-Langenecker SA. Influence of fluid therapy on the haemostatic system of intensive care patients. *Best Pract Res Clin Anaesthesiol.* 2009;23:225.
57. Bunn F, Trivedi D, Ashraf S. Colloid solutions for fluid resuscitation. *Cochrane Database Syst Rev.* 2011;(3):CD001319.
58. Perner A, Hasse N, Guttormsen, et al. Hydroxylethyl starch 130/0.42 versus Ringer's acetate in severe sepsis. *NEJM* 2012;367:124.
59. Zornow MH, Todd MM, Moore SS. The acute cerebral effects of changes in plasma osmolality and oncotic pressure. *Anesthesiology.* 1987;67:936.
60. Kaieda R, Todd MM, Warner DS. Prolonged reduction in colloid oncotic pressure does not increase brain edema following cryogenic injury in rabbits. *Anesthesiology.* 1989;71:554.
61. Warner DS, Boehland LA. Effects of iso-osmolal intravenous fluid therapy on post-ischemic brain water content in the rat. *Anesthesiology.* 1988;68:86.
62. Zornow MH, Scheller MS, Todd MM, et al. Acute cerebral effects of isotonic crystalloid and colloid solutions following cryogenic brain injury in the rabbit. *Anesthesiology.* 1988;69:180.
63. Drummond JC, Patel PM, Cole DJ, et al. The effect of the reduction of colloid oncotic pressure, with and without reduction of osmolality, on post-traumatic cerebral edema. *Anesthesiology.* 1998;88:993.
64. Velasco IT, Pontieri V, Rocha E et al. Hyperosmotic NaCl and severe hemorrhagic shock. *Am J Physiol.* 1980;239:H664.
65. Prough DS, Whitley JM, Taylor CL, et al. Regional cerebral blood flow following resuscitation from hemorrhagic shock with hypertonic saline: Influence of a subdural mass. *Anesthesiology.* 1991;75:319.
66. Prough DS, Whitley JM, Taylor CL, et al. Rebound intracranial hypertension in dogs after resuscitation with hypertonic solutions from hemorrhagic shock accompanied by an intracranial mass lesion. *J Neurosurg Anesthesiol.* 1999; 11:102.
67. Vassar MJ, Fischer RP, O'Brien PE, et al. A multicenter trial for resuscitation of injured patients with 7.5% sodium chloride. The effect of added dextran 70. *Arch Surg.* 1993;128: 1003.
68. Cooper DJ, Myles PS, McDermott FT, et al. Prehospital hypertonic saline resuscitation of patients with hypotension and severe traumatic brain injury: A randomized controlled trial. *JAMA.* 2004;291: 1350.
69. Chesnut RM. Avoidance of hypotension: conditio sine qua non of successful severe head-injury management. *J Trauma.* 1997;42:S4.
70. Zaloga GP, Hughes SS. Oliguria in patients with normal renal function. *Anesthesiology.* 1990;72:598.
71. Wong DH, O'Connor D, Tremper KK, et al. Changes in cardiac output after acute blood loss and position change in man. *Crit Care Med.* 1989;17:979.
72. Marik PE, Cavallazzi R, Vasu T, et al. Dynamic changes in arterial waveform derived variables and fluid responsiveness in mechanically ventilated patients: A systematic review of the literature. *Crit Care Med.* 2009;37:2642–2647.
73. Renner J, Scholz J, Bein B. Monitoring fluid therapy. *Best Pract Res Clin Anaesthesiol.* 2009;23:159.
74. Cannesson M, Manach YL, Hofer CK, et al. Assessing the diagnostic accuracy of pulse pressure variations for the prediction of fluid responsiveness. *Anesthesiology.* 2011;115;231-241.
75. Madan AK, Uy Barreta VV, Aliabadi-Wahle S, et al. Esophageal Doppler ultrasound monitor versus pulmonary artery catheter in the hemodynamic management of critically ill surgical patients. *J Trauma.* 1999;46:607.
76. Rivers E, Nguyen B, Havstad S, et al. Early goal-directed therapy in the treatment of severe sepsis and septic shock. *N Engl J Med.* 2001;345:1368.
77. Kern JW, Shoemaker WC. Meta-analysis of hemodynamic optimization in high-risk patients. *Crit Care Med.* 2002;30:1686.
78. Lobo SM, Lobo FR, Polachini CA, et al. Prospective, randomized trial comparing fluids and dobutamine optimization of oxygen delivery in high-risk surgical patients. *Crit Care.* 2006;10:R72.
79. Balogh Z, McKinley BA, Cocanour CS, et al. Supranormal trauma resuscitation causes more cases of abdominal compartment syndrome. *Arch Surg.* 2003; 138:637.
80. Wilson J, Woods I, Fawcett J, et al. Reducing the risk of major elective surgery: Randomised controlled trial of preoperative optimisation of oxygen delivery. *BMJ.* 1999;318:1099.
81. DiCorte CJ, Latham P, Greilich PE, et al. Esophageal Doppler monitor determinations of cardiac output and preload during cardiac operations. *Ann Thorac Surg.* 2000;69:1782.
82. Horowitz P, Kumar A. It's the colloid, not the esophageal Doppler Monitor. *Anesthesiology.* 2003;99:238.
83. Young WF. Primary aldosteronism: Renaissance of a syndrome. *Clin Endocrinol (Oxf).* 2007;66:607.
84. Karagiannis A, Tziomalos K, Papageorgiou A, et al. Spironolactone versus eplerenone for the treatment of idiopathic hyperaldosteronism. *Expert Opin Pharmacother.* 2008;9:509.
85. Kashyap AS. Hyperglycemia-induced hyponatremia: Is it time to correct the correction factor? *Arch Intern Med.* 1999;159:2745.
86. Gravenstein D. Transurethral resection of the prostate (TURP) syndrome: A review of the pathophysiology and management. *Anesth Analg* 1997;84:438.
87. Xu DL, Martin PY, Ohara M, et al. Upregulation of aquaporin-2 water channel expression in chronic heart failure rat. *J Clin Invest.* 1997;99:1500.
88. Fujita N, Ishikawa SE, Sasaki S, et al. Role of water channel AQP-CD in water retention in SIADH and cirrhotic rats. *Am J Physiol.* 1995;269:F926.
89. Ecelbarger CA, Nielsen S, Olson BR, et al. Role of renal aquaporins in escape from vasopressin-induced antidiuresis in rat. *J Clin Invest.* 1997;99:1852.
90. Moritz ML, Ayus JC. Hospital-acquired hyponatremia—why are hypotonic parenteral fluids still being used? *Nat Clin Pract Nephrol.* 2007;3:374.
91. Verbalis JG, Goldsmith SR, Greenberg A, et al. Hyponatremia treatment guidelines 2007: Expert panel recommendations. *Am J Med.* 2007;120:S1.
92. Katayama Y, Haraoka J, Hirabayashi H, et al. A randomized controlled trial of hydrocortisone against hyponatremia in patients with aneurysmal subarachnoid hemorrhage. *Stroke.* 2007;38:2373.
93. Fraser CL, Arieff AI. Fatal central diabetes mellitus and insipidus resulting from untreated hyponatremia: A new syndrome. *Ann Intern Med.* 1990;112:113.
94. Lien YH, Shapiro JI. Hyponatremia: Clinical diagnosis and management. *Am J Med.* 2007;120:653.
95. Steele A, Gowrishankar M, Abrahamson S, et al. Postoperative hyponatremia despite near-isotonic saline infusion: A phenomenon of desalination. *Ann Intern Med.* 1997;126:20.
96. Arieff AI. Postoperative hyponatraemic encephalopathy following elective surgery in children. *Paediatr Anesth.* 1998;8:1.
97. Karmel KS, Bear RA. Treatment of hyponatremia: A quantitative analysis. *Am J Kidney Dis.* 1994;21:439.
98. Kumar S, Rubin S, Mather PJ, et al. Hyponatremia and vasopressin antagonism in congestive heart failure. *Clin Cardiol.* 2007;30:546.
99. Decaux G. V2-antagonists for the treatment of hyponatraemia. *Nephrol Dial Transplant.* 2007;22:1853.
100. Cawley MJ. Hyponatremia: Current treatment strategies and the role of vasopressin antagonists. *Ann Pharmacother.* 2007;41:840.
101. Madias NE. Effects of tolvaptan, an oral vasopressin V2 receptor antagonist, in hyponatremia. *Am J Kidney Dis.* 2007;50:184.
102. Schrier RW, Gross P, Gheorghiade M, et al. Tolvaptan, a selective oral vasopressin V2-receptor antagonist, for hyponatremia. *N Engl J Med.* 2006;355:2099.
103. Sterns RH, Riggs JE, Schochet SS Jr. Osmotic demyelination syndrome following correction of hyponatremia. *N Engl J Med.* 1986;314:1535.
104. Adrogué HJ, Madias NE. Aiding fluid prescription for the dysnatremias. *Intensive Care Med.* 1997;23:309.
105. Biswas M, Davies JS. Hyponatraemia in clinical practice. *Postgrad Med J.* 2007; 83:373.
106. Esposito P, Piotti G, Bianzina S, et al. The syndrome of inappropriate antidiuresis: Pathophysiology, clinical management and new therapeutic options. *Nephron Clin Pract.* 2011;119:c62.
107. Loh JA, Verbalis JG. Disorders of water and salt metabolism associated with pituitary disease. *Endocrinol Metab Clin North Am.* 2008;37:213.
108. Ayus JC, Armstrong DL, Arieff AI. Effects of hypernatraemia in the central nervous system and its therapy in rats and rabbits. *J Physiol.* 1996;492:243.
109. Adrogué HJ, Madias NE. Hypernatremia. *N Engl J Med.* 2000;342:1493.
110. Liamis G, Kalogirou M, Saugos V, et al. Therapeutic approach in patients with dysnatraemias. *Nephrol Dial Transplant.* 2006;21:1564.
111. Adler SM, Verbalis JG. Disorders of body water homeostasis in critical illness. *Endocrinol Metab Clin North Am.* 2006;35:873.
112. Sood MM, Sood AR, Richardson R. Emergency management and commonly encountered outpatient scenarios in patients with hyperkalemia. *Mayo Clin Proc.* 2007;82:1553.
113. Gilligan P, Pountney A, Wilson B, et al. SOCRATES Episode II (synopsis of Cochrane reviews applicable to emergency services Episode II): The return of Series III. *Emerg Med J.* 2007;24:489.
114. Wahr JA, Parks R, Boisvert D, et al. Preoperative serum potassium levels and perioperative outcomes in cardiac surgery patients. *JAMA.* 1999;281:2203.
115. Suga SI, Phillips MI, Ray PE, et al. Hypokalemia induces renal injury and alterations in vasoactive mediators that favor salt sensitivity. *Am J Physiol Renal Physiol.* 2001;281:F620.
116. Lin SH, Halperin ML. Hypokalemia: A practical approach to diagnosis and its genetic basis. *Curr Med Chem.* 2007;14:1551.
117. Khosla N, Hogan D. Mineralocorticoid hypertension and hypokalemia. *Semin Nephrol.* 2006;26:434.
118. Furgeson SB, Chonchol M. Beta-blockade in chronic dialysis patients. *Semin Dial.* 2008;21:43.
119. Gronert GA. Succinylcholine hyperkalemia after burns. *Anesthesiology.* 1999;91:320.
120. Kim HJ, Han SW. Therapeutic approach to hyperkalemia. *Nephron.* 2002;92 (suppl 1):33.
121. Putcha N, Allon M. Management of hyperkalemia in dialysis patients. *Semin Dial.* 2007;20:431.
122. Shepard MM, Smith JW III. Hypercalcemia. *Am J Med Sci.* 2007;334:381.
123. Slomp J, van der Voort PHJ, Gerritsen RT, et al. Albumin-adjusted calcium is not suitable for diagnosis of hyper-and hypocalcemia in the critically ill. *Crit Care Med.* 2003;31:1389.
124. Brown EM, Pollak M, Hebert SC. The extracellular calcium-sensing receptor: Its role in health and disease. *Ann Rev Med.* 1998;49:15.
125. Brown EM, Pollak M, Seidman CE, et al. Calcium-ion-sensing cell-surface receptors. *N Engl J Med.* 1995;333:234.

126. Bushinsky DA, Monk RD. Calcium. *Lancet.* 1998;352:306.
127. Blair JM, Zheng Y, Dunstan CR. RANK ligand. *Int J Biochem Cell Biol.* 2007; 39:1077.
128. Dickerson RN. Treatment of hypocalcemia in critical illness—part 1. *Nutrition.* 2007;23:358.
129. Zivin JR, Gooley T, Zager RA, et al. Hypocalcemia: A pervasive metabolic abnormality in the critically ill. *Am J Kidney Dis.* 2001;37:689.
130. Guise TA, Mundy GR. Evaluation of hypocalcemia in children and adults. *J Clin Endocrinol Metab.* 1995;80:1473.
131. Sutters M, Gaboury CL, Bennett WM. Severe hyperphosphatemia and hypocalcemia: A dilemma in patient management. *J Am Soc Nephrol.* 1996;7:2055.
132. Mathru M, Rooney MW, Goldberg SA, et al. Separation of myocardial versus peripheral effects of calcium administration in normocalcemic and hypocalcemic states using pressure-volume (conductance) relationships. *Anesth Analg.* 1993;77:250.
133. Bilezikian JP. Management of acute hypercalcemia. *N Engl J Med.* 1992;326: 1196.
134. Zojer N, Ludwig H. Hematological emergencies. *Ann Oncol.* 2007;18(suppl 1): i45.
135. Ariyan CE, Sosa JA. Assessment and management of patients with abnormal calcium. *Crit Care Med.* 2004;32:S146.
136. Kane S, Borisov NN, Brixner D. Pharmacoeconomic evaluation of gastrointestinal tract events during treatment with risedronate or alendronate: A retrospective cohort study. *Am J Manag Care.* 2004;10:S216.
137. Miller RG, Bolognese M, Worley K, et al. Incidence of gastrointestinal events among bisphosphonate patients in an observational setting. *Am J Manag Care.* 2004;10:S207.
138. Valverde P. Pharmacotherapies to manage bone loss-associated diseases: A quest for the perfect benefit-to-risk ratio. *Curr Med Chem.* 2008;15:284.
139. Olszynski WP, Davison KS. Alendronate for the treatment of osteoporosis in men. *Expert Opin Pharmacother.* 2008;9:491.
140. Ogata H, Koiwa F, Ito H, et al. Therapeutic strategies for secondary hyperparathyroidism in dialysis patients. *Ther Apher Dial.* 2006;10:355.
141. Shahapuni I, Monge M, Oprisiu R, et al. Drug Insight: Renal indications of calcimimetics. *Nat Clin Pract Nephrol.* 2006;2:316.
142. Wuthrich RP, Martin D, Bilezikian JP. The role of calcimimetics in the treatment of hyperparathyroidism. *Eur J Clin Invest.* 2007;37:915.
143. Felsenfeld AJ, Levine BS. Milk alkali syndrome and the dynamics of calcium homeostasis. *Clin J Am Soc Nephrol.* 2006;1:641.
144. Peppers MP, Geheb M, Desai T. Hypophosphatemia and hyperphosphatemia. *Crit Care Clin.* 1991;7:201.
145. Giovannini I, Chiarla C, Nuzzo G. Pathophysiologic and clinical correlates of hypophosphatemia and the relationship with sepsis and outcome in postoperative patients after hepatectomy. *Shock.* 2002;18:111.
146. Brooks MJ, Melnik G. The refeeding syndrome: An approach to understanding its complications and preventing its occurrence. *Pharmacotherapy.* 1995;15:713.
147. Paleologos M, Stone E, Braude S. Persistent, progressive hypophosphataemia after voluntary hyperventilation. *Clin Sci (Lond).* 2000;98:619.
148. Rosen GH, Boullata JI, O'Rangers EA, et al. Intravenous phosphate repletion regimen for critically ill patients with moderate hypophosphatemia. *Crit Care Med.* 1995;23:1204.
149. Burke SK. Phosphate is a uremic toxin. *J Ren Nutr.* 2008;18:27.
150. Sprague SM. A comparative review of the efficacy and safety of established phosphate binders: Calcium, sevelamer, and lanthanum carbonate. *Curr Med Res Opin.* 2007;23:3167.
151. Topf JM, Murray PT. Hypomagnesemia and hypermagnesemia. *Rev Endocr Metab Disord.* 2003;4:195.
152. Gums JG. Magnesium in cardiovascular and other disorders. *Am J Health Syst Pharm.* 2004;61:1569.
153. Dube L, Granry JC. The therapeutic use of magnesium in anesthesiology, intensive care and emergency medicine: A review. *Can J Anaesth.* 2003;50:732.
154. Choi JH, Lee J, Park CM. Magnesium therapy improves thromboelastographic findings before liver transplantation: A preliminary study. *Can J Anaesth.* 2005; 52:156.
155. Lysakowski C, Dumont L, Czarnetzki C, et al. Magnesium as an adjuvant to postoperative analgesia: A systematic review of randomized trials. *Anesth Analg.* 2007;104:1532.
156. Van De Water JM, van den Bergh WM, Hoff RG, et al. Hypocalcaemia may reduce the beneficial effect of magnesium treatment in aneurysmal subarachnoid haemorrhage. *Magnes Res.* 2007;20:130.
157. van den Bergh WM, Algra A, Rinkel GJ. Electrocardiographic abnormalities and serum magnesium in patients with subarachnoid hemorrhage. *Stroke.* 2004; 35:644.
158. Sueta CA, Clarke SW, Dunlap SH, et al. Effect of acute magnesium administration on the frequency of ventricular arrhythmia in patients with heart failure. *Circulation.* 1994;89:660.
159. Redwood SR, Taggart PI, Sutton PM, et al. Effect of magnesium on the monophasic action potential during early ischemia in the in vivo human heart. *J Am Coll Cardiol.* 1996;28:1765.
160. Teo KK, Yusuf S, Collins R, et al. Effects of intravenous magnesium in suspected acute myocardial infarction: Overview of randomised trials. *BMJ.* 1991;303:1499.
161. Tzivoni D, Banai S, Schuger C, et al. Treatment of torsade de pointes with magnesium sulfate. *Circulation.* 1988;77:392.
162. Wilkes NJ, Mallett SV, Peachey T, et al. Correction of ionized plasma magnesium during cardiopulmonary bypass reduces the risk of postoperative cardiac arrhythmia. *Anesth Analg.* 2002;95:828.
163. Abbott LG, Rude RK. Clinical manifestations of magnesium deficiency. *Miner Electrolyte Metab.* 1993;19:314.
164. Elisaf M, Merkouropoulos M, Tsianos EV, et al. Pathogenetic mechanisms of hypomagnesemia in alcoholic patients. *J Trace Elem Med Biol.* 1995;9:210.
165. Soliman HM, Mercan D, Lobo SS, et al. Development of ionized hypomagnesemia is associated with higher mortality rates. *Crit Care Med.* 2003;31:1082.
166. Hebert P, Mehta N, Wang J, et al. Functional magnesium deficiency in critically ill patients identified using a magnesium-loading test. *Crit Care Med.* 1997; 25:749.

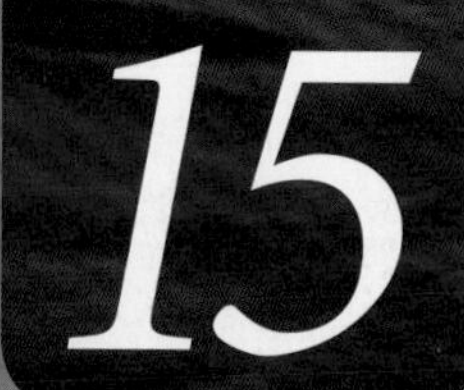

Autonomic Nervous System: Physiology and Pharmacology

LORETA GRECU

Key Points

1. The autonomic nervous system (ANS) includes that part of the central and peripheral nervous system concerned with involuntary regulation of cardiac muscle, smooth muscle, glandular and visceral functions.
2. The sympathetic and parasympathetic nervous systems (SNS, PNS) affect cardiac pump function in three ways: (1) by changing the rate (chronotropism), (2) by changing the strength of contraction (inotropism), and (3) by modulating coronary blood flow.
3. SNS nerves are by far the most important regulators of the peripheral circulation.
4. The ANS can be pharmacologically subdivided by the neurotransmitter secreted at the effector cell: Acetylcholine (ACh) released by the PNS, and the catecholamines epinephrine (EPI) and norepinephrine (NE), which are the mediators of peripheral SNS activity.
5. An agonist is a substance that interacts with a receptor to evoke a biologic response. An antagonist is a substance that interferes with the triggering of the response at a receptor site by an agonist.
6. The adrenergic receptors are termed adrenergic or noradrenergic, depending on their responsiveness to epinephrine (EPI) and norepinephrine (NE).
7. The numbers and sensitivity of adrenergic receptors can be influenced by normal, genetic, and developmental factors.
8. The autonomic nervous system reflex comprises (1) sensors, (2) afferent pathways, (3) CNS integration, and (4) efferent pathways to the receptors and efferent organs.
9. The clinical application of ANS pharmacology is based on the knowledge of ANS anatomy, physiology, and molecular pharmacology.
10. Clinically, anticholinesterase drugs may be divided into two types: the reversible and nonreversible cholinesterase inhibitors.
11. The net physiologic effect of a sympathomimetic agent is usually defined by the relative actions on the α, β, and dopaminergic receptors.
12. Dexmedetomidine is a more selective α_2 agonist than clonidine.
13. Drugs that bind selectively to α-adrenergic receptors block the action of endogenous catecholamines or moderate the effects of exogenous adrenergics.
14. Calcium channel blockers are not true pharmacologic antagonists of calcium. They interact with the cell membrane to control the intracellular concentration of calcium.

Multimedia

 Catecholamine Chemical Structures

 Renin Angiotensin

 Antimuscarinics

 Reversible Anticholinesterases

ANESTHESIA AND THE AUTONOMIC NERVOUS SYSTEM

Anesthesiology is the practice of autonomic medicine. Drugs that produce anesthesia may also have potent autonomic side effects. The greater part of our training and practice is spent acquiring skills in utilizing or averting the autonomic nervous system (ANS) side effects of anesthetic drugs under a variety of pathophysiologic conditions. The success of any anesthetic depends upon how well homeostasis is maintained. The anesthetic chart reflects ANS function.

1 The ANS includes that part of the central and peripheral nervous system concerned with involuntary regulation of cardiac muscle, smooth muscle, and glandular and visceral functions. ANS activity refers to visceral reflexes that function below the conscious level. The ANS is also responsive to changes in somatic motor and sensory activities of the body. The physiologic evidence of visceral reflexes as a result of somatic events is abundantly clear. The ANS is therefore not as distinct an entity as the term suggests. Neither somatic nor ANS activity occurs in isolation.[1] The ANS organizes visceral support for somatic behavior and adjusts body states in anticipation of emotional behavior or responses to the stress of disease. In brief, it organizes fight or flight responses.

Afferent fibers from visceral structures are the first link in the reflex arcs of the ANS, and may relay visceral pain or changes in vessel stretch. Most ANS efferent fibers are accompanied by sensory fibers that are now commonly recognized as components of the ANS. However, the afferent components of the ANS cannot be as distinctively divided as can the efferent nerves. ANS visceral sensory nerves are anatomically indistinguishable from somatic sensory nerves. The clinical importance of visceral afferent fibers is closely implicated in the management of chronic pain states.

FUNCTIONAL ANATOMY

The ANS falls into two divisions by anatomy, physiology, and pharmacology. Langley divided this nervous system into two parts in 1921. He retained the term "sympathetic" (sympathetic nervous system, SNS) introduced by Willis in 1665 for the first part, and introduced the term "parasympathetic" (parasympathetic nervous system, PNS) for the second. The term ANS was adopted as a comprehensive name for both. Table 15-1 lists the complementary

TABLE 15-1. HOMEOSTATIC BALANCE BETWEEN ADRENERGIC AND CHOLINERGIC EFFECTS

	Response	
Organ System	**Adrenergic**	**Cholinergic**
HEART		
Sinoatrial node	Tachycardia	Bradycardia
Atrioventricular node	Increased conduction	Decreased conduction
His-Purkinje	Increased automaticity and conduction velocity	Minimal
Myocardium	Increased contractility, conduction velocity, automaticity	Minimal decrease in contractility
Coronary vessels	Constriction (α_1) and dilation (β_1)	Dilation and constriction[a]
BLOOD VESSELS		
Skin and mucosa	Constriction	Dilation
Skeletal muscle	Constriction (α_1) > dilation (β_2)	Dilation
Pulmonary	Constriction	Dilation
BRONCHIAL SMOOTH MUSCLE	Relaxation	Contraction
GASTROINTESTINAL TRACT		
Gallbladder and ducts	Relaxation	Contraction
Gut motility	Decreased	Increased
Secretions	Decreased	Increased
Sphincters	Constriction	Relaxation
BLADDER		
Detrusor	Relaxes	Contracts
Trigone	Contracts	Relaxes
GLANDS		
Nasal	Vasoconstriction and reduced secretion	Stimulation of secretions
Lacrimal		
Parotid		
Submandibular		
Gastric		
Pancreatic		
SWEAT GLANDS	Diaphoresis (cholinergic)	None
APOCRINE GLANDS	Thick, odiferous secretion	None
EYE		
Pupil	Mydriasis	Miosis
Ciliary muscle	Relaxation for far vision	Contraction for near vision

[a]See "Interaction of Autonomic Nervous System Receptors."

ANATOMY AND PHYSIOLOGY

effects of SNS (adrenergic, sympathetic) and PNS (cholinergic, parasympathetic) activity of organ systems.

Central Autonomic Organization

Pure central ANS versus somatic centers are not known. Integration of ANS activity occurs at all levels of the cerebrospinal axis. Efferent ANS activity can be initiated locally and by centers located in the spinal cord, brain stem, and hypothalamus. The cerebral cortex is the highest level of ANS integration. Fainting at the sight of blood is an example of this higher level of somatic and ANS integration. ANS function has also been successfully modulated through conscious, intentional efforts demonstrating that somatic responses are always accompanied by visceral responses and vice versa.

The principal site of ANS organization is the *hypothalamus.* SNS functions are controlled by nuclei in the posterolateral hypothalamus. Stimulation of these nuclei results in a massive discharge of the sympathoadrenal system. PNS functions are governed by nuclei in the midline and some anterior nuclei of the hypothalamus. The anterior hypothalamus is involved with regulation of temperature. The supraoptic hypothalamic nuclei regulate water metabolism and are anatomically and functionally associated with the posterior lobe of the pituitary (see Interaction of Autonomic Nervous System Receptors). This hypothalamic–neurohypophyseal connection represents a central ANS mechanism that affects the kidney by means of antidiuretic hormone. Long-term blood pressure control, reactions to physical and emotional stress, sleep, and sexual reflexes are regulated through the hypothalamus.

The *medulla oblongata* and *pons* are vital centers of acute ANS organization. Together, they integrate momentary hemodynamic adjustments and maintain the sequence and automaticity of ventilation. Integration of afferent and efferent ANS impulses at this central nervous system (CNS) level is responsible for the tonic activity exhibited by the ANS. Tonicity holds visceral organs in a state of intermediate activity that can either be diminished or augmented by altering the rate of nerve firing. The nucleus tractus solitarius, located within the medulla, is the primary area for relay of afferent chemoreceptor and baroreceptor information from the glossopharyngeal and vagus nerves. Increased afferent impulses from these two nerves inhibits its peripheral SNS vascular tone, producing vasodilation; it also increases vagal tone, producing bradycardia. Studies of patients with high spinal cord lesions show that a number of reflex changes are mediated at the spinal or segmental level. ANS hyperreflexia is an example of spinal cord mediation of ANS reflexes without integration of function from higher inhibitory centers.[1]

Peripheral Autonomic Nervous System Organization

The peripheral ANS is the efferent (motor) component of the ANS and consists of the same two complementary parts: The SNS and the PNS. Most organs receive fibers from both divisions (Fig. 15-1). In general, activities of the two systems produce opposite but complementary effects (see Table 15-1). A few tissues, such as sweat glands and spleen, are innervated by only SNS fibers. Although the anatomy of the somatic and ANS sensory pathways is identical, the motor pathways are characteristically different. The efferent somatic motor system, like somatic afferents, is composed of a single (unipolar) neuron with its cell body in the ventral gray matter of the spinal cord. Its myelinated axon extends directly to the voluntary striated muscle unit. In contrast, the efferent (motor) ANS is a two-neuron (bipolar) chain from the CNS to the effector organ. The first neuron of both the SNS and PNS originates within the CNS but does not make direct contact with the effector organ. Instead, it relays the impulse to a second station known as an *ANS ganglion,* which contains the cell body of the second ANS (postganglionic) neuron. Its axon contacts the effector organ. Thus, the motor pathways of both divisions of the ANS are schematically a serial two-neuron chain consisting of a preganglionic neuron and a postganglionic effector neuron (Fig. 15-2).

Preganglionic fibers of both subdivisions are myelinated with diameters of less than 3 mm.[1] Impulses are conducted at a speed of 3 to 15 m/s. The postganglionic fibers are unmyelinated and conduct impulses at slower speeds of less than 2 m/s. They are similar to unmyelinated visceral and somatic afferent C fibers (Table 15-2). Compared with the myelinated somatic nerves, the ANS conducts impulses at speeds that preclude its participation in the immediate phase of a somatic response.

Sympathetic Nervous System

The efferent SNS is referred to as the thoracolumbar nervous system. Figure 15-1 demonstrates the distribution of the SNS and its innervation of visceral organs. The preganglionic fibers of the SNS (thoracolumbar division) originate in the intermediolateral gray column of the 12 thoracic (T1-12) and the first three lumbar segments (L1-3) of the spinal cord. The myelinated axons of these nerve cells leave the spinal cord with the motor fibers to form the white (myelinated) communicating rami (Fig. 15-3). The rami enter one of the paired 22 sympathetic ganglia at their respective segmental levels. Upon entering the paravertebral ganglia of the lateral sympathetic chain, the preganglionic fiber may follow one of three courses: (1) synapse with postganglionic fibers in

TABLE 15-2. CLASSIFICATION OF NERVE FIBERS

Description of Nerve Fibers	Group		Diameter (μm)	Conduction Velocity (m/s)
		Alpha α	20	120
		Beta β		
Myelinated somatic	A	Gamma γ		5–40 (pain fibers)
		Delta δ	3–4	5–40 (pain fibers)
		Epsilon ε	2	5
Myelinated visceral (Preganglionic autonomic)	B		<3	3–15
Unmyelinated somatic	C		<2	0.5–2 (pain fibers)

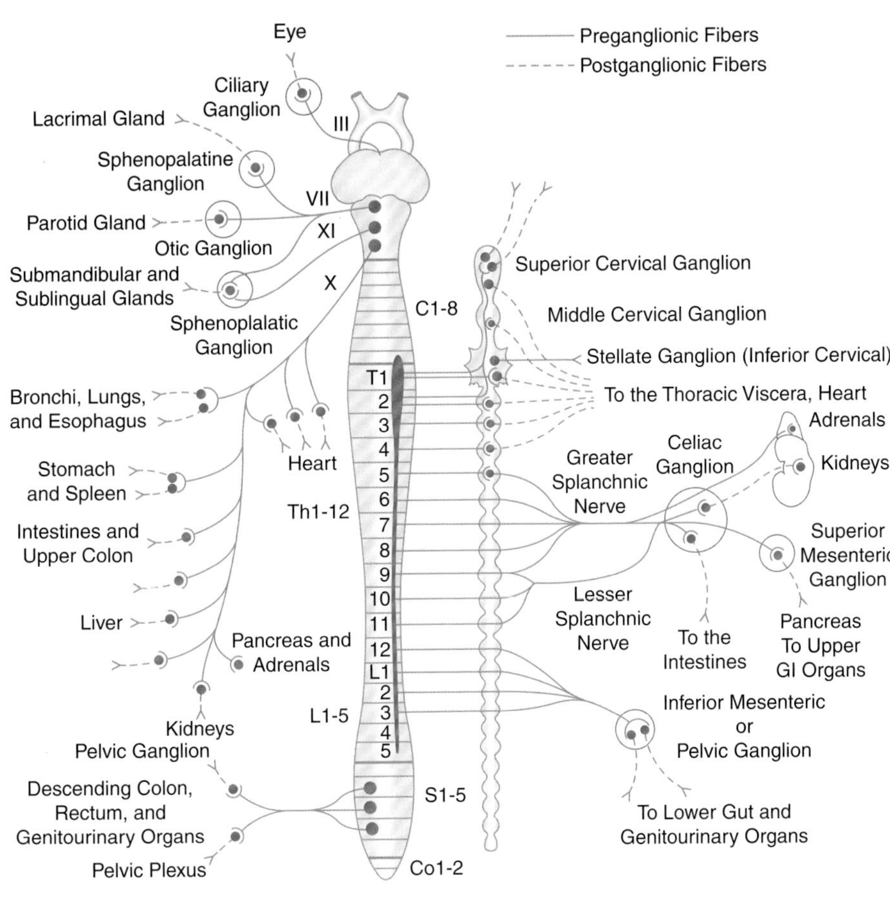

FIGURE 15-1. Schematic distribution of the craniosacral (parasympathetic) and thoracolumbar (sympathetic) nervous systems. Parasympathetic preganglionic fibers pass directly to the organ that is innervated. Their postganglionic cell bodies are situated near or within the innervated viscera. This limited distribution of parasympathetic postganglionic fibers is consistent with the discrete and limited effect of parasympathetic function. The postganglionic sympathetic neurons originate in either the paired sympathetic ganglia or one of the unpaired collateral plexuses. One preganglionic fiber influences many postganglionic neurons. Activation of the SNS produces a more diffuse physiologic response rather than a discrete, localized effect. GI, gastrointestinal.

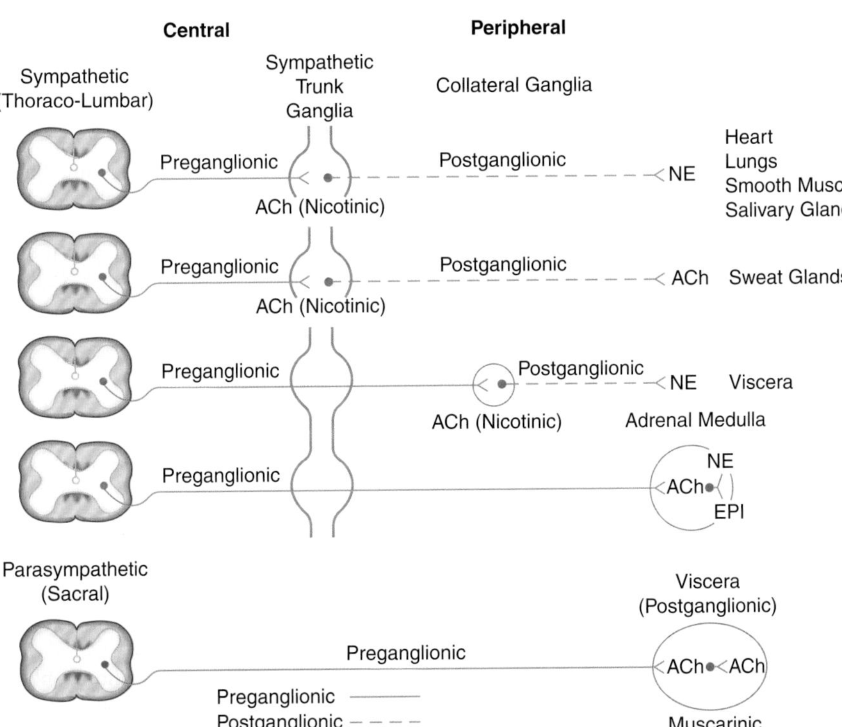

FIGURE 15-2. Schematic diagram of the efferent ANS. Efferent impulses are integrated centrally and sent reflexly to the adrenergic and cholinergic receptors. Sympathetic fibers ending in the adrenal medulla are preganglionic, and acetylcholine (ACh) is the neurotransmitter. Stimulation of the chromaffin cells, acting as postganglionic neurons, releases epinephrine (EPI) and norepinephrine (NE).

FIGURE 15-3. The spinal reflex arc of the somatic nerves is shown on the left. The different arrangements of neurons in the sympathetic system are shown on the right. Preganglionic fibers coming out through white rami may make synaptic connections following one of three courses: (1) synapse in ganglia at the level of exit, (2) course up or down the sympathetic chain to synapse at another level, or (3) exit the chain without synapsing to an outlying collateral ganglion.

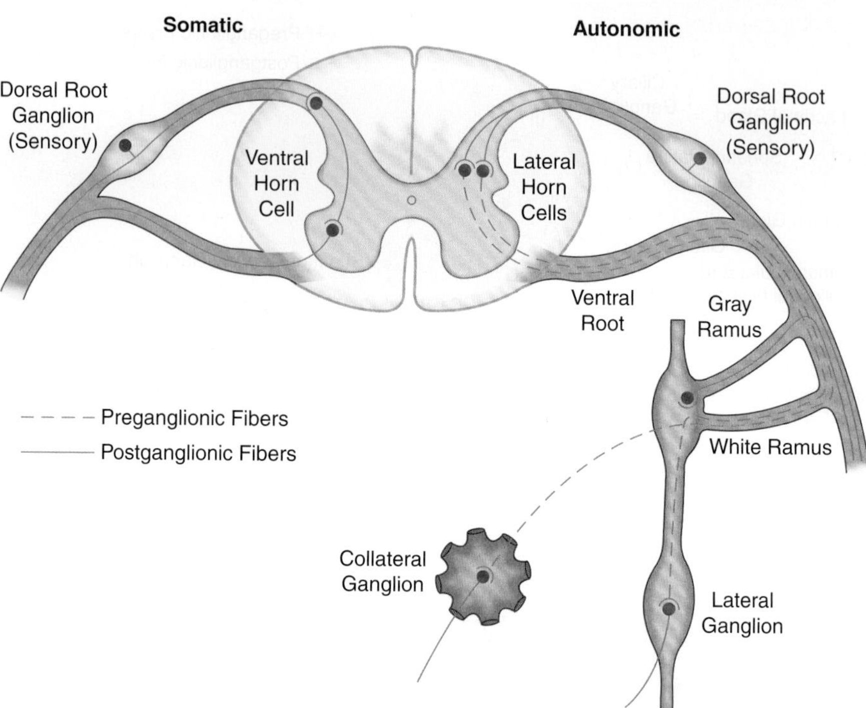

ganglia at the level of exit, (2) course upward or downward in the trunk of the SNS chain to synapse in ganglia at other levels, or (3) track for variable distances through the sympathetic chain and exit without synapsing to terminate in an outlying, unpaired, SNS collateral ganglion (Fig. 15-3). The adrenal gland is an exception to the rule. Preganglionic fibers pass directly into the adrenal medulla without synapsing in a ganglion (Fig. 15-2). The cells of the medulla are derived from neuronal tissue and are analogous to postganglionic neurons.

The sympathetic postganglionic neuronal cell bodies are located in ganglia of the paired lateral SNS chain or unpaired collateral ganglia in more peripheral plexuses. Collateral ganglia, such as the celiac and inferior mesenteric ganglia (plexus), are formed by the convergence of preganglionic fibers with many postganglionic neuronal bodies. SNS ganglia are almost always located closer to the spinal cord than to the organs they innervate. The sympathetic postganglionic neurons can therefore originate in either the paired lateral paravertebral SNS ganglia or one of the unpaired collateral plexus. The unmyelinated postganglionic fibers then proceed from the ganglia to terminate within the organs they innervate. Many of the postganglionic fibers pass from the lateral SNS chain back into the spinal nerves, forming the gray (unmyelinated) communicating rami at all levels of the spinal cord (Fig. 15-2). They are distributed distally to sweat glands, pilomotor muscle, and blood vessels of the skin and muscle. These nerves are unmyelinated C type fibers (Table 15-2) and are carried within the somatic nerves. Approximately 8% of the fibers in the average somatic nerve are sympathetic.

The first four or five thoracic spinal segments generate preganglionic fibers that ascend in the neck to form three special paired ganglia. These are the superior cervical, middle cervical, and cervicothoracic ganglia. The last is known as the stellate ganglion and is actually formed by the fusion of the inferior cervical and first thoracic SNS ganglia. These ganglia provide sympathetic innervation of the head, neck, upper extremities, heart, and lungs. Afferent pain fibers also travel with these nerves, accounting for chest, neck, or upper extremity pain with myocardial ischemia.

Activation of the SNS produces a diffuse physiologic response (mass reflex) rather than discrete effects. SNS postganglionic neurons outnumber the preganglionic neurons in an average ratio of 20:1 to 30:1.[2] One preganglionic fiber influences a larger number of postganglionic neurons, which are dispersed to many organs.

Parasympathetic Nervous System

The PNS, like the SNS, has both preganglionic and postganglionic neurons. The preganglionic cell bodies originate in the brain stem and sacral segments of the spinal cord. PNS preganglionic fibers are found in cranial nerves III (oculomotor), VII (facial), IX (glossopharyngeal), and X (vagus). The sacral outflow originates in the intermediolateral gray horns of the second, third, and fourth sacral nerves. Figure 15-1 shows the distribution of the PNS division and its innervation of visceral organs.

The vagus (cranial nerve X) nerve has the most extensive distribution of all the PNS, accounting for more than 75% of PNS activity. The paired vagus nerves supply PNS innervation to the heart, lungs, esophagus, stomach, small intestine, proximal half of the colon, liver, gallbladder, pancreas, and upper portions of the ureters. The sacral fibers form the pelvic visceral nerves, or nervi erigentes. These nerves supply the remainder of the viscera that are not innervated by the vagus. They supply the descending colon, rectum, uterus, bladder, and lower portions of the ureters and are primarily concerned with emptying. Various sexual reactions are also governed by the sacral PNS. The PNS is responsible for penile erection, but SNS stimulation governs ejaculation.

In contrast to the SNS division, PNS preganglionic fibers pass directly to the organ that is innervated. The postganglionic cell bodies are situated near or within the innervated viscera and generally are not visible. The proximity of PNS ganglia to or within the viscera provides a limited distribution of postganglionic fibers. The ratio of postganglionic to preganglionic fibers in many organs appears to be 1:1 to 3:1 compared with the 20:1 found in the SNS system. Auerbach's plexus in the distal colon is the exception, with a ratio of 8,000:1. The fact that PNS preganglionic fibers synapse with only a few postganglionic neurons is consistent with the discrete and limited effect of PNS function. For example, vagal bradycardia can occur without a concomitant change in intestinal motility or salivation. Mass reflex action is not a characteristic of the PNS. The effects of organ response to PNS stimulation are outlined in Table 15-1.

Autonomic Innervation

Heart

2 The heart is well supplied by the SNS and PNS. These nerves affect cardiac pump function in three ways: (1) by changing the rate (chronotropism), (2) by changing the strength of contraction (inotropism), and (3) by modulating coronary blood flow. The PNS cardiac vagal fibers approach the stellate ganglia and then join the efferent cardiac SNS fibers; therefore, the vagus nerve to the heart and lungs is a mixed nerve containing both PNS and SNS efferent fibers. The PNS fibers are distributed mainly to the sinoatrial and atrioventricular (AV) nodes and to a lesser extent to the atria. There is little or no distribution to the ventricles. Therefore, the main effect of vagal cardiac stimulation to the heart is chronotropic. Vagal stimulation decreases the rate of sinoatrial node discharge and decreases excitability of the AV junctional fibers, slowing impulse conduction to the ventricles. A strong vagal discharge can completely arrest sinoatrial node firing and block impulse conduction to the ventricles.[3]

The physiologic importance of the PNS on myocardial contractility is not as well understood as that of the SNS. Cholinergic blockade can double the heart rate (HR) without altering contractility of the left ventricle. Vagal stimulation of the heart can reduce left ventricular maximum rate of tension development (dP/dT) and decrease contractile force by as much as 10% to 20%. However, PNS stimulation is relatively unimportant in this regard compared with its predominant effect on HR. The SNS has the same supraventricular distribution as the PNS, but with stronger representation to the ventricles. SNS efferents to the myocardium funnel through the paired stellate ganglia. The right stellate ganglion distributes primarily to the anterior epicardial surface and the interventricular septum. Right stellate stimulation decreases systolic duration and increases HR. The left stellate ganglion supplies the posterior and lateral surfaces of both ventricles. Left stellate stimulation increases mean arterial pressure and left ventricular contractility without causing a substantial change in HR. Normal SNS tone maintains contractility approximately 20% above that in the absence of any SNS stimulation.[4] Therefore, the dominant effect of the ANS on myocardial contractility is mediated primarily through the SNS. Intrinsic mechanisms of the myocardium, however, can maintain circulation quite well without the ANS, as evidenced by the success of cardiac transplants (see Chapter 51 Transplant anesthesia). The heart and ANS are in perfect symbiosis. ANS via its components imprints the cardiac electrophysiology by potentially inducing significant dysrhythmias or electrocardiographic abnormalities, which in the end may lead to global cardiac dysfunction. The precise role of the ANS is unknown, specifically if it is an active component or just an accompaniment. Future research interests concern the modification of the autonomic cardiac innervation through pharmacology or using alternative approaches.[5] Early investigations, performed in anesthetized, open-chest animals, demonstrated that cardiac ANS nerves exert only slight effects on the coronary vascular bed; however, more recent studies on chronically instrumented, intact, conscious animals show considerable evidence for a strong SNS regulation of the small coronary resistance and larger conductance vessels[6,7] (see below Adrenergic Receptors).

Different segments of the coronary arterial tree react differently to various stimuli and drugs. Normally, the large conductance vessels contribute little to overall coronary vascular resistance (see Chapter 10 Cardiac Anatomy and Physiology). Fluctuations in resistance reflect changes in lumen size of the small, precapillary vessels. Blood flow through the resistance vessels is regulated primarily by the local metabolic requirements of the myocardium. The larger conductance vessels, however, can constrict markedly due to neurogenic stimulation. Neurogenic influence also assumes a greater role in the resistance vessels when they become hypoxic and lose autoregulation.

Peripheral Circulation

3 The SNS nerves are by far the most important regulators of the peripheral circulation. The PNS nerves play only a minor role in this regard. The PNS dilates vessels, but only in limited areas such as the genitalia. SNS stimulation produces both vasodilation and vasoconstriction, with vasoconstrictor effects predominating. The SNS effect on the vascular bed is determined by the type of receptors on which the SNS fiber terminates (see Adrenergic Receptors below). SNS constrictor receptors are distributed to all segments of the circulation. Blood vessels in the skin, kidneys, spleen, and mesentery have an extensive SNS distribution, whereas those in the heart, brain, and muscle have less SNS innervation.

Basal vasomotor tone is maintained by impulses from the lateral portion of the vasomotor center in the medulla oblongata that continually transmits impulses through the SNS, maintaining partial arteriolar and venular constriction. Circulating epinephrine (EPI) from the adrenal medulla has additive effects. This basal ANS tone maintains arteriolar constriction at an intermediate diameter. The arteriole, therefore, has the potential for either further constriction or dilation. If the basal tones were not present, the SNS could only affect vasoconstriction and not vasodilation.[8] The SNS tone in the venules produces little resistance to flow compared with the arterioles and the arteries. The importance of SNS stimulation of veins is to reduce or increase their capacity. By functioning as a reservoir for approximately 80% of the total blood volume, small changes in venous capacitance produce large changes in venous return and, thus, cardiac preload.

Lungs

The lungs are innervated by both the SNS and PNS. Postganglionic SNS fibers from the upper thoracic ganglia (stellate) pass to the lungs to innervate the smooth muscles of the bronchi and pulmonary blood vessels. PNS innervation of these structures is via the vagus nerve. SNS stimulation produces bronchodilation and pulmonary vasoconstriction.[9] Little else has been proven conclusively about the vasomotor control of the pulmonary vessels other than that they adjust to accommodate the output of the right ventricle. The effect of stimulation of the pulmonary SNS nerves on pulmonary vascular resistance is not ideal but may be important in maintaining hemodynamic stability during stress and exercise by balancing right and left ventricular output. Stimulation of the vagus nerve produces almost no vasodilation of the

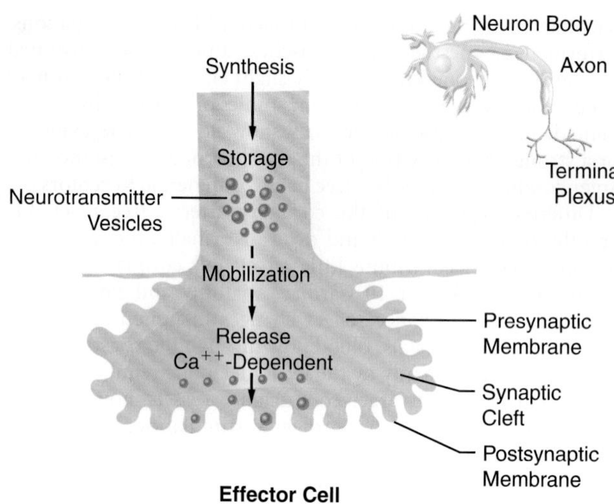

FIGURE 15-4. The anatomy and physiology of the terminal postganglionic fibers of sympathetic and parasympathetic fibers are similar.

pulmonary circulation. Hypoxic pulmonary vasoconstriction is a local phenomenon capable of providing a faster adjustment to the organism needs.

Both the SNS and the vagus nerve provide active bronchomotor control. SNS stimulation causes bronchodilation whereas vagal stimulation produces constriction. PNS stimulation may also increase secretions of the bronchial glands. Vagal receptor endings in the alveolar ducts also play an important role in the reflex regulation of the ventilation cycle. The lung has important non-ventilatory activity as well. It serves as a metabolic organ that removes local mediators such as norepinephrine (NE) from the circulation and converts others, such as angiotensin 1, to active compounds[10] (see below Interaction with Other Regulatory Systems).

Autonomic Nervous System Transmission

Transmission of excitation across the terminal junctional sites (synaptic clefts) of the peripheral ANS occurs through the mediation of released chemicals (Fig. 15-4). Transmitters interact with receptors on the end organ to evoke a biologic response.

4 The ANS can be pharmacologically subdivided by the neurotransmitter secreted at the effector cell. Pharmacologic parlance designates the SNS and PNS as adrenergic and cholinergic, respectively. The terminals of the PNS postganglionic fibers release acetylcholine (ACh). With the exception of sweat glands, NE is the principal neurotransmitter released at the terminals of the sympathetic postganglionic fibers (see Fig. 15-2). Co-transmission of adenosine triphosphate (ATP), neuropeptide Y (NPY), and NE has been demonstrated at vascular sympathetic nerve terminals in a number of different tissues including muscle, intestine, kidney, and skin (see below SNS Neurotransmission). The preganglionic neurons of both systems secrete ACh.

The terminations of the postganglionic fibers of both ANS subdivisions are anatomically and physiologically similar. The terminations are characterized by multiple branchings called terminal effector plexuses, or reticulae. These filaments surround the elements of the effector unit "like a mesh stocking".[8] Thus, one SNS postganglionic neuron, for example, can innervate ~25,000 effector cells, for example, vascular smooth muscle. The terminal filaments end in presynaptic enlargements called varicosities. Each varicosity contains vesicles, ~500 μm in diameter, in which the neurotransmitters are stored (Fig. 15-4). The rate of synthesis depends on the level of ANS activity and is regulated by local feedback. The distance between the varicosity and the effector cell (synaptic or junctional cleft) varies from 100 μm in ganglia and arterioles to as much as 20,000 μm in large arteries. The time for diffusion is directly proportional to the width of the synaptic gap. Depolarization on the nerve releases the vesicular contents into the synaptic cleft by exocytosis.

Parasympathetic Nervous System Transmission

Synthesis

ACh is considered the primary neurotransmitter of the PNS. ACh is formed in the presynaptic terminal by acetylation of choline with acetyl coenzyme A. This step is catalyzed by choline acetyl transferase (Fig. 15-5). ACh is then stored in a concentrated form in presynaptic vesicles. A continual release of small amounts of ACh, called quanta, occurs during the resting state. Each quantum results in small changes in the electrical potential of the synaptic end plate without producing depolarization. These are known as miniature end-plate potentials. Arrival of an action potential causes a synchronous release of hundreds of quanta, resulting in depolarization of the end plate. Release of ACh from the vesicles is dependent on influx of calcium (Ca^{2+}) from the interstitial space. ACh is not reused like NE; therefore, it must be synthesized constantly.

FIGURE 15-5. Synthesis and metabolism of acetylcholine.

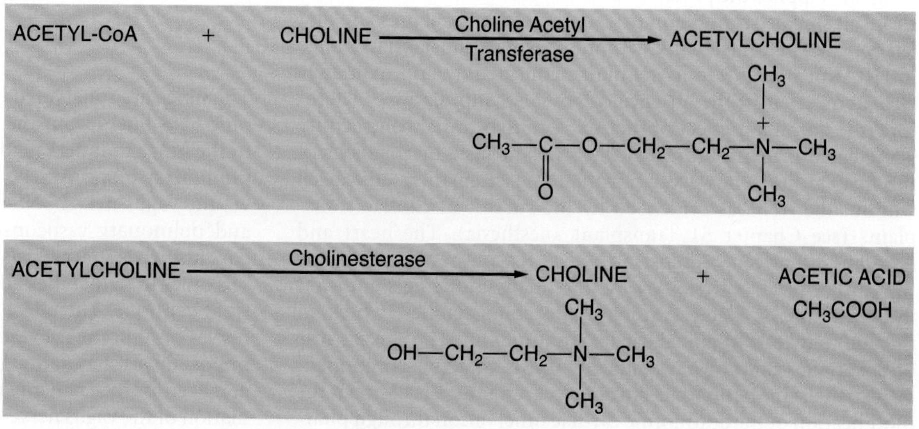

ACETYL-CoA + CHOLINE —Choline Acetyl Transferase→ ACETYLCHOLINE

$$CH_3-\underset{\underset{O}{\|}}{C}-O-CH_2-CH_2-\overset{+}{\underset{CH_3}{\overset{CH_3}{N}}}-CH_3$$

ACETYLCHOLINE —Cholinesterase→ CHOLINE + ACETIC ACID

$$OH-CH_2-CH_2-\underset{CH_3}{\overset{CH_3}{N}}-CH_3 \qquad CH_3COOH$$

Metabolism

The ability of a receptor to modulate function of an effector organ is dependent upon rapid recovery to its baseline state after stimulation. For this to occur, the neurotransmitter must be quickly removed from the vicinity of the receptor. ACh removal occurs by rapid hydrolysis by acetylcholinesterase (Fig. 15-5). This enzyme is found in neurons, at the neuromuscular junction, and in various other tissues of the body. A similar enzyme, pseudocholinesterase or plasma cholinesterase is also found throughout the body but only to a limited extent in neural tissue. It does not appear to be physiologically important in termination of the action of ACh. Both acetylcholinesterase and pseudocholinesterase hydrolyze ACh as well as other esters (such as the ester-type local anesthetics), and they may be distinguished by specific biochemical tests.[3]

Sympathetic Nervous System Transmission

Traditionally, the catecholamines EPI and NE are considered the main mediators of peripheral SNS activity. NE is released from localized presynaptic vesicles of nearly all postganglionic sympathetic nerves. Vascular SNS nerve terminals, however, also release ATP. Thus, ATP and NE are co-neurotransmitters. They are released directly to there site of action. Their postjunctional effects appear to be synergistic in tissues.

The SNS fibers ending in the adrenal medulla are preganglionic, and ACh is the neurotransmitter (see Fig. 15-2). It interacts with the chromaffin cells in the adrenal medulla, causing release of EPI and NE. The chromaffin cells take the place of the postganglionic neurons. Stimulation of the sympathetic nerves innervating the adrenal medulla, however, causes the release of large quantities of a mixture of EPI and NE into the circulation. The greater portion of this hormonal surge is normally EPI. EPI and NE, when released into the circulation, are classified as hormones in that they are synthesized, stored, and released from the adrenal medulla to act at distant sites.

Hormonal EPI and NE have essentially the same effects on effector cells as those caused by local direct sympathetic stimulation. The hormonal effects, although brief, last about 10 times as long as those caused by direct stimulation. EPI has a greater metabolic effect than NE. It can increase the metabolic rate of the body as much as 100%. It also increases glycogenolysis in the liver and muscle with glucose release into the blood. These functions are all necessary to prepare the body for fight or flight.

Catecholamines: The First Messenger

A catecholamine is any compound with a catechol nucleus (a benzene ring with two adjacent hydroxyl groups) and an amine-containing side chain. The chemical configuration of five of the more common catecholamines in clinical use is demonstrated in Figure 15-6. The endogenous catecholamines in humans are dopamine (DA), NE, and EPI. Dopamine is a neurotransmitter present in the CNS, primarily involved in coordinating motor activity in the brain. It is the precursor of NE. NE is synthesized and stored in nerve endings of postganglionic SNS neurons. It is also synthesized in the adrenal medulla and is the chemical precursor of EPI. Stored EPI is located chiefly in chromaffin cells of the adrenal medulla. About 80% to 85% of the catecholamine content of the adrenal medulla is EPI and 15% to 20% is NE. The brain contains both noradrenergic and dopaminergic receptors,

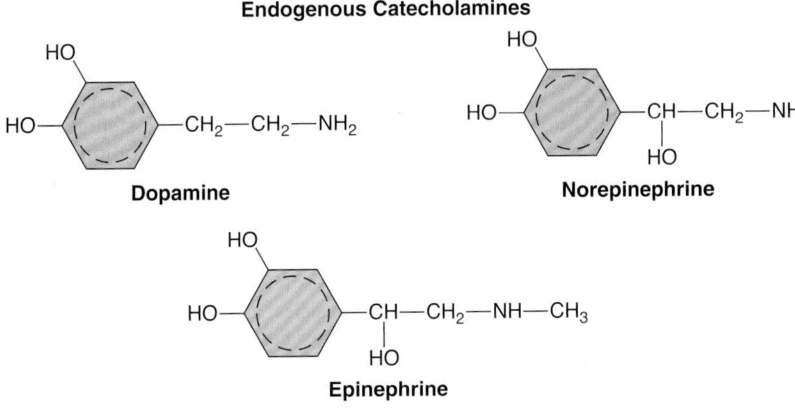

FIGURE 15-6. The chemical configurations of three endogenous catecholamines are compared with those of three synthetic catecholamines. Sympathomimetic drugs differ in their hemodynamic effects largely because of differences in substitution of the amine group on the catechol nucleus.

but circulating catecholamines do not cross the blood–brain barrier. The catecholamines present in the brain are synthesized there.

Catecholamines are often referred to as adrenergic drugs because their effector actions are mediated through receptors specific for the SNS. Sympathomimetics can activate these same receptors because of their structural similarity. For example, clonidine is an α_2-receptor agonist that does not possess a catechol nucleus and even has two ring systems that are aplanar to each other. However, clonidine enjoys a remarkable spatial similarity to NE that allows it to activate the α receptor. Drugs that produce sympathetic-like effects but lack basic catecholamine structure are defined as sympathomimetics. All clinically useful catecholamines are sympathomimetics, but not all sympathomimetics are catecholamines. The effects of endogenous or synthetic catecholamines on adrenergic receptors can be direct or indirect. Indirect-acting catecholamines (i.e., ephedrine) have little intrinsic effect on adrenergic receptors but produce their effects by stimulating release of the stored neurotransmitter from SNS nerve terminals. Some synthetic and endogenous catecholamines stimulate adrenergic receptor sites directly (e.g., phenylephirine), whereas others have a mixed mode of action. The actions of direct-acting catecholamines are independent of endogenous NE stores; however, the indirect-acting catecholamines are entirely dependent on adequate neuronal stores of endogenous NE.

Synthesis

The main site of NE synthesis is in or near the postganglionic nerve endings. Some synthesis does occur in vesicles near the cell body that pass to the nerve endings. Phenylalanine or tyrosine is taken up into the axoplasm of the nerve terminal and modified into either NE or EPI. Figure 15-7 demonstrates this synthesis cascade. Tyrosine hydroxylase catalyzes the conversion of tyrosine to dihydroxyphenylalanine. This is the rate-limiting step at which NE synthesis is controlled through feedback inhibition. Dopamine (DA) synthesis occurs in the cytoplasm of the neuron. The vesicles of peripheral postganglionic neurons contain the enzyme dopamine-b-hydroxylase, which converts dopamine to NE. The adrenal medulla additionally contains phenylethanolamine-N-methyltransferase, which converts NE to EPI. This reaction takes place outside the medullary vesicles, and the newly formed EPI then enters the vesicle for storage (Fig. 15-8). All the endogenous catecholamines are stored in presynaptic vesicles and released on arrival of an action potential. Excitation–secretion coupling in sympathetic neurons is Ca^{2+}-dependent.

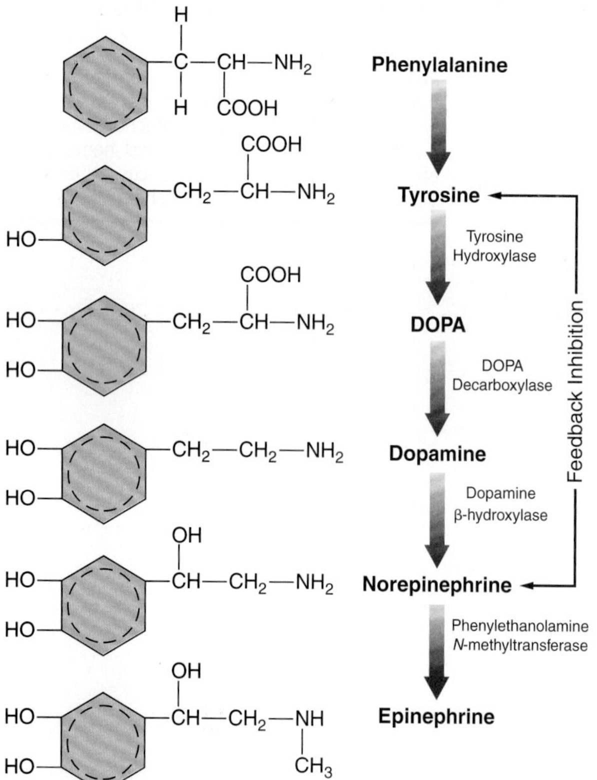

FIGURE 15-7. Schematic of the synthesis of catecholamines. The conversion of tyrosine to DOPA by tyrosine hydroxylase is inhibited by increased NE synthesis. Epinephrine is shown in these steps but is primarily synthesized in the adrenal medulla. DOPA, dihydroxyphenylalanine.

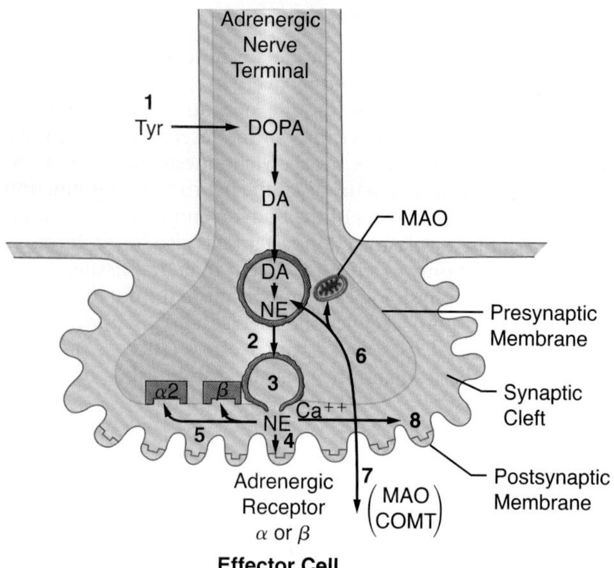

FIGURE 15-8. Schematic of the synthesis and disposition of NE in adrenergic neurotransmission. (1) Synthesis and storage in neuronal vesicles; (2) Action potential permits calcium entry with (3) exocytosis of NE into synaptic gap. (4) Released NE reacts with receptors on effector cell. NE (5) may react with presynaptic α-2 receptor to inhibit further NE release or with presynaptic β-receptor to enhance reuptake of NE (6) (uptake 1). Extraneuronal uptake (uptake 2) absorbs NE into effector cell (7) with overflow occurring systemically (8). MAO, monoamine oxidase; COMT, catechol-*O*-methyltransferase; Tyr, tyrosine; DOPA, dihydroxyphenylalanine; NE, norepinephrine.

Regulation

Increased SNS nervous activity, as in congestive heart failure or chronic stress, stimulates the synthesis of catecholamines. Glucocorticoids from the adrenal cortex stimulate an increase in phenylethanolamine-N-methyltransferase that methylates NE to EPI.

The release of NE is dependent upon depolarization of the nerve and an increase in calcium ion permeability. This release is inhibited by colchicine and prostaglandin E_2, suggesting a contractile mechanism. NE inhibits its own release by stimulating presynaptic (prejunctional) α_2 receptors. Phenoxybenzamine and phentolamine, α-receptor antagonists, increase the release of NE by blocking inhibitory presynaptic α_2 receptors (Fig. 15-9). Other receptors are also important in NE regulation (see below Other Receptors).

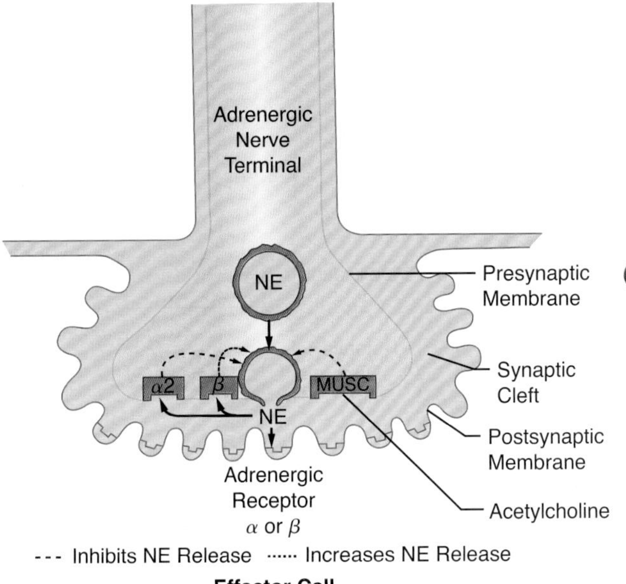

FIGURE 15-9. This schematic demonstrates just a few of the presynaptic adrenergic receptors thought to exist. Agonist and antagonist drugs are clinically available for these receptors (see Table 15-5). The α-2 receptors serve as a negative feedback mechanism whereby NE stimulation inhibits its own release. Presynaptic β-stimulation increases NE uptake, augmenting its availability. Presynaptic muscarinic (MUSC) receptors respond to ACh diffusing from nearby cholinergic terminals. They inhibit NE release and can be blocked by atropine. NE, norepinephrine.

Inactivation

The catecholamines are removed from the synaptic cleft by three mechanisms (Fig. 15-8). These are reuptake into the presynaptic terminals, extraneuronal uptake, and diffusion. Termination of NE action at the effector site is almost entirely by reuptake of NE into the terminals of the presynaptic neuron. This is an active, energy-requiring, and temperature-dependent process. The reuptake of NE in the presynaptic terminals is also a stereospecific process. Structurally similar compounds (guanethidine, metaraminol) may enter the vesicles and displace the neurotransmitter. Tricyclic antidepressants and cocaine inhibit the reuptake of NE, resulting in high synaptic NE concentrations and accentuated receptor response. In addition, evidence suggests that NE reuptake is mediated by a presynaptic β-adrenergic mechanism because β-blockade causes marked elevations of EPI and NE[11] (see Figs. 15-8 and 15-9). Extraneuronal uptake is a minor pathway for inactivating NE. Effector cells and other extraneuronal tissues take up NE. The NE that is taken up by the extraneuronal tissue is metabolized by monoamine oxidase (MAO) and by catechol-O-methyltransferase (COMT) to form vanillylmandelic acid. The minute amount of catecholamine that escapes these two mechanisms diffuses into the circulation, where it is metabolized by the liver and kidney. The same enzymes inactivate EPI. Reuptake is the predominant pathway for inactivation of the endogenous catecholamines, while metabolism by the liver and kidney is the predominant pathway for catecholamines given exogenously. This accounts for the longer duration of action of the exogenous catecholamines than that noted at the local synapse.

The final metabolic product of the catecholamines is vanillylmandelic acid. Vanillylmandelic acid constitutes the major metabolite (80% to 90%) of NE found in the urine. Less than 5% of released NE appears unchanged in the urine. The metabolic products excreted in the urine provide a gross estimate of SNS activity and can facilitate the clinical diagnosis of pheochromocytoma (see Chapter 46, Endocrine Function).

RECEPTORS

5 An agonist is a substance that interacts with a receptor to evoke a biologic response. ACh, NE, EPI, DA, and ATP are the major agonists of the ANS. An antagonist is a substance that interferes with the evocation of a response at a receptor site by an agonist. Receptors are therefore target sites that lead to a response by the effector cell when activated by an agonist. Receptors are protein macromolecules and are located in the plasma membrane. Several thousand receptors have been demonstrated in a single cell. The enormity of this network becomes apparent when one considers that ~25,000 single cells can be innervated by a single neuron.

Cholinergic Receptors

ACh is the neurotransmitter for three distinct classes of receptors. These receptors can be differentiated by their anatomic location and their affinity for various agonists and antagonists. ACh mediates the "first messenger" function of transmitting impulses within the PNS, the ganglia of the SNS, and the neuroeffector junction of striated, voluntary muscle (see Fig. 15-2). Cholinergic receptors are further subdivided into muscarinic and nicotinic receptors because muscarine and nicotine stimulate them selectively. However, both muscarinic and nicotinic receptors respond to ACh (see below Cholinergic Drugs). Muscarine activates cholinergic receptors at the postganglionic PNS junctions of cardiac and smooth muscle. Muscarinic stimulation is characterized by bradycardia, decreased inotropism, bronchoconstriction, miosis, salivation, gastrointestinal hypermotility, and increased gastric acid secretion (see Table 15-1). Muscarinic receptors can be blocked by atropine without effect on nicotinic receptors (see below Cholinergic Drugs). Muscarinic receptors are known to exist in sites other than PNS postganglionic junctions. They are found on the presynaptic membrane of sympathetic nerve terminals in the myocardium, coronary vessels, and peripheral vasculature (Fig. 15-9). These are referred to as adrenergic muscarinic receptors because of their location; however, ACh stimulates them also. Stimulation of these receptors inhibits release of NE in a manner similar to α_2-receptor stimulation. Muscarinic blockade removes the inhibition of NE release, augmenting SNS activity. Atropine, the prototypical muscarinic blocker, may produce sympathomimetic activity in this manner as well as vagal blockade. Neuromuscular blocking drugs that cause tachycardia are thought to have a similar mechanism of action. ACh acting on presynaptic adrenergic muscarinic receptors is a potent inhibitor of NE release.[11] The prejunctional muscarinic receptor may play an important physiologic role because several autonomically innervated tissues (e.g., the heart) possess ANS plexuses in which the SNS and PNS nerve terminals are closely associated. In these plexuses, ACh, released from the nearby PNS nerve terminals (vagus nerve), can inhibit NE release by activation of presynaptic adrenergic muscarinic receptors (Fig. 15-9).

Nicotinic receptors are found at the synaptic junctions of both SNS and PNS ganglia. Because both junctions are cholinergic, ACh or ACh-like substances such as nicotine will excite postganglionic fibers of both systems (see Fig. 15-2). Low doses of nicotine produce stimulation of ANS ganglia whereas high doses produce blockade. This dualism is referred to as the nicotinic effect (see below Ganglionic Drugs). Nicotinic stimulation of the SNS ganglia produces hypertension and tachycardia by causing the release of EPI and NE from the adrenal medulla. Adrenal hormone release is mediated by ACh in the chromaffin cells, which are analogous to postganglionic neurons (see Fig. 15-2). A further increase in nicotine concentration produces hypotension and neuromuscular weakness, as it becomes a ganglionic blocker. The cholinergic neuroeffector junction of skeletal muscle also contains nicotinic receptors, although they are not identical to the nicotinic receptors in ANS ganglia.

Adrenergic Receptors

6 The adrenergic receptors are termed adrenergic or noradrenergic, depending on their responsiveness to EPI or NE. The dissimilarities of these two drugs led Ahlquist in 1948 to propose two types of opposing adrenergic receptors, termed alpha (α) and beta (β). The development of new agonists and antagonists with relatively selective activity allowed subdivision the β-receptors into β_1 and β_2. α-receptors were subsequently divided into α_1 and α_2. These were later further subdivided using molecular cloning. The sympathomimetic adrenergic drugs in current use differ from one another in their effects largely because of differences in substitution on the amine group, which influences the relative α or β effect (see Fig. 15-6).

Another major peripheral adrenergic receptor specific for dopamine is termed the dopaminergic (DA) receptor. Further studies have revealed not only subsets of the α and β receptors but also the DA receptor. These DA receptors have been identified in the CNS and in renal, mesenteric, and coronary vessels. The physiologic importance of these receptors is a matter of controversy because there are no identifiable peripheral DA neurons. Dopamine measured in the circulation is assumed to result from spillover from the brain.

The function of dopamine in the CNS has long been known, but the peripheral dopamine receptor has been elucidated only within the past 25 years. The presence of the peripheral DA receptor was obscured because dopamine does not affect the DA receptor exclusively. It also stimulates α and β receptors in a dose-related manner. However, DA receptors function independently of α or β blockade and are modified by DA antagonists such as haloperidol, droperidol, and phenothiazines. Thus, there is a necessity for the addition of the DA receptor and its subsets (DA_1 and DA_2).

The distribution of adrenergic receptors in organs and tissues is not uniform and their function differs not only by their location but also in their numbers and/or distribution. Adrenergic receptors are found in two loci in the sympathetic neuroeffector junction. They are found in both the presynaptic (prejunctional) and postsynaptic (postjunctional) sites as well as extrasynaptic sites (Fig. 15-10). Table 15-3 is a review of the function and synaptic location of some of the clinically important receptors and their subtypes.

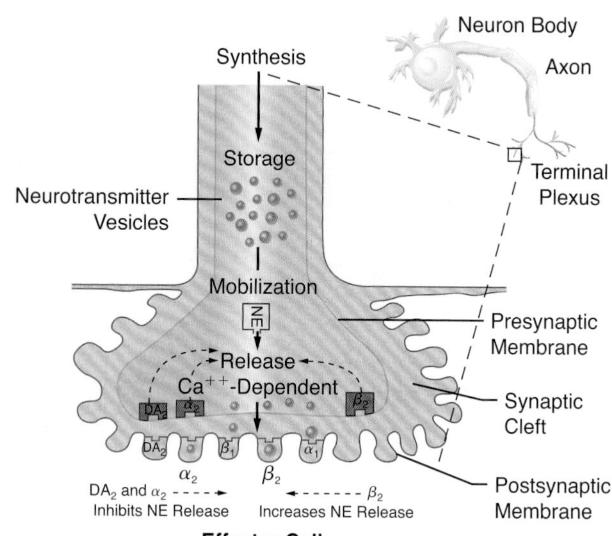

FIGURE 15-10. Location of several known adrenergic receptors. The presynaptic α-2 and DA receptors serve as a negative feedback mechanism, whereby stimulation of NE inhibits its own release. Presynaptic β-2 stimulation increases NE uptake, augmenting its availability. Postsynaptic α-2 and β-2 receptors are extrasynaptic and are considered noninnervated hormonal receptors. DA, dopamine; NE, norepinephrine.

Alpha-adrenergic Receptors

The alpha-adrenergic (α) receptors have been further subdivided into two clinically important classes, α_1 and α_2. This classification is based on their response to the α-antagonists yohimbine and prazosin. Prazosin is a more potent antagonist of α_1 receptors, whereas α_2 receptors are more sensitive to yohimbine. Recently, pharmacologic experiments have demonstrated the existence of two subtypes within the α_1 group, namely α_{1A} and α_{1B}, and at least two subtypes within the α_2 group respectively α_{2A} and α_{2B}. The importance of these subsets is still emerging, with evidence that the spleen and liver contain mainly α_{1B} receptors, and the heart, neocortex, kidney, vas deferens, and hippocampus contain equal amounts of α_{1A} and α_{1B} receptors. The α_1-adrenergic receptors are found in the smooth muscle cells of the peripheral vasculature coronary arteries, skin, uterus, intestinal mucosa, and splanchnic beds[12] (see Table 15-4). The α_1 receptors serve as postsynaptic activators of vascular and intestinal smooth muscle as well as of endocrine glands. Their activation results in either decreased or increased tone, depending upon the effector organ. The response in resistance and capacitance vessels is constriction, whereas in the intestinal tract it is relaxation. There is now a large body of evidence documenting the presence of postjunctional α_1 adrenoreceptors in the mammalian heart. α_1-adrenergic receptors have been shown to have a positive inotropic effect on cardiac tissues in most mammals studied, including humans. Experimental work strongly supports the concept that enhanced myocardial α_1 responsiveness plays a primary role in the genesis of malignant arrhythmias induced by catecholamines during myocardial ischemia and reperfusion. Drugs possessing potent α_1-antagonist activity such as prazosin and phentolamine provide significant antiarrhythmic activity. The clinical mechanism and significance of these findings are not yet clear. However, there is no doubt that α_1-adrenergic antagonists prevent catecholamine-induced ventricular arrhythmias.[13] In contrast, studies of the effects of β-antagonists in experimental and clinical myocardial infarction have provided conflicting results.

The discovery of presynaptic α-adrenoreceptors and their role in the modulation of NE transmission provided the stimulus for the subclassification of α receptors into α_1 and α_2 subtypes. Presynaptic α_1 receptors have not been identified receptors appear confined only to the postsynaptic membrane. On the other hand, α_2 receptors are found on both presynaptic and postsynaptic

TABLE 15-3. ADRENERGIC RECEPTORS: ORDER OF POTENCY OF AGONISTS AND ANTAGONISTS

Receptor		Agonists[a]	Antagonists	Location	Action
α_1	++++	Norepinephrine	Phenoxybenzamine[b]	Smooth muscle (vascular, iris, radial, ureter, pilomotor, uterus, trigone, gastrointestinal, and bladder sphincters)	Contraction Vasoconstriction
	+++	Epinephrine	Phentolamine[b]		
	++	Dopamine	Ergot alkaloids[b]		
	+	Isoproterenol	Prazosin		
			Tolazoline[b]	Brain	Neurotransmission
			Labetalol[b]	Smooth muscle (gastrointestinal)	Relaxation
				Heart	Glycogenolysis
				Salivary glands	Increased force,[c] glycolysis
				Adipose tissue	Secretion (K^+, H_2O)
				Sweat glands (localized)	Glycogenesis
				Kidney (proximal tubule)	Secretion
					Gluconeogenesis Na^+ reabsorption
α_2	++++	Clonidine	Yohimbine	Adrenergic nerve endings	Inhibition norepinephrine release
	+++	Norepinephrine	Piperoxan	Presynaptic—CNS	
	++	Epinephrine	Phentolamine[b]		
	++	Norepinephrine	Phenoxybenzamine[b]	Platelets	Aggregation, granule release
	+	Phenylephrine	Tolazoline[b]		
			Labetalol[b]	Adipose tissue	Inhibition lipolysis
				Endocrine pancreas	Inhibition insulin release
				Vascular smooth muscle—?	Contraction
				Kidney	Inhibition renin disease
				Brain	Neurotransmission
β_1	++++	Isoproterenol[b]	Acebutolol	Heart	Increased rate, contractility, conduction velocity
	+++	Epinephrine	Practolol		
	++	Norepinephrine	Propranolol[b]		Coronary vasodilation
	+	Dopamine	Alprenolol[b]	Adipose tissue	Lipolysis
			Metoprolol		
			Esmolol		
β_2	++++	Isoproterenol[a]	Propranolol[b]	Liver	Glycogenolysis, gluconeogenesis
	+++	Epinephrine	Butoxamine		
	+++	Norepinephrine	Alprenolol		
	+	Dopamine	Esmolol	Skeletal muscle	Glycogenolysis, lactate release
			Nadolol		
			Timolol	Smooth muscle (bronchi, uterus, vascular, gastrointestinal, detrusor, spleen capsule)	Relaxation
			Labetalol		
				Endocrine pancreas	Insulin secretion
				Salivary glands	Amylase secretion
DA_1	++++	Fenoldopam		Vascular smooth muscle	Vasodilation
	++	Dopamine	Haloperidol	Renal and mesentery	
	+	Epinephrine	Droperidol		
	+	Metoclopramide	Phenothiazines		
DA_2	++	Dopamine	Domperidone	Presynaptic—adrenergic nerve endings	Inhibits norepinephrine release
	+	Bromocriptine			

DA, dopamine.
[a]Listed in decreasing order of potency.
[b]Nonselective.
[c]β_1-adrenergic responses are greater.
Pluses indicate strength of potency.

TABLE 15-4. ADRENERGIC RECEPTORS

Receptor	Synaptic Site	Anatomic Site	Action	LV Function and Stroke Volume
α_1	Postsynaptic	Peripheral vascular smooth muscle	Constriction	Decreased
		Renal vascular smooth muscle	Constriction	
		Coronary arteries, epicardial	Constriction	
		Myocardium	Positive inotropism	Improved
		30–40% of resting tone		
		Renal tubules	Antidiuresis	
α_2	Presynaptic	Peripheral vascular smooth muscle release	Inhibit NE	
			Secondary vasodilation	Improved
		Coronaries		
		CNS	Inhibition of CNS activity	
			Sedation	
			Decrease MAC	
	Postsynaptic	Coronaries, endocardial	Constriction	Decreased
		CNS	Inhibition of insulin release	
			Decreased bowel motility	
			Inhibition of antidiuretic hormone	
			Analgesia	
		Renal tubule	Promotes Na^{2+} and H_2O excretion	
β_1	Postsynaptic NE sensitive	Myocardium	Positive inotropism and chronotropism	Improved
		Sinoatrial (SA) node		
		Ventricular conduction		
		Kidney	Renin release	
		Coronaries	Relaxation	
β_2	Presynaptic NE sensitive	Myocardium	Accelerates NE release	Improved
		SA node ventricular conduction vessels	Opposite action to presynaptic α_2 agonism	
			Constriction	
	Postsynaptic (extrasynaptic) (EPI sensitive)	Myocardium	Positive inotropism and chronotropism	
		Vascular smooth muscle	Relaxation	Improved
		Bronchial smooth muscle	Relaxation	Improved
		Renal vessels	Relaxation	Improved
DA_1	Postsynaptic	Blood vessels (renal, mesentery, coronary)	Vasodilation	Improved
		Renal tubules	Natriuresis	
			Diuresis	
		Juxtaglomerular cells	Renin release (modulates diuresis)	
		Sympathetic ganglia	Minor inhibition	
DA_2	Presynaptic	Postganglionic sympathetic nerves	Inhibit NE release	Improved
			Secondary vasodilation	
	Postsynaptic	Renal and mesenteric vasculature	? Vasoconstriction	

LV, left ventricular; NE, norepinephrine; MAC, EPI, epinephrine; DA, dopamine.

membranes of the adrenergic neuroeffector junction. Table 15-4 reviews these sites. Postsynaptic membranes contain a near equal mix of α_1 and α_2 receptors.

The α_2 adrenoreceptors may be subdivided even further into as many as four possible subtypes. The postsynaptic α_2 receptors have many actions, which include arterial and venous vasoconstriction, platelet aggregation, inhibition of insulin release, inhibition of bowel motility, stimulation of growth hormone release, and inhibition of antidiuretic hormone (ADH) release.

α_2 receptors can be found in cholinergic pathways as well as in adrenergic pathways. They can significantly modulate parasympathetic activity as well. Current research implies that α_2 stimulation of the parasympathetic pathways plays a role in the modulation of the baroreceptor reflex (increased sensitivity), vagal mediation of heart rate (bradycardia), bronchoconstriction, and salivation (dry mouth). However, cholinergic receptors can also be found in adrenergic pathways; thus, muscarinic and nicotinic receptors have been found in presynaptic and postsynaptic locations, where in turn they modulate sympathetic activity (see Fig. 15-9). There is speculation that the features that are so desirable to the anesthesiologist, such as sedation, anxiolysis, analgesia, and hypnosis, are mediated through this site.

Stimulation of presynaptic α_2 receptors mediates inhibition of NE release into the synaptic cleft, serving as a negative feedback mechanism. The central effects are primarily related to a reduction in sympathetic outflow with a concomitantly enhanced parasympathetic outflow (e.g., enhanced baroreceptor activity). This results in a decreased systemic vascular resistance, decreased cardiac output (CO), decreased inotropic state in the myocardium, and decreased HR. The peripheral presynaptic α_2 effects are similar, and NE release is inhibited in postganglionic neurons. However, stimulation of postsynaptic α_2 receptors, like the α_1 postsynaptic receptor, affects vasoconstriction. NE acts on both α_1 and α_2 receptors. Thus, NE not only activates smooth muscle vasoconstriction (postsynaptic α_1 and α_2 receptors) but also stimulates presynaptic α_2 receptors and inhibits its own release. Selective stimulation of the presynaptic α_2 receptor could produce a beneficial reduction of peripheral vascular resistance. Unfortunately, most known presynaptic α_2 agonists also stimulate the postsynaptic α_2 receptors, causing vasoconstriction. Blockade of α_2 presynaptic receptors, however, ablates normal inhibition of NE, causing vasoconstriction. Vasodilation occurs with the blockade of postsynaptic α_1 and α_2 receptors.

Alpha-adrenergic Receptors in the Cardiovascular System

Postsynaptic α_1 and α_2 receptors in the mammalian myocardium and coronary arteries mediate a number of responses.

CORONARY ARTERIES The presence of postsynaptic α_1 and α_2 receptors in mammalian models has been demonstrated. Sympathetic nerves cause coronary vasoconstriction, which is mediated predominately by postsynaptic α_2, more so than α_1 receptors. The larger epicardial arteries possess mainly α_1 receptors, whereas α_2 receptors and some α_1 receptors are present in the small coronary artery resistance vessels.[14] Epicardial vessels contribute only 5% to the total resistance of the coronary circulation; therefore, α_1 agonists such as phenylephrine have little influence on coronary resistance.[15,16] Myocardial ischemia has been shown to increase α_2 receptor density in the coronary arteries. Ischemia has also been shown to cause a reflex increase in sympathetic activity mediated by α mechanisms. This cascade may further increase coronary constriction. Postsynaptic α_1 receptors do not rely upon extracellular Ca^{2+} to constrict the vessel, whereas the α_2-constrictor response is highly dependent upon extracellular influx and exquisitely sensitive to calcium channel inhibitors.[17]

MYOCARDIUM The role of β receptors in mediating catecholamine-induced inotropism and arrhythmogenesis is well known (see below Beta-adrenergic Receptors). Studies have shown the presence of postsynaptic myocardial α_1 receptors, which also exert a major, facilatory, positive inotropic effect on the myocardium of several species of mammals including humans. Their contribution to malignant reperfusion arrhythmogenesis has also been recognized.

Phenylephrine, an α_1 agonist, can increase myocardial contractility two- to threefold compared with a six- to sevenfold increase produced by isoproterenol, a pure β agonist. Myocardial postsynaptic α_1 receptors mediate perhaps as much as 30% to 50% of the basal inotropic tone of the normal heart.

Postsynaptic myocardial α_1 receptors play a more prominent inotropic role in the failing heart by serving as a reserve to the normally predominant β_1 receptors. Although the response to both α_1 and β_1 agonists is reduced in the failing myocardium, the interaction between the two receptors is more apparent. Chronic heart failure is known to produce a reduced density (downregulation) of myocardial β_1 receptors as a result of high levels of circulating catecholamines. However, there is no evidence of downregulation of either α_1 or β_2 receptors in cardiac failure. The increase in density of myocardial α_1 adrenoreceptors is more pronounced with failure and myocardial ischemia.[18] Thus, enhanced myocardial α_1-receptor numbers and sensitivity may contribute to the positive inotropism seen during ischemia as well as to the malignant arrhythmias that occur with reperfusion. Intracellular mobilization of cytosolic Ca^{2+} by the activated α_1-myocardial receptors during ischemia appears to contribute to these arrhythmias. The α_1 receptor also increases the sensitivity of the contractile elements to Ca^{2+}. Drugs possessing potent α_1 antagonism such as prazosin and phentolamine have been shown to possess significant antiarrhythmic activity, but are of limited usefulness because of hypotension. Enhanced α_1 activity with myocardial ischemia may explain why the antiarrhythmic benefits of β antagonists in patients with acute myocardial infarction are far from certain. The contribution of β receptors to positive inotropism and arrhythmogenesis during ischemia and reperfusion may be overshadowed by the α receptors during acute failure and ischemia.

PERIPHERAL VESSELS Activation of the presynaptic α_2-vascular receptors produces vasodilation, whereas the postsynaptic α_1- and α_2-vascular receptors subserve vasoconstriction. Presynaptic vascular α_2 receptors inhibit NE release. This represents a negative feedback mechanism by which NE inhibits its own release via the prejunctional receptor. Presynaptic α_2 agonists, such as clonidine, inhibit NE release at the neurosympathetic junction producing vasodilatation. The effect of selective presynaptic α_2-receptor agonists to ameliorate coronary vasoconstriction in humans is unclear. Excitation of the inhibitory presynaptic α_2 receptors by endogenous or synthetic catecholamines also inhibits NE release. However, most sympathomimetics are nonselective α agonists that will excite equally presynaptic α_2 vasodilating receptors and vasoconstrictive postsynaptic α_1 and α_2 receptors. Postsynaptic α_1 and α_2 receptors coexist in both the arterial and venous sides of the circulation with the relative distribution of α_2 receptors being greater on the venous side.[12] This may explain why pure α_1 agonists, such as methoxamine, produce little venoconstriction, whereas many nonselective agonists such as phenylephrine produce significant venoconstriction. NE is the most potent venoconstrictor of all the catecholamines. Clinically, venoconstriction would have the effect of preloading by shifting venous capacitance centrally, whereas stimulation of arterial postsynaptic α_1 and α_2 receptors would affect afterloading by increasing arterial resistance.

Alpha-adrenergic Receptors in the Central Nervous System

All subtypes of the α, β, and DA receptors have been found in various regions of the brain and spinal cord. The functional role of the cerebral α and β receptors suggests a close association with blood pressure and HR control. Cerebral and spinal cord presynaptic α_2 receptors are also involved in inhibition of presynaptic NE release. Although the brain contains adrenergic and dopaminergic receptors, circulating catecholamines do not cross the blood–brain barrier. The catecholamines in the brain are synthesized there. Many actions have been attributed to the cerebral postsynaptic α_2 receptor. This includes inhibition of insulin release, inhibition of bowel motility, stimulation of growth hormone release, and inhibition of ADH release. Central neuraxial injections of α_2 agonists, such as clonidine, induce analgesia, sedation, and cardiovascular depression. The increased duration of epidural or intrathecal anesthesia by the addition of nonselective α agonists to the local anesthetic may produce additional analgesia through this mechanism.

Alpha Receptors in the Kidney

The kidney has an extensive and exclusive adrenergic innervation of the afferent and efferent glomerular arterioles, proximal and distal renal tubules, ascending loop of Henle, and juxtaglomerular apparatus. The greatest density of innervation is in the thick ascending loop of Henle, followed by the distal convoluted tubules and proximal tube. Both α_1 and α_2 subtypes are found in the kidney with the α_2 receptor dominating. The α_1 receptor is predominant in the renal vasculature and elicits vasoconstriction, which modulates renal blood flow. Tubular α_1 receptors enhance sodium and water reabsorption, leading to antinatriuresis, whereas tubular α_2 receptors promote sodium and water excretion.

Beta-adrenergic Receptors

The β-adrenergic receptors, like the α receptor, have been divided into subtypes. They are designated as the β_1 and β_2 subtypes. Recently, molecular cloning has demonstrated the existence of a third subtype, namely β_3 receptor. Activation of all these receptors subtypes induces the activation of adenylyl cyclase and increased conversion of ATP to cyclic adenosine-3′,5′-monophosphate (cAMP). β_1 receptors predominate in the myocardium, the sinoatrial node, and the ventricular conduction system. The β_1 receptors also mediate the effects of the catecholamines on the myocardium. These receptors are equally sensitive to EPI and NE, which distinguishes them from the β_2 receptors. Effects of β_1 stimulation are outlined in Table 15-4, which include their effects specifically on the cardiovascular system.

The β_2 receptors are located in the smooth muscles of the blood vessels in the skin, muscle, mesentery, and in bronchial smooth muscle. Stimulation produces vasodilation and bronchial relaxation. The β_2 receptors are more sensitive to EPI than NE. β receptors are found in both presynaptic and postsynaptic membranes of the adrenergic neuroeffector junction (Table 15-4). β_1 receptors are distributed to postsynaptic sites and have not been identified on the presynaptic membrane. Presynaptic β receptors are of the β_2 subtype. The effects of activation of the presynaptic β_2 receptor are diametrically opposed to those of the presynaptic α_2 receptor. The presynaptic β_2 receptor accelerates endogenous NE release, whereas blockade of this receptor will inhibit NE release. Antagonism of the presynaptic β_2 receptors produces a physiologic result similar to activation of the presynaptic α_2 receptor. The postsynaptic β_1 receptors are located on the synaptic membrane and respond primarily to neuronal NE. The postsynaptic β_2 receptors, like the postsynaptic α_2 receptor, respond primarily to circulating EPI.

Beta Receptors in the Cardiovascular System

MYOCARDIUM Myocardial β receptors were originally classified as β_1 receptors. Those in the vascular and bronchial smooth muscle were called the β_2 subtype. However, studies have confirmed the coexistence of β_1 and β_2 receptors in the myocardium.[19] Both β_1 and β_2 receptors are functionally coupled to adenylate cyclase, suggesting a similar involvement in the regulation of inotropism and chronotropism. Postsynaptic β_1 receptors are distributed predominantly to the myocardium, the sinoatrial node, and the ventricular conduction system. The β_2 receptors have the same distribution but are presynaptic. Activation of the presynaptic β_2 receptor accelerates the release of NE into the synaptic cleft. The β_2 receptor comprises 20% to 30% of the β receptors in the ventricular myocardium and up to 40% of the β receptors in the atrium.

The effect of NE on inotropism in the normal heart is mediated entirely through the postsynaptic β_1 receptor, whereas the inotropic effects of EPI are mediated through both the β_1- and β_2-myocardial receptors. The β_2 receptors may also mediate the chronotropic responses to EPI which explains why selective β_1 antagonists are less effective in suppressing induced tachycardia than the nonselective β_1 antagonist propranolol.

Peripheral Vessels

The postsynaptic vascular β receptors are virtually all of the β_2 subtype. The β_2 receptors are located in the smooth muscle of the blood vessels of the skin, muscle, mesentery, and bronchi. Stimulation of the postsynaptic β_2 receptor produces vasodilation and bronchial relaxation. Modest vasoconstriction occurs when subjected to blockade because the actions of the vascular postsynaptic β_2 receptors no longer oppose the actions of the α_1- and α_2-postsynaptic receptors.

Beta Receptors in the Kidney

The kidney contains both β_1 and β_2 receptors with the β_1 being predominant. Renin release from the juxtaglomerular apparatus is enhanced by β stimulation. The β_1 receptor evokes renin release in humans. Renal β_2 receptors also appear to regulate renal blood flow at the vascular level. They have been identified pharmacologically and mediate a vasodilatory response.

Dopaminergic Receptors

Dopamine, synthesized in 1910, was recognized in 1959 not only as a vasopressor and the precursor of NE and EPI, but also as an important central and peripheral neurotransmitter. Dopamine receptors (DA) are localized in the CNS, on blood vessels, and postganglionic sympathetic nerves (Table 15-4). Two clinically important types of DA receptors have been recognized: DA_1 and DA_2, while other subtypes such as DA_4 and DA_5 are still being investigated. The DA_1 receptors are postsynaptic, whereas the DA_2 receptors are both presynaptic and postsynaptic. The presynaptic DA_2 receptors, like the presynaptic α_2 receptor, inhibit NE release and can produce vasodilatation. The postsynaptic DA_2 receptor may subserve vasoconstriction similar to that of the postsynaptic α_2 receptor. This effect is opposite to that of the postsynaptic DA_1 renal vascular receptor. The zona glomerulosa of the adrenal cortex also contains DA_2 receptors, which inhibit the release of aldosterone.

Myocardium

Defining specific dopaminergic receptors has been difficult because dopamine also exerts effects on the α and β receptors. DA receptors have not been described in the myocardium. Effects of dopamine are those related to activation of β_1 receptors, which promote positive inotropism and chronotropism. β_2 activation may produce some systemic vasodilatation.

Peripheral Vessels

The greatest numbers of DA_1-postsynaptic receptors are found on vascular smooth muscle cells of the kidney and mesentery, but are also found in the other systemic arteries including coronary, cerebral, and cutaneous arteries. The vascular receptors are, like the β_2 receptors, linked to adenylate cyclase and mediate smooth muscle relaxation. Activation of these receptors produces vasodilatation, increasing blood flow to these organs. Concurrent activation of vascular presynaptic DA_2 receptors also inhibits NE release at presynaptic α_2 receptors, which may also contribute to peripheral vasodilatation. Higher doses of dopamine can mediate vasoconstriction via the postsynaptic α_1 and α_2 receptors. The constrictive effect is relatively weak in the cardiovascular system where the action of dopamine on adrenergic receptors is 1/35 and 1/50 as potent as that of EPI and NE, respectively.[20]

Central Nervous System

DA receptors have been identified in the hypothalamus where they are involved in prolactin release. They are also found in the basal ganglia where they coordinate motor function. Degeneration of dopaminergic neurons in the substantia nigra is the cause of Parkinson's disease. Another central action of dopamine is to stimulate the chemoreceptor trigger zone of the medulla, producing nausea and vomiting. Dopamine antagonists such as haloperidol and droperidol are clinically effective in countering this action.

Kidney and Mesentery

Apart from their effect on the vessels of the kidney and mesentery, DA receptors on the smooth muscle of the esophagus, stomach, and small intestine enhance secretion production and reduce intestinal motility.[20,21] Metoclopramide, a dopamine antagonist, is useful for aspiration prophylaxis by promoting gastric emptying. The distribution of DA receptors in the renal vasculature is well known, but DA receptors have other functions within the kidney. DA_1 receptors are located on renal tubules, which inhibit sodium reabsorption with subsequent natriuresis and diuresis. The natriuresis may be the result of a combined renal vasodilatation, improved CO, and tubular action of the DA_1 receptors. Juxtaglomerular cells also contain DA_1 receptors, which increase renin release when activated. This action modulates the diuresis produced by DA_1 activation of the tubules.

Dopamine has unique autonomic effects by activating specific peripheral dopaminergic receptors, which promote natriuresis and reduce afterload via dilatation of the renal and mesenteric arterial beds. Peripheral dopaminergic activity serves as a natural antihypertensive mechanism. Its actions are overshadowed by the opposite effect of its main biologic partner, NE. Plasma NE levels are known to increase with aging, likely the result of reduced clearance, while peripheral dopaminergic activity is known to diminish. Subtle changes in the DA–NE balance with aging may account for the diminished ability of the aged kidney to excrete a salt load.

Other Receptors

Adenosine Receptors

Adenosine produces inhibition of NE release. The effect of adenosine is blocked by caffeine and other methylxanthines. The physiologic function of these receptors may be the reduction of sympathetic tone under hypoxic conditions when adenosine production is enhanced. As a consequence of reduced NE release, cardiac work would be decreased and oxygen demand reduced. Adenosine has been effectively used to produce controlled hypotension.[22]

Serotonin

Serotonin (5-hydroxytryptamine) depresses the response of isolated blood vessels to SNS stimulation and decreases release of labeled NE in these preparations. Raising the external calcium ion concentration antagonizes this inhibitory action of serotonin. Thus, serotonin may inhibit neuronal NE release by a mechanism that limits the availability of calcium ions at the nerve terminal.

Prostaglandin E2, Histamine, and Opioids

Prostaglandin E2, histamine, and several opioids have been reported to act on prejunctional receptor sites to inhibit NE release in certain sympathetically innervated tissue. However, these inhibitory receptors are unlikely to play a physiologic role in limiting NE release since their direct antagonists, compounds such as inhibitors of cyclooxygenase, histamine antagonists, and naloxone do not increase a NE release.

Histamine acts in a manner similar to the neurotransmitters of the SNS. The cell membrane has specific receptors for histamine, with the individual response being determined by the type of cell being stimulated (see Chapter 12 The Allergic Response). Two receptors for histamine have been determined. These have been designated H_1 and H_2, for which it has been possible to develop specific agonists and antagonists. Stimulation of the H_1 receptors produces bronchoconstriction and intestinal contraction. The major role of the H_2 receptors is related to acid production by the parietal cells of the stomach; however, histamine is also present in relatively high concentrations in the myocardium and cardiac conducting tissue, where it exerts positive inotropic and chronotropic effects while depressing dromotropism. The positive inotropic and chronotropic effects of histamine are H_2 receptor effects that are not blocked by β antagonism. These effects are blocked by H_2 antagonists, such as cimetidine, which accounts for the occasional report of cardiovascular collapse following the use of cimetidine. The negative dromotropic effect and that of coronary spasm caused by histamine are H_1 receptor effects.

Adrenergic Receptor Numbers and Sensitivity

Receptors, once thought to be static entities, are now thought to be dynamically regulated by a variety of conditions and to be in a constant state of flux. Receptors are synthesized in the sarcoplasmic reticulum (SR) of the parent cell, where they may remain extrasynaptic or externalize to the synaptic membranes where they may cluster. Membrane receptors may be removed or internalized to intracellular sites for either dehydration or recycling.

7 The numbers and sensitivity of adrenergic receptors can be influenced by normal, genetic, and developmental factors. Changes in the number of receptors alter the response to catecholamines. Alteration in the number, or density of receptors is referred to as either upregulation or downregulation. As a rule, the number of receptors is inversely proportional to the ambient concentration of the catecholamines. Extended exposure of receptors to their agonists markedly reduces, but does not ablate, the biologic response to catecholamines. For example, increased adrenergic activity occurs in response to reduced perfusion as a result of acute or chronic myocardial dysfunction. Plasma catecholamines are increased. Subsequently, the myocardial postsynaptic β_1 receptors are "downregulated" (see Chapter 7 Basic

Principles of Clinical Pharmacology). This is thought to explain the diminished inotropic and chronotropic response to β_1 agonists and exercise in patients with chronic heart failure. However, calcium-induced inotropism is not impaired because extrasynaptic β_2-receptor numbers remain relatively intact. The β_2 receptors may account for up to 40% of the inotropism of the failing heart compared with 20% in the normal heart.[18,23] Tachyphylaxis to infused catecholamines is also thought to be the result of acute "downregulation" of receptors. There appears to be a reduction in numbers or sensitivity of β receptors in hypertensive patients who also have elevated plasma catecholamines. Downregulation is the presumptive explanation for the lack of correlation between plasma catecholamine levels and the blood pressure elevation in patients with pheochromocytoma. Chronic use of β agonists such as terbutaline, isoproterenol, or EPI for the treatment of asthma can result in tachyphylaxis because of downregulation. Even short-term use (1 to 6 hours) of β agonists may cause downregulation of receptor numbers. Downregulation is reversible on termination of the agonist. Chronic treatment of animals with nonselective β blockade causes a 100% increase in the number of β receptors. This accounts for the propranolol withdrawal syndrome in which the acute discontinuation of the β antagonist leaves the α receptors unopposed, in addition to an increased number of β receptors. Clonidine withdrawal can be explained by the same mechanism. Up- or downregulation of receptor numbers may not alter sensitivity of the receptor. Likewise, sensitivity may be increased or decreased in the presence of normal numbers of receptors. The pharmacologic factors affecting up- or downregulation of the α and β receptors are similar.

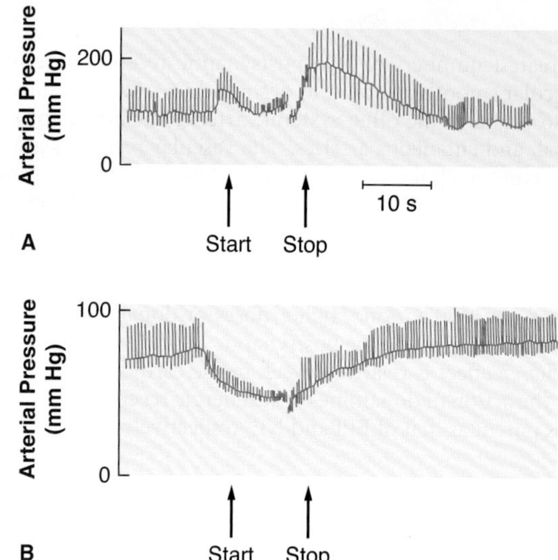

FIGURE 15-11. A: The normal blood pressure response to the Valsalva maneuver is demonstrated. Pulse rate moves in a reciprocal direction according to Marey's law of the heart. **B:** An abnormal Valsalva response is shown in a patient with C5 quadriplegia.

AUTONOMIC NERVOUS SYSTEM REFLEXES AND INTERACTIONS

8 The ANS reflex has been compared to a computer circuit. This control system, as in all reflex systems, has (1) sensors, (2) afferent pathways, (3) CNS integration, and (4) efferent pathways to the receptors and efferent organs. Fine adjustments are made at the local level through positive and negative feedback mechanisms. The baroreceptor is an example. The variable to be controlled (blood pressure) is sensed (carotid sinus), integrated (medullary vasomotor center), and adjusted through specific effector–receptor sites. Drugs or disease can interrupt this circuit at any point. β blockers may attenuate the effector response, whereas an α agonist such as clonidine may alter both the effector and the integrator functions of blood pressure control.

Baroreceptors

Several reflexes in the cardiovascular system help govern arterial blood pressure control cardiac output (CO), and heart rate (HR). The aim of the circulation is to provide blood flow to all the body organs (see Chapter 10 Cardiac Anatomy and Physiology). Yet, the most important controlled variable to which the sensors are attuned is blood pressure, a product of the blood flow and vascular resistance. Étienne Marey noted in 1859 that the pulse rate is inversely proportional to the blood pressure, and this is known as Marey's law. Subsequently, Hering, Koch, and others demonstrated that the alterations in HR evoked by changes in blood pressure are dependent on baroreceptors located in the aortic arch and the carotid sinuses. These pressure sensors react to alterations in stretch caused by blood pressure. Impulses from the carotid sinus and aortic arch reach the medullary vasomotor center by the glossopharyngeal and vagus nerves, respectively. Increased sensory traffic from the baroreceptors, caused by increased blood pressure, inhibits SNS effector traffic. The relative increase in vagal tone produces vasodilation, slowing of the HR, and a lowering of blood pressure. Real increases in vagal tone occur when blood pressure exceeds normal limits. The Valsalva maneuver can best demonstrate the arterial baroreceptor reflex (Fig. 15-11). The Valsalva maneuver raises the intrathoracic pressure by forced expiration against a closed glottis. The arterial blood pressure rises momentarily as the intrathoracic blood is forced into the heart (increased preload). Sustained intrathoracic pressure diminishes venous return, reduces the CO, and drops the blood pressure. Reflex vasoconstriction and tachycardia ensue. Blood pressure returns to normal with release of the forced expiration, but then briefly "overshoots" because of the vasoconstriction and increased venous return. A slowing of the HR accompanies the overshoot in pressure. The cardiovascular responses to the Valsalva maneuver require an intact ANS circuit from peripheral sensor to peripheral adrenergic receptors. The Valsalva maneuver has been used to identify patients at risk for anesthesia due to ANS instability (Fig. 15-11). This was once a major concern in patients receiving drugs that depleted catecholamines, such as reserpine. Dysfunction of the SNS is implicated if exaggerated and prolonged hypotension develops during the forced expiration phase (50% from resting mean arterial pressure). In addition, the overshoot at the end of the Valsalva maneuver is absent. Dysfunction of the PNS can be assumed if the HR does not respond appropriately to the blood pressure changes.

Venous baroreceptors may be more dominant in the moment-to-moment regulation of CO. Baroreceptors in the right atrium and great veins produce an increase in HR when stretched by increased right atrial pressure. Reduced venous pressure decreases HR. Unlike the arterial baroreceptors, venous sensors are not thought to alter vascular tone; however, venoconstriction is postulated to occur when atrial pressures decline. Stretch of the venous receptors produces changes in HR opposite to those produced when the arterial pressure sensors are stimulated. The arterial and venous pressure receptors are separately monitoring two of the four major determinants of CO: Afterload and preload, respectively. Venous baroreceptors sample preload by stretch of the atrium. Arterial baroreceptors survey resistance, or afterload, as reflected in the mean arterial pressure. Afterload and preload produce opposite effects on CO; thus, one should not be surprised that the venous and arterial baroreceptors produce opposing effects after a similar stretch stimulus, pressure.

Bainbridge described the venous baroreceptor reflex and demonstrated that it can be abolished by vagal resection. Numerous investigators have confirmed the acceleration of the HR in response to volume. However, the magnitude and direction of the HR response are dependent on the prevailing HR at the time of stimulation. The denervated, transplanted mammalian heart also accelerates in response to volume loading. HR, like CO, can apparently be adjusted to the quantity of blood entering the heart. The Bainbridge reflex relates to the characteristic but paradoxical slowing of the heart seen with spinal anesthesia. Blockade of the SNS levels of T1–4 ablates the efferent limb of the cardiac accelerator nerves. This source of cardiac deceleration is obvious, as the vagus nerve is unopposed. However, bradycardia during spinal anesthesia is more related to the development of arterial hypotension than to the height of the block. The primary defect in the development of spinal hypotension is a decrease in venous return. Theoretically, the arterial hypotension should reflexly produce a tachycardia through the arterial baroreceptors. Instead, bradycardia is more common. Greene suggests that in the unmedicated person, the venous baroreceptors are dominant over the arterial. A reduced venous pressure, therefore, slows HR.[24] In contrast, humorally mediated tachycardia is the usual response to hypotension or acidosis from other causes. In patients with difficult to control blood pressure, decreasing the sympathetic outflow seems to be beneficial in better regulating the blood pressure. Therefore, surgical interuption of renal efferent sympathetic outflow with radiofrequency ablation through femoral artery catheterization increases natriuresis and diuresis, and reduces renin production. Also, baroreflex sensitization through an implantable carotid sinus stimulator seems to be extremely promising in patients with refractory hypertension, with more research underway.[25]

Denervated Heart

Reflex modulation of the adrenergic agonists is best seen in the denervated transplant heart, which retains the recipient's innervated sinoatrial node and the donor's denervated sinoatrial node[26] (see Chapter 51 Transplant Anesthesia). NE infusion in the transplanted heart produces a slowing of the recipient's atrial rate through vagal feedback as the blood pressure rises. In the unmodulated donor heart, atrial rate increases. The baroreceptors are therefore not operant in the transplanted heart. Isoproterenol, a pure β agonist, increases the discharge rate of both the recipient and donor node by direct action, with the donor rate near doubling that of the recipient node. Atropine accelerates the recipient's atrial rate, whereas no effect is seen on the donor rate, which now controls HR.

β blockade produces comparable slowing of the sinoatrial node of both recipient and donor. The exercise capability of the denervated heart is conspicuously reduced by β blockade, presumably because of its reliance on circulating catecholamines. Propranolol has also been demonstrated to reduce the β response to chronotropic effects of NE and isoproterenol in the transplanted heart. The CO of the transplanted heart varies appropriately with changes in preload and afterload.

Interaction of Autonomic Nervous System Receptors

Strong interactions have been noted between SNS and PNS nerves in organs that receive dual, antagonistic innervation. Release of NE at the presynaptic terminal is modified by the PNS. For example, vagal inhibition of left ventricular contractility is accentuated as the level of SNS activity is raised. This interaction is termed accentuated antagonism and is mediated by a combination of presynaptic and postsynaptic mechanisms. The coronary arteries present an example of this phenomenon and deserve special attention.

The myocardium and coronary vessels are abundantly supplied with adrenergic and cholinergic fibers. Strong activity of both α and β receptors has been demonstrated in the coronary vascular bed. Selective stimulation of both the α_1 and postsynaptic α_2 receptors increases coronary vascular resistance, whereas selective α blockade eliminates this effect. Therefore, both β_1 and α_1 adrenoreceptors are present on coronary arteries and accessible to NE released by sympathetic nerves.[6,15]

The presynaptic adrenergic terminals of the myocardium and coronary vessels, like all blood vessels studied, contain muscarinic receptors.[11] Recent observations confirm that muscarinic agents and vagal stimulation, acting on the presynaptic, SNS muscarinic receptor, inhibit the release of NE in a manner similar to that of the presynaptic α_2 and DA_2 receptors (Fig. 15-9). Conversely, blockade of the muscarinic receptors with atropine markedly augments the positive inotropic responses to catecholamines.[6] Suppression of NE release explains, in part, vagal-induced attenuation of the inotropic response to strong SNS stimulation (accentuated antagonism) and only a weak negative inotropic effect of vagal stimulation when there is low background SNS activity. This may also explain why vagal activity reduces the vulnerability of the myocardium to fibrillation during infusions of NE.

ACh may cause coronary spasm during periods of high SNS tone.[6] Inhibition of NE release by presynaptic adrenergic muscarinic receptors of the smooth muscle of coronary vessels would lessen the coronary relaxation normally produced by NE on the β_1 receptor (Fig. 15-9). In anesthetized dogs, the rate of NE outflow into the coronary sinus blood, evoked by cardiac SNS stimulation, is markedly diminished by simultaneous vagal efferent stimulation.[27] This action is known to be prevented by atropine, which also causes coronary vasodilation.

Interaction with Other Regulatory Systems

The ANS is integrally related to several endocrine systems that ultimately summate to control blood pressure and regulate homeostasis. These include the renin–angiotensin system, ADH, glucocorticoids, and insulin (see Chapter 46 Endocrine Function). Both α and β receptors have been found in the endocrine pancreas and modulate insulin release (see Table 15-4). β stimulation increases insulin release, whereas α stimulation decreases it. The overall importance of this interaction is not entirely clear, but decreased tolerance to glucose and potassium has been noted in subjects taking β-blocking drugs. The renin–angiotensin system is a complex endocrine system that modulates both blood pressure and water–electrolyte homeostasis (Fig. 15-12). Renin is a proteolytic enzyme released by the cells of the juxtaglomerular apparatus of the renal cortex. Renin acts on plasma angiotensinogen to form angiotensin I. Angiotensin I is then converted to angiotensin II by a converting enzyme in the lung. Angiotensin II is a powerful direct arterial vasoconstrictor. It also acts

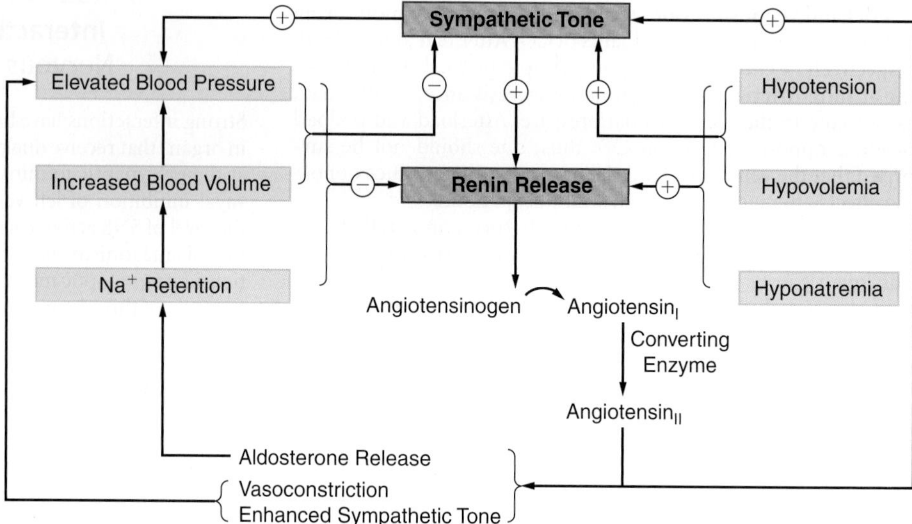

FIGURE 15-12. The interactions of the renin–angiotensin and SNS in regulating homeostasis are shown schematically along with the physiologic variables that modulate their function. Arrows with a plus sign (+) represent stimulation, and those with a minus sign (–) represent inhibition.

on the adrenal cortex to release aldosterone and on the adrenal medulla to release EPI. In addition to its direct effects on vascular smooth muscle, angiotensin II augments NE release via presynaptic receptors, thus enhancing peripheral SNS tone. Captopril, enalapril, and lisinopril inhibit the action of converting enzyme, thus preventing the conversion of angiotensin I to angiotensin II. Renin is released in response to hyponatremia, decreased renal perfusion pressure, and ANS stimulation via β receptors on juxtaglomerular cells. Changes in sympathetic tone may thus alter renin release and affect homeostasis in a variety of ways. The ANS is also intimately related to adrenocortical function. As outlined above, glucocorticoid release modulates phenylethanolamine-N-methyltransferase formation and thus synthesis of EPI. Glucocorticoids are also important in regulating the response of peripheral tissues to changes in SNS tone. Thus, the ANS is intimately related to other homeostatic mechanisms.

CLINICAL AUTONOMIC NERVOUS SYSTEM PHARMACOLOGY

9 The clinical application of ANS pharmacology is based on the knowledge of ANS anatomy, physiology, and molecular pharmacology. Drugs that modify ANS activity can be classified by their site of action, mechanism of action, or the pathology for which they are most commonly used. Antihypertensive drugs are an example of the third category. This classification is a matter of degree because considerable functional overlap occurs. An example of classification by site relates to the ganglionic agonists or blocking agents. ANS drugs can be further categorized as those that act at the prejunctional membrane and those acting postjunctionally. They can then be more specifically classified by the predominant receptor or receptors on which they act.

Mode of Action

ANS drugs may be broadly classified by mode of action according to their mimetic or lytic actions. This may also be termed agonist or antagonist. A sympathomimetic, such as ephedrine, mimics SNS sympathetic activity by stimulation of adrenergic receptor sites both directly and indirectly. Sympatholytic drugs cause dissolution of SNS activity at these same receptor sites. β receptor blockers are examples of sympatholytic drugs. Several modes of ANS drug action become evident when one follows the cascade of neurotransmission. Drugs that act on prejunctional membranes may therefore (1) interfere with transmitter synthesis (α-methyl paratyrosine), (2) interfere with transmitter storage (reserpine), (3) interfere with transmitter release (clonidine), (4) stimulate transmitter release (ephedrine), or (5) interfere with reuptake of transmitter (cocaine). Drugs may also (6) modify metabolism of the neurotransmitter in the synaptic cleft (anticholinesterase). Drugs acting at postjunctional sites may (7) directly stimulate postjunctional receptors and (8) interfere with transmitter agonist at the postjunctional receptor.

The ultimate response of an effector organ to an agonist or antagonist depends on (1) the drug, (2) its plasma concentration, (3) the number of receptors in the effector organ, (4) binding by the receptor, (5) the concurrent activities of other drugs and hormones, (6) the cellular metabolic status, and (7) reflex adjustments by the organism.

Ganglionic Drugs

SNS and PNS ganglia are pharmacologically similar in that the transmission through these ANS ganglia is effected by ACh (see Fig. 15-2). Most ganglionic agonists and antagonists are not selective and affect SNS and PNS ganglia equally. This nonselective property creates many undesirable and unpredictable side effects, which have limited the clinical usefulness of this category of drug.

Agonists

There are essentially no clinically useful ganglionic agonists. Nicotine is the prototypical ganglionic agonist. In low doses, it stimulates ANS ganglia and the neuromuscular junction of striated muscle. High doses produce ganglionic and neuromuscular blockade. The protean side effects of nicotinic stimulation render it useful only as an investigative tool.

Antagonists

Drugs that interfere with neurotransmission at ANS ganglia are known as ganglionic blocking agents. Nicotine, in high doses, is the prototypical ganglionic blocking agent also; however, early stimulatory nicotinic activity can be blocked both at the ganglia and at the muscle end plates with other ganglionic blockers and muscle relaxants, respectively, without blocking muscarinic effects. Ganglionic blockers produce their nicotinic effects by competing, mimicking, or interfering with ACh metabolism. Hexamethonium, trimethaphan, and pentolinium produce a selective nondepolarizing blockade of neurotransmission at ANS ganglia without producing nicotinic neuromuscular blockade. They compete with ACh in the ganglia without stimulating the receptors. The introduction of drugs that produce vasodilation directly or by action on the SNS vasomotor center has made the ganglionic blockers obsolete. d-tubocurare (dTC) produces a competitive nondepolarizing block of both motor end plates and ANS ganglia. The action of motor paralysis predominates, but the concomitant ganglionic blockade at higher doses explains part of the hypotensive effect often seen with the use of dTC for muscle relaxation. Anticholinesterase drugs may produce nicotinic type ganglionic blockade by competition with ACh as well as by persistent depolarization via accumulated ACh.

Trimethaphan produces blockade by competition with ACh for receptors, thus stabilizing the postsynaptic membrane. However, side effects and rapid onset tachyphylaxis have markedly reduced its use in anesthesia.[28] The patient's pupils become fixed and dilated during administration, which obscures eye signs, an important consideration for neurosurgery. In this regard, it is distinctly inferior to nitroprusside. The major advantage of trimethaphan is its short duration of action, which is the result of pseudocholinesterase hydrolysis.

Cholinergic Drugs

Muscarinic Agonists

The cholinomimetic muscarinic drugs act at sites in the body where ACh is the neurotransmitter of the nerve impulse. These drugs may be divided into three groups, the first two of which are direct muscarinic agonists. The third group acts indirectly. These groups are choline esters (ACh, methacholine, carbamylcholine, bethanechol), alkaloids (pilocarpine, muscarine), and anticholinesterases (physostigmine, neostigmine, pyridostigmine, edrophonium, echothiophate).

Direct Cholinomimetics

ACh has virtually no therapeutic applications because of its diffuse action and rapid hydrolysis by cholinesterase (see Fig. 15-5). One may encounter the use of topical ACh (1%) drops during cataract extraction when a rapid miosis is desired. Systemic effects

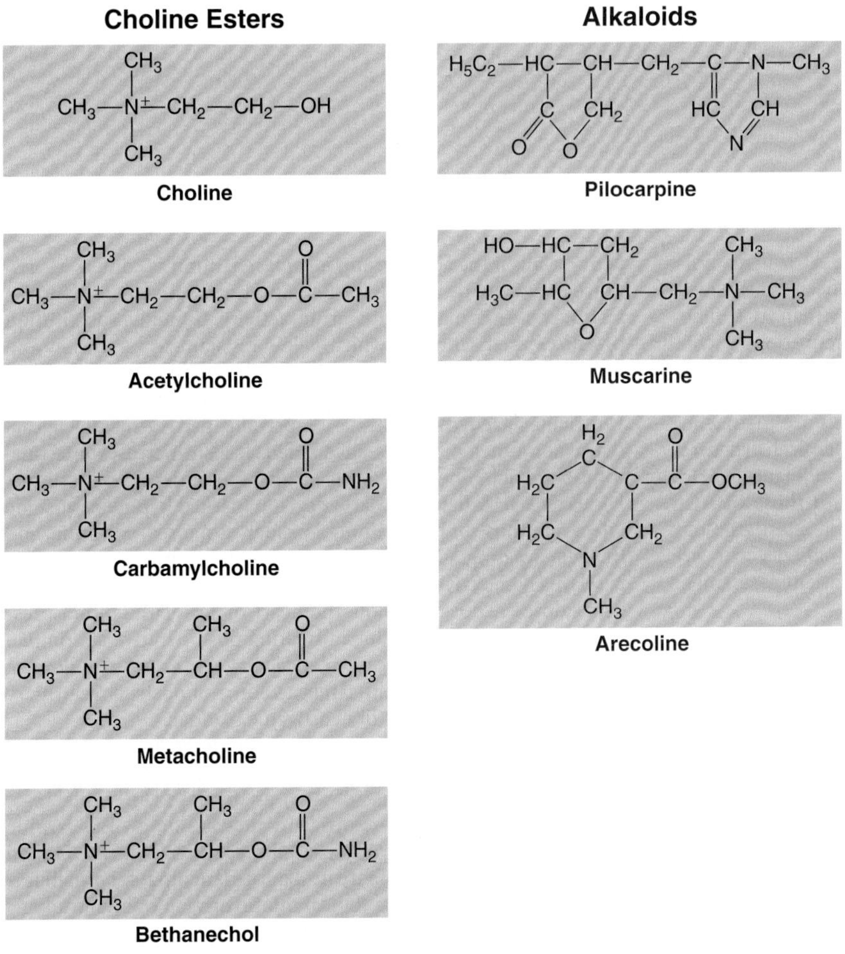

Choline Esters

Choline

Acetylcholine

Carbamylcholine

Metacholine

Bethanechol

Alkaloids

Pilocarpine

Muscarine

Arecoline

FIGURE 15-13. Chemical structures of direct-acting cholinomimetic esters and alkaloids.

TABLE 15-5. COMPARATIVE MUSCARINIC ACTIONS OF DIRECT CHOLINOMIMETIC AGENTS

			Systemic		
	Acetylcholine	Methacholine	Carbamylcholine	Bethanechol	Pilocarpine
Esterase Hydrolysis	+++	+	0	0	0
Eye (Topical)					
Iris	++	++	+++	+++	+++
Ciliary	++	++	+++	+++	++
Heart					
Rate	–	–	–	–	
Contractility	–	–	–	–	
Conduction	–	–	–	–	
Smooth Muscle					
Vascular	–	–	–	–	––
Bronchial	++	++	+	+	++
Gastrointestinal motility	++	++	+++	+++	++
Gastrointestinal sphincters	–	–	–	–	++
Biliary	++	++	+++	+++	++
Bladder					
Detrusor	++	++	+++	+++	++
Sphincter	–	–	–	–	–
Exocrine Glands					
Respiratory	+++	++	+++	++	++++
Salivary	++	++	++	++	+++++
Pharyngeal	++	++	++	++	++++
Lacrimal	++	++	++	++	++++
Sweat	++	++	++	++	+++++
Gastrointestinal acid and secretions	++	++	++	++	++++
Nicotinic Actions	+++	+	+++	–	+++

+, stimulation; –, inhibition.

are not usually seen because of the rapidity of ACh hydrolysis. Derivatives of ACh, other choline esters, have been synthesized, which possess more selective muscarinic activity than ACh. They differ from ACh in being more resistant to inactivation by cholinesterase and thus having a more prolonged and useful action. They also differ from ACh in their relative muscarinic and nicotinic activities. The best studied of these drugs are methacholine, bethanechol, and carbamylcholine. The chemical structures of ACh and these choline esters are shown in Figure 15-13. Their pharmacologic actions are compared with those of ACh in Table 15-5. These are not important drugs in anesthesiology practice but anesthesiologists may encounter patients who are receiving them. (See Chapter 22, Preoperative Patient Assessment and Management.)

ACh is a quaternary ammonium compound that interacts with postsynaptic receptors, causing conformational membrane changes. This results in increased permeability to small ions and, thus, depolarization. All the receptors translate the reversible binding of ACh into openings of discrete channels in excitable membranes, allowing Na^+ and K^+ ions to flow along their electrochemical gradients. Structure–activity relationships point to the presence of two important binding sites on the receptor, an esteratic site that binds the ester end of the molecule and an ionic site that binds the quaternary amine portion (see Fig. 15-5). Subtle changes in the structure of the compound can markedly alter the responses among different tissue groups. The degree of muscarinic activity falls if the acetyl group is replaced, but this confers a resistance to enzymatic hydrolysis. Bethanechol is resistant to hydrolysis but possesses mainly muscarinic activity. β-methyl substitution produces methacholine, which is less resistant to hydrolysis and is primarily a muscarinic agonist. Methacholine slows the heart and dilates peripheral blood vessels. It is used to terminate supraventricular tachydysrhythmias, especially paroxysmal tachycardia, when other measures have failed. It also increases intestinal tone. Methacholine should not be given to patients with asthma. Hypertensive patients may also develop marked hypotension. Side effects are those of PNS stimulation such as nausea, vomiting, and flushed sweating. Overdose is treated with atropine. Bethanechol is relatively selective for the gastrointestinal and urinary tracts. In usual doses it does not slow the heart or lower the blood pressure. Bethanechol is of value in treating postoperative abdominal distention (nonobstructive paralytic ileus), gastric atony following bilateral vagotomy, congenital megacolon, nonobstructive urinary retention, and some cases of neurogenic bladder.

Direct-acting cholinomimetic alkaloids include muscarine and pilocarpine. They act at the same sites as ACh, and their effects are similar to those of ACh as described in Table 15-5. There are no uses for these drugs in anesthesiology. Pilocarpine is the only drug of this group used therapeutically in the United States. Its sole use is for the treatment of glaucoma, for which it is the standard. It is used as a topical miotic drug in ophthalmologic practice to reduce intraocular pressure in glaucoma.

Muscarinic agonists are particularly dangerous in patients with myasthenia gravis (who are receiving anticholinesterases), bulbar palsy, cardiac disease, asthma, peptic ulcer, progressive muscular atrophy, or mechanical intestinal obstruction or urinary retention because they intensify these conditions.

Indirect Cholinomimetics

The indirect-acting cholinomimetic drugs are of greater importance to the anesthesiologist than are the direct-acting drugs. These drugs produce cholinomimetic effects indirectly as a result of inhibition or inactivation of the enzyme acetylcholinesterase, which normally destroys ACh by hydrolysis. They are referred to as cholinesterase inhibitors or anticholinesterases. Most of these drugs inhibit both acetylcholinesterase and pseudocholinesterase. Inhibition of acetylcholinesterase permits the accumulation of ACh transmitter in the synapse, resulting in intense PNS activity similar to that of the direct cholinomimetic agents. The accumulation of ACh by the anticholinesterases potentially can produce all of the following: (1) stimulation of muscarinic receptors at ANS effect organs, (2) stimulation followed by depression of all ANS ganglia and skeletal muscle (nicotinic), and (3) stimulation with later depression of cholinergic receptor sites in the CNS. All of these effects may be seen with lethal doses of anticholinesterase drugs, but therapeutic doses only produce the first two.

Actions of therapeutic significance of the anticholinesterase drugs to the anesthesiologist concern the eye, the intestine, and the neuromuscular junction. The effects of anticholinesterases are useful in the treatment of myasthenia gravis, glaucoma, and atony of the gastrointestinal and urinary tracts. Anticholinesterase drugs are used routinely in anesthesia to reverse nondepolarizing neuromuscular block. The most prominent pharmacologic effects of the anticholinesterase drugs are muscarinic. Their most useful actions are their nicotinic effects. Muscarinic activity is evoked by lower concentrations of ACh than are necessary to produce the desired nicotinic effect. For example, the anticholinesterase neostigmine reverses neuromuscular blockade by increasing ACh concentration at the muscle end plate, a nicotinic receptor. Nicotinic reversal of neuromuscular blockade can usually be produced safely only when the patient has been protected by atropine or other muscarinic blockers. This prevents the untoward muscarinic effects of bradycardia, hypotension, bronchospasm, or intestinal spasm. Reversal of neuromuscular blockade in patients who have had bowel anastomosis was at one time a major controversy. (See Chapter 20, Neuromuscular Agents.) Some thought that the muscarinic effects of anticholinesterase drugs (hypermotility) increased the risk of anastomotic leakage whereas others found no association between their use and subsequent breakdown. National experience has favored the latter opinion.

10 Clinically, anticholinesterase drugs may be divided into two types: The reversible and nonreversible cholinesterase inhibitors.[28] Reversible cholinesterase inhibitors delay the hydrolysis of ACh from 1 to 8 hours. Nonreversible drugs are so named because their inhibitory effects may last from days to weeks. The differences in duration of various anticholinesterases likely depend on whether they inhibit the anionic or esteratic site of acetylcholinesterase. Therefore, the anticholinesterase drugs have also been pharmacologically subdivided. Drugs that inhibit the anionic site are called competitive inhibitors. Their action is due to competition between the anticholinesterase and ACh for the anionic site. These drugs tend to be short-acting. Edrophonium is an example of this type. Drugs that inhibit the esteratic site are called acid-transferring inhibitors. These drugs include the longer acting neostigmine, pyridostigmine, and physostigmine.

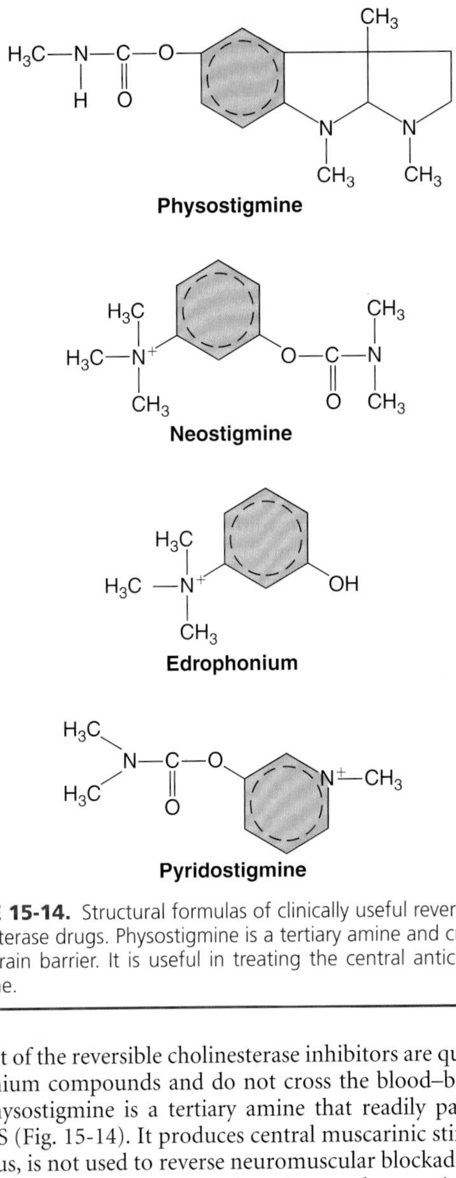

Physostigmine

Neostigmine

Edrophonium

Pyridostigmine

FIGURE 15-14. Structural formulas of clinically useful reversible anticholinesterase drugs. Physostigmine is a tertiary amine and crosses the blood–brain barrier. It is useful in treating the central anticholinergic syndrome.

Most of the reversible cholinesterase inhibitors are quaternary ammonium compounds and do not cross the blood–brain barrier. Physostigmine is a tertiary amine that readily passes into the CNS (Fig. 15-14). It produces central muscarinic stimulation and, thus, is not used to reverse neuromuscular blockade but can be used to treat atropine poisoning. Conversely, atropine is used to treat physostigmine poisoning. Physostigmine has also been found to be a specific antidote in the treatment of postoperative delirium (see below Central Anticholinergic Syndrome).[3]

The irreversible cholinesterase inhibitors are mostly organophosphate compounds. The organophosphate compounds are highly lipid-soluble, they readily pass into the CNS, and are rapidly absorbed through the skin. They are used as the active ingredient in potent insecticides and chemical warfare agents known as nerve gases (see Chapter 53, Emergency Preparedness for, and Disaster Management of, Casualties from Natural Disasters and Chemical , Biologic, Radiologic, Nuclear and High-Yield Explosive (CBRNE) Events). The only therapeutic drug of this group is echothiophate, which is available in the form of topical drops for the treatment of glaucoma. Its primary advantage is its prolonged duration of action. Topical absorption is variable but considerable. Echothiophate can remain effective for 2 or 3 weeks following cessation of therapy. A history of use of echothiophate is important in avoiding prolonged action of succinylcholine, which requires pseudocholinesterase for its hydrolysis. Organophosphate poisoning manifests all the signs and symptoms of excess ACh. The antidote cartridges dispensed to troops to counter the effects of anticholinesterase nerve gases contain only atropine, which would effectively counter the muscarinic effects of the gas; however, atropine does little to counter the high dose nicotinic muscle paralysis or the central ventilation depression that contributes to death from nerve gases. Treatment requires high doses of atropine, 35 to 70 mg/kg IV every 3 to 10 minutes until muscarinic symptoms abate. Lower doses at less frequent intervals may be required for several days. Central ventilatory depression and weakness require respiratory support and specific therapy of the cholinesterase lesion. Pralidoxime has been reported to reactivate cholinesterase activity by hydrolysis of the phosphate enzyme complex. It is particularly effective with parathion poisoning and is the only cholinesterase reactivator available in the United States.[28]

Muscarinic Antagonists

Muscarinic antagonist refers to a specific drug action for which the term anticholinergic is widely used. Any drug that interferes with the action of ACh as a transmitter can be considered an anticholinergic agent. The term anticholinergic refers to a broader classification that also includes the nicotinic antagonists.

Atropine-like Drugs

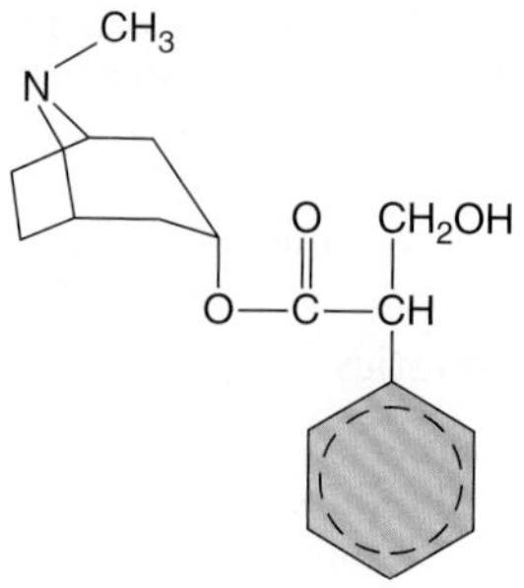

Atropine, scopolamine, and glycopyrrolate are the most commonly used muscarinic antagonists used in anesthesia (Fig. 15-15). The actions of these drugs include inhibition of salivary, bronchial, pancreatic, and gastrointestinal secretions and antagonize of the muscarinic side effects of anticholinesterases during reversal of muscle relaxants. Historically, atropine was introduced to anesthesia practice to prevent excessive secretions during ether anesthesia and to prevent vagal bradycardia during the administration of chloroform.[28] Antimuscarinic agents do not inhibit transmission equally, and there are marked variations in sensitivity at different muscarinic sites owing to differences in penetration and affinities of the various receptors. Differences in relative potency between the different antimuscarinics are outlined in Table 15-6. Atropine and scopolamine are tertiary amines (Fig. 15-15) and easily penetrate the blood–brain barrier and placenta. Glycopyrrolate is a quaternary amine that, like the reversible anticholinesterase drugs, does not easily penetrate these barriers. Glycopyrrolate, a synthetic antimuscarinic, has gained popularity because it avoids the central effects of the other two drugs. Clinical observations suggested that bradycardia associated with spinal anesthesia is refractory to the administration of glycopyrrolate, and that atropine and ephedrine are the drugs of choice in order to prevent a possible cardiac arrest. Nevertheless, recent date of only 69 parturients demonstrated that prophylactic administration of glycopyrrolate does prevent bradycardia associated with spinal anesthesia for cesarean delivery.[29] Atropine and scopolamine have notable CNS effects that are dissimilar. Scopolamine differs from atropine mainly in its central depressant effects, which produce sedation, amnesia, and euphoria. Such properties are widely used for premedication for cardiac patients in combination with morphine and a major tranquilizer. It also has been used to induce amnesia in patients who have a high risk for intraoperative awareness, such as trauma victims who are hemodynamically unstable and cannot receive adequate anesthesia. Atropine, as a premedicant, has slight effects on the CNS, including mild stimulation. Higher doses such as those given for reversal of muscle relaxants (1 to 2 mg) may produce restlessness, disorientation, hallucinations, and delirium (see below Central Anticholinergic Syndrome).

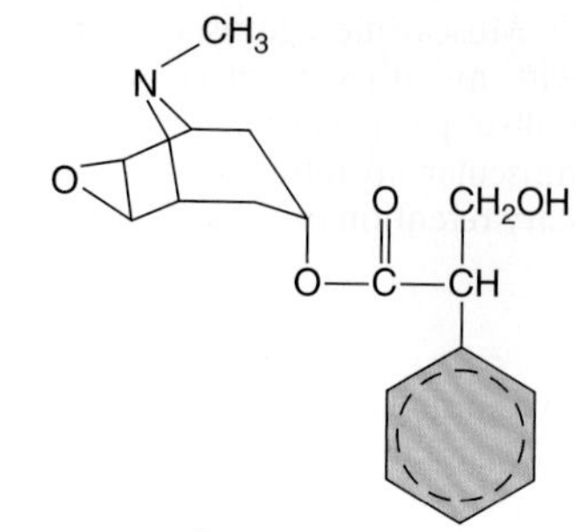

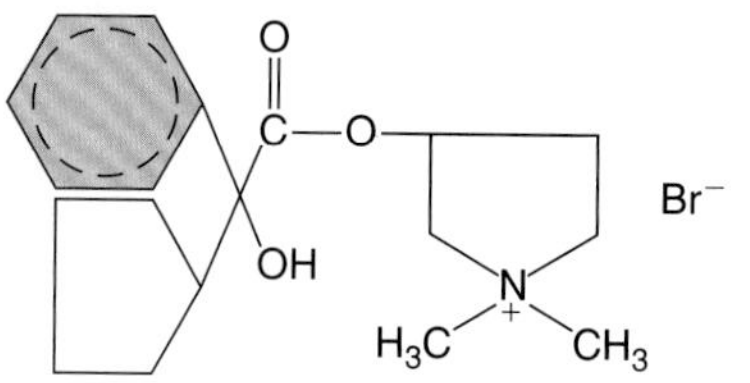

Atropine is useful in increasing CO when sinus bradycardia due to vagal stimulation is present. Atropine and scopolamine are noted to produce a paradoxical bradycardia when given in low doses. Scopolamine (0.1 to 0.2 mg) usually causes more slowing than atropine but also produces less cardiac acceleration at

Atropine

Scopolamine

Glycopyrrolate

FIGURE 15-15. Structural formulas of the clinically useful antimuscarinic drugs.

TABLE 15-6. COMPARISON OF ANTIMUSCARINIC DRUGS

	Duration						
	IV	IM (hr)	CNS	GI TONE	Gastric Acid	Airway Secretions[a]	Heart Rate
Atropine	15–30 min	2–4	++	–	–	–	+++[c]
Scopolamine	30–60 min	4–6	+++[b]	–	–	–	–0[c]
Glycopyrrolate	2–4 hr	6–8	0	–	–	–	+0

IV, intravenous; IM, intramuscular; GI, gastrointestinal.
[a]Secretions may be reduced by inspissations.
[b]CNS effect often manifest as sedation before stimulation.
[c]May decelerate initially.

higher doses. The usual intramuscular premedicant doses of scopolamine cause either a decrease or no change in HR. Atropine may also produce sympathomimetic effects by blocking presynaptic muscarinic receptors found on adrenergic nerve terminals.[30] ACh stimulation of these receptors inhibits NE release, and blockade by atropine releases this inhibition (see Cholinergic Receptors: Muscarinic). Atropine-like drugs that cross the blood–brain barrier also produce dilation of the pupil (mydriasis) and paralysis of accommodation (cycloplegia). Atropine-like drugs are widely used in ophthalmology as mydriatics and cycloplegics. Atropine is contraindicated in patients with narrow-angle glaucoma (see Chapter 48, Anesthesia for Ophthalmologic Surgery). Pupillary dilation thickens the peripheral part of the iris, which narrows the iridocorneal angle. This leads to impaired drainage of aqueous humor, and increase of the intraocular pressure. Doses of atropine used for premedication have little effect in this regard, whereas equal doses of scopolamine cause mydriasis. Prudence would dictate avoidance of either agent in patients with narrow-angle glaucoma. The need for antimuscarinic premedication is questionable in this situation.

Atropine and scopolamine also possess antiemetic action. Atropine, however, reduces the opening pressure of the lower esophageal sphincter, which theoretically increases the risk of passive regurgitation. The belladonna alkaloids (atropine and scopolamine) also block ACh transmission to sweat glands, which, although they are cholinergic, are innervated by the SNS. Antimuscarinic agents produce antinicotinic actions at higher doses and result in important actions on CNS transmission that are pharmacologically similar to the postganglionic cholinergic function. Atropine is best avoided where tachycardia would be harmful, as may occur in thyrotoxicosis, pheochromocytoma, or obstructive coronary artery disease. Atropine should be avoided in hyperpyrexial patients because it inhibits sweating.

Central Anticholinergic Syndrome

The belladonna alkaloids have long been known to produce undesirable side effects ranging from stupor (scopolamine) to delirium (atropine). This syndrome has been called postoperative delirium, atropine toxicity, and the central anticholinergic syndrome. Biochemical studies have demonstrated abundant muscarinic ACh receptors in the brain that can be affected by any drug possessing antimuscarinic activity and capable of crossing the blood–brain barrier. Hundreds of drugs exist that meet these criteria with which this syndrome has been associated. Table 15-7 lists some of those drugs.[3] High doses of atropinic alkaloids rapidly produce dryness of the mouth, blurred vision with photophobia (mydriasis), hot and dry skin (flushed), and fever. Mental symptoms range from sedation, stupor, and coma to anxiety, restlessness, disorientation, hallucinations, and delirium. Convulsions may occur if lethal poisoning has occurred. Although an alarming reaction may occur, fatalities are rare. Intoxication is usually short-lived and followed by amnesia. These reactions can be controlled by the intravenous injection of physostigmine. Physostigmine is an anticholinesterase that, by virtue of being a tertiary amine, readily passes into the CNS to counter antimuscarinic activity. It should be given slowly in 1 mg doses, not exceeding 3 mg, to avoid producing peripheral cholinergic activity. Neostigmine, pyridostigmine, and edrophonium are not effective because they cannot pass into the CNS. The duration of

TABLE 15-7. ANTIMUSCARINIC COMPOUNDS ASSOCIATED WITH CENTRAL ANTICHOLINERGIC SYNDROME

Belladonna Alkaloids
Atropine sulfate
Scopolamine hydrobromide

Synthetic and Natural Tertiary Amine Compounds
Dicyclomine antispasmodic with local anesthetic activity
Thiphenamil antispasmodic with local anesthetic activity
Procaine
Cocaine
Cyclopentolate mydriatic

Quaternary Derivatives of Belladonna Alkaloids
Methscopolamine bromide—antispasmodic
Homatropine methylbromide—sedative, antispasmodic
Homatropine hydrobromide—ophthalmic solution—mydriatic

Synthetic Quaternary Compounds
Methantheline bromide
Propantheline bromide

Antihistamines
Chlorpheniramine
Diphenhydramine

Plants
Deadly nightshade (atropine)
Bittersweet
Potato leaves and sprouts
Jimson or loco weed
Coca plant (cocaine)

Over-the-counter
Asthma-Dor—atropine-like
Compoz—scopolamine sedation
Sleep Eze—scopolamine sedation
Sominex—scopolamine sedation

Antiparkinson Drugs
Benztropine
Trihexphenidyl
Biperiden
Ethopropazine
Procyclidine

Antipsychotic Drugs
Chlorpromazine
Thioriazine
Haloperidol
Droperidol
Promethazine

Tricyclic Antidepressants
Amitriptyline
Imipramine
Desipramine

Synthetic Opioids
Meperidine
Methadone

physostigmine action may be shorter than that of the offending antimuscarinic agent and require repeated injection if symptoms recur. Physostigmine appears safe when used within dose recommendations and when indications are established. Central disorientation alone does not establish a diagnosis. Peripheral signs of antimuscarinic activity should be present in addition to a central anticholinergic syndrome.

Physostigmine has been reported to reverse the CNS effects of many of the drugs listed in Table 15-7, including antihistamines, tricyclic antidepressants, and tranquilizers. Reversal of the sedative effects of opioids and benzodiazepines has also been reported.[31] However, anticholinesterase agents potentiate cholinergic synaptic transmission and increase neuronal activity, even if no receptor antagonist is present. Thus, arousal may not be a function independent of its cholinesterase activity, and claims that physostigmine is a nonspecific CNS stimulant may not be warranted and could, in fact, be dangerous. These considerations, in association with possible significant bradycardia, made the use of physostigmine fairly scarce in the modern recovery rooms.

Sympathomimetic Drugs

The selection of vasoactive drugs requires knowledge of both the hemodynamic disturbance and the pharmacology of the available drugs. The catecholamines and sympathomimetic drugs continue to be the pharmacologic mainstay of cardiovascular support for the low-flow state. Sustained interest in the catecholamines is related to their predictable pharmacodynamics and favorable pharmacokinetic profiles. The half-life of most is short, ranging from 2 to 3 minutes. Undesirable side effects dissipate within minutes of lowering or stopping the infusion. Sympathomimetics, as a group, produce a wide range of hemodynamic effects and can be used in combination to achieve a yet wider spectrum of effects. As a result, one needs to become familiar with only a few agents to manage most clinical situations (Table 15-8).

The goal for managing the low output or high output shock syndrome is to establish and maintain adequate tissue perfusion. Sympathomimetics are not a substitute for volume, and are to be used in hypotensive emergencies, in order to preserve cerebral and coronary blood flow, that may be due to severe hemorrhage, spinal cord injury, antihypertensive overdose, or CNS depressant medication, just to name a few circumstances. Therefore, while intravascular volume is optimized, a vasoactive drug may be required to sustain CO. Aggressive fluid therapy will suffice in most instances. If, on the other hand, adequate fluid resuscitation has been achieved and hemodynamic status still requires sympathomimetics to maintain a normal arterial blood pressure, one must consider alternative causes for hypotension such as septic shock, and seek the most adequate therapy. The term "inodilator" entered our lexicon during the early 1990s to supplant the more archaic term vasopressor. This neologism reflects a change in philosophy in managing low-flow states, particularly those characterized by heart failure. The new synthetic sympathomimetics have been chemically engineered to obtain inotropism and vasodilation rather than for pressor effects. The potential for benefit or harm can best be understood in terms of receptor characteristics. For example, activation of the inotropic β_1 and β_2 receptors results in positive inotropism and chronotropism. Selective stimulation of the vascular β_2 receptors causes vasodilatation. Left ventricular outflow may improve as a function of afterload reduction and inotropism. However, chronotropism may not be a desirable feature in a patient with mitral (valvular) stenosis or coronary artery disease.

Catecholamine Receptor–Effector Coupling

11 The net physiologic effect of a sympathomimetic is usually defined as the algebraic sum of its relative actions on the α, β, and DA receptors. Most adrenergic drugs activate or block these receptors to varying degrees. Each catecholamine has a distinctive effect, qualitatively and quantitatively, on the myocardium and peripheral vasculature. Table 15-9 demonstrates the relative potency of the adrenergic amines on the various myocardial and vascular receptors. This relative potency is also dose-related, adding yet another variable. For many years, the emphasis on catecholamines was mainly on their actions on the myocardium and on the arteriolar resistance vessels. Changes in venous resistance contribute little to total vascular resistance and blood pressure. However, small changes in venous capacitance result in large changes in venous return because 60% to 70% of the circulating blood volume is the venous circulation.[4] The effect of the sympathomimetic amines on the venous circulation appears to be distributive meaning that acute venular constriction increases the central blood volume (preload), whereas dilatation decreases venous return by promoting peripheral pooling.[4] The distributive effect of a catecholamine may be as important as its inotropic action, and more important than its arteriolar effect.[11] Further definitions should elucidate some of the complex and confusing data in the literature generated from clinical observations that are limited solely to adrenergic effects on the myocardium and arteriolar vasculature.

Intravenous and intra-arterial infusions of EPI in humans have been shown to cause marked constriction of the veins. Arteriolar vasoconstriction may or may not precede venoconstriction; however, stroke volume (SV) does not increase until the onset of venoconstriction. The initial increase in CO seen with the infusion of EPI is more an effect of increased preload than an arteriolar or direct cardiac effect. NE produces a similar effect, but the onset of venoconstriction is slower. The peripheral receptors of both resistance and capacitance vessels subserve vasoconstriction, but with divergent effects on afterload and preload; therefore, the α_1 receptors have been subdivided into α_1 arterial (α_{1a}) and α_1 venous (α_{1v}). Dopamine has potent venoconstrictor (α_{1v}) effect at doses at which few α_{1a} or β_1 effects are noted.

Adverse Effects

The major adverse effects of the sympathomimetic amines are related to excessive α or β activity. The potential for harm can be understood in terms of receptor characteristics. Excessive β_1 activity may increase contractility but increase HR and myocardial oxygen consumption beyond supply. Severe dysrhythmias are a frequent companion of excess β_1 activity as a result of increased conduction velocity, automaticity, and ischemia. The β_2 activity has the potential to increase CO by reducing resistance (afterload) while reducing blood pressure. An excessive decrease in diastolic pressure, however, reduces coronary perfusion pressure and may further aggravate myocardial ischemia. Unfortunately, it is difficult to separate the inotropic, dromotropic, and chronotropic effects in the clinical setting. The characteristics of the ideal positive inotropic agent are listed in Table 15-9 for comparison with each drug as it is discussed.

Drugs with prominent α_1 agonist effects may produce an increase in blood pressure but at the same time can reduce total flow due to increases in arteriolar resistance (afterload). A more prominent α_1 venous constriction may improve CO by increasing preload or precipitate failure if preload exceeds the contractile limits of the myocardium. In general, the α effects of the sympathomimetics are of benefit only when used for specific indications

TABLE 15-8. DOSE SCHEDULE AND HEMODYNAMIC EFFECTS OF THE ADRENERGIC AGONISTS

Drug	Dosages		Site of Activity					Hemodynamics (↑ Increase; ↓ Decrease; – = No Change)					
Listed from α to β	IV Push adults	IV Infusion[a]	α_{1A}	α_{1V}	β_1	β_2	DA	CO	INOTROP	HR	VR	TPR	RBF
Phenylephrine	50–100 μg	a. 10 mg/250 mL	++++	+++++	0	0	0			Reflex			
		b. 40 μg/mL								Reflex			
		c. 0.15–0.75 μg/kg/min											
		d. 0.15 μg/kg/min											
Norepinephrine	N/R	a. 4 mg/250 mL	+++	+++	++++	?+	0	–↓	–	↓	↑↑↑	↑↑	––↓
		b. 16 μg/mL								Reflex			
		c. 0.01–0.1 μg/kg/min											
		d. 0.1 μg/kg/min											
Epinephrine	0.3–0.5 mL 1:1000	a. 1 mg/250 mL	+	+	++++	++++	0		↑–↓	↑	↑↑↑	↑↑↑	↓↓↓
	(0.3–0.5 mg)	b. 4 μg/mL	+++	+++	++++					Reflex			
	SC—Asthma IV—	0.01–0.03 μg/kg/min	+++++	+++++	++++								
	Anaphylaxis	c. 0.03–0.15 μg/kg/min	+	+									
	5 mL 1:10,000 (0.5	0.15–0.30 μg/kg/min											
	mg) cardiac arrest	d. 0.015 μg/kg/min											
	every 5 min												
Ephedrine	5–10 mg	N/R ++	+++	+++	++++	+++	↑↑	↑↑	↑	↑↑	↑	↑	↑
Dopamine[c]	N/R	a. 200 mg/250 mL				++	0	↑–	↑↑	↑↑	↑	↑↑	↓–
		b. 800 μg/mL					0	↑–↓	↑↑	↑	↑	↑↑↑	↓
		0.05–5 μg/kg/min						↑↑	↑↑	↑	↑	↑	↑
		c. 2–10 μg/kg/min						↑	↑				
		10 μg/kg/min[b]											
		d. 2 μg/kg/min									↑↑	↑	↑–↓
Dobutamine[c]	N/R	a. 250 mg/250 mL	+	++++	+++								
		b. 1,000 μg/mL	+++++	++++	+++++								
		c. 2–30μg/kg/min		++++									
		d. 5 μg/kg/min		++++									
Isoproterenol	0.004 mg	a. 1 mg/250 mL	0–+	?	++++	+++++	+++++	↑	↑	–	–	–↓	↑
	(0.2 mL of 0.2 mg/	b. 4 μg/mL					+++++	↑↑	↑↑	–↑	↑	–↑	↑
	mL solution)	c. 0.15 μg/kg/min to						↑–↓	–	↑↑	↑	↑↑	–↓
	Third-degree heart	desired effect						↑		–	↑		
	block	d. 0.015 μg/kg/min											

IV, intravenous; DA, dopamine; CO, cardiac output; Inotrop, contractility; HR, heart rate; VR, venous return (preload); TPR, peripheral resistance (afterload); RBF, renal blood flow; N/R, not recommended.

[a]a. Mixture
b. Concentration μg/mL.
c. Dose range μg/kg/min.
d. Standard rate infusion.

[b]"Rule of six."

[c]Dopamine and dobutamine employ the same doses. Dosage of either may quickly be calculated by multiplying patient's weight (kg) × 6 = mg added to 100 mL D5%W. The number of drops delivered through a calibrated infusor (60 drops = 1 mL) is the number of μg/kg/min infused into the patient. Example: 70 kg × 6 = 420; 420 mg/100 mL = 4,200 μg/kg or 70 μg gtt; 5 μg/kg/min = 5 gtt/min.

From: Lawson NW, Wallfisch HK. Cardiovascular pharmacology: A new look at the "pressors," Advances in Anesthesia. Edited by Stoelting RK, Barash PG, Gallagher TJ. Chicago, Year Book Medical Publishers, 1986, p 195, with permission.

TABLE 15-9. ACTIONS OF ADRENERGIC AGONISTS

Sympathomimetics	Receptors						Dose Dependence
	α_1	α_2	β_1	β_2	DA_1	DA_2	(α, β, or DA)
Phenylephrine	+++++	?	±	0	0		++
Norepinephrine	+++++	+++++	+++	0	0		+++
Epinephrine	+++++	+++	++++	++	0		++++
Ephedrine	++	?	+++	++	0		++
Dopamine	+ to +++++	?	++++	++	+++	?	+++++
Dobutamine	0 to +	?	++++	++	0		++
Isoproterenol	0	0	+++++	+++++	0		0

DA, dopamine.

such as significant vasodilation due to different mechanisms. Other measures like fluid resuscitation are usually more effective in improving flow and are indicated before a pressor should be used. Cardiopulmonary resuscitation is the primary example where a pressor effect is necessary to create diastolic coronary perfusion during closed or open heart massage. Any drug with strong α agonist properties seems equally effective in this regard. EPI, with its added β properties, has been the first-line agent for this situation. Vasopressin has recently been added as an important agent in cardiopulmonary resuscitation.[32]

Adrenergic Agonists (Tables 15-8 and 15-9)

Phenylephrine

Phenylephrine, considered a pure α drug, increases both venous constriction and arterial constriction in a dose-dependent manner. Venous constriction may be its most redeeming feature when compared with the purely arteriolar effect of methoxamine. One cannot discount the possibility of an inotropic effect now that α_1 receptors are known to exist in the myocardium. Acutely, venoconstriction favors venous return (preload), and even though arterial resistance (afterload) also increases, one may observe a rise in the arterial blood pressure. Due to the fact that phenylephrine does increase the venous return and stroke volume, but at the same time induces reflex bradycardia secondary to a vagal reflex, cardiac output may not be increased. Phenylephrine does not change CO in normal individuals but can cause decreased output in patients with ischemic heart disease.[33] Phenylephrine is useful in reversing right-to-left shunt in tetralogy of Fallot when patients are having "spells" during anesthesia. Phenylephrine has continued to be favored in operating rooms to increase blood pressure during cardiopulmonary bypass, in patients with critical aortic stenosis, tetralogy of Fallot, and hypotension during cesarean section, as well as vascular procedures its use is also common place to reverse the significant vasodilatory states related to regional blocks like spinal and epidural analgesia. Its efficacy, versatility (the fact that it can be used either as a bolus or as a peripheral infusion, make this drug one of the most commonly used medications in the operating room to reverse anesthetic hypotension due to a multitude of causes. Nevertheless, the lack of prospective data and the fact that it may significantly reduce cardiac output and increase the left ventricular afterload, makes it less than desirable in circumstances such as subarachnoid hemorrhage, traumatic brain injury, and septic shock (Thiele). While traditionally ephedrine was the vasopressor of choice in obstetric anesthesia practice, new evidence including the fact that ephedrine crosses the placenta more readily, and therefore worsens the fetal pH and base excess, making phenylephrine (even used as an infusion) the vasopressor of choice in most academic practices. The fact that it does not adversely affect the placental circulation, but only treats the maternal hypotension makes it an ideal agent, although it has a short half-life that may require the use of an infusion and may be associated with maternal bradycardia. Further studies are necessary to evaluate its effect in the parturient with compromised fetal–placental system. In the future it is possible that a combination of phenylephrine with ephedrine may prove to be best suited for handling complex circumstances such as these.[34–37]

Norepinephrine

NE is the naturally occurring mediator of the SNS and the immediate precursor of EPI. It produces direct-acting hemodynamic effects on the α and β receptors in a dose-related manner when given by infusion. NE produces increased CO and blood pressure when given in low doses (see Table 15-8). Higher doses reduce flow because α arteriolar constriction supersedes the β effects. Reflex baroreceptor–mediated bradycardia may occur despite active β stimulation. Increased plasma levels of the endogenous catecholamines NE and EPI are the sympathetic milieu in which exogenous sympathomimetics are ordinarily given. NE is the catecholamine standard against which other catecholamines are compared. Intravenous NE has received an unseemly reputation over the years that is not merited. Studies indicate that NE was being used in doses that are orders of magnitude greater than those necessary to obtain an optimal response. Complications such as tissue necrosis may be expected when NE is used. A resurgence of interest in this agent is noted and it has remained clinically useful because its predictable, prompt, and potent effects. Objections to the use of NE for the treatment of cardiogenic shock are based on two considerations: (1) vasoconstriction increases the pressure work of the left ventricle, with an adverse effect on the oxygen economy of the ischemic pump, and (2) these drugs cause further vasoconstriction and organ ischemia in a syndrome in which intense constriction may already have occurred. For management of cardiogenic shock, other drugs (dobutamine and milrinone) are more appropriate (see below Dobutamine and Milrinone). However, the predictability of NE pharmacologic effects makes it one of the most useful drugs when intense α activity is intended.

Reduced vascular tone states with or without cardiogenic shock, including separation from cardiopulmonary bypass, or situations when other vasopressors such as phenylephrine fail to maintain a steady hemodynamic state, render NE one of the most commonly used drugs.[11,38] Additional undesirable effects associated with NE include renal arteriolar constriction and oliguria. These effects are secondary to persistent and untreated hypovolemia. Clinicians managing oliguria in the intensive care units, after adequate fluid resuscitation to control prerenal causes, do use NE to maintain renal perfusion pressure, especially in cases of vasodilated hypotension.[39]

Norepinephrine should only be administered in a centrally placed IV to avoid tissue necrosis from extravasation. It can be used for its inotropic effect at low doses and titrated to effect while monitoring cardiac output. Monitoring of blood pressure alone, or titrating to a predetermined effect is often detrimental to cardiac output. Blood pressure increases are usually due to increased systemic vascular resistance (SVR) and excessive increase of the afterload can diminish forward flow and contribute to cardiac failure. Even moderate doses of norepinephrine may have a detrimental effect on end organ perfusion. This has given the drug an ill-deserved reputation when used to titrate to pressure rather than flow. However, in those clinical conditions characterized by high output, low-tone, states with a low perfusion pressure, norepinephrine has been shown to improve renal and splanchnic blood flow by increasing pressure provided the patient has been volume resuscitated and NE has become the first line of treatment of hypotension in septic patients.[38]

Epinephrine (EPI)

EPI is the prototypical endogenous catecholamine. It is synthesized, stored, and released from the adrenal medulla and is the key hormonal element in the fight-or-flight response. It is the most widely used catecholamine in medicine, and to date, it remains the drug of choice in cases of cardiac arrest. It is used to treat asthma, anaphylaxis, cardiac arrest, bleeding, and to prolong regional anesthesia. The cardiovascular effects of EPI, when given systemically, result from its direct stimulation of both α and β receptors. This effect is dose-dependent and is outlined in Table 15-8.

The effect of EPI on the peripheral vasculature is mixed. It has predominantly α-stimulating effects in some beds (skin, mucosa, and kidney) and β-stimulating actions in others (skeletal muscle). At therapeutic doses, β-adrenergic effects predominate in the peripheral vessels, and total resistance may be reduced. Constriction, however, is maintained in the renal and cutaneous areas because of its dominant α effect in these areas. An increase in CO with EPI may be due to a redistribution of blood to low resistance vessels in the muscle, but with further reduction in flow to vital organs. Cardiac dysrhythmias are a prominent concern, and the strong chronotropic effects of EPI have limited its use in the treatment of cardiogenic shock.

Epinephrine is commonly used in the perioperative period. It is often used to produce a bloodless field in dentistry, otolaryngology, and skin grafting either topically or in local and field blocks. Anesthesiologists often use it to prolong regional anesthesia (see Chapter 21 Local Anesthetics). The addition of epinephrine to arthroscopic infusions to attain a bloodless field is another area of increased epinephrine usage with the development of these techniques. The infusions are usually safe in maintaining a dry operative field because the solutions are very dilute at around 1:3,000,000. However, the large volumes infused, the unpredictable absorption of epinephrine offers the opportunity of exposure of the patient to an excessive amount of epinephrine over a short period of time. The dose of submucosally injected EPI necessary to produce ventricular cardiac dysrhythmia in 50% of patients anesthetized with a 1.25 MAC of a volatile anesthetic was 10.9, 10.9, and 6.7 μg/kg during administration of halothane, enflurane, and isoflurane, respectively.[40] The incidence of cardiac dysrhythmia is eliminated when this dose is halved in patients anesthetized with halothane or isoflurane. In contrast to adults, children seem to tolerate higher doses of subcutaneous EPI without developing cardiac dysrhythmia.[41] The current literature recommends the intramuscular route is the preferred method of administration for epinephrine in anaphylaxis and moderate to severe croup.[42] Epinephrine infusion maintains positive chronotropism in circumstances of symptomatic bradycardia, when single doses of atropine do not suffice.[43] At low doses, the use of epinephrine infusion may also induce a beneficial bronchodilation due to its effect on β_2 receptors. Epinephrine can also be used at higher doses, which induce a significant increase in the arterial blood pressure and cardiac output. Unfortunately, these relative high doses of EPI can result in increases in arrhythmogenic properties, including supraventricular and tachycardia, which impose an increase in the myocardial oxygen consumption, and therefore many clinicians find other alternatives.[43]

Ephedrine

Ephedrine is one of the most commonly used noncatecholamine sympathomimetic agents. It is used extensively for treating hypotension following spinal or epidural anesthesia. Ephedrine stimulates both α and β receptors by direct and indirect actions. It is predominantly an indirect-acting pressor, producing its effects by causing NE release. Tachyphylaxis develops rapidly and is probably related to the depletion of NE stores with repeated injection. The cardiovascular effects of ephedrine (see Table 15-8) are nearly identical to those of EPI but less potent. Its effects are sustained approximately 10 times longer than those of EPI. Ephedrine is now the second line of treatment for hypotension in obstetrics because although it improves uterine blood flow linearly with blood pressure, this drug is difficult to titrate, crosses the placenta and decreases the pH of the fetus[24,35–37] (see Chapter 40 Obstetrical Anesthesia). This effect is probably not related to its arteriolar vasoconstriction but rather to its venoconstrictive action. Ephedrine is a weak, indirect-acting sympathomimetic agent that produces venoconstriction to a greater degree than arteriolar constriction (see Table 15-10). This may be its most important and unappreciated effect. It causes a redistribution of blood centrally, improves venous return (preload), increases CO, and restores uterine perfusion. The mild β action restores HR simultaneously with improved venous return. An increased blood pressure is noted as a result rather than a cause of these events. Mild α_1-arteriolar constriction does occur, but the net effect of improving venous return and HR is increased CO. Uterine blood flow is spared. This response, however, depends on the patient's state of hydration.

Isoproterenol

Isoproterenol is a potent balanced β_1 and β_2 receptor agonist with no vasoconstrictor effects. It increases HR and contractility while decreasing systemic vascular resistance. Although it can increase CO, it is not useful in shock because it redistributes blood to nonessential areas by its preferential effect on the cutaneous and muscular vessels. As a result, it produces variable and unpredictable results on CO and blood pressure. Isoproterenol is a potent dysrhythmogenic drug and extends myocardial ischemic areas. Deleterious effects on an evolving cardiac ischemic process include cardiac dysrhythmias, tachycardia, and reduced diastolic

TABLE 15-10. COMPARISON OF RELATIVE A_1 CATECHOLAMINE RESPONSES ON PERIPHERAL RESISTANCE AND CAPACITANCE VESSELS[a]

	Vasoconstriction	
	α_1 Arterial (α_{1a})	α_1 Venous (α_{1v})
Norepinephrine	+++++	+++++
Phenylephrine	++++	+++++
Epinephrine	0/++++[b]	0/++++[b]
Dopamine	0/++++[c]	+++
Ephedrine	++	+++
Dobutamine	+/0	?
Isoproterenol	0	0

[a]Drugs are listed in descending order of potency within each vascular region.
[b]Dose-dependent; β effects of epinephrine predominate at low doses.
[c]Dose-dependent; dopamine and β effects predominate at low doses.
Reprinted with permission from: Lawson NW, Wallfisch HK. Cardiovascular pharmacology: A new look at the "pressors," Advances in Anesthesia. Edited by Stoelting RK, Barash PG, Gallagher TJ. Chicago, Year Book Medical Publishers, 1986, p 195.

coronary perfusion pressure and time. Increased myocardial oxygen demand makes it an unattractive drug for patients in cardiogenic shock. However, isoproterenol is helpful in managing cardiac failure associated with bradycardia, asthma, and cor pulmonale. It is also a useful chemical pacemaker in third degree heart block until an artificial pacemaker can be inserted or the cause can be removed, and may be one of the most important drugs used for denervated heart in cases of significant bradycardia (see above Denervated Heart, and Chapter 51 Transplant Anesthesia). Isoproterenol might be useful in treating both idiopathic and secondary pulmonary hypertension. It has also been reported as useful in improving the forward flow in patients with regurgitant aortic valvular disease, but it should not be used if there is an accompanying stenosis.

Dobutamine

Dobutamine (DBT) is a synthetic catecholamine modified from the classic inodilator isoproterenol. Isoproterenol was, in turn, synthesized from dopamine. Variations and similarities in structure can be seen in Figure 15-6. DBT has clear advantages over isoproterenol and dopamine in many clinical situations. It acts directly on β_1 receptors but exerts much weaker β_2 stimulation than isoproterenol. It does not cause NE release or stimulate DA receptors. DBT possesses weak α_1 agonism, which can be unmasked by β blockade as a prompt and dramatic increase in blood pressure. DBT increases HR more than EPI for a given increase in CO.[38,44]

DBT may decrease diastolic coronary filling pressure because of its vasodilation. However, it appears to produce coronary vasodilation in contrast to the constriction produced by dopamine. Dobutamine has been used effectively to improve coronary flow to differentiate, by echocardiography, responsive or unresponsive areas of dyskinesia in patients following myocardial infarction. DBT does not have any clinically important venoconstrictor activity. This is in contrast to dopamine which increases in ventricular filling pressure at low doses. Clinical studies suggest that DBT is less likely to increase HR than dopamine for a given dose, a major concern in the patient with coronary artery disease. DBT is a coronary artery dilator, whereas dopamine is not. Dopamine-induced tachycardia, however, may be of less concern in the septic patient who commonly has a misdistribution of volume, low vascular resistance, a preexisting refractory tachycardia, but a previously healthy heart. The empiric preference of dopamine in surgical units and DBT in coronary units has been observed and is perhaps well founded. Dopamine and DBT also have contrasting effects on the pulmonary vasculature. Dopamine has been noted to increase pulmonary artery pressure and does not inhibit the pulmonary hypoxic response. It is not recommended for patients in right heart failure. DBT does vasodilate the pulmonary vasculature and is helpful in treating right heart failure and cor pulmonale.[45,46] Dobutamine is highly controllable with a half-life of 2 minutes. Tachyphylaxis is rare but may be noted after 72 hours of administration. The net hemodynamic effects of DBT include an increase in CO, a decrease in left ventricular filling pressure, and a decrease in systemic vascular resistance without a significant increase in chronotropism at lower doses. It is the mainstay of inotropic therapy for septic shock in patients with myocardial dysfunction.[38,47,48]

Dopamine

Dopamine (DA) offers advantages over many sympathomimetics in treating the low output syndrome. It is a dose-related agonist to all three types of adrenoceptors, and the desired action can be selected by changing the infusion rate. The DA receptors are most sensitive followed by the β, and then α receptors. Dopamine dosage regimens have been traditionally, and arbitrarily, divided into low, medium, and high doses according to its dose-receptor sensitivity (Table 15-11). Renal and mesenteric vascular dilatation and tubular cell natriuresis are mediated through the DA receptors at low dose infusion rates of 0.5 to 2.0 μg/kg/min. This is often referred to as "renal dose dopamine" because of the purported enhanced renal blood flow and diuresis. However, the concept of "renal dose" DA is now considered outdated.[49,50] The hemodynamic effects of low dose DA are primarily related to vasodilatation by activation of the DA_1 and DA_2 receptors. Activation of presynaptic DA_2 adrenoceptors adds to the vasodilating effect of the DA_1 receptors by inhibiting presynaptic NE release in the renal and mesenteric vessels. The reduction of total systemic vascular resistance would be significant when one considers that 25% of the CO goes to the kidneys alone. A reduced diastolic blood pressure is often noted with a slight reflex tachycardia. Increasing the infusion rate of DA to 2 to 5 μg/kg/min begins to activate β receptors increasing the CO by increasing chronotropism and contractility with early venoconstriction (preload) and systemic vasodilatation (afterload reduction). Blood pressure may not increase despite significant increases in CO. This dose range would appear optimal for managing congestive heart and lung failure because it combines inotropism and afterload reduction with possible diuresis. However, inotropes without α activity are better utilized for this specific purpose. Further increases in dose activate α receptors, which will increase vascular resistance and blood pressure, but further improvements in CO may be attenuated. Infusion rates of greater than 10 μg/kg/min produce intense α activity, which may override any beneficial DA or β vasodilation effect on total flow. High dose dopamine behaves much like NE, and in fact, causes NE release at this dose range.

Despite the apparent dose-response divisions of DA, a wide variability of individual responses has been noted. The α-adrenergic effects can be seen in some individuals in doses as low as 5 μg/kg/min, whereas doses as high as 20 μg/kg/min may be required to obtain this effect in patients in shock. This wide

TABLE 15-11. β-ADRENERGIC BLOCKING DRUGS

Drug	Relative β_1 Selectivity	Membrane-stabilizing Activity	Intrinsic Sympathomimetic Activity	Plasma Half-life (hr)	Oral Availability (%)	Lipid Solubility	Elimination	Preparations
Propranolol	0	+	0	3–4	36	+++	Hepatic	Oral, IV
Metoprolol	++	0	0	3–4	38	+	Hepatic	
Atenolol	++	0	0	6–9	57	0	Renal	Oral, eye drops
Esmolol	++	0	0	0–16	–	?	RBC esterase	Oral
Timolol	0	0	0	4–5	50	+	Hepatic and renal	IV

RBC, red blood cells.
[a]Primarily hepatic, but active metabolites are formed that must be renally excreted.

variation in dose-response has led to a reexamination of DA as a primary adrenergic for patients in cardiogenic shock or failure. Increased venous return may not be desirable in this situation, but dopamine's hemodynamic versatility continues to be useful in cardiogenic shock when combined with other complementary catecholamines such as dobutamine. The venoconstriction, or distributive effects, of dopamine are useful in surgical patients in whom third space edema and sepsis are the most common abnormalities. Dopamine increases mean pulmonary arterial pressure and is not recommended for sole support in patients with right heart failure, adult respiratory distress syndrome, or pulmonary hypertension.

Combination Therapy

The studied use of adrenergic combinations in patients with cardiac failure has been proposed because pathophysiology cannot be approached with the attitude that β agonism is all good and α agonism is all bad. The objective is to increase coronary perfusion and CO while decreasing afterload. No single vasoactive agent can achieve this, but these conditions can be approached with combination therapy. Because of receptor summation during combination therapy, standard rates of infusion (as outlined in Table 15-8) no longer apply. Invasive hemodynamic monitoring is mandatory for success; otherwise, iatrogenic misadventures can be expected. Other conditions necessary for success with vasoactive drugs also require that the failing myocardium or vasculature have functional reserve, the reserve can be stimulated, and perfusion can be maintained. The adrenergic effects of combined sympathomimetics, appear to be additive and competitive for receptor sites. Summation is more consistent with current receptor pharmacology and can be used to advantage in avoiding unwanted side effects of one drug while supplementing its desired attributes with another. Because of summation, many combinations of vasoactive drugs have been found useful in making fine hemodynamic adjustments in the critically ill. The available sympathomimetic agents provide a wide range of hemodynamic effects particularly when combined with vasodilators. For example, if greater positive inotropic action and less vasoconstriction are desired, DBT could be added to dopamine. Also, nitroprusside could be added to dopamine or combined with any other appropriate inodilator.[51]

Dopamine and DBT are two of the most popular inodilators in use today. A comparison of these two drugs will underscore the importance of extracardiac side effects in selecting a drug either for use alone or in combination.[46] This comparison is particularly appropriate because dopamine and DBT are considered equipotent inotropic agents, and are effective in the same dose range of 2 to 15 μg/kg/min. Their differences can be compared at low (0.5 to 4 μg/kg/min), medium (5 to 9 μg/kg/min), and high (10 to 15 μg/kg/min) doses. This comparison will illustrate the divergent effects of two drugs on preload and afterload while sharing the property of inotropism. Although they share several clinical indications, these drugs are pharmacologically distinct and not interchangeable. Their divergent properties, do make them valuable when administered in combination. Although frequently combined previously, this combination therapy is falling out of favor since they act on the same receptors, and they have so many similarities of action. Therefore, most clinicians now combine an inotrope, such as dobutamine, or milrinone with the more potent α agonists phenylephrine, NE, or even epinephrine infusions. The goal is to compensate for the vasodilation induced by the inotropes, and to maintain an adequate perfusion pressure. DBT is a direct-acting catecholamine that produces a positive inotropic β_1 effect but with minimal changes in β_2 HR or vascular resistance (β_2, α_1 counteraction). Thus, DBT may not alter blood pressure even though CO is markedly improved (see Chapter 10 Cardiac Anatomy and Physiology).

Dobutamine, and milrinone (see below Milrinone) are the mainstay of treatment for decompensated cardiac failure. Although these agents do improve the CO, their use is associated with an increase in cardiac oxygen consumption, cardiac arrhythmias, and even mortality. Therefore, for patients with normal blood pressure and no evidence of hypoperfusion, there is little role for inotropic therapy. Nevertheless, in patients with evidence of impaired organ perfusion (hypotension, decreased renal function), and low output state, with or without congestion or pulmonary edema refractory to diuretics and vasodilators at optimal doses, there is a role for these agents, at least for short-term stabilization. Recently, a new class of drugs was developed, namely calcium-sensitizing agents (levosimendan; see below). These drugs are a unique class of positive inotropic agents that increase the sensitivity of the cardiomyocyte contractile apparatus to intracellular calcium. These may prove to be beneficial either alone or in combination with classical inotropes in management of decompensated heart failure. More studies are necessary to evaluate their overall benefit and long-term outcome.[52,53]

Fenoldopam

Fenoldopam, a *benzazepine* derivative, is a selective DA_1 agonist with no α or β receptor activity compared to dopamine[49] (see Chapter 55 Critical Care Medicine). Intravenous fenoldopam has direct natriuretic and diuretic properties and promotes an increase in creatinine clearance. It offers advantages in the acute resolution of severe hypertension compared to sodium nitroprusside particularly if the patient has preexisting renal impairment.[54] Preservation or augmentation of renal blood flow during blood pressure reduction presents a potential for use during several situations in the perioperative period. Fenoldopam has an elimination half-life of 5 minutes. Human studies have demonstrated that fenoldopam is a potent direct renal vasodilator. Intravenous fenoldopam may prove to be ideal for treating conditions in which renal vasoconstriction is an expected complication. Since it has renal vasodilatory effects, and it promotes increased urine output, fenoldopam has been employed in vascular anesthesia as a renal protector, especially in cases when renal arteries have been temporarily clamped. Its role in preventing the development of renal dysfunction is still debatable, since there are conflicting results in different studies. Stone et al. showed in a 315-patient population that fenoldopam was not useful in preventing further deterioration of the renal function after contrast administration. A large meta-analysis concluded that there is no pharmacologic intervention that is effective in treatment of patients with acute renal injury.[55,56] On the other hand, in a more recent and complete meta-analysis, Landoni et al. suggests that fenoldopam reduces the risk of acute tubular necrosis, the need for renal replacement therapy, and overall mortality in patients with acute kidney injury. Certainly under such circumstances of conflicting results, large randomized studies are necessary to reach a valid conclusion.[57] The onset of action with intravenous fenoldopam is about 5 minutes, reaching a steady state in approximately 20 minutes. The drug is rapidly metabolized in the liver and excreted in the urine. The elimination half-life is about 5 minutes. There has been no evidence of tolerance in reducing blood pressure for up to 24 hours. No rebound on withdrawal has been noted. The most common adverse effects of fenoldopam are related to vasodilation, which include hypotension, flushing, dizziness, headache tachycardia, nausea, and hypokalemia. It should be used cautiously in patients with glaucoma as it can increase intraocular pressure. No significant drug interactions have been reported. Concomitant use with β-blockers will reduce the effective dose of fenoldopam.

Fenoldopam is diluted in normal saline or 5% dextrose is given by continuous infusion without a bolus dose. The effective dosage range is 0.1 to 1.6 μg/kg/min. A reflex tachycardia may result. The dosage is titrated up every 15 minutes according to patient response. Any change in infusion rate response should be detectable within 15 minutes.

Clonidine

Clonidine is a centrally acting selective partial α_2 adrenergic agonist (220:1 α_2 to α_1). It is an antihypertensive drug due to its ability to decrease central sympathetic outflow. Stimulation of α_2 receptors in the vasomotor centers of the medulla oblongata is thought to produce this effect.[58] (It is not clear whether these are pre- or postsynaptic receptors, however, the end result is decreased SNS tone and enhanced vagal tone. Peripherally there is decreased plasma renin activity as well as decreased EPI and NE levels. This drug has been proven to be effective in the treatment of severe hypertension and renin-dependent hypertensive disease.

Clonidine is not available for intravenous use. The usual daily adult oral dose is 0.2 to 0.3 mg. A transdermal clonidine patch is available for use on a weekly basis for surgical patients unable to take oral medication. Clonidine is clinically useful in anesthesiology in other ways as well. It has been found to produce dose-dependent analgesia when introduced into the epidural or subarachnoid space in doses of 150 to 450 μg (see Chapter 56 Acute Pain Management). Clonidine can be added to local anesthetics for epidural, spinal, or regional blocks (more effective when used in blocks of upper limbs and when added to intermediate duration local anesthetics. It is useful even in cardiac patients, and it intensifies the anesthesia.[59,60] It can also be used postoperatively, since it reduces the dose of other regional anesthetic components, and subsequently lessens the possible side effects. One must be aware that clonidine can produce hypotension, bradycardia, and sedation.[61] Oral clonidine (5 μg/kg) when used as a premedicant enhances the postoperative analgesia provided by intrathecal morphine without adding to the side effects of the morphine. Other additional benefits noted from clonidine premedication include: (a) blunted reflex tachycardia for intubation, (b) reduction of vasomotor liability, (c) decreased plasma catecholamines, and (d) dramatic decreases in MAC for inhaled gases or injected drugs. Clonidine is rapidly absorbed by mouth and reaches peak plasma levels within 60 to 90 minutes. The elimination half-life is 9 to 12 hours. It is equally excreted in the liver and kidneys. The duration of the hypotensive effect after a single dose is about 8 hours. The transdermal administration of clonidine requires about 48 hours to achieve therapeutic levels. The decrease in systolic blood pressure is more prominent than the decrease in diastolic blood pressure. There seems to be no effects on glomerular filtration rate. The perioperative administration of clonidine either as an oral dose or as a patch for total of 4 days, has significantly reduced the incidence of myocardial ischemia and mortality up to 2 years postoperatively.

The most common side effects are sedation and a dry mouth. However, skin rashes are frequent with chronic use. Impotence may be seen occasionally, and orthostatic hypotension is a rare side effect. One of the more worrisome complications of chronic clonidine use is a withdrawal syndrome upon acute discontinuation of the drug. This usually occurs 18 hours after discontinuation. The symptoms are hypertension, tachycardia, insomnia, flushing, headache, apprehension, sweating, and tremulousness. It lasts for 24 to 72 hours and is most likely to occur in patients taking more than 1.2 mg/day of clonidine. The withdrawal syndrome has been noted postoperatively in patients who were withdrawn from clonidine before surgery. It can be confused with emergence symptoms following anesthesia particularly in a patient with uncontrolled hypertension.[62] Absent the availability of the oral route in the surgical patient, withdrawal can be treated with clonidine transdermally or more rapidly with rectal clonidine.

Dexmedetomidine

12 Dexmedetomidine is a more selective α_2 agonist than clonidine (see Chapter 55 Critical Care Medicine).[63] Compared to clonidine, dexmedetomidine is seven times more selective for $\alpha 2$ receptors 1,620:1 α_2 to α_1 and has a shorter half-life of 1.5 hours. The loading dose (1 μg/kg) is given over 10 minutes or longer. Then an infusion is begun at 0.2 to 0.7 μg/kg/hour. Due to hemodynamic side effects, some centers omit the loading dose and start the continuous infusion. It has a more rapid onset of action (less than 5 minutes). The time to peak effect is 15 minutes. It can be given intravenously and has many uses in anesthesiology. It provides excellent sedation, reduces blood pressure, HR, and profoundly decreases plasma

catecholamines. Little respiratory depression allows effective weaning from mechanical ventilation. It can be administered as a premedicant in cases of difficult intubations where awake fiberoptic intubation is employed, and has emerged as a valid alternative to other options for awake craniotomies due to its minimal respiratory effects and lack of impairment on electrophysiologic monitoring[64,65] (see Chapter 36 Anesthesia for Neurosurgery). In the intensive care unit (ICU), clonidine is used because of its sedating and analgesic effects without the respiratory depressive actions of other agents. There is concern for possible rebound hypertension, rebound hyperexcitability, and arrhythmias in infusions longer than 24 hours, and ultimately clinical trials are required to clarify these questions. In these patients it appears that dexmedetomidine is neuroprotective by reducing the number of delirium days and promoting a more physiologic sleep, all while being superior to benzodiazepines in reducing the number of ventilator days, delirium, and coma. There is even some preliminary data that suggests that by reduction of immunosuppression and opioid-sparing activity, dexmedetomidine may decrease mortality in septic patients.[66,67] A recent meta-analysis demonstrated a trend toward improved cardiac outcomes in noncardiac surgical patients that have been treated perioperatively with dexmedetomidine.[68] Dexmedetomidine has been shown to be an effective anxiolytic and sedative when used as premedication. Pretreatment with dexmedetomidine, like, clonidine, attenuates hemodynamic responses to intubation. Likewise, it decreases the MAC for volatile anesthetics from 35% to 50% but increases the likelihood of hypotension. Dexmedetomidine, like clonidine, increases the range of temperatures not triggering thermoregulatory defenses. It is likely to promote perioperative hypothermia but is also effective against shivering.

Non-adrenergic Sympathomimetic Agents

Non-adrenergic sympathomimetic drugs also act indirectly by influencing the cAMP-calcium cascade, exclusive of the receptors (see Fig. 15-10). The function of the second messenger (Ca^{2+}) nearly always goes together. This concept reinforces the recent appreciation of the homogeneity of action of a wide variety of drugs previously thought to be unrelated. Sympathomimetics have more pharmacologic similarities than differences.

Vasopressin

Vasopressin and its congener (desmopressin) are exogenous preparations of the endogenous ADH. ADH and oxytocin are the two principal hormones secreted by the posterior pituitary. Target sites for ADH are the renal collecting ducts, vascular smooth muscle, and cardiac myocytes. Water is passively reabsorbed from renal collecting ducts into extracellular fluid. Nonrenal actions include inotropism and intense vasoconstriction accounting for its alternative designation as vasopressin.[69] Arginine vasopressin (AVP) is the most potent form of ADH. Historically, vasopressin has been used for: (a) treatment of diabetes insipidus, (b) diagnosis of diabetes insipidus, (c) abdominal distention, (d) and as an adjunct in the treatment of gastrointestinal hemorrhage and esophageal varices. Recently, three new indications for the use of vasopressin have emerged. These are (1) pressure support for septic shock, (2) cardiac arrest secondary to ventricular fibrillation/ventricular tachycardia, or (3) pulseless electrical activity/asystole.[70–73] Animal studies have shown, both in open and closed chest models, vasopressin caused larger increases in SVR, cerebral perfusion pressure, and coronary perfusion pressure than EPI. Vasopressin is a more effective vasoconstrictor than EPI in the presence of hypoxia and acidosis. In contrast to EPI, vasopressin does not seem to increase mixed venous oxygen saturation (MVO_2) or lactate production.[73,74] The 2005 guidelines for ACLS of the American Heart Association recommend that vasopressin may be used to replace the first or second dose of EPI during the pulseless arrest algorithm[75] (see Chapter 58 Cardiopulmonary Resuscitation). EPI is class IIb recommendation, and vasopressin, which did not show any improvement in survival when compared with epinephrine, may be used instead of the first or the second dose of epinephrine, and is considered class indeterminate[43] (see Chapter 58 Cardiopulmonary Resuscitation). Vasopressin administered for cardiac arrest is known as "vasopressin injection USP." The dose in cardiac arrest is 40 IU in 40 mL intravenously as a single dose in a peripheral IV line. Extravasation may cause local tissue necrosis. Its use in vasodilated sepsis is by infusion pump starting at 0.04 IU/min. There are suggestions, that vasopressin may be useful in addition to potent α agonists for treatment of shock, especially due to relative sparing of the mesenteric vessels. These data are supported by rat studies.[76] Despite a theoretical advantage of using vasopressin to decrease the catecholamines dosage in septic patients, the use of vasopressin failed to decrease mortality when compared with norepinephrine.[70] In such circumstances, it seems that timing of initiation of therapy is the most important parameter for survival.[77,78]

Vasopressin antagonists such as Tolvaptan, Conivaptan, and Lixivaptan have been studied in patients with heart failure. While diuretics are a cornerstone of treatment of heart failure, they do not improve survival and may worsen hypotension, renal dysfunction, electrolyte abnormalities, and activation of the renin–angiotensin–aldosterone system. The vasopressin antagonists have been used with encouraging results with improving the symptomatology of heart failure, with effective diuresis without worsening of hyponatremia or renal function, but still failed to show an improvement in overall mortality.[79]

Adenosine

Adenosine, available for more than 50 years, has been recognized recently as a clinically useful drug. It is an endogenous nucleotide and is found in every cell in the body. It is composed of adenine and a pentose sugar. Production can be increased by stimuli such as hypoxia and ischemia. This ubiquitous nucleotide has potent electrophysiologic effects in addition to having a major role in regulation of vasomotor tone. Adenosine is believed to have a cardioprotective effect by regulating oxygen supply and demand (see Chapter 58 Cardiopulmonary Resuscitation). The receptors in the myocardial conduction system are the most sensitive and mediate SA node slowing and AV nodal conduction delay. Adenosine hyperpolarizes atrial myocytes and decreases their action potential duration via an increase in outward K^+ current. These are the acetylcholine-regulated K^+ channels. Adenosine mimics the effects of acetylcholine in many ways, including an extremely short plasma half-life of mere seconds. Adenosine also antagonizes the inward Ca^{2+} current produced by catecholamines. This antidysrhythmic mechanism of Ca^{2+} channel blockade is thought to be an indirect effect and important only when β stimulation is present. The primary antidysrhythmic effect of adenosine is to interrupt reentrant AV nodal tachycardia, which most likely relates to its K^+ current rather than Ca^{2+} current effects. The chief indication for adenosine is paroxysmal supraventricular tachycardia (PSVT), which it may terminate in a matter of seconds. Adenosine is the recommended as first line of treatment.[43,80] Adenosine is to be used only cautiously in patients with Wolf–Parkinson–White syndrome with narrow complex tachycardia, and should be avoided in Wolf–Parkinson–White syndrome with atrial fibrillation. The reason for this is that its use may increase the conduction via the atrioventricular node and induce ventricular fibrillation. One may use adenosine for reentrant tachycardias involving the AV node, as well as right ventricular tachycardias.[81] The same characteristics that make adenosine an effective therapeutic agent may also make it an ideal agent for diagnosing other types of dysrhythmia. The incidence of incorrect diagnosis of supraventricular dysrhythmia has been reported to be as high as 15% using conventional means. Approximately 10% of SVT do not involve AV nodal reentry. Adenosine will nevertheless slow AV nodal conduction in these cases, decrease the ventricular rate, and allow inspection of P waves. Thus, adenosine may be useful in unmasking atrial fibrillation, or flutter, when fast ventricular responses are noted. This significant slowing of the ventricular rate is useful clinically during deployment of endovascular stents, and should be used with caution. A number of side effects have been reported with the use of adenosine, including flushing, headache, dyspnea, bronchospasm, and chest pain. The majority of these are brief (seconds) and not clinically significant. Transient new dysrhythmia (65%) will be noted at the time of cardioversion, but these disappear during the half-life of the drug. Major hemodynamic changes are rare but consist of hypotension and bradycardia. Adenosine should be given by means of a rapid IV bolus with flush because of its extremely short half-life of less than 10 seconds. The initial adult dose is 6 mg in peripheral IVs and half this dose when administered via central circulation (100 to 150 μg/kg pediatrics), which can be followed by 12 mg within 1 to 2 minutes if the initial dose is without effect.[58] The 12 mg dose may be repeated once. The antidysrhythmic effect of adenosine occurs as soon as the drug reaches the AV node. Although both adenosine and verapamil are effective in treating PSVT one must be aware of side effects (more prominent hypotension when using verapamil) before choosing one versus the other.[82] Nevertheless, adenosine seems to be a better choice due to fewer side effects, a view that is upheld by the recent ACLS Guidelines. Recently, the use of adenosine in these circumstances has been expanded and now includes stable, narrow-complex tachycardias, unstable narrow-complex regular tachycardias while preparation for electrical cardioversion are being made, and stable, regular, monomorphic, wide-complex tachycardia as a therapeutic and diagnostic maneuver[43,83] (see Chapter 58 Cardiopulmonary Resuscitation).

Phosphodiesterase Inhibitors

Phosphodiesterase inhibitors have pharmacologic properties approaching the characteristics of the ideal inotropic agent.[84–86] They do not rely on stimulation of β and/or α receptors. These drugs combine positive inotropism with vasodilator activity by selectively inhibiting phosphodiesterase (PDE) III. PDE I and II hydrolyze all cyclic nucleotides, whereas PDE III acts specifically on cAMP. The PDE III inhibitors interact with PDE III at the cell membrane and impede the breakdown of cAMP. cAMP levels increase and protein kinase is activated to promote phosphorylation. In cardiac muscle, phosphorylation increases the slow inward movement of calcium current, promoting increased intracellular calcium stores. Thus, inotropism increases. In vascular smooth muscle, increased cAMP activity accounts for the vasodilation, decreased peripheral vascular resistance, and lusitropism. Amrinone (currently termed inamrinone) is the prototypical PDE III inhibitor, and like nitroprusside and nitroglycerin, promotes diastolic relaxation, which promotes ventricular filling.[87] Milrinone is currently the most popular PDE inhibitor released for clinical use in the United States. The degree of hemodynamic effect of these drugs depends on the dose, degree of inotropic reserve, and state of cAMP depletion.

Milrinone

Milrinone is a derivative of amrinone. (In most centers, milrinone has replaced amrinone; although in general their hemodynamic profiles are similar.) It has nearly 20 times the inotropic potency of the parent compound. Milrinone is active both intravenously and orally and has beneficial short-term hemodynamic effects in patients with severe refractory congestive heart failure. Improvement of CO appears to result from a combination of enhanced myocardial contractility and peripheral vasodilation. Treatment with oral milrinone for up to 11 months has been effective and well tolerated without evidence of fever, thrombocytopenia, or gastrointestinal effects. Milrinone has been approved for short-term IV therapy of congestive heart failure.[84–86] It is administered with a loading dose of 50 μg/kg over 10 minutes. The maintenance IV infusion rate ranges from a minimum of 0.375 μg/kg/min to a maximum of 0.75 mg/kg/min (not to exceed 1.13 mg/kg/day). Dosage must be adjusted in renal failure patients as milrinone is excreted in the urine primarily in unconjugated form. Peak response with an IV dose occurs after 5 minutes and reveals no evidence of tolerance over short-term trials (24 hours); it is compatible with other adrenergic agonists. It is an effective inotropic agent in patients receiving β blockers. Its efficacy in the patient who has been digitalized has been demonstrated. Milrinone and dobutamine have become the mainstay of treatment for decompensated heart failure patients who require intravenous vasodilators and positive inotropic agents. Nevertheless, the use of such agents significantly increases mortality.[88] One must be aware that these drugs may increase the risk of arrhythmias in these patients who may in fact require implantable cardioverter defibrillators.[89]

Glucagon

Glucagon is a single chain polypeptide of 29 amino acids that is secreted by pancreatic cells in response to hypoglycemia (see Chapter 46 Endocrine Function). The liver and kidney are responsible for its degradation. Known effects of this hormone in humans include the following: (1) inhibition of gastric motility, (2) enhanced urinary excretion of inorganic electrolytes, (3) increased insulin secretion, (4) hepatic glycogenolysis and gluconeogenesis, (5) anorexia, (6) inotropic and chronotropic cardiac effects, and (7) relaxation of smooth muscle (biliary, i.e., sphincters).[90] Little attention was given to glucagon until 1968, when it was demonstrated to produce positive inotropic and chronotropic effects in the canine heart. Glucagon enhances the activation of adenyl cyclase in a manner similar to that of NE, EPI, and isoproterenol. These cardiac actions of glucagon are not blocked by β blockade or catecholamine depletion. Glucagon, in contrast to the xanthines, rarely causes dysrhythmia, even in the face of ischemic heart disease, hypokalemia, and digitalis toxicity. Glucagon may possess antidysrhythmic activity in digitalis toxicity because it has been shown to enhance AV nodal conduction in patients with varying degrees of AV block. An IV dose of 1 to 5 mg of glucagon increases cardiac index, mean arterial pressure, and ventricular contractility, even in the presence of digitalis therapy. After a bolus dose, its action dissipates in approximately 30 minutes. Nausea and vomiting are common side effects in the awake patient, especially following a bolus dose. Hypokalemia, hypoglycemia, and hyperglycemia are also seen. Glucagon is also useful in treating insulin-induced hypoglycemia. Despite the obvious benefits of glucagon in cardiac patients, its use has not become popular. This pancreatic hormone may be of hemodynamic benefit when more conventional approaches have proved refractory in the following settings: (1) low CO syndrome following cardiopulmonary bypass, (2) low CO syndrome with myocardial infarction, (3) chronic congestive heart failure, and (4) excessive β-adrenergic blockade. In cases of anaphylactic shock with significant and refractory hypotension, glucagon is an extremely useful alternative agent in reversing the decreased blood pressure.[91]

Digitalis Glycosides

The most important actions of the digitalis glycosides are those affecting myocardial contractility, conduction, and rhythm. The glycoside most likely to be used by the anesthesiologist is digoxin. The principal uses of digoxin are for the treatment of congestive heart failure and to control supraventricular cardiac dysrhythmia such as atrial fibrillation. Digoxin is one of the few positive inotropes that does not increase HR. Digoxin enhances myocardial inotropism and automaticity but slows impulse propagation through the conduction tissues.[58] Despite nearly two centuries of use, its mechanism of action is only modestly certain. Digitalis reciprocally facilitates calcium entry into the myocardial cell by blocking the Na^+, K^+ adenosine triphosphatase pump. This calcium influx may account for its positive inotropic action because this inotropic response is not catecholamine- or β-receptor–dependent and is therefore effective in patients taking β-blocking drugs. The inhibition of this enzyme transport mechanism also results in a net K^+ loss from the myocardial cell. This contributes to digitalis toxicity with hypokalemia. Calcium potentiates the toxic effects of digitalis. Extreme caution should be observed when calcium is given to a patient taking digitalis or when digitalis administration is contemplated in the patient with hypercalcemia. Digitalis has been of little value in cardiogenic shock and has proved potentially injurious in patients with uncomplicated myocardial infarction because of its vasoconstrictive properties and effects on myocardial oxygen consumption in the absence of cardiomegaly. Care must be taken to rule out conditions in which the use of digitalis is of no benefit and is potentially harmful. These include mitral stenosis with normal sinus rhythm and constrictive pericarditis with tamponade. Signs and symptoms of idiopathic hypertrophic subaortic stenosis are often exacerbated by digitalis. With increased strength of contraction, the muscular obstruction can be markedly increased. The same is true for the use of digitalis in patients with infundibular pulmonic stenosis, as occurs with tetralogy of Fallot. Any augmentation of contractility may further reduce an already diminished pulmonary blood flow. Beware of digitalis toxic reactions in the older age group and in patients suffering from arterial hypoxemia, acidosis, renal compromise, hypothyroidism, hypokalemia, or hypomagnesemia as well as in patients receiving quinidine or calcium channel blockers.

When entertaining the possibility of perioperative digitalis administration, the following points must be considered.

1. Myocardial oxygen consumption is increased in the non-failing, non-dilated heart.
2. The therapeutic-to-toxic ratio of digitalis is narrow.
3. Inotropic drugs that are less toxic and reversible are readily available.
4. Verapamil or β blockers are more efficacious for supraventricular tachydysrhythmias not initiated by heart failure.
5. Digitalis may cause serious dysrhythmia in the unstable patient.
6. Serum potassium concentrations may fluctuate in the surgical patient.
7. Any cardiac dysrhythmia that occurs in the presence of digitalis must be considered a toxic phenomenon.
8. Digitalis-induced cardiac dysrhythmias are difficult to treat.
9. Renal compromise will result in toxic effects with standard maintenance doses.
10. Cardioversion may be dangerous after digitalis administration.
11. After initiation of digitalis therapy, the administration of alternative drugs becomes more complicated.

Digoxin, β-blockers and calcium channel blockers such as diltiazem and verapamil may be used in patients with heart failure and normal ejection fraction to control the heart rate, especially if patients do have supraventricular tachyarrhythmias such as atrial fibrillation. Nevertheless, digoxin is not recommended for patients with heart failure but with normal ejection fraction, since it may increase the left ventricular filling pressure, and subsequently aggravate their heart failure.[92]

Calcium Salts

Calcium is of great importance in the genesis of the cardiac action potential and is key to controlling intracellular energy storage and utilization. Movement of extracellular calcium across membranes also governs the function of uterine smooth muscle as well as the smooth muscle of the blood vessels. The sympathomimetic drugs promote the transmembrane influx of calcium, whereas the β blockers and calcium channel blockers inhibit such movement. The American Heart Association has recommended against the use of calcium during cardiac arrest except when hyperkalemia, hypocalcemia, or calcium channel blocker toxicity is present.[93] Subsequently, the indications for calcium use are now limited to only few clinical applications (see Chapter 58 Cardiopulmonary Resuscitation). Calcium chloride is often given at the termination of cardiopulmonary bypass to offset the myocardial depression associated with hypothermic potassium cardioplegia.[94] There is newer evidence that the use of calcium in the early post-bypass period may induce spasm of the coronaries, including the newly grafted internal mammary artery, also causes hypercontracture of the heart cells, and therefore increases the risk for myocardial ischemia, reperfusion injury, and even myocardial infarction.[95–97] The use of calcium salts is clearly indicated during rapid or massive transfusions of citrated blood.[94] Citrate binds calcium, and rapid infusion rates of citrated blood result in myocardial depression that is reversible by calcium. Two forms of calcium salts are commonly available: Calcium chloride and calcium gluconate. Traditionally, calcium gluconate has been preferred in pediatric patients and calcium chloride in adult patients. Previous data held that calcium chloride produced consistently higher and more predictable levels of ionized calcium.[98] Studies have shown, however, that ionization of any of the preparations is immediate and equally effective (see Chapter 14 Fluids, Electrolytes, and Acid-Base Physiology). Calcium chloride produces only transient increases in CO and blood pressure. Bolus doses of 2 to 10 mg/kg (1.5 mg/kg/min) of calcium chloride can produce moderate improvement in contractility. The rapid administration of calcium salts, if the heart is beating, can produce bradycardia and must be used cautiously in the patient who is digitalized because of the hazard of producing toxic effects. Calcium salts will precipitate as calcium carbonate if mixed with sodium bicarbonate.

Levosimendan is a calcium sensitizer that has both positive inotropic and vasodilatory effects, and appears to be cardioprotective. It is used as an alternative to other inotropes, or devices with very good results. For example, when compared with dobutamine levosimendan improved the left ventricular hemodynamic function in patients with cardiogenic shock, and reduced the intensive care unit stay, when compared to the usage of intra-arterial balloon pumps also reduced perioperative mortality and improved perioperative cardiac function in patients undergoing noncardiac surgeries. In patients with acute decompensated heart failure, levosimendan has favorable hemodynamic effects, while adverse effects and mortality are similar when compared to dobutamine.[99] It appears that levosimendan has cardioprotective effects shown by an attenuated rise in troponin associated with cardiopulmonary bypass, and it has become (in Europe) a viable treatment alternative for patients with decompensated cardiac failure. It also can be used in patients after myocardial infarction or after cardiac surgery who require higher doses of catecholamines associated with low cardiac output, especially since it appears that its safety, hospitalization rates, and mortality rates are superior to dobutamine, or placebo. One of the attractive features of this drug is the vasodilatory effects on the pulmonary circulation, thus decreasing the pulmonary vascular resistance, whilst improving the right ventricular performance in patients with decompensated heart failure. Nevertheless, it appears that in certain patients with nonvasoreactive pulmonary arterial hypertension, levosimendan does not decrease the vascular resistance, but is ineffective and increases the pulmonary pressures.[100–103]

Antidepressant Drugs

Monoamine Oxidase Inhibitors

Monoamine oxidase inhibitors (MAOIs) and the tricyclic antidepressants are used to treat psychotic depression. These drugs are not used in the practice of anesthesia but are a source of potentially serious anesthetic interactions in patients who are taking them chronically (see Chapter 22 Preoperative Patient Assessment and Management). Their use is rapidly declining as the nontricyclic antidepressants such as Prozac are more efficacious and produce fewer side effects. Few of the MAO inhibitors or tricyclic antidepressants will be encountered in an anesthesia practice today with the exceptions of phenelzine (Nardil) and amitriptyline (Amitril, Elavil). Their pharmacologic actions and side effects are a direct result of their effect on the cascade of catecholamine metabolism. MAOIs block the oxidative deamination of endogenous catecholamines into inactive vanillylmandelic acid. They do not inhibit synthesis. Thus, blockade of monoamine oxidase would produce an accumulation of NE, EPI, dopamine, and 5-hydroxytryptamine in adrenergically active tissues, including the brain. The action of sympathomimetic amines is potentiated in patients taking MAOIs. Indirect acting sympathomimetics (ephedrine, tyramine) produce an exaggerated response as they trigger the release of accumulated catecholamines. Foods containing a high tyramine content such as cheese, red Italian wine, and pickled herring can also precipitate hypertensive crises.[28] Meperidine has been reported to produce hypertensive crisis, convulsions, and coma with MAO inhibitors. Hepatotoxicity has been reported that does not seem to be related to dosage or duration of treatment. Its incidence is low but remains a factor in selecting anesthesia.

The anesthetic management of patients taking MAOIs remains controversial. Currently, recommendations for management include discontinuation of the drugs for at least 2 weeks before surgery; however, this recommendation is not based on controlled studies but rather is the result of limited case reports that suggest potent drug interactions.

Tricyclic Antidepressants

This group of antidepressant drugs is referred to as tricyclic antidepressants because of their structure. These drugs have almost replaced the MAOIs because of fewer side effects. All of these agents block uptake of NE into adrenergic nerve endings. Just as with the MAOIs, high doses of the tricyclic antidepressants can induce seizure activity that is responsive to diazepam. Neuroleptic drugs may potentiate the effects of tricyclic antidepressants by competition with metabolism in the liver. Chronic barbiturate use increases metabolism of the tricyclic antidepressants by microsomal enzyme induction. Other sedatives, however, potentiate the tricyclic antidepressants in a manner similar to that occurring with the MAOIs. Atropine also has an exaggerated effect because of the anticholinergic effect of tricyclic antidepressants. Prolonged sedation from thiopental has been reported. Ketamine may also be dangerous in patients taking tricyclic antidepressants by producing acute hypertension and cardiac dysrhythmia. Despite these serious interactions, discontinuation of these drugs before surgery is probably not necessary. The latency of onset of these drugs is from 2 to 5 weeks; however, the excretion of tricyclic antidepressants is rapid, with approximately 70% of a dose appearing in the urine during the first 72 hours. The long latency period for resumption of treatment militates against interrupted treatment. A thorough knowledge of the possible drug interactions and autonomic countermeasures now available obviates postponement.

Selective Serotonin Reuptake Inhibitors

Their mechanism of action appears to be the selective inhibition of neuronal uptake of serotonin. This potentiates the behavioral changes induced by the serotonin precursor, 5-hydroxytryptophan.[104] The availability of sympathetic antagonists for possible side effects during anesthesia weighs in favor of continuation of therapy versus the risk of exacerbation of a severe depression. Prozac (fluoxetine) is a popular oral nontricyclic antidepressant. The elimination half-life of Prozac is 1 to 3 days and can lead to significant accumulation of the drug. Prozac's metabolism, like that of other compounds including tricyclic antidepressants, phenobarbital, ethanol, and pentothal involves the P450 II D6 system, concomitant therapy with drugs also metabolized by this enzyme system may lead to drug interactions and prolongation of effect of the benzodiazepines. Wellbutrin® and Zyban® are the same drug, namely, bupropion hydrochloride. Zyban, however, is a sustained release drug. Wellbutrin is used as an antidepressant, whereas Zyban is marketed as a non-nicotine aid to smoking cessation. The neurochemical mechanism of the antidepressant effect of bupropion is not known. It does not inhibit monoamine oxidase and is a weak blocker of the neuronal uptake of serotonin and norepinephrine. It also inhibits the neuronal uptake of dopamine to some extent. No systematic data have been collected on the interactions of bupropion and other drugs. Duloxetine is a selective serotonin reuptake inhibitor (SSRI) that has been used as an antidepressant, but recently has been used for treatment of chronic pain due to its analgesic properties.[105] Patients with heart disease have emerged as a special category due to the finding that depression significantly affects the cardiovascular health. Several studies support the safety of SSRI's in these patients due to its association with a decrease in morbidity and mortality, and the need for continuous treatment, especially in the elderly. Nevertheless, there is some evidence although small that these drugs may increase the risk of bleeding. Since these patients may use concomitantly other antiplatelet/anticoagulation therapies, increased vigilance is mandatory.[106–109]

Adrenergic Antagonists–Sympatholytic Drugs

Alpha Antagonists

13 Drugs that bind selectively to α-adrenergic receptors block the action of endogenous catecholamines or moderate the effects

of exogenous adrenergics. The resultant effects may be ascribed together the blockade effect to α-adrenergic agonists or to unopposed β-adrenergic receptor activity. The effect is smooth muscle relaxation. The response to the vasculature may vary over a wide range in a single vascular bed depending on its intrinsic state of constriction. Vessels with higher initial tone have a greater response to α-blockade. Prominent clinical effects of α-blockers include hypotension, orthostatic hypotension, tachycardia and miosis, nasal stuffiness, diarrhea, and inhibition of ejaculation. The α-blockers may be classified according to binding characteristics. Phenoxybenzamine is an oral α-blocker that produces an irreversible blockade. It is a relatively nonselective α-blocker. Phentolamine, tolazoline, and prazosin are characterized by reversible binding and antagonism. When patients are taking these drugs chronically one should keep in mind that the normal autonomic response to stress, inhalation anesthetics, or extensive regional anesthesia may be blunted. Elevations of catecholamines will not reflexly increase peripheral vascular resistance and may actually decrease if vascular β receptors are unopposed. α-blockers are often used in combination with diuretics and other antihypertensives. Volume depletion may not be evident on preoperative examination but may become unmasked with the induction of anesthesia resulting in the onset of a marked hypotension. This hypotension is usually responsive to volume repletion and the temporary use of a direct acting α-agonist such as phenylephrine. There is no cause for discontinuation of these drugs before surgery but preloading with IV fluids is suggested to ensure adequate central volume.

Phentolamine

Phentolamine is used almost exclusively in the presurgical treatment of pheochromocytoma (see Chapter 46 Endocrine Function). It is a competitive antagonist at α_1 and α_2 receptors. Phentolamine may also have some antihistaminic and cholinomimetic activity. The cholinomimetic activity may result in abdominal cramping and diarrhea, both of which are blocked by atropine. Tachycardia and hypotension are also common side effects.

Intravenously, phentolamine produces peripheral vasodilatation and a decrease in systemic blood pressure within 2 minutes lasting from 10 to 15 minutes. Blood pressure reduction elicits baroreceptor reflexes and NE release. Cardiac arrhythmias and angina pectoris may accompany phentolamine administration. It can be given in doses of 30 to 70 μg/kg IV to produce a transient decrease in blood pressure. It can also be used as a continuous infusion to maintain blood pressure during resection of a pheochromocytoma.

Phenoxybenzamine

Phenoxybenzamine acts as a nonselective α-adrenergic antagonist (see Chapter 46 Endocrine Function). α-blockade is 100 times more potent on postsynaptic α_1 receptors than at α_2 receptors. Preoperatively in preparation for removal of a pheochromocytoma, the drug is administered orally starting at 10 mg BID.[110] The onset of α-blockade is slow. This is related to the time required for structural modification of the phenoxybenzamine molecule to become active. The elimination half-life is about 24 hours. Orthostatic hypotension is prominent especially in the presence of preexisting hypertension or hypovolemia. Cardiac output is often increased and renal blood flow is not greatly altered except in preexisting renal vasoconstriction or stenosis. Coronary and cerebral vascular resistance is not changed.

Prazosin

Prazosin is relatively selective for α_1 receptors, leaving the inhibiting effect of α_2 receptor activity on norepinephrine release intact. As a result, it is less likely than nonselective α-antagonists to evoke reflex tachycardia. The initial oral dose is 1 mg BID then titrated to effect. Prazosin dilates both arterioles and veins. Cardiovascular effects include total body reductions in systemic vascular resistance and venous return. When combined with a diuretic it is an effective antihypertensive drug. It should not be used with clonidine or α-methyldopa, as it appears to decrease their effectiveness. Prazosin may also cause bronchodilation.

Oral α_1-blockers have been found useful for benign prostatic hypertrophy (BPH) and hypertension. The anesthesiologist may encounter patients taking these medications on a chronic basis and must be aware of their possible interactions with anesthetics (see Chapter 22 Preoperative Patient Assessment and Management). Doxazosin is a long acting selective α_1-blocker used for treating BPH and hypertension. The most common side effect, as with all α-blockers is orthostatic hypotension and dizziness. Tamsulosin is another α-blocker that is used for BPH. It is not indicated for hypertension but it is capable of producing orthostatic hypotension.

Beta-antagonists (Beta-blockers)

β-adrenergic blockers were introduced in the 1960s. These sympatholytic agents have dominated cardiovascular pharmacology. They are among the most common drugs used in the treatment of cardiac disease and hypertension. A variety of drugs are available with β-blocking activity that may be distinguished by differing pharmacokinetic and pharmacodynamic properties. Examples of some of the drugs available and their diversity of actions are listed in Table 15-12. β-blockers can be classified according to whether they are selective or nonselective on the β_1- or β_2-receptor and whether they possess intrinsic sympathomimetic activity (ISA). For example, a β-blocker with selective properties for the β_1 receptor would bind to the cardiac receptors, whereas a nonselective β-blocker would bind to both β_1 (cardiac) and β_2 (vascular, bronchial smooth muscle, and metabolic) receptors. Nonselective β-antagonists are referred to as first generation β-blockers. These include propranolol, nadolol, sotalol, and timolol. Second generation drugs are those considered selective for β_1-adrenergic blockade. These include atenolol, esmolol, and metoprolol. Over the past decade, and because of their selectivity, the use of β-blockers has expanded to include the treatment of congestive heart failure (CHF). Recently, a new β-blockers subcategory has been developed, respectively, β-blocker with vasodilatory properties, such as in a new β-blocker, Nebivolol.[111] β-blockers are an important class of agents that are indicated for treatment of coronary artery disease, hypertension, heart failure, and tachyarrhythmias. They have a primary role in the treatment of patients after a myocardial infarction.[112] β-blockers have a direct effect on reducing the mortality in patients with heart failure due to left ventricular systolic dysfunction (bisoprolol, carvedilol, and metoprolol). Recently, a fourth agent has been used with similar favorable results, and this is nebivolol.[113,114] Nebivolol is a new β-blocker with an excellent β selectivity, and endothelium-dependent vasodilation secondary to L-arginine/NO pathway. Therefore, this novel drug has hemodynamic advantages and a better profile for side effects. Recent trials demonstrated a reduced morbidity and mortality in elderly patients with chronic heart failure, which makes this drug a very interesting option for the future treatment of cardiac disease, since for now it is available only in Europe.[111,115] Since there is data in the

TABLE 15-12. AUTONOMIC EFFECTS OF CALCIUM ENTRY BLOCKERS IN INTACT HUMANS

	Verapamil	Diltiazem	Nifedipine
Negative inotropic	+	0/+	0
Negative chronotropic	+	0/+	0
Negative dromotropic	++++	+++	0
Coronary vasodilation	++	+++	++++
Systemic vasodilation	++	++	++++
Bronchodilation	0/+		0/+

medical literature that β-blockers reduce the incidence of perioperative myocardial infarction, there is an increased interest in using these agents perioperatively in high risk patients undergoing vascular and other high risk surgical procedures[116] (see Chapter 39 Anesthesia for Vascular Surgery).

Selective β-blockade is of great benefit in treatment of patients with obstructive airway disease, diabetes, or peripheral vascular disease. However, it must be emphasized that specificity is a relative term and not absolute. Nonselective blocking effects may be seen in all tissues if higher blood levels are reached with "selective" drugs. For example, the use of β_1-selective blockers in patients with obstructive or reactive airway disease remains controversial. Patients with reactive airway disease may develop serious reductions in ventilatory function even with β_1-selective antagonists, but these circumstances are rare, so these drugs can be employed for large categories of patients. Other drugs are available for treatment of supraventricular arrhythmias and hypertension in asthmatics. Sympathetic activation generally results in increased circulating glucose levels secondary to enhanced glycogenolysis, lipolysis, and gluconeogenesis. Administration of β_2-blockers to insulin-dependent diabetics reduces their ability to recover from hypoglycemic episodes (see Chapter 46 Endocrine Function).

In patients receiving chronic β-blocker therapy, the drug should be continued throughout the perioperative and postoperative period[116] (see Chapter 39 Anesthesia for Vascular Surgery). Acute withdrawal of β-antagonists may produce a hemodynamic withdrawal syndrome and induce tachycardia.[28] HR is a major determinant of myocardial oxygen demands. Tachycardia is known to increase the risk of poor outcome in patients with ischemic heart disease; therefore, hemodynamic control of HR and BP (work) is important in reducing perioperative risk. Several studies have shown the benefits of prophylactic β-blockade with atenolol in patients at risk for ischemic cardiac disease.[117] The reduction in perioperative morbidity and mortality in these groups of patients was significant.[118–123] Recent data suggest that the use of β-blocker alone is not effective, unless tight heart rate control is present (less than 80 beats/min perioperatively). For this purpose a combination of drugs may be required; but further studies are underway which may indeed establish the best clinical practice.[119,124–128] The much anticipated POISE study proved that perioperative β-blockade does indeed reduce the risk of cardiac events but increased the risk of all-cause mortality and major strokes. Debated subjects regarding the concerning results included the dose of atenolol used, the value of blood pressure, the risk of perioperative anemia, and the value of acceptable blood pressure before administration of the next dose, still persist, and the use of β-blocker in the perioperative period became questionable for a brief period. While the European consensus accepts a systolic blood pressure of 100 mm Hg, the American College of Cardiology/American College of Cardiology Foundation Guidelines suggest that the next dose of β-blocker should be administered in the absence of hypotension. Clinicians have to decide what value is appropriate and individualized. Further larger study of 38,779 patients over a 12 year period by Wallace et al. showed that either starting of continuing the treatment with β-blocker does reduce the mortality in high risk patients at 30 days and 1 year, while withdrawal of the perioperative β-blockade in patients with known coronary artery disease, peripheral vascular disease, or with two risk factors for coronary artery disease including age over 60 years, diabetes, hypertension, hyperlipidemia, or smoking. Further studies are necessary to identify the best timing for treatment initiation and which class of β-blocker has more clinical impact.[129–131]

Several of the β-blockers listed in Table 15-12 also have a local anesthetic-like effect on myocardial membranes at high doses. This effect is similar to that of quinidine in that phase 0 of the cardiac action potential is depressed slowing conduction. This membrane stabilizing activity is caused by the D-isomer, whereas the L-isomer is responsible for β-blocking activity. The clinical significance of membrane-stabilizing activity is unclear.

Propranolol

Propranolol is the prototypical β-blocking drug against which all others are compared. It is nonselective and has no ISA but does have membrane-stabilizing activity at higher doses. It is available in both IV and oral forms. The IV dose is usually 0.5 to 1 mg repeated every 5 minutes up to a total of 5 mg with careful titration to effect.[58] It is highly lipophilic and is metabolized by the liver to more water-soluble metabolites, one of which, 17-OH propranolol, has weak β-blocking activity. There is a significant first-pass effect by the liver after oral administration of the drug. It is highly protein-bound, and the free drug level may be altered by other highly bound drugs. The elimination half-life is approximately 4 hours, but the pharmacologic half-life is around 10 hours. Hemodynamic effects include decreased HR and contractility. The major factors contributing to the decrease in blood pressure by propranolol are decreased CO and renin release. Systemic vascular resistance may increase upon acute administration owing to blockade of β_2 receptors in the peripheral vasculature. With chronic administration; however, peripheral vascular resistance decreases. This is thought to be secondary to decreased renin release and, possibly, decreased central SNS outflow. Complications with the use of propranolol include bradycardia, heart block, worsening of congestive heart failure, bronchospasm, and sedation.[132] During anesthesia with halothane, it may cause severe bradydysrhythmias. Due to the fact that it is not cardioselective, most clinicians are moving away from the routine use of propranolol, and instead using the selective alternatives such as metoprolol, or atenolol.

Metoprolol

Metoprolol is a relatively selective β-blocking drug with β-blocking effects at moderate and high doses. It has neither ISA nor membrane-stabilizing activity. It has a possible advantage in patients with reactive airway disease at oral doses up to 100 mg/day. The initial IV dose is 1.25 to 5 mg every 6 to 12 hours. For myocardial infarction the dose is 2 to 5 mg every 2 minutes for three doses, followed by 50 mg orally every 6 hours, with careful monitoring of the heart rate while the loading dose is being administered.[58] It is mostly metabolized in the liver, with only about 5% excreted unchanged in the urine. The elimination half-life is 3.5 hours. It is available in IV as well as oral form; therefore, it is commonly recommended prior to surgery and anesthesia.[113]

Atenolol

Atenolol is similar to metoprolol in that it is relatively cardioselective and has no ISA or membrane-stabilizing activity. It is less lipophilic, however, and is eliminated primarily by renal excretion. The starting dose is 5 mg over 5 minutes IV, and 25 to 50 mg/day oral administration.[58] The elimination half-life is 6 to 7 hours. The lack of first-pass metabolism results in more predictable blood levels after oral dosing. The main advantage of this drug is its once a day dosing.[117,133]

Esmolol

Esmolol has several uses in the perioperative period.[134] The most unique feature of the drug is the ester function incorporated into the phenoxypropanolamine structure. This allows for rapid degradation by esterases in the red blood cells and a resultant pharmacologic half-life of 10 to 20 minutes. Esmolol is cardioselective and appears to have little effect on bronchial or vascular tone at doses that decrease HR in humans. It has been used successfully in low doses in patients with asthma but caution is again advised when using β-blockers in these patients. The IV bolus dose is 0.25 to 0.5 mg/kg, and a continuous infusion loading dose is 500 μg/kg/min over 1 to 2 minutes, with a maintenance of 50 to 200 μg/kg/min.[58] Esmolol is metabolized rapidly in the blood by an esterase located in the red blood cell cytoplasm. It is different from the plasma cholinesterase and is not inhibited to a significant degree by physostigmine or echothiophate but is markedly inhibited by sodium fluoride. There are no apparent important clinical interactions between esmolol and other ester-containing drugs. At the highest infusion rates (500 μg/kg/min), esmolol does not prolong neuromuscular blockade by succinylcholine. Esmolol has proven to be useful in the perioperative period because it can be administered intravenously and its short half-life. This feature permits a trial of β-blockade in doubtful situations. Esmolol has been shown to blunt the response to intubation of the trachea and is moderately effective in treating postoperative hypertension.[135–137] Most reported studies in humans have used doses of 50 to 500 μg/kg/min. The most beneficial approach seems to be a loading dose of 500 μg/kg over 30 seconds, followed by continuous infusion of 50 to 300 μg/kg/min. Peak blockade appears to occur within 5 minutes. On discontinuation of the infusion, serum levels decline with an elimination half-life of 9 minutes.

Timolol

Timolol is also non-cardioselective with little ISA and no membrane-stabilizing activity. It is the only β-blocker used as the l-isomer rather than the racemic mixture. It is five to ten times as potent as propranolol. Hepatic metabolism accounts for approximately 66% of its elimination, and another 20% is found unchanged in the urine. The elimination half-life is 5.6 hours, and the pharmacologic half-life is approximately 15 hours. It was first used topically for treatment of glaucoma but is now used in hypertension and has been shown to decrease the risk of reinfarction and death following myocardial infarction. Its hemodynamic effects and side effects are similar to those of other β-blockers. The anesthesiologist should also be aware that timolol eye drops may be absorbed systemically and cause bradycardia and hypotension that are refractory to treatment with atropine.[138]

Other Beta-blockers

Other beta-blockers include drugs such as nadolol (non-cardioselective β-blocker), acebutolol (cardioselective β-blocker with ISA and membrane-stabilizing activity), pindolol (nonselective β-blocker with membrane-stabilizing activity and ISA), betaxolol (cardiac selective), penbutolol (nonselective with some intrinsic sympathetic activity), and carteolol (nonselective) are used for treatment of hypertension or heart rate control.

Mixed Antagonists

Labetalol

Labetalol is an antihypertensive drug with blocking activity at both α- and β-receptors. The relative α/β-blocking effects are dependent upon the route of administration. After oral administration, the ratio of α/β effectiveness is 1:3; however, when given intravenously, it is 1:7. The α effects are primarily on α_1-receptors, whereas the β effects on nonselective. Hemodynamic effects consist primarily of decreased peripheral resistance and decreased or unchanged HR with little change in CO. Serum renin activity is decreased. Maintenance of lower HRs in the presence of decreased systemic blood pressure is beneficial in controlling the myocardial oxygen supply/demand ratio and is a major benefit of labetalol in patients with coronary artery disease.

Labetalol is eliminated by hepatic glucuronide conjugation. The elimination half-life after IV administration is 5.5 hours and 6 to 8 hours after oral use. Elimination is not markedly prolonged in patients with hepatic or renal failure. Another advantage of the drug is the ability to convert from IV to oral forms of the same drug after the patient is stable. For treatment of hypertension when used as a bolus, the initial dose is 2.5 to 10 mg IV over 2 minutes, then repeat every 10 minutes to a total of 30 mg. When used as a continuous infusion, it is usually started at 0.5 to 2.0 mg/min and titrated to effect. Since there is an enhanced effect by inhalation anesthetics, these doses should be decreased when used intraoperatively.

Complications and contraindications are similar to those for the β-blockers. Labetalol should be used with caution in patients with compromised myocardial function because it may worsen heart failure. Also, owing to β-blocking activity, the drug may induce bronchospasm in asthmatics. As with other β-blockers, abrupt withdrawal is not recommended. Labetalol is favored by many anesthesiologists for use in the perioperative period, since it rapidly decreases both blood pressure, and to some extent also the heart rate, it can be used as a bolus, and ultimately achieves normotension within few minutes of initial administration.[139,140]

Calcium Channel Blockers

Calcium is regarded as the universal messenger in cells and plays a critical role in a number of biologic processes. It is involved in blood coagulation, a broad array of enzymatic reactions, metabolism of bone, neuromuscular transmission, electrical activation of various excitable membranes as well as endocrine secretion, and muscle contraction. Calcium initiates several physiologic events in the specialized automatic and conducting cells in the heart. It is involved in the genesis of the cardiac action potential, and it links excitation to contraction and controls energy stores and utilization. Movement of extracellular calcium across membranes also governs the function of smooth muscle in bronchi and in coronary, pulmonary, and systemic arterioles. Its roles in adrenergic effector response have been outlined in detail (see Molecular Pharmacology and Effector Response). Membrane calcium channels are known to provide a pathway for calcium influx across cell membranes that differ from calcium efflux movements associated with active pumps or exchange. The inward calcium channel exhibits two distinguishing properties: (1) selectivity in that they have the ability to distinguish between ion species and (2) excitability in that they have the property of responding to changes in membrane potential. Separate, ion-specific, channels for sodium and calcium influx exist. The status of these channels can vary to produce three kinetic states: Resting, activated, and inactivated.

Classification of calcium channel blockers has been difficult since their discovery. They were initially thought to be β-adrenergic blocking drugs because of their sympatholytic action. Later they were called calcium antagonists.

14 It is clear, however, that calcium antagonists are not true pharmacologic antagonists of calcium. Instead, they interact with the cell membrane to control the intracellular concentration of calcium. The correct terminology for this group of drugs appears to be calcium channel blockers. The molecular structures of three clinically useful calcium entry blockers are seen in Figure 15-16. These drugs produce vasodilatation, depress cardiac conduction velocity (dromotropism), depress contractility (inotropism), and decrease HR (chronotropism). All calcium channel blockers do this, but with varying degrees of potency in the intact human and in vitro (Table 15-11). Thus, despite their similarities, these drugs cannot be considered therapeutically interchangeable. The useful pharmacologic effects of the calcium channel blockers have been confined almost solely to the cardiovascular system.[123] The drugs are all absorbed via the gastrointestinal tract, but the extensive first-pass hepatic extraction of verapamil limits its bioavailability orally (Table 15-13). Onset of action is equivalent for all three drugs and is consistent with rapid membrane transport. All three drugs are extensively protein-bound and subject to the effect of changes in plasma protein concentration and competition from other protein-bound drugs and metabolites, but final elimination of verapamil and nifedipine is primarily renal. While its usage increases, so does the risk for toxicity and overdose, especially in patients with liver dysfunction or pediatric population. In case of overdose the hepatic enzymes may become saturated allowing for increased quantities of active drug to be present in circulation. Without a consistent antidote, signs of hypotension, bradycardia, even tachycardia, conduction abnormalities, altered mental status, seizures, respiratory depression, hyperglycemia, and metabolic acidosis should be watched for.[141]

Verapamil

Verapamil is a calcium channel blocker that is administered intravenously for terminating supraventricular tachydysrhythmias. Nearly all forms of supraventricular tachydysrhythmias are caused by reentry using either the sinoatrial or the AV node as part of the circuit. Verapamil terminates these cardiac dysrhythmias by decreasing nodal conductivity and converting the unidirectional block of reentry to a bi-directional block. Verapamil does not alter the action potential upstroke in fibers whose resting membrane potential is more negative than –60 mV, that is, fast action potentials. It does slow down or prevent depolarization in cardiac tissue with a resting membrane potential that is less negative than –50 mV, that is, calcium-dependent upstroke. Verapamil, therefore, has profound effects on pacemaker cells, which depend on the calcium current for depolarization. It depresses the rate of sinus discharge, reduces conduction velocity, and increases refractoriness of the AV node. A dose-dependent increase in the PR interval and AV interval is produced on the electrocardiogram. This has been described as a quinidine-like effect similar to that produced by Class IA antidysrhythmic drugs

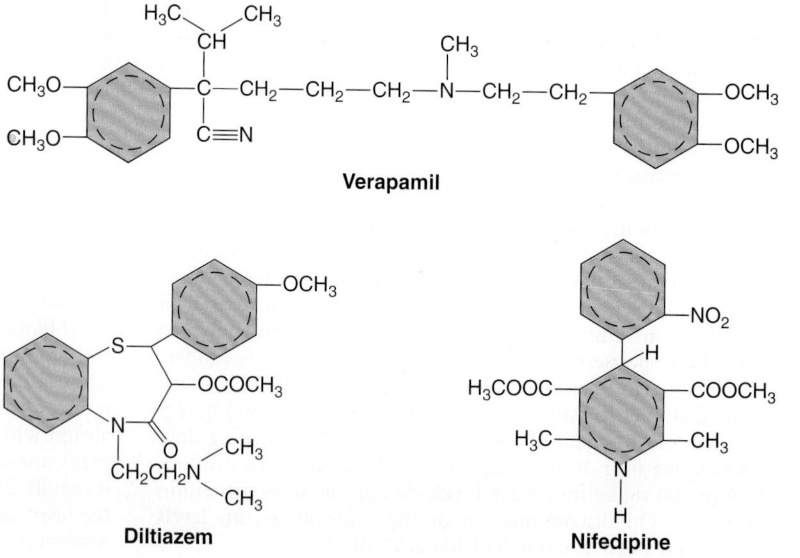

FIGURE 15-16. Structural formulas of the calcium entry blockers demonstrate dissimilar structures consistent with their dissimilar electrophysiologic and pharmacologic properties. They also share some similarities but cannot be considered therapeutically interchangeable. Nifedipine and nitrendipine are structurally similar and are both potent vasodilators.

TABLE 15-13. COMPARATIVE PHARMACOLOGY OF CALCIUM ENTRY BLOCKERS

	Verapamil	Diltiazem	Nifedipine
Dose			
Oral	80–160 mg tid	60–90 mg tid	10–20 mg tid
IV	75–150 μg/kg	75–150 μg/kg	5–15 μg/kg
Absorption			
Oral (%)	>90%	>90%	>90%
Bioavailability			
Oral (%)	<20%	? <20%	60–70%[a]
Onset			
Oral	15–20 min	20–30 min	15–20 min
IV	1 min	?	1 min
Sublingual	—	—	3 min
Peak Effect			
Oral	5 hr	30 min	1–2 hr
IV	5–30 min	?	1–3 hr
Elimination half-life	2–7 hr	4 hr	4–5 hr
Plasma protein binding	90%	80%	90%
Metabolism	70%	Deacetylated	80% to lactone
	First-pass hepatic		
Elimination			
Renal	75%	35%	70%
Gastrointestinal (liver)	15%	75%	<15%
Side effects	Constipation, headache, vertigo, hypotension, atrioventricular conduction disturbances	Headache, dizziness, flushing, atrioventricular conduction disturbances, constipation	Headache, hypotension, flushing, digital dysesthesias, leg edema

IV, intravenous.
[a]Light-sensitive.

(e.g., procainamide), which are also effective for supraventricular dysrhythmia. In contrast to procainamide, verapamil does not increase the QRS or Q–T interval because it lacks activity on the sodium-dependent action potentials.

Verapamil is a first-line drug for treatment of supraventricular tachydysrhythmias (Table 15-11) (see Chapter 58 Cardiopulmonary Resuscitation). The incidence of successful termination of paroxysmal atrial tachycardia with verapamil in adults has approached 90%. It is also effective in treating atrial fibrillation and atrial flutter by either converting to a sinus rhythm or slowing the ventricular response. The ventricular rate will slow down as a result of decreased conduction velocity through the AV node even when conversion is not produced. Caution must be exercised in treating patients when the underlying cause of the atrial tachycardia, atrial fibrillation, or atrial flutter is the Wolff–Parkinson–White syndrome.[43] Verapamil may terminate tachydysrhythmia by its specific depressant effects on the AV node, which is one limb of the reentrant pathway. It may also increase conduction velocity in the accessory tract, in which case the HR may increase. Verapamil has no adverse effects on bronchial asthma or obstructive lung disease, and may be selected over propranolol in patients with these conditions. It should be avoided in patients with sick sinus syndrome, AV block, and the presence of heart failure, unless the heart failure is the result of a supraventricular tachycardia. Verapamil has been effective in terminating ventricular tachycardias and premature depolarizations in about two-thirds of the treatment trials when other drugs have failed. It can be used also as an antihypertensive.[92,142] The important side effects of verapamil are directly related to its predominant pharmacologic action (see Table 15-11). It may produce unwanted AV conduction delays and bradycardia, resulting in cardiovascular collapse. Verapamil must be used carefully, if at all, in the presence of propranolol. The combined effect has produced complete heart block in animals and humans. It must be used carefully in digitalized patients for the same reason. No such interactions exist with nifedipine. The combination of β-blockade and nifedipine may be beneficial in patients with ischemic heart disease because the reflex tachycardia seen with nifedipine can be countered with β-blockade.

Nifedipine

Nifedipine is the most potent calcium entry blocker when tested in isolated tissue preparations. It is an equipotent cardiac depressant and vasodilator. Depression of inotropism and cardiac conduction, however, is not evident in the intact human. It does not affect baroreflex mechanisms and, as a result, the marked vasodilation is accompanied by increased SNS tone and afterload reduction (see Table 15-11).[28] A compensatory tachycardia may result, and CO may actually increase as a result of the afterload reduction. The most specific therapeutic application for nifedipine is coronary vasospasm (variant of Prinzmetal's angina) (see Chapter 38 Anesthesia for Cardiac Surgery). It has been more successful than nitroglycerin for this purpose because it produces a more profound and predictable coronary vasodilation. It has also been extremely useful in other types of ischemic heart disease ranging from unstable angina to myocardial infarction. The decrease in myocardial oxygen demand that results from the reduced afterload and reduced left ventricular volume appears to be the mechanism for the relief of angina. Coronary vasodilation is another factor, but it is not known if this is the antianginal effect in patients with coronary artery disease. The dilating effect may last only 5 minutes, but the antianginal effect may last more than 1 hour. As an antihypertensive the usual dosage is oral administration of 10 to 20 mg/day.[58]

Diltiazem

The hemodynamic effects of diltiazem lie somewhere between those of verapamil and nifedipine. It is less potent than either of these two agents. Diltiazem is a good coronary artery dilator but a poor peripheral vasodilator. It often produces bradycardia and delayed conduction, and reflex tachycardia is not a problem. It appears to be an effective oral drug for the treatment of coronary disease in which cardiac dysrhythmias are troublesome. Cardiac dysrhythmias are noticeably a part of the clinical picture in patients suffering from coronary spasm. Intravenous administration of diltiazem is effective therapy for supraventricular tachycardias including PSVT, atrial fibrillation, atrial flutter, and reentrant tachycardias. Like verapamil, diltiazem acts by prolonging AV nodal conduction. The peripheral vascular effects of diltiazem, though, are less severe, making it a more desirable therapeutic choice in most cases. A bolus dose of 0.25 mg/kg is administered over 2 minutes and may be repeated at 0.35 mg/kg if necessary after 15 minutes. An infusion of 5 to 15 mg/hr may be necessary to maintain the reduction of HR. The new 2005 ACLS Guidelines recommends the use of calcium channel blockers for a variety of supraventricular arrhythmias, and due to diminished peripheral vasodilation, which implies limited effect on the arterial blood pressure, diltiazem appears to be one of the best options for management of tachyarrhythmias[43] (see Chapter 58 Cardiopulmonary Resuscitation).

Nicardipine

Nicardipine hydrochloride is a calcium channel blocker that can be administered orally and intravenously. It is the only calcium channel blocker that can be titrated intravenously to be used as an antihypertensive agent, the usual dose being 1 to 2 μg/kg/min or 5 mg/hour.[58] Nicardipine is a smooth muscle relaxant producing vasodilation of peripheral and coronary arteries. It has a rapid onset of action, and the major effects last 10 to 15 minutes. Toxic metabolic products are not produced. It has minimal cardiodepressant effects and does not decrease the rate of the sinus node pacemaker or slow conduction through the AV node, but one should use it cautiously in patients having acute myocardial ischemia. Renal failure does not affect the dosage, but the dosage should be reduced in the elderly and those with hepatic dysfunction. It is compatible with most crystalloid solutions. Side effects of nicardipine include headache, lightheadedness, flushing, and hypotension. Reflex tachycardia is not a frequent finding with nicardipine, as is the case with nitroprusside, hydralazine, or nifedipine.[139,140,143]

Nimodipine

Nimodipine is highly lipophilic. It has a greater vasodilating effect on cerebral arteries than on vessels elsewhere because of its lipophilism, which promotes crossing the blood–brain barrier. Clinical studies demonstrate a favorable effect on the severity of neurologic deficits caused by cerebral vasospasm following subarachnoid hemorrhage. However, no radiographic evidence has been presented that nimodipine either prevents or relieves spasm of these arteries. The mechanism for clinical improvement is not known. It is an oral drug that is rapidly absorbed, with a T-terminal half-life of approximately 8 to 9 hours. The usual dose is 60 mg every 4 hours for 21 days.[58] Earlier elimination rates are much more rapid, which results in a need to redose every 4 hours. The bioavailability of an oral dose is only 13%. Dosage should be reduced in patients with hepatic dysfunction. The primary indication for nimodipine is for the improvement of neurologic deficits caused by vasospasm following subarachnoid hemorrhage from a ruptured cerebral aneurysm.[139,140,144]

Felodipine and Clevidipine

While felodipine is a daily drug that can be administered for blood pressure control, clevidipine is a new third generation ultra-short acting intravenous calcium channel blocker used for management of moderate to severe hypertension. The reason for the short duration of clevidipine is the ester hydrolysis by blood esterases to form inactive metabolites, which is independent of liver and renal function. Clevidipine has the potential to protect against organ reperfusion injury and may decrease the severity of low-flow myocardial ischemia, the infarct size, and maintain renal function.[145,146] Clevidipine is emerging as a novel alternative to nitroglycerin, sodium nitroprusside, and nicardipine in cardiac patients due to the fact that it is easily titratable, and short-acting. As shown in the Eclipse trial, it does not increase the risk for 30-day incidence of death, myocardial infarction, stroke, or renal dysfunction. Patients treated with clevidipine had a lower mortality rate at 30 days than those treated with nitroprusside.[147–149] Although expensive, due to the fact that it has to be discarded every 4 hours due to its lipid formulation, clevidipine demonstrates efficacy and safety in perioperative hypertension. More studies are necessary to evaluate its association with atrial fibrillation, hypotension, tachycardia, and renal failure.[150]

Calcium Channel Blockers and Anesthesia

Evidence indicates that halothane depresses slow channel kinetics. All of the potent inhalation anesthetics behave in a similar fashion in that they depress myocardial contractility and vascular tone in a dose-related manner. Most studies indicate that the calcium entry blockers and inhalation anesthetics exert additive effects on the inward calcium current.[151] Opioid anesthetics do not appear to add anything to the effects of the calcium entry blockers. Calcium channel blockers appear to augment the effects of both depolarizing and nondepolarizing muscle relaxants.[152] These observations serve as a word of caution because their clinical significance has not been defined. Prolonged apnea and relaxation have been reported when verapamil was used to treat a supraventricular tachycardia in a patient with Duchenne muscular dystrophy.[153] One must be aware that calcium channel blockers may have side effects such as hypotension, in cases of overdosage, headaches, facial flushing, dizziness, ankle edema, constipation, and may even induce angina, therefore their administration in perioperative period, when dehydration is a common occurrence should be closely monitored.[154] Calcium entry blockers should be continued until the time of surgery to maintain control of angina pectoris, hypertension, or cardiac dysrhythmia.[125] In addition, the use of calcium channel blockers in the perioperative period appears to induce a beneficial effect of decreasing cardiac complications unrelated to cardiac surgical procedures[155] (see Chapter 22 Preoperative Patient Assessment and Management). Verapamil may increase the toxicity of digoxin, the benzodiazepines, carbamazepine, oral hypoglycemics, and possibly quinidine and theophylline.[156] Cardiac failure, AV conduction disturbances, and sinus bradycardia may be more frequent with concurrent use of β-blockers. Severe hypotension and bradycardia may occur with bupivacaine. Decreased lithium effect and lithium neurotoxicity have both been reported with the concurrent use of verapamil.[157] The effects of verapamil may also be increased by cimetidine.

Vasodilators

Most antihypertensive drugs blunt the ANS or its effector organs or cause reflex increases in ANS outflow. Anesthetic agents may also inhibit ANS tone to some degree and might therefore have additive effects with antihypertensive drugs. In addition, patients with hypertension may exhibit greater lability in blood pressure intraoperatively and rebound hypertension in the postoperative period. A rational approach to their perioperative use includes decisions as to holding or continuing them preoperatively, possible interactions with anesthetic drugs, and resumption of treatment postoperatively.

Angiotensin-converting Enzyme Inhibitors (ACE-I)

The renin–angiotensin system is integrally related to the ANS in controlling blood pressure (see Fig. 15-12) (see Chapter 46 Endocrine Function). The central role of the renin–angiotensin–aldosterone system in the regulation of fluid balance and hemodynamics was not fully appreciated until the discovery and clinical application of inhibitors of the angiotensin-converting enzyme (ACE). Captopril, enalapril, and lisinopril inhibit the converting enzyme and thereby prevent the conversion of angiotensin I to the active angiotensin II. These drugs have been highly effective in the treatment of all levels of essential hypertension as well as renovascular and malignant hypertension. The cardiovascular effects normally involve only decreased peripheral vascular resistance. CO may remain normal or increase while the filling pressure remains unchanged. Thus, these drugs have been effective in the management of congestive heart failure as well.[47] There is usually no increase in SNS tone in response to the lowered blood pressure. ACE inhibition generally results in reductions in angiotensin–aldosterone, NE, and plasma antidiuretic hormone. This suppression is accompanied by a decrease in aldosterone and an improvement in cumulative plasma potassium levels, which are beneficial in both congestive heart failure and hypertension. It can be concluded that the major humoral responses to chronic congestive heart failure, even overlooking the effects of the diuretics, are affected by the release of angiotensin, aldosterone, and increased SNS tone. Captopril, the first orally active compound, has proven highly effective in the treatment of all levels of hypertension and congestive heart. Enalapril is a second-generation (non-sulfhydryl) ACE inhibitor. The omission of the sulfhydryl group possibly diminishes side effects. Both captopril and enalapril combine a high degree of clinical efficacy with a low rate of side effects. Both are eliminated via renal excretion and should be given in reduced doses to patients with renal dysfunction. Captopril has a shorter half-life and requires more frequent dosing than enalapril. Enalapril has to be converted by esterase in the liver and other tissues into the active compound enalaprilat. Lisinopril is one of these ACE inhibitors that is absorbed as the active form and is very long acting. The ACE inhibitors are associated with few side effects and are popular in treating hypertension. Captopril may produce reversible neutropenia, dermatitis, and angioedema. Enalapril produces syncope, headache, and dizziness in about 1% of elderly patients. All ACE inhibitors may cause hypotension in patients who are hypovolemic and taking diuretic therapy. The hypotensive effects are also enhanced by the concomitant use of calcium channel blockers. The ACE inhibitors blunt the hypokalemic effects of thiazide diuretics and may magnify the potassium-sparing effects of spironolactone, triamterene, and amiloride. In addition, nonsteroidal anti-inflammatory drugs, including aspirin, may magnify the potassium-retaining effects of ACE inhibitors. ACE-I are now a mainstay in treatment of patients with heart failure and decreased ejection fraction, since it increases their survival.[88] For patients with heart failure and normal left ventricular ejection fraction the first line of treatment are loop diuretics in combination with β-blockers and (ACE) inhibitors.[123] In the perioperative period, the ACE inhibitors have been associated with significant hypotension, which at times requires additional vasopressors to sustain systemic blood pressure,[158] such as when separating from cardiopulmonary bypass.

A new class of drugs, namely angiotensin–receptor blockers (ARBs) were developed by inhibiting directly the effects of the hormone angiotensin II. One could expect the same effectiveness, with less side effects like cough, angioneurotic edema, rash, etc.[159] On the other hand, there are data that this class of drugs may have some beneficial effects on decreasing the renal deterioration in diabetic patients. In patients with or without heart failure, the cardioprotective and renoprotective effects appear similar between the ARBs and ACE-I. In patients who cannot tolerate the ACE-I, especially patients with end-organ damage such as cardiovascular disease or diabetes mellitus, the use of ARBs is a valuable alternative.[160–162]

Hydralazine

Hydralazine is the most commonly used vasodilator. It can be given by the intramuscular, intravenous, and oral routes to achieve an optimum blood pressure control. It relaxes smooth muscle tone directly, without interacting with adrenergic or cholinergic receptors. The mechanism of action is unknown. It is most potent in coronary, splanchnic, renal, and cerebral vessels, causing increased blood flow in each of these organs. The decrease in cardiac afterload is beneficial, but, unfortunately, there is usually a concomitant reflex tachycardia that may be severe. It is commonly combined with a β-blocker such as propranolol. Hydralazine is metabolized by hepatic acetylation, and oral bioavailability may be low owing to first-pass metabolism. The elimination half-life is about 4 hours, but the pharmacologic half-life is much longer as a result of avid binding of the drug to smooth muscle. The effective half-life is approximately 100 hours. Side effects include a lupus-like syndrome, drug fever, skin rash, pancytopenia, and peripheral neuropathy. The IV dose for perioperative use is 5 to 10 mg in an IV bolus every 15 to 20 minutes until blood pressure control is achieved. It may also be given 10 to 40 mg intramuscularly, but the response is slower.[92,139,163]

Sodium Nitroprusside

Sodium nitroprusside is an extremely potent vasodilator that is available only for intravenous administration (see Chapter 38 Anesthesia for Cardiac Surgery). It acts directly on vascular smooth muscle, causing both arterial and venous dilation. The action of sodium nitroprusside on both venous and arterial sides of the circulation causes decreases in cardiac preload as well as afterload.[123,164] This results in decreased cardiac work; however, it has been suggested that sodium nitroprusside may further compromise ischemic myocardium in the presence of occlusive coronary artery disease by shunting blood away from the ischemic zone.[165] Other potential and deleterious side effects include pulmonary vasodilation with an increased ventilation–perfusion mismatch and with resultant hypoxia, and temporary decrease in platelet function.[166] Sodium nitroprusside is useful during the perioperative period. It lowers blood pressure within 1 to 2 minutes, with the effect dissipating within 2 minutes after infusion is stopped. It is extremely potent and should be administered through a central venous line by infusion pump while continuously monitoring arterial pressure. The starting dose is 0.25 to 0.5 μg/kg/min. It can be increased slowly as needed to control blood pressure, but chances for toxicity are greater if the dose of 2 μg/kg/min is exceeded. The dose required for steady state–induced hypotension is variable. The hypotensive effects of sodium nitroprusside may be potentiated by inhalation anesthetics and blood loss; therefore, close perioperative monitoring is essential. It is commonly used to induce hypotension for decreasing blood loss in patients predisposed to major hemorrhage.[139]

Chemically, sodium nitroprusside consists of a ferrous iron moiety bound with five cyanide molecules and one nitric group. The ferrous iron reacts with sulfhydryl groups in red blood cells and releases cyanide. Cyanide is reduced to thiocyanate in the liver and excreted in the urine. The half-life of thiocyanate is 4 days, and it accumulates in the presence of renal failure. Administration of high doses of sodium nitroprusside can result in cyanide toxicity. The cyanide molecule binds to cytochrome oxidase, interfering with electron transport and causing cellular hypoxia. Toxicity can be recognized by the triad of tachyphylaxis (increasing tolerance to the drug dose), elevated mixed venous PaO_2, and metabolic acidosis. The possible treatments of cyanide toxicity consist of (1) administration of amyl nitrate (by inhalation or directly into the anesthesia circuit), (2) infusion of sodium nitrite, and (3) administration of sodium thiosulfate.

Nitroglycerin

Nitroglycerin, or glyceril trinitrate is a venodilator used to treat myocardial ischemia (see Chapter 38 Anesthesia for Cardiac Surgery). Its predominant action is on venules, causing increased venous capacitance and decreased cardiac preload. Effects on the arterial side are minimal except at very high doses. The usual IV dose is 1 to 3 μg/kg/min. Upon IV administration effects can be seen within 2 minutes, and they usually resolve within 5 minutes of discontinuing the drug. Side effects are minimal, and there is no potential for cyanide toxicity as with nitroprusside. Use of nitroglycerin for control of perioperative hypertension has been reported but because of its relatively weak arteriolar action it is not as useful as other drugs as an antihypertensive agent.[123,164] In obstetric patients with preeclampsia; however, it may be chosen over nitroprusside to circumvent potential cyanide toxicity to the fetus.[167,168]

Nesiritide

Nesiritide is a recombinant form of a human B-type natriuretic peptide (BNP). It is identical with the endogenous hormone released by the ventricles in situations characterized by volume overload, and increase wall tension. Nesiritide acts on guanylate cyclase the same way as nitric oxide, and therefore has beneficial effects on hemodynamics by venous and arterial vasodilation, including coronary vasodilation. It is more effective than nitroglycerin in decreasing right atrial pressure, pulmonary capillary wedge pressure, systemic vascular resistance, ultimately improving the cardiac output. The possible side effects include hypotension, headache, and renal dysfunction. The dose is 2 μg/kg bolus, followed by continuous infusion of 0.01 μg/kg/min that may be increased to a maximum of 0.03 μg/kg/min, with the most significant side effect being hypotension. The biologic effects last longer than expected from the drug's half-life. Nesiritide is beneficial for rapid improvement of dyspnea, and can be used in patients with decompensated heart failure, in addition to diuretic therapy for rapid improvement of symptoms. It appears to have favorable effects on hemodynamics by reducing the right atrial pressure and pulmonary occlusion pressure, and improves coronary artery blood flow. It appears to increase urine output, and significantly blunt the creatinine rise in patients with decompensated cardiac failure undergoing cardiac surgery. Although relatively small, studies and meta-analyses suggest that treatment with nesiritide may decrease mortality when compared to milrinone and dobutamine; however, further studies are warranted to further study this effect.[34,47,164]

References

1. Guyton AC, Hall JE. The autonomic nervous system and the adrenal medulla. In: Guyton AC, Hall JE, eds. *Textbook of Medical Physiology*. 12th ed. Philadelphia, PA: Saunders/Elsevier; 2011:729–742.
2. Eisenhofer G,. Sympathetic nerve function–assessment by radioisotope dilution analysis. *Clin Auton Res*. 2005;15:264–283.
3. Flacke WE, Flacke JW. Cholinergic and anticholinergic agents. In: Smith NT, Corbascio AN, eds. *Drug Interactions in Anesthesia*. 2nd ed. Philadelphia, PA: Lea & Febiger; 1986:160–175.
4. Guyton AC, Hall JE. Cardiac output, venous return, and their regulation. In: Guyton AC, Hall JE, eds. *Textbook of Medical Physiology*. Philadelphia, PA: Saunders/Elsevier; 2006:229–242.
5. Kapa S, Venkatachalam KL, Asirvatham SJ. The autonomic nervous system in cardiac electrophysiology: An elegant interaction and emerging concepts. *Cardiol Rev*. 2010;18:275–284.
6. Ajani AE, Yan BP. The mystery of coronary artery spasm. *Heart Lung Circ*. 2007;16:10–15.
7. Kawano H, Ogawa H. Endothelial dysfunction and coronary artery spasm. *Curr Drug Targets Cardiovasc Haematol Disord*. 2004;4:23–33.
8. Bevan JA. Some bases of differences in vascular response to sympathetic activity. *Circ Res*. 1979;45:161–171.
9. O'Rourke ST, Vanhoutte PM. Adrenergic and cholinergic regulation of bronchial vascular tone. *Am Rev Respir Dis*. 1992;146:S11–S14.
10. Pearl RG, Maze M, Rosenthal MH. Pulmonary and systemic hemodynamic effects of central venous and left atrial sympathomimetic drug administration in the dog. *J Cardiothorac Anesth*. 1987;1:29–35.
11. Sinski M, Lewandowski J, Abramczyk P, et al. Why study sympathetic nervous system? *J Physiol Pharmacol*. 2006;57(Suppl 11):79–92.
12. Civantos Calzada B, Aleixandre de Artiñano A. Alpha-adrenoceptor subtypes. *Pharmacol Res*. 2001;44:195–208.
13. Aubry ML, Davey MJ, Petch B. Cardioprotective and antidysrhythmic effects of alpha 1-adrenoceptor blockade during myocardial ischaemia and reperfusion in the dog. *J Cardiovasc Pharmacol*. 1985;7(suppl 6):S93–102.
14. Cohen RA, Shepherd JT, Vanhoutte PM. Effects of the adrenergic transmitter on epicardial coronary arteries. *Fed Proc*. 1984;43:2862–2866.
15. Baumgart D, Haude M, Görge G, et al. Augmented alpha-adrenergic constriction of atherosclerotic human coronary arteries. *Circulation*. 1999;99:2090–2097.
16. Griggs DM Jr, Chilian WM, Boatwright RB, et al. Evidence against significant resting alpha-adrenergic coronary vasoconstrictor tone. *Fed Proc*. 1984;43:2873–2877.
17. Heusch G, Baumgart D, Camici P, et al. Alpha-adrenergic coronary vasoconstriction and myocardial ischemia in humans. *Circulation*. 2000;101:689–694.
18. Lymperopoulos A, Rengo G, Koch WJ. Adrenal adrenoceptors in heart failure: Fine-tuning cardiac stimulation. *Trends Mol Med*. 2007;13:503–511.
19. Vanhoutte PM. Endothelial adrenoceptors. *J Cardiovasc Pharmacol*. 2001;38:796–808.
20. Tobata D, Takao K, Mochizuki M, et al. Effects of dopamine, dobutamine, amrinone and milrinone on regional blood flow in isoflurane anesthetized dogs. *J Vet Med Sci*. 2004;66:1097–1105.
21. Hilberman JM, Maseda J, Stinson EB, et al. The diuretic properties of dopamine in patients after open-heart operation. *Anesthesiology*. 1984;61:489–494.
22. Owall A, Gordon E, Lagerkranser M, et al. Clinical experience with adenosine for controlled hypotension during cerebral aneurysm surgery. *Anesth Analg*. 1987;66:229–234.
23. Brodde OE. Beta-adrenoceptors in cardiac disease. *Pharmacol Ther*. 1993;60:405–430.
24. Pitkänen M. Spinal (subarahnoid) neural blockade. In: Cousins MJ, Carr DB, Horlocker TT, Bridenbaugh PO, eds. *Cousins & Bridenbaugh's Neural Blockade in Clinical Anesthesia and Pain Medicine*. 4th ed. Philadelphia, PA: Lippincott Williams & Wilkins, a Wolters Kluwer Business; 2009:213–240.
25. Krum H, Sobotka P, Mahfoud F, et al. Device-based antihypertensive therapy: Therapeutic modulation of the autonomic nervous system. *Circulation*. 2011;123:209–215.
26. Valantine H. Cardiac allograft vasculopathy after heart transplantation: Risk factors and management. *J Heart Lung Transpl*. 2004;23:S187–S193.

27. Levy MN, Blattberg B. Effect of vagal stimulation on the overflow of norepinephrine into the coronary sinus during cardiac sympathetic nerve stimulation in the dog. *Circ Res.* 1976;38:81–84.
28. Stoelting RK, Hillier SC. *Pharmacology & Physiology in Anesthetic Practice.* 4th ed. Philadelphia, PA: Lippincott Williams & Wilkins; 2006.
29. Chamchad D, Horrow JC, Nakhamchik L, et al. Prophylactic glycopyrrolate prevents bradycardia after spinal anesthesia for Cesarean section: A randomized, double-blinded, placebo-controlled prospective trial with heart rate variability correlation. *J Clin Anesth.* 2011;23:361–366.
30. Dampney RA, Coleman MJ, Fontes MA, et al. Central mechanisms underlying short- and long-term regulation of the cardiovascular system. *Clin Exp Pharmacol Physiol.* 2002;29:261–268.
31. Spaulding BC, Choi SD, Gross JB, et al. The effect of physostigmine on diazepam-induced ventilatory depression: A double-blind study. *Anesthesiology.* 1984;61:551–554.
32. Miano TA, Crouch MA. Evolving role of vasopressin in the treatment of cardiac arrest. *Pharmacotherapy.* 2006;26:828–839.
33. Rooke GA, Freund PR, Jacobson AF. Hemodynamic response and change in organ blood volume during spinal anesthesia in elderly men with cardiac disease. *Anesth Analg.* 1997;85:99–105.
34. Poole-Wilson PA, Opie LH. Digitalis, acute inotropes, and inotropic dilators. Acute and chronic heart failure: Positive inotropes, vasodilators and digoxin. In: Opie LH, Gersh BJ, eds. *Drugs for the Heart.* 7th ed. Philadelphia, PA: Saunders/Elsevier; 2009:160–199.
35. Ngan Kee WD. prevention of maternal hypotension after regional anaesthesia for caesarian section. *Curr Opin Anaesthesiol.* 2010;23:304–309.
36. Ngan Kee WD, Khaw KS. Vasopressor in obstetrics: What should we be using? *Curr Opin Anaesthesiol.* 2006;19:238–243.
37. Macarthur A, Riley ET. Obstetric anesthesia controversies: Vasopressor choice for postspinal hypotension during cesarean delivery. *Int Anesthesiol Clin.* 2007; 45:115–132.
38. Dellinger RP, Levy MM, Carlet JM, et al. International Surviving Sepsis Campaign Guidelines Committee, American Association of Critical-Care Nurses, American College of Chest Physicians, American College of Emergency Physicians, Canadian Critical Care Society, European Society of Clinical Microbiology and Infectious Diseases, European Society of Intensive Care Medicine, European Respiratory Society, International Sepsis Forum, Japanese Association for Acute Medicine, Japanese Society of Intensive Care Medicine, Society of Critical Care Medicine, Society of Hospital Medicine, Surgical Infection Society, World Federation of Societies of Intensive and Critical Care Medicine. Surviving Sepsis Campaign: International guidelines for management of severe sepsis and septic shock: 2008. *Crit Care Med.* 2008;36(1):296–327.
39. Sladen RN. Oliguria in the ICU. Systematic approach to diagnosis and treatment. *Anesthesiol Clin North Am.* 2000;18:739–752, viii.
40. Johnston RR, Eger EI II, Wilson C. A comparative interaction of epinephrine with enflurane, isoflurane, and halothane in man. *Anesth Analg.* 1976;55:709–712.
41. Karl HW, Swedlow DB, Lee KW, et al. Epinephrine-halothane interactions in children. *Anesthesiology.* 1983;58:142–145.
42. Walker DM. Update on epinephrine (adrenaline) for pediatric emergencies. *Curr Opin Pediatr.* 2009;21:313–319.
43. 2010 American Heart Association Guidelines for Cardiopulmonary Resuscitation and Emergency Cardiovascular Care. *Circulation.* 2010;122:S640–S747.
44. Butterworth JF 4th, Prielipp RC, Royster RL, et al. Dobutamine increases heart rate more than epinephrine in patients recovering from aortocoronary bypass surgery. *J Cardiothorac Vasc Anesth.* 1992;6:535–541.
45. Zamanian RT, Haddad F, Doyle RL, et al. Management strategies for patients with pulmonary hypertension in the intensive care unit. *Crit Care Med.* 2007;35:2037–2050.
46. Asfar P, Hauser B, Radermacher P, et al. Catecholamines and vasopressin during critical illness. *Crit Care Clin.* 2006;22:131–149, vi–vii.
47. Shin DD, Brandimarte F, De Luca L, et al. Review of current and investigational pharmacologic agents for acute heart failure syndromes. *Am J Cardiol.* 2007;99:4A–23A.
48. Holmes CL, Walley KR. Vasoactive drugs for vasodilatory shock in ICU. *Curr Opin Crit Care.* 2009;15:398–402.
49. Venkataraman R. Can we prevent acute kidney injury? *Crit Care Med.* 2008; 36:S166–S171.
50. Friedrich JO, Adhikari N, Herridge MS, et al. Meta-analysis: Low-dose dopamine increases urine output but does not prevent renal dysfunction or death. *Ann Intern Med.* 2005;142:510–524.
51. Banic A, Krejci V, Erni D, et al. Effects of sodium nitroprusside and phenylephrine on blood flow in free musculocutaneous flaps during general anesthesia. *Anesthesiology.* 1999;90:147–155.
52. Bayram M, De Luca L, Massie MB, et al. Reassessment of dobutamine, dopamine, and milrinone in the management of acute heart failure syndromes. *Am J Cardiol.* 2005;96:47G–58G.
53. Parissis J, Farmakis D, Nieminen M. Classical inotropes and new cardiac enhancers. *Heart Fail Rev.* 2007;12:149–156.
54. Petersen JW, Felker GM. Inotropes in the management of acute heart failure. *Crit Care Med.* 2008;36:S106–S111.
55. Feneck R. Drugs for the perioperative control of hypertension: Current issues and future directions. *Drugs.* 2007;67:2023–2044.
56. Stone GW, McCullough PA, Tumlin JA, et al. Fenoldopam mesylate for the prevention of contrast-induced nephropathy: A randomized controlled trial. *JAMA.* 2003;290:2284–2291.
57. Zacharias M, Gilmore IC, Herbison GP, et al. Interventions for protecting renal function in the perioperative period. *Cochrane Database Syst Rev.* 2005;(3)CD003590.
58. Landoni G, Biondi-Zoccai GG, Tumlin JA, et al. Beneficial impact of fenoldopam in critically ill patients with or at risk for acute renal failure: A meta-analysis of randomized clinical trials. *Am J Kidney Dis.* 2007;49:56–68.
59. Westfall TC, Westfall DP. Adrenergic agonists and antagonists. In: Brunton L, Chabner B, Knollman B, eds. *Goodman and Gilman's The Pharmacological Basis of Therapeutics.* 12th ed. New York, NY: McGraw-Hill Medical; 2011:277–334.
60. Nader ND, Li CM, Dosluoglu HH, et al. Adjuvant therapy with intrathecal clonidine improves postoperative pain in patients undergoing coronary artery bypass graft. *Clin J Pain.* 2009;25:101–106.
61. Axelsson K, Gupta A. Local anaesthetic adjuvants: Neuraxial versus peripheral. *Curr Opin Anaesthesiol.* 2009;22:649–654.
62. Buvanendran A, Kroin JS. Useful adjuvants for postoperative pain management. *Best Pract Res Clin Anaesthesiol.* 2007;21:31–49.
63. Wallace AW, Galindez D, Salahieh A, et al. Effect of clonidine on cardiovascular morbidity and mortality after noncardiac surgery. *Anesthesiology.* 2004;101:284–293.
64. Aantaa R, Kanto J, Scheinin M, et al. Dexmedetomidine, an alpha 2-adrenoceptor agonist, reduces anesthetic requirements for patients undergoing minor gynecologic surgery. *Anesthesiology.* 1990;73:230–235.
65. Frost EA, Booij LH. Anesthesia in the patient for awake craniotomy. *Curr Opin Anaesthsiol.* 2007;20:331–335.
66. Rozet I. Anesthesia for functional neurosurgery: The role of dexmedetomidine. *Curr Opin Anaesthsiol.* 2008;21:537–543.
67. Szumita PM, Baroletti SA, Anger KE, et al. Sedation and analgesia in the intensive care unit: Evaluating the role of dexmedetomidine. *Am J Health Syst Pharm.* 2007;64:37–44.
68. Mantz J, Josserand J, Hamada S. Dexmedetomidine: New insights. *Eur J Anaesthsiol.* 2011;28:3–6.
69. Biccard BM, Goga S, de Beurs J. Dexmedetomidine and cardiac protection for non-cardiac surgery: A meta-analysis of randomised controlled trials. *Anaesthesia.* 2008;63:4–14.
70. Lee CR, Watkins ML, Patterson JH, et al. Vasopressin: A new target for the treatment of heart failure. *Am Heart J.* 2003;146:9–18.
71. Russell JA. Vasopressin in septic shock. *Crit Care Med.* 2007;35:S609–S615.
72. Diamond LM. Cardiopulmonary resuscitation and acute cardiovascular life support–a protocol review of the updated guidelines. *Crit Care Clin.* 2007;23: 873–880, vii.
73. Russell JA, Walley KR, Singer J, et al. Vasopressin versus norepinephrine infusion in patients with septic shock. *N Engl J Med.* 2008;358:877–887.
74. Barrett LK, Singer M, Clapp LH, et al. Vasopressin: Mechanisms of action on the vasculature in health and in septic shock. *Crit Care Med.* 2007;35:33–40.
75. Craig RL, Michael LW, Patterson JH, et al. Vasopressin: A new target for the treatment of heart failure. *Am Heart J.* 2003;146:9–18.
76. Wyer PC, Perera P, Jin Z, et al. Vasopressin or epinephrine for out-of-hospital cardiac arrest. *Ann Emerg Med.* 2006;48:86–97.
77. Studer W, Wu X, Siegemund M, et al. Resuscitation from cardiac arrest with adrenaline/epinephrine or vasopressin: Effects on intestinal mucosal tonometer pCO(2) during the postresuscitation period in rats. *Resuscitation.* 2002;53: 201–207.
78. Parrillo JE. Septic shock–vasopressin, norepinephrine, and urgency. *N Engl J Med.* 2008;358:954–956.
79. Rivers E, Nguyen B, Havstad S, et al. Early goal-directed therapy in the treatment of severe sepsis and septic shock. *N Engl J Med.* 2001;345:1368–1377.
80. Oghlakian G, Klapholz M. Vasopressin and vasopressin receptor antagonists in heart failure. *Cardiol Rev.* 2009;17:10–15.
81. Delacretaz E. Clinical practice. Supraventricular tachycardia. *N Engl J Med.* 2006; 354:1039–1051.
82. Chiu C, Sequeira IB. Diagnosis and treatment of idiopathic ventricular tachycardia. *AACN Clin Issues.* 2004;15:449–461.
83. Delaney B, Loy J, Kelly AM. The relative efficacy of adenosine versus verapamil for the treatment of stable paroxysmal supraventricular tachycardia in adults: A meta-analysis. *Eur J Emerg Med.* 2011;18:148–152.
84. Holdgate A, Foo A. Adenosine versus intravenous calcium channel antagonists for the treatment of supraventricular tachycardia in adults. *Cochrane Database Syst Rev.* 2006; (4):CD005154.
85. Gillies M, Bellomo R, Doolan L, et al. Bench-to-bedside review: Inotropic drug therapy after adult cardiac surgery – a systematic literature review. *Crit Care.* 2005; 9:266–279.
86. McBride BF, White CM. Acute decompensated heart failure: A contemporary approach to pharmacotherapeutic management. *Pharmacotherapy.* 2003;23:997–1020.
87. Bristow MR, Shakar SF, Linseman JV, et al. Inotropes and beta-blockers: Is there a need for new guidelines? *J Cardiac Fail.* 2001;7:8–12.
88. Endoh M, Hori M. Acute heart failure: Inotropic agents and their clinical uses. *Expert Opin Pharmacother.* 2006;7:2179–2202.

89. Aronow WS. Treatment of heart failure with abnormal left ventricular systolic function in the elderly. *Heart Fail Clin.* 2007;3:423–436.
90. Rosen D, Decaro MV, Graham MG. Evidence-based treatment of chronic heart failure. *Compr Ther.* 2007;33:2–17.
91. Zaloga GP. Hormones: Vasopressin, Growth Hormone, Glucagon, Somatostatin, Prolactin, G-CSF, GM-CSF pages 700–714. In: Bart Chernow, ed.; D.Craig Brater, John W. Holaday, Gary P. Zaloga, Arno L. Zaritsky, Associate ed.; Lisa Daniel Sparks, Editorial Assistant. *The Pharmacologic Approach to the Critically Ill Patient.* 3rd ed. Baltimore: Williams & Wilkins, c1994.
92. Sampson HA, Munoz-Furlong A, Campbell RL, et al. Second symposium on the definition and management of anaphylaxis: Summary report–Second National Institute of Allergy and Infectious Disease/Food Allergy and Anaphylaxis Network symposium. *J Allergy Clin Immunol.* 2006;117:391–397.
93. Aronow WS. Treatment of heart failure with normal left ventricular ejection fraction. *Compr Ther.* 2007;33:223–230.
94. Ariyan CE, Sosa JA. Assessment and management of patients with abnormal calcium. *Crit Care Med.* 2004;32:S146–S154.
95. Aguilera IM, Vaughan RS, . Calcium and the anaesthetist. *Anaesthesia.* 2000;55: 779–790.
96. Shapira N, Schaff HV, White RD, et al. Hemodynamic effects of calcium chloride injection following cardiopulmonary bypass: Response to bolus injection and continuous infusion. *Ann Thorac Surg.* 1984;37:133–140.
97. Janelle GM, Urdaneta F, Martin TD, et al. Effects of calcium chloride on grafted internal mammary artery flow after cardiopulmonary bypass. *J Cardiothorac Vasc Anesth.* 2000;14:4–8.
98. Yellon DM, Hausenloy DJ. Myocardial reperfusion injury. *N Engl J Med.* 2007; 357:1121–1135.
99. White RD, Goldsmith RS, Rodriguez R, et al. Plasma ionic calcium levels following injection of chloride, gluconate, and gluceptate salts of calcium. *J Thorac Cardiovasc Surg.* 1976;71:609–613.
100. Sanchez CE, Richards DR. Contemporary in-hospital management strategies for acute decompensated heart failure. *Cardiol Rev.* 2011;19:122–129.
101. Cavusoglu Y, Beyaztas A, Birdane A, et al. Levosimendan and pulmonary hypertension. *J Cardiovasc Med.* 2010;11:478–480.
102. Russ MA, Prodzinsky R, Carter JM, et al. Right ventricular function in myocardial infarction complicated by cardiogenic shock; Improvement with levosimendan. *Crit Care Med.* 2009;37:3017–3023.
103. Falk S. Anesthetic consideration for the patient undergoing therapy for advanced heart failure. *Curr Opin Anesthesiol.* 2011;24:314–319.
104. Severi L, Lappa A, Landoni G, et al. Levosimendan versus intra-aortic ballon pump in high risk cardiac surgery patients. *J Cardiothor Vasc Anesth.* 2011; 25:632–636.
105. Bhatara VS, Magnus RD, Paul KL, et al. Serotonin syndrome induced by venlafaxine and fluoxetine: A case study in polypharmacy and potential pharmacodynamic and pharmacokinetic mechanisms. *Ann Pharmacother.* 1998;32: 432–436.
106. Bellingham GA, Peng PWH. Duloxetine: A review of its pharmacology and use in chronic pain management. *Reg Anesth Pain Med.* 2010;35:294–303.
107. Kok RM, Heeren TJ, Nolen WA. Continuing treatment of depression in the elderly: A systematic review and meta-analysis of double-blinded randomized controlled trials with antidepressants. *Am J Geriatr Psychiatry.* 2011;19:249–255.
108. Reeves RR, Wise PM, Cox SK. SSRIs & the risk of abnormal bleeding. *J Psychosoc Nurs Ment Health Serv.* 2007;45:15–21.
109. Roose SP, Miyazaki M. Pharmacologic treatment of depression in patients with heart disease. *Psychosom Med.* 2005;67(suppl 1):S54–S57.
110. Regan KL. Depression treatment with selective serotonin reuptake inhibitors for the postacute coronary syndrome population: A literature review. *J Cardiovasc Nurs.* 2008;23:489–496.
111. Pacak K. Preoperative management of the pheochromocytoma patient. *J Clin Endocrinol Metab.* 2007;92:4069–4079.
112. Weber MA. The role of the new beta-blockers in treating cardiovascular disease. *Am J Hypertens.* 2005;18:169S–176S.
113. Pratt CM. Three decades of clinical trials with beta-blockers: The contribution of the CAPRICORN trial and the effect of carvedilol on serious arrhythmias. *J Am Coll Cardiol.* 2005;45:531–532.
114. Effect of metoprolol CR/XL in chronic heart failure: Metoprolol CR/XL Randomised Intervention Trial in Congestive Heart Failure (MERIT-HF). *Lancet.* 1999;353:2001–2007.
115. Cleland JG, Loh H, Windram J. Are there clinically important differences between beta-blockers in heart failure? *Heart Fail Clin.* 2005;1:57–66.
116. Flather MD, Shibata MC, Coats AJ, et al. Randomized trial to determine the effect of nebivolol on mortality and cardiovascular hospital admission in elderly patients with heart failure (SENIORS). *Eur Heart J.* 2005;26:215–225.
117. Baxter AD, Kanji S. Protocol implementation in anesthesia: Beta-blockade in non-cardiac surgery patients. *Can J Anaesth.* 2007;54:114–123.
118. Wallace A, Layug B, Tateo I, et al. Prophylactic atenolol reduces postoperative myocardial ischemia. McSPI Research Group. *Anesthesiology.* 1998;88: 7–17.
119. Beattie WS, Wijeysundera DN, Karkouti K, et al. Does tight heart rate control improve beta-blocker efficacy? An updated analysis of the noncardiac surgical randomized trials. *Anesth Analg.* 2008;106:1039–1048.
120. Feringa HH, Bax JJ, Boersma E, et al. High-dose beta-blockers and tight heart rate control reduce myocardial ischemia and troponin T release in vascular surgery patients. *Circulation.* 2006;114:I344–I349.
121. London MJ. Beta blockers and alpha2 agonists for cardioprotection. *Best Pract Res Clin Anaesthesiol.* 2008;22:95–110.
122. London MJ. Quo vadis, perioperative beta blockade? Are you "POISE'd" on the brink? *Anesth Analg.* 2008;106:1025–1030.
123. Poldermans D, Boersma E. Beta-blocker therapy in noncardiac surgery. *N Engl J Med.* 2005;353:412–414.
124. Trujillo TC, Dobesh PP. Traditional management of chronic stable angina. *Pharmacotherapy.* 2007;27:1677–1692.
125. Fleisher LA. Perioperative beta-blockade: How best to translate evidence into practice. *Anesth Analg.* 2007;104:1–3.
126. Fleisher LA, Beckman JA, Brown KA, et al. ACC/AHA 2007 guidelines on perioperative cardiovascular evaluation and care for noncardiac surgery: Executive summary: A report of the American College of Cardiology/American Heart Association Task Force on Practice Guidelines (Writing Committee to Revise the 2002 Guidelines on Perioperative Cardiovascular Evaluation for Noncardiac Surgery). *Anesth Analg.* 2008;106:685–712.
127. Fleisher LA, Beckman JA, Brown KA, et al. ACC/AHA 2006 guideline update on perioperative cardiovascular evaluation for noncardiac surgery: Focused update on perioperative beta-blocker therapy: A report of the American College of Cardiology/American Heart Association Task Force on Practice Guidelines (Writing Committee to Update the 2002 Guidelines on Perioperative Cardiovascular Evaluation for Noncardiac Surgery): Developed in collaboration with the American Society of Echocardiography, American Society of Nuclear Cardiology, Heart Rhythm Society, Society of Cardiovascular Anesthesiologists, Society for Cardiovascular Angiography and Interventions, and Society for Vascular Medicine and Biology. *Circulation.* 2006;113:2662–2674.
128. Wetterslev J, Juul AB. Benefits and harms of perioperative beta-blockade. *Best Pract Res Clin Anaesthesiol.* 2006;20:285–302.
129. Poise Study Group. Effects of extended-release metoprolol succinate in patients undergoing non-cardiac surgery (POISE trial): A randomized controlled trial. *Lancet.* 2008;371:1839–1847.
130. Foëx P, Sear JW. Challenges of β-blockade in surgical patients. *Anesthesiology.* 2010;113:767–771.
131. Wallace AW, Au S, Cason BA. Peri-operative β-blockade. Atenolol is associated with reduced mortality when compared to metoprolol. *Anesthesiology.* 2011;114:824–836.
132. Wallace AW, Au S, Cason BA. Association of the pattern of use of peri-operative β-blockade and postoperative mortality. *Anesthesiology.* 2010;113:794–805.
133. Norbury WB, Jeschke MG, Herndon DN. Metabolism modulators in sepsis: Propranolol. *Crit Care Med.* 2007;35:S616–S620.
134. Mangano DT, Layug EL, Wallace A, et al. Effect of atenolol on mortality and cardiovascular morbidity after noncardiac surgery. Multicenter Study of Perioperative Ischemia Research Group.[Erratum appears in *N Engl J Med.* 1997;336(14):1039]. *N Engl J Med.* 1996;335:1713–1720.
135. Degoute CS. Controlled hypotension: A guide to drug choice. *Drugs.* 2007; 67:1053–1076.
136. Frakes MA. Rapid sequence induction medications: An update. *J Emerg Nurs.* 2003;29:533–540.
137. Frakes MA. Esmolol: A unique drug with ED applications. *J Emerg Nurs.* 2001; 27:47–51.
138. Tafreshi MJ, Weinacker AB. Beta-adrenergic-blocking agents in bronchospastic diseases: A therapeutic dilemma. *Pharmacotherapy.* 1999;19:974–978.
139. Nieminen T, Lehtimäki T, Mäenpää J, et al. Ophthalmic timolol: Plasma concentration and systemic cardiopulmonary effects. *Scand J Clin Lab Invest.* 2007; 67:237–245.
140. Ezzeddine MA, Suri MF, Hussein HM, et al. Blood pressure management in patients with acute stroke: Pathophysiology and treatment strategies. *Neurosurg Clin N Am.* 2006;17(suppl 1):41–56.
141. Mocco J, Zacharia BE, Komotar RJ, et al. A review of current and future medical therapies for cerebral vasospasm following aneurysmal subarachnoid hemorrhage. *Neurosurg Focus.* 2006;21:E9.
142. Arroyo AM, Kao LW. Calcium channel blocker toxicity. *Pediatr Emerg Care.* 2009;25:532–541.
143. Weck M. Treatment of hypertension in patients with diabetes mellitus: Relevance of sympathovagal balance and renal function. *Clin Res Cardiol.* 2007;96:707–718.
144. Curran MP, Robinson DM, Keating GM. Intravenous nicardipine: Its use in the short-term treatment of hypertension and various other indications. *Drugs.* 2006;66:1755–1782.
145. Pantoni L, del Ser T, Soglian AG, et al. Efficacy and safety of nimodipine in subcortical vascular dementia: A randomized placebo-controlled trial. *Stroke.* 2005;36:619–624.
146. Rhoney D, Peacock WF. Intravenous therapy for hypertensive emergencies, part 1. *Am J Health Syst Pharm.* 2009;66:1343–1352.
147. Rhoney D, Peacock WF. Intravenous therapy for hypertensive emergencies, part 2. *Am J Health Syst Pharm.* 2009;66:1448–1457.
148. Peacock FW 4th, Varon J, Ebrahimi R, et al. Clevidipine for severe hypertension in acute heart failure: A VELOCITY trial analysis. *Congest Heart Fail.* 2010;16: 55–59.

149. Kenyon KW. Clevidipine: An ultrashort-acting calcium channel antagonist for acute hypertension. *Ann Pharmacother.* 2009;43:1258–1265.
150. Aronson S, Dyke CM, Stierer KA, et al. The ECLIPSE trials: Comparative studies of clevidipine to nitroglycerin, sodium nitroprusside, and nicardipine for acute hypertension treatment in cardiac surgery patients. *Anesth Analg.* 2008;107: 1110–1121.
151. Ndefo UA, Erowelw GI, Ebiasah R, et al. Clevidipine: A new intravenous option for the management of acute hypertension. *Am J Health Syst Pharm.* 2010;67: 351–360.
152. Reves JG, Kissin I, Lell WA, et al. Calcium entry blockers: Uses and implications for anesthesiologists. *Anesthesiology.* 1982;57:504–518.
153. Carpenter RL, Mulroy MF. Edrophonium antagonizes combined lidocaine-pancuronium and verapamil-pancuronium neuromuscular blockade in cats. *Anesthesiology.* 1986;65:506–510.
154. Zalman F, Perloff JK, Durant NN, et al. Acute respiratory failure following intravenous verapamil in Duchenne's muscular dystrophy. *Am Heart J.* 1983;105: 510–511.
155. Opie LH. Calcium Channel Blockers (calcium antagonists). In: Opie LH, Gersh BJ, eds. *Drugs for the Heart.* 7th ed. Philadelphia, PA: Saunders/Elsevier; 2009: 59–87.
156. Wijeysundera DN, Beattie WS. Calcium channel blockers for reducing cardiac morbidity after noncardiac surgery: A meta-analysis. *Anesth Analg.* 2003;97: 634–641.
157. Zhou SF, Xue CC, Yu XQ, et al. Clinically important drug interactions potentially involving mechanism-based inhibition of cytochrome P450 3A4 and the role of therapeutic drug monitoring. *Ther Drug Monit.* 2007;29:687–710.
158. Price WA, Giannini AJ. Neurotoxicity caused by lithium-verapamil synergism. *J Clin Pharmacol.* 1986;26:717–719.
159. Tuman KJ, McCarthy RJ, O'Connor CJ, et al. Angiotensin-converting enzyme inhibitors increase vasoconstrictor requirements after cardiopulmonary bypass. *Anesth Analg.* 1995;80:473–479.
160. Cohn JN, Tognoni G; Valsartan Heart Failure Trial Investigators. A randomized trial of the angiotensin-receptor blocker valsartan in chronic heart failure. *N Engl J Med.* 2001;345:1667–1675.
161. Lewis EJ, Hunsicker LG, Clarke WR, et al. Renoprotective effect of the angiotensin-receptor antagonist irbesartan in patients with nephropathy due to type 2 diabetes. *N Engl J Med.* 2001;345:851–860.
162. Cantazaro DF, Frishman WH. Angiotensin receptor blockers for management of hypertension. *South Med J.* 2010;103:669–673.
163. Basile J, Toth PP. Angiotensin receptor blockers: Role in hypertension management, cardiovascular risk reduction, and nephropathy. *South Med J.* 2009; 102(suppl 1):S1–S12.
164. Vigil-De Gracia P, Ruiz E, Lopez JC, et al. Management of severe hypertension in the postpartum period with intravenous hydralazine or labetalol: A randomized clinical trial. *Hypertens Pregnancy.* 2007;26:163–171.
165. Elkayam U, Janmohamed M, Habib M, et al. Vasodilators in the management of acute heart failure. *Crit Care Med.* 2008;36:S95–105.
166. Chiariello M, Gold HK, Leinbach RC, et al. Comparison between the effects of nitroprusside and nitroglycerin on ischemic injury during acute myocardial infarction. *Circulation.* 1976;54:766–773.
167. Harris SN, Rinder CS, Rinder HM, et al. Nitroprusside inhibition of platelet function is transient and reversible by catecholamine priming. *Anesthesiology.* 1995;83:1145–1152.
168. Dufour P, Vinatier D, Puech F. The use of intravenous nitroglycerin for cervico-uterine relaxation: A review of the literature. *Arch Gynecol Obstet.* 1997;261: 1–7.

CHAPTER

16 Hemostasis and Transfusion Medicine

LOUANNE M. CARABINI • GLENN RAMSEY

Key Points

1. Perioperative blood component therapy accounts for at least 23% of transfusions.
2. Blood must not only be maintained as a fluid in normal circulation, but also be capable of forming a solid clot to stanch leaks in the vascular wall—and then dismantling the clot when the need has passed.
3. Clotting factors in the plasma are activated at sites of endothelial injury and assemble in enzymatic complexes to activate thrombin.
4. Fibrin clots must be broken down after their job is done, and fibrinolysis is a complex process with checks and balances.
5. The first screening test for hemostatic problems should always be the patient's medical history.
6. Platelet aggregation is the most detailed overall platelet function test.
7. A general oversight of plasma clotting factor activity is obtained by the *prothrombin time (PT)* for the intrinsic (tissue) pathway and the *activated partial thromboplastin time (aPTT)* for the extrinsic (contact) pathway.
8. Disseminated intravascular coagulopathy (DIC) describes unchecked coagulation initiated by pathologic systemic activation of the intrinsic clotting pathway.
9. The risk for venous thromboembolism is increased by intercurrent factors such as physical inactivity or immobilization, malignancy, oral contraceptives, estrogen therapy, and pregnancy.
10. Most anticoagulant therapies need ongoing or selective testing for assessment of therapeutic effect.
11. Leukoreduction to remove WBCs from RBCs and platelets reduces the risk of HLA alloimmunization, febrile nonhemolytic transfusion reactions, and CMV transmission in patients who require these precautions.
12. Plasma derivatives are proteins processed from plasma for therapeutic infusions.
13. Techniques have been developed to kill microbial pathogens in blood components.
14. Many years of effort have gone into the search for an oxygen-carrying substitute for RBCs.
15. Routine RBC compatibility testing includes ABO and RhD typing, an antibody screen for IgG non-ABO RBC antibodies, and an RBC cross-match.
16. Over the past decade, transfusion practices for medical and surgical patients shifted from a liberal strategy to more restrictive management with lower thresholds and careful consideration of the balance between transfusion risks and the physiologic consequences of anemia.

17 Oxygen delivery to the tissues (DO_2) is dependent on cardiac output (CO), regional blood flow, and oxygen-carrying capacity also known as the oxygen content (CaO_2) of blood.

18 Numerous recommendations provide guidance for the transfusion management of thrombocytopenia and acquired or inherited platelet disorders.

19 Cryoprecipitate is created by a controlled thaw of frozen plasma which allows for precipitation of large molecules.

20 Over the past few decades, the risk benefit ratio of blood product transfusion has been the subject of several studies and review articles.

21 Given the extensive use of more sensitive methods for screening and controlling the infectious risks of blood product transfusion, noninfectious complications have emerged as the major source of transfusion-related morbidity and mortality.

22 Transfusion-related acute lung injury (TRALI) is a clinical diagnosis that can be clouded by confounding comorbidities or patient acuity; therefore, TRALI tends to be underreported in the literature and is extremely difficult if not impossible to study with randomized prospective clinical trials.

23 Acute normovolemic hemodilution is the process of extracting multiple units of blood immediately before surgical incision while maintaining euvolemia with crystalloids or colloid supplementation.

24 Over the past decade, RBC salvage techniques have improved drastically and now offer an efficient, cost-effective, and safe method for perioperative blood conservation.

25 Disorders of hemostasis can be classified as those that cause a propensity for hemorrhage and those that facilitate inappropriate thrombosis.

26 Symptomatically disorders of primary hemostasis often present with superficial signs of bleeding on the skin or mucosa.

27 Von Willebrand disease (vWD) is the most common hereditary bleeding disorder with a prevalence of approximately 1% in the general population.

28 Hemophilia is a genetic disease that results from deficiencies or dysfunction of specific clotting factors.

29 Antiplatelet therapy is indicated for patients at risk of cerebral vascular accident, myocardial infarction, or other vascular thrombosis complications.

30 Heparin-induced thrombocytopenia (HIT) is a clinical disorder that develops after extended use of heparin therapy. It occurs in approximately 1% to 5% of patients receiving heparin and is associated with morbidity from thromboembolic complications.

31 Recombinant activated factor VII (rFVIIa) is now indicated for the treatment of acquired hemophilia and factor VII deficiency.

32 Prothrombin Complex Concentrates are now the drug of choice for emergent reversal of oral anticoagulants in place of rFVIIa and fresh frozen plasma.

33 Antifibrinolytic agents have been used to prevent and treat surgical blood loss for several decades.

Multimedia

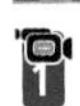

Cerebral Aneurysm Coiling

Formation and Lysis of Fibrin

INTRODUCTION

Over 23 million blood products were transfused throughout the United States during the year 2008 alone. This included over 15 million units of red blood cells (RBCs), about 2 million packs of platelets, over 4.4 million units of plasma, and approximately
1 1.1 million doses of cryoprecipitate. Perioperative blood component therapy accounts for at least 23% of these transfusions.[1] Consequently, it is imperative for the anesthesia provider to understand the treatment benefits, the rare and common adverse effects, and the specific therapeutic details of blood product preparation and delivery in order to best manage their patients.

This chapter begins with a review of primary and secondary hemostasis, fibrinolysis, and regulation of the coagulation pathway. We continue with a description of the most common coagulation profile tests followed by the method for blood product collection and storage. The therapeutic indications and risks associated with blood component therapy are discussed at length. The chapter also includes extensive clinical sections discussing congenital and acquired deficiencies in hemostasis and coagulation, as well as an up-to-date presentation of available pharmacologic treatment medications to maintain a balanced hemostatic mechanism.

HEMOSTASIS AND COAGULATION

Primary Hemostasis

2 Blood must not only be maintained as a fluid in normal circulation, but also be capable of forming a solid clot to staunch leaks in the vascular wall—and then dismantling the clot when the need has passed. This delicate equilibrium between anticoagulation and coagulation is maintained by a complex system of counterbalanced blood proteins and cells (platelets). Many congenital and acquired disorders can push the system toward either bleeding or thrombosis. The patient care team has a number of tests to evaluate the system and many therapeutic modalities to correct these imbalances.

Platelets adhere to sites of endothelial disruption, undergo activation to recruit more platelets and amplify the platelet response, and then cross-link with fibrin, the end product of the plasma clotting factor cascade, to form a platelet plug. *Primary hemostasis* (Fig. 16-1) describes the initiation of the platelet plug and clotting mechanism.

Adherence

When the endothelial lining is disrupted to expose the underlying matrix, platelets attach to collagen via surface integrin receptors—

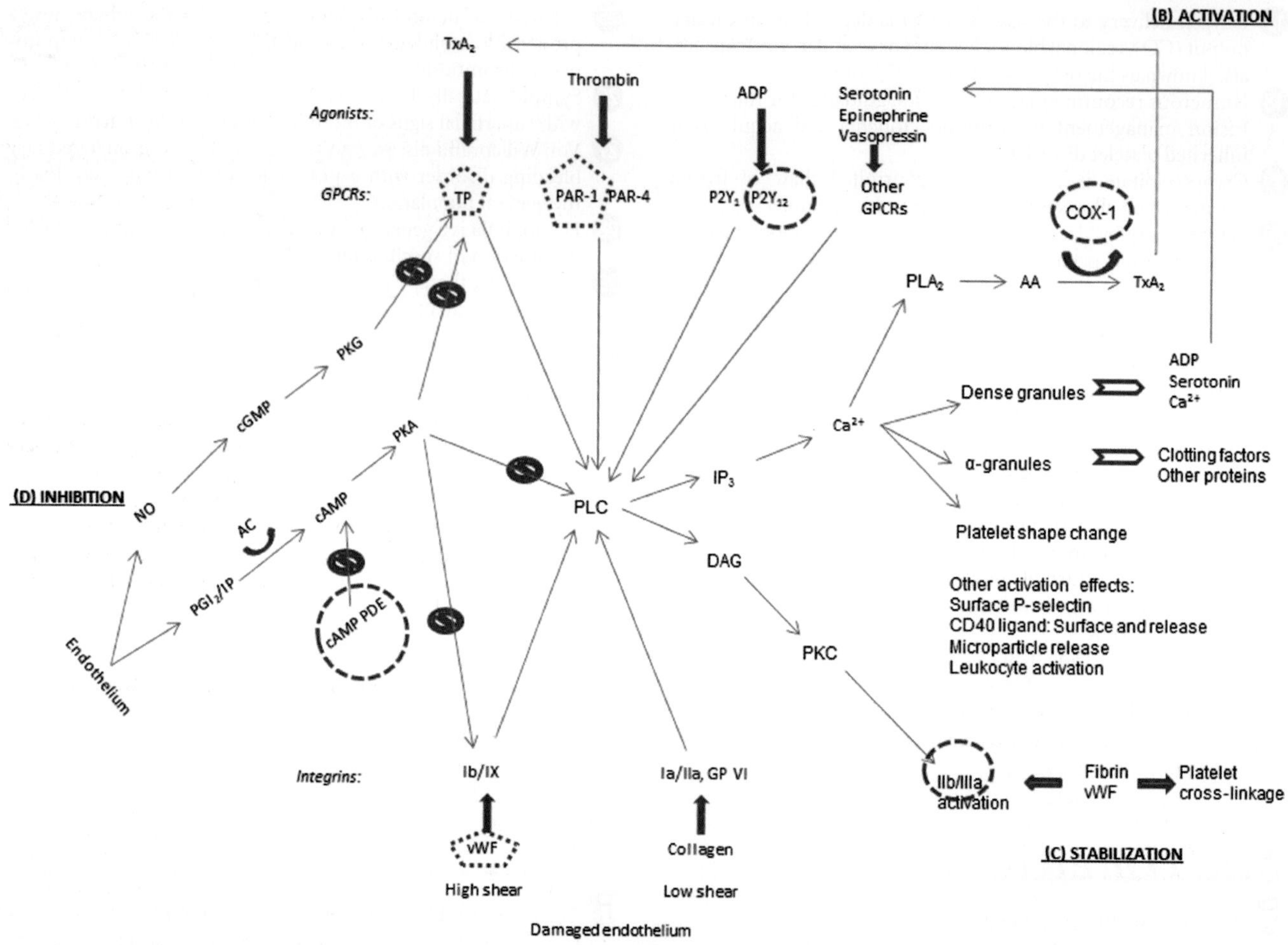

FIGURE 16-1. Overview of platelet pathways for adherence, activation, stabilization, and physiologic inhibition. *Thin arrows,* signaling pathways; *thick arrows,* ligand binding; *curved arrows,* catalysis; *clear arrows,* secretion; *slashed circles,* inhibitory signaling pathways; *round circles,* antiplatelet drug targets; *pentagons,* targets of antiplatelet drugs in development. **(A)** *Adherence:* vWF, von Willebrand factor. Glycoproteins Ib/IX, Ia/IIa, and VI. **(B)** *Activation:* Agonists: TxA_2, thromboxane A_2; ADP, adenosine diphosphate. Receptors: GPCR, G-protein–coupled receptor; TP, thromboxane prostanoid; PAR, protease-activated receptor. Intermediaries: PLC, phospholipase C; IP_3, inositol-1,4,5-triphosphate; DAG, diacylglycerol; PKC, protein kinase C; Ca^{2+}, calcium; PLA_2, phospholipase A_2; AA, arachidonic acid; COX, cyclooxygenase. **(C)** *Stabilization:* Glycoprotein IIb/IIIa. **(D)** *Inhibition:* NO, nitric oxide; PGI_2, prostaglandin I_2 (prostacyclin); IP, PGI_2 receptor; AC, adenylate cyclase; cAMP, cyclic adenosine monophosphate; PDE, phosphodiesterase; cGMP, cyclic guanosine monophosphate; PKA, protein kinase A; PKG, protein kinase G. Targets of antiplatelet drugs. COX-1: Aspirin and nonsteroidal antiinflammatory drugs (NSAIDs). $P2Y_{12}$: Clopidogrel, prasugrel, ticlopidine, and, in clinical trials, cangrelor, elinogrel, and ticagrelor. cAMP PDE: Dipyridamole and cilostazol. IIb/IIIa: Abciximab, eptifibatide, and tirofiban. Other drugs in clinical trials—TP: Terutroban; PAR-1: E5555, SCH 530348; vWF: AJW200, ARC1779.

glycoproteins (GP) Ia/IIa and GP VI (Fig. 16-1A). Collagen adherence is favored in low-shear conditions such as venous circulation.[2] In high-shear arterial blood flow, von Willebrand factor (vWF) from endothelial cells and from preexisting clot binds to integrin Ib/IX, the other major adherence anchor.[3] In capillary blood flow, platelets are pushed to the periphery by RBCs, so anemia lessens platelet contact and reduces platelet function.[2]

Activation

Platelet activation can be mediated by numerous signaling pathways from the platelet surface (Fig. 16-1B). In "outside-in" signaling, a central target is phospholipase C (PLC). The above adherence integrins trigger pathways to activate PLC.[2] Another set of surface receptors, G-protein–coupled receptors (GPCRs), are activated by an array of corresponding agonists, including thrombin from the factor clotting cascade, adenosine diphosphate (ADP), thromboxane A_2 (TxA_2), serotonin, epinephrine, and vasopressin. Each of these agonist–GPCR pairings set off activation pathways for PLC as well.[4]

Activated PLC leads to several structural changes in the platelets. Via inositol-1,4,5-triphosphate (IP_3), calcium (Ca^{2+}) is released from storage tubules. Calcium ions catalyze release of dense granules and α-granules at the platelet surface. These granules contain ADP, serotonin, and more Ca^{2+}, all of which can activate more platelets.[2] α-granules contain numerous proteins, including factor V, fibrinogen, and platelet factor 4 (PF-4), which promotes clotting by binding and neutralizing heparin-like compounds and heparin.[2] (This heparin–PF-4 complex is the target antigen for the antibodies causing heparin-induced thrombocytopenia [HIT], discussed in depth later in this chapter.) Calcium also facilitates rearrangement of the platelet microskeleton to change the platelet shape from round and discoid to flat and spiky. Furthermore, the Ca^{2+} helps activate phospholipase A_2 (PLA_2), which releases arachidonic acid (AA) from the platelet membrane. AA, as catalyzed by cyclooxygenase-1 (COX-1), is modified to TxA_2, which can then activate more platelets.[3] Activated platelets also have surface P-selectin and surface-bound and released CD40 ligand, and they release circulating microparticles and attract and activate leukocytes; these features further contribute to hemostasis and also play a role in inflammation.[2]

Stabilization

The activated PLC initiates "inside-out" signaling of GP IIb/IIIa via diacylglycerol (DAG) and protein kinase C (Fig. 16-1C). This changes the shape of GP IIb/IIIa, which permits it to better bind fibrin and vWF. These proteins can bridge to other activated platelets.[3] The fibrin binding can also enmesh the platelets, contributing to the formation of the platelet plug in the convergence of the platelet and clotting factor systems.

Inhibition

To maintain hemostatic balance, platelets are naturally inhibited in their endothelial environment. Endothelial cells secrete prostaglandin I_2 (PGI_2), which binds to a surface receptor to signal increased cyclic adenosine monophosphate (cAMP). Elevated cAMP activates protein kinase A (PKA), a multisite inhibitor of vWF adherence, TxA_2 activation, and PLC internal signaling. However, cAMP is metabolized by cAMP phosphodiesterase (PDE). Endothelial cells also secrete nitric oxide (NO), which at high levels initiates a signaling pathway leading to inhibition of the TxA_2 receptor.[4]

Mechanisms of Antiplatelet Medications

Figure 16-1 shows the sites of action for antiplatelet medications in use or in development. No drugs are available to counteract the first step, platelet adherence (Fig. 16-1A), although at least two compounds are under development to affect vWF's binding to GP Ib/IX. Aspirin and nonsteroidal antiinflammatory agents dampen the secretion of TxA_2 by inhibiting COX-1, the enzyme which converts AA into TxA_2 (Fig. 16-1B). Another agonist, ADP, has its $P2Y_{12}$ receptor blocked by clopidogrel and its analogues. Drugs are in development to block surface receptors for TxA_2 and thrombin. The formation and stabilization of the platelet plug is blocked by abciximab, eptifibatide, and tirofiban, which act at GP IIb/IIIa (Fig. 16-1C). Finally, the major inhibitory pathway mediated by endothelial PGI_2 is upregulated by dipyridamole and cilostazol (Fig. 16-1D). These medications are discussed further later in this chapter.

Secondary Hemostasis

3 Clotting factors in the plasma are activated at sites of endothelial injury and assemble in enzymatic complexes to activate thrombin. This *initiates* secondary hemostasis. Thrombin then *amplifies* production of itself by activating other more efficient enzymes which *propagate* a thrombin burst. Thrombin also converts fibrinogen to fibrin, which cross-links with activated platelets to form the platelet plug. Each of the three enzymatic complexes in the clotting process consists of four parts: An enzyme in the serine protease family, a cofactor, a plasma membrane phospholipid surface such as the platelet, and calcium ion (Ca^{2+}). The proteases convert other clotting factors from their inactive circulating configuration to an active form (termed [factor number]a).[5]

The extrinsic pathway (Fig. 16-2A–E). The process begins when endothelial disruption exposes tissue factor (TF) on underlying cell membranes (A), extrinsic to the circulation—

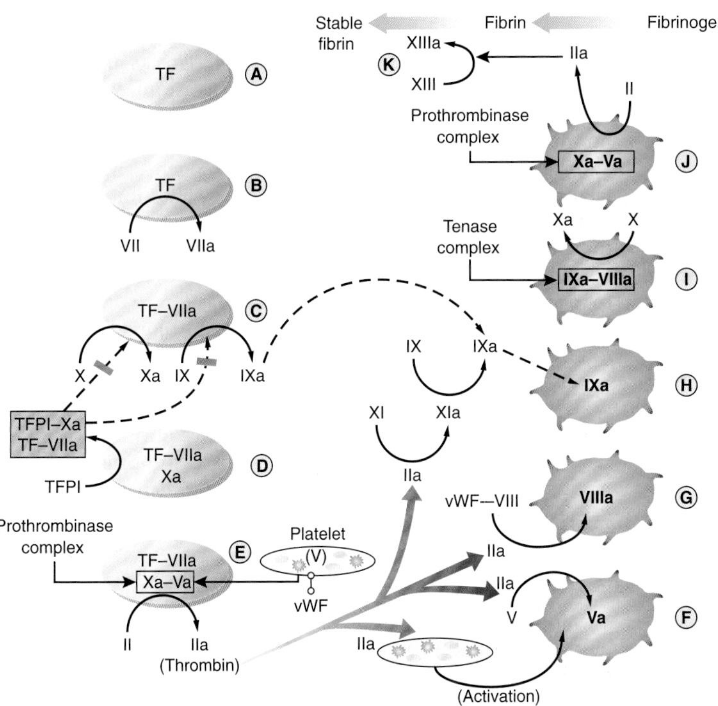

FIGURE 16-2. Summary of secondary hemostasis and the intrinsic, extrinsic, and common coagulation pathways. See text for details. TF, tissue factor; TFPI, tissue factor pathway inhibitor; vWF-VIII, circulating factor VIII bound to von Willebrand factor. (Reproduced with permission from: John C. Drummond, MD, and Charise T. Petrovitch, MD.)

hence the term "extrinsic pathway." TF binds both VII and VIIa, which circulates at low levels, and is a cofactor for the activation of factor VII (B). VIIa enzyme, TF cofactor, cell membrane phospholipid, and Ca^{2+} form the first complex, a low-efficiency extrinsic-pathway "tenase" which activates factor X and factor IX (C). Then Xa enzyme, its cofactor Va (derived in large part from factor V released from activated platelet α-granules), phospholipid, and Ca^{2+} assemble to form the second complex, a "prothrombinase," which converts prothrombin (II) to thrombin (IIa) (E).[5]

The intrinsic pathway (Fig. 16-2F–J). Thrombin has several central functions. It activates platelets via surface receptors PAR-1 and PAR-4 (see Primary Hemostasis), cleaves more V to Va (F), and initiates the "intrinsic" (intravascular) coagulation pathway by cleaving factor XI to XIa (G). XIa cleaves more IX to IXa (H). Thrombin also activates VIII to VIIIa (G). (VIII is carried and stabilized in the plasma by vWF until needed, and vWF deficiency results in low plasma VIII levels also.) The third complex is then formed: IXa enzyme, VIIIa cofactor, phospholipid, and Ca^{2+}. This is a high-efficiency intrinsic-pathway "tenase" (I) which provides many times more Xa for more prothrombinase complex (J). Ultimately, thrombin cleaves fibrinogen to fibrin monomers, which then polymerize extensively. Fibrin polymers are cross-linked by factor XIIIa (also activated by thrombin) to form the stable fibrin clot (K). Fibrin also cross-links activated platelets by their GP IIb/IIIa receptors to enmesh platelets and fibrin in the platelet plug (see Primary Hemostasis).[5]

All of these clotting factors are primarily produced in the liver, except for VIII, which is also released by endothelial cells and is well maintained in liver disease. The plasma half-life of most clotting factors is around 1.5 to 3 days, but those of the initiating factor VII (6 hours) and the cofactors V and VIII (8 to 12 hours) are much shorter. Four critical enzyme factors—VII in the extrinsic tenase, IX in the intrinsic tenase, X in the prothrombinase, and prothrombin (II)—must be carboxylated at multiple glutamic acid residues after translation, in order to interact with phospholipid and Ca^{2+}. Vitamin K in its reduced form is the cofactor for the glutamyl-carboxylase enzyme, and thus these factors are vitamin K–dependent.[5]

Inhibition of Clotting Factors

The clotting pathways have three main regulatory inhibitors: (1) TF pathway inhibitor (TFPI), (2) antithrombin-III (AT-III), and (3) protein C and its activation by the "protein C-ase" complex (Fig. 16-3).[1–5] (1) TFPI inhibits the external tenase complex by binding to the VIIa protease and to its Xa product. TFPI is produced in endothelial cells, from which its release is stimulated by heparin. Heparin in turn binds to and raises the inhibitory efficiency of TFPI. (2) AT-III is a serine protease inhibitor, or serpin. Serpins disrupt the active sites and increase the clearance of their target proteases. AT-III inhibits proteases in all clotting pathways: VIIa in intrinsic tenase, Xa in prothrombinase, XIa and IXa in the intrinsic tenase pathway, and thrombin. AT-III's inhibitory function is greatly increased when bound to heparin. (3) Protein C-ase is an enzymatic complex with the same structure as the coagulation complexes above: An enzyme, thrombin, its cofactor thrombomodulin, phospholipid, and Ca^{2+}. Thrombomodulin is expressed on endothelial cell membranes. In the protein C-ase complex, thrombin cleaves and activates protein C. Activated protein C (APC) brakes clotting by cleaving VIIIa and Va, the cofactors for the external tenase and the prothrombinase complexes. Protein C has a short half-life of 6 hours. Protein S is thought to be a cofactor for protein C; both are vitamin K–dependent.[5]

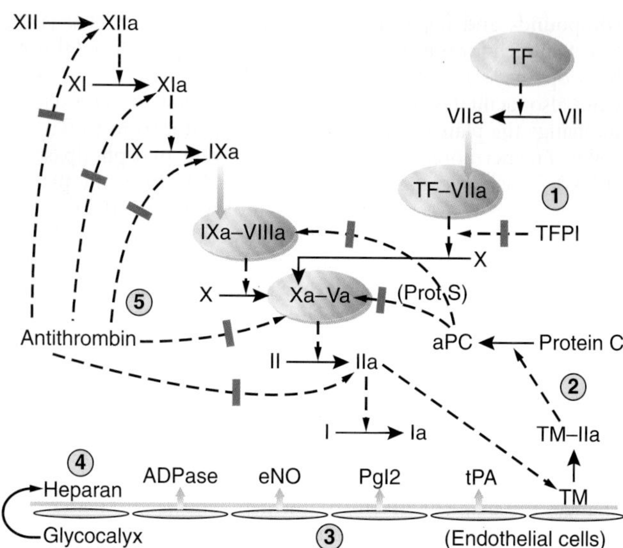

FIGURE 16-3. Depiction of the antithrombotic regulation of hemostasis. Five mechanisms serve to prevent unrestrained coagulation. (1) Tissue factor pathway inhibitor (TFPI) inhibits the initial activation of factor X by the extrinsic pathway. (2) A complex of thrombomodulin (TM) and thrombin (IIa) activates protein C, which, with protein S (Prot S) as a cofactor, inhibits activated factors V and VIII. (3) Intact vascular endothelium releases several substances that have a platelet-inhibiting or clot-lysing effect, including nitric oxide (eNO), prostacyclin (Pgl2), adenosine diphosphatase (ADPase), and tissue plasminogen activator (tPA). (4) In addition to TM, other coagulation-inhibiting substances including heparan sulfate and dermatan sulfate (latter not shown) are present in the intact glycocalyx. (5) Antithrombin-III binds, and thereby inhibits, several activated clotting factors (XIIa, XIa, IXa, Xa, and IIa). TF, tissue factor; aPC, activated protein C. (Reproduced with permission from: John C. Drummond, MD, and Charise T. Petrovitch, MD.)

Fibrinolysis

4 Fibrin clots must be broken down after their job is done, and fibrinolysis is also a complex process with checks and balances. In the end, plasminogen is activated to plasmin, which breaks down fibrin polymers (Fig. 16-4). Plasminogen activation has a minor and a major pathway. In the minor pathway, IXa, XIIa, and kallikrein can each activate plasminogen. The latter two factors are part of the "contact factors" which initiate in vitro clotting in the activated partial thromboplastin (activated partial thromboplastin time [aPTT]) test, but are not thought to take part in clotting in vivo. The minor pathway is thought to account for a small fraction of fibrinolysis.

The major activator of plasminogen in the blood is tissue plasminogen activator (tPA), which is secreted from endothelial cells. When associated with cross-linked fibrin, tPA becomes much more efficient. Once some plasmin is formed, it cleaves tPA to a more active form. tPA also directly cleaves fibrin polymers. In tissues, urokinase plasminogen activator is important in fibrinolysis. Urokinase is secreted from the endothelial cells and the kidney. Plasmin also activates urokinase to a more active form.

Inhibition of Fibrinolysis

Plasminogen activation inhibitor-1 (PAI-1) is a serpin which binds to tPA and urokinase and accelerates their clearance from plasma (Fig. 16-4). Activated platelets release PAI-1 from α-granules. Thrombin-activated fibrinolysis inhibitor (TAFI) is

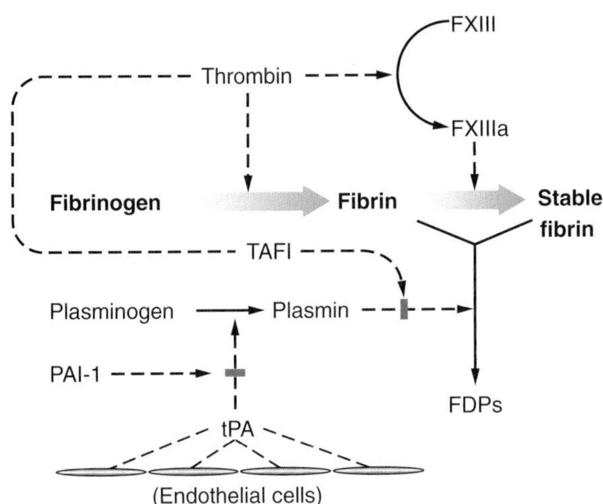

FIGURE 16-4. The mechanism and regulation of fibrinolysis. Fibrin is formed from fibrinogen by the action of thrombin (FIIa). Thrombin also converts factor XIII (FXIII) to activated factor XIII (FXIIIa), which in turn stabilizes the evolving fibrin clot by cross-linkage. Circulating plasminogen binds to fibrin and is converted to plasmin by tissue plasminogen activator (tPA) released from normal endothelium in areas remote from sites of vascular injury. Plasmin digests fibrin to its various degradation products (FDPs). The action of tPA can be inhibited by plasminogen activator inhibitor (PAI-1) released by endothelium and platelets. The action of plasmin is also inhibited by thrombin-activated fibrinolysis inhibitor (TAFI). (Reproduced with permission from: John C. Drummond, MD, and Charise T. Petrovitch, MD.)

activated by the thrombin–thrombomodulin protein C-ase complex. TAFI cleaves fibrin and fibrin polymers in a fashion which inhibits the action of tPA, and TAFI also inhibits the action of plasmin on fibrin. α_2-antiplasmin binds to plasmin and blocks its action, although this also slows the metabolism of plasmin.

LABORATORY EVALUATION OF HEMOSTASIS

5 The first screening test for hemostatic problems should always be the patient's medical history.[6] The nature of any abnormal bleeding is helpful; dermal or mucosal bleeding may suggest platelet dysfunction, whereas hemarthroses or soft tissue bleeding suggests factor deficiencies. Besides any direct past history of bleeding, thrombosis, or laboratory abnormalities, the patient's experience with hemostatic challenges such as surgery, dental procedures, and menstruation may help rule out clinical problems or suggest a lifelong congenital or more recent acquired disorder. The family history is helpful in diagnosing a congenital problem and the possible pattern of inheritance. Anticoagulants and antiplatelet medications, including over-the-counter drugs, should always be reviewed before ordering laboratory analysis.

Laboratory Evaluation of Primary Hemostasis

The normal automated platelet count in adults is approximately 150,000 to 400,000/μL. The peripheral blood smear should be examined in specimens with abnormal platelet counts or size. Microscopic review may reveal clotted specimens, artifactual platelet clumping in vitro, or abnormal platelet morphology. Large platelets are seen in some congenital disorders. One of the first platelet function tests (PFTs) was the template bleeding time, in which a standardized small cut is made on the subject's forearm and the bleeding duration timed. However, this test is invasive, labor-intensive, impractical to repeat frequently, poorly reproducible, and only modestly predictive for bleeding problems.

In vitro PFTs use various platelet agonists to activate and aggregate the patient's platelets.[7] For example, the PFA-100® device (Siemens, Munich, Germany) simulates capillary blood flow through a chamber after activation by collagen and either epinephrine or ADP. Prolonged "closure time" with collagen/epinephrine but not collagen/ADP suggests aspirin or other antiplatelet medications, whereas when both pairs are abnormal, other congenital or acquired platelet dysfunctions may be present. This type of testing is sometimes used as a screen in patients with a history suggesting platelet problems or von Willebrand disease (vWD). However, the sensitivity and specificity are low. False negatives are common, and abnormal results can also be caused by thrombocytopenia, uremia, or anemia. Several other devices test for specific antiplatelet medication effects from aspirin or P2Y12 inhibitors.[7]

6 Platelet aggregation is the most detailed overall PFT. Platelets are tested with multiple isolated agonists to assess their patterns of physical aggregation and, in turn, the platelets' own agonist release. Some uncommon congenital disorders lack responses to specific agonists in a characteristic fashion. More detailed testing may be needed for a specific diagnosis, such as electron microscopy for granule defects, flow cytometry for surface receptors and granule markers, or genetic testing.[8]

vWD is a factor deficiency which imparts clinical features of platelet dysfunction, due to the central role of vWF in cross-linking activated platelets to form the platelet plug.[9] Up to 1% of all patients have vWD, with a wide range of severity due to either quantitative or functional defects of vWF. Diagnostic testing is integral to deciphering the specific defect and type of vWD to ensure the appropriate treatment. Since vWF is the carrier for factor VIII (FVIII) in plasma, vWF protein levels usually correlate with FVIII levels. Initial testing for vWD should include the vWF antigen level, vWF activity level, and FVIII activity level for comparison with vWF. Blood group O persons have shorter plasma half-life and lower normal levels of vWF, so ABO blood typing may be needed to interpret a borderline vWF level. Type 1 vWD is a quantitative deficiency, with decreased antigen and activity. Type 2 vWD may have normal antigen levels, but decreased activity from a defective protein. Within type 2, there are several subtypes with different molecular defects, and specialized identification is needed in order to determine the best therapy. Type 3 vWD is a rare, very severe autosomal recessive deficiency.[9] The clinical features and management of vWD are discussed later in this chapter.

Laboratory Evaluation of Secondary Hemostasis and Coagulation

7 A general oversight of plasma clotting factor activity is obtained by the *prothrombin time (PT)* for the intrinsic (tissue) pathway and the *aPTT* for the extrinsic (contact) pathway (Fig. 16-2), with both tests completed through the common pathway.[6] These clotting tests are performed in blood specimens collected in a chelator (3.2% citrate) which binds Ca^{2+} to prevent clotting in the tube. The in vitro clotting test is activated by TF in the PT or negatively charged surfaces in the aPTT, using phospholipid as a platform (substituting for platelets). Ca^{2+} is then added to overcome the specimen chelation, and the time is measured

until complete fibrin clotting is observed. Representative normal ranges are around 12 to 15 seconds for the PT and 25 to 35 seconds for the aPTT, but are defined by each laboratory using its own equipment, reagents, and normal specimens. Testing is routinely performed at 37°C, but hypothermia in the patient impairs the enzymatic reactions of clot formation.

Clotting physiology is more complicated than the traditional diagrams of separate cascade pathways for these two tests. We have seen that thrombin from the intrinsic pathway activates the extrinsic pathway. In vitro, the aPTT clotting test is activated by synthetic contact materials which initiate via factor XII, so deficiencies of XII and other related contact factors cause a prolonged aPTT. However, deficiencies of these contact factors do not cause bleeding and may in fact be associated with impaired fibrinolysis and thrombosis. Fibrinogen activity is also a critical parameter. Most assays measure the functional conversion of fibrinogen to fibrin, although the fibrinogen protein level can also be measured for comparison to assess fibrinogen dysfunction. Normal fibrinogen levels are around 150 to 400 mg/dL.

Mixing Studies

To investigate unexpectedly elevated PT or aPTT values, the test should be repeated after mixing the patient's plasma with equal volumes of normal plasma. Even in severe factor deficiencies, the PT or aPTT shows substantial correction toward normal in a mixing study. However, if the patient's plasma contains an inhibitor or an anticoagulant, the normal plasma will also be affected and the PT or aPTT will not be correct.

Individual factor level activities are determined by the degree of correction which patient plasma gives when mixed with factor-deficient plasma. The classic congenital factor deficiencies are FVIII deficiency (hemophilia A) and factor IX deficiency (hemophilia B). Both are X-linked and thus nearly always in males. Factor XI deficiency is most often seen in persons of Ashkenazi Jewish descent. Acquired factor deficiencies usually involve multiple factors.[10] The vitamin K–dependent factors are II (thrombin), VII, IX, and X. In liver disease, all factor synthesis is deficient except FVIII, which also comes from endothelium. However, FVIII and other factors can be low in disseminated intravascular coagulation (DIC). As noted, FVIII may be low as part of vWD. Isolated factor X deficiency occurs in some patients with amyloidosis because the abnormal protein absorbs this factor. Performing a set of factors V, VII, and VIII may suggest a pattern to aid in the diagnosis of specific clinical syndromes.

Coagulation inhibitors are substances, usually antibodies, which block one or more clotting factors. Most do not cause bleeding; the most common examples are lupus anticoagulants (LAs), one type of antiphospholipid antibodies (APLA) discussed below in thrombosis tests. However, factor-specific inhibitor antibodies can block clotting in vivo and cause bleeding.[10] They are identified by their effect on the plasma factor's activity and semiquantified by assessing how much interference the patient's plasma gives to factor level measurements in normal plasma. Some severe hemophiliacs and other factor-deficient patients develop alloantibodies to therapeutic clotting factors, interfering with treatment and necessitating alternative factor therapies or immunosuppression. Bovine thrombin used for topical hemostasis can induce cross-reacting antibodies to the patient's own factor V. Autoantibodies to specific clotting factors, most commonly FVIII, can cause serious coagulopathy.

8 DIC describes unchecked coagulation initiated by pathologic systemic activation of the intrinsic clotting pathway. The specific pathophysiology of DIC is discussed later in this chapter, but diagnostic criteria require an inciting condition such as extensive tissue injury or a systemic inflammatory response secondary to infection, obstetrical complication, or malignancy. Intravascular platelet activation and fibrin formation lead to thrombocytopenia, hypofibrinogenemia, and RBCs sheared by fibrin strands (schistocytes). The results of coagulation profile tests vary, but often show prolonged PT and aPTT. In some patients, thrombosis is the most prominent clinical finding, but in most patients, the depletion of platelets and clotting factors with accompanying activation of fibrinolysis leads to diffuse consumptive coagulopathy. Fibrin formation followed by fibrinolysis generates the fibrin fragments called D-dimers, which when quantified in immunologic testing are a useful indicator of DIC.

Three other tests are commonly performed during surgery with whole-blood specimens: The *activated clotting time (ACT), ecarin clotting time (ECT),* and viscoelastic whole-blood clotting with thromboelastography. The ACT, a point of care test, assesses the intrinsic clotting pathway and is used mainly to monitor heparin anticoagulation and its protamine reversal during cardiopulmonary bypass or vascular surgery. The ECT also describes the intrinsic clotting function, but it is primarily used for measuring the clinical effects of direct thrombin inhibitors (DTIs) such as bivalirudin. These agents are often used for patients with HIT. The ACT and aPTT also reflect the clinical efficacy of DTIs, but at high doses required for cardiopulmonary bypass, ECT is more accurate.[11]

Thromboelastography

Whole-blood clotting and fibrinolysis can be assessed by viscoelastic testing in thromboelastography (TEG®, Haemoscope Corp., Niles, IL, USA) or rotation thromboelastometry (ROTEM®, Pentapharm GmBH, Munich, Germany). These tests measure the rate, strength, and lysis, if any, of clot formation. Numerous parameters can be measured with these tests; accordingly the TEG–ROTEM working group attempted to standardize the parameters obtained from both testing modalities in order to make them more clinically relevant. There are minor differences in the mechanisms for TEG versus ROTEM; however, both involve the use of whole blood in a heated cup with the addition of a sensor pin. The cup or the pin oscillates while the blood clots. The increasing resistance to oscillation is transmitted through the sensor pin and a graphic depiction of clot formation is displayed in the thromboelastogram.[12] The patterns obtained can implicate defects in factor levels, platelet function, fibrinogen concentration, and the presence of abnormal fibrinolysis, the latter which is difficult to measure rapidly otherwise. Testing can be performed in the presence of inhibitors of heparin or fibrinolysis to help judge whether these drugs would be effective. This test format has also been adapted to assess antiplatelet therapy in patients with ventricular assist devices.[13] Thromboelastography is helpful in determining the appropriate therapy, including platelets, plasma, fibrinogen replacement, or antifibrinolytics, as complex bleeding syndromes such as massive hemorrhage with consumptive or dilutional coagulopathy progress.

Diagnosis of Thromboembolic Disorders

9 The risk for DVT, PE, VTE, and other thromboses is increased by intercurrent factors such as physical inactivity or immobilization, malignancy, oral contraceptives, estrogen therapy, and pregnancy. However, in addition to or especially in the absence of such factors, laboratory testing often identifies an underlying congenital

or acquired predisposing abnormality which tips the hemostatic systems toward thrombosis. Discovery of one or more risk factors may influence the course of therapy and suggest benefit from family studies.

Congenital Risk Factors for Thrombosis

The most commonly tested congenital problems discussed below increase the risk of VTE.[14] Although arterial thrombosis may involve a few of these factors, platelets are more directly involved on the arterial side, and congenital contributions are less well defined. Some investigators have described a "sticky platelet syndrome," with hyperactive platelet aggregometry. Although severe congenital problems may present in childhood, they are rare; most thrombotic presentations are in adulthood over a lifetime of potential risk. Congenital problems are mostly categorized as deficiencies in antithrombotic pathways or hypercoagulable clotting factors.

Several congenital factors involve the protein C-ase complex and its function. The most common hypercoagulable mutation is factor V Leiden (FVL), in about 5% of Caucasians.[15] FV is the cofactor for factor X when the latter activates prothrombin to thrombin. APC is the natural brake on FV, by cleaving it at Arg506. FVL carries the autosomal dominant mutation Arg506Gln, rendering FV fairly resistant to APC. Thus FV is overactive and thrombin formation is favored. The FVL polymorphism is readily identified genetically. However, a small percentage of persons with resistance to APC have other mutations in FV or other conditions. Therefore, slightly more inclusive is the functional clotting test for APC resistance, which assesses plasma clotting time with and without reagent APC.

Protein C itself is functionally deficient in up to 0.5% of the population, with autosomal dominant inheritance. This leads to overactive FVIII and FV cofactors in their respective intrinsic tenase and prothrombinase complexes. Most have low activity and antigen (type I), but some have low activity with normal antigen levels (type II). Homozygous protein C deficiency is a very severe thrombotic disorder beginning in infancy. Protein S deficiency can lead to thrombosis because of its cofactor role to protein C. Around 1 in 700 persons has autosomal dominant deficiency. Protein S circulates partly bound to the complement C4 binding protein and partly as the unbound (free) active form. Nearly all cases of protein S deficiency can be identified by assaying the free antigen and then categorized as to whether the total antigen is low (type I) or normal (type II). Type II has low function but normal antigen levels, but this is rare. Both protein C and protein S are vitamin K–dependent, and therefore vitamin K deficiency or warfarin interferes with laboratory assessment of their activities. Warfarin-induced skin necrosis in protein C or S deficiencies is discussed in antithrombotic therapy testing below. In AT-III deficiency, the relative lack of its normal blocking function on the key enzymes VIIa, IXa, Xa, and XIa leads to thrombosis risk. Testing for AT-III activity will detect both quantitative and qualitative defects.

The best characterized congenital gain in function is the prothrombin mutation G20210A (guanine to adenine). This autosomal dominant condition is found in about 1 in 50 Caucasians, but is much less prevalent in African and Asian backgrounds. Persons with this variant have high circulating prothrombin levels as the reason for thrombosis risk. Genetic testing for the mutation is more definitive than prothrombin levels. Elevated FVIII levels may be a modest risk factor for thrombosis, but FVIII is an acute-phase reactant and rises in many intercurrent conditions. Whether there is an inherited element to persistently elevated FVIII levels is unclear.

Acquired Risk Factors for Thrombosis

Several factors increase the risk of thrombosis.[16] APLA are associated with both arterial and venous thrombosis risk. These antibodies bind to phospholipid–protein complexes. Several possible mechanisms for their in vivo effects have been proposed. They may bind to and activate endothelial cells, which in turn could directly tip off coagulation and/or cause vascular injury. They may interfere with phospholipids in the protein C-ase enzyme complex, leading to diminution of protein C's regulatory function. The various antigenic targets and mechanisms of APLA require multiple tests for their detection. Studies should include tests of clotting function, most notably LA tests, and tests of solid-phase binding to antigen targets, such as anticardiolipin antibodies (ACLA) and anti-β_2-glycoprotein-1 (AβGP). AβGP is a protein often present in the phospholipid–protein complex targeted by these antibodies.

LA antibodies are a common cause of prolonged aPTT which does not correct by mixing with normal plasma. It should be emphasized that the prolonged aPTT is a phenomenon of the in vitro test and is NOT associated with bleeding. However, not all LAs prolong the aPTT. Laboratories testing for LA should use at least two different tests to improve detection. One is usually a test based on the aPTT, but modified with phospholipid reagent selected to be sensitive to LA interference. A second clotting-based test is also recommended, such as the dilute Russell viper venom time (DRVVT), in which the snake venom activates factor X in the common pathway, leading to thrombin formation. This test's reagent phospholipid is adjusted by dilution to be LA-sensitive, but because the venom bypasses the usual initiating factors, the DVVRT is not affected by autoantibody inhibitors of FVIII or other upstream factors, a potential cause of confusion in the PTT-based assays.

ACLA and AβGP antibody tests usually employ enzyme immunoassays (EIA). AβGP may be more specific for physiologic thrombotic effect, by presenting an actual target of in vivo antibodies, whereas ACLA may develop in other conditions such as infections. For example, false-positive non-treponemal syphilis serology is sometimes seen with ACLA.

Hyperhomocysteinemia is a risk factor for venous and possibly arterial thrombosis. This amino acid is made from methionine and is then either converted back or processed to cysteine. The mechanism for thrombosis risk is unclear, but endothelial cell injury has been proposed. Fasting total homocysteine is the initial screening test. Hyperhomocysteinemia can be due to various congenital mutations in homocysteine's metabolic pathways or can be acquired via vitamin deficiencies affecting its metabolism (folate, B_{12}, B_6) or in many other medical conditions.

Monitoring Anticoagulation Therapeutic Agents

10 Most anticoagulant therapies need ongoing or selective testing for assessment of therapeutic effect. Appropriate monitoring ensures that these agents are maintained within the therapeutic range; otherwise patients are at risk of thromboembolism and bleeding complications both of which can have devastating consequences.

Warfarin Anticoagulation

Warfarin therapy must be monitored by the PT and its analogue for this purpose, the international normalized ratio (INR), in order to avoid under- or overcoagulation. PT methods and reagents can widely differ between laboratories, yielding varying PT values for the same degree of factor deficiency. However, each PT test vendor supplies a conversion parameter to express the PT as the INR in patients on warfarin. The INR is a normalized value which is intended to compare results across laboratories for evaluating combined deficiencies of factors II, VII, IX, and X, the warfarin-dependent factors. The INR's therapeutic range for warfarin anticoagulation is generally 2.0 to 3.0, except for mechanical heart valves and prevention of myocardial infarction (INR 2.5 to 3.5).[17]

When warfarin is started or stopped, the factors with the fastest plasma turnover, that is, the shortest half-lives, decline or rise the fastest, respectively. Thus, the inhibitor protein C, with a 6 hr half-life, declines faster than most clotting factors when warfarin takes effect, and this can cause an imbalance toward clotting during the initiation of warfarin therapy. Warfarin-induced skin necrosis is a thrombotic complication often occurring when previously unrecognized congenital protein C deficiency accentuates this imbalance.

Warfarin's pharmacology is affected by genetic variations in the metabolism of the drug (cytochrome P450, CYP2C9) or its counterbalancing vitamin K (vitamin K epoxide reductase complex subunit 1, VKORC1). Genetic polymorphism testing has been advocated for achieving more rapid therapeutic effect when initiating therapy or in assessing difficulty achieving the target INR, but indications for genetic testing are still under investigation. The INR is not calibrated to evaluate non-warfarin deficiencies such as liver disease, which affects most other clotting factors, and thus strictly speaking, the INR should not be used in other conditions including liver disease.

Heparin Anticoagulation Testing

The aPTT is used to assess heparin anticoagulation. Each laboratory determines its own therapeutic target range for heparin anticoagulation, typically on the order of 1.5 to 2.5 times the normal mean. The laboratory determines the exact range for their test system based on a functional enzymatic test for heparin action, the anti-factor Xa activity (aFXa). (This is a different test than the factor X activity level.) Using the aFXa assay, therapeutic target heparin levels of 0.3 to 0.7 aFXa units/mL are correlated with aPTT results for that range. aFXa testing can be helpful in assessing heparin resistance.

Low-molecular-weight heparin (LMWH) drugs and their analogue, synthetic pentasaccharide (e.g., fondaparinux), do not affect the aPTT assay, and coagulation testing is usually not needed. However, if necessary, the drugs' plasma activity levels can be assessed by the aFXa assay. This may be helpful in renal failure affecting drug excretion or in pregnant women, obese, and neonates for whom drug levels are less certain after subcutaneous injection. Like heparin, these agents inhibit factor Xa indirectly, that is, via their enhancing effect on antithrombin.

Heparin and to a lesser degree LMWH can stimulate the production of antibodies against the heparin–PF-4 complex. These antibodies can in turn cause HIT and/or activation of platelets to induce thrombosis.[18] If thrombocytopenia or thrombosis develops in a patient on these drugs, tests for HIT antibodies are available by EIA or by functional measures such as serotonin release. Patients with HIT must avoid heparin and LMWH.

Several newer anticoagulants have entered clinical practice, as alternatives to heparin in patients with HIT or as alternatives to warfarin. These are direct anticoagulants which are not mediated by antithrombin. The "xaban" class of drugs, including rivaroxaban and apixaban, directly inhibit factor Xa.[19] They prolong the PT and aPTT, but monitoring is not recommended and the INR should not be used. An aFXa-type assay adapted for these drugs is being researched.

DTIs also pose challenges for coagulation testing. These include hirudin from leeches, its recombinant "-rudin" mimicking molecules (bivalirudin, desirudin, lepirudin), and small synthetic molecules acting at the same site as hirudin on thrombin (argatroban, dabigatran). They all prolong the PT and aPTT and interfere with clot-based fibrinogen assays. There is no consensus on how to quantify the effect of these drugs. The ECT has been promulgated.[20] Ecarin, an enzyme in snake venom, cleaves prothrombin to a metabolic intermediate which is inhibited by hirudin and its analogues. However, the ECT is not widely available.

BLOOD COMPONENT PRODUCTION

Blood Collection

The production of blood components is highly controlled by regulations and accreditation requirements in the interests of donor and recipient safety and therapeutic efficacy. Blood donors are carefully screened and tested, and blood products are made in specialized laboratories and other facilities. Regional blood centers collect and provide most blood components for transfusion, although some hospitals collect blood or platelets to augment their supply. Virtually all blood components come from volunteer unpaid donors. Pharmaceutical companies process plasma into various derivatives or synthesize some desired proteins for infusion.

Blood donors undergo a confidential interview to screen for medical problems in their donation safety and for risks of disease transmission to their recipients.[21] They are questioned about risk factors, exposure, or signs of human immunodeficiency virus (HIV), hepatitis, and other infections. There are geographically based deferral criteria for tropical exposure to malaria and (in American donors) European exposure to variant Creutzfeldt–Jakob disease (vCJD). The donor's pulse, blood pressure, and hemoglobin/hematocrit level (US minimum 12.5 g/dL or 38%) are checked. Phlebotomy is performed with validated antiseptic measures to reduce the risk of bacterial contamination in the blood bags. In the United States, donors are deferred for 8 weeks after a whole-blood donation to avoid iron deficiency.

Table 16-1 shows the contents and storage parameters for blood components. In whole-blood donations, 450 to 500 mL of blood is collected into citrate anticoagulant and then separated by centrifugation into RBCs, platelets, and/or plasma. The RBC units usually have most plasma removed and replaced with preservative. In the United States, the plasma must be frozen within 6 hours of collection to be labeled fresh frozen plasma (FFP). A large proportion of plasma is now made as plasma frozen within 24 hours, with minimal effect on clotting factor content compared to FFP. Cryoprecipitate is made from barely thawed FFP, which has a precipitate enriched in fibrinogen; the precipitate is isolated by centrifugation and refrozen.[22] Five bags of "cryo" comprise a typical adult dose. Whole-blood–derived platelets (sometimes called "random-donor platelets") are derived from platelet-rich plasma in the United States and from the buffy-coat centrifugation layer in other countries.[23] Four to six units are pooled to yield one adult-sized dose of platelets. Traditionally, pooling was done at the hospital just before transfusion, but blood centers can now provide pre-pooled platelets to hospitals.

Blood components are also collected by apheresis, in which the donor's blood is processed by ex vivo centrifugation, the

TABLE 16-1. BLOOD COMPONENTS

Component	Average Volume	Storage Parameters
Packed red blood cells	300 mL	1–6°C for 21–35 days or 42 days with additive solution
Red blood cells, frozen	300 mL	<–65°C for 10 years
Platelets, whole-blood-derived	50 mL per bag, usual dose 4–6 bags	20–24°C for 5 days
Platelets, apheresis	300 mL	20–24°C for 5 days
Plasma, fresh frozen	250 mL	<–18°C for 1 year or <–65°C for 7 years
Plasma, frozen within 24 h	250 mL	<–18°C for 1 year
Cryoprecipitate	15 mL per bag, usual dose 4–6 bags	<–18°C for 1 year

desired component(s) are siphoned off into citrate anticoagulant, and the rest returned to the donor. Most platelets are produced by apheresis (sometimes called single-donor platelets). Plasma and RBCs can also be collected by apheresis, and if the donor's blood volume and cell counts permit, two doses of the desired component can be obtained in one collection session.

All donors are checked against files of deferred donors, and all donations are tested for blood-borne infectious agents. Tests for HIV, hepatitis B virus (HBV), and hepatitis C virus (HCV) are universally required.[24] The addition of sensitive nucleic acid testing (NAT; e.g., polymerase chain reaction) to routine serology shortens the window period in a recently infected donor down to 7 to 10 days for HIV and HCV and 1 month for HBV. The US FDA also requires testing for syphilis, human T-cell lymphotropic virus (HTLV), and West Nile virus (WNV). Also available for donors at risk is a test for *Trypanosoma cruzi* (Chagas disease). Cytomegalovirus (CMV) is mainly in WBCs; selected patients at risk for complications of infection from cellular components can receive either CMV-negative units or leukoreduced units.

At some centers, directed donations can be made by family or friends for a specific patient. These donations augment the overall supply of blood and donors, and could reduce the number of donor exposures by using the same donor(s) more than once. However, the infectious risk from these units is not considered any less than from community volunteer donors. Cellular components from blood relatives must be irradiated to prevent the risk of transfusion graft-versus-host disease (GVHD) from closely matched donor lymphocytes which are not rejected by the recipient.

Autologous donations by the patient can be made in advance of scheduled surgery, with physician approval. The usual minimum hemoglobin or hematocrit is 11 g/dL or 33%, respectively, which is lower than the minimum allowed for regular donors. Patients should be on erythropoietin or iron supplementation to support RBC replenishment. In order to achieve a net gain in RBC mass, donations should be scheduled with some lead time within the 6-week storage period to permit erythropoiesis before surgery. Erythropoietin assists with multiple donations. Autologous units are only used for the patient and cannot be given to anyone else, since they often have a lower RBC content than normal requirements, and surgical patients frequently have conditions disqualifying them for regular donation.

Component Processing and Storage

11 *Leukoreduction* (LR) to remove WBCs from RBCs and platelets reduces the risk of human leukocyte antigen (HLA) alloimmunization, febrile nonhemolytic transfusion reactions (FNHTRs), and CMV transmission in patients who require these precautions. LR is usually performed by filtration, although some apheresis collections have sufficiently precise cell separation to minimize WBC content. The WBC content is reduced from around 10^9 WBCs to $\leq 1 \times 10^6$ to 5×10^6 WBCs/unit.

In addition to the routine indications above, LR has been studied for the prevention of transfusion-related acute lung injury (TRALI) and so-called transfusion-related immunomodulation (TRIM), that is, possible immunosuppressive and pro-inflammatory effects mediated by donor WBCs. "Universal" LR of all cellular components is done in many countries, for this and other reasons. However, randomized controlled trials have been mostly inconclusive for benefit. Meta-analysis of available data has highlighted cardiac surgery as a setting in which there may be postoperative survival benefit associated with leukoreduced blood components, based on a small number of studies to date.[25]

Washing cellular components with saline is mostly done to remove plasma in patients with allergic transfusion reactions such as those who are IgA deficient. It does not affect the antigens on the cells and does not remove enough WBCs to prevent GVHD or HLA alloimmunization.

Irradiation of cellular components is performed to prevent transfusion GVHD from directed-donor units from blood relatives and in highly immunosuppressed patients at risk for this complication: Leukemia, lymphoma, hematopoietic stem cell transplants, congenital cellular immunodeficiencies.[26] The units are exposed to gamma irradiation (2,500 cGy) to damage donor WBC DNA and prevent a cellular immune proliferative response to the recipient's tissues. Irradiation is usually performed in cesium-137 blood irradiators. The blood units do not come in contact with the radioisotope and are not radioactive, but laboratory personnel must comply with radiation safety regulations. Blood units can also be irradiated by cobalt-60 beams in radiation therapy facilities, but in the United States, the FDA regulates this function closely. In recent years, X-ray generators which do not contain radioisotopes have been approved for blood components.

Platelets are stored at room temperature to preserve clotting function, but this increases the risk of bacterial growth in contaminated units, compared to other blood components. Accordingly, bacterial detection has become routine in many countries. Platelet testing must be done after a short period of storage in order to detect growing bacteria. Blood centers can take culture samples from plateletpheresis units and pre-pooled whole-blood–derived platelets before product release. However, culturing is not feasible from the small volumes of individual whole-blood–derived platelets when the transfusion service is pooling the units just before use. In this situation, bacterial antigen testing is available to transfusion services and is required by accrediting agencies in the United States.

RBC preservation solutions use CDPA—Citrate for anticoagulation, Phosphate as a buffer, Adenine, and 1 to 2 g of dextrose (D-glucose)—to maintain adenosine triphosphate (ATP) levels and RBC membrane integrity. However, despite preservatives, several metabolic changes occur during RBC storage. 2,3-Diphosphoglycerate (2,3-DPG) is depleted in the first 2 weeks, thus shifting the oxygen dissociation curve to the left and making hemoglobin more avid for O_2, although this reverses after transfusion. Furthermore, by the end of the 42-day shelf life of additive-solution RBCs, the pH is 6.5, the plasma K^+ is 50 mmol/L from RBC leakage and hemolysis, and 15% to 20% of the RBCs are nonviable.[27] RBC storage lesions could be involved in observations linking older units to adverse outcomes such as short-term mortality and multiple organ failure.[28] Randomized trials are underway to address this important question.

Plasma Derivatives

12 Plasma derivatives are proteins processed from plasma for therapeutic infusions. They include albumin, immunoglobulins (IGs), clotting factors, and other proteins. Derivatives are purified from plasma using physicochemical fractionation methods developed by Edwin J. Cohn in the 1930s. Donors for plasma derivatives are screened and tested just as blood component donors, and the separation techniques provide a degree of purification from microbial pathogens. However, the large numbers of donor units which must be pooled together for production of plasma derivatives introduce the possibility of contamination of an entire lot by a small number of infected donors. Such was the case in the early years of HIV when factor concentrates infected a large proportion of hemophiliacs before the risk was known. Because intact cells are not required, many derivatives can undergo purification and pathogen inactivation methods which are impractical for blood components.

Albumin is produced in large quantities for intravascular volume support and is pasteurized at 60°C for sterility. IGs are given for immune support or for immunomodulation to suppress native antibody production. IGs can also withstand robust pathogen inactivation processes, and in some cases are nanofiltered to remove viruses. To be given intravenously, IGs need extra processing to avoid reaction-provoking protein aggregates. Hyperimmune globulins are fractionated from the plasma of donors with high levels of antibody to specific antigens of interest, such as viruses (HBV, CMV, varicella zoster) or the Rh blood group D antigen (RhIG to prevent anti-D formation in RhD-negative women).

Factor concentrates for patients with congenital deficiencies are made with special techniques to ultrapurify factors VIII, IX, XIII, vWF, fibrinogen, and in some countries, factor XI—while also applying pathogen inactivation methods and viral filtration to remove microbes. However, plasma-free recombinant factors VIII and IX are also available to further allay concern about disease transmission, and recombinant activated factor VII (rFVIIa) is approved for rare VII-deficient patients. Some hemophiliacs develop inhibitory antibodies to the FVIII or factor IX they are missing. These inhibitor patients often need products which "bypass" their missing clotting step. The therapeutic potential of prothrombin complex concentrates (PCCs) containing multiple factors, or FVIIa to bypass secondary hemostasis and generate a thrombin burst is discussed later in this chapter. On the antithrombotic side of hemostasis, antithrombin concentrate is available.

Other plasma proteins which are purified for selected deficiencies are complement C1 esterase inhibitor (for hereditary angioedema) and α_1-antitrypsin.

Pathogen Inactivation

13 Techniques have been developed to kill microbial pathogens in blood components. This approach has the major advantage of protection against unrecognized infectious agents. None of these processes have been approved in the United States to date. The methods vary by blood component. In Europe and other countries, solvent-detergent and methylene blue treatments have been approved for plasma, and psoralen and riboflavin treatments for plasma and platelets. Cell-free plasma, either in pools or as individual units, can be treated with membrane-disrupting solvent-detergent treatments for enveloped viruses. Non-enveloped viruses, most prominently hepatitis A and parvovirus, are less susceptible, but NAT can be added to detect these agents.

More robust methods involve agents which damage nucleic acids. When methylene blue, psoralen, or riboflavin is added to the blood bag, they bind to nucleic acids. Then photoactivation is performed with specific wavelengths of light, cross-linking DNA and RNA to prevent microbial function. Not yet approved but under investigation is ultraviolet light treatment of platelets. RBC units are less amenable to photoactivation through the hemoglobin, although riboflavin is being explored. Certain alkylating agents have shown promising microbicidal activity, but modify the RBC membrane enough that subjects have formed antibodies against the treated RBCs.

The adverse effects that limit these techniques include the potential for reduced platelet count increments, alterations in plasma clotting factor levels, and potential toxicity from some of the added agents if they are not sufficiently removed after treatment.

RBC and Platelet Substitutes

14 Many years of effort have gone into the search for an oxygen-carrying substitute for RBCs. Oxygen-avid perfluorocarbon chemicals underwent international trials, but 100% O_2 administration was needed and clinical trials were unsuccessful (Castro). Several hemoglobin solutions have been made from pools of human or bovine hemoglobin, or from recombinant hemoglobin, all of which were chemically modified to facilitate extracellular O_2 offloading.[29] However, the potentially toxic effects of free hemoglobin, including intravascular binding of the vasodilator nitrous oxide (NO), are not sufficiently understood for regulatory approval. US clinical trials were unsuccessful in demonstrating clinical advantage in pre-hospital trauma management. None of these agents appear to hold much promise for clinical application in the near future. A more recent avenue of exploration is the possibility of "growing" RBCs in cell culture systems. They would be biocompatible and low in pathogen risk, and their RBC antigens could be engineered to some extent to maximize compatibility. The biology of cultivating mature normal RBCs in large scale is under investigation.

Platelets are so complex that it would be difficult to replace their functions fully. However, some early work has emerged on preserved platelets (e.g., freeze-dried or fixed) and on biocompatible platforms bearing hemostatic proteins, such as fibrinogen-coated albumin beads, which could supply some degree of platelet-like clotting function. Culturing platelets in vitro for therapeutic uses is also being pursued.[30]

BLOOD PRODUCTS AND TRANSFUSION THRESHOLDS

Compatibility Testing

15 Routine RBC compatibility testing includes ABO and RhD typing, an antibody screen for IgG non-ABO RBC antibodies, and an RBC cross-match. RBCs must be ABO-compatible to avoid intravascular hemolysis, and RhD-negative patients should receive D-negative RBCs to avoid anti-D alloimmunization. Rh, Kell, Kidd, Duffy, and some other non-ABO antibodies can also hemolyze transfused RBCs; 1% of all patients and 5% to 20% of heavily transfused patients have such antibodies. If no antibodies are present, the cross-match can be electronic; that is, RBC units are selected by the laboratory computer to be ABO- and RhD-compatible. But if hemolytic antibodies are detected or are on record, RBC units negative for the incompatible antigen(s) must be found, and a serologic cross-match of patient plasma versus donor RBCs is performed to confirm compatibility. Most hospitals have blood order schedules for their most common surgical procedures, which set forth a recommended number of RBC units to cover 80% to 90% of patients undergoing each procedure.

RBC compatibility testing takes 45 to 60 minutes, and much longer if antibodies are found. Hence, testing in advance of scheduled surgery is desirable. In emergencies, uncross-matched group O RBCs can be given, albeit with the risk of non-ABO antibody incompatibility. Group AB is the universal plasma which avoids transfusing anti-A or -B versus the patient's RBCs.

Red Blood Cells

16 Over the past decade, transfusion practices for medical and surgical patients shifted from a liberal strategy to more restrictive management with lower thresholds and careful consideration of the balance between transfusion risks and the physiologic consequences of anemia. The American Society for Anesthesiologists (ASA) *Practice Guidelines for Blood Component Therapy* state that "red blood cell transfusion is rarely indicated when the hemoglobin concentration is greater than 10 g/dL and is almost always indicated when it is less than 6 g/dL".[31] This leaves little guidance for the majority of anemic patients whose hemoglobin lies between 7 and 10 g/dL. In 1999, the Transfusion Requirements in Critical Care (TRICC) Investigators, Hebert et al., set a new precedent for the tolerance of hemoglobin levels as low as 7 g/dL without increasing morbidity or mortality.[32] The literature clearly supports a lower transfusion trigger for young healthy patients as evidence by trauma studies and case discussions of Jehovah's Witnesses.[33] However, the question of when to transfuse those at risk for tissue hypoxia such as patients with cardiovascular, cerebrovascular, or renal insufficiency remains controversial.

The original TRICC trial included critically ill but euvolemic patients in a large multicenter randomized control trial. The investigators compared the survival of patients transfused to hemoglobin levels greater than 10 g/dL in the liberal group with patients under a restrictive strategy who were not transfused until their hemoglobin fell to less than 7 g/dL. Overall survival for more than 800 patients did not differ between the groups.[32] Subsequent subgroup analysis of the TRICC trial and several meta-analysis and systematic reviews over the past 10 years not only confirmed these results, but established a possible morbidity and mortality risk associated with liberal transfusion management for a variety of different patient populations including those less than 55 years old, trauma patients, and those with stable cardiovascular disease.[33–36]

Traditionally, patients with cardiovascular disease and anemia were considered to be at significant risk of tissue ischemia and therefore thought to benefit from higher hemoglobin goals in the perioperative and critical care setting. These recommendations were based on two studies which showed an association between anemia in patients with cardiovascular disease and mortality that improved with transfusion.[37,38] Several retrospective studies and systematic reviews have since contradicted these findings by documenting the safety of hematocrits less than 24% during cardiac surgery with cardiopulmonary bypass.[34,39] The Transfusion Requirements After Cardiac Surgery (TRACS) trial randomized postcardiac surgery patients to restrictive (hematocrit >24%) versus liberal (hematocrit >30%) transfusion strategies and found no difference in 30-day mortality or severe morbidity. Furthermore, they found that transfusion was an independent risk factor for morbidity and mortality.[34,40] The most recent update to the Society of Thoracic Surgeons and the Society of Cardiovascular Anesthesiologists *Blood Conservation Clinical Practice Guidelines* recognizes that all cardiac surgery patients are at risk for tissue hypoxia and transfusion. These guidelines report that tissue oxygenation does not improve with transfusion for hemoglobin levels greater than 10 g/dL; and they state that "Transfusion is reasonable in most postoperative patients whose hemoglobin is less than 7 g/dL." For patients with hemoglobin levels between 7 and 10 g/dL the two societies recommend transfusion in patients with "critical noncardiac end-organ ischemia," active blood loss, or clinical indication of tissue hypoxia (low mixed venous oxygen saturation or electrocardiographic or echocardiographic evidence of myocardial ischemia).[41]

Patients with cerebrovascular disease or acute neurologic illness such as ischemic stroke, subarachnoid hemorrhage, and traumatic brain injury are at significant risk for secondary injury from tissue hypoxia. There are several studies and reviews devoted to the question of optimal brain tissue oxygen delivery during acute neurologic illness. Acute and chronic anemia initiates physiologic compensatory mechanisms discussed below as well as neuroprotective strategies for tolerating decreases in cerebral oxygen delivery; however, the hemoglobin level at which anemia induces detrimental patient outcomes remains unclear.[42] Evidence indicates that a hemoglobin level less than 9 g/dL is independently predictive of poor outcome especially in patients with cerebrovascular injury.[43,44] RBC transfusion perioperatively or during critical illness is also independently associated with morbidity and mortality.[43,45,46] This leaves the clinician with little guidance to decide when and who should be transfused. Clearly transfused RBCs do not function as well as endogenous erythrocytes and it remains unclear if transfused blood improves overall outcomes.

Physiologic Compensation for Anemia

There is ample evidence for the human tolerance of anemia both
17 acute and chronic. Oxygen delivery to the tissues (DO_2) is dependent on cardiac output (CO), regional blood flow, and oxygen-carrying capacity also known as the oxygen content (CaO_2) of blood.[42,47] The relationship between all of these variables is shown in Table 16-2. Hemoglobin plays an integral role in oxygen transport and delivery to the tissues. The clinical justification for RBC transfusion assumes that increasing the hemoglobin will improve oxygen-carrying capacity and therefore avoid tissue

TABLE 16-2. EQUATIONS FOR TISSUE OXYGENATION[42,47]

Parameter	Unit	Equation
Oxygen delivery (DO_2)	mL O_2/min	$DO_2 = CO\ (L/min) \times C_aO_2\ (mL/dL)$
Arterial oxygen content (C_aO_2)	mL O_2/dL	$C_aO_2 = 1.36 \times Hgb\ (g/dL) \times S_aO_2\ (\%) + [P_aO_2 \times 0.003]$
Venous oxygen content (C_vO_2)		$C_vO_2 = 1.36 \times Hgb\ (g/dL) \times S_vO_2\ (\%) + [P_vO_2 \times 0.003]$
Blood flow, cardiac output (CO)	L/min	Flow = $\pi r^4 \Delta P / 8 \eta L$ (r = radius, ΔP = change in pressure, η = viscosity, and L = length of the vessel)
Oxygen consumption (VO_2)	mL O_2/min	$VO_2 = CO\ (L/min) \times [C_aO_2 - C_vO_2]$
Oxygen extraction ratio (O_2EF)	%	$O_2EF = [C_aO_2 - C_vO_2]/C_aO_2 \times 100\%$ or $= VO_2/DO_2 \times 100\%$

Hgb, hemoglobin; P_aO_2, partial pressure of oxygen in arterial blood; P_vO_2, partial pressure of oxygen in venous blood.

hypoxia. However, given the ability of the body to compensate for anemia, it is unclear whether increasing hemoglobin in a stable anemic patient actually improves tissue oxygenation. There are several compensatory mechanisms for anemia, most notably (1) increased CO; (2) altered microcirculatory blood flow; and (3) improved tissue oxygen extraction from hemoglobin. These physiologic changes in conjunction with the detrimental impact of RBC storage limit the therapeutic effects of transfusion.[48]

1. *Increased CO.* There are several mechanisms for the increase in CO that occurs as compensation for isovolemic hemodilution. First of all, the heart rate increases secondary to a sympathetic surge initiated by anemia and hypoxia.[49–51] Secondly, higher stroke volume results from increased preload and decreased systemic vascular resistance and afterload. Isovolemic hemodilution occurs when acute blood loss is resuscitated with crystalloid or colloid fluids, thereby maintaining blood volume with lower hemoglobin. This decreases blood viscosity, one component of systemic vascular resistance, and decreases afterload by arterial vasodilation. The arterioles dilate as a result of the release of NO from endothelial cells. Lastly, tissue hypoxia will induce arteriovenous shunting and recruitment of new circulatory beds thereby increasing microcirculatory blood flow.[49]
2. *Altered Microcirculatory Blood Flow.* The decrease in blood viscosity associated with isovolemic hemodilution and chronic anemia improves blood flow especially through the microcirculation where lower shear force rates cause a pronounced vasodilation of capillary beds.[47,49,50] This improves venous return by lowering the resistance of venous beds and therefore increases preload and left ventricular filling. Patients with chronic anemia also increase angiogenesis and overall microcirculatory blood volume to compensate for the decreased oxygen-carrying capacity.[49] These mechanisms are extremely efficient. In fact, studies in anemic critically ill patients fail to show improvements in tissue oxygenation measures after transfusion.[48]
3. *Increased Tissue Oxygen Extraction.* Anemia causes the oxygen dissociation curve for oxyhemoglobin to shift to the right secondary to increased levels of 2,3-DPG in erythrocytes. This adaptive process is particularly influential for the physiologic compensation of chronic anemia and often the only mechanism necessary to maintain oxygen delivery. Isovolemic hemodilution to hematocrit levels less than 25% generates an increase in 2,3-DPG levels. Furthermore, acidemia associated with acute hemorrhage also shifts the oxygen dissociation curve to the right thereby decreasing the affinity of oxygen for hemoglobin at any partial pressure and improving the tissue oxygen extraction ratio.[49,50]

There continues to be controversy about RBC transfusion given the lack of evidence to support a universal transfusion threshold. Despite the wealth of literature documenting the potential harm, transfusion continues to be the mainstay of treatment for acute and chronic anemia. Healthy patients are most often able to compensate for anemia and tolerate critically low hemoglobin levels; however, the risk of tissue hypoxia in acute situations or in patients who are unable to compensate such as those with low cardiovascular reserve remains unclear. Each clinician must take into account the patient's comorbidities, the acuity of anemia, and their ability to compensate adequately without signs or symptoms of tissue hypoxia (Table 16-3).[52] Furthermore, it is important to measure the response to transfusion with follow-up hemoglobin levels in order to aid in the diagnosis of consumptive anemia, hemolysis, or ongoing bleeding as well as to guide further transfusions. In stable patients without ongoing bleeding, the hemoglobin should rise 1 g/dL with approximately 3% rise in hematocrit for each unit of packed RBCs given.[52]

The above discussion focuses on isovolemic hemodilution secondary to chronic anemia or acute hemorrhage post fluid resuscitation when compensatory mechanisms have had time to balance the detrimental effects of decreased hemoglobin levels. It is important to recognize that transfusion may be necessary

TABLE 16-3. CLINICAL INDICATIONS OF TISSUE HYPOXIA[52,53]

- Unstable vital signs
  - Tachycardia
  - Hypotension
  - Tachypnea or dyspnea
- Laboratory and invasive monitor indices
  - Mixed venous O_2 saturation (SV_mO_2) <50%
  - Central venous O_2 saturation (SV_cO_2) <60%
  - Increased O_2 extraction ratio (O_2ER) >50%
  - Lactic acidosis (metabolic acidemia with lactate >2 mmol/L)
- Signs of end-organ dysfunction
  - Electrocardiographic (ST changes, onset of arrhythmias) or echocardiographic indications of myocardial ischemia
  - Electroencephalographic indications of cerebral hypoperfusion
  - New onset oliguria (less than 0.5 mL/kg/h for >6 h)

prior to the availability of measured hemoglobin and hematocrit levels such as during acute hemorrhage, intraoperative bleeding, or trauma resuscitation. In the case of uncompensated blood loss, hemoglobin levels may be normal or misleadingly high. In these situations, the clinician must estimate blood loss from the patient's hemodynamic picture and assessment of the operative field in order to guide their transfusion management. Recent recommendations for intraoperative transfusion during massive bleeding focus on patients with class II hemorrhage (blood loss of 15% to 30% estimated blood volume) with preexisting anemia or cardiovascular disease and all patients with class III to IV hemorrhagic shock (blood loss of 30% to 40% estimated blood volume).[53] In these cases, the British Committee for Standards in Haematology guidelines for the management of massive transfusion recommend a goal hemoglobin over 8 g/dL.[54]

Platelets

18 Numerous recommendations provide guidance for the transfusion management of thrombocytopenia and acquired or inherited platelet disorders.[31,52,53,55–58] The indications for platelet transfusion depend on both quantitative and qualitative measures of platelet activity as well as the clinical setting. Table 16-4 outlines typical platelet thresholds for transfusion based on the clinical situation and patient history. For stable patients with severe thrombocytopenia, transfusion can be held until counts fall below 10,000 to 20,000/μL as long as they have no signs or symptoms of bleeding.[53,55,56,58] Prophylactic platelet transfusion is necessary for patient with severe thrombocytopenia <50,000/μL about to undergo major surgery or invasive procedures such as lumbar puncture, liver biopsy, neuraxial anesthesia, central venous catheterization, or endoscopy with biopsy.[56,57] In preparation for surgery on the eye or the central nervous system, the platelet count should be raised to >100,000/μL.[56,57]

Transfusion is not necessary for platelet counts >100,000/μL in clinically stable patients without suspicion of platelet dysfunction. Most patients with counts <50,000/μL and clinical bleeding require therapeutic transfusion.[31,55,56] There are several relative indications for transfusion of platelet counts between 50,000 and 100,000/μL. In particular, patients having surgery on vital organs such as the eye or central nervous system, or patients with multiple traumatic injuries, benefit from higher transfusion goals.[53,55,56] Furthermore, patients undergoing massive transfusion or hemorrhage with estimated blood loss of more than two blood volumes and ongoing bleeding should have a transfusion threshold of at least 75,000/μL to ensure the level does not fall below 50,000/μL.[53,54]

TABLE 16-4. INDICATIONS FOR PLATELET TRANSFUSION[31,53,55,57,58]

Indication	Threshold
Stable patients without evidence of bleeding or coagulopathy	<10,000/μL
Prophylaxis for invasive procedures such as lumbar puncture, neuraxial anesthesia, central venous catheterization, endoscopy with biopsy, liver biopsy, or major surgery	<50,000/μL
Stable patients with clinical evidence of bleeding or coagulopathy	<50,000/μL
Patients with DIC and signs of ongoing bleeding	<50,000/μL
Patients undergoing massive transfusion	<75,000/μL
Patients having surgery at critical sites such as the eye or central nervous system	<100,000/μL
Microvascular bleeding attributed to platelet dysfunction such as uremia, liver disease, post-cardiopulmonary bypass	Clinician judgment

DIC, disseminated intravascular coagulation.

TABLE 16-5. CAUSES OF ACQUIRED PLATELET DYSFUNCTION[57,59]

- Uremia
- Liver disease
- Paraproteinemia (multiple myeloma, Waldenström macroglobulinemia, monoclonal gammopathy, or polyclonal hypergammaglobulinemia)
- Myeloproliferative disease
- Myelodysplastic syndrome
- Disseminated intravascular coagulopathy
- Extracorporeal circulation (dialysis, cardiopulmonary bypass, plasmapheresis)
- Medications (aspirin, NSAIDS, thienopyridines, GP IIb/IIa antagonists, β-lactam antibiotics, antidepressants, phenothiazines)
- Herbal remedies (fish oil, flaxseed oil, ginger seed extract, *Ginkgo biloba,* garlic, turmeric)

NSAIDS, nonsteroidal antiinflammatory drugs; GP, glycoprotein.

Platelet transfusion should not be guided by platelet counts alone, but also by the clinical suspicion of platelet dysfunction which can be inherited or acquired. Qualitative dysfunction is often associated with systemic diseases such as uremia, liver failure, and disseminated intravascular coagulopathy. It also occurs after cardiopulmonary bypass, extracorporeal circulation such as dialysis or plasmaphoresis, and as a result of medication side effects[59] (Table 16-5). Regardless of the platelet count, if bleeding is out of proportion to the level of thrombocytopenia, qualitative deficiency should be suspected and treated.[53,56]

The average dose of platelets is one concentrate from apheresis donation or pools of five to eight concentrates from whole-blood or buffy-coat collections. These "units" generally contain about 3×10^{11} to 4×10^{11} platelets each.[53,55,56] Once platelets are given, a posttransfusion response should be followed to guide further therapy and to rule out ongoing consumptive pathophysiology. Refractoriness at 20 to 24 hours is generally associated with older platelets or increased consumption secondary to fever, infection, bleeding, or medications.[56] Adjunctive therapy for platelet dysfunction can be established with antifibrinolytics, DDAVP (1-deamino-8-D-arginine vasopressin, desmopressin), PCCs, or rFVIIa as discussed later in this chapter.[55,58]

Fresh Frozen Plasma

FFP is a blood component that contains all the factors involved in hemostasis. (As used here, "FFP" also includes plasma frozen within 24 hours.) The preparation and storage method discussed previously in this chapter involves either separation from whole

TABLE 16-6. INDICATIONS FOR THE USE OF FRESH FROZEN PLASMA[31,53,56,60,61]

- Correction of inherited factor deficiencies when there is no specific factor concentrate (e.g., factor V) and when the PT or aPTT is >1.5 times the mean control
- Correction of acquired multi-factor deficiencies with clinical evidence of bleeding or in anticipation of major surgery or an invasive procedure with PT or aPTT >1.5 times the control
  - Liver dysfunction with clinical signs of bleeding
  - DIC with clinical signs of bleeding
  - Microvascular bleeding associated with massive transfusion and estimated blood loss > one blood volume (when PT and aPTT are >1.5 times the control or cannot be obtained)
  - Reversal of vitamin K antagonists (warfarin)[a]
  - Heparin resistance secondary to antithrombin deficiency when AT concentrate is not available
- Treatment of thrombotic microangiopathies (thrombotic thrombocytopenic Purpura, HELLP syndrome, or hemolytic uremic syndrome)
- Treatment of hereditary angioedema when C1-esterase inhibitor is not available

[a]Prothrombin complex concentrates (II, VII, IX, X) are more effective than FFP.[41]

DIC, disseminated intravascular coagulation; PT, prothrombin time; aPTT, activated partial thromboplastin time; AT, antithrombin; HELLP, hemolytic anemia elevated liver enzymes and low platelet count.

blood or apheresis; both maintain normal levels of stable factors and at least 70% normal levels of labile factors such as FVIII and FV. Prior to use, each unit must be thawed at 30 to 37°C, but can be stored at 4 ± 2°C for up to 24 hours as thawed FFP or 5 days as thawed plasma.[53,56] FFP must be ABO-compatible with the recipient to avoid transfusion of donor anti-A and anti-B antibodies that may lead to hemolysis.[60]

FFP is indicated for the treatment of coagulopathy secondary to congenital or acquired factor deficiencies. The specific indications for FFP outlined in Table 16-6 are based on a compilation of guidelines from the ASA, the British Committee for Standards in Haematology, and the Italian Society of Transfusion Medicine and Immunohaematology (SIMTI).[31,53,56,60,61] The initial therapeutic dose of FFP averages 10 to 15 mL/kg in an attempt to obtain at least 30% factor activity. Repeat dosing should follow the results of serial diagnostic coagulation tests such as the PT and aPTT.[31,53,56,60,61] Although the guidelines for FFP continue to recommend prophylactic transfusions in patients at risk for bleeding, there is no evidence to support the efficacy of FFP reducing red cell transfusion, morbidity, or mortality, especially when given to patients with mild derangements in PT or aPTT and no clinical signs of bleeding.[61,62] The transfusion of plasma carries risks of several transfusion reactions, most notably TRALI, allergic reactions, and cardiopulmonary overload. The burden of adverse reactions in conjunction with limited prophylactic benefits and high frequency of inappropriate use makes FFP arguably the riskiest blood component transfused.[60,61,63,64]

Over the past decade there has been growing debate over formula-driven resuscitation protocols for trauma patients with major bleeding. Traditionally trauma patients were resuscitated first with fluid and red cell units only to receive FFP based on the results of coagulation tests.[54] This method perpetuates dilutional coagulopathy resulting in prolonged microvascular bleeding.[65] More recent studies show improved outcomes with higher ratios of red cell units to FFP (more than 3:2).[65,66] However, these findings are mostly retrospective and likely confounded by injury severity and the potential "survivor bias" that occurs when patients die of massive hemorrhage before FFP can be thawed and transfused.[66,67] The optimal management strategy for immediate resuscitation of trauma patients and those with acute massive hemorrhage is still under investigation. However, it is clear that coagulopathy driven by ongoing bleeding requires rapid response, and the best treatment strategies involve active management protocols to maintain intravascular volume, avoid platelet dysfunction, and facilitate hemoglobin and factor replacement.

Cryoprecipitate

19 Cryoprecipitate is created by a controlled thaw of frozen plasma which allows for precipitation of large molecules. It is then centrifuged with the final product containing fibrinogen, fibronectin, vWF, FVIII, and factor XIII.[68] One unit of plasma typically generates 10 to 20 mL of cryoprecipitate. These small concentrates are combined for a single adult dose of five bags and frozen at −20°C.[68,69] Current use of cryoprecipitate is limited to a few countries (United States and Canada) and generally only indicated for hypofibrinogenemia (Table 16-7). Compared to FFP, cryoprecipitate contains more fibrinogen per volume (15 vs. 2.5 g/L in FFP)[60] and therefore functions as a low-volume alternative for fibrinogen replacement especially during acquired hypofibrinogenemia states such as disseminated intravascular coagulopathy and massive hemorrhage. It carries similar transfusion risks as FFP and consequently has been replaced in several countries including Europe with fibrinogen concentrates, currently unavailable in the United States.[69]

Fibrinogen is primarily responsible for clot stabilization, but it also assists with platelet activation and aggregation and, at adequate concentrations, may compensate for low thrombin states.[69] Traditionally, the threshold for fibrinogen replacement has been levels less than 80 to 100 mg/dL.[31,60,68] However, a few studies of acquired hypofibrinogenemia with massive bleeding document the need for higher levels (150 to 200 mg/dL) to optimize clot stabilization.[70,71] A single dose of five pooled bags typically raises the fibrinogen concentration by 50 mg/dL.[68]

TABLE 16-7. INDICATIONS FOR THE USE OF CRYOPRECIPITATE[31,60,68–70]

- Microvascular bleeding with hypofibrinogenemia
  - DIC with fibrinogen <80–100 mg/dL
  - Hemorrhage or massive transfusion with fibrinogen <100–150 mg/dL
- Prophylaxis in patients with hemophilia A and vWD (if specific factor concentrates are unavailable or ineffective due to inhibitors)
- Prophylaxis for patients with congenital dysfibrinogenemias

DIC, disseminated intravascular coagulation; vWD, von Willebrand disease.

THE RISKS OF BLOOD PRODUCT ADMINISTRATION

20 Over the past few decades, the risk benefit ratio of blood product transfusion has been the subject of several studies and review articles. In the mid-1980s, the realization of transfusion-transmissible infections such as HIV and hepatitis initiated concerns about the infectious risks of blood product administration. Now that donor screening and product testing have drastically decreased the transmission of viral infections, nonviral risks of transfusion have gained emphasis and proven to be just as concerning if not associated with worse morbidity and mortality.

Infectious Risks of Blood Product Administration

Since the introduction of NAT for the major transfusion-transmittable viral infections (HCV in 2000, HIV in 2003, and HBV in 2006) the residual risk of infection from blood product transfusion has decreased substantially.[72] Prior to the institution of NAT, the blood supply was simply tested for the presence of viral antibodies leaving a long window period when the blood is infectious, but there was not sufficient time for the donor to mount a large enough antibody response to be detected by conventional testing. NAT increased the sensitivity of donor screening by testing for the presence of specific viral DNA. This significantly shortens the window period between when a donor gets infected and when the viral load is detectable. The residual risk of transfusion-transmitted infections depends mostly on the relative length of this window period determined by the reproductive rate of each virus and the prevalence of the disease. There is an additional risk of false negatives or mistaken release of quarantined blood products; however, these events account for less than 0.5% of the residual risk of transfusion-transmitted viral infection.[73]

The true risk of transfusion-transmittable infections is difficult if not impossible to accurately quantify given the variability of donor response to inoculation and the immune state of the recipient. However, the residual risk can be mathematically modeled from the prevalence of infection in donors and the known window period of each viral illness. The estimated residual risk of major viral infection and the viral-specific window periods are shown in Table 16-8 based on the reported incidence of infection in donors for the American Red Cross Blood Services.[73] These residual risks are likely overestimates since not all transfusions of known infected blood products result in recipient infection.[74,75] The mathematical modeling of residual risk assumes 100% infectivity with even one infectious unit of viral particles per blood bag. It also presumes that the collection and storage process is harmless to viral reproduction. Furthermore, viral infectivity will vary depending on the acute phase of infection when an immunocompetent recipient could resist transmission, or the chronic phase of infection when antibodies are present and reduce infectivity.[75]

Transfusion-transmitted viral infections have retained the most focus likely secondary to their associated morbidity and mortality. Despite increased awareness and public health initiatives, the incidence of HIV and HCV in the donor population continues to increase secondary to the prolonged survival of patients, making the prevalence of HIV and HCV in the general population higher. Contrary to HIV and HCV, the incidence of HBV has decreased since 1999 presumably due to the drastic rise in vaccination rates especially among the youth. Overall, given the static sensitivity of testing methods, the prevalence of disease in the general population is now the largest determinant of transfusion-transmittable infection risk.[73]

Human Immunodeficiency Virus

HIV is the retroviral etiology of the large epidemic that emerged in the early 1980s. As a retrovirus, it is transmitted as RNA and requires translation into DNA prior to replication. This virus was

TABLE 16-8. RESIDUAL RISK OF TRANSFUSION-TRANSMITTED INFECTIONS

Infection	Residual Risk	Window Period and Comments
Viral infections		
Human immunodeficiency virus (HIV)	1/1,860,800	9.1-day window
Hepatitis C (HCV)	1/1,657,700	7.4-day window
Hepatitis B (HBV)	1/366,500	38-day window
Human T-cell lymphotrophic virus (HTLV)	1/3,394,000	51-day window
West Nile virus (WNV)	Rare	11 cases reported from 2003–2010
Cytomegalovirus (CMV)—all donors	1–3%	
Leukoreduced products	0.023%	
Emerging infections	Rare	Incidence is too small to estimate
Chagas and malaria		Donor screening limits risk in the United States
Creutzfeldt–Jakob (vCJD)		Incubation for years
Dengue virus and *Babesia* species		Transient epidemics increase risks
Parvovirus (B19v)		May cause aplastic anemia in immunosuppressed patients
Bacterial contamination—all types	1/3,000	
Packed red blood cells	1/35,000	Lower risk than platelet concentrates
Platelets	1/15,000	Apheresis decreases risk

Data derived from several sources.[72–74,76–79]

highly transmittable in the US blood supply until sensitive NAT and donor screening became available. Incidence of transfusion transmission of HIV was as high as 1 in every 100 donation in the early 1980s and 1 in every 400,000 in 1997.[80] The residual risk of HIV has fallen to lower than 1 per 1.8 million blood product transfusions. Over the past few years, the prevalence of HIV has risen in the general population and therefore the residual risk of HIV transmission via blood supply has increased linearly; this is likely secondary to improved treatment and prolonged survival.[73,76]

Hepatitis C Virus

Although HCV is rarer than the other types of transmitted hepatitis and has a relatively benign acute phase, it progresses to chronic carrier state in up to 85% of infections and is associated with significant risk of fulminant hepatic failure, cirrhosis, hepatocellular carcinoma, and death.[74] Similar to HIV, the transfusion risk of HCV decreased drastically with the increased sensitivity of modern tests with NAT and donor screening. However, the incidence of donor HCV increased over the past 5 to 7 years secondary to increases in both incidence and prevalence in the general population. Recent reports have implicated higher infectivity rates in nonhospital-based health-care facilities and endoscopic procedures.[73,74] Furthermore, HCV infections become more aggressive and transmittable in patients coinfected with HIV secondary to the increased viral load that results from immunosuppression.[72]

Hepatitis B Virus

HBV is a common blood-borne pathogen with fairly high incidence of infection in the general population and over 300 million carriers worldwide.[74] The United States has a low prevalence rate of 2% compared to 8% to 15% in the Middle East, Africa, and parts of South America, and Asia.[72,74] The acute infection associated with contraction of HBV is asymptomatic in most patients or limited to mild constitutional signs and jaundice; however, rarely, it can progress to fulminant hepatic failure. The residual risk of transfusion-transmitted HBV remains high given the common prevalence of the disease and a long window period. This risk is now decreasing with substantial reductions in the incidence of HBV in the youth population likely secondary to the increasing availability and compliance with HBV vaccine.[73,74]

Human T-cell Lymphotropic Virus (HTLV)-1 and -2

HTLV-1 causes T-cell leukemia and lymphoma or HTLV-associated myelopathy in a small percentage of infected persons. HTLV-2 does not have any significant consequences for immunocompetent or even HIV coinfected patients.[72] Regardless of the relatively infrequent disease association with HTLV, the US blood supply is routinely tested for anti-HTLV antibodies indicative of previous infection.[73]

Cytomegalovirus

CMV is the most common transfusion-transmitted disease with an incidence of 1% to 3%.[73,77] In immune-competent recipients the infection is often asymptomatic or mild and self-limited. However, in immunocompromised patients, in particular, neonates, patients with HIV, and transplant recipients, the disease can be associated with severe multi-organ failure involving the liver, lungs, kidneys, hematologic system, gastrointestinal tract, and the central nervous system.[73,77] The CMV virus is carried by white blood cells and transmitted via CMV-seropositive cellular components. LR drastically decreases the infectivity of CMV-positive donor products, but has not completely eradicated the transfusion transmission of CMV.[77] Therefore, it is recommended that patients at risk for CMV infection receive leukoreduced blood products from CMV-seronegative–only donors.[73]

Emerging Infections

HIV remains the most noteworthy emergent microbial found to have infected the blood supply prior to clinical recognition. Since then several pathogens have also emerged through changes in ecologic and geographic factors such as travel, climate change, or new insect and animal vectors. The most recent example of a significant new transfusion-transmissible infection was the WNV, a mosquito-borne flavivirus which emerged in 1999. WNV causes only a mild febrile illness in healthy patients but it may progress to encephalitis or meningitis in immunosuppressed patients in 40% of infections.[72] Since the institution of widespread donor screening, the incidence of transfusion-transmitted WNV has dropped to only 11 reported cases from 2003 to 2010.[73] In order for a newly discovered pathogen to be concerning for transfusion transmission, it must pose a significant clinical risk, be transmissible via transfusion or transplantation, and it must be viable in collected and stored blood products.[78]

A few other pathogens have been red flagged by the American Association of Blood Banks (AABB) Transfusion-Transmitted Disease Committee as potential threats to the safety of the US blood supply including human vCJD, *Babesia* species, Parvovirus B19, dengue virus, Chagas disease, and *Plasmodium* species which cause malaria. vCJD is the human form of bovine spongiform encephalitis. It results in fatal degenerative neurologic disease secondary to prion proteins which precipitate an abnormal formation and structure of other proteins. It gained attention after an epidemic of cases in the 1980s to 1990s throughout the United Kingdom. Thus far, there have been three cases of confirmed transfusion-transmitted vCJD.[81] There are no known effective treatments and the incubation period is reported in years. Currently no testing regimens exist for diagnosis of prion disease in donors or collected blood, but donor deferral for those who resided in the United Kingdom during the epidemic has avoided any known cases within the United States.[78,81] The incidence and infectivity of other viral and parasitic pathogens is so rare, they do not warrant a careful discussion here; however, it is important to remember that there may be emerging infections that are unrecognized as of yet leaving the blood supply at constant risk.

Bacterial Contamination

Despite significant public concern for transfusion-transmitted viral disease, bacterial contamination of blood components marks the largest risk of transfusion-related infection by two or three orders of magnitude. It can progress to sepsis and has been reported to be one of the major causes of transfusion-associated fatality according to the FDA and the European Serious Hazards of Transfusion (SHOT) database.[79,82] Frequent pathogens implicated in bacterial contamination of blood products stem from skin flora, including *Staphylococcus, Corynebacterium, Bacillus,* and *Streptococcus* or secondary to Gram-negative species such as *Escherichia coli* and *Enterobacter cloacae.*[79] Platelet concentrates carry the highest risk of bacterial contamination since they are stored at 20 to 24°C, which provides a more suitable environment for bacterial replication, as opposed to red cell concentrates stored at 4°C or plasma which is frozen.[79]

Several methods aimed at reducing the risk of transfusion-transmitted bacterial infections have proven beneficial. Single-donor collections are associated with less contamination than platelet concentrates from pooled units likely secondary to fewer venipunctures and exposures to skin flora and collection processes. It is now standard practice to divert the first 20 to 40 mL of collected blood into a separate collection chamber to avoid contaminating the whole donation with blood and epidermal tissue from the initial venipuncture. Standards for skin preparation prior to blood donation and sterile techniques for collection and processing procedures have also decreased contaminants. Furthermore, all apheresis platelets are culture tested prior to storage.[79,83]

Bacterial sepsis continues to be a significant cause of transfusion morbidity and mortality especially as the incidence of transfusion-transmitted viral infections continues to decrease. Most fatal cases are secondary to Gram-negative species resulting from bacteremia that was asymptomatic at the time of donation.[79] Clinical signs of bacterial sepsis associated with transfusion include constitutional symptoms of fever, chills, dyspnea, and malaise that can progress to hemodynamic instability, organ dysfunction, and septic shock. Should bacterial contamination of blood components be considered after a transfusion, the blood bank should be notified immediately so they can culture the blood bag, quarantine other products derived from the same donor, and complete a full investigation.

Noninfectious Risks of Blood Product Administration

21 Given the extensive use of more sensitive methods for screening and controlling the infectious risks of blood product transfusion, noninfectious complications have emerged as the major source of transfusion-related morbidity and mortality. Table 16-9 summarizes the relative incidence and main features of the most common noninfectious risk of blood product administration.

Immune-mediated Transfusion Reactions

Febrile Non-Hemolytic Transfusion Reactions

Allergic and febrile reactions are the most common types of complications of transfused blood products although the incidence of both has decreased with the prominence of LR and single-donor apheresis platelet units.[88] FNHTRs classically present within 4 hours of transfusion with an increase in temperature of 1°C and may be associated with chills, rigors, anxiety, and headache.[89] They are often self-limited but can be prevented or treated with antiinflammatory or antipyretic medication. The pathophysiology of FNHTRs involves recipient alloimmunization to HLAs from donor white blood cells and the release of leukocyte-derived cytokines during product storage.[88,89] Subsequently the risk of

TABLE 16-9. **NONINFECTIOUS TRANSFUSION REACTIONS**

Adverse Reaction	Incidence	Notes
Immune-mediated reactions		
Febrile non-hemolytic transfusion reaction	0.03–2%	
Minor allergic reactions (urticaria, flushing)	1–3%	
Anaphylactic/toid reactions		IgA deficiency increases risk
Packed red blood cells	0.5/100,000	Washing may avoid reaction
Fresh frozen plasma and platelets	2–3/100,000	More prevalent with plasma-containing products[82]
Acute hemolytic transfusion reaction (AHTR)	1/80,000	
Delayed hemolytic transfusion reaction (DHTR)	1/1,500	Associated with alloantibodies to minor RBC antigens, Kidd, or Rh One-third have clinical reaction
Transfusion-related immunomodulation (TRIM)	100%	
Alloimmunization	2%	For all patients, risk increases with number of units transfused[84,85]
Transfusion-related acute lung injury (TRALI)	1/1,300–5,000	Varies with blood product component and patient population[86]
Graft-versus-host disease (TA-GVHD)	1/5,000	Related to immunosuppression; reduced risk with irradiation[82]
Posttransfusion purpura (PTP)	Rare	Attributed to antihuman platelet antigen-1a[82]
Reactions related to patient comorbidities or transfusion practice		
Transfusion-associated cardiovascular overload (TACO)	1–8%	Higher in critically ill patients[87]
Metabolic derangements		
Hyperkalemia		
Citrate toxicity		
Iron overload		
Hypothermia		
Infusion of microaggregate		

Frequencies are presented as percentages when >0.1% and otherwise as ratios.
IgA, immunoglobulin A.

febrile reactions increases with repetitive transfusions. Prior to the widespread institution of LR, the incidence of FNHTR was as high as 30%, but currently it decreased to a range between 0.03% and 2.18%.[88,89] Although these reactions are common, more serious adverse effects of transfusion, such as sepsis and hemolysis, may also present with fever and should be ruled out prior to diagnosing an FNHTR.

Allergic Reactions

Minor allergic reactions, a relatively common type of transfusion reaction, occur in about 1% to 3% of transfusions. Symptoms are most commonly described as urticaria, hives with or without pruritis, or angioedema.[88,89] The specific cause of allergic reactions is unclear but likely involves an immune response to recipient leukocyte antigens or transfused plasma proteins.[89] Major allergic reactions present as anaphylactoid or anaphylaxis with hemodynamic instability, bronchospasm, rash, and digestive upset.[82,88,90] These reactions are rare (Table 16-9), but can be fatal if unrecognized. Pathophysiologically, the donor mounts an immediate immune response to transfused plasma proteins or cellular antigens. The most commonly identified cause of transfusion-related anaphylaxis occurs in patients who are IgA deficient with anti-IgA antibodies. Classically anaphylaxis requires an immediate type I hypersensitivity IgE-mediated reaction; most major allergic responses to blood transfusions do not show laboratory evidence of IgE antibodies and are therefore technically anaphylactoid reactions.[90] These transfusion complications can be prevented in patients with known IgA deficiency by washing blood products prior to transfusion or by using products obtained from IgA-deficient donors.[89]

Acute hemolytic transfusion reactions (AHTRs) remain one of the leading causes of transfusion-related mortality. They occur with the transfusion of incompatible blood products when antibodies in recipient plasma complex with donor cellular antigens causing compliment activation and subsequent hemolysis. Classically AHTRs result from ABO incompatibility secondary to native anti-A or anti-B antibodies, and careful adherence to protocols for specimen phlebotomy and blood component administration is vital for prevention. However, growing evidence exists for the implication of other RBC antigens such as Kidd, Kell, and Duffy causing acute hemolytic reactions in patients with a history of transfusion exposure and alloimmunization.[89] Rarely, the transfusion of incompatible plasma (type O FFP to a patient with type A, B, or AB blood) has resulted in AHTRs as well.[82,89] These reactions are rare and have become less frequent with the institution of safety measures to reduce clerical error and improve the availability of cross-matched blood products. Recent data from national surveillance databases in the United States, the United Kingdom, and France report the risk of incompatible transfusions as 1/40,000 red cell units, and the risk of it causing AHTR is less than 1/80,000.[91]

AHTRs occur secondary to IgM-mediated antibody–antigen complexes that activate complement and result in hemolysis intravascularly and extravascularly in the spleen and liver. The release of bradykinin causes fever, hypotension, and hemodynamic instability while histamine release from mast cells leads to bronchospasm and urticaria as well as symptoms of dyspnea, flushing, and severe anxiety. Hemolysis results in the release of free hemoglobin which is bound by haptoglobin and plasma proteins but will also be eliminated by the kidney when these proteins are unavailable.[89,91] Severe hemolysis may lead to renal failure, disseminated intravascular coagulopathy, and death in 50% of cases.[91] General anesthesia can mask several of the presenting symptoms of AHTRs; therefore vigilance during transfusion of an anesthetized patient must remain high.

The diagnosis of hemolytic reactions is confirmed with laboratory analysis of free hemoglobin levels, low haptoglobin, bilirubin increases, direct antiglobulin (Coombs) test, and evidence of hematuria. Suspicion of a transfusion reaction should prompt immediate discontinuation of the transfusion and investigation into the donor and recipient blood type and antigen–antibody components. Treatment of AHTR involves supportive care for hemodynamic instability and microvascular bleeding as well as the maintenance of adequate urine output to avoid the renal failure associated with hematuria.

Delayed hemolytic transfusion reactions (DHTRs) result from alloantibodies to minor RBC antigens in the Rh, Kell, Kidd, Duffy, MNSs, and other blood groups. They generally present 3 to 10 days after transfusion of an apparent "compatible" blood component.[89] Typically the recipient has IgG alloantibodies to a particular RBC antigen and will mount an anamnestic immune response, but the pre-transfusion antibody levels are too low for serologic detection. Symptoms are much milder than AHTRs and rarely result in major morbidity or mortality because the hemolysis occurs extravascularly in the liver and spleen. Patients experience mild fever and possible rash with laboratory and clinical signs of hemolysis such as jaundice, hematuria, low haptoglobin, positive direct Coombs test, and decreasing hemoglobin levels.[89] The incidence of delayed hemolytic serologic reactions where there is serologic evidence of a hemolytic reaction occurs in 1 out of every 1,500 transfusions; however, only about a third of these result in clinical signs of DHTR. Symptoms are generally self-limited and treated supportively with hydration to protect the renal tubules during hemolysis and further compatible transfusions to support anemia as indicated.[89]

Transfusion-related Immunomodulation

Several decades ago in the 1970s, TRIM was discovered from improved survival of renal allografts for patients who had received a transfusion pre-transplant. This highlighted the potential immunosuppressant effects of stored allogeneic blood products. Immunosuppression associated with blood transfusion was further confirmed by the decreased rate of miscarriages for women with a history of recurrent spontaneous abortions and the reduced risk of recurrent Crohn's disease in patients who received transfusions. However, these beneficial effects are patient specific. Immunosuppression also proved to increase the recurrence of malignancies and possibly facilitate reactivation of latent infections such as CMV, HIV, and tuberculosis.[25] Since the landmark results of the TRICC trial by Hebert et al. documented detrimental effects of transfusions including TRALI, multi-organ system failure, and increased rates of infection, further studies have investigated a second source of immunomodulation involving pro-inflammatory mechanisms in addition to immunosuppression.[25,32,92,93]

Over the past 30 years, several investigators have tried to identify the exact mechanism for immunomodulation, but results point to a multifactorial pathophysiology that implicates the role of transfused WBCs, donor plasma HLA class 1 peptides, cytokines, and immune mediators released during blood product storage as well as the immune function of transfused RBCs within the microvasculature of the recipient.[25,92] Several experts propose a "two-insult" model for TRIM similar to the pathophysiologic mechanism for TRALI and acute respiratory distress syndrome.[92,94,95] Presumably most patients requiring blood products are suffering from a precondition that "primes" the immune system and vascular endothelium such as trauma, surgery, or acute

illness. This constitutes the first insult and causes active neutrophils to adhere to vascular endothelial cells and become hypersensitive to blood-bound immune mediators. The second insult occurs with the infusion of transfused blood products which contain WBCs with HLA class I antigens as well as soluble immune response modifiers in the form of cytokines, complement factors, and the breakdown products of lipid membranes.[25,92,94,95] Furthermore, RBC function within the microvasculature depends on their ability to retain deformability and shape. Alterations of the membrane surface proteins in stored RBCs result in decreased flexibility and increased aggregation and adhesion to the vascular endothelium that has previously been activated by a heightened systemic immune response.[92] Prestorage LR and post-storage 22
WBC filtration have been investigated as a means of limiting the deleterious effects of TRIM; however, results thus far are variable and unconvincing.[25] Nevertheless, the vast evidence collected over the past 30 years from clinical trials and animal studies supports the hypothesis that TRIM involves both pro-inflammatory mechanisms and systemic immunosuppression.

Alloimmunization

Alloimmunization refers to the induction of an immune response to allogenic antigen exposure. This process occurs occasionally through pregnancy, but the majority of alloimmunization results from transfusion of blood products containing immunogenic antigens on the surface of RBCs. Unlike classic ABO antigens which consist of carbohydrate chains, most of the non-ABO alloantigens (Kell, Kidd, Duffy, etc.) result from single amino acid polymorphisms between the recipient and donor.[84] AHTRs result in an immediate IgM-mediated immune response to ABO incompatibility with naturally occurring anti-A or anti-B antibodies. In contrast, alloimmunization prompts an amnestic IgG-mediated humoral immunity to foreign proteins and does not result in RBC destruction until the second antigen exposure.[84] Thus the clinical consequences of alloimmunization are rarely immediate or fatal, but the generation of antibodies may cause DHTRs and adds difficulty to subsequent cross-matched blood product availability.

The incidence of alloimmunization is approximately 1.8% to 8% depending on the patient's immunocompetency and the number of units transfused with incremental risks associated with higher number of transfusion exposures.[85] Adverse effects of alloimmunization become apparent with repeat transfusions as patients develop a risk of hemolytic transfusion reactions and become therapeutically refractory to blood products. This is especially evident for patients who require frequent platelet transfusion. Platelets carry significant levels of multiple human platelet antigens (HPA 1 to 15) which are also polymorphisms and result in the destruction of transfused platelets and subsequent refractory thrombocytopenia.[84] The use of single-donor apheresis units may limit the exposure to HPA and HLA but patients who receive one pooled unit of platelets have an 8% risk of alloimmunization to HPA.[84]

Transfusion-related Acute Lung Injury

Over the course of the past decade, the incidence of transfusion-transmissible infections has declined, leaving TRALI the leading cause of transfusion-associated mortality according to the United Kingdom's SHOT database and the most recent data from the United States Federal Drug Administration report.[96,97] Transfusion-related lung injury was first described in the 1950s, but it was not until 20 years later that an immunologic source was postulated. In the early 1980s, Popovsky reported five cases of TRALI with HLA antibody and antigen matches identified for three of the five cases. All of the patients had received products from multiparous female donors.[98] Recently a formal definition for the clinical diagnosis of TRALI was written and accepted. It was defined by the US National Heart, Lung, and Blood Institute as a new acute lung injury (ALI) within 6 hours of blood component therapy. Criteria for the diagnosis of ALI were published in 1994 by the North American-European Consensus Conference as non-cardiogenic pulmonary edema with acute bilateral infiltrates and hypoxemia ($PaO_2/FiO_2 \leq 300$ mm Hg or oxygen saturation ≤90% on room air and no evidence of left atrial hypertension).[86,99,100]

TRALI is a clinical diagnosis that can be clouded by confounding comorbidities or patient acuity; therefore, TRALI tends to be underreported in the literature and is extremely difficult if not impossible to study with randomized prospective clinical trials.[86,100] This leads to a wide range of incidence reports based mostly on observational studies and voluntary reporting to regulatory agencies. Furthermore, the incidence of TRALI varies with patient population and different blood product components depending on their degree of plasma volume, storage time, and collection process.[86] Previously published incidence rates for TRALI quote a risk of 1/5,408 units transfused or 1/625 patients transfused with any blood product, or 1/2,000 plasma-containing units.[86,100] However, this refers to early retrospective studies prior to the institution of a formal definition and diagnostic criteria. More recent data report an incidence of at least 1/1,323 units transfused with plasma-containing products. Random-donor platelets and FFP account for the vast majority of cases of TRALI.[86] According to the FDA report on TRALI fatalities from 2005 to 2010, FFP resulted in 43% of all fatal cases of TRALI while RBCs were only implicated in 28%.[97] The patient populations at the highest risk for TRALI include critical care patients, especially those receiving massive transfusion, and those with preexisting propensity for ALI such as sepsis, aspiration, burns, or patients who underwent cardiopulmonary bypass.[86,100,101] In a large prospective observational trial, Gajic et al. showed 8% incidence of TRALI in transfused critically ill patients.[101]

The pathophysiology of TRALI is complex and not yet fully understood. The clinical picture involves low-pressure pulmonary edema secondary to neutrophil activation and sequestration in the lungs. This results in endothelial injury and capillary leakage of proteinaceous fluid into the interstitium and intra-alveolar spaces.[98,102] There are two leading theories on the mechanism of lung injury, both with sound experimental and clinical evidence. The antibody-mediated model stems from evidence of antibody–antigen complexes in the plasma of transfusion recipients who suffered from TRALI.[98,99,102] These antibodies are mostly against HLAs (class I and II) and human neutrophil antigens (HNAs).[102,103] Antibodies form in the donor plasma after alloimmunization from pregnancy or prior transfusion or transplantation. Accordingly plasma donation from multiparous women has been implicated as one of the highest risks associated with TRALI.[99] Once the antibodies are transfused into the recipient, they complex with native WBC antigens on the surface of monocytes (HLA class II), endothelial cells (HLA class I), and neutrophils (HNAs and HLA class I) thereby activating the neutrophils to facilitate aggregation and release of cytotoxic mediators.[102,103] Subsequently, the endothelial lining of capillaries in the lung is damaged resulting in the extravasation of WBCs and the leakage of edema fluid.[98,102,103]

The second proposed mechanism of TRALI was termed the "Two-Hit Model" in the late 1990s by Silliman et al. when they discovered the role of biologic response modifiers in the pathophysiology. Stored blood components accumulate lipid degradation products, mostly phosphatidylcholine derivatives, which function to activate neutrophils primed and sequestered on the endothelial vascular lining of lung tissue.[94] Patients with the highest incidence of TRALI often suffer from a preexisting condition associated with a pro-inflammatory state such as active infection, trauma, surgery, or multiple transfusions.[99,102] Acute illness causes the immune system to be hyperreactive with polymorphonuclear leukocytes (PMNs) poised on the endothelial lining of microvasculature "primed" and ready to be activated by various biologic response modifiers, including cytokines, compliment, and leukotrienes.[94,102] The transfusion of stored blood products which accumulate reactive lipid particles, namely lysophosphatidylcholine derivatives, marks the second "hit" which activates primed PMNs and results in the destruction of the capillary lining of lung microvasculature.[94,102] The overall pathophysiology of TRALI likely involves both mechanisms of a preexisting primed immune system vulnerable to the transfusion of antibodies and biologic response modifiers present in stored blood products.

The management of TRALI focuses on supportive measures to limit lung injury and optimize oxygenation. This includes maximizing positive end expiratory pressures, avoiding volume overload, and low tidal volume strategies for mechanical ventilation in accordance with recommendations for ALI from any cause.[86] Furthermore, subsequent transfusions should be restricted as much as possible for patients with ALI and although there is little supportive evidence for the use of washed RBCs, all preventative measures should be encouraged for this high-risk population.[86] Several studies including the SHOT database from the UK and the FDA report of US transfusion-related fatalities have demonstrated decreased incidence of TRALI with the use of male-only plasma donation.[96,104] Male donors have fewer HLA antibodies than women, in particular those who have had previous pregnancies.[58,99] As discussed earlier, storage lesions of transfused blood components are also implicated in the pathophysiology of TRALI, and accordingly older transfusion products have been associated with increased incidence of TRALI. Furthermore the method of collection may impact the amount of antibodies in stored plasma. For instance, pooled platelets from multiple donors have a higher rate of causing TRALI than apheresis platelet units.[105] Lastly, the buffy-coat method of preparation of packed RBCs may decrease TRALI since it results in less plasma volume per unit of red cells.[98] Overall, prevention is the best treatment for TRALI and is currently a large focus of clinical and experimental study.

Transfusion-associated Graft-Versus-Host Disease

Transfusion-associated GVHD (TA-GVHD) is a rare but fulminant and fatal complication of blood products containing cellular components (platelets and packed RBCs). Mortality is more than 90% although incidence is decreasing across the globe secondary to preventative gamma irradiation and LR. It occurs when donor lymphocytes engraft in the recipient and attack host cells they recognize as foreign. Patients at risk for TA-GVHD include those immunocompromised from stem cell transplants, B-cell malignancies such as multiple myeloma, non-Hodgkin lymphoma, or acute lymphocytic leukemia, Hodgkin's disease, and congenital immunodeficiency syndromes.[106] Immunocompetent patients may also be at risk when transfused with directed donations from blood relations with similar HLA types because transfused donor lymphocytes are not recognized as foreign but still reject the recipient's tissue. TA-GVHD classically present 4 to 21 days after transfusion but clinical suspicion should exist for up to 6 weeks. Symptoms progress rapidly and generally affect the skin, hepatic, digestive, and hematopoietic organ systems causing fever, rash, liver dysfunction, diarrhea, and pancytopenia.[89,106]

Posttransfusion Purpura

Defined as severe thrombocytopenia with purpura occurring 5 to 10 days posttransfusion, posttransfusion purpura (PTP) is a very rare complication of transfusion (less than 300 reported cases), but associated with high morbidity and mortality.[82,89] Most patients have platelet-specific alloantibodies such as anti-HPA-1a, formerly termed anti-PL^{A1}. These antibodies are almost exclusively found in previously pregnant women and cause platelet destruction of both transfused and autologous platelets.[82,89] Intravenous IG is the first line of treatment, but plasmapheresis may be necessary to remove antibody and avoid bleeding complications.[89]

Nonimmune-mediated Transfusion Reactions

Transfusion-associated Cardiovascular Overload

Transfusion-associated cardiovascular overload (TACO) describes the occurrence of hydrostatic pulmonary edema after transfusion of blood component therapy. It differs from TRALI in that it is not immune mediated or associated with increased capillary permeability, and it responds rapidly to diuretic therapy and afterload reduction.[107] Similar to TRALI, TACO can be difficult to diagnose and is likely unreported in the literature. The diagnosis depends on clinical, radiographic, laboratory, or echocardiographic evidence of volume overload with left atrial hypertension after transfusion.[107] Studies explored the diagnostic utility of brain natriuretic peptide but the sensitivity and specificity are too low to be particularly helpful especially for critically ill patients or those with the suspicion of TRALI.[107] The overall incidence of TACO ranges from 1% to 8% of transfused patients and is more prevalent in critically ill patients with a history of cardiovascular disease and left ventricular dysfunction.[87] Other risk factors that predict TACO include the volume and rate of transfusion, especially plasma products, and overall fluid balance.[87] A few years ago, TACO was reported to be associated with transfusion-related fatalities and it continues to be implicated in lengthening hospital stay, but it is not significantly associated with decreased long-term survival; the original findings are likely secondary to patient comorbidities and acuity of illness.[108] Nevertheless, transfusion practices should be altered to reduce the risk of TACO by slowing infusion rates of blood products when possible and the use of low-volume alternatives to FFP.[87]

Metabolic Derangements

The metabolic derangements that occur as a consequence of transfusion are usually not evident unless patients received a large volume transfusion or rapid infusion rates, but these often include hyperkalemia, citrate toxicity, and hypothermia.[89] As storage time for blood products increases the cellular components leak potassium and metabolize glucose into lactate which can result in hyperkalemia and/or acidemia in the recipient especially with rapid transfusion.[89] The acidosis is quickly cleared by physiologic buffers and the elimination of carbon dioxide, but hyperkalemia can be of concern for patients at risk of cardiovascular complications such as neonates and patients with renal insufficiency.

Citrate is a common anticoagulant used in stored blood products and is generally metabolized by the liver and quickly eliminated. However, with rapid infusion rates, massive transfusion, or in patients with liver dysfunction, citrate accumulates in the plasma and chelates calcium resulting in hypocalcemia. Severe hypocalcemia leads to muscle weakness, tetany, arrhythmias, myocardial dysfunction, and acquired coagulopathy.[89]

Blood product transfusion can also lead to hypothermia especially during rapid infusion of previously cold or recently thawed blood products. The infusion of 1 unit of RBCs at 4°C can decrease the core body temperature by 0.25°C. Fluid warmers are standard of care for rapid transfusion; nevertheless hypothermia is commonly associated with massive transfusion and can result in platelet and coagulation factor dysfunction, arrhythmias, and myocardial depression. Several studies including a recent prospective randomized trial found mild hypothermia to be associated with increased blood loss, postoperative infections, cardiopulmonary morbidities, and longer hospitalization.[109]

Iron Overload

Packed RBCs contain approximately 250 mg of iron per unit which can accumulate in patients who require frequent transfusions for chronic anemia or hemoglobinopathies. Iron overload occurs when deposits in the liver, heart, and endocrine systems result in organ dysfunction.[89] Chelation therapy is the first line of treatment and prevention but difficult to administer secondary to the bioavailability and side effect profile of chelating agents. Exchange transfusion therapy decreases the iron load in comparison to traditional transfusion but it is expensive and associated with complications from central venous access and a larger amount of blood products.[89]

Microaggregate Administration

During storage, blood products collect microaggregates of cellular debris, platelets, fibrin composition, and even erythrocytes and WBCs. Standard 170 μm blood filters avoid aggregate infusion; however, it was traditionally taught that blood should not be diluted or flushed with calcium-containing fluids such as lactated Ringer, because theoretically, calcium could chelate the citrate anticoagulant preservative in stored blood products and result in blood clots prior to infusion.[110] Several studies have since negated this presumption and in fact confirmed the safety of ratios of more than 2:1 packed RBC to lactated Ringer's dilution fluid and flush without any clinical or experimental evidence of clot formation.[110]

BLOOD CONSERVATION STRATEGIES

Most healthy patients undergoing routine surgery will not require allogenic blood transfusion. However, there are some elective procedures such as liver resection, orthopedic surgery, cardiac surgery, and scoliosis correction where anticipated blood loss exceeds 30% of estimated blood volume increasing the possibility of needing red cell replacement. As discussed in detail earlier, blood component therapy is associated with significant morbidity and mortality for all patient populations. It is also a scarce resource and economically costly. This raises the focus on any methodology with the potential to conserve perioperative transfusion (Table 16-10).

TABLE 16-10. PERIOPERATIVE BLOOD CONSERVATION STRATEGIES

Technique	Comments
Preoperative autologous donation (PAD)	Increased transfusion requirement; lower preoperative hemoglobin
Acute normovolemic hemodilution (ANH)	Limited benefit; contains clotting factors and platelets
Intraoperative blood salvage (IOBS)	Cost-effective, low risk, and highly efficacious
Postoperative blood salvage (POBS)	Proven efficacious for orthopedic surgery
Pharmacologic agents	
Stimulants of erythropoiesis	Erythropoietin, vitamin B_{12}, folate
Prohemostatic agents	Vitamin K, DDAVP, antifibrinolytics, rFVIIa
Blood substitutes	Hemoglobin-based oxygen-carrying solutions

DDAVP, 1-deamino-8-D-arginine vasopressin; rFVIIa, recombinant activated factor VII.

Autologous Blood Transfusion

Autologous blood transfusion (ABT) first gained popularity because of the rising risk of transfusion-transmitted viral infections. All forms of ABT reduce the need for allogenic blood components; however, now that the incidence of infectious risks with allogenic blood has declined substantially, the utility of ABT is not as certain, especially when the process involves blood storage. ABT includes three separate processes: (1) preoperative autologous blood donation (PAD); (2) acute normovolemic hemodilution (ANH); and (3) perioperative blood cell salvage. Each method will be explored for its efficacy, indications, and disadvantages.

PAD summarizes the process of patients donating their own whole blood in the weeks preceding a planned surgical procedure to ensure that should red cell replacement be necessary, they receive autologous blood. PAD was initially popular in the 1980s when concern for transfusion-transmitted HIV was high; however, it has since become less useful given the reduced risk of transfusion-related infections and new realizations about the disadvantages of receiving stored blood. A recent meta-analysis showed a 63% reduced risk of allogenic blood transfusion with the use of PAD although total red cell transfusion (allogenic and autologous) requirements increased by 30%, and preoperative hemoglobin levels after blood donation prior to surgery decreased by more than 1 g/dL.[57,111–113] PAD eliminates the risk of viral infection and alloimmunization; however, it still requires blood collection and storage which carry risks of clerical error, cardiovascular overload, bacterial infection, and TRIM.

Current indications for PAD include patients in whom it would be difficult to find compatible blood products secondary to multiple antibodies or rare blood types, those who refuse to receive allogenic transfusion, and adolescent scoliosis surgery.[57,112–114] Typically each donation session collects 450 mL of whole blood not to exceed 6 mL/kg and can be repeated weekly until 72 hours prior to the scheduled procedure.[57] Patients are rarely able to donate more than 4 units because of the limited storage time and hemoglobin must remain above 11 g/dL before donation.[57] However, in the case of patients with multiple antibodies, donated units may be frozen. The timing and total amount for collection during PAD is controversial. The earlier the donation the more time a patient has to recover from iatrogenic anemia, but the effects of storage time on the functionality of transfused blood have yet to be clarified.[57,113] PAD is most effective when used in conjunction with preoperative erythropoietin which has been shown to increase the tolerance for repeat donations.[57,112,114] Iron supplementation is not indicated and generally not helpful in patients who are already iron replete; however, oral iron should be administered to patients known to be iron deficient prior to autologous donation and surgery.[57,111]

PAD should not be used unless the scheduled procedure is unlikely to be postponed so that the donated units are not wasted. Autologous donated units are not subjected to the same testing or deferral procedures as allogenic blood collection and therefore cannot be used by the general population if they are not retransfused into the patient. Wastage reports for PAD vary from 18% to over 50%.[113] However, avoiding wastage is not an indication for transfusion of autologous blood; patients should not be over-transfused simply because they have stored autologous units.[57,112,113] The contraindications for PAD include children under the age of 10 years, active infection or high risk of bacteremia, aortic stenosis, recent myocardial infarction, or cerebral vascular accident, congenital heart disease, and uncontrolled hypertension.[57,112] A history of coronary artery disease is not an absolute contraindication for PAD, especially if the patient is medically optimized and asymptomatic. As with any perioperative management plan, the advantages and disadvantages should be evaluated for individual circumstances of the patient's history, planned procedure, and physical state before implementing a PAD program.

23 *ANH* is the process of extracting multiple units of blood immediately before surgical incision while maintaining euvolemia with crystalloids or colloid supplementation. The withdrawn blood is high in hematocrit and contains clotting factors and functional platelets. After ANH, the patient loses blood with lower hemoglobin and fewer red cells. This process reduces the oxygen-carrying capacity of blood, but healthy patients maintain oxygen delivery with intact compensatory mechanisms such as increased CO and oxygen extraction.[112] At the end of surgery, the autologous units are reinfused thereby replacing RBCs, platelets, and plasma proteins including the factors active in hemostasis. This process eliminates the infectious and alloimmunization risks of allogenic transfusion and the immunomodulatory risks associated with blood storage. ANH was first used in the 1970s and several observational studies reported reduced rates of allogenic transfusion; however, a large meta-analysis documented no significant decrease in the need for allogenic blood products especially when the patient is managed with a transfusion protocol or other pharmacologic therapy for blood conservation.[53,112,115]

Procedurally, ANH involves the removal of a predetermined volume of blood after the induction of anesthesia but prior to surgical incision. Target hematocrit nadirs will vary based on individual patient history and baseline physiologic state, however, usually ranges from 25% to 30%.[112] The simple formula for allowable blood loss is used to calculate the volume to be removed. Volume to be removed = EBV × $[(Hct_i - Hct_t)/Hct_{ave}]$ where EBV is the estimated blood volume; Hct_i, the starting hematocrit; Hct_t, the target low hematocrit; Hct_{ave}, the average of Hct.[53,112] Euvolemia should be maintained with either crystalloids at a ratio of 3:1 with the volume of blood removed or colloids at a ratio of 1:1.[53] The blood must be stored at room temperature within the operating room for no longer than 6 hours.[53]

Given the limited evidence of benefit from ANH it is not recommended for routine use. However, it should be considered for patients undergoing surgical procedures where blood loss is anticipated to exceed 50% of the patient's circulating blood volume and when a patient has multiple antibodies or a rare blood type that creates difficulty with finding compatible products or for patients who do not consent to allogenic transfusion such as Jehovah's Witnesses.[53,112] The contraindications to ANH include preoperative anemia, significant cardiopulmonary comorbidity such as uncontrolled hypertension, aortic stenosis or recent myocardial infarction or cerebral vascular accident, or active infection.[112]

Perioperative Erythropoietin

Erythropoietin is the main regulator of erythropoiesis. Its endogenous release is stimulated by hematocrit levels below 30% or physiologic hypoxia.[53,112,113] It is generally indicated for refractory anemia in particular for patients with renal failure, but it has also been used to optimize patients with preoperative anemia or for those undergoing PAD. Conventional PAD programs keep hematocrit levels well above the threshold for endogenous erythropoietin release causing insufficient stimulation of erythropoiesis.[53,111–113] Several studies have shown a clear decrease in the requirements for allogenic blood transfusion especially when erythropoietin is used in conjunction with a PAD program for adolescent spine, orthopedic, or cardiac surgery.[53,111,112] However, the cost effectiveness of recombinant erythropoietin is not clear nor is the appropriate dosing regimen. For these reasons, routine use of erythropoietin is not recommended at this time, but further research may prove useful.

Perioperative Blood Salvage

RBC salvage was first attempted in the early nineteenth century for patients with postpartum hemorrhage. Not surprisingly, it was wrought with complications throughout its early development. It was not until the 1970s that commercial cell salvage devices became available for clinical use and yet there were still frequent complications such as hemolysis, air embolism, and
24 coagulopathy.[116] Over the past decade RBC salvage techniques have improved drastically and now offer an efficient, cost-effective, and safe method for perioperative blood conservation. In general, cell salvage involves the collection of shed blood, which is filtered and/or washed prior to reinfusion. This process can be carried out intraoperatively with direct suction of the surgical field or postoperatively in the case of orthopedic, cardiac, and thoracic surgery with the use of blood from wound drainage.

Intraoperative blood salvage (IOBS) requires the use of a double-lumen suction catheter with one port for aspiration from the surgical field and the other for the addition of an anticoagulant solution, usually heparin or citrate. Suctioned blood is then collected in a reservoir, filtered to remove large debris, and centrifuged resulting in red cell concentrates. The final step of washing clears the product of residual contaminants such as plasma, platelets, free hemoglobin, cellular fragments, WBCs, and the remaining heparin or citrate. The resultant red cells are resuspended in saline and ready for reinfusion. This is usually given back to the patient immediately through standard blood filters, but may be stored at 4°C for up to 6 hours with careful patient and product identification.[53,116] On average, IOBS yields a hematocrit ranging from 50% to 80%.[53,116] The efficiency depends on several factors including the volume of blood processed at a time, the length of time that blood remains in the wound, and the rate and precision of suctioning since increased turbulence from the surgical field adds shear stress which damages RBCs. Most modern-day cell savers, when used appropriately, provide red cell concentrates with a hematocrit of 60% to 70%.[53]

IOBS has proven benefits for reducing allogenic blood transfusion in major surgery, particularly orthopedics, spine fusion, and off-pump high-risk cardiac surgery when estimated blood loss is greater than 1,000 mL or 20% of the patient's blood volume is with anticipated recovery of 1.2 to 2 units of RBCs.[53,112,114,116] It is also indicated for patients with low preoperative hemoglobin who cannot tolerate PAD, in those unwilling to consent to allogenic transfusion, and for patients with preexisting bleeding risks or multiple alloantibodies.[53,112,114,116] Evidence shows that salvaged blood has better oxygen-carrying capacity and tissue oxygenation than stored blood secondary to the retained viability of red cell's biconcave disc shape and increased levels of 2,3-DPG and ATP.[116] There are very few studies directly comparing IOBS to ANH and PAD. One comparison for radical prostatectomy demonstrated that IOBS was as effective as PAD at reducing the requirement for allogenic transfusion. The patients in this study who underwent IOBS were less likely to receive any transfusion of stored blood and had significantly higher preoperative and postoperative hemoglobin levels.[117] Overall IOBS is cost-effective, convenient, and advantageous for emergency procedures when PAD is not feasible and when aggressive preoperative donation programs that provide adequate stimulus and time for erythropoiesis cannot be accomplished.[118]

The complications of IOBS are rare and mostly associated with the method of suctioning or contamination from the surgical field. Risks include nonimmunogenic hemolysis, fever, and contamination with various substances such as topical anticoagulants, urine, amniotic fluid, or bacteria. Washing the salvaged blood clears most contaminants and variable suction devices limit the sheer stress that causes hemolysis. Reinfusion of salvaged blood in volumes greater than 50% of the estimated blood volume can result in dilutional coagulopathy similar to the complication of massive transfusion of allogenic RBCs since neither contains clotting factors or platelets.[53,112,116] Lastly, IOBS can cause gas embolism when the reinfusion bag is connected in a continuous circuit with the patient.[112] Careful adherence to the recommended application of modern cell-saver devices effectively eliminates many of these concerns.

Traditionally, cell salvage was contraindicated in cancer surgery and operations where blood loss is contaminated by urine, anticoagulants, or amniotic fluid. However, several recent studies demonstrate the safety of cell salvage when blood is processed, washed, and administered through a leukodepletion filter.[116] Surgery for prostate cancer and gynecologic oncology, which often involves urine and malignant cells contaminating the field, has not shown significant increases in morbidity, mortality, or cancer recurrence. However, it is recommended that IOBS be filtered and irradiated when there is concern for malignancy and avoided completely when the tumor is ruptured causing an overwhelming concentration of cancer cells in shed blood.[112,116,117] The use of IOBS for obstetric cases raises concerns about amniotic fluid embolism recently termed "anaphylactoid syndrome of pregnancy." This syndrome is very rare and therefore it is difficult to establish the safety of a new technique; however, two systematic reviews of IOBS for caesarian delivery did not show any increase in amniotic fluid emboli.[116] Leukodepletion filters remove most of the amniotic fluid and debris although fetal RBCs cannot be differentiated from maternal red cells and may potentiate alloimmunization. This risk is already present during delivery and not exacerbated by the use of IOBS.[116] The only absolute contraindications to IOBS are microbial contamination of the surgical field and cancer surgery where tumor rupture or direct manipulation is likely.[116]

Postoperative blood salvage (POBS) involves the collection and reinfusion of blood shed into surgical wound drains in the immediate postoperative period. The recovered blood product can be processed in one of two ways: "Washed" POBS is centrifuged, washed, and resuspended as RBC concentrates, while "unwashed" POBS is filtered twice, once through a 100 to 200 μm filter to remove large debris and fibrin, then through the standard 40 μm filter to collect microaggregates.[52] The resultant hematocrit of unwashed POBS ranges from 20% to 30% and should not be expected to increase the patient's hemoglobin level, but rather it will avoid dilutional anemia associated with the fluid resuscitation for postoperative bleeding.[52] There are advantages and disadvantages to both techniques resulting in continued controversies over the safety and efficacy of postoperative cell salvage. Overall, POBS is indicated mainly for orthopedic procedures when postoperative blood loss is expected to exceed 750 to 1,500 mL.[119] Washed POBS has also been studied in post-cardiac surgery patients and shown to be efficacious at reducing the need for allogenic blood transfusion.[52,114,119]

Shed blood from surgical wounds differs from venous collected blood in that it contains inflammatory mediators, activated clotting factors, fibrin and fibrin split products, and the products of hemolysis such as free hemoglobin. These substances can precipitate renal damage, lung injury, or coagulopathy, and thus they are the source of controversy over POBS. Unwashed salvaged blood is not cleared of these bioactive contaminants but has yet to be associated with significant morbidity or mortality for orthopedic procedures.[52,119] POBS for cardiac surgery should be washed prior to reinfusion. There are increased levels of immune mediators and fat cells in blood shed from the thorax and mediastinum that are removed with washing, thus avoiding the hemostatic derangements associated with unwashed POBS in cardiac surgery.[52,119] As mentioned above, studies comparing washed and unwashed POBS for orthopedic procedures have yet to show significant differences in outcomes. Unwashed shed blood will have higher levels of free hemoglobin, but most patients free of preexisting liver and kidney disease have enough intravascular haptoglobin to bind the free hemoglobin thereby avoiding any renal damage.[119] Unwashed POBS is most commonly used for total knee arthroplasty; it is highly efficacious, is cost-effective, and requires little additional training in comparison to washed POBS. Theoretically washing the blood that is shed should lead to less hemostatic derangements and immunomodulation; however, meta-analysis and systemic reviews have yet to clearly show any benefit to washing POBS in orthopedic surgery and a few studies have questioned the viability of red cells after processing.[52,114,119]

POBS is a safe and efficacious means for reducing perioperative blood transfusion in orthopedic and cardiac surgery. The complications associated with both washed and filtered blood salvage are mostly theoretical and rare especially when the volume of blood reinfused is limited to less than 1,000 mls in the first six postoperative hours.[119] POBS is contraindicated for patients with preexisting hemoglobinopathies such as sickle cell disease and thalassemia.[52,119] Furthermore, similar to IOBS, blood should not be reinfused if it has been contaminated with microbials or drugs used topically in the surgical field that are not indicated for systemic use such as betadine, chlorhexidine, and topical antibiotics. Lastly, it is not recommended to use POBS from surgical sites with local infections or malignancy.[52,119]

Jehovah's Witnesses belong to an international well-established religious society that believes in a literal translation of the bible. Passages such as Leviticus 7 verse 25 which states "You must not eat the blood of any bird or animal" and Leviticus 17 verse 12, "None of you may eat blood," lead to a proscription against consenting to blood transfusion. Followers believe that once the blood has left the body it should not be returned to anyone. Receipt of a blood transfusion would be grounds for excommunication with no hope of eternal life.[120] Most Jehovah's Witnesses understand and accept the threat of death as a possible result of refusing therapeutic transfusion. Clearly this is challenging for treating physicians especially in the case of emergent hemorrhage. The best management for Jehovah's Witnesses is to have a well-prescribed perioperative management plan to maximize alternative blood conservation therapies and a clear conversation about the patient's individual concerns. Some patients consent to blood component therapy, factor concentrates derived from blood such as albumin or PCCs, or extracorporeal circulation which may include cardiopulmonary bypass, ANH, and intraoperative cell salvage if left in continuous circulation with the body.

Jehovah's Witnesses are one of the largest growing religious groups in the world with over 7 million congregants across over 230 countries.[120] Some of the most challenging questions arise with minors, emergencies, and unconscious patients when the physician is unable to have a clear conversation about the patient's specific beliefs. There is a great deal of individual variability within the religion and this can lead to drastically different management plans for bleeding and acute anemia. Often adult Jehovah's Witnesses will carry cards with an advance directive; however, if questions arise, physicians should seek the guidance of their hospital ethics committee and legal advisors and even an urgent application to the court system in the case of minors or unconscious patients where their wishes are unclear.

In preparation for elective surgery for a Jehovah's Witness, the use of prohemostatic medications such as antifibrinolytics, vitamin K, rFVIIa, and desmopressin should be considered and remain available perioperatively. In addition, the patients' preoperative hemoglobin should be optimized by stimulating erythropoiesis with recombinant erythropoietin, iron, and supplemental vitamin B_{12} and folate.[120] There is ongoing research into the clinical use of hemoglobin-based oxygen carriers which could revolutionize the treatment of not only Jehovah's Witnesses, but all patients given the significant risks of infectious and noninfectious adverse effects of blood transfusion. Several of these products are under investigation but have yet to be approved in the United States for concern of methemoglobinemia and toxicity including renal damage, liver dysfunction, and cardiovascular complications.[121]

DISORDERS OF HEMOSTASIS: DIAGNOSIS AND TREATMENT

As discussed in a previous section of this chapter, hemostasis is a complex mechanism of checks and balances that aims to control bleeding from sites of vascular injury while maintaining blood flow throughout the rest of the body. It involves countless proteins, enzymes, ligands, and molecules to serve as activators, cofactors, regulators, and inhibitors in hemostasis. When the equilibrium of this process is disrupted, it results in abnormal bleeding or clotting depending on the specific dysfunction
25 or deficiency. Accordingly, disorders of hemostasis can be classified as those that cause a propensity for hemorrhage and those that facilitate inappropriate thrombosis. The disorders are further separated by the involvement in primary hemostasis, the initial platelet plug, or secondary hemostasis including the clotting cascade and fibrin cross-linkage. Lastly, hemostatic disorders are pathologically caused by inherited genetic disease or acquired deficiencies.

26 Symptomatically disorders of primary hemostasis often present with superficial signs of bleeding on the skin or mucosa. Patients complain of petechia, mucosal bleeding, and easy bruising. They often suffer from prolonged bleeding from minor injury, frequent epistaxis, and menorrhagia secondary to deficient or dysfunctional platelet activity. In contrast, disorders of secondary hemostasis involve qualitative or quantitative dysfunction of clotting factors and cause more severe and deep tissue bleeding. These patients present with spontaneous hemarthroses, hematomas, and hemorrhage after traumatic injuries. Treatments depend on the specific cause of the disorder and often involve blood component therapy such as platelets, plasma, factor concentrates, or pharmacologic agents that enhance, inhibit, or bypass specific sites in the hemostatic process.

Disorders of Primary Hemostasis

Primary hemostasis involves the initial recruitment of platelets at the site of vascular injury to form a fragile platelet plug. Once platelets bind to the injured subendothelium, they become activated, thereby exposing additional receptor sites and releasing factors involved in further platelet recruitment, activation, aggregation, and the initiation of secondary hemostasis.

Hereditary disorders of platelets are rare and usually associated with defective receptor binding. Bernard–Soulier syndrome is an autosomal recessive disorder that results from an abnormality of the GP Ib receptor. This qualitative and quantitative dysfunction impairs platelet adhesion to exposed vWF at the site of vascular injury.[122] Glanzmann thrombasthenia occurs after a defect in the platelet integrin $\alpha IIb\beta 3$ receptor which, under normal circumstances, allows fibrinogen and other ligands to bind and facilitate platelet aggregation. It is also an autosomal recessive genetic disorder. Other inherited disorders of platelets generally involve ligand receptors or defects in the signaling cascade for the release of molecules involved in platelet activation such as thromboxane and adenine diphosphate.[122]

27 *vWD* is the most common hereditary bleeding disorder with a prevalence of approximately 1% in the general population.[123,124] The clinical features and severity of vWD vary immensely since it has several different types and classifications depending on the nature of the genetic mutation and its effect on the functionality of vWF (Table 16-11). vWF is a large multimeric protein with two different functions in hemostasis. There are several different genetic mutations that affect the various domains of vWF causing different quantitative and functional deficiencies. Each type of vWD presents differently, and in fact there are several complex laboratory evaluations necessary to classify the exact type of disease for each patient. It is still important to reach the correct diagnosis since appropriate treatment and prophylaxis differs for each class of the disorder.

vWF serves a central role in hemostasis. First of all, it functions in primary platelet adhesion and aggregation at the site of vascular injury through interaction with the GP Ib receptor on the platelet surface. Once exposed, vWF facilitates the interaction of platelets with collagen within the subendothelium and platelet–platelet interactions, both of which result in the initial platelet plug and subsequent platelet activation.[125] Secondly, it circulates as a complex with FVIII providing stability to the otherwise labile clotting factor until vWF binds to activated platelets via the GP IIb/IIIa receptor. This localizes FVIII to the site

TABLE 16-11. CLASSIFICATION OF INHERITED VON WILLEBRAND DISEASE[123]

Type	Pathophysiology	Comments
Type 1	Partial quantitative deficiency of vWF	Mildest; most common; responds to DDAVP
Type 2A	Dysfunction in platelet adhesion	May respond to DDAVP
Type 2M	Dysfunction in platelet adhesion	May respond to DDAVP
Type 2B	Increased platelet-binding affinity	Thrombocytopenia with DDAVP
Type 2N	Decreased F VIII-binding affinity	Often confused with hemophilia A
Type 3	Severe quantitative deficiency of vWF	Rarest; most severe; usually requires factor concentrates

vWF, von Willebrand factor; DDAVP, 1-deamino-8-D-arginine vasopressin; FVIII, factor VIII.

of injury.[124–126] The clinical features of vWD vary with differing levels of functionality that result from inherited disorders in protein synthesis, structure, function, and clearance. However, most types of vWD result from decreased levels or deficient function in primary hemostasis which presents with mucocutaneous bleeding such as epistaxis, menorrhagia, and prolonged bleeding from minor wounds and dental extractions. Frequently patients are not aware of the disorder until they undergo a bleeding questionnaire in anticipation of major surgery.[123]

There are three types of vWD. Types 1 and 3 result from quantitative deficiencies of vWF whereas type 2 occurs with various mutations causing qualitative dysfunction; it is further classified (A, B, M, and N) depending on the domain of the protein that is affected and the functional defect (Table 16-11).[123,124,126] Type 1 has an autosomal dominant inheritance pattern and results from a partial quantitative deficiency in vWF levels either from decreased synthesis and secretion from megakaryocytes and endothelial cells or from accelerated proteolysis and clearance. It is the most common and mildest type of vWD.[123] Type 3 is the most severe, but also the rarest; it has a recessive pattern of inheritance and results in significantly depressed levels of vWF. This is the only type likely to cause spontaneous hemorrhage in joints and soft tissues.[123] Type 2 has four subclassifications depending on the functional deficit. Types 2A and 2M result in deficiencies in platelet adhesion and decreased activity of vWF relative to the factor levels within the plasma. Type 2B involves increased affinity of vWF for the GP Ib receptor on the platelet surface. This causes spontaneous binding of vWF to platelets in circulation thereby increasing the cleavage and clearance of vWF. This type of vWD can be associated with thrombocytopenia and in fact, treatment with desmopressin commonly used to increase cleavage from FVIII and overall availability of vWF will precipitate thrombocytopenia.[123] Lastly, type 2N is characterized by decreased affinity for FVIII and deficiencies in secondary hemostasis. This type is often confused with hemophilia A given the depressed levels of FVIII associated with significantly decreased factor half-life.[123]

There are three primary criteria for the diagnosis of vWD including (1) a history of mucosal bleeding or prolonged bleeding after dental extractions, surgical procedures, or postpartum hemorrhage; (2) a family history of bleeding disorders although understandably this can be unreliable or unavailable; and (3) reduced activity of vWF demonstrated by various assays designed to test platelet adhesion, aggregation, and levels of vWF or FVIII complexes (e.g., vWF:factor antigen, vWF:ristocetin cofactor activity, and vWR:collagen-binding activity).[123,126] The laboratory diagnosis and classification of vWD is complex and often requires the expertise of a hematologist to correctly specify the type of disorder and consequently prescribe the appropriate prophylaxis regiment and treatment options. Overall, it is important to recognize that traditional coagulation profile tests such as PT and aPTT are often normal in patients with vWD. Specific diagnostic tests should be recommended for patients suspected of having vWD based on personal or family history of bleeding or positive validated bleeding questionnaires.[126]

There are two primary treatment options for patients with vWD including DDAVP and factor concentrates. DDAVP promotes the cleavage of vWF from FVIII and increases the availability of both; this is beneficial for most patients with type I partial deficiency and some type 2 subclassifications of vWD with the exception of type 2B as discussed above. DDAVP may not be therapeutic by itself for patients with type 3 and severely depressed levels of vWF. Often these patients require treatment with additional hemostatic medications such as antifibrinolytics and/or factor replacement with plasma-derived vWF/FVIII concentrates (Heamate P/Humate P).[127] These concentrates are only needed in approximately 20% of patients with vWD who do not respond to DDAVP and may vary in efficacy. Accordingly it is important to obtain the correct diagnosis in order to best manage each patient prophylactically before surgery and therapeutically in the event of uncontrolled bleeding.[127]

On rare occasions, vWD may be acquired in association with various disease processes such as lymphoproliferative or myeloproliferative disorders, autoimmune disease, cardiac dysfunction, mainly aortic stenosis and ventricular assist devices, or medication induced from quinolones, valproic acid, and hydroxyl ethyl starches. The pathophysiology of acquired vWD is multifactorial and may involve various mechanisms including immune-mediated clearance, binding or absorption into malignant cells or large molecules such as the starches, or enhanced proteolysis secondary to shear stress.[124,128] Treatment starts with discontinuation of the offending agent or management of the underlying condition; however, adjunctive therapeutic measures with DDAVP and/or antifibrinolytics to limit perioperative bleeding may be necessary. Treatment with factor concentrates, steroids, intravenous IG, or plasmapheresis is still under investigation.[128]

Disorders of Secondary Hemostasis

The Hemophilias

28 Hemophilia is a genetic disease that results from deficiencies or dysfunction of specific clotting factors. The most common form is hemophilia A which accounts for about 85% of the disease and stems from deficiencies of FVIII. Hemophilia B or the Christmas disease occurs in 14% of hemophiliacs and involves a defect in the production of factor IX. Both hemophilia A and B are X-linked recessive disorders and found almost exclusively in male patients.[129,130] Hemophilia was originally called the royal disease since Queen Victoria of England was a carrier of hemophilia B and

passed the disorder to the royal families of Spain, Germany, and Russia. Lastly, hemophilia C is very rare, only 1% of all hemophiliacs, and results from genetic mutations in factor XI; it is the only form that has an autosomal recessive inheritance pattern.

Hemophilia A affects approximately 1:5,000 males worldwide. Clinically, these patients suffer from spontaneous bleeding into their joints, muscles, and internal organs often requiring orthopedic surgery for long-term complications of hemarthroses. Central nervous system bleeding is rare, but can lead to severe disability and death.[131] Normal plasma concentrations of FVIII range between 100 and 200 ng/mL and the severity of disease varies depending on the residual factor activity. Patients with mild disease maintain factor levels between 5% and 30% and account for about 50% of patients with hemophilia A. Approximately 10% of patients have moderate disease with 2% to 5% of residual FVIII activity. The most severely affected patients account for about 40% of the disease prevalence and have less than 1% of normal factor activity.[131,132] Incidentally carrier females generally maintain about 50% of FVIII activity with no clinical signs of bleeding. Homozygous females may present with hemophilia, but this is rare and often associated with Turner's syndrome or X-chromosomal mosaicism.[131] Diagnosis starts with patients reporting a personal and/or family history of bleeding disorders among male relations. Confirmatory laboratory evidence includes prolonged aPTT and low factor activity levels. Typically the PT and bleeding times will be normal.[130,131]

Treatment for all hemophilia patients involves replacement of coagulation factor deficiencies which can be accomplished with plasma transfusion or factor concentrates. Historically hemophiliacs were exposed to several transfusion-related infectious risks prior to the availability of recombinant and virally inactivated factor concentrates. In the 1980s, more than 40% of patients with hemophilia suffered from AIDS.[131] Frequent transfusions for these patients are clearly associated with numerous infectious and noninfectious transfusion risks including the development of factor inhibitors and alloantibodies. Up to 30% of patients with severe hemophilia develop inhibitor antibodies to FVIII by the time they reach adulthood making them less responsive to factor concentrates.[133,134]

The goals of management of hemophilia continue to focus on prophylaxis against spontaneous bleeding as well as aggressive blood conservation strategies for anticipated invasive procedures. Patients with mild hemophilia A and hemophilia C often benefit from treatment with DDAVP which effectively raises the circulating availability of FVIII by increasing dissociation from vWF.[135] However, those with more severe disease require treatment of spontaneous and traumatic bleeding episodes as well as prophylaxis to avoid the long-term complications of hemarthroses. This is accomplished with transfusion of specific factor concentrates derived from virally inactivated plasma-derived or recombinant products.[130,132] Patients with inhibitors to FVIII or FIX often respond to rFVIIa or PCCs.[130–132] In anticipation of surgery or invasive procedures, the recommended dose of FVIII concentrates starts with 50 IU/kg ideal body weight in the average adult with severe disease. This should raise the factor activity to close to 100% (1 IU/mL plasma) and should be re-dosed every 8 to 12 hours until hemostasis is achieved.[130] The appropriate dosing regimen for prophylaxis is highly variable among patients given differing levels of disease severity and the impact of factor inhibitors. Titration of the dose of factor concentrates to trough levels of no less than 1 IU/dL (1% of normal) is recommended during long-term prophylaxis.[130,136]

Hemophilia B is clinically and pathophysiologically similar to hemophilia A, except it involves FIX and is much less common worldwide affecting roughly 1:25,000 males.[130] This form of hemophilia is treated with recombinant FIX concentrates but requires less frequent dosing regimens than FVIII concentrates due to a longer half-life (18 hours as opposed to 12 hours).[133] Luckily the development of factor inhibitors is much less prevalent in hemophilia B than in patients with hemophilia A and occurs in only 1% to 6% of severe patients. These patients are also generally responsive to bypass treatment with PCCs or rFVIIa in the case of urgent bleeding.[133]

Acquired hemophilia is a rare disease that usually develops in association with connective tissue disorders, pregnancy, or malignancy. It rarely occurs in young patients and stems from the development of antibodies to FVIII. The clinical symptoms of acquired hemophilia typically include subcutaneous bleeding episodes and soft tissue hematomas as opposed to the hemarthroses common to congenital hemophilia.[128] Diagnostically the aPTT is prolonged in conjunction with decreased FVIII activity levels, both due to the presence of inhibitors. The treatment for acquired hemophilia with acute bleeding depends on rFVIIa or PCCs to bypass FVIII, but some patients with mild disease will respond to adjunctive therapies such as DDAVP and antifibrinolytics. Once hemostasis is achieved, long-term management involves immunosuppression with steroids or cytotoxic agents. Remission occurs in approximately 70% of patients.[128]

Hereditary Hypercoagulability

The *FVL* genetic mutation causes resistance to the anticoagulant effects of APC on clotting factor V. It is the most common hereditary risk factor for hypercoagulability. Heterozygous patients have a fivefold increase in the risk of venous thromboembolism. This rises to 20- to 80-fold increased risk in homozygotes. Treatment involves lifelong therapeutic anticoagulation. The prevalence amongst Caucasians is approximately 5% throughout North America and Europe. Some investigators propose that the high prevalence in Caucasian stems from a protective genetic interplay against bleeding and mortality risk associated with hemophilia.[135]

Protein C and S deficiencies are autosomal dominant genetic diseases that result in increased risk of venous thromboembolism. Protein C inactivates factor V to curb the clotting cascade; it depends on protein S as a cofactor for appropriate function. Accordingly, deficiencies or dysfunction in either protein C or S result in a prothrombotic state.[137] Clinically, patients present with venous thromboembolism in early adulthood; arterial thrombosis is rare. Treatment of acute thrombosis requires therapeutic anticoagulation. Warfarin is indicated for long-term management but should be started slowly and only once the patient is therapeutic on heparin to avoid the risk of warfarin limb necrosis, a complication significantly associated with patients with protein C deficiency.[137]

Acquired Disorders of Hemostasis

Vitamin K Deficiency

Vitamin K is one of the essential fat-soluble vitamins required for the synthesis and final processing of several hemostatic factors, including factors II, VII, IX, X, and proteins C and S. Without vitamin K, these proteins do not undergo carboxylation and therefore cannot actively bind to the phospholipid membrane of platelets during secondary hemostasis. There are two sources of vitamin K; phylloquinone (K_1) is available in a number of foods such as leafy greens. The second type, menoquinone (K_2), is synthesized in the GI tract by intestinal bacteria and accounts for the bulk of vitamin K stored in the liver. The absorption of both types occurs in the small intestine and depends on the availability of bile salts. Accordingly, liver insufficiency and the sterile gut in newborns and patients undergoing oral antibiotic treatments are some of the leading causes of vitamin K deficiency.[138] Other causes include total parenteral nutrition, intestinal obstruction, or hyperperistalsis.[139]

Diagnostically vitamin K deficiency is typically demonstrated by prolonged PT and aPTT but can also be diagnosed with vitamin K blood levels or measures of non-carboxylated prothrombin.[138] It is treated with vitamin K replacement which can be administered parenterally, orally, or intramuscularly. Oral administration has the best bioavailability, but when rapid correction for a bleeding patient is needed, improvements in PT can be seen within 6 to 8 hours of intravenous or intramuscular treatment with doses ranging from 1 to 5 mg.[139]

Liver Disease

Patients with severe liver disease often present with bleeding complications perioperatively or spontaneously including central nervous system hemorrhage or gasterointestinal bleeding; and they are traditionally managed with prophylactic transfusions and adjunctive hemostatic medications in anticipation of surgical procedures or simply in response to high PT times. There are several etiologies related to the bleeding diathesis associated with liver disease including endothelial dysfunction, portal hypertension, thrombocytopenia, and the procoagulant imbalance discussed in the following section. However, the hemostatic system in chronic liver disease remains in balance, although fragile. Conventional laboratory tests such as the PT and aPTT overestimate the bleeding tendency of patients with liver disease and should not be used as the sole method for titrating plasma transfusion or treatment with hemostatic agents.[140]

Primary hemostasis which requires platelet adhesion and aggregation at the site of vascular injury was typically thought to be inefficient in chronic liver disease because of the propensity for thrombocytopenia. Unless severe, thrombocytopenia is often balanced with increased circulating levels of vWF that results from a reduced presence of ADAMTS 13, the protease that regulates plasma concentrations of vWF.[140] This balance remains fragile given that patients with severe liver disease and acute illness are also prone to endothelial and platelet dysfunction.

Secondary hemostasis involves the complex integration of procoagulant and anticoagulant factors several of which are synthesized by the liver. Liver disease results in deficiencies of factors II, V, VII, IX, X, and XI; this will cause profound prolongation of the PT and aPTT times in vitro. However, the liver is also responsible for the synthesis of protein C, protein S, and antithrombin which are integral anticoagulant factors.[140] Furthermore, these patients have increased circulating levels of FVIII in association with the increases in vWF mentioned above. Thus, the decreased levels of procoagulant factors are balanced by deficient amounts of anticoagulant factors and increased FVIII activity.[140] This maintains the balance of the secondary hemostatic mechanism.

Although hemostatic equilibrium is maintained with chronic liver disease the balance is not stable and often tipped in the direction of either hemorrhage or thrombosis by acute illness or any number of other morbidities associated with liver disease such as malnutrition, renal disease, infection, or medications. The use of laboratory tests to indicate the tendency for bleeding or thrombosis is difficult because conventional PT and aPTT conducted in vitro do not mimic the in vivo compensation mechanisms associated with chronic liver disease. Thrombin generation by procoagulant factors is regulated by the anticoagulant activity of protein C and its main activator, thrombomodulin.[140] In vitro thrombin generation is measured only by activation of procoagulant factors and will misrepresent the actual bleeding tendency of the patient.

Lastly, the balance of fibrinolysis is also maintained in chronic liver disease because although these patients suffer a deficiency of plasminogen, they are also found to have higher than normal levels of tPA secondary to lower levels of TAFI. This maintains the normal ratio of plasminogen to plasmin.[140] However, the balance of fibrinolysis and antifibrinolysis remains vulnerable especially in light of other risk factors such as infection, trauma, surgery, and medications common to the pathophysiologic course and medical management of chronic liver patients.

As mentioned above, conventional hemostatic tests such as PT and aPTT assays do not represent the bleeding or thrombotic tendencies of chronic liver disease. This is evident in patients with normal coagulation profiles who present with catastrophic gastrointestinal bleeding or in patients with prolonged PT times who still develop venous, arterial, and portal thrombosis. Theoretically the balance of prohemostatic and anticoagulant factors is maintained; however, these patients are at high risk for various physiologic and acquired circumstances to tip the equilibrium in favor of hemorrhage or thrombosis. The overall hemostatic state can be evaluated by measuring thrombin generation in the presence and absence of thrombomodulin. Alternatively, there is an assay available using snake venom extract (Protac, Pentapharm), in lieu of thrombomodulin to activate protein C in vitro.[140] These tests are still limited because they are conducted independent of platelets and they use an arbitrary amount of thrombomodulin. Nevertheless the circumstances of the test are more akin to the in vivo state of patients with liver disease than conventional PT and aPTT tests.[140] Accordingly, it is no longer recommended to prophylactically transfuse plasma in response to PT times or prior to minor procedures in a patient without clinical signs of bleeding. Furthermore, despite prolonged coagulation tests, patients with liver disease are still at significant risk for venous and arterial thrombosis and should be treated with appropriate prophylactic anticoagulation.[140]

Disseminated Intravacular Coagulopathy

Disseminated intravascular coagulopathy (DIC) is a disorder characterized by systemic activation of coagulation that results in an imbalance of hemostasis. It is always associated with a comorbid condition such as infection, inflammation, or malignancy which causes widespread activation of the coagulation cascade.[141] Table 16-12 lists the medical diseases and syndromes known to cause DIC. Clinically, DIC involves diffuse thrombosis that may lead to multi-organ system failure or consumptive coagulopathy and bleeding. Supportive care and treatment of the underlining disorder are the mainstays of management for DIC, but in severe cases of major hemorrhage or ischemic organ failure, DIC is treated with factor and fibrinogen replacement, anticoagulation, or pharmacologic therapies.

The exact pathophysiology of DIC depends on the causative condition, but primarily involves uncontrolled activation of hemostatic mechanisms for thrombin generation with simultaneous inhibition of fibrinolysis. Thrombin generation in DIC is initiated by TF and activated factor VII in the extrinsic pathway for coagulation.[141,142] The exposure of TF is facilitated by extensive vascular injury, expression on neoplastic cells, or the release of pro-inflammatory cytokines such as interleukin-6. DIC progresses as the regulation of thrombin generation is impaired secondary to decreased levels of natural occurring anticoagulants including AT-III, protein C, and TFPI.[141,142] Lastly, impaired fibrinolysis from an inappropriate increase in circulating levels of PAI-1 facilitates the progression of vascular microthrombi.[141]

DIC is estimated to be present in 1.72% of hospitalized patients, but the clinical features vary depending on the associated disease and the severity.[142] The complications of DIC include organ dysfunction and major bleeding. The kidneys and lungs are particularly vulnerable to ischemia from microthrombi and may develop acute renal failure and acute respiratory distress

TABLE 16-12. COMMON DISORDERS ASSOCIATED WITH DIC[141,142]

Disorder	Average Incidence of DIC	Comments
Sepsis	30–50%	Highest with Gram-negative bacilli
Trauma and burns	Rare	Associated with the degree of tissue injury
Malignancy	Up to 20%	Highest with adenocarcinoma or leukemia and lymphoma
Vascular disease	Rare	Higher with giant hemangiomas
Obstetric complication	Up to 50%	Including preeclampsia, placental abruption, or amniotic fluid embolism
Hemolysis	Rare	Higher with intravascular hemolysis
Severe organ dysfunction	Rare	Including pancreatitis, hepatitis, and end-stage renal failure

syndrome.[142] Furthermore, in severe DIC, widespread activation of hemostasis results in the consumption of coagulation factors and platelets which makes the patient vulnerable to bleeding at the site of tissue injury or spontaneous hemorrhage into the intracranial, intrathoracic, or intra-abdominal compartments.[141] DIC with severe thrombocytopenia or low AT-III levels is a poor prognostic indicator for hospital mortality.[141] However, major bleeding is rather infrequent with DIC and usually occurs only with platelets less than 50,000/μL or patients undergoing procedures. In fact, in a recent study of DIC with sepsis, transfusion for major bleeding was only required in 5% to 12% of patients.[141]

The diagnosis of DIC must consider the underlining disorder in conjunction with an abnormal hemostasis profile. Unfortunately, there is not a single laboratory finding indicative of DIC. High levels of fibrin split products are a sensitive marker, but carry very low specificity.[141,142] Rather, the compilation of prolonged PT and aPTT, thrombocytopenia, hypofibrinogenemia, and increasing fibrin degradation products in a patient with an associated condition leads to the clinical diagnosis of DIC. The International Society of Thrombosis and Hemostasis developed a scoring algorithm for the diagnosis of overt DIC which depends on these four laboratory findings[141,142] (Table 16-13). This algorithm was prospectively validated and found to have a sensitivity of 91% and a specificity of 97%.[141] Furthermore, low levels of AT-III and/or decreased concentration of individual clotting factors aid in the diagnosis.[141,142] Overall, DIC is a dynamic condition and is most accurately diagnosed with repeated measures of coagulation tests showing progression of thrombocytopenia and hypofibrinogenemia with increasing prolongation of PT and levels of fibrin degradation products.

The management for DIC primarily involves treatment of the causative condition and supportive measures to control progressive thrombosis and control any signs of hemorrhage. Consumptive coagulopathy and thrombocytopenia with clinical signs of bleeding should be treated with transfusion of plasma and platelets. However, prophylaxis for patients with abnormal laboratory findings and no signs of bleeding or planned procedures is not necessary. There is no evidence to support improved outcomes from prophylactic transfusion of plasma or platelets unless thrombocytopenia is severe (platelet counts <10,000 to 20,000/μL) or moderate (<50,000/μL) with clinical signs of bleeding or in preparation for invasive procedures.[141]

FFP is the mainstay of replacement therapy for consumption of clotting factors in DIC; however, it often requires large volumes of transfusion, 10 to 15 mL/kg, to correct the coagulopathy.[141,142] In the past, rFVIIa and PCCs have been used for patients with active bleeding and consumptive coagulopathy; however, the administration of active factor concentrates in the preparations of rFVIIa and PCCs can lead to progressive thrombosis in patients with overt DIC and is not recommended. Rather, the use of specific factor concentrations is preferred for measured factor deficiencies in patients with active bleeding.[141,142] Cryoprecipitate remains the product of choice for treatment of overt DIC with consumptive coagulopathy because it contains FVIII and fibrinogen which will treat progressive hypofibrinogenemia as well as factor deficiency with a low overall volume of transfusion.[141]

Arterial and venous thromboembolisms are more concerning than the risk of hemorrhage in patients with overt DIC. Anticoagulation is indicated to inhibit further activation of hemostasis in patients with signs of microthrombi such as organ dysfunction or diagnosed thromboembolism.[141] Studies of patients with DIC in sepsis proved the efficacy of heparin to halt thrombin generation, improve the coagulation profile, and reduce the risk of thrombosis. It is difficult to initiate therapeutic anticoagulation on a patient with signs or risks of bleeding; however, maintaining prophylaxis against venothromboembolism with heparin or LMWH is of utmost importance especially in patients with overt DIC and clinical signs of fibrin deposition and/or organ ischemia from microthrombi. Literature support is limited, but low-molecular-weight alternatives to unfractionated heparin (UFH) may provide better efficacy with lower bleeding risks.[141,142]

AT-III levels are reduced in DIC with impaired regulation of hemostasis. Several animal studies showed improved survival in

TABLE 16-13. SCORING ALGORITHM FOR THE DIAGNOSIS OF DIC[141,142]

Diagnostic Test	Score
Platelet count	>100,000/mm^3 = 0
	<100,000/mm^3 = 1
	<50,000/mm^3 = 2
Prothrombin time	<3 s = 0
	>3 s but <6 s = 1
	>6 s = 2
Fibrin degradation products	No increase = 0
	Moderate increase = 2
	Strong increase = 3
Fibrinogen level	>1 g/L = 0
	<1 g/L = 1

Score calculation:
- If ≥5, consistent with overt DIC.
- If <5, not likely overt DIC; repeat tests in 1 to 2 days.

Algorithm developed by the International Society of Thrombosis and Hemostasis.

DIC models after AT-III replacement. AT-III treatment has yet to be a standard of care for DIC management, but a few controlled trials in septic patients have showed improved coagulation test results and organ function.[142] Treatment with APC for septic patients with severe DIC was reported beneficial for morbidity and mortality especially in patients with multi-organ dysfunction. In 2009, the British Committee for Standards in Hematology recommended its use as standard treatment for patients with DIC in severe sepsis without preexisting risks of bleeding or thrombocytopenia. However, recent reviews of treatment with APC failed to show consistent survival benefits and have documented increased risks of bleeding complications. Consequently, just recently the British Committee changed its recommendation and the production company for APC concentrates removed the drug from the market.[143] Overall, the best therapy for overt DIC of any cause is to treat the underlining condition, continue to support organ function, and maintain control of hemostasis.

ANTICOAGULATION AND PHARMACOLOGIC THERAPY

Anticoagulation Regimens and Associated Anesthetic Concerns

29 *Antiplatelet therapy* is indicated for patients at risk of cerebral vascular accident, myocardial infarction, or other vascular thrombosis complications. There are several mechanisms for platelet dysfunction including COX inhibition, PDE inhibition, ADP receptor antagonism, and GP IIb/IIIa receptor antagonism.

Cyclooxygenase Inhibitors

Aspirin and nonsteroidal antiinflammatory (NSAID) agents are the most notable members of this class. There are two forms of the COX enzyme with variable distribution throughout the body. COX-1 plays an integral part in maintaining the integrity of the gastric lining, renal blood flow, and initiating the formation of TxA_2, an important molecule for platelet aggregation. Inhibition of COX-1 puts the patient at risk for bleeding as well as gastrointestinal and renal morbidity. COX-2 is primarily responsible for synthesizing the prostaglandin mediators of pain and inflammation. Aspirin is a noncompetitive and therefore irreversible inhibitor of both COX enzymes. Consequently, the effects of aspirin therapy last the lifetime of the affected platelets and can only be reversed with platelet transfusion.[144]

NSAID agents are competitive antagonists whose effects last only as long as the drug's time to elimination. Most NSAIDS (naprosyn and ibuprofen) are nonselective COX inhibitors. However, the development of selective COX-2 antagonists such as celecoxib aimed to provide pain relief without the gastrointestinal bleeding complications. Unfortunately, the initial benefits of COX-2 inhibitors were not sustained in long-term outcome studies, and the decreased incidence of gastrotoxicity is clinically insignificant when patients are simultaneously taking aspirin.[144] Recent clinical trials with selective COX-2 antagonists reported increased risks for cardiovascular complications likely secondary to impaired vascular endothelial function. The mechanism for cardiovascular risk is thought to be secondary to the unchecked inhibition of PGI_2 without antagonizing the synthesis of TxA_2 from COX-1 within platelets. This tips the balance in favor of a prothrombotic state.[144] The current recommendations from the American Heart Administration for the therapeutic use of COX-2 inhibitors, namely celecoxib, in patients with cardiovascular disease emphasize using the lowest effective dose in conjunction with a proton pump inhibitor and low-dose aspirin.[144]

Phosphodiesterase Inhibitors

PDE inhibitors are primarily used for stroke prophylaxis since they increase the production of cAMP, which is an active inhibitor of platelet aggregation. These medications are rarely the first-line drug of choice for patients with cerebrovascular disease, but rather used in conjunction with aspirin therapy. Dipyridamole is the prime therapeutic agent in this class, but caffeine, aminophylline, and theophylline also result in reversible platelet dysfunction.

ADP Receptor Antagonists

P2Y12 ADP receptor antagonists, such as clopidogrel, prasugrel, and ticlopidine, prevent the expression of GP IIb/IIIa on the surface of activated platelets, thereby inhibiting platelet adhesion and aggregation. These drugs are used for patients with coronary artery disease to prevent myocardial infarction, in-stent thrombosis, or for patients with cerebrovascular or peripheral artery disease to inhibit thromboembolism. Clopidogrel is the most commonly prescribed agent in this class and acts as a noncompetitive and irreversible antagonist. It is an inactive prodrug that requires oxidation to its active metabolite.[145] Recently, a genetic polymorphism was discovered that results in the inability to metabolize clopidogrel making it ineffective and putting patients at risk of cardiovascular morbidity and mortality. The FDA put a black box warning on the medication to remind clinicians to monitor the activity. Platelet function studies are insensitive and unreliable for clopidogrel, but tests are now available to measure the inhibition of the P2Y12 ADP receptor.[145]

GP IIb/IIIa Recptor Antagonists

GP IIb/IIIa receptor blockers inhibit the cross-linkage of fibrinogen, the final step in the common hemostatic pathway for platelet aggregation. They include abciximab (ReoPro), tirofiban (Aggrastat), and eptifibatide (Integrilin). These agents are administered only intravenously and primarily used for management of acute coronary syndrome. Their effects can be monitored with ACTs and are reversible with clearance of the drug. Most of these agents are renally excreted and have half-lives around 2.5 hours except for abciximab which has a significantly longer half-life (12 hours) and clinical effects that last for approximately 48 hours. All of these drugs cause thrombocytopenia, but the effect is strongest with abciximab with an incidence of about 2.5% as opposed to 0.5% with the other receptor antagonists.[146]

Vitamin K Antagonists

Warfarin is an oral anticoagulant therapy used as the first-line agent for management of hypercoagulable disorders, venous thromboembolism, and stroke prophylaxis for patients with atrial fibrillation or mechanical heart valves. Mechanistically, it competes with vitamin K for carboxylation-binding sites and inhibits the synthesis of vitamin K–dependent clotting factors, II, VII, IX, and X. Proteins C and S, natural anticoagulants, are also dependent on vitamin K for functionality and thus are subject to inhibition with warfarin therapy. In fact, patients may be hypercoagulable during the initial phase of treatment since proteins C and S have shorter half-lives than most clotting factors and will be inhibited first thereby leaving hemostasis and thrombin generation unregulated. Accordingly, patients at high risk for thromboembolism must be bridged with another anticoagulation regimen until the target INR is achieved.[147] Warfarin therapy is monitored with the INR (see section on laboratory interpretation); and therapeutic targets generally range between 2 and 3 although they will vary depending on the disease under treatment and the patient's bleeding risk.[147]

There is a significant risk of bleeding with any anticoagulation regimen; this demands appropriate protocols for reversal of the specific drug effects. The management protocol for warfarin reversal depends on the patient's symptoms and the state of urgency. As mentioned above, warfarin inhibits the synthesis of vitamin K–dependent clotting factors, II, VII, IX, and X; the most logical and appropriate reversal agent is replacement of vitamin K. Guidelines for the administration and reversal of warfarin were written and updated by the British Committee for Standards in Hematology in 2011.[147] For patients with INR >5.0 and no signs or symptoms of bleeding, warfarin administration should be held for one to two doses. Oral vitamin K should be administered if the INR is over 8.0. Patients who present with high INR and nonmajor bleeding should be reversed with 1 to 3 mg of intravenous vitamin K; this usually corrects the INR within 6 to 8 hours. Emergency reversal for patients with major bleeding or those who require immediate surgery can be achieved with a 25 to 50 units/kg dose of 4-factor PCCs which contain active factors II, VII, IX, and X. The 3-factor PCCs lack sufficient amounts of active factor VII to reliably reverse the effects of warfarin.[147] The half-life of most PCCs is short, and vitamin K should be given simultaneously for sustained results. Historically emergent reversal of warfarin was achieved with FFP; however, this requires large volumes of transfusion (10 to 15 mL/kg) and provides unreliable results. rFVIIa has also been used to reverse warfarin, but the supporting literature was retrospective and although it reliably corrects the INR, it does not consistently correct clinical bleeding likely secondary to the ongoing inhibition of other vitamin K–dependent clotting factors.[147] Consequently, the British Committee only recommends the use of FFP when PCCs are not available. rFVIIa is no longer an appropriate reversal agent for warfarin toxicity.

Anticoagulation regimens using oral vitamin K antagonists can be difficult to maintain within the desired target range. Warfarin has a long onset and offset of action, which puts patients at risk of thrombosis and bleeding especially in the perioperative period. It also has many food and drug interactions; and its metabolism is subject to pharmacogenomics that make dosing highly variable. Warfarin is hepatically metabolized by the P450 CYP2 enzymes and will interact with other commonly used medications such as antibiotics, barbiturates, phenytoin, and proton pump inhibitors. Alterations in dietary intake of vitamin K will also vary the clinical effect of maintenance dosages. Furthermore, there are genetic polymorphisms for the CYP2C2 and VKORC1 that decrease the metabolism of warfarin and put the patient at significant bleeding risk.[148] For these reasons, alternative oral anticoagulant agents have been pursued for many years with great potential in the new development of oral DTIs and factor Xa inhibitors.

New Oral Anticoagulants

Dabigatran (Pradaxa), a DTI, and the factor Xa inhibitors (rivaroxiban and apixaban) have completed phase III trials and passed FDA approval for stroke prophylaxis and therapeutic anticoagulation for patients with history of venous thromboembolism. Thrombin and factor X are at the end of the common pathway for clot formation and stabilization and play an integral part in the amplification of secondary hemostasis. Consequently, they are highly desirable targets for antagonism. Furthermore, these agents are significantly easier to manage than warfarin. They have short half-lives and rapid onset of action which negate the need for bridging therapy; and they are highly bioavailable with little interindividual variability. Thus coagulation monitoring is unnecessary. Lastly, they have few drug or dietary interactions. All three agents have a wide therapeutic window making dosing simple and universal. The only dosing concern with dabigatran in particular is renal excretion. The dose must be reduced for patients with decreased creatinine clearance (Table 16-14).[149]

The Re-Ly investigators, the ARISTOTLE group, and the EINSTEIN and ROCKET-AF trials, all compared dabigatran, apixaban, and rivaroxiban to warfarin, respectively, in large, multicenter, randomized controlled trials.[148,151–153] These trials were mostly noninferiority studies that documented that the new oral anticoagulants provide comparable clinical effects to warfarin and often with fewer hemorrhagic side effects. Their full clinical potential has yet to be examined, especially in the perioperative setting where further research is needed to determine the best way to manage bleeding tendencies with surgery and reinstitution of postoperative anticoagulation. Unfortunately there is currently no reliable coagulation test to monitor the clinical effects of these agents. They may prolong the aPTT, thrombin time, or the ecarin coagulation time, but these are not sensitive monitors for increased risk of bleeding.[148,149]

In the event of an emergency, there is no antidote or reliable regimen for drug reversal. Several therapies are currently being studied, including monoclonal antibodies and various blood

TABLE 16-14. ORAL ANTICOAGULATION MEDICATIONS[148,149,150]

	Warfarin	Dabigatran	Apixaban	Rivaroxiban
Target	Vitamin K	Thrombin	Factor Xa	Factor Xa
Time to peak (h)	72–96	1–2	3	2.5–4
Half-life (h)	40	9–13	8–15	7–11
Dose (mg)	2–10	150	5	20
Frequency	Daily or qod	Once or twice daily	Twice daily	Daily
Metabolism	None	Renal excretion	Hepatic	Hepatic
Drug interactions	CYP2C9	Few	CYP3A4	CYP3A4

qod, every other day.

products for transfusion. However, it makes the most sense to attempt reversal with PCCs. Dabigatran, rivaroxiban, and apixaban are competitive inhibitors of thrombin and factor Xa and most PCCs contain factors II, VII, IX, and X thereby overcoming the antagonistic effects. There are some reports that hemodialysis can eliminate dabigatran.[148,149] Perioperatively these agents should be discontinued 24 hours before minor surgery or diagnostic procedures and 48 hours before major surgery or procedures involving the eye, spine, and brain. The half-lives of these agents are all about 12 hours; thus assuming normal hepatic and renal function, more than four half-lives ensures almost 100% drug clearance.[149] However, further research is needed to document the best method for reversing the clinical effects of direct thrombin inhibition.

Heparin Therapy

Heparin therapy is one of the oldest and most common anticoagulation regimens. There are two main forms of heparin, UFH and LMWH. UFH indirectly inhibits thrombin and factor Xa by binding to AT-III causing a conformational shape change which significantly increases its activity. Although the use of UFH for prophylaxis against venous thromboembolism decreased in favor of alternatives such as LMWH and indirect factor Xa inhibitors, it is still used for emergent anticoagulation with acute coronary syndrome, pulmonary embolism, and during cardiopulmonary bypass or vascular surgery. The clinical effects of heparin therapy are monitored with the aPTT or ACT. Patients may be resistant to UFH if they have a hereditary insufficiency of AT-III or an acquired deficiency from prolonged heparin administration. AT-III is replenished with FFP transfusions. UFH is given parenterally and its clinical effects are fully reversible with protamine.[150] The main complication is HIT which is discussed below.

LMWH is a fractionated form of heparin which acts similarly, but with more specific inhibition of factor Xa. Several agents are currently available including enoxaparin, dalteparin, and reviparin. It is preferred over UFH for DVT prophylaxis and treatment because laboratory monitoring is unnecessary, and its longer half-life allows for once- or twice-daily dosing. Treatment can be monitored with factor Xa levels, but this is only necessary for obese patients and those with renal insufficiency which prolongs the elimination.[150] Reversal with protamine is unpredictable and not likely to completely resolve bleeding tendencies.

Indirect Factor Xa Antagonists

Fondaparinux is the principal agent used in this class. It is a highly specific antagonist for free factor Xa that also acts via binding with AT-III. Like LMWH, it is popular for DVT treatment and prophylaxis because it has a long half-life that requires only once-daily dosing, and highly reliable absorption that negates the need for coagulation monitoring. However, fondaparinux undergoes renal elimination necessitating a lower dose or coagulation monitoring with factor Xa levels in patients with renal insufficiency. There is no available antidote in the event of bleeding or the need for emergency procedures. Fortunately the incidence of HIT is relatively low for this class of agents, although they are not approved for use in patients with a history of HIT.[150]

Heparin-induced Thrombocytopenia

30 HIT is a clinical disorder that develops after extended use of heparin therapy. It occurs in approximately 1% to 5% of patients receiving heparin and is associated with morbidity from thromboembolic complications.[154–156] There are two types: HIT1 describes mild thrombocytopenia. It is benign and does not involve immune complexes. HIT2 is an immune-mediated response and carries a significant risk of hypercoagulability. IgG antibodies bind to heparin–PF-4 complexes on the surface of platelets thereby initiating primary hemostasis and thrombin generation.[155] HIT2 can occur in any patient receiving heparin therapy. Typically 5 to 10 days are required to mount a significant immune response, but patients who have recent exposure to heparin or a history of HIT can present with clinical symptoms immediately. Any form of heparin therapy can initiate HIT; however, UFH is more likely than LMWH to lead to immune complexes because the fractionated form is less antigenic with a weaker bond to PF-4.[155]

There are no specific laboratory tests for the clear diagnosis of HIT, and clinical signs can be clouded by alternative causes of thrombocytopenia and thrombosis. Diagnostic criteria begin with thrombocytopenia, defined as a fall in platelets to less than 150,000/μL or more than 50% from the patient's baseline. Thrombocytopenia typically occurs within 5 to 10 days of heparin initiation and will be seen in conjunction with signs of thrombosis. The clinical suspicion of HIT is then confirmed with laboratory tests for antibodies. The enzyme-linked immunosorbent assay (ELISA) is sensitive, but not as specific as the serotonin release assay, which is currently the gold standard with the highest sensitivity and specificity.[155,156] Unfortunately the serotonin assay is often delayed a few days during which patients must be treated with anticoagulation with the associated risk of bleeding complications. Patients suspected of having HIT should be managed with therapeutic anticoagulation and immediate discontinuation of all heparin therapy including heparin-coated indwelling catheters. The most commonly used agents are the parenteral DTIs such as bivalirudin, argatroban, and lepirudin. Oral vitamin K antagonists are contraindicated for HIT treatment because the decreased synthesis of proteins C and S enhances the patient's prothrombotic state. Furthermore, warfarin has been shown to cause gangrenous thrombosis of the limbs in patients with HIT.[154] Platelet transfusion should also be held unless the patient is severely thrombocytopenic (<20,000/μL) with signs of bleeding.

The diagnosis of HIT in patients who have undergone cardiac surgery is often complicated by preexisting or coexisting thrombocytopenia from other causes. According to guidelines from the American College of Chest Physicians, HIT should be suspected and treated in any patient who presents with more than 50% drop in platelets from baseline within 5 to 15 days after cardiac surgery especially if they show signs of thrombosis.[156] The clinical suspicion should be confirmed with ELISA and serotonin assays. The more pressing clinical question involves the need for anticoagulation for patients with a history of HIT who require cardiopulmonary bypass. This discussion will be covered in more depth in another chapter, but briefly, for non-emergent surgery, antibody titers should be measured with the possibility of administering a single dose of heparin for the time of bypass.[154,156] Otherwise, bivalirudin, a parenteral DTI with very short onset and half-life is an alternative agent for anticoagulation since it can be monitored with ACT and is easily titratable. However, there is currently no available reversal agent. Elimination is mostly enzymatic with a half-life of approximately 25 minutes.[150,154,156]

Parenteral Direct Thrombin Inhibitors

Lepirudin and desirudin are recombinant forms of hirudin, a naturally occurring anticoagulant. Argatroban and bivalirudin are synthetic agents in the same class. All four of these drugs directly inhibit thrombin in its free and fibrin-bound states. None of them are immunogenic and so there is no risk of HIT, although antibodies to lepirudin can cause bleeding complications.[150] The half-lives of these agents and their metabolism vary. Furthermore, there are currently no known antidotes to any of the DTIs and therefore, reversal depends upon their clearance. Clinical effects can be monitored with ACT or aPTT measurements. They are all approved for use in the United States, in particular for treatment of HIT.

Lepirudin and desirudin are largely metabolized by the kidney and will have prolonged effects in patients with renal insufficiency. Argatroban is metabolized by the liver with variable clearance in patients with hepatic dysfunction. It is commonly used for patients with HIT who often suffer from consequent renal failure. Argatroban will prolong the INR as well, which can complicate clinical titration of warfarin therapy for long-term anticoagulation. Bivalirudin is the shortest acting DTI with the quickest onset of action, as discussed above. It is metabolized by plasma proteases and renally excreted. Thus this is the drug of choice for patients with both renal and hepatic dysfunction, and its clinical versatility makes it a good agent for use with cardiopulmonary bypass in patients with HIT.[150]

Recombinant Activated Factor VII

rFVIIa (NovoSeven; Novo Nordisk) was originally FDA approved for prophylaxis and treatment of patients with hemophilia A or B
31 complicated by inhibitors to FVIII and factor IX concentrates. It is now also indicated for the treatment of acquired hemophilia and factor VII deficiency.[157] However, the majority of its use is "off-label" for the prevention and treatment of coagulopathy and major blood loss in patients with postpartum hemorrhage, trauma, reversal of various anticoagulants, and high-risk cardiothoracic, spinal, transplant, or vascular surgery.[157–159] The majority of supporting data for the use of rFVIIa as a hemostatic treatment stem from retrospective reports, observational studies, and case series. There are few randomized control trials showing improved clinical outcomes and no trials that report definitive mortality benefits.[158,159] In fact, a recent meta-analysis published by Levi et al. demonstrated an increased risk of arterial thromboembolism especially in elderly patients and high doses of rFVIIa (>120 μg/kg).[157] Phase III trials for rFVIIa treatment of warfarin-related intracerebral hemorrhage did not show significant benefit as a reversal agent.[158,160] These trials often document significant decreases in INR, but evidence of outcome improvement is lacking.[158,160] The true clinical benefits of rFVIIa remain unclear. Several randomized control trials have also shown a decrease in blood product transfusion and/or improved coagulation profile tests; however, it is difficult to randomize patients for indications of life-threatening hemorrhage and these studies are generally underpowered to show any true mortality benefit.[157,159,161,162] Overall, the lack of consistent dosing protocols or patient populations throughout the literature leaves one without a clear indication for the use of rFVIIa as a hemostatic agent for critical bleeding.

The hemostatic mechanism for rFVIIa remains unclear but likely involves more than the physiologic role of factor VII in secondary hemostasis. Theoretically, rFVIIa will only act with TF exposed from the vascular endothelial lining at a site of injury. However, certain hemorrhagic disorders such as DIC or poly-trauma can initiate systemic release of TF.[150,158] Furthermore, the clinical dosing of rFVIIa typically exceeds normal concentrations by 1,000-fold; at these doses, rFVIIa directly activates factor X and platelets generating a thrombin burst for procoagulant activity.[150,158,160] These mechanisms explain why arterial and venous thromboembolism are the major complications of concern with the use of rFVIIa, and why DIC or high risk for thromboembolism is the main contraindication.[150,158,160,163] Clinical doses for rFVIIa reported in the literature range from 20 μg/kg to over 200 μg/kg.[150,158–160,163] The only guidance for therapeutic dosing regimens is from its use in hemophilia which is typically treated with 80 to 90 μg/kg.[150,163] This is a supraphysiologic dose and likely more than necessary for patients without hemophilia. NovoSeven is a temporizing hemostatic agent used to improve the visual field during an operation, or to slow bleeding and provide time for resuscitation while the underlying cause of hemorrhage is controlled.[162] The half-life of rFVIIa is 2 to 2.5 hours, and the initial dose may require repeating until the bleeding is controlled.[157] It is important to recognize that the mechanism of action depends on platelet and fibrinogen function, both of which should be maintained before or during treatment with rFVIIa.[163] Overall, further research is needed to establish the appropriate dose and patient population while minimizing the risk of thromboembolism.

Prothrombin Complex Concentrates

PCCs have been available for treatment of patients with hemophilia B for several decades. It was first used as a source of factor IX in the 1970s prior to the advent of specific factor concentrates. Subsequently it provided bypass treatment for hemophiliacs with factor inhibitors. Over the years, the safety and efficacy of PCCs have improved dramatically, and now, although they are only FDA approved for use in hemophilia, they are mainly given for reversal of vitamin K antagonists and in the management of critical bleeding associated with major surgery, trauma, or liver failure.[164]

There are several commercially available formulations of PCCs containing varying amounts of three to four coagulation factors as well as one or more type of anticoagulant. The compositions include the vitamin K–dependent factors (II, VII, IX, and X) although not all products contain significant concentrations of factor VII. In fact, most of the PCCs available in the United States are 3-factor concentrates lacking factor VII (e.g., FEIBA, Baxter).[165] Most of the factors are administered in the inactive state which decreases the thrombogenic risks.[164] The anticoagulants are included to restore balance to the hemostatic mechanism. These vary from heparin to antithrombin or proteins C and S.[164]

32 PCCs are now the drug of choice for emergent reversal of oral anticoagulants in place of rFVIIa and FFP, the previous standard of care. As mentioned above, rFVIIa failed to show significant outcome improvements for treatment of warfarin-related intracerebral hemorrhage in phase III trials.[160] This is likely because it only replaces one of the vitamin K–dependent factors and although the INR and PT decrease, this did not translate to meaningful survival benefits. PCCs are now preferred over FFP as well, for several reasons. First of all, they provide faster correction of coagulopathy compared to FFP. The factors in plasma are relatively dilute and a large volume (10 to 15 mL/kg) is required for clinical reversal of oral anticoagulants. It takes extra time to match the patient's blood type and thaw the plasma putting the patient at risk of volume overload.[147,164] Furthermore, PCCs stem from human plasma, but they are treated with at least one viral reduction process, whereas transfusion of several units of FFP carries a significant risk of infectious and noninfectious transfusion reactions.[164] Although based on few randomized controlled trials, the current recommendations from the British and American guidelines for reversal of oral anticoagulants favor PCCs over both FFP and rFVIIa.[147,164,166] The hemostatic benefits of PCCs will likely translate to treatment of critical surgical bleeding, liver failure, and trauma, although the literature support for these indications is lacking.[165] It is important to remember that PCCs provide factor replacement for thrombin generation, their action still depends on adequate concentrations of platelets and fibrinogen.

The potential for PCCs to generate a significant thrombin burst puts the patients at risk for thrombotic complications. The exact pathogenesis for thrombosis remains unclear, but animal models indicate that the accumulation of prothrombin, inactive factor II, and/or factor X after PCC administration is correlated with thrombogenesis. Furthermore, this risk is associated with patients with thrombotic tendencies, such as those on anticoagulation and elderly patients who have a history of stroke. There are very few studies in trauma patients, but no significant reports of thrombotic complications in volunteers or those treated with PCCs for critical bleeding.[164]

The thrombotic risk can be minimized by avoiding repeat dosing. The factors within PCCs have varied half-lives with prothrombin remaining active in plasma for up to 60 hours and factor X present for 30 hours. This is in contrast to labile factor VII which only has a half-life of approximately 6 hours. Consequently, factors II and X, which are thought to be primarily responsible for thrombotic complications, have the potential to accumulate with repeat doses of PCCs. The need for repeat dosing can be avoided by the coadministration of vitamin K in patients treated for oral anticoagulant toxicity. This allows for increased synthesis of coagulation factors in balance with natural anticoagulants.[147,164,166] Furthermore, PCC dosing should be guided by the appropriate coagulation profile test. PT and INR only measure the procoagulant half of the hemostatic mechanism ignoring the presence of anticoagulant activity such as antithrombin or proteins C and S. In patients with severe liver disease or dilutional coagulopathy, the PT and INR times may be prolonged, but the concentrations of anticoagulants are also decreased leaving hemostasis balanced. Thrombin generation times or thromboelastography are more appropriate measures of the patient's risk of bleeding and better indicators of the efficacy of PCC. These tests should be considered before redosing since these patients may require simultaneous treatment with antithrombin, platelets, or fibrinogen. The only absolute contraindications to PCC administration are patients at high risk for thrombosis such as those in DIC or with active HIT.[164]

Desmopressin

Desmopressin (DDAVP) is a synthetic analog for the endogenous antidiuretic hormone, vasopressin. It acts at the V2 receptor which is found in the nephron and within endothelial cells. DDAVP was originally introduced for treatment of diabetes insipidus, but it was also found to improve hemostasis and platelet function. Consequently, it is one of the drugs of choice for treatment of mild bleeding in patients with vWD and mild hemophilia A as discussed earlier in this chapter.[167] Mechanistically it causes the release of FVIII and vWF from within vascular endothelial cells thereby improving platelet function. DDAVP does not increase the synthesis of these factors and therefore, tachyphylaxis occurs with frequent repeat dosing.[168] The appropriate dose for hemostasis is 0.3 μg/kg intravenously over 20 to 30 minutes. Levels of vWF and FVIII increase two- to fourfold within 30 minutes of administration. The effects last for approximately 6 to 8 hours.[167–169] Hypotension is the most commonly reported side effect presumably secondary to arterial vasodilation from the release of NO; it is best avoided with slower infusion rates. Hyponatremia and water retention are rare complications, but have been reported in pediatric patients.[168] As with all prothrombotic agents, DDAVP should be avoided in patients at high risk for thromboembolism, although the most recent meta-analysis did not report a significant incidence of thromboembolic complications.[168,169]

The hemostatic potential for DDAVP has been vastly studied for patients with critical bleeding from cardiac or spine surgery, uremia, antiplatelet agents, and liver disease. Several meta-analyses of randomized controlled trials report mild decreases in blood loss (80 mL per patient), but fail to translate into significant outcome improvements. There is no apparent effect on the number of patients transfused or the incidence of postoperative complications including reoperation. The only consistent clinical benefit of DDAVP is improved bleeding times for patients with congenital or acquired platelet dysfunction from cardiopulmonary bypass, chronic renal failure, or aspirin therapy.[168,169]

Antifibrinolytic Therapy

33 Antifibrinolytic agents have been used to prevent and treat surgical blood loss for several decades. There are two types, the lysine analogs, epsilon-aminocaproic acid (EACA) and tranexamic acid (TXA), and a serine protease inhibitor, aprotinin. Aprotinin was reported to have superior efficacy for reducing blood loss, minimizing transfusions, and preventing reoperations especially in cardiac surgery. It was removed from the market after several observational studies documented increased risk of renal failure, myocardial infarction, and death.[170,171] These findings were confirmed by the Canadian trial, Blood Conservation Using Antifibrinolytics in a Randomized Trial (BART), which was stopped early due to significantly higher mortality associated with aprotinin when compared to EACA and TXA.[168,172,173] However, aprotinin is now available in Canada and may be reintroduced in the United States in the near future. Both the lysine derivatives are widely used throughout the United States. Today, they are commonly administered as part of a multimodal approach to perioperative blood conservation strategies.

Aprotinin is a nonspecific serine protease inhibitor. It prevents the action of several proteins involved in coagulation and fibrinolysis including trypsin, plasmin, and kallikrein. It may also have an indirect effect on platelets to preserve their function especially during extracorporeal circulation.[174] The clinical efficacy of aprotinin to reduce perioperative blood loss, transfusions, and reoperations is clear from decades of research.[168,173,174] However, there is also an abundance of evidence reporting the negative association with renal failure and mortality. When compared to the lysine analogs in the BART randomized controlled trial as well as in several retrospective studies and meta-analyses, aprotinin shows reduced blood loss and transfusion requirements; however, the consistently higher mortality risk has changed the recommendations to favor the use of EACA and TXA for perioperative blood conservation.[170–173]

Lysine Analogs

EACA and TXA are synthetic derivatives of the amino acid, lysine. They competitively inhibit the binding site on plasminogen thereby preventing cleavage to plasmin and the resultant fibrinolysis.[168,174] Both agents are excreted by the kidney and may be administered intravenously or topically. Although there is more evidence to support the use of TXA, these agents appear to have equivalent efficacy and have been shown to moderately decrease perioperative blood loss in cardiac surgery as well as liver transplantation, orthopedic operations, and spine fusions.[173–177] Neither conclusively decreases rates of transfusion, reoperation, or mortality. The lysine analogs are inexpensive compared to aprotinin and there have been no reports of increased risk of thrombotic complications or renal failure.[168,173,174] The only documented adverse effects are mild nausea and vomiting with rapid infusion rates. Besides perioperative indications, antifibrinolytics were recently studied for their potential to minimize critical bleeding in trauma patients. The CRASH II multinational randomized controlled trial compared TXA with placebo in trauma patients with major hemorrhage and documented a reduced all-cause mortality and risk of death due to bleeding.[178] Overall, the lysine analogs are inexpensive and low-risk adjunctive agents that should be considered for use in major surgery or critical bleeding as part of a multimodal approach to blood conservation.

CONCLUSIONS

Clinical anesthesiology is a perioperative specialty that aims to maintain the patient's health and wellness throughout the course of surgery. This requires a clear understanding of how a person's preexisting comorbid status and anticipated surgical procedure can best be managed to gain the most therapeutic benefits from interventions with the least incurred risk. The anesthesiologist must remain vigilant in order to anticipate the possibility of derangements to coagulation and hemostasis that may occur with surgery, trauma, or critical illness. They must also know the best methods for avoiding hemorrhagic or thrombotic complications of surgery or treatment modalities to ensure the ability to treat any problems that arise, while limiting the risks of transfusion therapy and hemostatic pharmacologic agents.

Medicine is an evolving science with new treatments, medications, and procedures discovered every day, often presenting great challenges to the perioperative physician. For, example, new oral DTIs are replacing the use of warfarin for therapeutic anticoagulation; however, the appropriate reversal management is unclear as is the optimal timing for invasive procedures. Overall, understanding the hemostatic mechanism and the specifics of transfusion therapy is integral to the practice of anesthesia.

References

1. *The 2009 National Blood Collection and Utilization Survey Report.* Bethesda, MD: US Department of Health and Human Services and the American Association of Blood Banks; 2009.
2. Rivera J, Lozano ML, Navarro-Nunez L, et al. Platelet receptors and signaling in the dynamics of thrombus formation. *Haematologica.* 2009;94(5):700–711.
3. Brass L. Understanding and evaluating platelet function. *Hematology Am Soc Hematol Educ Program.* 2010;2010:387–396.
4. Li Z, Delaney MK, O'Brien KA, et al. Signaling during platelet adhesion and activation. *Arterioscler Thromb Vasc Biol.* 2010;30(12):2341–2349.
5. Mann KG. Thrombin generation in hemorrhage control and vascular occlusion. *Circulation.* 2011;124(2):225–235.
6. Godfrey EM, Godfrey AL, Perry DJ, et al. Don't be a clot: A radiologist's guide to haemostasis including novel antiplatelet and anticoagulant therapies. *Clin Radiol.* 2011;66(8):693–700.
7. Collet JP, Montalescot G. Platelet function testing and implications for clinical practice. *J Cardiovasc Pharmacol Ther.* 2009;14(3):157–169.
8. Lambert MP. What to do when you suspect an inherited platelet disorder. *Hematology Am Soc Hematol Educ Program.* 2011;2011:377–383.
9. James PD, Goodeve AC. von Willebrand disease. *Genet Med.* 2011;13(5):365–376.
10. Shander A, Walsh CE, Cromwell C. Acquired hemophilia: A rare but life-threatening potential cause of bleeding in the intensive care unit. *Intensive Care Med.* 2011;37(8):1240–1249.
11. Murphy GS, Marymont JH. Alternative anticoagulation management strategies for the patient with heparin-induced thrombocytopenia undergoing cardiac surgery. *J Cardiothorac Vasc Anesth.* 2007;21(1):113–126.
12. Chitlur M, Lusher J. Standardization of thromboelastography: Values and challenges. *Semin Thromb Hemost.* 2010;36(7):707–711.
13. Nair SC, Dargaud Y, Chitlur M, et al. Tests of global haemostasis and their applications in bleeding disorders. *Haemophilia.* 2010;16(suppl 5):85–92.
14. Middeldorp S. Is thrombophilia testing useful? *Hematology Am Soc Hematol Educ Program.* 2011;2011:150–155.
15. Kujovich JL. Factor V Leiden thrombophilia. *Genet Med.* 2011;13(1):1–16.
16. Previtali E, Bucciarelli P, Passamonti SM, et al. Risk factors for venous and arterial thrombosis. *Blood Transfus.* 2011;9(2):120–138.
17. Ng VL. Anticoagulation monitoring. *Clin Lab Med.* 2009;29(2):283–304.
18. Warkentin TE. How I diagnose and manage HIT. *Hematology Am Soc Hematol Educ Program.* 2011;2011:143–149.
19. Samama MM. The mechanism of action of rivaroxaban–an oral, direct Factor Xa inhibitor–compared with other anticoagulants. *Thromb Res.* 2011;127(6):497–504.
20. Lison S, Spannagl M. Monitoring of direct anticoagulants. *Wien Med Wochenschr.* 2011;161(3–4):58–62.
21. Eder A, ed. *Allogeneic and Autologous Blood Donor Selection, Technical Manual.* Bethesda, MD: American Association of Blood Banks; 2011.
22. Callum JL, Karkouti K, Lin Y. Cryoprecipitate: The current state of knowledge. *Transfus Med Rev.* 2009;23(3):177–188.
23. Stroncek DF, Rebulla P. Platelet transfusions. *Lancet.* 2007;370(9585):427–438.
24. Lindholm PF, Annen K, Ramsey G. Approaches to minimize infection risk in blood banking and transfusion practice. *Infect Disord Drug Targets.* 2011; 11(1):45–56.
25. Vamvakas EC, Blajchman MA. Transfusion-related immunomodulation (TRIM): An update. *Blood Rev.* 2007;21(6):327–348.
26. Dwyre DM, Holland PV. Transfusion-associated graft-versus-host disease. *Vox Sang.* 2008;95(2):85–93.
27. Lockwood WB, Leonard J, Liles SL, eds. *Storage, Monitoring, Pretransfusion Processing, and Distribution of Blood Components.* Bethesda, MD: American Association of Blood Banks; 2011.
28. Vamvakas EC. Meta-analysis of clinical studies of the purported deleterious effects of "old" (versus "fresh") red blood cells: Are we at equipoise? *Transfusion.* 2010;50(3):600–610.
29. Silverman TA, Weiskopf RB. Hemoglobin-based oxygen carriers: Current status and future directions. *Anesthesiology.* 2009;111(5):946–963.
30. Gekas C, Graf T. Induced pluripotent stem cell-derived human platelets: One step closer to the clinic. *J Exp Med.* 2010;207(13):2781–2784.
31. Practice guidelines for perioperative blood transfusion and adjuvant therapies. An updated report by the American Society of Anesthesiologists Task Force on Perioperative Blood Transfusion and Adjuvant Therapies. *Anesthesiology.* 2006;105(1):198–208.
32. Hebert PC, Wells G, Blajchman MA, et al. A multicenter, randomized, controlled clinical trial of transfusion requirements in critical care. Transfusion Requirements in Critical Care Investigators, Canadian Critical Care Trials Group. *N Engl J Med.* 1999;340(6):409–417.
33. Marik PE, Corwin HL. Efficacy of red blood cell transfusion in the critically ill: A systematic review of the literature. *Crit Care Med.* 2008;36(9):2667–2674.
34. Hajjar LA, Vincent JL, Galas FR, et al. Transfusion requirements after cardiac surgery: The TRACS randomized controlled trial. *JAMA.* 2010;304(14):1559–1567.
35. Hebert PC. The TRICC trial: A focus on the sub-group analysis. *Vox Sang.* 2002; 83(suppl 1):387–396.
36. Napolitano LM, Kurek S, Luchette FA, et al. Clinical practice guideline: Red blood cell transfusion in adult trauma and critical care. *Crit Care Med.* 2009;37(12):3124–3157.
37. Carson JL, Duff A, Poses RM, et al. Effect of anaemia and cardiovascular disease on surgical mortality and morbidity. *Lancet.* 1996;348(9034):1055–1060.
38. Hebert PC, Wells G, Tweeddale M, et al. Does transfusion practice affect mortality in critically ill patients? Transfusion Requirements in Critical Care (TRICC) Investigators and the Canadian Critical Care Trials Group. *Am J Respir Crit Care Med.* 1997;155(5):1618–1623.
39. von Heymann C, Sander M, Foer A, et al. The impact of an hematocrit of 20% during normothermic cardiopulmonary bypass for elective low risk coronary artery bypass graft surgery on oxygen delivery and clinical outcome–a randomized controlled study [ISRCTN35655335]. *Crit Care.* 2006;10(2):R58.
40. Surgenor SD, Kramer RS, Olmstead EM, et al. The association of perioperative red blood cell transfusions and decreased long-term survival after cardiac surgery. *Anesth Analg.* 2009;108(6):1741–1746.
41. Ferraris VA, Brown JR, Despotis GJ, et al. 2011 update to the Society of Thoracic Surgeons and the Society of Cardiovascular Anesthesiologists blood conservation clinical practice guidelines. *Ann Thorac Surg.* 2011;91(3):944–982.
42. Kramer AH, Zygun DA. Anemia and red blood cell transfusion in neurocritical care. *Crit Care.* 2009;13(3):R89.
43. Corwin HL, Gettinger A, Pearl RG, et al. The CRIT study: Anemia and blood transfusion in the critically ill–current clinical practice in the United States. *Crit Care Med.* 2004;32(1):39–52.
44. Naidech AM, Jovanovic B, Wartenberg KE, et al. Higher hemoglobin is associated with improved outcome after subarachnoid hemorrhage. *Crit Care Med.* 2007;35(10):2383–2389.
45. Bernard AC, Davenport DL, Chang PK, et al. Intraoperative transfusion of 1 U to 2 U packed red blood cells is associated with increased 30-day mortality, surgical-site infection, pneumonia, and sepsis in general surgery patients. *J Am Coll Surg.* 2009;208(5):931–937, 937.e1–937.e2, discussion 8–9.
46. Glance LG, Dick AW, Mukamel DB, et al. Association between intraoperative blood transfusion and mortality and morbidity in patients undergoing noncardiac surgery. *Anesthesiology.* 2011;114(2):283–292.
47. Wang JK, Klein HG. Red blood cell transfusion in the treatment and management of anaemia: The search for the elusive transfusion trigger. *Vox Sang.* 2010;98(1):2–11.
48. Yuruk K, Bartels SA, Milstein DM, et al. Red blood cell transfusions and tissue oxygenation in anemic hematology outpatients. *Transfusion.* 2012;52(3):641–646.
49. Metivier F, Marchais SJ, Guerin AP, et al. Pathophysiology of anaemia: Focus on the heart and blood vessels. *Nephrol Dial Transplant.* 2000;15(suppl 3):14–18.

50. Robertie PG, Gravlee GP. Safe limits of isovolemic hemodilution and recommendations for erythrocyte transfusion. *Int Anesthesiol Clin.* 1990;28(4):197–204.
51. Weiskopf RB, Feiner J, Hopf H, et al. Heart rate increases linearly in response to acute isovolemic anemia. *Transfusion.* 2003;43(2):235–240.
52. Liumbruno GM, Bennardello F, Lattanzio A, et al. Recommendations for the transfusion management of patients in the peri-operative period. III. The post-operative period. *Blood Transfus.* 2011;9(3):320–335.
53. Liumbruno GM, Bennardello F, Lattanzio A, et al. Recommendations for the transfusion management of patients in the peri-operative period. II. The intra-operative period. *Blood Transfus.* 2011;9(2):189–217.
54. Stainsby D, MacLennan S, Thomas D, et al. Guidelines on the management of massive blood loss. *Br J Haematol.* 2006;135(5):634–641.
55. British Committee for Standards in Haematology, Blood Transfusion Task Force. Guidelines for the use of platelet transfusions. *Br J Haematol.* 2003;122(1):10–23.
56. Liumbruno G, Bennardello F, Lattanzio A, et al. Recommendations for the transfusion of plasma and platelets. *Blood Transfus.* 2009;7(2):132–150.
57. Liumbruno GM, Bennardello F, Lattanzio A, et al. Recommendations for the transfusion management of patients in the peri-operative period. I. The pre-operative period. *Blood Transfus.* 2011;9(1):19–40.
58. Tosetto A, Balduini CL, Cattaneo M, et al. Management of bleeding and of invasive procedures in patients with platelet disorders and/or thrombocytopenia: Guidelines of the Italian Society for Haemostasis and Thrombosis (SISET). *Thromb Res.* 2009;124(5):e13–e18.
59. Shen YM, Frenkel EP. Acquired platelet dysfunction. *Hematol Oncol Clin North Am.* 2007;21(4):647–661, vi.
60. O'Shaughnessy DF, Atterbury C, Bolton Maggs P, et al. Guidelines for the use of fresh-frozen plasma, cryoprecipitate and cryosupernatant. *Br J Haematol.* 2004; 126(1):11–28.
61. Heim MU, Meyer B, Hellstern P. Recommendations for the use of therapeutic plasma. *Curr Vasc Pharmacol.* 2009;7(2):110–119.
62. Stanworth SJ, Walsh TS, Prescott RJ, et al. A national study of plasma use in critical care: Clinical indications, dose and effect on prothrombin time. *Crit Care.* 2011;15(2):R108.
63. Stanworth SJ, Grant-Casey J, Lowe D, et al. The use of fresh-frozen plasma in England: High levels of inappropriate use in adults and children. *Transfusion.* 2011;51(1):62–70.
64. Stanworth SJ, Hyde CJ, Murphy MF. Evidence for indications of fresh frozen plasma. *Transfus Clin Biol.* 2007;14(6):551–556.
65. Duchesne JC, Islam TM, Stuke L, et al. Hemostatic resuscitation during surgery improves survival in patients with traumatic-induced coagulopathy. *J Trauma.* 2009;67(1):33–37, discussion 7–9.
66. de Biasi AR, Stansbury LG, Dutton RP, et al. Blood product use in trauma resuscitation: Plasma deficit versus plasma ratio as predictors of mortality in trauma (CME). *Transfusion.* 2011;51(9):1925–1932.
67. Ho AM, Dion PW, Yeung JH, et al. Prevalence of survivor bias in observational studies on fresh frozen plasma: Erythrocyte ratios in trauma requiring massive transfusion. *Anesthesiology.* 2012;116(3):716–728.
68. Stanworth SJ. The evidence-based use of FFP and cryoprecipitate for abnormalities of coagulation tests and clinical coagulopathy. *Hematology Am Soc Hematol Educ Program.* 2007;2007:179–186.
69. Sorensen B, Bevan D. A critical evaluation of cryoprecipitate for replacement of fibrinogen. *Br J Haematol.* 2010;149(6):834–843.
70. Rossaint R, Bouillon B, Cerny V, et al. Management of bleeding following major trauma: An updated European guideline. *Crit Care.* 2010;14(2):R52.
71. Bolliger D, Szlam F, Molinaro RJ, et al. Finding the optimal concentration range for fibrinogen replacement after severe haemodilution: An in vitro model. *Br J Anaesth.* 2009;102(6):793–799.
72. Allain JP, Stramer SL, Carneiro-Proietti AB, et al. Transfusion-transmitted infectious diseases. *Biologicals.* 2009;37(2):71–77.
73. Zou S, Stramer SL, Dodd RY. Donor testing and risk: Current prevalence, incidence, and residual risk of transfusion-transmissible agents in US allogeneic donations. *Transfus Med Rev.* 2012;26(2):119–128.
74. Dwyre DM, Fernando LP, Holland PV. Hepatitis B, hepatitis C and HIV transfusion-transmitted infections in the 21st century. *Vox Sang.* 2011;100(1):92–98.
75. Kleinman SH, Lelie N, Busch MP. Infectivity of human immunodeficiency virus-1, hepatitis C virus, and hepatitis B virus and risk of transmission by transfusion. *Transfusion.* 2009;49(11):2454–2489.
76. Zou S, Musavi F, Notari EP, et al. Prevalence, incidence, and residual risk of major blood-borne infections among apheresis collections to the American Red Cross Blood Services, 2004 through 2008. *Transfusion.* 2010;50(7):1487–1494.
77. Wu Y, Zou S, Cable R, et al. Direct assessment of cytomegalovirus transfusion-transmitted risks after universal leukoreduction. *Transfusion.* 2010;50(4):776–786.
78. Stramer SL, Hollinger FB, Katz LM, et al. Emerging infectious disease agents and their potential threat to transfusion safety. *Transfusion.* 2009;49(suppl 2):1S–29S.
79. Liumbruno GM, Catalano L, Piccinini V, et al. Reduction of the risk of bacterial contamination of blood components through diversion of the first part of the donation of blood and blood components. *Blood Transfus.* 2009;7(2):86–93.
80. Shander A. Emerging risks and outcomes of blood transfusion in surgery. *Semin Hematol.* 2004;41(1 suppl 1):117–124.
81. Dorsey K, Zou S, Schonberger LB, et al. Lack of evidence of transfusion transmission of Creutzfeldt–Jakob disease in a US surveillance study. *Transfusion.* 2009;49(5):977–984.
82. Stainsby D, Jones H, Asher D, et al. Serious hazards of transfusion: A decade of hemovigilance in the UK. *Transfus Med Rev.* 2006;20(4):273–282.
83. Jenkins C, Ramirez-Arcos S, Goldman M, et al. Bacterial contamination in platelets: Incremental improvements drive down but do not eliminate risk. *Transfusion.* 2011;51(12):2555–2565.
84. Zimring JC, Welniak L, Semple JW, et al. Current problems and future directions of transfusion-induced alloimmunization: Summary of an NHLBI working group. *Transfusion.* 2011;51(2):435–441.
85. Zalpuri S, Zwaginga JJ, le Cessie S, et al. Red-blood-cell alloimmunization and number of red-blood-cell transfusions. *Vox Sang.* 2012;102(2):144–149.
86. Benson AB, Moss M, Silliman CC. Transfusion-related acute lung injury (TRALI): A clinical review with emphasis on the critically ill. *Br J Haematol.* 2009; 147(4):431–443.
87. Li G, Rachmale S, Kojicic M, et al. Incidence and transfusion risk factors for transfusion-associated circulatory overload among medical intensive care unit patients. *Transfusion.* 2011;51(2):338–343.
88. Marti-Carvajal AJ, Sola I, Gonzalez LE, et al. Pharmacological interventions for the prevention of allergic and febrile non-haemolytic transfusion reactions. *Cochrane Database Syst Rev.* 2010;6:CD007539.
89. Hendrickson JE, Hillyer CD. Noninfectious serious hazards of transfusion. *Anesth Analg.* 2009;108(3):759–769.
90. Sandler SG, Zantek ND. Review: IgA anaphylactic transfusion reactions. Part II. Clinical diagnosis and bedside management. *Immunohematology.* 2004;20(4):234–238.
91. Vamvakas EC, Blajchman MA. Transfusion-related mortality: The ongoing risks of allogeneic blood transfusion and the available strategies for their prevention. *Blood.* 2009;113(15):3406–3417.
92. Sparrow RL. Red blood cell storage and transfusion-related immunomodulation. *Blood Transfus.* 2010;8(suppl 3):s26–s30.
93. Vamvakas EC. White-blood-cell-containing allogeneic blood transfusion and postoperative infection or mortality: An updated meta-analysis. *Vox Sang.* 2007; 92(3):224–232.
94. Silliman CC. The two-event model of transfusion-related acute lung injury. *Crit Care Med.* 2006;34(5 suppl):S124–S131.
95. Wyman TH, Bjornsen AJ, Elzi DJ, et al. A two-insult in vitro model of PMN-mediated pulmonary endothelial damage: Requirements for adherence and chemokine release. *Am J Physiol Cell Physiol.* 2002;283(6):C1592–C1603.
96. Chapman CE, Stainsby D, Jones H, et al. Ten years of hemovigilance reports of transfusion-related acute lung injury in the United Kingdom and the impact of preferential use of male donor plasma. *Transfusion.* 2009;49(3):440–452.
97. *Fatalities Reported to FDA Following Blood Collection and Transfusion: Annual Summary for Fiscal Year 2010.* Silver Spring, MD: US Department of Health and Human Services, the Food and Drug Administration; 2010.
98. Saidenberg E, Petraszko T, Semple E, et al. Transfusion-related acute lung injury (TRALI): A Canadian blood services research and development symposium. *Transfus Med Rev.* 2010;24(4):305–324.
99. Gilliss BM, Looney MR. Experimental models of transfusion-related acute lung injury. *Transfus Med Rev.* 2011;25(1):1–11.
100. Toy P, Popovsky MA, Abraham E, et al. Transfusion-related acute lung injury: Definition and review. *Crit Care Med.* 2005;33(4):721–726.
101. Gajic O, Rana R, Winters JL, et al. Transfusion-related acute lung injury in the critically ill: Prospective nested case-control study. *Am J Respir Crit Care Med.* 2007;176(9):886–891.
102. Bux J, Sachs UJ. The pathogenesis of transfusion-related acute lung injury (TRALI). *Br J Haematol.* 2007;136(6):788–799.
103. Sachs UJ, Wasel W, Bayat B, et al. Mechanism of transfusion-related acute lung injury induced by HLA class II antibodies. *Blood.* 2011;117(2):669–677.
104. Wiersum-Osselton JC, Middelburg RA, Beckers EA, et al. Male-only fresh-frozen plasma for transfusion-related acute lung injury prevention: Before-and-after comparative cohort study. *Transfusion.* 2011;51(6):1278–1283.
105. Middelburg RA, Borkent B, Jansen M, et al. Storage time of blood products and transfusion-related acute lung injury. *Transfusion.* 2012;52(6):1386.
106. Neves JF, Marques A, Valente R, et al. Nonlethal, attenuated, transfusion-associated graft-versus-host disease in an immunocompromised child: Case report and review of the literature. *Transfusion.* 2010;50(11):2484–2488.
107. Li G, Daniels CE, Kojicic M, et al. The accuracy of natriuretic peptides (brain natriuretic peptide and N-terminal pro-brain natriuretic) in the differentiation between transfusion-related acute lung injury and transfusion-related circulatory overload in the critically ill. *Transfusion.* 2009;49(1):13–20.
108. Li G, Kojicic M, Reriani MK, et al. Long-term survival and quality of life after transfusion-associated pulmonary edema in critically ill medical patients. *Chest.* 2010;137(4):783–789.
109. Rajagopalan S, Mascha E, Na J, et al. The effects of mild perioperative hypothermia on blood loss and transfusion requirement. *Anesthesiology.* 2008;108(1):71–77.
110. Albert K, van Vlymen J, James P, et al. Ringer's lactate is compatible with the rapid infusion of AS-3 preserved packed red blood cells. *Can J Anaesth.* 2009;56(5):352–356.
111. Boulton FE, James V. Guidelines for policies on alternatives to allogeneic blood transfusion. 1. Predeposit autologous blood donation and transfusion. *Transfus Med.* 2007;17(5):354–365.
112. Cardone D, Klein AA. Perioperative blood conservation. *Eur J Anaesthesiol.* 2009;26(9):722–729.

113. Singbartl G. Pre-operative autologous blood donation: Clinical parameters and efficacy. *Blood Transfus.* 2011;9(1):10–18.
114. Munoz M, Garcia-Erce JA, Villar I, et al. Blood conservation strategies in major orthopaedic surgery: Efficacy, safety and European regulations. *Vox Sang.* 2009;96(1):1–13.
115. Segal JB, Blasco-Colmenares E, Norris EJ, et al. Preoperative acute normovolemic hemodilution: A meta-analysis. *Transfusion.* 2004;44(5):632–644.
116. Ashworth A, Klein AA. Cell salvage as part of a blood conservation strategy in anaesthesia. *Br J Anaesth.* 2010;105(4):401–416.
117. MacIvor D, Nelson J, Triulzi D. Impact of intraoperative red blood cell salvage on transfusion requirements and outcomes in radical prostatectomy. *Transfusion.* 2009;49(7):1431–1434.
118. Singbartl G, Schreiber J, Singbartl K. Preoperative autologous blood donation versus intraoperative blood salvage: Intraindividual analyses and modeling of efficacy in 1103 patients. *Transfusion.* 2009;49(11):2374–2383.
119. Munoz M, Slappendel R, Thomas D. Laboratory characteristics and clinical utility of post-operative cell salvage: Washed or unwashed blood transfusion? *Blood Transfus.* 2011;9(3):248–261.
120. Berend K, Levi M. Management of adult Jehovah's Witness patients with acute bleeding. *Am J Med.* 2009;122(12):1071–1076.
121. Mackenzie CF, Moon-Massat PF, Shander A, et al. When blood is not an option: Factors affecting survival after the use of a hemoglobin-based oxygen carrier in 54 patients with life-threatening anemia. *Anesth Analg.* 2010;110(3):685–693.
122. Israels SJ, El-Ekiaby M, Quiroga T, et al. Inherited disorders of platelet function and challenges to diagnosis of mucocutaneous bleeding. *Haemophilia.* 2010;16(suppl 5):152–159.
123. Federici AB. Classification of inherited von Willebrand disease and implications in clinical practice. *Thromb Res.* 2009;124(suppl 1):S2–S6.
124. Shetty S, Kasatkar P, Ghosh K. Pathophysiology of acquired von Willebrand disease: A concise review. *Eur J Haematol.* 2011;87(2):99–106.
125. Reininger AJ. Function of von Willebrand factor in haemostasis and thrombosis. *Haemophilia.* 2008;14(suppl 5):11–26.
126. Castaman G, Montgomery RR, Meschengieser SS, et al. von Willebrand's disease diagnosis and laboratory issues. *Haemophilia.* 2010;16(suppl 5):67–73.
127. Berntorp E. Prophylaxis in von Willebrand disease. *Haemophilia.* 2008;14(suppl 5): 47–53.
128. Collins P, Budde U, Rand JH, et al. Epidemiology and general guidelines of the management of acquired haemophilia and von Willebrand syndrome. *Haemophilia.* 2008;14(suppl 3):49–55.
129. Franchini M, Manzato F, Salvagno GL, et al. The use of desmopressin in congenital factor XI deficiency: A systematic review. *Ann Hematol.* 2009;88(10):931–935.
130. Lee JW. Von Willebrand disease, hemophilia A and B, and other factor deficiencies. *Int Anesthesiol Clin.* 2004;42(3):59–76.
131. Graw J, Brackmann HH, Oldenburg J, et al. Haemophilia A: From mutation analysis to new therapies. *Nat Rev Genet.* 2005;6(6):488–501.
132. Iorio A, Marchesini E, Marcucci M, et al. Clotting factor concentrates given to prevent bleeding and bleeding-related complications in people with hemophilia A or B. *Cochrane Database Syst Rev.* 2011;9:CD003429.
133. Giangrande P. Haemophilia B: Christmas disease. *Expert Opin Pharmacother.* 2005;6(9):1517–1524.
134. Goodeve AC, Rosen S, Verbruggen B. Haemophilia A and von Willebrand's disease. *Haemophilia.* 2010;16(suppl 5):79–84.
135. Franchini M, Lippi G. Factor V Leiden and hemophilia. *Thromb Res.* 2010; 125(2):119–123.
136. Richards M, Williams M, Chalmers E, et al. A United Kingdom Haemophilia Centre Doctors' Organization guideline approved by the British Committee for Standards in Haematology: Guideline on the use of prophylactic factor VIII concentrate in children and adults with severe haemophilia A. *Br J Haematol.* 2010;149(4):498–507.
137. Thomas RH. Hypercoagulability syndromes. *Arch Intern Med.* 2001;161(20):2433–2439.
138. Isarangkura P, Mahasandana C, Chuansumrit A, et al. Acquired bleeding disorders: The impact of health problems in the developing world. *Haemophilia.* 2004;10(suppl 4):188–195.
139. Wada H, Usui M, Sakuragawa N. Hemostatic abnormalities and liver diseases. *Semin Thromb Hemost.* 2008;34(8):772–778.
140. Tripodi A, Mannucci PM. The coagulopathy of chronic liver disease. *N Engl J Med.* 2011;365(2):147–156.
141. Levi M, Toh CH, Thachil J, et al. Guidelines for the diagnosis and management of disseminated intravascular coagulation. British Committee for Standards in Haematology. *Br J Haematol.* 2009;145(1):24–33.
142. Dalainas I. Pathogenesis, diagnosis, and management of disseminated intravascular coagulation: A literature review. *Eur Rev Med Pharmacol Sci.* 2008;12(1): 19–31.
143. Thachil J, Toh CH, Levi M, et al. The withdrawal of activated protein C from the use in patients with severe sepsis and DIC [amendment to the BCSH guideline on disseminated intravascular coagulation]. *Br J Haematol.* 2012;157(4):493–494.
144. Vardeny O, Solomon SD. Cyclooxygenase-2 inhibitors, nonsteroidal anti-inflammatory drugs, and cardiovascular risk. *Cardiol Clin.* 2008;26(4):589–601.
145. Smock KJ, Saunders PJ, Rodgers GM, et al. Laboratory evaluation of clopidogrel responsiveness by platelet function and genetic methods. *Am J Hematol.* 2011;86(12):1032–1034.
146. Kam PC, Egan MK. Platelet glycoprotein IIb/IIIa antagonists: Pharmacology and clinical developments. *Anesthesiology.* 2002;96(5):1237–1249.
147. Keeling D, Baglin T, Tait C, et al. Guidelines on oral anticoagulation with warfarin – fourth edition. *Br J Haematol.* 2011;154(3):311–324.
148. Bauer KA. Recent progress in anticoagulant therapy: Oral direct inhibitors of thrombin and factor Xa. *J Thromb Haemost.* 2011;9(suppl 1):12–19.
149. Augoustides JG. Advances in anticoagulation: Focus on dabigatran, an oral direct thrombin inhibitor. *J Cardiothorac Vasc Anesth.* 2011;25(6):1208–1212.
150. Levy JH, Key NS, Azran MS. Novel oral anticoagulants: Implications in the perioperative setting. *Anesthesiology.* 2010;113(3):726–745.
151. Connolly SJ, Ezekowitz MD, Yusuf S, et al. Dabigatran versus warfarin in patients with atrial fibrillation. *N Engl J Med.* 2009;361(12):1139–1151.
152. Granger CB, Alexander JH, McMurray JJ, et al. Apixaban versus warfarin in patients with atrial fibrillation. *N Engl J Med.* 2011;365(11):981–992.
153. Patel MR, Mahaffey KW, Garg J, et al. Rivaroxaban versus warfarin in nonvalvular atrial fibrillation. *N Engl J Med.* 2011;365(10):883–891.
154. Augoustides JG. Update in hematology: Heparin-induced thrombocytopenia and bivalirudin. *J Cardiothorac Vasc Anesth.* 2011;25(2):371–375.
155. Bambrah RK, Pham DC, Zaiden R, et al. Heparin-induced thrombocytopenia. *Clin Adv Hematol Oncol.* 2011;9(8):594–599.
156. Demma LJ, Winkler AM, Levy JH. A diagnosis of heparin-induced thrombocytopenia with combined clinical and laboratory methods in cardiothoracic surgical intensive care unit patients. *Anesth Analg.* 2011;113(4):697–702.
157. Levi M, Levy JH, Andersen HF, et al. Safety of recombinant activated factor VII in randomized clinical trials. *N Engl J Med.* 2010;363(19):1791–1800.
158. Karkouti K, Levy JH. Commentary: Recombinant activated factor VII: The controversial conundrum regarding its off-label use. *Anesth Analg.* 2011;113(4):711–712.
159. Lin Y, Stanworth S, Birchall J, et al. Use of recombinant factor VIIa for the prevention and treatment of bleeding in patients without hemophilia: A systematic review and meta-analysis. *CMAJ.* 2011;183(1):E9–E19.
160. Mayer SA, Brun NC, Begtrup K, et al. Efficacy and safety of recombinant activated factor VII for acute intracerebral hemorrhage. *N Engl J Med.* 2008;358(20): 2127–2137.
161. Dutton RP, Parr M, Tortella BJ, et al. Recombinant activated factor VII safety in trauma patients: Results from the CONTROL trial. *J Trauma.* 2011;71(1):12–19.
162. Hauser CJ, Boffard K, Dutton R, et al. Results of the CONTROL trial: Efficacy and safety of recombinant activated factor VII in the management of refractory traumatic hemorrhage. *J Trauma.* 2010;69(3):489–500.
163. Phillips LE, McLintock C, Pollock W, et al. Recombinant activated factor VII in obstetric hemorrhage: Experiences from the Australian and New Zealand Haemostasis Registry. *Anesth Analg.* 2009;109(6):1908–1915.
164. Sorensen B, Spahn DR, Innerhofer P, et al. Clinical review: Prothrombin complex concentrates–evaluation of safety and thrombogenicity. *Crit Care.* 2011; 15(1):201.
165. McSwain N Jr, Barbeau J. Potential use of prothrombin complex concentrate in trauma resuscitation. *J Trauma.* 2011;70(5 suppl):S53–S56.
166. Ansell J, Hirsh J, Hylek E, et al. Pharmacology and management of the vitamin K antagonists: American College of Chest Physicians Evidence-Based Clinical Practice Guidelines (8th edition). *Chest.* 2008;133(6 suppl):160S–198S.
167. Tuohy E, Litt E, Alikhan R. Treatment of patients with von Willebrand disease. *J Blood Med.* 2011;2:49–57.
168. Ozier Y, Bellamy L. Pharmacological agents: Antifibrinolytics and desmopressin. *Best Pract Res Clin Anaesthesiol.* 2010;24(1):107–119.
169. Crescenzi G, Landoni G, Biondi-Zoccai G, et al. Desmopressin reduces transfusion needs after surgery: A meta-analysis of randomized clinical trials. *Anesthesiology.* 2008;109(6):1063–1076.
170. Schneeweiss S, Seeger JD, Landon J, et al. Aprotinin during coronary-artery bypass grafting and risk of death. *N Engl J Med.* 2008;358(8):771–783.
171. Shaw AD, Stafford-Smith M, White WD, et al. The effect of aprotinin on outcome after coronary-artery bypass grafting. *N Engl J Med.* 2008;358(8):784–793.
172. Fergusson DA, Hebert PC, Mazer CD, et al. A comparison of aprotinin and lysine analogues in high-risk cardiac surgery. *N Engl J Med.* 2008;358(22):2319–2331.
173. Henry D, Carless P, Fergusson D, et al. The safety of aprotinin and lysine-derived antifibrinolytic drugs in cardiac surgery: A meta-analysis. *CMAJ.* 2009;180(2): 183–193.
174. Henry DA, Carless PA, Moxey AJ, et al. Anti-fibrinolytic use for minimising perioperative allogeneic blood transfusion. *Cochrane Database Syst Rev.* 2007; 4:CD001886.
175. Elgafy H, Bransford RJ, McGuire RA, et al. Blood loss in major spine surgery: Are there effective measures to decrease massive hemorrhage in major spine fusion surgery?*Spine.* 2010;35(9 Suppl):S47–S56.
176. Gurusamy KS, Pissanou T, Pikhart H, et al. Methods to decrease blood loss and transfusion requirements for liver transplantation. *Cochrane Database Syst Rev.* 2011;12:CD009052.
177. Kagoma YK, Crowther MA, Douketis J, et al. Use of antifibrinolytic therapy to reduce transfusion in patients undergoing orthopedic surgery: A systematic review of randomized trials. *Thromb Res.* 2009;123(5):687–696.
178. Shakur H, Roberts I, Bautista R, et al. Effects of tranexamic acid on death, vascular occlusive events, and blood transfusion in trauma patients with significant haemorrhage (CRASH-2): A randomised, placebo-controlled trial. *Lancet.* 2010;376(9734):23–32.

SECTION IV

Anesthetic Agents, Adjuvants, and Drug Interaction

CHAPTER

17 Inhaled Anesthetics

THOMAS J. EBERT • LARRY LINDENBAUM

Key Points

1. At equilibrium, the CNS partial pressure of inhaled anesthetics equals their arterial partial pressure, which in turn equals their alveolar partial pressure if cardiopulmonary function is normal.
2. The inspired concentration and the blood:gas solubility of an inhaled anesthetic are the major determinants of the speed of induction. Solubility alone determines the rate of elimination, provided there is normal cardiopulmonary function.
3. Isoflurane is the most potent of the volatile anesthetics in clinical use, desflurane is the least soluble, and sevoflurane is the least irritating to the airways.
4. Nitrous oxide (N_2O) can expand a pneumothorax to double or triple its size in 10 to 30 minutes, and washout of N_2O can lower alveolar concentrations of oxygen and carbon dioxide, a phenomenon called *diffusion hypoxia.*
5. Minimum alveolar concentration (MAC) is the alveolar concentration of an inhaled anesthetic at one atmosphere that prevents movement in response to a surgical stimulus in 50% of patients. Concentrations of inhaled anesthetics that provide loss of awareness and recall are about 0.4 to 0.5 MAC.
6. Excluding data in patients <1 year of age (where MAC is lower than in older children), MAC decreases approximately 6% per decade.
7. Volatile anesthetics depress cerebral metabolic rate and increase cerebral blood flow (CBF) in a dose-dependent manner. The latter effect may increase intracranial pressure in patients with a mass-occupying lesion of the brain.
8. Hypocapnia may blunt or abolish volatile anesthetic-induced increases in CBF depending on when the hypocapnia is produced and the nature of the cerebral disease process.
9. Volatile anesthetics produce dose-dependent depression of the electroencephalogram, sensory-evoked potentials, and motor-evoked potentials.
10. Volatile anesthetics in current use decrease arterial blood pressure, systemic vascular resistance, and myocardial function comparably and in a dose-dependent fashion.
11. Volatile anesthetics decrease tidal volume, decrease ventilatory response to hypercarbia and hypoxia, increase respiratory rate, and relax airway smooth muscle in a dose-dependent fashion.

12 Unlike halothane, volatile anesthetics in current use have minimal adverse effects on the liver and might afford some protection for hepatocytes from ischemic and/or hypoxic injury.

13 Volatile anesthetics are potent triggers for malignant hyperthermia in genetically susceptible patients.

14 CO_2 absorbents degrade sevoflurane, desflurane, and isoflurane to carbon monoxide when the normal water content of the absorbent (13% to 15%) is markedly decreased (<5%).

Multimedia

1 Inhaled Anesthetic Formulas

2 Inhaled Anesthetic Rate of Rise

Inhalation anesthetics are the most common drugs used for the provision of general anesthesia. Adding only a fraction of a volatile anesthetic to the inspired oxygen results in a state of unconsciousness and amnesia. When combined with intravenous adjuvants, such as opioids and benzodiazepines, a balanced technique is achieved that results in analgesia, further sedation/hypnosis, and amnesia. Inhaled anesthetics for surgical procedures are popular because of their ease of administration and the clinician's ability to reliably monitor their effects with both clinical signs and end-tidal concentrations. In addition, the volatile anesthetic gases are relatively inexpensive in terms of overall cost.

Sevoflurane, desflurane, and isoflurane are the most popular potent inhaled anesthetics used in adult surgical procedures (Fig. 17-1). In pediatric cases, sevoflurane is the most commonly employed. Although there are many similarities in terms of the overall effects of the volatile anesthetics (e.g., they all have a dose-dependent effect to decrease blood pressure [BP]), there are some unique differences that might influence the clinician's selection process depending on the patient's health and the surgical procedure. Discussion of these three most popular inhaled anesthetics provides the major emphasis of this chapter. For the sake of completeness and for historical perspective related to metabolism and toxicity, comments on halothane, enflurane, and methoxyflurane are also included.

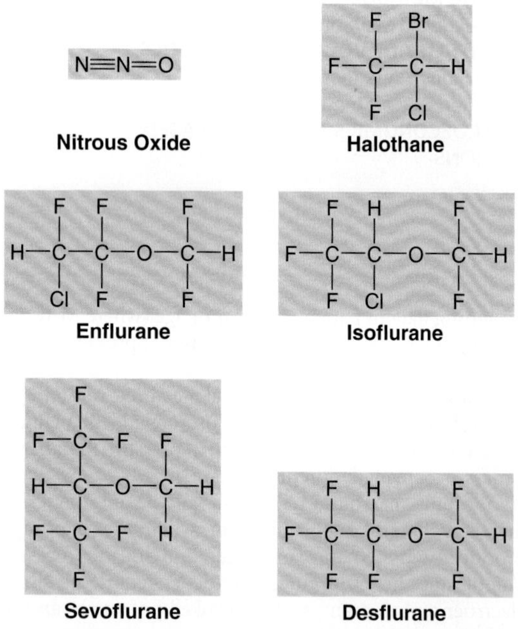

N≡N=O

Nitrous Oxide

Halothane

Enflurane

Isoflurane

Sevoflurane

Desflurane

FIGURE 17-1. Chemical structure of inhaled anesthetics. Halothane is an alkane, a halogen-substituted ethane derivative. It is no longer available commercially. Isoflurane and enflurane are isomers that are methyl ethyl ethers. Desflurane differs from isoflurane in the substitution of a fluorine for a chlorine atom and sevoflurane is a methyl isopropyl ether.

PHARMACOKINETIC PRINCIPLES

Kety in 1950 was the first to examine the pharmacokinetics of inhaled agents in a systematic fashion.[1] Eger accomplished much of the early research in the field, leading to his landmark text on the subject in 1974.[2] The inhaled anesthetics differ substantially from nearly all other drugs because they are gases given via inhalation. This makes their pharmacokinetics unique as well, and discussion of pharmacokinetic principles of currently used agents necessary for understanding and predicting their effects.

Drug pharmacology is classically divided into two disciplines, pharmacodynamics and pharmacokinetics. *Pharmacodynamics* can be defined as what drugs do to the body. It describes the desired and undesired effects of drugs, as well as the cellular and molecular changes leading to these effects. *Pharmacokinetics* can be defined as what the body does to drugs. It describes where drugs go, how they are transformed, and the cellular and molecular mechanisms underlying these processes.

Tissues are often grouped into hypothetical *compartments* based on perfusion. An important implication of different compartments and perfusion rates is the concept of redistribution. After a given amount of drug is administered, it reaches highly perfused tissue compartments first, where it can equilibrate rapidly and exert its effects. With time, however, compartments with lower perfusion rates receive the drug and additional equilibria are established between blood and these tissues. As the tissues with lower perfusion rates absorb the drug, maintenance of equilibria throughout the body requires drug transfer from highly perfused compartments back into the bloodstream. This lowering of drug concentration in one compartment by delivery into another compartment is called *redistribution.*

In discussions of the inhaled anesthetics, the absorption phase is usually called *uptake*, the metabolic phase is usually called *biotransformation*, and the excretion phase is usually called *elimination.*

Unique Features of Inhaled Anesthetics

Speed, Gas State, and Route of Administration

The inhaled anesthetics are among the most rapidly acting drugs in existence, and when administering a general anesthetic, this speed provides a margin of safety. The ability to quickly increase or decrease anesthetic levels as necessary can mean the difference between an anesthetic state and an anesthetic misadventure. Speed also means efficiency. Rapid induction and recovery may lead to faster operating room turnover times, shorter recovery room stays, and earlier discharges to home.

Technically, of the inhaled anesthetics only N_2O and xenon are true gases, while the so-called *potent agents* are the vapors of volatile liquids. But for simplicity, all of them are referred to as gases because they are all in the gas phase when administered via the lungs. As gases, none deviate significantly from ideal gas behavior. These agents are all nonionized and have low molecular weights. This allows them to diffuse rapidly without the need for facilitated diffusion or active transport from bloodstream to tissues. The other advantage of gases is that they can be delivered to the bloodstream via a unique route available in all patients: the lungs.

Speed, gaseous state, and route of administration combine to form the major beneficial feature of the inhaled anesthetics: The ability to decrease plasma concentrations as easily and as rapidly as they are increased.

Physical Characteristics of Inhaled Anesthetics

The physical characteristics of inhaled anesthetics are shown in Table 17-1. The goal of delivering inhaled anesthetics is to produce the anesthetic state by establishing a specific concentration of anesthetic molecules in the central nervous system (CNS). This is done by establishing the specific partial pressure of the agent in the lungs, which ultimately equilibrates with the brain and spinal
1 cord. At equilibrium, CNS partial pressure equals blood partial pressure, which in turn equals alveolar partial pressure:

$$P_{CNS} = P_{blood} = P_{alveoli} \quad (17\text{-}1)$$

where P is partial pressure. Equilibration is a result of three factors:

1. Inhaled anesthetics are gases rapidly transferred bidirectionally via the lungs to and from the bloodstream and subsequently to and from CNS tissues as partial pressures equilibrate.
2. Plasma and tissues have a low capacity to absorb the inhaled anesthetics relative to the amount we can deliver to the lungs, allowing us to quickly establish or abolish anesthetizing concentrations of anesthetic in the bloodstream and ultimately the CNS.
3. Metabolism, excretion, and redistribution of the inhaled anesthetics are minimal relative to the rate at which they are delivered or removed from the lungs. This permits easy maintenance of blood and CNS concentrations.

The so-called *permanent gases,* such as oxygen and nitrogen, exist only as gases at ambient temperatures. Gases such as N_2O can be compressed into liquids under high pressure at ambient temperature. Most *potent volatile anesthetics* are liquids at ambient temperature and pressure. If the system in which the volatile liquid resides is a closed container, molecules of the substance will equilibrate between the liquid and gas phases. At equilibrium, the pressure exerted by molecular collisions of the gas against the container walls is the *vapor pressure.* One important property of vapor pressure is that as long as *any* liquid remains in the container, the vapor pressure is independent of the volume of that liquid. As with any gas, however, vapor pressure is proportional to temperature.

For all of the potent agents, at 20°C the vapor pressure is below atmospheric pressure. If the temperature is raised, the vapor pressure increases. The *boiling point* of a liquid is the temperature at which its vapor pressure exceeds atmospheric pressure in an open container. Desflurane is bottled in a special container because its boiling point of 23.5°C makes it boil at typical room temperatures. Boiling does not occur within the bottle because it is countered by buildup of vapor pressure within the bottle, but once opened to air, the desflurane would quickly boil away. The bottle is designed to allow transfer of desflurane from bottle to vaporizer without exposure to the atmosphere.

Gases in Mixtures

For any mixture of gases in a closed container, each gas exerts a pressure proportional to its *fractional mass.* This is its *partial pressure.*

TABLE 17-1. PHYSIOCHEMICAL PROPERTIES OF VOLATILE ANESTHETICS

Property	Sevoflurane	Desflurane	Isoflurane	Enflurane	Halothane	N_2O
Boiling point (°C)	59	24	49	57	50	−88
Vapor pressure at 20°C (mm Hg)	157	669	238	172	243	38,770
Molecular weight (g)	200	168	184	184	197	44
Oil:gas partition coefficient	47	19	91	97	224	1.4
Blood:gas partition coefficient	0.65	0.42	1.46	1.9	2.50	0.46
Brain:blood solubility	1.7	1.3	1.6	1.4	1.9	1.1
Fat:blood solubility	47.5	27.2	44.9	36	51.1	2.3
Muscle:blood solubility	3.1	2.0	2.9	1.7	3.4	1.2
MAC in O_2 30–60 years, at 37°C P_B 760 (%)	1.8	6.6	1.17	1.63	0.75	104
MAC in 60–70% N_2O (%)	0.66	2.38	0.56	0.57	0.29	
MAC, >65 years (%)	1.45	5.17	1.0	1.55	0.64	—
Preservative	No	No	No	No	Thymol	No
Stable in moist CO_2 absorber	No	Yes	Yes	Yes	No	Yes
Flammability (%) (in 70% N_2O/30% O_2)	10	17	7	5.8	4.8	
Recovered as metabolites (%)	2–5	0.02	0.2	2.4	20	

MAC, minimum alveolar concentration; N_2O, nitrous oxide.

The sum of the partial pressures of each gas in a mixture of gases equals the total pressure of the entire mixture (Dalton's law).

$$P_{total} = P_{gas1} + P_{gas2} + \cdots + P_{gasN} \quad (17\text{-}2)$$

Another way to state this is that each gas in a mixture of gases at a given volume and temperature has a partial pressure that is the pressure it would have *if it alone* occupied the volume. The entire mixture behaves just as if it were a single gas according to the ideal gas law.

Gases in Solution

Partial pressure of a gas in solution is a bit complex because pressure can only be measured in the gas phase, while in solution the amount of gas is measured as a concentration. Partial pressure of a gas in solution refers to the pressure of the gas in the gas phase (if it were present) in equilibrium with the liquid. It is important to talk of partial pressures, however, because gases equilibrate based on partial pressures, not concentrations.

Gas molecules within a liquid interact with solvent molecules to a much larger extent than do molecules in the gas phase. *Solubility* is the term used to describe the tendency of a gas to equilibrate with a solution, hence determining its concentration in solution. Henry's law expresses the relationship of concentration of a gas in solution to the partial pressure of the gas with which the solution is in equilibrium:

$$C_g = kP_g \quad (17\text{-}3)$$

where C_g is concentration of gas in solution, k is a solubility constant, and P_g is the partial pressure of the gas. From Eq. 17-3 one can see that doubling the pressure of a gas doubles its concentration in solution. A more clinically useful expression of solubility is the solubility coefficient, λ:

$$\lambda = V_{dissolved\ gas}/V_{liquid} \text{ at } 37°C \quad (17\text{-}4)$$

where V = volume. This equation states that for any gas in equilibrium with a liquid, a certain volume of that gas dissolves in a given volume of liquid.

The principles of partial pressures and solubility apply in mixtures of gases in solution. That is, the concentration of any one gas in a mixture of gases in solution depends on two factors: (1) its partial pressure in the gas phase in equilibrium with the solution, and (2) its solubility within that solution.

The implications of these properties are that anesthetic gases administered via the lungs diffuse into blood until the partial pressures in alveoli and blood are equal. The concentration of anesthetic in the blood depends on the partial pressure at equilibrium and the blood solubility. Likewise, transfer of anesthetic from blood to target tissues also proceeds toward equalizing partial pressures, but at this interface there is no gas phase. A partial pressure still exists to force anesthetic molecules out of solution and into a gas phase but there is no gas phase because blood (outside the lungs) and tissues are like closed, liquid-filled containers. Remember the principle: The partial pressure of a gas in solution represents the pressure that the gas in equilibrium with the liquid *would have* if a gas phase existed in contact with the liquid phase.

The concentration of anesthetic in target tissue depends on the partial pressure at equilibrium and the target tissue solubility. Because inhaled anesthetics are gases, and because partial pressures of gases equilibrate throughout a system, *monitoring the alveolar concentration of inhaled anesthetics provides an index of their effects in the brain.*

In summary:

1. Inhaled anesthetics equilibrate based on their partial pressures in each tissue (or tissue compartment), *not* based on their concentrations.
2. The partial pressure of a gas in solution is defined by the partial pressure in the gas phase with which it is in equilibrium. Where there is no gas phase the partial pressure reflects a force to escape out of solution.
3. The concentration of anesthetic in a tissue depends on its partial pressure and tissue solubility.

Finally, the particular terminology used when referring to gases in the gas phase or absorbed in plasma or tissues is important. Inspired concentrations or fractional volumes of inhaled anesthetic are typically used rather than partial pressure. Partial pressure is expressed in millimeters of mercury (mm Hg) or torr (1 torr = 1 mm Hg) or kilopascals (kPa). For most drugs, concentration is expressed as mass (milligram [mg]) per volume (milliliter [mL]), but it can also be expressed in percent by weight or volume. Since volume of a gas in the gas phase is directly proportional to mass according to the ideal gas law, it is easier to express this fractional concentration as a percent by volume. In the gas phase, fractional concentration is equal to the partial pressure divided by ambient pressure, usually atmospheric, or:

$$\text{Fractional Volume} = P_{anesthetic}/P_{barometric} \quad (17\text{-}5)$$

Anesthetic Transfer: Machine to Central Nervous System

When the fresh gas flow and the vaporizer are turned on, fresh gas with a fixed fractional concentration of anesthetic leaves the fresh gas outlet and mixes with the gas in the circuit—the bag, tubing, absorbent canister, and piping. It is immediately diluted to a lower fractional concentration, then slowly rises as this compartment equilibrates with the fresh gas flow. With spontaneous patient ventilation by mask, the anesthetic gas passes from circuit to airways. The fractional concentration of anesthetic leaving the circuit is designated as F_I (fraction inspired). In the lungs the gas comprising the dead space in the airways (trachea, bronchi) and the alveoli further dilutes the circuit gas. The fractional concentration of anesthetic present in the alveoli is F_A (fraction alveolar). The anesthetic then passes across the alveolar–capillary membrane and dissolves in pulmonary blood according to the partial pressure of the gas and its blood solubility. It is further diluted and travels via bulk blood flow throughout the vascular tree. The anesthetic then passes via simple diffusion from blood to tissues as well as between tissues.

The vascular system delivers blood to three physiologic tissue groups: the vessel-rich group (VRG), the muscle group, and the fat group. The VRG includes the brain, heart, kidney, liver, digestive tract, and glandular tissues. The percent of body mass and perfusion of each group are shown in Table 17-2. The CNS tissues of the VRG are referred to as *tissues of desired effect.* The other tissues of the VRG that comprise the compartment are referred to as *tissues of undesired effects.* The tissues of the muscle and fat groups comprise the *tissues of accumulation.*

Anesthetic is delivered most rapidly to the VRG because of high blood flow. Here it diffuses according to partial pressure gradients. CNS tissue takes in the anesthetic according to the tissue solubility, and at a high enough tissue concentration,

TABLE 17-2. DISTRIBUTION OF CARDIAC OUTPUT BY TISSUE GROUP

Group	% Body Mass	% Cardiac Output	Perfusion (mL/min/100 g)
Vessel-rich	10	75	75
Muscle	50	19	3
Fat	20	6	3

unconsciousness and anesthesia are achieved. Increasing CNS tissue concentrations cause progressively deeper stages of anesthesia. As this is occurring, anesthetic is also distributing to other VRG tissues. Also coincident with delivery to the CNS, anesthetic is being delivered—albeit more slowly because of lower perfusion—to muscle and fat, where it accumulates and may affect the speed of emergence from the anesthetic. In reality, the fat solubilities provide little influence on emergence in cases lasting <4 hours since the delivery of anesthetic to fat tissue is extremely slow as a result of low blood flow. The concentration of inhaled anesthetic in a given tissue at a particular time during the administration depends not only on tissue blood flow, but also on tissue solubility, which governs how the inhaled anesthetics partition themselves between blood and tissue. Partitioning depends on the relative solubilities of the anesthetic for each compartment. These relative solubilities are expressed by a partition coefficient, δ, which is the ratio of dissolved gas (by volume) in two-tissue compartments at equilibrium. Some of the partition coefficients for the inhaled anesthetics are shown in Table 17-1.

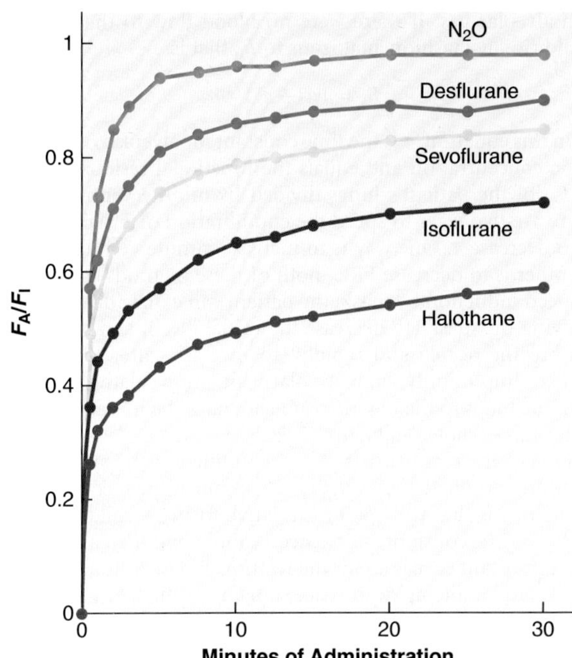

FIGURE 17-2. The rise in alveolar (F_A) anesthetic concentration toward the inspired (F_I) concentration is most rapid with the least soluble anesthetics, N_2O (nitrous oxide), desflurane, and sevoflurane. It rises most slowly with the more soluble anesthetics, such as halothane. All data are from human studies. (Adapted from: Yasuda N, Lockhart SH, Eger EI 2nd, et al. Comparison of kinetics of sevoflurane and isoflurane in humans. *Anesth Analg.* 1991;72:316; and Yasuda N, Lockhart SH, Eger EI 2nd, et al. Kinetics of desflurane, isoflurane, and halothane in humans. *Anesthesiology.* 1991;74:489.)

Uptake and Distribution

F_A/F_I

2 A simple, common way to assess anesthetic uptake is to follow the ratio of fractional concentration of alveolar anesthetic to inspired anesthetic (F_A/F_I) over time. Experimentally derived data for F_A/F_I versus time during induction are shown in Figure 17-2. The faster F_A rises relative to F_I, the faster the speed of induction since F_A is proportional to P_A ($F_A = P_A/P_{barometric}$) and $P_A = P_{blood} = P_{CNS}$; that is, the alveolar fraction is directly proportional to the partial pressure of anesthetic in the CNS.

As fresh gas carrying anesthetic begins to flow into the air-
2 filled circuit (assuming complete mixing), the concentration in the circuit (F_I) will rise according to first-order kinetics:

$$F_I = F_{FGO}(1 - e^{-T/\tau}) \quad (17\text{-}6)$$

F_{FGO} is the fraction of inspired anesthetic in the gas leaving the fresh gas outlet (i.e., the vaporizer setting), T is time, and τ is a time constant. The time constant is simply the volume or "capacity" of the circuit (V_C) divided by the fresh gas flow (FGF) or $\tau = V_C$/FGF. For example, if the bag, tubing, absorbent canister, and piping comprise 8 L, and the fresh gas flow is 2 L, the time constant $\tau = 8/2 = 4$. One of the characteristics of first-order kinetics is that 95% of maximum is reached after three time constants—in this case, $3 \times 4 = 12$ minutes.

Since 12 minutes is relatively long, starting with a higher F_{FGO} can increase the rate of rise of F_I. Using the earlier example with $\tau = 4$, by first-order kinetics 63% of maximum is reached after one time constant, or 4 minutes. To attain an F_I of 2% at 4 instead of 12 minutes, the F_{FGO} can be set to 3.2% (2% divided by 0.63) and then lowered to 2% at the 4-minute mark.

Other ways to speed the increase in F_I include increasing the fresh gas flow, thus decreasing τ. Furthermore, the rebreathing bag can be collapsed prior to starting the fresh gas flow, such that the capacity in the circuit (V_C) is less, which also decreases τ. Finally, at high flows (>4 L/min) there is far less mixing because fresh gas pushes "old" gas out of the circuit via the pop-off valve before complete mixing occurs, causing F_I to increase at a greater rate; this is the most important factor in rapidly increasing F_I to the desired concentration.

One factor that delays the rate of rise of F_I is that CO_2 absorbent can adsorb and decompose the inhaled anesthetics. From a practical standpoint, this does not affect the rate of rise in F_I to a significant extent compared with other factors. Another factor that delays the rate of rise of F_I is solubility of the inhaled anesthetics in some of the plastic and rubber parts of the anesthesia circuit. This absorption has been quantified, but plays only a small role in decreasing the rate of rise of F_I.

Rise in F_A in the Absence of Uptake

The rate of rise in F_I discussed earlier assumes that no anesthetic is mixing with gas in the patient's lungs. In reality, circuit gas mixes with exhaled gases from the lung with each breath, thus lowering F_I within the circuit. If high fresh gas flows (>4 L/min), which produce a high volume of gas at the desired concentration, are used, little mixing with exhaled air occurs and F_I is relatively fixed. In this situation, circuit gas enters the lungs where it mixes with alveolar gas. If there were no blood flow to the lungs, F_A would rise in a fashion analogous to F_I; that is:

$$F_A = F_I(1 - e^{-T/\tau}) \quad (17\text{-}7)$$

In this equation, τ is the time constant for alveolar rise in anesthetic concentration and equals the functional residual capacity (FRC) of the patient's lungs divided by minute ventilation, $\dot{V}_A$. There are two ways to speed the equilibration of F_A with F_I, that is, to decrease τ. One way is to increase minute ventilation, and the other is to decrease FRC. Both of these methods can be used to speed induction by mask; the patient can exhale deeply before applying the mask (to decrease the initial FRC), and the patient can breathe deeply and rapidly (to increase) after the mask is applied. Importantly, high alveolar ventilation relative to uptake from the lungs to the bloodstream generates the initial high slope to the curves shown in Figure 17-2.

One of the reasons that pediatric inductions by spontaneous breathing of inhaled anesthetics are so much quicker than adult inductions is that the low FRC relative to $\dot{V}_A$ of children makes for a low time constant, and hence a more rapid increase in F_A/F_I. One important caveat about the relationship of F_A to FRC is that FRC includes airway dead space; thus, in reality, F_A by Eq. 17-7 is not just the concentration of inhaled anesthetic in the alveoli but also the concentration in the entire lung. However, it is simply called the alveolar concentration because the dead space in the airways is relatively insignificant and only the alveolar gas is exchanging anesthetic with the blood.

Rise in F_A in the Presence of Uptake

Anesthetics *are* soluble in tissues, thus uptake of anesthetic from alveoli to blood is again characterized by first-order kinetics:

$$P_{bl}\,(\text{blood}) = P_A\,(\text{alveoli}) \times (1 - e^{-T/\tau}),$$

where

$$P_A = F_A \times P_B\,(\text{barometric}) \quad (17\text{-}8)$$

Here, P_B is the barometric pressure and the time constant, τ, equals "capacity" (volume of anesthetic dissolved in blood at the desired alveolar partial pressure) divided by flow (volume of anesthetic delivered per unit time). For any given flow of anesthetic into the system, this capacity for the more soluble halothane is greater than the capacity for the less soluble desflurane; thus, τ for halothane is greater than that for desflurane. The more soluble the inhaled anesthetic, the larger the capacity of the blood and tissues for that anesthetic, and the longer it takes to saturate at any given delivery rate.

The most important factor in the rate of rise of F_A/F_I is uptake of anesthetic from the alveoli into the bloodstream. The rate of rise of F_A/F_I (especially the position of the "knees" in the curves of Fig. 17-2) reflects the speed at which alveolar anesthetic (F_A) equilibrates with that being delivered to the lungs (F_I). Since there is uptake from alveoli to blood, F_A is not solely a function of F_I and time. The greater the uptake, the slower the rate of rise of F_A/F_I, and vice versa. Since uptake is proportional to tissue solubility, the less soluble the anesthetic (such as desflurane), the lesser its uptake and the faster it reaches equilibrium, $P_A = P_{blood} = P_{CNS}$.

Consider a hypothetical example. Suppose that halothane and desflurane are soluble in blood, but insoluble in all other tissues. Suppose further that total lung capacity and blood volume were both 5 L. If a fixed volume of anesthetic is delivered to the lungs (by asking the patient to take one deep breath and hold it), according to the blood:gas partition coefficients for halothane (2.5) and desflurane (0.42), 71.4% of the delivered halothane will be transferred to the blood while 28.6% remains in the alveoli (71.4/28.6 = 2.5). In contrast, 29.6% of the desflurane will be transferred to the blood while 70.4% remains in the alveoli (29.6/70.4 = 0.42). Therefore, 2.4 times (71.4/29.6) more halothane than desflurane (by volume or number of molecules) will be transferred from alveoli to bloodstream before partial pressures equilibrate. At equilibrium, the alveolar partial pressures of halothane and desflurane are 28.6% and 70.4% of their inhaled values, respectively. This means that F_A rises faster with desflurane than halothane, as does F_A/F_I.

Blood uptake of anesthetic is expressed by the equation:

$$\dot{V}_B = \delta_{b/g} * Q \times ((P_A - P_V)/P_B) \quad (17\text{-}9)$$

where $\dot{V}_B$ is blood uptake, $\delta_{b/g}$ is the blood:gas partition coefficient, Q is cardiac output, P_A is alveolar partial pressure of anesthetic, P_v is mixed venous partial pressure of anesthetic, and P_B is barometric pressure. This is the Fick equation applied to blood uptake of inhaled anesthetics. *The greater the value of $\dot{V}_B$, the greater the uptake from alveoli to blood, and the slower the rise in F_A/F_I.*

From the preceding paragraphs, the parameters that increase or decrease the rate of rise in F_A/F_I during induction can now be clearly delineated and these important factors have been substantiated in experimental models (Table 17-3).

TABLE 17-3. FACTORS THAT INCREASE OR DECREASE THE RATE OF RISE OF F_A/F_I

Increase	Decrease	
Low λ_B	High λ_B	The lower the blood:gas solubility, the faster the rise in F_A/F_I
Low Q	High Q	The lower the cardiac output, the faster the rise in F_A/F_I
High $\dot{V}_A$	Low $\dot{V}_A$	The higher the minute ventilation, the faster the rise in F_A/F_I
High $(P_A - P_v)$	Low $(P_A - P_v)$	At the beginning of induction, P_v is zero but rises rapidly (thus $[P_A - P_v]$ falls rapidly) and F_A/F_I increases rapidly. Later during induction and maintenance P_v rises more slowly and so F_A/F_I rises more slowly.
High F_I	Low F_I	A high F_I (high anesthetic concentration) speeds the rate of increase of F_A/F_I

λ_B = blood solubility; Q = cardiac output; $\dot{V}$ = minute ventilation; P_A, P_V = pulmonary arterial and venous blood partial pressures, respectively.

Distribution (Tissue Uptake)

The maximum F_A/F_I at a given inspired concentration of anesthetic, cardiac output, and minute ventilation depends entirely on the solubility of that drug in the blood as characterized by the blood:gas partition coefficient $\delta_{b/g}$. This can be seen in the time curves for the rise in F_A/F_I during induction for the various inhalation anesthetics shown in Figure 17-2. The first "knee" in each curve in Figure 17-2 represents the point at which the rapid rise in P_v begins to taper off; that is, when significant inhaled anesthetic concentrations begin to build up in the bloodstream because of distribution to and equilibration with the various tissue compartments.

As blood is equilibrating with alveolar gas, it also begins to equilibrate with the VRG, muscle, and, more gradually, the fat compartments based on perfusion. Muscle is not that different from the VRG, having partition coefficients that range from 1.2 (N_2O) to 3.4 (halothane), just under a threefold difference; and for each anesthetic except N_2O, the muscle partition coefficient is approximately double that for the VRG. Although both VRG and muscle are lean tissues, the muscle compartment equilibrates far more slowly than the VRG. The explanation comes in part due to the mass of the compartments relative to perfusion. The perfusion of the VRG is about 75 mL/min/100 g of tissue, whereas it is only 3 mL/min/100 g of tissue in the muscle (Table 17-2). This 25-fold difference in perfusion between VRG (especially brain) and muscle means that even if the partition coefficients were equal, the muscle would still take 25 times longer to equilibrate with blood.

Fat is perfused to a lesser extent than muscle and its time for equilibration with blood is considerably slower because the partition coefficients are so much greater. All of the potent agents are highly lipid-soluble. Partition coefficients range from 27 (desflurane) to 51 (halothane). On average, the solubility for these agents is about 25 times greater in fat than in the VRG group. Thus, fat equilibrates far more slowly with the blood and does not play a significant role in determining speed of induction. After long anesthetic exposures (>4 hours), the high saturation of fat tissue may play a role in delaying emergence.

Nitrous oxide represents an exception. Its partition coefficients are fairly similar in each tissue: It does not accumulate to any great extent and is not a very potent anesthetic. Its utility lies as an adjunct to the potent agents, and as a vehicle to speed induction.

Metabolism

Data suggest that enzymes responsible for biotransformation of inhaled anesthetics become saturated at less than anesthetizing doses of these drugs, such that metabolism plays little role in opposing induction. It may, however, have some significance to recovery from anesthesia, as discussed later.

Overpressurization and the Concentration Effect

There are several ways to speed uptake and induction of anesthesia with the inhaled anesthetics. The first is *overpressurization*, which is analogous to an intravenous bolus. This is the administration of a higher partial pressure of anesthetic than the alveolar concentration (F_A) actually desired for the patient. Inspired anesthetic concentration (F_I) can influence both F_A and the *rate of rise* of F_A/F_I. The greater the inspired concentration of an inhaled anesthetic, the greater the rate of rise. This concentration effect has two components: The concentrating effect and an augmented gas inflow effect.

For example, consider the administration of 10% anesthetic (10 parts anesthetic and 90 parts other gas) to a patient in whom 50% of the anesthetic in the alveoli is absorbed by the blood. In this case, five parts (0.5 × 10) anesthetic remain in the alveoli, five parts enter the blood, and 90 parts remain as other alveolar gas. The alveolar concentration is now 5/(90 + 5) = 5.3%. Consider next administering 50% anesthetic with the same 50% uptake. Now 25 parts anesthetic remain in alveoli, 25 parts pass into blood, and 50 parts remain as other alveolar gas. The alveolar concentration becomes 25/(50 + 25) = 33%. Giving five times as much anesthetic will lead to a 33%/5.3% = 6.2 times greater alveolar concentration. The higher the F_I, the greater the effect. Thus N_2O, typically given in concentrations of 50% to 70%, has the greatest concentrating effect. This is why the F_A/F_I versus time curve in Figure 17-2 rises the most quickly with N_2O, even though desflurane has a slightly lower blood:gas solubility.

This is not the complete picture; there is yet another factor to consider. As gas is leaving the alveoli for the blood, new gas at the original F_I is entering the lungs to replace that which is taken up by the blood. This other aspect of the concentration effect has been called *augmented gas inflow*. Again, take the example of 10% anesthetic delivered with 50% uptake into the bloodstream. The five parts anesthetic absorbed by the bloodstream are replaced by gas in the circuit that is still 10% anesthetic. The five parts anesthetic and 90 parts other gas left in the lungs mix with five parts replacement gas, or 5 × 0.10 = 0.5 parts anesthetic. Now the alveolar concentration is (5 + 0.5)/(100) = 5.5% (as compared to 5.3% without augmented inflow). For 50% anesthetic and 50% uptake, 25 parts of anesthetic removed from the alveoli are replaced with 25 parts of 50% anesthetic, giving a new alveolar concentration of (25 + 12.5)/(100) = 37.5% (as compared to 33% without augmented inflow). Thus, 5 times the F_I leads to 37.5/5.5 = 6.8 times greater F_A (compared to 6.2 times without augmented gas inflow). Of course, this cycle of absorbed gas being replaced by fresh gas inflow is continuous and has a finite rate, so our example is a simplification.

Second Gas Effect

A special case of concentration effect applies to administration of a potent anesthetic with N_2O, that is, two gases simultaneously. Along with the concentration of potent agent in the alveoli via its uptake, there is further concentration via the uptake of N_2O, a process called the *second gas effect*. The principle is simple (Figs. 17-3 and 17-4). Consider, for example, administering 2% of a potent anesthetic in 70% N_2O and 28% oxygen. In this case, N_2O, with its extremely high partial pressure (despite low solubility), partitions into the blood more rapidly than the potent anesthetic, decreasing the alveolar N_2O concentration by some amount (e.g., by 50%). Ignoring uptake of the potent anesthetic, the uptake of N_2O is 35 parts, leaving 35 parts N_2O, 28 parts O_2, and two parts potent agent in the alveoli. The anesthetic gas is now present in the alveoli at a concentration of 2/(2 + 35 + 28) = 3.1%. The potent agent has been concentrated and F_A is increased.

Ventilation Effects

As indicated by Figure 17-2 and Table 17-3, inhaled anesthetics with very low tissue solubility have an extremely rapid rise in F_A/F_I with induction. This suggests that there is very little room to

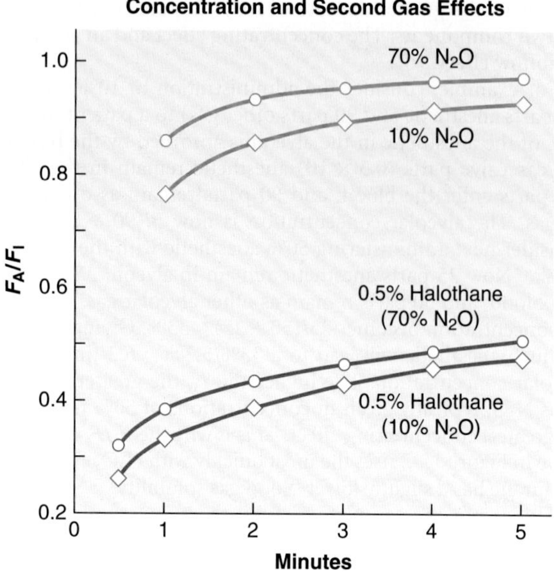

FIGURE 17-3. The concentration effect is demonstrated in the top half of the graph from dogs receiving N_2O (nitrous oxide). Administration of 70% N_2O produces a more rapid rise in the F_A/F_I ratio of N_2O than administration of 10% N_2O. The second gas effect is demonstrated in the lower graphs. The F_A/F_I ratio for 0.5% halothane rises more rapidly when given with 70% N_2O than when given with 10% N_2O. (Adapted from: Epstein RM, Rackow H, Salanitre E, et al. Influence of the concentration effect on the uptake of anesthetic mixtures: The second gas effect. *Anesthesiology.* 1964;25:364.)

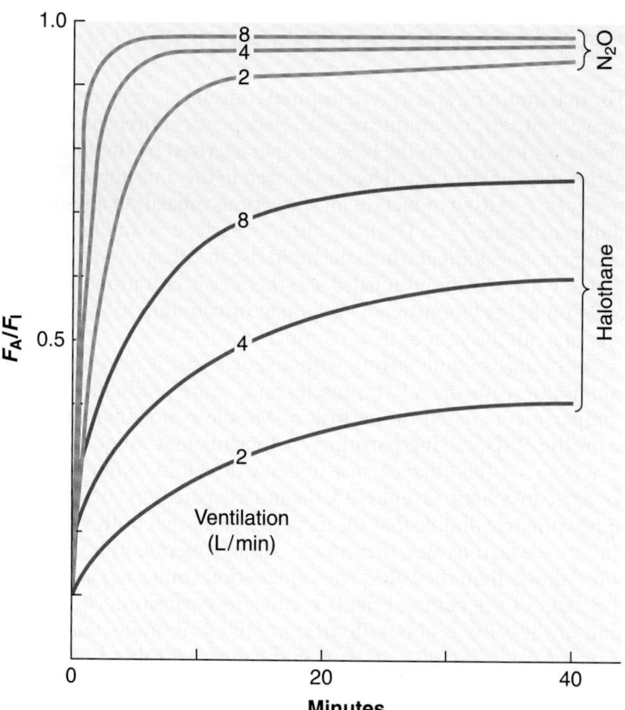

FIGURE 17-5. The F_A/F_I ratio rises more rapidly if ventilation is increased from 2 to 8 L/min. Solubility modifies this impact of ventilation; for example, the effect is greatest with the least-soluble anesthetic, N_2O (nitrous oxide; *top three lines*), and least with the more soluble anesthetic, halothane. (Adapted from: Eger EI 2nd. *Ventilation, circulation and uptake, Anesthetic Uptake and Action.* Baltimore, Williams & Wilkins, 1974, pp 122.)

improve this rate by increasing or decreasing ventilation, which is consistent with the experimental evidence shown in Figure 17-5. The greater the solubility of an inhaled anesthetic, the more rapidly it is absorbed by the bloodstream, such that anesthetic delivery to the lungs may be rate limiting to the rise in F_A/F_I. Therefore, for more soluble anesthetics, augmentation of anesthetic delivery by increasing minute ventilation also increases the rate of rise in F_A/F_I.

Spontaneous minute ventilation is not static, however, and to the extent that the inhaled anesthetics depress spontaneous ventilation with increasing inspired concentration, $\dot{V}_A$ will decrease and so will the rate of rise of F_A/F_I. This is demonstrated in Figure 17-5. This negative feedback should not be considered a

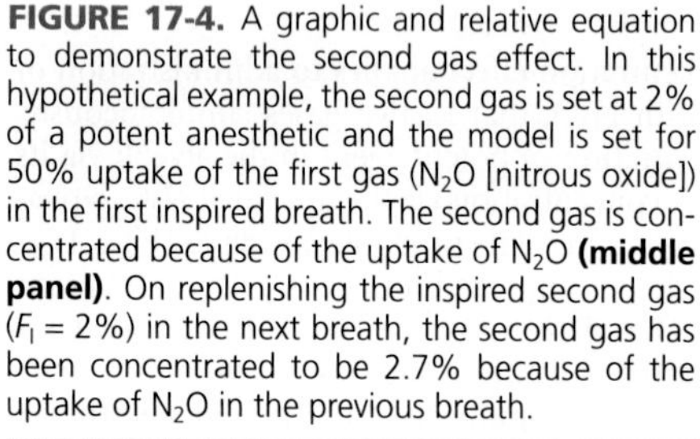

FIGURE 17-4. A graphic and relative equation to demonstrate the second gas effect. In this hypothetical example, the second gas is set at 2% of a potent anesthetic and the model is set for 50% uptake of the first gas (N_2O [nitrous oxide]) in the first inspired breath. The second gas is concentrated because of the uptake of N_2O **(middle panel)**. On replenishing the inspired second gas (F_I = 2%) in the next breath, the second gas has been concentrated to be 2.7% because of the uptake of N_2O in the previous breath.

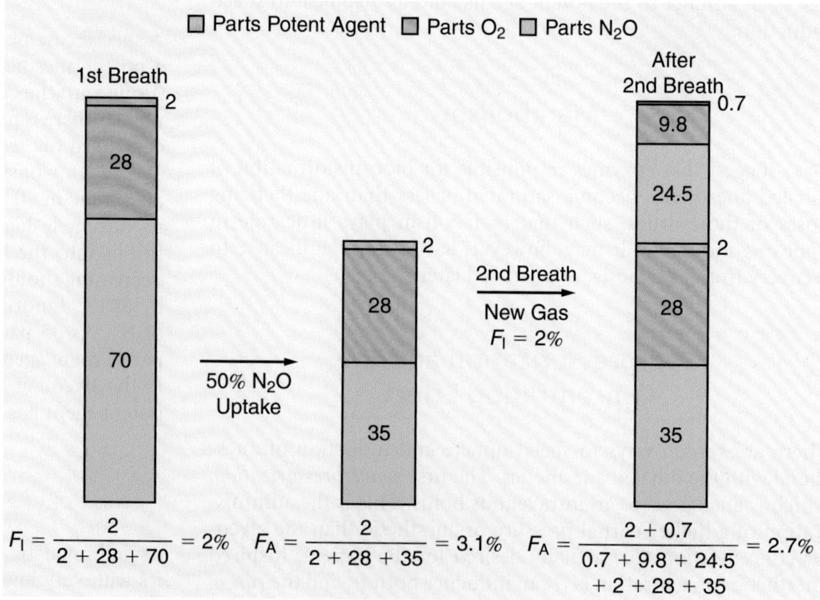

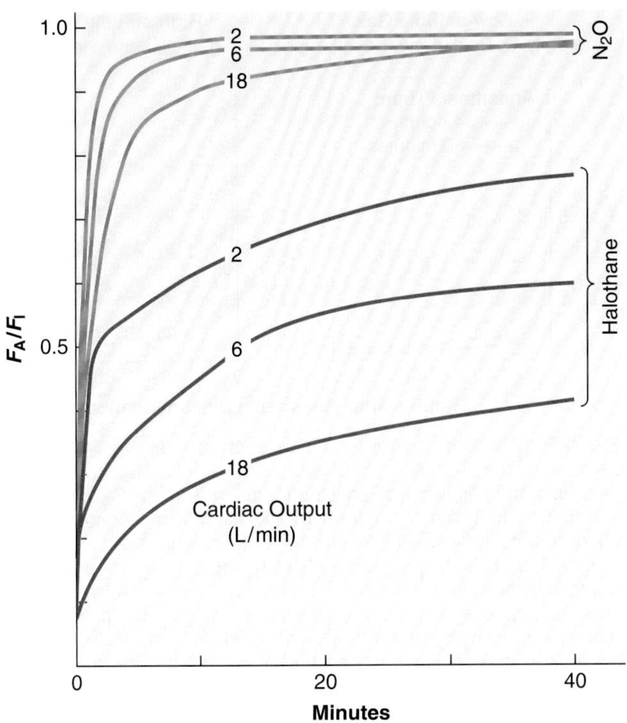

FIGURE 17-6. If ventilation is fixed, an increase in cardiac output from 2 to 18 L/min will decrease the alveolar anesthetic concentration by augmenting uptake, thereby slowing the rise of the F_A/F_I ratio. This effect is most prominent with the more soluble anesthetics (halothane) than with the less soluble anesthetics (N_2O [nitrous oxide]). (Adapted from: Eger EI II. *Ventilation, circulation and uptake, Anesthetic Uptake and Action.* Baltimore, Williams & Wilkins, 1974, p 131.)

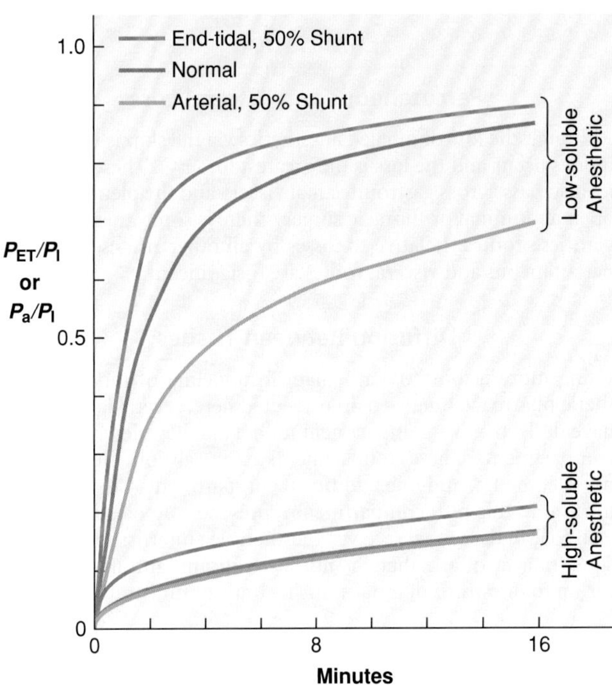

FIGURE 17-7. When no ventilation/perfusion abnormalities exist, the alveolar (P_A) or end-tidal (P_{ET}) and arterial (P_a) anesthetic partial pressures rise together (*blue lines*) toward the inspired partial pressure (P_I). When 50% of the cardiac output is shunted through the lungs, the rate of rise of the end-tidal partial pressure (*orange lines*) is accelerated while the rate of rise of the arterial partial pressure (*green lines*) is slowed. The greatest effect of shunting is found with the least soluble anesthetics. (Adapted from: Eger EI 2nd, Severinghaus JW. Effect of uneven pulmonary distribution of blood and gas on induction with inhalation anesthetics. *Anesthesiology.* 1964;25:620.)

drawback of the inhaled anesthetics because the respiratory depression produced at high anesthetic concentrations essentially slows the rise in F_A/F_I. This might arguably add a margin of safety in preventing an overdose. Controlled ventilation does not offer this margin of safety.

Perfusion Effects

As with ventilation, cardiac output is not static during the course of induction. For the less soluble agents, changes in cardiac output do not affect the rate of rise of F_A/F_I to a great extent, but for the more soluble agents the effect is noticeable, as seen in Figure 17-6. However, as inspired concentration increases, greater cardiovascular depression reduces anesthetic uptake and actually increases the rate of rise of F_A/F_I. This positive feedback can rapidly lead to profound cardiovascular depression. Figure 17-6 presents experimental data in which lower cardiac outputs lead to a much more rapid rise in F_A/F_I when $\dot{V}_A$ is held constant. This more rapid rise is greater than can be accounted for by concentration effect alone.

Ventilation–Perfusion Mismatching

Ventilation and perfusion are normally fairly well matched in healthy patients, such that P_A (alveolar partial pressure)/P_I and P_a (arterial partial pressure)/P_I are the same curve. However, if significant intrapulmonary shunt occurs, as in the case of inadvertent bronchial intubation, the rate of rise of alveolar and arterial anesthetic partial pressures can be affected. The effects, however, depend on the solubility of the anesthetic, as seen in Figure 17-7. Ventilation of the intubated lung is dramatically increased while perfusion increases slightly. The non-intubated lung receives no ventilation, while perfusion decreases slightly. For the less-soluble anesthetics, increased ventilation of the intubated lung cannot appreciably increase alveolar partial pressure relative to inspired concentration on that side, but alveolar partial pressure on the non-intubated side is essentially zero. Pulmonary mixed venous blood, therefore, comprises nearly equal parts of blood containing normal amounts of anesthetic and blood containing no anesthetic; that is, diluted relative to normal. Thus the rate of rise in P_a relative to P_I is significantly reduced. There is less total anesthetic uptake, so the rate of rise of P_A relative to P_I increases even though induction of anesthesia is slowed because CNS partial pressure equilibrates with P_a. For the more soluble anesthetics, increased ventilation of the intubated lung *does* increase the alveolar partial pressure relative to inspired concentration on that side. Pulmonary venous blood from the intubated side contains a higher concentration of anesthetic that lessens the dilution by blood from the non-intubated side. Thus, the rate of rise of P_a/P_I is not as depressed as that for the less soluble anesthetics, and induction of anesthesia is less delayed relative to normal.

Elimination

Percutaneous and Visceral Loss

Although the loss of inhaled anesthetics via the skin is very small, it does occur and the loss is the greatest for N_2O. These anesthetics also pass across gastrointestinal viscera and the pleura. During open abdominal or thoracic surgery there is some anesthetic loss via these routes. Relative to losses by all other routes, losses via percutaneous and visceral routes are insignificant.

Diffusion Between Tissues

Using more elaborate mathematical modeling of inhaled anesthetic pharmacokinetics than presented here, several laboratories have derived a five-compartment model that best describes tissue compartments. These compartments are the alveoli, the VRG, the muscle, the fat, and one additional compartment. Current opinion is that this fifth compartment represents adipose tissue adjacent to lean tissue that receives anesthetic via intertissue diffusion. This transfer of anesthetic is not insignificant, and may account for up to one-third of uptake during long administration.

Exhalation and Recovery

Recovery from anesthesia, like induction, depends on anesthetic solubility, cardiac output, and minute ventilation. Solubility is the primary determinant of the rate of fall of F_A (Fig. 17-8). The greater the solubility of inhaled anesthetic, the larger the capacity for absorption in the bloodstream and tissues. The "reservoir" of anesthetic in the body at the end of administration depends on tissue solubility (which determines the capacity) and the dose and duration of anesthetic (which determine how much of that capacity is filled). Recovery from anesthesia, or "washout," is usually expressed as the ratio of expired fractional concentration of anesthetic (F_A) to the expired concentration at time zero (F_{A0}) when the anesthetic was discontinued (or F_A/F_{A0}). Elimination curves of low- and high-soluble anesthetics are shown in Figure 17-9. The longer the duration of a highly soluble anesthetic, the greater the reservoir of anesthetic in the body, and the higher the curve seen in the right half of Figure 17-9. This effect is nearly absent with low-soluble agents such as N_2O, desflurane, and sevoflurane.[3]

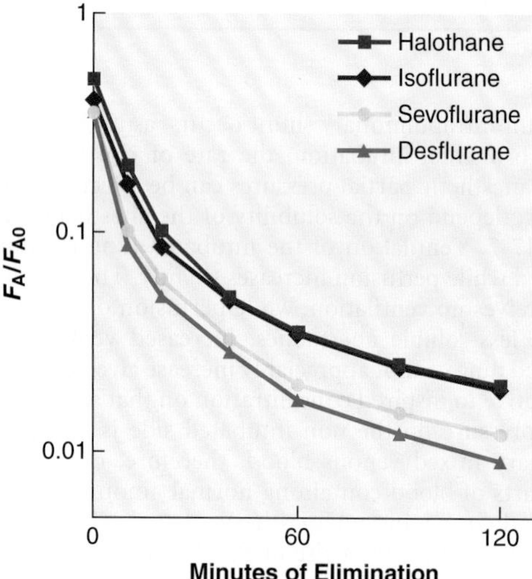

FIGURE 17-8. Elimination of anesthetic gases is defined as the ratio of end-tidal anesthetic concentration (F_A) to the last F_A during administration and immediately before the beginning of elimination (F_{A0}). During the 120-minute period after ending the anesthetic delivery, the elimination of sevoflurane and desflurane is 2 to 2.5 times faster than isoflurane or halothane (note logarithmic scale for the ordinate). (Adapted from: Yasuda N, Lockhart SH, Eger EI 2nd, et al. Comparison of kinetics of sevoflurane and isoflurane in humans. *Anesth Analg.* 1991;72:316; and Yasuda N, Lockhart SH, Eger EI 2nd, et al. Kinetics of desflurane, isoflurane, and halothane in humans. *Anesthesiology.* 1991;74:489.)

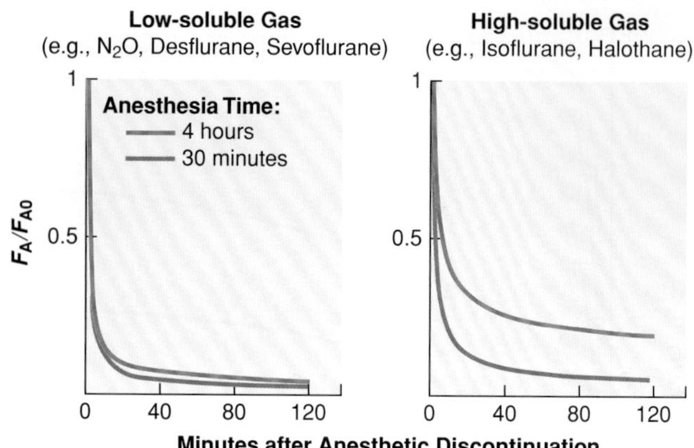

FIGURE 17-9. Both solubility and duration of anesthesia affect the decrease of the alveolar concentration (F_A) from its value immediately preceding the cessation of anesthetic administration (F_{A0}). A longer anesthetic time (from 15 minutes to 240 minutes) only slightly slows the decrease with low-soluble anesthetics **(left graph)**. An agent with a higher blood and tissue solubility **(right graph)** slows the elimination of the anesthetic and enhances the effect of duration. (Adapted from: Stoelting RK, Eger EI 2nd. The effects of ventilation and anesthetic solubility on recovery from anesthesia: An in vivo and analog analysis before and after equilibrium. *Anesthesiology.* 1969;30:290.)

There are two major pharmacokinetic differences between recovery and induction. First, whereas overpressurization can increase the speed of induction, there is no "underpressurization." Both induction and recovery rates depend on the P_A to P_v gradient, and P_A can never fall below zero. Second, whereas all tissues begin induction with zero anesthetic, each begins recovery with quite different anesthetic concentrations. The VRG tissues begin recovery with the same anesthetic partial pressure as that in alveoli, since $P_{CNS} = P_{blood} = P_{alveoli}$. The partial pressures in muscle and fat depend on the inspired concentration during anesthesia, the duration of administration, and the anesthetic tissue solubilities. As long as an arterial-to-tissue partial pressure gradient exists, these tissues will absorb anesthetic—especially fat, since it is a huge potential reservoir whose anesthetic partial pressures are typically low after hours of anesthesia. After discontinuation of anesthesia, muscle and fat may continue to absorb anesthetic, even hours later. The redistribution continues until blood/alveolar anesthetic partial pressure falls below tissue partial pressure. This redistribution causes the early rate of decline in alveolar anesthetic concentration during recovery to exceed its early rate of increase during induction.

Because VRG tissues are highly perfused and washout of anesthetic is mostly via elimination from these tissues early in recovery, all anesthetics, regardless of duration of administration, have approximately the same rate of elimination to 50% of F_{A0}. Unfortunately, halving the CNS concentration of anesthetic is rarely sufficient for waking the patient. More commonly, 80% to 90% of inhaled anesthetic must be eliminated before emergence. At these amounts of washout, the more soluble anesthetics are eliminated more slowly than less soluble agents.

Diffusion Hypoxia

During recovery from anesthesia, washout of high concentrations of N_2O can lower alveolar concentrations of oxygen and carbon dioxide, a phenomenon called *diffusion hypoxia.* The resulting alveolar hypoxia can cause hypoxemia, and alveolar hypocarbia can depress respiratory drive, which may exacerbate hypoxemia. It is therefore appropriate to initiate recovery from N_2O anesthesia with 100% oxygen rather than less concentrated O_2/air mixtures.

CLINICAL OVERVIEW OF CURRENT INHALED ANESTHETICS

Isoflurane

Isoflurane is a halogenated methyl ethyl ether that is a clear, nonflammable liquid at room temperature and has a high degree of pungency. It is the most potent of the volatile anesthetics in clinical use, has great physical stability, and undergoes essentially no deterioration during storage for up to 5 years or on exposure to sunlight. It has become the "gold standard" anesthetic since its introduction in the 1970s. There was a brief period of controversy concerning the use of isoflurane in patients with coronary disease because of the possibility for coronary "steal" arising from the
3 potent effects of isoflurane on coronary vasodilation. In clinical use, however, this has been, at most, a rare occurrence.

Desflurane

Desflurane is a fluorinated methyl ethyl ether that differs from isoflurane by just one atom: A fluorine atom is substituted for a chlorine atom on the α-ethyl component of isoflurane (Fig. 17-1). The process of complete fluorination of the ether molecule has several effects. It decreases blood and tissue solubility (the blood:gas solubility of desflurane equals that of N_2O), which results in a loss of potency (the MAC of desflurane is five times higher than isoflurane). It also results in a high vapor pressure owing to decreased intermolecular attraction, requiring the development of a new heated, pressurized vaporizer requiring electrical power to deliver a regulated concentration of desflurane as a gas. One of the advantages of desflurane is the near-absent metabolism to serum trifluoroacetate. This makes immune-mediated hepatitis a rare occurrence. Desflurane is the most pungent of the volatile anesthetics and, if administered via the face mask, results in coughing, salivation, breath holding, and laryngospasm. In extremely dry CO_2 absorbers, desflurane (and to a lesser extent isoflurane, enflurane, and sevoflurane) degrades to form carbon monoxide. Desflurane has the lowest blood:gas solubility of the potent volatile anesthetics; moreover, its fat solubility is roughly half that of the other volatile anesthetics. Thus, desflurane requires less downward titration in long surgical procedures to achieve a rapid emergence by virtue of decreased tissue saturation. This may be particularly advantageous in the morbidly obese patient.[4] Desflurane has been associated with tachycardia, hypertension, and, in select cases, myocardial ischemia when used in high concentrations or when rapidly increasing the inspired concentration (in the presence of minimal opioid adjuvants).

Sevoflurane

Sevoflurane is a sweet-smelling, completely fluorinated methyl isopropyl ether (Fig. 17-1). Its vapor pressure is roughly one-fourth that of desflurane and it can be used in a conventional vaporizer. The blood:gas solubility of sevoflurane is second only to desflurane in terms of potent volatile anesthetics. Sevoflurane is approximately half as potent as isoflurane, and some of the preservation of potency, despite fluorination, is because of the bulky propyl side chain on the ether molecule. Its minimal odor, lack of pungency, and potent bronchodilating characteristics make sevoflurane administration via the face mask for induction of anesthesia in both children and adults a reasonable alternative to IV anesthetics. Sevoflurane is half as potent a coronary vasodilator as isoflurane, but is 10 to 20 times more vulnerable to metabolism than isoflurane. The metabolism of sevoflurane results in inorganic fluoride; the increase in plasma fluoride after sevoflurane administration has not been associated with renal-concentrating defects. Unlike other potent volatile anesthetics, sevoflurane is not metabolized to trifluoroacetate; rather, it is metabolized to an acyl halide (hexafluoroisopropanol). This does not stimulate formation of antibodies associated with hepatitis.

Sevoflurane can form carbon monoxide during exposure to dry CO_2 absorbents, and can cause a canister fire via an exothermic reaction in dry absorbent. New generic versions of sevoflurane have the potential to break down to hydrogen fluoride when exposed to metal compounds because of their lack of adequate water in the formulation. Sevoflurane also breaks down in the presence of the carbon dioxide absorber to form a vinyl halide called *compound A.* Compound A has been shown to be a dose-dependent nephrotoxin in rats, but has not been associated with renal injury in human volunteers or patients, with or without renal impairment, even when fresh gas flows are 1 L/min or less.

Xenon

Xenon is an inert gas occurring naturally in air at 0.05 parts per million (ppm). Xenon has received considerable interest in the last few years because it has many characteristics approaching those of an "ideal" inhaled anesthetic.[5,6] It has a quick onset and offset, minimal effects on the cardiovascular and neural systems, and it is not a trigger for malignant hyperthermia (MH). It is not a pollutant or an occupational hazard, and does not add to global warming or the greenhouse gas effect. Its blood:gas partition coefficient is 0.115,[7] and unlike the other potent volatile anesthetics (except methoxyflurane), xenon provides some degree of analgesia. This action is likely due to *N*-Methyl-D-aspartate (NMDA) receptor inhibition. The MAC of xenon in humans is 71%, which might prove to be a limitation, although this is less than the MAC for N_2O. It is nonexplosive, nonpungent, and odorless, and thus can be inhaled with ease. In addition, it does not produce significant myocardial depression or alter coronary blood flow.[5,8] Because of its scarcity and high cost, new anesthetic systems are being developed to provide for recycling of xenon. If this proves to be too difficult from either a technical or patient safety standpoint, it may be necessary to use it in a very low, or closed, fresh gas flow system to reduce wastage.

Nitrous Oxide

4 Nitrous oxide is a sweet-smelling, nonflammable gas of low potency (MAC = 104%), and is relatively insoluble in blood. It is most commonly administered as an anesthetic adjuvant in

combination with opioids or volatile anesthetics during the conduct of general anesthesia. At room temperature it is a gas; its boiling point is –88.48°C (Table 17-1). It is stored in cylinders and condensed to 50 atmospheres, leading to a pressure of 745 psi. This pressure is maintained in the cylinders until no liquid remains. Only cylinder weight is a reliable indicator of the volume of N_2O in storage tanks. Although not flammable, N_2O will support combustion. Unlike the potent volatile anesthetics in clinical use, N_2O does not produce significant skeletal muscle relaxation, but it does have analgesic effects. Despite a long track record of use, controversy has surrounded N_2O in four areas: Its role in postoperative nausea and vomiting; its potential toxic effects on cell function via inactivation of vitamin B_{12}; its adverse effects related to absorption and expansion into air-filled structures and bubbles; and lastly, its effect on embryonic development. The one concern that seems most valid and most clinically relevant is the ability of N_2O to expand air-filled spaces because of its greater solubility in blood compared to nitrogen. This might explain the increased post-operative nausea and vomiting (PONV) associated with N_2O use since closed gas spaces reside in the middle ear and bowel. Other closed spaces may occur as a result of disease or surgery, such as a pneumothorax. Since nitrogen in air-filled spaces cannot be removed readily via the bloodstream, N_2O delivered to a patient diffuses from the blood into these closed gas spaces quite easily until the partial pressure equals that of the blood and alveoli. Compliant spaces will continue to expand until sufficient pressure is generated to oppose further N_2O flow into the space. The higher the inspired concentration of N_2O, the higher the partial pressure required for equilibration.

Seventy-five percent N_2O can expand a pneumothorax to double or triple its size in 10 and 30 minutes, respectively. Air-filled cuffs of pulmonary artery catheters and endotracheal tubes also expand with the use of N_2O, possibly causing tissue damage via increased pressure in the pulmonary artery or trachea, respectively.[9,10] Accumulation of N_2O in the middle ear can diminish hearing postoperatively[11] and is contraindicated for tympanoplasty because the increased pressure can dislodge a tympanic graft.

NEUROPHARMACOLOGY OF INHALED ANESTHETICS

Minimum Alveolar Concentration

5 Pharmacodynamic effects of anesthetics are based on the dose. In the case of inhaled agents we instead speak of the *minimum alveolar concentration* or MAC. MAC is the alveolar concentration of an anesthetic at one atmosphere (in volume %) that prevents movement in response to a surgical stimulus in 50% of patients. It is analogous to the ED_{50} expressed for intravenous drugs and can be used to compare anesthetic potency, that is, the lower the MAC the more potent the agent. A variety of surgical stimuli have been used to establish the MAC for each inhaled anesthetic, but the classic, defining, stimulus/response pairing is skeletal muscle movement in response to incision of the abdomen, though other responses have been used to establish MAC. Experimentally determined MAC values for humans for the inhaled anesthetics are shown in Table 17-1.

The 95% confidence ranges for MAC are approximately ±25% of the listed MAC values. Manufacturer's recommendations and clinical experience establish 1.2 to 1.3 times MAC as a dose that consistently prevents patient movement during surgical stimuli. Loss of consciousness typically precedes the absence of stimulus-induced movement by a wide margin. Although 1.2 to 1.3 MAC values do not *absolutely* ensure the defining criteria for brain anesthesia (the absence of self-awareness and recall), vast clinical experience suggests it is extremely unlikely for a patient to have awareness or recall of the surgical incision at these anesthetic concentrations, barring other conditions that increase MAC in that patient (Table 17-4).

TABLE 17-4. FACTORS THAT INCREASE MINIMUM ALVEOLAR CONCENTRATION

- Increased central neurotransmitter levels (monoamine oxidase inhibitors, acute dextroamphetamine administration, cocaine, ephedrine, levodopa)
- Hyperthermia
- Chronic ethanol abuse (determined in humans)
- Hypernatremia

Concentrations of inhaled anesthetics that provide loss of self-awareness and recall are about 0.4 to 0.5 MAC. Several lines of reasoning support the assertion. First, most patients receiving only 50% N_2O (approximately 0.4 to 0.5 MAC), as in a typical dentist's office, will have no recall of their procedure during N_2O administration. Second, various studies have shown that a shift in electroencephalogram (EEG) dominance to the anterior leads, that is, the shift from self-aware to non self-aware, accompanies loss of consciousness, and in primates, the EEG shift and loss of consciousness occur at 0.5 MAC.[12] Third, in dogs, loss of consciousness accompanies a sudden nonlinear fall in cerebral metabolic rate ($CMRO_2$) at approximately 0.5 MAC (Fig. 17-10).

MAC values can be established for any measurable response. For example, MAC-awake and MAC-BAR. MAC-awake is the alveolar concentration of anesthetic at which a patient opens his

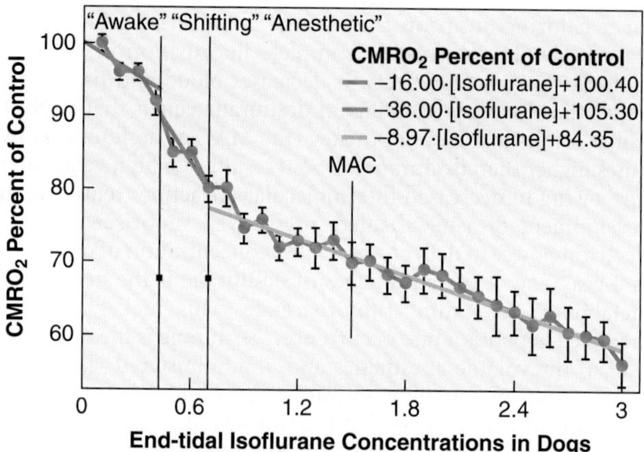

FIGURE 17-10. The effects of isoflurane on cerebral metabolic rate of oxygen consumption ($CMRO_2$) as a percentage of control ("awake"). $CMRO_2$ is plotted versus end-tidal isoflurane concentration. Regression lines for changes in $CMRO_2$ are drawn for each electroencephalogram-determined area. The pattern depicted here is characteristic of all of the anesthetics examined (enflurane, halothane, and isoflurane). MAC, minimum alveolar concentration. (Adapted from: Stullken EH Jr, Milde JH, Michenfelder JD, et al. The nonlinear responses of cerebral metabolism to low concentrations of halothane, enflurane, isoflurane and thiopental. *Anesthesiology.* 1977;46:28.)

or her eyes to command, and it varies from 0.15 to 0.5 MAC.[13] Interestingly, transition from awake to unconscious and back typically shows some hysteresis in that it quite consistently takes 0.4 to 0.5 MAC to lose consciousness, but less than that (as low as 0.15 MAC) to regain it. This may be because of the speed of alveolar wash-in versus wash-out.[14] MAC-BAR is the alveolar concentration of anesthetic that blunts adrenergic responses to noxious stimuli. It has been approximated at 50% higher than standard MAC. [15] MAC values also have been established for discreet levels of EEG activity, such as onset of burst suppression or isoelectricity.

Standard MAC values are roughly additive. Administering 0.5 MAC of a potent agent and 0.5 MAC of N_2O is equivalent to 1 MAC of potent agent in terms of preventing *patient movement,* although this does not hold over the entire range of N_2O doses. MAC effects for other response parameters are not necessarily additive. For example, combining 0.6 MAC of N_2O with 0.6 MAC of isoflurane produces less hypotension than 1.2 MAC of isoflurane alone because isoflurane is a more potent vasodilator and myocardial depressant at equivalent MAC than N_2O.

Various factors increase (Table 17-4) or decrease (Table 17-5) MAC. Unfortunately, no single mechanism explains these alterations, supporting the view that anesthesia is the net result of numerous and widely varying physiologic alterations. In general, those factors that increase CNS metabolic activity, neurotransmission, and CNS neurotransmitter levels increase MAC; upregulated CNS responses to chronically depressed neurotransmitter levels (as in chronic alcoholism) also seem to increase MAC. Conversely, those factors that decrease CNS metabolic activity, neurotransmission, and CNS neurotransmitter levels, as well as downregulated CNS responses to chronically elevated neurotransmitter levels all seem to decrease MAC. Many notable factors do not alter MAC, including duration of administration, gender, type of surgical stimulation, thyroid function, hypo- or hypercarbia, metabolic alkalosis, hyperkalemia, and magnesium levels. However, there may be a genetic component influencing MAC. Red-haired females have a 19% increase in MAC compared with dark-haired females.[16] These data suggest involvement of mutations of the melanocyte stimulating hormone receptor (*MC1R*) allele. Variants of the *MC1R* allele also have been implicated in altering analgesic responses to a κ opioid.[17] MAC also can vary in relationship to genotype and chromosomal substitutions as shown in rats.[18]

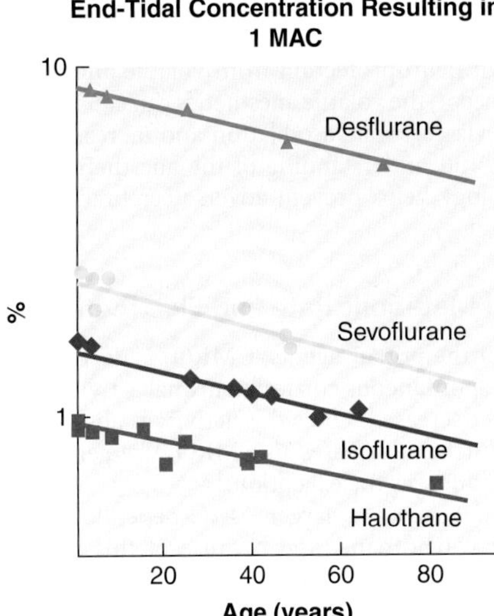

FIGURE 17-11. Effect of age on minimum alveolar concentration (MAC) is plotted. Regression lines are fitted to published values from separate studies. Data are from patients' ages 1 to 80 years. (Adapted from: Mapleson WW. Effect of age on MAC in humans: A meta-analysis. *Br J Anaesth.* 1996;76:179.)

TABLE 17-5. FACTORS THAT DECREASE MINIMUM ALVEOLAR CONCENTRATION

- Increasing age
- Metabolic acidosis
- Hypoxia (PaO_2, 38 mm Hg)
- Induced hypotension (mean arterial pressure <50 mm Hg)
- Decreased central neurotransmitter levels (α-methyldopa, reserpine, chronic dextroamphetamine administration, levodopa)
- α_2-agonists
- Hypothermia
- Hyponatremia
- Lithium
- Hypo-osmolality
- Pregnancy
- Acute ethanol administration[a]
- Ketamine
- Pancuronium[a]
- Physostigmine (10 times clinical doses)
- Neostigmine (10 times clinical doses)
- Lidocaine
- Opioids
- Opioid agonist-antagonist analgesics
- Barbiturates[a]
- Chlorpromazine[a]
- Diazepam[a]
- Hydroxyzine[a]
- Δ-9-Tetrahydrocannabinol
- Verapamil
- Anemia (<4.3 mL O_2/dL blood)

[a]Determined in humans.

The Effect of Age on MAC

The MAC for each of the potent anesthetic gases shows a clear,
6 age-related change (Fig. 17-11). MAC decreases with age and there are similarities between agents in the decline in MAC and age. Excluding patients <1 year of age (where MAC can be lower),[19] there is a linear model that describes a change in MAC of approximately 6% per decade, a 22% decrease in MAC from age 40 to 80 years, and a 27% decrease in MAC from age 1 to 40 years.[20]

Other Alterations in Neurophysiology

The modern potent anesthetics, isoflurane, desflurane, and sevoflurane, all have reasonably similar effects on a wide range of parameters including $CMRO_2$, the EEG, cerebral blood flow (CBF), and flow–metabolism coupling. There are notable differences in effects on intracerebral pressure (ICP), cerebrospinal fluid production and resorption, CO_2 vasoreactivity, CBF autoregulation, and cerebral protection. Nitrous oxide departs from the potent agents in several important respects, and is therefore discussed separately.

Although neuroprotection from volatile anesthetics is a well-defined concept, the volatile anesthetics can cause injury in certain conditions via cerebral vasodilation and increases in intracranial pressure. A full understanding of the anesthetic effects on cerebral physiology helps prevent adverse cerebral events in clinical practice.

Cerebral Metabolic Rate and Electroencephalogram

For most of the potent agents, $CMRO_2$ is decreased only to the extent that spontaneous cortical neuronal activity (as reflected on the EEG) is decreased. Once this activity is absent (an isoelectric EEG), no further decreases in $CMRO_2$ are generated. (Historically, halothane was the exception.)

Isoflurane causes a larger MAC-dependent depression of $CMRO_2$ than halothane, and because of this, can abolish EEG activity at clinical doses that are usually well tolerated from a hemodynamic standpoint.[21] Desflurane and sevoflurane both cause decreases in $CMRO_2$ similar to isoflurane.[22,23] Interestingly, while both desflurane and sevoflurane depress the EEG and abolish activity at clinically tolerated doses of approximately 2 MAC[22,23] in *dogs*, desflurane-induced isoelectric EEG reverts to continuous activity with time despite an unchanging MAC, a property unique to desflurane.[23]

7 Sevoflurane has no noteworthy adverse effects on cerebral physiology at normal CO_2 and BP.[24] During sevoflurane use combined with extreme hyperventilation to decrease cerebral blood flow by half, brain lactate levels can increase. High, long-lasting concentrations of sevoflurane (1.5 to 2.0 MAC), a sudden increase in cerebral sevoflurane concentrations, and/or hypocapnia can trigger EEG abnormalities that have resulted in increases in heart rate (HR) in both adults and children.[25–27] These data question the appropriateness of sevoflurane in patients with epilepsy,[28] but it remains uncertain if sevoflurane truly has a proconvulsant effect.

Cerebral Blood Flow, Flow–Metabolism Coupling, and Autoregulation

All of the potent agents increase CBF in a dose-dependent manner. Isoflurane, sevoflurane, and desflurane cause far less cerebral vasodilation per MAC-multiple than halothane (Fig. 17-12). Desflurane and sevoflurane both influence CBF in a manner similar to isoflurane, with minimal changes in CBF at concentrations less than 1.5 MAC.[22,23,29] An initial dose-dependent increase in CBF with halothane and isoflurane administration to animals subsequently recovers to preinduction levels in approximately 2 to 5 hours. The mechanism of this recovery is unclear.

The increase in CBF with increasing anesthetic dose occurs despite decreases in $CMRO_2$. This phenomenon has been called *uncoupling*, but from a mechanistic standpoint, true uncoupling of flow from metabolism may not occur. That is, as $CMRO_2$ is depressed by the volatile anesthetics, there still is a coupled decline in CBF opposed by a coincident direct vasodilatory effect on the cerebral blood vessels. The net effect on the cerebral vessels depends on the sum of indirect vasoconstricting and direct vasodilating influences.

Autoregulation is the intrinsic myogenic regulation of vascular tone. In normal brain, the mechanisms of autoregulation of CBF over a range of mean arterial pressures from 50 to 150 mm Hg are incompletely understood. Because the volatile anesthetics are direct vasodilators, all are considered to diminish autoregulation in a dose-dependent fashion such that at high anesthetic doses CBF is essentially pressure-passive. Sevoflurane preserves autoregulation up to approximately 1 MAC.[22] At 1.5 MAC, the

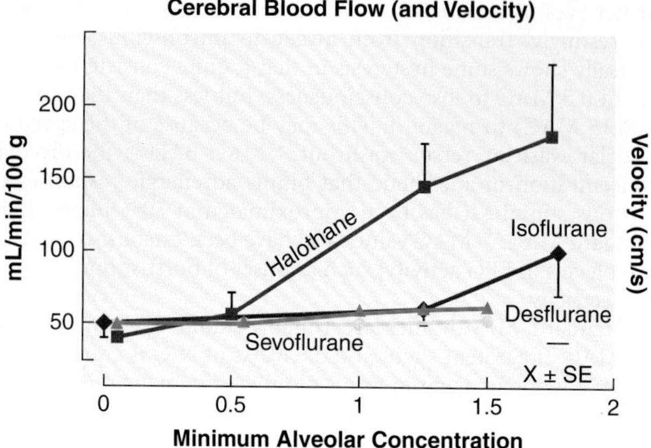

FIGURE 17-12. Cerebral blood flow (and velocity) measured in the presence of normocapnia and in the absence of surgical stimulation in volunteers receiving halothane or isoflurane. At light levels of anesthesia, halothane (but not isoflurane) increased cerebral blood flow. At 1.6 minimum alveolar concentration (MAC), isoflurane also increased cerebral blood flow. (Adapted from: Eger EI 2nd. *Isoflurane (Forane): A compendium and reference.* Madison, Ohio Medical Products, 1985.) Cerebral blood flow velocity measured before and during sevoflurane and desflurane anesthesia up to 1.5 MAC showed no change in cerebral blood flow and velocity. (Adapted from Bedforth NM, Hardman JG, Nathanson MH. Cerebral hemodynamic response to the introduction of desflurane: A comparison with sevoflurane. *Anesth Analg.* 2000;91:152.)

dynamic rate of autoregulation (change in middle cerebral artery blood flow after a rapid transient decrease in BP) is better preserved with sevoflurane than isoflurane (Fig. 17-13). This may be a result of less of a direct vasodilator effect of sevoflurane, preserving the ability of the vessel to respond to changes in BP at 1.5 MAC. Based on a similar model but a separate study of dynamic

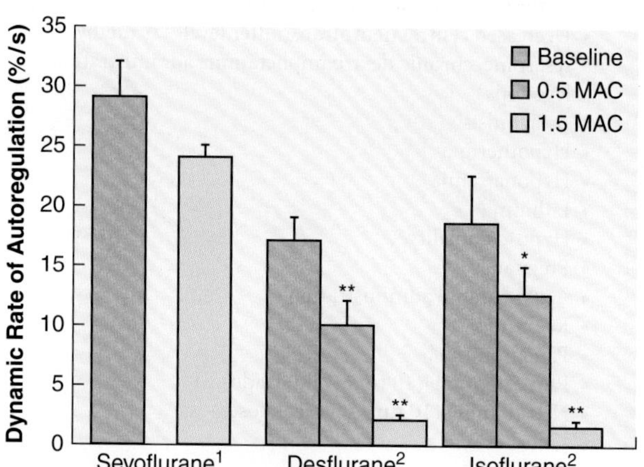

FIGURE 17-13. Dynamic rate of autoregulation (the change in middle cerebral artery blood flow after a rapid transient decrease in blood pressure) during awake (or fentanyl and N_2O baseline), 0.5, and 1.5 minimum alveolar anesthetic concentration (MAC) anesthesia. Values are mean ± SE (SD for sevoflurane). **P* <0.05 versus baseline, ***P* <0.001 versus baseline and sevoflurane. (Adapted from [1]Summors AC, Gupta AK, Matta BF. Dynamic cerebral autoregulation during sevoflurane anesthesia: A comparison with isoflurane. *Anesth Analg.* 1999;88:341–345; and [2]Strebel S, Lam AM, Matta B, et al. Dynamic and static cerebral autoregulation during isoflurane, desflurane, and propofol anesthesia. *Anesthesiology.* 1995;83:66–76.)

autoregulation of CBF, both desflurane and isoflurane reduced autoregulation in a dose-dependent manner (Fig. 17-13).

Intracerebral Pressure

For most anesthesiologists, the area of greatest clinical interest is the effect of volatile anesthetics on ICP. In general, ICP will increase or decrease in proportion to changes in CBF. Isoflurane increases ICP minimally in animals both with and without brain pathology, including those with an already elevated ICP.[30] In human studies there usually are mild increases in ICP with isoflurane administration that are blocked or blunted by hyperventilation or barbiturate coadministration.[31] There are some contradictory data, however. In one human study, hypocapnia did not prevent elevations in ICP with isoflurane administration in patients with space-occupying brain lesions.[32] However, isoflurane-induced increases in ICP tend to be of short duration, in one study only 30 minutes.[33]

Like isoflurane, both sevoflurane and desflurane >1 MAC produce mild increases in ICP, paralleling their mild increases in CBF.[22,23,34,35] One potential advantage of sevoflurane is that its lower pungency and airway irritation may lessen the risk of coughing and bucking and the associated rise in ICP as compared with desflurane or isoflurane. In fact, introduction of desflurane after propofol induction of anesthesia has led to significant increases in HR, mean arterial pressure, and middle cerebral artery blood flow velocity.[36] This may relate to the airway irritant effects of desflurane rather than a specific alteration in neurophysiology. However, several studies in both children and adults suggest that increases in ICP from desflurane are slightly greater than from either isoflurane or sevoflurane.[37,38] The bottom line is that all three potent agents may be used at appropriate doses, especially with adjunctive and compensatory therapies, in just about any neurosurgical procedure.

Cerebrospinal Fluid Production and Resorption

Isoflurane does not appear to alter CSF production,[33] but may increase, decrease, or leave unchanged the resistance to resorption depending on dose. Sevoflurane at 1 MAC depresses CSF production up to 40%.[39] Desflurane at 1 MAC leaves CSF production unchanged or increased.[37,40] In general, anesthetic effects on ICP via changes in CSF dynamics are clinically far less important than anesthetic effects on CBF.

Cerebral Blood Flow Response to Hypercapia and Hypocapia

Significant hypercapnia is associated with dramatic increases in CBF whether or not volatile anesthetics are administered. As discussed earlier, hypocapnia can blunt or abolish volatile anes-
8 thetic-induced increases in CBF depending on when the hypocapnia is produced. This vasoreactivity to CO_2 may be somewhat altered by the volatile anesthetics as compared with normal. Isoflurane does not abolish hypocapnic vasoconstriction.[41] Similarly, CO_2 vasoreactivity under desflurane anesthesia is normal up to 1.5 MAC,[30] and CO_2 vasoreactivity for sevoflurane is preserved at 1 MAC.[42]

Cerebral Protection

When isoflurane is used to lower BP and cerebral perfusion, tissue oxygen content is improved as compared to a similar BP effect created by other pharmacologic means. The improvement is most likely due to the beneficial effect of isoflurane to decrease $CMRO_2$.[43] Both sevoflurane and desflurane have been shown to improve neurologic outcome in comparison to N_2O-fentanyl after incomplete cerebral ischemia in a rat model.[44,45] In piglets undergoing low-flow cardiopulmonary bypass, desflurane improved neurologic outcome compared with a fentanyl/droperidol-based anesthetic.[46] In humans, desflurane has been shown to increase brain tissue PO_2 during administration, and to maintain PO_2 to a greater extent than thiopental during temporary cerebral artery occlusion during cerebrovascular surgery.[47] Neuroprotection and clinical outcome studies for sevoflurane and desflurane have not been published.

Postoperative Cognitive Dysfunction

Postoperative cognitive dysfunction (POCD) is defined as impairment to the mental processes of perception, memory, and information processing. These alterations have been shown to increase morbidity and mortality in the first year after surgery from causes such as decubiti, pneumonia, and deep vein thrombosis.[48] In the elderly in particular, subtle cognitive dysfunction can persist long after expected drug clearance. Despite the inhalational anesthetics being the most widely administered drugs in most operative settings, relatively few studies have investigated the effects of these medications on postoperative cognitive outcome.[49]

The effect of isoflurane on POCD has been more widely investigated than that of the other potent agents. As early as 1992, Tsai et al. reported that desflurane was superior to isoflurane in both emergence characteristics and the recovery of cognitive function.[50] Similar findings have been reported with the use of sevoflurane instead of isoflurane,[51,52] and these results were not influenced by the use of premedication, intraoperative opioids, and/or N_2O.[53] Chen et al.[54] have demonstrated that sevoflurane and desflurane have similar profiles when it comes to cognitive recovery, and multiple other studies have further confirmed this.[55] These results seem to be in conflict with those produced by Kanbak et al. who demonstrated in cardiopulmonary bypass patients that isoflurane promoted better neurocognitive function than either sevoflurane or desflurane.[49] It is clear from the wide variations in the results available in the literature that more research is required into this important topic. Further, while the mechanisms involved in the development of POCD are not well delineated, it seems clear that all modern anesthetics are associated with its development to one degree or another.[49–53,55–57]

As with the potent inhalational anesthetics, use of N_2O is also associated with POCD and delirium, and high doses of N_2O seem to be associated with interference with many cognitive functions.[58] Interestingly, the development of postoperative delirium after exposure to N_2O in a mixed anesthetic has a similar incidence to that when not exposed, suggesting that the mechanisms, while possibly different, are not additive.[59,60]

Processed Electroencephalograms and Neuromonitoring

9 All of the volatile anesthetics produce dose-dependent effects on the EEG, sensory-evoked potentials (SEPs), and motor-evoked potentials (MEPs). EEGs recorded on the scalp can be processed to quantify the amount of activity in each of four frequency bands: Delta (0 to 3 Hz), theta (4 to 7 Hz), alpha (8 to 13 Hz), and beta (>13 Hz). All three currently used agents at <1 MAC and N_2O at 30% to 70% can produce shifts to increasing frequencies. Between 1 and 2 MAC the potent agents produce shifts to decreasing frequencies and increases in amplitude. At >2 MAC, all of the potent agents can produce burst suppression or electrical silence. These are important factors to remember because EEG changes during administration of general anesthesia can also be caused by hypoxia, hypercarbia, and hypothermia. The EEG must always be interpreted within the appropriate clinical context.

All of the volatile agents cause a dose-dependent increase in latency and decrease in amplitude in all cortical SEP modalities. In subcortical modalities, such as brainstem auditory evoked potentials, these agents are associated with negligible effects. In general, visual evoked potentials are somewhat more sensitive to the effects of the volatile anesthetics than somatosensory evoked potentials. Like EEGs, these effects from anesthetics must be kept in mind when changes during SEPs occur, and appropriate doses of the volatile agents must be used. Sudden changes in the anesthetic regimen (>0.5 MAC) also seem to have greater effects on SEPs than more gradual changes.

MEPs evaluate the functional integrity of descending motor pathways. The evoked response is most commonly recorded as a muscle potential or a peripheral nerve signal. The trigger is typically transosseous activation via electrical or magnetic stimulation. MEPs are exquisitely sensitive to depression by volatile anesthetics, which are usually avoided in these cases.

Nitrous Oxide

The effects of N_2O on cerebral physiology are not clear. Both the MAC for N_2O and its effects on $CMRO_2$ vary widely depending on species. The difference in $CMRO_2$ effects may in part be accounted for by differences in MAC, but MAC-equivalent effects on $CMRO_2$ also differ. Several studies in dogs, goats, and swine found that N_2O increases $CMRO_2$ and CBF, while in rodents no such increases or only slight increases occur. In human studies, N_2O administration preserved CBF but decreased $CMRO_2$.[21]

Another problem is that N_2O is a co-anesthetic used to supplement potent agents, not a complete anesthetic in itself, and $CMRO_2$ effects may differ depending on the presence or absence of potent agent as well as the particular agent and dose. Addition of N_2O to 1 or 2.2 MAC isoflurane does not alter $CMRO_2$, but it does increase CBF at 1 MAC but not 2.2 MAC.

Barbiturates, narcotics, or a combination of the two appear to decrease or eliminate the increases in $CMRO_2$ and CBF produced by N_2O. The effect of pentobarbital/N_2O is dose-dependent, with preserved increases in $CMRO_2$ by N_2O at low-dose pentobarbital, and no changes in $CMRO_2$ at high-dose pentobarbital.[61] N_2O and benzodiazepine coadministration is particularly confusing. Midazolam/N_2O in dogs increased CBF but did not alter $CMRO_2$,[62] while the opposite was true in rats,[63] and both CBF and $CMRO_2$ declined in rats given diazepam/N_2O. N_2O administration increases ICP, but as is the case for $CMRO_2$ and CBF, changes in ICP are decreased or eliminated by a variety of co-anesthetics and, more importantly, by hypocapnia.

Nitrous oxide appears to have an antineuroprotective effect, as addition of N_2O to isoflurane during temporary ischemia is associated with greater tissue damage and worsened neurologic outcome.[63] In a study in mice, survival time after a hypoxic event was decreased by addition of N_2O.[64] Given the conflicting data on the effects of N_2O on $CMRO_2$, CBF, ICP, and the apparent antineuroprotective effect of this agent, avoidance or discontinuation of its use should be considered in surgical cases with a high likelihood of elevated ICP or significant cerebral ischemia.

THE CIRCULATORY SYSTEM

Hemodynamics

10 The cardiac, vascular, and autonomic effects of the volatile anesthetics have been defined through a number of studies carried out in human volunteers not undergoing surgery.[65–70] In general, the information from these volunteer studies has translated well to the patient population commonly exposed to these anesthetics during elective and emergent surgeries.

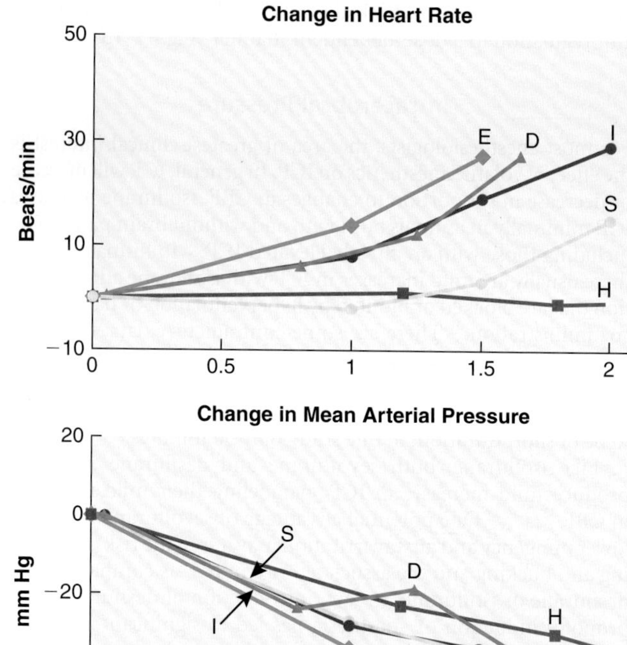

FIGURE 17-14. Heart rate and blood pressure changes (from awake baseline) in volunteers receiving general anesthesia with halothane (H), enflurane (E), isoflurane (I), desflurane (D), or sevoflurane (S). Halothane and sevoflurane produced little or no change in heart rate at <1.5 minimum alveolar concentration. All anesthetics caused similar decreases in blood pressure. (Adapted from: Malan TP Jr, DiNardo JA, Isner RJ, et al. Cardiovascular effects of sevoflurane compared with those of isoflurane in volunteers. *Anesthesiology.* 1995;83:918; Weiskopf RB, Cahalan MK, Eger EI 2nd, et al. Cardiovascular actions of desflurane in normocarbic volunteers. *Anesth Analg.* 1991;73:143; and Calverley RK, Smith NT, Prys-Roberts C, et al. Cardiovascular effects of enflurane anesthesia during controlled ventilation in man. *Anesth Analg.* 1978;57:619.)

A common effect of the potent volatile anesthetics has been to decrease BP in a dose-related fashion with essentially no differences noted between the volatile anesthetics at equianesthetic concentrations (Fig. 17-14). Their primary mechanism to decrease BP is via a potent effect to relax vascular smooth muscle leading to decreases in regional and systemic vascular resistance (Fig. 17-15). They have only minimal effects on cardiac output.

In volunteers, sevoflurane up to about 1 MAC does not change HR while enflurane, isoflurane, and desflurane result in 5% to 10% increases in HR from baseline (Fig. 17-14). Both desflurane and, to a lesser extent, isoflurane have been associated with transient and significant increases in HR during rapid increases in the inspired concentration of either anesthetic.[71,72] The mechanism(s) underlying these transient HR surges is likely due to the relative pungency of these anesthetics, which stimulates airway receptors to elicit a reflex tachycardia.[73] The tachycardia can be lessened with opioid or α_2-agonist pretreatment.[74–76]

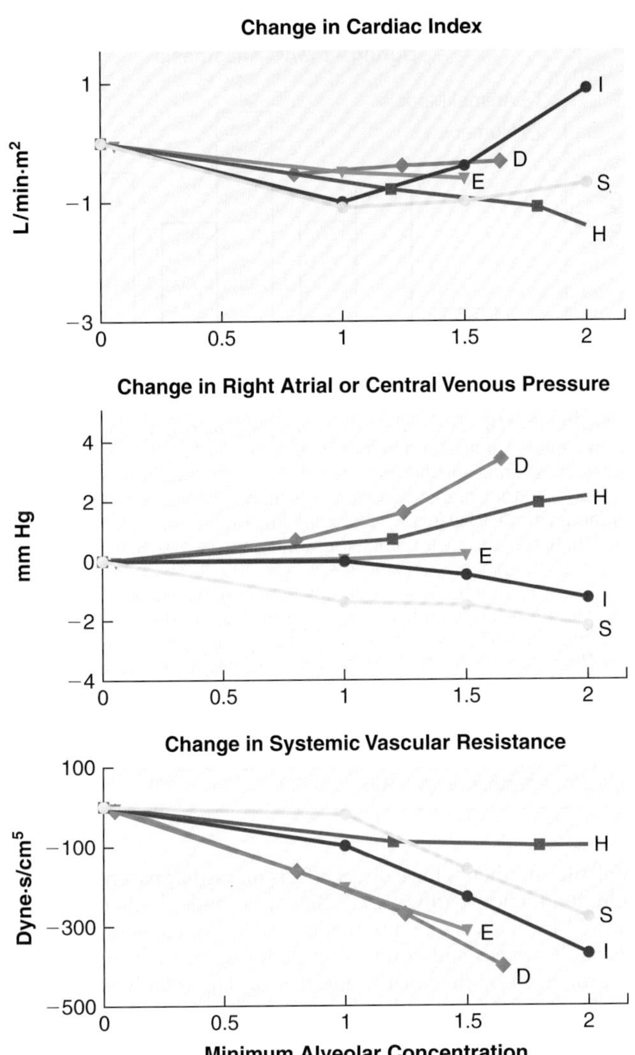

FIGURE 17-15. Cardiac index, central venous pressure (or right atrial pressure), and systemic vascular resistance changes (from awake baseline) in volunteers receiving general anesthesia with halothane (H), enflurane (E), isoflurane (I), desflurane (D), or sevoflurane (S). Increases in central venous pressure from halothane and desflurane might be due to different mechanisms. With halothane, the increase might be due to myocardial depression, whereas with desflurane, the increase is more likely due to venoconstriction. (Adapted from: Malan TP Jr, DiNardo JA, Isner RJ, et al. Cardiovascular effects of sevoflurane compared with those of isoflurane in volunteers. *Anesthesiology.* 1995;83:918; Weiskopf RB, Cahalan MK, Eger EI 2nd, et al. Cardiovascular actions of desflurane in normocarbic volunteers. *Anesth Analg.* 1991;73:143; and Calverley RK, Smith NT, Prys-Roberts C, et al. Cardiovascular effects of enflurane anesthesia during controlled ventilation in man. *Anesth Analg.* 1978;57:619.)

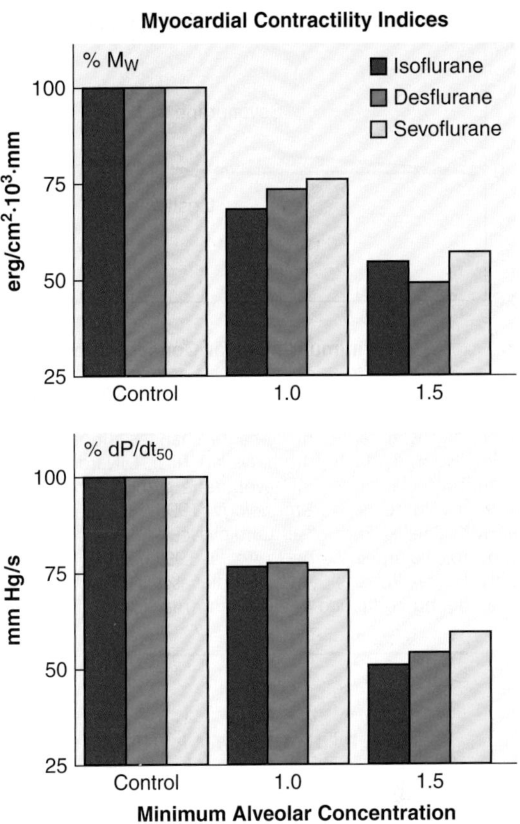

FIGURE 17-16. Myocardial contractility indices from chronically instrumented dogs. For these measurements, pharmacologic blockade of the autonomic nervous system was established to eliminate neural or circulating humoral influences on the inotropic state of the heart. The conscious control data were assigned 100%, and subsequent reductions in the inotropic state are depicted for both 1 and 1.5 minimum alveolar anesthetic concentrations of sevoflurane, desflurane, and isoflurane. There were no differences between these three volatile anesthetics. M_w, slope of the regional preload recruitable stroke work relationship; dP/dt_{50}, change in pressure per unit of time. (Adapted from: Pagel PS, Kampine JP, Schmeling WT, et al. Influence of volatile anesthetics on myocardial contractility in vivo: Desflurane versus isoflurane. *Anesthesiology.* 1991;74:900; and Harkin CP, Pagel PS, Kersten JR, et al. Direct negative inotropic and lusitropic effects of sevoflurane. *Anesthesiology.* 1994;81:156.)

Myocardial Contractility

Myocardial contractility indices have been directly evaluated in animals and indirectly evaluated in human volunteers during the administration of each of the volatile anesthetics. Isoflurane, desflurane, and sevoflurane produced similar dose-dependent reductions in indices of myocardial function in an autonomically denervated dog model (Fig. 17-16). Echocardiographic-determined indices of myocardial function in healthy humans, including the more noteworthy measurement of the velocity of circumferential fiber shortening (Fig. 17-17) have not been diminished by isoflurane, desflurane, or sevoflurane. However, in cardiac patients with ejection fractions above 40%, 1 MAC sevoflurane and desflurane reduced contractility, assessed as dp/dt_{max}. Despite the small reduction in baseline contractility, the anesthetics did not affect the ability of the myocardium to respond to an acute increase in cardiac preload. Thus, functional reserve of the heart was not impaired by the volatile anesthetics.[77] In addition, when comparing sevoflurane and desflurane to propofol in cardiac patients with impaired ventricular function after CABG surgery, the volatile anesthetics preserved and propofol worsened ventricular responses to acute increases in preload.[78]

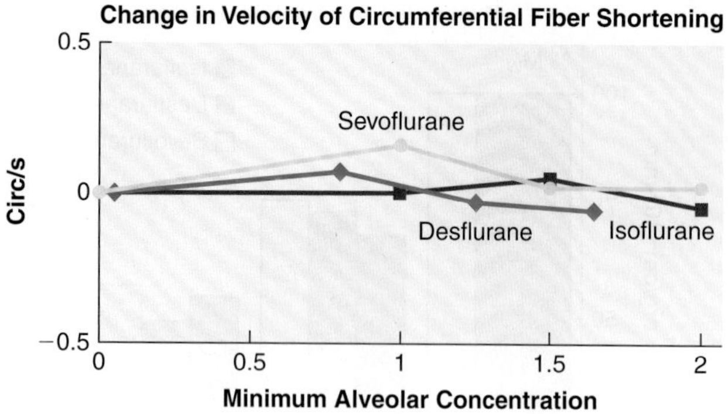

FIGURE 17-17. Noninvasive assessment of myocardial contractility with echocardiography during anesthesia in volunteers. Sevoflurane, desflurane, and isoflurane did not cause changes suggestive of myocardial depression. (Adapted from: Malan TP Jr, DiNardo JA, Isner RJ, et al. Cardiovascular effects of sevoflurane compared with those of isoflurane in volunteers. *Anesthesiology.* 1995;83:918; Weiskopf RB, Cahalan MK, Eger EI 2nd, et al. Cardiovascular actions of desflurane in normocarbic volunteers. *Anesth Analg.* 1991;73:143; and Calverley RK, Smith NT, Prys-Roberts C, et al. Cardiovascular effects of enflurane anesthesia during controlled ventilation in man. *Anesth Analg.* 1978; 57:619.)

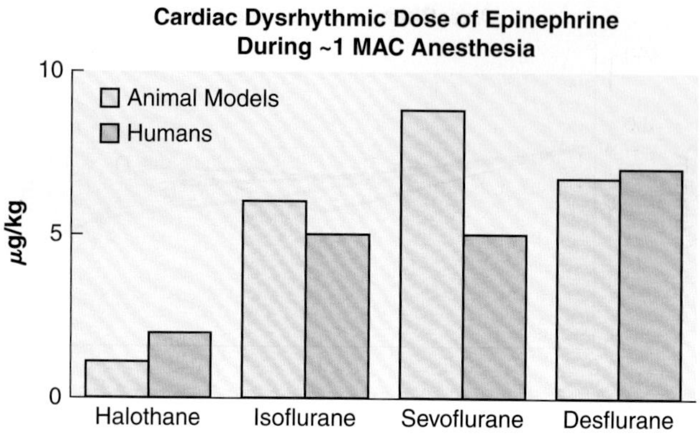

Cardiac Dysrhythmic Dose of Epinephrine During ~1 MAC Anesthesia
Animal Models
Humans
μg/kg
Halothane Isoflurane Sevoflurane Desflurane

FIGURE 17-18. The dose of epinephrine associated with cardiac arrhythmias in animal and human models was least with halothane. The ether anesthetics—isoflurane, desflurane, and sevoflurane—required three- to sixfold greater doses of epinephrine to cause arrhythmias. (Adapted from: Navarro R, Weiskopf RB, Moore MA, et al. Humans anesthetized with sevoflurane or isoflurane have similar arrhythmic response to epinephrine. *Anesthesiology.* 1994;80:545; Weiskopf RB, Eger EI 2nd, Holmes MA, et al. Epinephrine-induced premature ventricular contractions and changes in arterial blood pressure and heart rate during I-653, isoflurane, and halothane anesthesia in swine. *Anesthesiology.* 1989;70:293; Hayashi Y, Sumikawa K, Tashiro C, et al. Arrhythmogenic threshold of epinephrine during sevoflurane, enflurane, and isoflurane anesthesia in dogs. *Anesthesiology.* 1988;69:145; and Moore MA, Weiskopf RB, Eger EI 2nd, et al. Arrhythmogenic doses of epinephrine are similar during desflurane or isoflurane anesthesia in humans. *Anesthesiology.* 1993;79:943.)

Other Circulatory Effects

Most of the volatile anesthetics have been studied during both controlled and spontaneous ventilation.[67,69,79] The process of spontaneous ventilation reduces the high intrathoracic pressures from positive pressure ventilation. The negative intrathoracic pressure during the inspiratory phase of spontaneous ventilation augments venous return and cardiac filling and improves cardiac output and BP. Spontaneous ventilation is associated with higher $PaCO_2$, causing cerebral and systemic vascular relaxation. This contributes to an improved cardiac output via afterload reduction. Spontaneous ventilation in theory, would improve the safety of volatile anesthetic administration because the anesthetic concentration that produces cardiovascular collapse exceeds the concentration that results in apnea.

Nitrous oxide is commonly combined with potent volatile anesthetics to maintain general anesthesia. Nitrous oxide has unique cardiovascular actions. It increases sympathetic nervous system activity and vascular resistance when given in a 40% concentration.[65] When N_2O is combined with volatile anesthetics, systemic vascular resistance and BP are greater than when equipotent concentrations of the volatile anesthetics are evaluated without N_2O.[67,80] These effects might not be due solely to sympathetic activation from N_2O per se, but may be partially attributed to a decrease in the concentration of the coadministered potent volatile anesthetic required to achieve a MAC equivalent when using N_2O.

Oxygen consumption is decreased approximately 10% to 15% during general anesthesia.[81] The distribution of cardiac output also is altered by anesthesia. Blood flow to liver, kidneys, and gut is decreased, particularly at deep levels of anesthesia. In contrast, blood flow to the brain, muscle, and skin is increased or not changed during general anesthesia.[82] In humans, increases in muscle blood flow are noted with isoflurane, desflurane, and sevoflurane with minimal differences between anesthetics at equipotent concentrations.[83]

Isoflurane, sevoflurane, and desflurane do not sensitize the heart to the arrhythmogenic effects of epinephrine (Fig. 17-18). Volatile anesthetics have direct effects on cardiac pacemaker cells and conduction pathways.[84,85] Sinoatrial node discharge rate is slowed by the volatile anesthetics and conduction in the His–Purkinje system and conduction pathways in the ventricle also is prolonged by the volatile anesthetics. The volatile anesthetics prolong QT_c interval and in theory, especially with a baseline prolongation in myocardial repolarization, may predispose to ventricular tachyarrhythmias including torsade de pointes. Such an effect has been noted in a child with congenital prolonged QT syndrome.[86] In children studied at steady state 1 MAC, QT_c was more prolonged with desflurane than sevoflurane (Fig. 17-19).[87] When the effects of sevoflurane, propofol, and desflurane on QT interval dispersion and p dispersion were evaluated in adults, only desflurane prolonged intervals, although no increase in cardiac dysrhythmias were noted.[88]

Coronary Steal, Myocardial Ischemia, and Cardiac Outcome

Isoflurane (and most other potent volatile anesthetics) increases coronary blood flow many times beyond that of the myocardial oxygen demand, thereby creating potential for "steal." Steal is the diversion of blood from a myocardial bed with limited or inadequate perfusion to a bed with more adequate perfusion; especially one that has a remaining element of autoregulation.

Despite early worries that the potent vasodilation from isoflurane might cause coronary steal, clinical outcome studies have been unable to find an association between the use of isoflurane in patients undergoing CABG operations with an increased incidence of myocardial infarction or perioperative death.[89–91] This is in agreement with findings in a chronically instrumented dog model of multivessel coronary artery obstruction where neither

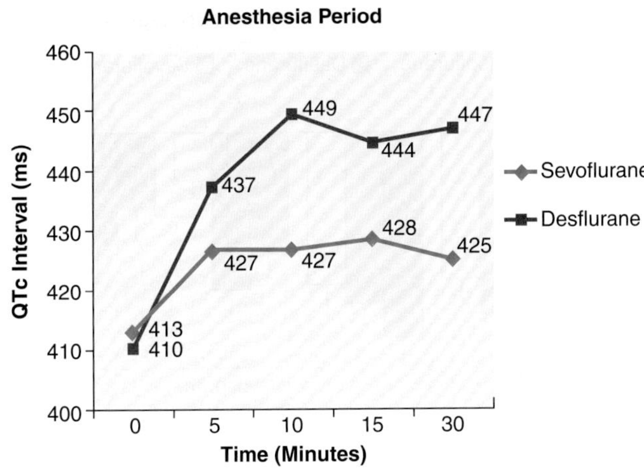

FIGURE 17-19. Mean QTc intervals in children, age 1 to 14 years, after inhalation of 2% sevoflurane or 6% desflurane, both in 66% N_2O/O_2. (Adapted from: Aypar E, Karagoz AH, Ozer S, Celiker A, Ocal T. The effects of sevoflurane and desflurane anesthesia on QTc interval and cardiac rhythm in children. *Pediatr Anaesth.* 2007;17:563–567.)

isoflurane, sevoflurane, or desflurane at concentrations up to 1.5 MAC resulted in abnormal collateral coronary blood flow redistribution (steal), whereas adenosine, a potent coronary vasodilator, clearly resulted in abnormal flow distribution.[92–95]

Several studies in patients with coronary artery disease either undergoing noncardiac or coronary artery bypass graft (CABG) surgery have demonstrated that myocardial ischemia and outcome from sevoflurane was no different from isoflurane.[96,97] Desflurane also appears to result in similar outcome effects as isoflurane in cardiac patients having CABG[98] with one exception. In a study in which desflurane was given without opioids to patients with coronary artery disease requiring CABG surgery, significant ischemia mandating the use of beta-blockers was noted.[99] Desflurane has not been evaluated in terms of ischemia and outcome in a patient population with coronary disease undergoing noncardiac surgery. Most studies would suggest that determinants of myocardial oxygen supply and demand, rather than the anesthetic, are of far greater importance to patient outcomes.

Cardioprotection from Volatile Anesthetics

A preconditioning stimulus such as brief coronary occlusion and ischemia initiates a signaling cascade of intracellular events that reduces ischemia and reperfusion myocardial injury. There is a memory effect from an ischemic stimulus that offers 2 to 3 hours of protection. The volatile anesthetics given before (preconditioning) or immediately after (postconditioning) mimic ischemic preconditioning and trigger a similar cascade of intracellular events resulting in reduced myocardial injury and myocardial protection that lasts beyond the elimination of the anesthetic.[100] Numerous factors may be involved in the protection, including the sodium:hydrogen exchanger, activation of opioid, bradykinin or adenosine receptors (particularly α_1 and α_2 subtypes), inhibitory G proteins, protein kinase C, tyrosine kinase, and potassium (K_{ATP}) channel opening. Pharmacologic blockade of these factors reduces or eliminates the cardioprotective effect of ischemic or volatile anesthetic preconditioning.[100,101] Alternatively, administration of certain drugs can mimic ischemic or volatile anesthetic preconditioning. These include adenosine, opioid agonists, and K_{ATP} channel openers.

Lipophilic volatile anesthetics diffuse through myocardial cell membranes and alter mitochondrial electron transport, leading to reactive oxygen species formation.[101] This may be the trigger for preconditioning via protein kinase C activation of K_{ATP} channel opening.[102,103] Approximately, 30% to 40% of the cardioprotection from the volatile anesthetics appears to be related to a reduced loading of calcium into the myocardial cells during ischemia. Preconditioned hearts may tolerate ischemia for 10 minutes longer than nonconditioned hearts.[104]

While these evolving data generally derive from animal models, there now is increasing evidence in cardiac patient populations that anesthetic cardioprotection lessens myocardial damage and improve cardiac outcomes during "on and off pump" cardiac surgery.[105,106] One meta analysis of 22 trials including nearly 2,000 patients undergoing CABG surgery found that sevoflurane and desflurane compared to a TIVA technique were associated with a 50% reduction in MI, reductions in cardiac troponin I peak levels, inotropic support, and all cause mortality, and shorter periods of mechanical ventilation and ICU stay.[107] Sulfonylurea oral hyperglycemic drugs close K_{ATP} channels, abolishing anesthetic preconditioning. They should be discontinued 24 to 48 hours prior to elective surgery in high-risk patients.[100] But hyperglycemia also prevents preconditioning, so insulin therapy should be started when holding oral agents.[108] Recent evidence suggests that volatile anesthetics including xenon, may protect other organs from ischemic injury, including kidney, liver, and brain.[109–112]

Autonomic Nervous System

The autonomic nervous system is modulated by baroreceptor reflex mechanisms. Studies have examined the behavior of the arterial baroreflex system during a hypotensive or hypertensive stimulus by evaluating changes in HR and sympathetic nerve activity in humans. Anesthetic mediated, dose-dependent decreases in reflex control mechanisms are evident (Figs. 17-20, 17-21).[113–116] These findings may useful in clinical practice. Low concentrations of volatile anesthetics result in only minimal impairment of reflex control mechanisms. Higher concentrations lead to greater reduction in the reflex responses to hypovolemia and perhaps an earlier recognition of the event because diminished reflex vasoconstriction and tachycardia to blood loss lead to hypotension, rather than masking the effect via reflex changes. Of note is a more rapid return of baroreflex function with the less soluble anesthetic sevoflurane versus isoflurane in the postoperative period.[117]

Desflurane has a unique and prominent effect on sympathetic outflow in humans, which is not apparent in animal models. With increasing steady state concentrations of desflurane, there is a progressive increase in resting sympathetic nervous system activity and plasma norepinephrine levels.[118] Despite this increase in tonic sympathetic outflow, BP decreases similarly to sevoflurane and isoflurane (Fig. 17-14). This raises the question as to whether desflurane has the ability to uncouple neuroeffector responses. In addition, desflurane can cause substantial activation of the sympathetic nervous system when the inspired concentration is increased, especially to concentrations above 5% to 6% (Fig. 17-22).[118] There is a transient surge in sympathetic outflow leading to both hypertension and tachycardia. In addition, the endocrine axis is activated as evidenced by 15- to 20-fold increases in plasma antidiuretic hormone and epinephrine and norepinephrine (Fig. 17-23). The hemodynamic response persists for 4 to 5 minutes and the endocrine response

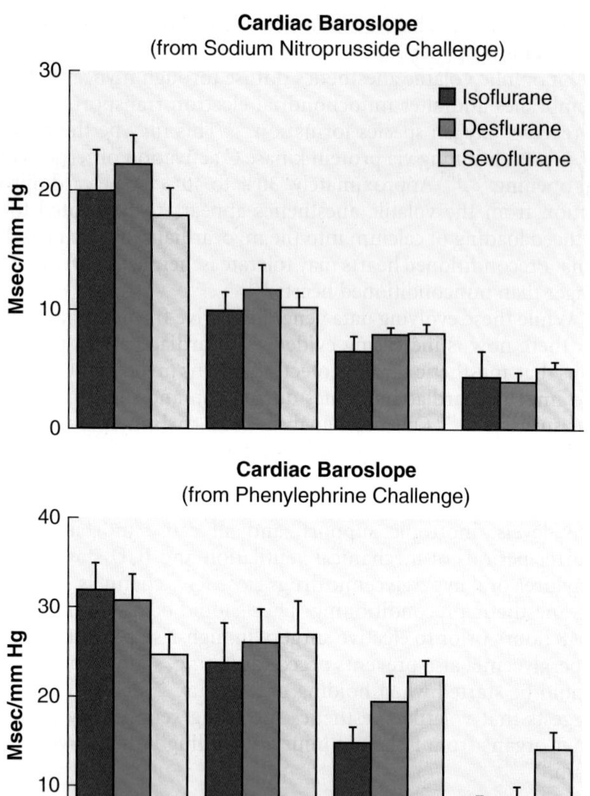

FIGURE 17-20. Summary data of the baroreflex regulation of heart rate (R–R interval) in response to a decreasing pressure stimulus (sodium nitroprusside) or in response to an increasing pressure stimulus (phenylephrine). These data were acquired in healthy volunteers who were randomized to receive isoflurane, desflurane, or sevoflurane. With increasing minimum alveolar anesthetic concentration, each of the volatile anesthetics led to a progressive reduction in the cardiac baroslope (an index of baroreflex sensitivity derived by relating changes in mean pressure to changes in R–R interval). There were no statistical differences between anesthetics. (Adapted from: Ebert TJ, Harkin CP, Muzi M. Cardiovascular responses to sevoflurane: A review. *Anesth Analg.* 1995;81:S11.)

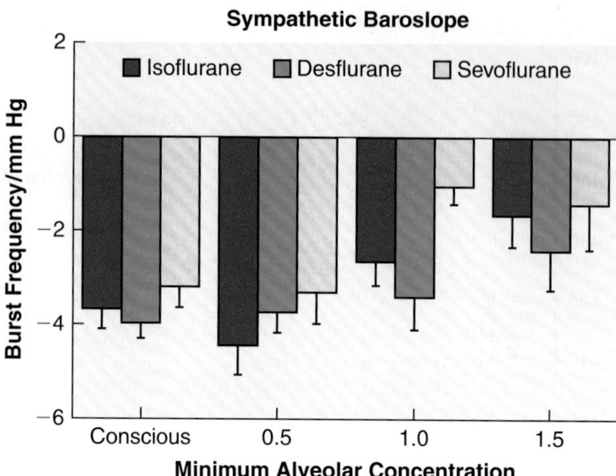

FIGURE 17-21. The sympathetic baroreflex function of healthy volunteers randomized to receive isoflurane, desflurane, or sevoflurane. The slope (sensitivity) is the relationship between decreasing diastolic pressure and increasing efferent sympathetic nerve activity. The reflex regulation of sympathetic outflow was fairly well preserved at 0.5 and 1.0 minimum alveolar anesthetic concentration (MAC) of anesthetic. At 1.5 MAC, there was a 50% decrease in the slope with all anesthetics. (Adapted from: Ebert TJ, Harkin CP, Muzi M. Cardiovascular responses to sevoflurane: A review. *Anesth Analg.* 1995;81:S11.)

persists for up to 30 minutes.[66,71,72] Adequate concentrations of opioids or clonidine given prior to increasing the concentration of desflurane have been shown to attenuate these responses.[74–76] The source of the neuroendocrine activation is likely from receptors in both the upper and lower airways that initiate the sympathetic activation.[73]

THE PULMONARY SYSTEM

General Ventilatory Effects

All volatile anesthetics decrease tidal volume and increase respiratory rate such that there are only minor effects on decreasing minute ventilation (Fig. 17-24). The ventilatory effects
11 are dose-dependent, with higher concentrations of volatile

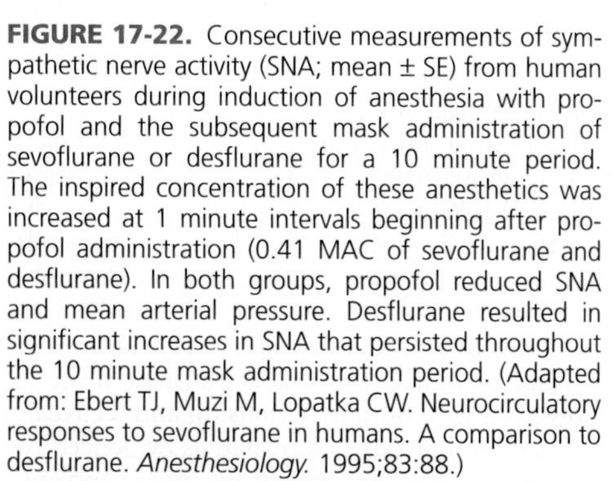

FIGURE 17-22. Consecutive measurements of sympathetic nerve activity (SNA; mean ± SE) from human volunteers during induction of anesthesia with propofol and the subsequent mask administration of sevoflurane or desflurane for a 10 minute period. The inspired concentration of these anesthetics was increased at 1 minute intervals beginning after propofol administration (0.41 MAC of sevoflurane and desflurane). In both groups, propofol reduced SNA and mean arterial pressure. Desflurane resulted in significant increases in SNA that persisted throughout the 10 minute mask administration period. (Adapted from: Ebert TJ, Muzi M, Lopatka CW. Neurocirculatory responses to sevoflurane in humans. A comparison to desflurane. *Anesthesiology.* 1995;83:88.)

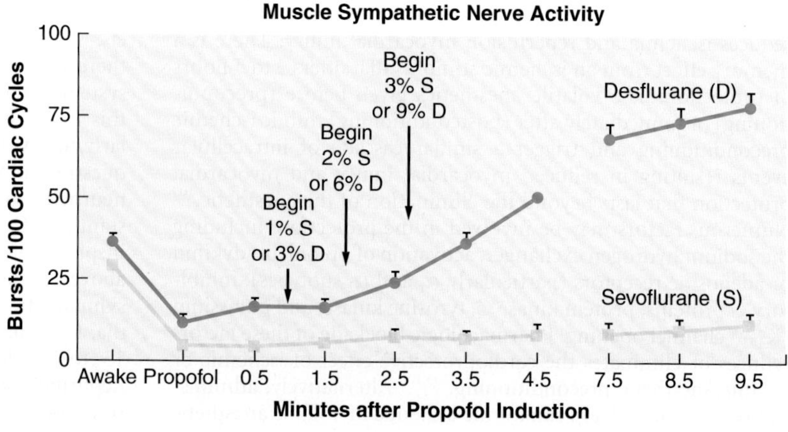

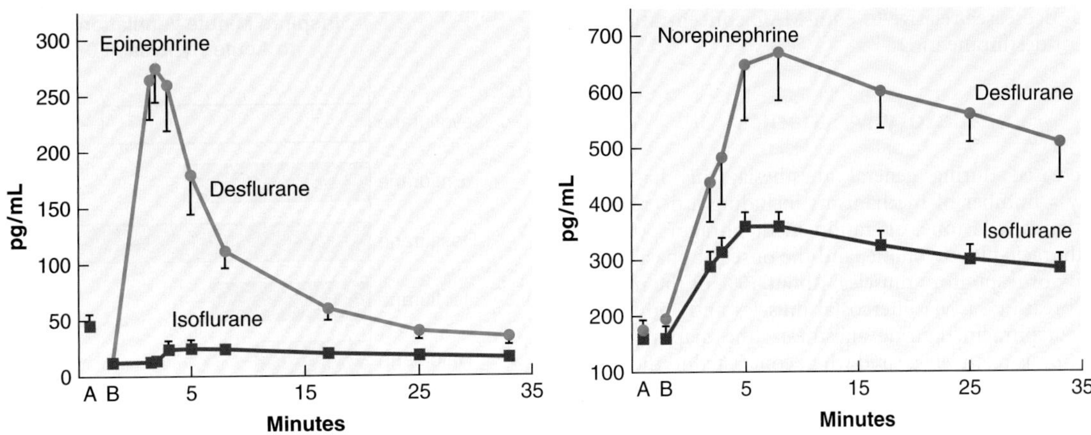

FIGURE 17-23. Stress hormone responses to a rapid increase in anesthetic concentration, from 4% to 12% inspired. Volunteers given desflurane showed a larger increase in plasma epinephrine and norepinephrine concentrations than when given isoflurane. Data are mean ± SE. A = awake value; B = value after 32 minutes of 0.55 minimum alveolar concentration; time represents minutes after the first breath of increased anesthetic concentration. (Adapted from: Weiskopf RB, Moore MA, Eger EI II, et al. Rapid increase in desflurane concentration is associated with greater transient cardiovascular stimulation than with rapid increase in isoflurane concentration in humans. *Anesthesiology.* 1994;80:1035.)

anesthetics resulting in greater decreases in tidal volume and greater increases in respiratory rate, with the exception of isoflurane, which does not increase respiratory rate above 1 MAC. Their net effect of a gradual decrease in minute ventilation has been associated with increasing resting P_aCO_2. The respiratory depression can be partially antagonized during surgical stimulation where respiratory rate and tidal volume have been shown to increase, resulting in a decrease in the P_aCO_2. Nitrous oxide increases respiratory rate as much or more than the inhaled anesthetics. When N_2O is added to sevoflurane or desflurane,

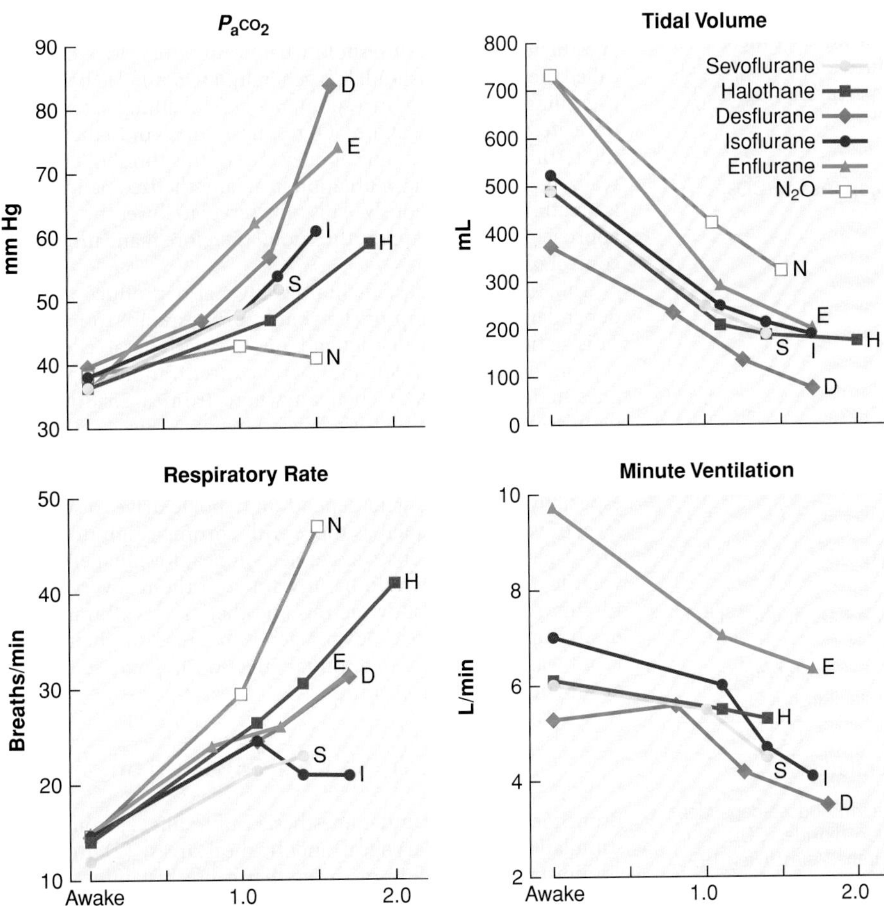

FIGURE 17-24. Comparison of mean changes in resting P_aCO_2, tidal volume, respiratory rate, and minute ventilation in patients anesthetized with either halothane, isoflurane, enflurane, sevoflurane, desflurane, or N_2O (N). Anesthetic-induced tachypnea compensates in part for the ventilatory depression caused by all volatile anesthetics (decrease in minute ventilation and tidal volume, and concomitant increase in P_aCO_2). Desflurane results in the greatest increase in P_aCO_2 with corresponding reductions in tidal volume and minute ventilation. Isoflurane, like all other inhaled agents, increases respiratory rate, but does not result in dose-dependent tachypnea. (Adapted from: Lockhart SH, Rampil IJ, Yasuda N, et al. Depression of ventilation by desflurane in humans. *Anesthesiology.* 1991;74:484; Doi M, Ikeda K. Respiratory effects of sevoflurane. *Anesth Analg.* 1987;66:241; Fourcade HE, Stevens WC, Larson CP Jr, et al. The ventilatory effects of Forane, a new inhaled anesthetic. *Anesthesiology.* 1971;35:26; and Calverley RK, Smith NT, Jones CW, et al. Ventilatory and cardiovascular effects of enflurane anesthesia during spontaneous ventilation in man. *Anesth Analg.* 1978;57:610.)

resting P_aCO_2 decreases relative to equi-MAC concentrations of sevoflurane or desflurane in O_2.

Ventilatory Mechanics

FRC is decreased during general anesthesia; this has been explained by a number of mechanisms including a decrease in the intercostal muscle tone, alteration in diaphragm position, changes in thoracic blood volume, and the onset of phasic expiratory activity of respiratory muscles. About 40% of the muscular work of breathing is via intercostal muscles and about 60% is from the diaphragm. During anesthesia, the diaphragmatic muscle function is relatively spared when contrasted to the parasternal intercostal muscles. However, inspiratory rib cage expansion is reasonably well maintained during anesthesia because of preserved activity of the scalene muscles. Expiration is generally considered a passive function mediated by the elastic recoil of the lung. The process of applying a resistance or load to expiration typically results in a slowing of respiration, but under anesthesia, further responses include a substantial asynchrony of the thoracic movements with respiration. This suggests that in patients with pulmonary disease associated with increased expiratory resistance, the act of spontaneous ventilation during general anesthesia might be poorly tolerated.

Response to Carbon Dioxide and Hypoxemia

In conscious humans, the central chemoreceptors respond vigorously to changes in arterial carbon dioxide tension such that minute ventilation increases 3 L/min per a 1 mm Hg increase in P_aCO_2. All of the inhaled anesthetics produce a dose-dependent depression of the ventilatory response to hypercarbia (Fig. 17-25).

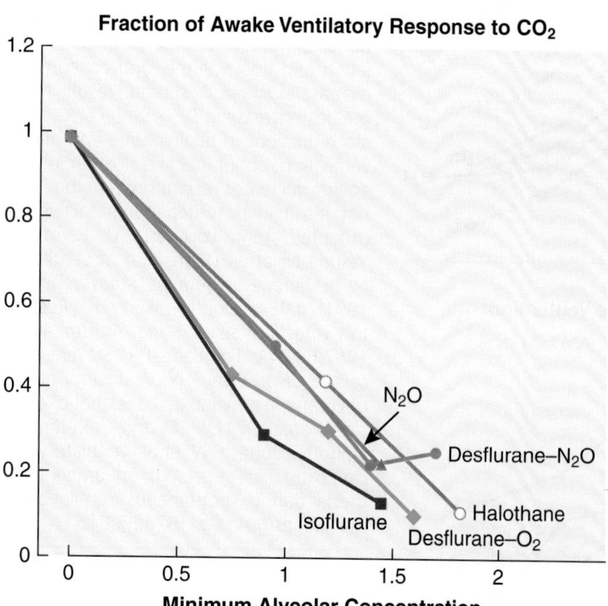

FIGURE 17-25. All inhaled anesthetics produce similar dose-dependent decreases in the ventilatory response to carbon dioxide (CO_2). N_2O, nitrous oxide. (Adapted from Eger EI 2nd. Desflurane. *Anesth Rev.* 1993; 20: 87; and Doi M, Ikeda K: Respiratory effects of sevoflurane. *Anesth Analg.* 1987;66: 241.)

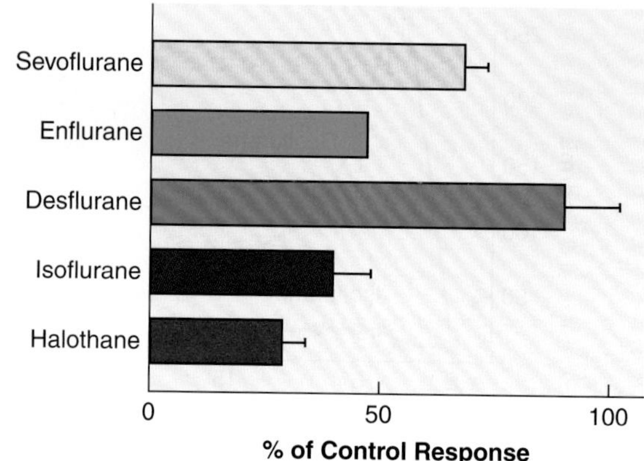

FIGURE 17-26. Influence of 0.1 minimum alveolar concentration (MAC) of five volatile anesthetic agents on the ventilatory response to a step decrease in end-tidal oxygen concentration. Values are mean ± SD. Subanesthetic concentrations of the volatile anesthetics, except desflurane and sevoflurane, profoundly depress the response to hypoxia. (Adapted from: Sarton E, Dahan A, Teppema L, et al. Acute pain and central nervous system arousal do not restore impaired hypoxic ventilatory responses during sevoflurane sedation. *Anesthesiology.* 1996;85:295.)

The addition of N_2O to a volatile anesthetic has been thought to diminish P_aCO_2 responses less than an equi-MAC dose of the anesthetic alone. The threshold where respiratory drive ceases is called the apneic threshold. It is generally 4 to 5 mm Hg below the prevailing resting P_aCO_2 in a spontaneously breathing patient. It is unrelated to the slope of the CO_2 response curves or to the level of the resting P_aCO_2. The clinical relevance of this threshold may be realized when assisting ventilation in an anesthetized patient who is breathing spontaneously. This only serves to lower the P_aCO_2 to approach that of the apneic threshold, therefore mandating more control of ventilation.

Inhaled anesthetics, including N_2O, also produce a dose-dependent attenuation of the ventilatory response to hypoxia. This action appears to depend on the peripheral chemoreceptors. In fact, even subanesthetic concentrations of volatile anesthetics (0.1 MAC) elicit anywhere from a 25% to 75% depression of the ventilatory drive to hypoxia (Fig. 17-26). The extreme sensitivity of the volatile anesthetics to inhibit ventilatory responses to hypoxia has important clinical implications, especially in patients who depend on hypoxic drive to set their level of ventilation, such as those with chronic respiratory failure or patients with obstructive sleep apnea. Residual effects of volatile anesthetics would be unwanted in the recovery room. In this regard, the short-acting anesthetics (sevoflurane and desflurane) may prove advantageous because of their more rapid washout and their minimal effect on hypoxic sensitivity at subanesthetic concentrations.

Bronchiolar Smooth Muscle Tone

Bronchoconstriction under anesthesia can result: (1) from direct stimulation of the laryngeal and tracheal areas, (2) from the administration of adjuvant drugs that cause histamine release, and (3) from noxious stimuli activating vagal afferent nerves. The reflex response to these stimuli may be greater in lightly versus

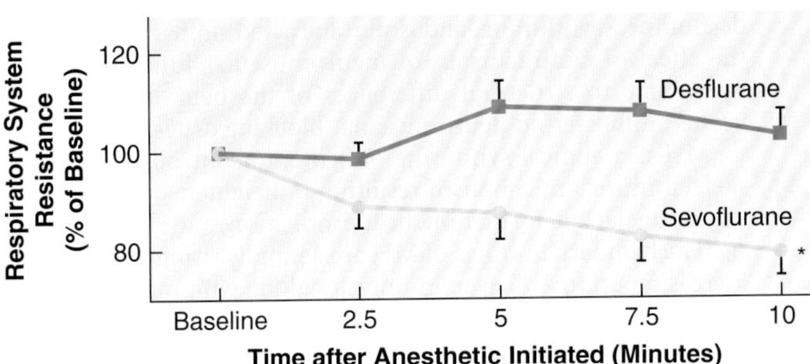

FIGURE 17-27. Changes in respiratory system resistance expressed as a percentage of the baseline recorded after tracheal intubation but prior to administration of sevoflurane or desflurane to the inspired gas mixture. Airway resistance responses to sevoflurane were significantly different from desflurane (* $p < 0.05$). (Adapted from: Goff MJ, Arain SR, Ficke DJ, et al. Absence of bronchodilation during desflurane anesthesia: A comparison to sevoflurane and thiopental. *Anesthesiology.* 2000;93:404.)

deeply anesthetized patients.[119] The response also is enhanced in patients with known reactive airway disease, including those requiring bronchodilator therapy or those with chronic smoking histories.

Airway smooth muscle extends as far distally as the terminal bronchioles and is under the influence of both parasympathetic and sympathetic nerves. The volatile anesthetics relax airway smooth muscle primarily by directly reducing smooth muscle tone and indirectly by inhibiting the reflex neural pathways.[120] Direct effects of the volatile anesthetics partially depend on an intact bronchial epithelium, suggesting that epithelial damage or inflammation secondary to asthma or a respiratory virus may lessen their bronchodilating effect.[121] In animal models studying 4th order bronchi, desflurane and sevoflurane were better bronchodilators than isoflurane.[121] The dilation was epithelium-dependent and mediated in part by a cyclooxygenase product and nitric oxide. In humans, early administration of desflurane after tracheal intubation and high concentrations (1.5 MAC) at steady state lessen the decrease in respiratory system resistance seen with sevoflurane (Fig. 17-27).[122,123] This may be attributed to a direct effect on bronchial smooth muscle from the pungency of desflurane. Volatile anesthetics have been used effectively to treat status asthmaticus when other conventional treatments have failed.[124,125]

Mucociliary Function

Ciliated respiratory epithelium extends from the trachea to the terminal bronchioles. Cells and glands in the tracheobronchial tree secrete mucus that captures surface particles for transport via ciliary action. There are a number of factors involved in diminished mucociliary function, particularly in the mechanically ventilated patient where dried, inspired gases impair ciliary movement, thicken the protective mucus, and reduce the ability of mucociliary function to transport surface particles out of the airway. Volatile anesthetics and N_2O reduce ciliary movement and alter the characteristics of mucus.[126] Smokers have impaired mucociliary function, and the combination of a volatile anesthetic in a smoker who is mechanically ventilated sets up a scenario for inadequate clearing of secretions, mucus plugging, atelectasis, and hypoxemia.

Pulmonary Vascular Resistance

Although systemic vascular smooth muscle is notably affected by the volatile anesthetics, the pulmonary vascular relaxation from clinically relevant concentrations of inhaled anesthetics is minimal. The small amount of pulmonary vasodilation from volatile anesthetics is offset by anesthetic-related decreases in cardiac output, resulting in little or no change in pulmonary artery pressures and pulmonary blood flow. Even N_2O, which has little effect on cardiac output and pulmonary blood flow, has at most a small effect to increase pulmonary vascular resistance. However, pulmonary vascular constriction from N_2O may be magnified in patients with resting pulmonary hypertension.[127]

Perhaps more important in terms of volatile anesthetics and pulmonary blood flow is their potential to attenuate hypoxic pulmonary vasoconstriction (HPV). During periods of hypoxemia, HPV reduces blood flow to underventilated areas of the lung, thereby diverting blood flow to areas of the lung with greater ventilation. The net effect is to improve the V/Q matching, resulting in a reduced amount of venous admixture and improved arterial oxygenation. Although all of the modern inhaled anesthetics in high concentrations have been shown to attenuate HPV in animal models, the situation is less clear in patient studies. This may reflect the multifactorial effects of the volatile anesthetics on factors involved in pulmonary blood flow, including their cardiovascular, autonomic, and humoral actions. Furthermore, nonpharmacologic variables impair HPV, including surgical trauma, temperature, pH, P_aCO_2, size of the hypoxic segment, and intensity of the hypoxic stimulus. One-lung ventilation (OLV) serves as a model where HPV should lessen the expected decrease in P_aO_2 and intrapulmonary shunt fraction (Qs/Qt). In patients undergoing OLV during thoracic surgery, volatile anesthetics have had minimal effects on P_aO_2 and Qs/Qt when changing from two-lung ventilation to OLV (Fig. 17-28).[128,129]

HEPATIC EFFECTS

12 Unlike most intravenous anesthetic drugs, modern-day volatile anesthetics undergo minimal liver metabolism, and because they are excreted primarily via the lungs, it is not surprising that they minimally affect hepatic function. The various factors that are known to affect drug metabolism, such as age, disease, genetics, and enzyme-inducing agents, have minor effects on the excretion of the volatile anesthetics.

There are two distinct mechanisms by which anesthetics have caused hepatitis; both discussed in Chapter 45 on hepatic anatomy function and physiology.

Another consideration is convincing evidence that volatile anesthetics can infer organ protection from ischemic injury (discussed earlier in the chapter). When sevoflurane was compared to propofol anesthesia in a prospective, randomized study of 320 patients undergoing CABG surgery, postoperative biochemical markers of hepatic dysfunction were lower after the sevoflurane-based anesthetic.[111]

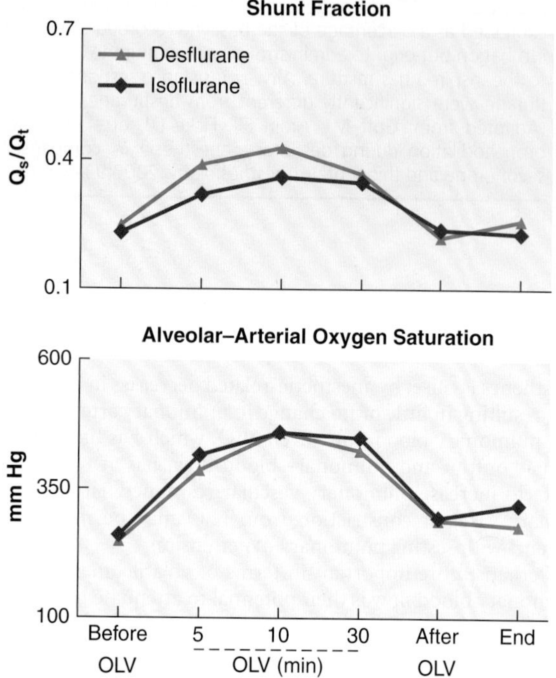

FIGURE 17-28. Shunt fraction **(top panel)** and the alveolar–arterial oxygen gradient **(bottom)** immediately before, during, and after one-lung ventilation (OLV) in patients anesthetized with desflurane or isoflurane. Data are means. (Adapted from: Pagel PS, Fu JL, Damask MC, et al. Desflurane and isoflurane produce similar alterations in systemic and pulmonary hemodynamics and arterial oxygenation in patients undergoing one-lung ventilation during thoracotomy. *Anesth Analg.* 1998;87:800.)

NEUROMUSCULAR SYSTEM AND MALIGNANT HYPERTHERMIA

The inhaled anesthetics have two important actions on neuromuscular function. They directly relax skeletal muscle and they potentiate the action of neuromuscular blocking drugs.[130,131] Nitrous oxide does not relax skeletal muscles. The direct effects of potent volatile anesthetics to relax skeletal muscle are most prominent above 1 MAC and an enhanced effect, by another 40% has been noted in patients with myasthenia gravis.[132]

Volatile anesthetic potentiation of neuromuscular blockade has been well documented. For example, the infusion rate of rocuronium required to maintain neuromuscular blockade is 30% to 40% less during isoflurane, desflurane, and sevoflurane compared with propofol.[133] A similar left shift in the dose-response relationship has been observed with cisatracurium during volatile anesthetic administration versus during intravenous anesthesia.[131] While the mechanism of volatile anesthetic potentiation of the neuromuscular blocking drugs is not entirely clear, it appears to be largely because of a postsynaptic effect at the nicotinic acetylcholine receptor located at the neuromuscular junction. Specifically, at the receptor level, the volatile anesthetics act synergistically with the neuromuscular blocking drugs to enhance their action.[134] The degree of enhancement is related to their aqueous concentration so that at equi-MAC concentrations, the less potent anesthetics (e.g., desflurane and sevoflurane vs. isoflurane) should have a greater inhibitory effect on neuromuscular transmission.[135] However, at equipotent concentrations, desflurane, sevoflurane, and isoflurane acted similarly to enhance the effect of cisatracurium on neuromuscular function.[131] This may relate to structural differences of the benzylisoquinolines versus aminosteroid neuromuscular blocking drugs.

MH is a clinical syndrome of acute, uncontrolled, increased
13 skeletal muscle metabolism resulting in heightened oxygen consumption, lactate formation, heat production, and rhabdomyolysis. The hallmark findings of MH are a rapidly rising temperature, increasing up to 1°C every 5 minutes along with increasing end-tidal CO_2, arrhythmias, and skeletal muscle rigidity. Susceptibility to MH is inherited and is transmitted as an autosomal dominant genetic disorder with reduced penetrance and variable expression. While N_2O and xenon are considered safe in MH-susceptible patients, all of the potent volatile anesthetics serve as triggers for MH in these patients.[136,137]

GENETIC EFFECTS, OBSTETRIC USE, AND EFFECTS ON FETAL DEVELOPMENT

The possibility of a health hazard from brief but chronic exposures to volatile anesthetics directly or as waste gases has been sought for several decades, and is probably nonexistent or at best minimal. The Ames test has been applied as a test for mutagenicity or carcinogenicity and has been negative for isoflurane, desflurane, sevoflurane, and N_2O. Genotoxicity can be inferred by demonstrating sister chromatid exchanges (SCE) in lymphocytes from peripheral blood. Desflurane but not sevoflurane transiently increased the frequency of SCE.[138,139] The clinical implications of these findings are not clear in relation to the negative Ames test. Nonetheless, the National Institute for Occupational Safety and Health has set exposure limits of 25 ppm for N_2O and 2 ppm for volatile anesthetics. Scavenging systems seem important in limiting anesthesia provider exposure. In a recent study evaluating anesthesia providers working in an unscavenged OR where average sevoflurane exposure was 9 ppm and N_2O exposure was 119 ppm, SCE were noted at nearly three times the control group, and the SCE effect was reversible after 2 months out of the OR.[140] In contrast, when a scavenging system was in place and exposures were limited to solely sevoflurane with a time weighted average of 0.2 ppm, only minor increases in SCE could be detected from lymphocytes.[141]

Volatile anesthetics can be teratogenic in animals,[142] but do not cause teratogenicity in humans. Mazze and Källén evaluated 5,405 surgeries in 2 million patients and found no increase in teratogenicity.[143] Nitrous oxide decreases the activity of vitamin B_{12}-dependent enzymes, methionine synthetase (MS) and thymidylate synthetase. The mechanism appears to be an irreversible oxidation of the cobalt atom of vitamin B_{12} by N_2O; for example, there is a 50% inactivation of MS after exposure to 46 minutes of 70% N_2O. This might affect the rapidly developing embryo/fetus because MS and thymidylate synthetase are involved in the formation of myelin and the formation of DNA, respectively. Megaloblastic changes in bone marrow are consistently observed in patients exposed to N_2O for 24 hours, and 4 days of exposure to N_2O has resulted in agranulocytosis. Furthermore, animals exposed to 15% N_2O for several weeks developed neurologic changes including spinal cord and peripheral nerve degeneration and ataxia. A sensory motor polyneuropathy that is often combined with signs of posterior lateral spinal cord degeneration has been described in humans who chronically inhale N_2O for recreational use.[144]

Uterine smooth muscle tone is diminished by volatile anesthetics in similar fashion to the effects of volatile anesthetics on vascular smooth muscle. There is a dose-dependent decrease in spontaneous myometrial contractility that is consistent among the volatile anesthetics. Desflurane and sevoflurane also inhibit the frequency and amplitude of myometrial contractions induced by oxytocin in a dose-dependent manner.[145] Uterine relaxation/atony can become problematic at concentrations of volatile anesthesia >1 MAC, and might delay the onset time of newborn respiration.[146] Consequently, a common technique used to provide general anesthesia for urgent cesarean sections is to administer low concentrations of the volatile anesthetic, such as 0.5 to 0.75 MAC, combined with N_2O. This decreases the likelihood of uterine atony and blood loss, especially at a time after delivery when oxytocin responsiveness of the uterus is essential. In some situations, uterine relaxation may be desirable, such as to remove a retained placenta. In this case, a brief, high concentration of a volatile anesthetic may be advantageous.

There has been an ongoing concern about the incidence of spontaneous abortions in operating room personnel chronically exposed to trace concentrations of inhaled anesthetics, especially N_2O.[147] Early epidemiologic studies suggested that operating room personnel had an increased incidence of spontaneous abortions and congenital abnormalities in offspring. However, subsequent analysis of the data suggests that inaccurate study design, confounding variables, and nonresponders might have led to flawed conclusions.[148] In prospective studies, no causal relationship has been shown between exposure to waste anesthetic gases and adverse health effects, regardless of the presence or absence of scavenging systems. Despite the unproven influence of trace concentrations of the volatile anesthetics on fetal development and spontaneous abortions, concerns for an adverse influence have resulted in the use of scavenging systems to remove anesthetic gases from the operating room and have led to the establishment of standards for waste gas exposure.

In terms of neonatal effects from general anesthesia, Apgar scores and acid–base balance are not affected by anesthetic technique, such as spinal versus general.[149] More sensitive measures of neurologic and behavioral function, such as the Scanlon Early Neonatal Neurobehavioral Scale and the Neurologic and Adaptive Capacities Score (NACS) indicate some transient depression of scores following general anesthesia that resolves at 24 hours after delivery.[149,150]

Neonatal brain development is a complicated yet intricate process of excess neuron generation followed by apoptosis (selective cell death). Recent studies have shown accelerated neuronal apoptosis in neonatal rat brains exposed to volatile anesthetics leading to behavioral anomalies. In a neonatal murine model, desflurane produced more neuroapoptosis than isoflurane and sevoflurane, and had a negative effect on working memory.[151] It is unclear if the findings in rodents can be extrapolated to humans, as the period of peak vulnerability with rapid synaptogenesis in rodents is very brief and easily exposed to an anesthetic. The equivalent period in humans extends from mid-gestation to several years after birth.[152,153]

ANESTHETIC DEGRADATION BY CARBON DIOXIDE ABSORBERS

Compound A

Sevoflurane undergoes base-catalyzed degradation in carbon dioxide absorbents to form a vinyl ether called *compound A*. The production of compound A is enhanced in low flow or closed circuit breathing systems and by warm or very dry CO_2 absorbents.[154,155]

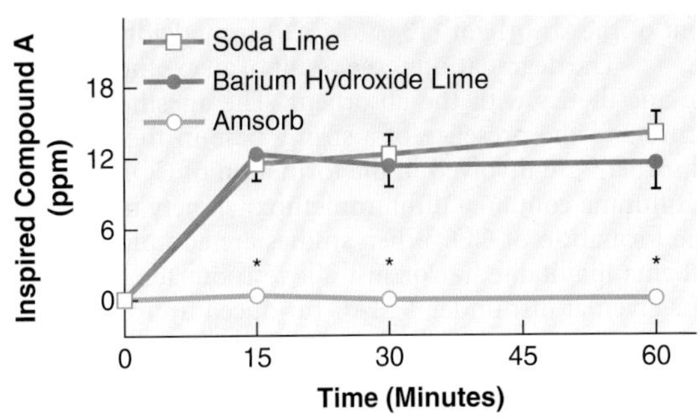

FIGURE 17-29. Compound A levels produced from three carbon dioxide absorbents during 1 minimum alveolar concentration sevoflurane anesthesia delivered to volunteers at 1 L/min fresh gas flow (mean ± SE). Gas samples were taken from the inspired limb of the anesthesia circuit. *Different from barium hydroxide lime or soda lime ($p < 0.05$). (Adapted from: Mchaourab A, Arain SR, Ebert TJ. Lack of degradation of sevoflurane by a new carbon dioxide absorbent in humans. *Anesthesiology.* 2001;94:1007.)

Barium hydroxide lime produces more compound A than soda lime and this can be attributed to slightly higher absorbent temperature during CO_2 extraction (Fig. 17-29).[156] Desiccated barium hydroxide lime also has been implicated in the heat and fires associated with sevoflurane, discussed later. This absorbent has been removed from the US market.

In patients and volunteers receiving sevoflurane in closed circuit or low-flow delivery systems, inspired compound A concentrations averaged 8 to 24 ppm and 20 to 32 ppm with soda lime and barium hydroxide lime, respectively.[157–160] Total exposures as high as 320 to 400 ppm·hr have had no clear effect on clinical markers of renal function.[161–163] In randomized and prospective volunteer and patient studies, no adverse renal effects from low-flow (0.5 to 1.0 L/min) or closed circuit sevoflurane anesthesia were detected using both standard clinical markers of renal function (serum creatinine and blood urea nitrogen concentrations) and experimental markers of renal function and structural integrity (proteinuria, glucosuria, and enzymuria).[158–160,162,164–166] In a prospective, multicenter, randomized study in patients with preexisting renal disease, there were no adverse renal effects of long duration, low-flow sevoflurane.[167,168] The majority of countries that have approved sevoflurane for clinical use have no flow restriction, perhaps because of the proven safety of sevoflurane in scientific studies. Pharmacovigilance supports the science; there has not been a single case report of renal injury directly attributable to sevoflurane after nearly two decades of use.

One explanation for the inconsistency between the early rat studies and human studies in terms of renal injury from compound A may be related to species differences in the metabolism of compound A. The biodegradation of compound A to cysteine conjugates and the further action of a renal enzyme called β-lyase on the conjugates can result in formation of a potentially toxic thiol. The β-lyase-dependent metabolism pathway in humans is far less extensive than the β-lyase pathway in rats (8–30 times less active).[169] Thus, compared with rats, humans (1) receive markedly lower doses of compound A, (2) metabolize a lower fraction of compound A via the renal β-lyase pathway, and (3) have not suffered renal injury.

Carbon Monoxide and Heat

14 Carbon dioxide (CO_2) absorbents degrade sevoflurane, desflurane, and isoflurane to carbon monoxide (CO) when the normal water

content of the absorbent (13% to 15%) is markedly decreased to <5%.[170–172] The degradation is the result of an exothermic reaction of the anesthetics with the absorbent. The anesthetic molecular structure and the presence of a strong base in the carbon dioxide absorbent are involved in the formation of CO.[171] Desflurane and isoflurane contain a difluoromethoxy moiety that is essential for the formation of CO. When studies are conducted with CO_2 absorbents maintained at or just above room temperature, desflurane given at just under 1 MAC produced up to 8,000 ppm of CO versus 79 ppm with nearly 2 MAC sevoflurane.[172] In desiccated barium hydroxide, CO production from desflurane was nearly threefold higher than with soda lime. In normal clinical use, CO_2 canister temperatures are 25°C to 45°C, but can be higher when employing a very low fresh gas flow. In a laboratory setting, when CO_2 canister temperature is not controlled and sevoflurane is administered to desiccated barium hydroxide, the exothermic reaction can substantially increase canister temperatures. If the canister temperature exceeds 80°C, significant CO production is noted with sevoflurane.[170] Instances of CO poisoning of patients have been reported in situations where the CO_2 absorbent has been presumably desiccated because an anesthetic machine had been left on with a high fresh gas flow passing through the CO_2 absorbent over an extended period of time.[173–176] In an experimental setting, overnight drying of barium hydroxide for 14 hours at 10 L/min fresh gas flow did not result in significant CO production from desflurane, whereas 24 to 66 hours of fresh gas flow drying produced significant CO production.[177]

Although desflurane produces the most CO with desiccated CO_2 absorbers, the reaction with sevoflurane produces the most heat.[178] The strong exothermic reaction has caused significant heat production, fires, and patient injuries.[179–181] Although sevoflurane is not flammable at <11%, formaldehyde, methanol, and formate have been identified,[182] and these alone or in combination with oxygen might be flammable at high canister temperatures. In experimental settings, long exposure of 1 MAC sevoflurane to desiccated barium hydroxide resulted in canister temperatures in excess of 300°C, which can be associated with smoldering, melting of plastic components, explosions, and fires.[170] Barium hydroxide has been removed from the US market.

There are newer CO_2 absorbents that do not degrade anesthetics (to either compound A or CO), and they should reduce exothermic reactions. "From a patient safety perspective, widespread adoption of a nondestructive CO_2 absorbent should be axiomatic."[183] Although the cost of these new CO_2 absorbents, Amsorb Plus (Armstrong Medical, Coleraine, UK) and DrägerSorb Free (Dräger, Lübek, Germany), is higher and the absorptive capacity may be lower than either barium hydroxide lime or soda lime, their benefit may be substantial. The use of a nondestructive absorbent eliminates all of the potential complications related to anesthetic breakdown and therefore minimizes the possibility of additional costs from those complications, including additional laboratory tests, hospital days, and medical/legal expenses. Adoption of these new absorbents into routine clinical practice is consistent with the patient safety goals of our anesthesia society.

Generic Sevoflurane Formulations

Generic formulations of sevoflurane were introduced into the clinical market in 2006. The methods for synthesizing sevoflurane differ between manufacturers.[184] Although the active ingredient of sevoflurane from different manufacturers is chemically equivalent, the water content in the formulations differs and this accounts for their different resistances to degradation to hydrogen fluoride when exposed to a Lewis acid (metal halides and metal oxides that are present in modern-day vaporizers). Adding water to the formulation inhibits the action of Lewis acids to degrade sevoflurane to hydrogen fluoride. The formulation of Abbott Labs was changed to contain 300 to 400 ppm of water, based on an early adverse experience with hydrogen fluoride formation from a lower water formulation in 1996. One generic formulation with a low water content has been shown in clinical and laboratory studies to degrade to toxic and corrosive hydrogen fluoride.[185] One report indicates that the Penlon Sigma Delta sevoflurane vaporizer can degrade a low-water formulation of sevoflurane, resulting in etching of the sight glass and corrosion of the plastic on the vaporizer and discoloration of the anesthetic.[186] Whether these differences in formulation lead to patient safety issues remains to be seen.

ANESTHETIC METABOLISM

Fluoride-induced Nephrotoxicity

The metabolism of enflurane can result in a well-described injury to renal collecting tubules.[187,188] The nephrotoxicity presents as a high-output renal insufficiency that is unresponsive to vasopressin and is characterized by dilute polyuria, dehydration, serum hypernatremia, hyperosmolality, elevated blood urea nitrogen, and creatinine. An association between increased plasma fluoride concentrations and metabolism led to a "fluoride hypothesis." This hypothesis has been reexamined recently in part because sevoflurane undergoes 5% metabolism leading to transient increases in serum fluoride concentrations without a renal-concentrating defect. The traditional hypothesis stated that both the duration of the high systemic fluoride concentrations (area under the fluoride-time curve) and the peak fluoride concentration (peaks above 50 μM appear to represent the toxic threshold) were related to nephrotoxicity (Fig. 17-30). The safety of sevoflurane with regard to fluoride concentrations may be the result of a rapid decline in plasma fluoride concentrations because of less availability of the anesthetic for metabolism from a faster washout compared with enflurane.[189] In addition, the potential for toxicity from relatively high plasma levels of fluoride following long exposure to sevoflurane is offset by the minimal amount of renal defluorination and this may explain its relative absence of renal-concentrating defects.[190]

CLINICAL UTILITY OF VOLATILE ANESTHETICS

For Induction of Anesthesia

The appeal of mask induction in the adult population centers on the potential safety and utility of this technique.[191–193] Sevoflurane is potent, poorly soluble in blood, nonpungent, and therefore inhaled easily. Spontaneous ventilation is preserved with a gas induction since patients essentially regulate their own depth of anesthesia (too much sevoflurane would suppress ventilation). Clinical studies indicate that stage two excitation is avoided with high concentrations of sevoflurane. The typical time to loss of consciousness is 60 seconds when delivering 8% sevoflurane via the face mask. Sevoflurane also has been administered by mask as an approach to the difficult adult airway because it preserves spontaneous ventilation and does not cause salivation.[194]

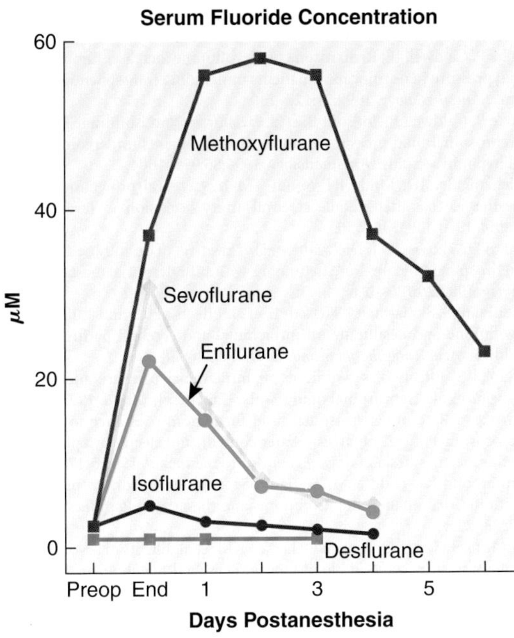

FIGURE 17-30. Plasma inorganic fluoride concentrations (mean ± SE) before and after 2 to 4 hours of methoxyflurane, enflurane, sevoflurane, isoflurane, and desflurane anesthesia. (Adapted from: Kharasch ED, Armstrong AS, Gunn K, et al. Clinical sevoflurane metabolism and disposition. II. The role of cytochrome P450 2E1 in fluoride and hexafluoroisopropanol formation. *Anesthesiology.* 1995;82:1379; Mazze RI. Metabolism of the inhaled anaesthetics: Implications of enzyme induction. *Br J Anaesth.* 1984;56:27S; and Sutton TS, Koblin DD, Gruenke LD, et al. Fluoride metabolites after prolonged exposure of volunteers and patients to desflurane. *Anesth Analg.* 1991;73:180.)

Laryngeal mask placement can be successfully achieved 2 minutes after administering 7% sevoflurane via the face mask.[193] The addition of N_2O to the inspired gas mixture does not add significantly to the induction sequence. The gas induction technique is improved by pretreatment with benzodiazepines and worsened with opioid pretreatment because of apnea.[192] Importantly, patient acceptance of this technique has been relatively high, exceeding 90%.[191]

For Maintenance of Anesthesia

The volatile anesthetics are clearly the most popular drug used to maintain anesthesia. They are easily administered via inhalation, they are readily titrated, they have a high safety ratio in terms of preventing recall, and the depth of anesthesia can be quickly adjusted in a predictable way while monitoring tissue levels via end-tidal concentrations. They are effective regardless of age or body habitus. They have some properties that prove beneficial in the operating room, including relaxation of skeletal muscle, preservation of cardiac output and cerebral blood flow, relatively predictable recovery profiles, and organ protection from ischemic injury. Some of the drawbacks to the use of the current volatile anesthetics are their absence of analgesic effects, their association with postoperative nausea and vomiting, their potential for carbon monoxide poisoning and hepatitis, their ability to induce neuroapoptosis leading to memory deficits in neonatal animal models, and their greenhouse gas effects adding to the potential for global warming.[195–197]

PHARMACOECONOMICS AND VALUE-BASED DECISIONS

In the current environment of cost containment, clinicians are constantly being pressured to use less expensive drugs, including volatile anesthetics. In terms of efficacy, all of the volatile anesthetics are reasonably similar; that is, they can be used to establish a state of anesthesia for surgical interventions and can be easily reversed. A common side effect of the volatile anesthetics is nausea and vomiting. The need for rescue medications to treat nausea and vomiting after volatile anesthesia needs to be considered in any legitimate cost analysis. Direct costs are not simply the cost per milliliter of liquid or cost per bottle of anesthetic. Rather, they reflect the combination of the potency of the drug to establish a MAC level, the fresh gas flow, and the cost of the anesthetic. Sevoflurane, isoflurane, and most recently, desflurane are generic products. Competition between manufacturers will drive down costs per bottle and costs per MAC-hr of use. The indirect costs are probably the most difficult to pinpoint, but may be the most important when evaluating the cost of using the new volatile anesthetics. Examples of indirect costs include costs associated with operating room time, time in the postanesthesia care unit versus bypassing the postanesthesia care unit to a step-down unit, labor costs, and outcome-related costs, such as time to resume normal activities.

One of the arguments for using sevoflurane and desflurane has been their relative speed in terms of emergence from anesthesia. This argument has been tempered somewhat by the basic knowledge that downward titration of volatile anesthetics can speed emergence times. Even the more soluble drug, isoflurane, can be titrated downward guided by clinical experience and/or a processed EEG monitor, permitting fast wake-ups regardless of the choice of anesthetic agent. However, there is strong evidence to support the use of the less-soluble (but more expensive) drugs in the longest surgical cases (Fig. 17-31).[198] In these cases the high direct cost of the anesthetic is balanced by the much improved recovery profile including a more rapid time to emergence and a more rapid discharge from the recovery room.

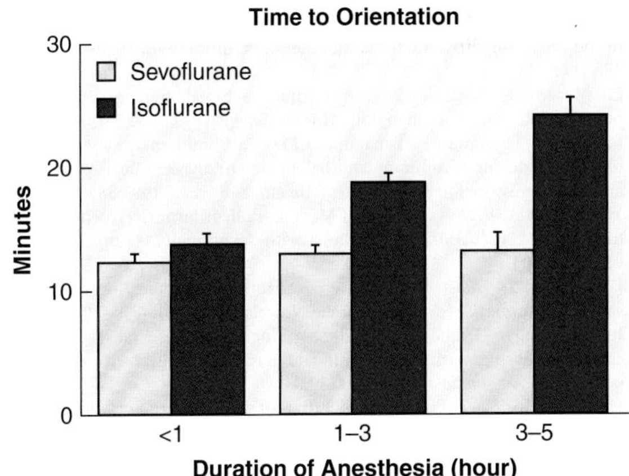

FIGURE 17-31. The recovery times to orientation after anesthesia of varying durations. With the less soluble anesthetic sevoflurane, the time to orientation was independent of the anesthetic duration. In contrast, long anesthetic durations with isoflurane were associated with delayed times to orientation. (Adapted from: Ebert TJ, Robinson BJ, Uhrich TD, et al. Recovery from sevoflurane anesthesia: A comparison to isoflurane and propofol anesthesia. *Anesthesiology.* 1998;89:1524.)

References

1. Kety SS. The physiological and physical factors governing the uptake of anesthetic gases by the body. *Anesthesiology.* 1950;11:517–526.
2. Eger EI. *Anesthetic Uptake and Action.* Baltimore: Williams & Wilkins; 1974:371.
3. Ebert TJ, Robinson BJ, Uhrich TD, et al. Recovery from sevoflurane anesthesia: A comparison to isoflurane and propofol anesthesia. *Anesthesiology.* 1998;89:1524–1531.
4. McKay RE, Malhotra A, Cakmakkaya OS, et al. Effect of increased body mass index and anaesthetic duration on recovery of protective airway reflexes after sevoflurane vs desflurane. *Br J Anaesth.* 2010;104:175–182.
5. Hettrick DA, Pagel PS, Kersten JR, et al. Cardiovascular effects of xenon in isoflurane-anesthetized dogs with dilated cardiomyopathy. *Anesthesiology.* 1998; 89:1166–1173.
6. Nakata Y, Goto T, Morita S. Comparison of inhalation inductions with xenon and sevoflurane. *Acta Anaesthesiol Scand.* 1997;41:1157–1161.
7. Goto T, Suwa K, Uezono S, et al. The blood-gas partition coefficient of xenon may be lower than generally accepted. *Br J Anaesth.* 1998;80:255–256.
8. Schaefer W, Meyer PT, Rossaint R, et al. Myocardial blood flow during general anesthesia with xenon in humans: A positron emission tomography study. *Anesthesiology.* 2011;114:1373–1379.
9. Kaplan R, Abramowitz MD, Epstein BS. Nitrous oxide and air-filled balloon-tipped catheters. *Anesthesiology.* 1981;55:71–73.
10. Stanley TH, Kawamura R, Graves C. Effects of nitrous oxide on volume and pressure of endotracheal tube cuffs. *Anesthesiology.* 1974;41:256–262.
11. Waun JE, Sweitzer RS, Hamilton WK. Effect of nitrous oxide on middle ear mechanics and hearing acuity. *Anesthesiology.* 1967;28:846–850.
12. Tinker JH, Sharbrough FW, Michenfelder JD. Anterior shift of the dominant EEG rhythm during anesthesia in the Java monkey: Correlation with anesthetic potency. *Anesthesiology.* 1977;46:252–259.
13. Gross JB, Alexander CM. Awakening concentrations of isoflurane are not affected by analgesic doses of morphine. *Anesth Analg.* 1988;67:27–30.
14. Katoh T, Suguro Y, Kimura T, et al. Cerebral awakening concentration of sevoflurane and isoflurane predicted during slow and fast alveolar washout. *Anesth Analg.* 1993;77:1012–1017.
15. Roizen MF, Horrigan RW, Frazer BM. Anesthetic doses blocking adrenergic (stress) and cardiovascular responses to incision–MAC BAR. *Anesthesiology.* 1981; 54:390–398.
16. Liem EB, Lin C, Suleman M, et al. Anesthetic requirement is increased in redheads. *Anesthesiology.* 2004;101:279–283.
17. Mogil JS, Wilson SG, Chesler EJ, et al. The nelanocortin-1 receptor gene mediates female-specific mechanisms of analgesia in mice and humans. *Proc Natl Acad Sci U S A.* 2003;100:4867–4872.
18. Stekiel TA, Contney SJ, Bosnjak ZJ, et al. Reversal of minimum alveolar concentrations of volatile anesthetics by chromosomal substitution. *Anesthesiology.* 2004;101:796–798.
19. LeDez KM, Lerman J. The minimum alveolar concentration (MAC) of isoflurane in preterm neonates. *Anesthesiology.* 1987;67:301–307.
20. Mapleson WW. Effect of age on MAC in humans: A meta-analysis. *Br J Anaesth.* 1996;76:179–185.
21. Smith AL, Wollman H. Cerebral blood flow and metabolism: Effects of anesthetic drugs and techniques. *Anesthesiology.* 1972;36:378–400.
22. Scheller MS, Nakakimura K, Fleischer JE, et al. Cerebral effects of sevoflurane in the dog: Comparison with isoflurane and enflurane. *Br J Anaesth.* 1990;65: 388–392.
23. Lutz LJ, Milde JH, Milde LN. The cerebral functional, metabolic, and hemodynamic effects of desflurane in dogs. *Anesthesiology.* 1990;73:125–131.
24. Fujibayashi T, Sugiura Y, Yanagimoto M, et al. Brain energy metabolism and blood flow during sevoflurane and halothane anesthesia: Effects of hypocapnia and blood pressure fluctuations. *Acta Anaesthesiol Scand.* 1994;38:413–418.
25. Yli-Hankala A, Vakkuri A, Särkelä M, et al. Epileptiform electroencephalogram during mask induction of anesthesia with sevoflurane. *Anesthesiology.* 1999; 91:1596–1603.
26. Jääskeläinen SK, Kaisti K, Suni L, et al. Sevoflurane is epileptogenic in healthy subjects at surgical levels of anesthesia. *Neurology.* 2003;61:1073–1078.
27. Julliac B, Guehl D, Chopin F, et al. Sharp increase in cerebral sevoflurane concentration during mask induction in adults is a major risk factor of spike wave occurrence. *Anesthesiology.* 2004:A-132.
28. Hisada K, Morioka T, Fukui K, et al. Effects of sevoflurane and isoflurane on electrocorticographic activities in patients with temporal lobe epilepsy. *J Neurosurg Anesthesiol.* 2001;13:333–337.
29. Algotsson L, Messeter K, Nordström CH, et al. Cerebral blood flow and oxygen consumption during isoflurane and halothane anesthesia in man. *Acta Anaesthesiol Scand.* 1988;32:15–20.
30. Lutz LJ, Milde JH, Milde LN. The response of the canine cerebral circulation to hyperventilation during anesthesia with desflurane. *Anesthesiology.* 1991;74: 504–507.
31. Adams RW, Cucchiara RF, Gronert GA, et al. Isoflurane and cerebrospinal fluid pressure in neurosurgical patients. *Anesthesiology.* 1981;54:97–99.
32. Grosslight K, Foster R, Colohan AR, et al. Isoflurane for neuroanesthesia: Risk factors for increases in intracranial pressure. *Anesthesiology.* 1985;63:533–536.
33. Artru AA. Isoflurane does not increase the rate of CSF production in the dog. *Anesthesiology.* 1984;60:193–197.
34. Talke P, Caldwell JE, Richardson CA. Sevoflurane increases lumbar cerebrospinal fluid pressure in normocapnic patients undergoing transsphenoidal hypophysectomy. *Anesthesiology.* 1999;91:127–130.
35. Talke P, Caldwell J, Dodsont B, et al. Desflurane and isoflurane increases lumbar cerebrospinal fluid pressure in normocapnic patients undergoing transsphenoidal hypophysectomy. *Anesthesiology.* 1996;85:999–1004.
36. Michenfelder JD, Milde JH, Sundt TM Jr. Cerebral protection by barbiturate anesthesia. Use after middle cerebral artery occlusion in Java monkeys. *Arch Neurol.* 1976:33: 3345–350.
37. Muzzi DA, Losasso TJ, Dietz NM, et al. The effect of desflurane and isoflurane on cerebrospinal fluid pressure in humans with supratentorial mass lesions. *Anesthesiology.* 1992;76:720–724.
38. Sponheim S, Skraastad Ø, Helseth E, et al. Effects of 0.5 and 1.0 MAC isoflurane, sevoflurane and desflurane on intracranial and cerebral perfusion pressures in children. *Acta Anaesthesiol Scand.* 2003;47:932–938.
39. Sugioka S. Effects of sevoflurane on intracranial pressure and formation and absorption of cerebrospinal fluid in cats. [Japanese]. *Masui.* 1992;41:1434–1442.
40. Artru AA. Rate of cerebrospinal fluid formation, resistance to reabsorption of cerebrospinal fluid, brain tissue water content, and electroencephalogram during desflurane anesthesia in dogs. *J Neurosurg Anesthesiol.* 1993;5:178–186.
41. Drummond JC, Todd MM, Toutant SM, et al. Brain surface protrusion during enflurane, halothane, and isoflurane anesthesia in cats. *Anesthesiology.* 1983; 59:288–293.
42. Bundgaard H, von Oettingen G, Larsen KM, et al. Effects of sevoflurane on intracranial pressure, cerebral blood flow and cerebral metabolism. *Acta Anaesthesiol Scand.* 1998;42:621–627.
43. Seyde WC, Longnecker DE. Cerebral oxygen tension in rats during deliberate hypotension with sodium nitroprusside, 2-chloroadenosine, or deep isoflurane anesthesia. *Anesthesiology.* 1986;64:480–485.
44. Engelhard K, Werner C, Reeker W, et al. Desflurane and isoflurane improve neurological outcome after incomplete cerebral ischaemia in rats. *Br J Anaesth.* 1999;83:415–421.
45. Werner C, Möllenberg O, Kochs E, et al. Sevoflurane improves neurological outcome after incomplete cerebral ischaemia in rats. *Br J Anaesth.* 1995;75:756–760.
46. Loepke AW, Priestley MA, Schultz SE, et al. Desflurane improves neurologic outcome after low-flow cardiopulmonary bypass in newborn pigs. *Anesthesiology.* 2002;97:1521–1527.
47. Hoffman WE, Charbel FT, Edelman G, et al. Thiopental and desflurane treatment for brain protection. *Neurosurgery.* 1998;43:1050–1053.
48. Engelhard K, Werner C. Postoperative cognitive dysfunction. *Anaesthesist.* 2005; 54:588–594.
49. Kanbak M, Saricaoglu F, Akinci SB, et al. The effects of isoflurane, sevoflurane, and desflurane anesthesia on neurocognitive outcome after cardiac surgery: A pilot study. *Heart Surg Forum.* 2007;10:E36–E41.
50. Tsai SK, Lee C, Kwan W, et al. Recovery of cognitive functions after anaesthesia with desflurane or isoflurane and nitrous oxide. *Br J Anaesth.* 1992;69:255–258.
51. Schwender D, End H, Daunderer M, et al. Sevoflurane and the nervous system. *Anaesthesist.* 1998;47(suppl 1):S37–S42.
52. el-Dawlatly AA. Sevoflurane vs isoflurane anaesthesia: A study of postoperative mental concentration and fine motor movements. *Middle East J Anesthesiol.* 2002;16:397–404.
53. Loscar M, Allhoff T, Ott E, et al. Awakening from anesthesia and recovery of cognitive function after desflurane or isoflurane. *Anaesthesist.* 1996;45:140–145.
54. Chen X, Zhao M, White PF, et al. The recovery of cognitive function after general anesthesia in elderly patients: A comparison of desflurane and sevoflurane. *Anesth Analg.* 2001;93:1489–1494.
55. Arain SR, Barth CD, Shankar H, et al. Choice of volatile anesthetic for the morbidly obese patient: Sevoflurane or desflurane. *J Clin Anesth.* 2005;17:413–419.
56. Dupont J, Tavernier B, Ghosez Y, et al. Recovery after anaesthesia for pulmonary surgery: Desflurane, sevoflurane and isoflurane. *Br J Anaesth.* 1999;82:355–359.
57. Mahajan VA, Ni Chonghaile M, Bokhari SA, et al. Recovery of older patients undergoing ambulatory anaesthesia with isoflurane or sevoflurane. *Eur J Anaesthesiol.* 2007;24:505–510.
58. Mahoney FC, Moore PA, Baker EL, et al. Experimental nitrous oxide exposure as a model system for evaluating neurobehavioral tests. *Toxicology.* 1988;49:449–457.
59. Leung JM, Sands LP, Vaurio LE, et al. Nitrous oxide does not change the incidence of postoperative delirium or cognitive decline in elderly surgical patients. *Br J Anaesth.* 2006;96:754–760.
60. El Otmani H, El Moutawakil B, Moutaouakil F, et al. Postoperative dementia: Toxicity of nitrous oxide. *Encephale.* 2007;33:95–97.
61. Sakabe T, Tsutsui T, Maekawa T, et al. Local cerebral glucose utilization during nitrous oxide and pentobarbital anesthesia in rats. *Anesthesiology.* 1985;63:262–266.
62. Fleischer JE, Milde JH, Moyer TP, et al. Cerebral effects of high-dose midazolam and subsequent reversal with Ro 15–1788 in dogs. *Anesthesiology.* 1988;68:234–242.
63. Hoffman WE, Miletich DJ, Albrecht RF. The effects of midazolam on cerebral blood flow and oxygen consumption and its interaction with nitrous oxide. *Anesth Analg.* 1986;65:729–733.
64. Hartung J, Cottrell JE. Nitrous oxide reduces thiopental-induced prolongation of survival in hypoxic and anoxic mice. *Anesth Analg.* 1987:66: 47–52.

65. Ebert TJ, Kampine JP. Nitrous oxide augments sympathetic outflow: Direct evidence from human peroneal nerve recordings. *Anesth Analg.* 1989;69:444–449.
66. Ebert TJ, Muzi M, Lopatka CW. Neurocirculatory responses to sevoflurane in humans. A comparison to desflurane. *Anesthesiology.* 1995;83:88–95.
67. Malan TP Jr, DiNardo JA, Isner RJ, et al. Cardiovascular effects of sevoflurane compared with those of isoflurane in volunteers. *Anesthesiology.* 1995;83:918–928.
68. Weiskopf RB, Cahalan MK, Eger EI 2nd, et al. Cardiovascular actions of desflurane in normocarbic volunteers. *Anesth Analg.* 1991;73:143–156.
69. Stevens WC, Cromwell TH, Halsey MJ, et al. The cardiovascular effects of a new inhalation anesthetic, Forane, in human volunteers at a constant arterial carbon dioxide tension. *Anesthesiology.* 1971;35:8–16.
70. Calverley RK, Smith NT, Prys-Roberts C, et al. Cardiovascular effects of enflurane anesthesia during controlled ventilation in man. *Anesth Analg.* 1978;57:619–628.
71. Ebert TJ, Muzi M. Sympathetic hyperactivity during desflurane anesthesia in healthy volunteers. A comparison with isoflurane. *Anesthesiology.* 1993;79:444–453.
72. Weiskopf RB, Moore MA, Eger EI 2nd, et al. Rapid increase in desflurane concentration is associated with greater transient cardiovascular stimulation than with rapid increase in isoflurane concentration in humans. *Anesthesiology.* 1994;80:1035–1045.
73. Muzi M, Ebert TJ, Hope WG, et al. Site(s) mediating sympathetic activation with desflurane. *Anesthesiology.* 1996;85:737–747.
74. Weiskopf RB, Eger EI 2nd, Noorani M, et al. Fentanyl, esmolol, and clonidine blunt the transient cardiovascular stimulation induced by desflurane in humans. *Anesthesiology.* 1994;81:1350–1355.
75. Yonker-Sell AE, Muzi M, Hope WG, et al. Alfentanil modifies the neurocirculatory responses to desflurane. *Anesth Analg.* 1996;82:162–166.
76. Pacentine GG, Muzi M, Ebert TJ. Effects of fentanyl on sympathetic activation associated with the administration of desflurane. *Anesthesiology.* 1995;82:823–831.
77. De Hert SG, Van der Linden PJ, ten Broecke PW, et al. Effects of desflurane and sevoflurane on length-dependent regulation of myocardial function in coronary surgery patients. *Anesthesiology.* 2001;95:357–363.
78. De Hert SG, Cromheecke S, ten Broecke PW, et al. Effects of propofol, desflurane, and sevoflurane on recovery of myocardial function after coronary surgery in elderly high-risk patients. *Anesthesiology.* 2003;99:314–323.
79. Weiskopf RB, Cahalan MK, Ionescu P, et al. Cardiovascular actions of desflurane with and without nitrous oxide during spontaneous ventilation in humans. *Anesth Analg.* 1991;73:165–174.
80. Cahalan MK, Weiskopf RB, Eger EI 2nd, et al. Hemodynamic effects of desflurane/nitrous oxide anesthesia in volunteers. *Anesth Analg.* 1991;73:157–164.
81. Theye RA, Michenfelder JD. Whole-body and organ VO2 changes with enflurane, isoflurane, and halothane. *Br J Anaesth.* 1975;47:813–817.
82. Crawford MW, Lerman J, Saldivia V, et al. Hemodynamic and organ blood flow responses to halothane and sevoflurane anesthesia during spontaneous ventilation. *Anesth Analg.* 1992;75:1000–1006.
83. Ebert TJ, Harkin CP, Muzi M. Cardiovascular responses to sevoflurane: A review. *Anesth Analg.* 1995;81:S11–S22.
84. Atlee JL 3rd, Bosnjak ZJ. Mechanisms for cardiac dysrhythmias during anesthesia. *Anesthesiology.* 1990;72:347–374.
85. Bosnjak ZJ, Kampine JP. Effects of halothane, enflurane, and isoflurane on the SA node. *Anesthesiology.* 1983;58:314–321.
86. Saussine M, Massad I, Raczka F, et al. Torsade de pointes during sevoflurane anesthesia in a child with congenital long QT syndrome. *Paediatr Anaesth.* 2006;16:63–65.
87. Aypar E, Karagoz AH, Ozer S, et al. The effects of sevoflurane and desflurane anesthesia on QTc interval and cardiac rhythm in children. *Paediatr Anaesth.* 2007;17:563–567.
88. Kazanci D, Unver S, Karadeniz U, et al. A comparison of the effects of desflurane, sevoflurane and propofol on QT, QTc, and P dispersion on ECG. *Ann Card Anaesth.* 2009;12:107–112.
89. Slogoff S, Keats AS, Dear WE, et al. Steal-prone coronary anatomy and myocardial ischemia associated with four primary anesthetic agents in humans. *Anesth Analg.* 1991;72:22–27.
90. O'Young J, Mastrocostopoulos G, Hilgenberg A, et al. Myocardial circulatory and metabolic effects of isoflurane and sufentanil during coronary artery surgery. *Anesthesiology.* 1987;66:653–658.
91. Tuman KJ, McCarthy RJ, Spiess BD, et al. Does choice of anesthetic agent significantly affect outcome after coronary artery surgery? *Anesthesiology.* 1989;70:189–198.
92. Hartman JC, Pagel PS, Kampine JP, et al. Influence of desflurane on regional distribution of coronary blood flow in a chronically instrumented canine model of multivessel coronary artery obstruction. *Anesth Analg.* 1991;72:289–299.
93. Hartman JC, Kampine JP, Schmeling WT, et al. Steal-prone coronary circulation in chronically instrumented dogs: Isoflurane versus adenosine. *Anesthesiology.* 1991;74:744–756.
94. Kersten JR, Brayer AP, Pagel PS, et al. Perfusion of ischemic myocardium during anesthesia with sevoflurane. *Anesthesiology.* 1994;81:995–1004.
95. Harkin CP, Pagel PS, Kersten JR, et al. Direct negative inotropic and lusitropic effects of sevoflurane. *Anesthesiology.* 1994;81:156–167.
96. Ebert TJ, Kharasch ED, Rooke GA, et al. Myocardial ischemia and adverse cardiac outcomes in cardiac patients undergoing noncardiac surgery with sevoflurane and isoflurane. Sevoflurane Ischemia Study Group. *Anesth Analg.* 1997;85:993–999.
97. Searle NR, Martineau RJ, Conzen P, et al. Comparison of sevoflurane/fentanyl and isoflurane/fentanyl during elective coronary artery bypass surgery. *Can J Anaesth.* 1996;43:890–899.
98. Thomson IR, Bowering JB, Hudson RJ, et al. A comparison of desflurane and isoflurane in patients undergoing coronary artery surgery. *Anesthesiology.* 1991;75:776–781.
99. Helman JD, Leung JM, Bellows WH, et al. The risk of myocardial ischemia in patients receiving desflurane versus sufentanil anesthesia for coronary artery bypass graft surgery. The S.P.I. Research Group. *Anesthesiology.* 1992;77:47–62.
100. Riess ML, Stowe DF, Warltier DC. Cardiac pharmacological preconditioning with volatile anesthetics: From bench to bedside? *Am J Physiol Heart Circ Physiol.* 2004;286:H1603–H1607.
101. Stowe DF, Kevin LG. Cardiac preconditioning by volatile anesthetic agents: A defining role for altered mitochondrial bioenergetics. *Antioxid Redox Signal.* 2004;6:439–448.
102. Novalija E, Kevin LG, Camara AK, et al. Reactive oxygen species precede the epsilon isoform of protein kinase C in the anesthetic preconditioning signaling cascade. *Anesthesiology.* 2003;99:421–428.
103. Kwok WM, Martinelli AT, Fujimoto K, et al. Differential modulation of the cardiac adenosine triphosphate-sensitive potassium channel by isoflurane and halothane. *Anesthesiology.* 2002;97:50–56.
104. Kevin LG, Katz P, Camara AK, et al. Anesthetic preconditioning: Effects on latency to ischemic injury in isolated hearts. *Anesthesiology.* 2003;99:385–391.
105. De Hert SG, Turani F, Mathur S, et al. Cardioprotection with volatile anesthetics: Mechanisms and clinical implications. *Anesth Analg.* 2005;100:1584–1593.
106. Yu CH, Beattie WS. The effects of volatile anesthetics on cardiac ischemic complications and mortality in CABG: A meta-analysis. *Can J Anaesth.* 2006;53:906–918.
107. Landoni G, Biondi-Zoccai GG, Zangrillo A, et al. Desflurane and sevoflurane in cardiac surgery: A meta-analysis of randomized clinical trials. *J Cardiothorac Vasc Anesth.* 2007;21:502–511.
108. Gu W, Pagel PS, Warltier DC, et al. Modifying cardiovascular risk in diabetes mellitus. *Anesthesiology.* 2003;98:774–779.
109. Clarkson AN. Anesthetic-mediated protection/preconditioning during cerebral ischemia. *Life Sci.* 2007;80:1157–1175.
110. Lee HT, Ota-Setlik A, Fu Y, et al. Differential protective effects of volatile anesthetics against renal ischemia-reperfusion injury in vivo. *Anesthesiology.* 2004;101:1313–1324.
111. Lorsomradee S, Cromheecke S, Lorsomradee S, et al. Effects of sevoflurane on biomechanical markers of hepatic and renal dysfunction after coronary artery surgery. *J Cardiothorac Vasc Anesth.* 2006;20:684–690.
112. Ma D, Lim T, Xu J, et al. Xenon preconditioning protects against renal ischemic-reperfusion injury via HIF-1alpha activation. *J Am Soc Nephrol.* 2009;20:713–720.
113. Muzi M, Ebert TJ. A randomized, prospective comparison of halothane, isoflurane and enflurane on baroreflex control of heart rate in humans. In: Bosnjak Z, Kampine JP, eds. *Advances in Pharmacology, Vol. 31: Anesthesia and Cardiovascular Disease.* San Diego: Academic Press; 1994:379–387.
114. Muzi M, Ebert TJ. A comparison of baroreflex sensitivity during isoflurane and desflurane anesthesia in humans. *Anesthesiology.* 1995;82:919–925.
115. Ebert TJ, Perez F, Uhrich TD, et al. Desflurane-mediated sympathetic activation occurs in humans despite preventing hypotension and baroreceptor unloading. *Anesthesiology.* 1998;88:1227–1232.
116. Tanaka M, Nishikawa T. Arterial baroreflex function in humans anaesthetized with sevoflurane. *Br J Anaesth.* 1999;82:350–354.
117. Tanaka M, Nishikawa T. Sevoflurane speeds recovery of baroreflex control of heart rate after minor surgical procedures compared with isoflurane. *Anesth Analg.* 1999;89:284–289.
118. Muzi M, Lopatka CW, Ebert TJ. Desflurane-mediated neurocirculatory activation in humans: Effects of concentration and rate of change on responses. *Anesthesiology.* 1996;84:1035–1042.
119. Hirshman CA, Bergman NA. Factors influencing intrapulmonary airway calibre during anaesthesia. *Br J Anaesth.* 1990;65:30–42.
120. Hirshman CA, Edelstein G, Peetz S, et al. Mechanism of action of inhalational anesthesia on airways. *Anesthesiology.* 1982;56:107–111.
121. Park KW, Dai HB, Lowenstein E, et al. Epithelial dependence of the bronchodilatory effect of sevoflurane and desflurane in rat distal bronchi. *Anesth Analg.* 1998;86:646–651.
122. Goff MJ, Arain SR, Ficke DJ, et al. Absence of bronchodilation during desflurane anesthesia: A comparison to sevoflurane and thiopental. *Anesthesiology.* 2000;93:404–408.
123. Nyktari V, Papaioannou A, Volakakis N, et al. Respiratory resistance during anaesthesia with isoflurane, sevoflurane, and desflurane: A randomized clinical trial. *Br J Anaesth.* 2011;107:454–461.
124. Mori N, Nagata H, Ohta S, et al. Prolonged sevoflurane inhalation was not nephrotoxic in two patients with refractory status asthmaticus. *Anesth Analg.* 1996;83:189–191.
125. Johnston RG, Noseworthy TW, Friesen EG, et al. Isoflurane therapy for status asthmaticus in children and adults. *Chest.* 1990;97:698–701.
126. Ledowski T, Manopas A, Lauer S. Bronchial mucus transport velocity in patients receiving desflurane and fentanyl vs. sevoflurane and fentanyl. *Eur J Anaesthesiol.* 2008;25:752–755.

127. Reiz S. Nitrous oxide augments the systemic and coronary haemodynamic effects of isoflurane in patients with ischaemic heart disease. *Acta Anaesthesiol Scand.* 1983;27:464–469.
128. Benumof JL, Augustine SD, Gibbons JA. Halothane and isoflurane only slightly impair arterial oxygenation during one-lung ventilation in patients undergoing thoracotomy. *Anesthesiology.* 1987;67:910–915.
129. Pagel PS, Fu JL, Damask MC, et al. Desflurane and isoflurane produce similar alterations in systemic and pulmonary hemodynamics and arterial oxygenation in patients undergoing one-lung ventilation during thoracotomy. *Anesth Analg.* 1998;87:800–807.
130. Kurahashi K, Maruta H. The effect of sevoflurane and isoflurane on the neuromuscular block produced by vecuronium continuous infusion. *Anesth Analg.* 1996;82:942–947.
131. Wulf H, Kahl M, Ledowski T. Augmentation of the neuromuscular blocking effects of cisatracurium during desflurane, sevoflurane, isoflurane or total i.v. anaesthesia. *Br J Anaesth.* 1998;80:308–312.
132. Nitahara K, Sugi Y, Higa K, et al. Neuromuscular effects of sevoflurane in myasthenia gravis patients. *Br J Anaesth.* 2007;98:337–341.
133. Bock M, Klippel K, Nitsche B, et al. Rocuronium potency and recovery characteristics during steady-state desflurane, sevoflurane, isoflurane or propofol anaesthesia. *Br J Anaesth.* 2000;84:43–47.
134. Paul M, Fokt RM, Kindler CH, et al. Characterization of the interactions between volatile anesthetics and neuromuscular blockers at the muscle nicotinic acetylcholine receptor. *Anesth Analg.* 2002;95:362–367.
135. Wright PM, Hart P, Lau M, et al. The magnitude and time course of vecuronium potentiation by desflurane versus isoflurane. *Anesthesiology.* 1995;82:404–411.
136. Ducart A, Adnet P, Renaud B, et al. Malignant hyperthermia during sevoflurane administration. *Anesth Analg.* 1995;80:609–611.
137. Allen GC, Brubaker CL. Human malignant hyperthermia associated with desflurane anesthesia. *Anesth Analg.* 1998;86:1328–1331.
138. Krause T, Scholz J, Jansen L, et al. Sevoflurane anaesthesia does not induce the formation of sister chromatid exchanges in peripheral blood lymphocytes of children. *Br J Anaesth.* 2003;90:233–235.
139. Akin A, Ugur F, Ozkul Y, et al. Desflurane anaesthesia increases sister chromatid exchanges in human lymphocytes. *Acta Anaesthesiol Scand.* 2005;49:1559–1561.
140. Eroglu A, Celep F, Erciyes N. A comparison of sister chromatid exchanges in lymphocytes of anesthesiologists to nonanesthesiologists in the same hospital. *Anesth Analg.* 2006;102:1573–1577.
141. Wiesner G, Schiewe-Langgartner F, Lindner R, et al. Increased formation of sister chromatid exchanges, but not of micronuclei, in anaesthetists exposed to low levels of sevoflurane. *Anaesthesia.* 2008;63:861–864.
142. Mazze RI, Wilson AI, Rice SA, et al. Fetal development in mice exposed to isoflurane. *Teratology.* 1985;32:339–345.
143. Mazze RI, Källén B. Reproductive outcome after anesthesia and operation during pregnancy: A registry study of 5405 cases. *Am J Obstet Gynecol.* 1989;161:1178–1185.
144. Layzer RB, Fishman RA, Schafer JA. Neuropathy following abuse of nitrous oxide. *Neurology.* 1978;28:504–506.
145. Yildiz K, Dogru K, Dalgic H, et al. Inhibitory effects of desflurane and sevoflurane on oxytocin-induced contractions of isolated pregnant human myometrium. *Acta Anaesthesiol Scand.* 2005;49:1355–1359.
146. Abboud TK, Zhu J, Richardson M, et al. Desflurane: A new volatile anesthetic for cesarean section. Maternal and neonatal effects. *Acta Anaesthesiol Scand.* 1995;39:723–726.
147. Lane GA, Nahrwold ML, Tait AR. Anesthetics as teratogens: Nitrous oxide is fetotoxic, xenon is not. *Science.* 1980;210:899–901.
148. McGregor DG. Occupational exposure to trace concentrations of waste anesthetic gases. *Mayo Clin Proc.* 2000;75:273–277.
149. Abboud TK, Nagappala S, Murakawa K, et al. Comparison of the effects of general and regional anesthesia for cesarean section on neonatal neurologic and adaptive capacity scores. *Anesth Analg.* 1985;64:996–1000.
150. Warren TM, Datta S, Ostheimer GW, et al. Comparisons of the maternal and neonatal effects of halothane, enflurane and isoflurane for cesarean delivery. *Anesth Analg.* 1983;62:516–520.
151. Kodama M, Satoh Y, Otsubo Y, et al. Neonatal desflurane exposure induces more robust neuroapoptosis than do isoflurane and sevoflurane and impairs working memory. *Anesthesiology.* 2011;115:979–991.
152. Cheek TG, Baird E. Anesthesia for nonobstetric surgery: Maternal and fetal considerations. *Clin Obstet Gynecol.* 2009;52:535–545.
153. Reitman E, Flood P. Anaesthetic considerations for non-obstetric surgery during pregnancy. *Br J Anaesth.* 2011;107(Suppl 1):i72–i78.
154. Ruzicka JA, Hidalgo JC, Tinker JH, et al. Inhibition of volatile sevoflurane degradation product formation in an anesthesia circuit by a reduction in soda lime temperature. *Anesthesiology.* 1994;81:238–244.
155. Fang ZX, Kandel L, Laster MJ, et al. Factors affecting production of compound A from the interaction of sevoflurane with Baralyme and soda lime. *Anesth Analg.* 1996;82:775–781.
156. Frink EJ Jr, Malan TP, Morgan SE, et al. Quantification of the degradation products of sevoflurane in two CO2 absorbents during low-flow anesthesia in surgical patients. *Anesthesiology.* 1992;77:1064–1069.
157. Ebert TJ, Arain SR. Renal responses to low-flow desflurane, sevoflurane, and propofol in patients. *Anesthesiology.* 2000;93:1401–1406.
158. Kharasch ED, Frink EJ Jr, Zager R, et al. Assessment of low-flow sevoflurane and isoflurane effects on renal function using sensitive markers of tubular toxicity. *Anesthesiology.* 1997;86:1238–1253.
159. Bito H, Ikeuchi Y, Ikeda K. Effects of low-flow sevoflurane anesthesia on renal function: Comparison with high-flow sevoflurane anesthesia and low-flow isoflurane anesthesia. *Anesthesiology.* 1997;86:1231–1237.
160. Bito H, Ikeda K. Closed-circuit anesthesia with sevoflurane in humans. Effects on renal and hepatic function and concentrations of breakdown products with soda lime in the circuit. *Anesthesiology.* 1994;80:71–76.
161. Eger EI 2nd, Koblin DD, Bowland T, et al. Nephrotoxicity of sevoflurane versus desflurane anesthesia in volunteers. *Anesth Analg.* 1997;84:160–168.
162. Ebert TJ, Frink EJ Jr, Kharasch ED. Absence of biochemical evidence for renal and hepatic dysfunction after 8 hours of 1.25 minimum alveolar concentration sevoflurane anesthesia in volunteers. *Anesthesiology.* 1998;88:601–610.
163. Eger EI 2nd, Gong D, Koblin DD, et al. Dose-related biochemical markers of renal injury after sevoflurane versus desflurane anesthesia in volunteers. *Anesth Analg.* 1997;85:1154–1163.
164. Groudine SB, Fragen RJ, Kharasch ED, et al. Comparison of renal function following anesthesia with low-flow sevoflurane and isoflurane. *J Clin Anesth.* 1999;11:201–207.
165. Bito H, Ikeda K. Renal and hepatic function in surgical patients after low-flow sevoflurane or isoflurane anesthesia. *Anesth Analg.* 1996;82:173–176.
166. Ebert TJ, Messana LD, Uhrich TD, et al. Absence of renal and hepatic toxicity after four hours of 1.25 minimum alveolar concentration sevoflurane anesthesia in volunteers. *Anesth Analg.* 1998;86:662–667.
167. Conzen PF, Kharasch ED, Czerner SF, et al. Low-flow sevoflurane compared with low-flow isoflurane anesthesia in patients with stable renal insufficiency. *Anesthesiology.* 2002;97:578–584.
168. Litz RJ, Hübler M, Lorenz W, et al. Renal responses to desflurane and isoflurane in patients with renal insufficiency. *Anesthesiology.* 2002;97:1133–1136.
169. Spracklin D, Kharasch ED. Evidence for the metabolism of fluoromethyl-1,1-difluoro-1-(trifluoromethyl)vinyl ether (Compound A), a sevoflurane degradation product, by cysteine conjugate beta-lyase. *Chem Res Toxicol.* 1996;9:696–702.
170. Holak EJ, Mei DA, Dunning MB 3rd, et al. Carbon monoxide production from sevoflurane breakdown: Modeling of exposures under clinical conditions. *Anesth Analg.* 2003;96:757–764.
171. Baxter PJ, Garton K, Kharasch ED. Mechanistic aspects of carbon monoxide formation from volatile anesthetics. *Anesthesiology.* 1998;89:929–941.
172. Fang ZX, Eger EI 2nd, Laster MJ, et al. Carbon monoxide production from degradation of desflurane, enflurane, isoflurane, halothane, and sevoflurane by soda lime and Baralyme. *Anesth Analg.* 1995;80:1187–1193.
173. Berry PD, Sessler DI, Larson MD. Severe carbon monoxide poisoning during desflurane anesthesia. *Anesthesiology.* 1999;90:613–616.
174. Woehlck HJ. Severe intraoperative CO poisoning: Should apathy prevail? *Anesthesiology.* 1999;90:353–354.
175. Woehlck HJ, Dunning M 3rd, Gandhi S, et al. Indirect detection of intraoperative carbon monoxide exposure by mass spectrometry during isoflurane anesthesia. *Anesthesiology.* 1995;83:213–217.
176. Woehlck HJ, Dunning M 3rd, Connolly LA. Reduction in the incidence of carbon monoxide exposures in humans undergoing general anesthesia. *Anesthesiology.* 1997;87:228–234.
177. Woehlck HJ, Dunning M 3rd, Raza T, et al. Physical factors affecting the production of carbon monoxide from anesthetic breakdown. *Anesthesiology.* 2001;94:453–456.
178. Wissing H, Kuhn I, Warnken U, et al. Carbon monoxide production from desflurane, enflurane, halothane, isoflurane and sevoflurane with dry soda lime. *Anesthesiology.* 2001;95:1205–1212.
179. Castro BA, Freedman LA, Craig WL, et al. Explosion within an anesthesia machine: Baralyme®, high fresh gas flows and sevoflurane concentration. *Anesthesiology.* 2004;101:537–539.
180. Wu J, Previte JP, Adler E, et al. Spontaneous ignition, explosion, and fire with sevoflurane and barium hydroxide lime. *Anesthesiology.* 2004;101:534–537.
181. Fatheree RS, Leighton BL. Acute respiratory distress syndrome after an exothermic Baralyme®-sevoflurane reaction. *Anesthesiology.* 2004;101:531–533.
182. Hanaki C, Fujii K, Morio M, et al. Decomposition of sevoflurane by sodalime. *Hiroshima J Med Sci.* 1987;36:61–67.
183. Kharasch ED. Putting the brakes on anesthetic breakdown. *Anesthesiology.* 1999;91:1192–1194.
184. Baker MT. Sevoflurane: Are there differences in products? *Anesth Analg.* 2007;104:1447–1451.
185. Kharasch ED, Subbarao GN, Cromack KR, et al. Sevoflurane formulation water content influences degradation by Lewis acids in vaporizers. *Anesth Analg.* 2009;108:1796–1802.
186. O'Neill B, Hafiz MA, De Beer DA. Corrosion of Penlon sevoflurane vaporisers. *Anaesthesia.* 2007;62:421.
187. Frink EJ Jr, Malan TP Jr, Isner RJ, et al. Renal concentrating function with prolonged sevoflurane or enflurane anesthesia in volunteers. *Anesthesiology.* 1994;80:1019–1025.
188. Mazze RI, Calverley RK, Smith NT. Inorganic fluoride nephrotoxicity: Prolonged enflurane and halothane anesthesia in volunteers. *Anesthesiology.* 1977;46:265–271.

189. Mazze RI. The safety of sevoflurane in humans. *Anesthesiology.* 1992;77:1062–1063.
190. Kharasch ED, Hankins DC, Thummel KE. Human kidney methoxyflurane and sevoflurane metabolism. Intrarenal fluoride production as a possible mechanism of methoxyflurane nephrotoxicity. *Anesthesiology.* 1995;82:689–699.
191. Thwaites A, Edmends S, Smith I. Inhalation induction with sevoflurane: A double-blind comparison with propofol. *Br J Anaesth.* 1997;78:356–361.
192. Muzi M, Colinco MD, Robinson BJ, et al. The effects of premedication on inhaled induction of anesthesia with sevoflurane. *Anesth Analg.* 1997;85:1143–1148.
193. Muzi M, Robinson BJ, Ebert TJ, et al. Induction of anesthesia and tracheal intubation with sevoflurane in adults. *Anesthesiology.* 1996;85:536–543.
194. Mostafa SM, Atherton AM. Sevoflurane for difficult tracheal intubation. *Br J Anaesth.* 1997;79:392–393.
195. Ryan SM, Nielsen CJ. Global warming potential of inhaled anesthetics: Application to clinical use. *Anesth Analg.* 2010;111:92–98.
196. Sulbaek Andersen MP, Nielsen OJ, Karpichev B, et al. Atmospheric chemistry of isoflurane, desflurane, and sevoflurane: Kinetics and mechanisms of reactions with chlorine atoms and OH radicals and global warming potentials. *J Phys Chem A.* 2012;116:5806–5820.
197. Sulbaek Andersen MP, Sander SP, Nielsen OJ, et al. Inhalation anaesthetics and climate change. *Br J Anaesth.* 2010;105:760–766.
198. Eger EI 2nd, Johnson BH. Rates of awakening from anesthesia with I-653, halothane, isoflurane, and sevoflurane: A test of the effect of anesthetic concentration and duration in rats. *Anesth Analg.* 1987;66:977–982.

CHAPTER

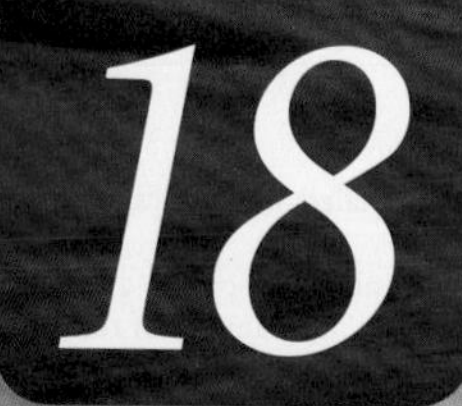

18 Intravenous Anesthetics

PAUL F. WHITE • MATTHEW R. ENG

Key Points

1. Low doses of IV anesthetics produce sedation, and high doses produce hypnosis (or unconsciousness)
2. All IV anesthetics are sedative–hypnotics and produce dose-dependent central nervous system (CNS) depression.
3. Dexmedetomidine is an α_2-agonist with sedative and opioid-sparing effects that is used as an anesthetic adjuvant in the operating room and intensive care unit.
4. With the exception of ketamine and dexmedetomidine, intravenous (IV) anesthetics lack intrinsic analgesic properties.
5. Compared to thiopental and propofol, methohexital produces less depression of electroencephalogram (EEG) activity.
6. IV anesthetics in combination with potent opioid analgesics and/or local anesthetics can be used to produce total intravenous anesthesia (TIVA).
7. Propofol possesses unique antiemetic and appetite-stimulating properties.
8. Midazolam possesses prominent amnestic and anxiolytic properties.
9. Etomidate produces less cardiovascular depression than the barbiturates and propofol.
10. Ketamine possesses both analgesic and psychomimetic properties.

Multimedia

 1 Drug Concentration and Effect

INTRODUCTION

1 In general, low doses of IV anesthetics produce sedation, and high doses produce hypnosis (or unconsciousness). The concept of intravenous (IV) anesthesia has evolved from primarily induction of general anesthesia to total IV anesthesia (TIVA).[1] TIVA has assumed increasing importance for therapeutic, as well as diagnostic, procedures in both adults and children.[2] IV anesthetic techniques are used for procedures in the operating room (OR) and in sites remote from the OR. In many centers in Europe and South America, TIVA has become more popular for general anesthesia than classic "balanced anesthesia" or volatile anesthetic-based techniques. For superficial surgical procedures, lower dosages of IV anesthetics are increasingly being used for sedation during local and regional anesthesia, so-called monitored anesthesia care (MAC) (see Chapter 29 Monitored Anesthesia Care).[2] This change has been a result of: (1) the development of rapid, short-acting IV hypnotic, analgesic, and muscle relaxant drugs; (2) the availability of pharmacokinetic and dynamic-based IV delivery systems; and (3) the development of the electroencephalogram (EEG)-based cerebral monitoring devices, which
2 measure the hypnotic component of the anesthetic state. All IV anesthetics are sedative–hypnotics and produce dose-dependent

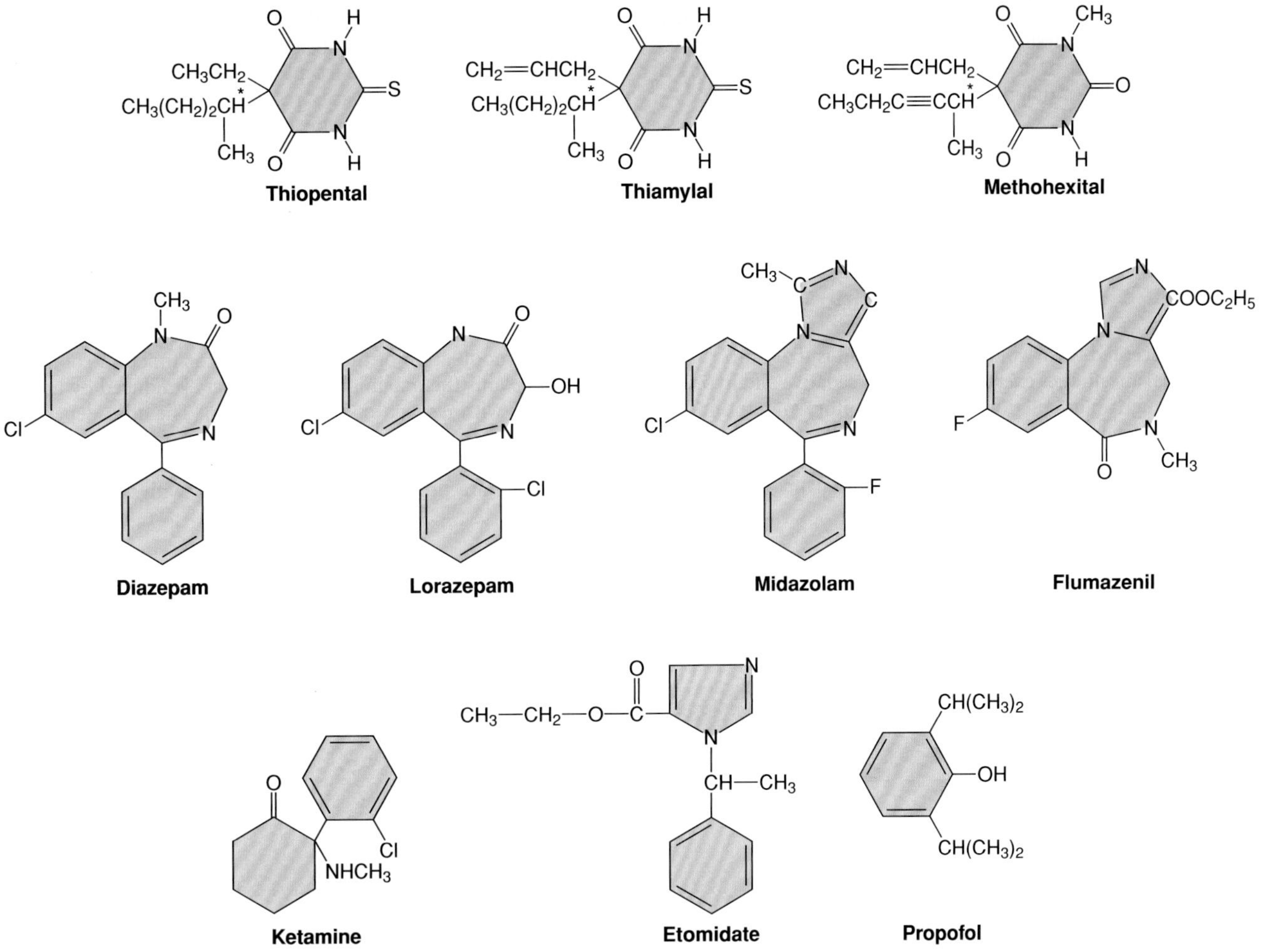

Thiopental Thiamylal Methohexital

Diazepam Lorazepam Midazolam Flumazenil

Ketamine Etomidate Propofol

FIGURE 18-1. Chemical structures of currently available nonopioid intravenous anesthetics.

central nervous system (CNS) depression. This chapter focuses on the pharmacologic properties and clinical uses of the currently available IV anesthetics.

Following its introduction into clinical practice, thiopental quickly became the gold standard of IV anesthetics against which all the newer IV drugs were compared. Many different hypnotic drugs are currently available for use during IV anesthesia (Fig. 18-1). Although propofol (currently the most widely used IV anesthetic) is both safe and effective, the "ideal" IV anesthetic is yet to be developed. The physical and pharmacologic properties that an ideal IV anesthetic would possess include the following:

1. Drug compatibility (water-solubility) and stability in solution.
2. Lack of pain on injection, veno-irritation, and local tissue damage following extravasation.
3. Low potential to release histamine or precipitate hypersensitivity reactions.
4. Rapid and smooth onset of hypnotic action without excitatory activity.
5. Rapid metabolism to pharmacologically inactive metabolites.
6. A steep dose-response relationship to enhance titratability and minimize tissue accumulation.
7. Lack of acute cardiovascular and respiratory depression.
8. Decreases in cerebral metabolism and intracranial pressure.
9. Rapid and smooth return of consciousness and cognitive skills with residual analgesia.
10. Absence of postoperative nausea and vomiting, amnesia, psychomimetic reactions, dizziness, headache, or prolonged sedation ("hangover" effects).

HISTORICAL PERSPECTIVE

Despite thiopental's proven clinical usefulness, safety, and widespread use over many decades of use, it has been supplanted by a variety of agents from different pharmacologic drug groups. The sedative–hypnotic drugs that have been more recently introduced into clinical practice (e.g., midazolam, ketamine, etomidate, propofol) have proven to be extremely valuable in specific clinical situations. These newer compounds combine many of the characteristics of the ideal IV anesthetic, but fail in aspects where the other drugs succeed. For some of these IV sedative–hypnotics, disadvantages have led to "restricted" indications (e.g., ketamine, etomidate). Although propofol is clearly the most popular of the sedative–hypnotic drug class, the optimal pharmacologic properties are not equally important in every clinical situation. Therefore, the anesthesiologist must make the choice of the IV anesthetic drug that best fits the needs of the individual patient and the operative (or diagnostic) procedure.

GENERAL PHARMACOLOGY OF INTRAVENOUS ANESTHETICS

Mechanism of Action

A widely accepted theory of anesthetic action is that both IV and inhalational anesthetics exert their primary sedative and hypnotic effects through an interaction with the inhibitory γ-aminobutyric acid (GABA) neurotransmitter system.[3] GABA is the principal inhibitory neurotransmitter within the CNS. The GABA and adrenergic neurotransmitter systems counterbalance the action of excitatory neurotransmitters. The GABA type A ($GABA_A$) receptor is a receptor complex consisting of up to five glycoprotein subunits. When the $GABA_A$ receptor is activated, transmembrane chloride conductance increases, resulting in hyperpolarization of the postsynaptic cell membrane and functional inhibition of the postsynaptic neuron. Sedative–hypnotic drugs interact with different components of the GABA-receptor complex (Fig. 18-2). However, the allosteric (structural) requirements for activation of the receptor are different for IV and volatile anesthetics.

Benzodiazepines bind to specific receptor sites that are part of the $GABA_A$-receptor complex. The binding of benzodiazepines to their receptor site increases the efficiency of the coupling between the GABA receptor and the chloride ion channel. The degree of modulation of the GABA-receptor function is limited, which explains the maximal "ceiling effect" produced by benzodiazepines with respect to CNS depression. The dose-dependent CNS depressant effect of benzodiazepines produce hypnosis, sedation, anxiolysis, amnesia, and anticonvulsant effects.[1] These CNS effects are presumed to be associated with stimulation of

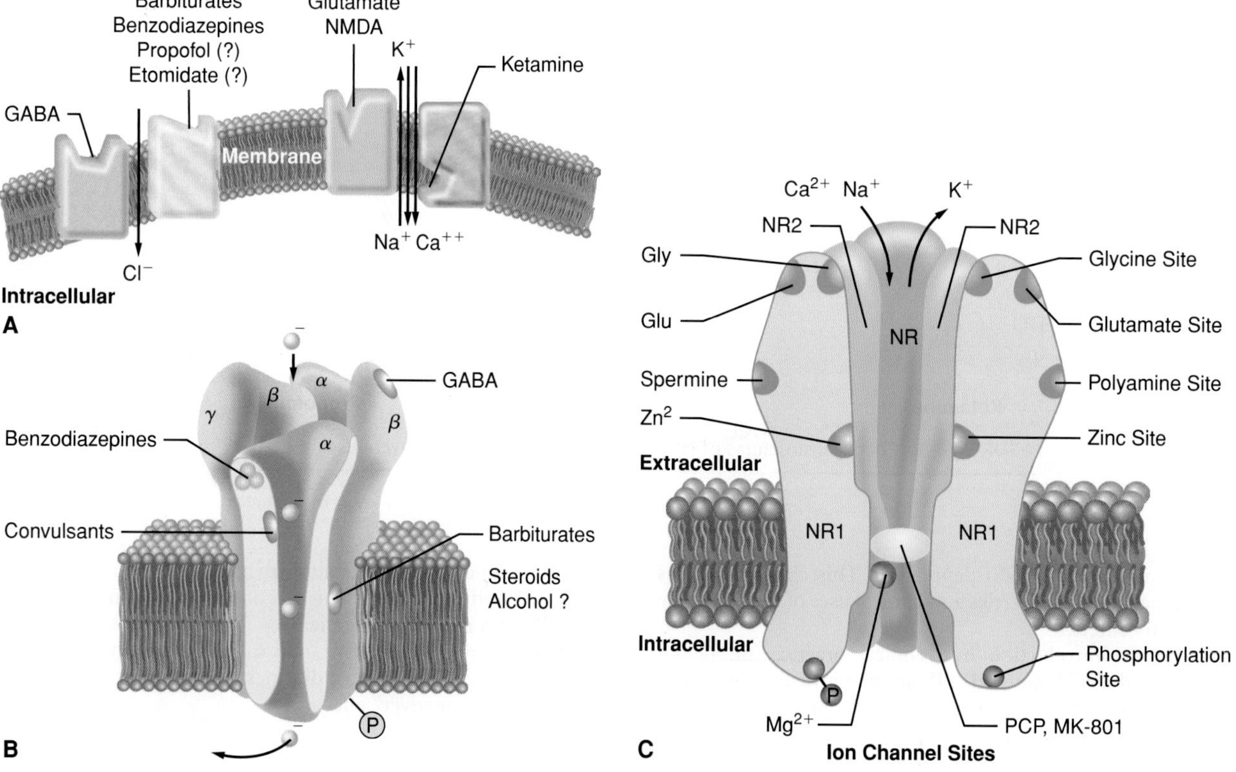

FIGURE 18-2. A: This model depicts the postsynaptic site of γ-aminobutyric acid (GABA) and glutamate within the central nervous system (CNS). GABA decreases the excitability of neurons by its action at the $GABA_A$-receptor complex. When GABA occupies the binding site of this complex, it allows inward flux of chloride ion, resulting in hyperpolarizing of the cell and subsequent resistance of the neuron to stimulation by excitatory transmitters. Barbiturates, benzodiazepines, propofol, and etomidate decrease neuronal excitability by enhancing the effect of GABA at this complex, facilitating this inhibitory effect on the postsynaptic cell. Glutamate and its analog N-methyl-D-aspartate (NMDA) are excitatory amino acids. When glutamate occupies the binding site on the NMDA subtype of the glutamate receptor, the channel opens and allows Na^+, K^+, and Ca^{2+} to either enter or leave the cell. Flux of these ions leads to depolarization of the postsynaptic neuron and initiation of an action potential and activation of other pathways. Ketamine blocks this open channel and prevents further ion flux, thus inhibiting the excitatory response to glutamate. (Reprinted with permission from: Van Hemelrijck J, Gonzales JM, White PF. Use of intravenous sedative agents. In: Rogers MC, Tinker JH, Covino BG, Longnecker DE, eds. *Principles and Practice of Anesthesiology.* Mosby: St. Louis; 1992:1131.) **B:** Schematic model of the $GABA_A$-receptor complex illustrating recognition sites for many of the substances that bind to the receptor. **C:** Model of the NMDA receptor showing sites for antagonist action. Ketamine binds to the site labeled PCP (phencyclidine). The pentameric structure of the receptor, composed of a combination of the subunits NR 1 and NR 2, is illustrated. (Altered with permission from: Leeson PD, Iversen LL. The glycine site on the NMDA receptor: Structure-activity relationships and therapeutic potential. *J Med Chem.* 1994;37:4053.)

different receptor subtypes and/or concentration-dependent receptor occupancy.[3] For example, it has been suggested that benzodiazepine receptor occupancy of 20% provides anxiolysis, while 30% to 50% receptor occupancy is associated with amnesia to sedation, and 60% receptor occupancy is required for hypnosis (or unconsciousness).[1]

The interaction of barbiturates and propofol with specific membrane structures appears to decrease the rate of dissociation of GABA from its receptor, thereby increasing the duration of the GABA-activated opening of the chloride ion channel (Fig. 18-2). Barbiturates can also mimic the action of GABA by directly activating the chloride channels. The proposed mechanism of action of thiopental relates to its ability to function as a competitive inhibitor at the nicotinic acetylcholine receptors in the CNS.[4] Etomidate augments GABA-gated chloride currents (i.e., indirect modulation) and at higher concentrations evokes chloride currents in the absence of GABA (i.e., direct activation). Although the mechanism of action of propofol is similar to that of the barbiturates (i.e., enhancing the activity of the GABA-activated chloride channel), it also possesses ion channel-blocking effects in cerebral cortex tissue and nicotinic acetylcholine receptors, as well as an inhibitory effect on lysophosphatidate signaling in lipid mediator receptors.[5]

Ketamine produces a functional dissociation between the thalamocortical and limbic systems, a state that has been termed *dissociative* anesthesia. Ketamine depresses neuronal function in the cerebral cortex and thalamus, while simultaneously activating the limbic system. The effect of ketamine on the medial medullary reticular formation may be involved in the affective component of its nociceptive activity. The CNS effects of ketamine appear to be primarily related to its antagonistic activity at the *N*-methyl-D-aspartate (NMDA) receptor (Fig. 18-2). Unlike the other IV anesthetics, ketamine does not interact with GABA receptors; however, it binds to non-NMDA glutamate receptors and nicotinic, muscarinic, monoaminergic, and even kappa-opioid receptors. In addition, it also inhibits neuronal sodium channels (producing a modest local anesthetic action) and calcium channels (causing cerebral vasodilatation).

3 The centrally active α_2-adrenergic receptor agonists, clonidine and dexmedetomidine, have potent sedative and opioid analgesic-sparing properties. These drugs also have significant effects on the peripheral α_2 receptors involved in regulating the cardiovascular system by inhibiting norepinephrine release. This class of anesthetic adjuvants can also reduce blood pressure and heart rate by decreasing the tonic levels of sympathetic outflow from the CNS and augmenting cardiac vagal activity, respectively.[6,7] However, dexmedetomidine failed to block the acute hyperdynamic response to electroconvulsive therapy (ECT) when administered as an adjuvant to methohexital anesthesia.[8] Earlier studies with clonidine demonstrated that this α_2 agonist–antagonist could also reduce the IV[9] and volatile[10] anesthetic requirements, as well as the postoperative opioid analgesic requirement.

Pharmacokinetics and Metabolism

An understanding of basic pharmacokinetic principles is integral to the understanding of the pharmacologic actions and interactions of IV anesthetic and adjunctive drugs, and will allow the anesthesiologist to develop more optimal dosing strategies when using IV techniques (see Chapter 7 Basic Principles of Clinical Pharmacology). Although lipid solubility facilitates diffusion of IV anesthetics across cellular membranes, including the blood–brain barrier, only the nonionized form of the compound is able to readily cross neuronal membranes. The ratio of the unionized-to-ionized fraction depends on the pKa of the drug and the pH of the body fluids.

The rapid onset of the CNS effect of most IV anesthetics can be explained by their high lipid solubility and the relatively high proportion of the cardiac output (20%) perfusing the brain. However, a variable degree of hysteresis exists between the blood concentration of the hypnotic drug and its onset of action on the CNS. The hysteresis is related in part to diffusion of these drugs into brain tissue and nonspecific CNS receptor binding. However, the number of CNS binding sites is usually saturable and only a small fraction of the available binding sites needs to be occupied to produce clinical effects. Although the total amount of drug in the blood is available for diffusion, the diffusion rate will be more limited for IV anesthetics with a high degree of plasma protein binding (90%) because only the "free" unbound drug can diffuse across membranes and exert central effects. When several drugs compete for the same binding sites, or when the protein concentration in the blood is decreased by preexisting disease (e.g., hepatic failure, malnutrition), a higher fraction of the unbound drug will be available to exert an effect on the CNS. Since only unbound drug is available for uptake and metabolism in the liver, highly protein-bound drugs may have a lower rate of hepatic metabolism as a result of their decreased hepatic extraction ratio (i.e., the fraction of the hepatic blood flow that is cleared of the drug).

The pharmacokinetics of IV hypnotics are characterized by rapid distribution and subsequent redistribution into several

TABLE 18-1. PHARMACOKINETIC VALUES FOR THE CURRENTLY AVAILABLE INTRAVENOUS SEDATIVE–HYPNOTIC DRUGS

Drug Name	Distribution Half-life (min)	Protein Binding (%)	Distribution Volume at Steady State (L/kg)	Clearance (mL/kg/min)	Elimination Half-life (h)
Thiopental	2–4	85	2.5	3.4	11
Methohexital	5–6	85	2.2	11	4
Propofol	2–4	98	2–10	20–30	4–23
Midazolam	7–15	94	1.1–1.7	6.4–11	1.7–2.6
Diazepam	10–15	98	0.7–1.7	0.2–0.5	20–50
Lorazepam	3–10	98	0.8–1.3	0.8–1.8	11–22
Etomidate	2–4	75	2.5–4.5	18–25	2.9–5.3
Ketamine	11–16	12	2.5–3.5	12–17	2–4

From: White PF. *Textbook of Intravenous Anesthesia*. Baltimore: Williams & Wilkins; 1997:27, 77.

hypothetical compartments (determined by their effect on blood flow to various tissues), followed by elimination (Table 18-1). The initial pharmacologic effects are related to the activity of the drug in the central compartment. The primary mechanism for terminating the central effects of IV anesthetics administered for induction of anesthesia is redistribution from the central highly perfused compartment (e.g., brain) to the larger, but less well perfused "peripheral" compartments (e.g., muscle, fat). Even for drugs with a high hepatic extraction ratio (e.g., propofol), elimination does not always play a major role in terminating the drug's sedative–hypnotic effects because elimination of the drug can occur only from the central compartment. The rate of elimination from the central compartment, the amount of drug present in the peripheral compartments, and the rate of redistribution from the peripheral compartments "back" into the central compartment determine the time necessary to eliminate the drug from the body and can directly influence intermediate and late recovery times.

Most IV anesthetic agents are eliminated via hepatic metabolism followed by renal excretion of more water-soluble metabolites. Some metabolites have pharmacologic activity and can produce prolonged drug effects (e.g., oxazepam, desmethyldiazepam, norketamine). Moreover, there is considerable interpatient variability in the clearance rates for commonly used IV anesthetic drugs. The elimination clearance is the distribution volume cleared of drug over time and is a measure of the efficacy of the elimination process. The slow elimination of some anesthetics is partly due to their high degree of protein binding that reduces their hepatic extraction ratio. Other drugs may have a high hepatic extraction ratio and elimination clearance despite extensive plasma protein binding (e.g., propofol), indicating that protein binding is not always a rate-limiting factor.

For most drugs, the hepatic enzyme systems are not saturated at clinically relevant drug concentrations, and the rate of drug elimination will decrease as an exponential function of the drug's plasma concentration (first-order kinetics). However, when high steady state plasma concentrations are achieved with prolonged infusions, hepatic enzyme systems can become saturated and the elimination rate becomes independent of the drug concentration
1 (zero-order kinetics). The elimination half-life ($t_{1/2}\beta$) is the time required for the anesthetic concentration to decrease by 50% during the terminal phase of the plasma decay curve. The $t_{1/2}\beta$ depends on the volume to be cleared (the distribution volume) and the efficiency of the metabolic clearance system. Because their volumes of distribution are similar, the wide variation in elimination half-life values for the IV anesthetics is a reflection of differences in their clearance values.

When a drug infusion is administered without a loading dose, at least three times the $t_{1/2}\beta$ value may be required to achieve a true "steady state" plasma concentration. The steady state concentration obtained during an anesthetic infusion depends on the rate of drug administration and its clearance rate. When an infusion is discontinued, the rate at which the plasma concentration decreases largely depends on the clearance rate (as reflected by the terminal $t_{1/2}\beta$ value). For drugs with shorter elimination half-lives, plasma concentration will decrease at a rate that allows for a more rapid recovery (e.g., propofol). Drugs with longer $t_{1/2}\beta$ values (e.g., thiopental and diazepam) are usually only administered by continuous IV infusion when the medical condition requires long-term treatment (e.g., elevated intracranial pressure [ICP] as a result of brain injury or prolonged sedation in the intensive care unit [ICU] because of respiratory failure).

Careful titration of an anesthetic drug to achieve the desired clinical effect is necessary to avoid drug accumulation and the resultant prolonged CNS effects after the infusion has been discontinued. Although the value of the $t_{1/2}\beta$ indicates how fast a drug is eliminated from the body, a more useful indicator of the acceptability of a hypnotic infusion for maintenance of anesthesia or sedation is the so-called context-sensitive half-time, a value derived from computer simulations of drug infusions.[11] The context-sensitive half-time is defined as the time necessary for the effect-compartment (i.e., effect site) concentration to decrease by 50% in relation to the duration of the infusion. The context-sensitive half-time becomes particularly important in determining recovery after prolonged infusions of sedative–hypnotic drugs. Drugs (e.g., propofol) may have a relatively short context-sensitive half-time despite the fact that a large amount of drug remains present in the "deep" (less well-perfused) tissue compartment. The slow return of the anesthetic from the deep compartment contributes little to the concentration of drug in the central compartment from which it is rapidly cleared. Therefore, the concentration in the central compartment rapidly declines below the hypnotic threshold after discontinuation of the infusion, contributing to short emergence times despite the fact that a substantial quantity of anesthetic drug may remain in the body.

Marked interpatient variability exists in the pharmacokinetics of IV sedative–hypnotic drugs. Factors that can influence anesthetic drug disposition include the degree of protein binding, the efficiency of hepatic and renal elimination processes, physiologic changes with aging, preexisting disease states, the operative site, body temperature, and drug interactions (e.g., coadministration of volatile anesthetics). For example, increased age, lean body (muscle) mass, and total body water decrease result in an increase in the steady state volume of distribution of most IV anesthetics. The increased distribution volume and decreased hepatic clearance leads to a prolongation of their $t_{1/2}\beta$ values. Moreover, a decrease of the volume of the central compartment may result in higher initial drug concentrations and can at least partially explain the decreased induction requirement in the elderly. Additionally, the slower redistribution from the vessel-rich tissues to intermediate compartments (e.g., muscles) also contributes to the age-related decrease in the induction dose requirements.[11] Although prolongation of the elimination half-time in the elderly does not provide an explanation for the decreased induction dose requirement, it is responsible for producing higher steady state plasma concentrations of IV anesthetics at any given infusion rate when administered for maintenance of general anesthesia or sedation, contributing to a slower recovery from the sub-hypnotic (residual) CNS depressant effects.

The hepatic clearance of IV anesthetics with a high (e.g., etomidate, propofol, ketamine) or intermediate (e.g., methohexital, midazolam) extraction ratio largely depends on hepatic blood flow, with most of the drug being removed from the blood as it flows through the liver (so-called perfusion-limited clearance). The elimination rate of drugs with low hepatic extraction ratios (e.g., thiopental, diazepam, lorazepam) depends on the enzymatic activity of the liver and is less dependent of hepatic blood flow (so-called capacity-limited clearance). Hepatic blood flow decreases during upper abdominal and laparoscopic surgery and, as a result, higher blood levels of drugs with perfusion-limited clearance are achieved at any given infusion rate. With aging, a decreased cardiac output and a redistribution of blood flow can partly explain the lower clearance rate for drugs with perfusion-limited clearance. Although concomitant administration of volatile anesthetics (which are known to decrease liver blood flow) has little influence on the elimination of thiopental, they can decrease the clearance of etomidate, ketamine, methohexital, and propofol. Other factors that decrease hepatic blood flow include hypocapnia, congestive heart failure, intravascular volume depletion, acute alcohol intoxication, circulatory collapse, increase intra-abdominal pressure, β-adrenergic blockade, and norepinephrine administration.

Hepatic disease can influence the pharmacokinetics of drugs by: (1) altering the plasma protein content and changing the degree of protein binding, (2) decreasing hepatic blood flow and producing intrahepatic shunting, and (3) depressing the metabolic enzymatic activity of the liver. Therefore, the influence of hepatic disease on pharmacokinetics and dynamics of IV anesthetics is difficult to predict. Renal disease can also alter the concentration of plasma and tissue proteins, as well as the degree of protein binding, thereby producing changes in free drug concentrations. Because IV anesthetic agents are primarily metabolized by the liver, renal insufficiency has little influence on their rate of metabolic inactivation or elimination of the primary compound.

Pharmacodynamic Effects

The principal pharmacologic effect of IV anesthetics is to produce progressively increasing sedation and ultimately hypnosis as a result of dose-dependent CNS depression. However, all sedative–hypnotics also directly or indirectly affect other major organ systems. The relationship between the dose of a sedative–hypnotic and its CNS effects can be defined by dose-response curves. Although most IV anesthetics are characterized by steep dose-response curves, the slopes of the curves are not always parallel (Fig. 18-3). However, the characteristics of a dose-response curve can only be interpreted in relation to the specific response for which it was constructed.

When steady state plasma concentrations are achieved, one can assume that the plasma concentration is in quasi-equilibrium with the effect-site concentration. Under these circumstances, it is possible to describe the relationship between drug and effect using a concentration-effect curve (Fig. 18-4). Because of the pharmacodynamic variability that exists among individuals, the plasma drug concentration necessary to obtain a particular effect is often described in terms of an effective concentration range, the so-called therapeutic window. Efficacy of an IV anesthetic relates to the maximum effect that can be achieved with respect to some measure of CNS function. Depending on the drug effect under consideration, the efficacy of sedative–hypnotics may appear to be <100%. Compared to thiopental and propofol, it is extremely difficult to produce an isoelectric [silent] EEG pattern with a benzodiazepine. Potency, on the other hand, relates to the quantity of drug necessary to obtain the maximum CNS effect. The relative potency of sedative–hypnotics also varies depending on the end point chosen. In the presence of an antagonist drug (e.g., flumazenil), the maximal response that can be obtained with a benzodiazepine agonist is further reduced because of competition for the same CNS receptor binding sites.

The influence of sedative–hypnotics on cerebral metabolism, cerebral hemodynamics, and ICP is of particular importance during neuroanesthesia. In patients with reduced cerebral compliance, a small increase in cerebral blood volume can cause a life-threatening increase in ICP. Most sedative–hypnotic drugs cause a proportional reduction in cerebral metabolism

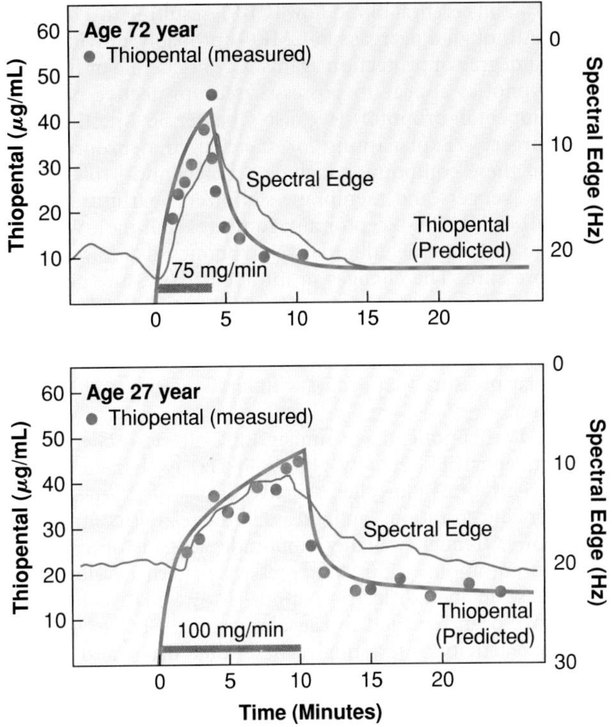

FIGURE 18-4. The concentration of thiopental versus time and spectral edge in an elderly patient **(top)** and in a younger patient **(bottom)**. *Solid horizontal bars* represent the length of thiopental infusion. *Filled circles* represent the measured thiopental concentration (linear scale), and the *solid line* next to them represents the fitted data from the pharmacokinetic model. The axis for spectral edge has been inverted for visual clarity. (Reprinted with permission from: Homer TD, Stanski DR. The effect of increasing age on thiopental disposition and anesthetic requirement. *Anesthesiology.* 1985;62:714.)

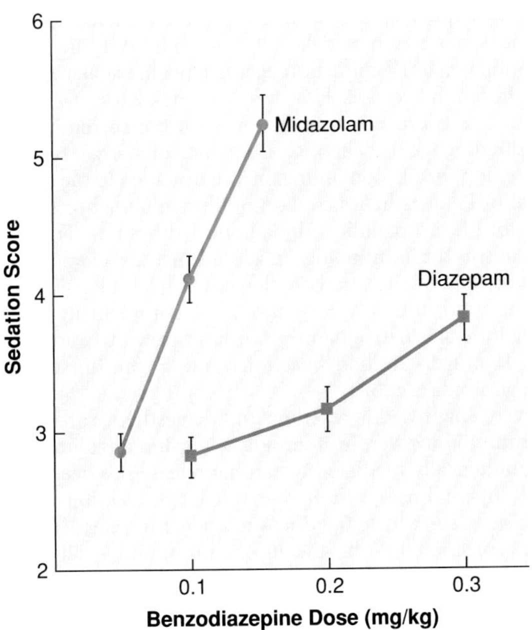

FIGURE 18-3. Dose-response relationships for sedation with midazolam (•) and diazepam (■). The level of sedation (2 = awake and alert to 6 = asleep and unarousable) was assessed 5 minutes after bolus doses of midazolam (0.05, 0.1, or 0.15 mg/kg) or diazepam (0.1, 0.2, or 0.3 mg/kg). Values represent mean values ± SEM. (Reprinted with permission from: White PF, Vasconez LO, Mathes SA, et al. Comparison of midazolam and diazepam for sedation during plastic surgery. *J Plast Reconstruct Surg.* 1988;81:703.)

($CMRO_2$) and cerebral blood flow (CBF), resulting in a decrease in ICP. Although a decrease in $CMRO_2$ probably provides only a modest degree of protection against CNS ischemia or hypoxia, some hypnotics appear to possess cerebroprotective potential (e.g., thiopental, propofol) (see also Chapter 36 Anesthesia for Neurosurgery). Explanations for the alleged neuroprotective effects of these compounds include a biochemical role as free radical scavengers and membrane stabilizers (barbiturates and propofol) or NMDA-receptor antagonists (ketamine). With the exception of ketamine, all sedative–hypnotics also lower intraocular pressure. The changes in intraocular pressure generally reflect the effects of the IV agent on systemic arterial pressure and intracranial hemodynamics. However, none of the available sedative–hypnotic drugs protect against the transient increase in intraocular pressure that occurs with laryngoscopy and tracheal intubation.

Most IV hypnotics have similar EEG effects. Activation of high-frequency EEG activity (15 to 30 Hz) is characteristic of low concentrations (so-called sedative doses) of IV anesthetics. At higher concentrations, an increase in the relative contribution of the lower frequency higher amplitude waves is observed. At high concentrations, a burst-suppressive pattern develops with an increase in the isoelectric periods. Most sedative–hypnotic drugs have been reported to cause occasional EEG seizure-like myoclonic activity. Interestingly, these same drugs also possess anticonvulsant properties.[12,13] When considering possible epileptogenic properties of CNS-depressant drugs, it is important to differentiate between true epileptogenic activity (e.g., methohexital) and myoclonic-like phenomena (e.g., etomidate, ketamine, propofol). Myoclonic activity is generally considered to be the result of an imbalance between excitatory and inhibitory subcortical centers, produced by an unequal degree of suppression of these brain centers by low concentrations of hypnotic drugs. Epileptic activity refers to a sudden alteration in CNS seizure-like activity resulting from a high-voltage electrical discharge at either cortical or subcortical sites, with subsequent spreading to the thalamic and brainstem centers. As a result of its vasoconstrictive effects on the cerebral vasculature, propofol may be useful for treatment of intractable migraine headaches.[14]

Although some induction drugs can increase airway sensitivity, coughing and airway irritation (e.g., bronchospasm) are usually a result of manipulation of the airway during "light" (inadequate) levels of IV anesthesia rather than to a direct drug effect. With the exception of ketamine (and to a lesser extent, etomidate), IV anesthetics produce dose-dependent respiratory depression, which is enhanced in patients with chronic obstructive pulmonary disease. The respiratory depression is characterized by a decrease in tidal volume and minute ventilation, as well as a transient rightward shift in the CO_2 response curve. Following the rapid injection of a large bolus dose of an IV anesthetic, transient apnea lasting 30 to 90 seconds is usually produced. Ketamine causes minimal respiratory depression when administered in the usual induction doses, while etomidate is associated with less respiratory depressant effects than the barbiturate compounds or propofol. The α_2-agonist dexmedetomidine has minimal depressant effects on respiratory function.[15] The sympatholytic effects of dexmedetomidine when administered for premedication may increase the incidence of intraoperative hypotension and bradycardia.[16]

Many different factors contribute to the hemodynamic changes associated with IV induction of anesthesia, including the patient's preexisting cardiovascular and fluid status, resting sympathetic nervous system tone, chronic cardiovascular drugs, preanesthetic medication, the speed of drug injection, and the onset of unconsciousness. In addition, cardiovascular changes can be attributed to the direct pharmacologic actions of anesthetic and analgesic drugs on the heart and peripheral vasculature. IV anesthetics can depress the CNS and peripheral nervous system responses, blunt the compensatory baroreceptor reflex mechanisms, produce direct myocardial depression, and lower peripheral vascular resistance (and/or dilate venous capacitance vessels), thereby decreasing venous return. Profound hemodynamic effects occur at induction of anesthesia in the presence of hypovolemia because a higher than expected drug concentration is achieved in the central compartment. Not surprisingly, the acute cardiocirculatory depressant effects of all IV anesthetics are accentuated in the elderly, as well as in the presence of preexisting cardiovascular disease (e.g., coronary artery disease, chronic hypertension).

The effects of IV anesthetics on neuroendocrine function are also influenced by the surgical stimuli. Surgery-induced increases in stress hormones (e.g., vasopressin [ADH], catecholamines) can result in increased peripheral vascular resistance, and a reduction of urine output. Similarly, glucose tolerance appears to be decreased by surgical stress, resulting in elevations in the glucose
4 concentration. Unlike ketamine and dexmedetomidine, most IV sedative–hypnotic drugs lack intrinsic analgesic activity. In fact, thiopental has been alleged to possess so-called antianalgesic activity (i.e., appearing to lower the pain threshold). Although propofol possesses dose-dependent effects on thalamocortical transfer of nociceptive information, pain-evoked cortical activity remains intact after loss of consciousness.[17]

Hypersensitivity (Allergic) Reactions

Allergic or hypersensitivity-type reactions to IV anesthetics are rare but can be severe and even life-threatening. IV drug administration bypasses the normal "protective barriers" against entrance of foreign molecules into the body. With the exception of etomidate, all IV induction agents have been alleged to cause some histamine release. However, the incidence of severe anaphylactic reactions is extremely low with the currently available IV induction agents. The high frequency of allergic reactions to the Cremophor EL–containing formulations led to the early withdrawal of IV anesthetics containing this solubilizing agent (e.g., propofol EL, propanidid, Alphadione [Althesin]). The possible mechanisms for immunologic reactions include: (1) direct action on mast cells, (2) classic complement activation after previous exposure and antibody formation, (3) complement activation through the alternative pathway without previous antigen exposure, (4) antigen-antibody reactions, and (5) the "mixed type" of anaphylactoid reactions.

Severe anaphylactic reactions to IV anesthetics are extremely uncommon; however, profound hypotension attributed to nonimmunologically mediated histamine release has been reported with thiopental use. Although anaphylactic reactions to etomidate have been reported, it does not appear to release histamine, and is considered to be the most "immunologically safe" IV anesthetic. Propofol does not normally trigger histamine release, but life-threatening anaphylactoid reactions have been reported in patients with a previous history of multiple-drug allergies. Barbiturates can also precipitate episodes of acute intermittent porphyria and their use is contraindicated in predisposed patients. Although benzodiazepines, ketamine, and etomidate are reported to be safe in humans, these drugs have been shown to be porphyrogenic in animal models. The most common causes of profound hypotension following IV induction of anesthesia are unexpected drug interactions and/or unrecognized hypovolemia.

COMPARATIVE PHYSICOCHEMICAL AND CLINICAL PHARMACOLOGIC PROPERTIES OF INTRAVENOUS AGENTS

Barbiturates

The most commonly used barbiturates are thiopental (5-ethyl-5-[1-methylbutyl]-2-thiobarbituric acid), methohexital (1-methyl-5-allyl-5-[1-methyl-2-pentanyl] barbituric acid), and thiamylal (5-allyl-5-[1-methylbutyl]-2-thiobarbituric acid). Thiopental (Pentothal) and thiamylal (Surital) are thiobarbiturates, while methohexital (Brevital) is an oxybarbiturate. Thiamylal is slightly more potent than thiopental but has a similar pharmacologic profile. Although the l-isomers of thiopental and thiamylal are twice as potent as the d-isomers, both hypnotics are commercially available as racemic mixtures. Because methohexital has two asymmetric centers, it has four stereoisomers. The β-l-isomer is 4 to 5 times more potent than the α-l-isomer, but it produces excessive motor responses. Therefore, methohexital is marketed as the racemic mixture of the two α-isomers.

All three barbiturates are available as sodium salts and must be dissolved in isotonic sodium chloride (0.9%) or water to prepare solutions of 2.5% thiopental, 1% to 2% methohexital, and 2% thiamylal. If refrigerated, solutions of the thiobarbiturates are stable for up to 2 weeks. Solutions of methohexital are stable for up to 6 weeks. When barbiturates are added to Ringer lactate or an acidic solution containing other water-soluble drugs, precipitation will occur and can occlude the IV catheter. Although the typical solution of thiopental (2.5%) is highly alkaline (pH 9) and can be irritating to the tissues if injected extravenously, it does not cause pain on injection and venoirritation is rare. In contrast, a 1% methohexital solution frequently causes discomfort when injected into small veins. Intra-arterial injection of thiobarbiturates is a serious complication as crystals can form in the arterioles and capillaries, causing intense vasoconstriction, thrombosis, and even tissue necrosis. Accidental intra-arterial injections should be treated promptly with intra-arterial administration of papaverine and lidocaine (or procaine), as well as a regional anesthesia-induced sympathectomy (stellate ganglion block, brachial plexus block) and heparinization.

Thiopental is metabolized in the liver to hydroxythiopental and the carboxylic acid derivative, which are more water soluble and have little CNS activity. When high doses of thiopental are administered, a desulfuration reaction can occur with the production of pentobarbital, which has long-lasting CNS-depressant activity. The low elimination clearance of thiopental (3.4 mL/kg/min) contributes to a long elimination half-life ($t_{1/2}\beta$ of 11 hours). Preexisting hepatic and renal disease result in decreased plasma protein binding, thereby increasing the free fraction of thiopental and enhancing its CNS and cardiovascular-depressant properties. During prolonged continuous administration of thiopental, the concentration in the tissues approaches the concentration in the central compartment, with termination of its CNS effects becoming solely dependent on elimination by nonlinear hepatic metabolism. Methohexital is metabolized in the liver to inactive hydroxyderivatives. The clearance of methohexital (11 mL/kg/min) is higher and more dependent on hepatic blood flow than thiopental, resulting in a shorter elimination half-life ($t_{1/2}\beta$ 4 hours).

The usual induction dose of thiopental is 3 to 5 mg/kg in adults, 5 to 6 mg/kg in children, and 6 to 8 mg/kg in infants. Because methohexital is approximately 2.7 times more potent than thiopental, a dose of 1.5 mg/kg is equivalent to 4 mg/kg of thiopental in adults. The dose of barbiturates necessary to induce anesthesia is reduced in premedicated patients, patients in early pregnancy (7 to 13 weeks' gestation), and those of more advanced American Society of Anesthesiologists physical status (III or IV). Geriatric patients require a 30% to 40% reduction in the usual adult dose because of a decrease of the volume of the central compartment and slowed redistribution of thiopental from the vessel-rich tissues to lean muscle.[18] When the calculation of the induction dose is based on the lean body mass rather than total body weight, dosage adjustments for age, sex, or obesity are not necessary. Thiopental infusion is seldom used to maintain anesthesia because of the long context-sensitive half-time and prolonged recovery period. Plasma thiopental levels necessary to maintain a hypnotic state range between 10 and 20 mg/mL. A typical infusion rate necessary to treat intracranial hypertension or intractable convulsions is 2 to 4 mg/kg/hr. The plasma concentration of methohexital needed to maintain hypnosis during anesthesia ranges between 3 and 5 mg/mL and can be achieved with an infusion rate of methohexital 50 to 120 μg/kg/min.

Barbiturates produce a proportional decrease in $CMRO_2$ and CBF, thereby lowering ICP. The maximal decrease in $CMRO_2$ (55%) occurs when the EEG becomes isoelectric (burst-suppressive pattern). An isoelectric EEG can be maintained with a thiopental infusion rate of 4 to 6 mg/kg/hr (resulting in plasma concentrations of 30 to 50 μg/mL). Because the decrease in systemic arterial pressure is usually less than the reduction in ICP, thiopental should improve cerebral perfusion and compliance. Therefore, thiopental is widely used to improve brain relaxation during neurosurgery and to improve cerebral perfusion pressure (CPP) after acute brain injury. Although barbiturate therapy is widely used to control ICP after brain injury, the results of outcome studies are no better than with other aggressive forms of cerebral antihypertensive therapy.

It has been suggested that barbiturates also possess "neuroprotective" properties secondary to their ability to decrease oxygen demand. Alternative explanations have been suggested, including a reverse steal ("Robin Hood effect") on CBF, free-radical scavenging, stabilization of liposomal membranes, as well as excitatory amino acid receptor blockade. On the basis of the evidence from experimental studies and a large randomized prospective multi-institutional study,[19] experts have concluded that barbiturates have no place in the therapy following resuscitation of a cardiac arrest patient. In contrast, barbiturates are frequently used for cerebroprotection during incomplete brain ischemia (e.g., carotid endarterectomy, temporary occlusion of cerebral arteries, profound hypotension, and cardiopulmonary bypass). By improving the brain's tolerance of incomplete ischemia in patients undergoing open heart surgery with cardiopulmonary bypass, barbiturates were alleged to decrease the incidence of postbypass neuropsychiatric disorders.[20] However, during valvular open heart cardiac surgery, a protective effect of barbiturate loading could not be demonstrated.[21] Given the lack of demonstrable neuroprotective effect, use of barbiturates during cardiac surgery is not recommended. Use of moderate degrees of hypothermia (33–34°C) might provide superior neuroprotection to the barbiturates without prolonging recovery.

Barbiturates cause predictable, dose-dependent EEG changes and possess potent anticonvulsant activity. Continuous infusions of thiopental have been used to treat refractory status epilepticus. However, low doses of thiopental may induce spike wave activity in epileptic patients. Methohexital has well-established epileptogenic effects in patients with psychomotor epilepsy. Low-dose methohexital infusions are frequently used to activate cortical

EEG seizure discharges in patients with temporal lobe epilepsy. 5 It is also the IV anesthetic of choice for electroconvulsive therapy[22] because, compared to thiopental and propofol, methohexital produces less depression of EEG activity. Since the frequency of epileptiform EEG activity during induction of anesthesia with methohexital is significantly less than that which occurs during normal periods of sleep in epileptic patients, this suggests that higher doses of methohexital produces anticonvulsant activity. Methohexital also causes myoclonic-like muscle tremors and other signs of excitatory activity (e.g., hiccoughing).

Barbiturates cause dose-dependent respiratory depression.[23] However, bronchospasm or laryngospasm following induction with thiopental is usually the result of airway manipulation in "lightly" anesthetized patients. Laryngeal reflexes appear to be more active after induction with thiopental than with propofol. The cardiovascular effects of thiopental and methohexital include decreases in cardiac output, systemic arterial pressure, and peripheral vascular resistance. The depressant effects of thiopental on cardiac output are primarily a result of a decrease in venous return caused by peripheral pooling, as well as a result of a direct myocardial depressant effect, which assumes increasing importance in the presence of hypovolemia and myocardial disease.[24] Use of appropriate doses can minimize the cardiodepressant effects of thiopental, even in infants.[25] An equipotent dose of methohexital produces even less hypotension than thiopental because of a greater tachycardic response to the blood pressure-lowering effects of the drug. If the blood pressure remains stable, the myocardial oxygen demand/supply ratio remains normal despite the increase in heart rate because of a concurrent decrease in coronary vascular resistance.

Propofol

Propofol (2,6-disopropylphenol), an alkylphenol compound, is virtually insoluble in aqueous solution. The initial Cremophor EL formulation of propofol was withdrawn from clinical testing because of the high incidence of anaphylactic reactions. Subsequently, propofol (10 mg/mL) was reintroduced as an egg lecithin emulsion formulation (Diprivan), consisting of 10% soybean oil, 2.25% glycerol, and 1.2% egg phosphatide. Microbial contamination of the original Diprivan formulation lead the manufacturer to add ethylenediaminetetraacetic acid (EDTA) to the propofol solution. With this formulation, injection pain occurs in 32% to 67% of patients when the drug is injected into small hand veins. This side effect can be minimized by injecting propofol into larger veins and by prior administration of either lidocaine or a potent opioid analgesic (e.g., fentanyl or remifentanil). A wide variety of drugs have been alleged to reduce pain on injection of propofol [e.g., metoprolol,[26] granisetron,[27] dolasetron,[28] and even thiopental[29]]. Diluting the formulation with additional solvent (Intralipid) or changing the lipid carrier (Lipofundin) also reduced propofol-induced injection pain, probably because of a decrease in the concentration of free propofol in the aqueous phase of the emulsion. A new propofol formulation with sodium metabisulphite (instead of EDTA) as an antimicrobial has been shown to be associated with less severe pain on injection.[30] Although the presence of the metabisulphite has raised concerns regarding its use in sulphite-allergic patients, this concern does not appear to be a clinically important problem. Of interest, a 2% formulation is available for long-term sedation to decrease the fluid (and lipid) volume.

A lower-lipid formulation of propofol (Ampofol) was introduced into clinical practice for both general anesthesia[31] and sedation.[32] The increased "free" fraction of propofol leads to increased pain when it is injected into small veins. Therefore, it is important to add lidocaine to the Ampofol formulation to minimize the pain on injection. A water-soluble prodrug of propofol, fospropofol (aka Aquavan or Lusedra), was approved by the FDA for use during local and regional anesthesia (e.g., conscious sedation and/or monitored anesthesia care [MAC]). This prodrug is rapidly hydrolyzed by plasma alkaline phosphatases in the circulation to release free propofol.[33] Therefore, it does not produce the typical pain on injection associated with propofol. However, it has a slower onset than propofol[34] and is frequently associated with a transient severe burning sensation in the perineal region immediately following IV injection. A microemulsion formulation of propofol (Aquafol) has been shown to be as effective and safe as the classical propofol formulation with similar pharmokinetics, but is associated with more severe and frequent injection pain.[35] A new lipid-free preparation of propofol has been developed containing the drug, sulfobutylether β-cyclodextrin and water.[36] Unfortunately, propofol in cyclodextrin (Captisol-enabled propofol) also produced significantly higher injection pain scores than the standard formulation.

Propofol's pharmacokinetics has been studied using single-bolus dosing and continuous infusions.[37] In studies using a two-compartment kinetic model, the initial distribution half-life is 2 to 4 minutes and the elimination half-life is 1 to 3 hours. Using a three-compartment model, the initial and slow distribution half-life values are 1 to 8 minutes and 30 to 70 minutes, respectively. The elimination half-life depends largely on the sampling time after discontinuing the administration of propofol and ranges from 2 to 24 hours. This long elimination half-life is indicative of the existence of a poorly perfused compartment from which propofol slowly diffuses back into the central compartment. Propofol is rapidly cleared from the central compartment by hepatic metabolism and the context-sensitive half-life for propofol infusions up to 8 hours is <40 minutes. Propofol is rapidly and extensively metabolized to inactive, water-soluble sulphate and glucuronic acid metabolites, which are eliminated by the kidneys. The clearance rate of propofol (20 to 30 mL/kg/min) exceeds hepatic blood flow, suggesting that an extrahepatic route of elimination (lungs) also contributes to its clearance. Nevertheless, changes in liver blood flow would be expected to produce marked alterations in the clearance rate of propofol. Surprisingly, few changes in propofol's pharmacokinetics have been reported in the presence of hepatic or renal disease.

The induction dose of propofol in healthy adults is 1.5 to 2.5 mg/kg, with blood levels of 2 to 6 μg/mL producing unconsciousness depending on the concomitant medications (e.g., opioid analgesics), the patient's age and physical status, and the extent of the surgical stimulation.[38] In the morbidly obese patient, the propofol induction and maintenance dosages should be calculated on the basis of patient's lean body weight.[39] In one of the first reports describing the use of propofol for induction and maintenance of anesthesia with nitrous oxide, an average infusion rate of 120 μg/kg/min was used.[40] The recommended maintenance infusion rate of propofol varies between 100 and 200 μg/kg/min for hypnosis and between 25 and 75 μg/kg/min for sedation. Awakening typically occurs at plasma propofol concentrations of 1 to 1.5 μg/mL.[41] Because a 50% decrease in the plasma propofol concentration is usually required for awakening, emergence following anesthesia is usually rapid even following more prolonged infusions (>3 hours).

Analogous to the barbiturates, children require higher induction and maintenance doses of propofol on a milligram per kilogram basis as a result of their larger central distribution volume and higher clearance rate. Elderly patients and those in poor health require lower induction and maintenance doses of propofol as a result of their smaller central distribution volume and decreased clearance rate. Although subhypnotic doses of propofol produce sedation and amnesia,[41] awareness has been reported even at higher infusion rates when propofol is used as the sole anesthetic.[42] Propofol often produces a subjective feeling of well-being (and even euphoria) on emergence, and it has been abused by health care professionals and others as a result of this CNS action.[43]

Propofol decreases $CMRO_2$ and CBF, as well as ICP.[44] However, when larger doses are administered, the marked depressant effect on systemic arterial pressure can significantly decrease CPP. Cerebrovascular autoregulation in response to changes in systemic arterial pressure and reactivity of the cerebral blood flow to changes in carbon dioxide tension are not affected by propofol. Evidence for a possible neuroprotective effect has been reported with *in vitro* preparations, and the use of propofol to produce EEG burst suppression has been proposed as a method for providing neuroprotection during aneurysm surgery. Its neuroprotective effect may at least partially be related to the antioxidant potential of propofol's phenol ring structure, which may act as a free radical scavenger, decreasing free radical–induced lipid peroxidation. A recent study reported that this antioxidant activity may offer many advantages in preventing the hypoperfusion–reperfusion phenomenon that can occur during major laparoscopic surgery.[45]
6 Although TIVA with propofol and an opioid analgesic is a safe and effective alternative to standard inhalation techniques (i.e., volatile anesthetic with nitrous oxide) for maintenance of anesthesia, concerns have been raised regarding the cost-effectiveness of this technique.[46]

Propofol produces cortical EEG changes that are similar to those of thiopental. However, sedative doses of propofol increase β-wave activity analogous to the benzodiazepines. Induction of anesthesia with propofol is occasionally accompanied by excitatory motor activity (so-called nonepileptic myoclonia). In a study involving patients without a history of seizure disorders, excitatory movements following propofol were not associated with EEG seizure activity.[47] Propofol appears to possess profound anticonvulsant properties.[48] Propofol has been reported to decrease spike activity in patients with cortical electrodes implanted for resection of epileptogenic foci and has been used successfully to terminate status epilepticus. The duration of motor and EEG seizure activity following ECT is significantly shorter with propofol than with other IV anesthetics. Propofol produces a decrease in the early components of somatosensory and motor-evoked potentials but does not influence the early components of the auditory-evoked potentials.

Propofol produces dose-dependent respiratory depression, with apnea occurring in 25% to 35% of patients after a typical induction dose. A maintenance infusion of propofol decreases tidal volume and increases respiratory rate. The ventilatory response to carbon dioxide and hypoxia is also significantly decreased by propofol. Propofol can produce bronchodilation in patients with chronic obstructive pulmonary disease and does not inhibit hypoxic pulmonary vasoconstriction.

The cardiovascular depressant effects of propofol are generally considered to be more profound than those of thiopental. Both direct myocardial depressant effects and decreased systemic vascular resistance have been implicated as important factors in producing cardiovascular depression. Direct myocardial depression and peripheral vasodilation are dose- and concentration-dependent. In addition to arterial vasodilation, propofol produces venodilation (caused both to a reduction in sympathetic activity and by a direct effect on the vascular smooth muscle), which further contributes to its hypotensive effect. The relaxation of the vascular smooth muscle may be because of an effect on intracellular calcium mobilization or because of an increase in the production of nitric oxide. Experiments in isolated myocardium suggest that the negative inotropic effect of propofol results from a decrease in intracellular calcium availability secondary to inhibition of transsarcolemmal calcium influx. A recent study in rats has suggested that an altered renin gene is responsible for enhanced sensitivity and hypotensive responses to propofol.[49]

Propofol also alters the baroreflex mechanism, resulting in a smaller increase in heart rate for a given decrease in arterial pressure.[50] The smaller increase in heart rate with propofol may account for the larger decrease in arterial pressure than with an equipotent dose of thiopental. Recent data suggest that induction of anesthesia with propofol attenuates desflurane-mediated sympathetic activation.[51] Age enhances the cardiodepressant response to propofol and a reduced dosage is required in studies of the elderly. Patients with limited cardiac reserve seem to tolerate the cardiac depression and systemic vasodilation produced by carefully titrated doses of propofol, and maintenance infusions are increasingly used at the end of cardiac surgery when early extubation is desired.

7 Propofol appears to possess antiemetic properties that contribute to a lower incidence of emetic sequelae after general anesthesia.[40] In fact, subanesthetic doses of propofol (10 to 20 mg bolus doses) have also been successfully used to treat nausea and emesis in the early postoperative period.[52] The postulated mechanisms include antidopaminergic activity, depressant effect on the chemoreceptor trigger zone and vagal nuclei, decreased release of glutamate and aspartate in the olfactory cortex, and reduction of serotonin concentrations in the area postrema. However, the ability of propofol to produce a sense of well-being may also contribute to its antiemetic action. Interestingly, propofol also decreases the pruritus produced by spinal opioids.

Propofol does not trigger malignant hyperthermia and may be considered the induction agent of choice in malignant hyperthermia-susceptible patients. The use of propofol infusions for sedation in the pediatric ICU has been linked to several deaths following prolonged administration because of lipid accumulation and hypotension. Although clinical doses of propofol do not affect cortisol synthesis or the response to adrenocorticotropic hormone stimulation, propofol has been reported to inhibit phagocytosis and killing of bacteria in vitro and to reduce proliferative responses when added to lymphocytes from critically ill patients.[53] Because fat emulsions are known to support the growth of microorganisms, contamination can occur as a result of dilution or fractionated use.[54]

In critically ill children and adults receiving high-dose infusions of propofol, some patients have been reported to experience so-called propofol infusion syndrome (PRIS), which is characterized by cardiac failure, rhabdomyolysis, metabolic acidosis, and renal failure and is often fatal.[55] Hyperkalemia, hypertriglyceridemia, and hepatomegaly are also key features. It is associated with high doses and long-term use of propofol (>4 mg/kg/hr for >24 hours). It occurs more commonly in children, and critically ill patients receiving catecholamines and glucocorticoids.

Benzodiazepines

The parenteral benzodiazepines include diazepam (Valium), lorazepam (Ativan), and midazolam (Versed), as well as the antagonist flumazenil (Romazicon). Diazepam and lorazepam are insoluble in water and their formulation contains propylene glycol, a tissue irritant that causes pain on injection and venous irritation. Diazepam is available in a lipid emulsion formulation, which does not cause pain or thrombophlebitis but is associated with a slightly lower bioavailability. Midazolam is a water-soluble benzodiazepine that is available in an acidified (pH 3.5) aqueous formulation that produces minimal local irritation after IV or intramuscular (IM) injection.[56] At physiologic pH, an intramolecular rearrangement occurs that changes the physicochemical properties of midazolam such that it becomes more lipid soluble.

Benzodiazepines undergo hepatic metabolism via oxidation and glucuronide conjugation. Oxidation reactions are susceptible to hepatic dysfunction and coadministration of other anesthetic drugs. Diazepam is metabolized to active metabolites (desmethyldiazepam, 3-hydroxydiazepam), which can prolong the residual sedative effects of diazepam because of their long $t_{1/2}\beta$ values. These metabolites undergo secondary conjugation to form inactive water-soluble glucuronide conjugates. Drugs that inhibit the oxidative metabolism of diazepam include the H_2-receptor blocking drug cimetidine. Severe liver disease reduces diazepam's protein-binding and hepatic-clearance rate, increases its volume of distribution, and thereby further prolongs the $t_{1/2}\beta$ value. Chronic renal disease decreases protein binding and increases the free drug fraction, resulting in enhanced hepatic metabolism and a shorter $t_{1/2}\beta$ value. In elderly patients, the clearance rate of diazepam is significantly decreased, with a $t_{1/2}\beta$ of 75 to 150 hours.

Lorazepam is directly conjugated to glucuronic acid to form pharmacologically inactive metabolites. Age and renal disease have little influence on the kinetics of lorazepam; however, severe hepatic disease decreases its clearance rate. Midazolam undergoes extensive oxidation by hepatic enzymes to form water-soluble hydroxylated metabolites, which are excreted in the urine. However, the primary metabolite, 1-hydroxymethylmidazolam, has mild CNS-depressant activity. The hepatic clearance rate of midazolam is five times greater than lorazepam and ten times greater than diazepam. Although changes in liver blood flow can affect the clearance of midazolam, age has relatively little influence on the elimination half-life of midazolam.

The benzodiazepines used in anesthesia are classified as either short (midazolam, flumazenil), intermediate (diazepam), or long acting (lorazepam). Since the distribution volumes are similar, the large difference in the elimination half-times is because of differences in their differing clearance rates (Table 18-1). The context-sensitive half-times for diazepam and lorazepam are very long; therefore, only midazolam should be used by continuous infusion to avoid excessive accumulation.

8 All benzodiazepines produce dose-dependent anxiolytic, anterograde amnestic, sedative, hypnotic, anticonvulsant, and spinally mediated muscle relaxant properties. Benzodiazepines differ in potency and efficacy with regard to their distinctive pharmacologic properties.[56] The dose-dependent pharmacologic activity implies that the CNS effects of various benzodiazepine compounds depend on the affinity for receptor subtypes and their degree of receptor binding. Although benzodiazepines can be used as hypnotics, they are primarily used as premedicants and adjuvant drugs because of their anxiolytic, sedative, and amnestic properties. For example, midazolam (0.02 to 0.04 mg/kg IV/IM) is the most commonly used premedicant. In addition, midazolam, 0.4 to 0.8 mg/kg administered orally 10 to 15 minutes before parental separation, is an excellent premedicant in children. In contrast to lorazepam, both diazepam and midazolam can be used to induce anesthesia because they have a relatively short onset time after IV administration. The half-life of equilibration between the plasma concentration of midazolam and its maximal EEG effect is only 2 to 3 minutes. The therapeutic window to maintain unconsciousness with midazolam is reported to be 100 to 200 ng/mL, with awakening occurring at plasma concentrations below 50 ng/mL. However, significant hypnotic synergism occurs when midazolam and opioid analgesics are administered in combination.

The usual induction dose of midazolam in premedicated patients is 0.1 to 0.2 mg/kg IV, with infusion rates of 0.25 to 1.0 μg/kg/min required to maintain hypnosis and amnesia in combination with inhalational agents and/or opioid analgesics. Higher maintenance infusion rates and prolonged administration will result in accumulation and prolonged recovery times. Lower infusion rates are sufficient to provide sedation and amnesia during local and regional anesthesia.[57] Patient-controlled administration of midazolam during procedures under local anesthesia is well accepted by patients and associated with few perioperative complications.[58]

Benzodiazepines decrease both $CMRO_2$ and CBF analogous to the barbiturates and propofol. However, in contrast to these compounds, midazolam is unable to produce a complete burst-suppressive (isoelectric) pattern on the EEG. Accordingly, there is a "ceiling" effect with respect to the decrease in $CMRO_2$ produced by increasing doses of midazolam. Midazolam produces a dose-related decrease in regional cerebral perfusion in the parts of the brain that subserve arousal, attention, and memory. Cerebral vasomotor responsiveness to carbon dioxide is preserved during midazolam anesthesia. In patients with severe head injury, a bolus dose of midazolam may decrease CPP with little effect on ICP. Although midazolam may improve neurologic outcome after incomplete ischemia in animal experiments, benzodiazepines have not been shown to possess neuroprotective activity in humans. Like the other sedative–hypnotic drugs, the benzodiazepines are potent anticonvulsants that are commonly used to treat status epilepticus.

Benzodiazepines produce dose-dependent respiratory depression. In healthy patients, the respiratory depression associated with benzodiazepine premedication is insignificant. However, the depressant effect is enhanced in patients with chronic respiratory disease, and synergistic depressant effects occur when benzodiazepines are coadministered with opioid analgesics. Benzodiazepines also depress the swallowing reflex and decrease upper airway reflex activity.

Both midazolam and diazepam produce decreases in systemic vascular resistance and blood pressure when large doses are administered for induction of anesthesia. However, the cardiovascular depressant effects of benzodiazepines are frequently "masked" by the stimulus of laryngoscopy and intubation. The cardiovascular depressant effects are directly related to the plasma concentration; however, a plateau plasma concentration appears to exist above which little further change in arterial blood pressure occurs. In the presence of heart failure, the decrease in preload and afterload produced by benzodiazepines may be beneficial in improving cardiac output. However, the cardiodepressant effect of benzodiazepines may be more marked in hypovolemic patients.

An investigational short-acting intravenous sedative, Ro 48–6791, is a water-soluble benzodiazepine that has full agonistic activity at CNS benzodiazepine receptors. Compared with midazolam, it is 2- to 2.5-fold more potent, has a higher plasma clearance rate, and has a similar onset and duration of action.[59] In a study involving outpatients undergoing endoscopy procedures, the times to ambulation and to recovery from psychomotor impairment were decreased compared to midazolam, although the later recovery end points (e.g., "fitness-for-discharge") were similar.[60]

In contrast to all other sedative–hypnotic drugs, there is a specific antagonist for benzodiazepines. Flumazenil, a 1,4-imidazobenzodiazepine derivative, has a high affinity for the benzodiazepine receptor but minimal intrinsic activity.[61] Flumazenil's molecular structure is similar to other benzodiazepines except for the absence of a phenyl group, which is replaced by a carbonyl group. It is water soluble and possesses moderate lipid solubility at physiologic pH. Flumazenil is rapidly metabolized in the liver, and its metabolites are excreted in the urine as glucuronide conjugates. Flumazenil acts as a competitive antagonist in the presence of benzodiazepine agonist compounds. The residual activity of the benzodiazepines in the presence of flumazenil depends on the relative concentrations of the agonist and antagonist drugs. As a result, it is possible to reverse benzodiazepine-induced anesthesia (or deep sedation) either completely or partially, depending on the dose of flumazenil (0.5–1 mg IV). Flumazenil is short acting, with an elimination half-life of ~1 hour.

Recurrence of the central effects of benzodiazepines (resedation) may occur after a single dose of flumazenil because of residual effects of the more slowly eliminated agonist drug.[62] If sustained antagonism is desired, it may be necessary to administer flumazenil as repeated bolus doses or a continuous infusion. In general, 45 to 90 minutes of antagonism can be expected following flumazenil 1 to 3 mg IV. However, the respiratory depression produced by benzodiazepines is not completely reversed by flumazenil.[63] Reversal of benzodiazepine sedation with flumazenil is not associated with adverse cardiovascular effects or evidence of an acute stress response.[64] Although flumazenil does not appear to change CBF or $CMRO_2$ following midazolam anesthesia for craniotomy, acute increases in ICP have been reported in head-injured patients receiving flumazenil.

Etomidate

Etomidate is a carboxylated imidazole-containing anesthetic compound (R-1-ethyl-1-[a-methylbenzyl] imidazole-5-carboxylate) 9
that is structurally unrelated to any other IV anesthetic. Only the d-isomer of etomidate possesses anesthetic activity. Analogous to midazolam (which also contains an imidazole nucleus), etomidate undergoes an intramolecular rearrangement at physiologic pH, resulting in a closed-ring structure with enhanced lipid solubility. The aqueous solution of etomidate (Amidate) is unstable at physiologic pH and is formulated in a 0.2% solution with 35% propylene glycol (pH 6.9), contributing to a high incidence of pain on injection, venoirritation, and hemolysis. A new lipid emulsion formulation (Etomidate-Lipuro) has been used in Europe for a number of years and appears to be associated with a lower incidence of side effects compared with the original propylene glycol formulation of etomidate.

The standard induction dose of etomidate (0.2 to 0.3 mg/kg IV) produces a rapid onset of anesthesia. Involuntary myoclonic movements are common during the induction period as a result of subcortical disinhibition and are unrelated to cortical seizure activity. The frequency of this myoclonic-like activity can be attenuated by prior administration of opioid analgesics, benzodiazepines, or small sedative doses (0.03 to 0.05 mg/kg) prior to induction of anesthesia.[65] Recently, remifentanil reduced etomidate-induced myoclonic activity without increasing side effects like apnea, emesis, or pruritus.[66] The notion of utilizing a priming dose to reduce the incidence of myclonus has recently been disproven.[67] Emergence time after etomidate anesthesia is dose-dependent but remains short even after administration of repeated bolus doses or continuous infusions. For maintenance of hypnosis, the target concentration is 300 to 500 ng/mL and can be rapidly achieved by administering a two- or three-stage infusion (e.g., 100 mg/kg/min for 10 minutes followed by 10 mg/kg/min or 100 mg/kg/min for 3 to 5 minutes, followed by 20 mg/kg/min for 20–30 minutes, and then 10 mg/kg/min). The pharmacokinetics of etomidate are optimally described by a three-compartment open model.[68] The high clearance rate of etomidate (18 to 25 mL/kg/min) is a result of extensive ester hydrolysis in the liver (forming inactive water-soluble metabolites). A significant decrease in plasma protein binding has been reported in the presence of uremia and hepatic cirrhosis. Severe hepatic disease causes a prolongation of the elimination half-life secondary to an increased volume of distribution and a decreased plasma clearance rate.

Analogous to the barbiturates, etomidate decreases $CMRO_2$, CBF, and ICP. However, the hemodynamic stability associated with etomidate will maintain adequate CPP. Etomidate has been used successfully for both induction and maintenance of anesthesia for neurosurgery. The well-known inhibitory effect of etomidate on adrenocortical synthetic function[69] limits its clinical usefulness for long-term treatment of elevated ICP. Although clear evidence for a neuroprotective effect in humans is lacking, etomidate is frequently used during temporary arterial occlusion and intraoperative angiography (for the treatment of cerebral aneurysms). Etomidate produces an EEG pattern that is similar to thiopental except for the absence of increased β-activity at lower doses. Etomidate has been alleged to produce convulsion-like EEG potentials in epileptic patients without the appearance of myoclonic or convulsant-like motor activity, a property that has been proven useful for intraoperative mapping of seizure foci. Analogous to methohexital, etomidate possesses anticonvulsant properties and has been used to terminate status epilepticus. Etomidate also produces a significant increase of the amplitude of somatosensory-evoked potentials while only minimally increasing their latency. Consequently, etomidate can be used to facilitate the interpretation of somatosensory-evoked potentials when the signal quality is poor.

Etomidate causes minimal cardiorespiratory depression even in the presence of cardiovascular and pulmonary disease.[70] The drug does not induce histamine release and can be safely used in patients with reactive airway disease. Consequently, etomidate is considered to be the induction agent of choice for poor-risk patients with cardiorespiratory disease, as well as in those situations in which preservation of a normal blood pressure is crucial (e.g., cerebrovascular disease). However, etomidate does not effectively blunt the sympathetic response to laryngoscopy and intubation unless combined with a potent opioid analgesic.

Etomidate is associated with a high incidence of postoperative nausea and emesis when used in combination with opioids for brief outpatient procedures. In addition, the increased mortality in critically ill patients sedated with an etomidate infusion has been attributed to its inhibitory effect on cortisol synthesis. Etomidate inhibits the activity of 11-β-hydroxylase, an enzyme necessary for the synthesis of cortisol, aldosterone, 17-hydroxyprogesterone, and corticosterone. Even after a single induction dose of etomidate,[71] adrenal suppression persists for 5 to 8 hours. Although the clinical significance of short-term blockade of cortisol synthesis is not known, the use of etomidate for maintenance of anesthesia has been questioned. Recently, etomidate has been reported to inhibit platelet function, resulting in prolongation of the bleeding time.[72] In spite of its side effect profile, etomidate remains a valuable induction drug for specific indications (e.g., in patients with severe cardiovascular and cerebrovascular disease).

Ketamine

Ketamine (Ketalar or Ketaject) is an arylcyclohexylamine that is structurally related to phencyclidine.[73] Ketamine is a water-soluble compound with a pKa of 7.5 and is available in 1%, 5%, and 10% aqueous solutions. The ketamine molecule contains a chiral center producing two optical isomers. The S(+) isomer of ketamine possesses more potent anesthetic and analgesic properties despite having a similar pharmacokinetic and pharmacodynamic profile as the racemic mixture (or the R[−] isomer).[74,75] Although the S(+)-ketamine has been in clinical use in Europe for many years, the most commonly used solution in the remainder of the world remains the racemic mixture of the two isomers. Ketamine is extensively metabolized by hepatic microsomal cytochrome P450 enzymes and its primary metabolite, norketamine, is one-third to one-fifth as potent as the parent compound. The metabolites of norketamine are excreted by the kidney as water-soluble hydroxylated and glucuronidated conjugates. Analogous to the barbiturates and propofol, ketamine has relatively short distribution and redistribution half-life values. Ketamine also has a high hepatic clearance rate (1 L/min) and a large distribution volume (3 L/kg), resulting in an elimination half-life of 2 to 4 hours. The high hepatic extraction ratio suggests that alterations in hepatic blood flow can significantly influence the clearance rate of ketamine.

10 Ketamine produces dose-dependent CNS depression leading to a so-called *dissociative anesthetic* state characterized by profound analgesia and amnesia, even though patients may be conscious and maintain protective reflexes. The proposed mechanism for this cataleptic state includes electrophysiologic inhibition of thalamocortical pathways and stimulation of the limbic system. Although it is most commonly administered parenterally, oral and intranasal administration of ketamine (6 mg/kg) has been used for premedication of pediatric patients. Following benzodiazepine premedication, ketamine 1 to 2 mg/kg IV (or 4 to 8 mg/kg IM) can be used for induction of anesthesia. The duration of ketamine-induced anesthesia is in the range of 10 to 20 minutes after a single induction dose; however, recovery to full orientation may require an additional 60 to 90 minutes. Emergence times are even longer following repeated bolus injections or a continuous infusion. S(+)-ketamine has a shorter recovery time compared with the racemic mixture. The therapeutic window for maintenance of unconsciousness with ketamine is between 0.6 and 2 μg/mL in adults and between 0.8 and 4 μg/mL in children. Analgesic effects are evident at subanesthetic doses of 0.1 to 0.5 mg/kg IV and plasma concentrations of between 85 and 160 ng/mL. Adjunctive use of a low-dose ketamine infusion (1 to 3 μg/kg/min IV) during the 24 to 48 hour period after major surgery produces significant opioid-sparing effects and decreases opioid-related gastrointestinal side effects.[76,77]

As a result of its NMDA-receptor blocking activity, ketamine should be highly effective for "preemptive" analgesia and opioid-resistant chronic pain states.[78] Unfortunately, a well-controlled study failed to demonstrate a preemptive effect when ketamine was administered prior to the surgical incision (vs. intraoperatively).[79] Nevertheless, other studies[80,81] described a beneficial opioid-sparing effect of small doses of ketamine (75 to 150 μg/kg IV) when administered as an adjuvant during surgery.

An important consideration in the use of ketamine anesthesia relates to the high incidence of psychomimetic reactions (namely, hallucinations, nightmares, altered short-term memory, and cognition) during the early recovery period. The incidence of these reactions is dose-dependent and can be reduced by coadministration of benzodiazepines, barbiturates, or propofol. Ketamine has been traditionally contraindicated for patients with increased ICP or reduced cerebral compliance because it increases $CMRO_2$, CBF, and ICP. However, there is recent evidence that IV induction doses of ketamine actually decrease ICP in traumatic brain injury patients during controlled ventilation with propofol sedation.[82] Prior administration of thiopental or benzodiazepines can blunt ketamine-induced increases in CBF. Because ketamine

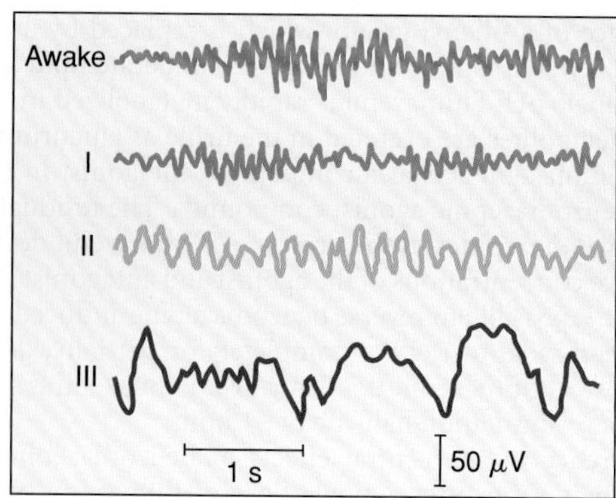

FIGURE 18-5. Progressive changes in the electroencephalogram (EEG) produced by ketamine. Stages I through III are achieved with racemic ketamine and its S(+)isomer. With R(−)ketamine, Stage II was the maximal EEG depression produced. (Reprinted with permission from: Shüttler J, Stanski DR, White PF, et al. Pharmacodynamic modeling of the EEG effect of ketamine and its enantiomers in man. *J Pharmacokinet Biopharm.* 1987;15:241.)

has antagonistic activity at the NMDA receptor, it may possess some inherent protective effects against brain ischemia. However, ketamine can adversely affect neurologic outcome in the presence of brain ischemia despite its NMDA-receptor blocking activity. Cortical EEG recordings following ketamine induction are characterized by the appearance of fast β activity (30 to 40 Hz) followed by moderate-voltage θ activity, mixed with high-voltage δ waves recurring at 3 to 4 second intervals. At higher dosages, ketamine produces a unique EEG burst-suppression pattern (Fig. 18-5).

Although ketamine-induced myoclonic and seizure-like activity has been observed in normal (nonepileptic) patients, ketamine appears to possess anticonvulsant activity.[12,13] Several studies have demonstrated the opioid-sparing effects of low-dose ketamine (75 to 200 μg/kg) when administered as an adjuvant during anesthesia.[80,81,83,84] Interestingly, small doses of ketamine have also been used in the treatment of severe depression in patients with chronic pain syndromes.[85,86] However, ketamine can produce adverse effects when administered in the presence of tricyclic antidepressants because both drugs inhibit norepinephrine reuptake and could produce severe hypotension, heart failure, and/or myocardial ischemia.[86,87]

Ketamine has well-characterized bronchodilatory activity. In the presence of active bronchospasm, ketamine is considered to be the IV induction agent of choice. Ketamine has been used in subanesthetic dosages to treat persistent bronchospasm in the OR and ICU. It is also used in combination with midazolam to provide sedation and analgesia for asthmatic patients. In contrast to the other IV anesthetics, protective airway reflexes are more likely to be preserved with ketamine. However, it must be emphasized that the use of ketamine does not obviate the need for tracheal intubation in the patient with a full stomach (because tracheal soiling has been reported in this situation). Ketamine causes minimal respiratory depression in clinically relevant doses and can facilitate the transition from mechanical to spontaneous ventilation after anesthesia. However, its ability to increase oral secretions can lead to laryngospasm during "light" anesthesia.

Ketamine has prominent cardiovascular-stimulating effects secondary to direct stimulation of the sympathetic nervous system. Ketamine is the only anesthetic that actually increases peripheral arteriolar resistance. As a result of its vasoconstrictive properties, ketamine can reduce the magnitude of redistribution hypothermia.[88] Induction of anesthesia with ketamine often produces significant increases in arterial blood pressure and heart rate. Although the mechanism of the cardiovascular stimulation is not entirely clear, it appears to be centrally mediated. There is evidence to suggest that ketamine attenuates baroreceptor activity via an effect on NMDA receptors in the nucleus tractus solitarius. Because of the increased cardiac work and myocardial oxygen consumption, ketamine negatively affects the balance between myocardial oxygen supply and demand. Consequently, its use is not recommended in patients with severe coronary artery disease. In contrast to the secondary cardiovascular stimulation, ketamine has intrinsic myocardial depressant properties that only become apparent in the seriously ill patient with depleted catecholamine reserves. Because ketamine can also increase pulmonary artery pressure, its use is contraindicated in adult patients with poor right ventricular reserve. Interestingly, the effect on the pulmonary vasculature seems to be attenuated in children.

The renewed interest in ketamine is related to the use of smaller doses (100 to 250 μg/kg) as an adjuvant during anesthesia.[83,84,89] The anesthetic (sedative) and opioid analgesic-sparing effects of ketamine can reduce ventilatory depression during monitored anesthesia care.[87,90,91] When used as an adjuvant to lidocaine for intravenous regional anesthesia, ketamine did not have any selective benefit compared to the same dose of ketamine administered systemically.[92] However, ketamine (0.5 mg/kg) at induction followed by a small intraoperative infusion of ketamine (0.3 mg/kg/hr) until the end of surgery can reduce remifentanil-induced postanesthetic shivering in the early recovery phase.[93] The availability of the stereoisomer of ketamine has increased the nonanesthetic adjunctive use of ketamine.[94] The anesthetic and analgesic potency of S(+)-ketamine is three times greater than R(–)-ketamine and twice that of the racemic mixture (Fig. 18-6), reflecting its fourfold greater affinity at the phencyclidine binding site on the NMDA receptor compared with the R(–) isomer. The therapeutic index of S(+)-ketamine is 2.5 times greater than both the R(–) and the racemic forms. In addition, hepatic biotransformation of S(+)-ketamine occurs 20% faster than that of the R(–) enantiomer, contributing to shorter emergence times and faster return of cognitive function. Both isomers produce similar cardiovascular-stimulating effects

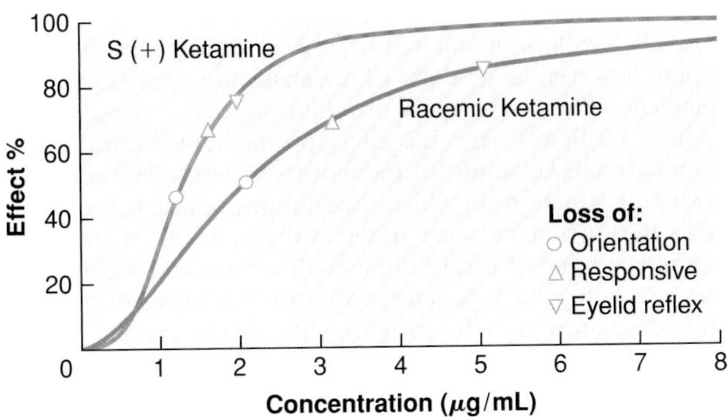

FIGURE 18-6. Concentration-response relationship for racemic ketamine and S(+)ketamine in relation to specific clinical end points. The slowing of the median electroencephalogram frequency was used as the effect (end point) and was related to the arterial blood concentrations of ketamine. (Reprinted with permission from: Schüttler J, Kloos S, Ihmsen H, et al. Pharmacokinetic-pharmacodynamic properties of S(+) ketamine versus racemic ketamine: A randomized double-blind study in volunteers. *Anesthesiology.* 1992;77:A330.)

and hormonal responses during surgery. Although the incidence of dreaming is similar with S(+)-ketamine and the racemic mixture, subjective mood and patient acceptance are higher with the S(+) isomer.[74,75]

Dexmedetomidine

Dexmedetomidine is a highly selective α_2-adrenoceptor agonist that has been approved by the FDA for the short-term (<24 hours) sedation of mechanically ventilated patients in the ICU setting, as well as for sedation during diagnostic and therapeutic procedures under MAC (e.g., neuroradiologic imaging procedures). In this setting it appears to offer some clinical advantages because it produces a unique type of sedation-analgesia with less ventilatory depression than the commonly used sedative–hypnotic and opioid analgesic drugs.[15]

When used for premedication prior to general anesthesia, dexmedetomidine produced preoperative sedation and anxiolysis comparable to midazolam.[16] However, its use led to an increased incidence of intraoperative hypotension and bradycardia compared with the commonly used benzodiazepine compound. When used for premedication prior to regional anesthesia, dexmedetomidine reduced patient anxiety, sympathoadrenal (stress) responses, and perioperative opioid analgesic requirements.[95] Hall et al.[96] also demonstrated the sedative, amnestic, and analgesic effects of low-dose infusions of dexmedetomidine (0.2 to 0.6 μg/kg/hr).

As an IV adjuvant during induction and/or maintenance of general anesthesia, dexmedetomidine will blunt the acute hemodynamic response to laryngoscopy and intubation.[97] It has also been used to facilitate awake fiberoptic intubation[98–100] and has most recently been utilized as part of a target-controlled technique.[101] When used as an anesthetic adjuvant during general anesthesia, dexmedetomidine has been reported to improve perioperative hemodynamic stability in vascular[102] and neurosurgical patients,[103,104] improve postoperative pain control after major surgery,[105–107] and may reduce postoperative nausea and vomiting after ambulatory surgery.[108] However, a study involving bariatric patients[109] failed to demonstrate any clinically significant improvements in patient outcomes after surgery despite producing both anesthetic and analgesic-sparing effects. Additionally, the use of dexmedetomidine as an adjuvant to propofol was associated with delayed emergence as compared to propofol alone.[110]

Dexmedetomidine is alleged to produce minimal respiratory depression during IV sedation. Although in one comparative study with propofol, arterial saturation was better preserved with dexmedetomidine,[111] another study reported similar respiratory rates and oxygen saturation values when propofol and dexmedetomidine infusions were utilized for IV sedation.[112] In a recent study utilizing an intraoperative infusion of dexmedetomidine as an adjuvant to inhalation anesthesia in children with obstructive sleep apnea undergoing tonsillectomy and adenoidectomy procedures, the α_2-agonist was reported to reduce desaturation events and emergence agitation in the PostAnesthesia Care Unit (PACU).[113]

Thus, dexmedetomidine appears to be a potentially useful adjuvant during local and regional anesthesia. It provides comparable sedation to midazolam[114] but has a slower onset and offset of sedation than propofol.[112] When administered as an adjuvant during IV regional anesthesia[115] it improved the quality of both intra- and postoperative analgesia. Because of its high cost, the cost-benefit ratio of dexmedetomidine as a routine IV adjuvant during general anesthesia clearly requires further investigation.

TABLE 18-2. INDUCTION CHARACTERISTICS AND DOSAGE REQUIREMENTS FOR THE CURRENTLY AVAILABLE SEDATIVE–HYPNOTIC DRUGS

Drug Name	Induction Dose (mg/kg)	Onset (s)	Duration (min)	Excitatory Activity	Pain on Injection	Heart Rate	Blood Pressure
Thiopental	3–6	<30	5–10	+	0–+	↑	↓
Methohexital	1–3	<30	5–10	++	+	↑↑	↓
Propofol	1.5–2.5	15–45	5–10	+	++	0–↓	↓↓
Midazolam	0.2–0.4	30–90	10–30	0	0	0	0/↓
Diazepam	0.3–0.6	45–90	15–30	0	+/+++	0	0/↓
Lorazepam	0.03–0.06	60–120	60–120	0	++	0	0/↓
Etomidate	0.2–0.3	15–45	3–12	+++	+++	0	0
Ketamine	1–2	45–60	10–20	+	0	↑↑	↑↑

0, none; +, minimal; ++, moderate; +++, severe; ↓, decrease; ↑, increase.
From: White PF. *Textbook of Intravenous Anesthesia*. Baltimore: Williams & Wilkins; 1997:27–46, 77–92.

CLINICAL USES OF INTRAVENOUS ANESTHETICS

Induction Agents

The induction characteristics and recommended dosages of the available IV anesthetic agents are summarized in Table 18-2. As a result of differences in pharmacokinetic (e.g., altered clearance and distribution volumes) and pharmacodynamic (altered brain sensitivity) variables, the induction dosages of all IV anesthetics need to be adjusted to meet the needs of individual patients. For example, advanced age, preexisting diseases (e.g., hypothyroidism, hypovolemia), premedication (e.g., benzodiazepines), and coadministration of adjuvant drugs (e.g., opioids, α_2-agonists) decrease the induction dose requirements. When there is concern regarding a possible abnormal response, assessing the effect of a small "test dose" (equal to 10% to 20% of the usual induction dose) will often identify those patients for whom a dosage adjustment is required. Before administering additional medication, adequate time should be allowed for the anesthetic to exert its effect, especially when using drugs with a slow onset of action (midazolam) or in the presence of a "slower" circulation time in elderly patients and those with congestive heart failure.

The clinical uses of propofol have expanded greatly since its introduction into clinical practice in 1989.[41] IV administration of propofol results in a rapid loss of consciousness (usually within one arm-to-brain circulation) that is comparable to that of the barbiturates. Although an induction dose of 2.5 mg/kg was initially recommended, the use of smaller induction doses of propofol (1 to 2 mg/kg) in combination with other IV adjuvants has minimized its acute cardiovascular and respiratory depressant effects. Recovery from the sedative–hypnotic effects of propofol is rapid with less residual sedation, fatigue ("hangover"), and cognitive impairment than with other available sedative–hypnotic drugs after short surgical procedures. Consequently, propofol has become the IV drug of choice for both outpatients undergoing ambulatory surgery, as well as for hospitalized patients with a stable cardiovascular status.

With benzodiazepines, there is wide variation in the dose-response relationships in unpremedicated elective surgery patients. Compared with midazolam, diazepam and lorazepam have slower onset times to achieve a peak effect and their dose-effect relationship is less predictable. As a result, diazepam and lorazepam are rarely used for induction of general anesthesia. In addition, the slow hepatic clearance of diazepam and lorazepam may contribute to prolonged residual effects (e.g., sedation, amnesia, fatigue) when they are used for premedication. Midazolam has a slightly more rapid onset and may be a useful induction agent for special indications (e.g., when nitrous oxide is contraindicated, or as part of a TIVA technique). However, when midazolam is used for induction and/or maintenance of anesthesia, return of consciousness takes substantially longer than with other sedative–hypnotic drugs. In spite of its extensive hepatic metabolism, recovery of cognitive function is still slower after midazolam compared with thiopental, methohexital, etomidate, or propofol.

In an effort to optimize the clinical use of midazolam during the induction period, it is used increasingly as a coinduction agent with other sedative–hypnotic drugs (e.g., propofol, ketamine). Midazolam 2 to 5 mg IV can provide for increased sedation, amnesia, and anxiolysis during the preinduction period. When midazolam is used in combination with propofol, 1.5 to 2 mg/kg IV,[116] or ketamine, 0.75 to 1 mg/kg IV,[117] it facilitates the onset of anesthesia and decreases the possibility of intraoperative recall without delaying emergence times. Midazolam also attenuates the cardiostimulatory response to ketamine, as well as its psychomimetic emergence reactions. Use of midazolam, 2 to 3 mg IV, with propofol reduces recall during the induction period; however, larger doses of midazolam (5 mg IV) will delay emergence after brief surgical procedures.

As a result of their side effect profiles, the clinical use of etomidate and ketamine for induction of anesthesia is restricted to specific situations in which their unique pharmacologic profiles offer advantages over other available IV anesthetics. For example, etomidate can facilitate maintenance of a stable blood pressure in high-risk patients with critical stenosis of the cerebral vasculature and in patients with severe cardiac impairment or unstable angina. Ketamine is a useful induction agent for patients with reactive airway disease, as well as for those situations where continued spontaneous ventilation is desirable during surgery.

Maintenance of Anesthesia

The continued popularity of volatile anesthetics for maintenance of anesthesia is primarily related to their rapid reversibility and ease of administration when using a conventional vaporizer delivery system. The availability of IV drugs with more rapid onset and shorter recovery profiles, as well as user-friendly infusion delivery systems, has facilitated the maintenance of anesthesia with continuous infusions of IV drugs, producing a TIVA state that compares favorably with the volatile anesthetics. In a comparison of the requirement of postoperative analgesics after inhalation and TIVA techniques, not surprisingly, postoperative pain was reduced after TIVA with a combination of propofol infusion supplemented with fentanyl bolus injections[118] because propofol has no significant analgesic properties.[119] TIVA techniques with propofol alone have been shown to have similar postoperative morphine requirements compared to inhalational techniques.[120] In addition, use of a TIVA technique for bariatric surgery in morbidly obese patients was associated with a similar recovery profile compared with a sevoflurane-based inhalation technique.[120] In pediatric patients undergoing rigid bronchoscopy, the use of sevoflurane-based inhalation technique was superior to TIVA technique with regard to hemodynamic stability, respiration rate, induction time, and emergence time.[121] In morbidly obese patients[122] and patients in the prone position,[123] TIVA technique utilizing propofol were associated with greater early impairment of postoperative lung function as compared to inhalational techniques.

The traditional intermittent bolus administration of IV drugs results in depth of anesthesia (and analgesia) that oscillates above and below the desired level.[124] Because of rapid distribution and redistribution of the IV anesthetics, the high peak blood concentration after each bolus is followed by a rapid decrease, producing fluctuating drug levels in the blood and hence the brain. The magnitude of the drug level fluctuation depends on the size of the bolus dose and the frequency of its administration. Wide variation in the plasma drug concentrations can result in hemodynamic and respiratory instability as a result of changes in the depth of anesthesia or sedation. By providing more stable blood (and brain) concentrations with a continuous IV infusion, it might be possible to improve anesthetic conditions and hemodynamic stability, as well as decreasing side effects and recovery times with IV anesthetics.[125] Administration of IV anesthetics by a variable-rate infusion is a logical extension of the incremental bolus method of drug titration, as a continuous infusion is equivalent to the sequential administration of infinitely small bolus doses.

Although an IV anesthetic can be titrated to achieve and maintain the desired clinical effect, knowledge of basic pharmacokinetic principles is helpful in more accurately predicting the optimal dosage requirements. The required plasma concentration depends on the desired pharmacologic effect (hypnosis, sedation), the concomitant use of other adjunctive drugs (opioid analgesics, muscle relaxants, cardiovascular drugs), the type of operation (superficial, intra-abdominal, intracranial), and the patient's sensitivity to the drug (age, drug history, preexisting diseases). Preexisting diseases (cirrhosis, congestive heart failure, renal failure) can markedly alter the pharmacokinetic variables of the highly protein-bound, lipophilic IV anesthetic drugs. In general, children have higher clearance rates, while the elderly have reduced clearance values and require lower propofol concentrations to maintain a hypnotic state.[126] Various intraoperative interventions (e.g., laryngoscopy, tracheal intubation, skin incision, entry into body cavities) transiently increase the anesthetic and/or analgesic requirements. Therefore, the infusion scheme should be tailored to provide peak drug concentrations during the periods of most intense stimulation. For specific surgical interventions, the so-called therapeutic window of an IV anesthetic is defined as the blood concentration range required to produce a given effect (Table 18-3). It must be emphasized that the therapeutic window for sedative–hypnotics is markedly influenced by the presence of adjunctive drugs (e.g., opioids, α_2-agonists, nitrous oxide).

The use of IV anesthetic techniques requires continuous titration of the drug infusion rate to the desired pharmacodynamic end point.[117] Most anesthesiologists rely on somatic and autonomic signs for assessing depth of IV anesthesia, analogous to the manner in which they titrate the volatile anesthetics. The most sensitive clinical signs of depth of anesthesia appear to be changes in muscle tone (i.e., electromyography [EMG]) and ventilatory rate and pattern.[127] However, if the patient has been given muscle relaxants, the anesthesiologist must rely on signs of autonomic hyperactivity (e.g., tachycardia, hypertension, lacrimation, diaphoresis). Unfortunately, the anesthetic drugs (ketamine), as well as adjunctive agents (α_2-agonists, beta-blockers, adenosine, calcium channel blockers), can directly influence the cardiovascular response to surgical stimulation. Although the cardiovascular signs of autonomic nervous system hyperactivity may be masked, other autonomic signs (e.g., diaphoresis) and purposeful movements may be more reliable indicators of depth of anesthesia than blood pressure because the latter depends on the ability of the heart to maintain the cardiac output in the face of acute changes in afterload. The heart rate response to surgical stimulation appears to be more useful than the blood pressure response in determining the need for additional analgesic medication. Moreover, it would appear that blood pressure and heart rate responses to surgical stimulation are a less useful guide with IV techniques than with volatile anesthetics. Interestingly, supplementation

TABLE 18-3. THERAPEUTIC BLOOD CONCENTRATIONS WHEN INTRAVENOUS ANESTHETICS ARE INFUSED FOR HYPNOSIS OR SEDATION

Drug Name	Major Surgery Procedures	Minor Surgery Procedures	Sedative Concentration	Awakening Concentration
Thiopental	10–20 μg/mL	10–20 μg/mL	4–8 μg/mL	4–8 μg/mL
Methohexital	6–15 μg/mL	5–10 μg/mL	1–3 μg/mL	1–3 μg/mL
Propofol	4–6 μg/mL	2–4 μg/mL	1–2 μg/mL	1–1.5 μg/mL
Midazolam	100–200 ng/mL	50–200 ng/mL	40–100 ng/mL	50–150 ng/mL
Etomidate	500–1000 ng/mL	300–600 ng/mL	100–300 ng/mL	200–350 ng/mL
Ketamine	1–4 μg/mL	0.6–2 μg/mL	0.1–1 μg/mL	NA

NA, not available.
From: White PF. *Textbook of Intravenous Anesthesia.* Baltimore: Williams & Wilkins; 1997:27, 77.

with a sedative–hypnotic (propofol) was as effective as a potent opioid analgesic in controlling acute autonomic responses during TIVA.[128]

The clinical assessment of anesthetic depth has become more challenging because IV anesthetic techniques involve a combination of hypnotics, opioids, muscle relaxants, and adjuvant drugs. The interactions between these drugs can result in additive, supra-additive, infra-additive, or even antagonistic effects. An ideal "depth of anesthesia" indicator would integrate the physiologic and neurologic information from all aspects of the anesthetic state. In the absence of a global cerebral function monitor, the depth of anesthesia device should provide an indication of one or more of the key components of general anesthesia (e.g., hypnosis, analgesia, amnesia, suppression of the stress response, or muscle relaxation). A simple, noninvasive monitor of the depth of anesthesia, which would reliably predict a patient's response to surgical stimulation, would be extremely valuable when using IV anesthetic techniques.

The EMG activity of the frontalis muscles increases significantly in patients who move in response to specific surgical stimuli.[127] However, EMG changes occur late and their interpretation is obscured by muscle relaxant drugs. The EEG changes depend largely on the type of anesthetic drugs used. Although a common EEG pattern can be recognized with increasing depression of CNS function by sedative–hypnotics and opioid analgesics, there is no characteristic EEG pattern associated with unconscious and amnestic states.[129] Univariate descriptors of EEG activity appear to be of limited clinical usefulness, and no meaningful correlation could be found between EEG spectral edge frequency and hemodynamic response to surgical stimuli during propofol anesthesia.[130] Although EEG variables (spectral edge frequency, median frequency) appear to be useful indicators of the CNS effects of anesthetic and analgesic drugs in the experimental setting, their usefulness in clinical practice is limited because of confounding factors (e.g., changing drug levels and surgical stimulation). The EEG-based bispectral index (BIS), patient state index, state entropy and response entropy, and cerebral state index all represent similar monitoring approaches that rely on sophisticated computerized algorithms to analyze the spontaneous EEG. These cerebral monitoring devices have proved to be a useful indicator of the hypnotic component of the anesthetic state. Several recent studies have demonstrated that the use of these indices can improve titration of IV anesthetics during surgery, thereby facilitating the recovery process.[131] Low intraoperative BIS values (<40 for greater than 5 minutes) have been associated with a higher risk of myocardial infarction and stroke, may lead to a worsening of long-term survival in the elderly.[132] However, a more recent study involving elderly patients[133] found no evidence that either cumulative BIS values below a threshold of 40 or 45 was injurious to patients. In fact, a lower processed value (median BIS value of 38) was recently reported to decrease the incidence of early postoperative cognitive dysfunction as compared to a higher average BIS value of 58.[134] Nevertheless, using EEG-based monitoring to improve titration of IV and inhalational anesthetics can reduce the time required to achieve fast-track eligibility and facilitate earlier discharge home after ambulatory surgery.[135,136]

An alternative to the spontaneous EEG involves the use of the evoked response of the EEG to sensory stimuli (e.g., auditory-evoked potential monitors). The ability to quantitatively assess the response of the body to varying levels of stimulation (sensory- or auditory-evoked responses) may be useful in improving the assessment of depth of anesthesia (see also Chapter 36 Anesthesia for Neurosurgery).[137] Although all sedative–hypnotic drugs affect the brainstem-evoked potentials, uncertainty still exists regarding the most useful evoked response(s) to measure. The complexity associated with recording evoked responses is much greater than recording the spontaneous EEG because the value is critically dependent on technical factors (e.g., stimulus intensity, stimulus rate, electrode position), body temperature, as well as the anesthetic drugs. Although most IV anesthetics produce dose-dependent changes in the somatosensory-evoked potentials, the correlation between the acute hemodynamic changes to surgical stimuli and the early auditory-evoked responses is poor. However, the early cortical (midlatency) auditory-evoked response might be useful in detecting awareness under anesthesia. Furthermore, the auditory-evoked potential index may be more discriminating than the spontaneous EEG-based devices in characterizing the transition from wakefulness to unresponsiveness.[138]

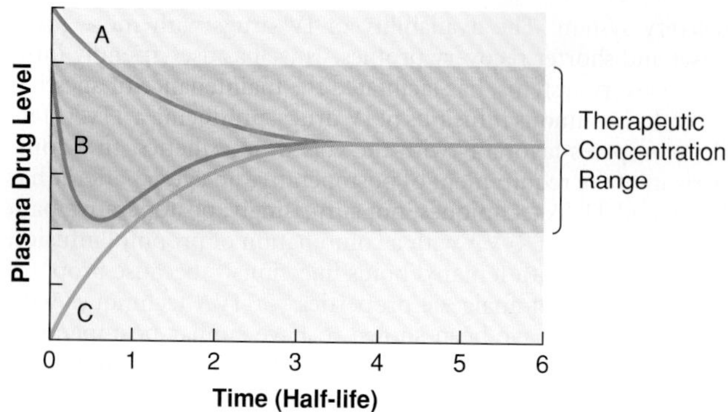

FIGURE 18-7. Simulated drug level curves when a constant infusion is administered following a "full" loading dose equal to [Cp] × Vd_{ss} (*Curve A*), a smaller loading dose equal to [Cp] × Vc (*Curve B*), or in the absence of a loading (*Curve C*). See text for details. (Reprinted with permission from White PF. Clinical uses of intravenous anesthetic and analgesic infusions. *Anesth Analg.* 1989;68:161.)

As a result of the availability of more rapid and shorter acting sedative–hypnotics, sophisticated computer technology, and new insights into pharmacokinetic–dynamic interactions, use of TIVA techniques has been steadily increasing throughout the world during the last decade. When using constant rate IV infusions, 4 to 5 half-lives may be required to achieve a steady state anesthetic concentration (Fig. 18-7). To more rapidly achieve a therapeutic blood concentration, it is necessary to administer a loading (priming) dose and to maintain the desired drug concentration using a maintenance infusion. The loading dose (LD) and initial maintenance infusion rate (MIR) can be calculated from previously determined population kinetic values using the following equations:

$$\text{LD} = \text{Cp (mg/mL)} \times \text{Vd (mL/kg)}$$

$$\text{MIR} = \text{Cp (mL/kg)} \times \text{Cl (mL/kg/min)}$$

where Cp = plasma drug concentration, Vd = distribution volume, and Cl = drug clearance.

The use of the smaller central volume of distribution (Vc) for the Vd component of the LD equation will underestimate the LD, whereas use of the larger steady state volume of distribution (Vd_{ss}) will result in drug levels that transiently exceed those that are desired. If a smaller LD is administered, a higher initial MIR will be required to compensate for the drug that is removed from the brain by both redistribution and elimination processes. As the redistribution phase assumes less importance, the MIR will decrease because it becomes solely dependent on the drug's elimination and the desired plasma concentration.

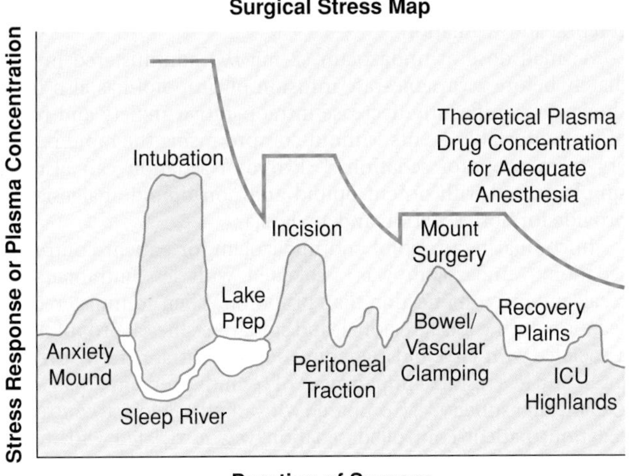

FIGURE 18-8. The "landscape" of surgical anesthesia. The surgical stimuli are not constant during an operation; therefore, the plasma concentration of an intravenous anesthetic should be titrated to match the needs of the individual patient. ICU, intensive care unit. (Reprinted with permission from: Glass PSA, Shafer SL, Jacobs JR, et al. *Intravenous drug delivery systems, Miller's Anesthesia,* 4th ed. New York: Churchill Livingstone; 1994:391.)

An alternative approach is to begin with a rapid loading infusion with a bolus-elimination transfer scheme that combines three functions, as shown in the following equation:

$$\text{Input} = V1 \cdot C_{ss} + Cl \cdot C_{ss} + V1 \cdot C_{ss}\,(k_{12} \cdot e^{-k21t})$$

where V1 = distribution volume of the central compartment, C_{ss} = steady state plasma concentration, Cl = drug clearance; k_{12} = distribution rate constant from the central to the rapid peripheral compartment, and k_{21} = redistribution rate constant from the rapid peripheral back into the central compartment. Implementation of the bolus-elimination transfer infusion scheme requires the use of a microprocessor-controlled pump. If a continuous infusion is to be used in an optimal manner to suppress responses to surgical stimuli, the MIR should be varied according to the individual patient responses (Fig. 18-8). Using an MIR large enough to suppress responses to the most intense surgical stimuli will lead to excessive drug accumulation, postoperative side effects, and a delayed recovery. Clinical signs of inadequate or excessive anesthesia can be treated by making 50% to 100% changes in the MIR. Abrupt increases in autonomic activity can be treated by giving a small bolus dose equal to 10% to 25% of the initial loading dose and increasing the MIR.

Despite the marked pharmacokinetic and pharmacodynamic variability that exists among surgical patients, computer programs have been developed that allow reasonable predictions of concentration-time profiles for IV anesthetics and analgesics. This new technology has led to the development of target-controlled infusions (TCI), whereby the anesthesiologist chooses a "target" blood or brain (effective site) drug concentration and the micropressor-controlled infusion pump infuses the drug at the rate needed to rapidly achieve and maintain the desired concentration based on population pharmacokinetic–dynamic data.[138] It is obvious that the targetted concentrations are only theoretical values and must be altered depending on the observed pharmacodynamic effect and the anticipated changes in surgical stimulation.

Closed-loop control based on plasma drug concentrations is not possible because there is no available method to obtain frequent measurements of drug concentrations in real time. A more advanced form of TCI uses a feedback signal generated by simulating a mathematical model of the control process. Clearly, the precision of control achievable with a model-based system is only as accurate as the model. An example of a model-based drug delivery system is the computer-assisted continuous infusion system. An ideal automatic anesthesia delivery device would titrate anesthetic to meet the needs of the individual patient using an acquired feedback signal that accurately reflects the effect site concentration of the drug. The most successful efforts at feedback control of anesthesia have used the BIS monitor[139,140] and cortical auditory-evoked responses to assess the pharmacodynamic end point.[137]

The rapid, short-acting sedative–hypnotics (e.g., methohexital, propofol) and opioids [e.g., alfentanil, remifentanil[141]] are better suited for continuous administration techniques than the more traditional anesthetic and analgesic agents because they can be more precisely titrated to meet the unique and changing needs of the individual patient. Traditionally, the elimination half-life of a particular drug has been used in attempting to predict the duration of drug action and the time to awakening after discontinuation of the anesthetic infusion. Using conceptual modeling techniques, it has been shown that the concept of context-sensitive half-time is more appropriate in choosing drugs for continuous IV administration (Fig. 18-9). Because none of the currently available IV drugs can provide for a complete anesthetic state without producing prolonged recovery times and undesirable side effects, it is necessary to administer a combination of IV drugs that provide for hypnosis, amnesia, hemodynamic stability, analgesia, and muscle relaxation. Selecting a combination of drugs with similar pharmacokinetics and compatible pharmacodynamic profiles should improve the anesthetic and surgical conditions. Sedative–hypnotics, opioids, sympatholytics, and muscle relaxants can be successfully administered using continuous

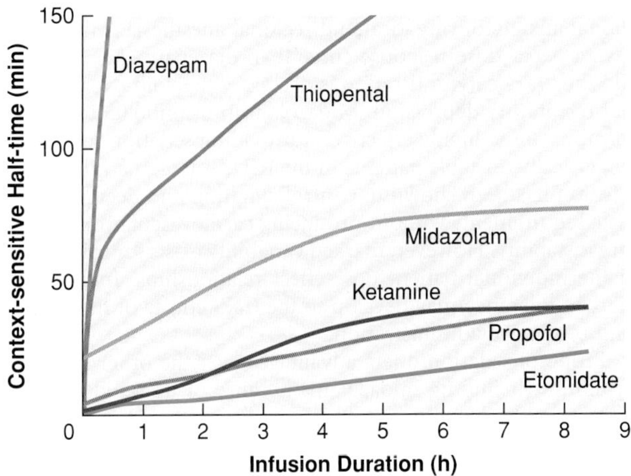

FIGURE 18-9. Context-sensitive half-time values as a function of infusion duration for intravenous anesthetics, including thiopental, midazolam, diazepam, ketamine, etomidate, and propofol. The context-sensitive half-time for thiopental and diazepam is significantly longer compared with etomidate, propofol, and midazolam, with an increasing infusion duration increase. (Reprinted with permission from: Hughes MA, Glass PSA, Jacobs JR. Context-sensitive half-time in multicompartment pharmacokinetic models for intravenous anesthesia. *Anesthesiology.* 1992;76:334.)

infusion TIVA techniques as alternatives to the volatile anesthetics and nitrous oxide.

Sedation in the Operating Room and Intensive Care Unit

The use of sedative–hypnotic drugs as part of a MAC technique in combination with local anesthetics is becoming increasingly popular.[116,142,143] During local or regional anesthesia, subhypnotic dosages of IV anesthetics can be infused to produce sedation, anxiolysis, and amnesia and enhance patient comfort. The optimum sedation technique achieves the desired clinical end points without producing perioperative side effects (e.g., respiratory depression, nausea, and vomiting).[2] In addition, it should provide for ease of titration to the desired level of sedation while providing for a rapid return to a "clear-headed" state on completion of the surgical procedure.

Sedation also constitutes an essential element in the management of patients in the ICU. The ideal sedative agent for critically ill patients would have minimal depressant effects on the respiratory and cardiovascular systems, would not influence biodegradation of other drugs, and would be independent of renal and hepatic function for its elimination. Recently, the BIS monitor has been used to monitor the depth of sedation in the ICU. The steady state BIS was demonstrated to have a statistically significant correlation to the Richmond Agitation Sedation Scale, additionally offering an objective and continuous measurement.[144] For patients undergoing cardiac surgery, rapid reversibility of the sedative state may result in earlier extubation and lead to a shorter stay in the ICU. Although intermittent bolus injections of sedative–hypnotic drugs (e.g., diazepam 2.5 to 5 mg, lorazepam 0.5 to 1 mg, midazolam 1.25 to 2.5 mg) have been administered during local anesthesia, continuous infusion techniques with propofol are becoming increasingly popular for maintaining a stable level of sedation in the OR and ICU settings.

Benzodiazepines, particularly midazolam, are still the most widely used for sedation in the ICU and for relief of acute situational anxiety during local and regional anesthesia. Midazolam has a steeper dose-response curve than diazepam (Fig. 18-3),[116] and therefore careful titration is necessary to avoid oversedation and respiratory depression. Midazolam infusion, 0.05 to 5.0 μg/kg/min, can be highly effective in providing sedation for hemodynamically unstable patients in the ICU.[145] Use of a midazolam infusion has been shown to control agitation and decrease analgesic requirements without producing cardiovascular or respiratory instability. However, marked variability exists for midazolam in the individual patient dose-effect relationships. In addition, marked tolerance may develop to the CNS effects of midazolam with prolonged administration.

Propofol sedation offers advantages over the other sedative–hypnotics (including midazolam) because of its rapid recovery and favorable side effect profile. In addition, the degree of sedation is readily changeable from "light" to "deep" levels by varying the MIR. Following a propofol loading dose of 0.25 to 0.5 mg/kg, a carefully titrated subhypnotic infusion of 25 to 75 μg/kg/min produces a stable level of sedation with minimal cardiorespiratory depression and a short recovery period. Because even low concentrations of propofol can depress the ventilatory response to hypoxia, supplemental oxygen should always be provided. Sedative infusions of propofol produce less perioperative amnesia than midazolam, and propofol-induced amnesia appears to be directly related to the infusion rate. Although midazolam and propofol when used for sedation produce equivalent decreases in cerebral flood flow, only midazolam is likely to improve dynamic cerebral autoregulation.[146]

A small dose of midazolam (2 mg IV) administered immediately before a variable-rate infusion of propofol has also been shown to significantly decrease intraoperative anxiety and recall of uncomfortable events without compromising the rapid recovery from propofol sedation.[143] Propofol sedation can also be supplemented with potent opioid and non-opioid analgesics to provide for both sedation and analgesia.

In comparing propofol and midazolam for patient-controlled sedation,[58] midazolam was associated with less intraoperative recall and pain on injection than propofol. When administered for sedation during local, regional, and spinal anesthesia, propofol was associated with a fivefold higher incidence of intraoperative dreaming[147] and less residual impairment of cognitive function than midazolam after surgery.[148] Compared with anesthesiologist-controlled sedation, patient-controlled sedation was associated with fewer propofol dosages, "lighter" levels of sedation, and reduced patient comfort.[149] Computer "target-controlled" sedation was also associated with more frequent "oversedation."[150] Finally, music can reduce the propofol dosage requirement during local and regional anesthesia.[151]

Compared with midazolam in the ICU setting, use of propofol sedation allowed for more rapid weaning of critically ill patients from artificial ventilation.[148] It has been suggested that the more rapid weaning after propofol sedation may be cost-saving compared with midazolam when only a limited period of sedation (<48 hours) is required.[152] Although a pharmacokinetic study yielded no evidence of a change in receptor sensitivity or drug accumulation over a 4-day study period, preliminary data suggest that tolerance to the CNS effects of propofol may develop with more prolonged administration (>1 week). Increasingly, dexmedetomidine infusions are being used in critically ill patients who require both sedation and analgesia.

Concerns have been raised about elevated lipid plasma levels in patients sedated with standard formulations of propofol over a period of several days, especially when high infusion rates (>6 mg/kg/hr) are used. Approximately 1% of critically ill patients receiving high-dose propofol infusions for >24 hours were observed to develop PRIS, which is manifested as a metabolic acidosis plus cardiac dysfunction, rhabdomyolysis, hypertriglyceridemia, and/or renal failure.[55] However, the availability of a propofol formulation with reduced lipid content (Ampofol) may decrease the risk of this problem in the future. Because of conflicting evidence regarding increased mortality as a result of myocardial failure when propofol was used for sedation in the neonatal ICU,[153–156] more safety data are needed to define the indications for the use of prolonged propofol infusions, especially in this patient population. Low-dose ketamine infusions (5 to 25 μg/kg/min) can also be used for sedation and analgesia during local or regional anesthetic procedures, as well as in the ICU setting.[74] Midazolam, 0.07 to 0.15 mg/kg infused over 3 to 5 minutes, followed by ketamine, 0.25 to 0.5 mg/kg IV over 1 to 3 minutes, produced excellent sedation, amnesia, and analgesia without significant cardiorespiratory depression.

Another alternative to propofol for sedation outside the OR is dexmedetomidine. The α_2-agonist can be infused at rates of 0.25 to 0.75 μg/kg/hr to produce sedation during gynecologic procedures[106] and in the ICU. Use of dexmedetomidine for sedation in the ICU has increased from 2% to 7.2% from 2001 to 2007.[157] With prolonged infusion in the ICU, dexmedetomidine was shown to have linear pharmacokinetics up to a dose of 2.5 μg/kg/hr.[158] Although the onset of sedation is slower than that of propofol, its opioid-sparing effects reduce the risk of ventilatory depression during procedures outside the OR and may facilitate weaning from mechanical ventilation in the ICU. In a recent study in healthy volunteers,[159] dexmedetomidine was shown to inhibit gastric emptying and prolong gastrointestinal transit—a potential issue that requires further investigation in ICU patients and surgical populations at risk to postoperative bowel dysfunction (e.g., elderly patients undergoing major abdominal surgery procedures). The relaxation of the lower esophageal sphincter during a dexmedetomidine infusion is similar to propofol, and unlikely to cause gastroesophageal reflux during sedation.[159] In the ambulatory setting, recovery from the sedative effects of dexmedetomidine is slower than with propofol.[159]

CONCLUSIONS

Despite the introduction of new IV anesthetic agents, it is obvious that many of the goals desirable in an ideal IV anesthetic have not been achieved with any of the currently available drugs. Nevertheless, each of these sedative–hypnotic drugs possesses characteristics that may be useful in specific clinical situations and when combined with an appropriate multimodal analgesic technique (e.g., opioids, nonsteroidal anti-inflammatory drugs, local anesthetics) can provide excellent anesthetic conditions. In situations in which a rapid recovery is not essential (e.g., inpatient procedures), thiopental may be the most cost-effective IV anesthetic. Although recovery from anesthesia with methohexital is more rapid than with thiopental (and compares favorably with propofol), excitatory side effects (e.g., myoclonus, hiccoughing) are more prominent than with thiopental or propofol. Methohexital remains the anesthetic of choice for ECT procedures.

Propofol is the IV drug of choice when a rapid and smooth recovery is essential (e.g., outpatient [ambulatory] anesthesia); increasingly, propofol has been used for all inpatient procedures because of the availability of less costly generic formulations. Recovery from propofol anesthesia is characterized by the absence of a "hangover effect" and reduced postoperative nausea and vomiting symptoms. The cardiovascular-depressant effects produced by propofol appear to be more pronounced than those of the other commonly used IV anesthetics, but can be minimized by careful titration and the use of a variable-rate infusion during the maintenance period. The ability to combine propofol with potent, rapid, and short-acting opioid analgesics (e.g., remifentanil) has facilitated the use of TIVA techniques. Improvements in the TCI delivery systems for IV anesthetics (propofol) and analgesics (remifentanil) and reduced cost of the devices and drugs will lead to a greater acceptance of TIVA techniques in the future.

When administered alone for induction of anesthesia, benzodiazepines are associated with a slower onset and more prolonged recovery profile. In the usual induction doses, benzodiazepines are associated with minimal cardiorespiratory depression and the reliable amnestic effect may be valuable during TIVA (e.g., for acute sedation prior to induction of anesthesia, for maintenance in the absence of nitrous oxide). When administered in smaller doses, midazolam can also be a valuable adjunct as part of a coinduction and/or maintenance technique. Other shorter-acting benzodiazepines may be developed in the future (e.g., Ro 48–6791).

Etomidate has minimal cardiovascular and respiratory depressant effects and is therefore an extremely useful induction agent in high-risk patients. It is also occasionally used as an alternative to methohexital for ECT procedures. The occurrence of pain on injection, excitatory phenomena, adrenocortical suppression, and a high incidence of postoperative nausea and vomiting have limited the use of etomidate to special situations in which its cardiovascular profile offers significant advantages over other available IV anesthetics. A new lipid formulation of etomidate is apparently associated with its fewer side effects and may allow this IV anesthetic to gain wider clinical acceptance in the future.

Ketamine is a unique IV anesthetic that produces a wide spectrum of pharmacologic effects including sedation, hypnosis, somatic analgesia, bronchodilation, and sympathetic nervous system stimulation. Induction of anesthesia can be rapidly achieved following IM injection, making ketamine a valuable alternative to an inhalation induction when IV access is difficult to establish. Ketamine is also indicated for induction of anesthesia in the presence of severe hypovolemic shock, acute bronchospastic states, right-to-left intracardiac shunts, and cardiac tamponade. The adverse hyperdynamic cardiovascular, cerebrodynamic, and psychomimetic effects of ketamine can be minimized by prior administration of a benzodiazepine (e.g., midazolam) or a sedative–hypnotic drug (e.g., thiopental, propofol). Ketamine is also useful as part of coinduction and maintenance anesthetic techniques when avoiding opioid analgesics is desirable. The introduction of the more potent S(+)-ketamine may increase use of ketamine in small doses or by continuous infusion as an IV adjuvant during general anesthesia because of its anesthetic and analgesic-sparing activity.

In summary, IV anesthesia has evolved from being used mainly for induction of anesthesia to providing unconsciousness and amnesia for surgical procedures performed under local, regional, and general anesthesia.[1] New insights into the pharmacokinetics and dynamics of IV anesthetics, as well as the development of computer technology to facilitate IV drug delivery (e.g., TCI) and monitoring of the sedative–hypnotic effects on the CNS, will further enhance the popularity of TIVA techniques. An increasingly important issue relates to the cost-benefit of IV anesthetic techniques compared to the traditional inhalation-based techniques with respect to both short-term and long-term outcomes.[160] While the search for the ideal IV anesthetic continues, the major challenge for anesthesiologists is to choose the sedative–hypnotic drug that most closely matches the individual patient's needs in a specific clinical situation.

References

1. White PF. *Textbook of Intravenous Anesthesia.* Baltimore: Williams & Wilkins; 1997:27, 77.
2. Sa Rego MM, Watcha MF, White PF. The changing role of monitored anesthesia care in the ambulatory setting. *Anesth Analg.* 1997;85:1020–1036.
3. Franks NP, Lieb WR. Molecular and cellular mechanisms of general anaesthesia. *Nature.* 1994;367:607–614.
4. Coates KM, Mather LE, Johnson R, et al. Thiopental is a competitive inhibitor at the human alpha7 nicotinic acetylcholine receptor. *Anesth Analg.* 2001;92:930–933.
5. Rossi MA, Chan CK, Christensen JD, et al. Interactions between propofol and lipid mediator receptors: Inhibition of lysophosphatidate signaling. *Anesth Analg.* 1996;83:1090–1096.
6. Shelly MP. Dexmedetomidine: A real innovation or more of the same? *Br J Anaesth.* 2001;87:677–678.
7. Ebert TJ, Hall JE, Barney JA, et al. The effects of increasing plasma concentrations of dexmedetomidine in humans. *Anesthesiology.* 2000;93:382–394.
8. Fu W, White PF. Dexmedetomidine failed to block the acute hyperdynamic response to electroconvulsive therapy. *Anesthesiology.* 1999;90:422–424.
9. Higuchi H, Adachi Y, Dahan A, et al. The interaction between propofol and clonidine for loss of consciousness. *Anesth Analg.* 2002;94:886–891.
10. Segal IS, Jarvis DJ, Duncan SR, et al. Clinical efficacy of oral-transdermal clonidine combinations during the perioperative period. *Anesthesiology.* 1991;74:220–225.
11. Hughes MA, Glass PS, Jacobs JR. Context-sensitive half-time in multicompartment pharmacokinetic models for intravenous anesthetic drugs. *Anesthesiology.* 1992;76:334–341.
12. Modica PA, Tempelhoff R, White PF. Pro- and anticonvulsant effects of anesthetics (Part II). *Anesth Analg.* 1990;70:433–444.

13. Modica PA, Tempelhoff R, White PF. Pro- and anticonvulsant effects of anesthetics (Part I). *Anesth Analg.* 1990;70:303–315.
14. Drummond-Lewis J, Scher C. Propofol: A new treatment strategy for refractory migraine headache. *Pain Med.* 2002;3:366–369.
15. Hsu YW, Cortinez LI, Robertson KM, et al. Dexmedetomidine pharmacodynamics: Part I: Crossover comparison of the respiratory effects of dexmedetomidine and remifentanil in healthy volunteers. *Anesthesiology.* 2004;101:1066–1076.
16. Scheinin H, Jaakola ML, Sjövall S, et al. Intramuscular dexmedetomidine as premedication for general anesthesia. A comparative multicenter study. *Anesthesiology.* 1993;78:1065–1075.
17. Hofbauer RK, Fiset P, Plourde G, et al. Dose-dependent effects of propofol on the central processing of thermal pain. *Anesthesiology.* 2004;100:386–394.
18. Avram MJ, Krejcie TC, Henthorn TK. The relationship of age to the pharmacokinetics of early drug distribution: The concurrent disposition of thiopental and indocyanine green. *Anesthesiology.* 1990;72:403–411.
19. Brain Resuscitation Clinical Trial (no authors listed). A randomized clinical study of cardiopulmonary-cerebral resuscitation: Design, methods, and patient characteristics. Brain Resuscitation Clinical Trial I Study Group. *Am J Emerg Med.* 1986;4(1):72–86.
20. Gunaydin B, Babacan A. Cerebral hypoperfusion after cardiac surgery and anesthetic strategies: A comparative study with high dose fentanyl and barbiturate anesthesia. *Ann Thorac Cardiovasc Surg.* 1998;4:12–17.
21. Newman MF, Croughwell ND, White WD, et al. Pharmacologic electroencephalographic suppression during cardiopulmonary bypass: A comparison of thiopental and isoflurane. *Anesth Analg.* 1998;86:246–251.
22. Ding Z, White PF. Anesthesia for electroconvulsive therapy. *Anesth Analg.* 2002; 94:1351–1364.
23. Blouin RT, Conard PF, Gross JB. Time course of ventilatory depression following induction doses of propofol and thiopental. *Anesthesiology.* 1991;75:940–944.
24. Vohra A, Thomas AN, Harper NJ, et al. Non-invasive measurement of cardiac output during induction of anaesthesia and tracheal intubation: Thiopentone and propofol compared. *Br J Anaesth.* 1991;67:64–68.
25. Bhutada A, Sahni R, Rastogi S, et al. Randomised controlled trial of thiopental for intubation in neonates. *Arch Dis Child Fetal Neonatal Ed.* 2000;82:F34–F37.
26. Asik I, Yorukoglu D, Gulay I, et al. Pain on injection of propofol: Comparison of metoprolol with lidocaine. *Eur J Anaesthesiol.* 2003;20:487–489.
27. Dubey PK, Prasad SS. Pain on injection of propofol: The effect of granisetron pretreatment. *Clin J Pain.* 2003;19:121–124.
28. Piper SN, R hm KD, Papsdorf M, et al. Dolasetron reduces pain on injection of propofol. *Anasthesiol Intensivmed Notfallmed Schmerzther.* 2002;37:528–531.
29. Agarwal A, Ansari MF, Gupta D, et al. Pretreatment with thiopental for prevention of pain associated with propofol injection. *Anesth Analg.* 2004;98:683–686.
30. Shao X, Li H, White PF, et al. Bisulfite-containing propofol: Is it a cost-effective alternative to Diprivan for induction of anesthesia? *Anesth Analg.* 2000;91: 871–875.
31. Song D, Hamza M, White PF, et al. The pharmacodynamic effects of a lower-lipid emulsion of propofol: A comparison with the standard propofol emulsion. *Anesth Analg.* 2004;98:687–691.
32. Song D, Hamza MA, White PF, et al. Comparison of a lower-lipid propofol emulsion with the standard emulsion for sedation during monitored anesthesia care. *Anesthesiology.* 2004;100:1072–1075.
33. Gibiansky E, Struys MM, Gibiansky L, et al. AQUAVAN injection, a water-soluble prodrug of propofol, as a bolus injection: A phase I dose-escalation comparison with DIPRIVAN (part 1): Pharmacokinetics. *Anesthesiology.* 2005;103:718–729.
34. Struys MM, Vanluchene AL, Gibiansky E, et al. AQUAVAN injection, a water-soluble prodrug of propofol, as a bolus injection: A phase I dose-escalation comparison with DIPRIVAN (part 2): Pharmacodynamics and safety. *Anesthesiology.* 2005;103:730–743.
35. Jung JA, Choi BM, Cho SH, et al. Effectiveness, safety, and pharmacokinetic and pharmacodynamic characteristics of microemulsion propofol in patients undergoing elective surgery under total intravenous anaesthesia. *Br J Anaesth.* 2010;104:563–576.
36. Wallentine CB, Shimode N, Egan TD, et al. Propofol in a modified cyclodextrin formulation: First human study of dose-response with emphasis on injection pain. *Anesth Analg.* 2011;113:738–741.
37. Shafer A, Doze VA, Shafer SL, et al. Pharmacokinetics and pharmacodynamics of propofol infusions during general anesthesia. *Anesthesiology.* 1988;69:348–356.
38. Sebel PS, Lowdon JD. Propofol: A new intravenous anesthetic. *Anesthesiology.* 1989;71:260–277.
39. Ingrande J, Brodsky JB, Lemmens HJ. Lean body weight scalar for the anesthetic induction dose of propofol in morbidly obese subjects. *Anesth Analg.* 2011; 113:57–62.
40. Doze VA, Westphal LM, White PF. Comparison of propofol with methohexital for outpatient anesthesia. *Anesth Analg.* 1986;65:1189–1195.
41. Smith I, White PF, Nathanson M, et al. Propofol. An update on its clinical use. *Anesthesiology.* 1994;81:1005–1043.
42. Glass PS. Prevention of awareness during total intravenous anesthesia. *Anesthesiology.* 1993;78:399–400.
43. Oxorn D, Orser B, Ferris LE, et al. Propofol and thiopental anesthesia: A comparison of the incidence of dreams and perioperative mood alterations. *Anesth Analg.* 1994;79:553–557.
44. Pinaud M, Lelausque JN, Chetanneau A, et al. Effects of propofol on cerebral hemodynamics and metabolism in patients with brain trauma. *Anesthesiology.* 1990;73:404–409.
45. Yagmurdur H, Cakan T, Bayrak A, et al. The effects of etomidate, thiopental, and propofol in induction on hypoperfusion-reperfusion phenomenon during laparoscopic cholecystectomy. *Acta Anaesthesiol Scand.* 2004;48:772–777.
46. Dolk A, Cannerfelt R, Anderson RE, et al. Inhalation anaesthesia is cost-effective for ambulatory surgery: A clinical comparison with propofol during elective knee arthroscopy. *Eur J Anaesthesiol.* 2002;19:88–92.
47. Reddy RV, Moorthy SS, Dierdorf SF, et al. Excitatory effects and electroencephalographic correlation of etomidate, thiopental, methohexital, and propofol. *Anesth Analg.* 1993;77:1008–1011.
48. Ebrahim ZY, Schubert A, Van Ness P, et al. The effect of propofol on the electroencephalogram of patients with epilepsy. *Anesth Analg.* 1994;78:275–279.
49. Stekiel TA, Contney SJ, Roman RJ, et al. Pharmacogenomic strain differences in cardiovascular sensitivity to propofol. *Anesthesiology.* 2011;115:1192–1200.
50. Sellgren J, Ejnell H, Elam M, et al. Sympathetic muscle nerve activity, peripheral blood flows, and baroreceptor reflexes in humans during propofol anesthesia and surgery. *Anesthesiology.* 1994;80:534–544.
51. Lopatka CW, Muzi M, Ebert TJ. Propofol, but not etomidate, reduces desflurane-mediated sympathetic activation in humans. *Can J Anaesth.* 1999;46:342–347.
52. Gan TJ, Glass PS, Howell ST, et al. Determination of plasma concentrations of propofol associated with 50% reduction in postoperative nausea. *Anesthesiology.* 1997;87:779–784.
53. Krumholz W, Endrass J, Hempelmann G. Propofol inhibits phagocytosis and killing of Staphylococcus aureus and Escherichia coli by polymorphonuclear leukocytes in vitro. *Can J Anaesth.* 1994;41:446–449.
54. Crowther J, Hrazdil J, Jolly DT, et al. Growth of microorganisms in propofol, thiopental, and a 1:1 mixture of propofol and thiopental. *Anesth Analg.* 1996; 82:475–478.
55. Vasile B, Rasulo F, Candiani A, et al. The pathophysiology of propofol infusion syndrome: A simple name for a complex syndrome. *Intensive Care Med.* 2003; 29:1417–1425.
56. Reves JG, Fragen RJ, Vinik HR, et al. Midazolam: Pharmacology and uses. *Anesthesiology.* 1985;62:310–324.
57. Urquhart ML, Klapp K, White PF. Patient-controlled analgesia: A comparison of intravenous versus subcutaneous hydromorphone. *Anesthesiology.* 1988;69: 428–432.
58. Ghouri AF, Taylor E, White PF. Patient-controlled drug administration during local anesthesia: A comparison of midazolam, propofol, and alfentanil. *J Clin Anesth.* 1992;4:476–479.
59. Dingemanse J, van Gerven JM, Schoemaker RC, et al. Integrated pharmacokinetics and pharmacodynamics of Ro 48–6791, a new benzodiazepine, in comparison with midazolam during first administration to healthy male subjects. *Br J Clin Pharmacol.* 1997;44:477–486.
60. Tang J, Wang B, White PF, et al. Comparison of the sedation and recovery profiles of Ro 48–6791, a new benzodiazepine, and midazolam in combination with meperidine for outpatient endoscopic procedures. *Anesth Analg.* 1999;89: 893–898.
61. Brogden RN, Goa KL. Flumazenil. A reappraisal of its pharmacological properties and therapeutic efficacy as a benzodiazepine antagonist. *Drugs.* 1991;42: 1061–1089.
62. Ghouri AF, Ruiz MA, White PF. Effect of flumazenil on recovery after midazolam and propofol sedation. *Anesthesiology.* 1994;81:333–339.
63. Flogel CM, Ward DS, Wada DR, et al. The effects of large-dose flumazenil on midazolam-induced ventilatory depression. *Anesth Analg.* 1993;77:1207–1214.
64. White PF, Shafer A, Boyle WA 3rd, et al. Benzodiazepine antagonism does not provoke a stress response. *Anesthesiology.* 1989;70:636–639.
65. Doenicke AW, Roizen MF, Kugler J, et al. Reducing myoclonus after etomidate. *Anesthesiology.* 1999;90:113–119.
66. Kelsaka E, Karakaya D, Sarihasan B, et al. Remifentanil pretreatment reduces myoclonus after etomidate. *J Clin Anesth.* 2006;18:83–86.
67. Nyman Y, von Hofsten K, Ritzmo C, et al. Effect of a small priming dose on myoclonic movements after intravenous anaesthesia induction with Etomidate-Lipuro in children. *Br J Anaesth.* 2011;107:225–228.
68. Van Hamme MJ, Ghoneim MM, Ambre JJ. Pharmacokinetics of etomidate, a new intravenous anesthetic. *Anesthesiology.* 1978;49:274–277.
69. Wagner RL, White PF, Kan PB, et al. Inhibition of adrenal steroidogenesis by the anesthetic etomidate. *N Engl J Med.* 1984;310:1415–1421.
70. Gooding JM, Weng JT, Smith RA, et al. Cardiovascular and pulmonary responses following etomidate induction of anesthesia in patients with demonstrated cardiac disease. *Anesth Analg.* 1979;58:40–41.
71. Wagner RL, White PF. Etomidate inhibits adrenocortical function in surgical patients. *Anesthesiology.* 1984;61:647–651.
72. Gries A, Weis S, Herr A, et al. Etomidate and thiopental inhibit platelet function in patients undergoing infrainguinal vascular surgery. *Acta Anaesthesiol Scand.* 2001;45:449–457.
73. White PF, Way WL, Trevor AJ. Ketamine–its pharmacology and therapeutic uses. *Anesthesiology.* 1982;56:119–136.
74. White PF, Ham J, Way WL, et al. Pharmacology of ketamine isomers in surgical patients. *Anesthesiology.* 1980;52:231–239.

75. White PF, Schüttler J, Shafer A, et al. Comparative pharmacology of the ketamine isomers. Studies in volunteers. *Br J Anaesth.* 1985;57:197–203.
76. Adriaenssens G, Vermeyen KM, Hoffmann VL, et al. Postoperative analgesia with i.v. patient-controlled morphine: Effect of adding ketamine. *Br J Anaesth.* 1999;83:393–396.
77. Guillou N, Tanguy M, Seguin P, et al. The effects of small-dose ketamine on morphine consumption in surgical intensive care unit patients after major abdominal surgery. *Anesth Analg.* 2003;97:843–847.
78. Rabben T, Skjelbred P, Oye I. Prolonged analgesic effect of ketamine, an N-methyl-D-aspartate receptor inhibitor, in patients with chronic pain. *J Pharmacol Exp Ther.* 1999;289:1060–6.
79. Dahl V, Ernoe PE, Steen T, et al. Does ketamine have preemptive effects in women undergoing abdominal hysterectomy procedures? *Anesth Analg.* 2000;90:1419–1422.
80. Suzuki M, Tsueda K, Lansing PS, et al. Small-dose ketamine enhances morphine-induced analgesia after outpatient surgery. *Anesth Analg.* 1999;89:98–103.
81. Menigaux C, Fletcher D, Dupont X, et al. The benefits of intraoperative small-dose ketamine on postoperative pain after anterior cruciate ligament repair. *Anesth Analg.* 2000;90:129–135.
82. Albanese J, Arnaud S, Rey M, et al. Ketamine decreases intracranial pressure and electroencephalographic activity in traumatic brain injury patients during propofol sedation. *Anesthesiology.* 1997;87:1328–1334.
83. Suzuki M. Role of N-methyl-D-aspartate receptor antagonists in postoperative pain management. *Curr Opin Anaesthesiol.* 2009;22:618–622.
84. Loftus RW, Yeager MP, Clark JA, et al. Intraoperative ketamine reduces perioperative opiate consumption in opiate-dependent patients with chronic back pain undergoing back surgery. *Anesthesiology.* 2010;113:639–646.
85. Berman RM, Cappiello A, Anand A, et al. Antidepressant effects of ketamine in depressed patients. *Biol Psychiatry.* 2000;47:351–354.
86. Kudoh A, Takahira Y, Katagai H, et al. Small-dose ketamine improves the postoperative state of depressed patients. *Anesth Analg.* 2002;95:114–118.
87. Mortero RF, Clark LD, Tolan MM, et al. The effects of small-dose ketamine on propofol sedation: Respiration, postoperative mood, perception, cognition, and pain. *Anesth Analg.* 2001;92:1465–1469.
88. Ikeda T, Kazama T, Sessler DI, et al. Induction of anesthesia with ketamine reduces the magnitude of redistribution hypothermia. *Anesth Analg.* 2001;93:934–938.
89. Kohrs R, Durieux ME. Ketamine: Teaching an old drug new tricks. *Anesth Analg.* 1998;87:1186–1193.
90. Badrinath S, Avramov MN, Shadrick M, et al. The use of a ketamine-propofol combination during monitored anesthesia care. *Anesth Analg.* 2000;90:858–862.
91. Deng XM, Xiao WJ, Luo MP, et al. The use of midazolam and small-dose ketamine for sedation and analgesia during local anesthesia. *Anesth Analg.* 2001;93:1174–1177.
92. Viscomi CM, Friend A, Parker C, et al. Ketamine as an adjuvant in lidocaine intravenous regional anesthesia: A randomized, double-blind, systemic control trial. *Reg Anesth Pain Med.* 2009;34:130–133.
93. Nakasuji M, Nakamura M, Imanaka N, et al. An intraoperative small dose of ketamine prevents remifentanil-induced postanesthetic shivering. *Anesth Analg.* 2011;113:484–487.
94. Sneyd JR. Recent advances in intravenous anaesthesia. *Br J Anaesth.* 2004;93:725–736.
95. Jaakola ML. Dexmedetomidine premedication before intravenous regional anesthesia in minor outpatient hand surgery. *J Clin Anesth.* 1994;6:204–211.
96. Hall JE, Uhrich TD, Barney JA, et al. Sedative, amnestic, and analgesic properties of small-dose dexmedetomidine infusions. *Anesth Analg.* 2000;90:699–705.
97. Yildiz M, Tavlan A, Tuncer S, et al. Effect of dexmedetomidine on haemodynamic responses to laryngoscopy and intubation : Perioperative haemodynamics and anaesthetic requirements. *Drugs R D.* 2006;7:43–52.
98. Scher CS, Gitlin MC. Dexmedetomidine and low-dose ketamine provide adequate sedation for awake fibreoptic intubation. *Can J Anaesth.* 2003;50:607–610.
99. Bergese SD, Khabiri B, Roberts WD, et al. Dexmedetomidine for conscious sedation in difficult awake fiberoptic intubation cases. *J Clin Anesth.* 2007;19:141–144.
100. Bergese SD, Patrick Bender S, McSweeney TD, et al. A comparative study of dexmedetomidine with midazolam and midazolam alone for sedation during elective awake fiberoptic intubation. *J Clin Anesth.* 2010;22:35–40.
101. Kunisawa T, Nagashima M, Hanada S, et al. Awake intubation under sedation using target-controlled infusion of dexmedetomidine: five case reports. *J Anesth.* 2010;24:789–792.
102. Huncke TK, Adelman M, Jacobowitz G, et al. A prospective, randomized, placebo-controlled study evaluating the efficacy of dexmedetomidine for sedation during vascular procedures. *Vasc Endovascular Surg.* 2010;44:257–261.
103. Tanskanen PE, Kyttä JV, Randell TT, et al. Dexmedetomidine as an anaesthetic adjuvant in patients undergoing intracranial tumour surgery: A double-blind, randomized and placebo-controlled study. *Br J Anaesth.* 2006;97:658–665.
104. Bekker A, Sturaitis M, Bloom M, et al. The effect of dexmedetomidine on perioperative hemodynamics in patients undergoing craniotomy. *Anesth Analg.* 2008;107:1340–1347.
105. Arain SR, Ruehlow RM, Uhrich TD, et al. The efficacy of dexmedetomidine versus morphine for postoperative analgesia after major inpatient surgery. *Anesth Analg.* 2004;98:153–158.
106. Gurbet A, Basagan-Mogol E, Turker G, et al. Intraoperative infusion of dexmedetomidine reduces perioperative analgesic requirements. *Can J Anaesth.* 2006;53:646–652.
107. Olutoye OA, Glover CD, Diefenderfer JW, et al. The effect of intraoperative dexmedetomidine on postoperative analgesia and sedation in pediatric patients undergoing tonsillectomy and adenoidectomy. *Anesth Analg.* 2010;111:490–495.
108. Salman N, Uzun S, Coskun F, et al. Dexmedetomidine as a substitute for remifentanil in ambulatory gynecologic laparoscopic surgery. *Saudi Med J.* 2009;30:77–81.
109. Tufanogullari B, White PF, Peixoto MP, et al. Dexmedetomidine infusion during laparoscopic bariatric surgery: The effect on recovery outcome variables. *Anesth Analg.* 2008;106:1741–1748.
110. Ohtani N, Kida K, Shoji K, et al. Recovery profiles from dexmedetomidine as a general anesthetic adjuvant in patients undergoing lower abdominal surgery. *Anesth Analg.* 2008;107:1871–1874.
111. Koroglu A, Teksan H, Sagir O, et al. A comparison of the sedative, hemodynamic, and respiratory effects of dexmedetomidine and propofol in children undergoing magnetic resonance imaging. *Anesth Analg.* 2006;103:63–67.
112. Arain SR, Ebert TJ. The efficacy, side effects, and recovery characteristics of dexmedetomidine versus propofol when used for intraoperative sedation. *Anesth Analg.* 2002;95:461–466.
113. Patel A, Davidson M, Tran MC, et al. Dexmedetomidine infusion for analgesia and prevention of emergence agitation in children with obstructive sleep apnea syndrome undergoing tonsillectomy and adenoidectomy. *Anesth Analg.* 2010;111:1004–1010.
114. Alhashemi JA. Dexmedetomidine vs midazolam for monitored anaesthesia care during cataract surgery. *Br J Anaesth.* 2006;96:722–726.
115. Memis D, Turan A, Karamanlioğlu B, et al. Adding dexmedetomidine to lidocaine for intravenous regional anesthesia. *Anesth Analg.* 2004;98:835–840.
116. White PF, Vasconez LO, Mathes SA, et al. Comparison of midazolam and diazepam for sedation during plastic surgery. *Plast Reconstr Surg.* 1988;81:703–712.
117. White PF. Comparative evaluation of intravenous agents for rapid sequence induction–thiopental, ketamine, and midazolam. *Anesthesiology.* 1982;57:279–284.
118. Kamata K, Nagata O, Iwakiri H, et al. Comparison of requirement for postoperative analgesics after inhalation and total intravenous anesthesia. *Masui.* 2003;52:1200–1203.
119. White PF. CON: Anesthesia versus analgesia: Assessing the analgesic effects of anesthetic drugs. *Anesth Analg.* 2010;111:88–89.
120. Fassoulaki A, Melemeni A, Paraskeva A, et al. Postoperative pain and analgesic requirements after anesthesia with sevoflurane, desflurane or propofol. *Anesth Analg.* 2008;107:1715–1719.
121. Liao R, Li JY, Liu GY. Comparison of sevoflurane volatile induction/maintenance anaesthesia and propofol-remifentanil total intravenous anaesthesia for rigid bronchoscopy under spontaneous breathing for tracheal/bronchial foreign body removal in children. *Eur J Anaesthesiol.* 2010;27:930–934.
122. Zoremba M, Dette F, Hunecke T, et al. A comparison of desflurane versus propofol: The effects on early postoperative lung function in overweight patients. *Anesth Analg.* 2011;113:63–69.
123. Tiefenthaler W, Pehboeck D, Hammerle E, et al. Lung function after total intravenous anaesthesia or balanced anaesthesia with sevoflurane. *Br J Anaesth.* 2011;106:272–276.
124. White PF. Use of continuous infusion versus intermittent bolus administration of fentanyl or ketamine during outpatient anesthesia. *Anesthesiology.* 1983;59:294–300.
125. White PF. Clinical uses of intravenous anesthetic and analgesic infusions. *Anesth Analg.* 1989;68:161–171.
126. Laalou FZ, Egard M, Guillot M, et al. Influence of preoperative cognitive status on propofol requirement to maintain hypnosis in the elderly. *Br J Anaesth.* 2010;105:342–346.
127. Chang T, Dworsky WA, White PF. Continuous electromyography for monitoring depth of anesthesia. *Anesth Analg.* 1988;67:521–525.
128. Monk TG, Ding Y, White PF. Total intravenous anesthesia: Effects of opioid versus hypnotic supplementation on autonomic responses and recovery. *Anesth Analg.* 1992;75:798–804.
129. Plourde G. Depth of anaesthesia. *Can J Anaesth.* 1991;38:270–274.
130. White PF, Boyle WA. Relationship between hemodynamic and electroencephalographic changes during general anesthesia. *Anesth Analg.* 1989;68:177–181.
131. White PF. Use of cerebral monitoring during anaesthesia: Effect on recovery profile. *Best Pract Res Clin Anaesthesiol.* 2006;20:181–189.
132. Leslie K, Myles PS, Forbes A, et al. The effect of bispectral index monitoring on long-term survival in the B-aware trial. *Anesth Analg.* 2010;110:816–822.
133. Kertai MD, Palanca BJ, Pal N, et al. Bispectral index monitoring, duration of bispectral index below 45, patient risk factors, and intermediate-term mortality after noncardiac surgery in the B-Unaware Trial. *Anesthesiology.* 2011;114:545–556.
134. An J, Fang Q, Huang C, et al. Deeper total intravenous anesthesia reduced the incidence of early postoperative cognitive dysfunction after microvascular decompression for facial spasm. *J Neurosurg Anesthesiol.* 2011;23:12–17.
135. Song D, van Vlymen J, White PF. Is the bispectral index useful in predicting fast-track eligibility after ambulatory anesthesia with propofol and desflurane? *Anesth Analg.* 1998;87:1245–1248.
136. White PF, Ma H, Tang J, et al. Does the use of electroencephalographic bispectral index or auditory evoked potential index monitoring facilitate recovery after desflurane anesthesia in the ambulatory setting? *Anesthesiology.* 2004;100:811–817.

137. Struys M, Versichelen L, Mortier E, et al. Comparison of spontaneous frontal EMG, EEG power spectrum and bispectral index to monitor propofol drug effect and emergence. *Acta Anaesthesiol Scand.* 1998;42:628–636.
138. Schraag S, Bothner U, Gajraj R, et al. The performance of electroencephalogram bispectral index and auditory evoked potential index to predict loss of consciousness during propofol infusion. *Anesth Analg.* 1999;89:1311–1315.
139. Hemmerling TM, Charabati S, Zaouter C, et al. A randomized controlled trial demonstrates that a novel closed-loop propofol system performs better hypnosis control than manual administration. *Can J Anaesth.* 2010;57:725–735.
140. Liu N, Chazot T, Hamada S, et al. Closed-loop coadministration of propofol and remifentanil guided by bispectral index: A randomized multicenter study. *Anesth Analg.* 2011;112:546–557.
141. Coskun D, Celebi H, Karaca G, et al. Remifentanil versus fentanyl compared in a target-controlled infusion of propofol anesthesia: Quality of anesthesia and recovery profile. *J Anesth.* 2010;24:373–379.
142. Milne SE, Kenny GN. Future applications for TCI systems. *Anaesthesia.* 1998; 53(suppl 1):56–60.
143. Taylor E, Ghouri AF, White PF. Midazolam in combination with propofol for sedation during local anesthesia. *J Clin Anesth.* 1992;4:213–216.
144. Ogilvie MP, Pereira BM, Ryan ML, et al. Bispectral index to monitor propofol sedation in trauma patients. *J Trauma.* 2011;71:1415–1421.
145. Shafer A, Doze VA, White PF. Pharmacokinetic variability of midazolam infusions in critically ill patients. *Crit Care Med.* 1990;18:1039–1041.
146. Ogawa Y, Iwasaki K, Aoki K, et al. The different effects of midazolam and propofol sedation on dynamic cerebral autoregulation. *Anesth Analg.* 2010;111:1279–1284.
147. Kim DK, Joo Y, Sung TY, et al. Dreaming in sedation during spinal anesthesia: A comparison of propofol and midazolam infusion. *Anesth Analg.* 2011;112:1076–1081.
148. White PF, Negus JB. Sedative infusions during local and regional anesthesia: A comparison of midazolam and propofol. *J Clin Anesth.* 1991;3:32–39.
149. Alhashemi JA, Kaki AM. Anesthesiologist-controlled versus patient-controlled propofol sedation for shockwave lithotripsy. *Can J Anaesth.* 2006;53:449–455.
150. Burns R, McCrae AF, Tiplady B. A comparison of target-controlled therapy with patient-controlled administration of propofol combined with midazolam for sedation during dental surgery. *Anaesthesia.* 2003;58:170–176.
151. Ayoub CM, Rizk LB, Yaacoub CI, et al. Music and ambient operating room noise in patients undergoing spinal anesthesia. *Anesth Analg.* 2005;100:1316–1319.
152. Aitkenhead AR, Pepperman ML, Willatts SM, et al. Comparison of propofol and midazolam for sedation in critically ill patients. *Lancet.* 1989;2:704–709.
153. Carrasco G, Molina R, Costa J, et al. Propofol vs midazolam in short-, medium-, and long-term sedation of critically ill patients. A cost-benefit analysis. *Chest.* 1993;103:557–564.
154. McFarlan CS, Anderson BJ, Short TG. The use of propofol infusions in paediatric anaesthesia: A practical guide. *Paediatr Anaesth.* 1999;9:209–216.
155. Parke TJ, Stevens JE, Rice AS, et al. Metabolic acidosis and fatal myocardial failure after propofol infusion in children: Five case reports. *BMJ.* 1992;305:613–616.
156. Martin PH, Murthy BV, Petros AJ. Metabolic, biochemical and haemodynamic effects of infusion of propofol for long-term sedation of children undergoing intensive care. *Br J Anaesth.* 1997;79:276–279.
157. Wunsch H, Kahn JM, Kramer AA, et al. Dexmedetomidine in the care of critically ill patients from 2001 to 2007: An observational cohort study. *Anesthesiology.* 2010;113:386–394.
158. Iirola T, Aantaa R, Laitio R, et al. Pharmacokinetics of prolonged infusion of high-dose dexmedetomidine in critically ill patients. *Crit Care.* 2011;15:R257.
159. Iirola T, Vilo S, Aantaa R, et al. Dexmedetomidine inhibits gastric emptying and oro-caecal transit in healthy volunteers. *Br J Anaesth.* 2011;106:522–527.
160. Sneyd JR, Holmes KA. Inhalational or total intravenous anaesthesia: Is total intravenous anaesthesia useful and are there economic benefits? *Curr Opin Anaesthesiol.* 2011;24:182–187.

CHAPTER

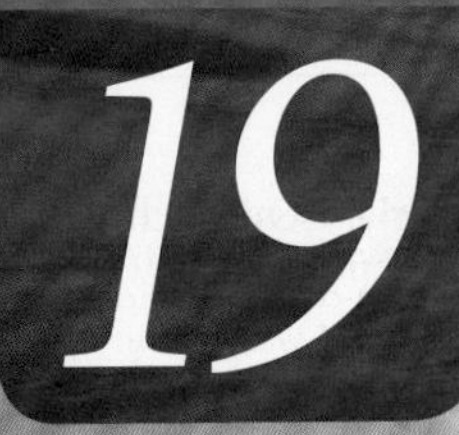

Opioids

ALBERT DAHAN • MARIEKE NIESTERS • ERIK OLOFSEN • TERRY SMITH • FRANK OVERDYK

Key Points

1. Opioids produce analgesia as well as serious side effects. All physicians who prescribe opioids for relief of acute or chronic pain need to know how to use these drugs safely. This requires an in-depth understanding of the pharmacokinetics and pharmacodynamics of opioids as well as the acquisition of sufficient clinical experience in their use.
2. Opioids act through specific opioid receptors on neuronal tissues such as peripheral nerves and neurons in the spinal cord and brain. The most important receptors include the μ-opioid receptor (MOR), δ-opioid receptor (DOR), and κ-opioid receptor (KOR). For anesthesia and pain relief, the MOR is most important. Opioids also act through non-neuronal pathways, such as those affecting the immune system, which may be of relevance in the treatment of inflammatory pain.
3. Opioids can be classified according to the strength or potency based on the plasma concentrations at which they exert their effects (C_{50} or the plasma concentration causing a 50% effect). Strong opioids include fentanyl, sufentanil, and remifentanil. Weak opioids include codeine and tramadol. An intermediate group includes morphine, methadone, oxycodone, and buprenorphine.
4. Endogenous opioid pathways are activated in cases of stress-induced analgesia, placebo-induced analgesia, and conditioning pain modulation (CPM). CPM occurs when pain arising from one focus is decreased by application of a second painful stimulus.
5. Opioid-induced hyperalgesia (OIH) is a paradoxical opioid effect whereby pain sensitivity increases during or following escalating opioid treatment. It is also observed postoperatively following the use of a remifentanil infusion during anesthesia. Greater and more frequent doses of morphine are required to treat postoperative pain. OIH may be treated and prevented by administration of a low dose of ketamine, an *N*-methyl-D-aspartate (NMDA) receptor antagonist.
6. The pharmacokinetic characteristics of a drug determine its behavior in the body of a patient. One important pharmacokinetic concept is that of context-sensitive half-time (CSt½). This is the time needed for the drug's plasma concentration to decrease by 50% from a steady-state concentration. For most opioids, this value is dependent on the duration of drug infusion. For example, for fentanyl the CSt½ increases rapidly with the infusion duration. In contrast, the CSt½ of remifentanil is independent of the infusion duration due to its rapid elimination from plasma. Thus it remains stable at about 2 minutes.
7. Opioid metabolism is affected by drugs that interfere with metabolizing cytochrome P450 enzymes, most importantly CYP3A4. Opioid metabolites can be active or inactive. Active metabolites need to be considered when treating patients. For example, the active metabolite of morphine, morphine-6-glucuronide, can accumulate in patients with renal impairment. Genetic variability in the CYP system can have important clinical implications, especially in case of variations in the copies of a gene coding for the metabolizing enzyme. An example is the enzyme CYP2D6 which catalyzes the conversion of codeine into morphine. Patients with multiple copies of the CYP2D6 gene and who receive codeine will have large plasma morphine concentrations with all related effects and side effects.
8. Opioid effects are variable among patients. Dosing is optimum when opioids are titrated to the effect. It is also important to take into account the delay between the administration of an opioid and its effect, which is defined as the blood–effect-site equilibration half-life or t½k_{e0}. This will allow proper and

timely dosing particularly when anticipating a stressful event (laryngoscopy, intubation, skin incision, etc.) and administering opioids to prevent the occurrence of a large hemodynamic response to these stimuli. The t½k_{e0} of morphine is 1 to 2 hours! Thus it is important to give an initial bolus dose or morphine 30 to 45 minutes before the end of surgery when using the drug for postoperative pain relief.

9 Opioids reduce the requirement of inhalational anesthetics and propofol during anesthesia, which makes rapid awakening from anesthesia possible. Using known pharmacokinetic and pharmacodynamic data it can be determined what doses and plasma concentrations will permit the shortest time to awakening. For example, termination of drug infusions at plasma concentrations of propofol 1.5 μg/mL and remifentanil 9.0 ng/mL will lead to patient awakening within 6.5 minutes.

10 Administration of opioids can potentially lead to life-threatening respiratory depression. The incidence of serious perioperative respiratory events is approximately 0.5% (1 in every 200 patients). Respiratory problems from opioids are more common in special patient populations including patients with obstructive sleep apnea (OSA), premature neonates, and very old or very ill patients. Careful, slow, infusion of opioids allows the gradual accumulation of arterial CO_2 which serves as a respiratory stimulant at the chemoreceptors and lowers the probability of apnea.

11 The nonspecific opioid receptor antagonist, naloxone, is the drug of choice to reverse opioid-induced respiratory depression. The required dose of naloxone depends on the pharmacokinetic and pharmacodynamic properties and the dose of the opioid that needs reversal. Postoperatively, when there is persistent apnea, opioid concentrations are often just above the threshold for respiratory depression. Intravenous administration of naloxone using incremental doses of 40 to 80 μg, to a cumulative dose of less than 400 μg, may be sufficient for breathing to resume.

12 Apart from respiratory depression, opioids cause a large number of side effects that require attention: Nausea with or without vomiting, smooth muscle spasms, skeletal muscle rigidity (fentanyl and congeners), histamine release (morphine, codeine, meperidine), itching (especially after spinal administration), miosis, sedation, and dizziness. The cardiovascular side effects of opioids include bradycardia and hypotension but are generally mild at usual clinical doses. However, when combined with anesthetics, even at usual clinical doses, or in severely ill patients, opioids may produce hemodynamic instability which requires treatment.

Multimedia

1 Dose-Effect Curves

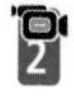 Drug Concentration and Effect

 Vomiting Pharmacology

INTRODUCTION

Administration of large doses of opioids has traditionally been restricted to anesthesiologists and other anesthesia providers because of their extensive experience and expertise in the use of these potent analgesics during anesthesia. Recently, however, there has been an exponential increase in the prescription of high-dose opioids by other healthcare providers for treatment of patients with chronic non-cancer pain (3% of adult US population).[1] This "epidemic" of opioid use by non-surgical patients, coupled with an emphasis on aggressive and effective postoperative pain management for patients undergoing surgery, has resulted in increasingly complex postoperative pain management problems for surgical patients and
1 an increase in opioid-related complications for patients with pain in general.[2,3] Consequently, expertise in the use of opioids is not only required in the operating room and postoperatively, but also when caring for patients with chronic pain in a nonsurgical setting. Certainly, knowledge on the safe use of opioids is a *conditio sine qua non* for all anesthesiologists and other anesthesia providers. An in-depth knowledge of the pharmacokinetics (PK), the pharmacodynamics (PD), and the side effect profile associated with different opioids, dosing regimens, and routes of administration is essential for their safe intra- and postoperative use. This chapter will review the endogenous opioid system, discuss the PK and PD properties of opioids relevant to perioperative dosing strategies, and delineate the associated side effect profiles of exogenous opioid analgesics.

Short History

Opium is among the oldest drugs in the world. Fossilized opium poppies have been found in Neanderthal excavation sites dating back to 30,000 BC. Many old civilizations, including the Sumerians, Egyptians, Greeks, Romans, and Chinese, used opium for nutritional, medicinal, euphoric, spiritual, and religious purposes. The first written reference to the medicinal use of the opium poppy is described in a Sumerian text dated near 4,000 BCE. Just over 200 years ago, the German pharmacist and chemist Friedrich Sertürner isolated a stable alkaloid crystal from the opium sap and named it morphine after the Greek god of dreams, Morpheus.[4,5] Morphine was 10-fold more potent than opium and soon replaced it not only for the treatment of severe pain, but also for a myriad of other purposes such as cough and diarrhea. After the invention of the hypodermic syringe in the 1850s, the Englishman Alexander Wood was the first to inject morphine in a controlled fashion into a patient producing more than a day's sleep (1853).[6] The first reported casualty from morphine occurred shortly thereafter when Wood injected his wife with morphine resulting in a fatal overdose from respiratory depression.[6] Morphine revolutionized the treatment of the wounded in battlefield medicine, but euphoric and addictive properties led to the addiction of thousands of soldiers to morphine during the American Civil War.

The synthesis of heroin in 1874 was based on the empirical finding that boiling morphine with specific acids caused the replacement of the two morphine –OH groups by –$OCOH_3$ producing diamorphine or heroin (Fig. 19-1).

After the structure of morphine was determined in the 1920s, the synthesis of new morphine-like opioid compounds was based

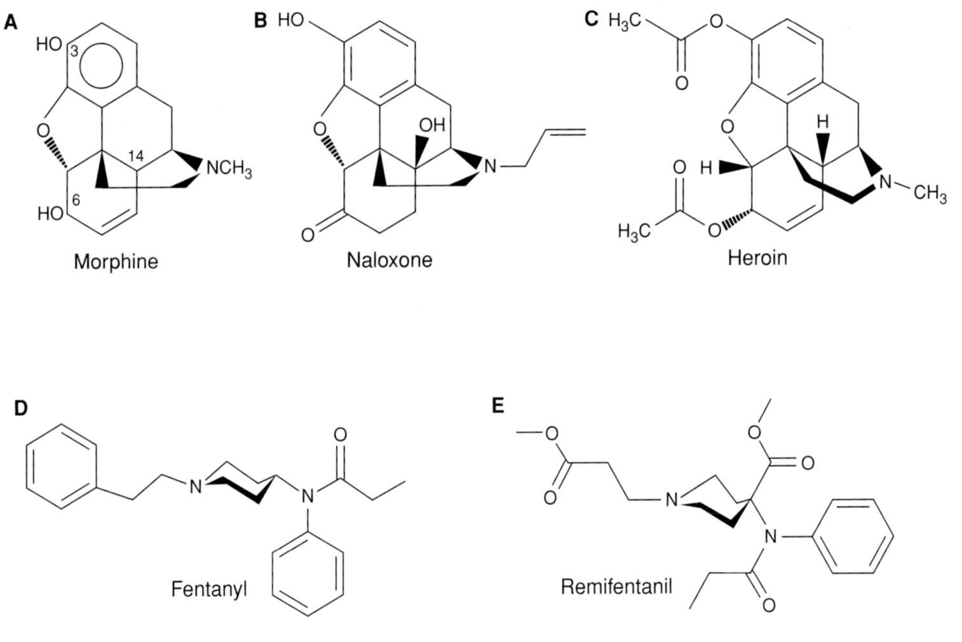

A Morphine B Naloxone C Heroin

D Fentanyl E Remifentanil

FIGURE 19-1. Chemical structures of common opioids.

on chemical principles rather than empirical discoveries. In 1937, meperidine (or pethidine) became the first synthetic opioid synthesized on the basis of the central structure of morphine. Since then many synthetic and semisynthetic opioids have been produced, including the clinically important opioid antagonists naloxone and naltrexone, by replacing the N-methyl substituent in morphine with allyl and cyclopropylmethyl groups, respectively (Fig. 19-1).[7]

For clinical use during anesthesia the most important opioids are the piperidines fentanyl, sufentanil, alfentanil, and remifentanil. These opioids produce potent analgesia and suppression of cardiovascular responses to noxious stimulation from surgery with predictable PK and PD. The latest potent opioid to be registered is tapentadol.[8,9] This molecule acts via activation of the opioid receptors at spinal and supraspinal sites and by inhibition of the reuptake of norepinephrine, activating α_2-adrenergic receptors in the spinal cord dorsal horn. This produces a synergistic analgesic effect with a more desirable gastrointestinal (GI) side effect profile. The continued development of opioids with complex simultaneous actions at opioid and non-opioid target sites is facilitated by new information gained about mechanisms involved in endogenous pain and analgesia as well as advances in pain-related pharmacology. Development of new opioids is also driven by concerns that the side effect profile of potent opioids, which presents a serious risk to patients, needs to be minimized.

The Endogenous Opioid System

A major breakthrough in the understanding of opioid pharmacology came from a series of discoveries of opioid receptors, endogenous opioid peptides, their encoding genes, and endogenous opioid alkaloids. The endogenous opioid system is composed of a family of structurally related endogenous peptides that act at a four-member opioid receptor family consisting of the μ-opioid receptor (MOR), κ-opioid receptor (KOR), δ-opioid receptor (DOR), and orphanin FQ/nociception (NOP) receptor.[10,11] This opioid system is involved in a variety of regulatory functions including important roles in nociceptive, stress, emotional, and hedonic responses and modulation of thermoregulation, breathing, neuroendocrine function, GI motility, and immune responses.

Various subtypes of opioid receptors have also been identified, with different pharmacologic functions. For example, at least three MOR subtypes have been described: μ_1 is predominantly involved in opioid analgesia, μ_2 is involved in opioid-induced respiratory depression, and μ_3 is involved in opioid-induced immune suppression.[12,13] Note, however, that the functional validation of most opioid receptor subtypes awaits the development of antagonists with sufficient selectivity to allow a clear differentiation by effect.

The endogenous opioid peptides include endorphins, enkephalins, and dynorphins, each of which display different affinities for the μ-, κ-, and δ-opioid receptors.[14] β-endorphins have a high affinity for the MOR, met- and leu-enkephalins for the KOR, and Dynorphin A for the DOR. The recently discovered nociceptin has been identified as a selective endogenous ligand of the NOP 2 receptor,[11,22] while endogenous morphine acts via the μ_3-receptor located on immune cells, such as human monocytes.[15]

Opioids act not only through central and peripheral neuronal pathways, but also via non-neuronal mechanisms, such as actions on the immune system.[16] Morphine and morphine-6-glucuronide (M6G), endogenously formed and stored in adrenal chromaffin cells and leukocytes, play an import role as modulators of non-neuronal responses in the immune system.[17] Our considerations of endogenous opioid systems, therefore, have expanded from an opioid peptide system present in the central nervous system (CNS) and peripheral nervous system to include various peptide and non-peptide ligands in neuronal and non-neuronal cells throughout the body.

Opioid receptors are linked to G proteins in the cell membrane and are hence members of the large G-protein–coupled receptor (GPCR) family.[18] GPCRs mediate a cascade of downstream signaling pathways leading to (i) the inhibition of adenyl cyclase and decreased cyclic AMP, (ii) activation of Ca^{2+} and K^+ channels, and (iii) activation of MAPK/ERK, PKC, and P13 K/Akt.[19] Interactions between opioid ligands and selective receptors have a number of important clinical effects. Morphine-induced analgesia and respiratory depression are both induced through activation of the MOR and subsequent activation of the adenylate cyclase/cyclic AMP pathway.[20] Recently, opioid-induced activation of alternate cell signaling pathways through interactions with many (opioid and non-opioid) receptor types have been shown to affect the growth and distribution of cancer cells.[19,21]

FIGURE 19-2. μ-, δ-, and κ-opioid receptor (MOR, DOR, and KOR, respectively) distribution in the brain of MOR knockout mice. The MOR is reduced in heterozygous MOR knockout mice and totally absent in homozygous knockout mice, while the other two receptor types remain present in both genotypes. +/+, wild-type mice; +/–, heterozygous MOR knockout mice; –/–, homozygous MOR knockout mice. Reprinted from: Matthes HWD, Maldonado R, Simonin F, et al. Loss of morphine-induced analgesia, reward effect and withdrawal symptoms in mice lacking the μ-opioid receptor gene. *Science.* 1996;383:819, with permission.

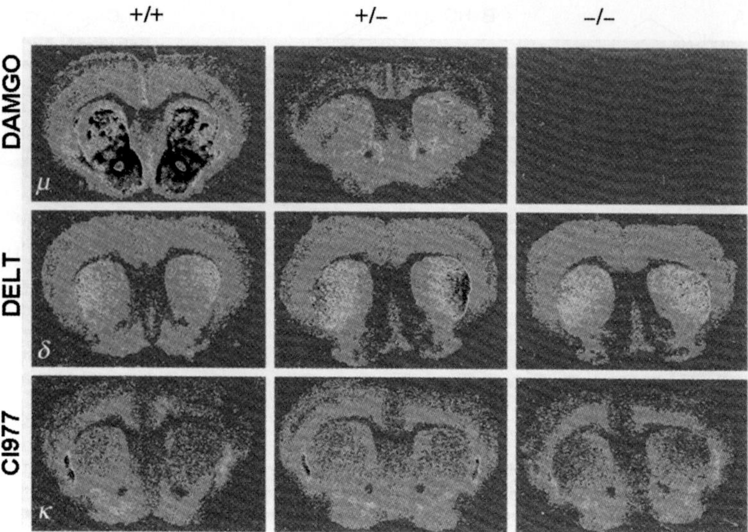

Opioid Receptor Knockout Mice

In the last decade a variety of mice lacking the various opioid receptors ("knockout mice") have been bred to understand the molecular targets of exogenous opioids (Fig. 19-2).[10] Inactivation of the μ-, κ-, and δ-opioid receptors, either separately or in combination, is not lethal. This suggests that the opioid receptor system is not crucial for development but is critical when experiencing stress or pain. For example, under conditions of fight or flight, recruitment of the endogenous opioid system will result in development of endogenous analgesia allowing the subject to respond to an acute body insult and consequently increases the chance of survival.

Studies indicate that morphine's action at the MOR gene produces its clinical effects. Mice lacking the MOR gene do not experience morphine-induced analgesia, respiratory depression, reward and withdrawal, inhibition of GI transit, immunosuppression, or an increase in steroid hormones (Fig. 19-3).[22–24] Analgesic responses after administration of other opioids, such as morphine's metabolite M6G, are also absent in MOR knockout mice.[25] These observations suggest the MOR is the target for both the desired and undesired effects of opioid analgesics and consequently designing a MOR activating drug that selectively produces desired effects such as analgesia, but not undesired effects such as life-threatening respiratory depression, is not possible.

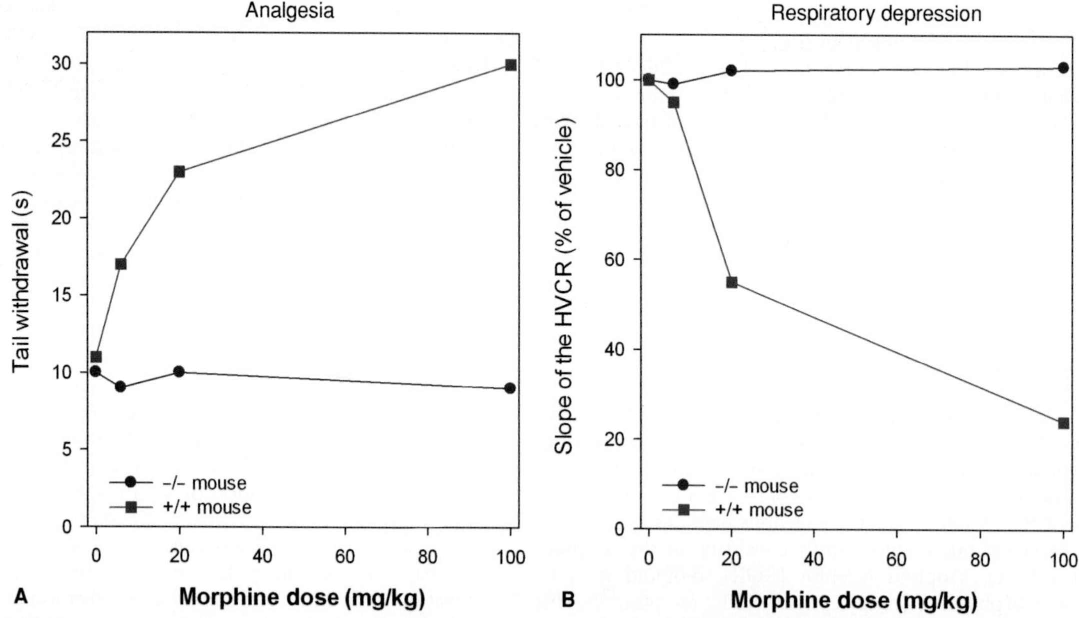

FIGURE 19-3. Effect of morphine in mice lacking the μ-opioid receptor (–/–, homozygous μ-opioid receptor knockout mice) and mice with intact receptors (+/+, wild-type mice) on analgesic responses [**(A)** tail flick test in two mice] and respiratory responses [**(B)** the hypercapnic ventilatory response (HCVR) in two mice]. Data adapted from: Romberg.

Classification of Exogenous Opioids

Opioids may be classified on the basis of their synthesis, chemical structure, potency, receptor binding, and effect at the opioid receptors. According to their synthesis opioids are subdivided into *natural* (morphine), *semisynthetic*, and *synthetic* opioids. Natural opioid alkaloids are known as opiates, while the term opioids is used for all opioids (endogenous opioid peptides, natural opioid alkaloids, semisynthetic opioids, and synthetic opioids).

Semisynthetic opioids are derived from the morphine molecule and include buprenorphine, codeine, etorphine, heroin, hydromorphone, oxycodone, and oxymorphone. The synthetic opioids comprise the piperidines (e.g., loperamide, meperidine, alfentanil, fentanyl, sufentanil, remifentanil) and the methadones (e.g., methadone, dextro-propoxyphene).

3 Opioid potency ranges from *weak opioids* such as codeine, dextro-propoxyphene, tramadol, and hydrocodone to *strong opioids*, which include etorphine, fentanyl, sufentanil, alfentanil, and remifentanil. Medium potency opioids include morphine, methadone, oxycodone, hydromorphone, and buprenorphine. Irrespective of the "strength" of these agents, all of these agents may potentially produce serious and potentially life-threatening side effects including sedation and respiratory depression, hypotension, and bradycardia. During surgery *strong* opioids are used in high doses while in the postoperative phase medium strength opioids such as morphine or methadone are used for treatment of acute pain. In 1986, the World Health Organization designed a stepwise approach for treatment of chronic cancer pain in which *weak* opioids are prescribed before *strong* opioids (http://www.who.int/cancer/palliative/painladder/en/).

Opioids may be *full agonists* which cause the maximum possible effect when activating their receptors. Opioid full agonists at the MOR include morphine, piperidines, and methadone. Opioid *partial agonists* activate their receptor but cause only a partial or reduced effect (Fig. 19-4). Buprenorphine acts as a partial agonist at the MOR while it is a full agonist at the NOP and DOR.[26] In clinical practice buprenorphine behaves as a full agonist with respect to pain relief yet its respiratory depressant effects are limited and display a "ceiling effect".[27] At the KOR buprenorphine acts as a competitive antagonist, which classifies this opioid also as a *mixed agonist–antagonist*. Naloxone and naltrexone are opioid *antagonists*.

A more practical classification of opioids is their subdivision into agents with a rapid onset and offset of action (e.g., remifentanil and alfentanil) and agents with a slow onset/offset of action (e.g., morphine and buprenorphine). The concept of onset/offset of action will be discussed below.

Opioids Acting at Opioid and Non-opioid Receptors

Most opioid analgesics act at multiple receptor systems with different affinities. For example, morphine acts with high affinity at the MOR and with lower affinities at the KOR and DOR. Various opioids including methadone, dextro-propoxyphene and ketobemidone are opioid analgesics and also antagonists at the *N*-methyl-D-aspartate (NMDA) receptor.[28,29] Of all opioids, methadone is the most potent NMDA receptor antagonist, being 6 to 18 times more potent than morphine in producing this effect. Antagonism of the NMDA receptor is clinically useful in reducing opioid tolerance and opioid-induced hyperalgesia (OIH) and in chronic pain states leading to pain hypersensitivity.[30]

Tramadol has both opioidergic and monoaminergic activity at dorsal horn spinal synapses of the nociceptive pathways.[31] The analgesic effect of tramadol is due to enhancement of spinal inhibition of 5-hydroxytryptamine (5HT) and norepinephrine reuptake, causing the accumulation of 5HT and norepinephrine in the dorsal spinal horn.

The latest "novel" opioid recently registered worldwide is tapentadol, a potent analgesic with reduced GI and CNS side effects.[8,9] Tapentadol has a dual mechanism of action. It is active at the MOR at spinal and supraspinal sites and as a norepinephrine reuptake inhibitor (NRI) in the spinal cord. The combination of these two mechanisms has been designated as the MOR–NRI concept. The affinity of tapentadol for the MOR is 50-fold lower than that of morphine. However, due to synergy between the two mechanisms of action, tapentadol produces potent analgesia and is useful in the treatment of moderate to severe acute and chronic pain. Tapentadol differs from tramadol due to its lack of serotonergic effects resulting in a lower incidence of nausea and vomiting. Tapentadol's low affinity for the MOR may limit its undesirable side effects although its respiratory side effects have not yet been fully studied.

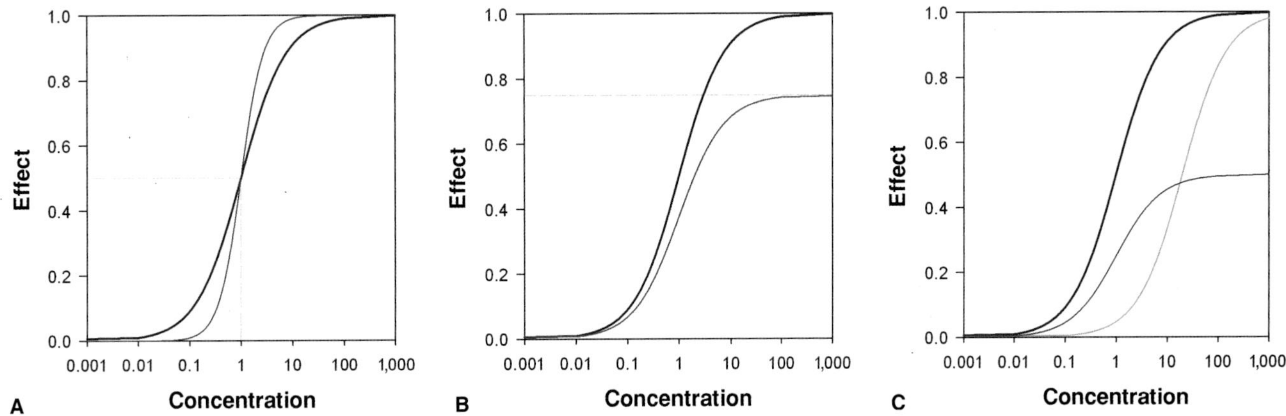

FIGURE 19-4. Sigmoid E_{max} relationships for **(A)** full opioid agonists with $C_{50} = 1$ and steepness parameter $\gamma = 1$ (*blue line*) and $\gamma = 2$ (*red line*), **(B)** full opioid agonist (*blue line* with $E_{max} = 1$) and a partial agonist (*green line* with $E_{max} = 0.75$), **(C)** the rightward shift (*gray line*) observed by adding a *competitive* antagonist (such as naloxone) on top of a full agonist (*blue line*) causing an increase in C_{50} and the downward shift of adding a *noncompetitive* antagonist (*purple line*) to the full agonist causing an effect similar to that observed in **(B)** (i.e., a partial agonistic effect).

Finally, non-opioids may also act at opioid receptors. An important example is ketamine, which is an NMDA receptor antagonist with affinity for multiple receptor systems including the opioid receptors.[32] Its anesthetic properties are related to its effect at the NMDA receptors while its analgesic effects are predominantly due to MOR activation.

OPIOID MECHANISMS

Mechanisms of Opioid Analgesia

Whereas nociception is the reception of signals in the CNS that have been triggered by noxious stimulation, pain is the subjective perception of that noxious stimulation. Opioids modify both nociception and the perception of a noxious stimulus (emotional coloring of pain).

Different types of peripheral sensory nociceptors, often free nerve endings, are stimulated by tissue damage and the resulting pain information is transmitted to the spinal cord by two types of small diameter peripheral afferent fibers: Slow conducting, unmyelinated C-fibers (which cause a dull burning pain) and faster, thinly myelinated Aδ fibers (which cause sharp, pricking pain). Both types of primary afferent fibers enter the dorsal horn of the spinal cord and terminate in its superficial layers (lamina I–II). Projection neurons from these laminae give rise to the ascending pathways of the spinothalamic tract. Thalamic nuclei receive the nociceptive inputs and pass the information to key brain pain reception sites such as the periaqueductal gray (PAG), amygdala, and somatosensory cortex. Activation of the MORs extensively located in these higher brain centers stimulates analgesia by activating *descending inhibitory pathways* from the PAG and rostroventral medulla (RVM) that inhibit nociceptive dorsal horn neuron firing in the spinal cord.[33,34] Opioids also exert actions in the cortex and limbic systems affecting cholinergic systems that lead to changes in arousal and pain perception.[35]

μ-opioid-induced analgesia and descending inhibitory pathways may be activated not only by exogenous opioids, but also by activation of endogenous opioid systems. Direct electrical stimulation of the PAG and RVM induces analgesia that may be reversed by opioid antagonists.[36] The electrically stimulated sites overlap with the opioid receptor sites and with opioid-containing interneurons, linking together the actions of exogenously applied analgesic stimuli and endogenous opioid systems. Three major examples of analgesia driven by the endogenous opioid system are (1) stress-induced analgesia[37]; (2) placebo-induced analgesia[38]; and (3) conditioning pain modulation (CPM).[39]

1. *Stress-induced analgesia.* The endogenous opioid system is activated under stressful conditions, as demonstrated by the delayed onset of pain by soldiers wounded in battle.[40] The same higher brain centers bearing MORs are involved in the implementation of stress-induced analgesia.
2. *Placebo-induced analgesia.* The endogenous opioid system also mediates placebo-induced analgesia, a reduction of pain
4 resulting from an expectation of pain relief. Studies using fMRI and PET show activation of the endogenous opioid systems and MORs in the brains of subjects receiving placebo described as an analgesic.[41–43] Placebo-induced analgesia may be used to enhance opioid-derived analgesia.
3. *CPM.* Formerly known as diffuse noxious inhibitory control, it is a condition in which pain arising from a noxious stimulus applied to one part of the body is decreased by application of a second remote noxious stimulus.[39,44,45] CPM is caused by the activation of descending inhibitory pathways.

Opioids may also act at spinal sites to induce analgesia. In the superficial laminae of the dorsal horn, local neuronal circuits process both ascending and descending pain pathways and are regulated by local endogenous opioid circuits.

Peripheral Opioid Analgesia

Opioids are also involved in peripheral analgesia by acting directly on sensory neurons (Aδ and C-fibers) to inhibit pain signal transmission. This is especially important in inflammatory pain. However, the immune system is also widely involved in peripheral analgesia.[46] Opioid receptors are located not only on neurons, but on immune cells, such as human leukocytes.[47] An insult to a peripheral tissue triggers the local release of many proinflammatory mediators that generate an inflammatory cascade, induce spontaneous nociceptor activity, and sensitize sensory neurons to induce spontaneous pain, allodynia (a non-painful stimulus is perceived as painful), and hyperalgesia (increased pain sensitivity). Early in the inflammatory process there is an influx of leukocytes into the inflamed area and these cells are a major source of opioid peptides to inflamed sites. Opioid peptides released locally interact with the opioid neuronal receptors to induce analgesia (Fig. 19-5).[48] The inflammatory process also stimulates further opioid receptor upregulation and thereby increases the antinociceptive action of opioid peptides released by immune cells. In aggregate, the inflammatory process not only promotes inflammation and its painful sequelae, but also initiates and sustains a counteracting analgesia driven by endogenous opioids.[49]

Opioid-induced Hyperalgesia (OIH) and Tolerance

Opioids can induce the paradoxical effect of OIH or an increase in pain sensitivity.[50] OIH may limit the analgesic effects of opioids. During long-term and/or high-dose opioid treatment, rapid opioid dose escalation, or administration of an opioid with rapid onset/offset (e.g., remifentanil), a paradoxical increase in pain accompanies the treatment escalation.[51,52] The MOR is not a prerequisite for OIH, as there is ample evidence from knockout mice
5 studies (devoid of MOR) or studies in mice treated with naloxone or naltrexone that OIH develops in response to exposure to high-dose opioids.[53–55] There may be various mechanisms for OIH, including activation of the central glutaminergic system, central nitric oxide production, and facilitation of descending pronociceptive systems.

Postoperative patients who have received remifentanil infusions intraoperatively can have a higher incidence of OIH and need greater doses of morphine for control of postoperative pain than patients receiving non-remifentanil–based anesthesia.[51] Although animal and human data indicate that all μ-opioids may cause OIH there seems to be a gradual difference in prevalence, with most observation of OIH following remifentanil treatment. This high incidence of OIH following remifentanil infusions may be related to its rapid offset of analgesia. In order to prevent severe pain responses following remifentanil-based anesthesia, administration of morphine (0.1 to 0.25 mg/kg) 45 to 60 minutes before the end of surgery is advisable, and adding a low-dose ketamine infusion may prevent the development of OIH (dose range: 10 to 30 mg/hr) due to ketamine's NMDA antagonistic properties.[52]

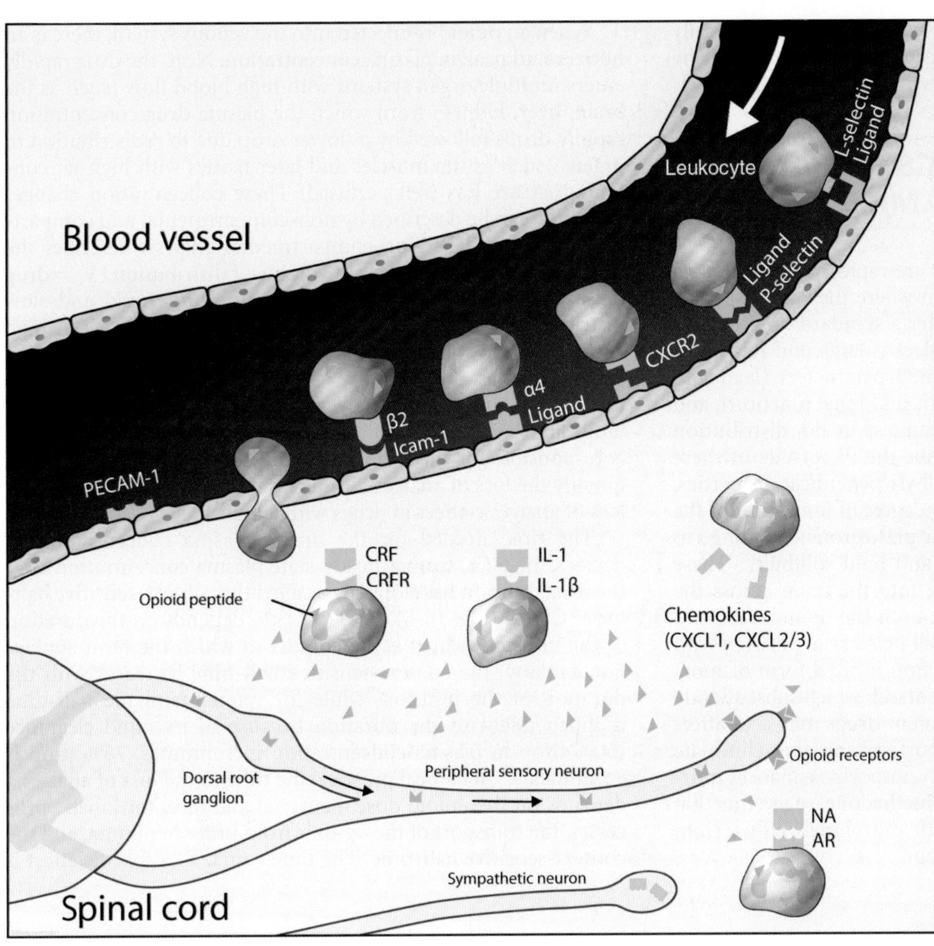

FIGURE 19-5. Schematic diagram illustrating the role of opioids in analgesia of peripheral inflammation. Opioid-containing leukocytes are attracted to inflamed tissue by various chemokines and cytokines. Specific upregulated protein facilitates leukocyte migration through the vascular endothelium. In the inflamed tissue leukocytes interact with releasing agents such as corticotropin-releasing factor (CRF), interleukin-1 (IL-1), and norepinephrine (NA) derived from postganglionic sympathetic neurons, to secrete opioid peptides. These bind to peripheral opioid receptors, synthesized in the dorsal root ganglia and transported to peripheral endings of sensory neurons, to mediate analgesia. AR, adrenergic receptor; CRFR, corticotropin-releasing factor receptor; PECAM-1, platelet endothelial adhesion molecule 1; Icam-1, intracellular adhesion molecule 1; CXCR2, chemokine (C-X-C motif) receptor 2; CXCL1, chemokine (C-X-C motif) ligand 1; CXCL2/3, chemokine (C-X-C motif) ligand 1/2.

OIH is not the same phenomenon as opioid tolerance.[50] *Acute opioid tolerance* due to tachyphylaxis requires increasing doses of the opioid to reach a specific analgesic end point during the initial hours of opioid treatment. *Chronic tolerance,* often seen in opioid abusers, occurs over days and manifests as a decreasing analgesic effect, resulting in dose escalation and increasing the likelihood of OIH. In contrast to OIH, opioid receptor–related and post-activation intracellular processes play an important role in the development of tolerance (including *β*-arrestin–dependent receptor desensitization and internalization, and G-receptor uncoupling).[56,57] Finally, *pseudo-tolerance* is a phenomenon seen in chronic pain patients due to progression of disease with an increase in the level of nociception often due to destruction of nerves in the tumor region, resulting in neuropathic pain, which is poorly responsive to opioid dose escalation.

ROUTES OF ADMINISTRATION

The most important and predictable route of administration of opioids perioperatively is the intravenous route, since the amount of drug entering the systemic circulation is precisely known. Non-intravenous administration routes (e.g., oral, subcutaneous, transdermal, inhalational, sublingual, oral transmucosal, intranasal, or rectal routes) are often more convenient for the patient although they come at the cost of more variable (and often slower) rates of absorption and bioavailability. Opioids given orally have bioavailabilities of 20% to 40% due to a rapid first-pass effect as a result of opioid metabolism in the liver.

Opioids given via epidural (e.g., patient-controlled epidural analgesia) and intrathecal routes need to diffuse into the surrounding nerve tissue and spinal cord to activate MORs. More lipophilic opioids (fentanyl, sufentanil) will penetrate faster and achieve higher concentrations into the spinal cord than hydrophilic opioids such as morphine and meperidine, yet they are also cleared from the spinal fluid more rapidly.[58] Thus the lipophilic opioids may cause an early-onset respiratory depression whereas morphine tends to cause late ventilatory depression due to its slow clearance from the spinal fluid. After the epidural administration of opioids, lipophilic drugs are rapidly absorbed into the systemic circulation resulting in plasma concentrations similar to those observed after low-dose intravenous injections.[58] The clinical effects of lipophilic opioids given epidurally are due to systemic, spinal, and supraspinal sites of action. It is important to note that epidurally administered opioids may exacerbate the risk of serious respiratory depression when coadministered with other parenteral opioids.

Intramuscular injections of opioids for treatment of postoperative pain should be avoided as there are superior alternatives such as the intravenous administration of opioids using patient-controlled analgesia (PCA) devices. Compared to IM injections intravenous PCA is associated with lower pain scores and greater patient satisfaction. PCA also does not require frequent painful injections. Under specific and exceptional circumstances, nurse-administered interval IM analgesia is acceptable, such as when the patient is unable to use the PCA device (mentally or physically incapacitated patients) or in case of fear of PCA by proxy.[59] The latter is the case when family members press the PCA button.

PHARMACOKINETICS (PK) AND PHARMACODYNAMICS (PD)

When injected intravenously opioids are rapidly transported to the heart and pulmonary vessels from where they are dispersed to the various organs and tissues. After a standard dose of opioid, the inter-patient variability of effect is large and related to various factors including weight-related parameters (lean and fat body mass), organ function (hepatic and renal function), and cardiac output. This variability is manifest in the distribution and elimination constants that describe the PK profile of these drugs, which is also related to their physicochemical properties, such as molecule size, pK_a (affects the degree of ionization of the molecule and depends on the plasma pH), protein binding (to albumin and α_1-acid glycoprotein), and lipid solubility. These factors affect the passage of the drug into the brain across the blood–brain barrier and hence affect both the opioid's PK and PD characteristics. For example, a small increase in pH seen with respiratory alkalosis will increase the non-ionized form of morphine, fentanyl, sufentanil, and remifentanil, which subsequently crosses the blood–brain barrier. Different drugs may also affect the blood–brain barrier active transport systems that eliminate opioids from the brain. For example, cyclosporine enhances morphine's analgesic effect but not that of methadone, suggesting that cyclosporine selectively interferes with morphine's efflux from the brain via specific transporter proteins.

When an opioid is injected into the venous system, there is an initial rapid peak in plasma concentration. Next, the drug rapidly enters multiple organ systems with high blood flow (such as the brain, liver, kidney) from which the plasma drug concentration rapidly drops followed by a slower drop due to redistribution to organs (such as the muscles and later tissues with high fat content) that are less well perfused. These concentration changes over time can be described by non-compartmental and compartmental PK models. Non-compartmental analysis describes the drug's PK behavior in terms of volume of distribution (V_D = drug dose/steady-state plasma drug concentration), rapid and slow distribution half-lives, and elimination half-life ($t½_{elim}$). A high V_D is observed for lipophilic opioids with low protein-binding affinity such as fentanyl (V_D = 300 L) but a low V_D is observed for remifentanil and alfentanil, due to a high clearance (remifentanil) and/or high protein binding. When V_D is small, clearance is responsible for the drop in plasma concentration and consequently the loss of analgesia, whereas redistribution accounts for loss of analgesic effect in drugs with a high V_D.

6 The time needed for the drug's plasma concentration to decrease by 50%, from a steady-state plasma concentration after the drug infusion has stopped, is called the context-sensitive half-time (CSt½) (Fig. 19-6).[60,61] The CSt½ depends on the duration of the infusion, which is the context to which the term applies. For fentanyl, the context-sensitive half-time increases with the duration of the infusion, while for remifentanil the half-time is independent of the duration because of its rapid clearance (50% drop in plasma concentration is 2 minutes, 75% drop is 8 minutes).[61] In clinical practice, the time to the loss of analgesia depends on the opioid dose, neuronal and receptor kinetic processes, the transport of the opioids from brain to plasma, and the context-sensitive half-time. The time course of a specific effect is

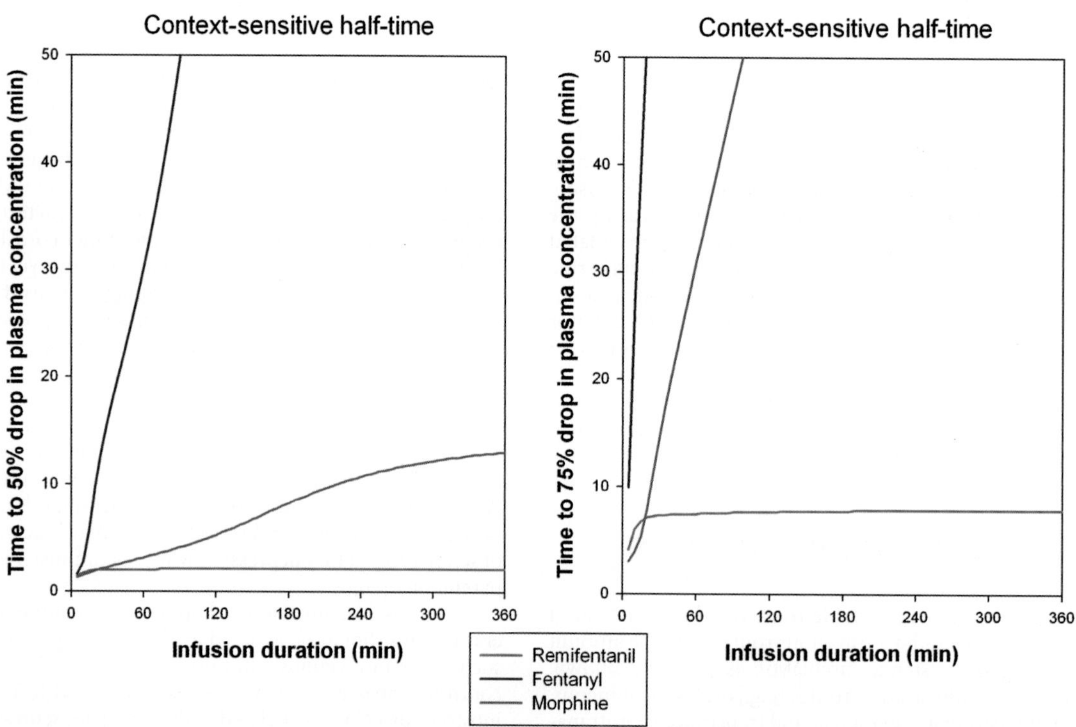

FIGURE 19-6. Context-sensitive half-times for remifentanil, fentanyl, and morphine. *Left:* Time to 50% drop in concentration versus infusion duration. *Right:* Time to 75% drop in concentration versus infusion duration.

difficult to predict for individual patients. For some side effects such as opioid-induced respiratory depression, the prediction of onset or offset of effect is even more complicated due to counteracting forces, such as the respiratory stimulant effects of increased arterial CO_2 and the presence of pain.[62]

Metabolism: Which Pathways and Metabolites are Clinically Relevant?

Most opioids are metabolized in the liver through either phase I (oxidative and reductive reactions catalyzed by the cytochrome P450 enzyme system) or phase II reactions (conjugation to a specific substrate). Metabolism may occur at other sites as well, such as in the enterocytes of the gastric tract, the kidney, or the brain. Excretion of the parent drug and/or metabolites occurs via the kidney and/or via the biliary tract into the gut where some opioids (morphine, buprenorphine) may undergo reuptake of the compound into the blood stream.

Three aspects of opioid metabolism have clinical importance:

1. Medications that inhibit or induce the CYP450 system may increase or decrease the clinical effect of opioids by interfering with their metabolism (Table 19-1).[63,64]
7 2. Opioid metabolites may either be active or inactive, which applies not only to their analgesic effect but also to their unwanted side effects.[65,66]
3. Genetic variability in the CYP system has clinical implications that are discussed in the section on *Pharmacogenetics.*

Morphine

Morphine undergoes rapid metabolism (by UGT2B7, a phase II reaction) in the liver and within minutes after its administration the two most important hydrophilic metabolites appear in plasma: Morphine-3-glucuronide (M3G) and M6G.[64–66] M3G is the major metabolite and about 60% of morphine is converted into M3G, while just 5% to 10% is converted to M6G. In humans M3G is without any analgesic or anti-analgesic action. M6G is a full MOR agonist but at the concentrations observed following morphine administration in a patient with normal renal function its contribution to the overall analgesic effect is minimal.[67] Due to its low lipophilicity, passage of M6G across the blood–brain barrier is slow and consequently limited. In the hepatocytes both M3G and M6G are transported back into the bloodstream while a small part is transported into the bile ducts.[68] In the gut both glucuronides are deglucuronidated and the resultant morphine molecule is partly absorbed by the enterocytes (Fig. 19-7). Enterocytes are able to metabolize morphine and transport the resultant M3G and M6G to the bloodstream (the enterohepatic cycle).

Since the morphine-glucuronides are excreted via the kidney, patients with renal failure are at risk for M6G-related side effects.[67] Since M6G is a full MOR agonist these side effects are typical of opioids and, most importantly, include sedation and respiratory depression. In patients with compromised renal function morphine treatment causes M6G to accumulate in high concentrations that may cause loss of consciousness and severe respiratory depression.[67,69] Attempts to market M6G as a potent opioid analgesic have failed, likely due to its slow onset/offset time ($t_{1/2}k_{e0}$ 4 to 6 hours) and low potency in humans.

Piperidines

Fentanyl, alfentanil, sufentanil, and remifentanil are lipophilic opioids that rapidly cross the blood–brain barrier. Fentanyl, alfentanil, and sufentanil are metabolized by the liver, catalyzed by the cytochrome P450 enzyme system.[64,70,71] *Fentanyl* has a high hepatic extraction ratio with clearance approaching liver blood flow (1.5 L/min). The major metabolite of fentanyl is the inactive compound norfentanyl. *Sufentanil* also has a high hepatic extraction ratio with a clearance of 0.9 L/min. *Alfentanil* is metabolized by CYP3A4 and 3A5 forming the inactive compounds noralfentanil and *N*-phenylpropionamide. The polymorphic expression of the CYP3A5 gene accounts for the great variability in alfentanil metabolism and clearance.[72] *Remifentanil* contrasts with the other piperidines in that it is not metabolized in the liver.[73] Remifentanil contains a methyl ester side chain (Fig. 19-1) that is metabolized by blood (within the erythrocyte) and tissue nonspecific esterases. This causes a rapid clearance of the drug (context sensitive half-life of 2 minutes) making it the most rapidly acting opioid currently available. Clearance of remifentanil is 3 to 5 L/min, which exceeds liver blood flow affirming its extrahepatic clearance. Remifentanil is usually administered as a continuous infusion since its plasma level decreases by 50% in as little as 40 seconds.[74–76]

TABLE 19-1. INHIBITORS AND INDUCERS OF CYP3A AND INHIBITORS OF CYP2D6

CYP3A Inhibitors	CYP3A Inducers	CYP2D6 Inhibitors
Antibiotics	**Antibiotics**	**Antidepressants**
Erythromycin, clarithromycin	Rifampicin	Clomipramine, fluoxetine, paroxetine
Calcium-channel blockers	**Anticonvulsants**	**Antipsychotics**
Diltiazem, verapamil	Carbamazepine, phenytoin, phenobarbital	Haloperidol
Anti-HIV agents	**Anti-HIV agents**	**Antidysrhythmics**
Delavirdine, indinavir, ritonavir, saquinavir	Efavirenz, nevirapine	Quinidine
Antifungal agents	**Others**	**Others**
Itraconazole, ketoconazole	St. John's wort Dexamethasone	Cimetidine
Others		
Grapefruit juice		

Data from: Wilkinson GR. Drug metabolism and variability among patients in drug response. *N Engl J Med.* 2005;352:2211.

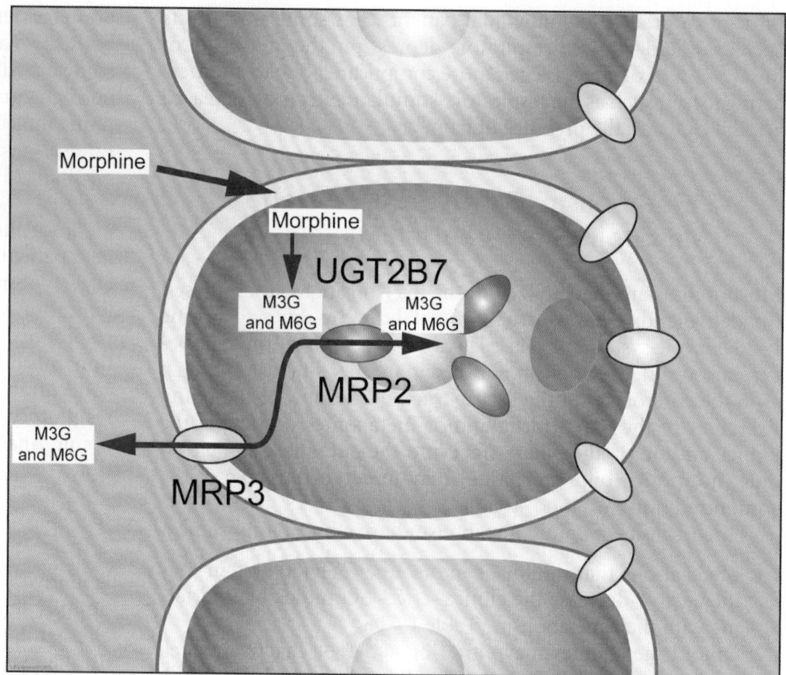

FIGURE 19-7. Morphine metabolism in the liver and transport of its metabolites into the bloodstream and bile system. Morphine enters the hepatocyte where it undergoes metabolism by UGT2B7 (a phase II reaction) into morphine-3-glucuronide (M3G) and morphine-6-glucuronide (M6G, not shown). These two glucuronides are transported via transporter proteins MRP3 (*yellow*) and MRP2 (*green*) back into the systemic circulation and into the biliary duct system.

Methadone

Methadone is extensively metabolized to an inactive form by CYP2B6, which is also affected by pharmacogenetic variability.[77,78] Methadone has a 60% to 95% bioavailability, high potency, and a long duration of action. Furthermore, there is considerable variation among recipients in the response to the drug. While methadone has properties which make it attractive for use intravenously as a perioperative analgesic, in a controlled and well-monitored environment, these same properties may prove hazardous when methadone is administered orally for treatment of patients with chronic pain. Large numbers of patient deaths have been attributed to the long, and often unpredictable, duration of action of methadone when administered orally.

Naloxone

Naloxone is the most valuable and popular nonspecific MOR antagonist.[79] Since it has a low and unpredictable bioavailability after oral intake due to an extensive (>95%) first-pass effect, naloxone is best given via the intravenous route.[79] The most important metabolic pathway of naloxone is glucuronidation into the inactive naloxone-3-glucuronide. Its duration of effect is short, ranging from 15 to 45 minutes, which requires it to be redosed or administered as a continuous infusion when antagonism is required for long-acting opioids or for patients experiencing an opioid overdose.

PKPD Models of Opioid Effect: Which End Point Serves the Clinician Best?

1 The PK of a drug describes the time course of dose to concentration; the PD describes the concentration to effect relationship;
2 the effect can be any of the desired or undesired drug effects. Pharmacokinetic–pharmacodynamic (PKPD) models are constructed for each drug to allow the clinician to understand and predict the clinical implication of a given dose to a desired effect.[80] These models allow dosing regimens to be constructed on the basis of patient characteristics such as total or lean body weight, gender, age, and other characteristics, making them particularly helpful when treating individual patients. The PK part of such models describes the drug distribution kinetics. This relates to both the parent drug and the possible metabolites. In compartmental models, the concentration–time profiles are described by drug transfer between interconnected hypothetical compartments, mimicking drug absorption, distribution, elimination, and metabolism. The PD part of the model describes the drug concentration–effect relationship. This hypothetical effect compartment is made infinitely small so that it does not influence the drug's disposition (PK) and is located at the drug's target organ, such as the muscle endplate for muscle relaxants and the brain for hypnotic drugs. For most opioid effects (such as analgesia, sedation, and respiratory depression) the effect site is located within the CNS while the effect site for constipation is the GI tract. The delay between the peak drug concentration in the plasma and the peak concentration at the effect site is described by the plasma–
8 effect-site equilibration constant k_{e0} (or its half-life $t½k_{e0} = \ln 2/k_{e0}$),[81–83] which is commonly referred to as hysteresis. For the analgesic and respiratory depressive effects of opioids, the hysteresis is determined by the drug's passage across the blood–brain barrier (the more lipophilic an opioid, the faster the transfer into the brain compartment), receptor kinetics, and neuronal dynamics. The effect-site concentration–effect relationship is described by a sigmoid E_{max} model[80–84]: Effect = $(C_E/C_{50})^{\gamma}/[1 + (C_E/C_{50})^{\gamma}]$, where C_E is the drug concentration in the hypothetical effect site, C_{50} is the measure of drug potency or the effect-site or steady-state concentration causing 50% of the effect, and γ is the Hill or steepness parameter (Fig. 19-4). In summary, any PKPD analysis using the above-mentioned descriptions yields PK parameters (volumes of distribution and clearances), as well PD parameters related to drug potency (C_{50}) and the onset/offset times of the drug ($t½k_{e0}$). It is important to understand that PK (volumes of distribution and rate constant) and PD (potency) values vary largely among patients. This is related to differences in physiology, underlying disease, age, weight, ethnicity, and other factors. Thus the clinician should choose a PK/PD set derived from a

TABLE 19-2. ESTIMATES OF THE t½k_{e0} FOR A VARIETY OF ANALGESICS DETERMINED FOR CLINICALLY RELEVANT END POINTS OF PAIN RELIEF AND RESPIRATORY DEPRESSION

Drug	t½k_{e0}	End Point Measured
Morphine	1.5 h	Postoperative analgesia
Ibuprofen	0.5 h	Postoperative analgesia
Acetaminophen	1 h	Postoperative analgesia
Morphine men	1.5 h	Relief of experimental pain
Morphine women	5 h	Relief of experimental pain
Fentanyl	20–40 min	Relief of experimental pain
Alfentanil	1–10 min	Relief of experimental pain
Remifentanil	1–1.5 min	Relief of experimental pain
Buprenorphine	2.5 h	Relief of experimental pain
S-ketamine	<1 min	Relief of experimental pain
Morphine	1.2 h	Respiratory depression
Buprenorphine	1.5 h	Respiratory depression
Fentanyl	15 min	Respiratory depression
Remifentanil	0.5 min	Respiratory depression
Naloxone	5–8 min	Relief of respiratory depression

Data from: Martini C, et al. Pharmacokinetic-pharmacodynamic modeling in acute and chronic pain: An overview of the recent literature. *Exp Rev Pharmacother* 2011;4:719.

population of subjects whose characteristics are most similar to the individual they are treating. For example, due to changes in PK and PD behavior, elderly patients display a greater opioid sensitivity[85]; patients with liver or renal insufficiency require adaptation to their dosing; and patients with certain genetic abnormalities may experience unusual responses to opioids (see later).[63,64]

For most opioids, the target effect when constructing PKPD models has traditionally been the slowing of the frequency components of the EEG, quantified by a shift in the 95th percentile of the power spectrum (95% spectral edge frequency).[86,87] The C_{50} and t½k_{e0} derived from these studies are useful to compare the potency and onset/offset of opioids. However, since the C_{50} for EEG effects occurs beyond the normal clinical dose range of opioids, more clinically useful C_{50} values would include those for the analgesic, respiratory depressive, and sedative effect of opioids. For alfentanil and fentanyl C_{50} values range from 75 and 1 ng/mL for sedation to 150 and 2 ng/mL for analgesia, respectively.[88,89] This indicates that these clinically relevant effects occur at lower doses than their effects on the EEG. For fentanyl it is of further interest that t½k_{e0} values for analgesia (20 to 40 minutes) and respiratory depression are much longer (15 minutes) than those observed for EEG-slowing (5 to 6 minutes). In Table 19-2 values of t½k_{e0} for the end points of pain relief and respiratory depression are given for various analgesics currently in use.

Pharmacodynamics: Dose Effect on Pain Relief

In postoperative patients following major orthopedic surgery under general anesthesia, it has been observed that some patients require a morphine dose of 0.02 mg/kg to obtain a visual analogue score of 30 mm or less while others require a dose 40 times as large (0.8 mg/kg).[90] Younger (<40 years) healthy volunteers of normal weight (BMI <25 kg/m²) had analgesic responses to a fixed dose of morphine that varied by a factor of 20 (Fig. 19-8).[91] This variability is not restricted to morphine but is observed for all opioids used for treatment of acute, perioperative, and chronic pain, including strong opioids such as fentanyl and remifentanil. These data suggest that the variability in opioid effect is related to both variability in PK-related parameters (which in turn are

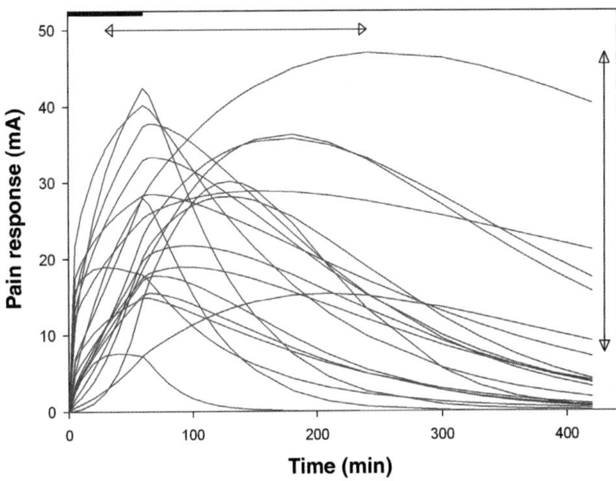

FIGURE 19-8. The variability observed in morphine analgesic effect. An intravenous infusion of 0.13 mg/kg was given to 10 healthy male (*green lines*) and female (*red lines*) volunteers. Their pain tolerance to a transcutaneous electrical stimulation (*y*-axis) was measured over a 7-hour period. The variability in magnitude of peak analgesia and time to peak effect are made visible by the *vertical and horizontal arrowed lines*. The *black bar* indicates the 1-hour morphine infusion. Data adapted from: Sarton E, Olofsen E, Romberg R, et al. Sex differences in morphine analgesia: An experimental study in healthy volunteers. *Anesthesiology*. 2000;93:1245.

attributable to differences in age, weight, body fat and muscle content, renal/liver function, cardiac output, genetic polymorphism in metabolic pathways, co-medication) and variability in PD-related parameters. These PD differences of opioid sensitivity and pain perception most likely have a genetic origin. To date, no clear genetic basis for variability in morphine or any other opioid PD effect has been demonstrated (for an exception see the section on *Pharmacogenetics*). These data indicate that the safest approach to opioid analgesia is one of careful titration to analgesic effect during surgery and in the postoperative period, with acute awareness of the undesirable dose-related side effects. This admonition to carefully titrate the administration of opioids is perhaps even more crucial when administering long-acting opioids orally for the treatment of chronic pain.

During surgery opioids are titrated in doses sufficient to dampen and prevent exaggerated hemodynamic responses to painful surgical stimuli. In the postoperative period (and in chronic pain patients) opioids are usually titrated in response to the patient's verbal response to pain. This requires not only a difference in administration approach but also requires a difference in vigilance with respect to opioid side effects. During surgery, potent high-dose piperidines (e.g., fentanyl, remifentanil) are the opioids of choice, while in the postoperative period medium strength opioids (morphine, methadone) are often chosen. During anesthesia one should be aware of hypotension and bradycardia, a common side effect of strong opioids, while in the postoperative period most important side effects to be avoided are respiratory depression and severe sedation, while other nonlife-threatening but important side effects in terms of patient satisfaction and health costs are nausea/vomiting and loss of bowel movement.

Morphine

In two studies on the postoperative effects of morphine following major surgery, the average iv dose of morphine to reach 50% pain relief was 20 mg resulting in a plasma concentration of 34 ng/mL and a $t\frac{1}{2}k_{e0}$ of about 2 hours (Fig. 19-9), although the initial onset of analgesia occurred between 15 and 30 minutes.[92,93] This means that there is a lag of hours between peak plasma morphine concentration and peak analgesic effect (i.e., hysteresis). Surprisingly, these parameters are not influenced by the patients' age, weight, and gender. Similar parameter values are observed in volunteers when studying the subject's response to an electrical cutaneous stimulus.[84,91] Given the long time to peak analgesia a practical strategy for dosing morphine in adults is to give an initial morphine bolus dose 20 to 45 minutes before the end of surgery followed by 2 mg bolus doses postoperatively until visual analog pain scores decrease to 3 or less (on a scale from 0 to 10) (Fig. 19-10).[84] At that point, the patient can be started on a PCA pump. Two considerations must accompany every postoperative acute pain plan. First, the postoperative analgesic regimen should be multimodal with morphine (or any other opioid) combined with opioid-sparing drugs such as acetaminophen and nonsteroidal antiinflammatory drugs such as diclofenac. Second, some patients require large doses of morphine and their pain appears unresponsive to morphine. Often it is not clear whether these patients are opioid tolerant or OIH accounts for their lack of pain relief. It is then wise not to continue dosing but to add an adjuvant such as one or two iv administrations of the NMDA receptor antagonist, ketamine (0.125 mg/kg) or an iv dose of an α_2-adrenergic receptor agonist, such as clonidine (75 μg). Both drugs are analgesics in their own right and enhance morphine's analgesic effect,[94,95] presumably by reducing OIH. A practical morphine PCA regimen may consist of a 1 mg dose, and 5-minute lockout with a maximum of 24 mg per 4 hours. It is important to follow the patient's pain assessment when titrating to effect, as nurses and physicians usually rate the pain 1 to 2 points lower than the patient (Fig. 19-11).

Other suitable opioids for postoperative pain relief are methadone, oxycodone, or piritramide.

Fentanyl

Fentanyl is about 100 times more potent than morphine. Like all opioids the analgesic response to iv fentanyl is highly variable. Fentanyl's lipophilic structure means it rapidly crosses the blood–brain barrier as is evident from a characteristic delta wave appearing on the EEG ($t\frac{1}{2}k_{e0}$ 6.5 minutes).[86,87] However, fentanyl's $t\frac{1}{2}k_{e0}$ for analgesic effect is longer with values ranging between 10 and 20 minutes (Figs. 19-9 and 19-12)[88]; fentanyl's potency (C_{50}) for analgesia ranges from 1 to 2 ng/mL.[88] Fentanyl is used during anesthesia to dampen cardiovascular responses to noxious stimulation from laryngoscopy, intubation, skin incision, and surgical stress.[96,97] On average, the requirements for inhalational anesthetics and propofol are reduced by about 50% when

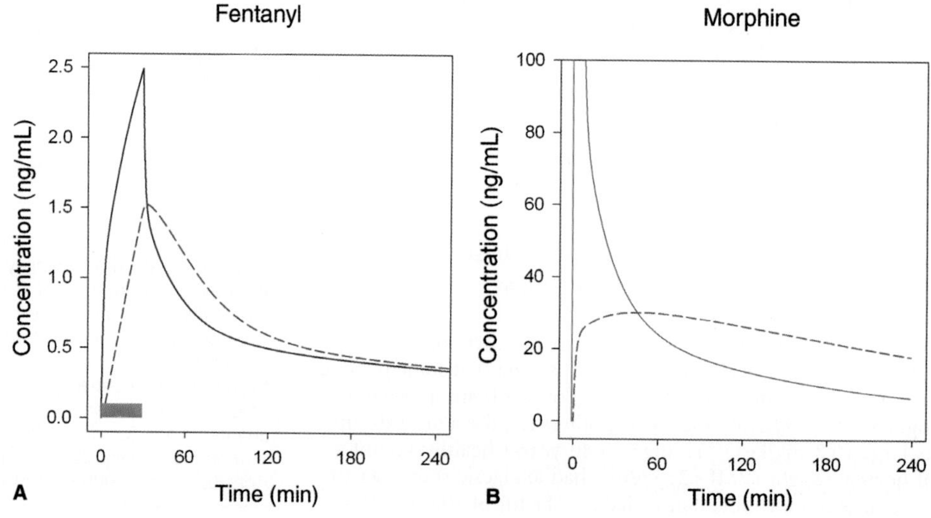

FIGURE 19-9. A: Pharmacokinetics of fentanyl following a 240 μg infusion given over 30 minutes (*yellow bar*). **B:** Pharmacokinetics of a single bolus of 20 mg morphine. The *continuous line* is the plasma concentration, the *broken line* the concentration in the effect site (the brain). The value for $t\frac{1}{2}k_{e0}$ of fentanyl here is 20 minutes and that of morphine 1 hour. These are the values observed for analgesia.

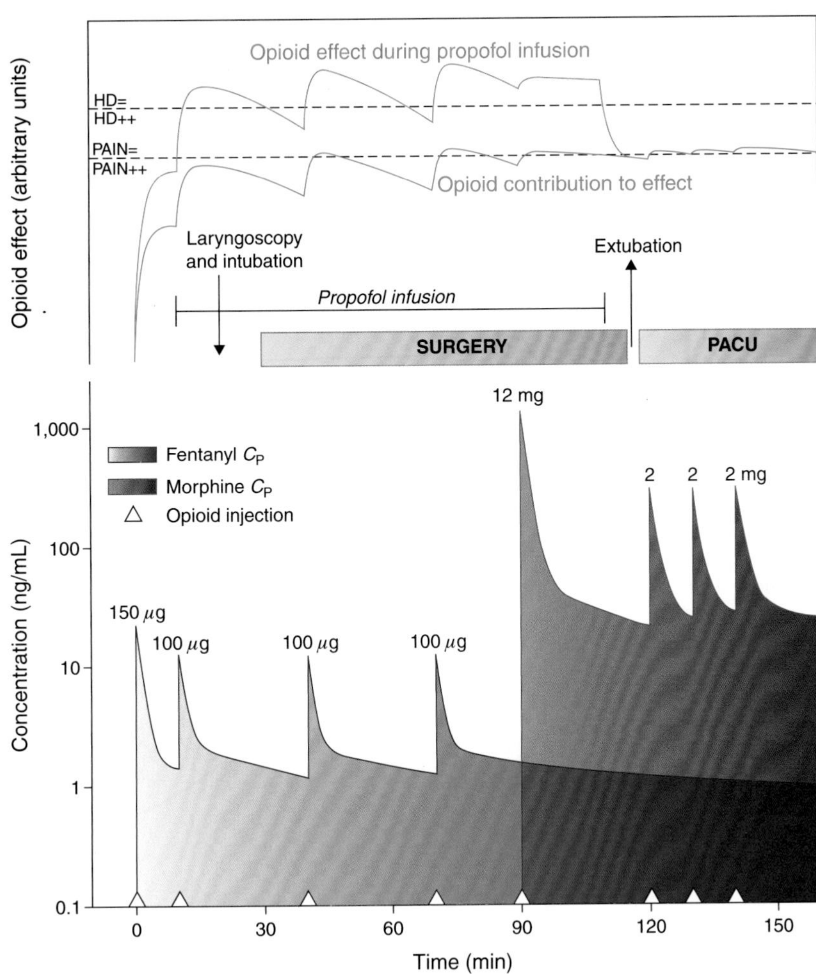

FIGURE 19-10. Simulated effect of multiple bolus doses of fentanyl (100 to 150 μg) during anesthesia and morphine during and following anesthesia, on the analgesic and hemodynamic state of the patient. An initial dose of morphine (12 mg) is given 30 minutes before the end of surgery followed by three 2 mg doses (at the end of this titration phase the patient can be set on PCA morphine). The *blue* and *red lines* are the simulated fentanyl and morphine plasma concentration (C_P). On *top* is the effect profile induced by the two opioids. During anesthesia fentanyl dosing is based predominantly on hemodynamic and other autonomic parameters; in the PACU morphine dosing is based on pain rating. During anesthesia, the combination of fentanyl and propofol provides greater analgesia than just the opioids (*orange line*). When propofol infusion is terminated the analgesic profile reverts to a lower level (from *orange* via *orange-green* to *green line*). HD= indicates that hemodynamic and other autonomic responses are in the normal range, HD++ indicates increased responses (such as high blood pressure, tachycardia, and sweating) due to the surgical stress; PAIN= indicates adequate analgesia, PAIN++ indicates pain. The *dotted lines* are the arbitrary divisions between adequate anesthesia and inadequate anesthesia, and adequate analgesia and inadequate analgesia.

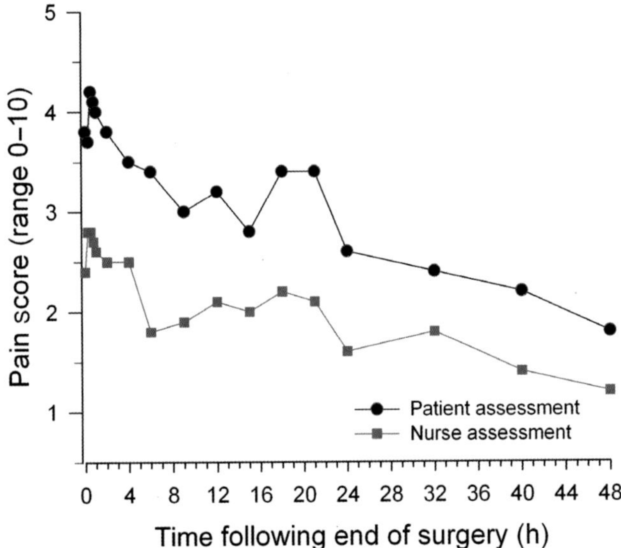

FIGURE 19-11. Comparison of mean pain scores during PCA morphine obtained from 30 patients and the nursing staff following major abdominal surgery (Dr. A. Dahan (2010), data on file).

administering 1.5 to 3 μg/kg iv fentanyl.[97–99] In fact, by combining fentanyl (or any other potent opioid) with propofol the requirement of both drugs to prevent movement and hemodynamic responses to laryngoscopy and surgical stress is reduced (Fig. 19-10).[97] Fentanyl dosing should be repeated at regular intervals in order to maintain a comfortable analgesic state (the dose and frequency are dependent on the patient's weight, dose, type of surgery, etc.). Be aware that a continuous infusion leads to the accumulation of the drug in the body as its 50% context-sensitive half-time increases rapidly with the duration of infusion (Fig. 19-6).[60] Similarly, frequent dosing of the drug may cause accumulation. Taking into account the drug's $t\frac{1}{2}k_{e0}$ fentanyl should be administered 5 to 10 minutes prior to an anticipated painful/stressful event such as laryngoscopy or skin incision (Fig. 19-10).

In the 1980s, high-dose fentanyl was often used in combination with nitrous oxide to provide both analgesia and suppression of consciousness. Although this provided excellent hemodynamic stability, it could not assure amnesia. Hence it is not surprising that this technique has been replaced by the technique of "balanced anesthesia" or total intravenous anesthesia (TIVA) where opioids are combined with sedatives, iv anesthetics, and muscle relaxants to assure amnesia, as well as analgesia.

Fentanyl is also used in the treatment of chronic pain. For example, the fentanyl patch is used in a large number of cancer and non-cancer chronic pain patients.[100] The transcutaneous

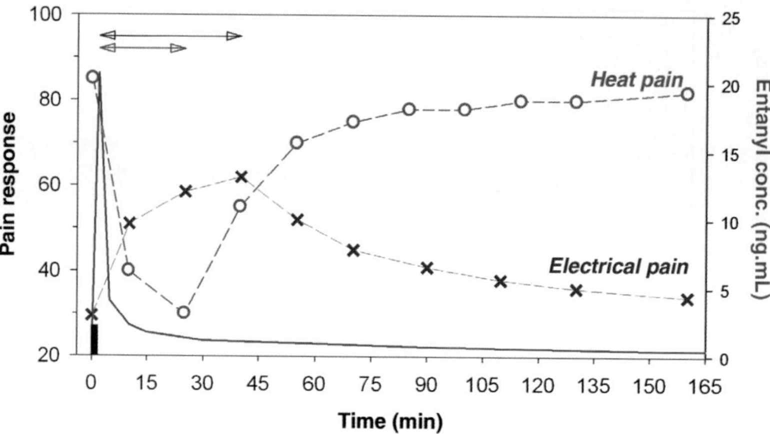

FIGURE 19-12. The delay in effect between peak fentanyl plasma concentration (*red line, right y-axis*) and peak analgesic response (*left y-axis*) as observed in one person following a bolus intravenous infusion of 3.25 μg/kg given at $t = 0$ minutes. The delays are given for the pain rating to a fixed heat stimulus to the skin (*blue line* and x's) and the tolerance responses to an electrical stimulus train (*green line* and o's). The delay for heat pain was 25 minutes (*green arrows*), the delay for electrical pain 40 minutes (*blue arrows*). These delays are much greater than that observed for EEG effects. The differences in delays may be explained by difference in processing of the different end points in the brain.

delivery of fentanyl ranges from 12 to 100 μg/hour, although absorption depends on a variety of factors such as skin thickness, subcutaneous fat layer, and subcutaneous perfusion. Peak analgesic effect is reached only after 10 to 12 hours and the effect of one patch lasts 3 to 4 days. Other methods of administration include intranasal fentanyl, sublingual fentanyl, fentanyl lozenges (a solid preparation in the form of a popsicle), mucosal patch (all four are used for treatment of breakthrough pain) and iontophoretic transdermal fentanyl applications. The home use of fentanyl in chronic pain patients comes with the danger of misuse and abuse by the patients or by family members or friends. This is a major concern as it leads to an increasing number of opioid fatalities.[101,102]

Remifentanil

Remifentanil, the newest piperidine available for use in humans, differs from the other strong opioids in its rapid onset/offset for all clinical effects including respiration (Fig. 19-13).[62] Indications for its use include anesthesia/surgery, patient controlled analgesia (PCA), analgesia and sedation in the ICU, diagnostic procedures, and the treatment of obstetric labor pain. The use of remifentanil in spontaneous breathing patients at relatively low infusion rates (<0.1 to 0.2 μg/kg/min) is feasible,[62,103] but requires adequate monitoring and skilled personnel to detect and overcome any possible respiratory event.

Remifentanil is 100 to 200 times more potent than morphine. Just like other opioids, remifentanil displays large variability in effect among patients. For example, Drover and Lemmens showed that the remifentanil plasma concentration causing a 50% probability (C_{P50}) of no clinical response to stimulation (laryngoscopy, intubation, skin incision, and skin closures) varies 50-fold, from 1.5 to 79 ng/mL, during abdominal surgery in patients anesthetized with a nitrous oxide and remifentanil combination.[104] In that study, a clear gender difference in potency of remifentanil was found (C_{P50} men 4.1 ng/mL, women 7.5 ng/mL). This difference can be accounted for by the difference in surgical stimulation of the prostatectomies versus hysterectomies. Different surgeries produce differences in nociception (i.e., pain) and hemodynamic stress responses and hence require different dosages to suppress pain and stress. The C_{P50} varied from 3.8 ng/mL for prostatectomies, 5.6 ng/mL for nephrectomies, and 7.5 ng/mL for abdominal hysterectomies. Like fentanyl, remifentanil causes a reduction of MAC and reduction in propofol requirement. Mertens et al.[105] showed that by increasing the remifentanil concentration from 0 to 2 ng/mL the mean propofol concentration required to obtain C_{P50} for laryngoscopy was reduced from 7 to 3 μg/mL, more than

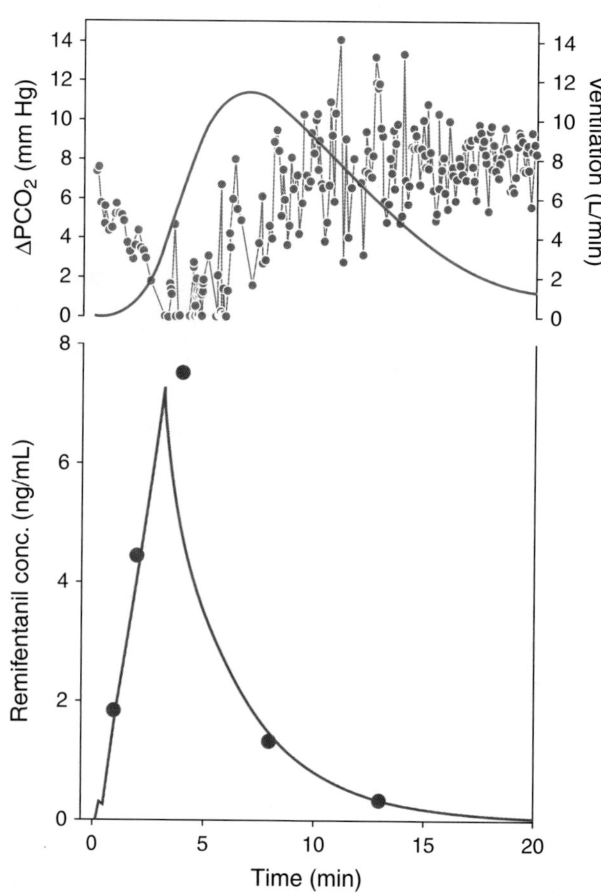

FIGURE 19-13. Effect of a short remifentanil infusion on breathing. Note the absence of a delay between the remifentanil plasma concentration and ventilation, and the short delay between the plasma concentration and the end-tidal PCO_2. *Top:* The increase in end-tidal PCO_2 (ΔPCO_2, *green line*), the measured inspired ventilation (*gray dots*, each dot is one breath). *Bottom:* The measured remifentanil plasma concentration (*red dots*) and the pharmacokinetic data fit (*red line*). The *black bar* indicates the infusion period. Data adapted from: Olofsen E, Boom M, Nieuwenhuijs D, et al. Modeling the non-steady-state respiratory effects of remifentanil in awake and propofol sedated healthy volunteers. *Anesthesiology*. 2010;212:1382.

60% reduction in dose requirement. When combining remifentanil with propofol (TIVA), the remifentanil effect remains variable. The remifentanil concentration added to a constant propofol plasma concentration of 2 μg/mL required for suppression of hemodynamic and movement responses during abdominal surgery varies from 3 to 15 ng/mL. Interestingly, at a higher propofol concentration of 4 μg/mL, the variability was reduced to 0 to 5 ng/mL. These data once again reinforce that opioid dosing, including remifentanil, requires titration to effect based on careful observation of the clinical response of the patient. Variations in the infusion rate should be based on an a priori knowledge of the PK and PD properties of the drug, patient characteristics, and, most importantly, hemodynamic responses and nociceptive input during surgery. Between intubation and surgical incision, when there is no stimulation, decreases of 30% to 40% in blood pressure and heart rate are not uncommon unless the remifentanil infusion is reduced during that period. Due to its rapid PK activity, the need for an initial remifentanil bolus is rather limited especially when there is ample time between the start of infusion and the first nociceptive stimulus (such as laryngoscopy). If a bolus is required a slow infusion (given in 1 to 2 minutes) of 0.5 to 1 μg/kg can be used.

The minimum alveolar concentration (MAC) reduction observed with remifentanil use[61,106] and its very short CSt½ (Fig. 19-6) make rapid awakening possible at the end of surgery. For example, after a 3-hour infusion of propofol and remifentanil for abdominal surgery, the shortest time to awakening (≈6.5 minutes) was observed after constant propofol and remifen-
9 tanil concentrations of 1.5 and 9.0 ng/mL, respectively.[105] At higher propofol but lower remifentanil concentrations the time to awakening increases. Note that all of these patients received morphine 0.1 mg/kg 30 minutes to the end of surgery to prevent overt pain responses upon awakening. The occurrence of postoperative pain following remifentanil "fast-track" anesthesia is frequently reported.[51] Postoperative pain scores are higher after a remifentanil-based anesthesia, and requirements for morphine are increased. This is due to the rapid decline in μ-opioid concentration causing a rapid decline in analgesic state combined with a persistence of OIH. Strategies to counteract this problem include starting morphine administration 30 to 45 minutes before the end of surgery, or a single fentanyl bolus of 50 μg or ketamine 0.125 mg/kg at the end of surgery.[52]

Pharmacogenetics

Pharmacogenetics describes the relationship between genetic variations and drug response.[63] Variations occur in genes that code for components of the metabolic pathways and transport of the drug across the blood–brain barrier (affecting PK behavior) and in genes that code for the opioid receptor or proteins in downstream signaling pathways (affecting PD behavior). The existence of a pharmacogenetic effect on PK is well established in opioid pharmacology, whereas an effect of genetic makeup on PD is less certain. For example, the literature on the significance of a specific mutation in the gene coding for MOR, *OPRM1:c.118 A > G* (dbSNP1799971), is equivocal.[69,107] Some examples of pharmacogenetic variations that influence opioid analgesia are given below.

The gene that codes for the melanocortin-1 receptor, the *MC1r* gene, is involved in the regulation of skin and hair pigmentation and immunomodulation. Sixty percent of redheads have at least two variant alleles of the gene and animal and human studies indicate that specific mutations in this gene cause a phenotype of red hair and a fair, freckled skin as well as an increase in μ-opioid analgesia.[108] The exact mechanism by which the *MC1r* gene influences pain pathways and interacts with the opioidergic system remains unknown. Possibly, the inactive MC1r causes a reflex increase in α-melanocyte–stimulating hormone (αMSH) and ACTH, which may act as the endogenous ligands to MC1r and which may induce neurobehavioral changes. Interestingly, redheads require more midazolam and inhalational anesthetics compared to otherwise pigmented (either blond or dark) individuals.[109]

While most CYP isoenzymes display polymorphisms, the genetic variability in the gene coding for CYP2D6 is clinically most important.[63,64] The CYP2D6 isoenzyme of the cytochrome P450 system is highly polymorphic with large variations between individuals in the number of gene copies in their DNA.[110] The rate of metabolism of opioids depends on the number of copies a subject expresses from ultrarapid metabolizing individuals with multiple copies of the *CYP2D6* gene to poor metabolizing individuals with two nonfunctional alleles of the gene (with some individuals demonstrating metabolism at a rate in-between extensive and intermediate individuals). The more copies of the gene the greater the metabolic power within the CYP2D6 pathway; the reverse is true for individuals without an active copy of the gene.[110] This is important for drugs that rely on CYP2D6 to convert an inactive precursor (prodrug), such as codeine, into the active component of pain therapy (for codeine this is morphine).[111] Patients without an active gene will have no benefit from treatment with codeine. Dangerous circumstances may occur when a patient is an extensive metabolizer and produces large amounts of the active component. There are multiple case reports showing codeine intoxication due to ultrarapid CYP2D6 metabolism.[111–113] A tragic example reported by Koren et al.[113] describes a normal full-term breastfed neonate that developed lethargy on postnatal day 7 and was found dead 6 days later. His mother had been prescribed 30 mg codeine combined with 500 mg acetaminophen for episiotomy pain (two tablets every 12 hours, reduced to 1 tablet per 12 hours after day 2 because of somnolence and constipation). Postmortem morphine plasma concentrations were 70 ng/mL (normal values for children breastfed by mothers receiving codeine is 0.2 to 2 ng/mL). The mother's milk contained 87 ng/mL morphine (typical mother milk concentrations after repeated codeine dosing is 2 to 20 ng/mL). Genotype analysis revealed that the mother had a 2 × 2 CYP2D6 gene duplication and was classified as an ultrarapid CYP2D6 metabolizer. The clinical picture is that of death due to morphine-induced respiratory depression.

Variations in the *ABCB1* gene, the gene coding for P-glycoprotein, a protein involved in the efflux of xenobiotics from the brain, cause variations in the toxicity of fentanyl. Park et al.[114] monitored the clinical effects (respiration rate) of 2.5 μg/kg intravenous fentanyl in patients under spinal anesthesia and assessed the influence of three single nucleotide polymorphisms in *ABCB1*. They observed an effect of the different genotypes on respiratory depression with an increased risk for a reduction in respiratory ratio in certain variant gene combinations. These data are best explained by a lesser efficacy of the variant P-glycoprotein to transport fentanyl from the brain.

OPIOID-INDUCED RESPIRATORY DEPRESSION

The incidence of respiratory depression from opioid treatment, acute or chronic, is poorly documented. The metrics in the literature defining respiratory depression are inconsistent, the data are predominantly retrospective, and most studies rely on intermittent sampling of data.[115] This is likely to miss a significant number of respiratory depression events from which the patient recovers spontaneously or is rescued by other means. A recent systematic review of the literature on postoperative opioid-induced respiratory depression estimates an average incidence of 0.5% with a range of 0.2% to 2%.[115] This would suggest that only one in 200 patients develops a respiratory event from opioids that requires an intervention such as the administration of naloxone. When the patient is examined more closely as in the case of randomized controlled trials in which morphine is used as positive control, the incidence of morphine-induced respiratory depression is many times higher with hypoventilation (defined by a respiratory rate <8 breaths/minute) occurring as frequent as in 30% of patients at one or more times during PCA morphine treatment.[116] This suggests that the respiratory depression from opioids frequently goes undetected and therefore is clearly underreported. The same applies to opioid treatment for chronic pain. Accidental deaths from opioids in chronic cancer pain patients are often falsely attributed to the progression of the underlying disease. Recently, there has been an alarming increase in reports of deaths from accidental opioid overdose among patients being treated for chronic non-cancer pain. Unfortunately, no valid data are available on the incidence of opioid-induced respiratory depression in chronic pain patients on strong opioids.

Various patient groups are at higher risk for development of opioid-related respiratory depression. These include obese
10 patients, patients with (central or peripheral) hypopneic and apneic periods during sleep, patients with neuromuscular disorders, (premature) neonates, chronic opioid users, and elderly patients.[115] Identification of these high-risk groups may be challenging. For instance, patients with undiagnosed sleep-related breathing disorders often present to the preoperative assessment clinic. A careful history (e.g., looking for daytime somnolence) and physical examination are required to uncover potential heightened opioid-associated respiratory risks. Furthermore specific questionnaires, such as the STOP-BANG questionnaire for obstructive sleep apnea, should be part of the screening routine in the obese and aging patient population.[117]

The respiratory depressant effects of opioids may be divided into two components: (1) suppression of the ventilatory drive (i.e., true respiratory depression from the inactivation of respiratory neurons in the brain stem) and (2) occlusion of the upper airways either from a direct suppression of neurons in the brainstem involved in maintaining the upper airway muscle tone or from the loss of muscle tone related to sedation.[118] While opioids clearly affect respiratory neurons in the brainstem, the direct effect of opioids on the upper airway musculature is less clear. Opioids combined with anesthetics do not increase the incidence of upper airway obstruction but do increase the number of central apneic events.[119] However, any dose of opioid that produces a generalized state of sedation and/or reduced muscle tone will give rise to upper airway collapse, even when the patient is considered awake.[120] Furthermore, depression of the chemo- and arousal reflexes by opioids will cause a delayed and less forceful response to upper airway obstruction.[121] This may lead to recurrent periods of hypoxemia in the first few postoperative nights. Recent data indicate that most patients receiving opioids, whether diagnosed with obstructive sleep apnea syndrome or not, develop both central and obstructive apneic events resulting in recurrent hypoxemia during the first three to five nights postoperatively.[122] Stone et al.[123] showed that patients on PCA morphine without supplemental oxygen develop recurrent and deep hypoxic events during the first few postoperative nights (Fig. 19-14). While supplemental oxygen results in fewer hypoxic events, it has a serious disadvantage as it masks hypoventilation and early detection

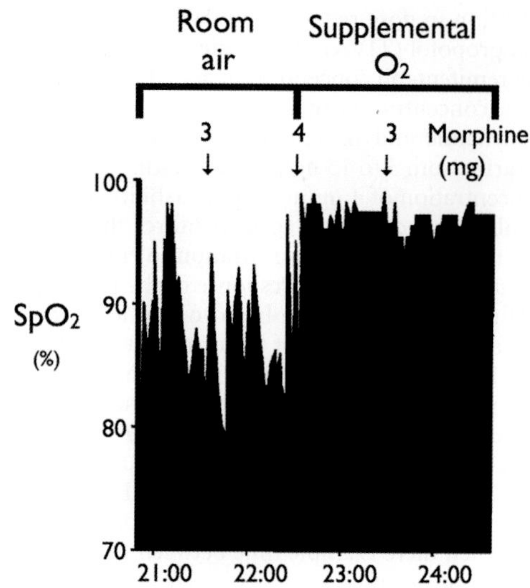

FIGURE 19-14. Effect of supplemental oxygen on pulse oximeter values in a postoperative patient on PCA morphine. Data from: Stone JG, Cozine KA, Wald A. Nocturnal oxygenation during patient-controlled analgesia. *Anesth Analg.* 1999;89:104, with permission.

of an obstructive respiratory event because the lungs are primed with supplemental oxygen.[124] Use of a pulse oximeter, especially in the presence of supplemental oxygen administration, is not a valid measure of the adequacy of ventilation.

Although the incidence of opioid-induced respiratory depression is low, fatalities do occur. Lötsch et al.[125] describe a case of a healthy 26-year, 51 kg, 165 cm, female treated with morphine after knee surgery under balanced anesthesia (sevoflurane 2% to 3%, 200 μg fentanyl). Following surgery she received four intravenous injections of morphine, with a total dose of 35 mg over 2 hours (almost 0.7 mg/kg). While the patient was comfortable and in no apparent distress directly after the last morphine dose, 40 minutes later the patient had "deep respiratory depression followed by a fatal cardiac arrest." At that time estimated brain concentrations were about 150 nM, which is above the toxic range for morphine. This case understates the need for a close understanding of the PK and PD of any opioid that is used in any patient. The physicians involved in this case did not take into account the very slow passage of morphine across the blood–brain barrier causing a peak in central effect 1 to 2 hours following peak plasma concentration. And while the onset of analgesic occurred relatively rapidly following the last dose, the fatal respiratory depression occurred 40 minutes later. Similar misunderstanding of the important role of PK by physicians prescribing oral methadone for treatment of chronic pain has led to patient deaths.

The drive to breathe is generated in multiple respiratory centers in the brainstem.[115,126] Respiratory neurons receive inputs from various sites in the CNS (cortex, limbic system, hypothalamus, spinal cord), a set of receptors located in the brainstem (central chemoreceptors), and in the carotid bodies (peripheral chemoreceptors). These sensors send information, changes in pH, PCO_2, and PO_2 of the CSF and arterial blood, to the brainstem respiratory centers, which appropriately adjust breathing rate and pulmonary tidal volume. For example, acidosis, hypercapnia, and hypoxia will cause hyperventilation, while hypocapnia and alkalosis will reduce minute ventilation. Opioid effects on MORs expressed on respiratory neurons cause a reduction in respiratory rate,[127] while a reduction in tidal volume is caused by the decreased input from the chemosensors. When an opioid is administered to a patient and the injection rate is sufficiently slow (over minutes) that the depression of the respiratory neurons in the brainstem coincides with the accumulation of arterial CO_2, the stimulatory effect of the increased CO_2 at the peripheral and central chemoreceptors will offset the decrease in tidal volume and reduced respiratory rate.[62] When just monitoring respiratory rate and oxygen saturation it appears that the opioid injected has no effect on the ventilatory system, but when also monitoring end-tidal (or arterial) CO_2 the opioid effect becomes visible. When injecting a strong opioid that rapidly crosses the blood–brain barrier, a rapid depression of respiratory neurons occurs and there will be no time for gradual CO_2 accumulation, resulting in an apneic patient. An example is given in Fig. 19-13, which shows that a rapid short-term infusion of remifentanil causes apnea and hypercapnia.[62] Breathing is restored by a high arterial CO_2 level combined with the rapid drop in brain (effect-site) remifentanil concentration. Slowing the speed of injection of this strong opioid allows the accumulation of arterial CO_2, and apnea will be prevented and the patient will continue to breathe albeit at a higher arterial PCO_2.

Similar to their analgesic PD properties, there is a large variation in the onset/offset times of the respiratory effect among the various opioids used perioperatively. Morphine has a slow onset/offset with $t½k_{e0}$ ranging between 1 and 2 hours[84]; fentanyl is faster with a value of 15 minutes,[88] while remifentanil is the fastest with a value of 1 to 2 minutes.[62] In general, when comparing opioid analgesics it is important to take into account not only their side effects (respiratory depression) but assess side effects relative to their analgesic properties. One way to compare opioids in this respect is by constructing the so-called safety or utility functions (UFos).[88,128,129] UFos are constructed by estimating *the difference* in probability of analgesia and respiratory depression from PKPD analyses. This is for various end points of effect, often analgesia ≥50%, and respiratory depression ≤50% (see Fig. 19-15). UFos are therefore context-sensitive and useful in tailoring opioids to specific patients. A negative UFo value indicates that the probability for respiratory depression is larger than the probability for analgesic efficacy. For low-dose morphine the probability for respiratory depression exceeds that of analgesia, whereas at higher doses resulting in a plasma concentration (C_P) >5 ng/mL the probability for analgesia is greater. At high morphine concentrations no difference in probability is apparent as the value of the UFo approaches zero. For fentanyl, an initial positive value at low doses (<0.5 ng/mL) is followed by a negative effect over the C_P range 0.5 to 3.0 ng/mL. For these reasons morphine is a better drug for postoperative PCA than fentanyl, when considering analgesia versus respiratory depression. These UFo curves are constructed from data in healthy volunteers. The curves of patients in pain will have a different form, more skewed to the left. However, since pain is not a constant in postoperative pain patients or chronic pain patients, these curves are still applicable to postoperative patients. Note that a positive value of the UFo does not mean that this opioid is without respiratory depression.

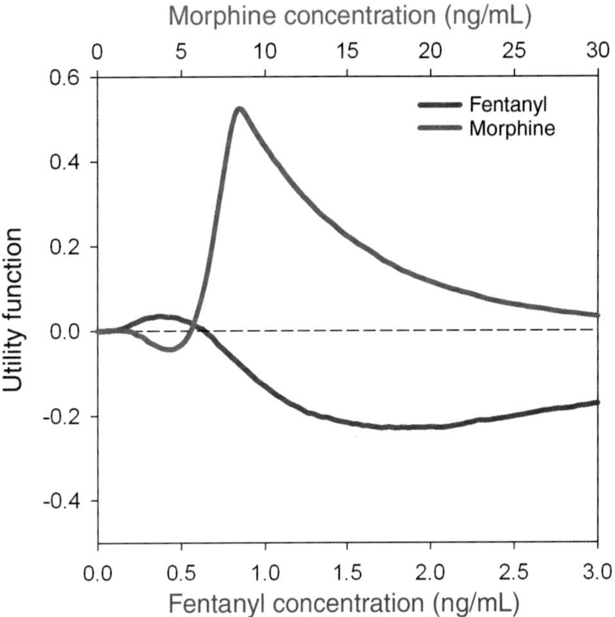

FIGURE 19-15. Safety or utility functions for morphine and fentanyl. The probability of an analgesic effect greater than 50% minus the probability of toxicity (in this case, respiratory depression) greater than 50% is given for the two opioids.

The drug of choice in case of life-threatening respiratory depression or the inability to resume spontaneous breathing is naloxone.[79] Naloxone is a competitive MOR antagonist causing a parallel rightward shift of the opioid dose–response relationship (Fig. 19-4). An oral MOR antagonist, naltrexone, is used in the treatment of alcoholism and opioid dependence.[79] Both antagonists are nonspecific, 11 meaning that they antagonize all pharmacologic effects of opioids. The magnitude and duration of reversal of respiratory depression by naloxone depends on (1) the PK and PD profile of the opioid that needs reversal and (2) the administration mode of naloxone (bolus injections vs. continuous infusion).[130] Naloxone's respiratory C_{50} (i.e., the concentration of naloxone that causes a 50% reversal of ventilation) is 2 nM, and the blood–effect-site equilibration half-life ($t½k_{e0}$) is 6.5 minutes, indicating that reversal is rapid. But the rate of decay of naloxone in plasma is relatively short ($t½_{elim}$ 30 minutes), resulting in "renarcotization" when used to reverse effects from opioids with a longer plasma half-life than naloxone.[130] However, opioid concentrations are often just above the threshold for respiratory depression, and intravenous titration of naloxone 40 to 80 μg bolus doses to cumulative doses of less than 400 μg is often sufficient to restore spontaneous breathing.[115] Respiratory depression from opioids occurs at higher receptor occupancy rates than analgesia. Therefore analgesia is not compromised with careful titration of naloxone to respiratory effect. Large doses of naloxone, as commonly used in resuscitation, will reverse analgesia immediately and may predispose patients to pain and catecholamine-associated hypertension and cardiac ischemia, if not monitored properly.[79] The naloxone titration opioid reversal approach is adequate for most opioids, with the exception of opioids with a high affinity for the MOR, such as buprenorphine.[131] In that case, a continuous naloxone infusion (2 to 4 mg/hr) will cause a slow but steady resumption of breathing activity. For remifentanil the use of bolus naloxone doses in case of respiratory depression is unnecessary. The termination of the infusion will provide a rapid return of spontaneous breathing.[132] When reversing apneic events due to an accidental opioid overdose (irrespective of the opioid taken), bolus doses are not sufficient and long-term infusions are required to prevent "renarcotization."

On the ward, patient monitoring is much less than in the operating room or post anesthesia care unit (PACU). Current methods for monitoring of the ECG and oxygen saturation and regular nurse visits are insufficient to predict the occurrence of life-threatening respiratory events. Significant drops in oxygen saturation and tachydysrhythmias do occur when the patient's breathing system has been compromised by recurrent central or obstructive apneas (or both) for an appreciable period and no arousal occurs.[123] Arousal is a wake-up from a state of sleep or sedation allowing the patient to open his or her throat and hyperventilate to overcome the period of

FIGURE 19-16. A: Breathing pattern in a patient with recurrent obstructive apneic events as might occur during sleep. SpO_2, oxygen saturation; $PaCO_2$, arterial carbon dioxide concentration; Ve, expired minute ventilation. **B:** Representation of recurrent activation of the saturation alarm in a patient with sleep apnea (alarm threshold set at 90%). This could possibly lead to alarm fatigue.[133] (*y*-axis = SpO_2.)

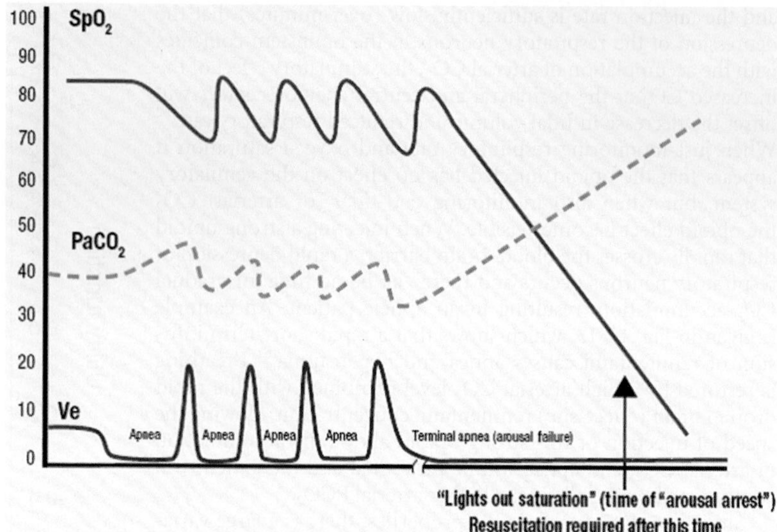

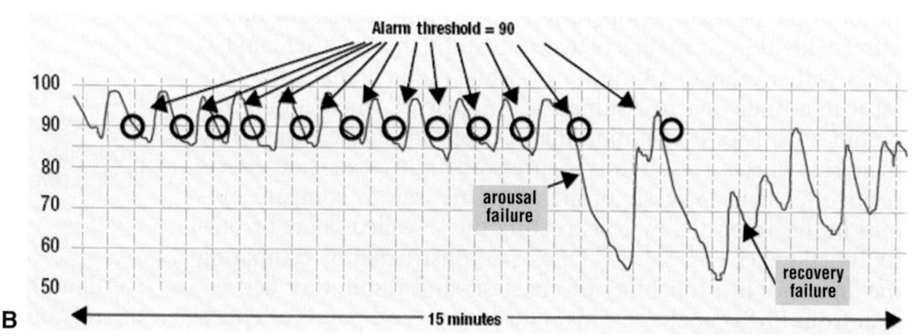

hypoxemia. Arousal is triggered by hypoxia. Arousal is depressed by opioids and sedatives.[121] Postoperative (nightly) respiratory events are often episodic with arousals and hyperventilation in-between events. This will cause repetitive triggering of the oxygen saturation monitoring alarm and possibly alarm fatigue of the nursing staff. When the alarm is then inactivated or unattended an arousal failure may occur which is potentially fatal (Fig. 19-16).[133] Alarms that give a direct indication of breathing activity are preferable. Examples are monitors that give an indirect measure of expiratory flow such as monitors at the mouth of end-tidal carbon dioxide and humidity. The latter device is a recent development that measures the exhaled water content and gives a reliable estimate of breathing frequency.[134] Both monitors will alarm in case of airway obstruction (flow rate is zero) or reduced breathing rates.

OTHER OPIOID-RELATED SIDE EFFECTS

12 Opioids case a large number of side effects, some causing great discomfort to the patient, others with potentially serious consequences. Opioid-induced respiratory depression has been discussed above.

Nausea and Vomiting

3 Postoperative nausea and vomiting (PONV) is a serious side effect from all opioids used in perioperative care. And although inhalation anesthetics contribute significantly to the problem, opioids are the major cause of PONV with an incidence of greater than 50% following balanced anesthesia.[135] Female patients seem more sensitive to opioid-induced PONV (see later). Patient distress from PONV is such that large numbers of patients would prefer being in pain than being nauseated.[136] Furthermore, retching and vomiting will induce severe pain from the stress it places on the wound. Opioids cause PONV due to their effects on the chemoreceptor trigger zone (CTZ) in the area postrema of the brainstem, as well as from direct effects on the GI tract.[137] Also movement effects (such as the transport of the patient from the operating room to the PACU) will contribute to PONV from effects via the vestibular system. Opioids cause an increased sensitivity of the vestibular system. The CTZ contains opioid, serotonin ($5HT_3$), histamine, dopamine (D_2), and muscarinic acetylcholine receptors.[137] The CTZ, vagal nerve, and vestibular organs project to the vomiting center in the medulla. Drugs used in the treatment of PONV include dopamine antagonists (e.g., droperidol), 5HT-antagonists (e.g., ondansetron) and steroids.[135,137] A better approach than treatment is the use of an adequate prevention strategy in patients with a known history of PONV or patients that will undergo surgeries with a known high incidence of PONV. This prevention approach includes the use of propofol rather than inhalation anesthetics, the use of epidural postoperative analgesia rather than iv opioids, and multimodal pharmacologic therapy, including a 5HT-antagonist, a dopamine antagonist, and a steroid (e.g., iv ondansetron 4 mg, droperidol 0.625 mg, and dexamethasone 4 mg) given prior to the end of surgery.

Smooth Muscle Effects

Opioid receptors are present in the enteric plexus within the smooth muscle layers of the GI tract. Opioids inhibit intestinal and pancreatic secretion, increase bowel tone, and decrease intestinal propulsive activity.[138] Consequently opioids cause delayed gastric emptying, constipation, bowel distension, and paralytic ileus. Although opioids affect GI motility from central sites as well, blockade of opioid receptors with opioid antagonists that do not cross the blood–brain barrier (such as methylnaltrexone) will have a favorable effect on GI motility.[139]

Due to spasms of the sphincter of Oddi and common bile duct, opioids may cause acute upper abdominal pain and colic-like complaints.[140] Opioids may also contribute to misinterpretation of perioperative cholangiograms. Naloxone or glucagon can be used for treatment as both cause relaxation of the sphincter muscle.

Activated opioid receptors present in the wall of the bladder and ureters can cause acute urine retention.[141] It is most often seen after epidural or spinal opioid administration with a higher incidence in men than women. Urine retention is related to the inability of the urethral sphincter muscle to relax while the bladder tone increases. Opioid-induced bladder dysfunction can be treated with naloxone or the peripherally acting methylnaltrexone.[142]

Skeletal Muscle Effects

Strong, high-dose opioids, especially when given rapidly, cause skeletal muscle rigidity, which includes thoracic, abdominal, and pharyngeal muscles.[143] Weak opioids may give rise to an increase in muscle tension in neck and thorax (some patients have the feeling that "an elephant sits on their chest" following 10 mg morphine iv). While the effect of weak opioids seems to wear off fairly rapidly (within 10 to 20 minutes), the effect of strong opioids requires muscle relaxation and intubation as ventilation may become compromised.

Histamine Release

High-dose morphine, codeine, and meperidine cause histamine release from mast cells, an effect that is non-opioid receptor related (naloxone does not prevent this effect).[144] This effect is not seen with piperidines (fentanyl and congeners). The consequence of histamine release is itching and redness of the skin and hives along the trajectory of the venous injection. Histamine may also cause a reduction in vascular resistance and systemic and pulmonary pressures.

Pruritus (Itch)

Animal research has shown the existence of itch-specific pathways that involve itch-specific (i.e., histamine-sensitive) neurons in the spinal cord dorsal horn that travel to the thalamus via the spinothalamic tract.[145] These neurons and pathways are distinct from pain-related neurons and pathways.[146] Painful stimuli such as scratching can abolish histamine-induced itch. Opioids commonly cause an itch typically of the nose, after systemic administration. After spinal opioid injections itching is very common and occurs in 60% to 90% of the patients. Opioid-induced itch serves possibly as a warning signal for the presence of exogenous μ-opioids (which are normally not present in the body). Not all opioids cause itching. For example, κ-opioids (e.g., pentazocine) are antipruritic. Treatment of opioid-induced itch is difficult and many treatments have been tried including MOR antagonists (e.g., naloxone, naltrexone, nalbuphine), histamine H_1 receptor antagonists, 5HT-antagonists (e.g., ondansetron), NSAIDs, prednisone, and a sub-hypnotic low-dose infusion of propofol.[147]

Pupil Effects

Opioids produce pupillary miosis.[148] Of all opioid effects, miosis occurs most rapidly and at lower doses than analgesia or respiratory depression (the fentanyl C_{50} for miosis is about half of that for analgesia).[88] The mechanism of pupil constriction is activation of MORs in the nucleus of Edinger–Westphal, which projects to the muscles of the iris via the oculomotor nerve.[149] Since the iris contains MORs a direct effect of opioids on the pupil diameter is possible.

Diffuse CNS Effects

There are a variety of CNS effects induced by opioids that can cause considerable discomfort to the patients, yet cannot be localized to a specific area of the CNS. These effects can occur after acute opioid treatment but are commonly seen in chronic pain patients on prolonged opioid treatment. These effects include dizziness, light headedness, sedation and drowsiness, euphoria, dysphoria, drug "high," cognitive dysfunction (e.g., memory loss), inability to concentrate or focus attention, hallucinations, and so on.[150] Some of these effects, such as dizziness, limit the use of opioids in the chronic pain setting, especially in elderly patients.[151]

Cardiovascular Effects

Opioids affect the cardiovascular system at central and peripheral sites.[152] Central effects include the activation of vagal nuclei and depression of vasomotor centers in the brainstem. Peripheral effects occur predominantly at high (supraclinical) doses and include direct myocardial depression and arterial and venous dilatation. Morphine may cause additional cardiovascular effects via the release of histamine (see above). The consequences are mild at clinical doses and include orthostatic hypotension, mild bradycardia, and a moderate reduction of systemic and pulmonary resistance. However, even at clinical doses, opioids can induce hemodynamic instability when combined with other drugs such as inhalation anesthetics, propofol, or benzodiazepines, and in severely ill patients (e.g., with sepsis). Treatment of hemodynamic instability includes the administration of atropine and vasopressors and moderate fluid therapy.

REMIFENTANIL FOR OBSTETRIC LABOR PAIN

The popularity of remifentanil PCA for treatment of obstetric labor pain has increased over the last years. The primary indication for this treatment modality is the presence of a condition which contraindicates epidural analgesia, or the unavailability of personnel to place an epidural. One approach is to use remifentanil at bolus doses of 30 μg with a 3-minute lockout period. In case of side effects (respiratory depression, nausea) the bolus dose may be reduced to 20 μg, while in case of insufficient pain relief the bolus dose may be increased to 40 μg. An infusion scheme of 40 μg bolus doses at 3-minute intervals results in plasma concentrations between 2 and 4 ng/mL, sufficient to relieve the pain of the uterine contraction. Clinical studies indicate that pain scores are not greatly reduced when compared to epidural analgesia but patient satisfaction is high.[153,154] Pain relief with epidural analgesia remains superior to PCA remifentanil or intramuscular meperidine.[153–155] Safety remains an important issue.[156] While in most studies oxygen saturation values do not seem to drop below 94% there are little data on the occurrence of short-term hypoxic and apneic events in the time following a contraction.[153] With appropriate monitoring from personnel present in the room with the patient, PCA remifentanil is a safe labor analgesic modality but it remains a secondary alternative to epidural analgesia.

GENDER DIFFERENCES

The first indications of the existence of important gender differences in opioid efficacy came from animal work. The resultant human literature is large with often conflicting results. A recent systematic review, however, gives valuable insights into the existence of gender differences in opioid efficacy in humans.[157] The largest evidence comes from morphine PCA studies following major abdominal or orthopedic surgery. Women have a greater analgesic effect from PCA than men and consequently consume less opioids postoperatively. With longer durations of PCA (>24 hours), the difference in effect between the sexes further increases. Interestingly, in the first minutes postoperatively, greater *morphine* opioid efficacy is observed in men, an effect that is reversed after 30 to 90 minutes. These data are best explained by a difference in morphine potency with greater potency in women, coupled to a slower onset/offset of the drug in women (i.e., greater value for $t½k_{e0}$ in women). The slower onset/offset times may be related to a slower passage across the blood–brain barrier, or differences in receptor distribution and kinetics in men and women.[91,158] As a consequence morphine will take longer to induce adequate analgesia in women, while a speedier effect is observed in men.[91] Due to the lower potency in men, they require multiple additional morphine administrations while women require fewer additional doses. The gender difference remains in older patients (>65 years), although in both sexes the opioid *requirements* for adequate analgesia are significantly reduced with age due to both PK and PD factors.[85] Similar to analgesia, there are gender-related differences in opioid-induced respiratory depression and nausea and vomiting, with greater effects observed in women compared to men.[159,160,161]

References

1. Dunn KM, Saunders KW, Rutter CM, et al. Opioid prescriptions for chronic pain and overdose: A cohort study. *Ann Int Med.* 2010;152:85.
2. Vila H Jr, Smith RA, Augustyniak MJ, et al. The efficacy of pain management before and after implementation of hospital-wide pain management standards: Is patient safety compromised by treatment solely based on numerical pain ratings? *Anesth Analg.* 2005;101:474.
3. Okie S. A flood of opioids, a rising tide of deaths. *N Engl J Med.* 2010;363:1981.
4. Sertürner F. Uber das Morphium, eine neue salzfähige Grundlage, und die Mekonsäure, als Hauptbestandtheile des Opiums. *Ann Physik.* 1917;5:56.
5. Huxtable RJ, Schwartz SK. The isolation of morphine. *Mol Interv.* 2001;1:189.
6. Bovill JG. Opium: A drug ancient and modern. In: Dahan A, van Kleef JW eds. *Advances in Anesthesia and Analgesia.* Leiden: University Medical Center; 2007; 1:13.
7. Garfield E. The 1982 John Scott Award goes to Jack Fishman and Harold Blumberg for synthesis and investigation of naloxone. *Essays Inform Sci.* 1983;6:121.
8. Tzschentke TM, Jahnel U, Kögel B, et al. Tapentadol hydrochloride: A next-generation, centrally acting analgesic with two mechanisms of action in a single molecule. *Drugs Today.* 2009;45:483.
9. Hatrick CT, Rozek RJ. Tapentadol in pain management: A μ-opioid receptor agonist and noradrenaline reuptake inhibitor. *CNS Drugs.* 2011;25:359.
10. Kieffer BL, Gavériaux-Ruff C. Exploring the opioid system by gene knockout. *Prog Neurobiol.* 2002;66:285.
11. Chiou LC, Liao YY, Fan PC, et al. Nociceptin/orphanin FQ peptide receptors: Implications' for pain and analgesia. *Curr Drug Targets.* 2007;8:117.
12. Pasternak GW. Pharmacological mechanisms of opioid analgesics. *Clin Neuropharmacol.* 1993;16:1.
13. Stefano GB. The μ_3 opiate receptor subtype. *Pain Forum.* 1999;8:206–209.
14. Alexander SPH, Mathie A, Peters JA. Guide to receptors and channels (GRAC), 4th Edn. *Br J Pharmacol.* 2009;158(suppl 1):S1.
15. Standifer KM, Pasternak GW. G proteins and opioid receptor-mediated signaling. *Cell Signal.* 1997;9:237.
16. Sacerdote P. Opioids and the immune system. *Pall Med.* 2006;20:s9–s16.
17. Glattard E, Muller A, Aunis D, et al. Rethinking the opiate system? Morphine and morphine 6 glucuronide as new endocrine and neuroendocrine mediators. *Med Sci Monit.* 2006;12:SR25.
18. Waldhoer M, Bartlett SE, Whistler JL. Opioid receptors. *Ann Rev Biochem.* 2004;73:953.
19. Chen YL, Law PY, Loh HH. The other side of the opioid story: Modulation of cell growth and survival signaling. *Curr Med Chem.* 2008;15:772.
20. Eguchi M. Recent advances in selective opioid receptor agonists and antagonists. *Med Res Rev.* 2004;24:182.
21. Bovill JG. Surgery for cancer: Does anesthesia matter? *Anesth Analg.* 2010;110:1524.
22. Matthes HWD, Maldonado R, Simonin F, et al. Loss of morphine-induced analgesia, reward effect and withdrawal symptoms in mice lacking the μ-opioid receptor gene. *Science.* 1996;383:819.
23. Kitchen I, Slowe SJ, Matthes HW, et al. Quantitative autoradiographic mapping of mu-, delta- and kappa-opioid receptors in knockout mice lacking the mu-opioid receptor gene. *Brain Res.* 1997;778:73.
24. Dahan A, Sarton E, Teppema L, et al. Anesthetic potency and influence of morphine and sevoflurane on respiration in μ-opioid receptor knockout mice. *Anesthesiology.* 2001;94:824.
25. Romberg R, Sarton E, Teppema L, et al. No difference between morphine and morphine-6-glucuronide on respiration in μ-opioid receptor deficient mice. *Br J Anaesth.* 2003;91:862.
26. Lutfy K, Eitan S, Bruyant CD, et al. Buprenorphine-induced antinociception is mediated by mu-opioid receptors and compromised by concomitant activation of opioid receptor-like receptors. *J Neurosci.* 2003;23:10331.
27. Dahan A, Yassen A, Romberg R, et al. Buprenorphine induces ceiling in respiratory depression but not in analgesia. *Br J Anaesth.* 2006;96:627.
28. Callahan RJ, Au JD, Paul M, Liu C, et al. Functional inhibition by methadone of N-methyl-D-aspartate receptors expressed in Xenopus oocytes: Stereospecific and subunit effects. *Anesth Analg.* 2004;98:653.
29. Dykstra LA, Fischer FB, Balter RE, et al. Opioid antinociception, tolerance and dependence: Interactions with the N-methyl-D-aspartate system in mice. *Behav Pharmacol.* 2011;22:540.
30. Kissin I, Bright CA, Bradley L. The effect of ketamine on opioid-induced acute tolerance: Can it explain reduction of opioid consumption with ketamine-opioid analgesic combinations? *Anesth Analg.* 2000;91:148.
31. Reeves RR, Burke RS. Tramadol: Basic pharmacology and emerging concepts. *Drugs Today.* 2008;44:827.
32. Sarton E, Teppema L, Olievier C, et al. Involvement of μ-opioid receptor in ketamine-induced respiratory depression and antinociception. *Anesth Analg.* 2001;93:1495.
33. Millan MJ. Descending control of pain. *Prog Neurobiol.* 2002;66:355f.
34. Ossipov MH, Dussor GO, Porreca F. Central modulation of pain. *J Clin Invest.* 2010;120:3779.
35. Brown EN, Purdon PL, Van Dort CJ. General anesthesia and altered states of arousal: A systems neuroscience analysis. *Ann Rev Neurosci.* 2011;34:601.
36. Fields HL. Pain modulation: Expectation, opioid analgesia and virtual pain. *Prog Pain Res.* 2000;122:245.
37. Butler RK, Finn DP. Stress-induced analgesia. *Prog Neurobiol.* 2009;88:184.
38. Eipert F, Bingel U, Schoell ED, et al. Activation of opioidergic descending pain control system underlies placebo analgesia. *Neuron.* 2009;63:533.
39. Pud D, Granovsky Y, Yarnitsky D. The methodology of experimentally-induced diffuse noxious inhibitory (DNIC)-line effects in humans. *Pain.* 2009;144:16.
40. Beecher HK. Pain in men wounded in battle. *Ann Surg.* 1946;123:96.
41. Zubieta J-K, Bueller JA, Jackson LR, et al. Placebo effects mediated by endogenous opioid activity on μ-opioid receptors. *J Neurosci.* 2005;25:7754.
42. Wager TD, Rilling JK, Smith EE, et al. Placebo-induced changes in FMRI in the anticipation and experience of pain. *Science.* 2004;303:1162.
43. Petrovic P, Kalso E, Petersson KM et al. Placebo and opioid analgesia – imaging a shared neuronal network. *Science.* 2002;295:1737.
44. Moont R, Pud D, Sprecher E, et al. "Pain inhibits pain" mechanisms: Is pain modulation simply due to distraction. *Pain.* 2010;150:113.

45. Niesters M, Dahan A, Swartjes M, et al. Effect of ketamine on endogenous pain modulation in healthy volunteers. *Pain.* 2010;152:656.
46. Scholz J, Woolf CJ. The neuropathic pain triad, neurons, immune cells and glia. *Nature Neurosci.* 2007;10:1361.
47. Kapitzke D, Vetter I, Cabot PJ. Endogenous opioid analgesia in peripheral tissues and the implications for pain control. *Ther Clin Risk Manag.* 2005;1:279.
48. Stein S, Halina M. Modulation of peripheral sensory information by the immune system: Implication for pain therapy. *Pharmacol Rev.* 2011;63:860.
49. Busch-Dienstfertig M, Stein C. Opioid receptors and opioid peptide-producing leucocytes in inflammatory pain – basic and therapeutic aspects. *Brain Beh Immun.* 2010;24:683.
50. Bekhit MH. Opioid-induced hyperalgesia and tolerance. *Am J Therapeut.* 2010;17:498.
51. Bruno G, Bossard AE, Coste C, et al. Acute opioid tolerance: Intraoperative remifentanil increases postoperative pain and morphine requirement. *Anesthesiology.* 2000;93:409.
52. Joly V, Richebe P, Guignard B, et al. Remifentanil-induced postoperative hyperalgesia and its prevention with small-dose ketamine. *Anesthesiology.* 2005;103:147.
53. van Dorp ELA, Kest B, Kowalczyk WJ, et al. Morphine-6-glucuronide rapidly increases pain sensitivity independently of opioid receptors in mice and humans. *Anesthesiology.* 2009;110:1356.
54. Juni A, Cai M, Stamkova M, et al. Sex-specific mediation of opioid-induced hyperalgesia by the melanocortin-1 receptor. *Anesthesiology.* 2010;112:181.
55. Waxman AR, Arout C, Caldwell M, et al. Acute and chronic fentanyl administration causes hyperalgesia independently of opioid receptor activity in mice. *Neurosci Lett.* 2009;468:68.
56. Bohn LM, Lefkowitz RJ, Gainetdinov RR, et al. Enhanced morphine analgesia in mice lacking beta-arrestin 2. *Science.* 1999;286:2495.
57. Zuo Z. The role of opioid receptor internalization and beta-arrestins in the development of opioid tolerance. *Anesth Analg.* 2005;101:728.
58. Narinder P. Opioids in acute pain. In: Stein C, ed. *Opioids in Pain Control, Basic and Clinical Aspects.* Cambridge, UK: Cambridge University Press; 1999:247.
59. Franson HE. Postoperative patient-controlled analgesia in the pediatric population: A literature review. *AANA J.* 2010;78:374.
60. Hughes MA, Glass PSA, Jacobs JR. Context-sensitive half-time in multicompartment: Pharmacokinetic models for intravenous anesthetic drugs. *Anesthesiology.* 1992;76:334.
61. Kapila A, Glass PSA, Jacobes JR, et al. Measured context-sensitive half-times of remifentanil and alfentanil. *Anesthesiology.* 1995;83:968.
62. Olofsen E, Boom M, Nieuwenhuijs D, et al. Modeling the non-steady-state respiratory effects of remifentanil in awake and propofol sedated healthy volunteers. *Anesthesiology.* 2010;212:1382.
63. Wilkinson GR. Drug metabolism and variability among patients in drug response. *N Engl J Med.* 2005;352:2211.
64. Smith HS. The metabolism of opioid agents and the clinical impact of their active metabolites. *Clin J Pain.* 2011;27:824.
65. Christrup LL. Morphine metabolites. *Acta Anaesthesiol Scand.* 1997;41:116.
66. van Dorp E, Romberg R, Sarton E, et al. Morphine-6-glucuronide: Morphine's successor for postoperative pain relief? *Anesth Analg.* 2006;102:1.
67. Romberg R, Olofsen E, Sarton E, et al. Pharmacokinetic/pharmacodynamic modeling of morphine-6-glucuronide-induced analgesia in healthy volunteers: Absence of sex differences. *Anesthesiology.* 2004;100:120.
68. Zelcer N, van de Wetering K, Hillebrand M, et al. Mice lacking multidrug resistance protein 3 show altered morphine pharmacokinetics and decreased antinociception by morphine-6-glucuronide. *Proc Natl Acad Sci USA.* 2005;102:7274.
69. Lötsch J, Zimmermann M, Darimont J, et al. Does the A118G polymorphism at the μ-opioid receptor gene protect against morphine-6-glucuronide toxicity? *Anesthesiology.* 2002;97:814.
70. Tateishi T, Krivoruk Y, Ueng YF, et al. Identification of liver cytochrome P-450 3 A as the enzyme responsible for fentanyl and sufentanil *N*-dealkylation. *Anesth Analg.* 1996;82:167.
71. Klees TM, Sheffels P, Dale O, et al. Metabolism of alfentanil by cytochrome P4503 A (CYP3 A) enzymes. *Drug Metab Dispos.* 2005;33:303.
72. Klees TM, Sheffels P, Thummel KE, et al. Pharmacogenetic determinants of human liver microsomal alfentanil metabolism and the role of cytochrome P450 3A5. *Anesthesiology.* 2005;102:550.
73. Scott LJ, Perry CM. Spotlight on remifentanil for general anesthesia. *CNS Drugs.* 2005;19:1069.
74. Minto CF, Schnider TW, Shafer SL. Pharmacokinetics and pharmacodynamics of remifentanil. II. Model application. *Anesthesiology.* 1997;86:24.
75. Minto CF, Schnider TW, Egan TD, et al. Influence of age and gender on the pharmacokinetics and pharmacodynamics of remifentanil. I. Model development. *Anesthesiology.* 1997;86:10.
76. Egan TD, Minto CF, Hermann DJ, et al. Remifentanil versus alfentanil: Comparative pharmacokinetics and pharmacodynamics in healthy adult male volunteers. *Anesthesiology.* 1996;84:821.
77. Totah RA, Sheffels P, Whittington D, et al. Role of CYP2B6 in stereoselective human methadone metabolism. *Anesthesiology.* 2008;108:363.
78. Kharasch E. Intraoperative methadone: Rediscovery, reappraisal and reinvigoration. *Anesth Analg.* 2011;112:13.
79. van Dorp E, Yassen A, Dahan A. Naloxone treatment in opioid addiction: The risks and benefits. *Exp Opin Drug Safe.* 2007;6:125.
80. Martini C, Olofsen E, Yassen A, et al. Pharmacokinetic-pharmacodynamic modeling in acute and chronic pain: An overview of the recent literature. *Exp Rev Pharmacother.* 2011;4:719.
81. Segre G. Kinetics of interaction between drugs and biological systems. *Farmaco Sci.* 1968;23:907.
82. Hull CJ. Pharmacokinetics and pharmacodynamic. *Br J Anaesth.* 1979;51:579.
83. Sheiner L, Stanski LB, Vozeh S, et al. Simultaneous modeling of pharmacokinetics and pharmacodynamics: Application to d-tubocurarine. *Clin Pharmacol Ther.* 1979;25:358.
84. Dahan A, Romberg R, Teppema L, et al. Simultaneous measurement and integrated analysis of analgesia and respiration after an intravenous morphine infusion. *Anesthesiology.* 2004;101:1201.
85. Aubrun F, Salvi N, Coriat P, et al. Sex- and age-related differences in morphine requirements for postoperative pain relief. *Anesthesiology.* 2005;103:156.
86. Scott JC, Cooke JE, Stanski DR. Electroencephalographic quantitation of opioid effect: Comparative pharmacodynamics of fentanyl and sufentanil. *Anesthesiology.* 1991;74:34.
87. Scott JC, Ponganis KV, Stanski DR. EEG quantitation of narcotic effect: The comparative pharmacodynamics of fentanyl and alfentanil. *Anesthesiology.* 1985;62:234.
88. Dahan A, Boom M, Olofsen E. Differences in onset/offset times for different end-points: Pain relief, pupil size and respiratory depression. *Anesthesiology.* 2011;A1569.
89. Olofsen E, Romberg R, Bijl H, et al. Alfentanil and placebo analgesia: Absence of sex differences. *Anesthesiology.* 2005;103:130.
90. Aubrun F, Langeron O, Quesnel C, et al. Relationships between measurement of pain using visual analog score and morphine requirements during postoperative intravenous morphine titration. *Anesthesiology.* 2003;98:1415.
91. Sarton E, Olofsen E, Romberg R, et al. Sex differences in morphine analgesia: An experimental study in healthy volunteers. *Anesthesiology.* 2000;93:1245.
92. Abou Hammoud H, Simon N, Urien S, et al. Intravenous morphine titration in immediate postoperative pain management: Population kinetic-pharmacodynamic and logistic regression analysis. *Pain.* 2009;144:139.
93. Mazoit JX, Btscher K, Samii K. Morphine in postoperative patients: Pharmacokinetics and pharmacodynamics of metabolites. *Anesth Analg.* 2007;105:70.
94. Tallarida RJ, Stone DJ, McCary JD, et al. Response surface analysis of synergism between morphine and clonidine. *J Phramacol Exp Ther.* 1999;289:8.
95. Schulte H, Sollevi A, Sgerdahl M. The synergistic effect of combined treatment with systematic ketamine and morphine on experimentally induced wind-up pain in humans. *Anesth Analg.* 2004;98:1574.
96. Daniel M, Weiskopf RB, Noorani M, et al. Fentanyl augments the blockade of the sympathetic response to incision (MAC-BAR) produced by desflurane and isoflurane. *Anesthesiology.* 1998;88:43.
97. Kazama T, Ikeda K, Morita K. The pharmacodynamic interaction between propofol and fentanyl with respect to suppression of somatic or hemodynamic responses to skin incision, peritoneum incision, and abdominal wall retraction. *Anesthesiology.* 1998;89:894.
98. Sebel PS, Glass PSA, Fletcher JE, et al. Reduction of the MAC of desflurane with fentanyl. *Anesthesiology.* 1992;88:43.
99. Katoh T, Ikeda K. The effects of fentanyl on sevoflurane requirements for loss of consciousness and skin incision. *Anesthesiology.* 1998;88:18.
100. Nelson L, Schwaner R. Transdermal fentanyl: Pharmacology and toxicology. *J Med Toxicol.* 2009;5:230.
101. Anonymous. Fentanyl patches: Preventable overdose. *Prescrire Int.* 2010;19:22.
102. Biedrzycki OJ, Bevan D, Lucas S. Fatal overdose due to prescription fentanyl patches in a patient with sickle cell/beta-thalassemia and acute chest syndrome: A case report and review of the literature. *Am J Forensic Med.* 2009;30:188.
103. Babenco HD, Conard PF, Gross JB. The pharmacodynamic effect of a remifentanil bolus on ventilatory control. *Anesthesiology.* 2000;92:393.
104. Drover D, Lemmens HJM. Population pharmacodynamics and pharmacokinetics of remifentanil as a supplement to nitrous oxide anesthesia for elective abdominal surgery. *Anesthesiology.* 1998;89:869.
105. Mertens M, Olofsen E, Engbers F, et al. Propofol reduces perioperative remifentanil requirements in a synergistic manner. Response surface modeling of perioperative remifentanil–propofol interactions. *Anesthesiology.* 2003;99:347.
106. Lang E, Kapila A, Schlugman D, et al. Reduction of isoflurane minimal alveolar concentration by remifentanil. *Anesthesiology.* 1996;85:721.
107. Klepstad P, Fladvad T, Skorpen F, et al. Influence from genetic variability on opioid use for cancer pain: A European genetic association study of 2294 pain patients. *Pain.* 2011;152:1139.
108. Mogil J, Ritchie J, Smith SB, et al. Melanocortin-1 receptor gene variants affect pain and mu-opioid analgesia in mice and humans. *J Med Genet.* 2005;42:583.
109. Liem EB, Lin CM, Suleman MI, et al. Anesthetic requirement is increased in redheads. *Anesthesiology.* 2004;101:279.
110. Weinshiliboum R. Inheritance and drug response. *N Engl J Med.* 2003;348:529.
111. Ciszkowski C, Madadi P, Phillips MS, et al. Codeine, ultrarapid-metabolism genotype, and postoperative death. *N Engl J Med.* 2009;361:827.
112. Gasche Y, Daali Y, Fahti M, et al. Codeine intoxication with ultrarapid CYP2D6 metabolism. *N Engl J Med.* 2004;351:2827.
113. Koren G, Cairns J, Gaedigk A, et al. Pharmacogenetics of morphine poisoning in a breastfed neonate of a codeine-prescribed mother. *Lancet.* 2006;368:704.

114. Park HJ, Shinn HK, Ryu SH, et al. Genetic polymorphism in the ABCB1 gene and the effects of fentanyl in Koreans. *Clin Pharmacol Ther.* 2007;81:539.
115. Dahan A, Aarts L, Smith TW. Incidence, reversal and prevention of opioid-induced respiratory depression. *Anesthesiology.* 2010;112:226.
116. Hanna MH, Elliott KM, Fung, M. Randomized, double-blind study of the analgesic efficacy of morphine-6-glucuronide *versus* morphine sulfate for postoperative pain in major surgery. *Anesthesiology.* 2005;102:815.
117. Chung F, Yegneswaran B, Liao P, et al. Stop questionnaire: A tool to screen for obstructive apnea. *Anesthesiology.* 2008;108:812.
118. Overdyk FJ, Hillman DR. Opioid modeling of central respiratory drive must take upper airway obstruction into account. *Anesthesiology.* 2011;114:219.
119. Bernards CM, Knowlton SL, Schmidt DF, et al. Respiratory and sleep effects of remifentanil in volunteers with moderate obstructive sleep apnea. *Anesthesiology.* 2009;110:41.
120. Wu A, Drummonmg GB. Sleep arousal after lower abdominal surgery and relation to recovery from respiratory obstruction. *Anesthesiology.* 2003;99:1295.
121. Dahan A. Influence of anesthesia and analgesia on the control of breathing. *Br J Anaesth.* 2003;91:40.
122. Chung F. http://anesthesiaandsleep.org/wp-content/uploads/2011/11/2011-Program-and-Speaker-Abstracts.pdf
123. Stone JG, Cozine KA, Wald A. Nocturnal oxygenation during patient-controlled analgesia. *Anesth Analg.* 1999;89:104.
124. Fu ES, Downs JB, Schweiger JW, et al. Supplemental oxygen impairs detection of hypoventilation by pulse oximetry. *Chest.* 2004;126:1552.
125. Lötsch J, Dudziak R, Freynhagen R, et al. Fatal respiratory depression after multiple intravenous morphine injections. *Clin Pharmacokinet.* 2006;45:1051.
126. Pattinson KTS. Opioids and the control of breathing. *Br J Anaesth.* 2008;106:347.
127. Smith JC, Ellenberger HH, Ballanyi K, et al. PreBötzinger complex: A brainstem region that may generate respiratory rhythm in humans. *Science.* 1991;254:726.
128. Cullberg M, Eriksson YGF, Wåhlander K, et al. Pharmacokinetics of ximelagatran and relationship to clinical response in acute deep vein thrombosis. *Clin Pharmacol Ther.* 2005;77:279.
129. Yassen A, Olofsen E, Dahan A, et al. Pharmacokinetic-pharmacodynamic modeling of the efficacy and safety of buprenorphine in rats. *Pharm Res.* 2008;25:183.
130. Olofsen E, van Dorp E, Teppema L, et al. Naloxone reversal of morphine and morphine-6-glucuronide-induced respiratory depression in healthy volunteers. *Anesthesiology.* 2010;112:1417.
131. van Dorp E, Yassen A, Sarton E, et al. Naloxone-reversal of buprenorphine-induced respiratory depression. *Anesthesiology.* 2006;105:51.
132. Amin HM, Sopchak AM, Esposito BF, et al. Naloxone-induced and spontaneous reversal of depressed ventilatory response to hypoxia during and after continuous infusion of remifentanil or alfentanil. *J Pharmacol Ther.* 1995;274:34.
133. Curry JP, Lynn LA. Threshold monitoring, alarm fatigue, and the patterns of unexpected hospital death. *APSF Newsletter.* 2011;26(Fall issue):32 (http://www.apsf.org/newsletters/html/2011/fall/07_threshold.htm).
134. Smith I, Mackay J, Fahrid N. Respiratory rate measurement: A comparison of methods. *Br J Healthcare Assistants* 2011;5:18.
135. Apfel CC, Korttila K, Abdalla M, et al. A factorial trial of six interventions for the prevention of postoperative nausea and vomiting. *N Engl J Med.* 2004;350:2441.
136. Macario A, Weinger N, Truong P, et al. Which clinical anesthesia outcomes are both common and important to avoid? *Anesth Analg.* 1999;88:1085.
137. Gan TJ. Mechanisms underlying postoperative nausea and vomiting and neurotransmitter receptor antagonist-based pharmacotherapy. *CNS Drugs.* 2007;21:813.
138. Panchal SJ, Müller-Schwefe P, Wurzelmann JI. Opioid-induced bowel dysfunction: Prevalence, pathophysiology and burden. *Int J Clin Pract.* 2007;61:1181.
139. Thomas J. Opioid-induced bowel dysfunction. *J Pain Symptom Manage.* 2008; 35:103.
140. Thompson DR. Narcotic analgesic effects on the sphincter of Oddi: A review of the data and therapeutic implications in treating pancreatitis. *Am J Gastroenterol* 2001;96:1266.
141. Verhamme KM, Sturkenboom MC, Stricker BH, et al. Drug-induced urinary retention: Incidence, management and prevention. *Drug Saf.* 2008;31:373.
142. Rosow CE, Gomery P, Chen TY, et al. Reversal of opioid-induced bladder dysfunction by intravenous naloxone and methylnaltrexone. *Clin Pharmacol Ther.* 2007;82:48.
143. Bennet JA, Abrams JT, Van Riper DF, et al. Difficult or impossible ventilation after sufentanil-induced anesthesia is caused primarily by vocal cord closure. *Anesthesiology.* 1997;87:1070.
144. Blunk JA, Schmelz M, Zeck S, et al. Opioid-induced mast cell activation and vascular responses is not mediated by mu-opioid receptors: An in vivo microdialysis study in human skin. *Anesth Analg.* 2004;98:364.
145. Schmelz M. A neural pathway for itch. *Nat Neurosci.* 2001;4:9.
146. Miayamoto T, Patapoutian A. Why does morphine make you itch? *Cell.* 2011; 147;261.
147. Ganesh A, Maxwell LG. Pathophysiology and management of opioid-induced pruritus. *Drugs.* 2007;67:2323.
148. Kharasch ED, Francis A, London A, et al. Sensitivity of intravenous and oral alfentanil and pupillary miosis as minimal and noninvasive probes for hepatic and first-pass CYP3 A induction. *Clin Phramacol Ther.* 2011;90:100.
149. Larson MD, Berry PD. Supraspinal papillary effects of intravenous and epidural fentanyl during isoflurane anesthesia. *Reg Anesth pain Med.* 2000;25:60.
150. Benyamin R, Trescott AM, Datta S, et al. Opioid complications and side effects. *Pain Physician.* 2008;11:S105.
151. Papaleontiou M, Henderson CR, Turner BJ, et al. Outcomes associated with opioid use in the treatment of chronic noncancer pain in older adults: A systematic review and meta-analysis. *J Am Geriatr Soc.* 2010;58:1353.
152. DeSouza G, Lewis MC, TerRiet MF. Severe bradycardia after remifentanil. *Anesthesiology.* 1997;87:1019.
153. Douma M, Middeldorp A, Dahan A, et al. A comparison of remifentanil patient-controlled analgesia with epidural analgesia during labour. *Int J Obstet Anesth.* 2011;20:118.
154. Volmanen PVE, Akural EI, Raudaskoski T, et al. Timing of intravenous patient-controlled remifentanil bolus during early labor. *Acta Anaesthesiol Scand.* 2011; 55:486.
155. Leong WL, Sng BL, Sia AT. A comparison between remifentanil and meperidine for labor analgesia; a systematic review. *Anesth Analg.* 2011;113:818.
156. Buehner U, Broadbent JR, Chesterfield B. Remifentanil patient-controlled analgesia for labour: A complete audit cycle. *Anaesth Intensive Care.* 2011;39:666.
157. Niesters M, Dahan A, Kest B, et al. Do sex differences exist in opioid analgesia? A systematic review and meta-analysis of human experimental and clinical studies. *Pain.* 2010;151:61.
158. Zubieta JK, Dannals RF, Frost JJ. Gender and age influences on human brain mu-opioid receptor binding measured by PET. *Am J Psychiatry.* 1999;156:842.
159. Dahan A, Sarton E, Olievier C. Sex-related differences in the influence of morphine on ventilatory control in humans. *Anesthesiology.* 1998;88:903.
160. Zun LS, Downey LV, Grossman W, et al. Gender differences in narcotic-induced emesis in the ED. *Am J Emerg Med.* 2002;20:151.
161. Cepeda MS, Farra JY, Baumgarten M, et al. Side effects of opioids during short-term administration: Effects of age, gender and race. *Clin Pharmacol Ther.* 2003; 74:102.

CHAPTER

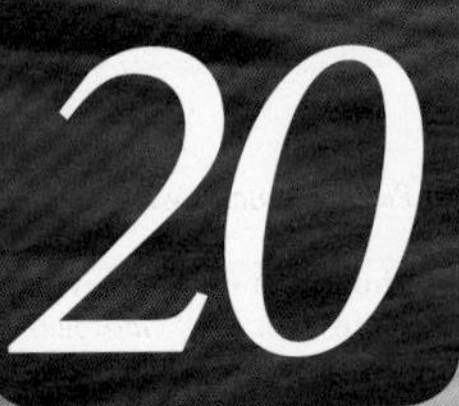

Neuromuscular Blocking Agents

FRANÇOIS DONATI

Key Points

1. Neuromuscular blocking agents are used to improve conditions for tracheal intubation, to provide immobility during surgery, and to facilitate mechanical ventilation.
2. Anticholinesterases inhibit breakdown of acetylcholine and help restore neuromuscular function after any nondepolarizing blocking agent, but their effect is limited so that their use does not rule out residual paralysis, defined as a train-of-four (TOF) ratio <0.9.
3. The main site of action of neuromuscular blocking agents (muscle relaxants) is on the nicotinic cholinergic receptor at the endplate of muscle. They also have effects at presynaptic receptors located on the nerve terminal.
4. The only depolarizing agent still in use is succinylcholine. All other drugs available are nondepolarizing. They compete with acetylcholine for the same binding sites.
5. Succinylcholine is a blocking agent that produces depolarization at the endplate and binds to extrajunctional receptors. In spite of many side effects, such as hyperkalemia, its rapid offset makes it the drug of choice for rapid sequence induction.
6. Fade in response to high frequency stimulation (e.g., TOF, 2 Hz for 2 seconds) is a characteristic of nondepolarizing blockade. The TOF fade is difficult to evaluate manually or visually during recovery when TOF ratio is >0.4.
7. When using mivacurium, reversal with anticholinesterases should be attempted only when all four twitches in response to TOF stimulation are visible at the adductor pollicis.
8. The upper airway is particularly sensitive to the effects of nondepolarizing blockade. Residual paralysis should be assumed to be present if TOF ratio at the adductor pollicis is <0.9.
9. Neuromuscular transmission can be restored by injection of sugammadex, an agent that binds specifically in a 1:1 molar ratio to rocuronium and vecuronium.
10. Sugammadex, if given in an appropriate dose, is effective at any depth of blockade.

Multimedia

1 Neuromuscular Blocking Agents

2 Fasciculations

3 Monitoring Nerve Block

It appears paradoxical that drugs having peripheral effects on neuromuscular transmission might have a role in anesthesia. If the patient is anesthetized, why provide agents to prevent movement? Yet, the introduction of muscle relaxants, more appropriately called *neuromuscular blocking agents,* into clinical practice in 1942 was an important milestone in the history of anesthesia.[1] While the usefulness of the new drugs became apparent, there were doubts regarding patient safety. In 1954, Beecher and Todd[2] claimed that anesthetic mortality increased sixfold when muscle relaxants were used. This situation was probably because of the suboptimal use of mechanical ventilation and reversal drugs, but other controversies have arisen in recent years for a variety
1 of reasons. Neuromuscular blocking agents are used to improve conditions for tracheal intubation, to provide immobility during surgery, and to facilitate mechanical ventilation.

For example, the incidence of awareness appears to be greater when neuromuscular blocking agents are used,[3] and some authors recommend restricting the use of these drugs whenever possible, as patient movement might be an indicator of consciousness. However, anesthetics act at the spinal cord level to produce immobility; thus, movement in response to a noxious stimulus indicates inadequate analgesia and does not necessarily mean that the patient is conscious.[4] Therefore, awareness does not occur because too much neuromuscular blocking agent has been given, but because too little anesthetic is administered. The controversy regarding neuromuscular blocking agents and awareness is complicated by the fact that neuromuscular blockade seems to affect the bispectral index (BIS), which is the most widely used measure of unconsciousness.[5] Reductions in BIS have been reported in awake individuals receiving succinylcholine and in mildly sedated patients given mivacurium.

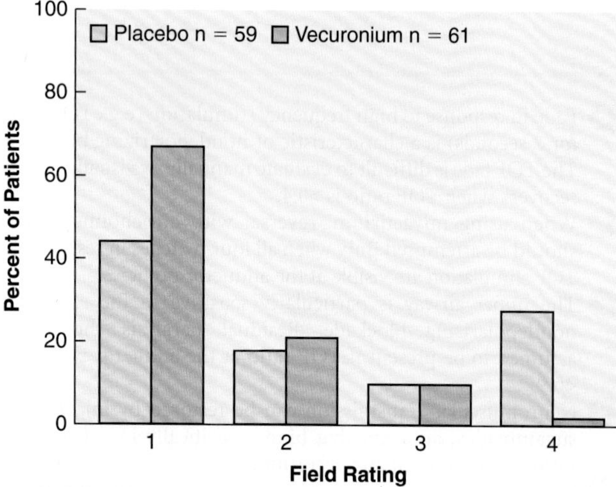

FIGURE 20-1. Surgeon's assessment of muscle relaxation during lower abdominal surgery. Rating goes from 1 (excellent) to 4 (poor). The incidence of poor rating was greater in patients not given vecuronium (29%) compared with those who received the drug (2%). (Redrawn from: King M, Sujirattanawimol N, Danielson DR, et al. Requirements for muscle relaxants during radical retropubic prostatectomy. *Anesthesiology.* 2000;93:1392.)

Complete paralysis is not required for the duration of all surgical procedures. However, neuromuscular blocking agents were found to make a difference in lower abdominal surgery, where surgical conditions were better in patients receiving vecuronium (Fig. 20-1).[6] In addition to providing immobility and better surgical conditions, neuromuscular blocking agents improve intubating conditions. The doses of opioids required for acceptable intubating conditions in the absence of muscle paralysis produce significant hypotension (Fig. 20-2).[7] Providing optimal intubating conditions is not a trivial objective. Poor intubating conditions may increase the incidence of laryngeal injury, as manifested by voice hoarseness and vocal cord damage (Fig. 20-3), and the best way to improve intubating conditions is to administer neuromuscular blocking agents.[10]

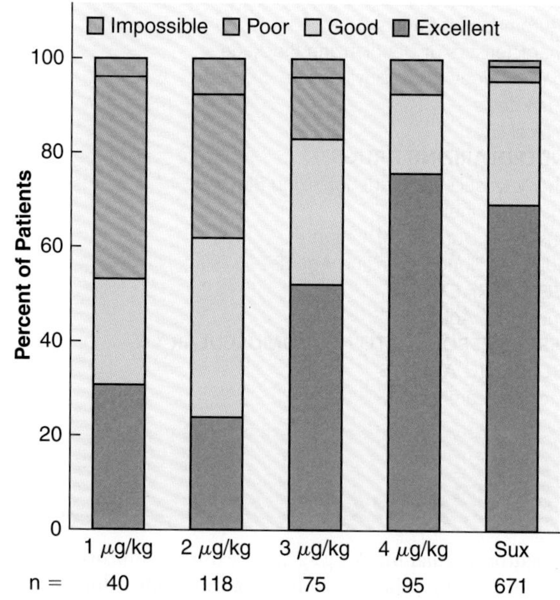

FIGURE 20-2. Neuromuscular blocking agents provide better intubating conditions than high doses of opioids, without hypotension. Hypnotic agent was propofol or thiopental. Intubating conditions are plotted against dose of remifentanil (in micrograms per kilogram). Results for succinylcholine (Sux), 1 mg/kg (with little opioid) are given for comparison. Hypotension was seen with remifentanil, 4 μg/kg. (Data obtained from references: McNeil IA, Culbert B, Russell I. Comparison of intubating conditions following propofol and succinylcholine with propofol and remifentanil 2 micrograms kg^{-1} or 4 micrograms kg^{-1}. *Br J Anaesth.* 2000;85:623–625; Naguib M, Samarkandi AH, El-Din ME, et al. The dose of succinylcholine required for excellent endotracheal intubating conditions. *Anesth Analg.* 2006;102:151–155; Andrews JI, Kumar N, van den Brom RH, et al. A large simple randomized trial of rocuronium versus succinylcholine in rapid-sequence induction of anaesthesia along with propofol. *Acta Anaesthesiol Scand.* 1999;43:4–8 ; Durmus M, Ender G, Kadir BA, et al. Remifentanil with thiopental for tracheal intubation without muscle relaxants. *Anesth Analg.* 2003;96:1336; Klemola UM, Mennander S, Saarnivaara L. Tracheal intubation without the use of muscle relaxants: Remifentanil or alfentanil in combination with propofol. *Acta Anaesthesiol Scand.* 2000;44:465; and Donati F. The right dose of succinylcholine. *Anesthesiology.* 2003;99:1037)

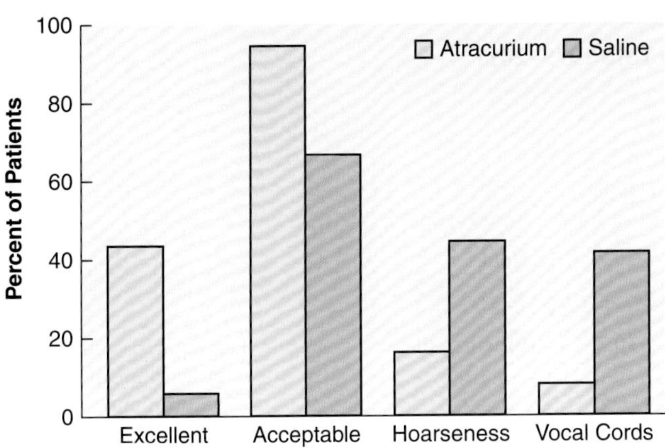

FIGURE 20-3. Neuromuscular blocking agents improve intubating conditions and reduce vocal cord sequelae. The graph depicts the incidence of excellent and acceptable (defined as good or excellent) intubating conditions after atracurium or saline. The percentage of patients who reported hoarseness and those with vocal cord lesions documented by stroboscopy is also shown. (Data from: Mencke T, Echternach M, Kleinschmidt S, et al. Laryngeal morbidity and quality of tracheal intubation: A randomized controlled trial. *Anesthesiology.* 2003;98:1049–1056.)

The effects of neuromuscular blocking drugs must have worn off or be reversed before the patient regains consciousness. Even with the introduction of shorter-acting neuromuscular blocking agents, reversal of blockade is required in most cases. However, residual paralysis is still a problem, more than 30 years after it was first described (Table 20-1), and in spite of the availability of shorter-acting neuromuscular blocking drugs and widespread use of neuromuscular monitoring.[21] Part of this might be related to the recognition that the threshold for complete neuromuscular recovery is a train-of-four (TOF) ratio of 0.9, instead of the tradi-
2 tional 0.7 (Fig. 20-4).[22] Sugammadex, a selective binding agent for

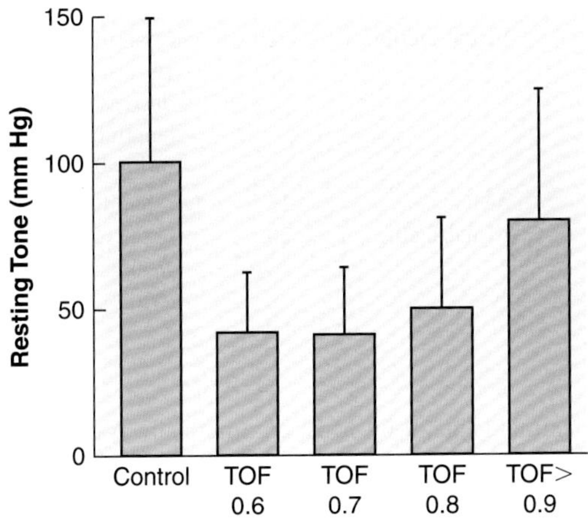

FIGURE 20-4. Upper esophageal resting tone in volunteers given vecuronium. Train-of-four (TOF) ratio was measured at the adductor pollicis muscle. Statistically significant decreases compared with control were found at all levels of paralysis until TOF ratio >0.9. (Redrawn from: Eriksson LI, Sundman E, Olsson R, et al. Functional assessment of the pharynx at rest and during swallowing in partially paralyzed humans: Simultaneous videomanometry and mechanomyography of awake human volunteers. *Anesthesiology.* 1997;87:1035.)

the neuromuscular blocking agents rocuronium and vecuronium, was created to address this problem. Thus, an understanding of the pharmacology of neuromuscular blocking agents and reversal drugs is essential.

PHYSIOLOGY AND PHARMACOLOGY

Structure

The cell bodies of motor neurons supplying skeletal muscle lie in the spinal cord. They receive and integrate information from the central nervous system. This information is carried via an elongated structure, the axon, to distant parts of the body. Each nerve cell supplies many muscle cells (or fibers) a short distance after branching into nerve terminals. The terminal portion of the axon is a specialized structure, the synapse, designed for the production and release of acetylcholine. The synapse is separated from the endplate of the muscle fiber by a narrow gap, called the *synaptic cleft,* which is approximately 50 nm in width (0.05 μm) (Fig. 20-5).[23–25] The nerve terminal is surrounded by a Schwann cell, and the synaptic cleft has a basement membrane and contains filaments that anchor the nerve terminal to the muscle.

The main site of action of neuromuscular blocking agents (muscle relaxants) is on the nicotinic cholinergic receptor at the
3 endplate of the muscle. They also have effects at presynaptic receptors located on the nerve terminal. The endplate is a specialized portion of the membrane of the muscle fiber where nicotinic acetylcholine receptors are concentrated. During development, multiple connections are made between nerve terminals and a single muscle fiber. However, as maturation continues, most of these connections atrophy and disappear, usually leaving only one connection per muscle fiber. This endplate continues to differentiate from the rest of the muscle fiber. The nerve terminal enlarges, and folds appear. The acetylcholine receptors cluster at the endplate, especially at the crests of the folds, and their density decreases to almost zero in extrajunctional areas.[23,25] Initially, the receptor density is of the order of 1,000/μm^2 of membrane surface. After maturation of the endplate, junctional receptor density increases to 10,000/μm^2 or more. Mammalian endplates usually have an oval shape with the short axis perpendicular to the fiber; their surface area is approximately 1,000 μm^2. The width of the endplate is sometimes as large as the diameter of the fiber, but is usually smaller. However, its length is only a small fraction of that of the fiber.

Nerve Stimulation

Under resting conditions, the electrical potential of the inside of a nerve cell is negative with respect to the outside (typically –90 mV). If this potential is made less negative (depolarization), sodium channels open and allow sodium ions to enter the cell. This influx of positive ions makes the potential inside the membrane positive with respect to the outside. This potential change, in turn, causes depolarization of the next segment of membrane, causing more sodium channels to open, and an electrical impulse, or action potential, propagates. The duration of the action potential is brief (<1 ms) because of rapid inactivation of sodium channels and activation of potassium channels. An action potential also triggers the opening of calcium channels, allowing calcium ions to penetrate the cell. This entry of calcium facilitates release of the neurotransmitter at the nerve terminal.

The sodium channels in the axon may be activated in response to electrical depolarization provided by a nerve stimulator. A

TABLE 20-1. SELECTED REPORTS OF RESIDUAL PARALYSIS 1979–2011

Study	Long-duration Drugs Used	Intermediate-duration Drugs Used	Reversal	TOF Threshold	Monitoring	Residual Paralysis (% of Patients)	Comments
Viby-Mogensen et al.,[11] 1979	*d*-tubocurarine Pancuronium Gallamine	—	Yes	0.7	None	42	—
Bevan et al.,[12] 1988	Pancuronium		Yes	0.7	Visual/tactile	36	Less paralysis with atracurium and vecuronium
		Atracurium	Yes	0.7		4	
		Vecuronium	Yes	0.7		9	
Fawcett et al.,[13] 1995		Atracurium/ vecuronium			Visual/tactile		More paralysis with infusions
		bolus	Yes	0.7		12	
		infusion	Yes	0.7		24	
Berg et al., 1997[14]	Pancuronium		Yes	0.7	Visual/tactile	26	More atelectasis when residual paralysis present
		Atracurium/ vecuronium	Yes	0.7		5	
Debaene et al.,[15] 2003		Atracurium/ Vecuronium rocuronium	No	0.7	None	16	Paralysis could be present even 4 h after injection
				0.9		45	
Murphy et al.,[16] 2003	Pancuronium		No	0.8	Optional	82	After cardiac surgery when ready to wean from ventilatory support
		Rocuronium	No	0.8		0	
Murphy et al.,[12] 2004	Pancuronium		Yes	0.7	Visual/tactile	47	More hypoxia and discharge delayed with pancuronium
				0.9		97	
		Rocuronium	Yes	0.7		7	
				0.9		33	
Baillard et al.,[17] 2005		Atracurium/ vecuronium/ rocuronium	No (94%)	0.9	None (98%)	63	Less paralysis when reversal and monitoring used
		Atracurium/ vecuronium/ rocuronium	No (58%)	0.9	None (40%)	3	
Murphy et al.,[18] 2008		Rocuronium	Yes	0.9	AMG	5	Less paralysis and fewer respiratory symptoms when AMG used
					Visual/tactile	30	
Butterly et al.,[19] 2010		Vecuronium/ cisatracurium	Yes	0.9	Visual/tactile	22	Less paralysis with cisatracurium; decreased PACU length of stay if TOF ratio >0.9
Murphy et al.,[20] 2011		Rocuronium	Yes	0.9	AMG	15	Less paralysis and fewer symptoms of weakness when AMG used
				0.9	Visual/tactile	50	

AMG, acceleromyography; TOF, train-of-four; PACU, postanesthesia care unit.

peripheral nerve is made up of a large number of axons, each of which responds in an all-or-none fashion to the stimulus applied. Thus, in the absence of neuromuscular blocking agents, the relationship between the amplitude of the muscle contraction and current applied is sigmoid. At low currents, the depolarization is insufficient in all axons. As current increases, more and more axons are depolarized to threshold and the strength of the muscle contraction increases. When the stimulating current reaches a certain level, all axons are depolarized to threshold and propagate an action potential. Increasing current beyond this point does not increase the amplitude of muscle contraction: The stimulation is supramaximal (Fig. 20-6). Most commercially available stimulators deliver impulses lasting 0.1 to 0.2 ms.

Release of Acetylcholine

Acetylcholine is synthesized from choline and acetate and packaged into 45 nm vesicles. Each vesicle contains 5,000 to 10,000 acetylcholine molecules. Some of these vesicles cluster near the cell membrane opposite the crests of the junctional folds of the endplate, in areas called *active zones* (Fig. 20-5).[23,24]

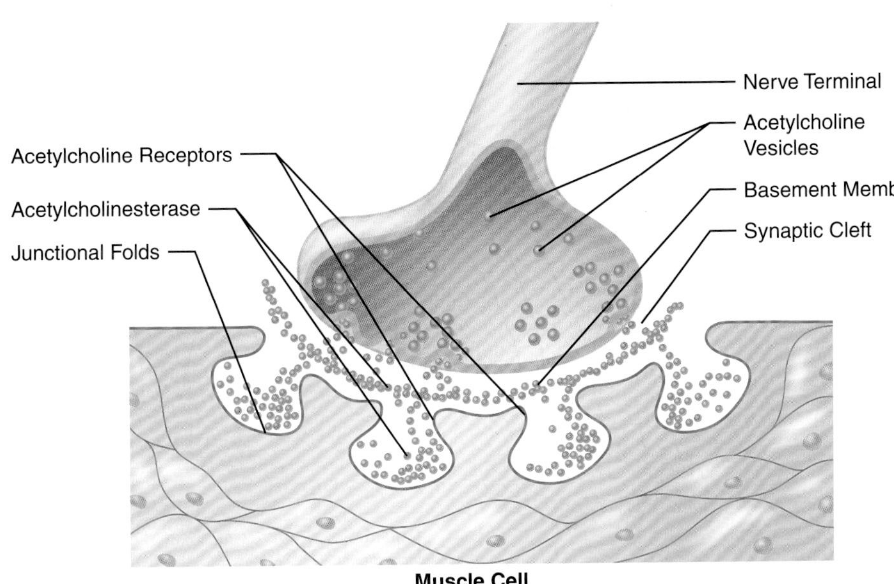

FIGURE 20-5. Schematic representation of the neuromuscular junction (not drawn to scale).

It is now widely accepted that acetylcholine is released in packets, or quanta, and that a quantum represents the contents of one vesicle. In the absence of nerve stimulation, quanta are released spontaneously, at random, and this is seen as small depolarizations of the endplate (miniature endplate potential). When an action potential invades the nerve terminal, approximately 200 to 400 quanta are released simultaneously, unloading approximately 1 to 4 million acetylcholine molecules into the synaptic cleft.[23,25] Calcium, which enters the nerve terminal through channels that open in response to depolarization, is required for vesicle fusion and release. Calcium channels are located near docking proteins, and this special geometric arrangement provides high intracellular concentrations of calcium to allow binding of specialized proteins on the vesicle membrane with docking proteins.[23,24] Binding produces fusion of the membranes and release of acetylcholine ensues. When the calcium concentration is decreased, or if the action of calcium is antagonized by magnesium, the release process is inhibited and transmission failure may occur. Other proteins regulate storage and mobilization of acetylcholine vesicles. It appears that a small proportion of vesicles is immediately releasable, while a much larger reserve pool can be mobilized more slowly. Each impulse releases 0.2% to 0.5% of the 75,000 to 100,000 vesicles in the nerve terminal. With repetitive stimulation, the amount of acetylcholine released decreases rapidly because only a small fraction of the vesicles is in a position to be released immediately. To sustain release during high-frequency stimulation, vesicles must be mobilized from the reserve pool.

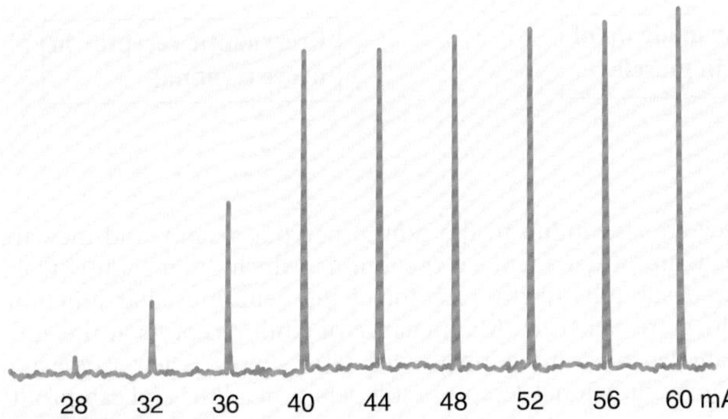

FIGURE 20-6. Example of increasing stimulating current in one patient. Current pulses, 0.2 ms duration, were delivered to the ulnar nerve at the wrist every 10 seconds. The force of contraction of the adductor pollicis muscle was measured and appears as spikes. No twitch was seen if the current was <28 mA. At current strengths of ≥40 mA, the current became supramaximal; increasing the current produced little change in force.

Postsynaptic Events

The receptors at the endplate are of the nicotinic cholinergic type. They are members of the class of Cys-loop ligand-gated ion channels, to which glycine, 5-HT_3, and GABA receptors belong.[26] These receptors are made up of five glycoprotein subunits arranged in the form of a rosette and lying across the whole cell membrane (Fig. 20-7). To date, 17 subtypes of the nicotinic receptor have been identified, and they differ by the type and arrangement of the subunits.[23] The nicotinic subtype present at the neuromuscular junction is made up of two identical subunits, designated α, and three others, called β, δ, and ε. There are two acetylcholine binding sites, each located on the outside part of the α subunit. When two acetylcholine molecules bind simultaneously to each binding site, an opening is created in the center of the rosette, allowing sodium ions to enter the cell and potassium ions to exit.[23,24] The inward movement of sodium is predominant because it is attracted by the negative voltage of the inside of the cell. This movement of sodium depolarizes the endplate; that is, its inside becomes less negative. There is a high density of sodium channels in the folds of synaptic clefts and in the perijunctional area.[24,25] These channels open when the membrane is depolarized beyond a critical point, allowing more sodium to enter the cell and producing further depolarization. This depolarization generates an action potential, which propagates by activation of sodium channels along the whole length of the muscle fiber. The muscle action potential has a duration of 5 to 15 ms and can be recorded as an electromyogram (EMG). It precedes the onset of contraction, or twitch, which lasts 100 to 200 ms. With high frequency (>10 Hz) stimulation, the muscle fiber does not have time

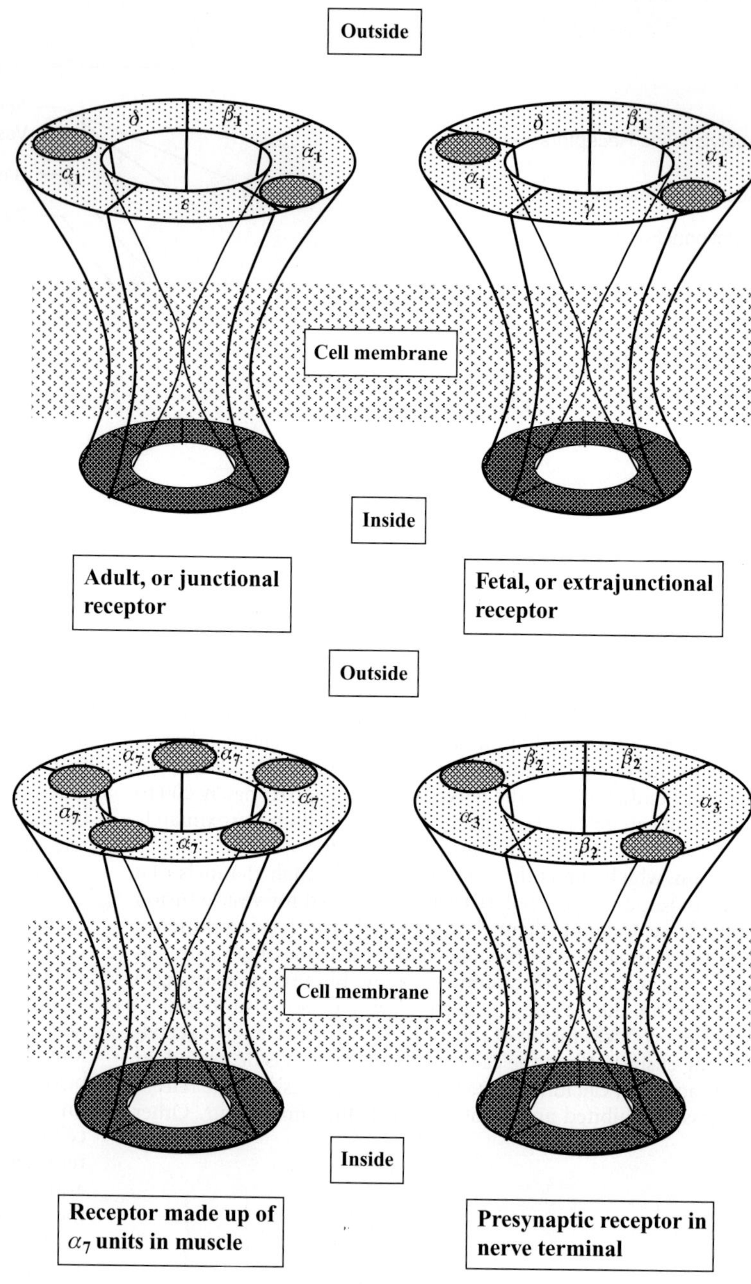

FIGURE 20-7. Four types of nicotinic receptors involved in neuromuscular transmission. All have five subunits. Postsynaptic adult receptors at the endplate have two α_1, one β_1, one δ, and one ε subunit. The immature, fetal or extrajunctional receptor has the same structure, except for a substitution of the ε by the γ subunits. It is distributed throughout the muscle membrane. Receptors made up of only α_7 subunits are also found in muscle. Presynaptic receptors, found in the nerve terminal are thought to be of the $\alpha_3\beta_2$ type. The acetylcholine binding sites are represented by a shaded oval area.

to relax before the next impulse, so contractions fuse and add up, and a tetanus is obtained.

Early in development, receptors are slightly different from those found at the adult endplate: They have a γ subunit instead of an ε subunit (Fig. 20-7), and they tend to be evenly distributed along the whole length of the muscle fiber.[23–25] The receptors with a γ subunit, are called *fetal* receptors. When the endplate develops, receptors tend to cluster at the neuromuscular junction and the density is low (typically 10/μm^2) in the extrajunctional areas.[25] As maturation continues, the γ subunit is substituted by an ε subunit, which is characteristic of the *adult* type, junctional receptor. In humans, the switch occurs in the third trimester of pregnancy. During development, neuronal $\alpha7$ receptors are also found in the muscle membrane. They are called neuronal because they are also found in the central nervous system, and they are made up of five identical α subunits, which differ slightly from the α subunits of the receptor at the neuromuscular junction, which are called $\alpha1$. Maintenance of adult receptors at the endplate depends on the integrity of nerve supply. A few γ-type and $\alpha7$ extrajunctional receptors still persist in adults and can proliferate in cases of denervation.[23]

The main action of nondepolarizing neuromuscular blocking drugs is to bind to at least one of the two α subunits of the postsynaptic receptor. This prevents access to the receptor by acetylcholine and does not produce opening of the receptor. Under normal circumstances, only a small fraction of available receptors must bind to acetylcholine to produce sufficient depolarization to trigger a muscle contraction. In other words, there is a wide

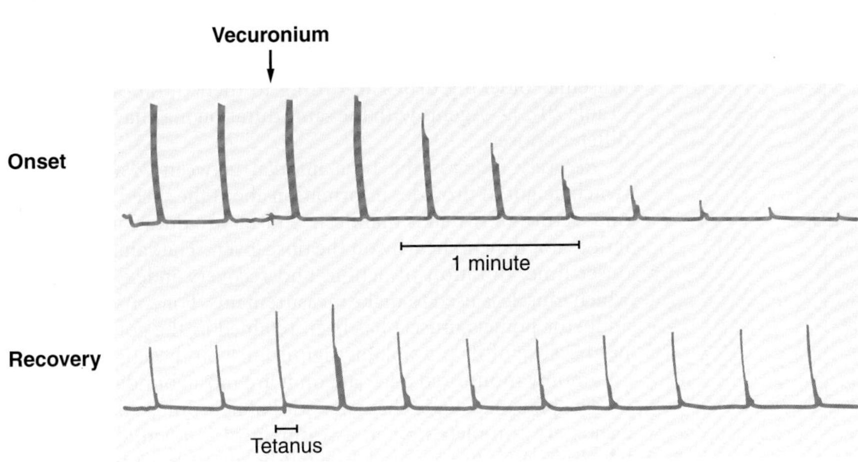

FIGURE 20-8. Characteristics of nondepolarizing blockade. Train-of-four (TOF) responses are equal before administration of vecuronium (*arrow*). For a given twitch depression, fade is less during onset (*top trace*) than recovery (*bottom trace*). A 50 Hz tetanus was applied during recovery, and the response is not sustained (tetanic fade). The TOF response immediately after the tetanus is enhanced, and progressively returns to its normal value within 1 to 2 minutes.

"margin of safety".[27] This redundancy implies that neuromuscular blocking drugs must be bound to a large number of receptors before any blockade is detectable. Animal studies suggest that 75% of receptors must be occupied before twitch height decreases in the presence of *d*-tubocurarine, and blockade is complete when 92% of receptors are occupied. The actual number depends on species and type of muscle, and humans might have a reduced margin of safety compared with other species.[27] So it is futile to correlate receptor occupancy data obtained in cats with certain clinical tests in humans, such as handgrip and head lift, which involve different muscle groups. However, the general concept that a large proportion of receptors must be occupied before blockade becomes detectable, and that measurable blockade occurs over a narrow range of receptor occupancy, remains applicable to clinical practice. Because it must overcome the margin of safety, the initial dose of neuromuscular blocking agent is greater than maintenance doses.

Acetylcholine is hydrolyzed rapidly by the enzyme acetyl cholinesterase, which is present in the folds of the endplate. It is also attached to stalks attached to the basement membrane in the synaptic cleft. The presence of the enzyme in the synaptic cleft suggests that not all the acetylcholine released reaches the endplate; some is hydrolyzed en route.[25,28]

Presynaptic Events

The release of acetylcholine normally decreases during high frequency stimulation because the pool of readily releasable acetylcholine becomes depleted faster than it can be replenished. Under normal circumstances, the reduced amount released is well above what is required to produce muscle contraction because of the high margin of safety at the neuromuscular junction. In addition, a positive feedback system involving activation of presynaptic receptors helps in the mobilization of acetylcholine vesicles.[23] There is some evidence that the presynaptic and postsynaptic receptors are of different subtypes, and that presynaptic receptors are most likely of the $\alpha_3\beta_2$ subtype, that is, they are made up of only α and β subunits.[29] This receptor contains α subunits that are slightly different from those found in postsynaptic receptors, thus the designation as α_3, instead of the α_1, and the β subunits (β_2) are also slightly different from the β_1 subunit found in postsynaptic receptors.

The putative role of the presynaptic receptors is to maintain the number of vesicles ready to be released. Nondepolarizing neuromuscular blocking drugs produce characteristic TOF and tetanic fade, probably by blocking presynaptic nicotinic receptors,[23,29] thus preventing mobilization of acetylcholine vesicles and leading to reduced acetylcholine release during high frequency stimulation. Succinylcholine has virtually no effect on these presynaptic receptors, which would explain the lack of fade observed with this drug. Presynaptic receptors may not be the only elements contributing to the fade phenomenon: They do not explain why fade is more prominent during onset than during recovery (Fig. 20-8), and why after sugammadex, TOF ratio is restored faster than first twitch.[30] Fade constitutes a key property of nondepolarizing neuromuscular blocking drugs and is useful for monitoring purposes.

NEUROMUSCULAR BLOCKING AGENTS

Neuromuscular blocking drugs interact with the acetylcholine receptor either by depolarizing the endplate (depolarizing agents) or by competing with acetylcholine for binding sites (nondepolarizing agents). The only depolarizing agent still in use is succinylcholine. All others are of the nondepolarizing type. 4

Pharmacologic Characteristics of Neuromuscular Blocking Agents

The effect of neuromuscular blocking drugs is measured as the depression of adductor muscle contraction (twitch) following electrical stimulation of the ulnar nerve. The value is compared with a control value, obtained before injection of the drug. Each drug has characteristic onset, potency, duration of action, and recovery index.

Potency of a drug is determined by constructing dose-response curves, which describe the relationship between twitch depression and dose (Fig. 20-9).[31] Then, the effective dose 50, or ED_{50}, which is the median dose corresponding to 50% twitch depression, is obtained. Because clinically useful relaxation is attained when twitch is abolished almost completely, the ED_{95}, corresponding to 95% block, is more commonly used. For example, the ED_{95} for vecuronium is 0.05 mg/kg, which means that half the patients will achieve at least 95% block of single twitch (compared with the pre-vecuronium value) with that dose, and half the subjects will reach <95% block. Rocuronium has an ED_{95} of 0.3 mg/kg. Therefore, it has one-sixth the potency of vecuronium. In other words, compared with vecuronium, six times as much rocuronium has to be given to produce the same effect. The ED_{95}

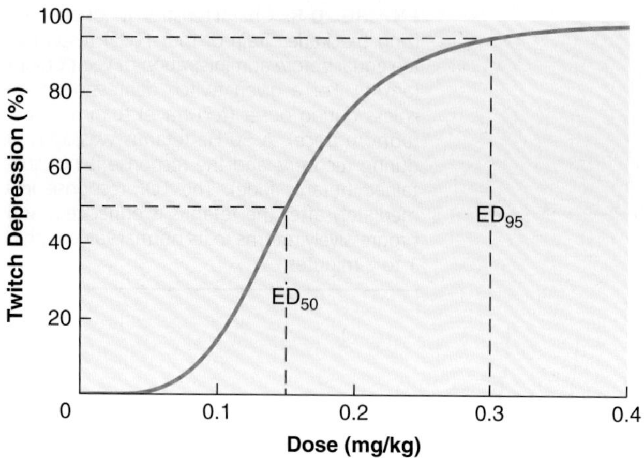

FIGURE 20-9. Example of a dose-response relationship. The actual numbers are approximately those for rocuronium. The ED_{50} is the dose corresponding to 50% blockade and ED_{95} is the dose corresponding to 95% blockade.

of known neuromuscular blocking agents vary over two orders of magnitude (Table 20-2).

Onset time, or time to maximum blockade, can be shortened if the dose is increased. When two or more drugs are compared, it is meaningful to compare only equipotent doses and usually clinically relevant doses ($2 \times ED_{95}$) are considered.[31]

Duration of action is the time from injection of the neuromuscular blocking agent to return of 25% twitch height (compared with control). Duration increases with dose, so it is usual to make comparisons between $2 \times ED_{95}$ doses, which are normal intubation doses. The 25% twitch height figure was chosen because rapid reversal can normally be achieved at that level. For nondepolarizing agents, the fourth twitch usually reappears when first twitch is close to 25%. Categories were proposed for neuromuscular blocking drugs according to their duration of action (Table 20-2).[31] Agents with the same duration may have markedly different onsets.

Recovery index is the time interval between 25% and 75% twitch height. It provides information about the speed of recovery once return of twitch is manifest. Contrary to duration of action, it does not depend heavily on the dose given. The values for ED_{95}, onset time, duration of action, and recovery index depend on which muscle is used to make measurements. For consistency, the adductor pollicis muscle has been retained as the gold standard, not because of its physiologic significance but because it is most commonly monitored and data on it are most abundant.

The pharmacologic characteristics of neuromuscular blocking agents are completed by an assessment of *intubating conditions,* which do not always parallel twitch height at the adductor pollicis muscle. Intubating conditions depend on paralysis of centrally located muscles, but also on the type and quantity of opioid and hypnotic drugs given for induction of anesthesia. To decrease variability between studies, criteria to grade intubating conditions as excellent, good, poor, or impossible in a scoring system were adopted by a group of experts who met in Copenhagen in 1994, and a revision of these standards was adopted at a later meeting in Stockholm in 2005.[32]

DEPOLARIZING DRUGS: SUCCINYLCHOLINE

Among drugs that depolarize the endplate, only succinylcholine
5 is still used clinically. In spite of a long list of undesired effects, succinylcholine remains popular because it is the only ultrarapid onset/ultrashort duration neuromuscular blocking drug currently available.

TABLE 20-2. POTENCY, ONSET TIME, DURATION, AND RECOVERY INDEX OF SELECTED NEUROMUSCULAR BLOCKING AGENTS

Agent	ED_{95} (mg/kg)	Onset Time (min)	Duration to 25% Recovery (min)	Recovery Index (25–75% recovery) (min)
Ultrashort-duration Agents				
Succinylcholine	0.3	1–1.5	6–8	2–4
Gantacurium[a]	0.19	1.7	6–8	2.5
Short-duration Agents				
Mivacurium[b]	0.08	3–4	15–20	7–10
Intermediate-duration Agents				
Atracurium	0.2–0.25	3–4	35–45	10–15
Cisatracurium	0.05	5–7	35–45	12–15
Rocuronium	0.3	1.5–3	30–40	8–12
Vecuronium	0.05	3–4	35–45	10–15
Long-duration Agents				
Doxacurium	0.025	5–10	40–120	30–40
d-tubocurarine[b]	0.5	2–4	60–120	30–45
Pancuronium	0.07	2–4	60–120	30–40

Typical values for the average young adult patient. Onset and duration data depend on dose. The values presented are the best estimates available for twice the ED_{95} and are measured at the adductor pollicis. Actual values may vary markedly from one individual to the next, and may be affected by age, other medications, and/or disease states. The categories under which the drugs are classified are somewhat arbitrary.

[a]Being investigated at the time of writing.

[b]No longer used or very limited use in North America.

Neuromuscular Effects

The effects of succinylcholine at the neuromuscular junction are not completely understood. The drug depolarizes postsynaptic and extrajunctional receptors. However, when the receptor is in contact with any agonist, including acetylcholine, for longer than a few milliseconds it ceases to respond to the agonist. Normally, this desensitization process does not occur with acetylcholine because of its rapid breakdown (<1 ms). However, succinylcholine remains at the endplate for much longer, so desensitization develops after a brief period of activation.[33] Another possible mechanism is the inactivation of sodium channels in the junctional and perijunctional areas, which occurs when the membrane remains depolarized.[33] This inactivation prevents the propagation of the action potential. Both desensitization of the receptor and inactivation of sodium channels might be present together.

1 Within 1 minute after succinylcholine injection and before paralysis is manifest, disorganized movements, or *fasciculations*,
2 are frequently observed. This activity probably reflects the agonist effect of succinylcholine, before desensitization takes place. Small doses of nondepolarizing drugs are effective in reducing the incidence of fasciculations.[34]

Succinylcholine has yet another neuromuscular effect. In some muscles, like the masseter and to a lesser extent the adductor pollicis, a sustained increase in tension that may last for several minutes can be observed. The mechanism of action of this tension change is uncertain but is most likely mediated by acetylcholine receptors because it is blocked by large amounts of nondepolarizing drugs.[35] The increase in masseteric tone, which is probably always present to some degree but is greater in some susceptible individuals, may lead to imperfect intubating conditions in a small proportion of patients. Masseter muscle spasm may be an exaggerated form of this response.

Characteristics of Depolarizing Blockade

After injection of succinylcholine, single-twitch height is decreased. However, the response to high frequency stimulation is sustained: Minimal TOF and tetanic fade is observed. The block is antagonized by nondepolarizing agents so that the ED_{95} is doubled if a small "defasciculating" dose of nondepolarizing drug is given prior to the intubating dose of succinylcholine, thus requiring an increased dose of succinylcholine.[36] Succinylcholine blockade is potentiated by inhibitors of acetyl cholinesterase, such as neostigmine and edrophonium. After administration of 7 to 10 mg/kg, or 30 to 60 minutes of exposure to succinylcholine, TOF and tetanic fade become apparent. Neostigmine or edrophonium can antagonize this block, which has been termed *nondepolarizing, dual,* or *phase II* block. The onset of phase II block coincides with tachyphylaxis, as more succinylcholine is required for the same effect.

Pharmacology of Succinylcholine

Succinylcholine is rapidly hydrolyzed by plasma cholinesterase (also called *pseudocholinesterase*), with an elimination half-life of <1 minute in patients.[37] Because of the rapid disappearance of succinylcholine from plasma, the maximum effect is reached quickly. Sub-paralyzing doses (up to 0.3 to 0.5 mg/kg) reach their maximal effect within approximately 1.5 to 2 minutes at the adductor pollicis muscle,[36] and within 1 minute at more central muscles, such as the masseter, the diaphragm, and the laryngeal muscles. With larger doses (1 to 2 mg/kg), abolition of twitch response can be reached even more rapidly (<1 minute).

The mean dose producing 95% blockade (ED_{95}) at the adductor pollicis muscle is 0.30 to 0.50 mg/kg.[36] These values are doubled if *d*-tubocurarine, 0.05 mg/kg, is given as a defasciculating agent.[36] The time until full recovery at the adductor pollicis is dose-dependent and reaches 10 to 12 minutes after a dose of 1 mg/kg (Fig. 20-10).[38] The diaphragm starts contracting and spontaneous breathing resumes after approximately 5 minutes.[39]

Side Effects

Cardiovascular

Sinus bradycardia with nodal or ventricular escape beats (or both) may occur, especially in children, and asystole has been described after a second dose of succinylcholine in both pediatric and adult patients. These effects can be attenuated with atropine or glycopyrrolate.[40] The mechanisms for the cardiovascular side effects of succinylcholine are not known because succinylcholine appears to have little effect on autonomic cholinergic receptors.[33] Succinylcholine increases catecholamine release, and tachycardia is seen frequently.

Anaphylaxis

Succinylcholine has been incriminated as the trigger of allergic reactions more often than any other drug used in anesthesia. Successive studies conducted in France indicate that the number of reported events is decreasing, corresponding to the gradual

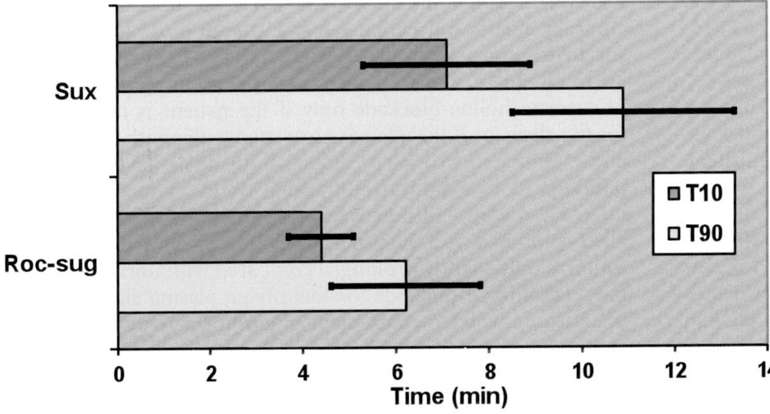

FIGURE 20-10. Duration of action of neuromuscular blockade with succinylcholine 1 mg/kg (Sux), and rocuronium 1.2 mg/kg followed 3 minutes later by sugammadex 16 mg/kg (Roc-sug). T10 and T90: Duration to 10% and 90% first twitch recovery, respectively. Bars indicate standard deviation. Data from: Lee C, Jahr JS, Candiotti KA, et al. Reversal of profound neuromuscular block by sugammadex administered three minutes after rocuronium. *Anesthesiology*. 2009;110:1020–1025.

replacement of succinylcholine by nondepolarizing drugs.[41] The incidence of anaphylactic reactions to succinylcholine is difficult to establish, but is probably of the order of 1:5,000 to 1:10,000.

Fasciculations

The prevalence of fasciculations is high (60% to 90%) after the rapid injection of succinylcholine, especially in muscular adults. This is a benign side effect of the drug, but many clinicians prefer to prevent fasciculations with a small dose of a nondepolarizing neuromuscular blocking drug is given 3 to 5 minutes before succinylcholine is effective.[34] When the drug was available, *d*-tubocurarine 0.05 mg/kg, or 3 mg, was used for this purpose. Rocuronium is an acceptable alternative, as long as appropriate doses (0.03 to 0.04 mg/kg, or 10% of the ED_{95}) are given.[42] A dose of 0.06 mg/kg leads to an unacceptably high incidence of symptoms of neuromuscular weakness, such as blurred vision, heavy eyelids, voice changes, difficulty swallowing, or even dyspnea, in the awake patient.[34,42,43] A meta-analysis shows that these side effects have been observed frequently,[34] but most of these data come from studies where large defasciculating doses of neuromuscular blocking agents, exceeding 10% of the ED_{95}, were given.[42] Atracurium, 0.02 mg/kg, is also effective. Pancuronium, vecuronium, cisatracurium, and mivacurium are not as effective as defasciculants. After these nondepolarizing drugs, the dose of succinylcholine must be increased from 1 mg/kg to 1.5 or preferably 2 mg/kg because of the antagonism between depolarizing and nondepolarizing drugs.[36] Other drugs, such as diazepam, lidocaine, fentanyl, calcium, vitamin C, magnesium, dantrolene, or a small dose of succinylcholine have all been used to prevent fasciculations. The results are no better than with nondepolarizing drugs and they may have undesirable effects of their own.

Muscle Pains

Generalized aches and pains, similar to the myalgia that follows violent exercise, are common 24 to 48 hours after succinylcholine administration. Their incidence is variable (1.5% to 89% of patients receiving succinylcholine) and are more common in young, ambulatory patients.[44] The intensity of muscle pains is not always correlated with the intensity of fasciculations, but the methods that have been shown effective to prevent fasciculations usually prevent muscle pains. For example, a precurarization dose of a nondepolarizing neuromuscular blocking agent is effective. Lidocaine (1 to 1.5 mg/kg), especially in conjunction with precurarization, has also been shown to be of value.[44] Calcium, vitamin C, benzodiazepines, magnesium, and dantrolene have been tried with inconclusive results.[44]

Intragastric Pressure

Succinylcholine increases intragastric pressure, and this effect is blocked by precurarization. However, succinylcholine causes even greater increases in lower esophageal sphincter pressure. Thus, succinylcholine does not appear to increase the risk of aspiration of gastric contents unless the lower esophageal sphincter is incompetent.

Intraocular Pressure

Intraocular pressure increases by 5 to 15 mm Hg after injection of succinylcholine, and this increase is still present after detachment of extraocular muscle, suggesting an intraocular etiology. Precurarization with a nondepolarizing blocker has little or no effect on this increase. This information has led to the widespread recommendation to avoid succinylcholine in open-eye injuries. However, it must be appreciated that inadequate anesthesia, elevated systemic blood pressure, and insufficient neuromuscular blockade during laryngoscopy and tracheal intubation might increase intraocular pressure more than succinylcholine. In addition, there is little evidence that the use of succinylcholine has led to blindness or extrusion of eye content.[45]

Intracranial Pressure

Succinylcholine may increase intracranial pressure, and this response is probably diminished by precurarization.[46] Again, laryngoscopy and tracheal intubation with inadequate anesthesia or muscle relaxation are likely to increase intracranial pressure even more than succinylcholine.

Hyperkalemia

Serum potassium increases by approximately 0.5 mEq/L a few minutes after injection of succinylcholine. This increase is not prevented completely by precurarization. In fact, only large doses of nondepolarizing blockers reliably abolish this effect.[47] Subjects with preexisting hyperkalemia, such as patients in renal failure, do not have a greater increase in potassium levels, but the absolute level might reach the toxic range. Succinylcholine is safe in normokalemic renal failure patients.[48] Severe hyperkalemia, occasionally leading to cardiac arrest, has been described in patients after major denervation injuries, spinal cord transection, peripheral denervation, stroke, trauma, extensive burns, and prolonged immobility with disease, and may be related to potassium loss via a proliferation of extrajunctional receptors.[47] Hyperkalemia has been reported with myotonia and muscle dystrophies, and cardiac arrests have been reported in children before the diagnosis of the disease was made.[47] Severe hyperkalemia after succinylcholine resulting in cardiac arrest has also been observed in acidotic hypovolemic patients.

Abnormal Plasma Cholinesterase

Plasma cholinesterase activity can be reduced by a number of endogenous and exogenous causes, such as pregnancy, liver disease, uremia, malnutrition, burns, plasmapheresis, and oral contraceptives. These conditions usually lead to a slight, clinically unimportant increase in the duration of action of succinylcholine. Plasma cholinesterase activity is reduced by the anticholinesterases neostigmine and pyridostigmine, but not edrophonium, so that the duration of succinylcholine given after neostigmine or pyridostigmine, but not after edrophonium, is increased.[49]

The cholinesterase gene is located on chromosome 3 at q26,[50] and over 20 mutations in the coding region of the plasma cholinergic gene have been identified. Many of these mutations are relatively frequent, like the K (13%) variants, but do not lead to clinically significant increases in the duration of blockade after succinylcholine. Other alleles, such as the A, F, or silent variant, are less frequent, and are associated with significant prolongation of succinylcholine blockade only if the patient is homozygous for the allele, or if the allele is associated with another abnormal allele. Only approximately 1:2,000 individuals have prolonged paralysis (2 to 6 hours) after usual doses of succinylcholine (1 to 1.5 mg/kg). In heterozygous patients with an abnormal allele combined with the usual allele (1:30 cases), the duration of action is only slightly prolonged compared with normal individuals. Traditional methods for identifying plasma cholinesterase phenotype involve measurement of enzyme activity with a substrate and inhibition with dibucaine, fluoride, and chloride. These tests are only capable of identifying some enzyme variants. The complete amino acid sequence of plasma cholinesterase has now been determined using molecular genetics techniques.[50] Whole blood or fresh-frozen plasma can accelerate succinylcholine metabolism in patients with low or absent plasma cholinesterase, but the best course of action is probably mechanical ventilation of the lungs and providing adequate sedation to the patient until full recovery of neuromuscular function can be demonstrated.

Clinical Uses

The main indication for succinylcholine is to facilitate tracheal intubation. In adults, a dose of 1.0 mg/kg yields 75% to 80% excellent intubation conditions within 1 to 1.5 minutes after an induction sequence that includes a hypnotic (propofol or thiopental) and a moderate opioid dose.[8,51] The dose must be increased to 1.5 to 2.0 mg/kg if a precurarizing dose of nondepolarizing blocker has been used.[36] Intubating conditions without precurarization are only marginally improved by increasing the dose to 2 mg/kg.[8]

Succinylcholine is especially indicated for "rapid sequence induction," when a patient presents with a full stomach and the possibility of aspiration of gastric contents. In this situation, manual ventilation of the lungs is avoided, if possible, to reduce the probability of aspiration because of excessive intragastric pressure caused by gas forced via the face mask. Thus, the ideal neuromuscular blocking agent has both a fast onset, to reduce the time between induction and intubation of the airway, and a rapid recovery, to allow return of normal breathing before the patient becomes hypoxic. The duration of action of succinylcholine, given at a dose of 1 mg/kg, is short enough so that the majority of properly preoxygenated patients resume respiratory efforts (5 to 6 minutes) before hypoxia can be detected.[38,39] It has been argued that this is valid only in relatively healthy subjects and not in all cases. As a result, a lower dose has been suggested. However, a dose of 0.5 to 0.6 mg/kg results in substantially fewer patients with excellent intubating conditions, and the decrease in duration is modest.[8] For maintenance of relaxation, typical infusion rates are approximately 50 to 100 μg/kg/min. However, the availability of short and intermediate nondepolarizing drugs makes succinylcholine infusions obsolete.

Children are slightly more resistant to succinylcholine than adults,[52] and doses of 1 to 2 mg/kg are required to facilitate intubation. In infants, 2 to 3 mg/kg may be required. Precurarization is not necessary in patients younger than 10 years because fasciculations are uncommon in this age group. Bradycardia is common in children unless atropine or glycopyrrolate is given.[40] Succinylcholine, at a dose of 4 mg/kg, is the only effective intramuscular neuromuscular blocking agent in children with difficult intravenous access and provides adequate intubating conditions in about 4 minutes. However, this route of administration should not be the method of choice.[53]

In obese individuals, the dose of succinylcholine, in milligrams per kilogram of actual body weight, is the same as in leaner patients. Calculating the dose per kilogram ideal body weight (IBW) might lead to underdosing and inadequate intubating conditions.[54] The volume of distribution, expressed per kilogram of actual body weight, of succinylcholine is probably decreased in obese individuals, but this is compensated by an increase in plasma cholinesterase activity.

NONDEPOLARIZING DRUGS

Nondepolarizing neuromuscular blocking drugs bind to the postsynaptic receptor in a competitive fashion, by binding to one of the α subunits of the receptor (Fig. 20-7).[24]

Characteristics of Nondepolarizing Blockade

6 The fade observed in response to high frequency stimulation is characteristic of nondepolarizing blockade.[29] With EMG recordings, fade increases with frequency in the range 0.1 Hz (every 10 seconds) until 2 Hz (every 0.5 second), and stays relatively stable between 2 and 50 Hz. At frequencies greater than 10 to 20 Hz, the individual contractile responses fuse, and the net result is called a tetanus. At 2 Hz, individual responses can be separated easily and fade is manifest. This is why the TOF mode of stimulation has been chosen. Mechanical fade is greater with 100 Hz than with 50 Hz.[55] Tetanic stimulation is followed by post-tetanic facilitation, which is an increased response to any stimulation applied soon after the tetanus. The intensity and duration of this effect depend on the frequency and duration of the tetanic stimulation. With a 50 Hz tetanus of 5-second duration (250 stimuli), twitch responses have been found to fall within 10% of their pre-tetanic values in 1 to 2 minutes[56] (Fig. 20-8).

Finally, nondepolarizing blockade can be antagonized with anticholinesterase agents like neostigmine. It is also antagonized by depolarizing agents such as succinylcholine provided that the nondepolarizing blockade is intense and that the succinylcholine dose is too small to produce a block of its own.

Pharmacokinetics

As is the case for other drugs used in anesthesia, the *elimination half-life* of neuromuscular blocking agents does not always correlate with duration of action because termination of action sometimes depends on redistribution instead of elimination. However, knowledge of the kinetics of the drug helps us understand the behavior of the drug in special situations (prolonged administration, disease of the organs of elimination, and so on).

Several mechanisms can explain the various categories of durations of action listed in Table 20-3:

1. All *long-duration* drugs have a long (1 to 2 hours) elimination half-life and depend on liver and/or kidney function for termination of action. Return of twitch height occurs during the elimination phase of the drug.
2. *Intermediate-duration* drugs either have an intermediate elimination half-life or long elimination half-lives but depend on redistribution rather than elimination for termination of effect. Atracurium and cisatracurium have intermediate elimination half-lives (20 to 25 minutes) and recovery of twitch height occurs during the elimination phase. Vecuronium and rocuronium have longer terminal half-lives (approximately 90 minutes), but their relatively short duration of action is due to extensive redistribution of the drug, so that recovery of twitch height occurs during redistribution, rather than during the elimination phase. Thus, durations of action of vecuronium, rocuronium, atracurium, and cisatracurium are similar.
3. *Short-duration* drugs have short elimination half-lives. The active isomers of mivacurium have elimination half-lives of a few minutes.
4. *Ultrashort-duration* drugs have a very short elimination half-life. Succinylcholine has an elimination half-life of less than 1 minute.

The *volume of distribution* of all these agents is approximately equal to extracellular fluid (ECF) volume (0.2 to 0.4 L/kg; Table 20-3). In infants, in whom the ECF volume as a proportion of body weight is increased, the volume of distribution of neuromuscular blocking drugs parallels ECF volume closely.

TABLE 20-3. TYPICAL PHARMACOKINETIC DATA FOR NEUROMUSCULAR BLOCKING AGENTS IN ADULTS, EXCEPT WHERE STATED

Drug	Volume of Distribution (L/kg)	Clearance (mL/kg/min)	Elimination Half-life (min)
Ultrashort-duration Agents			
Succinylcholine	0.04	37	0.65
Short-duration Agents			
Mivacurium			
Trans–trans	0.05	29	2.4
Cis–trans	0.05	46	2.0
Cis–cis	0.18	7	30
Intermediate-duration Agents			
Atracurium	0.14	5.5	20
Cisatracurium			
Adults	0.12	5	23
Intensive care	0.26	6.5	25
Rocuronium			
Adults	0.3	3	90
Intensive care	0.7	3	330
Vecuronium	0.4	5	70
Long-duration Agents			
Doxacurium	0.2	2.5	95
d-tubocurarine			
Adults	0.3	1–3	90
Elderly	0.3	0.8	270
Neonates	0.7	1.1	300
Infants	0.5	1.0	300
Children	0.3	1.5	90
Pancuronium	0.3	1.8	140

Onset and Duration of Action

Both onset time and duration of action depend on the dose given, but even at equipotent doses, different drugs may have different onset times and duration of action, because other factors play a role.

Onset time is determined by the time required for drug concentrations at the site of action to reach a critical level, usually that corresponding to 100% block. Onset time (2 to 7 minutes) is longer than time to peak plasma concentrations (<1 minute). This delay reflects the time required for drug transfer between plasma and neuromuscular junction and is represented quantitatively by a rate constant (k_{eo}). This rate constant corresponds to half-times of 5 to 10 minutes for most nondepolarizing drugs and is determined by all the factors that modify access of the drug to, and its removal from, the neuromuscular junction. These include cardiac output, distance of the muscle from the heart, and muscle blood flow. Thus, neuromuscular blockade usually occurs sooner at well-perfused centrally located muscles (diaphragm or vocal cords) than at peripheral locations (hand or foot). Also, if metabolism or redistribution is very rapid, for example, in the case of succinylcholine, the onset time is accelerated. Finally, potent drugs have a slower onset of action than less potent agents (Fig. 20-11).[57] This is because a large proportion of receptors must be occupied before blockade can be observed. Blockade of these receptors will occur faster, and onset will be more rapid, if more drug molecules

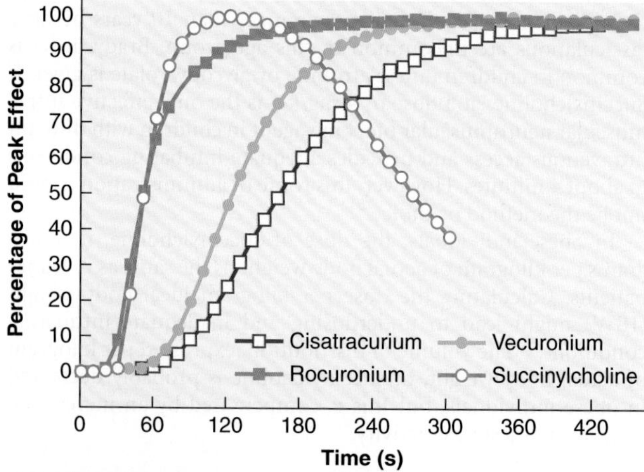

FIGURE 20-11. Neuromuscular blockade as a function of time for four neuromuscular blocking agents. Onset is faster for the less potent succinylcholine and rocuronium than for the more potent vecuronium and cisatracurium. (From: Kopman AF, Klewicka MM, Kopman DJ, et al. Molar potency is predictive of the speed of onset of neuromuscular block for agents of intermediate, short, and ultrashort duration. *Anesthesiology.* 1999;90:425, with permission.)

are available, that is, if potency is low. Table 20-2 shows that onset tends to be slower if a drug is potent, that is, if ED_{95} is small.

Duration of action is determined by the time required for drug concentrations at the site of action to decrease below a certain level, usually corresponding to 25% first twitch blockade. For a drug with rapidly decreasing plasma concentrations, duration of action tends to be short; for a drug that is eliminated slowly from plasma, duration of action will be long.

Individual Nondepolarizing Agents

Since 1942, nearly 50 nondepolarizing neuromuscular blocking agents have been introduced into clinical anesthesia. This section covers only those drugs currently available in North America and Europe, plus a few others of historical interest. The first agent to undergo clinical investigation was intocostrin, or *d*-tubocurarine, the purified and standardized product of curare obtained from the plant *Chondodendron tomentosum.*[1] *d*-tubocurarine has been completely replaced by more modern synthetic analogues.

d-tubocurarine

The dose of *d*-tubocurarine required to produce 95% twitch block at the adductor pollicis muscle, or ED_{95}, is 0.5 mg/kg. At that dose, the duration of action is typical of a long-duration agent (Table 20-2). The molecule undergoes minimal metabolism and is excreted in the kidney and in the bile. Like most other neuromuscular blocking drugs, it is not extensively (30% to 50%) protein bound. Hypotension frequently accompanies the administration of *d*-tubocurarine even at doses $<ED_{95}$. The mechanism involved is mainly histamine release, and skin flushing is frequently observed. Autonomic ganglionic blockade may also play a minor role.

Pharmacokinetics

d-tubocurarine was the first neuromuscular blocking agent whose concentration could be measured in plasma, and the pharmacokinetic studies conducted with this drug have led to the development of concepts that are helpful in understanding the behavior of all nondepolarizing agents in patients of different age groups and with disease of organs of elimination. The volume of distribution of the drug, expressed in mL/kg body weight, is greater in infants than in older children, young adults, and the elderly, but ED_{50} of *d*-tubocurarine, expressed in mg/kg body weight, does not vary markedly with age, from infancy to old age. These findings suggest that the *d*-tubocurarine concentration required for a given degree of blockade is less in infants than in older patients (Table 20-3).[58] This phenomenon has also been observed with other neuromuscular blocking agents. The decreased glomerular filtration rate in the very young and the very old results in an increased elimination half-life and prolonged duration of action.[58] The onset of action is more rapid in the young as a result of a more rapid circulation time.

Burns

Patients with massive burns demonstrate resistance to *d*-tubocurarine and other nondepolarizing drugs that depends on the size of the burn and the time since injury.[59] Higher concentrations of the free drug are required to produce a given degree of twitch depression compared with nonthermally injured patients. Compared with normal subjects, the number of acetylcholine receptors is increased in muscles close to the site of burn injury, but also, to a lesser extent, in more distant muscles.[60]

Clinical Use

The long duration and cardiovascular effects of *d*-tubocurarine have restricted its use. Drugs of intermediate duration with virtually no cardiovascular effects have almost eliminated the use of *d*-tubocurarine. When available, *d*-tubocurarine has been mainly confined to be used as a "precurarization" (3 mg/70 kg) before succinylcholine to reduce fasciculations and muscle pains. Rocuronium has largely replaced *d*-tubocurarine for this indication.

Atracurium

Atracurium is a bisquaternary ammonium benzylisoquinoline compound of intermediate duration of action. It is degraded via two metabolic pathways. One of these pathways is the Hofmann reaction, a nonenzymatic degradation with a rate that increases as temperature and/or pH increases. The second pathway is nonspecific ester hydrolysis. The enzymes involved in this metabolic pathway are a group of tissue esterases, which are distinct from plasma or acetyl cholinesterases.[61] The same group of enzymes is involved in the degradation of esmolol and remifentanil. It has been estimated that two-thirds of atracurium is degraded by ester hydrolysis and one-third by Hofmann reaction. Subjects with abnormal plasma cholinesterase have a normal response to atracurium.

The end products of the degradation of atracurium are laudanosine and acrylate fragments. Laudanosine has been reported as causing seizures in animals, but at doses largely exceeding the clinical range. No deleterious effect of laudanosine has been demonstrated conclusively in humans.[61] Laudanosine is excreted by the kidney. Acrylates have been shown to inhibit human cell proliferation in vitro.[62] However, the concentrations and exposure times required to obtain this effect are much greater than what is obtained normally in clinical practice.

Pharmacology

Atracurium is an intermediate-duration drug, with a terminal half-life of approximately 20 minutes. Termination of effect occurs during the elimination phase of the drug. Duration of action does not depend on age, renal function, or hepatic function. The ED_{95} of atracurium is 0.2 to 0.25 mg/kg. The onset of action is 3 to 5 minutes at $2 \times ED_{95}$ (0.5 mg/kg). Onset of atracurium can be shortened if the dose is increased, but it is not recommended to exceed 0.5 mg/kg because of hypotension and histamine release. The duration of action is also dose-related. The time to 25% first twitch recovery after 0.5 mg/kg is approximately 30 to 40 minutes.

Cardiovascular Effects

Like *d*-tubocurarine, atracurium releases histamine in a dose-related manner. If large doses (≥0.5 mg/kg) are administered, hypotension, tachycardia, skin flushing, and possibly bronchospasm may occur. These manifestations, which are observed in virtually every subject given a large enough dose, should not be confused with an anaphylactic reaction, which is a rare event seen in a few susceptible individuals, but could be triggered by a small dose. Anaphylactic reactions to atracurium have been described, but they do not appear to be more frequent than after other neuromuscular blocking drugs.[41]

Special Situations

Dosage requirements are similar in the elderly, younger adults, and children, presumably reflecting the organ independence of atracurium's elimination. Similarly, no dosage adjustment is required in individuals with renal or hepatic failure. As with other nondepolarizing agents, the dose must be increased in burn patients, partly because of increased protein binding and partly because of upregulation of receptors, causing resistance at the endplate. In the obese patient, the dose of atracurium, as for all neuromuscular blocking agents, should be calculated on the basis of lean body mass.

Clinical Uses

Atracurium has fallen into disfavor, probably because of its cardiovascular effects, in the United States, but remains popular in certain parts of Europe.[63] Intubating doses are 0.5 mg/kg, and laryngoscopy should be attempted only after 2 to 3 minutes. Cardiovascular manifestations of histamine release are often seen at that dose, and perfect intubating conditions are seen in only half the patients (Fig. 20-3).[10] For intubation, there has been a tendency to replace atracurium by agents with a shorter onset time and more cardiovascular stability, such as rocuronium. However, atracurium is convenient and versatile for maintenance of relaxation, either as a continuous infusion (5 to 10 μg/kg/min) or as intermittent injections (0.05 to 0.1 mg/kg every 10 to 15 minutes).

Cisatracurium

In an attempt to increase the gap between the neuromuscular blocking dose and the histamine-releasing dose, a potent isomer of atracurium, cisatracurium, was identified. Like atracurium, its cardiovascular effects are manifest only at doses exceeding 0.4 mg/kg, but its ED_{95} (0.05 mg/kg) is much lower. As a result, manifestations of histamine release are not seen in practice. The metabolism of cisatracurium is similar to that of atracurium, with Hofmann and ester hydrolysis both playing a role.[61]

Pharmacology

Because cisatracurium is a potent drug, its onset time is longer than that of atracurium and longer still than that of rocuronium. For example, equipotent doses of cisatracurium (0.046 mg/kg) and rocuronium (0.31 mg/kg) had onset times of 4.5 minutes and 1.7 minutes, respectively.[57] The elimination half-life (22 to 25 minutes) is similar to that of atracurium,[64] so the duration of action for $2 \times ED_{95}$ doses (0.1 mg/kg) is 30 to 45 minutes. However, in an attempt to accelerate onset, the recommended intubating dose is increased to 0.15 mg/kg. This dose is well below the threshold for histamine release, but the duration of action is prolonged to 45 to 60 minutes. Because the doses required to obtain paralysis are considerably less for cisatracurium than for atracurium, less laudanosine and less acrylate byproducts are produced.[61,62] Thus, the concerns raised by the potential toxic effects of these metabolites are virtually eliminated.

Special Situations

Like atracurium, there is no need to adjust dosage in the elderly, children, or infants, when compared with young adults. The experience in burn patients is limited, but the same principles that are valid for atracurium are expected to apply. In obese individuals, the dose of cisatracurium should be calculated on the basis of IBW.[65]

Side Effects

In contrast to atracurium, cisatracurium is devoid of histamine-releasing properties even at high doses ($8 \times ED_{95}$). It is also devoid of cardiovascular effects. However, anaphylactic reactions have been described.[41]

Clinical Use

Cisatracurium may be used to facilitate tracheal intubation at doses equivalent to 3 to 4 times the ED_{95} (0.15 to 0.2 mg/kg) when manual ventilation is possible after induction of anesthesia and when the duration of the procedure is expected to exceed 1 hour. Duration is shorter with lower doses, but onset time is prolonged and intubating conditions are less ideal. Neuromuscular blockade is easily maintained at a stable level by continuous intravenous infusion of cisatracurium (1 to 2 μg/kg/min) at a constant rate and does not change with time, suggesting the lack of a significant cumulative drug effect and lack of dependence on renal and/or hepatic clearance mechanisms.[66] The rate of recovery is independent of the dose of cisatracurium and the duration of the administration.

Since cisatracurium does not depend on end-organ function for its elimination, the drug appears suitable for administration in the intensive care unit (ICU). The infusion rates to keep patients paralyzed are greater than in the operating room (typically 5 μg/kg/min), with wide interindividual variability.[67] It is likely that prolonged exposure of the receptors to a neuromuscular blocking agent causes some upregulation, with a corresponding requirement for a higher dose.[59] Interestingly, patients with acute respiratory distress syndrome requiring respiratory support in the ICU randomized to cisatracurium had better survival than patients receiving placebo.[68]

Doxacurium

Doxacurium is a potent, long-acting benzylisoquinoline compound that is not degraded by Hofmann elimination or ester hydrolysis. Its elimination half-life is 1 to 2 hours and it depends on the kidney and the liver for its disposition. Thus, duration of action is prolonged in the elderly and in subjects with impaired renal or hepatic function. The ED_{95} for doxacurium is 25 μg/kg (Table 20-2).[69] Its cardiovascular stability is useful, but it has a limited place in clinical practice because of its very slow onset and long duration of action. It is unsuitable for facilitating tracheal intubation or for providing skeletal muscle relaxation during brief surgical procedures. When used in the ICU, recovery after stopping the infusion is prolonged when compared with cisatracurium.

Gantacurium and Other Chlorofumarates

Gantacurium was the first compound belonging to the class of asymmetric mixed-onium chlorofumarates to be investigated. It is a nondepolarizing drug and belongs to the class of asymmetric mixed-onium chlorofumarates. Its main degradation pathway involves cysteine in the plasma and is independent of plasma cholinesterase. The ED_{95} in humans is approximately 0.19 mg/kg.[70] Cardiovascular effects are observed at doses exceeding $3 \times ED_{95}$, and are most probably related to histamine release. At doses anticipated to be required for tracheal intubation (0.4 to 0.6 mg/kg), onset at the adductor pollicis muscle is 1.5 minutes and duration to 25% T_1 recovery is 8 to 10 minutes, comparable with that of succinylcholine.

Other compounds of the same class have also been synthesized, with the idea of developing a compound with more cardiovascular stability, longer duration of action, and the ability to be reversed by cysteine.[70] The most promising of these compounds is now CW002, for which the concept has been tested in dogs.[71]

Mivacurium

Mivacurium is a benzylisoquinoline derivative with a short duration of action that is hydrolyzed by plasma cholinesterase, like succinylcholine.[72] Contrary to succinylcholine, however, mivacurium produces nondepolarizing blockade. The drug is presented as a mixture of three isomers. Two of the isomers, the cis–trans and trans–trans, have short half-lives, but the cis–cis isomer has a much longer half-life (Table 20-3). The pharmacology of mivacurium is governed largely by the behavior of the trans–trans and cis–trans isomers, because the cis–cis isomer accounts for only 6% of the mixture and is less potent than the other two isomers. Mivacurium is no longer available in North America, but is used in many European countries.[63]

Pharmacology

The ED_{95} of mivacurium has been estimated in the range of 0.08 to 0.15 mg/kg (Table 20-2). At 0.2 or 0.25 mg/kg doses, intubating conditions are not as good as with succinylcholine. Onset time is surprisingly long for a drug whose active isomers have a terminal half-life of <2 minutes, with disappearance of the twitch taking as long as 2.5 to 4 minutes at 2 to 3 × ED_{95}.[72] This long onset time is probably the result of the high potency of mivacurium.[57] Recovery to 25% does not depend heavily on dose, being in the range of 15 to 25 minutes for doses of 0.15 to 0.25 mg/kg. The infusion rate to maintain blockade constant does not vary markedly with time, and recovery is as rapid after many hours of infusion than after a bolus dose.[72,73]

Side Effects

Like atracurium, mivacurium releases histamine in a dose-related fashion. Hypotension, tachycardia, and cutaneous signs, such as erythema and flushing, are seen frequently when doses exceed 0.2 mg/kg.

Pediatric Population

In infants and children the ED_{95} is approximately the same as in adults, but onset of block and recovery are more rapid. Cardiovascular effects are not as important as in adults, so doses up to 0.3 mg/kg have been used. The infusion rate required to maintain blockade is greater in children than in adults, and less in the elderly than in younger adults.

Burns

In burn patients, upregulation of the receptors, and to a lesser extent increased protein binding, causes a resistance to all nondepolarizing neuromuscular blocking agents. However, for mivacurium, the situation is different because plasma cholinesterase activity is decreased in burn patients. The net effect is either a normal or even an enhanced effect of usual doses.[74]

Reversal

Neostigmine has two opposing effects on mivacurium: It inhibits plasma cholinesterase,[49] thus interfering with the breakdown of mivacurium, but it also reverses nondepolarizing blockade. In fact, neostigmine has been shown to delay recovery if given during intense mivacurium neuromuscular block,[75] but to accelerate recovery if at least two twitches in the TOF are present. Edrophonium does not interfere with plasma cholinesterase activity[49] and was found to accelerate recovery, even when blockade is profound.[75] Mivacurium reversal has been suggested to be unnecessary because spontaneous recovery is rapid. However, residual block may be seen, particularly if large doses of mivacurium are used up to the end of anesthesia. Reversal with anticholinesterases
7 should be attempted only when all four twitches in response to TOF stimulation are visible at the adductor pollicis.

Plasma Cholinesterase

Mivacurium is metabolized by plasma cholinesterase somewhat more slowly than succinylcholine. The conditions associated with a decreased plasma cholinesterase activity known to affect succinylcholine metabolism also alter mivacurium duration of action.

Clinical Use

Mivacurium is well suited to surgical procedures requiring brief muscle relaxation, particularly those in which rapid recovery is required, such as ambulatory and laparoscopic surgery. However, it is not recommended for rapid-sequence induction. Cardiovascular effects may be avoided by administering the drug slowly or by splitting the dose into two injections, 30 seconds apart. Maintenance of relaxation is accomplished more easily by constant infusion (5 to 7 μg/kg/min in young and middle-aged adults) than by intermittent bolus injection. This infusion rate has to be increased in children and reduced in the elderly.

Pancuronium

Pancuronium belongs to a series of bisquaternary aminosteroid compounds. It is metabolized to a 3-OH compound, which has one-half the neuromuscular blocking activity of the parent compound. The ED_{95} of pancuronium is 0.07 mg/kg. The duration of action is long, being 1.5 to 2 hours after a 0.15 mg/kg dose. Clearance is decreased in renal and hepatic failure, demonstrating that excretion depends on both organs. The onset of action is more rapid in infants and children than in adults, and recovery is slower in the elderly.

Cardiovascular Effects

Pancuronium is associated with increases in heart rate, blood pressure, and cardiac output, particularly after large doses (2 × ED_{95}). The cause is uncertain but includes a vagolytic effect at the postganglionic nerve terminal, a sympathomimetic effect as a result of blocking of muscarinic receptors that normally exert some braking on ganglionic transmission, and an increase in catecholamine release. Pancuronium does not release histamine.

Clinical Use

The slow onset of action of pancuronium limits its usefulness in facilitating tracheal intubation. In cardiac anesthesia, pancuronium has enjoyed popularity because it counteracts the bradycardic effect of high doses of opioids. The use of pancuronium instead of rocuronium is associated with a higher incidence of muscular weakness after cardiac surgery,[16] and reversal in this setting should be considered seriously. In noncardiac patients, its use is associated with a high incidence of residual block in the postanesthesia care unit, even when reversal is given (Table 20-1).[21,76] Pancuronium neuromuscular block is more difficult to reverse than the block produced by intermediate duration agents.[12]

Rapacuronium

Rapacuronium is an aminosteroid compound that was introduced for clinical use in the United States in 1999 and was withdrawn in 2001 because of rare, but severe, cases of bronchospasm after intubation. This brief story needs to be mentioned for two reasons. First, the ED_{95} of rapacuronium was greater (0.75 mg/kg)[77] than that of any other neuromuscular blocking agent, and consequently it had a more rapid onset of action.[57] It could provide intubating conditions comparable to those afforded by succinylcholine. Second, the possibility of side effects is greater when large doses are utilized. Rapacuronium produced mild dose-related tachycardia and hypotension, but major concerns were voiced when severe increases in airway pressure and bronchospasm were observed in patients given rapacuronium. The mechanism for this effect is not an allergic or histamine-related reaction, but is most likely related to the effect of rapacuronium on M2 and M3 muscarinic receptors in the lung. Activation of the postsynaptic M3 receptors by acetylcholine produces bronchoconstriction, and the effect is terminated by presynaptic M2 receptors that counteract this effect. Rapacuronium blocks both receptors, but it has a greater affinity for the M2 receptor, so that clinical concentrations block the M2 receptor selectively. The net effect in susceptible individuals is that bronchoconstriction by activation of the M3 receptors is unopposed.[78] It appears that other neuromuscular blocking agents, such as mivacurium, vecuronium, rocuronium, and cisatracurium, are devoid of these airway effects, even at high doses.[78]

Rocuronium

Rocuronium is an aminosteroid compound with structural similarity with vecuronium and pancuronium. Its duration of action is comparable with that of vecuronium, but its onset is shorter.

Pharmacology

Plasma concentrations of rocuronium decrease rapidly after bolus injection because of hepatic uptake.[79] Thus, the duration of action of the drug is determined chiefly by redistribution, rather than by its rather long terminal elimination half-life (1 to 2 hours). Metabolism to 17-deacetylrocuronium is a very minor elimination pathway. Most of the drug is excreted unchanged in the urine, bile, or feces.[79]

With an ED_{95} of 0.3 mg/kg, rocuronium has one-sixth the potency of vecuronium, a more rapid onset, but a similar duration of action and similar pharmacokinetic behavior. With equipotent doses, rocuronium onset at the adductor pollicis muscle is much faster than that of cisatracurium, atracurium, and vecuronium (Fig. 20-11).[57] After doses of 0.6 mg/kg ($2 \times ED_{95}$) maximal block occurs in 1.5 to 2 minutes. In a multicenter study of 349 patients, intubating conditions at 60 seconds after 0.6 mg/kg rocuronium were good to excellent in 77% of cases. To obtain results similar to those after 1 mg/kg succinylcholine, the dose of rocuronium had to be increased to 1.0 mg/kg, which provided 92% good or excellent conditions.[9] However, the duration of action is longer than for succinylcholine, ranging between 30 and 40 minutes for a 0.6 mg/kg dose to approximately 60 minutes after 1 mg/kg in adults. Thus, rocuronium is an intermediate-duration drug.

As for other nondepolarizing agents, the onset of action of rocuronium is more rapid at the diaphragm and adductor laryngeal muscles than at the adductor pollicis muscle,[80–82] probably a result of a greater blood flow to centrally located muscles. Laryngeal adductor muscles are important in anesthesia because they close the vocal cords and insufficient relaxation prevents easy passage of the tracheal tube. Laryngeal adductor muscles are resistant to the effect of rocuronium, and the plasma concentration required for equivalent blockade is greater at the larynx than at the adductor pollicis muscle.[83] The same is true of the diaphragm, which is resistant to the effect of rocuronium and other neuromuscular blocking agents. Recovery is faster at the diaphragm and larynx than at the adductor pollicis muscle.[82]

Cardiovascular Effects

No hemodynamic changes (blood pressure, heart rate, or ECG) were seen in humans, and there were no increases in plasma histamine concentrations after doses of up to $4 \times ED_{95}$ (1.2 mg/kg).[84] Only slight hemodynamic changes are observed during coronary artery bypass surgery.

Allergy

See also Chapter 12 Immune Function and Allergic Response. Anaphylactic reactions have been described, and according to surveys conducted in France, these events seem to occur more frequently with rocuronium than with other neuromuscular blocking agents.[41] These findings have been criticized because up to 50% of the general population show a positive intradermal or pick test to the drug,[85] and many patients who were investigated for a possible anaphylactic reaction were falsely labeled allergic to the drug because of the high rate of false–positive tests. Overdiagnosis might have inflated the reported number of rocuronium anaphylaxis cases in Norway (29 cases in 150,000 administrations, or 1:5,000)[86] or in France,[41] while reports from other Nordic countries suggest a much lower incidence (7 cases in 800,000 administrations, or <1:100,000).[86] In the United States, the incidence of anaphylactic reactions to rocuronium and vecuronium may be as low as 1:1,000,000.[87] A recent US survey in an academic institution implicated neuromuscular blocking agents as causative agents of anaphylactic reaction in only 11% of events,[88] whereas they were incriminated in 58% of these events in France.[41] These, and other, data suggest marked variations in the geographical incidence of allergic reactions to neuromuscular blocking agents.

The possible factors for possible differences in anaphylactic reactions to neuromuscular blocking agents was first investigated in a study comparing subjects from Norway, where the number of reported anaphylactic cases is high, and Sweden, where those reports are virtually nonexistent.[89] It was found that a large proportion of Norwegians was sensitized to pholcodine, but this sensitization did not occur in Swedes.[89] Pholcodine is available as an antitussive in cough syrups in certain countries like Norway, France, Ireland, the United Kingdom, and Australia. It is not available in Sweden, Denmark, Germany, the United States, and Canada. It was later found that the rate of sensitization to pholcodine in different countries depends on national pholcodine consumption.[90] It is hypothesized that cross-sensitization may occur between pholcodine and neuromuscular blocking agents such as rocuronium and succinylcholine. Pholcodine exposure increases serum IgE against succinylcholine.[91] In 2007, pholcodine was withdrawn in Norway; the IgE antibody levels to pholcodine and succinylcholine have fallen within 1 to 2 years in sensitized patients, and the incidence of reported anaphylactic reactions to neuromuscular blocking agents has decreased.[92] However, pholcodine in the context may not be the only factor playing a role in the susceptibility to allergic reactions. The incidence of anaphylactic reactions to rocuronium remains very low, even in countries where pholcodine is available.

Special Situations

The potency of rocuronium has been reported to be slightly greater in women than in men, the ED_{95} being 0.27 and 0.39 mg/kg, respectively, with an increased duration in women.[93] Some ethnic groups are more sensitive to the drug. Chinese subjects living in Vancouver were found to be more sensitive than whites.[94] As with other nondepolarizing drugs, potency has been reported to vary according to geographical distribution. Most studies reported a greater potency in North America compared with Europe,[95] with one report showing a potency of rocuronium in mainland China as intermediate between European and American values.[95] Children (2 to 12 years old) require more rocuronium and the duration of action is less. Onset of action is shorter in the pediatric than in the adult population. For example, a dose of 1.2 mg/kg provides an onset time (39 seconds) comparable with that of succinylcholine, 2 mg/kg, and mean duration of action is 41 minutes.[96] Thus, the recommended doses are 0.9 to 1.2 mg/kg in this age group. Rocuronium is more potent in infants than in older children. Doses of 0.6 mg/kg have a longer duration in neonates (<1 month) than in infants (5 to 12 months), so a reduced dosage (0.45 mg/kg) is recommended.[97] In elderly patients, the ED_{95} is similar to that found in younger adults, but the duration of action is prolonged slightly.[98] Rocuronium has an increased terminal half-life in renal failure patients, probably because of its partial renal elimination, but this translates into only a slight prolongation of the block.[99] In hepatic disease, the slower uptake and elimination of rocuronium by the liver tends to prolong the duration of action of the drug, but this is compensated to some extent by the larger volume of distribution.[100]

Rapid Sequence Induction

Rocuronium is the drug of choice for rapid sequence induction if succinylcholine is contraindicated. Intubating conditions provided by rocuronium are excellent in approximately 80% of cases, and comparable to those offered by succinylcholine, at a dose of at least 1.0 mg/kg.[9] Doses corresponding to $2 \times ED_{95}$ or 0.6 mg/kg yield poorer intubating conditions. The major drawback of large rocuronium doses (≥1.0 mg/kg) is the long duration of action, which may exceed 1 hour. This problem can be circumvented if sugammadex is available.[38] In children, succinylcholine is relatively contraindicated because of the possible presence of undiagnosed muscle dystrophy in pediatric patients, especially in boys,[47] and duration of action of large doses (1.0 to 1.2 mg/kg) is shorter than in adults. Rocuronium is thus particularly indicated in this age group.

Clinical Use

The rapid onset and intermediate duration of action makes this agent a potential replacement for succinylcholine in conditions where rapid tracheal intubation is indicated. However, large doses (>1 mg/kg) are required, with the drawback being a prolonged duration of action. Contrary to succinylcholine, the option to wait for spontaneous breathing to resume before hypoxia is manifest does not exist with rocuronium, except if sugammadex is available. Clinicians should remember, however, that if they decide to depend on sugammadex in the case of a "can't intubate, can't ventilate" scenario, two issues should be considered: (1) the hypnotics and opioids given at induction may lead to respiratory depression and delay the recovery of breathing movements, irrespective of neuromuscular blockade; and (2) delays are likely in making the decision to administer sugammadex; drawing up the correct dose (16 mg/kg)[38]; injecting sugammadex; and waiting for the effect to be manifest.[101]

Rocuronium has gradually replaced vecuronium as an intermediate-duration neuromuscular blocking agent because of its more rapid onset. Initial doses of 0.6 mg/kg intravenously will usually produce acceptable intubating conditions within 90 seconds. Duration of action is 30 to 40 minutes. Smaller doses (typically, 0.45 mg/kg) have a shorter duration of action, but time to intubation must be increased. Subsequent doses of 0.1 to 0.2 mg/kg will provide clinical relaxation for 10 to 20 minutes. Alternatively, rocuronium might be given by continued infusion, titrated with the help of a nerve stimulator. Infusion rates are in the range 5 to 10 μg/kg/min.[66] Recovery after infusions is slower than after bolus doses.

To shorten the onset time, the "priming principle," which involves the administration of a small dose of rocuronium usually 3 minutes before induction, has been advocated. As with defasciculating doses before succinylcholine, it is not recommended to administer more than $0.1 \times ED_{95}$,[42] which, in the case of rocuronium, amounts to 0.03 mg/kg, much less than the typical intubating dose (0.6 mg/kg). Such a small dose has minimal effects on onset times of rocuronium, because it has a rather short time even without priming, and because the priming dose is only a tiny fraction of the total dose. Thus, the priming technique is not recommended. A "timing principle" has been described in which 0.6 mg/kg rocuronium is given *before* the induction agent, which is administered at the onset of ptosis. Considering that loss of consciousness does not occur immediately after injection of the induction agent, this technique is not recommended.

Rocuronium causes pain on injection, like propofol. Unlike propofol, however, rocuronium is normally given after the patient is anesthetized. Patient movement after injection of rocuronium is a sign of inadequate analgesia. Rocuronium and thiopental do not mix. They form a precipitate when they are in the same intravenous line. If thiopental is used for induction of anesthesia, the line must be flushed carefully before rocuronium is given. Such precipitates do not occur with propofol.

Vecuronium

Vecuronium is an intermediate-duration aminosteroid neuromuscular relaxant without cardiovascular effects. Its ED_{95} is 0.04 to 0.05 mg/kg. Its duration and recovery characteristics are comparable with those of rocuronium. However, its onset of action is slower.

Pharmacology

Vecuronium is a monoquaternary ammonium compound produced by demethylation of the pancuronium molecule. Vecuronium undergoes spontaneous deacetylation to produce 3-OH, 17-OH, and 3,17-$(OH)_2$ metabolites. The most potent of these metabolites, 3-OH vecuronium, with approximately 60% of the activity of vecuronium, is excreted by the kidney and may be responsible, in part, for prolonged paralysis in patients in the ICU. Like rocuronium, vecuronium has been found less potent and with a shorter duration of action in men than in women, probably because of a greater volume of distribution in men.

Duration of action of vecuronium, like that of rocuronium, is governed by redistribution, not by elimination. Attempts have been made to speed the onset of action by using the priming principle, that is, by administering a small, sub-paralyzing dose several minutes before the main dose is given. With the availability of rocuronium, which has a more rapid onset of action than that of vecuronium, "priming" becomes an obsolete practice.

Cardiovascular Effects

Vecuronium usually produces no cardiovascular effects with clinical doses. It does not induce histamine release. Bradycardia has been described with high-dose opioid anesthesia, and this might be the reflection of the opioid effect. Allergic reactions have been described, but no more frequently than after the use of other neuromuscular blocking drugs.[41]

Clinical Use

The cardiovascular neutrality and intermediate duration of action make vecuronium a suitable agent for use in patients with ischemic heart disease or those undergoing short, ambulatory surgery. As with rocuronium, care should be taken when vecuronium is administered immediately after thiopental because a precipitate of barbituric acid may be formed that may obstruct the intravenous cannula.

Large doses (0.1 to 0.2 mg/kg) can be used to facilitate tracheal intubation instead of succinylcholine. For maintenance of relaxation, vecuronium may be given using intermittent boluses, 0.01 to 0.02 mg/kg, or by continuous infusion at a rate of 1 to 2 μg/kg/min. However, the rate of spontaneous recovery of neuromuscular function is slower after administration by infusion than by intermittent boluses.[13] Vecuronium has now largely been replaced by the more rapid rocuronium.

DRUG INTERACTIONS

Many interactions between neuromuscular blocking drugs and several anesthetic and nonanesthetic drugs have been documented. Only some of the most clinically relevant interactions will be discussed here.

Anesthetic Agents

Inhalational Agents

The anesthetic vapors potentiate neuromuscular blockade in a dose-related fashion. Studies attempting to quantify the magnitude of this effect have led to conflicting results because the time factor is also important. The older halogenated agents, halothane, enflurane, and isoflurane may take 2 hours or more to equilibrate with muscle, so in practice the potentiating effect of these vapors might not be immediately apparent. At similar minimum alveolar concentration (MAC), enflurane appears to potentiate nondepolarizing blockade more than does isoflurane, which in turn potentiates to a greater extent than halothane. The newer agents, sevoflurane and desflurane equilibrate more rapidly with muscle, but the effect may be measurable only after 30 minutes or more. For example, the duration of action of a bolus dose of mivacurium given at induction of anesthesia is not altered by the presence of sevoflurane (1 MAC). However, the infusion rate required to maintain block decreases by 75% over the next 1.5 hours, compared with no change under propofol anesthesia.[73] The degree of potentiation increases with the concentration of sevoflurane. Recovery rate is longer in the presence of sevoflurane, even if the infusion rate of mivacurium was less. There is evidence that desflurane might have a greater potentiating effect on the neuromuscular junction than sevoflurane.[102] Nitrous oxide (70% inspired) has minimal effects on neuromuscular blockade, if any; it was found to decrease the ED_{50} of rocuronium by approximately 20%,[103] but had no effect of infusion requirement to maintain 90% block.[104]

The mechanism of action of potentiation by halogenated agents is uncertain, but it appears that they produce their effects at the neuromuscular junction. Isoflurane and sevoflurane inhibit current through the nicotinic receptor at the neuromuscular junction, and this inhibition is dose-dependent.[105]

Intravenous Anesthetics

Although some slight potentiation of neuromuscular blockade has been demonstrated with high doses of most intravenous induction agents in animals, clinical doses of drugs such as midazolam, thiopental, propofol, fentanyl, and ketamine have little or no neuromuscular effect in humans.

Local Anesthetics

Lidocaine, procaine, and other local anesthetic agents produce neuromuscular blockade in their own right as well as potentiating the effects of depolarizing and nondepolarizing neuromuscular blocking drugs. A longer duration of action of vecuronium was found in patients under general anesthesia with an epidural catheter injected with mepivacaine,[106] but not with levobupivacaine.[107] The exact mechanisms for this interaction are uncertain, and it is likely that the effect depends on the dose of local anesthetic.

Interactions Between Nondepolarizing Blocking Drugs

Combinations of two nondepolarizing neuromuscular blocking drugs are either additive or synergistic, depending on which two drugs are involved. Addition occurs when the total effect equals that of equipotent doses of each drug. For example, atracurium and cisatracurium have an additive interaction.[108] An ED_{95} of either atracurium (0.2 mg/kg) or cisatracurium (0.05 mg/kg) yields 95% blockade. Half the ED_{95} of atracurium (0.1 mg/kg) plus half the ED_{95} of cisatracurium (0.025 mg/kg) will also produce 95% block. However, some combinations are synergistic; that is, the combined effect of half the ED_{95} of each drug given together produces >95% block. For example, the ED_{95}s of cisatracurium and rocuronium are 0.05 and 0.3 mg/kg, respectively; if half these ED_{95}s are given in combination (0.025 and 0.15 mg/kg, respectively), the effect will be >95% twitch depression. To get 95% block, only one-fourth the ED_{95} of each drug needs to be given together; that is, cisatracurium, 0.0125 mg/kg, with rocuronium, 0.075 mg/kg.[108] The first such synergism was demonstrated for pancuronium–metocurine combinations, and the mixture was advocated for its lack of cardiovascular effects. With the availability of a variety of single drugs without cardiovascular effects at reasonable cost, there are few indications of synergistic drug mixtures.

Interactions of a different nature occur when administration of a nondepolarizing agent is followed by injection of another nondepolarizing agent with a different duration of action. Usually, the duration of action of the second agent is that of the first drug given. For example, if mivacurium, a short-acting agent, is given after the longer-acting rocuronium, it has a longer duration of action, much like that of rocuronium. On the contrary, if mivacurium is the first drug, rocuronium given as a top-up dose has a short duration of action.[109] Thus, switching to a shorter duration agent at the end of a case will not provide paralysis of a brief duration. The reason why the characteristics of the first agent given are determinant is that the size of the loading dose is greater than that of the maintenance dose, so that even when the second dose is given, the majority of receptors is still occupied by the first drug.

Nondepolarizing–Depolarizing Interactions

Depolarizing and nondepolarizing relaxants are mutually antagonistic. When *d*-tubocurarine or other nondepolarizing agents are given before succinylcholine to prevent fasciculations and muscle pain, the succinylcholine is less potent and has a shorter duration of action.[36] The response to a small dose of succinylcholine at the end of an anesthetic in which a nondepolarizing agent has been used is difficult to predict. It may either antagonize or potentiate the blockade, depending on the degree of nondepolarizing block. Antagonism is more likely if blockade is deep and potentiation if blockade is shallow. If an anticholinesterase agent has been given, then the effect of the succinylcholine is potentiated because of inhibition of plasma cholinesterase.[49]

Antibiotics

The older antibiotics neomycin, streptomycin, and the polymyxins have been found to depress neuromuscular function, but these drugs are no longer used frequently. Other aminoglycosides (e.g., gentamicin, netilmicin, tobramycin) and metronidazole have minor, if any, effects on nondepolarizing neuromuscular blockade.[110] The lincosamides, clindamycin and lincomycin, have prejunctional and postjunctional effects, but prolongation of blockade by clindamycin is unlikely to occur clinically unless large doses are used. The penicillins, cephalosporins, tetracyclines, and erythromycin are devoid of neuromuscular effects at clinically relevant doses.

Anticonvulsants

Acute administration of phenytoin produces augmentation of neuromuscular block,[111] but duration of pancuronium, metocurine, vecuronium, and rocuronium blockade is markedly shorter in patients receiving chronic anticonvulsant therapy with carbamazepine or phenytoin.[112,113] The requirements for atracurium, mivacurium, and cisatracurium are the same or increased slightly by chronic administration of anticonvulsant drugs.[114] The difference between benzylisoquinolines and aminosteroid drugs in this respect probably has a pharmacokinetic origin. Anticonvulsant drugs are strong enzyme inducers, which lead to a more rapid clearance of aminosteroids. In patients with chronic carbamazepine therapy, the clearance of vecuronium was found to be increased and its terminal half-life decreased.[112]

Cardiovascular Drugs

Beta-blocking drugs and calcium channel antagonists have been found to have neuromuscular effects in vitro, but in practice, the duration of action of neuromuscular blocking agents is not altered in patients taking these drugs chronically.[113] Ephedrine given at induction of anesthesia has been found to accelerate onset of action of rocuronium while esmolol prolongs onset time.[115] The mechanism for this effect is probably by alteration of drug delivery to the site of action by changes in cardiac output. It is possible to improve intubating conditions provided by rocuronium by giving ephedrine at induction of anesthesia.

Magnesium

Magnesium is used in anesthesia for its cardiovascular, neuroprotective, and antinociceptive effects.[116] Calcium is required for the release of acetylcholine,[23,24] and magnesium antagonizes this effect. Magnesium was found to decrease onset time of rocuronium and prolong duration of action of cisatracurium and rocuronium.[116] Previous administration of magnesium abolishes succinylcholine-induced fasciculations, but it does not prolong the duration of neuromuscular blockade.[116]

Miscellaneous

Metoclopramide inhibits plasma cholinesterase and thus prolongs the action of succinylcholine and mivacurium. Inconsistent interactions have been described for diuretics, digoxin, and corticosteroids, probably because these drugs induce chronic fluid and electrolyte shifts, the magnitude of which depends on the condition being treated.

ALTERED RESPONSES TO NEUROMUSCULAR BLOCKING AGENTS

Intensive Care Unit

Neuromuscular blocking agents are useful in the ICU to facilitate mechanical ventilation, and their use is frequent in patients requiring ventilation in the prone position, permissive hypercapnia, high positive end-expiratory pressure, and elevated airways pressure.[117] It is essential to provide sedation to patients who receive paralyzing agents, to prevent discomfort associated with the inability to move. There was considerable enthusiasm for the liberal use of neuromuscular blocking agents in the ICU a few decades ago, but the practice changed following several reports of critically ill patients who demonstrated residual weakness for unexpectedly long periods after discontinuation of a neuromuscular blocking agent. In some, recovery took several months.[118] Pancuronium and vecuronium were used most frequently in the earlier studies, and the aminosteroids were suspected of causing more myopathy than the benzylisoquinolines were. However, similar syndromes have been described after atracurium and cisatracurium, and it is unclear whether the frequency of reports of weakness reflects the relative usage of the drugs rather than a particular association with steroid-based compounds. Electromyographic studies have shown variable lesions from myopathy to axonal degeneration of motor and sensory fibers. The picture is complicated by the syndrome of "critical illness neuropathy," which occurs in patients with sepsis and multiorgan failure, even in individuals not given neuromuscular blocking agents. Administration of corticosteroids is also considered a risk factor.[117] Symptoms include failure to wean from mechanical ventilation, limb weakness, and impaired deep tendon reflexes, but sensory function is usually not affected. There are no controlled clinical studies to allow the several initiating factors to be identified and matched with particular syndromes.

In recent years, the indications for neuromuscular blocking agents in the ICU have been narrowed, and patients thus treated appeared to do better. In a recent study, patients with severe adult respiratory distress syndrome were randomized to cisatracurium for 48 hours or no neuromuscular blocking agent. Mortality at 28 days and ventilator-free days were reduced in the cisatracurium group.[68] The mechanisms for this beneficial effect of neuromuscular blockade are uncertain. In the absence of more definitive studies, it is recommended to administer neuromuscular blocking agents only to patients who cannot be managed otherwise, to limit the duration of administration to a few days or less, to use only the dose that is necessary, and to interrupt temporarily the administration of the neuromuscular blocking agent every day or so.[117]

Studies in ICU patients in whom the administration of a neuromuscular blocking agent was adjusted according to strict neuromuscular monitoring criteria have shown considerable variation in the requirement for neuromuscular blocking agent to maintain the same effect among patients and a wide within-patient pharmacokinetic variability.[67] Vecuronium and rocuronium have been associated with recovery times of several hours. With cisatracurium, this interval was shorter (approximately 1 hour) and less variable.[67] Drug requirement is variable from patient to patient, is usually greater than in the operating room, and tends to increase with time, probably because of upregulation of receptors.[59] The variability of response from patient to patient suggests the need for careful individualized monitoring of neuromuscular block in ICU patients, although the optimal method and level of block to be achieved are uncertain. Titrating neuromuscular blocking agents to the minimum infusion rate is probably best.

Myasthenia Gravis

Myasthenia gravis is an autoimmune disease in which circulating antibodies produce a functional reduction in the number of postsynaptic acetylcholine receptors.[119]

Diagnosis and Management

The hallmark of myasthenia gravis is fatigue. Presentation is extremely varied but typically, ocular symptoms, such as diplopia and ptosis, occur first. Bulbar involvement is usually seen next. Patients may proceed to have extremity weakness and respiratory difficulties.[119] The characteristic EMG finding in myasthenia gravis is a voltage decrement to repeated stimulation at 2 to 5 Hz. This finding is also characteristic of nondepolarizing blockade in non-myasthenic individuals. Edrophonium, 2 to 8 mg, produces brief recovery from myasthenia gravis and can be used as a diagnostic test. Finally, up to 80% of patients have an increased titer of the acetylcholine receptor antibody.

Treatment is largely symptomatic. Anticholinesterase agents such as pyridostigmine are used to increase neurotransmission at the neuromuscular junction. Corticosteroids and immunotherapy with azathioprine might produce long-term improvement. Plasmapheresis might be effective by eliminating the circulating antibody. Finally, many myasthenic patients have an associated thymoma, and surgical removal of the thymus may be indicated.[119]

Response to Neuromuscular Blocking Agents

Patients with myasthenia gravis are usually resistant to succinylcholine, with larger than usual doses required to produce complete blockade. This effect might be offset by the inhibition of plasma cholinesterase activity provided by pyridostigmine. Sensitivity to nondepolarizing neuromuscular blocking drugs is increased to a variable extent, depending on the severity of the disease. The ED_{95} of vecuronium was found to be decreased by more than half in myasthenic patients, and the response of the orbicularis oculi muscle is depressed even more than that of the adductor pollicis muscle, reflecting some degree of ocular involvement.[120]

Management of Anesthesia

Traditionally, neuromuscular blocking drugs have been avoided in the patient with myasthenia gravis by the use of inhalational vapors with or without local anesthesia. More recently, there have been several reports of the successful use of small, titrated doses of atracurium, mivacurium, vecuronium, or rocuronium, administered under careful neuromuscular monitoring.[119] The effect of reversal drugs might be less than expected because myasthenic patients already receive drugs that produce cholinesterase inhibition. Thus, it is preferable to continue mechanical ventilation until spontaneous recovery is manifest. After thymectomy, the need for mechanical support of ventilation can usually be predicted from preoperative lung function tests.

Myotonia

The myotonias are a group of diseases characterized by an abnormal delay in muscle relaxation after contraction. They are classified into dystrophic and nondystrophic myotonias. By far the two most common forms of dystrophic myotonia (DM), or myotonic dystrophy, are Steinert's disease (DM1) and proximal myotonic dystrophy (DM2). Both these conditions are autosomal dominant, and are characterized by a defect in gene replication and splicing, leading to repeats.[121] Onset of Steinert's disease (DM1) is variable but occurs commonly in adolescence or early adulthood. Inability to relax the hand after a handshake is common. Common features of the disease are baldness, cataracts, cardiac conduction defects, sleep apnea, and mental retardation. Proximal myotonic dystrophy (DM2) is less common. The nondystrophic myotonias include a group of rare diseases due to abnormalities in ionic channels, such as myotonia congenita (Thomsen's and Becker's diseases, which are due to a defect of chloride channels), hyperkalemic periodic paralysis, and paramyotonia congenita.[121]

Response to Neuromuscular Blocking Agents

The characteristic response to succinylcholine in patients with myotonia is a sustained, dose-related contracture that may make ventilation difficult for several minutes.[121] Muscle membrane fragility may be responsible for the exaggerated hyperkalemia that is produced after succinylcholine.[47] Most case reports suggest that the response to nondepolarizing drugs is normal.[121] However, myotonic responses have been observed after reversal with neostigmine.

Anesthesia

Succinylcholine is best avoided. Short- or intermediate-duration nondepolarizing agents may be used in usual doses with careful neuromuscular monitoring. Anticholinesterases are best avoided, and mechanical ventilation should be maintained until the effects of nondepolarizing agents have worn off completely. Sugammadex has been used successfully in patients with myotonia.

Muscular Dystrophy

The muscular dystrophies are a group of many diseases, with variability in presentation and typical age at onset of symptoms, characterized by muscle weakness. The most common of these is the Duchenne-type muscular dystrophy (DMD), an X-linked hereditary disease that usually becomes apparent in childhood. Other types of muscular dystrophy include Becker, limb-girdle, fasciohumeral, Emery–Dreifuss, nemaline rod, and oculopharyngeal dystrophy.[122]

Response to Neuromuscular Blocking Agents

There have been several reports of cardiac arrest after administration of succinylcholine in children with muscle dystrophy, often associated with hyperkalemia and rhabdomyolysis. In several instances the disease was latent. Resuscitation was found to be difficult, and several of these cases were fatal.[47,122] The most likely explanation for these adverse events is previously undiagnosed, latent, muscular dystrophy. In most case reports, the response to nondepolarizing agents, such as vecuronium, atracurium, and mivacurium, has been described as normal, although there have been sporadic instances of increased sensitivity. There are little data on the response to anticholinesterases. Patients with DMD are probably no more susceptible to malignant hyperthermia than the rest of the population.

Anesthesia

Succinylcholine should be avoided in patients with muscular dystrophy, especially if onset of symptoms occurred in childhood or adolescence. The possibility of latent or unrecognized DMD in young males (<10 years old) may be a reason to avoid succinylcholine in this patient population. Careful titration of short- or intermediate-duration nondepolarizing agents should be done. Anticholinesterases do not appear to be contraindicated and sugammadex would seem to be a good choice.

Upper Motor Neuron Lesions

Patients with hemiplegia or quadriplegia as a result of central nervous system lesions show an abnormal response to both depolarizing and nondepolarizing agents. Hyperkalemia and cardiac arrest have been described after succinylcholine, probably as a result of extrajunctional receptor proliferation. Hyperkalemia is typically seen if the drug is given from 1 week to 6 months after the lesion, but may be seen before and after that period.[47] There is resistance to nondepolarizing neuromuscular blocking drugs below the level of the lesion. In hemiplegic patients, monitoring of the affected side shows that the block is less intense and recovery is more rapid than on the unaffected side. However, the apparently normal side also demonstrates some resistance to nondepolarizing drugs. Similar findings have been reported after a stroke, with a greater resistance on the affected side.

Burns

As a result of the proliferation of extrajunctional receptors, succinylcholine produces severe hyperkalemia in patients with burns, and this may lead to cardiac arrest. The magnitude of the problem depends on the extent of the injury. It may appear as early as 24 to 48 hours after the burn injury and usually ends with healing.[47] Resistance to the effects of nondepolarizing neuromuscular blocking agents is manifest, even in muscles that are apparently not affected by the burn.[59,60,74]

Miscellaneous

Denervated muscle demonstrates potassium release after succinylcholine and resistance to nondepolarizing relaxants. Contractures in response to succinylcholine have also been observed in amyotrophic lateral sclerosis and multiple sclerosis. There have been isolated reports of hyperkalemia after succinylcholine in several neurologic diseases, including Friedrich's ataxia, polyneuritis, and Parkinson's disease.

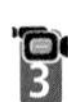

MONITORING NEUROMUSCULAR BLOCKADE

Why Monitor?

Deep levels of paralysis are usually desired during anesthesia to facilitate tracheal intubation and to obtain an immobile surgical field. However, complete return of respiratory function must be attained before the trachea is extubated. Administration of neuromuscular blocking drugs must be individualized because blockade occurs over a narrow range of receptor occupancy, and because there is considerable interindividual variability in response. Thus, it is important for the clinician to assess the effect of neuromuscular blocking drugs without the confounding influence of volatile agents, intravenous anesthetics, and opioids. One should remember, however, that monitoring is a tool, not a cure. Neuromuscular blocking agents have the same effects, whether or not monitoring is used. Some studies, but not all, found that careful monitoring is associated with a decrease in the incidence of residual paralysis, probably because the information obtained was treated differently in different studies.[21] To test the function of the neuromuscular junction, a peripheral nerve is stimulated electrically, and the response of the muscle is assessed.

Stimulator Characteristics

The response of the nerve to electrical stimulation depends on three factors: The current applied, the duration of the current, and the position of the electrodes. Stimulators should be able to deliver a maximum current in the range of 60 to 80 mA. Most stimulators are designed to provide constant current, irrespective of impedance changes due to drying of the electrode gel, cooling, decreased sweat gland function, and so forth. However, this constant current feature does not hold for high impedances (>5 kΩ). Thus, electrodes should be firmly applied to the skin. A current display monitor on the stimulator is an asset because accidental disconnection can be identified easily by a current approaching 0 mA. The duration of the current pulse should be long enough for all axons in the nerve to depolarize but short enough to avoid the possibility of exceeding the refractory period of the nerve. In practice, pulse durations of 0.1 to 0.2 ms are acceptable. At least one electrode should be on the skin overlying the nerve to be stimulated. If the negative electrode is used for this purpose, the threshold to supramaximal stimulation is less than that for the positive electrode. However, the difference is not large in practice. The position of the other electrode is not critical, but it should not be placed in the vicinity of other nerves. There is no need to use needle electrodes. Silver–silver chloride surface electrodes, used to monitor the electrocardiogram, are adequate for peripheral nerve stimulation, without the risk of bleeding, infection, and burns. In practice, applying these electrodes along the course of a nerve gives the best results (Fig. 20-12).

Monitoring Modalities

Different stimulation modalities were introduced into clinical practice to take advantage of the characteristic features of nondepolarizing neuromuscular blockade: Fade and post-tetanic facilitation with high frequency stimulation. Thus, the following discussion refers mostly to the nondepolarizing block.

Single Twitch

The simplest way to stimulate a nerve is to apply a single stimulus, at intervals of >10 seconds (frequency, <0.1 Hz). This interval is needed to allow the neuromuscular junction to recover if nondepolarizing agents are used. With shorter intervals, fade might be present. With depolarizing agents like succinylcholine, little fade occurs and a higher frequency, such as 1 Hz, may be used without concern for fade. The amplitude of response is compared with a control, pre-blockade twitch height. The single-twitch modality is useful to construct dose-response curves and to evaluate onset time. However, because a control value is required, the clinical usefulness of this mode of stimulation is limited.

Tetanus

When stimulation is applied at a frequency of ≥30 Hz, the mechanical response of the muscle is fusion of individual twitch

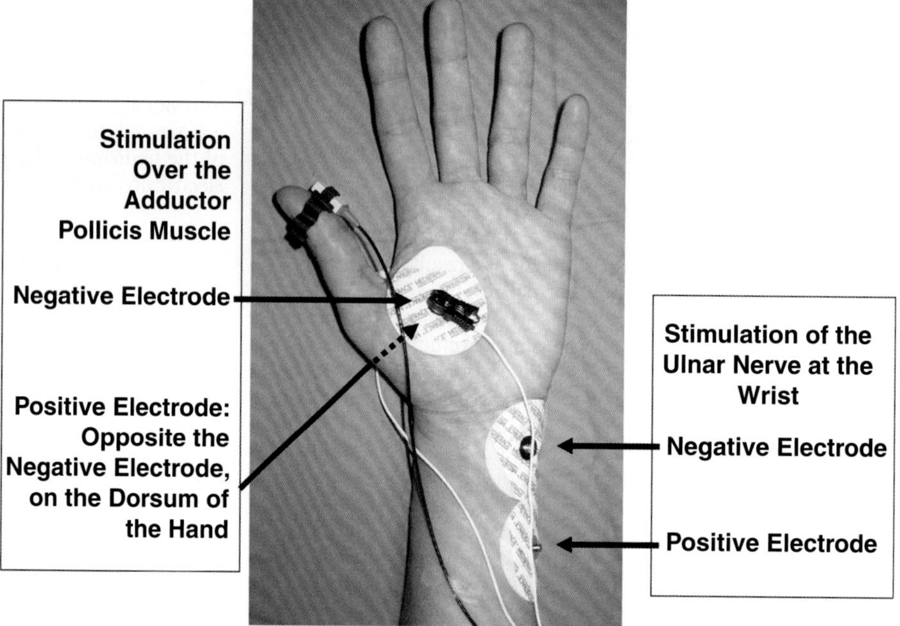

FIGURE 20-12. Electrode placement to obtain contraction of the adductor pollicis muscle. The traditional method is to apply the electrodes over the course of the ulnar nerve at the wrist, with the negative electrode distal (*right*). An alternate method is to position the electrodes over the adductor pollicis muscle (*left*), the negative electrode on the palm of the hand, the positive in the same location, but on the dorsum of the hand. The device fixed to the thumb is an accelerometer.

responses. In the absence of neuromuscular blocking drugs, no fade is present and the response is sustained. During nondepolarizing blockade, the mechanical response appears as a peak, followed by a fade (Fig. 20-8). The sensitivity of tetanic stimulation in the detection of residual neuromuscular blockade is greater than that of single twitch; that is, tetanic fade might be present while twitch height is normal. Most nerve stimulators provide a 5-second train at a frequency of 50 Hz. This frequency was adopted because at higher frequencies, some fade may be seen even in the absence of neuromuscular blocking drugs. However, more fade is seen with 100 Hz than 50 Hz frequencies, and 100 Hz, 5-second trains are most useful in the detection of residual block.[55,123] With tetanic stimulation, no control, pre-blockade response is required, as the degree of muscle paralysis can be assessed by the degree of fade following tetanic stimulation. However, the main disadvantage of this mode of stimulation is post-tetanic facilitation (Fig. 20-8), which is an enhanced response to any type of stimulation for a short period of time after the tetanus. The magnitude and duration of this facilitation depend on the frequency and duration of the tetanic stimulation. For a 50 Hz tetanus applied for 5 seconds, the duration of this interval appears to be at least 1 to 2 minutes.[56] If single-twitch stimulation is performed during that time, the response is spuriously exaggerated.

Train-of-four

With 2 Hz stimulation, the mechanical or electrical response decreases little after the fourth stimulus, and the degree of fade is similar to that found at 50 Hz. Thus, applying TOF stimulation at 2 Hz provides more sensitivity than single twitch and approximately the same sensitivity as tetanic stimulation at 50 Hz. In addition, this relatively low frequency allows the response to be evaluated manually or visually. Moreover, the presence of a small number of impulses (four) eliminates the problem of post-tetanic facilitation. Train-of-four stimulation can be repeated every 12 to 15 seconds. There is a fairly close relationship between single-twitch depression and TOF response, and no control is required for the latter. During recovery, the second twitch reappears at 80% to 90% single-twitch block, the third at 70% to 80%, and when blockade is 65% to 75%, all four twitches become visible.[124] Then, the TOF ratio, defined as the height of the fourth twitch to that of the first twitch, is linearly related to first twitch height when blockade is <70%. When single-twitch height has recovered to 100%, the TOF ratio is approximately 70%.

Post-tetanic Count

During profound neuromuscular blockade, there is no response to single-twitch, tetanic, or TOF stimulation. To estimate the time required before the return of a response, one may use a technique that depends on the principle of post-tetanic facilitation. A 50 Hz tetanus is applied for 5 seconds, followed by a 3-second pause and by a series of stimulations at 1 Hz. Facilitation produces a certain number of visible post-tetanic twitches (Fig. 20-13). The number of visible twitches correlates inversely with the time required for a return of single-twitch or TOF responses.[125] For intermediate-duration drugs, the time from a post-tetanic count (PTC) of 1 to reappearance of twitch is 15 to 30 minutes.

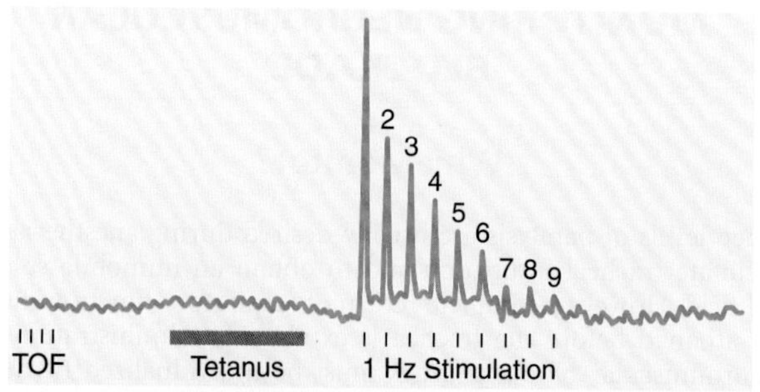

FIGURE 20-13. Post-tetanic count (PTC). During profound blockade, no response is seen to train-of-four (TOF) or tetanus. However, because there is post-tetanic facilitation, some twitches can be seen after tetanic stimulation. In this example, the PTC is 9.

Double-burst Stimulation

Train-of-four fade may be difficult to evaluate by visual or tactile means during recovery from neuromuscular blockade. Irrespective of experience, it is difficult for anesthesiologists to detect TOF fade when actual TOF ratio is 0.4 or greater, meaning that residual paralysis can go undetected.[123] This shortcoming can be overcome, to a certain extent, by applying two short tetanic stimulations (three impulses at 50 Hz, separated by 750 ms), and by evaluating the ratio of the second to the first response. The double-burst stimulation ratio correlates closely with the TOF ratio, but is easier to detect manually.[123] At least 12 to 15 seconds must elapse between two consecutive double-burst stimulations.

Recording the Response

The contractile response of a muscle following nerve stimulation can be assessed either with one's own senses (sight or touch), or with an instrument that measures force, electrical voltage, acceleration, movement, or sound generated by muscle activity. Visual and tactile assessment is qualitative, or subjective, because the response is assessed as present or absent, weak or strong; the other methods are called quantitative, or objective, because a number is associated with each response.[126]

Visual and Tactile Evaluation

The easiest and least expensive way to assess depth of paralysis is to observe or feel the contraction of the muscle following stimulation of the nerve. However, serious errors in assessment can be made when evaluating the response of the adductor pollicis muscle to ulnar nerve stimulation. The TOF count, or number of visible responses, can be made reliably during a surgical procedure,[124] but TOF fade is difficult to detect during recovery. Several investigations suggest that TOF ratios as low as 0.3[123] can be seen and felt as sustained. The detection rate for tetanic fade (50 Hz) is no better.[123] With double-burst stimulation, fade can be detected reliably up to TOF ratios in the range of 0.6 to 0.7.[123] With 100 Hz tetanic stimulation, fade might be detected at TOF ratios of 0.8 to 1.0[55,123] but it may be seen in individuals with no neuromuscular block.

Measurement of Force

A force transducer can overcome the shortcomings of one's senses. If applied correctly, force measurement, or mechanomyography (MMG), provides accurate and reliable responses, displayed as either a digital or an analog signal on a monitor. Force measurement can be measured after single-twitch, tetanus, TOF, double-burst, or post-tetanic stimulation. Unfortunately, MMG transducers are expensive, bulky, cumbersome, and can be applied to only one muscle, usually the adductor pollicis.[126]

Electromyography

It is possible to measure the electrical instead of the mechanical response of the muscle. One electrode should be positioned over the neuromuscular junction, which is usually close to the midportion of the muscle, and the other near the insertion of the muscle. A third, neutral electrode can be located anywhere else. Theoretically, any superficial muscle can be used for EMG recordings. In practice, such recordings are limited to the hypothenar eminence, the first dorsal interosseous, and the adductor pollicis muscles, which are all supplied by the ulnar nerve. Most EMG recording devices compute the area under the EMG curve during a specified time window after the stimulus is applied. There is usually good correlation between EMG and force of the adductor pollicis muscle if the EMG signal is taken from the thenar eminence.[126]

Accelerometry

According to Newton's law, acceleration is proportional to force if mass remains unchanged. Acceleromyography (AMG) devices are usually attached to the tip of the thumb (Fig. 20-12) and a digital readout is obtained. Contrary to MMG and EMG setups, the thumb must be free to move when AMG is measured. The setup is sensitive to inadvertent displacement of the thumb and, in the absence of neuromuscular blocking drugs, TOF ratios >100% can be obtained.[123,126] There have been attempts to reduce variability and TOF ratios >100% with the use of special soft splints or by holding the thumb with a small elastic band, with mixed results. In spite of these shortcomings, AMG monitors have become increasingly popular because they are easy to use, are less cumbersome, can be used on muscles other than the adductor pollicis, and are relatively inexpensive. The use of accelerometry is helpful in the diagnosis of residual paralysis, and in some instances may prevent the occurrence of the condition (Table 20-1).[18,20]

Displacement

A variety of instruments have been proposed that respond to motion or displacement, and thus qualify as kinemyography (KMG) devices. They usually consist of a flexible band placed between the thumb and the index finger.[126] A sensor supplies an electrical current when the band is bent. A thorough evaluation of these devices has not been made, but data indicate that there are slight but clinically insignificant differences between the results such displacement transducers and mechanomyography provide.[126] Contrary to AMG, KMG-measured TOF ratios do not normally exceed 100%.

Phonomyography

A contracting muscle emits low frequency sounds. TOF response and fade can be heard with a stethoscope placed over the adductor pollicis muscle. A quantitative response can be obtained with special microphones, and constitutes the basis for phonomyography, or PMG.[126] An excellent correlation exists between PMG and MMG has been found at several muscles, but at the time of writing, no commercial devices using PMG were available.

Choice of Muscle

Muscles do not respond in a uniform fashion to neuromuscular blocking drugs. After administration of a neuromuscular blocking agent, differences with respect to onset time, maximum blockade, and duration of action can be measured between muscles. It is not practical to monitor the muscles of physiologic importance, for example, the abdominal muscles during surgery, or the respiratory and upper airway muscles postoperatively. A better approach is to choose a monitoring site that has a response similar to the muscle of interest. For example, monitoring the response of the facial nerve around the eye is a good indicator of intubating conditions, and the use of the adductor pollicis muscle during recovery reflects upper airway muscle function. Another strategy is to stick to one monitoring site, such as the adductor pollicis muscle, and interpret the information provided from knowledge of the different responses between muscles (Fig. 20-14).

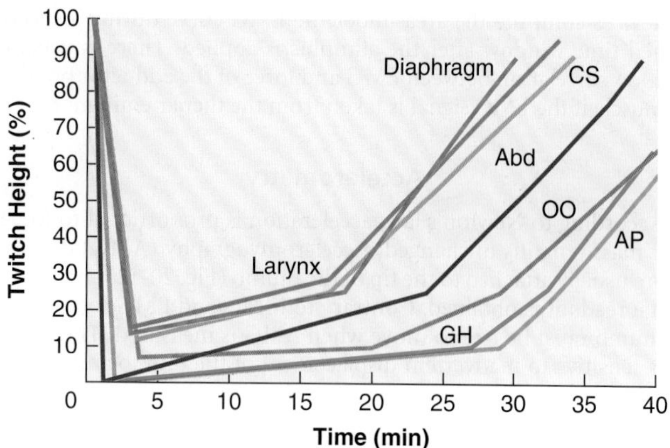

FIGURE 20-14. Approximate time course of twitch height after rocuronium, 0.6 mg/kg, at different muscles. Larynx, laryngeal adductors (vocal cords); CS, corrugator supercilii muscle (eyebrow); Abd, abdominal muscles; OO, orbicularis oculi muscle (eyelid); GH, geniohyoid muscle (upper airway); AP, adductor pollicis muscle (thumb). (Data are taken or inferred from references Plaud B, Debaene B, Donati F. The corrugator supercilii, not the orbicularis oculi, reflects rocuronium neuromuscular blockade at the laryngeal adductor muscles. *Anesthesiology.* 2001;95:96–101; Dhonneur G, Kirov K, Slavov V, et al. Effects of an intubating dose of succinylcholine and rocuronium on the larynx and diaphragm: An electromyographic study in humans. *Anesthesiology.* 1999;90:951–955; Kirov K, Motamed C, Ndoko SK, et al. TOF count at corrugator supercilii reflects abdominal muscles relaxation better than at adductor pollicis. *Br J Anaesth.* 2007;98:611–614; and Nepveu ME, Donati F, Fortier LP. Train-of-four stimulation for adductor pollicis neuromuscular monitoring can be applied at the wrist or over the hand. *Anesth Analg.* 2005;100:149–154.)

Adductor Pollicis Muscle

The adductor pollicis muscle is accessible during most surgical procedures. It is supplied by the ulnar nerve, which becomes superficial at the wrist where a negative electrode can be positioned. The positive electrode is applied a few centimeters proximally (Fig. 20-12). The force of contraction of the adductor pollicis muscle can be measured with transducers, and it has become a standard in research. After injection of a dose that produces less than 100% blockade, the time to maximal blockade is longer than in centrally located muscles.[129,130] The adductor pollicis muscle is relatively sensitive to nondepolarizing neuromuscular blocking drugs, so it recovers later than the diaphragm,[129] laryngeal adductors,[130] and abdominal muscles (Fig. 20-14).[127] Recovery of upper airway muscles such as the geniohyoid and the adductor pollicis occurs more or less simultaneously (Fig. 20-14), so that residual blockade the adductor pollicis indicates the possibility of upper airway obstruction.[131]

The adductor pollicis muscle can also be stimulated by applying electrodes directly over it, in the space lying between the base of the first and second metacarpals, on the palmar and dorsal aspects on the hand, respectively (Fig. 20-12). Such a stimulation avoids the confounding movement of hypothenar muscles. The current to obtain direct muscle stimulation with this electrode position is much higher than for nerve stimulation. Confirmation that direct muscle stimulation does not normally occur can be obtained when neuromuscular blocking agents abolish the response completely.[128] The ability to detect fade by visual or tactile means is the same, whether the stimulating electrodes are applied at the wrist or the hand.[123]

Other Muscles of the Hand

Ulnar nerve stimulation also produces flexion and abduction of the fifth finger, which usually recovers before the adductor pollicis muscle, the discrepancy in first twitch or TOF ratio being of the order of 15% to 20%.[132] Relying on the response of the fifth finger might overestimate recovery from blockade. Abduction of the index finger also results from stimulation of the ulnar nerve because of contraction of the first dorsal interosseous, the sensitivity of which is comparable with that of the adductor pollicis muscle. The hypothenar eminence (near the fifth finger) and the first dorsal interosseous are particularly well suited for EMG recordings.[132] Stimulation in the hand (Fig. 20-12) eliminates contraction of the hypothenar muscles, but may evoke movement of the first dorsal interosseous.

Muscles Surrounding the Eye

There are two important muscles around the eye, both supplied by the facial nerve, with major differences in response of muscles and these differences have introduced some confusion in the literature. The orbicularis oculi muscle essentially covers the *eyelid,* and its response to neuromuscular blocking agents is similar to that of the adductor pollicis muscle.[80] However, the muscle that moves the *eyebrow* is the corrugator supercilii, and recordings at that site are similar to that of the laryngeal adductors (Fig. 20-14), with a faster onset and more rapid recovery than at the adductor pollicis.[80] Thus, facial nerve stimulation with inspection of the response of the eyebrow is indicated to predict intubating conditions and to monitor profound blockade.[129] The facial nerve can be stimulated 2 to 3 cm posterior to the lateral border of the orbit. There is no need to use stimulating currents >20 to 30 mA.

Muscles of the Foot

The posterior tibial nerve can be stimulated behind the internal malleolus to produce flexion of the big toe by contraction of the flexor hallucis muscle. The response of this muscle is comparable with that of the adductor pollicis muscle. Stimulation of the external peroneal nerve produces dorsiflexion, but the sensitivity of the muscles involved has not been measured.

Clinical Applications

Interpretation of monitoring depends on the context during which neuromuscular blocking agents or reversal drugs are given. Typically, one needs monitoring to predict intubating conditions, to provide relaxation during the surgical procedure, and to assess readiness for, and effectiveness of, reversal agents. These situations are summarized in Table 20-4.

Monitoring Onset

The quality of intubating conditions depends chiefly on the state of relaxation of muscles of the jaw, pharynx, larynx, and respiratory system, where paralysis will occur sooner because of a greater blood flow than in the more peripheral muscles of the hand or foot. Among these centrally located muscles, the laryngeal adductors and the diaphragm are the most resistant to nondepolarizing agents, so both need a relatively large dose to be blocked completely, allowing easy passage of a tracheal tube through the vocal cords and absence of coughing. As a result of different sensitivities and onset times, blockade in laryngeal and hand muscles after a bolus dose of neuromuscular blocking agent might follow

TABLE 20-4. SUGGESTED MANAGEMENT OF NEUROMUSCULAR BLOCKADE ACCORDING TO MONITORING

Site	Modality	Response	Interpretation	Comments
Prediction of Tracheal Intubating Conditions				
Any site	Single twitch, TOF	Present	Adequate conditions not met	Deep blockade is required for intubation
Corrugator supercilii	Single twitch, TOF	Absent	Adequate conditions likely	Corrugator supercilii reflects vocal cords and diaphragm
Adductor pollicis	Single twitch, TOF	Absent	Adequate conditions likely only if high dose given	Adductor pollicis is more sensitive than vocal cords and diaphragm
Flexor hallucis (foot)	Single twitch, TOF	Absent	Adequate conditions likely only if high dose given	Foot muscles are sensitive and block late
Intraoperative Conditions				
Adductor pollicis	PTC	1–2	Very deep blockade	Return of diaphragm movements possible, no TOF response at adductor pollicis
Corrugator supercilii	TOF	1–2	Deep blockade	Return of abdominal tone possible, no TOF response at adductor pollicis
Adductor pollicis	TOF	1–2	Moderate blockade	Usually sufficient for most procedures
Corrugator supercilii	TOF	4, with or without fade	Moderate to shallow blockade	Difficult to interpret without adductor pollicis data
Adductor pollicis	TOF	4, with or without fade	Shallow blockade	Additional relaxation might be needed
Management of Recovery				
Adductor pollicis	PTC	0	Wait or sugammadex 16 mg/kg	Sugammadex after rocuronium or vecuronium only
Adductor pollicis	PTC	1–2	Wait or sugammadex 4 mg/kg	
Corrugator supercilii	TOF	1–2	Wait or sugammadex 4 mg/kg	
Adductor pollicis	TOF	2	Wait or sugammadex 2 mg/kg	
Corrugator supercilii	TOF	4 with or without fade	Wait or correlate with adductor pollicis or sugammadex 4 mg/kg	Corrugator supercilii recovers early. Correlation with adductor pollicis preferable
Hypothenar eminence (5th finger)	TOF	4 with or without fade	Observe thumb motion	Adductor pollicis recovers later
Adductor pollicis	TOF, visual or tactile	4 with fade	Wait or neostigmine 0.04–0.05 mg/kg or sugammadex 2 mg/kg	Neostigmine: After any nondepolarizing agent
Adductor pollicis	TOF, visual or tactile	4 without fade	Wait or neostigmine 0.020 mg/kg	
Adductor pollicis	DBS, visual or tactile	Fade	Wait or neostigmine 0.02–0.05 mg/kg	Less neostigmine needed if no TOF fade
Adductor pollicis	DBS, visual or tactile	No fade	Wait or neostigmine 0.020 mg/kg	DBS fade detected when TOF ratio = 0.6
Adductor pollicis	TOF, quantitative	TOF ratio <0.90	Wait or neostigmine	Neostigmine 0.04–0.05 mg/kg if TOF ratio <0.4; 0.02 mg/kg if TOF ratio >0.4
Adductor pollicis	100 Hz	No fade	No reversal necessary	100 Hz detected when TOF ratio = 0.8–0.9
Adductor pollicis	TOF, quantitative	TOF ratio ≥0.9	No reversal necessary	

TOF, train of four; PTC, post-tetanic count; DBS, double burst stimulation.
Actual management depends on patient, surgical procedure, and previous response to neuromuscular blocking agents.

one of three patterns. At relatively low doses (e.g., rocuronium, 0.3 mg/kg), onset time is slower at the adductor pollicis than at the laryngeal muscles, but blockade is incomplete at both muscles. If the dose is increased (e.g., rocuronium, 0.5 mg/kg), onset is faster at the adductor pollicis muscle because these doses produce 100% blockade at the adductor pollicis without blocking laryngeal muscles completely (Fig. 20-14).[81] Onset time decreases considerably in any muscle if the dose given is sufficient to reach 100%. Finally, if the dose is large enough (e.g., rocuronium, 1.0 mg/kg) to block the laryngeal muscles completely, onset time again becomes shorter at the larynx. It is not surprising that monitoring the adductor pollicis muscle predicts intubating conditions poorly. Facial nerve stimulation with visual observation of the response over the eyebrow gives better results because the response of the corrugator supercilii is close to that of the vocal cords. TOF fade takes longer to develop than single-twitch depression (Fig. 20-8), and during onset, TOF stimulation does not have any advantages over single-twitch stimulation at 0.1 Hz.

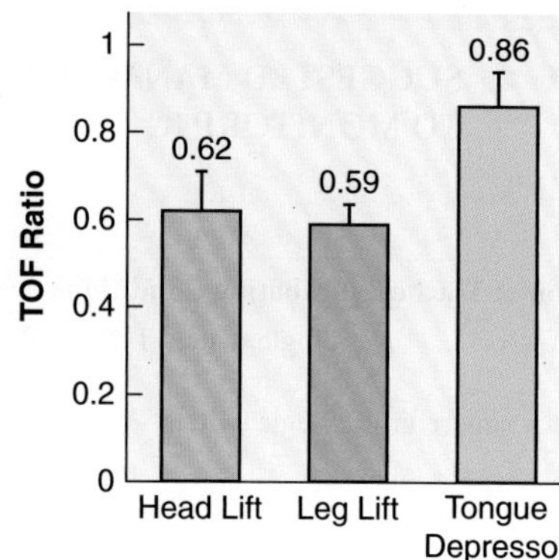

FIGURE 20-15. Correlation between train-of-four (TOF) responses at the adductor pollicis muscle and certain clinical tests of neuromuscular recovery. Volunteers were given mivacurium and were asked to lift their heads for 5 seconds (head lift), lift their legs for 5 seconds (leg lift), or hold a tongue depressor between their teeth against force (tongue depressor). The minimum TOF ratio (and SD) when each of these tests was passed is indicated. (Data from: Kopman et al.[134]).

Monitoring Surgical Relaxation

Adequate surgical relaxation is usually obtained when fewer than two or three visible twitches are observed at the adductor pollicis muscle, but this level might be insufficient in many cases. Diaphragmatic movements and abdominal tone may return earlier than the twitch response at the adductor pollicis.[129,127] Giving more neuromuscular blocking agent to deepen blockade will abolish these movements, but are not the only method to solve the problem. Administration of opioids, increasing the concentration of inhalational agents, and/or hyperventilation to decrease CO_2 might be indicated. An additional dose of neuromuscular blocking agent, especially if given toward the end of the procedure, might delay recovery, unless sugammadex reversal is planned. To monitor profound relaxation, the PTC can be used at the adductor pollicis muscle,[125] provided that this type of stimulation is not repeated more often than every 2 to 3 minutes. A suitable alternative is stimulation of the facial nerve with observation of the response over the eyebrow, which recovers at the same rate as such resistant muscles as the diaphragm.[129]

Monitoring Recovery

Complete return of neuromuscular function should be achieved at the conclusion of surgery before one proceeds with extubation. Traditionally, a TOF ratio of 0.7 was considered to be the threshold below which residual weakness of the respiratory muscles could be present. There is abundant evidence that significant weakness may occur up to TOF ratio values of 0.9, and that this is due to incomplete return of upper airway function.[18,22,133] Awake volunteers given mivacurium failed to perform the head-lift test when the TOF ratio at the adductor pollicis muscle decreased below 0.62, but needed a TOF ratio of at least 0.86 to hold a tongue depressor between their teeth (Fig. 20-15).[134] These data suggest that the head-lift test does not guarantee full recovery, and that the upper airway muscles used to retain a tongue depressor are very sensitive to the residual effects of neuromuscular blocking drugs. Furthermore, impairment in swallowing and laryngeal aspiration of a pharyngeal fluid was observed at TOF ratios as high as 0.9 in volunteers given vecuronium (Fig. 20-4).[22] Supraglottic area was reduced in volunteers who received a rocuronium infusion to a TOF of 0.8.[136] Whereas tidal volume and end-tidal CO_2 are preserved in awake patients receiving relatively high doses of neuromuscular blocking drugs, administration of small doses of vecuronium to maintain TOF at <0.9 leads to severe impairment of the ventilatory response to hypoxia (Fig. 20-16).[135] The response to hypercapnia is maintained, and this indicates that the response to hypoxia is not a result of respiratory muscle weakness.[135] In patients, airway obstruction, hypoxemia, and dyspnea are more likely to occur when TOF ratio is <0.9.[133] Taken together, the results of these investigations indicate that normal respiratory and upper airway function does not return to normal unless the TOF ratio at the adductor pollicis muscle is 0.9 or more.

Monitoring at the end of a surgical procedure is important to determine the type and dose of reversal agent required. Anticholinesterase agents should be given only when four twitches are visible at the adductor pollicis muscle,[126] which corresponds to a first-twitch recovery of >25%. Sugammadex may be given at deeper level of blockade, but the dose depends on the intensity of paralysis.[126] The presence of spontaneous breathing is not a sign of adequate neuromuscular recovery, because the diaphragm recovers earlier than the much more sensitive upper airway muscles, such as the geniohyoid, which recovers, on average, at the same time as the adductor pollicis muscle.[131] Therefore, the adductor pollicis muscle should be used to monitor recovery, instead of

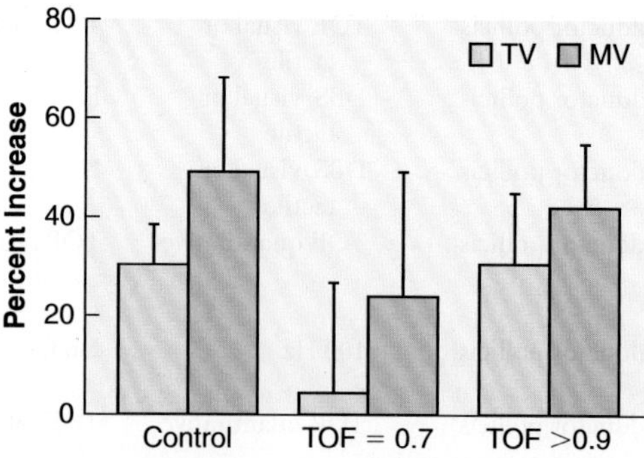

FIGURE 20-16. Response to hypoxia is impaired during recovery from vecuronium blockade. Normal response is an increase in minute volume (MV) or tidal volume (TV; control). These increases are decreased significantly when vecuronium produces a train-of-four ratio (TOF) of 0.7 at the adductor pollicis muscle. They return to near-normal values at a TOF >0.9. (Data from: Eriksson et al.[135]).

the more resistant muscles of the hypothenar eminence or those around the eye.

Human senses are poor at detecting fade when the TOF is >0.4, so the visual or tactile evaluation of TOF response is not reliable for ruling out residual blockade, defined as a TOF ratio of <0.9.[123] Compared with TOF, the ability to detect fade is not improved by using tetanic stimulation at 50 Hz for 5 seconds.[123] With double-burst stimulation, detection failures may occur at TOF ratios of 0.6 to 0.7.[123] However, fade can be detected visually at TOF ratios of 0.8 to 0.9 by using 100 Hz tetanic stimulation,[55,123] although this threshold may vary from patient to patient.[123] A 100 Hz stimulation is painful, and should not be applied to awake or lightly anesthetized patients. Traditionally, a 5-minute interval was recommended between a 50 and 100 Hz tetanus and subsequent stimuli, because of the presence of post-tetanic facilitation. But a 2-minute interval is probably sufficient.[56] Mechanographic and EMG equipments give reliable values of TOF ratio, but the use of this equipment is limited by size, cost, and convenience. Accelerometers are less bulky and cheaper, but they can overestimate the value of TOF ratio during recovery.[123,126] It has been suggested that a TOF ratio of 1.0 obtained by AMG must be obtained before neuromuscular function can be considered complete.[123] Monitoring devices based on the measurement of displacement may prove to have more reliable TOF ratios than AMG. Intraoperative monitoring using AMG has been shown to decrease the incidence of symptoms of residual paralysis.[18,20]

Quantitative monitoring is not available everywhere,[63] so the clinician should be aware of the shortcomings of qualitative monitoring. When only visual and tactile methods are available, it is recommended to wait until a TOF count of four is obtained before administering an anticholinesterase drug, and to be prepared to wait as long as 15 to 20 minutes for the full response of the anticholinesterase agent in some patients. Extubation may be performed before if the patient is not at risk of aspiration and if measures are taken to maintain the upper airway patent, such as the application of jaw thrust, the insertion of an oral or nasal airway, and/or positioning the patient in the most comfortable position (the lateral or upright position). Potential problems with neuromuscular recovery should be anticipated early by identifying patients at risk for postoperative upper airway obstruction (neck surgery, sleep apnea, obesity, respiratory disease, neuromuscular disease), frequent neuromuscular monitoring throughout the anesthetic to get a sense of how the individual patient responds to neuromuscular blocking drugs, and by refraining to administer too much neuromuscular blocking drug toward the end of the procedure.

Factors Affecting the Monitoring of Neuromuscular Blockade

Many drugs interfere with neuromuscular function and these are dealt with elsewhere (see "Drug Interactions"). However, certain situations make the interpretation of data on neuromuscular function difficult. Central hypothermia may slow the metabolism of neuromuscular blocking agents and prolong blockade in all muscles of the body.[137] If the extremity where monitoring is performed is cold, the degree of block will be accentuated. Thus, if only the monitored hand is cold, without central hypothermia, the degree of paralysis will appear deeper.[137] Resistance to nondepolarizing neuromuscular blocking drugs occurs with nerve damage, including peripheral nerve trauma, cord transection, and stroke. In this case, monitoring of the involved limb would tend to underestimate the degree of muscle paralysis. Depth of paralysis should also be adjusted for the type of patient, as well as the type of surgery. For example, it is not necessary to paralyze frail individuals or patients at the extremes of age to the same extent as young muscular adults. The same applies to patients with debilitating muscular diseases.

Neuromuscular monitoring by itself does not guarantee adequate relaxation during surgery and complete recovery postoperatively. The surgical field may be poor in spite of full paralysis of the hand because of a difference in response between muscles. Residual paralysis might occur because of excess neuromuscular blocking agents given, early administration of reversal, or an abnormal response of the patient. The effect of the neuromuscular blocking drug is the same whether or not monitoring is used. Neuromuscular monitoring can help in the diagnosis of inadequate skeletal muscle relaxation during surgery or insufficient recovery after surgery, but does not, in itself, treat these conditions.

REVERSAL OF NEUROMUSCULAR BLOCK

Residual Paralysis

In most circumstances, all efforts should be made to ensure that the patient leaves the operating room with unimpaired muscle strength. Specifically, respiratory and upper airway muscles must function normally so the patient can breathe, cough, swallow secretions, and keep his or her airway patent. Three strategies can be adopted to achieve this goal. The first is to titrate neuromuscular blocking agents carefully so that no residual effect is manifest at the end of surgery. The second is to accelerate recovery by giving an anticholinesterase agent. This second option gives the opportunity to maintain a deeper level of blockade until the end of surgery. A third possibility is selective binding of the neuromuscular blocking agent with specific cyclodextrin molecule to restore neuromuscular function. This last option was not available in North America at the time of writing. All three strategies involve careful monitoring of blockade.

Assessment of Neuromuscular Blockade

Spontaneous breathing can resume even if relatively deep degrees of paralysis are still present because of the relative diaphragm-sparing effect of neuromuscular blocking agents. Spontaneous ventilation, adequate to prevent hypercapnia, can be maintained despite considerable measurable skeletal muscle weakness if a patent airway is ensured. However, the weakest point in the respiratory system is the upper airway. When given vecuronium, swallowing was impaired and laryngeal aspiration occurred when the TOF was ≤0.9.[22] These problems are difficult to diagnose when a
8 tracheal tube is in place. Consequently, several indirect indices, which are easier to measure, have been correlated with the more specific tests of lung and upper airway function.

Clinical Evaluation

Several crude tests have been suggested, including head lift for 5 seconds, tongue protrusion, hand grip, and the ability to lift the legs off the bed to determine recovery of neuromuscular function.[133] There is good evidence that head lift and leg lift for 5 seconds are rather crude tests of recovery, as patients have the ability to perform these maneuvers when TOF ratio is as low as 0.6 (Fig. 20-15).[134] A more sensitive test is the ability to hold the jaws shut and prevent removal of a tongue depressor. This maneuver correlated with a TOF ratio measured at the adductor pollicis muscle of >0.86, whereas head lift and leg lift could be performed at more intense levels of paralysis (Fig. 20-15).[134] All subjects complained of visual symptoms until TOF ratio was >0.9. Pressure measurements in the upper esophagus have been shown to be decreased (Fig. 20-4) and laryngeal aspiration detected at a TOF ratio <0.9.[22] Thus, it appears that a normal head lift or leg lift is insufficient to guarantee normal upper airway function. The ability to resist removal of an object (such as a tongue depressor or a tracheal tube) from the mouth by closing the teeth probably correlates better with adequate upper airway function.

Evoked Responses to Nerve Stimulation

The clinical tests previously described are usually unobtainable in the patient recovering from anesthesia. Furthermore, it is preferable to assess the degree of recovery before emergence. Evoked responses to nerve stimulation are then appropriate. The target is a TOF ratio >0.9, considering that upper airway function does not recover completely until the TOF ratio at the adductor pollicis muscle is at least 0.9.

The decision to omit pharmacologic reversal of neuromuscular blockade must be made carefully because the presence of residual paralysis may be missed. A long time since the last dose of neuromuscular blocking agent is not a guarantee that recovery is complete. Residual paralysis has been found as long as 4 hours after an intubating dose of an intermediate-duration agent.[15] As mentioned earlier, visual and tactile evaluation of neuromuscular blockade by TOF or 50 Hz tetanic stimulation may fail to detect fade.[123] Double-burst stimulation is more sensitive, but becomes unreliable at TOF ratios in the range of 0.6 to 0.9.[123] The most sensitive test is the ability to maintain sustained contraction to 100 Hz tetanus for 5 seconds. Fade may be detected when TOF ratio is as high as 0.8 to 0.9.[55,123] Tetanic stimulation at 100 Hz is painful and must be performed only in adequately anesthetized patients.

Because of the limitations of the visual and tactile estimate of the TOF response during recovery, quantitative measurement has been advocated.[126] Acceleromyographic (AMG) or kinemyographic (KMG) methods are probably the most convenient. However, it must be appreciated that the TOF ratio obtained with AMG is greater than that measured with MMG and may exceed 1.0. An accelerographic TOF ratio of 1.0 has been proposed as the equivalent of a mechanomyographic TOF of 0.9.[123]

Residual Paralysis

Several studies have demonstrated that residual neuromuscular blockade is frequent in patients in the recovery room after surgery. In 1979, Viby-Mogensen et al.[11] found in 72 adult patients given long-acting agents that the TOF ratio was 0.7 in 30 (42%) patients, and that 16 of the 68 patients (24%) who were awake were unable to sustain head lift for 5 seconds. In that study, the patients received appropriate doses of neostigmine. Similar results have been obtained in other parts of the world (Table 20-1).[21,126] Early studies on the problem of residual paralysis used a TOF ratio of 0.7 for residual paralysis, which was the accepted threshold at the time. If the current 0.9 criterion had been applied in the study of Viby-Mogensen et al.,[11] 72% of patients would have been classified as having residual block. Residual paralysis, whether defined as TOF ratio of 0.7 or 0.9, is less frequent but not abolished if intermediate agents are substituted for the long-acting drugs and if reversal is given.[12,16,21] If intermediate-duration agents are used and neostigmine reversal is given, the TOF ratio is <0.7 in fewer than 10% of patients. However, as many as 40% of patients may have a TOF ratio <0.9, which indicates that residual paralysis is a significant problem.[21] Subjects emerging from anesthesia with a TOF ratio <0.9 are more likely to suffer episodes of oxygen desaturation, airway obstruction,[18] and muscle weakness,[20] and tend to stay longer in the postanesthesia care unit.[19]

The role of neuromuscular monitoring in the prevention of residual paralysis has been controversial. Naguib et al.[21] reviewed many studies and concluded that the use of a conventional nerve stimulator with qualitative evaluation did not reduce the incidence of residual paralysis. However, the number of studies was small, the results were heavily dependent on study design, and in most studies the total dose of neuromuscular blocking agent was the same in the monitored and the non-monitored groups. More recently, the use of AMG has been associated with a lower incidence of residual paralysis than the use of qualitative monitoring, in spite of similar doses of neuromuscular blocking agent in both groups.[18,20] However, the most important reason for high incidence of residual paralysis seems to be omission of reversal agents.[21] In one study, more systematic institution of pharmacologic reversal and neuromuscular monitoring was associated with a decrease in the incidence of residual paralysis (TOF >0.9) from 62% to 3%.[17]

Clinical Importance

Residual paralysis in the recovery room has been shown to be associated with significant morbidity. In 1997, Berg et al.[14] studied nearly 700 general surgical patients who randomly received pancuronium, vecuronium, or atracurium to produce surgical relaxation. In patients who had received pancuronium, the incidence of postoperative partial paralysis, defined by the then-accepted criterion of a TOF ratio <0.7, was five times that in patients receiving either of the two intermediate-acting drugs (26% vs. 5%). In addition, the incidence of atelectasis demonstrated on chest radiographs taken 2 days later was greater in patients who had received pancuronium and who had not attained a TOF ratio of 0.7 (16%) than in those who exceeded this threshold (4.8%).[14] In a study involving 246 patients, readiness for discharge from the postanesthesia care unit was found to be 224 minutes in patients with a TOF ratio <0.9, compared with only 149 minutes for those with no residual paralysis when admitted to the postanesthesia care unit.[19] In a large study involving over 800,000 patients, the adjusted odds ratio for 24-hour mortality was 10 times greater in patients not receiving reversal of neuromuscular blockade compared with those receiving it.[138] Although the cause and effect relationship cannot be established in this retrospective study, it is possible that unsuspected respiratory failure was involved in these cases.[138]

Anticholinesterase Agents

Acetylcholinesterase inhibitors, also called anticholinesterase agents, have been widely used to reverse the effect of neuromuscular blocking agents. The pharmacologic principle involved is inhibition of acetylcholine breakdown to increase its concentration of acetylcholine at the neuromuscular junction, thus tilting the competition for receptors in favor of the neurotransmitter. The traditional anticholinesterase drugs are neostigmine, edrophonium, and pyridostigmine. All three drugs have a similar duration of action (1 to 2 hours), and they differ by their onset of action. Peak action of edrophonium is reached within 1 to 2 minutes, but the drug appeared to be less effective than neostigmine when antagonizing moderate to deep blockade. Availability of edrophonium is limited. Pyridostigmine has fallen out of favor because of a longer onset of action than neostigmine. The most commonly used anticholinesterase agent worldwide is neostigmine. Other drugs such as suramin and 3–4 aminopyridine are not as effective, or more toxic, or both. The monopoly occupied by neostigmine is now challenged, at least in certain areas of the world, by the introduction of a selective binding agent, sugammadex. Although most of the following applies to edrophonium and pyridostigmine, the discussion that follows will focus on neostigmine.

Neostigmine: Mechanism of Action

Neostigmine is a reversible acetylcholinesterase inhibitor, but this may not be the only mechanism by which blockade is antagonized. This inhibition is present at all cholinergic synapses in the peripheral nervous system. Thus, neostigmine has potent parasympathomimetic activity, which is attenuated or abolished by the administration of an antimuscarinic agent, atropine or glycopyrrolate. Neostigmine, edrophonium, and pyridostigmine are quaternary ammonium compounds, which do not penetrate the blood–brain barrier well. Thus, although these agents have the ability to affect cholinergic function in the central nervous system, the concentrations in the brain are usually too small for such an effect. Physostigmine is an anticholinesterase that can cross the blood–brain barrier easily. For this reason, it is not used to reverse neuromuscular blockade. Donepezil, used in the management of Alzheimer's disease, also inhibits acetylcholinesterase and crosses the blood–brain barrier.

Inhibition of acetylcholinesterase results in an increased amount of acetylcholine reaching the receptor and in a longer time for acetylcholine to remain in the synaptic cleft. This causes an increase in the size and duration of the end plate potentials.[139] There is evidence that some of the effects of neostigmine are not the result of cholinesterase inhibition.[139] Anticholinesterases also have presynaptic effects. In the absence of neuromuscular blocking drugs, they potentiate the normal twitch response in a way similar to succinylcholine, probably as a result of the generation of action potentials that spread antidromically. A ceiling effect, that is, the inability for large doses to produce an increasing effect, has been demonstrated in vitro[140] and can be observed in patients.[141]

Neostigmine Block

Large doses of anticholinesterases, especially if given when neuromuscular block is absent, may produce evidence of neuromuscular dysfunction. For example, neostigmine given when neuromuscular function had recovered to a TOF ratio of 1.0 produced increased collapsibility of the upper airway and a reduced activity of the genioglossus muscle in volunteers when a negative pressure was applied.[142] The problem might be less when some degree of neuromuscular blockade is present before neostigmine is given. The mechanism involved is uncertain. There are no clinical reports of postoperative weakness attributed to reversal agents. Still, it appears prudent to reduce the dose of anticholinesterase agent if recovery from neuromuscular block is almost complete.

Potency

When considering the relationship between dose and response for anticholinesterase agents, several factors need to be taken into account. These drugs are normally given when a certain degree of blockade is present, and neuromuscular function is already recovering at a certain rate. To obtain the effect of the anticholinesterase agent alone, the level of neuromuscular block has to be maintained constant. This constant neuromuscular blockade can be accomplished *in vitro* in rat hemidiaphragms perfused with a constant concentration of a neuromuscular blocking agent. Bartkowski et al.[140] showed with a constant concentration of pancuronium, that edrophonium, neostigmine, and pyridostigmine produced dose-related reversal of twitch height, with the effect reaching a maximum when a certain dose was attained. For example, when

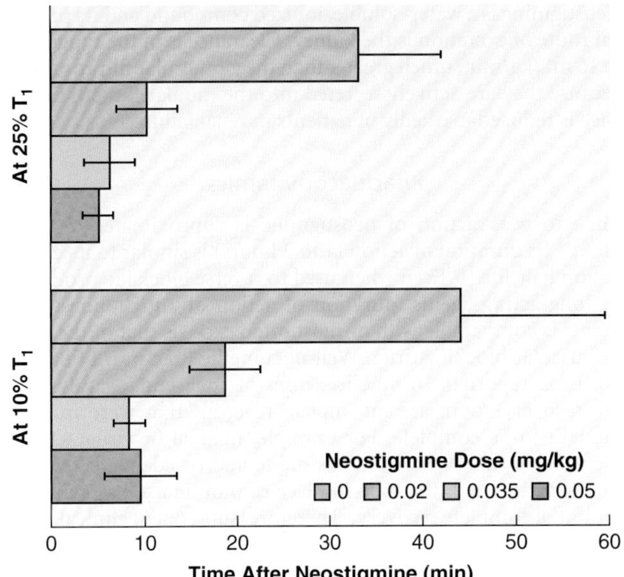

FIGURE 20-17. Neostigmine is more effective at greater degree of recovery from rocuronium blockade. Time to reach a train-of-four (TOF) ratio of 0.8 after various doses of neostigmine. This time is less if neostigmine is given at 25% than at 10% first-twitch recovery. Notice a ceiling effect for neostigmine at doses >0.035 mg/kg. A dose of 0 indicates no reversal given. (Data from: McCourt KC, Mirakhur RK, Kerr CM. Dosage of neostigmine for reversal of rocuronium block from two levels of spontaneous recovery. *Anaesthesia*. 1999;54:651–655.)

initial twitch height was 0.4 (60% block), large concentrations of neostigmine produced a TOF ratio of 0.95; when initial twitch height was 0.05 (95% block), the maximum neostigmine effect plateaued at a TOF ratio of 0.8. This ceiling effect was seen for all three anticholinesterase agents. A similar situation was created in patients, when a large dose of neostigmine (70 μg/kg) was given during a constant infusion of vecuronium adjusted to keep first twitch blockade at 95%. Peak effect was seen in approximately 5 minutes, but median TOF ratio was only 0.54, an indication that reversal of deep blockade with neostigmine is incomplete.[143] In practice, however, neostigmine is given when the effect of the neuromuscular blocking agent is wearing off. Not surprisingly, recovery was found to be more complete (TOF ratio approximately 0.9 after 15 minutes) with the intermediate acting agents than with the longer acting pancuronium (mean TOF ratio 0.76).[144] Neostigmine in this case was given at 25% twitch height recovery. If neostigmine is given at a deeper level of block (10% twitch height) time to complete recovery is increased (Figure 20-17).[141] Recovery time was also shown to depend on the dose of neostigmine, but a maximum effect was seen at high doses; recovery time was similar for 0.035 and 0.05 mg/kg, suggesting that the ceiling effect is present at doses commonly used clinically.[141] Taken together, these data indicate that anticholinesterase-assisted recovery is the sum of two components: (1) spontaneous recovery from the neuromuscular blocking agent itself, which is a reflection of the pharmacokinetic characteristics of the drug; and (2) assisted recovery, which depends on the dose and type of anticholinesterase agent given.

Pharmacokinetics

Following bolus intravenous injection, the plasma concentration of neostigmine decreases rapidly during the first 5 to 10 minutes and then more slowly. Its volume of distribution is in the range of 0.7 to 1.4 L/kg and the elimination half-life is 60 to 120 minutes.[143]

Neostigmine is a water-soluble, ionized compound and its principal route of excretion is the kidney. Clearance is in the range of 8 to 16 mL/kg/min, much greater than the glomerular filtration rate because they are actively secreted into the tubular lumen. Clearance is reduced markedly in patients in renal failure.

Pharmacodynamics

Time to peak action of neostigmine is approximately 5 minutes.[143] Its duration of action (1 to 2 hours) is similar to its elimination half-life.[143] Even when used to reverse blockade produced by long-acting agents, duration of action of anticholinesterase agents is comparable with or most often exceeds that of the neuromuscular blocking drug. Well-documented recurarization has not been reported. In practice, cases of apparent reparalysis in the recovery room are incomplete reversals that were initially thought to be complete. For example, manual or visual assessment using the TOF or tetanus mode and/or adequate respiratory function with the tube in place cannot be used as evidence for initial complete recovery. Therefore, subsequent clinical signs of weakness or upper airway obstruction after extubation are the result of persisting inadequate reversal, not reparalysis.

Factors Affecting Neostigmine Reversal

Several factors modify the rate of recovery of neuromuscular activity after reversal, such as intensity of block, dose, and drug interactions. Patient characteristics can also play a role.

Intensity of Block

The more intense the block at the time of reversal, the longer the recovery of neuromuscular activity (Fig. 20-17).[141] When neostigmine is administered after spontaneous recovery to ≥25% T_1 has occurred, which usually corresponds to the reappearance of the fourth twitch, recovery is rapid and the time from reversal to TOF >0.9 usually occurs within 15 minutes if an intermediate duration agent has been given.[145] If neostigmine is administered when the second twitch in the TOF reappears, mean time to a TOF ratio of 0.9 can vary between 9 and 19 minutes, with wide interindividual variations (Fig. 20-18).[144,146,147] If neostigmine is administered at deeper blockade, time to recovery to a TOF ratio of 0.9 may be extremely long (Fig. 20-18). The median time was 49 minutes when neostigmine 50 μg/kg was given at a PTC of 1 to 2.[148] Thus,

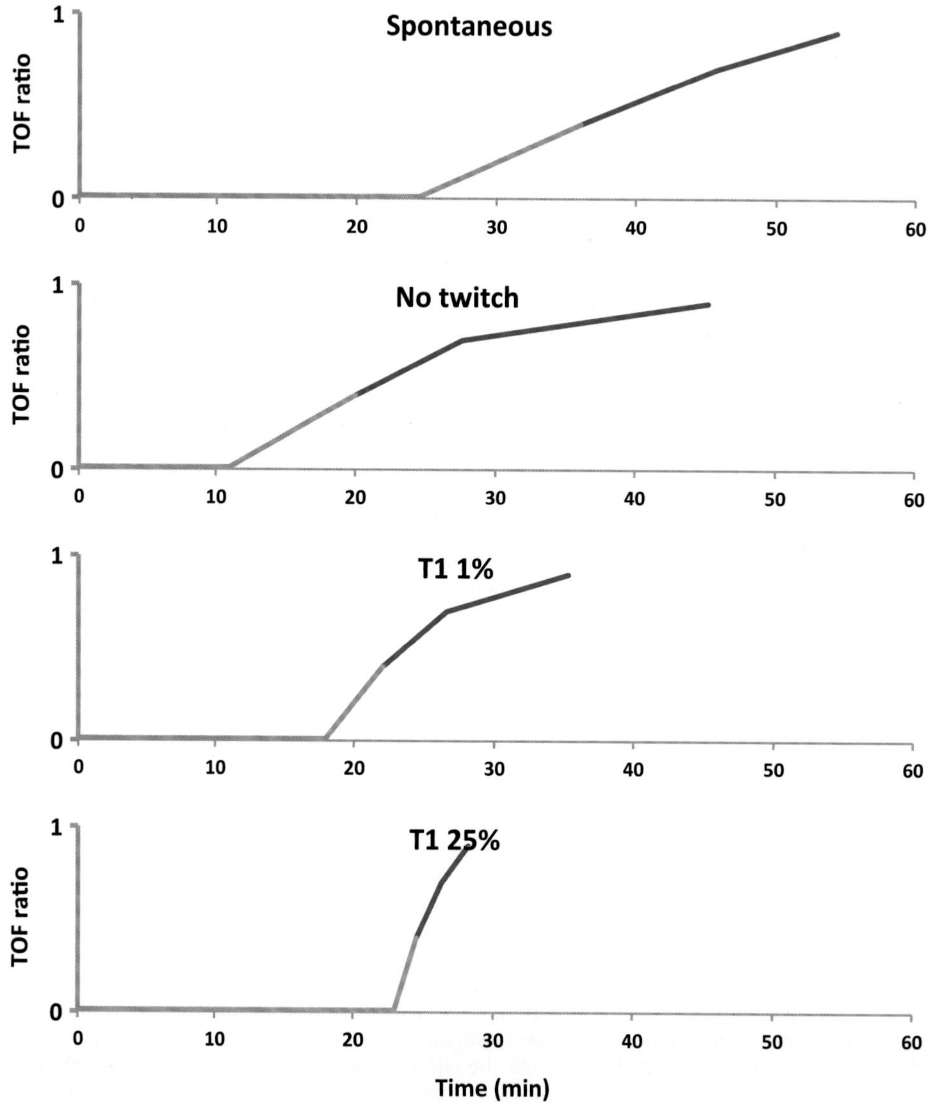

FIGURE 20-18. Time from injection of rocuronium until recovery to train-of-four ratio (TOF) of 0.9 in adults. Reversal with neostigmine was either not given (spontaneous) or given 5 minutes after rocuronium (No twitch), or at 1% twitch recovery (T1 1%), or at 25% twitch recovery (T1 25%). The Train-of-four (TOF) ratio is indicated against time until TOF ratio of 0.9 was reached (end of the line). Time is shortest when neostigmine is given at T1 25%, than is at reappearance of the fourth twitch response. This strategy also minimizes duration of blind paralysis (dark blue segment), when TOF ratio is between 0.4 and 0.9 and fade is difficult to detect by visual or tactile means. (Data from: Bevan et al.[149])

it is recommended that reversal should not be attempted until T_1 ≥25% when four twitches to TOF stimulation are visible.

One might argue that reversal can be attempted earlier, for instance when there is only one or no twitch visible following TOF stimulation, because one would otherwise spend time waiting for all four twitches to reappear. Several studies dealt with the problem of total time between injection of the neuromuscular blocking agent until complete recovery, with the reversal agent given at different levels of spontaneous recovery. All these studies show that early reversal, that is, when 0 to 2 twitches are present, does not shorten total time from administration of neuromuscular blocking agent to full recovery, compared with reversal given when 3 to 4 twitches are present. For example, Bevan et al.[149] administered large doses of neostigmine (0.07 mg/kg) after rocuronium and vecuronium and measured time until TOF ratio was 0.9. Neostigmine always decreased the time to recovery, no matter when it was given, compared with spontaneous recovery. However, time from injection to full recovery was longer when neostigmine was given 5 minutes after rocuronium (42.1 minutes) than at 25% recovery (28.2 minutes; Fig. 20-18).[149] In addition, giving the reversal agent too early leads to a period of "blind paralysis" because neostigmine-assisted recovery is characterized by an early, rapid phase, followed by slower recovery. As a result, the interval between a TOF ratio of 0.4 to 0.9, that is, the time when fade is difficult to detect, is likely to be much longer with early neostigmine administration. Thus, there is little advantage in attempting early reversal.

Dose

Over a certain dose range, the degree and rate of reversal depends directly on dose.[141] However, all anticholinesterase agents demonstrate a ceiling effect (Fig. 20-17). The maximum recommended dose of neostigmine is 0.07 mg/kg, and there is evidence that lower doses are just as effective. For example, time to complete recovery is similar with 0.035 and 0.05 mg/kg, but both these doses are more effective than 0.020 mg/kg.[141]

Choice of Neuromuscular Blocking Agent

Recovery of neuromuscular activity after reversal depends on the rate of spontaneous recovery as well as the acceleration induced by the reversal agent. Consequently, the overall recovery of intermediate-acting agents (atracurium, vecuronium, rocuronium) following the same dose of anticholinesterase is more rapid and more complete than after the long-acting pancuronium.[145] This difference is probably why residual paralysis is more frequent with longer-acting neuromuscular blocking agents. There are no major differences in recovery rate between individual intermediate-duration drugs (atracurium, vecuronium, rocuronium, cisatracurium). After prolonged infusions, recovery is slower than after intermittent bolus administration, probably because of differences in the rate of spontaneous recovery.[13]

Age

Recovery of neuromuscular activity occurs more rapidly with smaller doses of anticholinesterases in infants and children than in adults.[149] Residual weakness in the recovery room is found less frequently in children than in adults. The effectiveness of reversal has not been studied extensively in the elderly. Although the elimination of neostigmine is decreased in this age group, this reduction is counterbalanced by the tendency for neuromuscular blockade to wear off more slowly. This is especially true of steroidal neuromuscular blocking agents, such as vecuronium and rocuronium, which have a slower recovery index in the elderly.

Drug Interactions

Drugs that potentiate neuromuscular blockade can slow reversal or produce recurarization if given after anticholinesterase administration. Halogenated agents, when continued after neostigmine administration, prolong time to full reversal. Even when they are discontinued at the time of anticholinesterase drug administration, reversal time is not reduced significantly, probably because washout of the vapor from muscle tissue takes time. Care must be taken if aminoglycoside antibiotics or magnesium[116] must be given shortly after reversal agents.

Anticholinesterases: Other Effects

Cardiovascular

Anticholinesterase agents provoke profound vagal stimulation. The time course of the vagal effects parallels the reversal of block, and the bradycardia and bradyarrhythmias can be prevented with anticholinergic agents. Atropine has a rapid onset of action (1 minute), duration of 30 to 60 minutes, and crosses the blood–brain barrier. Given in combination with neostigmine, it gives rise to an initial tachycardia, reflecting its rapid onset of action, followed by a decrease in heart rate. With glycopyrrolate, onset is slower, but still faster than neostigmine, so that heart rate usually increases first, but not as much as with atropine, and then decreases. Because glycopyrrolate does not cross the blood–brain barrier, the incidence of memory deficits after anesthesia might be less than that after atropine. If atropine is given with neostigmine, the dose is approximately half that of neostigmine (atropine 0.020 mg/kg for neostigmine 0.040 mg/kg). Such a combination leads to an initial tachycardia followed by a slight bradycardia. With glycopyrrolate, the dose is one-fourth to one-fifth that of neostigmine (0.010 μg/kg for neostigmine 0.040 to 0.050 μg/kg), and the heart rate changes are less brisk than with atropine.

Other Cholinergic Effects

Anticholinesterases produce increased salivation and bowel motility. Although atropine blocks the former, it appears to have little effect on peristalsis. Some reports claim an increase in bowel anastomotic leakage after the reversal of neuromuscular blockade. There has been concern over the possible impact of anticholinesterase agents on postoperative nausea and vomiting (PONV). A meta-analysis, published in 1999, concluded that neostigmine had no effect on the overall incidence of PONV, but large doses (2.5 mg or more in adults) were associated with a higher incidence of PONV than no reversal, while lower doses led to less PONV.[150] A more recent meta-analysis reanalyzed the data and incorporated additional studies. It concluded that there was no relation between administration of neostigmine and PONV.[151] At any rate, possible nausea and vomiting is preferable to signs and symptoms of respiratory paralysis.

Respiratory Effects

Neostigmine may cause an increase in airway resistance, but anticholinergics reduce this effect. Several other factors, such as pain, the presence of an endotracheal tube, or light anesthesia, may predispose to bronchoconstriction at the end of surgery so that it is difficult to determine the role of reversal agents.

Clinical Use

Several strategies have been proposed to restore neuromuscular function at the end of surgery and anesthesia. One of them involves restricting the dose of nondepolarizing blocking agent at induction of anesthesia to what is necessary for the duration of the procedure, minimal additional doses and reliance of complete spontaneous recovery in an attempt to avoid reversal with anticholinesterase agents. This approach is not without dangers. Even relatively modest doses ($2 \times ED_{95}$) of atracurium, vecuronium, or rocuronium are associated with residual paralysis (TOF ratio <0.9) after as long as 4 hours after injection.[15] Visual or tactile monitoring with TOF, 50 Hz tetanus, or double-burst stimulation cannot eliminate some degree of residual paralysis.[123] Only a sustained response to a 100 Hz tetanus may rule out the presence of residual paralysis by tactile or visual means.[55,123] The use of objective monitoring, such as acceleromyography, is even better.[123] Still, pharmacologically assisted recovery is required in most cases, as it is illusory to aim for complete recovery only by careful titration of neuromuscular blocking agents. In a study examining anesthetic outcomes in the Netherlands, the use of reversal agents was found to be associated with a tenfold reduction in mortality.[138] Not surprisingly, the more systematic use of reversal agents in one institution led to a substantial decrease in residual paralysis.[17]

Administration of anticholinesterase agents will accelerate recovery, no matter when they are given in the course of recovery (Fig. 20-18). However, there are advantages in giving reversal agents when spontaneous recovery is well under way, preferably when four twitches are present after TOF stimulation. If neostigmine is given when deep blockade is present (no twitch or only one twitch present; Fig. 20-18), reversal takes longer than if four twitches are present. As a result, time from injection of rocuronium until full recovery (TOF ratio >0.9) is not reduced, and may in fact be increased, if neostigmine is given too early (Fig. 20-18). Furthermore, the patient might be more difficult to manage with early reversal: Duration of blind paralysis (from TOF ratio of 0.4, when TOF fade becomes undetectable, until TOF is 0.9) is longer with early reversal. This means that missing residual paralysis is more likely with hasty administration of anticholinesterase agents. Therefore, if four twitches are not visible after TOF stimulation, it is recommended to keep the patient anesthetized and mechanically ventilated until four twitches reappear and then administer anticholinesterases.

Intense blockade is not expected to be reversed effectively by increasing the dose of anticholinesterase (Fig. 20-17). In general, neostigmine doses of 0.04 to 0.05 mg/kg should be sufficient, and there is no advantage in exceeding 0.07 mg/kg because of the ceiling effect of the drug. Edrophonium is not recommended for intense block. Pyridostigmine has a slow onset of action and does not appear to accelerate reversal of short- and intermediate-duration drugs to a great extent.

When recovery appears almost complete—that is, when four seemingly equal twitches are seen after TOF stimulation—a reduced dose of neostigmine (0.01 to 0.02 mg/kg) is adequate. In patients given neostigmine when the AMG TOF ratio was 0.4, a level at which tactile or visual fade is not detected, median time to a TOF ratio of 0.9 was 6 minutes with both 0.010 and 0.020 mg/kg, and 4 minutes with 0.030 mg/kg, much shorter than with placebo (13 minutes).[152]

Sugammadex

A new method of reversing neuromuscular blockade has been available in many countries since 2009, but not in North America. Sugammadex leads to restoration of normal neuromuscular function not by interfering with acetylcholine, the nicotinic receptor or acetylcholinesterase, but by selectively binding to rocuronium, and to a lesser extent to vecuronium and pancuronium.[153,154] The compound is a gamma-cyclodextrin, made up of eight sugars arranged in a ring to make a center to accommodate the rocuronium molecule. Once bound, rocuronium is held in place by polar side chains attached to the ring. Because sugammadex does not bind to any known receptor, it is devoid of major cardiovascular or other side effects.[144] It does not bind neuromuscular blocking drugs that do not have a steroid nucleus. Block produced by succinylcholine or by any of the benzylisoquinolines, such as atracurium, cisatracurium and mivacurium, is unaffected by sugammadex.

Mechanism of Action

9 Neuromuscular transmission can be restored by injection of sugammadex, an agent that binds specifically in a 1:1 molar ratio to rocuronium and vecuronium. Sugammadex has a molecular weight of 2,178 daltons[153] and binds with rocuronium or vecuronium in a 1:1 molar ratio. The rocuronium molecule is less bulky (610 daltons), so 3.6 mg (or mg/kg) of sugammadex is required to bind 1.0 mg (or mg/kg) of rocuronium. Binding is tight, but not irreversible. This means that rocuronium–sugammadex complexes form while some others break up into their two constituents. The dissociation constant has been estimated to be 0.045 to 0.1 μmol/L with the most recent estimate at 0.055 μmol/L,[154] and it is not known whether it is affected by pH, temperature, type of fluid or tissue, or other factors. The dissociation constant for vecuronium is higher, 0.17 μmol/L,[154] implying that the binding is one-third as tight. The binding of hundreds of drugs, including corticosteroids, with sugammadex has been measured. Only the estrogen modulator toremifene, and the antibiotics flucloxacillin and fusidic acid have been found to have potential interactions with sugammadex at clinical concentrations.[154] Sugammadex also binds to pancuronium, but binding is not as tight as with rocuronium and vecuronium.[154]

After injection of sugammadex, evidence suggests that binding of rocuronium in plasma leads to a marked decrease in free (unbound) rocuronium concentration, leading to a large concentration gradient of free rocuronium between the neuromuscular junction and plasma. This favors movement of rocuronium from neuromuscular junction to plasma, down its concentration gradient, thus producing less neuromuscular block.

Pharmacology

In patients receiving rocuronium, return of a TOF ratio to 0.9 is accelerated by sugammadex in a dose-dependent manner. If sugammadex is given on return of the second twitch in the TOF, doses of 2 mg/kg result in the return of train-of-four ratio to 0.9 within approximately 2 to 4 minutes.[144,146,147,155] This interval is shorter than after either neostigmine reversal, when given at approximately the same level of recovery (Fig. 20-19).[144,146,147] With lower doses (0.5 to 1 mg/kg) recovery time is longer[156] and reparalysis may be observed.[157] Compared with rocuronium, vecuronium has less affinity for sugammadex, but there are fewer vecuronium molecules in circulation. As a result of these two opposing effects, the dose of sugammadex required for restoration of neuromuscular function is approximately the same for vecuronium and rocuronium (Fig. 20-19).[156]

10 Sugammadex is also effective when blockade is deep, but larger doses are required. When a PTC of 2 is present, which for rocuronium occurs 15 to 20 minutes before return of twitch, the required dose is 4 mg/kg (Fig. 20-19).[148] Sugammadex could also be used in the case of a failed intubation. If rocuronium 0.6 mg/kg was given, sugammadex 8 mg/kg might be effective as early as 3 minutes after rocuronium injection, and if the dose of rocuronium is doubled to 1.2 mg/kg, one might need 16 mg/kg of sugammadex (Fig. 20-10).[38] The

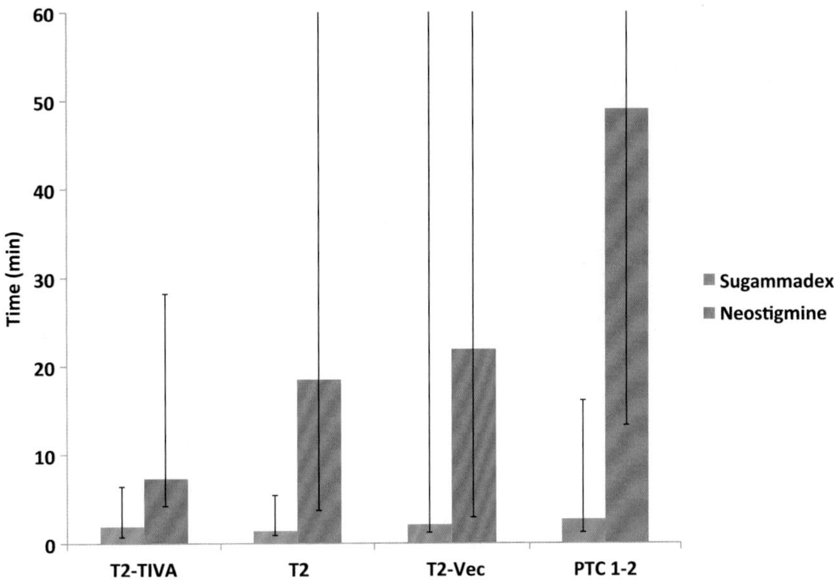

FIGURE 20-19. Median time to recovery to a train-of-four (TOF) ratio of 0.9 with neostigmine and sugammadex. Reversal was attempted at return of two visible twitches (T2) (three studies) or at a post-tetanic count (PTC) of 1 to 2 (one study). Background anesthetic in all studies was sevoflurane, except in one indicated by total intravenous anesthesia (TIVA). Rocuronium was used before sugammadex in all studies except the one indicated by Vec. Dose of sugammadex was 2 mg/kg for T2 studies and 4 mg/kg for the PTC study. Dose of neostigmine was 0.050 mg/kg in all studies except the one on PTC 1 to 2, where it was 0.070 mg/kg. Error bars indicate range. Data from: Flockton EA, Mastronardi P, Hunter JM, et al. Reversal of rocuronium-induced neuromuscular block with sugammadex is faster than reversal of cisatracurium-induced block with neostigmine. *Br J Anaesth.* 2008;100:622–630; Khuenl-Brady KS, Wattwil M, Vanacker BF, et al. Sugammadex provides faster reversal of vecuronium-induced neuromuscular blockade compared with neostigmine: A multicenter, randomized, controlled trial. *Anesth Analg.* 2010;110:64–73; Blobner M, Eriksson LI, Scholz J, et al. Reversal of rocuronium-induced neuromuscular blockade with sugammadex compared with neostigmine during sevoflurane anesthesia: Results of a randomised, controlled trial. *Eur J Anaesthesiol.* 2010;27:874—881; and Jones RK, Caldwell JE, Brull SJ, et al. Reversal of profound rocuronium-induced blockade with sugammadex. A randomized comparison with neostigmine. *Anesthesiology.* 2008;109:816–824, respectively.

availability of sugammadex might make succinylcholine somewhat obsolete for intubation.

Pharmacokinetics

In adults, sugammadex has a volume of distribution that is similar to ECF (20 L). Its terminal half-life is approximately 2 hours.[155] Both sugammadex and sugammadex–rocuronium complexes are excreted unchanged via the kidney. In patients receiving rocuronium, injection of sugammadex increases the total (free plus bound) plasma concentrations of rocuronium, which suggests that it causes sequestration of rocuronium in the plasma by drawing it from peripheral tissues. In patients with renal failure, clearance of sugammadex is decreased markedly and elimination half-lives of days have been measured.[158] Rocuronium–sugammadex complexes remain in the body for days.

Special Populations

In infants and children, the dose of sugammadex appears to be similar to that recommended for adults against rocuronium blockade.[159] Clearance decreases and terminal half-life increases with advancing age. In patients with age >75 years, clearance was found to be reduced by half and terminal half-life was 4.6 hours, compared with 2.4 hours in middle-aged adults.[155] Time to recovery to a TOF ratio of 0.9 increases with age, with mean times being 2.6 minutes in adults 18 to 64 years old and 3.8 in elderly patients >75 years old (Fig. 20-20).[155] This reduced clearance is related to decreased renal function in the elderly, and patients with no renal function have extremely long elimination half-lives.[158] In morbidly obese individuals, sugammadex produces slower recovery if dose is based on IBW rather than total body weight (TBW). However, calculating the dose by adding 40% to IBW provides as rapid a recovery as for TBW dosing.[160]

Clinical Use

Availability

An application was submitted to the Food and Drug Administration (FDA) in 2008 to introduce sugammadex into clinical practice. A similar application was filed with the European Union authorities at the same time, based on the same preclinical and clinical data. The drug was approved in Europe, but not in the United States. The FDA justified its decision by the occurrence of hypersensitivity reactions in volunteers receiving high doses and requested more studies.[70,161] These events were not considered allergic reactions, but case reports of sugammadex allergic reactions have been published. Another concern has been a transient effect on hemostasis following injection of sugammadex, with increases in prothrombin time (PT), which is mentioned

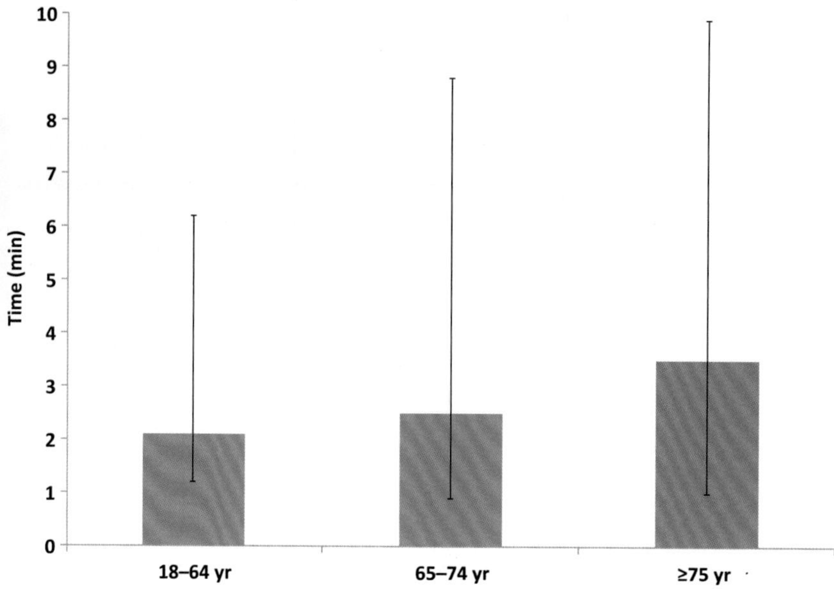

FIGURE 20-20. Median time to recovery to a train-of-four (TOF) ratio >0.9 in adult patients belonging to different age groups, when sugammadex 2 mg/kg was given at recovery of the second twitch in the TOF. Error bars indicate range. Data from: McDonagh DL, Benedict PE, Kovac AL, et al. Efficacy, safety, and pharmacokinetics of sugammadex for the reversal of rocuronium-induced neuromuscular blockade in elderly patients. *Anesthesiology*. 2011;114:318–329.

in the product monograph in many countries. Considering the marked superiority of sugammadex over neostigmine in its ability to restore neuromuscular blockade, it is hoped that the concerns raised by the FDA will be addressed soon and that the drug will be available soon in the North American market.

How much paralysis? Theoretically, sugammadex could make management of muscle relaxation quite simple: A large dose of rocuronium or vecuronium could be injected at induction of anesthesia, followed by a suitably large dose of sugammadex at the end of the case, with no need for monitoring or concern for residual paralysis. This evolution in practice could be considered as yielding some benefits: More profound relaxation provides better and faster intubating conditions, better surgical conditions, and less damage to the laryngeal structures; faster and more predictable recovery could diminish the incidence of residual paralysis and reduce turnaround time. But these benefits will come at a cost. First, sugammadex is expensive. The standard dose of 200 mg (slightly more than 2 mg/kg in most adult patients) costs approximately 100$, and provides reliable return of neuromuscular function provided that two twitches have returned. For deeper block, doses as high as 16 mg/kg might be required, with a corresponding increase in price. The indiscriminate use of large doses of rocuronium or vecuronium would mandate the systematic injection of large doses of sugammadex (at least 4 mg/kg and probably higher), and this would impact negatively on the costs of an anesthetic. The second reason why not to adopt this practice is to minimize problems if reparalysis is required, for example if a second surgery is indicated within minutes or hours of giving sugammadex. The problem has been addressed by Cammu et al., who found that rocuronium 1.2 mg/kg after sugammadex 4 mg/kg produces complete abolition of twitch response.[162] However, onset is typically longer and duration shorter even compared with rocuronium 0.6 mg/kg given without previous sugammadex. Prolongation of onset time and shortening of duration is more apparent if the interval between sugammadex and rocuronium is brief. For example, in Cammu et al.'s study, mean onset time for rocuronium 0.6 mg/kg was 1.25 minutes.[162] Sugammadex was given at a PTC of 1 to 2, followed, after a certain time interval, by rocuronium, 1.2 mg/kg. If this interval was 5 minutes, mean rocuronium onset time was 3.06 minutes; for sugammadex–rocuronium intervals >25 minutes, onset time was 1.73 minutes, but still longer than for the smaller initial rocuronium dose. Clinical duration of action ranged from 17.7 minutes for a 5-minute interval to 46 minutes for a 45-minute interval. The third reason for avoiding high doses of sugammadex if possible is avoidance of side effects. Although sugammadex has been associated with very few side effects, the problems of hypersensitivity and deficiencies in hemostasis appear to be dose-related.[161] Finally, there are probably disadvantages associated with the practice of abolishing all movement during surgery: An important sign of inadequate analgesia and anesthesia is lost. It is also unclear whether awareness can be totally avoided by the use of BIS monitoring, as large doses of neuromuscular blocking agents can depress BIS in certain circumstances.[5] Therefore, there seem to be valid reasons to avoid the systematic use of large doses.

Reparalysis

Using less than adequate doses of sugammadex can lead to delayed manifestations of residual blockade. If the dose of sugammadex is too small to bind most of the rocuronium molecules in the body, it may be enough to restore neuromuscular function because initially, it may be enough to bind most of the circulating rocuronium. However, as rocuronium is drawn from deeper compartments (rocuronium is redistributed extensively), reparalysis may occur if the quantity of sugammadex is not sufficient. Cases of reparalysis have been documented, especially with inadequate doses (0.5 to 1.0 mg/kg).[157] These cases respond to an additional dose of sugammadex.

Moderate to Profound Blockade

Sugammadex is particularly useful when blockade at the end of the surgical procedure is moderate to profound, defined as fewer than two twitches observed in response to TOF stimulation at the adductor pollicis, when the neuromuscular blocking agent is rocuronium or vecuronium. When two twitches are present, sugammadex 2 mg/kg restores neuromuscular transmission to a TOF ratio of 0.9 within 2 to 4 minutes, much faster than neostigmine (10 to 20 minutes). For deeper blockade, corresponding to a PTC of 1to 2,

4 mg/kg is be required for rapid (2 to 4 minutes) return of neuromuscular function.[148] The use of neostigmine at such deep levels of blockade is not recommended, because effective reversal may not obtained for 1 to 2 hours (Fig. 20-19). Therefore, sugammadex is particularly useful when profound relaxation is required until the end of the surgical procedure. Examples of such situations include certain laparoscopic procedures, major abdominal surgery, and procedures shorter than anticipated. Certain categories of patients might also require more muscle relaxation, such as obese individuals and muscular patients.[160]

Shallow to Moderate Blockade

When more than two twitches are visible after TOF stimulation, a 2 mg/kg dose of sugammadex will undoubtedly work, but it is unclear how effective a smaller dose might be. If four equal twitches are detected by visual or tactile means, that is if the measured TOF ratio is >0.9, one study suggests that as little 0.22 mg/kg is effective,[163] but no data are available for the more common situation when the TOF visibly fades.

Rapid Sequence Induction

With the possibility of using sugammadex at any depth of blockade, including shortly after rocuronium has been given, rocuronium might replace succinylcholine for rapid sequence induction, with sugammadex as backup. Succinylcholine 1 mg/kg was compared with rocuronium 1.2 mg/kg followed 3 minutes later by sugammadex 16 mg/kg in more than 100 patients. Total duration of blockade from injection of the neuromuscular blocking agent was actually shorter and more predictable with the rocuronium–sugammadex combination (Fig. 20-10).[38] Mean duration to 10% T1, which normally corresponds to return of breathing movements, was shorter with rocuronium–sugammadex (4.4 minutes) than with succinylcholine (7.1 minutes), with less interpatient variability. These data should not, however, encourage anesthesiologists to adopt a sloppy approach to airway management. First, some patients desaturate within a 4.4-minute interval. Second, although the diaphragm might have recovered to a certain extent, respiratory drive might be inhibited by hypnotic agents and opioids given at induction, and there might be incomplete recovery of key muscles, such as those of the upper airway. Finally, real life situations are not like well-rehearsed research protocols. To illustrate this, a failed intubation scenario was simulated by Bisschops et al.,[101] which demonstrates that when rocuronium is given and unexpected intubation difficulties are encountered, a decision has to be made to administer sugammadex, the correct dose has to be obtained, drawn up, and injected, and time is required to observe the full effect, all this before the patient becomes hypoxic. At the time of writing (end of 2011), rocuronium had been given for rapid sequence induction with sugammadex at the end of the case, for example, for cesarean delivery,[164] but no report of rescue sugammadex injection had been published.

CONCLUSION

Neuromuscular blocking agents are useful in anesthesia, but because they do not provide unconsciousness or analgesia, and because they can impair respiratory function, they must be used carefully. Monitoring should be used whenever neuromuscular blocking agents are given, to obtain optimal intubating conditions, adequate relaxation during surgery, and complete recovery before extubation. In recent years, new drug development has shifted from finding compounds with fast onset, short duration, and nondepolarizing properties to designing drugs that accelerate recovery.

References

1. Griffith HR, Johnson GE. The use of curare in general anesthesia. *Anesthesiology.* 1942;3:418–420.
2. Beecher HK, Todd DP. A study of the deaths associated with anesthesia and surgery: Based on a study of 599, 548 anesthesias in ten institutions 1948–1952, inclusive. *Ann Surg.* 1954;140:2–35.
3. Mashour GA, Orser BA, Avidan MS. Intraoperative awareness: From neurobiology to clinical practice. *Anesthesiology.* 2011;114:1218–1233.
4. Sonner JM, Antognini JF, Dutton RC, et al. Inhaled anesthetics and immobility: Mechanisms, mysteries, and minimum alveolar anesthetic concentration. *Anesth Analg.* 2003;97:718–740.
5. Ekman A, Stalberg E, Sundman E, et al. The effect of neuromuscular block and noxious stimulation on hypnosis monitoring during sevoflurane anesthesia. *Anesth Analg.* 2007;105:688–695.
6. King M, Sujirattanawimol N, Danielson DR, et al. Requirements for muscle relaxants during radical retropubic prostatectomy. *Anesthesiology.* 2000;93:1392–1397.
7. McNeil IA, Culbert B, Russell I. Comparison of intubating conditions following propofol and succinylcholine with propofol and remifentanil 2 micrograms kg^{-1} or 4 micrograms kg^{-1}. *Br J Anaesth.* 2000;85:623–625.
8. Naguib M, Samarkandi AH, El-Din ME, et al. The dose of succinylcholine required for excellent endotracheal intubating conditions. *Anesth Analg.* 2006;102:151–155.
9. Andrews JI, Kumar N, van den Brom RH, et al. A large simple randomized trial of rocuronium versus succinylcholine in rapid-sequence induction of anaesthesia along with propofol. *Acta Anaesthesiol Scand.* 1999;43:4–8.
10. Mencke T, Echternach M, Kleinschmidt S, et al. Laryngeal morbidity and quality of tracheal intubation: A randomized controlled trial. *Anesthesiology.* 2003;98:1049–1056.
11. Viby-Mogensen J, Jørgensen BC, Ording H. Residual curarization in the recovery room. *Anesthesiology.* 1979;50:539–541.
12. Bevan DR, Smith CE, Donati F. Postoperative neuromuscular blockade: A comparison between atracurium, vecuronium, and pancuronium. *Anesthesiology.* 1988;69:272–276.
13. Fawcett WJ, Dash A, Francis GA, et al. Recovery from neuromuscular blockade: Residual curarisation following atracurium or vecuronium by bolus dosing or infusions. *Acta Anaesthesiol Scand.* 1995;39:288–293.
14. Berg H, Roed J, Viby-Mogensen J, et al. Residual neuromuscular block is a risk factor for postoperative pulmonary complications. A prospective, randomised, and blinded study of postoperative pulmonary complications after atracurium, vecuronium and pancuronium. *Acta Anaesthesiol Scand.* 1997;41:1095–1103.
15. Debaene B, Plaud B, Dilly MP, et al. Residual paralysis in the PACU after a single intubating dose of nondepolarizing muscle relaxant with an intermediate duration of action. *Anesthesiology.* 2003;98:1042–1048.
16. Murphy GS, Szokol JW, Marymont JH, et al. Recovery of neuromuscular function after cardiac surgery: Pancuronium versus rocuronium. *Anesth Analg.* 2003;96:1301–1307.
17. Baillard C, Clec'h C, Catineau J, et al. Postoperative residual neuromuscular block: A survey of management. *Br J Anaesth.* 2005;95:622–626.
18. Murphy GS, Szokol JW, Marymont JH, et al. Intraoperative acceleromyographic monitoring reduces the risk of residual neuromuscular blockade and adverse respiratory events in the postanesthesia care unit. *Anesthesiology.* 2008;109:389–398.
19. Butterly A, Bittner EA, George E, et al. Postoperative residual curarization from intermediate-acting neuromuscular blocking agents delays recovery room discharge. *Br J Anaesth.* 2010;105:304–309.
20. Murphy GS, Szokol JW, Avram MJ, et al. Intraoperative acceleromyography monitoring reduces symptoms of muscle weakness and improves quality of recovery in the early postoperative period. *Anesthesiology.* 2011;115:946–954.
21. Naguib M, Kopman AF, Ensor JE. Neuromuscular monitoring and postoperative residual curarisation: A meta-analysis. *Br J Anaesth.* 2007;98:302–316.
22. Eriksson LI, Sundman E, Olsson R, et al. Functional assessment of the pharynx at rest and during swallowing in partially paralyzed humans: Simultaneous videomanometry and mechanomyography of awake human volunteers. *Anesthesiology.* 1997;87:1035–1043.
23. Martyn JA, Fagerlund MJ, Eriksson LI. Basic principles of neuromuscular transmission. *Anaesthesia.* 2009;64:(suppl 1)1–9.
24. Naguib M, Flood P, McArdle JJ, et al. Advances in neurobiology of the neuromuscular junction: Implications for the anesthesiologist. *Anesthesiology.* 2002;96:202–231.
25. Hughes BW, Kusner LL, Kaminski HJ. Molecular architecture of the neuromuscular junction. *Muscle Nerve.* 2006;33:445–461.
26. Zouridakis M, Zisimopoulou P, Poulas K, et al. Recent advances in understanding the structure of nicotinic acetylcholine receptors. *IUBMB Life.* 2009;61:407–423.
27. Wood SJ, Slater CR. Safety factor at the neuromuscular junction. *Prog Neurobiol.* 2001;64:393–429.

28. Rotundo RL. Expression and localization of acetylcholinesterase at the neuromuscular junction. *J Neurocytol.* 2003;32:743–766.
29. Jonsson M, Gurley D, Dabrowski M, et al. Distinct pharmacologic properties of neuromuscular blocking agents on human neuronal nicotinic acetylcholine receptors: A possible explanation for the train-of-four fade. *Anesthesiology.* 2006;105:521–533.
30. Staals LM, Driessen JJ, van Egmond J, et al. Train-of-four ratio recovery often precedes twitch recovery when neuromuscular block is reversed by sugammadex. *Acta Anesthesiol Scand.* 2011;55:700–707.
31. Donati F. Neuromuscular blocking drugs for the new millennium: Current practice, future trends—comparative pharmacology of neuromuscular blocking drugs. *Anesth Analg.* 2000;90:S2–S6.
32. Fuchs-Buder T, Claudius C, Stovgaard LT, et al. Good clinical research practice in pharmacodynamic studies of neuromuscular blocking agents II: The Stockholm revision. *Acta Anaesthesiol Scand.* 2007;51:789–808.
33. Jonsson M, Dabrowski M, Gurley DA, et al. Activation and inhibition of human muscular and neuronal nicotinic acetylcholine receptors by succinylcholine. *Anesthesiology.* 2006;104:724–733.
34. Schreiber JU, Lysakowski C, Fuchs-Buder T, et al. Prevention of succinylcholine-induced fasciculation and myalgia: A meta-analysis of randomized trials. *Anesthesiology.* 2005;103:877–884.
35. Smith CE, Saddler JM, Bevan JC, et al. Pretreatment with non-depolarizing neuromuscular blocking agents and suxamethonium-induced increases in resting jaw tension in children. *Br J Anaesth.* 1990;64:577–581.
36. Szalados JE, Donati F, Bevan DR. Effect of *d*-tubocurarine pretreatment on succinylcholine twitch augmentation and neuromuscular blockade. *Anesth Analg.* 1990;71:55–59.
37. Roy JJ, Donati F, Boismenu D, et al. Concentration-effect relation of succinylcholine chloride during propofol anesthesia. *Anesthesiology.* 2002;97:1082–1092.
38. Lee C, Jahr JS, Candiotti KA, et al. Reversal of profound neuromuscular block by sugammadex administered three minutes after rocuronium. *Anesthesiology.* 2009;110:1020–1025.
39. Hayes AH, Breslin DS, Mirakhur RK, et al. Frequency of haemoglobin desaturation with the use of succinylcholine during rapid sequence induction of anaesthesia. *Acta Anaesthesiol Scand.* 2001;45:746.
40. Lerman J, Chinyanga HM. The heart rate response to succinylcholine in children: A comparison of atropine and glycopyrrolate. *Can Anaesth Soc J.* 1983;30:377–381.
41. Mertes PM, Alla F, Tréchot P, et al. Anaphylaxis during anesthesia in France: An 8-year national survey. *J Allergy Clin Immunol.* 2011;128:366–373.
42. Donati F. Dose inflation when using precurarization. *Anesthesiology.* 2006;105:222–223.
43. Mencke T, Schreiber JU, Becker C, et al. Pretreatment before succinylcholine for outpatient anesthesia? *Anesth Analg.* 2002;94:573–576.
44. Wong SF, Chung F. Succinylcholine-associated postoperative myalgia. *Anaesthesia.* 2000;55:144–152.
45. Vachon CA, Warner DO, Bacon DR. Succinylcholine and the open globe. Tracing the teaching. *Anesthesiology.* 2003;99:220–223.
46. Minton MD, Grosslight K, Stirt JA, et al. Increases in intracranial pressure from succinylcholine: Prevention by prior nondepolarizing blockade. *Anesthesiology.* 1986;65:165–169.
47. Gronert GA. Cardiac arrest after succinylcholine: Mortality greater with rhabdomyolysis than receptor upregulation. *Anesthesiology.* 2001;94:523–529.
48. Thapa S, Brull SJ. Succinylcholine-induced hyperkalemia in patients with renal failure: An old question revisited. *Anesth Analg.* 2000;91:237–241.
49. Fleming NW, Macres S, Antognini JF, et al. Neuromuscular blocking action of suxamethonium after antagonism of vecuronium by edrophonium, pyridostigmine or neostigmine. *Br J Anaesth.* 1996;77:492–495.
50. Levano S, Ginz H, Siegemund M, et al. Genotyping the butyrylcholinesterase in patients with prolonged neuromuscular block after succinylcholine. *Anesthesiology.* 2005;102:531–535.
51. El-Orbany M, Connolly LA. Rapid sequence induction: Current controversy. *Anesth Analg.* 2010;110:1318–1325.
52. Meakin G, McKiernan EP, Morris P, et al. Dose-response curves for suxamethonium in neonates, infants and children. *Br J Anaesth.* 1989;62:655–658.
53. Donati F, Guay J. No substitute for the intravenous route. *Anesthesiology.* 2001;94:1–2.
54. Lemmens HJ, Brodsky JB. The dose of succinylcholine in morbid obesity. *Anesth Analg.* 2006;102:438–442.
55. Baurain MJ, Hennart DA, Godschalx A, et al. Visual evaluation of residual curarization in anesthetized patients using one hundred-hertz, five-second tetanic stimulation at the adductor pollicis muscle. *Anesth Analg.* 1998;87:185–189.
56. Brull SJ, Connelly NR, O'Connor TZ, et al. Effect of tetanus on subsequent neuromuscular monitoring in patients receiving vecuronium. *Anesthesiology.* 1991;74:64.
57. Kopman AF, Klewicka MM, Kopman DJ, et al. Molar potency is predictive of the speed of onset of neuromuscular block for agents of intermediate, short, and ultrashort duration. *Anesthesiology.* 1999;90:425–431.
58. Fisher DM, O'Keeffe C, Stanski DR, et al. Pharmacokinetics and pharmacodynamics of *d*-tubocurarine in infants, children, and adults. *Anesthesiology.* 1982;57:203.
59. Martyn JA, White DA, Gronert GA, et al. Up-and-down regulation of skeletal muscle acetylcholine receptors. Effects on neuromuscular blockers. *Anesthesiology.* 1992;76:822–843.
60. Ibebunjo C, Martyn JA. Thermal injury induces greater resistance to *d*-tubocurarine in local rather than in distant muscles in the rat. *Anesth Analg.* 2000;91:1243–1249.
61. Fodale V, Santamaria LB. Laudanosine, an atracurium and cisatracurium metabolite. *Eur J Anaesthesiol.* 2002;19:466–473.
62. Amann A, Rieder J, Fleischer M, et al. The influence of atracurium, cisatracurium, and mivacurium on the proliferation of two human cell lines in vitro. *Anesth Analg.* 2001;93:690–696.
63. Naguib M, Kopman AF, Lien CA, et al. A survey of current management of neuromuscular block in the United States and Europe. *Anesth Analg.* 2010;111:110–119.
64. Lien CA, Schmith VD, Belmont MR, et al. Pharmacokinetics of cisatracurium in patients receiving nitrous oxide/opioid/barbiturate anesthesia. *Anesthesiology.* 1996;84:300–308.
65. Leykin Y, Pellis T, Lucca M, et al. The effects of cisatracurium on morbidly obese women. *Anesth Analg.* 2004;99:1090–1094.
66. Miller DR, Wherrett C, Hull K, et al. Cumulation characteristics of cisatracurium and rocuronium during continuous infusion. *Can J Anaesth.* 2000;47:943–949.
67. Lagneau F, D'honneur G, Plaud B, et al. A comparison of two depths of prolonged neuromuscular blockade induced by cisatracurium in mechanically ventilated critically ill patients. *Intensive Care Med.* 2002;28:1735–1741.
68. Papazian L, Forel JM, Gacouin A, et al. Neuromuscular blockers in early acute respiratory distress syndrome. *N Engl J Med.* 2010;363:1107–1116.
69. Basta SJ, Savarese JJ, Ali HH, et al. Clinical pharmacology of doxacurium chloride. A new long-acting nondepolarizing muscle relaxant. *Anesthesiology.* 1988;69:478–486.
70. Naguib M, Brull SJ. Update on neuromuscular pharmacology. *Curr Opin Anaesthesiol.* 2009;22:483–490.
71. Savarese JJ, McGilvra JD, Sunaga H, et al. Rapid chemical antagonism of neuromuscular blockade by L-cysteine adduction to and inactivation of the olefinic (double-bonded) isoquilolinium diester compounds gantacurium (AV430A), CW 002, and CW 011. *Anesthesiology.* 2010;113:58–73.
72. Savarese JJ, Ali HH, Basta SJ, et al. The clinical neuromuscular pharmacology of mivacurium chloride (BW B1090U). A short-acting nondepolarizing ester neuromuscular blocking drug. *Anesthesiology.* 1988;68:723–732.
73. Motamed C, Donati F. Sevoflurane and isoflurane, but not propofol, decrease mivacurium requirements over time. *Can J Anaesth.* 2002;49:907–912.
74. Han TH, Martyn JAJ. Neuromuscular pharmacodynamics of mivacurium in adults with major burns. *Br J Anaesth.* 2011;106:675–679.
75. Kao YJ, Le ND. The reversal of profound mivacurium-induced neuromuscular blockade. *Can J Anaesth.* 1996;43:1128–1133.
76. Murphy GS, Szokol JW, Franklin M, et al. Postanesthesia care unit recovery times and neuromuscular blocking drugs: A prospective study of orthopedic surgical patients randomized to receive pancuronium or rocuronium. *Anesth Analg.* 2004;98:193–200.
77. Kopman AF, Klewincka MM, Ghori K, et al. Dose-response and onset/offset characteristics of rapacuronium. *Anesthesiology.* 2000;93:1017–1021.
78. Jooste E, Zhang Y, Emala CW. Neuromuscular blocking agents' differential bronchoconstrictive potential in Guinea pig airways. *Anesthesiology.* 2007;106:763–772.
79. Proost JH, Eriksson LI, Mirakhur RK, et al. Urinary, biliary and faecal excretion of rocuronium in humans. *Br J Anaesth.* 2000;85:717–723.
80. Plaud B, Debaene B, Donati F. The corrugator supercilii, not the orbicularis oculi, reflects rocuronium neuromuscular blockade at the laryngeal adductor muscles. *Anesthesiology.* 2001;95:96–101.
81. Wright PM, Caldwell JE, Miller RD. Onset and duration of rocuronium and succinylcholine at the adductor pollicis and laryngeal adductor muscles in anesthetized humans. *Anesthesiology.* 1994;81:1110–1115.
82. Dhonneur G, Kirov K, Slavov V, et al. Effects of an intubating dose of succinylcholine and rocuronium on the larynx and diaphragm: An electromyographic study in humans. *Anesthesiology.* 1999;90:951–955.
83. Plaud B, Proost JH, Wierda JM, et al. Pharmacokinetics and pharmacodynamics of rocuronium at the vocal cords and the adductor pollicis in humans. *Clin Pharmacol Ther.* 1995;58:185–191.
84. Levy JH, Davis GK, Duggan J, et al. Determination of the hemodynamics and histamine release of rocuronium (Org 9426) when administered in increased doses under N2O/O2-sufentanil anesthesia. *Anesth Analg.* 1994;78:318–321.
85. Dhonneur G, Combes X, Chassard D, et al. Skin sensitivity to rocuronium and vecuronium: A randomized controlled prick-testing study in healthy volunteers. *Anesth Analg.* 2004;98:986–989.
86. Laake JH, Røttingen JA. Rocuronium and anaphylaxis—a statistical challenge. *Acta Anaesthesiol Scand.* 2001;45:1196–1203.
87. Bhananker SM, O'Donnell JT, Salemi JR, et al. The risk of anaphylactic reactions to rocuronium in the United States is comparable to that of vecuronium: An analysis of food and drug administration reporting of adverse events. *Anesth Analg.* 2005;101:819–822.
88. Gurrieri C, Weingarten TN, Martin DP, et al. Allergic reactions during anesthesia at a large United States referral center. *Anesth Analg.* 2011;113:1202–1212.

89. Florvaag E, Johansson SG, Oman H, et al. Prevalence of IgE antibodies to morphine. Relation to the high and low incidences of NMBA anaphylaxis in Norway and Sweden, respectively. *Acta Anaesthesiol Scand.* 2005;49:437–444.
90. Johansson SGO, Florvaag E, Oman H, et al. National pholcodine consumption and prevalence of IgE-sensitization: A multicentre study. *Allergy.* 2010;65:498–502.
91. Harboe T, Johansson SGO, Florvaag E, et al. Pholcodine exposure raises serum IgE in patients with previous anaphylaxis to neuromuscular blocking agents. *Allergy.* 2007;62:1445–1450.
92. Florvaag E, Johansson SG, Irgens A, et al. IgE-sensitization of the cough suppressant pholcodine and the effects of its withdrawal from the Norwegian market. *Allergy.* 2011;66:955–960.
93. Xue FS, Tong SY, Liao X, et al. Dose-response and time course of effect of rocuronium in male and female anesthetized patients. *Anesth Analg.* 1997;85:667–671.
94. Collins LM, Bevan JC, Bevan DR, et al. The prolonged duration of rocuronium in Chinese patients. *Anesth Analg.* 2000;91:1526–1530.
95. Dahaba AA, Perelman SI, Moskowitz DM, et al. Geographic regional differences in rocuronium bromide dose-response relation and time course of action: An overlooked factor in determining recommended dosage. *Anesthesiology.* 2006;104:950–953.
96. Woolf RL, Crawford MW, Choo SM. Dose-response of rocuronium bromide in children anesthetized with propofol: A comparison with succinylcholine. *Anesthesiology.* 1997;87:1368–1372.
97. Rapp HJ, Altenmueller CA, Waschke C. Neuromuscular recovery following rocuronium bromide single dose in infants. *Paediatr Anaesth.* 2004;14:329–335.
98. Bevan DR, Fiset P, Balendran P, et al. Pharmacodynamic behaviour of rocuronium in the elderly. *Can J Anaesth.* 1993;40:127–132.
99. Szenohradszky J, Fisher DM, Segredo V, et al. Pharmacokinetics of rocuronium bromide (ORG 9426) in patients with normal renal function or patients undergoing cadaver renal transplantation. *Anesthesiology.* 1992;77:899–904.
100. Khalil M, D'Honneur G, Duvaldestin P, et al. Pharmacokinetics and pharmacodynamics of rocuronium in patients with cirrhosis. *Anesthesiology.* 1994;80:1241–1247.
101. Bisschops MM, Holleman C, Huitink JM. Can sugammadex save the patient in a simulated 'cannot intubate, cannot ventilate' situation? *Anaesthesia.* 2010;65:936–941.
102. Hemmerling TM, Schuettler J, Schwilden H. Desflurane reduces the effective therapeutic infusion rate (ETI) of cisatracurium more than isoflurane, sevoflurane, or propofol. *Can J Anaesth.* 2001;48:532–537.
103. Kopman AF, Chin WA, Moe J, et al. The effect of nitrous oxide on the dose-response relationship of rocuronium. *Anesth Analg.* 2005;100:1343–1347.
104. Illman H, Antila H, Olkkola KT. Quantitation of the effect of nitrous oxide on rocuronium infusion requirements using closed-loop feedback control. *Anesthesiology.* 2008;108:388–391.
105. Paul M, Fokt RM, Kindler CH, et al. Characterization of the interactions between volatile anesthetics and neuromuscular blockers at the muscle nicotinic acetylcholine receptor. *Anesth Analg.* 2002;95:362–367.
106. Suzuki T, Mizutani H, Ishikawa K, et al. Epidurally administered mepivacaine delays recovery of train-of-four ratio from vecuronium-induced neuromuscular block. *Br J Anaesth.* 2007;99:721–725.
107. Sahin SH, Colak A, Sezer A, et al. Effect of epidural levobupivacaine on recovery from vecuronium-induced neuromuscular block in patients undergoing lower abdominal surgery. *Anaesth Intensive Care.* 2011;39:607–610.
108. Kim KS, Chun YS, Chon SU, et al. Neuromuscular interaction between cisatracurium and mivacurium, atracurium, vecuronium or rocuronium administered in combination. *Anaesthesia.* 1998;53:872–878.
109. Kim DW, Joshi GP, White PF, et al. Interactions between mivacurium, rocuronium, and vecuronium during general anesthesia. *Anesth Analg.* 1996;83:818–822.
110. Cooper R, Maddineni VR, Mirakhur RK. Clinical interaction between rocuronium and some commonly used antimicrobial agents. *Eur J Anaesthesiol.* 1993;10:331–335.
111. Spacek A, Nickl S, Neiger FX, et al. Augmentation of the rocuronium-induced neuromuscular block by the acutely administered phenytoin. *Anesthesiology.* 1999;90:1551–1555.
112. Alloul K, Whalley DG, Shutway F, et al. Pharmacokinetic origin of carbamazepine-induced resistance to vecuronium neuromuscular blockade in anesthetized patients. *Anesthesiology.* 1996;84:330–339.
113. Loan PB, Connolly FM, Mirakhur RK, et al. Neuromuscular effects of rocuronium in patients receiving beta-adrenoreceptor blocking, calcium entry blocking and anticonvulsant drugs. *Br J Anaesth.* 1997;78:90–91.
114. Richard A, Girard F, Girard DC, et al. Cisatracurium-induced neuromuscular blockade is affected by chronic phenytoin or carbamazepine treatment in neurosurgical patients. *Anesth Analg.* 2005;100:538–544.
115. Szmuk P, Ezri T, Chelly JE, et al. The onset time of rocuronium is slowed by esmolol and accelerated by ephedrine. *Anesth Analg.* 2000;90:1217–1219.
116. Herroeder S, Schonherr ME, De Hert SG, et al. Magnesium–essentials for the anesthesiologist. *Anesthesiology.* 2011;114:971–993.
117. Arroliga A, Frutos-Vivar F, Hall J, et al. Use of sedatives and neuromuscular blockers in a cohort of patients receiving mechanical ventilation. *Chest.* 2005;128:496–506.
118. Fletcher SN, Kennedy DD, Ghosh IR, et al. Persistent neuromuscular and neurophysiologic abnormalities in long-term survivors of prolonged critical illness. *Crit Care Med.* 2003;31:1012–1016.
119. Hirsch NP. Neuromuscular junction in health and disease. *Br J Anaesth.* 2007;99:132–138.
120. Itoh H, Shibata K, Yoshida M, et al. Neuromuscular monitoring at the orbicularis oculi may overestimate the blockade in myasthenic patients. *Anesthesiology.* 2000;93:1194–1197.
121. Parness J, Bandschapp O, Girard T. The myotonias and susceptibility to malignant hyperthermia. *Anesth Analg.* 2009;109:1054–1064.
122. Gurnaney H, Brown A, Litman RS. Malignant hyperthermia and muscular dystrophies. *Anesth Analg.* 2009;109:1043–1048.
123. Capron F, Fortier LP, Racine S, et al. Tactile fade detection with hand or wrist stimulation using train-of-four, double-burst stimulation, 50-hertz tetanus, 100-hertz tetanus, and acceleromyography. *Anesth Analg.* 2006;102:1578–1584.
124. O'Hara DA, Fragen RJ, Shanks CA. Comparison of visual and measured train-of-four recovery after vecuronium-induced neuromuscular blockade using two anaesthetic techniques. *Br J Anaesth.* 1986;58:1300–1302.
125. Viby-Mogensen J, Howardy-Hansen P, Chraemmer-Jørgensen B, et al. Posttetanic count (PTC): A new method of evaluating an intense nondepolarizing neuromuscular blockade. *Anesthesiology.* 1981;55:458–461.
126. Brull S, Murphy GS. Residual neuromuscular block: Lessons unlearned. Part II: Methods to reduce the risk of residual weakness. *Anesth Analg.* 2010;111:129–140.
127. Kirov K, Motamed C, Ndoko SK, et al. TOF count at corrugator supercilii reflects abdominal muscles relaxation better than at adductor pollicis. *Br J Anaesth.* 2007;98:611–614.
128. Nepveu ME, Donati F, Fortier LP. Train-of-four stimulation for adductor pollicis neuromuscular monitoring can be applied at the wrist or over the hand. *Anesth Analg.* 2005;100:149–154.
129. Donati F, Meistelman C, Plaud B. Vecuronium neuromuscular blockade at the diaphragm, the orbicularis oculi, and adductor pollicis muscles. *Anesthesiology.* 1990;73:870–875.
130. Donati F, Meistelman C, Plaud B. Vecuronium neuromuscular blockade at the adductor muscles of the larynx and adductor pollicis. *Anesthesiology.* 1991;74:833–837.
131. D'Honneur G, Guignard B, Slavov V, et al. Comparison of the neuromuscular blocking effect of atracurium and vecuronium on the adductor pollicis and the geniohyoid muscle in humans. *Anesthesiology.* 1995;82:649–654.
132. Kopman AF. The relationship of evoked electromyographic and mechanical responses following atracurium in humans. *Anesthesiology.* 1985;63:208–211.
133. Murphy GS, Brull SJ. Residual neuromuscular block: Lessons unlearned. Part I: Definitions, incidence, and adverse physiologic effects of neuromuscular block. *Anesth Analg.* 2010;111:120–128.
134. Kopman AF, Yee PS, Neuman GG. Relationship of the train-of-four fade ratio to clinical signs and symptoms of residual paralysis in awake volunteers. *Anesthesiology.* 1997;86:765–771.
135. Eriksson LI, Lennmarken C, Wyon N, et al. Attenuated ventilatory response to hypoxaemia at vecuronium-induced partial neuromuscular block. *Acta Anaesthesiol Scand.* 1992;36:710–715.
136. Eikermann M, Vogt FM, Herbstreit F, et al. The predisposition to inspiratory upper airway collapse during partial neuromuscular blockade. *Am J Resp Crit Care Med.* 2007;175:9–15.
137. Heier T, Caldwell JE. Impact of hypothermia on the response to neuromuscular blocking drugs. *Anesthesiology.* 2006;104:1070–1080.
138. Arbous MS, Meursing AE, van Kleef JW, et al. Impact of anesthesia management characteristics on severe morbidity and mortality. *Anesthesiology.* 2005;102:257–268.
139. Fiekers JF. Concentration-dependent effects of neostigmine on the endplate acetylcholine receptor channel complex. *J Neurosci.* 1985;5:502–514.
140. Bartkowski RR. Incomplete reversal of pancuronium neuromuscular blockade by neostigmine, pyridostigmine, and edrophonium. *Anesth Analg.* 1987;66:594–598.
141. McCourt KC, Mirakhur RK, Kerr CM. Dosage of neostigmine for reversal of rocuronium block from two levels of spontaneous recovery. *Anaesthesia.* 1999;54:651–655.
142. Herbstreit F, Zigrann D, Ochterbeck C, et al. Neostigmine/glycopyrrolate administered after recovery from neuromuscular block increases upper airway collapsibility by decreasing genioglossus muscle activity in response to negative pharyngeal pressure. *Anesthesiology.* 2010;113:1280–1288.
143. Heier T, Clough D, Wright PM, et al. The influence of mild hypothermia on the pharmacokinetics and time course of action of neostigmine in anesthetized volunteers. *Anesthesiology.* 2002;97:90–95.
144. Flockton EA, Mastronardi P, Hunter JM, et al. Reversal of rocuronium-induced neuromuscular block with sugammadex is faster than reversal of cisatracurium-induced block with neostigmine. *Br J Anaesth.* 2008;100:622–630.
145. Baurain MJ, Hoton F, d'Hollander AA, et al. Is recovery of neuromuscular transmission complete after the use of neostigmine to antagonize block produced by rocuronium, vecuronium, atracurium and pancuronium? *Br J Anaesth.* 1996;77:496–499.
146. Khuenl-Brady KS, Wattwil M, Vanacker BF, et al. Sugammadex provides faster reversal of vecuronium-induced neuromuscular blockade compared

with neostigmine: A multicenter, randomized, controlled trial. *Anesth Analg.* 2010;110:64–73.

147. Blobner M, Eriksson LI, Scholz J, et al. Reversal of rocuronium-induced neuromuscular blockade with sugammadex compared with neostigmine during sevoflurane anesthesia: Results of a randomised, controlled trial. *Eur J Anaesthesiol.* 2010;27:874–881.
148. Jones RK, Caldwell JE, Brull SJ, et al. Reversal of profound rocuronium-induced blockade with sugammadex. A randomized comparison with neostigmine. *Anesthesiology.* 2008;109:816–824.
149. Bevan JC, Collins L, Fowler C, et al. Early and late reversal of rocuronium and vecuronium with neostigmine in adults and children. *Anesth Analg.* 1999;89:333–339.
150. Tramer MR, Fuchs-Buder T. Omitting antagonism of neuromuscular block: Effect on postoperative nausea and vomiting and risk of residual paralysis. A systematic review. *Br J Anaesth.* 1999;82:379–386.
151. Cheng CR, Sessler DI, Apfel CC. Does neostigmine administration produce a clinically important increase in postoperative nausea and vomiting? *Anesth Analg.* 2005;101:1349–1355.
152. Fuchs-Buder T, Meistelman C, Alla F, et al. Antagonism of low degrees of atracurium-induced neuromuscular blockade: Dose-effect relationship for neostigmine. *Anesthesiology.* 2010;112:34–40.
153. Naguib M. Sugammadex: Another milestone in clinical neuromuscular pharmacology. *Anesth Analg.* 2007;104:575–581.
154. Zwiers A, van den Heuvel M, Smeets J, et al. Assessment of the potential for displacement interactions with sugammadex. A pharmacokinetic-pharmacodynamic modeling approach. *Clin drug Investig.* 2011;31:101–111.
155. McDonagh DL, Benedict PE, Kovac AL, et al. Efficacy, safety, and pharmacokinetics of sugammadex for the reversal of rocuronium-induced neuromuscular blockade in elderly patients. *Anesthesiology.* 2011;114:318–329.
156. Suy K, Morias K, Cammu G, et al. Effective reversal of moderate rocuronium- or vecuronium-induced neuromuscular block with sugammadex, a selective relaxant binding agent. *Anesthesiology.* 2007;106:283–288.
157. Eleveld DJ, Kuizenga K, Proost JH, et al. A temporary decrease in twitch response during reversal of rocuronium-induced muscle relaxation with a small dose of sugammadex. *Anesth Analg.* 2007;104:582–584.
158. Staals LM, Snoeck MMJ, Driessen JJ, et al. Reduced clearance of rocuronium and sugammadex in patients with severe to end-stage renal failure: A pharmacokinetic study. *Br J Anaesth.* 2010;104:31–39.
159. Plaud B, Meretoja O, Hofmockel R, et al. Reversal of rocuronium-induced neuromuscular blockade with sugammadex in pediatric and adult surgical patients. *Anesthesiology.* 2009;110:284–294.
160. Van Lancker P, Dillemans B, Bogaert T, et al. Ideal versus corrected body weight for dosage of sugammadex in morbidly obese patients. *Anaesthesia.* 2011;66:721–725.
161. Peeters PAM, van den Heuvel M, van Heumen E, et al. Safety, tolerability and pharmacokinetics of sugammadex using single high doses (up to 96 mg/kg) in healthy adult subjects: A randomized, double-blind, crossover, placebo-controlled, single-centre study. *Clin Drug Investig.* 2010;30:867–874.
162. Cammu G, de Kam PJ, De Graeve K, et al. Repeat dosing of rocuronium 1.2 mg kg^{-1} after reversal of neuromuscular block by sugammadex 4.0 mg kg^{-1} in anaesthetized healthy volunteers: A modelling-based pilot study. *Br J Anaesth.* 2010;105:487–492.
163. Schaller SJ, Fink H, Ulm K, et al. Sugammadex and neostigmine dose-finding study for reversal of shallow residual neuromuscular block. *Anesthesiology.* 2010;113:1054–1060.
164. Pühringer FK, Kristen P, Rex C. Sugammadex reversal of rocuronium-induced neuromuscular block in Caesarean section patients: a series of seven cases. *Br J Anaesth.* 2010;105:657–660.

CHAPTER

21 Local Anesthetics

YI LIN • SPENCER S. LIU

Key Points

1. Local anesthetics provide anesthesia and analgesia by blocking the transmission of pain sensation along nerve fibers.
2. The key target of local anesthetics is the voltage-gated sodium channel. The binding is intracellular and is mediated by hydrophobic interactions.
3. The degree of nerve blockade depends on both drug concentration and volume.
4. Most clinically relevant agents contain a lipid-soluble benzene ring connected to an amide group and are categorized as either aminoesters or aminoamides, based on their chemical linkage.
5. Potency is related to hydrophobicity and physiochemical properties of the agent. In general, more potent agents are more lipid soluble.
6. Efficacy for clinical use of local anesthetics may be increased by addition of epinephrine, opioids, and α_2-adrenergic agonists. The value of alkalinization of local anesthetics appears to be debatable as a clinically useful tool to improve anesthesia.
7. The rate of local anesthetic system absorption depends on the site of injection, the dose, the drug's intrinsic pharmacokinetic properties, and the addition of a vasoactive agent.
8. Systemic toxicity from the clinical use of local anesthetics is an uncommon occurrence. Patients with cardiovascular collapse from bupivacaine, ropivacaine, and levobupivacaine may be especially difficult to resuscitate; however, intravenous lipid infusion is a promising new therapy.

Multimedia

 1 Peripheral Nerve Cross-section

 2 Ankle Block

1 Local anesthetics block the conduction of impulses in electrically excitable tissues. One of the important uses is to provide anesthesia and analgesia by blocking the transmission of pain sensation along nerve fibers. The molecular target of these agents is specific and the interaction has been extensively studied. Existing clinical applications are numerous and continue to expand. A comprehensive understanding of the mechanisms and the physiochemical properties of these agents would enable optimization of the therapeutic potential and avoid complications associated with inadvertent systemic toxicity.

MECHANISMS OF ACTION OF LOCAL ANESTHETICS

Anatomy of Nerves

Local anesthetics are used to block nerves in the peripheral nervous system (PNS) and central nervous system (CNS). In the PNS, nerves contain both afferent and efferent fibers, which

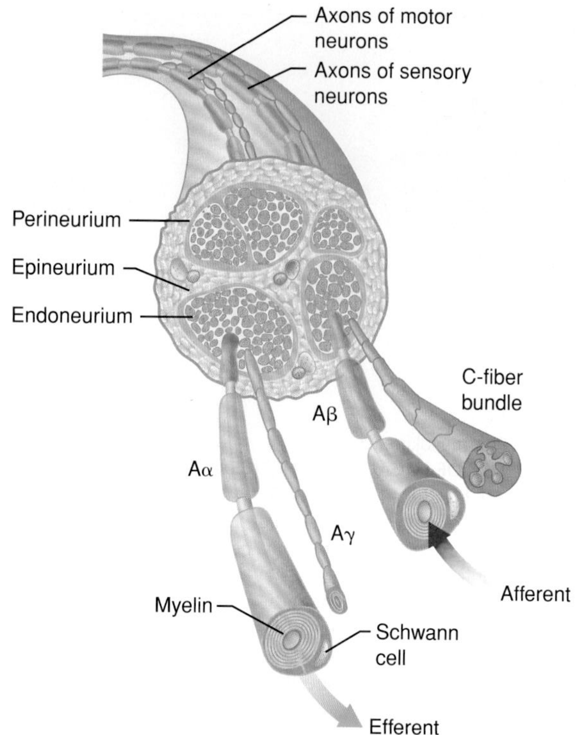

FIGURE 21-1. Schematic cross section of typical peripheral nerve. The epineurium, consisting of collagen fibers, is oriented along the long axis of the nerve. The perineurium is a discrete cell layer, whereas the endoneurium is a matrix of connective tissue. Both afferent and efferent axons are shown. Sympathetic axons (not shown) are also present in mixed peripheral nerves. (Adapted from: Strichartz GR. Neural physiology and local anesthetic action. In: Cousins MJ, Bridenbaugh PO, eds. *Neural Blockade in Clinical Anesthesia and Management of Pain.* Philadelphia, PA: Lippincott-Raven; 1998:35, with permission.)

are bundled into one or more fascicles and organized within three tissue layers.[1] Individual nerve fibers within each fascicle are surrounded by the *endoneurium,* a loose connective tissue containing glial cells, fibroblasts, and blood capillaries. A dense layer of collagenous connective tissue called the *perineurium* surrounds each fascicle. A final layer of dense connective tissue, the *epineurium,* encases groups of fascicles into a cylindrical sheath (Fig. 21-1). These layers of tissue offer protection to the surrounded nerve fibers and act as barriers to passive diffusion of local anesthetics.[2]

Nerves in both the CNS and PNS are differentiated by the presence or absence of myelin sheath. Myelinated nerve fibers are surrounded by Schwann cells in the PNS and by oligodendrocytes in the CNS. The cells form a concentrically wrapped lipid bilayer sheath around the axons that cover the length of the nerve.[3] The myelin sheath is interrupted at short, regular intervals by specialized regions called *nodes of Ranvier,* which contain densely clustered protein elements essential for transmission of neuronal signals[4] (Fig. 21-2). As electrical signals are renewed at each node, nerve impulses move in myelinated fibers by saltatory conduction. In contrast, there are no nodes of Ranvier in nonmyelinated nerve fibers. Although these nerve fibers are similarly encased in Schwann cells, the plasma membrane does not wrap around the axons concentrically. Several nerve fibers may be simultaneously embedded within a single Schwann cell[1] (Fig. 21-3).

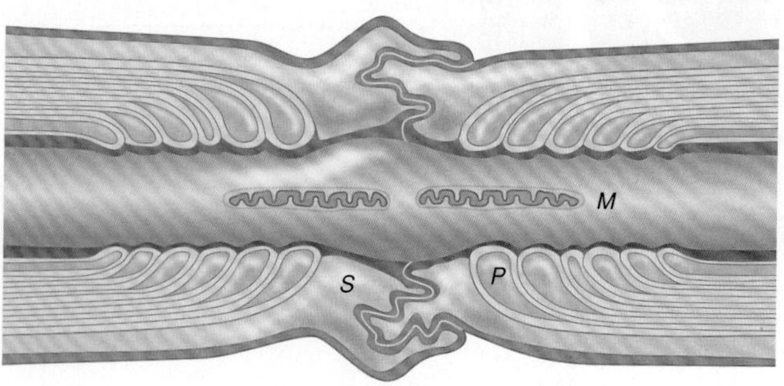

FIGURE 21-2. Diagram of node of Ranvier displaying mitochondria (*M*), tight junctions in paranodal area (*P*), and Schwann cell (*S*) surrounding node. (Adapted from: Strichartz GR. Mechanisms of action of local anesthetic agents. In: Rogers MC, Tinker JH, Covino BG, et al., eds. *Principles and Practice of Anesthesiology.* St. Louis, MO: Mosby Year Book; 1993:1197, with permission.)

Nerve fibers are commonly classified according to their size, conduction velocity, and function (Table 21-1). In general, nerve fibers with cross-sectional diameter greater than 1 μm are myelinated. Both a larger nerve size and the presence of myelin sheath are associated with faster conduction velocity.[5] Nerve fibers with large diameters have better intrinsic electric conductance. Myelin improves the electrical insulation of nerve fibers and permits more rapid impulse transmission via saltatory conduction. Large-diameter, myelinated fibers, many of which are classified as A fibers, are typically involved in motor and sensory functions in which speed of nerve transmission is critical. In contrast, small-diameter, nonmyelinated C fibers have slower conduction velocity and relay sensory information such as pain, temperature, and autonomic functions.

Electrophysiology of Neural Conduction and Voltage-gated Sodium Channels

Transmission of electrical impulses along the cell membrane forms the basis of signal transduction along nerve fibers. Energy necessary for the propagation and maintenance of the electric potential is maintained on the cell surface by ionic disequilibria across the semipermeable cell membrane.[6] The resting membrane potential, approximately −60 to −70 mV in neurons (the extracellular electric potential is, by convention, defined as zero, and the intracellular

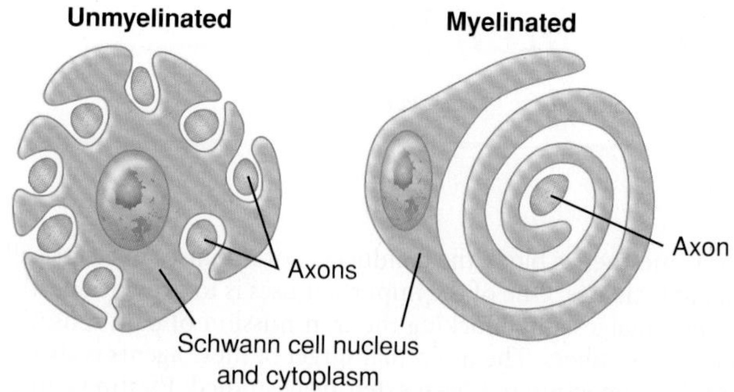

FIGURE 21-3. Schwann cells form myelin around one myelinated axon or encompass several unmyelinated axons. (Adapted from: Carpenter RL, Mackey DC. Local anesthetics. In: Barash PG, Cullen BF, Stoelting RF, eds. *Clinical Anesthesia.* 3rd ed. Philadelphia, PA: Lippincott-Raven; 1996:413, with permission.)

TABLE 21-1. CLASSIFICATION OF NERVE FIBERS

Classification	Diameter (μm)	Myelin	Conduction (m/s)	Location	Function
Aα, Aβ	6–22	+	30–120	Afferents/efferents for muscles and joints	Motor and proprioception
Aγ	3–6	+	15–35	Efferent to muscle spindle	Muscle tone
Aδ	1–4	+	5–25	Afferent sensory nerve	Pain Touch Temperature
B	<3	+	3–15	Preganglionic sympathetic	Autonomic function
C	0.3–1.3	–	0.7–1.3	Postganglionic sympathetic Afferent sensory nerve	Autonomic function Pain Temperature

potential is thus negative relative to it), is derived predominantly from a difference in the intracellular and extracellular concentrations of potassium and sodium ions. Neurons at rest are more permeable to potassium ions than sodium ions because of potassium leak channels; therefore membrane potential is closer to the equilibrium potential of potassium (E_K –80 mV) than that of sodium (E_{Na} +60 mV). The ion gradient is continuously regenerated by protein pumps, cotransporters, and channels via adenosine triphosphate–dependent process.

Electrical impulses are conducted along nerve fibers as action potentials. They are brief, localized spikes of positive charge, or depolarizations, on the cell membrane caused by rapid influx of sodium ions down its electrochemical gradient.[7] An action potential is initiated by local membrane depolarization, such as at the cell body or nerve terminal by ligand–receptor complex. When a certain charge threshold is reached, an action potential is triggered and further depolarization occurs in an "all-or-none" fashion.[8] The spike in membrane potential peaks around +50 mV, at which point the influx of sodium is replaced with an efflux of potassium, causing a reversal of membrane potential, or repolarization. The passive diffusion of membrane depolarization triggers other action potentials in either adjacent cell membrane in *nonmyelinated* nerve fibers or adjacent nodes of Ranvier in *myelinated* nerve fibers, resulting in a wave of action potential being propagated along the nerve. A short *refractory period* that ensues after each action potential prevents the retrograde spread of action potential on previously activated membranes.[7]

The flow of ions responsible for action potentials is mediated by a variety of channels and pumps, the most important of which are the voltage-gated sodium channels. They are essential for the influx of sodium ions during the rapid depolarization phase of the action potential and belong to a family of channel proteins that also includes voltage-gated potassium and voltage-gated calcium channels. Each voltage-gated sodium channel is a complex made up of one principal α-subunit and one or more auxiliary β-subunits.[9] The α-subunit is a single-polypeptide transmembrane protein that contains most of the key components of the channel function. They include four homologous α-helical domains (D1 to D4) that form the channel pore and control ion selectivity, voltage-sensing regions that regulate gating function and inactivation, and phosphorylation sites for modulation by protein kinases. β-subunits are short polypeptide proteins with a single transmembrane domain. They are linked to α-subunits by either noncovalent or disulfide bonds; although they are dispensable for channel activity, evidence suggests that they perhaps play a role in modulation of channel expression, localization, and function.

In the absence of a stimulus, voltage-gated sodium channels exist predominantly in the resting or closed state (Fig. 21-4). On membrane depolarization, positive charges on the membrane interact with charged amino acid residues in the voltage-sensing regions (S4).[10] This induces a conformational change in the channel, converting it to the open state. Sodium ions rush through the opened pore, which is lined with negatively charged residues. Ion selectivity is determined by these amino acid residues; changes in their composition can lead to increased permeability for other cations, such as potassium and calcium.[11] Within milliseconds after opening, channels undergo a transition to the inactivated state. Depending on the frequency and voltage of the initial depolarizing

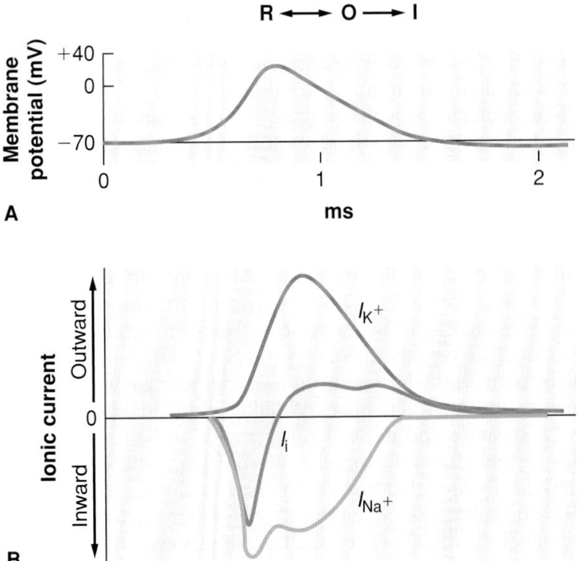

FIGURE 21-4. Illustration of dominant form of sodium channel during generation of an action potential. R, resting form; O, open form; I, inactive form. **(A)** The concurrent generation of an action potential as the membrane depolarizes from resting potential. **(B)** The concurrent changes in ion flux, as inward sodium current (I_{NA}+) and outward potassium current (I_K+) together yield the net ionic current across the membrane (I_i). (Adapted from: Strichartz GR. Neural physiology and local anesthetic action. In: Cousins MJ, Bridenbaugh PO, eds. *Neural Blockade in Clinical Anesthesia and Management of Pain*. Philadelphia, PA: Lippincott-Raven; 1998:35, with permission.)

TABLE 21-2. VOLTAGE-GATED SODIUM CHANNELS

Name	Tissue Expression	Tetrodotoxin	Associated Channelopathies
Na_V 1.1	CNS, heart	Sensitive	Inherited febrile epilepsy
Na_V 1.2	CNS nonmyelinated axons	Sensitive	Inherited febrile epilepsy
Na_V 1.3	Fetal DRG	Sensitive	None known
Na_V 1.4	Skeletal muscle	Sensitive	Hyperkalemic periodic paralysis, paramyotonia congenita
Na_V 1.5	Heart, embryonic neurons	Insensitive	Brugada syndrome, long QT syndrome
Na_V 1.6	Nodes of Ranvier	Sensitive	None known
Na_V 1.7	CNS, DRG, sympathetic neurons	Sensitive	Erythromelalgia, paroxysmal extreme pain disorder, congenital insensitivity to pain
Na_V 1.8	Small DRG neurons	Insensitive	None known
Na_V 1.9	Small DRG neurons	Insensitive	None known

CNS, central nervous system; DRG, dorsal root ganglion.
Data adapted from: Benarroch EE. Sodium channels and pain. *Neurology.* 2007:68:233; and Koopmann TT, Bezzina CR, Wilde AA. Voltage-gated sodium channels: Action players with many faces. *Ann Med.* 2006:38:472.

stimulus, the channel may undergo either fast or slow inactivation. Slow or fast inactivation refers to the duration in which the channel remains refractory to repeat depolarization before resetting to the closed state. Fast inactivation completes within a millisecond and is sensitive to the action of local anesthetics. It is mediated by a short mobile intracellular polypeptide loop connecting domains D3 and D4 that closes the channel from inside the cell via a hinge-lid mechanism.[12] A triad of highly hydrophobic amino acids (isoleucine, phenylalanine, and methionine [IFM]) appears to be an important structural determinant of fast activation; disrupting the loop or changing the hydrophobicity of the amino acids abrogates fast inactivation.[13,14] Slow activation, lasting seconds to minutes, is distinct from fast activation. It is resistant to the action of local anesthetics and its mechanism is less well understood. It often occurs after prolonged depolarization and is believed to be important in regulating membrane excitability.

Nine isoforms of voltage-gated sodium channels (Na_V 1.1 to Na_V 1.9) have been identified; each relates to a unique α-subunit subtype (Table 21-2). Each isoform varies slightly in its channel kinetics, such as threshold of activation and mode of inactivation, and its sensitivity to blocking agents like tetrodotoxins and local anesthetics. Cell and tissue expression of individual isoforms may be quite specific; for instance, Na_V 1.2 is found almost exclusively in the CNS, whereas Na_V 1.6 is restricted to nodes of Ranvier in both CNS and PNS.[15] Likewise, several isoforms could be present on a single cell type; both Na_V 1.8 and Na_V 1.9 have been found in small- to medium-sized neurons in dorsal root ganglions that are connected to Aδ and C fibers. Whether individual isoforms each have a separate and defined role remains to be seen; however, clues to their function may be inferred from studies of several inherited diseases that have been associated with sodium channelopathies. Hyperexcitability of Na_V 1.7 has been implicated in several painful disease states, such as primary erythromelalgia and paroxysmal extreme pain disorder.[16,17] Conversely, null mutation of Na_V 1.7 is linked to a rare genetic condition in which otherwise normal individuals have severely impaired perception to pain.[18,19]

Molecular Mechanisms of Local Anesthetics

2 Local anesthetics block the transmission of nerve impulses by targeting the function of voltage-gated sodium channels. Although several local anesthetics can bind to other receptors like voltage-gated potassium channels and nicotinic acetylcholine receptors and their amphipathic nature may enable them to interact with plasma membranes, it is widely accepted that they induce anesthesia and analgesia through direct interactions with the sodium channels. Other molecules with local anesthetic properties such as tricyclic antidepressants and anticonvulsants may likewise interact with voltage-gated sodium channels; however, it is unclear if they act through similar mechanisms. Therefore, the following discussion is limited to the "traditional" set of local anesthetic molecules.

Local anesthetics reversibly bind the intracellular portion of voltage-gated sodium channels (Fig. 21-5). Early experiments

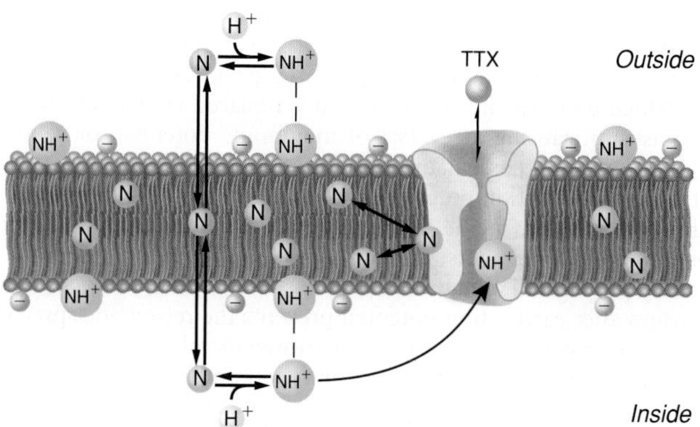

FIGURE 21-5. Diagram of bilayer lipid membrane of conductive tissue with sodium channel spanning the membrane. Tertiary amine local anesthetics exist as neutral base (N) and protonated, charged form (NH+) in equilibrium. The neutral base (N) is more lipid soluble, preferentially partitions into the lipophilic membrane interior, and easily passes through the membrane. The charged form (NH+) is more water soluble and binds to the sodium channel at the negatively charged membrane surface. Both forms can affect the function of the sodium channel. The N form can cause membrane expansion and closure of the sodium channel. The NH+ form will directly inhibit the sodium channel by binding with a local anesthetic receptor. The natural "local anesthetic" tetrodotoxin (*TTX*) binds at the external surface of the sodium channel and has no interaction with the clinically used local anesthetics. (Adapted from: Strichartz GR. Neural physiology and local anesthetic action. In: Cousins MJ, Bridenbaugh PO, eds. *Neural Blockade in Clinical Anesthesia and Management of Pain.* Philadelphia, PA: Lippincott-Raven; 1998:35, with permission.)

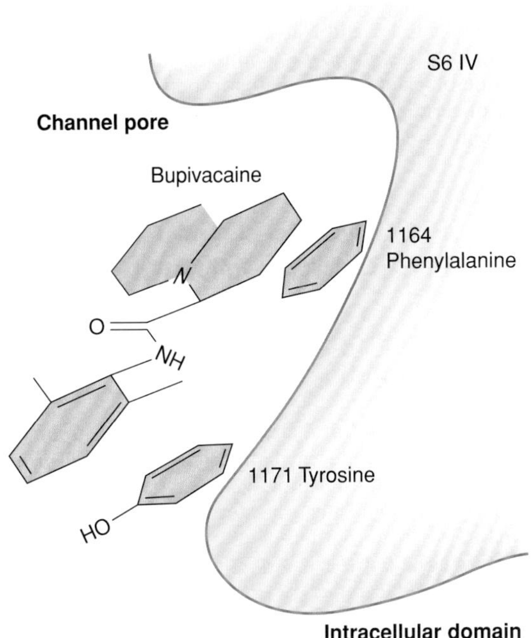

FIGURE 21-6. Diagram of local anesthetic–binding site, depicting a hydrophobic pocket within the channel pore. (Adapted from: Ragsdale DS, McPhee JC, Scheuer T, et al. Molecular determinants of state-dependent block of Na+ channels by local anesthetics. *Science.* 1994;265:1724, with permission.)

with giant squid axons demonstrated that a derivative of lidocaine with a permanent positive charge, QX314, which cannot cross the plasma membrane, blocks ion current through voltage-gated sodium channels only with intra-axoplasmic injections, but not with external application.[20] Subsequent mutational analyses have supported the observation and identified specific sites on the channel involved in drug recognition.[21] Several hydrophobic aromatic residues (a phenylalanine at position 1,764 and a tyrosine at position 1,771 in Na_V 1.2) located within an α-helix (S6) of domains 1, 3, and 4 are essential for drug binding (Fig. 21-6). They line an inner cavity within the intracellular portion of the channel pore and span a region about 11 Å apart, roughly the size of a local anesthetic molecule. Changes in either residue severely reduce the binding affinity. Another hydrophobic amino acid (an isoleucine at position 1,760), located near the outer pore opening, has similarly been found to influence the dissociation of local anesthetics from the channel by antagonizing the release of drugs through the channel pore.

Application of local anesthetics typically produces a concentration-dependent decrease in the peak sodium current.[22,23] Known as "tonic blockade," it reflects the reduction in the number of sodium channels for a given drug concentration present in the open state at equilibrium. In contrast, repetitive stimulation of the sodium channels often leads to a shift in the steady-state equilibrium, resulting in a greater number of channels being blocked at the same drug concentration. Termed *use-dependent blockade,* the exact mechanism is incompletely understood and has been the subject of many competing hypotheses. One popular theory, the *modulated-receptor theory,* proposes that local anesthetics bind to the open or the inactivated channels more avidly than the resting channels, suggesting that drug affinity is a function of a channel's conformational state. An alternate theory, the *guarded-receptor theory,* assumes that the intrinsic binding affinity remains essentially constant regardless of a channel's conformation; rather, the apparent affinity is associated with increased access to the recognition site resulting from channel gating. Experimental evidence so far has been inconclusive.

Mechanism of Nerve Blockade

Local anesthetics block peripheral nerves by disrupting the transmission of action potentials along nerve fibers. To get to its site of action, principally the voltage-gated sodium channels, local anesthetics have to reach the targeted nerve membrane. This entails the diffusion of drugs through tissues and the generation of a concentration gradient. Even with close proximity of deposition, only about 1% to 2% of injected local anesthetics ultimately penetrate into the nerve.[24] As discussed earlier, the perineural sheath encasing nerve fibers appears to be an important determinant; nerves that have been desheathed in vitro require about a hundred-fold lower local anesthetic concentration (in the 0.7 to 0.9 mM range for lidocaine) than nerves in vivo (the typical 2% lidocaine used clinically is equivalent to 75 mM concentration). Although it may vary with anatomic location and nerve physiology, functional block typically occurs within 5 minutes of injection in rat sciatic nerves, and this time course corresponds to the peak in the intraneural drug absorption.

3 The degree of nerve blockade depends on the local anesthetic concentration and volume. For a given drug, a minimal concentration is necessary to effect complete nerve blockade. It reflects the potency of the local anesthetics and the intrinsic conduction properties of nerve fibers, which in turn likely depend on the drug's binding affinity to the ion channels and the degree of drug saturation necessary to halt the transmission of action potentials. Accordingly, individual types of nerve fibers differ in their minimal blocking concentration, such that some A fibers are blocked by lower drug concentrations than C fibers.[25] Likewise, the pattern of stimulation (tonic vs. use-dependent blockade) influences the degree of conduction failure; repetitive stimulations, which can lead to a shift in steady-state equilibrium of blocked sodium channels, are associated with higher conduction failure than tonic stimulation at a given drug concentration.[26]

Of equal importance as drug concentration is the local anesthetic volume. A sufficient volume is needed to suppress the regeneration of nerve impulse over a critical length of nerve fiber. According to the model of decremental conduction (Fig. 21-7), as membrane depolarization from an action potential passively decays with distance along nerve fibers, the presence of local anesthetics decreases the ability of adjacent membrane or successive nodes of Ranvier to regenerate the impulse.[27] Transmission stops once the membrane depolarization falls below the threshold for action potential activation. Too short an exposure length allows impulses to "skip" over membranes or nodes that are blocked by even the highest drug concentration, whereas exposure of a long nerve segment to a relatively low drug concentration can still result in gradual extinction of impulses by decremental decay.

Not all sensory and motor modalities are blocked equally by local anesthetics. It has long been observed that application of local anesthetics produced an ordered progression of sensory and motor deficits, starting commonly with the disappearance of temperature sensation, followed by proprioception, motor function, sharp pain, and then light touch. Termed *differential blockade,* historically this had been thought to be related simply to the diameter of the nerve fibers, with the smaller fibers inherently more susceptible to drug blockade than larger fibers.[28]

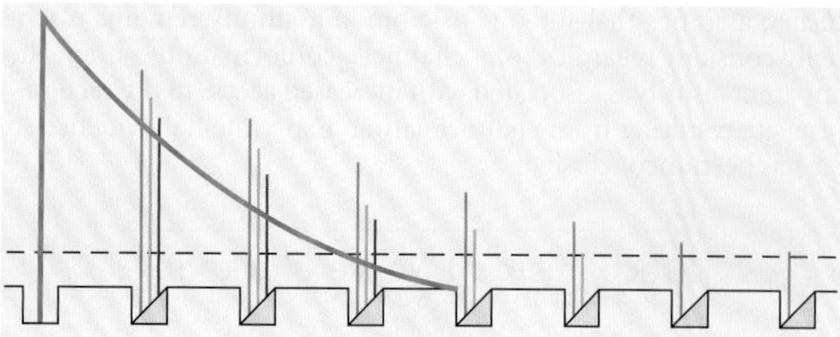

FIGURE 21-7. Diagram illustrating the principle of decremental conduction block by local anesthetic at a myelinated axon. The first node of Ranvier at left contains no local anesthetic and gives rise to a normal action potential (*solid curve*). If the nodes succeeding the first are occupied by a concentration of local anesthetic high enough to block 74% to 84% of the sodium conductance, then the action potential amplitudes decrease at successive nodes (amplitudes are indicated by *interrupted bars* representing three increasing concentrations of local anesthetic). Eventually, the impulse decays to below-threshold amplitude if the series of local anesthetic–containing nodes is long enough. Propagation of the impulse is then blocked by decremental conduction, even though none of the nodes are completely blocked. Concentrations of local anesthetics that block more than 84% of the sodium conductance at three successive nodes prevent any impulse propagation at all. (Adapted from: Fink BR. Mechanisms of differential axial blockade in epidural and spinal anesthesia. *Anesthesiology.* 1989;70:851, with permission.)

However, while the "size principle" of differential blockade is consistent with many experimental findings, it does not appear to be universally true. Larger, myelinated Aδ fibers (believed to mediate sharp pain) have been found to be blocked preferentially over small, nonmyelinated C fibers (dull pain). Furthermore, within the C fibers are fast and slow components of impulse transmission, each with distinct susceptibility to drug blockade.[29] These observations argue against a purely pharmacokinetic mechanism as the sole basis for explaining differential blockade. Instead, it may also likely depend on the intrinsic excitatory properties of the nerve fibers, namely, the patterned expression of voltage-gated sodium channels. Indeed, two channel isoforms, Na_V 1.7 and Na_V 1.8, both present on dorsal root ganglions, have been shown to possess different sensitivities to lidocaine blockade.[30] It remains to be seen how differential blockade of certain channels might translate into selective inhibition of pain and other sensory modalities.

PHARMACOLOGY AND PHARMACODYNAMICS

Chemical Properties and Relationship to Activity and Potency

4 Most clinically relevant local anesthetics are made up of a lipid-soluble, aromatic benzene ring connected to an amide group via either an amide or an ester moiety. The type of linkage divides them broadly into two categories, the *aminoesters* and the *aminoamides.* Aside from a difference in their metabolic pathways (aminoesters are hydrolyzed by plasma cholinesterases and aminoamides are degraded by hepatic carboxylesterase) and the incidence of allergic reactions attributed, their membership in either category offers little in distinction of their biophysical properties. Rather, the distinguishing physiochemical characteristics are associated with the alkalinity of the amide group, the lipophilicity conferred by the alkyl substitution on the amide group and the benzene ring, and the stereochemistry of related isomers.

The tertiary amide found in local anesthetics is capable of accepting a proton, albeit with low affinity; thus, these compounds are classified as weak bases. At physiologic pH, local anesthetics in solution are in equilibrium between the protonated, cationic form and the lipid-soluble, neutral forms. The ratio of the two forms depends on the pK_a or the dissociation constant of the local anesthetics and the surrounding pH (Table 21-3). A ratio with high concentration of the lipid-soluble form favors entry into the cell, as the main pathway for entry is by passive adsorption of lipid-soluble

TABLE 21-3. PHYSICOCHEMICAL PROPERTIES OF CLINICALLY USED LOCAL ANESTHETICS

Local Anesthetic	pK_a	Percent Ionized (at pH 7.4)	Partition Coefficient (Lipid Solubility)	Percent Protein Binding
Amides				
Bupivacaine[a]	8.1	83	3,420	95
Etidocaine	7.7	66	7,317	94
Lidocaine	7.9	76	366	64
Mepivacaine	7.6	61	130	77
Prilocaine	7.9	76	129	55
Ropivacaine	8.1	83	775	94
Esters				
Chloroprocaine	8.7	95	810	N/A
Procaine	8.9	97	100	6
Tetracaine	8.5	93	5,822	94

[a]Levobupivacaine has same physicochemical properties as racemate.
N/A, not available.
Data from: Liu SS. Local anesthetics and analgesia. In: Ashburn MA, Rice LJ, eds. *The Management of Pain.* New York: Churchill Livingstone; 1997:141.

TABLE 21-4. RELATIVE POTENCY OF LOCAL ANESTHETICS FOR DIFFERENT CLINICAL APPLICATIONS

	Bupivacaine	Chloroprocaine	Lidocaine	Mepivacaine	Prilocaine	Ropivacaine
Peripheral nerve	3.6	N/A	1	2.6	0.8	3.6
Spinal	9.6	1	1	1	1	N/A
Epidural	4	0.5	1	1	1	4

N/A, not available.

Data from: Camorcia M. Minimum local analgesic doses of ropivacaine, levobupivacaine, and bupivacaine for intrathecal labor analgesia. *Anesthesiology.* 2005;102:646; Faccenda KA. A comparison of levobupivacaine 0.5% and racemic bupivacaine 0.5% for extradural anesthesia for caesarean section. *Reg Anesth Pain Med.* 2003;28:394; McDonald SB. Hyperbaric spinal ropivacaine: A comparison to bupivacaine in volunteers. *Anesthesiology.* 1999;90:971; Marsan A. Prilocaine or mepivacaine for combined sciatic-femoral nerve block in patients receiving elective knee arthroscopy. *Minerva Anestesiol.* 2004;70:763; Casati A. Lidocaine versus ropivacaine for continuous interscalene brachial plexus block after open shoulder surgery. *Acta Anaesthesiol Scand.* 2003;47:35; Casati A. A double-blind study of axillary brachial plexus block by 0.75% ropivacaine or 2% mepivacaine. *Eur J Anaesthesiol.* 1998;15:549; Fanelli G. A double-blind comparison of ropivacaine, bupivacaine, and mepivacaine during sciatic and femoral nerve blockade. *Anesth Analg.* 1998;87:597; Yoos JR. Spinal 2-chloroprocaine: A comparison with small-dose bupivacaine in volunteers. *Anesth Analg.* 2005;100:566; Kouri ME. Spinal 2-chloroprocaine: A comparison with lidocaine in volunteers. *Anesth Analg.* 2004;98:75.

form through the cell membrane.[2] Clinically, alkalization of the
anesthetic solution increases the ratio of the lipid-soluble form to 6
cationic form, thereby facilitating cell entry. Once inside the cell, equilibrium is reestablished between the cationic and the neutral forms, and it appears that the cationic form is more potent of the two in its activity on sodium channels.[31]

Lipid solubility of local anesthetics is determined by the degree of alkyl group substitution on the amide group and the benzene ring. In the laboratory, it is measured by the partition coefficient in octanol, a hydrophobic solvent, and compounds with high octanol:buffer partition coefficients are more lipid soluble.[32] A positive correlation exists between the potency of the local anesthetics and their octanol:buffer partition coefficient; highly lipid-soluble agents are more potent and tend to have a longer duration of action than ones that are less lipid soluble.[33] This is consistent with experimental findings that show local anesthetics bind to a hydrophobic pocket within the sodium channels, suggesting that ligand binding may be mediated primarily by hydrophobic and van der Waals interactions[21] (Fig. 21-6).

5 Whereas the correlation between local anesthetic potency and hydrophobicity generally holds true in vitro, it may not be as exact in vivo. As opposed to setups with isolated nerves, other factors may influence the potency of local anesthetics on nerves in situ.[34] For example, highly lipid-soluble agents may be sequestered into surrounding adipose cells. Vasodilatory properties of local anesthetics may likewise alter drug redistribution into the neighboring tissues.[35,36] Relative potency of local anesthetics has been determined for different clinical applications and these values are listed in Table 21-4.

Finally, anesthetic activity and potency are affected by the stereochemistry of local anesthetics. Many older drugs exist as racemic mixtures; that is, enantiomeric stereoisomers differing in the arrangement at the asymmetric or chiral carbon atom are in equal proportion. Newer agents, namely, ropivacaine and levobupivacaine, are available as purely single enantiomers. They were initially developed as less cardiotoxic alternatives to bupivacaine. While the desired improvement in the safety index has been generally supported by clinical studies, it appears that, overall, this is at the expense of a slight decrease in potency and shorter duration of action compared with the racemic mixtures.[37,38] A theoretical basis for the difference between the enantiomeric stereoisomers can be readily hypothesized; however, little is known of the exact mechanisms involved. Likely, it may include subtle stereoselective preference in local anesthetic binding among the individual sodium channel isoforms.

Additives to Increase Local Anesthetic Activity

Epinephrine

Reported benefits of epinephrine include prolongation of local anesthetic block, increased intensity of block, and decreased systemic absorption of local anesthetic.[39] Epinephrine's vasoconstrictive effects augment local anesthetics by antagonizing inherent vasodilating effects of local anesthetics, decreasing systemic absorption and intraneural clearance, and perhaps by redistributing intraneural local anesthetic.[39,40]

Direct analgesic effects from epinephrine may also occur via interaction with α_2-adrenergic receptors in the brain and spinal cord,[41] especially because local anesthetics increase the vascular uptake of epinephrine.[42] The clinical effects of the use of epinephrine are listed in Table 21-5. The smallest dose is suggested because epinephrine combined with local anesthetics may have toxic effects on tissue,[43] the cardiovascular system,[44] peripheral nerves, and the spinal cord.[39]

Alkalinization of Local Anesthetic Solution

Local anesthetic solutions are alkalinized in order to hasten onset of neural block.[45] The pH of commercial preparations of local anesthetics ranges from 3.9 to 6.47 and is especially acidic if prepackaged with epinephrine.[46] As the pK_a of commonly used local anesthetics ranges from 7.6 to 8.9 (Table 21-3), less than 3% of the commercially prepared local anesthetic exists as the lipid-soluble neutral form. As previously discussed, the neutral form is believed to be important for penetration into the neural cytoplasm, whereas the charged form primarily interacts with the local anesthetic receptor within the sodium channel. Therefore, the rationale for alkalinization was to increase the ratio of local anesthetic existing as the lipid-soluble neutral form. However, clinically used local anesthetics cannot be alkalinized beyond a pH of 6.05 to 8 before precipitation occurs[46] and these pH values will only increase the neutral form to about 10%.

Clinical studies on the association between alkalinization of local anesthetics and hastening of block onset have shown an improvement of less than 5 minutes compared with commercial preparations.[45,47] Furthermore, results from a study in rats indicate that alkalinization of lidocaine may also decrease the duration of peripheral nerve blocks if the mixture contained no

TABLE 21-5. EFFECTS OF ADDITION OF EPINEPHRINE TO LOCAL ANESTHETICS

	Increase Duration	Decrease Blood Levels (%)	Dose/Concentration of Epinephrine
Nerve block			
Bupivacaine	+/–	10–20	1:200,000
Lidocaine	++	20–30	1:200,000
Mepivacaine	++	20–30	1:200,000
Ropivacaine	––	0	1:200,000
Epidural			
Bupivacaine	+/–	10–20	1:300,000–1:200,000
Levobupivacaine	+/–	10	1:200,000–1:400,000
Chloroprocaine	++		1:200,000
Lidocaine	++	20–30	1:600,000–1:200,000
Mepivacaine	++	20–30	1:200,000
Ropivacaine	––	0	1:200,000
Spinal			
Bupivacaine	+/–		0.2 mg
Lidocaine	++		0.2 mg
Tetracaine	++		0.2 mg

++, overall supported; ––, overall not supported; +/–, inconsistent.
Data from: Liu SS. Local anesthetics and analgesia. In: Ashburn MA, Rice LJ, eds. *The Management of Pain.* New York, NY: Churchill Livingstone; 1997:141; and Kopacz DJ. A comparison of epidural levobupivacaine 0.5% with or without epinephrine for lumbar spine surgery. *Anesth Analg.* 2001;93:755.

epinephrine.[48] Together, alkalinization of local anesthetics appears limited as a clinically useful adjuvant to improving anesthesia.

Opioids

Opioids have multiple central and peripheral mechanisms of analgesic action (see Chapter 19: Opioids). Spinal administration of opioids provides analgesia primarily by attenuating C-fiber nociception[49] and is independent of supraspinal mechanisms.[50] Coadministration of opioids with central neuraxial local anesthetics results in synergistic analgesia.[51] An exception to this analgesic synergy is chloroprocaine, which appears to decrease the effectiveness of opioids coadministered epidurally.[52] The reason is unclear but the mechanism does not seem to involve direct antagonism of opioid receptors.[53] Nonetheless, clinical studies support the practice of central neuraxial coadministration of local anesthetics and opioids for prolongation and intensification of analgesia and anesthesia.[51]

The discovery of peripheral opioid receptors initially generated much interest in the use of opioids as adjuvants to local anesthetics for peripheral nerve blockade.[54] However, while some studies have reported favorable outcome of such coadministration, others have failed to demonstrate any increased efficacy.[55] A problem that has plagued many studies is the lack of adequate controls for differentiating the analgesic effects of opioids acting peripherally versus a more central mechanism resulting from systemically absorbed opioids. Nonetheless, recent carefully designed trials have shown that some opioids, namely, buprenorphine, may enhance and prolong postoperative analgesia better than either local anesthetics alone or local anesthetics administered with intramuscular buprenorphine.[56,57] Finally, cumulative evidence does not support the use of intraarticular coadministration of local anesthetic and opioid for postoperative analgesia.[58]

α_2-adrenergic Agonists

α_2-adrenergic agonists can be a useful adjuvant to local anesthetics. α_2-specific agonists such as clonidine produce analgesia via supraspinal and spinal adrenergic receptors.[59] Clonidine also has direct inhibitory effects on peripheral nerve conduction (A and C nerve fibers).[60] Thus, addition of clonidine may have multiple routes of action depending on the type of application. Preliminary evidence suggests that coadministration of an α_2-agonist and local anesthetic results in central neuraxial and peripheral nerve analgesic synergy,[61] whereas systemic (supraspinal) effects are additive.[62] On average, clonidine improves the duration of analgesia by about 2 hours, regardless of whether an intermediate- or long-acting local anesthetic is used.[63] Overall, results from clinical trials indicate that clonidine can enhance local anesthetics when used for intrathecal and epidural anesthesia and peripheral nerve blocks.[63,64]

Steroids

Potent glucocorticoid injections have been widely used for the treatment of chronic low back pain caused by radiculopathy. Experiments in animals using extended-release preparations of local anesthetics have found that addition of dexamethasone to the mixture prolongs the conduction block after peripheral nerve application.[65,66] The duration of the blockade is associated with the potency of the glucocorticoid activity and appears to be steroid receptor dependent and locally mediated.[67] Clinical reports of the use of dexamethasone as an adjuvant to local anesthetics have shown similar prolongation of anesthesia after brachial plexus blockades[68,69] and intravenous regional anesthesia.[70] Combined with intermediate- to long-acting local anesthetics, dexamethasone extends the duration of analgesia by approximately 50% after utilization of the supraclavicular[68] or interscalene approach[69] to the brachial plexus block (Fig. 21-8). Although

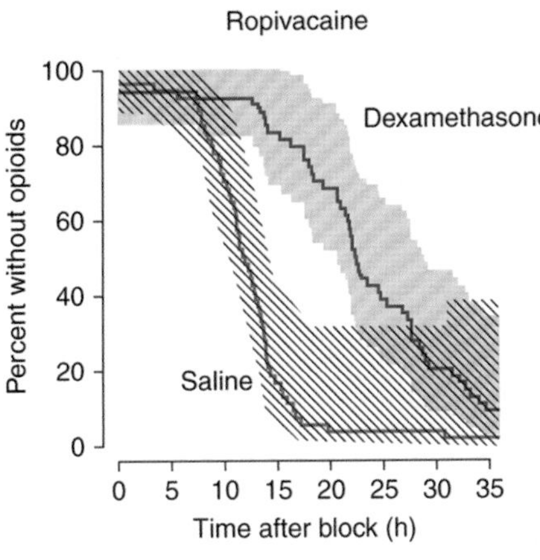

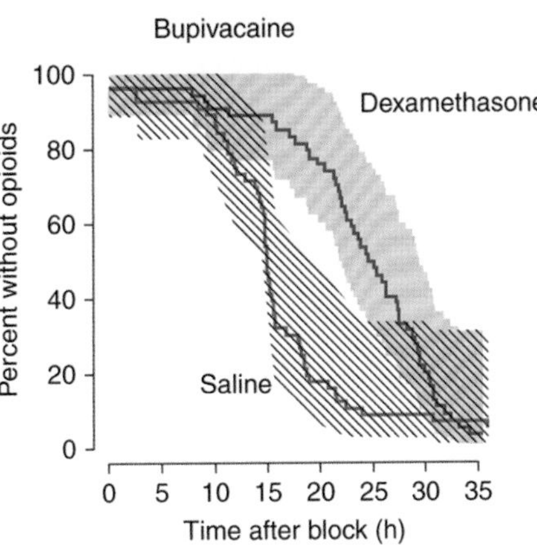

FIGURE 21-8. Addition of dexamethasone to either ropivacaine or bupivacaine increases the duration of analgesia after interscalene brachial plexus block. Data shown as the Kaplan–Meier survival density estimates with the shaded region representing the 95% confidence interval. (Reprinted from: Cummings KC, Napierkowski DE, Parra-Sanchez I, et al. Effect of dexamethasone on the duration of interscalene nerve blocks with ropivacaine or bupivacaine. *Br J Anaesth.* 2011;107:446, with permission.)

initial laboratory data show no evidence of increased neurotoxicity from use of dexamethasone as compared with other adjuvants, our current understanding of its mechanism of action and potential side effects remains incomplete.[71]

PHARMACOKINETICS OF LOCAL ANESTHETICS

Plasma concentration of local anesthetics is a function of the dose administered and the rates of systemic absorption, tissue distribution, and drug elimination. Elevated levels may produce unintended effects in other electric-sensitive systems, most importantly, the cardiovascular system and the CNS. Having a thorough understanding of the factors involved would enable one to maximize the local anesthetic potential while avoiding possible complications arising from systemic local anesthetic toxicity.

Systemic Absorption

Decreasing systemic absorption of local anesthetics increases their
7 safety margin in clinical uses. The rate and extent of systemic absorption depends on the site of injection, the dose, the drug's intrinsic pharmacokinetic properties, and the addition of a vasoactive agent. The vascularity of the tissue markedly influences the rate of drug absorption, such that deposition of local anesthetics in vessel-rich tissues results in higher peak plasma levels in a shorter period of time. Accordingly, the rate of systemic absorption is greatest with intercostal nerve blocks, and followed in decreasing order, by caudal and epidural injections, brachial plexus block, and femoral and sciatic nerve blocks (Table 21-6). Thus, the same amount of local anesthetics injected would result in unequal peak plasma levels, depending on the site of drug delivery.

For a given site of injection, the rate of systemic absorption and the peak plasma level are directly proportional to the dose of local anesthetic deposited. This relationship is nearly linear (Fig. 21-9) and independent of the drug concentration and the speed of injection.[72]

The rate of systemic absorption differs with individual local anesthetics. In general, more potent, lipid-soluble agents are associated with a slower rate of absorption than less lipid-soluble compounds (Fig. 21-10). Sequestration into lipid-rich compartments

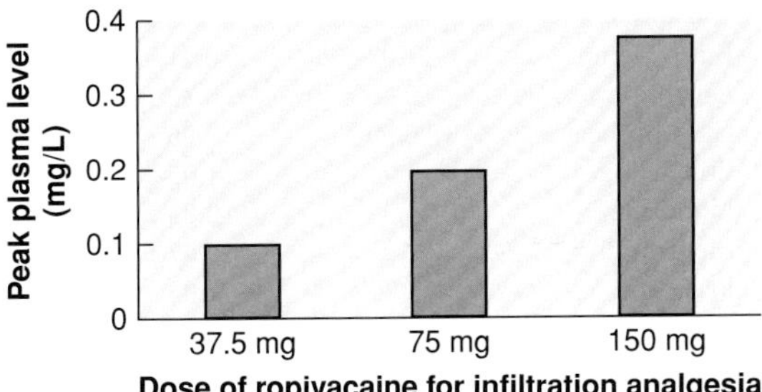

FIGURE 21-9. Increasing doses of ropivacaine used for wound infiltration result in linearly increasing maximal plasma concentrations (C_{max}). (Data from: Mulroy MF, Burgess FW, Emanuelsson B-M. Ropivacaine 0.25% and 0.5%, but not 0.125%, provide effective wound infiltration analgesia after outpatient hernia repair, but with sustained plasma drug levels. *Reg Anesth Pain Med.* 1999;24:136.)

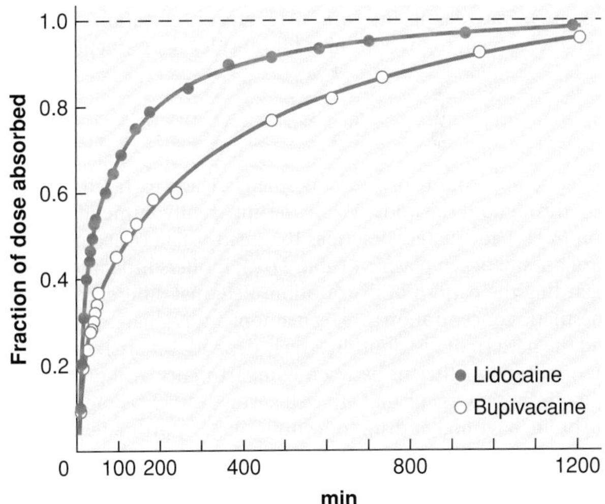

FIGURE 21-10. Fraction of dose absorbed into the systemic circulation over time from epidural injection of lidocaine or bupivacaine. Bupivacaine is a more lipid soluble, more potent agent with less systemic absorption over time. (Adapted from: Tucker GT, Mather LE. Properties, absorption, and disposition of local anesthetic agents. In: Cousins MJ, Bridenbaugh PO, eds. *Neural Blockade in Clinical Anesthesia and Management of Pain.* Philadelphia, PA: Lippincott-Raven; 1998:55, with permission.)

TABLE 21-6. TYPICAL C_{MAX} AFTER REGIONAL ANESTHETICS WITH COMMONLY USED LOCAL ANESTHETICS

Local Anesthetic	Technique	Dose (mg)	C_{max} (μg/mL)	T_{max} (min)	Toxic Plasma Concentration (μg/mL)
Bupivacaine	Brachial plexus	150	1.0	20	3
	Celiac plexus	100	1.50	17	
	Epidural	150	1.26	20	
	Intercostal	140	0.90	30	
	Lumbar sympathetic	52.5	0.49	24	
	Sciatic/femoral	400	1.89	15	
Levobupivacaine	Epidural	75	0.36	50	4
	Brachial plexus	250	1.2	55	
Lidocaine	Brachial plexus	400	4.00	25	5
	Epidural	400	4.27	20	
	Intercostal	400	6.8	15	
Mepivacaine	Brachial plexus	500	3.68	24	5
	Epidural	500	4.95	16	
	Intercostal	500	8.06	9	
	Sciatic/femoral	500	3.59	31	
Ropivacaine	Brachial plexus	190	1.3	53	4
	Epidural	150	1.07	40	
	Intercostal	140	1.10	21	

C_{max}, peak plasma levels; T_{max}, time until C_{max}.
Data from: Liu SS. Local anesthetics and analgesia. In: Ashburn MA, Rice LJ, eds. *The Management of Pain.* New York, NY: Churchill Livingstone; 1997:141; Berrisford RG. Plasma concentrations of bupivacaine and its enantiomers during continuous extrapleural intercostal nerve block. *Br J Anaesth.* 1993;70:201; Kopacz DJ. A comparison of epidural levobupivacaine 0.5% with or without epinephrine for lumbar spine surgery. *Anesth Analg.* 2001;93:755; Crews JC. Levobupivacaine for axillary brachial plexus block: A pharmacokinetic and clinical comparison in patients with normal renal function or renal disease. *Anesth Analg.* 2002;95:219.

may not be the only explanation. Local anesthetics exert direct effects on vascular smooth muscles in a concentration-dependent manner. At low concentrations, more potent agents appear to cause more vasoconstriction than less potent agents, thereby decreasing the rate of vascular absorption.[36] At high concentrations, vasodilatory effects seem to predominate for most local anesthetics.

Distribution

Systemic absorption of local anesthetics leads to rapid distribution throughout the body. While the apparent volume of distribution (VD_{ss}) adequately describes the steady-state concentration of local anesthetics in plasma (Table 21-7), it offers little information regarding the pattern of distribution. Regional differences in local anesthetic concentrations are seen among individual organ systems and the pattern of distribution largely depends on organ perfusion, the partition coefficient between compartments, and plasma protein binding.[73] Organs that are well perfused, such as the heart and the brain, have higher drug concentrations. Unfortunately, they are also the organs most seriously affected by local anesthetic toxicity.

Elimination

The metabolic pathway for clearance of local anesthetics is primarily determined by their chemical linkage. Aminoesters are hydrolyzed by plasma cholinesterases and aminoamides are transformed by hepatic carboxylesterases and cytochrome P450 enzymes. Severe liver disease may slow the clearance of aminoamide local anesthetics and significant drug levels may therefore accumulate.[74]

Clinical Pharmacokinetics

The primary benefit of understanding the systemic pharmacokinetics of local anesthetics is the ability to predict the peak plasma level (C_{max}) after the agents are administered, thereby avoiding

TABLE 21-7. PHARMACOKINETIC PARAMETERS OF CLINICALLY USED LOCAL ANESTHETICS

Local Anesthetic	VD_{ss} (L/kg)	CL (L/kg/h)	$T_{1/2}$ (h)
Bupivacaine	1.02	0.41	3.5
Levobupivacaine	0.78	0.32	2.6
Chloroprocaine	0.50	2.96	0.11
Etidocaine	1.9	1.05	2.6
Lidocaine	1.3	0.85	1.6
Mepivacaine	1.2	0.67	1.9
Prilocaine	2.73	2.03	1.6
Procaine	0.93	5.62	0.14
Ropivacaine	0.84	0.63	1.9

VD_{ss}, volume of distribution at steady state; CL, total body clearance; $T_{1/2}$, terminal elimination half-life.
Data from: Denson DD. Physiology and pharmacology of local anesthetics, In: Sinatra RS, Hord AH, Ginsberg B, et al. *Acute Pain. Mechanisms and Management.* St. Louis, MO: Mosby Year Book; 1992:124; and Burm AG, van der Meer AD, van Kleef JW, et al. Pharmacokinetics of the enantiomers of bupivacaine following intravenous administration of the racemate. *Br J Clin Pharmacol.* 1994;38:125.

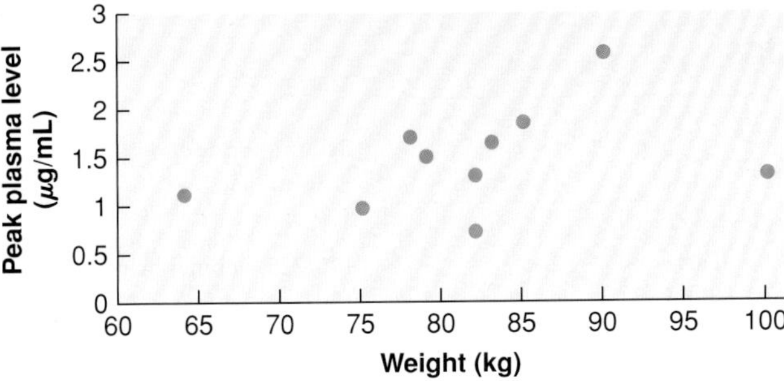

FIGURE 21-11. Lack of correlation between patient weight and peak plasma concentration after epidural administration of 150 mg of bupivacaine. (Data from: Sharrock NE, Mather LE, Go G, et al. Arterial and pulmonary concentrations of the enantiomers of bupivacaine after epidural injection in elderly patients. *Anesth Analg.* 1998;86:812.)

the administration of toxic doses (Tables 21-6, 21-8, and 21-9). Nonetheless, pharmacokinetics are difficult to predict in any given circumstance as both physical and pathophysiologic characteristics will affect the individual pharmacokinetics. There is some evidence for increased systemic plasma levels of local anesthetics in the very young and in the elderly owing to decreased clearance and increased absorption[75]; however, the correlation of systemic blood levels between the dose of local anesthetic and weight is often inconsistent (Fig. 21-11) (76). Effects of gender on clinical pharmacokinetics of local anesthetics have not been well defined,[77] although pregnancy may decrease clearance.[78] Pathophysiologic states such as cardiac and hepatic disease will alter expected pharmacokinetic parameters (Table 21-10), and lower doses of local anesthetics should be used for these patients. As expected, renal disease has little effect on pharmacokinetic parameters of local anesthetics (Table 21-10). All of these factors should be considered when using local anesthetics and minimizing systemic toxicity, the commonly accepted maximal dosages (Table 21-9) notwithstanding.

CLINICAL USE OF LOCAL ANESTHETICS

There are myriads of uses of local anesthetics in the modern practice of anesthesia. They all take advantage of their ability to attenuate or block pain and other noxious stimuli. When applied topically to the skin, a eutectic mixture of lidocaine and prilocaine reduces the sharp, painful sensation associated with needle insertion and intravenous catheter placement, particularly in the pediatric population.[79] In the awake patient, aerosolized benzocaine and viscous lidocaine directed at the mucosal surface can help blunt the reflexive response associated with airway instrumentation (Chapter 27: Airway Management). In addition, lidocaine can be given intravenously to decrease the incidence and the severity of pain associated with propofol administration (Chapter 30: Ambulatory Anesthesia). Likewise, intravenous lidocaine may also help to reduce the hemodynamic response to tracheal intubation and extubation.[80,81]

By far the most common application, local infiltration of the dermis, provides quick onset of anesthesia suitable for a broad variety of minor, superficial procedures. The clinical profile of some commonly used agents is listed in Table 21-9. For a wider and greater area of coverage, a regional anatomic approach to anesthesia and analgesia can be used. This can be accomplished either by intravenous administration of local anesthetics to a limb under pneumatic compression (Bier block) or by direct application of local anesthetics to a set of nerves (nerve blocks). Local anesthetics can be deposited centrally near the nerve roots, either intrathecally in the lumbar cistern or epidurally in the thoracic, lumbar, and caudal regions of the spine (Chapter 34: Epidural and Spinal Anesthesia). Alternatively, injections can be made peripherally at the plexus, such as at the brachial or lumbar plexus block, or on the nerve fibers (Chapter 35: Peripheral Nerve Blockade). The duration of the anesthesia and analgesia is dependent on the type of local anesthetics used, though it can be extended with continuous infusion through an indwelling catheter.

TABLE 21-8. RELATIVE POTENCY FOR SYSTEMIC CENTRAL NERVOUS SYSTEM TOXICITY BY LOCAL ANESTHETICS AND RATIO OF DOSAGE NEEDED FOR CARDIOVASCULAR SYSTEM:CENTRAL NERVOUS SYSTEM (CVS:CNS) TOXICITY

Agent	Relative Potency for CNS Toxicity	CVS:CNS
Bupivacaine	4.0	2.0
Levobupivacaine	2.9	2.0
Chloroprocaine	0.3	3.7
Etidocaine	2.0	4.4
Lidocaine	1.0	7.1
Mepivacaine	1.4	7.1
Prilocaine	1.2	3.1
Procaine	0.3	3.7
Ropivacaine	2.9	2.0
Tetracaine	2.0	

Data from: Liu SS. Local anesthetics and analgesia. In: Ashburn MA, Rice LJ, eds. *The Management of Pain.* New York, NY: Churchill Livingstone; 1997:141; and Groban L. Central nervous system and cardiac effects from long-acting amide local anesthetic toxicity in the intact animal model. *Reg Anesth Pain Med.* 2003;28:3.

TABLE 21-9. CLINICAL PROFILE OF LOCAL ANESTHETICS

Local Anesthetic	Concentration (%)	Clinical Use	Onset	Duration (h)	Recommended Maximum Single Dose (mg)
Amides					
Bupivacaine	0.25	Infiltration	Fast	2–8	175/225 + epinephrine
Levobupivacaine	0.25–0.5	Peripheral nerve block	Slow	4–12	150
	0.5–0.75	Epidural anesthesia	Moderate	2–5	150
	0.03–0.25	Epidural analgesia	N/A	N/A	N/A
	0.5–0.75	Spinal anesthesia	Fast	1–4	20
Etidocaine	0.5	Infiltration	Fast	2–8	300/400 + epinephrine
	0.5–1	Peripheral nerve block	Fast	3–12	300/400 + epinephrine
	1–1.5	Epidural anesthesia	Fast	2–4	300/400 + epinephrine
Lidocaine	0.5–1	Infiltration	Fast	1–4	300/500 + epinephrine
	0.25–0.5	IV regional anesthesia	Fast	0.5–1	300
	1–1.5	Peripheral nerve block	Fast	1–3	300/500 + epinephrine
	1.5–2	Epidural anesthesia	Fast	1–2	300/500 + epinephrine
	1.5–5	Spinal anesthesia	Fast	0.5–1	100
	4	Topical	Fast	0.5–1	300
Mepivacaine	0.5–1	Infiltration	Fast	1–4	400/500 + epinephrine
	1–1.5	Peripheral nerve block	Fast	2–4	400/500 + epinephrine
	1.5–2	Epidural anesthesia	Fast	1–3	400/500 + epinephrine
	2–4	Spinal anesthesia	Fast	1–2	100
Prilocaine	0.5–1	Infiltration	Fast	1–2	600
	0.25–0.5	IV regional anesthesia	Fast	0.5–1	600
	1.5–2	Peripheral nerve block	Fast	1.5–3	600
	2–3	Epidural	Fast	1–3	600
Ropivacaine	0.2–0.5	Infiltration	Fast	2–6	200
	0.5–1	Peripheral nerve block	Slow	5–8	250
	0.5–1	Epidural anesthesia	Moderate	2–6	200
	0.05–0.2	Epidural analgesia	N/A	N/A	N/A
Mixture					
Lidocaine + prilocaine	2.5/2.5	Skin topical	Slow	3–5	20 g
Esters					
Benzocaine	Up to 20	Topical	Fast	0.5–1	200
Chloroprocaine	1	Infiltration	Fast	0.5–1	800/1,000 + epinephrine
	2	Peripheral nerve block	Fast	0.5–1	800/1,000 + epinephrine
	2–3	Epidural anesthesia	Fast	0.5–1	800/1,000 + epinephrine
Cocaine	4–10	Topical	Fast	0.5–1	150
Procaine	10	Spinal anesthesia	Fast	0.5–1	1,000
Tetracaine	2	Topical	Fast	0.5–1	20
	0.5	Spinal anesthesia	Fast	2–6	20

IV, intravenous; N/A, not available.
Adapted from: Covino BG, Wildsmith JAW. Clinical pharmacology of local anesthetic agents. In: Cousins MJ, Bridenbaugh PO, eds. *Neural Blockade in Clinical Anesthesia and Management of Pain*. Philadelphia, PA: Lippincott-Raven; 1998:97, with permission.

TOXICITY OF LOCAL ANESTHETICS

Systemic Toxicity of Local Anesthetics

Central Nervous System Toxicity

Local anesthetics readily cross the blood–brain barrier and as a result, CNS toxicity can result from systemic absorption or inadvertent intravascular injections. The effects on the CNS are determined by the plasma concentration of the local anesthetics (Table 21-11). At low plasma concentration, mild disturbances to the sensory systems appear. As the plasma concentration increases, CNS excitatory and seizure activities predominate. If the plasma concentration is sufficiently large or the increase is rapid, the CNS excitation may progress to generalized CNS depression and coma, leading to respiratory depression and arrest.[82]

The potential for CNS toxicity correlates directly with the potency of local anesthetics (Tables 21-4 and 21-8).[82] Highly potent, lipid-soluble agents such as bupivacaine can cause CNS toxicity at doses that are a fraction of those of less potent agents. The potential for CNS toxicity is further modified by other factors. For example, a decrease in protein binding and clearance of local anesthetics, systemic acidosis, hypercapnia, and hypercarbia can all increase the risk for CNS toxicity. Conversely, coadministration of

TABLE 21-10. EFFECTS OF CARDIAC, HEPATIC, AND RENAL DISEASE ON LIDOCAINE PHARMACOKINETICS

	VD_{ss} (L/kg)	CL (mL/kg/min)	$T_{1/2}$ (h)
Normal	1.32	10.0	1.8
Cardiac failure	0.88	6.3	1.9
Hepatic disease	2.31	6.0	4.9
Renal disease	1.2	13.7	1.3

VD_{ss}, volume of distribution at steady state; CL, total body clearance; $T_{1/2}$, terminal elimination half-life.
Data from: Thomson PD. Lidocaine pharmacokinetics in advanced heart failure, liver disease, and renal failure in humans. *Ann Intern Med.* 1973;78:499.

CNS depressive agents, such as barbiturates and benzodiazepines, may decrease the likelihood for seizures.[83]

Clinical reports suggest CNS toxicity resulting from the use local anesthetics in regional anesthesia is uncommon. Surveys from France and the United States of over 280,000 cases involving regional anesthesia show an incidence of seizures approximately 1/10,000 with epidural injections and 7/10,000 with peripheral nerve blocks.[84,85] The higher incidence of CNS toxicity resulting from peripheral nerve blocks may be due to differences in practice or, perhaps, decreased clinical awareness. Nonetheless, in an analysis of closed malpractice claims in the United States from 1980 to 1999, epidural anesthesia (primarily obstetrical) constituted all of the cases of death or brain damage resulting from unintentional intravenous injection of local anesthetic.[86]

Cardiovascular Toxicity of Local Anesthetics

8 In general, systemic cardiovascular toxicity is seen at a plasma concentration far greater than that for CNS toxicity. The potential for cardiovascular toxicity, like that for CNS toxicity, correlates closely with the potency, or lipid solubility, of local anesthetics (Tables 21-4 and 21-8). However, while all local anesthetics can cause hypotension, dysrhythmias, and myocardial depression, more potent agents (bupivacaine, ropivacaine, and levobupivacaine) are predisposed to devastating outcomes such as fatal cardiovascular collapse and complete heart block (Fig. 21-12).[87]

TABLE 21-11. DOSE-DEPENDENT SYSTEMIC EFFECTS OF LIDOCAINE

Plasma Concentration (μg/mL)	Effect
1–5	Analgesia
5–10	Lightheadedness Tinnitus Numbness of tongue
10–15	Seizures Unconsciousness
15–25	Coma Respiratory arrest
>25	Cardiovascular depression

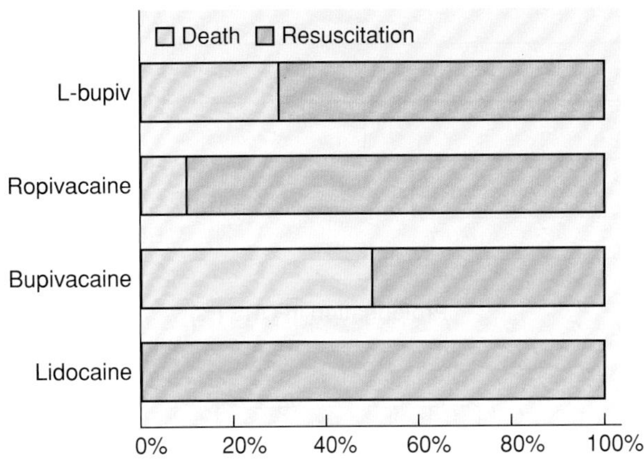

FIGURE 21-12. Success of resuscitation of dogs after cardiovascular collapse from intravenous infusions of lidocaine, bupivacaine, levobupivacaine (L-bupiv), and ropivacaine. Success rates were greater for lidocaine (100%), than ropivacaine (90%), levobupivacaine (70%), and bupivacaine (50%). Required doses to induce cardiovascular collapse were greater for lidocaine (127 mg/kg), than ropivacaine (42 mg/kg), levobupivacaine (27 mg/kg), and bupivacaine (22 mg/kg). (Data from: Groban L, Deal DD, Vernon JC, et al. Cardiac resuscitation after incremental overdosage with lidocaine, bupivacaine, levobupivacaine, and ropivacaine in anesthetized dogs. *Anesth Analg.* 2001;92:37.)

Among the potent long-acting agents, ropivacaine and levobupivacaine may have a safer cardiovascular toxicity profile than bupivacaine. In animal models, both ropivacaine and levobupivacaine appear to exhibit 30% to 40% less cardiovascular toxicity than bupivacaine on a milligram to milligram basis[32,82,88] (Fig. 21-13); however, in human studies, that difference appears less striking[89,90] (Fig. 21-14). Detailed electrophysiologic studies with isolated heart muscles and cultured cardiomyocytes support the view that *S*(−)-bupivacaine (levobupivacaine) is generally less potent than *R*(+)-bupivacaine in blocking the cardiac action potential[91] and binding of voltage-gated sodium channels during the inactivated stage.[92] Likewise for ropivacaine, evidence suggests that the propyl side chain renders it less cardiodepressive than the larger butyl side chain of bupivacaine.[93]

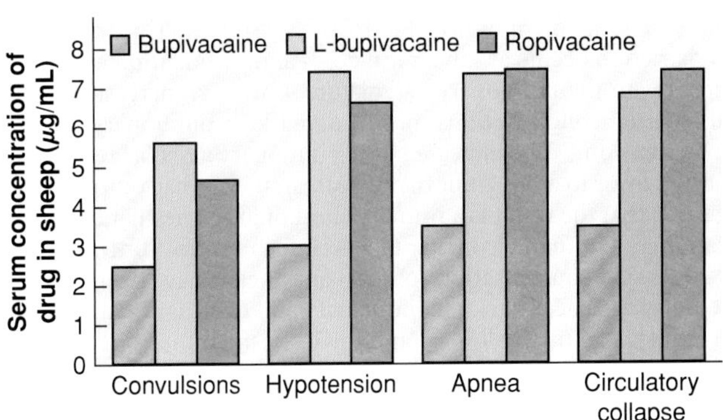

FIGURE 21-13. Serum concentrations in sheep at each toxic manifestation for bupivacaine, levo (L)-bupivacaine, and ropivacaine in sheep. Both levobupivacaine and ropivacaine required significantly greater serum concentrations than bupivacaine. (Data from: Santos AC, DeArmas PI. Systemic toxicity of levobupivacaine, bupivacaine, and ropivacaine during continuous intravenous infusion to nonpregnant and pregnant ewes. *Anesthesiology.* 2001;95:1256.)

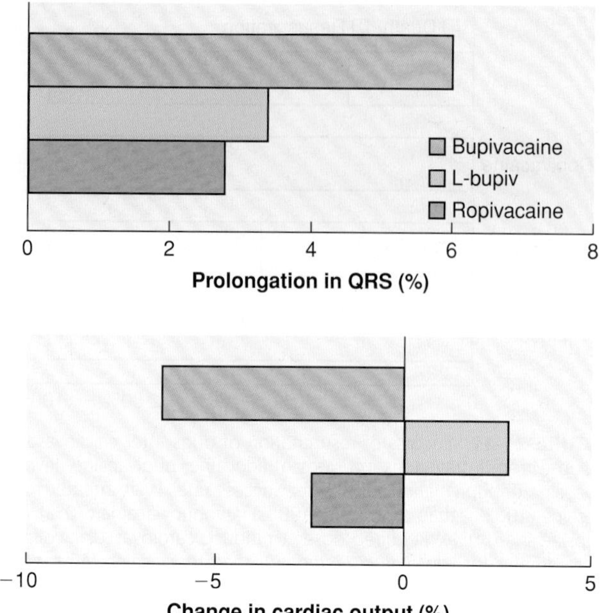

FIGURE 21-14. Mild prolongation in QRS interval and change in cardiac output after intravenous infusions of bupivacaine (103 mg), levobupivacaine (L-bupiv; 37 mg), and ropivacaine (115 mg) in healthy volunteers. (Data from: Knudsen K, Beckman Suurkula M, Blomberg S, et al. Central nervous and cardiovascular effects of i.v. infusions of ropivacaine, bupivacaine and placebo in volunteers. *Br Anaesth.* 1997;78:507; and Stewart J, Kellett N, Castro D. The central nervous system and cardiovascular effects of levobupivacaine and ropivacaine in healthy volunteers. *Anesth Analg.* 2003;97:412.)

The underlying pathophysiology responsible for local anesthetic–induced cardiovascular collapse has not been fully established. While local anesthetics undoubtedly cause major disturbances to the heart, their effects on other organ systems may also play a role. For example, systemic bupivacaine has been shown to impair regulation by the CNS of the cardiovascular system. Disruption to the arterial baroreflex in the brain stem by bupivacaine can lead to attenuation of the heart rhythm response to changes in blood pressure.[94,95] Local anesthetics also act on smooth muscle endothelium surrounding blood vessels. In the periphery, vasoconstriction occurs at subclinical doses and vasodilation at higher doses.[96] In the pulmonary vasculature, however, increasing local anesthetic concentrations produce marked pulmonary artery hypertension.[97] The increase in the pulmonary vascular resistance occurs prior to any significant decrease in the cardiac output, suggesting that the result is a primary effect of local anesthetic intoxication, rather than secondary to a decline in cardiac contractility.

Elevated concentrations of local anesthetics have been shown to delay cardiac electrical conductivity and decrease cardiac contractility. Although all local anesthetics disturb the cardiac conduction system via a dose-dependent block of sodium channels (seen clinically as a prolongation of the PR interval and duration of the QRS complex), several features unique to bupivacaine seem to potentiate its cardiotoxicity. First, bupivacaine has an inherently greater affinity for binding resting and inactivated sodium channels than lidocaine.[98] Second, although all local anesthetics bind sodium channels during cardiac systole and dissociate during diastole (Fig. 21-15), the dissociation of bupivacaine during diastole occurs more slowly than lidocaine. This slow rate of dissociation prevents a complete recovery of the channels at the end of each cardiac cycle (at the physiologic heart rate of 60 to 80 beats/minute), thereby leading to an accumulation and worsening of the conduction defect. In contrast, lidocaine fully dissociates from sodium channels during diastole and little accumulation of conduction delay occurs (Fig. 21-16).[98,99] Finally,

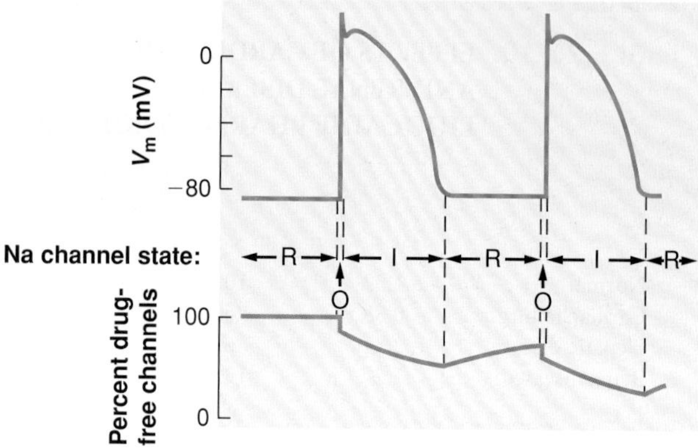

FIGURE 21-15. Diagram illustrating the relationship between cardiac action potential (*top*), sodium channel state (*middle*), and block of sodium channels by bupivacaine (*bottom*). R, resting form; O, open form; I, inactive form. Sodium channels are predominantly in the resting form during diastole, open transiently during the action potential upstroke, and are in the inactive form during the action potential plateau. Block of sodium channels by bupivacaine accumulates during the action potential (systole) with recovery occurring during diastole. Recovery of sodium channels is from dissociation of bupivacaine and is time-dependent. Recovery during each diastolic interval is incomplete and results in accumulation of sodium channel block with successive heartbeats. (Adapted from: Clarkson CW, Hondegham LM. Mechanisms for bupivacaine depression of cardiac conduction: Fast block of sodium channels during the action potential with slow recovery from block during diastole. *Anesthesiology.* 1985;62:396, with permission.)

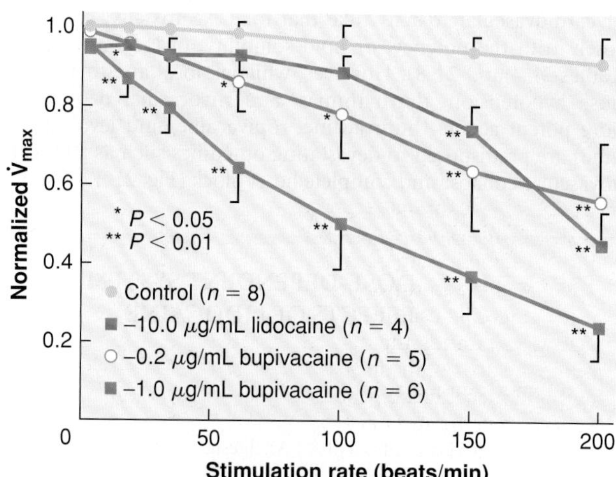

FIGURE 21-16. Heart rate–dependent effects of lidocaine and bupivacaine on velocity of the cardiac action potential ($\dot{V}_{max}$). Bupivacaine progressively decreases $\dot{V}_{max}$ at heart rates above 10 beats/minute because of accumulation of sodium channel block, whereas lidocaine does not decrease $\dot{V}_{max}$ until heart rate exceeds 150 beats/minute. (Adapted from: Clarkson CW, Hondegham LM. Mechanisms for bupivacaine depression of cardiac conduction: Fast block of sodium channels during the action potential with slow recovery from block during diastole. *Anesthesiology.* 1985;62:396, with permission.)

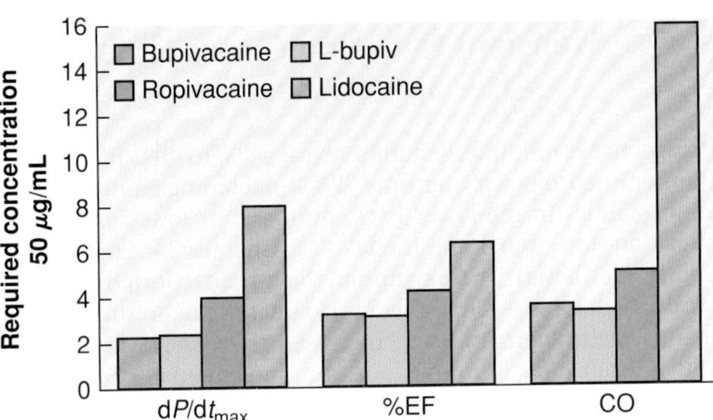

FIGURE 21-17. Plasma concentrations required to induce myocardial depression in dogs administered bupivacaine, levobupivacaine (L-bupiv), ropivacaine, and lidocaine. dP/dt_{max}, 35% reduction of inotropy from baseline measure; %EF, 35% reduction in ejection fraction from baseline measure; CO, 25% reduction in cardiac output from baseline measure. (Data from: Groban L, Deal DD, Vernon JC, et al. Does local anesthetic stereoselectivity or structure predict myocardial depression in anesthetized canines? *Reg Anesth Pain Med.* 2002;27:460.)

bupivacaine exerts a greater degree of direct myocardial depression than less potent agents (Fig. 21-17).[82,93]

Current understanding of the molecular mechanisms underlying local anesthetic cardiac toxicity is limited. It is widely accepted that local anesthetics bind and disrupt the normal function of the heart-specific voltage-gated sodium channel, Na_v 1.5, in cardiac myocytes; however, there appears to be other intracellular targets as well. Local anesthetics have been shown to antagonize the currents of other cations, primarily calcium and potassium.[98] The degree of antagonism between bupivacaine and less potent agents appears to differ and that difference may contribute to the severity in the disturbance of the cardiac membrane potentials. Lastly, individuals and experimental animal models with L-carnitine deficiency exhibit an increased susceptibility to local anesthetic–associated cardiac toxicity, suggesting that local anesthetics can affect mitochondrial function and fatty acid metabolism.[100,101]

Treatment of Systemic Toxicity from Local Anesthetics

The best practice for managing systemic local anesthetic intoxication starts with vigilance and prevention. Elevated plasmic levels of local anesthetics can occur by inadvertent intravascular injections or systemic absorption. The risk for intravascular injections can be reduced by using a local anesthetic test dose (about 3 mL), frequently aspirating the injectate for signs of blood return, and dividing the dose of the local anesthetics.[83,102] Understanding the drug's pharmacokinetic profile and having a good knowledge of the anatomy in the area of local anesthetic injection may help predict the rate of tissue absorption and thus avoid toxic systemic accumulation. Heart rate and rhythm, blood pressure, and oxygenation should be monitored at all times. Early CNS toxicity may be manifested by tinnitus or excessive sedation.

The treatment of suspected systemic local anesthetic toxicity is primarily supportive. Administration of local anesthetic should cease immediately. Oxygenation and ventilation should be maintained and the airway, if necessary, must be secured. This is necessary not only as a standard part of resuscitation, but also to prevent further exacerbation of local anesthetic toxicity by hypoxemia, hypercapnia, and acidemia.[83] In many cases, with proper airway management and reversal of acidosis, more serious complications of local anesthetic intoxication can be avoided, especially in cases involving less potent agents.

Local anesthetic–induced seizure activity can vastly increase the body's metabolism and the resultant metabolic acidosis may make resuscitation more difficult. Prolonged seizures should therefore be suppressed. Benzodiazepines, such as midazolam or diazepam, have been shown to raise the seizure threshold in animals and are the preferred agents for preventing and terminating seizures. Hypnotic agents, such as propofol and thiopental, may not be best suited for terminating local anesthetic–induced seizures, because at significant doses, they can potentiate the myocardial depression exerted by the causative agent.[102] If seizure activity is prolonged, succinylcholine or other neuromuscular blockers can be administered not only to facilitate pulmonary ventilation, but also to disrupt muscular activity and reduce the consequent metabolic demand. However, it is important to note that muscle relaxants do not reduce the electrical excitation in the CNS and cerebral metabolic stress may continue unabated.

Mild myocardial depression and systemic vasodilation can be corrected with sympathomimetic agents such as ephedrine or epinephrine. Pending cardiovascular collapse from severe cardiac dysrhythmias should prompt immediate initiation of cardiopulmonary resuscitation. For ventricular fibrillation and cardiac arrest, electrocardioversion and pharmacologic means should be attempted to restore sinus rhythm. Epinephrine, in small initial doses, and amiodarone, are the preferred agents. Calcium channel and β-adrenergic receptor blocking drugs can worsen myocardial function and are best avoided.[102]

Historically, emergent cardiopulmonary bypass was considered the only effective life-saving measure for otherwise fatal dysrhythmias and cardiac collapse resulting from local anesthetic cardiac toxicity.[103,104] However, evidence is accumulating to support the use of an intravenous infusion of lipid emulsion to hasten the return of normal cardiac function. Studies in animals have demonstrated efficacy of a lipid infusion in reversing bupivacaine-induced asystole.[105,106] Subsequent clinical reports have described successful resuscitation using lipid emulsions in individuals with local anesthetic–induced cardiac arrest.[107,108] The lipid emulsion may act as a plasma "sink" to absorb tissue-bound local anesthetics via partition principles.[109] Alternatively, the lipids may provide an usable energy source to bypass the impediment on the cardiac mitochondria.[110] The recommended dosing for lipid emulsion therapy is listed in Table 21-12.

TABLE 21-12. RECOMMENDED LIPID EMULSION DOSING FOR TREATMENT OF LOCAL ANESTHETIC CARDIOVASCULAR TOXICITY

1	Initiate intravenous bolus of 1.5 cc/kg of 20% lipid emulsion
2	Continue infusion at 0.25 cc/kg/min for at least 10 min after the return of cardiac function
3	If cardiovascular instability continues, consider repeating the bolus and increasing the infusion to 0.5 cc/kg/min
4	Up to 10 cc/kg over 30 min is the recommended upper limit for initial dosing

Adapted from: Weinberg GL. Treatment of local anesthetic systemic toxicity (LAST). *Reg Anesth Pain Med.* 2010;35:188.

Neural Toxicity of Local Anesthetics

In addition to their systemic effects, direct application of local anesthetics can result in histopathologic changes consistent with neuronal injury. The causative mechanisms remain speculative, but studies in animals and tissue cultures show evidence of demyelination, Wallerian degeneration, dysregulation of axonal transport, disruption of the blood–nerve barrier, decreased blood flow to the vasanervorum, and loss of cell membrane integrity.[111,112] The degree of neural injury appears to correlate with possible intraneural placement of local anesthetic, as well as the concentration, and the duration of exposure to the local anesthetics. Intrafascicular injections result in more histologic changes than either extrafascicular or extraneural placement, with the latter associated with the mildest damage.[113] In large concentrations, all clinically important local anesthetics can produce dose-dependent abnormalities in nerve fibers; however, in clinically relevant concentrations, they appear generally safe.[114,115]

The significance of these experimental findings is unclear as clinical injury is rare. A systematic review of approximately 2.7 million centrally administered local anesthetic neuraxial blocks determined an occurrence of radiculopathy at approximately 0.03% and of paraplegia at approximately 0.0008%.[116] Furthermore, direct intraneural injections of local anesthetics per se do not invariably lead to detectable neurologic symptoms.[117] Nonetheless, there have been clinical scenarios in which a greater propensity for nerve injury has been described. The use of microcatheters with high concentration of lidocaine for continuous spinal anesthesia has been associated with an increased incidence of radiculopathy and cauda equina syndrome.[118] Likewise, chloroprocaine, used until the early 1980s for epidural and intrathecal injections, has been linked to prolonged sensory and motor deficits, possibly due to toxic effects of the preservative, sodium bisulfite.[119] While the clinical use of local anesthetics appears to be safe, it behooves the practitioner to be mindful of their potential deleterious effects on nerves.

Transient Neurologic Symptoms After Spinal Anesthesia

Prospective, randomized studies reveal a 4% to 40% incidence of transient neurologic symptoms (TNS), including pain or sensory abnormalities in the lower back, buttocks, or lower extremities, after lidocaine spinal anesthesia[120,121] (Chapter 34: Epidural and Spinal Anesthesia). These symptoms have been reported with other local anesthetics as well (Table 21-13) but have not resulted in permanent neurologic injury.[121] Increased risk of TNS is associated with lidocaine, the lithotomy position, and ambulatory anesthesia, but not with baricity of solution or dose of local anesthetic.[120,121] The potential neurologic etiology of this syndrome coupled with known concentration-dependent toxicity of lidocaine led to concerns over a neurotoxic etiology for TNS from spinal lidocaine.

However, evidence for a direct linear relation between nerve toxicity and symptoms is scant. While the concentration of local anesthetics may be a strong factor for determining nerve injury, such as with cauda equina syndrome, there does not appear to be a dose relation in TNS. The incidence of TNS is similar when there is a 10-fold difference in the concentration of lidocaine utilized (0.5% and 5%).[122] Furthermore, a study comparing volunteers with and without TNS after lidocaine spinal anesthesia shows no abnormalities detectable by routine electrophysiologic testing, such as electromyography, nerve conduction, or somatosensory-evoked potentials. Finally, effective treatment for TNS includes nonsteroidal antiinflammatory agents and trigger point injections. These are regimens more effective for alleviating myofascial pain than for neuropathic pain.[120] Overall, there is little evidence to support a neurotoxic etiology for TNS.[120] Other potential etiologies for TNS include patient positioning, sciatic nerve stretch, muscle spasm, and myofascial strain.[120]

Myotoxicity of Local Anesthetics

As with neural toxicity, local anesthetics can also cause histopathologic changes in skeletal muscle. Myotoxicity can result from most local anesthetic agents in clinically relevant concentrations[123] and

TABLE 21-13. THE INCIDENCE OF TRANSIENT NEUROLOGIC SYMPTOMS (TNS) VARIES WITH TYPE OF SPINAL LOCAL ANESTHETIC AND SURGERY

Local Anesthetic	Concentration (%)	Type of Surgery	Approximate Incidence of TNS (%)
Lidocaine	2–5	Lithotomy position	30–36
	2–5	Knee arthroscopy	18–22
	0.5	Knee arthroscopy	17
	2–5	Mixed supine position	4–8
Mepivacaine	1.5–4	Mixed	23
Procaine	10	Knee arthroscopy	6
Bupivacaine	0.5–0.75	Mixed	1
Levobupivacaine	0.5	Mixed	1
Prilocaine	2–5	Mixed	1
Ropivacaine	0.5–0.75	Mixed	1

Data from Pollock JE. Transient neurologic symptoms: Etiology, risk factors, and management. *Reg Anesth Pain Med.* 2002;27:581; and Breebaart MB. Urinary bladder scanning after day-case arthroscopy under spinal anaesthesia: Comparison between lidocaine, ropivacaine, and levobupivacaine. *Br J Anaesth.* 2003;90:309.

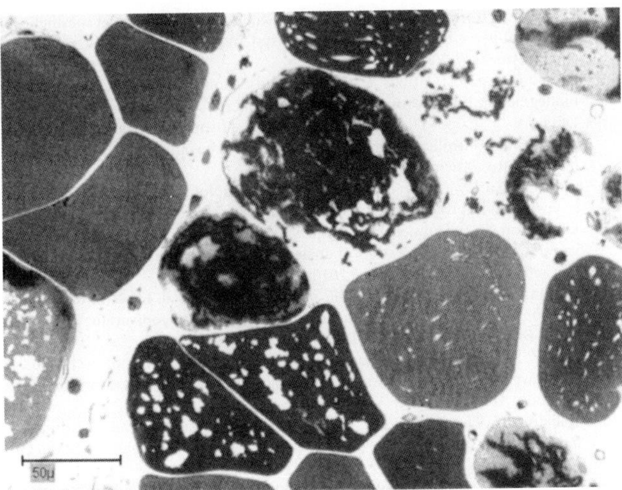

FIGURE 21-18. Skeletal muscle cross section with characteristic histologic changes after continuous exposure to bupivacaine for 6 hours. A whole spectrum of necrobiotic changes can be encountered, ranging from slightly damaged vacuolated fibers and fibers with condensed myofibrils to entirely disintegrated and necrotic cells. The majority of the myocytes are morphologically affected. In addition, a marked interstitial and myoseptal edema appears within the sections. However, scattered fibers remain intact. (Reprinted from: Zink W, Graf B. Local anesthetic myotoxicity. *Reg Anesth Pain Med.* 2004;29:333–340, with permission.)

manifest clinically as muscle pain and dysfunction. Histopathologic studies show hypercontracted myofibrils, followed by lytic degeneration of striated muscle sarcoplasmic reticulum, and diffuse myonecrosis (Fig. 21-18). The changes are drug-specific (tetracaine and procaine produce the least injury; bupivacaine the most) and dose duration dependent[124] and seem to affect the young more than the old.[125] Experimental evidence points to disturbances in the oxidative function of mitochondria and dysregulation of intracellular calcium homeostasis as possible subcellular pathomechanisms.[126] In cell cultures, these disruptions appear to be diminished with co-application with erythropoietin or *N*-acetylcysteine.[127,128] It remains to be seen if these agents may become clinically useful or necessary, as most myotoxic injuries are subclinical and appear entirely reversible.[124]

Allergic Reactions to Local Anesthetics (see also Chapter 12)

Untoward reactions to local anesthetics are relatively common, but true immunologic reactions are rare. The immune-mediated hypersensitivity reaction may be type I (immunoglobulin E) or type IV (cellular immunity). Type I hypersensitivity reactions can result in anaphylaxis and potentially be life-threatening, but fortunately, the incidence is estimated to be less than 1% of all reported cases. Type IV hypersensitivity reactions are delayed-type reactions mediated by T lymphocytes.[129,130] The symptoms can manifest within 12 to 48 hours of exposure and most commonly present as contact dermatitis (dermal erythema, pruritus, papules, and vesicles). The vast majority of reported hypersensitivity reactions have been associated with aminoester agents, likely due to their metabolism to *para*-aminobenzoic acid, which is a recognized allergen. Preservatives, such as methylparaben and metabisulfite, present in many local anesthetic preparations may also trigger allergic responses. Evaluation with skin-pricks, intradermal injections, or subcutaneous provocative dose challenges are recommended for individuals with suspected local anesthetic allergy.[131]

References

1. Wheater PR, Burkitt HG, Daniels VG. *Functional Histology.* 2nd ed. New York, NY: Churchill Livingstone; 1987:95.
2. Ritchie JM, Ritchie B, Greengard P. The effect of the nerve sheath on the action of local anesthetics. *J Pharmacol Exp Ther.* 1965;150:160.
3. Coggeshall RE. A fine structural analysis of the myelin sheath in rat spinal roots. *Anat Rec.* 1979;194:201.
4. Waxman SG, Ritchie JM. Organization of ion channels in the myelinated nerve fiber. *Science.* 1985;228:1502.
5. Koester J. *Passive membrane properties of the neuron.* In: Kandel ER, Schwartz JH, Jessell TM. *Principles of Neuroscience.* 3rd ed. New York, NY: Elsevier Science; 1991.
6. Hodgkin AL, Katz B. The effect of sodium ions on the electrical activity of the giant axon of the squid. *J Physiol.* 1949;108:37.
7. Hodgkin AL, Huxley AF. A quantitative description of membrane current and its application to conduction and excitation in nerve. *J Physiol.* 1952;117:500.
8. Sigworth FJ, Neher E. Single Na+ channel currents observed in cultured rat muscle cells. *Nature.* 1980;287:447.
9. Catterall WA. From ionic currents to molecular mechanisms: The structure and function of voltage-gated sodium channels. *Neuron.* 2000;26:13.
10. Hirschberg B, Rovner A, Lieberman M, et al. Transfer of twelve charges is needed to open skeletal muscle Na+ channels. *J Gen Physiol.* 1995;106:1053.
11. Heinemann SH, Terlau H, Stühmer W, et al. Calcium channel characteristics conferred on the sodium channel by single mutations. *Nature.* 1992;356:441.
12. Armstrong CM. Sodium channels and gating currents. *Physiol Rev.* 1981;61:644.
13. Stühmer W, Conti F, Suzuki H, et al. Structural parts involved in activation and inactivation of the sodium channel. *Nature.* 1989;339:597.
14. West JW, Patton DE, Scheuer T, et al. A cluster of hydrophobic amino acid residues required for fast Na(+)-channel inactivation. *Proc Natl Acad Sci USA.* 1992;89:10910.
15. Woods JN, Boorman JP, Okuse K, et al. Voltage-gated sodium channels and pain pathways. *J Neurobiol.* 2004;61:55.
16. Drenth JP, te Morsche RH, Guillet G, et al. SCN9A mutations define primary erythermalgia as a neuropathic disorder of voltage gated sodium channels. *J Invest Dermatol.* 2005;124:1333.
17. Fertleman CR, Baker MD, Parker KA, et al. SCN9A mutations in paroxysmal extreme pain disorder: Allelic variants underlie distinct channel defects and phenotypes. *Neuron.* 2006;52:767.
18. Cox JJ, Reimann F, Nicholas AK, et al. An SCN9A channelopathy causes congenital inability to experience pain. *Nature.* 2006;444:894.
19. Goldberg Y, Macfarlane J, Macdonald M, et al. Loss-of-function mutations in the Na(v) 1.7 gene underlie congenital indifference to pain in multiple human populations. *Clin Genet.* 2007;71:311.
20. Frazier DT, Narahashi T, Yamada M. The site of action and active form of local anesthetics. II. Experiments with quaternary compounds. *J Pharmacol Exp Ther.* 1970;171:45.
21. Ragsdale DS, McPhee JC, Scheuer T, et al. Molecular determinants of state-dependent block of Na+ channels by local anesthetics. *Science.* 1994;265:1724.
22. Scholz A. Mechanisms of (local) anaesthetics on voltage-gated sodium and other ion channels. *Br J Anaesth.* 2002;89:52.
23. Ulbricht W. Sodium channel inactivation: Molecular determinants and modulation. *Physiol Rev.* 2005;85:1271.
24. Popitz-Bergez FA, Leeson S, Strichartz GR, et al. Relation between functional deficit and intraneural local anesthetic during peripheral nerve block. A study in the rat sciatic nerve. *Anesthesiology.* 1995;83:583.
25. Fink BR, Cairns AM. Differential slowing and block of conduction by lidocaine in individual afferent myelinated and unmyelinated axons. *Anesthesiology.* 1984;60:111.
26. Fink BR, Cairns AM. Differential use-dependent (frequency-dependent) effects in single mammalian axons: Data and clinical considerations. *Anesthesiology.* 1987;67:477.
27. Fink BR. Mechanisms of differential axial blockade in epidural and subarachnoid anesthesia. *Anesthesiology.* 1989;70:851.
28. Gasser HS, Erlanger J. The role of fiber size in the establishment of a nerve block by pressure or cocaine. *Am J Physiol.* 1929;88:581.
29. Gokin AP, Philip B, Strichartz GR. Preferential block of small myelinated sensory and motor fibers by lidocaine: In vivo electrophysiology in the rat sciatic nerve. *Anesthesiology.* 2001;95:1441.
30. Chevrier P, Vijayaragavan K, Chahine M. Differential modulation of Nav 1.7 and Nav 1.8 peripheral nerve sodium channels by the local anesthetic lidocaine. *Br J Pharmacol.* 2004;142:576.
31. Chernoff DM, Strichartz GR. Tonic and phasic block of neuronal sodium currents by 5-hydroxyhexano-2 ,6 -xylide, a neutral lidocaine homologue. *J Gen Physiol.* 1989:93:1075.

32. Strichartz GR, Sanchez V, Arthur GR, et al. Fundamental properties of local anesthetics. II. Measured octanol:Buffer partition coefficients and pK_a values of clinically used drugs. *Anesth Analg.* 1990;71:158.
33. Bokesch PM, Post C, Strichartz G. Structure-activity relationship of lidocaine homologs producing tonic and frequency-dependent impulse blockade in nerve. *J Pharmacol Exp Ther.* 1986;237:773.
34. Gissen AJ, Covino BG, Gregus J. Differential sensitivity of fast and slow fibers in mammalian nerve. III. Effect of etidocaine and bupivacaine on fast/slow fibers. *Anesth Analg.* 1982;61:570.
35. Johns RA, DiFazio CA, Longnecker DE. Lidocaine constricts or dilates rat arterioles in a dose-dependent manner. *Anesthesiology.* 1985;62:141.
36. Johns RA, Seyde WC, DiFazio CA, et al. Dose-dependent effects of bupivacaine on rat muscle arterioles. *Anesthesiology.* 1986;65:186.
37. Foster RH, Markham A. Levobupivacaine: A review of its pharmacology and use as a local anaesthetic. *Drugs.* 2000;59:551.
38. McClellan KJ, Faulds D. Ropivacaine: An update of its use in regional anaesthesia. *Drugs.* 2000;60:1065.
39. Neal JM. Effects of epinephrine in local anesthetics on the central and peripheral nervous systems: Neurotoxicity and neural blood flow. *Reg Anesth Pain Med.* 2003;28:124.
40. Sinnott CJ, Cogswell III LP, Johnson A, et al. On the mechanism by which epinephrine potentiates lidocaine's peripheral nerve block. *Anesthesiology.* 2003; 98:181.
41. Curatolo M, Petersen-Felix S, Arendt-Nielsen L, et al. Epidural epinephrine and clonidine: Segmental analgesia and effects on different pain modalities. *Anesthesiology.* 1997;87:785.
42. Ueda W, Hirakawa M, Mori K. Acceleration of epinephrine absorption by lidocaine. *Anesthesiology.* 1985;63:717.
43. Magee C, Rodeheaver GT, Edgerton MT, et al. Studies of the mechanisms by which epinephrine damages tissue defenses. *J Surg Res.* 1977;23:126.
44. Hall JA, Ferro A. Myocardial ischaemia and ventricular arrhythmias precipitated by physiological concentrations of adrenaline in patients with coronary artery disease. *Br Heart J.* 1992;67:419.
45. Lambert DH. Clinical value of adding sodium bicarbonate to local anesthetics. *Reg Anesth Pain Med.* 2002;27:328.
46. Ikuta PT, Raza SM, Durrani Z. pH adjustment schedule for the amide local anesthetics. *Reg Anesth.* 1989;14:229.
47. Neal JM, Hebl JR, Gerancher JC, et al. Brachial plexus anesthesia: Essentials of our current understanding. *Reg Anesth Pain Med.* 2002;27:402.
48. Sinnott CJ, Garfield JM, Thalhammer JG. Addition of sodium bicarbonate to lidocaine decreases the duration of peripheral nerve block in the rat. *Anesthesiology.* 2000;93:1045.
49. Wang C, Chakrabarti MK, Galletly DC, et al. Relative effects of intrathecal administration of fentanyl and midazolam on A delta and C fibre reflexes. *Neuropharmacology.* 1992;31:439.
50. Niv D, Nemirovsky A, Rudick V. Antinociception induced by simultaneous intrathecal and intraperitoneal administration of low doses of morphine. *Anesth Analg.* 1995;80:886.
51. Walker SM, Goudas LC, Cousins MJ, et al. Combination spinal analgesic chemotherapy: A systematic review. *Anesth Analg.* 2002;95:674.
52. Karambelkar DJ, Ramanathan S. 2-chloroprocaine antagonism of epidural morphine analgesia. *Acta Anaesth Scand.* 1997;41:774.
53. Coda B, Bausch S, Haas M, et al. The hypothesis that antagonism of fentanyl analgesia by 2-chloroprocaine is mediated by direct action on opioid receptors. *Reg Anesth.* 1997;22:43.
54. Janson W, Stein C. Peripheral opioid analgesia. *Curr Pharm Biotechnol.* 2003; 4:270.
55. Picard PR, Tramer MR, McQuay HJ, et al. Analgesic efficacy of peripheral opioids (all except intra-articular): A qualitative systematic review of randomised controlled trials. *Pain.* 1997;72:309.
56. Candido KD, Winnie AP, Ghaleb AH, et al. Buprenorphine added to the local anesthetic for axillary brachial plexus block prolongs postoperative analgesia. *Reg Anesth Pain Med.* 2002;27:162.
57. Candido KD, Hennes J, Gonzalez S, et al. Buprenorphine enhances and prolongs the postoperative analgesic effect of bupivacaine in patients receiving infragluteal sciatic nerve block. *Anesthesiology.* 2010;113:419.
58. Rosseland LA. No evidence for analgesic effect of intra-articular morphine after knee arthroscopy: A qualitative systematic review. *Reg Anesth Pain Med.* 2005;30:83.
59. Eisenach JC, De Kock M, Klimscha W. Alpha(2)-adrenergic agonists for regional anesthesia: A clinical review of clonidine (1984–1995). *Anesthesiology.* 1996;85: 655.
60. Butterworth JF, Strichartz GR. The α_2-adrenergic agonists clonidine and guanfacine produce tonic and phasic block of conduction in rat sciatic nerve fibers. *Anesth Analg.* 1993;76:295.
61. Gaumann DM, Brunet PC, Jirounek P. Clonidine enhances the effects of lidocaine on C fiber action potential. *Anesth Analg.* 1992;74:719.
62. Pertovaara A, Hamalainen MM. Spinal potentiation and supraspinal additivity in the antinociceptive interaction between systemically administered α_2-adrenoreceptor agonist and cocaine in the rat. *Anesth Analg.* 1994;79:261.
63. Popping DM, Elia N, Marret, et al. Clonidine as an adjuvant to local anesthetics for peripheral nerve and plexus blocks. *Anesthesiology.* 2009;111:406.
64. Colin JL, McCartney ED, Apatu E. Should we add clonidine to local anesthetic for peripheral nerve blockade? A qualitative systematic review of the literature. *Reg Anesth Pain Med.* 2007;32:330.
65. Curley J, Castillo J, Hotz J, et al. Prolonged regional nerve blockade: Injectable biodegradable bupivacaine/polyester microspheres. *Anesthesiology.* 1996;84:140.
66. Drager C, Benziger D, Gao F, et al. Prolonged intercostal nerve blockade in sheep using controlled-release of bupivacaine and dexamethasone from polymer microspheres. *Anesthesiology.* 1998;89:969.
67. Castillo J, Curley J, Hotz, et al. Glucocorticoids prolong rat sciatic nerve blockade in vivo from bupivacaine microspheres. *Anesthesiology.* 1996;85:1157.
68. Parrington SJ, O'Donnell DO, Chan V, et al. Dexamethasone added to mepivacaine prolongs the duration of analgesia after supraclavicular brachial plexus blockade. *Reg Anesth Pain Med.* 2010;35:422.
69. Cummings KC, Napierkowski DE, Parra-Sanchez I, et al. Effect of dexamethasone on the duration of interscalene nerve blocks with ropivacaine or bupivacaine. *Br J Anaesth.* 2011;107:446.
70. Bigat Z, Boztug N, Hadimioglu N, et al. Does dexamethasone improve the quality of intravenous regional anesthesia and analgesia? A randomized, controlled clinical study. *Anesth Analg.* 2006;102:605.
71. Williams BA, Hough KA, Tsui B, et al. Neurotoxicity of adjuvants used in perineural anesthesia and analgesia in comparison with ropivacaine. *Reg Anesth Pain Med.* 2011;36:225.
72. Morrison LM, Emanuelsson BM, McClure JH, et al. Efficacy and kinetics of extradural ropivacaine: Comparison with bupivacaine. *Br J Anaesth.* 1994;72:164.
73. Tucker GT, Mather LE. Pharmacology of local anaesthetic agents. Pharmacokinetics of local anaesthetic agents. *Br J Anaesth.* 1975;47(suppl):213.
74. Thomson PD, Melmon KL, Richardson JA, et al. Lidocaine pharmacokinetics in advanced heart failure, liver disease, and renal failure in humans. *Ann Intern Med.* 1973;78:499.
75. Rosenberg PR, Veering BT, Urmey WF. Maximum recommended doses of local anesthetics: A multifactorial concept. *Reg Anesth Pain Med.* 2004;29:564.
76. Braid DP, Scott DB. Dosage of lignocaine in epidural block in relation to toxicity. *Br J Anaesth.* 1996;38:596.
77. Adinoff B, Devous Sr MD, Best SE, et al. Gender differences in limbic responsiveness, by SPECT, following pharmacologic challenge in healthy subjects. *Neuroimage.* 2003;18:697.
78. Tucker GT, Mather LE. Properties, absorption, and disposition of local anesthetic agents. In: Cousins MJ, Bridenbaugh PO, eds. *Neural Blockade in Clinical Anesthesia and Management of Pain.* 3rd ed. Philadelphia, PA: Lippincott-Raven Publishers; 1998:55.
79. Lander JA, Weltman BJ, So SS. EMLA and amethocaine for reduction of children's pain associated with needle insertion. *Cochrane Database Syst Rev.* 2006;3: CD004236.
80. Ugur B, Ogurlu M, Gezer E, et al. Effects of esmolol, lidocaine and fentanyl on haemodynamic responses to endotracheal intubation. A comparative study. *Clin Drug Investig.* 2007;27:269.
81. Adamzik M, Groeben H, Farahani R, et al. Intravenous lidocaine after tracheal intubation mitigates bronchoconstriction in patients with asthma. *Anesth Analg.* 2007;104:168.
82. Groban L. Central nervous system and cardiac effects from long-acting amide local anesthetic toxicity in the intact animal model. *Reg Anesth Pain Med.* 2003; 28:3.
83. Weinberg GL. Current concepts in resuscitation of patients with local anesthetic cardiac toxicity. *Reg Anesth Pain Med.* 2002;27:568.
84. Brown DL, Ransom DM, Hall JA, et al. Regional anesthesia and local anesthetic-induced systemic toxicity: Seizure frequency and accompanying cardiovascular changes. *Anesth Analg.* 1995;81:321.
85. Auroy Y, Benhamou D, Bargues L, et al. Major complications of regional anesthesia in France: The SOS Regional Anesthesia Hotline Service. *Anesthesiology.* 2002;97:1274.
86. Lee LA, Posner KL, Domino KB, et al. Injuries associated with regional anesthesia in the 1980s and 1990s: A closed claim analysis. *Anesthesiology.* 2004;101:143.
87. Butterworth JF. Models and mechanisms of local anesthetic cardiac toxicity. *Reg Anesth Pain Med.* 2010;35:167.
88. Mather LE, Copeland SE, Ladd LA. Acute toxicity of local anesthetics: Underlying pharmacokinetic and pharmacodynamic concepts. *Reg Anesth Pain Med.* 2005;30:553.
89. Knudsen K, Beckman Suurkula M, Blomberg S, et al. Central nervous and cardiovascular effects of i.v. infusions of ropivacaine, bupivacaine and placebo in volunteers. *Br J Anaesth.* 1997;78:507.
90. Stewart J, Kellett N, Castro D. The central nervous system and cardiovascular effects of levobupivacaine and ropivacaine in healthy volunteers. *Anesth Analg.* 2002;97:412.
91. Vanhoutte F, Vereecke J, Verbeke N, et al. Stereoselective effects of the enantiomers of bupivacaine on the electrophysiological properties of the guinea-pig papillary muscle. *Br J Pharmacol.* 1991;103:1275.
92. Valenzuela C, Snyders D, Bennett PB, et al. Stereoselective block of sodium channels by bupivacaine in guinea pig ventricular myocytes. *Circulation.* 1995;92:3014.
93. Groban L, Deal DD, Vernon JC, et al. Does local anesthetic stereoselectivity or structure predict myocardial depression in anesthetized canines? *Reg Anesth Pain Med.* 2002;27:460.

94. Pickering AE, Waki H, Headley PM, et al. Investigation of systemic bupivacaine toxicity using the in situ perfused working heart-brainstem preparation of the rat. *Anesthesiology.* 2002;97:1550.
95. Chang KSK, Yang M, Andresen MC. Clinically relevant concentrations of bupivacaine inhibit rat aortic baroreceptors. *Anesth Analg.* 1994;78:501.
96. Newton DJ, McLeod GA, Khan F, et al. Vasoactive characteristics of bupivacaine and levobupivacaine with and without adjuvant epinephrine in peripheral human skin. *Br J Anaesth.* 2005;94:662.
97. Liu P, Feldman HS, Covina BM, et al. Acute cardiovascular toxicity of intravenous amide local anesthetics in anesthetized ventilated dogs. *Anesth Analg.* 1982;61:317.
98. Guo XT, Castle NA, Chernoff DM, et al. Comparative inhibition of voltage-gated cation channels by local anesthetics. *Ann N Y Acad Sci.* 1991;625:181.
99. Clarkson CW, Hondegham LM. Mechanisms for bupivacaine depression of cardiac conduction: Fast block of sodium channels during the action potential with slow recovery from block during diastole. *Anesthesiology.* 1985;62:396.
100. Nouette-Gaulain K, Forestier F, Malgat M, et al. Effects of bupivacaine on mitochondrial energy metabolism in heart of rats following exposure to chronic hypoxia. *Anesthesiology.* 2002;97:1507.
101. Wong GK, Crawford MW. Carnitine deficiency increases susceptibility to bupivacaine-induced cardiotoxicity in rats. *Anesthesiology.* 2011;114:1417.
102. Weinberg GL. Treatment of local anesthetic systemic toxicity (LAST). *Reg Anesth Pain Med.* 2010;35:188.
103. Long WB, Rosenblum S, Grady IP. Successful resuscitation of bupivacaine-induced cardiac arrest using cardiopulmonary bypass. *Anesth Analg.* 1989;79:403.
104. Soltesz EG, van Pelt F, Byrne JG. Emergent cardiopulmonary bypass for bupivacaine cardiotoxicity. *J Cardiothorac Vasc Anesth.* 2003;17:357.
105. Weinberg GL, VadeBoncouer T, Ramaraju GA, et al. Pretreatment or resuscitation with a lipid infusion shifts the dose-response to bupivacaine-induced asystole in rats. *Anesthesiology.* 1998;99:1071.
106. Weinberg GL, Ripper R, Feinstein DL, et al. Lipid emulsion infusion rescues dogs from bupivacaine-induced cardiac toxicity. *Reg Anesth Pain Med.* 2003;28:198.
107. Rosenblatt MA, Abel M, Fischer GW, et al. Successful use of a 20% lipid emulsion to resuscitate a patient after a presumed bupivacaine-related cardiac arrest. *Anesthesiology.* 2006;105:217.
108. Litz RJ, Popp M, Stehr SN, et al. Successful resuscitation of a patient with ropivacaine-induced asystole after axillary plexus block using lipid infusion. *Anaesthesia.* 2006;61:800.
109. Weinberg GL, Ripper R, Murphy P, et al. Lipid infusion accelerates removal of bupivacaine and recovery from bupivacaine toxicity in the isolated rat heart. *Reg Anesth Pain Med.* 2006;31:296.
110. Weinberg GL, Palmer JW, VadeBoncouer TR, et al. Bupivacaine inhibits acylcarnitine exchange in cardiac mitochondria. *Anesthesiology.* 2000;92:523.
111. Kitagawa N, Oda M, Totoki T. Possible mechanism of irreversible nerve injury caused by local anesthetics and membrane disruption. *Anesthesiology.* 2004;100:962.
112. Kalichman MW. Physiologic mechanisms by which local anesthetics may cause injury to nerve and spinal cord. *Reg Anesth.* 1993;18:448.
113. Whitlock EL, Brenner MJ, Fox IK, et al. Ropivacaine-induced peripheral nerve injection injury in the rodent model. *Anesth Analg.* 2010;111:214.
114. Selander D. Neurotoxicity of local anesthetics: Animal data. *Reg Anesth.* 1993; 18:461.
115. Kroin JS, Buvanendran A, Williams DK, et al. Local anesthetic sciatic nerve block and nerve fiber damage in diabetic rats. *Reg Anesth Pain Med.* 2010;35:343.
116. Brull R, McCartney CJL, Chan VWS, et al. Neurological complications after regional anesthesia: Contemporary estimates of risk. *Anesth Analg.* 2007;104:965.
117. Bigeleisen PE. Nerve puncture and apparent intraneural injection during ultrasound-guided axillary block does not invariably result in neurologic injury. *Anesthesiology.* 2006;105:779.
118. Rigler M, Drasner K, Krejcie T, et al. Cauda equina syndrome after continuous spinal anesthesia. *Anesth Analg.* 1991;72:275.
119. Reisner L, Hochman B, Plumer M. Persistent neurologic deficit and adhesive arachnoiditis following intrathecal 2-chloroprocaine injection. *Anesth Analg.* 1980; 58:452.
120. Pollock JE. Transient neurologic symptoms: Etiology, risk factors, and management. *Reg Anesth Pain Med.* 2002;27:581.
121. Zaric D, Christiansen C, Pace NL, et al. Transient neurologic symptoms after spinal anesthesia with lidocaine versus other local anesthetics: A systematic review of randomized, controlled trials. *Anesth Analg.* 2005;100:1811.
122. Pollock JE, Liu SS, Neal JM, et al. Dilution of lidocaine does not decrease the incidence of transient neurologic symptoms. *Anesthesiology.* 1999;90:445.
123. Hogan Q, Dotson R, Erickson S, et al. Local anesthetic myotoxicity: A case and review. *Anesthesiology.* 1994;80:942.
124. Zink W, Bohl JRE, Hacke N, et al. The long term myotoxic effects of bupivacaine and ropivacaine after continuous peripheral nerve blocks. *Anesth Analg.* 2005;101:548.
125. Nouette-Gaulain K, Dadure C, Morau D, et al. Age-dependent bupivacaine-induced muscle toxicity during continuous peripheral nerve block in rats. *Anesthesiology.* 2009;111:1120.
126. Nouette-Gaulain K, Sirvent P, Canal-Raffin M, et al. Effects of intermittent femoral nerve injections of bupivacaine, levobupivacaine, and ropivacaine on mitochondrial energy metabolism and intracellular calcium homeostasis in rat psoas muscle. *Anesthesiology.* 2007;106:1026.
127. Nouette-Gaulain K, Bellance N, Prevost B, et al. Erythropoietin protects against local anesthetic myotoxicity during continuous regional anesthesia. *Anesthesiology.* 2009;110:648.
128. Galbes O, Bourret A, Nouette-Gaulain K, et al. N-acetylcysteine protects against bupivacaine-induced myotoxicity caused by oxidative and sarcoplasmic reticulum stress in human skeletal myotubes. *Anesthesiology.* 2010;113:560.
129. Boren E, Teuber SS, Naguwa SM, et al. A critical review of local anesthetic sensitivity. *Clin Rev Allergy Immunol.* 2007;32:119.
130. Phillips JF, Yates AB, Deshazo RD. Approach to patients with suspected hypersensitivity to local anesthetics. *Am J Med Sci.* 2007;334:190.
131. McClimon B, Rank M, Li J. The predictive value of skin testing in the diagnosis of local anesthetic allergy. *Allergy Asthma Proc.* 2011;32:95.

SECTION V

Preanesthetic Evaluation and Preparation

CHAPTER

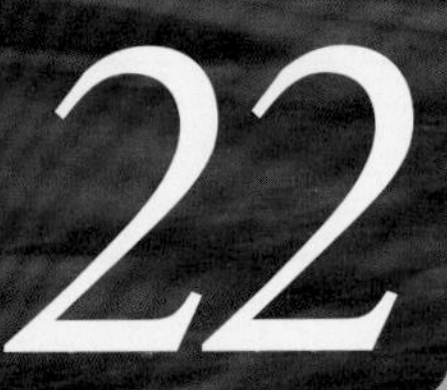

22 Preoperative Patient Assessment and Management

TARA M. HATA • J. STEVEN HATA

Key Points

1. The goals of a preoperative evaluation are to reduce patient risk and morbidity associated with surgery and coexisting diseases, promote efficiency and reduce costs, as well as to prepare the patient medically and psychologically for surgery and anesthesia.
2. The Joint Commission requires that all patients receive a preoperative anesthetic evaluation, and the American Society of Anesthesiologists (ASA) published a Practice Advisory for Preanesthesia Evaluation in 2002 and Approved Basic Standards for Preoperative Care, which were reaffirmed in 2010.
3. It is important for the evaluation to be complete, accurate, and clear, not only to allow the information to be relayed to others who may care for the patient perioperatively, but also for medicolegal purposes.
4. The preoperative evaluation serves as a screening tool to anticipate and avoid airway difficulties or problems with anesthetic drugs. In addition to the history and physical examination, previous anesthesia records should be reviewed. Contraindications to specific drugs, such as succinylcholine, nitrous oxide, or volatile agents, should be sought.
5. Review of the patient's allergies and medication list, including over-the-counter and herbal medications, should specifically screen for latex allergy and potential drug interactions. It should also alert the anesthesiologist to the need for steroid coverage.
6. When evaluating the patient with hypertension, diabetes mellitus, or obesity it is important to determine the presence of end-organ damage such as cardiovascular disease.
7. Exercise tolerance is the most important determinant of cardiac risk. Algorithms exist for preoperative evaluation of cardiac patients undergoing noncardiac surgery and are useful guides for further testing and evaluation.
8. Preoperative laboratory tests should be ordered on the basis of positive findings from the history and physical examination or anticipated physiologic disturbances during surgery such as blood loss.
9. Optimization of the patient's health status prior to surgery includes clear instruction regarding nothing by mouth times as well as which medications to administer immediately before surgery. In general, most medications for hypertension or cardiac disease should be continued, and consideration should be given to titrating an appropriate dose of beta-blocker in patients at risk. The need for subacute bacterial endocarditis prophylaxis should be anticipated. Likewise, drugs for asthma or chronic obstructive pulmonary disease should be continued or administered prophylactically. Medications taken for the treatment of reflux should be continued, or initiated for those patients with untreated symptoms. For diabetic patients, oral hypoglycemic agents should often be held, but patients requiring insulin will need to continue to take adjusted doses.
10. Although preoperative sedation is generally limited to drugs given immediately prior to anesthesia, the timing of administration must be planned when oral sedation is needed in children to allow optimal effect and avoid operating room delays.

Multimedia

1 Airway Exam

1 The goals of preoperative evaluation are to reduce patient risk and the morbidity of surgery, as well as to promote efficiency
2 and reduce costs. The Joint Commission requires that all patients receive a preoperative anesthetic evaluation. The American Society of Anesthesiologists (ASA) published on their web site an updated Practice Advisory for Preanesthesia Evaluation in 2003 and also reaffirmed the ASA Basic Standards for Preanesthetic Care in 2010, which outline the minimum requirements for a preoperative evaluation. The most recent ASA Practice Guidelines can be found at http://www.asahq.org. Conducting a preoperative evaluation is based on the premise that it will modify patient care and improve outcome. There is evidence, although not entirely convincing in all instances, that the preoperative evaluation will increase patient safety. That is, armed with knowledge preoperatively, the anesthesiologist can formulate and conduct an anesthetic plan that avoids dangers inherent in patient disease states. Furthermore, preoperative evaluations may reduce costs and cancellation rates, increasing resource utilization in the operating room (OR). This notion assumes that evaluations are done by anesthesiologists or other health-care providers familiar with anesthesia, surgery, and perioperative events.

The preoperative evaluation has several components and goals. One should review the available medical record, obtain a history, and perform a physical examination pertinent to the patient and contemplated surgery. On the basis of the history and physical examination, the appropriate laboratory tests and preoperative consultations should be obtained. Through these, one needs to determine whether the patient's preoperative condition may be improved prior to surgery. Guided by these factors, the anesthesiologist should choose the appropriate anesthetic and care plan. Finally, the process should be used to educate the patient about anesthesia and the perioperative period, answer all questions, and obtain informed consent.

The first part of this chapter outlines clinical risk factors pertinent to patients scheduled for anesthesia and surgery and the use of tests to confirm diagnoses. The second part discusses preoperative medication. The chapter provides only an overview of the preoperative management process; for more details, the reader is referred to chapters focusing on specific organ systems.

CHANGING CONCEPTS IN PREOPERATIVE EVALUATION

In the past, patients were admitted to the hospital at least a day prior to surgery. Currently, more and more patients are admitted to the hospital from the postanesthesia care unit. Older patients are scheduled for more complex procedures, and there is more pressure on the anesthesiologist to reduce the time between cases. The first time that the anesthesiologist performing the anesthetic sees the patient may be just prior to anesthesia and surgery. Others may have seen the patient previously in a preoperative evaluation clinic. Only a short time exists to engender trust and answer last-minute questions. It is often impossible to alter medical therapy immediately preoperatively. However, preoperative screening clinics are becoming more effective and clinical practice guidelines are becoming more prevalent. Information technology has helped the anesthesiologist in previewing the upcoming patients who will be anesthetized. Preoperative questionnaires and computer-driven programs have become alternatives to traditional information gathering. Finally, when anesthesiologists are responsible for ordering preoperative laboratory tests, cost saving occurs and cancellations of planned surgical procedures become less likely. In this setting it is important that there is communication between the preoperative evaluation clinic and the anesthesiologist performing the anesthetic.

APPROACH TO THE HEALTHY PATIENT

Standardization of best clinical practices may be enhanced by process control practices. In this regard, the preoperative evaluation form can serve as the basis for formulating the best anesthetic plan
3 tailored to the patient. It should aid the anesthesiologist in identifying potential complications, increase consistency in best care practices, as well as serve as a medicolegal document. The importance of the design has increased as it is more common today for the evaluation to be completed in a preoperative clinic by another physician or health professional who may not personally perform the anesthetic, but also because regulatory agencies such as Joint Commission on Accreditation of Healthcare Organizations (JCAHO) demand better documentation. Therefore, the information obtained needs to be complete, concise, and legible. In those hospitals that have electronic medical records, legibility is no longer an issue. A group from University of California, San Diego, studied the quality of preoperative evaluation forms across the United States and rated them in three categories: informational content, ease of use, and ease of reading.[1] Their results revealed that a surprisingly high percentage of forms are missing important information. While most anesthesiology departments will transition to electronic records, Figure 22-1 is an example of a preoperative evaluation form in paper format, which gives a concise view of the subjects that should be covered, with pertinent information listed in check boxes.

The approach to the patient should always begin with a thorough history and physical examination. These two evaluations alone may be sufficient (without additional routine laboratory tests).

Indication for the Surgical Procedure. This is part of the preoperative history because it will help determine the urgency of the surgery. True emergency procedures, which are associated with a recognized higher anesthetic morbidity and mortality, require a more abbreviated evaluation. A less defined area is the approach to urgent procedures. For example, ischemic limbs require surgery soon after presentation, but can usually be delayed for 24 hours for further evaluation. The indication for the surgical procedure may also have implications on other aspects of perioperative management. For example, the presence of a small bowel obstruction has implications regarding the risk of aspiration and the need for a rapid sequence induction. The extent of a lung resection will dictate the need for further pulmonary testing and perioperative monitoring. Patients undergoing carotid endarterectomy may require a more extensive neurologic examination, as well as testing to rule out coronary artery disease (CAD). The planned procedure also dictates patient positioning and often whether blood products

PRE-ANESTHETIC EVALUATION

Operation Proposed

Surgical Diagnosis

Age______ Gender______ Wt______ Ht______

BP P rr T

Allergies ☐ Latex allergy

Medications (Include Drugs, OTC and Herbals):

Anesthetic History ☐ Malignant hyperthermia

HEENT ☐ Hx of difficult airway

Teeth:

Class: I II III IV

Chin:

Neck:

Respiratory System ☐ WNL

☐ Asthma ☐ Bronchitis ☐ COPD ☐ Pneumonia

☐ TB ☐ Penumothorax ☐ Recent URI ☐ Dyspnea

☐ Cough ☐ RequiresO2 ☐ Steroids ☐ Snoring/Sleep Apnea

Tobacco:____ppd ____YR

Chest Exam:

CxR:

Anesthetic options / risks discussed________

☐ Risks discussed and patient/guardian understands.

Print Name/Signature Time Date

Patient Name

Cardiovascular System ☐ WNL

☐ CHD ☐ HTN ☐ CAD ☐ MI ☐ Valve disease

☐ Cardiomyopathy ☐ CHF ☐ RF ☐ Pacer ☐ Dysrrhythmia

☐ PVD ☐ Angina ☐ DOE ☐ Orthopnea ☐ Murmur

Exercise tolerance:

CV Exam:

EKG:

Echo/Cath:

Central Nervous System ☐ WNL

☐ CVA ☐ TIA ☐ LOC ☐ Seizures ☐ ↑ ICP

☐ HA ☐ NM disease ☐ Weakness ☐ Parethesias ☐ Psych disorder

☐ Altered MS/GCS ☐ Spinal cord injury

Renal ☐ WNL

☐ Insufficiency ☐ Failure ☐ Dialysis: last date ________

GI, Hepatic ☐ WNL

☐ Liver disease ☐ Hepatitis ☐ Bowel obstruction ☐ N/V ☐ Reflux

ETOH_drinks / ______

Endocrine, Metabolic, Infections, Other ☐ WNL

☐ Diabetes ☐ Thyroid disease ☐ RA ☐ Steroids

☐ Coagulopathy ☐ Chemotherapy ☐ Sickle Cell ☐ Pregnant

☐ Anemia ☐ HIV ☐ MRSA ☐ VRE

Additional Information / Interval History

☐ Advance directive(s) documented elsewhere

NPO Status:

Invasive monitors:

IV Access:

Pt Instructions:

Print Staff Name/Signature Time Date

Hospital Number

Lab Data

☐ Patient examined and chart reviewed. Patient approved for anesthesia.

☐ Potential post-op ICU admission

A/P:

Attending Signature Time Date

POSTANESTHETIC EVALUATION

PACU / ICU / Ward

☐ Extubated O2 sat______

☐ Satisfactory spont vent P______

☐ Protective reflexes BP______

☐ Follows commands IT______

☐ Report given T______

Signature Time Date

POSTANESTHETIC PROGRESS NOTE

☐ No anesthesia related adverse events

Signature Time Date

FIGURE 22-1. Example of preanesthetic evaluation form.

will be necessary. Frequently, further information will be required that necessitates contacting the surgeon. Perioperative care of the patient, as well as efficiency in the OR, is always enhanced by close communication with the surgeons.

4 *Response to Previous Anesthetics.* The ability to review previous anesthetic records is helpful in detecting the presence of a difficult airway, a history of malignant hyperthermia (MH), and the individual's response to surgical stress and specific anesthetics. The patient should be questioned regarding any previous difficulty with anesthesia or other family members having difficulty with anesthesia. A patient history relating an "allergy" to anesthesia should make one suspicious for MH. In those patients diagnosed with MH or as MH susceptible, not only will it affect the anesthetic regimen, but it should also bring into question the appropriateness of outpatient surgery.

Perhaps not life threatening, but persistent nausea and vomiting after a previous surgery may be the patient's most negative and lasting memory. There are multiple predictors for postoperative nausea and vomiting, including the type of surgical procedure, the anesthetic agents, as well as patient factors. A risk score for predicting postoperative nausea and vomiting after *inhalation* anesthesia identified four risk factors: female gender, prior history of motion sickness or postoperative nausea, nonsmoking, and the use of postoperative opioids. The investigators suggested prophylactic antiemetic therapy when two or more of the risk factors were present when using volatile anesthetics.[2,3] However, armed with this knowledge preoperatively, the anesthesiologist is able to tailor the anesthetic or possibly avoid general anesthesia and opioids altogether.

5 *Medications/Allergies.* The history should include a complete list of medications, including over-the-counter and herbal products (Table 22-1), to define a preoperative medication regimen, anticipate potential drug interactions, and provide clues to underlying disease. A complete list of drug allergies, including previous reactions, should be obtained, as well as an inquiry concerning reaction to latex.

If the patient presents on the day of surgery, the anesthesiologist should determine when the patient last ate, as well as note the sites of preexisting intravenous cannulae and invasive monitors. Once the general issues are completed, the preoperative history and physical examination can focus on specific systems.

Screening Patients Using a Systems Approach

Airway

At the forefront of every anesthesiologist's mind is the concern about the patient's airway. Questions to address include

TABLE 22-1. HERBAL/DIETARY SUPPLEMENTS AND DRUG INTERACTIONS

Brand Name	Common Uses	Pharmacologic Effects & Drug Interactions
Echinacea	Treat URI, UTI, wounds, and burns	Activation of cell-mediated immunity Allergic reactions, decreased effectiveness of immunosuppressants
Ephedra	Weight loss aid Bacteriostatic Antitussive	Increased HR and BP thru direct and indirect sympathomimetic effects Potential arrhythmias with digoxin or halothane, hypertension with oxytocin Enhanced sympathomimetic effects with other sympathomimetics or MAOIs
Feverfew	Migraine prophylaxis Antipyretic	Inhibit platelet activity and increase bleeding Rebound headache with sudden cessation
GBL, BD, GHB (Gamma-butyrolactone)	Bodybuilding Weight loss aid Sleep aid	Illegally distributed drugs Death, Seizures, unconsciousness Bradycardia, slowed respirations
Garlic	Inhibition of platelet aggregation Lipid lowering, BP lowering Antioxidant	Potential for increased bleeding
Ginger	Antinausea Antispasmodic	Potent inhibitor of thromboxane synthetase; may increase bleeding time
Ginkgo	Blood thinner	May enhance bleeding in patients on anticoagulant or antithrombotic therapy
Ginseng	Energy level enhancer Antioxidant	May inhibit platelet aggregation and increase bleeding Decreased blood glucose
Goldenseal	Diuretic Anti-inflammatory Laxative	Functions as an oxytocic Overdose (?) may cause paralysis May worsen edema and/or hypertension
Kava-kava	Anxiolytic	Potentiates sedative effects of anesthetics Potentiates ethanol effects May cause hepatotoxicity
Licorice	Treat gastritis/ulcers Treat cough/bronchitis	Glycyrrhizic acid in licorice may cause high blood pressure, hypokalemia, edema Contraindicated in many chronic liver conditions, renal insufficiency
St. John's wort	Treat depression, anxiety	May induce hepatic cytochromes P450, 3A4 and decrease drug levels (i.e. digoxin) May prolong effects of anesthesia (anecdotal reports)
Valerian	Mild sedative, anxiolytic	May potentiate sedative effects of anesthetics
Vitamin E	Slow aging Prevent stroke, pulmonary emboli Prevent atherosclerosis Promote wound healing	May increase bleeding, particularly in conjunction with other anti-coagulant and antithrombotic drugs. High doses may increase risk of death in patients with serious heart disease

Adapted from the ASA Physician Brochure: What You Should Know About Your Patients' Use of Herbal Medicines and Other Dietary Supplements, 2003 www. ASAhq.org

whether there is potential for difficulty in maintaining a patent airway with a mask and a laryngeal mask airway or in the ability to place an endotracheal tube when the patient is under general anesthesia. The ability to review previous anesthetic records is especially useful in uncovering an unsuspected "difficult airway" or to confirm previous uneventful intubations, noting whether the patient's body habitus has changed in the interim. Patients should be questioned about their ability to breathe through their nose, whether there is suspected or diagnosed obstructive sleep apnea (OSA), and whether they have orthopnea. Evaluation of the airway involves examination of the oral cavity including dentition, determination of the thyromental distance, assessment of the size of the patient's neck and scanning for tracheal deviation or masses, as well as evaluation of their ability to flex the base of the neck and extend the head. For trauma patients or patients with severe rheumatoid arthritis or Down syndrome, assessment of the cervical spine is critical. The presence of symptoms or signs of cervical cord compression should be assessed. In some instances, radiographic examination may also be required.

The Mallampati classification has become the standard for assessing the relationship of the tongue size relative to the oral cavity (Table 22-2),[4] although by itself the Mallampati classification has a low positive predictive value in identifying patients who are difficult to intubate.[5,6] Intubation involves multiple steps: Flexion of the neck, extension of the head, opening the mouth to insert the laryngoscope, and displacing the tongue forward and down into the submandibular space to expose the glottis. Therefore, a multifactorial approach to predict intubation difficulty as shown in Table 22-3 has proven more helpful. One must keep in

TABLE 22-2. MODIFIED MALLAMPATI AIRWAY CLASSIFICATION SYSTEM

Class	Direct Visualization, Patient Seated
I	Full view of soft palate, uvula, tonsillar pillars
II	Soft palate and upper portion of uvula
III	Soft palate
IV	Hard palate only

Modified from Mallampati RS, Gatt SP, Gugino LD, et al. A clinical sign to predict difficult tracheal intubation: A prospective study. *Can Anaesth Soc J.* 1985;32:429, with permission.

mind that factors that predict a difficult intubation are not necessarily the same factors that predict a difficult mask airway. For example, the absence of teeth clearly makes laryngoscopy less difficult, but at the same time can make maintaining a mask airway more challenging.

Pulmonary System

A screening evaluation should include questions regarding the history of tobacco use, dyspnea, exercise tolerance, cough, wheezing, inhaler use, recent upper respiratory tract infection, stridor, and snoring or sleep apnea. Physical examination should assess the respiratory rate as well as the chest excursion, use of accessory muscles, nail color, and the patient's ability to carry on a conversation or to walk without dyspnea. Auscultation should be used to detect decreased breath sounds, wheezing, stridor, or rales. For the patient with positive findings, see the section on the preoperative evaluation of the patient with pulmonary disease.

TABLE 22-3. COMPONENTS OF THE AIRWAY EXAMINATION WHICH SUGGEST DIFFICULTY WITH INTUBATION

1. Long upper incisors
2. A prominent "overbite"
3. The patient cannot protrude the mandibular incisors anterior to maxillary incisors.
4. Interincisor distance is less than 3 cm when mouth is fully opened.
5. Uvula is not visible when tongue is protruded with patient in sitting position.
6. Shape of palate is highly arched or very narrow.
7. Mandibular space is noncompliant.
8. Thyromental distance is less than three fingerbreadths.
9. Neck is short or thick.
10. Patient lacks normal range of motion of head and neck.

This table displays some findings of the airway physical examination that may suggest difficulty with intubation. Clinical context and judgment determine which of the components apply to a particular patient. The order of presentation in this table follows the "line of sight" that occurs during conventional oral laryngoscopy.
Modified from the Task Force on Difficult Airway Management: Practice guidelines for management of the difficult airway: An updated report by the American Society of Anesthesiologist Task Force on Management of the Difficult Airway. *Anesthesiology.* 2003;98:1269.

Cardiovascular System

6 When screening a patient for cardiovascular disease prior to surgery, the anesthesiologist is most interested in recognizing the signs and symptoms of uncontrolled hypertension and unstable cardiac disease such as myocardial ischemia, congestive heart failure, valvular heart disease, and significant cardiac dysrhythmias. Symptoms of cardiovascular disease should be carefully determined, especially the characteristics of chest pain, if present. Certain populations of patients, such as the elderly, women, or diabetics, may present with more atypical features. The presence of unstable angina has been associated with a high perioperative risk of myocardial infarction (MI).[7] The perioperative period is associated with a hypercoagulable state and surges in endogenous catecholamines, both of which may exacerbate the underlying process in unstable angina, increasing the risk of acute infarction. The preoperative evaluation can affect a patient's short- and long-term health by instituting treatment of unstable angina. Symptoms of clinically important valvular disease should be sought, such as angina, dyspnea, syncope, or congestive heart failure that would require further evaluation. Importantly, the anesthesiologist must identify patients who have undergone coronary artery stent or cardiac implantable device placement to be able to coordinate perioperative management with the cardiologist (see section on patient with cardiovascular disease).

The anesthesiologist should also be familiar with the American Heart Association (AHA) web site (http://www.heart.org/), which has links to the latest AHA statements and guidelines for health professionals. Here, one can find the most recent recommendations regarding which patients and procedures require subacute bacterial endocarditis prophylaxis.[8]

The examination of the cardiovascular system should include blood pressure evaluation, measuring both arms when appropriate. The anesthesiologist should take into account the effects of preoperative anxiety and may want a record of resting blood pressure measurements. However, Bedford and Feinstein[9] reported that the admission blood pressure was the best predictor of HR and BP response to laryngoscopy. Auscultation of the heart is performed, specifically listening for a murmur radiating to the carotids suggestive of aortic stenosis, abnormal rhythms, or a gallop suggestive of heart failure. The presence of bruits over the carotid arteries would warrant further workup to determine the risk of stroke. The extremities should be examined for the presence of peripheral pulses to exclude peripheral vascular disease or congenital cardiovascular disease.

Neurologic System

A screening of the neurologic system in the apparently healthy patient can be accomplished through simple observation. The patient's ability to answer health history questions practically ensures a normal mental status. Questions can be directed regarding a history of stroke and to exclude the presence of cerebrovascular disease, seizure history, preexisting neuromuscular disease, or nerve injuries. The neurologic examination may be cursory in healthy patients or extensive in patients with coexisting disease. Testing of strength, reflexes, and sensation may be important in

TABLE 22-4. AMERICAN SOCIETY OF ANESTHESIOLOGISTS (ASA) PHYSICAL STATUS (PS) CLASSIFICATION

ASA PS class 1	Normal healthy patient. No organic, physiologic, biochemical, or psychiatric disturbance
ASA PS class 2	Mild-to-moderate systemic disease that is well controlled and causes no organ dysfunction or functional limitation, that is, treated hypertension
ASA PS class 3	Severe systemic disease of at least one organ system that does cause functional limitation, that is, stable angina
ASA PS class 4	Severe systemic end-stage disease of at least one organ system that is life threatening with or without surgery, that is, congestive heart failure or renal failure
ASA PS class 5	Moribund patient who has little chance of survival but is submitted to surgery as a last resort (resuscitative effort), that is, ruptured aortic aneurysm
ASA PS class 6	A declared brain-dead patient whose organs are being removed for donor purposes
Emergency operation (E)	Any patient in whom an emergency operation is required

Modified from American Society of Anesthesiologists: New classification of physical status. *Anesthesiology* 1963;24:111.

patients if the anesthetic plan or surgical procedure may result in a change in the condition.

Endocrine System

Each patient should be questioned for symptoms that suggest endocrine diseases that may affect the perioperative course: diabetes mellitus, thyroid disease, parathyroid disease, endocrine-secreting tumors, and adrenal cortical suppression.

EVALUATION OF THE PATIENT WITH KNOWN SYSTEMIC DISEASE

Cardiovascular Disease

The preoperative evaluation of the patient with suspected cardiovascular disease has been approached in two ways: Clinical risk indices and preoperative cardiac testing. The goals are to define risk, determine which patients will benefit from further testing, form an appropriate anesthetic plan, and identify patients who will benefit from perioperative beta-blockade, interventional therapy, or even surgery. Clinical risk indices range from the physical status index of the ASA (Table 22-4) to the Goldman Cardiac Risk Index, which has recently been updated.

In an update of the Goldman Cardiac Risk Index, the investigators studied 4,315 patients aged 50 years and older who were undergoing elective, major noncardiac procedures.[10] Six independent predictors of complications were identified and included in a revised risk index: high-risk type of surgery, history of ischemic heart disease, history of congestive heart failure, history of cerebrovascular disease, preoperative treatment with insulin, and preoperative serum creatinine >2.0 mg/dL. Cardiac complications rose with an increase in the number of risk factors present. Rates of major cardiac complications with 0, 1, 2, or 3 of these factors were 0.5%, 1.3%, 4%, and 9%, respectively, in the derivation cohort and 0.4%, 0.9%, 7%, and 11%, respectively, among 1,422 patients in the validation cohort (Fig. 22-2).

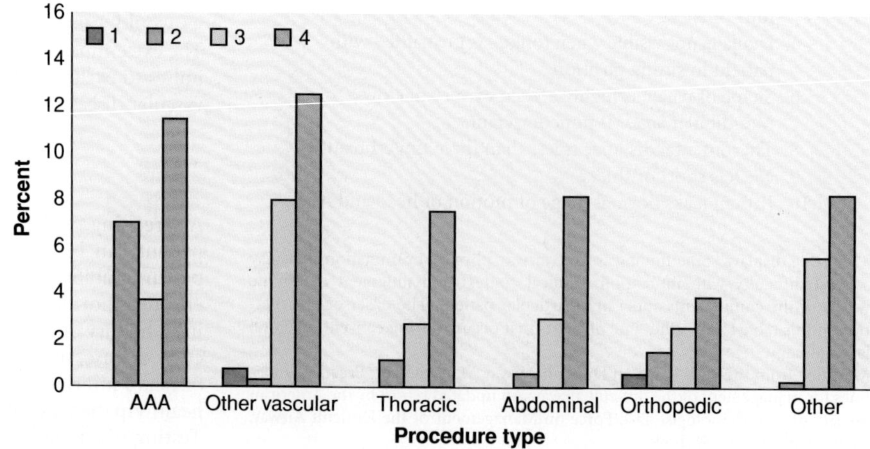

FIGURE 22-2. Cardiac risk index (CRI). Bars represent rate of major cardiac complications in entire patient population (both derivation and validation cohorts combined) for patients in revised CRI classes according to the type of procedure performed. Note that, by definition, patients undergoing abdominal aortic aneurysm (AAA), thoracic, and abdominal procedures were excluded from class I. In all subsets except patients undergoing AAA, there was a statistically significant trend toward greater risk with higher-risk class. See text for details. (Reproduced from Lee TH, Marcantonio ER, Mangione CM, et al. Derivation and prospective validation of a simple index for prediction of cardiac risk of major noncardiac surgery. *Circulation.* 1999;100:1043, with permission.)

While all of these indices provide information to assess the probability of complications and provide an estimate of risk, they do not prescribe perioperative management. In contrast, the anesthesiologist is most concerned with forming an anesthetic plan after defining the cardiovascular risk factors.

In patients with symptomatic coronary disease, the preoperative evaluation may reveal a change in the frequency or pattern of anginal symptoms. Certain populations of patients—for example, the elderly, women, or diabetics—may present with more atypical features. The presence of unstable angina has been associated with a high perioperative risk of MI.[7]

In virtually all studies, the presence of active congestive heart failure preoperatively has been associated with an increased incidence of perioperative cardiac morbidity.[11,12] Stabilization of ventricular function and treatment for pulmonary edema are important prior to elective surgery. Because the type of perioperative monitoring and treatments would be different, clarifying the cause of heart failure is important. Congestive symptoms may be a result of nonischemic cardiomyopathy or cardiac valvular insufficiency and/or stenosis.

Adults with a prior MI almost always have CAD. Traditionally, risk assessment for noncardiac surgery was based on the time interval between the MI and surgery. Multiple older studies have demonstrated an increased incidence of reinfarction if the MI was within 6 months of surgery.[13–15] With improvements in perioperative care, this difference has decreased. Therefore, the importance of the intervening time interval may no longer be valid in the current era of interventional therapy and risk stratification after an acute MI. Although many patients with an MI may continue to have myocardium at risk for subsequent ischemia and infarction, other patients may have their critical coronary stenoses either totally occluded or widely patent. For example, the use of percutaneous transluminal coronary angioplasty, thrombolysis, and early coronary artery bypass grafting (CABG) has changed the natural history of the disease.[16,17] Therefore, patients should be evaluated from the perspective of their risk for ongoing ischemia. The American Heart Association (AHA)/American College of Cardiology (ACC) Task Force on Perioperative Evaluation of the Cardiac Patient Undergoing Noncardiac Surgery has defined patient risk groups—based on clinical predictors (Table 22-5).[18]

Identifying Patients at Risk for Cardiac Disease

For those patients without overt symptoms or history, the probability of CAD varies with the type and number of atherosclerotic risk factors present. Peripheral arterial disease has been shown to be associated with CAD in multiple studies.[19]

Diabetes Mellitus

Diabetes mellitus is a common disease with a pathophysiology that affects multiple organ systems. Complications of diabetes

TABLE 22-5. CLINICAL PREDICTORS OF INCREASED PERIOPERATIVE CARDIOVASCULAR RISK (MYOCARDIAL INFARCTION, CONGESTIVE HEART FAILURE, DEATH)

Major

Unstable coronary syndromes
- Recent myocardial infarction[a] with evidence of important ischemic risk by clinical symptoms or noninvasive study
- Unstable or severe[b] angina (Canadian class III or IV)[c]

Decompensated congestive heart failure

Significant dysrhythmias
- High-grade atrioventricular block
- Symptomatic ventricular arrhythmias in the presence of underlying heart disease
- Supraventricular arrhythmias with uncontrolled ventricular rate

Severe valvular disease

Intermediate

Mild angina pectoris (Canadian class I or II)

Prior myocardial infarction by history or pathologic Q waves

Compensated or prior congestive heart failure

History of cerebrovascular disease

Diabetes mellitus

Renal insufficiency

Minor (markers for disease that have not been proven to increase perioperative risk independently)

Advanced age

Abnormal ECG (left ventricular hypertrophy, left bundle-branch block, ST-T abnormalities)

Rhythm other than sinus (e.g., atrial fibrillation)

Low functional capacity (e.g., inability to climb one flight of stairs with a bag of groceries)

Uncontrolled systemic hypertension

[a]The American College of Cardiology National Database Library defines recent myocardial infarction as >7 days but ≤1 month (30 days).

[b]May include "stable" angina in patients who are unusually sedentary.

[c]Campeau L. Grading of angina pectoris. *Circulation.* 1976;54:522.

ECG, electrocardiogram.

Modified and updated from Eagle K, Brundage B, Chaitman B, et al. Guidelines for perioperative cardiovascular evaluation of the noncardiac surgery. A report of the American Heart Association/American College of Cardiology Task Force on Assessment of Diagnostic and Therapeutic Cardiovascular Procedures. *Circulation.* 1996;93:1278, with permission.

mellitus are frequently the cause of urgent or emergent surgery, especially in the elderly. Diabetes accelerates the progression of atherosclerosis, so it is not surprising that diabetics have a higher incidence of CAD than nondiabetics. There is a high incidence of both silent MI and myocardial ischemia.[20] Eagle et al.[21] demonstrated that diabetes is an independent risk factor for perioperative cardiac morbidity. The duration of the disease and other associated end-organ dysfunction may alter the overall cardiac risk. Autonomic neuropathy has been reported as the best predictor of silent CAD.[22] Because these patients are at very high risk for a silent MI, an electrocardiogram (ECG) should be obtained to examine for the presence of Q waves.

Hypertension

Hypertension has also been associated with an increased incidence of silent myocardial ischemia and infarction.[20] Hypertensive patients who have left ventricular hypertrophy and are undergoing noncardiac surgery are at a higher perioperative risk than nonhypertensive patients.[23]

Investigators have suggested that the presence of a strain pattern on ECG suggests a chronic ischemic state.[24] Therefore, these patients should also be considered to have an increased probability of CAD and for perioperative morbidity.

There is controversy regarding a trigger to delay or cancel a surgical procedure in a patient with untreated or inadequately treated hypertension. Hypertension has been divided into three stages, with stage 3 denoting that which might be used as a cutoff (Table 22-6).[25] Aggressive treatment of blood pressure is associated with increased reduction in long-term risk, although the effect diminishes in all but diabetic patients as diastolic blood pressure is reduced below 90 mm Hg. Although there has been a suggestion in the literature that a case should be delayed if the diastolic pressure is >110 mm Hg, the study often quoted as the basis for this determination demonstrated no major morbidity in that small group of patients.[26] Other authors state that there is little association between blood pressures of <180 mm Hg systolic or 110 mm Hg diastolic and postoperative outcomes. However, such patients are prone to perioperative myocardial ischemia, ventricular dysrhythmias, and lability in blood pressure. It is less clear in patients with blood pressures above 180/110 mm Hg, although no absolute evidence exists that postponing surgery will reduce risk.[27,28] In the absence of end-organ changes, such as renal insufficiency or left ventricular hypertrophy with strain, the benefits of optimizing blood pressure must be weighed against the risks of delaying surgery.

TABLE 22-6. BLOOD PRESSURE

Category	Systolic (mm Hg)		Diastolic (mm Hg)
Optimal	<120	and	<80
Normal	<130	and	<85
High-normal	130–139	or	85–89
Hypertension			
Stage 1	140–159	or	90–99
Stage 2	160–179	or	100–109
Stage 3	≥180	or	≥110

Reproduced from Sixth report of the Joint National Committee on Prevention, Detection, Evaluation, and Treatment of High Blood Pressure. *Arch Intern Med.* 1997;157:2413, with permission.

Other Risk Factors

Several other factors associated with atherosclerosis have been used to suggest an increased probability of CAD. These include tobacco use and hypercholesterolemia. Although these risk factors increase the probability of developing CAD, they have not been shown to increase perioperative cardiac risk. When attempting to determine the overall probability of disease, the number of risk factors and severity of each are important.

Importance of Surgical Procedure

The surgical procedure influences the scope of preoperative evaluation required by determining the potential range of physiologic flux during the perioperative period. Few data exist defining the surgery-specific incidence of complications. Peripheral procedures, such as those included in a study of ambulatory surgery completed at the Mayo Clinic, are associated with an extremely low incidence of morbidity and mortality,[29] while major vascular procedures are associated with the highest incidence of complications. The AHA/American College of Cardiology guidelines describe risk stratification for noncardiac surgery as shown in Table 22-7.[18] Eagle et al.[30] published data on the incidence of perioperative MI and mortality by procedure for patients enrolled in the Coronary Artery Surgery Study. They determined the overall

TABLE 22-7. CARDIAC RISK[a] STRATIFICATION BASED ON THE SURGICAL PROCEDURE IN PATIENTS WITH KNOWN CORONARY ARTERY DISEASE

High	(Reported cardiac risk often >5%) • Emergent major operations, particularly in the elderly • Aortic and other major vascular open surgeries • Peripheral vascular surgery • Anticipated prolonged surgical procedures associated with large fluid shifts and/or blood loss
Intermediate	(Reported cardiac risk generally 1-5%) • Carotid endarterectomy • Head and neck surgery • Intraperitoneal and intrathoracic surgery • Orthopedic surgery • Prostate surgery
Low[b]	(Reported cardiac risk generally <1%) • Endoscopic procedures • Superficial procedures • Cataract surgery • Breast Ambulatory procedures

[a]Combined incidence of cardiac death and nonfatal myocardial infarction.
[b]Do not generally require further preoperative cardiac testing.
Modified and updated from Eagle K, Brundage B, Chaitman B, et al. Guidelines for perioperative cardiovascular evaluation of the noncardiac surgery. A report of the American Heart Association/American College of Cardiology Task Force on Assessment of Diagnostic and Therapeutic Cardiovascular Procedures. *Circulation.* 1996;93:1278, with permission.

TABLE 22-8. ESTIMATED ENERGY REQUIREMENT FOR VARIOUS ACTIVITIES

1 MET	Can you take care of yourself? Eat, dress, or use the toilet? Walk indoors around the house? Walk a block or two on level ground at 2–3 mph or 3.2–4.8 km/h? Do light work around the house, like dusting or washing dishes?	4 METs	Walk on level ground at 4 mph or 6.4 km/h? Run a short distance? Do heavy work around the house, like scrubbing floors or lifting or moving heavy furniture? Participate in moderate recreational activities like golf, bowling, dancing, doubles tennis, or throwing a baseball or football?
4 METs	Climb a flight of stairs or walk up a hill?	>10 METs	Participate in strenuous sports like swimming, singles tennis, football, basketball, or skiing

MET, metabolic equivalent.
Adapted from the Duke Activity Status Index and American Heart Association Exercise Standards. Reproduced from Eagle K, Brundage B, Chaitman B, et al. Guidelines for perioperative cardiovascular evaluation of the noncardiac surgery. A report of the American Heart Association/American College of Cardiology Task Force on Assessment of Diagnostic and Therapeutic Cardiovascular Procedures. *Circulation.* 1996;93:1278, with permission.

risk of perioperative morbidity in patients with known CAD treated either medically or with prior CABG. Their data differed slightly and found that high-risk procedures include major vascular, abdominal, thoracic, and orthopedic surgery.

Importance of Exercise Tolerance

7 Exercise tolerance is one of the most important determinants of perioperative risk and the need for further testing and invasive monitoring. An excellent exercise tolerance, even in patients with stable angina, suggests that the myocardium can be stressed without failing. If a patient can walk a mile without becoming short of breath, the probability of extensive CAD is small. Alternatively, if patients experience dyspnea associated with chest pain during minimal exertion, the probability of extensive CAD is high, which has been associated with greater perioperative risk. In addition, these patients are at risk for developing hypotension with ischemia and therefore may benefit from more extensive monitoring, coronary intervention therapy, or revascularization. Exercise tolerance can be assessed with formal treadmill testing or with a questionnaire that assesses activities of daily living (Table 22-8).[18]

Reilly et al.[31] have evaluated the predictive value of self-reported exercise tolerance for serious perioperative complications and demonstrated that a poor exercise tolerance (could not walk four blocks and climb two flights of stairs) independently predicted complications. The likelihood of a serious adverse event was inversely related to the number of blocks that could be walked. Therefore, there is good evidence to suggest that minimal additional testing is necessary if the patient is able to describe a good exercise tolerance.

Indications for Further Cardiac Testing

Multiple algorithms have been proposed to determine which patients require further testing. As described previously, the risk associated with the proposed surgical procedure influences the decision to perform further diagnostic testing and interventions. With the reduction in perioperative morbidity, it has been suggested that extensive cardiovascular testing is not necessary. However, until these findings can be confirmed, further testing may be warranted.

The algorithm to determine the need for testing proposed by the American College of Cardiology/American Heart Association Task Force updated in 2002 and again in 2007[32] is based on the available evidence and expert opinion that integrates clinical history, surgery-specific risk, and exercise tolerance. In the first step, the clinician evaluates the urgency of the surgery and the appropriateness of a formal preoperative assessment. Next, one should determine if the patient has undergone a recent revascularization procedure or coronary evaluation. Those patients with unstable coronary syndromes should be identified, and appropriate treatment instituted. Finally, the decision to undergo further testing depends on the interaction of the clinical risk factors, surgery-specific risk, and functional capacity. For patients at intermediate clinical risk, both exercise tolerance and the extent of the surgery are taken into account to determine the need for further testing. Importantly, no preoperative cardiovascular testing should be performed if the results will not change perioperative management.

Electrocardiogram

Preoperative 12-lead ECG can provide important information on the state of the patient's myocardium and coronary circulation. Abnormal Q waves in high-risk patients are highly suggestive of a past MI. Confirmation of active ischemia usually requires changes in at least two leads. It has been estimated that approximately 30% of MIs occur without symptoms ("silent infarctions") and can only be detected on routine ECGs, with the highest incidence occurring in patients with either diabetes or hypertension. The Framingham study showed that long-term prognosis is not improved by lack of symptoms.[20] The absence of Q waves on the ECG does not exclude the occurrence of a Q-wave MI in the past. Between 5% and 27% of Q waves disappeared over the 10-year period following an infarction during the 1970s.[33] Those patients in whom the ECG reverts to normal have improved survival compared with those with consistent abnormalities, with or without Q waves. The presence of Q waves on a preoperative ECG in a high-risk patient, regardless of symptoms, should alert the anesthesiologist to the increased perioperative risk and the possibility of active ischemia.

It has not been established that information obtained from the preoperative ECG affects clinical care. A review of clinical studies on the matter is inconclusive. In one retrospective review of adult patients undergoing ambulatory surgery, the preoperative ECG was not predictive of perioperative risk.[34] Although controversy exists, there are current recommendations for the need for a preoperative ECG. A preoperative resting 12-lead ECG is recommended for patients with at least one clinical risk factor who are undergoing vascular surgical procedures and for patients with known CAD, peripheral arterial disease, or cerebrovascular disease who are undergoing intermediate-risk surgical procedures. A perioperative ECG is reasonable in persons with no clinical risk factors who are about to undergo vascular surgical procedures and may be reasonable in patients with at least one clinical risk factor who are undergoing intermediate-risk operative procedures.[32]

Noninvasive Cardiovascular Testing

The exercise ECG has been the traditional method in the past for evaluating patients with suspected CAD. It represents the most cost-effective and least invasive method for detecting ischemia, with a sensitivity of 70% to 80% and a specificity of 60% to 75% for identifying CAD. A positive exercise stress test alerts the anesthesiologist that the patient is at risk for ischemia associated with increased heart rate, with the greatest risk in those who develop ischemia only after mild exercise. However, as discussed previously, the ability to exercise suggests that no further testing is necessary, and therefore stress electrocardiography is infrequently indicated.

A number of high-risk patients are either unable to exercise or have contraindications to exercise, for example, those with claudication. Therefore, pharmacologic stress testing and ambulatory electrocardiography have come into vogue, particularly as preoperative cardiovascular tests in patients scheduled for vascular surgery. Pharmacologic stress thallium imaging is useful in those patients who are unable to exercise. Dipyridamole or adenosine is administered as a coronary vasodilator to assess flow heterogeneity. The presence of a redistribution defect is predictive of postoperative cardiac events, especially in patients undergoing peripheral vascular surgery. Similarly, dobutamine can be used to increase myocardial oxygen demand, by increasing heart rate and blood pressure, in those patients who cannot exercise.

The ambulatory ECG (e.g., Holter monitoring) provides a means of continuously monitoring the ECG for significant ST segment changes preoperatively. One study demonstrated that the presence of silent ischemia is a strong predictor of outcome, while its absence is associated with a favorable outcome in 99% of the patients studied.[35] Other investigators have demonstrated the value of ambulatory ECG monitoring, although the negative predictive values have not been as high as reported by some.

Stress echocardiography is another preoperative test that may be of value in evaluating patients with suspected CAD. The appearance of either new or more severe regional wall motion abnormalities with exercise is considered a positive test. Either represents areas at risk for myocardial ischemia. The advantage of stress echocardiogram is that it is a dynamic assessment of ventricular function. Dobutamine echocardiography has also been studied and found to have among the best predictive values. It is generally accepted that the group at risk is composed of those who demonstrate regional wall motion abnormalities at low heart rates.

Several groups have published meta-analyses of preoperative diagnostic tests. One group of investigators demonstrated good predictive values using ambulatory ECG monitoring, radionuclide angiography, dipyridamole thallium imaging, or dobutamine stress echocardiography.[36] Shaw et al.[37] also demonstrated good predictive values of dipyridamole thallium imaging and dobutamine stress echocardiography. Both of these studies demonstrated the superior value of dobutamine stress echocardiography; however, there was significant overlap of the confidence intervals with other tests. The most important determinant with respect to the choice of preoperative testing is the expertise of the local institution.

Current recommendations are that patients with active cardiac conditions such as unstable angina, congestive heart failure, significant dysrhythmias, and severe valvular disease should undergo noninvasive stress testing before noncardiac surgery. Noninvasive stress testing for patients with multiple clinical risk factors and poor functional capacity (less than four metabolic equivalents) who require vascular surgery is reasonable if it will change management. Noninvasive testing in other patients about to go under intermediate-risk noncardiac surgery or vascular surgery is less clear.[32]

Assessment of Ventricular and Valvular Function

Both echocardiography and radionuclide angiography can assess cardiac ejection fraction at rest and under stress. Echocardiography is less invasive and able to assess regional wall motion abnormalities, wall thickness, valvular function, and valve area. Pulse-wave Doppler can be used to determine the velocity time integral. Ejection fraction can then be calculated by determining the cross-sectional area of the ventricle. Conflicting results exist with regard to the predictive value of ejection fraction using either echocardiographic or radionuclide measurements. It is reasonable for those with dyspnea of unknown origin and for those with current or prior heart failure with worsening dyspnea or other change in clinical status to have preoperative evaluations of left ventricular function. The benefits of reassessment of left ventricular function in clinically stable patients with previous cardiomyopathy are unknown.[32] Echocardiography can provide important information regarding valvular function, which may have important implications for either cardiac or noncardiac surgery, and is discussed more fully later in this text. Aortic stenosis has been associated with a poor prognosis in noncardiac surgical patients, and knowledge of valvular lesions may modify perioperative hemodynamic therapy.[11]

Coronary Angiography

Coronary angiography is currently the best method for defining coronary anatomy. In addition, information regarding ventricular and valvular function can also be assessed. Hemodynamic indices can be determined such as ventricular pressures and pressure gradients across valves. This information is routinely available in patients scheduled for CABG. Narrowing of the left main coronary artery and certain other lesions may be associated with a greater perioperative risk. Diffuse atherosclerosis in small vessels, as seen in diabetics, may lead to incomplete revascularization and a risk of developing ischemia despite CABG. Coronary angiography is used by cardiologists to determine whether coronary vascularization is an option.

Unlike the exercise or pharmacologic stress tests discussed earlier, coronary angiography provides anatomic, not functional, information. Although a critical coronary stenosis delineates an area of risk for developing myocardial ischemia, the functional response of that ischemia cannot be assessed by angiography alone. A critical stenosis may or may not be the underlying cause for a perioperative MI that occurs. In the ambulatory population, many infarctions are the result of acute thrombosis of a noncritical stenosis. Therefore, the value of routine angiography prior to noncardiac surgery depends on the identification of lesions that will cause morbidity and mortality.

Patients with restricted physical activity in whom functional capacity is difficult to determine may benefit from sophisticated imaging techniques such as cardiac computed tomography.[38]

Perioperative Coronary Interventions

Guidelines to reduce the perioperative risk of noncardiac surgery have recently been reviewed. There are several large studies that suggest that in patients who survive CABG, the risk of subsequent noncardiac surgery is low.[7,10] Although there is little data to support the notion of coronary revascularization solely for the purpose of improving perioperative outcome, it is true that for some patients scheduled for high-risk surgery, long-term survival may be enhanced by revascularization. Two studies used the Coronary Artery Surgery Study database and found that CABG significantly improved survival in those patients with both peripheral vascular disease and triple-vessel coronary disease, especially the group with depressed ventricular function.[39] After reviewing all available data, most clinicians believe the indication for CABG prior to noncardiac surgery remains the same as in other settings and is independent of the proposed noncardiac surgery.

The value of percutaneous transluminal coronary angioplasty is less well established. The current evidence does not support the use of percutaneous transluminal coronary angioplasty beyond established indications for nonoperative patients.

Patients with Coronary Artery Stents

Early surgery after coronary stent placement has been associated with adverse cardiac events. A significant incidence of perioperative death and of hemorrhage in patients after stent placement has been reported. The waiting period for surgery after bare metal stent placement is generally recognized as 1 month as a minimum, while the waiting period for drug-eluting stents is 12 months. This difference is because the incidence of stent thrombosis for the drug-eluting stents has been found to be similar to the bare metal stents in the early phase after placement, but less well defined over a longer period of time. Currently, patients are invariably taking aspirin and clopidogrel as antiplatelet therapy after stent placement. A thienopyridine (ticlopidine or clopidogrel) is generally continued with aspirin for 1 month after bare metal stenting and for 12 months after drug-eluting stent placement (Fig. 22-3). Perioperative management weighs the risk of bleeding versus a stent thrombosis. The decision must involve anesthesiologist, surgeons, cardiologists, and intensivists. For those patients who have a high risk for stent thrombosis, many advocate that at least aspirin be continued in the perioperative period. Also, the anesthesiologist must weigh the risk of regional versus general anesthesia when these patients are taking antiplatelet therapy. Surgery in patients with recent stent placement should probably only be considered in centers where 24-hour interventional cardiologists are available.[40–42]

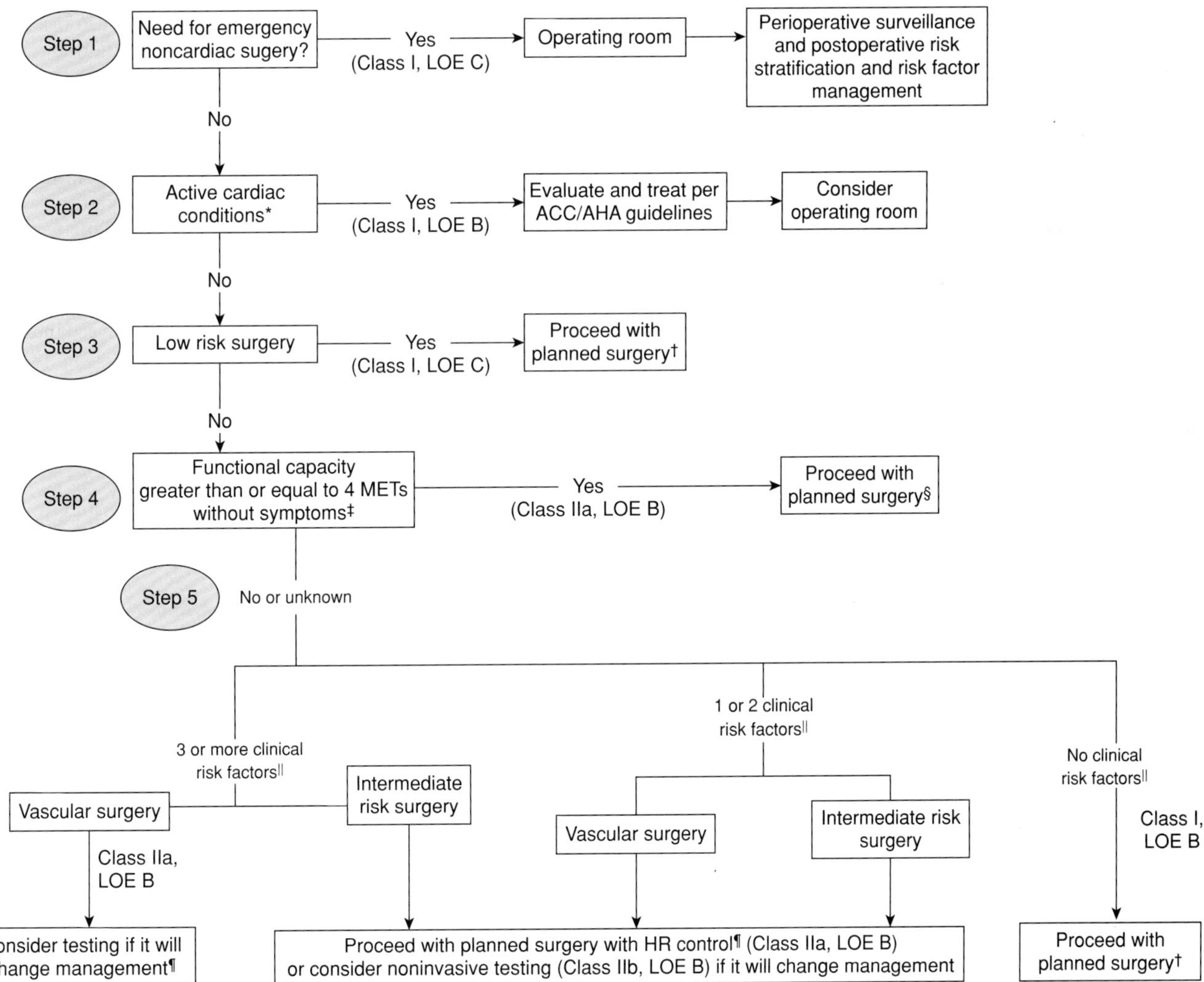

FIGURE 22-3. Cardiac evaluation algorithm for patients at least 50 years with cardiac risk factors undergoing non-cardiac surgery. || Clinical risk factors include ischemic heart disease, diabetes mellitus, cerebrovascular disease, renal insufficiency, compensated or history of congestive heart failure. AHA: American Heart Association; ACC: American College of Cardiology; HR; heart rate; LOE, level of evidence; MET: metabolic equivalent. (Used with permission from ACC/AHA 2007 Guidelines on Perioperative Cardiovascular Evaluation and Care for Noncardiac Surgery. *Circulation* 2007;116:e418–e500.

Patients with Cardiovascular Implantable Electronic Devices

With the increasing prevalence of patients treated with pacemakers and implantable defibrillators, the preoperative evaluation must address their management during the perioperative period. The function of these devices can be impaired by electromagnetic interference during surgery. Current guidelines for the management of these devices have been recently published.[43]

Pulmonary Disease

Pulmonary complications occur more frequently than cardiac complications, with an incidence of 5% to 10% in those having major noncardiac procedures. Perioperative pulmonary complications include aspiration, atelectasis, pneumonia, bronchitis, bronchospasm, hypoxemia, exacerbation of chronic obstructive pulmonary disease, and respiratory failure requiring mechanical ventilation.[44]

Postoperative respiratory failure is a major cause of morbidity and mortality, contributing to increased length of hospital stay and substantial economic cost. The risk of mortality with the development of respiratory failure is substantial, similar to perioperative MI. Understanding of clinical risk factors has increased substantially through the use of epidemiologic analyses of large clinical databases. Recent epidemiologic studies support that preoperative covariates can be used in models to predict patient groups at increased risk for respiratory failure.[44,45] Clinical guidelines from the American College of Physicians have been developed to assess both the preoperative risk and prevention strategies to limit the risk of respiratory failure.[46] Preoperative testing, such as pulmonary function testing and chest x-rays, is not recommended on a routine basis, as it appears to have limited benefit in predicting perioperative respiratory failure and complication rate. Although preoperative chest x-rays can identify structural lung abnormalities, these are not frequently associated with significant changes in clinical management for the general population. In contrast, laboratory studies identifying a reduction in serum albumin levels and increased levels of blood urea nitrogen (BUN) appear associated with an increased risk of perioperative pulmonary morbidity.[44]

Epidemiologic studies significantly support the relationship of the anatomic location of the surgery and pulmonary risk.[44] With regard to the surgical site, thoracic, open aortic, or upper abdominal surgery has been associated with the highest risk for postoperative pulmonary problems. Risk increases as the incision approaches the diaphragm.[44,47–49] Decreases in postoperative vital capacity, functional residual capacity, as well as diaphragmatic dysfunction can contribute to hypoxemia and atelectasis.[50] Functional residual capacity may take up to 2 weeks to return to baseline. Diaphragmatic dysfunction occurs despite adequate analgesia and is theorized to be caused by phrenic nerve inhibition.[51] Neurosurgery and neck surgery may be associated with perioperative aspiration pneumonia.

The need for emergency surgery and the need for general anesthesia are also associated with increased risk. Not only can the surgery affect pulmonary function, but general anesthesia also results in mechanical changes such as a decrease in the functional residual capacity and altered diaphragmatic motion leading to ventilation/perfusion abnormalities. General anesthesia also induces negative changes at the microscopic level causing inhibition of mucociliary clearance, increased alveolar–capillary permeability, inhibition of surfactant production, increased nitric oxide synthetase, and increased sensitivity of the pulmonary vasculature to neurohumoral mediators. Subanesthetic levels of intravenous or volatile agents have the ability to blunt the ventilatory response to hypoxemia and hypercarbia. Duration of anesthesia is a well-established risk factor for postoperative pulmonary complications, with morbidity rates increasing after 2 to 3 hours.[52] However, when considering laparoscopic surgery which is often longer in duration, the associated decrease in pulmonary complications compared with an open procedure usually outweighs the risk of increased anesthesia time.[53]

Atelectasis during the intraoperative and postoperative periods can contribute to the risk of perioperative respiratory failure. The preoperative assessment should address the following therapies: Epidural analgesia during the perioperative period, lung expansion methods, and deep venous thrombosis prophylaxis. Intraoperative measures to limit the risk of hospital-acquired pneumonia have been proposed, largely focused on reducing the risk of bacterial contamination of the lung during the perioperative period. For high-risk patient groups there are supportive studies of benefits of preoperative oral antiseptic decontamination before endotracheal intubation as well as the role of specialized endotracheal tubes to decrease the risk of nosocomial pneumonia.[54–56]

Preoperative evaluation of patients with preexisting pulmonary disease should include assessment of the type and severity of disease, as well as its reversibility (Table 22-9).

TABLE 22-9. POTENTIAL PATIENT-RELATED RISK FACTORS FOR POSTOPERATIVE PULMONARY COMPLICATIONS

Potential Risk Factor	Type of Surgery	Unadjusted Relative Risk Associated with Factor
Smoking	Coronary bypass	3.4
	Abdominal	1.4–4.3
ASA class > II	Unselected	1.7
	Thoracic or abdominal	1.5–3.2
Age >70 years	Unselected	1.9–2.4
	Thoracic or abdominal	0.9–1.9
Obesity	Unselected	1.3
	Thoracic or abdominal	0.8–1.7
COPD	Unselected	2.7–3.6
	Thoracic or abdominal	4.7

ASA, American Society of Anesthesiologists; COPD, chronic obstructive pulmonary disease.
Adapted from Smetana GW. Preoperative pulmonary evaluation. *N Engl J Med.* 1999;340:942.

Tobacco Use

Smoking is an important risk factor, but one that usually cannot be influenced. Even among smokers who have not developed chronic lung disease, smoking is known to increase carboxyhemoglobin levels, decrease ciliary function, and increase sputum production, as well as cause stimulation of the cardiovascular system secondary to nicotine. While cessation of smoking for 2 days can decrease carboxyhemoglobin levels, abolish the nicotine effects, and improve mucous clearance, prospective studies showed that smoking cessation for at least 4 to 8 weeks was necessary to reduce the rate of postoperative pulmonary complications.[57,58] Recent studies of nicotine transdermal patches used during the perioperative period have shown increased mortality and are best avoided.[59] Patients who smoke often show increased airway reactivity under general anesthesia, and it may be useful to administer a bronchodilator such as albuterol preoperatively.

Asthma

Asthma is one of the most common coexisting diseases that confront the anesthesiologist. During the patient interview it is important to elicit information regarding inciting factors, severity, reversibility, and current status. Frequent use of bronchodilators, hospitalizations for asthma, and requirement for systemic steroids are all indicators of the severity of the disease. After an acute exacerbation of asthma, airway hyperreactivity may persist for several weeks.[60] In addition to bronchodilators, perioperative steroids are worth considering as prophylaxis for the severe asthmatic, for example, hydrocortisone 100 mg intravenously every 8 hours on the day of surgery. The possibility of adrenal insufficiency is also a concern in those patients who have received more than a "burst and taper" of steroids in the previous 6 months. This group of patients should be administered "stress doses" of steroids perioperatively. Kabalin et al.[61] found there was a low complication rate for asthmatics treated with short-term steroids undergoing surgery. Significantly, they found no association with impaired wound healing or infections. For patients using inhaled steroids, they should be administered regularly, starting at least 48 hours prior to surgery for optimal effectiveness.

Obstructive Sleep Apnea

OSA is a syndrome defined by periodic obstruction of the upper airway during sleep, leading to episodic oxygen desaturation and hypercarbia. This episodic desaturation, in turn, causes episodic arousal, leading to chronic sleep deprivation with daytime hypersomnolence and even behavioral changes in children. Depending on the frequency and severity of events, it may lead to other changes such as chronic pulmonary hypertension and right heart failure. It is estimated to be present in 9% of women and 24% of men, with the great majority of these being undiagnosed. Factors commonly associated with an increased risk of sleep apnea include obesity (body mass index >35 kg/m^2 or 95th percentile for age), increased neck circumference, severe tonsillar hypertrophy, and anatomic abnormalities of the upper airway.

Because of their propensity for airway collapse and sleep deprivation, patients with OSA are especially susceptible to the respiratory depressant and airway obstructive effects of sedatives, narcotics, and inhaled anesthetics both intraoperatively and postoperatively. Preoperative identification of those patients at risk allows them to undergo a formal sleep study to determine the presence and severity of symptoms and also allows preoperative initiation of continuous positive airway pressure (CPAP). In 2006, the ASA published practice guidelines for the perioperative management of patients with OSA.[62] During the preoperative evaluation, specific questions should be directed toward the patient and family regarding the presence of symptoms and signs of OSA:

- Does the patient snore loudly enough to be heard through a door or snore frequently?
- Have you observed pauses in the patient's breathing during sleep?
- Does the patient have frequent arousals from sleep or awakenings with a choking sensation?
- Does the patient experience frequent daytime somnolence and fatigue or fall asleep easily in a non-stimulating environment?
- Does your child appear restless when sleeping or have difficulty with breathing?
- Is your child overly aggressive or does he/she have trouble concentrating?

If the patient has predisposing anatomy and/or signs or symptoms in two or more areas, he/she should be referred for a sleep study. If a sleep study is not possible, the patient should be managed as he/she has OSA. The risk of perioperative complications in patients with OSA increases with the severity of sleep apnea, the invasiveness of surgery, and the amount of postoperative opioids required. There is general consensus that preoperative initiation of nasal mask CPAP reduces perioperative risk, perhaps by decreasing the sleep deprivation and secondary hypersomnolence.[62] Importantly, OSA is also associated with difficult airway management, making it even more important to examine previous anesthesia records and to perform a thorough airway examination. Emergency airway equipment should be readily available at the surgical center.

There are multiple management decisions to make in coordination with the surgeon with respect to the OSA patient:

- Determine whether there are noninvasive ways of performing the operation that would decrease the need for opioids postoperatively.
- Discuss whether it is feasible to perform surgery under neuraxial, regional, or local anesthesia, decreasing the total amount of anesthesia or opioids needed.
- Determine whether nonsteroidal antiinflammatory agents are acceptable for postoperative analgesia.
- Discuss whether outpatient surgery is a safe option.
- Determine whether the patient will be able to use CPAP postoperatively.
- Determine whether postoperative admission to an intensive care unit or monitored unit is required for the patient who is a first-time user of CPAP.

The ASA practice guidelines for OSA recommend hospitalization after uvulopalatoplasty surgery and after tonsillectomy for OSA in children younger than 3 years. Postoperative hospitalization is also recommended for those OSA patients with other coexisting diseases. When procedures are performed on an outpatient basis, prolonged postoperative monitoring should be continued to ensure that the patient is able to maintain room air saturation without obstruction when left undisturbed in recovery. Recovery with the patient's head and thorax elevated is also recommended to optimize airway patency. The task force recommends continuous pulse oximetry during hospitalization, as well as supplemental oxygen until the patient can maintain their baseline oxygen saturation on room air.

Endocrine Disease

Diabetes Mellitus

Diabetes mellitus is the most common endocrinopathy, with the incidence of type 1 diabetes at 0.4% of the population and type

2 diabetes affecting approximately 8% to 10% of Americans, but projected to develop in >30% of Americans born after 2000, largely because of the rise in obesity.[63] Critical illness–induced hyperglycemia, defined as a blood glucose >200 mg/dL in the absence of known diabetes, occurs frequently, particularly in the elderly.[64] Diabetes mellitus has acute and chronic disease manifestations, making it more likely for diabetics to require surgery. The majority of diabetics develop secondary disease in one or more organ systems, which must be identified preoperatively so that an appropriate plan can be developed for perioperative management. While long-term, close control of glucose may limit some of the microvascular effects of diabetes (retinopathy, neuropathy, and nephropathy), macrovascular events such as myocardial ischemia or infarction or stroke may not be decreased. Diabetics have an increased risk of CAD, hypertension, congestive heart failure, and perioperative MI. The 2002 American College of Cardiology/AHA guidelines on perioperative cardiac assessment of patients undergoing noncardiac surgery place diabetics, especially those receiving insulin, at a minimum of intermediate risk.[65] They also state that most diabetic patients >65 years of age have significant CAD, with the incidence of silent ischemia increased due to associated diabetic autonomic neuropathy.

Diabetics are also more likely than the general population to have cerebral vascular, peripheral vascular, and renal vascular disease. Diabetes mellitus is the leading cause of renal failure requiring dialysis. Peripheral neuropathies and vascular disease make these patients more susceptible to positioning injuries during surgery as well as postoperatively. Autonomic neuropathy may predispose the patient to hemodynamic instability during anesthesia and theoretically increase the risk of pulmonary aspiration because of the associated gastroparesis. These deficits should be documented prior to anesthesia and the anesthetic plan adjusted accordingly. Stiff joint syndrome due to glycosylation of proteins and abnormal collagen cross-linking may significantly affect the temporomandibular, atlantooccipital, and cervical spine joints in patients with long-standing type 1 diabetes, resulting in difficulty with intubation. A thorough airway examination should be performed prior to anesthesia and a high index of suspicion maintained for a potentially difficult airway. Some suggest using the "prayer sign" as an evaluation tool: Patients who are unable to completely oppose their hands (with no space between) should be suspected of also having changes in other joints potentially impacting airway manipulation.

Regimens for perioperative glycemic control vary enormously, not only between type 1 and type 2 diabetics, but also within each group. Patients with type 1 diabetes have an absolute insulin deficiency usually due to destruction of pancreatic beta cells. These patients must receive insulin to prevent diabetic ketoacidosis. Home glucose management most often relies on a combination of short- and intermediate- or long-acting insulin regimens. Insulin pumps are increasingly common and are used to administer a continuous subcutaneous infusion of short-acting insulin, supplemented by boluses dictated by glucose levels, diet, and exercise. Type 2 diabetes accounts for the great majority of diabetics and is defined by variable degrees of insulin deficiency and resistance. Although most commonly associated with obesity, it may also be induced by corticosteroids or pregnancy. Ketoacidosis is uncommon in type 2 diabetes, and the stress of severe infection or illness is more likely to provoke a nonketotic hyperosmolar state, which is characterized by severe dehydration, hyperglycemia, and hyperosmolarity. In type 2 diabetics, glucose control is most commonly achieved with diet, exercise, and/or oral hypoglycemic drugs. These agents primarily work by increasing endogenous insulin release, increasing insulin sensitivity, and/or decreasing hepatic gluconeogenesis. These drugs fall under the main categories of sulfonylureas, biguanides, thiazolidinediones, and meglitinides. If glycemic control is unsuccessful, then insulin is generally added to the regimen.

Ideally, both type 1 and 2 diabetic patients should be evaluated by the preoperative clinic as well as the patient's endocrinologist 1 to 2 weeks before elective surgery. In addition to a thorough history and physical examination, a judicious laboratory investigation should include determination of blood glucose, hemoglobin A1c, serum electrolytes, creatinine, and an ECG. If the patient's glycemic control is inadequate based on a hemoglobin A1c being outside of the target range (7% to 9% for <5 years old; 6% to 8% for >5 years old), abnormal electrolytes, or ketonuria, then elective surgery should be delayed to allow optimization of preoperative glycemic control. Administration of perioperative beta-blockers should be considered in diabetic patients with CAD in an attempt to limit perioperative myocardial ischemia, as there is no evidence of worsened glucose intolerance or masking of hypoglycemic symptoms. However, the physician should be attentive to the possibility of precipitating heart failure.

Perioperative Glucose Management

Anesthesia and surgery interrupt the regular meal schedule and insulin administration in patients with diabetes mellitus. Perioperative stress may increase serum glucose concentrations secondary to the release of cortisol and catecholamines. The majority of available literature suggests that better glycemic control may limit morbidity (length of hospital/intensive care unit stay, infection rate, wound healing, outcomes after strokes/MIs) and mortality particularly in cardiac surgery patients, carotid endarterectomy patients, and the critically ill.[64,66–68] Although a randomized trial found an increase in the incidence of death and perioperative stroke in cardiac surgery patients where an attempt was made to maintain the glucose between 80 and 100 mg/dL,[69] recent systematic reviews have found a reduction in morbidity and mortality associated with better glycemic control, but recognize the increased risk of hypoglycemia.[70] More studies are needed to more closely define the target level for glucose control. There is general consensus that an attempt should be made to control the upper limit of glucose to <200 mg/dL, although some will argue that tighter control is warranted. Guidelines for ambulatory and hospitalized patients have been recently published.[71,72] The following recommendations can serve as a general guide:

- Plan with the surgeon to schedule the surgery as the first case of the day to prevent prolonged fasting.
- As a general rule, oral hypoglycemic agents are held on the day of surgery to avoid reactive hypoglycemia until oral intake is restarted.
- Insulin therapy should balance adequate glucose control with the avoidance of hypoglycemia. Insulin is usually continued through the evening before surgery.
- Schedule the patient to arrive in the early morning with an empty stomach and check blood glucose on arrival.
- If patients develop symptoms of or measurable hypoglycemia, they should be counseled to take a glucose tablet or clear juice.
- Type 1 diabetics should be continued on basal insulin administration even during preoperative fasting to prevent ketoacidosis. Administer half the usual morning dose of intermediate- or long-acting insulin after arrival to the surgery center where a maintenance IV can be started. Hold the usual dose of rapid- or short-acting insulin.
- Use the patient's own sliding scale to administer short-acting insulin subcutaneously prior to the scheduled surgery and during short operations.

- Patients on insulin pumps may be managed by continuing the pump for short operations or changing over to an intravenous insulin infusion for moderate or major operations.

This strategy, along with blood glucose determinations every 1 to 2 hours, may be all that is necessary for well-controlled diabetics undergoing short, noninvasive outpatient operations. In addition, it is important to prevent postoperative nausea and vomiting and to encourage the early resumption of diet, allowing return to their previous insulin regimen. For type 1 or 2 diabetics undergoing moderate or major surgery, insulin is generally administered in the form of an intravenous infusion of regular insulin. Discontinuing the patient's own insulin pump will avoid problems with insulin preparations and pump technology.

There are several methods of administering an insulin infusion, none of which has proved superior. Concurrent separate infusions of insulin and glucose are more easily adjusted and may provide better glycemic control than combined glucose/insulin/potassium infusions. To increase the safety, the insulin infusion (which is on a separate pump) is added via a side port to the same line delivering the glucose infusion. A separate nonglucose isotonic solution should be used to replace deficits and intraoperative fluid losses. All protocols rely on the frequent determination of a plasma glucose level at least every 1 to 2 hours to allow titration of insulin.[73–75]

Thyroid and Parathyroid Diseases

Thyroid and parathyroid diseases have clinical manifestations that are important to the preoperative evaluation (Table 22-10). Although thyroid function tests are more sensitive, thyroid disease is usually adequately evaluated by clinical history, and the evaluation should focus on evaluating for signs and symptoms of hypothyroidism and hyperthyroidism. Hypothyroidism can lead to the development of hypothermia, hypoglycemia, hypoventilation, and hyponatremia, as well as a susceptibility to depressant drugs. Anesthesiologists should be alert to the possibility of the hypermetabolic state of thyroid storm in patients with hyperthyroidism. A large thyroid mass may distort the upper airway, producing inspiratory stridor or wheezing, especially evident in the supine position. In these cases, a chest x-ray should be obtained looking for evidence of tracheal deviation or narrowing. A computed tomography scan of the upper airway and trachea will provide better detail of any airway compromise. Patients with hyperparathyroidism often have hypercalcemia, indicating the need for preoperative determination of a serum calcium level.

Adrenal Disorders

Classic findings in the patient with a *pheochromocytoma* include intermittent hypertension, headache, diaphoresis, and tachycardia. Patients with other endocrine tumors have a higher incidence of multiple endocrine neoplasia syndrome, and pheochromocytoma should be ruled out as the cause of unexplained hypertension. Over time, the mortality for surgical resection of a pheochromocytoma has decreased because of improvements in perioperative therapy for patients with the syndrome. A more important issue is to identify patients with a possible pheochromocytoma preoperatively before they are scheduled for other types of surgery.

Adrenal–cortical suppression is a more common disorder in patients presenting for surgery, and one should have a high index of suspicion in those patients taking long-term corticosteroids. Cushing syndrome is the most obvious manifestation of long-term high-dose steroid treatment, and the hallmark symptoms include moon facies, striations of the skin, truncal obesity, hypertension, easy bruisability, and hypovolemia. Preoperative preparation for patients with adrenal suppression includes correction of any fluid and electrolyte abnormalities, as well as steroid supplementation.

There is consensus that for patients taking corticosteroids for long periods, perioperative steroid supplementation is indicated to cover the stresses of anesthesia and surgery; however, in patients who have had only a short course of steroids within the 12 months prior to surgery, the use of steroid supplementation is controversial. It is impossible to identify the specific duration of therapy or dose of steroids that produces pituitary and adrenal suppression. Marked variability among patients exists. Certainly, more suppression may be expected with a higher dose and a longer duration of therapy. A conservative estimate is to consider treatment in any patient who has received corticosteroid therapy for at least 1 month in the past 6 to 12 months. The dose and duration of supplemental steroid administration depend on an estimate of the stress of the surgical procedure in the perioperative period. One regimen is to administer 25 mg of cortisol

TABLE 22-10. CLINICAL MANIFESTATIONS OF THYROID AND PARATHYROID DISEASES

	Hyperthyroidism	Hypothyroidism	Hyperparathyroidism
General	Weight loss; heat intolerance; warm, moist skin	Cold intolerance	Weight loss, polydipsia
Cardiovascular	Tachycardia, atrial fibrillation, congestive heart failure	Bradycardia, congestive heart failure, cardiomegaly, pericardial or pleural effusion	Hypertension, heart block
Neurologic	Nervousness, tremor, hyperactive reflexes	Slow mental function, minimal reflexes	Weakness, lethargy, headache, insomnia, apathy, depression
Musculoskeletal	Muscle weakness, bone resorption	Large tongue, amyloidosis	Bone pains, arthritis, pathologic fractures
Gastrointestinal	Diarrhea	Delayed gastric emptying	Anorexia, nausea, vomiting, constipation, epigastric pain
Hematologic	Anemia, thrombocytopenia		
Renal		Impaired free water clearance	Polyuria, hematuria

Adapted from Roizen MF. Anesthesia for the patient with endocrine disease, part 1. *Curr Rev Clin Anesth.* 1987;6:43.

TABLE 22-11. PERIOPERATIVE CORTICOSTEROID COVERAGE

For minor surgery	The patient should take 1.5–2 times his/her usual prednisone dosage on the morning of surgery. The following day the patient should take his/her normal prednisone dose (or parenteral equivalent if gut cannot be used). The surgeon and anesthesiologist should be aware that the patient is glucocorticoid-dependent and should be prepared to administer more "steroids" if the surgery becomes prolonged or more extensive.
For moderate surgery	The patient should be given 2 times his/her usual glucocorticoid dosage orally (if possible) on the morning of surgery and/or 25 mg hydrocortisone IV before the operation, then 75 mg hydrocortisone IV during the operation, and 50 mg hydrocortisone IV after the operation; then the dose should be rapidly tapered over 48 h to the usual dose—if the postoperative course is uncomplicated.
For major surgery	The patient should be given 2 times his/her usual glucocorticoid dosage orally (if possible) on the morning of surgery and/or 50 mg hydrocortisone IV before the operation, then 100 mg hydrocortisone IV during the operation. After the operation, 100 mg IV q8h × 24 h should be administered and then rapidly tapered (over 48–72 h) to the patient's usual glucocorticoid dosage—if the postoperative course is uncomplicated.

IV, intravenously.
Adapted from Brussel T, Chernow B. Perioperative management of endocrine problems: Thyroid, adrenal cortex, pituitary. *Am Soc Anesthesiol.* 1990;3:48.

preoperatively and then give an intravenous infusion of 100 mg of cortisol over the next 12 to 24 hours for adult patients. Another method is to administer 100 mg of hydrocortisone intravenously before, during, and after surgery. This dose is meant to equal the estimated maximum amount of steroid that the adrenal glands could produce during stress in a 24-hour period. When considering whether to administer steroids the anesthesiologist should keep in mind that the risk–benefit ratio is usually very small (Table 22-11).

Other Organ Systems

Renal disease has important implications for fluid and electrolyte management, as well as metabolism of drugs. In those patients with renal failure, the timing of their most recent dialysis will determine whether they are hyper- or hypovolemic and hyper- or hypokalemic. There will be patients who will require dialysis before coming for surgery. Because renal failure is also associated with anemia and qualitatively deficient platelets, there should be a lower threshold for determining these lab results preoperatively.

Liver disease is associated with altered protein binding and volume of distribution of drugs, as well as coagulation abnormalities. Coagulation disorders may discourage the choice of regional anesthesia. The anesthesiologist should inquire about bruising, bleeding, and the use of medications that influence platelet function such as nonsteroidal antiinflammatory drugs and anticoagulants. End-stage liver disease may also lead to esophageal varices, important information that allows the anesthesiologist to potentially avoid esophageal instrumentation. Ascites, a more obvious physical finding of liver failure, may significantly affect the patient's respiratory mechanics and make it difficult for them to lie flat.

Arthritis is becoming more prevalent in our aging population combined with our sedentary lifestyle. Osteoarthritis may result in difficulty positioning the head to facilitate tracheal intubation or difficulty in positioning for regional anesthesia. Rheumatoid arthritis is a multisystem disease, potentially leading to other derangements such as restrictive lung disease, pleural effusions, pericarditis, anemia, and atlantooccipital instability.

Finally, the anesthesiologist should inquire about infectious diseases that will dictate the need for increased protective measures for OR personnel and equipment.

PREOPERATIVE LABORATORY TESTING

Defining Normal Values

In attempting to determine the optimal choice of preoperative tests, it is important to understand the interpretation of the results. Ideally, tests would either confirm or exclude the presence of a disease; however, most tests only increase or decrease the probability of disease. In determining reference ranges for diagnostic tests, values that fall outside the 95% confidence intervals for normal individuals are considered abnormal. Therefore, up to 5% of normal individuals can have "abnormal" test results. To determine its clinical relevance, a test must be interpreted within the context of the clinical situation. Performing tests in patients with no risk for having the pathophysiologic process of interest can yield a high number of false-positive results. For example, a low potassium value (3.0 mg/dL) in an otherwise healthy individual is most likely a normal result. Interpreting this test as abnormal, and initiating treatment, could lead to harm without any benefit.

Risks and Costs versus Benefits

8 The ASA Statement on Routine Preoperative Laboratory and Diagnostic Screening (2008) states that preoperative tests, as a component of the preanesthesia evaluation, may be indicated for various purposes, including but not limited to (1) discovery or identification of a disease or disorder which may affect perioperative anesthetic care, (2) verification or assessment of an already known disease, disorder, and medical or alternative therapy which may affect perioperative anesthetic care, and (3) formulation of specific plans and alternatives for perioperative anesthetic care. No routine laboratory or diagnostic screening test is necessary for the preanesthetic evaluation of patients. Appropriate indications for ordering tests include the identification of specific clinical indicators or risk factors (e.g., age, preexisting disease, magnitude of the surgical procedure).

The use of medical testing is associated with significant cost, both in real dollars and in potential harm. Routine preoperative testing has been estimated to cost $3 billion annually. An "abnormal" test that is later determined to be a false result can lead to significant cost and real harm. For example, a positive exercise electrocardiographic stress test in a healthy 40-year-old woman may lead to coronary angiography. Coronary angiography is not a benign procedure and can lead to vascular injuries. On the basis of Bayesian analysis, a positive test result in this patient is most likely a false positive, and the test was inappropriately used. Therefore, the woman and her physician would gain no additional information, thousands of dollars in medical costs would accrue, and she may sustain morbidity.

Several studies have evaluated the implications of reduced testing. Golub et al.[76] retrospectively reviewed the records of 325 patients who had undergone preadmission testing prior to ambulatory surgery. Of these, 272 (84%) had at least one abnormal screening test result, while only 28 surgeries were delayed or canceled. The authors estimated that only three patients potentially benefited from preadmission testing, including a new diagnosis of diabetes in one and nonspecific ECG changes in two, one of whom had known ischemic heart disease.

In a study published in 1991, Narr et al.[77] at the Mayo Clinic demonstrated minimal benefits from routine testing and proposed that routine laboratory screening tests were not required in healthy patients. In a follow-up study published in 1997, a cohort of patients who had no preoperative testing during 1994 was reviewed and found to include no deaths or major perioperative morbidity.[78] The authors concluded that current anesthetic and medical practices rapidly identify indications for laboratory evaluation when necessary, and therefore routine testing was not indicated in this healthy cohort.

Even if testing better defines a disease state, the risks of any intervention based on the results may outweigh the benefit. Cardiovascular testing is a classic example. If a noninvasive test is positive, coronary angiography may be performed. A positive angiogram may then result in CABG prior to the planned noncardiac surgery. Although cardiovascular morbidity and mortality may be reduced in patients with significant CAD who have undergone coronary revascularization, the morbidity associated with both the testing and the revascularization procedure may be greater than any potential benefit. Roizen and Cohn[79] have suggested a protocol for screening tests based on the preoperative evaluation and proposed procedure using a risk–benefit analysis. The following protocol for laboratory testing is modified from their recommendations and the 2002 "ASA Practice Advisory for Preanesthetic Evaluation" (class C procedures are defined as highly invasive and commonly necessitate blood administration, invasive monitoring, and postoperative care in a critical care unit):

Recommended Laboratory Testing

Blood Count
- Neonates
- Physiologic age ≥75 years
- Malignancy
- Renal disease
- Anticoagulant use
- Bleeding/hematologic disorder
- Class C procedure

Coagulation Studies
- Chemotherapy
- Hepatic disease
- Bleeding disorder
- Anticoagulants

Electrolytes
- Renal disease
- Diabetes
- Diuretic, digoxin, or steroid use
- CNS disease
- Endocrine disorders

Blood Urea Nitrogen/Creatinine
- Physiologic age ≥75 years
- Cardiovascular disease
- Renal disease
- Diabetes
- Diuretic or digoxin use
- CNS disease
- Class C procedure

Blood Glucose
- Physiologic age ≥75 years
- Diabetes
- Steroid use
- CNS disease
- Class C procedure

Liver Function Tests
- Hepatic disease
- Hepatitis exposure
- Malnutrition

Chest X-Ray
- Cardiovascular disease
- Chronic obstructive pulmonary disease (COPD)
- Malignancy

ECG
- Physiologic age ≥75 years
- Cardiovascular disease
- Pulmonary disease
- Diabetes
- Digoxin use
- CNS disease
- Class C procedure

Pregnancy Test
- Possible pregnancy

Albumin
- Physiologic age ≥75 years
- Malnutrition
- Class C procedure

Type and Screen
- Physiologic age ≥75 years
- Hematologic disorder
- Coagulation abnormality
- Class C procedure

Complete Blood Count and Hemoglobin Concentration

A preoperative hemoglobin value has been suggested as the only test necessary in many patients prior to elective surgery; however, even this minimal standard has been questioned. Baron et al.[80] reviewed the records of 1,863 pediatric patients scheduled for elective outpatient procedures. In only 1.1% of patients was the hematocrit abnormal, and in none of these patients was the procedure canceled or the anesthetic plan modified. However, a baseline hematocrit is still indicated in any procedure with a risk of blood loss.

The standard regarding the lowest acceptable perioperative hematocrit and indication for a preoperative transfusion has changed during the past decade. The current recommendations of the National Blood Resource Education Committee are that a hemoglobin level of 7 g/dL is acceptable in patients without systemic disease. In patients with systemic disease, signs of inadequate systemic oxygen delivery (tachycardia, tachypnea) are an indication for transfusion.

Electrolytes, BUN/Creatinine

In the past, patients routinely received a chemistry panel prior to surgery. Because of technology issues, it may be cheaper to obtain a standard battery than to determine one particular test. However, testing rarely leads to any change in perioperative management.

There are numerous guidelines regarding the need for preoperative electrolytes. The only consensus is the lack of routine testing in asymptomatic adults, although a creatinine and glucose has been recommended in older patients. In patients with systemic diseases or on medications that affect the kidneys, electrolytes, BUN, and creatinine evaluation are indicated.

Coagulation Studies

Coagulation disorders can have significant impact on the surgical procedure and perioperative management. In patients with hemophilia or von Willebrand disease, abnormal laboratory studies even in the absence of clinical abnormalities require preoperative preparation of the patient. A prothrombin and partial thromboplastin time analysis is indicated in patients with a past history of prolonged bleeding following injuries or surgical procedures, as well as in patients with known or suspected liver disease, malabsorption, or malnutrition, and patients taking certain medications such as antibiotics and chemotherapeutic agents.

Pregnancy Testing

Routine pregnancy testing in women of childbearing potential is a subject of considerable debate. The rationale is that specific agents may be avoided, or surgery may be delayed. Information regarding the last menstrual period can help define the potential, but does not eliminate the possibility. A number of studies have evaluated the validity of history as a means of assessing pregnancy status in adolescents with conflicting results. Current practice varies dramatically among centers and among anesthesiologists and may be a function of the population served.

Chest X-rays

A preoperative chest x-ray can identify abnormalities that may lead to either delay or cancellation of the planned surgical procedure or modification of perioperative care. For example, identification of pneumonia, pulmonary edema, pulmonary nodules, or a mediastinal mass could all lead to modification of care. However, again, routine testing in the population without risk factors can lead to more harm than benefit. Roizen and Cohn[79] have demonstrated substantial harm from additional procedures based on an abnormal routine preoperative chest x-ray.

The American College of Physicians suggests that a chest x-ray is indicated in the presence of active chest disease or an intrathoracic procedure, but not on the basis of advanced age alone.[81] In a meta-analysis, Archer et al.[82] reviewed the published reports from 1966 to 1992 in the English, French, and Spanish literature. Twenty-one reports were identified with sufficient data to evaluate the use of testing. On average, abnormalities were reported in 10% of routine preoperative chest x-rays, of which only 1.3% were unexpected. These findings result in modification in management in only 0.1% of patients, with unknown influence on outcome. The authors estimated that each finding that influenced management would cost $23,000, concluding that routine chest x-rays without a clinical indication were not justified.

Pulmonary Function Tests

Consensus guidelines do not support routine use of pulmonary function studies to predict perioperative respiratory complications. Pulmonary function tests can be generally divided into two categories, spirometry and arterial blood gas. Spirometry can provide information on forced vital capacity (FVC), forced expiratory volume in 1 second (FEV_1), ratio of FEV_1/FVC, and average forced expiratory flow from 25% to 75% (FEF 25–75%). Although each of these measures has a sound physiologic basis, their practical assessment can vary greatly among healthy persons, and the tests rarely provide additional information beyond that obtained from history. For those patients considered for pulmonary resection, evaluation using spirometry, diffusion capacity measurements, radionucleotide lung perfusion scanning, and cardiopulmonary exercise testing may help to define those patients at high risk.[83]

With the availability of the pulse oximeter, the use of preoperative arterial blood gas sampling has become less important. It may still be indicated, since determining the baseline CO_2 is useful in managing postoperative ventilation settings and resting hypercapnia is associated with increased perioperative risk. One method of assessing the probability of CO_2 retention is evaluation of the serum bicarbonate. A normal serum bicarbonate will virtually exclude the diagnosis of chronic CO_2 retention.

SUMMARY OF THE PREOPERATIVE EVALUATION

There are multiple factors that are associated with increased perioperative risk, as discussed within this chapter. Clinical judgment is necessary and requires addressing the following fundamental questions:

1. Are the risk factors modifiable?
2. Will delaying the procedure add to perioperative risk or patient morbidity?
3. What interventions during the preoperative period can be implemented to reduce risk?
4. Has the patient been provided information regarding risk in order to make an informed decision?

An effective preoperative evaluation will address these concerns and recommend therapeutic interventions to limit risk. Finally, the anesthesiologist can play an important role in reducing inappropriate utilization of medical technology and in helping to coordinate the patient's care among the multiple physician specialties often required for patients with complex illnesses who require surgery.

9

PREPARATION FOR ANESTHESIA

Continuing Current Medications/ Treatment of Coexisting Diseases

It is the responsibility of the anesthesiologist to instruct patients regarding which medications to take and which to hold preoperatively. Occasionally, new medications will be prescribed or doses increased, such as steroids for adrenal insufficiency. Prescribed and over-the-counter mediations may affect the anesthetic, and anesthesiologists must be knowledgeable about their actions. As a general rule, patients may take their prescription medications with water on the day of surgery. Exceptions exist, particularly for the management of diabetes. See the section on Diabetes, Preoperative glucose management.

Beta-blockers

The role of beta-blockers during the perioperative period has evolved over the past decade based on clinical studies evaluating both effectiveness and the potential for risk. Historically, beta-blockers in this setting have been felt to reduce the incidence of mortality and nonfatal MI after surgery.[84] Current guidelines have recommended that beta-blockers be continued in those receiving beta-blockers to treat angina pectoris, symptomatic arrhythmias, and hypertension. Recent clinical studies, however, appear to support that decision for perioperative beta-blocker requires clinical judgment in evaluating the patient's risk factors for cardiovascular complications together with the type of surgery. The POISE trial, a large, multicenter, randomized controlled trial, compared preoperative beta-blocker therapy with placebo.[85] Patients receiving beta-blocker therapy had a lower risk of perioperative MI, but were at significantly *increased* risk for mortality and stroke. As potential mechanisms for the enhanced risk, perioperative hypotension and bradycardia were significantly increased in patients receiving beta-blocker. A meta-analysis evaluating perioperative beta-blockade in noncardiac surgery in 33 randomized, controlled trials with 12,306 patients found no difference in overall mortality, but decreased risk of perioperative MI.[86] Similar to the POISE trial, the risk of nonfatal stroke was increased with beta-blockade. Recognizing the previous referenced studies and others addressing the benefits and risks of perioperative beta-blocker therapy, national guidelines from the American College of Cardiology Foundation/American Heart Association (ACCF/AHA) have been updated.[87] The guidelines support, as a class I recommendation, the perioperative continuation of beta-blockers for patients receiving beta-blocker for appropriate conditions. They support the role for beta-blocker therapy *titrated to heart rate and blood pressure* for patients undergoing vascular procedures or intermediate-risk surgeries with CAD, cardiac ischemia identified by preoperative testing, or more than one high risk factor. The latter includes coronary heart disease, diabetes mellitus congestive heart failure, cerebrovascular disease, or renal insufficiency. Importantly, the ACCF/AHA guidelines stress the uncertainty for the role of beta-blockade for vascular or intermediate-risk surgery in patients with only one risk factor without ischemic heart disease or in patients without risk factors who have not taken beta-blocker therapy previously. On the basis of the results of the POISE trial, there appears increased potential for perioperative risk associated with fixed, high-dose beta-blocker therapy begun on the day of surgery. Perioperative titration of beta-blockade appears to offer a role in the reduction of risk for perioperative MI, but the optimal heart rate remains controversial.

Statins

Studies have shown that statins can reduce cardiovascular morbidity and mortality, have a lipid-lowering effect, enhance nitric-oxide–mediated pathways, reduce vascular inflammation, and have direct cardioprotective effects. There is a small risk of rhabdomyolysis with statin therapy.

Some have recommended these medications be given in the perioperative period for patients with coronary heart disease. Current guidelines recommend continuing statin therapy in the perioperative period for those already taking the medication. More studies are needed in regard to initiating statin therapy preoperatively in other patients. There is some evidence that this class of drugs may have benefit in those undergoing vascular surgery and in those with one clinical risk factor for myocardial ischemia about to undergo an intermediate-risk surgical procedure. If indeed statin therapy is effective preoperatively, the dose, timing of initiation of therapy, and length of therapy are yet to be determined.[88,89]

Prevention of Perioperative Pulmonary Aspiration

Many patients who present for anesthesia are considered to have an increased risk for aspiration. Extrapolating results from a study in monkeys led to the statement in 1974 that patients who had a 25 mL residual gastric volume of pH <2.5 were at risk. Using these guidelines in humans, some have estimated that 40% to 80% of patients scheduled for elective surgery may be at risk.[90,91] However, today, clinically significant pulmonary aspiration is very rare in healthy patients undergoing general anesthesia, quoted as occurring in 1 in 3,000 to 1 in 6,000 anesthetics. This increases to 1 in 600 for emergency anesthesia. Data presented on aspiration from the Australian Anaesthetic Incident Monitoring Study[92] found 133 cases of aspiration in 5,000 incidents reported. They rated the top 10 patient risk factors as shown in Table 22-12, although almost 25% of the patients had no risk factors. Errors in judgment, fault in airway management technique, and inadequate patient preparation were felt to be the most common factors contributing to the events.

ASA Fasting Guidelines

The ASA in 2011 published updated Practice Guidelines for Preoperative Fasting and Pharmacologic Intervention for the Prevention of Perioperative Aspiration.[93] The guidelines specifically deal with healthy patients of all ages scheduled for elective procedures where general anesthesia, regional anesthesia, or sedation will be administered. The purpose of the guidelines is to not only avoid prolonged fasting leading to dehydration, hypoglycemia, and patient dissatisfaction, but also avoid delaying procedures and potentially increasing the risk of pulmonary aspiration.

TABLE 22-12. TOP 10 FACTORS PREDISPOSING TO ASPIRATION

1	Emergency surgery
2	Inadequate anesthesia
3	Abdominal pathology
4	Obesity
5	Opioid medication
6	Neurologic deficit
7	Lithotomy
8	Difficult intubation/airway
9	Reflux
10	Hiatal hernia

Adapted from Kluger MT, Short TG. Aspiration during anaesthesia: A review of 133 cases from the Australian Anaesthetic Incident Monitoring Study (AIMS). *Anaesthesia.* 1999;54:19–26.

Recommendations for Clear Liquids: At Least 2 Hours

The primary support for the task force recommendations comes from a meta-analysis of randomized controlled trials comparing fasting times for clear liquids of 2 to 4 hours *versus* more than 4 hours. Adult patients fasting for 2 to 4 hours had *smaller* gastric volumes and higher gastric pH values compared to those fasting more than 4 hours. The differences in gastric volumes were equivocal in children. Therefore, the task force recommendations are unchanged for *healthy* patients. *Examples of clear liquids include, but are not limited to, water, fruit juices without pulp, carbonated beverages, clear tea, and black coffee (no alcohol).* They wrote that the type of liquid was more important than the volume.

Recommendations for Breast Milk: At Least 4 Hours

The fasting recommendations for breast milk are also unchanged, as the task force found only equivocal findings regarding gastric fluid volume and pH from observational studies in infants.[93]

Recommendations for Infant Formula, Nonhuman Milk, and Solids: At Least 6 Hours

Again, among the observational and randomized control studies, the task force found no evidence to support any change in the previous recommendations for at least a 6-hour fast before elective procedures.[93] They noted that the amount and type of food must be considered and recommended at least 8 hours before elective procedures for fried or fatty food that typically delays gastric emptying time.

For a summary of the fasting guidelines see Table 22-13.

Pharmacologic Agents to Reduce the Risk of Pulmonary Aspiration

Many different kinds of drugs have been used to decrease gastric fluid volume and increase the pH of gastric fluid in an effort to reduce the risk of aspiration pneumonitis: Histamine-2 receptor antagonists, proton pump inhibitors (PPIs), antacids, antiemetics, and gastrokinetic agents. The ASA Task Force reviewed the literature, as well as surveyed experts and ASA members to arrive at their 2011 recommendations for pharmacologic agents to reduce the risk of pulmonary aspiration. *They found uniformly that the literature is insufficient to evaluate or support the effect of administering any of the above classes of drugs on the perioperative incidence of emesis/reflux or pulmonary aspiration. Therefore, they could not recommend the routine preoperative use of such drugs for patients who have no apparent increased risk for pulmonary aspiration.*[93] However, the drugs were found to be effective for their intended use and are more cost effective when prescribed for patients with risk factors for pulmonary aspiration.

TABLE 22-13. SUMMARY OF FASTING RECOMMENDATIONS TO REDUCE THE RISK OF PULMONARY ASPIRATION

Ingested Material	Minimum Fasting Period, Applied to All Ages (h)
Clear liquids	2
Breast milk	4
Infant formula	6
Nonhuman milk	6

This summary applies only to healthy patients who are undergoing elective procedures and are not intended for women in labor. Following the guidelines does not guarantee complete gastric emptying. Examples of clear liquids are water, fruit juices without pulp, carbonated beverages, clear tea, and black coffee.
Adapted from Practice guidelines for preoperative fasting and the use of pharmacologic agents to reduce the risk of pulmonary aspiration: Application to healthy patients undergoing elective procedures: An updated report by the American Society of Anesthesiologists Committee on Standards and Practice Parameters. *Anesthesiology.* 2011;114:495–511.

Histamine-2 Receptor Antagonists

Meta-analyses of randomized, placebo-controlled trials support the efficacy of the H-2 receptor antagonists cimetidine, ranitidine, and famotidine in reducing gastric volume and acidity.[93] They block the ability of histamine to induce secretion of gastric fluid with a high hydrogen ion concentration. Multiple-dose regimens may be more effective in increasing gastric pH than a single dose before operation on the day of surgery.

CIMETIDINE. Cimetidine is usually administered in 150 to 300 mg doses orally or parenterally. Administration of 300 mg of cimetidine orally 1 to 1.5 hours before surgery has been shown to increase the gastric fluid pH above 2.5 in 80% of patients.[94,95] Cimetidine can be given intravenously for those unable to take oral medications. Cimetidine can cross the placenta, but adverse fetal effects are unproved. The gastric effects of cimetidine last as long as 3 or 4 hours, and therefore this drug is suitable for operations of that duration. Side effects of cimetidine include inhibition of the hepatic mixed-function oxidase enzyme system; therefore, it can prolong the half-life of many drugs, including diazepam, chlordiazepoxide, theophylline, propranolol, and lidocaine. The clinical significance of this after one or two preoperative doses of cimetidine is uncertain. Life-threatening cardiac dysrhythmias, hypotension, cardiac arrest, and central nervous system depression have been reported after cimetidine administration. These side effects may be especially likely to occur in critically ill patients after rapid intravenous administration. As discussed previously, cimetidine does not affect gastric fluid already present.

RANITIDINE. Ranitidine is more potent, specific, and longer acting than cimetidine. The usual oral dose is 150 mg. Ranitidine, 50 mg, given parenterally will decrease gastric fluid pH within 1 hour. It is as effective in reducing the number of patients at risk for gastric aspiration as cimetidine and produces fewer cardiovascular or central nervous system side effects. The effects of ranitidine last up to 9 hours. Thus, it may be superior to cimetidine at the conclusion of lengthy procedures in reducing the risk of aspiration pneumonitis during emergence from anesthesia and extubation of the trachea.

FAMOTIDINE. It is a third H-2 receptor blocker that has been given preoperatively to raise gastric fluid pH. Its pharmacokinetics are similar to those of cimetidine and ranitidine, with the exception of having a longer serum elimination half-life than the other two drugs. Famotidine in a dose of 40 mg orally 1.5 to 3 hours preoperatively has been shown to be effective in increasing gastric pH.

Antacids

Antacids are used to neutralize the acid in gastric contents. Randomized controlled trials demonstrate their effectiveness.[93] A single dose of antacid given 15 to 30 minutes before induction of anesthesia is almost 100% effective in increasing gastric fluid pH above 2.5. The nonparticulate antacid, 0.3 M sodium citrate, is commonly given before emergency operations. The nonparticulate antacids do not produce pulmonary damage themselves if aspiration should occur. Although colloid antacid suspension may be more effective than the nonparticulate antacids in increasing gastric fluid pH, aspiration of particulate antacids may cause significant and persistent pulmonary damage, such as pulmonary edema and arterial hypoxemia.

Withholding antacids because of concern about increasing gastric volume is not warranted, considering animal evidence documenting increased mortality after aspiration of low volumes of acidic gastric fluid (0.3 mL/kg, pH 1) compared with aspiration of large volumes of buffered gastric fluid (1 to 2 mL/kg, pH 1.8).[96] Complete mixing of the antacid with all gastric contents may be questionable in the immobile patient, and the effect of antacids on food particles within the stomach is unknown.

Proton Pump Inhibitors

PPIs suppress gastric acid secretion in a dose-dependent manner by binding to the proton pump of the parietal cell. Randomized controlled trials support their efficacy in reducing gastric volume and acidity.[93,97] For an adult patient, administering 40 mg of IV omeprazole 30 minutes before induction has been used. Oral doses of 40 to 80 mg must be given 2 to 4 hours before surgery to be effective. Effect on gastric pH may last as long as 24 hours.

Gastrokinetic Agents: Metoclopramide

Meta-analysis of randomized placebo-controlled trials support the efficacy of metoclopramide to reduce gastric volume and is equivocal regarding its effect on gastric acidity during the perioperative period.[93] Metoclopramide is a dopamine antagonist that stimulates upper gastrointestinal motility, increases gastroesophageal sphincter tone, and relaxes the pylorus and duodenum. It also has antiemetic properties. Metoclopramide speeds gastric emptying but has no known effect on acid secretion and gastric fluid pH. It may be administered orally or parenterally. A parenteral dose of 5 to 10 mg is usually given 15 to 30 minutes before induction. Administration intravenously over 3 to 5 minutes usually prevents the abdominal cramping that can occur from more rapid administration. An oral dose of 10 mg achieves onset within 30 to 60 minutes. The elimination half-life of metoclopramide is approximately 2 to 4 hours.

The clinical usefulness of the gastrokinetic agents is found in those patients who are likely to have large gastric fluid volumes, such as parturients, patients scheduled for emergency surgery, obese patients, trauma patients, and those with gastroparesis secondary to diabetes mellitus. However, it is not recommended for those patients diagnosed with bowel obstruction. The combination of metoclopramide with an H-2 receptor antagonist does not decrease the effect of either drug, and the effects may be additive.[93]

As reviewed above, the drugs used to decrease gastric fluid volume and acidity are effective and relatively free of side effects. The use of these agents is warranted in patients with decreased gastric emptying, reflux, and those presenting for emergency procedures. However, none of the drugs or combination of drugs is absolutely reliable in preventing the risk of aspiration in all patients all of the time. Therefore, their use does not eliminate the need for careful anesthetic techniques to protect the airway during induction, maintenance, and emergence from anesthesia.

PSYCHOLOGICAL/PHARMACOLOGICAL PREPARATION

Anesthetic management for patients begins with preoperative psychological preparation and, if necessary, preoperative medication. Specific pharmacologic actions should be kept in mind when these drugs are administered before operation, and they should be tailored to the needs of each patient. The anesthesiologist should assess the patient's mental and physical condition during the preoperative visit. Because it is actually the beginning of the anesthetic, choice of preoperative medication should be based on the same considerations as the choice of anesthesia, including considerations of the patient's medical problems, requirements of the surgery, and recovery goals. Satisfactory preoperative preparation and medication facilitate an uneventful perioperative course. Poor preparation may begin a series of problems and misadventures.

No consensus exists on the choice of preoperative medications, and historically their use was dominated by tradition. A significant decrease in preoperative sedation has been driven by the ever-increasing numbers of outpatient procedures performed. There is general agreement that most patients should enter the OR after anxiety has been relieved, and this should be accomplished without affecting patient safety or prolonging recovery time.

Preoperative medication involves not only sedation, but also physiologic preparation. The patient should be instructed regarding whether to take or withhold any prescribed medications on the day of surgery. It includes prescribing other mediations to prevent perioperative complications such as aspiration or allergic reactions in patients at risk.

Psychological Preparation

Psychological preparation of the patient involves preoperative visit and interview with the patient and family members. The anesthesiologist should explain anticipated events and the proposed anesthetic management in an effort to reduce anxiety and allay apprehension. Patients may perceive the day of surgery as the biggest, most threatening day in their lives; they do not wish to be treated impersonally in the OR. The anesthesiologist's first direct encounter with the patient may be in the immediate preoperative period. A growing number of patients receive their preanesthetic evaluations by others in preoperative evaluation clinics or just prior to surgery. Preoperative visits must be conducted efficiently, but they must also be informative and reassuring, answering all questions. Most of the anesthesiologist's time is spent with an unconscious or sedated patient; therefore, he/she must take time before the operation to earn the trust and confidence of that patient.

Most patients are anxious before surgery. Studies show that, depending on the intensity of inquiry, 40% to 85% of patients are apprehensive before surgery. Preoperative anxiety states are at a high level, and most patients expect apprehension to be relieved before they arrive in the OR. The classic study by Egbert et al.[98] showed that an average of 57% of patients felt anxious before operation. An informative and comforting preoperative visit may replace many milligrams of depressant medication. For example, the study by Egbert et al. showed that more patients were adequately prepared for surgery after a preoperative interview than after 2 mg/kg of pentobarbital given intramuscularly

TABLE 22-14. COMPARISON OF PREOPERATIVE VISIT (PERCENTAGE OF PATIENTS) AND PENTOBARBITAL (2 mg/kg IM)

	Felt Drowsy	Felt Nervous	Adequate Preparation
Control group	18	58	35
Pentobarbital group	30	61	48
Preoperative visit	26	40	65
Preoperative visit and pentobarbital	38	38	71

IM, intramuscularly.
Data from Egbert LD, Battit GE, Turndorf H, et al. The value of the preoperative visit by the anesthetist. *JAMA*. 1963;185:553.

1 hour before surgery (Table 22-14).[98] However, psychological preparation cannot accomplish everything and will not relieve all anxiety.

After the patient interview, the use of preoperative medication in selected patients serves to achieve amnesia or sedation, as well as provide any needed analgesia. Always remember that preoperative depressant drugs are not a substitute for a comforting and tactful preoperative visit.

Pharmacologic Preparation

The ideal drug or combination of drugs for preoperative pharmacologic preparation is as elusive as is the ideal anesthetic technique and is not based on a large body of data that is either definitive or persuasive. In selecting the appropriate drug and dose for preoperative medication, the patient's psychological condition, physical status, and age must be considered. The surgical procedure, expected duration, and whether it is an outpatient procedure are important factors as well. Finally, the anesthesiologist must know the patient's weight, prior response to depressant drugs, including unwanted side effects, and allergies.

The goals to be achieved for each patient with preoperative medication are intimately involved in the selection process. The desired goals may be multiple and should be tailored to the needs of each patient. Some of the goals, such as relief of anxiety and production of sedation, apply to almost every patient, whereas others, such as aspiration prophylaxis, are necessary only occasionally. Prophylaxis against allergic reactions, such as to latex, applies in only a few instances. Prevention of autonomic reflexes mediated through the vagus nerve or prevention of nausea may be better attempted immediately before the anticipated need.

Some patients should not receive depressant drugs before surgery. Those with little physiologic reserve, head injury, hypovolemia, or at the extremes of age may be harmed more than helped by many of the medications normally used before operation. In contrast, the conditions of others demand that attempts be made pharmacologically to reduce anxiety and provide analgesia or dry secretions in the airway to produce a safer perioperative course. For elective surgery, the anesthesiologist will, in most instances, want the patient to enter the OR free of anxiety and sedated, yet easily arousable and cooperative.

The timing and route of administration of the preoperative medications are important. Every attempt should be made to time the administration of the preoperative medications so that they achieve their full effect before the patient's arrival in the OR. As a general rule, oral tablets should be given to the patient 60 minutes before arrival in the OR. Intravenous agents, on the other hand, produce effects after a few circulation times. The drug(s), doses, route of administration, and effects should be recorded on the anesthetic record. A list of common preoperative medications is presented in Table 22-15.

TABLE 22-15. COMMON PREOPERATIVE MEDICATIONS, DOSES, AND ADMINISTRATION ROUTES

Medication	Administration Route	Dose
Lorazepam	Oral, IV	0.5–4 mg
Midazolam	IV	Titration of 1.0–2.5 mg doses
Fentanyl	IV	Titration of 25–50 μg doses
Morphine	IV	Titration of 1.0–2.5 mg doses
Meperidine	IV	Titration of 10–25 mg doses
Cimetidine	Oral, IV	150–300 mg
Ranitidine	Oral	50–200 mg
Metoclopramide	IV	5–10 mg
Atropine	IV	0.2–0.4 mg
Glycopyrrolate	IV	0.1–0.2 mg
Scopolamine	IV	0.1–0.4 mg

IV, intravenous.
Modified from Stoelting RK, Miller RD, eds. *Basics of Anesthesia*. New York: Churchill Livingstone; 1984.

TABLE 22-16. COMPARISON OF PHARMACOLOGIC VARIABLES OF BENZODIAZEPINES

	Diazepam	Lorazepam	Midazolam
Dose equivalent (mg)	10	1–2	3–5
Time to peak effect after oral dose (h)	1–1.5	2–4	0.5–1
Elimination half-time (h)	20–40	10–20	1–4
Clearance (mL/kg/min)	0.2–0.5	0.7–1.0	6.4–11.1
Volume of distribution (L/kg)	0.7–1.7	0.8–1.3	1.1–1.7

Adapted from Reves JG, Fragen RJ, Vinick HR, et al. Midazolam: Pharmacology and uses. *Anesthesiology.* 1985;62:310; Stoelting RK. *Pharmacology and Physiology in Anesthetic Practice.* Philadelphia, PA: JB Lippincott; 1987.

Benzodiazepines

Benzodiazepines are among the most popular drugs used for preoperative medication because they produce anxiolysis, amnesia, and sedation (Table 22-16). Because the site of action of benzodiazepines is located on the GABA receptor in the central nervous system (Fig. 22-4), there is relatively little depression of the ventilatory or cardiovascular systems with premedicant doses. Benzodiazepines have a wide therapeutic index and a low incidence of toxicity. Other than central nervous system depression, which can be of excessive duration especially with lorazepam, these drugs lack the side effects common to opioids, such as nausea and vomiting. Two caveats to keep in mind: These drugs are not analgesic agents, and benzodiazepines may not always produce a calming effect, but rarely can cause a paradoxical agitation, manifested as restlessness and delirium.

MIDAZOLAM. Midazolam has predominantly replaced the use of lorazepam and diazepam for preoperative medication and conscious sedation. It is common to administer sedative doses intravenously just prior to the trip to the OR. The physicochemical properties of the drug allow for its water solubility and rapid metabolism. As with other benzodiazepines, midazolam produces anxiolysis, sedation, and amnesia. It is 2 to 3 times as potent as diazepam because of its increased affinity for the benzodiazepine receptor. The usual dose is 1 to 2 mg titrated at a time intravenously. There is no irritation or phlebitis with injection of midazolam, as opposed to diazepam. The incidence of side effects after administration is low, although depression of ventilation and sedation may be greater than expected, especially in elderly patients or when the drug is combined with other central nervous system depressants. The onset after intravenous administration would be expected to occur after 1 to 2 minutes. In addition to quicker onset, more rapid recovery occurs after midazolam administration compared with diazepam. This more rapid onset is the result of the lipid solubility of midazolam and its rapid redistribution to the peripheral tissues and metabolic biotransformation. For these reasons, midazolam should usually be given within an hour of induction. Midazolam is metabolized by hepatic microsomal enzymes to essentially inactive hydroxylated metabolites. H-2 receptor antagonists do not interfere with its metabolism. The elimination half-life of midazolam is approximately 1 to 4 hours and may be extended in the elderly. Tests show that mental function usually returns to normal within 4 hours of administration, and amnesia may only last 20 to 30 minutes.[99] The properties of midazolam make it ideal for shorter procedures.

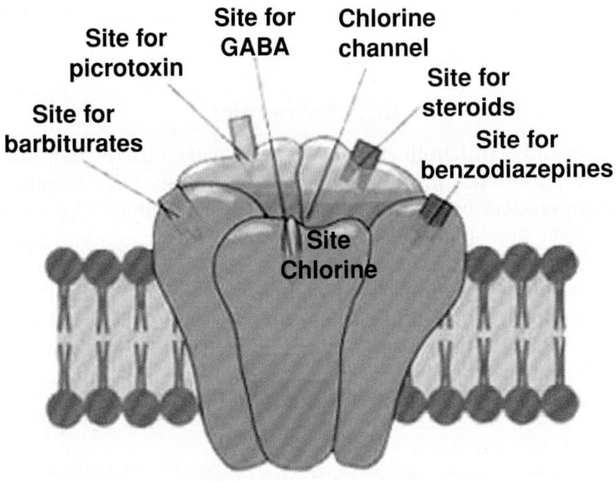

FIGURE 22-4. Schematic diagram of the benzodiazepine site on the GABA (γ-aminobutyric acid) receptor. (Reproduced with permission from Carlson N. *Foundations of Physiological Psychology.* 7th ed. Boston, MA: Pearson Education, Inc; 2007:115.)

LORAZEPAM AND DIAZEPAM. Lorazepam is 5 to 10 times as potent as diazepam and can produce profound amnesia, relief of anxiety, and sedation (Fig. 22-5).[100] Like diazepam, it has an extremely long half-life, but an even longer duration because of its affinity for the receptor.[101] Because of their duration, lorazepam and diazepam are not useful in instances in which rapid awakening is necessary, such as with outpatient anesthesia. Their use may be more suited for those patients already taking chronic benzodiazepines for anxiety and who may need the anxiolysis prior to arrival in the preoperative area.

Although lorazepam is insoluble in water and requires a solvent such as polyethylene glycol or propylene glycol, IV administration, unlike diazepam, is not associated with pain on injection or phlebitis. In addition to the intravenous route, lorazepam is reliably absorbed orally. Bradshaw et al.[102] demonstrated clinical effects 30 to 60 minutes after oral administration of lorazepam. Peak plasma concentrations may not occur until 2 to 4 hours after oral administration. Therefore, lorazepam must be ordered well before surgery so that the drug has time to be effective before the patient arrives in the OR. Lorazepam also may be given sublingually. The usual dose is about 25 to 50 μg/kg and should not exceed 4 mg.[100,101] With recommended doses, anterograde amnesia may

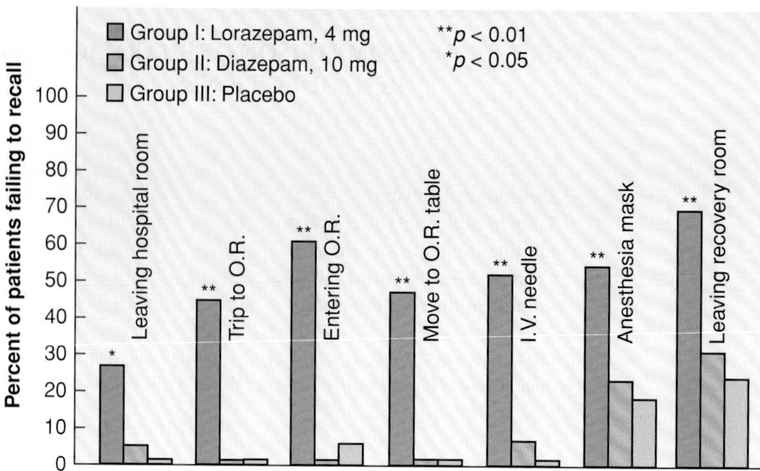

FIGURE 22-5. Percentage of patients in each group failing to recall specific events of the operative day. Medications were administered intramuscularly. O.R., operating room; I.V., intravenous. (Reprinted from Fragen RJ, Caldwell N. Lorazepam premedication: Lack of recall and relief of anxiety. *Anesth Analg.* 1976;55:792, with permission.)

be produced for as long as 4 to 6 hours without excessive sedation. Higher doses lead to prolonged and excessive sedation without more amnesia. There are no active metabolites of lorazepam; because its metabolism is not dependent on microsomal enzymes, there is less influence from age or liver disease. As with diazepam, little cardiorespiratory depression occurs with lorazepam.

Diphenhydramine

Diphenhydramine is a histamine-1 receptor antagonist, which blocks the peripheral effects of histamine. It also has sedative, anticholinergic, and antiemetic activity. A dose of 50 mg will last 3 to 6 hours in an adult. Diphenhydramine is not often used for preoperative sedation, but it is often used in combination with histamine-2 blockers and steroids for prophylaxis in patients with latex allergy, as well as for prophylaxis before chemotherapy and radiologic studies using contrast.

Opioids

Morphine and meperidine were historically the most frequently used opioids for intramuscular preoperative medication, during a time when the majority of patients were admitted the night before surgery. Currently, when analgesia is needed preoperatively, the administration of intravenous fentanyl with its rapid onset and shorter duration has become much more common. In a patient not experiencing pain, opioids may produce dysphoria. The opioids given in premedicant doses do not produce sedation or amnesia and are often combined with a benzodiazepine for these effects. Opioids are also useful to ameliorate the discomfort during regional anesthesia procedures or during the insertion of invasive monitoring catheters or large intravenous lines. The analgesic properties and respiratory depressant effects of opioids usually go hand in hand. The decrease in the carbon dioxide drive at the medullary respiratory center may be prolonged. Furthermore, there is a decrease in the responsiveness to hypoxia at the carotid body after injection of only low doses of opioids.[103] The anesthesiologist may wish to consider supplemental oxygen for the patient receiving opioid premedication. A common side effect of all opioids is nausea and vomiting, which are due to effects on the chemoreceptor trigger zone as well as the vestibular system.

Fentanyl is a synthetic opioid agonist structurally similar to meperidine. It is 75 to 125 times more potent than morphine in its analgesic characteristics. The lipid solubility of fentanyl is greater than that of morphine, which contributes to its rapid onset of action. Peak plasma concentrations occur within 6 to 7 minutes following intravenous administration and its elimination half-time is 3 to 6 hours. The drug's much shorter duration of action is attributed to redistribution to inactive tissues, such as the lungs, fat, and skeletal muscle. Metabolism occurs primarily by N-demethylation to norfentanyl, which is a less potent analgesic. In doses of 1 to 2 μg/kg intravenously, fentanyl may be used to provide preoperative analgesia. Fentanyl causes neither myocardial depression nor histamine release, but may be associated with ventilatory depression and profound bradycardia. Elderly and debilitated patients can be expected to have an increased sensitivity to its effects. Synergistic effects with benzodiazepines warrant close observation when this combination is given in the preoperative period.

Opioid-dependent Patients

Withdrawal produced by drug cessation is a preoperative issue in the patient who is taking methadone or is dependent on other opioids. There should be an attempt to maintain opioid use at the usual level by continuing methadone or substituting other appropriate agents for methadone. The anesthesiologist should be cautioned about using agonist–antagonist drugs in these patients in the preoperative period for fear of producing withdrawal.

Anticholinergics

Historically, anticholinergic drugs were widely used when inhalation anesthetics produced copious respiratory tract secretions and intraoperative bradycardia was a frequent danger. The advent of newer inhalation agents has markedly decreased the routine use of anticholinergic drugs for preoperative medication. Specific indications for an anticholinergic before surgery are (1) antisialagogue effect, (2) sedation and amnesia, and (3) vagolytic effect (Table 22-17). In the past, anticholinergics were also administered in an attempt to decrease gastric acid secretion, but research has shown them not to be effective for this purpose.[93]

Antisialagogue Effect

Anticholinergics have been prescribed in a selective fashion when drying of the upper airway is desirable. For example, when awake fiberoptic endotracheal intubation is a possibility or bronchoscopic exam is planned, the anesthesiologist will find the conditions more

TABLE 22-17. COMPARISON OF EFFECTS OF THREE ANTICHOLINERGIC DRUGS

	Atropine	Glycopyrrolate	Scopolamine
Increased heart rate	+++	++	+
Antisialagogue	+	++	+
Sedation	+	0	+++

0, no effect; +, small effect; + +, moderate effect; + + +, large effect.
Adapted from Stoelting RK. *Pharmacology and Physiology in Anesthetic Practice.* Philadelphia, PA: JB Lippincott; 1991.

satisfactory for visualization when an anticholinergic drug has been administered.[104] Anticholinergics are also felt to increase the effectiveness of topical anesthesia in the airway by preventing a dilutional effect from secretions and allowing contact of the local anesthetic with the mucosa. Surgeons may also request an antisialagogue for intraoral operations. Glycopyrrolate is the most potent antisialagogue, with less likelihood of increasing heart rate than atropine. Because glycopyrrolate is a quaternary amine, it does not easily cross the blood–brain barrier and does not produce sedation as seen with scopolamine, a tertiary amine.

Sedation and Amnesia

While midazolam has largely taken over as the preoperative sedative of choice, historically scopolamine was often given intramuscularly in combination with morphine. Scopolamine does not produce amnesia in all patients. It may not be as effective as lorazepam or diazepam in preventing recall. Scopolamine has an additive amnestic effect when combined with benzodiazepines. The study by Frumin et al.[105] showed that the combination of diazepam and scopolamine produced amnesia more often than did diazepam alone. The additive amnestic effect may be useful for the unstable patient who does not tolerate general anesthesia.

Vagolytic Action

Vagolytic action of the anticholinergic drugs is produced through the blockade of effects of acetylcholine on the sinoatrial node. Atropine given intravenously is more potent than glycopyrrolate in increasing heart rate. The vagolytic action of the anticholinergic drugs is useful in the prevention of reflex bradycardia that may result from traction on extraocular muscles or abdominal viscera, carotid sinus stimulation, or repeated doses of succinylcholine. As these bradycardic events occur in the OR, it is more effective to administer the drug during anesthesia.

Side Effects of Anticholinergic Drugs

CENTRAL NERVOUS SYSTEM TOXICITY. Scopolamine and atropine (tertiary amines) may cause central nervous system toxicity, the so-called central anticholinergic syndrome. This syndrome is most likely to occur after the administration of scopolamine, but can be seen after high doses of atropine. The symptoms of central nervous system toxicity resulting from anticholinergic drugs include delirium, restlessness, confusion, and obtundation. Elderly patients and patients with pain appear to be particularly susceptible, and the syndrome has been noted to be potentiated by inhalation anesthetics. The administration of 1 to 2 mg of physostigmine intravenously can successfully treat the syndrome.

INTRAOCULAR PRESSURE. Mydriasis and cycloplegia from anticholinergic drugs may place patients with glaucoma at risk for increased intraocular pressure. Atropine and glycopyrrolate may be less likely to increase intraocular pressure than scopolamine. In patients with glaucoma, most anesthesiologists feel safe in continuing medications for glaucoma up until the time of surgery and using atropine or glycopyrrolate when necessary.

HYPERTHERMIA. Sweat glands of the body are innervated by the sympathetic nervous system, but use cholinergic transmission. Therefore, administration of anticholinergic agents interferes with the sweating mechanism, which may cause body temperature to increase, especially when using active warming devices in the OR. The patient appears hot and dry. In children, one will typically find that the subsequent increase in temperature will drive the heart rate up further.

PSYCHOLOGICAL AND PHARMACOLOGIC PREPARATION FOR THE PEDIATRIC PATIENT

10 Compared with adults, preoperative preparation for children includes age-specific psychological preparation and an emphasis on oral medications when pharmacologic sedation is desired. What remains the same is the need to assess the needs of each child individually and to tailor the psychological preparation and preoperative medication accordingly.

Psychological Factors in Pediatric Patients

Hospital admission and major surgery can produce long-lasting psychological effects in some children. The hospital stay is stressful and full of apprehension for almost all children. The demeanor and communicative efforts of the anesthesiologist can make a difference to the child and family who are getting ready for a procedure under anesthesia.

Age is probably the most important aspect when psychological preparation of the pediatric patient is considered. A baby younger than 6 to 8 months of age is not emotionally upset when separated from his/her parent. Others in the health-care team can substitute very easily. Preoperative preparation in this age group is often directed toward educating and comforting the parents. However, toddler and preschool children are at an age when hospitalization may be the most upsetting and will become upset when separated from their parents or entering the OR. It is difficult to explain the forthcoming events to children in this age group. It is easier to communicate with patients from age 5 years to adolescence. The anesthesiologist can explain and offer reassurance about such issues as separation from parents and the home, OR events, and any of the patient's perceived fears of surgery and anesthesia. Adolescent patients may already be anxious and apprehensive. They may also be worried about loss of consciousness, have a fear of death, or be apprehensive about what they will do or say after preoperative sedation or during anesthesia. The more fearful child may be difficult to identify, but is usually the child who is quiet during the preoperative interview and appears nonchalant or even detached. If these patients can be identified before operation, they are often candidates for premedication.

For the previously mentioned reasons, a good preoperative visit and proper psychological preparation may be even more important in children than adults. The art of psychological preparation that is acquired by the anesthesiologist makes the preoperative visit a time of reassurance and explanation. It is an opportunity to connect with the child by becoming familiar with their favorite games, toys or cartoons, and to gain their trust. Most anesthesiologists will want to involve the parents when possible. Some hospitals have found brochures, motion pictures, and slide shows to be helpful in preparing pediatric patients for the OR but are not uniformly satisfactory. The child may want to bring a personal belonging, such as a stuffed animal or blanket, to the OR for security. When caring for any age child, but especially the toddler or preschooler, the most effective techniques are those using distraction, rather than reassurance. The school age child may wish to take an active role by doing such things as holding the face mask during inhalation induction of anesthesia. It may be helpful for a child with supportive parents to have them accompany the child to the OR after an explanation of events that may occur during induction. The emphasis is on support from the parent, rather than simply their presence.[106] It is common in some hospitals for a parent to go into the OR and stay until induction is complete.

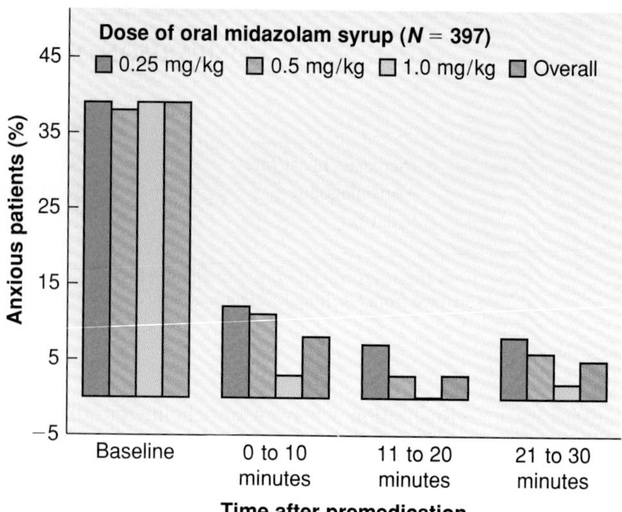

FIGURE 22-6. Percentage of patients exhibiting anxiety from baseline to time after oral midazolam. There was a positive association between dose and onset of anxiolysis ($p = 0.01$); a larger proportion of children achieved satisfactory anxiolysis within 10 minutes at the higher doses. (Reprinted from Coté CJ, Cohen IT, Suresh S, et al. A comparison of three doses of a commercially prepared oral midazolam syrup in children. *Anesth Analg.* 2002;94:37, with permission.)

Pharmacologic Preparation for Pediatric Patients

The discussion of pharmacologic preparation for the pediatric patient presumes proper psychological preparation, a satisfactory OR environment, and preparation for an efficient and timely induction of anesthesia. Premedication generally is not used before the infant has developed separation anxiety. In patients without IV access, oral premedication is useful to reduce apprehension, produce sedation and amnesia, and facilitate smooth induction of anesthesia when an inhalation method is planned. The use of preoperative medication is controversial in pediatric patients and may not be completely successful in as many as 20% of instances.[107] It has not been proved to reduce unwanted psychological outcome after surgery and anesthesia. Neither has it been shown that the uneventful induction of anesthesia is less likely to produce long-lasting psychological problems in children. There is emphasis on avoiding intramuscular injections in children, and the oral route is often preferred for preoperative medication.

Midazolam

Many different sedative–hypnotic drugs via different routes (oral, intranasal, intramuscular, and rectal) have been prescribed for children before operation. However, oral midazolam has become the most commonly used premedicant at a dose of 0.5 to 0.75 mg/kg (Fig. 22-6).[108,109] The cherry-flavored oral preparation is acceptable to most children, although it has a bitter aftertaste. It is effective in producing sedation and compliance, but not usually sleep, in about 15 minutes and lasts for 30 to 60 minutes. Intranasal midazolam is also very effective and has a faster onset, but has the disadvantage of causing nasal burning and bitter aftertaste. Using the concentrated parenteral formulation of midazolam (5 mg/mL), the usual intranasal dose is 0.2 to 0.3 mg/kg and it is administered most easily via a nasal atomizer.

Ketamine

Oral ketamine (5 to 10 mg/kg) has been prescribed 20 to 30 minutes before induction. Although often allowing smooth separation from parents, oral secretions and preoperative or postoperative delirium can be problems. Intramuscular ketamine (5 to 10 mg/kg) can be particularly helpful in the older or handicap patient who is extremely recalcitrant or combative. An antisialagogue is often used with ketamine to prevent copious secretions.

Both midazolam and ketamine, as well as barbiturates such as methohexital or pentobarbital, have been administered rectally to infant or toddler-age patients with success, although this has become increasingly rare.

Opioids

There is the occasional need for opioid premedication in children suffering from pain. When an IV catheter is not in place, transmucosal administration of fentanyl in the form of the Oral Transmucosal Fentanyl Citrate (OTFC) lollipop or the IV formulation (10 to 15 μg/kg) appears to be effective in producing sedation preoperatively, although the pharmacokinetics are highly variable.[110] Disadvantages of transmucosal fentanyl include a possible increase in gastric fluid volume and an increase in the incidence of rigidity, respiratory depression, pruritus, nausea, and vomiting. Fentanyl has also been administered by the intranasal route

(2 μg/kg), but again, postoperative nausea and vomiting, in addition to respiratory complications, have resulted in lack of enthusiasm for this technique.

For information on anesthesia for ambulatory surgery, see Chapter 30.

ANTIBIOTIC PROPHYLAXIS

Surgical antibiotic prophylaxis has become an outcome measure on which hospital and anesthesia performance are measured, and reimbursement or even accreditation may depend on properly timed and dosed administration. Anesthesiologists frequently administer antibiotics to patients prior to surgery for contaminated and clean-contaminated procedures, or for clean surgical procedures when infection would be catastrophic, such as for device implants. Other indications for the use of prophylactic antibiotics include the prevention of endocarditis and the prevention of infection in immunocompromised patients.

Cephalosporins are the most popular antibiotics because they cover skin microbes. For intestinal surgery anaerobic and Gram-negative coverage is needed. The National Surgical Infection Project recommends that antibiotics be administered within 1 hour prior to incision.[111] There are two exceptions to this policy: (1) Vancomycin should be given 2 hours prior to incision, and (2) when a tourniquet is used, the antibiotics should be administered prior to its inflation. Furthermore, if the surgical procedure is prolonged, it is recommended that the antibiotic be redosed when two half-lives have elapsed. For example, cefazolin has a half-life of 2 hours; therefore it should be redosed if the surgical procedure extends past 4 hours. Research on morbidly obese patients has shown that the dose required to achieve adequate tissue levels is twice that for normal weight patients.[112] Those allergic to penicillin, cephalosporins, and related compounds (beta-lactam allergy) may receive either vancomycin or clindamycin.

SUMMARY OF PATIENT PREPARATION

The anesthesiologist who takes the time to adequately prepare the patient medically and psychologically for anesthesia and surgery will find that their job of caring for the patient intraoperatively becomes easier, and they are more likely to have a positive outcome as well as a satisfied patient.

References

1. Takata MN, Benumof JL, Mazzei WJ. The preoperative evaluation form: Assessment of quality from one hundred thirty-eight institutions and recommendations for a high-quality form. *J Clin Anes.* 2001;13:345.
2. Apfel CC, Läärä E, Koivuranta M, et al. A simplified risk score for predicting postoperative nausea and vomiting. *Anesthesiology.* 1999;91:693.
3. Apfel CC, Korttila K, Abdalla M, et al. A factorial trial of six interventions for the prevention of postoperative nausea and vomiting. *N Engl J Med.* 2004;350:2441.
4. Mallampati RS, Gatt SP, Gugino LD, et al. A clinical sign to predict difficult tracheal intubation: A prospective study. *Can Anaesth Soc J.* 1985;32:429.
5. Frerk CM. Predicting difficult intubation. *Anaesthesia.* 1991;46:1005.
6. Savva D. Prediction of difficult tracheal intubation. *Br J Anaesth.* 1994;73:149.
7. Shah KB, Kleinman BS, Rao T, et al. Angina and other risk factors in patients with cardiac diseases undergoing noncardiac operations. *Anesth Analg.* 1990;70:240.
8. Wilson W, Taubert KA, Gewitz M, et al. Prevention of infective endocarditis: Guidelines from the American Heart Association: A Guideline from the American Heart Association Rheumatic Fever, Endocarditis, and Kawasaki Disease Committee, Council on Cardiovascular Disease in the Young, and the Council on Clinical Cardiology, Council on Cardiovascular Surgery and Anesthesia, and the Quality of Care and Outcomes Research Interdisciplinary Working Group. *Circulation.* 2007;116(15):1736–1754.
9. Bedford R, Feinstein B. Hospital admission blood pressure, a predictor for hypertension following endotracheal intubation. *Anesth Analg.* 1980;59:367.
10. Lee TH, Marcantonio ER, Mangione CM, et al. Derivation and prospective validation of a simple index for prediction of cardiac risk of major noncardiac surgery. *Circulation.* 1999;100:1043.
11. Goldman L, Caldera DL, Nussbaum SR, et al. Multifactorial index of cardiac risk in noncardiac surgical procedures. *N Engl J Med.* 1977;297:845.
12. Detsky A, Abrams H, McLaughlin J, et al. Predicting cardiac complications in patients undergoing non-cardiac surgery. *J Gen Intern Med.* 1986;1:211.
13. Tarhan S, Moffitt EA, Taylor WF, et al. Myocardial infarction after general anesthesia. *JAMA.* 1972;220:1451.
14. Rao TL, Jacobs KH, El-Etr AA. Reinfarction following anesthesia in patients with myocardial infarction. *Anesthesiology.* 1983;59:499.
15. Shah KB, Kleinman BS, Sami H, et al. Reevaluation of perioperative myocardial infarction in patients with prior myocardial infarction undergoing noncardiac operations. *Anesth Analg.* 1990;71:231.
16. Califf RM, Topol EJ, George BS, et al. One-year outcome after therapy with tissue plasminogen activator: Report from the thrombolysis and angioplasty in myocardial infarction trial. *Am Heart J.* 1990;119:777.
17. Rouleau JL, Talajic M, Sussex B, et al. Myocardial infarction patients in the 1990s—their risk factors, stratification and survival in Canada: The Canadian Assessment of Myocardial Infarction (CAMI) study. *J Am Coll Cardiol.* 1996; 27:1119.
18. Eagle K, Brundage B, Chaitman B, et al. Guidelines for perioperative cardiovascular evaluation of the noncardiac surgery. A report of the American Heart Association/American College of Cardiology Task Force on Assessment of Diagnostic and Therapeutic Cardiovascular Procedures. *Circulation.* 1996;93:1278.
19. Hertzer NR, Bevan EG, Young JR, et al. Coronary artery disease in peripheral vascular patients: A classification of 1000 coronary angiograms and results of surgical management. *Ann Surg.* 1984;199:223.
20. Kannel W, Abbott R: Incidence and prognosis of unrecognized myocardial infarction: An update on the Framingham study. *N Engl J Med.* 1984;311:1144.
21. Eagle KA, Coley CM, Newell JB, et al. Combining clinical and thallium data optimizes preoperative assessment of cardiac risk before major vascular surgery. *Ann Intern Med.* 1989;110:859.
22. Acharya DU, Shekhar YC, Aggarwal A, et al. Lack of pain during myocardial infarction in diabetics: Is autonomic dysfunction responsible? *Am J Cardiol.* 1991; 68:793.
23. Hollenberg M, Mangano DT, Browner WS, et al. Predictors of postoperative myocardial ischemia in patients undergoing noncardiac surgery. The study of perioperative ischemia research. *JAMA.* 1992;268:205.
24. Pringle SD, MacFarlane PW, McKillop JH, et al. Pathophysiologic assessment of left ventricular hypertrophy and strain in asymptomatic patients with essential hypertension. *J Am Coll Cardiol.* 1989;13:1377.
25. Sixth report of the Joint National Committee on Prevention, Detection, Evaluation, and Treatment of High Blood Pressure. *Arch Intern Med.* 1997;157:2413.
26. Goldman L, Caldera DL. Risks of general anesthesia and elective operation in the hypertensive patient. *Anesthesiology.* 1979;50:285.
27. Howell SJ, Sear JW, Foex P. Hypertension, hypertensive heart disease and perioperative cardiac risk. *Br J Anaesth.* 2004;92:570.
28. Wesker N, Klien M, Szendro G. The dilemma of immediate preoperative hypertension. *J Clin Anesth.* 2003;15:179.
29. Warner MA, Shields SE, Chute CG. Major morbidity and mortality within 1 month of ambulatory surgery and anesthesia. *JAMA.* 1993;270:1437.
30. Eagle KA, Rihal CS, Mickel MC, et al. Cardiac risk of noncardiac surgery: Influence of coronary disease and type of surgery in 3368 operations. CASS Investigators and University of Michigan Heart Care Program. *Circulation.* 1997;96: 1882.
31. Reilly DF, McNeely MJ, Doerner D, et al. Self-reported exercise tolerance and the risk of serious perioperative complications. *Arch Intern Med.* 1999;159:2185.
32. Fleisher LA, Beckman JA, Brown KA, et al. ACC/AHA 2007 guidelines on perioperative cardiovascular evaluation and care for noncardiac surgery: Executive summary. A report of the American College of Cardiology/American Heart Association Task Force on Practice Guidelines. *Circulation* 2007; 116:1971–1996.
33. Kalbfleisch JM, Shudaksharappa KS, Conrad LL, et al. Disappearance of the Q deflection following myocardial infarction. *Am Heart J.* 1968;76:193.
34. Gold BS, Young ML, Kinman JL, et al. The utility of preoperative electrocardiograms in the ambulatory surgical patient. *Arch Intern Med.* 1992;152:301.
35. Raby KE, Goldman L, Creager MA, et al. Correlation between perioperative ischemia and major cardiac events after peripheral vascular surgery. *N Engl J Med.* 1989;321:1296.
36. Mantha S, Roizen MF, Barnard J, et al. Relative effectiveness of four preoperative tests for predicting adverse cardiac outcomes after vascular surgery: A meta-analysis. *Anesth Analg.* 1994;79:422.
37. Shaw LJ, Eagle KA, Gersh BJ, et al. Meta-analysis of intravenous dipyridamole–thallium-201 imaging (1985 to 1994) and dobutamine echocardiography (1991 to 1994) for risk stratification before vascular surgery. *J Am Coll Cardiol.* 1996; 27:787.

38. Lavi R, Lavi S, Daghini E, et al. New frontiers in the evaluation of cardiac patients for noncardiac surgery. *Anesthesiology.* 2007;107:1018.
39. Caplan RA, Connis RT, Nickinovich DG, et al. Practice alert for the perioperative management of patients with coronary artery stents: A report by the American Society of Anesthesiologists Committee on Standards and Practice Parameters. *Anesthesiology.* 2009;110(1):22–23.
40. Dupuis JY, Labinaz M. Noncardiac surgery in patients with coronary artery stent: What should the anesthesiologist know? *Can J Anesth.* 2005;52:356.
41. Schouten O, Jeroen JB, Poldermans D. Management of patients with cardiac stents undergoing noncardiac surgery. *Curr Opin Anaesthesiol.* 2007;20:274–278.
42. Riddell JW, Chiche L, Plaud B, et al. Coronary stents and noncardiac surgery. *Circulation.* 2007;116:378.
43. Crossley GH, Poole JE, Rozner MA, et al. The Heart Rhythm Society (HRS)/ American Society of Anesthesiologists (ASA) expert consensus statement on the perioperative management of patients with implantable defibrillators, pacemakers and arrhythmia monitors: Facilities and patient management this document was developed as a joint project with the American Society of Anesthesiologists (ASA), and in collaboration with the American Heart Association (AHA), and the Society of Thoracic Surgeons (STS). *Heart Rhythm.* 2011;8(7):1114–1154.
44. Arozullah AM, Daley J, Henderson WG, et al. Multifactorial risk index for predicting postoperative respiratory failure in men after major noncardiac surgery. The National Veterans Administration Surgical Quality Improvement Program. *Ann Surg.* 2000;232(2):242–253.
45. Johnson RG, Arozullah AM, Neumayer L, et al. Multivariable predictors of postoperative respiratory failure after general and vascular surgery: Results from the patient safety in surgery study. *J Am Coll Surg.* 2007;204(6):1188–1198.
46. Qaseem A, Snow V, Fitterman N, et al. Risk assessment for and strategies to reduce perioperative pulmonary complications for patients undergoing noncardiothoracic surgery: A guideline from the American College of Physicians. *Ann Intern Med.* 2006;144(8):575–580.
47. Smetana GW. Preoperative pulmonary evaluation. *N Engl J Med.* 1999;340:937.
48. Arozullah AM, Khuri SF, Henderson WG, et al. Development and validation of a multifactorial risk index for predicting postoperative pneumonia after major noncardiac surgery. *Ann Intern Med.* 2001;135:847.
49. Smetana GW. Preoperative pulmonary evaluation: Identifying and reducing risks for pulmonary complications. *Clev Clin J Med.* 2006;73:3646.
50. Meyers JR, Lembeck L, O'Kane H, et al. Changes in functional residual capacity of the lung after operation. *Arch Surg.* 1975;110:576.
51. Dureuil B, Viires N, Cantineau JP, et al. Diaphragmatic contractility after upper abdominal surgery. *J Appl Physiol.* 1986;61:1775.
52. Fisher BW, Majumdar SR, McAlistar FA. Predicting pulmonary complications after nonthoracic surgery: A systematic review of blinded studies. *Am J Med.* 2002; 112:219.
53. Hall JC, Tarala RA, Hall JL. A case-control study of postoperative pulmonary complications after laparoscopic and open cholecystectomy. *J Laparoendosc Surg.* 1996;6:87.
54. Houston S, Hougland P, Anderson JJ, et al. Effectiveness of 0.12% chlorhexidine gluconate oral rinse in reducing prevalence of nosocomial pneumonia in patients undergoing heart surgery. *Am J Crit Care.* 2002;11(6):567–570.
55. Collard HR, Saint S, Matthay MA. Prevention of ventilator-associated pneumonia: An evidence-based systematic review. *Ann Intern Med.* 2003;138(6):494–501.
56. Kollef MH, Afessa B, Anzueto A, et al. Silver-coated endotracheal tubes and incidence of ventilator-associated pneumonia: The NASCENT randomized trial. *JAMA.* 2008;300(7):805–813.
57. Warner MA, Divertie MB, Tinker JH. Preoperative cessation of smoking and pulmonary complications in coronary artery bypass patients. *Anesthesiology.* 1984;60:609.
58. Rock P, Passannante A. Preoperative assessment: Pulmonary. *Anesthesiol Clin N Am.* 2002;22:77.
59. Paciullo CA, Short MR, Steinke DT, et al. Impact of nicotine replacement therapy on postoperative mortality following coronary artery bypass graft surgery. *Ann Pharmacother.* 2009;43(7):1197–1202.
60. Whyte MK, Choudry NB, Ind PW. Bronchial hyperresponsiveness in patients recovering from acute severe asthma. *Respir Med.* 1993;87:29.
61. Kabalin CS, Yarnold PR, Grammer LC. Low complication rate of corticosteroid-treated asthmatics undergoing surgical procedures. *Arch Intern Med.* 1995;155:1379.
62. Practice guidelines for the perioperative management of patients with obstructive sleep apnea (OSA): A report by the ASA Task Force. *Anesthesiology.* 2006; 104:1081.
63. Narayan KM, Boyle JP, Thompson TJ, et al. Lifetime risk for diabetes mellitus in the United States. *JAMA.* 2003;290:1884.
64. Coursin DB, Connery LE, Ketzler JT. Perioperative diabetic and hyperglycemic management issues. *Crit Care Med.* 2004;32(4 Suppl):S116.
65. Eagle KA, Berger PB, Calkins H, et al. ACC/AHA guideline update for perioperative cardiovascular evaluation for noncardiac surgery—executive summary a report of the American College of Cardiology/American Heart Association Task Force on Practice Guidelines (Committee to Update the 1996 Guidelines on Perioperative Cardiovascular Evaluation for Noncardiac Surgery). *Circulation.* 2002;105:1257.
66. Furnary AP, Wu Y: Clinical effects of hyperglycemia in the cardiac surgery population: The Portland Diabetic Project. *Endocr Pract.* 2006;12(Suppl 3):22.
67. McGirt MJ, Woodworth GF, Brooke BS, et al. Hyperglycemia independently increases the risk of perioperative stroke, myocardial infarction, and death after carotid endarterectomy. *Neurosurgery.* 2006;58:1066.
68. Blondet JJ, Beilman GJ: Glycemic control and prevention of perioperative infection. *Curr Opin Crit Care.* 2007;13:421.
69. Gandhi GY, Nuttall GA, Abel MD, et al. Intensive intraoperative insulin therapy versus conventional glucose management during cardiac surgery: A randomized trial. *Ann Intern Med.* 2007;146:233.
70. Gandhi GY, Murad MH, Flynn DN, et al. Effect of perioperative insulin infusion on surgical morbidity and mortality: Systematic review and meta-analysis of randomized trials. *Mayo Clin Proc.* 2008;83(4):418–430.
71. Joshi GP, Chung F, Vann MA, et al. Society for Ambulatory Anesthesia consensus statement on perioperative blood glucose management in diabetic patients undergoing ambulatory surgery. *Anesth Analg.* 2010;111(6):1378–1387.
72. Qaseem A, Humphrey LL, Chou R, et al. Use of intensive insulin therapy for the management of glycemic control in hospitalized patients: A clinical practice guideline from the American College of Physicians. *Ann Intern Med.* 2011; 154(4):260–267.
73. Furnary AP, Cheek DB, Holmes SC, et al. Achieving tight glycemic control in the operating room: Lessons learned from 12 years in the trenches of a paradigm shift in anesthetic care. *Semin Thorac Cardiovasc Surg.* 2006;18:339.
74. Robertshaw HJ, Hall GM. Diabetes mellitus: Anaesthetic management. *Anaesthesia.* 2006;61:1187.
75. Rhodes ET, Ferrari LR, Wolfsdorf JI, et al. Perioperative management of pediatric surgical patients with diabetes mellitus. *Anesth Analg.* 2005;101:986.
76. Golub R, Cantu R, Sorrento JJ, et al. Efficacy of preadmission testing in ambulatory surgical patients. *Am J Surg.* 1992;163:565.
77. Narr BJ, Hansen TR, Warner MA. Preoperative laboratory screening in healthy Mayo patients: Cost-effective elimination of tests and unchanged outcomes. *Mayo Clin Proc.* 1991;66:155.
78. Narr BJ, Warner ME, Schroeder DR, et al. Outcomes of patients with no laboratory assessment before anesthesia and a surgical procedure. *Mayo Clin Proc.* 1997; 72:505.
79. Roizen MF, Cohn S. Preoperative evaluation for elective surgery: What laboratory tests are needed? In: Stoelting RK, ed. *Advances in Anesthesia.* St Louis, MO: Mosby Year Book; 1993:25.
80. Baron MJ, Gunter J, White P. Is the pediatric preoperative hematocrit determination necessary? *South Med J.* 1992;85:1187.
81. Sox HCJ. *Common Diagnostic Tests: Use and Interpretation.* Philadelphia, PA: American College of Physicians; 1990.
82. Archer C, Levy AR, McGregor M. Value of routine preoperative chest x-rays: A meta-analysis. *Can J Anaesth.* 1993;40:1022.
83. Colice GL, Shafazand S, Griffin JP, et al. Physiologic evaluation of the patient with lung cancer being considered for resectional surgery: ACCP evidenced-based clinical practice guidelines (2nd edition). *Chest.* 2007;132(3 Suppl):161S–177S.
84. Feringa HH, Bax JJ, Poldermans D. Perioperative medical management of ischemic heart disease in patients undergoing noncardiac surgery. *Curr Opin Anaesth.* 2007;20:254.
85. Devereaux PJ, Yang H, Yusuf S, et al. Effects of extended-release metoprolol succinate in patients undergoing non-cardiac surgery (POISE trial): A randomised controlled trial. *Lancet.* 2008;371(9627):1839–1847.
86. Bangalore S, Wetterslev J, Pranesh S, et al. Perioperative beta blockers in patients having non-cardiac surgery: A meta-analysis. *Lancet.* 2008;372(9654):1962–1976.
87. Fleisher LA, Beckman JA, Brown KA, et al. 2009 ACCF/AHA focused update on perioperative beta blockade incorporated into the ACC/AHA 2007 guidelines on perioperative cardiovascular evaluation and care for noncardiac surgery. *J Am Coll Cardiol.* 2009;54(22):e13–e118.
88. Kersten JR, Fleisher LA. Statins: The next advance in cardioprotection? *Anesthesiology.* 2006;105:1079.
89. Hindler K, Shaw A, Samuels J, et al. Improved postoperative outcomes associated with preoperative statin therapy. *Anesthesiology.* 2006;105:1260.
90. Stoelting RK. Responses to atropine, glycopyrrolate and Riopan on gastric fluid pH and volume in adult patients. *Anesthesiology.* 1978;48:367.
91. Manchikanti L, Roush JR. The effect of preanesthetic glycopyrrolate and cimetidine in gastric fluid pH and volume in outpatients. *Anesth Analg.* 1984;63:40.
92. Kluger MT, Short TG. Aspiration during anaesthesia: A review of 133 cases from the Australian Anaesthetic Incident Monitoring Study (AIMS). *Anaesthesia.* 1999;54:19–26.
93. American Society of Anesthesiologists Committee. Practice guidelines for preoperative fasting and the use of pharmacologic agents to reduce the risk of pulmonary aspiration: Application to healthy patients undergoing elective procedures: An updated report by the American Society of Anesthesiologists Committee on Standards and Practice Parameters. *Anesthesiology.* 2011;114:495–511.
94. Stoelting RK. Gastric fluid pH in patients receiving cimetidine. *Anesth Analg.* 1978;57:675.
95. Maliniak K, Vahil AH. Pre-anesthetic cimetidine and gastric pH. *Anesth Analg.* 1979;58:309.

96. James CF, Modell JH, Gibbs CP, et al. Pulmonary aspiration: Effects of volume and pH in the rat. *Anesth Analg.* 1984;63:665.
97. Haskins DA, Jahr JS, Texidor M, et al. Single-dose oral omeprazole for reduction of gastric residual acidity in adults for outpatient surgery. *Acta Anaesthesiol Scand.* 1992;36:513.
98. Egbert LD, Battit GE, Turndorf H, et al. The value of the preoperative visit by the anesthetist. *JAMA.* 1963;185:553.
99. Reves JG, Fragen RJ, Vinick HR, et al. Midazolam: Pharmacology and uses. *Anesthesiology.* 1985;62:310.
100. Fragen RJ, Caldwell N. Lorazepam premedication: Lack of recall and relief of anxiety. *Anesth Analg.* 1976;55:792.
101. White PF. Pharmacologic and clinical aspects of preoperative medication. *Anesth Analg.* 1986;65:963.
102. Bradshaw EG, Ali AA, Mulley BA, et al. Plasma concentrations and clinical effects of lorazepam after oral administration. *Br J Anaesth.* 1981;53:517.
103. Weil JV, McCullough RE, Kline JS. Diminished ventilatory response to hypoxia and hypercapnia after morphine in man. *N Engl J Med.* 1975;292:1103.
104. Falick YS, Smiler BG. Is anticholinergic premedication necessary? *Anesthesiology.* 1975;43:472.
105. Frumin MJ, Herekar VR, Jarvik ME. Amnesic actions of diazepam and scopolamine in man. *Anesthesiology.* 1976;45:406.
106. Vetter TR. The epidemiology and selective identification of children at risk for preoperative anxiety reactions. *Anesth Analg.* 1993;77:96.
107. Kain ZN, MacLaren J, McClain BC, et al. Effects of age and emotionality on the effectiveness of midazolam administered preoperatively to children. *Anesthesiology.* 2007;107:545.
108. Weldon BC, Watcha MF, White PF. Oral midazolam in children: Effect of time and adjunctive therapy. *Anesth Analg.* 1992;75:51.
109. Coté CJ, Cohen IT, Suresh S, et al. A comparison of three doses of a commercially prepared oral midazolam syrup in children. *Anesth Analg.* 2002;94:37.
110. Wheeler M, Birmingham PK, Lugo RA, et al. The pharmacokinetics of the intravenous formulation of fentanyl citrate administered orally in children undergoing general anesthesia. *Anesth Analg.* 2004;99(5):1347–1351.
111. Bratzler DW, Houck PM. Antimicrobial prophylaxis for surgery: An advisory statement from the National Surgical Infection Prevention Project. *Am J Surg.* 2005;189:395.
112. Gorden SM. Antibiotic prophylaxis against postoperative wound infections. *Cleve Clin J Med.* 2006;73:S42–S45.

CHAPTER

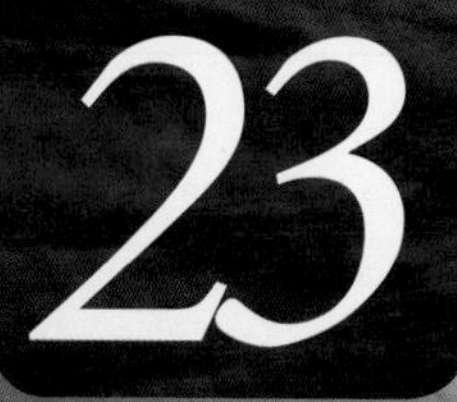

Rare Coexisting Diseases

STEPHEN F. DIERDORF • J. SCOTT WALTON • ANDREW F. STASIC

KeyPoints

1. The cytoskeleton of the muscle membrane in patients with muscular dystrophy is abnormal and susceptible to damage. Massive release of intracellular contents, including potassium, may occur after exposure to succinylcholine or halogenated, inhaled anesthetics.
2. Myotonic dystrophy produces cardiac conduction delay that can manifest as high-grade atrioventricular block.
3. Patients with myasthenia gravis are exquisitely sensitive to nondepolarizing muscle relaxants. Short-acting muscle relaxants and objective monitoring of neuromuscular function are indicated.
4. Many types of cancer, in addition to small cell cancer of the lung, can produce myasthenic syndrome.
5. Patients with multiple sclerosis should be advised that an exacerbation of their neurologic symptoms may occur during the perioperative period.
6. An unexpected increase in end-tidal carbon dioxide is the most sensitive sign of malignant hyperthermia.
7. Hypoglycemia and metabolic acidosis are a constant risk in patients with glycogen storage diseases.
8. Repeated episodes of sickling in patients with sickle cell disease cause pulmonary hypertension. Patients with sickle cell disease and pulmonary hypertension have increased perioperative mortality.
9. Rheumatoid arthritis is a multisystem disease that causes subclinical cardiac and pulmonary dysfunction.
10. Patients with rheumatoid arthritis can have significant degeneration of the cervical spine with few neurologic symptoms. Cervical manipulation during laryngoscopy and tracheal intubation requires special precautions.
11. Esophageal dysfunction in patients with scleroderma or dermatomyositis increases the risk of aspiration pneumonitis.
12. Patients with epidermolysis bullosa can have undiagnosed dilated cardiomyopathy.

Multimedia

1. Duchenne Muscular Dystrophy
2. Dantrolene Mixing
3. Removing Anesthetics from the Breathing Circuit
4. Raynauds
5. Scleroderma
6. Epidermolysis Bullosa
7. Pemphigus

Rare disorders may influence the conduct of anesthesia. Although the anesthesiologist may encounter such diseases only on rare occasions, he/she must recognize potential interactions between the disease and anesthesia. Advances in molecular medicine continue to clarify disease mechanisms and provide the basis for new therapies.

MUSCULOSKELETAL DISEASES

The cytoskeleton of the muscle membrane protects the integrity of the membrane and is composed of proteins such as dystrophin, merosin, utrophin, syntrophin, dystrobrevin, and sarcoglycans (Fig. 23-1). Insufficient quantities of normal proteins or the presence of abnormal proteins may weaken the membrane and make it more susceptible to damage.

Muscular Dystrophy

The muscular dystrophies are diseases associated with abnormalities of the muscle membrane and are characterized by progressive loss of skeletal muscle function (Table 23-1) (Fig. 23-2).[1] Dysfunctions of cardiac and smooth muscle are less evident but contribute significantly to morbidity and mortality.

TABLE 23-1. TYPES OF MUSCULAR DYSTROPHY

Duchenne
Becker
Emery–Dreifuss
Limb-girdle
Facioscapulohumeral
Oculopharyngeal
Congenital muscular dystrophy

Duchenne Muscular Dystrophy

Duchenne muscular dystrophy (DMD) is caused by the absence of dystrophin, a major component of the muscle membrane cytoskeleton. DMD is a sex-linked recessive trait most evident in boys and is characterized by painless degeneration and atrophy of skeletal muscle. Muscle weakness produces symptoms between the ages of 2 and 5 years and significant limitation by 12 years of age. Kyphoscoliosis may require surgical intervention for stabilization. Death is usually secondary to congestive heart failure or pneumonia. Aggressive treatment of cardiopulmonary dysfunction; however, has improved survival for many patients until the fourth decade of life. Serum creatine kinase levels parallel the course of the disease. In the patient's early years of life, the creatine kinase level is increased. Later, as significant amounts of muscle have degenerated, creatine kinase levels decrease.

Degeneration of cardiac muscle is evidenced by a progressive decrease in R-wave amplitude in the lateral precordial leads of the electrocardiogram. Serial echocardiograms provide important information about cardiac function. Loss of myocardial tissue results in cardiomyopathy, ventricular dysrhythmias, and mitral regurgitation. Treatment of cardiac dysfunction includes angiotensin-converting enzyme (ACE) inhibitors, β-adrenergic blockers, and dysrhythmia surveillance.[2]

Ineffective cough caused by diminished muscle strength results in retention of pulmonary secretions and pneumonia. Smooth muscle involvement causes intestinal hypomotility, gastroparesis, and delayed gastric emptying.

Although the genetic defect that causes DMD is known, specific gene therapy remains elusive. Current treatment is supportive and directed at improvement of cardiorespiratory function.

Becker Muscular Dystrophy

Dystrophin is present in patients with Becker muscular dystrophy (BMD) but is reduced in amount. The clinical course with respect to skeletal muscle function is milder in BMD patients when compared to patients with DMD. Cardiac involvement is, however, more prevalent in patients with BMD. Patients with BMD may also have epilepsy, macroglossia, and color blindness.[3] Female carriers of both DMD and BMD may also have cardiac abnormalities.

Emery–Dreifuss Muscular Dystrophy

Emery–Dreifuss muscular dystrophy is characterized by contractures of the elbow, ankles, spine, and humeropectoral weakness.

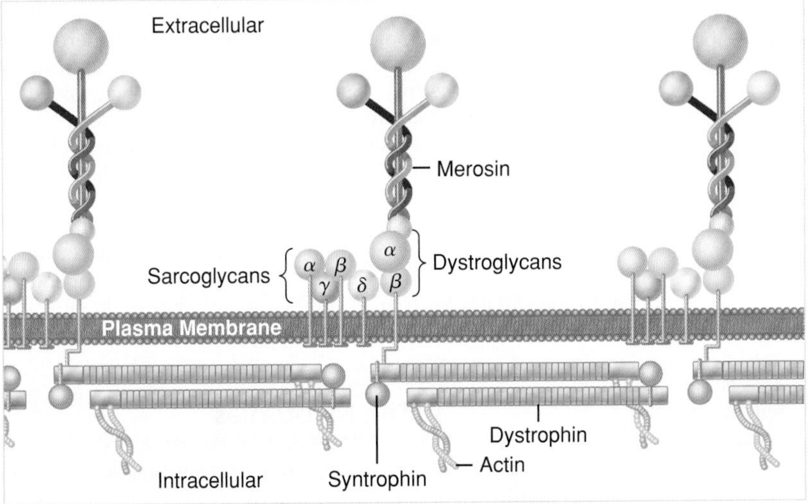

FIGURE 23-1. Muscle cell cytoskeleton. (Reprinted from: Duggan DJ, Gorospe JR, Fanin M, et al. Mutations in the sarcoglycan genes in patients with myopathy. *N Engl J Med.* 1997;336:618–624, with permission.)

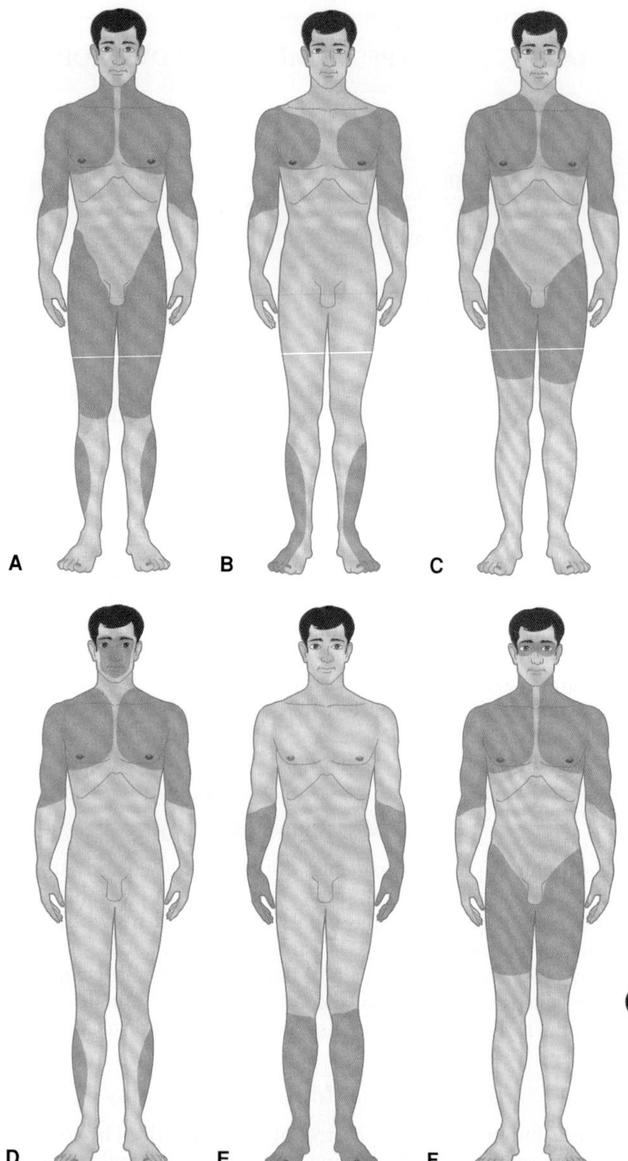

FIGURE 23-2. Distribution of predominant muscle weakness in different types of muscular dystrophy. **(A)** Duchenne-type and Becker-type. **(B)** Emery–Dreifuss. **(C)** Limb-girdle. **(D)** Facioscapulohumeral. **(E)** Distal. **(F)** Oculopharyngeal. (Reproduced from: BMJ Publishing Group. Emery AE. The muscular dystrophies. *BMJ.* 1998;317: 991–995.)

The skeletal muscle manifestations are usually mild, whereas cardiac conduction defects can be fatal. Implantable defibrillating cardiac pacemakers are often indicated.

Limb-girdle Muscular Dystrophy

Patients with limb-girdle muscular dystrophy exhibit weakness of the shoulder and pelvic girdles. Numerous genetic defects have been discovered that cause abnormalities in different muscle membrane proteins (e.g., calpain-3, dysferlin, and sarcoglycans). Cardiomyopathy and atrioventricular conduction defects can occur.

Facioscapulohumeral Muscular Dystrophy

Patients with this disease have diverse clinical manifestations such as weakness of the facial, scapulohumeral, anterior tibial, and pelvic girdle muscles. Associated abnormalities include retinal vascular disease, deafness, and neurologic dysfunction. Cardiac conduction defects and dysrhythmias may occur.

Oculopharyngeal Muscular Dystrophy

Oculopharyngeal muscular dystrophy (OPMD) presents in late adulthood with ptosis and dysphagia. Dysphagia is secondary to pharyngeal and esophageal muscle weakness. Weakness of the head, neck, and arms may also occur. Patients often require levator resection for ptosis or cricopharyngeal myotomy for dysphagia. Reported anesthesia experience for patients with OPMD is limited. Onset time for non-depolarizing muscle relaxants may be delayed although recovery appears to be normal.[4]

Congenital Muscular Dystrophy

Congenital muscular dystrophy is characterized by early onset (infancy) of hypotonia, developmental delay, feeding difficulties, and respiratory dysfunction. Included in this group of muscular dystrophies are merosin-deficient muscular dystrophy, Walker–Warburg syndrome, Ulrich disease, muscle–eye–brain disease, rigid spine muscular dystrophy, central core disease, myotubular dystrophy, and nemaline myopathy. Although respiratory dysfunction can be severe, cardiac involvement is not as prominent as in other muscular dystrophies.

Management of Anesthesia

The significant complications from anesthesia in patients with muscular dystrophy are secondary to the effects of anesthetic drugs on myocardial and skeletal muscle.[5] There are numerous case reports of rhabdomyolysis and/or cardiac arrest during
1 general anesthesia in patients with DMD and BMD. These cases are associated with rhabdomyolysis and hyperkalemia and have occurred with volatile anesthetics alone or in combination with succinylcholine. Halogenated volatile anesthetics may release intracellular calcium, damage the muscle membrane, and cause rhabdomyolysis. These rhabdomyolytic episodes (anesthesia-induced rhabdomyolysis [AIR]) are unpredictable and may depend upon the state of the muscle degeneration and regeneration that is occurring in the patient. The use of volatile anesthetics in patients with muscular dystrophy is controversial.[6] Although the rhabdomyolysis may resemble malignant hyperthermia, it is doubtful that muscular dystrophy patients are more prone to malignant hyperthermia.[7] Succinylcholine should be avoided in patients with muscular dystrophy and close monitoring for evidence of rhabdomyolysis during the perioperative period should be performed. Patients with muscular dystrophy may have a prolonged recovery from non-depolarizing muscle relaxants.

Degeneration of gastrointestinal smooth muscle with hypomotility of the intestine and delayed gastric emptying in conjunction with impaired swallowing increases the risk of perioperative aspiration of gastric contents. Vigorous respiratory therapy and mechanical ventilation may be required after surgery.

The Myotonias

Myotonia is the delayed relaxation of skeletal muscle after voluntary contraction. Electromyography demonstrates repetitive

TABLE 23-2. CLASSIFICATION OF MYOTONIC DYSTROPHY

Myotonic Dystrophy Type 1
Congenital
Childhood-onset
Adult-onset
Late-onset
Myotonic Dystrophy Type 2
Proximal myotonic dystrophy
Proximal myotonic myopathy
Proximal myotonic myopathy syndrome

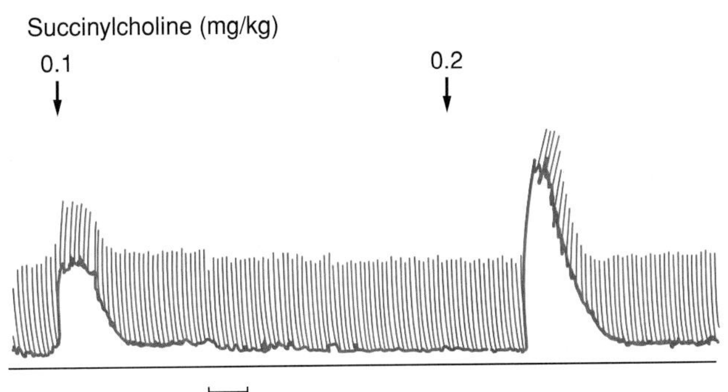

FIGURE 23-3. Administration of low doses of succinylcholine to a patient with myotonic dystrophy produces an exaggerated contraction of skeletal muscle. (Reprinted from: Mitchell MM, Ali HH, Savarese JJ. Myotonia and neuromuscular blocking drugs. *Anesthesiology.* 1978;49:44–48, with permission).

muscle fiber discharges that fluctuate. These abnormalities are caused by dysfunction of ion channels in the muscle membrane. There are two types of myotonic dystrophy caused by mutations in two distinct gene loci: Myotonic dystrophy type 1 and myotonic dystrophy type 2. The genetic alteration in type 1 is an unstable trinucleotide expansion (CTG) on chromosome 19q. Type 2 is caused by a quadnucleotide expansion (CCTG) on chromosome 3q. Both mutations produce RNA toxicity.

Myotonic dystrophy type 1 is the more common form and is subdivided by age of onset (Table 23-2). Type 1 is a multisystem disease that affects the musculoskeletal system, the heart, the respiratory system, central nervous system, and endocrine system.[8] Muscle weakness begins distally and progresses to proximal muscles and muscle wasting occurs over time. Pulmonary function studies demonstrate a restrictive pattern, mild arterial hypoxemia, and diminished ventilatory responses to hypoxia and hypercapnia. Respiratory muscle weakness diminishes the effectiveness of cough and may lead to pneumonia. Aspiration of gastric contents may occur because of gastric atony and pharyngeal muscle dysfunction. Myotonia of the respiratory muscles can produce intense dyspnea.

Cardiac manifestations include atrioventricular (AV) conduc-
2 tion delay, atrial tachydysrhythmias, diastolic dysfunction, cardiomyopathy, and mitral valve prolapse. Sudden death may be secondary to third degree atrioventricular block or ventricular dysrhythmias. Echocardiography may reveal subclinical evidence of left ventricular systolic and diastolic function.[9]

Other clinical features include cataracts, premature balding, diabetes mellitus, thyroid dysfunction, adrenal insufficiency, and gonadal atrophy. Pregnancy often produces an exacerbation of myotonic dystrophy and congestive heart failure is more likely to occur during pregnancy. Cesarean section is often required because of uterine smooth muscle dysfunction. Infants of mothers with myotonic dystrophy may develop congenital myotonic dystrophy that features hypotonia, feeding difficulty, and respiratory failure.

Until specific molecular therapies are available, treatment is directed at symptom management, such as pacemaker implantation for cardiac dysrhythmias or surgery for cataracts or gallbladder dysfunction.

Management of Anesthesia

Patients with type 1 myotonic dystrophy have far more perioperative complications than patients with type 2 myotonic dystrophy.[10,11] Considerations for anesthesia for patients with myotonic dystrophy include the presence of cardiac and respiratory muscle disease and abnormal responses to drugs used during anesthesia. Succinylcholine produces an exaggerated contracture and its use should be avoided (Fig. 23-3). The myotonic response to succinylcholine can be so severe that ventilation and tracheal intubation are difficult. Most patients with type 1 myotonic dystrophy develop a chronic myopathy and the response to nondepolarizing muscle relaxants may be enhanced. Reversal with neostigmine may provoke myotonia. The response to a peripheral nerve stimulator must be carefully evaluated because muscle stimulation may produce myotonia that could be misinterpreted as sustained tetanus when significant neuromuscular blockade still exists. Reversal of rocuronium with sugammadex would be an attractive alternative.

Patients with myotonic dystrophy are sensitive to the respiratory depressant effects of opioids, barbiturates, benzodiazepines, and inhaled anesthetics. Respiratory complications are more likely to occur in the early postoperative period after upper abdominal surgery or in those patients in whom preoperative upper extremity weakness was evident.[12]

No specific anesthetic technique has been shown to be superior for patients with myotonic dystrophy. Carefully controlled propofol infusions have been used successfully. Inhaled anesthetics may be used but close monitoring of cardiac rhythm and function is indicated. Postoperative mechanical ventilation should be employed until muscle strength and function return.[13] Regional anesthesia has been described for both children and adults with myotonic dystrophy.[14]

Skeletal muscle weakness and myotonia are exacerbated during pregnancy. Labor is typically prolonged and there is an increased incidence of postpartum hemorrhage from placenta accreta. Spinal and epidural anesthesia have been successfully used for pregnant patients.

Familial Periodic Paralysis

The familial periodic paralyses are a subgroup of diseases referred to as the hereditary skeletal muscle ion channelopathies. This group of diseases includes hyperkalemic and hypokalemic periodic paralysis, myotonia congenita, paramyotonia congenita, and the sodium channel myotonias. Alterations in the sodium, potassium, and calcium channels result in muscle membrane inexcitability and weakness.[15]

TABLE 23-3. CLINICAL FEATURES OF FAMILIAL PERIODIC PARALYSIS

Hypokalemic
Calcium channel defect
Potassium level <3 mEq/L during symptoms
Precipitating factors
- High glucose meals
- Strenuous exercise
- Glucose–insulin infusions
- Stress
- Hypothermia

Chronic myopathy with aging

Hyperkalemic
Sodium channel defect
Potassium level >5.5 mEq/L during symptoms
Precipitating factors
- Rest after exercise
- Potassium infusions
- Metabolic acidosis
- Hypothermia

Skeletal muscle weakness may be localized to tongue and eyelids

Hyperkalemic Periodic Paralysis

Hyperkalemic periodic paralysis is characterized by episodes of myotonia and muscle weakness that may last for several hours. Weakness can occur during rest after strenuous exercise, infusion of potassium, metabolic acidosis, or hypothermia (Table 23-3). The hyperkalemia is transient and occurs only at the time of weakness. Acute attacks can be fatal because of cardiac dysrhythmias or respiratory failure. A chronic myopathy frequently develops in older patients. Treatment consists of a low potassium diet and the administration of thiazide diuretics.

Hypokalemic Periodic Paralysis

Hypokalemic periodic paralysis is caused by a mutation in two skeletal muscle membrane cation channels. Paralysis can be produced by a decrease in serum potassium levels caused by strenuous exercise, infusion of glucose and insulin, or ingestion of carbohydrates and sodium rich food. Paralysis usually affects the limbs and trunk, but spares the diaphragm. Chronic muscle weakness occurs in most patients as they age.

Thyrotoxic hypokalemic periodic paralysis occurs with thyrotoxicosis in combination with hypokalemia. There is only rarely a family history and presentation is generally later in life. Treatment is directed at treatment of the hyperthyroidism.[16]

Management of Anesthesia

The primary goal with both forms of familial periodic paralysis is maintenance of normal potassium levels and avoidance of events that precipitate weakness. Any electrolyte abnormality should be corrected prior to surgery. These patients may be sensitive to nondepolarizing muscle relaxants, and short-acting muscle relaxants are preferred. Succinylcholine is best avoided as its administration may alter potassium levels. Metabolic changes (acidosis and alkalosis) or medications (glucose and insulin, diuretics) that reduce potassium levels may cause weakness or paralysis. Because changes in potassium levels precede the onset of weakness, serial measurement of potassium levels during prolonged surgical procedures and the early postoperative period should be considered. The ECG should be monitored for evidence of potassium-related dysrhythmias. Other recommendations include avoidance of carbohydrate loads, hypothermia, and excessive hyperventilation. Halogenated inhaled anesthetics and regional anesthesia have been administered without complication.

Myasthenia Gravis

Myasthenia gravis (MG) is an autoimmune disease with antibodies directed against acetylcholine receptors or other proteins in the postsynaptic membrane of the neuromuscular junction (NMJ). Eighty-five percent of patients with MG have identifiable antiacetylcholine receptor antibodies. Seventy percent of MG patients without AChR (AChR-MG) antibodies have autoantibodies against other NMJ proteins such as muscle specific tyrosine kinase (MuSK, MuSK-MG). It is likely that seronegative MG patients have low antibody titer levels that are not measurable by current assay techniques. The autoantibodies damage the muscle membrane by activation of complement, lysis of the postsynaptic membrane, and loss of postsynaptic folds.[17] The thymus may play a central role in the pathogenesis of MG as 90% of MG patients have histologic abnormalities such as thymoma, thymic hyperplasia, or thymic atrophy.

The clinical hallmark of MG is skeletal muscle weakness. The weakness is aggravated by repetitive muscle use and there are periods of exacerbation alternating with remission. Any skeletal muscle can be affected, although there is a predilection for muscles innervated by cranial nerves. Initial symptoms include diplopia, dysarthria, dysphagia, or limb muscle weakness. Myasthenic crises occur in 20% to 30% of MG patients and can be precipitated by poor control of MG, emotional stress, hyperthermia, or pulmonary infections. Myasthenic crisis is characterized by severe muscle weakness and respiratory failure. Cardiac manifestations of MG include focal myocarditis, atrial fibrillation, atrioventricular conduction delay, and left ventricular diastolic dysfunction.

Some pregnant patients have a remission during pregnancy while others (20% to 40%) have increased symptoms during gestation and postpartum respiratory failure can occur. Fifteen percent to twenty percent of neonates born to myasthenic mothers have transient myasthenia from passive transfer of acetylcholine receptor antibodies. Neonatal myasthenia begins 12 to 48 hours after birth and may persist for weeks. Babies from mothers with MuSK-MG have more severe neonatal myasthenia.

Disease classification is based on skeletal muscle groups affected as well as age of onset (Table 23-4). The Osserman staging system is based on the severity of the disease (Table 23-5).

No single test is definitive for the diagnosis of MG and the diagnosis is not always obvious. Serologic testing may detect anti-AChR or anti-MuSK antibodies. Single fiber electromyography is the most sensitive of the electrodiagnostic tests.[18]

Treatment includes the administration of cholinesterase inhibitors (pyridostigmine), corticosteroids, immunosuppressants, intravenous immunoglobulin (IVG), and plasmapheresis. Cholinesterase inhibitors increase the concentration of acetylcholine (ACh) at the postsynaptic membrane. Consistent control of MG with only pyridostigmine can, however, be quite challenging. Under-dosing will result in residual muscle weakness and over-dosing may produce a "cholinergic crisis" characterized by abdominal pain, salivation, bradycardia, and skeletal muscle weakness. Corticosteroids (prednisone) are nonspecific immunosuppressants used when pyridostigmine does not produce satisfactory control. Azathioprine is the most frequently prescribed

TABLE 23-4. DIFFERENT PRESENTATIONS OF MYASTHENIA GRAVIS

Type	Etiology	Onset	Sex	Thymus	Course
Neonatal myasthenia	Passage of antibodies from myasthenic mothers across the placenta	Neonatal	Both sexes	Normal	Transient
Congenital myasthenia	Congenital end-plate pathology, genetic autosomal recessive pattern of inheritance	0–2 yr	Male > female	Normal	Nonfluctuating compatible with long survival
Juvenile myasthenia	Autoimmune disorder	2–20 yr	Female > male (4:1)	Hyperplasia	Slowly progressive, tendency to relapse and remission
Adult myasthenia	Autoimmune disorder	20–40 yr	Female > male thymoma	Hyperplasia > within 3–5 yr	Maximum severity
Elderly myasthenia	Autoimmune disorder	>40 yr	Male > female	Thymoma (benign or locally invasive)	Rapid progress, higher mortality

Reproduced from Baraka A: Anesthesia and myasthenia gravis. *Can J Anaesth* 1992;39:476, with permission.

specific immunosuppressant for the treatment of MG. Other immunosuppressants under investigation include cyclosporine, tacrolimus, mycophenolate, cyclophosphamide, methotrexate, and rituximib. The administration of IVG and plasmapheresis are used when rapid treatment is required.[19]

The role of thymectomy for the treatment of MG remains controversial. Ten percent of MG patients have a thymoma and thymectomy is clearly indicated. Less invasive surgical techniques for thymectomy such as video-assisted thoracoscopic surgery (VATS) produce good results with a low incidence of perioperative complications.[20]

Management of Anesthesia

The primary concern for anesthesia is the potential interaction between the disease, treatment of the disease, and anesthetic 3 drugs that may exacerbate muscle weakness. The uncontrolled or poorly controlled myasthenic patient is exquisitely sensitive to non-depolarizing muscle relaxants (Fig. 23-4). Small doses of non-depolarizing relaxants can produce significant respiratory muscle weakness. An anesthetic technique that avoids the use of muscle relaxants would be preferred. Isoflurane, sevoflurane, and desflurane depress neuromuscular transmission and may provide adequate muscle relaxation for tracheal intubation.[21] If muscle relaxation is required, a small dose of a short-acting non-depolarizer should be used. The use of rocuronium with reversal with sugammadex is an attractive alternative to reversal with cholinesterase inhibitors. Although poorly controlled myasthenic patients are resistant to succinylcholine, a dose of 1.5 to 2 mg/kg will be adequate for rapid tracheal intubation. Pyridostigmine may, however, prolong the duration of action of succinylcholine. Close, objective monitoring of neuromuscular transmission and clinical effect is necessary. Patients with MG can be quite challenging to wean from mechanical ventilation.[22]

Exacerbations of MG should be anticipated during pregnancy. Epidural analgesia can be used during labor and delivery.[23] Amide local anesthetics may be better than ester local anesthetics as the metabolism of amides is not affected by cholinesterase activity.

TABLE 23-5. OSSERMAN STAGING SYSTEM FOR MYASTHENIA GRAVIS

Type I
Ocular weakness only

Type IIA
Generalized muscle weakness

Type IIB
Generalized moderate weakness and/or bulbar dysfunction

Type III
Acute, fulminant presentation and/or respiratory dysfunction

Type IV
Severe, generalized myasthenia

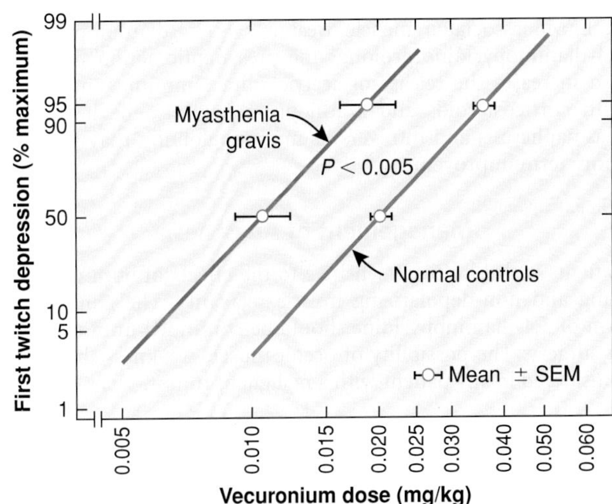

FIGURE 23-4. Dose-response for vecuronium in normal patients and patients with myasthenia gravis. (Reprinted from: Eisenkraft JB, Book WJ, Papatestas AE. Sensitivity to vecuronium in myasthenia gravis: A dose-response study. *Can J Anaesth.* 1990;37:301–306, with permission.)

TABLE 23-6. COMPARISON OF MYASTHENIC SYNDROME AND MYASTHENIA GRAVIS

	Myasthenic Syndrome	Myasthenia Gravis
Manifestations	Proximal limb weakness (arms > legs)	Extraocular, bulbar, and facial muscle weakness
	Strength improves with exercise	Fatigue with exercise
	Muscle pain common	Muscle pain uncommon
	Reflexes absent or decreased	Reflexes normal
Gender	Male > female	Female > male
Coexisting pathology	Small cell carcinoma of lung	Thymoma
Response to muscle relaxants	Sensitive to succinylcholine and nondepolarizing muscle relaxants	Resistant to succinylcholine
		Sensitive to nondepolarizing muscle relaxants
	Poor response to anticholinesterases	Poor response to anticholinesterases

Reprinted from Stoelting RK, Dierdorf SF, eds: *Anesthesia and Co-Existing Disease,* 3rd ed. New York, Churchill Livingstone, 1993, with permission.

Myasthenic Syndrome (Lambert–Eaton)

4 The Lambert–Eaton myasthenic syndrome (LEMS) is an autoimmune disease frequently associated with cancers and is categorized as a paraneoplastic syndrome.[24] Many tumors express onconeural antigens that resemble normal neural tissue components. Autoantibodies are produced that attack neural tissue. Patients with LEMS have autoantibodies directed against presynaptic voltage-gated calcium ion channels. This results in a decreased release of acetylcholine and subsequent muscle weakness. The muscle weakness often appears months to years before the diagnosis of the malignancy. Small cell lung cancer is most frequently associated with LEMS. The typical LEMS patient is a male older than 40 years of age with proximal muscle weakness (hip, shoulder) that affects gait and the ability to stand and climb stairs (Table 23-6). Autonomic dysfunction with dry mouth, constipation, erectile dysfunction, and reduced sweating often occurs. Paraneoplastic neurologic syndrome has also been reported with breast and ovarian cancers, lymphomas, testicular cancer, and neuroblastoma.

Treatment of the underlying neoplasm may improve the neurologic condition. The most effective drug for the treatment of LEMS associated muscle weakness is 3,4-diaminopyridine. 3,4-diaminopyridine prolongs the presynaptic action potential and increases the release of acetylcholine. Immunosuppression with corticosteroids and azathioprine may also be beneficial. Plasmapheresis and intravenous immunoglobulin may produce short-term improvement.[25]

Management of Anesthesia

Patients with LEMS are sensitive to the effects of both depolarizing and non-depolarizing muscle relaxants. The administration of 3,4-diaminopyridine should be continued until the time of surgery. The possibility of occult muscle weakness should be considered in any patient with a malignant tumor.

Guillain–Barré Syndrome (Polyradiculoneuritis)

Guillain–Barré syndrome (GBS) is the acute form of a group of disorders classified as the inflammatory neuropathies. Other diseases in this group include acute inflammatory demyelinating polyneuropathy (AIDP), acute motor axonal neuropathy (AMAN), acute motor-sensory axonal neuropathy, Miller-Fisher syndrome, and chronic inflammatory demyelinating polyneuropathy (CIDP).

GBS is an autoimmune disease triggered by a viral or bacterial infection and is an example of molecular mimicry and cross-reactivity. The infectious agent produces a substance that causes an immune reaction. Unfortunately, that substance resembles a neural component of the host and autoantibodies develop that attack the host. Patients with GBS develop antibodies to gangliosides in the peripheral nerves.[26] Most patients with GBS have a history of a respiratory or gastrointestinal infection within 4 weeks of the onset of neurologic symptoms. Infections with *Campylobacter jejuni, Haemophilus influenzae, Mycoplasma pneumoniae,* Epstein-Barr virus, and cytomegalovirus are most frequently associated with GBS. There are sporadic case reports of GBS or a GBS-like syndrome presenting after surgical procedures.

GBS is characterized by onset of skeletal muscle weakness or paralysis of the legs. Paresthesias may precede the weakness. The paralysis progresses cephalad to include muscles of the trunk and arms with maximal weakness developing 2 to 4 weeks after the onset. A plateau phase usually develops before recovery begins. The most serious problem is ventilatory insufficiency and 25% of patients with GBS will require mechanical ventilation. Although 85% of GBS patients achieve a good recovery, 3% to 5% develop a chronic, recurrent neuropathy.

Autonomic nervous system dysfunction can produce wide fluctuations in cardiovascular parameters. In a manner similar to autonomic hyperreflexia, physical stimulation can precipitate hypertension, tachycardia, and cardiac dysrhythmias.

Plasma exchange and the administration of intravenous immunoglobulin have been shown to be effective for patients with GBS.[27]

Management of Anesthesia

Autonomic nervous system dysfunction may cause hypotension secondary to postural changes, blood loss, or positive pressure ventilation. Noxious stimuli such as laryngoscopy and tracheal intubation may produce exaggerated increases in heart rate and blood pressure.

Succinylcholine should be avoided because of the danger of hyperkalemia. This risk may persist after clinical recovery from GBS.[28] A short-acting non-depolarizing muscle relaxant with minimal cardiovascular effects (cisatracurium, rocuronium) would be a useful choice. The sensitivity to non-depolarizing muscle relaxants may vary from extreme sensitivity to resistance, depending on the phase of the disease.[29] It is likely that mechanical ventilation may be required in the immediate postoperative period. Patients with GBS who have pronounced sensory disturbances may benefit from neuraxial opioids.

CENTRAL NERVOUS SYSTEM DISEASES

Multiple Sclerosis

The features of multiple sclerosis (MS) are inflammation and demyelination in the brain and spinal cord. Although circulating T cells cannot normally penetrate the blood–brain barrier, an environmental stimulus (virus) may activate T cells. The activated T cells cross the blood–brain barrier and initiate an inflammatory and immunologic attack on myelin.[30,31] Demyelination interferes with neural transmission and causes CNS dysfunction. The ability of neural tissue to repair itself during the early phases of the disease explains the relapsing nature of MS. There is also evidence that damage is not restricted to white matter and that gray matter is also affected.

The symptoms of MS depend on the sites of demyelination. Brainstem involvement can produce nystagmus, diplopia, trigeminal neuralgia, autonomic dysfunction, and alterations in ventilation that lead to hypoxemia and respiratory failure. Lesions of the spinal cord produce weakness and paresthesias. The legs are affected more than the arms. Bowel retention and urinary incontinence are frequent complaints. The course of MS is characterized by exacerbations of symptoms at unpredictable intervals over a period of years. Patients are classified during the early phases as either relapsing–remitting (85%) or primary progressive MS. Many patients with relapsing–remitting MS develop neurodegeneration and are categorized as secondary progressive MS. Patients with primary progressive MS are devoid of acute episodes, but develop progressive neurodegeneration. Pregnancy is associated with improvement of symptoms, but relapse often occurs within the first three postpartum months.

Clinical criteria for the diagnosis of MS include onset between 10 and 50 years of age, signs and symptoms of CNS white matter disease, two or more attacks separated by a month or more, and involvement of two or more non-contiguous anatomic areas. Elevated levels of IgG and albumin in the cerebrospinal fluid are characteristic of MS. Magnetic resonance imaging (MRI) is a sensitive diagnostic tool for MS and provides direct evidence of the location of demyelinated plaques in the CNS.[32]

Therapy for MS is directed at modulating the immunologic and inflammatory responses that damage the CNS. Current therapy for MS includes interferon preparations, glatiramer, mitoxantrone, and monoclonal antibodies. Interferon works by reducing T cell transit across the blood–brain barrier. Glatiramer is a mixture of polypeptides that mimic the structure of myelin and serve as a decoy for autoantibodies. Mitoxantrone is related to the antineoplastic drugs doxorubicin and may be cardiotoxic. Natalizumab prevents T cell migration but can produce a fatal leukoencephalopathy. The most recent therapeutic breakthrough in the treatment of MS has been the development of oral agents.[33] These include cladribine, fingolimod, laquinimod, teriflunomide, and dimethyl fumarate. Corticosteroids are still used for acute relapses that do not respond to other medications.

Many patients with MS experience chronic pain, including central neuropathic pain, paresthesias, trigeminal neuralgia, and spasticity. Symptomatic therapy includes diazepam, dantrolene, and baclofen for spasticity. Painful dysesthesias, tonic seizures, and ataxia can be treated with carbamazepine. Nonspecific measures include the avoidance of excessive fatigue, emotional stress, and hyperthermia. Demyelinated fibers are extremely sensitive to increases in temperature and hyperthermia can block impulse conduction.

Management of Anesthesia

The effect of surgery and anesthesia on the course of MS is controversial. Some reports have indicated that regional anesthesia and general anesthesia have been reported to exacerbate MS. Other reports, however, have found no correlation between anesthesia and the course of the disease. Factors other than anesthesia such as infection, hyperpyrexia, and emotional stress may contribute to an increased risk of an exacerbation. Preoperatively, the patient should be advised that surgery and anesthesia could produce a relapse despite a well-managed anesthetic.

Although the mechanism is not known, spinal anesthesia has been associated with a relapse of MS. It could be speculated that demyelinated areas of the spinal cord are more sensitive to the effects of local anesthetics, causing a relative neurotoxicity.
5 Evidence for this theory is found by the observation that higher concentrations of bupivacaine (0.25%) used for epidural analgesia were more likely to cause neurologic dysfunction than lower concentrations.[34] With such a precaution, epidural analgesia can be safely provided for women during labor.

Autonomic dysfunction may enhance the hypotensive effects of volatile anesthetics. Drug interactions that may be anticipated during the perioperative period include cardiotoxicity from immunosuppressants, and altered responses to muscle relaxants. Baclofen increases the sensitivity to nondepolarizing muscle relaxants and anticonvulsants produce resistance to nondepolarizing muscle relaxants. Succinylcholine could produce an exaggerated release of potassium. Respiratory muscle weakness and respiratory control dysfunction increase the likelihood of respiratory support during the immediate postoperative period.[35]

Epilepsy

A seizure is a common manifestation of many types of CNS disease and is the external manifestation of epilepsy. A seizure results from the excessive discharge of large numbers of neurons that become depolarized in a synchronous fashion. Epilepsy (idiopathic seizures) begins in childhood. The sudden onset of seizures in an adult may indicate focal brain disease (tumor). The onset of seizures after 60 years of age can be a result of cerebrovascular disease, head injury, tumor, infection, or a metabolic disturbance.

Although there are many antiseizure drugs, 30% of epileptic patients are poorly controlled and sudden death may occur in adults with epilepsy since childhood (Table 23-7).[36,37] The newer antiseizure drugs target ion channels, GABA receptors, amino acid receptors, and synaptic proteins.[38]

The most frequently encountered types of seizures are:

1. *Grand mal seizure:* A grand mal seizure is characterized by generalized tonic–clonic activity. All respiratory effort is arrested and a period of arterial hypoxemia ensures. The tonic phase lasts 20 to 40 seconds and is followed by the clonic phase. In the postictal period, the patient is lethargic and confused. Diazepam, thiopental, and propofol are effective for treatment of acute, generalized seizures. Epileptic patients resistant to drug therapy may benefit from surgical resection of a seizure focus or implantation of a vagal nerve stimulator (VNS).
2. *Focal cortical seizure:* Focal cortical seizures may be motor or sensory depending on the site of neuronal discharge. There

TABLE 23-7. ANTIEPILEPTIC DRUGS (AED) CLASSIFIED BY MECHANISM OF ACTION

Enhance GABAergic System
Barbiturates
Benzodiazepines
Primidone
Tiagibine
Vigabatrin
Affect Cation Channels
Phenytoin
Carbamazepine
Oxcarbazepine
Lamotrigine
Topiramate
Ethosuximide
Valproate
Retigabine
Zonisamide
Antagonists of Excitatory Amino Acids
Felbamate
Lacosamide
Talampanel
Unknown Mechanism of Action
Acetazolamide
Sulthiame
Gabapentin
Pregabalin
Levetiracetam
AEDs for Status Epilepticus
Propofol
Diazepam
Lorazepam
Midazolam
Fosphenytoin

is usually no loss of consciousness, although the focal seizure may induce a grand mal seizure.

3. *Absence seizure (petit mal):* Absence seizures are characterized by a brief loss of awareness (30 seconds). Additional manifestations include staring, blinking, and rolling of the eyes. Absence seizures typically occur in children and young adults.
4. *Akinetic seizure:* Akinetic seizures are a sudden, brief loss of consciousness and postural tone. These types of seizures usually occur in children and can result in a severe head injury from the fall.
5. *Status epilepticus:* Status epilepticus is defined as two consecutive tonic–clonic seizures without regaining consciousness, or seizure activity that is unabated for 30 minutes or more. Grand mal status epilepticus may last for more than 48 hours with a seizure frequency of 4 to 5 per hour and mortality can be as high as 20%. As the seizure progresses, skeletal muscle activity diminishes and seizure activity may only be evident on the EEG. Respiratory effects of status epilepticus include inhibition of respiratory centers, uncoordinated skeletal muscle activity that impairs ventilation and bronchoconstriction. Phenobarbital, phenytoin, benzodiazepines, thiopental, and propofol are good choices for initial therapy. On rare occasions, general anesthesia may be required.

Management of Anesthesia

Most inhaled anesthetics, including nitrous oxide, have been reported to produce seizure activity. Such activity during the administration of isoflurane and desflurane is extremely rare as these drugs produce a dose-dependent depression of EEG activity. Sevoflurane may be epileptogenic, although the clinical significance is uncertain.[39] Stimulation of hepatic microsomal enzymes by anticonvulsant drugs may increase the rate of biotransformation of halogenated anesthetics and increase the risk of organ damage. Ketamine may produce seizure activity and it would seem reasonable to avoid its use, as there are other suitable induction agents (e.g., thiopental, propofol, benzodiazepines). Potent opioids such as fentanyl, sufentanil, and remifentanil may produce myoclonic activity or chest wall rigidity that may be confused with seizure activity. Despite these concerns, the degree of preoperative seizure control may be a more important predictor of perioperative seizures.[40] Local anesthetics can decrease the seizure threshold but there is no evidence that regional anesthesia increases the risk of seizures.[41]

Side effects of antiseizure medications include leucopenia, anemia, hepatitis and hepatic failure, pancreatitis, coagulopathy, cardiotoxicity, hypothyroidism, and skin rash.[42] Complications of vagal nerve stimulators include vocal cord paralysis, facial palsy, bradycardia/asystole, and airway obstruction.[43] Appropriate airway resuscitation equipment and rapid-acting anticonvulsants such as barbiturates, propofol, and benzodiazepines should be readily available if a perioperative seizure occurs.

Alzheimer Disease

Alzheimer disease is the major cause of dementia in the United States and there are over 5 million people in the United States with the disease. The incidence is 5% in persons over the age of 65 years and 30% over the age of 85 years. Alzheimer disease is characterized by cognitive impairment, poor decision making, language deterioration, gait disturbances, seizures, agitation, and psychosis. A positive diagnosis can, however, only be made at autopsy. Imaging studies show hippocampal atrophy (MRI) and glucose hypometabolism (PET). The deposition of amyloid β peptides appears to be central to the degeneration and death of neurons. Deposition of amyloid β peptides produces amyloid plaques and neurofibrillary tangles and activates the apoptotic cell death cascade. There is no specific therapy for Alzheimer disease. Initial symptomatic therapy is with cholinesterase inhibitors (donepezil, rivastigmine, galantamine) and an NMDA receptor antagonist (memantine). Cholinesterase inhibitors improve the patient's ability to perform daily living activities and may improve cognition. Side effects of cholinesterase inhibitors include nausea, emesis, bradycardia, syncope, and fatigue. Antidepressants, anticonvulsants, and antipsychotics are used for neuropsychiatric symptoms as necessary. A large number of experimental therapies are directed at disease modifying pathways with immunotherapy, secretase inhibitors, amyloid aggregators, chelation, and Tau aggregation inhibitors.[44]

Management of Anesthesia

Animal studies have demonstrated that volatile, halogenated anesthetics produce neuronal changes that resemble the diseased neurons of patients with Alzheimer disease. These findings have caused significant controversy about the use of halogenated anesthetics in neonates and elderly patients.[45–47] Any clinical recommendations concerning the use of halogenated, inhaled anesthetics are, however, speculative. Postoperative cognitive dysfunction (POCD) is well known in elderly patients, but the causes remain elusive. Patients and their families should be advised that POCD can occur.

The selection of anesthetics and techniques will be influenced by the patient's physiologic condition and the degree of neurologic impairment. The patient's preoperative drug list should be reviewed for the possibility of interactions with anesthetics. Patients are likely to be confused and uncooperative because of dementia. Sedative premedication should be used with caution, if at all, as mental confusion may worsen. If an anticholinergic is required, glycopyrrolate, which does not cross the blood–brain barrier, is preferable to atropine or scopolamine. Patients receiving cholinesterase inhibitors may have a prolonged response to succinylcholine.

Parkinson Disease

Parkinson disease (PD) is a degenerative CNS disease caused by a loss of dopaminergic cells in the basal ganglia of the brain. The characteristic pathologic feature is the presence of Lewy bodies in the neurons of the substantia nigra. Lewy bodies are aggregations of damaged proteins. The etiology of PD is an interaction of a genetic predisposition and unidentified environmental factors. Other than the well-described postencephalitic PD, there is little evidence that PD is caused by a virus.[48]

The clinical effects of PD are caused by dopamine deficiency. The most characteristic features of PD are resting tremor, cogwheel rigidity of the extremities, bradykinesia, shuffling gait, stooped posture, and facial immobility. These features are secondary to diminished inhibition of the extrapyramidal motor system as a result of dopamine deficiency. Other clinical features include seborrhea, sialorrhea, orthostatic hypotension, bladder dysfunction, diaphragmatic spasm, oculogyric crisis, dementia, and mental depression.

Treatment is directed toward increasing dopamine levels in the brain, but preventing the adverse peripheral effects of dopamine. Levodopa is the single most effective drug for patients with PD. When administered orally, levodopa is converted to dopamine and causes side effects such as nausea, emesia, and hypotension. To avoid such side effects, levodopa is administered with carbidopa and entacopone. Carbidopa is a peripheral decarboxylase inhibitor and entacopone is a catechol-O-methyltransferase inhibitor that increases the bioavailability of levodopa. Other drugs that improve function are the monoamine oxidase-B inhibitors, selegiline and rasagiline. Dopamine receptor agonists such as bromocriptine, pramipexole, ropinirole, pergolide, and cabergoline can also be used for the treatment of PD. Pergolide and cabergoline are ergot-derived drugs that can cause cardiac valvular fibrosis and insufficiency. Implantation of deep-brain stimulators (DBS) may be quite effective for patients with advanced PD. The therapeutic regimen for patients with PD is complex and requires a skilled neurologist to individualize therapy.[49]

Management of Anesthesia

The patient's medications should be administered on the morning of surgery. The half-life of levodopa is short and interruption in therapy for more than 6 to 12 hours can result in severe skeletal muscle rigidity that interferes with ventilation. Consultation with the patient's neurologist and continuation of the patient's drug regimen may avert complications. Apomorphine is a dopamine agonist that can be administered subcutaneously or intravenously if oral levodopa cannot be given. Dopamine antagonists such as phenothiazines, droperidol, and metoclopramide should be avoided. Alfentanil and fentanyl may produce dystonic reactions when administered rapidly. The incidence of side effects from thiopental and propofol is low. Although ketamine could produce an exaggerated sympathetic nervous system response with resultant tachycardia and hypertension, it has been used without difficulty in patients with PD. There are no reports of adverse responses to isoflurane, sevoflurane, or desflurane. The likelihood of coexisting heart diseases in elderly patients with PD will influence the selection of anesthetics and monitoring techniques.[50]

Anesthetics administered to patients who are receiving monoamine oxidase-B inhibitors (selegiline, rasagiline) are generally uneventful. There are, however, reports of agitation, muscle rigidity, and hyperthermia in patients receiving selegiline and meperidine. Patients being treated with dopamine agonists may be at increased risk for neuroleptic malignant syndrome (NMS).

Anesthesia for PD patients undergoing implantation of deep brain stimulators (DBS) can be challenging. Awake techniques with sedation and local anesthesia are preferred as intraoperative testing of the stimulator can be performed. Agitated and uncooperative patients may, however, require general anesthesia. Hypertension, seizures, and interference with other devices can occur.[51]

Autonomic dysfunction is common. The most consistent cardiovascular finding is orthostatic hypotension that may be aggravated by the vasodilatory effects of anti-Parkinson drugs. Patients with PD are more likely to develop excessive decreases in blood pressure in response to inhaled anesthetics. Salivation and esophageal dysfunction are common and patients with PD are at increased risk for aspiration pneumonitis.

Perioperative respiratory complications are common.[52] Upper airway obstruction may be a result of poor coordination of upper airway muscles secondary to neurotransmitter imbalance. Some patients with upper airway obstruction may respond favorably to anti-Parkinson medications.

Patients with PD are susceptible to postoperative confusion and hallucinations. These alterations may not appear until 24 to 72 hours after surgery.

Huntington Disease

Huntington disease (HD) is an autosomal dominant inherited disease characterized by progressive neurodegeneration. HD is one of the trinucleotide repeat disorders. An increase in cytosine, adenine, and guanine (CAG) repeat sequences on chromosome 4 is the genetic defect that produces a mutant huntingtin protein. Huntingtin is found in all human cells, but most notably in brain cell. Neurons from patients with Huntington disease show abnormal inclusion bodies containing mutant huntingtin and polyglutamine. Associated with HD is atrophy of the caudate and putamen. Identification of the Huntington gene provides a reliable predictive test; however, the delayed nature of the clinical manifestations presents legal and ethical concerns about predictive testing.[53]

Clinical features include choreiform movements, depression, and dementia. Onset is typically between 35 and 40 years of age, but can be as late as 80 years. The disease continues to progress for several years and depression increases the possibility of suicide. Death occurs 17 to 20 years after diagnosis and is usually from malnutrition or aspiration pneumonitis. Hypothalamic atrophy can cause endocrine changes such as elevated cortisol levels, reduced testosterone levels, and diabetes.

There is no specific therapy for HD. Drugs used for the treatment of chorea include tetrabenzine, tiapride, olanzapine, pimozide, risperidone, and fluphenazine. Antidepressants are used to treat psychiatric symptoms.

Management of Anesthesia

The medical literature is sparse with regard to the anesthetic management of patients with HD. Many of the manifestations of HD are typical of patients with neurodegenerative disorders. As the disease progresses, the pharyngeal muscles become dysfunctional and the risk of aspiration pneumonitis increases.[54] As for any patient with a neurodegenerative disease, delayed emergence and an increased likelihood of respiratory complications must be anticipated after surgery.

Although there are no specific contraindications to the use of inhaled or intravenous anesthetics, recovery from propofol may be faster than with other intravenous hypnotics. Short-acting muscle relaxants are preferable to long-acting relaxants. Decreased plasma cholinesterase activity may prolong the response to succinylcholine. Spinal anesthesia has been successfully used in patients with HD.

Amyotrophic Lateral Sclerosis

Amyotrophic lateral sclerosis (ALS, Lou Gehrig's disease) is a degenerative disease of motor neurons (upper and lower) throughout the CNS. The cause of ALS is unknown and many hypotheses have been proposed, including glutamate-induced excitotoxicity and oxidative stress. Ten percent of ALS cases are familial and 90% are sporadic. Progression of the disease is relentless—50% of patients die within 30 months of the onset of symptoms. Twenty percent, however, may survive 5 to 10 years.

There are four patterns of clinical presentation: (1) limb onset, (2) bulbar onset, (3) pure upper motor neuron, and (4) progressive muscular atrophy.[55] Signs and symptoms are influenced by the affected neurons. Initial symptoms are skeletal muscle weakness and fasciculation. Dysarthria and dysphagia are a result of bulbar atrophy. Pulmonary function testing demonstrates a decrease in vital capacity and maximal voluntary ventilation. Respiratory failure eventually develops and ventilatory support may be required. The cause of death is respiratory failure or circulatory collapse. Patients with ALS have autonomic dysfunction as evidenced by resting tachycardia, orthostatic hypotension, and elevated circulating levels of epinephrine and norepinephrine.

Treatment is largely symptomatic and treatment coordinated by specialized ALS clinics improves survival. Riluzole, a glutamate release inhibitor, is the only specific drug for the treatment of ALS. Riluzole modestly improves survival by 3 to 6 months.

Management of Anesthesia

There is no evidence that a specific anesthetic technique is best for patients with ALS. Neuromuscular transmission is markedly abnormal and ALS patients can be very sensitive to nondepolarizing muscle relaxants. ALS patients should be considered to be at risk for succinylcholine-induced hyperkalemia. The need for postoperative ventilatory support is likely.

Creutzfeldt–Jakob Disease

Creutzfeldt–Jakob disease (CJD) is one of a group of diseases termed the transmissible spongiform encephalopathies. Pathologically, these diseases are characterized by vacuolation of brain cells and neuronal death. There are four types of CJD: Familial (*f*CJD), sporadic (*s*CJD), iatrogenic (*i*CJD), and variant (*v*CJD). CJD is an infection caused by a prion, a small protein devoid of nucleic acid. PrP^c is a naturally occurring protein concentrated in neurons. PrP^{sc} is a mutant protein with the same amino acid sequence as PrP^c, but with a different conformation. The structure of PrP^{sc} renders the protein resistant to conventional decontamination techniques. CJD is a very rare cause of dementia, but the discovery of transmission of a prion disease (bovine spongiform encephalopathy, mad cow disease) from cows to humans in 1996 catapulted CJD to prominence. This form is termed variant CJD (*v*CJD).[56]

The clinical characteristics of *s*CJD are subacute dementia, myoclonus, and EEG changes. The EEG pattern is relatively characteristic with diffuse slow activity and periodic complexes. Progressive loss of cognitive and neurologic function occurs. Patients with *v*CJD present with psychiatric features, such as dysphoria, withdrawal, anxiety, and insomnia. Neurologic features develop 1 to 2 months after the psychiatric changes commence. Transmission of *v*CJD is by ingestion of contaminated animal products. Iatrogenic transmission of *i*CJD has been linked to contaminated dural graft material, corneal transplants, contaminated surgical instruments, pooled human growth hormone, and blood. There is no specific treatment for CJD. Investigational therapies are aimed at preventing prion transmission from the periphery to the CNS and at neuron regeneration.

Management of Anesthesia

CJD is a transmissible disease and appropriate precautions must be observed when administering anesthesia. High-risk patient tissues include brain, spinal cord, cerebrospinal fluid, lymphoid tissue, and blood. Single-use anesthesia supplies, including face masks, breathing circuits, laryngoscopes, and tracheal tubes offer the highest degree of protection.[57]

Patients with degenerative neurologic diseases are prone to aspiration pneumonitis because they have impaired swallowing function and decreased laryngeal reflexes. Because lower motor neuron dysfunction occurs in patients with CJD patients, succinylcholine should be avoided. The autonomic and peripheral nervous systems are adversely affected and abnormal cardiovascular responses to anesthesia and vasoactive drugs can occur.

INHERITED DISORDERS

Malignant Hyperthermia

Malignant hyperthermia (MH) is a pharmacogenetic disease characterized by extreme hypermetabolism when a genetically susceptible individual is exposed to a triggering agent. The clinical features are a result of hypermetabolism and include an increase in end-tidal CO_2, tachycardia, tachypnea, metabolic acidosis, muscle rigidity, and possibly rhabdomyolysis. All potent, inhaled halogenated anesthetics and succinylcholine are triggering agents.[58] The history of MH and anesthesia is well known and considerable progress has been made in the elucidation of the pathophysiology and genetics of MH.[59] The genetics of human MH is, however, complex, and a simple, noninvasive test for susceptibility is not yet available.

The final common pathway that leads to MH is uncontrolled release and regulation of calcium in muscle sarcoplasm. The

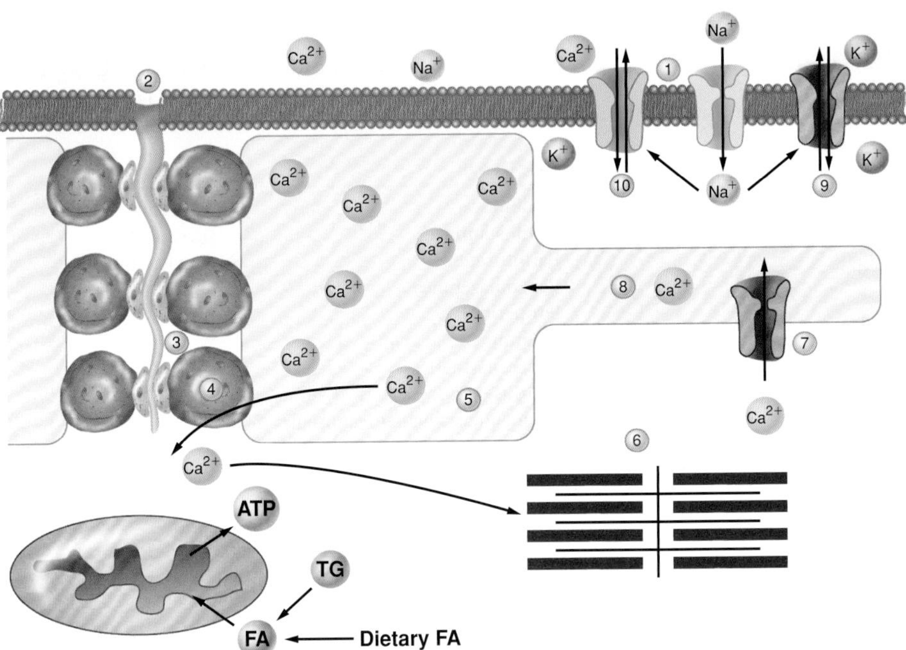

FIGURE 23-5. Excitation-contraction coupling and malignant hyperthermia. ATP, adenosine triphosphate; FA, fatty acids; TG, triglycerides.

calcium release channel in human muscle is the ryanodine receptor (RYR) and mutations in the receptor may cause MH in susceptible patients. Other mechanisms that influence skeletal muscle calcium control may also be defective in patients with MH (Fig. 23-5).[60]

The most effective treatment for an MH episode is dantrolene. Dantrolene may act at multiple sites, including the ryanodine receptor, to inhibit calcium release into the muscle sarcoplasm. The discovery that dantrolene was effective for the treatment of MH has dramatically reduced mortality from MH.

Management of the Acute Malignant Hyperthermia Episode

2 The key to the successful management of an acute MH episode is early recognition and prompt treatment with dantrolene. An 6 unexplained increase in expired CO_2, tachycardia, tachypnea, hyperthermia, and metabolic acidosis is highly suspicious for MH. Discontinuation of potential triggering agents and the administration of dantrolene (2.5 mg/kg) would be prudent. Serial arterial blood gas measurements are helpful for tracking metabolic acidosis and the response to therapy. Fulminant or unrecognized MH can cause rhabdomyolysis, hyperkalemia, myoglobinuria, disseminated intravascular coagulation, and cardiac arrest. Supportive treatment includes hyperventilation, treatment of acidosis, cardiac dysrhythmias, and hyperkalemia, active cooling, and maintenance of urinary output (Table 23-8).[61]

The diagnosis of MH is not always obvious. Intraoperative thyrotoxicosis and sepsis may mimic an MH episode. A clinical grading system can be used to objectively evaluate a suspected MH episode and aid in referral of patients for definitive testing (Table 23-9).

Management of the MH Susceptible Patient

The gold standard for the diagnosis of malignant hyperthermia susceptibility (MHS) is the caffeine–halothane contracture test. The biopsy and test should be performed at an MH diagnostic center. Molecular genetic testing can supplement the caffeine–halothane contracture test. Future research may permit the development of a noninvasive, definitive test for MH.

Anesthesia for the malignant hyperthermia susceptible patient (MHS) is based on avoidance of triggering agents such as halogenated, inhaled anesthetics and succinylcholine. Despite the avoidance of triggering agents, MHS patients still require vigilant

TABLE 23-8. TREATMENT OF AN ACUTE EPISODE OF MALIGNANT HYPERTHERMIA

Discontinue triggering agents
- Halogenated, inhaled anesthetics
- Succinylcholine

Hyperventilation with 100% oxygen

Administer dantrolene 2.5 mg/kg
- Titrate additional dantrolene to heart rate, temperature, and $PaCO_2$
- Serial monitoring of arterial blood gases

Correction of metabolic acidosis with $NaHCO_3$

Control of dysrhythmias
- Lidocaine
- *Avoid* calcium channel blockers

Active cooling
- Surface ice packs
- Body cavity lavage
- Cardiopulmonary bypass in severe cases
- Cease active cooling when core temperature reaches 38°C

Correction of hyperkalemia
- Glucose, insulin, bicarbonate, hyperventilation
- Calcium if hyperkalemia causes cardiac dysfunction

Measurement of renal function, liver function, and coagulation

After acute episode subsides, monitor for recrudescence of MH, disseminated intravascular coagulation (DIC), and myoglobinuria

TABLE 23-9. MALIGNANT HYPERTHERMIA CLINICAL GRADING SCALE

Process I: Muscle rigidity	
Generalized rigidity	15
Masseter rigidity	15
Process II: Myonecrosis	
Elevated CK >20,000 (after succinylcholine administration)	15
Elevated CK > 10,000 (without exposure to succinylcholine)	15
Cola-colored urine	10
Myoglobin in urine >60 mg/L	5
Blood/plasma/serum K^+ >6 mEg/L	3
Process III: Respiratory acidosis	
$Petco_2$ >55 with controlled ventilation	15
$Paco_2$ >60 with controlled ventilation	15
$Petco_2$ >60 with spontaneous ventilation	15
Inappropriate hypercarbia	15
Inappropriate tachypnea	10
Process IV: Temperature increase	
Rapid increase in temperature	15
Inappropriate temperature >38.8°C in perioperative period	10
Process V: Cardiac involvement	
Inappropriate tachycardia	3
Ventricular tachycardia or fibrillation	3

CK, creatine kinase.
See Larach, et al.[93] for full details of this scoring system. Briefly, a case may receive 15 points for the worst presentation in five of the first six categories. A Sum of more than 50 points is termed *D6*, almost certainly a case of malignant hyperthermia (MH). A sum of 35 to 49 points is *D5*, very likely to be a case of MH.

TABLE 23-10. SAFE VERSUS UNSAFE DRUGS IN MALIGNANT HYPERTHERMIA

Safe Drugs	Unsafe Drugs
Antibiotics	All halogenated inhaled anesthetics
Antihistamines	Succinylcholine
Barbiturates	
Benzodiazepines	
Droperidol	
Ketamine	
Local anesthetics	
Nitrous oxide	
Nondepolarizing neuromuscular blockers	
Opioids	
Propofol	
Propranolol	
Vasoactive drugs	

monitoring during the perioperative period as MH can present with a variety of clinical patterns. There are also rare reports of stress induced MH in humans.

The anesthesia machine requires preparation prior to use for MHS patients. Some institutions have maintained machines with no previous exposure to volatile anesthetics. The Malignant Hyperthermia Association of the United States (MHAUS) has recommendations for purging anesthesia machines to reduce trace concentrations of volatile anesthetics to acceptable levels. Insertion of activated charcoal filters into the inspiratory and expiratory limbs of the anesthesia circuit rapidly reduces the concentration of trace volatile anesthetics.[62]

Drugs considered safe for MHS patients include thiopental, propofol, midazolam, diazepam, opioids, cisatracurium, atracurium, rocuronium, vecuronium, pancuronium, neostigmine, and glycopyrrolate (Table 23-10). Regional anesthesia is also suitable for MHS patients. Dantrolene does not have to be administered preoperatively, but must be readily available.

Porphyria

There are eight disorders of heme synthesis in the group of diseases called porphyria. Heme is used for the synthesis of hemoglobin in erythropoietic cells and the production of cytochromes in the liver. The porphyrias are caused by defects in the synthetic pathway of heme that lead to the accumulation of toxic intermediates.[63] The three acute porphyrias that can produce clinically significant attacks that are of the most interest to anesthesiologists are: Acute intermittent porphyria, variegate porphyria, and coproporphyria.

Acute intermittent porphyria (AIP) is caused by a deficiency of porphobilinogen deaminase with the accumulation of delta-aminolevulinic acid. AIP typically occurs in the young adults and is more common in women. The clinical features of AIP are fever, tachycardia, nausea, emesis, abdominal pain, weakness, seizures, confusion, and hallucinations. Muscle weakness can be so severe that respiratory failure develops. Hyponatremia may occur secondary to inappropriate secretion of ADH. The mental changes that occur during an acute episode are often misdiagnosed as a primary psychiatric disease. Rarely, severe hypertension and encephalopathy develop. Attacks may last for 1 to 2 weeks. Skin lesions do not develop in patients with AIP. Attacks may be triggered by hormonal changes during the menstrual cycle, fasting, infections, and exposure to triggering drugs. Treatment consists of removal of triggering factors, avoidance of porphyrinogenic drugs, and resolution of underlying infection. Specific therapy for acute episodes is the intravenous infusion of human hemin solution that inhibits 5-aminolevulinic acid synthase and decreases excretion of porphobilinogen. Liver transplantation has been effective for patients with severe AIP.

Patients with variegate porphyria and hereditary coproporphyria may develop acute attacks. Skin lesions typically develop with variegate porphyria and occasionally with hereditary coproporphyria. Toxic metabolite levels are not as high as with AIP.

Management of Anesthesia

The main goals of anesthesia are to avoid triggering drugs in susceptible patients. Susceptible patients, however, are rarely identified preoperatively and the triggering potential of some drugs is unknown. More than 300 mutations in the heme synthesis pathway have been identified and many variations in clinical response may occur. A drug that may be non-triggering in one patient may serve as a trigger in another. Anesthesia drugs that should definitely be avoided are the barbiturates and etomidate (Table 23-11). Short-acting drugs that are rapidly eliminated

TABLE 23-11. DRUGS KNOWN TO PRECIPITATE PORPHYRIA

Sedatives	**Antibiotics**
Barbiturates	Sulfonamides
Etomidate	Chloramphenicol
Chlordiazepoxide	**Hypoglycemic Sulfonylureas**
Diazepam, lorazepam, midazolam	Tolbutamide
	Chlorpropamide
Glutethimide	**Toxins**
Analgesics	Lead
Pentazocine	Ethanol
Antipyrine	**Miscellaneous**
Aminopyridine	Ergot preparations
Ropivacaine	Amphetamines
Anticonvulsants	Methyldopa
Phenytoin	
Methsuximide	

are preferred. Propofol, isoflurane, sevoflurane, desflurane, fentanyl, morphine, and ketamine have been administered without apparent complications. Succinylcholine, cisatracurium, and rocuronium are acceptable for muscle relaxation. Regional anesthesia may be administered as well.

Cholinesterase Disorders

Plasma cholinesterase (pseudocholinesterase, butyrylcholinesterase) is an enzyme synthesized in the liver. This enzyme hydrolyzes succinylcholine, mivacurium, procaine, chloroprocaine, tetracaine, and cocaine. Individuals may exhibit prolonged duration of action with these drugs, especially succinylcholine. The most significant complication for the anesthesiologist is prolonged apnea after succinylcholine. The molecular genetics of cholinesterase inheritance is not simple, as 20 variants have been described. Some variants produce cholinesterase with very little activity and succinylcholine-induced paralysis may last for several hours. Individuals with other variants may have a prolongation of succinylcholine activity that is not clinically discernible. A few genetic variants produce a cholinesterase that accelerates the hydrolysis of succinylcholine, thereby producing a shorter duration of action. Individuals with genetically deficient plasma cholinesterase activity are not known to have other pathologic conditions. There is some evidence that plasma cholinesterase variants in some ethnic groups may impart a protective effect against atherosclerosis. 7

Acquired deficiencies of cholinesterase activity are most notably caused by liver disease. Other diseases associated with decreased cholinesterase activity include carcinomas, uremia, collagen vascular diseases, malnutrition, and myxedema. Plasma cholinesterase activity, however, must be decreased by more than 75% for there to be a clinically significant decrease in succinylcholine hydrolysis. Drugs that may interfere with succinylcholine metabolism include neostigmine, pyridostigmine, ecothiophate, cyclophosphamide, chlorpromazine, and organophosphate insecticides.

Management of Anesthesia

Preoperative knowledge of a plasma cholinesterase abnormality allows the anesthesiologist to avoid the use of drugs hydrolyzed by cholinesterase and the course of anesthesia will be uneventful. The usual clinical presentation, however, of a cholinesterase abnormality is prolonged apnea after succinylcholine. Apnea can be very prolonged if additional succinylcholine is administered after tracheal intubation or a non-depolarizing muscle relaxant is given followed by reversal with neostigmine. A prudent clinical practice is to be certain that recovery from the initial dose of succinylcholine has occurred before administering more muscle relaxant. Mechanical ventilation and adequate sedation should be continued until full recovery of neuromuscular function is assured.

If prolonged apnea after succinylcholine occurs, laboratory testing should be performed after the patient has fully recovered. Inheritance of atypical cholinesterase in most patients is classic and there are three genotypes: Normal (EuEu), heterozygous (EuEa), and homozygous abnormal (EaEa). The two tests that will provide the most information are a cholinesterase activity level and the dibucaine number (Table 23-12).

Glycogen Storage Diseases

The glycogen storage diseases (GSD) are inherited disorders caused by abnormalities of enzymes that regulate glycogen synthesis and breakdown. Glycogen is a complex storage form of glucose found in the liver and muscle. Glucose absorbed by the liver is phosphorylated by glucokinase and elongated into chains by glycogen synthetase for storage. During periods of fasting, hepatic glycogen phosphorylase and glucose-6-phosphatase cleave glucose from glycogen and release glucose into the circulation (Fig. 23-6).

The GSD are rare diseases (incidence 1:200,000–1:400,000) and there are several types with various manifestations. There are, however, three features common to all types of GSD:

1. Acidosis secondary to fat and protein metabolism
2. Risk of hypoglycemia secondary to the failure to metabolize glycogen to glucose
3. Cardiac and hepatic dysfunction secondary to destruction of normal tissue by accumulated glycogen.

TABLE 23-12. CLASSIC CHOLINESTERASE GENOTYPES

Genotype	Cholinesterase Activity	Dibucaine Number	Succinylcholine Apnea (min)
Normal (EuEu)	++++	78–86	5
Heterozygote (EuEa)	++	51–70	15
Homozygote (EaEa)	+	18–26	120–300

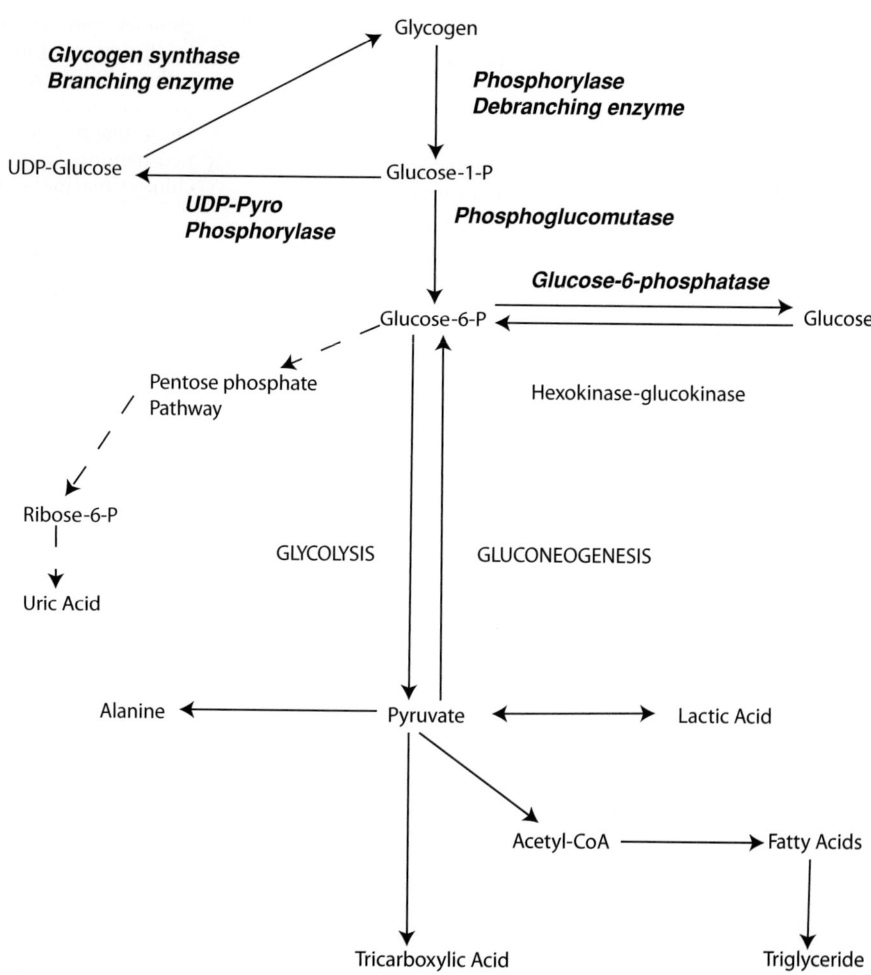

FIGURE 23-6. Simplified pathway of glycogen synthesis and degradation. (From: Ozen H. Glycogen storage diseases: New perspectives. *World J Gastroenterol.* 2007;13:2541–2553.)

Management of Anesthesia

Guidelines for anesthesia for patients with GSD include careful monitoring of glucose and provision of exogenous glucose during fasting periods and evaluation of cardiac and hepatic function. The degree of organ dysfunction varies among the different types of GSD.

Type I (von Gierke disease, glucose-6-phosphatase deficiency): These patients do not tolerate fasting and should have preoperative intravenous glucose fluid therapy. Hypoglycemia, acidosis, and seizures are common. Platelet dysfunction may occur. Cardiac dysrhythmias and cardiac arrest may occur secondary to lactic acidosis.

Type II (Pompe disease, lysosomal acid glucosidase deficiency): The infantile form has an extremely poor prognosis and cardiac arrest can occur during the perioperative period.[64,65] Regional anesthesia may be an attractive alternative to general anesthesia for infants with Pompe's disease. Glycogen infiltration of cardiac muscle causes concentric hypertrophy. Measurement of left ventricular mass by echocardiography provides a good estimate of left ventricular hypertrophy. Changes in preload, afterload, heart rate, and diastolic blood pressure can lead to cardiac arrest.

Type III (Forbes or Cori disease, glycogen debranching enzyme deficiency): Hepatomegaly, muscle weakness, and cardiomyopathy are common. Fasting causes ketotic hypoglycemia. Anesthetic considerations include macroglossia, hypotonia, increased sensitivity to non-depolarizing muscle relaxants, and hypertrophic cardiomyopathy.

Type IV (Andersen disease, branching enzyme deficiency): Glycogen accumulates in the liver, heart, muscle, and nerves. Clinical manifestations are diverse. The severe infantile form is characterized by hepatosplenomegaly, cirrhosis, hypotonia, and failure to thrive. Manifestations of progressive forms include cirrhosis, portal hypertension, esophageal varices, and dilated cardiomyopathy. A neuromuscular variant with sensory and motor deficits, weakness, and dementia has been described.

Type V (McArdle disease, muscle glycogen phosphorylase deficiency): Muscle cramping with exercise is characteristic of McArdle disease. Rhabdomyolysis and myoglobinuria can occur after exertion or succinylcholine administration. Rhabdomyolysis may occur after cardiopulmonary bypass. Tourniquets should be avoided.

Type VI (Hers disease, hepatic phosphorylase deficiency): Relatively benign disease with normal muscle and cardiac physiology. Symptoms improve with age.

Type VII (Tarui disease, muscle phosphofructokinase deficiency): Clinical manifestations with muscle cramps, exercise intolerance, and episodic myoglobinuria are similar to those of McArdle disease. No hepatic or cardiac involvement.

Type IX (hepatic glycogen phosphorylase kinase deficiency): Patients have short stature, hypotonia, muscle cramping, and exertional myoglobinuria.

Type XI (Fanconi–Bickel syndrome, glucose transporter enzyme deficiency): Patients have short stature, hepatomegaly, fasting hypoglycemia, and proximal renal tubular acidosis.

Type 0 (hepatic glycogen synthase deficiency): Type 0 is characterized by short stature, fasting hypoglycemia, seizures, and severe developmental delay. Preoperative fasting may cause severe ketotic hypoglycemia.

Mucopolysaccharidoses

The mucopolysaccharidoses (MPS) are the result of a deficiency of lysosomal enzymes that cleave mucopolysaccharides (glycosaminoglycans). An accumulation of mucopolysaccharides occurs in the brain, heart, liver, bone, cornea, and tracheobronchial tree. There are seven types and several subtypes of MPS (Table 23-13). The clinical manifestations may be severe and present in infancy or may be mild and become evident in adulthood.

The musculoskeletal manifestations are the most visible and include coarse facial features (gargoylism), stiff joints, chest deformity (thoracolumbar kyphoscoliosis), and dwarfism. Infiltration and opacification of the cornea causes visual impairment. Imaging of the cervical spine may reveal asymptomatic odontoid hypoplasia.

Deposition of mucopolysaccharides in cardiac valves, coronary arteries, and myocardium can cause valvular dysfunction, cardiac dysrhythmias, myocardial ischemia, dilated cardiomyopathy, and narrowing of the great vessels.[66] Echocardiography can provide useful information about valvular and ventricular function.

Upper airway abnormalities include macroglossia, epiglottic stiffness, tracheal compression, and bronchial narrowing. Obstructive sleep apnea secondary to adenotonsillar hypertrophy may require excision of tonsils and adenoids, uvulopalatoplasty, or tracheostomy.

There is no specific therapy for MPS. Enzyme replacement therapy, stem cell transplantation, and bone marrow transplantation have been employed with some success. Most therapy is directed at reducing the impact of mucopolysaccharide deposition on organ function.

TABLE 23-13. CLASSIFICATION OF MUCOPOLYSACCHARIDOSES

Type I (H)
Eponym: Hurler
Enzyme defect: α-L-iduronidase
Clinical features: Macrocephaly, coarse facies, short neck, odontoid hypoplasia, macroglossia, cardiomegaly, mitral regurgitation, coronary intimal thickening, cardiomegaly, mental retardation, death <14 years of age

Type I (S)
Eponym: Scheie
Enzyme defect: α-L-iduronidase
Clinical features: Normal intelligence, mild coarse facies, macroglossia, prognathia, short neck, aortic regurgitation

Type I (H/S)
Eponym: Hurler—Scheie
Enzyme defect: α-L-iduronidase
Clinical features: Macrocephaly, macroglossia, micrognathia, coarse facies, short neck, mitral and aortic regurgitation

Type II
Eponym: Hunter
Enzyme defect: Iduronidate-2-sulfatase
Clinical features: Variable course, survival to adulthood, +/– mental retardation, macrocephaly, coarse facies, short neck, hydrocephalus, ischemic cardiomyopathy

Type IIIA
Eponym: San Filippo
Enzyme defect: Heparan-N-sulfatase
Clinical features: Aggressive behavior, coarse facies, short stature, lumbar vertebral dysplasia, minimal to no cardiac effects

Type IIIB
Eponym: San Fillippo
Enzyme defect: α-N-acetyl-glucose-amidase
Clinical features: Progressive dementia, seizures, survival to second or third decade, mild coarse facies, stiff joints, gait disturbance, minimal to no cardiac effects

Type IIIC
Eponym: San Filippo
Enzyme defect: α-N-acetyl-glucose aminidase, N-acetyltransferase
Clinical features: Mild coarse facies, stiff joints, gait disturbance, minimal to no cardiac effects

Type IIID
Eponym: San Filippo
Enzyme defect: N-acetyl-glucosamine-6-sulfatase
Clinical features: Coarse hair, normal stature, mild coarse facies, stiff joints gait disturbance, minimal to no cardiac effects

Type IVA
Eponym: Morquio
Enzyme defect: N-acetyl-galastosamine-6-sulfatase
Clinical features: Trunk type dwarfism, skeletal dysplasia, short stature, mild coarse facies, joint laxity, odontoid hypoplasia, short neck,
C1-C2 subluxation, aortic regurgitation

Type IVB
Eponym: Morquio
Enzyme defect: β-galactosidase
Clinical features: same as type IVA

Type VI
Eponym: Maroteaux–Lamy
Enzyme defect: N-acetyl-galactosamine-4-sulfatase
Clinical features: Hurler appearance, normal intelligence, macrocephaly, coarse facies, macroglossia, odontoid hypoplasia, short stature, mitral and aortic regurgitation

Type VII
Eponym: Sly
Enzyme defect: β-glucuronidase
Clinical features: Macrocephaly, coarse facies, odontoid hypoplasia, stiff joints, short stature, mitral and aortic regurgitation, aortic dissection

Management of Anesthesia

Preoperative evaluation is focused on examination of the upper airway and assessment of cardiopulmonary function. Airway management can be quite challenging. Difficult laryngoscopy should be anticipated and the risk of airway complications including failed intubation and death are increased.[67] Laryngoscopy is complicated by thick, noncompressible soft tissue of the upper airway, macroglossia, copious airway secretions, and bony deformities of the head and neck. Overextension of the neck during laryngoscopy in patients with odontoid hypoplasia increases the risk of spinal cord compression. Variable success has been reported with supraglottic airways and videolaryngoscopes. All options for airway management should be readily available. Postobstructive pulmonary edema has been reported in patients with MPS.

TABLE 23-14. TYPES OF OSTEOGENESIS IMPERFECTA

Type 1
Inheritance: Autosomal dominant
Severity: Mild, nondeforming, long-term survival
Manifestations: Increased risk of fractures, short stature, blue sclerae, hearing impairment
Special anesthetic considerations: Abnormal dentition

Type II
Inheritance: Autosomal dominant
Severity: Death in utero or within first month of life
Manifestations: Multiple in utero fractures, micromelia, small thorax, respiratory failure
Special anesthetic considerations:

Type III
Inheritance: Autosomal dominant
Severity: Progressive deforming, death in the second to fourth decade of life
Manifestations: Multiple fractures, growth retardation, kyphoscoliosis, vertebral compression
Special anesthetic considerations: Airway anomalies

Type IV
Inheritance: Autosomal dominant
Severity: Moderately deforming, long-term survival
Manifestations: In utero fractures, fractures with minor trauma, bowing of lower extremities with weight bearing
Special anesthetic considerations: Abnormal dentition, midface and mandibular deformity

Type V
Inheritance: Autosomal dominant
Severity: Moderately deforming, long-term survival
Manifestations: In utero fractures, fractures with minor trauma, bowing of lower extremities with weight bearing
Special anesthetic considerations: Midface and mandibular deformity

Type VI
Inheritance: Autosomal recessive
Severity: Moderately to severely deforming, long-term survival
Manifestations: In utero fractures, fractures with minor trauma, bowing of lower extremities with weight bearing
Special anesthetic considerations: Midface and mandibular deformities

Cardiac involvement will influence the selection of anesthetic technique and choice of intraoperative monitors. Careful preoperative assessment of cardiac function is required for patients with certain types of MPS (e.g., Hurlers).

The variability of clinical abnormalities in patients with MPS requires individualized treatment of each patient. Some types of MPS produce severe airway and cardiac effects, while other types cause only minor dysfunction.

Osteogenesis Imperfecta

Osteogenesis imperfecta (OI) is a genetic disease that results from defective synthesis of type I collagen. Type I collagen is the primary component of the extracellular matrix of bone and skin. There are six types of OI and five of the six are inherited as autosomal dominants and one is autosomal recessive (Table 23-14). OI may produce only mild symptoms in some patients and can be fatal early in life in others. OI is a multisystem disease that manifests with brittle, easily fractured bones, osteoporosis, kyphoscoliosis, joint laxity, blue sclera, and tendon weakness. Cardiovascular abnormalities include mitral and aortic regurgitation, aortic dilation, and aortic dissection. Central nervous system manifestations such as headache, cranial nerve dysfunction, nystagmus, and quadriparesis can be secondary to craniovertebral instability, atlantoaxial subluxation, and hydrocephalus. Defective platelet aggregation can cause a coagulopathy.

Management of Anesthesia

Preoperative evaluation should focus on the airway and cervical range of motion. An echocardiogram may be indicated if there is a history or aortic dilation or valvular insufficiency. Megalocephaly and a short neck can make direct laryngoscopy difficult and alternative intubation techniques may be required. Great care must be taken with patient positioning to minimize the risk of bone fractures. Induction of anesthesia can be performed with inhalation or intravenous techniques. Regional anesthesia is generally avoided because of the risk of spinal damage; however, caudal analgesia has been used in selected patients.[68] Mild intraoperative temperature elevation can occur in OI patients. There is, however, no evidence that OI patients are at increased risk for malignant hyperthermia.[69]

ANEMIAS

Anemia is an absolute or relative deficiency in the concentration of circulating red blood cells. Anemias are classified as nutritional, hemolytic, and genetic (Table 23-15). Compensatory mechanisms develop to offset the decreased oxygen carrying capacity of the blood (Table 23-16). In a healthy patient, symptoms do not develop until the hemoglobin level decreases below 7 g/dL. Symptoms are variable and depend on concurrent disease processes. There is no universally accepted hematocrit that demands transfusion. The patient's physiologic condition and coexisting diseases must be factored into a subjective decision.

Nutritional Deficiency Anemias

The three primary causes of nutritional deficiency anemia are iron deficiency, vitamin B_{12} deficiency, and folic acid deficiency. Chronic illness, cancer, and poor dietary intake can result in

TABLE 23-15. TYPES OF ANEMIA

Nutritional
Iron deficiency
Vitamin B_{12} deficiency
Folic acid deficiency
Anemia of chronic illness
Hemolytic
Spherocytois
Glucose-6-phosphate dehydrogenase deficiency
Immune-mediated
Drug-induced ABO incompatibility
Hemoglobinopathies
Hemoglobin S (sickle cell)
Thalassemia major (Cooley's anemia)
Thalassemia intermedia
Thalassemia minor

nutritional anemia. Seventy-five percent of critically ill patients are anemic. Hepcidin, a peptide secreted by the liver, inhibits erythropoiesis by suppressing the release of iron.[70] Hepcidin production is increased during inflammation and can produce anemia in chronically ill patients. The development of hepcidin antagonists might be effective for correction of anemia in critically ill patients without transfusion.

Iron deficiency anemia produces a microcytic, hypochromic red blood cell (RBC). Iron deficiency anemia may be an absolute deficiency secondary to decreased oral intake or a relative deficiency caused by a rapid turnover of RBCs (e.g., chronic blood loss, hemolysis).

Megaloblastic anemia can be caused by vitamin B_{12} (cobalamin) deficiency, folate deficiency, or refractory bone marrow disease. Absorption of vitamin B_{12} by the gastrointestinal tract depends on the release of intrinsic factor, a glycoprotein secreted by gastric parietal cells. Atrophy of gastric mucosa causes vitamin B_{12} deficiency and megaloblastic anemia. Chronic gastritis and gastric atrophy may be caused by autoantibodies to gastric parietal cells. Vitamin B_{12} deficiency can also interfere with myelination and cause CNS dysfunction. The typical clinical presentation is a peripheral neuropathy with symmetric loss of proprioception and vibratory sensation in the lower extremities. These abnormalities are secondary to degeneration of the lateral and posterior spinal cord columns. Administration of parenteral vitamin B_{12} reverses both the hematologic and neurologic changes in adults. The neuropathy of vitamin B_{12} deficiency must be considered when regional or peripheral nerve blocks are performed. The clinical effect of nitrous oxide on vitamin B_{12} metabolism is controversial. Nitrous oxide inactivates the vitamin B_{12} component of methionine synthetase and prolonged exposure to nitrous oxide produces megaloblastic anemia and neurologic changes similar to pernicious anemia. In susceptible patients (chronic illness, elderly patients), there is also evidence that an exposure of short duration can cause megaloblastic red cell changes.[71] Whether nitrous oxide causes postoperative neurologic dysfunction is controversial; however, the number of case reports of neuropathy associated with nitrous oxide exposure has increased.

TABLE 23-16. COMPENSATORY MECHANISMS TO INCREASE OXYGEN DELIVERY WITH CHRONIC ANEMIA

Increased cardiac output
Increased RBC 2,3-diphosphoglycerate
Increased P-50
Increased plasma volume
Decreased blood viscosity

Folic acid deficiency also produces megaloblastic anemia. Peripheral neuropathy may occur, but is not as common as with vitamin B_{12} deficiency. Causes of folic acid deficiency include alcoholism, pregnancy, and malabsorption syndromes. Methotrexate and phenytoin are known to interfere with folic acid absorption.

Hemolytic Anemias

The life span of a normal erythrocyte is 120 days. Abnormalities in the erythrocyte may result in premature destruction and hemolysis of the cell. Causes of hemolytic anemia include structural erythrocyte abnormalities, enzyme deficiencies, and immune-mediated hemolysis.

Hereditary Spherocytosis

Spherocytosis, elliptocytosis, pyropoikilocytosis, and stomatocytosis are four types of hereditary membrane defects resulting in abnormally shaped red blood cells (RBC).

Spherocytosis is the most common of the RBC membrane defects and is caused by an abnormality in the proteins that form the skeleton of the RBC membrane. The RBC is rounded and more fragile than the normal biconcave RBC. The spleen destroys the abnormal RBCs and chronic anemia develops. Cholelithiasis from chronic hemolysis and elevation of the serum bilirubin occur. Hemolytic crises accompanied by anemia, emesis, and abdominal pain can be triggered by infection or folic acid deficiency.

Splenectomy has been the treatment of choice for patients with hereditary spherocytosis. Splenectomy is usually delayed until the patient is 6 years of age to decrease the risk of post-splenectomy infection. More recent evidence suggests that splenectomy carries a lifelong increased risk of infection and an increased risk of adverse vascular events such as myocardial infarction, stroke, pulmonary embolism, and portal vein thrombosis.

Glucose-6-phosphate Dehydrogenase Deficiency

Glucose-6-phosphate dehydrogenase (G6PD) is the most common enzymopathy in humans and afflicts 400 million people worldwide. G6PD deficiency may confer malarial resistance and the distribution of this variant parallels the distribution of malaria. African-Americans, Africans, Asians, Indians, and Mediterranean populations are susceptible to G6PD deficiency. G6PD initiates the pentose monophosphate shunt that begins the metabolism of glucose in the RBC. This pathway in which glucose is converted to pentoses and nicotinamide-adenine dinucleotide phosphate (NADPH) is abnormal and without NADPH, the RBC is vulnerable to damage by oxidation. A deficiency of G6PD results in decreased levels of glutathione when the RBC is exposed to oxidants. This increases the rigidity of the RBC membrane and accelerates clearance of the cell from the circulation. The biochemistry of G6PD deficiency is complex and more than 400 biochemical variants of G6PD have been identified.[72] There are five classes

TABLE 23-17. DRUGS THAT CAN PRODUCE HEMOLYSIS IN PATIENTS WITH GLUCOSE-6-PHOSPHATE DEHYDROGENASE DEFICIENCY

Phenacetin	Nalidixic acid
Aspirin (high doses)	Isoniazid
Penicillin	Primaquine
Streptomycin	Quinine
Chloramphenicol	Quinidine
Sulfacetamide	Doxorubicin
Sulfanilamide	Methylene blue
Sulfapyridine	Nitrofurantoin

of G6PD deficiency based on the G6PD enzyme activity: Class I: Severely deficient (chronic hemolytic anemia), Class II: 1% to 10% activity, Class III: 10% to 60% activity, Class IV: 60% to 150% activity, and Class V: >150% activity.

The primary clinical manifestation is acute hemolysis that can be triggered by conditions that place oxidative stress on RBCs: Infection, drug exposure, or ingestion of fava beans. Signs and symptoms include anemia, headache, substernal and abdominal pain, back pain, jaundice, tachycardia, and fatigue.

There are a number of drugs and chemicals (naphthalene) that enhance the destruction of RBCs in patients with G6PD deficiency (Table 23-17). Because of variation in G6PD deficiencies, the severity of clinical manifestations is also highly variable. Hemolysis typically begins 2 to 5 days after drug exposure. The hemolysis is self-limited as only the older RBCs are affected. Some drugs produce hemolysis only with high doses (e.g., aspirin). Patients with G6PD deficiency are unable to reduce methemoglobin produced by sodium nitrate; therefore, sodium nitroprusside and prilocaine should not be administered. Anesthetic drugs have not been implicated as hemolytic agents; however, early postoperative evidence of hemolysis might suggest a G6PD deficiency.[73]

Pyruvate Kinase Deficiency

Pyruvate kinase (PK) is a glycolytic enzyme in the Embden–Meyerhof pathway that produces pyruvate and adenosine triphosphate (ATP). A deficiency of PK results in potassium leakage from the RBC membrane, thereby increasing its rigidity and accelerating RBC destruction by the spleen.

Clinically, the PK deficient patient exhibits anemia, cholelithiasis, and splenomegaly. The degree of anemia varies from very mild to a severe, transfusion, dependent anemia. These clinical features are very similar to those in patients with spherocytosis. There are no special considerations for anesthesia other than those for any patient with chronic anemia.

Immune Hemolytic Anemia

The immune hemolytic anemias are characterized by immunologic alterations in the RBC membrane and are caused by infection, disease, or RBC sensitization. There are three types of immune hemolytic anemia: Autoimmune, drug-induced, and alloimmune (RBC sensitization). Mechanisms of immune hemolytic anemia can be complex and of many types. Autoimmune hemolytic anemia includes both warm and cold antibody hemolytic anemia. Cold autoimmune hemolytic anemia is of special concern to the anesthesiologist because of the likelihood that the cold operating room environment or hypothermia during cardiopulmonary bypass (CPB) may initiate hemolysis. Cold hemagglutinin disease is caused by IgM autoantibodies that react with I antigens of RBCs. Plasmapheresis to reduce the titer of cold antibody is recommended before hypothermic procedures such as CPB. Collagen vascular diseases, solid organ transplantation, blood transfusion, neoplasia, and infection can produce immune hemolysis by a variety of mechanisms including warm and cold antibody mediated hemolysis.

There are three types of drug-induced immune hemolysis: Autoantibody, hapten-induced, and immune complex.[74] Hemolysis induced by α-methyldopa is of the autoimmune type mediated by an IgG antibody that does not fix complement. The hapten-induced type is characteristic of a penicillin reaction. The immune complex type can occur after the administration of antimalarials, sulfonamides, isoniazid, phenacetin, acetaminophen, cephalosporins, tetracyclines, hydralazine, and hydrochlorothiazide.

The classic example of alloimmune hemolysis (RBC sensitization) is hemolytic disease of the newborn produced by Rh sensitization. An Rh-negative mother with Rh antibodies produces hemolysis in an Rh-positive fetus. Differences in fetal and maternal ABO groups may cause hemolysis. This is unusual, however, because A and B antibodies are of the IgM class and do not readily cross the placenta.

Treatment of immune hemolytic anemia is initially with corticosteroids. Splenectomy and rituximab are effective in some patients.

Hemoglobinopathies

Hemoglobinopathies are diseases cause by genetic errors in hemoglobin synthesis. Normal hemoglobin is composed of four globin subunits: Two alpha (α) globins, and an additional globin pair that can be beta (β), delta (δ), or gamma (γ). Table 23-18 lists the many types of hemoglobin that may occur.

Illness is caused by anemia, accumulation of inappropriate hemoglobin precursors, immunocompromise, tissue infarction, and inflammation.

Many hemoglobinopathies convey survival protection in endemic malaria areas by decreasing RBC life span and promoting RBC turnover. The most common hemoglobinopathies are sickle cell disease (SCD), hemoglobin C, and the thalassemias. SCD and thalassemia together represent the most common severe genetic disorders in the world. The incidence of SCD is 1 in 600 and 8% to 10% of African-Americans have sickle cell trait.

TABLE 23-18. TYPES OF HEMOGLOBIN

Hemoglobin	Structure	Clinical Setting
Hemoglobin A	$\alpha 2\beta 2$	Normal adult hgb
Hemoglobin A2	$\alpha 2\delta 2$	Normal adult hgb variant
Hemoglobin F	$\alpha 2\gamma 2$	Normal fetal hemoglobin
Hemoglobin S	$\alpha 2\beta S2$	Sickle cell hemoglobin
Hemoglobin C	$\alpha 2\beta C2$	Hemoglobin C
Hemoglobin E	$\alpha 2\beta E2$	Hemoglobin E
Hemoglobin Bart's	$\gamma 4$	β thalassemia
Hemoglobin H	$\beta 4$	α thalassemia

TABLE 23-19. MECHANISMS OF CELLULAR AND TISSUE INJURY IN SICKLE CELL DISEASE

Erythrocyte and platelet adhesion to endothelium
Activation of coagulation system with thrombosis and ischemia
Reperfusion injury
Leukocytosis and immune system activation
Free radical injury secondary to leukocyte superoxide release
Decreased nitric oxide secondary to leukocyte superoxide release
Activation of cytokine and inflammatory mediators
Hemolysis and release of free hemoglobin
Free radical injury secondary to free hemoglobin
Decreased nitric oxide due to uptake by free hemoglobin
Endothelial dysfunction secondary to inflammation and nitric oxide depletion
Excessive iron stores secondary to repeated erythrocyte transfusion

Sickle Cell Disease

A single amino acid (valine) is substituted for glutamic acid on the β globin chain. The effect of this amino acid substitution on hemoglobin is profound. The most striking alteration occurs when hemoglobin S is exposed to low concentrations of oxygen. The hemoglobin molecule becomes unstable and polymerizes with other hemoglobin S molecules to form a crystalline gel that deforms the RBC into the characteristic sickle shape. The damaged RBC is more prone to hemolysis and removal by the spleen. RBC life span in SCD is 12 to 17 days compared to 120 days for normal RBCs. Many of the clinical manifestations of SCD can be explained by obstruction of small blood vessels, tissue ischemia, and chronic anemia. Other more insidious mechanisms, however, cause significant physiologic derangements that are responsible for the long-term effects of SCD (Table 23-19).

Patients with SCD display remarkable variability in disease severity. Some patients are plagued by early and frequent complications culminating in death at an early age, while others experience few symptoms. The one factor that correlates with lower disease severity is an elevated level of fetal hemoglobin. SCD can produce manifestations in every organ system (Table 23-20). There are a number of acute, recurrent, and severe problems associated with SCD: Vaso-occlusive crisis, acute chest syndrome, sequestration crisis, aplastic crisis, asthma, and pulmonary hypertension.

Vaso-occlusive crisis (VOC): VOC is often the first and most frequent manifestation of SCD and is secondary to tissue ischemia and infarction. The pain of VOC may be mild requiring oral analgesics, hydration, and rest or can be severe requiring hospitalization, parenteral narcotics, intravenous hydration, supplemental oxygen, and regional anesthesia.[75] The incidence of VOC in the perioperative period is 10%.

Acute Chest Syndrome (ACS): ACS represents the single greatest threat to the patient with SCD as the mortality is 1% to 20%.

TABLE 23-20. CLINICAL MANIFESTATIONS OF SICKLE CELL DISEASE

Hematologic	**Pulmonary**	**Renal**
Hemolytic anemia	Acute chest syndrome	Papillary necrosis
Aplastic anemia	Hypoxemia	Glomerular sclerosis
Leukocytosis	Pulmonary infarction	Renal failure
Spleen	Fibrosis	**Psychosocial**
Infarction	Asthma	Depression
Hyposplenism	Sleep apnea	Anxiety
Splenic sequestration	Thromboembolism	Substance abuse
Central Nervous System	Pneumonia	Narcotic dependence
Stroke		**Genitourinary**
Hemorrhage		Priapism
Aneurysm		Infection
Meningitis		**Hepatobiliary**
Musculoskeletal		Jaundice
Painful crises		Hepatitis
Bone marrow hyperplasia		Cirrhosis
Avascular necrosis		Cholelithiasis
Osteomyelitis		Cholestasis
Bone infarcts		**Eye**
Skeletal deformity		Retinopathy
Growth retardation		Hemorrhage
Cutaneous ulceration		Visual loss
Cardiac		**Immune system**
Cardiomegaly		Immunosuppression
Pulmonary hypertension		Leukocytosis
Cor pulmonale		
Diastolic dysfunction		
Cardiomyopathy		

The diagnosis of ACS can be made when there are new lung infiltrates on a chest radiograph in the presence of any of the following: Chest pain, cough, dyspnea, wheezing, or hypoxemia. Proposed mechanisms of ACS are thrombosis, embolism (clot and fat), and infection. The incidence of ACS is higher in children and may be related to infection. The treatment of ACS is supportive. A severe and potentially fatal manifestation of ACS is plastic bronchitis. The bronchial cast that is characteristic of plastic bronchitis acts as a foreign, obstructive body and emergent bronchoscopy may be required. The frequency of ACS after abdominal surgery is 10% to 20%. Factors associated with ACS in the postoperative period include pain, splinting, narcotic analgesia, and hypoventilation. The incidence of postoperative ACS is reduced with preoperative transfusion and postoperative incentive spirometry.[76]

Sequestration crisis: Sequestration crisis occurs when the splenic removal of RBCs exceeds the rate of RBC production. Severe anemia and hemodynamic instability can occur. A history of sequestration crisis may be an indication for early splenectomy.

Aplastic crisis: Patients with SCD must maintain a high and continuous rate of production of RBCs. Even mild bone marrow suppression can cause the rapid onset of anemia. Aplastic crisis occurs when the production of RBCs is suppressed by a viral infection (parovirus B19).

8 *Asthma and pulmonary hypertension:* Asthma (incidence: 50%) and pulmonary hypertension (incidence: 10%) are common in patients with SCD. Mortality of patients with SCD is increased when asthma and pulmonary hypertension are present.

It is not uncommon for the sickle cell gene to be combined with other abnormal hemoglobin genes. In patients with combined hemoglobinopathies, symptoms of SCD are usually present but are less severe than patients with homozygous SCD.

Therapy for patients with SCD includes oral penicillin prophylaxis, hydroxyurea, and pneumococcal vaccination. Daily administration of penicillin reduces the likelihood of pneumococcal infection in children less than 5 years of age. Hydroxyurea therapy reduces the incidence and severity of VOC and ACS. Yearly assessment of stroke risk with transcranial Doppler is indicated. Those patients with elevated cerebral blood flow velocity should be placed on a program of regular blood transfusion to reduce the risk of stroke.

Management of Anesthesia

Patients with SCD frequently require anesthesia and surgery and preoperative evaluation is directed at identifying which organs have been damaged. A preoperative hemoglobin level should be obtained. Patients receiving hydroxyurea may have myelosuppression and a complete blood count may be helpful. A preoperative echocardiogram is indicated in patients with limited physical activity, hypoxemia, respiratory distress, frequent episodes of VOC or ACS, or symptoms consistent with cor pulmonale. Common echocardiographic findings in patients with SCD include left ventricular hypertrophy, right ventricular dilation, and atrial enlargement.[77]

The need for preoperative RBC transfusion is dependent on the severity of SCD and the type of proposed surgery. Most patients with SCD can be adequately prepared with simple transfusion. The typical hemoglobin level in patients with SCD is 5 to 8 g/dL and transfusion is performed to raise the hemoglobin level to 10 g/dL. Exchange transfusion is indicated when the baseline hemoglobin level is high. Intraoperative RBC transfusion is employed to replace significant intraoperative blood loss and maintain a hemoglobin level of 10 g/dL. Preoperative exchange transfusion is commonly used for cardiac surgical procedures, but simple transfusion is used in some institutions. Cell saver blood salvage has been used without complication in SCD patients.

Other objectives of the intraoperative management of SCD patients include maintenance of normothermia and hydration with intravenous fluids. Extremity tourniquets can be used if they are critical to the performance of the surgery. The incidence of complication with tourniquet use in SCD patients is 12%. Pain and narcotic induced hypoventilation have been implicated as causes of postoperative ACS and strategies to provide analgesia without narcotics may reduce the incidence of ACS. Regional analgesia may be central to this strategy.

Surgery and anesthesia in patients with sickle cell trait (Hgb SA) are generally uneventful. Sudden death after intense physical activity has, however, been reported in patients with Hgb SA. It is conceivable that SA patients undergoing excessive perioperative physiologic stress could develop complications.

Thalassemia

Thalassemia is the result of underproduction of α or β globin chains of the hemoglobin molecule. Alpha thalassemia is the result of underproduction of α chains and beta thalassemia results from a deficiency of β chains. Inheritance of thalassemia is typically autosomal recessive, but the genetics is complex and thalassemia produces a wide spectrum of clinical manifestations. The reduced globin synthesis results in anemia secondary to a reduced concentration of hemoglobin in the RBC and decreased RBC production. Disease severity ranges from death in utero to a normal life expectancy with minimal problems. There are three clinical types of thalassemia: Thalassemia major, thalassemia intermedia, and thalassemia minor. The patient with thalassemia major requires regular RBC transfusion to maintain an adequate hemoglobin level. Patients with thalassemia intermedia require occasional transfusion and patients with thalassemia minor rarely require transfusion.

There are many factors that cause physiologic dysfunction in thalassemia patients. Severe anemia stimulates bone marrow proliferation producing widespread skeletal abnormalities. Spinal cord compression from extramedullary erythropoiesis can occur. Regular RBC transfusion to maintain a level of 10 g/dL suppresses bone marrow hyperplasia. Frequent blood transfusion does; however, cause iron overload that can cause cardiac, hepatic, immune, and endocrine dysfunction. Manifestations of cardiac iron overload include dysrhythmias, pulmonary hypertension, and congestive heart failure.[78,79] Hepatic complications include fibrosis and cirrhosis and an increased risk of hepatitis. Hypogonadism, diabetes, hypothyroidism, hypoparathyroidism, hypopituitarism, and adrenal insufficiency also result from iron overload. Macrophage dysfunction often leads to an increased risk of infection. Iron chelation therapy (deferoxamine, defereridone, and deferasirox) is used prophylactically to minimize the risk of iron overload.

Successful bone marrow transplantation is curative for some patients with thalassemia. Bone marrow transplantation is typically used for children that develop early and severe complications from thalassemia.

Management of Anesthesia

Patients with thalassemia often require cholecystectomy, splenectomy, vascular access, and correction of skeletal abnormalities. The preoperative evaluation should include a hemoglobin level and an evaluation of cardiac, hepatic, and endocrine function. Perioperative risk depends upon the severity of organ dysfunction secondary to thalassemia and iron overload. There is a high incidence of alloimmunization and blood should be cross-matched in advance of anticipated need.

Facial dysmorphism from extramedullary erythropoiesis can complicate airway management and direct laryngoscopy. The possibility of extramedullary bone marrow deposition in the spinal canal may be a relative contraindication to neuraxial anesthesia. Spinal anesthesia has, however, been successfully used for cesarean section. Cell saver RBC salvage has been successfully used for patients with thalassemia.

COLLAGEN VASCULAR DISEASES

The four most common collagen vascular diseases are rheumatoid arthritis, systemic lupus erythematosus, systemic sclerosis (scleroderma), and the inflammatory myopathies (dermatomyositis/polymyositis). Although many patients may have a discrete disease, many others are considered to have overlap syndromes (mixed connective tissue diseases) with features of different collagen vascular diseases. The etiology of the collagen vascular diseases is unknown, although the immune system is clearly involved in the cascade of pathologic events that cause the clinical manifestations. Although all of these diseases have effects on joints, each has diffuse systemic effects as well. The alteration in joint function and the systemic effects will affect the management of anesthesia.

TABLE 23-21. EXTRA-ARTICULAR MANIFESTATIONS OF RHEUMATOID ARTHRITIS

Skin
Raynaud's phenomenon
Digital necrosis

Eyes
Scleritis
Corneal ulceration

Lung
Pleural effusions
Pulmonary fibrosis

Heart
Pericarditis
Cardiac tamponade
Coronary arteritis
Aortic insufficiency

Kidney
Interstitial fibrosis
Glomerulonephritis
Amyloid deposition

Peripheral Nervous System
Compression syndromes
Mononeuritis

Central Nervous System
Dural nodules
Necrotizing vasculitis

Liver
Hepatitis

Blood

Anemia
Leukopenia

Rheumatoid Arthritis

Rheumatoid arthritis (RA) is a chronic, autoimmune and inflammatory disease characterized by symmetric polyarthropathy and diverse clinical effects. Although the etiology is unknown, research continues to delineate the pathogenesis. There are interactions between environmental factors and genetic susceptibility that initiates the process that causes RA. Activated endothelial cells attract adhesion molecules that bind to proteins and initiate a sequence of events that stimulate T cells and B lymphocytes. The release of cytokines (tumor necrosis factor, interleukin-1, interleukin-6) accelerates the inflammatory cascade.[80] B lymphocytes produce autoantibodies (rheumatoid factor) that further increase cytokine production. Seventy-five percent of RA patients have measurable levels of rheumatoid factor. The pathologic changes of RA begin with cellular hyperplasia of the synovium followed by invasion of lymphocytes, plasma cells, and fibroblasts. Cartilage and articular surfaces are ultimately destroyed.

The hands and wrists are involved first, particularly the metacarpophalangeal and interphalangeal joints. The knee is the most frequently involved joint of the lower extremity. The upper cervical spine is affected in 80% of patients with RA. Instability of the cervical spine may manifest as atlantoaxial instability, cranial settling, and subaxial instability. Plain radiography and CT of the cervical spine will demonstrate the bony changes caused by RA. MRI is better suited to study the effects on the spinal cord. The degree of cord compression may not, however, correlate with the patient's symptoms. Although a very rare event, spinal cord damage after laryngoscopy and tracheal intubation has been reported.[81] Intradural cord compression secondary to rheumatoid nodules or pannus formation can also occur. RA commonly affects the joints of the larynx, resulting in limitation of vocal cord movement and edema of the laryngeal mucosa that can progress to airway obstruction. Arthritic changes in the temporomandibular joints can also occur. All of these abnormalities can complicate laryngoscopy and tracheal intubation.

Extra-articular and systemic manifestations of RA are diverse
9 (Table 23-21). Cardiovascular disease is a common cause of mortality and there is a high incidence of subclinical cardiac dysfunction.[82] Pericarditis occurs in one-third of RA patients and can produce constrictive pericarditis or cardiac tamponade. Other cardiovascular manifestations include coronary artery disease, myocarditis, diastolic dysfunction, aortitis (aortic root dilation, aortic valve insufficiency), dysrhythmias, and pulmonary hypertension. Pulmonary changes include interstitial lung disease, reduced oxygen diffusion capacity, obstructive and restrictive lung disease, pulmonary nodules, and pleural effusions. Several of the antirheumatic drugs can cause or accentuate pulmonary dysfunction. Renal failure is a common cause of death and may be secondary to vasculitis, amyloidosis, and antirheumatic drugs. Mild anemia is present in almost all patients with RA. The anemia may be secondary to decreased erythropoiesis or a side effect of drug therapy.

Neurologic complications of RA include peripheral nerve compression from joint destruction and noncompressive neuropathies (mononeuritis multiplex) secondary to vasculitis of blood vessels supplying affected nerves (vasa nervorum). Cervical myelopathy may be secondary to cervical spine degeneration. Rheumatoid vasculitis can affect cerebral blood vessels resulting in headache, hemiparesis, aphasia, and confusion.

The disease process of immunoinflammation that causes RA is complex and monotherapy is unlikely to be completely successful. There are three groups of antirheumatic drugs: Nonsteroidal anti-inflammatory drugs (NSAIDs), corticosteroids, and disease modifying antirheumatic drugs (DMARDS). NSAIDs reduce inflammation and pain; however, they do little to affect the ultimate course of the disease. Corticosteroids are effective but the side effects associated with long-term use limit their usefulness. DMARDs are now the first line of therapy for the early treatment of RA. Methotrexate has proven to be very effective and is often the initial drug of choice. Less commonly used DMARDs include leflunomide, cyclosporine, azathioprine, gold, sulfasalzine, and hydroxychloroquine. Biologic DMARDs are directed at interrupting the early phases of the inflammatory process by inhibition of tumor necrosis factor (TNF), blockade of interleukin-1 and interleukin-6, and inhibition of T cells and B lymphocytes.[83] Potential side effects of the biologic DMARDs include an increased susceptibility to infection and cancer. Kinase inhibitors directed at inhibition of the intracellular triggers of inflammation are under investigation. Surgical procedures such as synovectomy, tenolysis, and joint replacement are performed to relieve pain and restore joint function.

Management of Anesthesia

RA is a multisystem disease with diverse clinical manifestations. Although joint disabilities are obvious, less evident are the effects of RA on heart, lungs, kidneys, liver, and CNS. The type and severity of systemic dysfunction must be considered when planning an anesthetic for the patient with RA.[84]

Arthritic changes in the temporomandibular joints, cricoaryte-
10 noid joints, and the cervical spine can render rigid, direct laryngoscopy and tracheal intubation difficult. The incidence of atlantoaxial subluxation may exceed 40% in RA patients and flexion of the neck can compress the spinal cord. Intubation techniques that minimize neck manipulation may be indicated. Such techniques include the use of video laryngoscopes, flexible fiberscopes, or awake intubation. Many patients with RA are asymptomatic with respect to disease of the cervical spine (Fig. 23-7). Preoperative imaging studies (radiography, CT, MRI) may be indicated if the degree of cervical involvement is unknown. Cricoarytenoid arthritis produces edema of the larynx and may decrease the size of the glottic inlet, necessitating the use of a smaller than predicted tracheal tube.

The degree of cardiopulmonary involvement by the rheumatoid process will certainly influence the selection of anesthetics and monitors. The need for postoperative ventilatory support should be anticipated if severe pulmonary disease is present.

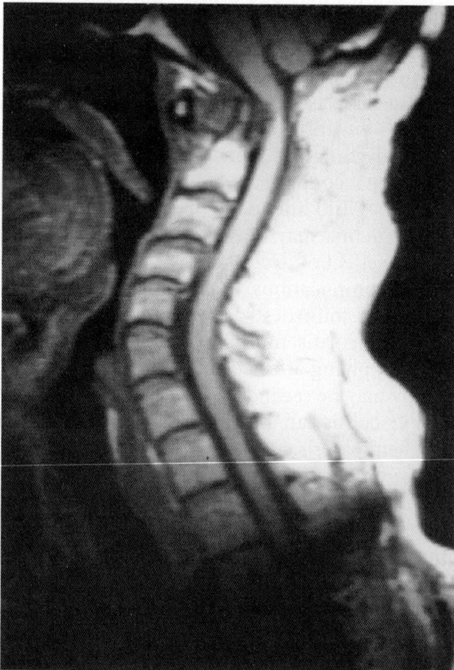

FIGURE 23-7. Magnetic resonance imaging of a cervical spine in a patient with rheumatoid arthritis. Although the patient had no neurologic symptoms, there is severe spinal stenosis in the upper cervical spine.

Perioperative corticosteroid supplementation may be necessary for patients receiving chronic steroid therapy. Aspirin and other anti-inflammatory drugs interfere with platelet function and clotting may be abnormal. Drug-induced anemia and hepatic and renal dysfunction may be present.

Restriction of joint mobility necessitates careful positioning of the patient during surgery. The extremities should be positioned to minimize the risk of neurovascular compression and further joint injury. Preoperative examination of joint motion will help determine how the extremities and neck should be positioned.

Systemic Lupus Erythematosus

Systemic lupus erythematosus (SLE) is an autoimmune disorder with diverse clinical and immunologic manifestations. The etiology of SLE is unknown, but appears to be a complex interaction between genetic susceptibility and hormonal and environmental influences. The typical patient with SLE is a female of childbearing age and of African or Asian ethnicity. Patients with SLE produce autoantibodies to DNA, RNA polymerase, cardiolipin, and ribosomal phosphoproteins. It has been speculated that cell apoptosis releases intracellular proteins that generate an antibody response in susceptible patients. Clinical manifestations in some patients can be the result of an autoantibody highly specific for one protein within an organ. Circulating antibodies may be present years before the onset of clinical symptoms.

The clinical manifestations of SLE are diverse and many can be life-threatening. The most common presenting features are polyarthritis and dermatitis. The arthritis is migratory and can involve any joint, including the joints of the cervical spine. The classic malar rash is present in only one-third of SLE patients. Renal disease is present in nearly 60% of SLE patients and is a common cause of morbidity and mortality. Dialysis or renal transplantation is required in 10% to 20% of SLE patients. Proteinuria, hypertension, and decreased creatinine clearance are the usual manifestations of lupus nephritis. CNS involvement occurs in 50% of SLE patients and is secondary to vasculitis. CNS manifestations include seizures, stroke, dementia, psychosis, myelitis, and peripheral neuropathy.

SLE produces a diffuse serositis that manifests as pleuritis and pericarditis. Although 60% of SLE patients have a pericardial effusion, cardiac tamponade is uncommon. Accelerated arteriosclerosis, cardiac conduction abnormalities, and ventricular dysfunction are other cardiac features of SLE. A noninfectious endocarditis (Libman–Sacks endocarditis) may cause mitral regurgitation. One-third of SLE patients have detectable antiphospholipid antibodies and may have thromboembolic complications. Pulmonary effects of SLE include pleural effusion, pneumonitis, pulmonary
4 hypertension, and pulmonary hemorrhage. There is a high incidence of pulmonary hypertension in SLE patients with Raynaud's phenomenon. Pulmonary function studies demonstrate a restrictive disease pattern and a decreased diffusion capacity. Hoarseness, stridor, and airway obstruction can be caused by cricoarytenoiditis. Gastrointestinal manifestations of SLE include esophageal dysmotility, peritonitis, pancreatitis, and bowel ischemia. An autoimmune hepatitis occurs in 10% of SLE patients.

Despite the diverse effects of SLE and the lack of specific therapy, current treatment regimens have improved survival. NSAIDs are used for mild arthritis. Antimalarials (hydroxychloroquine) control arthritis and dermatitis and have antithrombotic effects. Corticosteroids are effective for moderate and severe SLE. Immunosuppressants such as cyclophosphamide, azathioprine,

TABLE 23-22. ADVERSE EFFECTS OF DRUGS USED TO TREAT COLLAGEN VASCULAR DISEASES

Class of Drugs	Effects
Immunosuppressants	
Methotrexate	Hepatotoxicity, anemia, leucopenia
Azathioprine	Biliary stasis, leucopenia
Cyclosporine	Nephrotoxicity, hypertension, hypomagnesemia
Cyclophosphamide	Leucopenia, hemorrhagic cystitis, pseudocholinesterase inhibition
Leflunomide	Hepatotoxicity, weight loss, hypertension
Mycophenolate mofetil	Nausea, emesis, diarrhea
TNF Antagonists	
Etanercept	Infections, tuberculosis
Infliximab	Lymphoma, heart failure
Adalimumab	
Golimumab	
Certolizumab	
Interleukin-1 Antagonists	
Anakinra	Infection, skin irritation
Interleukin-6 Antagonists	
Tocilizumab	Infection, headache, stomatitis, fever
T-cell Inhibitors	
Abatacept	Infection
CD20 Monoclonal Antibody	
Rituximab	Infection, infusion reaction
Antimalarials	
Hydroxychloroquine	Myopathy, retinopathy
Corticosteroids	Hypertension, fluid retention, osteoporosis, infection, glucose intolerance
Aspirin	Platelet dysfunction, peptic ulcer, hypersensitivity
NSAIDs	Peptic ulcer, leucopenia, coronary artery disease
COX-2-inhibitors	Nephrotoxicity, cardiovascular dysfunction
Gold	Aplastic anemia, dermatitis, nephritis
Penicillamine	Glomerulonephritis, myasthenia, aplastic anemia

TNF, tumor necrosis factor; NSAIDs, nonsteroidal anti-inflammatory drugs; COX-2, cyclooxygenase-2.

methotrexate, and mycophenolate mofetil are effective and lower dosage requirements for corticosteroids. Immune-cell targeted therapy, interleukin inhibition, and TNF inhibitors are under investigation.[85] The potential for side effects from any of the SLE drugs is significant (Table 23-22).

More than 80 drugs have been reported to cause drug-induced lupus. Drug-induced lupus may be caused by drug metabolites that stimulate T cells. The most common agents are procaineamide, quinidine, hydralazine, methyldopa, enalapril, captopril, clonidine, isoniazid, and minocycline. The clinical features of drug-induced lupus are mild and include arthralgia, fever, anemia, and leucopenia. These effects resolve within weeks to months after drug discontinuation.

Management of Anesthesia

Careful preoperative evaluation of the SLE patient is necessary because of the diverse effects of the disease.[86] Preoperative chest radiography, echocardiography, or pulmonary function testing may be necessary if the clinical history suggests cardiopulmonary dysfunction. Myocardial dysfunction will certainly influence the choice of anesthetic and type of perioperative monitoring. Preoperative quantitation of renal function may be indicated. Although minor changes in hepatic function are often present, these changes are generally not significant. Patients with SLE are at increased risk for postoperative infections.

Arthritic involvement of the cervical spine is unusual and tracheal intubation is generally not difficult. The potential for laryngeal involvement and upper airway obstruction does, however, require clinical evaluation of laryngeal function. Should postextubation laryngeal edema or stridor occur, intravenous corticosteroids are effective.

Drugs for the treatment of SLE may influence the choice of anesthetics. Patients receiving corticosteroids will usually require the administration of corticosteroids during the perioperative period. Cyclophosphamide inhibits plasma cholinesterase and may prolong the response to succinylcholine.

Systemic Sclerosis (Scleroderma)

5

Systemic sclerosis (SSc) is characterized by changes in the microvasculature that lead to organ fibrosis. SSc is a multisystem disease that affects the skin, blood vessels, and internal organs. The cascade of events may begin with vasospasm and cell death. The release of cellular products initiates an autoimmune response with production of autoantibodies and activation of an inflammatory process that causes obliteration of small arteries with resultant fibrosis and atrophy of organs.[87]

The skin is swollen and thickened in the early phases of the disease. Eventually the skin becomes fibrotic and taut and joint motion is severely restricted. Raynaud's phenomenon is present in 85% of patients with SSc and is often the presenting symptom.

The same vasculopathy that affects the skin affects small vessels in other organs. The lung is affected in more than 80% of SSc patients and consists of interstitial fibrosis, pulmonary hypertension, and impaired diffusion capacity. These changes in conjunction with the effects of chronic aspiration pneumonitis produce restrictive lung disease. Myocardial fibrosis occurs in practically all SSc patients. The clinical manifestations of cardiac dysfunction, however, may be occult as only 25% of patients have symptoms. Echocardiography may reveal a decreased ejection fraction and impaired diastolic function. Degeneration of the cardiac conduction system may cause conduction delay and dysrhythmias. Pericardial effusion is common. Cardiac tamponade is rare.

Renal dysfunction is common and secondary to renal vasculopathy. Renal dysfunction can be so severe that a scleroderma renal crisis develops with hypertension, retinopathy, and a rapid deterioration in renal function.

Gastrointestinal motility is markedly decreased, especially in the esophagus. Frequent episodes of gastroesophageal reflux and aspiration pneumonitis exacerbate pulmonary dysfunction. Involvement of the small intestine and colon can cause pseudo-obstruction.

Therapy is directed at several pathways and may be organ specific. Corticosteroids are beneficial, but the likelihood of side effects is great. Cyclophosphamide is the immunosuppressant with the greatest effect. Vasodilators, ACE inhibitors and angiotensin receptor blockers, are used for the treatment of hypertension and cardiac dysfunction. Prostacyclin agonists, endothelin receptor blockers, cytokine inhibitors, and stem cell transplantation may also be used.

Management of Anesthesia

SSc, like other collagen vascular diseases, is a multisystem disease with many manifestations. There are no specific contraindications to any type of anesthesia. The anesthetic technique, however, must be guided by coexisting organ dysfunction.

Tracheal intubation can be quite difficult. Fibrotic and taut facial skin can markedly hinder active and passive motion of the temporomandibular joint. Awake, fiberoptic-assisted laryngoscopy may be required. Tracheostomy may be necessary in severely affected patients. Orotracheal intubation is preferred as the fragility of the nasal mucosa increases the risk of severe nasal hemorrhage from nasotracheal intubation.

Patients with SSc are at risk for aspiration pneumonitis dur-
11 ing induction of anesthesia because of esophageal dysmotility and gastroesophageal reflux. Chronic arterial hypoxemia is often present because of restrictive lung disease and impaired oxygen diffusion. Compromised myocardial function and coronary arteriosclerosis may necessitate the use of invasive cardiovascular monitors. Transesophageal echocardiography (TEE) can provide valuable information about cardiac function. Venous access can be challenging and central venous cannulation may be required. Myopathy is present in most patients with SSc and an increased sensitivity to muscle relaxants should be anticipated.

Regional anesthesia can be used, although the response to local anesthetics may be prolonged. The anesthesiologist is often consulted as to the efficacy of sympathetic blockade for the treatment of vasospasm secondary to Raynaud's phenomenon.

Inflammatory Myopathies (Dermatomyositis/Polymyositis)

Four diseases comprise the inflammatory myopathies: Dermatomyositis (DM), polymyositis (PM), inclusion body myositis, and autoimmune necrotizing myositis. Although the clinical features of the four diseases are diverse, severe muscle weakness and noninfectious muscle inflammation are present in all four.

Dermatomyositis (DM) is the most common of the four and is the result of an antibody-induced complement activation that lyses muscle capillaries and causes muscle necrosis. Common presenting features are proximal muscle weakness and a characteristic skin rash that may precede the onset of weakness. The skin rash consists of a purplish discoloration of the eyelids (heliotrope rash), periorbital edema, and scaly erythematous lesions on the knuckles (Gottron's papules). DM can occur in children and adults.[88] The presenting symptoms of polymyositis (PM) are muscle pain and proximal weakness that occur after the second decade of life. Fifty percent of DM and PM patients have pulmonary disease. The pulmonary manifestations are interstitial pneumonitis, alveolitis, and bronchopneumonia. Aspiration pneumonia is very common. Intrinsic lung disease and thoracic muscle weakness produce a restrictive pulmonary pattern and decreased oxygen diffusion capacity. Myocardial fibrosis can cause congestive heart failure and dysrhythmias. Patients with DM and PM are at increased risk for cancer.

Treatment of DM and PM is with corticosteroids, intravenous immunoglobulin, immunosuppressants, and immunomodulators.

Inclusion body myositis typically presents with weakness of the quadriceps and ankle dorsiflexors in men >50 years of age. There is no effective treatment.

Management of Anesthesia

The reported experience with anesthesia in patients with inflammatory myopathies is limited and generalizations from a few case reports must be interpreted with caution.

Patients with DM may have restriction of motion of the temporomandibular joints and decreased mouth opening that render rigid, direct laryngoscopy difficult. An awake, fiberoptic-assisted intubation may be required. Tracheal intubation is not usually difficult in patients with PM.

Dysphagia and gastroesophageal reflux are common and there is an increased risk of aspiration pneumonitis. Gastrointestinal perforations that require surgical intervention are common in patients with PM.

The degree of coexisting cardiopulmonary disease will influence the selection of anesthetics and monitors. Cardiac dysfunction may be subclinical and preoperative echocardiography may be beneficial.

It should be anticipated that variation in response to muscle relaxants will occur. It may be prudent to avoid succinylcholine as hyperkalemia may occur. Succinylcholine has, however, been administered to patients with DM without complication.[89] Short-acting non-depolarizing muscle relaxants would be a better choice. Postoperative mechanical ventilation may be required for patients with coexisting muscle weakness and lung disease.

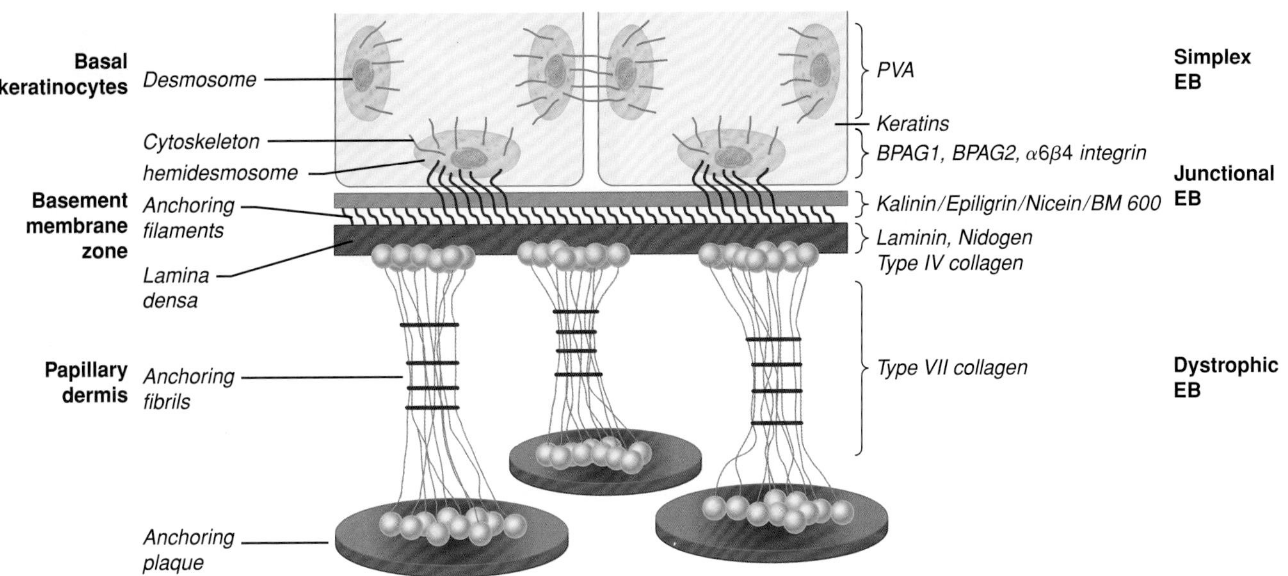

FIGURE 23-8. The ultrastructure of the zones of the skin. The diagram demonstrates where skin separation occurs in different types of epidermolysis bullosa (EB). (Reproduced from: Uitto J, Christiano AM. Molecular genetics of the cutaneous basement membrane zone. *J Clin Invest.* 1992;90:687–692, with permission.)

SKIN DISORDERS

Most primary diseases of the skin are localized and cause few systemic effects or complications during the administration of anesthesia. Two blistering skin diseases can result in perioperative complications: Epidermolysis bullosa and pemphigus.

Epidermolysis Bullosa

6 Epidermolysis bullosa (EB) is a rare skin disease that can be inherited or acquired. Patients with heritable forms have abnormalities in the anchoring systems of skin layers. The acquired forms are autoimmune disorders in which autoantibodies are produced that destroy the basement membrane of the skin and mucosa. The end result is the loss or absence of normal intercellular bridges and separation of skin layers, intradermal fluid accumulation, and bullae formation (Fig. 23-8). Lateral shearing forces applied to the skin are especially damaging; whereas, pressure applied perpendicular to the skin is not as hazardous. Although there are 30 subtypes of EB, these disorders can be classified into four groups depending on where the skin separation occurs: Epidermolysis simplex (EBS), junctional epidermolysis (JEB), epidermolysis bullosa dystrophica (DEB), and Kindler syndrome (mixed EB).[90] Although serious complications can occur with any form of epidermolysis, EBS is generally benign. Some types of JEB are lethal by 1 year of age and can have laryngeal involvement.

DEB is caused by a defect in type VII collagen. DEB produces severe scarring of the fingers and toes with pseudosyndactyly formation (Fig 23-9). Secondary infection of bullae and malignant 12
degeneration of the skin are common. The esophagus is commonly involved with resultant dysphagia, esophageal strictures, and poor nutrition. Dilated cardiomyopathy with a markedly decreased ejection fraction and formation of intracardiac thrombi can develop. Serial echocardiography may be indicated.[91] Glomerulonephritis may be secondary to streptococcal infection and is manifest by nephritis and albuminuria. Anemia is usually present as a result of poor nutrition and recurrent infection. Hypoplasia of tooth enamel causes carious degeneration of the teeth and the need for extensive dental restorations. Patients with DEB rarely survive beyond the third decade of life.

Medical therapy for DEB has not been very successful. Phenytoin, a collagenase inhibitor may produce short-term improvement. Gene therapy injection of fibroblasts and stem cell therapy are under investigation. Surgical therapy is directed at preservation and improvement of hand function.

Management of Anesthesia

It is critical that trauma to the skin and mucous membranes be minimized during the intraoperative period. Gel pads or needle electrodes can be used for ECG monitoring. The blood pressure cuff should be well padded with a loose cotton dressing, and intravascular catheters anchored with sutures or a gauze dressing rather than tape. Trauma from a face mask can be minimized by generous lubrication of the mask or the use of silicone-based padding at points of pressure application.[92] Frictional trauma to the oropharynx can result in the formation of large intraoral bullae, airway obstruction, and hemorrhage from denuded mucosa. All airway instruments should be well lubricated. Scarring of the oral cavity can cause microstomia and immobility of the tongue that increases the difficulty of tracheal intubation. Fiberoptic-assisted laryngoscopy may be required. Tracheal intubation is generally safe for patients with DEB.

Surgical procedures that are typically performed in patients with DEB include reconstructive hand procedures, dental restorations, esophageal dilation, and feeding gastrostomies. The possibility of an unrecognized cardiomyopathy and interactions with anesthetics must be considered. Many patients with DEB have decreased levels of physical activity from limb deformities and their history of exercise tolerance may be inaccurate. Ketamine may be useful for extremity procedures as it provides good

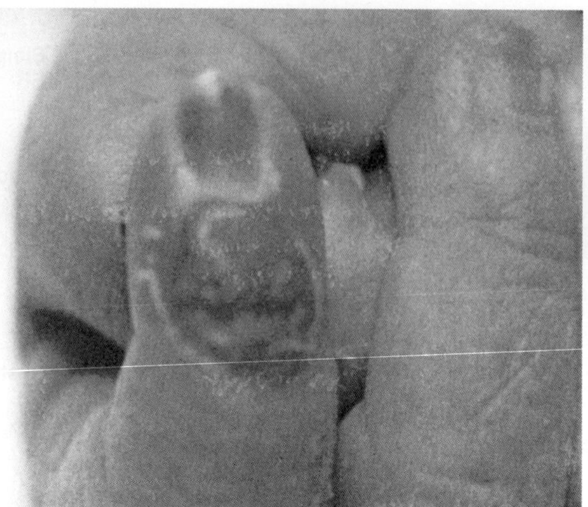
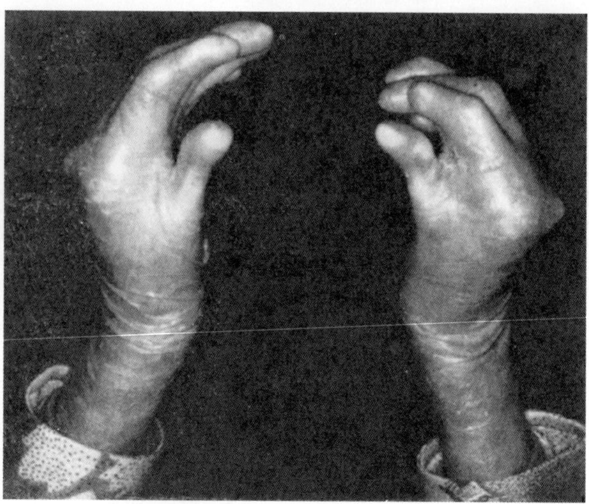

FIGURE 23-9. Epidermolysis bullosa. **(A)** Bullous lesion of the finger in a neonate with epidermolysis bullosa. **(B)** Hands of an older child with epidermolysis progression to produce severe scarring and pseudosyndactyly. (Courtesy of James E. Bennett, MD, Division of Plastic Surgery, Indiana University School of Medicine, Indianapolis, IN.)

analgesia and may not require supplementation with inhaled anesthetics. Regional anesthesia, including spinal, epidural, and brachial plexus anesthesia has been used successfully for patients with DEB.

Despite all the potential complications with anesthesia for patients with DEB, intraoperative management is associated with surprisingly few adverse effects. This is especially true when care is provided at a center experienced with the management of patients with DEB.[93]

Pemphigus

7 Pemphigus is an autoimmune vesiculobullous disease that involves extensive areas of the skin and mucous membranes. IgG autoantibodies attack desmosomal proteins, desmoglein 3 and desmoglein 1, leading to loss of cell adhesion and separation of epithelial layers. There are five types of pemphigus: Pemphigus vulgaris, pemphigus foliaceous, pemphigus erythematosus, drug-induced pemphigus, and paraneoplastic pemphigus. Drugs that have been implicated as causing pemphigus include penicillamine, cephalosporins, ACE inhibitors, phenobarbital, propranolol, levodopa, nifedipine, and NSAIDs.

Pemphigus vulgaris (PV) is the most common type and is of the most importance to the anesthesiologist because of the occurrence of oral lesions. Oral lesions develop in 50% to 70% of patients with PV. Lesions of the pharynx, larynx, esophagus, conjunctiva, urethra, cervix, and anus can develop. Oropharyngeal lesions can make eating so painful that malnutrition develops. Skin denudation and bullae formation can cause significant fluid and protein losses and increase the risk of secondary infection.[94] As with epidermolysis bullosa, lateral shearing force is more likely to produce bullae than pressure perpendicular to the skin surface. Systemic corticosteroids are the most effective treatment for PV. Improvement may be seen within days of corticosteroid therapy with full healing in 6 to 8 weeks. Immunosuppressants, immunomodulators, and intravenous immunoglobulin can be used to reduce corticosteroid doses.

Paraneoplastic pemphigus is associated with a number of malignant tumors, especially lymphomas and leukemias. IgG antibodies are produced that react to desmoglein 3 and 1. Oral and cutaneous lesions occur. Obstructive respiratory failure may result from inflammation and sloughing of tracheal tissue.

Management of Anesthesia

Preoperative drug therapy and the extreme fragility of the mucous membranes are the primary concerns for management of anesthesia for patients with PV. Corticosteroid supplementation will be necessary during the perioperative period if the patient's therapy includes steroids. Management of the airway and tracheal intubation should be performed as described for patients with DEB.

There are no specific contraindications to the use of any intravenous or inhaled anesthetic. Ketamine and regional anesthesia have been used for PV patients. Methotrexate may produce hepatorenal dysfunction and bone marrow suppression and cyclophosphamide can prolong the action of succinylcholine by inhibiting cholinesterase activity.

References

1. Emery AE. The muscular dystrophies. *Lancet*. 2002;359:687–695.
2. Spurney CF. Cardiomyopathy of Duchene muscular dystrophy: Current understanding and future directions. *Muscle Nerve*. 2011;44:8–19.
3. Finsterer J, Stöllberger C. Cardiac involvement in Becker muscular dystrophy. *Can J Cardiol*. 2008;24:786–792.
4. Caron M-J, Girard F, Girard DC, et al. Cisatracurium pharmacodynamics in patients with oculopharyngeal muscular dystrophy. *Anesth Analg*. 2005;100: 393–397.
5. Klingler W, Lehmann-Horn F, Jurkat-Rott K. Complications of anaesthesia in neuromuscular disorders. *Neuromuscul Disord*. 2005;15:191–206.
6. Veyckemans F. Can inhalation agent be used in the presence of a child with myopathy? *Curr Opin Anaesthesiol*. 2010;23:348–355.
7. Gurnaney H, Brown A, Litman RS. Malignant hyperthermia and muscular dystrophies. *Anesth Analg*. 2009;109:1043–1048.
8. Kaminsky P, Poussel M, Pruna L, et al. Organ dysfunction and muscular disability in myotonic dystrophy type 1. *Medicine (Baltimore)*. 2011;90:262–268.
9. Bhakta D, Groh MR, Shen C, et al. Increased mortality with left ventricular systolic dysfunction and heart failure in adults with myotonic dystrophy type 1. *Am Heart J*. 2010;160:1137–1141.
10. Weingarten TN, Hofer RE, Milone M, et al. Anesthesia and myotonic dystrophy type 2: A case series. *Can J Anaesth*. 2010;57:248–255.

11. Kirzinger L, Schmidt A, Kornblum C, et al. Side effects of anesthesia in DM2 as compared to DM1: A comparative retrospective study. *Eur J Neurol.* 2010;17: 842–845.
12. Mathieu J, Allard P, Gobeil G, et al. Anesthetic and surgical complications in 219 cases of myotonic dystrophy. *Neurol.* 1997;49:1646–1650.
13. Owen PM, Chu C. Emergency caesarean section in a patient with myotonic dystrophy: A case of failed postoperative extubation in a patient with mild disease. *Anaesth Intensive Care.* 2011;39:293–298.
14. White RJ, Bass SP. Myotonic dystrophy and paediatric anaesthesia. *Pediatr Anaesth.* 2003;13:94–102.
15. Jurkat-Rott K, Lehmann-Horn F. State of the art in hereditary muscle channelopathies. *Acta Myol.* 2010;29:343–350.
16. Raja Rayan DL, Hanna MG. Skeletal muscle channelopathies: Nondystrophic myotonias and periodic paralysis. *Curr Opin Neurol.* 2010;23:466–476.
17. Gomez AM, Van Den Broeck J, Vrolix K, et al. Antibody effector mechanisms in myasthenia gravis-pathogenesis at the neuromuscular junction. *Autoimmunity.* 2010;43:353–370.
18. Conti-Fine BM, Milani M, Kaminski HJ. Myasthenia gravis: Past, present, and future. *J Clin Invest.* 2006;116:2843–2854.
19. Kumar V, Kaminski HJ. Treatment of myasthenia gravis. *Curr Neurol Neurosci Rep.* 2011;11:89–96.
20. Zahid I, Sharif S, Routledge T, et al. Video-assisted thoracoscopic surgery or transsternal thymectomy in the treatment of myasthenia gravis? *Interact Cardiovasc Thorac Surg.* 2011;12:40–46.
21. Gritti P, Sgarzi M, Carrara B, et al. A standardized protocol for the perioperative management of myasthenia gravis patients. Experience with 110 patients. *Acta Anaesthesiol Scand.* 2012;56:66–75.
22. Dillon FX. Anesthesia issues in the perioperative management of myasthenia gravis. *Semin Neurol.* 2004;24:83–94.
23. Almeida C, Coutinho E, Moreira D, et al. Myasthenia gravis and pregnancy: Anesthetic management – a series of cases. *Eur J Anaesthesiol.* 2010;27:985–990.
24. Braik T, Evans AT, Telfer M, et al. Paraneoplastic neurological syndromes: Unusual presentations of cancer. A practical review. *Am J Med Sci.* 2010;340: 301–308.
25. Gilhus NE. Lambert–Eaton myasthenic syndrome; pathogenesis, diagnosis, and therapy. *Autoimmune Dis.* 2011;2011:973808 (Hindawi Publishing).
26. van Doorn PA, Ruts L, Jacobs BC. Clinical features, pathogenesis, and treatment of Guillain-Barré syndrome. *Lancet Neurol.* 2008;7:939–950.
27. van Doorn PA, Kuitwaard K, Walgaard C, et al. IVIG treatment and prognosis in Guillain-Barré syndrome. *J Clin Immunol.* 2010;30(suppl 1):S74–S78.
28. Feldman JM. Cardiac arrest after succinylcholine in a pregnant patient recovered from Guillain-Barré syndrome. *Anesthesiology.* 1990;72:942–944.
29. Fiacchino F, Gemma M, Bricchi M, et al. Hypo- and hypersensitivity to vecuronium in a patient with Guillain-Barré syndrome. *Anesth Analg.* 1994;78: 187–189.
30. Goverman JM. Immune tolerance in multiple sclerosis. *Immunol Rev.* 2011;241: 228–240.
31. Ontaneda D, Hyland M, Cohen JA. Multiple sclerosis: New insights in pathogenesis and novel therapeutics. *Annu Rev Med.* 2012;63:389–404.
32. Fillippi M, Rocca MA. MR imaging of multiple sclerosis. *Radiology.* 2011;259: 659–681.
33. Gawronski KM, Rainka MM, Patel MJ, et al. Treatment options for multiple sclerosis: Current and emerging therapies. *Pharmacotherapy.* 2010;30:916–927.
34. Bader AM, Hunt CO, Datta S, et al. Anesthesia for the patient with multiple sclerosis. *J Clin Anesth.* 1988;1:21–24.
35. Dorotta IR, Schubert A. Multiple sclerosis and anesthetic implications. *Curr Opin Anaesthesiol.* 2002;15:365–370.
36. Schmidt D. Drug treatment of epilepsy: Options and limitations. *Epilepsy Behav* 2009;15:56–65.
37. Devinsky O Sudden, unexpected death in epilepsy. *N Engl J Med.* 2011;365: 1801–1811.
38. Lason W, Dudra-Jastrebska M, Rejdak K, et al. Basic mechanisms of antiepileptic drugs and their pharmacokinetic/pharmacodynamic interactions: An update. *Pharmacol Rep.* 2011;63:271–292.
39. Jääskeläinen SK, Kaisti K, Suni L. Sevoflurane is epileptogenic in healthy subjects at surgical levels of anesthesia. *Neurology.* 2003;61:1073–1078.
40. Niesen AD, Jacob AK, Aho LE, et al. Perioperative seizures in patients with a history of seizure disorder. *Anesth Analg.* 2010;111:729–735.
41. Kopp SL, Wynd KP, Horlocker TT, et al. Regional blockade in patients with a history of seizure disorder. *Anesth Analg.* 2009;109:272–278.
42. Kofke WA. Anesthetic management of the patient with epilepsy or prior seizures. *Curr Opin Anaesthesiol.* 2010;23:391–399.
43. Ramani R. Vagus nerve stimulation therapy for seizures. *J Neurosurg Anesthesiol.* 2008;20:29–35.
44. Ballard C, Gauthier S, Corbett A, et al. Alzheimer's disease. *Lancet.* 2011;377: 1019–1031.
45. Bittner EA, Yue Y, Xie Z. Brief review: Anesthetic toxicity in elderly, cognitive dysfunction, and Alzheimer's disease. *Can J Anaesth.* 2011;58:216–223.
46. Fodale V, Santamaria LB, Schifilliti D, et al. Anaesthetic and postoperative dysfunction: A pathological mechanism mimicking Alzheimer's disease. *Anaesthesia.* 2010;65:388–395.
47. Davidson AJ. Anesthesia and neurotoxicity to the developing brain: The clinical relevance. *Paediatr Anaesth.* 2011;21:716–721.
48. Schapira AH, Jenner P. Etiology and pathogenesis of Parkinson's disease. *Mov Disord.* 2011;6:1049–1055.
49. Hickey P, Stacy M. Available and emerging treatments for Parkinson's disease: A review. *Drug Des Devel Ther.* 2011;5:241.
50. Kalenka A, Schwarz A. Anaesthesia and Parkinson's disease: How to manage with new therapies? *Curr Opin Anaesthesiol.* 2009;22:419–424.
51. Poon CC, Irwin MG. Anaesthesia for deep brain stimulation in patients with implanted neurostimulator devices. *Br J Anaesth.* 2009;103:152–165.
52. Gálvez-Jiménez N , Lang AE. The perioperative management of Parkinson's disease revisited. *Neurol Clin.* 2004;22:367–377.
53. Roos RA. Huntington's disease: A clinical review. *Orphanet J Rare Dis.* 2010;5:40.
54. Kivela JE, Sprung J, Southorn PA, et al. Anesthetic management of patients with Huntington disease. *Anesth Analg.* 2010;110:515–523.
55. Kiernan MC, Vucic S, Cheah BC, et al. Amyotrophic lateral sclerosis. *Lancet.* 2011;377:942–955.
56. Norrby E. Prions and protein-folding diseases. *J Intern Med.* 2011;270:1–14.
57. Telfer JM. Creutzfeldt–Jakob disease—implications for anaesthetists in New Zealand. *Anaesth Intensive Care.* 2009;37:386–391.
58. Hopkins PM. Malignant hyperthermia: Pharmacology of triggering. *Br J Anaesth.* 2011;107:48–56.
59. Nelson TE. Malignant hyperthermia: A pharmacogenetic disease of Ca^{++} regulating proteins. *Curr Mol Med.* 2002;2:347–369.
60. Hirshey Dirksen SJ, Larach MG, Rosenberg H, et al. Special Article: Future directions in malignant hyperthermia research and patient care. *Anesth Analg.* 2011;113:1108–1119.
61. Glahn KP, Ellis FR, Halsall PJ, et al. Recognizing and managing a malignant hyperthermia crisis: Guidelines from the European Malignant Hyperthermia Group. *Br J Anaesth.* 2010;105:417–420.
62. Kim TW, Nemergut ME. Preparation of modern anesthesia workstations for malignant hyperthermia-susceptible patients: A review of past and present practice. *Anesthesiology.* 2011;114:205–212.
63. Puy H, Gouya L, Deybach J-C. Porphyrias. *Lancet.* 2010;375:924–937.
64. Desena HC, Brumund MR, Superneau D, et al. Ventricular fibrillation in a patient with Pompe disease: A cautionary tale. *Congenit Heart Dis.* 2011;6: 397–401.
65. Wang LY, Ross AK, Li JS, et al. Cardiac arrhythmias following anesthesia induction in infantile-onset Pompe disease: A case series. *Pediatr Anesth.* 2007;17:738–748.
66. Braunlin EA, Harmatz PR, Scarpa M, et al. Cardiac disease in patients with mucopolysaccharidoses: Presentation, diagnosis, and management. *J Inherit Metab Dis.* 2011;34:1183–1197.
67. Ingelmo PM, Parini R, Grimaldi M, et al. Multidetector computed tomography (MDCT) for preoperative assessment in children with mucopolysaccharidoses. *Minerva Anestesiol.* 2011;77:774–780.
68. Stynowick GA, Tobias JD. Perioperative care of the patient with osteogenesis imperfecta. *Orthopedics.* 2007;30:1043–1049.
69. Bojanic K, Kivela JE, Gurrieri C, et al. Perioperative course and intraoperative temperatures in patients with osteogenesis imperfecta. *Eur J Anaesthesiol.* 2011; 28:370–375.
70. Lasocki S, Longrois D, Montravers P, et al. Hepcidin and anemia of the critically ill patient: Bench to bedside. *Anesthesiology.* 2011;114:688–694.
71. Myles PS, Leslie K, Sibert B, et al. A review of the risks and benefits of nitrous oxide in current anaesthetic practice. *Anaesth Intensive Care.* 2004;32:165–172.
72. Cappellini MD, Fiorelli G. Glucose-6-phosphate dehydrogenase deficiency. *Lancet.* 2008;371:64–74.
73. Elyassi AR, Rowshan HH. Perioperative management of the glucose-6-phosphate dehydrogenase deficient patient: A review of the literature. *Anesth Prog.* 2009;56: 86–91.
74. Garratty G. Immune hemolytic anemia associated with drug therapy. *Blood Rev.* 2010;24:143.
75. Firth PG. Anesthesia and hemoglobinopathies. *Anesthesiol Clin.* 2009;27:321–326.
76. Khoury RA, Musallam KM, Mroueh S, et al. Pulmonary complications of sickle cell disease. *Hemoglobin.* 2011;35:625–635.
77. Gladwin MT. Prevalence, risk factors and mortality of pulmonary hypertension defined by right heart catheterization in patients with sickle cell disease. *Expert Rev Hematol.* 2011;4:593–596.
78. Borgna-Pignatti C, Gamberini MR. Complications of thalassemia major and their treatment. *Expert Rev Hematol.* 2011;4:353–366.
79. Derchi G, Formisano F, Balocco M, et al. Clinical management of cardiovascular complications in patients with thalassemia major: A large observational multicenter study. *Eur J Echocardiogr.* 2011;12:242–246.
80. Cooles FAH, Isaacs JD. Pathophysiology of rheumatoid arthritis. *Curr Opin Rheumatol.* 2011;23:233–240.
81. Yaszemski MJ, Shepler TR. Sudden death from cord compression associated with atlantoaxial instability in rheumatoid arthritis. A case report. *Spine (Phila Pa 1976).* 1990;15:338–341.
82. Gabriel SE. Cardiovascular morbidity and mortality in rheumatoid arthritis. *Am J Med.* 2008;121:S9–S14.
83. Curtis JR, Singht JA. Use of biologics in rheumatoid arthritis: Current and emerging paradigms of care. *Clin Ther.* 2011;33:679–707.

84. Lisowska B, Rutkowska-Sak L, Maldyk P. Anaesthesiological problems in patients with rheumatoid arthritis undergoing orthopaedic surgeries. *Clin Rheumatol.* 2008;27:553–556.
85. Yildirim-Toruner C, Diamond B. Current and novel therapies in the treatment of systemic lupus erythematosus. *J Allergy Clin Immunol.* 2011;127:303–312.
86. Ben-Menachem E. Review article: Systemic lupus erythematosus: A review for anesthesiologists. *Anesth Analg.* 2010;111:665–676.
87. Mahoney WM, Fleming JN, Schwartz SM. A unifying hypothesis for scleroderma: Identifying a target cell for scleroderma. *Curr Rheumatol Rep.* 2011;13:28–36.
88. Mammen AL. Dermatomyositis and polymyositis: Clinical presentation, autoantibodies, and pathogenesis. *Ann N Y Acad Sci.* 2010;1184:134–153.
89. Brown S, Shupak RC, Patel C, et al. Neuromuscular blockade in a patient with active dermatomyositis. *Anesthesiology.* 1992;77:1031–1033.
90. Shinkuma S, McMillan JR, Shimizu H. Ultrastructure and molecular pathogenesis of epidermolysis bullosa. *Clin Dermatol.* 2011;29:412–419.
91. Sidwell RU, Yates R, Atherton D. Dilated cardiomyopathy in dystrophic epidermolysis bullosa. *Arch Dis Child.* 2000;83:59–63.
92. Goldschneider K, Lucky AW, Mellerio JE, et al. Perioperative care of patients with epidermolysis bullosa: Proceedings of the 5th international symposium on epidermolysis bullosa, Santiago Chile, December 4–6, 2008. *Pediatr Anesth.* 2010;20:797–804.
93. Gottschalk A, Venherm S, Vowinkel T, et al. Anesthesia for balloon dilation of esophageal strictures in children with epidermolysis bullosa dystrophica: From intubation to sedation. *Curr Opin Anaesthesiol.* 2010;23:518–522.
94. Venugopal SS, Murrell DF. Diagnosis and clinical features of pemphigus vulgaris. *Dermatol Clin.* 2011;29:373–380.

CHAPTER

24 The Anesthesia Workstation and Delivery Systems for Inhaled Anesthetics

KEVIN T. RIUTORT • JAMES B. EISENKRAFT

Key Points

1. The most important (but often overlooked) item in the pre-use checkout of the anesthesia workstation is to have immediately available, a functioning self-inflating resuscitation bag and a full auxiliary tank of oxygen.
2. The low-pressure circuit (LPC) is the "vulnerable area" of the anesthesia workstation because it is most subject to breakage and leaks. The LPC is located downstream from all anesthesia machine safety features except the oxygen analyzer (or, in some cases, the ratio controller), and it is the portion of the machine where a leak is most likely to go unrecognized if an inappropriate LPC leak test is performed. Leaks in the LPC can cause delivery of a hypoxic or sub-anesthetic mixture, leading to patient hypoxic injury or awareness during anesthesia.
3. Because some GE Healthcare/Datex-Ohmeda anesthesia machines have a one-way check valve in the low-pressure circuit (LPC), a negative-pressure leak test is required to detect leaks in the LPC. A positive-pressure leak test will not detect leaks in the LPC of a machine with an outlet check valve.
4. Internal vaporizer leaks can only be detected with the vaporizer turned to the "on" position. In the "off" position the vaporizer is excluded from the low-pressure circuit.
5. Before administering an anesthetic, the circle breathing system must be checked for leaks and for correct flow. To test for leaks, the circle system is pressurized to 30 cm water pressure, and the circle system airway pressure gauge is observed (static test). To check for appropriate flow to rule out obstructions and faulty

valves, the ventilator and a test lung (breathing bag) are used (dynamic test). In addition, the manual/bag circuit must be actuated by compressing the reservoir bag, in order to rule out obstructions to flow in the manual/bag mode.

6 Many new anesthesia workstation self-tests do not detect internal vaporizer leaks unless each vaporizer is individually turned on during repeated self-tests.

7 In the event of a gas pipeline crossover, two actions must be taken. The backup oxygen cylinder must be turned on (since the tank valve should always be turned off when not in use), and the wall/pipeline supply sources must be disconnected.

8 The oxygen failure cutoff valves (also known previously as "fail-safe" valves, "hypoxic guards," or "proportioning systems") help minimize the likelihood of delivery of a hypoxic gas mixture, but they are not foolproof. Delivery of a hypoxic mixture may still result from (1) the wrong supply gas, either in the cylinder or in the main pipeline; (2) a defective or broken safety device; (3) leaks downstream from the safety devices; (4) inert gas administration (for instance, helium may not be subject to the oxygen failure cutoff valve); and (5) dilution of the inspired oxygen concentration by high concentrations of inhaled anesthetics.

9 Because of desflurane's low boiling point (22.8°C) and high vapor pressure (669 mm Hg at 20°C), controlled vaporization of desflurane requires specially designed vaporizers, such as the GE Healthcare/Datex-Ohmeda Tec 6, the Dräger D-Vapor, and the GE Healthcare Aladin cassette vaporizing system.

10 Misfilling an empty variable bypass vaporizer with desflurane could theoretically be catastrophic, resulting in delivery of a hypoxic mixture and a massive overdose of inhaled desflurane anesthetic.

11 Inhaled anesthetics can interact with CO_2 absorbents and produce toxic compounds. During sevoflurane (only) anesthesia, compound A can be formed, particularly at low fresh gas flow rates. During desflurane>sevoflurane anesthesia, carbon monoxide can be produced, particularly with desiccated absorbents.

12 Desiccated strong base absorbents (particularly barium hydroxide lime, Baralyme) can react with sevoflurane, producing extremely high absorber temperatures and combustible decomposition products. These in combination with the oxygen- or nitrous oxide-enriched environment of the circle system have produced very high temperatures and fires within the breathing system. For this reason, Baralyme is no longer available in the United States.

13 Anesthesia ventilators with ascending bellows (bellows that ascend during the expiratory phase) were initially thought to be safer than descending bellows. This is because a breathing system disconnection would be obvious since the ascending bellows would not refill/rise during exhalation. Contemporary machines with descending bellows, however, have been carefully redesigned to address these initial limitations. Current descending bellows ventilators have featherlight bellows, an electric eye at the bottom of the bellows housing to detect bellows movement, and the bellows housing is subjected to PEEP, such that in case of a disconnect, the bellows would actually rise and stay up.

14 With older design machines, use of the oxygen flush valve during the inspiratory phase of mechanical ventilation could cause barotrauma, particularly in pediatric patients. The newer workstations have fresh-gas decouplers or peak-inspiratory pressure limiters that were designed to prevent these complications. Ventilators that use fresh gas decoupling technology virtually eliminate the possibility of barotrauma by oxygen flushing during the inspiratory phase because fresh gas flow and oxygen flush flow are diverted to the reservoir bag. However, if the reservoir bag has a large leak or is absent altogether, patient awareness under anesthesia and delivery of a lower-than-expected oxygen concentration could occur because of entrainment of room air.

15 With newer GE Healthcare/Datex-Ohmeda anesthesia ventilators such as the 7900 series SmartVent, both the patient circuit gas and the drive gas are scavenged, resulting in substantially increased volumes of scavenged gas. Thus, the scavenging system flow removal must be set appropriately high to accommodate the increased volume; otherwise, undesired PEEP and contamination of the operating room environment could result.

16 Modern ventilators compensate for the changes in fresh gas flow, respiratory rate, and I:E ratio so that the delivered tidal volume does not change from that set to be delivered. This compensation is achieved either by "fresh gas decoupling" (in Dräger Fabius, Tiro, and Apollo workstations) or by "fresh gas compensation" (in GE Healthcare/Datex-Ohmeda workstations).

Multimedia

1 Bourdon Tube
2 Circle System
3 Liquid Oxygen Storage Tank
4 E-Cylinder
5 Oxygen Proportioning Systems
6 Oxygen Flush Valve
7 Vaporizer Interlocking Mechanism
8 Desflurane
9 CO_2 Absorber
10 Rebreathing CO_2
11 Ventilator Bellows
12 Ascending Bellows Ventilator
13 Wire Anenometers
14 Scavenger System

INTRODUCTION

The anesthesia machine is, conceptually, a pump for delivering medical gases and inhalation agents to the patient's lungs. The function of the anesthesia machine is to (1) receive gases from the central supply and cylinders, (2) meter them and add anesthetic vapors, and finally, (3) deliver them to the patient breathing circuit.[1] This machine has evolved over the past 160 years from a rather simple ether inhaler to a complex device of valves, pistons, vaporizers, monitors, and electronic circuitry.

The "pump" in the modern anesthesia machine is either a mechanical ventilator or the lungs of the spontaneously breathing patient, or perhaps, a combination of the two. The anesthesia

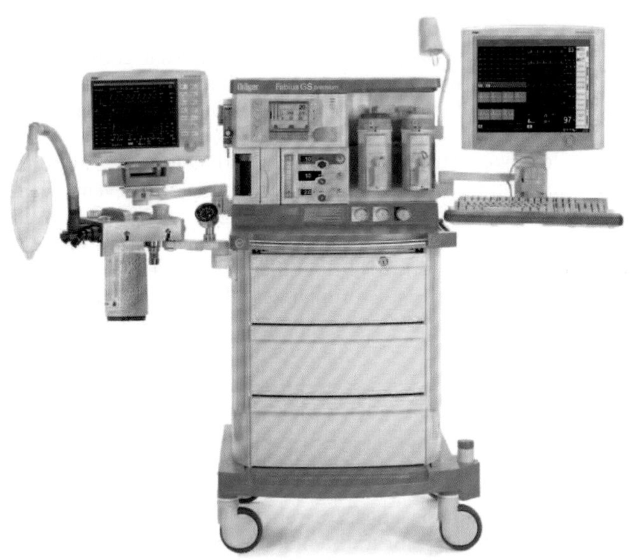

FIGURE 24-1. Dräger Medical Fabius GS anesthesia workstation. (Courtesy Dräger Medical AG.)

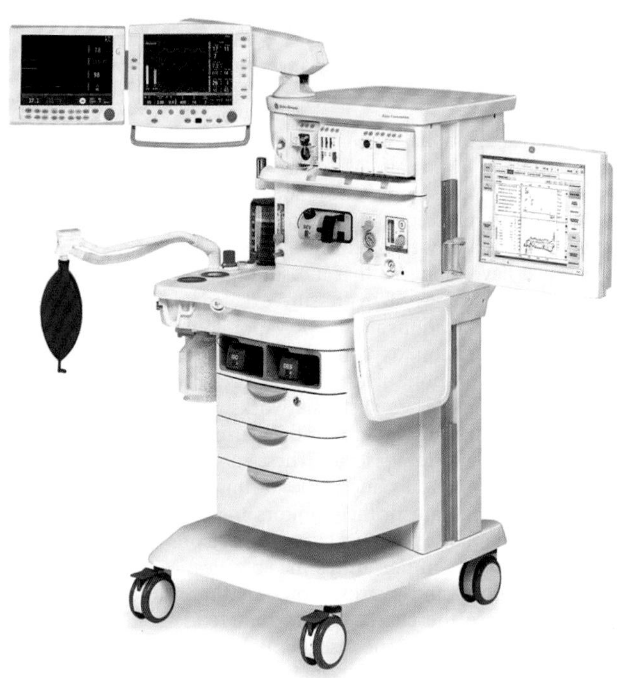

FIGURE 24-2. GE Healthcare Aisys Anesthesia Carestation. This workstation has electronic control of gas flows using a gas mixer and an electronically controlled Aladin vaporizing system for potent inhaled volatile anesthetics. (Courtesy GE Healthcare.)

pump has a supply system: medical gases from either a pipeline supply or a gas cylinder, alongside vaporizers delivering potent inhaled anesthetic agents that are mixed with the medical gases. The anesthesia pump also has an exhaust system, the waste gas scavenging system, which removes excess gases from the patient's breathing circuit. The breathing circuit is a series of hoses, valves, filters, switches, and regulators that interconnect the supply system, the patient, and the exhaust system.

Modern anesthesia machines (Figs. 24-1 and 24-2) are now more properly referred to as *anesthesia workstations.* The anesthesia workstation, as defined by the ASTM International (ASTM, originally known as the American Society for Testing and Materials), is a system for administering anesthetics to patients consisting of the *anesthesia gas supply device, the anesthesia ventilator, monitoring devices,* and *protection devices.*[2] The protection device is designed to prevent the patient from hazardous output due to incorrect delivery of energy or substances; for example, the adjustable pressure-limiting (APL) valve prevents barotrauma.

In this chapter, the anesthesia workstation is examined piece by piece. The normal operation, function, and integration of major anesthesia workstation subsystems are described. More importantly, the potential problems and hazards associated with the various components of the anesthesia delivery system, and the appropriate preoperative checks that may help to detect and prevent such problems, are illustrated.

ANESTHESIA WORKSTATION STANDARDS AND PRE-USE PROCEDURES

A few years ago, a fundamental knowledge of the basic anesthesia machine pneumatics would have sufficed for most anesthesia providers. Today, a detailed understanding of pneumatics, electronics, and even computer science is necessary to fully understand the capabilities and complexities of the anesthesia workstation. Along with the changes in the composition of the anesthesia workstation to include more complex ventilation systems and integrated monitoring, recently there has also been increasing divergence between anesthesia workstation designs from different manufacturers. In 1993, a joint effort between the American Society of Anesthesiologists (ASA) and the U.S. Food and Drug Administration (FDA) produced the 1993 FDA Anesthesia Apparatus Pre-Use Checkout Recommendations (Appendix A). This pre-use checklist was versatile and could be applied to most commonly available anesthesia machines equally well and did not require users to vary the pre-use procedure significantly from machine to machine.

Today, because of variations in fundamental anesthesia workstation design, the 1993 FDA pre-use checklist is no longer applicable to many contemporary workstations. Anesthesia providers must be aware of this limitation, and the original equipment manufacturer's recommended pre-use checklist should be followed. Some of the newer workstations have computer-assisted self-tests that automatically perform a part of the pre-use machine checkout procedure. The availability of such automated checkout features further adds to the complexity of constructing a uniform pre-use checklist such as the one utilized in the recent past. Ultimately, the responsibility of performing an adequate pre-use checkout of the anesthesia workstation falls to the individual operator: regardless of the level of his/her training and the quality of technical support. The anesthesia care provider has the ultimate responsibility for proper function of all anesthesia delivery equipment that he or she uses. The anesthesia provider of record must be aware of which anesthesia workstation components are checked out by the automated self-tests and which ones are not. Because of the number of workstations currently available and the variability among their self-testing procedures, the following discussion will be limited to general topics related to these systems.

STANDARDS FOR ANESTHESIA MACHINES AND WORKSTATIONS

The American National Standards Institute (ANSI) and the American Society for Testing and Materials (ASTM) define standards for anesthesia machines and workstations, and provide guidelines to manufacturers regarding their minimum performance, design characteristics, and safety requirements. Newly manufactured workstations must have monitors that measure the following parameters: continuous breathing system pressure, exhaled tidal volume, ventilatory CO_2 concentration, anesthetic vapor concentration, inspired oxygen concentration, oxygen supply pressure, arterial hemoglobin oxygen saturation, arterial blood pressure, and continuous electrocardiogram. The anesthesia workstation must have a prioritized alarm system that groups the alarms into three categories: high, medium, and low priority. These monitors and alarms may be enabled automatically and made to function by turning on the anesthesia workstation, or the monitors and alarms can be enabled manually and made functional by following a pre-use checklist.[2,3]

Perhaps just as important as the specifications for new anesthesia machines and workstations that are introduced into clinical care are the characteristics that render older machines obsolete. This is not an inconsequential issue, since the financial investment for replacing older machines is significant. The ASA document, "Guidelines for Determining Anesthesia Machine Obsolescence," addresses some of the absolute as well as relative criteria that can help institutions make a decision on when even otherwise functioning equipment should be replaced.[4]

FAILURE OF ANESTHESIA EQUIPMENT

An 11-year study of 1,000 anesthesia incidents in the United Kingdom revealed that the most common failure was due to an equipment leak (61/1,000).[5] The authors stated the most likely underlying cause of system leaks was due to "design weakness"; for example, push-on tapers in breathing circuits that can easily become disconnected. Poor equipment maintenance and setup were the second most common underlying causes of equipment failure. Equipment failure due to entrapped cables may result in the inability to ventilate (thus warranting careful attention to organization and tidiness of the anesthesia workstation environment by the anesthesia provider).[6–8] The authors found that the pulse oximeter alarm was the most common, principal monitor alerting the anesthesiologist to an equipment problem.

In a review of the ASA "Closed Claims" database, Caplan et al. found that although claims related to the medical gas-delivery system were rare, when they occurred, they were usually severe, 76% resulting in death or permanent brain injury. The most common malfunction in Caplan et al's review was the breathing circuit (39%), followed by vaporizers (21%), ventilators (17%), gas tanks or gas lines (11%), and the anesthesia machine itself (7%). Use error was judged to be the cause in 75% of the 72 gas delivery equipment claims reviewed, while pure failure of equipment was considered the cause in the remainder.[9]

SAFETY FEATURES OF NEWER ANESTHESIA WORKSTATIONS

Older conventional anesthesia machines have design limitations that limit their safety. For example, some machines may lack features to prevent barotrauma during oxygen flush, lack automated pre-use checkout, have multiple external connections, and have gas-driven ventilator bellows that do not fully empty and which may allow "breath stacking" as well as inaccurate tidal volume delivery.[10]

Modern workstations have designs that incorporate additional safety features such as fresh gas decoupling to prevent barotrauma during oxygen flush, have integrated, software-driven self-checkout routines, have limited external connections, and have electronic, piston-driven ventilators that deliver accurate tidal volumes.[10] Table 24-1 summarizes relevant safety features of newer anesthesia workstations.

CHECKOUT OF THE ANESTHESIA WORKSTATION

A complete anesthesia apparatus checkout procedure must be performed each day prior to the first use of the anesthesia workstation. An abbreviated checkout procedure should be performed before each subsequent case. The 1993 FDA Anesthesia Apparatus Checkout Recommendations (reproduced in Appendix A) remain applicable to the majority of older anesthesia machines in use worldwide.[11–15]

In 2008 the ASA published recommendations for pre-anesthesia checkout machines, taking into consideration newer workstations that perform automated checkout.[16] Since the design of newer workstations varies considerably, no single pre-use procedure is applicable. These guidelines present a template for individual departments and practitioners to design pre-anesthesia checkout procedures specific to their needs and equipment (Appendix B). Sample checkout procedures are published on the ASA website (http://www.asahq.org), and they encompass adult as well as pediatric equipment from major equipment manufacturers in the United States. The reader is strongly encouraged to review the checkout procedures reproduced in Appendices A and B and to understand the rationale for and importance of each step.

1 Perhaps the most important but often overlooked item in the pre-use checkout of the anesthesia workstation is to have immediately available a functioning (tested) self-inflating resuscitation bag (SIRB) and a full auxiliary tank of oxygen (Fig. 24-3). This is "plan B"—the backup plan. Many of the adverse outcomes associated with anesthesia equipment mishaps could have been averted if the SIRB had been used or used sooner. A recent study reported that the SIRB was the item most frequently missed in the pre-anesthesia setup.[17]

The next three most important preoperative checks are (1) oxygen analyzer calibration, (2) the low-pressure circuit leak test, and (3) the circle system test. These are discussed in the following sections. Additional details regarding these systems are presented briefly in subsequent sections describing the anatomy of the anesthesia workstation; for a more comprehensive review, the reader is encouraged to consult the operator's manual of their own equipment manufacturer. For a simplified diagram of a two-gas anesthesia machine and the components described in the following discussion, please refer to Figure 24-4. A comprehensive discussion of Figure 24-4 can also be found in the Anesthesia Workstation Pneumatics section.

Oxygen Analyzer Calibration

The oxygen analyzer is one of the most important monitors on the anesthesia workstation. It is the only machine safety device

TABLE 24-1. COMPARISON OF ANESTHESIA WORKSTATION FUNCTIONS

Anesthesia Workstation Function	Narkomed AV2+	Ohmeda 7800	Dräger Narkomed 6400	Dräger Julian[a]	Dräger Fabius GS 1.3	GE/Datex-Ohmeda Aestiva/5	GE/Datex-Ohmeda ADU	GE Aisys	Dräger Apollo
Increase in fresh gas flow (FGF) increases tidal volume (Vt)	Yes	Yes	No	No	No	Initially	No	No	No
Pre-use system leakage is measured	No	No	Yes	Yes	Yes	No	Yes	Yes	Yes
Proximal leak compensation	No	No	No	No	No	Yes	No	Yes	Yes
Leakage measurement during operation	No	No	Yes	Yes	No	No	No	Yes	No
Hose compliance compensation	No	No	Yes	Yes	Yes	No	Yes	Yes	Yes
System compliance compensation	No	No	Yes	Yes	Yes	Yes	Yes	Yes	Yes
The reported exhaled Vt is adjusted for hose compliance	No	No	Yes	No	Yes	No	No	Yes	Yes
The fresh gas inflow is distal to:	Absorber	Absorber	Absorber	Mid-absorber	Absorber	Absorber	Inspiratory valve	Absorber	Absorber
The fresh gas inflow is proximal to:	Inspiratory valve	Inspiratory valve	Decoupling valve	Mid-absorber	Decoupling valve	Inspiratory valve	Y-piece	Inspiratory valve	Decoupling valve
At low FGF, what gas fills the reservoir bag?	Exhaled	Exhaled	Scrubbed	Exhaled	Scrubbed	Exhaled	Exhaled	Exhaled	Exhaled
Mechanism of volume control ventilation (VCV)	Mechanical limit	Metered	Displacement	Metered	Displacement	Metered/servo	Metered/calculated	Metered, calculated	Metered
Limiting of pressure control ventilation (PCV)	Pressure limited	None	Flow/pressure limited	Flow/pressure limited	Flow/pressure limited	Pressure limited	Flow/pressure limited	Flow/pressure limited	Flow/pressure limited
FIO_2 compensated for volatile agent	No	No	No	No	No	No	Yes	Yes	No
Synchronized intermittent mechanical ventilation (SIMV)	No	No	Yes	No	No	No	Yes	Yes	Yes
The manufacturer specified minimum Vt	N/A	18	10	50	20	20	20	20	20
Fresh gas flow (FGF) control	Needle valve	Needle valve	Needle valve	Digital control	Needle valve	Needle valve	Needle valve	Digital control	Needle valve
Fresh gas flow (FGF) measurement	Flow tubes	Flow tubes	Flow tubes	Electronic	Electronic	Flow tubes	Electronic	Electronic	Electronic
Backup flow tube	N/A	N/A	N/A	No	Yes	N/A	Yes	Yes (fail-safe mode)	Yes
Integrated capnography	No	No	Yes	Yes	No	No	Yes	Yes	Yes

TABLE 24-1. COMPARISON OF ANESTHESIA WORKSTATION FUNCTIONS (*continued*)

Anesthesia Workstation Function	Narkomed AV2+	Ohmeda 7800	Dräger Narkomed 6400	Dräger Julian[a]	Dräger Fabius GS 1.3	GE/Datex-Ohmeda Aestiva/5	GE/Datex-Ohmeda ADU	GE Aisys	Dräger Apollo
Integrated anesthetic gas monitoring	No	No	Yes	Yes	No	No	Yes	Yes	Yes
Effect of lost oxygen pressure on FGF	No FGF	No FGF	No FGF	Auto air on	Air available	Air available	Air available	Air available	Air available
Sampled gas returned to circuit	No	No	No	No	No	No	Yes	No	Yes
Mechanical airway pressure gauge	Yes	Yes	No	No	Yes	Yes	No	No	Yes
Absorber removable during VCV	No	No	No	No	Yes	No	Yes	Yes (optional)	Yes (optional)
Room air entrained during a circuit leak	No	No	Yes	Yes	Yes	No	No	No	Yes
Room air entrained with inadequate FGF	No	No	No	No	Yes	No	No	No	No
Effect of O_2 flush during VCV inspiration	>Vt, held at press. limit	>Vt, end at press. limit	None	>Vt, held at press. limit	None	>Vt, end at press. limit	>Vt, end at press. release	>Vt, end at press. release	None
Fail-safe integrated with the ratio controller	No	No	No	Yes, electronic	Yes, pneumatic	No	Yes, electronic	Yes, electronic	Yes, electronic
Method to find a low-pressure/vaporizer leak	Positive pressure	Negative pressure	Automatic, vaporizer open	Automatic, vaporizer open	Automatic, vaporizer open	Negative pressure	Automatic	Automatic	Automatic, vaporizer open
Ventilator drive gas scavenging	No	No	N/A	Yes	N/A	Yes	No	Yes	N/A

Adapted from: Olympio MA. Modern anesthesia machines offer new safety features. *APSF Newsletter.* 2003;18:17.
[a]Not available in the United States.

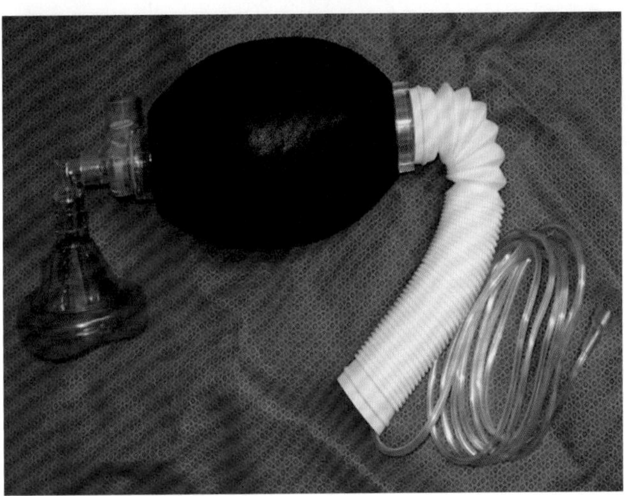

FIGURE 24-3. Self-inflating resuscitation bag (SIRB). Many of the adverse outcomes associated with anesthesia equipment mishaps could have been averted if a functional SIRB had been used sooner.

that evaluates the integrity of the low-pressure circuit in an ongoing fashion. Other machine safety devices, such as the oxygen failure cutoff ("fail-safe") valve, the oxygen supply failure alarm, and the proportioning system, are all upstream from the flow control valves. The only machine monitor that detects problems downstream from the flow control valves is the oxygen analyzer. Calibration of this monitor is described in Appendix A (Anesthesia Apparatus Checkout Recommendations, 1993, Step 9). The actual procedure for calibrating the oxygen analyzer has remained reasonably similar over the recent generations of the anesthesia workstations (Guideline for Designing Pre-Anesthesia Checkout Procedures, 2008, Item 10 in Appendix B). Generally, the oxygen concentration-sensing element (usually a fuel cell on traditional machines) must be exposed to room air (at sea level) for calibration to 21%. This may require manually setting a dial on older machines, but on newer ones, it usually only involves temporary removal of the sensor, selecting and then confirming that the oxygen calibration is to be performed from a set of menus on the workstation's display screen, and finally reinstalling the sensor. The function of the low oxygen concentration alarm should be verified by setting the alarm to trigger above the current oxygen reading. Newer workstations have automatic oxygen sensor calibration.

Low-Pressure Circuit Leak Test

2 The low-pressure circuit leak test checks the integrity of the anesthesia machine from the flow control valves to the common gas outlet. It evaluates the portion of the machine that is downstream from all safety devices except the oxygen analyzer. The components located within this area are *precisely* the ones most subject to breakage and leaks. Leaks in the low-pressure circuit can cause hypoxia or patient awareness.[18,19] Flow tubes, the most delicate pneumatic component of the machine, can crack or break. A typical three-gas anesthesia machine has 16 O-rings in the low-pressure circuit. Leaks can occur at the interface between the glass flow tubes.[20] and the manifold, and at the O-ring junctions between the vaporizer and its manifold. Loose filler caps on vaporizers are a common source of leaks, and these leaks can

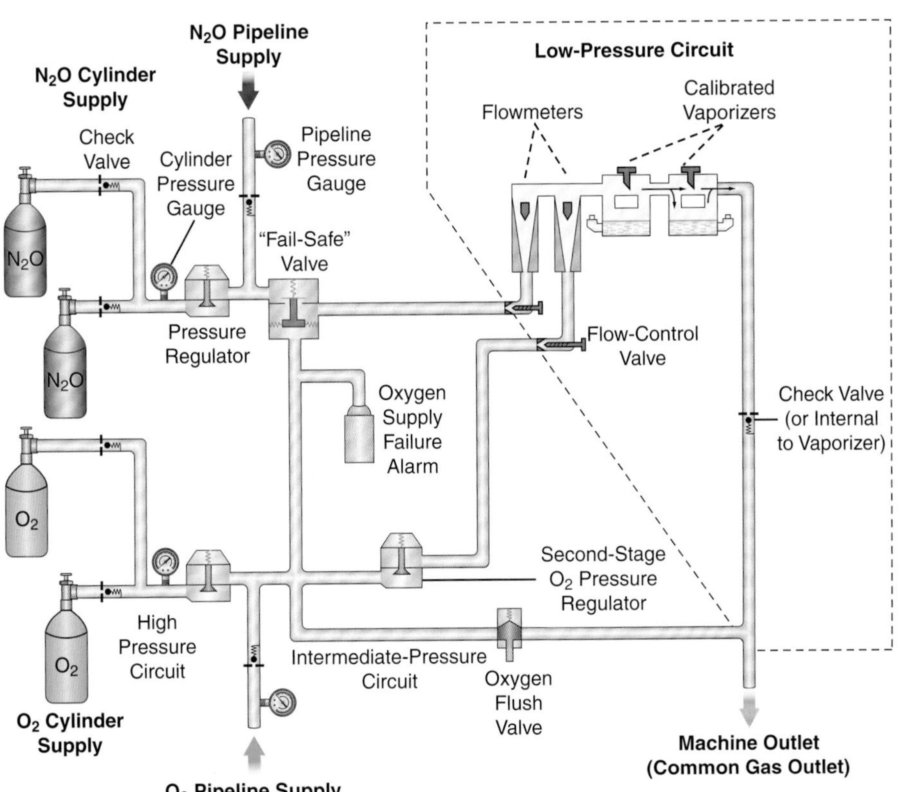

FIGURE 24-4. Diagram of a generic two-gas anesthesia machine. (Modified with permission from: *Check-Out, A Guide for Preoperative Inspection of an Anesthesia Machine.* Park Ridge, IL: American Society of Anesthesiologists; 1987.)

lead to delivery of sub-anesthetic doses of inhaled agents, causing patient awareness during general anesthesia.[18,21]

Several different methods have been used to check the low-pressure circuit for leaks. They include the oxygen flush test, the common gas outlet occlusion test, the traditional positive-pressure leak test, the North American Dräger positive-pressure leak test, the Ohmeda 8000 internal positive-pressure leak test, the Ohmeda negative-pressure leak test, the 1993 FDA universal negative-pressure leak test, and others. One reason for the large number of methods is that the internal design of various machines differs considerably. The most notable example is that many GE Healthcare/Datex-Ohmeda (hereafter referred to as Datex-Ohmeda) machines/workstations have a check valve near the common gas outlet, whereas Dräger Medical workstations do not. The presence or absence of the outlet check valve profoundly influences which pre-use check is indicated.

Several mishaps have resulted from application of the wrong
3 leak test to the wrong machine.[22–25] Therefore, it is mandatory to perform the appropriate low-pressure leak test each day. To do this, it is essential to understand the exact location and operating principles of the Datex-Ohmeda check valve. Many Datex-Ohmeda anesthesia workstations have a machine outlet check valve located in the low-pressure circuit (Table 24-1). The check valve is located downstream from the vaporizers and upstream from the oxygen flush valve (Fig. 24-4). It is open in the absence of back pressure. Gas flow from the manifold moves the rubber flapper valve off its seat and allows gas to proceed freely to the common gas outlet. The valve closes when back pressure is exerted.[12,26] Back pressure sufficient to close the check valve may occur with the following conditions: oxygen flushing, peak breathing circuit pressures generated during positive-pressure ventilation, or use of a positive-pressure leak test.

Generally speaking, the low-pressure circuit of anesthesia workstations without an outlet check valve can be tested using a positive-pressure leak test, and machines with outlet check valves must be tested using a negative-pressure leak test. When performing a positive-pressure leak test, the operator generates positive pressure in the low-pressure circuit using flow from the anesthesia machine or from a positive-pressure squeeze bulb to detect a leak. When performing a negative-pressure leak test, the operator creates negative pressure in the low-pressure circuit using a suction bulb to detect leaks. Two different low-pressure circuit leak tests are described below.

Oxygen Flush Positive-Pressure Leak Test

Historically, older anesthesia machines did not have check valves in the low-pressure circuit. Therefore, it was common practice to pressurize the breathing circuit and the low-pressure circuit with the oxygen flush valve to test for internal anesthesia machine leaks by observing the breathing system pressure gauge. Because many modern Datex-Ohmeda machines now have check valves in the low-pressure circuit, application of a positive-pressure leak test to these machines can be misleading or even dangerous (Fig. 24-5). Inappropriate use of the oxygen flush valve or the presence of a leaking flush valve may lead to inadequate evaluation of the low-pressure circuit for leaks. In turn, this can lead the workstation user into a false sense of security despite the presence of large leaks.[22–24,27,28] Positive pressure from the breathing circuit results in closure of the outlet check valve, and the value on the breathing system pressure gauge will fail to decrease. The system appears to be gas tight, but in actuality, only the circuitry downstream from the outlet check valve is leak-free.[29] Thus, a vulnerable area exists from the check valve back to the flow control valves because this area is not tested by a positive-pressure leak test.

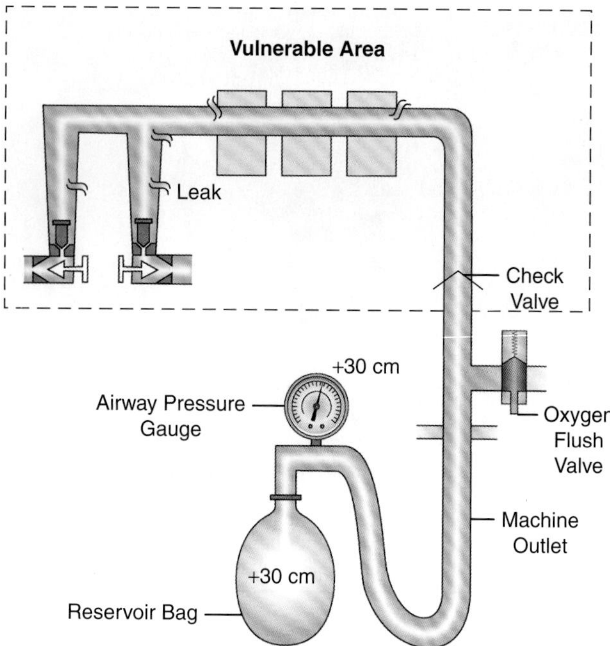

FIGURE 24-5. Inappropriate use of the oxygen flush valve to check the low-pressure circuit of an Ohmeda machine equipped with a check valve. The area within the rectangle is not checked by the inappropriate use of the oxygen flush valve. The components located within this area are *precisely* the ones most subject to breakage and leaks. Positive pressure within the patient circuit closes the check valve, and the value on the airway pressure gauge does not decrease despite leaks in the low-pressure circuit.

Verifying the Integrity of the Gas Supply Lines between the Flowmeters and the Common Gas Outlet

The 1993 FDA Universal negative-pressure leak test (Appendix A, Step 5) was named "universal" because at that time it could be used to check all contemporary anesthesia machines regardless of the presence or absence of an outlet check valve in the low-pressure circuit.[13] It remains applicable for many older anesthesia machines, but for many newer machines this "universal" test is not applicable. Table 24-1 describes how newer workstations are tested for low-pressure circuit and vaporizer leaks. Leaks in the gas supply lines between the flowmeters and the common gas outlet should be checked daily or whenever a vaporizer is changed (Appendix B, Item 8). The most thorough technique is to check each vaporizer individually by turning it on and then
4 evaluating the low-pressure system for leaks. It is important to note that automated checkout procedures may not necessarily evaluate leaks at the vaporizer, if the vaporizer is not turned on during testing. In addition, vaporizers should be adequately filled and filler ports should be tightly closed (Appendix B, Item 7). As mentioned previously, the ASA now recommends that individual institutions develop internal guidelines specific to their own equipment and needs.

The 1993 FDA low-pressure system leak check is based on the Datex-Ohmeda negative-pressure leak test (Fig. 24-6). It is performed using a negative-pressure leak testing device, which is a simple suction 15 cc volume bulb that when evacuated generates a negative pressure of 65 mm Hg. The machine main ON/OFF switch, the flow control valves, and the vaporizers are all turned off. The suction bulb is connected to the common gas outlet and

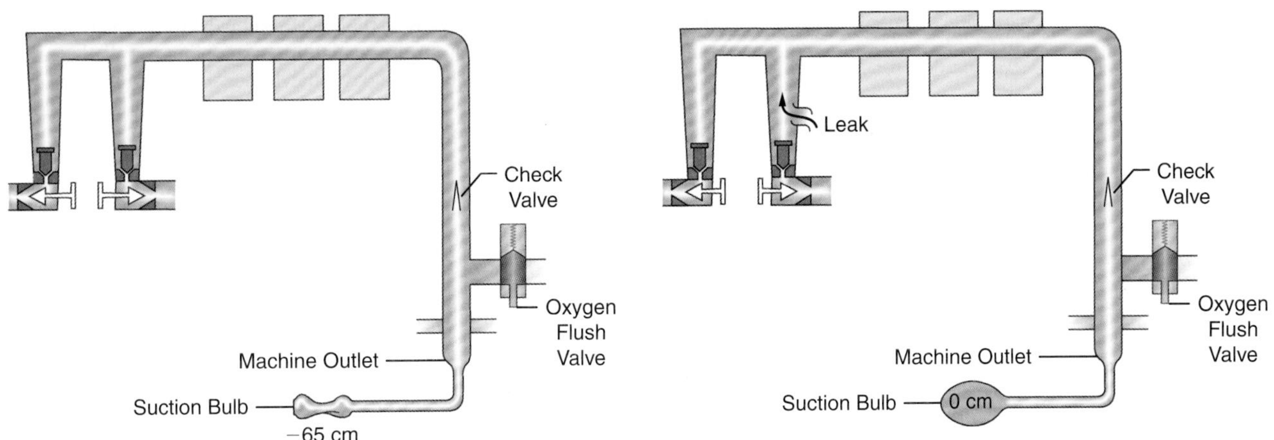

FIGURE 24-6. FDA negative-pressure leak test. **(Left)** A negative-pressure leak testing device is attached directly to the machine common gas outlet. Squeezing the bulb creates a vacuum in the low-pressure circuit and opens the check valve. **(Right)** When a leak is present in the low-pressure circuit, room air is entrained through the leak and the suction bulb inflates. (Reprinted with permission from: Andrews JJ. Understanding anesthesia machines. In: *1988 Review Course Lectures,* p 78. Cleveland: International Anesthesia Research Society, 1988.)

squeezed repeatedly until it is fully collapsed. This action creates a vacuum in the low-pressure system circuitry. The machine is considered leak-free if the suction bulb remains collapsed for at least 10 seconds. A leak is present if the bulb reinflates during this period. The test is repeated with each vaporizer individually turned to the on position because internal vaporizer leaks can be detected only when the vaporizer is turned on and becomes part of the low-pressure system. If the bulb reinflates in less than 10 seconds, a leak is present somewhere in the low-pressure circuit.

Evaluation of the Circle System

5 The circle system tests (Appendix B, Items 12–13) evaluate the integrity of the circle breathing system, which spans from the machine common gas outlet to the Y-piece (Fig. 24-7). The test has two components: (1) *breathing system pressure and leak testing* and (2) *verification that gas flows properly through the breathing circuit during both inspiration and exhalation.* To thoroughly check the circle system for leaks, valve integrity, and obstruction, both tests must be performed preoperatively. The ASA 2008 recommendations call for performing the breathing system test and leak test before starting each case, such that pressure can be developed in the system during both manual/bag and automatic/mechanical ventilation. Automated leak testing routines are implemented in modern workstations; system compliance is also calculated and used to adjust volume delivery during mechanical ventilation (Appendix B, Item 12). Because pressure and leak testing cannot identify all obstructions in the breathing circuit or confirm the function of the inspiratory and expiratory unidirectional valves, a test lung or second reservoir bag connected at the Y-piece can be used to confirm circuit integrity and function. Visual inspection of the unidirectional valves should be performed daily, though, because subtle damage to these valves is difficult to determine. Older 1993 FDA checkout procedures to identify valve incompetence that may not be visually obvious can be implemented, but are typically too complex for daily testing (Appendix B, Item 13).[30,31]

In the 1993 FDA Anesthesia Apparatus Checkout Recommendations, a *leak test* is performed by closing the APL (or pop-off) valve, occluding the Y-piece, and pressurizing the circuit to 30 cm water pressure using the oxygen flush valve. The value on the pressure gauge will not decrease if the circle system is leak-free, but this does not assure unidirectional valve integrity or function. The value on the pressure gauge will read 30 cm H_2O even if the unidirectional valves are stuck shut or are incompetent. In addition, a *flow test* checks the integrity of the unidirectional valves, and it detects obstruction in the circle system. It can be performed by removing the Y-piece from the circle system and breathing through the two corrugated hoses individually. The unidirectional valve leaflets should be present and should move appropriately. The operator should be able to inhale but not be able to exhale through the inspiratory limb. The operator should be able to exhale but not inhale through the expiratory limb. The flow test can also be performed by using the ventilator and a reservoir bag connected to the "Y" piece as described in the 1993 FDA

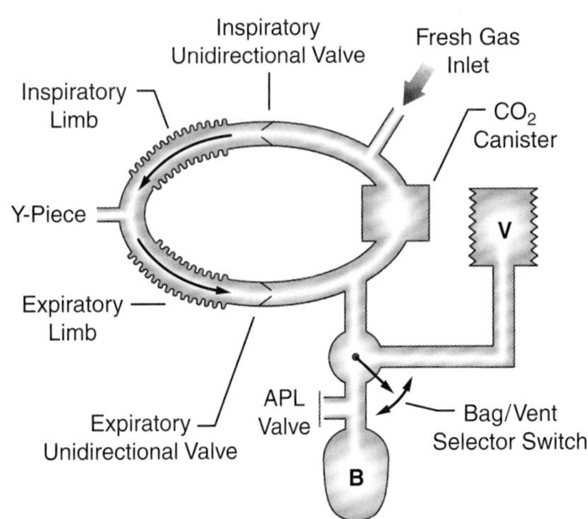

FIGURE 24-7. Components of the circle breathing system. B, reservoir bag; V, ventilator; APL, adjustable pressure-limiting (pop-off) valve. (Reproduced with permission from: Brockwell RC. Inhaled anesthetic delivery systems. In: Miller RD, ed. *Anesthesia.* 6th ed. Philadelphia, PA: Churchill Livingstone; 2004:295.)

Anesthesia Apparatus Checkout Recommendations (Appendix A, Steps 11–12).[13]

Workstation Self-Tests

Many new anesthesia workstations now incorporate technology that allows the machine to either automatically or manually guide the user through a series of self-tests to check for functionality of electronic, mechanical, and pneumatic components. Tested components commonly include the gas supply system, flow control valves, the circle system, ventilator, and integrated vaporizers. The comprehensiveness of these self-diagnostic tests varies from one model and manufacturer to another. If these tests are to be employed, users must be certain to read and strictly follow all manufacturer recommendations. Although a thorough understanding of what the particular workstation's self-tests include is very helpful, this information is often difficult to obtain and may vary greatly between devices.

6 One particularly important point of caution with self-tests should be noted on systems with manifold-mounted vaporizers such as the Dräger Apollo, Dräger Fabius GS and Narkomed 6000 series. A manifold-mounted vaporizer does not become a part of an anesthesia workstation's low-pressure system until its concentration control dial is turned to the "on" position. Therefore, to detect internal vaporizer leaks in this type of a system, the "leak test" portion of the self-diagnostic must be repeated with each individual vaporizer turned to the "on" position. If this precaution is not taken, large leaks that could potentially result in patient awareness, such as those from a loose filler cap or cracked fill indicator, could go undetected.

Anesthesia Workstation Pneumatics

The Anatomy of an Anesthesia Workstation

A simplified diagram of a generic two-gas anesthesia machine is shown in Figure 24-4. The pressures within the anesthesia workstation can be divided into three circuits: a high-pressure, an intermediate-pressure, and a low-pressure circuit. The *high-pressure circuit* is confined to the cylinders and the cylinder primary pressure regulators. For oxygen, the pressure range of the high-pressure circuit extends from a high of 2,200 pounds per square inch gauge (psig) to 45 psig, which is the regulated cylinder pressure. For nitrous oxide in the high-pressure circuit, pressures range from a high of 750 psig in the cylinder to a low of 45 psig. The *intermediate-pressure circuit* begins at the regulated cylinder supply sources at a pressure of 45 psig, includes the pipeline sources at 50 to 55 psig and extends to the flow control valves. Depending on the manufacturer and specific machine design, second-stage pressure regulators may be used to decrease the pipeline supply pressures to the flow control valves to even lower pressures such as 14 psig or 26 psig within the intermediate-pressure circuit.[32,33] Finally, the *low-pressure circuit* extends from the flow control valves to the common gas outlet. Therefore, the low-pressure circuit includes the flow tubes, vaporizer manifold, vaporizers, and the one-way outlet check valve on most GE Healthcare/Datex-Ohmeda machines.[33]

Both oxygen and nitrous oxide are supplied to the workstation from two sources: a pipeline supply source and a cylinder supply source. The pipeline supply source is the primary gas source for
3 the anesthesia workstation. The hospital pipeline supply system provides gases to the machine at approximately 50 psig, which is the normal working pressure of most machines. The cylinder supply source serves as a backup if the pipeline supply fails or acts as the primary supply if the anesthesia workstation is being used in a location without the availability of pipeline supplied gases. As previously described, the oxygen cylinder source is regulated from 2,200 psig to approximately 45 psig, and the nitrous oxide cylinder source is regulated from 745 psig to approximately 45 psig.[32–34]

A safety device traditionally referred to as the *fail-safe* valve (and currently more appropriately termed the "*oxygen failure cutoff valve*") is located downstream from the nitrous oxide supply source. It serves as an interface between the oxygen and nitrous oxide supply sources. This valve shuts off, or proportionally decreases, the supply of nitrous oxide (and other gases) if the oxygen supply pressure decreases. To meet ASTM standards, contemporary machines have an alarm device to monitor the oxygen supply pressure. A high-priority alarm is actuated when a decreasing oxygen supply pressure reaches a predetermined threshold, such as 30 psig.[32–34]

Many GE Healthcare/Datex-Ohmeda machines have a second-stage pressure regulator for oxygen that is located downstream from the oxygen supply source in the intermediate-pressure circuit. It is adjusted to a precise pressure level, such as 14 psig.[32] This regulator supplies a constant pressure to the oxygen flow-control valve regardless of fluctuating oxygen pipeline pressures. The flow from the oxygen flow-control valve will be constant provided that its oxygen supply pressure is >14 psig.

The flow control valves represent an important anatomic landmark within the anesthesia workstation because they separate the intermediate-pressure circuit from the low-pressure circuit. The low-pressure circuit is that part of the machine that lies downstream from the flow control valves. The operator regulates flow entering the low-pressure circuit by adjusting the flow control valves. The oxygen and nitrous oxide flow-control valves are linked mechanically or pneumatically by a proportioning system to help prevent unintended delivery of a hypoxic mixture. After leaving the flow tubes, the mixture of gases travels through a common manifold and may be directed to a concentration-calibrated vaporizer. Precise amounts of potent inhaled volatile anesthetic can be added, depending on vaporizer concentration control dial setting. The total fresh gas flow (FGF) plus the anesthetic vapor then flow toward the common gas outlet.[32,33]

Many Datex-Ohmeda anesthesia machines have a one-way check valve located between the vaporizers and the common gas outlet in the mixed-gas line. Its purpose is to prevent back flow into the vaporizer during positive-pressure ventilation, therefore minimizing the effects of downstream intermittent pressure fluctuations on inhaled anesthetic concentration (see Vaporizers: Intermittent Back Pressure section). The presence or absence of this check valve *profoundly* influences which preoperative leak test is indicated (see Checking Your Anesthesia Workstation). The oxygen flush connection joins the mixed-gas line between the one-way check valve (when present) and the machine common gas outlet. Thus, when the oxygen flush valve is activated the pipeline oxygen flows directly to the common gas outlet at a rate of 35 to 75 L/min and potentially at a pressure of 55 psig.

Pipeline Supply Source

Most hospitals today have a central piping system to deliver medical gases including oxygen, nitrous oxide, air, and carbon dioxide to outlets in the operating room. The central piping system must supply the correct gases at the appropriate pressure for the anesthesia workstation to function properly. Unfortunately, this does not always occur. Even as recently as 2002, a large medical center with a huge cryogenic bulk oxygen storage system was not immune to component failures that contributed to a critical oxygen pipeline supply failure.[35] In this case, a faulty joint ruptured at the bottom of the primary cryogenic oxygen storage tank, releasing 8,000 gallons of liquid oxygen to flood the streets in the surrounding area and compromised oxygen delivery to the medical center.

In a 1976 survey of approximately 200 hospitals, 31% reported difficulties with pipeline systems.[36] The most common problem was inadequate oxygen pressure, followed by excessive pipeline pressures. The most devastating reported hazard, however, was accidental crossing of oxygen and nitrous oxide pipelines, which has led to many deaths. This problem caused 23 deaths in a newly constructed wing of a general hospital in Sudbury, Ontario, during a 5-month period.[37] In 2002, two hypoxic deaths were reported in New Haven, Connecticut. These resulted from a medical gas system failure in which an altered oxygen flowmeter was connected to a wall supply source for nitrous oxide.[38]

7 In the event that a pipeline crossover is suspected, the workstation user must immediately take two corrective actions. First, the backup oxygen cylinder should be turned on. Then, the pipeline supply must be disconnected. This second step is mandatory because the machine will preferentially use the (potentially) inappropriate 50 psig pipeline supply source instead of the lower-pressure (45 psig) oxygen cylinder source if the wall supply is not disconnected. Recent publications suggest that many anesthesia providers may not appreciate the importance of or reasons for these actions.[39,40]

The wall outlet connections for pipeline gases are gas-specific. If they are "quick connect" fittings then they are gas-specific within the same manufacturer. For example, a wall oxygen outlet made by Ohmeda will not accept an oxygen connector made by Chemetron, even though the gas is the same. This can create problems if outlets and connectors by more than one manufacturer exist in the same facility.[41] Many institutions seeking to create uniformity are now using nationally standardized Diameter Index Safety System (DISS) threaded connections. The DISS provides threaded, noninterchangeable connections for medical gas lines, which minimizes the risk of misconnection. Regardless of which type of gas-specific connector (DISS or "quick connect") exists at the wall end of the hose conducting gas to the anesthesia machine, the gas enters the anesthesia machine through DISS inlet connections (see Fig. 24-4; arrows). A pressure gauge measures the pipeline gas pressure when the machine is connected to a pipeline supply. A check valve is located downstream from the inlet. It prevents reverse flow of gases from the machine to the pipeline or the atmosphere.

Cylinder Supply Source

Anesthesia workstations have E-cylinders for use when a pipeline supply source is not available or if the pipeline system fails. Anesthesia providers can easily become complacent and falsely assume that backup gas cylinders are, in fact, present on the anesthesia workstation, and further, if present, that they contain an adequate supply of compressed gas. The pre-use checklist should contain steps that confirm both.

Medical gases supplied in E-cylinders are attached to the anesthesia machine via the hanger yoke assembly. The hanger yoke assembly orients and supports the cylinder, provides a gas-tight seal, and ensures a unidirectional flow of gases into the machine.[33] Each hanger yoke is equipped with the Pin Index Safety System (PISS). The PISS is a safeguard introduced to eliminate cylinder interchanging and the possibility of accidentally placing the incorrect gas on a yoke designed to accommodate another gas. Two metal pins on the yoke assembly are arranged so that that they project into corresponding holes in the cylinder valve. Each gas or combination of gases has a specific and unique pin arrangement.[42,43] A failure of the pin index system, and medical staff to properly identify E-cylinder contents, was the cause of an intraoperative fire during laparoscopy.[44] A mixture of oxygen and CO_2 was utilized rather than 100% CO_2.

Once the cylinders are turned on, compressed gases may pass from their respective high-pressure cylinder sources into the anesthesia machine (see Fig. 24-4). A check valve is located downstream from each cylinder if a double-yoke assembly is used. This check valve serves several functions. First, it minimizes gas transfer from a cylinder at high pressure to one with a lower pressure. Second, it allows an empty cylinder to be exchanged for a full one while gas flow continues from the other cylinder into the machine with minimal loss of gas or supply pressure. Third, it minimizes leakage from an open cylinder to the atmosphere if one cylinder is absent.[32,33] A cylinder supply pressure gauge is located downstream from the check valves. The gauge will indicate the pressure in the cylinder having the higher pressure when two reserve cylinders of the same gas are opened at the same time.

Each cylinder supply source has a pressure-reducing valve known as the cylinder pressure regulator. It reduces the high and variable storage pressure present in a cylinder to a lower, more constant pressure suitable for use in the anesthesia machine. The oxygen cylinder pressure regulator reduces the oxygen cylinder pressure from a high of 2,200 psig to approximately 45 psig. The nitrous oxide cylinder pressure regulator receives pressure of up to 745 psig and reduces it to approximately 45 psig.[32,33]

The gas supply cylinder valves should be turned off when not in use, except during the preoperative machine pre-use checkout. If the cylinder supply valves are left open, the reserve cylinder supply can be silently depleted whenever the pressure inside the machine decreases to a value lower than the regulated cylinder pressure. For example, oxygen pressure within the machine can decrease below 45 psig with oxygen flushing or possibly even during the use of a pneumatically driven ventilator, particularly at high inspiratory flow rates. In addition, the pipeline supply pressures of all gases can fall to less than 45 psig if problems exist in the central piping system. If the cylinders are left open when this occurs, they will eventually become depleted and no reserve supply may be available if a complete central pipeline failure were to occur.[29,32]

The amount of time that an anesthesia machine can operate from the E-cylinder supply is important knowledge. This is particularly true now that anesthesia is being provided more frequently in office-based and in remote (outside the OR) hospital settings where pipeline oxygen may not be available. Oxygen can exist only in gaseous form at room temperature, and it obeys Boyle's law which states that for a fixed mass of gas at constant temperature, the product of pressure times volume is constant.[45] The volume of oxygen available from the cylinder is directly proportional to the cylinder pressure.

4 An E-cylinder has an internal volume of 4.8 L and when "full" is pressurized to 2,000 psig. Since psig is the pressure measured in excess of atmospheric pressure (14.7 psia, pounds per square inch absolute pressure), the cylinder pressure is 2,014.7 psia. Applying Boyle's Law:

$$2{,}014.7 \times 4.8 = 14.7 \times V2$$

Therefore, V2, the volume of oxygen in a "full" E-cylinder at 1 atm is

$$(2{,}014.7 \times 4.8)/14.7 = 658 \text{ L}$$

The following equation has been proposed to help estimate the remaining time that oxygen can be delivered at a given flow rate[46]:

$$\text{Approx. remaining time (hours)} \approx \frac{\text{Oxygen cylinder pressure (psig)}}{200 \times \text{Oxygen flow rate (L/min)}}$$

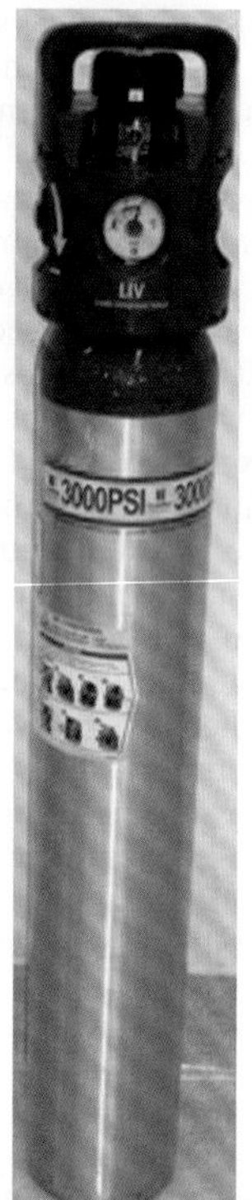

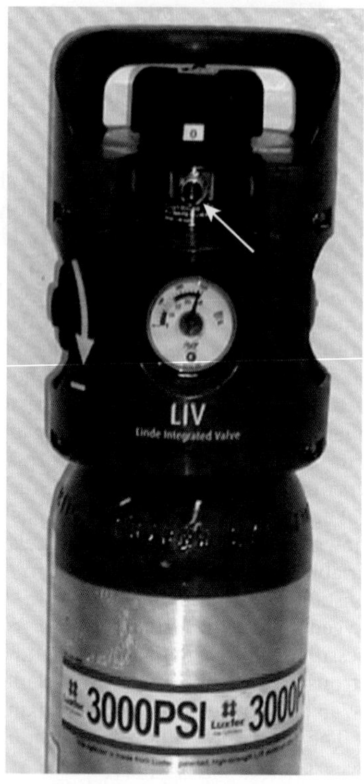

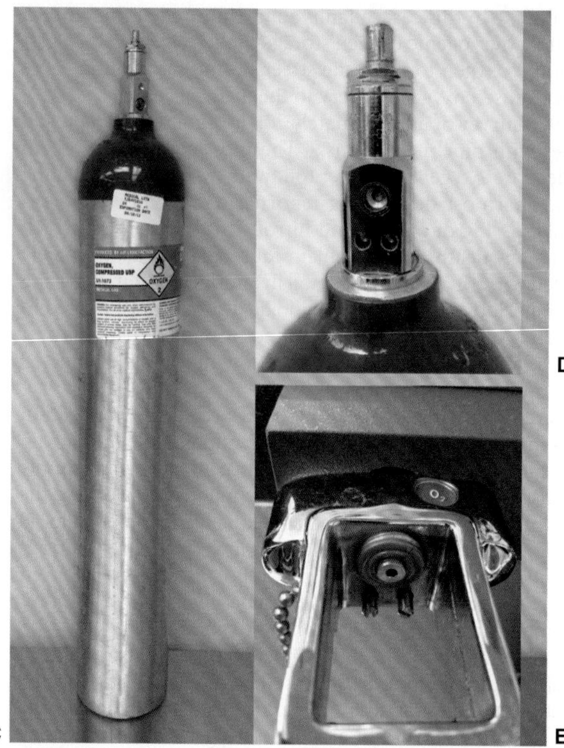

A B C D E

FIGURE 24-8. (A) 3,000 psig E-cylinder with Linde Integrated Valve LIV **(B)**, Linde Gas North America LLC that permits adjustable flows of ¼ to 25 L/min from the low-pressure nozzle (B-arrow). There is also a high-pressure regulator that can supply oxygen at 50 psig via a DISS connector. Standard E-cylinder **(C)** showing pin-index safety system **(D)** and mating yoke **(E)**.

For example, an E-cylinder of oxygen with a pressure of 1,000 psig, used at an oxygen flow rate of 5 L/min would be depleted in

$$[1{,}000/(200 \times 5)] \simeq 1 \text{ hour}$$

It should be noted that this calculation will provide only a gross estimate of remaining time and may not be exact. Furthermore, users should be cautioned that use of a pneumatically driven mechanical ventilator will dramatically increase oxygen utilization rates and decrease the remaining time until the cylinder is depleted. Uses of spontaneous or manual ventilation, with low FGF rates in a circle system with CO_2 absorption, will significantly reduce oxygen consumption from an E-cylinder if this is the only source of oxygen available.[7,8,35] Because electrically powered piston type anesthesia ventilators, such as found in the Dräger Fabius GS and Apollo workstations, do not impact oxygen usage rates they may be preferable to conventional gas-driven ventilators in practice settings where the supply of compressed gas cylinders may be limited.

A new regulator for E-cylinders of oxygen is available that permits controlled delivery of oxygen via a nozzle at flows of ≤25 L/min for patient transport (Fig. 24-8 A,B,C,D and E). The tank regulator also permits delivery of oxygen at 50 psig from a DISS connection (Fig. 26-9). If the oxygen hose from the anesthesia machine is connected to a central source (e.g., at the wall) via a DISS connector, and that central source becomes unavailable, then the machine hose can be easily connected to the tank's DISS connector and provide a backup supply of oxygen (Fig. 24-9 B). A conventional E cylinder with pin index safety system is shown in Fig. 24-8, C,D,E.

Nitrous Oxide

Nitrous oxide (N_2O) can be supplied to the anesthesia machine from the pipeline system at a pressure of approximately 50 psig or from a backup E-cylinder in the N_2O hanger yoke. N_2O has a molecular weight of 44 atomic mass units (AMU) and a boiling point of −88°C at 760 mm Hg (14.7 psia) pressure.[47] The critical temperature (CT) is the highest temperature at which a gas can exist in liquid form. The CT of N_2O is 36.5°C (critical pressure: 1,054 psig), therefore N_2O can exist as a liquid at room temperature (20°C). E-cylinders of N_2O are factory-filled to 90% to 95% capacity with liquid N_2O. Above the liquid in the tank is N_2O vapor. Because the liquid agent is in equilibrium with its vapor or gas phase, the pressure exerted by the gaseous N_2O is its saturated vapor pressure (SVP) at the ambient temperature. At 20°C, the SVP of N_2O is 750 psig.

A full E-tank of N_2O generates approximately 1,600 L of gas at 1 atm pressure at sea level (14.7 psia). As long as some liquid N_2O is present in the tank and the ambient temperature remains at 20°C, the pressure in the N_2O tank will remain at 750 psig, which is the SVP of N_2O at 20°C. The volume of N_2O gas available from a tank therefore cannot be determined by reference to the N_2O tank pressure gauge. It is determined by weighing the tank and subtracting the weight of the empty tank (tare weight) to determine the weight of the contained N_2O.

Once all the liquid N_2O has been used and the tank contains only gas, Boyle's law (i.e., $P1 \times V1 = P2 \times V2$) may be applied. When the tank pressure is ~750 psig (or 764.7 psia) from gas only, and the internal volume of the E-cylinder is 4.8 L, the

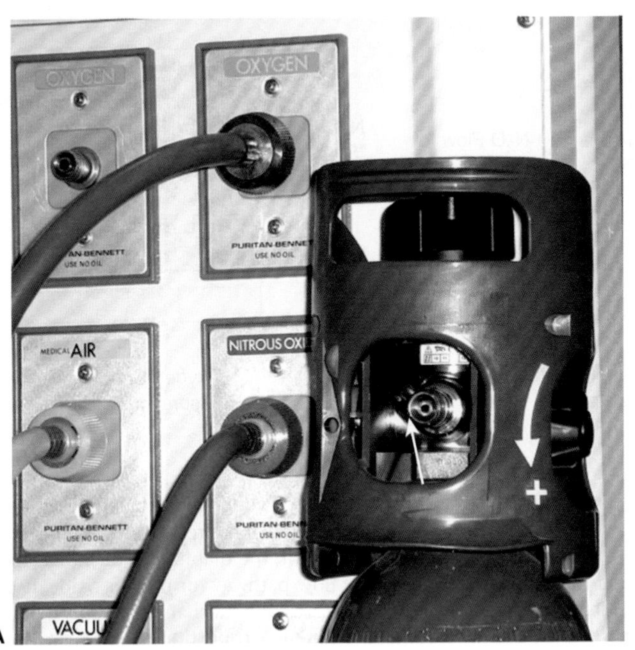

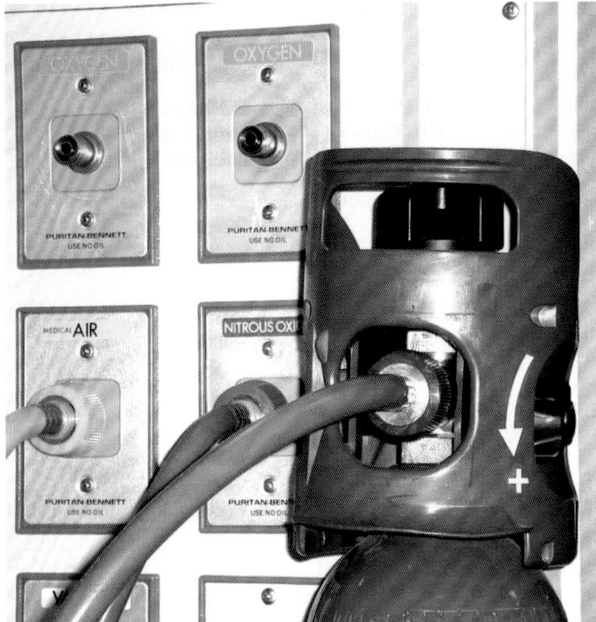

FIGURE 24-9. A. 3,000 psig E-cylinder valve showing 50 psig DISS connection (arrow) that **(B)** could be connected to the machine oxygen hose if wall oxygen supply fails.

volume of N_2O available at a pressure of 1 atm (i.e., 760 mm Hg or 14.7 psia) is 250 L. At this point the N_2O tank is 250/1,600, or ~16%, full. From then on, as N_2O continues to be utilized, the value on the tank pressure gauge will fall.

Nitrous oxide from the tank supply enters the N_2O hanger yoke at pressures of up to 750 psig (at 20°C) and then passes through a regulator that reduces this pressure to 40 to 45 psig (Fig. 38-2). The PISS is designed to ensure that only a N_2O tank may hang in a N_2O hanger yoke. As with oxygen, a check valve in each yoke prevents the back leakage of N_2O if no tank is hanging in the yoke.

The N_2O pipeline is supplied from a bulk storage container of liquid N_2O or from banks of large N_2O tanks, usually H cylinders. (Each H cylinder of N_2O evolves 16,000 L of gas at atmospheric pressure.) The pressure in the N_2O pipeline is regulated to approximately 50 psig to supply the outlets in the operating room. Having entered the anesthesia machine intermediate-pressure system, N_2O must flow past the "fail-safe" valve to reach the N_2O flow-control.

Machine Intermediate-Pressure System

Having entered the anesthesia machine's intermediate-pressure system from the pipeline supply at ~50 psig, or from the tank supply at 45 psig, oxygen can take several paths:

1. To the DISS auxiliary oxygen takeoff, which can be connected to a Sanders type jet ventilating system
2. To supply a pneumatically powered bellows ventilator
3. Via a regulator and an auxiliary oxygen flowmeter to be connected to a nasal cannula, self-inflating resuscitation bag, etc.
4. To the oxygen low-pressure alarm sensor
5. To the pressure sensitive shutoff ("fail-safe") valve
6. To the oxygen flush control valve
7. To the oxygen flowmeter (in some machines via a second-stage regulator)

Oxygen Supply Pressure Failure Safety Devices

The 2000 ASTM F1850-00 standard states, "The anesthesia gas supply device shall be designed so that whenever oxygen supply pressure is reduced to below the manufacturer specified minimum, the delivered oxygen concentration shall not decrease below 19% at the common gas outlet."[48] Contemporary anesthesia machines have a number of safety devices that act together in a cascade manner to minimize the risk of delivery of a hypoxic gas mixture as oxygen pressure decreases. Several of these devices are described in the following sections.

Pneumatic and Electronic Alarm Devices

Many older anesthesia machines have a pneumatic alarm device that provides an audible warning when the oxygen supply pressure decreases to a predetermined threshold value such as 30 psig. The 2000 ASTM F1850-00 standard mandated that a medium priority alarm be activated within 5 seconds when the oxygen pressure decreases below a manufacturer-specific pressure threshold.[48] Electronic alarm devices are now used to meet this guideline.

Oxygen Failure Cutoff ("Fail-Safe") Valves

8 An oxygen failure cutoff valve is present in the gas line supplying each of the flowmeters except oxygen. Controlled by oxygen supply pressure, the valve shuts off (or proportionally decreases) the supply pressure of all other gases (nitrous oxide, CO_2, helium, and in some machines, air) as the oxygen supply pressure decreases. Unfortunately, the misnomer "fail-safe" has led to the misconception that the valve prevents administration of a hypoxic mixture. This is not the case. Machines that are either not equipped with a N_2O/O_2 flow proportioning system (see Proportioning Systems

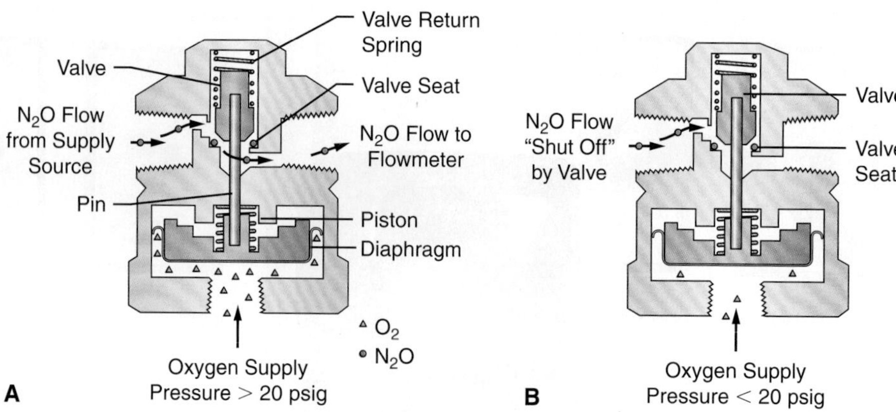

FIGURE 24-10. Pressure-sensor shutoff valve. The valve is open in **A** because the oxygen supply pressure is greater than the threshold value of 20 psig. The valve is closed in **B** because of inadequate oxygen pressure. (Redrawn with permission from: Bowie E, Huffman LM. *The Anesthesia Machine: Essentials for Understanding.* Madison, WI, Ohmeda, a division of BOC Health Care, Inc., 1985.)

section) or ones whose system may be disabled by the user can deliver a hypoxic mixture under normal working conditions. On such a system, the oxygen flow-control valve can be closed intentionally or accidentally. Normal oxygen pressure will keep other gas lines open so that a hypoxic mixture could result.[32,33]

Many Datex-Ohmeda machines are equipped with a fail-safe valve known as the pressure-sensor shutoff valve (Fig. 24-10). On older machines, this valve operates in a threshold manner and is either open or closed. Oxygen supply pressure opens the valve, and the valve return spring closes the valve. Figure 24-10 shows a nitrous oxide pressure-sensor shutoff valve with a threshold pressure of 20 psig. In Figure 24-10A, an oxygen supply pressure greater than 20 psig is exerted on the mobile diaphragm. This pressure moves the piston and pin upward and the valve opens. Nitrous oxide flows freely to the nitrous oxide flow-control valve. In Figure 24-10B, the oxygen supply pressure is less than 20 psig, and the force of the valve return spring completely closes the valve.[32] Nitrous oxide flow stops at the closed fail-safe valve, and it does not advance to the nitrous oxide flow-control valve.

In the GE Datex Aestiva/5, which is a more recent model machine, the "fail-safe " valve is not of an "open or closed" design, rather it is a variable valve in a balance regulator. The balance regulator works as follows. The second-stage pressure regulator for oxygen reduces the pressure to about 30 psig in the intermediate-pressure system. The oxygen pressure is then piloted to the balance regulator where it is applied to the oxygen side of the regulated diaphragm. If the pressure of oxygen is sufficient, the diaphragm pushes against a mechanism that opens the flow pathway for nitrous oxide. If the oxygen piloting pressure decreases, the mechanism begins to close off the pathway for nitrous oxide in proportion to the decrease in piloted oxygen pressure. The balance regulator for nitrous oxide closes completely when the pressure of oxygen falls to 0.5 psig. Balance regulators for heliox and CO_2 interrupt the flows of these gases when the piloted oxygen pressure falls below 10 psig.[26]

Dräger Medical uses a different fail-safe valve known as the Oxygen Failure Protection Device (OFPD) to interface the oxygen pressure with that of other gases, such as nitrous oxide or inert gases. Similar in principle to the balance regulator described in the previous paragraph, the OFPD is based on a proportioning principle rather than a threshold principle. The pressure of all gases controlled by the OFPD will decrease in proportion with the oxygen pressure. The OFPD consists of a seat-nozzle assembly connected to a spring-loaded piston (Fig. 24-11). The oxygen supply pressure in the left panel of Figure 24-11 is 50 psig. This pressure pushes the piston upward, forcing the nozzle away from the valve seat. Nitrous oxide and/or other gases advance toward the flow control valve at 50 psig. The oxygen pressure in the right panel is 0 psig. The spring is expanded and forces the nozzle

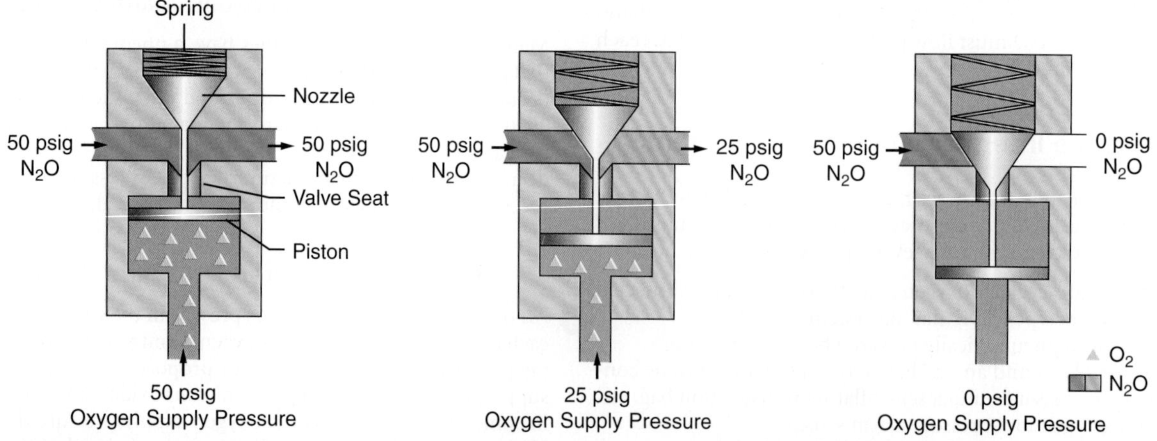

FIGURE 24-11. Oxygen Failure Protection Device/Sensitive Oxygen Ratio Controller (OFPD/S-ORC), which responds proportionally to changes in oxygen supply pressure. (Redrawn with permission from: *Narkomed 2A Anesthesia System: Technical Service Manual.* 6th ed. Telford, PA: North American Dräger; 1985.)

against the seat, preventing flow through the device. Finally, the center panel shows an intermediate oxygen pressure of 25 psig. The force of the spring partially closes the valve. The nitrous oxide pressure delivered to the flow control valve is 25 psig. There is a continuum of intermediate configurations between the extremes (0 to 50 psig) of oxygen supply pressure. These intermediate valve configurations are responsible for the proportional nature of the OFPD. An important concept to be understood with these particular fail-safe devices is that the older Datex-Ohmeda Pressure Sensor Shutoff Valve is threshold in nature (all-or-nothing), whereas the GE balance regulator and Dräger Oxygen Failure Protection Device are variable, flow type proportioning systems.

Second-Stage Oxygen Pressure Regulator

Most contemporary GE Datex-Ohmeda workstations have a second-stage oxygen pressure regulator set at a specific value, ranging from 12 to 19 psig. Output from the oxygen flowmeter is constant when the oxygen supply pressure exceeds the threshold (minimal) value. The pressure-sensor shutoff valve of older Datex-Ohmeda machines is set at a higher threshold value (20 to 30 psig) to ensure that oxygen is the last gas flowing if oxygen pressure failure occurs.

Flowmeter Assemblies

The flowmeter assembly (Fig. 24-12) precisely controls and measures gas flow to the common gas outlet. With traditional glass flowmeter assemblies, the flow control needle valve regulates the amount of flow that enters a tapered, transparent flow tube known as a Thorpe tube. The tube is tapered such that it has a small cross-sectional area at its lower (low flow) end, and a larger cross-sectional area at its upper (high flow) end. A mobile indicator float inside the flow tube indicates the amount of flow passing through the associated flow control valve. The quantity of flow is indicated on a scale associated with the flow tube.[32,33] Some newer anesthesia workstations have now replaced the conventional glass flow tubes with electronic flow sensors that measure the flow of the individual gases. The flow rate data are then presented in numerical format, graphical format, or a combination of the two. The integration of these "electronic flowmeters" is an essential step in the evolution of the anesthesia workstation if it is to become fully integrated with anesthesia data-capturing systems, such as computerized anesthesia record keepers (or AIMS: anesthesia information management systems).

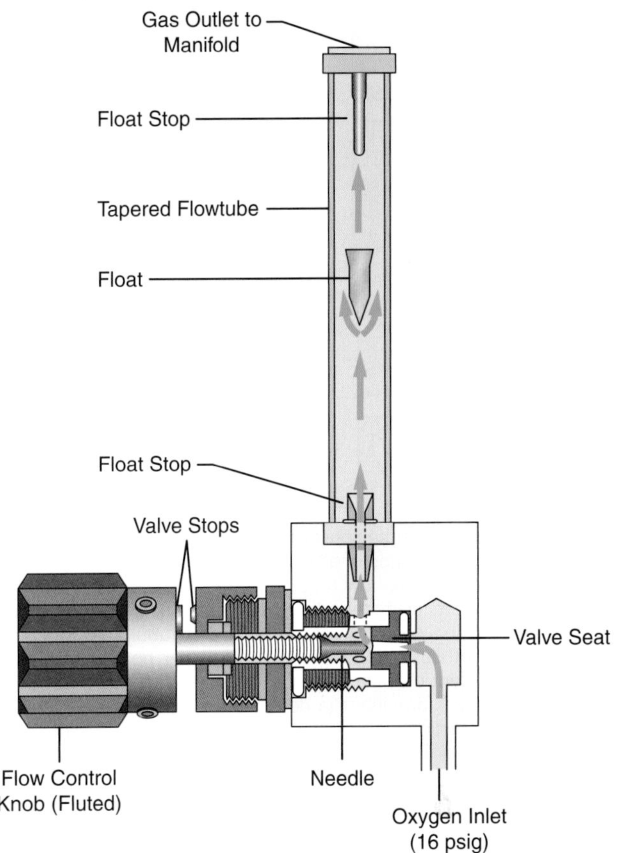

FIGURE 24-12. Oxygen flowmeter assembly. The oxygen flowmeter assembly is composed of the flow control valve assembly plus the flowmeter subassembly. Note that this is a GE Datex-Ohmeda design because in this figure oxygen is supplied to the flowmeter at 16 psig from a second-stage regulator. (Reproduced with permission from: Bowie E, Huffman LM. *The Anesthesia Machine: Essentials for Understanding*. Madison, WI: Ohmeda, a division of BOC Health Care, Inc., 1985.)

Operating Principles of Conventional Flowmeters

Opening the flow control needle valve allows gas to travel through the space between the float and the flow tube. This space is known as the annular space (Fig. 24-13). The indicator float hovers freely in an equilibrium position where the upward force resulting from gas flow equals the downward force on the float resulting from gravity at a given flow rate. The float moves to a new equilibrium position in the tube when flow is changed. These flowmeters are commonly referred to as *constant pressure variable orifice* flowmeters because the pressure decrease across the float remains constant for all positions in the tube.[33,49,50]

Flow tubes are tapered, with the smallest diameter at the bottom of the tube and the largest diameter at the top. The term *variable orifice* designates this type of unit because the annular space between the float and the inner wall of the flow tube varies with the position of the float. Flow through the constriction created by the float can be laminar or turbulent, depending on the flow rate (Fig. 24-14). The characteristics of a gas that influence its flow

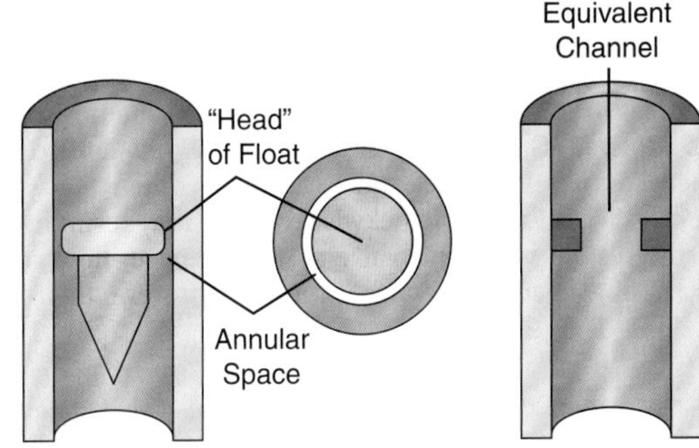

FIGURE 24-13. The annular space. The clearance between the head of the float and the flow tube is known as the annular space. It can be considered equivalent to a circular channel of the same cross-sectional area. (Redrawn with permission from: Macintosh R, Mushin WW, Epstein HG. *Physics for the Anaesthetist*. 3rd ed. Oxford: Blackwell Scientific Publications; 1963.)

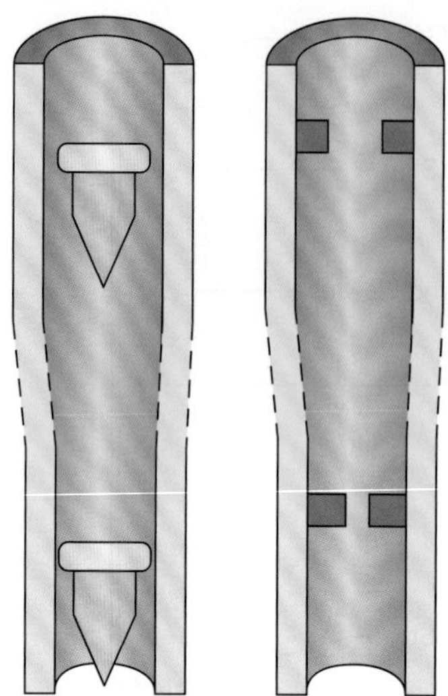

FIGURE 24-14. Flow tube constriction. The lower half of illustration represents the lower portion of a flow tube. The clearance between the head of the float and the flow tube is narrow. The equivalent channel is tubular because its diameter is less than its length. Viscosity is dominant in determining gas flow rate through this tubular constriction. The upper half of illustration represents the upper portion of a flow tube. The equivalent channel is orificial because its length is less than its width. Density is dominant in determining gas flow rate through this orificial constriction. (Redrawn with permission from: Macintosh R, Mushin WW, Epstein HG. *Physics for the Anaesthetist.* 3rd ed. Oxford: Blackwell Scientific Publications; 1963.)

rate through a given constriction are viscosity (laminar flow) and density (turbulent flow). Because the annular space is tubular, at low flow rates laminar flow is present and *viscosity* determines the gas flow rate. The annular space simulates an orifice at high flow rates, and turbulent gas flow then depends predominantly on the *density* of the gas.[32,33]

Components of the Flowmeter Assembly

Flow Control Valve Assembly

The flow control valve (see Fig. 24-10) assembly consists of a flow control knob, a needle valve, a valve seat, and a pair of valve stops.[32] The assembly can receive its pneumatic input either directly from the pipeline source (50 psig) or from a second-stage pressure regulator. The location of the needle valve in the valve seat changes to establish different orifices when the flow control valve is adjusted. Gas flow increases when the flow control valve is turned counterclockwise, and it decreases when the valve is turned clockwise. Extreme clockwise rotation may result in damage to the needle valve and valve seat. Therefore, flow control valves are equipped with valve "stops" to prevent this occurrence.[33]

SAFETY FEATURES. Contemporary flow-control valve assemblies have numerous safety features. The oxygen flow-control knob is physically distinguishable from other gas knobs. It is distinctively fluted, projects beyond the control knobs of the other gases, and is larger in diameter than the flow control knobs of other gases. All knobs are color coded for the appropriate gas, and the chemical formula or name of the gas is permanently marked on each. Flow control knobs are recessed or protected with a shield or barrier to minimize accidental change from a preset position. If a single gas has two flow tubes, the tubes are arranged in series and are controlled by a single flow-control valve.[48]

In many of the new anesthesia workstations, the flowmeters have been replaced by electronic control panels that contain "soft keys." In order to adjust any gas flow, the operator must perform the following steps: (1) select and press the "soft key" to identify the gas and anesthetic agent selected; (2) turn the selector knob to adjust the desired flow level; and (3) press the selector knob again to confirm the selected flow level and anesthetic agent (see Electronic Flowmeters section).

Flowmeter Subassembly

The flowmeter subassembly (see Fig. 24-12) consists of the flow tube, the indicator float with float stops, and the indicator scale.[33]

FLOW TUBES. Contemporary flow tubes are made of glass. Most have a single taper in which the inner diameter of the flow tube increases uniformly from bottom to top. Manufacturers provide double flow tubes for oxygen and nitrous oxide to provide better visual discrimination at low flow rates. A fine flow tube indicates flow from approximately 200 mL/min to 1 L/min, and a coarse flow tube indicates flow from approximately 1 mL/min to 10 or 12 L/min. The two tubes are connected in series and supplied from a single flow-control valve. The total gas flow is that shown on the higher flowmeter.

INDICATOR FLOATS AND FLOAT STOPS. Contemporary anesthesia machines use several different types of bobbins or floats, including plumb-bob floats, rotating skirted floats, and ball floats. Flow is read at the top of plumb-bob and skirted floats and at the center of the ball on the ball-type floats.[33] Flow tubes are equipped with float stops at the top and bottom of the tube. The upper stop prevents the float from ascending to the top of the tube and plugging the outlet. It also ensures that the float will be visible at maximum flows instead of being hidden in the manifold. The bottom float stop provides a central foundation for the indicator when the flow control valve is turned off.[32,33]

SCALE. The flowmeter scale can be marked directly on the flow tube or located to the right of the tube.[48] Gradations corresponding to equal increments in flow rate are closer together at the top of the scale because the annular space increases more rapidly than does the internal diameter from bottom to top of the tube. Rib guides are used in some flow tubes with ball-type indicators to minimize this compression effect. They are tapered glass ridges that run the length of the tube. There are usually three rib guides that are equally spaced around the inner circumference of the tube. In the presence of rib guides, the annular space from the bottom to the top of the tube increases almost proportionally with the internal diameter. This results in a nearly linear scale.[33] Rib guides are employed on many Dräger Medical flow tubes.

SAFETY FEATURES. The flowmeter subassemblies for each gas on the Datex-Ohmeda Modulus I, Modulus II, Modulus II Plus, CD, and Aestiva are housed in independent, color-coded, pin-specific modules. The flow tubes are adjacent to a gas-specific, color-coded backing. The flow scale and the chemical formula (or name of the gas) is permanently etched on the backing to the right of the flow tube. Flowmeter scales are individually hand-calibrated using the specific float to provide a high degree of accuracy. The tube, float, and scale make an inseparable unit. The entire set must be replaced if any component is damaged.

Dräger Medical does not use a modular system for the flowmeter subassembly. The flow scale, the chemical symbol, and the gas-specific color codes are etched directly onto the flow tube. The scale in use is obvious when two flow tubes for the same gas are used.

Problems with Flowmeters

Leaks

Flowmeter leaks are a substantial hazard because the flowmeters are located downstream from all machine safety devices except the oxygen analyzer.[51] Leaks can occur at the O-ring junctions between the glass flow tubes and the metal manifold or in cracked or broken glass flow tubes, the most fragile pneumatic component of the anesthesia machine. Even though gross damage to conventional glass flow tubes is usually apparent, subtle cracks and chips may be overlooked, resulting in errors of delivered flows.[52] The use of electronic flowmeters and the removal of conventional glass flow tubes from some newer anesthesia workstations (e.g., Datex-Ohmeda S/5 ADU and the Dräger Fabius) may help to eliminate these potential sources of leaks (see Electronic Flowmeters section).

Eger et al.[53] demonstrated that, in the presence of a flowmeter leak, a hypoxic mixture is less likely to occur if the oxygen flowmeter is located downstream from all other flowmeters. Figure 24-15 is an updated version of the figure in Eger's original publication. The unused airflow tube has a large leak. Nitrous oxide and oxygen flow rates are set at a ratio of 3:1. A potentially dangerous arrangement is shown in Figures 24-15A and 24-15B because the nitrous oxide flowmeter is located in the downstream position. A hypoxic mixture can result because a substantial portion of oxygen flow passes through the leak, and all nitrous oxide is directed to the common gas outlet. Safer configurations are shown in Figures 24-15C and 24-15D. The oxygen flowmeter is located in the downstream position. A portion of the nitrous oxide flow escapes through the leak, and the remainder goes toward the common gas outlet. A hypoxic mixture is less likely because all the oxygen flow is advanced by the nitrous oxide. On most Dräger workstations the flowmeters are arranged as in Figure 24-15C, and GE Datex-Ohmeda flowmeters are as in Figure 24-15D.

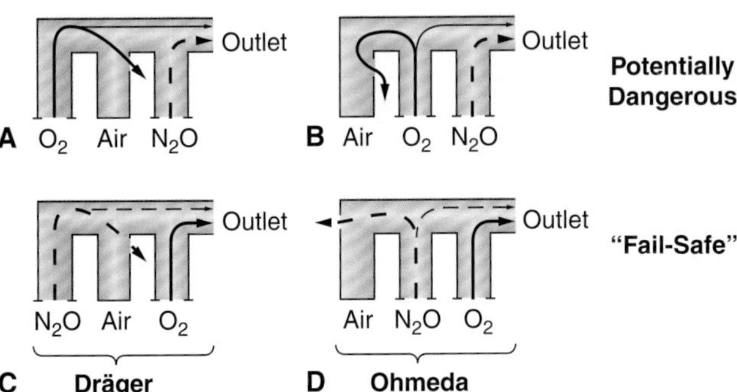

FIGURE 24-15. Flowmeter sequence—a potential cause of hypoxia. In the event of a flowmeter leak, a potentially dangerous arrangement exists when nitrous oxide is located in the downstream position (**A** and **B**). The safest configuration exists when oxygen is located in the downstream position (**C** and **D**). See text for details. (Modified with permission from: Eger EI 2nd, Hylton RR, Irwin RH, et al. Anesthetic flowmeter sequence—a cause for hypoxia. *Anesthesiology.* 1963;24:396.)

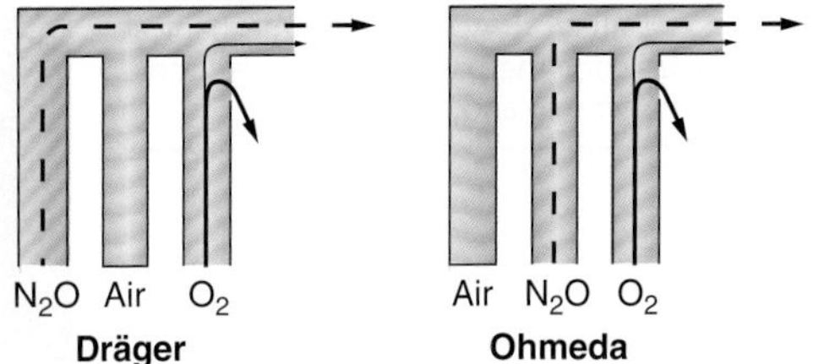

FIGURE 24-16. Oxygen flow tube leak. An oxygen flow tube leak can produce a hypoxic mixture regardless of flow tube arrangement. (Reproduced with permission from: Brockwell RC. Inhaled anesthetic delivery systems. In: Miller RD, ed. *Anesthesia.* 6th ed. Philadelphia, PA: Churchill Livingstone; 2004:281.)

A leak in the oxygen flow tube may result in creation of a hypoxic mixture even when oxygen is located in the downstream position (Fig. 24-16).[51,52] Oxygen escapes through the leak and nitrous oxide continues to flow toward the common outlet, particularly at high ratios of nitrous oxide to oxygen flow.

Inaccuracy

Flow measurement error can occur even when flowmeters are assembled properly with appropriate components. Dirt or static electricity can cause a float to stick, and the actual flow may be higher or lower than that indicated. Sticking of the indicator float is more common in the low flow ranges because the annular space is smaller. A damaged float can cause inaccurate readings because the precise relationship between the float and the flow tube is altered. Back pressure from the breathing circuit can cause a float to drop so that it reads less than the actual flow. Finally, if flowmeters are not aligned properly in the vertical position (plumb), readings can be inaccurate because tilting distorts the annular space.[24,33,52]

Ambiguous Scale

Before the standardization of flowmeter scales and the widespread use of oxygen analyzers, at least two deaths resulted from confusion created by ambiguous scales.[24,52,54] The operator read the float position beside an adjacent but erroneous scale in both cases. Today this error is less likely to occur because contemporary flowmeter scales are marked either directly onto the flow tube or immediately to the right of it.[48] The possibility of confusion is minimized when the scale is etched directly onto the tube.

Electronic Flowmeters

Newer anesthesia workstations such as the GE-Datex-Ohmeda S/5 ADU, the Dräger Fabius GS, and the Dräger Apollo (among others) have conventional flow control knobs and flow control valves, but have electronic flow sensors and digital displays rather than glass flow tubes (Fig. 24-17). The output from the flow control valve is represented graphically and/or numerically in liters per minute on the workstation's integrated user interface. These systems are dependent on electrical power to provide a precise display of gas flows. However, even when electrical power is totally interrupted, since the flow control valves themselves are mechanical (i.e., non-electronic), the set gas flows will continue uninterrupted. Since these machines do not have individual flow tubes that physically quantitate the flow of each gas, a small conventional pneumatic "fresh gas" or "total flow" indicator is also provided that

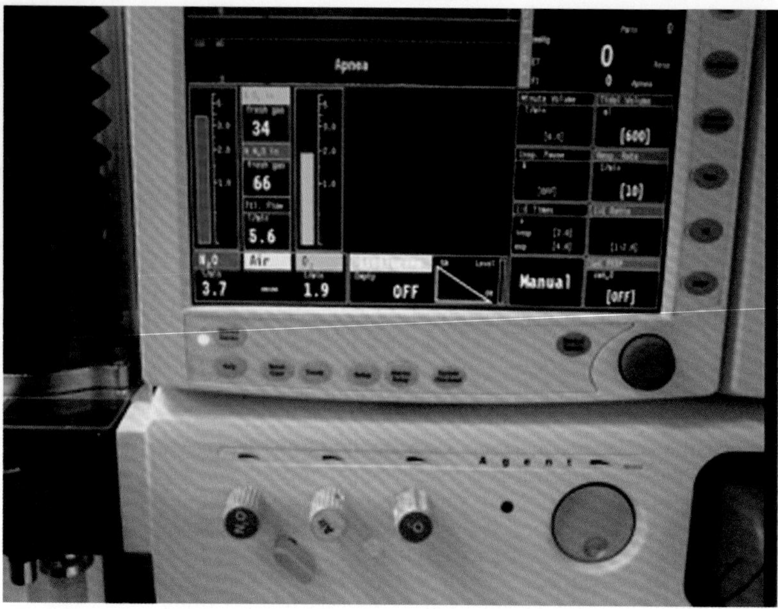

FIGURE 24-17. Datex S5/ADU. Note mechanical needle valve controls for the gas flows but electronic display of virtual flowmeter and digital readout.

gives the user an estimate of the total quantity of fresh gas flowing from all gas flow-control valves to the anesthesia workstation's common gas outlet, and is functional even in the event of a total power failure (Fig. 24-18).

In the GE Datex Aisys Carestation, the traditional needle valve gas flow controls and color-coded control knobs are replaced by an electronic control system that uses a gas mixer. In the GE Aisys Carestation, the second gas, either N_2O or air is first selected, followed by the desired inspired oxygen concentration (FIO_2) and total FGF. Total flow and FIO_2 selections are made by pressing soft keys on the control panel, adjusting the settings using a "com wheel," and then pressing the com wheel to "confirm."

In the Aisys Carestation, the controls to increase or decrease flows (or agent concentration) represent a departure from the traditional. The traditional needle valve gas flow controls were designed by mechanical engineers so that one turns the flow control knob counterclockwise to increase flow (by opening the valve wider). The same applies to increasing agent concentration on a variable bypass vaporizer. The Aisys Carestation controls are designed by electrical engineers where the standard is to increase the output by rotating the dial (com wheel) in a clockwise direction. Thus when learning to use the Aisys Carestation workstation, the operator must adapt to "clockwise to increase" and remember to confirm new settings, otherwise they are not implemented. In the event the gas mixer fails, the Aisys Carestation will switch to a backup system that permits delivery of oxygen to the breathing system via an Alternate Oxygen flowmeter, which is a traditional mechanical needle valve and rotameter flow tube.

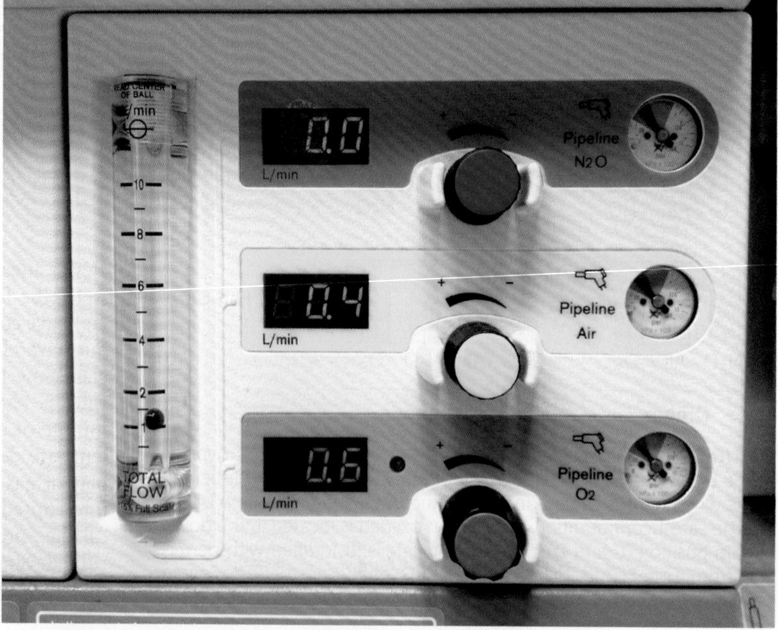

FIGURE 24-18. Dräger Fabius GS. Note needle valve controls, graphical and digital flow displays. The total gas flow rotameter continues to function if electrical power is lost.

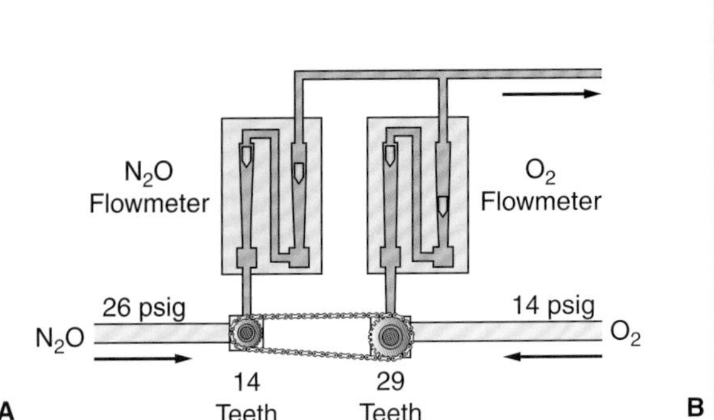

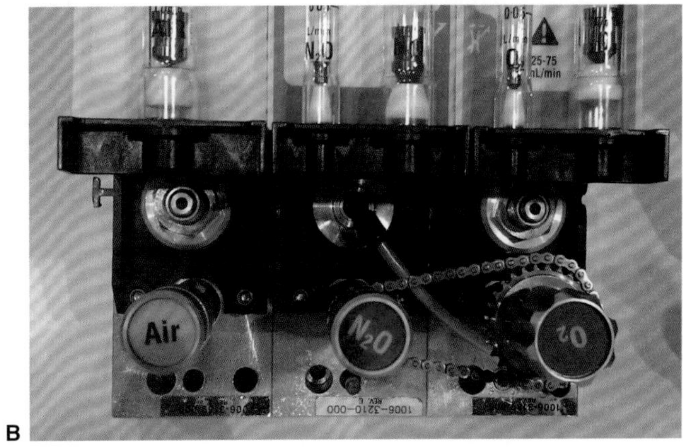

FIGURE 24-19. A. Schematic and **(B)** photo of Ohmeda Link-25 Proportion-Limiting Control System. See text for details.

Proportioning Systems

5 Manufacturers equip anesthesia workstations with N_2O/O_2 proportioning systems designed to prevent creation and delivery of a hypoxic mixture when nitrous oxide is administered. Nitrous oxide and oxygen are interfaced mechanically and/or pneumatically, or electronically (on the GE Aisys Carestation), so that the minimum oxygen concentration at the common gas outlet is between 23% and 25% depending on the manufacturer.

GE-Datex-Ohmeda Link-25 Proportion-Limiting Control System

Traditional GE-Datex-Ohmeda machines use the Link-25 System. The heart of the system is the mechanical integration of the nitrous oxide and oxygen flow-control valves. It allows independent adjustment of either valve, yet automatically intercedes to maintain a minimum 25% oxygen concentration with a maximum nitrous oxide–oxygen flow ratio of 3:1. The Link-25 automatically increases oxygen flow to prevent delivery of a hypoxic mixture.

Figure 24-19 illustrates the GE-Datex-Ohmeda Link-25 System. The nitrous oxide and oxygen flow-control valves are identical. A 14-tooth sprocket is attached to the nitrous oxide flow-control valve, and a 29-tooth sprocket is attached to the oxygen flow-control valve. A stainless steel chain physically links the sprockets. When the nitrous oxide flow-control valve is turned through 2.09 revolutions, or 29 teeth, the oxygen flow-control valve will revolve once because of the gear ratio. The final 3:1 flow ratio results because the nitrous oxide flow-control valve is supplied with nitrous oxide at a pressure of approximately 26 psig from a second-stage N_2O regulator, whereas the oxygen flow-control valve is supplied by a second-stage regulator at 14 psig. The combination of the mechanical and pneumatic aspects of the system yields the final minimum 25% oxygen concentration. The GE-Datex-Ohmeda Link-25 proportioning system *increases oxygen flow* when nitrous oxide flow would be excessive *by opening the O_2 needle valve more.* Conversely, if the oxygen flow is decreased such that the nitrous oxide flow would be excessive, it acts to *decrease the flow of N_2O by physically decreasing the opening of the nitrous oxide needle valve.*

Several reports have described failures of the Link-25 system.[54–57] The authors of these reports describe failures either that resulted in inability to administer oxygen without nitrous oxide or that allowed creation of a hypoxic mixture.

Dräger Oxygen Ratio Monitor Controller/ Sensitive Oxygen Ratio Controller System

Dräger's proportioning system, the Oxygen Ratio Monitor Controller (ORMC), is used on the North American Dräger Narkomed 2A, 2B, 3, and 4 machines. An equivalent system used on some more recent Dräger workstations such as the Fabius GS, Narkomed 6000 series, and the Apollo is known as the Sensitive Oxygen Ratio Controller (S-ORC). The ORMC and the S-ORC are pneumatic oxygen–nitrous oxide interlock systems designed to maintain a fresh gas oxygen concentration of at least 25 ± 3% when nitrous oxide is used. They control the fresh gas oxygen concentration to levels substantially greater than 25% when the oxygen flow rate is <1 L/min. The ORMC and S-ORC limit nitrous oxide flow to prevent delivery of a hypoxic mixture *by decreasing the supply pressure of* nitrous oxide *to its flow control needle valve.* This is unlike the Link-25 system, in which the gas supply pressure to the nitrous oxide needle valve is held constant (by the second-stage regulator) and gas flow changes are made by physically changing the size of the needle valve opening.

A schematic of the ORMC is shown in Figure 24-20. It consists of an oxygen chamber, a nitrous oxide chamber, and a nitrous oxide slave control valve. All are interconnected by a mobile horizontal shaft. The pneumatic input into the device is from the oxygen and the nitrous oxide flowmeters. These flowmeters are unique because they have specific resistors located downstream from the flow control valves. These resistors create back pressures directed to the oxygen and nitrous oxide chambers. The value of the oxygen flow tube resistor is 3 to 4 times that of the nitrous oxide flow tube resistor, and the relative value of these resistors determines the value of the controlled fresh gas oxygen concentration. The back pressures in the oxygen and nitrous oxide chambers are applied against rubber diaphragms attached to the mobile horizontal shaft. Movement of the shaft adjusts the opening of the nitrous oxide slave control valve, which in turn adjusts the feed pressure of the nitrous oxide flow control needle valve.

If the oxygen flow, and therefore back pressure, is proportionally higher than the nitrous oxide back pressure, the nitrous oxide slave control valve opens more widely, increasing the pressure of nitrous oxide upstream of the nitrous oxide flow-control needle valve, which results in an increase in nitrous oxide flow. As the nitrous oxide flow is increased manually, the nitrous oxide back pressure forces the shaft rightward toward the oxygen chamber. The nitrous oxide slave control valve opening becomes more

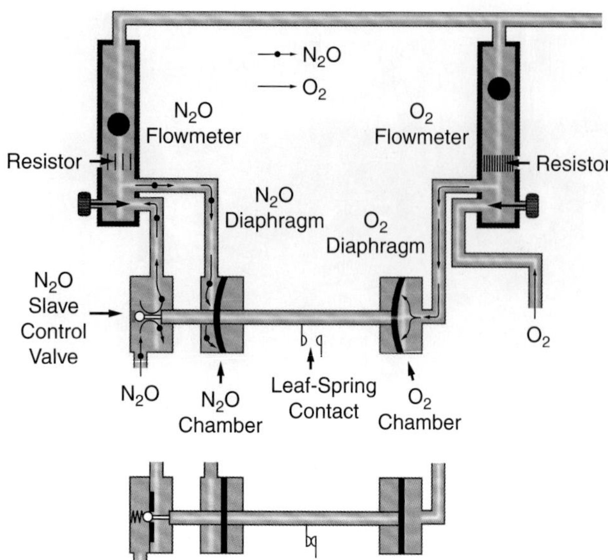

FIGURE 24-20. Dräger Oxygen Ratio Monitor Controller. See text for details. (Redrawn with permission from: Schreiber P. *Safety Guidelines for Anesthesia Systems.* Telford, PA: North American Dräger; 1984.)

restrictive and limits the nitrous oxide supply pressure to the flowmeter, which decreases the nitrous oxide flow.

Figure 24-20 illustrates the action of a single ORMC/S-ORC under different sets of circumstances. The back pressure exerted on the oxygen diaphragm, in the upper configuration is greater than that exerted on the nitrous oxide diaphragm. This causes the horizontal shaft to move to the left, opening the nitrous oxide slave control valve. Nitrous oxide is then able to proceed to its flow control valve and out through the flowmeter. In the lower configuration, the nitrous oxide slave control valve is closed because of inadequate oxygen back pressure.[34] To summarize, in contrast to the GE-Datex-Ohmeda Link-25 System which actively increases oxygen flow to maintain a fresh gas oxygen concentration ≥25%, the Dräger ORMC and S-ORC are systems that limit nitrous oxide flow to prevent delivery of a fresh gas mixture with an oxygen concentration ≤25%.

Limitations

N_2O/O_2 proportioning systems are not foolproof. Workstations equipped with these systems can still deliver a hypoxic mixture under certain conditions. Following is a description of some of the situations in which this may occur.

Wrong Supply Gas

Both the GE-Datex-Ohmeda Link-25 and the Dräger ORMC/S-ORC will be defeated if a gas other than oxygen is present in the oxygen pipeline and will allow delivery of hypoxic gas mixtures. In the Link-25 System, the nitrous oxide and oxygen flow-control valves will continue to be mechanically linked. Nevertheless, a hypoxic mixture can proceed to the common gas outlet. In the case of the Dräger ORMC or S-ORC, the rubber diaphragm for oxygen will reflect adequate supply pressure on the oxygen side even though the incorrect gas is present, and flow of both the wrong gas plus nitrous oxide will result. The oxygen analyzer is the only workstation monitor besides an integrated multigas analyzer that would detect this condition in either system.

Defective Pneumatics or Mechanics

Normal operation of the Datex-Ohmeda Link-25 and the Dräger ORMC/S-ORC is contingent on pneumatic and mechanical integrity.[58] Pneumatic integrity in the Datex-Ohmeda system requires properly functioning second-stage regulators. A nitrous oxide: xygen ratio other than 3:1 may result if the regulators are not precise. The chain connecting the two sprockets must be intact—if the chain is cut or broken, a 97% nitrous oxide concentration can result.[59] In the Dräger System, a functional OFPD is necessary to supply appropriate pressure to the ORMC. The mechanical aspects of the ORMC/S-ORC, such as the rubber diaphragms, the flow tube resistors, and the nitrous oxide slave control valve, must likewise be intact.

Leaks Downstream

The ORMC/S-ORC and the Link-25 function at the level of the flow control valves. A leak downstream from these devices, such as a broken oxygen flow tube (see Fig. 24-16), can result in delivery of a hypoxic mixture to the common gas outlet. In this situation, oxygen escapes through the leak and the predominant gas delivered is nitrous oxide. The oxygen monitor and/or integrated multigas analyzer are the only machine safety devices that can detect this problem.[51] For the majority of its products, Dräger Medical recommends a pre-use positive-pressure leak test to detect such a leak. However, in addition to this test, for many Dräger machines, application of the negative-pressure leak test as well may provide a more sensitive method to detect such a leak. Datex-Ohmeda almost universally recommends a pre-use negative-pressure leak test for its workstations, because of the frequently present check valve located at the common gas outlet (see Checking Your Anesthesia Workstation section).

Inert Gas Administration

Administration of a third inert gas, such as helium, nitrogen, or carbon dioxide, can cause a hypoxic mixture because contemporary proportioning systems link only nitrous oxide and oxygen.[60] Use of an oxygen analyzer to monitor the inspired oxygen concentration is mandatory (or a multigas analyzer when available) if the operator uses a third gas.

Dilution of Inspired Oxygen Concentration by Potent Inhaled Volatile Anesthetics

Volatile inhaled anesthetics are added to the mixed gases downstream from both the flowmeters and the proportioning system. Concentrations of less-potent inhaled anesthetics such as desflurane (MAC ~ 7%) may account for a larger percentage of the total fresh gas composition than more potent agents such as isoflurane (MAC ~ 1.2%). This can be seen when the maximum vaporizer concentration dial settings of the various volatile agents are examined (e.g., desflurane maximum dial setting of 18% vs. isoflurane maximum dial setting of 5%). Since significant percentages of these inhaled anesthetics may be added downstream of the proportioning system, the resulting gas/vapor mixture may contain an inspired oxygen concentration that is <21%. Awareness of this possibility, particularly when high concentrations of desflurane are used, is essential.

Oxygen Flush Valve

6 The oxygen flush valve allows direct communication between the oxygen intermediate-pressure circuit and the low-pressure circuit (see Fig. 24-4). Flow from the oxygen flush valve enters the

low-pressure circuit downstream from the vaporizers and, most importantly, downstream from any outlet check valve, if present. The spring-loaded oxygen flush valve remains closed until the operator opens it by depressing the oxygen flush button. Actuation of the valve delivers 100% oxygen at a flow of 35 to 75 L/min to the breathing circuit.[32]

The oxygen flush valve can provide a "high pressure" oxygen source that might be used for jet ventilation under the following circumstances: (1) the anesthesia machine is equipped with a one-way check valve positioned between the vaporizers and the oxygen flush valve; and (2) when a positive-pressure relief valve exists downstream from the vaporizers. The pressure relief valve must be upstream of the outlet check valve. Because the Ohmeda Modulus II has such a one-way check valve and its low-pressure system positive-pressure relief valve is upstream from the outlet check valve, the entire oxygen flow of 35 to 75 L/min is delivered to the common gas outlet at a pressure of 45 to 50 psig. On the other hand, the Ohmeda Modulus II Plus and some Ohmeda Excel machines are not capable of functioning as an appropriate oxygen source for jet ventilation. The Ohmeda Modulus II plus, which does not have the check valve, provides only 7 psig at the common gas outlet because much of the oxygen flows retrograde into the low-pressure circuit and out to atmosphere through an internal relief valve located upstream from the oxygen flush valve. The Ohmeda Excel 210, which does have a one-way check valve, also has a positive-pressure relief valve downstream from the check valve and therefore is unsuitable for jet ventilation. Older North American Dräger machines such as the Narkomed 2A (which also does not have the outlet check valve) produce a pressure of 18 psig at the common gas outlet because oxygen is vented to atmosphere through a pressure relief valve located in the Dräger Vapor vaporizers.[61]

It must be emphasized that use of the oxygen flush to drive a jet ventilation system connected at the machine's common gas outlet is an "off label" use of the machine, and is not recommended by the machine manufacturers. If jet ventilation is required, a purpose-built Sanders type system should be used, connected to a 50 psig oxygen source.

Several hazards have been reported with use of the oxygen flush valve. A defective or damaged valve can stick in the fully open position, resulting in barotrauma.[62] A valve sticking in a partially open position can result in patient awareness during general anesthesia, because the oxygen flow from the incompetent valve dilutes the inhaled anesthetic.[28] Improper use of normally functioning oxygen flush valves also can result in problems. Overzealous intraoperative oxygen flushing can dilute inhaled anesthetics. Oxygen flushing during the inspiratory phase of positive-pressure ventilation can produce barotrauma in patients if the anesthesia machine does not incorporate fresh gas decoupling or an appropriately adjusted inspiratory pressure limiter. Anesthesia systems (Dräger Narkomed 6000 series, Julian, Fabius GS, and Datascope Anestar) with fresh gas decoupling are inherently safer from the standpoint of minimizing the chance of producing barotrauma from inappropriate oxygen flush valve use. These systems physically separate the fresh gas inflow from either the flowmeters or the oxygen flush valve, from the delivered tidal volume presented to the patient's lungs (see Fresh Gas Decoupling section). With traditional anesthesia breathing circuits, excess volume cannot be vented during the inspiratory phase of mechanical ventilation because the ventilator pressure relief valve is closed and the APL valve is either out-of-circuit or closed.[63] An alternative solution to this problem is used in the GE-Datex-Ohmeda S/5 ADU and GE-Aestiva. The breathing systems on these machines utilize an integrated adjustable pressure limiter. If this device is properly adjusted, it functions like the APL (or pop-off) valve to limit the maximum airway pressure to a safe level, thereby reducing the possibility of barotrauma.

Some very old anesthesia systems made use of a freestanding vaporizer downstream from the common gas outlet; on these systems, oxygen flushing could rapidly deliver dangerously large quantities of inhaled anesthetic to the patient. Finally, inappropriate use of the oxygen flush to evaluate the low-pressure circuit for leaks can be misleading, particularly on GE Datex-Ohmeda machines with a one-way check valve at the common gas outlet.[27] Since back pressure from the breathing circuit closes the one-way check valve gas-tight, major low-pressure circuit leaks can go undetected with this leak test (see Checking Your Anesthesia Workstation section).

WEB-BASED ANESTHESIA SOFTWARE SIMULATION, THE VIRTUAL ANESTHESIA MACHINE

The advances in web-based application technology, as well as trends to incorporate simulation into anesthesia training and education, have generated development of online anesthesia simulation resources. The Virtual Anesthesia Machine (VAM) is a web-based anesthesia simulation environment (Fig. 24-21) that provides information on the function of anesthesia machines along with tutorials and operational scenarios, including failure modes of new and traditional anesthesia workstations.[64] It is available for use free of charge. The VAM allows the user to adjust most of the controls found on a modern anesthesia workstation: gas flows, ventilator settings, etc. The authors of the VAM, in collaboration with the Anesthesia Patient Safety Foundation (APSF), have created the Anesthesia Machine Workbook (AMW). The AMW provides additional information and tutorials covering six anesthesia machine subsystems: the high-pressure system, the low-pressure system, the breathing circuit, manual ventilation, mechanical ventilation, and the scavenging system.[65]

VAPORIZERS

As dramatically as the evolution of the anesthesia workstation has been in recent years, vaporizers have also changed from rudimentary ether inhalers and the "Copper Kettle" to the temperature-compensated, computer-controlled, and flow-sensing devices in use today. In 1993, with the introduction of desflurane to the clinical setting, an even more sophisticated vaporizer was introduced to handle the unique physical properties of this agent. Now, a new generation of anesthesia vaporizers blending traditional technology and "new" computerized control technology has emerged in the GE-Datex Aladin cassette vaporizer system. Before proceeding with a discussion of variable bypass vaporizers, the Datex-Ohmeda Tec 6 desflurane vaporizer and the Datex-Ohmeda Aladin cassette vaporizer, it is important to review certain physical principles to facilitate understanding of the operating principles, construction, and design of contemporary volatile anesthetic vaporizers.

Physics

Vapor Pressure

Contemporary inhaled volatile anesthetics exist in the liquid state at temperatures below 20°C. When a volatile liquid is in a closed container, molecules escape from the liquid phase to the vapor phase until the number of molecules in the vapor phase is constant. These molecules in the vapor phase bombard the wall of

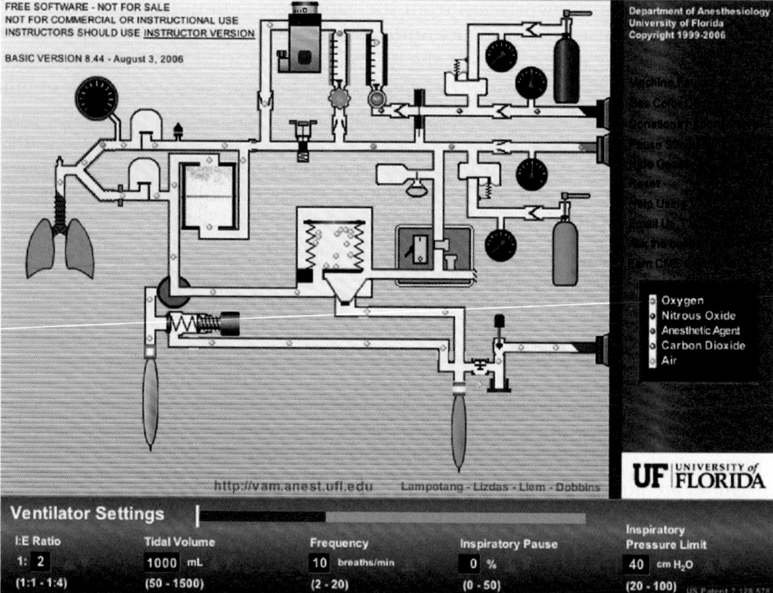

FIGURE 24-21. The Virtual Anesthesia Machine (VAM) simulator, an interactive model of an anesthesia machine. (With permission from: Lampotang S, Lizdas DE—see http://vam.anest.ufl.edu/)

the container and create a pressure known as the *saturated vapor pressure.* As the temperature increases, more molecules enter the vapor phase, and the vapor pressure increases (Fig. 24-22). Vapor pressure is independent of atmospheric pressure and is dependent only on the temperature and physical characteristics of the liquid. The *boiling point* of a liquid is defined as that temperature at which the vapor pressure equals atmospheric pressure.[49,66,67] At 760 mm Hg, the boiling points for desflurane, isoflurane, halothane, enflurane, and sevoflurane are approximately 22.8, 48.5, 50.2, 56.5, and 58.5°C, respectively. Unlike other contemporary inhaled anesthetics, desflurane boils at temperatures that may be encountered in particularly warm clinical settings such as pediatric and burn operating rooms. This unique physical characteristic alone mandates a special vaporizer design to control the delivery of desflurane. If agent-specific vaporizers are accidentally filled with incorrect liquid anesthetic agents, the resulting mixtures of volatile agents may demonstrate properties that differ from those of the individual component agents. The altered vapor pressure and other physical properties of the mixtures that result from the mixing of various agents may alter the output of the vaporizer (see Variable Bypass Vaporizers: Misfilling section).[68]

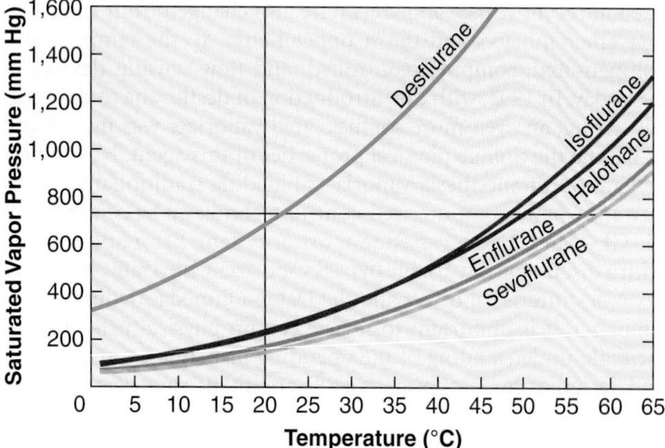

FIGURE 24-22. Saturated vapor pressure versus temperature curves for desflurane, isoflurane, halothane, enflurane, and sevoflurane. The vapor pressure curve for desflurane is both steeper and shifted to higher vapor pressures when compared with the curves for other contemporary inhaled anesthetics. (From inhaled anesthetic package insert equations and from Susay SR, Smith MA, Lockwood GG. The saturated vapor pressure of desflurane at various temperatures. *Anesth Analg.* 1996;83:864.)

Latent Heat of Vaporization

When a molecule is converted from a liquid to the gaseous phase, energy is consumed because the molecules of a liquid tend to cohere. The amount of energy that is consumed by a given liquid as it is converted to a vapor is referred to as the *latent heat of vaporization.* It is more precisely defined as the number of calories required to change 1 g of liquid into vapor without a temperature change. The thermal energy for vaporization must be derived from the liquid itself or from an external source. The temperature of the liquid itself will decrease during vaporization in the absence of an external energy source. This energy loss can lead to significant decreases in temperature of the remaining liquid and can greatly decrease subsequent vaporization.[49,66,69]

Specific Heat

The *specific heat* of a substance is the number of calories required to increase the temperature of 1 g of a substance by 1°C.[19,49,66] The substance can be a solid, liquid, or gas. The concept of specific heat is important to the design, operation, and construction of vaporizers because it is applicable in two ways. First, the specific heat value for an inhaled anesthetic is important because it indicates how much heat must be supplied to the liquid to maintain a constant temperature when heat is being lost during vaporization. Second, manufacturers select vaporizer component materials that have a high specific heat to minimize temperature changes associated with vaporization.

Thermal Conductivity

Thermal conductivity is a measure of the speed with which heat flows through a substance. The higher the thermal conductivity, the better the substance conducts heat.[66] Vaporizers are constructed of metals that have relatively high thermal conductivity, thus maintaining a uniform internal temperature.

Ambient Pressure Effects

These are discussed in the section entitled "GE-Datex-Ohmeda Tec 6 and Dräger D-Vapor Vaporizers for Desflurane: Factors that Influence Vaporizer Output: Varied Altitudes."

Variable Bypass Vaporizers

The GE-Datex-Ohmeda Tec 4, Tec 5, and Tec 7, as well as the Dräger Vapor 19.n and 2000 series, vaporizers are classified as variable bypass, flow-over, temperature-compensated, agent-specific, out-of-breathing circuit vaporizers.[66] *Variable bypass* refers to the method for regulating the anesthetic agent concentration output from the vaporizer. As fresh gas from the machine flowmeters enters the vaporizer inlet, the concentration control dial setting determines the ratio of incoming gas that flows through the bypass chamber to that entering the vaporizing chamber (sump). The gas channeled through the vaporizing chamber flows over a wick system saturated with the liquid anesthetic and subsequently also becomes saturated with vapor. Thus, *flow-over* refers to the method of vaporization and is in contrast to a *bubble-through* system that is used in now-obsolete measured flow vaporizers (e.g., Copper Kettle, Verni-Trol). The GE-Ohmeda Tec 4, Tec 5, and Tec 7, and the Dräger Vapor 19.n and Vapor 2000 series are further classified as *temperature compensated.* Each is equipped with an automated temperature-compensating device that helps maintain a constant vapor concentration output for a given concentration dial setting, and over a wide range of operating temperatures. These vaporizers are *agent specific* because each is designed to accommodate a single anesthetic agent, and *out-of-circuit,* that is, physically located outside of the breathing circuit. Variable bypass vaporizers are used to deliver halothane, enflurane, isoflurane, and sevoflurane, but not desflurane.

Basic Operating Principles

A diagram of a generic, variable bypass vaporizer is shown in Figure 24-23. In principle, it creates a saturated vapor concentration of the liquid agent in the vaporizing chamber and dilutes this to clinically usable concentrations by mixing it with fresh gas from the vaporizer bypass. (For example, the saturated vapor pressure of sevoflurane is 160 mm Hg at 20°C, at sea level this corresponds to a vapor concentration of 160 mm Hg/760 mm Hg × 100 = 21% which is too high for clinical use. Therefore, the vaporizer must dilute this 21% concentration to a clinical value indicated on the vaporizer dial.) Vaporizer components include the concentration control dial, the bypass chamber, the vaporizing chamber, the filler port, and the filler cap. Using the filler port, the operator fills the vaporizing chamber with liquid anesthetic. The maximum safe fill level is predetermined by the position of the filler port, which is designed to minimize the likelihood of overfilling. If a vaporizer is overfilled or tilted, liquid anesthetic can spill into the bypass via the inlet and outlet chambers. If this were to happen, both the vaporizing chamber flow and the bypass flow could potentially be carrying saturated anesthetic vapor, and an overdose would result. The concentration control dial is a variable restrictor, which is located either in the bypass or in the outlet of the vaporizing chamber. The function of the concentration control dial is to proportion fresh gas inflow between the bypass and the vaporizing chamber.

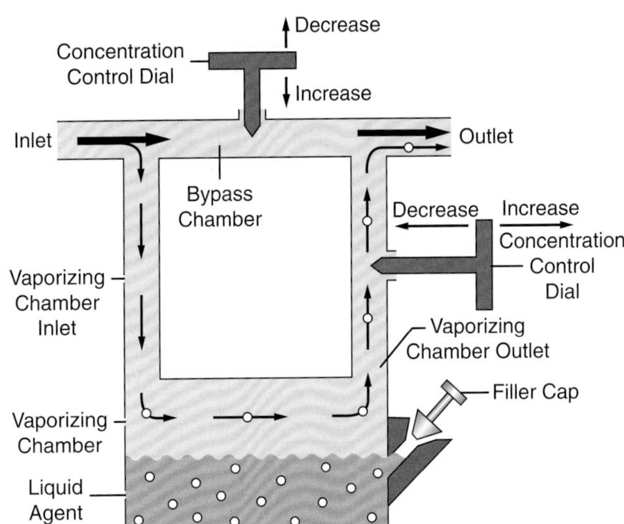

FIGURE 24-23. Generic variable bypass vaporizer. See text for details.

FGF from the machine's flowmeters enters the inlet of the vaporizer. Most of the flow passes straight through the bypass chamber to the vaporizer outlet. A smaller fraction of the fresh gas inflow is diverted to the vaporizing chamber. Depending on the temperature and vapor pressure of the particular inhaled anesthetic, the fresh gas entering the vaporizing chamber entrains a specific flow of the anesthetic agent saturated vapor. The mixture that exits the vaporizer outlet comprises flow through the bypass chamber, flow through the vaporizing chamber, and flow of entrained anesthetic vapor. The final concentration of inhaled anesthetic (in volumes percent) is the ratio of the flow of the entrained anesthetic vapor to the total gas flow.[66,70,71] The quantity (mL) of liquid volatile anesthetic agent used by a typical vaporizer is proportional to the FGF rate and the concentration set on the dial. It can be approximated from the following formula:

$$3 \times \text{FGF (L/min)} \times \text{vol\%} = \text{mL of liquid volatile anesthetic per hour.}$$ [72]

The saturated vapor pressure (SVP) of a potent volatile anesthetic depends on the ambient temperature (see Fig. 24-22). For example, at 20°C the SVP of isoflurane is 238 mm Hg, whereas at 35°C the SVP is almost double (450 mm Hg). Variable bypass vaporizers incorporate a mechanism to compensate for variations in ambient temperature. The temperature-compensating valve of the GE-Datex-Ohmeda Tec-type vaporizers is shown in Figure 24-24. At relatively high ambient temperatures, such as those commonly seen in operating rooms designated for the care of pediatric or burn patients, the SVP in the vaporizing chamber is high. To compensate for this, the bimetallic strip of the temperature-compensating valve leans to the right, decreasing the resistance to gas flow through the bypass chamber. This allows more flow to pass through the bypass chamber and less flow to pass through the vaporizing chamber. In contrast, in a cold environment, the SVP of the agent in the vaporizing chamber is decreased. To compensate for this decrease in SVP, the bimetallic strip leans to the left. This increases the resistance to flow through the bypass chamber, causing relatively more flow to pass through the vaporizing chamber and less flow to pass

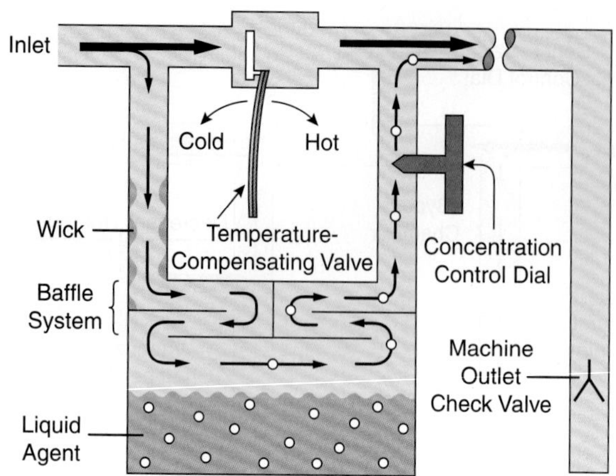

FIGURE 24-24. Simplified schematic of the GE-Ohmeda Tec Type Vaporizer. Note bimetallic strip temperature-compensating mechanism in the bypass chamber. See text for details.

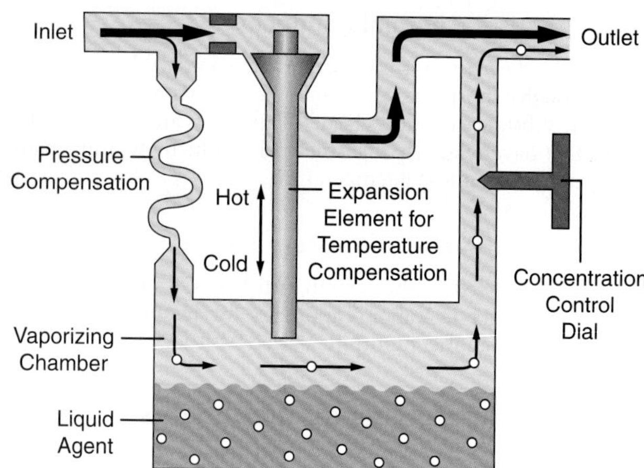

FIGURE 24-25. Simplified schematic of the Dräger Vapor 19.1 vaporizer. Here an expansion element performs the same function as the bimetallic strip in the previous figure. See text for details.

through the bypass chamber. The net effect in both situations is maintenance of relatively constant vapor output concentration.

Factors That Influence Vaporizer Output

If an ideal vaporizer existed, for a given concentration dial setting, its output would be constant regardless of changes in FGF rate, temperature, back pressure, and fresh gas mixture composition. Designing such a vaporizer is difficult because as ambient conditions change, the physical properties of gases and of the vaporizers themselves can change.[70] Contemporary vaporizers approach ideal but still have some limitations. Even though some of the most sophisticated vaporizer systems now available use computer-controlled components and multiple sensors, they have yet to become significantly more accurate than conventional mechanical flow-splitting (variable bypass) vaporizers. Several factors that affect vaporizer performance in general are described below.

Fresh Gas Flow Rate

With a fixed dial setting, vaporizer output can vary with the rate of gas flowing through the vaporizer. This variation is particularly notable at extremes of flow rates. The output of all variable bypass vaporizers is less than the dial setting at low flow rates (less than 250 mL/min). This results from the relatively high density of volatile inhaled anesthetic vapors. At low flow rates, insufficient turbulence is generated in the vaporizing chamber to advance the vapor molecules upwardly. At extremely high flow rates, such as 15 L/min, the output of most variable bypass vaporizers is less than the dial setting. This discrepancy is attributed to incomplete mixing and failure to saturate the carrier gas in the vaporizing chamber. In addition, the resistance characteristics of the bypass chamber and the vaporizing chamber can vary as flow increases. These variations can result in decreased output concentration.[70]

Temperature

Because of improvements in design, the output of contemporary temperature-compensated vaporizers is almost linear over a wide range of temperatures. Automatic temperature-compensating mechanisms in the bypass chamber maintain a constant vaporizer output with varying temperatures.[32] As previously described, a bimetallic strip (see Fig. 24-24) or in Dräger Vapor vaporizers, an expansion element (Fig. 24-25), directs a greater proportion of gas flow through the bypass chamber as temperature increases.[70] In addition, the wick systems are placed in direct contact with the metal wall of the vaporizer to help replace energy (heat) consumed during vaporization.

The materials from which vaporizers are constructed are chosen because they have a relatively high specific heat and high thermal conductivity. These factors help minimize the effect of cooling of the liquid anesthetic during vaporization. In addition, they should not react chemically with the liquid anesthetic agent.[73]

Intermittent Back Pressure

Intermittent back pressure that results from either positive-pressure ventilation or use of the oxygen flush valve may result in higher-than-expected vaporizer output. This phenomenon, known as the *pumping effect,* is more pronounced at low FGF rates, low concentration dial settings, and low levels of liquid anesthetic in the vaporizing chamber.[66,70,74,75] In addition, the pumping effect is increased by rapid respiratory rates, high peak inspired pressures, and rapid decreases in pressure during exhalation.[49,63,66,67,76] Newer variable bypass vaporizers such as the GE-Datex-Ohmeda Tec 4, Tec 5, and Tec 7, and Dräger Vapor 19.n and 20.n (Vapor 2000 series) are relatively immune from the pumping effect. One proposed mechanism for the pumping effect is dependent on retrograde pressure transmission from the patient circuit to the vaporizer during the inspiratory phase of positive-pressure ventilation. Gas molecules are compressed in both the bypass and vaporizing chambers. When the back pressure is suddenly released during the expiratory phase of positive-pressure ventilation, vapor exits the vaporizing chamber via both the vaporizing chamber outlet and retrograde through the vaporizing chamber inlet. This occurs because the output resistance of the bypass chamber is lower than that of the vaporizing chamber, particularly at low concentration dial settings. The increased output concentration results from the increments of vapor that flow in a retrograde direction to the bypass chamber.[70,74,75]

To decrease the pumping effect, the vaporizing chambers of contemporary variable bypass systems are smaller than those of older model vaporizers (e.g., Fluotec Mark II: vaporizing chamber volume 750 mL).[74] Consequently, no substantial volumes of vapor can be discharged from the vaporizing chamber into the bypass chamber during the expiratory phase of ventilation. The Dräger Vapor 19.1 and 20.n (see Fig. 24-25) have a long spiral tube that serves as the inlet to the vaporizing chamber. When the pressure in the vaporizing chamber is released, some of the vapor enters this tube but does not enter the bypass chamber because of the tube's length.[74] The Tec 4 (see Fig. 24-24) has an extensive baffle system in the vaporizing chamber, and a one-way check valve has been inserted at the common gas outlet (outlet check valve) to minimize the pumping effect. This check valve attenuates, but does not eliminate, the pressure increase because gas still flows from the flowmeters to the vaporizer during the inspiratory phase of positive-pressure ventilation.[77]

Fresh Gas Composition

Vaporizer output is influenced by the composition of the gas that flows through the vaporizer.[78] During experimental conditions, when the carrier gas is rapidly changed from 100% oxygen to 100% nitrous oxide, a sudden transient decrease in vaporizer output occurs, followed by a slow increase to a new steady-state value.[79] Because nitrous oxide is more soluble than oxygen in the anesthetic liquid in the vaporizer sump, when this change occurs the output from the vaporizing chamber is transiently decreased.[80] Once the anesthetic liquid is totally saturated with nitrous oxide, vaporizing chamber output increases somewhat, and a new steady state is established.

The explanation for the new steady-state output value is less well understood.[78–85] With contemporary vaporizers such as the Dräger Vapor 19.n and 20.n and the GE Tec-type vaporizers, the steady-state output value is less when nitrous oxide rather than oxygen is the carrier gas (see Fig. 24-26). Conversely, the output of some older vaporizers is increased when nitrous oxide is the carrier gas instead of oxygen.[82,85] The steady-state plateau is achieved more rapidly with increased FGF rates, regardless of the ultimate output value.[79,80] Factors that contribute to the characteristic steady-state response resulting when various carrier gases are used include the viscosity and density of the carrier gas (i.e., whether the flow is laminar or turbulent), the relative solubilities of the carrier gas in the anesthetic liquid, the flow-splitting characteristics of the specific vaporizer, and the concentration control dial setting.[84]

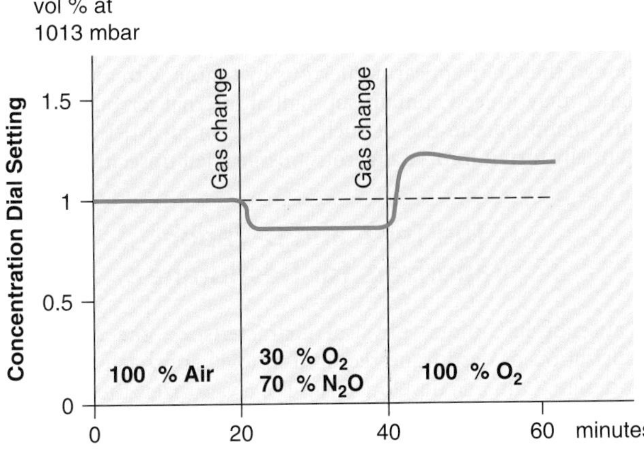

FIGURE 24-26. Influence of gas composition on delivered anesthetic concentration. A Dräger Vapor 2000 vaporizer is initially set at 1 vol% and 100% air. The concentration falls by 10% (not more than 0.4 vol%) of the set value after switching to a mixture of 30% O_2 and 70% N_2O. When 100% O_2 is used, the concentration rises by 10% of the set value (not more than 0.4 vol%) (From: Schreiber P. *Anaesthetic Equipment: Performance, Classification, and Safety*. New York: Springer; 1972).

Safety Features

Contemporary vaporizers (e.g., Dräger Vapor 19.n and Vapor 2000 series, and the GE-Datex-Ohmeda Tec 5, and Tec 7) have built-in safety features that have minimized or eliminated many of the hazards once associated with variable bypass vaporizers. Agent-specific, keyed filling devices help prevent filling a vaporizer with the wrong agent. Overfilling of vaporizers is minimized because the filler port is located at the maximum safe liquid level. Vaporizers are firmly secured to a vaporizer manifold on the anesthesia workstation and have anti-spill protection designs (e.g., "Transport" setting on Dräger Vapor 2000 series vaporizers) so that problems associated with vaporizer tipping are prevented. Contemporary interlock systems prevent simultaneous administration of more than one inhaled anesthetic.

Hazards

Despite many safety features, some hazards continue to be associated with contemporary variable bypass vaporizers.

Misfilling

Vaporizers not equipped with keyed fillers have been occasionally misfilled with the wrong anesthetic liquid. A potential for misfilling exists even on contemporary vaporizers equipped with keyed fillers.[86–88] When a vaporizer misfilling occurs, patients can be rendered inadequately, or excessively, anesthetized depending on which "incorrect" agent is in the vaporizer. The use of an anesthetic agent analyzer should alert the user to such a problem. In principle, if a vaporizer designed for an agent with a relatively low SVP (e.g., sevoflurane-160 mm Hg at 20°C) is erroneously filled with an agent that has a relatively high SVP (e.g., isoflurane-240 mm Hg at 20°C) the output concentration of isoflurane (in vol%) will be greater than that set on the concentration dial of the sevoflurane vaporizer. Conversely, an isoflurane vaporizer misfilled with sevoflurane will deliver a lower concentration of sevoflurane than that set on the concentration dial. In addition to considering the agent concentration output of a misfilled vaporizer, one must also consider the potency output. Thus, a sevoflurane vaporizer set to deliver 2% sevoflurane (1 MAC) that is misfilled with isoflurane will deliver >3% isoflurane which would be more than double the potency (MAC multiple) expected!

Contamination

Contamination of anesthetic vaporizer contents has occurred by filling an isoflurane vaporizer with a contaminated bottle of isoflurane. A potentially serious incident was avoided because the operator detected an abnormal acrid odor.[89]

Tipping

Tipping of a vaporizer can occur when they are incorrectly "switched out" or moved. However, tipping is unlikely when a vaporizer is secured to the anesthesia workstation manifold short of the entire machine being turned over. Excessive tipping can cause the liquid agent to enter the bypass chamber and can cause an output with extremely high agent vapor concentration.[90]

One milliliter of liquid anesthetic produces approximately 200 mL of anesthetic vapor at 20°C and 1 atm pressure so that even a small quantity of liquid anesthetic in the bypass can produce a large amount of vapor.[70,71] If a vaporizer has been tipped, it should not be used clinically until it has been purged for 20 to 30 minutes *using a high FGF rate* from the machine's flowmeters. During this procedure, the vaporizer concentration control *dial should be set at a high concentration* which maximizes bypass chamber flow as well as vaporizing chamber inlet and outlet flows. Purging should continue until all spilled liquid anesthetic has been cleared. Following this procedure the accuracy of the vaporizer output must be confirmed using an agent analyzer before placing the vaporizer back into clinical service. As mentioned above, the Dräger Vapor 20.n series vaporizers have a transport ("T") dial setting that prevents tipping-related problems. When the dial is set to this position, the vaporizer sump is isolated from the bypass chamber, thereby reducing the likelihood of spillage (and a possible accidental overdose). In order to remove a Vapor 2000 from the anesthesia workstation, the control dial must be set to the "T" position.

The design of the GE-Datex-Ohmeda Tec 6 and the Aladin cassette vaporizer systems has essentially eliminated the dangers of tipping. Since the Aladin vaporizer's bypass chamber is physically separated from the "cassette," and permanently resides in the anesthesia workstation, the possibility of tipping is virtually eliminated. Tipping of the Aladin cassettes themselves when they are not installed in the vaporizer is not problematic. Similarly, Dräger's D-Vapor (desflurane) vaporizer is hermetically tight and can be transported in any position before draining.

Overfilling

Improper filling procedures combined with failure of the vaporizer sight glass can cause overfilling and anesthetic overdose. When liquid anesthetic enters the bypass chamber up to 10 times the intended vapor concentration can be delivered to the common gas outlet.[91] Most modern vaporizers are now relatively immune to overfilling because of side-fill rather than top-fill designs.

Underfilling

Just as with overfilling, underfilling of anesthetic vaporizers may also be problematic. When a Tec 5 sevoflurane vaporizer is in a low-fill state and used under conditions of high FGF rates (>7.5 L/min) and high dial setting (such as seen during inhalational inductions), the vaporizer output may abruptly decrease to less than 2%. The causes of this problem are likely multifactorial. However, the combination of low vaporizer fill state (<25% full) in combination with the high vaporizing chamber flow, can result in a clinically significant and reproducible decrease in vapor output.[92]

Simultaneous Inhaled Anesthetic Administration

9 On some older anesthesia machines from Datex-Ohmeda that are equipped with the Select-a-Tec® three-vaporizer manifold that does not utilize a vapor-interlock system, two inhaled anesthetics can be administered simultaneously when the center vaporizer is removed. On such machines, either the left vaporizer or the right vaporizer should be moved to the center position if the middle vaporizer is removed (as indicated by the manifold warning label). Once this is done, the vaporizer's interlock system will allow only one agent to be administered at a time. More contemporary Select-a-Tec vaporizer manifolds have a built-in vapor-interlock or vapor-exclusion device that prevents this problem. On these newer three-vaporizer systems, a U-shaped plastic device links the vaporizer extension rods even when the vaporizers are not adjacent to one another on the manifold. On such a system, the manifold plus the vaporizers themselves constitute the vapor-interlock or vapor-exclusion system.

Leaks

Vaporizer leaks do occur frequently and can potentially result in patient awareness during anesthesia[18,23,75,93] or in contamination of the operating room environment. A loose filler cap is the most common source of vaporizer leaks. With some key-filled Penlon and Dräger vaporizers, a loose filler screw clamp allows escape of saturated anesthetic vapor.[18] Leaks can occur at the O-ring junctions between the vaporizer and its manifold. To detect a leak within a vaporizer, the concentration control dial must be in the "on" position. Even though vaporizer leaks in Dräger anesthesia systems can potentially be detected with a conventional positive-pressure low-pressure system leak test (because of the absence of an outlet check valve), a negative-pressure leak test is probably more sensitive. GE-Datex-Ohmeda recommends a negative-pressure leak testing device (suction bulb) to detect vaporizer leaks in the Modulus I, Modulus II, Excel, and the Aestiva workstations because of the check valve located just upstream of each machine's fresh gas outlet (see Checking Your Anesthesia Workstation section).

Many newer anesthesia workstations are capable of performing self-testing procedures that, in some cases, may eliminate the need for the conventional negative-pressure leak testing. However, it is of vital importance that anesthesia providers understand that these self-tests may not detect internal vaporizer leaks in systems with add-on vaporizers. For the self-tests to determine if an internal vaporizer leak is present, the leak test must be repeated for each vaporizer sequentially, while its concentration control dial is turned to the "on" position. Recall that when a vaporizer's concentration control dial is set in the "off" position, it may not be possible to detect even major internal leaks such as an absent or loose filler cap.

Anesthesia Vaporizers and Environmental Considerations

Today, more than ever, anesthetics are being administered to patients outside the operating room. One such location where it is sometimes difficult to work is the MRI suite. The presence of a powerful magnetic field, the significant noise pollution, and limited access to the patient during the procedure all complicate care in this setting. It is imperative that only nonferrous (MRI compatible) equipment be used in these settings. Some anesthesia vaporizers, although they may appear nonferrous by testing with a horseshoe magnet, may indeed contain substantial internal ferrous components. Inappropriate use of such a device in an MRI suite may potentially turn it into a dangerous missile if left unsecured.[94]

The Tec 6 and D-Vapor Vaporizers for Desflurane

8 Because of its unique physical characteristics, the controlled vaporization of desflurane required a novel approach to vaporizer design. Ohmeda developed the Tec 6 vaporizer, the first such system, and introduced it into clinical use in the early 1990s. The Tec 6 vaporizer is an electrically heated, pressurized device specifically designed to deliver desflurane.[95,96] The vapor pressure of desflurane is 3 to 4 times that of other contemporary inhaled anesthetics, and it boils at 22.8°C which is slightly above normal room temperature (see Fig. 24-22). Desflurane has a minimum alveolar anesthetic concentration (MAC) value of 6% to 7%.[97] It is valuable because it has a low blood:gas partition coefficient of 0.45 at 37°C, and recovery from anesthesia is more rapid than from other potent inhaled anesthetics.[97] In 2004, Dräger Medical

received FDA approval for its own version of the Tec 6 desflurane vaporizer, the D-Vapor. The operating principles described in the following discussion are applicable to both vaporizers although reference is made to the Tec 6 specifically.

Unsuitability of Contemporary Variable Bypass Vaporizers for Controlled Vaporization of Desflurane

Desflurane's high volatility and moderate potency preclude its use with contemporary variable bypass vaporizers such as GE-Datex-Ohmeda Tec 4, Tec 5, and Tec 7, or the Dräger Vapor 19.n or 20.n for two primary reasons[95]:

1. At 20°C the SVP of desflurane is 669 mm Hg (almost 1 atm pressure at sea level).
   The vapor pressures of sevoflurane, enflurane, isoflurane, halothane, and desflurane at 20°C are 160, 172, 240, 244, and 669 mm Hg, respectively (see Fig. 24-22).[97] Equal amounts of flow through a traditional vaporizer would vaporize many more volumes of desflurane than any other of these agents. For example, at 1 atm and 20°C, 100 mL/min passing through the vaporizing chamber would entrain 735 mL/min desflurane versus 25, 29, 46, and 47 mL/min of sevoflurane, enflurane, isoflurane, and halothane, respectively.[95] Under these same conditions, to produce 1% desflurane output the amount of bypass flow necessary to achieve sufficient dilution of the large volume of desflurane vapor would be approximately 73 L/min, compared to 5 L/min or less for the other four anesthetics. In addition, at temperatures ≥22.8°C at 1 atm, desflurane will boil. The amount of vapor produced would be uncontrolled and limited only by the heat energy available from the vaporizer.[95]
2. Contemporary variable bypass vaporizers lack an external heat source.
   The latent heat of vaporization for desflurane is approximately equal to those of the other potent agents but its MAC is 4 to 9 times higher. Thus, the absolute amount of desflurane liquid vaporized over a given time period is considerably greater than that of the other anesthetic agents. To deliver desflurane via a conventional vaporizer in higher (equivalent MAC) concentrations would lead to excessive cooling of the vaporizer and would significantly reduce its output. In the absence of an external heat source, temperature compensation using traditional mechanical devices would be almost impossible. Because of the broad range of temperatures seen in the clinical setting, and because of desflurane's steep SVP versus temperature curve (see Fig. 24-22), the delivery of desflurane in a conventional anesthetic vaporizer would be unpredictable.[95]

Operating Principles of the Tec 6 and D-Vapor

The Tec 6 was introduced in 1993. The physical appearance and operation of the Tec 6 are similar to contemporary vaporizers, but some aspects of the internal design and operating principles are radically different. The Tec 6 Plus represents a later version of the original Tec 6. The Tec 6 Plus has the same basic Tec 6 design, but also incorporates an enhanced audible alarm system.

Functionally, the Tec 6's operation is more accurately described as a dual-gas blender than as a vaporizer. A simplified schematic of the Tec 6 is shown in Figure 24-27. The vaporizer has two independent gas circuits arranged in parallel. The fresh gas circuit is shown in darker gray, and the vapor circuit in light gray. The FGF from the machine's flowmeters enters at the fresh gas inlet, passes through a fixed restrictor (R1), and exits at the vaporizer gas outlet. The vapor circuit originates at the desflurane sump, which is electrically heated and thermostatically controlled to 39°C, a temperature well above desflurane's boiling point at 1 atm. The heated sump assembly creates a reservoir of desflurane vapor. At 39°C, the vapor pressure in the sump is approximately 1,500 mm Hg, or 2 atm absolute (see Fig. 24-22). Just downstream from the sump is the shutoff valve. After the vaporizer has warmed up to working temperature, the shutoff valve fully opens when the concentration control valve is turned to the "on" position. A pressure-regulating valve located downstream from the shutoff valve regulates downward the pressure to approximately 1.1 atm absolute (74 mm Hg gauge) at a FGF rate of 10 L/min. The operator

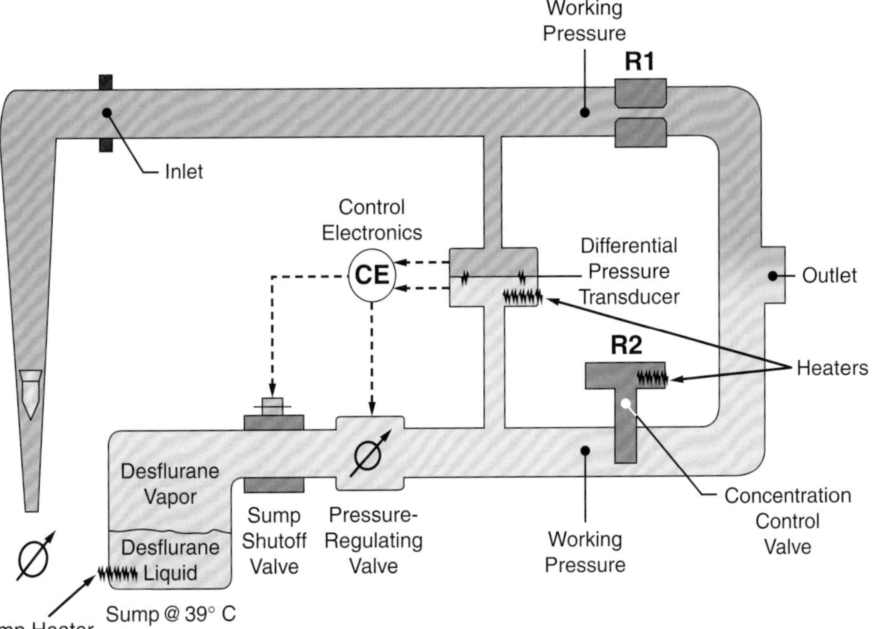

FIGURE 24-27. Simplified schematic of the Tec 6 desflurane vaporizer. (Modified from: Andrews JJ. *Operating Principles of the Ohmeda Tec 6 Desflurane Vaporizer: A Collection of Twelve Color Illustrations.* Washington, DC: Library of Congress, Copyright 1996, with permission.)

TABLE 24-2. FRESH GAS FLOW RATE VERSUS WORKING PRESSURE

Fresh Gas Flow Rate (L/min)	Working Pressure at R1 and R2 (Gauge) (Gas Inlet Pressure)		
	mbar	cm Water	mm Hg
1	10	10.2	7.4
5	50	51.0	37.0
10	100	102.0	74.0

Reprinted with permission from: Andrews JJ, Johnston RV Jr. The new Tec 6 desflurane vaporizer. *Anesth Analg.* 1993;76:1338.

TABLE 24-3. DIAL SETTING VERSUS FLOW THROUGH RESTRICTOR R2

Dial Setting (vol%)[a]	Fresh Gas Flow Rate (L/min)	Approximate Vapor Flow Rate Through R2 (mL/min)
1	1	10
6	1	64
12	1	136
18	1	220

Reprinted with permission from: Andrews JJ, Johnston RV Jr. The new Tec 6 desflurane vaporizer. *Anesth Analg.* 1993;76:1338.
[a] vol% = [(vapor flow rate)/(fresh gas flow rate + vapor flow rate)] × 100%.

controls desflurane output by adjusting the concentration control valve (R2), which is a variable restrictor.[95]

The vapor flow through R2 joins the FGF through R1 at a point downstream from the restrictors. Until this point, the two circuits are physically separated. They are interfaced pneumatically and electronically, however, through differential pressure transducers, a control electronics system, and a pressure-regulating valve. When a constant FGF encounters the fixed restrictor, R1, a specific back pressure, proportional to the FGF rate, pushes against the diaphragm of the control differential pressure transducer. The differential pressure transducer conveys the pressure difference between the fresh gas circuit and the vapor circuit to the control electronics system. The control electronics system regulates the pressure-regulating valve so that the pressure in the vapor circuit equals the pressure in the fresh gas circuit. This equalized pressure supplying R1 and R2 is the working pressure, and the working pressure is constant at a fixed FGF rate. If the operator increases the FGF rate, more back pressure is exerted upon the diaphragm of the control pressure transducer, and the working pressure of the vaporizer increases.[95]

Table 24-2 shows the approximate correlation between FGF rate and working pressure for a typical vaporizer. At a FGF rate of 1 L/min, the working pressure is 10 millibars, or 7.4 mm Hg gauge. At a FGF rate of 10 L/min, the working pressure is 100 millibars, or 74 mm Hg gauge. Therefore, there is a linear relationship between FGF rate and working pressure. When the FGF rate is increased 10-fold, the working pressure increases 10-fold.[95]

The following are two examples to demonstrate the operating principles of the Tec 6 (and D-Vapor).[95]

Example A: Constant FGF rate of 1 L/min, with an increase in the dial setting.

With a FGF rate of 1 L/min, the working pressure of the vaporizer is 7.4 mm Hg. That is, the pressure supplying R1 and R2 is 7.4 mm Hg. As the operator increases the dial setting, the opening at R2 becomes larger, allowing more vapor to pass through R2. Specific vapor flow rates at different dial settings are shown in Table 24-3.

Example B: Constant dial setting with an increase in FGF from 1 to 10 L/min.

At a FGF rate of 1 L/min, the working pressure is 7.4 mm Hg, and at a dial setting of 6% the vapor flow rate through R2 is 64 mL/min (see Tables 24-2 and 24-3). With a 10-fold increase in the FGF rate, there is a concomitant 10-fold increase in the working pressure to 74 mm Hg. The ratio of resistances of R2 to R1 is constant at a fixed dial setting of 6%. Because R2 is supplied by 10 times more pressure, the vapor flow rate through R2 increases 10-fold to 640 mL/min. Vaporizer output in volumes percent is constant because both the FGF and the vapor flow increase proportionally.

Factors That Influence Vaporizer Output

Varied altitude and carrier gas composition influence Tec 6 output. Each is discussed in the following sections.

Changes in Altitude

Changes in ambient pressure may significantly affect the output of older Tec-type vaporizers (i.e., those in which gas flow splitting occurs at the entrance to the vaporizing chamber) in terms of volumes percent (vol%, i.e., concentration), but the effect on anesthetic potency (i.e., partial pressure of agent) is minimal. This effect is illustrated using the example of isoflurane shown in Table 24-4. With a constant dial setting of 0.89%, at 1 atm (760 mm Hg), if perfectly calibrated, the vol% delivered would be 0.89% and the partial pressure of isoflurane would be 6.8 mm Hg. Maintaining the same dial setting and lowering ambient pressure to 0.66 atm or 502 mm Hg (roughly equivalent to 10,000 ft elevation) would result in an increase in the concentration output to 1.75% (almost double), but the partial pressure only increases to 8.77 mm Hg (only a 29% increase) because of the proportionate decrease in ambient pressure (Fig. 24-28).

It is generally considered that the partial pressure of the anesthetic agent in the central nervous system, not its concentration in

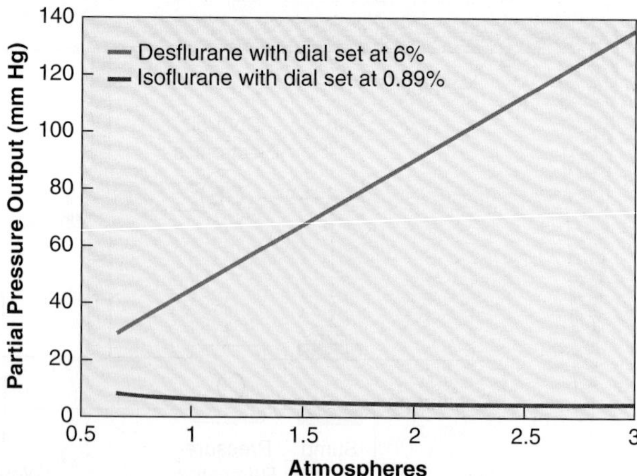

FIGURE 24-28. Performance of Tec type vaporizer versus the Tec 6 desflurane vaporizer at varying ambient atmospheric pressures (1 atm = 760 mm Hg).

TABLE 24-4. PERFORMANCE OF OLDER* TEC TYPE VAPORIZERS VERSUS THE TEC 6 DESFLURANE VAPORIZER AT VARYING AMBIENT PRESSURES

		Isoflurane Vaporizer with a Dial Setting of 0.89%			Tec 6 Desflurane Vaporizer with a Dial Setting of 6%
Atmospheres	Ambient Pressure (mm Hg)	Isoflurane Vapor Entrained by 100 cc O_2	Output Concentration	Partial Pressure Output (mm Hg)	Partial Pressure Output of Desflurane (mm Hg)
0.66 (2/3)	500 (10,000 ft)	91	1.753%	8.77	30
0.74	560	74	1.429%	8.0	33.6
0.80	608 (6,564 ft)	64.32	1.25%	7.6	36.5
1.0	760	46	0.89%	6.8	45.6
1.5	1,140	26.4	0.515%	5.87	68.4
2	1,520	19	0.36%	5.5	91.2
3	2,280	11.65	0.228%	5.198	136

The following were assumed: 5,000 cc bypass chamber flow, 100 cc vaporizing chamber flow—equivalent to an isoflurane dial setting of 0.89%.
*Variable bypass vaporizers in which the incoming gas flow is split before gas enters the vaporizing chamber.

vol%, is responsible for the anesthetic effect. To obtain a consistent depth of anesthesia when gross changes in barometric pressure occur, the concentration in vol% must be changed in inverse proportion to the barometric pressure.

In contemporary variable bypass vaporizers (e.g., GE Tec 5, Tec 7, Dräger Vapor 19.1 and Vapor 2000) the flow split occurs as gas leaves the vaporizing chamber, so that for any given dial setting and fresh gas flow, the volume of gas saturated with vapor that leaves the vaporizing chamber remains constant, to be diluted by the bypass flow. Assume that gas leaves the vaporizing chamber of an isoflurane vaporizer at 100 cc/min. At 1 atm (760 mm Hg) that gas would be 31.3% isoflurane by volume (238/760) and the partial pressure would be 31.3% × 760 = 238 mm Hg. At a barometric pressure of 500 mm Hg, the gas exiting the vaporizing chamber would be 47.6% isoflurane by volume (238/500) and the partial pressure would be 47.6% × 500 = 238 mm Hg. By splitting flow at the exit of the vaporizing chamber, these vaporizers become pressure compensated.

The above examples should be considered in stark contrast to the response of the Tec 6 desflurane vaporizer at varied altitudes (Fig. 24-28 and Table 24-4). One must remember this device is more accurately described as a dual gas "blender" than a vaporizer. Regardless of the ambient pressure, the Tec 6 will maintain a constant concentration of vapor output (vol%), not a constant partial pressure. This means that at high altitudes, the partial pressure of desflurane for any given dial setting will be decreased in proportion to the atmospheric pressure divided by the calibration pressure (normally 760 mm Hg) according to the following formula.

$$\text{Required Dial Setting} = \frac{\text{Normal Dial Setting (\%v/v} \times \text{760 mm Hg)}}{\text{Ambient Pressure (mm Hg)}}$$

For example at an altitude of 2,000 m (6,564 ft) where the ambient pressure is 608 mm Hg, the Tec 6 dial setting must be advanced from 10% to 12.5% to avoid underdosing that could potentially result in the patient having awareness. Conversely, the Tec 6's maintenance of a constant vol% output under hyperbaric conditions could produce significant increases in partial pressure output, and if not accounted for, the potential for anesthetic overdose. Therefore, in hyperbaric settings the Tec 6 dial setting would need to be decreased to maintain the desired partial pressure output of desflurane.

Carrier Gas Composition

Vaporizer output approximates the dial setting when oxygen is the carrier gas because the Tec 6 vaporizer is calibrated using 100% oxygen. At low flow rates when a carrier gas other than 100% oxygen is used, however, a clear trend toward reduction in vaporizer output emerges. This reduction parallels the proportional decrease in viscosity of the carrier gas. Nitrous oxide has a lower viscosity than oxygen, so the back pressure generated by resistor R1 (see Fig. 24-27) is less when nitrous oxide is the carrier gas, and the working pressure is reduced. At low flow rates using nitrous oxide as the carrier gas, vaporizer output is approximately 20% less than the dial setting. This suggests that, at clinically useful FGF rates, the gas flow across resistor R1 is laminar, and the working pressure is proportional to both the FGF rate and the viscosity of the carrier gas.[99]

Safety Features

10 Because desflurane's SVP at room temperature is near 1 atm, misfilling contemporary vaporizers with desflurane could theoretically result in both desflurane overdose and creation of a hypoxic gas mixture.[100] GE-Datex-Ohmeda has introduced a unique, anesthetic-specific filling system to minimize occurrence of this potential hazard. The agent-specific filler of the desflurane bottle known as the "Saf-T-Fill" adapter is intended to prevent its use with traditional vaporizers. The filling system also minimizes spillage of liquid or vapor anesthetic by maintaining a "closed system" during the filling process. Each desflurane bottle has a spring-loaded filler cap with an O-ring on the tip. The spring seals the bottle until it is engaged in the filler port of the vaporizer. Thus, this anesthetic-specific filling system interlocks the vaporizer and the dispensing bottle, preventing loss of anesthetic to the atmosphere. Despite these safety features designed to minimize filling errors, a case report described the misfilling of a Tec 6 desflurane vaporizer with sevoflurane. This error was possible because of similarities between a new type of keyed filler for sevoflurane and the desflurane Saf-T-fill adapter. In this case, however, the desflurane vaporizer detected this error and automatically shut itself off.[86]

Major vaporizer faults cause the shutoff valve located just downstream from the desflurane sump (see Fig. 24-27) to close,

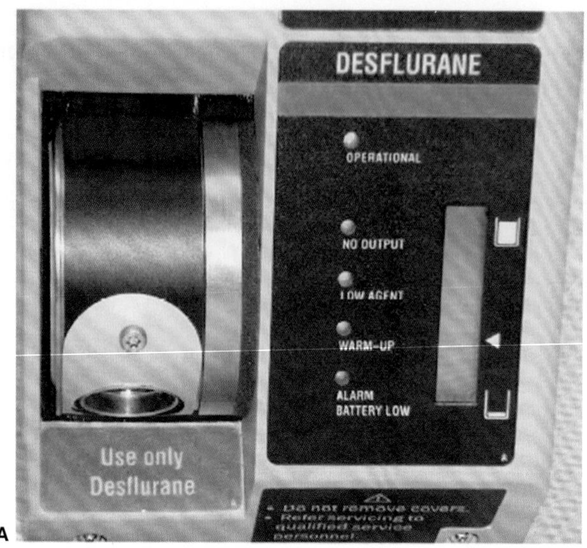

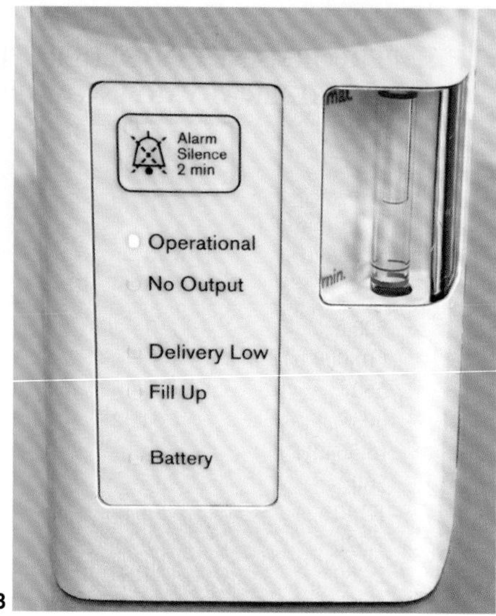

FIGURE 24-29. (A) Tec 6 desflurane vaporizer alarm indicators. **(B)** Dräger D-Vapor desflurane alarm indicators.

producing a no-output situation. The valve is closed and a "no-output" alarm is activated immediately if any of the following conditions occur: (1) the anesthetic level decreases to <20 mL; (2) the vaporizer is tilted; (3) a power failure occurs; or (4) there is a disparity between the pressure in the vapor circuit versus the pressure in the fresh gas circuit exceeding a specified tolerance. Note the alarm panel on the front of the Tec 6 vaporizer (Fig. 24-29A) showing "No Output," "Low Agent" "Warm Up," and "Alarm Battery Low" indicators.

The Dräger D-Vapor vaporizer has similar alarms (Fig. 24-29B). The "No Output" alarm (flashes red) indicates that the vaporizer is unable to deliver anesthetic (i.e., the vaporizer is warming up) or there is a device failure. The "Delivery Low" alarm (flashes red) triggers when the vaporizer is unable to supply the output set by the concentration dial (only with FGF > 1.5 L/min), the reservoir is empty, or if there is an apparatus fault. The "Fill Up" alarm (glows amber) indicates the reservoir level has dropped below the refill mark (the reservoir contains <40 mL). The "Battery" alarm will indicate (1) *amber glow* if the vaporizer is not able to operate without power, (2) *amber flashing* if the vaporizer is currently operating on battery backup, (3) *flashing amber plus "No Output" flashing red* if the vaporizer battery is depleted after operating on battery backup and another method of anesthesia is required. The vaporizer will also provide an audible alarm along with visual alarms. Medium priority alarms (amber glowing and flashing) may be silenced; high-priority alarms (red flashing) cannot be silenced.[101]

Summary

The Tec 6 vaporizer is an electrically heated, thermostatically controlled, constant-temperature, pressurized, electromechanically coupled dual circuit, gas–vapor blender. The pressure in the vapor circuit is electronically regulated to equal the pressure in the fresh gas circuit. At a constant FGF rate, the operator regulates vapor flow using a conventional concentration control dial. When the FGF rate increases, the working pressure increases proportionally. For a given concentration setting even when varying the FGF rate, the vaporizer output is constant because the amount of flow through each circuit remains in the same proportion.[95]

The GE-Datex-Ohmeda Aladin Cassette Vaporizer

The vaporizer system used in the GE-Datex-Ohmeda S/5 ADU and GE Aisys Carestation is unique in that the single electronically controlled vaporizer is designed to deliver five different inhaled anesthetics including halothane, isoflurane, enflurane, sevoflurane, and desflurane (Figs. 24-30 and 24-31). The vaporizer consists of a permanent internal control unit housed within the workstation and an interchangeable Aladin agent-specific cassette that contains anesthetic liquid. The Aladin agent cassettes are color coded for each anesthetic agent, and they are also magnetically coded so that the workstation can identify which anesthetic cassette has been inserted. The cassettes are filled using agent-specific fillers.[66]

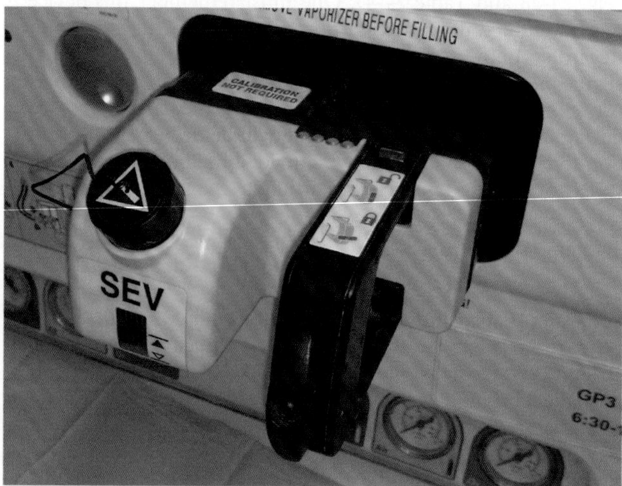

FIGURE 24-30. Aladin vaporizer sevoflurane cassette (GE Healthcare).

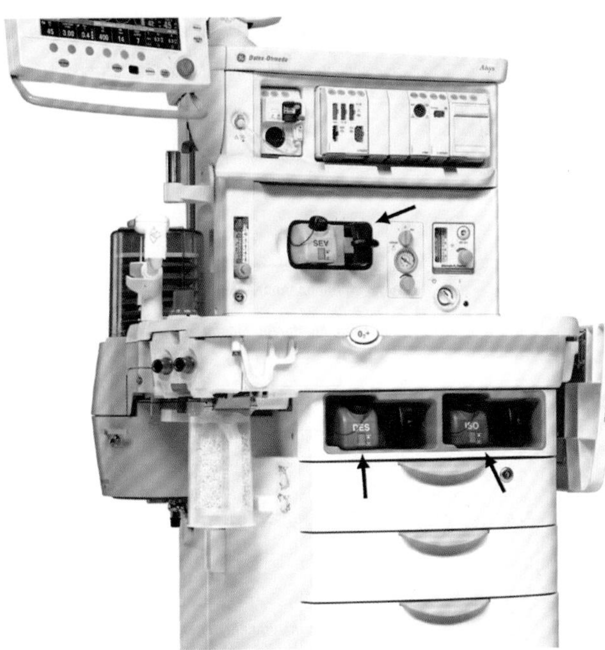

FIGURE 24-31. Aladin cassette vaporizers (arrows) on a GE Datex-Ohmeda Aisys Carestation. Upper cassette is in use, lower cassettes are stored on workstation.

Though very different in external appearance, the functional anatomy of the Aladin cassette vaporizer (Fig. 24-32) is very similar to that of the traditional variable bypass vaporizers because it is also made up of a bypass chamber and vaporizing chamber. A fixed restrictor is located in the bypass chamber, and flow measurement sensors are located both in the bypass chamber and in the outlet of the vaporizing chamber. The heart of the Aladin vaporizer is the electronically regulated flow control valve located in the vaporizing chamber outlet. This valve is controlled by a central processing unit (CPU). The CPU receives input from multiple sources including the concentration control dial, a pressure sensor located inside the vaporizing chamber (cassette), a temperature sensor located inside the vaporizing chamber, a flow measurement unit located in the bypass chamber, and a flow measurement unit located in the outlet of the vaporizing chamber. The CPU also receives input from the machine's flowmeters regarding the composition of the carrier gas. Using data from these multiple sources, the CPU is able to precisely regulate the flow control valve to attain the desired vapor concentration output. Appropriate electronic control of the flow control valve is essential to the proper function of this vaporizer.[66,102]

A fixed restrictor is located in the bypass chamber, and it causes flow from the vaporizer inlet to split into two flow streams (see Fig. 24-32). One stream passes through the bypass chamber, and the other portion enters the inlet of the vaporizing chamber and passes through a one-way check valve. The presence of this check valve is unique to the Aladin system. This one-way valve prevents retrograde flow of the anesthetic vapor back into the bypass chamber, and its presence is crucial when delivering desflurane if the room temperature is greater than the boiling point for desflurane (22.8°C). A precise amount of vapor-saturated carrier gas passes through the flow control valve, which is regulated by the CPU. This flow then joins the bypass flow and is directed to the outlet of the vaporizer.

As mentioned during the discussion of the Tec 6, the controlled vaporization of desflurane presents a unique challenge, particularly when the room temperature is greater than the boiling point of desflurane (22.8°C). At higher temperatures, the pressure inside the vaporizer sump increases, and the sump becomes pressurized. When the sump pressure exceeds the pressure in the bypass chamber, the one-way check valve located in the vaporizing chamber inlet closes preventing carrier gas from entering the vaporizing chamber. At this point, the carrier gas passes straight through the bypass chamber and its flow sensor. Under these conditions, the electronically regulated flow control valve simply meters in the appropriate flow of pure desflurane vapor needed to achieve the desired final concentration selected by the user. At least one case report has described a failure of the vaporizing

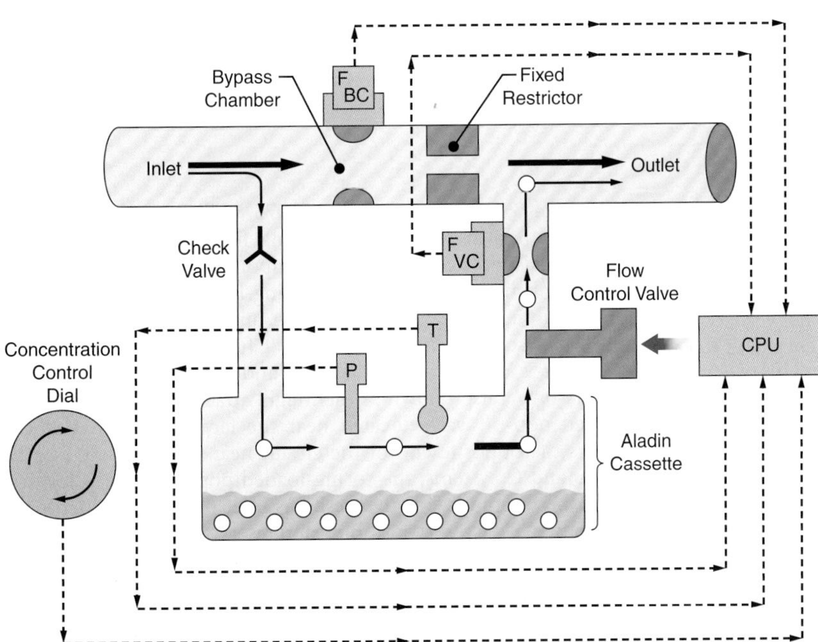

FIGURE 24-32. Simplified schematic of GE-Datex-Ohmeda Aladin Cassette Vaporizer. The *black arrows* represent flow from the flowmeters, and the *white circles* represent anesthetic vapor. The heart of the vaporizer is the electronically controlled flow control valve located in the outlet of the vaporizing chamber. CPU, central processing unit; F_{BC}, flow measurement unit, which measures flow through the bypass chamber; F_{VC}, flow measurement unit, which measures flow through the vaporizing chamber; P, pressure sensor; T, temperature sensor. (Modified from: Andrews, JJ. *Operating Principles of the Datex-Ohmeda Aladin Cassette Vaporizer: A Collection of Color Illustrations.* Washington, DC: Library of Congress; 2000.)

TABLE 24-5. VAPORIZER MODELS AND CHARACTERISTICS

Type of Vaporizer	Tec 4, Tec 5, SevoTec, Vapor 19.n, Vapor 2000, Aladin	Tec 6 (Desflurane), D-Vapor (Desflurane)
Carrier gas flow	Variable bypass	Dual circuit
Vaporization method	Flow-over	Gas/vapor blender
Temperature compensation	Automatic	Thermostatically controlled at 39°C
Calibration	Agent specific	Agent specific
Position	Out of circuit	Out of circuit
Fill capacity	Tec 4: 125 mL Tec 5: 300 mL Vapor 19.n: 200 mL Vapor 2000: 360 mL (dry wick) Aladin: 250 mL	Tec 6: 425 mL D-Vapor: 300 mL

chamber inlet check valve to function as designed. In this case, an anesthetic overdose occurred as a result of spill-over of desflurane from the vaporizing chamber in a retrograde fashion into the bypass chamber. This report reminds Aladin users to be cautious of this potential problem when desflurane is used.[102]

During operating conditions in which high FGF rates and/or high dial settings are used, large quantities of anesthetic liquid are rapidly vaporized. The temperature of the remaining liquid anesthetic and the vaporizer itself decreases as a result of energy consumption of the latent heat of vaporization. To offset this cooling effect, the workstation (GE ADU and Aisys) is equipped with a fan that forces warmed air from an "agent heating resistor" across the cassette (vaporizer sump) to raise its temperature when necessary. The fan is activated during two common clinical scenarios: (1) desflurane induction and maintenance, and (2) sevoflurane induction. A summary of the characteristics of various vaporizer models currently in use is found in Table 24-5.

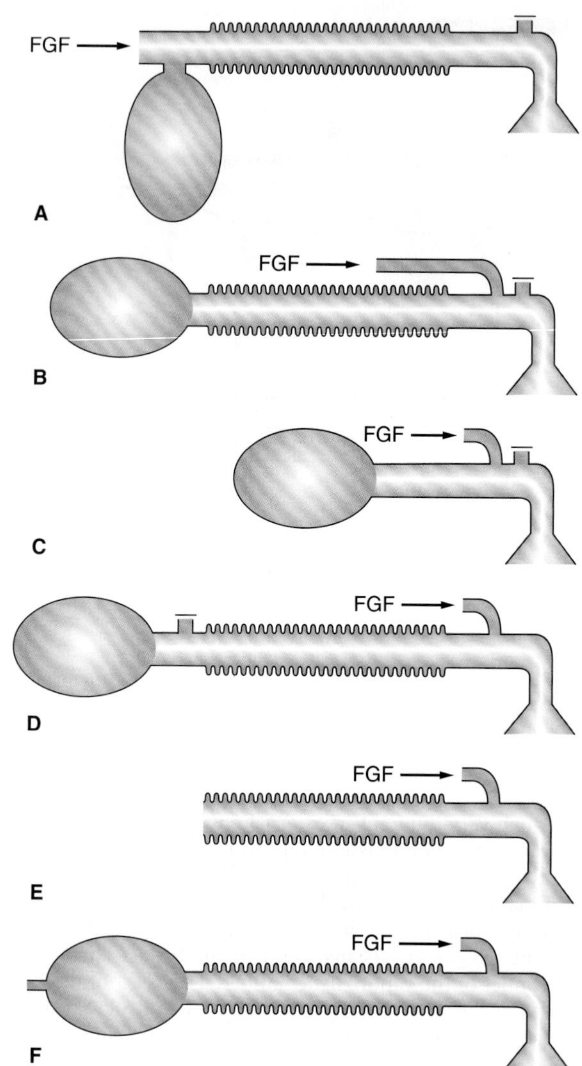

FIGURE 24-33. Mapleson breathing systems **(A–F)**. (Redrawn with permission from: Willis BA, Pender JW, Mapleson WW. Rebreathing in a T-piece: volunteer and theoretical studies of the Jackson-Rees modification of Ayre's T-piece during spontaneous respiration. *Br J Anaesth.* 1975;47:1239.)

ANESTHESIA BREATHING CIRCUITS

As the prescribed mixture of gases from the flowmeters and vaporizer exits the anesthesia workstation at the common gas outlet, it then enters an anesthetic breathing circuit. The function of the anesthesia breathing circuit is not only to deliver oxygen and anesthetic gases to the patient, but also to eliminate CO_2. Carbon dioxide can be removed either by washout with adequate fresh gas inflow or by the use of CO_2 absorbent media (e.g., soda lime absorption). The following discussion focuses on the semiclosed rebreathing circuits and the circle system.

Mapleson Systems

In 1954, Mapleson described and analyzed five different semiclosed anesthetic systems; these are now classically referred to as the Mapleson systems and are designated with letters A through E (Fig. 24-33).[103] Subsequently in 1975, Willis et al. described the F system that was added to the original five.[104] The Mapleson systems consist of several common components. These components commonly include a facemask, a spring-loaded pop-off valve, reservoir tubing, fresh gas inflow tubing, and a reservoir bag. Within the Mapleson systems, three distinct functional groups can be seen. They include the A, the B, C, and the D, E, F groups. The Mapleson A, also known as the Magill attachment, has a spring-loaded pop-off valve located near the facemask, and the FGF enters the opposite end of the circuit near the reservoir bag. In the B and C systems, the spring-loaded pop-off valve is located near the facemask, but the fresh gas inlet tubing is located near the patient. The reservoir tubing and reservoir bag serve as a blind limb where fresh gas, dead space gas, and alveolar gas can collect. Finally, in the Mapleson D, E, F group, or "T-piece" group, the fresh gas enters near the patient, and excess gas is released at the opposite end of the circuit.

Even though the components and component arrangements are simple, functional analysis of the Mapleson systems can be complex. The amount of CO_2 rebreathing associated with each system is multifactorial, and variables that dictate the ultimate CO_2 concentration include (1) the fresh gas inflow rate, (2) the patient's minute ventilation, (3) the mode of ventilation (spontaneous or controlled), (4) the tidal volume, (5) the respiratory rate, (6) the I:E ratio, (7) the duration of the expiratory pause, (8) the peak inspiratory flow rate, (9) the volume of the reservoir tube, (10) the volume of the breathing bag, (11) ventilation by mask, (12) ventilation through an endotracheal tube, and (13) the CO_2 sampling site.

The performance of the Mapleson systems is best understood by studying the expiratory phase of the respiratory cycle.[105] Illustrations of the various Mapleson system component arrangements are shown in Figure 24-33. During spontaneous ventilation, the Mapleson A has the best efficiency of the six systems requiring a fresh gas inflow rate of only one time the patient's minute ventilation to prevent rebreathing of exhaled CO_2. However, it has the least efficiency during controlled ventilation, requiring a FGF as high as 20 L/min to prevent rebreathing. Systems D, E, and F are slightly more efficient than systems B and C. To prevent rebreathing of CO_2, the D, E, and F systems require a FGF rate of approximately 2.5 times the minute ventilation, whereas the FGF rates required for B and C systems are somewhat higher.[106]

The following summarizes the relative efficiency of the different Mapleson systems with respect to prevention of rebreathing: during spontaneous ventilation, A > DFE > CB; during controlled ventilation, DFE > BC > A.[103,106] The Mapleson A, B, and C systems are rarely used today, but the D, E, F systems are still commonly employed. In the United States, the most popular representative from the D, E, F group is the Bain circuit.

Bain Circuit

The Bain circuit is a coaxial circuit and a modification of the Mapleson D system. The fresh gas flows through a narrow inner tube within the outer corrugated tubing. The inner fresh gas tubing enters the outer corrugated hose near the reservoir bag, but the fresh gas actually empties into the circuit at the patient end (Fig. 24-34). Exhaled gases enter the corrugated tubing and are vented through the expiratory valve near the reservoir bag. The Bain circuit may be used for both spontaneous and controlled ventilation. The fresh gas inflow rate necessary to prevent rebreathing is 2.5 times the minute ventilation.

The Bain circuit has many advantages over other systems. It is lightweight, convenient, and disposable. Scavenging of the waste gases from the "pop-off" valve is facilitated because the valve is located away from the patient. Exhaled gases in the outer reservoir tubing add warmth by countercurrent heat exchange to inspired fresh gases. The main hazards related to the use of the Bain circuit are either an unrecognized disconnection or kinking of the inner fresh gas hose. These problems can cause hypercarbia from inadequate gas flow or increased respiratory resistance. As with other circuits, an obstructed antimicrobial filter positioned between the Bain circuit and the tracheal tube can result in increased resistance in the circuit. This may produce hypoventilation and hypoxemia, and may even mimic the signs and symptoms of severe bronchospasm.[107]

The outer corrugated tube is transparent to allow ongoing inspection of the inner tube. The integrity of the inner tube can be assessed as described by Pethick.[108] With his technique, high-flow oxygen is fed into the circuit while the patient end is occluded until the reservoir bag is filled. The patient end is opened, and oxygen is flushed into the circuit. If the inner tube is intact, the Venturi effect occurs at the patient end. This causes a decrease in pressure within the circuit, and as a result, the reservoir bag deflates. Conversely, a leak in the inner tube allows the fresh gas to escape into the expiratory limb, and the reservoir bag will remain inflated. This test is recommended as a part of the preanesthesia check if a Bain circuit is used.

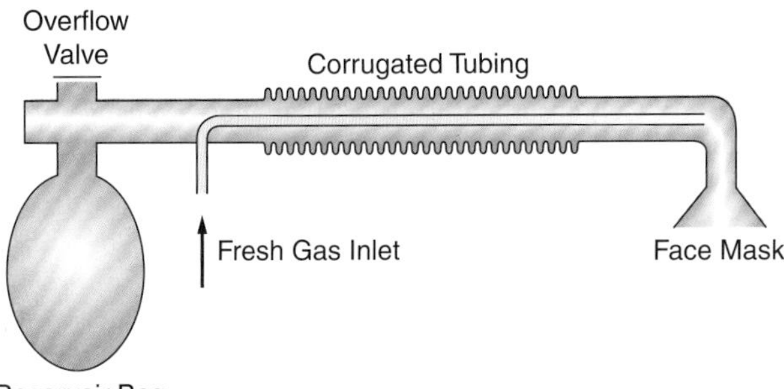

FIGURE 24-34. The Bain Circuit (Coaxial version of Mapleson D). (Redrawn with permission from: Bain JA, Spoerel WE. A streamlined anaesthetic system. *Can Anaesth Soc J.* 1972;19(4):426–435.)

Circle Breathing Systems

For many years, the overall design of the circle breathing system has changed among anesthesia workstation manufacturers. Both the individual components and the order in which they appeared in the circle system were consistent across major platforms. More recently, however, with the increasing technologic complexity of the anesthesia workstation, the circle system has gone through some major changes as well. These changes have resulted in part from an effort to improve patient safety (as in the integration of Fresh Gas Decoupling and Inspiratory Pressure Limiters), but have also allowed the deployment of new technologic advances. Examples of major new technologies include (1) a return to the application of single-circuit piston-type ventilators and (2) use of new spirometry devices that are located at the Y-connector instead of at the traditional location in the expiratory limb of the circuit. The following discussion first focuses on the traditional circle breathing system, and then is followed by a brief discussion of some variations in the designs of newer circle systems.

The Traditional Circle Breathing System

The circle system remains the most popular breathing system in the United States. It is so named because its components are arranged in a circular manner (see Fig. 24-7). A coaxial version of the traditional circle system, referred to as either a "Universal F" or a "single limb circuit," has increased in popularity over recent years. While these systems appear very different externally, they have the same overall functional layout as the traditional circle system and the following discussion is applicable to both the traditional circle system and the coaxial Universal F system.

The circle system prevents rebreathing of CO_2 by use of CO_2 absorbents, but allows partial rebreathing of other exhaled gases. The extent of rebreathing of the other exhaled gases depends on breathing circuit component arrangement and the FGF rate. A circle system can be semiopen, semiclosed, or closed, depending on the amount of FGF.[109] A *semiopen* system has no rebreathing and requires a very high FGF. A *semiclosed* system is associated with some rebreathing of exhaled gases and is the system that is most commonly used in the United States. A *closed* system is one in which the FGF exactly matches that being taken up, or consumed, by the patient. In a closed system, there is complete rebreathing of exhaled gases after absorption of CO_2, and the overflow (pop-off or APL) valve or ventilator pressure relief valve remains closed.

The circle system (Fig. 24-7) consists of seven primary components: (1) a fresh gas inflow source; (2) inspiratory and expiratory unidirectional valves; (3) inspiratory and expiratory corrugated tubes; (4) a Y-piece connector; (5) an overflow or pop-off valve, referred to as the adjustable pressure-limiting (APL) valve; (6) a reservoir bag; and (7) a canister containing CO_2 absorbent. The inspiratory and expiratory valves that are placed in the system to ensure gas flow through the corrugated hoses remains unidirectional. The fresh gas inflow enters the circle by a connection from the common gas outlet of the anesthesia machine.

Numerous variations of the circle arrangement are possible, depending on the relative positions of the unidirectional valves, the APL valve, the reservoir bag, the CO_2 absorber, and the site of fresh gas entry. However, to prevent rebreathing of CO_2 *in a traditional circle system*, three rules must be followed: (1) a unidirectional valve must be located between the patient and the reservoir bag on both the inspiratory and the expiratory limbs of the circuit; (2) the fresh gas inflow cannot enter the circuit between the expiratory valve and the patient; and (3) the overflow (pop-off) valve cannot be located between the patient and the inspiratory valve. If these rules are followed, any arrangement of the other components will prevent rebreathing of CO_2. Some newer anesthesia workstations now employ less traditional circle breathing systems. Two of these systems (the Datex-Ohmeda S/5 ADU breathing system and the Dräger Narkomed 6000 series and Fabius GS workstations breathing system) are discussed in greater detail (see the Anesthesia Workstation Variations section).

The most efficient circle system arrangement with the highest conservation of fresh gases is one in which the unidirectional valves are near the patient and the pop-off valve is located just downstream from the expiratory valve. This arrangement minimizes dead space gas and preferentially eliminates exhaled alveolar gases. A more practical arrangement, the one used on most conventional anesthesia machines (see Fig. 24-7), is somewhat less efficient because it allows alveolar and dead space gases to mix before they are vented.[110,111]

The main advantages of the circle system over other breathing systems include its (1) maintenance of relatively stable inspired gas concentrations; (2) conservation of respiratory moisture and heat; and (3) prevention of operating room atmosphere contamination by waste gases. In addition, the circle system can be used as a semiclosed system or as a closed system with very low fresh gas flows. The major disadvantage of the circle system stems from its complex design. Commonly, the circle system may have 10 or more different connections. These multiple connection sites set the stage for misconnections, disconnections, obstructions, and leaks. In an ASA "closed claims" analysis of adverse anesthetic outcomes arising from gas delivery equipment, more than one-third (25/72) of malpractice claims resulted from breathing circuit misconnections or disconnections.[9] Malfunction of the circle system's unidirectional valves can result in life-threatening problems. Rebreathing can occur if the valves stick in the open position, and total occlusion of the circuit can occur if they are stuck shut. If the expiratory valve is stuck in the closed position, breath-stacking and barotrauma or volutrauma can result. Obstructed filters located in the expiratory limb of the circle breathing system have caused increased airway pressures, hemodynamic collapse, and bilateral tension pneumothorax. Causes of circle system obstruction and failure include manufacturing defects, debris, patient secretions, and particulate obstruction from other odd sources such as albuterol nebulization.[112–115] Some systems, such as the Datex-Ohmeda 7900 SmartVent, use flow transducers located on both the inspiratory and the expiratory limbs of the circle system. In one report, cracks in the flow transducer tubing used by this system produced a leak in the circle system that was difficult to detect.[116]

CO_2 ABSORBENTS

In the early 2000s, there were several reports of adverse chemical reactions between CO_2 absorbent materials and anesthetic agents. Some of these undesirable interactions were quite dramatic, such as sevoflurane interacting with desiccated Baralyme®, resulting in fires within the breathing system and severe patient injury.[117,118] Although other sources of ignition and fire in the breathing system continue to be described, the Baralyme®-sevoflurane problem is somewhat unique in that nothing "unusual" is added to or removed from the breathing system for this to occur.[119] In August 2004, the manufacturer of Baralyme (Allied Healthcare Products) discontinued the sale of this absorbent. Other reactions between agents such as desflurane or sevoflurane and desiccated strong base absorbents can produce more insidious patient morbidity and potentially even death from the release of byproducts such as carbon monoxide or compound A.[120] Although absorbent materials may be problematic, they still represent an important component of the circle breathing system.

Different anesthesia breathing systems eliminate CO_2 with varying degrees of efficiency. The closed and semiclosed circle systems both *require* that CO_2 be absorbed from the exhaled gases to avoid hypercapnea. If one could design an ideal CO_2 absorbent, its characteristics would include lack of reactivity with common anesthetics, lack of toxicity, low resistance to gas flow, low cost, ease of handling, and efficiency in CO_2 absorption.

The Absorber Canister

On many anesthesia machines, the absorber canister (see Fig. 24-7) is composed of two clear plastic canisters arranged in series. The canisters can be filled either with loose bulk absorbent or with absorbent supplied by the factory in prefilled plastic disposable cartridges called prepacks. Free granules from bulk absorbent can create a clinically significant leak if they lodge between the clear plastic canister and the O-ring gasket of the absorber, or between other joints in the circuit.[121] Leaks have also been caused by defective prepacks, which were larger than factory specifications.[122] Prepacks can also cause total obstruction of the circle system if the clear plastic shipping wrapper is not removed prior to use.[123] Contemporary workstations from GE Healthcare and Dräger use proprietary CO_2 absorbent canisters that allow exchange of the canisters while maintaining the breathing circuit integrity.

Chemistry of Absorbents

Several formulations of CO_2 absorbents are available today, including soda lime, and calcium hydroxide lime (Amsorb®). Of these agents, the most commonly used is soda lime.[124] All serve to remove CO_2 from the breathing circuit with varying degrees of efficiency.

By weight, the approximate composition of "high moisture" soda lime is 80% calcium hydroxide, 15% water, 4% sodium hydroxide, and 1% potassium hydroxide (an activator). Small amounts of silica are added to produce calcium and sodium silicate. This addition produces a harder and more stable pellet and thereby reduces dust formation. The efficiency of the soda lime absorption varies inversely with the hardness; therefore, little silicate is used in contemporary soda lime.[125,126] Sodium hydroxide is the catalyst for the CO_2 absorptive properties of soda lime. Calcium hydroxide lime is one of the newest clinically available CO_2 absorbents. It consists primarily of calcium hydroxide and calcium chloride and contains two setting agents: calcium sulfate and polyvinylpyrrolidine. The latter two agents serve to enhance the hardness and porosity of the agent.[127] The most significant advantage of calcium hydroxide lime over other agents is its lack of the strong bases, sodium and potassium hydroxide. The absence of these chemicals eliminates the undesirable production of carbon monoxide, the potentially nephrotoxic substance known as compound A, and may reduce or eliminate the possibility of a fire in the breathing circuit.[128] The most significant disadvantages of calcium hydroxide lime are (1) less absorptive capacity, about 50% less than strong-base containing absorbents, and (2) generally higher cost per unit than other absorbents.[129,130]

The size of the actual absorptive granules has been determined over time by trial and error. The current size particles represent a compromise between resistance to gas flow and absorptive efficiency. The smaller the granule size, the greater the surface area that is available for absorption. However, as particle size decreases, resistance to gas flow increases. The granular size of soda lime used in clinical practice is between 4 and 8 mesh, a size at which absorptive surface area and resistance to flow are optimized. Mesh size refers to the number of openings per linear inch in a sieve through which the granular particles can pass. A 4-mesh screen means that there are four quarter-inch openings per linear inch. Likewise, an 8-mesh screen has eight per linear inch (i.e., granule size is >1/8 inch but <1/4 inch).[125] The absorption of CO_2 by absorbents such as soda lime occurs by a series of chemical reactions; it is not a physical process like soaking water into a sponge. CO_2 combines with water to form carbonic acid. Carbonic acid reacts with the hydroxides to form sodium (or potassium) carbonate and water. Calcium hydroxide accepts the carbonate to form calcium carbonate and sodium (or potassium) hydroxide. The equations for the reactions are as follows:

1. $CO_2 + H_2O \Leftrightarrow H_2CO_3$
2. $H_2CO_3 + 2NaOH(KOH) \Leftrightarrow Na_2CO_3(K_2CO_3) + 2H_2O + \text{Heat}$
3. $Na_2CO_3(K_2CO_3) + Ca(OH)_2 \Leftrightarrow CaCO_3 + 2NaOH(KOH)$

Some CO_2 may react directly with $Ca(OH)_2$, but this reaction is much slower.

Absorptive Capacity

The maximum amount of CO_2 that can be absorbed by soda lime is 26 L of CO_2 per 100 g of absorbent. The absorptive capacity of calcium hydroxide lime is significantly less and has been reported at 10.2 L per 100 g of absorbent.[127,129] However, as previously mentioned, absorptive capacity is the product of both available chemical reactivity and physical (granule) availability. As the absorbent granules stack up in the absorber canisters, small passageways inevitably form. These small passages channel gases preferentially through low resistance areas. Because of this phenomenon, functional absorptive capacity of either soda lime or calcium hydroxide lime may be substantially decreased. In practice, because of channeling, the efficiency of soda lime may be reduced to allow only 10 to 20 L or less of CO_2 to actually be absorbed per 100 g of absorbent.[131]

Indicators

Ethyl violet is the pH indicator added to soda lime to help assess the functional integrity of the absorbent. This compound is a substituted triphenylmethane dye with a critical pH of 10.3.[126] 9 Ethyl violet changes from colorless to violet in color when the pH of the absorbent decreases as a result of CO_2 absorption. When the absorbent is fresh, the pH exceeds the critical pH of the indicator dye, and it exists in its colorless form. However, as absorbent becomes exhausted, the pH decreases below 10.3, and ethyl violet changes to its violet form because of alcohol dehydration. This change in color indicates that the absorptive capacity of the material has been consumed. Unfortunately, in some circumstances ethyl violet may not always be a reliable indicator of the functional status of absorbent. For example, prolonged exposure of ethyl violet to fluorescent lights can produce photodeactivation of this dye.[132] When this occurs, the absorbent appears white even though it may have a reduced pH and its absorptive capacity has been exhausted.[132] Even in the absence of color changes, clinical signs that the CO_2 absorbent is exhausted include

1. Increased spontaneous respiratory rate (requires that no neuromuscular blocking drug be used)
2. Initial increase in blood pressure and heart rate, followed later by a decrease in both
3. Increased sympathetic drive: skin flushing, sweating, tachydysrhythmia, hypermetabolic state (increased CO_2 production; must rule out malignant hyperthermia)
4. Respiratory acidosis as evidenced by arterial blood gas analysis
5. Increased surgical bleeding—due to both hypertension and coagulopathy

Although a diagnosis of depletion of CO_2 absorbent capability can be made by observation of clinical signs, the most sensitive 10 indicator of this problem is capnography. If the end-expiratory level of exhaled CO_2 is increased, and the inspiratory level is greater than zero, then exhaustion of the CO_2 absorbent must be pursued as a possible cause.

Interactions of Inhaled Anesthetics with Absorbents

11 It is important and desirable to have CO_2 absorbents that neither release toxic particles or fumes nor produce toxic compounds when exposed to common anesthetics. Soda lime and Amsorb generally fit this description, but inhaled anesthetics do interact with all absorbents to some extent.

Sevoflurane has been shown to produce degradation products upon interaction with CO_2 absorbents.[120,133,134] The major degradation product produced is an olefin compound known as fluoromethyl-2, 2-difluoro-1-(trifluoromethyl) vinyl ether, or compound A. During sevoflurane anesthesia, factors apparently leading to an increase in the concentration of compound A include (1) low flow or closed circuit anesthetic techniques; (2) the use of Baralyme® (now no longer available) rather than soda lime; (3) higher concentrations of sevoflurane in the anesthetic circuit; (4) higher absorbent temperatures; and (5) fresh absorbent.[133–136] Interestingly, the dehydration of Baralyme® increased the concentration of compound A, but the dehydration of soda lime decreases the concentration of compound A.[137,138] Apparently, the degradation products released during clinical conditions do not commonly result in adverse effects in humans even during low flow anesthesia.[139–141] Hepatorenal function biomarkers using

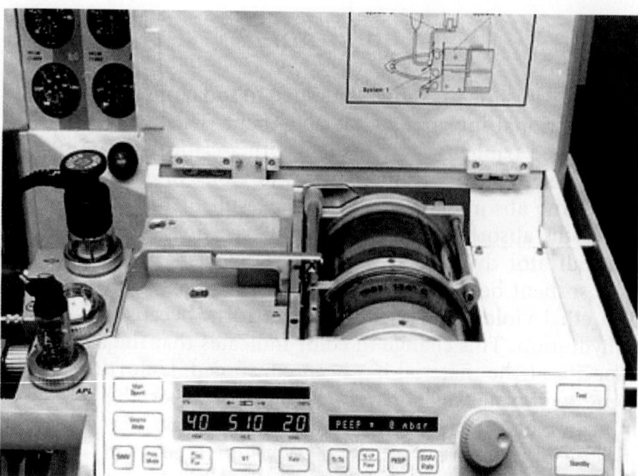

FIGURE 24-35. The Dräger Medical Narkomed 6000 with its single-circuit ventilator. The *horizontal arrow* indicates the piston cylinder unit of the Divan Ventilator. The *vertical arrow* indicates the rectangular valve manifold for fresh gas decoupling.

sevoflurane are unchanged in patients during low flow anesthesia when compared to high flow anesthesia.[142]

Desiccated strong-base absorbents can also degrade contemporary inhaled anesthetics to clinically significant concentrations of carbon monoxide (CO) as well as trifluoromethane, which can interfere with anesthetic gas monitoring.[120] Under certain conditions, this process can produce very high carboxyhemoglobin concentrations, reaching 35% or more.[143] Higher levels of carbon monoxide are more likely after prolonged contact between absorbent and anesthetics, and after disuse of an absorber for at least 2 days, especially over a weekend.[144] Thus, case reports describing carbon monoxide poisoning have been most common in patients 12
anesthetized on Monday morning, presumably because continuous flow from the anesthesia machine desiccated the absorbents over the weekend. FGF rates of 5 L/min or more through the breathing system and absorbent (without a patient connected) are sufficient to cause critical drying of the absorbent material. This is even worse when the reservoir bag is left off the breathing circuit. Absence of the reservoir bag facilitates retrograde flow through the circle system (Fig. 24-35).[143] Because the inspiratory valve leaflet produces some resistance to flow, the FGF takes the retrograde path of least resistance through the absorbent and out to atmosphere via the 22 mm reservoir bag mount.

Several factors appear to increase the production of carbon monoxide and result in increased carboxyhemoglobin levels. They include (1) the inhaled anesthetic used (for a given MAC multiple, the magnitude of CO production from greatest to least is desflurane ≥ enflurane > isoflurane >> halothane = sevoflurane); (2) the absorbent dryness (completely dry absorbent produces more CO than hydrated absorbent); (3) the type of absorbent (at a given water content, Baralyme® produced more CO than does soda lime); (4) the temperature (increased temperature increases CO production); (5) the anesthetic concentration (more CO is produced from higher anesthetic concentrations)[145]; (6) low FGF rates; and (7) reduced experimental animal (patient) size per 100 g of absorbent.[120,146]

Several interventions have been suggested to reduce the incidence of carbon monoxide exposure in patients undergoing general anesthesia.[25] These interventions include (1) educating anesthesia personnel regarding the etiology of CO production; (2) turning off the anesthesia machine at the conclusion of the last case of the day to eliminate FGF that dries the absorbent; (3) changing CO_2 absorbent if fresh gas was found flowing during the morning machine pre-use check; (4) rehydrating desiccated absorbent by adding water; (5) changing the chemical composition of soda lime to reduce or eliminate potassium hydroxide (such products now available include Drägersorb® 800 plus, Sofnolime®, and Spherasorb®); and (6) using absorbent materials such as calcium hydroxide lime that are free of both sodium and potassium hydroxides. The elimination of sodium and potassium hydroxides from desiccated soda lime diminishes or eliminates degradation of desflurane to carbon monoxide and sevoflurane to compound A, but does not compromise CO_2 absorption.[128,147] Because of the increasing evidence that exposure of volatile anesthetics to desiccated CO_2 absorbents, the APSF convened in 2005 a conference entitled, "Carbon Dioxide Absorbent Desiccation: APSF Conference on Safety Considerations." The consensus statement following this conference included two broad recommendations: (a) the use of CO_2 absorbents that, when exposed to volatile anesthetics, do not result in significant degradation; and (b) institutions have in-place policies that address prevention of CO_2 desiccation if conventional CO_2 absorbents are used. In circumstances where absorbents that degrade volatile anesthetics are used (such as the strong base absorbents), the APSF conference experts agreed with the following recommendations[124]:

1. Turn off all gas flow when the machine is not in use
2. Change absorbents regularly (on Monday mornings, since the absorbent may have become desiccated over the weekend)
3. Change absorbent whenever the color change indicates exhaustion
4. Change BOTH canisters in a 2-canister system
5. Change absorbent whenever the FGF has been left on for an extensive or indeterminate period of time
6. If compact canisters are used, consider changing them more frequently

One extremely rare but potentially life-threatening complication related to CO_2 absorbent use is the development of fires within the breathing system. Specifically, this can occur as the result of interactions between the strong-base absorbents (particularly with the now obsolete Baralyme®) and the inhaled anesthetic, sevoflurane. In August 2003, Abbott Laboratories changed the package insert for sevoflurane to describe this rare phenomenon and the conditions under which it could occur. Almost 1 year later, in the fall of 2004, several case reports describing patient injuries related to this problem were published (all involving Baralyme®). When desiccated strong-base absorbents are exposed to sevoflurane, absorber temperatures of several hundred degrees may result from their interaction. The build-up of very high temperatures, the formation of combustible degradation byproducts (formaldehyde, methanol, and formic acid), plus the oxygen- or nitrous oxide-enriched environment provide all the substrates necessary for a fire to occur.[120]

ANESTHESIA VENTILATORS

The ventilator on the modern anesthesia workstation serves as a mechanized substitute for the manual squeezing of the reservoir bag of the circle system, the Bain circuit, or another breathing system. As recently in the late 1980s, anesthesia ventilators were mere adjuncts to the anesthesia machine. Today, in newer anesthesia workstations, they have attained a prominent central role. In addition to the near ubiquitous role of the anesthesia ventilator in today's anesthesia workstation, many advanced ICU-style ventilation features have also been integrated into anesthesia ventilators (see Fig. 24-35). Although many similarities exist between today's anesthesia ventilator and ICU ventilator, some fundamental differences in ventilation parameters and control systems remain. The following discussion focuses on the classification, operating principles, and hazards associated with use of contemporary anesthesia ventilators.

Classification

Ventilators can be classified according to their power source, drive mechanism, cycling mechanism, and bellows type.[148,149]

Power Source

The power source required to operate a mechanical ventilator is provided by compressed gas, electricity, or both. Older pneumatic 13 ventilators required only a pneumatic power source to function properly. Contemporary electronic ventilators from Dräger Medical, Datex-Ohmeda, and others require either an electrical only or both an electrical and a pneumatic power source.

Drive Mechanism and Circuit Designation

Double-circuit ventilators (in which one circuit contains patient gas and the other circuit contains drive gas) are used most commonly in modern anesthesia workstations. Generally, these conventional ventilators are pneumatically driven. In a double-circuit ventilator, a driving force—pressurized gas—compresses a component analogous to the reservoir bag known as the ventilator bellows. The bellows then in turn delivers ventilation to the patient. The driving gas in the GE-Datex-Ohmeda ventilators is 100% oxygen. In the North American Dräger AV-E and AV-2+, a Venturi device mixes oxygen and air. Some newer pneumatic anesthesia workstations have the ability for the user to select whether compressed air or oxygen is used as the driving gas.

More recently, with the introduction of circle breathing systems that integrate fresh gas decoupling, resurgence has been seen in the utilization of mechanically driven anesthesia ventilators. These "piston"-type ventilators utilize a computer-controlled stepper motor instead of compressed drive gas to actuate gas movement in the breathing system. In these systems, rather than having dual circuits, a single patient gas circuit is present. Thus, they are classified as piston-driven, single-circuit ventilators. The piston operates much like the plunger of a syringe to deliver the desired tidal volume or airway pressure to the patient breathing circuit. Sophisticated computerized controls are able to provide advanced types of ventilatory support such as synchronized intermittent mandatory ventilation (S-IMV), pressure-controlled ventilation (PCV), and pressure support–assisted ventilation, in addition to the conventional volume and pressure control. Since the patient's mechanical breath is delivered without the use of compressed gas to actuate a bellows, these systems consume dramatically less compressed gas during ventilator operation than traditional pneumatic ventilators. This improvement in efficiency may have clinical significance when the anesthesia workstation is used in a setting where no pipeline gas supply is available (e.g., remote locations or office-based anesthesia practices).

Cycling Mechanism

Most anesthesia machine ventilators are time cycled and provide ventilator support in the control mode. Inspiratory phase is initiated by a timing device. Older pneumatic ventilators use a fluidic (fluid logic) timing device. Contemporary electronic ventilators use a solid-state electronic timing device and are thus classified as time cycled and electronically controlled. More advanced ventilation modes such as S-IMV, PCV, and modes that utilize a pressure-support option have an adjustable threshold pressure trigger as well. In these modes, pressure sensors provide feedback to the ventilator control system to allow it to determine when to initiate and/or terminate the respiratory cycle.

Bellows Classification

The direction of bellows movement during the expiratory phase
11 determines the bellows classification. *Ascending (standing) bellows* ascend during the expiratory phase (Fig. 24-36B, right), whereas
12 *descending (hanging) bellows* descend during the expiratory phase. Older pneumatic ventilators and some new anesthesia workstations use weighted descending bellows, while most contemporary electronic ventilators have an ascending bellows design. Of the two configurations, the ascending bellows is generally thought to be safer. An ascending bellows will not fill if a total disconnection occurs. However, the bellows of a descending bellows ventilator will continue its upward and downward movement despite a patient disconnection. The driving gas pushes the bellows upward during the inspiratory phase. During the expiratory phase, room air is entrained into the breathing system at the site of the disconnection because gravity acts on the weighted bellows. The disconnection pressure monitor and the volume monitor may be fooled even if a disconnection is complete (see Problems and Hazards section). Some contemporary anesthesia workstation designs have returned to the descending bellows to integrate fresh gas decoupling (Dräger Julian and Datascope Anestar). An essential safety feature on any anesthesia workstation that utilizes a descending bellows is an integrated CO_2 apnea alarm that cannot be disabled while the ventilator is in use.

Operating Principles of Ascending Bellows Ventilators

Contemporary examples of ascending bellows, double-circuit, electronic ventilators include the Dräger Medical AV-E, AV-2+, the GE-Datex-Ohmeda 7000, 7800, and 7900 series. A generic ascending bellows ventilator is illustrated in Figure 24-36. It may be viewed as a reservoir bag (bellows) located within a clear plastic box. The bellows physically separates the driving gas circuit from the patient gas circuit. The driving gas circuit is located outside the bellows, and the patient gas circuit is inside the bellows. During the inspiratory phase (Fig. 24-36A, left) the driving gas enters the bellows chamber, causing the pressure within it to increase. This increase in pressure is responsible for two events. First, the ventilator relief valve closes, preventing anesthetic gas from escaping into the scavenging system. Second, the bellows is compressed, and the anesthetic gas within the bellows is delivered to the patient's lungs. This compression action is analogous to the hand of the anesthesiologist squeezing the breathing bag.[63]

During the expiratory phase (see Fig. 24-36B), the driving gas exits the bellows housing. This produces a decrease to atmospheric pressure within both the bellows housing and the pilot line to the ventilator relief valve. The decrease in pressure to the ventilator relief valve causes the "mushroom valve" portion of the assembly to open. Exhaled patient gases refill the bellows before any scavenging can begin. The bellows refill first because a weighted ball [like those used in ball-type positive end-expiratory

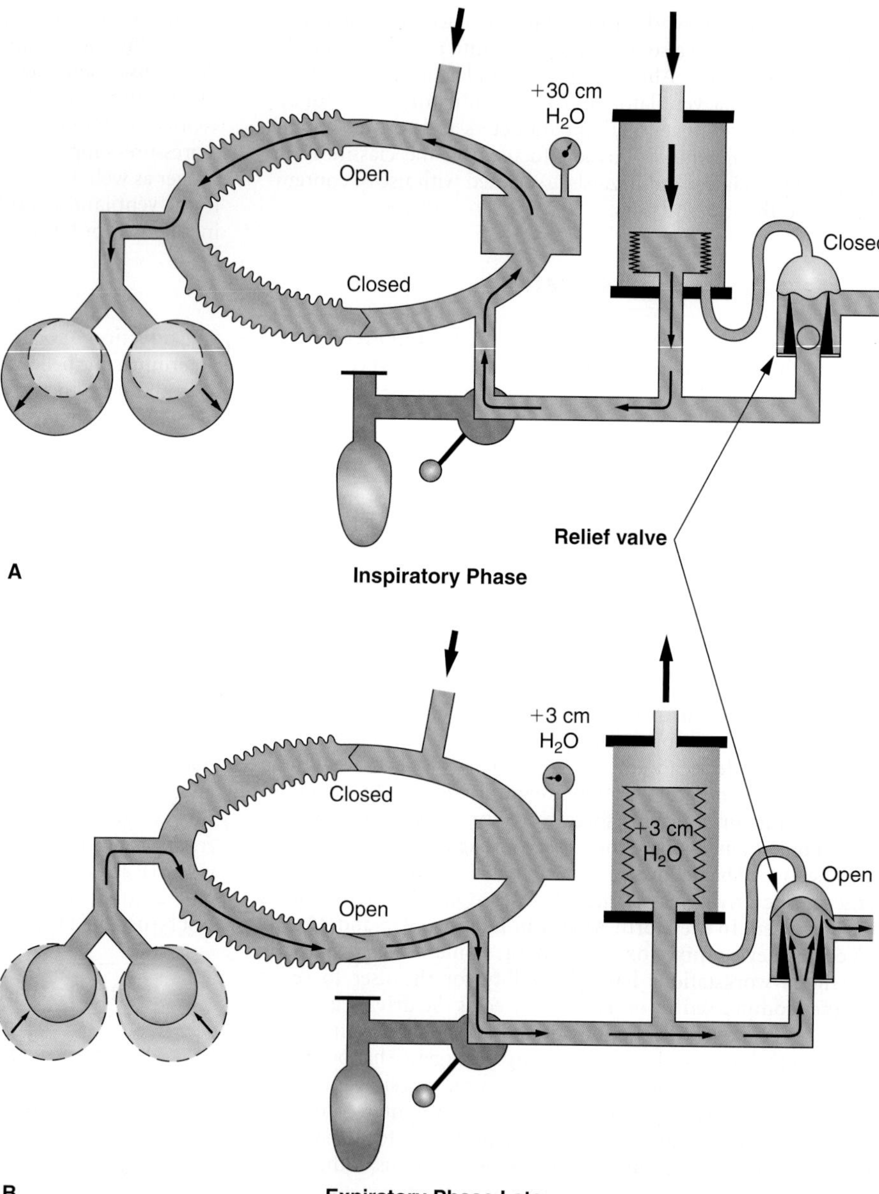

FIGURE 24-36. Inspiratory **(A)** and expiratory **(B)** phases of gas flow in a traditional circle system with an ascending bellows ventilator. The bellows physically separates the driving-gas circuit from the patient gas circuit. The driving-gas circuit is located outside the bellows, and the patient gas circuit is inside the bellows. During inspiratory phase **(A)**, the driving gas enters the bellows chamber, causing the pressure within it to increase. This causes the ventilator relief valve to close, preventing anesthetic gas from escaping into the scavenging system, and the bellows to compress, delivering anesthetic gas within the bellows to the patient's lungs. During expiratory phase **(B)**, pressure within the bellows chamber and the pilot line decreases to zero, causing the mushroom portion of the ventilator relief valve to open. Gas exhaled by the patient refills the bellows before any scavenging occurs, because a weighted ball is incorporated into the base of the ventilator relief valve. Scavenging occurs only during the expiratory phase, because the ventilator relief valve is only open during expiration. (Reprinted with permission from: Andrews JJ. *The Circle System. A Collection of 30 Color Illustrations.* Washington, DC: Library of Congress; 1998.)

pressure (PEEP) valves] or similar device is incorporated into the base of the ventilator relief valve. This ball produces 2 to 3 cm water of back pressure; therefore, flow to scavenging occurs only after the bellows fills completely and the pressure inside the bellows exceeds the pressure threshold of the "ball valve." This design causes all ascending bellows ventilators to produce 2 to 3 cm water pressure of PEEP within the breathing circuit when the ventilator is in use. Scavenging occurs only during the expiratory phase, as the ventilator relief valve is open only during expiration.[63]

14 It is important to understand that on most older anesthesia workstations, gas flow from the anesthesia machine into the breathing circuit is continuous and independent of ventilator activity. During the inspiratory phase of mechanical ventilation, the ventilator relief valve is closed (see Fig. 24-36A), and the breathing system's APL (pop-off) valve is most commonly out of circuit. Therefore, the patient's lungs receive the volume from the bellows plus that entering the circuit from the flowmeters during the inspiratory phase. Factors that influence the relationship between set tidal volume and exhaled tidal volume include the FGF settings, the inspiratory time, the compliance of the breathing circuit, external leakage, and the location of the tidal volume sensor. Usually, the volume gained from the flowmeters during inspiration is counteracted by the volume lost to compliance of the breathing circuit, and set tidal volume generally approximates the exhaled tidal volume. However, certain conditions such as inappropriate activation of the oxygen flush valve during the inspiratory phase can result in barotrauma and/or volutrauma to the patient's lungs because excess pressure and volume may not be able to be vented from the circle system.

Problems and Hazards

Numerous hazards are associated with anesthesia ventilators. These include problems with the breathing circuit, the bellows assembly, and the control assembly.

Traditional Circle System Problems

Breathing circuit misconnections and disconnection are a leading cause of critical incidents in anesthesia.[9,150] The most common disconnection site is at the Y-piece. Disconnections can be complete or partial (leaks). In the past, a common source of leaks with older absorbers was failure to close the APL (or pop-off) valve upon initiation of mechanical ventilation. On today's anesthesia workstations, the bag/ventilator selector switch has virtually eliminated this problem, as the APL valve is usually out of circuit when the ventilator mode is selected. Preexisting undetected leaks can exist in compressed, corrugated, disposable anesthetic circuits. To detect such a leak preoperatively, the circuit must be fully expanded before it is checked for leaks.[151] As previously mentioned, disconnections and leaks are made more obvious with the ascending bellows ventilator systems because they result in a situation in which the bellows will not refill.[51]

Several breathing system disconnection monitors exist, although none should replace the anesthesia provider's vigilance. Monitoring of breath sounds and observation of chest wall excursion should continue despite use of both mechanical (spirometers and pressure sensors) and physiologic monitors.

Pneumatic and electronic pressure monitors are helpful in detecting disconnections. Factors that influence monitor effectiveness include the disconnection site, the pressure sensor location, the threshold pressure alarm limit, the inspiratory flow rate, and the resistance of the disconnected breathing circuit.[152,153] Various anesthesia workstations and ventilators have different locations for the airway pressure sensor and different values for the threshold pressure alarm limit. The threshold pressure alarm limit may be preset at the factory or adjustable. An audible or visual alarm is actuated if the peak inspiratory pressure of the breathing circuit does not exceed the threshold pressure alarm limit. When an adjustable threshold pressure alarm limit is available, such as on many workstations from Dräger Medical and GE Healthcare, the operator should set the pressure alarm limit to within 5 cm water of the peak inspiratory pressure. On systems that have an "autoset" feature, when activated, the threshold limit is automatically set at 3 to 5 cm water pressure below the current peak inspiratory pressure. On such systems, failure to reset the threshold pressure alarm limit may result in either an "Apnea Pressure" or "Threshold Low" alert. Figure 24-37 illustrates how a partial disconnection (leak) may be unrecognized by the low-pressure monitor if the threshold pressure alarm limit is set too low or if the factory preset value is relatively low.

13

Respiratory volume monitors are useful in detecting disconnections. Volume monitors may sense exhaled tidal volume, inhaled tidal volume, minute volume, or all three. The user should bracket the high and low threshold volumes slightly above and below the exhaled volumes. For example, if the exhaled minute volume of a patient is 10 L/min, reasonable alarm limits would be 8 to 12 L/min. Many of the older Datex-Ohmeda ventilators are equipped with volume monitor sensors that use infrared light/turbine technology. These volume sensors are usually located in the expiratory limb of the breathing circuit and thus measure exhaled tidal volume. In the case of the Datex-Ohmeda S/5 ADU, a special attachment known as the D-Lite® spirometry connector is placed in the breathing circuit between the Y-piece and the patient's airway (i.e., tracheal tube connector, LMA). This device permits measurement of both inhaled and exhaled volumes and pressures (see Anesthesia Workstation Variations section). With the older infrared type sensors, exposure to a direct beam of light from the overhead surgical lighting could cause erroneous volume readings as the surgical beam interfered with the infrared sensor. Other types of expiratory volume sensors can be seen in systems such as the Datex-Ohmeda Aestiva, Aespire, and other workstations that incorporate the 7100 ventilator or 7900 SmartVent. These systems generally utilize differential pressure transduction technology to determine inhaled and exhaled volumes and to measure airway pressures. The Dräger Medical Narkomed 6000 series, 2B and GS workstations commonly use an ultrasonic flow sensor located in the expiratory limb. Still other systems from Dräger measure exhaled volume using "hot wire" sensor technology. With this type of sensor, a tiny array of two platinum wires is electrically heated to a high temperature. As gas flows past the heated wires, they tend to be cooled. The amount of energy required to maintain the temperature of the wire is proportional to the volume of gas flowing past it. This system, however, has been associated in at least one report of accidental fire in the breathing circuit.[154]

Capnographs (CO_2 monitors) are probably the best devices for revealing circuit disconnections. CO_2 concentration is measured near the Y-piece either directly (mainstream) or by continuous aspiration of a gas sample to the analyzer instrument (sidestream). Either a sudden change in the differences between the inspiratory and end-tidal CO_2 concentrations or the acute absence of measured CO_2 indicates a disconnection, a nonventilated patient, or other problems.[51] Importantly, an absence of exhaled CO_2 can also be an indication of low (or no) cardiac output rather than a mechanical equipment problem.

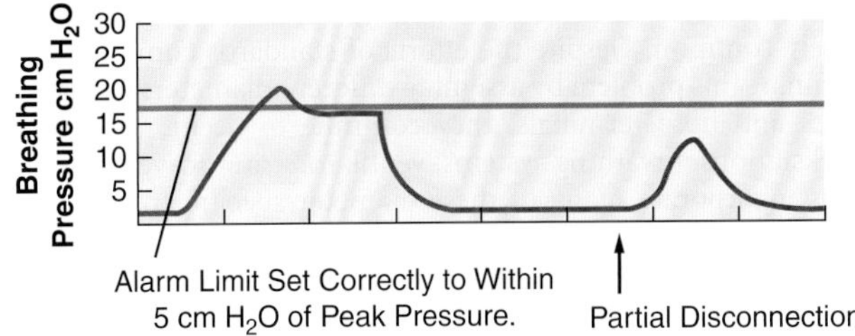

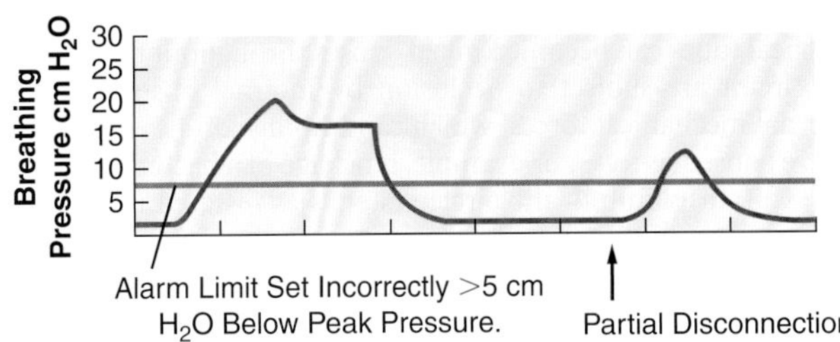

FIGURE 24-37. Threshold pressure alarm limit. **(Top)** The threshold pressure alarm limit (*dotted line*) has been set appropriately. An alarm is actuated when a partial disconnection occurs (*arrow*) because the threshold pressure alarm limit is not exceeded by the breathing circuit pressure. **(Bottom)** A partial disconnection is unrecognized by the pressure monitor because the threshold pressure alarm limit has been set too low. (Redrawn with permission from: *Baromed Breathing Pressure Monitor: Operator's Instruction Manual.* Telford, PA: North American Dräger; 1986.)

Misconnections of the breathing system are unfortunately relatively common. Despite the efforts of standards committees to eliminate this problem by assigning different diameters to various hoses and hose terminals, they continue to occur. Anesthesia workstations, breathing systems, ventilators, and scavenging systems incorporate many of these diameter-specific connections. The "ability" of anesthesia providers to outwit these "foolproof" systems has led to various hoses being cleverly adapted or forcefully fitted to inappropriate terminals and even to various other solid cylindrically shaped protrusions of the anesthesia machine.[51]

Occlusion (obstruction) of the breathing circuit may occur. Tracheal tubes can become kinked. Hoses throughout the breathing circuit are subject to occlusion by internal obstruction or external mechanical forces, which can impinge on flow and have severe consequences. For example, blockage of a bacterial filter in the expiratory limb of the circle system has resulted in bilateral tension pneumothorax.[113] Incorrect insertion of flow direction–sensitive components can result in a no-flow state.[51] Examples of these components include some PEEP valves and cascade humidifiers. Depending on the location of the occlusion relative to the pressure sensor, a high-pressure alarm may (or may not) alert the practitioner to the problem.

Excess inflow to the breathing circuit from the anesthesia machine during the inspiratory phase can cause barotrauma. The best example of this phenomenon is oxygen flushing. Excess volume cannot be vented from the system during inspiration because the ventilator relief valve is closed and the APL valve is out of circuit.[63] A high-pressure alarm, if present, may be activated when the pressure becomes excessive. With many Dräger Medical systems, both audible and visual alarms are actuated when the high-pressure threshold is exceeded. In the Ohmeda Modulus II Plus System, the GE-Datex-Ohmeda 7810 ventilator automatically switches from the inspiratory to the expiratory phase when the adjustable peak pressure threshold is exceeded.

On workstations equipped with adjustable inspiratory pressure limiters such as the GE-Datex-Ohmeda S/5 ADU, Aestiva and Aisys, and Dräger Medical's Narkomed 6000 series, 2B, 2C, GS, Fabius GS and Apollo maximal inspiratory pressure may be set by the user to a desired peak airway pressure. An adjustable pressure relief valve will open when the predetermined user-selected pressure threshold is exceeded. This should prevent generation of excessive airway pressure. Unfortunately, this feature is dependent on the user having preset the appropriate "pop-off" pressure. If the setting is too low, insufficient pressure for ventilation may be generated, resulting in inadequate minute ventilation; if set too high, the excessive airway pressure may still occur, resulting in barotrauma. The piston-driven ventilator in the Dräger Fabius GS and Apollo, as well as others may also include a factory preset peak inspiratory pressure safety valve that opens at a preset airway pressure such as 75 cm of water pressure to minimize the risk of barotrauma.

Bellows Assembly Problems

Leaks can occur in the bellows assembly. Improper seating of the plastic bellows housing can result in inadequate ventilation because a portion of the driving gas leaks to the atmosphere. A hole in the bellows can lead to alveolar hyperinflation and possibly barotrauma in some ventilators because high-pressure driving gas can enter the patient circuit. The oxygen concentration of the patient gas may increase when the driving gas is 100% oxygen, or it may decrease if the driving gas is composed of an air–oxygen mixture.[155]

The ventilator relief valve can cause problems. Hypoventilation occurs if the valve is incompetent because the anesthetic gases are delivered to the scavenging system instead of to the patient during the inspiratory phase. Gas molecules preferentially exit into the scavenging system because it represents the path of least resistance, and the pressure within the scavenging system can be subatmospheric. Ventilator relief valve incompetency can result from a disconnected pilot line, a ruptured valve, or from a damaged flapper valve.[156,157] A ventilator relief valve stuck in the closed or partially closed position can produce either barotrauma or undesired PEEP.[158] Excessive suction from the scavenging system can draw the ventilator relief valve to its seat and close the valve during both the inspiratory and expiratory phases.[51] In this case, breathing circuit pressure increases because excess anesthetic gas cannot be vented. It is worthwhile to note that during the expiratory phase, some newer machines from GE-Datex-Ohmeda (S/5 ADU, 7100 and 7900 SmartVent) scavenge both excess patient gases and the exhausted ventilator drive gas. That is, when the ventilator relief valve opens, and waste anesthetic gases are vented from the breathing circuit, the drive gas from the bellows housing joins with it to enter the scavenging system. Under certain conditions, the large volume of exhausted gases could overwhelm the scavenging system, resulting in contamination of the operating room atmosphere with waste anesthetic gases (see Scavenging Systems section). Other mechanical problems that can occur include leaks within the system, faulty pressure regulators, and faulty valves. Unlikely problems such as an occluded muffler on the Dräger AV-E ventilator can result in barotrauma. In this case, obstruction of driving gas outflow closes the ventilator relief valve, and excess patient gas cannot be vented.[159]

Control Assembly and Power Supply Problems

The control assembly can be the source of both electrical and mechanical problems. Electrical failure can be total or partial; the former is the more obvious. As anesthesia workstations are becoming increasingly dependent on integrated computer-controlled systems, power supply interruptions become more significant. Battery backup systems are designed to continue operation of essential electronics during brief outages. However, even with these systems, in the event of a failure, some time may be required to reboot a computerized system after an electrical outage has occurred. During this time the availability of certain workstation features such as manual or mechanical ventilation can be variable. One cluster of electrical failures that could have potentially resulted in operating room fires was reported early on after the release of the Dräger Medical Narkomed 6000. Problems with the workstation's power supply printed circuit boards prompted a corrective recall action in November 2002.[160]

ANESTHESIA WORKSTATION VARIATIONS

With the introduction of new technology, often comes the need for adaptation of current technology to successfully allow its integration into existing systems. Otherwise, a more comprehensive redesign of an entire anesthesia system "from the ground up" could be necessary. One such example of adaptation in the anesthesia workstation can be seen with two new design variations of the circle breathing system. The first of these is found on the GE-Datex-Ohmeda S/5 ADU, and the second is incorporated into the Dräger Fabius GS and Apollo workstations. Since use of the circle system is fundamental to the day-to-day practice for most anesthesiologists, a comprehensive understanding of these new systems is crucial for their safe use.

Datex-Ohmeda S/5 ADU and GE Healthcare Aisys Carestation

15 The Datex-Ohmeda S/5 ADU debuted as the AS/3 ADU in 1998. Along with its more comprehensive safety features and integrated design that eliminated glass flow tubes and conventional anesthesia vaporizers in exchange for a computer screen with digital FGF scales and the built-in Aladin Cassette vaporizer system, the machine had a radically different appearance in general. It is not until closer inspection that the other unique properties of the ADU begin to stand out. The principal difference in the ADU's circle system lies in the incorporation of the patented "D-Lite" flow and pressure transducer fitting into the circle at the level of the Y-connector. The D-Lite spirometry module was redesigned to accommodate low-flow anesthesia and is currently a design feature of the GE Healthcare Aisys workstation. On most traditional circle systems, exhaled tidal volume is measured by a spirometry sensor located in proximity to the expiratory valve. The placement of the D-Lite fitting at the Y-connector provides a better location to perform exhaled volume measurement and allows airway gas composition and pressure monitoring to be done with a single adapter instead of with multiple fittings added to the breathing circuit. In addition, it provides the ability to assess both inspiratory and expiratory gas flows and therefore generation of complete flow-volume spirometry. The relocation of the spirometer sensor to the Y-connector also makes it necessary to move the location of the fresh gas inlet to the "patient" side of the inspiratory unidirectional valve without adversely affecting accuracy of exhaled tidal volume measurement. On the other hand, placement of the D-Lite sensor near the patient adds bulk and weight to the breathing circuit and may interfere with mask ventilation.

This atypical circle system arrangement with the fresh gas entering on the patient side of the inspiratory valve is advantageous for several reasons. It is likely to be more efficient in delivering fresh gas to the patient, while preferentially eliminating exhaled gases. It is also less likely to cause desiccation of the CO_2 absorbent (see Interactions of Inhaled Anesthetics with Absorbents section). Other notable changes on the S/5 ADU circle system include a compact proprietary CO_2 absorbent canister design that can be changed during ventilation without loss of circle system integrity, and the reorientation of the inspiratory and expiratory unidirectional valves from a horizontal position to a vertical position on the "compact block" assembly just below the absorbent canister. The reorientation of the unidirectional valves reduces the breathing circuit resistance encountered by a spontaneously breathing patient. The vertically oriented unidirectional valves only have to be tipped away from the vertical position to be opened, unlike conventional horizontal valve discs, which have to be physically lifted off from the valve seat against gravity to be opened.

In the newest GE workstations (e.g., Aisys, Aespire, Avance) that use the Advanced Breathing System, the inspiratory and expiratory check valves are oriented horizontally and the circle system arrangement is such that fresh gas enters the circuit upstream from the inspiratory unidirectional valve.

The GE SmartVent 7900 is an electronically controlled, pneumatically driven ventilator. Sensors in the breathing circuit allow the ventilator to compensate for compression losses, fresh gas contribution, and small leaks. Delivered tidal volume is determined by differential pressure, variable orifice flow sensors on both the inspiratory and expiratory sides of the breathing circuit. The inspiratory flow sensor is located downstream of the gas system inspiratory check valve. Feedback from this sensor is used to calculate supply tidal volume corrections for FGF and circuit compression losses. The expiratory flow sensor is located at the input to the gas system expiratory check valve. Breathing rate and expiratory tidal volume are determined by this sensor. Excess fresh gas from the bellows and ventilator drive gas is transferred to the scavenging system.

The Dräger Medical Narkomed 6000 Series, Fabius GS and Apollo Workstations

Several important differences exist between the traditional circle breathing systems and those utilized in the newest Dräger products. At first glance, the most notable difference lies in the appearance and design of the ventilators used with these systems. From the inconspicuous horizontally mounted Divan piston ventilator of the Narkomed 6000 to the vertically mounted and visible piston ventilator of the Fabius GS with its electronic FGF indicators (virtual flowmeters displayed on the screen), these systems appear drastically different from traditional anesthesia systems. The piston ventilators of the Dräger Narkomed 6000 (Divan ventilator) and Fabius series (E-Vent ventilator) anesthesia systems are classified as "electrically powered, piston driven, single circuit, electronically controlled with fresh gas decoupling." The ventilator found on the Dräger Apollo workstation, the E-Vent plus, is an electrically driven and electronically controlled, fresh gas decoupled, high-speed piston ventilator that requires no drive gas (unlike the traditional bellows ventilators). The E-Vent plus ventilator offers modes of ventilation previously found only on intensive care unit ventilators: including synchronized volume mode with adjustable flow trigger, and pressure support.

16 The circle breathing systems utilized by these Dräger (and Datascope Anestar) workstations incorporate a feature known as Fresh Gas Decoupling (FGD). The incorporation of this patient safety enhancing technology has required a significant redesign of the traditional circle system. A functional schematic of a circle system similar to the one used by the Dräger Fabius GS series mechanical ventilation can be seen in Figure 24-38. To understand the operating principles of FGD, it is important to have a good understanding of gas flows in a traditional circle system both during inspiratory and expiratory phases of mechanical ventilation. A complete discussion of this was presented earlier in the section entitled Operating Principles of Ascending Bellows Ventilators.

The key concept of the FGD breathing system can be illustrated during the inspiratory phase of mechanical ventilation. With the traditional circle system, several events are occurring: (1) continuous fresh gas flow from the flowmeters and/or the oxygen flush valve is entering the circle system at the fresh gas inlet; (2) the ventilator is delivering the prescribed tidal volume to the patient's lungs; and (3) the ventilator relief valve (ventilator exhaust valve) is closed, so no gas is escaping the circle system except into the patient's lungs.[161] In a traditional circle system, when these events coincide and fresh gas inflow is coupled directly into the circle system, the total volume delivered to the patient's lungs is the sum of the volume delivered by the ventilator, plus the volume of gas that enters the circle via the fresh gas inlet minus the volume lost to breathing system compliance (usually 2 to 3 mL/cm H_2O pressure). In contrast, when FGD is used, during the inspiratory phase (see Fig. 24-38) the fresh gas coming from the anesthesia workstation flowmeters via the fresh gas inlet is diverted into the reservoir bag by a decoupling valve that is located between the fresh gas source and the ventilator circuit. The reservoir (breathing) bag serves as an accumulator for fresh gas until the expiratory phase begins. During expiratory phase, the decoupling valve

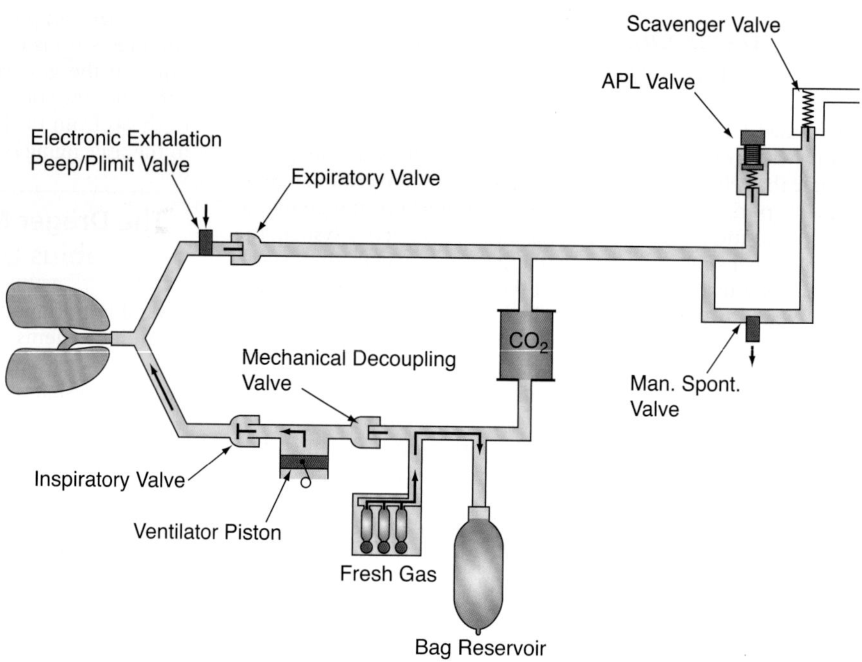

FIGURE 24-38. Dräger Fabius GS fresh gas decoupled breathing system during inspiratory phase of mechanical ventilation. The figure demonstrates the path of fresh gas (and O_2 flush) into the reservoir bag during upstroke of the ventilator piston. Note the requirement here for a mechanical decoupling valve and electronic exhalation/PEEP/Plimit valve. A man/spont valve is electronically opened during CMV, so that excess gas can escape through the low-pressure scavenger valve, which also allows preferential filling of the reservoir bag during the inspiratory phase. (Olympio MA, 2003, reproduced with permission.)

opens, allowing the accumulated fresh gas in the reservoir bag to be drawn into the circle system to refill the piston ventilator chamber (or descending bellows in the Datascope Anestar). Since the ventilator exhaust valve also opens during the expiratory phase, excess fresh gas and exhaled patient gases are allowed to escape to the scavenging system.

Contemporary fresh gas decoupled systems are designed with either piston-type (Dräger) or descending bellows–type ventilators. Since the bellows in either of these types of systems refills under slight negative pressure, it allows the accumulated fresh gas from the reservoir bag to be drawn into the ventilator for delivery to the patient during the next ventilator cycle.

The advantages of circle systems using FGD include more accurate delivery of the set tidal volume and decreased risk of barotrauma and volutrauma. With a traditional circle system, increases in fresh gas flow from the flowmeters or from inappropriate use of the oxygen flush valve may contribute directly to tidal volume, which if excessive, may result in pneumothorax or other injuries. Since systems with FGD isolate fresh gas coming into the system from the patient while the ventilator exhaust valve is closed, the risk of barotrauma is greatly reduced.

Possibly the greatest disadvantage to the new anesthesia circle systems that utilize FGD is the possibility of entraining room air into the patient gas circuit. As previously discussed, in a fresh gas decoupled system the bellows or piston refills under slight negative pressure. If the volume of gas contained in the reservoir bag plus the returning volume of gas exhaled from the patient's lungs is inadequate to refill the bellows or piston chamber, negative patient airway pressures could develop. To prevent this, a negative-pressure relief valve is placed in the breathing system (see Fig. 24-38). If breathing system pressure falls below a preset value such as –2 cm H_2O, then the relief valve opens and ambient air is entrained into the patient gas circuit. If this goes undetected, the entrained atmospheric gases could lead to dilution of the inhaled anesthetic agents, the enriched oxygen mixture (resulting in a lowering of the enriched oxygen concentration toward 21%), or both. If unnoticed, this dilution of patient gases could lead to intraoperative patient awareness or hypoxia. High-priority alarms with both audible and visual alerts should notify the user that fresh gas flow is inadequate and room air is being entrained.

Another potential problem with an FGD system such as seen on the Narkomed 6000 series lies in its reliance on the reservoir bag to accumulate the incoming fresh gas. If the reservoir bag is removed during mechanical ventilation, or if it has a significant leak from poor fit on the bag mount or a perforation, room air may enter the breathing circuit as the ventilator piston unit refills during expiratory phase. This may also result in dilution of the inhaled anesthetic agents, the enriched oxygen mixture, or both. Furthermore, this type of a disruption could lead to significant contamination of the operating room atmosphere with anesthetic gases as fresh gases would be allowed to escape into the atmosphere.

WASTE GAS SCAVENGING SYSTEMS

14 Scavenging is the collection and the subsequent removal of waste anesthetic gases from the operating room.[162] In most cases, the amount of gas used to anesthetize a patient for a given anesthetic far exceeds the minimal amount needed. Therefore, scavenging minimizes operating room contamination by removing this excess of gases. In 1977, the National Institute for Occupational Safety and Health (NIOSH) published a document entitled "Criteria for a Recommended Standard: Occupational Exposure to Waste Anesthetic Gases and Vapors."[163] Although it was maintained that a minimal safe level of exposure could not be defined, NIOSH made the recommendations shown in Table 24-6.[163] It should be remembered that the 2 parts per million (ppm) ceiling for volatile anesthetics was established in 1977, before desflurane and sevoflurane were introduced into clinical practice. However, this limit is likely to be similarly applicable for the newer volatile anesthetics.[164] The NIOSH recommendations have never promulgated into law and therefore are not enforceable by the Occupational Safety and

TABLE 24-6. NIOSH RECOMMENDATIONS FOR MAXIMUM LEVELS FOR EXPOSURE OF PERSONNEL TO TRACE ANESTHESIA GASES AND VAPORS

Anesthetic Gas	Maximum TWA[a] Concentration (ppm)
Halogenated agent alone	2
Nitrous oxide	25
Combination of halogenated agent plus nitrous oxide	
Halogenated agent	0.5
Nitrous oxide	25
Dental facilities (nitrous oxide alone)	50

Reprinted with permission from: US Department of Health, Education, and Welfare. Criteria for a recommended standard: occupational exposure to waste anesthetic gases and vapors. March ed, Washington, DC; 1977.
Note: Despite being in clinical use for more than 15 years, isoflurane, desflurane, and sevoflurane have not been tested for maximum recommended trace gas levels.
[a]TWA, time-weighted average. Time-weighted average sampling, also known as time-integrated sampling, is a sampling method that evaluates the average concentration of anesthetic gas over a prolonged period of time, such as 1 to 8 hours.

Health Administration (OSHA). In 1991, the ASTM released the ASTM F1343-91 standard entitled "Standard Specification for Anesthetic Equipment–Scavenging Systems for Anesthetic Gases."[165] The document provided guidelines for devices that safely and effectively scavenge waste anesthetic gases to reduce contamination in anesthetizing areas.[165] Because of lack of safety data on exposure to the newer halogenated anesthetic agents (isoflurane, desflurane, and sevoflurane), NIOSH has requested comments and information relevant to the evaluation of health risks associated with occupational exposure to these agents in order to establish recommended maximum exposure levels (REL).[166] In 1999, the ASA Task Force on Trace Anesthetic Gases developed a booklet entitled "Waste Anesthetic Gases: Information for Management in Anesthetizing Areas and the Postanesthesia Care Unit." This ASA publication addresses analysis of the literature, the role of regulatory agencies, scavenging and monitoring equipment, and recommendations.[167]

The two major causes of waste gas contamination in the operating room are the anesthetic technique employed and equipment issues.[167,168] Regarding the anesthetic technique, the following factors cause operating room atmosphere contamination: (1) failure to turn off gas flow control valves at the end of an anesthetic; (2) poorly fitting masks, flushing the circuit; (3) filling anesthetic vaporizers; (4) use of uncuffed tracheal tubes; and (5) use of breathing circuits such as the Jackson-Rees (modification of Ayre's T-piece/Mapleson E rebreathing circuit), which are difficult to scavenge. Equipment failure or lack of understanding of proper equipment use can also contribute to operating room contamination. Leaks can occur in the high-pressure hoses, the nitrous oxide tank mounting, the high-pressure circuit and low-pressure circuit of the anesthesia machine, or in the circle system, particularly at the CO_2 absorber assembly. The anesthesia provider must be certain that the scavenging system is operational and adjusted properly to ensure adequate scavenging. If sidestream CO_2 or multigas analyzers are used, the analyzed gas (withdrawn from the circuit at a rate of 50 to 250 cc/min) must be directed to the scavenging system or returned to the breathing system to prevent contamination of the operating room atmosphere.[167,168]

Components

Scavenging systems generally consist of five components (Fig. 24-39): (1) the gas-collecting assembly, (2) the transfer means, (3) the scavenging interface, (4) the gas-disposal assembly tubing, and (5) an active or passive gas-disposal assembly.[163] An "active system" uses a central evacuation (vacuum) system to remove waste gases. The "weight" or pressure of the waste gas itself produces flow through a "passive system."

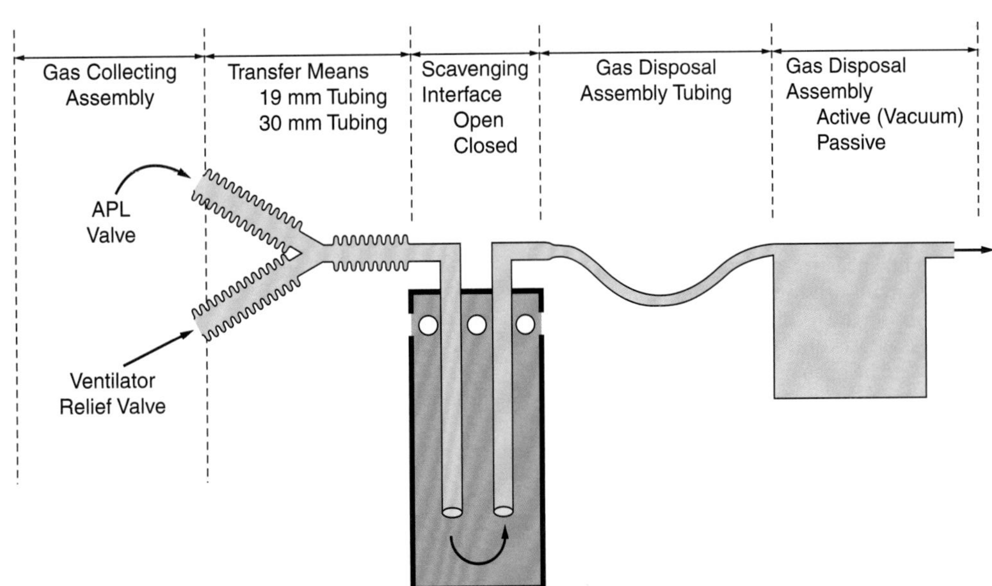

FIGURE 24-39. Components of a scavenging system. APL, adjustable pressure-limiting valve.

Gas-Collecting Assembly

The gas-collecting assembly captures excess anesthetic gas and delivers it to the transfer tubing.[148] Waste anesthetic gases are vented from the anesthesia system either through the APL valve or through the ventilator relief valve. All excess patient gas either is vented into the room (e.g., from a poor facemask fit or tracheal tube leak) or exits the breathing system through one of these valves. Gas passing through these valves accumulates in the gas-collecting assembly and is directed to the transfer means. In some newer GE Healthcare systems (e.g., S5/ADU workstation) and others that incorporate either the 7100 or 7900 ventilators, the ventilator drive gas is also exhausted into the scavenging system. This is significant, because under conditions of high fresh gas flows and high minute ventilation, the gases flowing into the scavenging interface may overwhelm the evacuation system. If this occurs, waste anesthetic gases may overflow the system via the positive-pressure relief valve (closed systems) or through the atmospheric vents (open systems) into the operating room atmosphere. In contrast, most other pneumatic ventilators from both Datex-Ohmeda and Dräger exhaust their drive gas (oxygen or an oxygen/air mixture) into the operating room through a small vent on the back of the ventilator control housing.

Transfer Means

The transfer means carries excess gas from the gas-collecting assembly to the scavenging interface. The tubing diameter must be either 19 mm or 30 mm, as specified by the ASTM F1343-91 standard.[165] The tubing should be sufficiently rigid to prevent kinking, and as short as possible to minimize the chance of occlusion. Some manufacturers color code the transfer tubing with yellow bands to distinguish it from 22 mm diameter breathing system tubing. Many machines have separate transfer tubes for the APL valve and for the ventilator relief valve. The two tubes usually merge into a single hose before they enter the scavenging interface. Occlusion of the transfer means can be particularly problematic since it is upstream from the pressure-buffering features of the scavenging interface. If the transfer means is occluded, baseline breathing circuit pressure will increase and barotrauma can occur.

Scavenging Interface

The scavenging interface is the most important component of the system because it protects the breathing circuit or ventilator from excessive positive or negative pressures.[162] The interface should limit the pressures immediately downstream from the gas collecting assembly to between –0.5 and +10 cm H_2O with normal working conditions.[165] Positive-pressure relief is mandatory, irrespective of the type of disposal system used, to vent excess gas in case of occlusion downstream from the interface. If the disposal system is an "active system," negative-pressure relief is necessary to protect the breathing circuit or ventilator from excessive subatmospheric pressure. A reservoir is highly desirable with active systems, since it stores waste gases until the evacuation system can remove them. Interfaces can be open or closed, depending on the method used to provide positive- and negative-pressure relief.[162]

Open Interfaces

An open interface contains no valves and is open to the atmosphere, allowing both positive- and negative-pressure relief. Open interfaces should be used only with active disposal systems that use a central evacuation system. Open interfaces require a reservoir because waste gases are intermittently discharged in surges, whereas flow from the evacuation system is continuous.[162]

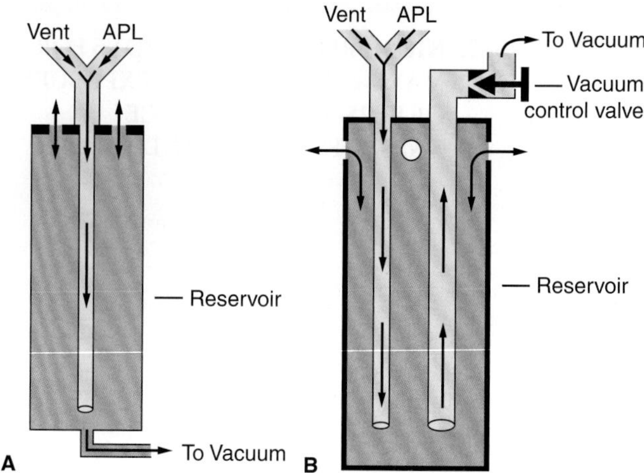

FIGURE 24-40. (**A** and **B**) Two open reservoir scavenging interfaces. Each requires an active disposal system. APL, adjustable pressure-limiting valve. See text for details. (Modified with permission from: Dorsch JA, Dorsch SE. Controlling trace gas levels. In: Dorsch JA, Dorsch SE eds. *Understanding Anesthesia Equipment.* 4th ed. Baltimore, MD: Williams & Wilkins; 1999:355.)

Many contemporary anesthesia machines are equipped with open interfaces like those in Figures 24-40A and 24-40B.[169] An open canister provides reservoir capacity. The canister volume should be large enough to accommodate a variety of waste gas flow rates. Gas enters the system at the top of the canister and travels through a narrow inner tube to the canister base. Gases are stored in the reservoir between breaths. Positive- and negative-pressure relief is provided by holes in the top of the canister. The open interface shown in Figure 24-40A differs somewhat from the one shown in Figure 24-40B. The operator can regulate the vacuum by adjusting the vacuum control valve shown in Figure 24-40B.[169]

The efficiency of an open interface depends on several factors. The vacuum flow rate per minute must equal or exceed the volume of excess gases to prevent spillage. The volume of the reservoir and the flow characteristics within the interface are important. Spillage will occur if the volume of a single exhaled breath exceeds the capacity of the reservoir. The flow characteristics of the system are important because gas leakage can occur long before the volume of waste gas equals the reservoir volume if significant turbulence occurs within the interface.[170]

Closed Interfaces

A closed interface communicates with the atmosphere through valves. All closed interfaces must have a positive-pressure relief valve to vent excess system pressure if obstruction occurs downstream from the interface. A negative-pressure relief valve is mandatory to protect the breathing system from subatmospheric pressure if an active disposal system is used.[162] Two types of closed interfaces are commercially available. One has positive-pressure relief only; the other has both positive- and negative-pressure relief. Each type is discussed in the following sections.

POSITIVE PRESSURE RELIEF ONLY. This interface (Fig. 24-41, left) has a single positive-pressure relief valve and is designed to be used only with passive disposal systems. Waste gas enters the interface at the waste gas inlets. Transfer of the waste gas from the interface to the disposal system relies on the "weight" or pressure of the waste gas itself since a negative-pressure evacuation system is

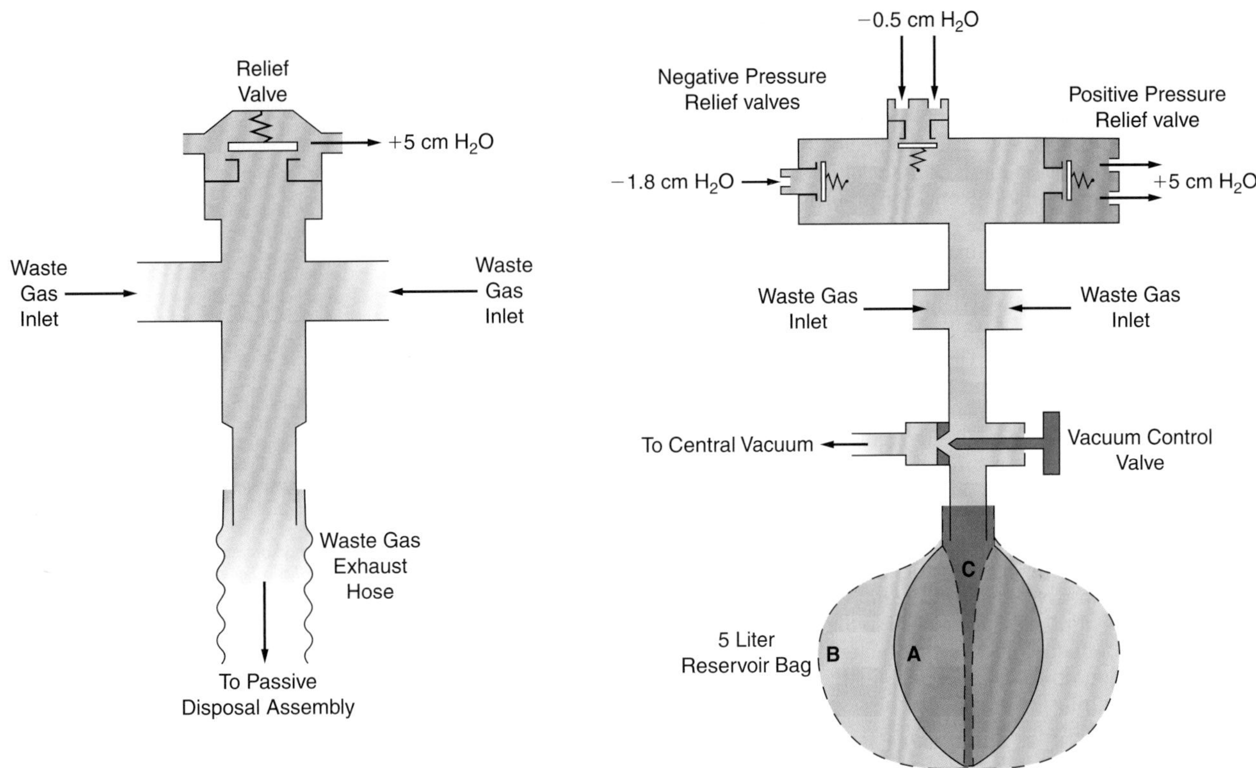

FIGURE 24-41. Closed scavenging interfaces. **(Left)** Interface used with a passive disposal system. **(Right)** Interface used with an active system. See text for details. (Modified with permission from: **(Left)** *Scavenger Interface for Air Conditioning: Instruction Manual.* Telford, PA: North American Dräger; 1984. **(Right)** *Narkomed 2A Anesthesia System: Technical Service Manual.* Telford, PA: North American Dräger; 1985.)

not used. The positive-pressure relief valve opens at a preset value such as 5 cm water if an obstruction between the interface and the disposal system occurs.[171] On this type of system, a reservoir bag is not required.

POSITIVE AND NEGATIVE PRESSURE RELIEF. This interface has a positive-pressure relief valve, and at least one negative-pressure relief valve, in addition to a reservoir bag. It is used with active disposal systems. Figure 24-41 (right) is a schematic of Dräger Medical's closed interface for suction systems. A variable volume of waste gas intermittently enters the interface through the waste gas inlets. The reservoir intermittently accumulates excess gas until the evacuation system eliminates it. The operator should adjust the vacuum control valve so that the reservoir bag is properly inflated (A), not over-distended (B), or completely deflated (C). Gas is vented to the atmosphere through the positive-pressure relief valve if the system pressure exceeds +5 cm water. Room air is entrained through the negative-pressure relief valve if the system pressure is more negative than –0.5 cm H_2O. On some systems, a backup negative-pressure relief valve opens at −1.8 cm H_2O if the primary negative-pressure relief valve becomes occluded.

The effectiveness of a closed system in preventing spillage depends on the rate of waste gas inflow, the evacuation flow rate, and the size of the reservoir. Leakage of waste gases into the atmosphere occurs only when the reservoir bag becomes fully inflated and the pressure increases sufficiently to open the positive-pressure relief valve. In contrast, the effectiveness of an open system to prevent spillage depends not only on the volume of the reservoir but also on the flow characteristics within the interface.[170]

Gas-Disposal Assembly Conduit

The gas-disposal assembly conduit (see Fig. 24-39) conducts waste gas from the scavenging interface to the gas-disposal assembly. It should be collapse-proof and should run overhead, if possible, to minimize the chances of accidental occlusion.[165]

Gas-Disposal Assembly

The gas-disposal assembly ultimately eliminates excess waste gas (see Fig. 24-40). There are two types of disposal systems: active and passive.

The most common method of gas disposal is the active assembly, which uses a central evacuation system. A vacuum pump serves as the mechanical flow-inducing device that removes the waste gases usually to the outside of the building. An interface with a negative-pressure relief valve is mandatory because the pressure within the system is negative. A reservoir is very desirable, and the larger the reservoir, the lower the suction flow rate needed.[162,170]

A passive disposal system does not use a mechanical flow-inducing device. Instead, the "weight" or pressure from the heavier-than-air anesthetic gases produces flow through the system. Positive-pressure relief is mandatory, but negative-pressure relief and a reservoir are unnecessary. Excess waste gases can be eliminated from the surgical suite in a number of ways. Some include venting through the wall, ceiling, floor, or to the room exhaust grill of a non-recirculating air conditioning system.[162,170]

Hazards

Scavenging systems minimize operating room atmosphere contamination, yet they add complexity to the anesthesia system. A scavenging system functionally extends the anesthesia circuit all the way from the anesthesia machine to the ultimate disposal site. This extension increases the potential for problems. Obstruction of scavenging pathways can cause excessive positive pressure in the breathing circuit, and barotrauma can occur. Excessive vacuum applied to a scavenging system can result in undesirable negative pressures within the breathing system.

In 2004, another unusual problem that resulted from waste gas scavenging was reported.[172] The authors reported cases of fires in engineering equipment rooms that house the vacuum pumps used for waste anesthetic gas evacuation. It seems that in some hospitals, waste gases are not directly vented outside, but may be vented into machine rooms that have vents that open to the outside. Since some anesthesia machines are designed such that ventilator drive gas is also scavenged. This gas is 100% oxygen in most cases and is added to gas from the breathing system. As a result, the environment in these machine rooms may become highly enriched with oxygen gas. The result of this has been the production of fires in these spaces outside the operating room. These sites may contain equipment or materials such as petroleum distillates (pumps/oil/grease) that in the presence of an oxygen-enriched atmosphere could be excessively combustible and present a severe fire hazard.

References

1. Lampotang S, Lizdas DE, Liem EB, et al. The Anesthesia Patient Safety Foundation Anesthesia Machine Workbook v1.1a. 2011; http://vam.anest.ufl.edu/members/workbook/apsf-workbook-english.html
2. American Society for Testing and Materials. *Standard Specification for Particular Requirements for Anesthesia Workstations and Their Components (ASTM F1850-00, reapproved).* Philadelphia, PA: American Society for Testing and Materials West Conshohocken; 2005.
3. American National Standards Institute. *Minimum Performance and Safety Requirements for Components and Systems of Continuous Flow Anesthesia Machines for Human Use (ANSI Z79.8-1979).* New York: American National Standards Institute; 1979.
4. American Society of Anesthesiologists. *Manual for Anesthesia Department Organization and Management*; 2007. http://www.asawebapps.org/docs/madomfile.htm
5. James RH. 1000 anaesthetic incidents: experience to date. *Anaesthesia.* 2003; 58(9):856–863.
6. Kibelbek MJ. Cable trapped under Dräger Fabius automatic pressure limiting valve causes inability to ventilate. *Anesthesiology.* 2007;106(3):639–640; author reply 640.
7. Klemenzson GK, Perouansky M. Contemporary anesthesia ventilators incur a significant "oxygen cost." *Can J Anaesth.* 2004;51(6):616–620.
8. Taenzer AH, Kovatsis PG, Raessler KL. E-cylinder-powered mechanical ventilation may adversely impact anesthetic management and efficiency. *Anesth Analg.* 2002;95(1):148–150.
9. Caplan RA, Vistica MF, Posner KL, et al. Adverse anesthetic outcomes arising from gas delivery equipment. *Anesthesiology.* 1997;87:741–748.
10. Olympio MA. Modern anesthesia machines offer new safety features. *APSF Newsletter.* 2003;18(2):17.
11. Cooper JB. Toward prevention of anesthetic mishaps. *Int Anesthesiol Clin.* 1984; 22:167–183.
12. Emergency Care Research Institute. Avoiding anesthetic mishaps through pre-use checks. *Health Devices.* 1982;11:201.
13. Food and Drug Administration. *FDA Anesthesia Apparatus Checkout Recommendations.* 8th ed. Rockville, MD: Food and Drug Administration; 1986.
14. Food and Drug Administration. *Anesthesia Apparatus Checkout Recommendations.* Rockville, MD: Food and Drug Administration; 1993.
15. Spooner RB, Kirby RR. Equipment related anesthetic incidents. *Int Anesthesiol Clin.* 1984;22(2):133–147.
16. American Society of Anesthesiologists. *Guideline for Designing Pre-Anesthesia Checkout Procedures.* Park Ridge, IL; 2008. http://www.asahq.org/For-Members/Clinical-Information/2008-ASA-Recommendations-for-PreAnesthesia-Checkout.aspx
17. Demaria S Jr, Blasius K, Neustein SM. Missed steps in the preanesthetic set-up. *Anesth Analg.* 2011;113(1):84–88.
18. Lewis SE, Andrews JJ, Long GW. An unexpected penlon sigma elite vaporizer leak. *Anesthesiology.* 1999;90:1221–1224.
19. Myers JA, Good ML, Andrews JJ. Comparison of tests for detecting leaks in the low-pressure system of anesthesia gas machines. *Anesth Analg.* 1997;84:179–184.
20. Eng TS, Durieux ME. Automated machine checkout leaves an internal gas leak undetected: the need for complete checkout procedures [case report]. *Anesth Analg.* 2012; 114(1):144–146.
21. Dorsch JA, Dorsch SE. Hazards of anesthesia machines and breathing systems. In: Dorsch JA, Dorsch SE, eds. *Understanding Anesthesia Equipment.* 5th ed. Baltimore, MD: Williams & Wilkins; 2007:404.
22. Comm G, Rendell-Baker L. Back pressure check valves a hazard. *Anesthesiology.* 1982;56:327–328.
23. Peters KR, Wingard DW. Anesthesia machine leakage due to misaligned vaporizers. *Anesth Rev.* 1987;14:36.
24. Rendell-Baker L. Problems with anesthetic and respiratory therapy equipment. *Int Anesthesiol Clin.* 1982;20:1–258.
25. Yasukawa M, Yasukawa K. Hypoventilation due to disconnection of the vaporizer and negative-pressure leak test to find disconnection. *Masui.* 1992;41(8):1345–1349.
26. Datex-Ohmeda. *Explore the Anesthesia System.* Madison, WI: GE Healthcare; 2003.
27. Dodgson BG. Inappropriate use of the oxygen flush to check an anaesthetic machine. *Can J Anaesth.* 1988;35:436–437.
28. Mann D, Ananian J, Alston T. Oxygen flush valve booby trap. *Anesthesiology.* 2004; 101:558.
29. Dorsch JA, Dorsch SE. Equipment checkout and maintenance. In: Dorsch JA, Dorsch SE, eds. *Understanding Anesthesia Equipment.* 5th ed. Baltimore, MD: Williams & Wilkins; 2007:931.
30. Weigel WA, Murray WB. Detecting unidirectional valve incompetence by the modified pressure decline method. *Anesth Analg.* 2005;100(6):1723–1727.
31. Eappen S, Corn SB. The anesthesia machine valve tester: a new device and method for evaluating the competence of unidirectional anesthetic valves. *J Clin Monit..* 1966;12(4):305–309.
32. Bowie E, Huffman LM. *The Anesthesia Machine: Essentials for Understanding.* Madison, WI: Ohmeda, The BOC Group Inc; 1985.
33. Dorsch JA, Dorsch SE. The anesthesia machine. In: Dorsch JA, Dorsch SE, eds. *Understanding Anesthesia Equipment.* 5th ed. Baltimore, MD: Williams & Wilkins; 2007:83.
34. Cicman JH, Jacoby MI, Skibo VF, et al. Anesthesia systems. Part 1: Operating principles of fundamental components. *J Clin Monit.* 1992;8(4):295–307.
35. Schumacher SD, Brockwell RC, Andrews JJ, et al. Bulk liquid oxygen supply failure. *Anesthesiology.* 2004;100(1):186–189.
36. Feeley TW, Hedley-Whyte J. Bulk oxygen and nitrous oxide delivery systems: design and dangers. *Anesthesiology.* 1976;44:301–305.
37. Pelton DA. Non-flammable medical gas pipeline systems. In: Wyant GM, ed. *Mechanical Misadventures in Anesthesia.* 1st ed. Toronto: University of Toronto Press; 1978:8.
38. Stassou A. Two die in hospital mix-up. *WTNH News.* New Haven, CT, 2002.
39. Mudumbai SC, Fanning R, Howard SK, et al. Use of medical simulation to explore equipment failures and human-machine interactions in anesthesia machine pipeline supply crossover. *Anesth Analg.* 2010;110(5):1292–1296.
40. Lorraway PG, Savoldelli GL, Joo HS, et al. Management of simulated oxygen supply failure: is there a gap in the curriculum? *Anesth Analg.* 2006;102(3):865–867.
41. Ellett AE, Shields JC, Ifune C, et al. A near miss: a nitrous oxide-carbon dioxide mix-up despite current safety standards. *Anesthesiology.* 2009;110(6):1429–1431.
42. Adriani J. Clinical application of physical principles concerning gases and vapor to anesthesiology. In: Adriani J, ed. *The Chemistry and Physics of Anesthesia.* 2nd ed. Springfield, IL: Charles C Thomas; 1962:58.
43. Manual of the Compressed Gas Association: Standards for Compressed Cylinder Valve Outlet and Inlet Connections 1994, Washington, DC.
44. Greilich PE, Greilich NB, Froelich EG. Intraabdominal fire during laparoscopic cholecystectomy. *Anesthesiology.* 1995;83(4):871–874.
45. Partbrook GD, Davis PD, Parbrook EO. *Basic Physics and Measurement in Anesthesia.* 2nd ed. Norwalk, CT: Appleton Century Crofts; 1986.
46. Atlas G. A method to quickly estimate remaining time for an oxygen E-cylinder. *Anesth Analg.* 2004;98(4):1190.
47. Davis PD, Parbrook GD, Kenny GNC. *Basic Physics and Measurement in Anesthesia.* 4th ed. Boston, MA: Butterworth-Heinemann; 1995.
48. American Society for Testing and Materials. *Standard Specification for Particular Requirements for Anesthesia Workstations and Their Components (ASTM F1850-00).* Philadelphia, PA: American Society for Testing and Materials West Conshohocken; 2000.
49. Adriani J. Principles of physics and chemistry of solids and fluids applicable to anesthesiology. In: Adriani J, ed. *The Chemistry and Physics of Anesthesia.* 2nd ed. Springfield, IL: Charles C. Thomas; 1962:7.
50. Macintosh R, Mushin WW, Epstein HG, eds. *Physics for the Anaesthetist.* 3rd ed. Oxford: Blackwell Scientific Publications; 1963:196.
51. Schreiber P. *Safety Guidelines for Anesthesia Systems.* Telford, PA: North American Dräger; 1984.
52. Eger EI, II, Epstein RM. Hazards of anesthetic equipment. *Anesthesiology.* 1964; 24:490–504.

53. Eger EI, II, Hylton RR, Irwin RH, et al. Anesthetic flowmeter sequence—a cause for hypoxia. *Anesthesiology.* 1963;24:396.
54. Mazze RI. Therapeutic misadventures with oxygen delivery systems: the need for continuous in-line oxygen monitors. *Anesth Analg.* 1972;51:787–792.
55. Cheng CJ, Garewal DS. A failure of the chain link mechanism of the Ohmeda Excel 210 anesthetic Machine. *Anesth Analg.* 2001;92:913–914.
56. Kidd AG, Hall I. Fault with an Ohmeda Excel 210 anesthetic machine [letter and response]. *Anaesthesia.* 1994;49:83.
57. Lohman G. Fault with an Ohmeda Excel 410 machine [letter and response]. *Anaesthesia.* 1991;46:695.
58. Richards C. Failure of a nitrous oxide–oxygen proportioning device. *Anesthesiology.* 1989;71(6):997–998.
59. Abraham ZA, Basagoitia B. A potentially lethal anesthesia machine failure. *Anesthesiology.* 1987;66:589–590.
60. Neubarth J. Another hazardous gas supply misconnection [letter]. *Anesth Analg.* 1995;80(1):206.
61. Gaughan SD, Benumof JL, Ozaki GT. Can an anesthesia machine flush valve provide for effective jet ventilation?. *Anesth Analg.* 1993;76:800–808.
62. Anderson CE, Rendell-Baker L. Exposed O_2 flush hazard. *Anesthesiology.* 1982; 56(4):328.
63. Andrews J. Understanding your anesthesia machine and ventilator. *International Anesthesia Research Society 63rd Congress.* Lake Buena Vista, FL: International Anesthesia Research Society; 1989;59.
64. Lampotang S, Lizdas DE, Liem EB. The Virtual Anesthesia Machine website. 2007; http://vam.anest.ufl.edu/
65. Lampotang S, Lizdas D, Liem E, et al. *The Anesthesia Patient Safety Foundation Anesthesia Machine Workbook* v1.1a. 2007; http://vam.anest.ufl.edu/members/workbook/apsf-workbook-english.html
66. Dorsch JA, Dorsch SE. Vaporizers. In: Dorsch JA, Dorsch SE, eds. *Understanding Anesthesia Equipment.* 5th ed. Baltimore, MD: Williams & Wilkins; 2007:121.
67. Macintosh R, Mushin WW, Epstein HG, eds. *Physics for the Anaesthetist.* 3rd ed. Oxford: Blackwell Scientific Publications; 1963:68.
68. Korman B, Richie IM. Chemistry of halothane–enflurane mixtures applied to anesthesia. *Anesthesiology.* 1985;63:152–156.
69. Macintosh R, Mushin WW, Epstein HG, eds. *Physics for the Anaesthetist.* 3rd ed. Oxford: Blackwell Scientific Publications; 1963:26.
70. Schreiber P. *Anaesthetic Equipment: Performance, Classification, and Safety.* New York: Springer; 1972.
71. Eisenkraft JB. Anesthesia vaporizers. In: Eisenkraft JB, Ehrenwerth J, eds. *Anesthesia Equipment: Principles and Applications.* St. Louis: Mosby; 1993.
72. Dräger Medical. *Dräger Vapor 2000 Anesthetic Vaporizer Operating Instructions.* Telford, PA; 2001;62.
73. Kharasch ED, Subbarao GN, Cromack KR, et al. Sevoflurane formulation water content influences degradation by Lewis acids in vaporizers. *Anesth Analg.* 2009; 108(6):1796–1802.
74. Hill DW. The design and calibration of vaporizers for volatile anaesthetic agents. *Br J Anaesth.* 1968;40:648.
75. Hill DW, Lowe HJ. Comparison of concentration of halothane in closed and semi-closed circuits during controlled ventilation. *Anesthesiology.* 1962;23:291–298.
76. Anonymous. Internal leakage from anesthesia unit flush valves. *Health Devices.* 1981;10.
77. Morris LE. Problems in the performance of anesthesia vaporizers. *Int Anesthesiol Clin.* 1974;12:199–219.
78. Diaz PD. The influence of carrier gas on the output of automatic vaporizers. *Br J Anaesth.* 1976;48:387–391.
79. Palayiwa E, Sanderson MH, Hahn CEW. Effects of carrier gas composition on the output of six anaesthetic vaporizers. *Br J Anaesth.* 1983;55:1025–1038.
80. Gould DB, Lampert BA, MacKrell TN. Effect of nitrous oxide solubility on vaporizer aberrance. *Anesth Analg.* 1982;61:938–940.
81. Lin CY. Assessment of vaporizer performance in low-flow and closed-circuit anesthesia. *Anesth Analg.* 1980;59:359–366.
82. Nawaf K, Stoelting RK. Nitrous oxide increases enflurane concentrations delivered by ethrane vaporizers. *Anesth Analg.* 1979;58:30–32.
83. Prins L, Strupat J, Clement J, et al. An evaluation of gas density dependence of anaesthetic vaporizers. *Can Anaesth Soc J.* 1980;27:106–110.
84. Scheller MS, Drummond JC. Solubility of N_2O in volatile anesthetics contributes to vaporizer aberrancy when changing carrier gases. *Anesth Analg.* 1986;65:88–90.
85. Stoelting RK. The effect of nitrous oxide on halothane output from Fluotec Mark 2 vaporizers. *Anesthesiology.* 1971;35:215–218.
86. Broka SM, Gourdange PA, Joucken KL. Sevoflurane and desflurane confusion. *Anesth Analg.* 1999;88:1194.
87. George TM. Failure of keyed agent-specific filling devices. *Anesthesiology.* 1984; 61:228–229.
88. Riegle EV, Desertspring D. Failure of the agent-specific filling device [letter]. *Anesthesiology.* 1990;73.353–354.
89. Lippmann M, Foran W, Ginsburg R, et al. Contamination of anesthetic vaporizer contents. *Anesthesiology.* 1993;78:1175–1177.
90. Munson WM. Cardiac arrest: a hazard of tipping a vaporizer. *Anesthesiology.* 1965;26:235.
91. Sinclair A, van Bergen J. Vaporizer overfilling. *Can J Anaesth.* 1993;40:1–3.
92. Seropian MA, Robins B. Smaller than expected sevoflurane concentrations using the SevoTec 5 vaporizer at low fill states and high fresh gas glows. *Anesth Analg.* 2000;91:834–836.
93. Meister GC, Becker KE, Jr. Potential fresh gas flow leak through Dräger Vapor 19.1 vaporizer with key-index fill port. *Anesthesiology.* 1993;78:211–212.
94. Zimmer C, Janssen M, Treschan T, et al. Near-miss accident during magnetic resonance imaging by a "flying sevoflurane vaporizer" due to ferromagnetism undetectable by handheld magnet. *Anesthesiology.* 2004;100:1329–1330.
95. Andrews JJ, Johnston RV, Jr. The new Tec 6 desflurane vaporizer. *Anesth Analg.* 1993;76:1338–1341.
96. Weiskopf RB, Sampson D, Moore MA. The desflurane (Tec 6) vaporizer: design, design considerations and performance evaluation. *Br J Anaesth.* 1994;72: 474–479.
97. Eger EI 2nd. New inhaled anesthetics. *Anesthesiology.* 1994;80:906–922.
98. Susay SR, Smith MA, Lockwood GG. The saturated vapor pressure of desflurane at various temperatures. *Anesth Analg.* 1996;83:864–866.
99. Johnston RV Jr, Andrews JJ, Deyo DJ, et al. The effects of carrier gas composition on the performance of the Tec 6 desflurane vaporizer. *Anesth Analg.* 1994;79:548–552.
100. Andrews JJ, Johnston RV Jr, Kramer GC. Consequences of misfilling contemporary vaporizers with desflurane. *Can J Anaesth.* 1993;40:71–76.
101. Dräger Medical. *D-Vapor Desflurane Vaporizer Instructions for Use.* Telford, PA; 2005.
102. Hendrickx JF, Carette RM, Deloof T, et al. Severe ADU desflurane vaporizing unit malfunction. *Anesthesiology.* 2003;99:1459–1460.
103. Mapleson WW. The elimination of rebreathing in various semiclosed anaesthetic systems. *Br J Anaesth.* 1954;26:323–332.
104. Willis BA, Pender JW, Mapleson WW. Rebreathing in a T-piece: volunteer and theoretical studies of the Jackson-Rees modification of Ayre's T-piece during spontaneous respiration. *Br J Anaesth.* 1975;47:1239–1246.
105. Sykes MK. Rebreathing circuits: a review. *Br J Anaesth.* 1968;40(9):666–674.
106. Froese AB, Rose DK. A detailed analysis of T-piece systems. In: Steward, ed. *Some Aspects of Paediatric Anaesthesia:* Elsevier North-Holland Biomedical Press; Amsterdam, The Netherlands 1982:101.
107. Aarhus D, Søredie E, Holst-Larsen H. Mechanical obstruction in the anaesthesia delivery-system mimicking severe bronchospasm. *Anaesthesia.* 1997;52:992–994.
108. Pethick SL. Letter to the editor. *Can Anaesth Soc J.* 1975;22:115.
109. Moyers J. A nomenclature for methods of inhalation anesthesia. *Anesthesiology.* 1953;14:609–611.
110. Eger EI II. Anesthetic systems: construction and function. In: Eger EI II, ed. *Anesthetic Uptake and Action.* Baltimore, MD: Williams & Wilkins; 1974:206.
111. Eger EI II, Ethans CT. The effects of inflow, overflow and valve placement on economy of the circle system. *Anesthesiology.* 1968;29:93–100.
112. Chacon AC, Kuczkowski KM, Sanchez RA. Unusual case of breathing circuit obstruction: plastic packaging revisited [letter to the editor]. *Anesthesiology.* 2004;100:753.
113. McEwan AI, Dowell L, Karis JH. Bilateral tension pneumothorax caused by a blocked bacterial filter in an anesthesia breathing circuit. *Anesth Analg.* 1993; 76:440–442.
114. Smith CR, Otworth JR, Kaluszyk GSW. Bilateral tension pneumothorax due to a defective anesthesia breathing circuit filter. *J Clin Anesth.* 1991;3:229–234.
115. Walton JS, Fears R, Burt N, et al. Intraoperative breathing circuit obstruction caused by albuterol nebulization. *Anesth Analg.* 1999;89:650–651.
116. Dhar P, George I, Mankad A, et al. Flow transducer gas leak detected after induction. *Anesth Analg.* 1999;89:1587.
117. Kanno T, Aso C, Saito S, et al. A combustive destruction of expiration valve in an anesthetic circuit. *Anesthesiology.* 2003;98:577–579.
118. Laster M, Roth P, Eger E II. Fires from the interaction of anesthetics with desiccated absorbent. *Anesth Analg.* 2004;99:769–774.
119. Laudanski K, Schwab WK, Bakuzonis CW, et al. Thermal damage of the humidified ventilator circuit in the operating room: an analysis of plausible causes. *Anesth Analg.* 2010;111(6):1433–1436.
120. Holak EJ, Mei DA, Dunning MB III, et al. Carbon monoxide production from sevoflurane breakdown. *Anesth Analg.* 2003;96:757–764.
121. Kummar P, Korula G, Kumar S, et al. Unusual cause of leak in Datex Aisys. *Anesth Analg.* 2009;109(4):1350–1351; discussion 1351–1352.
122. Kshatri AM, Kingsley CP. Defective carbon dioxide absorber as a cause for a leak in a breathing circuit. *Anesthesiology.* 1996;84:475–476.
123. Norman PH, Daley MD, Walker JR, et al. Obstruction due to retained carbon dioxide absorber canister wrapping. *Anesth Analg.* 1996;83:425–426.
124. Olympio MA. Carbon dioxide absorbent desiccation safety conference convened by APSF. *APSF Newsletter.* 2005;20(2):25–29.
125. Adriani J. Carbon dioxide absorption. In: Adriani J, ed. *The Chemistry and Physics of Anesthesia.* 2nd ed. Springfield, IL: Charles C. Thomas; 1962:151.
126. Dewey Almy Chemical Division. *The Sodasorb Manual of CO_2 Absorption.* New York: W.R. Grace & Co; 1962.
127. Murray JM, Renfrew CW, Bedi A, et al. A new carbon dioxide absorbent for use in anesthetic breathing systems. *Anesthesiology.* 1999;91:1342–1348.
128. Versichelen LF, Bouche MP, Rolly G, et al. Only carbon dioxide absorbents free of both NaOH and KOH do not generate compound-A during in vitro closed system sevoflurane. *Anesthesiology.* 2001;95:750–755.

129. Higuchi H, Adachi Y, Arimura S, et al. The carbon dioxide absorption capacity of Amsorb is half that of soda lime. *Anesth Analg.* 2001;93:221–225.
130. Sosis MB. Why not use Amsorb alone as the CO_2 absorbent and avoid any risk of CO production? [letter to the editor]. *Anesthesiology.* 2003;98(5):1299.
131. Brown ES. Performance of absorbents: continuous flow. *Anesthesiology.* 1959; 20:41–44.
132. Andrews JJ, Johnston RV Jr, Bee DE, et al. Photodeactivation of ethyl violet: a potential hazard of Sodasorb. *Anesthesiology.* 1990;72:59–64.
133. Kharasch ED, Powers KM, Artru AA. Comparison of Amsorb, sodalime, Baralyme® degradation of volatile anesthetics and formation of carbon monoxide and compound A in swine in vivo. *Anesthesiology.* 2002;96:173–182.
134. Morio M, Fujii K, Satoh N, et al. Reaction of sevoflurane and its degradation products with soda lime. *Anesthesiology.* 1992;77:1155–1164.
135. Fang ZX, Kandel L, Laster MJ, et al. Factors affecting production of compound-A from the interaction of sevoflurane with Baralyme® and soda lime. *Anesth Analg.* 1996;82:775–781.
136. Frink EJ Jr, Malan TP, Morgan SE, et al. Quantification of the degradation products of sevoflurane in two CO2 absorbents during low-flow anesthesia in surgical patients. *Anesthesiology.* 1992;77:1064–1069.
137. Eger EI 2nd, Ionescu P, Laster MJ, et al. Baralyme dehydration increases and soda lime dehydration decreases the concentration of compound A resulting from sevoflurane degradation in a standard anesthetic circuit. *Anesth Analg.* 1997; 85:892–898.
138. Steffey EP, Laster MJ, Ionescu P, et al. Dehydration of Baralyme® increases compound A resulting from sevoflurane degradation in a standard anesthetic circuit used to anesthetize swine. *Anesth Analg.* 1997;85:1382–1386.
139. Bito H, Ikeuchi Y, Ikeda K. Effects of low-flow sevoflurane anesthesia on renal function: comparison with high-flow sevoflurane anesthesia and low-flow isoflurane anesthesia. *Anesthesiology.* 1997;86:1231–1237.
140. Eger EI 2nd, Koblin DD, Bowland T, et al. Nephrotoxicity of sevoflurane versus desflurane anesthesia in volunteers. *Anesth Analg.* 1997;84:160–168.
141. Kharasch ED, Frink EJ Jr., Zager R, et al. Assessment of low-flow sevoflurane and isoflurane effects on renal function using sensitive markers of tubular toxicity. *Anesthesiology.* 1997;86:1238–1253.
142. Fukuda H, Kawamoto M, Yuge O, et al. A comparison of the effects of prolonged (>10 hour) low-flow sevoflurane, high-flow sevoflurane, and low-flow isoflurane anaesthesia on hepatorenal function in orthopaedic patients. *Anaesth Intensive Care.* 2004;32(2):210–218.
143. Berry PD, Sessler DI, Larson MD. Severe carbon monoxide poisoning during desflurane anesthesia. *Anesthesiology.* 1999;90:613–616.
144. Woehlck HJ, Dunning M 3rd, Connolly LA. Reduction in the incidence of carbon monoxide exposures in humans undergoing general anesthesia. *Anesthesiology.* 1997;87(2):228–234.
145. Fang ZX, Eger EI 2nd, Laster MJ, et al. Carbon monoxide production from degradation of desflurane, enflurane, isoflurane, halothane, and sevoflurane by soda lime and Baralyme®. *Anesth Analg.* 1995;80:1187–1193.
146. Bonome C, Belda J, Alvarez-Refojo F, et al. Low-flow anesthesia and reduced animal size increase carboxyhemoglobin levels in swine during desflurane and isoflurane breakdown in dried soda lime. *Anesth Analg.* 1999;89:909–916.
147. Neumann MA, Laster MJ, Weiskopf RB, et al. The elimination of sodium and potassium hydroxides from desiccated soda lime diminishes degradation of desflurane to carbon monoxide and sevoflurane to compound A but does not compromise carbon dioxide absorption. *Anesth Analg.* 1999;89:768–773.
148. McPherson SP, Spearman CB. In: McPherson SP, Spearman CB, eds. *Respiratory Therapy Equipment.* 3rd ed. St. Louis: C.V. Mosby; 1985:230.
149. Spearman CB, Sanders HG. Physical principles and functional designs of ventilators. In: Kirby RR, Smith RA, Desautels DA, eds. *Mechanical Ventilation.* New York: Churchill Livingstone; 1985:59.
150. Cooper JB, Newbower RS, Kitz RJ. An analysis of major errors and equipment failures in anesthesia management: considerations for prevention and detection. *Anesthesiology.* 1984;60:34–42.
151. Reinhart DJ, Friz R. Undetected leak in corrugated circuit tubing in compressed configuration. *Anesthesiology.* 1993;78:218.
152. Raphael DT, Weller RS, Doran DJ. A response algorithm for the low-pressure alarm condition. *Anesth Analg.* 1988;67:876–883.
153. Slee TA, Pavlin EG. Failure of low pressure alarm associated with use of a humidifier. *Anesthesiology.* 1988;69:791–793.
154. Fatheree RS, Leighton BL. Acute respiratory distress syndrome after an exothermic Baralyme-sevoflurane reaction. *Anesthesiology.* 2004;101:531–533.
155. Feeley TW, Bancroft ML. Problems with mechanical ventilators. *Int Anesthesiol Clin.* 1982;20:83–93.
156. Khalil SN, Gholston TK, Binderman J, et al. Flapper valve malfunction in an Ohio closed scavenging system. *Anesth Analg.* 1987;66:1334–1336.
157. Sommer RM, Bhalla GS, Jackson JM, et al. Hypoventilation caused by ventilator valve rupture. *Anesth Analg.* 1988;67:999–1001.
158. Bourke D, Tolentino D. Inadvertent positive end-expiratory caused by a malfunctioning ventilator relief valve. *Anesth Analg.* 2003;97:492–493.
159. Roth S, Tweedie E, Sommer RM. Excessive airway pressure due to a malfunctioning anesthesia ventilator. *Anesthesiology.* 1986;65:532–534.
160. Usher A, Cave D, Finegan B. Critical incident with Narkomed 6000 anesthesia system [letter to the editor]. *Anesthesiology.* 2003;99:762.
161. Dorsch JA, Dorsch SE. Anesthesia ventilators. In: Dorsch JA, Dorsch SE, eds. *Understanding Anesthesia Equipment.* 5th ed. Baltimore, MD: Williams & Wilkins; 2007:310.
162. Dorsch JA, Dorsch SE. Controlling trace gas levels. In: Dorsch JA, Dorsch SE, eds. *Understanding Anesthesia Equipment.* 5th ed. Baltimore, MD: Williams & Wilkins; 2007:373.
163. US Department of Health Education and Welfare. *Criteria for a Recommended Standard: Occupational Exposure to Waste Anesthetic Gases and Vapors.* March ed. Washington, DC: US Department of Health Education and Welfare; 1977.
164. Sessler DI, Badgwell JM. Exposure of postoperative nurses to exhaled anesthetic gases. *Anaesth Analg.* 1998;87:1083–1088.
165. American Society for Testing and Materials. *Standard Specification for Anesthetic Equipment-Scavenging Systems for Anesthetic Gases (ASTM F1343-91).* Philadelphia, PA: American Society for Testing and Materials; 1991.
166. Hall A. Request for information on waste halogenated anesthetic agents: isoflurane, desflurane, and sevoflurane. *Fed Regist.* 2006;71:8859–8860.
167. ASA Task Force on Trace Anesthetic Gases. *Waste Anesthetic Gases: Information for Management in Anesthetizing Areas and the Postanesthesia Care Unit.* Park Ridge, IL: American Society of Anesthesiologists; 1999.
168. Kanmura Y, Sakai J, Yoshinaka H, et al. Causes of nitrous oxide contamination in operating rooms. *Anesthesiology.* 1999;90:693–696.
169. Open Reservoir Scavenger. *Operator's Instruction Manual.* Telford, PA: North American Dräger; 1986.
170. Gray WM. Symposium on anaesthetic equipment. Scavenging equipment. *Br J Anaesth.* 1985;57:685–695.
171. Brockwell RC, Andrews JJ. *Understanding Your Anesthesia Machine, ASA Refresher Courses.* In: Schwartz AJ, ed. Philadelphia, PA: Lippincott Williams & Wilkins; 2002.
172. Allen M, Lees DE. Fires in medical vacuum pumps: do you need to be concerned? *ASA Newsletter.* 2004;68(10):22.

APPENDIX A

FDA 1993 Anesthesia Apparatus Checkout Recommendations[14]

This checkout, or a reasonable equivalent, should be conducted before administration of anesthesia. These recommendations are only valid for an anesthesia system that conforms to current and relevant standards and includes an ascending bellows ventilator and at least the following monitors: Capnograph, pulse oximeter, oxygen analyzer, respiratory volume monitor (spirometer), and breathing system pressure monitor with high- and low-pressure alarms. This is a guideline that users are encouraged to modify to accommodate differences in equipment design and variations in local clinical practice. Such local modifications should have appropriate peer review. Users should refer to the operator's manual for the manufacturer's specific procedures and precautions, especially the manufacturer's low-pressure leak test (Step 5).

Emergency Ventilation Equipment

1. ***Verify Backup Ventilation Equipment is Available and Functioning**

High-Pressure System

2. ***Check Oxygen Cylinder Supply**
   a. Open O_2 cylinder and verify at least half full (about 1,000 psi)
   b. Close cylinder
3. ***Check Central Pipeline Supplies**
   a. Check that hoses are connected and pipeline gauges read about 50 psi

Low-Pressure System

4. ***Check Initial Status of Low-Pressure System**
   a. Close flow control valves and turn vaporizers off
   b. Check fill level and tighten vaporizers' filler caps
5. ***Perform Leak Check of Machine Low-Pressure System**
   a. Verify that the machine master switch and flow control valves are OFF
   b. Attach "Suction Bulb" to common (fresh) gas outlet
   c. Squeeze bulb repeatedly until fully collapsed
   d. Verify bulb stays fully collapsed for at least 10 seconds
   e. Open one vaporizer at a time and repeat "c" and "d" as above
   f. Remove suction bulb and reconnect fresh gas hose
6. ***Turn on Machine Master Switch** and all other necessary electrical equipment
7. ***Test Flowmeters**
   a. Adjust flow of all gases through their full range, checking for smooth operation of floats and undamaged flow tubes
   b. Attempt to create a hypoxic O_2/N_2O mixture and verify correct changes in flow and/or alarm

Scavenging System

8. ***Adjust and Check Scavenging System**
   a. Ensure proper connections between the scavenging system and both APL (pop-off) valve and ventilator relief valve
   b. Adjust waste gas vacuum (if possible)
   c. Fully open APL valve and occlude Y-piece
   d. With minimum O_2 flow, allow scavenger reservoir bag to collapse completely and verify that absorber pressure gauge reads about zero
   e. With the O_2 flush activated, allow the scavenger reservoir bag to distend fully and then verify that absorber pressure gauge reads $<$10 cm H_2O

Breathing System

9. ***Calibrate O_2 Monitor**
   a. Ensure monitor reads 21% in room air
   b. Verify low O_2 alarm is enabled and functioning
   c. Reinstall sensor in circuit and flush breathing system with O_2
   d. Verify that monitor now reads greater than 90%
10. **Check Initial Status of Breathing System**
    a. Set selector switch to "Bag" mode
    b. Check that breathing circuit is complete, undamaged, and unobstructed
    c. Verify that CO_2 absorbent is adequate
    d. Install the breathing circuit accessory equipment (e.g., humidifier, PEEP valve) to be used during the case
11. **Perform Leak Check of the Breathing System**
    a. Set all gas flows to zero (or minimum)
    b. Close APL (pop-off) valve and occlude Y-piece
    c. Pressurize breathing system to about 30 cm H_2O with O_2 flush
    d. Ensure that pressure remains fixed for at least 10 seconds
    e. Open APL (pop-off) valve and ensure that pressure decreases

Manual and Automatic Ventilation Systems

12. **Test Ventilation Systems and Unidirectional Valves**
    a. Place a second breathing bag on Y-piece
    b. Set appropriate ventilator parameters for next patient
    c. Switch to automatic ventilation (Ventilator) mode
    d. Turn ventilator ON and fill bellows and breathing bag with O_2 flush
    e. Set O_2 flow to minimum, other gas flows to zero
    f. Verify that during inspiration bellows deliver appropriate tidal volume and that during expiration bellows fill completely
    g. Set fresh gas flow to about 5 L/min

h. Verify that the ventilator bellows and simulated lungs fill and empty appropriately without sustained pressure at end expiration
i. Check for proper action of unidirectional valves
j. Exercise breathing circuit accessories to ensure proper function
k. Turn ventilator OFF and switch to manual ventilation (bag/APL) mode
l. Ventilate manually and assure inflation and deflation of artificial lungs and appropriate feel of system resistance and compliance
m. Remove second breathing bag from Y-piece

Monitors

13. Check, Calibrate, and/or Set Alarm Limits of All Monitors
a. Capnometer
b. Oxygen Analyzer
c. Pressure monitor with High- and Low-Airway Pressure Alarms
d. Pulse Oximeter
e. Respiratory Volume Monitor (Spirometer)

Final Position

14. Check Final Status of Machine
a. Vaporizers off
b. APL valve open
c. Selector switch to "Bag"
d. All flowmeters to zero (or minimum)
e. Patient suction level adequate
f. Breathing system ready to use

*If an anesthesia provider uses the same machine in successive cases, these steps need not be repeated or may be abbreviated after the initial checkout.

APPENDIX B

Recommendations for Pre-Anesthesia Checkout Procedures (2008)[16]

Sub-Committee of ASA Committee on Equipment and Facilities

Guidelines for Pre-Anesthesia Checkout Procedures

Background

Improperly checking anesthesia equipment prior to use can lead to patient injury and has also been associated with an increased risk of severe postoperative morbidity and mortality.[1,2] In 1993, a pre-anesthesia checkout (PAC) was developed and widely accepted to be an important step in the process of preparing to deliver anesthesia care.[3] Despite the accepted importance of the PAC, available evidence suggests that the current version is neither well understood nor reliably utilized by anesthesia providers.[4–6] Furthermore, anesthesia delivery systems have evolved to the point that one checkout procedure is not applicable to all anesthesia delivery systems currently on the market. For these reasons, a new approach to the PAC has been developed. The goal was to provide guidelines applicable to all anesthesia delivery systems so that individual departments can develop a PAC that can be performed consistently and expeditiously.

General Considerations

The following document is intended to serve not as a PAC itself, but rather as a template for developing checkout procedures that are appropriate for each individual anesthesia machine design. When using this template to develop a checkout procedure for systems that incorporate automated checkout features, items that are not evaluated by the automated checkout need to be identified, and supplemental manual checkout procedures included as needed.

Simply because an automated checkout procedure exists does not mean it can completely replace a manual checkout procedure or that it can be performed safely without adequate training and a thorough understanding of what the automated checkout accomplishes. An automated checkout procedure can be incomplete and/or misleading. For example, the leak test performed by some current automated checkouts does not test for leaks at the vaporizers. As a result, a loose vaporizer filler cap, or a leak at the vaporizer mount, could easily be missed.

Ideally automated checkout procedure should clearly reveal to the user the functions that are being checked, any deficient function that is found and recommendations to correct the problem. Documentation of the automated checkout process should preferably be in a manner that can be recorded on the anesthesia record.

Operator's manuals, which accompany anesthesia delivery systems, include extensive recommendations for equipment checkout. While these recommendations are quite extensive and typically not utilized by anesthesia providers, they are nevertheless important references for developing machine-specific and institution-specific checkout procedures.

Personnel Performing the PAC

The previously accepted Anesthesia Apparatus Checkout Recommendation placed all of the responsibility for pre-use checkout on the anesthesia provider. Sole reliance on one individual to complete the checkout process may increase the likelihood that one or more steps will be omitted or performed improperly. This guideline identifies those aspects of the PAC that could be completed by a qualified anesthesia and/or biomedical technician. Utilizing technicians to perform some aspects of the PAC may improve compliance with the PAC. Steps completed by a technician may be part of the morning pre-use check or part of a procedure performed at the end of each day. Critical checkout steps (e.g., availability of backup ventilation equipment) will benefit from intentional redundancy (i.e., having more than one individual responsible for checking the equipment). **Regardless of the level of training and support by technicians, the anesthesia care provider is ultimately responsible for proper function of all equipment used to provide anesthesia care.**

Adaptation of the PAC to local needs, assignment of responsibility for the checkout procedures, and training are the responsibilities of the individual anesthesia department. Training procedures should be documented. Proper documentation should include records of completed coursework (e.g., a manufacturer course) or for in-house training, a listing of the competency items taught and records of successful completion by trainees.

Objectives for a New PAC

- Outline the essential items that need to be available and functioning properly before delivering every anesthetic.
- Identify the frequency with which each of the items needs to be checked.
- Suggest which items may be checked by a qualified anesthesia technician, a biomedical technician, or a manufacturer-certified service technician.

Basic Principles

- The anesthesia care provider is ultimately responsible for ensuring that the anesthesia equipment is safe and ready for use. This responsibility includes adequate familiarity with the equipment, following relevant local policies for performing and documenting the PAC and being knowledgeable about those procedures.
- Depending upon the staffing resources in a particular institution, anesthesia technicians and/or biomedical technicians can participate in the PAC. Biomedical technicians are often trained and certified by manufacturers to perform on-site maintenance of anesthesia delivery systems and therefore can be a useful resource for completing regular checkout procedures. Anesthesia technicians are not commonly trained to perform checkout procedures. Involving the anesthesia technicians is intended to enhance compliance with the PAC. Each department should decide whether or not the available technicians can or should be trained.
- Critical items will benefit from redundant checks to avoid errors and omissions.
- When more than one person is responsible for checking an item, all parties should perform the check if intentional redundancy is deemed important, or either party may be acceptable, depending upon the available resources.
- Whoever conducts the PAC should provide documentation of successful performance. The anesthesia provider should include this documentation on the patient chart.
- Whenever an anesthesia machine is moved to a new location, a complete beginning-of-the-day checkout should be performed.
- Automated checks should clearly distinguish the components of the delivery system that are checked automatically from those which require manual checkout.
- Ideally, the date, time, and outcome of the most recent check(s) should be recorded and the information made accessible to the user.
- Specific procedures for pre-use checkout cannot be prescribed in this document since they vary with the delivery systems. Clinicians must learn how to effectively perform the necessary pre-use check for each piece of equipment they use.
- Each department or healthcare facility should work with the manufacturer(s) of their equipment to develop pre-use checkout procedures that satisfy both the following guidelines and the needs of the local department.
- Default settings for ventilators, monitors, and alarms should be checked to determine if they are appropriate.
- These checkout recommendations are intended to replace the preexisting FDA-approved Anesthesia Apparatus Checkout Recommendations. They are not intended to be a replacement for required preventive maintenance.
- The PAC is essential to safe care but should not delay initiating care if the patient needs are so urgent that time taken to complete the PAC could worsen the patient's outcome.

ASA 2008 Guidelines for Developing Institution-Specific Checkout Procedures Prior to Anesthesia Delivery[16]

These guidelines describe a basic approach to checkout procedures and rationale which will ensure that these priorities are satisfied. They should be used to develop institution-specific checkout procedures designed for the equipment and resources available. (Examples of institution-specific procedures for current anesthesia delivery systems are published on the ASA website.)

Requirements for Safe Delivery of Anesthesia Care

- Reliable delivery of oxygen at any appropriate concentration up to 100%
- Reliable means of positive-pressure ventilation
- Backup ventilation equipment available and functioning

- Controlled release of positive pressure from the breathing circuit
- Anesthesia vapor delivery (if intended as part of the anesthetic plan)
- Adequate suction
- Means to conform to standards for patient monitoring[7,8]

Specific Items

The following items need to be checked as part of a complete PAC. The intent is to identify what to check, the recommended frequency of checking and the individual(s) who could be responsible for the item. For these guidelines, the responsible party would fall into 1 of 4 categories: Provider, Technician, Technician or Provider, or Technician and Provider. The designation "Technician and Provider" means that the provider must perform the check whether or not it has been completed by a technician. It is not intended to make the use of technician checks mandatory. The intent is not to specify how an item needs to be checked, as the specific checkout procedure will depend upon the equipment being used.

Item #1: Verify auxiliary oxygen cylinder and self-inflating manual ventilation device are available and functioning

Frequency: Daily

Responsible Parties: Provider and technician

Rationale: Failure to be able to ventilate is a major cause of morbidity and mortality related to anesthesia care. Because equipment failure with resulting inability to ventilate the patient can occur at any time, a self-inflating manual ventilation device (e.g., AMBU bag) should be present at every anesthetizing location for every case and should be checked for proper function. In addition, a source of oxygen separate from the anesthesia machine and pipeline supply, specifically an oxygen cylinder with regulator and a means to open the cylinder valve, should be immediately available and checked. After checking the cylinder pressure, it is recommended that the main cylinder valve be closed to avoid inadvertent emptying of the cylinder through a leaky or open regulator.

Item #2: Verify patient suction is adequate to clear the airway

Frequency: Prior to each use

Responsible Parties: Provider and technician

Rationale: Safe anesthetic care requires the immediate availability of suction to clear the airway if needed.

Item #3: Turn on anesthesia delivery system and confirm that AC power is available

Frequency: Daily

Responsible Parties: Provider or technician

Rationale: Anesthesia delivery systems typically function with backup battery power if AC power fails. Unless the presence of AC power is confirmed, the first obvious sign of power failure can be a complete system shutdown when the batteries can no longer power the system. Many anesthesia delivery systems have visual indicators of the power source showing the presence of both AC and battery power. These indicators should be checked and connection of the power cord to a functional AC power source should be confirmed.

Desflurane vaporizers require electrical power and recommendations for checking power to these vaporizers should also be followed.

Item #4: Verify availability of required monitors and check alarms

Frequency: Prior to each use

Responsible Parties: Provider or technician

Rationale: Standards for patient monitoring during anesthesia are clearly defined.[7,8] The ability to conform to these standards should be confirmed for every anesthetic. The first step is to visually verify that the appropriate monitoring supplies (BP cuffs, oximetry probes, etc.) are available. All monitors should be turned on and proper completion of power-up self-tests confirmed. Given the importance of pulse oximetry and capnography to patient safety, verifying proper function of these devices before anesthetizing the patient is essential. Capnometer function can be verified by exhaling through the breathing circuit or gas sensor to generate a capnogram, or verifying that the patient's breathing efforts generate a capnogram before the patient is anesthetized. Visual and audible alarm signals should be generated when this is discontinued. Pulse oximeter function, including an audible alarm, can be verified by placing the sensor on a finger and observing for a proper recording. The pulse oximeter alarm can be tested by introducing motion artifact or removing the sensor.

Audible alarms have also been reconfirmed as essential to patient safety by ASA, AANA, APSF, and JCAHO.[i] Proper monitor functioning includes visual and audible alarm signals that function as designed.

Item #5: Verify that pressure is adequate on the spare oxygen cylinder mounted on the anesthesia machine

Frequency: Daily

Responsible Parties: Provider and technician

Rationale: Anesthesia delivery systems rely on a supply of oxygen for various machine functions. At a minimum, the oxygen supply is used to provide oxygen to the patient. Pneumatically powered ventilators also rely on a gas supply. Oxygen cylinder(s) should be mounted on the anesthesia delivery system and determined to have an acceptable minimum pressure. The acceptable pressure depends on the intended use, the design of the anesthesia delivery system and the availability of piped oxygen.

[i]ASA, American Society of Anesthesiologists; AANA, American Association of Nurse Anesthetists; APSF, Anesthesia Patient Safety Foundation; JCAHO, Joint Commission on the Accreditation of Healthcare Organizations.

- Typically, an oxygen cylinder will be used if the central oxygen supply fails
- If the cylinder is intended to be the primary source of oxygen (e.g., remote site anesthesia), then a cylinder supply sufficient to last for the entire anesthetic is required. If a pneumatically powered ventilator that uses oxygen as its driving gas will be

used, a full "E" oxygen cylinder may provide only 30 minutes of oxygen. In that case, the maximum duration of oxygen supply can be obtained from an oxygen cylinder if it is used only to provide fresh gas to the patient in conjunction with manual or spontaneous ventilation. Mechanical ventilators will consume the oxygen supply if pneumatically powered ventilators that require oxygen to power the ventilator are used. Electrically powered ventilators do not consume oxygen so that the duration of a cylinder supply will depend only on total fresh gas flow.

- The oxygen cylinder valve should be closed after it has been verified that adequate pressure is present, unless the cylinder is to be the primary source of oxygen (i.e., piped oxygen is not available). If the valve remains open and the pipeline supply should fail, the oxygen cylinder can become depleted while the anesthesia provider is unaware of the oxygen supply problem.

Other gas supply cylinders (e.g., Heliox, CO_2, Air, N_2O) need to be checked only if that gas is required to provide anesthetic care.

Item #6: Verify that piped gas pressures are ≥50 psig

Frequency: Daily
Responsible Parties: Provider and technician
Rationale: A minimum gas supply pressure is required for proper function of the anesthesia delivery system. Gas supplied from a central source can fail for a variety of reasons. Therefore, the pressure in the piped gas supply should be checked at least once daily.

Item #7: Verify that vaporizers are adequately filled and, if applicable, that the filler ports are tightly closed

Frequency: Prior to each use
Responsible Parties: Provider; technician if redundancy desired
Rationale: If anesthetic vapor delivery is planned, an adequate supply is essential to reduce the risk of light anesthesia or recall. This is especially true if an anesthetic agent monitor with a low agent alarm is not being used. Partially open filler ports are a common cause of leaks that may not be detected if the vaporizer control dial is not open when a leak test is performed. This leak source can be minimized by tightly closing filler ports. Newer vaporizer designs have filling systems that automatically close the filler port when filling is completed.

High and low anesthetic agent alarms are useful to help prevent over- or under-dosage of anesthetic vapor. Use of these alarms is encouraged and they should be set to the appropriate limits and enabled.

Item #8: Verify that there are no leaks in the gas supply lines between the flowmeters and the common gas outlet

Frequency: Daily and whenever a vaporizer is changed
Responsible Parties: Provider or technician
Rationale: The gas supply in this part of the anesthesia delivery system passes through the anesthetic vaporizer(s) on most anesthesia delivery systems. In order to perform a thorough leak test, each vaporizer must be turned on individually to check for leaks at the vaporizer mount(s) or inside the vaporizer. Furthermore, some machines have a check valve between the flowmeters and the common gas outlet, requiring a negative pressure test to adequately check for leaks. Automated checkout procedures typically include a leak test but may not evaluate leaks at the vaporizer especially if the vaporizer is not turned on during the leak test. When relying upon automated testing to evaluate the system for leaks, the automated leak test would need to be repeated for each vaporizer in place. This test should also be completed whenever a vaporizer is changed. The risk of a leak at the vaporizer depends upon the vaporizer design. Vaporizer designs where the filler port closes automatically after filling can reduce the risk of leaks.

Technicians can provide useful assistance with this aspect of the machine checkout since it can be time consuming.

Item #9: Test scavenging system function

Frequency: Daily
Responsible Parties: Provider or technician
Rationale: A properly functioning scavenging system prevents room contamination by anesthetic gases. Proper function depends upon correct connections between the scavenging system and the anesthesia delivery system. These connections should be checked daily by a provider or technician. Depending upon the scavenging system design, proper function may also require that the vacuum level is adequate which should also be confirmed daily. Some scavenging systems have mechanical positive and negative pressure relief valves. Positive and negative pressure relief is important to protect the patient circuit from pressure fluctuations related to the scavenging system. Proper checkout of the scavenging system should ensure that positive and negative pressure relief is functioning properly. Due to the complexity of checking for effective positive and negative pressure relief, and the variations in scavenging system design, a properly trained technician can facilitate this aspect of the checkout process.

Item #10: Calibrate, or verify calibration of, the oxygen monitor and check the low oxygen alarm

Frequency: Daily
Responsible Parties: Provider or technician
Rationale: Continuous monitoring of the inspired oxygen concentration is the last line of defense against delivering hypoxic gas concentrations to the patient. The oxygen monitor is essential for detecting adulteration of the oxygen supply. Most oxygen monitors require calibration once daily, although some are self-calibrating. For self-calibrating oxygen monitors, they should be verified to read 21% when sampling room air. This is a step that is easily completed by a trained technician. When more than one oxygen monitor is present, the primary sensor that will be relied upon for oxygen monitoring should be checked.

The low oxygen concentration alarm should also be checked at this time by setting the alarm above the measured oxygen concentration and confirming that an audible alarm signal is generated.

Item #11: Verify carbon dioxide absorbent is not exhausted

Frequency: Prior to each use
Responsible Parties: Provider or technician

Rationale: Proper function of a circle anesthesia system relies on the absorbent to remove carbon dioxide from rebreathed gas. Exhausted absorbent as indicated by the characteristic color change should be replaced. It is possible for absorbent material to lose the ability to absorb CO_2 yet the characteristic color change may be absent or difficult to see. Some newer absorbents do change color when desiccated. Capnography should be utilized for every anesthetic and, when using a circle anesthesia system, rebreathing carbon dioxide as indicated by an inspired CO_2 concentration >0 can also indicate exhausted absorbent (See Note 2 in Appendix).

Item #12: Breathing system pressure and leak testing

Frequency: Prior to each use
Responsible Parties: Provider and technician
Rationale: The breathing system pressure and leak test should be performed with the circuit configuration to be used during anesthetic delivery. If any components of the circuit are changed after this test is completed, the test should be performed again. Although the anesthesia provider should perform this test before each use, anesthesia technicians who replace and assemble circuits can also perform this check and add redundancy to this important checkout procedure. Proper testing will demonstrate that pressure can be developed in the breathing system during both manual and mechanical ventilation and that pressure can be relieved during manual ventilation by opening the APL valve. Automated testing is often implemented in the newer anesthesia delivery systems to evaluate the system for leaks and also to determine the compliance of the breathing system. The compliance value determined during this testing will be used to automatically adjust the volume delivered by the ventilator to maintain a constant volume delivery to the patient. It is important that the circuit configuration that is to be used be in place during the test.

Item #13: Verify that gas flows properly through the breathing circuit during both inspiration and exhalation

Frequency: Prior to each use
Responsible Parties: Provider and technician
Rationale: Pressure and leak testing does not identify all obstructions in the breathing circuit or confirm proper function of the inspiratory and expiratory unidirectional valves. A test lung or second reservoir bag can be used to confirm that flow through the circuit is unimpeded. Complete testing includes both manual and mechanical ventilation. The presence of the unidirectional valves can be assessed visually during the PAC. Proper function of these valves cannot be visually assessed since subtle valve incompetence may not be detected. Checkout procedures to identify valve incompetence which may not be visually obvious can be implemented but are typically too complex for daily testing. A trained technician can perform regular valve competence tests. (See Note 4 in Appendix.) Capnography should be used during every anesthetic and the presence of carbon dioxide in the inspired gases can help to detect an incompetent valve.

Item #14: Document completion of checkout procedures

Frequency: Prior to each use
Responsible Parties: Provider and technician
Rationale: Each individual responsible for checkout procedures should document completion of these procedures. Documentation gives credit for completing the job and can be helpful if an adverse event should occur. Some automated checkout systems maintain an audit trail of completed checkout procedures that are dated and timed.

Item #15: Confirm ventilator settings and evaluate readiness to deliver anesthesia care (ANESHESIA TIME OUT)

Frequency: Immediately prior to initiating the anesthetic
Responsible Parties: Provider
Rationale: This step is intended to avoid errors due to production pressure or other sources of haste. The goal is to confirm that appropriate checks have been completed and that essential equipment is indeed available. The concept is analogous to the "time out" used to confirm patient identity and surgical site prior to incision. Improper ventilator settings can be harmful especially if a small patient is following a much larger patient or vice versa. Pressure limit settings (when available) should be used to prevent excessive volume delivery from improper ventilator settings.

Items to check:

- Monitors functional?
- Capnogram present?
- Oxygen saturation by pulse oximetry measured?
- Flowmeter and ventilator settings proper?
- Manual/ventilator switch set to manual?
- Vaporizer(s) adequately filled?

SUMMARY OF CHECKOUT RECOMMENDATIONS BY FREQUENCY AND RESPONSIBLE PARTY

To Be Completed Daily

Item to Be Completed		Responsible Party
Item #1:	Verify auxiliary oxygen cylinder and self-inflating manual ventilation device are available and functioning	Provider and Tech
Item #2:	Verify patient suction is adequate to clear the airway	Provider and Tech
Item #3:	Turn on anesthesia delivery system and confirm that ac power is available	Provider or Tech
Item #4:	Verify availability of required monitors, including alarms	Provider or Tech
Item #5:	Verify that pressure is adequate on the spare oxygen cylinder mounted on the anesthesia machine	Provider and Tech
Item #6:	Verify that the piped gas pressures are ≥50 psig	Provider and Tech
Item #7:	Verify that vaporizers are adequately filled and, if applicable, that the filler ports are tightly closed	Provider or Tech
Item #8:	Verify that there are no leaks in the gas supply lines between the flowmeters and the common gas outlet	Provider or Tech
Item #9:	Test scavenging system function	Provider or Tech
Item #10:	Calibrate, or verify calibration of, the oxygen monitor and check the low oxygen alarm	Provider or Tech
Item #11:	Verify carbon dioxide absorbent is not exhausted	Provider or Tech
Item #12:	Breathing system pressure and leak testing	Provider and Tech
Item #13:	Verify that gas flows properly through the breathing circuit during both inspiration and exhalation	Provider and Tech
Item #14:	Document completion of checkout procedures	Provider and Tech
Item #15:	Confirm ventilator settings and evaluate readiness to deliver anesthesia care (ANESTHESIA TIME OUT)	Provider

To Be Completed Prior to Each Procedure

Item #2:	Verify patient suction is adequate to clear the airway	Provider and Tech
Item #4:	Verify availability of required monitors, including alarms	Provider or Tech
Item #7:	Verify that vaporizers are adequately filled and if applicable that the filler ports are tightly closed	Provider
Item #11:	Verify carbon dioxide absorbent is not exhausted	Provider or Tech
Item #12:	Breathing system pressure and leak testing	Provider and Tech
Item #13:	Verify that gas flows properly through the breathing circuit during both inspiration and exhalation	Provider and Tech
Item #14:	Document completion of checkout procedures	Provider and Tech
Item #15:	Confirm ventilator settings and evaluate readiness to deliver anesthesia care (ANESTHESIA TIME OUT)	Provider

References to Appendix B

1. Cooper JB, Newbower RS, Kitz RJ. An analysis of major errors and equipment failures in anesthesia management: considerations for prevention and detection. *Anesthesiology.* 1984;60:34–42.
2. Arbous MS, Meursing AE, van Kleef JW, et al. Impact of anesthesia management characteristics on severe morbidity and mortality. *Anesthesiology.* 2005;102:257–268.
3. Anesthesia Apparatus Checkout Recommendations, 1993. http://www.fda.gov/cdrh/humfac/anesckot.html
4. March MG, Crowley JJ. An evaluation of anesthesiologists' present checkout methods and the validity of the FDA checklist. *Anesthesiology.* 1991;75:724–729.
5. Lampotang S, Moon S, Lizdas DE, et al. Anesthesia machine pre-use check survey—preliminary results [abstracted]. *Anesthesiology.* 2005;A1195.
6. Larson ER, Nuttall GA, Ogren BD, et al. A prospective study on anesthesia machine fault identification. *Anesth Analg.* 2007;104(1):154–156.
7. American Society of Anesthesiologists. *Standards for Basic Anesthetic Monitoring.* October 25, 2005. http://www.asahq.org/publicationsAndServices/standards/02.pdf
8. Scope and Standards for Nurse Anesthesia Practice. In: *The Professional Practice Manual for the Certified Registered Nurse Anesthetist.* Park Ridge, IL: American Association of Nurse Anesthetists; 2006.

ADDITIONAL NOTES TO APPENDIX B

1. *Testing the flowmeters:* This step is present in the 1993 Checkout Recommendation and is intended to check the oxygen/nitrous oxide proportioning system. It has been eliminated from the Pre-anesthesia Checkout in these guidelines because proper function is verified during the preventive maintenance and failures of this system in a properly maintained delivery system are rare.
2. *Desiccated carbon dioxide absorbent:* Carbon dioxide absorbents which contain sodium, potassium or barium hydroxide may become dangerous when desiccated, producing carbon monoxide and/or excessive heat leading to fires. Unfortunately, it is not possible to reliably identify when the absorbent material has been desiccated. Some departments elect to change all absorbent material on Monday morning to eliminate the possibility of using absorbent exposed to continuous fresh gas flow throughout the weekend. Other departments elect to use absorbent materials that do not pose a risk when desiccated. It is important to have a strategy to prevent the hazards related to using absorbents containing the problematic hydroxides that have desiccated. There are no steps that could be included in the checkout recommendation that can reliably identify desiccated absorbent. If a department uses absorbent that may be hazardous when desiccated, it may be prudent to change the absorbent material whenever the duration of time exposure to high fresh gas flow cannot be determined and is likely to have been prolonged. A protocol for preventing absorbent hazards should be part of every department's risk management strategy.
3. *Anesthesia information systems and automated record keepers:* These systems are being adopted by an increasing number of anesthesia departments and are the mainstay of the recordkeeping process in those departments. Reliably functioning systems is therefore important to the conduct of an anesthetic, although not essential to patient safety in the same fashion as the anesthesia delivery system and patient monitors. For departments that rely upon these systems, it would be prudent to have a protocol for checking connections and the proper functioning of the associated computers, displays and network function.
4. *Testing circle system valve competence:* As part of the test Item 13 (Verify that gas flows properly through the breathing circuit during both inspiration and exhalation), the inspiratory and expiratory valves are visually observed for proper cycling (opening and closing fully). Visual inspection will also detect a missing valve leaflet. Ascertaining full closure of the valve is subjective. Incompetence of the valve may also be detected during test Item 13 through spirometry at the expiratory limb. For expiratory valve malfunction, a spirometer with reverse flow detection will alarm when gas flows retrograde in the expiratory limb. For inspiratory valve malfunction, the measured exhaled tidal volume will be less than the expected value. Capnography may also help to detect incompetence of the unidirectional valves. Intraoperatively, an inspiratory valve malfunction may not be indicated by an elevation of the inspired CO_2 baseline. If the delivered tidal volume exceeds the volume of gas in the inspiratory limb containing CO_2, rebreathing will appear on the capnogram as a gradual, instead of sharp, downstroke. An expiratory valve malfunction is indicated by an elevated CO_2 baseline as there is typically a large volume of exhaled gas containing CO_2 that can return to the patient.

SECTION VI

Anesthetic Management

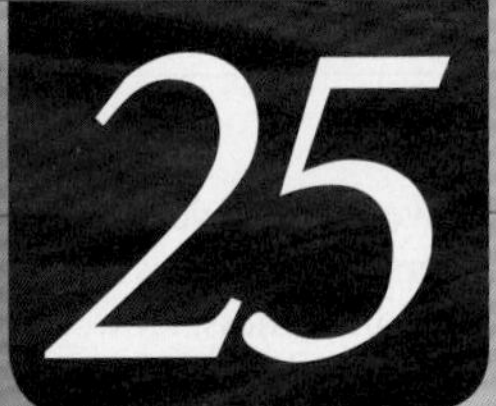
CHAPTER 25

Commonly Used Monitoring Techniques

CHRISTOPHER W. CONNOR

Key Points

1. The purpose of monitoring equipment is to augment the situational awareness of the anesthesiologist by providing clinical data either more rapidly than can be achieved manually or more precisely than can be achieved by direct examination of the patient. The value of any particular monitoring technique lies in its ability to inform the practice of the anesthesiologist so that the patient's physiologic condition can be maintained within satisfactory parameters. No monitoring technique, however sophisticated, can substitute for the judgment of the anesthesiologist.
2. It is mandatory to measure inspired oxygen concentration for patients receiving general anesthesia to prevent the inadvertent administration of a hypoxic gas mixture. However, inspired oxygen concentration monitoring cannot reliably detect disconnection of the circuit, nor does it guarantee adequate arterial oxygenation.
3. Pulse oximetry provides a noninvasive means to detect the onset of hypoxemia rapidly. Modern pulse oximeters are noninvasive, continuous, autocalibrating, have quick response times and are suitable for use during transport. However, pulse oximetry is

a poor indicator of adequate ventilation; desaturation is a late sign of apnea or respiratory insufficiency.

4 Monitoring of expired carbon dioxide is now recommended for procedures involving moderate to deep sedation, in addition to procedures performed under general anesthesia. Advances in infrared absorption spectroscopy have led to the production of conveniently portable devices for expired gas analysis.

5 During direct invasive arterial pressure monitoring, the fidelity of the system is optimized when the catheter and tubing are stiff, the mass of the fluid is small, and the length of the connecting tubing is not excessive.

6 Automated noninvasive blood pressure monitors use the oscillometric method to estimate arterial blood pressure. Pulsatile flow generates oscillations in the internal pressure of an inflated blood pressure cuff; these oscillations are greatest when the cuff is inflated to mean arterial pressure. During prolonged surgical cases, it may be prudent to relocate the blood pressure cuff every few hours to reduce the risk of neurapraxia or cutaneous injury.

7 On the basis of available evidence, it is difficult to draw meaningful conclusions regarding the effectiveness of pulmonary artery catheter (PAC) monitoring in reducing morbidity and mortality in critically ill patients. Expert opinion suggests that perioperative complications may be reduced if PACs are used in the appropriate patients and settings, and if clinicians interpret and apply the data provided by the PAC correctly. New, noninvasive devices have been developed to generate similar cardiac output parameters to the PAC, as well as potentially to be able to predict fluid responsiveness. However, certain common comorbidities can impair the accuracy of these devices; the PAC thermodilution technique remains the clinical gold standard for measuring cardiac output.

8 Clinical studies have demonstrated that patients in whom intraoperative hypothermia develops are at a higher risk for development of postoperative myocardial ischemia and wound infection compared with patients who are normothermic in the perioperative period. Although liquid crystal skin temperature strips are convenient to apply, they do not correlate well with core temperature measurements.

9 Although the algorithms used by processed EEG monitors are proprietary, the general features of the EEG that they use are well described. Processed EEG monitors have not been demonstrated to be superior to end-tidal agent concentration monitoring in the prevention of awareness under anesthesia, although neither technique is sufficient to avoid awareness with complete reliability.

10 The advent of "smarter" and more technically sophisticated monitoring devices does not relieve the anesthesiologist of their obligation to employ their clinical judgment wisely. On the contrary, it requires the anesthesiologist to understand the operation of these devices intimately so that they can be used safely, accurately, and appropriately.

Multimedia

1 Oximetry
2 Galvanic Oxygen Analyzers
3 Capnogram
4 Cardiac Oscillation
5 Arterial Line Tracing
6 Arterial Line Insertion
7 Ultrasound Guided Radial Artery Cannulation
8 Transducer
9 Arterial Line Infection
10 Arterial Line Complications
11 NIBP Oscillations
12 Swan Pressure Tracing
13 Swan Real Life
14 CVP Waveforms
15 Ultrasound Guided IJ Insertion
16 Thermodilution Cardiac Output
17 Respiratory Variation

INTRODUCTION

Historically, the foundation of anesthesia practice has been vigilance and ongoing clinical examination of the patient. The development of modern monitoring equipment does not replace these responsibilities. Automated monitoring equipment provides the anesthesiologist with the ability to acquire clinical information either more rapidly or frequently than can be achieved through manual techniques, or in a more quantitatively precise manner than can be achieved by physical examination alone. The purpose of monitoring equipment, then, is to augment the situational awareness of the anesthesiologist so that clinical problems can
1 be recognized and addressed in a timely manner, and to guide treatment. The value of any particular monitoring technique lies in its ability to inform the practice of the anesthesiologist so that the patient's physiologic condition can be maintained within satisfactory parameters. The term itself is derived from *monere*, which in Latin means to warn, remind, or admonish.

This chapter discusses the methods and biomedical devices through which anesthesiologists monitor the physiologic state of the patient during anesthesia care. The principles of operation for each of these devices are explained. These explanations are, by necessity, simplified as the actual design of a biomedical device involves significant engineering complexity. However, the explanations are intended to be sufficient to allow the anesthesiologist to understand how the device acquires its clinical data, and to understand how that process might be compromised and the data made erroneous; to understand how the device works, and how it may fail. There is little high-grade evidence that electronic monitors, by themselves, reduce morbidity and mortality. There is also controversy regarding the need for specific monitors in certain clinical situations, particularly where use of the monitor in question may add significant cost, or where the invasiveness of the monitoring technique may place the patient at risk of iatrogenic complications. Against these costs and risks, the anesthesiologist must balance the likely benefit from a particular monitoring technique, when used and interpreted correctly. Therefore, alongside the science and engineering aspects of monitoring, there is also the clinical art of choosing how a patient should best be monitored intraoperatively. For each of the monitoring techniques, relative indications, contraindications, and common technical problems are discussed.

Standards for basic anesthetic monitoring have been established by the American Society of Anesthesiologists (ASA). Since 1986, these standards have emphasized the evolution of technology and practice. The current standards (which became effective on July 1, 2011) emphasize the importance of regular and frequent measurements, integration of clinical judgment and experience, and the potential for extenuating circumstances that can influence the applicability or accuracy of monitoring systems.[1]

Standard I requires qualified personnel to be present in the operating room during general anesthesia, regional anesthesia, and monitored anesthesia care to monitor the patient continuously and modify anesthesia care based on clinical observations and the responses of the patient to dynamic changes resulting from surgery or drug therapy. Standard II focuses attention on continually evaluating the patient's oxygenation, ventilation, circulation, and temperature. Standard II specifically mandates the following:

1. Use of an inspired oxygen analyzer with a low concentration limit alarm during general anesthesia.
2. Quantitative assessment of blood oxygenation during any anesthesia care.
3. Continuously ensuring the adequacy of ventilation by physical diagnostic techniques during all anesthesia care. Continual identification of expired carbon dioxide is performed unless precluded by the type of patient, procedure, or equipment. Quantitative monitoring of tidal volume and capnography is strongly encouraged in patients undergoing general anesthesia.
4. When administering regional anesthesia or local anesthesia, sufficient ventilation should be assessed by qualitative clinical signs. During moderate or deep sedation, ventilation shall be evaluated by continual assessment of qualitative clinical signs, and also monitoring for the presence of exhaled carbon dioxide unless precluded by the type of patient, procedure, or equipment.
5. Ensuring correct placement of an endotracheal intubation or laryngeal mask airway requires clinical assessment and qualitative identification of carbon dioxide in the expired gas.
6. When using a mechanical ventilator, use of a device that is able to detect a disconnection of any part of the breathing system.
7. The adequacy of circulation should be monitored by the continuous display of the electrocardiogram, and by determining the arterial blood pressure and heart rate at least every 5 minutes. During general anesthesia, circulatory function is to be continually evaluated by at least one of the following: Palpation of a pulse, auscultation of heart sounds, monitoring of a tracing of intra-arterial pressure, ultrasound peripheral pulse monitoring, or pulse plethysmography or oximetry.
8. During all anesthetics, the means for continuously measuring the patient's temperature must be available. Every patient receiving anesthesia shall have temperature monitored when clinically significant changes in body temperature are intended, anticipated, or suspected.

MONITORING OF INSPIRED OXYGEN CONCENTRATION

Principles of Operation

Oxygen is a highly reactive chemical species, providing many chemical and physical opportunities to detect its presence. Three main types of oxygen analyzers are seen in clinical practice: Paramagnetic oxygen analyzers, galvanic cell analyzers, and polarographic oxygen analyzers.

1 Paramagnetic gases are attracted to magnetic energy because of unpaired electrons in their outer shell orbits. Oxygen is a highly paramagnetic gas. Differential paramagnetic oximetry has been incorporated into a variety of operating room monitors. These instruments detect the change in sample line pressure resulting from the attraction of oxygen by switched magnetic fields. Signal changes during electromagnetic switching correlate with the oxygen concentration in the sample line.[2]

Galvanic cell analyzers meet the performance criteria necessary for operative monitoring. These analyzers measure the current produced when oxygen diffuses across a membrane and is reduced to molecular oxygen at the anode of an electrical circuit.[3] The electron flow (current) is proportional to the partial pressure of oxygen in the fuel cell. Galvanic cell analyzers require regular replacement of the galvanic sensor capsule. In the sensor, the electric potential for the reduction of oxygen results from a chemical reaction. Over time, the reactants require replenishment.[4]

Polarographic oxygen analyzers are commonly used in anesthesia monitoring. In this electrochemical system, oxygen diffuses through an oxygen-permeable polymeric membrane and participates in the following reaction: $O_2 + 2H_2O + 4e^- \rightarrow 4OH^-$. The current change is proportional to the number of oxygen molecules surrounding the electrode. Polarographic oxygen sensors are versatile and are important components of gas machine oxygen analyzers, blood gas analyzers, and transcutaneous oxygen analyzers.[5]

Proper Use and Interpretation

2 The concentration of oxygen in the anesthetic circuit must be measured. Anesthesia machine manufacturers place oxygen sensors on the inspired limb of the anesthesia circuit to detect and alarm in the event that hypoxic gas mixtures are delivered to the patient. Carbon dioxide may reduce the usable lifetime of a galvanic oxygen sensor, so it is preferable to place the oxygen sensor on the inspired limb. Oxygen monitors require a fast response time (2 to 10 seconds), accuracy (±2% of the actual level), and stability when exposed to humidity and inhalation agents.

The removable, external oxygen sensors seen commonly on anesthesia machines such as the Narkomed and Drager Fabius are of the galvanic type. These devices should be calibrated against room air ($FiO_2 = 0.21$) daily, and also after 8 hours of use. These devices may also infrequently require calibration against $FiO_2 = 1$. As part of the preoperative checkout of the anesthesia machine, the clinician must confirm that the alarm limits of the inspired oxygen analyzer are set appropriately to alert to the presence of hypoxic mixtures. Inspired oxygen alarms cannot be relied upon to detect disconnection of the circuit.

Indications

According to the ASA Standards for Basic Anesthesia Monitoring,[1] Standard 2.2.1 states "During every administration of general anesthesia using an anesthesia machine, the concentration of oxygen in the patient breathing system shall be measured by an oxygen analyzer with a low oxygen concentration limit alarm in use."

The careful monitoring of the inspired oxygen concentration is of particular significance during low-flow anesthesia, in which the anesthesiologist attempts to minimize the fresh gas flow to the amount of oxygen necessary to replace the patient's metabolic utilization. The gas mixture within the breathing circuit may become hypoxic if insufficient fresh gas flow is supplied, even if the fresh gas flow itself comprises pure oxygen.

Contraindications

This requirement to monitor inspired oxygen concentration may be waived by the responsible anesthesiologist under extenuating circumstances. There are no clinical contraindications to monitoring inspired oxygen concentration.

Common Problems and Limitations

Adequate inspiratory oxygen concentration does not guarantee adequate arterial oxygen concentration.[6] Consequently, ASA[1] Standard 2.2.2 mandates additional monitoring for blood oxygenation, including the provision of adequate lighting and exposure to assess the patient's color by direct observation.

MONITORING OF ARTERIAL OXYGENATION BY PULSE OXIMETRY

Principles of Operation

Pulse oximeters measure pulse rate and estimate the oxygen saturation of hemoglobin (Hb; Spo_2) on a noninvasive, continuous basis.[7] The oxygen saturation of hemoglobin (as a percentage) is related to the oxygen tension (as a partial pressure, mm Hg) by the oxyhemoglobin dissociation curve. On the steep part of the curve, a predictable correlation exists between arterial oxyhemoglobin saturation (Sao_2) and partial pressures of oxygen (PaO_2). In this range, the Sao_2 is a good reflection of the extent of hypoxemia and the changing status of arterial oxygenation. For PaO_2 greater than 75 mm Hg, the Sao_2 reaches a plateau and no longer reflects changes in PaO_2. Coexisting medical conditions, such as hypercapnia, acidosis, and hyperthermia, cause the oxyhemoglobin dissociation curve to shift to the right and decrease the affinity of hemoglobin for oxygen (Fig. 25-1). This favors the unloading of oxygen from hemoglobin to peripheral tissues.

Pulse oximetry is based on the following premises:

1. The color of blood is a function of oxygen saturation.
2. The change in color results from the optical properties of hemoglobin and its interaction with oxygen.
3. The ratio of oxyhemoglobin (HbO_2) and hemoglobin (Hb) can be determined by absorption spectrophotometry.

Oxygen saturation is determined by spectrophotometry, which is based on the Beer–Lambert law. At a constant light intensity and hemoglobin concentration, the intensity of light transmitted through a tissue is a logarithmic function of the oxygen saturation of Hb. Two wavelengths of light are required to distinguish HbO_2 from Hb. Light-emitting diodes in the pulse sensor emit red (660 nm) and near infrared (940 nm) light. The percentage

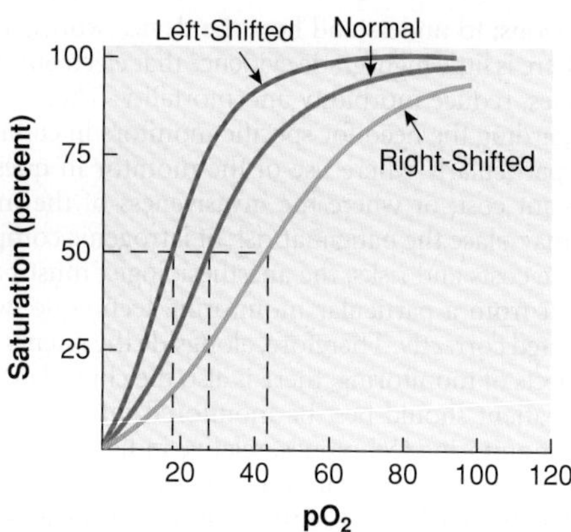

FIGURE 25-1. The oxyhemoglobin dissociation curve. The relationship between arterial saturation of hemoglobin and oxygen tension is represented by the sigmoid-shaped oxyhemoglobin dissociation curve. When the curve is left-shifted, the hemoglobin molecule binds oxygen more tightly. (Reproduced from: Brown M, Vender JS. Noninvasive oxygen monitoring. *Crit Care Clin* 1988;4:493–509.)

of HbO_2 is determined by measuring the ratio of infrared and red light sensed by a photodetector. Pulse oximeters perform a plethysmographic analysis to differentiate the pulsatile "arterial" signal from the nonpulsatile signal resulting from "venous" absorption and other tissues such as skin, muscle, and bone. The absence of a pulsatile waveform during extreme hypothermia or hypoperfusion can limit the ability of a pulse oximeter to calculate the Spo_2.

The Spo_2 measured by pulse oximetry is not the same as the arterial saturation (Sao_2) measured by a laboratory co-oximeter. Pulse oximetry measures the "functional" saturation, which is defined by the following equation:

$$Spo_2 = \frac{HbO_2}{HbO_2 + Hb} \times 100\%$$

Laboratory co-oximeters use multiple wavelengths to distinguish other types of Hb, such as carboxyhemoglobin (COHb) and methemoglobin (MetHb) by their characteristic absorption. Co-oximeters measure the "fractional" saturation, which is defined by the following equation:

$$S_aO_2 = \frac{HbO_2}{HbO_2 + Hb + COHb + MetHb} \times 100\%$$

In clinical circumstances where other Hb moieties are present, the Spo_2 measurement may not correlate with the actual Sao_2 reported by the blood gas laboratory. For example, MetHb absorbs red and infrared wavelengths of light in a 1:1 ratio corresponding to an Spo_2 of approximately 85%. Therefore, increases in MetHb produce an underestimation when $Spo_2 > 70\%$ and an overestimation when $Spo_2 < 70\%$. Similarly, COHb also produces artificially high and misleading results; one study showed that at 70% COHb, the Spo_2 still measured 90%. In most patients, MetHb and COHb are present in low concentrations so that the functional saturation approximates the fractional value.[9]

Proper Use and Interpretation

The assessment of arterial oxygenation is an integral part of anesthesia practice. Early detection and prompt intervention may limit serious sequelae of hypoxemia. The clinical signs associated with hypoxemia (e.g., tachycardia, altered mental status, cyanosis) are often masked or difficult to appreciate during anesthesia.

The appropriate use of pulse oximetry necessitates an appreciation of both physiologic and technical limitations. Despite the numerous clinical benefits of pulse oximetry, other factors affect its accuracy and reliability. Factors that may be present during anesthesia care and that affect the accuracy and reliability of pulse oximetry include dyshemoglobins, dyes (methylene blue, indocyanine green, and indigo carmine), nail polish, ambient light, light-emitting diode variability, motion artifact, and background noise. Electrocautery can interfere with pulse oximetry if the radiofrequency emissions are sensed by the photodetector. Surgical stereotactic positioning systems that make use of infrared position sensors may interfere with the infrared signals used by the pulse oximeter. Reports of burns or pressure necrosis exist but are infrequent. Inspecting the digits during monitoring can reduce these complications.

Recent developments in pulse oximetry technology reportedly may permit more accurate measurements of Spo_2 during patient movement, low-perfusion conditions, and in the presence of dyshemoglobins. Some of these instruments use complex signal processing of the two wavelengths of light to improve the signal-to-noise ratio and reject artifact. Studies in volunteers suggest that the performance of pulse oximeters incorporating this technology is superior to conventional oximetry during motion of the hand, hypoperfusion, and hypothermia.[10,11] Other pulse oximetry devices incorporate eight wavelengths of light to more accurately measure COHb and MetHb.[9]

Indications

Pulse oximetry has been used in all patient age groups to detect and prevent hypoxemia. The clinical benefits of pulse
3 oximetry are enhanced by its simplicity. Modern pulse oximeters are noninvasive, continuous, and autocalibrating. They have quick response times and their battery backup provides monitoring during transport. The clinical accuracy is typically reported to be within ±2% to 3% at 70% to 100% saturation and ±3% at 50% to 70% saturation. Published data from numerous investigations support accuracy and precision reported by instrument manufacturers. Quantitative assessment of arterial oxygen saturation is mandated by the ASA monitoring standards,[1] and the convenience and safety of pulse oximetry has supplanted earlier techniques such as heated transcutaneous pO_2 electrodes.[12]

Pulse oximetry has wide applicability in many hospital and nonhospital settings. However, there are no definitive data demonstrating a reduction in morbidity or mortality associated with the advent of pulse oximetry. An older large randomized trial did not detect a significant difference in postoperative complications when routine pulse oximetry was used.[13] However, a reduction of anesthesia mortality, as well as fewer malpractice claims from respiratory events, coincident with the introduction of pulse oximeters suggests that the routine use of these devices may have been a contributing factor.

Contraindications

There are no clinical contraindications to monitoring arterial oxygen saturation with pulse oximetry.

Common Problems and Limitations

Arterial oxygen monitors do not ensure adequacy of oxygen delivery to, or utilization by peripheral tissues and should not be considered a replacement for arterial blood gas measurements or mixed central venous oxygen saturation when more definitive information regarding oxygen supply and utilization is required.

Unless the patient is in breathing room air, pulse oximetry is a poor indicator of adequate ventilation; patients who have been breathing 100% FiO_2 may be apneic for several minutes before desaturation is detected by the pulse oximeter. Once the P_AO_2 has fallen sufficiently to cause a detectable decrease in Spo_2, further desaturation may occur precipitously once the steep part of the HbO_2 dissociation curve is reached.

MONITORING OF EXPIRED GASES

Principles of Operation

The patient's expired gas is likely to be composed of a mixture of oxygen (O_2), nitrogen (N_2), carbon dioxide (CO_2), and anesthetic gases such as nitrous oxide (N_2O) and highly potent halogenated agents (sevoflurane, isoflurane, or desflurane). Anesthesiologists have long sought to measure the composition of expired gases noninvasively and in real time; these measurements can provide vital information regarding the patient's respiratory condition and assist in the titration of volatile anesthetic agents.

In 1972, White and Wardley-Smith[14] described the construction of a simple detector of anesthetic gases. Anesthetic gases will tend to partition into silicone rubber, changing the elastic properties of the rubber. A mechanical device can be constructed to maintain silicone rubber strips under light tension; this device is attached to the expiratory limb of the anesthesia circuit so that the strips are exposed to the patient's expired gases. As the concentration of anesthetic gas rises, the length of the strips will change proportionally, and a mechanical linkage to a pointer on a gauge can display this change. Although the practical shortcomings of such a device are obvious from a contemporary viewpoint, this is only evidence of how much biomedical engineering sophistication has been applied to this important problem in the intervening 40 years. For instance, the response time of this simple device would be expected to be very slow. However, if piezoelectric crystals are coated with a layer of lipid, the concentration of anesthetic gases can be detected by changes in the resonant frequency of the crystal as anesthetic gases partition into the lipid coating. This idea makes use of the same physical behavior of anesthetic gases, but evolved in its implementation so that the response time is now sufficient to detect inspired, expired, and breath-to-breath changes in anesthetic gas concentrations.[15] Nevertheless, this new device is still significantly limited by its inability to identify the gas it is detecting and by its inability to work with mixtures of different gases.

Mass spectrometry systems and Raman scattering devices addressed these shortcomings. Mass spectroscopy systems obtain a sample of expired gas, and bombard this gas mixture with electrons, creating ion fragments of a predictable mass and charge. These fragments are accelerated in a vacuum. A sample of this mixture enters a measurement chamber, where the fragment stream is subjected to a high magnetic field. The magnetic field separates the fragments by their mass and charge. The fragments are deflected onto a detector plate, and each gas has a specific landing site on the detector plate. The ion impacts are proportional to the concentration of the parent gas or vapor. The processor section of the mass spectrometer system calculates the concentration of the gases of interest. Mass spectrometers are large devices and were often multiplexed—that is, connected to multiple patients, taking expired gas samples from each in turn.[16]

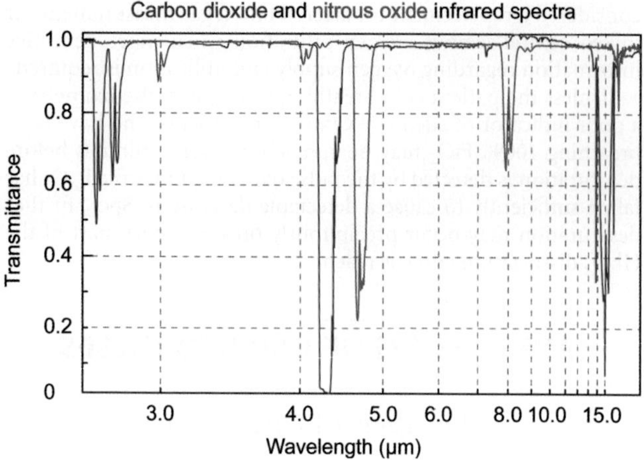

FIGURE 25-2. Gaseous phase infrared transmission spectrum for carbon dioxide and nitrous oxide. Modified from the National Institute of Standards and Technology (http://www.nist.gov); and Craver CD, Coblentz Society. The Coblentz Society desk book of infrared spectra. 2nd ed. Kirwood, MO (P.O. Box 9952, Kirkwood 63122): The Society; 1982.

Raman scattering results when photons generated by a high-intensity argon laser collide with gas molecules. The scattered photons are measured as peaks in a spectrum that determine the concentration and composition of respiratory gases and inhaled vapors. O_2, N_2, N_2O, CO_2, H_2O vapors and inhaled anesthetic agents are all simultaneously measurable using Raman scattering.[17]

Infrared absorption spectrophotometry (IRAS) gas analysis devices have now supplanted all of these earlier measurement techniques in clinical practice. Asymmetric, polyatomic molecules like CO_2 absorb infrared light at specific wavelengths. By transmitting light through a pure sample of a gas over the range of infrared frequencies, a unique infrared transmission spectrum (like a fingerprint) can be created for the gas (Fig. 25-2).

CO_2 strongly absorbs infrared light with a wavelength of 4.3 microns. At this wavelength there is minimal interference from other gases that may also be present, such as water vapor, oxygen, nitrous oxide, and inhaled anesthetic agents. Infrared light at this wavelength can be passed through a sample of gas to an infrared detector. As the concentration of carbon dioxide increases, the intensity of the light that reaches the detector decreases, in accordance with the Beer–Lambert law.

IRAS devices have five components: A multiple-wavelength infrared light source, a gas sampler, an optical path, a detection system, and a signal processor. Operating room IRAS devices can detect CO_2, N_2O, and the potent inhaled anesthetic agents as mixed together in a sample of the patient's expired gas. The gas mixture is passed through the optical path of multiple infrared beams whose wavelengths are chosen to correspond to key features in the transmission spectra of the gases of interest. By analyzing the combination of absorption of infrared light at these wavelengths, the presence and concentrations of all of these gases can be determined simultaneously.[19] The use of multiple wavelengths allows the gases to be identified automatically. Older IRAS devices used a hot electrical element to generate radiant infrared light over a broad range of wavelengths. An optical filter wheel was then used to cut out all but the desired wavelengths. Contemporary devices make use of small lasers and filters, designed such that they emit only at the desired wavelengths. This approach consumes much less electrical power, is physically less heavy and

TABLE 25-1. DETECTION OF CRITICAL EVENTS BY IMPLEMENTING GAS ANALYSIS

Event	Gas Measured by Analyzer
Error in gas delivery	O_2, N_2, CO_2, agent analysis
Anesthesia machine malfunction	O_2, N_2, CO_2, agent
Disconnection	CO_2, O_2, agent analysis
Vaporizer malfunction or contamination	Agent analysis
Anesthesia circuit leaks	N_2, CO_2 analysis
Endotracheal cuff leaks	N_2, CO_2
Poor mask or LMA fit	N_2, CO_2
Hypoventilation	CO_2 analysis
Malignant hyperthermia	CO_2
Airway obstruction	CO_2
Air embolism	CO_2, N_2
Circuit hypoxia	O_2 analysis
Vaporizer overdose	Agent analysis

LMA, laryngeal mask airway.
Modified from: Knopes KD, Hecker BR. Monitoring anesthetic gases, In: Lake CL, ed. *Clinical Monitoring*. Philadelphia, PA, WB Saunders; 1990, p 24, with permission.

has led to the development of conveniently portable handheld gas analyzers.[20]

Proper Use and Interpretation

Expired gas analysis allows the clinician to monitor inspired and expired concentrations of carbon dioxide and anesthetic gases simultaneously. These measurements require separate clinical interpretation. Critical events that can be detected by the analysis of respiratory gases and anesthetic vapors are listed in Table 25-1.

Interpretation of Inspired and Expired Carbon Dioxide Concentrations

Capnometry is the measurement and numeric representation of the CO_2 concentration during inspiration and expiration. A capnogram is a continuous concentration–time display of the CO_2 concentration sampled at a patient's airway during ventilation. The capnogram is divided into four distinct phases (Fig. 25-3).

The first phase (A–B) represents the initial stage of expiration. Gas sampled during this phase occupies the anatomic dead space

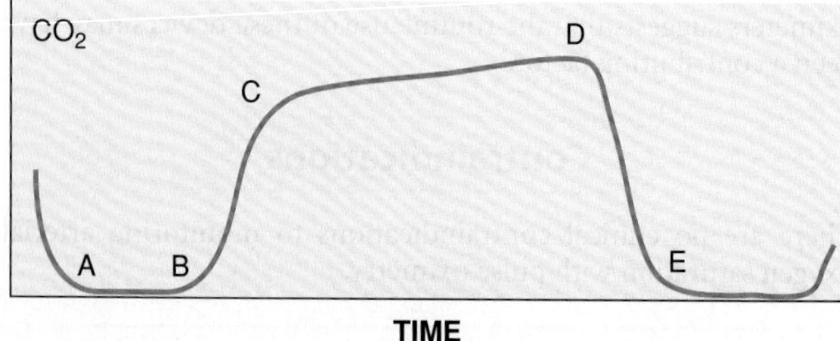

FIGURE 25-3. The normal capnogram. Point D delineates the end-tidal CO_2 ($ETCO_2$). $ETCO_2$ is the best reflection of the alveolar CO_2 partial pressure. See text for discussion of the curve.

and is normally devoid of CO_2. At point B, CO_2-containing gas presents itself at the sampling site, and a sharp upstroke (B–C) is seen in the capnogram. The slope of this upstroke is determined by the evenness of expiratory ventilation and alveolar emptying. Phase C–D represents the alveolar or expiratory plateau. At this phase of the capnogram, alveolar gas is being sampled. Normally, this part of the waveform is almost horizontal. However, when ventilation and perfusion are mismatched, Phase C–D may take an upward slope. Point D is the highest CO_2 value and is called the end-tidal CO_2 ($ETCO_2$). $ETCO_2$ is the best reflection of the alveolar CO_2 (P_ACO_2). As the patient begins to inspire, fresh gas is entrained and there is a steep downstroke (D–E) back to baseline. Unless rebreathing of CO_2 occurs, the baseline approaches zero. If the P_ACO_2–$PaCO_2$ gradient is constant and small, capnography provides a noninvasive, continuous, real-time reflection of ventilation. The $ETCO_2$–$PaCO_2$ gradient typically is around 5 mm Hg during routine general anesthesia in otherwise healthy, supine patients.

The size and shape of the capnogram waveform can provide additional clinical information.[21] A slow rate of rise of the second phase (B–C) is suggestive of either chronic obstructive pulmonary disease or acute airway obstruction as from bronchoconstriction (asthma) secondary to mismatch in alveolar ventilation and alveolar perfusion. A normally shaped capnogram with an increase in $ETCO_2$ suggests alveolar hypoventilation or an increase in CO_2 production. Transient increases in $ETCO_2$ are often observed during tourniquet release, aortic unclamping, or the administration of bicarbonate.

Capnography is an essential element in determining the appropriate placement of endotracheal tubes. The presence of a stable $ETCO_2$ for three successive breaths indicates that the tube is not in the esophagus. A continuous, stable CO_2 waveform ensures the presence of alveolar ventilation but does not necessarily indicate that the endotracheal tube is properly positioned in the trachea. An endobronchial intuition, in which the tip of the tube is located in a main stem bronchus, cannot be ruled out until breath sounds are auscultated bilaterally. A continuous CO_2 tracing also does not guarantee that the endotracheal tube is placed securely; an endotracheal tube placed proximally to the vocal cords may still produce an otherwise satisfactory tracing until it becomes dislodged.

A sudden drop in $ETCO_2$ to near zero followed by the absence of a CO_2 waveform heralds a potentially life-threatening problem that could indicate malposition of an endotracheal tube into the pharynx or esophagus, sudden severe hypotension, massive pulmonary embolism, a cardiac arrest, or a disconnection or disruption of sampling lines. When a sudden drop of the $ETCO_2$ occurs, it is essential to quickly verify that there is pulmonary ventilation and to identify physiologic and mechanical factors that might account for then $ETCO_2$ of zero. During life-saving cardiopulmonary resuscitation, the generation of adequate circulation can be assessed by the restoration of the CO_2 waveform.

Whereas abrupt decreases in the $ETCO_2$ are often associated with an altered cardiopulmonary status (e.g., embolism or hypoperfusion), gradual reductions in $ETCO_2$ more often reflect decreases in $PaCO_2$ that occur when there exists an imbalance between minute ventilation and metabolic rate (i.e., CO_2 production), as commonly occurs during anesthesia at a fixed minute ventilation. Increases in $ETCO_2$ can be expected when CO_2 production exceeds ventilation, such as in hyperthermia or when an exogenous source of CO_2 is present. Capnographic waveforms that do not return to zero during inspiration indicate rebreathing of carbon dioxide. This can occur if the carbon dioxide absorber in an anesthesia machine is chemically exhausted if a valve in the ventilator circuit is not functioning properly, or if the flow of fresh gas is insufficient. An elevated baseline can also be seen if the device is calibrated incorrectly.

TABLE 25-2. FACTORS THAT MAY CHANGE END-TIDAL CO_2 ($ETCO_2$) DURING ANESTHESIA

Increases in $ETCO_2$	Decreases in $ETCO_2$
Elements that Change CO_2 Production	
Increases in metabolic rate	**Decreases in metabolic rate**
Hyperthermia	Hypothermia
Sepsis	Hypothyroidism
Malignant hyperthermia	
Shivering	
Hyperthyroidism	
Elements that Change CO_2 Elimination	
Hypoventilation	Hyperventilation
Rebreathing	Hypoperfusion
	Pulmonary embolism

Alterations in ventilation, cardiac output (CO), distribution of pulmonary blood flow and metabolic activity influence $ETCO_2$ concentration and the capnogram obtained during quantitative expired gas analysis. Table 25-2 summarizes the common elements that may be reflected by changes in $ETCO_2$ during anesthesia care.

Interpretation of Inspired and Expired Anesthetic Gas Concentrations

Monitoring the concentration of expired anesthetic gases assists the anesthesiologist in titrating those gases to the clinical circumstances of the patient. At high fresh gas flow rates, the concentration of an anesthetic gas in a circle breathing system will approximate the concentration set on the vaporizer. However, high fresh gas flow rates leads to wasteful use of anesthetic vapor. As the fresh gas flow rate is lowered, the concentration within the circuit and the concentration set at the vaporizer can become more decoupled. Inspired and expired gas concentration monitoring allows the anesthesiologist to maintain satisfactory and well-controlled agent levels in the circuit even when extremely low fresh gas flows are used. In an ideal, leak-free anesthesia system, the fresh gas flow can be minimized to only the amount of pure oxygen necessary to replace the patient's metabolic utilization—a practice known as "closed-circuit anesthesia." This practice makes the most economic use of anesthetic vapor.[22]

Anesthetic gases have differing potencies, and so their concentrations are often normalized against the concentration of that agent required to produce a predetermined clinical endpoint. The most commonly used endpoint is the MAC value, defined as the end-tidal gas concentration that when maintained constant for 15 minutes at a pressure of 1 atmosphere inhibits movement in response to a midline laparotomy incision in 50% of patients.[23,24] Historically, MAC is an acronym of *minimum alveolar concentration*, although it is more accurately a median constant end-tidal partial pressure. Monitoring of end-tidal gas concentrations performed with reference to MAC values helps to prevent the occurrence of intraoperative awareness and in some studies was superior to the use of processed EEG monitors.[25]

Indications

4 Monitoring of the partial pressure of expiratory CO_2 has evolved into an important physiologic and safety monitor. Capnography

is the standard of care for monitoring the adequacy of ventilation in patients receiving general anesthesia. It is also now mandated for use to monitor ventilation during procedures performed while the patient is under moderate or deep sedation.[1]

Contraindications

There are no contraindications to the use of capnography, provided that the data obtained are evaluated in the context of the patient's clinical circumstances. It is generally safe to use capnography for the monitoring of all patients.

Monitoring of expired anesthetic gases is only informative if detectable gases are used to maintain anesthesia. Infrared spectroscopy cannot detect Xenon, and is not informative if anesthesia is maintained using a total intravenous technique.

4 Common Problems and Limitations

The sampling lines or water traps of expired gas analyzers may become occluded with condensed water vapor during prolonged use. Disconnecting the sampling line and flushing it with air from a syringe can sometimes clear it, but it may be necessary to replace these components. Elevating the sidestream sampling line above the ventilator circuit helps prevent the entry of condensed water. A humidity barrier is also useful, although this will increase the response time of the capnogram.

Although mass spectroscopy and Raman scattering are no longer seen in clinical practice, these technologies are able to detect the concentration of N_2 directly. Nitrogen monitoring provides quantification of washout during preoxygenation. A sudden rise in N_2 in the exhaled gas indicates either introduction of air from leaks in the anesthesia delivery system or venous air embolism. Infrared gas analyzers do not detect N_2 directly, and its concentration must be inferred as the amount remaining after other measurable gases are accounted for.

Although capnography provides a quantitative measurement of $ETCO_2$, it is not as accurate as blood gas analysis for the assessment of the partial pressure of arterial carbon dioxide. A gradient exists between the partial pressure of arterial carbon dioxide and $ETCO_2$; this gradient increases as the dead-space volume increases. In disease states characterized by increased dead space and ventilation–perfusion mismatch, such as emphysema or pulmonary embolism, or in iatrogenic single lung ventilation, an arterial blood gas analysis is necessary for an accurate determination of the partial pressure of arterial carbon dioxide.

INVASIVE MONITORING OF SYSTEMIC BLOOD PRESSURE

Principles of Operation

5 Indwelling arterial cannulation permits the opportunity to monitor arterial blood pressure continuously and to have vascular access for arterial blood sampling. Intra-arterial blood pressure monitoring uses fluid-filled tubing to transmit the force of the pressure pulse wave to a pressure transducer that converts the displacement of a silicon crystal into voltage changes. These electrical signals are amplified, filtered, and displayed as the arterial pressure trace. Intra-arterial pressure transducing systems are subject to many potential errors based on the physical properties of fluid motion and the performance of the catheter–transducer–amplification system used to sense, process, and display the pressure pulse wave.

The behavior of transducers, fluid couplings, signal amplification, and display systems can be described by a complex second-order differential equation. Solving the equation predicts the output and characterizes the fidelity of the system's ability to faithfully display and estimate the arterial pressure over time. The fidelity of fluid-coupled transducing systems is constrained by two properties: *Damping* (ζ) and *natural frequency* (f_n). Zeta (ζ) describes the tendency for fluid in the measuring system to extinguish motion, and f_n describes the frequency at which the measuring system is most prone to resonance. The fidelity of the transduced pressure depends on optimizing ζ and f_n so that the system can respond appropriately to the range of frequencies contained in the pressure pulse wave. Analysis of high-fidelity recordings of arterial blood pressure indicates that the pressure trace contains frequencies from 1 to 30 Hz. The "fast flush" test is a method used at the bedside to determine the natural frequency and damping characteristics of the transducing system. This test examines the characteristics of the resonant waves recorded after the release of a flush. Damping is estimated by the amplitude ratio of the first pair of resonant waves and the natural frequency is estimated by dividing the tracing speed by the interval cycle.[26]

Proper Use and Interpretation

Multiple arteries can be used for direct measurement of blood pressure, including the radial, brachial, axillary, femoral, and dorsalis pedis arteries (Table 25-3). The radial artery remains the most popular site for cannulation because of its accessibility and the presence of a collateral blood supply. In the past, assessment of the patency of the ulnar circulation by performance of an Allen test has been recommended before cannulation. An Allen test is performed by compressing both radial and ulnar arteries while

TABLE 25-3. ARTERIAL CANNULATION AND DIRECT BLOOD PRESSURE MONITORING

Arterial Cannulation Site	Clinical Points of Interest
Radial artery	Preferred site for monitoring Nontapered catheters preferred
Ulnar artery	Complication similar to radial Primary source of hand blood flow
Brachial artery	Insertion site medial to biceps tendon Median nerve damage is potential hazard Can accommodate 18-gauge cannula
Axillary artery	Insertion site at junction of pectoralis and deltoid muscles Specialized kits available
Femoral artery	Easy access in low-flow states Potential for local and retroperitoneal hemorrhage Longer catheters preferred
Dorsalis pedis artery	Collateral circulation = posterior tibial artery Higher systolic pressure estimates

the patient tightens his or her fist. Releasing pressure on each respective artery determines the dominant vessel supplying blood to the hand. The prognostic value of the Allen test in assessing the adequacy of the collateral circulation has not been confirmed.[27,28]

6 Three techniques for cannulation are common: Direct arterial puncture, guidewire-assisted cannulation (Seldinger technique), and the transfixion–withdrawal method.[29] A necessary condition for percutaneous placement is identification of the arterial pulse, which may be enhanced by a Doppler flow detection device in
7 patients with poor peripheral pulses.[30] Ultrasound imaging with Doppler color flowmetry can provide valuable further assistance when the pulse is difficult to locate or the caliber of the vessel appears to be small.[31]

Arterial blood pressure transduction systems must be "zeroed"
8 before use. The transducer is positioned at the same level as the right atrium, the stopcock is opened to the atmosphere so that pressure-sensing crystal senses only atmospheric pressure, and the "Zero Sensor" (or equivalent) option is selected on the monitoring equipment. This procedure establishes the calibration of the sensor and establishes the level of the right atrium as the datum reference point. For neurosurgical procedures in which the patient may be positioned in an upright or beach-chair position, it is a common practice to zero the transducer at the level of the Circle of Willis so that the arterial pressure tracing provides a reading that is adjusted for the height of the fluid column between the heart and the brain; it represents the arterial pressure at the base of the brain.

Direct arterial pressure monitoring requires constant vigilance. The data displayed must correlate with clinical conditions before therapeutic interventions are initiated. Sudden increases in the transduced blood pressure may represent a hydrostatic error because the position of the transducer was not adjusted after change in the operating room table's height. Sudden decreases often result from kinking of the catheter or tubing. Before initiating therapy, the transducer system should be examined quickly and the patency of the arterial cannula verified. This ensures the accuracy of the measurement and avoids the initiation of a potentially dangerous medication error.

9 Traumatic cannulation has been associated with hematoma formation, thrombosis, and damage to adjacent nerves. Abnormal radial artery blood flow after catheter removal occurs frequently. Studies suggest that blood flow normalizes in 3 to 70 days. Radial artery thrombosis can be minimized by using small catheters, avoiding polypropylene-tapered catheters, and reducing the duration of arterial cannulation. Flexible guidewires may reduce the potential trauma associated with catheters negotiating tortuous vessels. After arterial cannulation has been performed, the tissues that are perfused by that artery should be examined intermittently for signs of thromboembolism or ischemia. During cannula removal, the potential for thromboembolism may be diminished by compressing the proximal and distal arterial segment while aspirating the cannula during withdrawal.

Indications

The standards for basic monitoring[1] stipulate that arterial blood pressure shall be determined and recorded at least every 5 minutes. This standard is usually met by intermittent, noninvasive blood pressure monitoring. However, continuous monitoring may be indicated by patient comorbidities or by the nature of the surgery to be performed. 10

Arterial catheters provide continuous monitoring of blood pressure and convenient vascular access to obtain blood samples for laboratory assays, including blood gas analysis to assess respiratory function. Placement of an arterial catheter can therefore be indicated by the need to meet any of these contingencies:

1. **Rapid changes in blood pressure or extremes of blood pressure are anticipated.**
   High-risk vascular surgeries, trauma surgeries, neurosurgical procedures, intrathoracic and cardiac procedures are associated with the risk of sudden blood loss and rapid changes in blood pressure. These procedures may also involve periods of deliberate hypotension or hypertension.
2. **The ability of the patient to tolerate hemodynamic instability is impaired.**
   Patients with clinically significant cardiac disease, such as coronary artery disease, valvular disease, or heart failure may require continuous monitoring in order to allow treatment for hypotension to be implemented rapidly and minimize the risk of coronary ischemia. Similar concerns apply to patients with a history of cerebrovascular disease. Procedures that involve potential compromise to the vascular supply of the spinal cord indicate the use of an arterial catheter to maintain adequate perfusion and decrease the risk of postoperative paraplegia from spinal cord infarction.[32]
   Critically ill patients may already be hemodynamically unstable at the time of presentation, and require the administration of inotropes and vasopressors. Continuous blood pressure monitoring is indicated to manage the titration of these agents.
3. **Compromise of the patient's respiratory function, oxygenation or ventilation is anticipated.**
   Mismatch between pulmonary ventilation and perfusion will impair the ability of $ETCO_2$ to predict P_ACO_2. This may arise iatrogenically during procedures that require single lung ventilation. Patients may present with pulmonary comorbidities such as ARDS, pulmonary embolism, and pulmonary hypertension with consequent ventilation–perfusion mismatch and impaired alveolar diffusion. Arterial catheters provide a means to obtain arterial blood gas samples frequently to assess changes in respiratory function.
4. **Metabolic derangements are anticipated.**
   Surgical procedures that are anticipated to produce large volume fluid shifts may indicate the placement of an arterial catheter to enable laboratory samples to be drawn frequently and to allow electrolyte and acid–base disturbances to be detected and corrected.

Contraindications

Arterial cannulation is regarded as an invasive procedure with documented morbidity. Ischemia after radial artery cannulation resulting from thrombosis, proximal emboli, or prolonged shock has been described.[33] Contributing factors include severe atherosclerosis, diabetes, low CO, and intense peripheral vasoconstriction. Ischemia, hemorrhage, thrombosis, embolism, cerebral air embolism (retrograde flow associated with flushing), aneurysm formation, arteriovenous fistula formation, skin necrosis, and infection have reportedly occurred as the direct result of arterial cannulation, arterial blood sampling, or high-pressure flushing. Patients with compromised collateral arterial supply, such as those with Reynaud's phenomenon or thromboangiitis obliterans (Buerger's disease), are at increased risk for ischemic complications.[29]

Common Problems and Limitations

5 The fidelity of the transducer system is optimized when catheters and tubing are stiff, the mass of the fluid is small, the number of

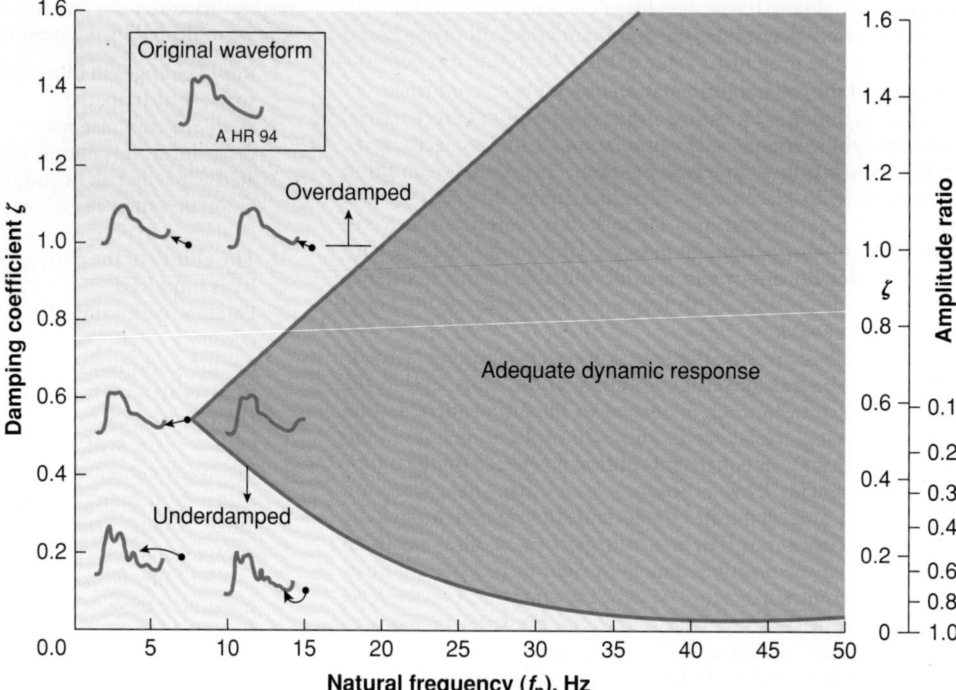

FIGURE 25-4. The relationship between the frequency of fluid-filled transducing systems and damping (ζ). The shaded area represents the appropriate range of damping for a given natural frequency (f_n). The size of the wedge also depends on the steepness of the arterial pressure trace and heart rate. (Reproduced from: Gardner RM. Direct blood pressure measurement–dynamic response requirements. *Anesthesiology* 1981;54: 227–236.)

stopcocks is limited, and the connecting tubing is not excessive. Figure 25-4 demonstrates the effect of damping on the character of the arterial pressure trace. In clinical practice, under-damped transducer systems tend to overestimate the systolic pressure by 15 to 30 mm Hg and amplify artifacts. Likewise, excessive increases in ζ reduce fidelity and underestimate systolic pressure.

Continuous-flush devices are incorporated into disposable transducer kits and infuse at 3 to 6 mL/hr. In neonates, the infusion volume may contribute to fluid overload. Continuous-flush devices have little effect on the blood pressure measurement. However, pressurized flush systems may serve as a source of an air embolism. Removing air from the pressurized infusion bag, stopcocks, and tubing minimizes the potential for air embolism.

A satisfactory Allen test does not rule out the possibility of formation of thrombus on the catheter and subsequent distal embolic complications. Although an intact palmar arch will provide some collateralization of arterial blood supply to the hand, this does not protect against emboli to the distal digital arteries.[35]

INTERMITTENT NONINVASIVE MONITORING OF SYSTEMIC BLOOD PRESSURE

Principles of Operation

The simplest method of blood pressure determination estimates systolic blood pressure by palpating the return of an arterial pulse while a more proximal occluding cuff is deflated. Modifications of this technique include the observance of the return of Doppler sounds, the transduced arterial pressure trace, or a photoplethysmographic pulse wave as produced by a pulse oximeter.

Auscultation of the Korotkoff sounds permit estimation of both systolic (SP) and diastolic (DP) blood pressures. Korotkoff sounds result from turbulent flow within an artery created by the mechanical deformation from the blood pressure cuff. Systolic blood pressure is signaled by the appearance of the first Korotkoff sound. Disappearance of the sound or a muffled tone signals the diastolic blood pressure. The mean arterial pressure (MAP) can be calculated using an estimating equation:

$$MAP = DP + \frac{SP - DP}{3}$$

In contemporary practice, automated noninvasive blood pressure monitors (also known as automated sphygmomanometers) employ the oscillometric method[36] to estimate the arterial blood pressure. The oscillometric method uses an occluding cuff to measure the pressure fluctuations that occur
6 due to arterial pulsations. The systolic blood pressure is estimated using the maximum cuff pressure at which pressure oscillations can be perceived. The MAP is estimated by the cuff pressure at which the amplitude of the oscillations is greatest. The diastolic pressure is estimated using the minimum cuff pressure at which pressure fluctuations can be perceived. Some automated noninvasive blood pressure monitors refine these estimates using proprietary, empirical formulae,[37] and so results may not be consistent from device to device.[38] The operation of automated blood pressure cuffs is covered by US[39] and international[40] standards.

Proper Use and Interpretation

In the anesthetized patient, automated oscillometry is usually accurate and versatile. A variety of cuff sizes make it possible to use oscillometry in all age groups. Different strategies of cuff inflation and deflation may be used to obtain blood pressure measurements. A common approach is for the cuff to be

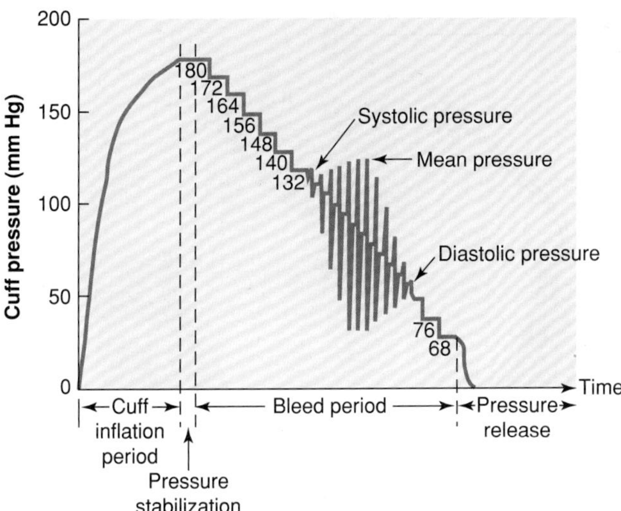

FIGURE 25-5. Sequence of oscillometric blood pressure determination. The pressure oscillations increase in magnitude, then decrease. The oscillations are analyzed to determine systolic, mean, and diastolic pressures as shown. (Modified from: Dorsch JA, Dorsch SE. *Understanding Anesthesia Equipment.* 4th ed. Baltimore: Williams & Wilkins; 1999.)

rapidly inflated to a predetermined initial pressure expected to be above systolic blood pressure. A sensor checks to ensure that pressure fluctuations are not present. The cuff is then decrementally deflated. At each interval, the sensor measures the magnitude of oscillations that are present in the cuff pressure. Once the cuff pressure falls below the point at which oscillations can be detected, the cuff is rapidly and completely deflated (Fig. 25-5).

Another common strategy involves the opposite approach of incrementally inflating the cuff. Once the cuff pressure has increased above the systolic blood pressure, the sensor no longer perceives oscillations, and the cuff is rapidly and completely deflated.

Indications

ASA[1] Standard 4.2.2 mandates that "Every patient receiving anesthesia shall have arterial blood pressure and heart rate determined and evaluated at least every five minutes." The use of an oscillometric noninvasive blood pressure cuff usually provides a straightforward method for satisfying this requirement for those patients whose medical comorbidities do not require continuous monitoring of blood pressure.

Contraindications

Noninvasive blood pressure cuffs apply force to the encircled limb that is sufficient to occlude blood flow. Contraindications to their use therefore exist in circumstances where the patient is likely to sustain traumatic injury from this repeated mechanical process. Examples include local bone fracture (such as a humeral fracture), open injuries to the extremity, local presence of an arteriovenous dialysis fistula or indwelling PICC (peripherally inserted central catheter) line. The site of measurement should also be carefully chosen in patients who have undergone axillary lymph node dissection as these patients may have impaired lymphatic drainage from the associated limb and be susceptible to limb edema from repeated vascular occlusion.

Noninvasive blood pressure cuffs can potentially become a source of iatrogenic injury even in normal use on a healthy limb. The repeated cycling of the blood pressure cuff during very prolonged surgical cases may lead to local skin abrasion or contusion; applying a light dressing underneath the cuff may mitigate these side-effects. The radial nerve describes a spiraling path around the humerus and is also potentially susceptible to neurapraxia from mechanical compression.[42,43] During very prolonged surgical cases, it may be prudent to relocate the blood pressure cuff every few hours.

Common Problems and Limitations

The American Heart Association recommends that the bladder width for indirect blood pressure monitoring should approximate 40% of the circumference of the extremity. Bladder length should be sufficient to encircle at least 80% of the extremity. Falsely high estimates result when cuffs are too small, when cuffs are applied too loosely, or when the extremity is below heart level. Falsely low estimates result when cuffs are too large, when the extremity is above heart level, or after quick deflations.[44]

The detection of changes in Korotkoff sounds is subjective and prone to errors based on deficiencies in sound transmission or hearing. Cuff deflation rate also influences accuracy; quick deflations underestimate blood pressure. Noninvasive blood pressure cuffs are also subject to significant wear-and-tear from repeated use in the operating room. The development of a small air leak in the hose or cuff will often prevent the device from following its inflation strategy and render it inoperative.[45]

Palpation, auscultatory, and oscillometric techniques require pulsatile blood flow and may be unreliable during conditions of low flow, patients with nonpulsatile left ventricular assist devices, or if the arterial walls are sufficiently sclerotic or stiffened such that pulsations are not readily transmitted.

Automated oscillometry has been demonstrated to correlate well with direct intra-arterial measurement of MAP and diastolic blood pressure.[46–48] Oscillometry does require additional signal processing to smooth out pronounced respiratory variations or motion artifacts, but these events tend to occur at frequencies that are distinct from pulsatile variations in pressure. Cuff movement, erratic pulse transmission, arrhythmias and inadvertent occlusion of the pressure tubing may influence accuracy. Periods of significant hemodynamic variability may require more frequent measurement of blood pressure to guide optimal intraoperative management.[49] This problem can be approached statistically by assessing the ability of a blood pressure measurement to predict the next blood pressure measurement, and hence the ability of the anesthesiologist to infer and intervene upon unacceptable trends in the blood pressure. Although Standard 4.2.2 mandates that blood pressure be measured only every 5 minutes, some evidence exists that this predictive ability may begin to decline for measurement intervals of greater than 3 minutes.[50]

Automated noninvasive blood pressure cuffs are usually placed around the upper arm, but it is usually acceptable to place the cuff around the forearm, wrist or ankle if the upper arm is inaccessible or if the patient's body habitus is otherwise unfavorable.[51–53] As the site of measurement is moved more peripherally, the measured systolic pressure tends to increase, and the diastolic pressure tends to decrease. An exception is the parturient undergoing cesarean section; the correlation between calf and upper arm blood pressures was found to be poor in this patient population.[54]

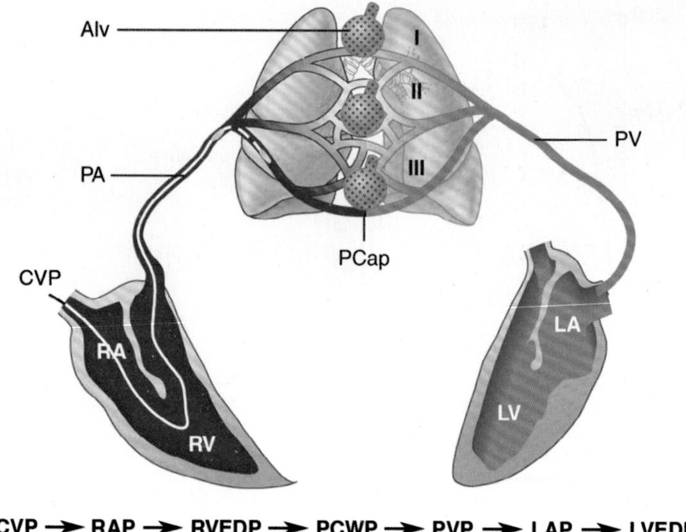

FIGURE 25-6. The progression of intracardiac pressures from central venous pressure to end-diastolic left ventricular pressure. The anatomic position of a pulmonary artery catheter in the pulmonary artery is shown. The dashed line shows the position of the inflated pulmonary artery catheter balloon in the "wedged" position. CVP, central venous pressure; RA, right atrium; RV, right ventricle; PA, pulmonary artery; Alv, alveolus; PCap, pulmonary capillary; PV, pulmonary vein; LA, left atrium; LV, left ventricle. I, II, and III characterize the relationship of $P_{alveolar}$, $P_{arterial}$, and P_{venous} as described by West et al.[55] The bottom of the figure shows a progressive correlation of vascular pressures. (Reproduced from Vender JS. Invasive cardiac monitoring. *Crit Care Clin* 1988;4:455–477.)

MONITORING OF CENTRAL VENOUS AND RIGHT HEART PRESSURES

Principles of Operation

Central venous cannulas are important portals for intraoperative vascular access and for the assessment of changes in vascular volume. Central venous cannulas permit the rapid administration of fluids, insertion of pulmonary artery catheters (PACs) or central venous O_2 ($S_{cv}O_2$) catheters, insertion of transvenous electrodes, monitoring of central venous pressure (CVP), and a site for observation and treatment of venous air embolism. The main value of monitoring central venous and right heart pressures lies in their ability to approximate or trend in conjunction with the left ventricular end-diastolic volume (LVEDV) because left ventricular end-diastolic pressure (LVEDP) predicts left-ventricular filling (i.e., LVEDV) through the Frank–Starling mechanism.

12 Figure 25-6 demonstrates the progression of pressures from CVP through to the pulmonary artery occlusion pressure (PAOP) 13 which reflects LVEDP. Ideally, all proximal pressures reflect changes in LVEDP. The CVP is the easiest to measure as it does not require that any portion of the catheter to be placed within the heart. The CVP is essentially equivalent to right atrial pressure and serves as a reflection of right ventricular preload.[57] The output of the right ventricle and the output of the left ventricle must be approximately the same in a structurally normal cardiopulmonary system, not withstanding a small amount of physiologic shunt caused by the bronchial arteries. However, it has been well demonstrated that right-sided pressures in the heart often are poor indicators of left ventricular filling, either as absolute numbers or in terms of the direction of change in response to therapy. The correlation of these pressures as estimates of LVEDP (and, by extension, LVEDV) is directly related to their proximity to the left ventricle and the status of ventricular compliance. PACs therefore provide more clinical information than central venous monitoring alone; PACs are able to separate the behavior of the right side of the heart, the lung parenchyma, and the left side of the heart. Pulsatile pressures in the pulmonary artery provide an assessment of right ventricular function. The *pulmonary capillary occlusion pressure* (PCOP) provides the closest approximation to LVEDP. The PAC is allowed to "wedge" (i.e., occlude the pulmonary artery in which it resides), with the balloon inflated, in the pulmonary vasculature. During end-diastole, there is cessation of forward blood flow, and a static fluid column is presumed to exist from the left ventricle to the PAC tip with no pressure drop (Fig. 25-6).

The measurement of right heart pressures can therefore indirectly assess left ventricular preload, diagnose the existence of pulmonary hypertension, or differentiate cardiac and noncardiac causes of pulmonary edema.

Proper Use and Interpretation

Careful leveling and zeroing of the pressure transducers is essential, as described earlier for invasive arterial pressure monitoring. 14 The normal CVP waveform consists of three peaks (a, c, and v waves) and two descents (x, y), each resulting from the ebb and flow of blood in the right atrium. The character of the CVP trace depends on many factors, including heart rate, conduction disturbances, tricuspid valve function, normal or abnormal intrathoracic pressure changes, and changes in right ventricular compliance. In patients with atrial fibrillation, a waves are absent. When resistance to the emptying of the right atrium is present, large a waves are often observed. Examples include tricuspid stenosis, right ventricular hypertrophy as a result of pulmonic stenosis, or acute or chronic lung disease associated with pulmonary hypertension. Large a waves may also be observed when right ventricular compliance is impaired.

Tricuspid regurgitation typically produces giant v waves that begin immediately after the QRS complex. Large v waves are often observed when right ventricular ischemia or failure is present or when ventricular compliance is impaired by constrictive pericarditis or cardiac tamponade. A prominent v wave during CVP monitoring may suggest right ventricular papillary muscle ischemia and tricuspid regurgitation. When right ventricular compliance decreases, the CVP often increases with prominent a and v waves fusing to form an *m* or *w* configuration (Fig. 25-7).

CVP monitoring can be unreliable for estimating left ventricular filling pressures, especially when cardiac or pulmonary

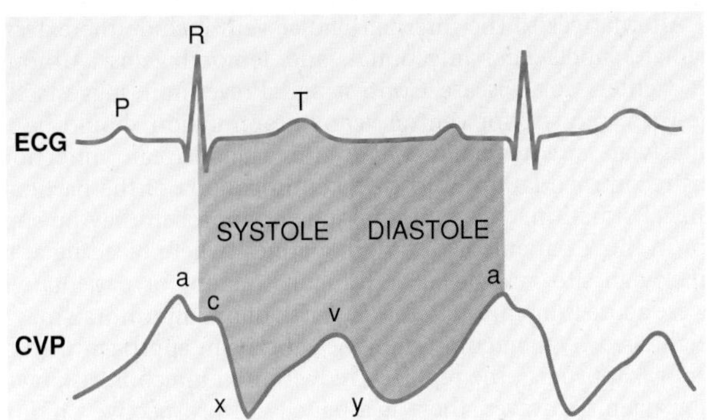

FIGURE 25-7. The normal central venous pressure (CVP) trace. ECG, electrocardiogram. (Redrawn from Mark JB. Central venous pressure monitoring: Clinical insights beyond the numbers. *J Cardiothorac Vasc Anesth.* 1991;5:163–173.)

parenchymal disease processes alter the normal cardiovascular pressure–volume relationships. However, CVP monitoring is less invasive and less costly than pulmonary artery monitoring and offers an understanding of right-sided hemodynamic events and the status of vascular volume. The validity of PAC monitoring depends on a properly functioning pressure monitoring system, correctly identifying the "true" PCOP, and integration of the various factors that affect the relationship of PAOP, and the other cardiac pressures and volumes that are determinants of ventricular function. Figure 25-8 depicts the transduced pressure 7 waves observed as a PAC is floated to the wedged position. Catheter placement is most commonly performed by observing the pressure waves as the catheter is floated from the CVP position through the right heart chambers into the pulmonary artery.

West et al.[55] described a gravity-dependent difference between ventilation and perfusion in the lung. The variability in pulmonary blood flow is a result of differences in pulmonary artery

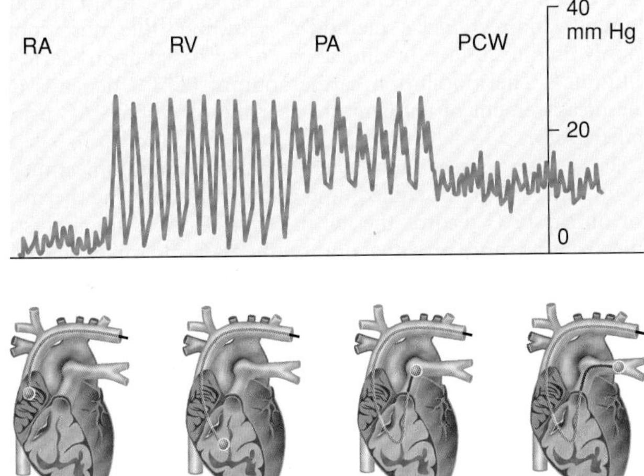

FIGURE 25-8. Pressure tracing observed during the flotation of a pulmonary artery catheter. RA, right atrium; RV, right ventricle; PA, pulmonary artery; PCW, pulmonary capillary wedge pressure. (Reproduced from Dizon CT, Barash PG. The value of monitoring pulmonary artery pressure in clinical practice. *Conn Med* 1977;41:622–625.)

(P_A), alveolar (P_{alv}), and venous pressures (P_V) and is categorized into three distinct zones, as shown in Figure 25-6. Only Zone III ($P_A > P_V > P_{alv}$) meets the criteria for uninterrupted blood flow and for a continuous communication via a static fluid column with distal intracardiac pressures. Flow-directed PACs usually advance to gravity-dependent areas of highest blood flow. However, increases in alveolar pressure, decreases in perfusion, or changes in the position of the patient can convert areas of zone III into either zone II or I. The following characteristics suggest that the PAC tip is not in zone III: PAOP > PAEDP (pulmonary artery end-diastolic pressure), nonphasic PAOP tracing, and inability to aspirate blood from the distal port when the catheter is wedged.

Indications

Even without the monitoring of pressures, central venous access may be indicated to provide a route of administration for vasoactive drugs, for parenteral nutrition, for higher-concentration electrolyte solutions, for prolonged vascular access, or for a temporary pacemaker.

CVPs correlate well with right ventricular preload and so provide a quantitative, direct means of assessing the volumetric status of a patient. CVP monitoring may be indicated in cases in which there are expected to be rapid or large shifts in intravascular volume. CVP monitoring may also be useful in assessing volumetric status when other clinical signs of volumetric status, such as urine output, may be inaccurate or unavailable due either to the procedure or to the patient's comorbidities.

PACs have not been shown to improve outcomes.[59] The decision to place a PAC therefore requires careful individualization of patient care. There must be a specific question regarding the patient's management that can only be addressed with the data that the catheter will provide. This question should be of sufficient importance that the plan of management will potentially be altered depending on the results of PAC monitoring. The information that PACs provide may be particularly informative in the management of patients with severe pulmonary hypertension, or to help differentiate noncardiogenic and cardiogenic shock.

Contraindications

Obstruction at the mitral valve from mitral stenosis, atrial myxoma, or clot can interfere with the ability of left atrial pressure to reflect LVEDP. Similarly, mitral regurgitation, a noncompliant left atrium, or left-to-right intracardiac shunting often is associated with large v waves. Decreases in left ventricular compliance, aortic regurgitation, or premature closure of the mitral valve may reverse the left atrial pressure–LVEDP gradient. When these comorbidities occur, PAOP is not a valid reflection of LVEDP.

Central venous access represents an invasive process with inherent risks, some of which are rare but are potentially life-threatening. Adverse effects from CVP or PAC monitoring can be a result of accessing the central venous circulation, the catheterization procedure, or from use or presence of the catheter after placement. Unintentional puncture of nearby arteries, bleeding, neuropathy, and pneumothorax may result from needle insertion into adjacent structures. Air embolism may occur if a cannula is open to the atmosphere and air is entrained during or after catheter placement. Dysrhythmias are common during the catheterization procedure, with a reported incidence of 4.7% to 68.9%. Ventricular tachycardia or fibrillation may be induced during catheter advancement. Catheter advancement has been

TABLE 25-4. ADVERSE EFFECTS ASSOCIATED WITH PULMONARY ARTERY MONITORING

Complication	Reported Incidence (%)
Central venous access	
Arterial puncture	0.1–13
Postoperative neuropathy	0.3–1.1
Pneumothorax	0.3–4.5
Air embolism	0.5
Flotation of pulmonary artery catheter (PAC)	
Minor dysrhythmias	4–68.9
Ventricular tachycardia or fibrillation	0.3–62.7
Right bundle-branch block	0.1–4.3
Complete heart block (prior left bundle-branch block)	0–8.5
Complications associated with catheter residence	
Pulmonary artery rupture	0.03–1.5
Positive cultures from catheter tip	1.4–34.8
Sepsis secondary to catheter resistance	0.7–11.4
Thrombophlebitis	6.5
Venous thrombosis	0.5–66.7
Pulmonary infarction	0.1–5.6
Mural thrombus	28–61
Valvular or endocardial vegetations	2.2–100
Deaths attributed to pulmonary artery catheter	0.02–1.5

From: American Society of Anesthesiologists Task Force on Pulmonary Artery C. Practice guidelines for pulmonary artery catheterization: An updated report by the American Society of Anesthesiologists Task Force on Pulmonary Artery Catheterization. *Anesthesiology* 2003;99:988–1014.

associated with right bundle-branch block and may precipitate complete heart block in patients with pre-existing left bundle-branch block. The most dreaded complication associated with PAC monitoring is pulmonary artery rupture. Pulmonary hypertension, coagulopathy, and heparinization are often present in patients who have died of pulmonary artery rupture. Perforations and subsequent hemorrhage can be avoided by restricting "overwedging," minimizing the number of balloon inflations, and using proper technique during balloon inflations. Table 25-4 summarizes the adverse effects as reported by the ASA Task Force on pulmonary artery catheterization.[60]

Common Problems and Limitations

The right internal jugular vein is the most common site for cannulation by anesthesiologists because it is accessible from the head of the operating table, has a predictable anatomy, and has a high success rate in both adults and children.[61] The left-sided internal jugular vein is also available but is less desirable because of the potential for damaging the thoracic duct or difficulty in maneuvering catheters through the jugular–subclavian junction. 15 Accidental carotid artery puncture is a potential problem with either location. Use of an ultrasound-guided technique is now strongly recommended to reduce complications and improve first-attempt success rates.[62]

Alternatives to the internal jugular vein include the external jugular, subclavian, antecubital, and femoral veins. Although the Centers for Disease Control and Prevention suggests that the preferred site for central venous cannulation should be the subclavian site to potentially reduce bloodstream infections, this recommendation must be taken in context of the particular clinical situation.[62] The internal jugular approach may be superior in those patients with coagulopathies (where bleeding at the subclavian site may be more difficult to stop) or patients with severe acute lung injury (where the risk of pneumothorax may be heightened). When comparing the subclavian approach with the femoral approach, the reported reduction in infection risk favors subclavian. However, there is a paucity of prospective randomized data when comparing subclavian to internal jugular.[63] Infection is a potential complication of the continued use of CVP and PAC catheters, although ongoing research suggests that this complication may be preventable with scrupulous attention to sterile technique.[64]

MONITORING OF CARDIAC OUTPUT BY PULMONARY ARTERIAL CATHETER

Principles of Operation

Provided that the heart is structurally normal, without septal defects and without a patent ductus, so that no intracardiac recirculation or shunting of blood can occur, the time-averaged flow of blood through the right ventricular outflow tract (RVOT) will accurately approximate the CO. A small amount of venous return to the left side of the heart from the bronchial circulation and thebesian veins is ignored. Time averaging suppresses the effects of beat-to-beat pulsatility.

A properly positioned PAC passes through the RVOT. CO monitoring using a PAC therefore depends on assessing the rate of blood flow through the right side of the heart and using this as a measure of CO. Techniques to measure the flow rate are based upon the idea of measuring the dilution by the passing blood flow of some known quantity of an indicator.[65] This indicator could be a dye, or oxygen content (Fick's method), or carbon dioxide content (indirect Fick's method).[66] However, the most commonly used technique in clinical practice is based upon thermo-16 dilution.[67] Thermodilution cardiac output (TCO) depends on the measurement of temperature near the tip of the PAC using a thermistor.

CO can be assessed intermittently by using a bolus injection of room-temperature or chilled fluid as the indicator. The thermistor on the PAC records the fall in temperature as this bolus is injected via a more proximal port on the PAC and mixes with the surrounding blood flow. The total flow through the RVOT, and hence the CO, can be estimated from the area under this blood temperature curve, combined with knowledge of the specific heat capacity and gravity of blood and the injectate, the volume of the injectate, and the size of the catheter. When performed properly, TCO measurements correlate well with direct Fick or dye dilution estimates of CO.[68]

Continuous CO monitoring offers the potential to identify acute changes in ventricular performance as they occur. Pulsed thermodilution uses a coiled filament that applies a low-power heating signal within the right atrium and ventricle in a cyclical manner based on a proprietary, pseudorandom sequence. The thermistor at the tip of the PAC detects these changes in blood temperature and sends the temperature information to a microcomputer that uses stochastic analysis to create a thermodilution curve. CO is then computed in a similar fashion to the bolus technique, using a conservation of heat equation, although effectively using a warmed bolus rather than a chilled bolus.[69] Another technique applies heat to a thermistor located at the tip of a PAC. The blood flow through the RVOT subsequently cools the tip, and the temperature changes registered are proportional to the rate of blood flow. Although a time lag can exist, continuous CO monitoring compares favorably with bolus CO measurements, even under conditions of varying patient temperature and CO.

Proper Use and Interpretation

TCO estimates can vary with the respiratory cycle. Performing measurements at peak inspiration or end expiration can reduce this variability. Ensuring that the rate of injection and the volume are constant enhances precision. Most TCO computers require that repeat measurements be delayed for 30 to 90 seconds to stabilize the thermal environment of the PAC thermistor. The TCO computer displays the CO directly in L/min.

TCO measurements depend on the assumption that changes in thermal energy are carried forward to the thermistor, and so the measurements depend on the correct positioning of the catheter. If the catheter is insufficiently advanced such that the port through which a bolus injectate is administered is still within the introducer sheath, then there will be reflux of the injectate within the introducer sheath. This will result in some of the change in thermal energy being "lost" into the sheath. A smaller-than-expected change in temperature will then be seen at the thermistor, appearing as if the injectate had been injected into a larger volume of blood flow. The TCO computer will interpret and present this as an erroneously high CO. Similarly erroneous readings may be produced if the catheter is advanced too far, such that the heating filament of a continuous TCO catheter lies beyond the pulmonic valve. Hypothermia and the rapid concurrent administration of unwarmed intravenous fluids may affect the accuracy of TCO measurements.

Indications

Measurement of CO is required to determine physiologic factors such as the rate of oxygen delivery to peripheral tissues, possible clinical indications include severe sepsis, cardiogenic shock, and dependence on inotropes. An additional technologic refinement of the PAC is the *oximetric* PAC, which uses reflectance spectrophotometry to identify the saturation of the mixed venous blood surrounding the tip of the PAC, $S_{\bar{v}}O_2$. Three-wavelength in vivo systems correlate well with simultaneous samples measured by co-oximetry.[70] Knowledge of the $S_{\bar{v}}O_2$ allows the rate of extraction of oxygen by peripheral tissues ($\dot{\psi}o_2$) to be calculated. Neglecting the small amount of oxygen dissolved in blood:

$$\dot{\psi}o_2 = 13.8 \times [\text{Hgb}] \times CO \times (S_\alpha O_2 - S_v O_2)$$

Where [Hb] is the concentration of hemoglobin, the amount of O_2 carried by 100% saturated Hb is 13.8 mL O_2/unit Hb and is the oxygen-carrying capacity of hemoglobin, CO is the cardiac output in L/min and $(S_\alpha O_2 - S_v O_2)$ is the difference between the arterial and mixed venous oxygen saturations.

The use of PACs in practice has diminished over the last 5 years,[71] and this may partly be due to the greater use of techniques such as transesophageal echocardiography and arterial waveform analysis that can estimate CO in a less-invasive manner. However, thermodilution via a PAC remains the clinical gold standard for the determination of CO and should be considered when knowledge of the CO is necessary for the patient's management and when other comorbidities would render less invasive techniques inaccurate.

Contraindications

Measurement of CO requires a PAC that is designed for the purpose. Other than contraindications to the PAC, there are no additional contraindications for CO monitoring.

Common Problems and Limitations

The intermittent TCO technique assumes that there is adequate mixing of the cooled injectate with the surrounding blood flow. It is necessary that the temperature of the injectate be distinct from the temperature of the blood in order to generate a change in the distal temperature measurement. Improved measurements can be obtained by using a cooler injectate, producing a greater temperature change to detect and hence an improved signal-to-noise ratio.[72]

The presence of intracardiac shunts or significant tricuspid regurgitation can invalidate the assumptions underlying TCO. Intracardiac shunts allow accessory blood flow paths, such that flow through the RVOT may no longer approximate CO accurately. Significant tricuspid regurgitation can compromise thermodilution methods by permitting retrograde blood flow, invalidating the assumption that all changes in thermal energy caused by the indicator are carried forward to the detecting thermistor.

ANESTHETIC MANAGEMENT

17

MONITORING OF CARDIAC OUTPUT BY ARTERIAL WAVEFORM ANALYSIS

Principles of Operation

The use of a PAC remains the gold standard for the determination of CO, but the use of PACs in the management of patients requiring intensive care has not been demonstrated to be associated with reduced mortality.[73] PACs can be associated with a high rate of iatrogenic complications,[74] and the ASA recommends that only clinicians with regular, ongoing experience of the procedure[60] should place pulmonary catheters. Nevertheless, the determination of CO allows more accurate assessment of the hemodynamic status of a critically ill patient than can be obtained by clinical assessment alone. This notion has created increasing interest in biomedical devices that can estimate CO in a less invasive manner; arterial waveform analysis is one such technique.[75]

There are presently three well-established arterial waveform devices on the market: FloTrac (Edwards Lifesciences, Irvine, CA), PiCCO (PULSION Medical Systems AG, Munich, Germany), and LiDCOrapid (LiDCO Ltd., London, England).[76] These devices attach to a peripheral arterial line and measure the fluctuations in arterial pressure, measuring the heart rate (HR) and estimating the beat-to-beat variation in stroke volume (SV). The CO is given by the product of the heart rate and stroke volume (CO = HR × SV).

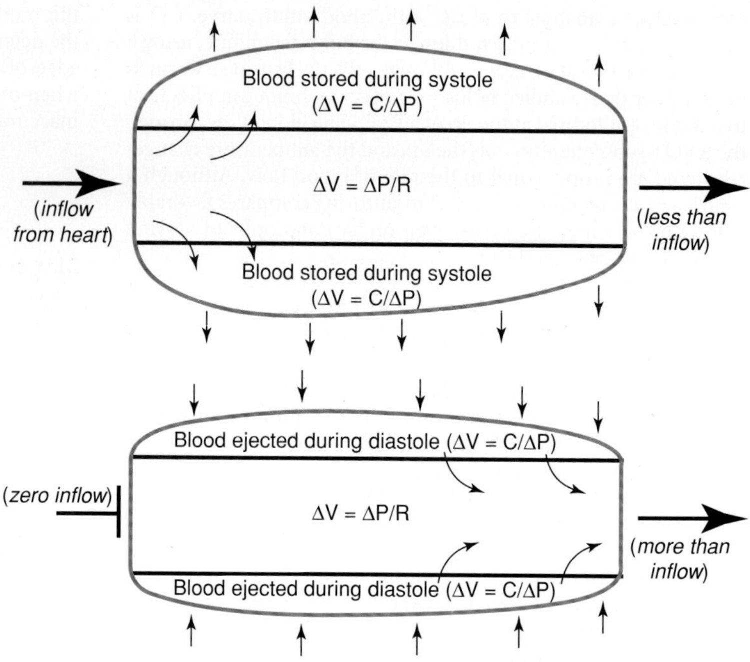

FIGURE 25-9. Depiction of blood flow into and out of a prototypical "Windkessel artery." Several points are to be noted: First, during systole, inflow into the artery is less than outflow, because some of the blood is stored in the expanding, compliant vessel. Second, during diastole, inflow into the artery is zero and outflow is enhanced by the contracting vessel. (Reproduced from: Thiele RH, Durieux ME. Arterial waveform analysis for the anesthesiologist: Past, present, and future concepts. *Anesth Analg* 2011;113:766–776.)

It is a straightforward matter to measure HR from an arterial waveform tracing; it is the estimation of beat-to-beat SV that presents the technical challenge. The first modern mathematical description of the shape of the arterial waveform was described by Otto Frank,[77] and gave rise to the "Windkessel" (German: *Air chamber*) model for arterial behavior. Usually when considering the flow of an incompressible fluid, such as blood, in a section of tube, the assumption is made that the volume of the fluid entering the tube is the same as the volume of the fluid leaving the tube. This assumption allows a *continuity equation* to be created, from which models of fluid flow can be derived. The basis of the Windkessel model is the realization that, although blood is incompressible, the artery itself is distensible and so the volumes of blood entering and leaving an arterial segment at any given moment may be different. There is storage of blood and distension of the artery during systole, and ejection of blood and relaxation of the artery during diastole. The volumes of blood entering and leaving are only the same when averaged over the cardiac cycle (Fig. 25-9).

This behavior is mathematically similar to that seen in the modeling of a compressible fluid, such as air, when flowing in rigid vessels, hence the name the "Windkessel" model. The air may store and release energy through changes in pressure and compression. In arterial waveform analysis, it is the fluid that is incompressible, and it is the nonrigid arterial vessel that may store and release energy by elastic deformation. The behavior of the artery is dependent on its resistance to flow *R* and its compliance *C* and, from cadaveric studies of the human aorta,[78] these values are known to be predictable.

The total stroke volume SV must be equal to the forward flow in systole (Q_s) plus the forward flow in diastole (Q_d), assuming the aortic valve is competent.

$$SV = Q_s + Q_d$$

At the beginning of diastole, there is no further inflow into the aorta, and so Q_d is proportional to the difference between the pressure in the aorta and the pressure in the arterial beds. This is described as the end-systolic mean distending pressure P_{md}, equivalent to the idea of a "pressure head." Therefore:

$$Q_d = k \times P_{md}$$

where *k* is a constant of proportionality dependent on the properties of resistance and compliance as described above. As the peripheral vascular resistance should not change over a single cardiac cycle, the values of Q_s and Q_d should be proportional to A_s and A_d, the areas under the pressure curve during systole and diastole respectively. Therefore:

$$Q_s/A_s = Q_d/A_d \quad \text{or, alternatively} \quad Q_s = Q_d\frac{A_s}{A_d}$$

Rearranging these model equations:

$$SV = Q_d\left(1+\frac{A_s}{A_d}\right) \quad \text{and so} \quad SV = kP_{md}\left(1+\frac{A_s}{A_d}\right)$$

This model (Fig. 25-10) demonstrates how, in principle, a beat-to-beat estimate of stroke volume SV can be generated from measurements of the arterial waveform. The algorithms used by actual clinical devices are more complex and proprietary. Although the analysis above is necessarily simplified, it nevertheless illustrates the fundamental principles and requirements of these devices. For instance, the model depends on an additional value *k*, which has to be determined either by calibrating the prediction of this model to another measurement of stroke volume (such as TEE [transesophageal echocardiogram] or thermodilution) or in an uncalibrated manner by estimating its value from biophysical models based on variables such as the patient's age, sex, height, and weight.[80] The PiCCO device makes use of an external calibration reading, whereas the FloTrac and LiDCOrapid devices use an uncalibrated, biophysical model approach.

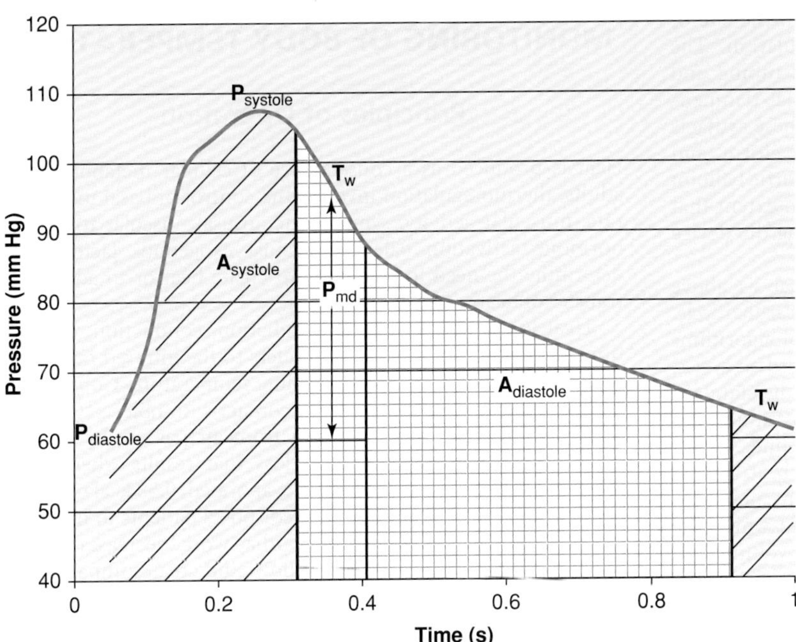

FIGURE 25-10. A graphical depiction of the components of the arterial waveform used by the Windkessel-based area under the curve method. Note that P_{md} represents the increment in mean pressure over the whole arterial bed at the end of systole[79] and that T_w represents the transmission time (from the aorta to the periphery). (Reproduced from: Thiele RH, Durieux ME. Arterial waveform analysis for the anesthesiologist: Past, present, and future concepts. *Anesth Analg* 2011;113:766–776.)

Proper Use and Interpretation

Arterial Waveform CO monitors make use of standard equipment for arterial cannulation. A stiff arterial line, flushed from a pressurized fluid source, is attached to the arterial cannula in the usual fashion. However, in place of the usual piezoelectric pressure sensor with a single electrical connection, a specialized sensor is used with two connectors so that pressure information can be supplied simultaneously to the anesthesia monitor and to the CO monitor. The arterial line is zeroed in the usual fashion. The display of arterial pressures by the anesthesia monitor is unaffected by the presence of the CO monitor. It is possible to transduce arterial pressures alone, without connecting the CO monitor. Uncalibrated devices, such as the FloTrac and LiDCOrapid, require information about the patient such as age, height, weight, and sex in order to estimate the physiologic properties of the patient's arterial system and estimated body surface area. The device may require a brief interval of time to gather initial arterial pressure data, but will shortly begin to report CO and other indices such as cardiac index, stroke volume, stroke volume variation, and stroke volume index. These indices represent various combinations of stroke volume, heart rate, and body surface area. Further, user intervention is not generally required. These values, in the manner estimated by the device, are most useful for assessing relative volume status and for assessing the response to fluid resuscitation.[81–84] The ability of the device to respond to changes in CO caused by inotropes or vasopressors.[81,85] is uncertain; the limits of its reliability, accuracy, and utility in this setting are the subject of ongoing research and algorithmic refinement.

Indications

The use of an arterial waveform CO monitor is not mandated, and so the indications for use are at the discretion of the practitioner. The device is likely to be most helpful to the clinician in cases where there are expected to be large fluid shifts and in which the patient's volemic status may become difficult to determine by clinical assessment and usual monitoring techniques. It may be preferable, and less invasive, to guide fluid resuscitation with arterial waveform CO measurements rather than placing a central venous catheter or a PAC. This approach is particularly attractive if the patient already requires an arterial line for other indications, or if the patient's comorbidities relatively contraindicate the placement of a central line or PAC. The FloTrac device has been demonstrated to show excellent concordance with TEE in measuring CO under conditions of changing fluid preload.[81]

It is possible to extract other indices from analysis of the arterial waveform, and measurements such as systolic pulse variation (SPV) and stroke volume variation (SVV) may also be useful in predicting responsiveness to fluid resuscitation.[86,87]

Contraindications

Devices such as the FloTrac and LiDCOrapid that do not require additional calibration are no more invasive than the arterial line to which they are attached. The same contraindications that apply to arterial lines, such as poor or absent collateralization of arterial supply to the extremity, also apply to these devices.

Devices that estimate CO from the arterial waveform do so based upon a number of physiologic assumptions that were touched upon during the derivation of the simplified model above. There are many disease states, some common, which violate these assumptions and can significantly compromise the accuracy of the device; these are discussed below.

Common Problems and Limitations

All arterial waveform CO monitors are dependent on accurate, high fidelity measurement of arterial pressures. Satisfactory operation depends upon good arterial perfusion to the site of measurement and good peripheral arterial cannulation. The pressure transducer system must use appropriate tubing and be flushed and zeroed correctly so that bias, signal dampening, or flail are not seen in the arterial waveform. These artifacts corrupt the frequency spectrum of the arterial waveform, and impair accurate measurement. The use of an intra-aortic balloon pump may distort the arterial waveform to such an extent that the resulting waveform is uninterpretable, rendering the device inoperative.[88]

The simplified model of arterial waveform analysis above made use of information obtained from only a single cardiac cycle. Unlike this, all of the current monitors make use of algorithms that depend on information obtained over many cardiac cycles. The FloTrac monitor depends, for example, upon the standard deviation, skewness, and kurtosis of the statistical distribution of arterial pressures obtained over the preceding 20 seconds.[80] This implicitly assumes that the CO remains relatively beat-to-beat constant over the sampling interval. This assumption can be violated in the presence of irregular heart rhythms, in which the preload of the left ventricle and hence the stroke volume can demonstrate significant beat-to-beat variability. Arterial waveform CO monitors are therefore known to be prone to inaccuracy in the setting of atrial fibrillation.[89]

In the simplified model above, the properties of systemic vascular resistance (SVR) and arterial compliance (C) were subsumed into the parameter *k*, and it was proposed that *k* might be obtained from a population-based biophysical model. However, in the presence of sepsis[85,90] or some other high-output state such as liver transplantation surgery,[84] the deviation of these values from the expected population norms can cause inaccuracy when compared to the measurement of CO by PAC. With ongoing research and refinement of the devices and their algorithms, this situation appears to be improving.[83] However, a similar problem applies to the iatrogenic reduction of the compliance of arterial vessels through the administration of vasopressors. Arterial waveform CO devices appear to be reliable at assessing changes in CO caused by fluid resuscitation, of some utility at detecting changes caused by inotropes,[81] but poor at assessing changes caused by alteration in vascular tone by agents such as phenylephrine[81] or norepinephrine.[82]

Finally, arterial waveform analysis depends upon the assumption that there is no further inflow into the arterial system at the end of systole, as used in the analysis based on the parameter P_{md} above. This assumption is violated in the setting of aortic insufficiency, in which there is negative, regurgitant flow to the left ventricle. Arterial waveform analysis is expected to demonstrate inaccuracy in this presentation.[88] Conversely, aortic stenosis does not appear to impair the accuracy of measurement of CO.

In summary, arterial waveform analysis has been demonstrated in many studies to provide a reasonable estimate of CO, in reasonable approximation to more invasive techniques. The degree to which a new monitoring technique must agree with the "gold standard" to be clinically useful is a matter of clinical judgment and not a question that can be definitively addressed by statistics alone. Presently, the devices appear to be most useful as a guide to fluid resuscitation, rather than as a guide to the administration of inotropes or vasopressors. There are a number of relatively common clinical scenarios in which the accuracy of these devices can be anticipated to be impaired, based upon violation of the underlying physiologic assumptions on which their algorithms depend, and the clinician must exercise caution in interpreting the measurements of CO obtained under those circumstances.

MONITORING OF BODY TEMPERATURE

Principles of Operation

Heat is produced as a consequence of cellular metabolism. In adults, thermoregulation involves the control of basal metabolic rate, muscular activity, sympathetic arousal, vascular tone, and hormone activation balanced against exogenous factors that determine the need for the body to create heat or to adjust the transfer of heat to the environment.

Heat losses may result from radiation, conduction, convection, and evaporation. Radiation refers to the infrared rays emanating from all objects above absolute temperature. Conduction refers to the transfer of heat from contact with objects. Convection refers to the transfer of heat from air passing by objects. Evaporation represents the heat loss that results when water vaporizes. For every gram of water evaporated, 0.58 kcal of heat is lost. Perioperative hypothermia predisposes patients to increases in metabolic rate (shivering) and cardiac work, decreases in drug metabolism and cutaneous blood flow, and creates impairments of coagulation. Anesthesiologists frequently monitor temperature and attempt to maintain central core temperature at near-normal values in all patients undergoing anesthesia.

Temperature is usually measured using electrical probes containing calibrated thermistors or thermocouples that serve as temperature transducers. Thermistors respond to temperature changes by changing their electrical resistance. Thermocouples are constructed by passing current through a circuit where the electrodes are made of two dissimilar metals. The current measured is directly proportional to the temperature difference between the two metal junctions. Thermocouple temperature probes maintain one junction at a known temperature and place the second junction on the temperature probe tip. Skin temperature can also be monitored using liquid crystal thermometry.

Proper Use and Interpretation

Central core temperatures can be estimated using probes that can be placed into the bladder, distal esophagus, ear canal, trachea, nasopharynx, or rectum.[91] Pulmonary artery blood temperature is also a good estimate of central core temperature. Thermoregulatory responses are based on a physiologically weighted average reflecting changes in the mean body temperature. Mean body temperature is estimated by the following equation:

$$T_{\text{mean body}} = 0.85T_{\text{core}} + 0.15T_{\text{skin}}$$

Indications

Humans maintain their core temperature by balancing heat production from metabolism and the many environmental factors that supply heat or cool the body. Regional temperature information from the skin, muscle, body cavities, spinal cord, and brain are integrated in the central nervous system. Conceptually, thermoregulation involves the integration of "set points," which, when exceeded, trigger temperature-dissipating, temperature-conserving, or heat-producing mechanisms. Both general and regional anesthesia inhibit afferent and efferent control of thermoregulation.[92,93] In addition, the operating room environment and surgical exposure often contribute to excessive heat losses. Heat

loss is common during surgery because the surgical environment transfers heat from the patient, and anesthesia reduces heat production and diminishes the capability of patients to monitor and
8 maintain thermoregulation. Clinical studies have demonstrated that patients in whom intraoperative hypothermia develops are at a higher risk for development of postoperative myocardial ischemia and wound infection compared with patients who are normothermic in the perioperative period.[94,95]

The ability to monitor body temperature is a standard of anesthesia care.[1] The continual observation of temperature changes in anesthetized patients allows for the detection of accidental heat loss or malignant hyperthermia.

Contraindications

There are no absolute contraindications to temperature monitoring. In patients whose thermoregulatory responses are intact, such as conscious patients or patients receiving light or moderate sedation, continuous temperature monitoring is usually uninformative.

Common Problems and Limitations

Skin temperature monitoring has been advocated to identify peripheral vasoconstriction but is not adequate to determine alterations in mean body temperature that may occur during surgery. Core temperature sites have been established as reliable indicators of changes in mean temperature. During routine noncardiac surgery, temperature differences between these sites are small. When anesthetized patients are being cooled, changes in rectal temperature often lag behind those of other probe locations, and the adequacy of rewarming is best judged by measuring temperature at several locations.

Although liquid crystal skin temperature strips are convenient to apply, they do not correlate with core temperature measurements.[96]

MONITORING OF PROCESSED EEG SIGNALS

Principles of Operation

EEG monitoring initially entered anesthetic practice as a highly sensitive and moderately specific means of monitoring for cerebral ischemia, and as such found use in carotid surgery. Occlusion of one of the carotid arteries for surgery makes the ipsilateral side of the brain dependent on perfusion from the contralateral carotid artery via the Circle of Willis, creating a risk of ipsilateral ischemia. In this form, a dedicated technician usually performs intraoperative EEG monitoring.

More recently, EEG monitoring has begun to gain acceptance as a means of estimating depth of anesthesia. Statistical signal-processing techniques have been developed and embodied as biomedical devices that are able to take an ensemble of EEG data and, in real-time, display an estimate of "anesthetic depth." The two most commonly used processed EEG monitors are the BIS (Covidien) and SedLine (Masimo), and the operation of these devices is similar. After first cleaning the patient's forehead, a single-use set of small, adhesive electrical sensors are applied. The sensors are positioned to enable the device to detect EEG activity in the frontal lobes of the brain. The sensors are attached to the main device via a single connector. The device checks the quality of the electrical connection to the sensors, and checks that each of the sensors has made a good electrical contact with the patient's forehead, and that the sensors are not in inadvertent electrical connection with each other. In the event that the configuration of the sensors is unacceptable, the device displays a pictorial indication of the problem so that the practitioner can attempt to remedy the problem. If the electrical connection between the sensor and the skin is poor, signal reception will be impaired and the device will warn that the sensor impedance (i.e., its electrical resistance) is too high. The sensors make use of a conductive electrical gel, and so this can often be remedied by applying firm but careful pressure to the affected sensor to produce a better electrical contact. However, too much pressure may cause the gel to leak out from under the sensor and cause a "gel bridge," an inadvertent direct electrical connection to a neighboring electrode. In this case, the surplus gel may be wiped away, or a new set of sensors may be required. When all the electrical connections are satisfactory, the device will begin to acquire and process EEG data.

9 Although the algorithms used by processed EEG monitors are proprietary, the general features of the EEG that they use are well described.[97] Processed EEG monitors make use of the following statistical measures:

- Zero crossing frequency (ZXF). An estimate of the "average" frequency of the EEG, obtained by calculating the number of times the EEG voltage crosses the zero voltage level per second.[98]
- Burst suppression ratio (BSR). During periods of deep anesthesia, the EEG may demonstrate periods of low voltage or even zero (isoelectric) voltage, and bursts of higher voltage activity are no longer seen. Suppressed states are defined as those periods for which the EEG demonstrates a voltage of less than 5 mV for a period of at least 0.5 seconds, and the BSR is defined as the ratio of that time fraction to the overall EEG recording. Profoundly burst suppressed (isoelectric) states are sometimes induced as part of neuroanesthesia,[99] as they may provide some protection against cerebral ischemia by reducing cellular metabolic demand. Burst suppression is also seen in unanesthetized comatose patients, although in these patients it carries a grave prognosis.[100]
- Median power frequency (MPF) and spectral edge frequency (SEF). The EEG signal can be converted to a frequency spectrum using the fast Fourier transform,[101] making it possible to describe the amount of signal power present at various frequencies. The MPF is the frequency at which the power in the signal can be split into two equal frequency bands, above and below. The SEF is the frequency below which 95% of the total signal power can be found.[97]
- Beta (β) power ratio. The β power ratio describes the relative amount of β_2 wave activity in the EEG signal (signal power between 30 to 47 Hz) compared to the amount of β wave activity (signal power between 11 to 20 Hz). Changes in this ratio appear to correlate clinically with the onset of light sedation.
- Bispectrum. The bispectrum is a second-order property of the frequency spectrum of the EEG signal.[102] The bispectrum can be used to calculate bicoherence, a mathematical property that describes the similarity in phase between signals at three different frequencies, f_1, f_2, and $f_1 + f_2$. A high level of bicoherence is suggestive that the signals may be generated from a common underlying rhythm. As sedation is increased, local cortical activity becomes suppressed and the EEG activity begins to demonstrate a greater underlying cortical synchronization, which can be detected as increased bicoherence in the EEG signal.

Proper Use and Interpretation

Both the BIS and SedLine devices display a unitless number in the range of 0 to 100, which is derived from the measured EEG data by the device's proprietary algorithms. A value of 0 corresponds to an absence of any discernable electrical activity. A value of 100 corresponds to the EEG activity seen in a fully awake and alert individual. The algorithms used in the devices specify a differing "optimal range" for general anesthesia; for the BIS it is defined as between 40 and 60, for the SedLine it is 25 to 50.

The algorithms used in the devices appear to correlate best with clinical assessment of the depth of anesthesia when anesthetic agents such as volatile gases or propofol are used. Although, increasing concentrations of these agents do not always reliably lower the reported number further[103–105] if the patient is already deeply anesthetized. This relationship between concentration and effect is not seen for all anesthetic agents (Fig. 25-11).

Dissociative intravenous agents such as ketamine can actively confound processed EEG monitors through paradoxical cortical excitation; the monitor tends to misread the increased cortical activity as a sign of lessened anesthesia.[106] Lower doses of ketamine may be desirable as part of an overall anesthetic plan to reduce opioid administration; appropriate quantities of ketamine can be infused more slowly without apparently affecting the processed EEG reading.[107] Propofol and remifentanil are often used in combination for total intravenous anesthesia (TIVA), but processed EEG monitors can be insensitive to the administration of even high concentrations of opioids.[108] The monitor may therefore reflect mostly the action of the propofol on the anesthetic state.

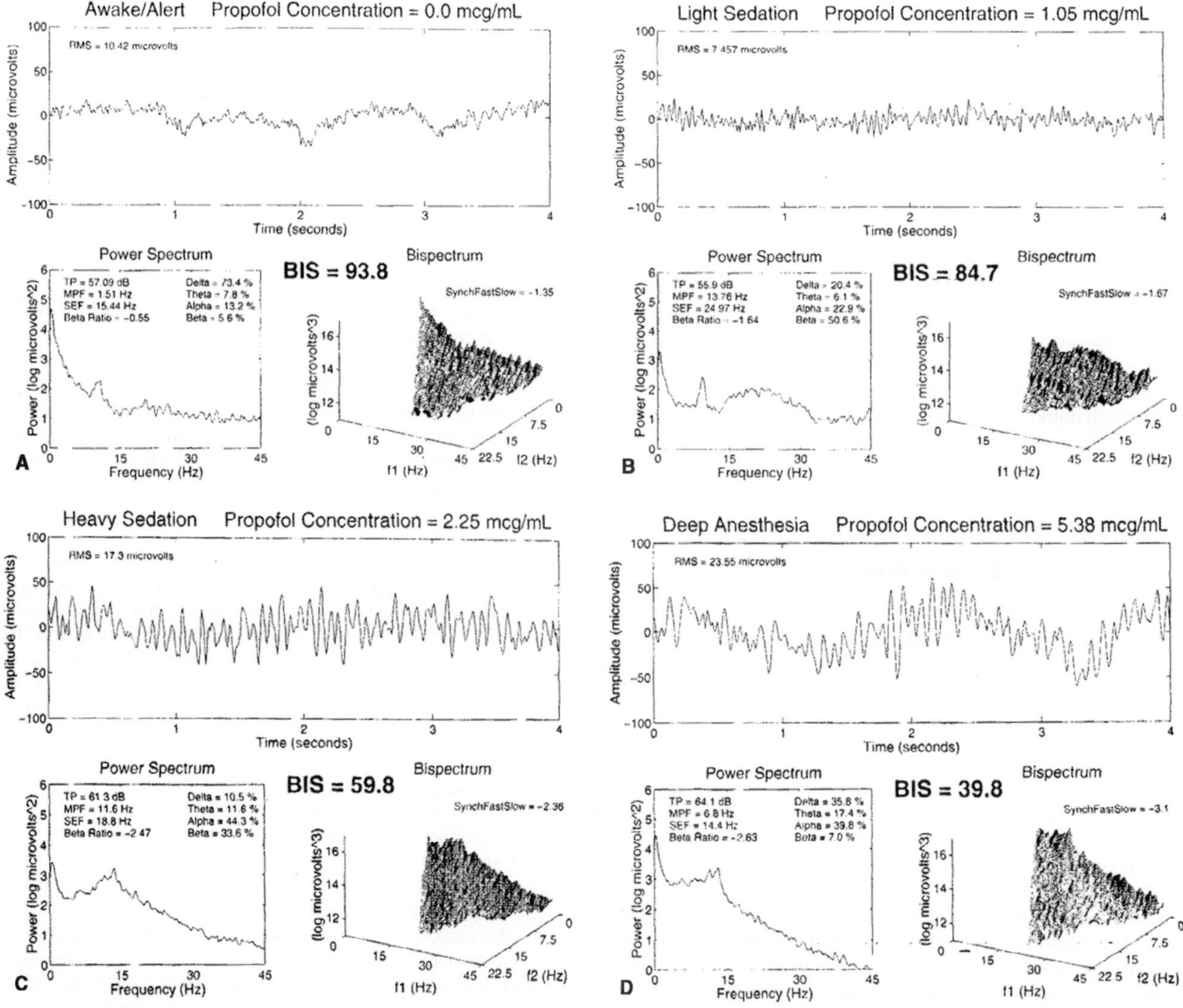

FIGURE 25-11. Representative data from a single human volunteer demonstrating changes in EEG with increasing serum concentrations of propofol. In each of the four concentrations, 4 seconds of raw EEG data is plotted in the top half of the figure. In the lower left is the corresponding power spectrum and spectral parameters computed from the same EEG epoch. The lower right quadrant displays the bispectrum for the same raw data. The final BIS score is shown. Modified from: Rampil IJ. A primer for EEG signal processing in anesthesia. *Anesthesiology.* 1998;89:980–1002, Figure 16.

Indications

The use of processed EEG monitors is not mandated, and so the indications for use are at the discretion of the practitioner. Processed EEG monitors have not been demonstrated to be superior to end-tidal agent concentration monitoring in the prevention of awareness under anesthesia. However, the use of end-tidal agent concentration monitoring assumes that volatile anesthetic gases are used, and that their end-tidal concentrations provide a reasonable surrogate for their action on consciousness. Processed EEG monitoring may be useful as a guide when a total intravenous anesthetic approach is planned, since it can provide some degree of feedback on the current pharmacodynamics effects of the administered agents when there is no end-tidal agent concentration to measure.

Patients with pre-existing cognitive deficits, sensory impairment,[109] or known risk of post-operative delirium may benefit from the administration of less anesthesia than would be indicated by end-tidal agent monitoring alone.[110] Processed EEG monitoring may be useful in satisfactorily titrating their anesthetic plan to permit faster recovery from anesthesia.[111]

For types of emergent surgery, such as cesarean sections under GA,[112] trauma laparotomies, or surgery in the critically ill hemodynamically unstable patient, it may not be physiologically possible to administer the usual quantities of anesthesia, placing these patients at a greater risk of intraoperative awareness. Processed EEG monitoring may provide some assistance in titrating anesthesia in these vulnerable patients, and some reassurance that explicit recall will be unlikely. A prior history of intraoperative awareness may therefore also be an indication.

Mechanically ventilated patients in the intensive care unit are usually assessed clinically for their level of sedation, but the use of the standard Sedation–Agitation Scale or the Richmond Agitation–Sedation Scale may be impossible in some patients due to therapeutic neuromuscular paralysis. Processed EEG monitors may provide some guidance to sedation management under these circumstances.[113,114]

Contraindications

Use of a processed EEG device may be contraindicated in a patient with significant craniofacial trauma, such that the physical pressure required to place the sensors cannot be safely applied. Placement may also be relatively contraindicated in patients with existing superficial injury to the forehead in the region where the sensors will be applied.

The use of processed EEG sensors for patients who will be in prone position for surgery is controversial, and may be a relative contraindication. In prone position, the patient's head may rest such that excessive continuous pressure is applied to the skin underneath the sensors. Disfiguring injury to the forehead has been reported,[115] perhaps related to a combination of pressure and irritation from the conductive gel on the sensors. This can lead to a dilemma: Prolonged spinal surgery performed using somatosensory or motor evoked potential monitoring can relatively contraindicate the use of volatile gases and neuromuscular blockers, and make a propofol–remifentanil TIVA technique attractive. This anesthetic technique provides an indication for processed EEG monitoring, but the prolonged prone positioning provides a relative contraindication. Prone positioning requires vigilant attention to facial features such as the eyes and nose to avoid injury by pressure and impingement. Therefore, if it is determined that processed EEG monitoring is to be applied to a prone patient, it is recommended that equally vigilant attention be paid to the condition of the forehead.

Common Problems and Limitations

It has been suggested that processed EEG monitoring devices may reduce the risk of intraoperative awareness.[116] However, subsequent studies have either failed to demonstrate a reduction[117] in intraoperative awareness or even, conversely, have found an increase in intraoperative awareness[25] when compared to anesthetic practice guided by the end-tidal agent concentrations[19] of anesthetic gases.[24]

Cases of intraoperative awareness were found when using either end-tidal agent concentration monitoring or processed EEG monitoring; neither technique was sufficient to avoid awareness with complete reliability. This difficulty may relate to our lack of understanding of what "anesthetic depth" even means.[110,118] Intraoperative awareness as a phenomenon is dependent on the interaction of consciousness, memory, and the biologic action of anesthetic agents. These, even taken individually, are complex and incompletely understood processes.[119–121] It should not therefore be surprising that any device or algorithm that seeks to reduce these processes to a single numerical readout may prove to be fallible.

FUTURE TRENDS IN MONITORING

Anesthesiologists have been at the forefront of the incorporation of innovative biomedical devices and technologies into their practice. We will continue to adapt our practice to make use of new technologies to enhance patient safety. There are three trends in device design that appear most likely to lead to further improvements in our practice: Greater automated marshaling of monitoring and clinical data, the dissemination of our current devices into wider hospital use, and the development of devices with greater algorithmic sophistication to obtain clinical data less invasively.

Anesthesia information management systems (AIMS) will continue to become more interconnected with patient monitoring devices, and also with drug delivery systems such as infusion pumps and vaporizers. AIMS will also begin to interface more deeply with hospital-wide computerized provider order entry (CPOE) systems, allowing patient clinical data and documentation to be available immediately to the anesthesiologist. The safety of the administration of intravenous medications will be enhanced by the routine use of machine-readable labels, whether by barcoding or RFID (Radio frequency Identification), so that the intended administration of a medication will be known to the AIMS system prior to the actual administration. AIMS will make use of this information to alert to the potential for drug interactions and allergies during the case itself, immediately prior to administration. The automatic availability of this data will allow the AIMS to provide decision support to the anesthesiologist, tracking the administration of intravenous medications and providing predictions of plasma and effect-site concentrations to improve dose titration. Overall, improvements in the automated marshaling and display of patient data will assist the anesthesiologist with situational awareness, involving more intelligent alarm systems to decrease false positive alerts and more accurately guide the anesthesiologist to aspects of the patient's management that require attention. The sophistication of AIMS user interfaces will continue to improve, so that the interaction between the anesthesiologist and the tasks of computer-based monitoring and charting will become smooth, fast, natural, and efficient.

In the recent revision of the ASA Standards for Basic Monitoring,[1] the indications for capnography have been broadened to include the evaluation of ventilation during moderate or deep sedation. Moderate sedation may be performed by clinicians untrained in the practice of anesthesia, and so the effect of this standard will be the dissemination of capnographic equipment previously used only by anesthesiologists to the wider care environment. Anesthesiologists should be at the forefront of educational efforts to ensure that our medical colleagues use these devices appropriately, enhancing patient safety.

A trend in the development of biomedical devices is toward devices that use complex algorithmic models to infer clinical data in a less invasive or more rapid manner. Examples are arterial waveform CO monitors that produce an estimate of CO from the arterial pressure tracing alone, noninvasive hemoglobin monitors that estimate serum hemoglobin from infrared pulse oximetry, target-controlled infusion pumps which make use of population pharmacokinetic and pharmacodynamic data to estimate the redistribution and effect of a medication, and processed EEG monitors which attempt to reduce an ensemble of EEG data to a quantitated endpoint of consciousness. These devices are examples of incredible biomedical sophistication, usually the product of decades of scientific research and subsequent engineering refinement. However, the algorithms that these devices use are generally derived from the responses of healthy volunteers. The protocols used for the development of the algorithms are often seemingly simplistic or artificial when compared to the complexity of actual anesthetic practice. The result is that, during their initial introduction to practice, the functionality of the devices in the sickest of patients is not necessarily well characterized or understood. To put it more briefly: It may work, but does it *really* work? It is our sickest patients who have the most to gain from devices that allow us to assess their clinical condition more rapidly and less invasively, but it is our sickest patients who are the most vulnerable should the devices tend to become inaccurate
10 under just those clinical conditions. The limits of the reliability and clinical applicability of these devices must be a matter of concern for the practicing anesthesiologist. Though devices are becoming "smarter," it will not excuse us of the knowledge to know how to employ them wisely.

References

1. American Society of Anesthesiologists. Basic Anesthetic Monitoring, Standards for (Effective July 1, 2011).
2. Merilainen PT. A differential paramagnetic sensor for breath-by-breath oximetry. *J Clin Monit.* 1990;6:65–73.
3. Roe PG, Tyler CK, Tennant R, et al. Oxygen analysers. An evaluation of five fuel cell models. *Anaesthesia.* 1987;42:175–181.
4. Meyer RM. Oxygen analyzers: Failure rates and life spans of galvanic cells. *J Clin Monit.* 1990;6:196–202.
5. Bageant RA. Oxygen analyzers. *Respir Care.* 1976;21:410–416.
6. Barker L, Webb RK, Runciman WB, et al. The Australian incident monitoring study. The oxygen analyser: Applications and limitations–an analysis of 200 incident reports. *Anaesth Intensive Care.* 1993;21:570–574.
7. Ortega R, Hansen CJ, Elterman K, et al. Videos in clinical medicine. Pulse oximetry. *N Engl J Med.* 2011;364:e33.
8. Brown M, Vender JS. Noninvasive oxygen monitoring. *Crit Care Clin.* 1988; 4:493–509.
9. Barker SJ, Curry J, Redford D, et al. Measurement of carboxyhemoglobin and methemoglobin by pulse oximetry: A human volunteer study. *Anesthesiology.* 2006; 105:892–897.
10. Barker SJ. "Motion-resistant" pulse oximetry: A comparison of new and old models. *Anesth Analg.* 2002;95:967–972, table of contents.
11. Nishiyama T. Pulse oximeters demonstrate different responses during hypothermia and changes in perfusion. *Can J Anaesth.* 2006;53:136–138.
12. Eberhard P, Severinghaus JW. Measurement of heated skin O2 diffusion conductance and PO_2 sensor induced O_2 gradient. *Acta Anaesthesiol Scand Suppl.* 1978;68:1–3.
13. Moller JT, Johannessen NW, Espersen K, et al. Randomized evaluation of pulse oximetry in 20,802 patients: II. Perioperative events and postoperative complications. *Anesthesiology.* 1993;78:445–453.
14. White DC, Wardley-Smith B. The "narkotest" anaesthetic gas meter. *Br J Anaesth.* 1972;44:1100–1104.
15. Westenskow DR, Silva FH. Laboratory evaluation of the vital signs (ICOR) piezoelectric anesthetic agent analyzer. *J Clin Monit.* 1991;7:189–194.
16. Jee GI, Roy RJ. Adaptive control of multiplexed closed-circuit anesthesia. *IEEE Trans Biomed Eng.* 1992;39:1071–1080.
17. Westenskow DR, Smith KW, Coleman DL, et al. Clinical evaluation of a Raman scattering multiple gas analyzer for the operating room. *Anesthesiology.* 1989;70: 350–355.
18. Craver CD, Coblentz Society. *The Coblentz Society Desk Book of Infrared Spectra.* 2nd ed. Kirkwood, MO (P.O. Box 9952, Kirkwood 63122): The Society; 1982.
19. Walder B, Lauber R, Zbinden AM. Accuracy and cross-sensitivity of 10 different anesthetic gas monitors. *J Clin Monit.* 1993;9:364–373.
20. Colman Y, Krauss B. Microstream capnograpy technology: A new approach to an old problem. *J Clin Monit Comput.* 1999;15:403–409.
21. Williamson JA, Webb RK, Cockings J, et al. The Australian incident monitoring study. The capnograph: Applications and limitations–an analysis of 2000 incident reports. *Anaesth Intensive Care.* 1993;21:551–557.
22. Lockwood GG, White DC. Measuring the costs of inhaled anaesthetics. *Br J Anaesth.* 2001;87:559–563.
23. Eger EI 2nd, Saidman LJ, Brandstater B. Minimum alveolar anesthetic concentration: A standard of anesthetic potency. *Anesthesiology.* 1965;26:756–763.
24. Eger EI 2nd. Age, minimum alveolar anesthetic concentration, and minimum alveolar anesthetic concentration-awake. *Anesth Analg.* 2001;93:947–953.
25. Avidan MS, Jacobsohn E, Glick D, et al. Prevention of intraoperative awareness in a high-risk surgical population. *N Engl J Med.* 2011;365:591–600.
26. Kleinman B, Powell S, Kumar P, et al. The fast flush test measures the dynamic response of the entire blood pressure monitoring system. *Anesthesiology.* 1992; 77:1215–1220.
27. Slogoff S, Keats AS, Arlund C. On the safety of radial artery cannulation. *Anesthesiology.* 1983;59:42–47.
28. McGregor AD. The Allen test—an investigation of its accuracy by fluorescein angiography. *J Hand Surg Br.* 1987;12:82–85.
29. Tegtmeyer K, Brady G, Lai S, et al. Videos in Clinical Medicine. Placement of an arterial line. *N Engl J Med.* 2006;354:e13.
30. Maher JJ, Dougherty JM. Radial artery cannulation guided by Doppler ultrasound. *Am J Emerg Med.* 1989;7:260–262.
31. Levin PD, Sheinin O, Gozal Y. Use of ultrasound guidance in the insertion of radial artery catheters. *Crit Care Med.* 2003;31:481–484.
32. Hobai IA, Bittner EA, Grecu L. Perioperative spinal cord infarction in nonaortic surgery: Report of three cases and review of the literature. *J Clin Anesth.* 2008;20:307–312.
33. Vender JS, Watts DR. Differential diagnosis of hand ischemia in the presence of an arterial cannula. *Anesth Analg.* 1982;61:465–468.
34. Gardner RM. Direct blood pressure measurement–dynamic response requirements. *Anesthesiology.* 1981;54:227–236.
35. Mangano DT, Hickey RF. Ischemic injury following uncomplicated radial artery catheterization. *Anesth Analg.* 1979;58:55–57.
36. Ng KG, Small CF. Survey of automated noninvasive blood pressure monitors. *J Clin Eng.* 1994;19:452–475.
37. Ramsey M 3rd. Blood pressure monitoring: Automated oscillometric devices. *J Clin Monit.* 1991;7:56–67.
38. Kaufmann MA, Pargger H, Drop LJ. Oscillometric blood pressure measurements by different devices are not interchangeable. *Anesth Analg.* 1996;82:377–381.
39. Institute ANS. *Manual, Electronic or Automated Sphygmomanometers.* New York, NY: American National Standard Institute; 2002.
40. IEC 60601-2-30. Particular requirements for the safety, including essential performance, of automatic cycling non-invasive blood pressure monitoring equipment. Geneva, Switzerland: International Electrotechnical Commission; 1999.
41. Dorsch JA, Dorsch SE. *Understanding Anesthesia Equipment.* 4th ed. Baltimore, MD: Williams & Wilkins; 1999.
42. Swei SC, Liou CC, Liu HH, et al. Acute radial nerve injury associated with an automatic blood pressure monitor. *Acta Anaesthesiol Taiwan.* 2009;47:147–149.
43. Lin CC, Jawan B, de Villa MV, et al. Blood pressure cuff compression injury of the radial nerve. *J Clin Anesth.* 2001;13:306–308.
44. Jones DW, Appel LJ, Sheps SG, et al. Measuring blood pressure accurately: New and persistent challenges. *JAMA.* 2003;289:1027–1030.
45. Webb RK, Russell WJ, Klepper I, et al. The Australian incident monitoring study. Equipment failure: An analysis of 2000 incident reports. *Anaesth Intensive Care.* 1993;21:673–677.
46. Loubser PG. Comparing direct and indirect arterial blood pressures. *Anesthesiology.* 1985;63:566–567.
47. Nystrom E, Reid KH, Bennett R, et al. A comparison of two automated indirect arterial blood pressure meters: With recordings from a radial arterial catheter in anesthetized surgical patients. *Anesthesiology.* 1985;62:526–530.

48. van Egmond J, Hasenbos M, Crul JF. Invasive vs. non-invasive measurement of arterial pressure. Comparison of two automatic methods and simultaneously measured direct intra-arterial pressure. *Br J Anaesth.* 1985;57:434–444.
49. Derrick JL, Bassin DJ. Sampling intervals to record severe hypotensive and hypoxic episodes in anesthetised patients. *J Clin Monit Comput.* 1998;14:347–351.
50. Harrison MJ, Connor CW. Statistics-based alarms from sequential physiological measurements. *Anaesthesia.* 2007;62:1015–1023.
51. Emerick DR. An evaluation of non-invasive blood pressure (NIBP) monitoring on the wrist: Comparison with upper arm NIBP measurement. *Anaesth Intensive Care.* 2002;30:43–47.
52. Singer AJ, Kahn SR, Thode HC Jr, et al. Comparison of forearm and upper arm blood pressures. *Prehosp Emerg Care.* 1999;3:123–126.
53. Block FE, Schulte GT. Ankle blood pressure measurement, an acceptable alternative to arm measurements. *Int J Clin Monit Comput.* 1996;13:167–171.
54. Zahn J, Bernstein H, Hossain S, et al. Comparison of non-invasive blood pressure measurements on the arm and calf during cesarean delivery. *J Clin Monit Comput.* 2000;16:557–562.
55. West JB, Dollery CT, Naimark A. Distribution of blood flow in isolated lung; relation to vascular and alveolar pressures. *J Appl Physiol.* 1964;19:713–724.
56. Vender JS. Invasive cardiac monitoring. *Crit Care Clin.* 1988;4:455–477.
57. Mark JB. Central venous pressure monitoring: Clinical insights beyond the numbers. *J Cardiothorac Vasc Anesth.* 1991;5:163–173.
58. Dizon CT, Barash PG. The value of monitoring pulmonary artery pressure in clinical practice. *Conn Med.* 1977;41:622–625.
59. Shah MR, Hasselblad V, Stevenson LW, et al. Impact of the pulmonary artery catheter in critically ill patients: Meta-analysis of randomized clinical trials. *JAMA.* 2005;294:1664–1670.
60. American Society of Anesthesiologists Task Force on Pulmonary Artery C. Practice guidelines for pulmonary artery catheterization: An updated report by the American Society of Anesthesiologists Task Force on Pulmonary Artery Catheterization. *Anesthesiology.* 2003;99:988–1014.
61. Ortega R, Song M, Hansen CJ, et al. Videos in clinical medicine. Ultrasound-guided internal jugular vein cannulation. *N Engl J Med.* 2010;362:e57.
62. O'Grady NP, Alexander M, Burns LA, et al. Summary of recommendations: Guidelines for the prevention of intravascular catheter-related infections. *Clin Infect Dis.* 2011;52:1087–1099.
63. Hamilton HC, Foxcroft DR. Central venous access sites for the prevention of venous thrombosis, stenosis and infection in patients requiring long-term intravenous therapy. *Cochrane Database Syst Rev.* 2007;18:CD004084.
64. Pronovost P, Needham D, Berenholtz S, et al. An intervention to decrease catheter-related bloodstream infections in the ICU. *N Engl J Med.* 2006;355:2725–2732.
65. Stewart GN. Researches on the circulation time and on the influences which affect it. *J Physiol.* 1897;22:159–183.
66. Hamilton WF, Riley RL, Attyah AM, et al. Comparison of the Fick and dye injection methods of measuring the cardiac output in man. *Am J Physiol.* 1948;153:309–321.
67. Fegler G. Measurement of cardiac output in anaesthetized animals by a thermodilution method. *Q J Exp Physiol Cogn Med Sci.* 1954;39:153–164.
68. Branthwaite MA, Bradley RD. Measurement of cardiac output by thermal dilution in man. *J Appl Physiol.* 1968;24:434–438.
69. Mihm FG, Gettinger A, Hanson CW 3rd, et al. A multicenter evaluation of a new continuous cardiac output pulmonary artery catheter system. *Crit Care Med.* 1998;26:1346–1350.
70. Scuderi PE, MacGregor DA, Bowton DL, et al. A laboratory comparison of three pulmonary artery oximetry catheters. *Anesthesiology.* 1994;81:245–253.
71. Koo KK, Sun JC, Zhou Q, et al. Pulmonary artery catheters: Evolving rates and reasons for use. *Crit Care Med.* 2011;39:1613–1618.
72. Pearl RG, Rosenthal MH, Nielson L, et al. Effect of injectate volume and temperature on thermodilution cardiac output determination. *Anesthesiology.* 1986;64:798–801.
73. Connors AF Jr, Speroff T, Dawson NV, et al. The effectiveness of right heart catheterization in the initial care of critically ill patients. SUPPORT Investigators. *JAMA.* 1996;276:889–897.
74. Harvey S, Harrison DA, Singer M, et al. Assessment of the clinical effectiveness of pulmonary artery catheters in management of patients in intensive care (PAC-Man): A randomised controlled trial. *Lancet.* 2005;366:472–477.
75. Thiele RH, Durieux ME. Arterial waveform analysis for the anesthesiologist: Past, present, and future concepts. *Anesth Analg.* 2011;113:766–776.
76. Critchley LA. Validation of the MostCare pulse contour cardiac output monitor: Beyond the Bland and Altman plot. *Anesth Analg.* 2011;113:1292–1294.
77. Sagawa K, Lie RK, Schaefer J. Translation of Otto Frank's paper "Die Grundform des Arteriellen Pulses" Zeitschrift fur Biologie 37: 483–526 (1899). *J Mol Cell Cardiol.* 1990;22:253–254.
78. Langewouters GJ, Wesseling KH, Goedhard WJ. The static elastic properties of 45 human thoracic and 20 abdominal aortas in vitro and the parameters of a new model. *J Biomech.* 1984;17:425–435.
79. Warner HR, Swan HJ, Connolly DC, et al. Quantitation of beat-to-beat changes in stroke volume from the aortic pulse contour in man. *J Appl Physiol.* 1953;5:495–507.
80. Maus TM, Lee DE. Arterial pressure-based cardiac output assessment. *J Cardiothorac Vasc Anesth.* 2008;22:468–473.
81. Meng L, Tran NP, Alexander BS, et al. The impact of phenylephrine, ephedrine, and increased preload on third-generation Vigileo-FloTrac and esophageal doppler cardiac output measurements. *Anesth Analg.* 2011;113:751–757.
82. Monnet X, Letierce A, Hamzaoui O, et al. Arterial pressure allows monitoring the changes in cardiac output induced by volume expansion but not by norepinephrine. *Crit Care Med.* 2011;39:1394–1399.
83. Biancofiore G, Critchley LA, Lee A, et al. Evaluation of a new software version of the FloTrac/Vigileo (version 3.02) and a comparison with previous data in cirrhotic patients undergoing liver transplant surgery. *Anesth Analg.* 2011;113:515–522.
84. Biais M, Nouette-Gaulain K, Cottenceau V, et al. Cardiac output measurement in patients undergoing liver transplantation: Pulmonary artery catheter versus uncalibrated arterial pressure waveform analysis. *Anesth Analg.* 2008;106:1480–1486, table of contents.
85. Monnet X, Anguel N, Naudin B, et al. Arterial pressure-based cardiac output in septic patients: Different accuracy of pulse contour and uncalibrated pressure waveform devices. *Crit Care.* 2010;14:R109.
86. Michard F. Changes in arterial pressure during mechanical ventilation. *Anesthesiology.* 2005;103:419–428; quiz 49–45.
87. Biais M, Nouette-Gaulain K, Cottenceau V, et al. Uncalibrated pulse contour-derived stroke volume variation predicts fluid responsiveness in mechanically ventilated patients undergoing liver transplantation. *Br J Anaesth.* 2008;101:761–768.
88. Lorsomradee S, Cromheecke S, De Hert SG. Uncalibrated arterial pulse contour analysis versus continuous thermodilution technique: Effects of alterations in arterial waveform. *J Cardiothorac Vasc Anesth.* 2007;21:636–643.
89. Opdam HI, Wan L, Bellomo R. A pilot assessment of the FloTrac cardiac output monitoring system. *Intensive Care Med.* 2007;33:344–349.
90. Slagt C, Beute J, Hoeksema M, et al. Cardiac output derived from arterial pressure waveform analysis without calibration vs. thermodilution in septic shock: Evolving accuracy of software versions. *Eur J Anaesthesiol.* 2010;27:550–554.
91. Yamakage M, Kawana S, Watanabe H, et al. The utility of tracheal temperature monitoring. *Anesth Analg.* 1993;76:795–799.
92. Sessler DI. Central thermoregulatory inhibition by general anesthesia. *Anesthesiology.* 1991;75:557–559.
93. Ozaki M, Kurz A, Sessler DI, et al. Thermoregulatory thresholds during epidural and spinal anesthesia. *Anesthesiology.* 1994;81:282–288.
94. Kurz A, Sessler DI, Lenhardt R. Perioperative normothermia to reduce the incidence of surgical-wound infection and shorten hospitalization. Study of wound infection and temperature group. *N Engl J Med.* 1996;334:1209–1215.
95. Frank SM, Fleisher LA, Breslow MJ, et al. Perioperative maintenance of normothermia reduces the incidence of morbid cardiac events. A randomized clinical trial. *JAMA.* 1997;277:1127–1134.
96. Vaughan MS, Cork RC, Vaughan RW. Inaccuracy of liquid crystal thermometry to identify core temperature trends in postoperative adults. *Anesth Analg.* 1982;61:284–287.
97. Rampil IJ. A primer for EEG signal processing in anesthesia. *Anesthesiology.* 1998;89:980–1002.
98. Burch NR, Nettleton WJ Jr., Sweeney J, et al. Period analysis of the electroencephalogram on a general-purpose digital computer. *Ann N Y Acad Sci.* 1964;115:827–843.
99. Doyle PW, Matta BF. Burst suppression or isoelectric encephalogram for cerebral protection: Evidence from metabolic suppression studies. *Br J Anaesth.* 1999;83:580–584.
100. Brenner RP, Schwartzman RJ, Richey ET. Prognostic significance of episodic low amplitude or relatively isoelectric EEG patterns. *Dis Nerv Syst.* 1975;36:582–587.
101. Cooley JW, Tukey JW. An algorithm for machine calculation of complex Fourier series. *Math Comp.* 1965;19:297–301.
102. Proakis JG. *Advanced Digital Signal Processing.* New York, Toronto: Macmillan; Maxwell Macmillan Canada; Maxwell Macmillan International; 1992.
103. Kreuer S, Bruhn J, Larsen R, et al. Comparison of BIS and AAI as measures of anaesthetic drug effect during desflurane–remifentanil anaesthesia. *Acta Anaesthesiol Scand.* 2004;48:1168–1173.
104. Whitlock EL, Villafranca AJ, Lin N, et al. Relationship between bispectral index values and volatile anesthetic concentrations during the maintenance phase of anesthesia in the B-Unaware trial. *Anesthesiology.* 2011;115:1209–1218.
105. Tirel O, Wodey E, Harris R, et al. Variation of bispectral index under TIVA with propofol in a paediatric population. *Br J Anaesth.* 2008;100:82–87.
106. Hans P, Dewandre PY, Brichant JF, et al. Comparative effects of ketamine on bispectral index and spectral entropy of the electroencephalogram under sevoflurane anaesthesia. *Br J Anaesth.* 2005;94:336–340.
107. Faraoni D, Salengros JC, Engelman E, et al. Ketamine has no effect on bispectral index during stable propofol-remifentanil anaesthesia. *Br J Anaesth.* 2009;102:336–339.
108. Yufune S, Takamatsu I, Masui K, et al. Effect of remifentanil on plasma propofol concentration and bispectral index during propofol anaesthesia. *Br J Anaesth.* 2011;106:208–214.
109. Brandes IF, Stuth EA. Use of BIS monitor in a child with congenital insensitivity to pain with anhidrosis. *Paediatr Anaesth.* 2006;16:466–470.
110. Crosby G. General anesthesia–minding the mind during surgery. *N Engl J Med.* 2011;365:660–661.

111. Gan TJ, Glass PS, Windsor A, et al. Bispectral index monitoring allows faster emergence and improved recovery from propofol, alfentanil, and nitrous oxide anesthesia. BIS utility study group. *Anesthesiology.* 1997;87:808–815.
112. Chin KJ, Yeo SW. A BIS-guided study of sevoflurane requirements for adequate depth of anaesthesia in Caesarean section. *Anaesthesia.* 2004;59:1064–1068.
113. Fraser GL, Riker RR. Bispectral index monitoring in the intensive care unit provides more signal than noise. *Pharmacotherapy.* 2005;25:19S–27S.
114. Vivien B, Di Maria S, Ouattara A, et al. Overestimation of bispectral index in sedated intensive care unit patients revealed by administration of muscle relaxant. *Anesthesiology.* 2003;99:9–17.
115. Pousman RM, Eilers WA 3rd, Johns B, et al. Irritant contact dermatitis after use of bispectral index sensor in prone position. *Anesth Analg.* 2002;95:1337–1338, table of contents.
116. Myles PS, Leslie K, McNeil J, et al. Bispectral index monitoring to prevent awareness during anaesthesia: The B-Aware randomised controlled trial. *Lancet.* 2004; 363:1757–1763.
117. Avidan MS, Zhang L, Burnside BA, et al. Anesthesia awareness and the bispectral index. *N Engl J Med.* 2008;358:1097–1108.
118. Sleigh JW. Depth of Anesthesia: Perhaps the patient isn't a submarine. *Anesthesiology.* 2011;115:1149–1150.
119. Dehaene S, Changeux JP. Experimental and theoretical approaches to conscious processing. *Neuron.* 2011;70:200–227.
120. Kandel ER. The biology of memory: A forty-year perspective. *J Neurosci.* 2009; 29:12748–12756.
121. Brown EN, Lydic R, Schiff ND. General anesthesia, sleep, and coma. *N Engl J Med.* 2010;363:2638–2650.

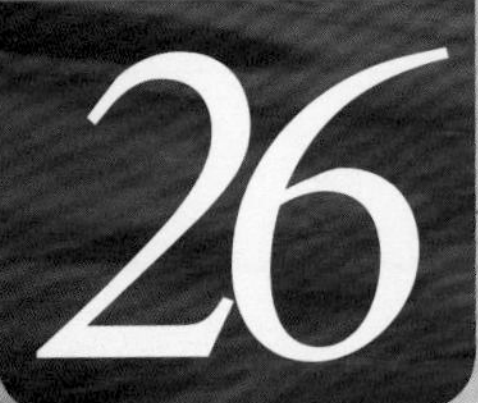

CHAPTER 26

Echocardiography

ALBERT C. PERRINO JR • WANDA M. POPESCU • NIKOLAOS J. SKUBAS

Key Points

1. Understanding the principles of ultrasound and echocardiographic instrumentation is essential in optimizing image quality.
2. Performing a comprehensive echocardiographic examination ensures that important pathologies are recognized.
3. Two-dimensional and Doppler techniques have complementary roles in the assessment of cardiovascular function.
4. Global left ventricular systolic function is influenced by load and contractility alterations; regional wall motion grading is based on systolic endocardial excursion and myocardial thickening.
5. Transmitral flow and pulmonary vein flow Doppler along with tissue Doppler imaging provide accurate diastolic function assessment.
6. Severity of aortic stenosis is estimated based on the aortic valve area calculated by continuity equation.
7. The ratio of the width of the regurgitant jet to the diameter of the left ventricular outflow tract is useful in assessing the severity of aortic insufficiency. Diastolic flow reversal in the descending thoracic aorta is significant for severe aortic insufficiency.
8. Mitral regurgitation can be of structural or functional etiology. The vena contracta of the regurgitant jet and the effective regurgitant orifice area by proximal isovelocity surface area method help grade severity.
9. Aortic atheromas larger than 4 mm are harbingers of thromboembolic events.
10. The false lumen of aortic dissection does not have diastolic flow.

Multimedia

1. TEE Probe Movements
2. ME Ascending Aortic LAX and SAX
3. ME AV SAX
4. ME AV LAX
5. ME Bicaval
6. ME RV Inflow–outflow
7. ME Four Chamber
8. ME Two Chamber
9. ME Commissural View
10. ME LAX
11. TG Mid SAX
12. TG Basal SAX
13. TG Two Chamber
14. TG LAX
15. Deep TG LAX
16. Desc Aortic SAX and LAX
17. UE Aortic Arch SAX
18. UE Aortic Arch LAX

Echocardiography is the first imaging technique to enter the mainstream of intraoperative patient monitoring. A remarkably versatile tool, real-time echocardiography provides a comprehensive evaluation of myocardial, valvular, and hemodynamic performances. These capabilities attracted the attention of anesthesiologists and surgeons challenged by the unique difficulties of perioperative cardiovascular management. Over the 30 years following the first report of intraoperative echocardiography to assess ventricular function by Barash and colleagues in 1978, echocardiography has emerged as the technique of choice for a wide variety of intraoperative case challenges.[1]

The benefit of intraoperative echocardiography in both cardiac and noncardiac surgical populations is supported by several case series.[2–8] Applications range from guiding the placement of intracardiac and intravascular catheters and devices, to the assessment of the severity of valve pathology and immediate evaluation of a surgical intervention, to the rapid diagnosis of acute hemodynamic instability and directing appropriate therapies.[9–11] Consequently, expertise in intraoperative echocardiography is highly desired among anesthesiology practitioners. The National Board of Echocardiography has established a certification pathway in perioperative transesophageal echocardiography (TEE), http://www.echoboards.org/certification/certexpl.html. The American Society of Anesthesiologists in conjunction with the National Board of Echocardiography has established a second certification pathway in basic perioperative echocardiography, http://www.asahq.org/publicationsAndServices/standards/TEE.pdf and, www.echoboards.org/content/basic-pteexam. These efforts are unique in intraoperative monitoring and attest to the critical role that accurate and thorough echocardiographic interpretation plays in current anesthetic practice.

PRINCIPLES AND TECHNOLOGY OF ECHOCARDIOGRAPHY

Echocardiography generates dynamic images of the heart from the reflections of sound waves. The echocardiography system transmits a brief pulse of high-frequency sound (i.e., ultrasound) that propagates through and is subsequently reflected from the cardiac structures encountered. The ultrasound transducer records the time delay and signal intensity for each
1 returning reflection. Since the speed of sound in tissue is constant, the time delay allows the echo system to precisely calculate the location of cardiac structures and thereby create an image map of the heart.

Physics of Sound

Sound is the vibration of a physical medium. In clinical echocardiography, a mechanical vibrator, known as the *transducer,* is placed in contact with the esophagus (TEE), skin (transthoracic echocardiography [TTE]), or the heart (epicardial echocardiography) to create tissue vibrations. The resulting tissue vibrations create a longitudinal wave with alternating areas of *compression* and *rarefaction* (Fig. 26-1).

The *amplitude* of a sound wave represents its peak pressure and is appreciated as loudness. The level of sound energy in an area of tissue is referred to as *intensity.* The intensity of the sound signal is proportional to the square of the amplitude and is an important factor regarding the potential for tissue damage with ultrasound. Since levels of sound pressure vary over a large range, it is convenient to use the logarithmic decibel (dB) scale:

$$\text{Decibel (dB)} = 10 \log_{10} I/Ir = 10 \log_{10} A^2/A_r^2 = 20 \log_{10} A/A_r$$

where A is the measured sound amplitude and A_r is a standard reference sound level; I is the intensity and I_r is a standard reference intensity. The Food and Drug Administration limits the intensity output of cardiac ultrasound systems to be <720 W/cm^2 because of concerns of potential tissue injury.[12]

Sound waves are also characterized by their *frequency* (f), or pitch, expressed in cycles per second, or Hertz (Hz), and by their *wavelength* (λ). These attributes significantly impact the depth of penetration of a sound wave in tissue and the image resolution of the ultrasound system.

The propagation *velocity* of sound (v) is determined solely by the medium through which it passes. In soft tissue, the speed of sound is approximately 1,540 m/s. As the product of wavelength and frequency equals velocity: $V = \lambda \times f$, it becomes apparent that the wavelength and frequency are inversely related: $\lambda = v \times 1/f$ and that $\lambda = (1{,}540 \text{ m/s})f$. High-frequency, short-wavelength ultrasound is more easily focused and directed to a specific target location. Image resolution also increases with short-wavelength

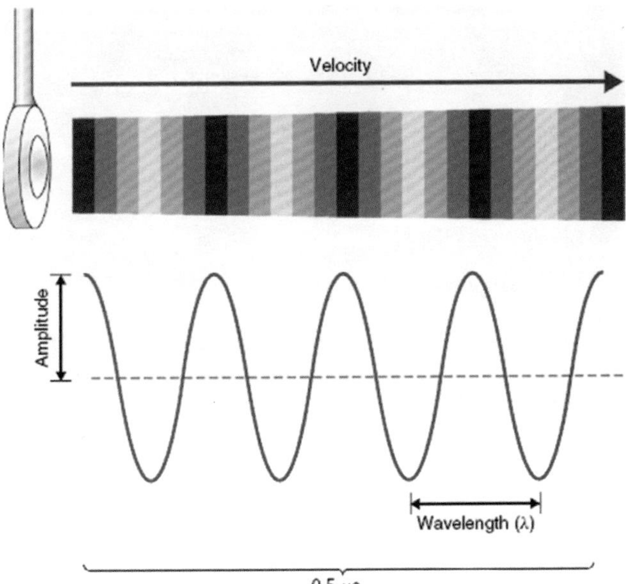

FIGURE 26-1. Sound wave. Vibrations of the ultrasound transducer create cycles of compression and rarefaction in the adjacent tissue. The ultrasound energy is characterized by its amplitude, wavelength, frequency, and propagation velocity. In this example, four sound waves are shown in a period of 0.5 μs. The frequency can be calculated as four cycles divided by 0.5 μs and equals 8 MHz.

sound waves; for these reasons, ultrasonic frequencies of 2 to 10 MHz are preferred in clinical echocardiography.

Properties of Sound Transmission in Tissue

The propagation of a sound wave through the body is markedly affected by its interactions with the various tissues encountered. These interactions result in reflection, refraction, scattering, and attenuation of the ultrasound signal and determine the resulting appearance of the two-dimensional image.

Echocardiographic imaging relies on the transmission and subsequent reflection of ultrasound energy back to the transducer. A sound wave propagates smoothly through uniform tissue until it encounters the interface between two tissues varying in acoustic impedance (a property largely related to the *density* [ρ] of the tissue and the speed that ultrasound travels). A large interface oriented perpendicular to the sound beam will produce a mirror-like reflection of sound back toward the transducer with only a portion of the signal passing through the interface. Since cardiac structures are detected by their reflected echocardiography signal, echocardiographers adjust the position of the TEE transducer so that the direction of its beam is perpendicular to the cardiac structure of interest.

Refraction causes a change in direction of propagating sound and occurs when an interface lies oblique to the sound beam. Refraction is an important factor in the formation of artifacts as the transducer mistakenly interprets a reflection from the refracted beam as originating from a cardiac structure located within the *intended* scanning field.

Scattering reflections occur when an ultrasound beam encounters small or irregularly shaped surfaces, such as red blood cells. These reflectors scatter ultrasound energy in all directions, so that far less energy is reflected back to the transducer. This type of reflection is the basis of the Doppler analysis of blood flow (see following).

Even when traveling through uniform tissue, sound undergoes a steady loss (i.e., *attenuation*) in intensity as a consequence of dispersion and absorption. Attenuation results in less energy returning to the transducer and low-quality images with poor signal-to-noise ratios. To combat attenuation, echocardiographers select better penetrating low-frequency signals (e.g., 2.5 instead of 7.5 MHz) and choose an imaging window that is close to the structure of interest. Adjusting the gain controls to amplify the weak returning signals makes their appearance brighter on the display. Unfortunately, this increases the brightness of artifactual noise, which negatively impacts the image appearance.

Instrumentation

Transducers

Ultrasound transducers use piezoelectric crystals to create a brief pulse of ultrasound. Alternating electrical current stimulates polarized particles within the crystal's matrix to rapidly vibrate, generating ultrasound. Conversely, when a sound reflection strikes the crystal, the impact vibrates the polarized particles and generates an electric current. This property allows the piezoelectric crystal to function as both a transmitter and a receiver of ultrasound.

The shorter the length of the sound pulses, the better the axial resolution of the system. High-resolution imaging transducers emit sound pulses of just two to four cycles of short-wavelength, high-frequency sound.

Beam Shape

The ultrasound transducer emits a three-dimensional ultrasound beam similar to a movie projection (Fig. 26-2). The beam is narrow in the near field and then diverges into the far field zone. Focusing of the beam is used to improve spatial resolution by narrowing the ultrasound beam at the desired depth. The dense, narrow beam is preferred because it provides improved spatial resolution, produces high-intensity reflections, and reduces artifact. Echocardiographers adjust focal depth and focus to optimize the image resolution.

Resolution

Three parameters are evaluated when assessing the resolution of an ultrasound system: The resolution of objects lying along the axis of the ultrasound beam (*axial resolution*), the resolution of objects horizontal to the beam's orientation (*lateral resolution*), and the resolution of objects lying vertical to the beam's orientation (*elevational resolution*).

Short pulses of high-frequency ultrasound offer the greatest axial resolution but have a decreased tissue penetration. As resolution is highest along the axial plane, echocardiographic measurements are most precise when taken parallel to the beam's axis. Accordingly, echocardiographers select transmitted frequency based on the particular imaging need.

Beam size determines the lateral and elevational resolution. Broad beams produce a "smeared" image of two nearby objects, whereas narrow beams can identify each object individually. Beam size is reduced by selecting high-signal frequencies and minimizing imaging depth.

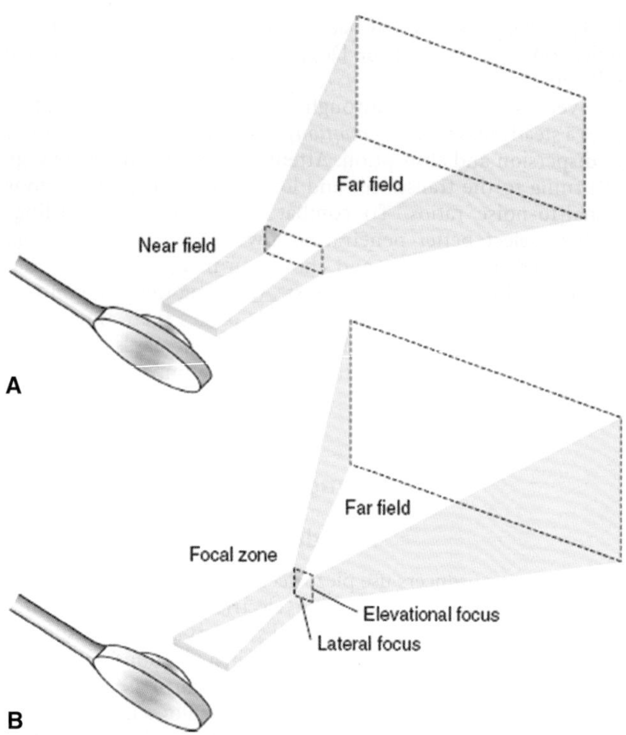

FIGURE 26-2. Three-dimensional beam. The ultrasound probe projects a three-dimensional beam. The dimensions of this projection have important effects on the imaging resolution and artifact. Typically, a narrow profile is preferred. **A:** Unfocused beam. The beam is narrow in the near field and then diverges in the far field. **B:** Focused beam. Focusing has resulted in a narrower beam in both the lateral and elevational planes, so that the imaging resolution of structures in the focal zone is improved. Distal to the focal zone, the beam rapidly diverges, and the images of structures in this area will be of lower quality.

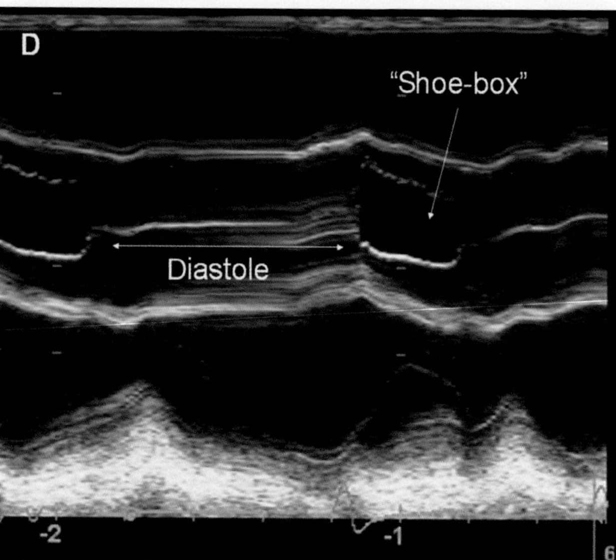

FIGURE 26-3. Method-mode (M-mode) echocardiography of a normal aortic valve. The M-mode cursor is placed at the center of the aortic valve and the motion of the aortic cusps over time is shown. During diastolic coaptation the aortic valve cusps appear as a thick, bright white line (*long arrow*), while in systolic apposition they form a "shoe-box" (*short arrow*).

Signal Processing

To convert echoes into images, the returning ultrasound pulses are received, electronically processed, and displayed. The oscillator repeatedly cycles the transducer from a brief transmission to a relatively long receive mode. During the receive phase, the reflected echocardiography signals are captured and converted to electrical signals by the piezoelectric crystal. The echocardiography system employs a series of controls including system gain, time gain compensation, compression, and postprocessing settings (not unlike those available with digital imaging software) to optimize the signal for display. Adjustments are used, for example, to emphasize edge detection versus tissue texture, or to improve the delineation of weaker reflectors. The choice of settings is dictated by the examination and the preferences of the echocardiographer.

Image Display

Ultrasonic imaging is based on the amplitude and time delay of the reflected signals. Since the velocity in tissue is a relatively constant 1,540 m/s, only the distance of the structure from the transducer alters the time required for the ultrasound wave to travel to and from the reflected structure. So by timing the interval between transmission and return of the reflections, the echocardiography system can precisely calculate the distance of a structure from the transducer.

Current imaging is based on brightness mode or *B-mode technology*. With B-mode, the amplitude of the returning echoes from a single pulse determines the display brightness of the representative pixels. *M-mode* or motion mode adds temporal information to B-mode by displaying a series of sequentially collected B-mode images. M-mode echocardiography provides a one-dimensional, single-beam view through the heart but updates the B-mode images at a very high rate, providing dynamic real-time imaging. M-mode remains the best technique for examining the timing of cardiac events (Fig. 26-3).

Two-dimensional (2-D) echocardiography is a modification of B-mode echocardiography and the mainstay of the echocardiographic examination. Instead of repeatedly firing ultrasound pulses in a single direction, the transducer in 2-D echocardiography sequentially directs the ultrasound pulses across a sector of the cardiac anatomy. In this way, 2-D imaging displays a tomographic section of the cardiac anatomy, and unlike M-mode, reveals the shape and lateral motion (Fig. 26-4).

Two-dimensional scanning is achieved using phased array technology, which sequentially activates each crystal in the array and thereby steers the beam without the transducer itself being moved. The two commonly used electronic scanning systems in medical ultrasound are the linear scanners and sector scanners.

The *linear scanner* uses a long linear array. Groups of crystals are activated sequentially from one end of the transducer to the other. The firing of each group of crystals creates an image of the structures directly in front of them. With sequential firing, the anatomic features from one end of the transducer to the other are imaged (Fig. 26-5). The disadvantage of this approach is that the transducer face must be large to cover a broad anatomic area. The linear array is commonly used to guide vascular access and regional anesthetic procedures.

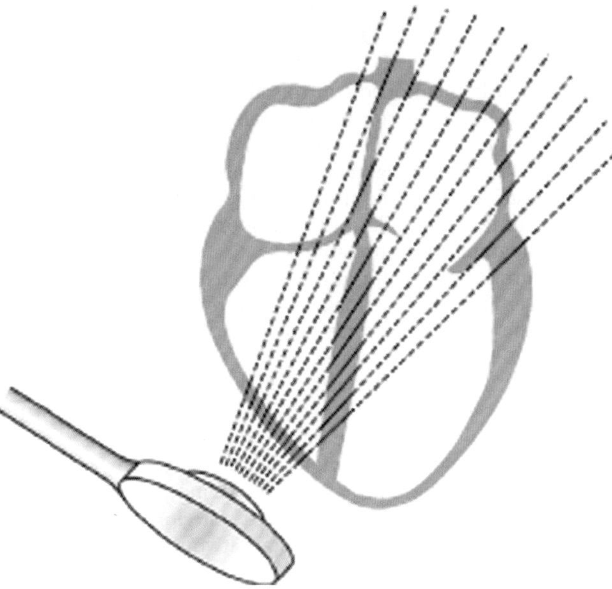

FIGURE 26-4. Scan lines. Illustration of the arced sector from a phased array two-dimensional echocardiogram. Each dotted line represents an individual brightness mode scan line. Any structure that interacts with a scan line will create reflections (*dark highlight*); however, structures that lie between the scan lines are not interrogated, and the echocardiography system averages the neighboring signals to fill in this defect. Accordingly, the closer the scan lines, the better the image quality.

The phased array *sector scanner* is the most commonly used in echocardiography. Here the ultrasound scan is sequentially directed in a fan-like arc. The resulting sector image known as a *frame* is similar in shape to that covered by a windshield wiper. The 2-D scanner then repeats the entire process to update the image and capture motion.

Spatial Versus Dynamic Image Quality

Expert echocardiographers select machine settings to optimize particular image qualities for the examination at hand. As discussed in the following sections, these selections will determine whether sector size, spatial resolution, or dynamic motion is best displayed.

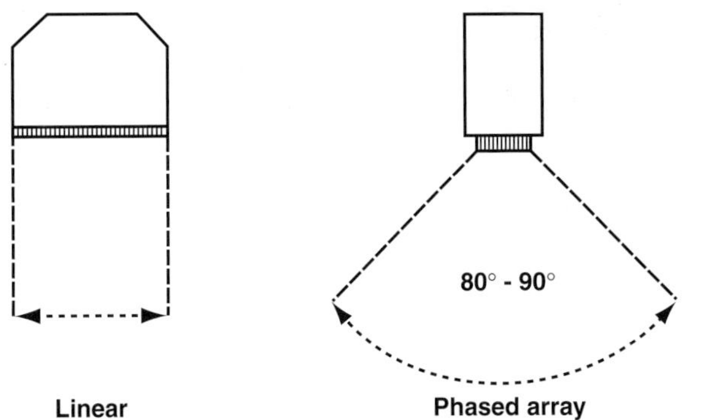

FIGURE 26-5. Linear scanners image a rectangular section of the anatomy compared with the arced sector imaged with phased array scanners.

The *pulse repetition frequency* is the rate at which sound pulses are triggered. The greater the pulse repetition frequency, the greater the number of scan lines that are emitted in a given period of time. This enhances motion display. Unfortunately, sector depth must be reduced because pulse repetition frequency is inversely related to the sector depth as a longer period of time is required for the ultrasound to travel the increased distances.

The *frame rate* is the frequency at which the sector is rescanned. A high frame rate improves the capture of movement. Typically, frame rates >30 per second are desired. The frame rate is critically dependent on the sector depth, which determines the time required for each scan line to be received, and the sector width, which increases the number of scan lines that must be transmitted. Consequently, increases in sector size and depth come at the cost of a decreased frame rate and poor motion imaging.

The number of scan lines per degree of the sector (*scan line density*) greatly affects the image resolution. Doubling the scan lines essentially doubles the lateral resolution. However, the cost is a decrease in the frame rate and motion imaging.

The echocardiographer must thoughtfully select among settings that will often have opposing effects between the size of the imaging field, the imaging resolution, and the frame rate. A common approach is to focus each part of the examination on a given structure of interest and select the imaging plane that best delineates the structure in the near field. Motion display can then be enhanced without costs in lateral resolution by decreasing the sector angle and depth. In situations in which the maximal frame rate is desired, M-mode is chosen.

TWO-DIMENSIONAL AND THREE-DIMENSIONAL TRANSESOPHAGEAL ECHOCARDIOGRAPHY EXAMINATION

TEE is the favored approach to intraoperative echocardiography. Compared with TTE, TEE offers additional "windows" to view the heart, often with improved image quality from the anatomic proximity of the esophagus and heart. In the operating room (OR), TEE is useful because the probe does not interfere with the operative field and can be left in situ, providing continuous, real-time hemodynamic information used to diagnose and manage critical cardiac events. TEE is also useful in situations in which the transthoracic examination is limited by various factors (obesity, emphysema, surgical dressings, and prosthetic valves) and for examining cardiac structures not well visualized with TTE (left atrial appendage).

This section is designed to introduce TEE image orientation and the diagnostic utility of each view. In addition, examination sequences useful for obtaining a comprehensive or targeted examination are provided. Readers are referred to *A Practical Approach to Transesophageal Echocardiography.*[13] for a more detailed description of the TEE examinations described in this section.

Probe Insertion

1 The TEE probe is inserted in the anesthetized patient in a manner similar to insertion of an orogastric tube. For improved image quality, the stomach is emptied of gastric contents and air prior to probe insertion. The jaw is lifted with the left hand and the TEE probe, well lubricated, is inserted with the right hand by applying gentle but constant pressure. If significant

resistance is encountered, additional force should be strictly avoided as oropharyngeal or esophageal injury may result. Rather, a decrease in neck extension and/or use of a laryngoscope to visualize the oropharyngeal structures often will allow easy passage of the probe. The TEE probe is advanced beyond the larynx and the cricopharyngeal muscle (around 25 to 30 cm from teeth) until a loss of resistance is appreciated. At this point, the TEE probe lies in the upper esophagus and the first cardiovascular images are seen. Extrinsic compression of the esophagus (e.g., osteophytes or an aortic aneurysm) may impede probe placement.[9,10]

Transesophageal Echocardiography Safety

TEE is a semi-invasive procedure. When performed by qualified operators, TEE has a low incidence of complications. A retrospective study performed on 846 patients who underwent TEE described the following complications: Three patients with pharyngeal abrasions, one patient with a chipped tooth, and few patients with transient vocal cord paresis.[14] Another retrospective study performed on a large case series of 7,200 patients showed that the morbidity associated with TEE placement is 0.2% and the mortality is 0%.[15] The most common complaint (0.1%) was postoperative odynophagia. Various studies have suggested an association between swallowing dysfunction after cardiac surgery and the use of intraoperative TEE.[16,17] This fact is important as postoperative swallowing dysfunction is associated with pulmonary complications.[16]

Contraindication to Transesophageal Echocardiography Probe Placement

To maintain the safety profile of TEE, each patient should be evaluated before the procedure for signs, symptoms, or history of esophageal pathology. Amongst the most feared complications of TEE are esophageal or gastric perforation.[18] For skilled practitioners, this complication is extremely rare. Patients with extensive esophageal and gastric diseases are at highest risk of perforation. Contraindications to TEE probe placement are represented by esophageal stricture, rings or webs, esophageal masses (especially malignant tumors), recent bleeding of esophageal varices, Zenker's diverticulum, status post radiation to the neck, and recent gastric bypass surgery.[13,18] In the rare case in which TEE is essential and is the only alternative, placement of the TEE probe can be performed under direct visualization with a combined gastroscopic and echocardiographic examination.[13]

Probe Manipulation

Image acquisition depends on precise manipulation of the TEE probe. By advancing the shaft of the probe, the probe position can be moved from the upper esophagus to the midesophagus and into the stomach. The shaft can also be manually rotated to the left or to the right. By using the large knob on the probe handle, the head of the probe can be anteflexed (turning the knob clockwise) and retroflexed (turning the knob counter clockwise). The smaller knob, located on top of the large knob, is used to tilt the head of the probe to the right or to the left. Using the electronic switch on the probe handle, the operator can rotate the ultrasound beam from 0 (transverse plane) to 180 degrees in 1-degree increments.

Orientation

The previously mentioned controls allow the experienced echocardiographers to perform comprehensive cardiac imaging. However, the diversity of imaging planes can confuse the less experienced echocardiographers, leaving them unable to recognize the various anatomic structures presented. Thus, an understanding of the basic rules of imaging orientation is essential to echocardiographic interpretation.

The ultrasound beam is always directed perpendicular to the probe face. The 2-D TEE image is displayed as a sector scan. The apex of the sector is in close proximity to the TEE probe and the structures seen in this area will be the posterior ones (e.g., left atrium). The arc of the sector will display the more distal and thereby more anterior structures. The angle of rotation of the imaging array determines the right and left orientations. An easy way to understand this orientation is to place your right hand in front of your chest with the palm facing down, the thumb oriented left and the fingers oriented anterior right. The scan lines that generate the TEE image start at your fingers and sweep toward the thumb. Consequently, the right anatomic structures will be displayed on the left side of the monitor (similar to chest x-ray orientation; Fig. 26-6). Increasing the imaging plane angle produces clockwise rotation of the sector scan. This can be visualized by rotating your hand in a clockwise fashion. For example, at the 90-degree imaging plane the left side of the screen now displays posterior structures (note position of fingers) and the right side of the screen anterior structures (note the position of the thumb; Fig. 26-7).

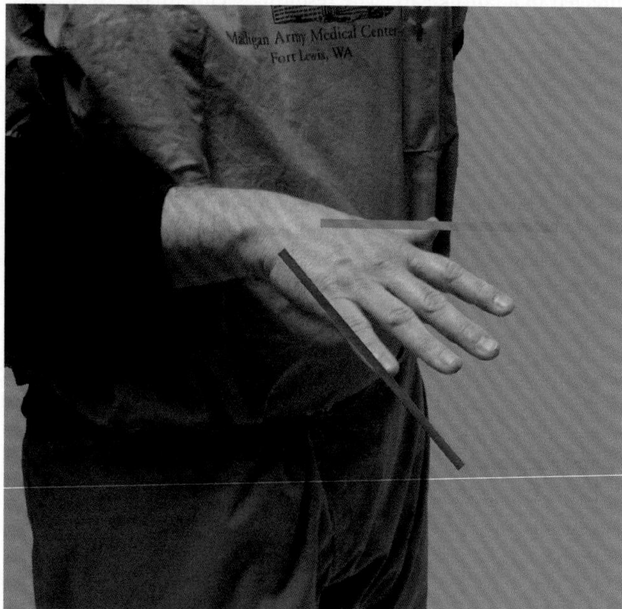

FIGURE 26-6. Orientation of the hand, as described in the text, for an imaging plane of 0 degree. The imaging plane is projected like a wedge anteriorly through the heart. The image is created by multiple scan lines traveling back and forth from the patient's left (*green line*) to the patient's right (*red line*). The resulting image is displayed on the monitor as a sector with the green edge (*green line*) on the right side of the monitor and the red edge (*red line*) on the left.

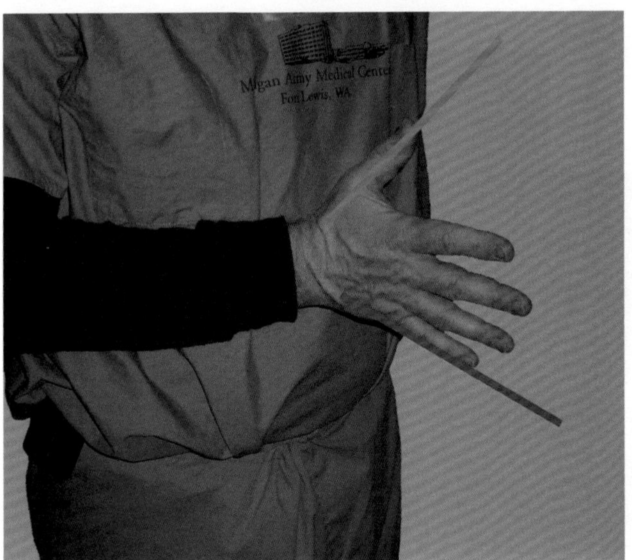

FIGURE 26-7. Orientation of the hand, as described in the text, for an imaging plane of 90 degrees. The imaging sector is rotated so that the green edge (*green line*) has moved clockwise and is now cephalad and the red edge is now caudad. As previously described, the green edge is displayed on the right side of the monitor and the red edge on the left.

Goals of the Two-dimensional Examination

2 Each TEE examination is performed with the goal that no important diagnosis is missed. For this reason, a comprehensive evaluation is preferred with each cardiac chamber and valve imaged in at least two orthogonal planes. However, in an emergency situation, such examination may not be possible. In these cases, most echocardiographers will focus the TEE examination to those views most likely to provide a diagnosis, that is, in a hypotensive patient the transgastric short-axis view of the left ventricle is examined for diagnosing hypovolemia, coronary ischemia, or acute heart failure.

To achieve the goals of the intraoperative TEE examination, the Society of Cardiovascular Anesthesiologists together with the American Society of Echocardiography has published guidelines for performing a comprehensive intraoperative TEE examination.[19] These guidelines include 20 standardized 2-D echocardiographic views. Each TEE examination should be recorded (video tapes or digital media) along with a detailed report of the examination. Miller et al.[20] proposed a shortened version of the comprehensive examination that would meet the goals established by these guidelines for basic intraoperative TEE proficiency and is particularly useful when time constraints preclude a more extensive examination. The sequence in which the views are acquired differs among echocardiographers. In the following section, we detail the acquisition and anatomic features of the most commonly used intraoperative views.

1. The midesophageal ascending aorta short-axis view.
   This view is obtained by advancing the probe slightly from the upper esophagus until the ascending aorta (AA) is seen and then rotating the multiplane angle from 0 to 45 degrees to obtain a true short axis. This "great vessel view" images the AA in short axis and the main pulmonary artery (PA) with its bifurcation and right PA in long axis and the superior vena cava in short axis (Fig. 26-8). If the multiplane angle is advanced by ~90 degrees, then the midesophageal AA long-axis view is obtained, in which the AA is visualized in a longitudinal cut and the right PA is visualized as a circular cross-sectional cut (Fig. 26-9). The main uses of the midesophageal ascending aorta short-axis view are to:
   a. Measure the AA dimensions and evaluate the presence of dissection flaps
   b. Evaluate the PA (position of catheter or rule out thrombus)
   c. Align the Doppler beam parallel to the blood flow in the main PA
2. The midesophageal aortic valve short-axis view.
   This view is obtained from the previous view by advancing the probe until the aortic valve (AV) is visible, and then rotating the multiplane angle between 30 and 60 degrees. In

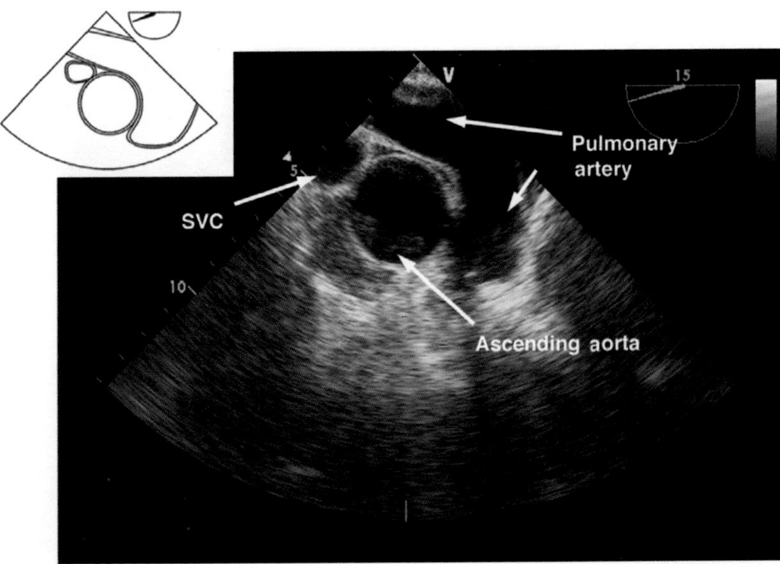

FIGURE 26-8. Midesophageal ascending aortic short-axis view. SVC, superior vena cava.

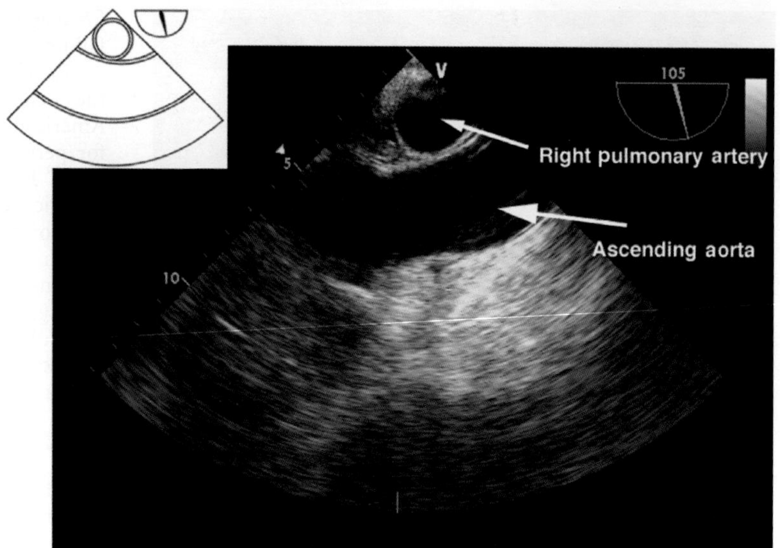

FIGURE 26-9. Midesophageal ascending aortic long-axis view.

the closed position, the three cusps of the AV form what is known as the "Mercedes Benz" sign (Fig. 26-10). This view is used to:

a. Evaluate the size, number, appearance and motion of AV cusps
b. Measure the area of the AV orifice (planimetry)
c. Evaluate the presence of aortic insufficiency (AI) or aortic stenosis (AS) by applying color flow Doppler (CFD)
d. Assess the interatrial septum for patent foramen ovale (PFO) or atrial septal defect (ASD)

3. The midesophageal aortic valve long-axis view.
This view is obtained from the previous view by rotating the multiplane angle to 120 to 160 degrees (Fig. 26-11). The view is used to assess:
   a. The AV annulus, sinus of Valsalva, sinotubular junction, and AA dimensions
   b. AI by using CFD
   c. Vegetations or masses attached to the AV
   d. Left ventricular outflow tract (LVOT) pathology (e.g., hypertrophic septum with possible LVOT obstruction)
   e. The presence of calcification or dissection flaps in the proximal AA
4. The midesophageal bicaval view.
This view is obtained from the previous view by turning the probe shaft to the patient's right and decreasing the multiplane angle to ~110 degrees (Fig. 26-12). The view is used to:
   a. Assess the interatrial septum (aided by CFD) to detect a PFO or ASD. Evaluate the passage of agitated saline across the interatrial septum following release of a Valsalva maneuver
   b. Guide placement of catheters, wires, and cannulae
   c. Examine for the presence of thrombus or tumors

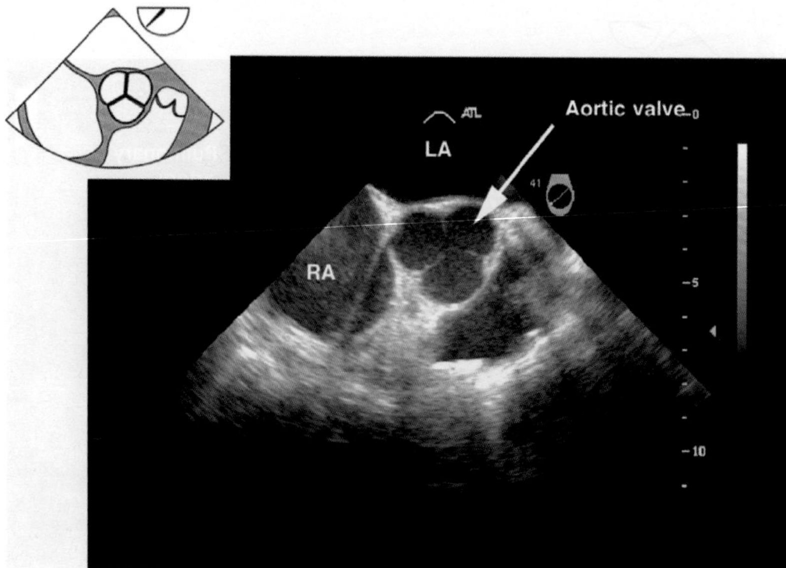

FIGURE 26-10. Midesophageal aortic valve short-axis view. RA, right atrium; LA, left atrium.

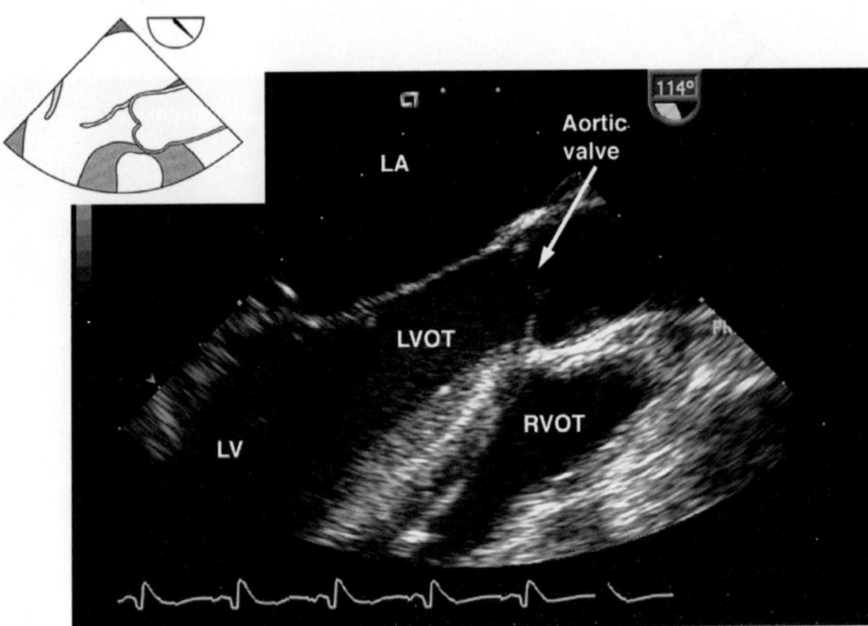

FIGURE 26-11. Midesophageal aortic valve long-axis view. LA, left atrium; LV, left ventricle; LVOT, left ventricular outflow tract; RVOT, right ventricular outflow tract.

6 5. The midesophageal right ventricular inflow–outflow view. This view is obtained from the previous view by decreasing the multiplane angle to approximately 60 to 90 degrees (Fig. 26-13). The main uses of the view are to evaluate the:

a. Pulmonary valve (PV) by measuring the pulmonary annulus and to detect pulmonary insufficiency by applying CFD
b. RV and right ventricular outflow tract (RVOT) structure and function
c. Tricuspid valve (TV) anatomy and function by aligning the Doppler beam with the RV diastolic blood inflow or a systolic regurgitation
d. Passage of a PAC across the RV to the PA

7 6. The midesophageal four-chamber view.
This view is obtained from the previous view by returning the multiplane angle between 0 and 20 degrees and slightly advancing the probe to the level of the mitral valve (MV). In this view, the four cardiac chambers and the TV and MV are visualized

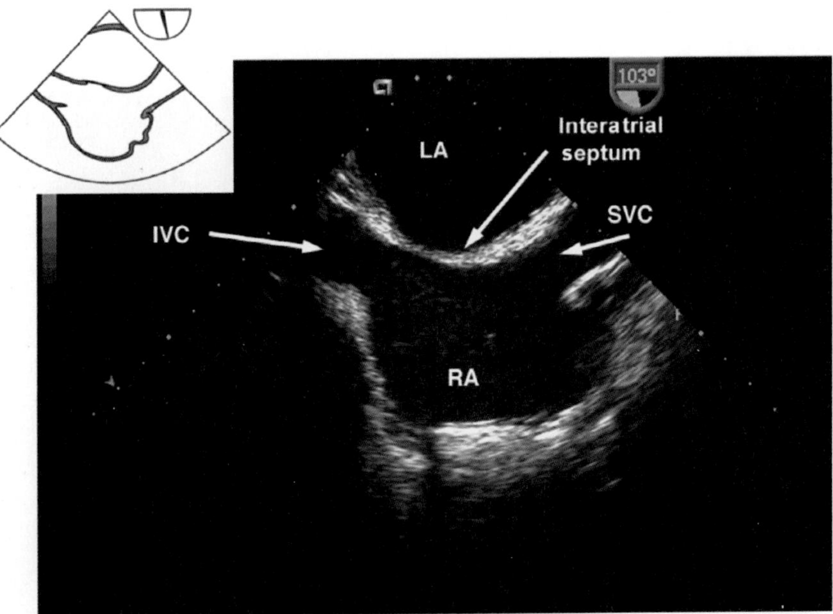

FIGURE 26-12. Midesophageal bicaval view. IVC, inferior vena cava; LA, left atrium; SVC, superior vena cava; RA, right atrium.

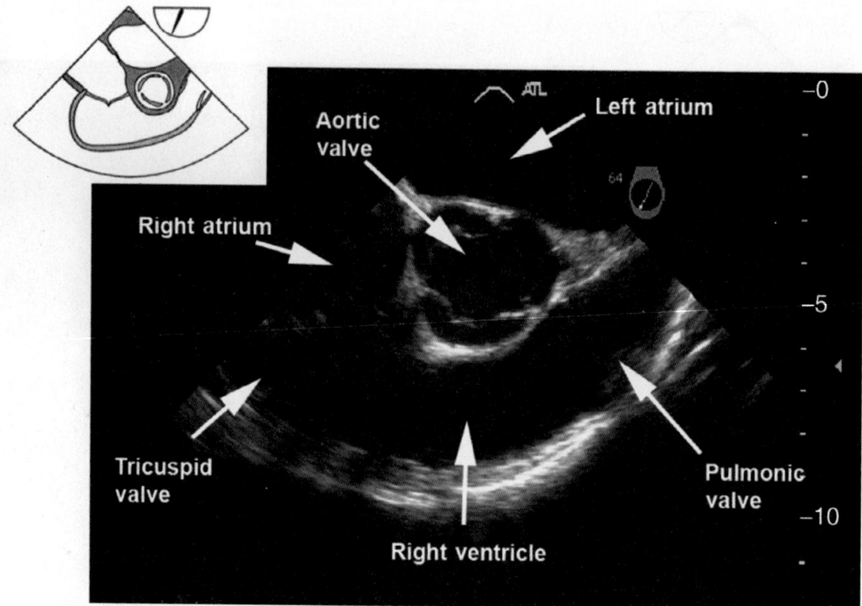

FIGURE 26-13. Midesophageal right ventricular inflow–outflow view.

(Fig. 26-14). Slight withdrawal or anteflexion of the probe will visualize the LVOT and AV and represents the midesophageal five-chamber view. The midesophageal four-chamber view is one of the most recognizable and valuable diagnostic views. Its main uses are to evaluate the:

a. Left atrium, right atrium, RV, and the LV (inferoseptal and anterolateral walls) size and function
b. TV and MV structure and function; CFD will detect valvular pathology
c. Diastolic function
d. The presence of atrial or ventricular septal defect

7. The midesophageal two-chamber view.
This view is obtained from the previous view by rotating the multiplane angle to 90 degrees. In this view, the left atrial appendage is examined for the presence of thrombus. Slight retroflexion is used to avoid a foreshortened view of the LV so as to visualize the LV apex (Fig. 26-15). If the multiplane angle is rotated to just 60 degrees, then the midesophageal mitral commissural view is obtained (Fig. 26-16). The main uses of the midesophageal two-chamber view are to evaluate the:
a. LV anterior and inferior wall function
b. LV apex as well as to diagnose apical thrombus

8. The midesophageal long-axis view.
This view is obtained from the previous view by rotating the multiplane angle to 120 to 135 degrees (Fig. 26-17). The main uses of the midesophageal long-axis view are to evaluate the:
a. LV anteroseptal and posterior wall function
b. LV outflow tract pathology
c. MV anatomy and function

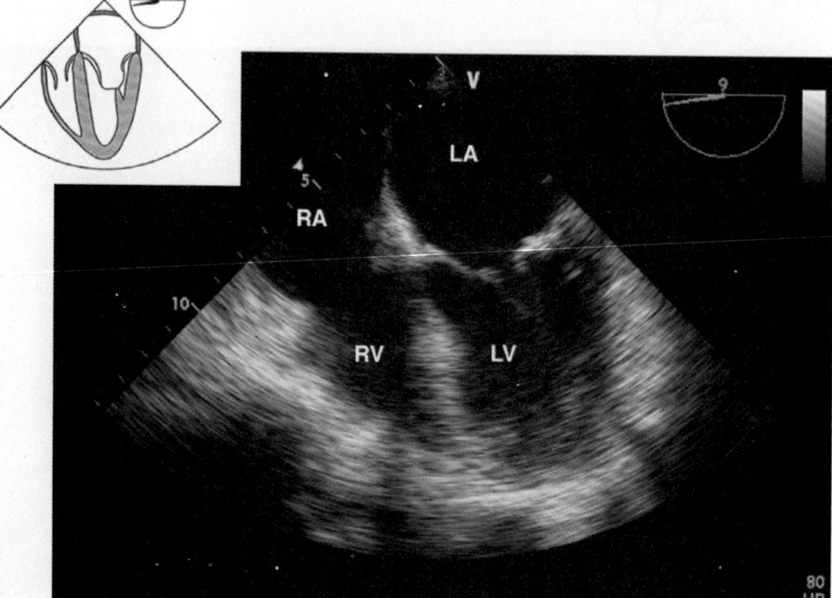

FIGURE 26-14. Midesophageal four-chamber view. RA, right atrium; RV, right ventricle; LA, left atrium; LV, left ventricle.

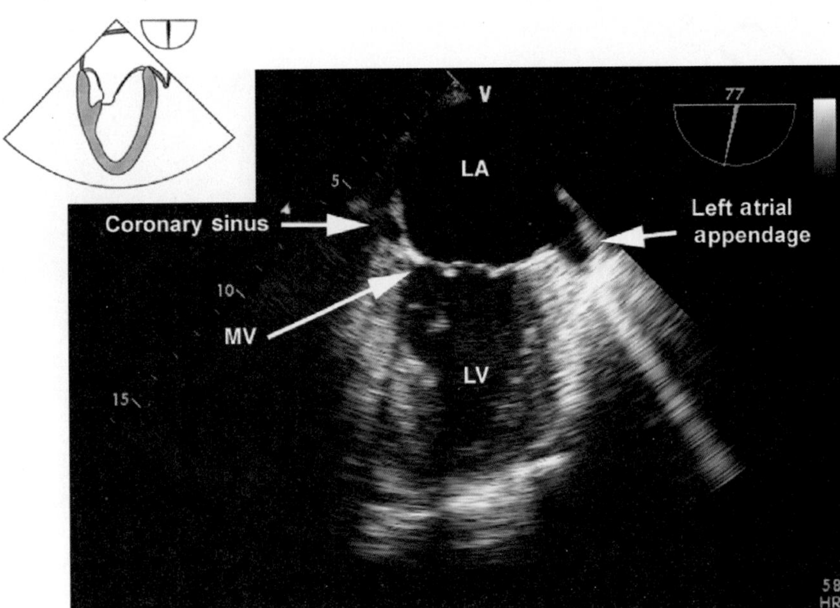

FIGURE 26-15. Midesophageal two-chamber view. LA, left atrium; MV, mitral valve; LV, left ventricle.

9. The transgastric midpapillary short-axis view.
 The view is obtained by advancing the TEE probe from the midesophageal four-chamber view into the stomach, anteflexing and then withdrawing until contact is made with the gastric wall. The LV is visualized as a doughnut in cross-section and both papillary muscles should be seen (Fig. 26-18). Additional anteflexion obtains the transgastric basal short-axis view (Fig. 26-19), which allows for inspection of the anterior and posterior mitral valve leaflets. Advancement of the probe allows visualization of the LV apex in cross-section. The transgastric midpapillary short-axis view is unique in that it visualizes LV walls perfused by each of the three major coronary arteries. The view is considered to be the most useful one in situations of intraoperative hemodynamic instability as it allows immediate diagnosis of hypovolemic state, contractile failure, or coronary ischemia.

 The primary uses of the transgastric midpapillary short-axis view include assessment of the:
 a. LV size (enlargement, hypertrophy) and cavity volume
 b. Global ventricular systolic function and regional wall motion
10. The transgastric two-chamber view.
 This view is obtained from the previous one by rotating the multiplane angle to 90 degrees. The LV is visualized in a longitudinal section with the apex at the left of the display and MV at the right (Fig. 26-20). The primary use of this view is to:
 a. Assess function of the LV anterior and inferior walls
 b. Evaluate the anatomy and function of the MV and chordae tendineae

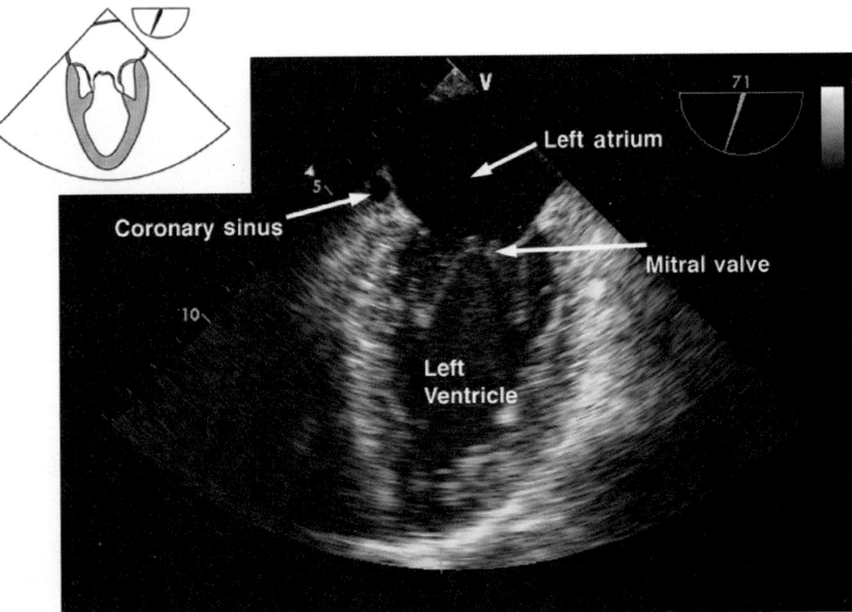

FIGURE 26-16. Midesophageal commissural view.

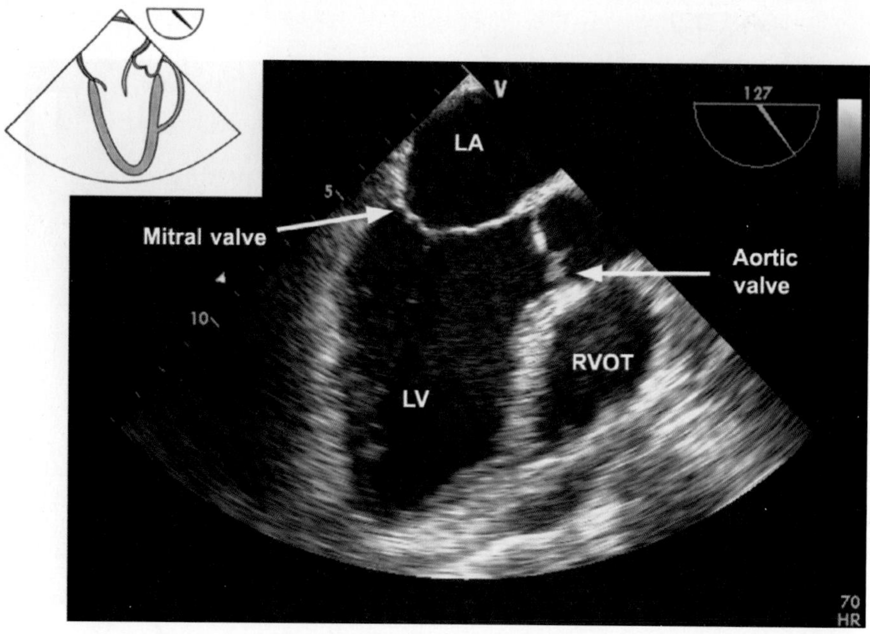

FIGURE 26-17. Midesophageal long-axis view. LA, left atrium; LV, left ventricle; RVOT, right ventricular outflow tract.

14
11. The transgastric long-axis view.
    This view is obtained from the previous view by rotating the multiplane angle to 120 degrees (Fig. 26-21). The main uses of the view are to:
    a. Position the Doppler beam parallel to blood flow across the LVOT and AV
    b. Assess systolic function of the anteroseptal and inferolateral LV walls

15
12. The deep transgastric long-axis view.
    This view is obtained by advancing the probe deep in the stomach, toward the LV apex, and then anteflexing and slightly withdrawing the probe (Fig. 26-22). The main use of the view is:
    a. Doppler assessment of LVOT and aortic blood velocities
    b. Evaluation of AV function with CFD

16
13. Descending aortic short- and long-axis views.
    The descending aortic short-axis view is obtained from the midesophageal four-chamber view by turning the TEE probe to the left until the descending aorta in cross-section is seen as a circular structure (Fig. 26-23). Rotating the multiplane angle to 90 degrees visualizes the descending aorta in a longitudinal section as a tubular vascular structure (Fig. 26-24).

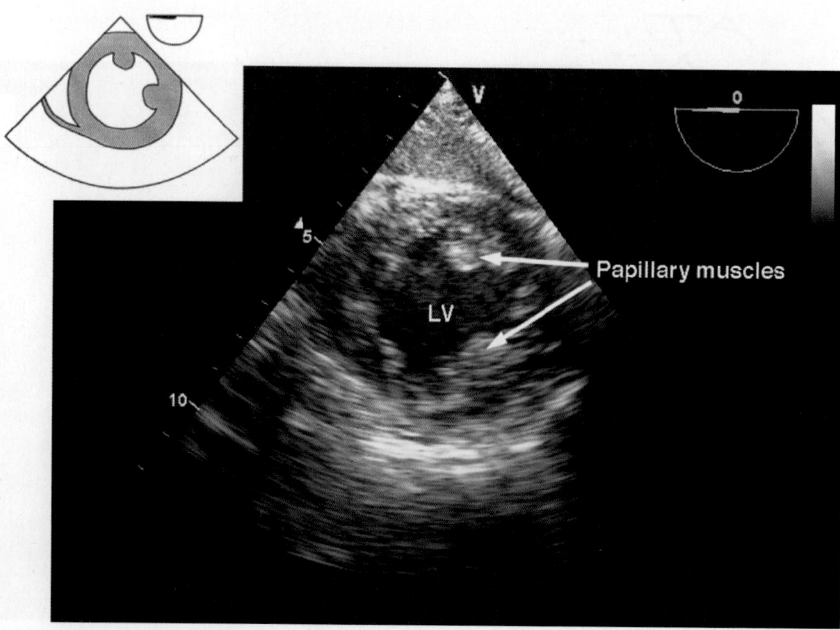

FIGURE 26-18. Transgastric short-axis view. LV, left ventricle.

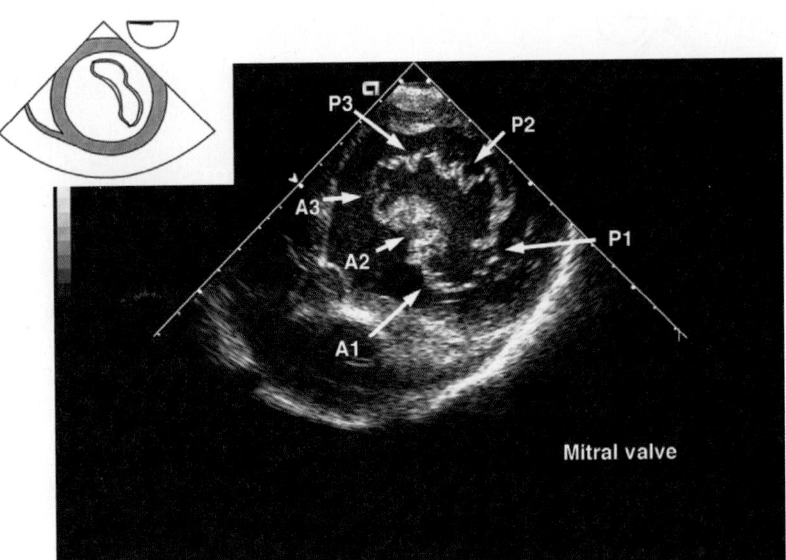

FIGURE 26-19. Transgastric basal short-axis view. A1–3, anterior leaflet of mitral valve, scallops 1–3; P1–3, posterior leaflet of mitral valve, scallops 1–3.

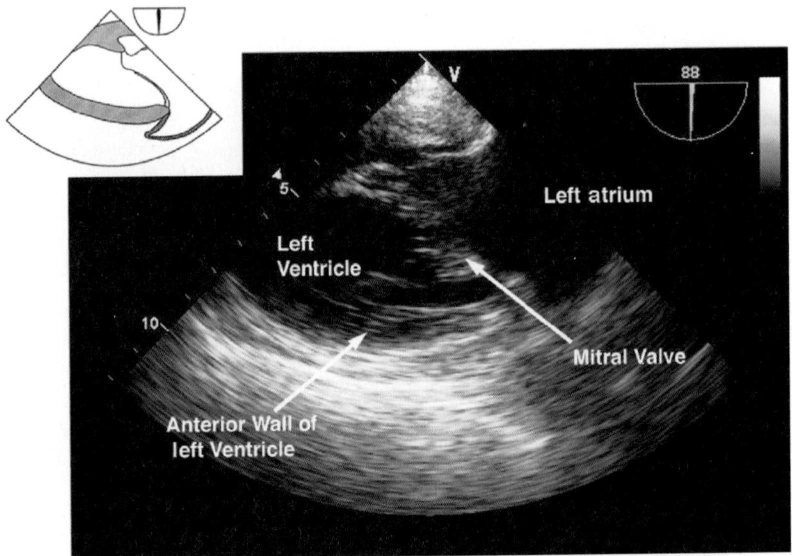

FIGURE 26-20. Transgastric two-chamber view.

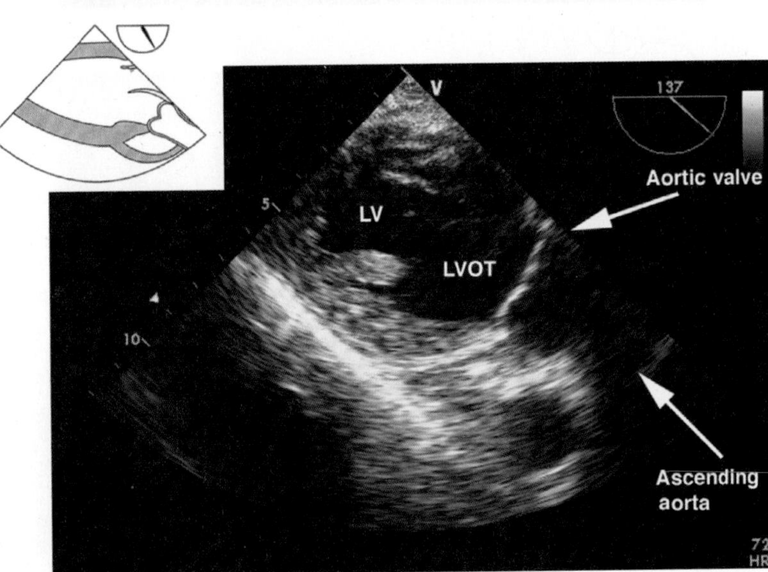

FIGURE 26-21. Transgastric long-axis view. LV, left ventricle; LVOT, left ventricular outflow tract.

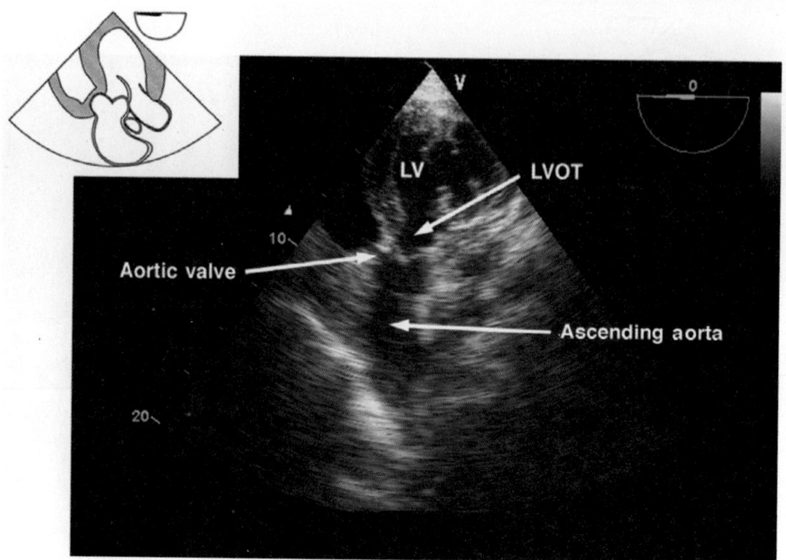

FIGURE 26-22. Deep transgastric long-axis view. LV, left ventricle; LVOT, left ventricular outflow tract.

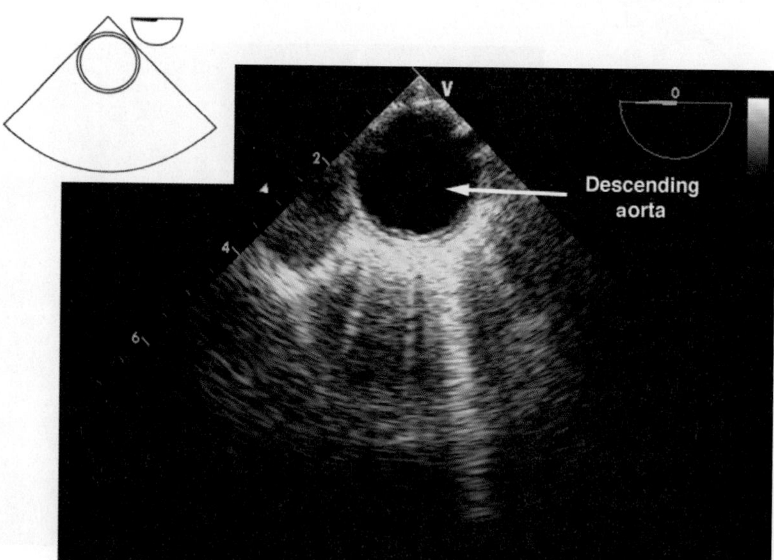

FIGURE 26-23. Descending aortic short-axis view.

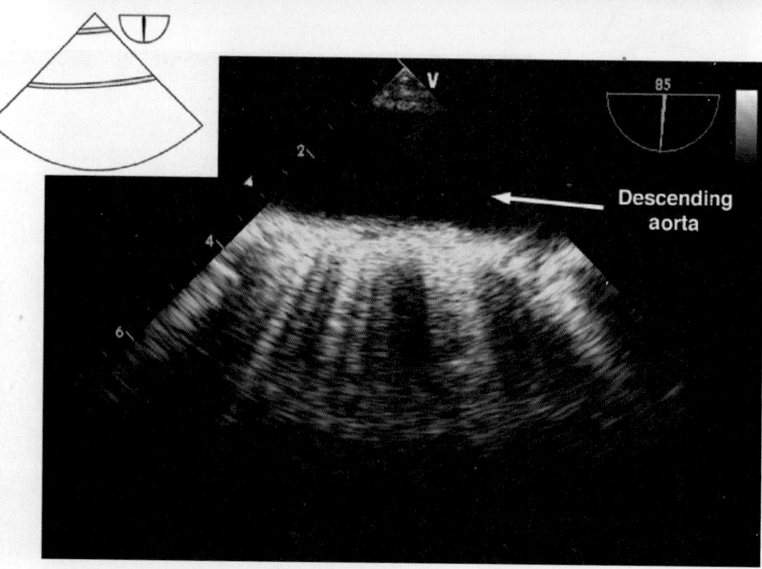

FIGURE 26-24. Descending aortic long-axis view.

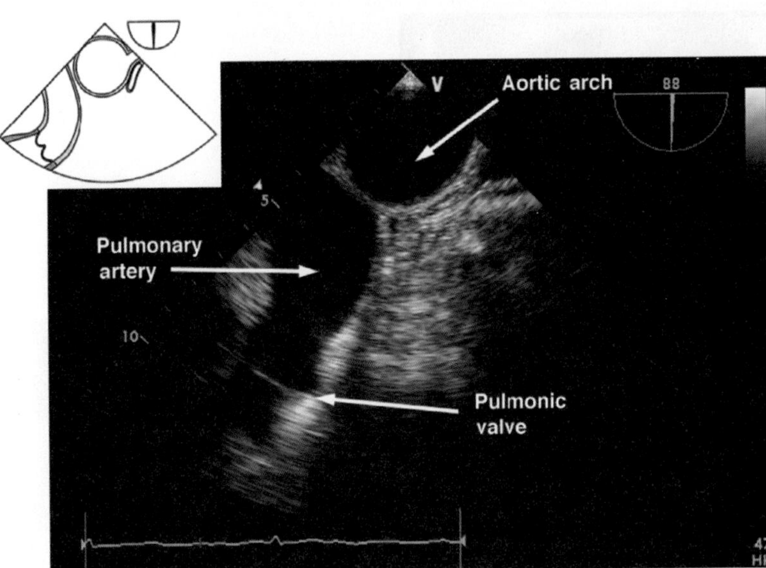

FIGURE 26-25. Upper esophageal aortic arch short-axis view.

In order to examine the entire descending aorta, the probe is gradually advanced and withdrawn in the esophagus. These views are used to: 18

a. Identify pathology of the descending aorta (atheroma, hematoma, dissection flaps, aneurysm)
b. Assist with placement of guide wires and cannulae (intra-aortic balloon pump [IABP], aortic cannula)

17 14. Upper esophageal aortic arch short-axis view.
The view is obtained from the descending aortic long-axis view by withdrawing the probe in the upper esophagus and turning it to the right until the tubular structure transforms into a circular one (Fig. 26-25). The view is used to assess the presence of pathology in the distal aortic arch and Doppler assessment of pulmonary artery blood velocities. If the multiplane angle is rotated back to 0 degree, the upper esophageal aortic arch long-axis view is obtained (Fig. 26-26).

Three-dimensional Echocardiography

In order to better conceptualize the morphology and pathology of the heart, three-dimensional (3-D) image presentation has been developed. The recent introduction of a real-time 3-D TEE probe makes this goal a reality for intraoperative echocardiographers. This technology is capable of acquiring full volumes of the left ventricle, of visualizing heart valves in three dimensions (Fig. 26-27), and assessing the synchrony of LV contraction.[21]

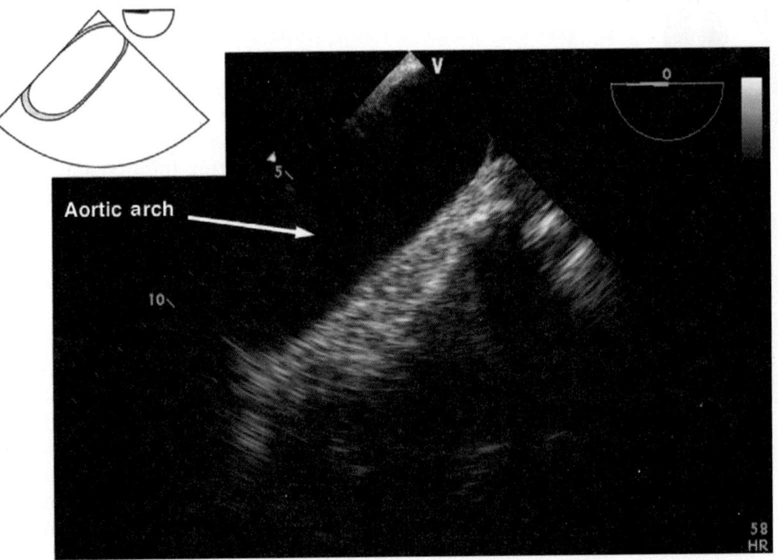

FIGURE 26-26. Upper esophageal aortic arch long-axis view.

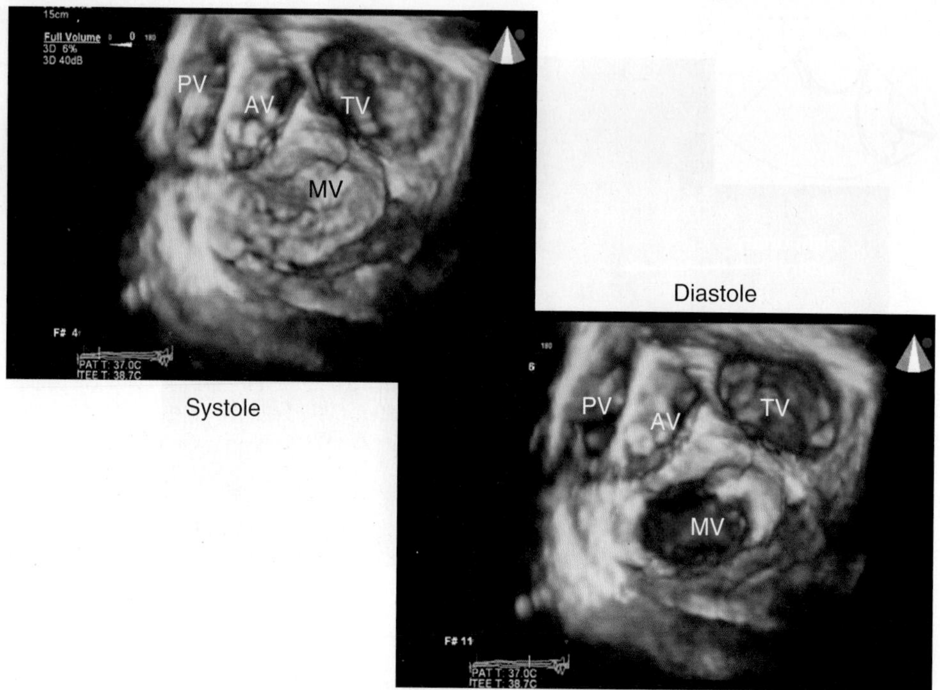

FIGURE 26-27. Three-dimensional transesophageal echocardiographic imaging of the base of the heart with the atria removed, in systole and diastole. AV, aortic valve; MV, mitral valve; PV, pulmonic valve; TV, tricuspid valve.

Uses of 3-D TEE are just emerging. The utility of 3-D imaging of the MV for an MV repair surgery is of particular interest (Fig. 26-28).[22] The capacity of this probe to assess LV contraction synchrony in patients undergoing resynchronization therapy with biventricular pacing may offer a means to maximize their cardiac output. Additional intraoperative applications have emerged, involving percutaneous procedures (transcutaneous aortic valve insertion, noninvasive mitral repair, repair of paraprosthetic leaks, closure of ASD) and open surgical procedures. Guidelines on the use of 3-D echocardiography have also been published.[23]

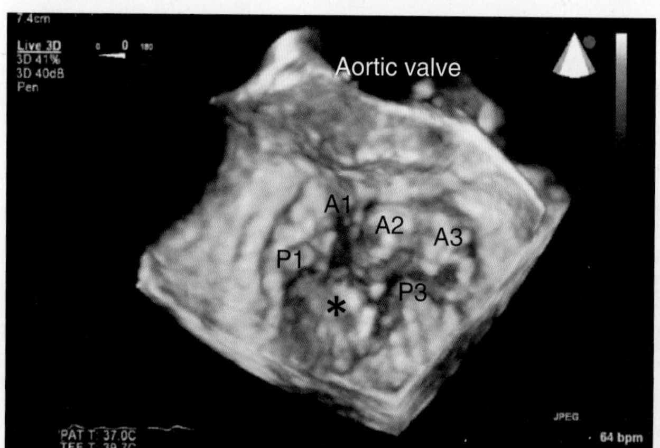

FIGURE 26-28. Three-dimensional imaging of prolapsing middle scallop of the posterior mitral valve leaflet (asterisk). A1–3, lateral, middle and medial scallops of the anterior mitral valve leaflet; P1, lateral scallop of the posterior mitral valve leaflet; P3, medial scallop of the posterior mitral valve leaflet.

DOPPLER ECHOCARDIOGRAPHY AND HEMODYNAMICS

The use of 2-D echocardiography captures high-fidelity motion images of cardiac structures, but not blood flow. Blood flow indices such as blood velocities, stroke volume, and pressure gradients are the domain of Doppler echocardiography. Unlike 2-D imaging, which relies on the time delay and amplitude of reflected ultrasound, Doppler technologies are based on the change in frequency that occurs when ultrasound interacts with moving objects. Reflections from red blood cells are used to determine blood flow velocity and calculate hemodynamic parameters. The combination of 2-D images and quantitative Doppler measure-
3 ments create a uniquely powerful diagnostic tool. Accordingly, Doppler assessments are an essential element of the echocardiographic examination.[24]

The motion of an object causes a sound wave to be compressed in the direction of the motion and expanded in the direction opposite to the motion. This alteration in frequency is known as the *Doppler effect.* By monitoring the frequency pattern of reflections of red blood cells, Doppler echocardiography can determine the speed, direction, and timing of blood flow. The *Doppler equation* describes the relationship between the alteration in ultrasound frequency and blood flow velocity (Fig. 26-29)

$$\Delta f = v \times \cos\theta \times 2f_t/c$$

where Δf is the difference between transmitted frequency (f_t) and received frequency, v is blood velocity, c is the speed of sound in blood (1,540 m/s), and θ is the angle of incidence between the ultrasound beam and blood flow. Conceptually, the equation is simplified by observing that the change in ultrasound frequency is related to just two variables: Blood velocity and cos θ. For this reason the Doppler signal is shifted *only* by the component of the blood velocity that is in the direction of the beam path (i.e., v cos θ).

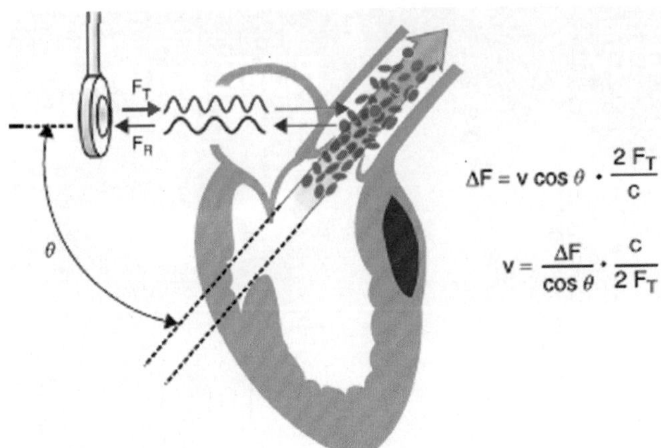

FIGURE 26-29. Calculating blood flow velocity: The Doppler equation. The Doppler equation calculates blood flow velocity based on two variables: The Doppler frequency shift (ΔF) and the cosine (cos) of the angle of incidence between the ultrasound beam and the blood flow. The Doppler frequency shift is measured by the echocardiographic system, but cos θ is unknown, and manual entry by the echocardiographer is required for its estimation. v, flood flow velocity; F_T, transmitted signal frequency; F_R, reflected signal frequency; ΔF, difference between F_R, and F_T; c, speed of sound in tissue; θ, angle of incidence between the orientation of the ultrasound beam and that of the blood flow.

When the beam angle divergence is >30 degrees the value of cos θ decreases rapidly and the Doppler system will markedly underestimate blood velocity. The requirement of near-parallel orientation ($\cos 0 = 1$) for Doppler examinations contrasts with the near-perpendicular orientation preferred for 2-D imaging. Consequently, the preferred imaging planes for Doppler will differ from those used for 2-D imaging.

Spectral Doppler

Two Doppler techniques, *pulsed wave* (PW) and *continuous wave* (CW), are commonly used to evaluate blood flow. A thorough understanding of the advantages and disadvantages of each technique is critical in selecting the one most appropriate for the clinical setting at hand.[25,26] In clinical practice, PW and CW Dopplers are frequently used in conjunction with 2-D imaging. The 2-D image is used to identify the area of interest and guide the echocardiographer in precisely localizing the sampling volume in a PW study or in directing the beam in a CW study.

Pulsed-wave Doppler

PW Doppler offers the echocardiographer the ability to sample blood flow velocity from a particular location. The PW transducer uses a single crystal as both the emitter and the receiver of ultrasound waves. Like the pulsed echocardiography system described for 2-D imaging, the PW Doppler system transmits a short burst of ultrasound toward the target and then switches to receive mode to interpret the returning echoes. Since the speed of sound (c) in tissue is constant, the time delay for a signal to reach its target and return to the transducer depends solely on the distance (d) to the target. Consequently, reflected signals from locations more distant from the transducer return after a greater time interval. By *time gating*, the electronic circuitry of the PW transducer interprets returning echoes only after a predetermined time delay following the transmission of an ultrasound pulse. In this way, only those signals associated with a location, referred to as the *sample volume*, are selected for evaluation.

The pulsed-Doppler system uses a repeating pattern of ultrasound transmission and reception. The rate at which the device repeatedly generates sound bursts is known as the *pulse repetition frequency*. Since the speed of sound through tissue is a constant, the pulse repetition frequency is directly related to the depth of the sample volume. The pulse repetition frequency is analogous to the frame rate of a movie camera. Like the multiple frames on a roll of movie film, each ultrasound pulse interacts with the blood flow for a brief period of time, and just as a series of movie frames display motion, a series of pulsed cycles are consecutively analyzed to determine the blood flow. The Doppler data is frequently presented as a velocity–time plot known as the *spectral display* (Fig. 26-30B).

Since the pulsed-Doppler data are collected intermittently, the maximal frequency and blood flow velocity that can be accurately measured by PW Doppler are limited. The maximal frequency, which equals one-half the pulse repetition frequency, is known as the *Nyquist limit*. At blood velocities above the Nyquist limit, analysis of the returning signal becomes ambiguous, with the velocities appearing to be in the opposite direction. A similar effect is seen in movie animation, in which a rapidly spinning wheel appears to spin backward because of the slow frame rate. The ambiguous signal from frequencies above the Nyquist limit produces *aliasing*, and the velocity signal may appear on the other side of the zero velocity baseline, hence the term *wraparound*. The Nyquist limitation has led to an alternative approach for the assessment of high-velocity blood flows, namely CW Doppler.

Continuous-wave Doppler

The CW Doppler technique avoids the maximal velocity limitation of PW systems by using two crystals, one continuously transmitting and the other continuously receiving the reflected ultrasound signal. With continuous reception of the Doppler signal, the Nyquist limit is not applicable, and blood flows with very high velocities are recorded accurately. The CW mode receives reflected signals from blood flow throughout its beam path because it is not time-gated like the PW technique (Fig. 26-30A). The inability to select blood flow from a specific location favors the selection of CW Doppler primarily for the detection of the highest velocities along the beam path, which is useful in applications such as determining the high velocity jet of aortic stenosis.

Color-flow Doppler

CFD provides a dramatic display of both blood flow and cardiac anatomy by combining 2-D echocardiography and Doppler (Fig. 26-31). The PW Doppler used for CFD differs from that previously discussed in two important ways. CFD performs *multiple* sample volume recordings along each scan line as the beam is swept through the sector. This approach provides flow data at each location in the sector, which can be overlaid on the structural data obtained by 2-D imaging. The Doppler velocity data from each sample volume are color-coded and superimposed on top of the gray scale 2-D image. In the most widely accepted color code, red hues indicate flow toward the transducer and blue hues indicates flow away from the transducer. The ability to provide a real-time, integrated display of flow and structural information makes CFD useful for assessing valvular function, aortic dissection, and congenital heart abnormalities. However, an important caveat to its use in the clinical setting must be noted. Since it relies on PW Doppler measurements, CFD is susceptible to alias artifacts. Aliasing in the color flow map is illustrated in Figure 26-32. This alias pattern

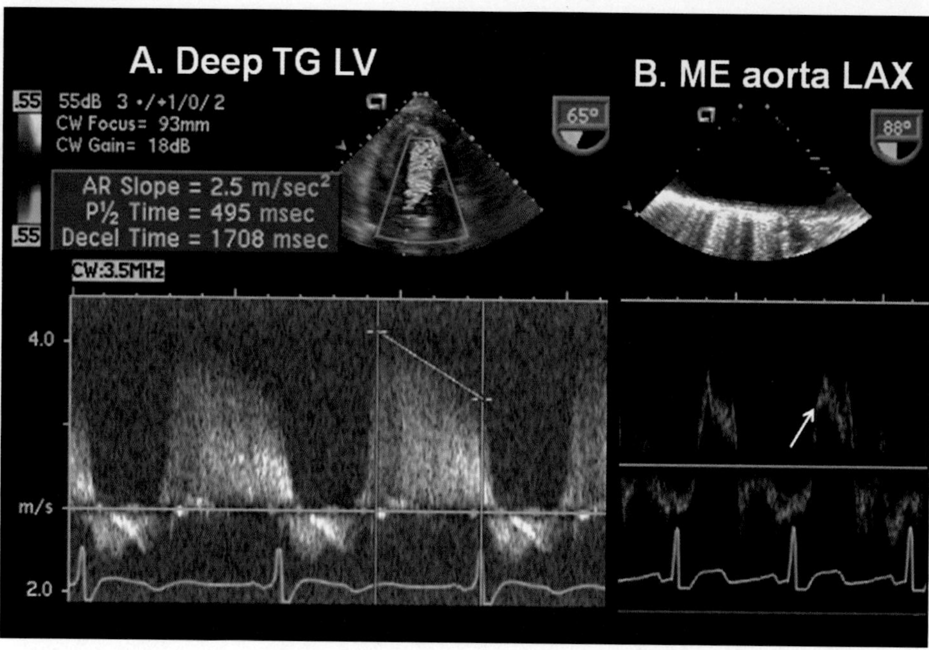

FIGURE 26-30. Doppler echocardiography in aortic insufficiency. **A:** The deep transgastric (deep TG) long-axis view is displayed. A color-Doppler sector is placed over the aortic valve and LV outflow tract and the aortic insufficiency (AI) jet is imaged. The continuous-wave (CW) Doppler cursor is positioned at the center of the AI flow and the spectral display of the AI jet is shown against time. The slope of the AI jet is used to calculate the pressure half time (P½ Time). A short P½ time is associated with severe AI. **B:** The descending aorta is imaged in long axis. The sample volume of pulsed-wave Doppler is placed upstream. There is a systolic wave above the baseline, as the blood moves toward the transesophageal echocardiography transducer, and a diastolic wave (*arrow*), indicating reversal of aortic flow because of severe AI. Decel, deceleration.

can be useful to calculate blood flow in mitral valve disease using the proximal isovelocity surface area (PISA) method (Fig. 26-32).

Hemodynamic Assessments

Doppler echocardiography's ability to quantitatively measure blood velocity yields a wealth of information on the hemodynamic state. Stroke volume, chamber pressures, valvular disease, pulmonary vascular resistance, ventricular function (systolic and diastolic), and anatomic defects are commonly assessed with perioperative Doppler echocardiography.[27]

Volumetric Flow Assessments

Measurements such as stroke volume and cardiac output express the volume of blood ejected by the heart over time. Volumetric parameters are calculated using the principle that volumetric flow (Q) equals blood flow velocity (v) times the cross-sectional area (CSA) of the conduit, that is $Q = v \times CSA$. To determine volumetric

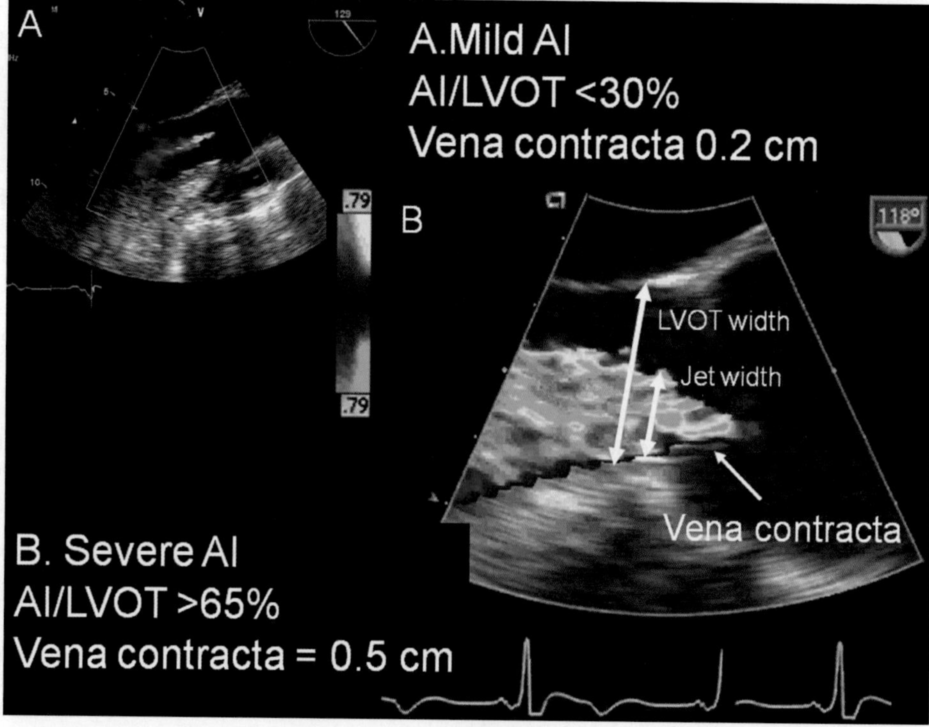

FIGURE 26-31. Evaluation of aortic insufficiency (AI). Color-flow Doppler of the aortic valve (AV) in the midesophageal long-axis view. AI is graded using (*1*) the relative ratio of the AI jet thickness to the diameter of left ventricular outflow tract (LVOT); both measurements are performed at the same site, usually within 0.5 to 1 cm proximal to the AV plane; and (*2*) the width of the AI jet as it crosses the AV cusps (vena contracta).

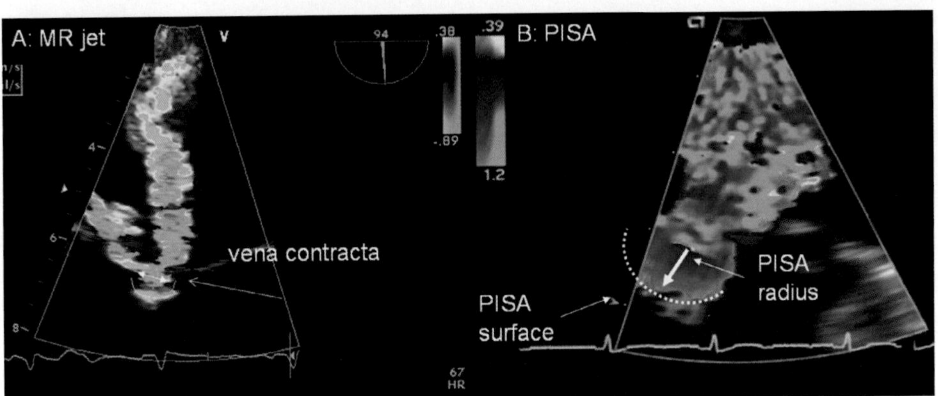

FIGURE 26-32. Doppler evaluation of mitral regurgitation (MR) severity. MR severity is evaluated using color Doppler. **A:** MR jet is imaged with color-flow Doppler (midesophageal two-chamber view). The Nyquist limit is moved upward to demonstrate flow acceleration inside the left ventricle and the neck (vena contracta) of the MR jet. **B:** Zoom of the proximal MR jet allows measurement of the proximal isovelocity surface area (PISA) radius and calculation of the incompetent mitral valve orifice.

flows with echocardiography, a Doppler measurement of the blood flow velocities and a 2-D measurement of the CSA are recorded.

Stroke Volume and Cardiac Output

To calculate stroke volume, the instantaneous velocities during systole are traced from the spectral display and the echocardiographic system's software package calculates the time–velocity integral (VTI, in centimeters). In effect, the VTI represents the distance ($v \times t = d$) blood traveled during systole (i.e., stroke distance). By multiplying the VTI by the CSA (in square centimeters) of the conduit (e.g., aorta, MV, PA) through which the blood traveled, the stroke volume (in cubic centimeters) is obtained: SV = VTI × CSA (Fig. 26-33).[28–30] Cardiac output, which expresses volumetric flow in cubic centimeters per minute, is estimated from the product of SV and heart rate: CO = VTI × CSA × HR. Figure 26-34 demonstrates calculation of cardiac output and stroke volume from the LVOT.

Valve Area

The Continuity Equation. The principle of conservation of mass is the basis of the *continuity equation,* which is commonly used to measure the aortic valve area.[31] The continuity equation simply states that the volume of blood passing through one site in the heart (e.g., the LVOT) is equal to the mass or volume of blood passing through another site (e.g., the aortic valve).

Volumetric Flow_1 = Volumetric Flow_2; therefore

$$CSA_1 \times VTI_1 = CSA_2 \times VTI_2 \text{ and}$$

$$CSA_1 = CSA_2 \times VTI_2/VTI_1$$

Figure 26-35 demonstrates calculation of AV area using this approach.

Pressure Assessment

The Bernoulli Equation. Pressure gradients are used to estimate intracavitary pressures and to assess conditions such as valvular disease (e.g., aortic stenosis), septal defects, outflow tract obstruction, and major vessel pathology (e.g., coarctation). As blood flows across a narrowed or stenotic orifice, blood flow velocity increases. The increase in velocities relates to the degree of narrowing. In the clinical situation, the *simplified Bernoulli equation* describes the relation between the increases in blood flow velocity and the pressure gradient across the narrowed orifice:[11] $\Delta P = 4V_{max}^2$ where ΔP in millimeters of mercury is the pressure gradient across the narrowed orifice and V_{max}^4 in meters per second is the maximum velocity across that orifice measured by Doppler.

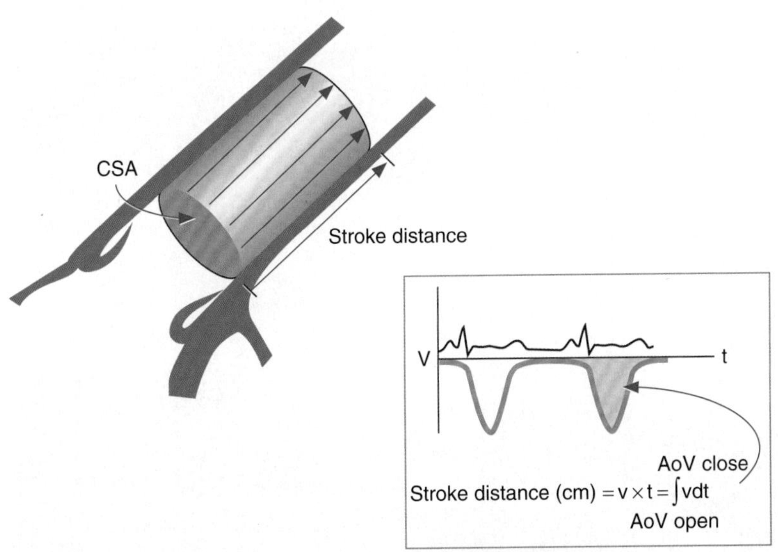

FIGURE 26-33. Determination of stroke volume. Volumetric flow can be determined from a combination of area and velocity measurements. In this example, the flow through the ascending aorta is used to determine the stroke volume. Integrating the Doppler-derived flow velocities over time (known as the time–velocity integral) during a single cardiac cycle calculates the stroke distance. The cross-sectional area measurement is obtained by two-dimensional echocardiography. The product of these two measurements, conceptualized as a cylinder, is the stroke volume. CSA, cross-sectional area; AoV, aortic valve.

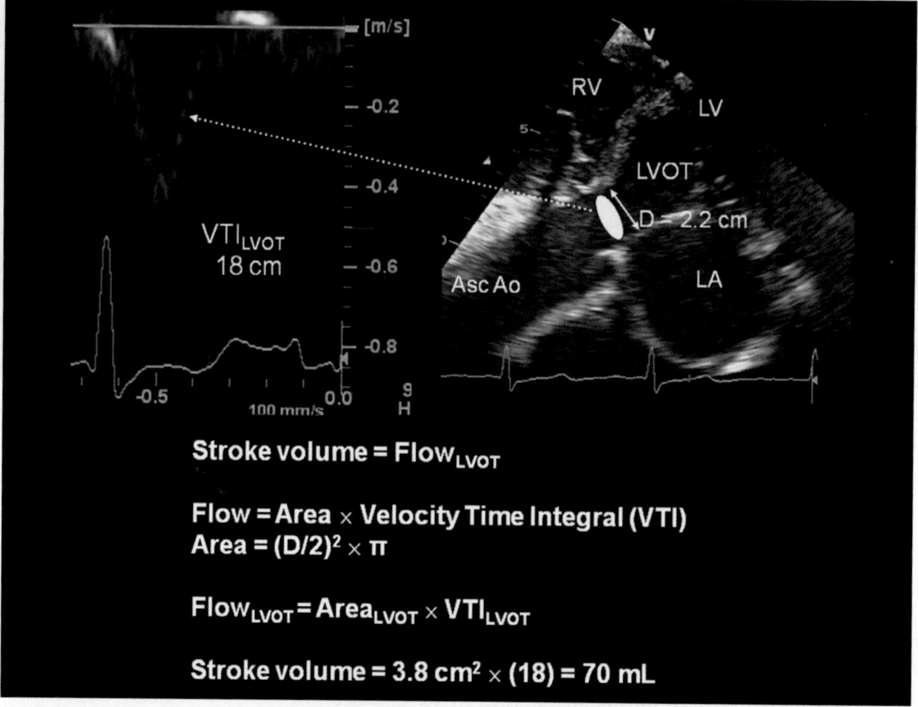

FIGURE 26-34. Stroke volume calculation. Stroke volume is equal to the blood flow crossing the left ventricular outflow tract (LVOT). In the deep transgastric long-axis view, the LVOT orifice (*large oval*) can be calculated from the LVOT diameter (D). The blood flow velocity across the LVOT is measured with pulsed Doppler, and the velocity time integral (VTI) by tracing the velocity envelope. RV, right ventricle; LA, left atrium.

Thus in clinical echocardiography, pressure gradient is obtained by the straightforward process of measuring the peak velocity of blood flow across the lesion of interest.[32,33] The measured peak velocity is then entered into the simplified Bernoulli equation to estimate the pressure gradient.

The Bernoulli equation is commonly employed to measure the pressure gradient across a stenotic valve. In addition, the rate of decline in the pressure gradient across the valve is related to the severity of the disease.[34,35] This *pressure half-time* is the time required for the peak transvalvular pressure gradient to decrease by 50%. Typically, a larger orifice will have a shorter pressure half-time as pressures equalize faster.

Measurement of Intracavitary Pressures

Intracavitary and pulmonary arterial pressures are estimated from the pressure gradient across two adjacent chambers. The pressure gradient is defined as the difference in pressure from the "driving"

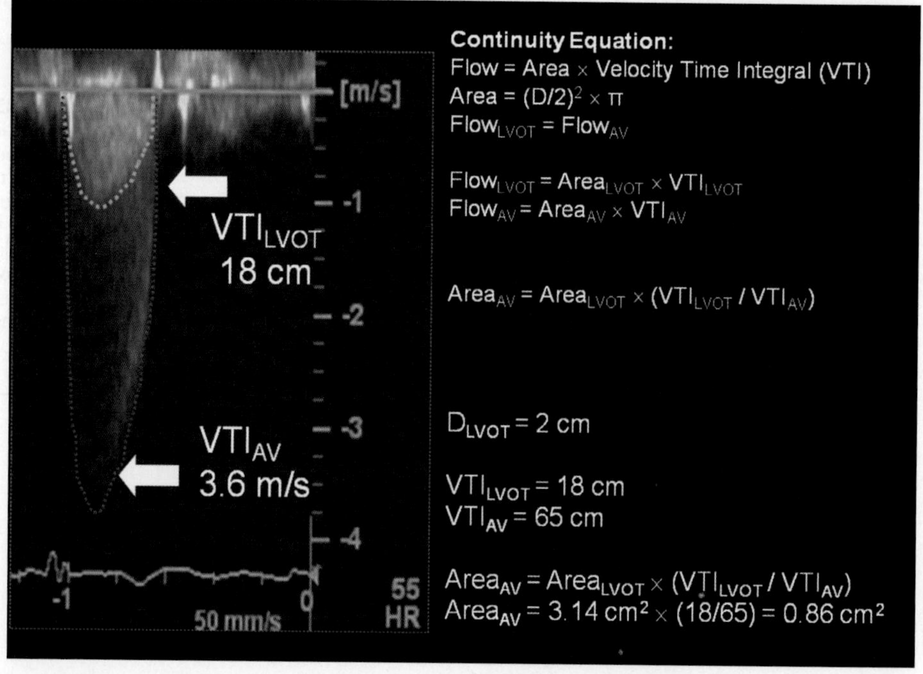

FIGURE 26-35. Evaluation of aortic stenosis. Calculation of aortic valve area using the "double envelope" technique. The cursor of continuous-wave Doppler is placed in the middle of the blood flow traversing the stenosed aortic valve, and two envelopes are identified. The one with the slower velocity is from the left ventricular outflow tract (LVOT) and the one with the fastest is from the aortic valve (AV). The envelopes of the velocities are traced to derive the respective velocity time integrals (VTI). The aortic valve area is calculated using the continuity equation. D, diameter.

TABLE 26-1. CALCULATION OF CARDIOPULMONARY PRESSURES

Pressure	Equation
RVSP or PASP	$= 4(V_{TR})^2 + RAP$
PAMP	$= 4(V_{early}\ PI)^2 + RAP$
PADP	$= 4(V_{late}\ PI)^2 + RAP$
LAP	$= SBP - 4(V_{MR})^2$
LVEDP	$= DBP - 4(V_{AI\ end})^2$

RVSP, right ventricular systolic pressure; PASP, pulmonary artery systolic pressure; v, peak velocity; TR, tricuspid regurgitation; RAP, right atrial pressure; PAMP, pulmonary artery mean pressure; PI, pulmonic valve insufficiency; PADP, pulmonary artery diastolic pressure; LAP, left atrial pressure; SBP, systolic blood pressure; MR, mitral regurgitation; LVEDP, left ventricular end-diastolic pressure; DBP, diastolic blood pressure; AI, aortic insufficiency.

chamber to the "receiving" chamber. Echocardiographically, the pressure gradient is calculated from the Doppler-derived velocities of the regurgitant jet into the receiving chamber.[36–38] Table 26-1 provides calculations of intracardiac and PA pressures.

ECHOCARDIOGRAPHIC EVALUATION OF SYSTOLIC FUNCTION

Evaluation of LV systolic function is a primary component of every echocardiographic examination. Information about global as well as regional LV performance is accomplished by assessing the size, shape and LV contractile function. Both qualitative assessments (which are inherently subjective) and quantitative techniques (which produce hard numerical estimates) are useful: 2-D and motion mode (M-mode) image the LV walls and cavity and Doppler echocardiography measures the velocity of blood flow and moving tissue.

Left Ventricular Walls

The LV cavity and walls at the basal, mid, and apical levels are evaluated in the midesophageal and transgastric views. From the midesophageal position, the TEE imaging array is rotated electronically in a clockwise fashion to scan the entire circumference of the LV cavity and walls in a longitudinal orientation. Further advancement of the TEE probe to the transgastric position combined with anterior flexion (anteflexion) of the probe sequentially images the LV short axis from its base to apex. The echocardiographic imaging of blood and myocardium is based on their different acoustic properties: Muscle tissue is reflective and imaged in shades of gray, while ultrasound easily propagates through blood, resulting in the LV cavity appearing dark. Their interface is the endocardial surface, which typically produces the brightest signal. The evaluation focuses on the shape, size, and motion of LV walls.

Shape

The LV's longitudinal shape is evaluated in the midesophageal views (Fig. 26-36). It appears bullet-shaped with the mitral annulus and leaflets comprising its broad base, and the walls tapering toward its apex. In the midesophageal view at 0-degree rotation (midesophageal four-chamber, midesophageal five-chamber) the inferolateral wall of the LV appears on the right of the TEE monitor screen and the inferoseptal wall on the left. Clockwise rotation of the multiplane angle to about 90 degrees (midesophageal two-chamber) will image the long axis of the LV, with the anterior and inferior walls presented on the right and left sides of the monitor, respectively. Further rotation to approximately 135 degrees will image the LV anteroseptal and inferolateral walls on the right and left sides of the screen.

The echocardiographer must be careful to image the LV along the true long axis in the midesophageal views. Often, in the midesophageal four-chamber view, the imaging plane may cut obliquely in an anterior direction, which causes an increase in the apparent wall thickness and foreshortens the LV cavity. This is avoided by confirming that the LV long-axis measurement approximates that of the LV length (as measured from the mitral annular plane to the apex, typically in the midesophageal two-chamber view). In many cases slight retroflection or rotation of the multiplane angle from 0 to 20 degrees is helpful to achieve the best alignment. The LV walls are divided into three segments each—basal, mid, and apical—as defined by lines drawn perpendicular to the LV long axis at the tips and base of the papillary muscles.

From the transgastric position, the LV is seen along its short axis, and its shape resembles a doughnut. The basal segments are imaged in short axis with the TEE probe in the distal esophagus or very high up inside the stomach. At this depth, the mitral leaflets (base of heart) are seen "enface" (Fig. 26-19). Gradual advancement of the TEE probe into the stomach images the mid LV segments (Fig. 26-18). Here, the anatomic landmark is the body of the papillary muscles at 2 o'clock (posteromedial) and 5 o'clock (anterolateral). Further advancement of the TEE probe will image the LV apex, much thicker and with smaller cavity. In either midesophageal or transgastric imaging planes, the LV walls thicken in systole and thin in diastole. As seen in the midesophageal views, the LV base descends toward the LV apex and ascends at diastole.

Aneurysms

Aneurysms appear as a dilated part of the LV perimeter with thinned wall(s) and decreased motion. Aneurysms are always pathologic and usually due to ischemia-related necrosis and weakening of the LV wall. Aneurysms are separated into true and false. If all myocardial layers (epi-, mid-, and endocardium) are present in the wall of the aneurysm, it is called a *true aneurysm*. The "neck" of a true aneurysm is usually wide, and the aneurysmal cavity shallows with a smooth transition from normal to aneurysmal walls. An aneurysm is called *false* or "pseudo" if the LV wall contains only some of the myocardial layers (usually the epicardium and part of the midwall). False aneurysms are caused by necrosis of the LV wall, usually from myocardial infarction. Sometimes, the wall of a false aneurysm consists only of the attached pericardium. False aneurysms have a narrower neck and the transition between healthy and diseased wall segments is abrupt. A false aneurysm is prone to rupture and is treated surgically. Blood flow is sluggish within aneurysms. Red blood cells clump together, which increases echogenicity and creates spontaneous echocardiography contrast, a smoke-like appearance inside the LV cavity. Thrombus, appearing with brightness similar to that of myocardium but clearly separated from the LV wall, can also develop in aneurysms.

Texture

The *texture* of the LV walls may offer additional information in patients with infiltrative cardiomyopathies, such as amyloid, where the thickened myocardium has a speckled appearance.

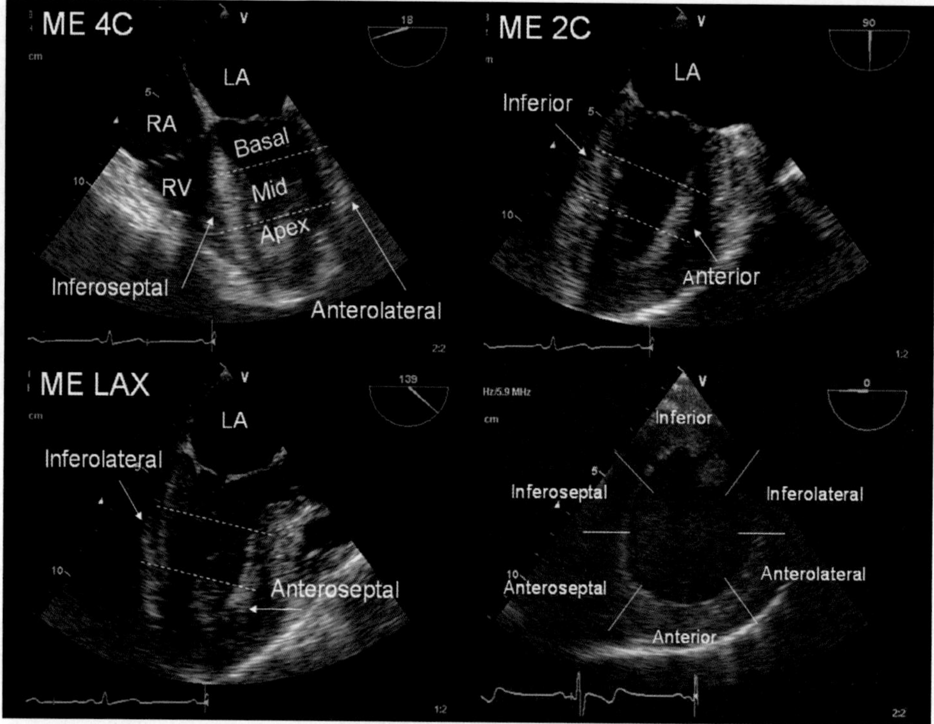

FIGURE 26-36. Left ventricular (LV) walls. In the esophagus, the transesophageal echocardiography (TEE) probe is rotated clockwise from 0 to 140 degrees to obtain the midesophageal (ME) views. Advancement of the TEE probe inside the stomach obtains the transgastric (TG) midpapillary short-axis view. In the ME views, the LV is divided in basal, mid, and apical segments. 4C, four-chamber; 2C, two-chamber; LA, left atrium; RA, right atrium; RV, right ventricle.

Wall Thickness

LV hypertrophy is termed *concentric* if the cavity is not increased (usually resulting from increased pressure work) and *eccentric* when there is LV dilation (usually resulting from increased volume work). The diagnosis is made by summing the end-diastolic (ED) wall thickness of the anteroseptal and inferolateral LV segments in the basal transgastric short-axis view, just at the tips of the papillary muscles (Fig. 26-37). Normal values are 18 ± 2 mm (men) and 15.5 ± 1.5 mm (women).

Segments and Regional Function

Abnormal myocardial wall systolic thickening is a sensitive marker of myocardial ischemia that appears earlier than electrocardiographic and hemodynamic changes.[39–41] Regional LV systolic function reflects the regional myocardial blood flow.[42] The association of the regional LV wall motion with the underlying coronary artery distribution is used to diagnose local perfusion defects. The LV is divided into 17 regional segments[43] (Fig. 26-36). Along the longitudinal plane each wall is divided into basal, mid, and apical levels. The basal and mid levels are further divided into anterior, inferior, two septal (anteroseptal and inferoseptal), and two lateral (anterolateral and inferolateral) segments. The apical level is divided into four segments (anterior, inferior, septal, and lateral) and the apical cap is the seventeenth segment. To limit misdiagnosis, evaluation of each segment is done in at least two different views, ensuring that both endocardium and epicardium are visible. A midesophageal or transgastric view is digitally stored and played over time. The segmental (or regional) function is evaluated by noticing the presence or absence of endocardial excursion (toward the LV cavity) and degree of systolic wall thickening during one or two consecutive cardiac cycles (Fig. 26-37). The electrocardiogram is used to define systole and diastole. The function of each wall segment is scored as shown in Table 26-2.[44] The wall motion score index is the sum of all scores divided by the number of segments evaluated. The evaluation of segmental wall motion to detect ischemia is not error-free. In addition to being a subjective assessment, wall motion may be affected by tethering, regional loading conditions, and stunning.[45] Epicardial pacing of the free wall of the right ventricle (RV) (as in the post-bypass period) produces a left bundle block and induces septal wall motion abnormalities. Interobserver reproducibility is better for normally contracting segments than for dysfunctional segments.[46] Because of these issues, wall thickening is a more reliable marker of regional function.

4

Left Ventricular Cavity

Diameters

The LV cavity is defined by its long and short axes. The LV major (or long) axis dimension is measured in the midesophageal two-chamber view, from the base of the mitral annulus to the LV apex (Fig. 26-38) while the minor (or short) axis dimension is measured in either the midesophageal or transgastric two-chamber views, perpendicular to the long axis, at the height of the papillary muscle tips. The minor axis is equal to one-half of the long-axis measurement. Proper measurement of the LV minor axis is used to quantify the LV end-diastolic (ED) volume. Normal LV ED dimensions (EDDs) are 4.2 to 5.9 cm (men) and 3.9 to 5.3 cm (women). An increased LV EDD denotes LV dilation and volume overload, while a decreased LV EDD denotes hypovolemia and inadequate preload.

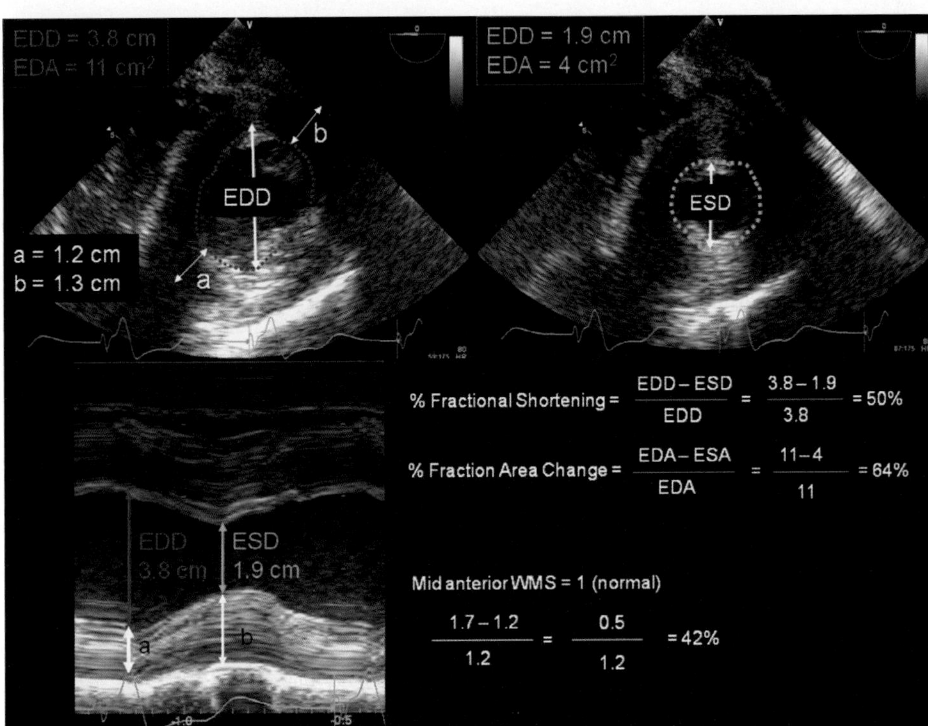

FIGURE 26-37. Two-dimensional evaluation of left ventricular (LV) global and regional functions. Regional and global evaluation of the LV using the transgastric short-axis view at the midpapillary level. Measurements are performed at end-diastole (ED) and end-systole (ES). **Top panels:** Measurement of diameters (D), areas (A), and wall thickness. Wall thickness is measured at ED in the anteroseptal and inferolateral wall segments. **Bottom panel:** Diameter and wall thickness measured using method mode with the cursor crossing the middle of inferior **(top)** and anterior **(bottom)** segments. The percent change of wall thickness of the midanterior wall segment can be used to grade its regional function. In this example, wall motion score (WMS) is 1 **(normal)** because the segment thickens >30%.

Global Systolic Function

Systolic function is responsible for delivering a sufficient amount of blood to the vessels at a high enough pressure to perfuse the tissues adequately. A variety of echocardiographic measurements are used to evaluate the components (preload, afterload, and contractility), which collectively define LV global systolic function. The techniques for LV evaluation are described in detail in references.[47,48]

Percent Fractional Shortening (%FS)

FS measures the relative change of the LV short axis diameter between ED and end-systole (ES; Fig. 26-37). FS is a one-dimensional, unitless measurement of systolic function. Measurements are done in the transgastric midpapillary short-axis view, just above the papillary muscles. A larger number occurs when the LV has normal or increased systolic function. FS is not a substitute for ejection fraction (EF) and may overestimate systolic function if there is LV dilation or abnormal wall motion at another level. %FS = (LV EDD − LV ESD)/(LV EDD) × 100 and is normally 27% to 45%.

TABLE 26-2. GRADING OF WALL FUNCTION

Regional Function	Grade	Inward Radial Motion (Systolic Wall Thickening)
Normal	1	>30% (marked)
Hypokinetic	2	>10% to <30% (reduced)
Akinetic	3	<10% (negligible)
Dyskinetic	4	Paradoxical systolic motion (systolic thinning)
Aneurysmal	5	Diastolic deformation

Volumes

LV volume measurements are used to calculate preload (ED volume [EDV]) as well as stroke volume (SV) and EF. The ED and ES LV volumes can be derived from manually tracing the endocardial border in ED and ES, respectively.

LV volume is commonly measured using the modified Simpson or the area length method. The biplane method of discs (or modified Simpson' rule) conceives a series of disks inside the LV cavity, which have equal thickness and are stacked like coins along the LV long-axis dimension (Fig. 26-38). The diameter of each disk is the short-axis dimension as defined from the LV endocardium tracing. Measurements are performed in the mid-esophageal four- and two-chamber views. Alternatively, the area length method can be used to calculate LV volume: LV volume = 5/6 × [(area) × (length)]. This approach is performed in one of the previous views and calculates the LV volume using the endocardial-enclosed area and the LV major axis (Fig. 26-38). In most adults, an ED area <12 cm^2 indicates hypovolemia.[49] Reliable and correct visualization of the endocardial border is paramount for accurate measurement of LV volumes with either method. The methods underestimate LV volume when the LV cavity is "foreshortened."

Percent Fractional Area Change (FAC)

FAC is the percent difference between ED and ES LV areas (Fig. 26-37). The LV area is measured by manually tracing the endocardial border in the transgastric midpapillary short-axis view in ED and in ES. The papillary muscles are not traced. Unlike LVEF

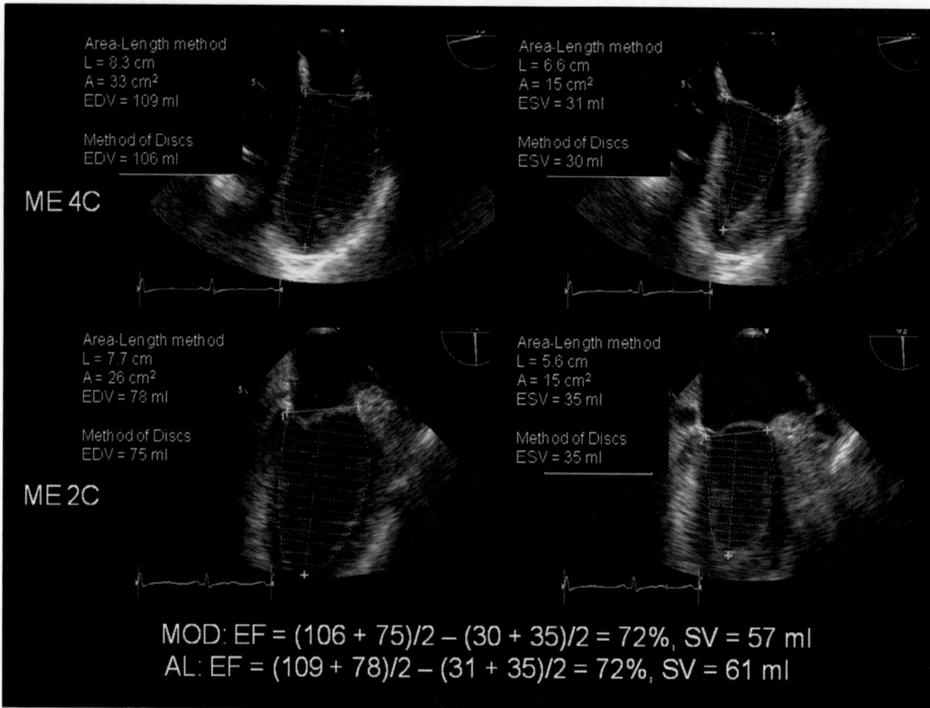

FIGURE 26-38. Quantitation of left ventricular (LV) systolic function. The midesophageal (ME) LV four-chamber (ME 4C) and two-chamber (ME 2C) views are obtained. The images are examined in end-diastole (ED) and end-systole (ES). The LV endocardium is traced. This automatically defines the LV area (A) and long axis (L). The system software will calculate LV volumes using either the method of discs (MOD) or the area–length method (AL). EF, ejection fraction; EDV, end-diastolic volume; ESV, end-systolic volume; SV, stroke volume.

measurements, FAC does not take into account the presence of wall motion abnormalities at a different level; for example, the function of the LV apex, which is frequently involved in coronary artery disease. Therefore, caution is advised when interpreting FAC. Normal values are 56% to 65%.[50]

Visual Estimation of FAC

The most frequently used technique to evaluate global LV function as well as preload is visual estimation of FAC, often referred to as the *eyeball* EF. Although highly subjective, it is practiced widely and is accurate in experienced echocardiographers, especially in normally contracting ventricles.[51] With LV dysfunction, visual evaluations of FAC become less reproducible among different observers.[46]

Ejection Fraction

EF is the most frequently used estimate of LV systolic function. The evaluation of EF provides prognostic information about mortality and morbidity.[52] EF and stroke volume are affected by factors such as preload, afterload, and heart rate, and thus are not always indicators of intrinsic systolic function. Typical clinical scenarios in which EF does not represent LV systolic function include the hypercontractile LV in mitral regurgitation (where more than half of ED volume may regurgitate inside the left atrium) or the hypocontractile LV in aortic stenosis (where LV systolic performance is poor despite preserved contractility).

Stroke Volume

Stroke volume is calculated as the difference between EDV and ESV, and percent EF is calculated as %EF = SV/EDV × 100 = (EDV – ESV)/EDV × 100. Normal values are: EDV, 67 to 155 mL (men), 56 to 104 mL (women); ESV, 22 to 58 mL (men) and 19 to 49 mL (women); %EF, >55%.

Associated Findings

Sluggish flow will clump together red blood cells, producing spontaneous echocardiography contrast, which is imaged as "smoke." Thrombus is also found if there is blood stasis, such as inside an aneurysm or at the LV apex. These findings are often present when LV function is depressed.

Tissue Echocardiography—Myocardial Velocity

Tissue Doppler imaging (TDI) measures the velocity of myocardial motion along the longitudinal axis and is a sensitive measurement of regional and global functions and outcome.[53] The myocardial velocity is measured from the basal LV segments with the sample volume placed next to the mitral annulus. The velocities are comprised of a systolic (S′) followed by, in the opposite direction, two diastolic waves, one early (E′) and one following atrial contraction (A′). A reduced, or delayed S′ velocity is associated with development of regional ischemia (Fig. 26-39).[54]

EVALUATION OF LEFT VENTRICULAR DIASTOLIC FUNCTION

An increased recognition of the impact of LV diastolic function on the overall cardiac function and outcome has driven efforts to both monitor and optimize diastolic performance in the perioperative period. The presence of preoperative asymptomatic ventricular dysfunction, in patients undergoing vascular surgery, is associated

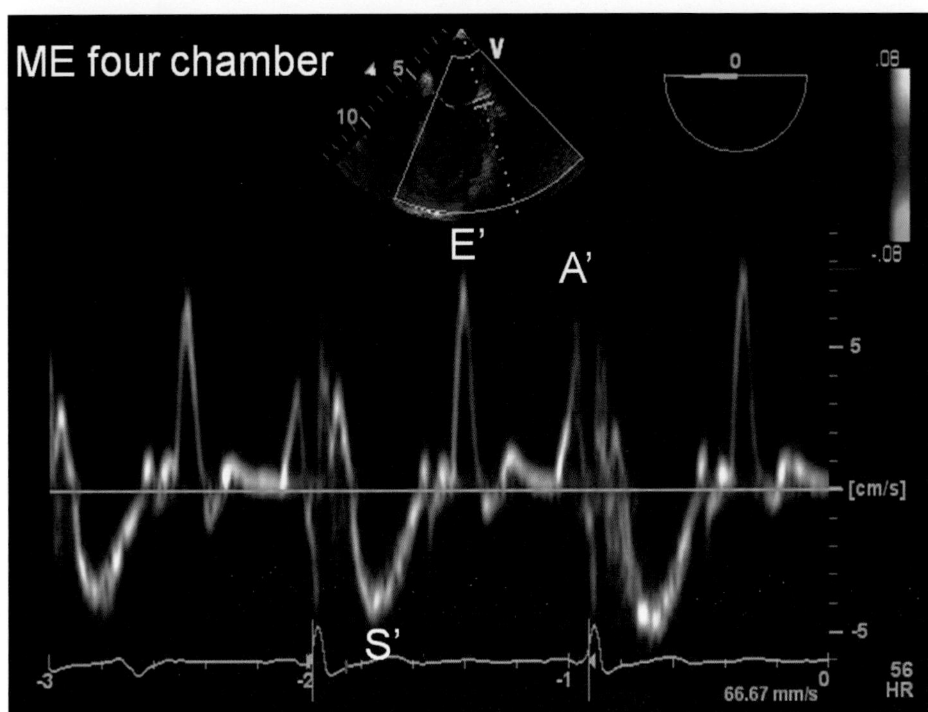

FIGURE 26-39. Tissue Doppler imaging. Myocardial velocity of basal anterolateral segment of left ventricle is measured with pulsed-wave tissue Doppler. ME, midesophageal; S′, systolic velocity; E′, early diastolic velocity; A′, late diastolic velocity.

with increased short- and long-term morbidity and mortality.[55] Furthermore, there is a significant association between the presence of perioperative diastolic dysfunction and postoperative heart failure as well as increased hospital length of stay.[56] Several echocardiographic studies have suggested that patients with diastolic dysfunction presenting for cardiac surgery may be prone to intraoperative hemodynamic instability and worse outcomes.[57,58] These reasons support diastolic function assessment as part of the comprehensive perioperative echocardiographic examination.[59] Doppler echocardiography is the preferred technique to assess diastolic performance and grade the severity of the disease process.

Diastolic dysfunction is defined as the inability of the LV to fill at normal left atrial (LA) pressures and is characterized by a decrease in relaxation and/or LV compliance. Diastolic dysfunction may be present in the absence of clinical symptoms of heart failure. When these symptoms occur in the presence of diastolic dysfunction, then the diagnosis of diastolic heart failure is made.

Diastolic Physiology

Traditionally, the cardiac cycle has been divided into two phases: Systole, comprising isovolumic contraction and ejection, and diastole, comprising isovolumic relaxation, rapid filling, diastasis, and atrial contraction. Rather than a passive phase of the cardiac cycle when filling of the heart occurs, diastole is currently regarded as being intimately coupled and interdependent with systole. In this respect, Nishimura and Tajik.[60] have proposed dividing the cardiac cycle into three phases: Contraction, relaxation, and filling. Contraction encompasses the isovolumic contraction and the first half of ejection. The critical insight into the proposal of Nishimura and Tajik is that relaxation begins during the second part of *ejection,* and then continues during the isovolumic relaxation and rapid filling phases, illustrating the interdependency of systole and diastole. The filling phase consists of the early rapid filling phase, diastasis, and atrial contraction. The early filling phase coincides with and depends on the continuation of relaxation.

Ventricular filling is affected by load factors (preload and afterload) as well as mechanical factors such as ventricular relaxation and compliance, ventricular contraction, atrial contraction and MV dynamics, viscoelastic forces of the myocardium, and pericardial restraint.

The early manifestation of diastolic dysfunction is characterized by an impaired relaxation, implying that the rate and duration of decrease in LV pressure after systolic contraction is prolonged. This results in an inability of the LV to fill adequately during the rapid filling phase. A compensatory increase in filling occurs with atrial contraction. This stage of disease is known as *grade I diastolic dysfunction.* In more advanced stages of disease, grades II and III of diastolic dysfunction, a decrease in LV compliance ensues. Compliance is defined as a change of volume with respect to a change in pressure. Thus, a decrease in LV compliance will lead to a disproportionate increase in LV pressures and, ultimately, LA pressures.

Echocardiographic Assessment of Left Ventricular Diastolic Function

Echocardiography has become the diagnostic modality of choice for patients with diastolic dysfunction. Echocardiographic assessments have been validated by cardiac catheterization and correlate with clinical presentation.[61] The American Society of Echocardiography has issued recommendations for evaluating and grading the left ventricular diastolic function using a combination of 2-D echocardiography, pulsed-wave Doppler, M-mode color Doppler, and tissue Doppler.[62,59] This section is limited to the discussion of
5 the two most commonly used methods: Pulsed-wave Doppler of transmitral and pulmonary vein flows (PVFs) and TDI.

Imaging Views and Techniques

The echocardiographic acquisition of the diastolic parameters is best done when integrated in a standard examination. The typical view used for both transmitral flow Doppler (TMF) as well as for the TDI is the midesophageal four-chamber view. Interrogation of the pulmonary vein is usually performed in the midesophageal commissural or midesophageal two-chamber views. The interrogation volume sample should be placed at the tips of the MV for TMF assessment and 1 to 2 cm inside the pulmonary vein for the PVF assessment. For TDI of myocardial velocity profiles, the sample volume is typically placed at the junction of the mitral annulus and the lateral wall.

Interpretation of Pulsed-wave Doppler Flow Velocity Curves

Relaxation, the active phase of diastole, commences with the dissociation of actin–myosin cross-bridges and a lowering of the intracellular calcium. LV pressure begins to fall and eventually becomes lower than ascending aortic pressure, resulting in closure of the AV. As the ventricle continues to relax, the LV pressure falls below LA pressure, reaching its nadir, and promotes opening of the MV. At this point, the pressure gradient between the LA and LV is maximal and early rapid filling phase of the LV occurs. This phase is responsible for 80% to 90% of LV filling. As the ventricle fills, the LV pressure gradually rises and equates the pressure in the LA; thus, minimal flow or diastasis occurs. With commencement of the atrial contraction phase, the pressure gradient between the LA and LV rises once again and blood flows from the LA to the LV. At the end of the LA systole, the pressure in the LV rises above the LA pressure and promotes closure of the MV (Fig. 26-40).

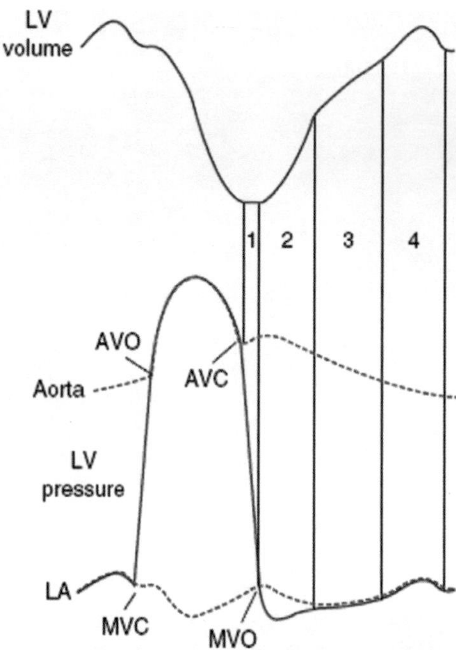

FIGURE 26-40. Diastolic phase of the cardiac cycle. During isovolumic relaxation (*1*) left ventricular (LV) pressure falls rapidly following aortic valve closure (AVC). When LV pressure decreases below left atrial (LA) pressure, the mitral valve opens (MVO), initiating early, rapid LV filling (*2*). Equilibration of LV and LA pressures results in diminished transmitral flow during diastasis (*3*) until atrial contraction (*4*). Diastole terminates with mitral valve closure (MVC). (Reproduced from Plotnick GD. Changes in diastolic function—difficult to measure, harder to interpret. *Am Heart J* 1989;118:637, with permission.)

Doppler assessment of the TMF and PVF velocities reflects the instantaneous pressure gradient (see previous discussion of the Bernoulli principle). Therefore, the displayed velocity waveforms parallel the changes in pressure gradient occurring in the left heart. The TMF profile consists of two waves, the "E" and "A" waves. The peak E wave represents the peak early filling velocity. The rate of decrease of velocity following the peak E velocity is known as the *deceleration time* (DT). The DT depends on how fast the pressure rises in LV during the rapid filling phase and represents a direct measure of ventricular compliance. Thus, if the ventricular compliance decreases, the DT shortens. The peak A wave represents the peak blood velocity during atrial contraction. In a normal individual, the E wave is slightly larger than the A wave and the DT is 200 ± 40 msec (Fig. 26-41).

Similar events take place in the LA. Ventricular contraction lowers the MV annulus creating a suction effect and promoting blood flow from the pulmonary veins to the LA. Filling of the LA decreases the pressure gradient between the pulmonary veins and LA and blood flow plateaus. As the MV opens, an open conduit forms between the pulmonary veins, LA, and LV; thus, additional forward flow to the LA occurs. Subsequently, atrial contraction raises LA pressure above pulmonary vein pressure and promotes backward blood flow into them. A normal PVF velocity curve consists of systolic forward flow representing the "S" wave, diastolic forward flow representing the "D" wave, and a reversal of velocity during atrial contraction representing the "a" wave (Fig. 26-41).

As diastolic dysfunction develops, the patterns of the flow velocity curves change in concordance with the pressure gradient changes in the pulmonary vein—LA–LV system. In grade I diastolic dysfunction, as the LV is incompletely relaxed when early ventricular filling occurs, the pressure gradient, and thus E wave velocity, is less than normal. The delayed relaxation prolongs LV filling late into diastole, and therefore the DT is prolonged. A compensatory increase in TMF during atrial contraction, due to the higher residual atrial preload, generates a high A wave velocity. Thus, the TMF curve of an individual with abnormal relaxation is represented by a low E, high A, and prolonged DT. The increased residual atrial preload generates a smaller pressure gradient between the pulmonary veins and LA; thus, less flow to the LA occurs during the early filling phase. This is represented on the PVF curves as a higher S/D ratio as compared to normal (Fig. 26-41).

Progression of diastolic disease leads to grade II diastolic dysfunction, which is marked by decreases in LV compliance. LA pressure rises as a compensatory mechanism to normalize the pressure gradient across the MV. In this scenario, the TMF velocities resemble the normal curve; thus, this stage is known as *pseudonormal.* Because of the high LA pressure, less flow from the pulmonary veins occurs during ventricular systole, generating a lower S wave on the PVF curves, and thus a lower S/D ratio. During atrial contraction, a larger amount of blood is pushed back in the pulmonary veins, represented by a deeper a wave (Fig. 26-41).

Grade III diastolic dysfunction, known as the *restrictive phase,* is characterized by a significantly decreased LV compliance. The high LA–LV pressure gradient produces a fast acceleration of blood flow in the LV. This is represented by a high E velocity on the TMF curve. LV pressure increases rapidly during filling because of the increased LV stiffness resulting in a short DT. The forward filling velocity at atrial contraction is low (small A wave) because of the decreased compliance. The elevated LA

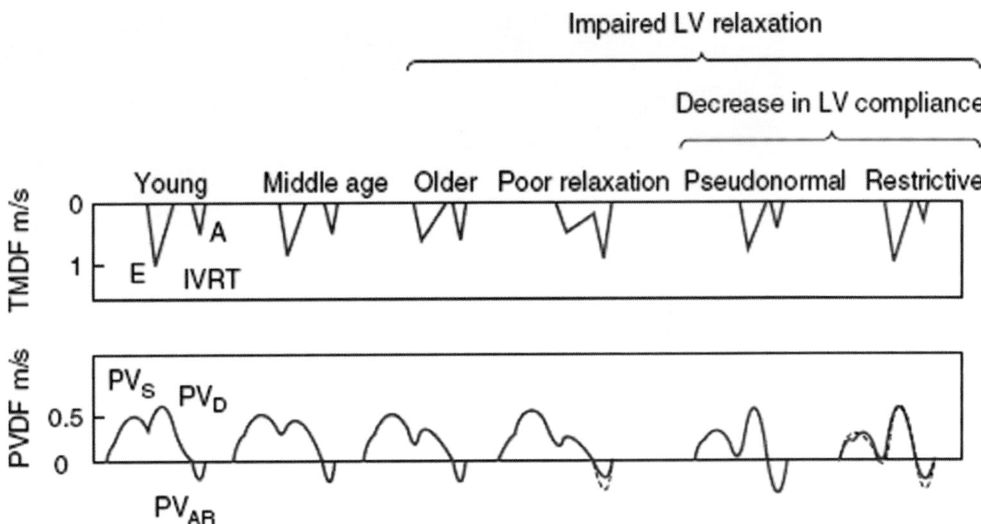

FIGURE 26-41. The impact of progressive left ventricular (LV) diastolic dysfunction on transmitral Doppler flow (TMDF) and pulmonary venous Doppler flow (PVDF). The transmitral pressure gradient is initially elevated in normal, young individuals because of vigorous LV relaxation and elastic recoil, before diminishing when relaxation becomes impaired and finally increasing again when left atrial pressure increases from an elevated LV end-diastolic pressure in the restrictive pattern of LV diastolic dysfunction. Respective changes are noted in pulmonary vein (PV) profile. E, E-wave; A, A-wave; IVRT, left ventricular isovolumic relaxation time; PV_{AR}, late diastolic retrograde velocity; PV_{S1}, first systolic component; PV_{S2}, second systolic component; PV_D, diastolic component.

pressures inhibit blood flow from the pulmonary veins to the LA during ventricular systole, and the PVF curves show a decreased S/D ratio (Fig. 26-41). One of the important caveats to assessing diastolic function using pulsed-wave Doppler is that the flow patterns depend on pressure gradients and therefore are affected by both preload and afterload. In settings in which the load conditions vary at a fast pace, such as the operating room, changes in TMF or PVF velocities may be difficult to interpret. TDI, which directly measures myocardial velocities, provides a more load-independent method of diastolic function assessment.[63]

The normal mitral annular TDI profile has a biphasic diastolic component: The early diastolic wave E′ related to the early filling and the late diastolic wave A′ related to atrial contraction (Fig. 26-39). In a healthy patient, the TDI pattern mirrors the TMF pattern, except with lower velocities. E′ reflects LV relaxation and values <8 cm/s are considered a sign of diastolic dysfunction.[64] Thus, in patients with pseudonormal or restrictive disease, in whom normal or elevated E wave TMF velocities occur despite advanced pathology, the TDI E′ wave remains reduced, making it a useful approach to diagnosis.

Pericardial Disease: Constrictive Pericarditis and Pericardial Tamponade

Diastolic filling is also impacted by pericardial restraint. Pericardial pathologies, such as constrictive pericarditis or pericardial tamponade, impede diastolic flow.[65] On TMF Doppler profiles these diseases resemble the diastolic restrictive filling pattern. Two-dimensional echocardiography can be helpful in differentiating among these pathologies. In constrictive pericarditis the pericardium appears thick, fibrotic, calcified, and thus echogenic; the inferior vena cava is dilated and the ventricular septum has an abnormal motion.

Pericardial effusions can be global, surrounding the entire heart, or loculated, as seen mostly after cardiac surgery (Fig. 26-42). Since the intrapericardial volume is constant, cardiac chambers are compressed when at their lowest pressure (atria in systole, ventricles in diastole). Pericardial tamponade is characterized by the presence of a large pericardial effusion seen as an echo-free (black) space, a "swinging motion" of the heart, early diastolic RV collapse, and late diastolic right atrium (RA) collapse.

In summary, diastolic filling is an active process and a major component of effective cardiac performance. The presence of diastolic dysfunction, whether resulting from loss in fluid volume, LV disease, or pericardial restraint, is associated with potential deleterious surgical outcomes. Doppler echocardiography, in particular TDI, provides the anesthesiologist the means to rapidly diagnose and guide therapy of such patients in the perioperative period.

EVALUATION OF VALVULAR HEART DISEASE

Two-dimensional echocardiography and Doppler are complementary methods in valve assessment. The 2-D echocardiography provides evaluation of valve anatomy and function and Doppler assesses the physiologic consequences and severity of the lesion.

Aortic Stenosis

Two-dimensional and M-mode Echocardiography

The normal aortic valve (AV) has three cusps, which open without restriction in systole, yielding an AV area 3 to 4 cm^2. The appearance of the valve and the systolic excursion of its cusps are imaged with 2-D and M-mode echocardiography. The AV is

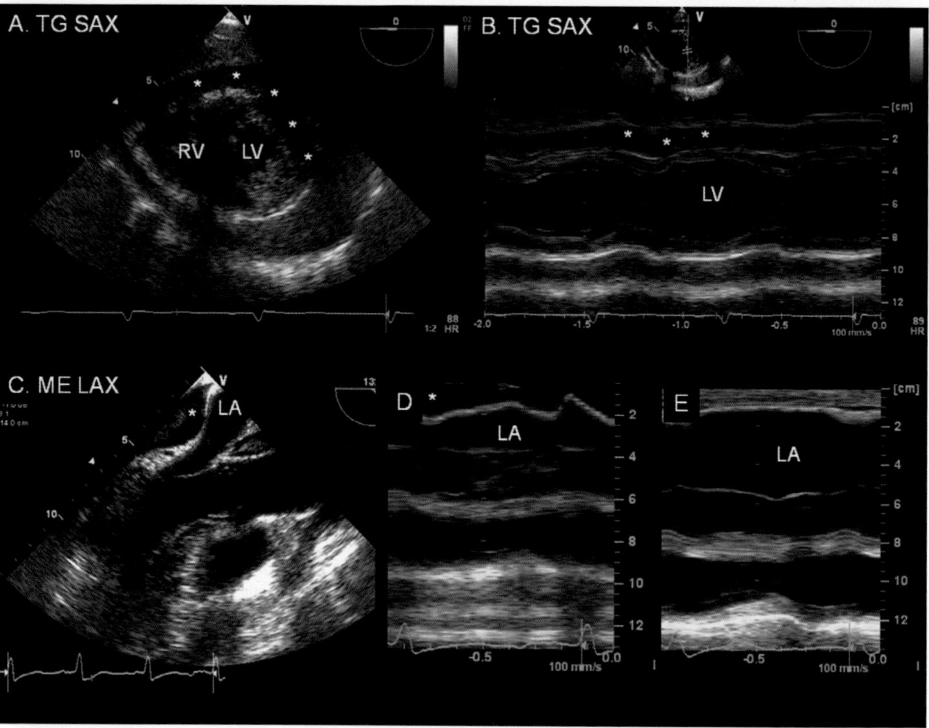

FIGURE 26-42. Echocardiographic findings in pericardial effusion. **A:** Global pericardial effusion (asterisks) surrounding both right ventricle (RV) and left ventricle (LV). Transgastric short-axis (TG SAX) view. **B:** M-mode echocardiography demonstrates separation of the epicardium from the pericardium (asterisks) from pericardial effusion. **C:** Regional pericardial effusion (asterisks) compressing the left atrium (LA), seen in the mid-esophageal long-axis (ME LAX) view. **D:** M-mode echocardiography reveals systolic compression (asterisk) of LA. **E:** After evacuation of the fluid collection, the LA size increases.

imaged enface in the midesophageal aortic valve short-axis view and its profile in the midesophageal aortic valve long-axis view (Figs. 26-10 and 26-11). With the TEE probe inside the stomach, the AV is imaged in the deep transgastric long axis and transgastric long-axis views (Figs. 26-21 and 26-22). Owing to the increased afterload, associated findings may include concentric hypertrophy of the LV, decreased EF, as well as mitral regurgitation and left atrial dilatation.

Doppler Echocardiography

Jet Velocity, Transvalvular Pressure Gradient. The transvalvular pressure gradient can be calculated from the CWD-measured velocity (V) using the modified Bernoulli equation: $\Delta P = 4 \times V^2$.[66] The mean gradient, calculated from the VTI tracing is commonly reported as it correlates well with the angiographically determined pressure gradient.[67] However, for any given valve area, the flow velocity and pressure gradient vary with changes in stroke volume and cardiac output. An LV with normal function will generate a large pressure gradient across a critically stenosed AV, and a dysfunctional LV will not.[68]

Valve Area

Using the continuity equation, the flow across the LVOT equals the flow across the stenosed AV or $VTI_{LVOT} \times Area_{LVOT} = VTI_{AV} \times Area_{AV}$. By rearranging the equation, $Area_{AV} = (VTI_{LVOT} \times Area_{LVOT})/(VTI_{AV})$. The $Area_{LVOT}$ is calculated using the LVOT diameter at the site of the Doppler measurement (Fig. 26-35). An error in the LVOT diameter measurement is geometrically increased as $Area_{LVOT} = \pi \times (D/2)^2$). The VTI_{LVOT}/VTI_{AV} ratio is often calculated to avoid this error as flow changes will be reflected proportionally across both the AV and LVOT (Doppler dimensionless index). An index value <0.25% indicates an AV
6 area <0.75 cm^2. The echocardiographic cut-off values for grading aortic stenosis are shown in Table 26-3.[69]

TABLE 26-3. GRADING OF AORTIC STENOSIS

	Aortic Sclerosis	Mild	Moderate	Severe	
Peak AV velocity (m/s)	<=2.5	2.6–2.9	3.0–4.0	>4	>4.0
LVOT/AV velocity ratio		>0.5	0.25–0.5	<0.25	
Mean transvalvular gradient (mm Hg)		<20	20–40	>4	>40
AVA (cm^2)		>1.5	1.5–1.0	<1	<1.0

AV, aortic valve; AVA, AV area.

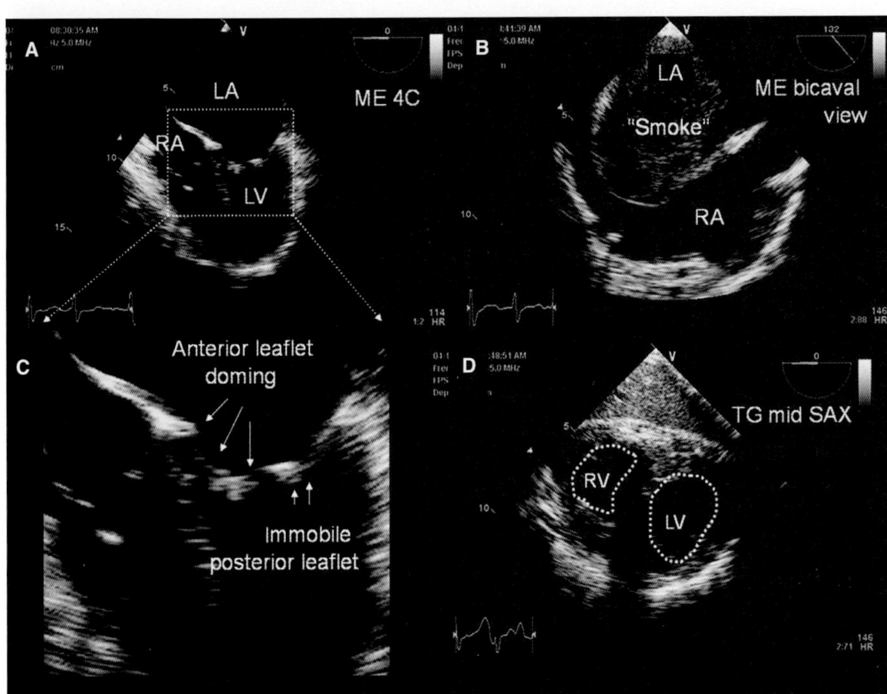

FIGURE 26-43. Two-dimensional echocardiographic findings in mitral stenosis. **A:** In the midesophageal four-chamber (ME 4C) view, echocardiographic signs of mitral stenosis include a dilated left atrium (LA) with a rightward displacement of the interatrial septum (indicating the elevated LA pressure), and a small left ventricle (LV). **B:** In the midesophageal bicaval view, red blood cell clumping creates spontaneous echocardiography contrast. Note the rightward displacement of the interatrial septum toward the right atrium (RA). **C:** A zoom image of the mitral valve and neighboring structures in midesophageal four-chamber view. The anterior mitral leaflet exhibits diastolic doming while the posterior mitral leaflet is immobile. **D:** In the transgastric midpapillary short-axis (TG mid SAX) view, the LV cavity is relatively small, as compared with the right ventricle (RV), and interventricular septum appears thickened.

Mitral Stenosis

Two-dimensional Echocardiography

The MV is imaged in the midesophageal views and in the basal transgastric short-axis views. The leaflets can appear thickened and calcified (thus, strongly echogenic), while there may be fusion of the chordae and papillary muscles. The major and most striking finding in mitral stenosis (MS) is the inability of the two mitral leaflets to separate from each other in diastole. Instead, their tips remain opposed while the body of the leaflets bows toward the LV cavity because of the incoming blood (Fig. 26-43). The area of the MV orifice can be traced by planimetry in the transgastric basal short-axis view.[70] Associated findings in MS are a dilated left atrium and left atrial appendage (because of increased pressure), and the presence of thrombus or spontaneous echocardiographic contrast due to low flow in the LA. The LV cavity appears small, with a thickened and immobile interventricular septum. The right ventricle may be dilated and/or hypertrophied, with thickened walls, because of increased pressure work (Fig. 26-43 and Table 26-4).

TABLE 26-4. GRADING OF MITRAL STENOSIS

	Mild	Moderate	Severe
Mean pressure gradient (mm Hg)	<6	5–10	>10
Pressure half time (ms)	≤100	100–220	>220
Mitral valve area (cm^2)	>1.5	1.0–1.5	<1.0
Systolic pulmonary artery pressure (mm Hg)	<30	30–50	>50

Doppler Echocardiography

Transvalvular Pressure Gradient. The increased diastolic pressure gradient is measured with continuous Doppler in the midesophageal four-chamber or long-axis view.[66] The early diastolic velocity of the transmitral flow (E wave) is increased (usually >1.5 m/s). This is not specific to MS, as E velocity will also be elevated in the presence of increased blood flow, as in severe mitral regurgitation.[71] In severe MS, the mean pressure gradient is >10 mm Hg (Fig. 26-44).

Pressure Half-time (PHT)

The deceleration of E velocity is decreased, because in MS the equalization of transmitral valve pressures takes a longer time. PHT is the time required for the peak pressure to decrease to half its value. The decaying velocity is traced on the CWD signal obtained from across the MV in diastole and the analysis package calculates the PHT (Fig. 26-44B). MV area (MVA) is calculated as 220/PHT. A prolonged PHT >220 ms is related to severe MS (calculated MVA <1 cm^2) as smaller MV orifices will prolong the pressure decay across the valve.[72] When LV compliance is decreased or there is coexisting aortic regurgitation, the increased LV pressure results in a faster pressure equilibration across the stenosed MV. In such cases, PHT will be shortened, and the calculated MVA may be erroneously overestimated.[73]

Associated Findings

CFD will display a "rising sun" pattern of diastolic velocities inside the LA, indicating the high velocity (and increased pressure gradient) across the stenosed MV that exceeds the limits of the color scale (Fig. 26-44A). Associated findings include pulmonary insufficiency due to pulmonary hypertension and tricuspid regurgitation.

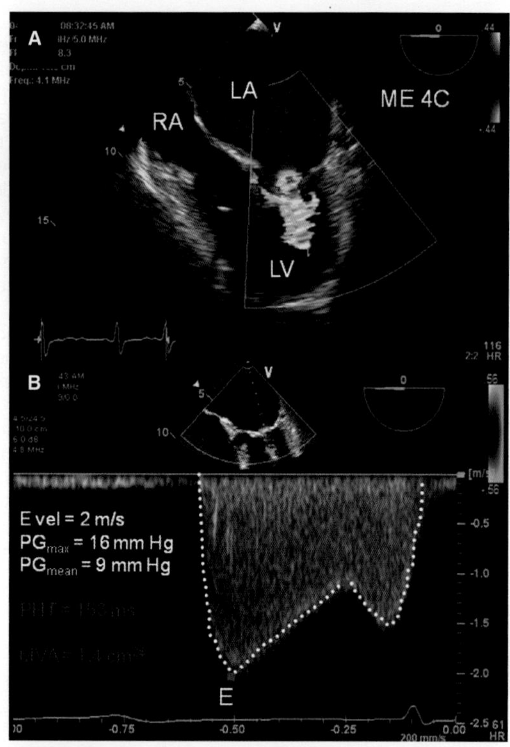

FIGURE 26-44. Doppler echocardiography findings in mitral stenosis. **A:** Diastolic blood acceleration upstream of the mitral valve is seen with color-flow Doppler ("rising sun"). **B:** Spectral display of the diastolic velocity decay is imaged with a pulsed-wave Doppler sample volume placed at the tips of the mitral valve. Tracing of the velocity envelope (*white dots*) calculates the maximum and mean pressure gradient (PG). The pressure half-time (PHT) is calculated from the deceleration of the peak velocity (Evel) (*red dots*). The mitral valve area (MVA) is derived from the empiric formula: MVA = 220/PHT.

Aortic Regurgitation

Two-dimensional and M-mode Echocardiography

The AV is imaged in the same views used for the assessment of aortic stenosis. Associated findings may include dilated aortic root (Marfan's syndrome), endocarditis lesions, dilated ascending aorta, calcified AV, aortic dissection (may be associated with acute aortic insufficiency [AI]), fluttering of the anterior mitral leaflet and restricted diastolic opening of the MV from the AI jet, or a dilated LV in chronic AI (Table 26-5).

Doppler Echocardiography

Color Flow. In either of the midesophageal or the transgastric views of the AV, a CFD sector over the AV and the LVOT will demonstrate the presence or absence of the AI regurgitant jet. CFD reveals the characteristics of the AI jet as it enters the LVOT in diastole. The following techniques are used to grade the severity of AI.

Ratio of Jet Height to LVOT Diameter

The maximal height of the AI jet (within <1 cm from the AV plane) is compared with the LVOT diameter at the same point.

TABLE 26-5. GRADING OF AORTIC INSUFFICIENCY (AI)

	Mild	Moderate	Severe
AI jet height/ LVOT diameter (%)	<25	25–64	>65
Vena contracta (mm)	<0.3–	–0.3–0.6	>6
PHT (ms)	>500	200–500	<200
Aortic diastolic flow reversal	—	—	Holodiastolic

LVOT, left ventricular outflow tract; PHT, pressure half-time.

The recommended view is the midesophageal aortic valve long-axis view. A central jet usually is caused by aortic root dilation, whereas an eccentric jet implies an AV cusp lesion. The propagation of the jet into the LV does not correlate well with the angiographic degree of AI, and should not be used to grade AI (Fig. 26-31).[74]

Vena Contracta

Vena contracta is the narrowest "neck" of the AI jet as it traverses the AV plane, usually best appreciated in the midesophageal aortic valve long-axis view. The largest diameter of the vena
7 contracta in diastole is selected (Fig. 26-31). The size of vena contracta is relatively load-independent and provides a reliable way to quantitate AI intraoperatively, in the presence of fluctuating hemodynamics.[74]

Pressure Half-time

PHT of the AI jet is recorded in the transgastric long axis or deep transgastric long-axis view. PHT expresses the pressure equilibration of the diastolic blood pressure ("driving" pressure) and the diastolic LV pressure ("resistance" pressure). A short PHT (<200 ms) is associated with severe AI. Factors associated with decreased LV compliance (e.g., LV failure with restrictive filling pattern) will cause the transaortic pressure gradient to dissipate faster and will overestimate the severity of AI (Fig. 26-30).

Aortic Diastolic Flow Reversal

Retrograde diastolic flow in the descending and abdominal aorta is sensitive and specific for severe AI. This is imaged with PWD in the midesophageal long-axis view of the distal descending aorta (Fig. 26-30).[75]

Other Findings

Severe AI rapidly elevates LV diastolic pressure and shortens the early transmitral flow velocity, resulting in a *restrictive LV filling pattern.* The *regurgitant volume* is calculated using the continuity equation and equals the difference between LVOT flow and the diastolic transmitral flow. Values >60 mL are consistent with severe AI.

Mitral Regurgitation

Two-dimensional Echocardiography

The normal MV anatomy consists of two leaflets (anterior and posterior), their coaptation surface, the fibrous mitral annulus, the subvalvular apparatus with the two papillary muscles (anterolateral and posteromedial), and their chordae tendineae, which attach to the underside of the mitral leaflets. The competency of the MV depends on adequate coaptation between the D-shaped anterior leaflet and the crescent-shaped posterior leaflet. Common causes of mitral regurgitation (MR) are myxomatous valve degeneration, endocarditis, and ischemic, rheumatic and congenital heart disease (CHD).

The required TEE views for imaging of the MV include the midesophageal four-chamber, midesophageal commissural, midesophageal two-chamber, midesophageal aortic valve long-axis view, and the basal transgastric short-axis and two-chamber views (Figs. 26-14–26-20).[76] Echocardiographic findings may include any of the following: Abnormal texture of leaflets (myxomatous degeneration), flail and/or prolapsing leaflet, ruptured chordae, papillary muscle dysfunction or rupture (secondary to ischemia), mitral annulus calcification, or endocarditis lesions. The leaflet motion is commonly reported using Carpentier's classification as described in Table 26-6.

Doppler Echocardiography

Color-flow Doppler. CFD is commonly used as a screening tool for the detection of MR. It provides an easy, qualitative technique but additional tests are advised to grade the severity of MR (Fig. 26-45). If the MR jet is >40% of the LA area, often times severe MR is present.[77] There are several limitations to this technique. It is difficult to visualize the entire LA with TEE. Secondly, eccentric jets that are in contact with the LA walls are underestimated (Coandă effect).[78] Third, machine settings such as frame rate and color Doppler scale influence the appearance of the MR jet. Fourth, despite its appearance, the color area associated with MR is not equivalent to regurgitant volume. CFD simply shows the area within the LA where blood has abnormal velocity and is dependent on the systolic pressure gradient between the LV (adequate LV systolic function) and the LA (chamber compliance). In acute MR, for example, the MR jet velocities are low because MR occurs in a noncompliant chamber.

TABLE 26-6. CARPENTIER CLASSIFICATION OF MITRAL REGURGITATION (MR)

Carpentier Type	Motion Leaflet	Jet Direction
1	Normal	Central
2	Excessive (prolapse, flail)	Away from lesion
3a	Restricted, structure is abnormal	Variable
3b	Restricted, structure is normal	

Proximal Isovelocity Surface Area

During systole, blood inside the LV cavity accelerates as it converges toward the orifice of the incompetent MV (Fig. 26-32). This velocity pattern resembles concentric hemispheres, whose surfaces have the same velocity at a given distance (radius, R) from the MV orifice. Such an isovelocity surface is called *PISA*. Its velocity can be determined by the color Doppler system's aliasing

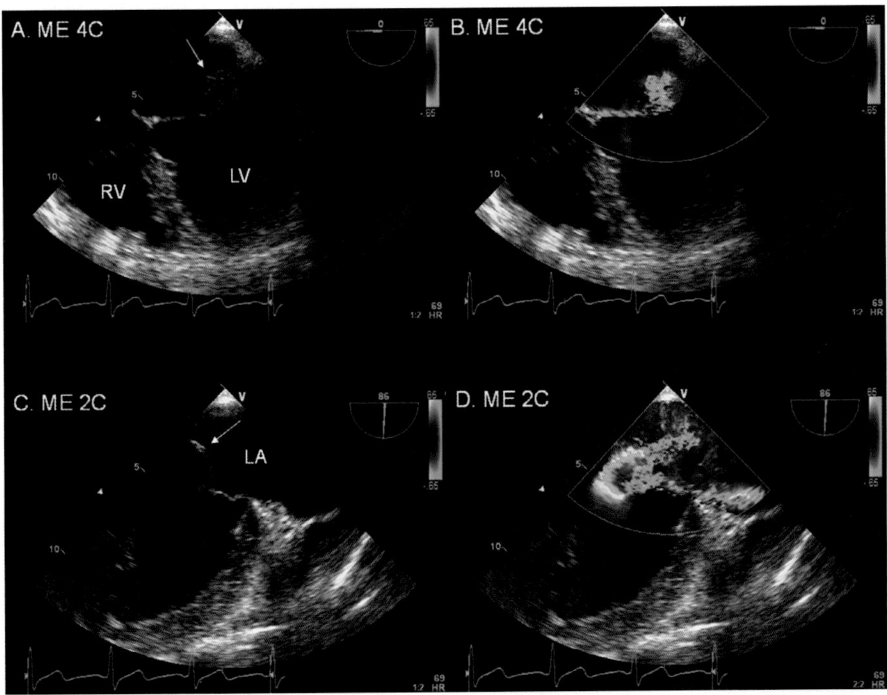

FIGURE 26-45. Mitral regurgitation. The anatomy of mitral valve (MV) is depicted with two-dimensional **(A** and **C)** echocardiographic imaging, and the presence of mitral regurgitation (MR) is imaged with color Doppler **(B** and **D).** The MV is incompetent because of posterior leaflet prolapse inside the left atrium (LA) during systole (*arrows left* in **A** and **C**). Left ventricular (LV) systolic contraction generates and anterior-directed MR jet, away from the MV lesion area. ME 4C, midesophageal four-chamber view; ME 2C, midesophageal two-chamber view.

velocity.[79] Based on the principle of conservation of mass (continuity equation), the flow through the MR orifice is the same as the flow of the PISA surface:

$$\text{MR flow} = \text{PISA flow},$$

$$\text{MR orifice} \times \text{MR velocity} = 2\pi(R^2) \times \text{Aliasing Velocity}.$$

$$\text{MR orifice} = 6.28(R^2) \times \text{Aliasing Velocity/MR Velocity}.$$

A simplified PISA equation yields MR orifice = (PISA radius)^2/2, provided the Nyquist limit is set at 40 cm/s and that the MR jet has a velocity of 5 m/s.[80] Most significantly, a small error in measuring the PISA radius (R^2) will be squared in the equation.

Vena Contracta

Vena contracta is the narrowest part of the MR jet, and reflects
8 the effective or physiologic area of the MR jet (Fig. 26-32). MR is severe if vena contracta is ≥7 mm.

Pulmonary Vein Inflow Pattern

The increased volume inside the LA will augment the transmitral diastolic pressure gradient and will produce a restrictive filling pattern in severe MR (E to A wave ratio >2). For the same reasons, the systolic filling of the LA via the pulmonary veins (S wave) will be decreased, in moderate and severe MR (Table 26-7).

Tricuspid Regurgitation

The tricuspid valve (TV) is evaluated concomitant with the right ventricle, using the midesophageal four-chamber, midesophageal right ventricular inflow–outflow, midesophageal bicaval, and transgastric RV long-axis views. The TV plane is closer to the cardiac apex than the MV plane. Tricuspid regurgitation (TR) is most commonly secondary to pulmonary hypertension from left-sided cardiac pathology, while endocarditis, carcinoid, Ebstein's anomaly, and rheumatic heart disease are less frequent causes of TR.

Two-dimensional Echocardiography

The TV anatomy is examined for abnormal appearance (annular dilation, endocarditis vegetations, and thrombus) and motion (prolapsing or flailing leaflets). Structures proximal (inferior vena cava, right atrium, and interatrial septum) and distal (right ventricle and interventricular septum) to the TV are examined for signs of volume and pressure overload.

Doppler Echocardiography

CFD is applied to detect the presence, size, and direction of a TR jet, its vena contracta, and the PISA inside the RV. CWD is used to measure the TR jet velocity and calculate the RV and PA systolic pressure. PWD is used to record the hepatic vein flow pattern. Grading of severity of TR is shown in Table 26-8.

Pulmonic Valve Regurgitation

Pulmonic valve regurgitation (PR) is evaluated in the midesophageal right ventricular inflow–outflow, the upper esophageal aortic arch short axis, and in the modified deep transgastric RV views (approximately 60 to 70 degrees). PR is often an incidental finding. PR can develop because of right-sided endocarditis, or

TABLE 26-7. GRADING OF MITRAL REGURGITATION

	Mild	Moderate	Severe
Qualitative Findings			
Jet area/LA area	<20%	—	>40%
Density of CW signal	—	—	Dense, complete envelope
Pulmonary blood flow	—	S blunted (S/D < 1)	S reversed (S < 0)
Quantitative Measurements			
Vena contracta (mm)	<3	3–7	≥7
EROA (cm^2)	<0.20	0.20–0.40	≥0.40
Regurgitant volume (mL)	<30	30–60	≥60
Regurgitant fraction (%)	<30	30–50	≥50

LA, left atrium; CW, continuous wave; S, S wave; S/D, Systolic wave of pulmonary vein flow to diastolic wave of pulmonary vein flow ratio; EROA, effective regurgitant orifice area

TABLE 26-8. GRADING OF TRICUSPID REGURGITATION

Echocardiographic Parameter	Mild	Severe
TV morphology	Normal	Prolapse, malcoaptation, endocarditis lesion, mass
IVC/RA/RV size	Normal	Dilated/increased
TR jet area (cm^2)	<5	>10
Vena contracta width (mm) (Nyquist limit 50–60 cm/s)	—	>7
PISA radius (mm) (Nyquist limit ~28 cm/s)	<6	>9
TR jet features	Soft, parabolic	Dense, triangular, early peak
Hepatic vein flow pattern	S > D	Systolic wave below baseline

TV, tricuspid valve; IVC, inferior vena cava; RA, right atrium; RV, right ventricle; PISA, proximal isovelocity surface area; TR, tricuspid regurgitation; S, Systolic wave of hepatic view flow; D, diastolic wave of hepatic vein flow.

TABLE 26-9. GRADING OF PULMONARY REGURGITATION

Parameter	Mild	Severe
PV morphology	Normal	Abnormal
RV size	Normal	Dilated
PR jet size	Length <1 cm, narrow origin	Large, wide origin
PR jet features	Soft, slow deceleration	Dense, rapid deceleration

PV, pulmonary vein; RV, right ventricle; PR, pulmonary regurgitation.

secondary to pulmonary hypertension. Grading of severity of PR is described in Table 26-9.

DISEASES OF THE AORTA

The evaluation of the aorta is an important part of perioperative TEE. In routine cases such as coronary artery bypass surgery, evaluation of the aorta may reveal previously unknown, significant atheromatous disease of the aorta and alter the surgical plan (off-pump bypass, alternative sites for cannulation). In emergencies, the diagnosis of aortic pathology (dissection, aneurysm, transsection) may prove life-saving.

Two-dimensional and Motion-mode Echocardiography

The entire thoracic aorta can be imaged with TEE, apart from the distal ascending and proximal arch segments, where the interposition of the left main bronchus between the esophagus and the left atrium prohibits the propagation of ultrasound. This blind spot can be imaged using epiaortic scanning.[81] The normal aorta has a smooth endothelial surface, and blood flow is laminar. Atherosclerotic plaques are irregularly shaped, sometimes mobile protrusions, inside the aortic lumen. The search for atheromas should be done by imaging the entire circumference of the aortic lumen (short-axis views). Once a particular lesion is found, scanning in long-axis view should be performed
9 (Fig. 26-46). Plaques thicker than 4 mm are more likely to cause an embolic event.[82,83]

Aortic aneurysm is a dilatation of the aorta, usually >4 cm. Once the aneurysm is >5.5 cm, the probability of rupture increases (Fig. 26-47A, B). Dissection is a separation between the intimal and medial layers of the aortic wall, creating a false lumen for
10 blood flow[84] (Figs. 26-47C, D and 26-48). Both the true and false lumens fill with blood during systole, but only the true lumen has blood during diastole. Intramural hematoma is considered a precursor of dissection and should be treated similarly.[85] Compared with an atheroma, an intramural hematoma has a smooth surface.

CARDIAC MASSES

Cardiac tumors can either originate from the heart or are metastases from other sites. They can embolize, cause arrhythmias, or cause heart failure. The most common primary tumor is myxoma,

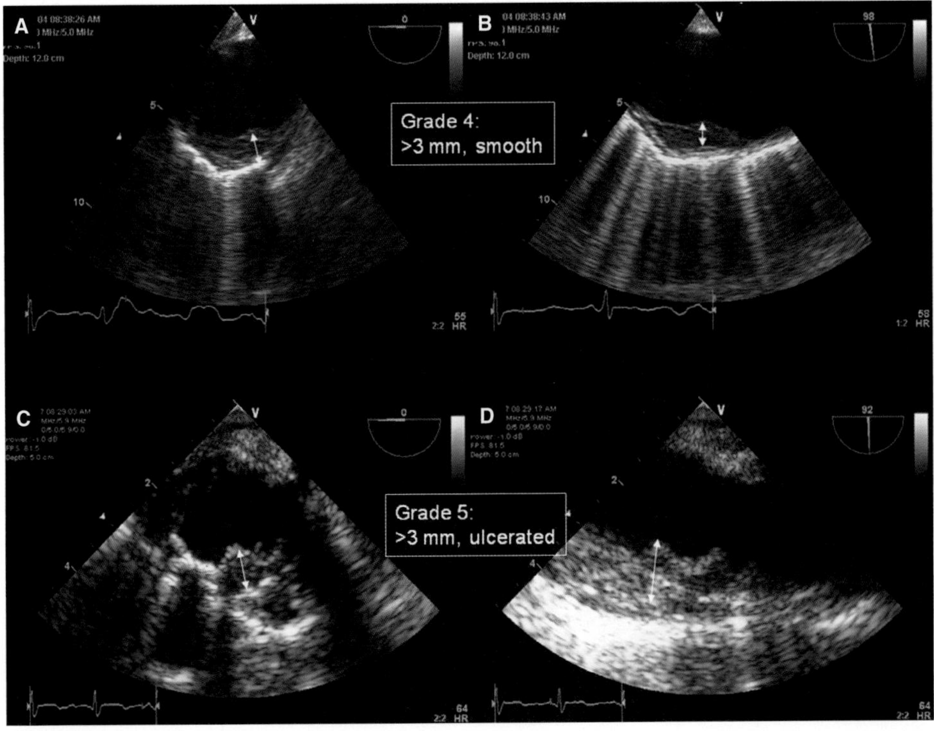

FIGURE 26-46. Aortic atheromas imaged in descending thoracic aorta short **(A** and **C)** and long **(B** and **D)** axis views.

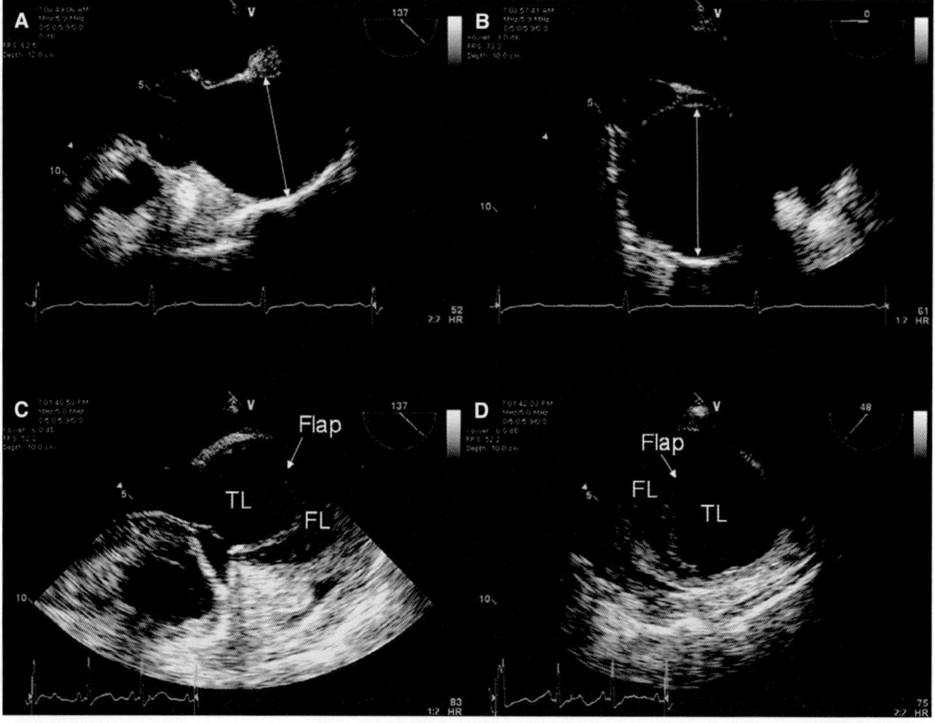

FIGURE 26-47. Aortic disease. Ascending aorta aneurysm distal to the sinotubular junction (midesophageal ascending aorta long **(A)** and short **(B)** axis views). The diameter of the aorta is 5 cm. **C:** Ascending aorta dissection (Stanford type A) originating from the sinotubular junction. The true lumen (TL) expands in systole and the flap is convex toward the false lumen (FL). **D:** Descending aorta dissection (DeBakey type III).

which is located most frequently at the interatrial septum. The potential of myxomas to obstruct the inflow or outflow region of a ventricle is demonstrated with Doppler echocardiography. The next most frequent tumor is fibroma of the ventricular wall. Fibromas are usually calcified, and can decrease the ventricular volume. Renal cell tumors often extend into the inferior vena cava and right atrium (Fig. 26-49). Pacemaker wires, thrombus, and normal anatomic structures that mimic the appearance of pathology (Eustachian valve, crista terminalis, Chiari network, or "Coumadin" ridge) should be differentiated from tumors.

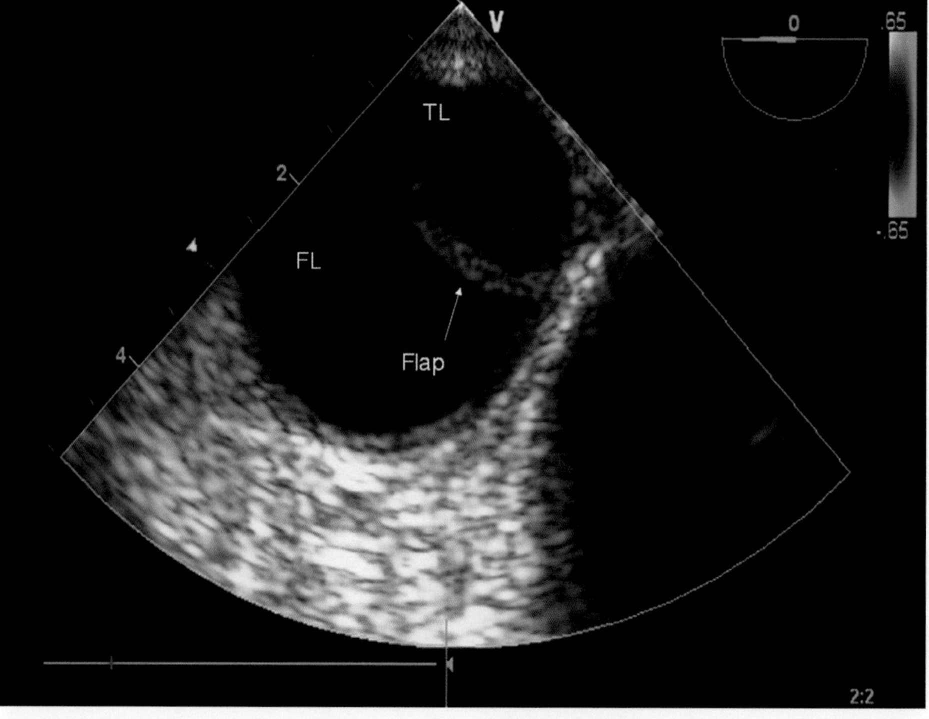

FIGURE 26-48. Aortic dissection. The descending aorta is seen in short axis. The aortic true lumen (TL) contains the aortic endothelium and has a smooth endoluminal surface. The intimal flap usually bows toward the false lumen (FL). Color-flow Doppler demonstrates blood flow inside the true lumen (which expands in systole) and the absence of flow inside the false lumen.

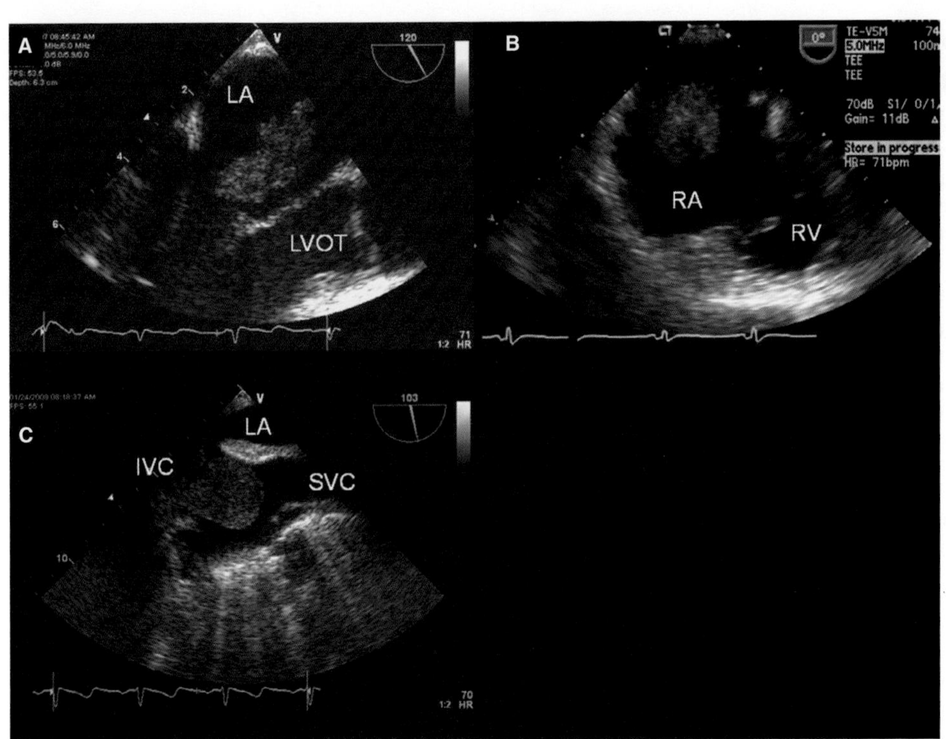

FIGURE 26-49. Cardiac masses. **A:** Left atrial (LA) myxoma seen in the midesophageal long-axis view. **B:** Right atrial (RA) myxoma seen inside the right atrium (RA) in the midesophageal four-chamber view. **C:** Renal cell tumor occupying the inferior vena cava (IVC) and extending inside the RA. LVOT, left ventricular outflow tract; RV, right ventricle; SVC, superior vena cava.

CONGENITAL HEART DISEASE

The spectrum of CHD seen in adults varies widely. Echocardiography is the primary imaging modality for diagnostic assessment of CHD. Advances in surgery have increased the survival rate of children with repaired CHD and, as a consequence, adults with repaired CHD are increasingly common in the OR. Common lesions evaluated with TEE include ASD, ventricular septal defect, patent ductus arteriosus, coarctation of the aorta, bicuspid AV, and repaired tetralogy of Fallot (Fig. 26-50).[86]

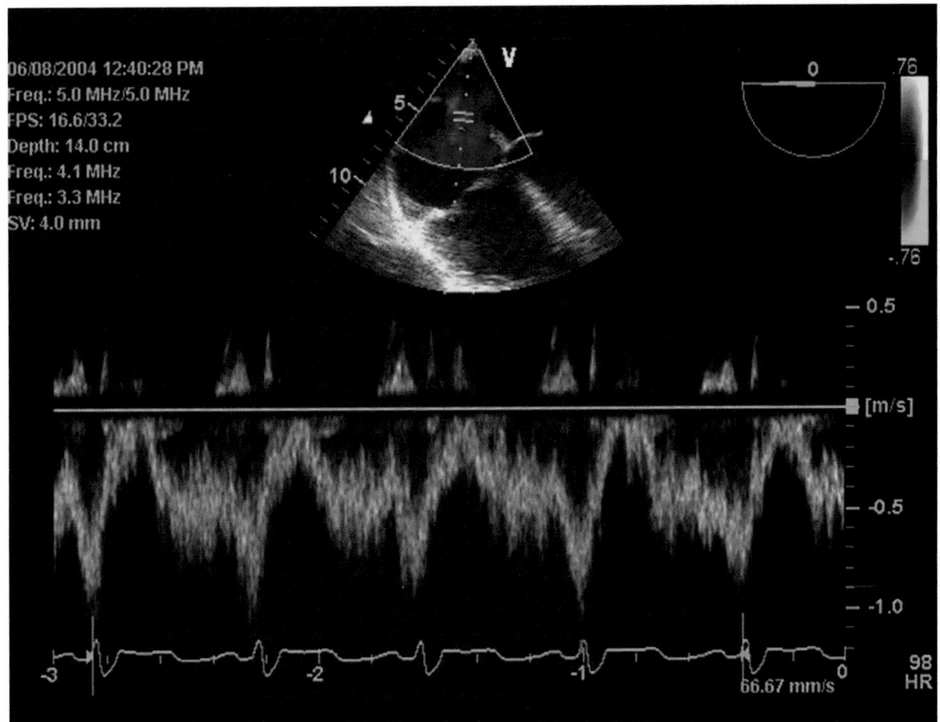

FIGURE 26-50. Atrial septal defect (ASD). In the midesophageal four-chamber view, a color-Doppler sector is positioned over the interatrial septum. An ASD with a left-to-right communication is shown in blue color, as the blood moves away from the transducer **(top panel)**. Pulsed-wave Doppler interrogation of the ASD measures a peak velocity gradient of 1 m/s.

ECHOCARDIOGRAPHY-ASSISTED PROCEDURES

In addition to its role in diagnostics, echocardiography is also employed to assist various procedures such as the placement of central venous catheter, IABP catheter, coronary sinus (CS) cannula, and guide wires for other venous or arterial cannulae.

Ultrasound-guided Central Vein Cannulation

The placement of central venous catheters is associated with complications including injury to vascular structures (carotid artery), pleura, nerve bundles, lymphatic system, and even the spinal canal. Historically, anatomic landmarks guided needle orientation during central venous access. However, multiple studies have demonstrated that the anatomic relationship between the internal jugular vein and the carotid artery varies, and that even experienced physicians encounter complications.[87] Visual guidance by ultrasound provides real-time feedback, reducing the complication rate and the procedure time.[88] For patient safety reasons the National Institute for Clinical Excellence, as well as the Society of Cardiovascular Anesthesiologists, have recommended that internal jugular central lines be placed under guidance of 2-D ultrasound imaging.[89,90]

A linear array hand-held transducer with high frequencies (7.5 to 12 MHz) is preferred for ultrasound-guided central line placement. The technique relies on placing the transducer over the traditional anatomic landmarks and identifying the internal jugular vein (IJ) and carotid artery (CA) in short axis and their anatomic relationship (Fig. 26-51). The 2-D criteria of differentiating the CA from the IJ vein are distensibility (the IJ increases in size with the Valsalva maneuver and the Trendelenburg position) and compressibility (the IJ will decrease in size with pressure applied over it by the transducer). Applying CFD with the transducer oriented slightly caudad displays the CA with red pulsating flow and the IJ with a continuous blue flow (Fig. 26-51). Note that if the transducer is oriented cephalad the colors are reversed. The needle insertion and venous puncture is performed under ultrasound guidance. The longitudinal view (Fig. 26-52A) is then used to view the wire's placement in the vessel. TEE can confirm the guide wire's position in the superior vena cava (Fig. 26-52B).

For PAC placement, TEE is useful in guiding the catheter through the right heart and confirming proper position in the PA. In the midesophageal right ventricular inflow–outflow view, the PAC can be followed from the RA, passing the TV into the RV, and then passing the PV into the PA. The midesophageal ascending aortic short-axis view may be used to position the PAC so that its tip lies in the right PA (if that is the desired position; some clinicians prefer positioning the PAC in the main PA).

Although ultrasound can be a valuable tool in decreasing the number of complications associated with central vein cannulation and PAC placement, it does not eliminate the risks.

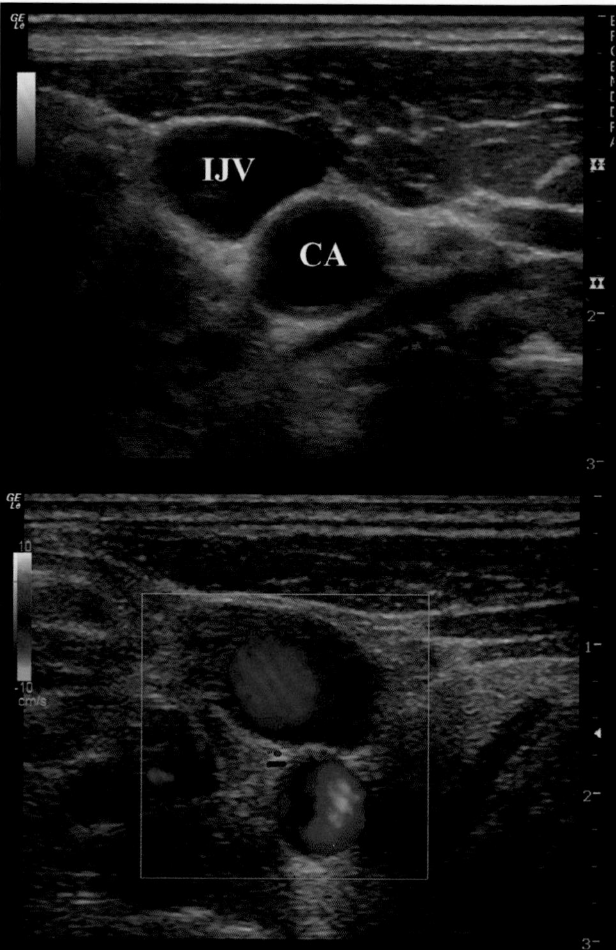

FIGURE 26-51. Internal jugular vein (IJV) and carotid artery (CA) and their anatomic relationship. **Top panel:** Two-dimensional examination, using a linear scanner, showing the IJV lateral to the CA. **Bottom panel:** Color-flow Doppler is applied showing continuous blue flow in the IJV and pulsating red flow in the CA (transducer oriented caudad).

Intra-aortic Balloon Pump Placement

The use of TEE during IABP placement allows positioning of the catheter to the preferred location, just distal to the left subclavian artery. Prior to its insertion, the echocardiographer should assess the descending thoracic aorta for the presence of mobile atheroma or aortic dissections. These situations may represent contraindications to catheter placement. During cannulation, the presence of the guide wire in the descending aorta should be confirmed with TEE. Optimal function of the IABP requires that the tip lies 1 to 10 cm distal to the left subclavian artery. The exact position of the IABP catheter tip is best visualized using the descending aortic long-axis view.[91]

Coronary Sinus Cannulation

TEE is helpful to guide the placement of the cannula and to check for proper position. Improper insertion of the cannula can result in injury to the interatrial septum or to the crux of the heart, the fragile area joining the atria and ventricles. View of the coronary sinus (CS) is obtained from the midesophageal four-chamber view by retroflexing the probe (Fig. 26-53). After the cannula is positioned in the CS, the multiplane angle should be rotated to 90 degrees and the CS will be seen in cross section. The tip of the cannula will be displayed as a small echo-dense dot in the middle of the CS. This view will assure that the cannula is positioned at an appropriate depth.

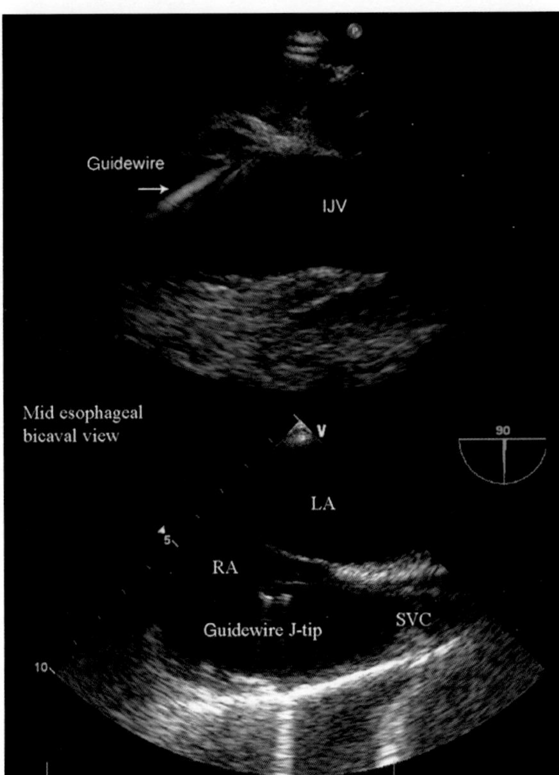

FIGURE 26-52. Top: Ultrasound confirmation of guide wire position. A sector scanner transducer is used to visualize the internal jugular vein (IJV) in long axis. The guide wire is seen as a thin echo-dense linear structure positioned in the lumen of the vein. **Bottom:** Transesophageal echocardiographic confirmation of guide wire position. The mid-esophageal bicaval view is used. The guide wire is seen in the superior vena cava (SVC), with the tip in the right atrium (RA); LA, left atrium.

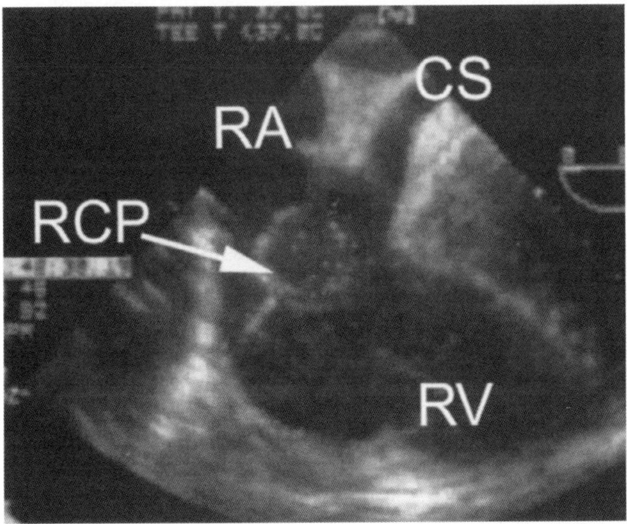

FIGURE 26-53. Probe retroflexion from the midesophageal four-chamber view is used to visualize the coronary sinus (CS). The *arrow* points to the balloon of the retrograde cannula (RCP), right atrium (RA), and right ventricle (RV).

Other Cannulation Techniques

TEE is useful in verifying the position of various other cannulae. For example, when femoral artery–femoral vein bypass is instituted, the venous cannula can be visualized as it advances in the inferior vena cava up to the level of the RA. Proper position of guide wires used for aortic cannulation can be confirmed with TEE.

EPICARDIAL AND EPIAORTIC ECHOCARDIOGRAPHY

Epicardial Echocardiography

During surgeries performed via sternotomy or thoracotomy, epicardial echocardiography can be performed and is particularly valuable in those cases in which the TEE probe cannot be placed or is contraindicated. The epicardial views are similar to the ones obtained via TTE. The American Society of Echocardiography in collaboration with the Society of Cardiovascular Anesthesiologists has recently issued guidelines for the performance of epicardial echocardiography.[92] The epicardial probe uses high-frequency transducers (5 to 12 MHz) that may require a standoff device and/or saline in the mediastinum for best imaging. Epicardial imaging offers superior image quality as well as a better window to the anterior cardiac structures (aorta and AV, PA and PV).

Epiaortic Examination

Because of the interposition of the left bronchus, the distal AA and the proximal aortic arch cannot be visualized with TEE. The ascending aortic and proximal aortic arches are of particular interest during cardiac surgeries as they represent sites for aortic cannulation. Epiaortic scanning for atheroma is performed using a small footprint, linear array transducer. Guidelines for intraoperative epiaortic examination have been published.[81]

ECHOCARDIOGRAPHY OUTSIDE THE OPERATING ROOM

An understanding of echocardiography is also relevant to anesthesiologists in that many patients with a history of heart disease will have undergone an echocardiographic examination prior to surgery. The echocardiography report from a preoperative examination is useful for assessing surgical risk and developing the anesthetic plan. Echocardiography has also established itself as particularly valuable in the assessment of postoperative hemodynamic instability. It offers rapid diagnosis by differentiating among the potential complications faced in postoperative care, such as hypovolemia, pericardial tamponade (Fig. 26-42), aortic dissection, myocardial infarction, endocarditis, and pulmonary embolism.

References

1. Barash PG, Glanz S, Katz JD, et al. Ventricular function in children during halothane anesthesia: An echocardiographic evaluation. *Anesthesiology.* 1978;49:79.
2. Click RL, Abel MD, Schaff HV. Intraoperative transesophageal echocardiography: 5-year prospective review of impact on surgical management. *Mayo Clin Proc.* 2000;75:241.

3. Couture P, Denault AY, McKenty S, et al. Impact of routine use of intraoperative transesophageal echocardiography during cardiac surgery. *Can J Anaesth.* 2000; 47:20.
4. Schmidlin D, Bettex D, Bernard E, et al. Transesophageal echocardiography in cardiac and vascular surgery: Implications and observer variability. *Br J Anaesth.* 2001;86:497.
5. Perrino AC, Reeves ST. Echocardiographic assessment during non-cardiac surgery. In: Savage RM, Aronson S, eds. *Comprehensive Textbook of Intraoperative TEE.* Philadelphia, PA: Lippincott Williams & Wilkins; 2004.
6. Suriani RJ, Neustein S, Shore-Lesserson L, et al. Intraoperative transesophageal echocardiography during noncardiac surgery. *J Cardiothorac Vasc Anesth.* 1998; 12:274.
7. Kolev N, Brase R, Swanvelder M, et al. The influence of transesophageal echocardiography on intra-operative decision making. *Anaesthesia.* 1998;53:767.
8. Denault AY, Couture P, McKenty S, et al. Perioperative use of transesophageal echocardiography by anesthesiologists: Impact in noncardiac surgery and in the intensive care unit. *Can J Anaesth.* 2002;49:287.
9. American Society of Anesthesiologists and the Society of Cardiovascular Anesthesiologists Task Force on Transesophageal Echocardiography. Practice guidelines of perioperative transesophageal echocardiography. *Anesthesiology.* 1996;84: 986.
10. American Society of Anesthesiologists, Society of Cardiovascular Anesthesiologists Task Force. Practice guidelines for perioperative transesophageal echocardiography: An update report by the American Society of Anesthesiologists and the Society of Cardiovascular Anesthesiologists Task Force on Transesophageal Echocardiography. *Anesthesiology.* 2010;112:1084.
11. Cheitlin MD, Armstrong WF, Aurigemma GP, et al. ACC. AHA. ASE. ACC/AHA/ASE 2003 Guideline Update for the Clinical Application of Echocardiography: Summary article. A report of the American College of Cardiology/American Heart. *Circulation.* 2003;108:1146–1162.
12. Center for Devices and Radiological Health: Revised 510(k) Diagnostic Ultrasound Guidance for 1993. Rockville, MD: US Food and Drug Administration; 1993.
13. Miller JP. Two-dimensional examination. In: Perrino AC, Reeves S, eds. *A Practical Approach to Transesophageal Echocardiography.* 2nd ed. Philadelphia PA: Lippincott, Williams & Wilkins; 2007:24.
14. Rafferty T, LaMantia KR, Davis E, et al. Quality assurance for intraoperative transesophageal echocardiography monitoring: A report of 846 procedures. *Anesth Analg.* 1993;76:228.
15. Kallameyer IJ, Collard CD, Fox JA, et al. The safety of intraoperative transesophageal echocardiography: A case series of 7200 cardiac surgical patients. *Anesth Analg.* 2001;92:1126.
16. Hogue CW, Lappas GD, Creswell LL, et al. Swallowing dysfunction after cardiac operations. *J Thorac Cardiovasc Surg.* 1995;110:517.
17. Rousou JA, Tighe DA, Garb JL, et al. Risk of dysphagia after transesophageal echocardiography during cardiac operations. *Ann Thorac Surg.* 2000;69:486.
18. Hilberath JN, Oakes DA, Shernan SK, et al. Safety of transesophageal echocardiography. *J Am Soc Echocardiogr.* 2010;23:1115.
19. Shanewise JS, Cheung AT, Aronson S, et al. ASE/SCA guidelines for performing a comprehensive intraoperative multiplane transesophageal echocardiographic examinations: Recommendations of the American Society of Echocardiography Council for Intraoperative Echocardiography and the Society of Cardiovascular Anesthesiologists Task Force for Certification in Perioperative Transesophageal Echocardiography. *Anesth Analg.* 1999;89:870.
20. Miller JP, Lambert AS, Shapiro WA, et al. The adequacy of basic intraoperative transesophageal echocardiography performed by experienced anesthesiologists. *Anesth Analg.* 2001;92:1103.
21. Meineri M, Vegas A. Three-dimensional transesophageal echocardiography is a major advance for intraoperative clinical management of patients undergoing cardiac surgery: A core review. *Anesth Analg.* 2010;110:1548.
22. Ahmed S, Nanda NC, Miller AP, et al. Usefulness of transesophageal three-dimensional echocardiography in the identification of individual segment/scallop prolapse of the mitral valve. *Echocardiography.* 2003;20:203.
23. Lang RM, Badano LP, Tsang W, et al. EAE/ASE Recommendations for image acquisition and display using three-dimensional echocardiography. *J Am Soc Echocardiogr.* 2012;25:3.
24. Perrino AC. Doppler technology and technique. In: Perrino AC, Reeves S, eds. *A Practical Approach to Transesophageal Echocardiography.* 2nd ed. Philadelphia, PA: Lippincott, Williams & Wilkins; 2007:109.
25. Quiñones MA, Otto CM, Stoddard M, et al. Recommendations for quantification of Doppler echocardiography: A report from the Doppler Quantification Task Force of the Nomenclature and Standards Committee of the American Society of Echocardiography: *J Am Soc Echocardiogr.* 2002;15:167.
26. Nishimura RA, Miller FA, Callahan MJ, et al. Doppler echocardiography: Theory, instrumentation, technique, and application. *Mayo Clin Proc.* 1985;60:321.
27. Maslow A, Perrino AC. Quantitative Doppler and hemodynamics. In: Perrino AC, Reeves S, eds. *A Practical Approach to Transesophageal Echocardiography.* 2nd ed. Philadelphia, PA: Lippincott, Williams & Wilkins; 2007:127.
28. Perrino AC, Harris SN, Luther MA. Intraoperative determination of cardiac output using multiplane transesophageal echocardiography: A comparison to thermodilution. *Anesthesiology.* 1998;89:350.
29. Harris SN, Luther MA, Perrino AC. Multiplane transesophageal echocardiography acquisition of ascending aortic flow velocities: A comparison with established techniques. *J Am Soc Echocardiogr.* 1999;12:754.
30. Muhiudeen IA, Kuecherer HF, Lee E, et al. Intraoperative estimation of cardiac output by transesophageal pulsed Doppler echocardiography. *Anesthesiology.* 1991;74:9.
31. Otto CM, Pearlman AS, Comess KA, et al. Determination of the stenotic aortic valve area in adults using Doppler echocardiography. *J Am Coll Cardiol.* 1986; 7:509.
32. Currie PJ, Seward JB, Reeder GS, et al. Continuous-wave Doppler echocardiographic assessment of severity of calcific aortic stenosis: a simultaneous Doppler-catheter correlative study in 100 adult patients. *Circulation.* 1985;71:1162.
33. Hatle L, Brubakk A, Tromsdal A, et al. Noninvasive assessment of pressure drop in mitral stenosis by Doppler ultrasound. *Br Heart J.* 1978;40:131.
34. Stamm RB, Martin RP. Quantification of pressure gradients across stenotic valves by Doppler ultrasound. *J Am Coll Cardiol.* 1983;2:707.
35. Teague SM, Heinsimer JA, Anderson JL, et al. Quantification of aortic regurgitation utilizing continuous wave Doppler ultrasound. *J Am Coll Cardiol.* 1986; 8:592.
36. Lee RT, Lord CP, Plappert T, et al. Prospective Doppler echocardiographic evaluation of pulmonary artery diastolic pressure in the medical intensive care unit. *Am J Cardiol.* 1989;64:1366.
37. Gorcsan J III, Snow FR, Paulsen W, et al. Noninvasive estimation of left atrial pressure in patients with congestive heart failure and mitral regurgitation by Doppler echocardiography. *Am Heart J.* 1991;11:858.
38. Nishimura RA, Tajik AJ. Determination of left-sided pressure gradients by utilizing Doppler aortic and mitral regurgitation signals: Validation by simultaneous dual catheter and Doppler studies. *J Am Coll Cardiol.* 1988;11:317.
39. Leung JM, O'Kelly BF, Mangano DT. Relationship of regional wall motion abnormalities to hemodynamic indices of myocardial oxygen supply and demand in patients undergoing CABG surgery. *Anesthesiology.* 1990;73:802.
40. Hauser AM, Gangadharan V, Ramos RG, et al. Sequence of mechanical, electrocardiographic and clinical effects of repeated coronary artery occlusion in human beings: Echocardiographic observations during coronary angioplasty. *J Am Coll Cardiol.* 1985;5:193.
41. Battler A, Froelicher VF, Gallagher KP, et al. Dissociation between regional myocardial dysfunction and ECG changes during ischemia in the conscious dog. *Circulation.* 1980;62:735.
42. Ross J Jr. Myocardial perfusion-contraction matching: Implications for coronary artery disease and hibernation. *Circulation.* 1991;83:1076.
43. Cerqueira MD, Weissman NJ, Dilsizian V, et al. Standardized myocardial segmentation and nomenclature for tomographic imaging of the heart. A statement for healthcare professionals from the cardiac imaging committee of the Council on Clinical Cardiology of the American Heart Association. American Heart Association Writing Group on myocardial segmentation and registration for cardiac imaging. *Circulation.* 2002;105:539.
44. Lang RM, Bierig M, Devereux RB, et al. Recommendations for chamber quantification: A report from the American Society of Echocardiography's Guidelines and Standards Committee and the Chamber Quantification Writing group, developed in conjunction with the European Association of Echocardiography, a branch of the European Society of Cardiology. *J Am Soc Echocardiogr.* 2005; 18:1440.
45. Lieberman AN, Weiss JL, Jugdutt BI, et al. Two-dimensional echocardiography and infarct size: Relationship of regional wall motion and thickening to the extent of myocardial infarction in the dog. *Circulation.* 1981;63:739.
46. Bergquist BD, Leung JM, Bellows WH. Transesophageal echocardiography in myocardial revascularization: I. Accuracy of intraoperative real-time interpretation. *Anesth Analg.* 1996;82:1132.
47. Odell DH, Cahalan MK. Assessment of left ventricular global and segmental systolic function with transesophageal echocardiography. *Anesthesiol Clin.* 2006; 24:755.
48. London MJ. Assessment of left ventricular global systolic function by transesophageal echocardiography. *Ann Card Anaesth.* 2006;9:157.
49. Cheung AT, Savino JS, Weiss SJ, et al. Echocardiographic and hemodynamic index of left ventricular preload in patients with normal and abnormal ventricular function. *Anesthesiology.* 1994;81:376.
50. Skarvan K, Lambert A, Filipovic M. Reference values for left ventricular function in subjects under general anesthesia and controlled ventilation assessed by two-dimensional transesophageal echocardiography. *Eur J Anaesthesiol.* 2001; 18:713.
51. Swenson JD, Bull D, Stringham J. Subjective assessment of left ventricular preload using transesophageal echocardiography: corresponding pulmonary artery occlusion pressures. *J Cardiothorac Vasc Anesth.* 2001;15:580.
52. Ditooe N, Stultz D, Schwartz BP, et al. Qualitative left ventricular systolic function: From chamber to myocardium. *Crit Care Med.* 2007;35:S330.
53. Skubas N. Intraoperative Doppler tissue imaging is a valuable addition to the cardiac anesthesiologists' armamentarium: A core review. *Anesth Analg.* 2009; 108:48–66.
54. Derumeaux G, Ovize M, Loufoua J, et al. Doppler tissue imaging quantitates regional wall motion during myocardial ischemia and reperfusion. *Circulation.* 1998;97:1970.

55. Flu WJ, van Kujik JP, Hoeks SE, et al. Prognostic implications of asymptomatic left ventricular dysfunction in patients undergoing vascular surgery. *Anesthesiology.* 2010;112:1316.
56. Matyal R, Hess PE, Subramaniam B, et al. Perioperative diastolic dysfunction during vascular surgery and its association with postoperative outcome. *J Vasc Surg.* 2009;50:70.
57. Bernard F, Denault A, Babin D, et al. Diastolic dysfunction is predictive of difficult weaning from cardiopulmonary bypass. *Anesth Analg.* 2001;92:291.
58. Swaminathan M, Nicoara A, Phillips-Bute B, et al. Utility of a simple algorithm to grade diastolic dysfunction and predict outcome after bypass graft surgery. *Ann Thorac Surg.* 2011;91:1844.
59. Matyal R, Skubas NJ, Shernan SK, et al. Perioperative assessment of diastolic dysfunction. *Anesth Analg.* 2011;113:449.
60. Nishimura RA, Tajik AJ. Evaluation of diastolic filling of left ventricle in health and disease: Doppler echocardiography is the clinician's Rosetta stone. *J Am Coll Cardiol.* 1997;30:8.
61. Gilman G, Nelson TA, Hansen WH. Diastolic function: A sonographer's approach to the essential echocardiographic measurements of left ventricular diastolic function. *J Am Soc Echocardiogr.* 2007;20:199.
62. Nagueh SF, Appleton CP, Gillebert TC, et al. Recommendations for the evaluation of left ventricular diastolic function by echocardiography. *J Am Soc Echocardiogr.* 2009;22:107.
63. Sutherland GR, Stewart MJ, Groundstroem KW, et al. Color Doppler myocardial imaging: A new technique for the assessment of myocardial function. *J Am Soc Echocardiogr.* 1994;7:441.
64. Pirracchio R, Cholley B, De Hert S, et al. Diastolic heart failure in anesthesia and critical care. *Br J Anaesth.* 2007;98:707.
65. Shernan SK. In: Perrino AC, Reeves S, eds. *A Practical Approach to Transesophageal Echocardiography.* 2nd ed. Philadelphia, PA: Lippincott, Williams & Wilkins; 2007:146.
66. Baumgartner H, Hung J, Bermejo J, et al. Echocardiographic assessment of valve stenosis: EAE/ASE recommendations for clinical practice. *J Am Soc Echocardiogr.* 2009;22:1.
67. Baumgartner H, Stefenelli T, Niederberger J, et al. "Overestimation" of catheter gradients by Doppler ultrasound in patients with aortic stenosis: A predictable manifestation of pressure recovery. *J Am Coll Cardiol.* 1999;33:1655.
68. Burwash IG, Dickinson A, Teskey RJ. Aortic valve area discrepancy by Gorlin equation and Doppler echocardiography continuity equation: Relationship to flow in patients with valvular aortic stenosis. *Can J Cardiol.* 2000;16:985.
69. Bonow RO, Carabello BA, Chatterjee KA, et al. ACC/AHA 2006 guidelines for the management of patients with valvular heart disease: A report of the American College of Cardiology/American Heart Association task force on practice guidelines. *Circulation.* 2006;114:e84.
70. Henry WL, Griffith JM, Michaelis LL. Measurement of mitral orifice area in patients with mitral valve disease, by real-time, two-dimensional echocardiography. *Circulation.* 1975;51:827.
71. Bruce CJ, Nishimura RA. Clinical assessment and management of mitral stenosis, valvular heart disease. *Cardiol Clin.* 1998;16:375.
72. Libanoff AJ, Roadbard S. Atrioventricular pressure half-time: Measure of mitral valve orifice area. *Circulation.* 1968;38:144.
73. Braverman AC, Thomas JD, Lee R. Doppler echocardiographic estimation of mitral valve area during changing hemodynamic conditions. *Am J Cardiol.* 1991;68:1485.
74. Perry GJ, Helmecke F, Nanda NC. Evaluation of aortic insufficiency by Doppler color flow mapping. *J Am Coll Cardiol.* 1987;9:952.
75. Takenaka K, Sakamoto T, Dabestani A. Pulsed Doppler echocardiographic detection of regurgitant blood flow in the ascending, descending and abdominal aorta of patients with aortic regurgitation. *J Cardiol.* 1987;17:301.
76. Lambert AS, Miller JP, Merrick SH. Improved evaluation of the location and mechanism of mitral valve regurgitation with a systemic transesophageal echocardiography examination. *Anesth Analg.* 1999;88:1205.
77. Helmcke F, Nanda NC, Hsiung MC. Color Doppler assessment of mitral regurgitation orthogonal planes. *Circulation.* 1987;75:175.
78. Schiller NB, Foster E, Redberg RF. Transesophageal echocardiography in the evaluation of mitral regurgitation. The twenty-four signs of severe mitral regurgitation. *Cardiol Clin.* 1993;11:399.
79. Simpson IA, Shiota T, Gharib M. Current status of flow convergence for clinical applications: Is it a leaning tower of "PISA"? *J Am Coll Cardiol.* 1996;27:504.
80. Pu M, Prior DL, Fan X, et al. Calculation of mitral regurgitation orifice area with use of a simplified proximal convergence method: Initial clinical application. *J Am Soc Echocardiogr.* 2001;14:180.
81. Glas KE, Swaminathan M, Reeves ST, et al. Guidelines for the performance of a comprehensive intraoperative epiaortic ultrasonographic examination: Recommendations of the American Society of Echocardiography and the Society of Cardiovascular Anesthesiologists; endorsed by the Society of Thoracic Surgeons. *J Am Soc Echocardiogr.* 2007;20:1227.
82. Massachusetts Medical Society. Atherosclerotic disease of the aortic arch as a risk factor for recurrent ischemic stroke. The French study of aortic plaques in stroke groups. *N Engl J Med.* 1996;334:1216.
83. Weber A, Jones EF, Zavala JA, et al. Intraobserver and interobserver variability of transesophageal echocardiography in aortic arch atheroma measurement. *J Am Soc Echocardiogr.* 2008;21:127.
84. Vignon P, Spencer KT, Rambaud G, et al. Differential transesophageal echocardiographic diagnosis between linear artifacts and intraluminal flap of aortic dissection or disruption. *Chest.* 2001;119:1778.
85. Hiratzka LF, Bakris GL, Beckman JA, et al. 2010 ACCF/AHA/AATS/ACR/ASA/SCA/SCAI/SIR/STS/SVM Guidelines for the diagnosis and management of patients with thoracic aortic disease: Executive summary. *Anesth Analg.* 2010;111:279.
86. Russell IA, Rouine-Rapp K, Stratmann G, et al. Congenital heart disease in the adult: A review with Internet-accessible transesophageal echocardiographic images. *Anesth Analg.* 2006;102:694.
87. Denys BG, Uretsky BF. Anatomical variations of internal jugular vein location: Impact on central venous access. *Crit Care Med.* 1991;19:1516.
88. Karakitsos D, Labropoulos N, De Groot E, et al. Real-time ultrasound-guided catheterization of the internal jugular vein: A prospective comparison with the landmark technique in critical care patients. *Crit Care.* 2006;10:R162.
89. National Institute for Clinical Excellence (NICE). *Guidance on the Use of Ultrasound Locating Devices for Placing Central Venous Catheters.* London, UK: National Institute for Clinical Excellence; 2002.
90. Troianos CA, Hartman GS, Glas KE, et al. Guidelines for performing ultrasound guided vascular cannulation: Recommendations of the American Society of Anesthesiologists and the Society of Cardiovascular Anesthesiologists. *J Am Soc Echocardiogr.* 2011;24:1291.
91. Klopman MA, Chen EP, Sniecinski RM. Positioning an intraaortic balloon pump using transesophageal echocardiogram guidance. *Anesth Analg.* 2011;113:40.
92. Reeves ST, Glass KE, Eltzschig H, et al. Guidelines for performing a comprehensive intraoperative epicardial echocardiography examination: Recommendations of the American Society of Echocardiography and the Society of Cardiovascular Anesthesiologists. *J Am Soc Echocardiogr.* 2007;20:427.

CHAPTER

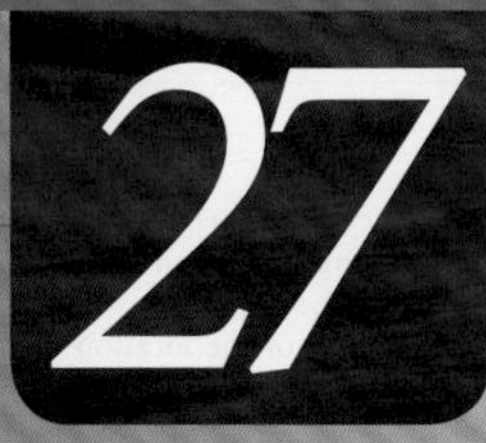

Airway Management

WILLIAM H. ROSENBLATT • WARIYA SUKHUPRAGARN

Key Points

1. Management of the airway is paramount to safe perioperative care. Following a series of evaluation procedures affects outcomes in a favorable way.
2. The anatomically complex airway undergoes growth and development and significant changes in its size, shape, and relation to the cervical spine between infancy and childhood.
3. A thorough airway-relevant history and physical examination must be obtained during the preoperative evaluation.
4. Preoxygenation (also commonly termed *denitrogenation*) should be practiced in all cases when time permits.
5. The advent of the laryngeal mask airway (LMA), as well as other supraglottic airways (SGAs), has led some to question the relative safety of tracheal intubation.
6. Successful laryngoscopy involves the distortion of the normal anatomic planes of the SGA to produce a line of direct visualization from the operator's eye to the larynx.
7. The technique of rapid-sequence induction is performed to gain control of the airway in the shortest period of time after the ablation of protective airway reflexes with the induction of anesthesia.
8. The period of extubation may be far more treacherous than that of induction and intubation.
9. Awake intubation is usually successful if approached with care and patience.
10. Awake airway management remains a mainstay of the American Society of Anesthesiologists' difficult airway algorithm.
11. An ever-increasing number of airway management devices are commercially available.
12. When access to the airway from the mouth or nose fails, emergency access via the extrathoracic trachea is a feasible alternative.

Multimedia

1 Indirect Laryngoscopy
2 Airway Evaluation
3 Vocal Chord Polyp
4 Preoxygenation
5 Preoxygenation Errors
6 ETT LMA Pressures
7 LMA
8 Laryngoscopy Pitfalls
9 Laryngoscopy
10 Right Endotracheal Intubation
11 Colorimetric CO_2 Detection
12 Airway Trans-Illumination
13 GlideScope
14 Channel Scopes—Airtraq
15 Rapid-Sequence Intubation
16 Aspiration
17 Loose Teeth
18 Endotracheal Extubation Procedure
19 Tracheostomy
20 O_2 Dissociation Curve
21 Nasal Intubation
22 FOB
23 Esophageal Intubation
24 Bougie
25 Jet Ventilation

Dedication: To the late Andranik Ovassapian, MD—his contributions appear so often in this chapter that he must be considered a co-author.

PERSPECTIVES ON AIRWAY MANAGEMENT

In the more than two decades since the publication of the first edition of this text, the field of airway management has undergone a vigorous revolution. Although the airway manager of today may still employ many of the devices available in 1988, the array of devices, algorithms, and pharmaceuticals in the modern airway armamentarium can be daunting. Fortunately, expertise in a limited, albeit complementary, number of tools as well as careful thought given to planning suffices in most cases. Although the final decade of the last century saw a resolute swing toward the application of supraglottic ventilation, a more recently introduced generation of devices reflects the application of imaging technology in the realm of tracheal intubation. The role of supraglottic airways (SGAs) is firmly established in routine anesthetic care as well as airway rescue, but the widespread adoption of video and optical laryngoscopy promises to remove many of the failings of a technique that has been in use for more than 200 years, that is direct laryngoscopy.

Techniques and practices in airway management have long been an important concern of the American Society of Anesthesiologists (ASA), as illustrated by the publication of original and revised difficult airway guidelines.[1] Analysis of the Society's closed claims database, in the periods before and after the 1993 publication of the ASA difficult airway guidelines, reveals both encouraging as well as disturbing trends.[2] A significant decrease in claims related to death/brain death at the induction of anesthesia is not matched with a decrease during emergence and the postoperative period. Although the closed claims data are useful, it has significant limitations, including its retrospective and nonrandom nature, and the lack of a denominator.[2]

1 Management of the airway is paramount to safe perioperative care. Difficult and failed airway management account for 2.3% of anesthetic deaths in the United States[3] and the following steps become necessary to favorably affect the outcome: (1) a thorough airway history and physical examination; (2) consideration of the ease of rapid tracheal intubation, by direct or indirect laryngoscopy; (3) formation of management plans for the use of a supraglottic means of ventilation (e.g., face mask, SGA); (4) weighing the risk of aspiration of gastric contents; and (5) estimating the relative risk to the patient of failed airway maneuvers.[4] This chapter will reflect the need to consider these five factors when approaching any patient who requires or may require airway control. This text will focus on routine and rescue airway management techniques. Specialty-specific techniques (e.g., elective suspension laryngoscopy, jet ventilation) are not included.

TABLE 27-1. ANATOMIC DIFFERENCES BETWEEN THE PEDIATRIC AND ADULT AIRWAYS

Proportionately smaller infant/child larynx
Narrowest portion: Cricoid cartilage in infant/child; vocal folds in adult
Relative vertical location: C3–C5 in infant/child; C4–C6 in adult
Epiglottis: Longer, narrower, and stiffer in infant/child
Aryepiglottic folds closer to midline in infant/child
Vocal folds: Anterior angle with respect to perpendicular axis of larynx in infant/child
Pliable laryngeal cartilage in infant/child
Mucosa more vulnerable to trauma in infant/child

Review of Airway Anatomy

The term *airway* refers to the upper airway—consisting of the nasal and oral cavities, pharynx, larynx, trachea, and principal bronchi. The airway in humans is primarily a conducting pathway. Because the oroesophageal and nasotracheal passages cross each other, anatomic and functional complexities have evolved for protection of the sublaryngeal airway against aspiration of
2 food that passes through the pharynx. The anatomically complex airway undergoes growth and development and significant changes in its size, shape, and relationship to the cervical spine between infancy and childhood.[5] As are other bodily systems, the airway is not immune from the influence of genetic, nutritional, and hormonal factors. Table 27-1 illustrates the anatomic differences in the larynx of infants and adult.

The laryngeal skeleton consists of nine cartilages (three paired and three unpaired); together, these house the vocal folds, which extend in an anterior–posterior plane from the thyroid cartilage to the arytenoid cartilages. The shield-shaped thyroid cartilage acts as the anterior "protective housing" of the vocal mechanism (Fig. 27-1). Movements of the laryngeal structures are controlled by two groups of muscles: The extrinsic muscles, which move the larynx as a whole; and the intrinsic muscles, which move the various cartilages in relation to one another. The larynx is innervated by two branches of each vagus nerve: The superior laryngeal and recurrent laryngeal nerves. Because the recurrent laryngeal nerves supply all of the intrinsic muscles of the larynx (with the exception

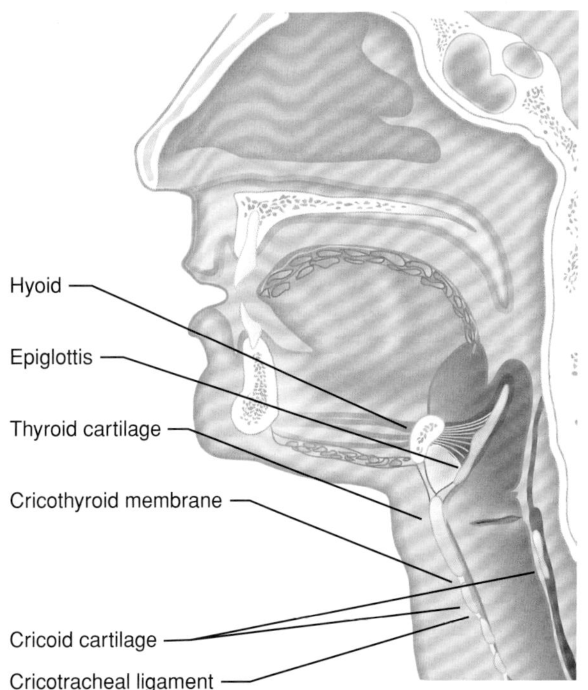

FIGURE 27-1. The major landmarks of the airway mechanism. Note that the cricoid cartilage is <1 cm in height in its anterior aspect, but may be 2 cm in height posteriorly.

of cricothyroid muscle), trauma to these nerves can result in vocal cord dysfunction. As a result of unilateral nerve injury, airway function is usually unimpaired, although the protective role of larynx in preventing aspiration may be compromised.

An important, externally identifiable structure is the membrane joining the superior aspect of the cricoid cartilage and the inferior edge of the thyroid cartilage. The cricothyroid membrane (CTM) is typically 8 to 12 mm in width and 10.4 to 13.7 mm in height in the adult, and it is composed of a yellow elastic tissue that lies directly beneath the skin and a fascial layer. It can be identified 1 to 1.5 fingerbreadths below the laryngeal prominence (thyroid notch).[6] The membrane has a central portion known as the *conus elasticus* and two lateral thinner portions. Directly beneath the membrane is the laryngeal mucosa. Because of anatomic variability in the course of veins and arteries and the membrane's proximity to the vocal folds (which may be 0.9 cm above the ligaments' upper border), it is suggested that any incisions or needle punctures to the CTM be made in its inferior third and be directed posteriorly (a posterior probing needle will strike the back side of the ring-shaped cricoid cartilage). Identification of an appropriate incision or puncture site may be difficult. Elliot et al.[7] found that only 30% of anesthesiologists were able to correctly identify the skin over the CTM, in a controlled situation. It should be noted that the ASA Difficult Airway Guidelines suggest that every patient be evaluated for difficult surgical airway—this should prompt the clinician to include examination of the laryngeal structures in every patient.[1]

At the base of the larynx, suspended by the underside of the CTM, is the signet ring–shaped cricoid cartilage. This cartilage is approximately 1 cm in height anteriorly, but almost 2 cm in height in its posterior aspect as it extends in a cephalad direction (Fig. 27-1). Inferiorly, the trachea is suspended from the cricoid cartilage by the cricotracheal ligament. The trachea measures approximately 15 cm in adults and is circumferentially supported by 17 to 18 C-shaped cartilages, with a membranous posterior aspect overlying the esophagus.

In the adult, the first tracheal ring is anterior to the sixth cervical vertebrae. The tracheal cartilages are interconnected by fibroelastic tissue, which allows for expansion of the trachea both in length and in diameter with inspiration/expiration and flexion/extension of the thoracocervical spine. The trachea ends at the carina (opposite the fifth thoracic vertebra), where it bifurcates into the principal bronchi. The right principal bronchus is larger in diameter than the left and deviates from the plane of the trachea at a less acute angle. Aspirated materials, as well as a deeply inserted endotracheal tube (ETT), tend to gain entry into the right principal bronchus, although left-sided positioning cannot be excluded. Cartilaginous rings support the first seven generations of the bronchi.

History of Airway Management

Obstruction of the airway was a poorly understood phenomenon prior to 1874. Opening the mouth with a wooden screw and drawing the tongue forward with a forceps or a steel-gloved finger was the height of airway management.[8] Recognition that the base of the tongue falling against the posterior pharyngeal wall accounted for most airway obstruction did not occur until 1880. Credit for the first use of a true SGA is given to Joseph Thomas Clover (1825–1882),[9] although it is possible that devices were used toward the end of the first millennium. Clover used a nasopharyngeal tube for the delivery of chloroform anesthesia. The O'Dwyer tube was introduced in 1884. This device consisted of a curved metal conduit, with a conical end that could seal the laryngeal inlet when placed into the oropharynx. Although it was designed for the treatment of narcotic overdose, it was later modified to be used with volatile anesthetics. Over the next 50 years, several modifications of the basic oropharyngeal airway were described. In the 1930s, Ralph Waters introduced the now-familiar flattened tube oral airway. Guedel modified Waters' concept by fitting his airway within a stiff rubber envelope in an attempt to reduce mucosal trauma.

Tracheal intubation was first described in 1788 as a means of resuscitation of the "apparently dead",[10] but it was not used for the delivery of anesthesia until almost 100 years later. The forerunner of the modern ETT was designed by the German otolaryngologist, Dr. Franz Kuhn (1866–1929). Kuhn developed a flexo-metallic tube that resisted kinking and could be shaped to the patient's upper airway anatomy. It was inserted using a rigid stylet, and the hypopharynx was sealed with oiled gauze packing. Sir Ivan Magill and Stanley Rowbotham are credited with the initial development of modern tracheal intubation. Performing anesthesia for reconstructive facial surgery (during World War I), they developed a two-tube nasal system. One narrow tube (gum elastic design) was passed through the nares and guided into the larynx using a surgical laryngoscope. The other tube was blindly passed into the pharynx to provide for the escape of gases. During use of this "Magill" tube, the exhaust lumen would occasionally pass blindly into the larynx, leading Sir Ivan to describe "blind nasal intubation."[11]

Cuffed SGAs were initially described in the early part of the 20th century. Three factors led to the development of these devices: (1) the introduction of cyclopropane (which was explosive and required an airtight circuit for appropriate gas containment), (2) the fact that blind and laryngoscopic-guided tracheal intubation remained a difficult task, and (3) a recognized need for protection of the lower airway from blood and surgical debris in the upper airway.[9] The Primrose cuffed oropharyngeal tube, the Shipway airway (a Guedel oropharyngeal airway fitted with a cuff, and a circuit connector designed by Sir Ivan Magill), and the Lessinger airway were predecessors of the modern supraglottic devices. In 1937, Leech introduced a "pharyngeal bulb gasway" with a noninflatable cuff that fits snuggly into the hypopharynx.

The use of SGAs remained dominant until the introduction of curare in 1942, and the mass training of anesthesiologists in tracheal intubation in anticipation of casualties during World War II. The description by Mendelson[12] of gastric-content aspiration in obstetric cases (66 of 44,016 patients, with 2 deaths) furthered the shift toward tracheal intubation in most surgical procedures. Within a few years, proficiency in direct laryngoscopy and tracheal intubation became a mark of professionalism. The advent of succinylcholine (1951) furthered the dominance of tracheal intubation by providing rapid and profound muscle relaxation.

By 1981, two types of airway management prevailed: Tracheal intubation or the anesthesia face mask/Guedel airway. Although both were time-tested, each had its failings (apart from airway failure in a small number of patients). Tracheal intubation was associated with dental and soft tissue injury as well as cardiovascular stimulation, and mask ventilation often required a hands-on-the-airway technique. These difficulties led to the reconsideration of SGAs.

In 1981, Dr. Archie Brain conceived the idea of fitting a mask-like structure over the larynx. The first prototypes of the laryngeal mask airway (LMA) were built from a Goldman dental mask, fitted with a tracheal tube. The motivation behind his early concepts and the evolution of his designs was the belief that airway control could be achieved less traumatically than tracheal intubation and more reliably than face mask ventilation. The LMA Classic was introduced into practice in the United Kingdom in 1989, and approved by the U.S. Food and Drug Administration in 1991. A variety of advanced models followed (e.g., intubation capable, gastric drainage), as will be discussed later in this chapter. With the expiration of several patents, as well as the introduction of other design concepts (e.g., noninflated masks), several devices applying the supraglottic ventilation concept were subsequently introduced.

Parallel to the development of SGA devices, the concept of indirect laryngoscopy was being increasingly considered. Although fiberoptic devices were applied to the problem of difficult tracheal intubation in the late 1960s, this technology was expensive, required a unique skill set, and was not readily available. It was not until the late 1980s that technical skill in flexible fiberoptic airway management was considered a critical anesthetic skill.[13] Bullard introduced the use of a fiberoptic bundle to the rigid laryngoscope. The Bullard laryngoscope incorporated optical and light-transmitting fiberoptic bundles into an anatomically shaped blade. A detachable stylet held the tracheal tube near the optic objective, which could be placed proximal to the larynx with minimal movement of the head and neck. Though less commonly used today, the Bullard laryngoscope can be considered the vanguard of the modern video laryngoscopes and optical and video stylets.[14] Fiberoptic elements were also incorporated into standard laryngoscope blades such as the Storz Endovision Video-Macintosh blade.

With the advent of inexpensive and miniaturized light-sensitive computer chip devices (i.e., CMOS), the era of video laryngoscopy was born in the first years of the 21st century. The GlideScope was the first of a generation of laryngoscopic devices to use CMOS technology to indirectly visualize the larynx. The GlideScope's acutely angled blade placed the clinician's point of vision around the base of the tongue without the need to establish a direct line of site from the operator's eye to the larynx. Difficulty in placement of the ETT led to the introduction of both specialized stylets and the channeled-type laryngoscope in the late 2000s. Each of the advents will be discussed in the following text.

Limitations of Patient History and Physical Examination

Airway management always begins with evaluation and planning. 3 A thorough airway-relevant history must be obtained whenever possible including a search for documentation to confirm or dismiss manifest problems. It is becoming common practice for a dedicated difficult airway "note" to be incorporated into electronic medical records and for a "difficult airway letter" to be given to patients describing critical and nonanticipated events. In the absence of such documentation, the clinician should seek the anesthetic records of past surgical visits. In particularly difficult cases, this may involve contacting other institutions. In cases where this information is not available, adopting a low threshold for using the safest approach to airway management (e.g., awake intubation) will mitigate risk. This assumes that a clinician skilled in this technique is available. It is not unusual for a patient to be referred to a different facility or practitioner because of airway management issues. Signs and symptoms related to the airway should be sought (Table 27-2). Many congenital and acquired syndromes are associated with difficult airway management (Table 27-3).

Over the last two decades, several physical evaluation measures have become popularized, although their reproducibility and predictability have been disputed. The difficulty in developing the

TABLE 27-2. SIGNS, SYMPTOMS, AND DISORDERS WITH AIRWAY MANAGEMENT IMPLICATIONS

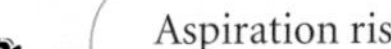

Aspiration risk
- History of voice changes
- History of vocal cord polyps
- History of frequent pneumonias
- Coughing after eating/drinking
- Acute narcotic therapy
- Acute trauma
- Intensive care unit admission (current)
- Pregnancy (gestational age ≥12 weeks)
- Immediate postpartum (before second postpartum day)
- Systemic disease associated gastroparesis: Diabetes mellitus, postvagotomy, collagen vascular disease, Parkinson disease, thyroid dysfunction, liver disease, CNS tumors, chronic renal insufficiency

Difficult laryngoscopy/SGA ventilation
- History of surgical manipulation in or around the airway
- History of radiation therapy of the head/neck
- Various congenital and acquired syndromes (Table 29-3)

Obstructive sleep apnea
- Body mass index >35 kg/m^2 (indicative)
- Loud snoring
- Pauses in breathing during normal sleep
- Sleep interruption (with choking)
- Daytime somnolence/napping
- Airway affecting craniofacial abnormalities

Lingual tonsil hyperplasia/supraglottic cyst or tumors
- Chronic sore throat
- Globus sensation
- Voice change
- Dysphagia
- Obstructive sleep apnea
- History of tonsillectomy (controversial)[18]

Thyroglossal duct cyst
- Asymptomatic anterior cervical mass that moves with deglutination
- Complications: Cysts infection, fistula, spontaneous rupture, voice change, dysphagia, dyspnea, and snoring

Signs and symptoms related to the airway
- Snoring
- Changes in voice
- Dysphagia
- Stridor
- Bleeding
- Cervical spine pain or limited range of motion
- Upper extremity neuropathy
- Temporomandibular joint pain or dysfunction

Sequelae of previous intubation
- Chipped teeth
- Significant prolonged sore throat/mandible after a previous anesthetic

TABLE 27-3. SYNDROMES ASSOCIATED WITH DIFFICULT AIRWAY MANAGEMENT

Pathologic Condition	Principal Pathologic Clinical Features Pertaining to Airway
Congenital	
Pierre Robin syndrome	Micrognathia, macroglossia, glossoptosis, cleft soft palate
Treacher Collins syndrome	Auricular and ocular defects; malar and mandibular hypoplasia, microstomia, choanal atresia
Goldenhar syndrome	Auricular and ocular defects; malar and mandibular hypoplasia; occipitalization of atlas
Down syndrome	Poorly developed or absent bridge of the nose; macroglossia, microcephaly, cervical spine abnormalities
Klippel–Feil syndrome	Congenital fusion of a variable number of cervical vertebrae; restriction of neck movement
Alpert syndrome	Maxillary hypoplasia, prognathism, cleft soft palate, tracheobronchial cartilaginous anomalies
Beckwith syndrome	Macroglossia
Cherubism	Tumorous lesion of mandibles and maxillae with intraoral masses
Cretinism	Absent thyroid tissue or defective synthesis of thyroxine; macroglossia, goiter, compression of trachea, deviation of larynx/trachea
Cri du chat syndrome	Microcephaly, micrognathia, laryngomalacia, stridor
Meckel syndrome	Microcephaly, micrognathia, cleft epiglottis
von Recklinghausen disease	Increased incidence of pheochromocytoma; tumors may occur in the larynx and right ventricle outflow tract
Hurler/Hunter syndrome	Stiff joints, upper airway obstruction due to infiltration of lymphoid tissue; abnormal tracheobronchial cartilages
Pompe disease	Muscle deposits, macroglossia
Acquired	
Infections	
Supraglottitis	Laryngeal edema
Croup	Laryngeal edema
Abscess (intraoral, retropharyngeal)	Distortion and stenosis of the airway and trismus
Papillomatosis	Chronic viral infection forming obstructive papillomas
Ludwig angina	Distortion and stenosis of the airway and trismus
Arthritis	
Rheumatoid arthritis	Temporomandibular joint ankylosis, cricoarytenoid arthritis, deviation of larynx, restricted mobility of cervical spine
Ankylosing spondylitis	Ankylosis of cervical spine; less commonly ankylosis of temporomandibular joints; lack of mobility of cervical spine
Benign Tumors	
Cystic hygroma, lipoma, adenoma, goiter	
Stenosis or distortion of the airway	
Malignant Tumors	
Carcinoma of tongue/larynx/thyroid	Stenosis or distortion of the airway; fixation of larynx or adjacent tissues (e.g., infiltration or fibrosis from irradiation)
Trauma	
Head/facial/cervical spine	Cerebrospinal rhinorrhea, edema of the airway; hemorrhage; unstable fracture(s) of the maxillae and mandible; intralaryngeal damage
Miscellaneous Conditions	
Morbid obesity	Short, thick neck, and large tongue are likely to be present
Acromegaly	Macroglossia; prognathism
Acute burns	Edema of airway

perfect airway evaluation tool lies in two interrelated areas: Simplicity and interdependency. Simple bedside evaluation tools are useful, but adequate evaluation may require endoscopic, radiologic, or other currently uncommon examinations.[15,26,17] Interdependency refers to the predictive value of one airway examination measure based on the findings of another. This is discussed later in "Direct Laryngoscopy," under the topic of functional airway assessment (FAA). Details of the various examinations and their interdependency are discussed in that section.

Historically, airway assessment has been synonymous with evaluation for the ease of direct laryngoscopy (DL), the end point being the anticipated degree of visualization of the larynx. The changing landscape of laryngoscopy (i.e., the rapid proliferation of indirect techniques including video laryngoscopy [VL]) may make many evaluation indexes obsolete or irrelevant. Efforts to define attributes that identify the difficult DL patient have been only modestly successful. Shiga et al.[18] performed a meta-analysis of studies of the physical predictors of difficult DL. They concluded

TABLE 27-4. SUMMARY OF POOLED SENSITIVITY AND SPECIFICITY OF COMMONLY USED METHODS OF AIRWAY EVALUATION

Examination	Sensitivity (%)	Specificity (%)
Mallampati classification	49	86
Thyromental distance	20	94
Sternomental distance	62	82
Mouth opening	46	89

Data derived from Mendelson CL. The aspiration of stomach contents into the lungs during obstetric anesthesia. *Am J Obstet Gynecol.* 1946;52:191.

that when interpreted as individual test, currently used techniques of evaluation have only modest discriminative power (Tables 27-4 and 27-5).

Despite the disappointing usefulness of these individual indexes in identifying the difficult to intubate patient (by DL), other authors have recognized that combinations of tests can provide improved predictability. El-Ganzouri et al.[19] designed a statistical model for stratifying risk of difficult DL in a large population. This multivariate index assigned relative weights to each physical examination or historical finding based on the odds of a high-grade laryngeal view being achieved on DL. The authors noted that with increasing multivariate index scores, positive predictive value increased, but sensitivity decreased (i.e., higher multivariate index scores occur when there are more positive physical findings, but not all difficult laryngoscopy patients will manifest multiple findings). Compared with the Mallampati classification alone, the multivariate composite index had improved positive predictive and specificity values at equal sensitivity. Of course, some pathology will only present with the induction of anesthesia and/or attempts at laryngoscopy.[20,21] Other groups have used similar regimens to increase the predictability of multivariate indexes by incorporating imaging technologies.[22] In a small population of patients, Naguib et al.[22] were able to achieve high predictive accuracy (90% or higher) when physical examination and imaging scores were weighted. A simplified scoring system, studied on a multi-institution population of 3,763 patients,

TABLE 27-5. TECHNIQUES OF COMMON AIRWAY INDEXES MEASUREMENT

Thyromental distance: Measured along a straight line from tip of mentum to thyroid notch in neck-extended position

Mouth opening: Interincisor distance (or interalveolus distance when edentulous) with the mouth fully opened[19]

Mallampati score (see Fig. 27-7)

Head and neck movement: The range of motion from full extension to full flexion[20]

Ability to prognath: Capacity to bring the lower incisors in front of the upper incisors[19]

TABLE 27-6. SIMPLIFIED RISK SCORE FOR DIFFICULT INTUABTION

Number of Risk Factor[a]	Incidence of Difficult Intubation
0	0
1	2%
2	4%
3	8%
4 or 5	17%

[a]Presence of upper front teeth, History of a difficult intubation, Mallampati >1, Mallampati of 4, mouth opening <4 cm.

recognized both the difficulty of constructing a complex analysis in the preoperative holding area and the failure of any model to be completely predictive.[23] Accepting a discriminating power of 70%, this model found five attributes that could be used to predict difficult laryngoscopy (Table 27-6).

Because it is a relatively new area, specific information is not yet complete on the external airway findings that may indicate failure of indirect laryngoscopy. Studies comparing DL with a Macintosh laryngoscope and video laryngoscopy with the GlideScope (Verathon, Bothell, WA) indicate that though no single examination finding may distinguish the success or failure with each device, the failure to visualize the larynx with the GlideScope was characterized by higher multivariate risk scores of the same clinical finding.[24] Others have found that the following preoperative findings contribute to failure of VL: Scarring, radiation, masses or thickness of the neck, thyromental distance of <6 cm, limited cervical motion, and operator experience.[25]

In general, tracheal intubation should be considered nonroutine under the following conditions: (1) The presence of equally important priorities to the management of the airway (such as a full stomach or open globe), (2) abnormal airway anatomy, (3) an emergency, or (4) direct injury to the upper airway and larynx and/or trachea. Although the finding of abnormal anatomy is not necessarily synonymous with the difficult airway, it should kindle a heightened level of suspicion. Several investigators have identified anatomic features as having unfavorable influences on the mechanics of DL; these are explainable on the basis of inability to create a line of site from the operator's eye to the aperture of the larynx.

Few studies have objectively determined those findings that identify the difficult-to-mask ventilate patient. This basic airway maneuver was examined in a control study by Langeron et al.[26] Of 1,502 patients (excluding planned rapid-sequence induction or emergency cases), 5% of patients were characterized as difficult to ventilate. Only one patient in the series was unable to be ventilated by a face mask. Table 27-7 describes the criteria for defining difficult mask ventilation and the five independent clinical predictors found by Langeron et al.[26] The presence of two predictors indicated a high likelihood of difficult mask ventilation. Kheterpal et al.[27] investigating 53,041 patients and, using different criteria, found an impossible-to-mask ventilate incidence of 0.15%. In addition to the criteria used by Langeron et al., these authors found that a finding of a high Mallampati score, poor mandibular protrusion, a history of radiation therapy to the neck, and male gender improved the prediction of difficult mask ventilation.

Ultrasonography (US) currently has limited application in airway evaluation. Ezri et al.[28,29] showed that obese patients who

TABLE 27-7. ASSESSMENT AND PREDICTABILITY OF DIFFICULT MASK VENTILATION[31,32]

Criteria for Difficult Mask Ventilation	
Inability for one anesthesiologist to maintain oxygen saturation >92%	
Significant gas leak around face mask	
Need for ≥4 L/min gas flow (or use of fresh gas flow button more than twice)	
No chest movement	
Two-handed mask ventilation needed	
Change of operator required	
Independent Risk Factors for Difficult Mask Ventilation	**Odds Ratio**
Presence of a beard	3.18
Body mass index >26 ng/m^2	2.75
Lack of teeth	2.28
Age >55 yrs	2.26
History of snoring	1.84

were difficult to intubate by direct laryngoscopy had increased pretracheal adipose (28(±2.7) mm vs. 17(±1.8) mm), mirroring Brodsky's finding regarding neck circumference in this population. Bedside US has proven useful in other areas of airway management, including confirmation of tracheal intubation, exclusion of esophageal intubation, lung excursion (and assuring bilateral ventilation), verifying ventilation in the absence of CO_2 detection, and identifying the cricoid membrane. The availability of US technology is widespread, portable to the bedside, and provides rapid, real-time, and dynamic images. These characteristics make it desirable to use in the operating room, and the promise of airway evaluation is enticing. Linear high-frequency transducers image within 2 to 3 cm of the skin surface and are the most useful probe for airway examination. Although it may be possible to examine the upper airway for changes such as hypertrophic lingual tonsils, its clinical relevancy (e.g., impact on laryngoscopy) has not been studied.[29] Subglottic hemangiomas, laryngeal stenosis and cysts, and papillomas have been identified by US. Correct tracheal tube size including double-lumen tubes can be estimated based on the US image.

Predicting difficulty in DL remains, in a large part, an enigma. As previously illustrated, the commonly used indexes may not only be less predictive than originally thought, but they may also be misleading. The advent of video laryngoscopy may make these deficits irrelevant; new criteria will need to be explored.

CLINICAL MANAGEMENT OF THE AIRWAY

4

Preoxygenation

4 Preoxygenation (also commonly termed *denitrogenation*) should be practiced in all cases when time allows.[30] This procedure entails the replacement of the nitrogen volume of the lung (as much as 95% of the functional residual capacity) with oxygen in order to provide a reservoir for diffusion into the alveolar capillary blood after the onset of apnea. Preoxygenation with 100% O_2 via a tight-fitting face mask for several minutes in a spontaneously breathing patient can furnish up to 8 or more minutes of oxygen reserve following apnea (in a patient without significant cardiopulmonary disease and with a normal oxygen consumption). In one study of healthy, nonobese patients who were allowed to breathe 100% O_2 preoperatively, subjects sustained an oxygen saturation of >90% for 6 ± 0.5 minutes, whereas obese patients experienced oxyhemoglobin desaturation to <90% in 2.7 ± 0.25 minutes.[30] Under ideal conditions, the patient breathing room air (F_{IO_2} = 0.21) will experience oxyhemoglobin desaturation to a level of <90% after approximately 1 to 2 minutes of apnea. Patients with pulmonary disease, or with conditions affecting metabolism or lung volumes, frequently evidence desaturation sooner, owing to increased O_2 extraction, decreased functional residual capacity, or right-to-left transpulmonary shunting. The most common reason for not achieving a maximum alveolar oxygen store during preoxygenation is a loose-fitting mask, allowing the entrainment of room air.[30]

Time-sparing methods of preoxygenation have also been described. Using a series of four vital capacity breaths of 100% O_2 over a 30-second period, a high arterial Pa_{O_2} (339 mm Hg) can be achieved, but the time to desaturation is consistently shorter as compared with traditional techniques.[30] A modified vital capacity technique, wherein the patient is asked to take eight deep breaths in a 60-second period, shows promise in terms of prolonging the time to desaturation.[30] The authors of the current chapter prefer the technique of applying a tight-fitting mask for 5 minutes or more of tidal volume breathing; the mask is placed immediately after the patient has been made comfortable on the operating room table, and it remains in place during intravenous catheter insertion and the application of monitors. Fresh gas flow into the mask should be a minimum of 10 to 12 L/min. Pharyngeal insufflation of oxygen has been described to delay the onset of oxyhemoglobin desaturation (<90%) during apnea.[30] In this technique, oxygen is insufflated at a rate of 3 L/min via a catheter passed through the nares. This technique relies on the phenomenon of apneic oxygenation, a process by which gases are entrained into the alveolar space during apnea, in the presence of a patent airway. In the obese patient, bilevel positive airway pressure as well as the head-up position (approximately 25 degrees) have been advocated to both reach maximal preinduction arterial oxygenation and to delay oxyhemoglobin desaturation.[30] Surprisingly, the head-up position may not improve the efficacy of preoxygenation in the pregnant patient.

5 Some circumstances can serve to decrease the effectiveness of preoxygenation. For example, the patient who experiences claustrophobia with the anesthesia face mask (which can almost always be overcome by patients holding the mask themselves) or the use of self-inflating breathing bags (which do not deliver an F_{IO_2} of 100% during spontaneous breathing) can decrease effectiveness of preoxygenation. Likewise, leaks between the face mask and patient's facial contours allow entrainment of air, thereby reducing the F_{IO_2}. Leaks as small as 4 mm (cross-sectional) can cause significant reductions in the inspired oxygen content.[31]

Support of the Airway with the Induction of Anesthesia

With the induction of anesthesia and the onset of apnea, ventilation and oxygenation must be supported by the anesthesiologist. Traditional methods include the anesthesia face mask and the ETT. During the last two decades, several SGA devices have been introduced into worldwide clinical practice. Although older data suggest that 35% or more of general anesthetics in the United States are performed with these devices, more recent data from the United Kingdom imply a 56% incidence.[32,33]

The Anesthesia Face Mask

The anesthesia face mask is the device most commonly used to deliver anesthetic gases and oxygen as well as to ventilate the patient who has been made apneic. The skillful use of a face mask may be challenging and, despite the many advances in airway management, remains a mainstay in the delivery of anesthesia and in resuscitation. When the induction of anesthesia is initiated, the patient's level of consciousness changes from the awake state, with a competent and protected airway, to the unconscious state, with an unprotected and potentially obstructed airway. This drug-induced central ventilatory depression and relaxation of the musculature of the upper airway can rapidly lead to hypercapnia and hypoxia. Face mask ventilation is minimally invasive, virtually universal, and requires the least sophisticated equipment, thus making it critical to management of the airway.

The mask is gently held on the patient's face with the left hand, leaving the right hand free for other tasks (Fig. 27-2). Air leak around the edges of the mask is prevented by downward pressure. Most modern masks can be distorted by the operator's fingers in order to seal around the facial contours. Elastic "mask straps" may be used to help secure the mask in the awake or anesthetized patient who is breathing spontaneously and without obstruction, or to complement the left-hand grip. The mask straps can be particularly helpful for the clinician with short fingers. During a preoxygenation phase of anesthetic induction, gas leaks should be avoided; during inspiration, the patient may entrain air, limiting the efficacy of the preoxygenation maneuver.

In preparation for using the face mask for positive-pressure ventilation (once apnea is induced), appropriate positioning of the patient is paramount. With the patient in the supine position, the head and neck are placed in the *sniffing* position, which is discussed extensively later. This position improves mask ventilation by anteriorizing the base of the tongue and the epiglottis.

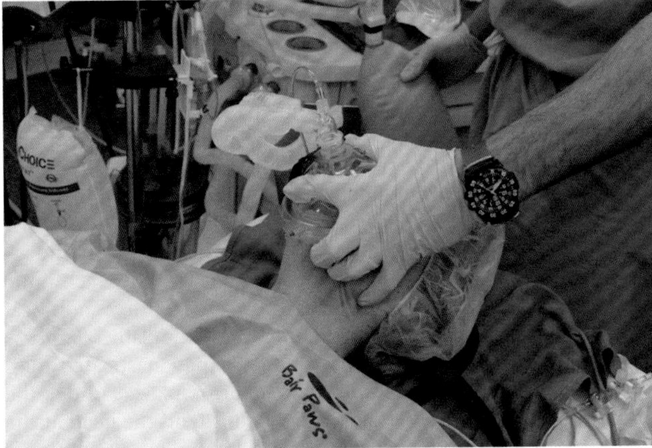

FIGURE 27-2. Holding the anesthesia mask on the face. The thumb and the first finger grip the mask in such a fashion that the anesthesia circuit (or Ambu bag) connection abuts the web between these digits. This allows the palm of the hand to apply pressure to the left side of the mask, while the tips of these two digits apply pressure over the right. The third finger helps to secure under the mentum, and the fourth finger is under the angle of the mandible or along the lower mandibular ridge. Mask straps (on pillow) may be used to complement the hand grip by securing the right side of the mask.

This has been demonstrated in endoscopic studies in anesthetized patients.[34]

After induction of anesthesia, a tight fit of the face mask is achieved by downward displacement of the mask between the thumb and the first finger with concurrent upward displacement of the mandible with the remaining fingers. This latter maneuver, commonly known as a *jaw thrust,* raises the soft tissues of the anterior airway off the pharyngeal wall and allows for improved ventilation. In patients who are obese, edentulous, or bearded, two hands or a mask strap may be required to ensure a tight-fitting mask seal. When two hands are required for holding the face mask, a second operator obviously will be required in order to squeeze the reservoir bag. If necessary, the second operator can lend a third hand to the mask fitting, providing for both jaw-thrust and chin lift.

One useful, albeit poorly characterized, maneuver that can aid in face mask ventilation is the *expiratory chin drop.* When positive-pressure inspiration is successful, but is not followed by passive gas escape during expiration, allowing phasic head flexion and reducing chin/jaw lifting will often improve gas egress.

When a patient has presented with removable dentures, leaving the prosthetics in place can aid face mask ventilation.[35]

The patient with normal lung compliance should require no more than 20 to 25 cm H_2O pressure to inflate the lungs. If more pressure than this is required, the clinician should re-evaluate the adequacy of the airway, adjust the mask fit, seek the aid of a second operator in order to perform two- or three-handed mask holds, and/or consider other devices that aid in the creation of an open passage for air flow through the upper airway (e.g., oral airway, SGA). Both rigid oral airways and soft nasal airways create an artificial passage to the hypopharynx. A variety of oral and nasal airways are available, but they will not be discussed in detail in this text. Nasal airways are less likely to stimulate cough, gag, or vomiting in the lightly anesthetized patient, but the risk of epistaxis must always be weighed. Nasal manipulation, including use of a nasal airway is avoided in patients at risk for epistaxis (e.g., iatrogenic or pathologic coagulopathy, pregnancy, Hereditary Hemorrhagic Telangiectasia, uncontrolled hypertension). The nasal airway is inserted along the floor of the nose, in a directly anterior–posterior direction, and should always be lubricated to reduce trauma to the nasal turbinates. Resistance to insertion should prompt repositioning of the airway bevel, reassessment of the direction of insertion forces, or change to the contralateral nare. The airway should be long enough to reach from the nare to the thyroid notch when placed alongside the face of the patient. Oral airways should likewise reach from the teeth (or alveolar ridge) to the mandibular angle. The typical rounded oral airway is placed with its longitudinal concavity rotated in a rostrad direction. Once the distal end of the airway has been inserted to the level of the oropharynx, the device is rotated 180 degrees as insertion continues, to reach its ultimate position. This maneuver avoids displacement of the tongue into the hypopharynx. A small oral aperture, an intrapharyngeal mass or foreign body, intact gag reflex or otherwise light anesthesia may prevent its placement. As will be discussed later, some intubating oral airways are large and have a rectangular cross section. These tend to be too large for intraoral rotation. They are inserted with the concavity facing caudad while the tongue is stabilized by a tongue depressor or held by the operator.

Obstruction to mask ventilation may be caused by laryngospasm, a reflex closure of the vocal folds. Laryngospasm occurs from local stimulation by a foreign body (e.g., oral or nasal airway), saliva, blood, or vomitus touching the glottis, or even a light plane of anesthesia. Hypoxia as well as noncardiogenic pulmonary edema can result if there is continued spontaneous ventilation against closed vocal cords (or other obstruction). Treatment of laryngospasm includes removal of an offending stimulus (if it can be identified), removal of secretions, continuous positive airway pressure, deepening of the anesthetic state, and the use of a rapid-acting muscle relaxant.

If there are no contraindications (e.g., a full stomach or other aspiration risk), mask ventilation can be the technique employed for the duration of anesthesia maintenance. Otherwise, it is commonly used to administer anesthetic gases until the anesthetic state is adequate for use of another means of airway support (e.g., SGA, ETT). This decision is made after careful consideration of the patient's coexisting diseases and surgical requirements.

Supraglottic Airways

The LMA ushered in the first major use of SGAs in the United States. However, by the time of its initial introduction in 1989 and approval by the U.S. Food and Drug Administration in 1991, it was being used in more than 500 hospitals in the United Kingdom. Although initially approved for use as a substitute for face mask ventilation, and when tracheal intubation was not achievable, it soon enjoyed wide use in surgical cases traditionally managed with tracheal intubation.[32] SGAs are associated with lower incidence of sore throat, coughing and laryngospasm on emergence as compared to tracheal intubation.[36]

The US patents on the original LMA design expired in 2002 ushering in a proliferation of similar devices. A wealth of information exists on the LMA and its subsequent iterations (all by the original inventor, Dr. Archie Brain). Much of this knowledge may be applied to newer devices. This chapter devotes a considerable amount of text to the family of LMAs. This is not meant to infer preference, but rather the availability of information. Although similar data are not available in the United States, the LMA accounts for 87% of SGA use in the United Kingdom.[37]

5 The advent of the LMA as well as other SGAs has led some to question the relative safety of tracheal intubation.[38] This, along with the ASA closed claims database information, lends support to the search for safe alternatives to tracheal intubation whenever possible.[39] Similarly, pharyngeal mucosal (traumatic) changes, as a result of SGA use, appear to be markedly delayed when compared with the effects of the ETT in the trachea. In one animal study, mucosal injury from the LMA ProSeal (The Laryngeal Mask Company, Jersey, UK) did not occur until more than 9 hours of continuous use.[40]

The LMA Classic. The LMA is composed of a small "mask" designed to sit in the hypopharynx, with an anterior surface aperture overlying the laryngeal inlet (Fig. 27-3). The rim of the mask is composed of an inflatable cuff that fills the hypopharyngeal space, creating a seal that allows positive-pressure ventilation with up to 20 cm H_2O pressure. The adequacy of the seal depends on correct placement and appropriate size. It is less dependent on the cuff filling pressure or volume. Attached to the posterior surface of the mask is a barrel (airway tube) that extends from the mask's central aperture through the mouth and can be connected to a self-inflating resuscitation bag or anesthesia circuit. Although the original mask was constructed of silicone, the single-use model, the LMA Unique (Laryngeal Mask Airway-North America, San Diego, CA), is more ubiquitous today.

LMA size selection is critical to its successful use and to the avoidance of minor as well as more significant complications. Neonatal to large adult sizes are available. The manufacturer recommends that the clinician choose the largest size that will fit comfortably in the oral cavity, which is then inflated to the minimum pressure that allows ventilation to 20 cm H_2O without an air leak. The intracuff pressure should never exceed 60 cm H_2O
6 (and should be periodically monitored if nitrous oxide is used as part of the anesthetic). When an adequate seal cannot be obtained with 60 cm H_2O cuff pressure, the LMA may be malpositioned and/or sizing should be re-evaluated. Light anesthesia may also contribute to poor seal or partial or complete laryngospasm.

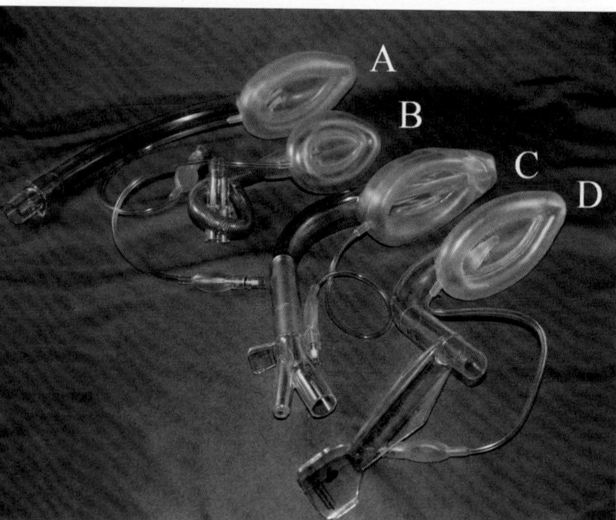

FIGURE 27-3. The family of laryngeal mask airways (from top): **(A)** Unique, **(B)** flexible, **(C)** supreme, **(D)** fastrach.

The insertion of the LMA as described by its inventor, Dr. Archie J. I. Brain, has been modified by a number of writers. Discussion of these various alternatives is beyond the scope of this text. To understand the insertion technique, we review the processes of deglutination, which the procedure mimics: Lubrication with saliva; formation of a flat oval food bolus by the tongue; initiation of the swallowing reflex by stimulation of the palate; upward pressure by the tongue flattening the food bolus against the palate; directing of the food bolus toward the posterior pharyngeal wall and into the hypopharynx by the shape of the palate and pharyngeal wall; head extension and neck flexion, which enlarges the space behind the tongue to allow passage of the food bolus into the hypopharynx; and finally, opening of the upper esophageal sphincter to allow esophageal entry of the food bolus. These functions allow the food bolus to reach its mark blindly while avoiding the anterior pharyngeal structures and avoiding reflex responses meant to protect the airway.

The currently recommended insertion technique is illustrated in Figure 27-4, and has 98% success rate. The principles of LMA insertion can be applied to all other SGAs, though the manufacturer's recommendations should be sought. In this technique the palatal surface of the mask is lubricated with a nonlocal anesthetic–containing lubricant (simulating the saliva), and is fully deflated to form a thin, flat wedge shape (masticated food bolus). The operator's nondominant hand is placed under the occiput to flex the neck on the thorax and extend the head at the atlanto-occipital joint (creating a space behind the larynx; this action also tends to open the mouth).[41] The index finger of the dominant hand is placed in the cleft between the mask and barrel. The hard palate is visualized and the superior (nonaperture) surface of the mask is placed against it. Force is applied by the index finger in an upward direction toward the top of the patient's head. This will cause the mask to flatten out against the palate and follow the shape of the palate as it slides into the pharynx and hypopharynx. The index finger continues along this arc, continually applying an outward pressure until the resistance of the upper

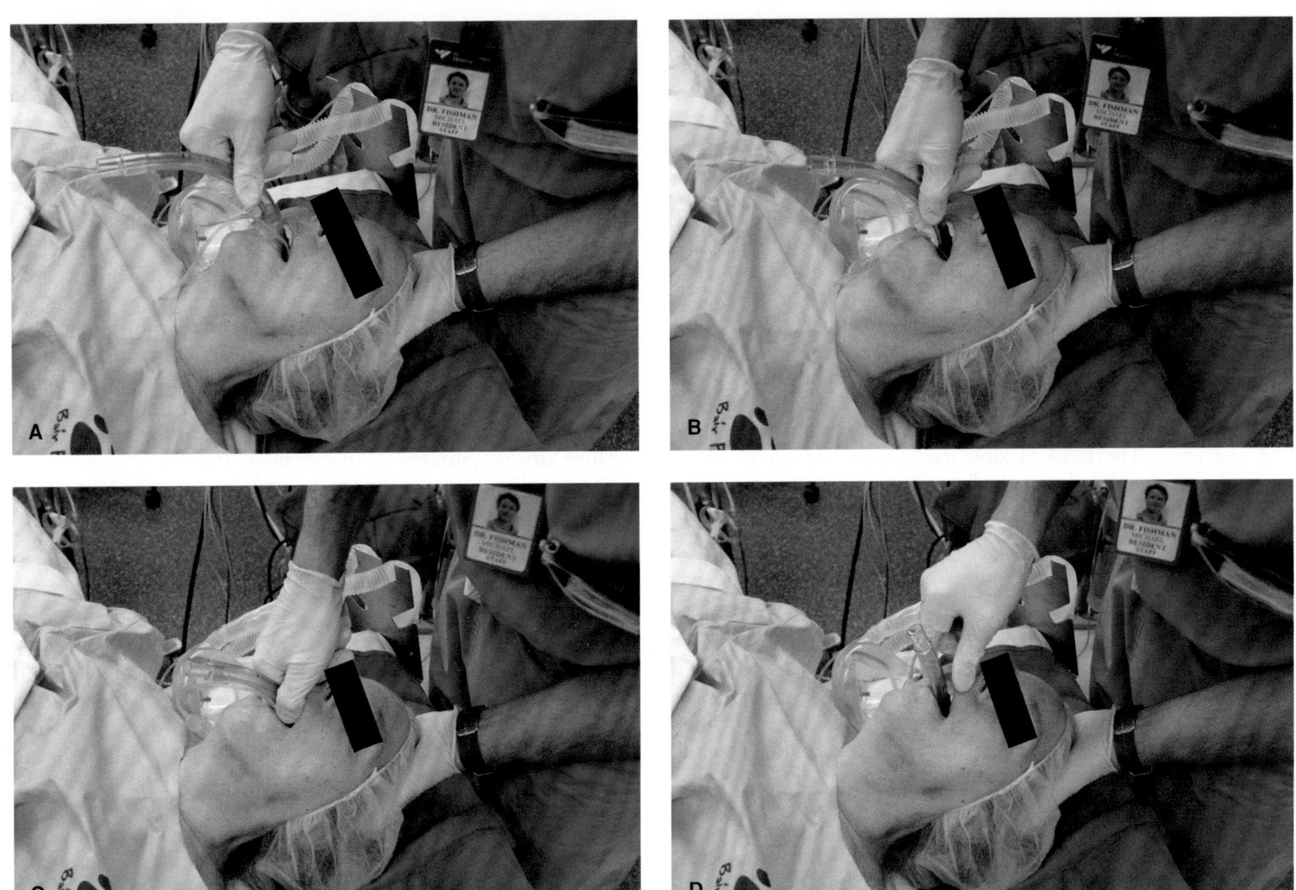

FIGURE 27-4. Insertion of the laryngeal mask airway (LMA). The LMA is inserted with the index finger of the dominant hand pressing with a force vector against the hard palate (**A** and **B**). The outward force vector is continued from the hard palate to the pharynx and hypopharynx **(C)** until the index finger meets resistance against the upper esophageal sphincter and is removed **(D)**.

esophageal sphincter is met. The most common error made by
7 clinicians is applying pressure with a posterior vector. This tends to catch the tip of the LMA on the posterior pharyngeal wall, causing folding with resultant misplacement and trauma.

Once insertion is complete, removal of the inserting hand is facilitated by gentle stabilization of the LMA barrel with the non-dominant hand. Prior to attachment of the anesthesia circuit, the LMA is inflated with the minimum amount of gas to form an effective seal. Sixty centimeters of H_2O pressure is the maximum suggested pilot valve pressure. Accompanying the inflation, one should be able to observe a rising of the cricoid and thyroid cartilages and lifting of the barrel out of the mouth by approximately 1 cm as the mask is lifted off the upper esophageal sphincter. If a midline position is not possible owing to the nature of the patient position or surgical procedure, a flexible LMA (discussed later) should be considered. A bite block is recommended to prevent biting and occlusion of the LMA barrel.

Although the distal tip of the LMA mask sits in the esophageal inlet, it does not reliably seal it. The LMA was not designed to protect against the aspiration of gastric contents. Despite this, when used in patients at low risk for regurgitation, the rate of aspiration during LMA use is similar to that in all non-LMA general anesthetics (approximately 2 in 10,000 cases), although the incidence of gastroesophageal reflux may be increased when compared with use of the face mask.[42]

If regurgitated gastric contents are noted in the LMA barrel, maneuvers similar to those applied when using an ETT should be instituted: Patient in Trendelenburg position, administer 100% oxygen, leave the LMA in place and use a flexible suction device down the barrel, and if necessary, deepen the anesthetic.

When populations of patients considered to have a full stomach are studied (in controlled trials, prospective series, or anecdotally), there is a low incidence of aspiration noted with elective or emergency LMA use. Reports have included patients who are morbidly obese or experience frequent gastroesophageal reflux, those undergoing elective cesarean section or airway rescue during labor, and those presenting to emergency departments or paramedic crews.[43,44] During cardiopulmonary resuscitation, the incidence of gastroesophageal regurgitation is four times greater with a bag-valve mask than with the LMA.[45]

Although first introduced for use with spontaneous ventilation, the LMA has proved useful for cases in which positive-pressure ventilation is either desired or preferred.[46] Contrary to initial impression, positive-pressure ventilation can be safely accomplished with the LMA.[47] There is no difference found in gastric inflation with positive pressure (<17 cm H_2O) when comparing the LMA and the ETT.[48] When using the LMA Classic, one should limit tidal volumes to 8 mL/kg and airway pressure to 20 cm H_2O. LMA use has been described with supine, prone, lateral, oblique, Trendelenburg, and lithotomy positions. Although the manufacturer recommends use for a maximum of 2 to 3 hours, reports of use for more than 24 hours can be found.[49] Although no studies have examined histologic changes in the mucosa with prolonged LMA use, Goldmann et al. [50] saw no evidence of mucosal changes with up to 9 hours of ProSeal LMA use, though damage was consistently evident after 12 hours.

The LMA Flexible. The introduction of the LMA Flexible (The Laryngeal Mask Company, Jersey, UK) (Fig. 27-3) has permitted extension of LMA use to a variety of cases in which the airway is shared with the surgical team (e.g., otolaryngologic surgery) or within the surgical field (e.g., ophthalmologic surgery). The LMA Flexible differs from the original design by virtue of a thin-walled, small-diameter, wire-reinforced (kink-resistant) barrel, which can be positioned out of the midline without affecting the hypopharyngeal position of the mask. It was designed to be used with a tonsillar mouth gag employed in surgery on the mouth and pharynx.[51] The LMA Flexible has also proved useful when heavy drapes are placed over the head and airway (e.g., mastoidectomy, ophthalmic procedures), when there is movement of the head position during surgery (e.g., tympanostomy tubes), or when the LMA barrel cannot be secured in the midline (e.g., mid or lateral facial surgery). The use of this mask in surgery above the level of the hypopharynx, including tonsillectomy, affords a number of clinically important advantages over tracheal intubation (Table 27-8). When correctly placed, the LMA mask serves to better block the airway from blood, secretions, and surgical debris above the level of the mask, as compared with the tracheal tube, which is known to not protect the trachea from liquids instilled into the pharynx.[47]

The SGA and Bronchospasm. SGAs appear to be well suited to the patient with a history of bronchospasm. SGAs present a unique opportunity for the clinician to conveniently and effectively control the airway without having to introduce a foreign body into the trachea. Thus, it may be an ideal airway tool in the asthmatic patient who is not at risk for reflux and aspiration.[52] Because the halogenated inhaled anesthetics are potent bronchodilators, it is at the time of emergence, when the anesthetic is discontinued, that the patient at risk for bronchospasm is most likely to wheeze. In the patient managed with an SGA, there is no foreign body in the sensitive bronchorespiratory tree and the patient can be fully emerged prior to removal of the device. In the event that uncontrollable bronchospasm does occur intraoperatively (e.g., from vagal stimuli such as traction on the peritoneum), intubation can be performed through many SGAs or after removal. When tracheal intubation is mandatory (for the surgical procedure) yet concerns regarding bronchospasm exist, the Bailey maneuver is employed.[53] In this maneuver, the deflated LMA is placed behind the *in situ* ETT. The ETT is removed and the LMA is inflated. The patient is then emerged on the LMA.

TABLE 27-8. ADVANTAGES OF THE LARYNGEAL MASK AIRWAY IN SUPRAGLOTTIC SURGERY

- Improved protection of the airway from blood and surgical debris
- Reduced cardiovascular responses
- Reduced coughing on emergence
- Reduced laryngospasm after airway device removal
- Improved oxygen saturation after airway device removal
- Ability to administer oxygen until complete restoration of airway reflexes

SGA Removal. Timing of the removal of SGAs at the end of surgery is critical.[54] SGAs should be removed either when the patient is deeply anesthetized or after protective reflexes have returned and the patient is able to open the mouth on command. Removal during excitation stages of emergence can be accompanied by coughing and/or laryngospasm. Many clinicians remove the LMA fully inflated; thus, it acts as a "scoop" for secretions above the mask, bringing them out of the airway.[55] This has been particularly useful in otolaryngologic surgery.

Contraindications to SGA Use. The primary contraindication to elective use of the SGA is a risk of gastric-content aspiration (e.g., full stomach, hiatus hernia with significant gastroesophageal reflux, intestinal obstruction, delayed gastric emptying, poor history). Other contraindications include poor lung compliance or high airway resistance, glottic or subglottic airway obstruction, and limited mouth opening (<1.5 cm).[56]

SGA Use Complications. Apart from gastroesophageal reflux and aspiration, reported complications have included laryngospasm, coughing, gagging, retching, bronchospasm, and other events characteristic of airway manipulation. The incidence of SGA-induced postoperative sore throat varies from 4% to 50% and is highly dependent on the study methods. No single device shows a consistently lower rate of dysphagia, though all appear to be better than tracheal intubation in this regard with expected rates of 30% to 70%.[57] SGAs may cause transient changes in vocal cord function. This is possibly related to cuff overinflation during prolonged procedures.

There have been rare reports of nerve injury associated with SGA use, including recurrent hypoglossal, lingual, and inferior alveolar nerves. The injuries are typically manifest from emergence to 48 hours after surgery and the majority resolved spontaneously in 1 hour to 18 months. Predisposing factors include the use of small masks, nitrous oxide, lidocaine lubrication, cuff overinflation, difficult or alternate insertion techniques, and cervical bone or joint disease.[58] Pressure neuropraxia from the tube or cuff is the most common cause.

The Laryngeal Tube (VBM Medizintechnik, GmbH, Sulz, Germany) consists of a single-lumen tube with an approximately 130-degree midshaft angle and two (distal and proximal) low-pressure cuffs (Fig. 27-5A). An oval aperture between the cuffs serves as a ventilation orifice. The distal cuff encloses the distal end of the tube. When inserted correctly, the proximal cuff seals the oral and nasal pharynx, whereas the distal cuff sits within the upper esophageal sphincter. Ventilation (spontaneous or positive pressure) occurs via an anterior surface orifice midway between the cuffs. The cuffs are inflated via a common pilot valve. The original Laryngeal Tube is available in single-use or reusable models, requires a mouth opening of at least 2.3 cm, and is inserted either blindly or with the aid of a laryngoscope. The Laryngeal Tube Suction is a modification of the Laryngeal Tube, with the addition of a second lumen for suction and gastric drainage (the orifice of which is at the distal aspect of the esophageal cuff). Six sizes (0 to 5) are suitable for neonates to large adults. Using the Laryngeal Tube in children under 10 years old is less effective than the LMA during spontaneous or assisted ventilation and for fiberoptic evaluation of the airway.[59] The Laryngeal Tube is not recommended for children weighing <10 kg because of technical difficulties and inadequate ventilation. A successful use of the Laryngeal Tube Suction was reported in an emergency airway situation in a pregnant woman with history of gastroesophageal reflux who underwent cesarean section but could not be intubated. The device improved oxygen saturation and drained gastric contents during the patient's emergence from rapid-sequence intubation.[60]

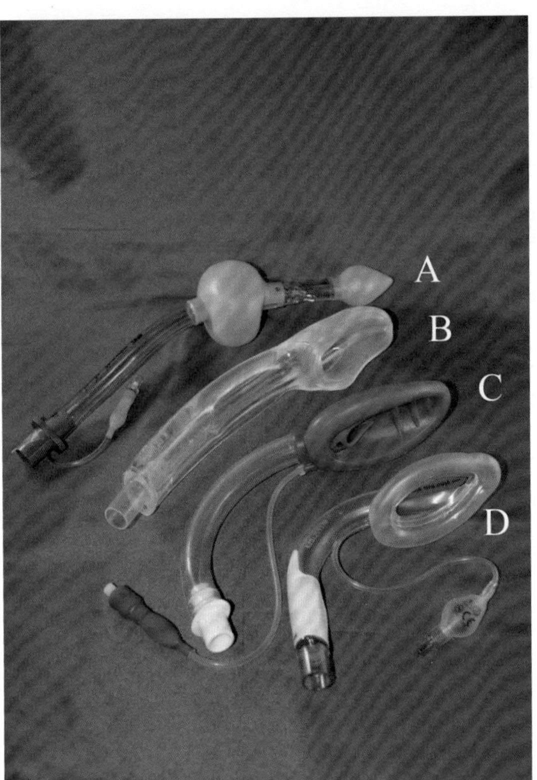

FIGURE 27-5. **(A)** The laryngeal tube, **(B)** I-Gel, **(C)** Air-Q, **(D)** Aura-I.

TABLE 27-9. FEATURES OF THE LARYNGEAL MASK AIRWAY PROSEAL

Feature	Clinical Impact
Gastric drain	Position confirmation Suprasternal notch test[a67] No gas leak via gastric drain[66] Successfully passing gastric tube Active gastric emptying Passive gastric emptying Protection from gastric-content aspiration
Posterior cuff	Increased seal pressure
Bite block	Prevents patient biting, obstruction Position confirmation 50% or more of the bite block should be within the oral cavity[67]
Wire-reinforced airway barrel	Reduced overall size Decreased ability to tracheally intubate
Large barrel/bite block	First insertion less successful than LMA classic Confers rotational stability Size choice: Size down from LMA classic

LMA, laryngeal mask airway.
[a]When a small amount of lubricant is used to occlude the gastric drain, gentle pressure on the suprasternal notch is reflected in movement of the lubricant meniscus.

A study in 15 fresh cadavers showed that mucosal pressures in the lateral pharynx, the base of tongue, and the posterior pharynx were similar between Laryngeal Tube and LMA ProSeal, but pressure on the posterior hypopharynx was always higher with the Laryngeal Tube. The investigators expressed concern that pressure from the Laryngeal Tube might impede pharyngeal perfusion more than LMA ProSeal.[61] A case of acute tongue and uvula ulceration after using the Laryngeal Tube for hysteroscopy has been reported.[62]

Cookgas Air-Q Airway. Developed by Dr. Daniel Cook (Cookgas LLC, St Louis, MO), the Air-Q perilaryngeal airway functions as an elective SGA, or as a conduit for blind or fiberoptic-aided intubation of the trachea (Fig. 27-5C). The barrel of the airway is precurved and of wide diameter, and will accept a tracheal tube from 5- to 8-mm internal diameter (ID). The keyhole-shaped airway outlet is designed to steer the ETT toward the larynx. A cuff, grossly the shape of the LMA cuff, seals the perilaryngeal space. The device is inserted (cuff deflated) by a technique similar to that recommended for the LMA (see the previous discussion). If, after insertion, the airway is obstructed, an up–down motion of the barrel will often realign the epiglottis. Blind tracheal intubation should be undertaken only if the airway is clear and the patient is muscle relaxed and/or sufficiently anesthetized. Airway seal pressures are similar to that of the ProSeal LMA.[63] The ETT cuff is completely deflated and lubricated. It is inserted 12 to 15 cm into the device barrel. Advancement past this point will be into the larynx. If resistance is met, the device can be repositioned. Once tracheal intubation is assured, the device can be removed with the help of a specialized stylet marketed by the manufacturer. In a study comparing like devices, the Fastrach LMA had a higher blind intubation rate as compared to the Air-Q, although all patients could be intubated with the addition of fiberoptic guidance.[64]

The Double-lumen SGAs. The LMA Proseal was developed by Dr. Brain as the first double-lumen SGA. The original intent of the LMA Proseal's gastric drain was to aid the clinician in the diagnosis of SGA malposition—if not placed correctly with the device's distal tip within the opening of the esophagus, an air leak would be detected. Several tests were developed to verify positioning with the LMA Proseal (Table 27-9).[65–68] The LMA ProSeal also increases the maximum airway seal during positive-pressure ventilation as compared with other LMA devices (≥40 cm H_2O), and allows passive (regurgitation) and active (gastric tube insertion) emptying of the stomach.[66–68] The advanced capabilities of the LMA Proseal allowed its use in the care of obese patients, patients undergoing intra-abdominal procedures, and in airway resuscitation.[41,69,70] A single-use version of the double-lumen LMA, the LMA-Supreme also incorporated a fixed curvature replicating the insertion ease of the LMA Fastrach (Fig. 27-3C). This device also allowed inspiratory pressures of >35 cm H_2O, and has been used for intra-abdominal procedures.[71]

The Laryngeal Tube Suction is a modification of the Laryngeal Tube, with the addition of a second lumen for suction and gastric drainage (the orifice of which is at the distal aspect of the esophageal cuff). Six sizes (0 to 5) are suitable for neonates to large adults. Using the Laryngeal Tube in children under 10 years old is less effective than the LMA during spontaneous or assisted ventilation and for fiberoptic evaluation of the airway.[59] The Laryngeal Tube is not recommended for children weighing <10 kg because of technical difficulties and inadequate ventilation.

The I-Gel. This SGA innovates a new concept in design with the advent of a solid, elastomer gel body, mounted on a plastic barrel, with no inflatable cuff.[72] A drain tube runs the length of the device from the distal tip, which sits over the esophageal inlet, to an outlet lateral to the airway circuit connector. A gastric tube may be placed into the stomach via this drain, which also serves as a passage for passively regurgitated gastric contents. The gastric drain is relatively small, the largest size accommodating a 14-French tube. (Fig. 27-5B). Airway leak pressures have been reported as ranging from 24 to 30 cm of water in adults, and may be, according to some studies, superior to the seal of the classic LMA when used in children. Sore throat occurs at rates similar to the LMA (10% to 12%), although some reports note a lower rate of visible blood on the device at removal. Success rates (first-time insertion, adequate seal pressure, etc.) are comparable to the LMA and PLMA. Contrary to a widely held belief, the solid mask of the I-Gel does not change the shape as it is warmed by the pharyngeal mucosa (personal communication, Muhammed Nasir, MD).

Tracheal Intubation

6 **Direct Laryngoscopy.** Successful laryngoscopy involves the distortion of the normal anatomic planes of the upper airway to produce a line of direct visualization from the operator's eye to the larynx; this requires the creation of a new (nonanatomic) visual axis, through maximal alignment of the axes of the oral and pharyngeal cavities, and displacement of the tongue. Unanticipated failure of DL is primarily a problem of tongue displacement (inability to align the axes can be anticipated by physical examination).[10] As pointed out in the ASA Difficult Airway Practice Guidelines, no one measure may be adequate to determine difficulty of DL, and multiple measures must be integrated in order to make sensible airway management decisions.[1] Shiga et al.[18] published a meta-analysis of studies regarding airway physical examination scores and cautioned on the poor sensitivity and only modest specificity of all routine tests.

In 1944, Bannister and MacBeth proposed a three-axis model to explain the anatomic relationships involved airway axis alignment, thereby elucidating the rationale of the intubation sniffing position (SP) described by Sir Ivan Magill.[11] In the SP, the neck is flexed by 35 degrees and the head extended by 15 degrees. This is achieved by placing a support (around 7 cm in the adult) under the head in patients who were easy to intubate by DL. Others have suggested positing the patient so that the external auditory meatus is level with the sternal notch (EAM-SN position). This is helpful, especially in the obese patient.[73] The three-axis explanation has been challenged by Adnet et al.[74] who noted that, although extension at the atlanto-occipital joint maximally facilitated an oral cavity/pharyngeal alignment, no significant improvement was achieved with flexion of the cervical spine on the thorax. Chou and Wu[75] refined this approach by noting that laryngeal axis alignment is unnecessary. The end point of the effort to create an in-line space for tracheal intubation is the glottic aperture. These authors propose a two-axis/tongue-displacement model. This model does not depend on the alignment of all axes to create an in-line view of the larynx, but rather maximizes the spaces between the alveolar ridge and the laryngeal aperture through oropharyngeal alignment and tongue displacement. This concept can be used to not only understand the problems that may hinder DL, but also why common indexes of airway assessment fail in their predictive power. This concept has been described previously as FAA.[76]

FAA is a method of examining the functional nature of each of the anatomic correlates of the commonly used assessment indices. FAA places an emphasis on the interdependence of these anatomic characteristics rather than on their individual size or functional integrity. As explained by Chou and Wu,[75] when the head and neck are in the neutral position, the oral and pharyngeal axes are perpendicular to each other. With maximal extension of a normal atlanto-occipital joint, 35 degrees or more of motion is attained (Fig. 27-6). This brings the angle between the oral and pharyngeal axes to 125 degrees. Although it is an improvement, it is certainly not the 180 degrees required for creation of a line of site to the glottis. A different space must be created. This space is created by displacement of the tongue with the laryngoscope. Although atlanto-occipital extension cannot by itself allow direct laryngeal vision, it does provide anterior displacement of the mass of the tongue and brings up the alveolar ridge into improved position relative to the tongue and larynx. The extension of the atlanto-occipital point also provides an advantage in mouth opening. Calder et al.[41] have shown that the maximal mouth opening is 26% greater in full atlanto-occipital extension as compared with the neutral head position. Temporomandibular jaw function also contributes to the displacement of the tongue away from the required visual axis. Rotation and translation of the temporomandibular joint result in a relaxation of the

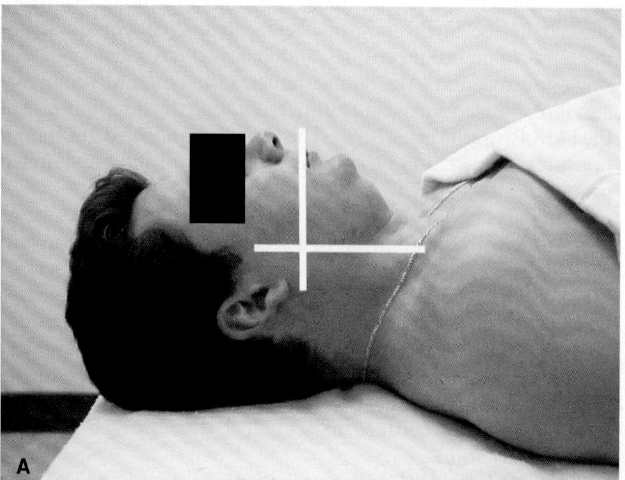

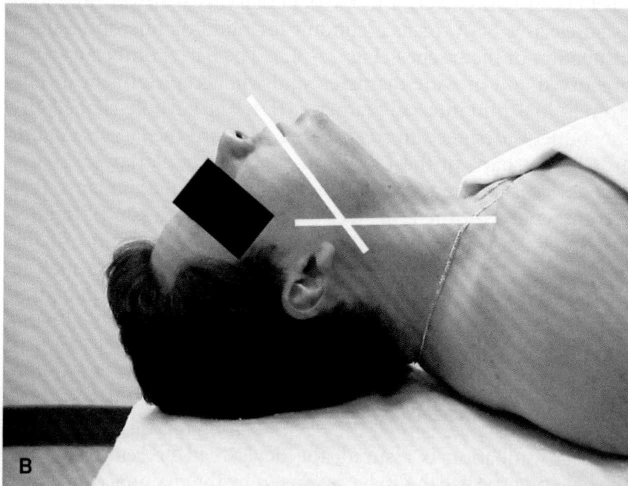

FIGURE 27-6. A: With the patient supine, the oral and pharyngeal axes do not overlap. **B:** Extension at the atlanto-occipital joint maximally overlaps the oral and pharyngeal axes.

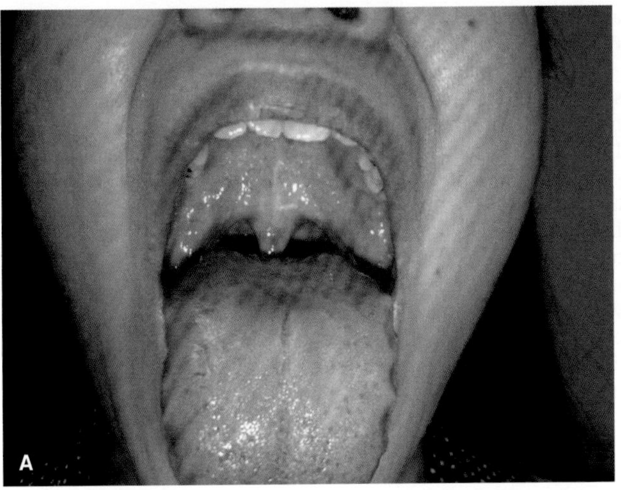

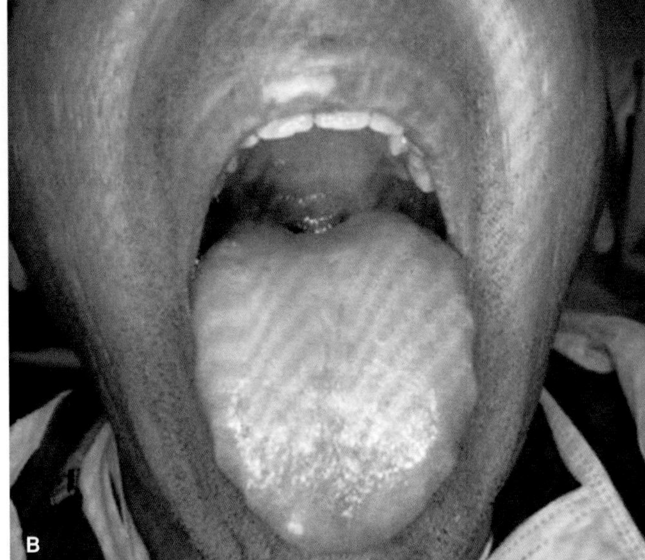

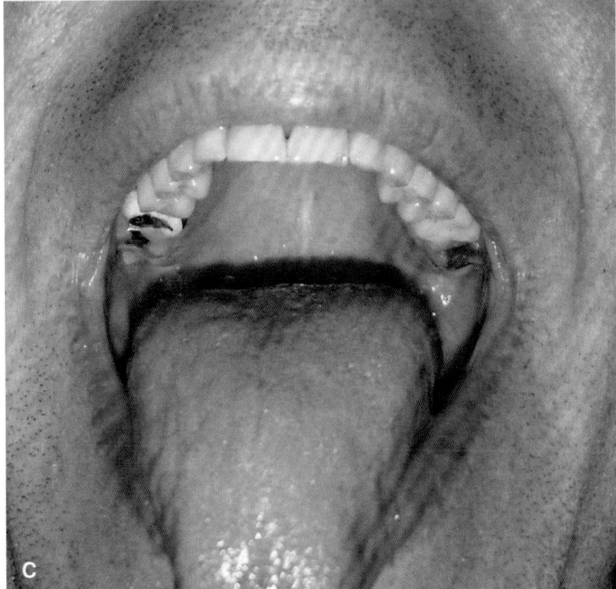

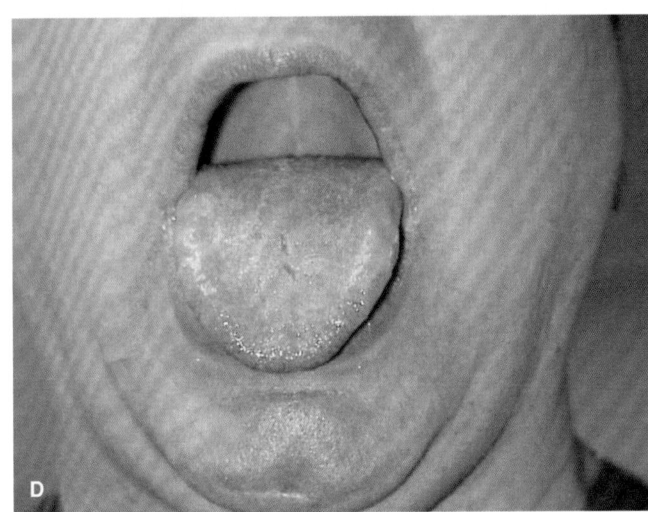

FIGURE 27-7. Mallampati/Samsoon–Young classification of the oropharyngeal view.[77] **A:** Class I: uvula, faucial pillars, soft palate visible. **B:** Class II: Faucial pillars, soft palate visible. **C:** Class III: Soft and hard palate visible. **D:** Class IV: Hard palate visible only (added by Samsoon and Young).

tongue insertion as well as creation of the aperture width needed for instrumentation.

Using the FAA approach to airway evaluation also helps to explain the value of the popular yet highly criticized Mallampati and thyromental distance indices.[77] These two measures have historically been considered important because they approximate the relative mass of the tongue (Mallampati) and the anterior–posterior borders of space into which it will be displaced by the laryngoscope (Fig. 27-7). As noted elsewhere, these indices have shown to have poor and/or variable predictive power. Two groups have considered the interrelated nature of these measures in a way that reveals why they perform poorly when considered individually. Ayoub et al.[78] found a high Mallampati score to be predictive of a difficult DL when the thyromental distance was <4 cm. When the thyromental distance was >4 cm, relative tongue size (as determined by the Mallampati classification) was not predictive. Iohom et al.[6] found similar results using a thyromental distance cutoff of 6 cm. The finding that the predictive power of the Mallampati improves when the mandible is short is consistent with the concept of FAA: When the mandibular space is restricted, tongue size is important. When the space is large, a tongue of any nonpathologic size should be accommodated. An exception to this may be hypopharyngeal tongue, as described by Chou and Wu;[79] although according to those authors, measurement of the mandibular hyoid distance should help in diagnosing this.

As noted above, a common cause of difficulty in DL is a pathologic increase in tongue size. Ovassapian et al.[16] have identified lingual tonsil hyperplasia as the most commonly undiagnosed cause of unanticipated difficult DL. They reviewed the cases of unanticipated difficult DL in their institution from 1999 to 2000. Thirty-three patients were identified. All patients were found to have lingual tonsil hyperplasia on fiberoptic examination (Fig. 27-8).

Devices that aid in placing the patient in a sniffing position have become available. These include the sniff position pillow

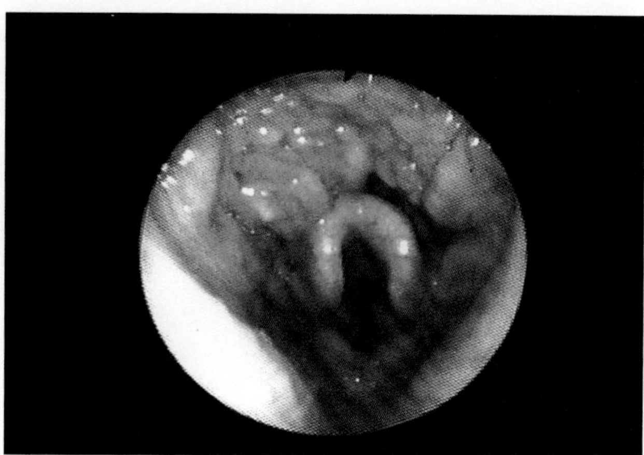

FIGURE 27-8. Lingual tonsil hyperplasia: The vallecula is filled with hyperplastic lymphoid tissue in a patient who had an unanticipated difficult direct laryngoscopy.

(Popitz Pillow, Alimed, Dedham, MA) and Pi's Pillow (American Eagle Medical, Holbrook, NY), which can be configured for the awake (comfortable) then asleep (functional position) patient.

The obese patient may need further positioning to move the mass of the chest away from the plane across which the laryngoscope handle will sweep as it is manipulated into the mouth, as well as compensate for the increased anterior–posterior diameter of the chest. This may require placing a wedge-shaped lift (e.g., the Troop Elevation Pillow, Mercury Medical, Clearwater, FL; under the scapula, shoulders, and nape of neck, raising the head and neck above the thorax and providing a grade in order to allow gravity to pull the pannus' weight away from the airway, as well as producing an EAM-SN position.[73]

After the head and neck have been positioned, the mouth is opened by one of two techniques. The first method encourages extension of the atlanto-occipital joint by the use of the dominant hand under the occiput. This maneuver leads to passive opening of the mouth, and can be accentuated by using the fourth finger of the nondominant hand (holding the laryngoscope) to apply pressure over the chin in a caudad direction. In the second technique, which tends to be more effective but requires contact of the (gloved) hand with the teeth and/or gum, caudad pressure is applied with the thumb of the dominant hand on the mandibular canine/bicuspids on the patient's same side while the first finger, crossed below the thumb, applies cephalad pressure to the ipsilateral maxillary canine/bicuspid. The ultimate goal of both techniques is rotation and translation of the temporomandibular joint in order to achieve the widest interincisor gap, and relaxation of the mandibular space. The patient, whether conscious or not, is now ready for laryngoscopy.

8 **Use of the Direct Laryngoscope Blade.** Proper use of the laryngoscope blade is vital to the success of this basic airway management technique. Two blade types are commonly available and
9 each is applied in a unique manner. Many other blades have been described but will not be discussed here; the reader is directed to some excellent reviews.[80]

The curved (Macintosh) blade is used to displace the epiglottis out of the line of sight by tensing the glossoepiglottic ligament, whereas the straight blade (Miller) compresses the epiglottis against the base of the tongue. Both blades include a flange along the left side of their length, which is used to sweep the tongue to the left side of the mouth. Blades with a right-sided flange are available for the left-handed practitioner, but they are not commonly found in practice.

In most available systems, the blade incorporates the light source, either a bulb placed near the distal blade aspect or a rigid fiberoptic cable that transmits light produced within the handle. In either case, these blades must be long enough to achieve their respective applications. Therefore, blade size needs to be chosen appropriately and, on occasion, exchanged after a failed attempt at DL. As a generalization, the Macintosh blade is regarded as advantageous whenever there is little room to pass an ETT (e.g., small mouth), whereas the Miller blade is considered better in the patient who has a small mandibular space, large incisor teeth, or a large epiglottis.[81] The straight-against-the-tongue nature of the Miller blade affords maximal transfer of workforce from the operator's elbow and shoulder onto the surface of the tongue in order to displace it into a small mandibular space.

With the left hand holding the laryngoscope handle, the blade is inserted into the right side of the mouth, with care taken not to compress the upper lip against the teeth. As the blade is advanced toward the epiglottis, it is swept leftward, using the flange to displace the tongue to the left as the blade compresses it into the mandibular space. After reaching the base of the tongue (the Macintosh blade tip in the vallecula, or the Miller blade compressing the epiglottis

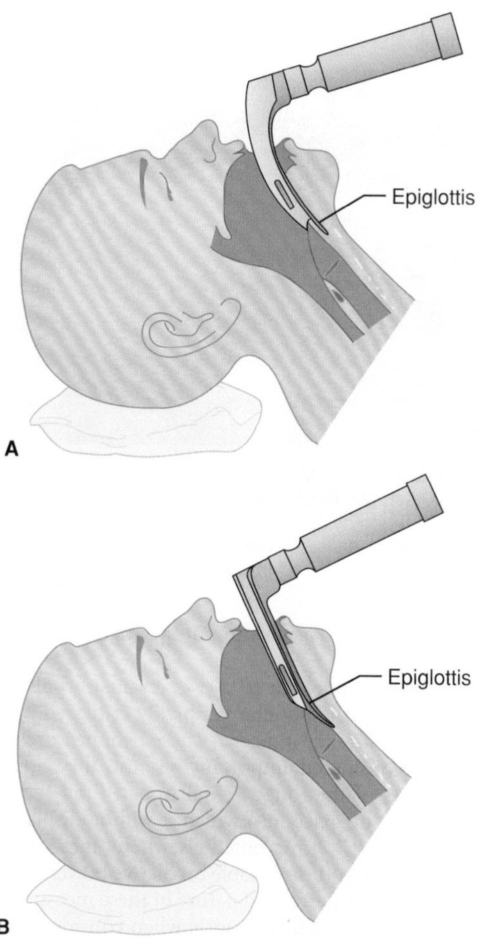

FIGURE 27-9. A: When a curved laryngoscope blade is used, the tip of the blade is placed in the vallecula, the space between the base of the tongue and the pharyngeal surface of the epiglottis. **B:** The tip of a straight blade is advanced beneath the epiglottis.

against the base of the tongue), the operator's arm and shoulder lift in an anterior–caudad direction (Fig. 27-9).

Importantly, the laryngoscopist must strive to avoid rotating the wrist and the laryngoscope handle in a cephalad direction, bringing the blade against the upper incisor teeth. Extending either blade style too deeply can bring the tip of the blade to rest under the larynx itself so that forward pressure lifts the entire airway from view.

Special considerations apply to the technique of laryngoscopy and intubation in the infant and child. Because of the relatively larger size of the occiput in children, producing an anatomic sniffing position, elevation of the head (as done in the adult) is not required.[81] On occasion, one may need to elevate the thorax instead. The relatively short neck gives the impression of an anterior position of the larynx. Posterior cricoid pressure is often required to place the laryngeal inlet into view. A straight blade is more helpful in displacing the stiff, omega-shaped, and high epiglottis. Because the cricoid cartilage is the narrowest aspect of the airway until 6 to 8 years of age, the intubator must be sensitive to resistance to advancement of the ETT that has easily passed the vocal folds. Hyperextension at the atlanto-occipital joint, as done in adults, may cause airway obstruction from the relative pliability of the trachea. In the child, there is a higher risk of endobronchial intubation or accidental extubation with head movement owing to the short length of the trachea.

10

With laryngoscopy, the view of the larynx may be complete, partial, or impossible. A laryngeal view scoring system that has won general acceptance was developed by Cormack and Lehane[82] who described four grades of laryngeal view. Grade 1 includes visualization of the entire glottic aperture, grade 2 includes visualization of only the posterior aspects of the glottic aperture, grade 3 is visualization of the tip of the epiglottis, and grade 4 is visualization of no more than the soft palate (Fig. 27-10). A Cormack–Lehane grade 3 or 4 is expected in 1.5% to 8.5% of adult laryngoscopies.[83]

This system has proved useful not only as a means of recording the laryngeal view on individual patients, but also as a clinical end point in the evaluation of preoperative airway assessments tools. A modification of the Cormack and Lehane score has been proposed by Koh et al.[84] who noted that when a partial vocal cord view ("2A") is achieved, tracheal intubation was significantly easier than when only the arytenoids and epiglottis were visualized ("2B").

Another view scoring system is based on the clinician's estimate of the percent of glottic opening (POGO) seen during laryngoscopy (e.g., 0% to 100% of the span from anterior

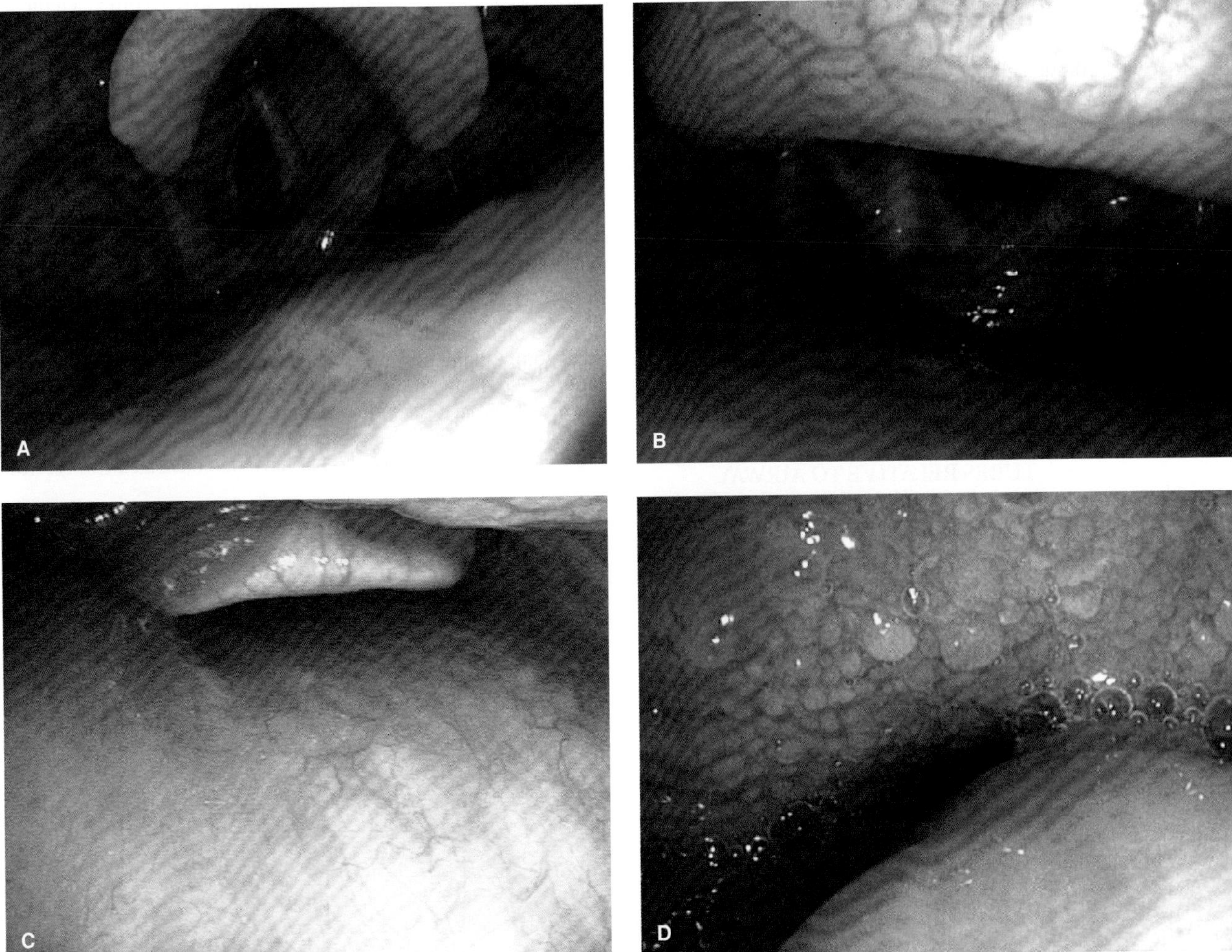

FIGURE 27-10. The Cormack–Lehane laryngeal view scoring system: Grade 1 **(A)**, grade 2 **(B)**, grade 3 **(C)**, and grade 4 **(D)**.

commissure to the interarytenoid notch). The POGO score was found to have improved interexaminer reliability when compared to the Cormack and Lehane system, and has been adopted by many researchers in the comparative evaluation of video laryngoscopy.[85]

If during laryngoscopy, a satisfactory laryngeal view is not achieved, the backward–upward–rightward pressure (BURP) maneuver may aid in improving the view. In this maneuver, a second operator displaces the larynx (B) backward against the cervical vertebrae, (U) superiorly as possible and (R) slightly laterally to the right, using external pressure over the cricoid cartilage. The BURP maneuver has been shown to improve the laryngeal view, decreasing the rate of difficult intubation in a study of 1,993 patients from 4.7% to 1.8%.[86] When a left-handed operator is using a left-handed laryngoscope blade, the lateral external pressure should displace the larynx to the left. Similarly, Benumof and Cooper describe "optimal external laryngeal manipulation," which consists of pressing posteriorly and cephalad over the thyroid, hyoid, and cricoid cartilages.[87]

Once the larynx is visualized with a left-side–flanged blade, the tracheal tube is inserted from the right-hand side, care being taken not to obstruct the view of the vocal cords. Whenever possible, the action of the ETT passing through the vocal cords should be witnessed by the laryngoscopist. The tracheal tube should be inserted to a depth of at least 2 cm after the disappearance of the tracheal tube cuff into the larynx in order to approximate placement in the midtrachea. This should present the 21- and 23-cm external markings at the teeth for the typical adult female and male, respectively.[88] Although allowances should be made for individual circumstances, a size 7 to 8 ID tracheal tube is used in the adult female, and size 8 to 9 tracheal tube used in the adult male. The larger tracheal tubes may be desirable if pulmonary toilet or diagnostic or therapeutic bronchoscopy is to be part of the clinical course. Pediatric laryngoscope blades and tracheal tube sizes are presented in detail in Table 27-10 (see also Chapter 45).

An alternative approach to DL has been described by Henderson.[88] In this approach to tongue displacement, a straight-bladed laryngoscope is introduced into the right side of the mouth. The blade is advanced between the tongue and palatine tonsil. The blade passes below the epiglottis, which is then elevated. This approach subjects the tongue to less compressive forces. It has been suggested that this technique may improve the view of the larynx in the presence of lingual tonsil hyperplasia.

TABLE 27-10. SIZE AND LENGTH OF TRACHEAL TUBES RELATIVE TO AIRWAY ANATOMY

Age	Internal Diameter (mm)	Distance from Lips to Midtrachea[a] (cm)
Premature	2.5	8
Full term	3	10
1–6 mo	3.5	11
6–12 mo	4	12
2 yrs	4.5	13
4 yrs	5	14
6 yrs	5.5	15
8 yrs	6.5	16[b]
10 yrs	7	17–18[c]
12 yrs	7.5	18–20
14 yrs	8–9	20–22

[a]Add 2 to 3 cm for nasal tubes.
[b]Females.
[c]Males.

Verification of successful tracheal tube placement is made by a variety of methods. The gold standards for confirmation of 11 placement include visualization of placement through the vocal folds and sustained detection of exhaled carbon dioxide as measured with capnography or a disposable chemical colorimetric device such as the Easy Cap II. Other portable techniques include auscultation over the chest and abdomen, visualization of the 12 chest excursion, observation of condensation in the ETT, use of a self-inflating bulb (TubeChek-B, Ambu, Linthicum, MD), lighted stylets, standard and dedicated fiberoptic devices used to identify the tracheal rings and carina (Foley Flexible Airway Stylet, Clarus Medical, Golden Valley, MN), and ultrasound or chest X-ray.[89]

Although DL remains the most used method for tracheal intubation, it is far from successful in all cases and not always benign when successful. DL may be difficult or impossible in 8.5% and 1.8% of attempts, respectively.[90] The analysis of Domino et al.[39] of the ASA Closed Claims Database reveals that claims for laryngeal injury during DL arise more often in "easy" as opposed to difficult laryngoscopies. Among the 4,460 cases in the ASA Closed Claim Database, 87 instances of laryngeal trauma were recorded. Of these, 80% occurred during routine (nondifficult) tracheal intubation, in which no injury was suspected. This has led some to question whether routine tracheal intubation is as safe as assumed.[38]

Image-guided laryngoscopy promises to quickly dominate the science and art of tracheal intubation. The first decade of the 21st century saw a proliferation of optical and video-transmitting devices, primarily as the result of the availability of inexpensive CMOS technology. The unifying characteristics of these laryngoscopes are the nonaxial-dependent view required of direct laryngoscopy. A large variety of devices, employing optical or video transmission of the laryngeal image are now available.

Optical Stylets. A new generation of fiberoptic devices is focused on simplicity and portability by incorporating optical and light source elements into a single stylet-like stainless steel sheath. The lack of a tongue-displacing blade and a suction/oxygen channel are potential disadvantages. Both the Shikani Seeing Stylet and the Bonfils Intubation Fiberscope (BIF) (Karl Storz Endoscopy, Tuttingen, Germany; Fig. 27-11) have demonstrated less cervical

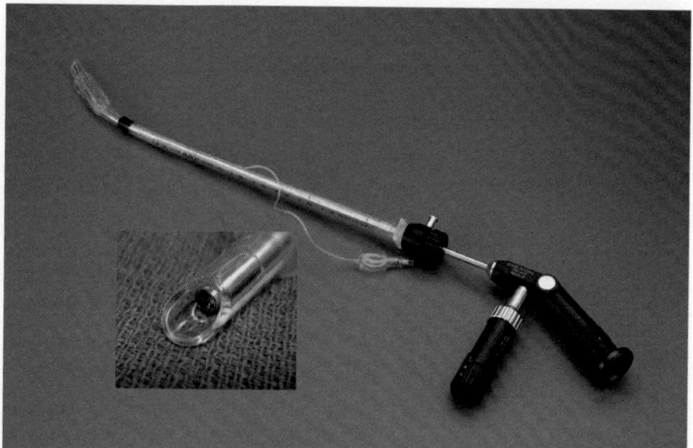

FIGURE 27-11. The Bonfils (Karl Storz Endoscopy, Culver City, CA). Inset: Objective end within tracheal tube.

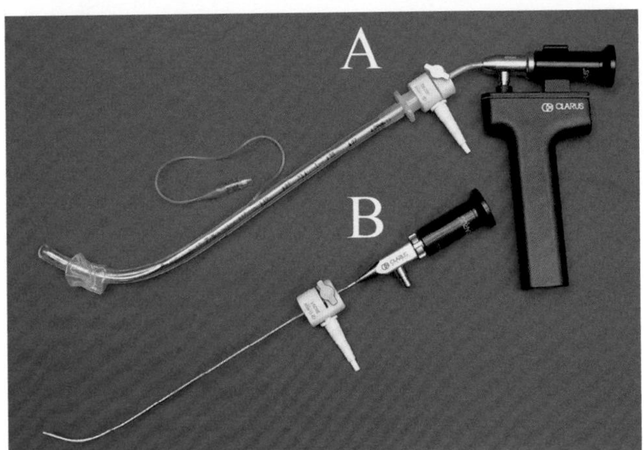

FIGURE 27-12. **A:** The Shikani Seeing Optical Stylet (*Clarus* Medical, LLC, Minneapolis, MN). **B:** The Levitan FPS.

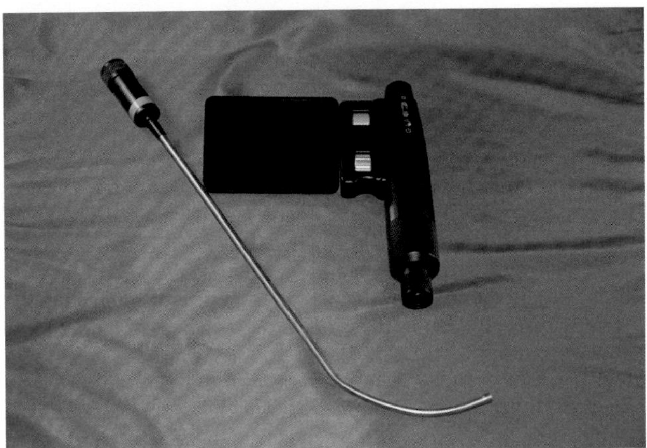

FIGURE 27-13. The Clarus Video System (*Clarus* Medical, LLC, Minneapolis, MN).

spine motion when compared to direct laryngoscopy.[91,92] The BIF is a long, rigid tubular device with conventional optical and light-transmitting fiberoptic elements.[93] A proximal-end eyepiece (with adjustable diopter) can be used with the naked eye or fitted with a standard endoscopy camera. A cable (or battery-powered attachment) brings illumination from an external light source. The distal end has a 40-degree angulation. The objective lens allows a 100-degree field of view. Sizes with external diameters of 2, 3.5, and 5 mm are available. Suction may be applied through a working channel. The technique of use replicates the paraglossal approach of laryngoscopy discussed previously in this chapter.

The Shikani Seeing Optical Stylet (SOS) (*Clarus* Medical, LLC, Minneapolis, MN) has a similar configuration to the BIF, with the exception that the distal half of the stylet is malleable (Fig. 27-12). The light source may be self-contained (a proprietary powered handle or a green line [Rusch Medical, Duluth, GA] laryngoscope handle), or cabled. The adult Shikani can accommodate a 5.5-mm ID tracheal tube or larger. The pediatric model can be fitted with a 2.5-mm ID tracheal tube or larger. Unlike the Bofils, a midline approach is recommended. Although the Shikani can be used as an independent intubating device, it can also be employed as an adjunct to direct laryngoscopy when a high Cormack and Lehane score is archived. Although it is primarily an oral intubation device, the SOS has also been used for nasal intubation.

Levitan First Pass Success Scope (*Clarus* Medical, LLC, Minneapolis, MN), a shorter (30-cm) version of the SOS, is designed to be used during DL when a high laryngeal view score is encountered (Fig. 27-12B). The shorter length allows more ergonomic positioning by the laryngoscopist.[94] A 6-mm ID tracheal tube or larger may be used. Because of its short length, a standard tracheal tube should be trimmed in length so that the objective lens is within the bevel.[95] The hypothetical benefit of this practice is the reduction of unanticipated difficult intubations and the maintenance of alternative technique skills by incorporating this or similar devices into daily practice.[96]

The Clarus Video System (*Clarus* Medical, LLC, Minneapolis, MN) (Fig. 27-13) replicates the malleable stylet concept of the SOS with the incorporation of CMOS technology. A 4-inch LED adjustable angle screen is mounted on the handle. The screen has a proprietary video-out port. A setting on the controls illuminates a distal, anteriorly positioned red diode, which may be visible through the skin when the objective is in the larynx.

13

Video Laryngoscopes. The GlideScope (Verathon, Bothell, WA; Fig. 27-14C) provides an electronically projected image on a video monitor emanating from a video chip set at the distal end of a conventional-like laryngoscope blade, but with a more acute (60 degrees) distal angulation.[97] Illumination is likewise generated at the distal position. This configuration affords several advantages: (1) It may be handled with a skill set similar to that

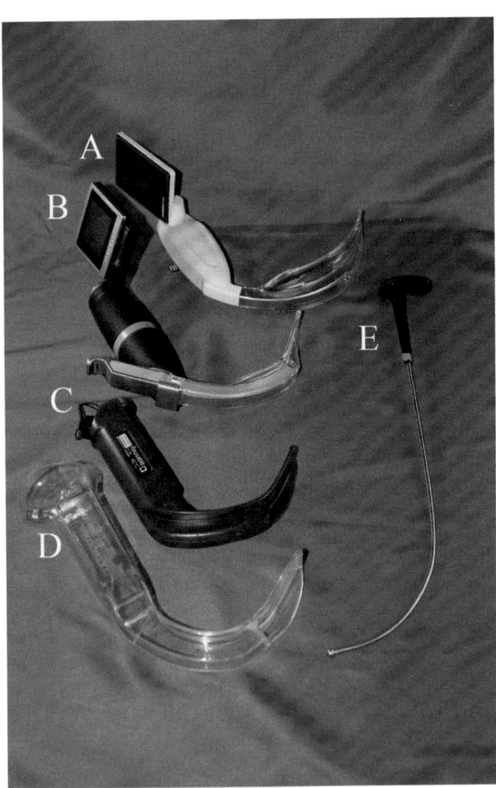

FIGURE 27-14. **(A)** McGrath Mac and **(B)** Mcgrath Series 5 (McGrath Medical, UK), **(C)** GlideScope Multiuse blade and **(D)** GlideScope Cobalt single-use blade (Verathon, Bethel, WA), **(E)** Gliderite rigid stylet (Verathon, Bethel, WA).

used with conventional DL. (2) The operator's point of sight (e.g., the video apparatus) is positioned close to the distal blade aspect. (3) The video apparatus is a charged coupled-like device (thereby eliminating fragile fiberoptic elements). The operator, therefore, "sees" at a position behind the tongue, and displacement as with conventional DL is not necessary in most cases. Similarly, lingual tonsil hyperplasia should not affect the visual axis as it does with conventional DL. (4) The video image of the airway is displayed on a lightweight portable screen, and allows for visualization by more than one individual (e.g., aid, mentor, student). (5) Less stress may be imposed on the airway by virtue of reduced compressive force directed to the tongue. (6) An external light source is not required.

When used by inexperienced operators the GlideScope provides better glottic exposure as compared with DL (Cormack–Lehane grade 1 view in 85.7% vs. 48.9%) and can obtain Cormack–Lehane grade 1 or 2 in 77% of patients in whom no glottic exposure was achieved by DL.[97] A large prospective, nonrandomized study of 1,755 patients showed a 98% intubation success rate, including 96% success in patients predicted to be difficult by DL, and a 94% failed-DL rescue rate.[98] In one study, placement of the ETT required an additional 16 seconds (on average) when compared to DL.[97,99]

The classic GlideScope insertion technique follows the midline approach. After the uvula is visualized, the blade is advanced midline into the vallecula or can be passed posterior to the epiglottis.[97] For patients with a limited mouth aperture, an alternative insertion has been described in which the blade is inserted like a Guedel airway; that is, the GlideScope blade concavity facing rostrad and rotated 180 degrees counterclockwise once the distal tip is in the oropharynx. This maneuver displaces the tongue to the left and minimizes neck movements.

Although achieving a good laryngeal view with the GlideScope appears relatively easy, ETT manipulation into the larynx may be more difficult because of the acute blade angulation. The use of a stylet is advised to deliver the ETT.[100,101] Different authors have suggested stylet shaping with a bend of 60 degrees, 90 degrees, a dynamic stylet, J, or "gear shift" shape. Reverse loading technique or use of a gum elastic bougie has also been described.[102] There is one study that evidenced that the angle of the ETT had greater impact on time to intubation than the Cormack and Lehane grade of the image.[103] A dedicated, nonmalleable stylet, the GlideScope reusable stylet (Verathon), has been introduced. This stylet has a 90-degree bend, and may be used with various video laryngoscopes. The GlideScope has also been used to facilitate nasotracheal intubation with a reduced time to intubation when compared with DL and a high first-time success rate.

The 60-degree angulation of the GlideScope reduces cervical spine motion by 50% at the C2 to C5 segments compared with Macintosh laryngoscopy. Theoretically, the airway axes do not need to be aligned to affect a good view, but manipulation of the GlideScope to the position to achieve an adequate image can cause cervical segment extension. It has been successfully used to achieve tracheal intubation in patients with limited cervical spine movement because of ankylosing spondylitis and cervical spine arthritis, but it may be difficult to use in patients with limited oral aperture.[104,105]

Control studies have shown no significant advantage of the GlideScope in preventing hemodynamic responses to orotracheal intubation as compared with the Macintosh direct laryngoscope, although others have shown cardiovascular responses similar to intubation with a flexible fiberoptic bronchoscope.[106]

Traumatic complications associated with the use of the GlideScope video laryngoscope have been related to blind manipulation of the ETT as it enters the airway but is not yet visualized on the perilaryngeal image. Traumatic events, which appear to be more likely with the use of a rigid stylet, are primarily reported to involve the soft palate, palatoglossal arch, right palatopharyngeal arch, and right anterior tonsillar pillar;[107–111] (Fig. 27-15). Steps to avoid soft tissue trauma include (1) assuring that the stylet is within the bevel of the ETT, (2) focusing the operator's attention on the tracheal tube as it enters the mouth (attention is turned to the video image only when the distal ETT becomes visible), and (3) maintaining a midline ETT position.

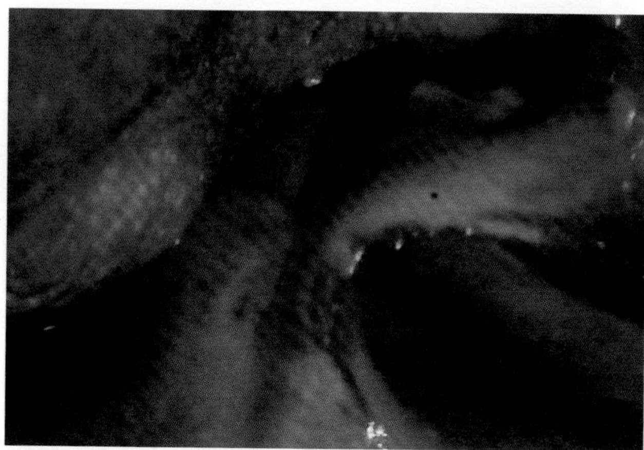

FIGURE 27-15. Passage of a tracheal tube through the right palatoglossal arch due to blind spot created with video laryngoscopy.

The C-Mac (Karl Storz Endovision, Culver City, CA; Fig. 27-16) consists of a conventional-appearing laryngoscope handle and blade fitted with illumination and image fiberoptics. Although the image projected from the CMAC closely resembles that seen with the naked eye, ETT placement is facilitated because the operator does not need to maintain an unobstructed line of sight (by using the video monitor). Use of the C-Mac is identical to standard

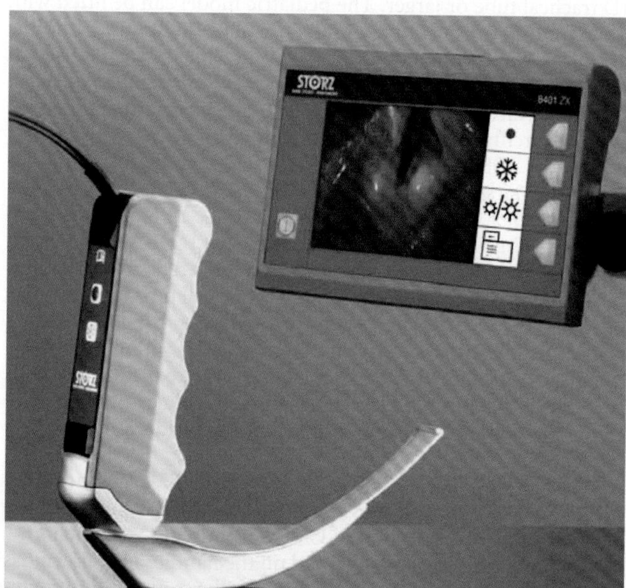

FIGURE 27-16. The C-Mac (Karl Storz Endovision, Culver City, CA).

DL, making the video facility uniquely valuable during supervised instruction. A comparison study of direct and video-assisted views of the larynx revealed significant improvement of the glottic view with the CMAC.[112] In controlled trials, the VM facilitated tracheal intubation in bariatric and thoracic surgery patients.[113]

The McGrath Series 5 video laryngoscope (Aircraft Medical, Edinburgh) was introduced to clinical practice in 2007 (Fig. 27-14A). The unique features of the McGrath are (1) a self-contained unit including laryngoscopic blade, handle, power source (1.5 V batteries), and a 3.3- × 2.2-cm liquid crystal display (LCD) screen; (2) an acute distal angle blade; (3) adjustable blade length; and (4) a disposable patient contact blade. As with the GlideScope, the acute angle blade improves the Cormack and Lehane grade of the laryngeal view by affording the operator an oblique line of sight around the base of the tongue. In one uncontrolled series, tracheal intubation was successful in 98% of 150 elective surgery patients.[114] As with the GlideScope, because McGrath video laryngoscopy does not involve creation of a direct line of sight to the larynx, tracheal tube placement may be awkward. Use of a semi or nonmalleable stylet is advisable with both devices, with a 60- to 90-degree upward bend of the distal tracheal tube. Because the angle of the distal ETT-stylet is anterior as it enters the larynx, a 1- to 2-cm withdrawal of the stylet at this juncture facilitates advancement. Concerns regarding the intubation "blind spot" are similar to those with the GlideScope.

The McGrath Mac (Aircraft Medical, Edinburgh, UK) is the newer-generation McGrath video laryngoscope with a reduced blade curvature and slimmer blade design (11.9 mm). The "blind spot" noted with the GlideScope and McGrath Series 5 is reduced. A 2.5-inch improved screen allows shared viewers. The reduced blade curve allows improved direct laryngoscopic use as compared to the more acutely angled blade of the Series 5. Although there may be less concern for soft tissue trauma, the cautions mentioned above should be applied.

The Airtraq optical laryngoscope (Prodol Meditec S.A., Vizcaya, Spain; Fig. 27-17B) is a single-use, anatomically shaped laryngoscope optical prism, "channel" device, with a lateral guiding channel that holds and guides the ETT through the vocal cords. Whereas DL is used to displace the anterior airway structures, and VLs place the operators point of vision around the tongue, the channel devices replicate the near 90-degree relationship of the oral and pharyngeal axes, much like an earlier device, the Bullard laryngoscope. The Airtraq has a built-in antifog system and a low-temperature light. A tracheal tube is secured within the guiding channel. With the patient in a neutral position, the Airtraq is guided around the oral and pharyngeal axes. The distal blade can be guided above or below the epiglottis. Once the larynx is centered in the visual field, the tracheal tube is slid down the channel (without rotation) and observed to enter the larynx. Unlike the classic video laryngoscopes described above, the tracheal tube distal end can be visualized throughout its course reducing the opportunity for soft tissue trauma.

14

The Airtraq has been successfully used as a rescue device in patients after failed intubation with DL.[115] Reports of its use in awake patients, patients with cervical spine disease, and after failed DL have been published.[116] One study showed the need for fewer maneuvers to improve glottic exposure and fewer alterations in blood pressure and heart rate when compared with DL.[117] Reduced cervical spine movement in patients with midline axial stabilization has been demonstrated.

The Airway Scope (Pentax AWS, AWS-S100; Hoya- Pentax, Tokyo, Japan) is a reusable channel device that uses CMOS imaging technology on a camera cord fitted into a single-use blade (Fig. 27-17A). A 2.4-inch LCD monitor is integrated into the handle. The monitor has a wide viewing angle and is readily visible from behind and from the side of the Airway Scope. The angle of the monitor can be adjusted for easier viewing. The disposable blade accepts ETTs with outside diameters between 8.5 mm and 11 mm, and incorporates a working channel for injection of lidocaine, a small suction catheter, or oxygen insufflation. In one small, nonblinded, noncrossover study the AWS had a higher success rate than the GlideScope (100% vs. 96%) in patients predicted to be difficult by DL (84%).[118] The AWS also produced less of a hemodynamic response. As with other channel scopes, the AWS had a higher success rate than the GlideScope in normal volunteers with restricted neck mobility.[98]

Although the Airtraq and AWS use a similar axes-following design in carrying the tracheal tube into the hypopharynx, ETT presentation to the larynx appear different.[119] The Airtraq manufacturers recommend that the blade tip should enter the vallecula (though lifting the epiglottis from a "Miller" position will also lead to successful intubation). The AWS manufacturer recommends using the blade to lift the epiglottis and, in practice, placing the blade in the vallecula often leads to failure of intubation. The difference in the use and success of these two very similar devices appears to be a much closer positioning of the ETT to the AWS blade as it is extended out of the channel.[119]

The King Vision Video Laryngoscope (King systems, Noblesville, IN) includes a reusable, battery-operated OLED display and disposable channeled and nonchanneled blades. The device can, therefore, be used as a classic VL or a channel scope.

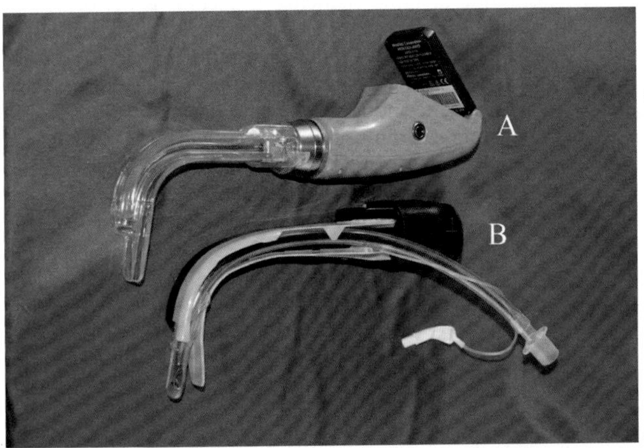

FIGURE 27-17. (A) The Pentax Airway Scope, **(B)** The Airtraq laryngoscope (Prodol Meditec S.A., Vizcaya, Spain).

15

NPO Status and Rapid-sequence Induction

Prevention of the pulmonary aspiration of gastric contents is one of the primary concerns of the airway manager. Anesthetic induction profoundly depresses intrinsic reflexes that protect the airway from the entrance of foreign bodies, including regurgitated material. Many routine patients will present in situations where aspiration is a significant risk (e.g., urgent procedures soon after food ingestion). Rapid-sequence induction, as described, is practiced. In situations where a difficult airway patient presents similarly, awake intubation is often chosen, as described in this chapter (see Airway Approach Algorithm). In both cases and in other situations with varying degrees of concern, pharmacologic therapy can help to mitigate risk. The goal of this therapy is to reduce both the volume and acidity of the gastric contents (Table 27-11). Obesity by itself, long taught as a risk factor for gastric-content aspiration,

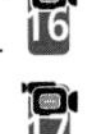
16 17

TABLE 27-11. PULMONARY ASPIRATION (A) PATIENTS AT RISK FOR ASPIRATION, (B) ASA RECOMMNENDED FASTING GUIDELEINES, (C) METHODS TO REDUCE RISK

(A) Patients at risk for aspiration
Full stomach (recent ingestion)
Diabetes mellitus (with peripheral neuropathy)
Gastroesophageal reflux/hiatal hernia
Pregnancy
Acute pain/acute opioid therapy renal colic
Bowel obstruction/intra-abdominal process

(B) Summary of fasting recommendations (WR-BB)

Ingested material	Minimum fasting period
Clear liquids	2 h
Breast milk	4 h
Infant formula	6 h
Nonhuman milk	6 h
Light meal	6 h

(C) Methods to reduce risk
Minimize intake, adequate preoperative fasting, clear liquids only if necessary
Increase gastric emptying, prokinetics (e.g., metoclopramide)
Reduce gastric volume and acidity, Nasogastric tube, nonparticulate antacid (e.g., sodium citrate), H_2-receptor antagonists (e.g., famotidine), proton pump inhibitors (e.g., lansoprazole)
Airway management and protection, cricoid pressure, cuffed endotracheal intubation

may not be a risk in this regard.[120] Although initial studies touted the increased volume of (more) acid secretions in the obese fasting patient, as compared with the lean control, others have refuted this claim.[121,122]

Control of Gastric Contents

Control of gastric contents involves (1) minimizing intake, (2) increasing gastric emptying with prokinetics, and (3) reducing gastric volume and acidity with a nasogastric tube, antacids, H_2-receptor antagonists, and proton pump inhibitors (PPIs). Clear liquids can be administered to children and adults up to 2 and 3 hours, respectively, prior to anesthesia without increased risk for regurgitation and aspiration.[123] Gastric emptying is slower for milk than for clear liquids. Human breast milk is cleared more rapidly than other milk products.[124] Altered physiologic states (e.g., pregnancy and diabetes mellitus) and gastrointestinal pathology (e.g., bowel obstruction and peritonitis) adversely affect the rate of gastric emptying, thereby increasing aspiration risk. The extent of delayed gastric emptying with diabetes mellitus correlates well with the presence of autonomic neuropathy, but not with age, duration of disease, preprandial HbA_{1C}, or peripheral neuropathy. The time difference in the delay between diabetic and healthy patients ranges from 30 minutes to 2 hours.[125] The ASA recommends a fasting period of 4 hours for breast milk, 6 hours for both nonhuman milk and infant formula, and also 6 hours for a light solid meal.[123]

Reduction of gastric acidity can be achieved with the aid of H_2-receptor antagonists and PPIs, which also reduce gastric volume. Famotidine effectively reduces gastric volume and increases gastric pH better than ranitidine given a few hours before surgery.[126] The PPIs rabeprazole, lansoprazole, and omeprazole are most effective when given in two successive doses, in the evening before and on the morning of anesthesia.[127,128] When given in a single dose, rabeprazole and lansoprazole should be administered on the morning of anesthesia, as they are not sufficiently effective when given the previous night. Single-dose therapy with omeprazole is best given the previous night.[127,128,129] Sodium citrate, best administered within 1 hour preoperatively in a dose of 15 to 30 mL, increases gastric pH to >2.5, and when combined with metoclopramide (10 mg IV), it reduces gastric contents to <25 mL. A nasogastric (NG) tube can be used to reduce gastric volume prior to induction of anesthesia in an emergency situation, as well as in elective patients with a high risk of regurgitation and aspiration. The presence of an NG tube does not guarantee an empty stomach and may impair the function of the LES and UES. An *in situ* NG tube does not diminish the effectiveness of cricoid pressure.[130] The NG tube also provides a passage for passive drainage of gastric contents and is best left in place and open to freely drain during induction of anesthesia.

7 The technique of rapid-sequence induction is performed to gain control of the airway in the shortest amount of time after the ablation of protective airway reflexes with the induction of anesthesia. In the rapid-sequence technique, the administration of an intravenous anesthetic induction agent is immediately followed by a rapidly acting neuromuscular blocking drug. Laryngoscopy and intubation are performed as soon as muscle relaxation is confirmed. Cricoid pressure (Sellick maneuver) is applied by an assistant from the beginning of induction until confirmation of ETT placement. Cricoid pressure entails the downward displacement of the cricoid cartilage against the vertebral bodies. In this manner, it was presumed that the lumen of the esophagus is ablated, while the completely circular nature of the cricoid cartilage maintains the tracheal lumen. Early cadaveric studies showed that correctly applied cricoid pressure was effective in preventing gastric fluids from leaking into the pharynx. Unfortunately, the esophagus is laterally displaced in a majority of normal patients.[131] Because cricoid pressure further lateralizes the esophagus, the adequacy of esophageal ablation has been questioned. Cricoid pressure is contraindicated with active vomiting

(risk of esophageal rupture), cervical spine fracture, and laryngeal fracture. Historically face mask ventilation is not undertaken for the 40 to 90 seconds required to achieve adequate neuromuscular relaxation. This practice is based on minimal data and has recently been questioned. Many clinicians do practice face mask ventilation during the apneic period.[132]

If during rapid-sequence induction there are difficulties in securing the airway and oxyhemoglobin desaturation occurs, gentle positive-pressure ventilation may be used while maintaining cricoid pressure. This positive pressure should require <25 cm H_2O pressure. Some authors argue that because cricoid pressure is of dubious efficacy and may distort the laryngoscopist view, it should be released if difficulties are encountered during the intubation attempt.[133]

The Intubating Supralaryngeal Airways. Blind, fiberoptic-aided, stylet-guided, and laryngoscopy-directed tracheal intubation via SGAs has been widely reported in adults and children. Many limitations to this technique have been described. In an effort to overcome these limitations, Brain et al.[134] introduced a version of the LMA with a large-diameter (13-mm ID), short-length (14-cm), and rigid stainless steel barrel curved to align the mask aperture to the glottic vestibule (Fig. 27-3D). Other manufacturers have introduced similar devices including the Aura-I (Ambu Corporation, Denmark) (Fig. 27-5D) and the Air-Q (Cookgas LLC, St. Louis, MO) (Fig. 27-5C).

The mask of the LMA Fastrach (Laryngeal Mask Company, Jersey, UK) differs from Dr. Brain's original LMA design with the incorporation of a vertically oriented, semirigid bar fixed at the proximal end of the bowl aperture and positioned to sit beneath the epiglottis in the average-sized adult. A handle at the proximal end of the barrel is used for insertion, repositioning, and removal. Originally made of stainless steel and silicone, a plastic single-use version is available. The LMA Fastrach barrel can accommodate up to an 8-mm ID-cuffed ETT, which can be inserted blindly or over a fiberscope or other flexible stylet device. The LMA Fastrach is designed to be used with a straight tracheal tube manufactured in both single- and multiple-use models (Euromedics, Kedah, Malaysia), although standard or Parker Flex-Tip (Parker Medical, Englewood, CO) polyvinyl chloride tracheal tubes have been used.[135]

The LMA Fastrach is available in adult sizes with cuffs equivalent to the size 3, 4, and 5 LMAs. Experience has suggested that most adults between 40 and 70 kg are best managed with a size 4 LMA Fastrach; larger persons require the size 5.

A large study has shown the utility of the LMA Fastrach in patients who were anticipated as well as unanticipated to be difficult to intubate. Ferson et al.[136] successfully intubated 234 patients over a 3-year period using the LMA Fastrach. Studied patients included those with normal-appearing airways on routine examination whose airways were unexpectedly difficult to manage, patients with a Cormack and Lehane laryngeal view grade 4 on laryngoscopic examination, patients with immobilized or traumatized cervical spines, and patients with airway tumors, prior airway surgery, or radiation. Successful blind intubation via the LMA Fastrach occurred in 97% of patients; the remaining patient intubations were facilitated with adjunct use of a fiberoptic intubation scope. A design of the LMA Fastrach, the CTrach (introduced in 2004 but no longer available), incorporated a fiberoptic cable and monitor into the LMA Fastrach design.

The LMA Fastrach is inserted with the head in a neutral position. It can be used in the unconscious or awake patient (with the use of topical anesthetics). The mask of the LMA Fastrach cuff is tested, deflated, and lubricated as described for the LMA. It is inserted into the mouth so that the mask lies flat against the palate. Gentle pressure on the handle and barrel reproduces the palatal pressure described for insertion of the LMA Classic. A smooth backward rotation of the handle toward the top of the head seats the tip of the mask in the hypopharynx, posterior to the cricoid cartilage. Once seated, the mask of the LMA Fastrach is inflated via the pilot cuff. An Ambu bag or anesthesia circuit is attached to the proximal end of the LMA Fastrach barrel and ventilation is attempted. By using the LMA Fastrach handle, the position of the device can be optimized by lateral and anterior–posterior manipulation. This action is termed the *Chandy maneuver* (after Dr. Chandy Verghese, Redding, United Kingdom). A seemingly common cause of airway obstruction with the LMA Fastrach is the down-folding of the epiglottis. This can be relieved with a smooth rotational movement of the inflated LMA Fastrach out of the airway (6 cm along the axis of the insertion), and immediate replacement (the up–down maneuver).

After adequate ventilation is achieved, the ETT is advanced though the barrel. As the ETT exits the bowl aperture of the LMA Fastrach, the semirigid elevating bar is pushed anteriorly, carrying the epiglottis out of the way of the airway. If positioned correctly, the ETT can freely enter the glottis.

The second part of the Chandy maneuver may facilitate blind tracheal intubation. In this maneuver, the handle is used to gently lift (without rotation) the LMA Fastrach anteriorly, sealing the bowl against the larynx.

When blind intubation fails (esophageal insertion or obstruction), several maneuvers are undertaken.[136] Early obstruction is typically caused by a down-folded epiglottis. An up–down maneuver, as described earlier, can be employed and tracheal intubation attempts repeated. Early resistance may also signify vallecular entrapment secondary to too large an LMA Fastrach size. The operator may remove the LMA Fastrach and place a smaller-sized one. Later obstruction may signify entrapment or too small a device, and again, a change is indicated.

When intubation fails despite the Chandy or up–down maneuvers or a change in the device size, the clinician should recall that intubating SGAs are first and foremost ventilation devices. Typically, ventilation will be adequate despite failure to intubate. At this juncture, the clinician can (1) continue with short surgical procedures using the intubating SGA as a simple SGA (procedures longer than 15 minutes may be ill advised because of the pressure exerted by the LMA Fastrach on tissues), (2) change to another SGA device, (3) diagnose the intubation impediment with the aid of another device (e.g., fiberoptic bronchoscope or Foley Flexible Airway Stylet), (4) remove the SGA and employ another technique of tracheal intubation, or (5) in the resuscitative situation, perform a surgical airway while continuing ventilation with the SGA. This last procedure may be an underappreciated facility of all the SGAs. These devices may serve as a bridge while invasive airway procedures are performed.

Once intubation is achieved and confirmed by physical examination (e.g., auscultation, chest wall rise, and fall) and capnography, an intubating SGA may be removed. Although this is a typical requirement of the rigid devices, some intubating SGAs may be left *in situ*. The ETT circuit adapter is removed and the intubating SGA is withdrawn over the ETT. During this removal procedure, the ETT is stabilized by one of two methods. A stabilizing rod (supplied by the manufacturer) can be held against the ETT as the LMA Fastrach is retreated out of the mouth. In the second technique, described by Rosenblatt et al.,[138] a Magill forceps is used to hold the proximal tip of the ETT while the LMA Fastrach is removed. In the midremoval position, a finger is placed in the mouth to identify and stabilize the ETT, while the Magill forceps is removed and the LMA Fastrach is fully retreated.

The precurve Aura-I intubating SGA lacks the rigid components as well as the epiglottic lifting bar concept of the LMA

Fastrach. It can be left *in situ* after intubation, or used for long periods as a simple SGA. When using for tracheal intubation, a flexible fiberscope should be used (Fig. 27-5D).

The Air-Q SGA also forgoes the rigid components and epiglottic lifting bar. Unlike the devices discussed above, it lacks the 90-degree precurvature of the barrel (Fig. 27-5C). The Air-Q is designed primarily as a routine-use SGA device with intubating capabilities. Unlike the other intubating SGAs, a range of pediatric sizes are available. As a routine SGA, leak pressures of 25 to 30 cm H_2O are obtained.[137] In adults, there is a 92% intubation success rate when coupled with the use of a flexible fiberscope. In infants, intubation success rates of 95% have been achieved.[139]

Extubation of the Trachea

Although a wealth of literature is focused on the field of tracheal intubation, few reviews have intensely contemplated the area of extubation after completion of surgery or prolonged ventilatory
8 support.[140] Indeed, the period of extubation may be far more treacherous than that of intubation (Table 27-12, Section A).

TABLE 27-12. TRACHEAL EXTUBATION

(A) Causes of ventilatory compromise during tracheal extubation
Residual anesthetic
Poor central respiratory effort
Decreased respiratory rate
Decreased respiratory drive in response to CO_2
Decreased respiratory drive in response to O_2
Reduced tone of upper airway musculature
Reduced gag and swallow reflex
Decreased threshold to laryngospasm
Surgical airway compromise
Surgical airway edema
Vocal cord paralysis
Arytenoid cartilage dislocation
Supraglottic edema with airway obstruction by the epiglottis
Retro arytenoid edema with limited vocal fold abduction
Subglottic edema
Tracheomalacia (from long-standing tracheal intubation)
Bronchospasm
(B) Complications of tracheal extubation
Respiratory drive failure
Hypoxia (e.g., atelectasis)
Upper airway obstruction (e.g., edema, residual anesthetic)
Vocal fold–related obstruction (e.g., vocal cord paralysis)
Tracheal obstruction (e.g., subglottic edema)
Bronchospasm
Aspiration
Hypertension
Increased intracranial pressure
Increased pulmonary artery pressure
Increased bronchial stump pressure (e.g., after pulmonary resection)
Increased ocular pressure
Increased abdominal wall pressure (e.g., risk of wound dehiscence)

Routine Extubation

Extubation of the trachea must not be considered a benign pro-
18 cedure. It is not simply the elimination or reversal of tracheal intubation. Extubation is fraught with its own set of potential complications (Table 27-12, Section B). Appropriately trained personnel and proper equipment should be immediately avail-
19 able at the time of extubation. This may range from a postanesthetic care unit nurse or respiratory therapist with a set of laryngoscopes to a surgeon prepared to perform an emergency tracheostomy.

Most adult patients are extubated after the return of consciousness and spontaneous respiration, the resolution of neuromuscular block, and the ability of the patient to follow simple commands (Table 27-13). The patient is asked to open the mouth, and a suction catheter is used to remove excessive secretions and/or blood. The head of the bed may be placed in a 10-degree Trendelenburg position. The airway pressure is allowed to rise to 5 to 15 cm of H_2O to facilitate a "passive cough," and the ETT is removed after the cuff (if present) is deflated.[81] If coughing or straining is contraindicated or hazardous (e.g., increased intracranial pressure), extubation may be performed while the patient is in a surgical plane of anesthesia and breathing spontaneously. In patients at risk for gastric content aspiration (e.g., full stomach) or upper airway obstruction, the clinician needs to assess the relative risk of each potential morbidity (e.g., coughing vs. obstruction vs. aspiration).

Laryngospasm at the time of extubation accounts for 23% of all critical postoperative respiratory events in adults.[81] Laryngospasm may be triggered by respiratory secretions, vomitus, blood, or a foreign body in the airway; pain in any part of the body; and pelvic or abdominal visceral stimulation. The cause of airway obstruction during laryngospasm is the contraction of the lateral cricoarytenoids, the thyroarytenoid, and the cricothyroid muscles. Management of laryngospasm consists of the immediate removal of the offending stimulus (if identifiable),

TABLE 27-13. CRITERIA FOR ROUTINE "AWAKE" EXTUBATION

Subjective clinical criteria
Follows commands
Clear oropharynx/hypopharynx (e.g., no active bleeding, secretions cleared)
Intact gag reflex
Sustained head lift for 5 s, sustained hand grasp
Adequate pain control
Minimal end expiratory concentration of inhaled anesthetics
Objective criteria
Vital capacity: ≥10 mL/kg
Peak voluntary negative inspiratory pressure: >–20 cm H_2O
Tidal volume >6 cc/kg
Sustained tetanic contraction (5 s)
T_1/T_4 ratio >0.7
Alveolar–arterial $Pa{O_2}$ gradient (on $F{IO_2}$ of 1): <350 mm Hg[a]
Dead space to tidal volume ratio: ≤0.6[a]

[a]Used during weaning from mechanical ventilation in the intensive care setting.

administration of oxygen with continuous positive airway pressure, and if other maneuvers are unsuccessful, the use of a small dose of short-acting muscle relaxants.[81]

Patients who are not fully recovered from neuromuscular relaxation are at risk of airway obstruction and aspiration at the time of extubation.[141] The soft palate (especially in the obstructive sleep apnea patient), tongue, and epiglottis may all contribute to obstruction. Murphy et al.[142] found that standard clinical criteria for adequacy of neuromuscular reversal such as 5-second head lift or hand grip, eye opening on command, negative inspiratory force more than –20 cm H_2O, or vital capacity breath of >15 cc/kg does not always signify acceptable neuromuscular recovery. Fifty-eight percent of patients in whom standard clinical criteria were achieved had a train-of-four ratio of <0.7 and 88% had a train-of-four ratio of <0.9. Though cholinesterase antagonists are historically used to reverse nondepolarizing neuromuscular blockers, a new class of agents have been introduced.[143] Cyclodextrins are hollow-structure molecules capable of trapping other molecules within their core. The lipohillic core of the agent Sugammadex (Merck & Co) traps the Rocurimium or Vecuronium molecule in one of the tightest cyclodextrin-target bonds known. Sugammadex can remove blocking agents that are bound to the neuromuscular junction. The trapped neuromuscular blocker is unavailable to bind to the neuromuscular junction and is excreted in the urine. This is discussed more thoroughly in Chapter 20.

Airway obstruction may be a cause of extubation failure. Edema of the uvula, soft palate, tongue, and structures of the glottis may also contribute to obstruction. Direct trauma from both intubation, and surgical devices, as well as impaired lymphatic and venous drainage may contribute. Palatopharyngeal edema associated with anterior cervical spine procedures as well as hematomas (e.g., following endarterectomy) contributes to postextubation airway failure. Lingual edema may be caused by surgical mouth gags and extreme neck flexion. Bilateral vocal cord paralysis may result from trauma to the recurrent laryngeal nerves causing unopposed adduction. Not only may this occur following neck or intrathoracic surgery, but also after internal jugular line placement or endotracheal intubation. Misplacement of the tracheal tube cuff, so that it produces pressure on the thyroid cartilage, as well as overpressurization with excessive inflation or nitrous oxide diffusion has also been noted as contributing factors. Transient vocal cord and swallowing dysfunction have been demonstrated in the absence of injury, making normal patients at risk of aspiration after general anesthesia.

Pharmacologic agents used during the maintenance and emergence phases of the anesthetic may affect the success of extubation. Though low concentrations of potent inhalation anesthetics (e.g., 0.5 Minimal Alveolar Concentration) do not alter the respiratory response to CO_2, they may blunt hypoxic drive. The opioid-receptor agonist and, to a lesser extent, benzodiazepine affect both hypercarbic and hypoxic respiratory drives. Some nondepolarizing muscle relaxants also reduce the hypoxic ventilatory drive secondary to their effect on cholinergic receptors in the carotid body.[140,141]

Identification of Patients at Risk for Complications at Extubation

A number of well-known clinical situations may place patients at increased risk for complication at the time of extubation (Table 27-14). However, the clinician should evaluate every

TABLE 27-14. CLINICAL SITUATIONS PRESENTING INCREASED RISK FOR COMPLICATIONS AT EXTUBATION[a]

Paradoxical vocal cord motion (pre-existing)	Poorly understood mechanism
Thyroid surgery	4.3% recurrent laryngeal nerve injury
Local edema	
Tracheomalacia (e.g., from long-standing goiter)	
Laryngoscopy (diagnostic)	Edema, laryngospasm, especially with biopsy
Uvulopalatoplasty	Palatal and oropharyngeal edema
Obstructive sleep apnea syndrome (uncorrected, postoperative)	
Carotid endarterectomy	Wound hematoma, glottic edema, nerve palsies
Maxillofacial trauma	Laryngeal fracture, reduced level of consciousness, requirements for mandibular/maxillary wires
Cervical vertebrae decompression/fixation	Supraglottic and hypopharyngeal edema
Parkinson disease	
Rheumatoid arthritis	
Generalized edema	Laryngotracheal narrowing
Angioneurotic edema	Laryngotracheal narrowing
Anaphylaxis	Laryngotracheal narrowing
Hypopharyngeal infections	Laryngotracheal narrowing
Hypoventilation syndromes[a]	
Hypoxemic syndromes[b]	
Inadequate airway-protective reflexes	Aspiration risk

[a]Residual anesthetic or preoperative medications (including alcohol and illicit drugs), central sleep apnea, carotid endarterectomy, poliomyelitis, Guillain–Barré syndrome, myasthenia gravis, botulism, thoracic skeletal deformity, severe pain (with diaphragmatic splinting), morbid obesity, severe chronic obstructive pulmonary disease.

[b]Hypoventilation, ventilation–perfusion mismatch, intracardiac or intrapulmonary shunting, increased oxygen consumption, severe anemia, impaired alveolar oxygen diffusion.

patient in terms of potential for problems, in the same manner that the anesthesiologist prepares for the unanticipated difficult intubation.

Approach to the Difficult Extubation

When there is a suspicion that a patient may have difficulty with oxygenation or ventilation after tracheal extubation, the clinician may choose from a number of management strategies. These may range from the preparation of standby reintubation equipment to the active establishment of a bridge or guide for reintubation and/or oxygenation. When the patient's intubation is without difficulty and there is no substantial reason to believe that an interim insult to the airway has occurred, extubation may be accomplished in a routine fashion, with a heightened state of readiness for reintubation.

A popular test used to predict postextubation airway competency is the detection of a leak on deflation of the ETT cuff. A recent investigation has cast doubt on the reliability of this test as a predictor of airway incompetence: The absence of an airway leak on cuff deflation was not predictive of subsequent ventilatory failure after extubation.[144] Patients with a reduced cuff leak volume are at risk for postextubation stridor.[84] In trauma patients, the cuff-leak test was found to be especially unreliable.

A randomized control trial in 2007 revealed that multiple-dose dexamethasone effectively reduced incidence of postextubation strider in adult patients at high risk for postextubation laryngeal edema while single-dose injection of dexamethasone given 1 hour before extubation did not reduce the number of patients requiring reintubation.[145]

A fiberoptic bronchoscope may be used to view the tracheal structures during the removal of the ETT. If extubation is tolerated, the fiberoptic bronchoscope can be slowly withdrawn into the subglottic region. If secretions do not obstruct the objective lens, the vocal folds and other structures may be visualized and evaluated.

A number of obturators are available for use in trial extubation. These devices may be left in place in the airway for extended periods. These devices are generally referred to as airway exchange catheters (AECs). Mort found that the success of first-pass reintubation was significantly higher, and the incidence of hypoxia lower, in patients with a retained tracheal tube exchange catheter.[146]

It is beyond the scope of this text to describe all the commercially available AECs. The Cook Airway Exchange Catheters (Cook Critical Care, Bloomington, IN) are manufactured with external diameters of 2.7, 3.7, 4.7, and 6.33 mm. The smallest diameter catheter (which can fit within a 3-mm ID ETT) is 45 cm long, whereas the others are 83 cm long. They all have a central lumen and rounded, atraumatic ends. The catheters are graduated from the distal end. The proximal end is fitted with either a 15-mm or a Luer-lock Rapi-Fit adapter, which can be quickly removed and replaced for ETT removal or exchange. With these adapters in place an oxygen source can be used to provide insufflated or jet-ventilated oxygen if the patient fails extubation and/or if reintubation over the catheter fails.

The CardioMed endotracheal ventilation catheter (Gromley, ON) designed by Richard Cooper, MD, a Canadian anesthesiologist, is 85 cm in length and has inner and outer diameters of either 3 or 4 mm, respectively. An integral Luer-lock fitting adapter is found at the proximal end, whereas the blunted distal end incorporates eight helically arranged side holes in addition to the distal end hole. The arrangement of these holes is meant to center the catheter during oxygen insufflation and prevent traumatic "whipping" within the trachea. The use of this catheter for ETT exchange, tracheal reintubation, oxygen insufflation, jet oxygenation, and end-tidal CO_2 detection after extubation has been documented by the inventor.[81]

AECs have been associated with significant morbidity including loss of airway control, mucosal trauma, pneumothorax, esophageal intubation, and death.[147] Complication rates of up to 60% have been reported.[148] Pneumothorax in the absence of gas insufflation via the AEC has been reported.[147]

Specific cautions are often exercised to reduce complications with AECs, though little empiric literature is available. First, prior to placement of an AEC, the patient should both meet extubation criteria, and, in most cases, should have been breathing 100% oxygen in an effort to maximize alveolar reserve. Second, an AEC with an external diameter closest to the internal diameter of the *in situ* ETT should be available and lubricated. Using an appropriately sized AEC will reduce the chance of "Murphy eye" passage and the potential for mucosal trauma. This size congruency will also facilitate reintubation by reducing "hang-up," and reduce accidental esophageal intubation due to ETT dislodgement of the AEC position. Third, when the patient is ready for extubation, the anesthesia circuit is removed and the AEC distal end is placed to the depth of the tracheal tube bevel. Common AECs are graduated and these marks may be matched with the markings on the ETT (Fig. 27-18). If care had been taken with the initial tracheal tube positioning, this would result in a midtracheal positioning of the AEC, reducing the chance of endobronchеal placement. Fourth, careful attention is paid to maintaining AEC position as the ETT is removed. If tracheal reintubation is required, an ETT with the internal diameter matching the AEC external diameter should be employed. This will reduce size discrepancy–created clefts, which can entrap airway tissues, causing trauma and hindering reintubation (Fig. 27-19). If the ETT will not pass into the glottis, lifting the tongue with a laryngoscope may facilitate reintubation. A 2- or 3-cm withdrawal of the ETT, counterclockwise tracheal tube rotation (90 degrees), and reinsertion will often overcome "hang-up" tissue entrapment. If jet insufflation of oxygen via the AEC is deemed required at any time, the following precautions are best observed: The patient should be flaccid or muscle relaxed to prevent glottic closure, an oral airway or other device should be used to maintain an open upper airway, and careful inspiratory pressure and duration must be titrated to observed chest expansion and recoil.

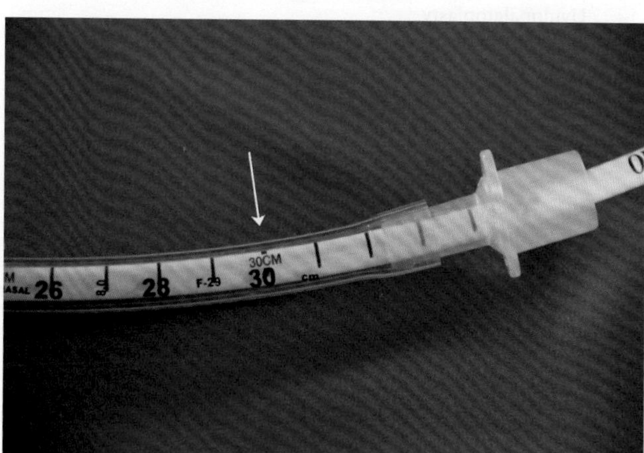

FIGURE 27-18. Marking of an airway exchange catheter (AEC) are aligned with the markings on the *in situ* tracheal tube. By aligning these marks as the AEC is inserted prevents bronchial trauma.

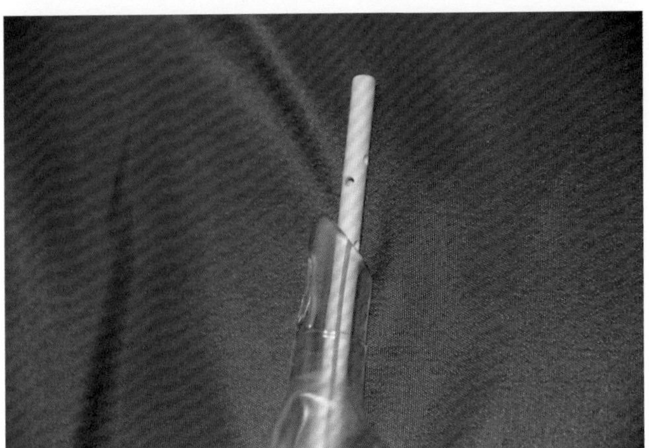

FIGURE 27-19. Size discrepancy between an airway exchange catheter and a re-inserted tracheal tube can create clefts which can trap tissues and hinder intubation.

THE DIFFICULT AIRWAY

The Difficult Airway Algorithm

In 1993, the ASA Task Force on the Difficult Airway first published an algorithm that has become a staple of management for clinicians. This algorithm was reissued in 2003.[1] As will be discussed, the most dramatic change in the ASA Difficult Airway Algorithm (ASA–DAA) was the repositioning of the LMA from the emergency to the routine management pathway (Fig. 27-20B). The ASA[1] defines the difficult airway as the situation in which the "conventionally trained anesthesiologist experiences difficulty with intubation, mask ventilation, or both."

As well as being an important standard for the anesthesiologist, the ASA algorithm is widely accepted as a model for the approach to the difficult airway for nurse anesthetists, emergency medicine physicians, and prehospital personnel. Although the algorithm largely speaks for itself, its salient features are discussed here. One statement in this document summarizes the difficulty of writing and recommending practices in the difficult airway management: "The difficult airway represents a complex interaction between patient factors, the clinical setting, and the skills of the practitioner."[1] It should be well recognized that though the ASA–DAA is a staple in the United States and much of the world, several groups worldwide have written their own airway algorithms emphasizing techniques and approaches native to their practice. The reader is encouraged to explore these important alternative approaches.[83,149–153] Entry into the algorithm begins with the evaluation of the airway. Although there is some debate as to the value of particular evaluation methods and indices, the clinician must use all available data and his or her own clinical experience to reach a general impression as to the difficulty of the patient's airway in terms of laryngoscopy (DL or video) and intubation, supraglottic ventilation techniques, aspiration risk, or apnea tolerance.

This evaluation should direct the clinician to enter the ASA–DAA at one of its two root points: Awake intubation (Fig. 27-20A) or intubation attempts after the induction of general anesthesia (Fig. 27-20). The decision to enter the algorithm via either approach is a preoperative one. Box A is chosen when difficulty is anticipated that will place the patient at jeopardy, whereas box B is for the situation in which there may be anticipated difficulty with either ventilation or tracheal intubation, but an uncorrectable situation is not expected. This has been further delineated into a preoperative decision tree by Rosenblatt,[4] the AAA. Figure 27-21 outlines the AAA, which is a simple one-pathway algorithm for entering into the ASA–DAA. Branch choice, like the previously noted statement from the ASA practice guidelines, is highly dependent on the clinician's skill and

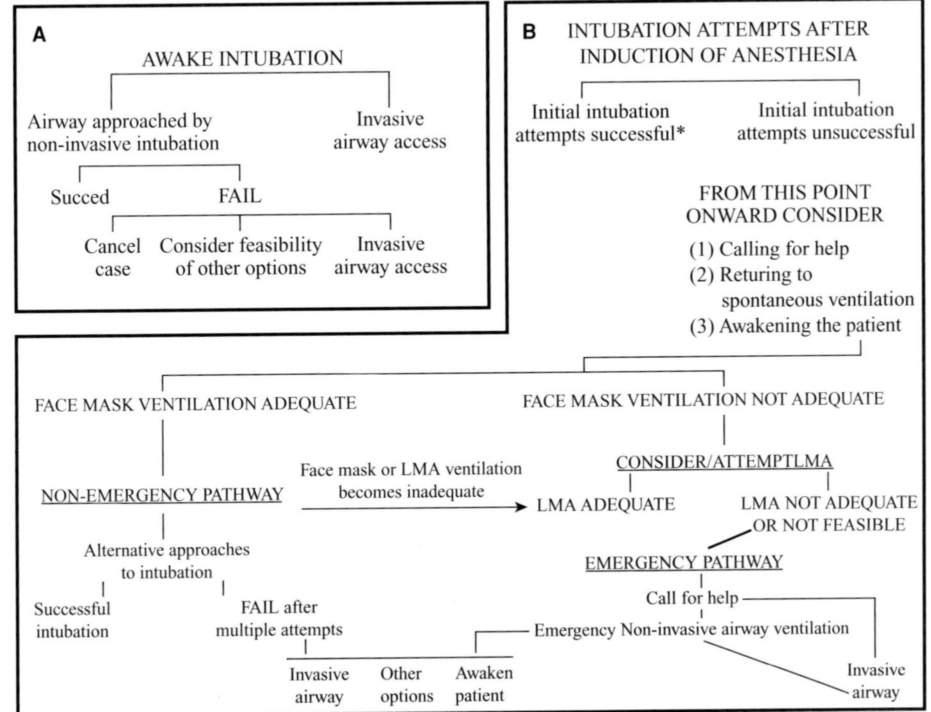

FIGURE 27-20. The American Society of Anesthesiologists Difficult Airway Algorithm. **A:** Awake intubation. **B:** Intubation attempts after induction of anesthesia.

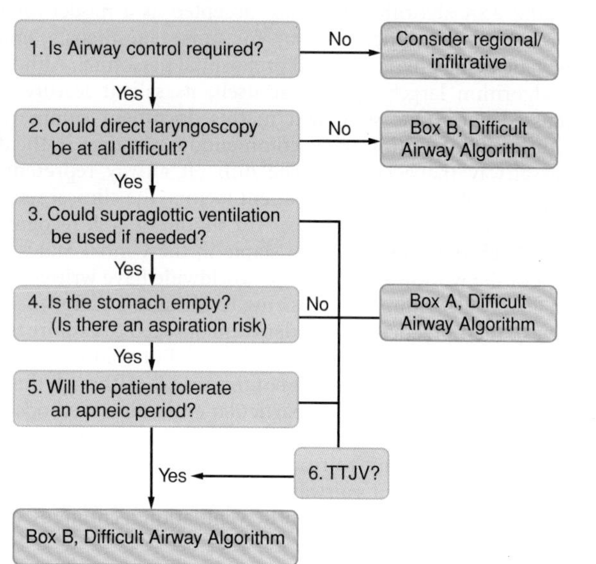

FIGURE 27-21. The Airway Approach Algorithm: A decision tree approach to entry into the American Society of Anesthesiologists Difficult Airway Algorithm. TTJV, transtracheal jet ventilation.

experience. Details of the AAA can be found elsewhere and are summarized here.[4,154]

1. **Is airway control necessary?** No matter, however, routine sedation or general anesthesia become, whether or not to make a patient apneic should always be considered seriously and alternatives should be contemplated. Periodic analysis of the closed claims database illustrates that a plan for airway control is always needed independent of the choice of anesthetic technique.[31]
2. **Could tracheal intubation be (at all) difficult?** If there is no indication that rapid tracheal intubation (e.g., by DL, video laryngoscopy or other means familiar to the operator) will be difficult, the clinician may proceed as clinically appropriate. If there is an indication, based on history or physical examination, that there may be difficulty with rapid tracheal intubation, the AAA is followed to the next question. By choosing to continue down the algorithm, the clinician is not assuming tracheal intubation difficulty, rather he or she is anticipating the viability of rescue maneuvers should difficultly occur.
3. **Can SGA ventilation be used if needed?** If the clinician identifies a reason that SGA ventilation (by face mask, LMA, or other device) could be difficult, he or she is projecting the possibility that a juncture of "cannot intubate (Question 2)—cannot ventilate (Question 3)" could be reached. Because this is a preoperative algorithm, box A (awake intubation) of the ASA–DAA may be the preferred root entry point.
4. **Is there an aspiration risk?** As discussed earlier, the patient at risk for aspiration is not a candidate for elective SGA use. Because the AAA is a preoperative algorithm, and therefore allows the luxury of discretionary paths, the juncture of "cannot intubate/should not ventilate" can be avoided by entering the ASA–DAA at box A.
5. **Will the patient tolerate an apneic period?** Question 3 is difficult to answer and is highly dependent on the skills and experience of the clinician. Should intubation fail, and SGA ventilation is inadequate, the patient's ability to sustain oxygen saturation will dictate the ability to tolerate an apneic period. Factors such as age, pregnancy, pulmonary status, abnormal oxygen consumption (e.g., fever), and choice of induction agents will influence this. If time to oxyhemoglobin desaturation is limited, box A may be prophylactically chosen.
6. **Can hypoxia be rapidly corrected through other means?** Transtracheal jet oxygenation will be discussed later in this
20 chapter. The question that arises here is in regards to access to the patient's larynx, the availability of equipment and knowledgeable personnel, and the experience of the operator. For example, if an error in judgment is made and the operator finds himself or herself in a "cannot intubate/cannot ventilate" scenario, will these conditions allow for using transtracheal jet ventilation (TTJV) to temporize the situation? All conditions may be right, but if the patient is morbidly obese or has had scarring or radiation changes over the larynx/trachea, this option may not be available. These factors have been discussed in detail elsewhere.[4,154]

The exception to the AAA occurs with the patient who is unable to cooperate owing to mental retardation, intoxication, anxiety, depressed level of consciousness, or age. This patient may still be approached by box A (Fig. 27-20A), but awake intubation may need to be modified in favor of techniques that maintain spontaneous ventilation (e.g., inhalation induction, titrated intravenous agents such as dexmedetomidine).

Preparation of the patient for awake intubation is dis-
9 cussed later. In most instances, awake intubation is successful if approached with care and patience. When awake intubation fails, the clinician has a number of options. First, one can consider cancellation of the surgical case. In this situation, specialized equipment or personnel can be assembled for a return to the operating room. Where cancellation is not an option, regional anesthetic techniques can be considered, or if demanded by the situation, a surgical airway (e.g., tracheostomy) may be called for.

The decision to proceed with regional anesthesia because the airway cannot be assessed or has been proven to be difficult to manage must be considered in terms of risks and benefits (Table 27-15). The ASA Closed Claims Database project has identified failure in regional anesthesia as a source of serious error when no airway strategy was prophylactically considered.[2]

The ASA–DAA becomes truly useful in the unanticipated difficult airway (box B in Fig. 27-20, unable to intubate by DL after the induction of anesthesia). When induction agents (with or without muscle relaxants) have been administered and the airway cannot be controlled, vital management decisions must be made rapidly. Typically, the clinician has attempted direct or video laryngoscopy and tracheal intubation after successful or failed anesthesia mask ventilation. Even if the patient's oxygen saturation remains adequate throughout these efforts, the number of laryngoscopy attempts should be limited to three.[155] Significant soft tissue trauma can result from multiple laryngoscopies, thereby worsening the situation. First, mask ventilation should be instituted. If face mask ventilation is adequate, the ASA–DAA nonemergency pathway is entered. The clinician may then turn to the most convenient and/or appropriate technique for establishing tracheal intubation, if needed. This might include, but is not limited to video laryngoscopy, intubation facilitated by a fiberoptic bronchoscope, SGA, intubating SGA, bougie, lighted stylet, or a retrograde wire. A surgical airway will sometimes be the most appropriate approach. (The most widely applied of these procedures, as well as new techniques, will be discussed within the clinical scenarios presented later.) When mask ventilation fails,

TABLE 27-15. FACTORS TO CONSIDER IN PROCEEDING WITH REGIONAL ANESTHESIA (RA) AFTER THE PATIENT HAS BEEN JUDGED TO HAVE A DIFFICULT AIRWAY

May Consider RA	Should not Consider RA
Superficial surgery	Cavity-invading surgery
Minimal sedation needed	Significant sedation needed
Local infiltration adequate	Extensive neuroaxial/local anesthetic required or risk of intravascular injection/absorption is high
Access to the airway	Poor access to the airway
Surgery can be halted at any time	Surgery cannot be stopped once started

the algorithm suggests supraglottic ventilation via an SGA. If successful, the nonemergency pathway of the ASA–DAA has again been entered and alternative techniques of tracheal intubation may be used, if needed.

Should SGA ventilation fail to sustain the patient adequately, the emergency pathway is entered. The ASA–DAA suggests use of an esophageal–tracheal Combitube, rigid bronchoscopy, transtracheal oxygenation, or a surgical airway.

At any juncture, the decision to awaken the patient should be considered based on the adequacy of ventilation, the risk of aspiration, and the risk of proceeding with intubation attempts or the surgical procedure.

Awake Airway Management

10 Awake airway management remains a mainstay of the ASA's difficult airway algorithm. The awake state provides maintenance of spontaneous ventilation in the event that the airway cannot be secured rapidly, increased size and patency of the pharynx, relative forward placement of the base of the tongue, posterior placement of the larynx, and a cooperative patient.[156] The effect of sedatives and general anesthetics on airway patency may be secondary to direct effects on motoneurons and on the reticular activating system. The sleep apnea patient may be particularly prone to obstruction with minimal sedation. In addition, the awake state confers some maintenance of upper and lower esophageal sphincter tone, thus reducing the risk of reflux. In the event that reflux occurs, the patient can close the glottis and/or expel aspirated foreign bodies by cough to the extent that these reflexes have not been obtunded by local anesthesia.[157] Lastly, patients at risk for neurologic sequelae (e.g., patients with unstable cervical spine pathology) may undergo active sensory–motor testing immediately after tracheal intubation. In an emergent situation, there may be cautions (e.g., cardiovascular stimulation in the presence of cardiac ischemia or ischemic risk, bronchospasm, increased intraocular pressure, increased intracranial pressure) but no absolute contraindications to awake intubation. Contraindications to elective awake intubation include patient refusal or inability to cooperate (e.g., child, profound mental retardation, dementia, intoxication) or allergy to local anesthetics.

Once the clinician has decided to proceed with awake airway management, the patient must be prepared both physically and psychologically. Most adult patients will appreciate an explanation of the need for an awake airway examination and will be more cooperative once they realize the importance of, and rationale for, any uncomfortable procedures. Patients understand safety and the discussion should emphasize the anesthesiologist's concerns. Once the airway has been prepared, patients will realize that they should experience little further discomfort during the intubation.

Apart from appropriate explanation, medication can also be used to allay anxiety. If sedatives are to be used, the clinician must keep in mind that producing obstruction or apnea in the difficult airway patient can be devastating and an overly sedated patient may not be able to protect the airway from regurgitated gastric contents, or cooperate with procedures. Although almost any sedative agent can be used, some rules should apply to all: Judicious dosing, avoid polypharmacy (try to use no more than two agents), and have reversal agents at hand. Small doses of benzodiazepines (e.g., diazepam, midazolam, lorazepam) are commonly used to alleviate anxiety without producing significant respiratory depression. These drugs may be given in intravenous or oral forms and may be reversed with specific antagonists (e.g., flumazenil). Opioid receptor agonists (e.g., fentanyl, alfentanil, remifentanil) can also be used in small, titrated doses for their sedative and antitussive effects, although caution must be exercised. A specific antagonist (e.g., naloxone) should always be immediately available. Ketamine, droperidol, and dexmedetomidine have also been popular among clinicians. Dexmedetomidine, a highly selective centrally acting α_2-adrenergic agonist, has been used for sedation and analgesia without respiratory depression in patients who underwent awake intubation because of difficult airways, cervical spine problems, and inability to cooperate with awake intubation.[158] Combined with topical anesthesia, dexmedetomidine sedation provided for a smooth intubation. A loading dose of dexmedetomidine is 1 μg/kg intravenously over 10 minutes, and maintenance infusion dose is 0.2 to 0.7 μg/kg/h.[81] Dexmedetomidine may cause hypotension, which can be corrected by phenylephrine or ephedrine. Deep sedation with dexmedetomidine should not be confused with awake intubation, during which the clinician strives to maintain airway-protective reflexes and patient responsiveness to verbal commands and cooperation.

Administration of antisialagogues is important to the success of awake intubation techniques. Clearing of airway secretions is essential to the use of indirect optical instruments (e.g., flexible or rigid fiberoptic laryngoscope, video laryngoscope) because small amounts of any liquid can obscure the objective lens. The commonly used drugs atropine (0.5 to 1 mg intramuscularly or intravenously) and glycopyrrolate (0.2 to 0.4 mg intramuscularly or intravenously) have other significant effects: By reducing saliva production, these drugs increase the effectiveness of topically applied local anesthetics by removing a barrier to mucosal contact and by reducing drug dilution. The clinician must wait until the patient reports the drying activity of the injected antisialagogue.

Vasoconstriction of the nasal passages is required if there is to be instrumentation of this part of the airway. Oxymetazoline is a potent and long-lasting vasoconstrictor. In the authors' experience the nasal passages should always be included in the preparation for awake intubation. First, if during the course of the awake intubation, the plan is changed from the oral to nasal route, preparation is complete. Second, much of the preparation of the nose with local anesthesia (see later discussion), which can occur prior to the peak onset of the desiccant, will affect the pharyngeal airway. If the patient is at risk for gastric regurgitation and aspiration, prophylactic measures should be undertaken. It is also prudent to supply supplemental oxygen to the patient by nasal cannula (which can be placed over the nose or mouth).

Local anesthetics are a cornerstone of awake airway control techniques (see Chapter 21). The airway, from the base of the tongue to the bronchi, comprises an undeniably sensitive series of structures. Topical anesthesia and injected nerve block techniques have been developed to blunt the protective airway reflexes as well as to provide analgesia. As is well known to the anesthetic practitioner, local anesthetics are both effective and potentially dangerous drugs. The clinician should have a thorough understanding of the mechanism of action, metabolism, toxicities, and acceptable cumulative doses of the drugs that he or she chooses to employ in the airway. Because much of the agent used will be within the tracheal–bronchial tree and can travel to the alveoli, there is potential for significant intravascular absorption with some techniques. In a human study on lidocaine toxicity, 400 or 800 mg was topically applied to the upper airway. Serial blood lidocaine levels were measured peaking 60 minutes later at 0.5 and 1.28 μg/mL, respectively. Toxic levels of lidocaine are considered to be 4 μg/mL.[159] In a recent study using the same dose of lidocaine administered by nebulizer, serum levels of 2.8 and 6.5 μg/mL were measured within 10 minutes of dose completion, respectively.[160]

Despite the myriad of local anesthetics available, only those most commonly used in airway preparation will be discussed here. In reality, the choice of local anesthetic employed has little to do with success of the technique of awake intubation; ignoring the other aspects of preparation outlined here leads to failure just as readily.[154]

Among otolaryngologists, cocaine is a popular topical agent. Not only is it a highly effective local anesthetic, but it is also the only local anesthetic that is a potent vasoconstrictor. It is commonly available in a 4% solution. The total dose applied to the mucosa should not exceed 200 mg in the adult. Cocaine should not be used in patients with known cocaine hypersensitivity, hypertension, ischemic heart disease, preeclampsia, or those taking monoamine oxidase inhibitors. Because cocaine is metabolized by pseudocholinesterase, it is contraindicated in patients who are deficient in this enzyme.

Lidocaine, an amide local anesthetic, is available in a wide variety of preparations and doses. Topically applied, peak onset is within 15 minutes.

Tetracaine is an amide local anesthetic with a longer duration of action than either cocaine or lidocaine. Solutions of 0.5%, 1%, and 2% are available. Absorption of this drug from the respiratory and gastrointestinal tracts is rapid, and toxicity after nebulized application has been reported with doses as low as 40 mg, although the acceptable safe dose in adults is 100 mg by other routes of application.[161]

Benzocaine is popular among some clinicians because of its very rapid onset (<1 minute) and short duration (approximately 10 minutes). It is available in 10%, 15%, and 20% solutions. It has been combined with tetracaine in some preparations to prolong the duration of action. A 0.5-second aerosol administration of Benzocaine can deliver as much as 30 mg of benzocaine, the toxic dose being 100 mg. Another common preparation is to combine benzocaine with tetracaine, butyl aminobenzoate, benzalkonium chloride, and cetyldimethylethyl ammonium bromide. Benzocaine may produce methemoglobinemia, which is treated by the administration of methylene blue (1 to 2 mg intravenously over several minutes).[162]

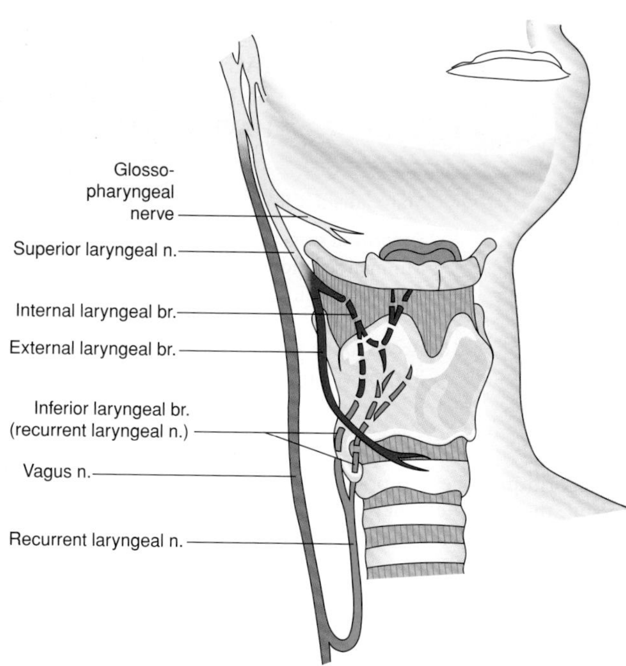

FIGURE 27-22. Laryngeal innervation.

There are three anatomic areas to which the clinician directs local anesthetic therapy: The nasal cavity/nasopharynx, the pharynx/base of tongue, and the hypopharynx/larynx/trachea (Fig. 27-22). The nasal cavity is innervated by the greater and lesser palatine nerves (innervating the nasal turbinates and most of the nasal septum) and the anterior ethmoid nerve (innervating the nares and anterior third of the nasal septum). The two palatine nerves arise from the sphenopalatine ganglion, located posterior to the middle turbinate. Two techniques for nerve block have been described. The ganglion can be approached through a noninvasive nasal approach: Cotton-tipped applicators soaked in local anesthetic are passed along the lower border of the middle turbinate until the posterior wall of the nasopharynx is reached. They are left in place for 5 to 10 minutes. In the oral approach, a needle is introduced into the greater palatine foramen, which can be palpated in the posterior lateral aspect of the hard palate, 1 cm medial to the second and third maxillary molars. Anesthetic solution (1 to 2 mL) is injected with a spinal needle inserted in a superior/posterior direction at a depth of 2 to 3 cm. Care must be taken not to inject into the sphenopalatine artery. The anterior ethmoid nerve can be blocked by cotton-tipped applicators soaked in local anesthetic placed along the dorsal surface of the nose until the anterior cribriform plate is reached. The applicator is left in place for 5 to 10 minutes.

The oropharynx is innervated by branches of the vagus, facial, and glossopharyngeal nerves. The glossopharyngeal nerve travels anteriorly along the lateral surface of the pharynx, its three branches supplying sensory innervation to the posterior third of the tongue, the vallecula, the anterior surface of the epiglottis

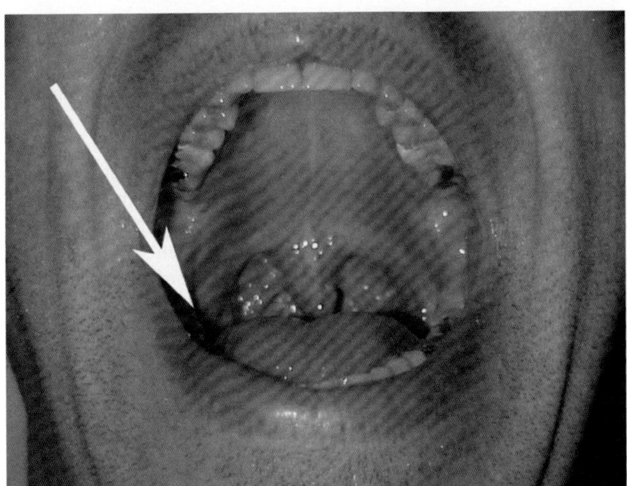

FIGURE 27-23. The palatoglossal arch (*arrow*) is a soft tissue fold that is a continuation of the posterior edge of the soft palate to the base of the tongue. A local anesthetic-soaked swab placed in the gutter along the base of the tongue is left in contact with the fold for 5 to 10 minutes.

(lingual branch), the walls of the pharynx (pharyngeal branch), and the tonsils (tonsillar branch). A wide variety of techniques may be used to anesthetize this part of the airway. The simplest techniques involve aerosolized local anesthetic solution, or a voluntary "swish and swallow." Some patients may require a glossopharyngeal nerve block, especially when topical techniques do not adequately block the gag reflex. The branches of this nerve are most easily accessed as they transverse the palatoglossal folds. These folds are seen as soft tissue ridges that extend from the posterior aspect of the soft palate to the base of the tongue, bilaterally (Fig. 27-23). A noninvasive technique employs anesthetic-soaked cotton-tipped applicators that are positioned against the inferior most aspect of the folds, and left in place for 5 to 10 minutes. When the noninvasive technique proves inadequate, local anesthetic can be injected. Standing on the side contralateral to the nerve to be blocked, the operator displaces the extended tongue to the contralateral side and a 25-gauge spinal needle is inserted into the fold near the floor of the mouth. An aspiration test is performed. If air is aspirated, the needle has passed through-and-through the membrane. If blood is aspirated, the needle tip is redirected more medially. The lingual branch is most readily blocked in this manner, but retrograde tracking of the injectate has also been demonstrated.[157] Even though it provides a reliable block, this technique is reported to be painful and may result in a bothersome and persistent hematoma.[163] A posterior approach to the glossopharyngeal nerve has been described in the otolaryngologic literature (for tonsillectomy). It may be difficult to visualize the site of needle insertion as it is behind the palatopharyngeal arch where the nerve is in close proximity to the carotid artery. Because of the risk for arterial injection and bleeding, the technique will not be described here; however, the reader is referred to a more authoritative text.[81]

The internal branch of the superior laryngeal nerve, which is a branch of the vagus nerve, provides sensory innervation to the base of the tongue, epiglottis, aryepiglottic folds, and arytenoids. The branch originates from the superior laryngeal nerve lateral to the cornu of the hyoid bone. It then pierces the thyrohyoid membrane and travels under the mucosa in the pyriform recess. The remaining portion of the superior laryngeal nerve, the external branch, supplies motor innervation to the cricothyroid muscle. Several blocks of the internal branch have been described. In many instances topical application of anesthetics in the pharyngeal/hypopharyngeal cavities will provide adequate analgesia. An external block is performed with the patient supine with the head extended and the clinician standing on the side ipsilateral to the nerve to be blocked. The clinician identifies the superior cornu of the hyoid bone beneath the angle of the mandible. Using one hand, medially directed pressure is applied to the contralateral hyoid cornu, displacing the ipsilateral hyoid cornu toward the clinician. Caution must be taken to locate the carotid artery and displace it if necessary. The needle can be inserted directly over the hyoid cornu and then "walked" off the cartilage in an anterior–caudad direction until it can be passed through the ligament to a depth of 1 to 2 cm. Before the injection of local anesthetic, an aspiration test should be performed to ensure that one has not entered the pyriform sinus or a vascular structure. Local anesthetic (1.5 to 2 mL) is injected in the space between the thyrohyoid membrane and the pharyngeal mucosa. The superior laryngeal nerve can also be blocked with a noninvasive internal technique. The patient is asked to open the mouth widely, and the tongue is grasped using a gauze pad or tongue blade. A right-angled forceps (e.g., Jackson-Krause forceps) with anesthetic-soaked cotton swabs is slid over the lateral tongue and into the pyriform sinuses bilaterally. The cotton swabs or sponge are held in place for 5 minutes.

Sensory innervation of the vocal folds and the trachea is provided by the recurrent laryngeal nerve. Transtracheal injection of local anesthetic can easily be performed to produce adequate analgesia. A syringe fitted with a fine needle and filled with a local anesthetic solution (e.g., 2 to 4 mL of 2% or 4% lidocaine) is inserted through the CTM, perpendicular to the plane of the cervical spine. In this orientation, the needle is likely to impact the posterior aspect of the cricoid cartilage if advanced too far, and not puncture the esophagus. In addition, this angle will help to avoid trauma to the near-lying vocal folds. Constant retraction on the syringe plunger reveals free air aspiration when the trachea is entered.

After the percutaneous puncture is made and the trachea is identified by free air aspiration, the anesthetic agent is injected. Coughing is likely to occur, and the needle should be stabilized to prevent mucosal abrasions.

An effective and noninvasive technique of tracheal and vocal cord topical analgesia uses the working channel of the fiberoptic bronchoscope. A disadvantage of this technique is that solutions leaving the working channel can obscure the objective lens. This can be overcome by use of an epidural catheter, inserted through the working channel, as described by Ovassapian.[164] Not only does this prevent the obscuring of the view, but also allows specific "aiming" of the anesthetic stream. Multiorifice catheters should be trimmed in length so only the distal orifice exists.

Clinical Difficult Airway Scenarios

The clinician approaching the patient with a difficult airway has a vast armamentarium of techniques and instruments that can be applied to securing and maintaining oxygenation and ventilation.[165] Although this array can be confusing, textbook authors cannot dictate specific approaches in every situation; moreover, the variability of patient presentation makes specific recommendations difficult. Thus, in order to discuss management, the following section presents a number of brief clinical scenarios and the authors' own approach. The major alternative airway management techniques are discussed in this manner. All of the clinical cases described herein have been managed by the authors or a colleague. Other techniques that might be applied in each situation are also discussed. In these cases, as in actual practice, the first technique applied may not have been the best one. The principle of flexibility (and a keen eye to the need to change course quickly) will be emphasized repeatedly. In view of the critical importance of the act of airway control, the clinician must be prepared to alter his or her approach as the situation demands.

Unfortunately, clinicians rarely employ alternative techniques until a difficult situation arises. Heidegger et al.[96] introduced a simple algorithm for incorporating flexible fiberoptic-aided tracheal intubation into daily practice as a routine alternative to DL. Their incidence of difficult intubation was 6 in 1,324 cases, or 0.049%, markedly lower than reported previously.

Case 1: Preoperative Endoscopy

A 52-year-old man presents for direct laryngoscopy, esophagoscopy, and biopsy of a base of tongue tumor. The patient had sought otolaryngologic consultation after the discovery of a left neck mass on routine physical examination. He had experienced no change in voice, but, over the past 6 months had experienced progressive difficulty in swallowing and the sensation of fullness in his throat. The patient had no other medical problems, including gastroesophageal reflux disease, but did have sleep apnea requiring nightly use of CPAP. The surgeon's examination notes describe a 3 cm base of tongue mass. In the holding area oxymetazoline was applied to both nares, followed by 50 mg of 2% lidocaine viscous solution. A few minutes later a 3.2-mm diameter flexible intubation scope was inserted via one nare. The scope's objective was positioned in the nasopharynx, and on flexion, the epiglottis, and glottis could be visualized. The patient was taken to the operating room, anesthesia was induced and the trachea intubated with a video laryngoscope.

Preoperative endoscopic airway examination (PEAE) has recently been described.[17] Based upon the office airway examination used by otolaryngologists during office consultations, PEAE can be used to gather information about the airway to help guide airway management decisions. In the case described, pathology of the hypopharyngeal airway could affect the success of airway management. By visualizing the intact airway the decision could be made to proceed with routine induction of anesthesia. PEAE was studied in 148 patients presenting for intra-airway related surgery. In 24% of patients, PEAE resulted in a modification of the clinically decided airway plan. Though clinical assessment dictated awake intubation in 44 patients, only 16 were judged to need awake intubation after PEAE. More importantly, 8 of 94 patients who were to be induced prior to airway control underwent awake intubation after PEAE. For these patients PEAE revealed an unexpectedly affected airway, resulting in a critical change in the airway plan. During PEAE, which requires <5 minutes to complete, the clinician evaluates three aspects of the airway. First, is there an obstruction to rapid intubation of the trachea; second, is there a lesion which could interfere with the placement or function of a supraglottic airway; and third, is there any anterior lesion which routine laryngoscopy (direct or indirect) might dislodge or otherwise traumatize? An affirmative answer to any one of these questions encourages awake intubation. As noted above, PEAE most often serves to reassure the clinician that lesions, otherwise invisible on physical examination, are not a hindrance to routine airway management. But likewise, PEAE can often reveal unexpectedly compromising lesions for which the clinician might have otherwise been ill prepared.

Case 2: Flexible Fiberoptic-aided Intubation

A 50-year-old man with symptomatic cervical vertebrae disk herniation presents for disk resection and spinal fixation. He has a history of tobacco use, alcohol consumption, and gastroesophageal reflux. In the preoperative holding area, 0.4 mg of intravenous glycopyrrolate is injected, and oxymetazoline is administered to the nasal cavity (commercial preparation: Afrin spray). Swabs of 5% lidocaine ointment (50 mg) are applied into the nose. Fifteen minutes later, when the patient states that his oral secretions are minimized, topical anesthesia is administered to the remaining airway, as described. The patient receives 4 mg of intravenous midazolam. An intubating oral airway is placed without eliciting a gag reflex and a flexible fiberoptic bronchoscope is advanced into the airway. The vocal ligaments are visualized, and 4 mL of 4% lidocaine solution are injected through the accessory lumen of the fiberscope (using the Ovassapian catheter technique), being seen to bathe the laryngeal and sublaryngeal structures.[164] The distal end of the fiberscope is advanced into the larynx, and a 7-ID ETT, which had been threaded onto the insertion shaft of the fiberscope, is advanced into the trachea. The fiberscope is removed while the structures of the carina, trachea, and finally the tracheal tube are observed. The anesthesia circuit is attached to the tracheal tube and a steady output of carbon dioxide is detected by capnography. A brief sensory and motor neurologic examination is performed by the attending surgeon and general anesthesia is induced.

Use of the Fiberoptic Bronchoscope in Airway Management

The fiberoptic bronchoscope is a ubiquitous instrument in anesthesia, being available to 99% of surveyed active ASA members.[165] The technique of fiberoptic-aided intubation was first performed using a choledochoscope in a patient with Still's disease (idiopathic, adult-onset arthritis).[166] By the late 1980s it was recognized that the use of the flexible fiberoptic bronchoscope represented such a significant advancement in the management of the patient with a difficult airway that experts stated that no anesthesiologist could afford not to be facile with this technique.[167] It is now generally accepted that for a variety of clinical situations, the fiberoptic bronchoscope is a critical tool in the armamentarium of the anesthesiologist dealing with the awake or unconscious patient who is, or appears to be, difficult to intubate.[157] The fiberoptic bronchoscope has proven to be the most versatile tool available in this regard.[165]

There is no true or firm indication for fiberoptic bronchoscope-aided intubation. There are, however, many clinical situations in which the fiberoptic bronchoscope can be of unparalleled aid in securing the airway, especially if the clinician has made an effort to master the necessary skills by using it in routine endotracheal intubations.[96,164] These include anticipated difficult intubation by history or physical examination findings, unanticipated difficult intubation (in which other techniques have failed), lower and upper airway obstruction, unstable or fixed cervical spine disease, mass effect in the upper or lower airways, dental risk or damage, and awake intubation.[164] Unlike the other devices used to intubate the trachea, the fiberoptic bronchoscope can also serve to visualize structures below the level of the vocal folds. For example, it can identify the placement of the tracheal tube or aid in placement of a double-lumen tracheal tube. It may be helpful in diagnosis within the trachea and bronchial tree or in pulmonary toilet (Fig. 27-24).

Contraindications to fiberoptic bronchoscope-aided intubation are relative (Table 27-16).

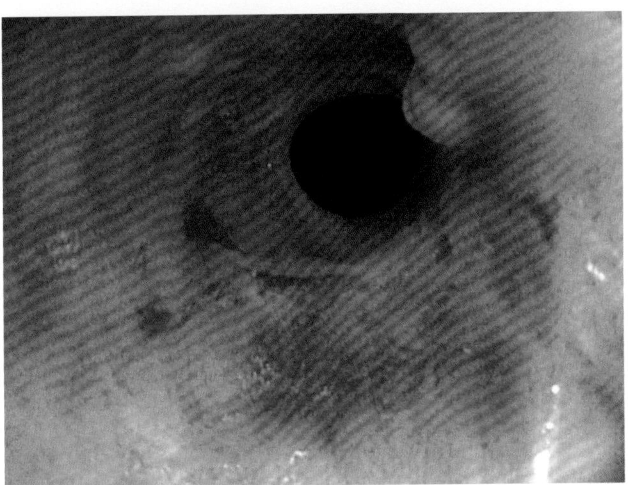

FIGURE 27-24. The fiberoptic bronchoscope may be useful for diagnosis and therapy below the level of the vocal ligaments, including bronchial segments examination and toilet. Laryngeal web is shown here.

Because the optical elements are small (the objective lens is typically 2 mm in diameter or smaller), minute amounts of airway secretions, blood, or traumatic debris can hinder visualization. Care must be taken to remove these obstacles from the airway beforehand; application of intramuscular or intravenous antisialagogues (e.g., glycopyrrolate, 0.2 to 0.4 mg; atropine, 0.5 to 1 mg) will produce a drying effect within 15 minutes, but caution should be taken in patients who may not be able to tolerate an increase in heart rate. Vasoconstriction of the nose using topical oxymetazoline, phenylephrine, or cocaine reduces the chances of bleeding if this route is chosen. If an awake intubation is planned using the fiberoptic bronchoscope, the patient must be able to cooperate—a "quiet" airway, with little motion of the head, neck, tongue, and larynx, is vital to success. Finally, because fiberoptic bronchoscope-aided intubation of the trachea can require significant time, especially if the clinician is not facile with the device, hypoxia or impending airway loss is a contraindication, and a more rapid method of securing an airway (e.g., LMA or surgical airway) should be considered.

Elements of the Fiberoptic Bronchoscope

The fiberoptic bronchoscope is a fragile device with optical and nonoptical elements. The fundamental element consists of a glass–fiber bundle. Each fiber is 8 to 12 *microns* in diameter, and is coated with a secondary glass layer termed the *cladding*. The cladding aids in maintaining the image within each fiber as the light is reflected off the sidewall at a rate of 10,000 times per meter as it moves from the objective lens to the eyepiece lens in the operator's handle. The typical intubating fiberoptic bronchoscope has 10,000 to 30,000 such fibers encased in a 60 cm, water-impermeable insertion cord, with gradation marks every 10 cm. Although the fibers are allowed to rotate over each other throughout the length of the cord, they are fused together at the two ends in a coherent pattern; that is, the arrangement of the fibers at the eyepiece end is identical to the arrangement at the objective lens, where a diopter ring allows focusing. Therefore, one might envision that the image before the objective lens (i.e., the objective) is divided into 10,000 individual and unique pixels, which independently travel down an unwieldy cord to be reassembled in front of the eyepiece lens. Broken fibers, which may occur because of bending of the insertion cord, entrapping the cord in other equipment, and dropping the fiberoptic bronchoscope, are readily apparent and are generally no more than a nuisance until the number of broken fibers interferes with the visual field.

TABLE 27-16. CONTRAINDICATIONS TO FIBEROPTIC BRONCHOSCOPY

Hypoxia
Heavy airway secretions not relieved with suction or antisialagogues
Bleeding from the upper or lower airway not relieved with suction
Local anesthetic allergy (for awake attempts)
Inability to cooperate (for awake attempts)

Newer technologies promise to make fiber breakage an obsolete problem. The advent of the charge-coupled device technology was embraced in the manufacture of endoscopes used for diagnostic purposes. These devices produce high-resolution images in order to detect small lesions or perform delicate procedures (e.g., venous dissection). Manufactures were slow to incorporate this costly technology into intubating flexible scopes, which work in a macro environment, not requiring the same micro resolution. Although some manufactures have produced these devices for the anesthesia market, CMOS technology, which may be produced at far lower costs, promises to increase the number of available devices.

The insertion cord also contains an *accessory lumen* ("working channel"): A lumen, up to 2 mm in diameter, which travels from the distal tip to the handle. It can be used for applying suction, or oxygen, and instilling lavaging fluids or drugs (e.g., local anesthetics). There is one report of gastric rupture attributed to the insufflation of oxygen through the working channel when the fiberoptic bronchoscope was within the esophagus.[168] In general, fiberoptic bronchoscopes that are <2 mm in external diameter (e.g., pediatric) do not have a working channel.

Two wires traveling from a lever in the handle down the length of the insertion cord control the movement of the distal tip in the sagittal plane. The entire insertion cord is protected by a metal "wrap" until the level of the distal tip, which is hinged for movement. Coronal plane movement is accomplished by a combined use of the control lever and rotation of the entire fiberoptic bronchoscope from handle to distal end. Because the fibers are able to move over one another, except for where they are fused at the extreme ends of the optic cord, rotational control is maximized by reducing any curves in the fiberoptic bronchoscope insertion cord.

The final element of the fiberoptic bronchoscope is the light source. Illumination of the objective is provided by one or two noncoherent bundles of glass fibers that transmit light from the handle to the distal tip. The light is provided either by a "universal" cord that emerges from the handle and is inserted into a medical-grade endoscopic light source, or may be provided by a battery-operated light source on the handle.

Use of the Fiberoptic Bronchoscope

The fiberoptic bronchoscope is held in the nondominant hand, the thumb over the control lever and the index finger poised over the working channel valve. The dominant hand will be used to steady and hold the insertion cord as it is manipulated in the patient. Many operators are tempted to "switch" hands, but the thumb of the nondominant hand should be capable of controlling the gross movement of the control lever. Any experienced endoscopist will recognize that the fine control required to hold the shaft of the endoscope steady, advance the objective end into the airway, and make directional adjustments is where the art of endoscopy lies.

The insertion shaft is lubricated with a medical grade lubricant and it is threaded through the lumen of an ETT, the objective end emerging from the main ETT orifice. A clinically appropriate ETT should be chosen, but the larger the ratio between the internal diameter of the ETT and the external diameter of the insertion shaft, the greater the risk of "hang-up" on airway structures, as occurs in 20% to 30% of attempts.[164]

Hang-up occurs when a cleft exists between these two devices because of the differential sizes. Hang-up may involve entrapment of the epiglottis, corniculate/arytenoid cartilages, the aryepiglottic folds, or the vocal folds, and can occur with any number of stylet-guided techniques (e.g., fiberoptic, retrograde wire, lighted stylet), although it is most thoroughly described with fiberoptic-aided intubation.[168,169] The orientation of the tracheal tube bevel is important in this regard. In orotracheal intubation, the bevel cleft is likely to entrap the right arytenoid cartilage when the ETT is in its typical concavity-anterior position. Rotation of the ETT 90 degrees counterclockwise places the bevel cleft anteriorly and improves passage. During nasotracheal intubation, the epiglottis may be entrapped, and a bevel-up position (rotation of the ETT 90 degrees clockwise) may facilitate passage.[171]

Tracheal tube design may also affect passage. It has been suggested that the Parker Flex-Tip may pass the airway structures more easily than a standard ETT bevel.[171] The use of soft-tipped ETTs, asking the patient to inspire deeply during the ETT advancement, and the "double setup" ETT, which uses a small ETT (e.g., 5 ID) within a clinically adequate ETT (e.g., 7.5 ID) to overcome the clefts caused by size differentials have been described.[169]

The clinician chooses the route of intubation, either oral or nasal, based on clinical requirements, surgical needs, operator experience, and other intubation techniques available should fiberoptic bronchoscope-aided intubation fail. This last factor is important because should an attempt at nasal intubation fail, there may be significant bleeding, which may hinder other indirect visualization techniques. The nasal route is considered easier by many clinicians, although other cautions apply: Vasoconstrictors should be applied to reduce bleeding; the turbinates (lateral walls) may obstruct ETT passage, bleed, be avulsed, or be painful when traumatized; small, lubricated, and softened (bathed in warm water) ETT should be employed.

A variety of intubating oral airways are commercially available. Their chief function is to provide a clear visual path from the oral aperture to the hypopharynx, keep the bronchoscope and tracheal tube in the airway midline, prevent the patient from biting the insertion cord, and provide a clear airway for the spontaneously or mask-ventilated patient. The common characteristic of all intubating oral airways is a channel along the length of the airway large enough to allow the passage of the tracheal tube. The Ovassapian airway provides two sets of semicircular, incomplete flexible flanges that stabilize the ETT (up to size 9 ID) in the midline but allow its removal from the airway after intubation has been accomplished so that the intubating oral airway can be removed from the mouth. The flat lingual surface of the airway gives it good lateral and rotational stability. The Patil–Syracuse endoscopic airway and the Luomanen oral airway were also designed for fiberoptic-aided intubation. Each has a central groove, open at the lingual (Patil–Syracuse) or palatal (Luomanen) aspect, which allows easy removal of the ETT. The flat lingual surface provides good stability. Although this style of intubating oral airway provides superb access to the pharynx, it is larger than other airways and is often uncomfortable for the patient. The Williams airway and the Berman airway were both designed for blind oral intubation. Both are molded plastic with a complete circular internal lumen that guides the ETT toward the larynx. These airways have a small profile and are often better tolerated by the awake patient, but tend to be less stable on the tongue. Because the internal lumen is a complete circle, the Williams airway must be retreated off the ETT if it is going to be removed after intubation. This may pose difficulty if the ETT in use has a fused circuit adapter. The Berman airway solves this problem by being split along the length of one side. The plastic of the opposite side is thin and malleable. If the interincisor gap is adequate, the airway can be opened laterally to allow removal from the ETT.

After successful navigation through the oral airway, the endoscopist visualizes the vocal folds. If glottic closure, gag, or coughing occurs as the fiberoptic bronchoscope's distal tip stimulates the structures of the larynx, the operator can choose to apply local anesthetic through the working channel, administer more sedation, or withdraw the scope and reinforce preparatory procedures. The clinician might also decide to advance the fiberoptic bronchoscope into the larynx without further preparation. The actions taken must be dictated by the individual clinical situation; in the elective scenario, for example, there may be time for reinforced airway analgesia, whereas in the face of impending respiratory arrest, patient discomfort may need to be tolerated. Once the larynx is entered, the operator may choose a structure, such as the tracheal carina, to serve as an identifying landmark as the ETT is advanced. Simply because the fiberoptic bronchoscope has entered the trachea, there is no guarantee that the intubation will be successful. Ten percent of ETT advancements are accompanied by hang-up. Therefore, a patient with a critical airway should not be induced with a general anesthetic with the assumption that the ETT will be easy to pass.

The primary literature contains a number of variations and adjuncts to fiberoptic bronchoscope-aided intubation. Table 27-17 which is not meant to be exhaustive, lists several of these techniques.

Although fiberoptic bronchoscope-aided intubation is a versatile and vital technique, there are several pitfalls, most of which have been discussed. Table 27-18 lists the most common reasons for failure of fiberoptic bronchoscope-aided intubation.

Flexible fiberoptic-aided intubation is a technology-intense technique. Apart from the delicate fiberoptic device, there are cameras, recorders, light sources, and a variety of disposable adjuncts that are typically required. Dedicated wheeled carts, designed to carry required and optional equipment in a functional arrangement, are available.

Case 3: Failed Rapid-sequence Induction and the SGA

A 39-year-old man presents for elective uvulopharyngopalatoplasty. He has no previous surgical history. His maximal incisor gap is 5 cm, thyromental distance is 7 cm, and his oropharyngeal view is a Samsoon–Young class 2. There is no limitation in head and neck flexion and extension. During a sleep apnea study, he had 15 apneic events each hour. The patient has a significant history of gastroesophageal reflux, and rapid-sequence induction is planned. After the administration of a hypotic, succinylcholine, and cricoid pressure (Sellick maneuver), DL with a Macintosh number 3 laryngoscope blade reveals a large epiglottis obscuring the view of the vocal folds (Cormack–Lehane grade 3).[82] Significant hyperplasia of

TABLE 27-17. AIDS TO FIBEROPTIC-AIDED INTUBATION

Technique	Advantage
Endoscopy mask	Controlled ventilation maintained during or between attempts at FOB-aided intubation
Laryngeal mask	Excellent view of the larynx and ability to ventilate during or between attempts at FOB-aided intubation
Fiberoptic-aided retrograde intubation	Guiding of the FOB with a wire known to be entering the trachea
Retrograde fiberoptic intubation	Changing a tracheostomy to an oral or nasal tracheal tube when antegrade intubation is difficult or impossible
FOB-aided intubation with the aid of a rigid laryngoscope	Helpful with an obstructing mass or large epiglottis

FOB, fiberoptic bronchoscope.

the base of the tongue, which prevents its full displacement, is also noted. The BURP maneuver does not improve the view.[86] A Macintosh 4 and Miller 3 blades are used and do not improve the view. Oxygen saturation, which was 100% prior to induction, is now 92%, and face mask ventilation is initiated with the Sellick maneuver in place. Complete obstruction to ventilation is encountered, despite chin and/or jaw lift, two-person ventilation, and a reduction in the degree of cricoid pressure. The oxygen saturation falls to 85% and a size 5 LMA (which had been prepared prior to the induction of anesthesia) is inserted with the technique as described by the inventor, Dr. Archie Brain. Immediately, a clear airway is established and the Sellick pressure remains in place. A second dose of hypnotic is administered, and the patient is intubated by the blind passage of a 7-ID ETT via the LMA. The LMA is then removed using a Cook airway exchange catheter as a stylet, and the surgical case proceeds.

The SGA in the Failed Airway

One clear advantage of SGA use is in the failed airway. There have been many reported (and unreported) cases of failed intubation and failure to ventilate by face mask in which the airway was rescued with an LMA, Laryngeal Tube, Cobra PLA, or another SGA.[172,173]

Parmet et al.[174] estimate that 1 in 800,000 patients cannot be managed with an LMA, providing an 80-fold increase in margin of safety over the oft-noted 1 in 10,000 patients who cannot be ventilated by mask nor intubated by traditional means. Likewise, a wealth of literature describes the use of the various SGAs in elective difficult airway management in awake and unconscious patients, in anticipated and unanticipated situations, in cervical spine injury, and in pediatric dysmorphic syndromes.[69,70,146]

The characteristics of the SGAs that underlie their superiority as a tool in the difficult airway armamentarium are that they are well tolerated by the patient, simulating the natural distension of the hypopharyngeal tissues by food, and that its insertion follows an intrinsic pathway, requiring no tissue distortion (as with laryngoscopy), which may not be possible in all patients. Finally, it is a blind technique not hindered by blood, secretions, debris, and edema from previous attempts at laryngoscopy.[175] Because most of the ease of insertion of the SGA does not depend on anatomy that can be assessed on routine physical examination, typical airway assessment measures do not apply to its application.[176] The major disadvantage of the SGAs in resuscitation is the lack of mechanical protection from regurgitation and aspiration.[177,178]

Lower rates of regurgitation during cardiopulmonary resuscitation with an LMA (3.5%) than with the bag-valve-mask ventilation (12.4%) have been shown.[179] Even in the face of regurgitation, pulmonary aspiration is a rare event.[180] Unfortunately, the use of the Sellick maneuver may prevent proper seating of the LMA in a minority of instances.[181] This may require the brief removal of the cricoid pressure until the LMA has been properly seated. Cricoid pressure is effective with an LMA *in situ*. Had it been available, the LMA Fastrack would also have been an ideal device in this case scenario.

TABLE 27-18. COMMON REASONS FOR FAILURE DURING FIBEROPTIC-AIDED INTUBATION

Lack of experience: Not practicing on routine intubations
Failure to adequately dry the airway: Underdose or rushed technique
Failure to adequately anesthetize the airway of the awake patient: Secretions not dried; rushed technique
Nasal cavity bleeding: Inadequate vasoconstriction; rushed technique; forcible ETT insertion
Obstructing base of tongue or epiglottis: Poor choice of intubating airway; require chin lift/jaw thrust
Inadequate sedation of the awake patient
Hang-up: ETT too large
Fogging of the FOB: Suction or oxygen not attached to working channel; cold bronchoscope

ETT, endotracheal tube; FOB, fiberoptic bronchoscope.

Case 4: Deviation from the Difficult Airway Algorithm

Thirteen hours after admission to the intensive care unit, a 76-year-old woman who had sustained trauma to the face, head, and neck in a motor vehicle accident is noted to have progressive decline in her level of consciousness and respiratory effort. On examination, there appears to be an adequate interincisor gap and thyromental distance. The oropharyngeal view and range of motion of the head and neck cannot be evaluated. Because of the inability to fully evaluate the airway with respect to ease of intubation, an awake procedure is chosen. Fiberoptic devices are not considered usable because of the presence of fresh and clotted blood in the mouth as a result of continued epistaxis. Other airway techniques that require significant patient preparation are not considered because of the rapid progression of the patient's respiratory failure. In addition, the presence of fresh blood in the oral and pharyngeal cavities will hinder adequate drying and analgesia. Blind nasal intubation is considered contraindicated based on the obvious facial trauma and the risk of cribriform plate disruption. Neither equipment for retrograde intubation nor the tracheal esophageal Combitube is readily available. A lighted stylet intubation guide is available, but no clinician present is experienced with this technique. Although the mental status change is believed to reflect an intracranial process (e.g., intracranial hypertension), the risk of complete loss of the airway is judged to be the primary clinical hazard. Awake DL is attempted with manual in-line stabilization of the neck. After clearing fresh blood from the pharynx with a Yankauer suction catheter, a Cormack–Lehane grade 3 laryngeal view is obtained, but because of patient resistance (biting on the laryngoscope and movement), tracheal intubation is not achieved. The decision is made to proceed with rapid-sequence induction and intubation, with preparations made for an emergency tracheostomy. After surgical preparation of the neck and preoxygenation, intravenous succinylcholine and etomidate are administered, DL is undertaken, the larynx is easily visualized, and the trachea is intubated.

Muscle Relaxants and Direct Laryngoscopy

23 In the case described, the use of muscle relaxants significantly improved the ability to visualize the larynx. In one study, the use of muscle relaxants during a DL increased the success rate of intubation and was associated with fewer incidents of airway trauma, intubation attempts, esophageal intubations, aspiration, and even death.[182] Intubating conditions with and without muscle relaxation have been investigated in few well-controlled trials because the superior intubating conditions achieved with muscle relaxants have discouraged inclusion of control groups.[183] The effects of muscle relaxation that improve laryngoscopic view include allowing complete temporomandibular joint relaxation and opening, anterior movement of the epiglottis, and widening of the laryngeal vestibule and laryngeal sinus.[184] In addition, the finding that laryngoscopic stimulation of the pharyngeal musculature causes the upper airway lumen to appear small is offset by the use of relaxants.

Leaving the Algorithm

The situation described in case 4 is unusual in that rapid-sequence induction was attempted because the clinical situation had deviated from the ASA–DAA owing to the progressive nature of the airway compromise. The situation was more akin to the "crash" airway described by Walls.[185] In this case, the institution of muscle relaxation, which might be considered contraindicated in the apparently difficult-to-intubate patient, allowed for full visualization of the larynx. Knowing that failure to intubate in this case would result in probable loss of the airway, the clinician was prepared for cricothyroidotomy. Although the ASA–DAA is a valuable tool in the process of managing the difficult airway, the clinician must always be prepared for the case that does not fit the mold. As stated earlier, adaptability in a rapidly changing clinical situation is critical to the success of airway management. Also of interest in this case was the availability of a lighted stylet for use in similar difficult airway scenarios. Although this device may have been useful in the current case, no clinician present was familiar with its operation. A critical situation is not an occasion for trying an unfamiliar technology.

Other Devices

11 An ever-increasing number of airway management devices are commercially available. Although encyclopedic coverage of these tools is beyond the scope of this chapter, a review of the more established equipment follows.

Combitube

The Esophageal Tracheal Combitube (Combitube) was developed by Dr. Michael Frass, a critical care physician in Vienna, Austria, in 1986. Its design was meant to improve and replace the esophageal obturator airway, which was a rescue airway introduced in 1968. The Combitube is a double-lumen device, the distal end of which is meant to be blindly placed into the esophagus. One lumen begins at this distal point with a large orifice, and travels to outside the patient where it opens to the atmosphere. This lumen serves as a gastric drain. The second lumen travels from outside the patient to a point in the hypopharynx. This lumen has a multiorifice opening that faces the larynx and acts as the airway. The Combitube has two cuffs, one within the esophagus and a second at the oral cavity/pharynx juncture. The Combitube is functional if introduced into the esophagus (ventilation being achieved through the pharyngeal lumen, via the hypopharyngeal perforations) or in the trachea (ventilation being achieved through the gastric drain, via the distal aperture). In either case, the proximal balloon seals both the oral and nasal passages, and the distal cuff isolates the respiratory system from the gastrointestinal system. The device is available in two sizes: The 41-French size is used for larger adults (height >168 cm) and the 37-French size is used for adults 122 to 183 cm (Fig. 27-25).

24 Airway Bougie

Airway bougies encompass a series of solid or hollow, semimalleable stylets that may be blindly manipulated into the larynx. An

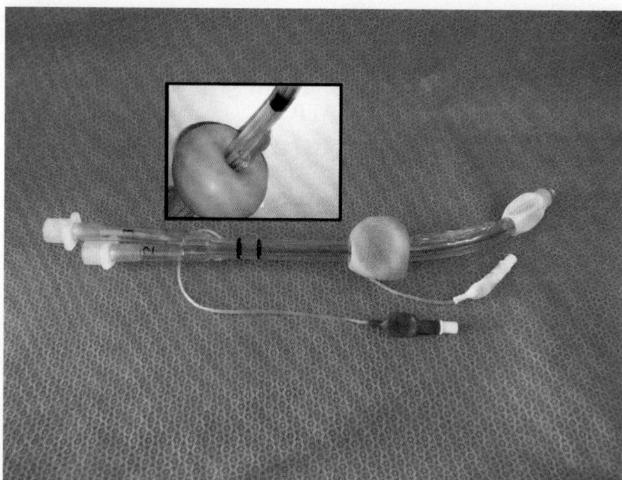

FIGURE 27-25. The esophageal tracheal Combitube. Inset: The fiberoptic port of the Easy Tube.

ETT is then "threaded" over the bougie and into the trachea. These bougies are generally low cost and highly portable. The Eschmann introducer (Eschmann Health Care, Kent, England) was introduced in 1949. It is 60 cm long, 15 French, and angled 40 degrees 3.5 cm from its distal end. It is constructed from a woven polyester base, which is malleable. It can be very helpful when the larynx cannot be visualized with laryngoscopy. The introducer (also known as the *gum elastic bougie*) can be manipulated under the epiglottis, its angled segment directed anteriorly toward the larynx. Once it has entered the larynx and trachea, a distinctive "clicking" feel is elicited as the tip passes over the cartilaginous structures. A similar device, the Frova Intubating Introducer (Cook Critical Care, Bloomington, IN) is disposable, has an optional "stiffening" stylet and a hollow bore. The internal lumen allows for the insufflation of oxygen, the detection of carbon dioxide, and the use of a self-inflating bulb to detect inadvertent esophageal placement.

Minimally Invasive Transtracheal Procedures

12 When access to the airway from the mouth or nose fails, is unavailable or particularly difficult (e.g., maxillofacial, pharyngeal, or laryngeal trauma, pathology, or deformity), access via the extrathoracic trachea is a feasible route to the airway. The clinician must be familiar with these alternative techniques of intubation, oxygenation, and ventilation for both elective and emergency airway access. Though the noninvasive tools of the modern airway armamentarium can manage most situations, the clinician may consider training in elective minimally invasive techniques (e.g., retrograde wire-aided intubation), but must be facile with at least one of the techniques of emergency oxygenation. Although surgical tracheostomy and cricothyroidotomy are beyond the scope of this chapter, percutaneous techniques will be considered.

Retrograde Wire-aided Tracheal Intubation

Retrograde wire intubation (RWI) involves the antegrade pulling or guiding of an ETT into the airway using a wire that has been passed into the larynx via a percutaneous puncture through the cricothyroid or cricotracheal membrane, and blindly passed retrograde into the hypopharynx, pharynx, and out of the mouth or nose. In 1993, the technique was included in the ASA's Difficult Airway Algorithm. The basic equipment used in the retrograde intubation technique is listed in Table 27-19.

RWI has been described in a number of clinical situations as a primary intubation technique (elective or urgent) and after failed attempts at DL, fiberoptic-aided intubation, and LMA-guided intubation.[81] The most common indications are inability to visualize the vocal folds owing to blood, secretions, or anatomic variations, unstable cervical spine, upper airway malignancy, and mandibular fracture. Contraindications include lack of access to the CTM or the cricotracheal ligament (because of severe neck deformity, obesity, mass), laryngotracheal disease (stenosis, malignancy, infection), coagulopathy, and overlying skin infection.

The anatomic relationships to be considered in RWI have been described elsewhere in this chapter. Common complications reported with RWI include bleeding, subcutaneous emphysema, pneumomediastinum, pneumothorax, breath-holding, caudal traveling catheter, and trigeminal nerve trauma. The readers are referred to early editions of this text or to other authoritative texts for a complete description.

TABLE 27-19. EQUIPMENT FOR RETROGRADE WIRE INTUBATION

18 gauge or larger angiocatheter
Luer-lock syringe, 3 mL or larger
Guide wire:
- Preferably J-type end
- Length: At least 2.5 times the length of a standard ETT (typically 110–120 cm)
- Diameter: Capable of passing via angiocatheter being chosen

Other: Scalpel blade, nerve hook, Magill forceps, 30 inch silk suture, epidural catheter

ETT, endotracheal tube.

Cricothyrotomy

Cricothyroidotomy, cricothyrotomy, coniotomy, and minitracheostomy are synonyms for establishing an air passage through the CTM. The CTM is a fibroelastic membrane, lying over the tracheal mucosa. It is attached to the inferior border of the thyroid cartilage and superior edge of the cricoid cartilage. Although cricothyrotomy is the procedure of choice in an emergency situation, it may also apply to an elective situation when there is limited access to the trachea (e.g., severe cervical kyphoscoliosis). Cricothyrotomy is contraindicated in neonates and children younger than 6 years of age, and in patients with laryngeal fractures. Otolaryngologists and other surgical services prefer intratracheal airway access whenever feasible because of the high incidence of long-term complications after surgical cricothyrotomy.

25 **Percutaneous translaryngeal jet ventilation (PTJV),** as a form of cricothyroidotomy, is the most familiar to anesthesiologists. The ASA–DAA lists PTJV as an option in the "cannot mask ventilate/cannot intubate" situation. PTJV is a simple and relatively safe means to sustain the patient's life in this critical situation.[81] A body of literature exits detailing the gerry-rigging of conveyance systems for PTJV and the use of intravenous catheters for transtracheal puncture. These systems have proven faulty, inadequate, and dangerous.[186] Experts in the field recommend that all anesthetizing positions have access to both manufactured, high-pressure oxygen conveyance devices, and specifically designed translaryngeal catheters.

Before contemplating PTJV the location of the CTM will need to be identified. Elliot et al. have cast doubt on the ability of anesthesiologists to locate the CTM in elective, let alone, emergency situations.[187] Obesity, cervical kyphosis, female gender, therapeutic radiation, surgical, or traumatic scarring may hinder CTM location. A careful reading of the ASA–DAA should lead the airway manager to seek to identify the CTM in every patient. Applying this examination in all instances should improve familiarity with the surface landmarks. (1) Bedside ultrasound in the sagittal plane can reveal the CTM as a lucent shadow between opaque cartilaginous structures, and may be useful in emergency situations if immediately available.[188]

When performing PTJV, a large-bore translaryngeal catheter, (14 gauge or larger) attached to a 5 mL or larger empty or fluid-filled (saline or local anesthetic) syringe, should be used to enter the airway. The patient is positioned supine, with the head midline or extended on the neck and thorax (if not contraindicated by the clinical situation). After aseptic preparation, local anesthetic may be injected over the CTM (if the patient is awake and time permits). The right-handed clinician stands on the left side of the patient. The clinician can use his or her nondominant hand to stabilize the larynx. The catheter-needle is advanced at right

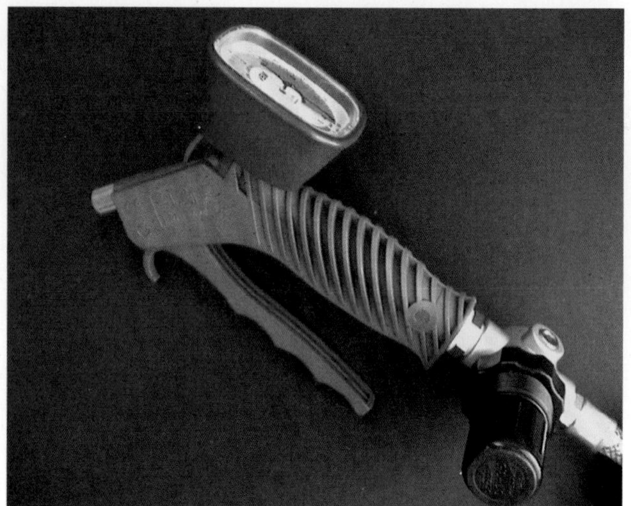

FIGURE 27-26. System for regulation of a high-pressure oxygen source for transtracheal jet ventilation.

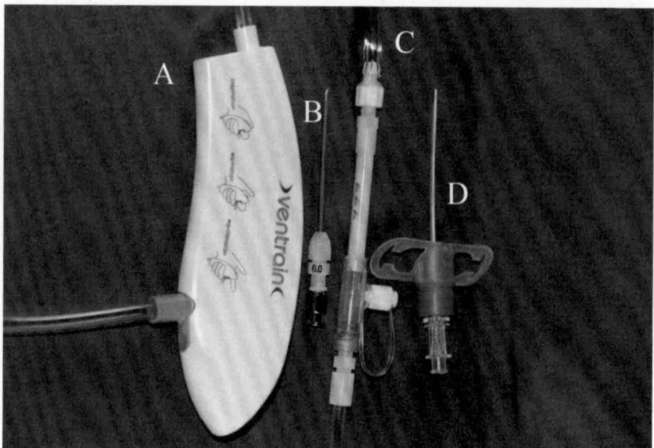

FIGURE 27-27. (A) Ventrain (B) Cook transtracheal needle (C) Enk flow modulator (D) Ravussin needle.

angles to the plane of the cervical spine in the caudad third of the membrane. From the moment of skin puncture, there should be constant aspiration on the syringe plunger. Free aspiration of air confirms entrance into the trachea but does not indicate the direction that the catheter travels in the larynx; cephalad extension will not provide adequate oxygenation. Unless there is significant pulmonary fluid (e.g., blood, aspirated gastric contents, or water from drowning), the aspiration of tracheal air should be incontrovertible. The needle–catheter assembly should be advanced slightly, and subsequently the catheter advanced fully into the airway. Dedicated devices made of kink-resistant materials and with accessory ports are available such as the Cook TTJV catheter (Cook Critical Care, Bloomington, IN). Catheters designed for intravenous infusion have long been shown to kink in the airway.[186]

Once the catheter has been successfully placed in the airway, an oxygen source is attached. The clinician may have several options in this regard, but due to the high resistance of the catheter, availability of a high-pressure source is mandatory. A 50 psi source with a metered and adjustable hand-controlled valve (Fig. 27-26) and a Luer-lock connector is down-regulated to 15 to 30 psi of oxygen (central hospital supply or regulated cylinder) is delivered directly through the catheter, with insufflations of 1 to 1.5 seconds at a rate of 12 insufflations per minute. Insufflation and expiration ratios and driving pressure are adjusted to provide visible chest excursion and recoil. If a 14-gauge catheter has been placed, this system will deliver a tidal volume of 400 to 700 mL. Low-pressure systems cannot provide enough flow to expand the chest adequately for oxygenation and ventilation (e.g., Ambu bag, 6 psi; anesthesia machine common gas outlet, 20 psi). Critically, systems delivering pressurized oxygen require a path for gas egress. Standard high-pressure regulating valves as described above are one-way only, and generally contraindicated with a completely obstructed upper airway. Fortunately, this tends to be an uncommon situation. In any case, the clinician employing any type of translaryngeal oxygenation must strive to maintain any upper airway patency (oral or nasal airway, supraglottic airway, etc.).

Alternatively, low-flow oxygen delivery meters common in the hospital environment can also be used for PTLV. These systems are capable of delivering constant flow of 15 L/min and have been shown effective for resuscitation. Generally, this gas source is applied using "flow interruption," that is, during the inspiratory phase flow is directed to the patient, and diverted in expiration. As discussed above, gerry-rigged devices are often suspect in function—for example, using a standard three-way stopcock as a flow diverter has been shown to be potentially hazardous because forward flow (inspiration) is never fully stopped.[189] The Enk flow modulator (Cook Critical Care, Bloomington, IN) is a simple, inexpensive, hand-operated flow diverter which not only stops forward gas flow during the expiratory phase, but has also been shown to act as an expiratory flow pathway. (Fig. 27-27C).[190] The Enk flow modulator has been used successfully in models of near and complete upper airway obstruction. A new concept in PTLV is expiratory ventilatory assistance.[189] Using a venturi-like valve, the Ventrain (Dolphys Medical, Denmark) is capable of active gas removal from the rescue catheter during the expiratory phase of PTLV. The device has been shown to be effective in oxygenation and carbon dioxide removal in two large animal models via a 75 mm long, 2-mm ID transtracheal catheter for 15 minutes (unpublished) (Fig. 27-27A).

Specialized percutaneous cricothyroidotomy systems have been developed that improve the ease of this technique. These devices generally provide a large-bore access that is adequate for oxygenation and ventilation with low-pressure systems. The Melker emergency cricothyroidotomy catheter set (Cook Critical Care, Bloomington, IN) uses a Seldinger—catheter-over-a-wire—technique familiar to most anesthesia practitioners. The set comes in a variety of cannula sizes (3.5-, 4-, and 6-mm ID, cuffed and uncuffed). Preparation and positioning of the patient are the same as with needle cricothyroidotomy. A 1- to 1.5-cm vertical incision of the skin only is made over the lower third of the CTM. Aiming 45 degrees caudad, a percutaneous puncture of the subcutaneous tissue and CTM is made with the provided 18-gauge needle–catheter assembly and syringe. After air is aspirated, the catheter is advanced into the trachea. The provided guidewire is inserted through the catheter and into the trachea. The catheter is removed and the tracheal cannula, fitted internally with a curved dilator, is threaded onto the wire. The dilator is advanced through the membrane using firm pressure. Significant resistance to its advancement may indicate that the skin incision needs to be extended. Once the cannula–dilator has been fully inserted, the dilator and wire are removed. The 15-mm circuit adapter end of the cannula is now attached to an Ambu bag or anesthesia circuit.

Other percutaneous systems include Nu-trake (Weiss Emergency Airway System; International Medical Devices) and the

Quicktrach transtracheal catheter (VBM Medizintechnik). Non-needle puncture techniques are beyond the current discussion.

Severe complications of PTLV are related to barotraumas such as cervicomediastinal emphysema, pneumothorax, or tension pneumothorax. Causes of insufflation of air into the paratracheal spaces include a misplaced cannula, multiple tracheal punctures or migration due to coughing. Bilateral tension pneumothorax with jet ventilation has been reported.[191]

CONCLUSIONS

Apart from monitoring, the management of the "routine" patient airway is the most common task of the anesthesiologist—even during the administration of regional anesthesia, the airway must be monitored and possibly supported. Unfortunately, routine tasks often become neglected as the clinician becomes distracted. But the consequences of a lost airway are so devastating that the clinician can never afford a lackadaisical approach.

Although the ASA's Task Force on the Difficult Airway has given the medical community an immensely valuable tool in the approach to the patient with the difficult airway, the Task Force's algorithm must be viewed as a starting point only. Judgment, experience, clinical situation, and available resources all affect the appropriateness of the chosen pathway through, or divergence from, the algorithm. The clinician does not need to be expert in all the equipment and techniques currently available. Rather, a broad range of approaches should be mastered so that the failure of one does not present a roadblock to airway management and emergency rescue.

Whereas one may argue that the last decade of the 20th century was the decade of the SGA, the first decades of the 21st century are witnessing the application of the imaging technology to airway management. A balance between supraglottic ventilation and video-assisted intubation is the challenge of the coming years.

The medical manufacturing community, and the far-sighted clinicians who supply it with concepts for airway management products, has supplied a vast array of devices. Many represent redundancy in concept, and each has its supporters and detractors. No one device can be considered superior to another when considered in isolation. It is the clinician and his or her resources (both equipment and personnel) and judgment that determine the effectiveness of any technique. In the management of the difficult airway, flexibility, and not rigidity, prevails.

References

1. Practice guidelines for the management of the difficult airway. An updated report by the American Society of Anesthesiologists Task Force on Management of the Difficult Airway. *Anesthesiology.* 2003;98:1269.
2. Peterson GN, Domino KB, Caplan RA, et al. Management of the difficult airway: A closed claims analysis. *Anesthesiology.* 2005;103:33.
3. Li G, Warner M, Lang BH, et al. Epidemiology of anesthesia-related mortality in the United States, 1999–2005. *Anesthesiology.* 2009;110:759.
4. Rosenblatt W. The airway approach algorithm. *J Clin Anesth.* 2004;16:312.
5. Westhorpe RN. The position of the larynx in children and its relationship to the ease of intubation. *Anaesth Intensive Care.* 1987;15:384.
6. Iohom G, Ronayne M, Cunningham AJ. Prediction of difficult tracheal intubation. *Eur J Anaesthesiol.* 2003;20:31.
7. Elliott DS, Baker PA, Scott MR, et al. Accuracy of surface landmark identification for cannula cricothyroidotomy. *Anaesthesia.* 2010;65:889.
8. Sykes WS. *Essays on the First Hundred Years of Anesthesia.* London: Churchill Livingstone; 1982.
9. Brimacombe JR, ed. *Laryngeal Mask Anesthesia: Principles and Practice.* Philadelphia, PA: Saunders; 2005.
10. Brandt L. The first reported oral intubation of the human trachea. *Anesth Analg.* 1987;66:1198.
11. Magill IW. Technique in endotracheal anaesthesia. *Proc R Soc Med.* 1928;22:83.
12. Mendelson CL. The aspiration of stomach contents into the lungs during obstetric anesthesia. *Am J Obstet Gynecol.* 1946;52:191.
13. Ovassapian A, Yelich SJ, Dykes MH, et al. Learning fibreoptic intubation: Use of simulators v. traditional teaching. *Br J Anaesth.* 1988;61:217–220.
14. Kaplan MB, Ward DS, Berci G. A new video laryngoscope—an aid to intubation and teaching. *J Clin Anesth.* 2002;14:620.
15. Breitmeier D, Wilke N, Schulz Y, et al. The lingual tonsillar hyperplasia in relation to unanticipated difficult intubation: Is there any relationship between lingual tonsillar hyperplasia and tonsillectomy? *Am J Forensic Med Pathol.* 2005; 26:131.
16. Ovassapian A, Glassenberg R, Randel GI, et al. The unexpected difficult airway and lingual tonsil hyperplasia – a case series and a review of the literature. *Anesthesiology.* 2002;97:124.
17. Rosenblatt W, Ianus AI, Sukhupragarn W, et al. Preoperative endoscopic airway examination (PEAE) provides superior airway information and may reduce the use of unnecessary awake intubation. *Anesth Analg.* 2011;112:602.
18. Shiga T, Wajima Z, Inoue T, et al. Predicting difficult intubation in apparently normal patients: A meta-analysis of bedside screening test performance. *Anesthesiology.* 2005;103:429.
19. El-Ganzouri AR, McCarthy RJ, Tuman KJ, et al. Preoperative airway assessment: Predictive value of a multivariate risk index. *Anesth Analg.* 1996;82:1197.
20. Wilson ME, Spiegelhalter D, Robertson J, et al. Predicting difficult intubation. *Br J Anaesth.* 1988;61:211.
21. Patel SK, Whitten CW, Ivy R 3rd, et al. Failure of the laryngeal mask airway: An undiagnosed laryngeal carcinoma. *Anesth Analg.* 1998;86:438.
22. Naguib M, Malabarey T, AlSatli RA, et al. Predictive models for difficult laryngoscopy. A clinical, radiologic and three dimensional computer imaging study. *Can J Anesth.* 1999;46:748.
23. Eberhart LH, Arndt C, Aust HJ, et al. A simplified risk score to predict difficult intubation: Development and prospective evaluation in 3763 patients. *Eur J Anaesthesiol.* 2011;27(11):935.
24. Cortellazzi P, Minati L, Falcone C, et al. Predictive value of the El-Ganzouri multivariate risk index for difficult tracheal intubation; a comparison of Glidescope videolaryngoscopy and conventional Macintosh laryngoscopy. *Br J Anaesth.* 2007; 99:906.
25. Aziz MF, Healy D, Kheterpal S, et al. Routine clinical practice effectiveness of the Glidescope in difficult airway management: An analysis of 2,004 Glidescope intubations, complications, and failures from two institutions. *Anesthesiology.* 2011; 114(1):34–41.
26. Langeron O, Masso E, Huraux C, et al. Prediction of difficult mask ventilation. *Anesthesiology.* 2000;92:1229.
27. Kheterpal S, Martin L, Shanks AM, et al. Prediction and outcomes of impossible mask ventilation: A review of 50,000 anesthetics. *Anesthesiology.* 2009;110:891.
28. Ezri T, Gewürtz G, Sessler DI, et al. Prediction of difficult laryngoscopy in obese patients by ultrasound quantification of anterior neck soft tissue. *Anaesthesia.* 2003;58:1111.
29. Kristensen MS. Ultrasonography in the management of the airway. *Acta Anaesthesiol Scand.* 2011;55:1155.
30. Tanoubi I, Drolet P, Donati F. Optimizing preoxygenation in adults. *Can J Anesth.* 2009;56:449.
31. Kwei P, Matzelle S, Wallman D, et al. Inadequate preoxygenation during spontaneous ventilation with single patient use self-inflating resuscitation bags. *Anaesth Intensive Care.* 2006;34:685.
32. Rosenblatt WH, Ovassappian A, Eige S. *Use of the Laryngeal Mask Airway in the United States: A Randomized Survey of ASA Members.* ASA Annual Meeting, Orlando, Florida; 1998.
33. Ezri T, Szmuk P, Warters RD, et al. Difficult airway management practice patterns among anesthesiologists practicing in the United States: Have we made any progress? *J Clin Anesth.* 2003;15:418.
34. Isono S, Tanaka A, Ishikawa T, et al. Sniffing position improves pharyngeal airway patency in anesthetized patients with obstructive sleep apnea. *Anesthesiology.* 2005;103:489.
35. Conlon NP, Sullivan RP, Herbison PG, et al. The effect of leaving dentures in place on bag-mask ventilation at induction of general anesthesia. *Anesth Analg.* 2007;105:370.
36. Halaseh BK, Sukkar ZF, Hassan LH, et al. The use of ProSeal laryngeal mask airway in caesarean section–experience in 3000 cases. *Anaesth Intensive Care.* 2010; 38:1023.
37. Woodall NM, Cook TM. National census of airway management techniques used for anaesthesia in the UK: First phase of the Fourth National Audit Project at the Royal College of Anaesthetists. *Br J Anaesth.* 2011;106:266.
38. Maktabi MA, Smith RB, Todd MM. Is routine endotracheal intubation as safe as we think or wish? (Editorial). *Anesthesiology.* 2003;99:24.
39. Domino KB, Posner KL, Caplan RA, et al. Airway injury during anesthesia—a closed claims analysis. *Anesthesiology.* 1999;91:1703.
40. Goldmann K, Dieterich J, Roessler M. Laryngopharyngeal mucosal injury after prolonged use of the ProSeal TM LMA in a porcine model: A pilot study. *Can J Anaesth.* 2007;54:822.

41. Calder I, Picard J, Chapman M, et al. Mouth opening: A new angle. *Anesthesiology.* 2003;99:799.
42. Brimacombe JR, Berry A. The incidence of aspiration associated with the laryngeal mask airway: A meta-analysis of published literature. *J Clin Anesth.* 1995;7:297.
43. Yardy N, Hancox D, Strang TSO. A comparison of two airway aids for emergency use by unskilled personnel: The Combitube and laryngeal mask. *Anaesthesia.* 1999;54:181.
44. Han TH, Brimacombe JR, Lee EJ, et al. The laryngeal mask airway is effective (and probably safe) in selected healthy parturients for elective Cesarean section: A prospective study of 1067 cases. *Can J Anaesth.* 2001;48:1117.
45. Stone BJ, Chantler PJ. The incidence of regurgitation during cardiopulmonary resuscitation: A comparison between the bag valve mask and laryngeal mask airway. *Resuscitation.* 1998;38:3.
46. Verghese C, Brimacombe J. Survey of laryngeal mask airway usage in 11,910 patients: Safety and efficacy for conventional and nonconventional usage. *Anesth Analg.* 1996;82:129.
47. Idrees A, Khan FA. A comparative study of positive pressure ventilation via laryngeal mask airway and endotracheal tube. *J Pak Med Assoc.* 2000;50:333.
48. Brimacombe JR, Brain AI, Berry AM, et al. Gastric insufflation and the laryngeal mask. *Anesth Analg.* 1998;86:914.
49. Brimacombe J, Shorney N. The laryngeal mask airway and prolonged balanced regional anaesthesia. *Can J Anaesth.* 1993;40:360.
50. Goldmann K, Dieterich J, Roessler M. Laryngopharyngeal mucosal injury after prolonged use of the ProSeal LMA in a porcine model: A pilot study. *Can J Anaesth.* 2007;54:822.
51. Williams PJ, Bailey PM. Comparison of the reinforced laryngeal mask airway and tracheal intubation for adenotonsillectomy. *Br J Anaesth.* 1993;70:30.
52. Kim ES, Bishop MJ. Endotracheal intubation, but not laryngeal mask airway insertion, produces reversible bronchoconstriction. *Anesthesiology.* 1999;90:391.
53. Nair I, Bailey PM. Use of the laryngeal mask for airway maintenance following trachea extubation [letter]. *Anaesthesia.* 1995;50:174.
54. Goldmann K, Kuhlmann S, Gerlach M, et al. Removal of the laryngeal mask airway in the post-anesthesia care unit : A means of process optimization. *Anaesthestist.* 2011;60:1002.
55. Deakin CD, Diprose P, Majumdar R, et al. An investigation into the quantity of secretions removed by inflated and deflated laryngeal mask airways. *Anaesthesia.* 2000;55:478.
56. Brimacombe JR. Advanced uses: Clinical situations. In: Brimacombe JR, Brain AIJ, eds. *The Laryngeal Mask Airway. A Review and Practical Guide.* London: WB Saunders; 2004:138.
57. Turkstra TP, Smitheram AK, Alabdulhadi O, et al. The Flex-Tip™ tracheal tube does not reduce the incidence of postoperative sore throat: A randomized controlled trial. *Can J Anaesth.* 2011;58:1090.
58. Brimacombe J, Clarke G, Keller C. Lingual nerve injury associated with the ProSeal laryngeal mask airway: A case report and review of the literature. *Br J Anaesth.* 2005;95:420.
59. Bortone L, Ingelmo PM, De Ninno G, et al. Randomized controlled trial comparing the laryngeal tube and the laryngeal mask in pediatric patients. *Paediatr Anaesth.* 2006;16:251.
60. Zand F, Amini A. Use of the laryngeal tube-S for airway management and prevention of aspiration after a failed tracheal intubation in a parturient. *Anesthesiology.* 2005;102:481.
61. Keller C, Brimacombe J, Kleinsasser A, et al. Pharyngeal mucosal pressures with the laryngeal tube airway versus ProSeal laryngeal mask airway. *Anasthesiol Intensivmed Notfallmed Schmerzther.* 2003;38:393.
62. Banchereau F, Delaunay F, Herve Y, et al. Oropharyngeal ulcers following anaesthesia with the laryngeal tube S. *Ann Fr Anesth Reanim.* 2006;25:884.
63. Galgon RE, Schroeder KM, Han S, et al. The air-Q(®) intubating laryngeal airway vs the LMA-ProSeal(TM): A prospective, randomised trial of airway seal pressure. *Anaesthesia.* 2011;66:1093.
64. Erlacher W, Tiefenbrunner H, Kästenbauer T, et al. CobraPLUS and Cookgas air-Q versus Fastrach for blind endotracheal intubation: A randomised controlled trial. *Eur J Anaesthesiol.* 2011;28:181.
65. O'Connor CJ, Borromeo CJ, Stix MS. Assessing proseal laryngeal mask position: The suprasternal notch test. *Anesth Analg.* 2002;94:1374.
66. Brain AIJ, Verghese C, Strube PJ. The LMA Proseal—a laryngeal mask with an oesophageal vent. *Br J Anaesth.* 2000;84:650.
67. Stix MS, O'Connor CJ. Depth of insertion of the proseal laryngeal mask airway. *Br J Anesth.* 2003;90:235.
68. Brimacombe J, Keller C, Fullkrug B, et al. A multicenter study comparing the proseal and classic laryngeal mask airway in anesthetized, non-paralyzed patients. *Anesthesiology.* 2002;96:289.
69. Rosenblatt WH. The use of the LMA-proseal in airway resuscitation. *Anesth Analg.* 2004;97:1773.
70. Awan R, Nolan JP, Cook TM. Use of the proseal laryngeal mask for airway maintenance during emergency cesarean section of the failed tracheal intubation. *Br J Anaesth.* 2004;92:144.
71. Beleña JM, Gracia JL, Ayala JL, et al. The Laryngeal Mask Airway Supreme for positive pressure ventilation during laparoscopic cholecystectomy. *J Clin Anesth.* 2011;23:456.
72. Beringer RM, Kelly F, Cook TM, et al. A cohort evaluation of the paediatric i-gel(™) airway during anaesthesia in 120 children. *Anaesthesia.* 2011;66:1121.
73. El-Orbany M, Woehick H, Salem MR. Head and neck position for direct laryngoscopy. *Anesth Anal.* 2011;113:103.
74. Adnet F, Borran SW, Lapostalle F, et al. The three axis alignment theory and the sniffing position: Perpetuation of an anatomic myth? *Anesthesiology.* 1999; 91:1964.
75. Chou HC, Wu TL. Rethinking the three axis alignment theory for direct laryngoscopy. *Acta Anaesthesiol Scand.* 2001;45:261.
76. Rosenblatt WH. Preoperative planning of airway management in critical care patients. *Crit Care Med.* 2004;32(4 suppl):186.
77. Mallampati SR, Gatt SP, Gugino LD, et al. A clinical sign to predict difficult tracheal intubation: A prospective study. *Can Anaesth Soc J.* 1985;32:429.
78. Ayoub C, Baraka A, el-Khatib M, et al. A new cut-off point of thyromental distance for prediction of difficult airway. *Middle East J Anesthesiol.* 2000;15:619.
79. Chou HC, Wu TL. Thyromental distance and anterior larynx: Misconceptional and misname? *Anesth Analg.* 2003;96:1526.
80. Levitan RM. Advanced concepts in laryngoscope blade design. In: Levitan RM, ed. *The Airway Cam Guide to Intubation and Practical Emergency Airway Management.* Pennsylvania, PA: Exton; 2004:185.
81. Hagberg CA, ed. *Benumof's Airway Management: Principles and Practice.* Philadelphia, PA: Mosby; 2007.
82. Cormack RS, Lehane J. Difficult tracheal intubation in obstetrics. *Anaesthesia.* 1984;39:1105.
83. Crosby ET, Cooper RM, Douglas MJ, et al. The unanticipated difficult airway with recommendations for management. *Can J Anaesth.* 1998;45:757.
84. Koh LK, Kong CE, Ip-Yam PC. The modified Cormack-Lehane score for the grading of direct laryngoscopy: Evaluation in the Asian population. *Anaesth Intensive Care.* 2002;30:48.
85. Ochroch EA, Hollander JE, Kush S, et al. Assessment of laryngeal view: Percentage of glottic opening score vs Cormack and Lehane grading. *Can J Anaesth.* 1999;46:987.
86. Ulrich B, Listyo R, Gerig HJ, et al. The difficult intubation: The value of BURP and 3 predictive tests of difficult intubation. *Anaesthesist.* 1998;47:45.
87. Benumof JL, Cooper SD. Quantitative improvement in laryngoscopic view by optimal external laryngeal manipulation. *J Clin Anesth.* 1996;8:136.
88. Henderson JJ. The use of the paraglossal straight blade laryngoscopy in difficult tracheal intubation. *Anaesthesia.* 1997;52:552.
89. Cardoso MM, Banner MJ, Melker RJ, et al. Portable devices used to detect endotracheal intubation during emergency situations: A review. *Crit Care Med.* 1998;26:957.
90. Rose DK, Cohen MM. The airway: Problems and predictions in 18,500 patients. *Can J Anaesth.* 1994;41:372.
91. Turkstra TP, Pelz DM, Shaikh AA, et al. Cervical spine motion: A fluoroscopic comparison of Shikani Optical Stylet® vs Macintosh laryngoscope. *Can J Anaesth.* 2007;54:441.
92. Rudolph C, Schneider JP, Wallenborn J, et al. Movement of the upper cervical spine during laryngoscopy: A comparison of the Bonfils intubation fibrescope and the Macintosh laryngoscope. *Anaesthesia.* 2005;60:668.
93. Halligan M, Charters P. A clinical evaluation of the Bonfils intubation fiberscope. *Anaesthesia.* 2003;58:1087.
94. Greenland KB, Liu G, Tan H, et al. Comparison of the Levitan FPS Scope and the single-use bougie for simulated difficult intubation in anaesthetised patients. *Anaesthesia.* 2007;62:509.
95. Levitan R. Design rationale and intended use of a short optical stylet for routine fiberoptic augmentation of emergency laryngoscopy. *Ann Emerg Med.* 2006;24:490.
96. Heidegger T, Gerig HJ, Ulrich B, et al. Validation of a simple algorithm for tracheal intubation: Daily practice is the key to success in emergencies and analysis of 13,248 intubations. *Anesth Anal.* 2001;92:517.
97. Cooper RM, Pacey JA, Bishop MJ, et al. Early clinical experience with a new videolaryngoscope (GlideScope) in 728 patients. *Can J Anaesth.* 2005;52:191.
98. Aziz M, Healy D, Kheterpal S, et al. Routine clinical practice effectiveness of the Glidescope in difficult airway management. *Anesthesiology.* 2011;14:1.
99. Sun DA, Warriner CB, Parsons DG, et al. The GlideScope video laryngoscope: Randomized clinical trial in 200 patients. *Br J Anaesth.* 2005;94:381.
100. Kramer DC, Osborn IP. More maneuvers to facilitate tracheal intubation with the GlideScope. *Can J Anaesth.* 2006;53:737.
101. Doyle DJ, Zura A, Ramachandran M. Video laryngoscopy in the management of the difficult airway. *Can J Anaesth.* 2004;51:95.
102. Dow WA, Parsons DG. 'Reverse loading' to facilitate Glidescope intubation. *Can J Anaesth.* 2007;54:161.
103. Jones PM, Turkstra TP, Armstrong KP, et al. Effect of stylet angulation and endotracheal tube camber on time to intubation with the GlideScope. *Can J Anaesth.* 2007;54:21.
104. Turkstra TP, Craen RA, Pelz DM, et al. Cervical spine motion: A fluoroscopic comparison during intubation with lighted stylet, GlideScope, and Macintosh laryngoscope. *Anesth Analg.* 2005;101:910.
105. Gunaydin B, Gungor I, Yigit N, et al. The Glidescope for tracheal intubation in patients with ankylosing spondylitis. comment. *Br J Anaesth.* 2007;98:408.
106. Xue FS, Zhang GH, Li XY, et al. Comparison of hemodynamic responses to orotracheal intubation with the GlideScope(R) video laryngoscope and the Macintosh direct laryngoscope. *J Clin Anesth.* 2007;19:245.

107. Cross P, Cytryn J, Cheng KK. Perforation of the soft palate using the GlideScope(R) videolaryngoscope. *Can J Anaesth.* 2007;54:588.
108. Hirabayashi Y. Pharyngeal injury related to GlideScope video laryngoscope. Otolaryngol. *Head Neck Surg.* 2007;137:175.
109. Cooper RM. Complications associated with the use of the GlideScope video laryngoscope. *Can J Anaesth.* 2007;54:54.
110. Choo MK, Yeo VS, See JJ. Another complication associated with video laryngoscopy. *Can J Anaesth.* 2007;54:322.
111. Malik AM, Frogel JK. Anterior tonsillar pillar perforation during GlideScope video laryngoscopy. *Anesth Analg.* 2007;104:1610.
112. Kaplan MB, Hagberg CA, Ward DS, et al. Comparison of direct and video-assisted views of the larynx during routine intubation. *J Clin Anesth.* 2006;18:357.
113. Kaplan MB, Ward D, Hagberg CA, et al. Seeing is believing: The importance of video laryngoscopy in teaching and in managing the difficult airway. *Surg Endosc.* 2006;20(suppl 2):S479.
114. Skippey B, Ray D, McKeown D. The McGrath video laryngoscope—an initial clinical evaluation. *Can J Anesth.* 2007;54:307.
115. Maharaj CH, Costello JF, McDonnell JG, et al. The Airtraq as a rescue airway device following failed direct laryngoscopy: A case series. *Anaesthesia.* 2007; 62:598.
116. Suzuki A, Toyama Y, Iwasaki H, et al. Airtraq for awake tracheal intubation. *Anaesthesia.* 2007;62:746.
117. Maharaj CH, Buckley E, Harte BH, et al. Endotracheal intubation in patients with cervical spine immobilization: A comparison of Macintosh and Airtraq laryngoscopes. *Anesthesiology.* 2007;107:53.
118. Malik MA, Subramaniam R, Maharaj CH et al: Randomized controlled trial of the Pentax AWS® Glidescope® and Macintosh laryngoscopies in predicted difficult intubation. *Br J Anaesth* 2009;103:761
119. Suzuki A, Abe N, Sasakawa T, et al. Pentax-AWS (Airway Scope) and Airtraq: Big difference between two similar devices. *J Anesth.* 2008;22:1–2.
120. Kristensen S. Airway management and morbid obesity. *Eur J Anaesth.* 2010; 27:923.
121. Juvin P, Fevre G, Merouche M, et al. Gastric residue is not more copious in obese patients. *Anesth Analg.* 2001;93:162.
122. Harter RL, Kelly WB, Kramer MG, et al. A comparison of the volume and pH of gastric contents of obese and lean surgical patients. *Anesth Analg.* 1998;86:147.
123. Practice Guidelines for Preoperative Fasting and the Use of Pharmacologic Agents to Reduce the Risk of Pulmonary Aspiration. Application to healthy patients undergoing elective procedures. *Anesthesiology.* 2011;114:495.
124. Van Den Driessche M, Peeters K, Marien P, et al. Gastric emptying in formula-fed and breast-fed infants measured with 13C-octanoic acid breath test. *J Pediatr Gastroenterol Nutr.* 1999;29:46.
125. Merio R, Festa A, Bergmann H, et al. Slow gastric emptying in Type I diabetes: Relation to autonomic and peripheral neuropathy, blood glucose, and glycemic control. *Diabetes Care.* 1997;20:419.
126. Kulkarni PN, Batra YK, Wig J. Effects of different combinations of H2 receptor antagonist with gastrokinetic drugs on gastric fluid pH and volume in children—a comparative study. *Int J Pharmacol Ther.* 1997;35:561.
127. Nishina K, Mikawa K, Takao Y, et al. A comparison of rabeprazole, lansoprazole and ranitidine for improving preoperative gastric fluid property in adults undergoing elective surgery. *Anesth Analg.* 2000;90:717.
128. Nishina K, Mikawa K, Maekawa N, et al. A comparison of lansoprazole, omeprazole and ranitidine for reducing preoperative gastric secretion in adult patients undergoing elective surgery. *Anesth Analg.* 1996;82:832.
129. Escolano F, Castano J, Lopez R, et al. Effects of omeprazole, ranitidine, Famotidine and placebo on gastric secretion in patients undergoing elective surgery. *Br J Anaesth.* 1992;69:404.
130. Vanner RG, Asai T. Safe use of cricoid pressure. *Anaesthesia.* 1999;54:1.
131. Smith KJ, Dombranowski J, Yip G, et al. Cricoid pressure displaces the esophagus: An observational study using magnetic resonance imaging. *Anesthesiology.* 2003;99:60.
132. Brown JPR. Bag valve mask ventilation in rapid sequence induction. *Anaesthesia.* 2004;69:784.
133. Alstrom HB, Belhage B. Cricoid pressure in rapid sequence intubation? *Ugeskr Laeger.* 2007;169:2305.
134. Brain AI, Verghese C, Addy EV, et al. The intubating laryngeal mask. I: Development of a new device for intubation of the trachea. *Br J Anaesth.* 1997;79:699.
135. Kundra P, Sujata N, Ravishankar M. Conventional tracheal tubes for intubation through the intubating laryngeal mask airway. *Anesth Analg.* 2005;100:284.
136. Ferson DZ, Rosenblatt WH, Johansen MJ, et al. Use of the intubating LMA-Fastrach in 254 patients with difficult-to-manage airways. *Anesthesiology.* 2001; 95:1175.
137. Joffe AM, Liew EC, Galgon RE et al: The second-generation air-Q intubating laryngeal mask for airway maintenance during anaesthesia in adults: a report of the first 70 uses. 2011;39:40
138. Rosenblatt WH, Murphy M. The intubating laryngeal mask: Use of a new ventilating intubating device in the emergency department. *Ann Emerg Med.* 1999; 33:234.
139. Sinha R, Chandralekha B, Ray R. Evaluation of air-Q(TM) intubating laryngeal airway as a conduit for tracheal intubation in infants – a pilot study. *Paed Anaesth.* 2011;22:156.
140. Miller KA, Harkin CP, Bailey PL. Postoperative tracheal extubation. *Anesth Analg.* 1995;80:149.
141. Murphy GS, Brull SJ. Residual neuromuscular block: Lessons unlearned. Part I: Definitions, incidence, and adverse physiologic effects of residual neuromuscular block. *Anesth Analg.* 2010;111:120.
142. Murphy GS, Szokol JW, Marymont JH, et al. Residual paralysis at the time of tracheal extubation. *Anesth Analg.* 2005;100:1840.
143. Gaszynski T, Szewczyk T, Gaszynski W. Randomized comparison of sugammadex and neostigmine for reversal of rocuronium-induced muscle relaxation in morbidly obese undergoing general anaesthesia. *Br J Anaesth.* 2012;108: 236.
144. Shin SH, Heath K, Reeds S, et al. The cuff leak test is not predictive of successful extubation. *Am Surg.* 2008;74:1182.
145. Lee CH, Peng MJ, Wu CL. Dexamethasone to prevent post extubation airway obstruction in adults: A prospective, randomized, double-blind, placebo-controlled study. *Crit Care.* 2007;11:R72.
146. Mort TC. Continuous airway access for the difficult extubation: The efficacy of the airway exchange catheter. *Anesth Analg.* 2007;105:1357.
147. Harris K, Chalhoub M, Maroun R, et al. Endotracheal tube exchangers: Should we look for safer alternatives? *Heart Lung.* 2012;41:67.
148. Mort TC, Meisterling EM, Waberski WM. Exchanging a tracheal tube in the ICU patient: A comparison of two exchangers with direct laryngoscopy. *Anesthesiology.* 1997;87:240A.
149. Daucourt V, Michel P, Avargues P, et al. Guidelines on difficult intubation in anesthesia: Evaluation of 2 information diffusion methods. *Rev Epidemiol Sante Publique.* 1999;47:353.
150. Kroesen G. Guidelines for the advanced management of the airway and ventilation during resuscitation. A statement by the airway and ventilation management working group of the European Resuscitation Council, 1996. *Resuscitation.* 1997;35:89.
151. Petrini F, Accorsi A, Adrario E, et al. Gruppo di Studio SIAARTI Vie Aeree Difficili; Recommendations for airway control and difficult airway management. *Minerva Anestesiol.* 2005;71:617.
152. Henderson J, Popat M, Latto P, et al. Difficult airway society guidelines. *Anaesthesia.* 2004;59:1242.
153. Schalte G, Rex S, Henzler D. Airway management. *Anaesthesist.* 2007;56:837.
154. Rosenblatt WH. Awake intubation made easy! ASA refresher courses in anesthesiology. 2009;37:167.
155. Mort TC. Emergency tracheal intubation: Complications associated with repeated laryngoscopic attempts. *Anesth Analg.* 2004;99:607.
156. Nandi PR, Charlesworth CH, Taylor SJ, et al. Effect of general anaesthesia on the pharynx. *Br J Anaesth.* 1991;66:157.
157. Benumof JL. Management of the difficult adult airway: With special emphasis on awake tracheal intubation. *Anesthesiology.* 1991;75:1087.
158. Madhere M, Vanguar D, Saidov A. Dexmedetomidine as sole agent for awake fiberoptic intubation in a patient with local anesthetic allergy. *J Anesth.* 2011; 25:592.
159. Nydahl PA, Axelsson K. Venous blood concentration of lidocaine after nasopharyngeal application of 2% lidocaine gel. *Acta Anaesthesiol Scand.* 1988; 32:135.
160. Wieczorek PM, Schricker T, Vinet B, et al. Airway topicalisation in morbidly obese patients using atomised lidocaine: 2% compared with 4%. *Anaesthesia.* 2007; 62:984.
161. Weisel W, Tella RA. Reaction to tetracaine used as topical anesthetic in bronchoscopy: A study of 1000 cases. *JAMA.* 1951;147:218.
162. AHFS Drug Information 2007. In: McEvoy GK, ed. *Methylene Blue.* Bethesda, MD: American Society of Health-System Pharmacists; 2007:3664.
163. Sitzman BT, Rich GF, Rockwell JJ, et al. Local anesthetic administration for awake direct laryngoscopy. Are glossopharyngeal nerve blocks superior? *Anesthesiology.* 1997;86:34.
164. Ovassapian A, ed. *Fiberoptic Endoscopy and the Difficult Airway.* Philadelphia, PA: Lippincott-Raven; 1996:47.
165. Rosenblatt WH, Wagner PJ, Ovassapian A, et al. Practice patterns in managing the difficult airway by anesthesiologists in the United States. *Anesth Analg.* 1998;87:153.
166. Murphy P. A fibre-optic endoscope used for nasal intubation. *Anaesthesia.* 1967; 22:489.
167. Ovassapian A, Yelich SJ, Dykes MH, et al. Learning fibreoptic intubation: Use of simulators vs. traditional teaching. *Br J Anaesth.* 1988;61:217.
168. Hershey MD, Hannenberg AA. Gastric distention and rupture from oxygen insufflation during fiberoptic intubation. *Anesthesiology.* 1996;85:1479.
169. Rosenblatt WH. Overcoming obstruction during bronchoscope-guided intubation of the trachea with the double setup endotracheal tube. *Anesth Analg.* 1996; 83:175.
170. Ovassapian A, Yellich J, Dykes MHM, et al. Fiberoptic nasotracheal intubation: Incidence and causes of failure. *Anesth Analg.* 1983;62:692.
171. Kristensen MS. The Parker flex-tip tube versus a standard tube for fiberoptic orotracehal intubation: Randomized double blind study. *Anesthesiology.* 2003; 98:334.
172. Martin SE, Ochsner MG, Jarman RH, et al. Laryngeal mask airway in air transport when intubation fails: Case report. *J Trauma.* 1997;42:333.

173. Brimacombe JR, De Maio B. Emergency use of the laryngeal mask airway during helicopter transfer of a neonate. *J Clin Anesth.* 1995;7:689.
174. Parmet JL, Colonna-Romano P, Horrow JC, et al. The laryngeal mask airway reliably provides rescue ventilation in cases of unanticipated difficult tracheal intubation along with difficult mask ventilation. *Anesth Analg.* 1998;87:661.
175. Asai T, Latto P. Role of the laryngeal mask in patients with difficult tracheal intubation and difficult ventilation. In: Latto IP, Vaughan RS, eds. *Difficulties in Tracheal Intubation.* London: WB Saunders; 1997:177.
176. Brimacombe JR, Berry AM. Mallampati grade and laryngeal mask placement. *Anesth Analg.* 1996;82:1112.
177. Cook TM, Lee G, Nolan JP. The ProSeal laryngeal mask airway: A review of the literature. *Can J Anaesth.* 2005;52:739.
178. Agro F, Frass M, Benumof JL, et al. Current status of the Combitube: A review of the literature. *J Clin Anesth.* 2002;14:307.
179. Verghese C, Prior Willeard PFS. Immediate management of the airway during cardiopulmonary resuscitation in a hospital without a resident anaesthesiologist. *Eur J Emerg Med.* 1994;1:123.
180. Keller C, Brimacombe J, Bittersohl J, et al. Aspiration and laryngeal mask airway: Three cases and a review of the literature. *Br J Anaesth.* 2004;93:579.
181. Aoyama K, Takenaka I. Cricoid pressure impedes positioning and ventilation through the laryngeal mask. *Can J Anaesth.* 1996;43:1035.
182. Gnauck K, Lungo JB, Scalzo A, et al. Emergency intubation of the pediatric medical patient: Use of anesthetic agents in the emergency department. *Ann Emerg Med.* 1994;23:1242.
183. Li J, Murphy-Lavoie H, Bugas C, et al. Complications of emergency intubation with and without paralysis. *Am J Emerg Med.* 1999;17:141.
184. Sivarajan M, Joy JV. Effects of general anesthesia and paralysis on upper airway changes due to head position in humans. *Anesthesiology.* 1996;85:787.
185. Walls RM. Management of the difficult airway in the trauma patient. *Emerg Med Clin North Am.* 1998;16:45.
186. Hamaekers AEW, Borg PAJ, Enk D. A bench study of ventilation via two self-assembled jet devices and the oxygen flow modulator in simulated upper airway obstruction. *Anaesthesia.* 2009;64:1353.
187. Elliott DSJ, Baker PA, Scott MR, et al. Accuracy of surface landmark identification for cannula cricothyroidotomy. *Anaesthesia.* 2010;65:889.
188. Kristensen MS. Ultrasonography in the management of the airway. *Acta Anaesthesiol Scand.* 2011;55:1155.
189. Hamaekers A, Borg P, Enk D. The importance of flow and pressure release in emergency jet ventilation devices. *Paed Anaesth.* 2009;19:452.
190. Lenfant F, Péan D, Brisard L, et al. Oxygen delivery during transtracheal oxygenation: A comparison of two manual devices. *Anesth Analg.* 2010;111:922.
191. Bellemain A, Ghimouz A, Goater P, et al. Bilateral tension pneumothorax after retrieval of transtracheal jet ventilation catheter. *Ann Fr Anesth Reanim.* 2006;25:401.

CHAPTER

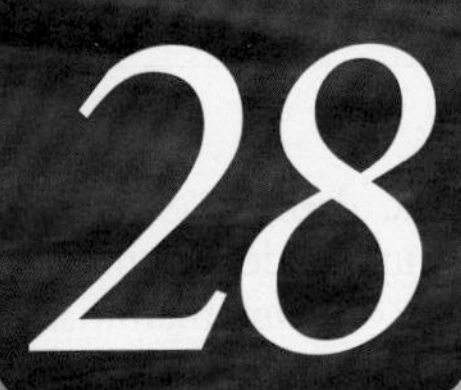

Patient Positioning and Potential Injuries

MARY E. WARNER

Key Points

1. Sedated or anesthetized patients should be placed in positions that are comfortable while they are awake.
2. Padding provided by any number of different materials (e.g., gel or foam pads, blankets) should be used to widely disperse point pressure on body parts and soft tissues.
3. The etiologies of peripheral neuropathies are often not clear. While there are potential anatomic and neurophysiologic reasons, recent data suggest that general inflammatory reactions may be important etiologic factors.
4. Positioning-related perioperative vision loss has been catastrophic for patients undergoing extensive spine procedures while positioned prone. Recent data suggest that it may be related to venous congestion in the optic canal. Measures to reduce the frequency and severity of this problem are presented.
5. Excessive flexion or extension of the spine in anesthetized patients who are placed in unique surgical positions may contribute to spinal cord ischemia and catastrophic neurologic damage.

Multimedia

1. Brachial Plexus Injury
2. Upper Extremity Neuropathy
3. Ulnar Nerve Compression
4. Ventilation and Perfusion in the Lateral Position
5. Prone Position Facial
6. Prone Position

1 Positioning a patient for a surgical procedure is frequently a compromise between what the anesthetized patient can tolerate, both structurally and physiologically, and what the surgical team requires for access to its anatomic target. Establishment of the intended surgical posture may need to be modified to match the patient's tolerance. This chapter presents the significance of various positions in which a patient may be placed during an operation, briefly describes the techniques of establishing the positions, and discusses the potential complications of each posture. It also will present recent data that suggest perioperative inflammatory responses to play an important role in the development of peripheral and, potentially, central neuropathies.

It is very important for clinicians to understand the physiologic and potential pathologic consequences of patient positioning. A number of studies of large surgical populations have provided information on the frequency and natural history of rare perioperative events such as neuropathies and vision loss. However, these studies frequently have provided insufficient data to allow speculation as to potential mechanisms of injury. Based on the findings of these studies, investigators are seeking to confirm mechanisms of injury and the efficacy of novel interventions to decrease the frequency of these perioperative events. Until these investigations are complete, the etiologic mechanisms for many potential positioning-related complications remain unknown.

The lack of solid scientific information on basic mechanisms of positioning-related complications often leads to medicolegal entanglements. Notations on anesthesia and operating room records may be absent or uninformative. Careful descriptive notations about positions used during anesthesia and surgery, as well as brief comments about special protective measures such as eye care and pressure-point padding, are useful to include on the anesthesia record. In potentially complicated or contentious circumstances, a separate brief description of care documented in the patient's record is advisable. Only in this manner can subsequent inquiries be properly answered on behalf of either the patient or the anesthesiologist. When credible, expanded knowledge that further delineates mechanisms of positioning-related complications is available, these issues and the care of patients will be improved.

GENERAL PRINCIPLES

2 Without doubt, direct compression of neural and soft tissue may result in ischemia and tissue damage. Many efforts have been directed at provider education over the years to reduce direct tissue trauma from compression. Most anesthesia providers are taught from the start of their training that various maneuvers, pads, and positioning devices are useful to reduce point pressure on neural and soft tissues. Despite these efforts, neuropathies and soft tissue damage still occur. Is it a failure of education, the incorrect application of this information, or other issues that contribute to the continued presence of perioperative positioning injuries? Or perhaps, are there etiologic mechanisms at work that we do not yet understand?

3 Recent work by Staff et al.[1] at Mayo Clinic suggests that we do not yet fully understand the etiologic mechanisms of positioning issues. The authors reported inflammatory neuropathies in 33 patients who had severe postsurgical peripheral neuropathies, with most involving the ulnar nerve and motor components of it. Surprisingly, the majority of these patients had widespread microvasculitic neuropathies, and many were responsive to immunologic modulation with high doses of corticosteroids. The inflammatory response may be dramatically altered in the postoperative period, and microvasculitic neuropathy appears to be a previously unrecognized cause of peripheral neuropathy. Large epidemiologic studies will eventually help determine the role that this new etiology plays in the origin of perioperative neuropathies of all sorts. In the meantime, this report serves as evidence that a number of perioperative neuropathies may, in fact, have no relationship to intraoperative positioning or management of physiologic factors.[2]

Viruses have been associated with central as well as peripheral neuropathies that develop in the perioperative period. As noted above, immunosuppression is present in a fairly significant proportion of patients undergoing major surgical procedures. Anesthetics, blood products, and even antibiotics have been shown to result in varying degrees of immunosuppression.[3] This immunosuppression may provide opportunities for existing viruses or newly introduced viruses to activate, particularly in neural tissues. For example, the onset of shingles may be more frequent in surgical compared to general populations.[4]

Positioning can, of course, cause tissue damage. Stretch of neural tissue may be an important factor in the development of peripheral and central neuropathies. Stretch of many mammalian nerves to 5% greater than their normal resting length has been shown repeatedly to lead to ischemia by reducing both arteriole and venule blood flow. The kinking of the arterioles and venules associated with neuronal stretch leads to ischemia. If the ischemia is prolonged, it may result in permanent neural damage. The impact of stretch on other soft tissues is less well documented and would be highly dependent on the type of tissue and amount of stretch.

Point pressure on any soft tissue may reduce local blood flow and cause ischemia. There are many ways to reduce point pressure, but the most commonly used involve padding. While there may be distinct differences in mechanical properties of various padding materials (e.g., gels, foam, textiles, and others), none have been proven to be significantly better than the others in reducing the frequency or severity of nerve or soft tissue damage perioperatively. The basic principle is to use any of these materials to protect nerves and soft tissues from point pressure.

SUPINE POSITIONS

Variations of Supine Positions

Supine

Horizontal

In the traditional supine position, the patient lies on his or her back with a small pillow beneath the head (Fig. 28-1). The arms are either comfortably padded and restrained alongside the trunk or abducted on well-padded arm boards. Either arm (or both) may be extended ventrally and the flexed forearm secured to an elevated frame in such a way that perfusion of the hand is not compromised, no skin-to-metal contact exists to cause electrical burns if a cautery is used, and the brachial neurovascular bundle is neither stretched nor compressed at the axilla. The lumbar spine may need padded support to prevent a postoperative backache (see "Complications of Supine Positions"). Bony contact points at the occiput, elbows, and heels should be padded. Fortunately, most modern surgical tables have mattress pads that are sufficiently buoyant and thick to allow dispersion of point pressure.

Although the horizontal supine posture has a long history of widespread use, it does not place hip and knee joints in neutral positions and is poorly tolerated for prolonged periods by an immobilized, awake patient.

Contoured

A contoured supine posture (Fig. 28-2) has been termed the *lawn chair position*. It is established by arranging the surface of the operating table so that the trunk–thigh hinge is angulated approximately 15 degrees and the thigh–knee hinge is angulated a similar amount in the opposite direction. Alternatively, a rolled towel, pillow, or blanket can be placed beneath the patient's knees to keep them flexed. The patient of average height then lies comfortably with hips and knees flexed gently.

Lateral Uterine or Abdominal Mass Displacement

With a patient in the supine position, a mobile abdominal mass, such as a very large tumor or a pregnant uterus, can rest on the great vessels of the abdomen and compromise circulation. This is known as the *aortocaval syndrome* or the *supine hypotensive*

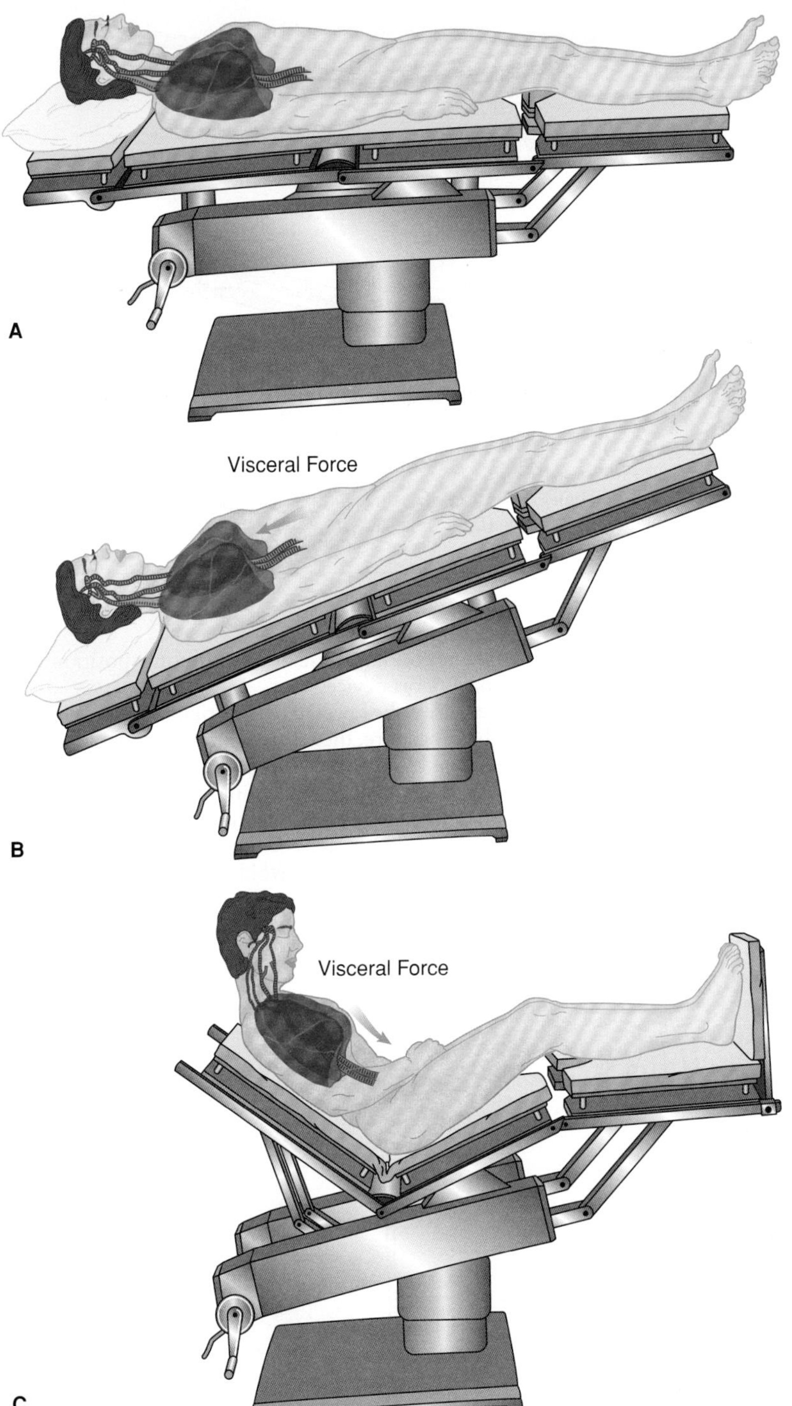

FIGURE 28-1. A: Supine adult with minimal gradients in the horizontal vascular axis. Pulmonary blood volume is greatest dorsally. Viscera displace the diaphragm cephalad. Cerebral circulation is slightly above heart level if the head is on a small pillow. **B:** Head-down tilt aids blood return from lower extremities but encourages reflex vasodilation, congests vessels in the poorly ventilated lung apices, and increases intracranial blood volume. **C:** Elevation of the head shifts abdominal viscera away from the diaphragm and improves ventilation of the lung bases. According to the gradient above the heart, pressure in arteries of the head and neck decreases; pressure in accompanying veins may become subatmospheric.

syndrome. A significant degree of perfusion can be restored if the compressive mass is rolled toward the left hemiabdomen by leftward tilt of the tabletop or by a wedge under the right hip.

Lithotomy

Standard

In the standard lithotomy position (Fig. 28-3), the patient lies supine, typically with one or both arms extended laterally to <90 degrees on arm boards. Each lower extremity is flexed at the hip and knee, and both limbs are simultaneously elevated and separated so that the perineum becomes accessible to the surgeon. For many gynecologic and urologic procedures, the patient's thighs are flexed approximately 90 degrees on the trunk and the knees are bent sufficiently to maintain the lower legs nearly parallel to the floor. More acute flexion of the knees or hips can threaten to angulate and compress major vessels at either joint. In addition, hip flexion to >90 degrees on the trunk has been shown to increase stretch of the inguinal ligaments.[5] Branches of the lateral

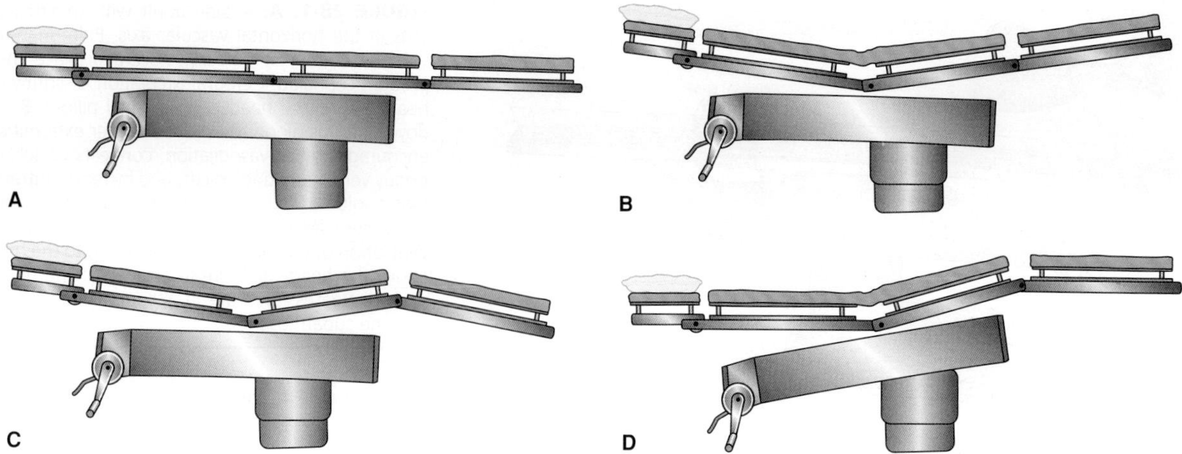

FIGURE 28-2. Establishment of the contoured supine ("lawn chair") position. **(A)** Traditional flat supine tabletop. **(B)** Thighs flexed on trunk. **(C)** Knees gently flexed in final body position. **(D)** Trunk section leveled to stabilize floor-supported arm board.

femoral cutaneous nerves often pass directly through these ligaments and can be impinged and become ischemic within the stretched ligament.

Numerous devices are available to hold legs that are elevated during obstetric delivery or perineal operations. Each device should be fitted to the stature of the individual patient. Care should be taken to ensure that angulations or edges of the padded holder do not compress the popliteal space or the upper dorsal thigh. Compartment syndromes of one or both lower extremities have resulted from prolonged use of the lithotomy position with various types of support devices.

When the legs are to be lowered to the original supine position at the end of the procedure, they should first be brought together at the knees and ankles in the sagittal plane and then lowered slowly together to the tabletop. This minimizes torsion stress on the lumbar spine that would occur if each leg were lowered independently. It also permits gradual accommodation to the increase in circulatory capacitance, thereby avoiding sudden hypotension.

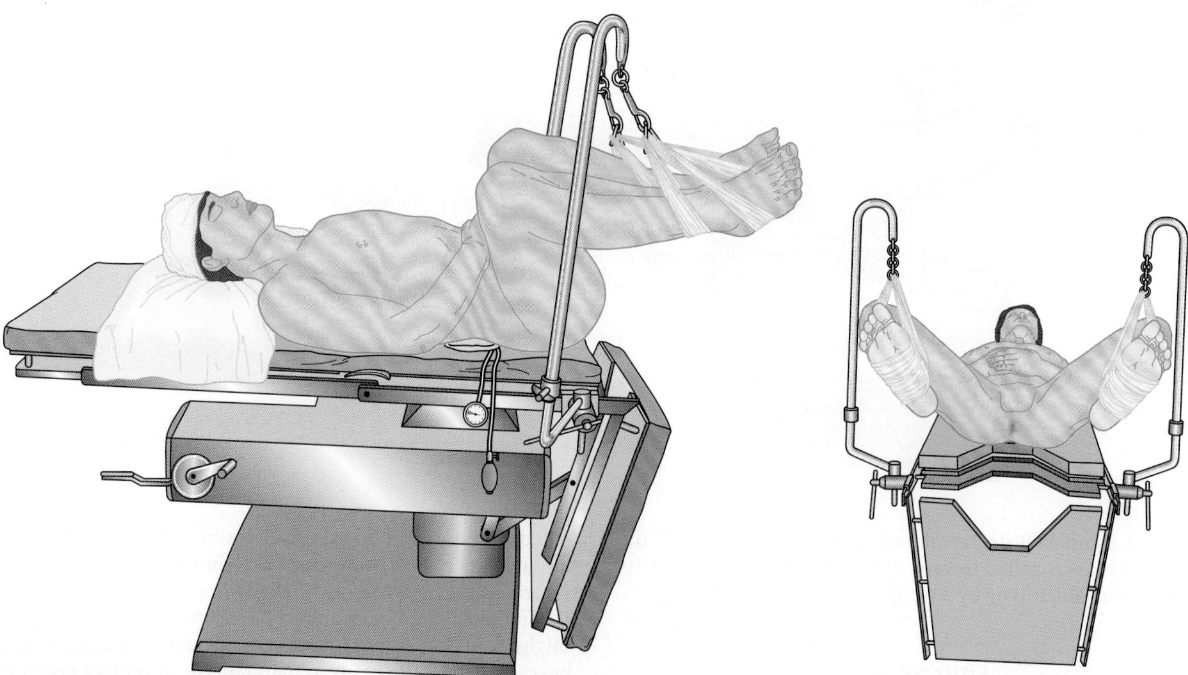

FIGURE 28-3. Standard lithotomy position with "candy cane" extremity support. Thighs are flexed approximately 90 degrees on abdomen; knees are flexed enough to bring lower legs grossly parallel to the torso section of the tabletop. Arms are retained on boards, crossed on the abdomen, or snugged at the sides of patient.

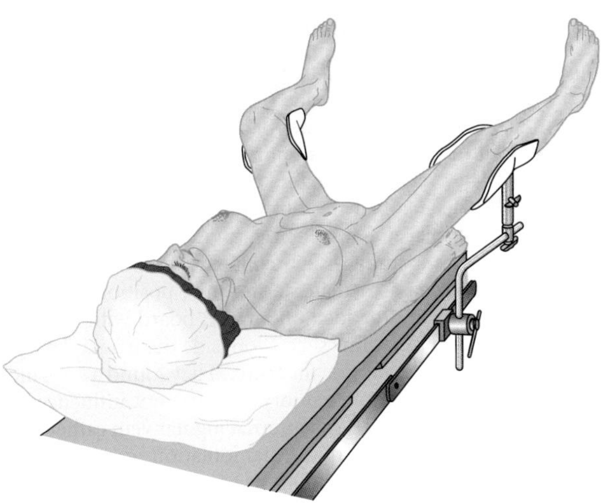

FIGURE 28-4. Low lithotomy position for perineal access, transurethral instrumentation, or combined abdominoperineal procedures.

Low

For most urologic procedures and for many procedures that require simultaneous access to the abdomen and perineum, the degree of thigh elevation in the lithotomy position is only approximately 30 to 45 degrees (Fig. 28-4). This reduces perfusion gradients to and from the lower extremities and improves access to a perineal surgical site for members of the operating team who may need to stand at the lateral aspect of either leg.

High

Some surgeons prefer to improve access to the perineum by suspending the patient's feet from high poles. The effect is to have the patient's legs almost fully extended on the thighs (Fig. 28-5) and the thighs flexed 90 degrees or more on the trunk. The posture produces a significant uphill gradient for arterial perfusion into the feet, requiring careful avoidance of systemic hypotension. There is considerable variation in lower extremity perfusion pressure in volunteers placed in high lithotomy positions; however, they all tend to have low perfusion pressures.[6,7] Less mobile patients may tolerate this posture poorly because of angulation and compression of the contents of the femoral canal by the inguinal ligament (Fig. 28-5A), or stretch of the sciatic nerve (Fig. 28-5B), or both.

Exaggerated

Transperineal access to the retropubic area requires that the patient's pelvis be flexed ventrally on the spine, the thighs almost forcibly flexed on the trunk, and the lower legs aimed skyward so they are out of the way (Fig. 28-6). The result places the long axis of the symphysis pubis almost parallel to the floor. This exaggerated

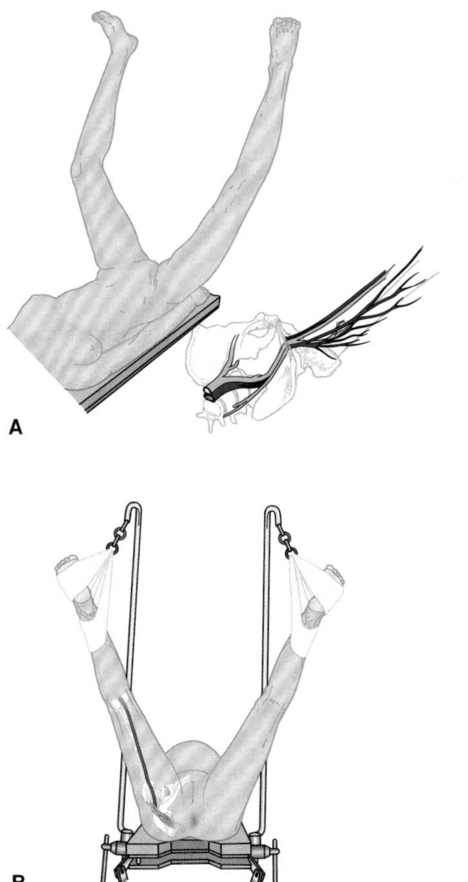

FIGURE 28-5. High lithotomy position. Note potential for angulation and compression/obstruction of contents of femoral canal (**A**, *inset*) or stretch of sciatic nerve **(B)**. Reproduced from: McLeskey CH, ed. *Geriatric Anesthesiology.* Baltimore, MD: Williams & Wilkins; 1997:146, with permission.

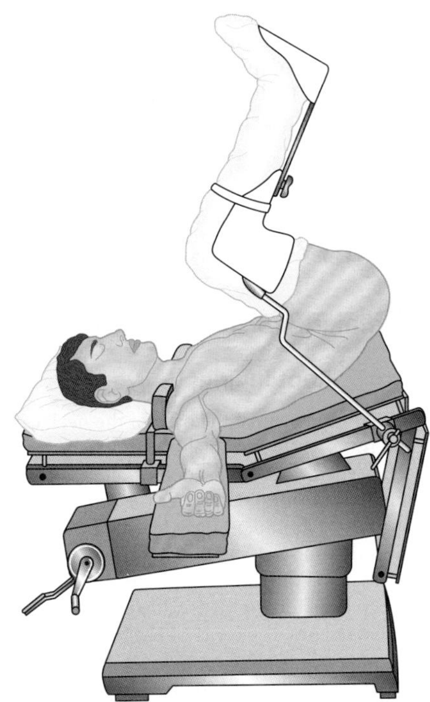

FIGURE 28-6. The exaggerated lithotomy position. Shoulder support may be needed to stabilize the torso. If used, it should be placed over the acromioclavicular area to minimize compression of the brachial plexus and adjacent vessels.

lithotomy position stresses the lumbar spine, produces a significant uphill gradient for perfusion of the feet, and may restrict ventilation because of abdominal compression by bulky thighs. It can be tolerated under anesthesia but rarely can be assumed by an awake patient. Control of ventilation is usually necessary. If pre-existing painful lumbar spine disease is present, an alternative surgical position may need to be chosen beforehand to avoid severely accentuating the lumbar distress after surgery. This position has been associated with a very high frequency of lower extremity compartment syndrome.[8] Maintenance of adequate perfusion pressure in the legs is important.

Complications of Supine Positions

Pressure Alopecia

Prolonged compression of hair follicles can produce hair loss. Abel and Lewis [9] described patients who had pain, swelling, and exudation where the occiput had been supporting the weight of the head for long periods in a head-down position. Alopecia occurred between the 3rd and 28th postoperative day; regrowth was complete within 3 months. Use of tight head straps to hold anesthetic face masks and prolonged hypotension and hypothermia have also been associated with compression alopecia.[10] Frequently turning the patient's head during long operations[11] and use of padded, soft head supports are recommended to reduce the risks of this complication.

Pressure-point Issues

Weight-bearing bony prominences can produce ischemic necrosis of overlying tissue unless proper padding is applied. Hypothermia and vasoconstrictive hypotension may enhance the process. The heels, the elbows, and the sacrum are particularly vulnerable. The use of a variety of pads (e.g., foam or gel) may disperse point pressure if used for protection. Although their use may protect against skin and soft tissue compression and ischemia, there are no studies that have proven their use to be beneficial in reducing peripheral neuropathies in the perioperative period.

BRACHIAL PLEXUS AND UPPER EXTREMITY NEUROPATHIES

Brachial Plexus Neuropathy

Root Injuries

1 Shoulder braces placed tight against the base of the neck can compress and injure the roots of the brachial plexus when steep head-down positions are used. Braces, if needed at all, are considered less harmful when placed more laterally over the acromioclavicular joint. In general, the use of shoulder braces should be discouraged.

Supine positions do not usually threaten structures in the patient's neck unless considerable lateral displacement of the head occurs or if steep head-down tilt is added. When lateral displacement of the head occurs, the roots of the brachial plexus on the side of the obtuse head–shoulder angle can be stretched and damaged. If the upper extremity is fixed at the wrist (e.g., by wrist wrap or a sheet or towel used to tuck the arm), the stretch injury
2 of the plexus can be accentuated as the head moves laterally away from the anchoring point of the wrist. Similarly, exaggerated rotation of the head away from an extended arm may be associated with a brachial plexus injury.

Sternal Retraction

Frequently, the patient undergoing a median sternotomy has both arms padded and secured alongside the torso. An alternative is to have both arms abducted.[12] Vander Salm et al.[13,14] described first rib fractures and brachial plexus injuries associated with median sternotomies. They related the extent of the injury to the amount of retractor displacement of the rib, with the most severe injury being caused by displacement sufficient to produce a first rib fracture. Roy et al.,[15] in a study of 200 consecutive adults scheduled for cardiac surgery via a median sternotomy, positioned the left arm either abducted and padded on an arm board with the palm supinated or secured by a draw sheet alongside the trunk; the right arm was always placed alongside the trunk. They found a 10% incidence of upper extremity nerve injury that was not influenced by internal mammary artery harvest, internal jugular vein catheterization, or left arm position. Surgical manipulation was more contributory than extremity positioning in producing trauma to the brachial plexus. Jellish et al.[12] reported that there is less slowing of somatosensory evoked potentials (SSEPs) of the ulnar nerve during sternotomy when both arms are abducted instead of tucked at the sides. However, they found no differences in perioperative symptoms between patients in the arm-abducted versus arm-at-side groups.

Long Thoracic Nerve Dysfunction

A number of lawsuits have centered on postoperative serratus anterior muscle dysfunction and winging of the scapula (Fig. 28-7) alleged to be the result of position-related injuries to the long thoracic nerve, a nerve arising from nerve roots C5, C6, and C7. Because C5 and C6 fibers of the nerve course through the middle scalene muscle and emerge from its lateral border to join the fibers from C7, it has been proposed that neuropathies of the long thoracic nerve are traumatic in origin.[16] Because the nerve is not routinely involved in a stretch injury of the brachial plexus and because the plexus is not routinely involved when long thoracic nerve dysfunction occurs, the relationship between postoperative long thoracic neuropathy and patient positioning remains speculative. Based on the evidence of Foo and Swann[17] plus data from various litigations, Martin[18] concluded that in the absence of demonstrable trauma, postoperative dysfunctions of the long thoracic nerve were quite likely the result of coincidental neuropathies, possibly of viral origin.

Axillary Trauma Associated with the Humeral Head

Abduction of the arm on an arm board to >90 degrees may thrust the head of the humerus into the axillary neurovascular bundle. This bundle typically lies on the flexion side of the shoulder joint. However, when the arm is abducted to >90 degrees, the bundle is now on the extension side of the joint. The bundle is both compressed and stretched at that point, and its neural structures may be damaged. In the same manner, vessels can be compressed or occluded and perfusion of the extremity can be jeopardized.

Radial Nerve Compression

The radial nerve, arising from roots C6 to C8 and T1, passes dorsolaterally around the middle and lower portions of the humerus

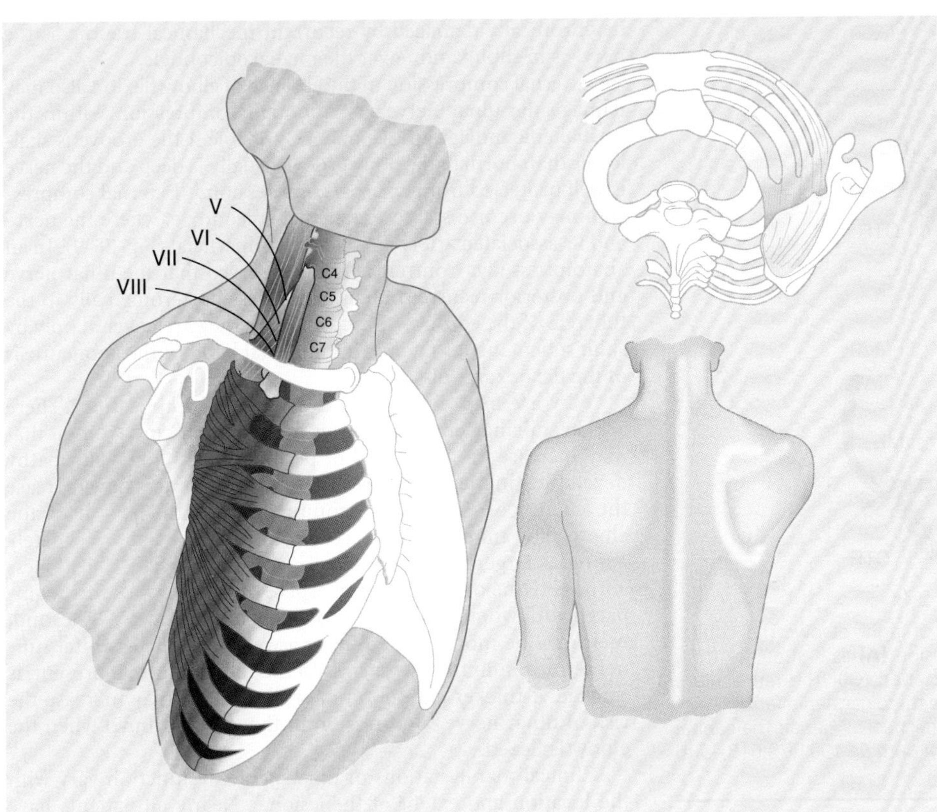

FIGURE 28-7. Scapular winging. The serratus anterior muscle (*upper right*) is supplied solely by the long thoracic nerve that branches immediately from C5, C6, C7, and sometimes C8 (*left figure*). Arising on the lateral ribs and inserting on the deep surface of the scapula, the muscle keeps the shoulder girdle approximated to the dorsal rib cage. Long thoracic nerve palsy allows dorsal protrusion of the scapula (*lower right*). See text for details.

in the musculospiral groove. At a point on the lateral aspect of the arm, approximately three fingerbreadths proximal to the lateral epicondyle of the humerus, the nerve can be compressed against the underlying bone and injured. Pressure from the vertical bar of an anesthesia screen or a similar device against the lateral aspect of the arm, excessive cycling of an automatic blood pressure cuff, and compression at the midhumerus level by restrictive sheets or towels used to tuck the arms have been implicated in causing damage to the radial nerve. Other support devices, including arm boards and slings used when patients are positioned laterally, can directly compress the radial nerve as it wraps around the musculospiral groove.

Median Nerve Dysfunction

Isolated perioperative injuries to the median nerve are uncommon and the mechanism is usually obscure.[19,20] A potential source of injury is iatrogenic trauma to the nerve during access to vessels in the antecubital fossa, as might occur during venipuncture. Anecdotally, this problem appears to occur primarily in men 20 to 40 years of age who cannot easily extend their elbows completely. Forced elbow extension after administration of muscle relaxants and while positioning the arms, with resultant stretch of the median nerve, has been suggested as one potential mechanism for this problem.

Ulnar Neuropathy

Improper anesthetic care and patient malpositioning have been implicated as causative factors in the development of ulnar neuropathies since reports by Büdinger[21] and Garriques[22] in the 1890s. These factors likely play an etiologic role for this problem in some surgical patients. Other factors, however, may contribute to the development of postoperative ulnar neuropathies. In a series of 12 inpatients with newly acquired ulnar neuropathy, Wadsworth and Williams[23] determined that external compression of an ulnar nerve during surgery was a factor in only two patients. Ulnar neuropathies develop in medical as well as surgical patients.[24] The mechanisms of ulnar neuropathy are unclear.

Typically, anesthesia-related ulnar nerve injury is thought to be associated with external nerve compression or stretch caused by malpositioning during the intraoperative period. Although this implication may be true for some patients, three findings suggest that other factors may contribute. First, patient characteristics (e.g., male sex, high body mass index, and prolonged postoperative bed rest) are associated with these ulnar neuropathies.[25] Various reports suggest that 70% to 90% of patients who have this problem are men.[19,20,23–25] Second, many patients with perioperative ulnar neuropathies have a high frequency of contralateral ulnar nerve conduction dysfunction.[26] This finding suggests that many of these patients likely have asymptomatic but abnormal ulnar nerves before their anesthetics, and these abnormal nerves may become symptomatic during the perioperative period. Finally, many patients do not notice or complain of ulnar nerve symptoms until >48 hours after their surgical procedures.[25,26] A prospective study of ulnar neuropathy in 1,502 surgical patients found that none of the patients had symptoms of the neuropathy during the first 2 postoperative days.[27] It is not clear whether the onset of symptoms indicates the time that an injury has occurred to the nerve. Prielipp et al.[28] found that 8 of 15 awake volunteers who had notable alterations in their ulnar nerve SSEP signals from direct ulnar nerve pressure did not perceive a paresthesia, even when the SSEP waveforms decreased as much as 72%.

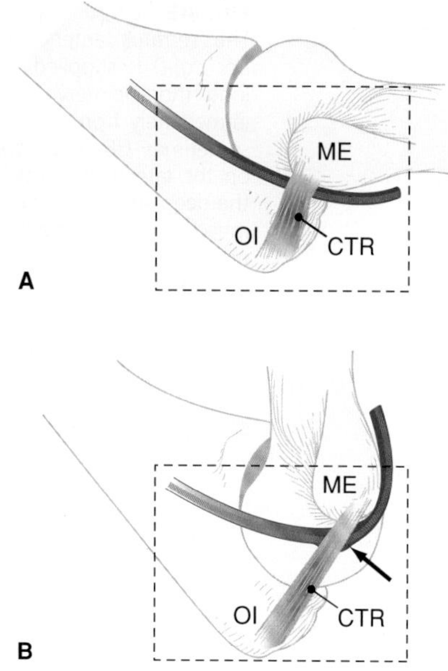

FIGURE 28-8. Medial-to-lateral view of right elbow. The cubital tunnel retinaculum (CTR) is lax in extension **(A)** as it stretches from the medial epicondyle (ME) to the olecranon (Ol). The retinaculum tightens in flexion **(B)** and can compress the ulnar nerve (*arrow*). Reprinted from: O'Driscoll SW, Horii E, Carmichael SW, et al. The cubital tunnel and ulnar neuropathy. *J Bone Joint Surg Br.* 1991;73:613, with permission.

Elbow flexion can cause ulnar nerve damage by several mechanisms. In some patients, the ulnar nerve is compressed by the aponeurosis of the flexor carpi ulnaris muscle and cubital tunnel retinaculum when the elbow is flexed by >110 degrees[29,30] (Fig. 28-8). In other patients, this fibrotendinous roof of the cubital tunnel is poorly formed and can lead to anterior subluxation or dislocation of the ulnar nerve over the medial epicondyle of the humerus during elbow flexion. This displacement has been observed in approximately 16% of cadavers in whom the flexor muscle aponeurosis and supporting tissues have not been dissected.[31,32] Ashenhurst[32] has speculated that the ulnar nerve may be chronically damaged by recurrent mechanical trauma as the nerve is in subluxation over the medial epicondyle.

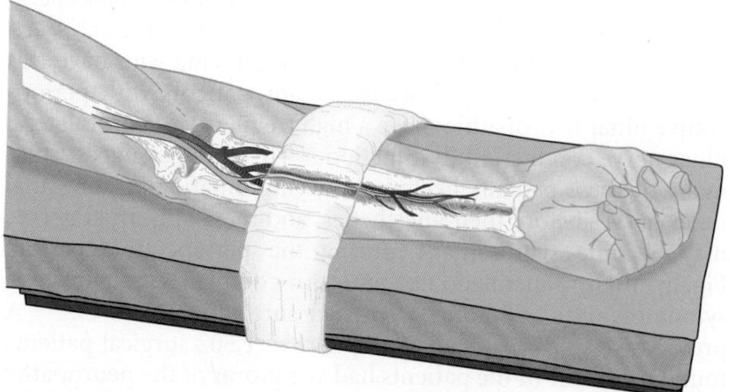

FIGURE 28-9. Arm restraint, if excessively tight, can compress the anterior interosseous nerve and vessel against the interosseous membrane in the volar forearm to produce an ischemic neuropathy. Reproduced from: McLeskey CH, ed. *Geriatric Anesthesiology.* Baltimore, MD: Williams & Wilkins; 1997:155, with permission.

External compression in the absence of elbow flexion also may damage the ulnar nerve.[33,34] Although compression within the medial epicondylar groove may be possible if the groove is shallower than normal, the bony groove usually is deep and the nerve is well protected from external compression.[35] External compression may occur distal to the medial epicondyle, where the nerve and its associated artery are relatively superficial (Fig. 28-9). In an anatomic study, Contreras et al.[36] observed that the ulnar nerve and posterior recurrent ulnar artery pass posteromedially to the tubercle of the coronoid process, where they are covered only by skin, subcutaneous fat, and a thin distal band of the aponeurosis of the flexor carpi ulnaris.

Why are men more likely to have this complication? There are several anatomic differences between men and women that may increase the likelihood of perioperative ulnar neuropathy developing in men. First, two anatomic differences may increase the chance of ulnar nerve compression in the region of the elbow. The tubercle of the coronoid process is approximately 1.5 times larger in men than women.[36] In addition, there is less adipose tissue over the medial aspect of the elbow of men compared with women of similar body fat composition.[36–38] Second, men may be more likely to have a well-developed cubital tunnel retinaculum than women, and the retinaculum, if present, is thicker. A thicker cubital tunnel retinaculum may increase the risk of ulnar nerve compression in the cubital tunnel when the elbow is flexed.

Clinical manifestations of ulnar nerve dysfunction vary with the location and extent of the lesion.[39] Nearly all patients have numbness, tingling, or pain in the sensory distribution of the ulnar nerves once they become symptomatic. However, there can be considerable ulnar nerve dysfunction before symptoms appear. Prielipp et al.[28] found that only 8 of 15 male volunteers with significant ulnar nerve conduction slowing noted any symptoms. More studies are needed to better understand the mechanism and natural history of ulnar neuropathy.

Perioperative ulnar neuropathy is relatively common.[19,20,27] Also, a significant proportion of patients have symptoms of bilateral ulnar nerve dysfunctions both before and after surgery.[27] Therefore, some have speculated that it might be helpful during the preanesthetic interview to inquire about a history of ulnar neuropathies ("crazy bone" problems) or previous surgery at the elbow. If such a history is indicated, the finding must be recorded and a discussion with the patient or family should present the possibility of a postoperative recurrence despite special precautions of padding and positioning.

The time of recognition of digital anesthesia associated with ulnar nerve dysfunction may be quite important in establishing the origin of the postoperative syndrome. If ulnar hypesthesia or anesthesia is noted promptly after the end of anesthesia, as in the recovery facility, the condition is likely to be associated with events that occurred during anesthesia or surgery. If the recognition is delayed for many hours, the likelihood of cause shifts from the intra-anesthetic period to postoperative events. In a review of closed claims, Kroll et al.[19] commented that postoperative ulnar dysfunction can occur as a result of events in the postanesthetic period and that nerve injury may develop in certain susceptible patients "despite conventionally accepted methods of positioning and padding."

Opioids may mask postoperative dysesthesias and pain, but even strong analgesics do not appear to mask a loss of sensation as a result of nerve dysfunction. It may be helpful to assess ulnar nerve function and record these observations before discharging the patient from the recovery room.

OTHER SUPINE POSITION PROBLEMS

Arm Complications

Arm boards should be securely attached to the operating table to prevent accidental release. An arm that is not properly secured can slip over the edge of the table or arm board, resulting in injury to the capsule of the shoulder joint by excessive dorsal extension of the humerus, fracture of the neck of an osteoporotic humerus, or injury to the ulnar nerve at the elbow. Conversely, in the unlikely event that the retaining strap or other holding device or cloth is excessively tight across the supinated forearm (Fig. 28-9), the potential exists for pressure to compress the anterior interosseous nerve, a branch of the median nerve in the upper forearm that courses with its artery along the volar surface of the tough interosseous membrane. The result is an ischemic injury to the distribution of the nerve and artery that resembles a compartment syndrome in the lower extremity and may require prompt surgical decompression.[40–42]

Backache and Paraplegia

Lumbar backache can be worsened by the ligamentous relaxation that occurs with general, spinal, or epidural anesthesia. Loss of normal lumbar curvature in the supine position is apparently the issue. Padding placed under the lumbar spine before the induction of anesthesia may help retain lordosis and make a patient with known lumbar distress more comfortable. Hyperlordosis should be avoided, however. Hyperextension of the lumbar spine, especially to an angulation of >10 degrees at the L2 to L3 apex of the lumbar spine, may result in ischemia of the spinal nerves.[43] Multiple patients undergoing pelvic procedures have been reported to have developed paraplegia. In these patients, hyperlordosis was induced by retroflexing the operating room tables maximally, elevating kidney restfully, and adding padding (e.g., towels, rolls, pillows, and even liter bags of crystalloid) under the lumbar spine to maximize hyperlordosis.

Perineal Crush Injury

The supine patient who is placed on a fracture table for repair of a fractured femur usually has the pelvis retained in place by a vertical pole at the perineum (Fig. 28-10), with the foot of the injured extremity fixed to a mobile rest. An auger gear on the rest lengthens the distance between the foot and the pelvis so that the bone fragments can be distracted and realigned. Unless the pole is well padded, severe pressure can be exerted on the pelvis, and damage can occur to the genitalia and the pudendal nerves. Complete loss of penile sensation has been reported after use of the fracture table.[44,45] The correct position for the pole is against the pelvis between the genitalia and the uninjured limb.[44]

Compartment Syndrome

If, for whatever reason, perfusion to an extremity is inadequate, a compartment syndrome may develop. Characterized by ischemia, hypoxic edema, elevated tissue pressure within fascial compartments of the leg, and extensive rhabdomyolysis, the syndrome produces extensive and potentially lasting damage to the muscles and nerves in the compartment.

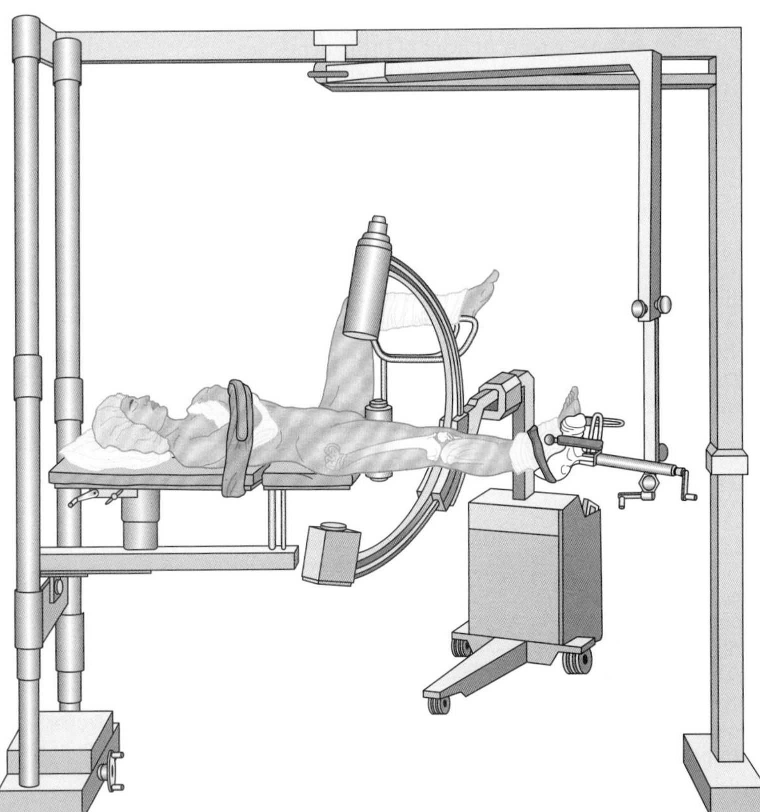

FIGURE 28-10. Traction table with perineal post stabilizing patient while leg is elongated to reposition bone ends. Elevated leg risks hypoperfusion; pelvic post threatens genitalia and perineum.

Causes of a compartment syndrome that may be associated with positioning factors while a patient is in any of the dorsal decubitus positions include (1) systemic hypotension and loss of driving pressure to the extremity (augmented by elevation of the extremity); (2) vascular obstruction of major leg vessels by intrapelvic retractors, by excessive flexion of knees or hips, or by undue popliteal pressure from a knee crutch; and (3) external compression of the elevated extremity by straps or leg wrappings that are too tight, by the inadvertent pressure of the arm of a surgical assistant, or by the weight of the extremity against a poorly supportive leg holder. A tight strap on an arm as well as tight "draw sheets" for maintaining arms at the patient's sides may compress the anterior interosseous neurovascular bundle and may be associated with an anterior interosseous neuropathy or a forearm or a hand compartment syndrome.[41,42]

Several clinical characteristics seem to be associated with perioperative compartment syndrome. Prolonged lithotomy posture in excess of 5 hours has been a common factor in literature anecdotes of postlithotomy compartment syndromes. For lengthy procedures in the lithotomy position, well-padded holders that immobilize the limb by supporting the foot without compressing the calf or popliteal fossa seem to be the least threatening choice. There is considerable variability in the perfusion pressure of the lower extremity in elevated legs. Halliwill et al.[6] and Pfeffer et al.[7] found significant blood pressure variation at the ankle in volunteers placed in various lithotomy positions. Several volunteers had mean pressures of <20 mm Hg when positioned in the high lithotomy position. This pressure is less than intracompartment pressures commonly measured in many lithotomy positions.

Warner et al.[46] have shown that perioperative compartment syndromes occur in patients in positions other than lithotomy. The frequency of this problem appears to occur as often (approximately 1 in 9,000 patients studied retrospectively) in anesthetized patients who are positioned laterally as in similar patients who are positioned in lithotomy. The difference between compartment syndromes in these two groups is that patients in a lateral decubitus position tend to have compartment syndromes of either arm, while those in a lithotomy position have compartment syndromes of the lower extremities.

Finger Injury

Amputation of fingers has been reported when they were caught between the leg and thigh sections of the operating table as the leg section was returned to the horizontal position at the termination of an operation performed in the lithotomy position.[47] A towel used to create a boxing glove-like wrap on the hands of lithotomized patients or carefully removing the patient's hands from the risk position before raising the foot of the table may prevent such a tragic misadventure.

LATERAL POSITIONS

There are several general positioning concepts to consider when placing a patient into a lateral decubitus position. Wrapping the legs and thighs in compressive bandages has been commonly used to combat venous pooling. Marked flexion of the lower extremities at knees and hips can partially or completely obstruct venous return to the inferior vena cava either by angulation of vessels at the popliteal space and inguinal ligament or by thigh compression against an obese abdomen. A small support placed just caudad of the downside axilla can be used to lift the thorax enough to relieve pressure on the axillary neurovascular bundle and prevent disturbed blood flow to the arm and hand. However, this chest support (inappropriately called an *axillary roll* by some) has not been proven to reduce the frequency of ischemia, nerve damage, or compartment syndrome to the downside upper extremity. It may, however, decrease shoulder discomfort postoperatively. Any padding should support only the chest wall and it should be periodically observed to ensure that it does not impinge on the neurovascular structures of the axilla.

Variations of Lateral Positions

Standard Lateral Position

In the standard lateral position (Fig. 28-11), the patient is rolled onto one side on a flat table surface and stabilized in that posture by flexing the downside thigh. The downside knee is bent to retain the leg on the table and improve the stabilization of the trunk. The common peroneal nerve of that side is padded to minimize compression damage caused by the weight of the legs. The upside thigh and leg are extended comfortably, and pillows are placed between the lower extremities. The head is supported by pillows or a headrest so that the cervical and thoracic spines are properly aligned. A small pad, thick enough to raise the chest wall and prevent excessive compression of the shoulder or entrapment/compression of the neurovascular structures of the axilla, is placed just caudad to the downside axilla. This padding may support adequate perfusion of the downside hand and minimize circumduction of the dependent shoulder, which might stretch its suprascapular nerve.

Arms may be extended ventrally and retained on a single arm board with suitable padding between them, or they may be individually retained on a padded two-level arm support that can also help to stabilize the thorax. An alternate method of arm arrangement is to flex each elbow and place the arms on suitable padding on the table in front of the patient's face.

The patient is stabilized in the lateral position by the use of one or more retaining tapes or straps stretched across the hip and fixed to the underside of the tabletop. Care must be taken to see that the hip tapes or straps lie safely between the iliac crest and the head of the femur rather than over the head of the femur. An

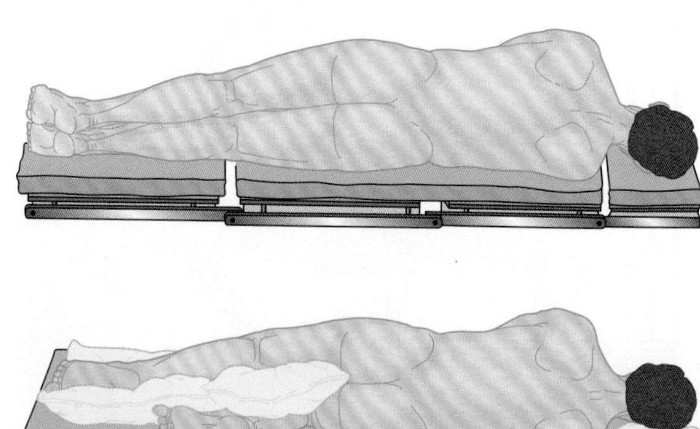

FIGURE 28-11. The standard lateral decubitus position. Proper head support, axillary roll, and leg pillow arrangement are shown on *lower figure*. Downside leg is flexed at hip and knee to stabilize torso. Retaining straps and pad for downside peroneal nerve are not shown.

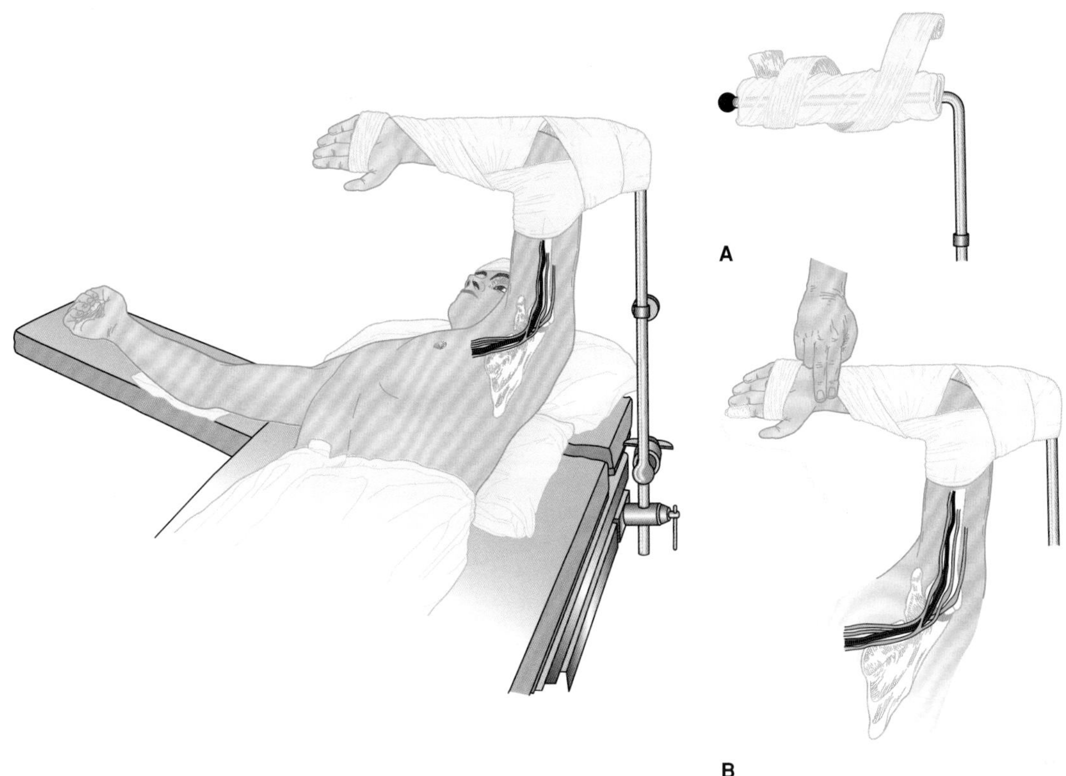

FIGURE 28-12. The semisupine position with dorsal pads supporting the torso, the extended arm padded at the elbow, and the elevated arm restrained on a well-cushioned, adjustable overhead bar **(A)**. Axillary contents are not under tension and are not compromised by the head of the humerus **(B)**. A pulse oximeter provides assurance that the digital circulation is likely not compromised. The position is safe only if the arm does not become a hanging mechanism to support the torso. Reproduced from: Collins VJ, ed. *Principles of Anesthesiology.* 3rd ed. Philadelphia, PA: Lea & Febiger; 1993:176, with permission.

additional restraining tape or strap may be used across the thorax or shoulders if needed. Other methods such as the use of "*bean bag*" or vacuum-supported retention devices are commonly used. As with any such devices, it is essential to ensure that point pressure on bony prominences is minimized and body structures are appropriately supported.

Semisupine and Semiprone

Semilateral postures are designed to allow surgeons to reach anterolateral (semisupine) and posterolateral (semiprone) structures of the trunk. In the semisupine position, the upside arm must be carefully supported so that it is not hyperextended and no traction or compression is applied to the brachial and axillary neurovascular bundles (Fig. 28-12). The supporting bar should be well wrapped to prevent electrical grounding contact (Fig. 28-12A). Sufficient noncompressible padding should be placed under the torso (Fig. 28-12, *large figure*) and hip to prevent the patient from rolling supine and stretching the anchored extremity. The pulse of the restrained wrist should be checked to ensure adequate circulation in the elevated arm and hand (Fig. 28-12B).

Flexed Lateral Positions

Lateral Jackknife

The lateral jackknife position places the downside iliac crest over the hinge between the back and thigh sections of the table (Fig. 28-13). The tabletop is angulated at that point to flex the thighs on the trunk laterally. After the patient has been suitably positioned and restrained, the chassis of the table is tipped so that the uppermost surface of the patient's flank and thorax becomes essentially horizontal. As a result, the feet are below the level of the heart, and significant amounts of blood may pool in distensible vessels in each leg.

The lateral jackknife position is usually intended to stretch the upside flank and widen intercostal spaces as an asset to a thoracotomy incision. However, in terms of lumbar stress, restriction by the taut flank of upside costal margin motion, and pooling of blood in depressed lower extremities, the position has the potential to impose a significant physiologic insult. Actually, its usefulness to the surgeon is brief, and its use should be limited. Once the rib-spreading retractor is placed in the incision, the position has reduced value for the rest of the operation.[48]

Kidney

The kidney position (Fig. 28-14) resembles the lateral jackknife position, but it adds the use of an elevated rest (the *kidney rest*) under the downside iliac crest to increase the amount of lateral flexion and improve access to the upside kidney under the overhanging costal margin. Unlike the lateral jackknife position, the kidney position does not have a useful alternative for a flank approach to the kidney. Thus, the physiologic insults associated with the posture need to be limited by vigilant anesthesia and,

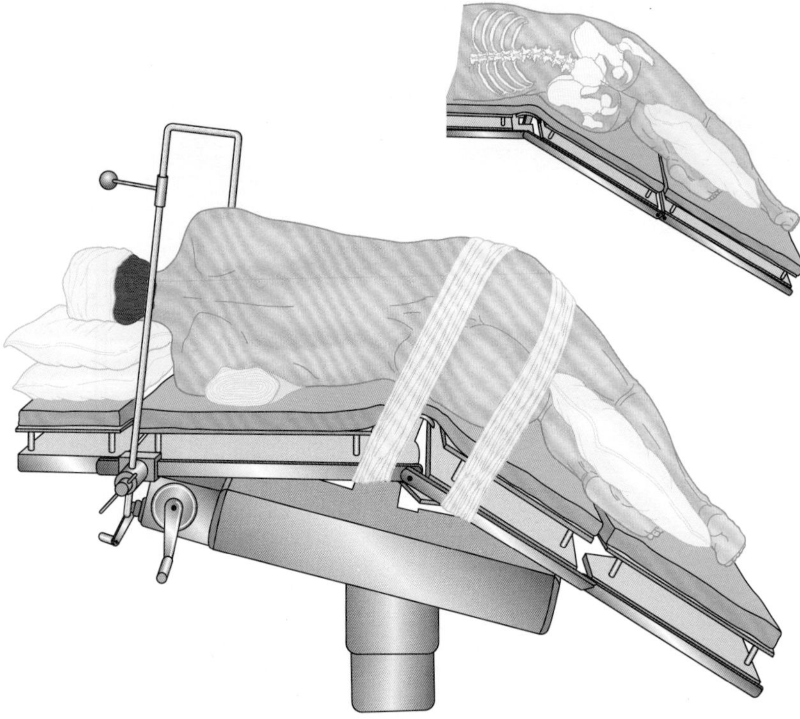

FIGURE 28-13. The lateral jackknife position, intended to open intercostal spaces. Note the properly placed restraining tapes (*large figure*) thrusting cephalad to retain the iliac crest at the flexion point of the table and prevent caudad slippage, which compresses the downside flank (*inset*).

hopefully, rapid surgery. Strict stabilizing precautions should be taken to prevent the patient from subsequently shifting caudad on the table in such a manner that the elevated rest relocates into the downside flank and becomes a severe impediment to ventilation of the dependent lung.

Complications of Lateral Positions

Eyes and Ears

Injuries to the dependent eye are unlikely if the head is properly supported during and after the turn from the supine to the lateral position. If the patient's face turns toward the mattress, however, and the lids are not closed or the eyes otherwise protected, abrasions of the ocular surface can occur. Direct pressure on the globe can displace the crystalline lens, increase intraocular pressure or, particularly if systemic hypotension is present, can cause ischemia.

In the lateral position, the weight of the head can press the downside ear against a rough or wrinkled supporting surface. Careful padding with a pillow or a foam sponge usually provides sufficient protection against contusion of the ear. The external ear (pinna) should also be palpated to ensure that it has not been folded over in the process of placing support beneath the head.

Neck

Lateral flexion of the neck is possible when the head of a patient in the lateral position is inadequately supported. If the cervical spine is arthritic, postoperative neck pain can be troublesome. Pain from a symptomatic protrusion of a cervical disk can be intensified unless the head is carefully positioned so that lateral or ventral flexion, extension, or rotation is avoided.

Suprascapular Nerve

Ventral circumduction of the dependent shoulder can rotate the suprascapular notch away from the root of the neck (Fig. 28-15). Because the suprascapular nerve is fixed both paravertebrally and at the notch, circumduction can stretch the nerve and produce troublesome, diffuse, dull shoulder pain. The diagnosis is established by blocking the nerve at the notch and producing pain relief. Treatment may require resecting the ligament over the notch to decompress the nerve. A supporting pad placed under the thorax caudad of the axilla and thick enough to raise the chest off the shoulder may prevent a circumduction stretch injury to the nerve.

Long Thoracic Nerve

Instances of postoperative "winging" of the scapula have followed use of lateral positions.[18] Although coincidental viral neuropathies of the long thoracic nerve may play an etiologic role in postoperative appearances of scapular winging in patients for whom only a supine position was used, the possibility of trauma to the nerve while establishing the lateral position is difficult to refute. Lateral flexion of the neck may stretch the long thoracic nerve in the obtuse angle of the neck.

PRONE POSITIONS

Variations of Prone Positions

Full Prone

In the so-called *full prone position* (Fig. 28-16), the requirement to elevate the trunk off the supporting surface so that the ventral abdominal wall is freed of compression almost always results

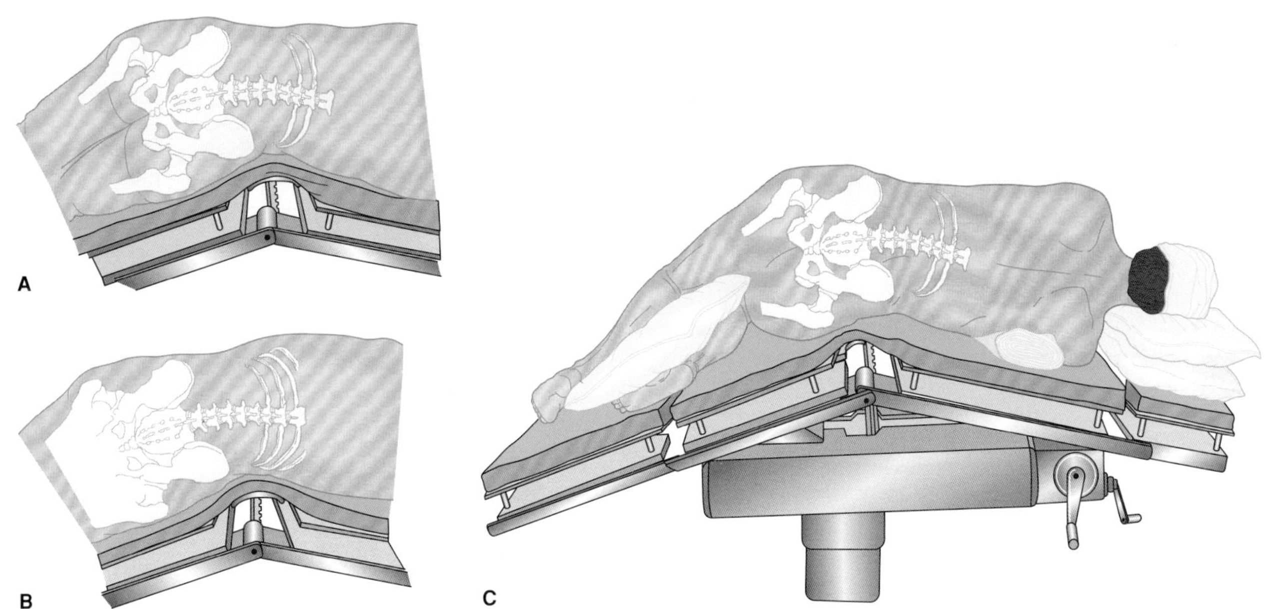

FIGURE 28-14. The flexed lateral (kidney) position. Upper panels show improper locations of the elevated transverse rest, the flexion point of the table, in the flank **(A)** or at the lower costal margin **(B)** to impede ventilation of the downside lung. The iliac crest at the proper flexion point **(C)**, allowing the best possible expansion of the downside lung. Restraining tapes deleted for clarity.

in the head and lower extremities being below the level of the spine. If the tabletop is angulated at the trunk–thigh hinge to remove the lumbar lordosis and separate the lumbar spinous processes, and if the chassis is then rotated head-up sufficiently to level the patient's back, a significant perfusion gradient may develop between the legs and the heart.[49] Wrapping the legs in compressive bandages, or the use of full-length elastic hosiery, minimizes pooling of blood in distensible vessels and supports venous return.

When this position results in the head being lower than the heart, the pressure gradient can result in venous and lymphatic stasis in the head. This position may result in facial and airway edema, making extubation of intubated patients challenging, especially after prolonged procedures such as spine fusions. In addition, over the past decade or two, long spine surgical procedures have resulted in a surprising number of patients who experience severe vision loss. This vision loss is primarily related to ischemic optic neuropathy. While the etiology of the ischemic optic neuropathy is not entirely clear, recent work by Lee et al.[50] suggests that prone positions with the head lower than the heart may lead to venous and lymphatic congestion in the optic canal. This congestion, added to the effect of gravity on the suspended globe of the eye, can result in optic nerve stretch and possibly the development of ischemic neuropathy (see Complications of Prone Positions, Blindness).[51]

Various pelvic, abdominal, and chest supports, including parallel rolls of tightly packed sheets, gels, padded and adjustable metal frames, and four-pillar frames, have been devised to free the abdomen from compression. Each has merit, and no specific unit has been shown to be better than the others for hemodynamic or respiratory maintenance. However, the use of frames may produce more opportunities for point pressure, and if they are used, careful padding of contact points should be considered. The choice of equipment should be based on the physique of the patient, the requirements of the surgical procedure, and the availability.

Pronated patients with limited mobility of the neck, a history of postural neck pain, or a history suggesting a symptomatic cervical disk should have their heads retained in the sagittal plane, either with a skull-pin head clamp or with a face rest. Face rests have fluctuating popularity. Excessive periocular pressure must be considered and avoided if a face rest is used. If the neck is pain-free and its mobility is satisfactory, the head can be turned laterally and supported to prevent pressure

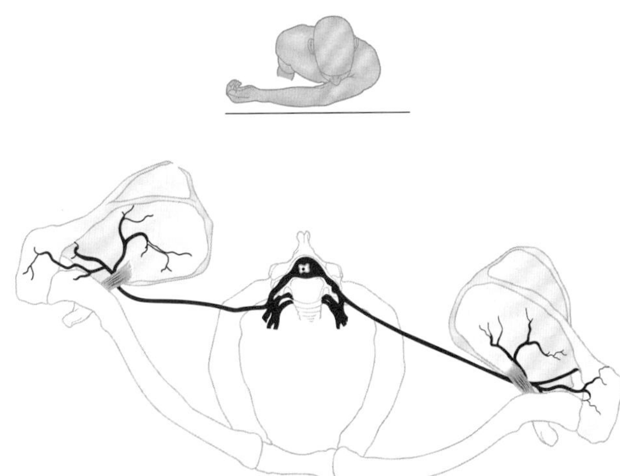

FIGURE 28-15. Circumduction of the arm displacing the scapula and stretching the suprascapular nerve between its anchoring points at the cervical spine and the suprascapular notch.

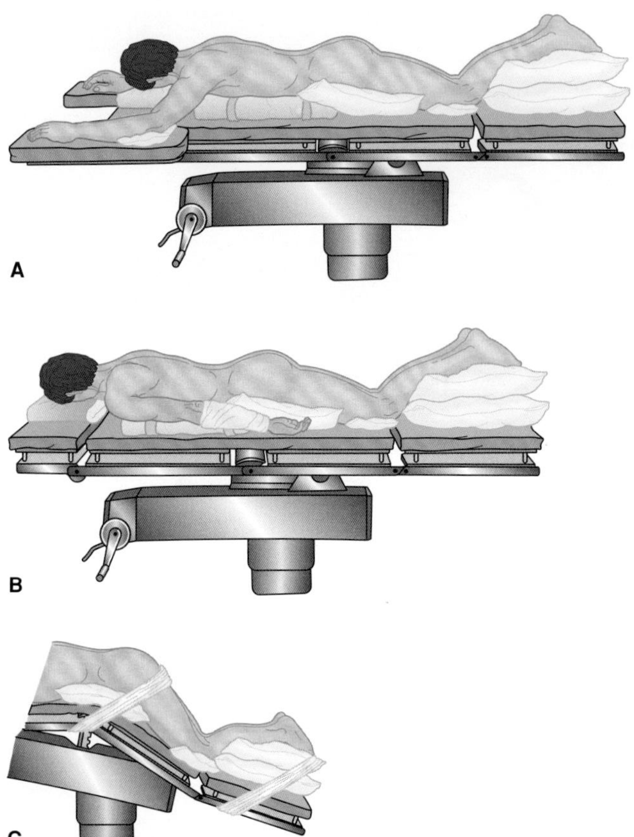

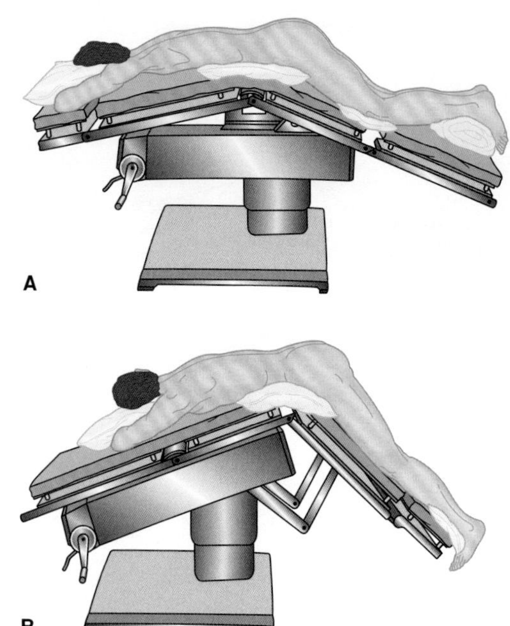

FIGURE 28-17. The prone jackknife positions. **(A)** Low jackknife position with the trunk–thigh hinge of the table used as the flexion position and augmented by a pillow under the pelvis. **(B)** Full jackknife position with the thigh–leg hinge of the table used as the flexion point to achieve more acute angulation of the hips on the torso.

FIGURE 28-16. The classic prone position. **(A)** Flat table with relaxed arms extended alongside patient's head. Parallel chest rolls extended from just caudad of clavicle to just beyond inguinal area, with pillow over pelvic end. Elbows and knees are padded, and legs are bent at the knees. Head is turned onto a C-shaped pad, gel, or foam sponge that frees the downside eye and ear from compression. **(B)** Same posture with arms snugly retained alongside torso. **(C)** Table flexed to reduce lumbar lordosis; subgluteal area straps placed after the legs are lowered to provide cephalad thrust and prevent caudad slippage.

on the downside eye and ear. However, forced rotation of the pronated head should be carefully avoided lest it induces postoperative neck pain or cervical nerve root or vascular compression.

When a patient is scheduled to be pronated after induction of anesthesia, it is worthwhile during the preanesthetic interview to obtain and record information about any limitations that may exist in his or her ability to raise the arms overhead during work or sleep. If the patient is symptomatic, it may be prudent to place the arms alongside the torso after pronation (see "Thoracic Outlet Syndrome"). If the arms are placed alongside the head (i.e., extended ventrally at the shoulder, flexed at the elbow, and abducted onto arm boards; the "surrender" position), the musculature about the shoulders should be under no tension, neither humeral head should stretch nor compress its axillary neurovascular bundle (i.e., shoulders should be abducted <90 degrees), ulnar nerves at the elbow should be padded, and the pulses at the wrists should remain full. Anterior (forward) flexion of the shoulders may reduce tension on the neurovascular structures of the axilla.

Prone Jackknife

The prone jackknife posture is used to provide access to the sacral, perianal, and perineal areas as well as to the lower alimentary canal (Fig. 28-17). The thighs are flexed on the trunk more than is usual in the full prone position, with the table surface hinges determining the degree of flexion achievable.

Prone Kneeling

Kneeling positions have been used to improve operative conditions in the lumbar and cervicooccipital areas (Fig. 28-18). Numerous frames have been constructed to support the weight of a kneeling patient, and their usefulness again depends on the physique of the patient. If the vertebral column is unstable, kneeling frames are not as useful as parallel longitudinal supports because kneeling risks application of shearing forces at the fracture site, with the potential for damage of the contents of the spinal canal. In massively obese patients who must be operated on in the prone position, kneeling frames tend to prevent pressure on the abdomen more successfully than longitudinal frames. However, prolonged kneeling can be fraught with hazards such as compartment syndrome and soft tissue problems. It appears that the use of prone kneeling positions is less frequent today than in the past.

Complications of Prone Positions

Eyes and Ears

The eyes and ears may sustain injury in the prone position. The eyelids should be closed, and each eye should be protected in some manner so that the lids cannot be accidentally separated

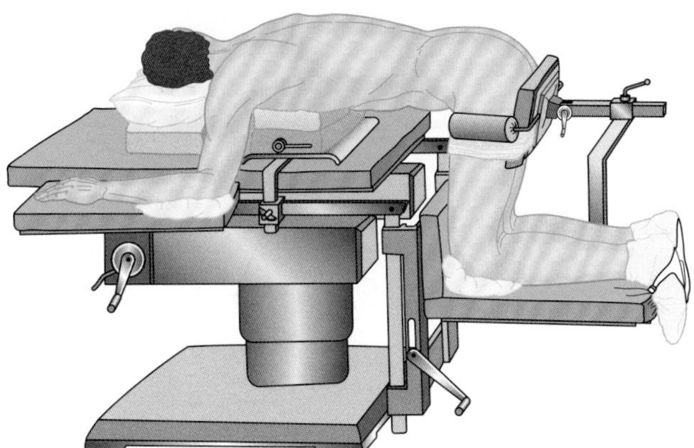

FIGURE 28-18. The Andrews kneeling frame with Wiltse's thoracic frame in use.

and the cornea scratched. Instillation of lubrication in the eyes should be considered, although the value of this treatment is debated. The eyes should also be protected against the head turning after positioning and pressure being exerted on the globe. Monitoring wires and intravenous tubing should be checked after
5 pronation to see that none has migrated beneath the head. If the head is retained in the sagittal plane, the eyes should be checked after positioning to ensure that they are safe from compression by any headrest.

Conjunctival edema usually occurs in the eyes of the pronated patient if the head is at or below the level of the heart. It is usually transient, inconsequential, and requires only re-establishment of the normal tissue perfusion gradients of the supine position, or of a slight amount of head-up tilt, to be redistributed. There does not appear to be any connection between this edema and the occurrence of posterior ischemic optic neuropathy.

Blindness

4 Permanent loss of vision can occur after nonocular surgical procedures, especially those performed in a prone position.[50] The occurrence of this devastating complication is particularly associated with extensive surgical procedures done in the prone position, such as reconstructive spine surgery, where there is associated blood loss, anemia, and hypotension.

The Postoperative Visual Loss Study Group has recently used data from the American Society of Anesthesiologists Postoperative Visual Loss Registry to study ischemic optic neuropathy in spine fusion patients.[50] Using a 1:4 case-control methodology, the authors found six risk factors, half of which strongly support their speculation that acute venous congestion of the optic canal is a potential etiology of ischemic optic neuropathy in this setting. The use of a Wilson surgical bed frame with its elevated curvature resulting in the head being lower than the heart, obesity with its potential elevation of intra-abdominal pressure in prone-positioned patients, and long anesthetic durations can all contribute to elevated venous congestion in the optic canal and potentially reduce optic nerve perfusion pressure. The authors also found that increased estimated blood loss, male gender, and lower percent of colloid administration were independently associated with the development of ischemic optic neuropathy after spinal fusion surgery.

These results suggest that the ASA's 2012 Practice Advisory on this issue is relevant.[51] Basically, it is prudent to attempt to reduce venous congestion in the optic canal. That is, prone positioning should allow the patients' heads to be level with or higher than their hearts. It may be helpful to use colloids as well as crystalloids to maintain intravascular volume. Intraoperative positioning that helps reduce intra-abdominal pressure and, therefore, venous congestion, may be useful. The use of the Wilson frame and other positioning devices should be assessed carefully, with a goal to reduce pressure on the abdomen and to keep the head level with or higher than the heart. Since the authors found duration of anesthesia to be an independent risk factor for ischemic optic neuropathy in this population, it may be prudent to work with spine surgeons to determine if there is merit to limiting the duration of surgeries that are anticipated to be prolonged, especially six hours or longer. Staging these procedures may be helpful.

Neck Problems

Anesthesia impairs reflex muscle spasm that protects the skeleton against motion that would be painful if the patient were alert. Lateral rotation of the head and neck of an anesthetized, pronated patient, particularly one with an arthritic cervical spine, can stretch relaxed skeletal muscles and ligaments and injure articulations of cervical vertebrae. Postoperative neck pain and limitation of motion can result. The arthritic neck is usually best managed by keeping the head in the sagittal plane when the patient is prone.

Extremes of head and neck rotation can also interfere with flow in either the ipsilateral or contralateral vessels to and from the head. Excessive head rotation can reduce flow in both the carotid[52] and vertebral systems.[53] Impaired cerebral perfusion is the obvious consequence.

Brachial Plexus Injuries

Stretch injuries to the roots of the brachial plexus (Fig. 28-19A) on the side contralateral to the turned face are possible if the contralateral shoulder is held firmly caudad by a wrist restraint. If an arm is placed on an arm board alongside the head, care must be taken to ensure that the head of the humerus is not stretching and compressing the axillary neurovascular bundle (Fig. 28-19B,C).

When an arm is placed on an arm board alongside the head, the forearm naturally pronates. As a result, the ulnar nerve, lying in the cubital tunnel (the groove between the olecranon process and the medial epicondyle of the humerus), is vulnerable to being compressed by the weight of the elbow (Fig. 28-19D). Consequently, the medial aspect of the elbow must be well padded and its weight borne across a large area to avoid point pressure.

Asking patients about their ability to work or sleep with arms elevated overhead may identify patients with *thoracic outlet obstruction*. A useful preoperative test if the history is in question is to have the patient clasp hands behind the occiput during the interview (Fig. 28-20). If the patient describes dysesthesias, it may be prudent to keep the arms alongside the trunk in the prone position. Agonizing, debilitating, and unremitting postoperative pain has been known to follow overhead arm placement in pronated patients who have had prior discomfort in their arms in that position.

Breast Injuries

The breasts of a pronated woman, if forced laterally or medially by chest and abdominal wall supports, can be stretched and injured along their sternal borders. Direct pressure on breasts (particularly if breast prostheses are present) can cause ischemia to breast tissue and should be avoided. Multiple cases of breast tissue ischemia have been reported, often resulting in mastectomy and the need for reconstruction.

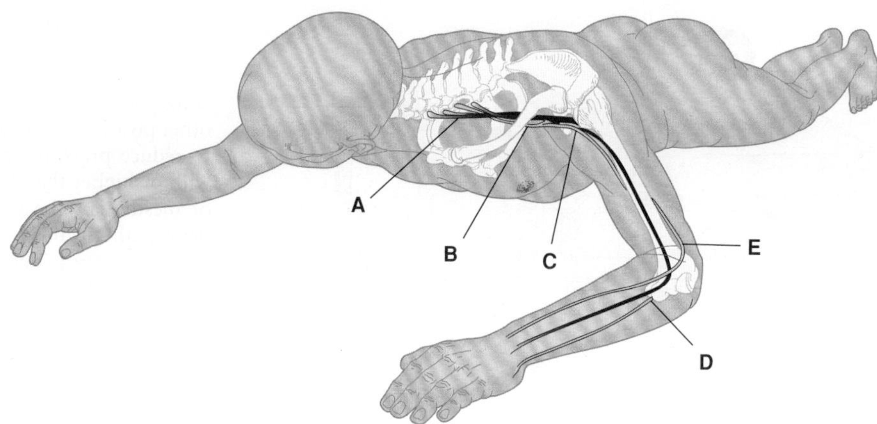

FIGURE 28-19. Sources of potential injury to the brachial plexus and its peripheral components when the patient is in the prone position. **(A)** Neck rotation, stretching roots of the plexus. **(B)** Compression of the plexus and vessels between the clavicle and first rib. **(C)** Injury to the axillary neurovascular bundle from the head of the humerus. **(D)** Compression of the ulnar nerve before, beyond, and within the cubital tunnel. **(E)** Area of vulnerability of the radial nerve to lateral compression proximal to the elbow.

Abdominal Compression

Compression of the abdomen by the weight of the prone patient's trunk can cause viscera to force the diaphragm cephalad enough to impair ventilation. If intra-abdominal pressure approaches or exceeds venous pressure, return of blood from the pelvis and lower extremities is reduced or obstructed. Because the vertebral venous plexuses communicate directly with the abdominal veins, increased intra-abdominal pressure is transmitted to the perivertebral and intraspinal surgical field in the form of venous distention and increased difficulty with hemostasis. The various available supportive pads and frames, when properly used, are designed to remove pressure from the abdomen and avoid these problems.

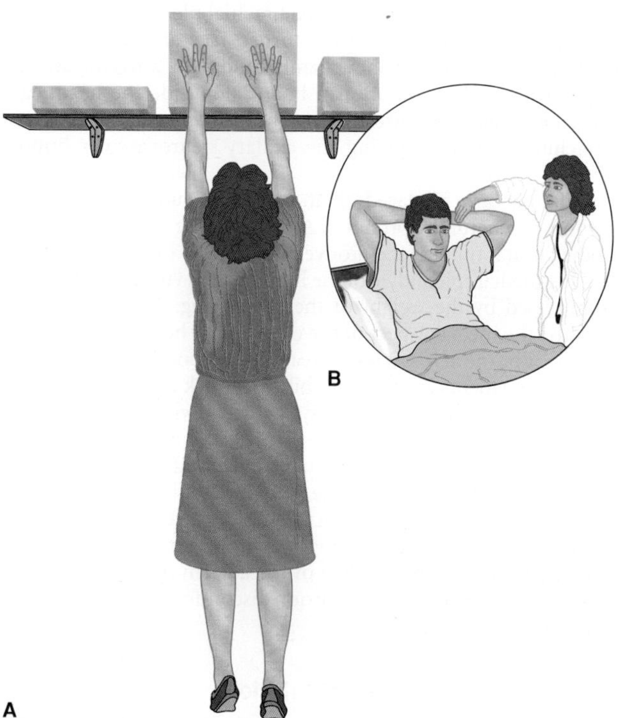

FIGURE 28-20. Assessment of a potential thoracic outlet syndrome. **(A)** This patient has a history of distress when trying to work or sleep with arms overhead. **(B)** Interview carried out with this patient's hands clasped on occiput and radial pulses checked for damping. Reproduced from: McLeskey CH, ed. *Geriatric Anesthesiology.* Baltimore, MD: Williams & Wilkins; 1997:186, with permission.

Stoma and Genitals

Stoma that drains visceral contents through the abdominal wall is at risk in the prone position if they lie against a part of any supporting frame or pad. Compressive ischemia of the stomal orifice
6 can cause it to slough. The same issue is present for genitals, especially the penis and scrotum of men turned prone.

HEAD-ELEVATED POSITIONS

Variations of Head-elevated Positions

Sitting

The classic *sitting position* for surgery places the patient in a semireclining posture on an operating table, with the legs elevated to approximately the level of the heart and the head flexed ventrally on the neck (Fig. 28-21). Head flexion should not be sufficient to force the chin into the suprasternal notch (see "Midcervical Tetraplegia"). Elastic stockings or compressive wraps around the legs reduce pooling of blood in the lower extremities. The head often is held in place by some type of a face rest or by a three-pin skull fixation frame.

Supine—Tilted Head Up

A supine recumbent position with the head of the patient elevated is used for many operations involving the ventral and lateral aspects of the head (Fig. 28-22) and neck, and occasionally with the neck flexed, for transcranial access to the top of the brain. Its purpose is to improve access to the surgical target for the operating team as well as to drain blood and irrigation solutions away from the wound. The back section of the surgical table can be elevated as needed to produce a low sitting position (Fig. 28-22A), or the entire table can be rotated head high with the patient's extended legs supported by a foot rest (Fig. 28-22B). Although the degree of tilt typically is not great, small pressure gradients are created along the vascular axis that can pool blood

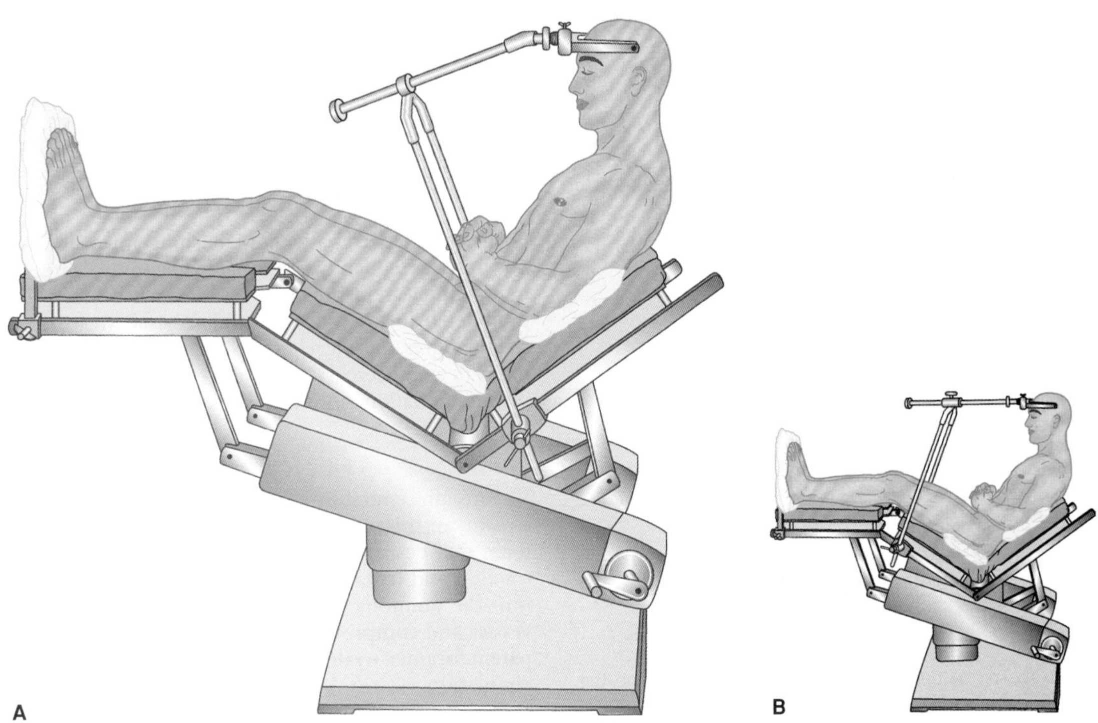

FIGURE 28-21. A: Conventional neurosurgical sitting position. The legs are at approximately the level of the heart and gently flexed on the thighs; the feet are supported at right angles to the legs; subgluteal padding protects the sciatic nerve. The frame of the head holder is *properly* clamped to the side rails of the back section in the event of hemodynamically significant air embolism. **B:** *Improper* attachment of the head frame to the table side rails at the thigh section. In this position, the patient's head could not be quickly lowered because it would require disengaging the skull clamp.

in the lower extremities or entrain air in patulous vessels that are incised above the level of the heart.

For operations around the shoulder joint, the patient may be placed in a head-elevated semisupine position (Fig. 28-23). The upper trunk typically is moved laterally until the raised surgical shoulder extends beyond the edge of the operating table. The torso is supported so that the hips are on the table, the surgical shoulder is off and above the table edge, and the head rests on either a pillow (Fig. 28-23A) or a headrest (Fig. 28-23B). Access is thereby provided to both the dorsal and ventral aspects of the shoulder girdle. The surgical arm remains on the front of the torso and is prepared and draped to be mobile in the surgical field.

Lateral—Tilted Head Up

The lateral position with the head somewhat elevated, a means of access to occipitocervical lesions, has also been referred to as the *park bench position.* All the stabilizing requirements needed for the usual lateral position apply. The head may be held firmly in a three-pin skull fixation holder, which can be readjusted as needed during surgery, or supported by pillows or padding. Although the degree of head elevation used typically is <15 degrees, the position does not completely remove the threat of venous air embolization. The anesthesiologist has good access to the patient's face and thorax for purposes of monitoring, manipulation, and resuscitation. Considerable attention should be directed to avoid compression of neck veins, which can lead to an increase in intracranial pressure and to edema of the tongue.

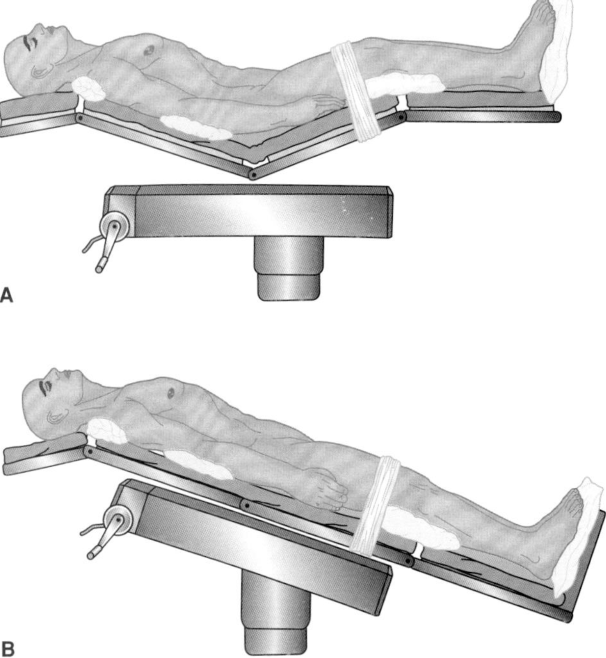

FIGURE 28-22. Head-elevated positions often used for operations about the ventral and ventrolateral aspects of the head, face, neck, and cervical spine. **(A)** The legs are at approximately heart level and the gradient into the head is appreciable but slight. **(B)** The flat table and foot rest are useful when a thyroidectomy is planned under regional anesthesia.

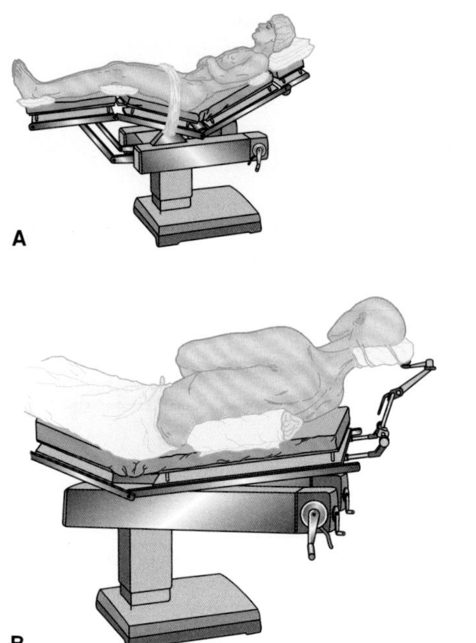

FIGURE 28-23. **A:** The barber chair position for surgery around the shoulder joint. **B:** The upper torso is rotated toward the nonsurgical shoulder and supported with a firm roll or pad.

Prone—Tilted Head Up

The prone posture with the table rotated head high (Fig. 28-24) can be used to access dorsal structures of the head and neck. Usually the perceived advantage of this position compared with a sitting position is the avoidance of air embolization. Although the pressure gradients for air entrainment into patulous veins are less than in the full sitting position, the hazard is not eliminated. As a result of the positive-pressure inflation cycle of passive ventilation, a bothersome recurrent flux of cerebrospinal fluid into and out of the exposed wound may be encountered. The posture also restricts resuscitative access to the thorax.

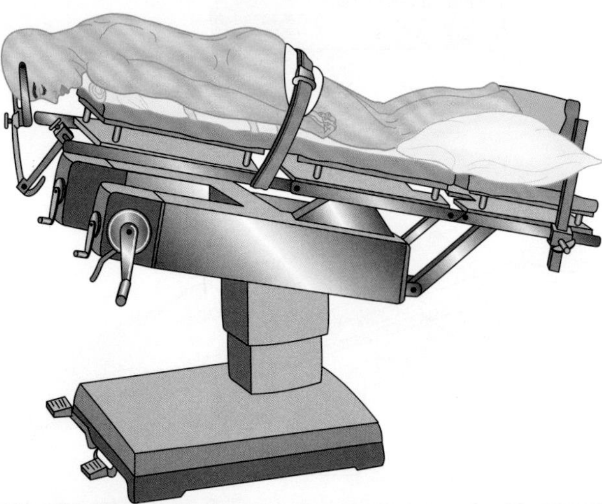

FIGURE 28-24. The skull-pin headrest used to stabilize a patient in the head-elevated prone position. Note the chest rolls used to free the abdomen from compression and the gluteal strap to minimize caudad slippage after head-up tilt.

Complications of Head-elevated Positions

Postural Hypotension

In the anesthetized patient, establishing any of the head-elevated positions is frequently accompanied by some degree of reduction in systemic blood pressure. The normal protective reflexes are inhibited by drugs used during anesthesia. Measuring mean arterial pressures at the level of the circle of Willis is recommended by many to assess cerebral perfusion pressures more accurately. This recommendation, however, is controversial.[54–58]

Air Embolus

Venous air embolization is potentially lethal. In the bloodstream, air migrates to the heart, where it creates a compressible foam that destroys the propulsive efficiency of ventricular contraction and irritates the conduction system. Air can also move into the pulmonary vasculature, where bubbles obstruct small vessels and compromise gas exchange, or it can cross through a patent foramen ovale to the left side of the heart and the systemic circulation.

The potential for venous air embolization increases with the degree of elevation of the operative site above the heart. Although the occurrence of air emboli is a relatively frequent phenomenon in head-elevated positions, most of the emboli are small in volume, clinically silent, and recognizable only by sophisticated Doppler detection or echocardiographic (e.g., transesophageal) techniques. Nevertheless, the potential for dangerous accumulations of entrained air requires immediate detection of the embolization, a careful search for its portal of entry, and prompt treatment of its clinical effects (see Chapter 36).

Edema of the Face, Tongue, and Neck

Severe postoperative macroglossia, apparently because of venous and lymphatic obstruction, can be caused by prolonged, marked neck flexion. Postoperative need for a tracheostomy has been reported. Try to avoid placing the patient's chin firmly against the chest and use an oral airway to protect the endotracheal tube. Extremes of neck flexion, with or without head rotation, have been widely used to gain access to structures in the posterior fossa and cervical spine, but their potential for damage should be understood and excessive flexion–rotation avoided if possible. Moore et al.[59] have suggested that the primary mechanism may be neurologically determined rather than being the result of either vascular obstruction or local trauma. This problem also has been described with the use of transesophageal echocardiography probes.

Midcervical Tetraplegia

This devastating injury occurs after hyperflexion of the neck, with
5 or without rotation of the head, and is attributed to stretching of the spinal cord with resulting compromise of its vasculature in the midcervical area. An element of spondylosis or a spondylotic bar may be involved.[60,61] The result is paralysis below the general level of the fifth cervical vertebra. Although most reports in the literature have described the condition as occurring after the use of the sitting position, midcervical tetraplegia has also occurred after prolonged, nonforced head flexion for intracranial surgery in the supine position.

Sciatic Nerve

Stretch injuries of the sciatic nerve can occur in some seated patients if the hips are markedly flexed without bending the knees. Prolonged compression of the sciatic nerve as it emerges from the pelvis is possible in a thin, seated patient if the buttocks are not suitably padded. Foot drop may be the result of injuries to either the sciatic nerve or the common peroneal nerve and can be bilateral.

HEAD-DOWN POSITIONS

The introduction of robotic procedures has resulted in an increased use of head-down positions. The great majority of robotic procedures early in the introduction of the technology have involved prostatectomies, colorectal, and gynecologic procedures. Thus, most of these initial procedures and the experience gained with robotic procedures have been performed in the pelvis and lower abdomen. As with any introduction of new technology, there is a steep learning curve for the operators. Typically, early adopters of robotic technology have requested steep head-down positions of supine patients. These steep head-down positions have resulted in a variety of complications that challenge anesthesia providers and patients.

Complications of Head-down Positions

Head and Neck Injury

During the early years of the introduction of robotic surgery technique, several patients have suffered severe injury and have even died from body shifts on operating room tables that have been tilted severely head-down. There are several anecdotes from medicolegal actions involving patients who slid off operating tables with resulting neck injuries. In one instance, a patient in a supine and very steep head-down position apparently somersaulted heels over head off the operating room table and subsequently died from a massive intracranial bleed. Steep head-down tilt is not often warranted and should be actively discouraged when appropriate. Skilled operators often find that they need less steep head-down tilt as they gain experience and expertise with robotic procedures.

Brachial Plexopathy

A risk of brachial plexus injuries associated with cephalad movement of the patient while the arms or shoulders are secured to the table with retention materials or shoulder braces is often present in this position. Cephalad movement when arms are fixated or when shoulder restraints with either braces, tape, "bean bag" devices, or other torso restraints are used may result in stretch of the middle and lower divisions of the brachial plexus. If the cephalad movement results in a relative hyperabduction of the shoulder to >90 degrees, the brachial plexus can be stretched as it courses distally around the hyperabducted head of the humerus.

Depending on the degree of head depression, the addition of tilt to the lithotomy position combines the worst features of both the lithotomy and the head-down postures. The weight of abdominal viscera on the diaphragm adds to whatever abdominal compression is produced by the flexed thighs of an obese patient or of one placed in an exaggerated lithotomy position. Ventilation should be assisted or controlled. Because elevation of the lower extremities above the heart produces an "uphill" perfusion gradient, systemic hypotension and compressive leg wrapping may limit perfusion to the periphery, and both can be factors in the development of compartment syndromes in the legs of patients in the lithotomy position.[5] This perfusion gradient often is unpredictable and exaggerated, potentially increasing the risk of compartment syndrome.[6,7]

Cephalad displacement of the diaphragm and obstruction of its caudad inspiratory stroke accompany a head-down position because of gravity-shifted abdominal viscera. Consequently, the work of spontaneous ventilation is increased for an anesthetized patient in a posture that already worsens the ventilation–perfusion ratio by gravitational accumulation of blood in the poorly ventilated lung apices. During controlled ventilation, higher inspiratory pressures are needed to expand the lung.

Cranial vascular congestion and increased intracranial pressure can be expected to result from head-down tilt. For patients with known or suspected intracranial disease, the position should be used only in those rare instances in which a surgically useful alternate posture cannot be found. Maintenance of the position should then be as brief as possible.

Steep head-down tilt positions (e.g., 30 to 45 degrees of head-down tilt) may require some means of preventing the patient from sliding cephalad out of position. The use of bent knees is a satisfactory method for retaining position for the tilted patient (Fig. 28-25) if the flexed knee joints are placed sufficiently caudad

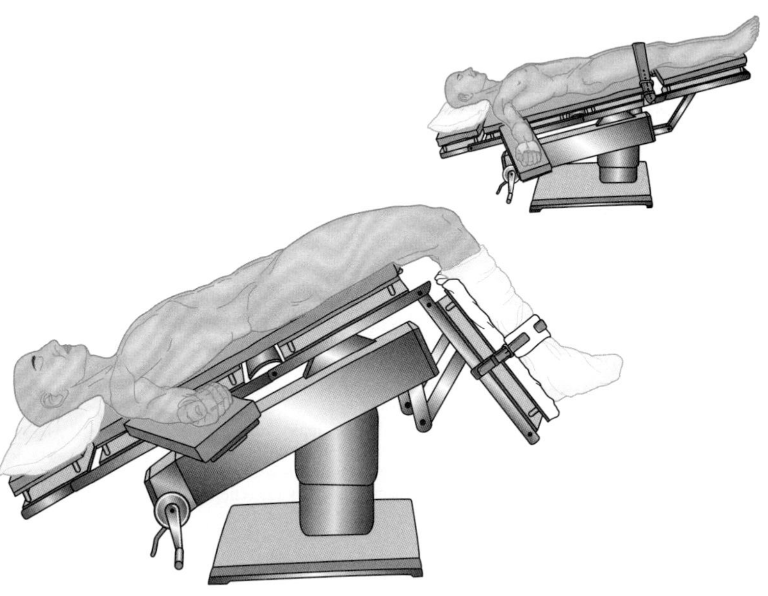

FIGURE 28-25. Head-down tilt. *Lower figure* shows traditional steep (30- to 45-degree) tilt. Leg restraints and knee flexion stabilize the patient, avoiding the need for wristlets or shoulder braces that threaten the brachial plexus. *Upper figure* shows 10 to 15 degrees of head-down tilt.

ANESTHETIC MANAGEMENT

of the leg–thigh hinge of the tabletop so that the adjacent firm edge of the depressed leg section of the table cannot indent either proximal calf or obstruct structures in the popliteal space. Compressive ischemia and phlebitis or a compartment syndrome may result if either of them occurs.

Historically, shoulder braces also have been used to prevent cephalad sliding in steep head-down tilt positions. These braces are best tolerated if placed over the acromioclavicular joints, but care must be taken to see that the shoulder is not forced sufficiently caudad to trap and compress the subclavian neurovascular bundle between the clavicle and the first rib. If the braces are placed medially against the root of the neck, they may easily compress neurovascular structures that emerge from the area of the scalene musculature. For these and other reasons, the use of shoulder braces has waned in popularity and should not be used if possible.

For many of these reasons, steep head-down positions should be used only when a unique surgical issue requires it for optimal exposure and only as long as needed for that exposure.

SUMMARY

There are many ways that patients can be injured during surgical procedures. Careful consideration of intraoperative and postoperative positioning may help reduce the frequency and severity of perioperative positioning-related events. Although many problems that appear to be related to perioperative positioning may seem simple and preventable, the etiologic mechanisms of many of these problems are often not readily apparent. Much work still remains to determine the roles of other potential etiologies such as perioperative inflammatory responses, immunosuppression, and virus activation on the development of these problems.

References

1. Staff NP, Engelstad J, Klein CJ, et al. Post-surgical inflammatory neuropathy. *Brain.* 2010;133:2866–2880.
2. Lanier WL, Warner MA. In reply. *Anesthesiology.* 2011;115:1135–1137.
3. Warner MA. Cracking open the door on perioperative visual loss. *Anesthesiology.* 2012;116:1–2.
4. Gilden DH, Katz RI. Surgical induction of zoster in a contralateral homologous dermatomal distribution. *Arch Neurol.* 2003;60:616–617.
5. Martin JT. 1992–Compartment syndromes: Concepts and perspectives for the anesthesiologist. *Anesth Analg.* 1992;75:275–283.
6. Halliwill JR, Hewitt SA, Joyner MJ, et al. Effects of various lithotomy positions on lower extremity blood pressures. *Anesthesiology.* 1999;89:1373–1376.
7. Pfeffer SD, Halliwill JR, Warner MA. Effects of lithotomy position and external compression on lower leg muscle compartment pressure. *Anesthesiology.* 2001; 95:632–636.
8. Angermeier KW, Jordan GH. Complications of the exaggerated lithotomy position: a review of 177 cases. *J Urol.* 1994;151:866–868.
9. Abel RR, Lewis GM. Postoperative alopecia. *Arch Dermatol.* 1960;81:34–42.
10. Gormley T, Sokoll MD. Permanent alopecia from pressure of a headstrap. *JAMA.* 1967;199:747–748.
11. Lawson NW, Mills NL, Ochsner JL. Occipital alopecia following cardiopulmonary bypass. *J Thorac Cardiovasc Surg.* 1976;71:342–347.
12. Jellish WS, Blakeman B, Warf P, et al. Hands-up positioning during asymmetric sternal retraction for internal mammary artery harvest: a possible method to reduce brachial plexus injury. *Anesth Analg.* 1997;84:260–265.
13. Vander Salm TJ, Cereda JM, Cutler BS. Brachial plexus injury following median sternotomy. *J Thorac Cardiovasc Surg.* 1980;80:447–452.
14. Vander Salm TJ, Cutler BS, Okike ON. Brachial plexus injury following median sternotomy: Part II. *J Thorac Cardiovasc Surg.* 1982;83:914–917.
15. Roy RC, Stafford MA, Charlton JE. Nerve injury and musculoskeletal complaints after cardiac surgery: influence of internal mammary artery dissection and left arm position. *Anesth Analg.* 1988;67:277–279.
16. Gregg JR, Labosky D, Harty M, et al. Serratus anterior paralysis in the young athlete. *J Bone Joint Surg Am.* 1979;61:825–832.
17. Foo CL, Swann M. Isolated paralysis of the serratus anterior. *J Bone Joint Surg Br.* 1983;65:552–556.
18. Martin JT. Postoperative isolated dysfunction of the long thoracic nerve: a rare entity of uncertain etiology. *Anesth Analg.* 1989;69:614–619.
19. Kroll DA, Caplan RA, Posner K, et al. Nerve injury associated with anesthesia. *Anesthesiology.* 1990;73:202–207.
20. Cheney FW, Domino KB, Caplan RA, et al. Nerve injury associated with anesthesia. *Anesthesiology.* 1999;90:1062–1069.
21. Büdinger K. Ueber Lähmungen nach Chloroform-Narkosen. *Archiv für Klinische Chiruque.* 1894;47:121.
22. Garriques HJ. Anaesthesia-paralysis. *Am J Med Sci.* 1897;113:81–89.
23. Wadsworth TG, Williams JR. Cubital tunnel external compression syndrome. *BMJ.* 1973;1:662–666.
24. Warner MA, Warner DO, Harper CM, et al. Ulnar neuropathy in medical patients. *Anesthesiology.* 2000;92:613–615.
25. Warner MA, Warner ME, Martin JT. Ulnar neuropathy. Incidence, outcome, and risk factors in sedated or anesthetized patients. *Anesthesiology.* 1994;81: 1332–1340.
26. Alvine FG, Schurrer ME. Postoperative ulnar-nerve palsy. Are there predisposing factors? *J Bone Joint Surg Am.* 1987;69:255–259.
27. Warner MA, Warner DO, Matsumoto JY, et al. Ulnar neuropathy in surgical patients. *Anesthesiology.* 1999;90:54–59.
28. Prielipp RC, Morell RC, Walker FO, et al. Ulnar nerve pressure: influence of arm position and relationship to somatosensory evoked potentials. *Anesthesiology.* 1999;91:345–354.
29. Campbell WW, Pridgeon RM, Riaz G, et al. Variations in anatomy of the ulnar nerve at the cubital tunnel: pitfalls in the diagnosis of ulnar neuropathy at the elbow. *Muscle Nerve.* 1991;14:733–738.
30. O'Driscoll SW, Horii E, Carmichael SW, et al. The cubital tunnel and ulnar neuropathy. *J Bone Joint Surg Am.* 1991;73:613–617.
31. Childress HM. Recurrent ulnar nerve dislocation at the elbow. *J Bone Joint Surg.* 1956;38:978–984.
32. Ashenhurst EM. Anatomical factors in the etiology of ulnar neuropathy. *Can Med Assoc J.* 1962;87:159–163.
33. Macnicol MF. Extraneural pressures affecting the ulnar nerve at the elbow. *Hand.* 1982;14:5–11.
34. Morell RC, Prielipp RC, Harwood TN, et al. Men are more susceptible than women to direct pressure on unmyelinated ulnar nerve fibers. *Anesth Analg.* 2003;97:1183–1188.
35. Pechan J, Julis I. The pressure measurement in the ulnar nerve. A contribution to the pathophysiology of the cubital tunnel syndrome. *J Biomech.* 1975;8:75–79.
36. Contreras MG, Warner MA, Charboneau WJ, et al. The anatomy of the ulnar nerve at the elbow: potential relationship of acute ulnar neuropathy to gender differences. *Clin Anat.* 1998;11:372–378.
37. Shimokata H, Tobin JD, Muller DC, et al. Studies in the distribution of body fat: I. Effects of age, sex, and obesity. *J Gerontol.* 1989;44:M66–M73.
38. Hattori K, Numata N, Ikoma M, et al. Sex differences in the distribution of subcutaneous and internal fat. *Hum Biol.* 1991;63:53–63.
39. Chusid JG. *Correlative Neuroanatomy and Functional Neurology.* Los Altos, CA: Lange Medical Publications; 1985:149.
40. Hill NA, Howard FM, Huffer BR. The incomplete anterior interosseous nerve syndrome. *J Hand Surg Am.* 1985;10:4–16.
41. Kies SJ, Danielson DR, Dennison DJ, et al. Perioperative compartment syndrome of the hand. *Anesthesiology.* 2004;101:1232–1234.
42. Contreras MG, Warner MA, Carmichael SW, et al. Perioperative anterior interosseous neuropathy. *Anesthesiology.* 2002;96:243–245.
43. Amoiridis G, Wöhrle JC, Langkafel M, et al. Spinal cord infarction after surgery in a patient in the hyperlordotic position. *Anesthesiology.* 1996;84:228–230.
44. Hofmann A, Jones RE, Schoenvogel R. Pudendal nerve neuropraxia as a result of traction on the fracture table. *J Bone Joint Surg Am.* 1982;64:136–138.
45. Lindenbaum SD, Fleming LL, Smith DW. Pudendal nerve palsies associated with closed intramedullary femoral fixation. *J Bone Joint Surg Am.* 1982;64:934–938.
46. Warner ME, LaMaster LM, Thoeming AK, et al. Compartment syndrome in surgical patients. *Anesthesiology.* 2001;94:705–708.
47. Courington FW, Little DM Jr. The role of posture in anesthesia. *Clin Anesth.* 1968;3:24–54.
48. Lawson NW, Meyer DJ Jr. The lateral decubitus position. In: Martin JT, Warner MA, eds. *Anesthesiologic Considerations, Positioning in Anesthesia and Surgery.* 3rd ed. Philadelphia, PA: WB Saunders; 1997:127.
49. Edgcombe H, Carter K, Yarrow S. Anaesthesia in the prone position. *Br J Anaesth.* 2008;100:165–183.
50. The Postoperative Visual Loss Study Group. Risk factors associated with ischemic optic neuropathy after spinal fusion surgery. *Anesthesiology.* 2012;116:15–24.
51. American Society of Anesthesiologists Committee on Standards and Practice Parameters. Practice advisory for perioperative visual loss associated with spine surgery. *Anesthesiology.* 2012;116:274–285.
52. Sherman DD, Hart RG, Easton JD. Abrupt change in head position and cerebral infarction. *Stroke.* 1981;12:2–6.

53. Toole JF. Effects of change of head, limb and body position on cephalic circulation. *N Engl J Med.* 1968;279:307–311.
54. Cullen DJ, Kirby RR. Beach chair position may decrease cerebral perfusion. *APSF Newsletter.* 2007;22:25.
55. Cucchiara RF. Hazards of beach chair position explored. *APSF Newsletter.* 2008;22:8.
56. Munis J. The problems of posture, pressure, and perfusion. *APSF Newsletter.* 2008;22:82.
57. Drummond JC, Hargens AP, Patel PM. Hydrostatic gradient is important – blood pressure should be corrected. *APSF Newsletter.* 2009;24:6.
58. Lanier WL. Cerebral perfusion: err on the side of caution. *APSF Newsletter.* 2009;24:1.
59. Moore JK, Chaudhri S, Moore AP, et al. Macroglossia and posterior fossa disease. *Anaesthesia.* 1988;43:382–385.
60. Hitselberger WE, House WF. A warning regarding the sitting position for acoustic tumor surgery. *Arch Otolaryngol.* 1980;106:69.
61. Wilder BL. Hypothesis: the etiology of midcervical quadriplegia after operation with the patient in the sitting position. *Neurosurgery.* 1982;11:530–531.

CHAPTER

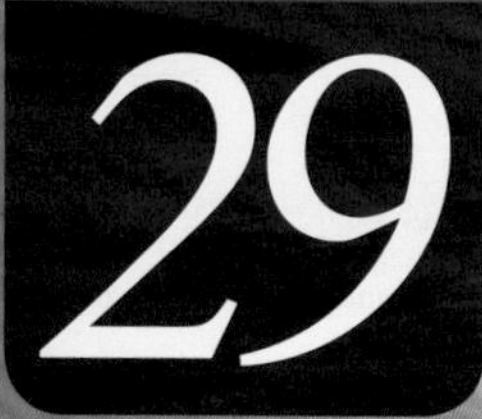

Monitored Anesthesia Care

SIMON C. HILLIER • MICHAEL S. MAZUREK • JEANA E. HAVIDICH

Key Points

1. The standards for preoperative evaluation, intraoperative monitoring, and the continuous presence of a member of the anesthesia care team are no different from those for general or regional anesthesia.
2. As a general principle, to avoid excessive levels of sedation, drugs should be titrated in small increments or by adjustable infusions rather than administered in larger doses according to predetermined notions of efficacy.
3. The context-sensitive half-time describes the time required for the plasma drug concentration to decline by 50% after terminating an infusion of a particular duration.
4. At the present time, no single drug can provide all the components of monitored anesthesia care (i.e., analgesia, anxiolysis, and hypnosis) with an acceptable margin of safety or ease of titratability.
5. During monitored anesthesia care, the maximum benefit of opioid supplementation, in terms of potentiation of other administered sedatives, will accrue when the opioid is used in the analgesic dose range. Within this dose range there is great potential for adverse cardiorespiratory interaction.
6. The important mechanisms whereby respiratory function may be compromised during monitored anesthesia care include the effects of sedatives and opioids on respiratory drive, upper airway patency, and protective airway reflexes.
7. If anesthesiologists are not willing or able to provide these services, others, who are less qualified, are prepared to assume that role.

Multimedia

1 Continuous Infusion

During monitored anesthesia care, the continuous attention of the anesthesiologist is directed at optimizing patient comfort and safety. Monitored anesthesia care usually involves the administration of drugs with anxiolytic, hypnotic, analgesic, and amnestic properties, either alone or as a supplement to a local or regional technique.

TERMINOLOGY

It is important to distinguish between "monitored anesthesia care" and "sedation/analgesia." In October 2004, the American Society of Anesthesiologists (ASA) House of Delegates approved a statement entitled "Distinguishing Monitored Anesthesia Care from Moderate Sedation/Analgesia."[1] *Sedation/analgesia* is the term currently used by the ASA in their recently published *Practice Guidelines for Sedation and Analgesia by Non-Anesthesiologists.*[2] *Monitored anesthesia care* implies the potential for a deeper level of sedation than that provided by sedation/analgesia and is always
1 administered by an anesthesiologist provider. The standards for preoperative evaluation, intraoperative monitoring, and the continuous presence of a member of the anesthesia care team are no different from those for general or regional anesthesia.[3]

Conceptually, monitored anesthesia care is attractive because it should invoke less physiologic disturbance and allow a more rapid recovery than general anesthesia. It is instructive to review the ASA position statement that defines monitored anesthesia care:[3]

Monitored anesthesia care is a specific anesthesia service for a diagnostic or therapeutic procedure. Indications for monitored anesthesia care include the nature of the procedure, the patient's clinical condition, and/or the potential need to convert to a general or regional anesthetic.

Monitored anesthesia care includes all aspects of anesthesia care—a preprocedure visit, intraprocedure care, and postprocedure anesthesia management. During monitored anesthesia care, the anesthesiologist provides or medically directs a number of specific services, including but not limited to:

- *Diagnosis and treatment of clinical problems that occur during the procedure*
- *Support of vital functions*
- *Administration of sedatives, analgesics, hypnotics, anesthetic agents, or other medications as necessary for patient safety*
- *Psychological support and physical comfort*
- *Provision of other medical services as needed to complete the procedure safely.*

Monitored anesthesia care may include varying levels of sedation, analgesia, and anxiolysis as necessary. The provider of monitored anesthesia care must be prepared and qualified to convert to general anesthesia when necessary. If the patient loses consciousness and the ability to respond purposefully, the anesthesia care is a general anesthetic, irrespective of whether airway instrumentation is required.

Monitored anesthesia care is a physician service provided to an individual patient. It should be subject to the same level of payment as general or regional anesthesia. Accordingly, the ASA Relative Value Guide provides for the use of proper base procedural units, time units, and modifier units as the basis for determining payment.

The ASA also states that monitored anesthesia care should be requested by the attending physician and be made known to the patient, in accordance with accepted procedures of the institution. In addition, the ASA states that the service must include the following:

1. Performance of a preanesthetic examination and evaluation.
2. Prescription of anesthetic care.
3. Personal participation in, or medical direction of, the entire plan of care.
4. Continuous physical presence of the anesthesiologist or, in the case of medical direction, of the resident or nurse anesthetist being medically directed.
5. Proximate presence, or in the case of medical direction, availability of the anesthesiologist for diagnosis and treatment of emergencies.

Furthermore, the ASA states that all institutional regulations pertaining to anesthesia services shall be observed, and all the usual services performed by the anesthesiologist shall be furnished, including but not limited to:

1. Usual noninvasive cardiocirculatory and respiratory monitoring.
2. Oxygen administration, when indicated.
3. Administration of sedatives, tranquilizers, antiemetics, narcotics, other analgesics, beta-blockers, vasopressors, bronchodilators, antihypertensives, or other pharmacologic therapy as may be required in the judgment of the anesthesiologist.

PREOPERATIVE ASSESSMENT

The preoperative evaluation is an essential prerequisite to monitored anesthesia care and should be as comprehensive as that performed prior to any general or regional anesthetic (see Chapter 22). However, in addition to the usual evaluation for the patient who is scheduled to undergo general anesthesia, there are additional considerations unique to the monitored anesthesia care that may ultimately determine the success or failure of the procedure. It is important to evaluate the patient's ability to remain motionless and, if necessary, actively cooperate throughout the procedure. Thus, it is important to evaluate the patient's psychological preparation for the planned procedure. It is also important to elicit the presence of coexisting sensorineural or cognitive deficits. These factors or the inability to communicate with the patient may occasionally make general anesthesia a more appropriate alternative. Verbal communication between physician and patient is very important for three reasons: (1) as a monitor of the level of sedation and cardiorespiratory function, (2) as a means of explanation and reassurance for the patient, and (3) as a mechanism of communication when the patient is required to actively cooperate. Although cardiorespiratory disease is often cited as an indication to perform a procedure using monitored anesthesia care rather than general anesthesia, there are occasions when cardiorespiratory disease may reduce the utility of monitored anesthesia care. For example, the presence of a persistent cough may make it very difficult for the patient to remain immobile, which can be particularly dangerous during ophthalmologic or awake neurosurgical procedures. Attempts to attenuate coughing with sedation techniques are likely to be unsuccessful and potentially harmful because a significant level of anesthesia is required to abolish the cough reflex. Similarly, some patients with significant cardiovascular or pulmonary disease may be unable to lie flat for an extended period.

TECHNIQUES OF MONITORED ANESTHESIA CARE

A variety of medications are commonly administered during monitored anesthesia care with the desired end points to provide patient comfort, maintain cardiorespiratory stability, improve operating conditions, and prevent recall of unpleasant perioperative events. It is helpful to delineate and individualize the goals for each patient in order to formulate an appropriate regimen, which frequently involves the administration of either individual or combinations of analgesic, amnestic, and hypnotic drugs. There should be a minimal incidence of side effects, such as cardiorespiratory depression, nausea and vomiting, delayed emergence, and dysphoria, and there should be a rapid and complete recovery. Ideally, the patient should be able to communicate during the procedure. Clinical experience suggests that a level of sedation that allows verbal communication is optimal for the patient's comfort and safety. If the level of sedation is deepened to the extent that verbal communication is lost, the risks of the technique approach those of general anesthesia with an unprotected and uncontrolled airway. However, because monitored anesthesia care is provided by anesthesiologists, the range of sedation may include deeper sedation techniques than those provided by nonanesthesiologists during sedation/analgesia.

The preanesthetic evaluation and plan should identify specific causes of and provide specific therapy for pain, anxiety, and agitation. Pain may be treated by local or regional analgesia, systemic analgesics, or removal of the painful stimulus. Anxiety may be reduced by the use of an anxiolytic such as a benzodiazepine and reassurance by the anesthesiologist. Patient agitation may be a result of pain or anxiety or life-threatening factors such as hypoxia, hypercarbia, impending local anesthetic toxicity, and cerebral hypoperfusion. Other causes of pain and agitation include a distended bladder, hypothermia, hyperthermia, pruritus, nausea, positional discomfort, uncomfortable oxygen masks and nasal cannulae, intravenous (IV) cannulation site infiltration, a member of the surgical team leaning on the patient, and prolonged pneumatic tourniquet inflation.

Pharmacologic Basis of Monitored Anesthesia Care Techniques—Optimizing Drug Administration

The ability to predict the effects of the drugs in our armamentarium demands an understanding of their pharmacokinetic and pharmacodynamic properties. This understanding is a fundamental prerequisite for the design of an effective sedation regimen and greatly increases the probability of producing the desired therapeutic effect. Context-sensitive half-time, effect–site equilibration time, and anesthetic/sedative drug interactions are fundamental concepts that are particularly useful in the context of monitored anesthesia care and will be discussed in some detail.

The ultimate objective of any dosing regimen is to deliver a therapeutic concentration of drug to its site of action, which is determined by the unique pharmacokinetic properties of that drug in that particular patient. The therapeutic response to a particular drug concentration is described by the pharmacodynamics of that particular patient–drug combination. There is a large degree of pharmacokinetic and pharmacodynamic variability, producing a significant variability in the dose-response relationship in clinical practice. Excessive sedation may result in cardiac or respiratory depression. Inadequate sedation may result in patient discomfort

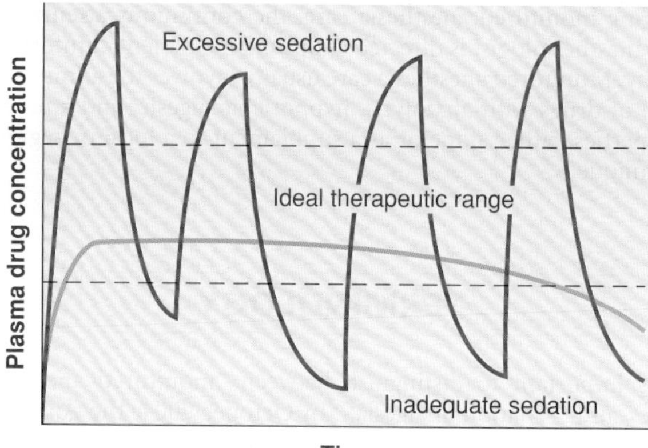

FIGURE 29-1. The changes in drug concentration during differing administration techniques. The *green line* represents a continuous infusion of a drug. In this situation the drug is maintained within the therapeutic range for most of the procedure. The *orange line* represents the drug concentration resulting from intermittent bolus administration. The drug concentration is significantly above or below the desired therapeutic level for most of the procedure.

2 and potential morbidity from lack of cooperation. As a general principle, to avoid excessive levels of sedation, drugs should be titrated in small increments or by adjustable infusions rather than administered in larger doses according to predetermined notions of efficacy.[4] In an ideal dosing regimen, an effective concentration of drug is achieved and then adjusted according to the magnitude of the noxious stimulus. If the noxious stimulus is increased or decreased, the concentration is increased or decreased accordingly. By the end of the procedure, the drug concentration should have decreased to a level compatible with rapid recovery. This approach requires the easily titratable drugs such as propofol. When using drugs such as propofol, adjustable-rate continuous infusions are the most logical method of maintaining a desired therapeutic concentration. When the traditional method of intermittent bolus administration is used, significant fluctuations in drug concentration occur. Under these circumstances, the plasma concentrations are either above or below the desired therapeutic range for a significant proportion of the procedure (Fig. 29-1). Continuous infusions are superior to intermittent bolus dosing because they produce less fluctuation in drug concentration, thus reducing the number of episodes of inadequate or excessive sedation. Administration of drugs by continuous infusion rather than by intermittent dosing also reduces the total amount of drug administered and facilitates a more prompt recovery.[5]

Distribution, Elimination, Accumulation, and Duration of Action

Following the administration of IV anesthetic drugs, the immediate distribution phase causes a brisk decrease in plasma levels as the drug is transported to the rapidly equilibrating vessel-rich group of tissues. There is a simultaneously occurring distribution of drug to the less well-perfused tissues such as muscle and skin. Over time, the drug is also distributed to the poorly perfused tissues such as bone and fat. Although the latter compartments are poorly perfused, they may accumulate significant amounts of lipophilic drugs during prolonged administration. This peripheral depot may contribute to a delayed recovery when the drug is eventually released back into the central compartment after its administration is discontinued. Redistributive factors are important determinants of drug effect and influence the plasma concentration of a drug in a time-dependent fashion.

The Elimination Half-life

Until recently, the elimination half-time was the predominant pharmacokinetic parameter used as the predictor of an anesthetic drug's duration of action. In everyday clinical practice, however, this parameter has not greatly enhanced our ability to predict anesthetic drug disposition. Only in single-compartment models does the elimination half-time actually represent the time required for a drug to reach half of its initial concentration after administration. In a single-compartment model, elimination is the only process that can alter drug concentration. Intercompartmental distribution cannot occur because there are no other compartments for the drug to be distributed to and fro. Most drugs in the anesthesiologist's armamentarium are lipophilic and are, therefore, more suited to multicompartmental modeling than single-compartment modeling. Similarly, other pharmacokinetic parameters, such as distribution half-time, distribution volume, intercompartmental rate constants, and so forth, do not provide us with a practical means of predicting drug disposition. In multicompartmental models, the metabolism and excretion of some IV anesthetic drugs may have only a minor contribution to the changes in plasma concentration when compared with the effects of intercompartmental distribution.

Context-sensitive Half-time

The concept of context-sensitive half-time was developed to improve the description and understanding of anesthetic drug disposition.[6] This concept has greatly improved our understanding of anesthetic drug disposition and is clinically applicable. The effect of distribution on plasma drug concentration varies in magnitude and direction over time and depends on the drug concentration gradients that exist between the various compartments. For example, during the early part of an infusion of a lipophilic drug, distributive factors will tend to decrease plasma concentrations as the drug is transported to the unsaturated peripheral tissues. Later, after the infusion is discontinued, drug will return from the peripheral tissues and re-enter the central circulation. The relative effect on plasma concentrations of distributive processes versus elimination varies over time and from drug to drug. 3 The context-sensitive half-time describes the time required for the plasma drug concentration to decline by 50% after terminating an infusion of a particular duration.[7] This parameter is calculated by using computer simulation of multicompartmental models of drug disposition (Fig. 29-2). The context-sensitive half-time reflects the combined effects of distribution and metabolism on drug disposition. There are several interesting aspects of these data. First, the data confirm the clinical impression that as the infusion duration increases, the context-sensitive half-time of all the drugs increases; this phenomenon is not described in any way by the elimination half-life. The increase in context-sensitive half-time is particularly marked with fentanyl and thiopental. In the case of fentanyl, drug that is irreversibly eliminated from the plasma by hepatic clearance is immediately replaced by drug returning from the peripheral compartments. Thus, although fentanyl has a shorter elimination half-life than that of sufentanil (462 vs. 577 minutes), its context-sensitive half-time is much greater than that of sufentanil after an infusion of longer than 2 hours. The storage and later release of fentanyl from peripheral binding sites delay the decline in plasma concentration that would otherwise occur. The context-sensitive half-times of all the drugs bear no constant relationship to their elimination half-times. Compare also the context-sensitive half-times of propofol and thiopental (Fig. 29-2). Although the context-sensitive half-times of propofol and thiopental are comparable following a brief infusion, the context-sensitive half-time of thiopental increases rapidly following all but the shortest infusions. This finding confirms the clinical impression that thiopental is not an ideal drug for continuous infusion during ambulatory procedures. The context-sensitive half-time of propofol is prolonged to a minimal extent as the infusion duration increases. After an infusion of propofol, the drug that returns to the plasma from the peripheral compartments is rapidly cleared by metabolic processes and is, therefore, not available to retard the decay in plasma levels. This difference between thiopental and propofol is attributable to (1) the high metabolic clearance of propofol compared with thiopental, and (2) the relatively slow rate at which propofol returns to the plasma from peripheral compartments.

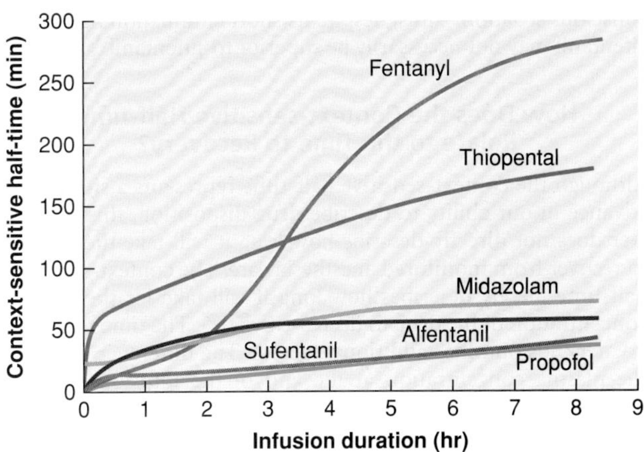

FIGURE 29-2. Context-sensitive half-time as a function of infusion duration. These data were generated from the computer model of Hughes et al.[5] It can be seen that the context-sensitive half-time of propofol demonstrates a minimal increase as the duration of the infusion increases. Also note that for infusions of short duration, sufentanil has a shorter half-time than alfentanil. (Reproduced from Hughes MA, Glass PSA, Jacobs JR. Context-sensitive half-time in multicompartment pharmacokinetic models for intravenous anesthetic drugs. *Anesthesiology* 1992;76:334, with permission.)

Alfentanil is the opioid that has, until recently, been most frequently studied, described, and promoted in the context of ambulatory techniques. Alfentanil has a very short elimination half-time, one-fifth that of sufentanil (111 vs. 577 minutes). However, despite the longer elimination half-time of sufentanil, its context-sensitive half-time is actually less than that of alfentanil for infusions up to 8 hours in duration. This phenomenon is explained in part by the huge distribution volume of sufentanil. After termination of a sufentanil infusion, the decay in plasma drug concentrations is accelerated not only by elimination but also by the continued redistribution of sufentanil into peripheral compartments. On the other hand, the small distribution volume of alfentanil equilibrates rapidly; therefore, peripheral distribution of drug away from the plasma is not a significant contributor to the decay in plasma concentration after an infusion. The data derived from computer simulation by Hughes et al.[5] show that the plasma decay of alfentanil is slower than that of sufentanil following infusions of similar duration to those used during conscious sedation. Thus, despite its short elimination half-time, alfentanil may not necessarily be superior to sufentanil.[8]

How Does the Context-sensitive Half-time Relate to the Time to Recovery?

Although the context-sensitive half-time represents a significant advance in our ability to describe drug disposition, this parameter does not directly describe how long it will take the patient to recover from monitored anesthesia care. The context-sensitive half-time merely describes how long it will take for the plasma concentration of the drug to decrease by 50%. The time to recovery depends on other additional factors. The difference between the plasma concentration at the end of the infusion and the plasma concentration below which awakening can be expected is an obvious factor in determining time to recovery. For example, if the drug concentration is maintained at a level just above that required for awakening, the time to recovery will be more rapid than after an infusion during which the drug concentration is much greater than that required for awakening (Fig. 29-3). Furthermore, although context-sensitive half-time is a reflection of plasma drug decay, awakening from anesthesia is actually a function of effect–site (i.e., brain) concentration decay. Changes in effect–site concentration demonstrate a variable time lag behind changes in plasma drug concentration. Effect–site equilibration is a concept that is particularly relevant to IV sedation. When a drug is administered intravenously by bolus or infused rapidly, there is a delay before the onset of clinical effect. This delay occurs because the plasma is not usually the site of action but is merely the route by which the drug reaches its effect site. If some parameter of drug effect can be measured (e.g., power spectrum electroencephalographic [EEG] analysis in the case of opioids), the half-time of equilibration between drug concentration in the blood and the drug effect can then be determined.[9] This parameter is abbreviated $t_{1/2}k_{e0}$. Drugs with a short $t_{1/2}k_{e0}$ will equilibrate rapidly with the brain and have a shorter delay in onset than drugs that have a longer $t_{1/2}k_{e0}$. Thiopental, propofol, and alfentanil have short $t_{1/2}k_{e0}$ values compared with midazolam, sufentanil, and fentanyl.

The $t_{1/2}k_{e0}$ allows predictions to be made of the time course of equilibration of the drug between the blood and the brain. A distinct time lag between the peak serum fentanyl concentration and the peak EEG slowing can be seen. In contrast, following alfentanil administration, the EEG changes closely parallel serum concentrations. The $t_{1/2}k_{e0}$ for fentanyl is 6.4 minutes compared with a $t_{1/2}k_{e0}$ of 1.1 minutes for alfentanil. If an opioid is required to blunt the response to a single brief stimulus, alfentanil might represent a logical choice over fentanyl. The $t_{1/2}k_{e0}$ is an important determinant of bolus spacing when titrating drugs to clinical effect. In the case of drugs like midazolam and propofol, boluses of drug should be spaced far enough apart to allow the full peak effect to be clinically appreciated before further drug administration in order to avoid inadvertent overdosing.[10–12] For example, even if the shortest quoted equilibration half-time for midazolam (0.9 minutes) is used, it will take 2.7 minutes for effect–site concentrations to be 87.5% equilibrated. Other factors are also important determinants of bolus size and spacing. For example, a low cardiac output will markedly delay drug arrival at the site of action. If sufficient time is not given for the drug to take effect before giving additional drug increments, significant cardiorespiratory compromise may occur. Furthermore, the effects of initial doses of most drugs in anesthetic practice are terminated by redistribution, which depends on blood flow to redistribution sites. If there is reduced blood flow to redistribution sites because of preexisting and iatrogenic decreases in cardiac output, the dangerous adverse effects of these drugs are likely to be both delayed and markedly prolonged. An example of this scenario is the patient with a hemodynamic compromise caused by a tachydysrhythmia who requires sedation for cardioversion. Careful, well-spaced, small boluses of drug should be given to induce the appropriate level of sedation, bearing in mind that it may take several minutes for the full effect of a small bolus dose to become apparent.

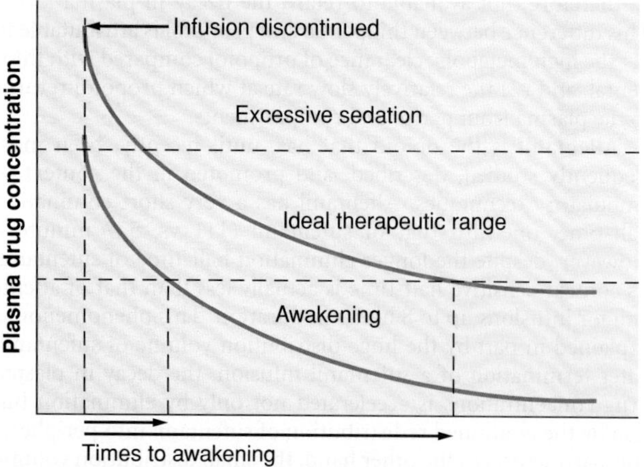

FIGURE 29-3. The context-sensitive half-time is not the sole determinant of the time it takes for the patient to awaken. This parameter merely reflects the time taken for the plasma concentration of a drug to decrease by 50%. The time to awakening is determined in addition by the difference in concentration at the end of the procedure and the concentration below which awakening will occur.

DRUG INTERACTIONS IN MONITORED ANESTHESIA CARE

4 At the present time, no single drug can provide all the components of monitored anesthesia care (i.e., analgesia, anxiolysis, and hypnosis) with an acceptable margin of safety or ease of titratability. Therefore, patient comfort is usually maintained with a combination of drugs. By acting synergistically, combinations of drugs enable reductions in the dose requirements of individual drugs. For example, the combination of propofol and fentanyl by infusion has been shown to produce a more rapid recovery and better stress response abolition than the use of propofol alone.[13–15] In addition, lower doses of each drug may reduce the untoward side effects associated with higher doses leading to increased patient satisfaction and decreased times to discharge. However, synergistic interaction may also extend to the undesirable interactions of the drugs such as cardiorespiratory depression.

Drug interactions may have both a pharmacodynamic and a pharmacokinetic basis and may vary depending on the combination of drugs being coadministered, the dose range over which these drugs are administered, and the specific clinical effect that is measured. For example, because fentanyl is primarily an analgesic rather than a hypnotic, it reduces propofol requirements for suppression of response to skin incision to a much greater degree than it reduces propofol requirements for induction of anesthesia.[16] On the other hand, because midazolam has significant hypnotic properties, it displays significant synergism with propofol or thiopental when used to induce hypnosis.[17–19]

The plasma concentration of a drug at steady state that is required to abolish purposeful movement at skin incision in 50%

of patients ($Cp_{ss}50$) is a measure of potency that is analogous to the familiar parameter of minimum alveolar concentration (MAC) of the volatile inhaled anesthetics. IV anesthetic interactions may be evaluated by their effect on the $Cp_{ss}50$ in a manner analogous to the expression of the effects of opioids on volatile anesthetic requirements in terms of MAC reduction.[20] For example, during general anesthesia, opioid requirements to suppress the responses to noxious stimuli are tenfold higher when used as the sole agent compared with when they are used in conjunction with a nitrous oxide/potent inhaled vapor technique. This interaction persists at the lighter levels of anesthesia encountered during monitored anesthesia care. Therefore, it is likely that a rapid recovery would be facilitated by using opioids in combination with other agents (e.g., propofol/midazolam) rather than as the sole drug.

Drug interactions are dose dependent. For example, when fentanyl is combined with isoflurane, the greatest reduction in isoflurane MAC occurs within the analgesic concentration range of fentanyl (i.e., 1 to 2 ng/mL). At a fentanyl concentration of 1.7 ng/mL, the MAC of isoflurane is reduced by 50%.[21] Once the fentanyl concentration is increased beyond 3 ng/mL, there appears to be minimal further reduction with a maximum MAC reduction of 80%. Likewise, the MAC of desflurane is reduced by approximately 50% 25 minutes after a 3-μg/kg IV bolus of fentanyl.[22] However, when the fentanyl bolus is increased to 6 μg/kg, there is no significant further decrease in the MAC of desflurane. Studies with other opioids have yielded similar results.[23–25] The interactions between propofol and opioids are important because these agents are frequently used during monitored anesthesia care. When analgesic concentrations of fentanyl (0.6 ng/mL) are used in combination with propofol for anesthesia, the $Cp_{ss}50$ of propofol is reduced by 50% compared with when propofol is used as the sole agent.[17] However, when the dose of fentanyl is increased, there is no significant further reduction of the $Cp_{ss}50$ for propofol beyond a fentanyl concentration of 3 ng/mL.

Although the data presented here pertain to patients under general anesthesia, these findings have important implications for monitored anesthesia care. These studies demonstrate that the potentiating effects of opioids on coadministered sedatives are pronounced within the dose range commonly used during monitored anesthesia care. Furthermore, the data suggest that the dose-response curve is likely to be steep within this dose range, thus supporting the clinical impression that significant increases in depth of sedation can occur with only modest increments in opioid or hypnotic/sedative dosage. The following clinical recom-
5 mendations can be made: During monitored anesthesia care, the maximum benefit of opioid supplementation, in terms of potentiation of other administered sedatives, will accrue when the opioid is used in the analgesic dose range. Within this dose range there is great potential for adverse cardiorespiratory interaction.

Opioid and benzodiazepine combinations are frequently used to achieve the components of hypnosis, amnesia, and analgesia. This drug combination displays marked synergism in producing hypnosis. Approximately 25% of the median effective dose for each individual drug is required in combination to induce hypnosis in 50% of patients.[26] If the combination were simply additive, hypnosis would be induced in only approximately 25% of patients. Even subanalgesic doses of alfentanil (3 μg/kg) produce a profound reduction in midazolam requirements for hypnosis.[27] This synergism also extends to the unwanted effects of these drugs, producing the life-threatening complications of respiratory and cardiac depression. Several fatalities have been reported after the use of midazolam, the majority of these being related to adverse respiratory events.[28] In many of these cases, midazolam was used in combination with an opioid. The effects of midazolam and fentanyl on respiratory function in healthy volunteers have been examined by Bailey et al.[29] Whereas midazolam produced no significant respiratory effects alone, and fentanyl alone produced hypoxemia (oxyhemoglobin saturation 95%) in half of the subjects, the combination of midazolam 0.05 μg/kg and fentanyl 2 μg/kg resulted in hypoxemia in 11 of 12 subjects and apnea (no spontaneous respiratory effort for 15 seconds) in 6 of 12 subjects. The combination of midazolam and fentanyl places patients at high risk for developing hypoxemia and apnea. The respiratory depressant effects of this drug combination are likely to be even more significant in the patient with coexisting respiratory or central nervous system disease or at the extremes of age. In clinical practice, the clinical advantages of the synergy between opioids and benzodiazepines for the maintenance of patient comfort should be carefully weighed against the disadvantages of the potentially adverse effect of this drug combination on the cardiovascular and respiratory systems.

SPECIFIC DRUGS USED FOR MONITORED ANESTHESIA CARE

Propofol

Over the past 30 years, propofol has become a popular choice for monitored anesthetic care due to its side effect profile and ease of titratability. Propofol has many of the ideal properties of a sedative–hypnotic for use in monitored anesthesia care. Its pharmacokinetic profile, that is, a context-sensitive half-time that remains short even after infusions of prolonged duration and a short effect–site equilibration time makes it an easily titratable drug with an excellent recovery profile. The quality of recovery and the low incidence of nausea and vomiting make propofol particularly well suited to ambulatory monitored anesthesia care procedures. A significant body of experience with the use of propofol for monitored anesthesia care has emerged. Propofol has significant advantages compared with benzodiazepines when used as the hypnotic component of a monitored anesthesia care technique. Although midazolam has a relatively short elimination half-time, its context-sensitive half-time is approximately twice that of propofol. Whereas propofol is noted for the rapid return to clear-headedness midazolam is often associated with prolonged postoperative sedation and psychomotor impairment, particularly in the elderly. Propofol in typical monitored anesthesia care doses (25 to 75 μg/kg/min) has minimal analgesic properties although propofol use during anesthesia has been associated with less postoperative pain and narcotic use when compared to isoflurane.[30] However, the unique advantages of propofol can be exploited to the maximum when propofol is used to provide sedation when the analgesic component is provided by a local or regional analgesic technique. The use of propofol (50 to 70 μg/kg/min) to provide sedation (defined as sleep with preservation of the eyelash reflex and purposeful reaction to verbal or mild physical stimulation) as an adjunct to spinal anesthesia for lower limb surgery has been examined.[31–33] After termination of infusions of approximately 100 minutes, patients regained consciousness in approximately 4 minutes. The authors also noted the ease with which general anesthesia could be induced if necessary by increasing the propofol infusion. The same group also compared propofol (60.5 μg/kg/min) with midazolam (4.3 μg/kg/min) as an adjunct to spinal anesthesia. The propofol group had faster immediate recovery than the midazolam group (2.3 vs. 9.2 minutes to spontaneous eye opening). Furthermore, psychomotor function was comparable with baseline values following propofol

TABLE 29-1. PUBLISHED STRATEGIES FOR REDUCING THE PAIN ON INTRAVENOUS INJECTION OF PROPOFOL

Using larger veins in antecubital fossa
Decreasing the speed of injection
Injection into a fast-running intravenous line
Diluting with 5% glucose or 10% intralipid
Adding lidocaine to propofol
Pretreating with lidocaine and venous occlusion
Pretreatment with opioid
Pretreatment with pentothal
Cooling propofol to 4°C prior to injection
Injecting cooled saline (4°C) prior to injection
Discontinuing intravenous fluid administration during injection

sedation but did not return to baseline until 2 hours after midazolam administration. Several studies comparing propofol and midazolam sedation for local and regional anesthesia demonstrated that propofol produced less postoperative sedation, drowsiness, confusion, and clumsiness than midazolam but that discharge times varied.[34,35]

General anesthesia with propofol is generally associated with less nausea and vomiting than most other anesthetic techniques.[36–41] There is growing evidence that even subhypnotic doses of propofol also possess direct antiemetic properties particularly when combined with an antiemetic in patients at risk for nausea and vomiting.[42–45] Thus, it is likely that the beneficial effects of propofol upon nausea and vomiting will be a feature of monitored anesthesia care techniques using this drug. On the other hand, even during low-dose infusions used for sedation, pain during injection of propofol may be troublesome in 33% to 50% of patients.[35,46] Several strategies for reducing the pain of propofol administration are described in Table 29-1.[47]

Fospropofol

In December 2008, fospropofol, a prodrug of propofol, was approved by the FDA for use during monitored anesthetic care, but at this time, it has not been extensively studied. This phosphate ester prodrug is metabolized by endothelial cell alkaline phosphatases to intermediate metabolites of propofol, formaldehyde, and phosphate.[48–50] Recent publications on the pharmacodynamics and pharmacokinetics of fospropofol were retracted due to an error discovered in the analytical propofol assay.[51–53] It is known that the active metabolite of propofol has a Cmax value of 4 minutes which is longer than the lipid-based fospropofol formulation. Information obtained from the manufacturer's website listed the terminal phase elimination half-life ($t_{1/2}$) of fospropofol as 0.81 ± 0.08 and 0.88 ± 0.08 hours in healthy subjects and patients, respectively. In healthy subjects, the apparent total body clearance of liberated propofol was 1.95 ± 0.345 L/hr/kg and $t_{1/2}$ was 2.06 ± 0.77 hours. In patients, clearance of fospropofol was 0.31 ± 0.14 L/hr/kg, and clearance for propofol was 2.74 ± 0.80 L/hr/kg and is similar to that observed in healthy subjects. Pharmacokinetics of fospropofol does not appear to be affected by patients with mild to moderate renal insufficiency. At this time, it has not been studied in patients with hepatic impairment.

The standard dosing regimen recommended by the manufacturer Eisai is an initial IV bolus dose of 6.5 mg/kg followed by supplemental doses of 1.6 mg/kg as needed. No initial dose should exceed 16.5 mL; no supplemental bolus should exceed 4 mL. If patients are greater than 65 years of age or classified as ASA physical status 3 or 4, a modified dosing regimen (a 25% reduction of the standard dose), should be administered. Supplemental doses should only be administered after patients can demonstrate movement upon command (verbal or tactile stimulation) and not more frequently than every 4 minutes (accessed from Eisai website January 2012 URL http://us.eisai.com/product.asp?ID=274).

At the time of this writing, there are limited numbers of clinical control trials to evaluate the safety and efficacy of fospropofol for short procedures requiring monitored anesthesia care. Cohen et al.[54] conducted a randomized controlled multicenter trial of 127 ASA PS range from 1 to 4 undergoing colonoscopy. The investigators randomized patients into two main treatment arms (fospropofol vs. midazolam). The fospropofol group was further randomized into one of four treatment arms of increasing doses of fospropofol (2 mg/kg, 5 mg/kg, 6.5 mg/kg, or 8 mg/kg). All patients were pretreated with 50 μg of fentanyl. They concluded that the optimal dose to provide moderate sedation was 6.5 mg/kg. The higher dose of 8 mg/kg met the criteria for deep sedation and was not necessary in order to complete the procedure. The most common adverse effects reported included paresthesias described as a burning sensation in the perineal and perianal area, pruritus, hypoxemia, hypotension, and abdominal pain. An additional follow-up publication by the same investigators analyzed 314 patients and concluded that the appropriate dose for moderate sedation was 6.5 mg/kg. At this dosage, they reported a 4% incidence of deep sedation.[55]

Fospropofol was also studied as the sedative agent for patients undergoing bronchoscopy. This study is a multicentered double blinded randomized controlled study of 252 patients classified as ASA P1 to P4 undergoing flexible bronchoscopy. All patients received 50 μg of fentanyl prior to the administration of either 2 mg/kg or 6.5 mg/kg fospropofol. The investigators reported a higher success rate with the higher dose of 6.5 mg/kg compared to 2 mg/kg (88.7 vs. 27.5% respectively; $p < 0.001$). The most common adverse events reported included paresthesias (47.6%), pruritus (14.7%), hypoxemia (14.3%), and hypotension (3.2%). Approximately one-third of patients who received the 6.5 mg/kg dose required some form of airway support. There was a higher satisfaction rate of both physician and patient when the 6.5 mg/kg dose was administered.

It should be noted that these studies were fully sponsored by the manufacturer and conducted by nonanesthesiologists. One of the investigators is a consultant for the manufacturer MGI/Eisai corporation. The manufacturer attempted to obtain FDA approval for nonanesthesiologists to provide fospropofol for monitored anesthesia care; however, this request was later denied. The Drug Enforcement Administration listed fospropofol as a class IV controlled substance.

Benzodiazepines

Benzodiazepines are commonly used during monitored anesthesia care for their anxiolytic, amnestic, and hypnotic properties. Patients presenting for diagnostic and surgical procedures frequently request some form of anxiolytic. Midazolam is usually administered prior to the start of the surgical or diagnostic procedures to facilitate amnesia and reduce the patient's level of anxiety. Compared to other benzodiazepines, midazolam's relatively

TABLE 29-2. COMPARISON OF THE IMPORTANT PROPERTIES OF MIDAZOLAM AND DIAZEPAM

Midazolam	Diazepam
Water-soluble, does not require propylene glycol for solubilizing	Lipid-soluble, requires propylene glycol for solubilizing
Nonvenoirritant, usually painless	Venoirritant, pain on injection
Thrombophlebitis rare	Thrombophlebitis common
Short elimination half-time (1–4 h)	Long elimination half-time (>20 h)
Clearance unaffected by H_2 antagonists	Clearance reduced by H_2 antagonists
Inactive metabolites (1-hydroxymidazolam)	Active metabolites (desmethyldiazepam, oxazepam)
Resedation unlikely	Resedation more likely

short elimination half-life and decreased likelihood of concomitant drug interactions makes this a superior choice to other benzodiazepines. The important differences between midazolam and diazepam are listed in Table 29-2.[56] Although midazolam has a short elimination half-time, there is often significant and prolonged psychomotor impairment following sedation techniques using midazolam as a significant component. With the recent availability of propofol, midazolam may be better used in a modified role by using lower doses prior to the start of a propofol infusion to provide the specific amnestic and perhaps anxiolytic component of a "balanced" sedation technique rather than as the major hypnotic component.[57] A study in healthy volunteers demonstrated that propofol reduced the distribution and clearance of midazolam in a concentration-dependent manner. The group reported increased plasma levels of midazolam ranging from 5% (±14.7%) to 26% (±9.4%) during increasing doses of propofol for monitored anesthesia care. This strategy allows the more evanescent and titratable propofol to provide the desired level of deep sedation in an adjustable manner according to the specific stimulus. The analgesic component, if required, of a balanced monitored anesthesia care technique may be provided by regional/local techniques or opioids. Again, when using opioids with benzodiazepines, the potential for significant respiratory impairment should be considered.

Age of the patient should be taken into consideration when administering benzodiazepines. The dose of a particular benzodiazepine required to reach a desired clinical end point is reduced in elderly compared with younger patients.[58] This difference in dosing requirements in elderly patients is mainly related to pharmacodynamic factors. As demonstrated by the threefold decrease in plasma concentration of midazolam, 50% of patients would be expected not to respond to verbal command (Cp50) in an 80-year-old patient compared with a 40-year-old patient (Fig. 29-4).[59]

Benzodiazepines are valuable components of monitored anesthesia care techniques because they enhance patient comfort, improve operating conditions, and provide amnesia. However, recovery of psychomotor and cognitive function may be significantly prolonged following benzodiazepine sedation, especially when compared with sedative–hypnotic techniques using propofol as the major component.[60] The specific benzodiazepine antagonist flumazenil provides the potential to improve the recovery profile of benzodiazepines by permitting the active termination of their sedative and amnestic effects without invoking adverse side effects. However, the potential for resedation remains an obstacle to the routine use of benzodiazepine reversal, particularly in patients undergoing ambulatory procedures. The effects of midazolam may recur up to 90 minutes following the administration of flumazenil.[46] Thus it is possible that patients could be discharged prematurely to a less well-monitored area, or even out of the hospital in the case of ambulatory surgery, and later experience recurrence of benzodiazepine effects. An important additional issue is that of cost. The routine use of flumazenil-antagonized benzodiazepine sedation has a significant cost disadvantage. Ghouri et al.[46] demonstrated that flumazenil-antagonized midazolam sedation was more expensive than propofol sedation ($68.67 vs. $27.80). Typical dose requirements for use of flumazenil are listed in Table 29-3.

Opioids

Opioids are administered in the context of monitored anesthesia care to provide the specific analgesic component of a "balanced" technique. Opioids are indicated when regional or local anesthetic techniques are inappropriate or ineffective and are typically administered immediately prior to the painful or invasive

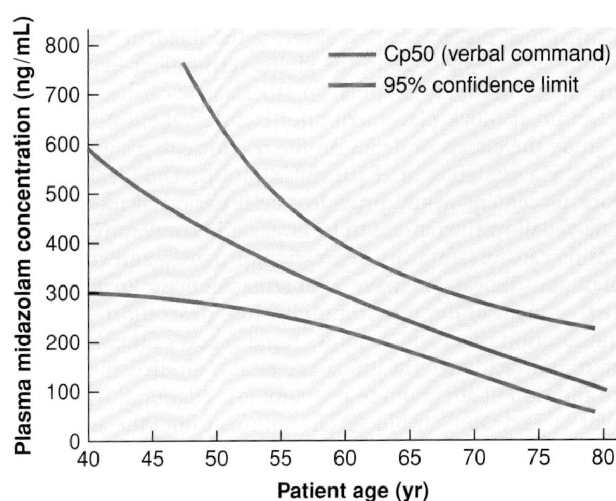

FIGURE 29-4. Midazolam Cp50 (the concentration at which 50% of subjects will fail to respond to a verbal command) as a function of age. There is a marked decrease in midazolam requirements as patient age increases. (Reproduced from Jacobs JR, Reves JG, Marty J, et al. Aging increases pharmacodynamic sensitivity to the hypnotic effects of midazolam. *Anesth Analg* 1995;80:143, with permission.)

TABLE 29-3. RECOMMENDED REGIMEN FOR THE USE OF FLUMAZENIL TO ANTAGONIZE BENZODIAZEPINE EFFECTS

Initial recommended dose of 0.2 mg
If desired level of consciousness is not achieved in 45 s, repeat 0.2-mg dose
0.2-mg doses may need to be repeated every 60 s until a maximum of 1 mg is administered
Be aware of the potential for resedation

portion of the procedure. In addition, opioids may be indicated to blunt untoward hemodynamic and physiologic responses, a desirable effect in patients with significant cardiac disease. Pain relief may be required for factors other than the procedure itself, such as uncomfortable positioning, propofol injection, pneumatic tourniquet pain, or other pain not relieved by the local anesthetic technique. The choice of a particular opioid depends on several factors including cost, availability, time of onset, duration, and potential side effects. Opioids frequently administered during monitored anesthesia care include alfentanil, fentanyl, and remifentanil. Their adverse effects include respiratory depression, muscle rigidity, and nausea and vomiting, all of which are undesirable in the spontaneously breathing patient with an unprotected airway. A complicating issue is that the ability to predict the effect of a given dose of opioid in a particular patient is limited by significant interpatient pharmacokinetic and pharmacodynamic variability. Furthermore, the coadministration of sedative agents increases the risk of serious adverse events, particularly respiratory arrest. This problem is usually overcome in practice by the cautious incremental administration of small, carefully titrated boluses or by titrating infusions to the desired effect.

An example in which the patient must briefly cooperate and remain motionless is during the placement of a retrobulbar block prior to ophthalmic procedures. Patient movement during block placement may increase the incidence of complications such as damage to the globe, retrobulbar hemorrhage, optic nerve injury, total spinal anesthesia, and cardiac arrest.[61,62] Retrobulbar block placement affords an excellent opportunity to study the effects of drugs on the response to a standardized, ethically acceptable, brief painful stimulus. The ideal drug for block placement would provide a brief period of intense analgesia yet allow the patient to be awake and cooperative without causing cardiorespiratory depression or nausea and vomiting.[36] Alfentanil appears to have a pharmacokinetic advantage for the treatment of discrete stimuli because of its short effect–site equilibration time, which allows rapid access of the drug to the brain and facilitates titration. Yee et al.[63] studied the effect of the addition of alfentanil to propofol for sedation during placement of a retrobulbar block. The authors found the addition of alfentanil improved the conditions of block placement although increased doses of alfentanil were associated with oxygen desaturation. In addition, the total amount of propofol for sedation decreased proportional to the increasing concentration of alfentanil. Other opioids, including fentanyl and remifentanil, have been successfully administered for ophthalmic surgery without significant side effects.[64–66] In a study conducted by Ahmad et al.,[67] a bolus of 1 μg/kg of remifentanil over 30 seconds was administered 90 seconds prior to block placement. More than three-quarters of patients receiving remifentanil did not report any pain during subsequent block placement. However, 15% of the patients given a single bolus alone had significant respiratory depression (respiratory rates <8 breaths per minute), and 19% of those given a bolus followed by an infusion had significant respiratory depression. The group also noted that remifentanil provided superior analgesia compared to alfentanil administered at a dose of 7 μg/kg.

The well-described phenomenon of patient awareness and subsequent recall of intraoperative events following high-dose opioid anesthesia is taken as evidence that opioids lack significant amnestic properties. However, when the effects of low-dose fentanyl on memory were specifically examined in volunteers, it was found that although the subjects appeared to be awake during the fentanyl infusion, there was significant memory impairment.[68] In this study, the degree of stimulation was probably less than that experienced by a patient undergoing a painful surgical procedure. Recall for a painful stimulus during an invasive procedure may not be impaired to the same degree as recall for the less noxious stimuli experienced by the subjects of this study. Aydin et al.[69] noted the addition of fentanyl to local anesthesia during cataract surgery provided a significant difference in sedation levels, however, it was of brief duration. If amnesia is desired as part of a balanced technique, a sedative–hypnotic agent should be administered and the dose of both agents decreased to avoid any cardiorespiratory events.

Remifentanil

Remifentanil is a potent, ultrashort acting opioid used during monitored anesthesia care to provide analgesia during brief, painful procedures. Remifentanil is typically administered by a bolus to achieve therapeutic analgesia followed by a continuous infusion. If the situation permits, the bolus should be avoided to decrease the incidence of adverse cardiorespiratory effects. It has been suggested that the administration of continuous infusions during monitored anesthesia care improves the operative conditions for the proceduralist.[70,71]

Remifentanil has pharmacodynamic properties similar to those of other potent μ-opioid receptor agonists such as fentanyl and alfentanil. However, remifentanil is predominantly metabolized by nonspecific esterases generating an extremely rapid clearance and termination of effect making it an attractive choice for patients with significant hepatic or renal disease.[72,73] Another major advantage is the intense analgesia of limited duration, which is advantageous to prevent respiratory depression after the stimulating portion of the procedure is completed. The context-sensitive half-time of remifentanil is consistently short, 3 to 5 minutes, increasing to a minimal degree with the duration of the infusion.[74,75] Furthermore, remifentanil has a short effect–site equilibration time ($t_{1/2}k_{e0}$) of 1 to 1.5 minutes. This $t_{1/2}k_{e0}$ is slightly longer than that of alfentanil (0.6 to 1.2 minutes) but much shorter than that of fentanyl (4 to 5 minutes) and morphine (approximately 20 minutes), and makes the onset of effect after drug administration very rapid, thus facilitating titration of effect during monitored anesthesia care.

In clinical practice, remifentanil has been used successfully as the analgesic component of sedation techniques for regional and local anesthesia. Its unique pharmacokinetic profile makes it well suited for monitored anesthesia care techniques. Published experience with the use of remifentanil suggests that it is possible to titrate remifentanil administration to provide effective analgesia with minimal respiratory depression. The published data can be used to generate some practical clinical guidelines,[76] which are discussed here.

1. The most desirable therapeutic end point for remifentanil administration is effective analgesia and patient comfort rather than sedation. Sedative drugs such as propofol or midazolam can be used in combination with remifentanil to provide the hypnotic–amnestic component of the sedation technique, remembering that the concomitant administration of midazolam decreases remifentanil dose requirements by up to 50%.[77]
2. Published data suggest that bolus administration of remifentanil is associated with an increased incidence of respiratory depression and chest wall rigidity. Because these side effects are likely to be related to high peak concentrations of drugs, it is recommended that remifentanil boluses be administered slowly (over 30 to 90 seconds) or avoided completely by using a pure infusion technique. If respiratory depression is promptly recognized and the remifentanil administration is reduced or discontinued, it should resolve within approximately 3 minutes. Despite the pharmacokinetic advantages of remifentanil, the level of vigilance required for its administration should be no different from that for any other potent opioid. Although the offset time of remifentanil is rapid, it still requires the recognition of respiratory depression to trigger a downward adjustment in dosage. Similarly, the short $t_{1/2}k_{e0}$ of remifentanil suggests that sudden respiratory depression may occur in response to upward adjustments in dosage. Despite the potential for respiratory depression, the efficacy of remifentanil boluses during monitored anesthesia care has been investigated by several groups.[66,78–80]
3. The effects of coadministration of benzodiazepines and opioids are well documented. The addition of midazolam to provide the anxiolytic–sedative and amnestic components of a sedation technique has been shown to increase patient satisfaction and significantly reduce remifentanil dose requirements. The combination of remifentanil with midazolam significantly reduces patient anxiety when compared with the use of the opioid alone.[42] Even relatively low-dose midazolam (2 mg IV) produces significant reductions in remifentanil requirements and patient anxiety. During breast or lymph node biopsy, remifentanil infusion requirements were 0.065 μg/kg/min when preceded by midazolam compared with 0.123 μg/kg/min when used alone.[77] The advantages of coadministration of small doses of midazolam include increased patient satisfaction, increased amnesia, decreased nausea and vomiting, and decreased anxiety. The disadvantages include a tendency toward increased respiratory depression, apnea, and excessive sedation.
4. Because most painful stimuli are of unpredictable duration and because the risk of adverse respiratory events is increased following bolus administration, the most logical method for the administration of remifentanil during monitored anesthesia care is by an adjustable infusion. This should ideally be preceded by a small bolus of midazolam. Most investigators have used infusion rates that start at 0.1 μg/kg/min approximately 5 minutes prior to the first painful stimulus. This initial "loading" infusion is then weaned to approximately 0.05 μg/kg/min to maintain patient comfort. The maintenance infusion is adjusted upward in response to pain or hemodynamic response or downward in response to excessive sedation, respiratory depression, or apnea. A typical incremental change in infusion rate is 0.025 μg/kg/min. The use of remifentanil infusions of 0.2 μg/kg/min is associated with an increased incidence of respiratory depression that is not necessarily associated with superior analgesia. As in the case of propofol administration, inadvertent interruption of remifentanil administration will result in abrupt offset of effect, which may result in patient discomfort, hemodynamic instability, and even morbidity due to patient movement. It is therefore very important to ensure that the drug delivery system is monitored carefully during the procedure. Remifentanil is supplied as a powder that must be reconstituted prior to use. It is particularly important when administering this drug to patients with an unsecured airway to ensure that there are no errors in drug dilution that would result in inadvertent dosing errors.

Typical adult dose recommendations for opioids and other drugs discussed in the text are listed in Table 29-4.

Ketamine

Ketamine, a phencyclidine derivative, is an intense analgesic frequently used as a component of pediatric sedation techniques and is rapidly gaining popularity in the adult population.[81–83] When used in small doses (0.25 to 0.5 mg/kg), its use is associated with minimal respiratory and cardiovascular depression. Ketamine produces a dissociative state in which the eyes remain open with a nystagmic gaze. However, as the dose of ketamine increases, or when used in combination with other sedatives, a state of deep sedation and/or general anesthesia may be inadvertently achieved. Increased oral secretions make laryngospasm more likely. The fear of laryngospasm is the underlying rationale for the frequent administration of an antisialagogue such as atropine or glycopyrrolate. Ketamine is frequently combined with a benzodiazepine to reduce the incidence of hallucinations associated with its use. However, this practice is controversial.[84] There are increasing reports in the emergency medicine literature of replacing benzodiazepines and/or opioids with propofol when ketamine is administered for sedation. Advantages of the administration of "ketofol" are predominately due to the ability of these drugs to balance the negative side effects of the other. For example, the analgesic effect of ketamine reduces the dosage of propofol required in order to complete an invasive or painful procedure. Frequent advantages cited included preserved hemodynamic stability, decreased nausea and vomiting, improved procedural conditions, and decreased airway complications.[85–89] Problems may arise when repeated doses or prolonged administration of the drug combinations are required due to differences in half-life. The effect of ketamine may outlast the effects of propofol under these conditions. Patient movement may make ketamine less than ideal for procedures requiring a completely motionless patient. Ketamine can elevate intracranial and intraocular pressure and is thus relatively contraindicated in patients with increased intracranial pressure and with glaucoma or open-globe injuries.[90] Although it has been suggested that airway reflexes are relatively preserved with ketamine, there is no convincing evidence to support this notion.

Ketamine can be administered orally, intramuscularly, or intravenously. The oral dose of ketamine is 4 to 6 mg/kg. The onset of action typically occurs within 20 to 30 minutes and the duration of effect is between 60 and 90 minutes. The intramuscular dose is 2 to 4 mg/kg with an onset of action of 5 to 10 minutes and typically has a duration of effect of 30 to 120 minutes. When administered via the IV route, ketamine should be given in small (0.25 to 1 mg/kg) increments, titrating to effect with an onset of action of 1 to 2 minutes and an approximate duration of 20 to 60 minutes.

TABLE 29-4. TYPICAL DOSE RANGES OF SEDATIVE, HYPNOTIC, AND ANALGESIC DRUGS

Drug	Typical Adult Intravenous Dose Range (Titrated to Effect in Small Increments)
Benzodiazepines	
Midazolam	1–2 mg prior to propofol or remifentanil infusion
	2–8 mg as major component
Diazepam	2.5–10 mg
Opioid Analgesics	
Alfentanil	5–20 μg/kg bolus 2 min prior to stimulus
Fentanyl	0.5–2-μg/kg bolus 2–4 min prior to stimulus
Remifentanil	Infusion 0.1 μg/kg/min 5 min prior to stimulus
	Wean to 0.05 μg/kg/min as tolerated
	Adjust up or down in increments of 0.025 μg/kg/min
	Reduce dose accordingly when coadministered with midazolam or propofol
	Avoid boluses
Hypnotics	
Propofol	250–500-μg/kg boluses
	25–75 μg/kg/min infusion
Dexmedetomidine	Loading infusion: 0.5–1 μg/kg over 10–20 min
	Maintenance infusion: 0.2–0.7–1 μg/kg/h

Dexmedetomidine

Dexmedetomidine is a selective α_2 receptor agonist that depresses central sympathetic function and produces sedation and analgesia. The α_2 agonists potentiate opioid-induced analgesia, benzodiazepine-induced hypnosis, and have potent MAC-sparing effects when administered with volatile agents.

Compared with other sedative and analgesic drugs, dexmedetomidine appears to have relatively minor effects on respiratory function when used in the typical dose range.[91–93] Of note, unlike during opioid-induced sedation, the hypercapnic arousal response, a feature of natural sleep, appears to be preserved during dexmedetomidine sedation. However, airway intervention to relieve obstruction and apnea may be required during dexmedetomidine administration, particularly when used in combination with other respiratory depressants.[94] Dexmedetomidine has been used for sedation during instrumentation of the difficult airway. Patients undergoing fiberoptic intubation sedated with dexmedetomidine are generally comfortable yet cooperative.[95–99] Administration of α_2 agonist is associated with a reduction of sympathetic outflow and an increase in cardiac vagal activity; therefore, it is not surprising that hypotension and bradycardia may occur during dexmedetomidine administration. Clinically significant episodes of bradycardia and sinus arrest have been associated with dexmedetomidine administration in young, healthy volunteers with high vagal tone, particularly during rapid IV or bolus administration.[100,101] The α_2 agonists do have peripheral vasoconstrictive effects that can occasionally precipitate hypertension. Despite this phenomenon, the incidence of hypertensive episodes requiring intervention is lower when compared with an equivalent propofol-based technique.[102]

Dexmedetomidine has been used successfully in both adult and pediatric patients for monitored anesthesia care during the awake portions of craniotomies requiring patient cooperation for cortical speech mapping.[103,104] Dexmedetomidine has been used as sedative supplementation to regional anesthesia during carotid endarterectomy. Under these circumstances, there were fewer fluctuations from the desired sedation level when compared with the combination of midazolam, fentanyl, and propofol.[105] Dexmedetomidine tends to decrease cerebral blood flow both directly via α_2-mediated constriction of cerebral blood vessels and indirectly via its effect on systemic pressure. However, there appears to be a concomitant decrease in cerebral metabolic rate.[106] To add further reassurance, the use of dexmedetomidine does not appear to be associated with an increase in the need for intracarotid shunting in patients undergoing awake carotid endarterectomy.[107]

The lack of pain on injection and its analgesic and minimal adverse respiratory properties would seem to make dexmedetomidine a useful alternative to propofol in certain circumstances. However, when compared with propofol, the target sedation level takes longer to achieve with dexmedetomidine (25 vs. 10 minutes).[108] Furthermore, if loading boluses of dexmedetomidine are used to accelerate the onset of sedation, bradycardia and hypotension may occur. Although the use of dexmedetomidine may result in greater sedation, lower blood pressure, and improved analgesia in the recovery room when compared with propofol, the time to postanesthesia care unit discharge is not significantly different.[109] Dexmedetomidine is most often delivered as an initial bolus followed by a continuous infusion. Initial bolus doses range from 0.5 to 1 μg/kg over 10 to 20 minutes, followed by a continuous infusion of 0.2 to 0.7 μg/kg/hr.

Two large retrospective observational studies from a single children's hospital suggest that dexmedetomidine may be used for sedation for pediatric magnetic resonance imaging and computed tomography studies.[109,110] In these studies, the loading dose of dexmedetomidine was 2 to 3 μg/kg over 10 minutes, followed by an infusion of between 1 and 2 μg/kg/hr. However, approximately 15% of patients required a second bolus in order to achieve satisfactory conditions to complete the scan. The analgesic properties of dexmedetomidine may make it a useful alternative to the use of propofol as a sole agent during painful procedures. However, the time taken to deliver the loading dose, the occasional

TABLE 29-5. A COMPARISON OF SOME IMPORTANT PROPERTIES OF PROPOFOL AND DEXMEDETOMIDINE

	Propofol	Dexmedetomidine
Pain on injection	Yes	Minimal
Analgesic properties in subhypnotic doses	Minimal	Yes
Amnestic properties in subhypnotic doses	Significant	Insignificant
Time of onset with typical administration	Rapid	5–10 min
Restrictive regulations on use by nonanesthesia-trained providers	Yes	No
Potential for significant bradycardia	Minimal	Significant

need to rebolus, hypotension, bradycardia, and the relatively long recovery time may limit the utility of dexmedetomidine for very brief procedures such as computed tomography studies. On the other hand, the pain on injection of propofol and the legislative constraints on the administration of propofol by nonanesthesia-trained providers may make dexmedetomidine advantageous in certain circumstances.

Amnesia During Sedation with Dexmedetomidine or Propofol

Drugs with sedative–hypnotic properties reduce attention to stimuli as a direct consequence of depression of consciousness. Therefore, all sedative–hypnotics have the potential to impair memory formation because attention to stimuli is a crucial element of explicit memory formation. However, like benzodiazepines, propofol has significant amnestic effects at subhypnotic doses, suggesting an additional amnestic mechanism that is separate from its sedative effect.[111] In the case of propofol, drug-induced amnesia appears to be a consequence of lack of retention of information that was already successfully stored into long-term memory.[112] In contrast to propofol and benzodiazepines, it is unlikely that dexmedetomidine has amnestic properties at subhypnotic doses.[113] If amnesia is desired for a procedure performed during dexmedetomidine administration, loss of consciousness would be necessary if dexmedetomidine is used as the sole agent. Alternatively, amnestic doses of propofol or a benzodiazepine may be used to supplement dexmedetomidine. The properties of propofol and dexmedetomidine are compared in Table 29-5.

Patient-controlled Sedation and Analgesia

Techniques that allow the direct patient control of the level of sedation may positively affect patient satisfaction.[114] The degree of sedation desired by the patient varies significantly and the individual response to drugs is variable. Patient-controlled sedation appears to be an attractive solution to this problem. One approach to patient-controlled sedation has been to use a conventional patient-controlled analgesia (PCA) delivery system set to deliver 0.7-mg/kg boluses of propofol with a 3-minute lockout period.[115] Other approaches include fixed-dose combinations of 0.5-mg midazolam and 25-μg fentanyl with a 5-minute lockout interval between doses.[116] The pharmacokinetic profile of alfentanil is ideal for the treatment of short, discrete episodes of pain. These properties have been exploited during vaginal ovum retrieval procedures, when ultrasonically guided needles are passed through the vaginal wall under monitored anesthesia care. Zelcer et al.[117] used a PCA delivery system to allow self-administration of alfentanil during this procedure. After midazolam premedication and a loading dose of alfentanil, patients received 5-μg/kg boluses of alfentanil via the PCA pump with a mandatory 3-minute lockout period. Patient acceptability, alfentanil dosage, respiratory variables, and pain scores were similar to those obtained with physician-controlled analgesia. From the limited data that are available, intraoperative PCA during monitored anesthesia care appears to be an effective alternative to physician-administered analgesia.

RESPIRATORY FUNCTION AND SEDATIVE–HYPNOTICS

During monitored anesthesia care, there is significant potential for respiratory compromise mediated via several important mechanisms. These include adverse effects on respiratory drive, either directly as a result of sedative–hypnotic or opioid administration or indirectly as a consequence of brain stem hypoperfusion resulting from hypotension. There may also be a marked increase in the work of breathing because of increased upper airway resistance.[118] During sedation, it is likely that protective airway reflexes will be attenuated. On the other hand, sedative doses of benzodiazepines appear to have variable effects on respiratory system mechanics, either decreasing, increasing, or having no effect on functional residual capacity.[119,120]

Sedation and Upper Airway Patency

The upper airway is located outside the thorax. During normal inspiration, the pressure within the upper airway is subatmospheric; thus, there is a tendency for the upper airway to collapse under the influence of the surrounding atmospheric pressure. However, in the normal subject this tendency for airway collapse is opposed by upper airway dilator muscle tone. These muscles probably both increase the diameter and reduce the compliance of the upper airway. An increase in upper airway dilator muscle tone occurs during inspiration, commencing just prior to diaphragmatic contraction.[121] Several studies have confirmed the importance of coordinated activation of the diaphragmatic and upper airway respiratory muscles in maintaining airway patency. Upper airway dilator muscle control appears to be extremely sensitive to sedative–hypnotic drug administration.[122] For example, sedative doses of midazolam have been reported to increase inspiratory subglottic airway resistance by three- to fourfold.[123] Sedative doses of diazepam selectively suppress genioglossal muscle activity to a greater degree than diaphragmatic activity; furthermore, this effect is exaggerated in elderly patients. In all these examples, the increased upper airway resistance markedly increased the work of breathing. The response to this obstruction is a significant increase in intercostal and accessory muscle activity. However, this response is only partially effective because the increase in inspiratory force will further decrease intraluminal upper airway pressure, predisposing to further airway collapse. It is likely that these effects will be of greatest significance in patients with pre-existing respiratory compromise, such as elderly patients or those with chronic obstructive pulmonary disease. These patients often have limited respiratory reserve and are unable to increase their respiratory muscle activity in response to the increased work of breathing induced by sedation and may become hypercarbic, acidotic, and hypoxic.

Sedation and Protective Airway Reflexes

Competent laryngeal and upper airway reflexes are required to protect the lower airway from aspiration. Protective laryngeal and pharyngeal reflexes are depressed by anesthesia and sedation. Furthermore, it is also well documented that protective airway reflexes are compromised by advanced age and debilitation. Therefore, it is likely that significant depression of airway reflexes could occur during sedation in the elderly or debilitated patient. Aspiration of gastric contents could occur either in the operating room or during recovery, particularly if oral intake is allowed before the return of adequate upper airway protective reflexes. The time required for the return of protective reflexes varies considerably. Complete recovery of the swallowing reflex occurs approximately 15 minutes after the return of consciousness following propofol anesthesia.[124,72] However, the IV administration of 15 mg of diazepam has been shown to depress the swallowing reflex for up to 4 hours.[125] The swallowing reflex is significantly depressed for up to 2 hours following the administration of midazolam despite the return to a normal state of consciousness.[126] In otherwise healthy adult male volunteers, the inhalation of 50% nitrous oxide was associated with marked depression of the swallowing reflex.[127]

It is apparent from the sources previously quoted that the protective airway reflexes alone cannot be relied on to protect the lower airway from aspiration during sedation. Thus, patients who are deemed to be at risk from aspiration of gastric contents should be maintained at the lightest level of sedation possible. Ideally, the patient should be awake enough to recognize the regurgitation of gastric contents and be able to protect his or her own airway. If the ability of the patient to protect his or her own airway cannot be reliably guaranteed and regurgitation/aspiration is thought to be a significant risk, placement of a cuffed endotracheal tube under general anesthesia should be seriously considered.

Sedation and Respiratory Control

Clinical experience would lead most anesthesiologists to predict that the administration of sedative–hypnotic drugs is associated with the depression of respiratory drive. However, the findings of scientific studies in this area are often conflicting and confusing. On occasion they show minimal effects of sedative drugs, if any, on ventilatory responsiveness. However, it is important to note that in many cases the methods used to measure respiratory drive may affect the outcome of the study by stimulating the subject, thus attenuating the negative effect of the drug on respiratory drive. In clinical practice, it is likely that during regional anesthesia there is a degree of deafferentation that will potentiate the respiratory depressant effects of sedative–hypnotic drugs.[128] Most studies have demonstrated that opioids depress the ventilatory response to hypercapnia and hypoxia.[129–132] Reports of the effects of sedative doses of benzodiazepines on carbon dioxide responsiveness have shown variable results, including no significant effect and clinically significant depression.[132–136] However, when opioids and benzodiazepines are used in combination, there appears to be a consistent and marked negative effect on respiratory responsiveness.[28,137] Although the addition of sedative doses of propofol to opioids showed little potentiation of the respiratory effects of opioids, caution is still warranted when combinations of sedative–hypnotics are used.

SUPPLEMENTAL OXYGEN ADMINISTRATION

Hypoxia as a result of alveolar hypoventilation is a relatively common occurrence following the administration of sedatives, analgesics, and hypnotics. In the absence of significant lung disease, the administration of only modest concentrations of supplemental oxygen is frequently effective in restoring the patient's oxygen saturation to an acceptable level. This concept is well illustrated by reference to the familiar alveolar gas equation. An extreme example illustrates the point: An otherwise healthy adult male breathing room air receives a dose of an opioid that causes marked alveolar hypoventilation such that his alveolar PCO_2 is increased to 80 mm Hg. The alveolar gas equation predicts that his arterial PO_2 will fall to approximately 40 mm Hg as shown here:

$$P_{AO_2} = P_{IO_2} - P_{ACO_2}/R$$

$$P_{IO_2} = F_{IO_2} \times (P_B - P_{H_2O})$$

$$P_{IO_2} = 0.21 \times (760 - 47) = 150 \text{ mm Hg}$$

$$P_{AO_2} = 150 - 80/0.8$$

$$P_{AO_2} = 50 \text{ mm Hg}$$

where P_{AO_2} is alveolar partial pressure of oxygen, P_{IO_2} is inspired partial pressure of oxygen, P_{ACO_2} is alveolar partial pressure of carbon dioxide, R is respiratory quotient, P_B is barometric pressure, and P_{H_2O} is water vapor pressure at body temperature.

Assuming a normal alveolar to arterial (A–a) gradient, his P_{AO_2} will be 40 mm Hg, corresponding to an arterial oxygen saturation of 75%. If while initiating definitive therapy for hypoventilation this patient were to receive only a modest increase in inspired oxygen, a marked improvement in arterial saturation would be achieved:

$$F_{IO_2} \text{ increased to } 28\%$$

$$P_{IO_2} = 0.28 \times (760 - 47) = 200 \text{ mm Hg}$$

$$P_{AO_2} = 200 - 80/0.8$$

$$P_{AO_2} = 100 \text{ mm Hg}$$

This theoretical example serves to highlight an important point. First, in isolated hypoventilation modest increases in inspired oxygen are remarkably effective at restoring oxygen saturation to acceptable levels. However, a patient who is receiving minimal supplemental oxygen and has an acceptable oxygen saturation may have significant undetected alveolar hypoventilation. The necessity to administer oxygen supplementation is controversial. Deitch et al.[138] reported use of supplemental oxygen (2 L/min) during sedation with midazolam and fentanyl did not reduce the occurrence of hypoxia compared to patients on room air. The investigators conducted a similar study evaluating the effect of 3 L/min of oxygen in patients receiving propofol and reported that patients on oxygen had a lower incidence of desaturations compared to patients on room air (18% vs. 28%, respectively) although it was not found to be significant.[139] The authors claimed physician recognition and correction of an obstructed airway was of greater significance than supplemental oxygen. It should be noted that the data from the ASA closed claims analysis shows that respiratory depression associated with monitored anesthesia care accounted for over one-third of closed-claim injuries in remote locations.[140] We recommend that before discharging patients, it is useful to measure their oxygen saturation while breathing room air.

MONITORING DURING MONITORED ANESTHESIA CARE

American Society of Anesthesiologists Standards

The ASA standards for basic anesthetic monitoring are applicable to all levels of anesthesia care, including monitored anesthesia care. It is useful to review the components of the ASA standards that are pertinent to monitored anesthesia care as approved by the House of Delegates on October 20, 2010 with an effective day of July 1, 2011.[141] (See Chapter 25 Commonly Used Monitoring Techniques for the current ASA standards.)

Communication and Observation

A conscientious and well-trained anesthesia caregiver is the single most vital monitor in the operating room. However, his or her effectiveness will be markedly enhanced by the use of the basic quantitative and qualitative monitoring devices, which should be readily available in all operating rooms. It is important that the anesthesiologist continually evaluates the patient's response to verbal stimulation to effectively titrate the level of sedation and to allow the earlier detection of neurologic or cardiorespiratory dysfunction. Continuous visual, tactile, and auditory assessment of physiologic function should include observation of the rate, depth, and pattern of respiration; palpation of the arterial pulse; and assessment of peripheral perfusion by extremity temperature and capillary refill. In addition, the patient should be continually observed for diaphoresis, pallor, shivering, cyanosis, and acute changes in neurologic status.

Auscultation

Auscultation of heart and breath sounds has long been a vital component of monitoring during anesthesia. Placement of a precordial stethoscope near the sternal notch of a nonintubated patient provides important information concerning upper airway patency as well as a continuous monitor of heart sounds and ventilation. Continuous precordial auscultation is an inexpensive, effective, and essentially risk-free process that serves as an additional important purpose by bringing the anesthesia care provider closer to the patient. If access to the patient is limited during the procedure, FM wireless or infrared remote transmission systems are now commercially available.

Pulse Oximetry

No monitor of oxygen transport has had a greater impact on the practice of anesthesiology than the pulse oximeter.[142] Pulse oximetry is noninvasive, safe, and comfortable to the awake patient; it is also technically simple to apply and interpret, and allows continuous real-time monitoring of arterial oxygenation. The use of a quantitative measure of oxygenation is specifically mandated by the ASA standards for intraoperative monitoring.
6 The important mechanisms whereby respiratory function may be compromised during monitored anesthesia care include the effects of sedatives and opioids on respiratory drive, upper airway patency, and protective airway reflexes. Additional important risk factors for arterial desaturation include obesity, pre-existing upper airway obstruction and respiratory disease, increased metabolic rate, general anesthesia, the extremes of age, surgical site and patient positioning.[143–145] The fundamental importance of monitoring oxygenation during monitored anesthesia care can be appreciated from the closed-claim study of Caplan et al.[128] who examined 14 cases of sudden cardiac arrest in otherwise healthy patients who received spinal anesthesia. These major anesthetic mishaps occurred before the routine adoption of pulse oximetry. One of the major findings of this study was that cyanosis frequently heralded the onset of cardiac arrest, suggesting that unappreciated respiratory insufficiency may have played an important role. Further support for the use of pulse oximetry comes from the ASA Committee on Professional Liability analysis of closed anesthesia claims, which reveals that respiratory events constitute the single largest source of adverse outcome. Furthermore, review of these cases suggests that pulse oximetry in combination with capnometry would have prevented the adverse outcome in most cases.

Capnography

Although capnography is most effective in the intubated patient, useful information may be obtained from a spontaneously breathing, nonintubated patient. Capnography may be used to monitor respiratory rate and aid in the detection and management of airway obstruction. There are numerous methods to monitor end-tidal carbon dioxide. In addition, it may be able to detect hypoventilation during the administration of supplemental oxygen.[146] Sidestream capnographs have been adapted for use with face masks, nasal airways, and nasal cannulae and have been used successfully during monitored anesthesia care.[83–86,147,148] Nasal cannulae for oxygen delivery have been modified to provide an integral port for respiratory gas sampling and are available commercially. Alternatively, capnograph sampling lines can be attached to shortened IV catheters and inserted inside nasal oxygen probes. There is growing evidence that capnography may reduce risk associated with sedation/analgesia or monitored anesthesia care in both the pediatric and adult population.[146,149,150] Waugh et al.[151] conducted a meta-analysis to determine if the addition of capnography identified more respiratory complications than standard monitoring alone. They reported that cases of respiratory depression were 17.6 times more likely to be detected if monitored with capnography. Currently, capnography is not a standard of care; however, because of the low cost and enhanced patient safety, we recommend routine use for all patients receiving sedation/analgesia or monitored anesthesia care.

Cardiovascular System

At a minimum, the electrocardiogram must be continually displayed and the blood pressure measured and recorded at least every 5 minutes during monitored anesthesia care. The pulse should be monitored by palpation, oximetry, or auscultation. The selection of additional hemodynamic monitoring is usually determined more by the cardiovascular status of the patient than the magnitude of the procedure. Most procedures performed under monitored anesthesia care do not involve major hemorrhage, fluid shifts, or major physiologic trespass. Decisions concerning choice of monitoring for myocardial ischemia and other adverse hemodynamic events will need to be individualized on a case-by-case basis.

Temperature Monitoring and Management During Monitored Anesthesia Care

The value of temperature monitoring is well established during general anesthesia, the perioperative period being frequently complicated by hypothermia and hyperthermia. Although sedation techniques used during monitored anesthesia care do not generally trigger malignant hyperthermia, there is potential for significant inadvertent hypothermia, particularly during neuraxial anesthesia. Even monitored anesthesia care techniques unaccompanied by regional anesthesia are associated with hypothermia at the extremes of age, both the old and very young having impaired thermoregulatory mechanisms. The elderly also have markedly reduced muscle mass and therefore basal heat production. Although the anesthesiologist may be able to exert some control over the ambient temperature in the operating room, he or she may be unable to influence the temperature at remote anesthetizing locations. Radiology suites are often maintained at lower temperatures to accommodate the computer systems that are used to reconstruct images. Radiant heating lamps, forced-air heaters, fluid warmers, or warming blankets, all common items in operating rooms, may be unavailable and unsuitable for use at remote locations. Forced-air heating has been shown to be an effective means of maintaining normothermia, and can be combined with IV fluid warming.[152,153] Even mild perioperative hypothermia (i.e., 1° to 2°C) accompanying general anesthesia is associated with adverse myocardial outcomes, increased bleeding tendency and transfusion requirements, wound infections, and delayed wound healing and hospital discharge.[154–159] At this time, there is no evidence suggesting that the morbidity associated with perioperative hypothermia is any less during monitored anesthesia care than during general anesthesia. The morbidity associated with perioperative hypothermia is well described in high-risk patients; this is a group of patients who are very likely to undergo procedures under monitored anesthesia care. When hypothermia is significant, shivering may interfere with the planned procedure and markedly increase oxygen requirements and predispose susceptible patients to myocardial ischemia or respiratory insufficiency. The major thermoregulatory defenses against hypothermia include vasoconstriction, shivering, and behavior. Vasoconstriction and shivering are impaired during major conduction anesthesia. Behavioral thermoregulation is impaired even in the conscious patient. Regional anesthesia has major effects on thermoregulation.[160] Lower extremity vasodilatation causes central cooling via a redistribution of heat from the core to the periphery. Afferent input to the hypothalamus from the warm peripheral compartment counteracts conflicting input from the cooling central compartment, thus delaying the initiation of compensatory thermoregulation. In the absence of reliable temperature monitoring, it is possible that the first indication of hypothermia would be the onset of shivering, by which time considerable central cooling may have occurred.

Frank et al.[161] have examined the issue of temperature monitoring and management during neuraxial anesthesia and found that temperature monitoring is significantly underused, with only one-third of patients being monitored. Furthermore, the method that was most frequently used to monitor temperature may not accurately reflect core temperature, the most important determinant of thermoregulatory response and perioperative morbidity. Forehead skin surface was the most commonly monitored site. The accuracy of these devices for perioperative temperature monitoring remains controversial; they do not reliably detect malignant hyperthermia and are not sufficiently accurate for fever screening purposes in children.[162] Sessler[163] recommends the use of a properly positioned axillary probe or intermittent oral temperature monitoring during neuraxial anesthetics.

Patients will frequently complain of feeling too warm when covered by heavy drapes. Although malignant hyperthermia is rare during monitored anesthesia care, hyperthermia is still possible as a result of thyroid storm or malignant neuroleptic syndrome. The subjective sensation of hyperthermia may also be the first indicator of important adverse events in evolution such as hypoxia, hypercarbia, cerebral ischemia, local anesthetic toxicity, and myocardial ischemia.

Bispectral Index Monitoring During Monitored Anesthesia Care

The bispectral index (BIS) is a processed EEG parameter that was developed specifically to evaluate patient response during drug-induced anesthesia and sedation. Sedation monitoring is attractive because of the potential to titrate drugs more accurately, avoiding the adverse effects of both over- and under-dosing. BIS monitoring has some potential advantages over conventional intermittent techniques of patient assessment. Conventional assessment involves patient stimulation at frequent intervals to determine the level of consciousness, requires patient cooperation, and is subject to testing fatigue. An example of a conventional assessment tool is the Observer's Assessment of Alertness/Sedation Scale (Table 29-6).[164] The BIS has been shown to be a useful monitor of drug-induced sedation and recall in volunteers and has been shown to correlate with Observer's Assessment of Alertness/Sedation Scale scores during propofol-induced sedation in patients undergoing surgery with regional anesthesia.[165] An increasing depth of sedation was associated with a predictable decrease in the BIS. Absence of recall was associated with BIS values below 80. These findings correspond with those of Kearse et al.[166] who found no intraoperative recall at BIS values below 79 during midazolam-, isoflurane-, and propofol-induced sedation. However, the inability to recall a nonnoxious stimulus such as a picture, as used in the previously mentioned studies, may not necessarily correspond to amnesia to noxious events such as surgical stimulation. Despite this caveat, Liu et al.[165] suggest that using a combination of propofol and midazolam to achieve a BIS value below 80 will minimize the possibility of intraoperative recall. Although the use of BIS to monitor sedation is appealing, conventional assessment of sedation is an important mechanism whereby continuous patient contact is maintained. Ideally, BIS monitoring will be employed in the future as an adjunct to clinical evaluation rather than as the primary monitor of consciousness.

TABLE 29-6. OBSERVER'S ASSESSMENT OF ALERTNESS/SEDATION SCALE

Responsiveness	Speech	Facial Expression	Eyes	Composite Score
Responds readily to name spoken in normal tone	Normal	Normal	Clear, no ptosis	5 (alert)
Lethargic response to name spoken in normal tone	Mild slowing or thickening	Mild relaxation	Glazed or mild ptosis (less than half the eye)	4
Responds only after name is called loudly or repeatedly	Slurring or prominent slowing	Marked relaxation (slack jaw)	Glazed and marked ptosis (half the eye or more)	3
Responds only after mild prodding or shaking	Few recognizable words			2
Does not respond to mild prodding or shaking				1 (asleep)

Preparedness to Recognize and Treat Local Anesthetic Toxicity

Monitored anesthesia care is often provided in the context of regional or local anesthetic techniques. It is vitally important that the anesthesiologist responsible for the patient have a high index of suspicion and be fully prepared to recognize and treat local anesthetic toxicity immediately (see Chapter 21). This point deserves special emphasis, particularly in view of the fact that monitored anesthesia care is often provided to the elderly or debilitated patient who has been deemed "unfit" for general anesthesia; these are the patients most likely to suffer adverse reactions to local anesthetic drugs. Even if the anesthesiologist does not perform the block personally, he or she is in a unique position to fulfill an important "preventive" role by advising the surgeon about the most appropriate volume, concentration, and type of local anesthetic drug or technique to be used.

Systemic local anesthetic toxicity occurs when plasma concentrations of drug are excessively high. Plasma concentrations will increase when the rate of entry of drug into the circulation exceeds the rate of drug clearance from the circulation. The clinically recognizable effects of local anesthetics on the central nervous system are concentration dependent. At low concentrations, sedation and numbness of the tongue and circumoral tissues and a metallic taste are prominent features. As concentrations increase, restlessness, vertigo, tinnitus, and difficulty focusing may occur. Higher concentrations result in slurred speech and skeletal muscle twitching, which often herald the onset of tonic–clonic seizures.

The conduct of monitored anesthesia care may modify the individual's response to the potentially toxic effects of local anesthetic administration and adversely affect the margin of safety of a regional or local technique. For example, a patient with compromised cardiovascular function may experience a further decline in cardiac output during sedation. The resultant reduction in hepatic blood flow will reduce the clearance of local anesthetics that are metabolized by the liver and have a high hepatic extraction ratio, thereby increasing the likelihood of achieving toxic plasma concentrations. A patient receiving sedation may experience respiratory depression and a subsequent increase in arterial carbon dioxide concentration. Hypercarbia adversely affects the margin of safety in several ways. By increasing cerebral blood flow, hypercarbia will increase the amount of local anesthetic that is delivered to the brain, thereby increasing the potential for neurotoxicity. By reducing neuronal axoplasmic pH, hypercarbia increases the intracellular concentration of the charged, active form of local anesthetic, thus also increasing its toxicity. In addition, hypercarbia, acidosis, and hypoxia all markedly potentiate the cardiovascular toxicity of local anesthetics. Furthermore, the administration of sedative–hypnotic drugs may interfere with the patient's ability to communicate the symptoms of impending neurotoxicity. However, the anticonvulsant properties of benzodiazepines and barbiturates may attenuate the seizures associated with neurotoxicity. In both of these circumstances, it is possible that the symptoms of cardiotoxicity will be the first evidence that an adverse reaction has occurred. Thus, appropriate treatment is delayed or inadvertent intravascular injection is continued because of the absence of any clinical evidence of neurotoxicity. Cardiovascular toxicity usually occurs at a higher plasma concentration than neurotoxicity, but when it does occur, it is usually much more difficult to manage than neurotoxicity. Although cardiotoxicity is usually preceded by neurotoxicity, it may occur de novo when bupivacaine is being used.

Sedation and Analgesia by Nonanesthesiologists

Although anesthesiologists have specific training and expertise to provide sedation and analgesia, in clinical practice these services are frequently provided by nonanesthesiologists. The specific reasons for nonanesthesiologist involvement differ from institution to institution and from case to case and include convenience, availability, and scheduling issues; perceived lack of anesthesiologist enthusiasm; perceived increased cost; and a perceived lack of benefit concerning patient satisfaction and safety when sedation and analgesia are provided by anesthesiologists. Despite our frequent noninvolvement in these cases, anesthesiologists are indirectly involved in the care of these patients by being required to participate in the development of institutional policies and procedures for sedation and analgesia. To assist anesthesiologists in this process, an ASA task force has developed practice guidelines for sedation and analgesia by nonanesthesiologists.[2]

Four levels of sedation are defined in the ASA practice guidelines and include minimal sedation, moderate sedation, deep sedation, and general anesthesia. The practice guidelines emphasize that sedation and analgesia represent a continuum of sedation wherein patients can easily pass into a level of sedation deeper than intended. The ASA House of Delegates issued a statement on this continuum of depth of sedation originally in October 1999, and most recently amended it in October 2004. This statement

TABLE 29-7. CONTINUUM OF DEPTH OF SEDATION

	Minimal Sedation	Moderate Sedation	Deep Sedation	General Anesthesia
Responsiveness	Normal response to verbal stimulation	Purposeful response to verbal or tactile stimulation	Purposeful response following repeated or painful stimulation	Unarousable, even with a painful stimulus
Airway	Unaffected	No intervention required	Intervention may be required	Intervention often required
Spontaneous ventilation	Unaffected	Adequate	May be inadequate	Frequently inadequate
Cardiovascular function	Unaffected	Usually maintained	Usually maintained	May be impaired

Adapted from ASA House of Delegates. Continuum of depth of sedation, www.asahq.org 2004.

contains a chart representing the clinical progression along this continuum (Table 29-7).[167] When monitoring a sedated patient during a procedure, it is important to recognize when a patient becomes more deeply sedated than intended so that the care team can act appropriately to prevent cardiorespiratory compromise.

The guidelines emphasize the importance of preprocedure patient evaluation, patient preparation, and appropriate fasting periods. The importance of continuous patient monitoring is discussed—in particular, the response of the patient to commands as a guide to the level of sedation. The appropriate monitoring of pulmonary ventilation, oxygenation, and hemodynamics is also discussed, and recommendations are made for the contemporaneous recording of these parameters. The task force strongly suggests that an individual other than the person performing the procedure be available to monitor the patient's comfort and physiologic status. Education and training of providers is recommended. Specific educational objectives include the potentiation of sedative-induced respiratory depression by concomitantly administered opioids, adequate time intervals between doses of sedative/analgesics to avoid cumulative overdosage, and familiarity with sedative/analgesic antagonists. The routine administration of supplemental oxygen is recommended. At least one person with advanced life support skills should be present during the procedure. This individual should have the ability to recognize airway obstruction, establish an airway, and maintain oxygenation and ventilation. The practice guidelines recommend that appropriate patient-size emergency equipment be readily available, specifically including equipment for establishing an airway and delivering positive pressure ventilation with supplemental oxygen, emergency resuscitation drugs, and a working defibrillator. The presence of reliable intravenous access until the patient is no longer at risk for cardiorespiratory depression will improve safety. Adequate postprocedure recovery care with appropriate monitoring must be provided until discharge. Certain high-risk patient groups (e.g., uncooperative patients, extremes of age, severe cardiac, pulmonary, hepatic, renal, or central nervous system disease, morbid obesity, sleep apnea, pregnancy, and patients who abuse drug or alcohol) will be encountered, and the guidelines recommend that preprocedure consultation with anesthesiologists, cardiologists, pulmonologists, and so forth be performed *before* administration of sedation and analgesia by nonanesthesiologists.

Controversy exists regarding the level of training required for nonanesthesiologists to be credentialed to provide moderate and deep sedation. The ASA released a statement in October 2005, amended in 2011, suggesting a framework for granting privileges that will help ensure competence of individuals who administer or supervise the administration of moderate sedation.[168] This statement suggests that the practitioner should complete formal training in (1) the safe administration of sedative and analgesic drugs used to establish a level of moderate sedation, and (2) rescue of patients who exhibit adverse physiologic consequences of a deeper-than-intended level of sedation. The ASA released an advisory in October 2010 on granting privileges for deep sedation to nonanesthesiologist sedation practitioners.[169]

Recently, the Centers for Medicare and Medicaid Services (CMS) published a revised hospital anesthesia services interpretive guidelines requiring hospitals to establish policies and procedures that address whether specific clinical situations involve "anesthesia" versus "analgesia" services. The CMS document places general anesthesia, monitored anesthesia care, deep sedation, and regional anesthesia under "anesthesia" services. These "anesthesia" services must be provided by: A qualified anesthesiologist; a doctor of medicine or osteopathy, a dentist, oral surgeon, or podiatrist who is qualified to administer anesthesia under state law; an appropriately supervised Certified Registered Nurse Anesthetist or Anesthesia Assistant, all who are separate from the practitioner performing the procedure. Moderate sedation and minimal sedation fall under "analgesia" services.[170]

Finally, it is instructive to review an excerpt from the joint statement released in 2004, amended in 2009 by the American Association of Nurse Anesthetists and the ASA[171]:

> *Whenever propofol is used for sedation/anesthesia, it should be administered only by persons trained in the administration of general anesthesia, who are not simultaneously involved in these surgical or diagnostic procedures. This restriction is concordant with specific language in the propofol package insert, and failure to follow these recommendations could put patients at increased risk of significant injury or death.*

CONCLUSION

Through the use of monitored anesthesia care, an often terrifying and painful procedure can be made safe and comfortable for the patient. Monitored anesthesia care presents an opportunity for our patients to observe us at work. For the anesthesiologist, monitored anesthesia care presents an opportunity to provide a more prolonged and intimate level of care and reassurance to our patients that is in contrast to the more limited exposure that occurs during and after general anesthesia. Our airway management skills and our daily practice of applied pharmacology make

us uniquely qualified to provide this service. Monitored anesthesia care presents us with an opportunity to display these skills and increase our recognition in areas outside the operating room. The availability of drugs with a more favorable pharmacologic profile allows us to tailor our techniques to provide the specific components of analgesia, sedation, anxiolysis, and amnesia with minimal morbidity and to facilitate a prompt recovery. As the population ages, increasing numbers of patients will become candidates for monitored anesthesia care. Significant advances in nonsurgical fields (e.g., interventional radiology) will increase the number of procedures that are ideally performed under monitored anesthesia care. It is our responsibility to clearly demonstrate to our nonanesthesia colleagues that anesthesiologist-provided monitored anesthesia care contributes to the best outcome for
7 our patients. If anesthesiologists are not willing or able to provide these services, others, who are less well qualified, are prepared to assume that role.

References

1. American Society of Anesthesiologists. Distinguishing monitored anesthesia care ("MAC") from moderate sedation/analgesia (Conscious sedation). www.asahq.org 2009.
2. American Society of Anesthesiologists. Practice guidelines for sedation and analgesia by non-anesthesiologists. *Anesthesiology.* 2002;96:1004–1017.
3. American Society of Anesthesiologists. Position on monitored anesthesia care. www.asahq.org 2008.
4. Miner JR, Huber D, Nichols S, et al. The effect of the assignment of a pre-sedation target level on procedural sedation using propofol. *J Emerg Med.* 2007;32:249–255.
5. Ausems ME, Vuyk J, Hug CC, et al. Comparison of a computer-assisted infusion versus intermittent bolus administration of alfentanil as a supplement to nitrous oxide for lower abdominal surgery. *Anesthesiology.* 1988;68:851–861.
6. Hughes MA, Glass PS, Jacobs JR. Context-sensitive half-time in multicompartment pharmacokinetic models for intravenous anesthetic drugs. *Anesthesiology.* 1992;76:334–341.
7. Bailey JM. Context-sensitive half-times: What are they and how valuable are they in anaesthesiology? *Clin Pharmacokinet.* 2002;41:793–799.
8. Shafer SL, Varvel JR. Pharmacokinetics, pharmacodynamics, and rational opioid selection. *Anesthesiology.* 1991;74:53–63.
9. Scott JC, Ponganis KV, Stanski DR. EEG quantitation of narcotic effect: the comparative pharmacodynamics of fentanyl and alfentanil. *Anesthesiology.* 1985; 62:234–241.
10. Avramov MN, White PF. Use of alfentanil and propofol for outpatient monitored anesthesia care: Determining the optimal dosing regimen. *Anesth Analg.* 1997;85:566–572.
11. Mandema JW, Sansom LN, Dios-Vièitez MC, et al. Pharmacokinetic-pharmacodynamic modeling of the electroencephalographic effects of benzodiazepines. Correlation with receptor binding and anticonvulsant activity. *J Pharmacol Exp Ther.* 1991;257:472–478.
12. Newson C, Joshi GP, Victory R, et al. Comparison of propofol administration techniques for sedation during monitored anesthesia care. *Anesth Analg.* 1995;81:486–491.
13. Smith C, McEwan AI, Jhaveri R, et al. The interaction of fentanyl on the Cp50 of propofol for loss of consciousness and skin incision. *Anesthesiology.* 1994;81:820–828; discussion 26A.
14. Kazama T, Ikeda K, Morita K. Reduction by fentanyl of the Cp50 values of propofol and hemodynamic responses to various noxious stimuli. *Anesthesiology.* 1997;87:213–227.
15. Kazama T, Ikeda K, Morita K. The pharmacodynamic interaction between propofol and fentanyl with respect to the suppression of somatic or hemodynamic responses to skin incision, peritoneum incision, and abdominal wall retraction. *Anesthesiology.* 1998;89:894–906.
16. Smith C, McEwan AI, Jhaveri R, et al. Reduction of propofol Cp50 by fentanyl. *Anesthesiology.* 1992;77:A340.
17. Short TG, Plummer JL, Chui PT. Hypnotic and anaesthetic interactions between midazolam, propofol and alfentanil. *Br J Anaesth.* 1992;69:162–167.
18. Short TG, Chui PT. Propofol and midazolam act synergistically in combination. *Br J Anaesth.* 1991;67:539–545.
19. Teh J, Short TG, Wong J, et al. Pharmacokinetic interactions between midazolam and propofol: An infusion study. *Br J Anaesth.* 1994;72:62–65.
20. Simon CH. Achieving control of anesthetic administration: The infusion pump versus the vaporizer. *Anesthesiol Clin North America.* 1996;14:265–280.
21. McEwan AI, Smith C, Dyar O, et al. Isoflurane minimum alveolar concentration reduction by fentanyl. *Anesthesiology.* 1993;78:864–869.
22. Sebel PS, Glass PSA, Fletcher JE, et al. Reduction of the MAC of desflurane with fentanyl. *Anesthesiology.* 1992;76:52–59.
23. Lang E, Kapila A, Shlugman D, et al. Reduction of isoflurane minimal alveolar concentration by remifentanil. *Anesthesiology.* 1996;85:721–728.
24. Westmoreland CL, Sebel PS, Gropper A. Fentanyl or alfentanil decreases the minimum alveolar anesthetic concentration of isoflurane in surgical patients. *Anesth Analg.* 1994;78:23–28.
25. Brunner MD, Braithwaite P, Jhaveri R, et al. MAC reduction of isoflurane by sufentanil. *Br J Anaesth.* 1994;72:42–46.
26. Vinik HR, Bradley EL, Kissin I. Midazolam-alfentanil synergism for anesthetic induction in patients. *Anesth Analg.* 1989;69:213–217.
27. Kissin I, Vinik HR, Castillo R, et al. Alfentanil potentiates midazolam-induced unconsciousness in subanalgesic doses. *Anesth Analg.* 1990;71:65–69.
28. Administration FD. Black Box Warning. *Drug Bulletin.* 1988;18:15–16.
29. Bailey PL, Pace NL, Ashburn MA, et al. Frequent hypoxemia and apnea after sedation with midazolam and fentanyl. *Anesthesiology.* 1990;73:826–830.
30. Cheng SS, Yeh J, Flood P. Anesthesia matters: Patients anesthetized with propofol have less postoperative pain than those anesthetized with isoflurane. *Anesth Analg.* 2008;106:264–269.
31. Mackenzie N, Grant IS. Propofol for intravenous sedation. *Anaesthesia.* 1987; 42:3–6.
32. Wilson E, David A, Mackenzie N, et al. Sedation during spinal anaesthesia: Comparison of propofol and midazolam. *Br J Anaesth.* 1990;64:48–52.
33. Wilson E, Mackenzie N, Grant IS. A comparison of propofol and midazolam by infusion to provide sedation in patients who receive spinal anaesthesia. *Anaesthesia.* 1988;43:91–94.
34. Smith I, Monk TG, White PF, et al. Propofol infusion during regional anesthesia. *Anesth Analg.* 1994;79:313–319.
35. White PF, Negus JB. Sedative infusions during local and regional anesthesia: a comparison of midazolam and propofol. *J Clin Anesth.* 1991;3:32–39.
36. Gecaj-Gashi A, Hashimi M, Sada F, et al. Propofol vs isoflurane anesthesia-incidence of PONV in patients at maxillofacial surgery. *Adv Med Sci.* 2010;55:308–312.
37. Gauger PG, Shanks A, Morris M, et al. Propofol decreases early postoperative nausea and vomiting in patients undergoing thyroid and parathyroid operations. *World J Surg.* 2008;32:1525–1534.
38. Tan T, Bhinder R, Carey M, et al. Day-surgery patients anesthetized with propofol have less postoperative pain than those anesthetized with sevoflurane. *Anesth Analg.* 2010;111:83–85.
39. Vari A, Gazzanelli S, Cavallaro G, et al. Post-operative nausea and vomiting (PONV) after thyroid surgery: A prospective, randomized study comparing totally intravenous versus inhalational anesthetics. *Am Surg.* 2010;76:325–328.
40. Apfel CC, Korttila K, Abdalla M, et al. A factorial trial of six interventions for the prevention of postoperative nausea and vomiting. *N Engl J Med.* 2004;350:2441–2451.
41. Tramèr M, Moore A, McQuay H. Propofol anaesthesia and postoperative nausea and vomiting: Quantitative systematic review of randomized controlled studies. *Br J Anaesth.* 1997;78:247–255.
42. Fujii Y, Itakura M. Comparison of propofol, droperidol, and metoclopramide for prophylaxis of postoperative nausea and vomiting after breast cancer surgery: A prospective, randomized, double-blind, placebo-controlled study in Japanese patients. *Clin Ther.* 2008;30:2024–2029.
43. Fujii Y, Itakura M. Low-dose propofol to prevent nausea and vomiting after laparoscopic surgery. *Int J Gynaecol Obstet.* 2009;106:50–52.
44. Arslan M, Demir ME. Prevention of postoperative nausea and vomiting with a small dose of propofol combined with dexamethasone 4 mg or dexamethasone 8 mg in patients undergoing middle ear surgery: a prospective, randomized, double-blind study. *Bratisl Lek Listy.* 2011;112:332–336.
45. Borgeat A, Wilder-Smith OHG, Saiah M, et al. Subhypnotic doses of propofol possess direct antiemetic properties. *Anesth Analg.* 1992;74:539–541.
46. Ghouri AF, Ramirez Ruiz MA, White PF. Effect of flumazenil on recovery after midazolam and propofol sedation. *Anesthesiology.* 1994;81:333–339.
47. Smith I, White PF, Nathanson M, et al. Propofol. An update on its clinical use. *Anesthesiology.* 1994;81:1005–1043.
48. Moore GD, Walker AM, MacLaren R. Fospropofol: A new sedative-hypnotic agent for monitored anesthesia care. *Ann Pharmacother.* 2009;43:1802–1808.
49. Levitzky BE, Vargo JJ. Fospropofol disodium injection for the sedation of patients undergoing colonoscopy. *Ther Clin Risk Manag.* 2008;4:733–738.
50. Garnock-Jones KP, Scott LJ. Fospropofol. *Drugs.* 2010;70:469–477.
51. Struys MMRF, Fechner J, Schuttler J, et al. Erroneously published fospropofol pharmacokinetic-pharmacodynamic data and retraction of the affected publications. [Retraction of Fechner J, Ihmsen H, Hatterscheid D, Schiessl C, Vornov JJ, Burak E, Schwilden H, Schuttler J. Anesthesiology. 2003 Aug;99(2):303–13; PMID: 12883403]. [Retraction of Fechner J, Ihmsen H, Hatterscheid D, Jeleazcov C, Schiessl C, Vornov JJ, Schwilden H, Schuttler J. Anesthesiology. 2004 Sep;101(3):626–39; PMID: 15329587]. [Retraction of Shah A, Mistry B, Gibiansky E, Gibiansky L. Anesthesiology. 2008 Nov;109(5):937; discussion 937; PMID: 18946316]. [Retraction of Struys MM, Vanluchene AL, Gibiansky E, Gibiansky L, Vornov J, Mortier EP, Van Bortel L. Anesthesiology. 2005 Oct;103(4):730–43; PMID: 16192765]. [Retraction of Gibiansky E, Struys MM, Gibiansky L, Vanluchene AL, Vornov J, Mortier EP, Burak E, Van Bortel L. Anesthesiology. 2005 Oct;103(4):718–29; PMID: 16192764]. *Anesthesiology.* 2010;112:1056–1057.

ANESTHETIC MANAGEMENT

52. Shah A, Mistry B, Gibiansky E, et al. Fospropofol assay issues and impact on pharmacokinetic and pharmacodynamic evaluation. [Erratum appears in Anesthesiology. 2008 Nov;109(5):940]. [Retraction in Struys MM, Fechner J, Schuttler J, Schwilden H. Anesthesiology. 2010 Apr;112(4):1056–7; PMID: 20177373]. *Anesthesiology.* 2008;109:937; discussion
53. Shah A, Mistry B, Gibiansky E, et al. Fospropofol assay issues and impact on pharmacokinetic and pharmacodynamic evaluation. *Anesth Analg.* 2009;108:382; author reply 383.
54. Cohen LB. Clinical trial: A dose-response study of fospropofol disodium for moderate sedation during colonoscopy. *Aliment Pharmacol Ther.* 2008;27:597–608.
55. Cohen LB, Cattau E, Goetsch A, et al. A randomized, double-blind, phase 3 study of fospropofol disodium for sedation during colonoscopy. *J Clin Gastroenterol.* 2010;44:345–353.
56. Stoelting RKHS. *Benzodiazepines, Pharmacology and Physiology in Anesthetic Practice.* 4th ed. Philadelphia, PA: JB Lippincott; 2006.
57. Taylor E, Ghouri AF, White PF. Midazolam in combination with propofol for sedation during local anesthesia. *J Clin Anesth.* 1992;4:213–216.
58. Ekstein M, Gavish D, Ezri T, et al. Monitored anaesthesia care in the elderly: Guidelines and recommendations. *Drugs Aging.* 2008;25:477–500.
59. Jacobs JR, Reves JG, Marty J, et al. Aging increases pharmacodynamic sensitivity to the hypnotic effects of midazolam. *Anesth Analg.* 1995;80:143–148.
60. Pratila MG, Fischer ME, Alagesan R, et al. Propofol versus midazolam for monitored sedation: A comparison of intraoperative and recovery parameters. *J Clin Anesth.* 1993;5:268–274.
61. Tognetto D, di Lauro M, Fanni D, et al. Iatrogenic retinal traumas in ophthalmic surgery. *Graefes Arch Clin Exp Ophthalmol.* 2008;246:1361–1372.
62. Hamilton RC. *Complications of ophthalmic regional anesthesia. In:* Finucane BT, ed.*Complications of Regional Anesthesia.* New York, NY: Springer; 2007:87–101.
63. Yee JB, Burns TA, Mann JM, et al. Propofol and alfentanil for sedation during placement of retrobulbar block for cataract surgery. *J Clin Anesth.* 1996;8: 623–626.
64. Inan ÜÜ, Sivaci RG, Ermis SS, et al. Effects of fentanyl on pain and hemodynamic response after retrobulbar block in patients having phacoemulsification. *J Cataract Refract Surg.* 2003;29:1137–1142.
65. McHardy FE, Fortier J, Chung F, et al. A comparison of midazolam, alfentanil and propofol for sedation in outpatient intraocular surgery. *Can J Anaesth.* 2000;47:211–214.
66. Ryu J-H, So Y-M, Hwang J-W, et al. Optimal target concentration of remifentanil during cataract surgery with monitored anesthesia care. *J Clin Anesth.* 2010;22:533–537.
67. Ahmad S, Leavell ME, Fragen RJ, et al. Remifentanil versus alfentanil as analgesic adjuncts during placement of ophthalmologic nerve blocks. *Reg Anesth Pain Med.* 1999;24:331–336.
68. Veselis RA, Reinsel RA, Feshchenko VA, et al. Impaired memory and behavioral performance with fentanyl at low plasma concentrations. *Anesth Analg.* 1994;79:952–960.
69. Aydın ON, Ugur B, Kir E, et al. Effect of single-dose fentanyl on the cardiorespiratory system in elderly patients undergoing cataract surgery. *J Clin Anesth.* 2004;16:98–103.
70. Akcaboy ZN, Akcaboy EY, Albayrak D, et al. Can remifentanil be a better choice than propofol for colonoscopy during monitored anesthesia care? *Acta Anaesthesiol Scand.* 2006;50:736–741.
71. Keidan I, Berkenstadt H, Sidi A, et al. Propofol/remifentanil versus propofol alone for bone marrow aspiration in paediatric haemato-oncological patients. *Paediatr Anaesth.* 2001;11:297–301.
72. Glass PSA, Hardman D, Kamiyama Y, et al. Preliminary pharmacokinetics and pharmacodynamics of an ultra-short-acting opioid. *Anesth Analg.* 1993; 77:1031–1040.
73. Westmoreland CL, Hoke JF, Sebel PS, et al. Pharmacokinetics of remifentanil (GI87084B) and its major metabolite (GI90291) in patients undergoing elective inpatient surgery. *Anesthesiology.* 1993;79:893–903.
74. Egan TD, Lemmens HJ, Fiset P, et al. The pharmacokinetics of the new short-acting opioid remifentanil (GI87084B) in healthy adult male volunteers. *Anesthesiology.* 1993;79:881–892.
75. Kapila A, Glass PSA, Jacobs JR, et al. Measured context-sensitive half-times of remifentanil and alfentanil. *Anesthesiology.* 1995;83:968–975.
76. Servin F, Desmonts JM, Watkins WD. Remifentanil as an analgesic adjunct in local/regional anesthesia and in monitored anesthesia care. *Anesth Analg.* 1999; 89:S28–S32.
77. Avramov MN, Smith I, White PF. Interactions between midazolam and remifentanil during monitored anesthesia care. *Anesthesiology.* 1996;85:1283–1289.
78. Ryu J-H, Kim J-H, Park K-S, et al. Remifentanil-propofol versus fentanyl-propofol for monitored anesthesia care during hysteroscopy. *J Clin Anesth.* 2008;20:328–332.
79. Sa Rego MM, Inagaki Y, White PF. Remifentanil administration during monitored anesthesia care: Are intermittent boluses an effective alternative to a continuous infusion? *Anesth Analg.* 1999;88:518–522.
80. Smith I, Avramov MN, White PF. A comparison of propofol and remifentanil during monitored anesthesia care. *J Clin Anesth.* 1997;9:148–154.
81. Green SM. Research advances in procedural sedation and analgesia. *Ann Emerg Med.* 2007;49:31–36.
82. Green SM, Klooster M, Harris T, et al. Ketamine sedation for pediatric gastroenterology procedures. *J Pediatr Gastroenterol Nutr.* 2001;32:26–33.
83. McCarty E, Mencio G, Green N. Anesthesia and analgesia for the ambulatory management of fractures in children. *J Am Acad Orthop Surg.* 1999;7:81–91.
84. Sherwin TS, Green SM, Khan A, et al. Does adjunctive midazolam reduce recovery agitation after ketamine sedation for pediatric procedures? A randomized, double-blind, placebo-controlled trial. *Ann Emerg Med.* 2000;35:229–238.
85. Akin A, Esmaoglu A, Guler G, et al. Propofol and propofol-ketamine in pediatric patients undergoing cardiac catheterization. *Pediatr Cardiol.* 2005;26:553–557.
86. Akin A, Guler G, Esmaoglu A, et al. A comparison of fentanyl-propofol with a ketamine-propofol combination for sedation during endometrial biopsy. *J Clin Anesth.* 2005;17:187–190.
87. Aouad MT, Moussa AR, Dagher CM, et al. Addition of ketamine to propofol for initiation of procedural anesthesia in children reduces propofol consumption and preserves hemodynamic stability. *Acta Anaesthesiol Scand.* 2008;52:561–565.
88. Erden IA, Pamuk AG, Akinci SB, et al. Comparison of two ketamine-propofol dosing regimens for sedation during interventional radiology procedures. *Minerva Anestesiol.* 2010;76:260–265.
89. Phillips W, Anderson A, Rosengreen M, et al. Propofol versus propofol/ketamine for brief painful procedures in the emergency department: Clinical and bispectral index scale comparison. *J Pain Palliat Care Pharmacother.* 2010;24:349–355.
90. Nagdeve NG, Yaddanapudi S, Pandav SS. The effect of different doses of ketamine on intraocular pressure in anesthetized children. *J Pediatr Ophthalmol Strabismus.* 2006;43:219–223.
91. Hsu Y-W, Cortinez LI, Robertson KM, et al. Dexmedetomidine pharmacodynamics: part I: Crossover comparison of the respiratory effects of dexmedetomidine and remifentanil in healthy volunteers. *Anesthesiology.* 2004;101:1066–1076.
92. Shukry M, Miller JA. Update on dexmedetomidine: Use in nonintubated patients requiring sedation for surgical procedures. *Ther Clin Risk Manag.* 2010; 6:111–121.
93. Ebert TJ, Hall JE, Barney JA, et al. The effects of increasing plasma concentrations of dexmedetomidine in humans. *Anesthesiology.* 2000;93:382–394.
94. Ho AM-H, Chen S, Karmakar MK. Central apnoea after balanced general anaesthesia that included dexmedetomidine. *Br J Anaesth.* 2005;95:773–775.
95. Ramsay MA, Luterman DL. Dexmedetomidine as a total intravenous anesthetic agent. *Anesthesiology.* 2004;101:787–790.
96. Jooste EH, Ohkawa S, Sun LS. Fiberoptic intubation with dexmedetomidine in two children with spinal cord impingements. *Anesth Analg.* 2005;101:1248.
97. Maroof M, Khan R, Jain D, et al. Dexmedetomidine is a useful adjunct for awake intubation. *Can J Anaesth.* 2005;52:776–777.
98. Stamenkovic DM, Hassid M. Dexmedetomidine for fiberoptic intubation of a patient with severe mental retardation and atlantoaxial instability. *Acta Anaesthesiol Scand.* 2006;50:1314–1315.
99. Abdelmalak B, Makary L, Hoban J, et al. Dexmedetomidine as sole sedative for awake intubation in management of the critical airway. *J Clin Anesth.* 2007; 19:370–373.
100. Videira RLR, Ferreira RMV. Dexmedetomidine and asystole. *Anesthesiology.* 2004;101:1479.
101. Ingersoll-Weng E, Manecke GRJ, Thistlethwaite PA. Dexmedetomidine and cardiac arrest. *Anesthesiology.* 2004;100:738–739.
102. Talke P, Richardson CA, Scheinin M, et al. Postoperative pharmacokinetics and sympatholytic effects of dexmedetomidine. *Anesth Analg.* 1997;85:1136–1142.
103. Bekker AY, Kaufman B, Samir H, et al. The use of dexmedetomidine infusion for awake craniotomy. *Anesth Analg.* 2001;92:1251–1253.
104. Ard J, Doyle W, Bekker A. Awake craniotomy with dexmedetomidine in pediatric patients. *J Neurosurg Anesthesiol.* 2003;15:263–266.
105. Bekker AY, Basile J, Gold M, et al. Dexmedetomidine for awake carotid endarterectomy: Efficacy, hemodynamic profile, and side effects. *J Neurosurg Anesthesiol.* 2004;16:126–135.
106. Drummond JC, Dao AV, Roth DM, et al. Effect of dexmedetomidine on cerebral blood flow velocity, cerebral metabolic rate, and carbon dioxide response in normal humans. *Anesthesiology.* 2008;108:225–232.
107. Bekker A, Gold M, Ahmed R, et al. Dexmedetomidine does not increase the incidence of intracarotid shunting in patients undergoing awake carotid endarterectomy. *Anesth Analg.* 2006;103:955–958.
108. Arain SR, Ebert TJ. The efficacy, side effects, and recovery characteristics of dexmedetomidine versus propofol when used for intraoperative sedation. *Anesth Analg.* 2002;95:461–466.
109. Mason KP, Zgleszewski SE, Prescilla R, et al. Hemodynamic effects of dexmedetomidine sedation for CT imaging studies. *Paediatr Anaesth.* 2008;18: 393–402.
110. Mason KP, Zurakowski D, Zgleszewski SE, et al. High dose dexmedetomidine as the sole sedative for pediatric MRI. *Paediatr Anaesth.* 2008;18:403–411.
111. Veselis RA, Reinsel RA, Feshchenko VA, et al. Information loss over time defines the memory defect of propofol: A comparative response with thiopental and dexmedetomidine. *Anesthesiology.* 2004;101:831–841.
112. Robert AV. Memory: A guide for anaesthetists. *Best Pract Res Clin Anaesthesiol.* 2007;21:297–312.
113. Veselis RA, Reinsel RA, Feshchenko VA, et al. The comparative amnestic effects of midazolam, propofol, thiopental, and fentanyl at equisedative concentrations. *Anesthesiology.* 1997;87:749–764.

114. Perry F, Parker RK, White PF, et al. Role of psychological factors in postoperative pain control and recovery with patient-controlled analgesia. *Clin J Pain.* 1994;10:57–63; discussion 82–85.
115. Rudkin GE, Osborne GA, Finn BP, et al. Intra-operative patient-controlled sedation. *Anaesthesia.* 1992;47:376–381.
116. Park WY, Watkins PA. Patient-controlled sedation during epidural anesthesia. *Anesth Analg.* 1991;72:304–307.
117. Zelcer J, White PF, Chester S, et al. Intraoperative patient-controlled analgesia. *Anesth Analg.* 1992;75:41–44.
118. Morel DR, Forster A, Bachmann M, et al. Effect of intravenous midazolam on breathing pattern and chest wall mechanics in human. *J Appl Physiol.* 1984; 57:1104–1110.
119. Prato F, Knill R. Diazepam sedation reduces functional residual capacity and alters the distribution of ventilation in man. *Can J Anaesth.* 1983;30:493–500.
120. Cohen M. Phrenic and recurrent laryngeal discharge patterns and the Hering-Breuer reflex. *Am J Physiol.* 1975;228:1489–1496.
121. Gottfried SB, Strohl KP, Van de Graaff W, et al. Effects of phrenic stimulation on upper airway resistance in anesthetized dogs. *J Appl Physiol.* 1983;55:419–426.
122. Leiter JC, Knuth SL, Krol RC, et al. The effect of diazepam on genioglossal muscle activity in normal human subjects. *Am Rev Respir Dis.* 1985;132:216–219.
123. Montravers P, Dureuil B, Desmonts JM. Effects of I.V. midazolam on upper airway resistance. *Br J Anaesth.* 1992;68:27–31.
124. Rimaniol JM, D'Honneur G, Duvaldestin P. Recovery of the swallowing reflex after propofol anesthesia. *Anesth Analg.* 1994;79:856–859.
125. Groves ND, Rees JL, Rosen M. Effects of benzodiazepines on laryngeal reflexes. *Anaesthesia.* 1987;42:808–814.
126. Lambert Y, D'Honneur G, Abhay K, et al. Depression of swallowing reflex two hours after midazolam. *Anesthesiology.* 1991;75:A891.
127. Nishino T, Takizawa K, Yokokawa N, et al. Depression of the swallowing reflex during sedation and/or relative analgesia produced by inhalation of 50% nitrous oxide in oxygen. *Anesthesiology.* 1987;67:995–998.
128. Caplan RA, Ward RJ, Posner K, et al. Unexpected cardiac arrest during spinal anesthesia: A closed claims analysis of predisposing factors. *Anesthesiology.* 1988;68:5–11.
129. Weil JV, McCullough RE, Kline JS, et al. Diminished ventilatory response to hypoxia and hypercapnia after morphine in normal man. *N Engl J Med.* 1975; 292:1103–1106.
130. Santiago TV, Johnson J, Riley DJ, et al. Effects of morphine on ventilatory response to exercise. *J Appl Physiol.* 1979;47:112–118.
131. Rigg JRA. Ventilatory effects and plasma concentration of morphine in man. *Br J Anaesth.* 1978;50:759–765.
132. Pattinson KTS. Opioids and the control of respiration. *Br J Anaesth.* 2008;100: 747–758.
133. Power SJ, Morgan M, Chakrabarti MK. Carbon dioxide response curves following midazolam and diazepam. *Br J Anaesth.* 1983;55:837–842.
134. Alexander CM, Gross JB. Sedative doses of midazolam depress hypoxic ventilatory responses in humans. *Anesth Analg.* 1988;67:377–382.
135. Jordan C, Lehane JR, Jones JG. Respiratory depression following diazepam: Reversal with high-dose naloxone. *Anesthesiology.* 1980;53:293–298.
136. Yaster M, Nichols DG, Deshpande JK, et al. Midazolam-fentanyl intravenous sedation in children: Case report of respiratory arrest. *Pediatrics.* 1990;86:463–467.
137. White JM, Irvine RJ. Mechanisms of fatal opioid overdose. *Addiction.* 1999; 94:961–972.
138. Deitch K, Chudnofsky CR, Dominici P. The utility of supplemental oxygen during emergency department procedural sedation and analgesia with midazolam and fentanyl: A randomized, controlled trial. *Ann Emerg Med.* 2007;49:1–8.
139. Deitch K, Chudnofsky CR, Dominici P. The utility of supplemental oxygen during emergency department procedural sedation with propofol: A randomized, controlled trial. *Ann Emerg Med.* 2008;52:1–8.
140. Metzner J, Posner KL, Domino KB. The risk and safety of anesthesia at remote locations: The US closed claims analysis. *Curr Opin Anaesthesiol.* 2009;22: 502–508.
141. American Society of Anesthesiologists. Standards for basic anesthesia monitoring. www.asahq.org 2011.
142. KK BST. *Pulse Oximetry, Anesthetic Equipment: Principles and Applications.* St. Louis: Mosby; 1993:249.
143. Moller JT, Johannessen NW, Berg H, et al. Hypoxaemia during anaesthesia—an observer study. *Br J Anaesth.* 1991;66:437–444.
144. Motoyama EK, Glazener CH. Hypoxemia after general anesthesia in children. *Anesth Analg.* 1986;65:267–272.
145. Xue FS, Li BW, Zhang GS, et al. The influence of surgical sites on early postoperative hypoxemia in adults undergoing elective surgery. *Anesth Analg.* 1999;88: 213–219.
146. Lightdale JR, Goldmann DA, Feldman HA, et al. Microstream capnography improves patient monitoring during moderate sedation: A randomized, controlled trial. *Pediatrics.* 2006;117:e1170–e1178.
147. Bowe EA, Boysen PG, Broome JA, et al. Accurate determination of end-tidal carbon dioxide during administration of oxygen by nasal cannulae. *J Clin Monit Comput.* 1988;5:105–110.
148. Pressman MA. A simple method of measuring ETCO2 during MAC and major regional anesthesia. *Anesth Analg.* 1988;67:905–906.
149. Soto RG, Fu ES, Vila H, et al. Capnography accurately detects apnea during monitored anesthesia care. *Anesth Analg.* 2004;99:379–382.
150. Vargo JJ, Zuccaro G Jr, Dumot JA, et al. Automated graphic assessment of respiratory activity is superior to pulse oximetry and visual assessment for the detection of early respiratory depression during therapeutic upper endoscopy. *Gastrointest Endosc.* 2002;55:826–831.
151. Waugh JB, Epps CA, Khodneva YA. Capnography enhances surveillance of respiratory events during procedural sedation: A meta-analysis. *J Clin Anesth.* 2011; 23:189–196.
152. Kurz A, Kurz M, Poeschl G, et al. Forced-air warming maintains intraoperative normothermia better than circulating-water mattresses. *Anesth Analg.* 1993;77:89–95.
153. Hynson JM, Sessler DI. Intraoperative warming therapies: A comparison of three devices. *J Clin Anesth.* 1992;4:194–199.
154. Kurz A, Sessler DI, Lenhardt R. Perioperative normothermia to reduce the incidence of surgical-wound infection and shorten hospitalization. *N Engl J Med.* 1996;334:1209–1216.
155. Sessler DI. Complications and treatment of mild hypothermia. *Anesthesiology.* 2001;95:531–543.
156. Frank SM, Fleisher LA, Breslow MJ, et al. Perioperative maintenance of normothermia reduces the incidence of morbid cardiac events. *JAMA.* 1997;277:1127–1134.
157. Frank SM, Higgins MS, Breslow MJ, et al. The catecholamine, cortisol, and hemodynamic responses to mild perioperative hypothermia: A randomized clinical trial. *Anesthesiology.* 1995;82:83–93.
158. Schmied H, Reiter A, Kurz A, et al. Mild hypothermia increases blood loss and transfusion requirements during total hip arthroplasty. *Lancet.* 1996;347:289–292.
159. Lenhardt R, Marker E, Goll V, et al. Mild intraoperative hypothermia prolongs postanesthetic recovery. *Anesthesiology.* 1997;87:1318–1323.
160. Arkiliç CF, Akça O, Taguchi A, et al. Temperature monitoring and management during neuraxial anesthesia: An observational study. *Anesth Analg.* 2000;91:662–666.
161. Frank SM, Nguyen JM, Garcia CM, et al. Temperature monitoring practices during regional anesthesia. *Anesth Analg.* 1999;88:373.
162. Scholefield JH, Gerber MA, Dwyer P. Liquid crystal forehead temperature strips: A clinical appraisal. *Am J Dis Child.* 1982;136:198–201.
163. Sessler DI. Temperature monitoring and management during neuraxial anesthesia. *Anesth Analg.* 1999;88:243.
164. Chernik DA, Gillings D, Laine H, et al. Validity and reliability of the observer's assessment of alertness/sedation scale: Study with intravenous midazolam. *J Clin Psychopharmacol.* 1990;10:244–251.
165. Liu J, Singh H, White PF. Electroencephalographic bispectral index correlates with intraoperative recall and depth of propofol-induced sedation. *Anesth Analg.* 1997;84:185–189.
166. Kearse LA, Manberg P, Chamoun N, et al. Bispectral analysis of the electroencephalogram correlates with patient movement to skin incision during propofol/nitrous oxide anesthesia. *Anesthesiology.* 1994;81:1365–1370.
167. American Society of Anesthesiologists. Continuum of depth of sedation, definition of general anesthesia and levels of sedation/analgesia. www.asahq.org 2009.
168. American Society of Anesthesiologists. Statement on granting privileges for administration of moderate sedation to practitioners who are not anesthesia professionals. www.asahq.org 2011.
169. American Society of Anesthesiologists. Advisory for granting privileges for administration of moderate sedation to practitioners who are not anesthesia professionals. www.asahq.org 2010.
170. Centers for Medicare and Medicaid Services. Revised hospital anesthesia interpretive guidelines. www.asahq.org 2011.
171. American Society of Anesthesiologists. Statement of the safe use of propofol. www.asahq.org 2009.

CHAPTER

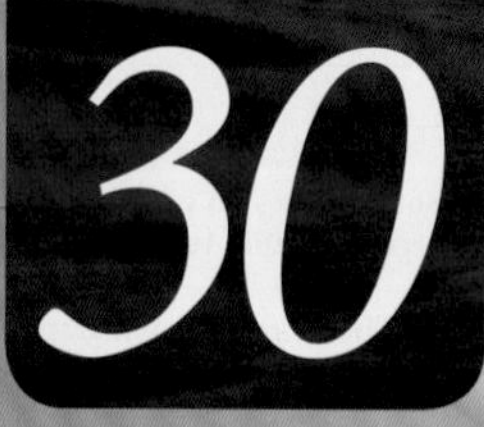

Ambulatory Anesthesia

J. LANCE LICHTOR

Key Points

1. Procedures appropriate for ambulatory surgery are those associated with postoperative care that is easily managed at home and with low rates of postoperative complications that require intensive physician or nursing management.
2. Whatever their age, ambulatory surgery is not restricted to patients of ASA physical status I or II. Patients of ASA physical status III or IV are appropriate candidates, providing their systemic diseases are medically stable.
3. In the 2006 ASA guidelines, the authors state that for patients with OSA, if a procedure is typically performed as an outpatient procedure and local or regional anesthesia is used, that the procedure can also be performed as an ambulatory procedure.
4. For adults, airflow obstruction has been shown to persist for up to 6 weeks after viral respiratory infections. For that reason, surgery should be delayed if an adult presents with a URI until 6 weeks have elapsed.
5. In 2011, the ASA updated practice guidelines for preoperative fasting. The guidelines allow a patient to have a light meal up to 6 hours before an elective procedure and support a fasting period for clear liquids of 2 hours for all patients.
6. Time until discharge from ambulatory surgery is no different after peripheral nerve, central neuraxial blocks or general anesthesia.
7. Postoperative pain control is best with regional techniques.
8. Nerve blocks using catheters can be placed before surgery that can be used to provide analgesia after the operation.
9. After induction doses of propofol or thiopental, impairment after thiopental can be apparent for up to 5 hours, but only for 1 hour after propofol.
10. Although many factors affect the choice of agents for maintenance of anesthesia, two primary concerns for ambulatory anesthesia are speed of wake-up and incidence of postoperative nausea and vomiting.
11. It is important to distinguish between wake-up time and discharge time. Patients may emerge from anesthesia with desflurane and nitrous oxide significantly faster than after propofol or sevoflurane and nitrous oxide, though the ability to sit up, stand, and tolerate fluids and the time to fitness for discharge may be no different.
12. Nausea, with or without vomiting, is probably the most important factor contributing to a delay in discharge of patients and an increase in unanticipated admissions of both children and adults after ambulatory surgery.
13. In addition to the PACU, most ambulatory surgery centers in the United States have Phase II Recovery, which may be located in a different space than the PACU, but may also be conducted in the PACU space. Patients remain in Phase II Recovery until they are able to tolerate liquids, walk, and (depending on the operation) void.

Multimedia

1 Vomiting Pharmacology

PLACE, PROCEDURES, AND PATIENT SELECTION

Ambulatory surgery occurs in a variety of settings. Some centers are within a hospital or in a freestanding satellite facility that is either part of or independent from a hospital. The independent facilities are often for-profit and not located in rural or inner-city areas. Some private companies acquire or build ambulatory facilities and then work usually with local surgeons who become the company's affiliated staff. Physician's office may also serve procedures (see Chapter 31 Office-based Anesthesia). Freestanding, independent facilities will continue to grow in number and popularity, although some consumers prefer care in units affiliated with hospitals.

A major concern of freestanding ambulatory surgery growth is that the surgery centers may force some hospitals out of business. This issue can be particularly problematic in areas in which population density or median income is low. Hospitals usually are nonprofit and care for patients who both can and cannot pay. Freestanding ambulatory facilities may also be nonprofit but usually do not provide charity care.

Some surgeons may work exclusively in a freestanding facility and not be on the staff of a hospital. A requirement for hospital staff privileges frequently is that a physician provides coverage for the hospital's emergency department. Hospitals may try to expand emergency department coverage, but are pressured by some specialist surgeons. Some hospitals have lost emergency department coverage for an entire surgical specialty because that surgical specialty works exclusively in a freestanding facility.

Costs are lower for ASCs. Scheduling can be more predictable because the variety of cases is low. Turnaround times are usually also lower. The profits, particularly for freestanding facilities, do not have to subsidize more expensive areas of the hospital, such as ICUs. They also tend to serve only well-insured patients. Medicare also pays ASCs at a lower percent than what they pay hospitals for the same procedure. Medicare can then save money, though the payment system may force some ambulatory facilities to decide whether they accept Medicare patients.

1 Procedures appropriate for ambulatory surgery are those associated with postoperative care that are easily managed at home and with low rates of postoperative complications that require intensive physician or nursing management. Establishing a low rate of postoperative complication depends on the relative aggressiveness of the facility, surgeon, patient, and payer. For example, procedures that postoperatively result in intense pain may be treated with continuous regional techniques that are continued at home whereas in other settings, these procedures are limited to inpatients.

Scoring systems have been developed to help determine the likelihood of hospital admission after ambulatory surgery. One system is based on patients who were hospitalized after ambulatory surgery[1] (Table 30-1).

Many facilities set a 4-hour limit as a criterion for performing a procedure. Patients undergoing longer procedures should have their operations earlier in the day, primarily because in most freestanding facilities, the anesthesiologist cannot leave until the last patient is discharged. The need for transfusion is also not a contraindication for ambulatory procedures. Some patients undergoing outpatient liposuction, for example, are given autologous blood. Because of blood banking issues, though, ambulatory procedures that require the use of a blood bank are more commonly performed in larger facilities. Freestanding dialysis facilities commonly receive blood shipped from a blood bank located elsewhere and the same can be set up with freestanding ambulatory surgery facilities. The key is to have proper procedures established.

TABLE 30-1. INDEX SCORING SYSTEM TO HELP IDENTIFY PATIENTS AT HIGHER RISK FOR HOSPITAL ADMISSION AFTER OUTPATIENT SURGERY

Assign 1 point each for
65 years or greater
Operating time longer than 120 min
Cardiac diagnoses
Peripheral vascular disease
Cerebrovascular disease
Malignancy
HIV-positive status
Use of regional anesthesia
Use of general anesthesia (2 points)

Patients with a score of 3 have 21 times odds of developing PONV than those with a score of 0 or 1.
Patients with a score >3 have 32 times odds of developing PONV than those with a score of 0 or 1.
Data from: Fleisher L, Pasternak L, Lyles A: A novel index of elevated risk of inpatient hospital admission immediately following outpatient surgery. *Arch Surg* 2007;142: 263–268.

Some have wondered about the safety office-based procedures, following reports of deaths in Florida (see Chapter 31 Office-based Anesthesia). In one series from Florida that reviewed office surgical incidents from January of 2000 to January of 2006 that resulted in death, injury, or hospital transfer, 46 deaths were identified.[2] Thrombophlebitis was the cause of death in the majority of patients. In a survey of 7,010 patients undergoing abdominal liposuction, the incidence of deep vein thrombosis was 0.04% and that of pulmonary embolus was 0.02%.[3] It is hoped that organizations will soon provide better guidelines for stratifying risk and strategies to prevent venous thromboembolism after liposuction surgery.

Infants whose postconceptual age is <46 weeks, or whose actual age is <60 weeks should be monitored for 12 hours after their procedure because they are at risk of developing apnea even without a history of apnea (Fig. 30-1).[4] Infants older than 46 weeks and <60 weeks without disease should be monitored for 6 hours after their procedures. In one series of 127 premature patients who underwent inguinal hernia surgery, though, none had postoperative apnea.[5] Some have found that spinal anesthesia without the use of other drugs intraoperatively or postoperatively is not associated with apnea; although in one study of 62 premature and former-premature infants who underwent surgery using spinal anesthesia, postoperative apnea was seen in 5 of

<46 weeks ⟶ 12-h monitoring
46–60 weeks: Comorbidity (chronic lung disease, continuing apnea, neurologic disease, or Hct < 30%) ⟶ 12-h monitoring
No comorbidity: ⟶ 6-h monitoring

FIGURE 30-1. Guide to determine length of monitoring for former preterm infants with a postconceptual age <60 weeks. Modified from: Walther-Larsen S, Rasmussen L. The former preterm infant and risk of postoperative apnoea: recommendations for management. *Acta Anaesthesiol Scand.* 2006;50:888–893.

55 premature infants.[6] Intravenous caffeine, 10 mg/kg, may help prevent apnea in infants, though the use of caffeine in the care of ambulatory patients at risk for apnea has not been studied.

At the other extreme of life, advanced age alone is not a reason to disallow surgery in an ambulatory setting. In a study of 89 patients who were 65 years and older randomized to receive either inpatient or outpatient care before undergoing inguinal hernia repair, all patients who were randomized to receive care as an outpatient were discharged on the day of surgery.[7] Up to 2 weeks later, outcome was no different between groups. Increasing age, however, does affect the pharmacokinetics of drugs (see Chapter 7 Basic Principles of Clinical Pharmacology). Even short-acting drugs such as midazolam and propofol have decreased clearance in older individuals. In addition, as mentioned above, increased age may be a factor that affects the likelihood of unanticipated admission.

Admission, by itself, is not necessarily bad if it results in a better quality of care or uncovers the need for more extensive surgery. With proper patient selection for ambulatory procedures, which are usually elective, the incidence of readmission should be very low. Most medical problems that older individuals may experience after ambulatory procedures are not related to patient age, but to specific organ dysfunction. For that reason, all individuals, whether young or old, deserve a careful preoperative history and physical examination.

2 Whatever their age, ambulatory surgery is no longer restricted to patients of American Society of Anesthesiologists (ASA) physical status I or II. Patients of ASA physical status III or IV are appropriate candidates, providing their systemic diseases are medically stable. In a review of ASA III patients who were compared with ASA I or II patients undergoing outpatient surgery, no significant increase in unplanned admissions, unplanned contact with health professionals, and postoperative complications was found.[8] Certainly, not all life-threatening diseases have been studied as to how appropriate such patients with these diseases might be if they were to undergo ambulatory surgery. Yet, of those patients with such diseases who have been studied, the disease label itself does not seem to preclude an ambulatory surgical procedure.

Patients who are obese represent a special situation. They are not more likely to have adverse outcomes, although they have a higher incidence of obstructive sleep apnea (OSA). In a review of 235 obese patients (body mass index [BMI] >40) who underwent outpatient surgery and were matched with control patients, unplanned admissions did not differ between groups.[7,9] In a study of obstructive sleep apnea in patients undergoing ambulatory surgery, undiagnosed OSA was relatively common, and there was no relationship between OSA and unplanned hospital admission. Patients with OSA, though, had a higher likelihood of difficult intubation, needed more pressors, and needed more oxygen management in the PACU.[10] Some feel that patients who need more narcotics may be at greater risk for apnea and should be observed for a longer period after their procedure. The ASA published practice guidelines for the perioperative
3 management of patients with OSA.[11] In those guidelines, the authors state that for patients with OSA, if a procedure is typically performed as an outpatient procedure and local or regional anesthesia is used, the procedure can also be performed as an ambulatory procedure. Yet for patients who are at increased risk for perioperative complications, the procedure should not be performed in a freestanding ambulatory surgery facility. Table 30-2 presents a more complete list of recommended ambulatory procedures for patients with OSA, based on the ASA guidelines.

Patients who undergo ambulatory surgery should have an adult take them home and stay with them afterward to provide care. Before the procedure, the patient should receive information about the procedure itself, where it will be performed, laboratory studies that will be ordered, and dietary restrictions. The patient must understand that he or she will be going home on the day of surgery. The patient, or some responsible person, must ensure all instructions are followed. Once at home, the patient must be able to tolerate the pain from the procedure, assuming adequate pain therapy is provided. The majority of patients are satisfied with early discharge, although a few prefer a longer stay in the facility. Patients for certain procedures such as laparoscopic cholecystectomy or transurethral resection of the prostate should live close to the ambulatory facility because postoperative complications may require their prompt return. "Reasonable" distance and time for the patient to get care if problems arise are not easily defined. This issue must be addressed by each facility and by each patient, and also depends on the type of surgery to be performed.

TABLE 30-2. CONSULTANT OPINIONS REGARDING PROCEDURES THAT MAY BE PERFORMED SAFELY ON AN OUTPATIENT BASIS FOR PATIENTS AT INCREASED PERIOPERATIVE RISK FROM OBSTRUCTIVE SLEEP APNEA

Type of Surgery/Anesthesia	Consultant Opinion
Superficial surgery/local or regional anesthesia	Agree
Superficial surgery/general anesthesia	Equivocal
Airway surgery (adult, e.g., UPPP)	Disagree
Tonsillectomy in children <3 years old	Disagree
Tonsillectomy in children >3 years old	Equivocal
Minor orthopaedic surgery/local or regional anesthesia	Agree
Minor orthopaedic surgery/general anesthesia	Equivocal
Gynecologic laparoscopy	Equivocal
Laparoscopic surgery, upper abdomen	Disagree
Lithotripsy	Agree

From: Gross JB, Bachenberg KL, Benumof JL, et al. Practice guidelines for the perioperative management of patients with obstructive sleep apnea: A report by the American Society of Anesthesiologists Task Force on Perioperative Management of patients with obstructive sleep apnea. *Anesthesiology.* 2006;104:1081–1093; quiz 1117–1118, with permission.

PREOPERATIVE EVALUATION AND REDUCTION OF PATIENT ANXIETY

Each outpatient facility should develop its own method of preoperative screening to be conducted before the day of surgery. The patient may visit the facility, or the staff members may telephone to obtain necessary information about the patient, including a complete medical history of the patient and family, the medications the patient is taking, and the problems the patient or the patient's family may have had with previous anesthetics. Screened patients may be less likely to cancel surgery. The screening may uncover the need for transportation to the facility or the need for child care. The process also provides the staff with an opportunity to remind patients of arrival time, suitable attire, and dietary restrictions (e.g., when to stop eating and drinking, no jewelry or makeup). Staff members can determine whether a responsible person is available to escort the patient to and from the facility and care for the patient at home after surgery. The screening is the ideal time for the anesthesiologist to talk to the patient, but if that is not possible, the anesthesiologist may review the screening record to determine whether additional evaluation by other consultants is necessary and whether laboratory tests must be obtained. Patients who do not show up for their clinic appointment may be more likely not to show up for their operation.[12]

Automated history-taking may also prove beneficial during the screening of a patient. Computerized questionnaires or checklists with plastic overlays automate the acquisition of patient histories, flag problem areas, and suggest laboratory tests to be ordered. Such devices can also be used in a surgeon's office, both to guide the surgeon in the selection of laboratory tests and to serve as a medical summary for the anesthesiologist. Such devices are particularly useful to control the cost of preoperative testing. They enable test ordering based on information obtained from a patient's responses to health questions, thus eliminating requests for tests that are not warranted by history or physical examination.

Upper Respiratory Tract Infection

4 For adults, airflow obstruction has been shown to persist for up to 6 weeks after viral respiratory infections. For that reason, surgery should be delayed if an adult presents with an upper respiratory infection (URI) until 6 weeks have elapsed. In the case of children, whether surgery should be delayed for that length of time is questionable. In a year-long survey of almost 10,000 children who underwent surgery, URI was associated with an increased risk for perioperative respiratory adverse events only when symptoms were present or had occurred within the 2 weeks before the procedure.[13] Although a case may be cancelled because a child is symptomatic, the child may develop another URI when the procedure is rescheduled. In children, URI has not been shown to be associated with an increased length of stay in the hospital after a procedure. Independent risk factors for adverse respiratory events in children with URIs include use of an endotracheal tube (versus use of a laryngeal mask airway [LMA] or face mask), history of prematurity, history of reactive airway disease, history of parental smoking, surgery involving the airway, presence of copious secretions, and nasal congestion. Generally, if a patient with a URI has a normal appetite, does not have a fever or an elevated respiratory rate, and does not appear toxic, it is probably safe to proceed with the planned procedure.

Restriction of Food and Liquids Prior to Ambulatory Surgery

To decrease the risk of aspiration of gastric contents, patients are routinely asked not to eat or drink anything (*non per os* [NPO] or "nothing by mouth") for at least 6 to 8 hours before surgery. Prolonged fasting could be detrimental to a patient. Yet in one study, where patients fasted from under 2 hours to more than 21 hours, there were minimal differences in blood pressure after propofol bolus for anesthesia induction.[14] No trial has shown that a shortened fluid fast increases the risk of aspiration. Fluids actually empty quickly from the stomach. In one study of children 6 to 14 years who fasted overnight and then drank 7 mL/kg, median half-life for gastric emptying as assessed using MRI, was 24 minutes, though there was considerable individual variation.[15] Admittedly, the majority of studies have not been specifically performed in individuals who are at an increased risk for aspiration.

5 In 2011, the ASA revised practice guidelines for preoperative fasting[16] (Table 30-3A and B). The guidelines allow a patient to have a light meal up to 6 hours before an elective procedure and support a fasting period for clear liquids of 2 hours for all patients. Coffee and tea are considered clear liquids. Coffee and tea drinkers should follow fasting guidelines but should be encouraged to drink coffee prior to their procedure because physical signs of withdrawal (e.g., headache) can easily occur. It is not clear if the guidelines should apply to patients with diabetes or dyspepsia. There is some evidence that shorter periods of preoperative fasting are accompanied by less postoperative nausea and vomiting (PONV). Yet, it is unclear whether rehydration during surgery is equivalent to a shorter fast before surgery in relation to PONV.

To ensure patients are optimally medically managed before their outpatient surgery, given the fact that clear liquids can be taken up to 2 hours before surgery, patients should be encouraged to take their chronic medications.

Anxiety Reduction

Clearly, some patients scheduled to undergo surgery are anxious, and they are probably anxious long before they come to the outpatient area. Indeed, anxiety probably begins as soon as the surgeon states the patient needs an operation and may not end even after discharge from the outpatient facility. Reasons for anxiety may include concerns about family, worry about pain after the procedure, and fear of complications.[17] Preoperative reassurance from nonanesthesia staff and providing booklets with information about the procedure also reduce preoperative anxiety. However, use of booklets is less effective than a preoperative visit by the anesthesiologist. Audiovisual instructions also reduce preoperative anxiety. However, not all outpatients are anxious. Indeed, physicians often tend to overestimate the level of anxiety that patients are actually experiencing.[18] Some operations can certainly generate more anxiety than others. If in doubt about patient anxiety, ask the patient.

Like adults, children should have some idea of what to expect during a procedure. But much of a child's anxiety before surgery concerns separation from a parent or parents. A child is more likely to demonstrate problematic behavior from the time of separation from parents to induction of anesthesia if the procedure has not been explained preoperatively. Parents and children need to be involved in some preoperative discussions together so the anxiety of the parents is not transmitted to the child. The transmission of anxiety is at least as problematic as is the separation itself (e.g., experiences of children being left with babysitters). If the parents are calm and can effectively manage the physical transfer to a warm and playful anesthesiologist or nurse, premedication is not necessary. Semisedation may be awkward, and recovery after premedication may be prolonged.

If a child is accompanied by a parent during the induction of anesthesia, the child's anxiety can be reduced. Some parents can become upset when they see their anesthetized child, who appears to be dead, albeit breathing and with a beating heart. Separation

TABLE 30-3. SUGGESTED GUIDELINES TO REDUCE THE RISK OF PULMONARY ASPIRATION

A. Foods

Type of Food	Time to Fast	Examples	Notes
Clear liquids	At least 2 h	Water, fruit juice without pulp, carbonated beverage, clear tea, black coffee	Alcohol not included
Breast milk	At least 4 h		
Infant formula	At least 6 h		
Light meal or nonhuman milk	At least 6 h		Consider amount and type of food
Fried or fatty foods	At least 8 h		

B. Medications

Medication	Recommendation
GI stimulants, e.g., metoclopramide	No routine use
Gastric acid secretion blockers, i.e., histamine-2 receptor antagonists	No routine use
Antacids, e.g., sodium citrate, sodium bicarbonate or magnesium trislicate	No routine use
Antiemetics, e.g., droperidol or ondansetron	No routine use
Anticholinergics, e.g., atropine, scopolamine or glycopyrrolate	No use
Multiple agents	No routine use

Based on: American Society of Anesthesiologists Committee: Practice guidelines for preoperative fasting and the use of pharmacologic agents to reduce the risk of pulmonary aspiration: application to healthy patients undergoing elective procedures: an updated report by the American Society of Anesthesiologists Committee on Standards and Practice Parameters. *Anesthesiology.* 2011;114:495–511.

anxiety on the part of the parents is probably no different if the child is awake or asleep. Those children who have preoperative instructions and coaching (child life specialist) both for themselves and their families, and their parent/s present during induction have less anxiety preoperatively, less postoperative delirium, shortened discharge time after surgery, and reduced analgesic consumption after surgery.[19] In addition, the patients had less severe emergence delirium symptoms, needed less fentanyl postoperatively, and were discharged earlier. Two important components of this technique are having the child practice with the anesthesia mask at home and use of distraction on the day of surgery.[20]

MANAGING THE ANESTHETIC: PREMEDICATION

The outpatient is not that different from the inpatient undergoing surgery. In both, premedication is useful to control anxiety, postoperative pain, nausea and vomiting, and to reduce the risk of aspiration during induction of anesthesia. Because the outpatient is going home on the day of surgery, the drugs given before anesthesia should not hinder recovery afterward. Most premedicants do not prolong recovery when given in appropriate doses for appropriate indications, although drug effects may be apparent even after discharge.

Benzodiazepines

Although historically many classes of drugs (e.g., barbiturates, antihistamines) have been used to reduce anxiety and induce sedation, benzodiazepines are currently the drugs most commonly used. Midazolam is the benzodiazepine most commonly used preoperatively. It can be used intravenously and orally. In adults, it can be used to control preoperative anxiety and, during a procedure alone or in combination with other drugs, for intravenous sedation. For children, oral midazolam in doses as small as 0.25 mg/kg produces effective sedation and reduces anxiety.[21] With this dose, most children can be effectively separated from their parents after 10 minutes and satisfactory sedation can be maintained for 45 minutes. Some children, particularly younger and more anxious children, even when they receive midazolam 0.5 mg/kg, show signs of distress.[22] Discharge may be delayed when midazolam is given before a short procedure. Oral diazepam is useful to control anxiety in adult patients, either the day before surgery or the day of surgery and before an intravenous line has been inserted.

Fatigue associated with the effects of anxiolytics may delay or prevent the discharge of patients on the day of surgery, although more frequently patients are not discharged because of the effects of the operation. With regard to anesthesia effects, patients normally stay in the facility not because they are too sleepy but because they are nauseous. In adults, particularly when midazolam is combined with fentanyl, patients can remain sleepy for up to 8 hours (Fig. 30-2).[23] Although children may be sleepier after oral midazolam, discharge times are not affected.

At proper doses, neither midazolam nor diazepam place patients at any additional risk for cardiovascular and respiratory depression. Decreased oxygen saturation has been reported after injection of midazolam. Routine administration of supplemental oxygen with or without continuous monitoring of arterial oxygenation is recommended whenever benzodiazepines are given intravenously. This precaution is important not only when midazolam is given as a premedicant but also when it is used alone or with other drugs for conscious sedation. The potential for amnesia after premedication is another concern, especially

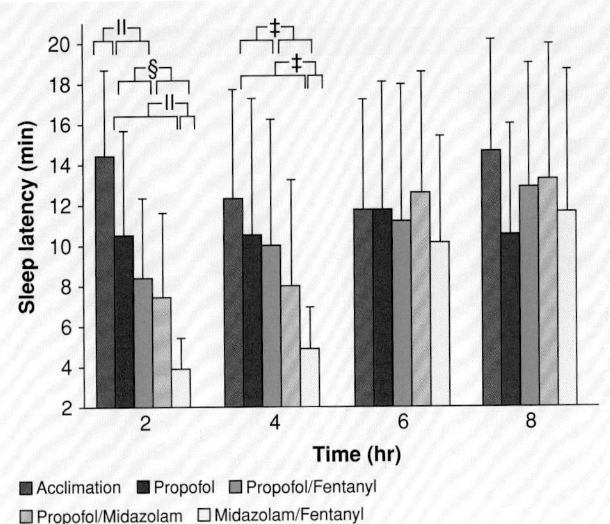

FIGURE 30-2. Patients can remain sleepy after receiving midazolam and fentanyl, even 8 hours after drug administration. The abscissa represents time (hours) after sedation. The ordinate represents sleep latency (i.e., time to fall asleep). Data are the mean time to fall asleep. An individual is sleepier if less time is required to fall asleep. Subjects receiving the midazolam and fentanyl combination were much sleepier than the same subjects receiving other types of sedation. Although not seen in the figure, up to 8 hours after sedation, some subjects were still sleepier than before they received drug. Reprinted from: Lichtor JL, Alessi R, Lane BS. Sleep tendency as a measure of recovery after drugs used for ambulatory surgery. *Anesthesiology.* 2002;96:878–883, with permission.

for patients undergoing ambulatory surgery. Anterograde amnesia certainly occurs. Although benzodiazepines facilitate retrograde amnesia, in one study there was no immediate retrograde amnesia after intravenous midazolam, 2 to 10 mg.[24] For benzodiazepines, the effects on memory are separate from the effects on sedation. In addition, amnesia is not simply an effect of drug administration but, among other factors, it is also a function of stimulus intensity.

Opioids and Nonsteroidal Analgesics

Opioids can be administered preoperatively to sedate patients, control hypertension during tracheal intubation, and decrease pain before surgery. Meperidine (but not morphine or fentanyl) is sometimes helpful in controlling shivering in the OR or the postanesthesia care unit (PACU), although treatment is usually instituted at the time of shivering and not in anticipation of the event.

Opioids are useful in controlling hypertension during tracheal intubation. Opioid premedication prevents increases in systolic pressure in a dose-dependent fashion. After tracheal intubation, systolic, diastolic, and mean arterial blood pressures sometimes decrease below baseline values.

It would seem that preoperative administration of opioids or nonsteroidal anti-inflammatory drugs (NSAIDs) may be useful for controlling pain in the early postoperative period. Indeed, in a study where patients undergoing laparoscopic cholecystectomy received oxycodone preoperatively, they had lower pain scores, required less rescue analgesic consumption, and had shorter time to discharge from the recovery room.[25] In another study, though, pain management for major plastic surgery procedures after celecoxib given before, during and after surgery, was no better than celecoxib given the day after surgery.[26] Ibuprofen or acetaminophen can be given rectally to children around the time of induction. In children, time to rescue analgesia is longer if rectal as opposed to intravenous acetaminophen is used.[27] In children, an initial loading dose of 40 mg/kg is appropriate. And, when preoperative rectal acetaminophen is combined with a nonsteroidal anti-inflammatory drug, particularly for more painful procedures, postoperative pain is less than when either drug is given individually.[28]

Preoperative sedation is not needed for every patient. The following is our practice when patients require drugs to relieve anxiety. For the patient who has been seen at least 24 hours before a scheduled procedure and expresses a desire for medication to relieve anxiety or has anxiety that cannot be relieved with comforting, oral diazepam, 2 to 5 mg per 70 kg body weight, is prescribed for the night before and at 6 am on the day of surgery (even if surgery is scheduled for 1 pm or later). For patients seen for the first time in the preoperative holding area who seem to need medication, midazolam, 0.01 mg/kg, is administered intravenously, or the patient is brought into the OR and propofol, 0.7 mg/kg, is injected intravenously. For children, when necessary, oral midazolam, 0.25 mg/kg, is administered in the preoperative holding area. When the child is asleep, acetaminophen, 40 mg/kg rectally, and ketorolac, 0.5 mg/kg intravenously, are administered prior to initiation of surgery.

INTRAOPERATIVE MANAGEMENT: CHOICE OF ANESTHETIC METHOD

There are several choices among anesthetic methods: General anesthesia, regional anesthesia, and local anesthesia. Regional and local anesthesia can be used with or without sedation. Except for obstetric cases, for which regional anesthesia may be safer than general anesthesia, all three types are otherwise equally safe. However, even for experienced anesthesiologists, there is a failure rate associated with regional anesthesia.

Certainly, some procedures are possible only with a general anesthetic. For others, the preference of patients, surgeons, or anesthesiologists may determine selection. The cost of sedation is usually less than the cost of a general or regional anesthetic. In a comparison of costs for patients undergoing inguinal hernia surgery in ten hospitals in Sweden, for example, intraoperative and postoperative costs were least in patients who received local anesthesia.[29] Those patients who received local anesthesia also spent less time in the OR, had less postoperative pain, and the least problems with urination. The three types of anesthesia, though, are not an option for all operations. In another study that compared groin hernia repair after either general, regional or local infiltration, medical complications were more common after regional versus general anesthesia and urologic complications were more common after regional versus local infiltration.[30] Less cost, then, may not always also be accompanied by improved quality. Where spinal anesthesia was compared to general anesthesia for patients undergoing hip or knee replacement procedures, costs for drugs and supplies were less for spinal anesthesia; recovery costs were also less due to less cost for pain management.[31]

Time to recovery may also influence the choice of anesthetic method. In a study of patients undergoing prostate biopsy, discharge after general anesthesia was faster than after spinal anesthesia.[32] Conversely, in a study of patients undergoing upper limb trauma surgery, pain in the PACU and time to meet criteria for hospital discharge was less than for patients who underwent

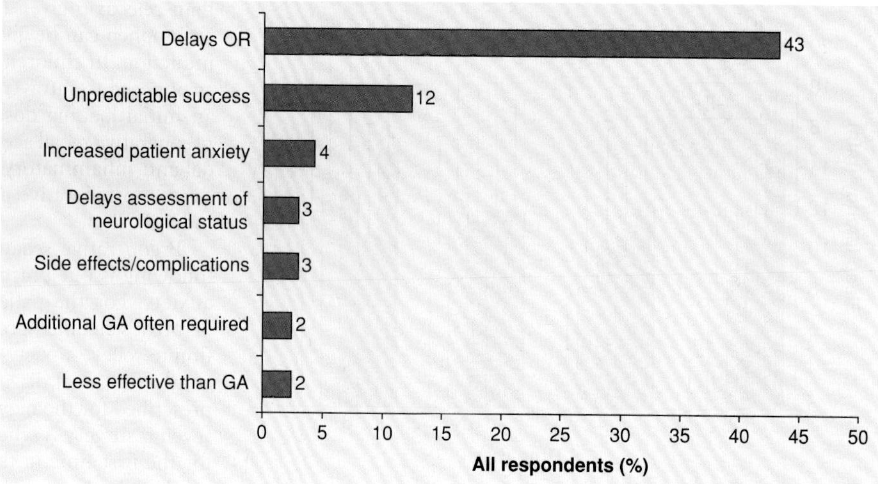

FIGURE 30-3. Operating room (OR) delays are the major reasons orthopedic surgeons do not favor regional anesthesia. GA, general anesthesia. Reprinted from: Oldman M, McCartney CJ, Leung A, et al. A survey of orthopedic surgeons' attitudes and knowledge regarding regional anesthesia. *Anesth Analg.* 2004;98:1486–1490, with permission.

6 general anesthesia for the procedure.[33] In a meta-analysis of peripheral nerve and central neuraxial blocks compared with general anesthesia, time until discharge from the ambulatory surgery unit was no different for the three groups.[34] Interestingly also, postoperative nausea in the central neuraxial block group was not different from the general anesthesia group. In a study of patients undergoing spinal or general anesthesia for knee surgery, recovery times were equivalent, but after spinal anesthesia, postoperative side effects were fewer.[35] In a study of stop-flow perfusion, a chemotherapeutic technique, where spinal anesthesia and general anesthesia were compared, anesthesia preparation was 5 minutes longer for spinal anesthesia, though using the study's standards for PACU admission, only patients receiving general anesthesia needed PACU admission.[36] Also, pain and PONV were greater in the general anesthesia group. When applying studies of regional anesthesia to everyday practice, remember that the studies come from centers where the authors are experienced in performing regional anesthesia and that might not be the case in other practices.

For some procedures such as arthroscopy, patients might prefer a regional anesthetic simply because they are curious and want to watch the surgery.[37] Postoperative pain is less after regional anesthesia, which is discussed in more detail later in this section. Also, with regional anesthesia or sedation, some of the side effects of general anesthesia can be avoided, although no form of medical care is without side effects. Whenever drugs are given that affect memory, patients might complain that they do not remember events that occur after the procedure. Although with regional anesthesia more time is required to place a block than it takes to induce a general anesthetic, a meta-analysis of several studies showed this increased time to be on average no more than 8 to 9 minutes.[34] In one survey of orthopedic surgeons, the majority of surgeons who direct their patients' choice of anesthetic choose regional anesthesia, although the potential delay in establishing a block and perceived unpredictable success detracted from their enthusiasm with regional anesthesia (Fig. 30-3).[38] For patients, the distinction between general anesthesia and regional anesthesia is probably less important than the fact the patient needs to undergo a procedure.[39]

One adverse effect associated with spinal anesthesia is headache, but headaches are also experienced by patients after general anesthesia. The incidence of headache after either technique may be similar especially when smaller spinal needles are used. Patients may experience backache after spinal anesthesia, although sore throat and nausea are higher after general anesthesia than spinal type. Larger studies of patients undergoing ambulatory surgery are needed that compare sedation with regional and general anesthesia.

Regional Techniques

Local anesthesia and regional anesthesia have long been used for ambulatory surgery. As early as 1963, for example, 56% of ambulatory procedures were performed with the use of these techniques.[40] Regional techniques commonly used for ambulatory surgery, in addition to spinal and epidural anesthesia, include local infiltration, brachial plexus and other peripheral nerve blocks, and intravenous regional anesthesia. General anesthesia can also be supplemented with regional nerve blocks.

Performing a block takes longer than inducing general anesthesia, and the incidence of failure is higher. Unnecessary delays can be obviated by performing the block beforehand in a preoperative holding area. As illustrated above, the increased setup time for a regional anesthetic may be associated with a shorter
7 time to discharge. Postoperative pain control is best with regional techniques.

An occasional patient may experience syncope when the needle for the regional block is inserted. In the experience of oral and maxillofacial surgeons in Massachusetts, 1 of 160 patients fainted when local anesthesia was injected, though a few patients who received general anesthesia fainted after the procedure.[41] When sedation accompanies local anesthesia injection, the incidence of syncope is reduced. Patients usually experience less postoperative pain when local or regional anesthesia has been used. Patients may still have a numb extremity (e.g., after a brachial plexus block) but otherwise meet all criteria for discharge. In such instances, the extremity must be well protected (e.g., with a sling for an upper extremity procedure) and patients must be cautioned to protect against injury because they are without normal sensations that would warn them of vulnerability. Reassurance that sensation will return should be provided.

Spinal Anesthesia

Children

Spinal anesthesia is used in some centers in particular for children undergoing inguinal hernia repair. One group described a series of >1,000 patients where spinal anesthesia was used for children aged 6 months to 14 years for procedures on the lower part of the body.[42] Muscle relaxation with the technique was excellent. In this series, all children left the OR awake and pain-free. The anesthesiology team used 0.5% hyperbaric bupivacaine at a dose of 0.2 mg/kg. In another single institution series of 505 patients 28 to 120 weeks of age at the time of surgery, spinal anesthesia with 0.5% hypobaric bupivacaine was also used.[43] The block was successful in 481 patients; the average number of attempts was 1.4; bloody taps were seen in 12% of cases; in 5 patients the anesthesia was converted to general, all due to surgery duration; and high spinal block occurred in 3 patients.

Adults

The use of spinal needles with pencil point, noncutting tips has prompted a resurgence of spinal anesthesia for ambulatory surgery in adults, though these needles were actually discovered more than 100 years ago.[44] Spinal anesthesia is suitable for pelvic, lower abdominal, and lower extremity surgery. One group described use of spinal anesthesia for ambulatory laparoscopic cholecystectomy with spinal needle insertion at T10, although even these authors recommended their technique not be used routinely because of the potential for direct contact of neural tissue by the spinal needle.[45] Certainly, patients with pre-existing spinal pathology have a higher incidence of complications after neuraxial blockade.[46]

Motor block of the legs may delay a patient's ability to walk. However, the use of a short-acting local anesthetic will minimize this problem. Nausea is much less frequent after epidural or spinal anesthesia than after general anesthesia.

Different drugs and drug concentrations have been used for spinal anesthesia. Lidocaine and mepivacaine are ideal for ambulatory surgery because of their short duration of action, although lidocaine use has been problematic because of transient neurologic symptoms. Transient neurologic symptoms can be seen after other local anesthetics, but the risk is 7 times more after intrathecal lidocaine than after bupivacaine, prilocaine, or procaine.[47]

Chloroprocaine spinal anesthesia has rapid onset and offset. Discharge times when using 2-chloroprocaine for spinal anesthesia are more than 60 minutes faster compared with the use of 0.75% hyperbaric bupivacaine.[48] Both ropivacaine and bupivacaine have been used for ambulatory surgical procedures, but recovery time is relatively long. In a study comparing 7.5 mg bupivacaine and 15 mg ropivacaine for spinal anesthesia for knee arthroscopy, time to ambulation for both drugs was about 5 hours.[49] The relative potencies of the drugs are different: In a study of intrathecal bupivacaine, levobupivacaine, or ropivacaine for lower limb surgery, the ED (50) for bilateral T12 sensory block to cold and successful surgery for at least 50 minutes was 5.50 mg for bupivacaine, 5.68 mg for levobupivacaine, and 8.41 mg for ropivacaine.[50]

Although headache is a common complication of lumbar puncture, smaller-gauge needles result in a lower incidence of postdural puncture headache. For those patients who do receive spinal anesthesia, it is incumbent on the anesthesiologist and the facility to have follow-up with telephone calls to ensure no disabling symptoms of headache have developed (see also Chapter 34 Epidural and Spinal Anesthesia). If the headache does not respond to bed rest, analgesics, and oral hydration, the patient must return to hospital for a course of intravenous caffeine therapy or an epidural blood patch.

Spinal anesthesia should not be avoided in ambulatory surgery patients simply because they may be more active postoperatively than inpatients. Bed rest does not reduce the frequency of headache. Indeed, early ambulation may decrease the incidence. Further study is needed to assess the relative risk–benefit ratio of spinal anesthesia as a technique for the ambulatory surgery patient.

Epidural and Caudal Anesthesia (see Chapter 34 Epidural and Spinal Anesthesia)

Epidural anesthesia takes longer to perform than spinal anesthesia. Onset with spinal anesthesia is more rapid, although recovery may be the same with either technique. In one study of patients undergoing knee arthroscopy, spinal anesthesia with small-dose lidocaine and fentanyl was compared with 3% 2-chloroporcaine administered in the epidural space: Intraoperative conditions, discharge characteristics and times, and recovery profiles were similar.[51] Also, failure rates for the two techniques, although low, were the same. Some studies suggest that bicarbonate can be added to solutions for faster onset of epidural anesthesia. An advantage of the epidural block is that it can be performed outside the OR, and after the surgical procedure is completed, the problem of postdural puncture headache is usually avoided.

Caudal anesthesia is a form of epidural anesthesia commonly used in children before surgery below the umbilicus as a supplement to general anesthesia and to control postoperative pain. Bupivacaine, 0.175% to 0.25%, or ropivacaine, 0.2%, in a volume of 0.5 to 1 mL/kg, may be used; a safe maximal dose is 2.5 mg/kg. Epinephrine, 1:200,000, when added to the anesthetic solution, may allow earlier detection of intravenous, rather than epidural, injection. Other useful albeit controversial additives for increasing duration of caudal blockade include opioids, ketamine, clonidine, and neostigmine.[52] In one survey of caudal anesthesia practice in Great Britain and Ireland, the most popular local anesthetics used were bupivacaine (43.4%) and levobupivacaine (41.7%) and the most common additives were clonidine (42.3%) and ketamine (37.5%).[53] The block may be more difficult in children, particularly those who weigh >10 kg and are obese, if landmarks for the block are difficult to locate. The block is usually administered while the child is anesthetized. After injection, the depth of general anesthesia can be reduced. Because of better pain control after a caudal block, children can usually ambulate earlier and be discharged sooner than without a caudal block. Pain control and discharge times are no different whether the caudal block is placed before surgery or after it is completed.

Nerve Blocks (see Chapter 35 Peripheral Nerve Blockade)

In a survey mailed to members of the Society for Ambulatory Anesthesia in 2001, there was shown to be widespread use of axillary and interscalene blocks for surgery in the upper extremity, and of ankle and femoral blocks for lower extremity surgery.[54] Nerve blocks are even popular in office-based settings.[55] Nerve blocks improve postoperative patient satisfaction—PONV and postoperative pain are less. Costs are also less. In a meta-analysis comparing regional with general anesthesia for ambulatory surgical procedures, central and peripheral nerve blocks increased anesthesia induction time by 8 to 9 minutes, though they were associated with decreased pain scores in the PACU and a decreased need for PACU analgesics.[56] Patients who received central nerve blocks, compared to those receiving general anesthesia did not stay in the PACU for a shorter period of time, did not have less nausea and stayed 35 minutes longer in the ambulatory surgery unit. More patients who received peripheral nerve blocks could bypass PACU; those who went to the PACU stayed 24 minutes

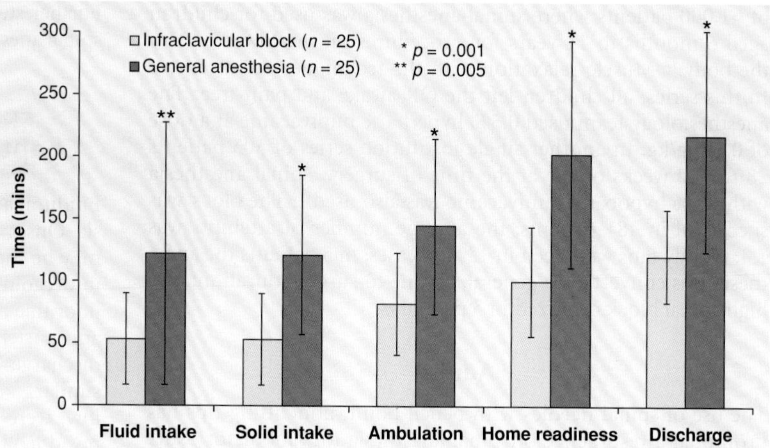

FIGURE 30-4. Recovery was faster when an infraclavicular brachial plexus block with a short-acting local anesthetic was used, compared with general anesthesia and wound infiltration for outpatients undergoing hand and wrist surgery. Times are calculated from the end of anesthesia. Reprinted from: Hadzic A, Arliss J, Kerimoglu B, et al. A comparison of infraclavicular nerve block versus general anesthesia for hand and wrist day-case surgeries. *Anesthesiology.* 2004;101:127–132, with permission.

less; and nausea was less. One nonrandomized study of outpatients in a university setting showed that PACU admissions, hospital cost, and unexpected hospital admission were all reduced when nerve block was used for anterior cruciate ligament repair reconstruction.[57] In a comparison of patients who underwent either infraclavicular brachial plexus block or general anesthesia for upper extremity surgery, after brachial plexus block more patients were able to bypass phase I PACU care, had less pain on PACU arrival, and were discharged much sooner (Fig. 30-4).[58]

Certain procedures can be quite painful, and hospitalization 8 may be required to control pain. Nerve blocks using catheters that can be used to provide analgesia after the operation can be placed before surgery. Paravertebral somatic nerve block can be used for breast surgery, followed by a continuous perineural infusion of local anesthetic at home for 24 to 48 hours.[59] Perineural catheters in the sciatic nerve through the popliteal fossa can be used to control pain after foot surgery for both adults and children.[60,61] Femoral nerve catheters left in for about 2 days after anterior cruciate ligament reconstruction surgery after patients were discharged have been shown to decrease postoperative pain up to 4 days after surgery.[62] Interscalene perineural catheters, kept in for 4 days after surgery, have been used for patients undergoing moderately painful shoulder surgery.[63] Compared with patients who have regional anesthesia for surgery and then treatment afterward with narcotics, patients who go home with the interscalene perineural catheters attached to an infusion pump with ropivacaine can leave the hospital earlier the day after surgery, and once home have less pain and require less narcotics (Fig. 30-5). Continuous cervical paravertebral block may also be useful for analgesia after shoulder surgery.[64] Popliteal catheters have been used for lower extremity surgery such as hallux valgus surgery.[65]

Patients who go home with catheters inserted must be taught about pump function, understand signs of local anesthesia toxicity, and have someone else at home who can provide assistance. Patients must be able to communicate with someone by phone. There should also be a catheter removal protocol.[66] The number of patients who have been sent home with catheters is increasing but is not large. More study is needed in order to demonstrate patient safety.

Sedation and Analgesia

Many patients who undergo surgery with local or regional anesthesia prefer to be sedated and to have no recollection of the procedure. Sedation is important, in part, because injection with local anesthetics can be painful and lying on a hard OR table can be uncomfortable. Levels of sedation vary from light, during which a patient's consciousness is minimally depressed, to very deep, in which protective reflexes are partially blocked and response to physical stimulation or verbal command may not be appropriate. When patients are unsuitable for outpatient general anesthesia, surgery can often be performed if local or regional anesthesia is supplemented with conscious sedation. However, serious risk, such as death, is probably no different after sedation than after general anesthesia. Children who have surgery usually will not remain immobile unless they are deeply sedated or receive general anesthesia.

For adults, the proper dose might be selected by having the patient control the dosage. Yet, at least for ambulatory surgical procedures, patient-controlled sedation is not popular. This may be because a member of the anesthesia care team must be continuously present anyway.

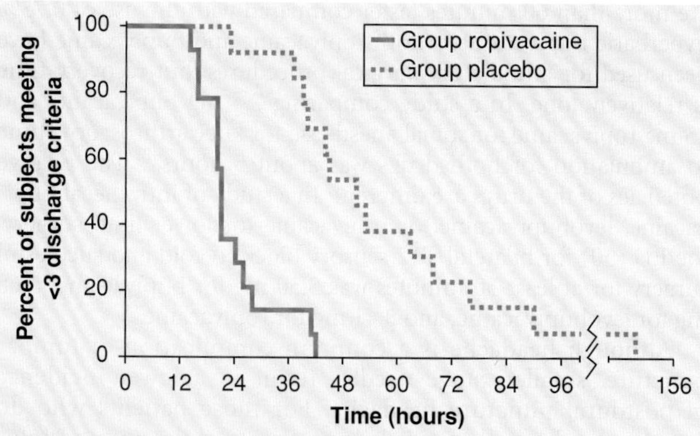

FIGURE 30-5. Patients who continued to receive an interscalene infusion of ropivacaine after surgery could be discharged home much earlier compared with patients who received postoperative narcotics. Discharge criteria included adequate analgesia, independence from intravenous opioids, and the ability to tolerate at least 50% of passive shoulder motion targets during physical therapy. Reprinted from: Ilfeld, BM, Vandenborne, K, Duncan, PW, et al. Ambulatory continuous interscalene nerve blocks decrease the time to discharge readiness after total shoulder arthroplasty: A randomized, triple-masked, placebo-controlled study. *Anesthesiology.* 2006;105:999–1007, with permission.

General Anesthesia

The drugs selected for general anesthesia determine how long patients stay in the PACU after surgery, and for some patients, whether they can be discharged to go home.

Induction

The popularity of propofol as an induction agent for outpatient surgery in part relates to its half-life: The elimination half-life of propofol is 1 to 3 hours, shorter than that of methohexital (6 to 8 hours) or thiopental (10 to 12 hours). Although the effect of drugs given for induction seems to be transient, these drugs can depress psychomo-
9 tor performance for several hours. After induction doses of propofol or thiopental, impairment after thiopental can be apparent for up to 5 hours, but only for 1 hour after propofol.

Pain on injection can be a problem with propofol. Pain is more likely on injection into dorsal hand veins and is minimized if forearm or larger antecubital veins are used. Some individuals, though, experience pain if the drug is injected into proximal larger veins. Nonetheless, thrombophlebitis does not appear to be a problem after intravenous administration of this agent. Such techniques as ketamine, 0.1 mg/kg, immediately before propofol injection or lidocaine, 20 mg, plus metoclopramide, 10 mg have been tried.[67,68] When more than 20 mg lidocaine is mixed with 20 mL propofol, oil droplets may coalesce and then embolize.[69] Many patients who experience pain during anesthesia induction when propofol is injected do not have recall of that pain after surgery.[70]

Most children and some adults prefer not to have an intravenous catheter inserted before the start of anesthesia. Sevoflurane has a relatively low blood–gas partition coefficient and the speed of induction is similar to, albeit somewhat slower than, that of propofol. Induction with sevoflurane can be hastened when the patient is told to breathe out to residual volume, take a vital capacity breath through a primed anesthesia circuit, and then hold the breath.

For short procedures, some patients may not require neuromuscular-blocking drugs; others may need brief paralysis (e.g., with succinylcholine) to facilitate tracheal intubation. Nondepolarizing drugs can be used to facilitate intubation and also during the procedure. Nondepolarizing drugs such as rocuronium have rapid onset times that are similar to those with succinylcholine. Of course, paralysis is not needed to insert an endotracheal tube; drug combinations such as propofol, alfentanil or remifentanil, with or without lidocaine obviate the need for paralysis.[71] Succinylcholine should be used with caution in children because of the possibility of cardiac arrest related to malignant hyperthermia or unsuspected muscular dystrophy, particularly Duchenne disease. Based on one study, patients would be willing to pay $33 out of pocket to avoid a drug like succinylcholine that is associated with postoperative myalgia.[72]

Maintenance

10 Although many factors affect the choice of agents for maintenance of anesthesia, two primary concerns for ambulatory anesthesia are speed of wake-up and incidence of PONV.

Anesthesia Maintenance and Wake-up Times

Time to recovery may be measured by various criteria; however, for an ambulatory center, a patient may be considered awake when he or she is able to leave the center. Actual discharge from an ambulatory center, though, may depend on administrative issues such as a written order from a surgeon or anesthesiologist. The time necessary before a patient can be taken from the OR after completion of surgery, or a patient's ability to skip the PACU and go directly to Phase II recovery (see Chapter 54 Postanesthesia Recovery), may be directly related to the anesthetic and may result in cost savings for an institution. Does choice of maintenance agent affect recovery after anesthesia? Propofol, desflurane, and sevoflurane have characteristics that make them ideal for maintenance of anesthesia for ambulatory surgery. Propofol has a short half-life and, when used as a maintenance agent, results in rapid recovery and few side effects. Desflurane and sevoflurane, halogenated ether anesthetics with low blood–gas partition coefficients, seem to be ideal for general anesthesia for ambulatory surgery. Sevoflurane, unlike desflurane, facilitates a smooth inhalation induction of anesthesia, the preferred technique to ensure rapid recovery of children in ambulatory surgery centers.

11 It is important to distinguish between wake-up time and discharge time. Patients may emerge from anesthesia with desflurane and nitrous oxide significantly faster than after propofol or sevoflurane and nitrous oxide, although the ability to sit up, stand, and tolerate fluids and the time to fitness for discharge may be no different. When the bispectral index (BIS) or other guide of anesthetic depth is used, the difference between drugs and wake-up times may not be as great.[73] Conversely, if fast wake-up times can translate to bypass of phase I, there may be cost savings.

Intraoperative Management of Postoperative Nausea and Vomiting

12 Nausea, with or without vomiting, is probably the most important factor contributing to a delay in discharge of patients and an increase in unanticipated admissions of both children and adults after ambulatory surgery. Patients hate vomiting. Studies have been performed in which patients are asked how much they would pay to avoid PONV or postoperative pain. Patients are willing to pay the most to prevent either of these outcomes, although the actual amount is a function, in part, on patient income.[74] Women, especially those who are pregnant, have a higher incidence of PONV. Other risk factors include a previous history of motion sickness or postanesthetic emesis, surgery within 1 to 7 days of the menstrual cycle, not smoking, and procedures such as laparoscopy, lithotripsy, major breast surgery, and ear, nose, or throat surgery (Table 30-4). The greater the number of risk factors, the greater the risk for nausea or vomiting after surgery.

TABLE 30-4. RISK OF PONV ACCORDING TO PATIENT, PROCEDURE, AND TYPE OF ANESTHESIA

Patient
Women, particularly if pregnant
History of motion sickness or PONV
Surgery within 1–7 d of menstrual cycle
Nonsmokers
Genetics
Procedure
Laparoscopy
Lithotripsy
Major breast surgery
Ear, nose, or throat surgery
Strabismus and other eye surgery
Anesthesia
Inhalation agents
Opioid analgesics
Nitrous oxide

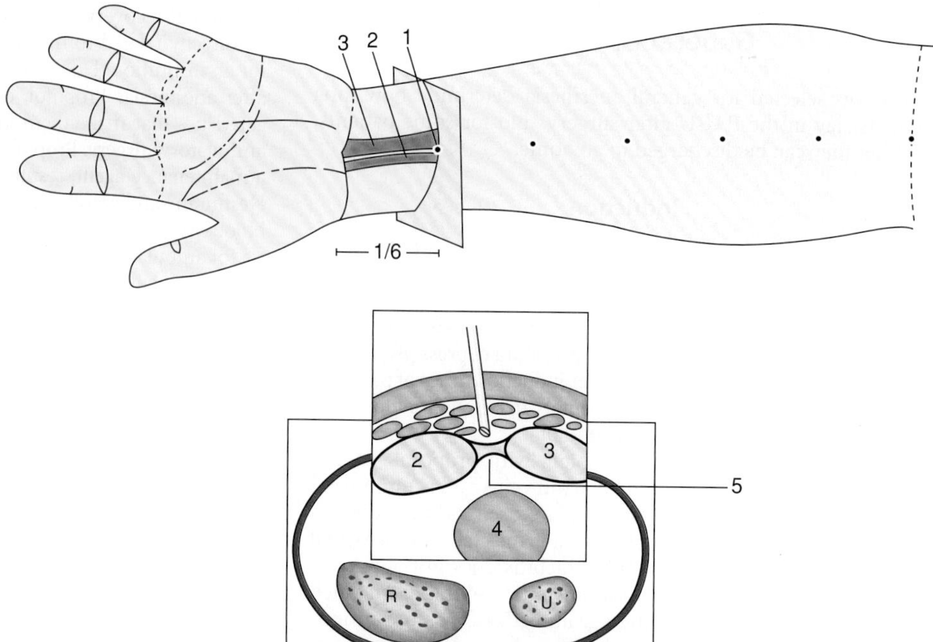

FIGURE 30-6. The P6 acupuncture point in relation to other hand structures is illustrated.[77] (1) P6 acupuncture point, (2) palmaris long tendon, (3) flexor carpi radialis tendon, (4) median nerve, and (5) palmar aponeurosis. Reprinted from: Wang SM, Kain ZN. P6 acupoint injections are as effective as droperidol in controlling early postoperative nausea and vomiting in children. *Anesthesiology.* 2002;97:359–366, with permission.

Inhalation agents are associated with an increased risk of PONV, particularly in the early stages of recovery; postoperative narcotic use is associated with PONV >2 hours after surgery.[75] There are also specific genotypes that are associated with more susceptibility to PONV.[76]

PONV treatment has been based on sites and pathways in the brain that are associated with PONV. Receptor antagonists, specifically selective serotonin antagonists (ondansetron, dolasetron, and granisetron), have been shown to have similar efficacy to help alleviate nausea and vomiting. Dopamine antagonists, antihistamines, and anticholinergic drugs are useful and are generally less expensive, but are associated with extensive side effects. Neurokinin (NK1) receptor antagonists may also be useful to control PONV. Therapies useful in controlling PONV include acupuncture or acupressure (Fig. 30-6),[78] supplemental fluid therapy,[79] (though type of fluid does not seem to be important)[80] clonidine (perhaps in part because it decreases anesthesia requirement),[81] and dexamethasone.[82] Whether acupressure is used before or after surgery is unclear,[83] though if, intraoperatively, leads to monitor patient paralysis are placed at the P6 acupuncture point and tetanus monitoring is used as the neuromuscular monitoring mode, PONV is reduced.[84]

Combination therapy is probably the most effective way to control PONV. Therapy includes avoidance of nitrous oxide; avoidance of inhalation agents; avoidance of muscle relaxant reversal, if clinically indicated; avoidance of narcotics; fluid hydration; and administration of a 5-HT3 antagonist, an antiemetic from a different drug class, and dexamethasone. Risk, of course, is a function of other factors, as previously described. In one study in which combination therapy was used, PONV incidence was <10% and postdischarge PONV was <20%.[82]

Because of its ability to decrease PONV, propofol is the best maintenance general anesthetic for ambulatory anesthesia. For example, in a study of 5,161 patients, propofol, compared with a volatile anesthetic, reduced nausea and vomiting by 19%; and nitrogen compared with nitrous oxide reduced the incidence by 12% (Fig. 30-7).[85] Propofol is now generic so the decision to use the drug should not be based on cost.

The use of nitrous oxide for ambulatory anesthesia is an issue because the incidence of emesis may be greater after nitrous oxide than after potent inhalation agents. Although many studies have shown that nitrous oxide can be used successfully for ambulatory anesthesia, there is evidence that nitrous oxide should be avoided, except for inhalation induction of anesthesia. In one study of patients undergoing major, albeit not ambulatory, surgery, avoidance of nitrous oxide reduced postoperative complications, including postoperative fever, wound infection, pneumonia,

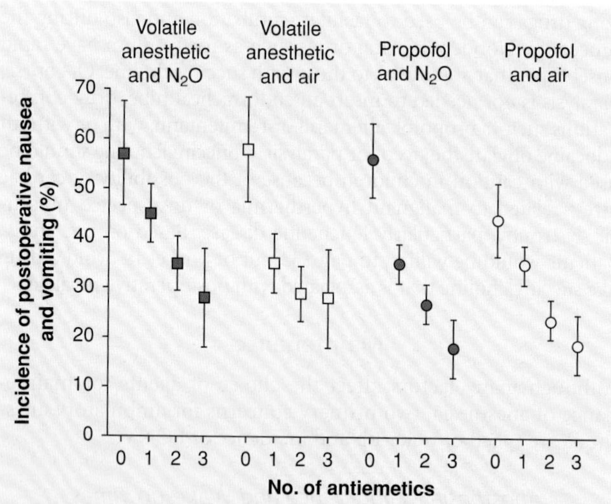

FIGURE 30-7. Postoperative nausea and vomiting (PONV) is least after a propofol anesthetic with air. Illustrated is the incidence of PONV when different anesthetics and different numbers of prophylactic antiemetic treatments are administered. Reprinted from: Apfel CC, Korttila K, Abdalla M, et al. A factorial trial of six interventions for the prevention of postoperative nausea and vomiting. *N Engl J Med.* 2004; 350:2441–2451, with permission.

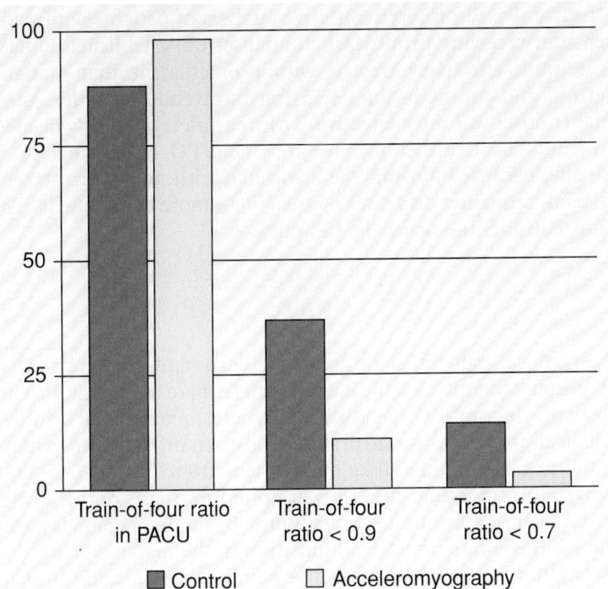

FIGURE 30-8. Patients who are monitored intraoperatively with accelerometry in the PACU have higher train-of-four ratio, and fewer patients with train-of-four ratio <0.9 and 0.7 (all significant). Modified from: Murphy GS, Szokol JW, Avram MJ, et al. Intraoperative acceleromyography monitoring reduces symptoms of muscle weakness and improves quality of recovery in the early postoperative period. *Anesthesiology.* 2011;115:946–954, with permission.

pulmonary atelectasis, and severe nausea or vomiting.[86] In another study, use of nitrous oxide resulted in higher patient costs due to PONV, wound infection, pneumonia, and atelectasis.[87] Whether the changes found in these two studies would be as dramatic in ambulatory patients is not clear. Yet, many would argue that nitrous oxide is no longer needed except for inhalation induction of anesthesia.

Not all intraoperative tachycardia and hypertension is due to pain. In one study, when esmolol was included with an alfentanil infusion for patients undergoing laparoscopic cholecystectomy, PONV was less due to less opioid use intraoperatively.[88] When minimizing opioid use with drugs not known to decrease pain, we must be certain that a patient's pain is adequately treated.

Paralysis

Muscle paralysis for ambulatory anesthesia extends beyond the time of paralysis for intubation, particularly when nondepolarizing drugs are used. The duration of action of rocuronium, vecuronium, rapacuronium, and atracurium ranges from 25 to 40 minutes. Reversal agents must be used unless there is no doubt that muscle relaxation has been fully reversed. The need for reversal is less when acceleromyography is used intraoperatively to monitor extent of paralysis. In one study of patients undergoing elective procedures, postoperative residual paralysis and symptoms of weakness were less and quality of recovery was higher when acceleromyography was used[89] (Fig. 30-8).

Intraoperative Management of Postoperative Pain

Opioids, when given intraoperatively, are useful to supplement both intraoperative and postoperative analgesia. Fentanyl is probably the most popular drug, although all other available narcotics have been tried. All narcotics can cause nausea, sedation, and dizziness, which can delay a patient's discharge. Nonsteroidal analgesics are not effective as supplements during general anesthesia, although they are useful in controlling postoperative pain, particularly when given before skin incision. To control postoperative pain, combination therapy is most useful. (See also the previous discussion on opioids and nonsteroidal analgesics in this chapter: "Opioids and Nonsteroidal Analgesics.")

Depth of Anesthesia

Use of BIS, and entropy, or auditory-evoked potential monitors can decrease anesthesia requirement without sacrificing amnesia during general anesthesia. Because less anesthesia is used, titration of anesthesia with these monitors results in earlier emergence from anesthesia. In a meta-analysis of BIS monitoring for ambulatory anesthesia, BIS monitoring was shown to reduce anesthetic use by 19%, with more modest decreases in PACU duration (4 minutes) and PONV (6%).[90] Results are even more modest, albeit mixed, in terms of later recovery end points. Sympatholytic drugs, instead of anesthesia, can be used to control autonomic responses to anesthesia. In fact, recovery is faster and side effects are fewer in ambulatory patients whose blood pressure is controlled by sympatholytics instead of inhalation agents.[91] In a study of almost 5,000 patients who underwent general anesthesia and who were paralyzed and/or were intubated, awareness was significantly reduced in the group of patients who were monitored with a BIS compared with the group who were not monitored with the BIS.[92] To be fair, not all agree that the use of depth of anesthesia monitoring decreases awareness: One group, in fact, found that when an inhalation agent was used for maintenance of anesthesia for patients with a high risk of recall, that recall, amount of anesthesia used, and postoperative adverse outcomes were no different if BIS or end-tidal anesthesia was used to monitor depth of anesthesia.[93] Entropy, auditory-evoked potential, and cerebral state monitors are similar to BIS. Because these monitors result in less use of anesthesia, there is the possibility that intraoperative awareness and myocardial ischemia might be increased.

Airways

The use of an LMA, or similar type of airway, provides several advantages for allowing a patient to return to baseline status quickly. Muscle relaxants required for intubation can be avoided. Coughing is less than with tracheal intubation. Anesthetic requirements are reduced. Hoarseness and sore throat are also reduced. Overall, cost savings result with the use of LMAs. Because of gastric insufflation, though, nausea and vomiting may be greater. The use of the LMA has been described for laparoscopic procedures, although the potential for aspiration exists because of an inflated abdomen during laparoscopy.

MANAGEMENT OF POSTANESTHESIA CARE (see also Chapter 54 Postanesthesia Recovery)

Many recovery challenges are part of patient selection and perioperative management and must be considered before the patient enters the PACU. Managing common problems in the PACU quickly and effectively is as important as appropriate patient selection and choice of anesthetic technique if the patient is to return home on the day of surgery. The three most common reasons for delay in patient discharge from the PACU are drowsiness, nausea and vomiting, and pain. All three are a function of intraoperative management, but nausea, vomiting, and pain also can be treated in the PACU.

Reversal of Drug Effects

Reversal of muscle relaxants is not unique to the ambulatory surgery patient and is not discussed here (see Chapter 20 Neuromuscular Blocking Agents). Reversal of opioids may sometimes be necessary. Flumazenil, a benzodiazepine receptor antagonist, has primarily been used to reverse the effects of sedation after endoscopy and spinal anesthesia. Reversal of psychomotor impairment with flumazenil is not complete, and the subjective experience of sedation is not necessarily attenuated. Reversal of amnesia with flumazenil is only partial, and the duration of the reversal effect may not be long enough to be clinically significant. Flumazenil should not be used routinely as a benzodiazepine antagonist, but may be used when sedation appears to be excessive. In addition, reversal of benzodiazepine-induced sedation by flumazenil should not replace appropriate ventilatory assistance and, if necessary, placement of an endotracheal tube.

Nausea and Vomiting

Nausea and vomiting are the most common reasons both children and adults have protracted stays in the PACU or unexpected hospital admission due to anesthesia. Nausea and vomiting are also the most common adverse effect in patients in the PACU. Much research has been undertaken to study prophylactic treatment of this problem before surgery, as well as techniques in the OR that can minimize nausea and vomiting in the PACU. The treatment of this problem, once it occurs in the PACU, has not received as much study. Yet, there are a variety of drugs that are effective in treating the problem. The 5-HT3 antagonists seem particularly effective. For example, in one study of children who underwent strabismus surgery and were then nauseous during the first 3 hours after recovery from anesthesia, emesis-free episodes were greater after granisetron, 40 μg/kg (88%), compared with droperidol, 50 μg/kg (63%), or metoclopramide, 0.25 mg/kg (58%).[94] In adults, granisetron, 40 μg/kg; metoclopramide, 0.2 mg/kg; or hydroxyzine, 25 mg, are also effective. Dexamethasone, 8 mg, given with other antiemetics can enhance treatment of established PONV in the PACU.[82]

All seratonin antagonists seem to be equally effective in treating PONV. Anticholinergics, particularly transdermal scopolamine is also effective. In one study, premedication with transdermal scopolamine was as effective as ondansetron or droperidol in preventing early and late PONV and postdischarge nausea and vomiting though it was associated with dry mouth.[95]

Midazolam and propofol, although more commonly used for sedation, have antiemetic effects that are longer in duration than their effects on sedation. For example, when patients in the PACU were nauseous and then received either propofol, 15 mg, or midazolam, 1 or 2 mg, subsequent nausea was no different than with ondansetron, 4 mg.[96] Though use of midazolam to treat PONV might seem odd, indeed, patients who have received midazolam preoperatively also have less PONV.[97] Acupressure bands or acupressure stimulation in the region of the P6 acupuncture point can help reduce PONV. When a ReliefBand (Neurowave Medical Technologies, Chicago, IL) acustimulation device was compared with ondansetron for patients who were nauseous in the PACU after receiving metoclopramide or droperidol and undergoing laparoscopic surgery, nausea was most effectively treated with both the ReliefBand and ondansetron, although both therapies were equally effective individually in treating PONV.[98] If patients have already received ondansetron prophylaxis in the OR, and then are nauseous in the PACU, another repeat dose might not be effective. Based on a retrospective analysis of patients with nausea after receiving prophylactic ondansetron, established PONV was more effectively treated with promethazine than ondansetron; and promethazine, 6.25 mg intravenously, rather than higher doses was most effective.[99] More work is obviously needed to study effective therapies for treatment PONV in the PACU. Finally, because pain may be associated with nausea, treatment of pain frequently decreases nausea. For a more complete discussion, consider the review by Le and Gan.[100]

Pain

Postsurgical pain must be treated quickly and effectively. It is important for the practitioner to differentiate postsurgical pain from the discomfort of hypoxemia, hypercapnia, or a full bladder. Medications for pain control should be given in small intravenous doses (e.g., 1 to 3 mg/70 kg morphine or 10 to 25 μg/70 kg fentanyl). Intramuscular injection of opioid for pain control in the PACU is probably not necessary. Onset of action of drugs is faster after intravenous catheter administration than after oral administration. Control of postoperative pain may include administration of opioid analgesics or NSAIDs, which are not associated with respiratory depression, nausea, or vomiting. Fentanyl is the narcotic frequently used to control postoperative pain that ambulatory surgery patients experience, although the effects of morphine and hydromorphone last longer. Patients who receive fentanyl for pain control may require additional injections and go home no sooner compared with patients who receive morphine. Oral tramadol/paracetamol (TP 37.5/325 mg) given after surgery and then as 1 tablet 4 times daily for 48 hours is an effective fixed drug combination for treating pain after a patient leaves after surgery.[101] Nonsteroidal medications, such as ketorolac or ibuprofen, can also effectively control postoperative pain[102] and, compared with narcotics, can give pain relief for a longer period and are associated with less nausea and vomiting. NSAIDs can increase bleeding, although there is no evidence at this time of such a danger for most ambulatory surgery procedures. When swelling and pain are problematic postoperatively, NSAIDs can be more effective than opioids in relieving both.

We manage pain in both adults and children initially either with a short-acting opioid analgesic such as fentanyl (25 μg/70 kg), or with an injection of ketorolac, 30 to 60 mg/70 kg intramuscularly or intravenously. Fentanyl is repeated at 5-minute intervals until pain is controlled. For children, we also use an elixir of acetaminophen containing codeine (120 mg acetaminophen and 12 mg codeine, in each 5 mL of solution). Five milliliters is administered to children between the ages of 3 and 6, and 10 mL to children between the ages of 7 and 12. Children are returned to parental care as soon as they are awake. We find frequently that infants younger than 6 months of age usually need to be reunited with their mothers for nursing or bottle feeding after a procedure not associated with severe pain. For older infants and young children in the PACU, acetaminophen, 60 mg per year of age (given orally or rectally), is commonly used to relieve mild pain. Intravenous fentanyl (up to a dose of 2 μg/kg) is preferred for more severe pain. Meperidine (0.5 mg/kg) and codeine (1 to 1.5 mg/kg) can be given intramuscularly if an intravenous route has not been established.

Preparation for Discharging the Patient

13 In addition to the PACU, most ambulatory surgery centers in the United States have Phase II Recovery, which may be located

in a different space than the PACU, but may also be conducted in the PACU space. Patients remain in Phase II Recovery, until they are able to tolerate liquids, walk, and/or (depending on the operation) void. With the anesthetics that are typically used in ambulatory surgery ORs, patients who are awakened in the OR and are evaluated as 9 or 10 according to the modified Aldrete scoring system (see Chapter 54 Postanesthesia Recovery) may be transferred directly to Phase II Recovery from the OR. Patients who undergo procedures under monitored anesthesia care can usually go straight to Phase II Recovery from the OR. After procedures using sedation, fast-tracking should take place and usually does not only because of departmental policy or personnel who are unaware of policy.[103] After general anesthesia, LMA use and pain control using nonopioid analgesics facilitates fast-tracking. In one study, 35% to 53% of patients who underwent laparoscopic gynecologic surgery were able to bypass the PACU.[104] In that study, residual sedation was the most common reason the PACU was not bypassed. In another study of patients who underwent outpatient knee surgery bypassed the PACU and were in Phase II Recovery, 31% required nursing interventions and were 3 times more likely to need a nursing intervention, compared with 16% who required a nursing intervention who first went to the PACU. Yet, discharge times were faster and unplanned hospital admissions were fewer if patients were able to bypass the PACU.[105] In a similar study, those authors found that even though direct transfer to Phase II Recovery may decrease time spent in the facility, nursing workload was no different than if patients first went to phase I (PACU) recovery.[106]

Some criteria for discharge to home were created without scientific basis. One criterion is the ability to tolerate liquids before being discharged. Postoperative nausea may be greater if patients are required to drink liquids prior to discharge. Even though it is warranted after spinal or epidural anesthesia, the requirement that low-risk patients void before discharge may only lengthen stay in the hospital, particularly if patients are willing to return to a medical facility if they are unable to void. Practical criteria for patient discharge from the OR, from the PACU, and from Phase II Recovery are needed such that there is no compromise in patient safety. The value of psychomotor tests to measure different phases of recovery (except for research purposes) is questionable.

Although scoring systems may be used to guide transfer from the PACU to the Phase II Recovery and from Phase II Recovery to home, they do little to test higher levels of function, such as the ability to use one's hands, to drive a car, or to remain alert long enough to drive. Patients may feel fine after they leave the hospital, but they should be advised against driving for at least 24 hours after a procedure. Patients and responsible parties should be reminded that the patient should not operate power tools or be involved in major business decisions for up to 24 hours. Once the patient leaves the medical facility, supervision may not be as good as it was in the hospital. Therefore, before a patient is discharged, dressings should be checked. It is wise to include the responsible person in all discharge instructions, which are best made available on printed forms.

Patients should also be informed that they may experience pain, headache, nausea, vomiting, or dizziness and, if succinylcholine was used, muscle aches and pains apart from the incision for at least 24 hours. A patient will be less stressed if the described symptoms are expected in the course of a normal recovery. Written instructions are important. The addition of written and oral education techniques at discharge has a significant impact on improving compliance.

When discussing discharge planning, it is also important to consider where a patient should return in case of a problem. Unlike a hospital, most ambulatory centers are not open around the clock. As ambulatory procedures are becoming more prevalent, patients are traveling farther distances.[107] Whether this is associated with increased risk is yet to be determined.

For patients with a language barrier, consent forms, procedural explanation, and discharge information may have to be written in languages other than English and the services of an interpreter may be necessary. Nursing staff should assess the adult who will take the patient home to determine whether he or she is a responsible person. A responsible person is someone who is physically and intellectually able to take care of the patient at home. Facilities should develop a method of follow-up after the patient has been discharged. At some facilities, staff members telephone the patient the next day to determine the progress of recovery; others use follow-up postcards.

Whenever we become innovative in the management of our outpatients, we must assess how a cost-effective, "no frills" approach to care affects patient safety. We must determine what we can do for the patient who lives alone, for the patient whose responsible person is unable to manage his or her needs, for the patient without means of transportation, and for the patient with limited insurance coverage. Hospital beds can be set aside for patients who require observation. Patients in these beds after an ambulatory surgical procedure are still considered outpatients. They are charged for the hours spent in the observation area. Some hospitals have joined with management firms to build a hospital hotel or medical motel close to the hospital itself. The hotel, usually a nonmedical facility, offers the outpatient a comfortable, inexpensive, and convenient place to recuperate while being cared for by family or nurses. Home health care nursing may be appropriate after surgical procedures such as reduction mammoplasty, abdominoplasty, vaginal hysterectomy, and major open ligament repairs of the knee. The various services for management and/or observation of outpatients after surgery stand today where techniques for management of outpatients during surgery stood in the health care delivery system 20 years ago. Prospective studies are needed to assess the quality of care and the effect that these innovative approaches have on patient safety.

Patient, procedure, availability and quality of aftercare, and anesthetic technique must be individually and collectively assessed to determine acceptability for ambulatory surgery. A delicate balance must be maintained between the physical status of the patient, the proposed surgical procedure, and the appropriate anesthetic technique, to which must be added the expertise level of the anesthesiologist caring for a patient.

Anesthesia for ambulatory surgery is a rapidly evolving specialty. Patients who were once believed to be unsuitable for ambulatory surgery are now considered to be appropriate candidates. Operations once believed unsuitable for outpatients are now routinely performed in the morning, so patients can be discharged in the afternoon or evening. The appropriate anesthetic management before these patients come to the OR, during their operation, and then afterward is the key to success. The availability of both shorter-acting anesthetics and longer-acting analgesics and antiemetics enables us to care for patients in ambulatory centers effectively.

ACKNOWLEDGMENTS

Yale University, Department of Anesthesiology

References

1. Fleisher L, Pasternak L, Lyles A. A novel index of elevated risk of inpatient hospital admission immediately following outpatient surgery. *Arch Surg.* 2007;142:263–268.
2. Clayman M, Seagle B. Office surgery safety: the myths and truths behind the Florida moratoria–six years of Florida data. *Plast Reconstr Surg.* 2006;118:777–785; discussion 786–787.
3. Matarasso A, Swift R, Rankin M. Abdominoplasty and abdominal contour surgery: a national plastic surgery survey. *Plast Reconstr Surg.* 2006;117:1797–1808.
4. Walther-Larsen S, Rasmussen L. The former preterm infant and risk of postoperative apnoea: recommendations for management. *Acta Anaesthesiol Scand.* 2006;50:888–893.
5. Lee SL, Gleason JM, Sydorak RM. A critical review of premature infants with inguinal hernias: optimal timing of repair, incarceration risk, and postoperative apnea. *J Pediatr Surg.* 2011;46:217–220.
6. Shenkman Z, Hoppenstein D, Litmanowitz I, et al. Spinal anesthesia in 62 premature, former-premature or young infants–technical aspects and pitfalls. *Can J Anaesth.* 2002;49:262–269.
7. Mattila K, Vironen J, Eklund A, et al. Randomized clinical trial comparing ambulatory and inpatient care after inguinal hernia repair in patients aged 65 years or older. *Am J Surg.* 2011;201:179–185.
8. Ansell G, Montgomery J. Outcome of ASA III patients undergoing day case surgery. *Br J Anaesth.* 2004;92:71–74.
9. Hofer RE, Kai T, Decker PA, et al. Obesity as a risk factor for unanticipated admissions after ambulatory surgery. *Mayo Clin Proc.* 2008;83:908–916.
10. Stierer TL, Wright C, George A, et al. Risk assessment of obstructive sleep apnea in a population of patients undergoing ambulatory surgery. *J Clin Sleep Med.* 2010;6:467–472.
11. Gross JB, Bachenberg KL, Benumof JL, et al. Practice guidelines for the perioperative management of patients with obstructive sleep apnea: a report by the American Society of Anesthesiologists Task Force on Perioperative Management of patients with obstructive sleep apnea. *Anesthesiology.* 2006;104:1081–1093; quiz 1117–1118.
12. Basson MD, Butler TW, Verma H. Predicting patient nonappearance for surgery as a scheduling strategy to optimize operating room utilization in a veterans' administration hospital. *Anesthesiology.* 2006;104:826–834.
13. von Ungern-Sternberg BS, Boda K, Chambers NA, et al. Risk assessment for respiratory complications in paediatric anaesthesia: a prospective cohort study. *Lancet.* 2010;376:773–783.
14. Morley AP, Nalla BP, Vamadevan S, et al. The influence of duration of fluid abstinence on hypotension during propofol induction. *Anesth Analg.* 2010;111: 1373–1377.
15. Schmitz A, Kellenberger CJ, Liamlahi R, et al. Gastric emptying after overnight fasting and clear fluid intake: a prospective investigation using serial magnetic resonance imaging in healthy children. *Br J Anaesth.* 2011;107:425–429.
16. American Society of Anesthesiologists Committee. Practice guidelines for preoperative fasting and the use of pharmacologic agents to reduce the risk of pulmonary aspiration: application to healthy patients undergoing elective procedures: an updated report by the American Society of Anesthesiologists Committee on Standards and Practice Parameters. *Anesthesiology.* 2011;114:495–511.
17. Jawaid M, Mushtaq A, Mukhtar S, et al. Preoperative anxiety before elective surgery. *Neurosciences (Riyadh).* 2007;12:145–148.
18. Fekrat F, Sahin A, Yazici K, et al. Anaesthetists' and surgeons' estimation of preoperative anxiety by patients submitted for elective surgery in a university hospital. *Eur J Anaesthesiol.* 2006;23:227–233.
19. Kain Z, Caldwell-Andrews A, Mayes L, et al. Family-centered preparation for surgery improves perioperative outcomes in children: a randomized controlled trial. *Anesthesiology.* 2007;106:65–74.
20. Fortier MA, Blount RL, Wang SM, et al. Analysing a family-centred preoperative intervention programme: a dismantling approach. *Br J Anaesth.* 2011;106:713–718.
21. Cote C, Cohen I, Suresh S, et al. A comparison of three doses of a commercially prepared oral midazolam syrup in children. *Anesth Analg.* 2002;94:37–43.
22. Kain ZN, MacLaren J, McClain BC, et al. Effects of age and emotionality on the effectiveness of midazolam administered preoperatively to children. *Anesthesiology.* 2007;107:545–552.
23. Lichtor JL, Alessi R, Lane BS. Sleep tendency as a measure of recovery after drugs used for ambulatory surgery. *Anesthesiology.* 2002;96:878–883.
24. Bulach R, Myles PS, Russnak M. Double-blind randomized controlled trial to determine extent of amnesia with midazolam given immediately before general anaesthesia. *Br J Anaesth.* 2005;94:300–305.
25. Fanelli G, Ghisi D, Berti M, et al. Preoperative administration of controlled-release oxycodone as a transition opioid for total intravenous anaesthesia in pain control after laparoscopic cholecystectomy. *Surg Endosc.* 2008;22:2220–2228.
26. Sun T, Sacan O, White PF, et al. Perioperative versus postoperative celecoxib on patient outcomes after major plastic surgery procedures. *Anesth Analg.* 2008; 106:950–958.
27. Capici F, Ingelmo PM, Davidson A, et al. Randomized controlled trial of duration of analgesia following intravenous or rectal acetaminophen after adenotonsillectomy in children. *Br J Anaesth.* 2008;100:251–255.
28. Ong CK, Seymour RA, Lirk P, et al. Combining paracetamol (acetaminophen) with nonsteroidal antiinflammatory drugs: a qualitative systematic review of analgesic efficacy for acute postoperative pain. *Anesth Analg.* 2010;110:1170–1179.
29. Nordin P, Zetterstrom H, Carlsson P, et al. Cost-effectiveness analysis of local, regional and general anaesthesia for inguinal hernia repair using data from a randomized clinical trial. *Br J Surg.* 2007;94:500–505.
30. Bay-Nielsen M, Kehlet H. Anaesthesia and post-operative morbidity after elective groin hernia repair: a nation-wide study. *Acta Anaesthesiol Scand.* 2008;52:169–174.
31. Gonano C, Leitgeb U, Sitzwohl C, et al. Spinal versus general anesthesia for orthopedic surgery: anesthesia drug and supply costs. *Anesth Analg.* 2006;102:524–529.
32. Nishikawa K, Yoshida S, Shimodate Y, et al. A comparison of spinal anesthesia with small-dose lidocaine and general anesthesia with fentanyl and propofol for ambulatory prostate biopsy procedures in elderly patients. *J Clin Anesth.* 2007;19:25–29.
33. O'Donnell BD, Ryan H, O'Sullivan O, et al. Ultrasound-guided axillary brachial plexus block with 20 milliliters local anesthetic mixture versus general anesthesia for upper limb trauma surgery: An observer-blinded, prospective, randomized, controlled trial. *Anesth Analg.* 2009;109:279–283.
34. Liu S, Strodtbeck W, Richman J, et al. A comparison of regional versus general anesthesia for ambulatory anesthesia: a meta-analysis of randomized controlled trials. *Anesth Analg.* 2005;101:1634–1642.
35. Korhonen A, Valanne J, Jokela R, et al. A comparison of selective spinal anesthesia with hyperbaric bupivacaine and general anesthesia with desflurane for outpatient knee arthroscopy. *Anesth Analg.* 2004;99:1668–1673.
36. Carron M, Freo U, Innocente F, et al. Recovery profiles of general anesthesia and spinal anesthesia for chemotherapeutic perfusion with circulatory block (stop-flow perfusion). *Anesth Analg.* 2007;105:1500–1503.
37. Pelinka L, Pelinka H, Leixnering M, et al. Why patients choose regional anesthesia for orthopedic and trauma surgery. *Arch Orthop Trauma Surg.* 2003;123:164–167.
38. Oldman M, McCartney C, Leung A, et al. A survey of orthopedic surgeons' attitudes and knowledge regarding regional anesthesia. *Anesth Analg.* 2004;98:1486–1490.
39. Webster F, Bremner S, McCartney CJ. Patient experiences as knowledge for the evidence base: a qualitative approach to understanding patient experiences regarding the use of regional anesthesia for hip and knee arthroplasty. *Reg Anesth Pain Med.* 2011;36:461–465.
40. Cohen D, Dillon J. Anesthesia for outpatient surgery. *JAMA.* 1966;196:1114–1116.
41. D'eramo E, Bookless S, Howard J. Adverse events with outpatient anesthesia in Massachusetts. *J Oral Maxillofac Surg.* 2003;61:793–800.
42. Puncuh F, Lampugnani E, Kokki H. Use of spinal anaesthesia in paediatric patients: a single centre experience with 1132 cases. *Paediatr Anaesth.* 2004; 14:564–567.
43. Kachko L, Simhi E, Tzeitlin E, et al. Spinal anesthesia in neonates and infants - a single-center experience of 505 cases. *Paediatr Anaesth.* 2007;17:647–653.
44. Calthorpe N. The history of spinal needles: getting to the point. *Anaesthesia.* 2004;59:1231–1241.
45. van Zundert A, Stultiens G, Jakimowicz J, et al. Laparoscopic cholecystectomy under segmental thoracic spinal anaesthesia: a feasibility study. *Br J Anaesth.* 2007; 98:682–686.
46. Hebl JR, Horlocker TT, Kopp SL, et al. Neuraxial blockade in patients with preexisting spinal stenosis, lumbar disk disease, or prior spine surgery: efficacy and neurologic complications. *Anesth Analg.* 2010;111:1511–1519.
47. Zaric D, Christiansen C, Pace N, et al. Transient neurologic symptoms after spinal anesthesia with lidocaine versus other local anesthetics: a systematic review of randomized, controlled trials. *Anesth Analg.* 2005;100:1811–1816.
48. Lacasse MA, Roy JD, Forget J, et al. Comparison of bupivacaine and 2-chloroprocaine for spinal anesthesia for outpatient surgery: a double-blind randomized trial. *Can J Anaesth.* 2011;58:384–391.
49. Boztug N, Bigat Z, Karsli B, et al. Comparison of ropivacaine and bupivacaine for intrathecal anesthesia during outpatient arthroscopic surgery. *J Clin Anesth.* 2006;18:521–525.
50. Lee YY, Ngan Kee WD, Fong SY, et al. The median effective dose of bupivacaine, levobupivacaine, and ropivacaine after intrathecal injection in lower limb surgery. *Anesth Analg.* 2009;109:1331–1334.
51. Pollock J, Mulroy M, Bent E, et al. A comparison of two regional anesthetic techniques for outpatient knee arthroscopy. *Anesth Analg.* 2003;97:397–401.
52. Lonnqvist P. Adjuncts to caudal block in children–Quo vadis? *Br J Anaesth.* 2005;95:431–433.
53. Menzies R, Congreve K, Herodes V, et al. A survey of pediatric caudal extradural anesthesia practice. *Paediatr Anaesth.* 2009;19:829–836.
54. Klein S, Pietrobon R, Nielsen K, et al. Peripheral nerve blockade with long-acting local anesthetics: a survey of the Society for Ambulatory Anesthesia. *Anesth Analg.* 2002;94:71–76.
55. Hausman LM, Eisenkraft JB, Rosenblatt MA. The safety and efficacy of regional anesthesia in an office-based setting. *J Clin Anesth.* 2008;20:271–275.
56. Liu SS, Strodtbeck WM, Richman JM, et al. A comparison of regional versus general anesthesia for ambulatory anesthesia: a meta-analysis of randomized controlled trials. *Anesth Analg.* 2005;101:1634–1642.
57. Williams B, Kentor M, Vogt M, et al. Economics of nerve block pain management after anterior cruciate ligament reconstruction: potential hospital cost savings via

associated postanesthesia care unit bypass and same-day discharge. *Anesthesiology.* 2004;100:697–706.
58. Hadzic A, Arliss J, Kerimoglu B, et al. A Comparison of Infraclavicular Nerve Block versus General Anesthesia for Hand and Wrist Day-case Surgeries. *Anesthesiology.* 2004;101:127–132.
59. Buckenmaier C3, Klein S, Nielsen K, et al. Continuous paravertebral catheter and outpatient infusion for breast surgery. *Anesth Analg.* 2003;97:715–717.
60. Zaric D, Boysen K, Christiansen J, et al. Continuous popliteal sciatic nerve block for outpatient foot surgery–a randomized, controlled trial. *Acta Anaesthesiol Scand.* 2004;48:337–341.
61. Dadure C, Bringuier S, Nicolas F, et al. Continuous epidural block versus continuous popliteal nerve block for postoperative pain relief after major podiatric surgery in children: a prospective, comparative randomized study. *Anesth Analg.* 2006;102:744–749.
62. Williams B, Kentor M, Vogt M, et al. Reduction of verbal pain scores after anterior cruciate ligament reconstruction with 2-day continuous femoral nerve block: a randomized clinical trial. *Anesthesiology.* 2006;104:315–327.
63. Ilfeld B, Vandenborne K, Duncan P, et al. Ambulatory continuous interscalene nerve blocks decrease the time to discharge readiness after total shoulder arthroplasty: a randomized, triple-masked, placebo-controlled study. *Anesthesiology.* 2006;105:999–1007.
64. Boezaart A, De Beer J, Nell M. Early experience with continuous cervical paravertebral block using a stimulating catheter. *Reg Anesth Pain Med.* 2003;28:406–413.
65. Capdevila X, Dadure C, Bringuier S, et al. Effect of patient-controlled perineural analgesia on rehabilitation and pain after ambulatory orthopedic surgery: a multicenter randomized trial. *Anesthesiology.* 2006;105:566–573.
66. Ilfeld BM. Continuous peripheral nerve blocks: a review of the published evidence. *Anesth Analg.* 2011;113:904–925.
67. Koo S, Cho S, Kim Y, et al. Small-dose ketamine reduces the pain of propofol injection. *Anesth Analg.* 2006;103:1444–1447.
68. Fujii Y, Nakayama M. A lidocaine/metoclopramide combination decreases pain on injection of propofol. *Can J Anaesth.* 2005;52:474–477.
69. Masaki Y, Tanaka M, Nishikawa T. Physicochemical compatibility of propofol-lidocaine mixture. *Anesth Analg.* 2003;97:1646–1651.
70. Kaur B, Ng WL, Leslie K. Audit of recall of propofol injection pain. *J Clin Anesth.* 2011;23:592–593.
71. Jabbour-Khoury S, Dabbous A, Rizk L, et al. A combination of alfentanil-lidocaine-propofol provides better intubating conditions than fentanyl-lidocaine-propofol in the absence of muscle relaxants. *Can J Anaesth.* 2003;50:116–120.
72. Allen TK, Habib AS, Dear GL, et al. How much are patients willing to pay to avoid postoperative muscle pain associated with succinylcholine? *J Clin Anesth.* 2007;19:601–608.
73. Pauls RJ, Dickson TJ, Kaufmann AM, et al. A comparison of the ability of the EEGo and BIS monitors to assess emergence following neurosurgery. *Can J. Anaesth.* 2009;56:366–373.
74. Macario A, Fleisher L. Is there value in obtaining a patient's willingness to pay for a particular anesthetic intervention? *Anesthesiology.* 2006;104:906–909.
75. Apfel C, Kranke P, Katz M, et al. Volatile anaesthetics may be the main cause of early but not delayed postoperative vomiting: a randomized controlled trial of factorial design. *Br J Anaesth.* 2002;88:659–668.
76. Janicki PK, Vealey R, Liu J, et al. Genome-wide Association study using pooled DNA to identify candidate markers mediating susceptibility to postoperative nausea and vomiting. *Anesthesiology.* 2011;115:54–64.
77. Wang SM, Kain ZN. P6 acupoint injections are as effective as droperidol in controlling early postoperative nausea and vomiting in children. *Anesthesiology.* 2002;97:359–366.
78. Lee A, Fan LT. Stimulation of the wrist acupuncture point P6 for preventing postoperative nausea and vomiting. *Cochrane Database Syst Rev.* 2009;(2):CD003281.
79. Magner J, McCaul C, Carton E, et al. Effect of intraoperative intravenous crystalloid infusion on postoperative nausea and vomiting after gynaecological laparoscopy: comparison of 30 and 10 ml kg-1. *Br J Anaesth.* 2004;93:381–385.
80. Haentjens LL, Ghoundiwal D, Touhiri K, et al. Does infusion of colloid influence the occurrence of postoperative nausea and vomiting after elective surgery in women? *Anesth Analg.* 2009;108:1788–1793.
81. Oddby-Muhrbeck E, Eksborg S, Bergendahl H, et al. Effects of clonidine on postoperative nausea and vomiting in breast cancer surgery. *Anesthesiology.* 2002;96:1109–1114.
82. Ormel G, Romundstad L, Lambert-Jensen P, et al. Dexamethasone has additive effect when combined with ondansetron and droperidol for treatment of established PONV. *Acta Anaesthesiol Scand.* 2011;55:1196–1205.
83. Frey UH, Funk M, Lohlein C, et al. Effect of P6 acustimulation on post-operative nausea and vomiting in patients undergoing a laparoscopic cholecystectomy. *Acta Anaesthesiol Scand.* 2009;53:1341–1347.
84. Kim YH, Kim KS, Lee HJ, et al. The efficacy of several neuromuscular monitoring modes at the P6 acupuncture point in preventing postoperative nausea and vomiting. *Anesth Analg.* 2011;112:819–823.
85. Apfel C, Korttila K, Abdalla M, et al. A factorial trial of six interventions for the prevention of postoperative nausea and vomiting. *N Engl J Med.* 2004;350:2441–2451.
86. Myles P, Leslie K, Chan M, et al. Avoidance of nitrous oxide for patients undergoing major surgery: a randomized controlled trial. *Anesthesiology.* 2007;107:221–231.
87. Graham AM, Myles PS, Leslie K, et al. A cost-benefit analysis of the ENIGMA trial. *Anesthesiology.* 2011;115:265–272.
88. Ozturk T, Kaya H, Aran G, et al. Postoperative beneficial effects of esmolol in treated hypertensive patients undergoing laparoscopic cholecystectomy. *Br J Anaesth.* 2008;100:211–214.
89. Murphy GS, Szokol JW, Avram MJ, et al. Intraoperative acceleromyography monitoring reduces symptoms of muscle weakness and improves quality of recovery in the early postoperative period. *Anesthesiology.* 2011;115:946–954.
90. Liu S. Effects of Bispectral Index monitoring on ambulatory anesthesia: a meta-analysis of randomized controlled trials and a cost analysis. *Anesthesiology.* 2004; 101:311–315.
91. White P, Wang B, Tang J, et al. The effect of intraoperative use of esmolol and nicardipine on recovery after ambulatory surgery. *Anesth Analg.* 2003;97:1633–1638.
92. Ekman A, Lindholm M, Lennmarken C, et al. Reduction in the incidence of awareness using BIS monitoring. *Acta Anaesthesiol Scand.* 2004;48:20–26.
93. Avidan MS, Jacobsohn E, Glick D, et al. Prevention of intraoperative awareness in a high-risk surgical population. *N Engl J Med.* 2011;365:591–600.
94. Fujii Y, Tanaka H, Ito M. Treatment of vomiting after paediatric strabismus surgery with granisetron, droperidol, and metoclopramide. *Ophthalmologica.* 2002; 216:359–362.
95. White PF, Tang J, Song D, et al. Transdermal scopolamine: an alternative to ondansetron and droperidol for the prevention of postoperative and postdischarge emetic symptoms. *Anesth Analg.* 2007;104:92–96.
96. Unlugenc H, Guler T, Gunes Y, et al. Comparative study of the antiemetic efficacy of ondansetron, propofol and midazolam in the early postoperative period. *Eur J Anaesthesiol.* 2004;21:60–65.
97. Riad W, Altaf R, Abdulla A, et al. Effect of midazolam, dexamethasone and their combination on the prevention of nausea and vomiting following strabismus repair in children. *Eur J Anaesthesiol.* 2007;24:697–701.
98. Coloma M, White P, Ogunnaike B, et al. Comparison of acustimulation and ondansetron for the treatment of established postoperative nausea and vomiting. *Anesthesiology.* 2002;97:1387–1392.
99. Habib A, Reuveni J, Taguchi A, et al. A comparison of ondansetron with promethazine for treating postoperative nausea and vomiting in patients who received prophylaxis with ondansetron: a retrospective database analysis. *Anesth Analg.* 2007;104:548–551.
100. Le TP, Gan TJ. Update on the management of postoperative nausea and vomiting and postdischarge nausea and vomiting in ambulatory surgery. *Anesthesiol Clin.* 2010;28:225–249.
101. Alfano G, Grieco M, Forino A, et al. Analgesia with paracetamol/tramadol vs. paracetamol/codeine in one day-surgery: a randomized open study. *Eur Rev Med Pharmacol Sci.* 2011;15:205–210.
102. White PF, Tang J, Wender RH, et al. The effects of oral ibuprofen and celecoxib in preventing pain, improving recovery outcomes and patient satisfaction after ambulatory surgery. *Anesth Analg.* 2011;112:323–329.
103. Twersky RS, Sapozhnikova S, Toure B. Risk factors associated with fast-track ineligibility after monitored anesthesia care in ambulatory surgery patients. *Anesth Analg.* 2008;106:1421–1426, table of contents.
104. Coloma M, Zhou T, White P, et al. Fast-tracking after outpatient laparoscopy: reasons for failure after propofol, sevoflurane, and desflurane anesthesia. *Anesth Analg.* 2001;93:112–115.
105. Williams B, Kentor M, Williams J, et al. PACU bypass after outpatient knee surgery is associated with fewer unplanned hospital admissions but more phase II nursing interventions. *Anesthesiology.* 2002;97:981–988.
106. Song D, Chung F, Ronayne M, et al. Fast-tracking (bypassing the PACU) does not reduce nursing workload after ambulatory surgery. *Br J Anaesth.* 2004;93:768–774.
107. Neuman MD, David G, Silber JH, et al. Changing access to emergency care for patients undergoing outpatient procedures at ambulatory surgery centers: evidence from Florida. *Med Care Res Rev.* 2011;68:247–258.
108. Tait A, Malviya S, Voepel-Lewis T, et al. Risk factors for perioperative adverse respiratory events in children with upper respiratory tract infections. *Anesthesiology.* 2001;95:299–306.

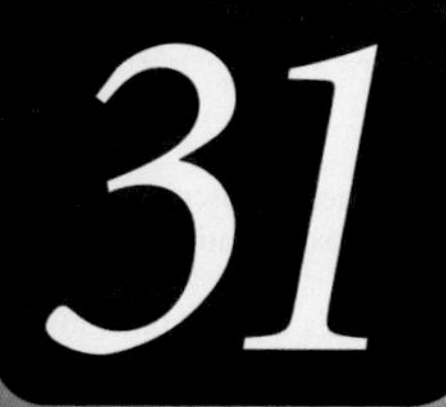

CHAPTER 31

Office-Based Anesthesia

LAURENCE M. HAUSMAN • MEG A. ROSENBLATT

Key Points

1. An office-based anesthetic is defined as an anesthetic that is performed in an outpatient venue such as an office or procedure room that is not accredited as either an ambulatory surgery center (ASC) or as a hospital.
2. Along with providing safe anesthetics across the spectrum of healthy to medically challenged patients undergoing increasingly complex procedures, the anesthesiologist must understand office safety and policy, legal and financial issues such as anti-trust laws, and billing and collection issues.
3. Advantages of an office-based procedure include cost containment, patient and surgeon convenience, decreased patient exposure to nosocomial infections, and both improved patient privacy and continuity of care.
4. It has been reported that there may, in fact, be an increased risk of injury during an office-based anesthetic secondary to the remote location of an office.
5. The ideal patient for an office-based procedure has an ASA physical status of 1 or 2.
6. The anesthesiologist should function as a zealous patient advocate in assuring that an anesthetic is performed only in a safe anesthetizing location, thus perioperative monitoring must adhere to the ASA standards.
7. It is recommended that there be at least one ACLS/PALS-certified member of the health-care team present until the last patient has left the office.
8. Each office must have a plan in place delineating the responsibilities of each staff member, in the event of an occurrence.
9. Governmental oversight of office-based surgery varies among states; currently regulations exist in many states and others are following.
10. It is in the anesthesia provider's best interest to seek legal counsel and create a valid business model before embarking on a career in OBA.

Multimedia

 Levels of Sedation

Office-based anesthesia (OBA) is a subset of both nonoperating room anesthesia (NORA; see Chapter 32) and ambulatory anesthesia (see Chapter 30). NORA refers to any anesthetic that takes place outside of the traditional operating room but usually within a fully licensed hospital. Examples of NORA locations include an endoscopy suite, an invasive radiology suite, a magnetic resonance imaging (MRI) machine or an area in which electroconvulsive therapy (ECT) takes place. Alternatively, an ambulatory anesthetic is one in which the patient arrives to the surgical venue the day of the procedure, is anesthetized, and is discharged home later that same day.

1 An office-based anesthetic is defined as an anesthetic that is performed in an outpatient venue such as an office or procedure room that is not accredited as either an ambulatory surgery center (ASC) or as a hospital. In contrast to an ASC, the office provides practitioners with the space for other activities such as consultation with new patients, the performance of routine history and physicals, and office administration. In addition, while ASCs are often multidisciplinary, office-based practices are generally confined to one specialty such as urology, gastroenterology, plastic surgery, or dentistry.[1,2]

Although an OBA practice may be an exciting alternative to the traditional hospital-based one, it requires the anesthesiologist to expand his or her role within the health-care delivery sys-
2 tem. Along with providing safe anesthetics across the spectrum of healthy to medically challenged patients undergoing increasingly complex procedures, the anesthesiologist must understand office safety and policy, legal and financial issues such as antitrust laws, and billing and collection issues.[3] These are relatively new responsibilities for the anesthesiologist, who has previously worked as a member within a hospital department either in a private or academic setting. A further challenge to the office-based practitioner is that presently there is little to no training in OBA within the anesthesia residency curriculum.[4]

BRIEF HISTORICAL PERSPECTIVE OF OBA

There have been reports of office-based surgery and anesthesia since the mid-nineteenth century. In 1856, John Snow documented his experience in providing anesthesia with chloroform for 867 dental patients, and approximately 3,021 teeth were extracted in private dental offices under his care.[5] Throughout history, the family physician performed house calls and numerous small surgical procedures such as the lancing of boils and repair of wounds were conducted within the comfort of the patient's home. The physician's private medical office was, likewise, utilized in the service of this type of surgical care.

As surgery became more invasive, the need for intensive perioperative physiologic monitoring became increasingly necessary. The capacity to administer blood products and the development of an extensive array of pharmaceutical agents began to play a role in patient care, fostering the growth of larger health-care delivery teams to assist in patient care. Thus, over time, the inpatient hospital became the primary setting in which surgery would be performed.

Over the past several decades, as a result of both surgical and anesthetic advances, the surgical experience has again changed. Through innovations such as laparoscopic techniques, surgery has become increasingly less invasive and less painful. In addition, newer anesthetics have the benefit of "fast-acting" profiles (associated with quick onsets and rapid termination of effect) and with fewer hemodynamic side effects, lending increasing number of procedures to be suitable for the performance in outpatient venues.[6,7]

During the 1970s, less than 10% of all surgical and diagnostic procedures were performed on an ambulatory basis and of these, virtually all were performed in hospitals. By 1987, approximately 25 million, or 40% of all procedures, were performed as ambulatory. In the United States, between 1984 and 1990, the number of office-based procedures increased from 400,000 to 1.2 million, and by 1994, 8.5% of all procedures were performed in offices.[8] In 1994, a landmark survey of the membership of the American Society of Plastic Surgeons (ASPS), revealed that 55% of the respondents performed the majority or all of their procedures in an office.[9] In the year 2000, approximately 75% of all procedures were performed on an outpatient basis; 17% in freestanding ASCs, and 14% to 25% (approximately 8 to 10 million) in physicians' offices.[10–12] By 2005, the American Hospital Association reported that while 82% of all procedures were performed on an ambulatory basis, 16% of all these ambulatory procedures were performed in private offices.[13]

ADVANTAGES/DISADVANTAGES

3 There are many advantages to an office-based procedure when compared to a traditional hospital-based one, and the most obvious of these advantages is cost containment. Several components make up the actual cost of a given surgical procedure. In addition to the professional fees of both the proceduralist and the anesthesiologist (which are usually negotiated prior to an elective procedure), there is a facility fee charged by the hospital or ASC. This fee generally covers the associated costs to the hospital/ASC, and includes overhead such as maintenance, equipment, and staffing. It often constitutes a large component of the patient's overall charge. In an office, this amount can easily be predicted and is often minimal when compared to that in a hospital. The reason for this discrepancy is that while the overhead costs in a small office are usually quite reasonable and managed, the comparable costs in a large tertiary care hospital can be both enormous and unpredictable.[10,11,14]

In 1994, Schultz determined the cost of an in-hospital laparoscopic inguinal hernia repair to be $5,494. When the same procedure was performed in an office, the price was decreased to $1,533.84. Similarly, the average cost of an in-hospital open inguinal hernia repair was found to be $2,237, while the same procedure performed in a private office cost $894.79.[15] In addition, Bartamian[16] reported that office-based ocular surgery, performed under monitored anesthesia care (MAC), can cost 70% less than similar procedures performed in a hospital. Some insurance companies now offer incentives to surgeons who utilize an office location as their surgical venue.[17]

Other clear advantages of office-based procedures include ease of scheduling (often with less paperwork), patient and surgeon convenience, decreased patient exposure to nosocomial infections, and both improved patient privacy and continuity of care (since an office is usually staffed by a small consistent group of personnel).[3,11,18,19]

There are potential disadvantages to an office-based procedure which relate to issues regarding patient safety and peer review.[20] In some parts of the country, no regulations governing office-based surgery and OBA exist. Therefore, there may be little to no oversight regarding the certification/qualification of either the surgeon or anesthesiologist to perform the intended procedures, the surgical office's policy regarding peer review, performance improvement, documentation, general policies and procedures,

TABLE 31-1. STATES WHICH HAVE REGULATIONS REGARDING OFFICE-BASED SURGERY AND ANESTHESIA

Alabama	Mississippi
Arizona	New Jersey
California	New York
Colorado	North Carolina
Connecticut	Ohio
District of Columbia	Oklahoma
Florida	Oregon
Illinois	Pennsylvania
Indiana	Virginia
Kansas	South Carolina
Kentucky	Tennessee
Louisiana	Texas
Massachusetts	Washington

and the reporting of adverse outcomes. However, the number of such states without regulation and oversight is rapidly decreasing[21] (Table 31-1).

OFFICE SAFETY

Media reports and newspaper articles raised the earliest questions regarding the safety of office-based procedures.[22] These exposes
4 in the lay press may be legitimate. It has been reported that there may, in fact, be an increased risk of injury during an office-based anesthetic secondary to the remote location of an office.[23]

Data reveal that injuries and deaths occurring in offices are often multifactorial in causation. Reasons include over-dosages of local anesthetics, prolonged surgery with occult blood loss, pulmonary embolism, accumulation of multiple anesthetics resulting in over-sedation, hypovolemia, hypoxemia, and the use of reversal drugs with short half lives.[24–26] Both the American Society of Anesthesiologists (ASA)and the Anesthesia Patient Safety Foundation[27,28] have emerged as leaders in the field of OBA safety and have advocated that the quality of care in office-based practice be no less than that of a hospital or ASC. Thus, it is imperative to ensure that all safety precautions one may take for granted in a hospital be present in the surgical office.

In 1990, the mortality rate from anesthesia was approximately 1/100,000. By the year 2000, the rate had decreased to 1/250,000 in hospitals and 1/400,000 in free-standing ASCs.[29] Although the interpretation of these figures is open to debate, the decrease in mortality can be attributed, in part, to improvements in the training of the anesthesia providers, the safety profiles of the newer anesthetics, improved perioperative monitoring capabilities and intrinsic safety mechanisms in place within the anesthetizing location. Since the majority of office-based patients are young and healthy, one would expect that an anesthetic performed there would be at least equally as safe as an anesthetic performed in a hospital, if not safer. However, reports of morbidity and mortality within office-based practices exist (and vary dramatically). In 1997, Morello et al. conducted a survey querying 418 accredited plastic surgeons' offices. They had a 57% response rate and found that over a 5-year period, 400,675 office procedures were conducted: 63.2% cosmetic and 36.8% reconstructive. Several outcomes were reviewed including hemorrhage, hypertension, hypotension, wound infection, need for hospital admission, and reoperation. There was an overall complication rate of 0.24%, and seven mortalities, which were both surgery and anesthesia related. They included two myocardial infarctions (one following augmentation mammoplasty, the other 4 hours after rhinoplasty) one case of cerebral hypoxia during abdominoplasty, one tension pneumothorax during breast augmentation, one cardiac arrest during carpal tunnel surgery, one stroke 3 days following rhytidectomy and brow lift, and one unexplained death.[30] These reports represent an overall mortality rate of 1 in 57,000! A report by Hoefflin et al.,[31] however, found no complications after 23,000 plastic surgical procedures that occurred in a single office under general anesthesia (GA). Similarly, Sullivan and Tattini retrospectively reviewed the results in an office performing over 5,000 surgical procedures by five independent plastic surgeons. The primary anesthetic technique during this time period consisted of deep sedation in conjunction with local anesthesia or regional block, and was performed by an anesthesiologist supervising a certified registered nurse anesthetist (CRNA). No mortalities occurred over the 5-year period.[32] Bitar et al. retrospectively studied adverse outcomes in 3,615 consecutive patients undergoing 4,778 plastic surgery procedures in offices between 1995 and 2000. The anesthetics were MAC with midazolam, propofol, and an opioid, and no deaths were reported. Dyspnea occurred in 0.05% of patients, nausea and vomiting 0.2%, and there was a 0.05% rate of hospital admissions.[33] When analyzing these outcomes, one must appreciate that, since the mortality rate from anesthesia is so low, an extremely large cohort group would be necessary to provide real data regarding the relative risk of an office-based anesthetic. Recent data even suggest a 10-fold increased risk of morbidity and mortality associated with an office-based anesthetic when compared to one performed in a free-standing ASC.[24]

Other studies also reveal a significant risk associated with an office-based procedure. Rao et al. reported that according to closed malpractice claims in Florida, 830 deaths and 4,000 injuries were associated with OBA between 1990 and 1999. These claims accounted for 30% of all malpractice claims in that state.[34] In a hospital operating room, the risks of an anesthetic are usually primarily related to the underlying medical condition of the patient, whereas in an office they may be increased risks secondary to factors such as inadequate standards and safeguards. More recent data from Florida have shown that office-based morbidity and mortality are usually the results of inadequate perioperative patient monitoring, over sedation and thromboembolitic events.[23,25,35] The challenge of acquiring accurate morbidity and mortality data for OBA is complicated by the fact that many offices are not required to report adverse events. In addition, although an anesthesiologist may not even be administering the anesthetic in an office, many complications may still be reported as anesthetic related.

Traditional credentialing procedures, such as board certification and the granting or renewing of hospital privileges based on competency and proof of continuing medical education, may not be required or enforced in an office. Within and among offices, providers of anesthesia may also have varying degrees of both education and expertise. The provider may be an anesthesiologist, a nurse anesthetist, a dental anesthetist, or a surgeon with little or no training in anesthesia. Furthermore, safety within an anesthetizing location also depends on the perioperative patient-monitoring capabilities. Although hospital patients are mandated by the accrediting organizations to have defined standards of care for monitoring in the operating rooms and postanesthesia care units (PACUs), these may be lacking in an inadequately prepared and nonaccredited surgical offices.[33] There have been patients' injuries reported during office-based procedures resulting from the use of obsolete and/or malfunctioning anesthesia machines, as well as from alarms that have not been serviced and/or are not functioning properly.[4] The ASA created guidelines for defining obsolete anesthesia machines, which prohibit the use of any anesthesia machine that lacks essential safety features (e.g., oxygen ratio device, oxygen pressure failure alarm), has the presence of unacceptable features (e.g., copper kettles, or vaporizers with rotary concentration dials that increase vapor concentration when the dial is turned clockwise), or for which routine maintenance is no longer possible.[36]

A review of ASA Closed Claims Project data, which incorporates information from the 35 liability insurers that indemnify approximately 50% of the practicing anesthesiologists in the United States, reveals safety concerns in office-based practices are more than theoretical.[24,37] As of 2001, there were 753 (13.7%) claims for ambulatory procedures and 14 (0.26%) for office-based ones. This small number of claims most likely due to the 3- to 5-year time lag in reporting to the database.[29] ASA physical status 1 or 2 females who had undergone elective surgery under GA make up the majority of claims filed. This statistic parallels the profiles of trends seen in operating rooms and free-standing ASCs. The injuries that occur in offices tend to be of greater severity than those that occur in ASCs. Twenty-one percent of the reported injuries sustained in offices were temporary and nondisabling in nature and 64% were permanent or led to death, while 62% of the injuries sustained in ASCs were temporary and nondisabling and only 21% were permanent or led to death.[29] A study by Coté et al.[38,39] concluded that the causes for injuries in an office ranged from human error to machine and equipment malfunction (Table 31-2).

The Closed Claims Project database reveals that injuries during office-based procedures occur throughout the perioperative period, and are multifactorial in etiology. The majority, 64%, occurred intraoperatively, while 14% occurred in the PACU and 21% after discharge.[29] Half of these adverse events were respiratory in nature and included airway obstruction, bronchospasm, inadequate oxygenation and ventilation, and unrecognized esophageal intubation. The second most common group of events were considered to be drug related, occurring 25% of the time. These included incorrect agent or dosage, allergy and malignant hyperthermia (MH). Cardiovascular injuries and equipment-related injuries each occurred in 8% of incidents.[29]

TABLE 31-2. CAUSES OF INJURY IN THE OFFICE-BASED PRACTICE. DATA FROM COTÉ ET AL.[38,39]

1. Inadequate resuscitation equipment
2. Inadequate monitoring
   a. Most commonly no pulse-oximetry
3. Inadequate preoperative or postoperative evaluation
4. Human error
   a. Slow recognition of an event
   b. Slow response to an event
   c. Lack of experience
   d. Drug over-dosage

An important point to consider when looking at adverse events is whether or not they were preventable. Again, according to the information in the Closed Claims Project database, only 13% of the events that occurred in ASCs were considered preventable, whereas 46% of the office-based ones were deemed so. Furthermore, all of the adverse respiratory events that occurred in the PACUs of offices would have been prevented, had pulse oximetry and capnography been used. Care was considered to be substandard in 50% of OBA claims and in 34% of ASC ones. In 2001, Claims originating from an office-based procedure resulted in a monetary award 92% of the time, with a median payment of $200,000 (ranging between $10,000 and $2,000,000), whereas claims originating from ASC-based procedures were compensated only 59% of the time with a median payout of $85,000 (ranging between $34 and $14,700,000).[29]

Ensuring office-based practice safety is critical. After several highly publicized office liposuction injuries and deaths in August 2000, the State of Florida attempted to address this problem by placing a 90-day moratorium on all office-based procedures that utilized anesthetic depths greater than conscious sedation. During that time a safety panel comprising of surgeons, anesthesiologists, and other health-care professionals was formed and charged with the task of developing recommendations to improve the safety record of office-based procedures. The panel's recommendations focused on factors including patient selection, preoperative evaluation and testing, procedures to be excluded, surgeon qualification and facility standards.[19,40] Other major organizations that have played a leading role in developing standards for the office-based practitioner include the ASA, the ASPS, the American Association of Nurse Anesthetists (AANA), and the American Medical Association (AMA).[27,40–42]

PATIENT SELECTION

Before presenting for an office-based procedure, the patient's medical condition should be optimally managed.[43] He or she should have a preoperative history and physical examination documented within 30 days prior to the procedure, and all pertinent laboratory tests as well as any medically indicated specialist consultation(s) must be readily available. Consent for the procedure and the anesthetic must also be in the chart. The anesthesiologist should have access to all of this information preoperatively and, when possible, contact the patient prior to the scheduled procedure. If a patient is an ASA physical status 1 or 2, the surgeon's office should arrange the surgery as per office protocol. However, if a patient has significant comorbid conditions, a preoperative anesthesiology consultation should be obtained before scheduling the patient for surgery.

Patient selection remains a controversial topic among practicing office-based anesthesiologists because little morbidity and mortality data exist to support the inclusion or exclusion of specific populations. A study by Meridy in 1982[44] concluded that patients should not be excluded from undergoing ambulatory procedures based solely on their age, the type of procedure, or the duration of the planned procedure. Similar data are yet to exist regarding office-based practices; however, some recom-
5 mendations have been made. The ASPS has acknowledged that the ideal patient for an office-based procedure has an ASA physical status of 1 or 2. They recommended that ASA physical status 3 patients undergo an office-based procedure only after an anesthesia consultation and only have an office-based procedure performed under local anesthesia without sedation. The ASA also has developed recommendations regarding patient selection.[45] It is

TABLE 31-3. POOR CANDIDATES FOR OFFICE-BASED PROCEDURES

1. Poorly controlled diabetes
2. History of substance abuse
3. Seizure disorder
4. Malignant hyperthermia susceptibility
5. Potential difficult airway
   a. Morbid obesity
   b. Obstructive sleep-apnea syndrome
6. NPO less than 8 h
7. No escort
8. Previous adverse outcomes from anesthesia
9. Significant drug allergies
10. Aspiration risk

important to realize that the office is often remote and the anesthesiologist may be unable to get assistance should it be required. Thus, groups of patients in whom anticipated anesthetic problems may develop should be avoided (Table 31-3). Individual anesthesiologists should therefore consider excluding certain patients with significant comorbid conditions in order to avoid unanticipated problems.

Morbidly obese patients and those with obstructive sleep apnea syndrome (OSAS) present unique and increasingly frequent challenges to the office-based practitioner.[46] Indeed, they are usually the same population, with estimates of 60% to 90% of all obstructive sleep apnea patients being obese (body mass index greater than or equal to 30 kg/m^2).[47,48] Confounding this problem is that the majority of the patients with OSAS have yet to be formally diagnosed.[49,50] These patients are likely to cause major anesthetic problems throughout the perioperative period.[51] There may be failure to intubate, or ventilate, they may have respiratory distress soon after extubation or suffer from respiratory arrest with preoperative sedation or postoperative analgesia.[49] These patients tend to be exquisitely sensitive to the respiratory depressant effects of even small dosages of sedation or analgesics.[51] Furthermore, respiratory depression may not be reversible with pharmacologic antagonism.[52] One of the first steps in the ASA algorithm for management of the difficult airway is to call for help. In an office, this is usually not possible. It has been recommended that a postoperative observational unit with close monitoring of oxygen saturation or an intensive care unit setting be used for monitoring the OSAS patient postoperatively.[53] It may, thus, be prudent to avoid performing general anesthetics on patients with OSAS in all outpatient setting especially locations as remote as an office-based practice.

Pulmonary embolism is a significant cause of perioperative morbidity and mortality from an office-based surgical procedure.[54,55] Reinisch found that 0.39% (37/9,493) of patients who underwent rhytidectomy developed a deep vein thrombosis (DVT). Of these, 40.5% (15/37) went on to form a pulmonary embolism. Although GA had only accounted for only 43% of the anesthetic techniques used for the procedure, 83.7% of the embolic events were associated with the patient having undergone a general anesthetic.[56] Risk factors for the development of DVT appear in Table 31-4.[57] The ASPS recommends that patients be stratified according to risk and the prophylactic treatment be directed by risk (Table 31-5).

TABLE 31-4. RISK FACTORS FOR THE DEVELOPMENT OF DEEP VEIN THROMBOSIS (DVT)

- Age greater than 40
- Anti-thrombin III deficiency
- Central nervous system disease
- Family history of DVT
- Heart failure
- History of a DVT
- Hypercoagulable states
- Lupus anticoagulant
- Malignancy
- Obesity
- Oral contraceptive use
- Polycythemia
- Previous miscarriage
- Radiation therapy for pelvic neoplasms
- Severe infection
- Trauma
- Venous insufficiency

As more subspecialists begin to perform office-based procedures, older and sicker patients will present. The anesthesiologist must be the patient's advocate in the matter of safety. This advocacy can only result from a true understanding of how to adequately select appropriate patients for this unique surgical venue.

TABLE 31-5. RECOMMENDED TREATMENT FOR PREVENTION OF DEEP VEIN THROMBOSIS IN PATIENTS, STRATIFIED BY RISK[56,57]

Cohort	Treatment
Low Risk	
• No risk factors	• Comfortable position
• Uncomplicated surgery	• Knees flexed at 5 degrees
• Short duration	• Avoid constriction and external pressure
Moderate Risk	
• Age >40 with no other risks	• Proper positioning
• Procedure >30 min	• Intermittent pneumatic compression of calf or ankle (prior to sedation and continued until patient is awake and moving)
• Oral contraceptive use	• Frequent alterations of the OR table
High Risk	
• Age >40 with concomitant risk factors	• Treatment as per patients with moderate risk
• Procedure >30 min	• Preoperative hematology consultation with consideration of perioperative antithrombotic therapy

SURGEON SELECTION

The relationship between the surgeon and the anesthesiologist must be one of mutual trust and understanding. Since the surgeon performing the procedure may also own the office, he or she must not put pressure on the anesthesiologist to perform an anesthetic if the anesthesiologist believes that the patient or procedure is not appropriate.

The surgeon must have a valid medical license, registration and Drug Enforcement Administration (DEA) certificate. He or she should be either board eligible or board certified by a recognized member of the American Board of Medical Specialties, and either have privileges to perform the proposed procedure in a local hospital, or have training and documented competency comparable to a practitioner who does have such privileges in a hospital. Although this requirement may sound intuitive, there have been cases reported of surgeons performing procedures for which they have little or no training.[11] In addition, the surgeon must have adequate liability insurance, at least equal to that carried by the anesthesiologist. If a lawsuit should arise and the surgeon is inadequately insured, the anesthesiologist may be held financially responsible, and become the "deep pocket." Similarly, the facility itself should have adequate liability insurance.

In addition, there should be a system in place for monitoring continuing medical education as well as peer review and performance improvement, for the surgeon/proceduralist, anesthesiologist, and nursing staff. This is often not the case in an office-based practice.[11] If an anesthesia group provides care at more than one office, an overall peer review for the practice may be used; it need not be specific to each individual office site. Solo anesthesia practitioners should not be exempt from this process. Anesthesiologists should only align themselves with the offices which have ongoing processes, or help to organize one. The peer review committee should include surgeons, anesthesiologists, and nursing staff. It should meet regularly and maintain a written record of minutes and recommendations. Similarly, continuing medical education should also be documented and at a minimum should be sufficient to meet relicensing requirements.

When formulating a quality assurance program, there should be random chart reviews as well as key sentinel events that trigger a case review (Table 31-6). It is imperative that this review be an open forum to ensure continued quality improvement of care, and not be biased or hindered by fear of litigation. Legal counsel should be sought to determine whether information disclosed at these meetings is discoverable in a court of law, should a malpractice claim arise.

OFFICE SELECTION AND REQUIREMENTS

6 The anesthesiologist should function as a zealous patient advocate in assuring that an anesthetic only be performed in a safe anesthetizing location. The office needs to be appropriately equipped, stocked, and maintained to perform a general anesthetic (GA) (Table 31-7). All supplies must be age and size appropriate for the patient population. If an anesthesia machine or ventilator is present, it must be regularly serviced and calibrated. If potent inhaled volatile agents or N_2O are used, there must be a functioning waste gas scavenging system. This system may be exhausted via a window or roof vent. However, the exhaust must not be vented back into the office or into any other inhabited space and

TABLE 31-6. SENTINEL EVENTS THAT SHOULD TRIGGER A CASE REVIEW AND BE PRESENTED AT A PERFORMANCE IMPROVEMENT/QUALITY ASSURANCE MEETING

1. Dental injury
2. Corneal abrasion
3. Perioperative MI or stroke
4. Aspiration
5. Reintubation
6. Return to the operating room
7. Peripheral nerve injury
8. Adverse drug reaction
9. Uncontrolled pain or nausea/vomiting
10. Unexpected hospital admission
11. Cardiac arrest
12. Death
13. Incomplete charts
14. Controlled substance discrepancy
15. Patient complaints
16. Neurologic injury

TABLE 31-7. SAFE DELIVERY OF OBA REQUIRES THE AVAILABILITY OF THE FOLLOWING EQUIPMENT

- Monitors
  - Noninvasive blood pressure with an assortment of cuff sizes
  - Heart Rate/ECG
  - Pulse oximeter
  - Temperature
  - Capnography
- Airway Supplies
  - Nasal cannulae
  - Oral airways
  - Face masks
  - Self-inflating bag-mask ventilation device
  - Laryngoscopes multiple sizes and styles (Mac and Miller)
  - Handles
  - Various sizes of tracheal tubes
  - Stylettes
- Emergency airway equipment (LMA's, cricothyrotomy kit, trans-tracheal jet ventilation equipment)
- Suction catheters and suction equipment
- Cardiac defibrillator
- Emergency drugs
  - ACLS drugs
  - Dantrolene and malignant hyperthermia supplies
- Anesthetic drugs
- Vascular cannulation equipment

TABLE 31-8. EMERGENCIES WHICH REQUIRE CONTINGENCY PLANS

1. Fire
2. Bomb/bomb threat
3. Power loss
4. Equipment malfunction
5. Loss of oxygen supply pressure
6. Cardiac or respiratory arrest in the waiting room, OR, or PACU
7. Earthquake
8. Hurricane
9. External disturbance such as a riot
10. Malignant hyperthermia
11. Massive blood loss
12. Emergency transfer of patient to a hospital

be in accordance with Occupational Safety and Health Administration (OSHA) standards. There are also portable scavenging systems available in the market that can be safely used. Air testing should be done on a regular basis. In an office without an exhaust system, total intravenous anesthesia (TIVA) techniques should be employed.

All offices, even those without ventilators or anesthesia machines, require a means to deliver positive pressure ventilation to the patient's lungs. This can be achieved by using a self-inflating resuscitation device. An adequate supply of compressed oxygen must be present as well as a back-up supply for use in an emergency. In offices that do not have a pipeline supply of oxygen, H cylinders are usually used and several E cylinders should be kept in reserve. A policy must be in place describing the transport, storage, and disposal of medical gases, consistent with state and local laws. All equipment described in the ASA algorithm for management of the difficult airway should be present.[58] A readily available means to create an emergency surgical airway and jet ventilation capability may be lifesaving.

Perioperative monitoring must adhere to the ASA standards for basic anesthetic monitoring.[59,60] These include continuous monitoring of heart rate and oxygen saturation, intermittent noninvasive blood pressure monitoring, end-tidal CO_2 ($EtCO_2$) monitoring, and the capacity for both temperature monitoring and continuous ECG. Monitors must be routinely serviced, calibrated, and repaired as necessary. All monitors should have a back-up battery supply and there should be an extra monitor available for an emergency.

All emergency drugs appearing on the American Heart Association Advanced Cardiac Life Support (ACLS) protocol should be available. The expiration dates for these agents should be checked on a regular basis, and outdated drugs replaced as necessary. A cardiac defibrillator with a battery backup must be immediately available and routinely checked, as should a source of suction including a pharyngeal suction catheter. The office-based anesthesiologist should be familiar with the signs and symptoms of MH and be prepared to begin the initial treatment if any triggering agents are stocked. This treatment would include ice, cold saline, insulin, calcium, and sodium bicarbonate. In addition, it would require having at least 12 bottles of dantrolene. A complete listing of MH supplies is available online at www.mhaus.org.[61] The office staff should undergo MH drills at least annually.

A protocol for the delivery and secure storage of controlled substances must be in place. A licensed anesthesiologist may supply these drugs in accordance with DEA regulations, as may any licensed physician with a current DEA registration certificate. Instead of transporting drugs, it is often more convenient to store them in the surgical office. In this situation, they must be stored in a double-locked storage cabinet installed in a secure location, in accordance with state and local regulations. The office in which the controlled substances will be dispensed must also be properly registered with the DEA. Drug accounting must be performed in accordance with state and federal regulations. Individual states have different provisions and regulations regarding the dispensing of controlled substances, and it is the responsibility of the dispensing physician to assure that the office-based practice is in compliance.

A medical director and a governing body, responsible for overall operations and ensuring high-quality patient care, should be identified for every office. There must also be a Policy and Procedures manual that outlines the responsibilities of each staff member including nurses (circulating/scrub and postop), physician assistants, surgical technicians, and office staff and administrators. The manual should include a description of the infection control policy as well as anesthesia policies. All nurses should be licensed by the state and have training and education consistent with their responsibilities. Basic cardiac life support (BLS) certification should be mandatory and ACLS certification is preferable. In addition, either the anesthesiologist or the physician who supervises the anesthesia care provider must be ACLS or pediatric advanced life support (PALS) certified, depending on the patient
7 population. There should always be at least one member of the health-care team with ACLS/PALS certification present in the office until the last patient has been discharged.

Emergencies can, and do, occur in an office-based setting
8 (Table 31-8). Each office must have a plan in place delineating the responsibilities of each staff member, in the event of such an occurrence. The physical structure of the office is an important consideration. There should be a clear egress that would easily accommodate a stretcher carrying a mechanically ventilated patient. Adequate clearance and room for transport in an elevator must also be considered.

Destinations for a patient in need of hospital admission must be identified. Developing an office–hospital relationship is challenging, as hospitals may be reluctant to be involved in office mishaps. However, it is of utmost importance to have a formal written arrangement. Telephoning the emergency services number (911) is an acceptable plan for transportation, provided the response time is rapid. If 911 is unavailable in a specific city, or has a slow response time, the office should have a contractual agreement with a local ambulance company.

The office must be prepared for an intraoperative fire. The ASA has recently published an advisory on the prevention and management of such an emergency.[62] Fire requires three components known as the "fire triad": An oxidizer (oxygen and nitrous oxide), an ignition source (electrocautery, laser, drill, etc.), and fuel (sponges, drapes, endotracheal tubes, solutions containing alcohol or other volatile compounds, etc.). The modern operating room contains all three in great supply. The first step in fire prevention is education. All members of the surgical and anesthesia team must be educated on how fires are started, sustained, and prevented. There must be regularly scheduled fire drills that include all employees, even those with nonclinical duties. These drills should highlight the responsibilities of each staff member.

Fire prevention is of the utmost importance. The ASA recommends that if flammable materials are used to prep the skin they should be allowed to completely dry before draping the surgical field. The field should then be draped in a manner that does not allow for oxygen to accumulate. This is important because these accumulated pockets of oxygen may flow into the surgical field where there is a source of ignition such as electrocautery. There must be communication between the surgeon and anesthesiologist when an oxygen-rich environment is being created near a surgical site. This scenario is common during facial plastic surgery. The surgeon and anesthesiologist must decide upon the depth of sedation required throughout different points of the procedure, and the need for supplemental oxygen must be determined. The inspiratory oxygen flow rate should be kept at a minimum, as guided by the oxygen saturation, and nitrous oxide (N_2O) should be avoided. The surgeon must be made aware of the inspiratory oxygen concentration, and the anesthesiologist must keep the oxygen concentration as low as clinically possible. Medical air insufflation or suctioning can be used to reduce oxygen accumulation. When using an ignition source in an oxygen-rich environment, the ASA recommends reducing the oxygen flow as low as possible without creating hypoxia, and waiting several minutes to allow the oxygen to dissipate.[57]

The management of a fire will require recognizing the early signs, stopping the procedure and ignition source, extinguishing the fire, and delivering care to the patient. It may even be necessary to evacuate the building. In any case, it is imperative that all these steps be reviewed regularly and drills performed. The office should have at least a 1-hour firewall present to help prevent the spread of fire.

There must be contingency plans in the event of a power-supply interruption or electrical failure. Each office should have an emergency generator capable of running necessary equipment and monitors; monitors should have battery backup power that is routinely checked. Battery reserve power will usually last for one and a half hours, but this needs to be verified for each piece of electrically powered equipment.

The office should keep patient records (including anesthesia records) in accordance with local laws, which is usually for a minimum of 5 years. Similarly, the anesthesiologist should maintain his or her own records, which include the preanesthesia history and physical, informed consent, intraoperative documentation and postoperative care record, as well as discharge orders.

Accreditation

One way to objectively evaluate an office is to have it accredited by a nationally recognized accrediting agency. The ASA has developed a classification of offices that stratifies them by the level of anesthetic depth that may be administered (Table 31-9).[45]

TABLE 31-9. ASA CLASSIFICATION OF SURGICAL PROCEDURES[45]

Class A
- Minor surgical procedures
- Local, topical, or infiltration of local anesthetic
- No sedation preoperatively or intraoperatively

Class B
- Minor or major surgical procedures
- Sedation via oral, rectal, or intravenous sedation
- Analgesic or dissociative drugs

Class C
- Minor or major surgical procedures
- General anesthesia
- Major conduction block anesthesia

Presently many states require offices to be accredited and more are following suit (Table 31-1). In states that do not require accreditation, there are benefits to voluntarily obtaining it. Often, accreditation will allow the facility fee to be reimbursed by a third-party payer in medically necessary procedures.[63] In addition, the patient may feel more comfortable undergoing a procedure in an office that has been accredited. Finally, as more states require accreditation, if a surgeon's office proactively becomes accredited in a state that subsequently requires it, there would be no interruption of services.

Currently there are three major accrediting bodies for office-based surgery offices, although several other agencies are also recognized. The Accreditation Association for Ambulatory Health Care (AAAHC) was the first major accrediting body, offering certification since 1998. The American Association for Accreditation of Ambulatory Surgical Facilities (AAAASF), originally the Accreditation Association for Ambulatory Plastic Surgical Facilities (AAAPSF), was the second, followed by The Joint Commission (TJC). To date, the most active organization is the AAAASF. Its requirements are simpler than those of AAAHC and TJC and accreditation is less expensive; however, changes are underway to allow AAAHC and TJC to be more competitive.[3] Each agency has different criteria for eligibility and different accreditation cycles pertaining to the time limit of a certificate.[64] The agencies deal with the entire perioperative spectrum of running a surgical office, ranging from physical office design to patient issues (Table 31-10).

TABLE 31-10. FACTORS CONSIDERED IN ACCREDITING AN OFFICE FOR SURGICAL PROCEDURES. A COMPLETE LISTING OF CRITERIA CAN BE OBTAINED FROM THE INDIVIDUAL AGENCIES

1. Physical layout of the office
2. Environmental safety/infection control
3. Patient and personnel records
4. Surgeon qualification
   a. Training
   b. Local hospital privileges (surgical and admission)
5. Office administration
6. Anesthesiologist requirements
7. Staffing intraoperatively and postoperatively
8. Monitoring capabilities both intraoperatively and postoperatively
9. Ancillary care
10. Equipment
11. Drugs (emergency, controlled substances, routine medications)
12. BLS, ACLS/PALS certification
13. Temperature
14. Neuromuscular functioning
15. Patient positioning
16. Pre- and postanesthesia care/documentation
17. Quality assurance/peer review
18. Liability insurance
19. PACU evaluation
20. Discharge evaluation
21. Emergency preparedness (fire/admission/transfer, etc.)

In addition, the AAAHC can accredit not only the surgical office, but also an anesthesia group that provides OBA.

The accrediting agencies were developed, in part, to reduce some of the variability that exists among offices in regard to safety issues. Several professional societies are encouraging their members to perform procedures only in accredited facilities. The Society for Aesthetic Plastic Surgeons mandates that all of its members perform procedures only in offices that have been accredited by one of the nationally recognized accrediting agencies, or have been certified to participate in the Medicare program under title XVIII, or are licensed by the state. The actual improvement in safety conferred by performing surgery in an accredited office has yet to be determined, and there are those who suggest that it provides no advantage.[65] As long as there is no mandatory reporting system in place, it will be impossible to determine the true incidence of morbidity associated with office-based practice. Clearly though, safety in an office depends upon more than just accreditation; there must be constant vigilance by all members of the health-care team.

PROCEDURE SELECTION

Early in the development of office-based surgery, procedures were generally noninvasive and of short duration. However, as newer surgical and anesthetic techniques have evolved, longer and more invasive procedures have been successfully performed.[66–73] Suitable office-based procedures range the gamut from superficial incision and drainage of abscesses to more invasive microlaparoscopies.

Duration of procedure has long been correlated with the need for hospital admission, with procedures lasting more than 1 hour being associated with a higher incidence of unplanned admission.[74] Other data have shown that longer procedures are also often associated with an increased incidence of postoperative nausea and vomiting (PONV), postoperative pain, and bleeding,[75,76] which may warrant hospital admission. For these reasons the ASPS has recommended that procedures be limited to 6 hours and be completed by 3 p.m. (15:00 hours), thus allowing for a full patient recovery with maximum office staffing.[40] In addition, when determining the suitability of a procedure, one must consider the possibility of hypothermia, blood loss, or significant fluid shifts.[40]

Specific Procedures

Liposuction

Liposuction is the most commonly performed cosmetic procedure, and is performed primarily by plastic surgeons and dermatologists.[77,78] It is accomplished by inserting hollow rods into small incisions in the skin, and suctioning subcutaneous fat into an aspiration canister. Superwet and tumescent techniques, introduced in the mid-1980s, utilize large volumes (1 to 4 cc) of infiltrate solution (0.9% saline or Ringer lactate with epinephrine 1:1,000,000 and lidocaine 0.025% to 0.1%) for each 1 cc of fat to be removed. Blood loss is generally 1% of the aspirate with these techniques.[79] The peak serum levels of lidocaine occur 12 to 14 hours after injection and decline over the subsequent 6 to 14 hours.[80,81] Although the maximum dose of lidocaine has been traditionally limited to 7 mg/kg, 35 to 55 mg/kg doses have been used safely because the tumescent technique results in a single compartment clearance similar to that of a sustained-release medication.[81,82]

Liposuction is not a benign procedure.[83] In 2000, a census survey of the 1,200 members of the American Society of Aesthetic Plastic Surgeons (ASAPS), revealed an overall mortality rate of 19.1 per 100,000 liposuction procedures, with pulmonary embolism diagnosed in 23.1% of deaths. Other etiologies of mortality included abdominal viscous perforation, anesthesia causes, fat embolism, infection, and hemorrhage. Also, 28.5% of all deaths in this study were reported as of unknown or confidential etiology.[84] Risk factors identified included the use of multiliter wetting solution infiltration, mega-volume aspiration causing massive third spacing, multiple concurrent procedures, anesthetic sedative effects yielding hypoventilation, and permissive discharge policies. The management of the postoperative period, with attention to fluid and electrolyte balance and pain control, is critical to an optimal outcome after liposuction. The patient's fluid deficit, maintenance, intraoperative loss, and third spacing should guide fluid management throughout the perioperative period. Generally, an office liposuction should be limited to 5,000 mL of total aspirant which includes supernatant fat and fluid.[40] It is also recommended that large-volume liposuction not be performed in conjunction with other procedures.

Iverson et al.[19,40] developed the following considerations and recommendations regarding office-based liposuction.

1. Plastic surgeons should follow the current ASA Guidelines for Sedation and Analgesia.
2. GA can be used safely in the office setting.
3. GA has advantages for more complex liposuction procedures that include precise dosing of sedatives, controlled patient movement, and airway management.
4. Epidural and spinal anesthesia in the office setting are discouraged because of the possibility of vasodilatation, hypotension, and fluid overload.
5. Moderate sedation/analgesia augments the patient's comfort and is an effective adjunct to the anesthetic infiltrate solutions.

In 2002, 261 respondents to a survey sent to the membership of The American Society for Dermatologic Surgery reported no mortalities among 66,570 liposuction procedures performed in hospitals, ASCs and offices. The authors reported adverse events, which mirrored those in the ASAPS. They found that serious adverse events occurred more frequently with procedures performed in hospital and ASCs than those in offices. This finding may be due to the fact that in hospitals liposuction is performed on sicker patients or that the procedures are associated with removal of a larger amount of fat. Interestingly, 71% of the offices surveyed were nonaccredited. Further, the authors reported that morbidity correlated better with the area of the body suctioned (abdomen and buttocks as compared to extremities), than the facility in which the procedure took place.[85]

Aesthetics

Many facial aesthetic procedures such as blepharoplasty, rhinoplasty, and meloplasty are routinely performed in offices, usually under varying depths of MAC, but occasionally with GA. Facial plastic procedures that require use of a laser, or even routine electrocautery, pose a problem for the anesthesiologist. Supplemental nasal oxygen in patients receiving sedation is a fire hazard. Any supplemental oxygen must be turned off during periods of laser or electrocautery use about the face, and this requires vigilance by the anesthesiologist who must be in constant communication with the surgeon. Methods for delivering supplemental oxygen to a patient having a facial procedure include nasal cannula, an oxygen hood, or placement of oxygen tubing in an oral/nasal airway. The latter usually requires a deeper level of sedation. The avoidance of supplemental oxygen when medically appropriate is ideal.

Breast

Procedures such as breast biopsy or augmentation, implant exchange, and completion of transverse rectus abdominal muscle (TRAM) flap (i.e., nipple construction or revisions) are routinely performed in office settings. Breast augmentation entails separating the pectoralis muscles from the chest wall, which is painful and usually requires GA and can be accomplished by using either a laryngeal mask airway (LMA), or tracheal tube. The use of regional anesthesia with paravertebral nerve blocks has also been reported.[86] Breast surgery has a high incidence of PONV, thus it is likely that patients undergoing breast surgery will require antiemetic medication in addition to postoperative analgesics.[87]

Gastrointestinal Endoscopy

Procedures performed by gastroenterologists include esophageal, gastric, and duodenal endoscopies (EGD) and colonoscopies. This patient population tends to be older, with significant comorbid conditions. Upper GI procedures rarely require endotracheal intubation because, although many of these patients have gastroesophageal reflux, the stomach is emptied under direct visualization. The endoscopist requires patient participation to aid in insertion of the endoscope, which can usually be accomplished, with sedation using small doses of propofol with or without midazolam.

Colonoscopy is painful secondary to the insertion and manipulation of the endoscope, and may be associated with cardiovascular effects, including dysrhythmia, bradycardia, hypotension, hypertension, myocardial infarction, and death. The mechanism of these cardiovascular effects is not known, but there is evidence that they may be mediated by the autonomic nervous system when stimulated by anxiety or discomfort.[88] Adding an opioid to midazolam during colonoscopy has been shown to improve patient tolerance of the procedure and decrease pain without increasing the frequency of respiratory events.[89] Interestingly, anesthetic techniques consisting of midazolam,[90] remifentanil/propofol, and fentanyl/propofol/midazolam[91] potentiate the low-frequency components of heart rate variability which reflects sympathetic activation as seen on continuous electrocardiography, and may contribute to the number of cardiovascular events that occur during colonoscopy.

Recently the gastroenterology community has sought to be able to provide moderate or even deep sedation with propofol without the assistance of a trained anesthesiologist.[92] However, due to safety concerns, propofol may still only be given by an anesthesiologist as indicated in the product insert. In addition, the Institute for Safe Medical Practices has indicated that propofol may only be administered by individuals who are "trained in the administration of drugs that cause deep sedation and GA" as well as only providing the sedation (not also performing the procedure) and be proficient at tracheal intubation.[93] The AAAASF has likewise indicated that anesthesia professionals are best qualified to administer propofol sedation.

Dentistry/Oral and Maxillofacial Surgery (OMS)

Nitrous oxide (N_2O) has been used for most of the world's office-based dental anesthetics since 1884, when Horace Wells, himself a dentist, had N_2O administered for a wisdom-tooth extraction by a colleague. It was Harry Langa, another dentist, who pioneered the concept of using lower concentrations of N_2O in combination with local anesthetics. This idea of "relative analgesia" was the forbearer of "conscious sedation".[94]

The American Association of Oral and Maxillofacial Surgeons studied a prospective cohort study of patients who underwent OMS surgery between January and December 2001. Of the 34,191 patients included, 71.9% received deep sedation/GA, 15.5% conscious sedations, and 12.6% local anesthesia. The operating surgeon provided anesthesia services in 96% of cases, and anesthesia-specific hospitalization rate was 4 per 100,000, with no reported mortalities. The authors attributed this safety level to the use of pulse oximetry, blood pressure and ventilation monitoring, as well as administration of supplemental oxygen.[95] As anesthesiologists increase their presence in the dental/OMS arena, one can expect an increased utilization of nontraditional agents for procedures.

Orthopedics/Podiatry

The orthopedic office provides an excellent location for the anesthesiologist who practices regional anesthesia. While knee arthroscopies can be performed with intraarticular local anesthesia and MAC, a three-in-one block of the lumbar plexus with bupivacaine or ropivacaine, supplementing the intra-articular local anesthetic in an arthroscopically assisted anterior cruciate ligament (ACL) repair will provide long-acting postoperative analgesia. Interscalene and axillary regional anesthetics avoid airway manipulations in patients undergoing upper extremity procedures, while ankle blocks or blocks of the sciatic nerve in the popliteal fossa provide anesthesia for operations on the lower extremity. All of these blocks can be supplemented with short-acting anxiolytic agents.

Spinal anesthetics in the office-based setting must be of short duration, secondary to limited PACU space. Lidocaine, which provides reliable short-acting analgesia, may be associated with an increased risk of transient neurologic symptoms (TNS) in the ambulatory patient population,[96] whereas using procaine–fentanyl spinals are associated with nausea and vomiting as well as pruritus.[97] When the neuraxial anesthetic wears off, issues of postoperative pain management arise; therefore, the patient must be discharged with oral analgesics as well as contact information for both the surgeon and the anesthesiologist.

Gynecology/Genitourinary

Many procedures, such as dilation and curettage, vasectomy, and cystoscopy have been routinely performed in offices.[98] Recently there has been an increase in more invasive procedures such as mini-laparoscopies, ovum retrieval, prostate biopsies, and lithotripsy, necessitating an anesthesiologist's expertise.[99] A variety of anesthetic options are available for these procedures and the anesthetic choice depends on the surgeon, patient, and anesthesiologist's preferences.

Ophthalmology/Otolaryngology

Ophthalmologic procedures suitable for the office include cataract extractions, lacrimal duct probing, and ocular plastics. Topical anesthesia and, periorbital or retrobulbar blocks are frequently used to provide analgesia. Supplemental sedation may be required. Otolaryngology procedures include endoscopic sinus surgery, turbinate resection, septoplasty, and myringotomy.[100] Again, combinations of topical and regional nerve blocks with supplemental sedation are commonly employed, but occasionally GA is used.[101,102]

Pediatrics

Although no minimum age requirement for a child to undergo an office-based anesthetic has been established, patients greater than 6 months of age and ASA physical status 1 or 2 may be reasonable candidates.[14] Appropriate OBA pediatric cases are usually dental, and chloral hydrate with N_2O has historically been the anesthetic choice of many dentists. However, the use of these agents is associated with significant morbidity. Ross et al.[14] found that in children between the ages of 1 and 9 years, 70 mg/kg of chloral hydrate with 30% N_2O resulted in hypoventilation in 94% of patients, which increased to 97% of patients when the chloral hydrate was combined with 50% N_2O. This increase is significant in view of the findings of Coté et al. who reviewed 95 adverse sedation-related events in pediatric patients. In the 93% of these cases that resulted in permanent neurologic injury or death, the anesthetic was delivered by either an oral surgeon, periodontist, or CRNA supervised by a dentist.[38,39]

There are increasing numbers of ophthalmologic (examination under anesthesia, lacrimal duct probing), otolaryngology (myringotomy), cast/dressing changes, and minor plastic procedures being performed on children in offices. The American Academy of Pediatrics, Section on Anesthesiology has developed guidelines for the pediatric perioperative environment, which should be adhered to in the OBA setting (Table 31-11).[103]

TABLE 31-11. GUIDELINES FOR THE PEDIATRIC PERIOPERATIVE ANESTHESIA ENVIRONMENT INCLUDE THE FOLLOWING CONSIDERATIONS

- Patient care facility and medical staff policies
  - Designation of operative procedures
  - Categorization of pediatric patients undergoing anesthesia
  - Annual minimal case volume to maintain clinical competence
- Clinical privileges of anesthesiologists
  - Regular privileges
  - Special clinical privileges
  - Pain management
- Patient care units
  - Preoperative evaluation and preparation units
  - Operating room
  - Anesthesiologists
  - Other health-care providers involved in perioperative care
  - Clinical laboratory and radiologic services availability and capabilities
  - Pediatric anesthesia equipment and drugs including resuscitation cart
- PACU
  - Nursing staff
  - Anesthesiologist/physician staff
  - Pediatric anesthesia equipment and drugs
- Postoperative intensive care

ANESTHETIC TECHNIQUES

The ASA recommends that anesthetics be provided or supervised by a fully licensed anesthesiologist.[45] If an anesthesiologist is directing anesthesia care, he or she must be immediately available throughout the entire perioperative period. Regulations in several states have questioned the need for this level of anesthesia training in the delivery of OBA. Some states allow for an anesthetic to be performed by a nonphysician anesthesia provider supervised by a licensed physician. In this situation, the supervising physician must be qualified to perform a preanesthetic focused history and physical examination as well as be immediately available throughout the perioperative period. He or she must know how to handle anesthetic-related emergencies and complications. The supervising physician must be ACLS certified.

OBA requires many levels of anesthesia ranging from sedation through regional and GA.[104] Anesthesia is, however, a continuum and it is often impossible to predict how a patient will react. The ASA has developed definitions regarding depths of anesthesia (Table 31-12). Patients will routinely drift between the anesthetic depths, thus it is imperative that the anesthesia provider or supervisor be able to rescue a patient from a deeper level of anesthetic than was anticipated.

TABLE 31-12. DEFINITIONS OF LEVELS OF SEDATION/ANALGESIA BY THE ASA (FROM: ASA: OCT. 13, 1999 BY HOUSE OF DELEGATES)

1. Minimal sedation (anxiolysis)
   a. Drug-induced sedation
   b. Patient responds normally to verbal commands
   c. Cognitive and motor function may be impaired
   d. Ventilatory and cardiovascular functions maintained normally
2. Moderate sedation/analgesia (conscious sedation)
   a. Drug-induced sedation
   b. Patient responds purposefully to verbal commands either alone or with light tactile stimulation
   c. Patient maintains a patent airway and spontaneous ventilation
   d. Cardiovascular function maintained
3. Deep sedation/analgesia
   a. Drug-induced sedation
   b. Patient cannot be easily aroused but can respond purposefully to repeated or painful stimulation
   c. Ventilatory function may be impaired, requiring assistance in maintaining a patent airway, and spontaneous ventilation may be inadequate
   d. Cardiovascular function is usually maintained
4. General anesthesia
   a. Drug-induced loss of consciousness
   b. Patients are not aroused by painful stimulation
   c. Ventilatory function is often impaired; patient may require assistance in maintaining a patent airway
   d. Spontaneous ventilation may be impaired as well as neuromuscular functioning
   e. Positive pressure ventilation is often required
   f. Cardiovascular function may be impaired.

TABLE 31-13. CLOSED CLAIMS REPORTED DISTRIBUTION OF PATIENT INJURIES DURING MAC REPORTED IN CLOSED CLAIMS[106]

Injury	%
1. Death	34%
2. Brain damage	19%
3. Nerve damage	7%
4. Eye damage	12%
5. Myocardial infarction	4%
6. Stroke	4%
7. Burn	4%
8. Emotional distress	4%
9. Aspiration	4%

When formulating an anesthetic plan, one must consider that all agents and techniques used should be short acting, and patients should be ready for discharge home soon after the completion of the procedure. Furthermore, any agents used should have a high safety profile as well as be cost effective. In choosing sedation over GA, one must not be under the false impression that sedation is inherently safer than GA. In 1988, Cohen et al.[105] reviewed the data from 100,000 anesthetics. They found that the group with the greatest number of mortalities had undergone procedures with sedation, whereas sedation constituted only 2% of all cases. The complication rate related to MAC anesthetics is increasing, as its use expands.

The Closed Claims Project database reveals that in the 1970s, sedation (often referred to as MAC) cases accounted for 1.6% of the claims, in the 1980s, 1.9%, and by the 1990s, 6% of the cases were MAC. The injuries sustained in patients receiving MAC ranged from emotional distress to death (Table 31-13). The percentage of claims resulting from mortality was identical for both MAC and GA cases. In the 1990s, when injuries other than death occurred during MAC anesthetics, they were more likely to be permanent, whereas injuries occurring during GA were more frequently temporary.[106] MAC anesthetics also tend to lead to litigation. Suits were filed in 90% of the MAC claims; 65% were settled, 20% went to judgment, and 15% were discontinued. The range of payout was $2,000 to $6,300,000 with a median of $75,000.[106]

Anesthetic Agents

Intravenous sedation (propofol, barbiturates, midazolam, fentanyl) is the most commonly used anesthetic technique in the OBA setting. When selecting an anesthetic for an office-based procedure, one must consider factors such as duration of action, cost effectiveness, and safety profile. The drugs should have a short half-life, be inexpensive, and not be associated with undesirable side effects such as nausea and vomiting.

Because of its desirable pharmacokinetics and pharmacodynamics (see Chapter 7 Pharmacologic Principles), propofol, a di-isopropyl phenol molecule, has long been a mainstay of ambulatory anesthesia. It has a rapid onset (approximately 1 arm–brain circulation time), and because of rapid redistribution, has a short clinical duration of action (approximately 15 minutes). Because of its short, context-sensitive half-time, propofol's clinical effect is terminated relatively quickly even after relatively long infusion times (8 hours).[107] In addition to its hypnotic properties, it has an intrinsic antiemetic effect. Propofol may cause a burning sensation on injection or illicit an allergic reaction. It is also associated with bradycardia, respiratory depression, and supports microbial growth. Propofol can be used alone or in combination with other agents by intermittent boluses or continuous infusion.

Fentanyl has long been the gold standard for short-acting narcotics, but recently the use of remifentanil has also increased in popularity. Remifentanil, an ultra–short-acting opioid, when combined with propofol for conscious sedation, has been shown to provide discharge readiness within 15 minutes after colonoscopy. This timeframe is a marked reduction from 48 to 80 minutes reported after the traditional meperidine/midazolam technique.[108] Remifentanil is also an ideal drug for use during many office-based procedures such as facial cosmetic procedures, which can be quite painful while the local anesthetic is being injected after which it is relatively painless. An important caveat to the use of remifentanil is that it may cause nausea and vomiting as well as apnea. In addition, it often requires the use of an infusion pump.

Ketamine, a phencyclidine derivative, has experienced a resurgence in popularity over the past several years in the OBA practice. The use of ketamine–propofol sedation has been described as an excellent way to provide a relaxed surgical field in a quiet, immobile patient, often eliminating the need for supplemental oxygen.[109] Ketamine functions as both an anesthetic and an analgesic. It does not depress respiration, and will increase laryngeal reflexes, thus decreasing the risk of aspiration. Furthermore, it is not associated with nausea and vomiting. Ketamine can, however, cause an increase in secretions as well as cause hallucinations. The latter can be decreased or eliminated by adding propofol and midazolam.[110–113] Glycopyrrolate can be used as an antisialagogue. Another advantage of ketamine is that it is relatively inexpensive.

Clonidine has been found to be useful in an office. Since it is an alpha-2 agonist, clonidine will help control blood pressure throughout the perioperative period, thus potentially minimizing blood loss.[114,115] In addition, it may decrease the total propofol usage.[113] However, its use may precipitate hypotension and oversedation.

Any type of anesthesia from sedation through GA and regional anesthesia can be administered in an office setting safely but it is vital that the office be adequately equipped and staffed to rescue a patient from a deeper stage of anesthesia. Thus if MAC is planned, GA must be anticipated.

TIVA is a common choice for non-OR anesthetics. This technique usually consists of propofol as the hypnotic component used in conjunction with either fentanyl, remifentanil, or ketamine as the analgesic component. All of these drugs can be given by intermittent bolus or infusion. Mathews et al.[116] found that remifentanil 0.085 μ/kg/min can substitute for N_2O 66%. Advantages of TIVA over inhalation anesthesia include avoidance of the need for gas scavenging and a reduced incidence of PONV. Since the availability of the newer less soluble inhalation agents (e.g., desflurane and sevoflurane), many authors have compared recovery times from these agents with the recovery time after a total intravenous anesthetic using a propofol infusion.[117,118] Recently, Gupta conducted a meta-analysis of all such publications and reported an overall faster recovery from desflurane when compared to either isoflurane- or propofol-based anesthetics. Recovery was also found to be faster from sevoflurane when compared to isoflurane. However, there was more PONV as well as postdischarge nausea and vomiting in the isoflurane groups compared to the propofol ones; for these considerations isoflurane may not be the best choice of inhalation agent in non-OR locations. Overall, the inhalation agent groups required more antiemetic treatment than the propofol groups.[119]

Depth of anesthesia monitoring has been shown to decrease the time to extubation and discharge readiness.[120–122] A depth of anesthesia monitor has been described as useful in the office during MAC procedures, with a possible decrease in total propofol usage.[123] Whether this type of monitoring will prove to be cost effective in the office-based situation remains to be seen.

Post-anesthesia Care Unit (PACU)

Following an office-based procedure, the patient should be able to sit in a chair, or ambulate to an examination room to dress, almost immediately postoperatively free of pain and PONV. A formal PACU may not be present, and the patient may be required to recover in the surgical suite. Regardless of where the patient recovers, it is important to adhere to all the ASA standards for monitoring and documentation throughout the postoperative period. Staffing in the recovery area must be adequate, and the use of a pulse oximeter is imperative.[124] It is recommended that there be at least one ACLS/PALS certified member of the healthcare team present until the last patient has left the office.

Since PACU space in an office is often limited, the anesthesiologist may have multiple locations to attend in a single day, and patient satisfaction a priority, prevention of PONV and pain are paramount. The effect of these physiologic occurrences are not limited to the patient and anesthesiologist, but may also have a profound economic impact on an office surgical unit.[125] It is imperative that every anesthetic administered be designed to maximize postoperative patient alertness and mobility and minimize the risks of the need for a prolonged PACU stay. It is recommended that a post anesthesia discharge scoring system and the clinical discharge criteria used in a traditional ambulatory surgery center, also be utilized in the office-based setting.[126] Interestingly, there is a trend to discharge patients, particularly after colonoscopy, without escorts. This practice has been sanctioned in some states. In New York, regulations require that all patients undergoing a procedure with anesthesia be "discharged in the company of a responsible adult, unless exempted by a physician".[127] Specific data confirming the safety of this practice do not exist.

Local anesthesia alone, minimal to moderate and deep sedation supplemented by wound infiltration with local anesthetics, or peripheral nerve blocks, often forms the basis for a multimodal strategy for postoperative pain management. These effective pain-relief techniques not only decrease the anesthetic and analgesic requirements during surgery, but also reduce the need for opioid analgesics in the postoperative period, thus facilitating the recovery process.[128] Nonopioid analgesics (e.g., acetaminophen) and nonsteroidal anti-inflammatory drugs (e.g., ketorolac) are routinely used. Ketorolac decreases the incidence of PONV and patients tolerate oral fluids and meet discharge criteria earlier than those receiving opioids.[129] In an effort to minimize the potential for postoperative bleeding and risk of gastrointestinal complications, more specific COX-2 inhibitors are being increasingly used as nonopioid adjuvants for minimizing postoperative pain.[130]

An optimal antiemetic regimen for OBA has yet to be established, but since the etiology of PONV is multifactorial, combination therapies may be more beneficial in high-risk patients.[131] Many traditional first-line therapies are associated with sedation, drowsiness, and extrapyramidal side effects, and have been supplanted by 5-HT_3 antagonists such as ondansetron, dolasetron, and granisetron.[132] Dexamethasone has been shown to improve the efficacy of both 5-HT_3 antagonists[133] as well as dopamine antagonists.[134] Routine prophylaxis, though, has not been shown to offer any advantage over symptomatic treatment[135] and has associated costs. However, prophylaxis should be considered for all patients with a high risk of PONV. Such patients include young women having breast or gynecologic surgery, nonsmokers, or patients with a history of PONV. Ensuring adequate hydration (up to 20 mL/kg), to avoid orthostatic hypotension and thus prevent the release of emetogenic chemicals by decreased blood flow to the midbrain emetic centers is an intervention that may be useful in the prevention of PONV.[129]

REGULATIONS

9 Governmental oversight of office-based surgery varies among states; currently regulations exist in many states and others are following. Whereas accreditation is often a voluntary certification of an office, regulations are governmental mandates imposed by the local or state government. It is imperative that anesthesiologists embarking on an office-based practice familiarize themselves with any rules and regulations that govern practice in their particular state.

In 1994, California was the first state to adopt legislation regarding OBA, followed by New Jersey. A closer look at these two states provides an example of the varied requirements being enforced by states throughout the country. California's regulations pertain to patients undergoing a GA, and do not address procedures performed under local, peripheral nerve block or sedation/anxiolysis administered in doses that do not affect a patient's life-preserving reflexes.[136] The regulations deal with issues ranging from office policy and mandatory reporting of adverse outcomes, to surgeon and anesthesia-provider qualifications.[137] California Health and Safety Code 1248–1248.85 mandates that surgical procedures occur only in offices that have been accredited or have been certified to participate in the Medicare Program under Title XVIII (42 U.S.C. Sec. 1395 et seq.) with very few exceptions.[138] In addition, the office must have a written plan in place that deals with issues regarding emergency admissions. The surgeon must have admitting privileges at a local licensed or accredited acute-care hospital or have a written transfer agreement with a physician who have such privileges. The office must have an agreement with the hospital for the admission, in accordance with the hospital's system of quality assurance and peer review. California law also requires that offices have adequate patient monitoring throughout the perioperative period, and have a system in place for the storage and maintenance of patient records. An office that fails to comply with the regulations in place risks sanctions ranging from reprimand with or without monetary penalties through criminal prosecution.

New Jersey's administrative Code 13:35–4A.1–13:35–4A.18 develops criteria for patient selection. Only ASA physical status 1 and 2 patients may undergo general or regional anesthesia. ASA physical status 3 patients can undergo only conscious sedation. The provider of GA must be credentialed to do so by a hospital, and only an appropriately credentialed physician may supervise a CRNA. New Jersey law establishes guidelines regarding mandatory monitoring, emergency supplies that must be present, physician credentialing and peer review. In contrast to California, New Jersey's regulations pertain to all patients undergoing a surgical procedure regardless of the anesthetic depth. However, similar to California, violations may result in fines ranging from reprimand to license revocation and criminal prosecution.[139]

Although many states have regulations in place regarding office-based surgical procedures, some still have none. Consequently, any physician who holds a valid medical license in an unregulated state may perform any procedure, he/she so chooses, within an office. A surgeon may perform a procedure for which he or she may have had little to no training, and may sedate a patient without any training in anesthesia or airway management. In fact, there have been reported cases of patients undergoing a procedure without a preoperative evaluation, pertinent labs, informed consent, intraoperative or postoperative monitoring or operative report, and without regard for sterile technique.[11] It is therefore imperative that the anesthesiologist continues to maintain the role of a zealous patient advocate, and help to educate the surgeon as to what constitutes a safe anesthetizing location.

Business and Legal Aspects

10 It is in the anesthesia provider's best interest to seek legal counsel and create a valid business model before embarking on a career in OBA. This model must consider the overhead costs associated with staffing and running a safe surgical office as well as the potential and probable case load and patient insurance mix. An OBA division within a department may provide benefits to an academic practice in addition to the monetary ones. There may be an intangible benefit to the community it serves, as well as enhancing the anesthesia-training program.[4] However, it would become necessary to involve the American Board of Anesthesiology (ABA) as well as the American College of Graduate Education (ACGME) to ensure that any resident rotation outside the ACGME-approved hospital setting is acceptable.

Many OBA groups have formed either professional corporations or limited-liability companies. Although not eliminating the need for liability insurance, both of these arrangements serve to protect the private assets of the anesthesiologist in the case of a malpractice claim.[3] Legal counsel may also prove to be beneficial in creating business plans that follow all state and federal laws regarding billing/collection and antitrust.[140]

It is imperative to have an aboveboard and legal relationship with every office in which a patient is sedated. Billing strategies must be legal and ethical. In this complex environment of third-party payers, it is quite easy to make legal errors. Ignorance of the law offers no protection or excuse, and one should seek the advice of expert billing agencies even if one chooses not to outsource this responsibility. In calculating pricing, one must include all overhead charges such as drugs, equipment, time, and business expenses including malpractice insurance. A pricing structure with the surgeon must exist before embarking on a business relationship. One must outline specifically what will be provided by the office (e.g., intravenous equipment, antibiotics, monitors) and what the anesthesiologist will supply. These decisions take on further legal implications when the office is charging a facility fee.

Conclusions

OBA continues to rapidly expand and pose unique challenges to anesthesiologists, who must not only provide medical care in remote environments, but also have a good business sense and an understanding of operating-room management. It is imperative that, although regulations have not kept pace with the growth of OBA, anesthesia providers make it their responsibility to help ensure that every possible safety measure is afforded to their patients. Decisions about appropriate patient/procedure selection and equipping anesthetizing locations must be made in conjunction with the surgeon. All clinical decisions and anesthetic techniques must take into consideration the need for rapid turnover and limited PACU availability. Any depth of anesthesia from minimal sedation through regional and GA may be delivered as long as the proper safeguards are in place.

The many advantages afforded by office-based surgery are fuelling its evolution and as more complex procedures are conducted on patients with increasing numbers of comorbidities, the anesthesiologist's role as patient advocate is vital.

References

1. Twersky R. Office-based anesthesia: Challenges and success. Available at: http://www.csaol.cn/img/2007asa/RCL_src/204_Twersky.pdf
2. Maurer W. Office-based anesthesia: A critical look. Available at: http://cms.clevelandclinic.org/body.cfm?wyzpdqabs=o&id=227&action=detail&ref=640
3. Koch ME, Dayan S, Barinholtz D. Office-based anesthesia: An overview. *Anesthesiol Clin North America.* 2003;21:417.
4. Hausman LM, Levine AI, Rosenblatt MA. A survey evaluating the training of anesthesiology residents in office-based anesthesia. *J Clin Anesth.* 2006;18:499.
5. Snow J. *On Chloroform and Other Anesthetics.* London, England: John Churchill; 1858:314–315.
6. Tang J, White PF, Wender RH, et.al. Fast-track office-based anesthesia: A comparison of propofol versus desflurane with antiemetic prophylaxis in spontaneously breathing patents. *Anesth Analg.* 2001;92(1):95–99.
7. White PF, Song D. New criteria for fast-tracking after outpatient anesthesia: A comparison with the modified Aldrete's scoring system. *Anesth Analg.* 1999; 88(5):1069–1072.
8. Lazarov SJ. Office-based surgery and anesthesia: Where are we now? *World J Urol.* 1998;16:384.
9. Courtiss EH, Goldwyn RM, Joffe JM, et al. Anesthetic practices in ambulatory surgery. *Plast Reconstr Surg.* 1994;93:792.
10. Wetchler BV. Online shopping for ambulatory surgery: Let the buyer beware! *Ambul Surg.* 2000;8:111.
11. Quattrone MS. Is the physician office the wild, wild west of health care? *J Ambul Care Manage.* 2000;23:64.
12. Laurito CE. Report of educational meeting: The Society for Office-Based Anesthesia, Orlando, Florida, March 7, 1998. *J Clin Anesth.* 1998;10:445.
13. http://www.aha.org/research/reports/tw/twjuly2006migration.pdf
14. Ross AK, Eck JB. Office-based anesthesia for children. *Anesthesiol Clin North America.* 2002;20:195.
15. Schultz LS. Cost analysis of office surgery clinic with comparison to hospital outpatient facilities for laparoscopic procedures. *Int Surg.* 1994;79:273.
16. Bartamian M, Meyer DR. Site of service, anesthesia, and postoperative practice patterns for oculoplastic and orbital surgeries. *Ophthalmology.* 1996;103:1628.
17. Way JC, Culham BA. Establishment and cost analysis of an office surgical suite. *Can J Surg.* 1996;39:379.
18. Anello S. Office-based anesthesia: Advantages, disadvantages and the nurse's role. *Plast Surg Nurs.* 2002;22:107.
19. Iverson RE, Lynch DJ. ASPS Task Force on Patient Safety in Office-Based Surgery Facilities: Patient safety in office-based surgery facilities: II. Patient selection. *Plast Reconstr Surg.* 2002;110:1785.
20. Metzner J, Posner KL, Domino KB. The risk and safety of anesthesia at remote locations: The US closed claims analysis. *Curr Opin Anesthesiol.* 2009;22: 502–508.
21. American Association for the Accreditation of Ambulatory Surgical Facilities. State laws and regulations for office-based surgery. http://www.fsmb.org/pdf/grpol_regulation_office_based_surgery.pdf. Accessed December 5, 2007.
22. Arens J. Anesthesia for office-based surgery: Are we paying too high a price for access and convenience? *Mayo Clin Proc.* 2000;75:225.
23. Missant C, Velde M. Morbidity and mortality related to anesthesia outside the operating room. *Curr Opin Anaesthesiol.* 2004;17:323–327.
24. Vila H, Soto R, Cantor AB, et al. Comparative outcomes analysis of procedures performed in physician offices and ambulatory surgery centers. *Arch Surg.* 2003; 138;991.
25. Clayman MA, Caffee HH. Office surgery safety and the Florida moratoria. *Ann Plast Surg.* 2006;56:78.
26. Melloni C. Morbidity and mortality related to anesthesia outside the operating room. *Minerva Anestesiol.* 2005;71:325–334.
27. American Society of Anesthesiologists. *Directory of Members.* Park Ridge, IL: ASA, 2000;480.
28. Anesthesia Patient Safety Foundation. Office based anesthesia growth provokes safety fears. *APSF.* 2000;15:1.
29. Domino KB. Office-based anesthesia: Lessons learned from the closed-claims project. *ASA Newsl.* 2001;65:9.
30. Morello DC, Colon GA, Fredricks S, et al. Patient safety in accredited office surgical facilities. *Plast Reconstr Surg.* 1997;99:1496.
31. Hoefflin SM, Bornstein JB, Gordon M. General anesthesia in an office-based plastic surgical facility: A report on more than 23,000 consecutive office-based procedures under general anesthesia with no significant anesthetic complications. *Plast Reconstr Surg.* 2001;107:243.
32. Sullivan PK, Tattini CD. Office-based operatory experience: An overview of anesthetic technique, procedures and complications. *Med Health R I.* 2001;84:392.
33. Bitar G, Mullis W, Jacobs W, et al. Safety and efficacy of office-based surgery with monitored anesthesia care/sedation in 4778 consecutive plastic surgery procedures. *Plast Reconstr Surg.* 2003;111:150.
34. Rao RB, Ely SF, Hoffman RS. Deaths related to liposuction. *N Engl J Med.* 1999; 340:1471.
35. McDevitt NB. Deep vein thrombosis prophylaxis. *Plast Reconstr Surg.* 1999;104: 1923–1928.

36. American Society of Anesthesiologists Committee on Equipment and Facilities. Guidelines for determining anesthesia machine obsolescence. http://www.asahq.org/publicationsAndServices/machineobsolescense.pdf. Accessed December 5, 2007.
37. Robbertze R, Posner KL, Domino K. Closed claims review of anesthesia for procedures outside the operating room. *Curr Opin Anesthesiol.* 2006;19:436–442.
38. Coté CJ, Karl HW, Notteman DA, et al. Adverse sedation events in pediatrics: Analysis of medications used for sedation. *Pediatrics.* 2000;106:663.
39. Coté CJ, Notteman DA, Karl HW, et al. Adverse sedation events in pediatrics: A critical incident analysis of contributing factors. *Pediatrics.* 2000;105:8–15.
40. Iverson R. ASPS Task Force on Patient Safety in Office-Based Surgery Facilities: Patient safety in office-based surgery facilities: I. Procedures in the office-based surgery setting. *Plast Reconstr Surg.* 2002;110:1337.
41. Tunajek SK. Office based procedure standards. *AANA J.* 1999;67:115.
42. American Medical Association House of Delegates at the I-01 Meeting. Office-based surgery core principles. *American Society of Anesthesiologists Newsletter.* 2004;68:14.
43. Haeck PC, Swanson JA, Iverson RE, et.al. Evidence-based patient safety advisory: Patient selection and procedures in ambulatory surgery. *Plast Reconstr Surg.* 2009;124:6S–38S.
44. Meridy HW. Criteria for selection of ambulatory surgical patients and guidelines for anesthetic management: A retrospective of 1553 cases. *Anesth Analg.* 1982;61:921.
45. American Society of Anesthesiologists Committee on Ambulatory Surgical Care and the American Society of Anesthesiologists Task Force on Office-Based Anesthesia. *Office-based anesthesia: Considerations for anesthesiologists in setting up and maintaining a safe office anesthesia environment.* Park Ridge, IL, American Society of Anesthesiologists, 2000.
46. Haeck PC, Swanson JA, Iverson RE, et.al. Evidence-based patient safety advisory: Patient assessment and prevention of pulmonary side effects in surgery. Part 1-obstructive sleep apnea and obstructive lung disease. *Plast Reconstr Surg.* 2009;124S:45S–56S.
47. Benumof JL. Obstructive sleep apnea in the adult obese patient: Implications for airway management. *J Clin Anesth.* 2001;13:144.
48. Boushra NN. Anaesthetic management of patients with sleep apnea syndrome. *Can J Anaesth.* 1996;43:599.
49. Benumof JL. Policies and procedures needed for sleep apnea patients. *APSF Newsletter.* 2002;17:57.17.
50. Young T, Evans L, Finn L, et al. Estimation of the clinically diagnosed proportion of sleep apnea syndrome in middle-aged men and women. *Sleep.* 1997;20:705.
51. Lofsky A. Sleep apnea and narcotic postoperative pain medication: A morbidity and mortality risk. *APSF Newsletter.* 2002;17:24.
52. Samuels SI, Rabinov W. Difficulty reversing drug-induced coma in a patient with sleep apnea. *Anesth Analg.* 1986;65:1222.
53. Benumof JL. Creation of observational unit may decrease sleep apnea risk. *APSF Newsletter.* 2002;17:39.
54. Coldiron B, Shreve E, Balkrishnan R. Patient injuries from surgical procedures performed in medical offices: Three years of Florida data. *Dermatol Surg.* 2004;30:1435.
55. Claymen MA, Seagle BM. Office surgery safety: The myths and truths behind the Florida moratoria-Six years of Florida data. *Plast Reconstr Surg.* 2006;118:777.
56. Reinisch JF, Russo RF, Bresnick SD. Deep vein thrombosis and pulmonary embolism following face lift: A study of incidence and prophylaxis. *Plastic Surg Forum.* 1998;21:159.
57. Davison SP, Venturi ML, Attinger CE, et al. Prevention of venous thromboembolism in the plastic surgery patient. *Plast Reconstr Surg.* 2004;114;43e.
58. American Society of Anesthesiologists: Practice guidelines for the management of the difficult airway. *Anesthesiology.* 2003;98:1269.
59. American Society of Anesthesiologists: Standards for basic anesthetic monitoring. *ASA Directory of Members, 2001. (last amended October 21, 1998)* Park Ridge, IL: American Society of Anesthesiologists; 2001, 493.
60. American Society of Anesthesiologists: Standards for postanesthesia care. *American Society of Anesthesiologists: Standards for basic anesthetic monitoring. ASA Directory of Members, 2001 (last amended October 19 1994).* Park Ridge, IL: American Society of Anesthesiologists; 2001, 494.
61. Gurunluoglu R, Swanson JA, Haeck PC, et al. Evidence-based patient safety advisory: Malignant hyperthermia. *Plast Reconstr Surg.* 2009;124:68S–81S.
62. American Society of Anesthesiologists Task Force on Operating Room Fires. Practice advisory for the prevention and management of operating room fires. *Anesthesiology.* 2008;108:786–801.
63. Moss E. MD office regs stalled in New Jersey. *APSF Newsletter.* 1997;37.
64. Yates JA. American Society of Plastic Surgeons: Office-based surgery accreditation crosswalk. *Plastic Surg Nurs.* 2002;22:125.
65. Coldiron B. Office surgical incidents: 19 months of Florida data. *Dermatol Surg.* 2002;28:710.
66. Bing J, McAuliffe MS, Lupton JR. Regional anesthesia with monitored anesthesia care for dermatologic laser surgery. *Dermatol Clin.* 2002;20:123.
67. Morris KT, Pommier RF, Vetto JT. Office-based wire-guided open breast biopsy under local anesthesia is accurate and cost effective. *Am J Surg.* 2000;179:422.
68. Jones JS, Streem SB. Office-based cystoureteroscopy for assessment of the upper urinary tract. *J Endourol.* 2002;16:307.
69. Friedman O, Deutsch ES, Reilly JS, et al. The feasibility of office-based laser-assisted tympanic membrane fenestration with tympanostomy tube insertion: The DuPont Hospital experience. *Int J Pediatr Otorhinolaryngol.* 2002;62:31.
70. Jones JS, Oder M, Zippe CD. Saturation prostate biopsy with periprostatic block can be performed in the office. *J Urol.* 2002;168:2108.
71. Goldrath MH, Sherman AI. Office hysteroscopy and suction curettage: Can we eliminate the hospital diagnostic dilatation and curettage? *Am J Obstet Gynecol.* 1985;152:220.
72. Armstrong M. Office-based procedures in rhinosinusitis. *Otolaryngol Clin N Am.* 2005;38:1327–1338.
73. Siegel GJ, Seiberling KA, Aguado AS. Office CO2 laser turbinoplasty. *Ear Nose Throat J.* 2008;87:386–391.
74. Mingus ML, Bodian CA, Bradford CN, et al. Prolonged surgery increases the likelihood of admission of scheduled ambulatory surgery patients. *J Clin Anesth.* 1997;9:446.
75. Fortier J, Chung F, Su J. Unanticipated admission after ambulatory surgery—A prospective study. *Can J Anaesth.* 1997;45;612.
76. Gold BS, Kitz DS, Lecky JH, et al. Unanticipated admission to the hospital following ambulatory surgery. *JAMA.* 1989;262:3008.
77. American Society of Plastic Surgeons: 2007 quick facts: Cosmetic and reconstructive plastic surgery trends. http://www.plasticsurgery.org/media/statistics/loader.cfm?url=/commonspot/security/getfile.cfm&pageID=29285
78. American Society for Aesthetic and Plastic Surgery. Top 5 surgical and nonsurgical cosmetic procedures. http://www.surgery.org
79. Iverson RE, Lynch DJ. American Society of Plastic Surgeons Committee on Safety: Practice advisory on liposuction. *Plast Reconstr Surg.* 2004;113:1478.
80. Fodor PB, Watson JP. Wetting solutions in ultra-sound assisted lipoplasty: A review. *Clin Plast Surg.* 1999;26:289.
81. Klein JA. Tumescent technique for regional anesthesia permits lidocaine doses of 35 mg/kg. *J Dermatol Surg Oncol.* 1990;16:248.
82. Ostad A, Kageyama N, Moy RL. Tumescent anesthesia with lidocaine dose of 55 mg/kg is safe for liposuction. *Dermatol Surg.* 1996;22:921.
83. Martinez MA, Ballesteros S, Segura LJ, et.al. Reporting a fatality during tumescent liposuction. *Forensic Sci Int.* 2008;178:e11–e16.
84. Grazer FM, deJong RH. Fatal outcome from liposuction: Census survey of cosmetic surgeons. *Plast Reconstr Surg.* 2000;105:436.
85. Housman TS, Lawrence N, Mellen BG, et al. The safety of liposuction: Results of a national survey. *Dermatol Surg.* 2002;28:971.
86. Conveney E, Weltz CR, Greengrass R, et al. Use of paravertebral block anesthesia in the surgical management of breast cancer. Experience in 156 cases. *Ann Surg.* 1998;227:496.
87. Jaffe SM, Campbell P, Bellman M, et al. Postoperative nausea and vomiting in women following breast surgery: An audit. *Eur J Anaesthesiol.* 2000;17:261.
88. Vawter M, Vicaroi MD, Moorthy K, et al. Electrocardiographic monitoring during colonoscopy. *Am J Gastroenterol.* 1975;63:115.
89. Radaelli F, Meucci G, Terruzzi V, et al. Single bolus of midazolam versus bolus midazolam plus meperidine for colonoscopy: A prospective, randomized trial. *Gastrointest Endosc.* 2003;57:329.
90. Ristikankare M, Julkunen R, Laitinen T. Effect of conscious sedation on cardiac autonomic regulation during colonoscopy. *Scand J Gastroenterol.* 2000;9:990.
91. Petelenz M, Gonciarz M, Macfarlane P, et al. Sympathovagal balance fluctuates during colonoscopy. *Endosc.* 2004;36:508.
92. Chutkan J, Cohen M, Abedi M, et al. Training guideline for use of propofol in gastrointestinal endoscopy. *Gastrointest Endosc.* 2004;60:167.
93. Institute for Safe Medication Practices. Propofol sedation: Who should administer? http://www.ismp.org/Newsletters/acutecare/articles/20051103.asp. Accessed Nov 5, 2011.
94. Finder RL. The art and science of office-based anesthesia in dentistry: A 150-year history. *Int Anesthesiol Clin.* 2003;41:1.
95. Perrott DH, Yuen JP, Andresen RV, et al. Office-based ambulatory anesthesia: Outcomes of clinical practices of oral and maxillofacial surgeons. *J Oral Maxillofac Surg.* 2003;61:938.
96. Freedman JM, Li DK, Drasner K, et al. Transient neurologic symptoms after spinal anesthesia: An epidemiologic study of 1,873 patients. *Anesthesiology.* 1998;89:633.
97. Mulroy MF, Larkin KL, Siddiqui A. Intrathecal fentanyl-induced pruritus is more severe in combination with procaine than with lidocaine or bupivacaine. *Reg Anesth Pain Med.* 2001;26:252.
98. Sardo ADS, Bettocchi S, Spinelli M, et.al. Review of new office-based hysteroscopic procedures 2003–2009. *J Minim Invasive Gynecol.* 2010;17:436–448.
99. Wortman M. Instituting an office-based surgery program in the gynecologists office. *J Minim Invasive Gynecol.* 2010;17;673–683.
100. Jourdy DN, Kacker A. Regional anesthesia for office-based procedures in otorhinolaryngology. *Anesthesiol Clin.* 2010;28:457–468.
101. Woo P. Office-based laryngeal procedures. *Otolaryngol Clin N Am.* 2006;39:111–133.
102. Lan MC, Hsu YB, Chang SY, et al. Office-based treatment of vocal cord polyp with flexible laryngovideostroboscopic surgery. *J Otolaryngol Head Neck Surg.* 2010;39:90–95.
103. Hackel A, Badgwell JM, Binding RR, et al. Guidelines for the pediatric perioperative environment. American Academy of Pediatrics Section on Anesthesiology. *Pediatrics.* 1999;103:572.

104. Tang J, Chen L, White PF, et al. Use of propofol for office-based anesthesia: Effect of nitrous oxide on recovery. *J Clin Anesth.* 1999;11:226.
105. Cohen MM, Duncan PG, Tate RB. Does anesthesia contribute to operative mortality? *JAMA.* 1988;260:2859.
106. Domino KB. Trends in anesthesia litigation in the 1990's: Monitored anesthesia care claims. *ASA Newsletter.* 1997;61:17.
107. Hughes MA, Glass PS, Jacobs JR. Context sensitive half-time in multicompartment pharmacokinetic models for intravenous anesthetic drugs. *Anesthesiology.* 1992;76:334–341.
108. Rudner R, Jalowiecki P, Kawecki P, et al. Conscious analgesia/sedation with remifentanil and propofol versus total intravenous anesthesia with fentanyl, midazolam, and propofol for outpatient colonoscopy. *Gastrointest Endosc.* 2003; 57:657.
109. Friedberg BL. Facial laser resurfacing with the propofol-ketamine technique: Room air, spontaneous ventilation (RASV) anesthesia. *Dermatol Surg.* 1999; 25:569.
110. Friedberg BK. Propofol-ketamine technique: Dissociative anesthesia for office surgery (a five year review of 1,264 cases). *Aesthetic Plast Surg.* 1999;23:70.
111. Friedberg BL. Propofol-ketamine technique. *Aesthetic Plast Surg.* 1993;17:297.
112. Friedberg BL. Hypnotic doses of propofol block ketamine-induced hallucinations. *Plast Reconstr Surg.* 1993;91:196.
113. Friedberg BL, Sigl JC. Clonidine premedication decreases propofol consumption during bispectral index (BIS) monitored propofol-ketamine technique for office-based surgery. *Dermatol Surg.* 2000;26:848.
114. Man D. Premedication with oral clonidine for facial rhytidectomy. *Plast Reconstr Surg.* 1994;94:214.
115. Baker TM, Stuzin JM, Baker TJ, et al. What's new in aesthetic surgery? *Clin Plast Surg.* 1996;23:16.
116. Mathews DM, Gaba V, Zaku B, et al. Can remifentanil replace nitrous oxide during anesthesia for ambulatory orthopedic surgery with desflurane and fentanyl? *Anesth Analg.* 2008;106:101–108.
117. Nathan N, Peyclit A, Lahrimi A, et al. Comparison of sevoflurane and propofol for ambulatory anaesthesia in gynaecological surgery. *Can J Anaesth.* 1998;45:1148–1150.
118. Song D, Joshi GP, White PF. Fast-track eligibility after ambulatory anesthesia: A comparison of desflurane, sevoflurane and propofol. *Anesth Analg.* 1998;86: 267–273.
119. Gupta A, Stierer T, Zuckerman R, et al. Comparison of recovery profile after ambulatory anesthesia with propofol, isoflurane, sevoflurane and desflurane: A systematic review. *Anesth Analg.* 2004;98:632–641.
120. Drover DR, Lemmens JH, Pierce ET, et al. Patient state index: Titration of delivery and recovery from propofol, alfentanil, and nitrous oxide anesthesia. *Anesthesiology.* 2002;97:82.
121. Gan TJ, Glass PS, Windsor A, et al. Bispectral index monitoring allows faster emergence and improved recovery from propofol, alfentanil, and nitrous oxide anesthesia. *Anesthesiology.* 1997;87:805.
122. Song D, Joshi GP, White PF. Titration of volatile anesthetics using bispectral analysis index facilitates recovery after ambulatory anesthesia. *Anesthesiology.* 1997; 87:842.
123. Friedberg B, Sigl JC. Bispectral index (BIS) monitoring decreases propofol usage during propofol-ketamine office based anesthesia. *Anesth Analg.* 1999;88 (S54):54.
124. Singer R, Thomas PE. Pulse oximeter in the ambulatory aesthetic surgical facility. *Plast Reconstr Surg.* 1988;82:111.
125. Tang J, Chen X, White PF, et al. Antiemetic prophylaxis for office-based surgery-are the 5-HT3 receptor antagonists beneficial? *Anesthesiology.* 2003;98:293.
126. Chung FF, Chan VW, Ong D. A postanesthetic discharge scoring system for home readiness after ambulatory surgery. *J Clin Anesth.* 1995;7:500.
127. Title 10 NYCRR, Section 755.6.f; Volume D.
128. White PF. The role of non-opioid analgesic techniques in the management of pain after ambulatory surgery. *Anesth Analg.* 2002;94:577.
129. Ding Y, White PF. Comparative effects of ketorolac, dezocine and fentanyl as adjuvants during outpatient anesthesia. *Anesth Analg.* 1992;75:566.
130. Desjardins PJ, Shu VS, Recker DP, et al. A single preoperative oral dose of valdecoxib, a new cyclooxygenase-2 specific inhibitor, relieves post-oral surgery or bunionectomy pain. *Anesthesiology.* 2002;97:565.
131. Gan TJ, Meyer TA, Apfel CC, et al. Society for ambulatory anesthesia guidelines for the management of postoperative nausea and vomiting. *Anesth Analg.* 2007;105:1615–1628.
132. Kovac AL. Prevention and treatment of postoperative nausea and vomiting. *Drugs.* 2000;59:213.
133. Henzi I, Walder B, Tramer MR. Dexamethasone for prophylaxis of postoperative nausea and vomiting: A quantitative systematic review. *Anesth Analg.* 2000;90:186.
134. Eberhart LH, Morin AM, Georgieff M. Dexamethasone for prophylaxis of postoperative nausea and vomiting. A meta-analysis of randomized controlled studies. *Anaesthesist.* 2000;49:713.
135. Scuderi PE, James RL, Harris L, et al. Antiemetic prophylaxis does not improve outcomes after outpatient surgery when compared to symptomatic treatment. *Anesthesiology.* 1999;90:360.
136. California Codes, Business & Professions Code, Division 2. Healing Arts, Chapter 5. Medicine Article 11.5. Surgery in certain outpatient settings, § 2216. Restrictions on use of anesthesia. 2003.
137. California Codes Business & Professions Code, Division 2. Healing Arts. Chapter 5. Medicine: Article 11.5. *Surgery in certain outpatient settings.* § 2215–2240, 2003.
138. California Health and Safety Code, Division 2. Licensing Provisions, Chapter 1.3. Outpatient settings: §1248.1. Required Settings, 2003.
139. New Jersey Administrative Code: Title 13. Law and public safety: Chapter 35. Board of medical examiners: Subchapter 4A. Surgery, special procedures, and anesthesia services performed in an office setting. 2003.
140. Manchikanti L, McMahon EB. Physician refer thyself: Is stark II, Phase III the final voyage? *Pain Physician.* 2007;10:725–741.

CHAPTER

32 Nonoperating Room Anesthesia (NORA)

KAREN J. SOUTER • ANDREW J. PITTAWAY

Key Points

1. Nonoperating room (NOR) locations are remote from a hospital's main operating room sites.
2. A significant number of the procedures performed in NOR locations require anesthesia or sedation.
3. A three-step approach that considers the patient, the procedure, and the environment is useful in considering any nonoperating room anesthetic.
4. Patient considerations include whether the patient will tolerate sedation or require general anesthesia, the ASA classification, significant comorbidities, and the level of monitoring.
5. Procedural considerations are both general (e.g., duration, position, and level of discomfort) and specific to individual specialties.
6. The American Society of Anesthesiologists (ASA) has defined guidelines to be applied to the administration of anesthesia at nonoperating room locations.
7. Patients should receive the same standard of care at a NOR site as they do in the operating room.
8. The anesthetic and monitoring equipment used for NORA must meet the same standards as equipment provided in the operating room.
9. Following NORA, the patient should be transported to an appropriate postanesthesia care unit, accompanied and monitored by anesthesia-trained personnel.
10. Environmental considerations include hazards such as radiation and the side effects of intravenous contrast agents.

Multimedia

Anesthesia in Remote Locations

GENERAL PRINCIPLES

1 Nonoperating Room Anesthesia (NORA) refers to anesthesia that is provided at locations remote from the familiar territory of the traditional operating room. These locations include radiology departments, endoscopy suites, magnetic resonance imaging (MRI) scanners, or dental clinics. This chapter will consider these locations. Discussion of anesthesia for surgical procedures performed in stand-alone ambulatory centers, or offices, is addressed in Chapters 30 and 31. Anesthesia and analgesia provided for
2 labor and delivery is in Chapter 40. Nonoperating room (NOR) cases account for a significant proportion of the procedural work of hospitals. Increasingly, the patients and/or the proceduralists require or request anesthesia or sedation to facilitate these procedures.

THE THREE-STEP APPROACH TO NORA

3 Away from the operating room, the anesthesiologist may lack familiar equipment and staff experienced in the care of the anesthetized patient. NORA; therefore, presents unique challenges and a systematic approach using the simple three-step paradigm "the PATIENT, the PROCEDURE, and the ENVIRONMENT" is recommended (Fig. 32-1).

The Patient

Patients may require sedation or anesthesia to tolerate NOR procedures for a number of reasons (Table 32-1). Children are more likely to require sedation or anesthesia for diagnostic and therapeutic procedures. Patients who are too ill to tolerate a major surgical procedure, but who may be able to undergo a palliative, less-invasive procedure also represent a challenge for
4 the NOR anesthesiologist. All patients presenting for NORA require a thorough preanesthetic assessment and the development of a sound anesthetic plan with appropriate levels of monitoring.

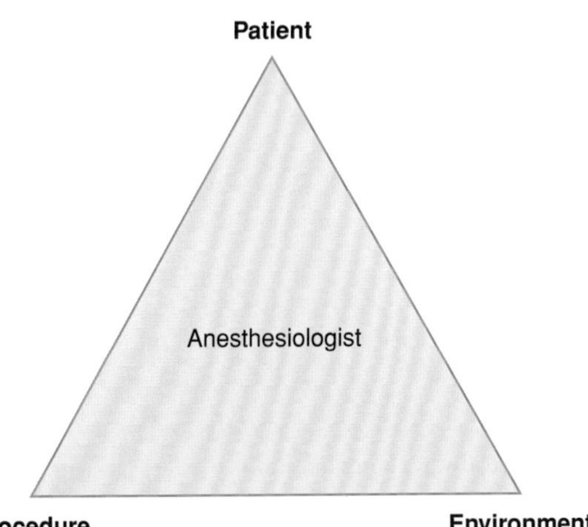

FIGURE 32-1. A three-step paradigm for NORA.

TABLE 32-1. PATIENT FACTORS REQUIRING SEDATION OR ANESTHESIA FOR NONOPERATING ROOM PROCEDURES

Claustrophobia, anxiety and panic disorders
Cerebral palsy, developmental delay and learning difficulties
Seizure disorders, movement disorders and muscular contractures
Pain, both related to the procedure and other causes
Acute trauma with unstable cardiovascular, respiratory, or neurologic function
Raised intracranial pressure
Significant comorbidity and patient frailty (ASA grades III, IV)
Child age, especially children <10 yrs

The Procedure

Common NOR procedures for which the patient may require anes-
5 thesia or sedation are listed (Table 32-2). The anesthesiologist must understand the nature of the procedure, including the position of the patient, how painful the procedure will be, and how long it will last. The optimum anesthesia plan provides safe patient care and facilitates the procedure. Discussions with the proceduralist must include contingencies for emergencies and adverse outcomes.

The Environment

6 The American Society of Anesthesiologists (ASA) has developed standards for NORA.[1] Prior to the anesthetic, the presence and proper functioning of all equipment needed for safe patient care must be established; this is described in Table 32-3. The location of immediately available resuscitation equipment should be noted and protocols developed with the local staff for dealing with emergencies, including cardiopulmonary resuscitation and the management of anaphylaxis.

Anesthesia Equipment and Monitors

In some NOR locations, anesthesia machines and monitors are provided; in others, it may be necessary to bring anesthesia equipment to the location. Small, portable anesthesia machines and monitors are available and recommended in these situations. Anesthesia machines and monitors that remain in a NOR location need to undergo routine maintenance. Infrequent use may result in degradation of equipment and the use of preprocedural checks, preferably with a standardized checklist, cannot be overemphasized before embarking on NORA. If more advanced monitors (e.g., an arterial line, central venous pressure, or intracranial pressure [ICP] monitoring) are required, these devices should be readily available. A preprepared cart containing essential equipment that is checked and restocked after each case is recommended.

PATIENT SAFETY IN NONOPERATING ROOM ANESTHESIA

Patient safety is of utmost importance in all types of anesthesia, not least NORA.

TABLE 32-2. COMMON NONOPERATING ROOM ANESTHESIA PROCEDURES

Radiologic imaging	Computed tomography (CT) Magnetic resonance imaging (MRI) Positron emission tomography (PET)
Diagnostic and therapeutic interventional radiology	Various vascular imaging, stenting, and embolization procedures Radiofrequency ablation (RFA) Transjugular intrahepatic portosystemic shunt (TIPS)
Diagnostic and therapeutic interventional neuroradiology	Occlusive ("closing") procedures • Embolization of cerebral aneurysm/AVM/vascular tumors Opening procedures • Angioplasty/stenting/thrombolysis in stroke cerebral atherosclerosis or cerebral vasospasm
Radiotherapy	Radiation therapy Intraoperative radiotherapy
Diagnostic and therapeutic interventional cardiology	
Cardiac catheterization laboratory	Diagnostic cardiac catheterization Percutaneous coronary interventions (PCI) Interventional techniques for management of structural heart disease (Transcatheter aortic valve implantation [TAVI]) Placement of left ventricular cardiac assist devices for hemodynamic support
Electrophysiology laboratory (EPL)	Electrophysiology studies and radiofrequency ablation Implantation of biventricular pacing systems and cardioverter defibrillators
Other Procedures	Cardioversion and Transesophageal echocardiography
Diagnostic and therapeutic interventional gastroenterology	Upper gastroenterology endoscopy Esophageal dilatation or stenting Percutaneous endoscopic gastrostomy tube placement Endoscopic retrograde cholangiopancreatography (ERCP) Colonoscopy Liver biopsy
Psychiatry	Electroconvulsive therapy (ECT)
Dentistry	Dental extractions Restorative dentistry

TABLE 32-3. ASA STANDARDS FOR NONOPERATING ROOM ANESTHETIZING LOCATIONS[1]

1. Oxygen-reliable source and full backup E-cylinder
2. Suction-adequate and reliable
3. Scavenging system if inhalational agents are administered
4. Anesthetic equipment
   - Backup self-inflating bag capable of delivering at least 90% oxygen by positive-pressure ventilation
   - Adequate anesthetic drugs and supplies
   - Anesthesia machine with equivalent function to those in the operating rooms and maintained to the same standards
   - Adequate monitoring equipment to allow adherence to the ASA standards for basic monitoring[4]
5. Electrical outlets
   - Sufficient for anesthesia machine and monitors
   - Isolated electrical power or ground fault circuit interrupters if "wet location"
6. Adequate illumination of patient, anesthesia machine, and monitoring equipment

Battery-operated backup light source

7. Sufficient space for:
   - Personnel and equipment
   - Easy and expeditious access to patient, anesthesia machine, and monitoring equipment
8. Resuscitation equipment immediately available
   - Defibrillator/emergency drugs/cardiopulmonary resuscitation equipment
9. Adequately trained staff to support the anesthesiologist and a reliable means of two-way communication
10. All building and safety codes and facility standards should be observed
11. Postanesthesia care facilities
    - Adequately trained staff to provide postanesthesia care
    - Appropriate equipment to allow safe transport to main postanesthesia care unit

Adverse Events

Significant adverse events occur infrequently in NOR locations, although the large multicenter studies needed to determine their true incidence are lacking.[2] The comparative safety of sedation administered by anesthesiology versus nonanesthesiology trained providers is not known.[2] Adverse events occurring during NORA have been investigated using the ASA closed claims database.[3] In this analysis, NORA was associated with a higher number of deaths compared to anesthesia conducted in the operating room and 50% of these were associated with monitored anesthesia care (MAC). Respiratory depression secondary to over-sedation was the most common type of adverse event in the closed claims study.[3] This is consistent with the findings from other studies where the majority of adverse events related to sedation in NORA are due to the airway and respiratory insufficiencies.[2] Capnography provides an earlier monitor of impending respiratory depression during sedation and is suggested as an important addition to pulse oximetry.[4,5,6]

Preprocedural Checklists

The use of checklists and pre- and postprocedural team briefings has been broadly embraced in operating room practice and emerging evidence points toward improved patient outcomes when checklists are employed.[7] Similar systems should be adopted in NOR sites and recently a checklist has been proposed for use in interventional radiology suites.[8]

Standards of Care for Nonoperating Room Anesthesia

7 The ASA has published a number of guidelines and standards of care for preanesthesia[9] and postanesthesia care,[10] basic monitoring stan-
8 dards,[4] and MAC.[11] These standards apply to patients being cared for in all NOR sites in the same way as they do in the operating rooms.

At the conclusion of the NOR procedure, the patient should be transported to a recovery area by a member of the anesthesia team who must provide a full verbal report to the recovery nursing staff.[10] The recovery area should be equipped to the same
9 standards as for postoperative patients.

Patient Transfer

Sick, unstable patients may be transferred back and forth between the intensive care unit, the operating rooms and NOR locations for imaging or diagnostic procedures. During transport the patient should be accompanied by a member of the anesthesia team to evaluate, monitor, and support the patient's medical condition. These patients are often mechanically ventilated and receiving a number of drug infusions for both sedation and hemodynamic support. Portable ventilators are useful for transport; these are often oxygen powered, and adequate supplies of oxygen must be available for the transfer. A manual self-inflating bag is essential in the event of ventilator failure. Infusion pumps and portable monitors should have adequate battery power for transit. The anesthesiologist should carry spare anesthetic and emergency drugs, equipment for intubation or reintubation, portable suction, and if the patient's condition requires, a portable defibrillator. It is vital to notify the destination area that the patient is in transit; so appropriate preparations to receive the patient can be made in advance. It is also useful to send personnel ahead to secure the elevators to prevent delays during transfer.

SEDATION AND ANESTHESIA

Definition of Sedation and Anesthesia

Many NOR procedures are performed under "sedation" or "MAC". A consistent definition of these terms is essential for clear communications between the various stakeholders involved in provision of NORA. On January 14, 2011, the Centers for Medicare and Medicaid Services (CMS) issued a revision to Interpretive Guideline (IG) for Hospitals No. 482.52 concerning anesthesia services.[12] This revised guideline places the responsibility and oversight for all anesthesia services under the direction of one suitably qualified individual, the "director of anesthesia services." IG 482.52 defines anesthesia as *"the administration of a medication to produce a blunting or loss of, pain perception (analgesia); voluntary and involuntary movements; autonomic function; and memory and/or consciousness."*

The Continuum of Anesthesia

Anesthesia exists along a continuum and the transition from minimal sedation to general anesthesia is not clear-cut[6,11] (Table 32-4). As sedation deepens, it is important to recognize the progressive blunting and loss of airway reflexes and patency, together with depression of spontaneous ventilation and cardiovascular function. The individual responsiveness of patients to different sedative agents varies, as do the levels of stimulation during the course of a procedure. Consequently, during the course of a NOR procedure under sedation, the patient may drift to a deeper level than the one intended, including transitioning into general anesthesia with

TABLE 32-4. DEFINITION OF GENERAL ANESTHESIA AND LEVELS OF SEDATION/ANALGESIA[6]

	Minimal Sedation (*Anxiolysis*)	Moderate Sedation/ Analgesia (*Conscious Sedation*)	Deep Sedation/Analgesia	General Anesthesia
Responsiveness	Normal response to verbal stimulation	Purposeful response to verbal or tactile stimulation	Purposeful response after repeated or painful stimulation	Unarousable, even with painful stimulus
Airway	Unaffected	No intervention required	Intervention may be required	Intervention often required
Spontaneous ventilation	Unaffected	Adequate	May be inadequate	Frequently inadequate
Cardiovascular function	Unaffected	Usually maintained	Usually maintained	May be impaired

loss of the airway. In any circumstances where a particular level of sedation is being provided, services must be immediately available to rescue a patient from a deeper than intended level of sedation or general anesthesia.[6,11,12]

ENVIRONMENTAL CONSIDERATIONS FOR NONOPERATING ROOM ANESTHESIA

X-rays and Fluoroscopy

When electrons are accelerated by means of a high voltage to a high velocity in a vacuum tube, a current is created that collides with a metal target producing X-rays. In medical X-ray tubes, the target is usually tungsten or a more crack-resistant alloy of rhenium (5%) and tungsten (95%). X-ray production is determined by, and directly proportional to, the tube current and the voltage. Fluoroscopy is a technique used to obtain real-time moving images of the internal structures. The patient is positioned between the X-ray source and a fluorescent screen; by coupling the fluoroscope to an X-ray image intensifier and a video camera, the images can be recorded and played on a monitor. Fluoroscopy is widely used in many NOR locations including interventional radiology, cardiac catheterization, and electrophysiologic procedures and in the gastroenterology suite. Large, C-shaped, mobile fluoroscopy devices (C-arms) are used to provide images in multiple dimensions. The C-arm moves back and forth around the patient during the procedure, taking up large amounts of space, limiting access to the patient and serving as a means of dislodging intravenous lines and endotracheal tubes (Fig. 32-2).

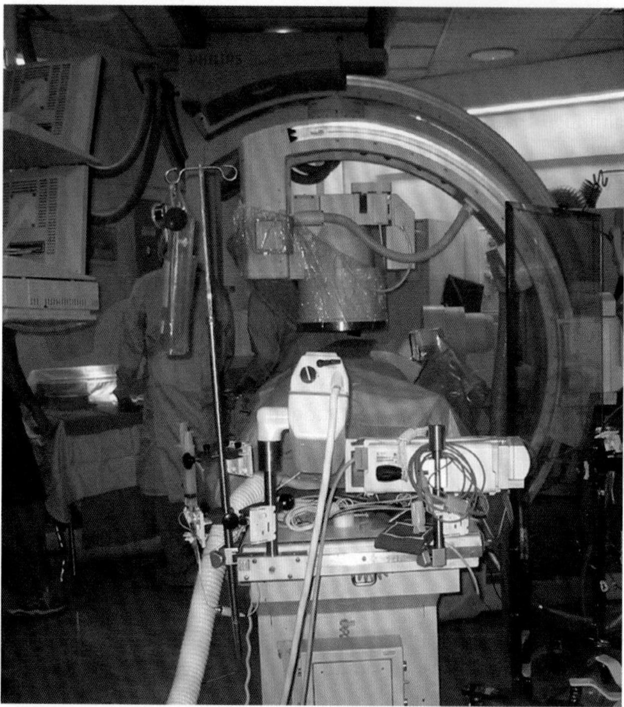

FIGURE 32-2. A radiology suite showing a C-arm and the high density of equipment that may separate the anesthesiologist from the patient.

Hazards of Ionizing Radiation

The use of fluoroscopy for both diagnostic and interventional procedures continues to increase and with it the risks exposure of patients and staff to the effects of ionizing radiation. Radiation exposure for patients varies depending on the type of procedure as well as patient and operator-related factors.[13,14] Occupational exposure for staff including anesthesiologists working in radiology suites is an important consideration. The Cardiovascular and Interventional Society of Europe (CIRSE) Standards of Practice Committee and the Society of Interventional Radiology (SIR) Safety and Health Committee have recently published guidelines on occupational protection from radiation.[15] A number of terms are used to define exposure to radiation; these are summarized in Table 32-5. Exposure from fluoroscopy is between 100 and 1,000 greater than from simple X-rays. For example, exposure from a simple chest X-ray is 0.02 mSv while pulmonary angiography produces 20 to 40 mSv.[16]

The effects of ionizing radiation on biologic tissues are classified as deterministic (dose related causing cell death and tissue damage) and stochastic (development of cancer from direct DNA ionization or the creation of hydroxyl radicals from X-ray

TABLE 32-5. COMMON TERMS USED IN RADIATION EXPOSURE[14]

Term	Units	Definition	Notes
Exposure	Roentgen (R)	Quantity of X-radiation or gamma radiation required to produce an amount of ionization	Measurements may be in exposure rate, i.e., amount of exposure per unit time e.g., fluoroscopy is measured in R/min
Absorbed dose	Rad (radiation absorbed dose) or Gray	Amount of ionizing radiation absorbed by the body	Depends on exposure to X-ray beam and the tissue type
Dose equivalent	Sievert (Sv)	Absorbed dose multiplied by a radiation quality factor specific for the type of radiation	Measures the "harmfulness" of any radiation-absorbed dose
Effective dose	Sievert (Sv)	Dose equivalent to the entire body caused by irradiating only a localized area. Calculated by multiplying the dose equivalent by a weighting factor specific for the irradiated organ	Takes into account the differing radiosensitivity of different organs Estimate of cancer risk

interactions with water molecules). Protective measures to reduce patient exposure to radiation should always be taken. 10 Staff, including the anesthesiologists must be aware of the hazards of occupational exposure to ionizing radiation.[15] Exposure to ionizing radiation may come from direct exposure and scatter. Patients are subjected to direct exposure where the beam enters the skin. Staff working in fluoroscopy suites are more at risk from scattered radiation, and as a general rule the exposure to staff is 1/1,000th the entrance skin exposure at 1 m from the fluoroscopy tube. Staff exposure to radiation can be minimized by[14]:

1. *Limiting the time of exposure to radiation.*
2. *Increasing the distance from the source of radiation.* (Dose rates increase or decrease according to the inverse square of the distance from the source.)
3. *Using protective shielding* (lead-lined garments or fixed and movable shields).
   Lead aprons, thyroid shields, and leaded eyeglasses are bulky and significantly increase staff fatigue. Recent studies have demonstrated that anesthesiologists are at equal risk of developing cataracts as neuroradiologists, and that the radiation may even be directed away from the neuroradiologists and toward the anesthesiologist.[17] Anesthesiologists must use appropriate leaded eye protection to minimize this risk. Anesthesiology staff should use movable or fixed lead-lined glass shields so that they can gain easy access to their patients while at the same time protect themselves from radiation.
4. *Using dosimeters.*
   National organizations set standards that limit the exposure of personnel to radiation doses, all personnel working in sites where there may be exposure to radiation should wear dosimeters to monitor their exposure. The International Commission on Radiological Protection (ICRP) recommends that staff must wear two dosimeters, one under the apron and one at collar level above the lead apron.[18] In the United States, the National Council on Radiation Protection and Measurements (NCRP) recommends an occupational limit of 50 mSv in any 1 year and a lifetime limit of 10 mSv multiplied by the individual's age in years.[19] Anesthesiologists who are involved in NOR cases that involve exposure to ionizing radiation must wear dosimeters and be included in the institution's radiation safety section or medical physics service regular monitoring to ensure that dose limits are not exceeded.[15]

Intravenous Contrast Agents

Intravenous contrast agents are commonly used in radiologic and MRI to enhance vascular imaging.[20] Radiologic contrast media are iodinated compounds classified according to their osmolarity (high, low, or iso-osmolar) and their ionicity (ionic or nonionic). Nonionic contrast agents cause less discomfort on injection and have a lower incidence of adverse reactions. MRI contrast agents are also divided into ionic and nonionic compounds. They are chelated metal complexes containing gadolinium, iron, or manganese.

Adverse reactions to contrast agents may be divided into renal adverse reactions and hypersensitivity reactions.

Renal Adverse Reactions

Contrast agents are eliminated via the kidneys, and contrast-induced nephropathy (CIN) occurs with an incidence of 7% to 15%[21]; intra-arterial injection is associated with a higher incidence of CIN than intravenous route.[20] CIN is defined as an increase in serum creatinine of 0.5 mg/dL or a 25% increase from the baseline within the first 24 hours, peaking at 5 days. It is the third leading cause of hospital-acquired acute renal failure.[22] Risk factors for CIN include history of renal disease, prior renal surgery, proteinuria, diabetes mellitus, hypertension, gout, and use of nephrotoxic drugs.[20] In the setting of CIN, metformin can cause lactic acidosis and should be discontinued prior to the patient receiving intravenous contrast agents. Iso-osmolar agents have the lowest risk of CIN and iodixanol has the lowest incidence of CIN in patients with renal impairment.[23] Preventative measures to avoid CIN include adequate hydration, maintaining a good urine output, and using sodium bicarbonate infusions to improve elimination of the contrast agent. The efficacy of N-acetylcysteine and other agents such as fenoldopam, dopamine, calcium-channel blockers, atrial natriuretic peptide, and L-arginine in mitigating CIN has not been proven.[21]

Hypersensitivity Reactions

Hypersensitivity reactions to contrast media are divided into immediate (<1 hour) and nonimmediate (>1 hour) reactions.[24] Mild immediate reactions occur in about 0.5% to 3% and severe reactions occur in 0.01% to 0.04%. Fatal hypersensitivity reactions may occur in about 1 per 100,000 contrast administrations.[24] The frequency of nonimmediate reactions is much more variable (0.5% to 23%) related partly to difficulty in determining whether symptoms relate to contrast agents or not.[24] The clinical manifestations of various hypersensitivity reactions to contrast media are outlined in Table 32-6.[25] Although widely used, the effectiveness of corticosteroids and antihistamines in preventing hypersensitivity reactions to contrast agents in unselected patients is doubtful.[26] Treatment of severe hypersensitivity reactions includes discontinuing the causative agent and supportive therapy; oxygen, airway securement, cardiovascular support with fluids, vasopressors, and inotropes, and if required, bronchodilators. Reactions to gadolinium-based contrast agents used for MRI are less

TABLE 32-6. CLINICAL MANIFESTATIONS OF IMMEDIATE AND NONIMMEDIATE HYPERSENSITIVITY REACTIONS TO RADIOCONTRAST AGENTS (MOST FREQUENT ARE UNDERLINED)[25]

Immediate Reactions	Nonimmediate Reactions
<u>Pruritus</u>	<u>Pruritus</u>
<u>Urticaria</u>	<u>Exanthema (mostly macular or maculopapular drug eruption)</u>
Angioedema/facial edema	Urticaria, angioedema
Abdominal pain, nausea, diarrhea	Erythema multiforme minor
Rhinitis (sneezing, rhinorrhea)	Fixed drug eruption
Hoarseness, cough	Stevens–Johnson syndrome
Dyspnea (bronchospasm, laryngeal edema)	Toxic epidermal necrolysis
Respiratory arrest	Graft-versus-host reaction
Hypotension, cardiovascular shock	Drug-related eosinophilia with systemic symptoms (DRESS)
Cardiac arrest	Symmetrical drug-related intertriginous and flexural exanthema (SDRIFE)
	Vasculitis

frequent than to iodinated contrast agents with hypersensitivity to gadolinium-containing agents occurring in 5.9 per 10,000 injections. The rate is higher (13 per 10,000) in patients undergoing abdominal MRI examinations. Severe reactions occur 1:10,000 to 1:40,000 and the mortality rate is 1 in a million injections.[27] Gadolinium-containing compounds have been associated with nephrogenic systemic fibrosis (NSF) in patients with renal insufficiency.[28]

SPECIFIC NONOPERATING ROOM PROCEDURES

Diagnostic and Interventional Radiology

Angiography

Angiography causes minimal discomfort and may be performed under local anesthesia with or without light sedation. Patients are required to remain completely motionless during these procedures, which may be lengthy, particularly spinal angiography. Neurologic disorders such as recent subarachnoid hemorrhage, stroke, and depressed level of consciousness or raised ICP may necessitate anesthesia with formal airway protection. Angiography is usually performed via the femoral artery; the femoral vein may also be accessed when imaging arteriovenous malformations (AVMs) or dural venous abnormalities. Liberal use of local anesthetic at the puncture site precludes the need for intravenous analgesia. The injection of contrast media into the cerebral arteries may cause discomfort, burning, or pruritus around the face and eyes. Hypotension and bradycardia may also occur. During angiography and other interventional radiologic procedures, the patient is placed on a moving gantry and the radiologist positions the patient to track catheters as they pass from the groin into the vessels of interest. It is vital to have extensions on all anesthesia breathing circuits, infusion lines, and monitors to prevent these from being accidentally dislodged as the radiologist swings the X-ray table back and forth. Care should be taken with positioning of radiopaque pieces of equipment. The electrocardiogram electrodes and metallic coils in the cuffs of endotracheal tubes may cause interesting and annoying artifacts if they lie over the area being imaged.

Interventional Neuroradiology

Interventional neuroradiology is an emerging specialty viewed as a hybrid of traditional neurosurgery and neuroradiology and recently defined as the *"treatment by endovascular access for the purpose of delivering therapeutic drugs and devices"*.[29] A variety of neurosurgical conditions especially neurovascular diseases are effectively managed by interventional neuroradiology (Table 32-2).

Cerebral aneurysms and AVMs are particularly amenable to occlusive endovascular treatments. A commonly employed technique is to insert detachable platinum coils into the abnormal vessel(s). Other occlusive agents include cyanoacrylates, "Onyx liquid embolic system" (Microtherapeutics Inc., USA) a biocompatible liquid embolic agent, and polyvinyl alcohol particles. These particles may also be used to produce temporary occlusion of blood vessels for preoperative embolization of vascular tumors such as meningiomas. A large multicenter study, the International Subarachnoid Aneurysm Trial (ISAT), recently reported a better outcome in patients with World Federation of Neurosurgical Societies (WFNS) grades 1 and 2 (good grades) presenting with anterior circulation aneurysms undergoing interventional neuroradiology compared to surgical clipping[30–32] In poor WFNS grade cerebral aneurysms and elderly patients, the superiority of one treatment or the other has not been clearly established for these patients.[33,34] Interventional neuroradiology is the standard treatment for posterior circulation aneurysms especially basilar artery tip aneurysms.

Procedural and Anesthetic Technique Considerations in Interventional Neuroradiology

For most interventional neuroradiologic procedures, arterial access is gained using a 6 or 7 French gauge sheath via the femoral or, rarely, the carotid or axillary artery. The umbilical vessels are an alternative route in neonates. Anticoagulation is required during and up to 24 hours after interventional radiologic procedures to prevent thromboembolism. Heparin, between 3,000 and 5,000 U (70 IU/kg) followed by an infusion is used to keep the activated clotting time (ACT) between 1.5 and 2.5 times the patient's baseline.[35] General anesthesia and conscious sedation are both suitable techniques for interventional neuroradiology depending on the complexity of the procedure, the need for blood pressure manipulation, and the need for intraprocedural assessment of neurologic function.[29,33] General anesthesia is usually conducted with endotracheal intubation and intermittent positive-pressure ventilation, although the laryngeal mask airway (LMA) is a suitable alternative in selected cases.[36] Sedation techniques vary; propofol infusions are widely used, as are combinations of a benzodiazepine (usually midazolam) and opioid (usually fentanyl). More recently, dexmedetomidine has been evaluated as a sedative agent that does not cause significant respiratory depression in patients requiring neurologic testing.[37] Dexmedetomidine has many advantages as a sedative agent; however, one study demonstrated impairment of cognitive testing in patients undergoing endovascular embolization of cerebral AVMs with dexmedetomidine as the sedative agent.[38] The anesthesiologist may facilitate the neuroradiologist in a number of ways by manipulating systemic blood pressure and controlling end-tidal carbon dioxide tension. Controlled hypotension is often requested to facilitate embolization of AVMs; beta-blockers and hydralazine are commonly used. Moderate hypertension may help reduce cerebral ischemia by maintaining cerebral perfusion; in this case, phenylephrine is the agent of choice. Certain procedures require patients to be awake for part of the procedure. The Wada test is used to determine the dominant side for cognitive functions such as speech and memory by injecting sodium amobarbital or methohexital into the carotid artery. This procedure may be used prior to surgery for nonlife-threatening conditions such as epilepsy. The superselective anesthesia functional examination (SAFE), is an extension of the Wada test[39] performed prior to therapeutic embolization to ensure that the catheter tip has not been placed in a vessel that supplies an eloquent area of the brain or spinal cord.

Major complications of interventional neuroradiology are hemorrhagic, such as aneurysm rupture, intracranial vessel injury or dissection; occlusive, such as displacement or fragmentation of embolic materials or vasospasm; or non-CNS complications, such as contrast hypersensitivity, anaphylaxis, CIN, and hemorrhage at the peripheral vessel puncture site causing groin or retroperitoneal hematoma.[29]

Computed Tomography

Computed tomography (CT) scanners obtain a cross-sectional image in a few seconds, and spiral scanners can image a slice of the body in <1 second, minimizing problems with motion artifacts. The procedure is painless and most adults do not require sedation or anesthesia. There is an absolute requirement for the patient to remain motionless while the study is being performed and children or adults with psychological or neurologic disorders preventing immobility may require sedation or anesthesia (Table 32-1). Contrast agents for CT imaging may be administered orally and the anesthesiologist needs to be aware of the possibility of a full stomach. CT scanning may be employed to facilitate invasive procedures such as abscess localization and drainage, ablation of bony metastases, and radiofrequency ablation (RFA) of malignancies. Patients with acute thoracic, abdominal, and cerebral trauma often require urgent imaging to facilitate diagnosis. These patients may develop hemorrhagic shock, raised ICP, depression of consciousness, and cardiac arrest in the CT scanner and must be adequately resuscitated and stabilized before transportation to the radiology department.

Radiofrequency Ablation

Percutaneous RFA is carried out in the radiology suite for treatment of primary and metastatic tumors in the liver, lung, adrenal gland, breast, thyroid, prostate, kidney, and spleen. A high-frequency alternating current is used to generate a localized heat source directly into the tumor causing coagulative necrosis and tumor cell death while avoiding the surrounding tissues. The majority of these procedures are tolerated without sedation. If an anesthesiologist does become involved in the care of these patients, careful evaluation is required; patients may be in the later stages of their disease, have often failed surgical treatment, and may well have undergone extensive radiation therapy and/or chemotherapy. Recently, high frequency jet ventilation (HFJV) has been used for patients undergoing anesthesia for RFA of liver tumors.[40] Positioning of the probe is critical and excursions of the diaphragm in ventilated or spontaneously ventilating patients may cause excessive movement; HFJV minimizes liver motion during these procedures.

Transjugular Intrahepatic Portosystemic Shunt

The transjugular intrahepatic portosystemic shunt (TIPS) is created via a catheter inserted in the internal jugular vein and directed into the liver. It connects the right or left portal vein through the liver parenchyma to one of the three hepatic veins.[41] The TIPS functions to decompress the portal circulation in patients with portal hypertension and is often performed in patients who have failed to respond to medical therapy.[42] The TIPS has been found to be effective in the secondary prophylaxis of bleeding varices and control of refractory cirrhotic ascites.[43] It may also be used as a bridge to transplant in patients with poor liver function. The procedure causes minimal stimulation, lasts between 2 and 3 hours, and may be performed under sedation or general anesthesia.[44] Patients presenting for a TIPS procedure, in general, have significant hepatic dysfunction, and require careful preoperative assessment and intraoperative management. The considerations are outlined in Table 32-7 (see also Chapter 45).

TABLE 32-7. CONSIDERATIONS IN PATIENTS PRESENTING FOR THE TRANSJUGULAR INTRAHEPATIC PORTOSYSTEMIC SHUNT PROCEDURE

Airway—risk of aspiration	Recent gastrointestinal bleeding Raised intragastric pressure due to ascites Decreased level of consciousness due to hepatic encephalopathy
CNS	Hepatic encephalopathy Altered mental status Variable response to anesthetic agents
Respiratory system	Decreased functional residual capacity due to ascites Pleural effusion Intrapulmonary shunts Pneumonia
Cardiovascular system	Associated alcoholic cardiomyopathy Altered volume status Acute hemorrhage from esophageal varices Intraperitoneal hemorrhage
Hematologic system	Coagulopathy Thrombocytopenia
Fluid balance	Ascites Risk of hepatorenal syndrome
Endocrine system	Tendency to hypoglycemia
Pharmacokinetics	Increased volume of distribution Decreased protein binding, drug metabolism, and elimination

Magnetic Resonance Imaging

Physical Principles

The physical principles of MRI are described in depth elsewhere.[45] Briefly, when atoms with an odd number of protons in their nuclei, notably hydrogen, are subjected to a powerful static magnetic field, they align themselves with the magnetic field. If they are then intermittently exposed to a radiofrequency wave, the nuclei change their alignment. As the radiofrequency pulses are discontinued, the protons return to their original alignment (i.e., they "relax") within the original magnetic field and, as they do, they release energy. The release of energy over time (the relaxation time) is specific for given tissues and is used to generate the MRI signal. The magnetic field strengths are expressed in Gauss (G) and Tesla (T; 1 T = 10,000 G). The earth's magnetic field is approximately 0.3 to 0.7 G. MRI scanners used for clinical purposes generate a field of 1.5 to 3 T, and machines generating magnetic fields from 4 to 9.4 T are used in research.

Hazards of MRI

MRI is devoid of the risks related to ionizing radiation; however, peripheral nerve stimulation (PNS) has been reported in biologic tissues exposed to radiofrequencies greater than 60 Hz. PNS results in sensory phenomena ranging from mild tingling to intolerable pain. MRI workers may experience transient vertigo-related symptoms and a metallic taste in the mouth when working in high (>3 T) magnetic fields.[46] Ferromagnetic implantable medical devices may move in the magnetic field with disastrous consequences. This is a particular concern in patients with cardiac pacemakers, which may malfunction, and cerebral aneurysm clips, which may move.[47] Before entering the vicinity of the magnet, patients and staff need to complete a rigorous checklist to ensure that they have no ferrometallic objects in their bodies.

The magnetic field takes several days to establish and is constantly present. It decreases in strength with distance from the center of the magnet. Ferromagnetic equipment such as IV poles, gas cylinders, laryngoscopes, and pens become potentially lethal projectiles if brought too close; a number of near-miss incidents and fatalities have been documented.[48] Considerable noise is generated by the rapidly alternating currents of the MRI scanner; this may exceed the occupational exposure limits, defined as a weekly average exposure of 99 dB and peak exposure of 140 dB.[49] Patients and staff should wear ear protection and staff should minimize time spent in the scanner. Cables and wires should not be wound in loops as this may cause induction-heating effects. Thermal injury may also occur in skin with large tattoos especially if these contain ferromagnetic inks. Patient monitors, ventilator equipment, and electrical infusion pumps may all malfunction when they come too close to the magnetic field. The electrocardiogram is sensitive to the changing magnetic signals, and it is nearly impossible to eliminate all artifacts. The electrodes should be placed close together and toward the center of the magnetic field. The leads should be insulated from the patient's skin to avoid causing thermal injury. MRI-compatible devices have been developed; however, in the absence of MRI-compatible monitors, tube extensions can be used to keep standard infusion pumps and monitors at a distance.[45] An MRI sequence takes upward of 30 minutes and many patients find it difficult to stay still for long periods. It may become very warm within the coil of the magnet, often reaching 80° F, adding to patient discomfort. A rise in body temperature is of particular concern in children who should have temperature monitored. Once a scan sequence is initiated, no one may enter or leave the scan room. In the case of an emergency, the MRI technicians should be notified, the scan sequence stopped, and the patient rapidly removed. Resuscitation attempts should take place outside the scanner because equipment such as laryngoscopes, oxygen cylinders, and cardiac defibrillators cannot be taken close to the magnet. Recent advances in technology have led to MRI being used continuously or intermittently during neurosurgical procedures in hybrid operating rooms/interventional suites.[50]

Anesthetic Technique

Thirty percent of adult patients experience some degree of anxiety during MRI scanning[51] and up to ten percent experience severe panic and claustrophobia. Four percent of adult patients will terminate the procedure prematurely[52] and fourteen percent require some form of sedation to tolerate MRI scanning.[53] Recently a three-fold reduction in claustrophobia has been reported with the use of short, conical-shaped MRI scanners with acoustic noise reduction.[54] Sedation for MRI may be provided as either oral sedation with benzodiazepines or minimal intravenous sedation. Anesthesiologists may become involved with more complex patients such as those with obesity, obstructive sleep apnea, raised ICP, movement disorders, developmental delay, and the potential for a difficult airway.

Pediatric Sedation and Anesthesia for MRI and CT Scans

In children, a combination of incomprehension, separation anxiety and fear can result in noncooperation and intolerance of relatively brief periods of immobility. Most children younger than 5 years and some as old as 11 years, particularly those with developmental delay, require sedation or general anesthesia for successful acquisition of MRI or CT images.[55,56] There is ongoing debate about the optimal care and techniques for these cases.[57] The benefits of a "sedation-only" approach include ease of medication administration (oral, rectal, or sometimes intravenous), lower cost (a sedation-trained nurse rather than an anesthesiologist), and more rapid wakening and discharge home. Disadvantages include a higher failure rate than general anesthesia, airway complications arising from over-sedation, unpredictable onset of enteral sedatives causing schedule delays, and inadequate analgesia during painful procedures. The choice of sedation or general anesthesia for a particular child is multifactorial and has been obfuscated in the past by the use of imprecise terms to describe the different clinical states.[58] In 2006, the acronym "SOAPME" was coined as a safety checklist before embarking upon any pediatric sedation or anesthetic (Suction, Oxygen, Airway equipment, appropriate Pharmaceuticals, Monitoring, and special Equipment).[59]

As with all NORA, the standards of care for pediatric patients undergoing sedation and/or general anesthesia for MRI and CT imaging are the same as those in the operating room[60] Adverse events related to pediatric sedation for CT and MRI include a 2.9% incidence of oxygen desaturation and failure of or inadequate sedation in 7% and 16% of cases respectively.[61] These events are more common in children with developmental delay[56] or higher ASA classification undergoing sedation. Careful screening of suitable candidates, rigorous oversight and a multidisciplinary team approach can reduce the incidence of failed and inadequate sedation.[62] Oral sedation techniques, if appropriately administered, can have a success rate as high as 93%.[55,61] The incidence of adverse events is considerably lower in children who undergo general anesthesia for scans (<0.7%).[55,61] Some institutions have a default general anesthesia policy for pediatric MRI and CT scans to avoid the relatively high failure rate, scheduling difficulties and risks of adverse events associated with sedation.[63] General anesthesia with formal airway management should be considered in cases where patency of the airway during sedation cannot be guaranteed (e.g., with obstructive sleep apnea or symptomatic gastroesophageal reflux disease). General anesthesia is also recommended in small (especially ex-premature) infants who are more sensitive to the respiratory depressant effects of sedative medications and prone to periods of apnea (see Chapter 41 Neonatal Anesthesia). Anesthesia can be induced and safely maintained via the inhalational or intravenous routes,[64–66] ideally either in (CT) or adjacent to (MRI) the scanner location. Nasal cannulas delivering low-flow oxygen (1 to 2 L/min) are typically used for sedated patients. Due to limited patient access and visibility, capnography is particularly useful for monitoring respiration in unintubated patients and mandatory in those with an advanced airway device.[4]

Sedative Agents

Oral chloral hydrate is a popular agent for sedation by nonanesthesiologists with an onset time of 30 minutes and duration of 1 to 2 hours.[67] It is particularly effective for children younger than 3 years of age, although with higher doses (75 to 100 mg/kg) there is risk of apnea and oxygen desaturation.[68] Chloral hydrate can cause excessive sedation, agitation, nausea and vomiting, and respiratory depression. Chloral hydrate failure rates of 20% in neurologically impaired children[69] and 14% in infants[70] undergoing MRI have been reported. A popular technique for otherwise healthy neonates is "feed, wrap, and scan" avoiding sedation or anesthesia altogether. The infant is swaddled in blankets after feeding and once asleep, placed (usually prone) onto the scanner table. When compared with oral chloral hydrate (50 mg/kg) this technique has a similar failure rate of 50%.[71]

Benzodiazepines such as midazolam administered either orally (0.25 to 0.75 mg/kg) or intravenously (0.05 to 0.15 mg/kg) are commonly used for premedication. The brief duration of action of midazolam; however, may mitigate against its use as sedation for prolonged MRI examinations. Other suitable agents for intravenous sedation include pentobarbital, ketamine and recently, dexmedetomidine.[60] Combination therapy with different categories of agents may be associated with a higher incidence of adverse airway events.[72]

Positron Emission Tomography

Positron emission tomography (PET) scanning is a newer imaging modality using radiolabeled isotopes to measure tissue glucose uptake thereby estimating tumor extent. Anesthesia concerns are those for CT; studies typically take longer to complete which may affect choice of technique/agent. Patients are typically exposed to greater ionizing radiation from both isotope and CT sources.[45]

Radiation Therapy

External beam radiation is a common treatment for children with malignancies. Adults typically tolerate the treatment and can lie still without sedation. It relies upon either highly tissue-targeted or total body irradiating (TBI) doses of X-rays. Proton beam therapy is a newer modality of this therapy, which has less potential for collateral injury to adjacent or beam-traversed tissues; a factor of utmost importance in pediatric patients at risk of long-term complications of radiation exposure.[73,74] Radiosensitive malignancies occurring in children are shown in Table 32-8. Tumors commonly involve vital structures such as the airway, thorax, mediastinum, heart, and central nervous system (CNS). Thorough preoperative assessment is essential, including assessment for raised ICP in children with CNS tumors. Many children receive concurrent cytotoxic or immunosuppressive chemotherapy and are at increased risk of sepsis, thrombocytopenia, and anemia. The challenges of anesthesia for children undergoing radiation therapy have recently been reviewed.[74,75,76] Patients are typically scheduled for a series of daily treatments, which can last upward of 45 minutes, over a 6-week period. Radiation doses are high, in the range of 180 to 250 cGy per treatment, and all personnel must leave the shielded room during the treatment. Direct observation of the patient is not possible and an interfaced system of closed-circuit television and telemetric microphones is used with standard monitoring.[75] In the event of a problem, shutdown of the radiation beam and immediate access to the patient (within 20 to 30 seconds) is crucial. Radiation therapy suites are often located remote from children's hospitals requiring daily transfer of patient and personnel to and from the site. Children older than 6 or 7 years can sometimes tolerate repeated treatment sessions without sedation or anesthesia using behavioral techniques.[76] Most children; however, require general anesthesia or deep sedation techniques with propofol.[77,78] Absence of any movement is crucial, particularly if X-ray images are obtained at the beginning to confirm treatment beam accuracy or if multiple position changes of either patient or linear accelerator are required. Immobilization devices, especially those applied to the face and head, are unpleasant for the child and may cause airway concerns for the anesthesiologist. Most children will have indwelling central venous access, avoiding the need for repeated intravenous puncture or inhalational induction.

TABLE 32-8. COMMON RADIOSENSITIVE TUMORS IN CHILDREN

Primary CNS tumor—neuroblastoma, medulloblastoma
Acute leukemia—CNS leukemia
Radiosensitive ocular tumors—retinoblastoma
Intra-abdominal tumors—Wilms' tumor
Rhabdomyosarcoma
Other tumors—Langerhans cell histiocytosis

Interventional Cardiology

There has been a significant increase in interventional cardiology procedures in the last decade resulting in an increased demand by cardiologists for the services of an anesthesiologist; in many cases a cardiac trained anesthesiologist.[79,80] Diagnostic and therapeutic interventional procedures are carried out in the cardiac catheterization laboratory and the electrophysiology laboratory (EPL).[81,82] These procedures are described in Table 32-2. Many patients will manage with light or moderate sedation supervision of the cardiologist; however, general anesthesia is becoming more widely practiced, particularly as procedures become longer and more complex and patient comorbidity increases. Transesophageal echocardiography (TEE) is increasingly used during these procedures and the input of an anesthesiologist during airway manipulation is advantageous.[82]

Cardiac Catheterization Procedures

Diagnostic cardiac catheterization procedures and percutaneous coronary interventions are commonly performed with conscious sedation. Percutaneous left ventricular assist devices (balloon pumps) are placed for patients in cardiogenic shock and these high-risk patients will benefit from the presence of a cardiac anesthetist to provide anesthesia and invasive monitoring. Percutaneous valve replacement procedures are often performed on patients with critical disease such as transcatheter aortic valve implantation (TAVI).[83] These patients suffer from numerous associated comorbidities and are too sick for surgical repair. Significant hemodynamic disturbances occur during the procedure, including periods of rapid ventricular pacing to allow placement of the implanted valve. The presence of a cardiac anesthetist is essential to care for these high-risk patients. The facility to move rapidly to the operating room and the availability of cardiopulmonary bypass are essential backups for any procedure carried out in the cardiac catheterization laboratory.

Electrophysiologic Procedures

Electrophysiologic studies and ablation of abnormal conduction pathways are performed for the treatment of dysrhythmias caused by aberrant conduction pathways. Once identified, the abnormal conduction pathways are ablated using radiofrequency techniques. The volatile anesthetic agents and propofol have been shown not to interfere with cardiac conduction during these procedures.[84] Electrophysiologic studies are lengthy (commonly 6 to 8 hours) and can cause discomfort. The cardiologist provokes the dysrhythmia they wish to ablate, thus the patient's antidysrhythmic therapy is stopped prior to the procedure. Intraoperative dysrhythmias are terminated using overdrive pacing via the cardiac catheters or, if unsuccessful, by external cardioversion. External defibrillation pads should be applied before the procedure. One study identified that 40% of patients undergoing electrophysiologic procedures require airway interventions and strongly recommended the involvement of anesthesia providers during these procedures.[85]

Nonoperating Room Pediatric Cardiac Procedures

Cardiac catheterization is performed in children with congenital heart disease for both hemodynamic assessment and interventional procedures.[86] Closure of atrial and ventricular septal defects and patent ductus arteriosus via the transcatheter route is increasingly replacing the surgical approach, while percutaneous treatments of aortic coarctation, pulmonary artery stenosis, and valvular disorders are on the horizon.[86] Careful cardiac assessment is essential and the presence of a pediatric anesthesiologist is desirable. The utilization of general anesthesia for pediatric cardiac catheterization has been reported as varying between institutions from 28% to 99% in a recent multicenter study.[87] Children undergoing RFA experience a high incidence of nausea and vomiting,[88] which may be reduced using a propofol infusion technique rather than volatile anesthesia. Children older than 10 years may tolerate RFA without anesthesia.[89] Patients often present with cyanosis, dyspnea, congestive heart failure, and intracardiac shunts. Hypoxia, hypercarbia, and sympathetic stimulation as a result of anxiety may exacerbate cardiopulmonary abnormalities. In patients with a patent ductus arteriosus, high oxygen tension can lead to premature closure and should be avoided. Prostaglandin infusions are often used to maintain duct patency. One must pay meticulous attention to preventing air bubbles entering intravenous lines because they may cross to the arterial circulation via a right-to-left shunt. The use of intravenous sedation and anesthesia, provided by appropriately trained and credentialed providers is increasingly the standard of care for pediatric NOR cardiac procedures.[90,91] A variety of anesthetic agents may be used including combinations of propofol–ketamine and dexmedetomidine–propofol infusions[92] as well as standard inhalational techniques and propofol infusions. The incidence of adverse events in children undergoing cardiac catheterization is reported to be between 5% and 18%, with a higher incidence (20%) in interventional cases compared to diagnostic (10%) or biopsy (4%) cases.[87]

Cardioversion

Atrial fibrillation (AF) is associated with a number of conditions; hypertension, chronic heart failure, valvular and ischemic heart diseases, and is a frequent sequela of cardiothoracic surgery. Transthoracic DC cardioversion is an accepted, often used treatment for atrial dysrhythmias including AF and atrial flutter. In patients with chronic AF, there is an increased risk of thromboembolic events (0.7% to 0.8%). This risk is almost 10 times greater (5% to 7%) if the patient is inadequately anticoagulated. Current guidelines require anticoagulation with warfarin to achieve an INR (International Normalized Ratio) of 2 to 3 for 3 weeks before cardioversion and continued for 4 weeks afterward if AF has been present longer than 48 hours.[93] Unstable patients needing urgent cardioversion should be heparinized. Alternatively TEE may be used to determine if thrombus is present in the left atrium. In the absence of thrombus, immediate cardioversion and short-term anticoagulation with heparin or warfarin is considered a safe approach.[93] The new oral anticoagulant Dabigatran, a reversible direct thrombin inhibitor with a rapid onset of effect is currently being evaluated as an alternative to standard longer term warfarin therapy in patients with AF.[94] Cardioversion takes a few seconds; however, it is distressing, and deep sedation or general anesthesia is preferable except in life-threatening situations. A small bolus of intravenous induction agent is usually sufficient to render the patient sufficiently unconscious for cardioversion. All currently available induction agents are effective. Etomidate produces less hypotension than propofol making it a better choice in patients with significant cardiac disease, although hypotension can be attenuated by using smaller doses of propofol (1 mg/kg).[95,96] When TEE is performed prior to cardioversion, the procedure takes longer and requires more sedation. Thorough airway evaluation is important prior to TEE; in most cases nasal cannulas are sufficient to provide supplemental oxygenation while the patient maintains his or her own airway. A technique using deep propofol sedation together with a laryngeal mask to support the airway and allow ventilation has also been described.[97] Occasionally tracheal intubation may be the most prudent approach. Before TEE, local anesthetic (either 4% lidocaine or 20% benzocaine) is sprayed into the oropharynx to allow less stimulating passage of the TEE probe. A bite block is inserted to prevent the patient from biting down on the probe, damaging both his/her teeth and the probe.

Gastroenterology

Procedures commonly performed in the gastrointestinal (GI) endoscopy suite are described in Table 32-2. The American Gastroenterological Association reports that 98% of patients for upper and lower endoscopies receive sedation.[98] Of these, over one-third are performed in ambulatory surgery centers and only 29% of these procedures involve anesthesia care providers.[98,99]

A degree of controversy surrounds the administration of sedation for GI procedures both in the United States[98] and world-wide.[100] A wide variety of sedation techniques are used for GI endoscopy and gastroenterologists are increasingly using propofol sedation techniques (nurse administered propofol sedation "NAPS"). With appropriately trained personnel, NAPS appears to be effective and safe,[101,102] although the use of propofol by those without expert airway skills is highly controversial in the anesthesiology community. Gastroenterologists do however, universally agree that patients in ASA classes III or IV, for complex procedures, or with histories of adverse or inadequate responses to sedation require the involvement of an anesthesiologist.[103]

Upper Gastrointestinal Endoscopy

Upper GI endoscopy is performed for diagnostic procedures, such as biopsy, and for therapeutic procedures, such as retrieval of foreign bodies, treatment of esophageal varices with sclerotherapy or band ligation, dilation of esophageal strictures, and placement of a percutaneous endoscopic gastrostomy. Patients may have a number of comorbidities, or a risk of gastroesophageal reflux, hepatic dysfunction, coagulopathy, and ascites. With general anesthesia, patients usually require tracheal intubation to protect the airway and facilitate passage of the endoscope. The LMA has also been used successfully[104] as an alternative device for airway management. Local anesthetic is sprayed into the oropharynx to facilitate passage of the endoscope; this can abolish the gag reflex, increasing the risk of aspiration. A bite block is inserted to prevent the patient from biting down on the endoscope and damaging both the teeth and the endoscope. Procedures are performed in the prone or semiprone position with the patient's head rotated to the side. This position makes the airway less accessible. Care and attention should also be paid to pressure areas, particularly the eyes, lips, and teeth. Extreme rotation of the neck should be avoided. Most procedures are brief, lasting 10 to 30 minutes, and are generally painless.

Endoscopic Retrograde Cholangiopancreatography

Endoscopic retrograde cholangiopancreatography (ERCP) is important in the diagnosis and treatment of both biliary and pancreatic diseases. During the procedure, the biliary and pancreatic duct systems are identified, instrumented, and therapeutic maneuvers such as the passage of stents or removal of stones carried out. Patients usually experience discomfort during ERCP and general anesthesia or deep sedation techniques are recommended for the procedure, which usually lasts between 20 and 80 minutes.[105] The airway and patient positioning considerations are similar to those for GI endoscopy. Sphincter of Oddi manometry may be performed in which case drugs that affect sphincter pressure such as atropine, glycopyrrolate, glucagon, and various opioids should be avoided. Patients presenting for ERCP may have significant comorbidities,[105] including acute cholangitis with septicemia, jaundice with liver dysfunction and coagulopathy, bleeding from esophageal varices resulting in hypovolemia, or biliary stricture following major hepatobiliary surgery, including liver transplantation. Transient bacteremia may occur during endoscopy, and antibiotic prophylaxis is recommended for patients with cardiac valvular abnormalities. Gastroenterologists frequently use antispasmodics such as glucagon and intravenous hyoscyamine to reduce duodenal motility and improve operating conditions during endoscopy,[106] sinus tachycardia may occur.

Electroconvulsive Therapy

Electroconvulsive therapy (ECT) has had an important role in the management of depression, mania, and affective disorders since the 1930s.[107] Typically it is performed 3 times per week for 6 to 12 treatments, followed by weekly or monthly maintenance therapy to prevent relapses.[108]

Physiologic Response to Electroconvulsive Therapy

The physiologic response to ECT includes generalized motor seizures and an acute cardiovascular response. The seizure usually lasts several minutes and minimum seizure duration of 25 seconds is recommended to ensure adequate antidepressant efficacy.[109] The cardiovascular response includes transient bradycardia and occasional asystole giving way to more prominent hypertension and tachycardia. Increased cerebral blood flow, raised ICP and cardiac dysrhythmias, myocardial ischemia, infarction, or neurologic vascular events may be precipitated. Short-term memory loss is also common following ECT. Other sequelae include myalgias, fracture/dislocations (if muscle relaxants are not properly deployed), headache, emergence agitation, status epilepticus, and sudden death.

Anesthetic Considerations for ECT

Scalp electrodes are placed to monitor the electroencephalogram and a blood pressure cuff is applied to an extremity and inflated before the muscle relaxant is administered to monitor the seizure. Patients presenting for ECT are often elderly, with a number of coexisting conditions. Antidepressant medications include tricyclic antidepressants, monoamine oxidase inhibitors, and selective serotonin-reuptake inhibitors; of these the monoamine oxidase inhibitors have the most significant interactions with anesthetic agents. The anesthetic requirements for ECT include amnesia, airway management, prevention of seizure-related injuries, control of hemodynamic responses, and a smooth, rapid emergence[108] Most of the intravenous induction agents have been used for ECT. Methohexital (1 to 1.5 mg/kg) is considered the "gold standard".[108] Etomidate (0.15 to 0.3 mg/kg) is generally associated with longer seizure duration and is the preferred agent of some psychiatrists, despite a slightly longer recovery and associated myoclonus.[110,111] Propofol (an anticonvulsant) is more effective at attenuating the acute hemodynamic responses than etomidate and in small doses (0.75 mg/kg) seizure duration is usually acceptable.[110] Short-acting opioids, such as remifentanil, can be used to decrease the dose of induction agent and prolong seizure duration without reducing the depth of anesthesia.[112] Muscle relaxants (succinylcholine, 0.75 to 1.5 mg/kg) are used to prevent fractures or dislocations occurring during the seizure.[108] Moderate hypocapnia improves the quality and duration of seizures;[113] mask ventilation is usually adequate although the LMA may be useful to improve ventilation.[114] Before administering the electricity, a bite guard is placed to protect the teeth. In younger patients, 15 to 30 mg of intravenous ketorolac helps to reduce ECT-induced myalgia. Older patients, or those in whom ketorolac is contraindicated, may receive aspirin or acetaminophen orally before their treatment. The parasympathetic effects of ECT, (salivation, transient bradycardia, and asystole) can be prevented by premedication with glycopyrrolate or atropine. Labetalol, esmolol, and the calcium channel antagonists nifedipine, diltiazem, and nicardipine all attenuate the hemodynamic responses to ECT. More recently, dexmedetomidine (1 μg/kg administered over 10 minutes just before induction of anesthesia) has been shown to be effective in controlling blood pressure without affecting seizure duration.[115]

Dental Surgery

Most dental procedures are performed in the office with no sedation and only local anesthesia. General anesthesia may be required during more complicated, painful, or prolonged procedures and when patient factors dictate (Table 32-1). A number of genetic diseases result in cognitive impairment, psychiatric morbidity, and behavioral abnormalities, which may place the patient or provider at risk. These patients usually require sedation or general anesthesia to tolerate dental procedures.[116] Congenital diseases are frequently associated with medical comorbidity, often involving the cardiovascular system and the airway (e.g., mucopolysaccharidoses).[117] Down's syndrome (trisomy of chromosome 21) is one of the more commonly encountered conditions, and the anesthesiologist should be aware of associated cardiac conduction and structural abnormalities, risk of atlanto-occipital instability, and a variety of potential airway problems (including macroglossia, hypoplastic maxilla, palatal abnormalities, and mandibular protrusion).

Profound hypotension may occur as a result of vasodilation and the myocardial-depressant effects of anesthetics being compounded by dependent pooling of blood when semirecumbent in the dental chair. Patients with neuromuscular diseases may have a history of aspiration and episodes of chronic recurrent pneumonitis that must be addressed before dental surgery. Induction of anesthesia in an unwilling patient is often challenging. Ketamine is a useful induction agent in this context; it may be given alone by a variety of routes (orally [5 to 10 mg/kg], intravenously [1 to 2 mg/kg], or most usefully, intramuscularly [2 to 4 mg/kg]).[118] The rectal and intranasal routes have also been used. Ketamine is also advantageous in that it does not abolish upper airway reflexes. Atropine and midazolam may be used in conjunction with ketamine to reduce side effects. Oral midazolam is also popular; a dose of 0.3 to 0.5 mg/kg oral suspension has an onset of 15 to 20 minutes. Its bitter taste may be disguised by adding a small amount of clear apple juice, or by encouraging the recipient to take the dose "in one go." The timely use of topical local anesthetic facilitates the painless placement of intravenous lines in needle-phobic children and adults. Alternatively, an inhalation induction may be attempted. During and after dental surgery, blood, saliva, and dental debris are present in the upper airway. A throat pack is used to help protect the airway and must be removed at the end of surgery. Retained throat packs are a cause of upper airway obstruction in the postanesthesia care unit (PACU) and can be rapidly lethal. Tracheal intubation, often via the nasal route, is required to protect the airway, although the LMA has been used successfully for both adults[119] and children[120] undergoing dental surgery. Anesthesia can be maintained with intravenous infusions or inhalation anesthesia. Patients need close observation during emergence and recovery. The immediate postoperative complications include bleeding, airway obstruction, and laryngospasm; later ones include drowsiness, nausea and vomiting, and pain.[121]

SUMMARY

The number and complexity of NOR procedures is steadily increasing. This increase has resulted in an expansion of anesthesia services in areas remote from the operating room that may not be familiar to anesthesia providers. In preparing to administer anesthesia or sedation in a NOR site, a simple three-step approach can be followed. This approach involves giving careful consideration to the evaluation and the needs of the *patient,* the particular challenges posed by the *procedure,* and the hazards and limitations of the *environment.* In all cases, the standards of anesthesia care and monitoring should be no different than those provided in the conventional operating room.

References

1. Statement on Nonoperating Room Anesthetizing Locations. Committee of Origin: Standards and Practice Parameters (Approved by the ASA House of Delegates on October 15, 2003 and amended on October 22, 2008); http://www.asahq.org/For-Members/Standards-Guidelines-and-Statements.aspx. Last viewed September 27, 2012.
2. Metzner J, Domino KB. Risks of anesthesia or sedation outside the operating room: The role of the anesthesia care provider. *Curr Opin Anaesthesiol.* 2010;23:523–531.
3. Metzner J, Posner KL, Domino KB. The risk and safety of anesthesia at remote locations: The US closed claims analysis. *Curr Opin Anaesthesiol.* 2009;22:502–508.
4. Standards for Basic Anesthetic Monitoring. Committee of Origin: Standards and Practice Parameters (Approved by the ASA House of Delegates on October 21, 1986, and last amended on October 20, 2010 with an effective date of July 1, 2011); http://www.asahq.org/For-Members/Standards-Guidelines-and-Statements.aspx. Last viewed September 27, 2012.
5. Waugh JB, Epps CA, Khodneva YA. Capnography enhances surveillance of respiratory events during procedural sedation: A meta-analysis. *J Clin Anesth.* 2011;23:189–196.
6. Practice guidelines for sedation and analgesia by non-anesthesiologists. An updated report by the American Society of Anesthesiologists task force on sedation and analgesia by non-anesthesiologists. *Anesthesiology.* 2002;96:1004–1017.
7. Semel ME, Resch S, Haynes AB, et al. Adopting a surgical safety checklist could save money and improve the quality of care in U.S. hospitals. *Health Aff (Millwood).* 2010;29:1593–1599.
8. Lee MJ, Fanelli F, Haage P, et al. Patient safety in interventional radiology: A CIRSE IR checklist. *Cardiovasc Intervent Radiol.* 2012;35:244–246.
9. Basic Standards for Preanesthesia Care. Committee of Origin: Standards and Practice Parameters (Approved by the ASA House of Delegates on October 14, 1987, and last affirmed on October 20, 2010); http://www.asahq.org/For-Members/Standards-Guidelines-and-Statements.aspx. Last viewed September 27, 2012.
10. Standards for Postanesthesia Care. Committee of Origin: Standards and Practice Parameters (Approved by the ASA House of Delegates on October 27, 2004, and last amended on October 21, 2009); http://www.asahq.org/For-Members/Standards-Guidelines-and-Statements.aspx. Last viewed September 27, 2012.
11. Position on Monitored Anesthesia Care. Committee of Origin: Economics (Approved by the House of Delegates on October 21, 1986, amended on October 25, 2005 and last updated on September 2, 2008); http://www.asahq.org/For-Members/Standards-Guidelines-and-Statements.aspx. Last viewed September 27, 2012
12. Department of Health and Human Services. Centers for Medicare and Medicaid Services Revised Hospital Anesthesia Services Interpretive Guidelines—State Operations Manual (SOM) Appendix A Ref: S&C—10-09-Hospital. Revised 2-05-2010. Available at: http://www.asahq.org/For-Members/Advocacy/Federal-Legislative-and-Regulatory-Activities/Interpretive-Guidelines.aspx. Last viewed September 29, 2012.
13. Miller DL. Overview of contemporary interventional fluoroscopy procedures. *Health Phys.* 2008;95:638–644.
14. Mitchell EL, Furey P. Prevention of radiation injury from medical imaging. *J Vasc Surg.* 2011;53:22S–27S.
15. Miller DL, Vañó E, Bartal G, et al. Occupational radiation protection in interventional radiology: A joint guideline of the Cardiovascular and Interventional Radiology Society of Europe and the Society of Interventional Radiology. *Cardiovasc Intervent Radiol.* 2010;33:230–239.
16. Semelka RC, Armao DM, Elias J Jr, et al. Imaging strategies to reduce the risk of radiation in CT studies, including selective substitution with MRI. *J Magn Reson Imaging.* 2007;25:900–909.
17. Anastasian ZH, Strozyk D, Meyers PM, et al. Radiation exposure of the anesthesiologist in the neurointerventional suite. *Anesthesiology.* 2011;114:512–520.
18. International Commission on Radiological Protection. Avoidance of radiation injuries from medical interventional procedures. ICRP Publication 85. *Ann ICRP.* 2000;30:7–67.
19. National Council on Radiation Protection and Measurements. Limitation of exposure to ionizing radiation. 1993; NCRP Report No. 116: National Council on Radiation Protection and Measurements, Bethesda, MD.
20. Thomsen HS. Contrast media safety—An update. *Eur J Radiol.* 2011;80:77–82.
21. McCullough PA. Radiocontrast-induced acute kidney injury. *Nephron Physiol.* 2008;109:61–72.
22. Nash K, Hafeez A, Hou S. Hospital-acquired renal insufficiency. *Am J Kidney Dis.* 2002;39:930–936.
23. Solomon R. The role of osmolality in the incidence of contrast-induced nephropathy: A systematic review of angiographic contrast media in high-risk patients. *Kidney Int.* 2005;68:2256–2263.
24. Brockow K, Christiansen C, Kanny G, et al. Management of hypersensitivity reactions to iodinated contrast media. *Allergy.* 2005;60:150–158.
25. Brockow K. Immediate and delayed reactions to radiocontrast media: Is there an allergic mechanism? *Immunol Allergy Clin N Am.* 2009;29:453–468.
26. Tramèr MR, von Elm E, Loubeyre P, et al. Pharmacological prevention of serious anaphylactic reactions due to iodinated contrast media: Systematic review. *BMJ.* 2006;333:675–678.
27. Prince MR, Zhang H, Zou Z, et al. Incidence of immediate gadolinium contrast media reactions. *Am J Roentgenol.* 2011;196:W138–W143.
28. Zou Z, Zhang HL, Roditi GH, et al. Nephrogenic systemic fibrosis review of 370 biopsy-confirmed cases. *JACC Cardiovasc Imaging.* 2011;4:1206–1216.
29. Varma MK, Price K, Jayakrishnan V, et al. Anaesthetic considerations for interventional neuroradiology. *Br J Anaesth.* 2007;99:75–85.
30. Molyneux A, Kerr R, Stratton I, et al. International subarachnoid aneurysm trial (ISAT) of neurosurgical clipping versus endovascular coiling in 2143 patients with ruptured intracranial aneurysms: A randomized trial. *Lancet.* 2002;360:1267–1274.
31. Molyneux A, Kerr R, Birks J, et al. Risk of recurrent subarachnoid, death or dependence and standardised mortality ratios after clipping or coiling of an intracranial aneurysm in the international subarachnoid aneurysm trial (ISAT): Long-term follow up. *Lancet Neurol.* 2009;8:427–433.
32. Molyneux A, Kerr R, Yu L, et al. International subarachnoid aneurysm trial(ISAT) of neurosurgical clipping vs. endovascular coiling in 2143 patients with intracranial aneurysms: A randomized comparison of effects on survival, dependency, seizures, rebleeding, subgroups and aneurysm occlusion. *Lancet.* 2005;366:809–817.
33. Schulenburg E, Matta B. Anaesthesia for interventional neuroradiology. *Curr Opin Anaesthesiol.* 2011;24:426–432.

34. Ryttlefors M, Enblad P, Kerr RS, et al. International sub-arachnoid aneurysm trial of neurosurgical clipping versus endovascular coiling: Subgroup analysis of 278 elderly patients. *Stroke.* 2008;39:2720–2726.
35. Kubalek R, Berlis A, Schwab M, et al. Activated clotting time or activated partial thromboplastin time as the method of choice for patients undergoing neuroradiological intervention. *Neuroradiology.* 2003;45:325.
36. See JJ, Manninen PH. Anesthesia for neuroradiology. *Curr Opin Anaesthesiol.* 2005;18:437.
37. Hall JE, Uhrich TD, Barney JA, et al. Sedative, amnesia and analgesic properties of small-dose dexmedetomidine infusions. *Anesth Analg.* 2000;90:699–705.
38. Bustillo MA, Lazar RM, Finck AD, et al. Dexmedetomidine may impair cognitive testing during endovascular embolization of cerebral arteriovenous malformations: A retrospective case report series. *J Neurosurg Anesthesiol.* 2002;14:209–212.
39. Rauch RA, Vinuela F, Dion J, et al. Preembolization functional evaluation in brain arteriovenous malformations: The ability of superselective Amytal test to predict neurologic dysfunction before embolization. *Am J Neuroradiol.* 1992;13:309–314.
40. Raiten J, Elkassabany N, Gao W, et al. Medical intelligence article: Novel uses of high frequency ventilation outside the operating room. *Anesth Analg.* 2011; 112:1110–1113.
41. Ong JP, Sands M, Younossi ZM. Transjugular intrahepatic portosystemic shunts (TIPS): A decade later. *J Clin Gastroenterol.* 2000;30:14–28.
42. Monescillo A, Martinez-Lagares F, Ruiz-del-Arbol L, et al. Influence of portal hypertension and its early decompression by TIPS placement on the outcome of variceal bleeding. *Hepatology.* 2004;40:793–801.
43. Zheng M, Chen Y, Bai J, et al. Transjugular intrahepatic portosystemic shunt versus endoscopic therapy in the secondary prophylaxis of variceal rebleeding in cirrhotic patients: Meta-analysis update. *J Clin Gastroenterol.* 2008;42:507–516.
44. Kelhoffer ER, Osborn IP. The gastroenterology suite and TIPS. *Int Anesthesiol Clin.* 2003;41:51–61.
45. Veenith T, Coles JP. Anesthesia for magnetic resonance imaging and positron emission tomography. *Curr Opin Anesthesiol.* 2011;24:451–458.
46. Institute of Physics. MRI and the Physical agents (EMF) directive. Institute of Physics Report 2008; http://www.iop.org/publications/iop/2008/file_38215.pdf. Last viewed December 9, 2011.
47. Farling PA, Flynn PA, Darwent G, et al. Safety in magnetic resonance units: An update. *Anaesthesia.* 2010;65:766–770.
48. Chaljub G, Kramer LA, Johnson RF 3rd, et al. Projectile cylinder accidents resulting from the presence of ferromagnetic nitrous oxide or oxygen tanks in the MR suite. *Am J Roentgenol.* 2001;177:27–30.
49. US Department of Health and Human services, Food and Drug Administration. Center for Devices and Radiological Health of 99 and 140dB, respectively; http://www.fda.gov/downloads/MedicalDevices/DeviceRegulationandGuidance/GuidanceDocuments/UCM072688.pdf. Last viewed December 15, 2011.
50. Senft C, Franz K, Ulrich CT, et al. Low field intraoperative MRI-guided surgery of gliomas: A single center experience. *Clin Neurol Neurosurg.* 2010;112:237–243.
51. Melendez JC, McCrank E. Anxiety-related reactions associated with magnetic resonance imaging examinations. *JAMA.* 1993;270:745–747.
52. Flaherty JA, Hoskinson K. Emotional distress during magnetic resonance imaging. *N Engl J Med.* 1989;320:467–468.
53. Murphy KJ, Brunberg JA. Adult claustrophobia, anxiety and sedation in MRI. *Magn Reson Imaging.* 1997;15:51–54.
54. Dewey M, Schink T, Dewey CF. Claustrophobia during magnetic resonance imaging: Cohort study in over 55,000 patients. *J Magn Reson Imaging.* 2007;26: 1322–1327.
55. Keengwe IN, Hegde S, Dearlove O, et al. Structured sedation programme for magnetic resonance imaging examination in children. *Anaesthesia.* 1999;54: 1069–1072.
56. Kannikeswaran N, Mahajan PV, Sethuraman U, et al. Sedation medication received and adverse events related to sedation for brain MRI in children with and without developmental disabilities. *Paediatr Anaesth.* 2009;19:250–256.
57. Krauss B, Green SM. Training and credentialing in procedural sedation and analgesia in children: Lessons from the United States model. *Paediatr Anaesth.* 2008;18:30–35.
58. Coté CJ. Round and round we go: Sedation – what is it, who does it, and have we made things safer for children? *Paediatr Anaesth.* 2008;18:3–8.
59. Coté CJ, Wilson S. Guidelines for monitoring and management of pediatric patients during and after sedation for diagnostic and therapeutic procedures: An update. *Pediatrics.* 2006;118:2587–2602.
60. Schulte-Uentrop L, Goepfert M. Anesthesia or sedation for MRI in children. *Curr Opin Anesthesiol.* 2010;23:513–517.
61. Malviya S, Voepel-Lewis T, Eldevik OP, et al. Sedation and general anaesthesia in children undergoing MRI and CT: Adverse events and outcomes. *Br J Anaesth.* 2000;84:743–748.
62. Hatch DJ, Sury MR. Sedation of children by non-anaesthetists. *Br J Anaesth.* 2000; 84:713–714.
63. Allen JG, Sury MR. Sedation of children undergoing magnetic resonance imaging. *Br J Anaesth.* 2007;98:548–549.
64. Cravero JP, Beach ML, Blike G, et al. The incidence and nature of adverse events during pediatric sedation/anesthesia with propofol for procedures outside the operating room: A report from the Pediatric Sedation Research Consortium. *Anesth Analg.* 2009;108:795–780.
65. Machata AM, Willschke H, Kabon B, et al. Propofol-based sedation regimen for infants and children undergoing ambulatory magnetic resonance imaging. *Br J Anaesth.* 2008;101:239–243.
66. Bryan YF, Hoke LK, Taghon TA, et al. A randomized trial comparing sevoflurane and propofol in children undergoing MRI scans. *Paediatr Anaesth.* 2009;19: 672–681.
67. Krauss B, Green SM. Procedural sedation and analgesia in children. *Lancet.* 2006;367:766–780.
68. Litman RS, Soin K, Salam A. Chloral hydrate sedation in term and preterm infants: An analysis of efficacy and complications. *Anesth Analg.* 2010;110:739–746.
69. Cortellazzi P, Lamperti M, Minati L, et al. Sedation of neurologically impaired children undergoing MRI: A sequential approach. *Paediatr Anaesth.* 2007;17:630–636.
70. Low E, O'Driscoll M, MacEneaney P, et al. Sedation with oral chloral hydrate in children undergoing MRI scanning. *Ir Med J.* 2008;101:80–82.
71. Beauve B, Dearlove O. Sedation of children under 4 weeks of age for MRI examinations. *Paediatr Anaesth.* 2008;18:892–893.
72. Green SM, Roback MG, Krauss B, et al. Predictors of airway and respiratory adverse events with ketamine sedation in the emergency department: An individual-patient data meta-analysis of 8282 children. *Ann Emerg Med.* 2009;54:158–168.
73. Alonso-Basanta M, Lustig RA, Kennedy DW. Proton beam therapy in skull base pathology. *Otolaryngol Clin North Am.* 2011;44:1173–1183.
74. Chalabi J, Patel S. Radiation therapy in children. *Int Anesthesiol Clin.* 2009;47:45–53.
75. McFadyen GJ, Pelly N, Orr RJ. Sedation and anesthesia for the pediatric patient undergoing radiotherapy. *Curr Opin Anaesthesiol.* 2011;24:433–438.
76. Harris EA. Sedation and anesthesia options for pediatric patients in the radiation oncology suite. *Int J Pediatr.* 2010;2010:870921. Epub 2010 May 13.
77. Buehrer S, Immoos S, Frei M, et al. Evaluation of propofol for repeated prolonged deep sedation in children undergoing proton radiation therapy. *Br J Anaesth.* 2007;99:556–560.
78. Anghelescu DL, Burgoyne LL, Liu W, et al. Safe anesthesia for radiotherapy in pediatric oncology: St. Jude Children's Research Hospital Experience, 2004–2006. *Int J Radiat Oncol Biol Phys.* 2008;71:491–497.
79. Mahajan A, Chua J. Pro: A cardiovascular anesthesiologist should provide services in the catheterization and electrophysiology laboratory. *J Cardiothorac Vasc Anesth.* 2011;25:553–556.
80. Reddy K, Jaggar S, Gillbe C. The anaesthetist and the cardiac catheterisation laboratory. *Anaesthesia.* 2006;61:1175–1186.
81. Shook DC, Gross W. Offsite anesthesiology in the cardiac catheterization lab. *Curr Opin Anaesthesiol.* 2007;20:352–358.
82. Faillace, RT, Kaddaha R, Bikkina R, et al. The role of the out-of-operating room anesthesiologist in the care of the cardiac patient. *Anesthesiol Clin.* 2009;27:29–46.
83. Billings FT, Kodali SK, Shanewise JS. Transcatheter aortic valve implantation: Anesthetic considerations. *Anesth Analg.* 2009;108:1453–1462.
84. Lavoie J, Walsh EP, Burrows FA, et al. Effects of propofol or isoflurane anesthesia on cardiac conduction in children undergoing radiofrequency catheter ablation for tachydysrhythmias. *Anesthesiology.* 1995;82:884–887.
85. Trentman TL, Fassett SL, Mueller JT, et al. Airway interventions in the cardiac electrophysiology laboratory: A retrospective review. *J Cardiothorac Vasc Anesth.* 2009;23:841–845.
86. Mertens L, Budts W. New developments in the transcatheter treatment of congenital heart disease. *Curr Opin Anaesthesiol.* 2004;17:329–334.
87. Bergersen L, Marshall A, Gauvreau K, et al. Adverse event rates in congenital cardiac catheterization – a multi-center experience. *Catheter Cardiovasc Interv.* 2010;75:389–400.
88. Erb TO, Hall JM, Ing RJ, et al. Postoperative nausea and vomiting in children and adolescents undergoing radiofrequency catheter ablation: A randomized comparison of propofol- and isoflurane-based anesthetics. *Anesth Analg.* 2002;95:1577–1581.
89. Joung B, Lee M, Sung JH. Pediatric radiofrequency catheter ablation: Sedation methods and success, complication and recurrence rates. *Circ J.* 2006;70:278–284.
90. Bernath MA, Sekarski N. Management of paediatric patients undergoing diagnostic and invasive cardiology procedures. *Curr Opin Anaesthesiol.* 2001;14: 441–446.
91. Cravero JP, Havidich JE. Pediatric sedation – evolution and revolution. *Paediatr Anaesth.* 2011;21:800–809.
92. Koruk S, Mizrak A, Kaya Ugur B, et al. Propofol/dexmedetomidine and propofol/ketamine combinations for anesthesia in pediatric patients undergoing transcatheter atrial septal defect closure: A prospective randomized study. *Clin Ther.* 2010;32:701–709.
93. Fuster V, Ryden LE, Cannom DS, et al. ACC/AHA/ESC 2006 guidelines for the management of patients with atrial fibrillation. *Circulation.* 2006;114: e257–e354.
94. Nagarakanti R, Ezekowitz MD, Oldgren J, et al. Dabigatran versus warfarin in patients with atrial fibrillation: An analysis of patients undergoing cardioversion. *Circulation.* 2011;123:131–136.
95. Herregods LL, Bossuyt GP, De Baerdemaeker LE, et al. Ambulatory electrical external cardioversion with propofol or etomidate. *J Clin Anesth.* 2003;15:91.
96. Parlak M, Parlak I, Erdur B, et al. Age effect on efficacy and side effects of two sedation and analgesia protocols on patients going through cardioversion: A randomized clinical trial. *Acad Emerg Med.* 2006;13:493.

97. Ferson D, Thakar D, Swafford J, et al. Use of deep intravenous sedation with propofol and the laryngeal mask airway during transesophageal echocardiography. *J Cardiothorac Vasc Anesth.* 2003;17:443.
98. Cohen LB, Wecsler JS, Gaetano JN, et al. Endoscopic sedation in the United States: Results from a nationwide survey. *Am J Gastroenterol.* 2006;101:967–974.
99. Goulson DT, Fragneto RY. Anesthesia for gastrointestinal endoscopic procedures. *Anesthesiology Clin.* 2009;27:71–85.
100. Werner C, Smith A, Van Aken H. Guidelines on non-anaesthesiologist administration of propofol for gastrointestinal endoscopy: A double-edged sword. *Eur J Anaesthesiol.* 2011;28:553–555.
101. Byrne MF, Baillie J. Nurse-assisted propofol sedation: The jury is in! *Am J Gastroenterol.* 2005;129:1781.
102. Jensen JT, Vilmann P, Horsted T, et al. Nurse-administered propofol sedation for endoscopy: A risk analysis during an implementation phase. *Endoscopy.* 2011;43: 716–722.
103. Cohen LB, Ladas SD, Vargoà JJ, et al. Sedation in digestive endoscopy: The Athens international position statements. *Aliment Pharmacol Ther.* 2010;32: 425–442.
104. Osborn IP, Cohen J, Soper RJ, et al. Laryngeal mask airway—A novel method of airway protection during ERCP: Comparison with endotracheal intubation. *Gastrointest Endosc.* 2002;56:122.
105. Martindale SJ. Anaesthetic considerations during endoscopic retrograde cholangiopancreatography. *Anaesth Intens Care.* 2006;35:302.
106. Lynch CR, Khandekar S, Lynch SM, et al. Sublingual L-hyoscyamine for duodenal antimotility during ERCP: A prospective randomized double-blinded study. *Gastrointest Endosc.* 2007;66:748–752.
107. UK ECT Review Group. Efficacy and safety of electroconvulsive therapy in depressive disorders: A systematic review and meta-analysis. *Lancet.* 2003;361: 9799–808.
108. Ding Z, White PF. Anesthesia for electroconvulsive therapy. *Anesth Analg.* 2002;94:1351.
109. American Psychiatric Association. *The Practice of Electroconvulsive Therapy: Recommendations for Treatment, Training and Privileging.* Washington, DC: American Psychiatric Press; 2000.
110. Patel AS, Gorst-Unsworth C, Venn RM, et al. Anesthesia and electroconvulsive therapy: A retrospective study comparing etomidate and propofol. *J ECT.* 2006;22:179.
111. Datto C, Rai AK, Ilivicky HJ, et al. Augmentation of seizure induction in electroconvulsive therapy: A clinical reappraisal. *J ECT.* 2002;18:118.
112. Chen ST. Remifentanil: A review of its use in electroconvulsive therapy. *J ECT.* 2011;274:323–327.
113. Sawayama E, Takahashi M, Inoue A. Moderate hyperventilation prolongs electroencephalogram seizure duration of the first electroconvulsive therapy. *J ECT.* 2008;24:195–198.
114. Nishihara F, Ohkawa M, Hiraoka H, et al. Benefits of the laryngeal mask for airway management during electroconvulsive therapy. *J ECT.* 2003;19:211.
115. Begec Z, Toprak HI, Demirbilek S, et al. Dexmedetomidine blunts acute hyperdynamic responses to electroconvulsive therapy without altering seizure duration. *Acta Anaesthesiol Scand.* 2008;52:302.
116. Courtman SP, Mumby D. Children with learning disabilities. *Peds Anesth.* 2008;18:198–207.
117. Butler MG, Hayes BG, Hathaway MM, et al. Specific genetic diseases at risk for sedation/anesthesia complications. *Anesth Analg.* 2000;91:837.
118. Bergman SA. Ketamine: Review of its pharmacology and its use in pediatric anesthesia. *Anesth Prog.* 1999;46:10.
119. Todd DW. A comparison of endotracheal intubation and use of the laryngeal mask airway for ambulatory oral surgery patients. *J Oral Maxillofac Surg.* 2002;60:2.
120. Dolling S, Anders NR, Rolfe SE. A comparison of deep vs. awake removal of the laryngeal mask airway in paediatric dental daycase surgery. A randomised controlled trial. *Anaesthesia.* 2003;58:1224.
121. Enever GR, Nunn JH, Sheehan JK. A comparison of post-operative morbidity following outpatient dental care under general anaesthesia in paediatric patients with and without disabilities. *Int J Paediatr Dent.* 2000;10:120.

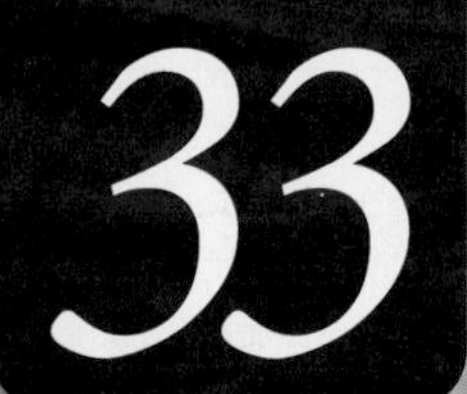

CHAPTER 33

Anesthesia for the Older Patient

G. ALEC ROOKE

Key Points

1. The aging of America presents a medical and economic challenge to the entire health care system as older patients present for surgery in ever-increasing numbers.
2. The aging process affects connective tissue and cellular function, including the mitochondria, and inevitably leads to decreased function and, ultimately, frailty.
3. The rate at which diminished function and frailty develop is highly variable and lends credence to the concept of physiologic age.
4. Decreased organ reserve and increased sensitivity to anesthetic agents result from generalized body composition changes such as connective tissue stiffening and decreased muscle mass, plus impaired autonomic reflexes, and increased sensitivity to drugs.
5. Preoperative preparation will more often involve evaluation of how best to enhance recovery of function after surgery, and discussions surrounding informed consent, living wills, and ethical treatment of the older patient.
6. Intraoperative management must take into account the increased sensitivity to drugs in the elderly patient, as well as an increased likelihood of hemodynamic, pulmonary, and thermoregulatory instability.
7. Analgesia is an important component of postoperative care, but is made more difficult by the increased likelihood of adverse consequences from the analgesic regimen.
8. Perioperative complications, most notably pulmonary, cardiac, and central nervous system complications such as delirium or cognitive decline, occur more commonly in the elderly patient because of an interaction between comorbid disease and the decreased physiologic reserve of aging.

Multimedia

 Age-Related Changes in Body Composition

 Cardiovascular Response to Orthostasis

Age is not a particularly interesting subject. Anyone can get old. All you have to do is live long enough.

—*Don Marquis*

The above quote suggests that aging is dull. To many medical practitioners, it is far worse than "dull." It is frustrating from its complexity of care, and discouraging in its monetary reimbursement. To those concerned with the federal budget, medical care for the aged threatens to bankrupt the nation. Nevertheless, the impact of aging on the practice of medicine is far-reaching and profound, and therefore cannot be ignored. Just as children are not "little adults," the older patient is truly different from the younger adult counterpart. All caregivers, including anesthesiologists, should be knowledgeable of at least some aspects of aging in order to provide intelligent deviation from their standard practice. Basic information is more available than ever before, much of it electronically from the American Society of Anesthesiologists (www.asahq.org), the Society for the Advancement of Geriatric Anesthesia (www.sagahq.org), and the American Geriatrics Society (www.americangeriatrics.org). In reality, caring for an older patient is rarely dull, if for no other reason than their diverse and fascinating lives. Anyone with a passing interest in physiology should enjoy the application of aging physiology to anesthetic management. Yes, their care is often time-consuming, stressful, and requires extra effort, but more often than not it provides the anesthesia caregiver the opportunity to truly practice medicine and make a positive impact on a vulnerable patient's life.

DEMOGRAPHICS AND ECONOMICS OF AGING

I advise you to go on living solely to enrage those who are paying your annuities. It is the only pleasure I have left.

—*Voltaire*

When Social Security was initiated in 1935, only 6.1% of the US population was older than 65 years.[a] By 2010 that percentage had grown to 13% and represented 40 million people. By 2030 it is expected to be nearly 20% of the US population and represent 71 million people. The percentage of the US population older than 85 is expected to double from 2010 (1.9%) to 2040 (estimated 3.7%). The growth of the US population and its older subgroups is shown in (Fig. 33-1). The impact of these statistics is enormous with respect to medical care. In 2007, patients over 65, 13% of the population, accounted for 43% of the total US 165 million inpatient days, a rate per capita 5 times greater than those under 65.[1] Upon examination of the 2006 inpatient and ambulatory procedure data, there were found to be an estimated 73 million surgical and nonsurgical procedures performed in the United States after exclusion of procedures that were unlikely to have involved anesthesia services.[2,3] Of these, 28% were on patients older than 65 years. Thus it appears that people over age 65 have surgery 2.7 times more often than people under age 65.

Federal spending for Medicare in 2011 was $498 billion or
1 13.5% of the federal budget.[b] This amount is more than 2.5 times what was spent in 2000, and represents a 2.2-fold increase per enrollee.[b,c] As impressive as Medicare expenditures may be, federal spending grossly underestimates the total cost of all health care spending for people over age 65. It is estimated that people over age 65 account for nearly half of the nation's health care costs. For 2011, total US health costs are estimated at $2.7 trillion, or approximately 17.7% of the gross national product.[d] In consequence, there is considerable pressure to contain health care costs in this country, including physician reimbursement, by both private insurance companies and the federal government. Unfortunately, federal reimbursement to anesthesiologists is especially poor. In 2004, Medicare reimbursed anesthesia care at approximately 33% of what commercial insurance companies paid.[e] This percentage is in sharp contrast to all other specialties, for which Medicare reimbursement is approximately 83% of commercial rates.[e] The average conversion factor has improved considerably in the last few years. Nevertheless, the 2011 national average value of $21.05 has barely matched inflation since the nadir of $16.60 in 2002.[f] Although Medicare will reimburse at the 50% level for up to four concurrent medically directed procedures, academic programs had been at a disadvantage since faculty are not permitted to staff more than two procedures simultaneously if residents were involved. Fortunately, as of 2010, Medicare reimburses academic institutions at 100% for two concurrent cases.

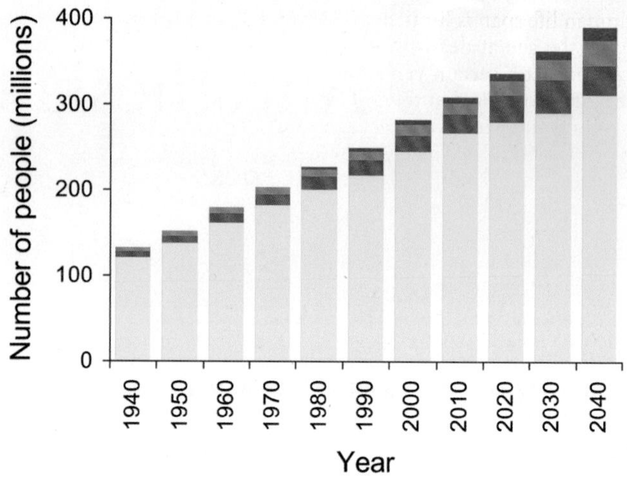

FIGURE 33-1. The actual and estimated US population from 1940 to 2040 is shown broken down by age range. Yellow bar, age <65; purple bar, age 65 to 74; green bar, age ≥75 for years 1940 to 1970, and age 75 to 84 from 1980 on; red bar, age ≥85. Data source: Statistical Abstract of the United States (www.census.gov).

THE PROCESS OF AGING

You can't help getting older, but you don't have to get old.

—*George Burns*

There are many theories of aging, and it is possible that each plays a role in the physiologic changes of aging and the inevitability of death. Some theories of programmed aging suggest that there are genetic codes that dictate how long a cell (and the organism as a whole) will live. This "killer gene" theory would have to confer an advantage to species survival for evolution to result in programmed death. Although this phenomenon does occur in nature (e.g., females of certain species of octopi), there is little evidence that such a mechanism applies to mammals. Another theory of limited cell viability is the attractive hypothesis of telomere shortening. Each time a cell divides, a telomere is cleaved off the DNA. When the DNA runs out of telomeres, the cell cannot divide and will eventually die.[4] Such limited cell division occurs in cultured mammalian cells, and although species life span correlates roughly with the number of allowable cell divisions, there is little evidence that telomere shortening affects human life span. Furthermore, aging involves more than just the death of the organism.

Mammalian aging clearly involves a gradual, cumulative process of damage and deterioration. The question could be posed: Why is such a process allowed in nature? Teleologic reasoning would suggest that once offspring have been raised, there is no further need for continued survival of the individual. Protective mechanisms against aging are costly to the organism, so the "disposable soma" theory of aging states that antiaging mechanisms only need to be good enough to give the next generation the best opportunity to reproduce. In fact, most of the gains in average human life span have been as the result of reducing those factors that cause premature death: Predation, accidents, and disease. The inability to thwart aging completely implies that the average

[a]www.census.gov, accessed Nov. 27, 2011.
[b]http://www.gpoaccess.gov/usbudget/fy11/pdf/hist.pdf, accessed Nov. 29, 2011.
[c]http://www.gpoaccess.gov/usbudget/fy05/pdf/hist.pdf, accessed Nov. 29, 2011.
[d]https://www.cms.gov/NationalHealthExpendData/downloads/proj2010.pdf, accessed Nov. 29, 2011.
[e]http://www.gao.gov/new.items/d07463.pdf.
[f]https://www.cms.gov/center/anesth.asp.

human life span is limited, and that if everyone died only of "old age," the age at death would end up being a bell-shaped curve centered at a certain value, probably around age 85.[5] Nevertheless, it is possible that the bell-shaped curve could be shifting to a higher value, but how far it can be shifted is unclear.

A variety of deleterious processes continually attack DNA,
2 proteins, and lipids. The primary culprits are free radicals and nonenzymatic glycosylation of sugars and amines. Free radicals are a by-product of oxidative metabolism, whereas glycosylation is enhanced by elevated glucose levels. Many of the changes associated with aging are the result of damage to protein. Collagen becomes stiffer from aromatic ring cleavage and by cross-linking to other collagen molecules. Elastin, once damaged and removed, is usually replaced by the stiffer collagen. In the cardiovascular system, arteries, veins, and the myocardium all stiffen with age. In contrast, lung parenchyma becomes less stiff because of loss of elastin without collagen substitution. DNA damage occurs as well and, curiously, mitochondrial DNA suffers more damage than nuclear DNA. In fact, one hypothesis of terminal aging and death is that we run out of energy as the mitochondria become less able to produce ATP. Damage to lipids also appears to play a major role in senescence and life span.[6] Caloric restriction, well documented to increase life span in small mammals, probably does so by decreasing the rate of oxidative damage.

Functional Reserve and the Concept of Frailty

Old age is no place for sissies.

—*Bette Davis*

Functional reserve represents the degree to which organ function can increase above the level necessary for basal activity. For healthy individuals, reserve peaks at approximately age 30, gradually declines over the next several decades, and then experiences more rapid decline beginning around the eighth decade. Assessment of reserve is something anesthesiologists perform all the time. For example, the ability to achieve a minimum of four metabolic equivalents appears to confer enough cardiovascular reserve to tolerate the stress of most surgical procedures.[7] Even without formal assessment, an intuitive sense of reserve is often obtained through simple observation. A person who looks and acts old presumably has suffered more from the aging process, regardless of chronologic age. The loss of subcutaneous tissue, unsteady or slowed gait, decreased cognition or memory, a stooped body habitus, and minimal muscle mass all contribute to the impression of frailty. It turns out that some of these traits may well correlate with reserve. For example, sarcopenia is a serious problem for the very old, and when severe enough, can lead to an accelerated deterioration with further weight loss, mental and physical decline, and increased mortality.[8] Indexes of frailty have been constructed and found to not only correlate with disability and mortality in community dwelling elderly, but also correlate with postoperative complications, especially the likelihood of discharge to a skilled or assisted living facility.[9,10]

Physiologic Age

If you didn't know how old you were, how old would you be?

—*James Hubert 'Eubie' Blake*

3 The aging process is highly variable from one individual to the next. The older we get, the more different we become. Ideally, an index of physiologic age would be available that would quantify functional reserve. One interesting approach to this objective that is available to the lay public is to quantify many of the known modifiable and nonmodifiable factors that influence life expectancy.[g] By plugging one's individual data into the program, a measure of how old you are relative to your chronologic age is provided, plus tips on how you can improve your health status and "lower" your age. Such an approach may be useful for promoting a healthy lifestyle, but does not address the ultimate goal of being able to quantify the reserve of each organ system, including the brain, and predict the risk of common perioperative complications.

THE PHYSIOLOGY OF ORGAN AGING

"If I'd known I was going to live this long, I'd have taken better care of myself."

—*James Hubert 'Eubie' Blake, age 100*

Defining what constitutes "normal aging" is difficult. Is it what happens under the best of circumstances, or what happens to the "average" person? Comparisons of young and elderly subjects may not strictly reflect aging, as the elderly subjects may have experienced a much different diet, lifestyle, and environmental exposure than what the young group will experience by the time they become old. Following a group of healthy subjects over a long period is more likely to define the effects of aging, but not all available data come from such longitudinal studies. Studies that examine only the very old persons may actually underestimate the typical effects of aging because individuals generally do not achieve old age unless there is something intrinsically robust about them. Lastly, the reader is reminded that, as with the discussion of physiologic age, the effects of aging apply in varying degrees to any given patient, and that disease will interact with aging to further diminish functional organ reserve.

Changes in Body Composition, and Liver and Kidney Aging

I have everything I had twenty years ago, only it's all a little bit lower.

—*Gypsy Rose Lee*

Changes in body composition are primarily characterized by a gradual loss of skeletal muscle and an increase in body fat, although
1 the latter is more prominent in women (Fig. 33-2). Basal metabolism declines with age, with most of the decline accounted for by the change in body composition.[11] There is a reduction in total
4 body water that reflects the reduction in cellular water that is associated with a loss of muscle and an increase in adipose tissue.[12] Aging causes a small decrease in plasma albumin levels; however, there is a small increase in α_1 acid glycoprotein.[13] The effect of these changes on drug protein binding and drug delivery, however, appear to be minimal.

Liver mass decreases with age, and accounts for most, but not all, of the 20% to 40% decrease in liver blood flow.[14] There is also a modest reduction in phase I drug metabolism and bile secretion with age. Other than the effect of aging on drug metabolism, liver reserve should be more than adequate even in the very old in the absence of disease.

Renal cortical mass also decreases by 20% to 25% with age, but the most prominent effect of aging is the loss of up to half of the

[g]www.RealAge.com, accessed Dec. 5, 2011.

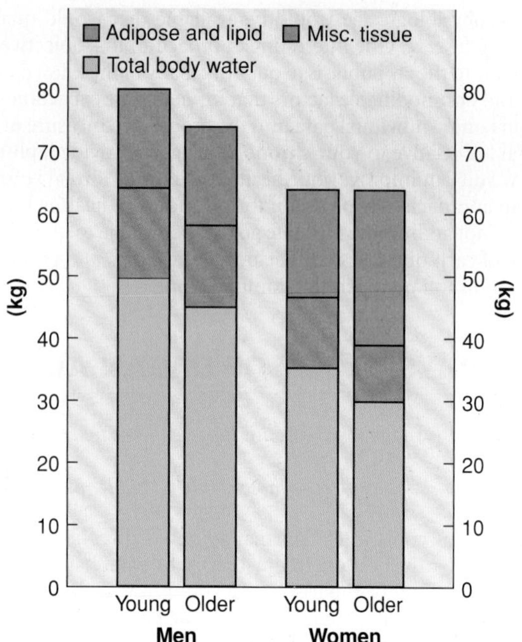

FIGURE 33-2. Age-related changes in body composition are gender-specific. In women, total body mass remains constant because increases in body fat (*upper shaded segment*) offset bone loss (*middle segment*) and intracellular dehydration (*lower shaded segment*). In men, body mass declines despite maintenance of body lipid and skeletal tissue elements because accelerating loss of skeletal muscle and other components of lean tissue mass produces marked contraction of intracellular water (*lower shaded segment*).

glomeruli by age 80.[15] The decrease in the glomerular filtration rate of approximately 1 mL/min/yr after age 40 typically reduces renal excretion of drugs to a level where drug dosage adjustment becomes a progressively important consideration beginning at approximately age 60. Nevertheless, the degree of decline in glomerular filtration rate is highly variable and is likely to be much less than predicted in many individuals, especially those who avoid excessive dietary protein.[16]

The aged kidney does not eliminate or retain sodium when necessary as effectively as that of a young adult.[16] Part of the failure to conserve sodium when appropriate may be because of reduced aldosterone secretion. Similarly, the aged kidney does not retain or eliminate free water as rapidly as young kidneys when challenged by water deprivation or free water excess. Lastly, the sensation of thirst declines with age. In short, fluid and electrolyte homeostasis is more vulnerable in the older patient, particularly when an older patient suffers acute injury or disease and eating and drinking becomes more of a chore.

For the most part, functional endocrine decline does not interact with anesthetic management to any significant degree. However, aging is associated with decreased insulin secretion in response to a glucose load, and also increased insulin resistance, particularly in skeletal muscle.[17] Thus, even healthy elderly patients may require insulin therapy more often perioperatively than young adults. Aging also results in decreases in testosterone, estrogen, and growth hormone production.[18] The use of hormonal therapy to reduce sarcopenia, frailty in general, and cognitive decline and dementia is the subject of considerable current investigation, but has no current application to anesthetic management.

Central Nervous System Aging

By the time you're eighty years old you've learned everything. You only have to remember it.

—*George Burns*

Brain mass begins to decrease slowly beginning at approximately age 50 and declines more rapidly later, such that an 80-year-old brain has typically lost 10% of its weight.[19] Neurotransmitter functions suffer more significantly, including dopamine, serotonin, γ-aminobutyric acid, and especially the acetylcholine system.[20] The latter is especially important because of its connection to Alzheimer's disease. Response times increase, and learning is more difficult, but vocabulary, "wisdom," and past knowledge are better preserved.[19] Nevertheless, of those individuals aged 85 and older, nearly half have significant cognitive impairment. In addition, some degree of atherosclerosis appears to be inevitable. Fortunately, and contrary to prior belief, the aged brain does make new neurons and is capable of forming new dendritic connections.[21]

Perhaps the best-known effect of brain aging as it applies to anesthesia is the approximately 6% decrease in MAC (minimum alveolar concentration) per decade after age 40.[22] This effect of aging is relatively simple to deal with in the clinical arena. Much more difficult is the potential interaction of anesthesia, the stress of surgery, and a brain with minimal reserve. Age is a major risk factor for postoperative delirium and/or cognitive decline (see "Perioperative Complications"). The other pertinent brain aging phenomenon is pharmacodynamic.

Drug Pharmacology and Aging

I don't do alcohol anymore – I get the same effect just standing up fast.

—*Author Unknown*

Drugs typically have a more pronounced effect in an older patient. The cause can be either pharmacodynamic, in which case the target organ (often the brain) is more sensitive to a given drug tissue level, or the cause can be pharmacokinetic, in which case a given dose of drug commonly produces higher blood levels in older patients.

Most intravenous anesthetic drugs are highly lipid soluble and so begin to enter tissue even before fully mixed in the blood. The rate of transfer depends on the rate of delivery (concentration times blood flow per gram of tissue), the concentration gradient of the drug between the blood and the tissue (obviously a high gradient initially), the ease with which the drug crosses the blood and tissue membranes, and the solubility of the drug in the tissue. Thus, the vessel-rich group (brain, heart, kidney, muscle) will acquire drug much more rapidly than the vessel-poor group (fat, bone). Protein binding may affect transfer, with drugs that are highly protein-bound having a lower free concentration and a slower rate of transfer.

Given the preceding, there are many ways for a drug bolus to have a more pronounced initial effect on older patients. During the drug redistribution phase the blood concentration typically is higher in older patients, partly because of a mildly contracted blood volume and partly because the reduction in muscle mass slows removal of the drug from blood. By keeping drug blood levels higher for a longer time, more drug will be driven into the other organs of the vessel-rich group such as brain (often the target organ) or heart. A prime example of this phenomenon is sodium pentothal, and to a lesser degree, propofol.[23]

Despite the fact that drugs typically have a greater effect on older patients, there is a general impression that bolus drugs take longer to achieve that greater effect. It is not entirely clear why this is so. Slower circulation is sometimes hypothesized, but total blood flow to any organ does not appear to decrease beyond that expected from the decrease in organ mass. Another possibility is a slower rate of transfer into the target organ. Drug effects are the result of tissue, not plasma concentrations. Brain–plasma equilibration is not instantaneous, and for at least some drugs (e.g., remifentanil), the equilibration half-life is prolonged in older brains.[24] Why crossing the blood–brain barrier should take longer with age is not understood.

Ultimately, though, the drug will distribute throughout the body based on tissue mass and solubility. Because most intravenous drugs used in anesthesia are highly lipid-soluble, most of the drug will end up in fat. How completely the drug is dispersed out of the blood and into the tissue is reflected by Vd_{ss}, the drug's volume of distribution at steady state. This variable is expressed as the liters of plasma that would be necessary to dilute the amount of drug administered down to the concentration observed in the plasma. As such, drugs that are very fat-soluble can have a value for Vd_{ss} that is several times greater than total body water. After the initial redistribution into vessel-rich group tissue, the drug will slowly diffuse back into the plasma as it continues to be absorbed into fat. In so doing, the target organ (e.g., brain) drug level will fall because the target organ is always in the vessel-rich group. Once a single therapeutic dose of a drug has fully distributed throughout the body, the blood and target organ drug levels are typically too low to have a meaningful clinical effect. However, very large doses, repeated doses, or infusions will eventually deliver enough drug to yield residual drug levels that produce therapeutic effects. At this point, the only way to decrease blood and target organ levels and eliminate the drug's effects is through metabolism. The elimination or metabolic half-life of a drug in the blood equals the volume of distribution at steady state (Vd_{ss}) divided by the clearance, where clearance represents the amount of blood from which drug is eliminated per minute.

The most prominent and consistent pharmacokinetic effect of aging is a decrease in drug metabolism, typically due to both a decrease in clearance and an increase in Vd_{ss} (Fig. 33-3). The increase in Vd_{ss} with age is likely due to the increase in body fat. Clearance decreases with age for any drug metabolized by the liver or kidney. When drug metabolism is via the liver, decreased

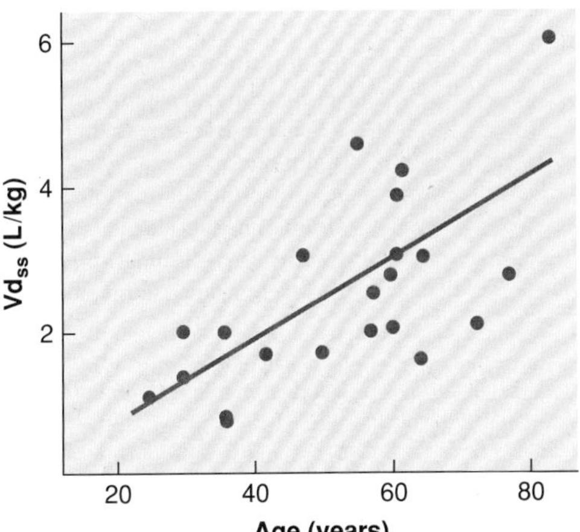

FIGURE 33-3. The effect of age on the volume of distribution at steady state (Vd_{ss}) for pentothal in women. (Reprinted from: Jung D, Mayersohn M, Perrier D, et al. Thiopental disposition as a function of age in female patients undergoing surgery. *Anesthesiology*. 1982;56:263, with permission.)

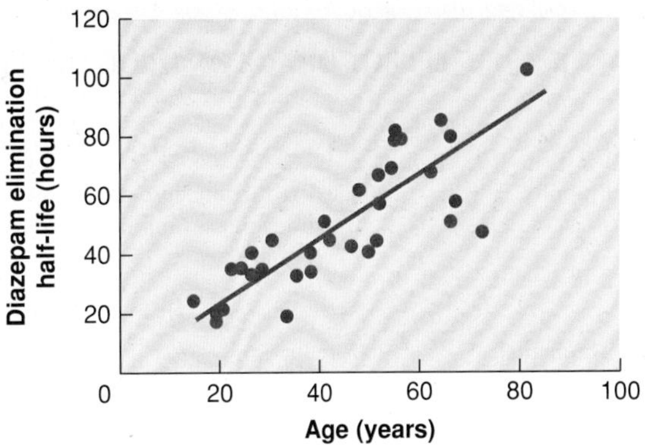

FIGURE 33-4. The effect of age on the elimination half-life of diazepam. The half-life in hours is equal to approximately the patient's age in years. (Reprinted from: Klotz U, Avant GR, Hoyumpa A, et al. The effects of age and liver disease on the disposition and elimination of diazepam in adult men. *J Clin Invest*. 1975;55:347, with permission.)

liver mass and blood flow will decrease clearance for both high and low extraction drugs. In addition, elderly patients are often on a host of chronic medications, a setup for drug interactions as well as for inhibition of drug metabolism. Drugs with primarily renal elimination will experience decreased metabolism because of reductions in glomerular filtration rate with aging. The net effect on drug metabolism is typically a doubling of the elimination half-life between old and young adults. However, with some drugs, the effect on half-life can be dramatic. In the case of diazepam, the half-life in hours is roughly equal to the patient's age (Fig. 33-4).[25] For a 72-year-old person, it would therefore require 3 days to metabolize half of a dose of diazepam. Such pharmacokinetics clearly illustrate why there is no place in modern medicine for the chronic use of diazepam and other drugs with similar half-lives when the desired effect is supposed to be transient (e.g., as a sleeping aid).

When dealing with infusions—or for that matter a series of bolus injections—the time it takes to decrease the blood and target organ drug levels to below the therapeutic threshold will depend on many factors. This is where the concept of the context-sensitive half-time proves useful; that is, the time necessary for a 50% (or any desired percent) decrease in plasma concentration following termination of an infusion. At one extreme, if the residual level produced by the cumulative drug administration is still very low, and only a modest decrease in blood level is necessary to reverse the drug effect, then the rapid redistribution of the most recently administered drug will lead to a rapid decrease in the blood level and termination of effect. At the other extreme, if there has been significant accumulation of drug in the body, and/or the maintenance blood level was high, then a long time may be required to decrease the drug levels enough to terminate the drug effect. As a general rule, the time to decrease the effect-site drug concentration is increased most dramatically by aging when a large percentage decrease in plasma level is necessary to dip below the therapeutic threshold.[26]

Review of the literature can yield a confusing picture when trying to sort out what pharmacologic variable is responsible for a given clinical effect. Fortunately, one does not need to know such details in order to use anesthetic drugs in an intelligent fashion with older patients. Table 33-1 summarizes some of this information for many of the common anesthetic drugs.[26–29] The effect of aging on sedative–hypnotic agents variably involves both pharmacodynamic and pharmacokinetic changes (Table 33-1).

TABLE 33-1. EFFECT OF AGE ON DRUG DOSING

Drug	Bolus Administration	Multiple Boluses or Infusion	Comments[a]
Propofol	20–60% reduction, dose on lean body mass, 1 mg/kg in very old	50% reduction, infusions beyond 50 min progressively increase the time required to decrease the blood level by 50% (but effect-site levels may decrease faster in elderly)	↑ brain sensitivity (by some reports), decreased V_{cen}, slowed redistribution
Thiopental	20% reduction	20% reduction	= brain sensitivity, decreased V_{cen}, slowed redistribution
Etomidate	25–50% reduction	—	= brain sensitivity
Midazolam	Compared to age 20, modest reduction at age 60, 75% reduction at age 90	Similar to bolus (metabolic $t_{½}$ longer, but not meaningful unless very large doses are used)	↑↑ brain sensitivity
Morphine	Probably 50% reduction. Peak morphine effect is 90 min (though half of peak effect at 5 min)	Long effect-site equilibration time translates into very slow reduction in effect on termination of infusion (4 h for 50% reduction)	Metabolite morphine-6-glucoronide build-up requires prolonged morphine use, but its renal excretion will make it very long-acting
Fentanyl	50% reduction	50% reduction	↑ brain sensitivity, minimal changes in pharmacokinetics; delayed absorption from fentanyl patch
Alfentanil, sufentanil	50% reduction	50% reduction	Probably ↑ brain sensitivity, minimal changes in pharmacokinetics
Remifentanil	50% reduction	50% reduction	Slower blood–brain equilibration, suggesting slower onset and offset, modest decreased V_{cen}
Hydromorphone	No studies on aging exist, but assume increased potency in elderly	Assume 50% reduction	Compared with morphine, no active metabolite, faster onset
Methadone	No studies on aging exist, but assume increased potency in elderly	Assume 50% reduction	—
Meperidine	Use only for postoperative shivering	Do not use	Toxic metabolite normeperidine, whose renal excretion decreases with age
Vecuronium	Slower onset (≈33%)	Slower recovery times	Slightly greater liver metabolism than renal, age nearly doubles metabolic $t_{½}$
Mivacurium	Equally fast onset in young and old	Modest dose reduction for infusion, longer recovery time on repeated bolus	Elimination by plasma cholinesterase, modest prolongation of metabolic $t_{½}$ by age
Cisatracurium	Slower onset (≈33%)	No significant changes with age	Mostly Hoffmann elimination, modest prolongation of metabolic $t_{½}$ by age
Rocuronium	Minimally slower onset	—	Liver metabolism slightly greater than renal, modest increase in metabolic $t_{½}$ by age
Pancuronium	—	—	Primarily renal elimination, aging doubles metabolic $t_{½}$
Pipecuronium	Slower onset (≈50%), elderly may be *less* sensitive	—	Primarily renal elimination, no apparent change in metabolic $t_{½}$
Succinylcholine	Slower onset (≈40%)	—	
Edrophonium	Similar dosing and onset	—	↑ V_{cen}, primarily renal elimination, modest increase in metabolic $t_{½}$ by age
Neostigmine	Despite pharmacokinetic changes, some studies indicate need for increased dose with age	—	↑ V_{cen}, hepatic elimination, modest increase in metabolic $t_{½}$ by age

[a]V_{cen}, central volume of distribution or initial volume of distribution. Although V_{cen} does not have an anatomic correlate, a smaller V_{cen} will increase initial plasma levels and enhance transfer of the drug in the target organ (e.g., brain, muscle).

For the opioids, the older brain appears to be more sensitive than that of young adults, whereas the pharmacokinetics of opioids are largely unaffected by age.

Despite the loss of muscle and motor neurons with age, muscle relaxants do not appear to be more potent in the older patient when steady-state blood levels for a given level of paralysis are compared. Muscle relaxants often have a decreased initial volume of distribution, but this pharmacokinetic change does not seem to translate into smaller doses. For drugs eliminated by the liver or kidney, and where the effect of a bolus is eliminated primarily by redistribution, multiple doses will result in drug accumulation, and each subsequent dose will have a more prolonged effect. This phenomenon will be exaggerated in elderly patients because of decreased metabolic elimination, and will be most prominent with the long-acting agents. Given the risk of residual neuromuscular blockade with long-acting drugs such as pancuronium, coupled with the muscle and nervous system changes of aging that increase the risk of ventilatory failure or aspiration postoperatively, it can be argued that long-acting neuromuscular blocking agents should be used very carefully in an older patient, if at all.

Cardiovascular Aging

A man is as old as his arteries.

—*Thomas Sydenham*

Virtually all components of the cardiovascular system are affected by the aging process. The major changes include (1) decreased response to β-receptor stimulation; (2) stiffening of the myocardium, arteries, and veins; (3) changes in the autonomic nervous system with increased sympathetic activity and decreased parasympathetic activity; (4) conduction system changes; and (5) defective ischemic preconditioning. Although atherosclerosis appears to affect everyone by virtue of the fact that the mechanisms of aging contribute to the development of atherosclerosis, it is not clear that it inevitably leads to functional impairment or disease.

With age, increased sympathetic activity is present at rest and there is typically an exaggerated response to stimuli that increase sympathetic activity.[30] Although there is some evidence of decreased responsiveness of α-receptors with age, it apparently is not enough to prevent changes in vascular resistance from making a significant contribution to the lability in blood pressure observed during anesthesia or contribute to the decrease in blood pressure when anesthesia removes that sympathetic tone.[31,32]

The efficacy of baroreflex control of blood pressure decreases with age.[33] The mechanism is primarily a decrease in the heart rate response and not a decrease in the baroreflex control of vascular tone. The decreased heart rate response to changes in blood pressure is in part due to lesser vagal tone at rest but the major mechanism is a decrease in the cardiac response to β-receptor stimulation.[32] The mechanism does not appear to be a downregulation of β-receptors on the heart, but a defect in the intracellular coupling. Both heart rate and contractility increase less in response to endogenous release or exogenous administration of catecholamines. The increase in heart rate with exercise is therefore also diminished, as is maximal heart rate (often quoted as 220 minus age), and the decrement contributes to the decreased exertional capacity with age, even in trained individuals. The decrease in resting vagal tone may limit the increase in heart rate after administration of atropine or glycopyrrolate.

Conductance artery (aorta to arterioles) stiffening typically leads to systolic hypertension via two mechanisms.[34,35] First, much of the stroke volume is stored in the thoracic aorta during ejection. Pressure must increase more to stretch out a stiffened aorta to accommodate that volume. Secondly, generalized arterial stiffening causes the pressure wave to transmit more rapidly. In everyone, the pressure wave reflects off the arterial walls and branch points and returns to the thoracic aorta, but the reflected waves return more rapidly in an older person. In young people, the reflected waves do not reach the heart until after ejection is complete. These waves are responsible for the modest bump in pressure in the aortic root just after the dicrotic notch. But in older people, the reflected waves return to the heart by late ejection and increase the pressure against which the left ventricle must pump to complete the stroke volume. At the end of ejection the ventricular contraction weakens, so ideal coupling would have the ventricle pushing against an ever-decreasing pressure. Since in the older person the ventricle must now pump against a higher pressure, this increased stress to the muscle stimulates hypertrophy.

Hypertrophy in and of itself stiffens the ventricle, but even worse, hypertrophy slows diastolic relaxation that, in turn, impairs ventricular filling in early diastole. The left ventricle now becomes more dependent on the atrial kick and requires an increase in left atrial pressure in order to preserve diastolic filling. The increase in atrial pressure is present at rest, but can be quite dynamic with acute increases during stress such as tachycardia. This phenomenon, termed *diastolic dysfunction,* increases in severity with age. The majority of cases of congestive heart failure in very old persons are due to diastolic dysfunction and occur in the absence of clinically significant systolic dysfunction.[32,36]

Adequate ventricular filling becomes more critical with age. The decreased response to β-receptor stimulation requires the ventricles to depend more on an adequate end-diastolic volume to generate enough contractile strength via the length–tension (Frank–Starling) relationship. The diastolic dysfunction requires an increase in central and pulmonary venous pressure to maintain that end-diastolic volume. The range in acceptable filling pressures ends up becoming narrower with age because too low a pressure results in inadequate filling. Since the normal pressure is already elevated, any further increase is that much closer to a pressure that results in fluid extravasation and adverse consequences such as pulmonary edema.

Unfortunately, aging also decreases the ability to maintain filling pressures in the acceptable range. In everyone, the veins serve as a reservoir for blood and serve to buffer changes in blood volume in order to maintain central blood volume and ventricular filling at an appropriate level. However, veins stiffen with age.[37] Venous stiffening impairs this buffering capacity and creates a situation where modest changes in venous blood volume may produce more dramatic changes in venous pressures and cardiac filling. In short, the system has become inherently more unstable as illustrated by the development of postural hypotension in elderly persons but not in young adults with mild hypovolemia (Fig. 33-5).[38]

Rhythm disturbances may develop with age. Fibrosis of the conduction system may lead to conduction blocks, and loss of sinoatrial node cells may make the older patient more prone to sick sinus syndrome. The prevalence of atrial fibrillation exponentially climbs with age, perhaps in part because of atrial enlargement with age.

Aging appears to diminish or even eliminate any protective effect of ischemic preconditioning, a phenomenon whereby a brief period of myocardial ischemia will lessen the adverse effects of a subsequent, more prolonged ischemic event. "Warm-up angina" is the ability to achieve a higher level of exertion after first exercising to the point of angina. Starting around age 65 the increment in the level of exertion progressively diminishes with age.[32] In younger adults, death or heart failure is a less frequent complication of a myocardial infarction if the patient had been

ANESTHETIC MANAGEMENT

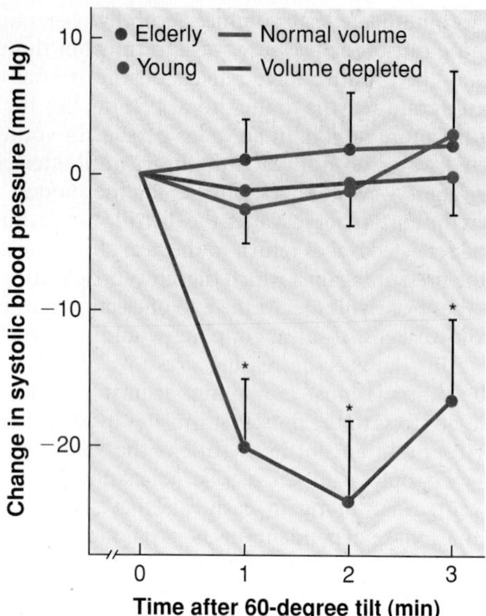

FIGURE 33-5. Young and elderly adults are subjected to a passive tilt test in their euvolemic state and after an approximate 2 kg of water and 100 mEq of sodium loss. With tilt, blood pools in the legs. Although young subjects tolerate tilt under both circumstances, the combination of hypovolemia and tilt exceeds the compensatory mechanisms of the older subjects. (Reprinted from: Shannon RP, Wei JY, Rosa RM, et al. The effect of age and sodium depletion on cardiovascular response to orthostasis. *Hypertension.* 1986;8:438, with permission.)

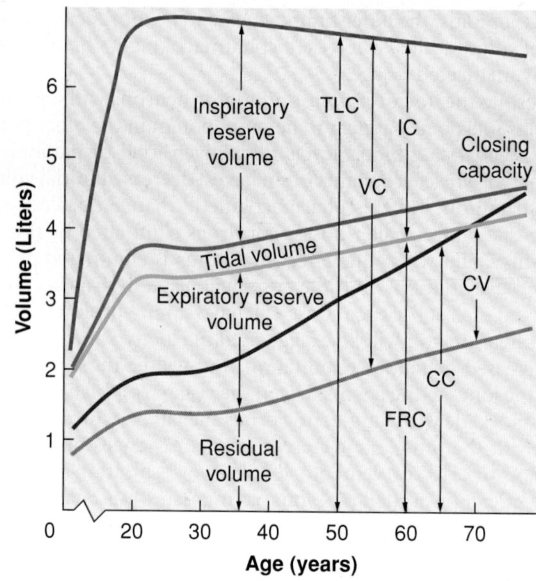

FIGURE 33-6. Effect of aging on lung volumes. With age, inspiratory capacity (IC) is compromised because of the combined effect of modest decreases in total lung capacity (TLC) and modest increase in functional residual capacity (FRC). Vital capacity (VC) decreases because of the decrease in IC and the increase in residual volume. However, the most dramatic change with aging is the increase in closing volume (CV) and closing capacity (CC) such that in very old persons, closing capacity exceeds functional residual capacity. (Reprinted from: Smith TC. Respiratory system: Aging, adversity, and anesthesia. In: McLeskey CH, ed. *Geriatric Anesthesiology.* 1st ed. Baltimore, MD: Williams & Wilkins; 1997:85, with permission.)

experiencing angina within 2 weeks of the myocardial infarction. This protective effect of angina is not present in older adults.[32]

This section began with a quote from Thomas Sydenham. Evidence is mounting that the quote is truly prophetic: Arterial stiffening may indeed be a marker of physiologic age. One of the manifestations of arterial stiffening is a widened pulse pressure. Once the difference between the systolic and the diastolic pressure reaches 80 mm Hg or more, there is a clear association with all-cause mortality, cardiovascular mortality, and a variety of morbidities including stroke, coronary disease, and renal failure.[34,39] Increased pulse pressure is also associated with increased morbidity and mortality after coronary artery bypass grafting.[34]

Pulmonary Aging

The most prominent effects of aging on the pulmonary system are increased stiffness of the chest wall and a decreased stiffness of the lung parenchyma.[40,41] Chest wall stiffening increases the work of breathing and also produces a more barrel-shaped thorax that leads to flattening of the diaphragm. Less diaphragmatic curvature provides a mechanical disadvantage for the generation of negative pressure in the intrapleural space. The stiffened chest wall, flattened diaphragm, and the loss of muscle mass from aging all combine to make the older patient more prone to fatigue when challenged by an increase in minute ventilation, and thus more likely to experience respiratory failure.

The decrease in lung tissue stiffness is due to a loss of elastin with age. Unlike elsewhere in the body, the elastin is not replaced with collagen and so the lungs become easier to inflate. There are several adverse effects of this increase in compliance. Small airways do not have enough inherent stiffness and so depend on tethering by the surrounding tissue to remain open. The degree of outward pull by the tissue depends on the stiffness of the tissue and the degree of stretch of the tissue. As the tissue loses its springiness, greater lung inflation is needed to produce the same amount of outward pull on the airways. The need for greater lung inflation to prevent small airway collapse is reflected by the increase in closing capacity with age (Fig. 33-6). Closing capacity typically exceeds functional residual capacity in the mid-60s, and will eventually exceed the tidal volume at some later age. Decreased lung tissue stiffness also increases ventilation–perfusion mismatch as each piece of lung tissue is less tethered to its neighbor, making ventilation less uniform. These changes, plus a modest reduction in alveolar surface area with age, contribute to a modest decline in resting Pa_{O_2} with age.[42]

Less-effective small airway tethering also leads to greater limitations during forced exhalation such as is present during exercise. At all ages, forced exhalation produces positive pressures in the intrapleural space that tend to compress intrathoracic airways. Only the airway connective tissue and lung tissue tethering oppose that compression. With less lung tissue tethering, airways compress at a larger lung volume in older subjects and produce a limitation in air flow during exhalation over a much larger percentage of the exhaled tidal volume (e.g., the last 45% in a 70-year-old person) than in a younger subject (e.g., 20% in a 30-year-old person).[43]

Changes within the nervous system further influence the respiratory system. Aging leads to an approximate 50% decrease in the ventilatory response to hypercapnia, and an even greater decrease in the response to hypoxia, especially at night.[44] Generalized loss of muscle tone with age applies to the hypopharyngeal and genioglossal muscles and predisposes elderly persons to upper airway obstruction. A high percentage, perhaps even 75%, of people over age 65 have sleep-disordered breathing, a phenomenon that may or may not be the same as sleep apnea, but certainly places the elderly people at increased risk of hypoxia postoperatively.[45] Aging also results in less-effective coughing and impaired swallowing. Aspiration is a significant cause of community-acquired pneumonia and may well play a role in the development of postoperative pneumonia.[46]

Thermoregulation and Aging

In the past decade or so, there has been heightened awareness of the adverse consequences of perioperative hypothermia as well as improved methods to prevent hypothermia. Even outside the operating room, elderly individuals are prone to hypothermia when stressed by modestly cold environments that would not affect younger individuals. The initial response to a cold environment is vasoconstriction, and if that response is insufficient and the subject becomes colder, then shivering is the second response. Both mechanisms are triggered by decreases in core and/or skin temperature. The two temperatures interact such that a decrease in skin temperature of 1 degree will initiate vasoconstriction or shivering at a core temperature approximately 0.2 degrees higher than would have otherwise occurred.[47] Although there is great variability among the elderly over the degree to which vasoconstriction and shivering are impaired, one should anticipate that elderly patients will have impaired vasoconstriction and metabolic heat production.[48]

At all ages, both inhalational and some intravenous agents (e.g., propofol and alfentanil but not midazolam) alter the regulatory thresholds such that body temperature must fall by as much as 4°C (7°F) before initiation of vasoconstriction or shivering. Aging further impairs the thresholds, by approximately 1°C (2°F), not only during general anesthesia but during spinal anesthesia as well.[47]

Given the impaired temperature regulation and decreased heat production of the elderly, it is not surprising that hypothermia occurs more frequently in older patients.[49] The risks of hypothermia include myocardial ischemia, surgical wound infection, coagulopathy with increased blood loss, and impaired drug metabolism.[47] Shivering places a significant metabolic stress on a patient and may not be well tolerated by a patient with borderline cardiac or pulmonary reserve. The prevention and treatment of hypothermia in an elderly patient does not appear to be any different than for younger adults.

CONDUCT OF ANESTHESIA

We've put more effort into helping folks reach old age than into helping them enjoy it.

—Frank A. Clark

The Preoperative Visit

The preoperative visit can be extremely important in the care of the elderly patient. Although the goals of the visit are no different than for any other patient, there are issues more common among the elderly population that should be raised. For example, will the patient's living situation provide the support necessary for a successful recovery? An aged spouse may not be physically capable of helping the patient dress, bath or perform some other activity of daily living (ADL) that the surgery temporarily prevents the patient from performing. Furthermore, elderly patients may require a long time to return to their preoperative level of function, assuming full recovery is even possible. For example, after major abdominal surgery, most older patients require at least 3 months for activities of daily living (ADLs) and independent ADLs to return to baseline.[50] Persistent disability at 6 months varies with the task. Although there is only a 9% incidence of persistent ADL deficits, there is a 19% incidence of deficit in independent ADLs, and a 52% incidence of diminished grip strength.

5 Older patients often recognize that the end of their lives is no longer the theoretical consideration of youth, so they are more likely to have living wills, health care proxies, and health care directives in place at the time of surgery. The older patient's expectations from surgery may be much different than that of their younger counterparts, and medical practitioners must be careful not to judge a patient's decision making based on the practitioner's values or expectations. This is particularly important when questions of competence arise and the physician could be tempted to question competence if the patient's decision does not coincide with the opinion of the physician.[51] A discussion of risks and benefits needs to include the probable degree of functional recovery and the speed with which that recovery is likely to occur. If health care directives prohibit various life-sustaining or resuscitative procedures, the patient/proxy and anesthesiologist must come to a mutual understanding of what will or will not be performed if an untoward event occurs in the perioperative period.

Polypharmacy and drug interactions are a huge problem for the elderly. As much as 30% of ambulatory older adults require medical care for adverse drug events, and upward of 30% of hospitalizations in the elderly are related to drug effects.[52] In fact, one of the major goals of geriatric consult services to surgical patients is to pare down those medications whenever possible. The anesthesiologist can help by alerting the primary care team to this issue and suggest a geriatric consult. In the very old, dehydration, elder abuse, and malnutrition are all more common than generally appreciated. In the case of malnutrition, the deficit may be limited to isolated deficiencies such as vitamin D or B_{12}, or it may be more global and include inadequate caloric intake from poor oral hygiene or the "anorexia of aging," in which neuroendocrine changes lead to early satiety and diminished sense of taste.[53] Nutritional status is an underappreciated risk factor for surgery. In fact, the Veterans Affairs National Surgical Quality Improvement Program found albumin to be as sensitive an index for mortality or morbidity as any other single indicator, including the American Society of Anesthesiologists status.[54]

Intraoperative Management

6 There is no simple cookbook on how to administer anesthesia to an older patient. Drug effects on any given patient are highly variable, and leaves a certain amount of guesswork for at least what the initial dose should be. Basic principles of drug use include smaller doses than with young adults, and the efficacy of using less drug becomes more apparent if the practitioner is patient enough to allow more time for the drug to achieve its peak effect. As with any tenuous patient, the art of anesthesia is an essential component of good care.

For induction, a given blood level of propofol causes a greater decrease in brain activity in an older patient, but the decrease in blood pressure is even more dramatic in comparison to the decrease observed in young adults.[55] Many strategies can be used to minimize the decrease in blood pressure, but most attempt to reduce the amount of propofol with the use of adjuncts such as opioids, or combining small doses of propofol with etomidate.

ANESTHETIC MANAGEMENT

Some advocate induction with a propofol infusion of 400 μg/kg/min to lessen the risk of overdose.[28] Etomidate has been observed to produce less hypotension than propofol in older patients.[56] Nevertheless, almost any standard technique is safe if performed carefully. Hypo- or hypertension, or both, may occur during induction, intubation, and the postintubation–preincision period. Cycling the blood pressure cuff every minute should alert the practitioner to these changes sooner than would less frequent cycling. Although swings in blood pressure may not be desirable, there is no evidence that even major, but brief, changes in blood pressure lead to adverse outcomes.

Whether general or neuraxial anesthesia is used, induction and maintenance of anesthesia will commonly result in a significant decrease in systemic blood pressure, more so than typically occurs in younger patients.[57] Although decreases in both systemic vascular resistance and cardiac output likely occur, the decrease in vascular resistance is probably the largest contributor, although this observation has really been confirmed only during spinal anesthesia.[31] Figure 33-7 demonstrates this dramatic decrease in vascular resistance and further shows that venous pooling is responsible for a decrease in preload that in turn decreases cardiac output. Because vascular resistance contributes significantly to the decrease in blood pressure during anesthesia, it has been argued that the use of α-agonists is an appropriate therapy and may be more effective than volume alone.[31] α-agonists also tend to promote venoconstriction, thereby shifting blood back to the central circulation and presumably reducing the need for at least some volume administration. Although no one would advocate vasoconstriction as a treatment for hypovolemia (except as a stopgap measure), the ventricle can only get so big; therefore, it is impossible for volume administration alone to raise cardiac output enough to compensate for a large decrease in vascular resistance. Furthermore, when sympathetic nervous system activity returns postoperatively, blood will shift from the periphery to the central circulation. Excess peripheral volume now becomes excess central volume and could push an elderly heart into diastolic heart failure. In short, volume administration to an older patient may be problematic, with a very fine line between too much and too little, and what was "just right" at one point may become "too much" later on.

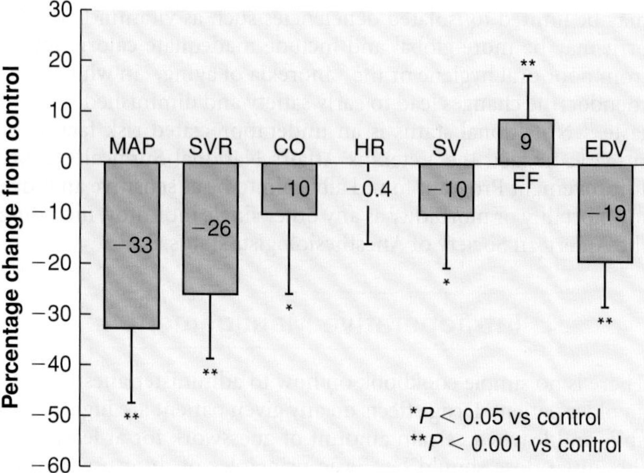

FIGURE 33-7. The response to total sympathectomy from spinal anesthesia is illustrated in older men with cardiac disease. Over 70% of the decrease in mean arterial blood pressure (MAP) was due to a decrease in systemic vascular resistance (SVR). Cardiac filling (EDV, end-diastolic volume) was markedly diminished, but its effect on stroke volume (SV) and cardiac output (CO) was ameliorated by an increase in ejection fraction (EF). Although heart rate (HR) increased in some subjects and decreased in others, the overall effect was no change. (Reprinted from: Rooke GA, Freund PR, Jacobson AF. Hemodynamic response and change in organ blood volume during spinal anesthesia in elderly men with cardiac disease. *Anesth Analg.* 1997;85:99, with permission.)

Postoperative Care

The goals of emergence and the immediate postoperative period are no different for an elderly than for a young patient, they are just more difficult to achieve. Analgesia is a major goal, and it should be stated up front that there is no evidence that pain is any less severe or any less detrimental in an older patient than in young patients. Less drug may be required (or not), but given that the standard approach to analgesia is to titrate to the desired effect, the outcome should be good pain relief for patients of any age. However, there are impediments to achieving adequate analgesia in an older patient.[58] Elderly patients sometimes underreport their pain level and may be more tolerant of their acute pain, perhaps partly because of the existence of chronic pain in their life. Older patients have more difficulty with visual analog scoring systems than verbal or numeric systems. If the patient is cognitively impaired, communication of pain is further impaired; indeed, demented patients often experience severe pain after hip surgery, but even mild cognitive impairment can lead to problems with pain assessment or with use of a patient-controlled analgesia machine.

7 Failure to achieve adequate levels of analgesia is associated with numerous adverse outcomes, including sleep deprivation, respiratory impairment, ileus, suboptimal mobilization, insulin resistance, tachycardia, and hypertension. The apparent paradox of adequate analgesia is that opioids are the mainstay of postoperative analgesia, and opioids are capable of producing many of those same adverse outcomes. Therefore, as with all medical care of elderly patients, good judgment, caution, and frequent monitoring of analgesia and adverse effects are essential. Adjunctive medications such as nonsteroidal anti-inflammatory drugs have been shown to reduce opioid requirements and some of the opioid adverse effects, but often carry their own risks such as renal damage or gastrointestinal toxicity.[58] Epidural analgesia is well known to provide analgesia that is superior to intravenous therapy, a finding that has been specifically replicated in the elderly.[59,60] Although improved cardiopulmonary outcomes were equivocal, more rapid return of bowel function, earlier mobilization, and nutritional status were better with epidural analgesia.

Although many aspects of postoperative care are more likely to be the purview of the surgeon or the internist, there are some things that the anesthesiologist could and probably should be watchful for when performing a postoperative visit on an older patient. If a patient had a surgery with major fluid requirements, it is important to look for signs of fluid overload, including rales, dyspnea, tachypnea, and orthopnea, particularly around postoperative day two when third space fluid tends to mobilize. A timely administration of a diuretic may prevent the patient from more florid pulmonary edema and the accompanying escalation of therapy and risk. Feel the pulse: Atrial fibrillation is often intermittent and the more often someone looks for it, the more likely it will be detected. Delirium often goes undetected in older patients, in part because it may come and go. Take the time to chat with the patient for a few minutes. It should not be difficult to become suspicious if the patient demonstrates waxing and waning alertness, is inattentive or distractible, displays rambled or incoherent speech, is disoriented, or has perceptual disturbances. It has been demonstrated that overall recovery and avoidance of complications, including delirium, pneumonia, uncontrolled pain, infection, and length of stay, can be enhanced by comprehensive evaluation and management of each patient's risk factors.[61,62] Anesthesiologists should be prepared to support such programs as much as possible.

PERIOPERATIVE COMPLICATIONS

My diseases are an asthma and a dropsy and, what is less curable, seventy-five.

—*Samuel Johnson*

The older patient is at increased risk for complications in the perioperative period, in part from comorbid disease and in part from the reduction in organ system reserve due to the aging process. Whether the aging process can be thought of as mere decreased reserve or subclinical disease is a matter of semantics. The result is the same: The elderly are at increased risk for almost every possible perioperative complication including cardiovascular, pulmonary, renal, central nervous system, wound infection, and death.[63,64]

8 Because the mechanisms of aging contribute not only to normal aging but to the development and severity of disease, one might expect that age and disease would interact in their contribution to perioperative risk. Confirmation of such a hypothesis is provided by a prospective survey of nearly 200,000 anesthetics in France.[65] Both age and the number of chronic diseases are associated with an increased rate of complications, but what is particularly interesting is an apparent interaction of these two factors. Figure 33-8 demonstrates that, for any given age group, the number of complications increases with the number of comorbid diseases. To be young and sick likely represents a special case as suggested by the point representing the ≤34-year-old group with three or more comorbid diseases. Ignoring that outlier, connecting the dots of equal number of comorbid disease reveals a modest increase in risk with age for patients with zero comorbid disease, but examination of points for one, two, or three or more diseases reveals an effect of age that becomes increasingly larger. In other words, age appears to interact with comorbid disease to increase risk.

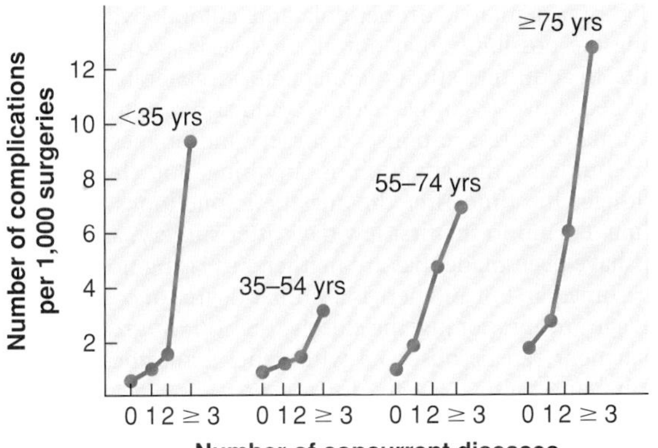

FIGURE 33-8. Details the interaction between age and comorbid disease. For each age bracket, as comorbid disease increases, so does the rate of complications. The effect of age on the complication rate is best visualized by examining points of equal comorbid disease. At zero disease, only a modest increase in complications is observed with increasing age. At ever-increasing degrees of comorbid disease, however, the increase in complications with age becomes more and more pronounced. (Reprinted from: Tiret L, Desmonts JM, Hatton F, et al. Complications associated with anaesthesia: A prospective survey in France. *Can Anesth Soc J.* 1986;33:336, with kind permission from Springer Science and Business Media.)

TABLE 33-2. EFFECT OF AGE ON SELECTED PERIOPERATIVE COMPLICATIONS AND ASSOCIATED MORTALITY[a]

	Complication Rate		Mortality Rate from the Complication	
Complication	Age <80	Age ≥80	Age <80	Age ≥80
Myocardial infarction	0.4	1	37.1	48
Cardiac arrest	0.9	2.1	80	88.2
Pneumonia	2.3	5.6	19.8	29.2
>48 h on ventilator	2.1	3.5	30.1	38.5
Required reintubation	1.6	2.8	32.3	44
Cerebrovascular accident	0.3	0.7	26.1	39.3
Coma >24 h	0.2	0.3	65.9	80.9
Prolonged ileus	1.2	1.7	9.2	16

[a]All differences between patients less than 80 vs. 80 and older are significant at $p < 0.001$, except for coma mortality ($p = 0.004$).
Modified from: Hamel MB, Henderson WG, Khuri SF, et al. Surgical outcomes for patients aged 80 and older: Morbidity and mortality from major noncardiac surgery. *J Am Geriat Soc.* 2005;53:424, with permission.

Complications of the cardiovascular and pulmonary systems are associated with the greatest perioperative mortality. The best database is provided by the Veterans Affairs National Surgical Quality Improvement Project, and much of the database involves examination of patients older than 80 (Table 33-2).[64] Although the perioperative complications of myocardial infarction or cardiac arrest carry higher associated mortality rates than pneumonia, prolonged intubation, or reintubation, the higher incidences of the pulmonary complications suggest that greater mortality results from pulmonary complications than from cardiac complications. That pulmonary complications are so significant underscores the need for a better understanding of the mechanism of postoperative pneumonia, particularly the likely contribution of silent aspiration.[66]

Central nervous system complications are also a major source of morbidity and mortality. The most burdensome problems appear to be stroke, postoperative delirium, and postoperative cognitive decline. All have the potential to cause debilitating morbidity and an adverse impact on the patient's quality of life, their families and the cost of medical care. Postoperative cognitive dysfunction (POCD) is a highly controversial topic in geriatric anesthesia, primarily because of the concern that general anesthesia may play an etiologic role.

In a nonsurgical elderly population, there is an annual stroke incidence of approximately 1%. The incidence of stroke in the older general surgical population is approximately 0.5% (Table 33-2).[64,67–69] Risk factors include age, atrial fibrillation (odds ratio 2), history of a prior stroke or TIA (odds ratio at least 1.6), recent myocardial infarction, COPD or current smoking, acute renal dysfunction or chronic dialysis, the type of surgery and a variety of comorbid diseases including diabetes and renal or cardiovascular disease.[67–71] A particularly interesting risk factor, at least for cardiac surgery patients, is an elevated arterial pulse pressure.[72] This finding supports the concept that age-related changes can influence perioperative risk just as it appears to influence morbidity in the general population. The POISE study raised the issue of perioperative beta-blockade increasing the risk of stroke, but when chronic, less intense beta-blockade is used such that risk is not present.[73,74] Strokes typically occur well after surgery, on average 7 days later, although upward of half occur within 24 hours.[67,69] Most perioperative strokes are ischemic and presumably from thromboembolism originating in the heart or arteries. The contribution of hypotension to focal stroke is questionable.[69] Mortality after a perioperative stroke is approximately twice that of a stroke in the general population, and overall mortality from perioperative stroke is at least 20%.[67,71] The continued use of aspirin throughout the perioperative period has been advocated.

Postoperative delirium is an acute confusional state manifested by an acute onset (hours to days) and vacillating levels of attention and cognitive skill.[75–77] Disorientation, perceptual disturbances (from situational misinterpretation to overt hallucinations), disorganized thinking, and problems with memory may be manifested. Emergence delirium alone does not qualify as postoperative delirium, but may be a risk factor.[78] Although most often short-lived (24 hours), delirium can be persistent and extend beyond hospital discharge.[75]

Delirium is most often diagnosed using Confusion Assessment Method, at least in research studies.[75,79] The mini-mental state examination can also be helpful, but its utility is higher for the identification of patients with pre-existing dementia. The risk of postoperative delirium after major surgery in older patients is approximately 10%; however, the risk varies with the surgical procedure.[76] Highest risk is emergent hip surgery, with an incidence of some 35%. The etiology of delirium is multifactorial. Risk factors include age, baseline low cognitive function (including dementia), depression, overall frailty, and general debility including dehydration or visual/auditory impairment.[75,77,80,81] The more risk factors present, the less perioperative stress seems to be required to push the patient over the edge to delirium.[76] That additional stress can include virtually any drug with central nervous system effects may contribute, including narcotics (especially meperidine), benzodiazepines (especially lorazepam), and drugs that possess anticholinergic properties (except perhaps glycopyrrolate). Other factors that likely contribute to delirium include sleep deprivation, being in an unfamiliar environment, and perioperative blood loss.

Narcotic administration represents a fine line between too much and too little, as inadequate pain control is also associated with delirium.[82] Analgesia with meperidine should be avoided, except perhaps in small doses for shivering, as it is clearly a risk factor for delirium, but there appears to be no superior choice among fentanyl, hydromorphone, and morphine.[83] Nevertheless, multimodal analgesia to reduce opiate use is considered a rational approach. Disappointingly, the selection of epidural analgesia over IV opioid analgesia does not appear to reduce the incidence of delirium.[83] Similarly, the use of regional instead of general anesthesia does not seem to reduce delirium, but this result may be due to the use of inappropriate drugs and/or heavy sedation in conjunction with the regional technique. Controlled sedation along with regional anesthesia does appear to reduce the incidence of delirium.[76,84] This is an important concept, as patients with diminished cognitive function have lower drug requirements for the same level of sedation.[85] Dexmedetomidine may be a better choice than benzodiazepines for ICU sedation.[75,86]

Delirium often goes undiagnosed in the elderly patient as it is typically hypoactive. The patient does not demonstrate behavior that draws attention. This characteristic is unfortunate because delirium is associated with an increased duration of hospitalization and its attendant costs, poorer long-term functional recovery, and increased mortality.[75,76,87] Outcomes are worst when the delirium is persistent. Once detected, management focuses on reversible risk factors such as current medications, pain management, and a better sleep environment. Special care programs designed to limit the reversible risk factors appear to reduce the incidence of delirium by up to 50%.[62,88] In the event the delirium is agitated, haloperidol in doses no greater than 1.5 mg can be helpful.[75] Haloperidol may be useful prophylactically in high risk surgeries as it appears to reduce the severity and duration of delirium but not its incidence.[89]

POCD is characterized by a long-term decrease in mental abilities after surgery. Other than the rare patient who suffers obvious impairment, POCD is inherently more difficult to diagnose than delirium because it usually requires sophisticated neuropsychological testing, including baseline tests prior to surgery. Selection of tests, their timing, and what deficits are required to qualify as cognitive decline have proven problematic in the literature.[77]

The seminal work not only examined surgical patients before and after surgery, but included control subjects who were tested over time as well. At 3 months after surgery, a 10% incidence of POCD was observed, in comparison to a 3% incidence in the nonsurgical control group.[90] Risk factors for POCD at 3 months after surgery include age, lower levels of education, prior history of stroke even in the absence of residual deficit, and POCD at hospital discharge.[91] Increased mortality at 1 year is associated with patients who demonstrate cognitive decline at both hospital discharge and at 3 months postoperatively.[91] Interestingly, postoperative delirium has not been found to be a risk factor for cognitive dysfunction at 3 months.[80]

Animal studies provide the most evidence for anesthetic CNS toxicity. Many studies of animals (typically mice) exposed to volatile anesthesia demonstrate impaired memory and diminished learning ability that persists for at least months after exposure.[92] Volatile anesthesia increases brain production of β-amyloid and abnormal tau protein (leads to neurofibrillatory tangles), both of which are associated with Alzheimer's disease, and also cell apoptosis.[92,93] However, other studies found that memory impairment and CNS chemical change only occurred in animals that had surgery plus anesthesia. Anesthesia without surgery was no different than control animals.[92] Curiously, the anesthetic in these latter studies was fentanyl, droperidol, and chloral hydrate, thereby raising the possibility that not all anesthesia agents yield similar results. In addition to the potential neurodegenerative mechanism described above, cognitive decline could also result from a neuroinflammatory stress response to surgery and/or anesthesia.[94]

In humans, the situation is anything but clear, especially the longer the time after the anesthetic one looks for cognitive decline. For up to the first few days after surgery, a few observations have been made that are neither surprising nor particularly worrisome. First of all, there is a similar degree of cognitive deficit in all age groups, not just the elderly.[95] Secondly, greater cognitive impairment can be observed with general anesthesia than with regional anesthesia.[96] Lastly, for the first few days the choice of general anesthesia makes a difference with propofol < desflurane < sevoflurane in degree of cognitive decline.[97,98]

By 3 months, however, the presence of POCD is almost exclusively a problem in older patients.[95] Furthermore, no differences can be detected between general and regional, or among the general anesthetic options.[96–98] By 1 year, even the best controlled studies suggest little or no demonstrable cognitive decline.[77,99] A longitudinal analysis of an Alzheimer's disease database of patients who started with none to mild dementia showed the same overall rate of cognitive decline whether or not they had surgery or suffered a major illness.[100] Using before and after neuropsychological testing, the incidence of POCD was compared for patients who underwent either coronary angiography, total hip arthroplasty or coronary artery bypass grafting.[101] At 1 week postoperatively, POCD was documented in 43% of the bypass graft patients and 17% for the hip replacement patients (angiography patients not tested at 1 week). At 3 months postprocedure, the incidence of POCD was 16% for both surgical groups and 21% for the angiography group (differences not significant). These two studies suggest there is no overall long-term adverse cognitive impact on patients, and that it is not the anesthetic which is to blame for whatever changes do occur.

So what do we tell our patients about stroke, delirium, and POCD? This is not an easy question to answer, especially for cognitive decline, but my experience has been that patients are satisfied to know the facts and are willing to accept the unknown, including the fact that there does not seem to be any clear evidence that basic anesthetic techniques differ in their impact on outcome.

Nevertheless, there are a few specific points about the conduct of anesthesia that can be made. Besides the obvious caveats ("avoid hypotension and hypoxia"), the basic approach to an anesthetic for an elderly patient can be described as cautious. Since stroke is likely a thromboembolic phenomenon, there may be little that can be done beyond standard, good anesthetic care. However, it is not clear that antiplatelet therapy needs to be discontinued for surgery as much as currently occurs. Perhaps it should be initiated in some patients if not already in use. The efficacy of statins has also not been adequately assessed. As previously discussed, drug choices and dose have a potentially major impact on delirium. Pain control with multimodal therapy to reduce opioid consumption is probably a good thing, but poor pain control may be almost as bad as too much opioid. Finally, it is not clear what the relationship is between anesthesia and cognitive decline, if there is one at all. Given that unsatisfactory statement, it seems reasonable to choose the anesthetic technique based on the other factors germane to the patient and surgery.

THE FUTURE

I will never be an old man. To me, old age is always 15 years older than I am.

—*Francis Bacon*

Improvements in surgical and anesthetic techniques that reduce the overall stress to the patient are permitting more surgeries to be performed on older and sicker patients than ever before. Nevertheless, the older patient will continue to experience the majority of perioperative adverse outcomes. Much remains to be accomplished in the quest to find ways to decrease the incidence and severity of those adverse outcomes.[66] The most pressing issues are arguably the prevention of postoperative delirium, cognitive decline, pneumonia, respiratory failure, and cardiovascular complications. Improved pain-control techniques that also diminish side effects, especially to the brain and bowels, would be welcome. However, other realms of care are just in their infancy, most notably whether the functional status of frail patients can be improved prior to surgery. For example, can short courses of better nutrition, exercise regimens, or even medications reduce complications or speed recovery and improve functional recovery? When caring for the elderly, especially the frail elderly, the overriding goal should be to produce as little stress to the patient as possible during both surgery and the subsequent hospitalization and recovery. Complete care will be multidisciplinary of necessity. No single specialty possesses the total perspective, and the anesthesiologist's expertise is an important component of that care.

References

1. Hall MJ, DeFrances CJ, Williams SN, et al. National hospital discharge survey: 2007 summary. *Natl Health Stat Report.* 2010;(29):1–20, 24.
2. Buie VC, Owings MF, DeFrances CJ, et al. National hospital discharge survey: 2006 summary. National Center for Health Statistics. *Vital Health Stat.* 2010; 13(168).
3. Cullen KA, Hall MJ, Golosinskiy A. Ambulatory surgery in the United States, 2006.2009;(11):1–25.
4. Ahmed A, Tollefsbol T. Telomeres and telomerase: Basic science implications for aging. *J Am Geriatr Soc.* 2001;49:1105.
5. Fries JF. Aging, natural selection, and the compression of morbidity. *N Engl J Med.* 1980;303:130.
6. Hulbert AJ, Pamplona R, Buffenstein R, et al. Life and death: Metabolic rate, membrane composition, and life span of animals. *Physiol Rev.* 2007;87:1175.
7. Fleisher LA, Beckman JA, Brown KA, et al. AHA/ACC 2007 guidelines on perioperative cardiovascular evaluation and care for noncardiac surgery. *J Am Coll Cardiol.* 2007;50:1707.
8. Vanitallie TB. Frailty in the elderly: Contributions of sarcopenia and visceral protein depletion. *Metabolism.* 2003;52(suppl 2):22.
9. Ensrud KE, Ewing SK, Cawthon PM, et al. A comparison of frailty indexes for the prediction of falls, disability, fractures, and mortality in older men. *J Am Geriatr Soc.* 2009;57:492.
10. Makary MA, Segev DL, Pronovost PJ, et al. Frailty as a predictor of surgical outcomes in older patients. *J Am Coll Surg.* 2010;210:901.
11. Fukagawa NK, Bandini LG, Young JB. Effect of age on body composition and resting metabolic rate. *Am J Physiol.* 1990;259:E233.
12. Doherty T. Invited review: Aging and sarcopenia. *J Appl Physiol.* 2003;95:1717.
13. Grandison MK, Boudinot FD. Age-related changes in protein binding of drugs: Implications for therapy. *Clin Pharmacokinet.* 2000;38:271.
14. Schmucker DL. Age-related changes in liver structure and function: Implications for disease? *Exp Gerontol.* 2005;40:650.
15. Muhlberg W, Platt D. Age-dependent changes of the kidneys: Pharmacologic implications. *Gerontology.* 1999;45:243.
16. Epstein M. Aging and the kidney. *J Am Soc Nephrol.* 1996;7:1106.
17. Scheen AJ. Diabetes mellitus in the elderly: Insulin resistance and/or impaired insulin secretion? *Diabetes Metab.* 2005;31:5S27.
18. Paganelli R, Di Iorio A, Cherubini A, et al. Frailty of older age: The role of the endocrine-immune interaction. *Curr Pharm Des.* 2006;12:3147.
19. Drachman DA. Aging of the brain, entropy, and Alzheimer disease. *Neurology.* 2006;67:1340.
20. Mrak RE, Griffin ST, Graham DI. Aging associated changes in human brain. *J Neuropathol Exp Neurol.* 1997;56:1269.
21. Shors TJ, Miesegaes G, Beylin A, et al. Neurogenesis in the adult is involved in the formation of trace memories. *Nature.* 2001;410:372.
22. Mapleson WW. Effect of age on MAC in humans: A meta-analysis. *Br J Anaesth.* 1996;76:179.
23. Jung D, Mayersohn M, Perrier D, et al. Thiopental disposition as a function of age in female patients undergoing surgery. *Anesthesiology.* 1982;56:263.
24. Minto CF, Schnider T, Egan T, et al. Influence of age and gender on the pharmacokinetics and pharmacodynamics of remifentanil: I. Model development. *Anesthesiology.* 1997;86:10.
25. Klotz U, Avant GR, Hoyumpa A, et al. The effects of age and liver disease on the disposition and elimination of diazepam in adult man. *J Clin Invest.* 1975;55:347.
26. Shafer SL. Pharmacokinetics and pharmacodynamics of the elderly. In: McLeskey CH, ed. *Geriatric Anesthesiology.* 1st ed. Baltimore, MD: Williams & Wilkins; 1997:123.
27. Shafer SL, Flood P. The pharmacology of opioids. In: Silverstein JH, Rooke GA, Reves JG, et al., eds. *Geriatric Anesthesiology.* 2nd ed. New York, NY: Springer; 2008:209.
28. McEvoy MD, Reves JG. Intravenous hypnotic anesthetics. In: Silverstein JH, Rooke GA, Reves JG, et al., eds. *Geriatric Anesthesiology.* 2nd ed. New York, NY: Springer; 2008:229.
29. Lien CA, Suzuki T. Relaxants and their reversal agents. In: Silverstein JH, Rooke GA, Reves JG, et al., eds. *Geriatric Anesthesiology.* 2nd ed. New York, NY: Springer; 2008:266.
30. Folkow B, Svanborg A. Physiology of cardiovascular aging. *Physiol Rev.* 1993; 73:725.
31. Rooke GA, Freund PR, Jacobson AF. Hemodynamic response and change in organ blood volume during spinal anesthesia in elderly men with cardiac disease. *Anesth Analg.* 1997;85:99.
32. Rooke GA. Cardiovascular aging and anesthetic implications. *J Cardiothorac Vasc Anesth.* 2003;17:512.
33. Ebert TJ, Morgan BJ, Barney JA, et al. Effects of aging on baroreflex regulation of sympathetic activity in humans. *Am J Physiol.* 1992;263:H798.
34. Barodka VM, Joshi BL, Berkowitz DE, et al. Implications of vascular aging. *Anesth Analg.* 2011;112:1048.
35. Nichols WW, O'Rourke MF, Avolio AP, et al. Effects of age on ventricular-vascular coupling. *Am J Cardiol.* 1985;55:1179.
36. Lakatta EG. Cardiovascular aging in health. *Clin Geriatr Med.* 2000;16:419.

37. Bouissou H, Julian M, Pieraggi M-Th, et al. Structure of healthy and varicose veins. In: Vanhoutte PM, ed. *Return Circulation and Norepinephrine: An Update.* Paris: John Libbey Eurotext; 1991:139.
38. Shannon RP, Wei JY, Rosa RM, et al. The effect of age and sodium depletion on cardiovascular response to orthostasis. *Hypertension.* 1986;8:438.
39. Domanski MJ, Davis BR, Pfeffer MA, et al. Isolated systolic hypertension – prognostic information provided by pulse pressure. *Hypertension.* 1999;34:375.
40. Crapo RO. The aging lung. In: Mahler DA, ed. *Pulmonary Disease in the Elderly Patient.* New York, NY: Marcel Dekker; 1993:1.
41. Wahba WM. Influence of aging on lung function—clinical significance of changes from age twenty. *Anesth Analg.* 1983;62:764.
42. Zaugg M, Lucchinetti E. Respiratory function in the elderly. *Anesthesiol Clin North America.* 2000;18:47.
43. DeLorey DS, Babb TG. Progressive mechanical ventilatory constraints with aging. *Am J Respir Crit Care Med.* 1999;160:169.
44. Kronenberg RS, Drage CW. Attenuation of the ventilatory and heart rate responses to hypoxia and hypercapnia with aging in normal men. *J Clin Invest.* 1973;52:1812.
45. Ancoli-Israel S, Coy T. Are breathing disturbances in elderly equivalent to sleep apnea syndrome? *Sleep.* 1994;17:77.
46. Marik PE, Kaplan D. Aspiration pneumonia and dysphagia in the elderly. *Chest.* 2003;124:328.
47. Sessler DI. Perioperative thermoregulation. In: Silverstein JH, Rooke GA, Reves JG, et al., eds. *Geriatric Anesthesiology.* 2nd ed. New York, NY: Springer; 2008:107.
48. Kenney WL, Munce TA. Invited review: Aging and human temperature regulation. *J Appl Physiol.* 2003;95:2598.
49. Vaughan MS, Vaughan RW, Cork RC. Postoperative hypothermia in adults: Relationship of age, anesthesia, and shivering to rewarming. *Anesth Analg.* 1981;60:746.
50. Lawrence VA, Hazuda HP, Cornell JP, et al. Functional independence after major abdominal surgery in the elderly. *J Am Coll Surg.* 2004;199:762.
51. Rosenthal RA, Kavic SM. Assessment and management of the geriatric patient. *Crit Care Med.* 2004;32(suppl):S92.
52. Fick DM, Cooper JW, Wade WE, et al. Updating the Beers criteria for potentially inappropriate medication use in older adults. *Arch Intern Med.* 2003;163:2716.
53. Rosenthal RA. Nutritional concerns in the older surgical patient. *J Am Coll Surg.* 2004;199:785.
54. Gibbs J, Cull W, Henderson W, et al. Preoperative serum albumin level as a predictor of operative mortality and morbidity. *Arch Surg.* 1999;134:36.
55. Kazama T, Ikeda K, Morita K, et al. Comparison of the effect-site k_{eo}s of propofol for blood pressure and EEG bispectral index in elderly and younger patients. *Anesthesiology.* 1999;90:1517.
56. Reich DL, Hossain S, Krol M, et al. Predictors of hypotension after induction of general anesthesia. *Anesth Analg.* 2005;101:622.
57. Forrest JB, Rehder K, Cahalan MK, et al. Multicenter study of general anesthesia. III. Predictors of severe perioperative adverse outcomes. *Anesthesiology.* 1992;76:3.
58. Aubrun F. Management of postoperative analgesia in elderly patients. *Reg Anesth Pain Med.* 2005;30:363.
59. Mann C, Pouzeratte Y, Bocarra G, et al. Comparison of intravenous or epidural patient-controlled analgesia in the elderly after major abdominal surgery. *Anesthesiology.* 2000;92:433.
60. Carli F, Phil M, Mayo N, et al. Epidural analgesia enhances functional exercise capacity and health related quality of life after colonic surgery. Results of a randomized trial. *Anesthesiology.* 2002;97:540.
61. Harari D, Hopper A, Dhesi J, et al. Proactive care of older people undergoing surgery ('POPS'): Designing, embedding, evaluating and funding a comprehensive geriatric assessment service for older elective surgical patients. *Age Ageing.* 2007;36:190.
62. Marcantonio ER, Flacker JM, Wright RJ, et al. Reducing delirium after hip fracture: A randomized trial. *J Am Geriatr Soc.* 2001;49:516.
63. Turrentine FE, Wang H, Simpson VB, et al. Surgical risk factors, morbidity, and mortality in elderly patients. *J Am Coll Surg.* 2006;203:865.
64. Hamel MB, Henderson WG, Khuri SF, et al. Surgical outcomes for patients aged 80 and older: Morbidity and mortality from major noncardiac surgery. *J Am Geriat Soc.* 2005;53:424.
65. Tiret L, Desmonts JM, Hatton F, et al. Complications associated with anaesthesia—a prospective survey in France. *Can Anesth. Soc J.* 1986;33:336.
66. Cook DJ, Rooke GA. Priorities in perioperative geriatrics. *Anesth Analg.* 2003; 96:1823.
67. Kam PCA, Calcroft RM. Perioperative stroke in general surgical patients. *Anaesthesia.* 1997;52:879.
68. Bateman BT, Schumacher HC, Wang S, et al. Perioperative acute ischemic stroke in noncardiac and nonvascular surgery. *Anesthesiology.* 2009;110:231–238.
69. Ng JLW, Chan MTV, Gelb AW. Perioperative stroke in noncardiac, nonneurosurgical surgery. *Anesthesiology.* 2011;115:879.
70. Kaatz S, Douketis JD, Zhou H, et al. Risk of stroke after surgery in patients with and without chronic atrial fibrillation. *J Thromb Haemost.* 2010;8:884.
71. Mashour GA, Shanks AM, Kheterpal S. Perioperative stroke and associated mortaility after noncardiac, nonneurologic surgery. *Anesthesiology.* 2011;114:1289.
72. Benjo A, Thompson RE, Fine D, et al. Pulse pressure is an age-independent predictor of stroke development after cardiac surgery. *Hypertension.* 2007;50:630.
73. Poise Study Group. Effects of extended-release metoprolol succinate in patients undergoing non-cardiac surgery (POISE trial): A randomized controlled trial. *Lancet.* 2008;371:1839.
74. van Lier F, Schouten O, Hoeks SE, et al. Impact of prophylactic β-blocker therapy to prevent stroke after noncardiac surgery. *Am J Cardiol.* 2010;105:43.
75. Rudolph JL, Marcantonio ER. Postoperative delirium: Acute change with long-term implications. *Anesth Analg.* 2011;112:1202.
76. Sieber FE. Postoperative delirium in the elderly surgical patient. *Anesthesiol Clin.* 2009;27:451.
77. Silverstein JH, Timberger M, Reich DL, et al. Central nervous system dysfunction after noncardiac surgery and anesthesia in the elderly. *Anesthesiology.* 2007;106:622.
78. Sharma PT, Sieber FE, Zakriya KJ. Recovery room delirium predicts postoperative delirium after hip-fracture repair. *Anesth Analg.* 2005;101:1215.
79. Inouye SK, van Dyck CH, Alessi CA, et al. Clarifying confusion: The confusion assessment method. *Ann Intern Med.* 1990;113:941.
80. Jankowski C, Trenerry MR, Cook DJ, et al. Cognitive and functional predictors and sequelae of postoperative delirium in elderly patients undergoing elective joint arthroplasty. *Anesth Analg.* 2011;112:1186.
81. Leung JM, Tsai TL, Sands LP. Preoperative frailty in older surgical patients is associated with early postoperative delirium. *Anesth Analg.* 2011;112:1199.
82. Vaurio LE, Sands LP, Wang Y, et al. Postoperative delirium: The importance of pain and pain management. *Anesth Analg.* 2006;102:1267.
83. Fong HK, Sands LP, Leung JM. The role of postoperative analgesia in delirium and cognitive decline in elderly patients: A systematic review. *Anesth Analg.* 2006; 102:1255.
84. Sieber FE, Zakriya KJ, Gottschalk A, et al. Sedation depth during spinal anesthesia and the development of postoperative delirium in elderly patients undergoing hip fracture repair. *Mayo Clin Proc.* 2010;85:18.
85. Laalou FZ, Egard M, Guillot M, et al. Influence of preoperative cognitive status on propofol requirement to maintain hypnosis in the elderly. *Brit J Anaesth.* 2010;105(3):342–346.
86. Riker RR, Shehabi Y, Bokesch PM, et al. Dexmedetomidine vs midazolam for sedation of critically ill patients: A randomized trial. *JAMA.* 2009;301:489.
87. Zakriya K, Sieber FE, Christmas C, et al. Brief postoperative delirium in hip fracture patients affects functional outcome at three months. *Anesth Analg.* 2004; 98:1798.
88. Bjorkelund KB, Hommel A, Thorngren KG, et al. Reducing delirium in elderly patients with hip fracture: A multi-factorial intervention study. *Acta Anaesthesiol Scand.* 2010;54:678.
89. Kalisvaart KJ, de Jonghe JF, Bogaards MJ, et al. Haloperidol prophylaxis for elderly hip-surgery patients at risk for delirium: A randomized placebo-controlled study. *J Am Geriatr Soc.* 2005;53:1658.
90. Moller JT, Cluitmans P, Rasmussen LS, et al. Long-term postoperative cognitive dysfunction in the elderly: ISPOCD1 study. *Lancet.* 1998;351:857.
91. Monk TG, Weldon BC, Garvan CW, et al. Predictors of cognitive dysfunction after major noncardiac surgery. *Anesthesiology.* 2008;108:18.
92. Bittner EA, Yun Yue Y, Xie Z. Brief review: Anesthetic neurotoxicity in the elderly, cognitive dysfunction and Alzheimer's disease. *Can J Anesth.* 2011;58:216.
93. Tang J, Eckenhoff MF, Eckenhoff, RG. Anesthesia and the old brain. *Anesth Analg.* 2010;110:421.
94. Hudson AE, Hemmings HC Jr. Are anaesthetics toxic to the brain? *Br J Anaesth.* 2011;107:30.
95. Crosby G, Culley DJ. Surgery and anesthesia: Healing the body but harming the brain? *Anesth Analg.* 2011;112:999.
96. Wu CL, Wesley Hsu W, Richman JM, et al. Postoperative cognitive function as an outcome of regional anesthesia and analgesia. *Reg Anesth Pain Med.* 2004;29:257.
97. Royse CF, Andrews DT, Newman SN, et al. The influence of propofol or desflurane on postoperative cognitive dysfunction in patients undergoing coronary artery bypass surgery. *Anaesthesia.* 2011;66:455.
98. Rörtgen D, Kloos J, Fries M, et al. Comparison of early cognitive function and recovery after desflurane or sevoflurane anaesthesia in the elderly: A double-blinded randomized controlled trial. *Br J Anaesth.* 2010;104:167.
99. Ancelin ML, de Roquefeuil G, Scali J, et al. Long-term post-operative cognitive decline in the elderly: The effects of anesthesia type, apolipoprotein E genotype, and clinical antecedents. *J Alzheimers Dis.* 2010;22:105.
100. Avidan MS, Searleman AC, Storandt M, et al. Long-term cognitive decline in older subjects was not attributable to noncardiac surgery or major illness. *Anesthesiology.* 2009;111:964.
101. Evered L, Scott DA, Silbert B, et al. Postoperative cognitive dysfunction is independent of type of surgery and anesthetic. *Anesth Analg.* 2011;112:1179.

CHAPTER

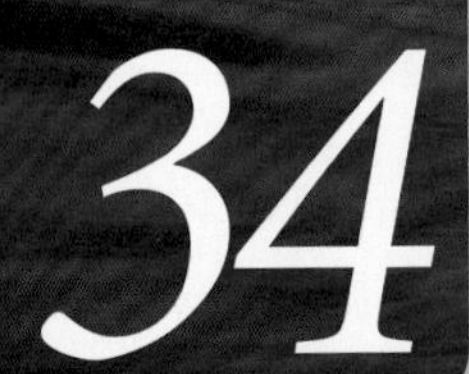

Epidural and Spinal Anesthesia

CHRISTOPHER M. BERNARDS • LUCY S. HOSTETTER

Key Points

1. Clinicians must develop a three-dimensional mental picture of the spinal anatomy so that when they contact bony structures during attempted epidural or spinal needle placement, they can redirect the needle in a reasoned and systematic manner and not subject the patient to random needle "pokes" in an effort to place the block.
2. The epidural fat and the epidural venous plexus do not form a continuous cylinder surrounding the spinal cord, as is often depicted. Rather, the epidural fat lies in discrete pockets in the posterior and lateral epidural space and the epidural veins travel primarily in the anterior and lateral epidural space and are normally absent in the posterior epidural space.
3. Serious systemic toxicity during attempted epidural block is almost always the result of inadvertent local anesthetic injection directly into the vasculature. Consequently, an appropriate test dose designed to identify intravascular injection is critical.
4. Physical characteristics (e.g., height, weight, cerebrospinal fluid volume) and age do have an effect on spinal and epidural block characteristics. However, the magnitude of the effects is relatively small and of such low predictive power that these characteristics are not useful predictors of local anesthetic dose in any individual patient.
5. The risk of hemodynamic complications of epidural and spinal anesthesia increases with increasing block height.
6. Lidocaine appears to be worse than other local anesthetics in terms of the risk of neurologic toxicity (i.e., cauda equina syndrome and transient neurologic symptoms).
7. Human studies suggest that the preservative-free formulation of chloroprocaine may offer a viable alternative to lidocaine for short-duration spinal anesthesia.
8. Administration of drugs that impair coagulation can put patients at increased risk of spinal hematoma. Our understanding of the relative risk of different classes of drugs affecting the clotting system is constantly evolving. Clinicians are directed to the consensus statement from the American Society for Regional Anesthesia and Pain Medicine for the most recent recommendations.

Multimedia

1 Dermatomes
2 Subarachnoid Block

3 Continuous Spinal
4 Hanging Drop
5 Paresthesias Spinal

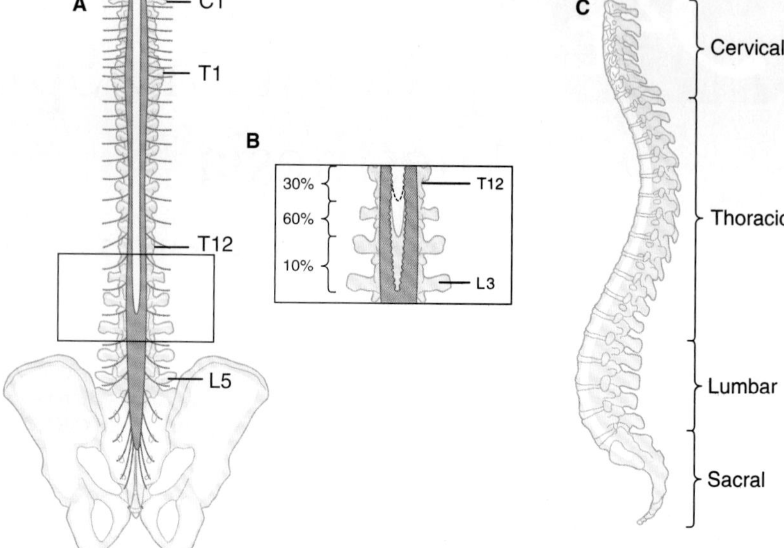

FIGURE 34-1. Posterior **(A)** and lateral **(C)** views of the human spinal column. Note the inset **(B)**, which depicts the variability in vertebral level at which the spinal cord terminates.

There are no absolute indications for spinal or epidural anesthesia. However, there are clinical situations in which patient preference, patient physiology, or the surgical procedure makes central neuraxial block the technique of choice. There is also evidence that these techniques may improve outcome in selected situations. Spinal and epidural anesthesia have been shown to blunt the "stress response" to surgery,[1] to decrease intraoperative blood loss,[2,3] to lower the incidence of postoperative thromboembolic events,[2–5] and to decrease morbidity and mortality in high-risk surgical patients.[6,7] In addition, both spinal and epidural techniques can be used to extend analgesia into the postoperative period, where their use has been shown to provide better analgesia than can be achieved with parenteral opioids.[8] In addition, central neuraxial analgesia has become an indispensable technique to provide analgesia to nonsurgical patients. Thus, these techniques are an indispensable part of modern anesthetic practice, and every anesthesiologist should be adept at performing them.

ANATOMY

1 Proficiency in spinal and epidural anesthesia requires a thorough understanding of the anatomy of the spine and spinal cord. The anesthesiologist must be familiar with the surface anatomy of the spine but must also develop a mental image of the three-dimensional anatomy of deeper structures. In addition, one must appreciate the relationship between the cutaneous dermatomes, the spinal nerves, the vertebrae, and the spinal segment from which each spinal nerve arises.

Vertebrae

The *spine* consists of 33 *vertebrae* (7 cervical, 12 thoracic, 5 lumbar, 5 fused sacral, and 4 fused coccygeal; Fig. 34-1). With the exception of C1, the cervical, thoracic, and lumbar vertebrae consist of a *body* anteriorly, two *pedicles* that project posteriorly from the body, and two *laminae* that connect the pedicles (Fig. 34-2). These structures form the *vertebral canal,* which contains the spinal cord, spinal nerves, and epidural space. The laminae give rise to the *transverse processes* that project laterally and the *spinous process* that projects posteriorly. These bony projections serve as sites for muscle and ligament attachments. The pedicles contain a superior and inferior *vertebral notch* through which the spinal nerves exit the vertebral canal. The superior and inferior *articular processes* arise at the junction of the lamina and pedicles and form joints with the adjoining vertebrae. The first cervical vertebra ("atlas") differs from this typical structure in that it does not have a body or a spinous process.

The five sacral vertebrae are fused together to form the wedge-shaped *sacrum,* which connects the spine with the iliac wings of the pelvis (Fig. 34-1). The fifth sacral vertebra is not fused posteriorly, giving rise to a variably shaped opening known as the *sacral hiatus.* Occasionally, other sacral vertebrae do not fuse posteriorly, giving rise to a much larger sacral hiatus. The *sacral cornua*

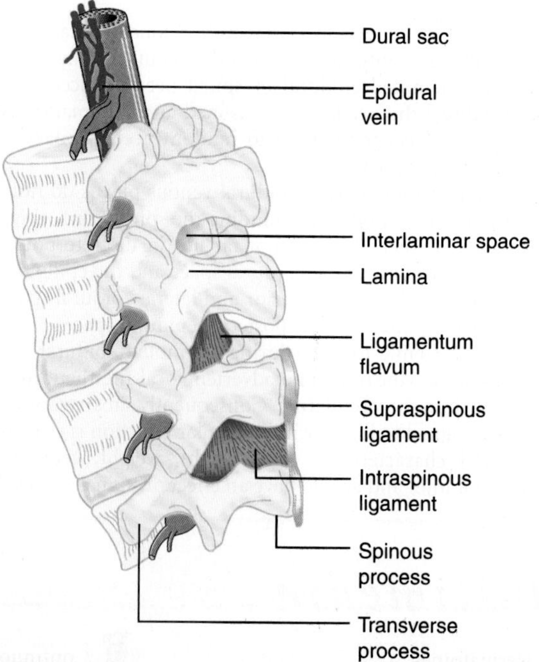

FIGURE 34-2. Detail of the lumbar spinal column and epidural space. Note that the epidural veins are largely restricted to the anterior and lateral epidural space.

are bony prominences on either side of the hiatus and aid in identifying it. The sacral hiatus provides an opening into the sacral canal, which is the caudal termination of the epidural space. The four rudimentary coccygeal vertebrae are fused together to form the *coccyx*, a narrow triangular bone that abuts the sacral hiatus and can be helpful in identifying it. The tip of the coccyx can often be palpated in the proximal gluteal cleft, and by running one's finger cephalad along its smooth surface, the sacral cornu can be identified as the first bony prominence encountered.

Identifying individual vertebrae is important for correctly locating the desired interspace for epidural and spinal blockade. The C7 and T1 spinous processes are the most prominent and are easily palpated while running the hand down the back of the neck. The twelfth thoracic vertebra can be identified by palpating the twelfth rib and tracing it back to its attachment to T12. A line drawn between the iliac crests crosses the body of L5 or the L4 to L5 interspace.

Ligaments

The vertebral bodies are stabilized by five ligaments that increase in size between the cervical and lumbar vertebrae (Fig. 34-2). From the sacrum to T7, the *supraspinous ligament* runs between the tips of the spinous processes. Above T7, this ligament continues as the *ligamentum nuchae* and attaches to the occipital protuberance at the base of the skull. The *interspinous ligament* attaches between the spinous processes and blends posteriorly with the supraspinous ligament and anteriorly with the ligamentum flavum. The *ligamentum flavum* is a tough, wedge-shaped ligament composed of elastin. It consists of right and left portions that span adjacent vertebral laminae and fuse in the midline to varying degrees.[7,8] The ligamentum flavum is thickest in the midline, measuring 3 to 5 mm at the L2 to L3 interspace of adults. The distance between the ligamentum flavum and the spinal meninges is also greater in the midline, measuring 4 to 6 mm at the L2 to L3 interspace.[9] As a result, midline insertion of an epidural needle is least likely to result in unintended meningeal puncture. The anterior and posterior *longitudinal ligaments* run along the anterior and posterior surfaces of the vertebral bodies.

Epidural Space

The epidural space is the space that lies between the spinal meninges and the sides of the vertebral canal (Fig. 34-3). It is bounded cranially by the foramen magnum, caudally by the sacrococcygeal ligament covering the sacral hiatus, anteriorly by the posterior longitudinal ligament, laterally by the vertebral pedicles, and posteriorly by both the ligamentum flavum and the vertebral lamina. The epidural space is not a closed space but communicates with the paravertebral space by way of the intervertebral foramina.[10] The epidural space is shallowest anteriorly where the dura may in some places fuse with the posterior longitudinal ligament. The space is deepest posteriorly, although the depth varies because the space is intermittently obliterated by contact between the dura mater and the ligamentum flavum or vertebral lamina. Contact between the dura mater and the pedicles also interrupts the epidural space laterally. Thus, the epidural space is composed of a series of discontinuous compartments that become continuous when the potential space separating the compartments is opened up by injection of air or liquid. A rich network of valveless veins (Batson plexus) courses through the anterior and lateral portions of the epidural space and only very rarely in the posterior epidural space (Fig. 34-2).[11] The epidural veins anastomose freely with extradural veins, including the pelvic veins, azygous system, and intracranial veins. The epidural space also contains lymphatics and segmental arteries running between the aorta and the spinal cord.

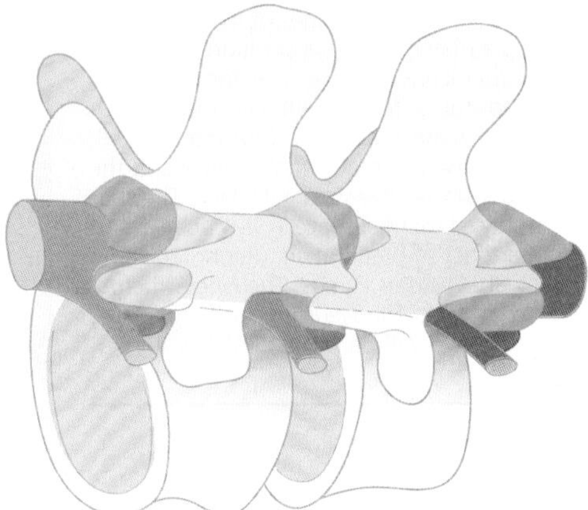

FIGURE 34-3. The compartments of the epidural space (*pink areas*) are discontinuous. Areas where no compartments are indicated represent a potential space where the dura mater normally abuts the sides of the vertebral canal. (Reprinted from: Hogan Q. Lumbar epidural anatomy: A new look by cryomicrotome section. *Anesthesiology.* 1991;75: 767, with permission.)

Epidural Fat

The most ubiquitous material in the epidural space is fat, which is principally located in the posterior and the lateral epidural
2 space (Fig. 34-3).[10] Interestingly, the epidural fat appears to have clinically important effects on the pharmacology of epidurally and intrathecally administered drugs. For example, using a pig model, Bernards et al.[12] showed that there is a linear relationship between an opioid's lipid solubility and its terminal elimination half-time in the epidural space, its mean residence time in the epidural space, and its concentration in epidural fat. In addition, net transfer of opioid from the epidural space to the intrathecal space was greatest for the least lipid-soluble opioid (morphine) and least for highly lipid-soluble opioids (fentanyl, sufentanil). In effect, increasing lipid solubility resulted in opioid "sequestration" in epidural fat, thereby reducing the bioavailability of drug in the underlying subarachnoid space and spinal tissue.

Epidural fat also appears to play a role in the pharmacokinetics of epidurally administered local anesthetics. Specifically, sequestration in epidural fat likely explains why a highly lipid-soluble local anesthetic like etidocaine is only approximately equipotent with lidocaine in the epidural space despite the fact that etidocaine is roughly seven times more potent than lidocaine in vitro. Because of its much greater lipid solubility, etidocaine is more likely than lidocaine to be sequestered in epidural fat, thereby reducing the amount of drug available to produce block in the spinal nerve roots and spinal cord. Consistent with this hypothesis, Tucker and Mather[13] showed that after administering 80 mg of etidocaine and 50 mg of lidocaine into the epidural space of sheep, the amount of etidocaine still present in epidural fat 12 hours later was more than 100 times greater than the amount of lidocaine. Thus, sequestration in epidural fat appears to play an important role in the pharmacokinetics of local anesthetics just as it does for epidural opioids.

Meninges

The spinal meninges consist of three protective membranes (dura mater, arachnoid mater, and pia mater), which are continuous with the cranial meninges (Fig. 34-4).

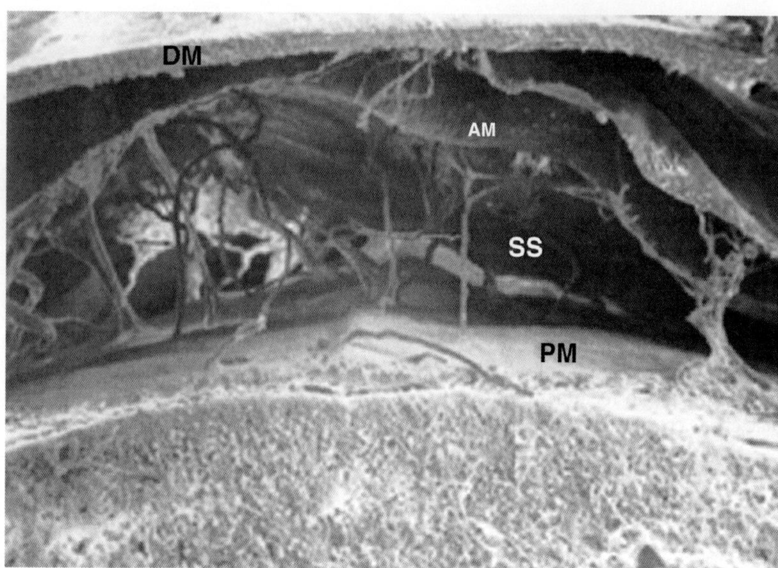

FIGURE 34-4. The spinal meninges of the dog, demonstrating the pia mater (PM) in apposition to the spinal cord, the subarachnoid space (SS), the arachnoid mater (AM), trabeculae (fibers stretching from arachnoid mater to pia mater), and the dura mater (DM). The separation between the arachnoid mater and the dura mater demonstrates the subdural space. The subdural space is only a potential space in vivo but is created here as an artifact of preparation. (Reprinted from: Peters A, Palay SL, Webster H, eds. *The Fine Structure of the Nervous System: The Neurons and Supporting Cells.* Philadelphia, PA: WB Saunders; 1976, with permission.)

Dura Mater

The dura mater is the outermost and thickest meningeal tissue. The spinal dura mater begins at the foramen magnum where it fuses with the periosteum of the skull, forming the cephalad border of the epidural space. Caudally, the dura mater ends at approximately S2, where it fuses with the filum terminale. The dura mater extends laterally along the spinal nerve roots and becomes continuous with the connective tissue of the epineurium at approximately the level of the intervertebral foramina. The dura mater is composed of randomly arranged collagen fibers and elastin fibers arranged longitudinally and circumferentially.[14] The dura mater is largely acellular except for a layer of cells that forms the border between the dura mater and the arachnoid mater. Despite the lack of cellular elements, the inner edge of the dura mater is highly vascular, which likely results in the dura mater being an important route of drug clearance from both the epidural space and the subarachnoid space.[15]

There is controversy regarding the existence and clinical significance of a dorsal midline connective tissue band, the *plica mediana dorsalis,* running from the dura mater to the ligamentum flavum. Anatomic studies using epiduroscopy and epidurography have demonstrated the presence of the plica mediana dorsalis and have led to speculation that this tissue band may on occasion be responsible for difficulty in inserting epidural catheters and for unilateral epidural block.[16,17] However, using cryomicrotome sections to investigate the epidural space, Hogan[10] failed to find evidence of a substantial connection between the dura mater and the ligamentum flavum. He speculated that the injection of either air or contrast required for the earlier studies may have compressed epidural contents (e.g., fat) and produced an artifact mimicking a connective tissue band. In addition, Hogan[18] has shown in a clinical study that there is no significant impediment to spread of injectate across the midline. Thus, the plica mediana dorsalis does not appear to be clinically relevant with respect to clinical epidural anesthesia.

The inner surface of the dura mater abuts the arachnoid mater. There is a potential space between these two membranes called the *subdural space* (Fig. 34-4). Occasionally, a drug intended for either the epidural space or the subarachnoid space is injected into the subdural space.[19] Subdural injection has been estimated to occur in 0.82% of intended epidural injections.[20] The radiology literature suggests that the incidence of subdural injection during intended subarachnoid injection for myelography may be as high as 10%.[21]

Arachnoid Mater

The arachnoid mater is a delicate, avascular membrane composed of overlapping layers of flattened cells with connective tissue fibers running between the cellular layers. The arachnoid cells are interconnected by frequent tight junctions and occluding junctions. These specialized cellular connections likely account for the fact that the arachnoid mater is the principal anatomic barrier for drugs moving between the epidural space and the spinal cord.[22]

In the region where the spinal nerve roots traverse the dura and arachnoid membranes, the arachnoid mater herniates through the dura mater into the epidural space to form arachnoid granulations. As with the cranial arachnoid granulations, the spinal arachnoid granulations serve as a site for material in the subarachnoid space to exit the central nervous system (CNS). Although some have postulated that the arachnoid granulations are a preferred route for drugs to move from the epidural space to the spinal cord, the available experimental data suggest that this is not the case.[23]

The *subarachnoid space* lies between the arachnoid mater and the pia mater and contains the cerebrospinal fluid (CSF). The spinal CSF is in continuity with the cranial CSF and provides an avenue for drugs in the spinal CSF to reach the brain. In addition, the spinal nerve roots and rootlets run in the subarachnoid space.

Pia Mater

The spinal pia mater is adherent to the spinal cord and is composed of a thin layer of connective tissue cells interspersed with collagen. Trabeculae connect the pia mater with the arachnoid mater and the cells of these two meninges blend together along the trabeculae. Unlike the arachnoid mater, the pia mater is fenestrated in places so that the spinal cord is in direct communication with the subarachnoid space. The pia mater extends to the tip of the spinal cord where it becomes the *filum terminale,* which anchors the spinal cord to the sacrum. The pia mater also gives rise to the dentate ligaments, which are thin connective tissue bands extending from the side of the spinal cord through the arachnoid mater to the dura mater. These ligaments serve to suspend the spinal cord within the meninges.

Cerebrospinal Fluid

CSF is a complex solution made up of 99% water and containing an array of molecules including electrolytes, proteins, glucose, neurotransmitters, neurotransmitter metabolites, cyclic nucleotides, amino acids, among many others. The CSF volume is approximately 100 to 160 mL in adult humans and it is produced at the rate of 20 to 25 mL/hr. Consequently, the entire CSF volume is replaced roughly every 6 hours.

According to the traditional view of CSF hydrodynamics, CSF is produced by plasma ultrafiltration in the choroid plexus within the cerebral ventricles. It then "flows" or "circulates" unidirectionally through the subarachnoid space to finally be absorbed by the arachnoid villi in the superior sagittal sinus and/or into lymphatics via perineural sheaths of cranial and spinal nerves. Several recent investigations, however, contradict this widely held view. Bulat et al.[24] hypothesized that CSF is formed by water filtration across arterial capillary walls in the CNS. The filtration of water from arterial capillaries generates an osmotic counterpressure that drives water reabsorption into cerebral microvessels (i.e., venous capillaries and postcapillary venules). Using radiolabeled water, they demonstrated that CSF does not flow through subarachnoid spaces and that the bulk removal of CSF occurred primarily via absorption into cerebral microvessels. Klarica et al.[25] further demonstrated that occlusion of the aqueduct of Sylvius does not alter isolated cerebral ventricle pressures, suggesting that the formation and absorption of CSF are in balance with one another.

In addition, the development of cine-magnetic resonance imaging and cine-computed tomography techniques have also shown that CSF does not circulate, rather it oscillates in the cephalocaudal axis with a frequency equal to the heart rate.[26,27] CSF oscillates because cerebral expansion during systole displaces CSF caudally into the spinal canal and cerebral contraction during diastole causes the CSF displaced into the spinal canal to retreat back into the cranial vault. Net CSF movement is estimated at 0.04% per oscillation.

The clinical significance of this understanding of CSF motion is that CSF cannot be relied on to distribute drugs in the subarachnoid space. This is of little importance in single-shot spinal anesthesia because the kinetic energy of the injection and the baricity of the solution serve to distribute the drug. However, the lack of significant net CSF motion explains why drug distribution during the very slow infusions used for chronic intrathecal analgesia results in very limited drug distribution.[28]

Spinal Cord

In the first-trimester fetus, the spinal cord extends from the foramen magnum to the end of the sacrum. Thereafter, the vertebral column lengthens more than the spinal cord so that at birth the spinal cord ends at about the level of the third lumbar vertebra. In the adult, the caudad tip of the spinal cord typically lies at the level of the first lumbar vertebra. However, in 30% of individuals the spinal cord may end at T12, while in 10% it may extend to L3 (Fig. 34-1).[29] A sacral spinal cord has been reported in an adult.[29] Flexion of the vertebral column causes the tip of the spinal cord to move slightly cephalad.

The spinal cord gives rise to 31 pairs of *spinal nerves,* each composed of an *anterior motor root* and a *posterior sensory root.* The nerve roots are in turn composed of multiple rootlets. The portion of the spinal cord that gives rise to all of the rootlets of a single spinal nerve is called a *cord segment.* The skin area innervated by a given spinal nerve and its corresponding cord segment is called a *dermatome* (Fig. 34-5). The intermediolateral gray matter of the T1 through L2 spinal cord segments contains the cell bodies of the *preganglionic sympathetic neurons.* These sympathetic neurons run with the corresponding spinal nerve to a point

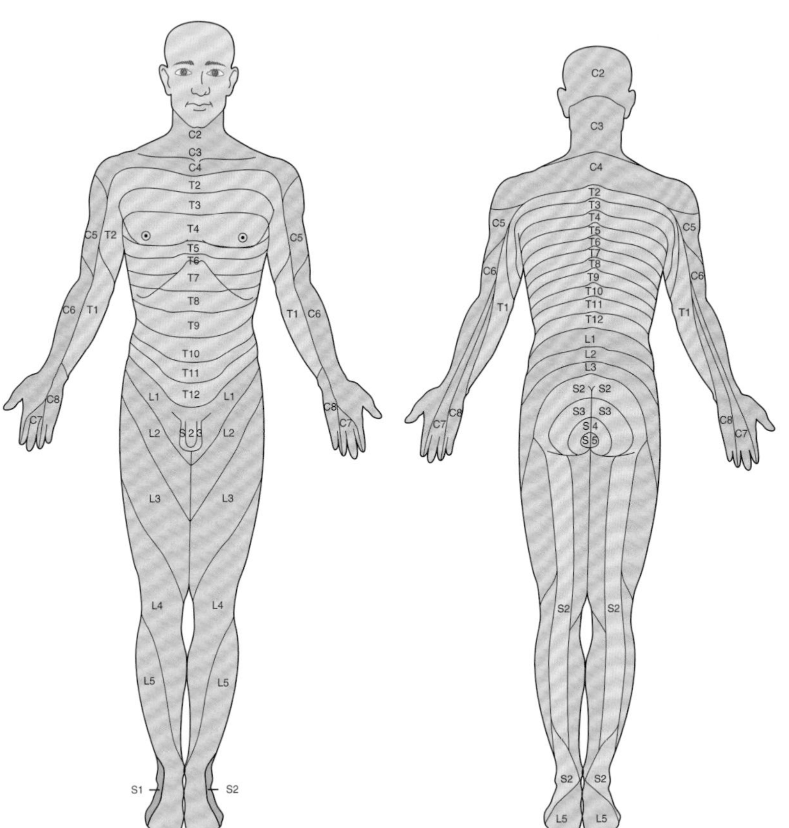

FIGURE 34-5. Human sensory dermatomes.

just beyond the intervertebral foramen where they exit to join the sympathetic chain ganglia.

The spinal nerves and their corresponding cord segments are named for the intervertebral foramen through which they run. In the cervical region, the spinal nerves are named for the vertebra forming the caudad half of the intervertebral foramen; for example, C4 emerges through an intervertebral foramen formed by C3 and C4. In the thoracic and lumbar regions, the nerve roots are named for the vertebrae forming the cephalad half of the intervertebral foramen; for example, L4 emerges through an intervertebral foramen formed by L4 and L5. Since the spinal cord usually ends between L1 and L2, the thoracic, lumbar, and sacral nerve roots run increasingly longer distances in the subarachnoid space to get from their spinal cord segment of origin to the intervertebral foramen through which they exit. Those nerves that extend beyond the end of the spinal cord to their exit site are collectively known as the *cauda equina* (Fig. 34-1).

TECHNIQUE

Spinal and epidural anesthesia should be performed only after appropriate monitors are applied and in a setting where equipment for airway management and resuscitation are immediately available. Before positioning the patient, all equipment for spinal block should be ready for use; for example, local anesthetics mixed and drawn up, needles uncapped, skin antiseptic solution available, and so on. Preparing all equipment ahead of time will minimize the time required to perform the block and thereby enhance patient comfort.

Needles

Spinal and epidural needles are classified by the design of their tips (Fig. 34-6). The Whitacre, Eldor, Marx, and Sprotte spinal needles have a "pencil-point" tip with one or two (Eldor) aperture(s) on the side of the shaft proximal to the tip. The Greene, Atraucan, and Quincke needles have beveled tips with cutting edges. The pencil-point needles require more force to insert than the bevel-tip needles but provide a better tactile "feel" of the various tissues encountered as the needle is inserted. In addition, the bevel has been shown to cause the needle to be deflected from the intended path as it passes through tissues while the pencil-point needles are not deflected.[30] Epidural needles have a larger diameter than spinal needles to facilitate the injection of fluid or air when using the "loss of resistance" technique to identify the epidural space. In addition, the larger diameter allows for easier insertion of catheters into the epidural space. The Tuohy epidural needle has a curved tip to help control the direction that the catheter moves in the epidural space. The Hustead needle tip is also curved, although somewhat less than the Tuohy needle. The Crawford needle tip is straight, making it less suitable for catheter insertion.

The outside diameter of both epidural and spinal needles is used to determine their gauge. Larger gauge (i.e., smaller diameter) spinal needles are less likely to cause postdural puncture headaches (PDPH), but are more readily deflected than smaller gauge needles. Epidural needles are typically sized 16G to 19G and spinal needles 22G to 29G. Spinal needles smaller than 22G are often easier to insert if an introducer needle is used. The introducer is inserted into the interspinous ligament in the intended direction of the spinal needle and the spinal needle is then inserted through the shaft of the introducer. The introducer prevents the spinal needle from being deflected or bent as it passes through the interspinous ligament.[30] Needles of the same outside diameter may have different inside diameters. This is important because inside diameter determines how large a catheter can be inserted through the needle and determines how rapidly CSF will appear at the needle hub during spinal needle insertion. All spinal and epidural needles come with a tight fitting stylet. The stylet prevents the needle from being plugged with skin or fat and, importantly, prevents dragging skin into the epidural or subarachnoid spaces, where the skin may grow and form dermoid tumors.

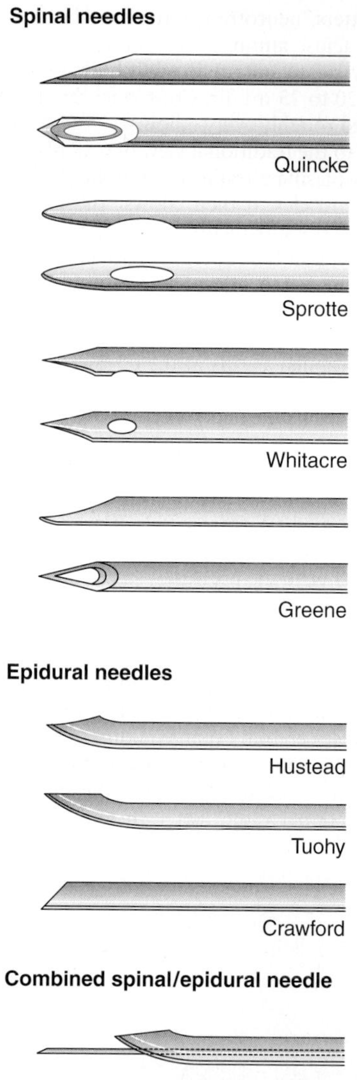

Spinal needles

Quincke

Sprotte

Whitacre

Greene

Epidural needles

Hustead

Tuohy

Crawford

Combined spinal/epidural needle

FIGURE 34-6. Some of the commercially available needles for spinal and epidural anesthesia. Needles are distinguished by the design of their tips.

Sedation

If the patient desires, light sedation is appropriate before placement of spinal or epidural block. Generally, the patient should not be heavily sedated because successful spinal and epidural anesthesia requires patient participation to maintain good position, evaluate block height, and to enable communication with the anesthesiologist should a paresthesia occur when the needle contacts neural elements. In addition, patient cooperation is required to properly evaluate an epidural test dose; sedation with as little as 1.5 mg of midazolam plus 75 μg of fentanyl has been shown to reduce the reliability of patient reports of subjective symptoms of intravenous (IV) local anesthetic injection.[31] Once the block is placed and adequate block height assured, the patient can be sedated as deemed appropriate.

Spinal Anesthesia

Position

Careful attention to patient positioning is critical to successful spinal puncture. Poor positioning can turn an otherwise easy spinal anesthetic into a challenge for both the anesthesiologist and the patient. Spinal needles are often inserted with the patient in the lateral decubitus position and this technique is described in detail later. However, both the prone jackknife and sitting positions offer advantages under specific circumstances. The sitting position is sometimes used in obese patients because it is often easier to identify the midline with the patient sitting. In addition, the sitting position allows one to restrict spinal block to the sacral dermatomes (*saddle block*) when using hyperbaric local anesthetic solutions. Spinal block is generally performed in the prone jackknife position only when this is the position to be used for surgery. The use of hypobaric local anesthetic solutions with the patient in the prone jackknife position produces sacral block for perirectal surgery.

In the lateral decubitus position, the patient lies with the operative side down when using hyperbaric local anesthetic solutions and with the operative side up when using hypobaric solutions, thus assuring that the earliest and most dense block occurs on the operative side. The back should be at the edge of the table so that the patient is within easy reach. The patient's shoulders and hips are both positioned perpendicular to the bed to help prevent rotation of the spine. The knees are drawn to the chest, the neck is flexed, and the patient is instructed to actively curve the lumbar spine outward toward the anesthesiologist. This will spread the spinous processes apart and maximize the size of the interlaminar foramen. It is useful to have an assistant who can help the patient maintain this position. Using the iliac crests as a landmark (a line drawn between the iliac crests crosses the body of L5 or the L4 to L5 interspace), the L2 to L3, L3 to L4, and L4 to L5 interspaces are identified and the desired interspace chosen for needle insertion. Interspaces above L2 to L3 are avoided to decrease the risk of hitting the spinal cord with the needle. Some find it helpful to mark the spinous processes flanking the desired interspace with a skin marker. This obviates the need to reidentify the intended interspace after the patient is prepared and draped.

The skin is prepared with an appropriate antiseptic solution and draped. All antiseptic solutions are neurotoxic, and care must be taken not to contaminate spinal needles or local anesthetics with the antiseptic solution. Chlorhexidine–alcohol antiseptic prevents colonization of percutaneous catheters better than does 10% povidone–iodine. Consequently, the American Society of Regional Anesthesia currently recommends chlorhexidine for skin antisepsis prior to regional anesthesia procedures.[a] How one drapes is a matter of personal preference, but clear plastic fenestrated drapes offer the important advantage of permitting visualization of the entire back, which makes it easier to identify a rotated or inadequately flexed spine.

[a]See http://www.asra.com/publications-infectious-complications-2004.php.

Midline Approach

For the midline approach to the subarachnoid space, the skin overlying the desired interspace is infiltrated with a small amount of local anesthetic to prevent pain when inserting the spinal needle. One should avoid raising too large a skin wheal because this can obscure palpation of the interspace, especially in obese patients. Additional local anesthetic (1 to 2 mL) is then deposited along the intended path of the spinal needle to a depth of 1 to 2 inches. This deeper infiltration provides additional anesthesia for spinal needle insertion and helps identify the correct path for the spinal needle. Infiltrating local anesthetic lateral to the midline is painful and generally unnecessary.

The spinal needle or introducer needle is inserted in the middle of the interspace with a slight cephalad angulation of 10 to 15 degrees (Fig. 34-7). The needle is then advanced, in order, through the subcutaneous tissue, supraspinous ligament, interspinous ligament, ligamentum flavum, epidural space, dura mater, and finally arachnoid mater. The ligaments produce a characteristic "feel" as the needle is advanced through them, and the anesthesiologist should develop the ability to distinguish a needle that is advancing through the high-resistance ligaments from one that is advancing through lower-resistance paraspinous muscle. This will allow early detection and correction of needles that are not advancing in the midline. Penetration of the dura mater often produces a subtle "pop" that is most easily detected with the pencil-point needles. Detection of dural penetration will prevent inserting the needle all the way through the subarachnoid space and contacting the vertebral body. In addition, learning to detect dural penetration will allow one to insert the spinal needle quickly without having to stop every few millimeters and remove the stylet to look for CSF at the needle hub.

Once the needle tip is believed to be in the subarachnoid space, the stylet is removed to see if CSF appears at the needle hub. With small diameter needles (26G to 29G) this generally

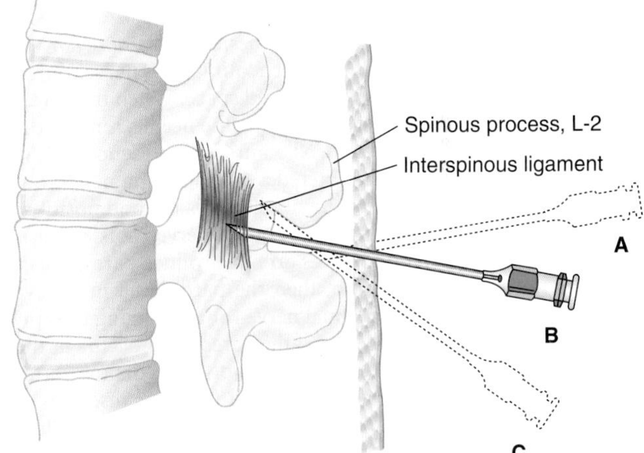

FIGURE 34-7. Midline approach to the subarachnoid space. The spinal needle is inserted with a slight cephalad angulation and should advance in the midline without contacting bone **(B)**. If bone is contacted, it may be either the caudad **(A)** or the cephalad spinous process **(C)**. The needle should be redirected slightly cephalad and reinserted. If bone is encountered at a shallower depth, the needle is likely walking up the cephalad spinous process. If bone is encountered at a deeper depth, the needle is likely walking down the inferior spinous process. If bone is repeatedly contacted at the same depth, the needle is likely off the midline and walking along the lamina. (Reprinted from: Mulroy MF. *Regional Anesthesia: An Illustrated Procedural Guide*. Boston: Little Brown; 1989, with permission.)

requires 5 to 10 seconds, but may require ≥1 minute in some patients. Gentle aspiration may speed the appearance of CSF. If CSF does not appear, the needle orifice may be obstructed by a nerve root and rotating the needle 90 degrees may result in CSF flow. Alternatively, the needle orifice may not be completely in the subarachnoid space and advancing an additional 1 to 2 mm may result in brisk CSF flow. This is particularly true of pencil-point needles, which have their orifice on the side of the needle shaft proximal to the needle tip. Finally, failure to obtain CSF suggests that the needle orifice is not in the subarachnoid space and the needle should be reinserted.

If bone is encountered during needle insertion, the anesthesiologist must develop a reasoned, systematic approach to redirecting the needle. Simply withdrawing the needle and repeatedly reinserting it in different directions is not appropriate. When contacting bone, the depth should be immediately noted and the needle redirected slightly cephalad. If bone is again encountered at a greater depth, then the needle is most likely walking down the inferior spinous process and it should be redirected more cephalad until the subarachnoid space is reached. If bone is encountered again at a shallower depth, then the needle is most likely walking up the superior spinous process and it should be redirected more caudad. If bone is repeatedly encountered at the same depth, then the needle is likely off the midline and walking along the vertebral lamina (Fig. 34-7).

When redirecting a needle it is important to withdraw the tip into the subcutaneous tissue. If the tip remains embedded in one of the vertebral ligaments, attempts at redirecting the needle will simply bend the shaft and will not reliably change needle direction. When using an introducer needle, it also must be withdrawn into the subcutaneous tissue before being redirected. Changes in needle direction should be made in small increments because even small changes in needle angle at the skin may result in fairly large changes in position of the needle tip when it reaches the spinal meninges at a depth of 4 to 6 cm. Care should be exercised when gripping the needle to ensure that it does not bow. Insertion of a curved needle will cause it to veer off course.

If the patient experiences a paresthesia, it is important to determine whether the needle tip has encountered a nerve root in the epidural space or in the subarachnoid space. When the paresthesia occurs, immediately stop advancing the needle, remove the stylet, and look for CSF at the needle hub. The presence of CSF confirms that the needle encountered a cauda equina nerve root in the subarachnoid space and the needle tip is in good position. Given how tightly packed the cauda equina nerve roots are, it is surprising that all spinal punctures do not produce paresthesias. If CSF is not visible at the hub, then the paresthesia may have resulted from contact with a spinal nerve root traversing the epidural space. This is especially true if the paresthesia occurs in the dermatome corresponding to the nerve root that exits the vertebral canal at the same level that the spinal needle is inserted. In this case, the needle has most likely deviated from the midline and should be redirected toward the side opposite the paresthesia. Occasionally, pain experienced when the needle contacts bone may be misinterpreted by the patient as a paresthesia and the anesthesiologist should be alert to this possibility.

Once the needle is correctly inserted into the subarachnoid space, it is fixed in position and the syringe containing local anesthetic is attached. CSF is gently aspirated to confirm that the needle is still in the subarachnoid space and the local anesthetic slowly injected (≤0.5 mL/sec). After completing the injection, a small volume of CSF is again aspirated to confirm that the needle tip remained in the subarachnoid space while the local anesthetic was deposited. This CSF is then reinjected and the needle, syringe, and any introducer removed together as a unit. If the surgical procedure is to be performed in the supine position, the patient is helped onto his or her back. To prevent excessive cephalad spread of hyperbaric local anesthetic, care should be taken to ensure that the patient's hips are not raised off the bed as they turn.

Once the block is placed, strict attention must be paid to the patient's hemodynamic status with blood pressure and/or heart rate supported as necessary. Block height should also be assessed early by pin prick or temperature sensation. Temperature sensation is tested by wiping the skin with alcohol, and may be preferable to pin prick because it is not painful. If, after a few minutes, the block is not rising high enough or is rising too high, the table may be tilted as appropriate to influence further spread of hypobaric or hyperbaric local anesthetics.

Paramedian Approach

The paramedian approach to the epidural and subarachnoid spaces is useful in situations where the patient's anatomy does not favor the midline approach, such as inability to flex the spine or heavily calcified interspinous ligaments. This approach can be used with the patient in any position and is probably the best approach for the patient in the prone jackknife position.

The spinous process forming the lower border of the desired interspace is identified. The needle is inserted approximately 1 cm lateral to this point and is directed toward the middle of the interspace by angling it approximately 45 degrees cephalad with just enough medial angulation (approximately 15 degrees) to compensate for the lateral insertion point. The first significant resistance encountered should be the ligamentum flavum. Bone encountered prior to the ligamentum flavum is usually the vertebral lamina of the cephalad vertebra and the needle should be redirected accordingly. An alternative method is to insert the needle perpendicular to the skin in all planes until the lamina is contacted. The needle is then walked off the superior edge of the lamina and into the subarachnoid space. The lamina provides a valuable landmark that facilitates correct needle placement; however, repeated needle contact with the periosteum can be painful.

Lumbosacral Approach

The lumbosacral (or Taylor) approach to the subarachnoid and epidural spaces is simply a paramedian approach directed at the L5 to S1 interspace, which is the largest interlaminar space. This approach may be useful when anatomic constraints make other approaches unfeasible. The patient may be positioned laterally, prone, or sitting, and the needle inserted at a point 1 cm medial and 1 cm inferior to the posterior superior iliac spine. The needle is angled cephalad 45 to 55 degrees and just medial enough to reach the midline at the level of the L5 spinous process. As with the paramedian approach, the interspinous ligament is bypassed and the first significant resistance felt should be the ligamentum flavum.

Continuous Spinal Anesthesia

3

Inserting a catheter into the subarachnoid space increases the utility of spinal anesthesia by permitting repeated drug administration as often as necessary to extend the level or duration of spinal block. A common and reasonable recommendation for subsequent dosing or "topping up" of continuous spinal blocks is to administer half the original dose of local anesthetic when the block has reached two thirds of its expected duration.

The technique is similar to that described for "single-shot" spinal anesthesia except that a needle large enough to accommodate the desired catheter must be used. After inserting the needle and obtaining free-flowing CSF, the catheter is simply threaded into the subarachnoid space a distance of 2 to 3 cm. It is often easier to insert the catheter if it is directed cephalad or caudad instead of laterally. If the catheter does not easily pass beyond the needle tip, rotating the needle 180 degrees may be helpful or another interspace may be used. Once the catheter is advanced beyond the needle tip, the catheter should not be withdrawn back into the needle shaft due to the risk of shearing the catheter off into the subarachnoid space.

A variety of catheters and needles are available for continuous spinal anesthesia. Commonly, 18G epidural needles and 20G catheters are used. However, needles and catheters this size carry a higher risk of PDPH, especially in young patients. Because of this risk, smaller needle and catheter combinations have been developed with catheters ranging in size from 24G to 32G. Although smaller catheters decrease the risk of PDPH, they have also been associated with multiple reports of neurologic injury, specifically, cauda equina syndrome (see "Complications"). For this reason, the United States Food and Drug Administration has advised against using any catheter smaller than 24G for continuous spinal anesthesia.

Epidural Anesthesia

For the novice, correct placement of an epidural needle can be technically more challenging than spinal needle placement because there is less room for error. However, with experience, epidural needle placement is often easier than spinal needle placement because the larger gauge needles used for epidural anesthesia are less likely to be deflected from their intended path and they produce much better tactile feel of the interspinous and flaval ligaments. In addition, the loss of resistance technique provides a much clearer end point when entering the epidural space than does the subtle "pop" of a spinal needle piercing the dura mater.

Patient preparation, positioning, monitors, and needle approaches for epidural anesthesia are the same as for spinal anesthesia. Unlike spinal anesthesia, epidural anesthesia may be performed at any intervertebral space. However, at vertebral levels above the termination of the spinal cord, the epidural needle may accidentally puncture the spinal meninges and damage the underlying spinal cord. To prevent accidental meningeal puncture, the anesthesiologist must learn to identify the interspinous ligaments and the ligamentum flavum by their feel. In addition, epidural needles must be advanced slowly and, most importantly, under control.

After proper positioning, sterile skin preparation, and draping, the desired interspace is identified and a local anesthetic skin wheal is raised at the point of needle insertion. Because epidural needles are relatively blunt, it is sometimes helpful to pierce the skin with a ≥18G hypodermic needle before inserting the epidural needle. For epidural anesthesia using the midline approach, the epidural needle is inserted through the subcutaneous tissue and into the interspinous ligament. The interspinous ligament has a characteristic "gritty" feel, much like inserting a needle into a bag of sand. This is especially true of younger patients. If the interspinous ligament is not clearly identified, then one should be suspicious that the needle is not in the midline. After engaging the interspinous ligament, the needle is advanced slowly through it until an increase in resistance is felt. This increased resistance represents the ligamentum flavum.

The epidural needle must now traverse the ligamentum flavum and stop within the epidural space before puncturing the spinal meninges. Numerous techniques for identifying the epidural space have been used successfully; however, the loss of resistance to fluid has the advantage of simplicity, reliability, and, most importantly, a higher success rate when compared to the use of air for loss of resistance.[32] In addition, use of fluid instead of air for loss of resistance decreases the risk of PDPH in the event of accidental meningeal puncture.[33]

A glass syringe or a specially designed low-resistance plastic syringe is filled with 2 to 3 mL of saline and a small (0.1 to 0.3 mL) air bubble. The syringe is attached to the epidural needle and the plunger is pressed until the air bubble is visibly compressed. If the needle tip is properly embedded within the ligamentum flavum, it should be possible to compress the air bubble without injecting fluid. In this way the air bubble serves as a gauge of the appropriate amount of pressure to exert on the syringe plunger. If the air bubble cannot be compressed without injecting fluid, then the needle tip is most likely not in the ligamentum flavum. In this case, the needle tip may still be in the interspinous ligament, or it may be off the midline in the paraspinous muscles. To differentiate between these possibilities, one can carefully advance the needle and syringe a few millimeters in an effort to engage the ligamentum flavum. If it is still not possible to compress the air bubble, withdraw the needle into the subcutaneous tissue and reinsert it.

Once the ligamentum flavum is identified, the needle is slowly advanced with the nondominant hand while the dominant hand maintains constant pressure on the syringe plunger (Fig. 34-8). Do not advance the needle with the hand compressing the plunger because this does not allow for adequate control of needle movement. As the needle tip enters the epidural space, there will be a sudden and dramatic loss of resistance as the saline is rapidly injected. Saline injection into the epidural space can be moderately painful and patients should be forewarned. If the needle is advancing obliquely through the ligamentum flavum, it is possible to enter into the paraspinous muscles instead of the epidural space. In this case the loss of resistance will be less dramatic. To

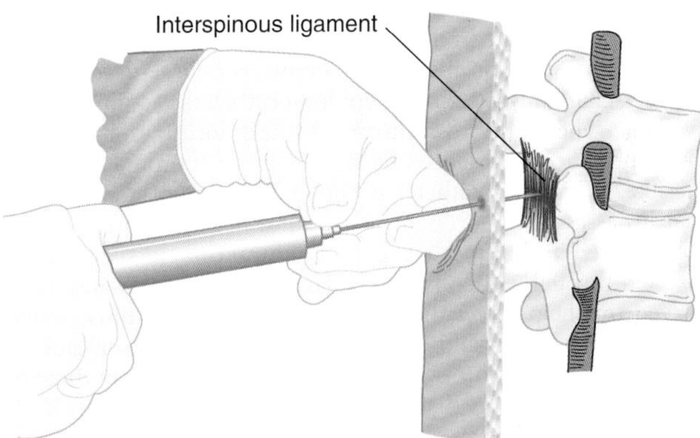

FIGURE 34-8. Proper hand position when using the loss-of-resistance technique to locate the epidural space. After embedding the needle tip in the ligamentum flavum, a syringe with 2 to 3 mL of saline and an air bubble is attached. The left hand rests securely on the back and the fingers of the left hand grasp the needle firmly. The left hand advances the needle slowly and under control by rotating at the wrist. The fingers of the right hand maintain constant pressure on the syringe plunger but do not aid in advancing the needle. If the needle tip is properly engaged in the ligamentum flavum, it should be possible to compress the air bubble without injecting the saline. As the needle tip enters the epidural space, there will be a sudden loss of resistance and the saline will be suddenly injected. (Reprinted from: Mulroy MF. *Regional Anesthesia: An Illustrated Procedural Guide*. Boston: Little Brown; 1989, with permission.)

help verify that the needle has entered the epidural space, 0.5 mL of air can be drawn into the syringe and injected. There will be virtually no resistance to air injection in the epidural space, while in the paraspinous muscles air injection will encounter demonstrable resistance.

After entering the epidural space, stop advancing the needle. Because the dura mater abuts the ligamentum flavum in many places, the dura may now be tented over the needle tip and advancing the needle any farther than necessary heightens the risk of accidental meningeal puncture, that is, "*wet tap.*" When the syringe is disconnected from the needle, it is common to have a small amount of fluid flow from the needle hub. This is usually the saline flowing back out of the epidural space but it could be CSF if the needle accidentally entered the subarachnoid space. CSF can often be distinguished by the fact that CSF will usually flow out in a volume greatly exceeding that used for the loss of resistance, CSF will be warm compared with saline, and CSF will test positive for glucose.

If a single-shot technique is to be used, then a local anesthetic test dose should be administered to help rule out undetected subarachnoid or IV needle placement. After a negative test dose, the desired volume of local anesthetic should be administered in small increments (e.g., 5 mL) at a rate of 0.5 to 1 mL/sec. Slow, incremental injection decreases the risk of pain during injection and allows detection of adverse reactions to accidental IV or subarachnoid placement before the entire dose is administered.

Continuous Epidural Anesthesia

Use of a catheter for epidural anesthesia affords much greater flexibility than the single-shot technique because the catheter can be used to prolong a block that is too short, to extend a block that is too low, or to provide postoperative analgesia. On the downside, catheters may migrate into an epidural vein, into the subarachnoid space, or out an intervertebral foramen. Catheter use is also more likely to result in unilateral epidural block, a clinical fact shown to result from catheter tips that end up in the anterior epidural space or migrate out an intervertebral foramina.[18,34] An ever-changing selection of epidural catheters is commercially available. They differ in diameter, stiffness, location of injection holes, presence or absence of a stylet, construction material, and the like. Whichever catheter is chosen, it is important to verify that it passes easily through the epidural needle before the needle is placed in the epidural space. Epidural catheters are usually inserted through either Tuohy or Hustead needles because their curved tips help direct the catheter away from the dura mater. The needle bevel should be directed either cephalad or caudad, although the direction of the bevel does not guarantee that the catheter will travel in that direction. The catheter will typically encounter resistance as it reaches the curve at the tip of the needle, but steady pressure will usually result in passage into the epidural space. If the catheter will not pass beyond the needle tip, it is possible that the needle opening is not completely in the epidural space or that some structure in the epidural space is preventing catheter insertion (e.g., epidural fat). In this instance, the needle can be carefully advanced 1 to 2 mm more or rotated 180 degrees and the catheter reinserted. Although either of these maneuvers may result in successful catheter placement, they also increase the risk of accidental meningeal puncture. Alternatively, the procedure can be repeated at another interspace or with a different needle approach, for example, paramedian. Occasionally a catheter will advance only a short distance past the needle tip. This raises the possibility that the needle tip is not in the epidural space and needs to be repositioned. In this case, the catheter should not be withdrawn back into the epidural needle because of the risk that the catheter tip will be sheared off by the bevel's sharp edge. Rather, the needle and catheter should be pulled out in tandem and the procedure repeated. An alternative explanation for the inability to thread an epidural catheter is that the tip of the epidural needle was bent during bony contact and now partially occludes the needle lumen.

The catheter should be advanced only 3 to 5 cm into the epidural space. Placing a longer length of catheter in the epidural space increases the risk that it will form a knot,[35,36] enter an epidural vein, puncture the spinal meninges, exit an intervertebral foramen, wrap around a nerve root, or wind up in some other disadvantageous location. Once the catheter is appropriately positioned in the epidural space, the needle is slowly withdrawn with one hand as the catheter is stabilized with the other. After the needle is removed, the length of the catheter in the epidural space is confirmed by subtracting the distance between the skin and the epidural space from the length of the catheter below the skin. Documenting this distance is important when trying to determine if catheters used in the postoperative period have been dislodged.

An epidural test dose must be administered through the catheter to test for IV or subarachnoid placement before incrementally delivering the entire epidural drug dose. In addition, because of the risk of undetected IV or subarachnoid migration of the catheter over time, additional test doses must be administered before each top-up dose is given through the catheter. As with continuous spinal anesthesia, a reasonable guideline for top-up doses is to administer half the initial local anesthetic dose at an interval equal to two thirds the expected duration of the block.

Epidural Test Dose

The epidural test dose is designed to identify epidural needles or catheters that have entered an epidural vein or the subarachnoid space. Failure to perform the test may result in IV injection of toxic doses of local anesthetic or total spinal block. Aspirating the
3 catheter or needle to check for blood or CSF is helpful if positive, but the incidence of false-negative aspirations is too high to rely on this technique alone.[37]

The most common test dose is 3 mL of local anesthetic containing 5 μg/mL of epinephrine (1:200,000). The dose of local anesthetic should be sufficient that subarachnoid injection will result in clear evidence of spinal anesthesia. Intravenous injection of this dose of epinephrine typically produces an average 30 beats per minute heart rate increase between 20 and 40 seconds after injection.[38,39] Heart rate increases may not be as evident in some patients taking beta-blocking drugs; reflex bradycardia often occurs in these patients.[38,40] In beta-blocked patients, a systolic blood pressure increase of ≥20 mm Hg may be a more reliable indicator of IV injection.[38,40]

Importantly, the sensitivity of the standard 15-μg epinephrine test dose has been shown to be markedly diminished by pre-existing high thoracic epidural anesthesia and/or concurrent general anesthesia.[41] Larger epinephrine doses may be effective at detecting IV injection in these settings, but that has not been shown experimentally.

Isoproterenol has also been used to detect intravascular injection.[42] In addition, air injection combined with a precordial Doppler to detect the characteristic murmur has been used successfully to test for IV placement of epidural catheters.[37] These techniques have been developed for the use in laboring women in whom the sensitivity of epinephrine as a test dose is disturbingly low because maternal heart rate increases during contractions are often as large as those produced by epinephrine.[43] The clinical indications for these alternative tests of IV injection await additional larger studies.

Combined Spinal–Epidural Anesthesia

Combined spinal–epidural anesthesia (CSEA) is a useful technique by which a spinal block and an epidural catheter are placed simultaneously. This technique is popular because it combines the rapid onset, dense block of spinal anesthesia with the flexibility afforded by an epidural catheter. There are special epidural needles with a separate lumen to accommodate a spinal needle available for CSEA (Fig. 34-6). However, the technique is easily performed by first placing a standard epidural needle in the epidural space and then inserting an appropriately sized spinal needle through the shaft of the epidural needle and into the subarachnoid space. The desired local anesthetic is injected into the subarachnoid space, the spinal needle is removed, and a catheter placed in the epidural space via the epidural needle. The catheter can then be used to extend the height or duration of intraoperative block or can be used to provide postoperative epidural analgesia.

An interesting pharmacologic aspect of CSEA is the observation that after the peak spinal block height is established, both saline and local anesthetic injected into the epidural space are effective at pushing the block level higher.[44–46] This observation has been interpreted to indicate that the mechanism by which the epidural "top-up" increases block height is by a volume effect (i.e., compression of the spinal meninges forcing CSF cephalad) as well as a local anesthetic effect.

A potential risk of this technique is that the meningeal hole made by the spinal needle may allow dangerously high concentrations of subsequently administered epidural drugs to reach the subarachnoid space. Anecdotal case reports and in vitro animal studies suggest that this may be a legitimate concern.[43,47–49] Although CSEA is advantageous in some circumstances, additional prospective studies are necessary to identify the relative risks and limitations of the technique.

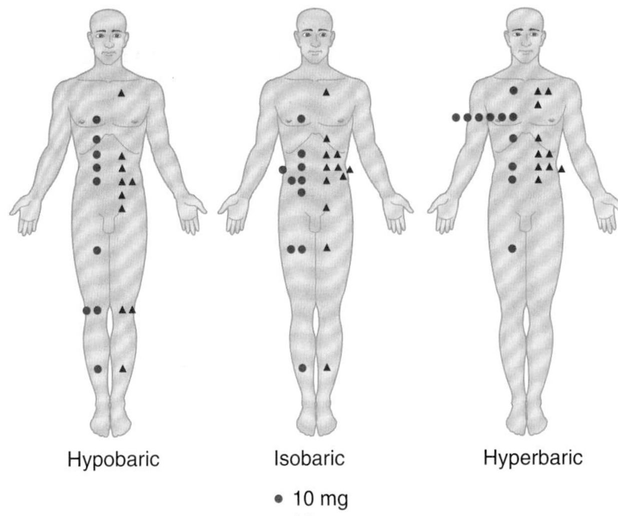

FIGURE 34-9. Peak spinal block height following 10- and 15-mg doses of hypobaric, isobaric, and hyperbaric tetracaine solutions injected at L3 to L4 with patients in the lateral horizontal position. Note that dose has no influence on block height and that there is considerable interindividual variability in peak block height, especially with the hypobaric solution. (Adapted from: Brown DT, Wildsmith JA, Covino BG, et al. Effect of baricity on spinal anaesthesia with amethocaine. *Br J Anaesth.* 1980;52:589, with permission.)

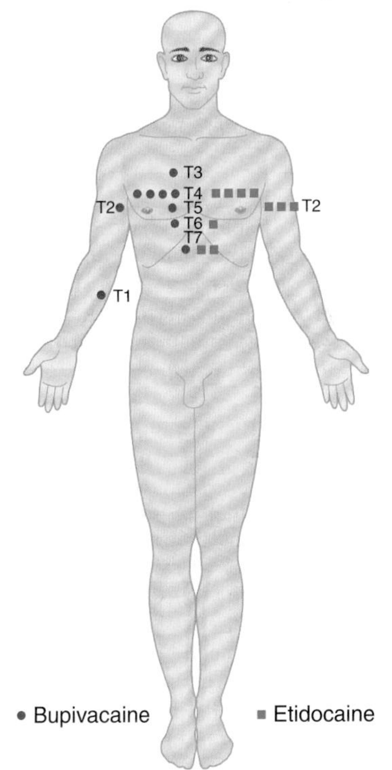

FIGURE 34-10. Peak epidural block height following 20 mL of 0.75% bupivacaine or 1.5% etidocaine injected via a catheter at the L1 to L2 interspace. Note that despite a well-controlled technique, the interindividual variability in block height is considerable and demonstrates the difficulty in accurately predicting block height in an individual patient. (Adapted from: Sinclair CJ, Scott DB. Comparison of bupivacaine and etidocaine in extradural blockade. *Br J Anaesth.* 1984;56:147, with permission.)

PHARMACOLOGY

Successful spinal or epidural anesthesia requires a block that is high enough to block sensation at the surgical site and last for the duration of the planned procedure. However, variability between patients is considerable (Figs. 34-9 and 34-10), reliably predicting the height and duration of central neuraxial block that will result from a particular local anesthetic dose is difficult. Thus, recommendations regarding local anesthetic choice and dose must be viewed as approximate guidelines. The clinician must understand the factors governing spinal and epidural block height and duration to individualize local anesthetic choice and dose for each patient and procedure.

Spinal Anesthesia

Block Height

Table 34-1 lists some common surgical procedures that are readily performed under spinal anesthesia and the block height that is usually sufficient to ensure patient comfort. Also listed are techniques that are appropriate to achieve the desired block height. The rationale for these recommendations is explained in the following section.

TABLE 34-1. REPRESENTATIVE SURGICAL PROCEDURES APPROPRIATE FOR SPINAL ANESTHESIA

Surgical Procedure	Suggested Block Height	Technique	Comments
Perianal Perirectal	L1–L2	Hyperbaric solution/ sitting position Hypobaric solution/ jackknife position Isobaric solution/ horizontal position	Patients must remain in relative head-up or head-down position when using hypobaric and hyperbaric solutions to maintain restricted spread during the procedure
Lower extremity Hip Transurethral resection of the prostate Vaginal/cervical	T10	Isobaric solution	Hypobaric and hyperbaric solutions are also suitable but may produce higher blocks than necessary
Herniorrhaphy Pelvic procedures Appendectomy	T6–T8	Hyperbaric solution/ horizontal position	Isobaric solutions injected at L2–L3 interspace may also be suitable
Abdominal Cesarean section	T4–T6	Hyperbaric solution/ horizontal position	Upper abdominal procedures usually require concomitant general anesthesia to prevent vagal reflexes and pain from traction on diaphragm, esophagus, and the like

Baricity and Patient Position

The height of spinal block is thought to be determined by the cephalad spread of local anesthetic within the CSF. Table 34-2 lists some of the many variables that have been proposed to influence the spread of local anesthetics within the subarachnoid space. Many of these variables have been shown to be of negligible clinical importance. Of those factors that do exert significant influence on local anesthetic spread, the baricity of the local anesthetic solution relative to patient position is probably the most important. *Baricity* is defined as the ratio of the density (mass/volume) of the local anesthetic solution divided by the density of CSF, which averages 1.0003 ± 0.0003 g/mL at 37°C. Solutions that have the same density as CSF have a baricity of 1 and are termed *isobaric.* Solutions that are denser than CSF are termed *hyperbaric,* whereas solutions that are less dense than CSF are termed *hypobaric.*

Table 34-3 lists the baricity of local anesthetic solutions commonly used for spinal anesthesia. For practical purposes, solutions with a baricity <0.9990 can be expected to reliably behave hypobarically in all patients. Hypobaric solutions are typically prepared by mixing the local anesthetic solution with distilled water. Solutions with a baricity of ≥1.0015 can be expected to reliably behave hyperbarically. Hyperbaric solutions are typically prepared by mixing the local anesthetic in 5% to 8% dextrose. The baricity of the resultant solution depends on the amount of dextrose added; however, dextrose concentrations between 1.25% and 8% result in equivalent block heights.[50,51] Lower dextrose concentrations have been shown to have a concentration-dependent effect on block height, with 0.33% producing a block to T9.5 on average, 0.83% producing a block to T7.2, and 8% producing a block to T3.6.[52]

TABLE 34-2. FACTORS THAT HAVE BEEN SUGGESTED AS POSSIBLE DETERMINANTS OF SPREAD OF LOCAL ANESTHETIC SOLUTIONS WITHIN THE SUBARACHNOID SPACE

Characteristics of the Local Anesthetic Solution
Baricity
Local anesthetic dose
Local anesthetic concentration
Volume injected

Patient Characteristics
Age
Weight
Height
Gender
Pregnancy
Patient position

Technique
Site of injection
Speed of injection
Barbotage
Direction of needle bevel
Addition of vasoconstrictors

Diffusion

Adapted from: Greene NM. Distribution of local anesthetic solutions within the subarachnoid space. *Anesth Analg.* 1985;64:715, with permission.

TABLE 34-3. BARICITY OF SOLUTIONS COMMONLY USED FOR SPINAL ANESTHESIA

	Baricity[a]
Hyperbaric	
Tetracaine: 0.5% in 5% dextrose	1.0133
Bupivacaine: 0.75% in 8.25% dextrose	1.0227
Lidocaine: 5% in 7.5% dextrose	1.0265
Procaine: 10% in water	1.0104
Isobaric[b]	
Tetracaine: 0.5% in normal saline	0.9997
Bupivacaine: 0.75% in saline	0.9988
Bupivacaine: 0.5% in saline	0.9983
Lidocaine: 2% in saline	0.9986
Hypobaric	
Tetracaine: 0.2% in water	0.9922
Bupivacaine: 0.3% in water	0.9946
Lidocaine: 0.5% in water	0.9985

[a]Measured at 37°C, except for hypobaric 0.5% lidocaine measured at 25°C. At 37°C, this solution's baricity is less.
[b]These solutions are slightly hypobaric but are used clinically as if they were isobaric.
Data from: Horlocker TT, Wedel DJ. Density, specific gravity, and baricity of spinal anesthetic solutions at body temperature. *Anesth Analg.* 1993;76:1015; Lambert D, Covino B. Hyperbaric, hypobaric and isobaric spinal anesthesia. *Resident Staff Physician.* 1987;33:79; Greene NM. Distribution of local anesthetic solutions within the subarachnoid space. *Anesth Analg.* 1985;64:715; and Bodily N, Carpenter R, Owens B. Lidocaine 0.5% spinal anaesthesia: A hypobaric solution for short-stay perirectal surgery. *Can J Anaesth.* 1992;39:770.

Baricity is important in determining local anesthetic spread and thus block height because gravity causes hyperbaric solutions to flow downward in CSF to the most dependent regions of the spinal column, whereas hypobaric solutions tend to rise in CSF. In contrast, gravity has no effect on the distribution of truly isobaric solutions. Thus, the anesthesiologist can exert considerable influence on block height by choice of anesthetic solution and proper patient positioning. Spinal block can be restricted to the sacral and low lumbar dermatomes (*"saddle block"*) by administering a hyperbaric local anesthetic solution with the patient in the sitting position[53] or by administering a hypobaric solution with the patient in the prone jackknife position. Similarly, high thoracic to midcervical levels of anesthesia can be reached by administering hyperbaric solutions with the patient in the horizontal and Trendelenburg positions[54,55] or by administering hypobaric solutions with the patient in a semisitting position. However, this use of hypobaric solutions is not recommended because the high block achieved and the diminished venous return associated with the upright posture can lead to significant cardiovascular compromise.

The sitting, Trendelenburg, and jackknife positions have marked influences on the distribution of hypobaric and hyperbaric solutions because these positions accentuate the effect of gravity. However, most spinal anesthetics are administered as hyperbaric solutions injected while patients are in the horizontal lateral position, after which they are turned to the horizontal supine position. In this situation the influence of gravity is more subtle because the dependent areas of the spinal column do not deviate as much from the horizontal. While the patient is turned laterally, gravity has a small but measurable effect on local anesthetic distribution in that hyperbaric solutions will produce a denser, longer-lasting block on the dependent side, while hypobaric solutions will have the opposite effect.[56] This makes hypobaric solutions ideal for unilateral procedures performed in the lateral position when the operative side is nondependent (e.g., hip surgery). Hyperbaric solutions can be used to advantage for unilateral procedures performed in the supine position if the operative side is dependent during drug injection and the patient is left in the lateral position for at least 6 minutes.[56] However, despite differences in block density and duration, peak block height will be comparable between the dependent and nondependent sides.

When the patient is turned supine following hyperbaric drug injection in the lateral position, the normal spinal curvature will influence subsequent movement of the injected solution. Hyperbaric solutions injected at the height of the lumbar lordosis will tend to flow cephalad to pool in the thoracic kyphosis and caudad to pool in the sacrum (Fig. 34-11). Pooling of hyperbaric local anesthetic solutions in the thoracic kyphosis has been evoked to explain the clinical observation that hyperbaric solutions tend to produce blocks with an average height in the midthoracic region (Fig. 34-9). In addition, hyperbaric solutions have also been observed to produce blocks with a bimodal distribution; that is, one group of patients with blocks centered in the low thoracic region and a second group of patients with blocks centered in the high thoracic region.[57,58] The presumed explanation for this observation is that the lumbar lordosis produces "splitting" of the local anesthetic solution with some portion flowing caudad toward the sacrum and the remainder flowing cephalad into the thoracic kyphosis. The cephalad extent of the block then depends on what fraction of the injected drug flows cephalad. Consistent with this hypothesis is the fact that eliminating the lumbar lordosis by maintaining the hips flexed has been shown to significantly reduce[58] or eliminate[57] the bimodal distribution of blocks without affecting maximal block height.

Obviously, gravity influences the distribution of hyperbaric and hypobaric solutions only until they are sufficiently diluted in CSF so that they become isobaric. At this point, the local anesthetic solution no longer moves in response to changes in patient position and the block is said to be "fixed." Interestingly, the time required for a local anesthetic solution to become fixed may be considerable. Povey et al.[53,54] showed that hyperbaric bupivacaine

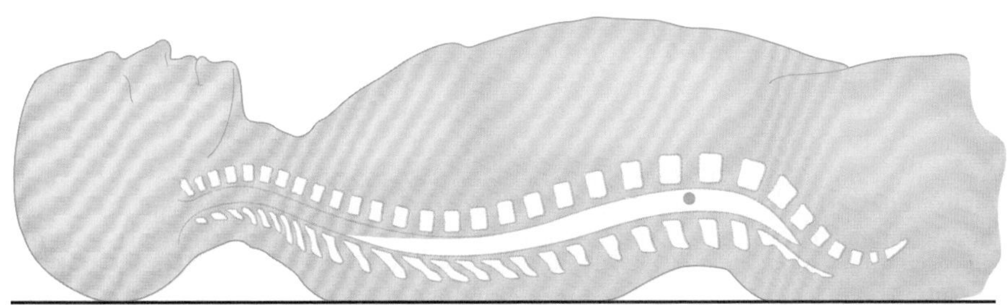

FIGURE 34-11. In the horizontal supine position, hyperbaric local anesthetic solutions injected at the height of the lumbar lordosis (*circle*) flow down the lumbar lordosis to pool in the sacrum and in the thoracic kyphosis. Pooling in the thoracic kyphosis is thought to explain the fact that hyperbaric solutions produce blocks with an average height of T4 to T6.

ANESTHETIC MANAGEMENT

injected in the sitting position produces a saddle block that is restricted to the lumbar segments for as long as the subjects remained sitting. However, even 60 minutes after bupivacaine injection the block spread to midthoracic levels after turning the patients supine. Similarly, Bodily et al.[59] found that hypobaric lidocaine administered in the jackknife position rose as many as six dermatomes when patients were allowed to sit upright in the recovery room as long as 60 minutes after lidocaine injection. Whether it is also possible to affect spread so long after injecting hyperbaric or hypobaric solutions in the horizontal position is unclear. Nonetheless, these findings demonstrate that in some situations it may be possible to exert influence on block height by adjusting patient position for at least 60 minutes after local anesthetic injection.

In contrast to the situation with hyperbaric solutions, patient position has no effect on the distribution of isobaric solutions because these solutions are not influenced by gravity. Consequently, isobaric solutions tend not to spread as far from the site of injection and produce blocks with an average height in the low thoracic region (Fig. 34-9).[51,60] The obvious caveat is that the local anesthetic solution must be truly isobaric in the patient in whom it is used. Because of the variability in CSF density among patients, it is difficult to produce reliably isobaric local anesthetic solutions. Nonetheless, as indicated in Table 34-3, several local anesthetic solutions are used as if they were isobaric. It is noteworthy that while isobaric solutions produce an average block height that is lower than comparable hyperbaric solutions,[51,60–62] the "isobaric" solutions produce blocks with a much greater variability in height.[63–65] Logan et al.[63] have termed plain bupivacaine "an unpredictable spinal anesthetic agent." The greater variability in spread may stem in part from the fact that these solutions are actually slightly hypobaric and their spread has been shown to be affected by patient position.[66,67] Temperature-related changes in baricity may also play a role in the variability in distribution of these nearly isobaric solutions. For example, Stienstra and van Poorten[68] have shown that the distribution of plain bupivacaine is significantly altered by changes in temperature of the injected solution, with greater spread found with warmer injectate. In addition, McClure et al.[69] have shown that increasing the volume and decreasing the concentration of isobaric tetracaine also increases the variability in block height. These and other unknown factors may play a role in the unpredictability of these nearly isobaric solutions. Although unpredictability is cause for concern, it should be pointed out that the lower average block height achieved offers potential advantages for surgical procedures below the umbilicus because of the decreased incidence of cardiovascular side effects associated with lower blocks. The isobaric solution that has been shown to most reliably produce a low thoracic block is 10 mg of tetracaine crystals diluted in 1- or 2-mL room temperature saline and injected in the horizontal position.[69]

Dose, Volume, and Concentration

Studies aimed at determining the effect of these three interdependent variables on block height are difficult to conduct and interpret because it is not possible to change one variable without simultaneously changing another. Nonetheless, it is possible to draw some conclusions regarding the effect of these variables on block height. Several studies with isobaric tetracaine and bupivacaine solutions have found that neither injected volume nor drug concentration affects block height when dose is held constant.[69–73] Drug dose does appear to play a small role in determining block height with isobaric bupivacaine. Two studies have found that 10 mg of isobaric bupivacaine results in significantly lower blocks than does 15 or 20 mg, but there is no difference in block height between the two higher doses.[74,75] In contrast, two studies that examined the effect of different doses of isobaric tetracaine found that doses between 5 and 15 mg had no effect on block height, producing blocks with an average height of T9 to T10.[60,76]

Drug dose and volume appear to be relatively unimportant in predicting the spread of hyperbaric local anesthetic solutions injected in the horizontal position. Increasing the dose and volume of hyperbaric tetracaine, while holding concentration constant, does not affect block height when doses between 7.5 and 15 mg are used.[60,76,77] Similarly, increasing the dose and volume of hyperbaric 0.5% bupivacaine does not increase block height when doses between 10 and 20 mg are used.[78,79] However, doses of hyperbaric 0.5% bupivacaine <10 mg have been shown to result in blocks that are approximately two and one-half dermatomes lower than those achieved with doses >10 mg.[78] The fact that bupivacaine dose affects block height only at the extreme low end of the usual dose range is consistent with the experience with isobaric bupivacaine reported earlier. The fact that drug dose is relatively unimportant in determining block height with hyperbaric solutions likely results from an overwhelming effect of baricity and patient position in determining spread of these solutions.

Injection Site

The site of injection can have an important effect on block height in some situations. In particular, sensory block height resulting from isobaric 0.5% bupivacaine is reduced by two dermatomes per interspace when comparing different groups of patients who received injections at the L2 to L3, L3 to L4, or L4 to L5 interspaces.[80,81] In an even more convincing study, this group of investigators performed repeated blocks in the same patient and found that by moving from the L3 to L4 to the L4 to L5 interspace means block height could be reduced from T6 to T10 when using isobaric 0.5% bupivacaine.[82] In contrast, Sundnes et al.[78] found no relationship between injection site and block height when using a hyperbaric bupivacaine solution, presumably because of the overwhelming effect of gravity and patient position on distribution of hyperbaric local anesthetics. Whether isobaric and hyperbaric solutions of other local anesthetics will behave similarly is not clear.

Patient Characteristics

4 In young adults, it was determined that the most important variable governing block height with hyperbaric local anesthetic solutions may be lumbosacral CSF volume.[83] However, it is unclear if these findings can be extrapolated to other local anesthetics or patient ages.

Higuchi et al.[84] performed a detailed examination of the effect of lumbar CSF volume, CSF density, lumbar CSF motion, patient age, weight, height, and body mass index (BMI) on spinal block with isobaric bupivacaine. Multiple linear regression demonstrated that neither patient age nor height correlated with any clinical characteristic of spinal block. However, CSF volume and weight were correlated with peak block height. CSF volume was the only variable to correlate with time to voiding. BMI was the only significant predictor of time to onset of complete sensory block.

Although these variables were statistically significant predictors of several important aspects of spinal block, the coefficients of determination (R^2) were generally small (average, 0.23; range, 0.08 to 0.46), indicating that these variables account for a relatively small amount of the variability in each of the block outcomes examined. Clearly, other factors contribute significantly to the clinical characteristics of spinal block with isobaric bupivacaine.

Although these studies are mechanistically important, their clinical application is necessarily limited by the difficulty in determining an individual patient's CSF volume, CSF density, and velocity of CSF movement.

Importantly, several investigators have found that patient age, weight, BMI, and height are either not predictive of clinical characteristics of spinal block[85–89] or are of such low predictive power as to be unreliable predictors in any individual patient.[65,80,90–92]

Onset

Most patients can sense the onset of spinal block within a very few minutes after drug injection regardless of the local anesthetic used. However, there is a significant difference among drugs in the time to reach peak block height. Lidocaine and mepivacaine tend to reach peak block height between 10 and 15 minutes, whereas tetracaine and bupivacaine may require >20 minutes before peak block height is reached.

Duration

Spinal blocks do not end abruptly after a fixed period of time. Rather, they recede gradually from the most cephalad dermatome to the most caudad. As a result, surgical anesthesia lasts significantly longer at sacral levels than at thoracic levels. Therefore, when discussing the duration of spinal block it is necessary to distinguish between duration at the surgical site and the time required for the block to completely resolve. The former is important for providing adequate surgical anesthesia, and the latter is important for assuring a timely recovery. A thorough understanding of the factors that govern block duration is necessary if the clinician is to choose techniques that result in an appropriate duration of spinal blockade.

Local Anesthetic

The principal determinant of spinal block duration is the local anesthetic drug employed. Procaine is the shortest-acting local anesthetic for subarachnoid use, lidocaine and mepivacaine are agents of intermediate duration, and bupivacaine and tetracaine are the longest-acting drugs. Table 34-4 lists the range of times required for sensory block to regress two dermatomes and to completely resolve with the local anesthetics most commonly used for spinal anesthesia. Although drug choice is the principal determinant of block duration, other variables are responsible for the wide range of block duration found in Table 34-4.

Drug Dose

Increasing local anesthetic dose clearly increases the duration of spinal block.[74,75,77,93,94] For example, Brown et al.[60] demonstrated that the duration of sensory block at L1 following 15 mg of tetracaine was approximately 20% greater than following 10 mg. Sheskey et al.[75] demonstrated an approximate 40% increase in block duration at L2 when comparing 10 mg of bupivacaine with 15 mg. Similarly, Axelsson et al.[93] found that the duration of sensory block at L2 was nearly doubled when comparing 10 mg of bupivacaine with 20 mg.

Block Height

If drug dose is held constant, higher blocks tend to regress faster than lower blocks.[94] Consequently, isobaric local anesthetic solutions will generally produce longer blocks than hyperbaric solutions using the same dose. The conventional wisdom is that greater cephalad spread results in relatively lower drug concentration in the CSF and spinal nerve roots. As a result, it takes less time for local anesthetic concentration to decrease below the minimally effective concentration.

Adrenergic Agonists

Adrenergic agonists, such as epinephrine, phenylephrine, and clonidine, are added to local anesthetics in an effort to prolong the duration of spinal anesthesia. Their effectiveness depends on the local anesthetic with which they are combined. In addition, they are more effective at prolonging block in the lumbar and sacral dermatomes than in thoracic dermatomes.

Epinephrine is typically administered in doses of 0.2 to 0.3 mg and phenylephrine in doses of 2 to 5 mg. There is evidence to

TABLE 34-4. DOSE AND DURATION OF LOCAL ANESTHETICS USED FOR SPINAL ANESTHESIA

		Duration of Sensory Block		
Drug	Dose (mg)[a]	Two-dermatome Regression (min)[b]	Complete Resolution (min)[b]	Prolongation by Adrenergic Agonists (%)[c]
Procaine	50–200	30–50	90–120	30–50
Chloroprocaine	30–100	30–50	70–150	NR
Lidocaine	25–100	40–100	140–240	20–50
Bupivacaine	5–20	90–140	240–380	20–50
Tetracaine	5–20	90–140	240–380	50–100

[a]The lowest doses are used primarily for very restricted blocks (e.g., saddle block), lest they become too dilute to be effective.
[b]Duration is influenced by dose and block height. The duration of surgical anesthesia will obviously depend on the surgical site.
[c]The effect of adrenergic agonists depends on the dose and choice of agonist. Prolongation is greatest at lumbar and sacral dermatomes and least at thoracic dermatomes.
NR: Not recommended; see text for explanation.

suggest a relationship between the dose of vasoconstrictor added and the duration of spinal anesthesia; however, the relationship is not strong.[95–98] At the maximal doses used clinically, phenylephrine (5 mg) prolongs spinal block to a greater degree than epinephrine (0.5 mg).[99,100] At lower doses, epinephrine (0.2 to 0.3 mg) and phenylephrine (2 to 3 mg) appear to be equally effective in prolonging spinal block.[98,101] Thus, both choice of adrenergic agonist and dose administered appear to play a role in determining block duration. Clonidine, most commonly in a dose of 75 to 150 mg, is at least as effective as moderate doses of phenylephrine and epinephrine at prolonging sensory block but has been associated with greater decreases in blood pressure in some[102] but not all studies.[103] Interestingly, clonidine also prolongs spinal block when administered orally.[104–106]

Tetracaine is the local anesthetic that is most dramatically prolonged by addition of adrenergic agonists. The duration of tetracaine spinal block may be increased 70% to 100% at lumbar and sacral dermatomes by the addition of phenylephrine. Epinephrine may prolong tetracaine spinal anesthesia by 40% to 60%. Clonidine prolongs tetracaine spinal block by 50% to 70%, with the larger effect occurring at lumbar dermatomes.

Bupivacaine spinal block is also prolonged by adrenergic agonists, although the effect is somewhat less than that seen with tetracaine (Table 34-4). Epinephrine in doses of 0.2 mg prolongs bupivacaine spinal block by 20% to 30%, but only in lumbar dermatomes. Larger doses of epinephrine (0.3 to 0.5 mg) prolong sensory block in thoracic dermatomes as well by 30% to 50%. Clonidine prolongs bupivacaine spinal block by 30% to 50% as well.

The effect of adrenergic agonists on the duration of lidocaine spinal block is controversial. Some clinical studies have demonstrated that adrenergic agonists clearly prolong lidocaine spinal block,[96,107–109] whereas others have concluded that adrenergic agonists do not produce clinically useful prolongation.[110,111] This discrepancy may be explained, in part, by the fact that spinal block duration is so variable that studies using small numbers of patients may lack sufficient statistical power to detect real differences in mean block duration between groups. This problem was obviated in an interesting study by Chiu et al.,[112] who used a crossover study design to demonstrate that 0.2 mg of epinephrine significantly prolonged lidocaine sensory block in lumbar and sacral dermatomes. Thus, the available data suggest that adding epinephrine to lidocaine will result in a somewhat longer block, at least in lumbar and sacral dermatomes, than would be achieved if epinephrine were not added.

The mechanism by which adrenergic agonists prolong spinal block is not clear. Originally, epinephrine and phenylephrine were added to local anesthetics with the intent of reducing local spinal cord blood flow and thereby slowing the rate of drug elimination from the spinal cord and CSF. There are animal studies that support this mechanism[113,114] and others that do not.[115,116] Animal studies with clonidine indicate that it does reduce regional spinal cord blood flow.[117] There are no human studies that have investigated the effect of intrathecal adrenergic agonists on spinal cord blood flow. However, there are human studies that demonstrate that epinephrine decreases the rate of local anesthetic clearance from the CSF[118,119] and also slows the rate at which subarachnoid local anesthetic appears in the plasma.[107] These findings have been interpreted as evidence of a vasoconstrictor-mediated decrease in drug clearance from the spinal cord; however, they are not proof that this is the only, or even the principal, mechanism by which adrenergic agonists prolong spinal anesthesia. Alternatively, Kozody et al.[120] have shown that intrathecal epinephrine decreases blood flow in the dura mater without altering spinal cord blood flow, a finding most consistent with decreased drug clearance via the dural vasculature.

Adrenergic agonists are potent analgesic agents in their own right when administered into the subarachnoid space.[121] Analgesia results from inhibition of nociceptive afferents, an effect that is mediated by stimulation of α-adrenergic receptors in the spinal cord dorsal horn. In addition, large intrathecal doses of α-adrenergic agonists have been shown to produce flaccidity in animal models by hyperpolarizing motor neurons.[122] Thus, prolongation of motor and sensory block by adrenergic agonists may be partly because of direct inhibitory effects of these drugs on sensory and motor neurons.

Epidural Anesthesia

Any procedure that can be performed under spinal anesthesia can also be performed under epidural block and requires the same block height (Table 34-1). As with spinal anesthesia, there is a great deal of variability among patients in spread (Fig. 34-10) and duration of epidural block (Table 34-5). Therefore, to choose the most appropriate local anesthetic and dose for a particular clinical situation, the anesthesiologist must be familiar with the variables that affect spread and duration of epidural anesthesia.

TABLE 34-5. LOCAL ANESTHETICS USED FOR SURGICAL EPIDURAL BLOCK

	Duration of Sensory Block		
Drug[a]	Two-dermatome Regression (min)	Complete Resolution (min)	Prolongation by Epinephrine (%)
Chloroprocaine 3%	45–60	100–160	40–60
Lidocaine 2%	60–100	160–200	40–80
Mepivacaine 2%	60–100	160–200	40–80
Ropivacaine 0.5–1%	90–180	240–420	No
Etidocaine 1–1.5%	120–240	300–460	No
Bupivacaine 0.5–0.75%	120–240	300–460	No

[a]These concentrations are recommended for surgical anesthesia; more dilute concentrations are appropriate for epidural analgesia.

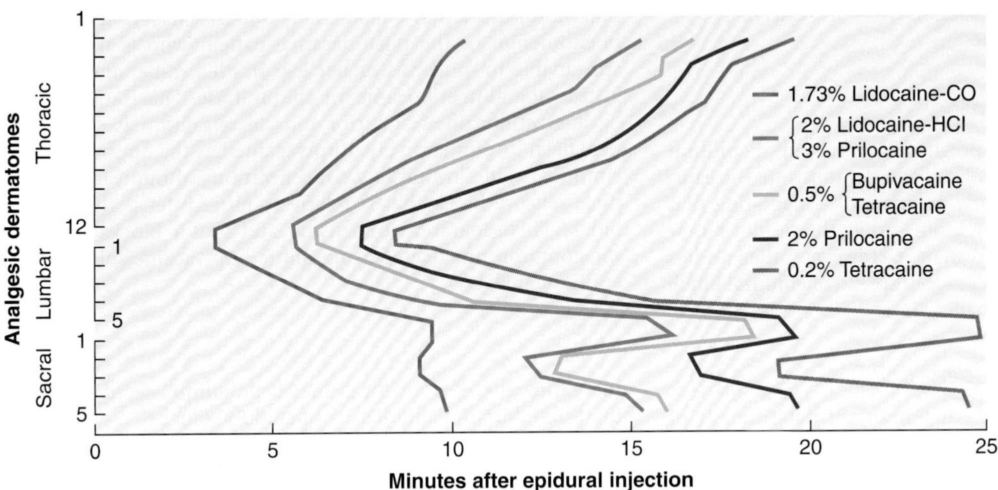

FIGURE 34-12. Spread of epidural sensory block over time following injection of various local anesthetic solutions at the L2 to L3 interspace. All solutions contained epinephrine 1:200,000. Sensory block spreads both cephalad and caudad from the site of injection with time. Note the delay in onset of block at the L5 and S1 dermatomes with all solutions tested. (Reprinted from: Bromage PR. *Epidural Analgesia.* Philadelphia, PA: WB Saunders; 1978, with permission.)

Block Spread

Injection Site

Unlike spinal anesthesia, epidural anesthesia produces a segmental block that spreads both caudally and cranially from the site of injection (Fig. 34-12). Thus, injection site is arguably the most important determinant of the spread of epidural block. *Caudal* epidural blocks are largely restricted to sacral and low lumbar dermatomes. Low thoracic levels can be reached with caudal injections if large volumes are used (e.g., 30 mL). However, the block at thoracic dermatomes tends to be patchy and short-lived following caudal injection.[123] *Lumbar* local anesthetic injections with volumes of 10 mL often extend caudad to include all sacral dermatomes, although the onset of block in the L5 and S1 roots is often delayed and may be patchy.[124] Twenty-milliliter volumes produce better-quality sacral anesthesia following lumbar injection. The slow onset at L5 and S1 is thought to result from their larger diameter and consequent slower drug penetration. Lumbar injections can be extended to midthoracic levels (T4 to T6) when 20-mL volumes of local anesthetic are used. *Thoracic* injections produce a symmetric segmental band of anesthesia, the width of which depends on the dose of local anesthetic administered. When using a mid-to-upper thoracic injection site, it is prudent to reduce the local anesthetic doses by approximately 30% to 50% relative to lumbar doses to prevent excessive cephalad spread. It is generally not feasible to produce surgical anesthesia in low lumbar and sacral dermatomes with midthoracic or higher injection sites. Thoracic epidural block is ideally suited for anesthesia of the chest and abdomen.

Dose, Volume, and Concentration

Within the range typically used for surgical anesthesia, drug concentration is relatively unimportant in determining block spread. However, drug dose and volume are important variables determining both spread and quality of epidural block. If drug concentration is held constant, increasing the volume of local anesthetic (and thereby the dose) will result in significantly greater average spread and greater block density. However, the relationship is nonlinear. For example, doubling the volume and dose of 1.5% lidocaine or 0.75% bupivacaine from 10 to 20 mL has been shown to increase spread by only three to four spinal segments.[124,125] Volume appears to be important in determining block spread independent of drug dose, but again the relationship is nonlinear. Erdemir et al.[126] showed that tripling the injected volume of lidocaine from 10 to 30 mL while holding the dose constant (300 mg) increased the cephalad extent of block by only 4.3 dermatomes. This tendency toward greater spread is thought to be explained by the observation that increasing the volume of solution injected into the epidural space increases cephalad distribution.[127]

Position

When using a single-shot technique, maintaining patients in the lateral position during and after epidural injection of surgical doses of local anesthetics does not seem to have a clinically important effect on spread of the block from side to side.[128] Similarly, studies examining the effect of patient position on cephalad spread of epidural block have generally found that the effect of posture on spread is not clinically important.[129] Interestingly, Ponhold et al.[130] demonstrated that maintaining a 30-degree head-up position significantly increased the frequency of adequate block at the L5 and S1 nerve roots even though there was no effect on the cephalad extent of anesthesia.

Patient Characteristics

Age

Most,[124,125,131–134] but not all,[135] studies that have examined the effect of age on epidural block have demonstrated greater spread in older patients. However, the effect of age is probably clinically significant only when comparing adults whose ages differ by ≥3 decades. Even so, the difference in block height is not likely to be more than three or four dermatomes. Greater spread in older patients is thought to be related to a less-compliant epidural space and diminished ability for epidural solutions to leak out of intervertebral foramina.[127,136] Both of these age-related changes would be expected to result in more extensive spread of solutions within the epidural space.

Height and Weight

The correlation between patient height[124,125,134,135] or weight[134,135] and spread of epidural block is weak and of little clinical significance except perhaps in patients who are extremely tall, extremely short, or morbidly obese.

Pregnancy

Studies examining the effect of pregnancy on spread of epidural block are conflicting. Some studies have demonstrated greater spread at term[137] and during early pregnancy,[131] suggesting that greater spread during pregnancy is not simply the result of anatomic changes associated with pregnancy. However, other studies have not found a significant difference in spread of epidural block between pregnant and nonpregnant women.[138–140]

Atherosclerosis

Atherosclerosis was suggested as an important determinant of the spread of epidural block[137]; however, subsequent studies have failed to confirm this relationship.[125,131,141]

Given the myriad factors that have some effect on spread of epidural anesthesia, how should anesthesiologists choose an appropriate local anesthetic dose for a single-shot epidural block? A useful recommendation is to assume that a 20-mL volume of all local anesthetics intended for surgical anesthesia will produce a midthoracic block on average after lumbar injection. If there are multiple reasons to expect that the block may spread excessively in an individual patient (e.g., advanced age, obesity, very short stature, high injection site) or if the procedure does not require a high block, then reduce the dose accordingly. If there are multiple reasons to expect that the spread may be reduced from the average, then increase the volume accordingly. Obviously, choice of the appropriate local anesthetic dose is obviated if an epidural catheter is used. In this situation, begin with a lower dose than one anticipates will be needed and administer additional local anesthetic as necessary to extend the block to the desired level.

Onset

The onset of epidural block with all local anesthetics can usually be detected within 5 minutes in the dermatomes immediately surrounding the injection site. The time to peak effect differs somewhat among local anesthetics. Shorter-acting drugs generally reach their maximum spread in 15 to 20 minutes, whereas longer-acting drugs require 20 to 25 minutes. Increasing the dose of local anesthetic speeds the onset of both motor and sensory blocks.

Duration

Local Anesthetic

As with spinal anesthesia, choice of local anesthetic is the most important determinant of the duration of epidural block. Chloroprocaine is the shortest-duration drug used for epidural anesthesia; lidocaine and mepivacaine provide blocks of intermediate duration; and bupivacaine, ropivacaine, and etidocaine produce the longest-lasting epidural block. Table 34-5 lists local anesthetics commonly used for epidural block and approximate duration of surgical anesthesia. Of note, tetracaine and procaine are not generally used for epidural block because of the poor quality block that these drugs produce.

Importantly, when used epidurally some local anesthetics exhibit considerable separation in both the intensity and duration of sensory and motor blocks. Etidocaine produces the most intense motor block and is unusual among local anesthetics in that motor block may considerably outlast sensory block.[142] The phenomenon of the postoperative patient who is in pain yet still unable to move his or her legs has led some anesthesiologists to abandon etidocaine for epidural use. This is unfortunate because etidocaine's superior muscle relaxation is sometimes beneficial intraoperatively. Bupivacaine has the opposite sensorimotor profile in that low concentrations of bupivacaine produce sensory block that is relatively more intense than motor block. This separation of sensory and motor blocks underlies the common practice of using dilute bupivacaine solutions for epidural analgesia.

Dose

Increasing the dose of local anesthetic administered results in increased duration and density of epidural block.[124,143–145]

Age

Studies that have evaluated the effect of age on epidural block duration are inconclusive. Veering et al.[133] found that duration of epidural block with plain bupivacaine was not significantly affected by age. Nydahl et al.[132] found that epidural block using bupivacaine with epinephrine was actually shorter in older patients. In contrast, Park et al.[131] found that epidural block using lidocaine with epinephrine was slightly but significantly longer in older patients. Additional studies are necessary to clarify the effect of age on duration of epidural block.

Adrenergic Agonists

Epinephrine, in a concentration of 5 μg/mL (1:200,000), is the most common adrenergic agonist added to epidural local anesthetics. It has been shown to prolong the duration of lidocaine and mepivacaine epidural block by as much as 80%.[146] Block is prolonged by decreased drug clearance from the epidural space,[147] probably as a result of reduced blood flow in the dura mater. As discussed earlier for spinal anesthesia, prolongation of motor and sensory blocks may be partly due to direct inhibitory effects of epinephrine on sensory and motor neurons.

Epinephrine does not significantly prolong the duration of anesthesia when added to concentrated solutions of bupivacaine,[148,149] etidocaine,[144,149] or ropivacaine[150] that are generally used for surgical anesthesia, probably because the inherent duration of these drugs exceeds the duration of epinephrine's effects. However, epinephrine does appear to prolong analgesia and improve the quality of block when added to more dilute solutions of these local anesthetics, such as those used for labor analgesia.[151–153]

Summary

The extent and duration of both spinal and epidural blocks are influenced by a number of variables, some of which are under the control of the anesthesiologist. Understanding the impact of these variables will allow the anesthesiologist to rationally select the most appropriate drug and dose for any clinical situation. However, even the most experienced anesthesiologist will still have blocks that are not adequate for the planned procedure. The frequency of failed blocks can be kept to a minimum if the clinician aims to produce blocks that are a little higher and a little longer than seems necessary. It is often easier to deal with a block that is too high or too long than to cover up for a block that is too low or too brief.

PHYSIOLOGY

Neurophysiology

The physiology of local anesthetic neural blockade is discussed in detail in Chapter 21. This section briefly presents aspects of the physiology of neural blockade that are unique to spinal and epidural anesthesia.

Site of Action

The site of action of spinal and epidural anesthesia is not precisely known. Following epidural administration, local anesthetic is found in the spinal nerves within the epidural space, in spinal nerve rootlets within the CSF, and in the spinal cord. Similarly, following intrathecal administration in animals, local anesthetic is found in all sites between the spinal nerve rootlets and the interior of the spinal cord.[154,155] Thus, neural blockade can potentially occur at any or all points along the neural pathways extending from the site of drug administration to the interior of the spinal cord.

In an interesting study in humans, Boswell et al.[156] demonstrated that patients are able to feel paresthesias during direct electrical stimulation of the spinal cord under spinal anesthesia. Cortical evoked potentials from direct spinal cord stimulation were also maintained under spinal anesthesia, although amplitudes were decreased. In contrast, paresthesias and cortical evoked potentials from tibial nerve stimulation were abolished by spinal anesthesia. These investigators concluded that neural pathways within the spinal cord were largely intact during spinal anesthesia and that the spinal nerve rootlets were the principal site of neural blockade.

The site of epidural block is less well localized. Monkey studies suggest that epidural block occurs largely at sites within the spinal meninges, including the cauda equina nerve roots, dorsal root entry zone, and the long tracts of spinal cord white matter.[157] However, these findings are not entirely consistent with the segmental onset of epidural anesthesia (Fig. 34-12) or with the limited segmental blocks that can be produced with small doses of lumbar epidural local anesthetics in humans. These clinical observations are most readily explained by block of the segmental spinal nerves as they traverse the epidural or paravertebral spaces. In reality, epidural block likely occurs at both extradural and subdural sites with extradural radicular block predominating early and subdural spinal block predominating later. This supposition is consistent with human studies by Urban,[158] who rigorously examined the anatomic pattern of analgesia that occurred during onset and regression of epidural block. He concluded that local anesthetics initially acted on radicular structures followed later by actions within the spinal cord.

Interestingly, human studies demonstrate that somatosensory evoked potentials are maintained during epidural anesthesia, although amplitudes are decreased and latencies are increased. This contrasts with spinal block in which evoked potentials are completely eliminated and supports the clinical impression that epidural block is generally less dense than that achieved with spinal anesthesia.

Differential Nerve Block

Differential block refers to a clinically important phenomenon in which nerve fibers subserving different functions display varying sensitivity to local anesthetic blockade. Sympathetic nerve fibers appear to be blocked by the lowest concentration of local anesthetic followed in order by fibers responsible for pain, touch, and motor function. This observation has led to the widely held belief that differences in sensitivity to local anesthetic blockade is explained solely by differences in fiber diameter, with smaller diameter neurons exhibiting greater sensitivity than larger diameter neurons. Although the mechanism for differential block in spinal and epidural anesthesia is not known, it is clear that fiber diameter is not the only, or perhaps not even the most important, factor contributing to differential block.[159,160]

Differential block occurs with both peripheral nerve blocks and central neuraxial blocks. In the peripheral nervous system, differential block is a temporal phenomenon with sympathetic block occurring first followed in time by sensory and motor blocks. In contrast, with spinal and epidural anesthesia differential block is manifest as a spatial separation in the modalities blocked. This is seen most clearly with spinal anesthesia in which sympathetic block may extend as many as two to six dermatomes higher than pin-prick sensation,[161] which in turn extends two to three dermatomes higher than motor block. This spatial separation is believed to result from a gradual decrease in local anesthetic concentration within the CSF as a function of distance from the site of injection. With epidural anesthesia, similar zones of differential sensory and sympathetic blocks are found.[162]

Perhaps the most troublesome consequence of differential block is the occasional patient who has intact touch and proprioception at the surgical site despite adequate blockade of pain sensation. Even the most stoic patients are likely to find this unpleasant and may lie in fear that the procedure will soon become painful. In no instance should the anesthesiologist downplay the distress this may cause patients. Reassurance and judicious sedation as necessary are usually sufficient to overcome this problem.

Another important neurophysiologic aspect of central neuroaxial block is that it produces sedation,[163] potentiates the effect of sedative hypnotic drugs,[164–166] and markedly decreases minimum alveolar concentration of volatile anesthetics.[167] The mechanism(s) underlying these effects is not known but *deafferentation* (the loss of ascending sensory input to the brain) is commonly invoked as causative.

Cardiovascular Physiology

5 Cardiovascular side effects, principally hypotension and bradycardia, are arguably the most important and most common physiologic changes during spinal and epidural anesthesia. Understanding the homeostatic mechanisms responsible for control of blood pressure and heart rate is essential for understanding and treating the cardiovascular changes associated with spinal and epidural anesthesia.

Spinal Anesthesia

Blockade of sympathetic efferents is the principal mechanism by which spinal anesthesia produces cardiovascular derangements. As would be expected, the incidence of significant hypotension or bradycardia is generally related to the extent of sympathetic blockade, which in turn parallels block height.[168,169] However, the severity of cardiovascular changes has been shown not to correlate with peak block height in one study[170] and to correlate poorly in another (Fig. 34-13).[168] Additional risk factors associated with hypotension include age >40 to 50 years, concurrent general anesthesia, obesity, hypovolemia, and addition of phenylephrine to the local anesthetic.[168,171]

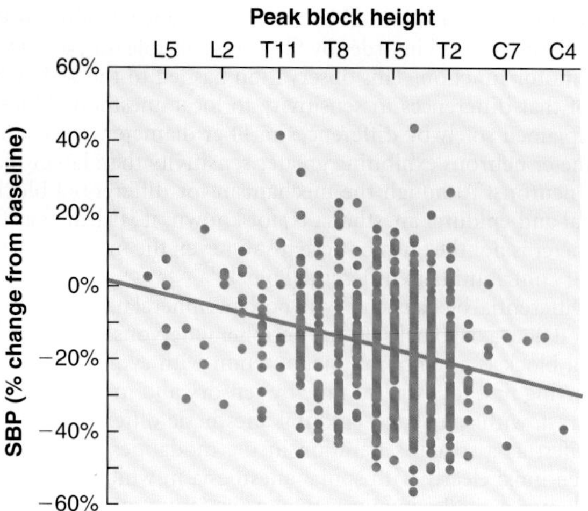

FIGURE 34-13. The relationship between peak block height and change in systolic blood pressure (SBP) during spinal anesthesia. Although there is a statistically significant correlation between block height and decrease in systolic blood pressure, the interindividual variability is so great that the relationship has little predictive value. This is reflected in the R^2 of 0.07 for the linear regression line. (From: Carpenter RL, Caplan RA, Brown DL, et al. Incidence and risk factors for side effects of spinal anesthesia. *Anesthesiology.* 1992;76:906, with permission.)

Hypotension during spinal anesthesia is the result of both arterial and venodilation. Venodilation increases volume in capacitance vessels, thereby decreasing venous return and right-sided filling pressures.[170,172–174] This fall in preload is thought to be the principal cause of decreased cardiac output during high spinal anesthesia. Arterial dilation during spinal anesthesia results in significant decreases in total peripheral resistance (Fig. 34-14).[173,175] Thus, the hypotension that accompanies 30% to 40% of spinal anesthetics may be the result of reductions in afterload, reductions in cardiac output, or both (Fig. 34-14). Human and animal studies indicate that an intact renin–angiotensin system helps to offset the hypotensive effects of sympathetic blockade.[176,177] This suggests extra caution when administering central neuraxial block to patients taking antihypertensives that impair the angiotensin system (e.g., angiotensin converting enzyme inhibitors or angiotensin II receptor blockers) and recognition that exogenous andiuretic hormone (vasopressin) may be necessary to induce peripheral vasoconstriction with refractory hypotension.

Heart rate does not change significantly during spinal anesthesia in most patients (Fig. 34-14). However, clinically significant bradycardia occasionally occurs with a reported incidence of 10% to 15%. As with hypotension, the risk of bradycardia increases with increasing block height.[168] Additional risk factors associated with bradycardia include age younger than 50 years, American Society of Anesthesiologists 1 physical status, and concurrent use of beta-blockers.[168,171] The mechanism responsible for bradycardia is not clear. Blockade of the sympathetic cardioaccelerator

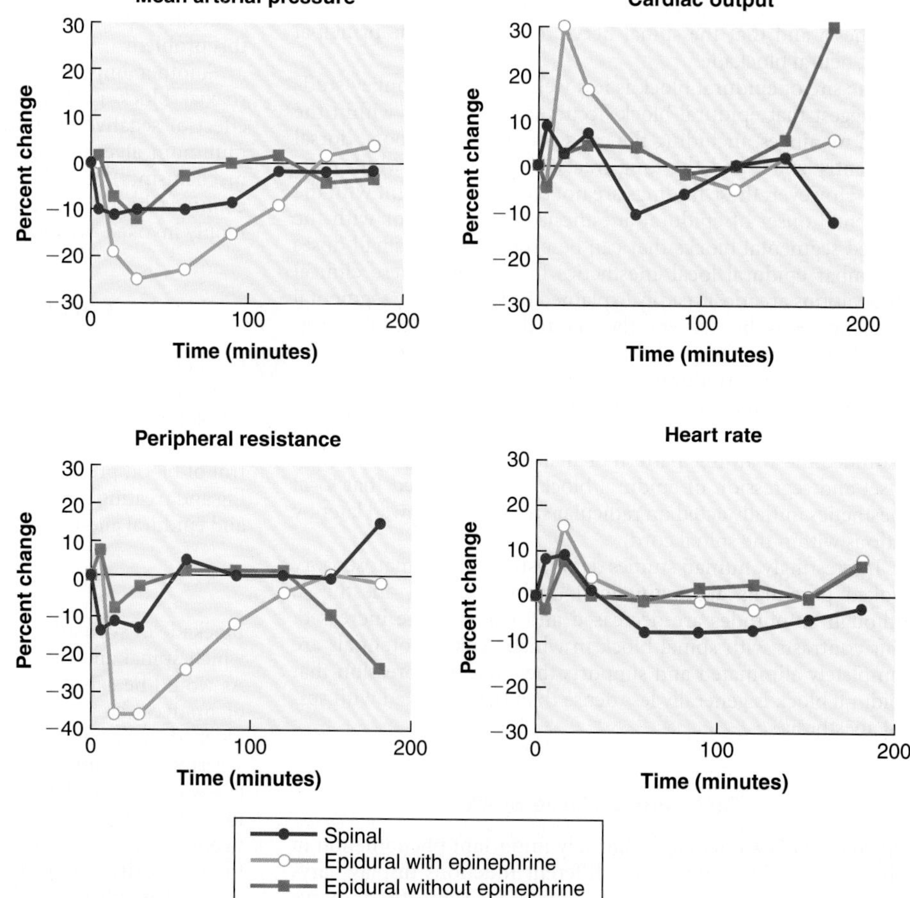

FIGURE 34-14. The cardiovascular effects of spinal and epidural anesthesia in volunteers with T5 blocks. The effects of spinal anesthesia and epidural anesthesia without epinephrine were generally comparable and are both qualitatively and quantitatively different from the effects of epidural anesthesia with epinephrine. (Modified from: Bonica JJ, Kennedu WF Jr, Ward RJ, et al. A comparison of the effects of high subarachnoid and epidural anesthesia. *Acta Anaesthesiol Scand.* 1966;23(suppl):429.)

fibers originating from T1 to T4 spinal segments is often suggested as the cause. The fact that bradycardia is more common with high blocks supports this mechanism. However, significant bradycardia sometimes occurs with blocks that are seemingly too low to block cardioaccelerator fibers. Diminished venous return has also been proposed as a cause of bradycardia during spinal anesthesia. Intracardiac stretch receptors have been shown to reflexively decrease heart rate when filling pressures fall (the Bezold–Jarisch reflex).[178] Consistent with this mechanism, Jacobsen et al.[179] demonstrated a significant reduction in left ventricular volumes and heart rate during hypotensive episodes in two patients during epidural anesthesia. They concluded that central volume depletion elicited a vagally mediated reflex slowing of heart rate. Similarly, Baron et al.[180] demonstrated that vagal activity is enhanced by decreased venous return during epidural anesthesia. However, this mechanism does not operate at all times in all patients. Anzai and Nishikawa[174] demonstrated significant heart rate increases in 40 patients who had their filling pressures suddenly decreased by body tilt during spinal anesthesia. In reality, both blockades of cardioaccelerator fibers and decreased filling pressures as well as other unrecognized factors likely contribute to bradycardia during spinal anesthesia.

Although bradycardia is usually of moderate severity and well tolerated, there have been reports of sudden, unexplained, severe bradycardia and asystole during both spinal and epidural anesthesia.[181,182] In addition, multiple case reports document that spinal anesthesia can also produce second- and third-degree heart blocks[183–185] and that pre-existing first-degree block may be a risk factor for progression to higher grade blocks during spinal anesthesia.[183] These reports document the need for continued vigilance with prompt and, if needed, aggressive treatment of the cardiovascular changes that accompany central neuraxial blockade.

Epidural Anesthesia

The hemodynamic changes produced by epidural anesthesia are largely dependent on whether or not epinephrine is added to the local anesthetic solution (Fig. 34-14).[186] High epidural block with local anesthetic solutions that do not contain epinephrine results in decreased stroke volume, cardiac output, total peripheral resistance, and arterial pressure. The magnitude of these changes is generally less than that seen with comparable levels of spinal block.[186] As with spinal anesthesia, these hemodynamic changes are believed to result from venous and arterial dilation induced by sympathetic blockade. In contrast, when epinephrine-containing solutions are used for epidural anesthesia, stroke volume, and cardiac output increase significantly (Fig. 34-14).[186] However, peripheral resistance falls dramatically, resulting in a decrease in arterial pressure greater than that seen with nonepinephrine-containing solutions. β_2-adrenergic–mediated vasodilatation produced by low doses of absorbed epinephrine accounts for the greater decrease in peripheral vascular resistance and blood pressure. Decreased peripheral resistance may also contribute to the marked increase in cardiac output. However, epinephrine-induced venoconstriction with a resultant increase in venous return may also play an important role in increasing cardiac output.[187]

Treating Hemodynamic Changes

Treatment of hypotension secondary to spinal and epidural blocks must be aimed at the root causes: Decreased cardiac output and/or decreased peripheral resistance. Bolus crystalloid administration has often been advocated to restore venous return and thus cardiac output during central neuraxial blockade. The effectiveness of this therapy in normovolemic patients, however, is controversial. Prehydrating patients with 500 to 1,500 mL of crystalloid does not reliably prevent hypotension, but has been shown to decrease the incidence of hypotension during spinal anesthesia in some,[188] but not all, studies.[169,189] Rapid crystalloid fluid administration increases atrial naturietic peptide release with subsequent vasodilator and diuretic effects.[190] Further, crystalloid fluid is rapidly redistributed from the intravascular compartment after administration. Ueyama et al.[191] demonstrated that after the administration of a 1,500-mL crystalloid preload, only 28% of the crystalloid remained intravascular after 30 minutes and the crystalloid preload did not significantly increase cardiac output or effectively prevent hypotension after spinal anesthesia. Thus, although judicious crystalloid preloading before central neuraxial blocks may benefit some, it cannot be relied on to prevent clinically significant hypotension in most patients. Colloid solutions that remain in the intravascular compartment longer offer an interesting alternative to crystalloids for preloading before central neuraxial blocks. Marhofer et al.[192] showed that 500 mL of 6% hetastarch actually increases systemic vascular resistance index in elderly patients having spinal anesthesia, whereas 1,500 mL of crystalloid significantly decreases systemic vascular resistance index. In contrast, Tamilselvan et al.[193] demonstrated increased cardiac output after 500- and 1,000-mL preload with 6% hetastarch but found no significant decrease in the incidence of hypotension compared to 1,500-mL crystalloid preload. Thus, while prophylactic colloid preload may increase cardiac output, this may not be sufficient to compensate for arterial blood pressure reduction after spinal anesthesia.

Vasopressors are a more reliable approach to treating hypotension secondary to central neuraxial blockade. Drugs with both α- and β-adrenergic activities have been shown to be superior to pure α-agonists for correcting the cardiovascular derangements produced by spinal and epidural anesthesia.[194,195] Ephedrine is the drug most commonly used to treat hypotension. Ephedrine boluses of 5- to 10-mg increase blood pressure by restoring cardiac output and peripheral vascular resistance. Dopamine, in low-to-moderate doses, has also been shown to correct the hemodynamic changes induced by central neuraxial block.[196,197] Dopamine may be preferable to ephedrine for long-term infusion because tachyphylaxis can develop with repeated ephedrine boluses. Pure α-adrenergic agonists, most commonly phenylephrine, are also used to correct hypotension during spinal anesthesia. However, α-agonists increase blood pressure largely by increasing systemic vascular resistance, sometimes at the expense of further decreasing cardiac output.[195] In addition, phenylephrine boluses have been shown to produce transient left ventricular dysfunction during epidural anesthesia with nonepinephrine-containing local anesthetics.[198] A potential, but as yet unstudied, role for α-agonists may be to treat hypotension that occurs during epidural anesthesia with epinephrine-containing local anesthetics. Because the principal derangement in this situation is a marked decrease in systemic vascular resistance, α-agonists may be an appropriate choice for treating hypotension in this setting. In addition, for patients who are taking medication that disrupts the renin–angiotensin system, vasopressin may be the optimal drug choice for restoration of adequate blood pressure.

Deciding *when* to treat hemodynamic derangements during spinal and epidural anesthesia is perhaps more difficult than deciding *how* to treat them. Currently no studies clearly define the lower limit of acceptable blood pressure or heart rate for any group of patients. In the absence of such data, several authors have recommended treating blood pressure if it decreases more than 25% to 30% below baseline or in normotensive patients, if systolic pressure falls below 90 mm Hg. Recommendations regarding bradycardia suggest initiating treatment if heart rate falls below 50 to 60 beats per minute. These recommendations are reasonable, although not universally applicable. Ultimately, anesthesiologists must decide what is an acceptable blood pressure and heart rate for an individual patient based on that patient's underlying medical condition.

Respiratory Physiology

Spinal and epidural blocks to midthoracic levels have little effect on pulmonary function in patients without pre-existing lung disease. Drugs used perioperatively for sedation during spinal or epidural block likely have a larger impact on pulmonary function than the block per se. In particular, lung volumes, resting minute ventilation, dead space, arterial blood gas tensions, and shunt fraction show little or no change during spinal or epidural anesthesia. Interestingly, the ventilatory response to hypercapnia is actually increased by spinal and epidural blocks.[199,200]

High blocks associated with abdominal and intercostal muscle paralysis can impair ventilatory functions requiring active exhalation. For example, expiratory reserve volume, peak expiratory flow, and maximum minute ventilation may be significantly reduced by high spinal and epidural blocks. The negative impact of high blocks on active exhalation suggests caution when using spinal or epidural anesthesia in patients with obstructive pulmonary disease, who need to cough to clear sputum, or who otherwise rely on their accessory muscles of respiration to maintain a clear airway and/or adequate ventilation.

Patients with high spinal or epidural blocks may complain of dyspnea despite normal or elevated minute ventilation. This likely results from the patient's inability to feel the chest wall move while breathing. This is understandably frightening to the patient, but reassurance is usually effective in alleviating the fear. The anesthesiologist must be alert to the possibility that the complaint of dyspnea stems from incipient respiratory failure secondary to respiratory muscle paralysis. A normal speaking voice, as opposed to a faint gasping voice, suggests ventilation is normal.

Gastrointestinal Physiology

The gastrointestinal effects of spinal and epidural anesthesia are largely the result of sympathetic blockade. The abdominal organs derive their sympathetic innervation from T6 to L2. Blockade of these fibers results in unopposed parasympathetic activity by way of the vagus nerve. Consequently, secretions increase, sphincters relax, and the bowel becomes constricted. Some surgeons believe this improves surgical exposure. Nausea is a common complication of spinal and epidural anesthesia. The etiology is unknown but an increased incidence of nausea during spinal anesthesia is associated with blocks higher than T5, hypotension, opioid premedication, and a history of motion sickness.[168,171]

Endocrine–Metabolic Physiology

Surgery produces numerous endocrine and metabolic changes, including increased protein catabolism and oxygen consumption as well as increases in circulating concentrations of catecholamines, growth hormone, renin, angiotensin, thyroid-stimulating hormone, β-endorphin, glucose, and free fatty acids, among others.[1] These endocrine–metabolic changes have collectively been termed the *surgical stress response*.

The mechanisms responsible for the stress response are complex and incompletely understood. However, afferent sensory information from the surgical site plays an important role in initiating and maintaining these changes.[1] Not surprisingly, spinal and epidural anesthesia have been shown to inhibit many of the endocrine–metabolic changes associated with the stress response. The inhibitory effect is greatest with lower abdominal and lower extremity procedures and least with upper abdominal and thoracic procedures. The salutary effect of spinal and epidural anesthesia is believed to result from blockade of the afferent sensory information that helps initiate the stress response.

Although some aspects of the surgical stress response may be beneficial, it is generally viewed as maladaptive and possibly a contributor to postoperative morbidity and mortality.[1] Despite the ability of central neuraxial block to decrease the stress response, there is as yet no clear evidence that this results in decreased morbidity or mortality.

COMPLICATIONS

Backache

Although postoperative backache occurs following general anesthesia, it is more common following epidural and spinal anesthesia.[201] Compared with spinal anesthesia, back pain following epidural anesthesia is more common (11% vs. 30%) and of longer duration.[202] Importantly, back pain has been cited in one study as the most common reason for patients to refuse future epidural block.[202] The etiology of backache is not clear, although needle trauma, local anesthetic irritation, and ligamentous strain secondary to muscle relaxation have been offered as explanations.

Postdural Puncture Headache

PDPH is a common complication of spinal anesthesia with a reported incidence as high as 25% in some studies. The risk of PDPH is less with epidural anesthesia, but it occurs in up to 50% of young patients following accidental meningeal puncture with large diameter epidural needles. The headache is characteristically mild or absent when the patient is supine, but head elevation rapidly leads to a severe fronto-occipital headache, which again improves on returning to the supine position. Occasionally, cranial nerve symptoms (e.g., diplopia, tinnitus) and nausea and vomiting are also present. The headache is believed to result from the loss of CSF through the meningeal needle hole, resulting in decreased CSF pressure without an accompanying decrease in intravenous pressure. This pressure difference causes cerebral venous dilation and is likely the cause of the resultant headache.

The incidence of PDPH decreases with increasing age (Fig. 34-15) and with the use of small diameter spinal needles with noncutting tips.[203,204] Inserting cutting needles with the bevel aligned parallel to the long axis of the meninges has also been shown to decrease the incidence of PDPH.[204,205] Some authors have suggested that parallel insertion spreads dural fibers, whereas perpendicular insertion cuts the fibers, resulting in a larger meningeal hole. However, the collagen fibers of the dura mater are arranged randomly; therefore, as many fibers will be cut with parallel insertion as with perpendicular insertion. A more likely explanation arises from the fact that the dura mater is under longitudinal tension. Thus, a slit-like hole oriented perpendicular to this longitudinal tension will tend to be pulled open, whereas a hole oriented parallel to this tension will be pulled closed. Some

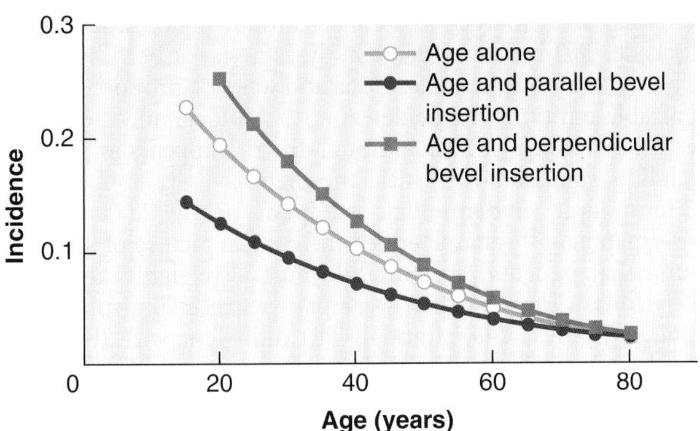

FIGURE 34-15. The incidence of postdural puncture headache decreases as patient age increases. When using beveled needles, the incidence is higher than average at any given age if the needle is inserted perpendicular to the spinal meninges and lower if inserted parallel to the spinal meninges. (Modified from: Lybecker H, Møller JT, May O, et al. Incidence and prediction of postdural puncture headache: A prospective study of 1021 spinal anesthesias. *Anesth Analg.* 1990;70:389.)

studies have suggested that women are at greater risk of developing PDPH. However, if age differences are accounted for, there does not appear to be a gender difference in the incidence of PDPH.[204] Folklore aside, remaining supine following meningeal puncture does not decrease the incidence of PDPH. Finally, the use of fluid, instead of air for loss of resistance during attempted epidural anesthesia does not alter the risk of accidental meningeal puncture, but does markedly decrease the risk of subsequently developing PDPH as intrathecal air may contribute to the headache.[33] PDPH usually resolves spontaneously in a few days to a week for most patients. However, there are reports of PDPH persisting for months following meningeal puncture. Initial treatment is appropriately conservative if this meets the patient's needs. Bed rest, hydration, and analgesics as necessary are the mainstay of conservative treatment. Cerebral vasoconstrictors such as caffeine, sumatriptan, and oral methergine may also produce short-term symptomatic relief.[206–208]

Epidural Blood Patch

Patients who are unable or unwilling to await spontaneous resolution of PDPH should be offered epidural blood patch. Ten to twenty milliliters of autologous blood is aseptically injected into epidural space at or near the interspace at which the meningeal puncture occurred. This is effective in relieving symptoms within 1 to 24 hours in 85% to 95% of patients; and approximately 90% of patients who fail an initial blood patch will respond to a second patch. Epidural blood patch is believed to compress the thecal space and increase subarachnoid pressure thereby forcing the CSF cephalad. In addition, clot formation over the meningeal hole prevents further CSF leak while the meningeal rent heals and provides a sustained therapeutic effect. The most common side effects of blood patch are backache and radicular pain, although transient bradycardia and cranial nerve palsies have also been reported.

The timing of epidural blood patch has been controversial. Some studies have shown that prophylactic blood patch is effective in preventing PDPH in patients in whom the meninges were accidentally punctured during attempted epidural anesthesia.[209,210] However, Scavone et al.[211] demonstrated that while prophylactic epidural blood patch shortened the duration of PDPH, it did not decrease the incidence of PDPH nor the need for therapeutic epidural blood patch. Further, recent evidence suggests a benefit to delaying epidural blood patch for 24 hours after symptoms develop. In a study of 504 patients who underwent epidural blood patch, Safa-Tisseront et al.[212] demonstrated complete symptomatic resolution in 75% of patients with PDPH who underwent epidural blood patch and only a 7% failure rate. The two predictive factors of epidural blood patch failure were increased needle diameter (<20G) and decreased time interval between dural puncture and epidural blood patch. Thus, these studies suggest that routine prophylactic blood patch is not appropriate for most patients and that epidural blood patch is best performed only after an initial 24-hour observation period with conservative treatment. However, it may be prudent to consider prophylactic epidural blood patch for the high-risk outpatients for whom a return trip to the hospital would be extremely difficult.

Hearing Loss

Hearing loss in the low-frequency range after spinal anesthesia has been reported. The incidence of hearing loss after spinal anesthesia varies greatly from 0.2% to 92%.[213,214] It is associated with PDPH and the use of larger gauge needles and it is thought to be due to CSF loss through the spinal puncture hole which results in decreased intracranial and intracochlear pressures. Onset of hearing loss occurs from 24 hours to 8 days following spinal anesthesia and usually resolves within 6 months. Lamberg et al.[215] demonstrated that a transient (1 to 3 days) mild decrease in hearing acuity (>10 dB) is common after spinal anesthesia, with an incidence of roughly 40% and a 3:1 female-to-male predominance. Some studies suggest that epidural volume expansion with normal saline may prevent the occurrence of postspinal hearing loss,[216] though more studies are necessary to understand the etiology and appropriate prevention or treatment of this side effect of spinal anesthesia.

Systemic Toxicity

Systemic toxicity of local anesthetics is discussed in detail in Chapter 21. Systemic toxicity does not occur with spinal anesthesia because the drug doses used are too low to cause toxic reactions even if injected intravenously. Both CNS and cardiovascular toxicity may occur during epidural anesthesia. CNS toxicity may result from local anesthetic absorption from the epidural space but more commonly occurs following accidental intravascular injection of local anesthetic. In contrast, cardiovascular toxicity from local anesthetics can probably only occur from unintended intravascular injection because the plasma concentrations of local anesthetics required to produce serious cardiovascular toxicity are very high. An adequate IV test dose and incremental injection of local anesthetics are the most important methods to prevent both CNS and cardiovascular toxicity during epidural anesthesia.

Total Spinal Anesthesia

Total spinal anesthesia occurs when local anesthetic spreads high enough to block the entire spinal cord and occasionally the brainstem during either spinal or epidural anesthesia. Profound hypotension and bradycardia are common secondary to complete sympathetic blockade. Respiratory arrest may occur as a result of respiratory muscle paralysis or dysfunction of brainstem respiratory control centers. Management includes vasopressors, atropine, and fluids as necessary to support the cardiovascular system, plus oxygen and controlled ventilation. If the cardiovascular and respiratory consequences are managed appropriately, total spinal block will resolve without sequelae.

Neurologic Injury

5 Serious neurologic injury is a rare but widely feared complication of epidural and spinal anesthesia. Multiple large series of spinal and epidural anesthesia report that neurologic injury occurs in approximately 0.03% to 0.1% of all central neuraxial blocks, although in most of these series the block was not clearly proven to be causative.[217] Persistent paresthesias and limited motor weakness are the most common injuries, although paraplegia and diffuse injury to cauda equina roots (*cauda equina syndrome*) do occur rarely. Injury may result from direct needle trauma to the spinal cord or spinal nerves, from spinal cord ischemia, from accidental injection of neurotoxic drugs or chemicals, from introduction of bacteria into the subarachnoid or epidural space, or very rarely from epidural hematoma.[217]

6 Importantly, local anesthetics intended for epidural and intrathecal use can themselves be neurotoxic in concentrations used clinically.[218] In particular, hyperbaric 5% lidocaine has been implicated as a cause of multiple cases of cauda equina syndrome following subarachnoid injection through small-bore ("microspinal") catheters during continuous spinal anesthesia.[219] Hyperbaric solutions injected through these high-resistance catheters have been shown to produce very little turbulence and thus poor mixing of the local anesthetic within CSF.[220] Nerve injury is believed to result from pooling of toxic concentrations of undiluted lidocaine around dependent cauda equina nerve roots. Consequently, the U.S. Food and Drug Administration has banned the use of these small-gauge catheters for continuous spinal anesthesia. Although the combination of microspinal catheters and high concentrations of lidocaine have clearly been implicated in causing cauda equina syndrome, this complication has also occurred when using larger (20G) catheters,[219] 2% lidocaine,[221] and 0.5% tetracaine.[219] A common thread in all of these reports has been the apparent maldistribution of the local anesthetic within the CSF. Maldistribution should be suspected whenever spinal block is unexpectedly restricted, and maneuvers such as altering patient position or drug baricity should be employed to improve drug distribution before additional drug is injected through a continuous spinal catheter. If these maneuvers fail to improve drug distribution, an alternative anesthetic technique should be employed.

The mechanism by which local anesthetics produce cauda equina syndrome is not yet clear; however, in vitro evidence suggests that local anesthetics can produce excitotoxic damage by depolarizing neurons and increasing intracellular calcium concentrations.[222] Other studies demonstrate that local anesthetics can cause neuronal injury by damaging neuronal plasma membranes through detergent-like actions[223,224] or by activation of phospholipase-C.[225] It is also unclear as yet whether adjuncts added to local anesthetics (e.g., epinephrine) contribute to cauda equina syndrome. However, based on animal studies, it has been argued that epinephrine should not be added to intrathecal lidocaine.[226] Rather, if a prolonged duration of spinal anesthesia is necessary, then a longer-acting drug like bupivacaine should be used.

Transient Neurologic Symptoms

In addition to cauda equina syndrome, the occurrence of *transient neurologic symptoms* (TNS) or *transient radicular irritation* (TRI) has also emerged as a concern following central neuraxial blockade. TRI is defined as pain, dysesthesia, or both, in the legs or buttocks after spinal anesthesia and was first proposed as a recognizable entity by Schneider et al.[227] All local anesthetics have been shown to cause TRI, although the risk appears to be greater with lidocaine than other local anesthetics.[228–234]

In a large epidemiologic study of nearly 2,000 patients, Freedman et al.[235] characterized the clinical picture of TRI. They found that patients receiving lidocaine were significantly more likely to develop TRI than were patients receiving spinal tetracaine or bupivacaine, although TRI did occur with these latter two drugs as well. Other risk factors for TRI include addition of phenylephrine to 0.5% tetracaine, surgery in the lithotomy position or with the leg flexed at the knee (as for meniscectomy), and outpatient status.[236,237] Evron et al.[238] reported the use of a double-orifice pencil-point needle was shown to significantly reduce the risk of TRI compared with a single-orifice needle. Variables shown not to increase the risk of TRI included lidocaine dose, addition of epinephrine to lidocaine, presence of dextrose, paresthesia, hypotension, and blood-tinged CSF among others.

Pain from TRI is not trivial, with the majority of patients rating it as moderate (visual analogue scale = 4 to 7/10). The pain usually resolves spontaneously within 72 hours, but a few patients have required up to 6 months.[235]

The mechanism responsible for TRI is unknown; however, it is not simply a milder manifestation of cauda equina syndrome. Differences in clinical presentation and risk factors suggest that these are not simply two points along a continuum of the same process.

Chloroprocaine

7 Chloroprocaine was introduced into clinical practice in 1951, and was used for spinal anesthesia beginning that year. In the early 1980s; however, clinicians reported multiple cases of neurologic injury following intrathecal injection of chloroprocaine. Importantly, the chloroprocaine solution available at the time contained either methylparaben as an antimicrobial or bisulfite as an antioxidant. Subsequent animal studies aimed at determining the mechanism for spinal injury have been confusing, with some authors reporting that chloroprocaine itself does not cause neurologic injury but that bisulfite does, and others reporting that chloroprocaine can cause neurologic injury but that bisulfite is neuroprotective.[239–241] Nonetheless, concern about the potential for chloroprocaine-mediated neurotoxicity led to its nearly complete abandonment as a spinal anesthetic, in large part because lidocaine was perceived as a safer alternative.

However, we now recognize that lidocaine is not without risk of neurologic toxicity; in fact, it may be the most neurotoxic spinal anesthetic. This observation, coupled with the fact that a preservative-free chloroprocaine formulation is now available, has led to a re-evaluation of chloroprocaine as a short-acting spinal anesthetic. In 2004, Kouri and Kopacz[242] compared the block characteristics of 40 mg of plain 2% lidocaine with 40 mg of plain 2% preservative-free chloroprocaine in humans using a double-blind, randomized crossover study design. They found that both drugs produced identical average block heights (T8), but that chloroprocaine resulted in more rapid resolution of sensory block (103 ± 13 vs. 126 ± 16 minutes) and faster attainment of discharge criteria (104 ± 12 vs. 134 ± 14 minutes). In addition, seven of eight volunteers experienced TNS following intrathecal lidocaine and none experienced TNS following 2% chloroprocaine. In other studies from the same research group, chloroprocaine spinal block height and duration were shown to be positively correlated with chloroprocaine dose[243] and addition of dextrose was shown not to alter spinal block characteristics, except that it increased postvoid bladder volume.[244] This group also performed studies to determine the effect of epinephrine and fentanyl as block-prolonging adjuvants to spinal chloroprocaine. Vath and Kopacz[245] found that the addition of 20 μg of fentanyl to 40 mg of chloroprocaine increased average peak block height (T5 vs. T9), prolonged the time for sensory block regression to L1 (78 ± 7 vs. 53 ± 19 minutes), and modestly increased the time to complete regression (104 ± 7 vs. 95 ± 9 minutes). Interestingly, Smith et al.[243] found that epinephrine (0.2 mg) increased chloroprocaine block duration but that its use was associated with a high incidence of myalgia, arthralgia, malaise, and anorexia that lasted up to 48 hours. The authors had no explanation for the epinephrine-associated side effects, but recommended against its use with intrathecal chloroprocaine. In a retrospective review of their experience with spinal chloroprocaine in 600 patients, Hejtmanek and Pollock[246] reported comparable clinical pharmacology, and no neurologic complications.

Thus, these studies, coupled with concerns about the potential for lidocaine-mediated neurotoxicity, raise the possibility that chloroprocaine will re-enter the mainstream as a spinal anesthetic, especially for ambulatory anesthesia.

Importantly, as of this writing, chloroprocaine is not specifically indicated for spinal anesthesia; therefore, its use is "off-label." But then, so is the use of multiple drugs that are routinely administered intrathecally, including plain bupivacaine, plain lidocaine, hydromorphone, fentanyl, and sufentanil, among others.

Spinal Hematoma

Spinal hematoma is a rare but potentially devastating complication of spinal and epidural anesthesia, with an incidence estimated to be <1 in 150,000. Patients most commonly present with numbness or lower extremity weakness, a fact that can make early detection difficult in patients receiving perioperative spinal local anesthetics for pain control. Early detection is critical because a delay of more than 8 hours in decompressing the spine reduces the odds of good recovery.[247]

8 Coagulation defects are the principal risk factor for epidural hematoma. This raises the legitimate question as to how to treat patients who are or who will be anticoagulated. This issue has been addressed in a Consensus Statement from the American Society for Regional Anesthesia and Pain Medicine[248] and the recommendations presented here are taken from this consensus statement. In brief, patients taking nonsteroidal anti-inflammatory drugs with antiplatelet effects (e.g., cyclooxygenase-1 inhibitors) or receiving subcutaneous unfractionated heparin for deep vein thrombosis prophylaxis are not viewed as being at increased risk of spinal hematoma.

In contrast, other classes of antiplatelet drugs, like thienopyridine derivatives (e.g., ticlopidine, clopidogrel) and glycoprotein IIb/IIIa antagonists (e.g., abciximab, eptifibatide, tirofiban) have a more potent effect on platelet aggregation, and neuraxial block should generally not be performed in patients taking these or similar medications. Further, the consensus statement recommends that ticlopidine be discontinued for 2 weeks and clopidogrel for 1 week before performing central neuraxial blocks. The glycoprotein IIb/IIIa antagonists have a shorter duration of action; thus, it is recommended that abciximab should be discontinued 24 to 48 hours before central neuraxial block, and eptifibatide and tirofiban should be discontinued 4 to 8 hours beforehand.

In patients receiving intravenous heparin, heparinization should be delayed for at least 1 hour after central neuraxial block. Further, neuraxial catheters should be removed at least 2 to 4 hours after the last intravenous dose. Patients receiving fractionated low-molecular-weight heparin (e.g., enoxaparin, dalteparin, tinzaparin) are considered to be at increased risk of spinal hematoma. Patients receiving these drugs preoperatively at thromboprophylactic doses should have the drug held for 12 hours before central neuraxial block. At higher doses, such as those used to treat established deep vein thrombosis, central neuraxial block should be delayed for 24 hours after the last dose. For patients in whom low-molecular-weight heparin is begun after surgery, single-shot central neuraxial blocks are not contraindicated provided that the first low-molecular-weight heparin dose is not administered until 24 hours postoperatively if using a twice-daily dosing regimen and 6 to 8 hours if using a once-daily dosing regimen. If an indwelling central neuraxial catheter is in place, it should not be removed until 10 to 12 hours after the last low-molecular-weight heparin dose, and the subsequent doses should not begin until at least 2 hours after catheter removal.

Patients who are "fully anticoagulated" (i.e., have elevated prothrombin time or partial thromboplastin time) or who are receiving thrombolytic or fibrinolytic therapy are considered to be at increased risk of spinal hematoma. These patients should not receive central neuraxial block except in very unusual circumstances when other options are not viable.

Importantly for those patients who may have an epidural or intrathecal catheter placed, its removal is nearly as great a risk for spinal hematoma as its insertion, and the timing of removal and anticoagulation should be coordinated. Also, drugs/regimens not considered to put patients at increased risk of neuraxial bleeding when used alone (e.g., minidose unfractionated heparin and nonsteroidal anti-inflammatory drugs) may in fact increase risk when combined.

CONTRAINDICATIONS

The only absolute contraindication to spinal or epidural anesthesia is patient refusal. However, several pre-existing conditions increase the relative risk of these techniques and the anesthesiologist must carefully weigh the expected benefits before proceeding. Some conditions that increase the apparent risk of central neuraxial block include the following:

1. Hypovolemia or shock increases the risk of hypotension.
2. Increased intracranial pressure increases the risk of brain herniation when CSF is lost through the needle, or if a further increase in intracranial pressure follows injection of large volumes of solution into the epidural or subarachnoid spaces.
3. Coagulopathy or thrombocytopenia increases the risk of epidural hematoma.
4. Sepsis increases the risk of meningitis.
5. Infection at the puncture site increases the risk of meningitis.

Pre-existing neurologic disease, particularly diseases that wax and wane (e.g., multiple sclerosis), have been considered a contraindication to central–neuraxial block by some authors. Unfortunately, there are no well-controlled studies that answer the question as to whether spinal or epidural anesthesia alters the course of any pre-existing neurologic disease. However, Hebl et al.[249] conducted an uncontrolled retrospective chart review of 567 patients with pre-existing sensorimotor neuropathy or diabetic polyneuropathy who underwent spinal anesthesia. Two of these patients (0.4%; confidence interval: 0.1% to 1.3%) developed significant and persistent new neurologic symptoms: Painful exacerbation of diabetic neuropathy and lumbar plexopathy superimposed on pre-existing sensorimotor neuropathy. In both cases, the role of spinal anesthesia in the patient's new symptoms was unknown; thus, it is difficult to use these data to inform the decision whether or not to use central neuraxial block in patients with pre-existing peripheral neuropathy. Until more and better data are available, it is prudent to inform patients that there may be a small risk that their neuropathy may worsen so that they can consider that when discussing their anesthetic choice.

SPINAL OR EPIDURAL ANESTHESIA?

Spinal and epidural anesthesia each have advantages and disadvantages that may make one or the other technique better suited to a particular patient or procedure. Controlled studies comparing both techniques for surgical anesthesia have consistently found that spinal anesthesia takes less time to perform, produces more rapid onset of better-quality sensorimotor block, and is associated with less pain during surgery. Despite these important advantages of spinal anesthesia, epidural anesthesia offers advantages too. Chief among them are the lower risk of PDPH, less hypotension if epinephrine is not added to the local anesthetic, the ability to prolong or extend the block via an indwelling catheter, and the option of using an epidural catheter to provide postoperative analgesia.

References

1. Kehlet H. The stress response to surgery: Release mechanisms and the modifying effect of pain relief. *Acta Chir Scand Suppl.* 1988;550:22.
2. Modig J, Borg T, Karlström G, et al. Thromboembolism after total hip replacement: Role of epidural and general anesthesia. *Anesth Analg.* 1983;62:174.
3. Thornburn J, Louden J, Vallance R. Spinal and general anesthesia in total hip replacement: Frequency of deep vein thrombosis. *Br J Anaesth.* 1980;52:1117.
4. Christopherson R, Beattie C, Frank SM, et al. Perioperative morbidity in patients randomized to epidural or general anesthesia for lower extremity vascular surgery. *Anesthesiology.* 1993;79:422.
5. Rosenfeld B, Beattie C, Christopherson R, et al. The effects of different anesthetic regimens on fibrinolysis and the development of postoperative arterial thrombosis. *Anesthesiology.* 1993;79:435.
6. Yeager M, Glass D, Neff R, et al. Epidural anesthesia and analgesia in high-risk surgical patients. *Anesthesiology.* 1987;66:729.
7. Moraca RJ, Sheldon DG, Thirlby RC. The role of epidural anesthesia and analgesia in surgical practice. *Ann Surg.* 2003;238:663.
8. Block BM, Liu SS, Rowlingson AJ, et al. Efficacy of postoperative epidural analgesia: A meta-analysis. *JAMA.* 2003;290:2455.
9. Zarzur E. Anatomic studies of the human lumbar ligamentum flavum. *Anesth Analg.* 1984;63:499.
10. Hogan Q. Lumbar epidural anatomy. A new look by cryomicrotome section. *Anesthesiology.* 1991;75:767.
11. Meijenhorst GC. Computed tomography of the lumbar epidural veins. *Radiology.* 1982;145:687.
12. Bernards CM, Shen DD, Sterling ES, et al. Epidural, cerebrospinal fluid, and plasma pharmacokinetics of epidural opioids (part 1): Differences among opioids. *Anesthesiology.* 2003;99:455.
13. Tucker G, Mather L. Properties, absorption, and disposition of local anesthetic agents. In: Cousins M, Bridenbaugh P, eds. *Neural Blockade in Clinical Anesthesia and Management of Pain.* 2nd ed. Philadelphia, PA: JB Lippincott; 1988:47.
14. Fink BR, Walker S. Orientation of fibers in human dorsal lumbar dura mater in relation to lumbar puncture. *Anesth Analg.* 1989;69:768.
15. Kerber CW, Newton TH. The macro and microvasculature of the dura mater. *Neuroradiology.* 1973;6:175.
16. Blomberg R. The dorsomedian connective tissue band in the lumbar epidural space of humans: An anatomical study using epiduroscopy in autopsy cases. *Anesth Analg.* 1986;65:747.
17. Savolaine ER, Pandya JB, Greenblatt SH, et al. Anatomy of the human lumbar epidural space: New insights using CT-epidurography. *Anesthesiology.* 1988;68:217.
18. Hogan Q. Epidural catheter tip position and distribution of injectate evaluated by computed tomography. *Anesthesiology.* 1999;90:964.
19. Manchada V, Murad S, Shilyansky G, et al. Unusual clinical course of accidental subdural local anesthetic injection. *Anesth Analg.* 1983;62:1124.
20. Lubenow T, Keh-Wong E, Kristof K, et al. Inadvertant subdural injection: A complication of epidural block. *Anesth Analg.* 1988;67:175.
21. Jones M, Newton T. Inadvertent extra-arachnoid injections in myelography. *Radiology.* 1963;80:818.
22. Bernards C, Hill H. Morphine and alfentanil permeability through the spinal dura, arachnoid and pia mater of dogs and monkeys. *Anesthesiology.* 1990;73:1214.
23. Bernards C, Hill H. The spinal nerve root sleeve is not a preferred route for redistribution of drugs from the epidural space to the spinal cord. *Anesthesiology.* 1991;75:827.
24. Bulat M, Lupret V, Oreskovic D, et al. Transventricular and transpial absorption of cerebrospinal fluid into cerebral microvessels. *Coll Antropol.* 2008;32(suppl 1):43.
25. Klarica M, Oreskovic D, Bozic B, et al. New experimental model of acute aqueductal blockage in cats: Effects on cerebrospinal fluid pressure and the size of brain ventricles. *Neurosci.* 2009;158:1397.
26. Henry-Feugeas MC, Idy-Peretti I, Baledent O, et al. Origin of subarachnoid cerebrospinal fluid pulsations: A phase-contrast MR analysis. *Magn Reson Imaging.* 2000;18:387.
27. Loth F, Yardimci MA, Alperin N. Hydrodynamic modeling of cerebrospinal fluid motion within the spinal cavity. *J Biomech Eng.* 2001;123:71.
28. Bernards CM. Cerebrospinal fluid and spinal cord distribution of baclofen and bupivacaine during slow intrathecal infusion in pigs. *Anesthesiology.* 2006;105:169.
29. Reiman A, Anson B. Vertebral level of termination of the spinal cord with report of a case of sacral cord. *Anat Rec.* 1944;88:127.
30. Drummond G, Scott D. Deflection of spinal needles by the bevel. *Anaesthesia.* 1980;35:854.
31. Moore JM, Liu SS, Neal JM. Premedication with fentanyl and midazolam decreases the reliability of intravenous lidocaine test dose. *Anesth Analg.* 1998;86:1015.
32. Evron S, Sessler D, Sadan O, et al. Identification of the epidural space: Loss of resistance with air, lidocaine, or the combination of air and lidocaine. *Anesth Analg.* 1999;99:245.
33. Aida S, Taga K, Yamakura T, et al. Headache after attempted epidural block: The role of intrathecal air. *Anesthesiology.* 1998;88:76.
34. Asato F, Goto F. Radiographic findings of unilateral epidural block. *Anesth Analg.* 1996;83:519.
35. Brichant JF, Bonhomme V, Hans P. On knots in epidural catheters: A case report and a review of the literature. *Int J Obstet Anesth.* 2006;15:159.
36. Gabopoulou Z, Mavrommati P, Chatzieleftheriou A, et al. Epidural catheter entrapment caused by a double knot after combined spinal–epidural anesthesia. *Reg Anesth Pain Med.* 2005;30:588.
37. Leighton BL, Norris MC, DeSinome CA, et al. The air test as a clinically useful indicator of intravenously placed epidural catheters. *Anesthesiology.* 1990;73:610.
38. Mackie K, Lam A. Epinephrine-containing test dose during beta-blockade. *J Clin Monit.* 1991;7:213.
39. Moore D, Batra M. The components of an effective test dose prior to epidural block. *Anesthesiology.* 1981;55:693.
40. Guinard J, Mulroy M, Carpenter R, et al. Test doses: Optimal epinephrine content with and without acute beta-adrenergic blockade. *Anesthesiology.* 1990;73:386.
41. Liu SS. Hemodynamic responses to an epinephrine test dose in adults during epidural or combined epidural-general anesthesia. *Anesth Analg.* 1996;83:97.
42. Leighton B, DeSimone C, Norris M, et al. Isoproterenol is an effective marker of intravenous injection in laboring women. *Anesthesiology.* 1989;71:206.
43. Leighton BL, Norris MC, Sosis M, et al. Limitations of epinephrine as a marker of intravascular injection in laboring women. *Anesthesiology.* 1987;66:688.
44. Takiguchi T, Okano T, Egawa H, et al. The effect of epidural saline injection on analgesic level during combined spinal and epidural anesthesia assessed clinically and myelographically [see comments]. *Anesth Analg.* 1997;85:1097.
45. Stienstra R, Dahan A, Alhadi BZ, et al. Mechanism of action of an epidural top-up in combined spinal epidural anesthesia. *Anesth Analg.* 1996;83:382.
46. Stienstra R, Dilrosun-Alhadi BZ, Dahan A, et al. The epidural "top-up" in combined spinal–epidural anesthesia: The effect of volume versus dose. *Anesth Analg.* 1999;88:810.
47. Myint Y, Bailey P, Milne B. Cardiorespiratory arrest following combined spinal epidural anaesthesia. *Anaesthesia.* 1993;48:684.
48. Bernards C, Kopacz D, Michel M. Effect of needle puncture on morphine and lidocaine flux through the spinal meninges of the monkey. *Anesthesiology.* 1994;80:853.
49. Hodgkinson R, Husain FJ. Obesity, gravity, and spread of epidural anesthesia. *Anesth Analg.* 1981;60:421.
50. Lee A, Ray D, Littlewood D, et al. Effect of dextrose concentration on the intrathecal spread of amethocaine. *Br J Anaesth.* 1988;61:135.
51. Chambers WA, Edstrom HH, Scott DB. Effect of baricity on spinal anaesthesia with bupivacaine. *Br J Anaesth.* 1981;53:279.
52. Bannister J, McClure JH, Wildsmith JA. Effect of glucose concentration on the intrathecal spread of 0.5% bupivacaine. *Br J Anaesth.* 1990;64:232.
53. Povey HM, Jacobsen J, Westergaard-Nielsen J. Subarachnoid analgesia with hyperbaric 0.5% bupivacaine: Effect of a 60-min period of sitting. *Acta Anaesthesiol Scand.* 1989;33:295.
54. Povey HM, Olsen PA, Pihl H. Spinal analgesia with hyperbaric 0.5% bupivacaine: Effects of different patient positions. *Acta Anaesthesiol Scand.* 1987;31:616.

55. Sinclair CJ, Scott DB, Edström H. Effect of the Trendelenburg position on spinal anaesthesia with hyperbaric bupivacaine. *Br J Anaesth.* 1982;54:497.
56. Martin-Salvaj G, Van Gessel E, Forster A, et al. Influence of duration of lateral decubitus on the spread of hyperbaric tetracaine during spinal anesthesia: A prospective time-response study. *Anesth Analg.* 1994;79:1107.
57. Smith T. The lumbar spine and subarachnoid block. *Anesthesiology.* 1968;29:60.
58. Logan MR, Drummond GB. Spinal anesthesia and lumbar lordosis. *Anesth Analg.* 1988;67:338.
59. Bodily M, Carpenter R, Owens B. Lidocaine 0.5% spinal anaesthesia: A hypobaric solution for short-stay perirectal surgery. *Can J Anaesth.* 1992;39:770.
60. Brown DT, Wildsmith JA, Covino BG, et al. Effect of baricity on spinal anesthesia with amethocaine. *Br J Anaesth.* 1980;52:589.
61. Cummings GC, Bamber DB, Edstrom HH, et al. Subarachnoid blockade with bupivacaine. A comparison with cinchocaine. *Br J Anaesth.* 1984;56:573.
62. Møller IW, Fernandes A, Edström HH. Subarachnoid anaesthesia with 0.5% bupivacaine: Effects of density. *Br J Anaesth.* 1984;56:1191.
63. Logan MR, McClure JH, Wildsmith JA. Plain bupivacaine: An unpredictable spinal anaesthetic agent. *Br J Anaesth.* 1986;58:292.
64. McKeown DW, Stewart K, Littlewood DG, et al. Spinal anesthesia with plain solutions of lidocaine (2%) and bupivacaine (0.5%). *Regional Anesth.* 1986;11:68.
65. Cameron AE, Arnold RW, Ghorisa MW, et al. Spinal analgesia using bupivacaine 0.5% plain. Variation in the extent of the block with patient age. *Anaesthesia.* 1981;36:318.
66. Kalso E, Tuominen M, Rosenberg PH. Effect of posture and some c.s.f. characteristics on spinal anaesthesia with isobaric 0.5% bupivacaine. *Br J Anaesth.* 1982;54:1179.
67. Tuominen M, Kalso E, Rosenberg P. Effects of posture on the spread of spinal anaesthesia with isobaric 0.75% or 0.5% bupivacaine. *Br J Anaesth.* 1982;54:313.
68. Stienstra R, van Poorten JF. The temperature of bupivacaine 0.5% affects the sensory level of spinal anesthesia. *Anesth Analg.* 1988;67:272.
69. McClure JH, Brown DT, Wildsmith JA. Effect of injected volume and speed of injection on the spread of spinal anaesthesia with isobaric amethocaine. *Br J Anaesth.* 1982;54:917.
70. Van Zundert AA, De Wolf AM. Extent of anesthesia and hemodynamic effects after subarachnoid administration of bupivacaine with epinephrine. *Anesth Analg.* 1988;67:784.
71. Nielsen TH, Kristoffersen E, Olsen KH, et al. Plain bupivacaine: 0.5% or 0.25% for spinal analgesia? *Br J Anaesth.* 1989;62:164.
72. Bengtsson M, Malmqvist LA, Edström HH. Spinal analgesia with glucose-free bupivacaine—Effects of volume and concentration. *Acta Anaesthesiol Scand.* 1984;28:583.
73. Blomqvist H, Nilsson A, Arweström E. Spinal anaesthesia with 15 mg bupivacaine 0.25% and 0.5%. *Regional Anesth.* 1988;13:165.
74. Mukkada TA, Bridenbaugh PO, Singh P, et al. Effects of dose, volume, and concentration of glucose-free bupivacaine in spinal anesthesia. *Regional Anesth.* 1986; 11:98.
75. Sheskey MC, Rocco AG, Bizzarri-Schmid M, et al. A dose-response study of bupivacaine for spinal anesthesia. *Anesth Analg.* 1983;62:931.
76. Wildsmith J, McClure J, Brown D, et al. Effects of posture on the spread of isobaric and hyperbaric amethocaine. *Br J Anaesth.* 1981;53:273.
77. Pflug AE, Aasheim GM, Beck HA. Spinal anesthesia: Bupivacaine versus tetracaine. *Anesth Analg.* 1976;55:489.
78. Sundnes KO, Vaagenes P, Skretting P, et al. Spinal analgesia with hyperbaric bupivacaine: Effects of volume of solution. *Br J Anaesth.* 1982;54:69.
79. Chambers WA, Littlewood DG, Scott DB. Spinal anesthesia with hyperbaric bupivacaine: Effect of added vasoconstrictors. *Anesth Analg.* 1982;61:49.
80. Taivainen T, Tuominen M, Rosenberg PH. Influence of obesity on the spread of spinal analgesia after injection of plain 0.5% bupivacaine at the L3–4 of L4–5 interspace. *Br J Anaesth.* 1990;64:542.
81. Tuominen M, Kuulasmaa K, Taivainen T, et al. Individual predictability of repeated spinal anaesthesia with isobaric bupivacaine. *Acta Anaesthesiol Scand.* 1989;33:13.
82. Tuominen M, Taivainen T, Rosenberg PH. Spread of spinal anaesthesia with plain 0.5% bupivacaine: Influence of the vertebral interspace used for injection. *Br J Anaesth.* 1989;62:358.
83. Carpenter RL, Hogan QH, Liu SS, et al. Lumbosacral cerebrospinal fluid volume is the primary determinant of sensory block extent and duration during spinal anesthesia [see comments]. *Anesthesiology.* 1998;89:24.
84. Higuchi H, Hirata J, Adachi Y, et al. Influence of lumbosacral cerebrospinal fluid density, velocity, and volume on extent and duration of plain bupivacaine spinal anesthesia. *Anesthesiology.* 2004;100:106.
85. Pargger H, Hampl KF, Aeschbach A, et al. Combined effect of patient variables on sensory level after spinal 0.5% plain bupivacaine. *Acta Anaesthesiol Scand.* 1998;42:430.
86. Veering BT, Burm AG, van Kleef JW, et al. Spinal anesthesia with glucose-free bupivacaine: Effects of age on neural blockade and pharmacokinetics. *Anesth Analg.* 1987;66:965.
87. Pitkänen M, Haapaniemi L, Tuominen M, et al. Influence of age on spinal anaesthesia with isobaric 0.5% bupivacaine. *Br J Anaesth.* 1984;56:279.
88. Norris M. Height, weight, and the spread of subarachnoid hyperbaric bupivacaine in the term parturient. *Anesth Analg.* 1988;67:555.
89. Norris MC. Patient variables and the subarachnoid spread of hyperbaric bupivacaine in the term parturient. *Anesthesiology.* 1990;72:478.
90. Wildsmith JA, Rocco AG. Current concepts in spinal anesthesia. *Regional Anesth.* 1985;10:119.
91. McCulloch WJ, Littlewood DG. Influence of obesity on spinal analgesia with isobaric 0.5% bupivacaine. *Br J Anaesth.* 1986;58:610.
92. Pitkänen MT. Body mass and spread of spinal anesthesia with bupivacaine. *Anesth Analg.* 1987;66:127.
93. Axelsson KH, Edström HH, Sundberg AE, et al. Spinal anaesthesia with hyperbaric 0.5% bupivacaine: Effects of volume. *Acta Anaesthesiol Scand.* 1982;26:439.
94. Bengtsson M, Edström HH, Löfström JB. Spinal analgesia with bupivacaine, mepivacaine and tetracaine. *Acta Anaesthesiol Scand.* 1983;27:278.
95. Racle J, Benkhadra A, Poy J, et al. Effect of increasing amounts of epinephrine during isobaric bupivacaine spinal anesthesia in elderly patients. *Anesth Analg.* 1987;66:882.
96. Vaida GT, Moss P, Capan LM, et al. Prolongation of lidocaine spinal anesthesia with phenylephrine. *Anesth Analg.* 1986;65:781.
97. Egbert LD, Deas TC. Effect of epinephrine upon the duration of spinal anesthesia. *Anesthesiology.* 1960;21:345.
98. Concepcion M, Maddi R, Francis D, et al. Vasoconstrictors in spinal anesthesia with tetracaine—A comparison of epinephrine and phenylephrine. *Anesth Analg.* 1984;63:134.
99. Meagher RP, Moore DC, DeVries JC. Phenylephrine: The most effective potentiator of tetracaine spinal anesthesia. *Anesth Analg.* 1966;45:134.
100. Caldwell C, Nielsen C, Baltz T, et al. Comparison of high-dose epinephrine and phenylephrine in spinal anesthesia with tetracaine. *Anesthesiology.* 1985;62:804.
101. Park WY, Balingit PE, Macnamara TE. Effects of patient age, pH of cerebrospinal fluid, and vasopressors on onset and duration of spinal anesthesia. *Anesth Analg.* 1975;54:455.
102. Fukuda T, Dohi S, Naito H. Comparisons of tetracaine spinal anesthesia with clonidine or phenylephrine in normotensive and hypertensive humans. *Anesth Analg.* 1994;78:106.
103. Bonnet F, Brun-Buisson V, Saada M, et al. Dose-related prolongation of hyperbaric tetracaine spinal anesthesia by clonidine in humans. *Anesth Analg.* 1989;68:619.
104. Dobrydnjov I, Samarutel J. Enhancement of intrathecal lidocaine by addition of local and systemic clonidine. *Acta Anaesthesiol Scand.* 1999;43:556.
105. Ota K, Namiki A, Ujike Y, et al. Prolongation of tetracaine spinal anesthesia by oral clonidine. *Anesth Analg.* 1992;75:262.
106. Ota K, Namiki A, Iwasaki H, et al. Dosing interval for prolongation of tetracaine spinal anesthesia by oral clonidine in humans. *Anesth Analg.* 1994;79:1117.
107. Axelsson K, Widman B. Blood concentration of lidocaine after spinal anaesthesia using lidocaine and lidocaine with adrenaline. *Acta Anaesthesiol Scand.* 1981;25:240.
108. Leicht CH, Carlson SA. Prolongation of lidocaine spinal anesthesia with epinephrine and phenylephrine. *Anesth Analg.* 1986;65:365.
109. Moore DC, Chadwick HS, Ready LB. Epinephrine prolongs libocaine spinal: Pain in the operative site is the most accurate method of determining local anesthetic duration. *Anesthesiology.* 1987;67:416.
110. Chambers WA, Littlewood DG, Logan MR, et al. Effect of added epinephrine on spinal anesthesia with lidocaine. *Anesth Analg.* 1981;60:417.
111. Spivey DL. Epinephrine does not prolong lidocaine spinal anesthesia in term parturients. *Anesth Analg.* 1985;64:468.
112. Chiu AA, Liu S, Carpenter RL, et al. The effects of epinephrine on lidocaine spinal anesthesia: A cross-over study. *Anesth Analg.* 1995;80:735.
113. Kozody R, Swartz J, Palahniuk RJ, et al. Spinal cord blood flow following subarachnoid lidocaine. *Can Anaesth Soc J.* 1985;32:472.
114. Kozody R, Palahniuk RJ, Cumming MO. Spinal cord blood flow following subarachnoid tetracaine. *Can Anaesth Soc J.* 1985;32:23.
115. Kozody R, Ong B, Palahniuk RJ, et al. Subarachnoid bupivacaine decreases spinal cord blood flow in dogs. *Can Anaesth Soc J.* 1985;32:216.
116. Denson DD, Bridenbaugh PO, Turner PA, et al. Neural blockade and pharmacokinetics following subarachnoid lidocaine in the rhesus monkey. I. Effects of epinephrine. *Anesth Analg.* 1982;61:746.
117. Crosby G, Russo M, Szabo M, et al. Subarachnoid clonidine reduces spinal cord blood flow and glucose utilization in conscious rats. *Anesthesiology.* 1990;73:1179.
118. Converse JG, Landmesser CM, Harmel MH. The concentration of pontocaine hydrochloride in the cerebrospinal fluid during spinal anesthesia, and the influence of epinephrine in prolonging the sensory anesthetic effect. *Anesthesiology.* 1954;15:1.
119. Mörch ET, Rosenberg MK, Truant AT. Lidocaine for spinal anesthesia. A study of the concentration in the spinal fluid. *Acta Anaesthesiol Scand.* 1957;1:105.
120. Kozody R, Palahniuk RJ, Wade JG, et al. The effect of subarachnoid epinephrine and phenylephrine on spinal cord blood flow. *Can Anaesth Soc J.* 1984;31:503.
121. Reddy SV, Maderdrut JL, Yaksh TL. Spinal cord pharmacology of adrenergic agonist-mediated antinociception. *J Pharmacol Exp Ther.* 1980;213:525.
122. Phillis J, Tebecis A, York D. Depression of spinal motoneurons by noradrenalin, 5-hydroxytryptamine and histamine. *Eur J Pharmacol.* 1968;4:471.
123. Park W, Massengale M, Macnamara T. Age, height, and speed of injection as factors determining caudal anesthetic level and occurrence of severe hypertension. *Anesthesiology.* 1979;51:81.

124. Park WY, Hagins FM, Rivat EL, et al. Age and epidural dose response in adult men. *Anesthesiology.* 1982;56:318.
125. Grundy EM, Ramamurthy S, Patel KP, et al. Extradural analgesia revisited. *Br J Anaesth.* 1978;50:805.
126. Erdemir HA, Soper LE, Sweet RB. Studies of factors affecting peridural anesthesia. *Anesth Analg.* 1965;44:400.
127. Burn JM, Guyer PB, Langdon L. The spread of solutions injected into the epidural space. *Br J Anaesth.* 1973;45:338.
128. Apostolou GA, Zarmakoupis PK, Mastrokostopoulos GT. Spread of epidural anesthesia and the lateral position. *Anesth Analg.* 1981;60:584.
129. Park WY, Hagins FM, Massengale MD, et al. The sitting position and anesthetic spread in the epidural space. *Anesth Analg.* 1984;63:863.
130. Ponhold H, Kulier A, Rehak P. 30 degree trunk elevation of the patient and quality of lumbar epidural anesthesia. Effects of elevation in operations on the lower extremities. *Anaesthetist.* 1993;42:788.
131. Park WY, Massengale M, Kim SI, et al. Age and the spread of local anesthetic solutions in the epidural space. *Anesth Analg.* 1980;59:768.
132. Nydahl PA, Philipson L, Axelsson K, et al. Epidural anesthesia with 0.5% bupivacaine: Influence of age on sensory and motor blockade. *Anesth Analg.* 1991; 73:780.
133. Veering BT, Burm AG, van Kleef JW, et al. Epidural anesthesia with bupivacaine: Effects of age on neural blockade and pharmacokinetics. *Anesth Analg.* 1987;66:589.
134. Hirabayashi Y, Saitoh K, Fukuda H, et al. Effect of age on dose requirement for lumbar epidural anesthesia. *Masui.* 1993;42:808.
135. Duggan J, Bowler GM, McClure JH, et al. Extradural block with bupivacaine: Influence of dose, volume, concentration and patient characteristics. *Br J Anaesth.* 1988;61:324.
136. Hirabayashi Y, Shimizu R, Matsuda I, et al. Effect of extradural compliance and resistance on spread of extradural analgesia. *Br J Anaesth.* 1990;65:508.
137. Bromage P. Spread of analgesic solutions in the epidural space and their site of action: A statistical study. *Br J Anaesth.* 1962;34:161.
138. Fagraeus L, Urban BJ, Bromage PR. Spread of epidural analgesia in early pregnancy. *Anesthesiology.* 1983;58:184.
139. Grundy EM, Zamora AM, Winnie AP. Comparison of spread of epidural anesthesia in pregnant and nonpregnant women. *Anesth Analg.* 1978;57:544.
140. Kalas DB, Senfield RM, Hehre FW. Continuous lumbar peridural anesthesia in obstetrics. IV: Comparison of the number of segments blocked in pregnant and nonpregnant subjects. *Anesth Analg.* 1966;45:848.
141. Sharrock NE. Lack of exaggerated spread of epidural anesthesia in patients with arteriosclerosis. *Anesthesiology.* 1977;47:307.
142. Axelsson K, Nydahl PA, Philipson L, et al. Motor and sensory blockade after epidural injection of mepivacaine, bupivacaine, and etidocaine—A double-blind study. *Anesth Analg.* 1989;69:739.
143. Kerkkamp HE, Gielen MJ, Wattwil M, et al. An open study comparison of 0.5%, 0.75% and 1.0% ropivacaine, with epinephrine, in epidural anesthesia in patients undergoing urologic surgery. *Regional Anesth.* 1990;15:53.
144. Buckley FP, Littlewood DG, Covino BG, et al. Effects of adrenaline and the concentration of solution on extradural block with etidocaine. *Br J Anaesth.* 1978; 50:171.
145. Scott DB, McClure JH, Gaisi RM, et al. Effects of concentration of local anaesthetic drugs in extradural block. *Br J Anaesth.* 1980;52:1033.
146. Bromage PR, Burfoot MF, Crowell DE, et al. Quality of epidural blockade. I: Influence of physical factors. *Br J Anaesth.* 1964;36:342.
147. Bernards CM, Shen DD, Sterling ES, et al. Epidural, cerebrospinal fluid, and plasma pharmacokinetics of epidural opioids (part 2): Effect of epinephrine. *Anesthesiology.* 2003;99:466.
148. Kier L. Continuous epidural analgesia in prostatectomy: Comparison of bupivacaine with and without adrenaline. *Acta Anaesthesiol Scand.* 1974;18:1.
149. Sinclair CJ, Scott DB. Comparison of bupivacaine and etidocaine in extradural blockade. *Br J Anaesth.* 1984;56:147.
150. Cederholm I, Anskär S, Bengtsson M. Sensory, motor, and sympathetic block during epidural analgesia with 0.5% and 0.75% ropivacaine with and without epinephrine. *Regional Anesth.* 1994;19:18.
151. Abboud T, Sheik-ol-Eslam A, Yanagi T, et al. Safety and efficacy of epinephrine added to bupivacaine for lumbar epidural analgesia in obstetrics. *Anesth Analg.* 1985;64:585.
152. Eisenach JC, Grice SC, Dewan DM. Epinephrine enhances analgesia produced by epidural bupivacaine during labor. *Anesth Analg.* 1987;66:447.
153. Finucane B, McCraney J, Bush D. Double-blind comparison of lidocaine and etidocaine during continuous epidural anesthesia for vaginal delivery. *South Med J.* 1978;71:667.
154. Cohen E. Distribution of local anesthetic agents in the neuroaxis of the dog. *Anesthesiology.* 1968;29:1002.
155. Post C, Freedman J, Ramsay C, et al. Redistribution of lidocaine and bupivacaine after intrathecal injection in mice. *Anesthesiology.* 1985;63:410.
156. Boswell M, Iacono R, Guthkelch A. Sites of action of subarachnoid lidocaine and tetracaine: Observations with evoked potential monitoring during spinal cord stimulator implantation. *Reg Anesth.* 1992;17:37.
157. Cusick J, Myklebust J, Abram S. Differential neural effects of epidural anesthetics. *Anesthesiology.* 1980;53:299.
158. Urban B. Clinical observations suggesting a changing site of action during induction and recession of spinal and epidural anesthesia. *Anesthesiology.* 1973;39:496.
159. Fink BR. Mechanisms of differential axial blockade in epidural and subarachnoid anesthesia. *Anesthesiology.* 1989;70:851.
160. Fink BR, Cairns AM. Lack of size-related differential sensitivity to equilibrium conduction block among mammalian myelinated axons exposed to lidocaine. *Anesth Analg.* 1987;66:948.
161. Chamberlain D, Chamberlain B. Changes in skin temperature of the trunk and their relationship to sympathetic block during spinal anesthesia. *Anesthesiology.* 1986;65:139.
162. Brull SJ, Greene NM. Zones of differential sensory block during extradural anaesthesia. *Br J Anaesth.* 1991;66:651.
163. Gentili M, Huu PC, Enel D, et al. Sedation depends on the level of sensory block induced by spinal anaesthesia. *Br J Anaesth.* 1998;81:970.
164. Ben-David B, Vaida S, Gaitini L. The influence of high spinal anesthesia on sensitivity to midazolam sedation [see comments]. *Anesth Analg.* 1995;81:525.
165. Tverskoy M, Shagal M, Finger J, et al. Subarachnoid bupivacaine blockade decreases midazolam and thiopental hypnotic requirements. *J Clin Anesth.* 1994; 6:487.
166. Tverskoy M, Shifrin V, Finger J, et al. Effect of epidural bupivacaine block on midazolam hypnotic requirements. *Reg Anesth.* 1996;21:209.
167. Hodgson P, Liu S, Gras T. Does epidural anesthesia have general anesthetic effects? A prospective, randomized, double-blind, placebo-controlled trial. *Anesthesiology.* 1999;91:1687.
168. Carpenter RL, Caplan RA, Brown DL, et al. Incidence and risk factors for side effects of spinal anesthesia. *Anesthesiology.* 1992;76:906.
169. Coe AJ, Revanäs B. Is crystalloid preloading useful in spinal anaesthesia in the elderly? *Anaesthesia.* 1990;45:241.
170. Phero JC, Bridenbaugh PO, Edström HH, et al. Hypotension in spinal anesthesia: A comparison of isobaric tetracaine with epinephrine and isobaric bupivacaine without epinephrine. *Anesth Analg.* 1987;66:549.
171. Tarkkila P, Isola J. A regression model for identifying patients at high risk of hypotension, bradycardia and nausea during spinal anesthesia. *Acta Anesthesiol Scand.* 1992;36:554.
172. Shimosato S, Etsten BE. The role of the venous system in cardiocirculatory dynamics during spinal and epidural anesthesia in man. *Anesthesiology.* 1969; 30:619.
173. Kennedy WF Jr, Bonica JJ, Akamatsu TJ, et al. Cardiovascular and respiratory effects of subarachnoid block in the presence of acute blood loss. *Anesthesiology.* 1968;29:29.
174. Anzai Y, Nishikawa T. Heart rate responses to body tilt during spinal anesthesia. *Anesth Analg.* 1991;73:385.
175. Ward RJ, Bonica JJ, Freund FG, et al. Epidural and subarachnoid anesthesia. Cardiovascular and respiratory effects. *JAMA.* 1965;191:275.
176. Carp H, Vadhera R, Jayaram A, et al. Endogenous vasopressin and renin-angiotensin systems support blood pressure after epidural block in humans. *Anesthesiology.* 1994;80:1000–1007; discussion 27A.
177. Peters J, Schlaghecke R, Thouet H, et al. Endogenous vasopressin supports blood pressure and prevents severe hypotension during epidural anesthesia in conscious dogs. *Anesthesiology.* 1990;73:694.
178. Pathak CL. Autoregulation of chronotropic response of the heart through pacemaker stretch. *Cardiology.* 1973;58:45.
179. Jacobsen J, Søfelt S, Brocks V, et al. Reduced left ventricular diameters at onset of bradycardia during epidural anaesthesia. *Acta Anaesthesiol Scand.* 1992;36: 831.
180. Baron JF, Decaux-Jacolot A, Edouard A, et al. Influence of venous return on baroreflex control of heart rate during lumbar epidural anesthesia in humans. *Anesthesiology.* 1986;64:188.
181. Caplan RA, Ward RJ, Posner K, et al. Unexpected cardiac arrest during spinal anesthesia: A closed claims analysis of predisposing factors. *Anesthesiology.* 1988;68:5.
182. Mackey DC, Carpenter RL, Thompson GE, et al. Bradycardia and asystole during spinal anesthesia: A report of three cases without morbidity. *Anesthesiology.* 1989;70:866.
183. Bernards CM, Hymas NJ. Progression of first degree heart block to high-grade second degree block during spinal anaesthesia. *Can J Anaesth.* 1992;39:173.
184. Jordi EM, Marsch SC, Strebel S. Third degree heart block and asystole associated with spinal anesthesia. *Anesthesiology.* 1998;89:257.
185. Shen CL, Hung YC, Chen PJ, et al. Mobitz type II AV block during spinal anesthesia. *Anesthesiology.* 1990;90:1477.
186. Bonica JJ, Kennedy WF Jr, Ward RJ, et al. A comparison of the effects of high subarachnoid and epidural anesthesia. *Acta Anaesthesiol Scand.* 1966;23:429.
187. Kerkkamp HE, Gielen MJ. Hemodynamic monitoring in epidural blockade: Cardiovascular effects of 20 ml 0.5% bupivacaine with and without epinephrine. *Regional Anesth.* 1990;15:137.
188. Venn PJ, Simpson DA, Rubin AP, et al. Effect of fluid preloading on cardiovascular variables after spinal anaesthesia with glucose-free 0.75% bupivacaine. *Br J Anaesth.* 1989;63:682.
189. Rout CC, Rocke DA, Levin J, et al. A reevaluation of the role of crystalloid preload in the prevention of hypotension associated with spinal anesthesia for elective cesarean section. *Anesthesiology.* 1993;79:262.

190. Pouta AM, Karinen J, Vuolteenaho OJ, et al. Effect of intravenous fluid preload on vasoactive peptide secretion during Caesarean section under spinal anaesthesia. *Anaesthesia.* 1996;51:128.
191. Ueyama H, He YL, Tanigami H, et al. Effects of crystalloid and colloid preload on blood volume in the parturient undergoing spinal anesthesia for elective cesarean section. *Anesthesiology.* 1999;91:1571.
192. Marhofer P, Faryniak B, Oismuller C, et al. Cardiovascular effects of 6% hetastarch and lactated Ringer's solution during spinal anesthesia. *Reg Anesth Pain Med.* 1999;24:399.
193. Tamilselvan P, Fernando R, Bray J, et al. The effects of crystalloid and colloid preload on cardiac output in the parturient undergoing planned cesarean delivery under spinal anesthesia: A randomized trial. *Anesth Analg.* 2009;109:1916.
194. Butterworth J, Piccione W, Berrizbeitia L, et al. Augmentation of venous return by adrenergic agonists during spinal anesthesia. *Anesth Analg.* 1986;65:612.
195. Ward RJ, Kennedy WF, Bonica JJ, et al. Experimental evaluation of atropine and vasopressors for the treatment of hypotension of high subarachnoid anesthesia. *Anesth Analg.* 1966;45:621.
196. Lundberg J, Norgren L, Thomson D, et al. Hemodynamic effects of dopamine during thoracic epidural analgesia in man. *Anesthesiology.* 1987;66:641.
197. Butterworth JF 4th, Austin JC, Johnson MD, et al. Effect of total spinal anesthesia on arterial and venous responses to dopamine and dobutamine. *Anesth Analg.* 1987;66:209.
198. Goertz AW, Seeling W, Heinrich H, et al. Effect of phenylephrine bolus administration of left ventricular function during high thoracic and lumbar epidural anesthesia combined with general anesthesia. *Anesth Analg.* 1993;76:541.
199. Sakura S, Saito Y, Kosaka Y. Effect of lumbar epidural anesthesia on ventilatory response to hypercapnia in young and elderly patients. *J Clin Anesth.* 1993;5:109.
200. Steinbrook R, Concepcion M, Topulos G. Ventilatory responses to hypercapnia during bupivacaine spinal anesthesia. *Anesth Analg.* 1988;67:247.
201. Dahl JB, Schultz P, Anker-Møller E, et al. Spinal anaesthesia in young patients using a 29-gauge needle: Technical considerations and an evaluation of postoperative complaints compared with general anaesthesia. *Br J Anaesth.* 1990;64:178.
202. Seeberger MD, Lang ML, Drewe J, et al. Comparison of spinal and epidural anesthesia for patients younger than 50 years of age. *Anesth Analg.* 1994;78:667.
203. Halpern S, Preston R. Postdural puncture headache and spinal needle design. *Anesthesiology.* 1994;81:1376.
204. Lybecker H, Møller JT, May O, et al. Incidence and prediction of postdural puncture headache. A prospective study of 1021 spinal anesthesias. *Anesth Analg.* 1990;70:389.
205. Flaatten H, Thorsen T, Askeland B, et al. Puncture technique and postural postdural puncture headache. A randomised, double-blind study comparing transverse and parallel puncture. *Acta Anaesthesiol Scand.* 1998;42:1209.
206. Camann WR, Murray RS, Mushlin PS, et al. Effects of oral caffeine on postdural puncture headache. A double-blind, placebo-controlled trial. *Anesth Analg.* 1990; 70:181.
207. Connelly NR, Parker RK, Rahimi A, et al. Sumatriptan in patients with postdural puncture headache. *Headache.* 2000;40:316.
208. Hakim S, Khan RM, Maroof M, et al. Methylergonovine maleate (methergine) relieves postdural puncture headache in obstetric patients. *Acta Obstet Gynecol Scand.* 2005;84:100.
209. Cheek TG, Banner R, Sauter J, et al. Prophylactic extradural blood patch is effective. *Br J Anaesth.* 1988;61:340.
210. Colonna-Romano P, Shapiro BE. Unintentional dural puncture and prophylactic epidural blood patch in obstetrics. *Anesth Analg.* 1989;69:522.
211. Scavone BM, Wong CA, Sullivan VT, et al. Efficacy of a prophylactic epidural blood patch in preventing post dural puncture headache in parturients after inadvertent dural puncture. *Anesthesiology.* 2004;101:1422.
212. Safa-Tisseront V, Thormann F, Malassine P, et al. Effectiveness of epidural blood patch in the management of postdural puncture headache. *Anesthesiology.* 2001;95:334.
213. Yildiz TS, Solak M, Iseri M, et al. Hearing loss after spinal anesthesia: The effect of different infusion solutions. *Otolaryngol Head Neck Surg.* 2007;137:79.
214. Schaffartzik W, Hirsch J, Frickmann F, et al. Hearing loss after spinal and general anesthesia: A comparative study. *Anesth Analg.* 2000;91:1466.
215. Lamberg T, Pitkanen MT, Marttila T, et al. Hearing loss after continuous or single-shot spinal anesthesia. *Reg Anesth.* 1997;22:539.
216. Tyagi A, Gupta U, Kumar A, et al. Role of repeated epidural injections in preventing post-spinal hearing loss. *J Clin Anesth.* 2010;22:587.
217. Kane R. Neurologic deficits following epidural or spinal anesthesia. *Anesth Analg.* 1981;60:150.
218. Lambert LA, Lambert DH, Strichartz GR. Irreversible conduction block in isolated nerve by high concentrations of local anesthetics. *Anesthesiology.* 1994;80:1082.
219. Rigler M, Drasner K, Krejcie T, et al. Cauda equina syndrome after continuous spinal anesthesia. *Anesth Analg.* 1991;72:275.
220. Ross B, Coda B, Heath C. Local anesthetic distribution in a spinal model: A possible mechanism of neurologic injury after continuous spinal anesthesia. *Reg Anesth.* 1992;17:69.
221. Drasner K, Rigler M, Sessler D, et al. Cauda equina syndrome following intended epidural anesthesia. *Anesthesiology.* 1992;77:582.
222. Gold MS, Reichling DB, Hampl KF, et al. Lidocaine toxicity in primary afferent neurons from the rat. *J Pharmacol Exp Ther.* 1998;285:413.
223. Johnson ME, Saenz JA, DaSilva AD, et al. Effect of local anesthetic on neuronal cytoplasmic calcium and plasma membrane lysis (necrosis) in a cell culture model. *Anesthesiology.* 2002;97:1466.
224. Kitagawa N, Oda M, Totoki T. Possible mechanism of irreversible nerve injury caused by local anesthetics: Detergent properties of local anesthetics and membrane disruption. *Anesthesiology.* 2004;100:962.
225. Raucher D, Sheetz MP. Phospholipase C activation by anesthetics decreases membrane-cytoskeleton adhesion. *J Cell Sci.* 2001;114:3759.
226. Drasner K. Lidocaine spinal anesthesia: A vanishing therapeutic index? [editorial; comment]. *Anesthesiology.* 1997;87:469.
227. Schneider M, Ettlin T, Kaufmann M, et al. Transient neurologic toxicity after hyperbaric subarachnoid anesthesia with 5% lidocaine [see comments]. *Anesth Analg.* 1993;76:1154.
228. Hiller A, Rosenberg PH. Transient neurological symptoms after spinal anaesthesia with 4% mepivacaine and 0.5% bupivacaine. *Br J Anaesth.* 1997;79:301.
229. Liguori GA, Zayas VM, Chisholm MF. Transient neurologic symptoms after spinal anesthesia with mepivacaine and lidocaine [see comments]. *Anesthesiology.* 1998;88:619.
230. Martinez-Bourio R, Arzuaga M, Quintana JM, et al. Incidence of transient neurologic symptoms after hyperbaric subarachnoid anesthesia with 5% lidocaine and 5% prilocaine [see comments]. *Anesthesiology.* 1998;88:624.
231. Hampl KF, Heinzmann-Wiedmer S, Luginbuehl I, et al. Transient neurologic symptoms after spinal anesthesia: A lower incidence with prilocaine and bupivacaine than with lidocaine [see comments]. *Anesthesiology.* 1998;88: 629.
232. Salmela L, Aromaa U. Transient radicular irritation after spinal anesthesia induced with hyperbaric solutions of cerebrospinal fluid-diluted lidocaine 50 mg/ml or mepivacaine 40 mg/ml or bupivacaine 5 mg/ml. *Acta Anaesthesiol Scand.* 1998;42:765.
233. Axelrod EH, Alexander GD, Brown M, et al. Procaine spinal anesthesia: A pilot study of the incidence of transient neurologic symptoms. *J Clin Anesth.* 1998;10:404.
234. Bergeron L, Girard M, Drolet P, et al. Spinal procaine with and without epinephrine and its relation to transient radicular irritation. *Can J Anaesth.* 1999;46: 846.
235. Freedman JM, Li DK, Drasner K, et al. Transient neurologic symptoms after spinal anesthesia: An epidemiologic study of 1,863 patients [published erratum appears in Anesthesiology 89(6) 1614, 1998]. *Anesthesiology.* 1998;89:633.
236. Sakura S, Sumi M, Sakaguchi Y, et al. The addition of phenylephrine contributes to the development of transient neurologic symptoms after spinal anesthesia with 0.5% tetracaine [see comments]. *Anesthesiology.* 1997;87:771.
237. Pollock JE, Neal JM, Stephenson CA, et al. Prospective study of the incidence of transient radicular irritation in patients undergoing spinal anesthesia [see comments]. *Anesthesiology.* 1996;84:1361.
238. Evron S, Gurstieva V, Ezri T, et al. Transient neurological symptoms after isobaric subarachnoid anesthesia with 2% lidocaine: The impact of needle type. *Anesth Analg.* 2007;105:1494.
239. Gissen A, Datta S, Lambert D. The chloroprocaine controversy: II. Is chloroprocaine neurotoxic? *Regional Anesthesia.* 1984;9:135.
240. Ravindran RS, Turner MS, Muller J. Neurologic effects of subarachnoid administration of 2-chloroprocaine-CE, bupivacaine, and low pH normal saline in dogs. *Anesth Analg.* 1982;61:279.
241. Taniguchi M, Bollen AW, Drasner K. Sodium bisulfite: Scapegoat for chloroprocaine neurotoxicity? *Anesthesiology.* 2004;100:85.
242. Kouri ME, Kopacz DJ. Spinal 2-chloroprocaine: A comparison with lidocaine in volunteers. *Anesth Analg.* 2004;98:75.
243. Smith KN, Kopacz DJ, McDonald SB. Spinal 2-chloroprocaine: A dose-ranging study and the effect of added epinephrine. *Anesth Analg.* 2004;98:81.
244. Warren DT, Kopacz DJ. Spinal 2-chloroprocaine: The effect of added dextrose. *Anesth Analg.* 2004;98:95.
245. Vath JS, Kopacz DJ. Spinal 2-chloroprocaine: The effect of added fentanyl. *Anesth Analg.* 2004;98:89.
246. Hejtmanek M, Pollock J: Chloroprocaine for spinal anesthesia: a retrospective analysis. *Acta Anaesthesiol Scand.* 2011;55:267.
247. Vandermeulen EP, Van Aken H, Vermylen J. Anticoagulants and spinal-epidural anesthesia. *Anesth Analg.* 1994;79:1165.
248. Horlocker TT, Wedel DJ, Rowlingson JC, et al. Regional anesthesia in the patient receiving antithrombotic or thrombolytic therapy: American Society of Regional Anesthesia and Pain Medicine Evidence-based Guidelines (third edition). *Reg Anesth Pain Med.* 2010;35:64.
249. Hebl JR, Kopp SL, Schroeder DR, et al. Neurologic complications after neuraxial anesthesia or analgesia in patients with preexisting peripheral sensorimotor neuropathy or diabetic polyneuropathy. *Anesth Analg.* 2006;103:1294.

SECTION VII

Anesthesia for Surgical Subspecialties

CHAPTER

35 Peripheral Nerve Blockade

BAN C.H. TSUI • RICHARD W. ROSENQUIST

Key Points

1. Peripheral nerve blocks provide effective anesthesia and analgesia in a site-specific manner with the potential for long-lasting effects.
2. Accurate identification of target nerves and precise and adequate placement of local anesthetic are critical for performing safe and successful peripheral nerve blocks.
3. Ultrasound imaging has renewed interest in peripheral nerve blocks because it allows visualization of needle movement toward nerve structure(s) in real time, minimizing the risk of needle contact with critical structures and potentially reducing complications. Although highly desirable as an aid to the performance of regional anesthesia, this technology requires considerable training and thorough knowledge of the equipment and cross-sectional regional nerve block anatomy.
4. Peripheral nerve stimulators are useful tools to facilitate nerve blocks, but they do not eliminate the risk of nerve injury. In the adult patient, maintenance of responsiveness may allow reporting of nerve contact or pain during injection.
5. Nerve blocks associated with bony or vascular landmarks are more reliable and easy to perform than those dependent on surface landmarks alone.
6. Larger volumes of local anesthetic may increase the potential success of peripheral nerve blocks, but the total milligram dosage must be limited to avoid systemic toxicity. Higher concentrations of local anesthetics increase the degree of motor block. Ultrasound imaging, through more accurate nerve localization and visualization of local anesthetic spread, may enable successful blocks to be performed with reduced volumes of local anesthetics, but this has yet to be proven.

Multimedia

1. Neck Anatomy
2. Brachial Plexus Block
3. Interscalene Block
4. Supraclavicular Block
5. Sensory Innervation of the Hand
6. TAP Block
7. Penile Block
8. Femoral Nerve Block
9. Ultrasound-Guided Saphenous Nerve Block
10. Ultrasound-Guided Popliteal Nerve Block
11. Ankle Block

INTRODUCTION

1 Regional anesthesia enables site-specific, long-lasting, and effective anesthesia and analgesia. It is suitable for many surgical patients and can improve analgesia,[1] reduce morbidity, mortality, and the need for reoperation after major surgical procedures.[2] Peripheral nerve blocks (PNB) can be used alone as the sole "surgical" anesthetic; as a supplement to provide analgesia and muscle relaxation together with general anesthesia; or as the initial step in providing prolonged postoperative analgesia, as with brachial plexus blocks or continuous peripheral nerve catheters. Compared to parenteral analgesics, single-shot or continuous PNB can provide superior analgesia and reduce the incidence of side effects.[3–5] Optimal pain relief and minimal side effects (e.g., nausea and vomiting) following surgery have a major impact on patient outcome, including patient satisfaction and earlier mobilization, as well as fulfilling the need for streamlined surgical services with lower costs.[6] Nevertheless, the safety and success of
2 PNB techniques are highly dependent on accurate delivery of the correct dose of local anesthetic; even in experienced hands, there is an inherent failure rate associated with regional anesthesia[7] with the potential—albeit rare—for systemic toxicity, infection, bleeding, permanent nerve injury, or other physical injury. In addition to the benefits of PNB, advances in knowledge (e.g., physiologic characteristics of solutions during electrical nerve stimulation) and technology (e.g., the introduction of anatomically based ultrasound imaging) have encouraged many anesthesiologists and surgeons to use PNB on a more frequent basis.

Advancements in medical knowledge and techniques are constantly being made and, while new advancements provide an opportunity for improved patient care, they need to be studied and compared to currently accepted techniques to evaluate their safety and utility. In contrast, anatomic structures are static, and an understanding of basic anatomy cannot be replaced by excellent technical skills and knowledge of the technique when performing regional anesthesia. Thus, this chapter provides an in-depth discussion of regional anatomy, while providing an overview of today's two most up-to-date techniques for nerve localization and block performance: Nerve stimulation (NS) and ultrasound (US) imaging. Specific techniques that are practically useful for the anesthesiologist are described in sections grouped by body location.

GENERAL PRINCIPLES AND EQUIPMENT

Regional anesthesia has long been regarded as an "art" and real success with these techniques was confined to a small number of gifted individuals. The introduction of NS some 30 years ago was the first step toward transforming regional anesthesia into a "science." This technique relies on physiologic responses of neural structures to electrical impulses. There is considerable interindividual variation in physiologic responses to NS. Furthermore, several other factors influence responses to NS, including injectates, physiologic solutions (e.g., blood), and disease. Despite these limitations, NS was one of the first objective methods available in regional anesthesia to place a needle in close proximity to a target nerve with some reliabil-
3 ity. One of the most exciting recent advances in regional anesthesia technology has been the introduction of anatomically based US imaging. This is the first time since the beginning of regional anesthesia practice that the target nerve can actually be visualized. This is a quantum leap in technology for those interested in this pursuit, and the realization of its potential benefits may encourage many anesthesiologists who had previously abandoned these techniques to resume or increase their use of regional anesthesia. However, despite initial excitement over this advancement, US images are subject to individual interpretation depending on experience, training, and where that experience and training was obtained. There is a substantial learning curve associated with US-guided regional anesthesia, and not all practitioners are skilled in interpreting US images. Consequently, in many situations, it is prudent to combine the two technologies of NS and US imaging together in order to achieve the goal of 100% success with all regional blocks. US alone may allow good visualization of the needle and nerve as well as a reasonable estimate of the spread of the full dose of the local anesthetic, yet the correct identity of the nerve may be unknown, especially for novice ultrasonographers.[8] By stimulating the nerve, its identity may be objectively determined by observing the motor response to NS.

Patient monitoring and other factors related to optimizing patient care and prevention of complications are similar to those for general anesthesia, with some important differences. Safe and successful performance of PNB requires careful selection of patients and administration of an appropriate type and dose of local anesthetic in the correct location. In addition, the patient must be monitored during the procedure and prior to discharge, and ambulatory patients with home going catheters should be monitored remotely with either telephone follow-up or home health care team visits until the catheter has been removed and the block has completely regressed.

Setup and Monitoring

Setup

Although regional blocks can be performed in the operating room setting just like general anesthesia, it is preferable and desirable to perform these techniques in a designated room or area outside the immediate operating room environment (Fig. 35-1). This is a consequence of what is commonly referred to as "soak time," which is the time it takes for local anesthetics to cross the cell membrane, block action potentials, and produce either analgesia or surgical anesthesia. The designated area must contain the necessary equipment for safe monitoring and resuscitation but must also contain all of the supplies and equipment to perform common and sophisticated regional block techniques. Some important considerations for this "block room" are described below:

- All supplies located in this area must be readily identifiable and accessible to the anesthesiologist.
- The area should be of ample size to allow block performance, monitoring, and resuscitation of patients.
- There should be equipment for oxygen delivery, emergency airway management and suction, and the area should have sufficient lighting.
- A practically organized equipment storage cart (Fig. 35-1) is desirable and should contain all of the necessary equipment (including that required for emergency procedures), supplies, local anesthetics, needles, nerve stimulators, block trays, dressings, and resuscitation drugs. A US machine should also be present.
- It is ideal to have a prepared specialty tray that includes items for sterile skin preparation and draping, a marking pen and ruler for landmark identification, needles and syringes for skin infiltration, and specific block needles and catheters.
- A selection of sedatives, hypnotics, and intravenous anesthetics should be immediately available to prepare patients for regional anesthesia. These drugs should be titrated to maximize benefits and minimize adverse effects (high therapeutic index); short-acting drugs with a high safety margin are desirable.

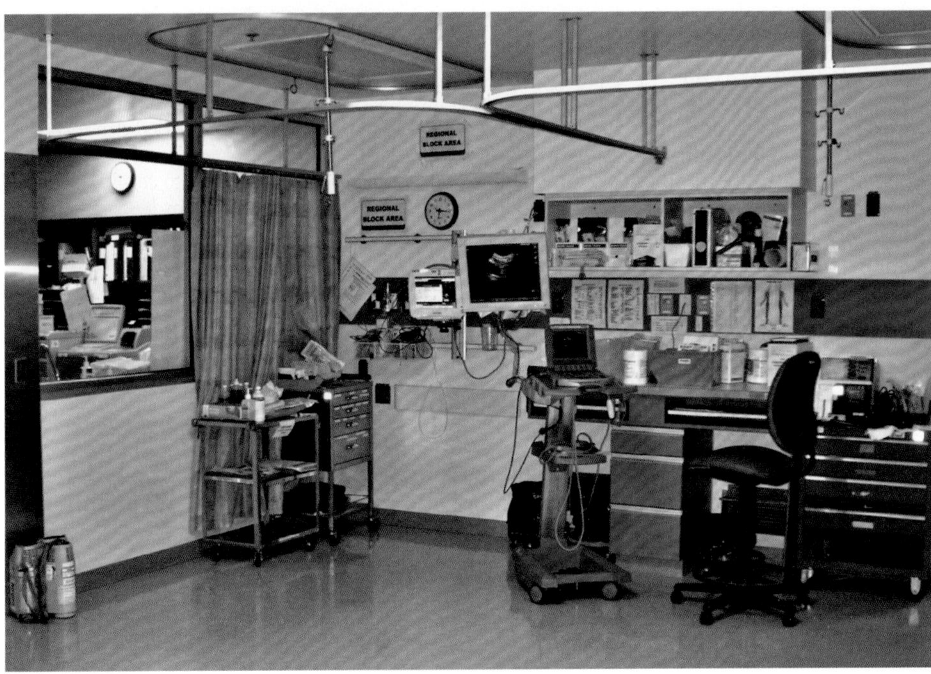

FIGURE 35-1. Designated regional block room with labeled storage cart.

- Emergency drugs should include atropine, epinephrine, phenylephrine, ephedrine, propofol, midazolam, succinylcholine, and intralipid. In addition, guidelines for resuscitation in the setting of local anesthetic toxicity should be laminated and kept with the intralipid.

Monitoring

When performing regional anesthesia, it is vital to have skilled personnel monitor the patient at all times. At minimum, standard monitoring should include electrocardiogram (ECG), noninvasive blood pressure (NIBP), and pulse oximetry. In addition, the patient's level of consciousness should be gauged frequently using verbal contact since vasovagal episodes are common during many regional procedures. At present, there are no practical or effective devices that detect rising blood levels of local anesthetic; however, this can be done indirectly by adding pharmacologic markers, such as epinephrine, in appropriate concentrations to the local anesthetics. Close observation for systemic toxicity secondary to rapid intravenous injection (within 2 minutes) as well as delayed (~20 minutes) absorption is essential. The patient should be monitored for at least 30 minutes following the procedure.

- Standard ECG and pulse oximetry are essential monitors when performing regional anesthesia.
- Careful monitoring of the patient's heart rate (along with ECG measurement) is important to detect tachycardia seen with epinephrine when it is included in a test dose. It is also useful as an indicator of systemic toxicity with bupivacaine and other potent local anesthetics.
- Before performing blocks with significant sympathetic effects, a baseline blood pressure reading should be obtained. Once the regional anesthesia procedure is complete, the monitors should remain attached. In conscious patients, end-tidal carbon dioxide monitoring is not required; however, there are special nasal prongs available for monitoring patients when this is considered necessary.
- At minimum, stable vital signs must be present following regional anesthesia to fulfill discharge criteria from the recovery area. If the block has not begun to regress, appropriate protection for the anesthetized limb and complete instructions should be provided to the patient and their family before discharge. For inpatients, appropriate orders should be written to assure limb protection.
- Patients receiving perineural local anesthetic infusions should be visited regularly by a qualified physician postoperatively (i.e., Acute Pain Service) with ongoing documentation of their condition in the medical record.

Common Techniques: Nerve Stimulation and Ultrasound Imaging

Nerve Stimulation

Basics of Technique and Equipment

Electrical stimulation of nerve structures was introduced to regional anesthesia in the middle of the 20th century.[9,10] A low-current electrical impulse applied to a peripheral nerve produces stimulation of motor fibers and theoretically identifies proximity to the nerve without actual needle contact or related patient discomfort. When NS techniques are used, it is unnecessary to make actual contact with the nerve (in contrast to the paresthesia method). This theoretically infers that the risk of nerve injury should be less when using NS methods, although this theory has not been proven. Stimulating catheters have recently been introduced and have increased our ability to accurately advance catheters over greater distances along nerve structures.[11,12]

4 Using motor responses to NS as a primary nerve localization technique has drawbacks. The main limitations with NS are related to the technique's inconsistent results[13,14] and the variance in electrical properties of different nerve stimulators.[15] Many variables affect the ability to stimulate nerves, including conductive area of the electrode (needle or stimulating catheter tip), electrical impedance of the tissues, electrode-to-nerve distance, current flow, and pulse duration.[16] Ultimately, the technique relies on the physiologic responses of neural structures to the stimulating current, which is subject to considerable interindividual variation.

Today's nerve stimulators have features to improve ease-of-use and success, such as maintaining a constant current with adjustable frequency, pulse width, and current intensity (milliamperes; mA). This enables a stable current output (an important safety feature) in the presence of varied resistances from the needle, tissues, and connectors. A clear digital display indicating the actual current delivery is important, as is regular calibration and testing. Some nerve stimulators are equipped with low (up to 6 mA) and high (up to 80 mA) current output ranges. The lower range is primarily for localizing peripheral nerves, while the higher range is mainly used for monitoring neuromuscular blockade. Recently, higher ranges have been utilized for transcutaneous NS techniques[17] (2 to 5 mA) including percutaneous electrode guidance[18] and surface nerve mapping,[11,19] and the epidural stimulation test (1 to 10 mA).[20,21] Most nerve stimulators deliver an electrical pulse width of 100 or 200 μs for stimulating motor nerves. Similar to current amplitude, the length of time over which the current is delivered (pulse width) is usually considered important, as shorter duration currents can selectively stimulate motor components of mixed nerves while sparing the discomfort caused by stimulation of sensory components. Some sophisticated devices allow variable pulse widths from 50 μs to 1 ms in an attempt to provide such selective stimulation. The general rule is to use short-duration current of ≤100 μs for peripheral NS, although there is some evidence that duration does not impact patient discomfort[22] and that intensity (mA) of the stimulation is perhaps the most important variable.[23]

Practical Guidelines

During initial advancement of the needle, the nerve stimulator should be set to deliver a current of 1 to 2 mA in order to gauge the approximate distance to the nerve. Depolarization of the nerve can also be improved by using the positive (anode; red) pole of the stimulator as the ground (reference or surface electrode) electrode and the negative (cathode; black) lead as the connection to the needle itself (known as cathodal preference). The actual location of the ground is of little importance with the use of constant-current nerve stimulators.[23] Generally, the needle is in close proximity to the nerve when the threshold for motor response is between 0.3 and 0.5 mA; placing the needle to the point where a motor response only requires 0.1 to 0.2 mA may increase the chance of intraneural injection and should be avoided.[24] Once a low threshold response is obtained, 2 to 3 mL of local anesthetic is injected and the operator watches for disappearance of the motor twitch, which is a signal to inject the remainder of the proposed dose in divided aliquots. This "Raj test"[25] was originally thought to result from physical displacement of the targeted nerve by the injectate, but this response has recently also been attributed to a change in the electrical field at the needle-tissue interface. Electrically conducting solutions (e.g., local anesthetic or saline) reduce the current density at the needle tip, thereby increasing the current threshold for motor response, whereas nonconducting solutions (e.g., dextrose 5% in water; D5W) increase the current density and maintain or augment the twitch response (Fig. 35-2).[26]

After nerve localization using a stimulating needle, introduction of a stimulating catheter with continuous stimulation of the nerve is suitable to provide continuous analgesia. Similar current thresholds are applicable with the use of stimulating catheters. If an attempt to dilate the perineural space is undertaken, injection of D5W is preferable in order to maintain the motor response to stimulation.[27] The reader is referred to the section on Other Related Equipment for optimal features of stimulating catheters.

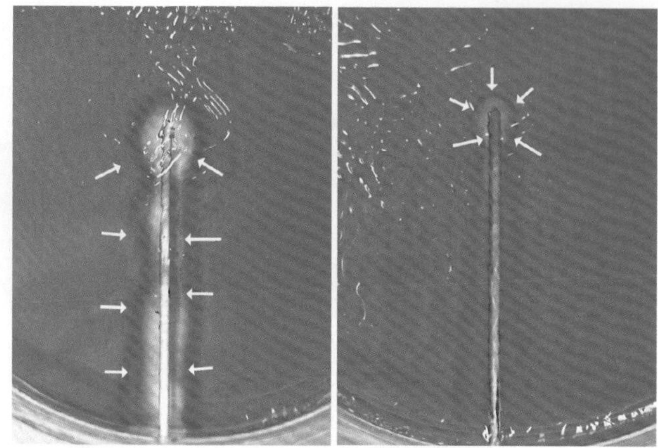

FIGURE 35-2. The current density is localized to the needle tip when using nonconducting solutions (e.g., D5W), thereby maintaining the motor response to the threshold current level during nerve stimulation.

Ultrasound Imaging

Basics of Technique and Equipment

US imaging is rapidly emerging as a very promising regional anesthesia tool since the size, depth and precise location of many nerves in their surrounding environment can be determined with correct interpretation of the visual image. Visualization of the moving needle, once inserted at an appropriate angle and within the plane of the US probe, as well as the spread of local anesthetic, provides valuable assistance to the anesthesiologist performing regional anesthesia. With US-guided PNB techniques, the operator can adjust needle or catheter placement under direct vision (i.e., US imaging), which may lead to fewer needle attempts and ultimately improved motor and sensory blocks. Furthermore, visibility of vital structures (e.g., blood vessels and pleura) is advantageous in order to avoid complications. Today, technologic advances have led to the development of US systems that can deliver high frequency (10 MHz or higher) sound waves offering the high axial resolution required for visualization of nerves and the ability to distinguish them from the surrounding anatomical structures (e.g., tendons, muscles). The proposed benefits of US guidance, as compared to NS, for upper extremity blocks include improved block success[28] and completeness,[29] reduced block performance and onset times,[28–31] prolonged duration of blocks,[30] and reduction in complications.[32] While the cumulative evidence may appear convincing, many of the studies show conflicting results for certain parameters, and the large variability in trial methodologies and application of different outcome measures account for many of the discrepancies. Indeed, the various endpoints used during research in regional anesthesia may bias outcomes when comparing multiple regional techniques. Recently, Marhofer et al.[33,34] published an excellent review of the current status of US and its use in regional anesthesia. They emphasize that adequate training in US-guided techniques is essential and suggest that education and proper technique can help ensure safe blocks. In addition, current advantages of using US in regional anesthesia, including direct visualization of subcutaneous structures, identification of anatomic variation, ability to use less local anesthetic, and improvement in block quality and patient satisfaction, are also discussed.

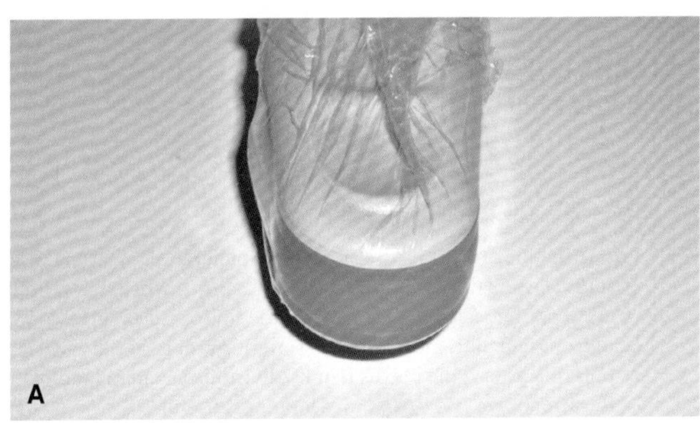

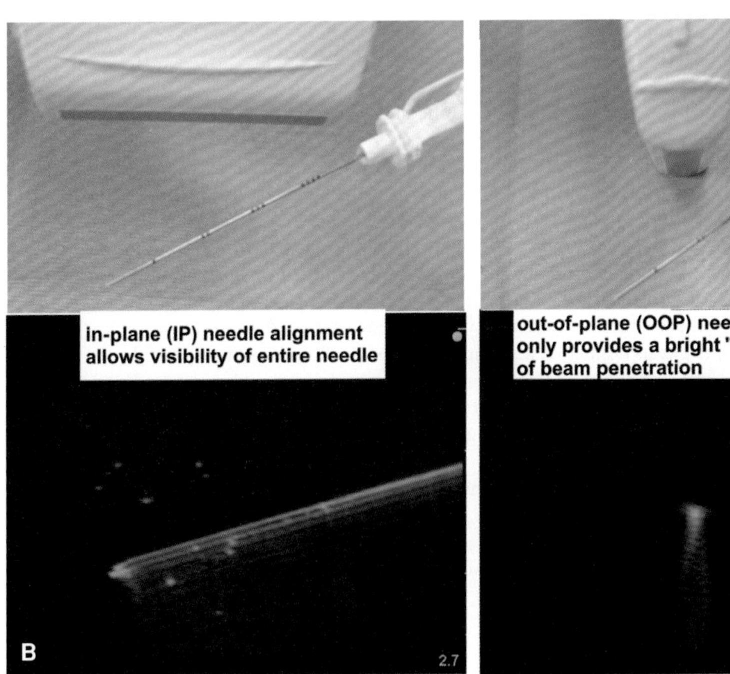

FIGURE 35-3. A: Probe sterility using a sterile transparent dressing (e.g., Tegaderm; 3M Health Care, St Paul, MN) without the full cover of a sterile sleeve. Other dressings may create multiple small wells over the probe surface due to adhesive pockets and lead to poor image quality.[36] **B:** In-plane and out-of-plane needle alignment and subsequent visibility of the needle.

US is defined as any sound with a frequency >20 kHz, although medical imaging generally requires between 3 and 15 MHz. Within the body, US scanners emit sound waves that produce an echo when they encounter a tissue interface. Therefore, US images reflect contours, including those of anatomic structures, based on differing acoustic impedances of tissue or fluids. Significant reflection of sound waves occurs at interfaces between substances of different acoustic impedance, resulting in good contour definition between different tissues. High US beam reflection, from high impedance/dense structures (e.g., bone, connective tissue), results in a bright (hyperechoic) image, often with dorsal shadowing underneath; low impedance structures reflect beams to a smaller extent and appear gray (hypoechoic); minimal impedance structures/spaces (e.g., fluid in vessels) appear black (anechoic).

Higher frequencies offer the best spatial resolution at superficial locations (e.g., brachial plexus at supraclavicular fossa), while lower frequencies are often required for structure delineation at deep locations (e.g., sciatic nerve in the subgluteal region). Block location and depth of target nerve structures determine which transducer offers the best imaging and resolution. Several functions of the US system are important to have familiarity with, including field and gain functions as well as Doppler effect. Doppler effect is very useful for identifying blood vessels during nerve localization using US guidance, since many nerves are situated in close proximity to vascular structures.

Practical Guidelines

Both the probe and the skin of the patient should be prepared for maximum sterility and optimal imaging. Probe sterility is paramount if performing real-time, or dynamic, US guidance during block performance. This can be maintained by standard sleeve covers but these can be expensive and cumbersome. For single-shot blocks, it is practical to use a sterile transparent dressing (e.g., Tegaderm; 3M Health Care, St Paul, MN) without the full cover of a sterile sleeve (Fig. 35-3A).[35] An issue when using standard long covers is the potential for air to track between the probe and the skin, which reduces image quality. The target area should be surveyed (scanned) using a generous amount of US gel (water soluble conductivity gel is optimal) prior to sterile preparation. One of the most common reasons for poor visualization is lack of sufficient gel for skin-probe contact.

5 For nerve localization during US-guided PNB, it is helpful to first identify one or more reliable anatomical landmarks (bone or vessel) with a known relationship to the nerve structure. The operator can then localize the nerve at a location near the landmark, and

TABLE 35-1. USEFUL ANATOMICAL LANDMARKS FOR LOCALIZING NERVES DURING COMMON ULTRASOUND-GUIDED PERIPHERAL NERVE BLOCKS

Peripheral Nerve Block Location	Anatomical Landmark(s)	Approach for Ultrasound Imaging
Interscalene	Subclavian artery and scalene muscles	Locate the plexus trunks/divisions superolateral to the artery at the supraclavicular fossa, and trace proximally to where the roots/trunks lie between the scalenus anterior and medius muscles (Fig. 35-18).
Supraclavicular	Subclavian artery	Scan from lateral to medial on the superior aspect of the clavicle to locate the pulsatile artery; the plexus trunks/divisions lie lateral and often superior to the artery (Fig. 35-19). Color Doppler is useful.
Infraclavicular	Subclavian/axillary artery and vein	Place the artery at the center of the field and locate the brachial plexus cords surrounding the artery (Fig. 35-20).
Axillary	Axillary artery	The terminal nerves surround the artery (Fig. 35-21).
Peripheral nerves		
Median nerve at antecubital fossa	Brachial artery	The large anechoic artery lies immediately lateral to the nerve (Fig. 35-24).
Radial nerve at anterior elbow	Humerus at spiral groove and deep brachial artery	To confirm the nerve's identity at the elbow, trace the nerve proximally and posteriorly toward the spiral groove of the humerus, just inferior to the deltoid muscle insertion. The nerve is located here adjacent to the deep brachial artery and can be followed back to the anterior elbow. (Fig. 35-22)
Ulnar at medial forearm	Ulnar artery	Scan at the anteromedial surface of the forearm approximately at the junction of its distal third and proximal two-thirds, to capture the ulnar nerve as it approaches the ulnar artery on its medial aspect (Fig. 35-25).
Lumbar plexus	Transverse processes	The plexus lies between and just deep to the lateral aspect (tips) of the processes (Fig. 35-33).
Femoral	Femoral artery	The nerve lies lateral to the artery (vein most medial) (Fig. 35-35). Insert the needle above the branching of the deep femoral artery.
Sciatic		
Classical/Labat	Ischial bone and inferior gluteal or pudendal vessels	The nerve lies lateral to the thinnest aspect of the ischial bone. The inferior gluteal artery generally lies medial to and at the same depth as the nerve (Fig. 35-39).
Subgluteal	Greater trochanter and ischial tuberosity	The nerve lies between the two bone structures (Fig. 35-40).
Popliteal	Popliteal artery	Trace the tibial and common peroneal nerves from the popliteal crease to where they form the sciatic nerve. At the crease, the tibial nerve lies adjacent to the popliteal artery. Scanning proximally to the sciatic bifurcation, the artery becomes deeper and at a greater distance from the nerve (Fig. 35-41).
Ankle		
Tibial (posterior tibial)	Posterior tibial artery	Nerve lies posterior to the artery (Fig. 35-43).
Deep peroneal	Anterior tibial artery	Nerve lies lateral to the artery (Fig. 35-44).

proceed to follow along, or "trace" the nerve to the optimal block location (Table 35-1).[36,37] Generally, nerve structures are most visible when the angle of incidence is approximately 90 degrees to the US beam. Obtaining a transverse axis view of the nerve usually allows the best appreciation of the anatomical relationship of the nerve with its surrounding structures. To obtain the best possible view of the shaft and tip of the needle, it is imperative to align the needle shaft to the longitudinal axis ("in-plane"; IP) of the US transducer (probe) (Fig. 35-3B). The nerve structure is often placed at the edge of the US screen to ensure adequate viewing distance for the needle shaft. An alternative approach uses a transverse or tangential ("out-of-plane"; OOP) alignment, which only allows appreciation of the needle in cross section and usually only during movement (Fig. 35-3B). The nerve structure is often placed in the center of the screen to guarantee that aligning the needle puncture with the center of the probe will ensure close needle tip-nerve alignment. This approach can be beneficial in certain block locations (compact areas) and for inserting catheters (e.g., at the subgluteal area), but should never be used in areas where needle tip visibility in relation to vital structures is critical (e.g., supraclavicular fossa near the pleura).

After the needle is seen to be close to the nerve(s), a 1- to 2-mL test dose of local anesthetic or D5W can be injected to visualize the spread and perform a "Raj test" if a stimulating needle is being used. The solution will be seen as a hypoechoic expansion and will often illuminate the surrounding area, enabling better visibility of the nerves and block needle. If NS is being used to confirm nerve identity, it is useful to administer D5W in order to maintain accurate motor responses.[27] This will be especially important during catheter introduction and advancement. If the test shows undesired injection near or within vessels or cavities, subsequent injection of local anesthetic should be postponed until better needle localization is achieved. If suboptimal spread of injectate is observed, the needle can be repositioned to allow another injection.

There can be a lengthy learning curve for US-guided nerve blocks, and techniques to improve needle and catheter visibility during advancement are important in order to improve training for this technology. Two such approaches have been described experimentally:

The "walk-down" approach to facilitate needle tip identification during OOP needling.[37,38] This technique involves calculating the required depth of puncture (with measurement to the desired neural structure recorded using US prior to the block) and using trigonometry with the shaft angle and length to calculate a "reasonable" location to place the initial needle puncture site. The initial shallow puncture will be easily seen as a bright dot on the screen, and the needle tip can be followed as it is "walked down" to the final calculated depth. For example, if the final depth of penetration for the block is 2 cm, the needle will ultimately obtain a 45-degree angle if the initial puncture site is 2 cm from the probe and the needle is incrementally angled to this level.

A method of needle-probe alignment using a laser attachment for the probe has been reported; the laser line will project onto both the needle shaft and the midline of the probe, indicating an IP position.[37,39] Aligning the visible optical laser line with the longitudinal axis of the US probe will mimic the "invisible" beam from the US probe and allow improvements with IP needle alignment. With the laser-unit attachment, any misalignment of the needle to the US beam can be easily detected and adjusted in real-time. Recently, commercially available GPS guidance systems intended to guide the needle tip location have been developed, but the merit of these devices remains to be determined.

Other Related Equipment

Needles

Needles used for regional techniques are often modified from standard injection needles. Although reports may speculate that needle design is a determinant of nerve or other tissue injury, there is insufficient evidence to fully substantiate this claim. For PNB, the "short bevel" (i.e., 30 to 45 degrees) or "B bevel" is often used to reduce the potential for injury to nerves.[40] Other modifications, such as the "pencil-point" needle, have been introduced in attempts to reduce nerve injury. Single-shot PNB techniques generally require using 22- to 24-gauge insulated needles with short bevels. If superficial and field blocks are performed, smaller gauge (e.g., 25 to 26 gauge) sharp needles can be utilized. Continuous blocks require larger-bore needles to facilitate catheter introduction (e.g., 18-gauge needles for 20-gauge catheters). Blunt-tipped Tuohy needles are commonly used for continuous PNB with success.[41] Short-bevel and Tuohy needles offer more resistance and give a better "feel" when traversing different tissues. Desired needle length will depend on each specific block and individual patient characteristics. Clear markings throughout the entire length of the needle are important for measuring depth of penetration, particularly for correspondence to US measurements.

Practical Tips

Techniques and devices have been proposed to limit injection pressure, since there is considerable variation among anesthesiologists in the amount of pressure they apply during injections[42] and high-pressure injections into the nerve (especially intrafascicular) have been associated with damage in animals.[43,44] Disposable, in-line injection pressure monitors are available, although their ability to prevent long-term injury is not well documented. Alternatively, a compressed air injection technique (CAIT) has been described to limit the generation of excessive pressure during injection. With this method, air is drawn into the syringe and compressed by 50% during the entire injection to maintain pressures of approximately 760 mm Hg (Boyle's law: Pressure × volume = constant).[45]

Catheters

Continuous-infusion catheter kits suitable for PNB are available that include a standard polyamide catheter, such as those previously used for epidural analgesia, combined with an insulated Tuohy needle with NS capability. Recently, catheters have been advanced to the point of making them amenable to stimulation (an electrode is placed into the catheter tip). This may enable more accurate advancement of catheters for substantial distances to provide continuous analgesia. Some studies have suggested that it may be helpful to inject a solution to dilate the perineural compartment to facilitate the advancement of catheter. The reader is referred to the discussion of practical guidelines of NS in the section Common Techniques: Nerve Stimulation and Ultrasound Imaging for discussion of injection solutions for perineural dilation. There are a number of continuous-infusion devices now available for both inpatient and outpatient use, which allow delivery of dilute local anesthetic concentrations for as long as 72 hours after surgery. Standard precautions are required to maintain sterility of the catheter and the insertion site, but complications have been rare with these techniques and new devices.

Avoiding Complications

In general, regional anesthesia has an excellent safety record. Complication rates are as low as 8 per 10,000 for seizures[2] and <0.1% to 1% for nerve injury,[7,46] and only rare cases of severe chronic pain syndromes following regional anesthesia have been reported.[47] Nevertheless, the incidence of some complications is often higher in PNB than other regional anesthesia/analgesia techniques, and results can be devastating. Choosing a suitable patient and applying the right dose of local anesthetic in the correct location are the primary considerations. Careful attention to any unusual responses or report of pain during block performance as well as follow-up prior to and after discharge is equally important, although often overlooked.

Patient Selection

Patient selection is a critical element for the performance of safe and effective PNB. Not all patients are suitable candidates for PNB. In general, patients scheduled for extremity, thoracic, abdominal, or perineal surgery should be considered potential candidates for peripheral regional anesthetic techniques. Adamant refusal of regional anesthesia by a patient is a contraindication to the procedure.

Other contraindications include local infection, systemic anticoagulation, and severe systemic coagulopathy. In most cases, schizophrenic patients should only receive regional techniques if general anesthesia is also performed. The presence of pre-existing neurologic disease is a controversial topic and, while a limited amount of data is available in the case of spinal anesthesia, the safety of PNB is unclear. One must be cognizant of the potential to compound existing neurologic deficit; therefore, clear documentation of the deficits prior to the procedure and a careful discussion of the potential risks and benefits are critical. For every clinical situation, the use of regional anesthesia must be carefully evaluated as a matter of risk versus benefit. It is imperative to follow applicable national and international guidelines, such as those set by the American Society of Anesthesiologists (ASA) for patient monitoring and those in place for anticoagulated patients, as provided by the American Society of Regional Anesthesia and Pain Medicine (ASRA).

Local Anesthetic Drug Selection, Toxicity, and Doses

This section will provide an overview of drug selection and toxicity during PNB. For a more detailed discussion of the pharmacology and toxicity of local anesthetics, the reader is referred to Chapter 21.

6 Rates of systemic and local toxicity and nerve injury with PNB are generally low, but the use of available methods to reduce inadvertent intravascular and intraneural injections is clearly warranted. It is important to note that lower concentrations of local anesthetic (e.g., 1% to 1.5% lidocaine, 0.125% to 0.5% bupivacaine) compared to those used for epidural anesthesia are appropriate for peripheral nerves. Neural toxicity of these anesthetics appears to be concentration dependent.[48] The use of highly concentrated solutions may be useful to increase motor block, but increases the total milligram dose of local anesthetic. To limit total drug dose, lower concentrations are usually indicated when larger volumes are required to anesthetize poorly localized peripheral nerves or to block a series of nerves. Nevertheless, there is no clinical evidence that prolonged exposure (as with continuous PNB) of nerves to local anesthetic solutions of appropriate concentration predisposes to neurotoxic injury.[49]

Systemic toxicity is most often related to accidental intravascular injection, and rarely to the administration of an excessive quantity of local anesthetic to an appropriate site. The risk of systemic toxic reactions is often related to the drug used. Ropivacaine (generally at 0.5%) is a recent example of a drug introduced into clinical practice in order to reduce central nervous system and cardiovascular toxicity through its physiochemical and stereoselective properties.[50,51] Despite this, there are examples of ropivacaine toxicity during PNB.[52–55] One strategy to potentially reduce the volume and concentration of local anesthetic solution required to produce a successful block is the use of US imaging to more accurately position the needle in close proximity to the nerve and to visualize the spread of solution to ensure adequate exposure.[56,57] Of greatest importance is the ability to avoid intravascular injection. This risk may be reduced when using US, especially if combined with color Doppler for vessel localization.

The degree of systemic drug absorption and the duration of anesthesia can also vary depending on the site of injection (i.e., level of vascularization) and addition of vasoconstrictors. The highest blood levels of local anesthetic occur after intercostal blocks, followed by caudal, epidural, brachial plexus, intravenous regional, and lower extremity blocks. Equivalent doses of local anesthetic may produce only 3 to 4 hours of anesthesia when placed in the epidural space, but 12 to 14 hours in the arm, and 24 to 36 hours when injected along the sciatic nerve. Many believe that the addition of epinephrine (1:200,000 to 1:400,000) is advantageous in prolonging the duration of block and in reducing systemic blood levels of local anesthetic, although this has more relevance to local anesthetics like lidocaine and less to ones like bupivacaine. Its use is not appropriate in the vicinity of "terminal" blood vessels, such as in the digits, penis, or ear or when using an intravenous regional technique. Using significant quantities of local anesthetic during PNB should not be performed unless oxygen, suction, and appropriate resuscitation equipment is immediately available. However, even small doses of local anesthetic may produce significant side effects when injected into susceptible regions such as the neck. When performing PNB, a test dose of an epinephrine-containing solution and small incremental injections are recommended to reduce the risk of unrecognized intravascular injection. Toxicity can also occur from peripheral absorption of excessive doses of local anesthetic. Patients should be observed carefully for at least 30 minutes following injection because peak blood levels may occur at this time.

Animal studies[58] and recent case reports[59,60] have shown successful resuscitation from local anesthetic toxicity by intravenous administration of intralipid (20% lipid; not the 10% lipid of propofol), using one or more boluses (each of 1 to 2 mL/kg or 100 mL) followed by a 30-minute infusion (0.5 mL/kg/min). It is important to use this strategy as an acute resuscitation agent, only after standard measures have proven ineffective.

Nerve Damage and Other Complications

Peripheral nerve injury in humans may result from intraneural injection[61,62] or direct needle trauma,[63] although there are other causes, including those related to the surgical procedures (e.g., patient positioning, proximity of nerve to surgical site, and tourniquet application).[64] Needle-related trauma without injection may result in injury of lesser magnitude than that from injection injury.[65] In animal studies, nerve injury appears to occur when high injection pressures are applied intrafascicularly and particularly when highly concentrated local anesthetic solutions or their preservatives are used.[43,44,66] One major sequela from intrafascicular injection is endoneural ischemia.[67] While in some cases these syndromes resolve uneventfully, full recovery of some peripheral injuries may never occur or may require several months, a result of slow regeneration of injured peripheral nerves.[61]

Other minor complications that have been reported following PNB include pain at the site of injection and local hematoma formation, but these are self-limited side effects and are best dealt with by communication with the patient and reassurance by the anesthesiologist. A hematoma around a peripheral nerve is not of the same significance or risk as that occurring in the epidural or subarachnoid space. It is important to address concerns expressed by patients and to make every effort to relieve any pain or discomfort resulting from various interventions.

Discharge Criteria

Stable vital signs must be present in order to fulfill criteria for discharge from the recovery area. In some cases, acceptable evidence of regressing sensory and motor blocks should be present. However, if a long-lasting local anesthetic was used to perform the block or a continuous catheter with an infusion of local anesthetic is present, the block may not show evidence of regression at the time of discharge. Postoperative follow-up is important to confirm that neurologic function has returned to normal. If a deficit is suspected, early neurologic assessment is critical to determine the appropriate course of management.

Patients should have well-controlled pain upon discharge. Incorporating a standard level of pain relief (e.g., on a verbal rating scale) prior to discharge home or to the ward is prudent. Specific common risks for certain blocks should be discussed with the patient prior to discharge. When discharging patients from postanesthesia care units while an extremity is still anesthetized (e.g., the block was performed to provide extended analgesia), it is absolutely necessary to provide in-depth instruction related to the risks and their prevention (e.g., risk of burns to anesthetized areas will require avoidance of certain forms of cooking; potential for developing pressure neuropathies). A clear understanding of the information provided is important for both the patient and their caregivers. Written instructions including expected course, common side effects, and 24-hour contact information should be provided.

Premedication and Sedation

The best preparation for a regional technique is careful patient selection and ensuring that the patient is adequately educated and informed about the anesthetic and surgical procedures. Supplemental medication is often helpful. Appropriate sedation and analgesia is an essential part of successful regional anesthesia in order to produce maximum benefit with minimal side effects. Effective sedation can be achieved with a variety of medications, including but not limited to propofol, midazolam, fentanyl, ketamine, remifentanil, alfentanil, or a combination of these drugs. The dosages should be titrated to reach an appropriate level of sedation for the individual patient, specific nerve block procedure and length of surgery. Some examples are listed below.

Bolus

- Midazolam 1 to 2 mg (titrated up to 0.07 mg/kg)
- Fentanyl 0.5 to 1 μg/kg
- Alfentanil 7 to 10 μg/kg
- Ketamine 0.1 to 0.5 mg/kg

In addition to the general comments about premedication discussed in earlier chapters, regional anesthesia techniques have special requirements. Sedation must be adjusted to the required level of patient cooperation. In the case of elicitation of a paresthesia (as during several blocks in the head and neck region) or electrical stimulation techniques, the level of sedation must be sufficient to allow the patient to identify and report nerve contact. Although a low dose of opioid (50 to 100 μg of fentanyl or equivalent) will help ease the discomfort of nerve localization, patient responsiveness must be maintained. This does not preclude the use of an amnestic agent; small doses of propofol or midazolam may provide excellent amnesia while maintaining levels of consciousness that still allow cooperation.

CLINICAL ANATOMY

Anatomical descriptions of major nerve structures, including plexuses and terminal/peripheral nerves are discussed in this section. The section is divided on the basis of regions of the body and includes the head and neck, spine, upper extremity, trunk, and lower extremity.

Head and Neck

Trigeminal Nerve

Sensory and motor innervation of the face is provided by the branches of the fifth cranial (trigeminal) nerve. The roots of this nerve arise from the base of the pons and send sensory branches to the large semilunar (trigeminal or Gasserian) ganglion, which lies on the dorsal surface of the petrous bone. Its anterior margin

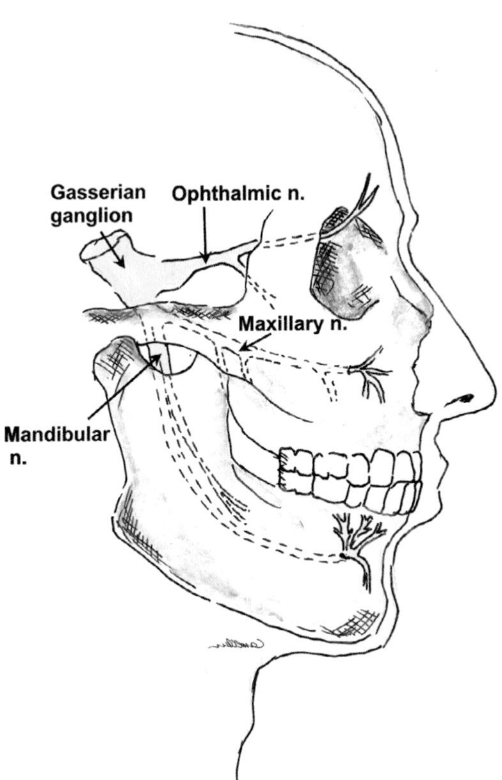

FIGURE 35-4. Major branches of the trigeminal nerve. The roots of this nerve arise from the pons and form the large Gasserian (or semilunar) ganglion. The three major branches have separate exits from the skull. The main terminal fibers of the ophthalmic nerve—the frontal nerve—terminate as the supraorbital and supratrochlear nerves and exit their respective foramen. The maxillary and mandibular branches emerge from the skull medial to the lateral pterygoid plate. The maxillary nerve terminates as the infraorbital nerve (through such named foramen), and the mandibular nerve provides the inferior alveolar nerve (as well as motor branches), which exits at the mental foramen as the mental nerve.

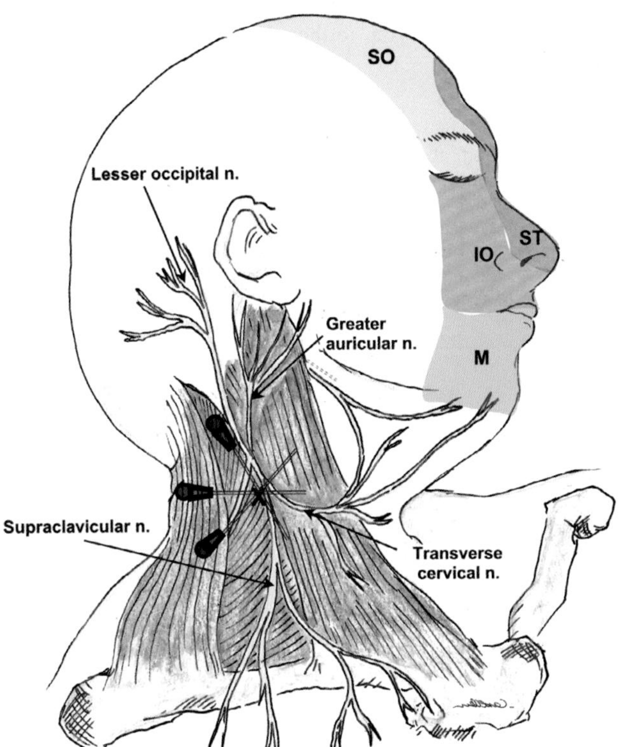

FIGURE 35-5. Lateral view of the surface of the head, showing the cutaneous innervation of the superficial/distal trigeminal nerve branches to the face and the anatomy and block needle insertion angles to perform a superficial cervical plexus block. The needle is initially inserted perpendicular to the skin at the midpoint of the lateral border of the sternocleidomastoid muscle (where it is crossed by the external jugular vein). Subsequently, the needle can be inserted in superior and inferior angulations to reach the entire cervical plexus. SO, supraoribtal nerve; ST, supratrochlear nerve; IO, infraorbital nerve; M, mental nerve.

gives rise to three main branches: The ophthalmic, maxillary, and mandibular nerves (Fig. 35-4). A smaller motor fiber nucleus lies behind the main trigeminal ganglion and sends motor branches to one terminal nerve, the mandibular. The three major branches of the trigeminal nerve each have a separate exit from the skull:

- The uppermost ophthalmic branch passes through the sphenoidal fissure into the orbit. The main terminal fibers of this sensory nerve, the *frontal nerve,* run to behind the center of the orbital cavity and bifurcate into the supratrochlear and supraorbital nerves. The *supratrochlear* branch traverses the orbit along the superior border and exits on the front of the face in the easily palpated supraorbital notch; the *supraorbital nerve* runs in a medial direction toward the trochlea (Fig. 35-5).
- The *maxillary* nerve contains only sensory fibers. It exits the skull through the round foramen (foramen rotundum), passes beneath the skull anteriorly, and enters the sphenopalatine fossa. At this point, it lies medial to the lateral pterygoid plate on each side. At the anterior end of this channel, it again moves superiorly to re-enter the skull in the infraorbital canal in the floor of the orbit. It branches to form the zygomatic nerve, which extends to the orbit, the short sphenopalatine (pterygopalatine) nerves, and the posterior dental branches. The anterior dental nerves arise from the main trunk as it passes through the infraorbital canal. The terminal infraorbital nerve penetrates through the inferior orbital fissure to the base of the orbit, to the infraorbital groove and canal (just below the eye and lateral to the nose), and reaches the facial surface of the maxilla. It then divides into the palpebral (lower eyelid), nasal (wing of the nose), and labial nerves (upper lip).
- The *mandibular* nerve is the third and largest branch of the trigeminal, and the only one to receive motor fibers. It exits the skull posterior to the maxillary nerve through the oval foramen (foramen ovale), forms a short thick trunk, and then divides into an anterior trunk, mainly motor, and a posterior trunk, which is mostly sensory. The main branch (posterior trunk) continues as the inferior alveolar nerve medial to the ramus of the mandible and innervates the molar and premolar teeth. This nerve curves anteriorly to follow the mandible and exits as a terminal branch (mental nerve) through the mental foramen. The *mental* nerve provides sensation to the lower lip and chin. Other terminal nerves include the lingual nerve (floor of mouth and anterior two-thirds of tongue) and the auriculotemporal nerve (ear and temple).

Cervical Plexus

Sensory and motor fibers of the neck and posterior scalp arise from the anterior rami (branches) of the first four cervical (C1–C4) spinal nerves. The cervical plexus is unique in that it divides early into cutaneous branches (penetrating the cervical fascia) (Fig. 35-6) and muscular branches (deeper branches that

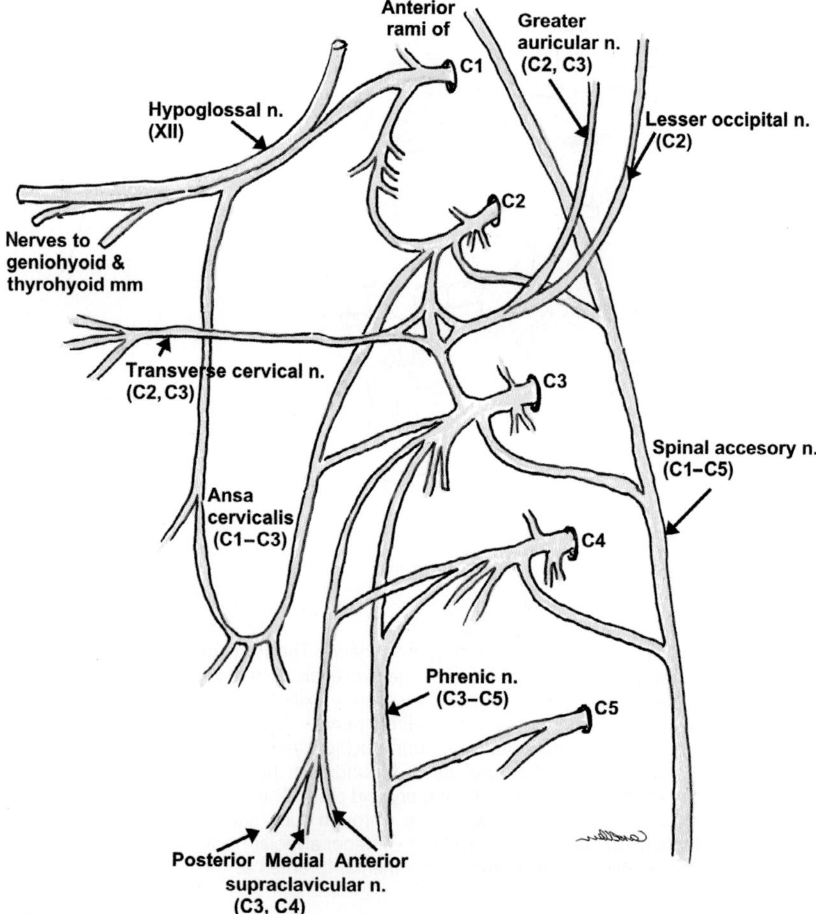

FIGURE 35-6. Schematic of the cervical plexus, which arises from the anterior primary rami of C2–C4. The motor branches (including the phrenic nerve) curl anteriorly around the anterior scalene muscle and travel caudally and medially to supply the deep muscles of the neck. The sensory branches exit at the lateral border of the sternocleidomastoid muscle to supply the skin of the neck and the shoulder.

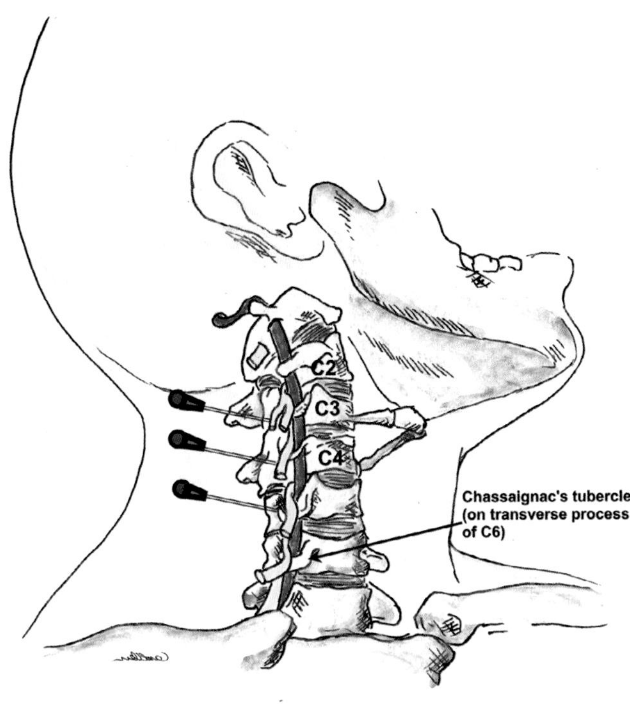

FIGURE 35-7. Needle insertion points and angles for the deep cervical plexus blockade. The nerve roots exit the vertebral column via the troughs formed by the transverse processes. The needle is inserted to make contact with the articular pillars of C2–C4 using a caudad and posterior direction.

innervate the muscles and joints), which can be blocked separately (Fig. 35-7). The dermatomes of the cervical nerves C2–C4 are illustrated in Figure 35-8.

- Classic cervical plexus anesthesia along the tubercles of the vertebral body produces both motor and sensory blockade. The transverse processes of the cervical vertebrae form peculiar elongated troughs for the emergence of their nerve roots. These troughs lie immediately lateral to a medial opening for the cephalad passage of the vertebral artery (Fig. 35-7). The trough at the terminal end of the transverse process divides into an anterior and a posterior tubercle, which can often be easily palpated.
- These tubercles also serve as the attachments for the anterior and middle scalene muscles, which form a compartment for the cervical plexus as well as the brachial plexus immediately below. The compartment at this level is less developed than the one formed around the brachial plexus.
- The deep muscular branches curl anteriorly around the lateral border of the anterior scalene and then proceed caudally and medially. Many branches serve the deep anterior neck muscles, but other branches include the inferior descending cervical nerve, the trapezius branch of the plexus, and the phrenic nerve, which give anterior branches to the sternocleidomastoid muscle as they pass behind it.
- The sensory fibers emerge behind the anterior scalene muscle but separate from the motor branches and continue laterally to emerge superficially under the posterior border of the sternocleidomastoid muscle. The branches, including the lesser occipital nerve, great auricular nerve, transverse cervical nerve, and the supraclavicular nerves (anterior, medial, and posterior branches), innervate the anterior and posterior skin of the neck and shoulder.

Occipital Nerve

The ophthalmic branch of the trigeminal nerve provides sensory innervation to the forehead and anterior scalp; the remainder of the scalp is innervated by fibers of the greater and lesser occipital nerves (Fig. 35-9).

- The *lesser occipital nerve* arises from the superficial (cutaneous) cervical plexus (Fig. 35-6) and traverses cephalad from the posterior edge of the sternocleidomastoid muscle toward the top of the head, dividing into several branches. The *greater occipital nerve* arises from the posterior ramus of the second cervical spinal nerve (the cervical plexus arises from the anterior rami) and travels in a cranial direction to reach the skin in the area of the superior nuchal line while giving branches to supply the head and laterally toward the ear.
- These nerves can be blocked by superficial injection at the point on the posterior skull where they emerge from below the muscles of the neck.

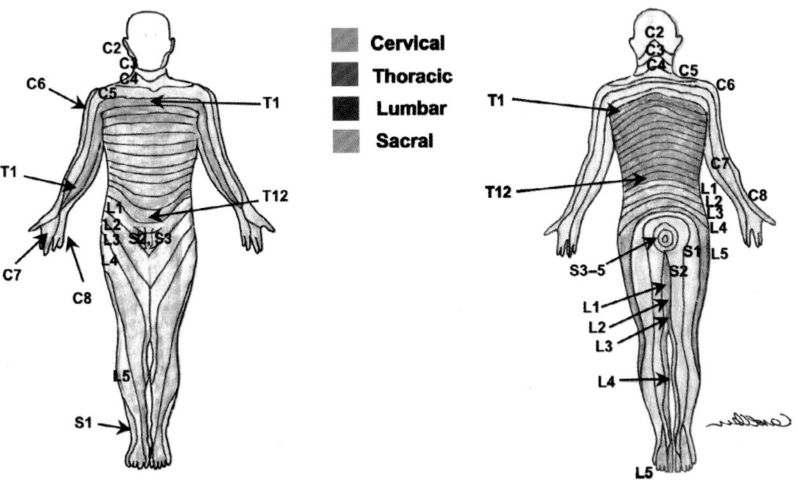

FIGURE 35-8. The cervical, thoracic, lumbar and sacral dermatomes of the body.

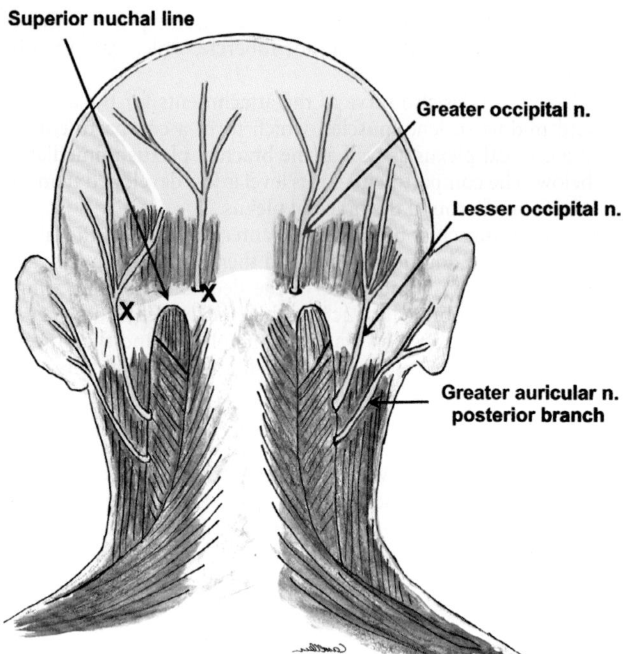

FIGURE 35-9. Greater and lesser occipital nerve distributions, supply, and block needle insertion sites.

Spine

Spinal/epidural anesthesia is not discussed in this chapter, but a basic description of the spinal nerves as well as vertebral structures is provided, given their relevance to the performance of other regional blocks.

Spinal Nerves

The spinal nerves are part of the peripheral nervous system, along with the cranial and autonomic nerves and their ganglia. There are 31 pairs of spinal nerves—8 cervical (C1–C8), 12 thoracic (T1–T12), 5 lumbar (L1–L5), 5 sacral (S1–S5), and 1 coccygeal.

- The spinal nerves are formed by the union of the ventral (anterior) and dorsal (posterior) spinal roots and consist of both motor and sensory fibers. In addition, all spinal nerves contain sympathetic fibers for supplying blood vessels, smooth muscle, and glands in the skin.
- The nerves give off sympathetic branches immediately after leaving the intervertebral foramen. Gray and white rami communicantes connect the spinal nerves to the sympathetic chain ganglia to allow preganglionic sympathetic fibers leaving the spinal cord (T1–L2/L3) to enter the chain and leave it again to be distributed with spinal nerves at all levels.
- Soon after exiting the intervertebral (spinal) foramina, each spinal nerve in turn divides into a larger ventral and a smaller dorsal ramus (branches). The ventral rami course laterally and anteriorly to supply the muscles, subcutaneous tissues (superficial fascia) and skin of the neck, trunk, and the upper and lower extremities (see the dermatomes of the body in Fig. 35-8). The dorsal rami course posteriorly and supply the paravertebral muscles, subcutaneous tissues, and skin of the back close to the midline.
- It is important to realize that the first cervical (C1) nerve leaves the spinal cord and courses above the atlas (C1 vertebra). Hence the cervical nerves are numbered corresponding to the vertebrae inferior to them. From this point on, all the spinal nerves are named corresponding to the vertebral level above. For example, the T3 and L4 spinal nerves exit below the T3 and L4 vertebrae, respectively.

Paravertebral Space

The paravertebral space is a bilateral wedge-shaped area between the individual vertebrae, on either side of and extending the entire length of the vertebral column. The spinal nerves pass through this space, giving off their sympathetic branch and a small dorsal sensory branch before exiting from the intervertebral foramina. In the thoracic region, its boundaries are as follows:

- Medially: The vertebral body, intervertebral disc and foramen, and spinous processes (angulation decreases from T1 to L4/L5);
- Anterolaterally: The parietal pleura; and
- Posteriorly: The costotransverse process, approximately 2.5 cm from the tip of the spinous process, often in a slightly caudad orientation.

The intervertebral foramina at each level lie between the transverse processes and approximately 1 to 2 cm anterior to the plane formed by the transverse processes in their associated fasciae. At this point, the sympathetic ganglia lie close to the somatic nerves, and coincidental sympathetic blockade is usually attained.

Orientation of the Vertebral Body Processes

There are variations in the anatomy of the vertebral column that should be considered when determining the desired location for needle insertion during blocks of the trunk.

- The spinous processes lie in the midline, with T7 at the distal tips of the scapulae and L4 at the level of the iliac crests.
- The transverse processes lie approximately 2.5 cm lateral to the spinous processes: At T1, the transverse process is directly lateral to its corresponding spinous process, but subsequent transverse processes are extended to increasingly cephalad locations (i.e., T7 transverse process is lateral to T6 spinous process).
- In the lumbar region, the spinous processes are straight, and the transverse processes lie opposite their own respective spinous process.

Upper Extremity

Brachial Plexus

The brachial plexus (Fig. 35-10) classically arises from the anterior primary rami of C5–C8 and T1 spinal nerves. The plexus consists of five *roots,* three *trunks,* six *divisions* (two per trunk), three *cords,* and five major terminal nerves.

- The C5–T1 nerve roots emerge from their corresponding intervertebral foramina and then travel along the grooves between the anterior and posterior tubercles of the corresponding transverse process. They finally emerge between the scalenus anterior and medius muscles, above the second part of subclavian artery and posterior to vertebral artery.
- The C5 and C6 nerve roots unite to form the *upper (superior) trunk,* C7 continues as the *middle trunk,* and C8 and T1 converge into the *lower (inferior) trunk.*
- Fibrous sheaths (as part of the prevertebral fascia) surround the anterior and posterior parts of the plexus and continue to

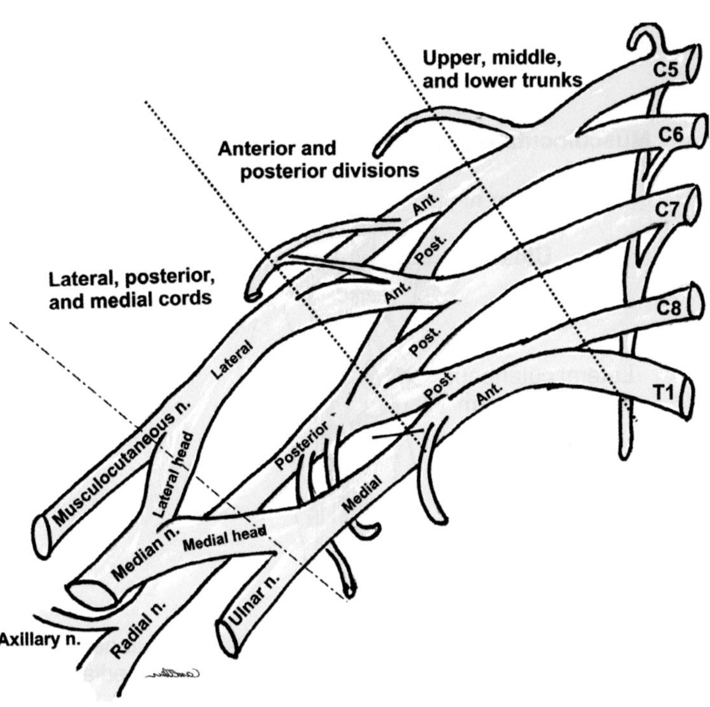

FIGURE 35-10. Schematic of the brachial plexus. Many branches, including the medial cutaneous nerves of the forearm and arm, which arise from the medial cord are not shown here.

envelope the plexus between the scalene muscles more distally (called the *interscalene fascial sheath* proximally and the *axillary sheath* distally).

- The three trunks travel inferolaterally and cross the base of the posterior triangle of the neck (superficial) and the first rib (upper and middle trunks above the subclavian artery and lower trunk behind or below the artery). At the lateral border of first rib, each trunk bifurcates into *anterior* and *posterior* divisions.
- Approximately at the level where the nerves course under the pectoralis minor muscle, the divisions converge to form three *cords: Lateral cord*—anterior divisions of upper and middle trunks (C5–C7); *medial cord*—anterior division of lower trunk (C8, T1); *posterior cord*—posterior divisions of all three trunks (C5–T1).
- The cords are grouped around the second part of the axillary artery (within 2.5 cm from its center).[68] There are three parts of the axillary artery named for their positions above (medial to), behind, and below (lateral to) the pectoralis minor muscle. Typically, with a US probe placed to view the transverse axis of the cords, the medial cord lies inferior, the lateral cord superior, and the posterior cord posterior to the first part of the axillary artery.
- Immediately beyond the pectoralis minor muscle, the three cords diverge into the terminal branches; these include the median, ulnar, radial, axillary, and musculocutaneous nerves.
- The phrenic nerve normally descends anterior to the scalenus anterior muscle and crosses the muscle from lateral to medial as it descends and passes under the clavicle and through the superior thoracic aperture into the superior mediastinum, just medial to the external jugular vein. However, there is anatomic variation of the course of the phrenic nerve and it is not always anterior to the scalenus anterior muscle.

Terminal Nerves of the Brachial Plexus

The anatomy of the peripheral nerves is outlined here, although the clinically related innervation patterns are included in the discussion of each block's technique. Figure 35-11 illustrates the courses of these nerves within the upper extremity. Figure 35-12 illustrates the cutaneous innervation of the terminal nerves of the upper extremity. The axillary nerve is an additional terminal nerve of the upper extremity, but the anatomy and blocking of this nerve will not be discussed here.

Radial Nerve (Originates from C5–C8 and T1 Roots, Upper and Middle Trunks, Posterior Divisions, and Posterior Cord)

- This nerve originates deep (often posteromedial)[69] to the axillary artery, descends within the axilla (giving off branches to long head of the triceps brachii), passes between the medial and lateral heads of the triceps, and then descends obliquely across the posterior aspect of the humerus along the spiral (radial) groove at the level of the deltoid insertion.
- The nerve travels posterior and medial to the deep brachial artery of the arm and reaches the lateral margin of the humerus 5 to 7 cm above the elbow before crossing over the lateral epicondyle and entering the anterior compartment of the arm.
- In front of the elbow, the nerve divides and continues as the superficial radial (sensory) and the deep posterior interosseous (motor) nerves.

Median Nerve (Originates from C5–C8, T1, All Trunks, and Lateral and Medial Cords)

- In the axilla, this nerve often lies anterolateral to the axillary artery.[69,70] The nerve descends along the medial aspect of the arm lateral to the brachial artery and crosses the artery, usually anteriorly, at the midpoint of the arm at the insertion of the coracobrachialis muscle.
- The nerve crosses the elbow lying medially on the brachialis muscle and just medial to the brachial artery and vein (all of these are medial to the biceps brachii tendon).
- Distal to the antecubital fossa, the nerve gives off the anterior interosseous nerve and cutaneous sensory branches.

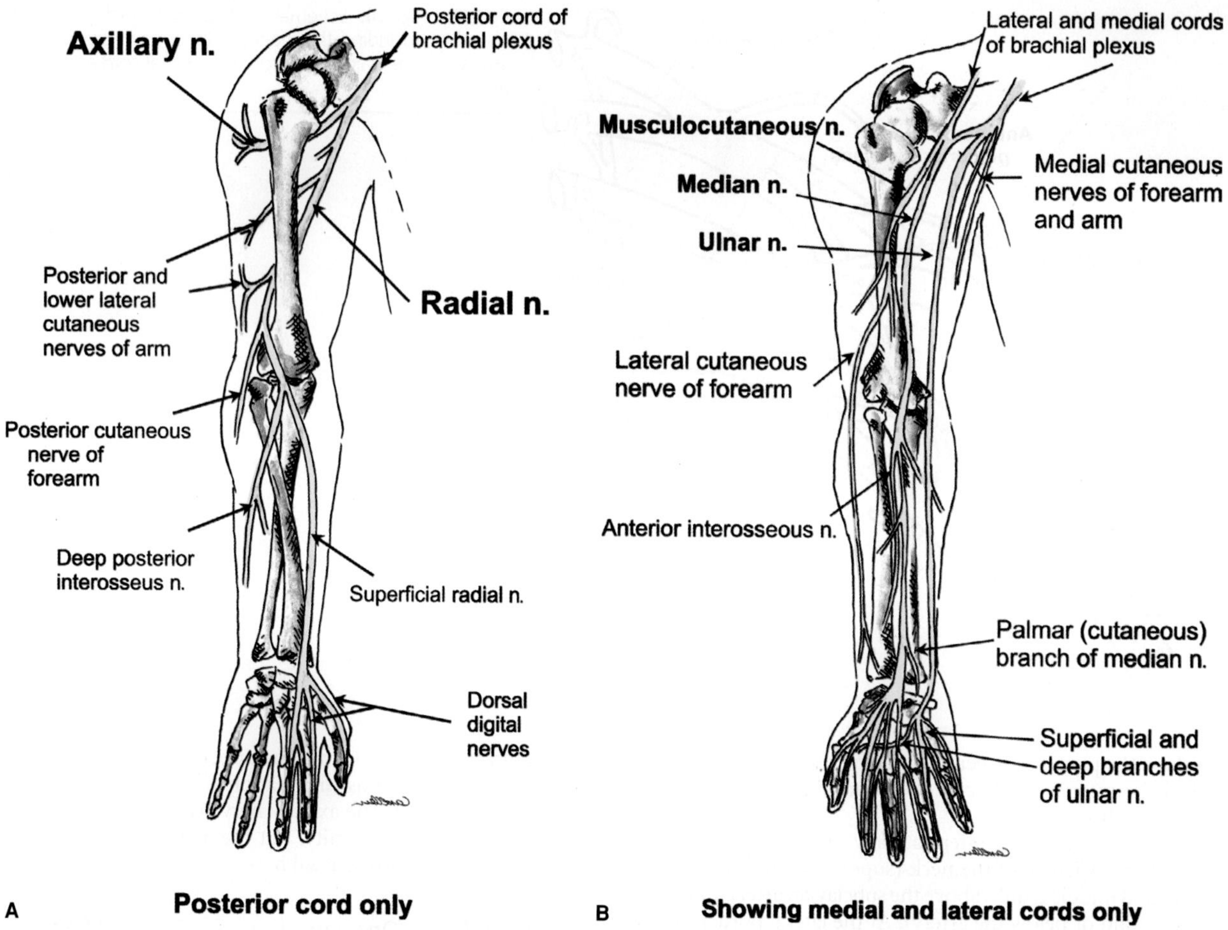

FIGURE 35-11. Courses of the terminal nerves of the upper extremity. The posterior view **(A)** illustrates the branches from the posterior cord (axillary and radial nerves) while the anterior view **(B)** illustrates the branches from the lateral (musculocutaneous and median nerves) and medial (median and ulnar nerves) cords.

Musculocutaneous Nerve (Originates from C5–C7 Roots, Upper and Middle Trunks, Anterior Divisions, Lateral Cord)

- This nerve leaves the fascial sheath of the plexus approximately at the level of the coracoid process; thus, the infraclavicular location for brachial plexus block is the most distal block for this nerve.
- Just distal (2 to 3 cm) to the pectoralis major muscle attachment, the nerve usually pierces the coracobrachialis muscle, after which it exits and comes to lie between the coracobrachialis muscle and the short and long heads of the biceps brachii muscle.

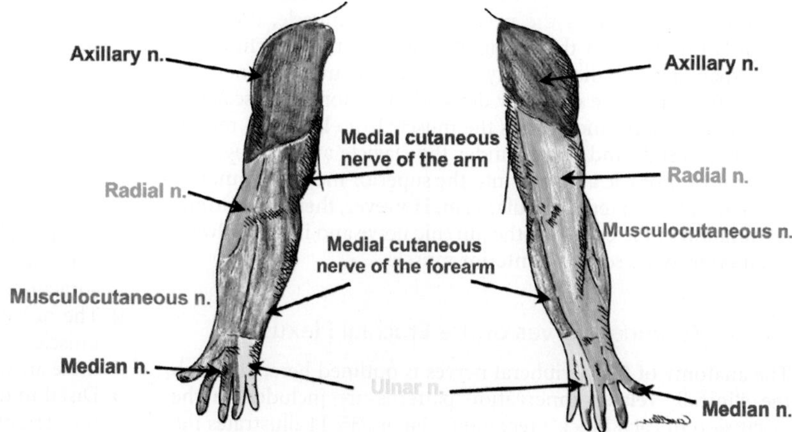

FIGURE 35-12. Cutaneous innervation of the upper extremity nerves.

- Although it is difficult to observe using US, the nerve continues as the lateral cutaneous nerve of the forearm at the antecubital fossa and courses along the lateral aspect of the forearm providing subsequent anterior and posterior branches.

Ulnar Nerve (Originates from C7–C8, T1 Roots, Lower Trunk, Anterior Division, Medial Cord)

- Initially, the nerve often courses between the axillary artery and vein (it may lie anteromedial to the artery and vein) and then along the medial aspect of the brachial artery to the midpoint of the humerus before passing posteriorly and following the anterior surface of the medial head of the triceps.
- The nerve then passes behind the medial epicondyle of the humerus (in the condylar groove), divides between the humeral and ulnar heads of the flexor carpi ulnaris, and lies on the medial aspect of the elbow joint.
- During its descent through the forearm, the nerve courses anteriorly, to approach the ulnar artery directly anterior to the ulna at the junction of the lower third and upper two-thirds of the forearm.
- At the wrist, it crosses superficial to the flexor retinaculum and divides into superficial and deep branches; the ulnar artery lies anterolateral to the nerve at the wrist.

Anatomic Variation

There are many variations in the anatomy of the brachial plexus[71] and in the course of the terminal nerves and vascular elements. Some of these variations may contribute to difficulty when performing PNB, since there may be unexpected NS responses (e.g., if two nerves are conjoined) or poor localization by NS or by US imaging (e.g., if the nerve follows a substantially different path). Some examples are described below:

- The plexus may include anterior rami from C4 to C8 ("prefixed") or, less commonly, from C5 to T2 ("postfixed").
- The existence and/or characteristics of the connective tissue sheath that invests the plexus at various regions are controversial. A continuous, tubular sheath has been shown unlikely, especially in the axillary region. A more convoluted and septated structure may be the cause of nonuniform distribution of local anesthetic in many cases, which supports the findings that multiple injection techniques may be superior.[72] US guidance can be valuable in this location to ensure circumferential spread of local anesthetic around the nerves.
- The interscalene groove may have variation in the relationship between the plexus roots and trunks and the muscles. For example, the C5 and/or C6 nerve roots may traverse either through or anterior to the anterior scalene muscle.[73]
- In many cadaver specimens, no inferior trunk exists.[74] A single cord or a pair of cords may develop. It has been observed that no discrete posterior cord forms in some cases, with the posterior divisions diverging to form terminal nerves.[71]
- The terminal nerves may lie in various relations to the axillary vessels. The use of combined NS- and US-guided technique to both confirm the nerve localization (NS) and obtain circumferential spread of local anesthetic around each of the nerves (US) may improve block success.[8] The musculocutaneous nerve may fuse to or have communications with the median nerve, which can result in the absence of the former from within the coracobrachialis muscle.[75,76] Communication between the median and ulnar nerves in the forearm are common, with the median nerve replacing the innervation to various muscles normally supplied by the ulnar nerve.[77]
- There may also be variations with respect to the vessels within the arm, with aberrant formations including double axillary veins, high origin of the radial artery, and double brachial arteries.[78–80]

Trunk

Intercostal Nerves and Articulations

Intercostal Nerves

- At the thoracic level, each anterior primary ramus enters a neurovascular bundle with its respective artery and vein and travels along the intercostal groove on the ventral caudad surface of each rib.
- The fasciae of the internal and external intercostal muscles provide interior and external borders of the intercostal groove.
- As the intercostal nerves travel beyond the midaxillary line, they give off a lateral sensory branch, while the main trunk continues on to the anterior abdominal wall to provide sensory and motor innervation for the trunk and abdomen down to the level of the pubis.
- The intercostal groove becomes much less well defined anterior to the midaxillary line, and the nerves begin to move away from their protected position. The lowermost intercostal nerve (subcostal; the 12th) is much less proximal to its accompanying rib and is not as easy to identify and anesthetize using a classic intercostal blockade technique.

Costovertebral Articulations

- The ribs articulate through two synovial joints with the vertebral column, each enclosed in fibrous capsules that are reinforced by ligaments:
  - *Costovertebral joint* is a synovial articulation of the head of the rib with the demi-facets on the adjacent thoracic vertebral bodies and the corresponding intervertebral disc of the upper vertebral joint (except for 1st, 10th, 11th, and 12th ribs, which articulate with a single vertebral facet).
  - *Costotransverse joint* is a synovial joint between the articular facets on the tubercles of the ribs and the transverse processes of the thoracic vertebrae (the 11th and 12th ribs lack this articulation since they do not possess tubercles). Penetration of the costotransverse ligament may occur during paravertebral block.

Lumbar Spinal Nerves and Plexus

The spinal nerves at the lumbar level follow the same course as those of the thoracic level when leaving the intervertebral foramen, yet the anterior (ventral) rami form the lumbar plexus instead of continuing as intercostal nerves. The lumbar plexus (Fig. 35-13) is formed by the union of the anterior primary rami of L1–L3 and part of L4.

- The upper nerve roots emerge from their foramina into a compartment lined by the fasciae of muscles anterior and posterior to it. In this case, the quadratus lumborum is posterior, while the posterior fascia of the psoas muscle provides the anterior border of the compartment before the nerves move into the body of the muscle.
- The lumbar plexus supplies the skin and muscles of the lower part of the anterior abdominal wall (including the external genitalia) and the skin and muscles of the anterior and medial

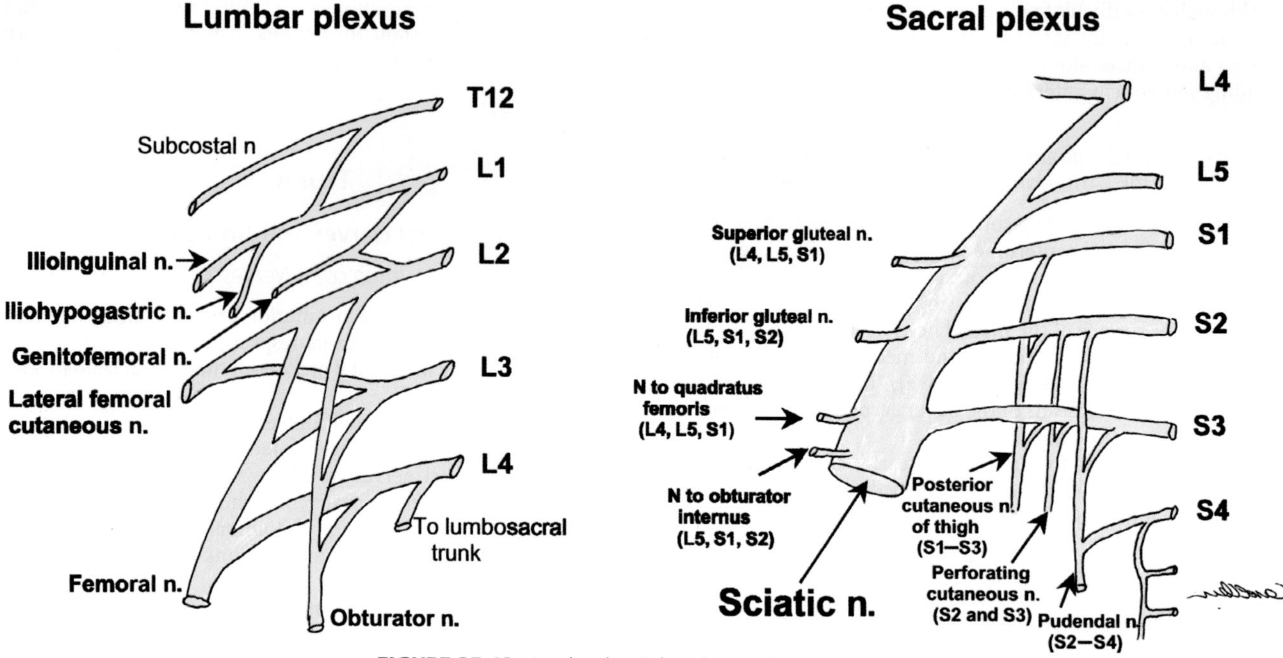

FIGURE 35-13. Lumbar (L1–L4) and sacral (L4–S4) plexuses.

compartments of the thigh. L1 bifurcates into an *upper* part (iliohypogastric and ilioinguinal nerves) and *a lower* part, which joins with a branch from L2 to form the genitofemoral nerve. L3, with portions of L2 and L4, divides into *anterior* and *posterior divisions;* the anterior division forms the obturator (L2–L4) and accessory obturator (L3, L4, when present) nerves, and the posterior division forms the lateral (femoral) cutaneous nerve of the thigh (L2–L3) and the femoral nerve (L2–L4).

In anatomic relation to the psoas major muscle, the obturator (L2–L4) and accessory obturator nerves emerge from its medial border, the genitofemoral (L1, L2) pierces the muscle to lie on its anterior surface, and all others emerge from its lateral border.

Terminal nerves of the lumbar plexus are discussed in the Lower Extremity section.

Inguinal Nerves

The iliohypogastric nerve penetrates the transverse abdominis muscle just above the iliac crest, supplies it, and divides into anterior and lateral cutaneous branches:

- The anterior branch pierces and supplies the internal oblique muscle just 2 cm medial to the anterior superior iliac spine. It then courses deep to the external oblique muscle and superior to the inguinal canal and pierces the external oblique aponeurosis about 2 to 3 cm above the superficial inguinal ring, terminating subcutaneously in the skin of the suprapubic region.
- The lateral cutaneous branch supplies the anterolateral portion of the gluteal skin after piercing both the oblique muscles. The ilioinguinal nerve pierces and supplies the internal oblique muscle and then enters the inguinal canal, in which it traverses outside the spermatic cord to emerge through the superficial (external) inguinal ring (the external oblique aponeurosis), where it provides cutaneous innervation to the skin of the scrotum (or labium majus) and adjacent thigh.

Lower Extremity

Together, the lumbar and sacral plexuses (Fig. 35-13) supply the lower limb. The formation of the lumbar plexus is discussed in the section above. Important landmarks that contain the plexus during its course include the psoas compartment, bordered posteriorly by the quadratus lumborum muscle and anteriorly by the posterior fascia of the psoas muscle, and, more distally, the substance of the psoas major muscle. The anatomy of the terminal nerves is examined below, as are the formation and branches of the sacral plexus. The cutaneous innervation in the lower extremity is shown in Figure 35-14. The lower extremity dermatomes are shown in Figure 35-8.

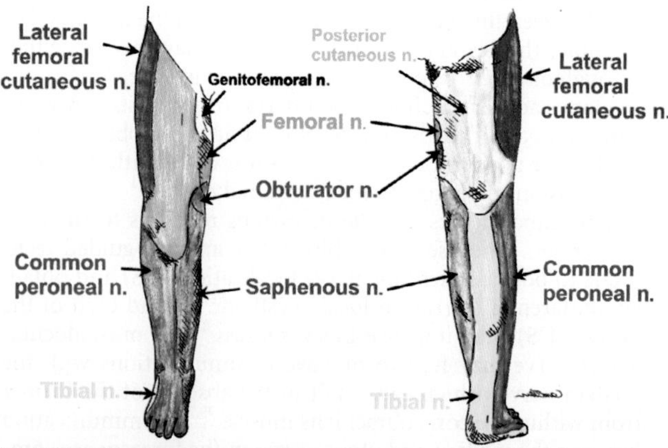

FIGURE 35-14. Cutaneous innervation from the terminal nerves of the lower extremity.

Sacral Plexus: Formation and Branches

At the medial border of the psoas major muscle, the lumbosacral trunk is formed by the union of a branch of L4 and the anterior ramus of L5. After exiting through the anterior sacral foramina, the anterior primary rami of S1–S4 join the lumbosacral trunk to form the sacral plexus (Fig. 35-13). The nerves of the plexus converge toward the greater sciatic foramen anterior to the piriformis muscle on the posterior pelvic wall. The main terminal nerves are the sciatic nerve (continuation of the plexus) and the pudendal nerves ("terminal branches"). Several other small branches are given off, including muscular branches (e.g., inferior and superior gluteal nerves and nerves to the quadratus femoris, piriformis, obturator internus, and external sphincter muscles), cutaneous branches (e.g., posterior cutaneous nerve of the thigh), and visceral branches (pelvis splanchnic nerves). The gluteal vessels (superior and inferior) generally follow the course of the sacral nerves in the anterior plane and can be used to help identify the sciatic nerve at its proximal course. Additional vascular structures that may be identified under US imaging are the pudendal vessels, which pass from the greater to lesser sciatic foramen between the sciatic and pudendal nerves.

Sciatic, Tibial, and Common Peroneal Nerves

The sciatic nerve—the largest nerve of the body—is usually the conjunction of two trunks initially enveloped in a common sheath: A lateral trunk (L4–S2), which eventually emerges as the common peroneal nerve and a medial trunk (L4–S3), which later becomes the tibial nerve. These combined nerves exit through the sciatic notch and pass anteriorly to the piriformis muscle to then lie between the ischial tuberosity and the greater trochanter of the femur. They curve caudally and descend in the posterior thigh adjacent to the femur. At a variable distance within the posterior thigh (often high in the popliteal fossa), the sciatic nerve bifurcates into the tibial and common peroneal nerves. The common peroneal nerve descends along the medial border of the biceps femoris muscle and then on the lateral border of the gastrocnemius muscle. At the fossa it gives off the lateral sural nerve, which forms the lateral sural cutaneous nerve by joining the medial sural nerve supplied by the tibial nerve. It winds around neck of the fibula and terminates as the deep and superficial peroneal nerves. In the posterior thigh, the tibial nerve is covered medially by the semitendinosus and semimembranosus muscles and laterally by the biceps femoris muscle. Beyond the knee joint, it is covered by both heads of the gastrocnemius muscle and then deep to the soleus muscle, before coming to an end on the tibialis posterior muscle and finally on the posterior surface of the tibial shaft medial to the medial malleolus. Within the fossa, it gives off muscular branches (gastrocnemius, soleus, popliteus, and plantaris muscles) as well as the medial sural nerve (to join its lateral counterpart from the common peroneal nerve). In the lower leg and foot, it gives off muscular, articular (ankle), and cutaneous branches and terminates as the medial and lateral plantar nerves. The nerve is often called the posterior tibial nerve in the lower leg.

Terminal Nerves of the Lumbar Plexus

Genitofemoral Nerve (L1, L2)

This nerve leaves the lumbar plexus at the lower border of the L3 vertebra. It pierces and then lies anterior to the psoas major muscle before descending subperitoneally and behind the ureter, where it divides into two branches (genital and femoral) at a variable distance above the inguinal ligament. The genital branch crosses the external iliac artery and traverses the inguinal canal. It supplies the cremaster muscle and skin over the scrotum and adjacent thigh (males) or the skin over anterior part of labium majus and mons pubis (females). The femoral branch descends lateral to the external iliac artery, passes under the inguinal ligament, enters the femoral sheath lateral to the femoral artery, and pierces the anterior layer of the femoral sheath and fascia lata. It innervates the skin immediately below the crease of the groin anterior to the upper part of the femoral triangle.

Lateral Cutaneous Nerve of Thigh (aka, Lateral Femoral Cutaneous Nerve) (L2, L3)

This nerve passes obliquely from the lateral border of the psoas major muscle over the iliacus to enter the thigh below or through the inguinal ligament, variably medial to the anterior superior iliac spine (Fig. 35-15). On the right side of the body, the nerve passes posterolateral to the cecum, and on the left it traverses behind the lower part of the descending colon. The nerve lies on top of the sartorius muscle before dividing into anterior (supplies skin over the anterolateral aspect of the thigh) and posterior (supplies skin on the lateral aspect of thigh from the greater trochanter to the midthigh) branches. Occasionally, this nerve is a branch of the femoral nerve rather than its own nerve.

Femoral Nerve (L2–L4)

The femoral nerve is the largest nerve of this plexus, supplying muscles and skin on the anterior aspect of the thigh. It descends through the psoas major muscle and emerges low at its lateral border, coursing inferiorly between the iliacus and psoas major muscles to enter the thigh under the inguinal ligament (Fig. 35-15). At the inguinal ligament (line running between anterior superior iliac spine and the medial pubic tubercle) and just distal to it (in the femoral triangle), the nerve lies slightly deeper (0.5 to 1 cm) and lateral (approximately 1.5 cm) to the femoral artery; the vein is medial to the artery ("VAN" is the mnemonic for the anatomical relationship, starting medially). At the femoral (inguinal) crease (a few centimeters caudad to the inguinal ligament), the nerve lies underneath the fascia iliaca (iliopectineal fascia), deep to the fascia lata. Beyond the femoral triangle, the nerve branches into anterior (quite proximally) and posterior divisions. The anterior division gives muscular branches to the pectineus and sartorius muscles and cutaneous branches (intermediate and medial cutaneous nerves of thigh) to the skin on the anterior aspect of the thigh. The posterior division sends muscular branches to the quadriceps femoris muscle and gives rise to the *saphenous nerve*, its largest cutaneous branch. The saphenous nerve follows the femoral artery, lying lateral to it within the adductor (Hunter's, subsartorial) canal and then crossing it anteriorly to lie medial to the artery. Distal to the canal, the saphenous nerve leaves the artery to lie superficial at the medial aspect of the knee; the nerve then continues inferiorly (subcutaneously) with the long (great) saphenous vein along the medial aspect of the leg down to the tibial aspect of the ankle. The saphenous branch supplies the skin on the medial aspect of the leg below the knee and on the medial aspect of the foot; it provides articular branches to the hip, knee and ankle joints.

Obturator Nerve (L2–L4)

The obturator nerve emerges from the medial border of the psoas major muscle at the pelvic brim to pass behind the common iliac vessels and lateral to the internal iliac vessels. It then courses inferiorly and anteriorly along the lateral wall of the pelvic cavity on the obturator internus muscle toward the obturator canal,

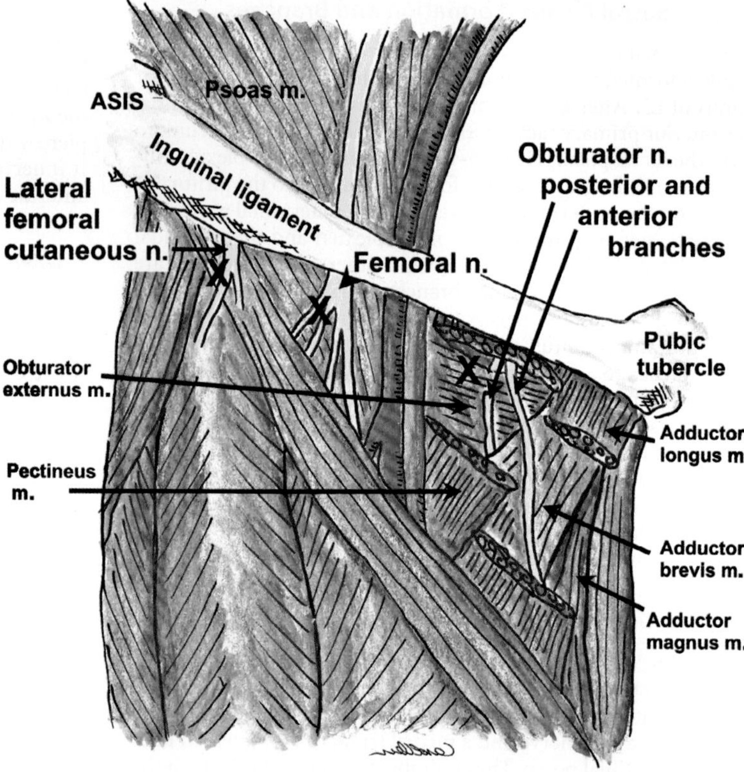

FIGURE 35-15. Illustration of the anterior thigh showing neuromuscular anatomy and needle insertion sites ("X") along the inguinal crease to block the major branches of the lumbar plexus. ASIS, anterior superior iliac spine.

through which it enters the upper part of the medial aspect of the thigh above and anterior to the obturator vessels. The nerve divides into its anterior and posterior branches near the obturator foramen (Fig. 35-15); the anterior branch passes into the thigh anterior to the obturator externus, descends in front of the adductor brevis, and behind the pectineus and adductor longus muscle, with its terminal cutaneous branches emerging as it courses alongside the femoral artery. It supplies the adductor longus, gracilis, adductor brevis (usually), and pectineus (often) muscles. Cutaneous branches supply the skin on the medial aspect of the thigh and perhaps to the medial knee. The nerve's posterior branch pierces the obturator externus muscle anteriorly and supplies it, then passes behind the adductor brevis muscle (sometimes supplies it) to descend on the anterior aspect of the adductor magnus muscle (medial to the anterior branch), which it supplies. There is no apparent cutaneous supply from this nerve. It then traverses the adductor canal with the femoral artery and vein to enter the popliteal fossa, where it terminates as an articular branch to the back of the knee joint capsule (oblique popliteal ligament).

Accessory Obturator Nerve (L3, L4)

This nerve is present in about 30% of individuals. It descends along the medial border of the psoas major muscle, crosses the superior pubic ramus behind the pectineus muscle, supplies it, and gives articular branches to the hip joint.

Nerves at the Ankle

By the time the femoral, tibial, and common peroneal nerves reach the ankle, there are five branches that cross this joint to provide innervation for the skin and muscles of the foot.

Deep Peroneal Nerve (L5, S1)

This nerve lies anterior to the tibia and interosseus membrane and lateral to the anterior tibial artery and vein at the ankle. It travels deep to and between the tendons of the extensor hallucis longus and extensor digitorum longus muscles. Beyond the extensor retinaculum, it branches into medial and lateral terminal branches; the medial branch passes over the dorsum of the foot and supplies the first web space through two terminal digital branches, and the lateral branch traverses laterally and terminates as the second, third, and fourth dorsal interosseus nerves.

Tibial Nerve (aka, Posterior Tibial Nerve; S1–S3)

On the posterior aspect of the knee joint, the tibial nerve joins the posterior tibial artery and then runs deep through to the lower third of the leg where it emerges at the medial border of the calcaneal tendon (Achilles tendon). Behind the medial malleolus it lies beneath several layers of fascia and is separated from the Achilles tendon only by the tendon of the flexor hallucis longus muscle. The nerve is posteromedial to the posterior tibial artery and vein, which are, in turn, posteromedial to the tendons of the flexor digitorum longus and tibialis posterior muscles. Just below the medial malleolus, the nerve divides into the lateral and medial plantar nerves. The nerve innervates the ankle joint through its articular branches and the skin over the medial malleolus, the inner aspect of the heel (including Achilles tendon), and the dorsum of the foot (through the medial and lateral plantar nerves) with its cutaneous branches.

Superficial Peroneal Nerve

The superficial peroneal nerve lies lateral to the deep peroneal nerve in the upper leg. In the anterolateral aspect of lower leg, it becomes superficial about 7 to 8 cm above the lateral malleolus and divides into medial and lateral dorsal cutaneous nerves to supply the dorsum of the foot.

Sural Nerve

This nerve arises from tibial (medial sural nerve) and common peroneal (lateral sural nerve) nerves. It emerges to the superficial compartment at a similar but posterior level to the superficial peroneal nerve, 7 to 8 cm above the lateral malleolus. It then curves around the malleolus at some distance (1 to 1.5 cm) to enter and innervate the lateral aspect of the dorsal surface of the foot.

Saphenous Nerve

The saphenous nerve is the superficial terminus of the femoral nerve, which supplies the skin over the lower medial leg (Fig. 35-14). It leaves the femoral nerve proximally in the femoral triangle (Scarpa's triangle), descends within the adductor canal, and courses beneath the sartorius muscle with the femoral artery (beginning lateral of the vessel at first and then crossing to the medial side superior to the artery just proximal of the lower end of the adductor magnus muscle). Further distally, the femoral artery departs away from the sartorius muscle, traveling deep to continue as the popliteal artery at the adductor hiatus. At this location, the saphenous nerve continues its course under the sartorius muscle, traveling adjacent to the saphenous branch of the descending genicular artery. It runs superficial at the medial surface of the lower leg and in front of the heel.

SPECIFIC TECHNIQUES

The remainder of this chapter is devoted to the procedural details of specific blocks, arranged, similar to the above section on anatomy, by regions of the body. In the sections for Upper Extremity, Trunk, and Lower Extremity, details for using NS and US imaging during the blocks are included. The nerve stimulator is set to deliver variable currents with a frequency of 2 Hz and pulse width of 0.1 ms unless stated otherwise. The volumes of local anesthetic included are those suggested for blocks during which NS was used for nerve localization; US guidance may reduce the required volume in some instances. The figures in these sections will focus predominantly on using combined US and NS-guided technique, although procedures for blind techniques using NS are also described. It is important to note that the figures illustrating technique in humans are representative of the clinical scenario, but without all of the sterile preparation required so as to facilitate observation of proper probe and needle handling. The description of each technique is accompanied by practical tips and evidence-based recommendations. In addition, most of the suggestions related to volume of local anesthetic are based on conventional technique. Although it is not yet well established, many experts speculate that the use of US guidance may reduce the volume of local anesthetic required to achieve adequate blockade.

Head and Neck

Regional anesthesia for the head and neck is diverse, and many head and neck surgical procedures are amenable to some form of regional block. A regional technique may be the sole mode of anesthesia or may be incorporated into a balanced general anesthetic offering optimal postsurgical analgesia. Blocks can be used for ophthalmic, neurologic, ENT, plastic, and endocrine surgeries. Regional anesthesia techniques, such as trigeminal or occipital nerve block, may also be used for diagnostic and therapeutic purposes in acute and chronic pain syndromes. Block techniques range from local infiltration to field block to specific nerve blocks. Since intraoperative airway control can be challenging, the absence of definitive airway control is a frequent source of concern with regional techniques.

Regional anesthesia of the head and neck depends primarily on local infiltration and/or specific nerve blocks placed with reliable anatomical landmarks. Elicitation of a paresthesia is the mainstay of nerve localization, while neither NS nor US imaging have been performed or reported to any extent for these blocks. Therefore, the description of techniques in this section will deviate from other areas where there is greater reliance on nerve localization modalities using NS and US imaging.

Trigeminal Nerve Blocks

For every procedure, prepare the needle insertion site and other applicable skin areas with an antiseptic solution and use sterile equipment. All of the blocks described below use the extraoral route, although alternative intraoral routes may be suitable in many cases.

Semilunar (Gasserian) Ganglion Block

The most comprehensive blockade of the trigeminal nerve targets the central ganglion (Fig. 35-4). This block is usually performed by neurosurgeons under fluoroscopic guidance for treatment of disabling trigeminal neuralgia. Few anesthesiologists perform this technically difficult block and it will not be described in detail here.

Superficial Trigeminal Nerve Branch Block

Trigeminal block can be easily performed by injection of the three individual terminal superficial branches (supraorbital, infraorbital, mental nerves). Each nerve is closely associated with their respective foramina, and all foramina lie in the same sagittal plane on each side of the face (approximately 2.5 cm lateral to the midfacial line passing through the pupil) (Fig. 35-16) and are easily located by US.[81] These foramina are readily palpable, and these nerves can be blocked with superficial injections of small quantities of local anesthetic. The bony landmarks are usually sufficient themselves for routine anesthetic purposes. However, paresthesias are desirable when performing neurolytic blocks with alcohol. An additional block of the supratrochlear nerve is required if the field of anesthesia is to cross the midline (Fig. 35-5). Generally, fine, short needles (e.g., 24 to 26 gauge, 25 to 40 mm) and small syringes (1 to 5 mL) will be suitable for these blocks. The block is usually performed with the patient in the supine position.

PROCEDURE

- Supraorbital nerve (terminal nerve of ophthalmic branch). The supraorbital notch is easily palpated at the medial upper angle of the orbit or located by US as shown in Figure 35-16. The needle is inserted and local anesthetic (see Comments) is slowly injected after aspiration, slightly outside the notch, and produces anesthesia of the ipsilateral forehead.
- Supratrochlear nerve (terminal nerve of ophthalmic branch). Anesthesia of the supratrochlear nerve is obtained with

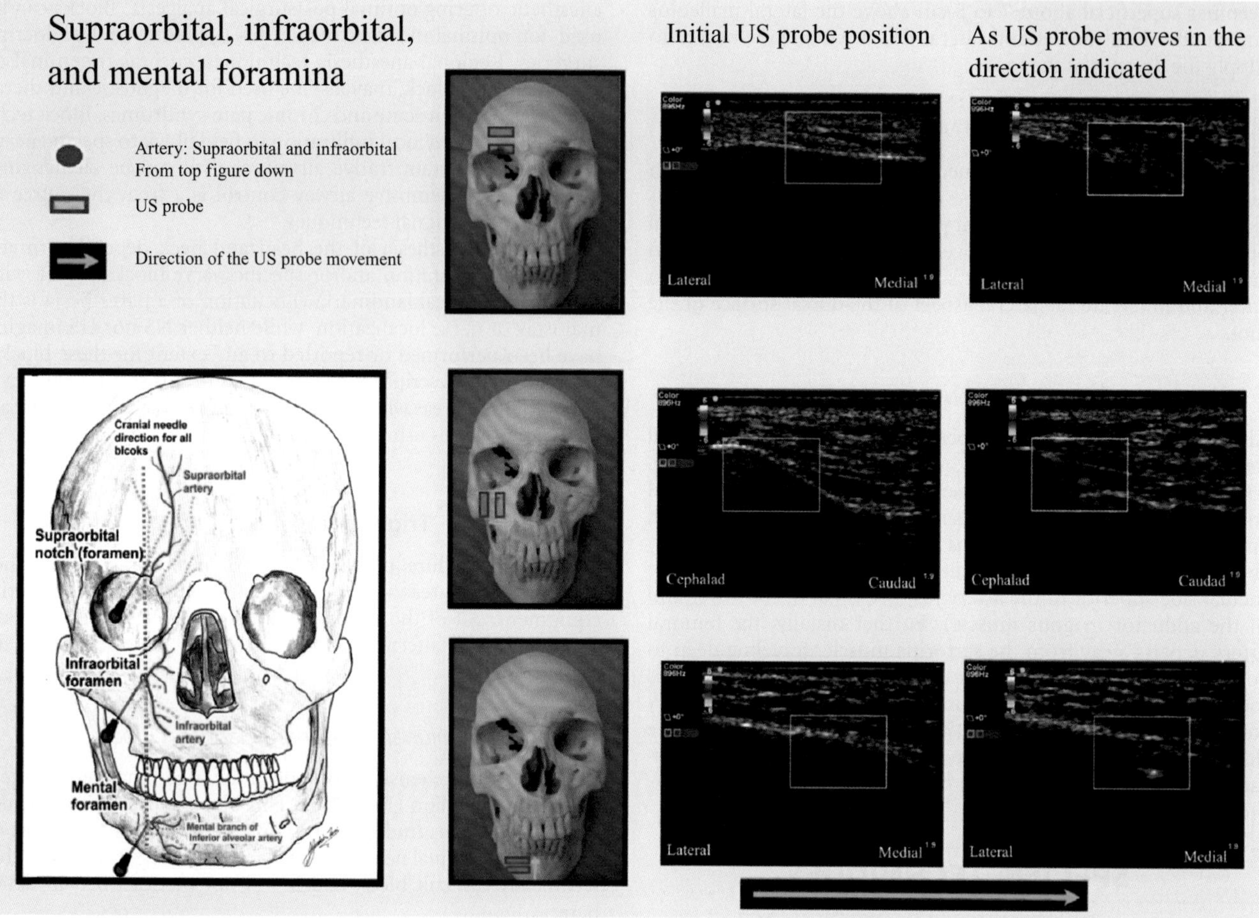

FIGURE 35-16. US showing the supraorbital, infraorbital, and mental foramena. The discontinuation of the hyperechoic bony line indicates a gap along the bone surface which is the foramen.

superficial infiltration of the upper internal angle of the orbital rim. This is needed if the field of anesthesia is to cross the midline.

- Infraorbital nerve (terminal branch of maxillary nerve). The infraorbital foramen lies about 1 cm below the middle of the lower orbital margin. If the foramen cannot be palpated directly, it can be identified by locating the discontinuity of the hyperechoic line on US[81] (Fig. 35-16). The needle should be introduced in a cranial direction through a skin wheal approximately 0.5 cm below the expected opening. After making contact with the bone and withdrawing slightly, injection of a small quantity of local anesthetic is performed. This block produces anesthesia of the middle third of the ipsilateral face.
- Mental nerve (sensory terminal branch of mandibular nerve). The mental nerve emerges from its foramen, which lies inferior to the outer lip at the level of the second premolar, midway between the upper and lower borders of the mandible. The mental canal angles medially and inferiorly; in this case, therefore, needle insertion should start approximately 0.5 cm above and 0.5 cm lateral to the anticipated location of the orifice if it cannot be palpated directly. Again, the use of US can aid identification of the foramen (Fig. 35-16). Slow injection after aspiration at the opening of the canal produces anesthesia of the mandibular area. Injection directly into the canal should be avoided to reduce the risk of neural injury.

COMMENTS

- Choice of local anesthetic for all blocks will depend on the purpose of the block and the duration of anesthesia required (e.g., 1% mepivacaine for shorter procedures and 0.75% ropivacaine for longer procedures). For surgical anesthesia, 2 to 5 mL of local anesthetic may be used, while diagnostic or therapeutic volumes will be much smaller (0.5 to 1 mL).
- The blocks should be followed by local compression to prevent hematoma formation.
- PNB of the terminal branches of the trigeminal nerve offers a safe and effective alternative to local infiltration for soft-tissue injury of the face. Despite this, local infiltration is often required to rectify incomplete anesthesia, especially of the supraorbital and infraorbital nerves.[82]
- Infraorbital nerve block may be performed for postoperative analgesia after cleft lip repair. Palpating anatomic landmarks for this block can be difficult in the neonate, due to the developing facial configuration.
- Skull nerve blocks can be used for craniotomy procedures and are also recommended to attenuate postoperative pain.[83] The nerves blocked to achieve successful anesthesia for craniotomy include the supraorbital and supratrochlear nerves, the greater and lesser occipital nerves, the auriculotemporal nerves and the greater auricular nerves.
- Supraorbital nerve blocks have been associated with a high requirement for supplementation, perhaps due to the anatomic

variation of the nerve. The nerve may exit the skull undivided or its medial and lateral branches may exit separately. For frame pin placement during stereotactic neurosurgery, failure to block the lateral branch may account for inadequate coverage.[84]

- During mental nerve block in older patients, resorption of the superior margin of the mandible will make the foramen appear to lie more superiorly along the ramus.

Maxillary Nerve Block

This block should be performed by practitioners with related and adequate experience. It is required when superficial block of the infraorbital nerve does not produce adequate anesthesia or when anesthesia of the more proximal superior dental nerves is required. This can be performed by a lateral approach to the sphenopalatine fossa.

PROCEDURE

- The patient either sits with the mouth slightly open, or lies supine with a small towel under the occiput and the head turned slightly away from the side to be blocked.
- Above the zygomatic arch: The center of the upper zygomatic arch is marked. A 60- to 90-mm needle is introduced at 45 degrees, caudally and medially, toward the contralateral molar teeth. After a paresthesia is elicited at the nostril, upper lip and cheek, slow incremental injection of local anesthetic is performed after slight needle withdrawal and with frequent aspiration.
- Below the zygomatic arch (Fig. 35-17): The zygomatic arch is marked along its course, and the patient is asked to open and close the mouth slowly so that the curved upper border of the mandible can be identified. The mandibular fossa is palpated between the condylar and coronoid processes. The lowest point of the mandibular notch is palpated, and an "X" is marked at this spot, which is usually at the midpoint of the zygoma. A local anesthetic skin wheal is raised at the "X" after appropriate skin preparation.
- With the patient's jaw in the open position, a 60- to 90-mm needle is introduced through the "X" at a 45-degree angle toward the dorsal part of the eyeball (cephalad and slightly anterior).
- The needle should contact the lateral portion of the pterygoid process (pterygoid plate) at a depth of 4 to 5 cm. It is then withdrawn and redirected slightly cephalad and anteriorly until it passes beyond the pterygoid plate and enters the pterygopalatine fossa at an additional depth of no more than 1 cm. A paresthesia in the nose or the upper teeth confirms nerve localization. The pterygopalatine fossa is highly vascular, so care must be exercised to avoid intravascular injection.
- Anesthesia can be achieved by injecting 5 mL into the pterygopalatine fossa, either on obtaining the paresthesia or blindly by advancing 1 cm beyond the plate.

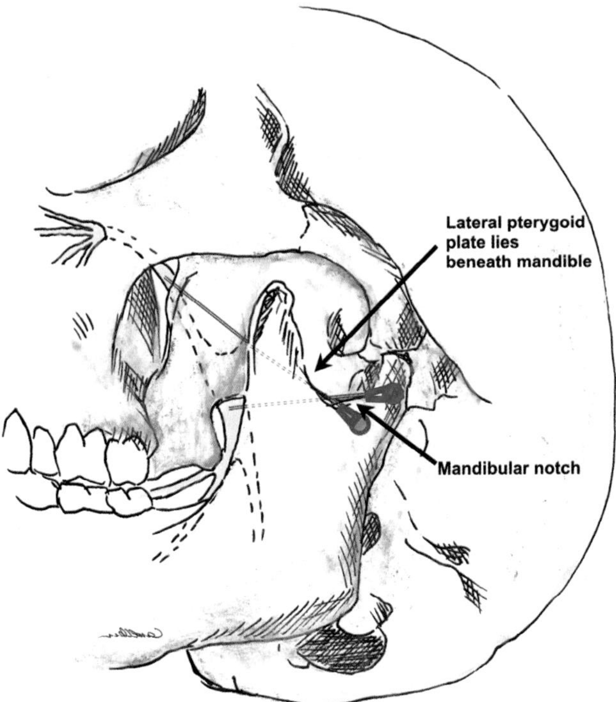

FIGURE 35-17. Lateral view of the skull showing the bony landmarks and final needle insertion angles for the maxillary (red needle) and mandibular (blue needle) nerves. Each block procedure involves first reaching the lateral pterygoid plate (see text for details).

COMMENTS

- One concern during this block is spread of local anesthetic to adjacent structures, especially to the nerves in the orbit. If pain occurs in the region of the orbit during the procedure, the injection should be stopped and the needle should be withdrawn.
- Although the mainstay of treatment for trigeminal neuralgia continues to be pharmacologic or neuroabalative, maxillary nerve block with extraoral mandibular nerve block has been reported to provide relief in some settings.[85]

Mandibular Nerve Block

This nerve can be blocked for dental and maxillary surgery or for inferior dental pain, trigeminal neuralgia in the third branch, or temporomandibular joint dysfunction. It is the only branch of the trigeminal nerve where anesthesia carries the risk of loss of motor (mastication) function.

PROCEDURE

- The patient lies supine with the face in profile. Landmarks for location of the mandibular fossa are the same as those described for maxillary nerve blockade.
- A 60- to 90-mm needle is introduced through the skin wheal and directed perpendicularly to the skin, without the cephalad angulation required for maxillary nerve anesthesia.
- When the pterygoid plate is contacted, the depth should be noted. The needle is then redirected posteriorly until it passes beyond the pterygoid plate. It should contact the nerve 0.5 to 1 cm deep from the point where the pterygoid plate was contacted (Fig. 35-17).
- Paresthesia of the lower jaw, lower lip, and lower incisors at a depth of approximately 4 to 4.5 cm confirms proximity to the nerve. Gentle exploration in a cephalad and caudad direction, from the initial point where the needle passes posterior to the plate, may be required. After slight needle withdrawal, 5 to 10 mL of solution is injected incrementally with repeated aspiration to avoid intravascular injection. As with maxillary blockade, paresthesias can be painful to the patient.

COMMENTS

- Anesthesia of the auriculotemporal nerve is often delayed.
- Facial nerve anesthesia can occasionally be seen when large volumes are injected to block the mandibular nerve. This is of little consequence unless neurolytic agents are used.

- A more serious complication is the possibility of intravascular injection in this highly vascularized area. Injection should be performed incrementally with small quantities and there should be constant observation for signs of toxicity.
- For patients with abnormal anatomy or accessory innervation to the mandible, alternatives to the standard mandibular block include the Gow-Gates and Akinosi-Vazirani blocks.[86]

Cervical Plexus Blocks

Anesthesia of either the deep or superficial cervical plexus or both can be used for procedures of the lateral or anterior neck such as parathyroidectomy and carotid endarterectomy. During carotid surgery, local infiltration of the carotid bifurcation may be necessary to block reflex hemodynamic changes associated with glossopharyngeal stimulation.

Deep Cervical Plexus Block

PROCEDURE

- The patient is placed supine with a small towel under the head, which is turned 45 degrees to the opposite side with slight neck extension.
- Landmarks include the posterior edge of the sternocleidomastoid muscle, the caudal portion of the mastoid process, the angle of the jaw, and the transverse processes of cervical vertebrae C2–C5 (about 1.5 cm apart). If all transverse processes cannot be palpated, the most prominent tubercle of C6 (Chassaignac's) is marked. A line is drawn from the mastoid process along the sternocleidomastoid muscle to reach the transverse process of C6. Each transverse process of C2–C5 is marked approximately 0.5 to 1 cm behind the line; the transverse process of C2 lies about 1.5 cm inferior to the mastoid process.
- Skin infiltration is carried out at the "X" marks of C2–C4, and three needles (22 gauge, 3.5 to 5 cm) are introduced perpendicular to the skin and advanced about 30 degrees caudally with a slight posterior orientation (Fig. 35-7).
- After confirming contact with the transverse process, the needle is withdrawn slightly and a syringe is connected to the needle. Two to three milliliters of local anesthetic solution is injected per segment for therapeutic or diagnostic purposes, while 5 to 10 mL per segment may be sufficient for surgical block (limiting the total to approximately 20 mL if superficial blocks are also performed).

COMMENTS

- The deep block may be performed by single injection at C3 or C4 as originally described by Winnie et al.[87] or by a standard three-injection technique.
- A recent anatomical study demonstrated that the longus capitis muscle is a suitable landmark for US-guided deep cervical plexus block[88]; with this approach, both the deep cervical plexus and sympathetic trunk can be blocked.
- Paresthesia occurring during these blocks has been associated with more effective anesthesia.[89]
- Anesthesia for carotid endarterectomy may involve performing combined superficial and deep cervical plexus blocks, yet the benefit of combined over superficial block alone has been questioned.[90,91] There appears to be no difference between these two approaches in the amount of supplemental local anesthesia required.
- There are several life-threatening complications that may arise from deep cervical plexus block. Injection may occur into the vertebral artery, and subarachnoid or epidural injections are possible if the needle is advanced too far medially into the vertebral foramen. This is more likely in the cervical region because of the longer dural sleeves that accompany these nerve branches. Careful monitoring of the patient should continue for 60 minutes after the block has been performed.
- Phrenic nerve palsy leading to hemidiaphragmatic paresis is a common occurrence with deep cervical plexus block.[92,93] This block is not indicated in any patient who depends on the diaphragm for tidal ventilation, nor is bilateral blockade ever recommended.
- Other well-described side effects include Horner's syndrome (if the superior cervical or cervicothoracic ganglion is blocked),[94] stellate ganglion block,[95] and hoarseness due to recurrent laryngeal nerve block.

Superficial Cervical Plexus Block

This block is performed in a position similar to deep cervical plexus block and results in anesthesia only of the sensory fibers of the plexus.

PROCEDURE

- An "X" is made at the midpoint of the posterior border of the sternocleidomastoid muscle (Fig. 35-5).
- Local skin infiltration is performed with a fan-like injection using 10 to 20 mL of local anesthetic along the posterior border of the sternocleidomastoid muscle 4 cm above and below the level of the midpoint.

COMMENTS

- The most common approach for minimally invasive parathyroidectomy (involving a small unilateral incision rather than bilateral neck exploration) includes a combination of C2–C4 superficial cervical plexus block, infiltration along the incision line and infiltration of the upper thyroid pedicle.[96] This approach can result in shorter anesthetic and operative times, leading to earlier hospital discharge, as well as significantly better postoperative pain relief.[96,97]
- Initial studies of US-guided superficial cervical plexus block showed no added benefit over the blind technique;[98] although US guidance may be helpful in emergency situations.[99]
- Using a modified surgical approach, thyroid surgery has been performed under superficial cervical plexus block in combination with anterior field block.[100]
- Minimally invasive surgery may require conversion to general anesthesia when there is difficulty ensuring adequate protection of the recurrent laryngeal nerve or when intraoperative diagnosis of parathyroid carcinoma or multiglandular parathyroid hyperplasia occurs.
- Phrenic nerve paralysis leading to diaphragmatic dysfunction,[89] vagus nerve block with resultant recurrent nerve paralysis,[101] and inadvertent intravascular injection[102] have all been reported.

Occipital Nerve Blocks

The greater and lesser occipital nerves can be blocked by superficial injection at the points on the posterior skull where they emerge from below the muscles of the neck. This block is rarely used for surgical procedures and is more often applied as a diagnostic step in evaluating head and neck pain complaints.

Procedure

- The patient sits with their head tilted forward slightly to expose the prominent nuchal ridge of bone at the posterior base of the skull.

- The inferior nuchal line is palpated at one-third of the distance between the external occipital protuberance and the foramen magnum. A mark is placed on the nuchal line at the lateral border of the insertion of the erector muscles of the neck, usually 2.5 cm from the midline. At this point, the branches of the greater occipital nerve usually pass laterally from behind the muscle to cross the nuchal line. The nerve is located directly lateral to the easily palpated occipital artery. During its ascent along the posterior skull, the lesser occipital nerve can be located an additional 2.5 cm away from the greater occipital nerve along the inferior nuchal line; a mark should be placed here as well (Fig. 35-9).
- A short, fine needle (e.g., 25 mm, 25 gauge) is introduced with a slight cranial angulation at each mark to the depth of the skull itself. After slight withdrawal, local anesthetic is injected (e.g., 0.5 to 1 mL of 1% lidocaine for diagnostic procedures or 1 to 3 mL of 0.75% ropivacaine for therapeutic procedures). Paresthesias are occasionally encountered but are not essential for obtaining simple skin anesthesia.
- If more anterior anesthesia of the scalp is required, the lesser occipital nerve branches can also be blocked by advancing the needle subcutaneously from this point in an anterior direction toward the mastoid process. A band of anesthetic solution is deposited along the line between skin entry and the mastoid process using 2 to 3 mL of local anesthetic.

Comments

- Blocking the lesser occipital and great auricular nerves (both blocked by subcutaneous injection from the angle of the mandible to the mastoid process) have been successful in providing postoperative analgesia after otoplasty.[103] Reducing the requirement for opioid analgesia (with its associated nausea and vomiting) is essential due to the high incidence of pain and vomiting on the first postoperative day related to the surgical procedure alone.
- The greater occipital nerve block is commonly used for primary headache syndromes. For chronic syndromes, the anterior region involving the trigeminal nerve is also blocked.[104] It has been reported for use with cervicogenic headache, occipital neuralgia, migraine, and cluster headache.[105]
- Complications with this technique are rare. Care must be taken not to advance the needle anteriorly under the skull, as the foramen magnum might be entered unintentionally with a long needle. Local hematoma may be produced with superficial injection, but this is only a temporary problem.

Upper Extremity

Although many approaches to the brachial plexus have been described, there are traditionally four anatomic locations where local anesthetics are placed: (1) the interscalene groove near the cervical transverse processes, (2) the subclavian sheath at the first rib, (3) near the coracoid process in the infraclavicular fossa, and (4) surrounding the axillary artery in the axilla. The introduction of US imaging has greatly increased the use of blocks at the supraclavicular fossa, as visualization of the subclavian artery and lung make these critical structures easier to avoid. It is important to stress that clear visibility of the needle is essential for this block (and generally for all blocks of the brachial plexus). The appropriate choice of approach depends not only on the patient's anatomy but on the site of surgery and the localization method.

The terminal branches of the brachial plexus can also be anesthetized by local anesthetic injection along their peripheral course as they cross joint spaces, where they lie in close proximity to easily identifiable structures (Table 35-1), or by injection of a dilute local anesthetic solution intravenously below a pneumatic tourniquet on the upper arm ("intravenous regional" or Bier block). The use of US may increase the number of locations where the terminal nerves can be successfully blocked. For example, the ulnar nerve can be blocked effectively at the medial surface of the midforearm, which may reduce the risk of ulnar nerve palsy posed by block at the elbow near the cubital tunnel. As stated in the introduction to Specific Techniques, the use of combined US- and NS-guided technique is stressed in the figures, and the use of all necessary sterile precaution was not included for simplicity of viewing.

Brachial Plexus Block

Interscalene Block

This block, as described by Winnie in 1970,[106] is indicated mostly for surgical anesthesia to the shoulder, upper arm, and forearm but is often insufficient for the hand. It frequently spares the lowest branches of the plexus, the C8 and T1 fibers, which innervate the caudad (ulnar) border of the forearm. Nevertheless, recent reports provide evidence that a low interscalene block (below C6, just superior to the clavicle) may provide sufficient anesthesia and analgesia for procedures on the lower arm.[107,108] The patient is positioned supine, with their head faced slightly to the contralateral side. The main surface landmark (sternocleidomastoid muscle) used for this block can be accentuated by asking the patient to reach for the ipsilateral knee and by rotating the head approximately 45 degrees to the nonoperative side. The head should also be slightly elevated, and the patient should be instructed to take a deep breath, since contraction of the scalenus muscles accentuates the interscalene groove. This groove lies immediately behind the lateral border of the clavicular head of the sternocleidomastoid muscle at the level of the cricoid cartilage (C6). As for all procedures of the upper extremity, prepare the needle insertion site and other applicable skin areas with an antiseptic solution and, if using US imaging, ensure sterility of the US probe with a standard sleeve cover or transparent dressing (not shown). Please refer to the accompanying video clip for a demonstration of continuous interscalene block.

PROCEDURE USING NERVE STIMULATION TECHNIQUE

- Landmarks: Using the maneuvers described above, the interscalene groove is palpated by rolling the fingers posteriorly off the lateral border of the sternocleidomastoid muscle; mark the groove as high as possible. After the patient relaxes, the prominent transverse process of C6 can often be felt directly in the groove and should be marked.
- Needling: A skin wheal is raised in the interscalene groove at the level of the cricoid. A 22-gauge, 35- to 50-mm insulated needle is introduced through the wheal. The needle is directed medially, caudally, and slightly posteriorly in the direction of the C6 transverse process. The caudad tilt of the needle is important to avoid either entering the neural foramen or injection into the dural nerve root sheath, and thus high-spinal anesthesia or spinal cord injury.[109] Avoiding medial placement, by using a mostly caudad and posterior direction, may reduce the risks even more. The superficial structures of the plexus have been shown to be located at an average, shallow depth of 5.5 mm.[110]
- Nerve localization: Applying an initial current of 0.8 mA is sufficient for stimulation of the plexus (usually at a depth of 1 to 3 cm), and the current is reduced to aim for a threshold current of 0.4 mA before injection after obtaining an appropriate

ANESTHESIA FOR SURGICAL SUBSPECIALTIES

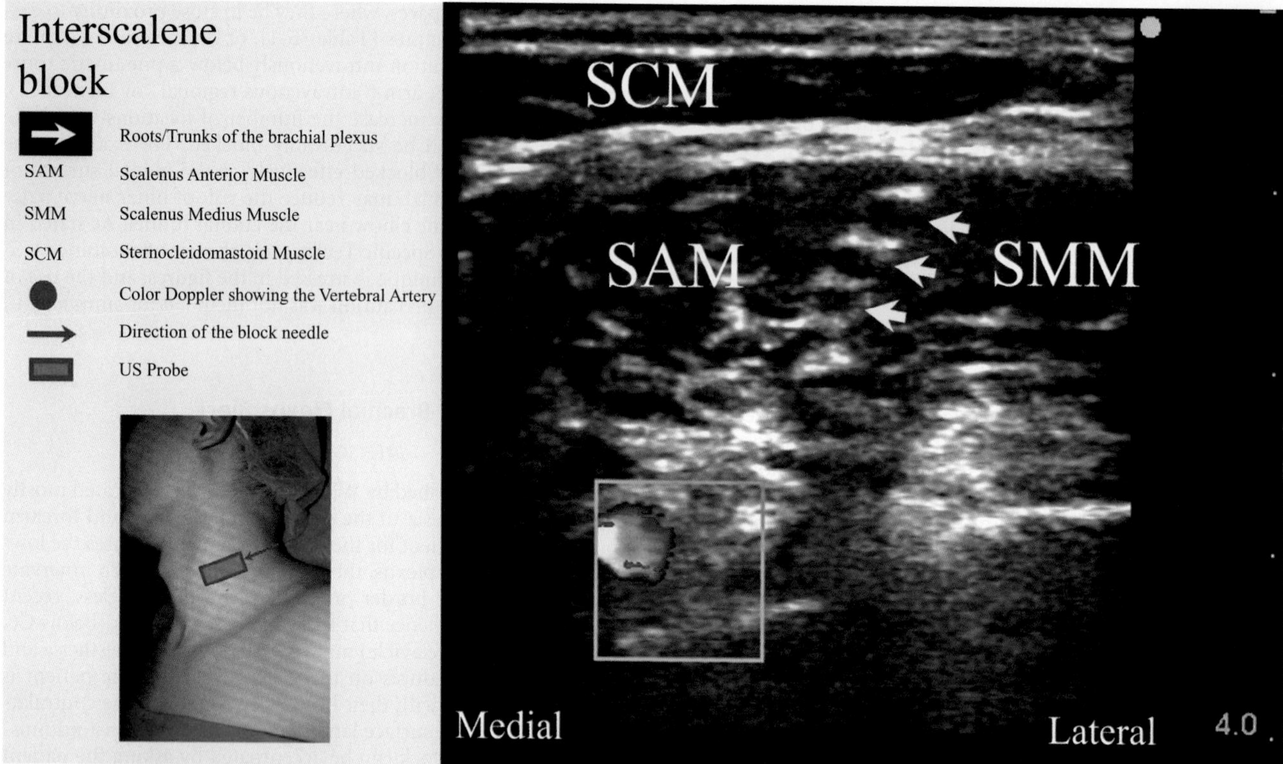

FIGURE 35-18. Ultrasound-guided interscalene block using an IP needle alignment to a linear high frequency probe. The needle is directed from lateral to medial with a slight caudal angle to avoid the intervertebral foramen. The roots/trunks of the plexus are usually seen as three or more round or oval-shaped hypoechoic structures sandwiched between the scalenus anterior and medius muscles in the interscalene groove. Note that the vertebral artery lies medial and deep to the brachial plexus.

motor response. Diaphragmatic or trapezius twitches should be avoided, as they are associated with cervical plexus stimulation; a diaphragmatic response indicates that the phrenic nerve is being stimulated and that the needle is too anterior.

- Injection: After careful aspiration, 25- to 30-mL local anesthetic is injected in small increments to detect intraneural or intravascular placement of the needle.

PROCEDURE USING ULTRASOUND GUIDANCE (FIG. 35-18)

- Scanning: Two scanning techniques are recommended for viewing the brachial plexus at the interscalene level: (1) beginning anteriorly at the cricoid cartilage level (C6) with movement from anterior and medial to posterior and lateral toward the interscalene groove, and (2) scanning proximally from the supraclavicular fossa to the interscalene location.
- Appearance: At the supraclavicular fossa, the brachial plexus (trunks/divisions) can be seen in short axis as a tightly enclosed cluster (i.e., honeycomb-like), superior and lateral to the subclavian artery (Fig. 35-19). After tracing the nerves in a proximal fashion toward the interscalene groove, the nerve structures (roots/trunks) are visualized in a sagittal oblique section as three (usually) or up to five round or oval-shaped hypoechoic (see Common Techniques: Nerve Stimulation and Ultrasound Imaging section) structures, sometimes with few internal punctate echoes, lying between the scalenus anterior and medius muscles. C8 and T1 roots may be difficult to identify because of their depth.[111,112]
- Needling: After infiltration of local anesthetics to the skin at the anticipated needle puncture site, a 22-gauge, 50-mm needle (insulated is recommended) is introduced either OOP (see Common Techniques section) or IP to the probe (Fig. 35-18) and advanced to a maximum of 3 cm for most patients. For OOP needle insertion technique, the clinician stands beside or cephalad to the probe and places the initial needle puncture site cranial to the probe. The needle is typically angled somewhat caudally toward the US beam plane. For IP needle insertion technique, the needle is moved from lateral to medial (still slightly caudad) and will first penetrate the scalenus medius muscle before entering the interscalene groove. It is recommended to use NS to enable further nerve localization.
- Local anesthetic spread: A test injection of D5W is recommended and will help confirm nerve localization and estimate the pattern of local anesthetic spread. Local anesthetic should be deposited in the midst of the neural structures so that it spreads to surround the nerves circumferentially. Local anesthetic distention in this compartment can be seen by US as a hypoechoic (fluid) expansion.

COMMENTS

- The use of long-acting local anesthetics may provide analgesia for 12 to 14 hours. For longer analgesia, insertion of a continuous catheter is effective for procedures such as total shoulder replacement, although securing the catheters in the mobile neck tissues is a challenge.
- Equal success has been achieved when any of the appropriate muscle responses is elicited as a positive stimulating test. Palpation of the muscle may confirm the motor response.
- Despite the fact that subarachnoid or intraneural injection can occur even when the threshold current is >0.4 mA, it is

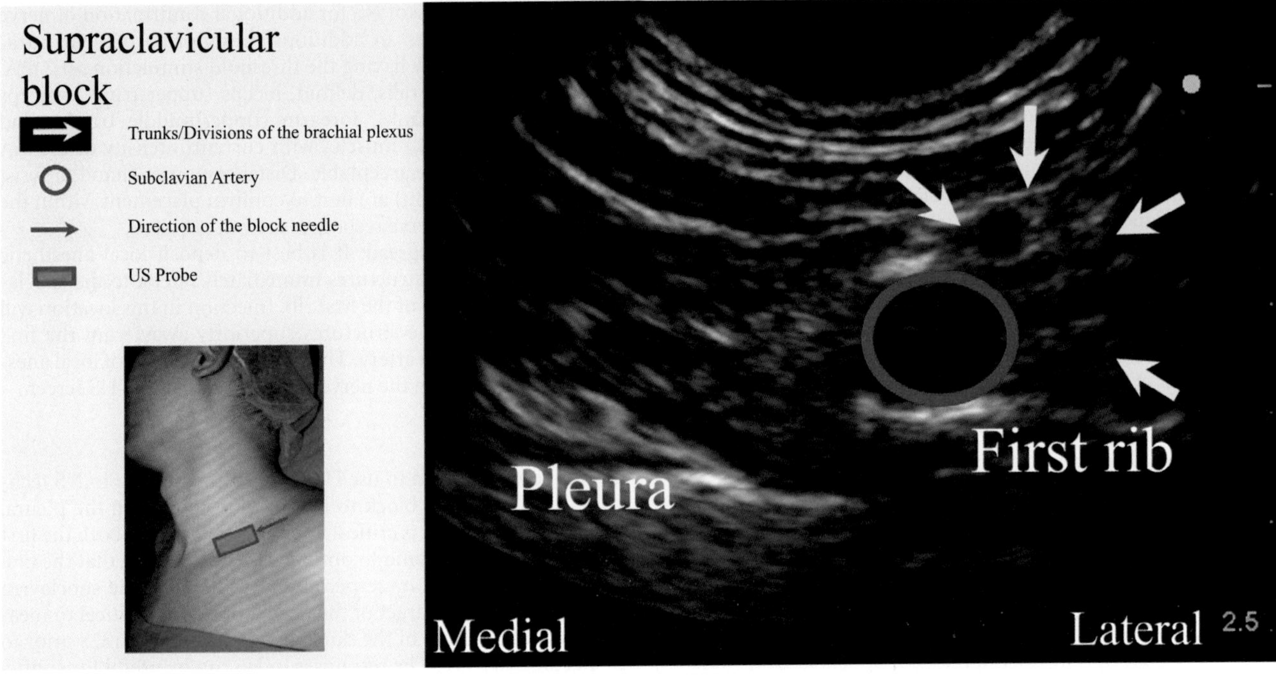

FIGURE 35-19. Ultrasound-guided supraclavicular block using IP needle alignment to a small footprint curved probe, and directing the needle from lateral to medial in a slightly sagittal plane. Color Doppler can also be valuable to locate the subclavian artery quickly in order to locate the plexus trunks/divisions immediately superolateral to the vessel.

advisable to avoid injecting when the current responses are less than 0.4 mA.

- If a continuous block is indicated, the needle entry point may be moved a centimeter cephalad for the OOP approach, making the corresponding angle of insertion a little steeper and more tangential to the course of the plexus. The bevel of the introducing needle should be directed laterally. Placement of a stimulating catheter may be aided by dilating the perineural space with D5W, which will allow the user to monitor the catheter's advancement to a location where motor response is maintained at <0.5 mA.
- Securing catheters in the freely mobile neck is a challenge. Some prefer to secure the catheter by tunneling 3 to 4 cm below the skin by passing it back through an intravenous catheter that has been introduced subcutaneously near the entry site.
- During OOP US-guided technique, angling the needle more than 45 degrees should be avoided as the needle may be inserted too deep and directed toward the spinal cord.
- Complications from this approach are related to the structures located in the vicinity of the tubercle. The cupola of the lung is close, particularly on the right side, and can be contacted if the needle is directed too far caudally. Pneumothorax should be considered if cough or chest pain is produced while exploring for the nerve. If the needle is allowed to pass directly medially, it may enter the intervertebral foramen, and injection of local anesthetic may produce spinal or epidural anesthesia. The vertebral artery passes posteriorly at the level of the sixth vertebra to lie in its canal in the transverse process that can be seen as a pulsatile structure deep to the plexus; direct injection into this vessel can rapidly produce central nervous system toxicity and convulsions. Careful aspiration and incremental injections are important to help avoid both of these potential problems.
- Even with appropriate injection, local anesthetic solution can spread to contiguous nerves. It may produce cervical plexus block, including motor fibers to the diaphragm, which may be a problem in patients with respiratory insufficiency. A case report described an optimal spread of local anesthetic and the possibility of using saline dilution technique should phrenic nerve block occur.[113]
- Horner's syndrome is common because of spread to the sympathetic chain on the anterior vertebral body.
- Neuropathy of the C6 root is a potential problem because the needle may unintentionally pin the nerve root against the tubercle and predispose to intraneural injection. The needle should be withdrawn slightly if the first injection produces the characteristic "crampy" pain sensation.
- An alternative technique for blocking the roots of the brachial plexus is to perform a cervical paravertebral block,[114] which can utilize the bony landmarks of the vertebral column. This is a high quality block and is readily performed using US guidance. A lateral US view of the brachial plexus at the level of C6 allows visualization of the needle as it passes lateral to the C6 transverse process and into the interscalene space. This view avoids the challenges of attempting to view the brachial plexus from a posterior approach in which the bony structures may obscure the view of the needle and plexus.

Supraclavicular Block

The supraclavicular block targets the trunks and/or divisions of the brachial plexus, depending on the location of the injection site and the patient's anatomy. Similar to the interscalene block, the patient is positioned supine with the head turned approximately 45 degrees to the contralateral side. Prepare the needle insertion site and other applicable skin areas with an antiseptic solution and ensure sterility of the US probe with a standard sleeve cover or transparent dressing. (Please refer to the accompanying video clip for a demonstration of the supraclavicular block.)

4

PROCEDURE USING NERVE STIMULATION TECHNIQUE (PLEASE NOTE THAT MOST CLINICIANS PREFER TO PERFORM THIS BLOCK UNDER US GUIDANCE TO MINIMIZE POTENTIAL COMPLICATIONS; SOME MAY USE NS AS AN ADJUNCT METHOD WITH US.)

- Landmarks: The outline of the clavicle is drawn on the skin and the midpoint of the clavicle is marked. An "X" is placed posterior to this midpoint in the interscalene groove, usually 1 cm behind the clavicle. The subclavian artery pulse serves as a reliable landmark in thinner individuals, as the plexus lies immediately cephaloposterior to the subclavian artery.
- Needling: Local infiltration is performed at the site of the nerve and a 2.5- to 5-cm, 22-gauge needle is introduced in the parasagittal plane at the superior border of the clavicle at the lateral edge of the sternocleidomastoid muscle insertion. An initial insertion angle of 45 degrees cephalad is recommended, with subsequent reductions in angle as necessary,[115] although an angle of <20 degrees may lead to the needle contacting the pleura and/or subclavian vein prior to the plexus. The rib may be contacted, with subsequent anteroposterior needle adjustment to contact the plexus, but avoiding rib contact may be most prudent. Careful lateral or medial exploration may be needed, but probing too medially increases the risk of contacting the pleura.
- Nerve localization: The responses to NS can be very useful for confirmation of needle proximity to the separate trunks. Twitches of pectoralis, deltoid, biceps (upper trunk), triceps (upper/middle trunk), forearm (upper/middle trunk), and hand (lower trunk) muscles with current intensity of 0.4 mA (0.1 to 0.3 ms) are acceptable. Distal responses (hand or wrist flexion or extension) are best to confirm placement within the fascia. Multiple nerve responses are not required.
- Injection: If a nerve response is produced during the course of exploration, the anesthetic solution can be injected while the needle is fixed in position. Twenty-five to forty milliliters of local anesthetic will produce adequate analgesia.

PROCEDURE USING ULTRASOUND IMAGING (FIG. 35-19)

- Scanning: The probe is first placed in a coronal oblique plane at the lateral end of and just above the upper border of the clavicle. It is then moved medially until an image of the subclavian artery appears on the screen. Some dorsal and ventral rotations of the probe may be necessary. With the subclavian artery in the middle of the screen, the plexus is located superolateral to the artery and the neurovascular structures lie above the first rib.
- Appearance: The subclavian artery is anechoic, hypodense, pulsatile and round; its identity can be further confirmed by color Doppler. Trunks/divisions of the brachial plexus appear as a cluster of hypoechoic "grape-like" structures consisting of usually three (more as one moves distally) hypoechoic nodules, all surrounded by a hyperechoic lining (presumably the connective tissues). With the probe in a coronal oblique plane, the plexus depth has been shown with MRI to equal 1.65 cm in males and 1.45 cm in females.[115,116] Medial and deep to the artery, the rib may be seen as a hyperechoic line with dorsal shadowing. The anechoic subclavian vein may be seen inferomedial to the artery.
- Needling: The selected needle insertion site is often more lateral with the US-guided technique than when using NS techniques. The skin is infiltrated with local anesthetic and a 22-gauge, 50-mm (or less) needle (insulated is recommended) is introduced with IP needle alignment to a curved, small footprint (Fig. 35-19) or linear probe. The needle is inserted immediately above the clavicle in a lateral-to-medial direction with a slight cephalad angle. It is recommended to have the concurrent use of NS for additional confirmation of nerve localization and as an additional monitor to prevent intraneural injection by having the threshold stimulation >0.2 mA. Twitches of pectoralis, deltoid, biceps (upper trunk), triceps (upper/middle trunk), forearm (upper/middle trunk), and hand (lower trunk) muscles with current intensity of 0.4 mA (0.1 to 0.3 ms) are acceptable. Distal responses (hand or wrist flexion or extension) are best to confirm placement within the fascia. Multiple nerve responses are not required.
- Local anesthetic spread: It is best to deposit local anesthetic next to the nerve structures immediately lateral to the subclavian artery on top of the first rib. Injection in this location will often lift the nerve structures superiorly away from the first rib and subclavian artery. The hypoechoic spread of local anesthetic surrounding the nerves may be seen on the US screen.

COMMENTS

- It is recommended to use US imaging in addition to NS technique during this block to help avoid puncturing the pleura. When using US, it is critical to be able to visualize both the first rib and the pleura and to optimize the image such that the first rib covers the pleura, especially just lateral to the subclavian artery where the target of the needle tip is. It is critical to measure and be aware of the skin-pleura distance with US prior to needle insertion. The responses to NS can be useful for confirmation of needle proximity to the separate trunks.
- The major challenge with US imaging in this region is the presence of a bony prominence (clavicle) and curved soft tissue contour that can interfere with imaging of the brachial plexus in short axis. Despite the disadvantages of commercially available low to moderate frequency curved array probes (e.g., C11, Titan or MicroMaxx, Sonosite Inc., Bothell, WA), a curved array probe with a small footprint is extremely useful in this compact area.
- The lateral-to-medial IP needle approach will ensure that the needle approaches the nerve structures before reaching the subclavian artery (i.e., less chance of inadvertent vascular puncture). However, using a slightly sagittal plane (Fig. 35-19) may reduce the risk of pleural puncture. The needle should be viewed at all times when using a lateral-to-medial approach.
- The greatest risk when using this technique is pneumothorax, as the cupola of the lung lies just medial to the first rib, not far from the plexus. The risk of pneumothorax is greater on the right side as the cupola of the lung is higher on that side. The risk is also greater in tall, thin patients.
- This method of brachial plexus PNB does not introduce any more complications than other methods of brachial plexus block.

Infraclavicular Block

Infraclavicular block targets the cords of the brachial plexus, and the nerves can be blocked next to the second part of the axillary artery at the level of the coracoid process. Brachial plexus block in the infraclavicular area offers excellent analgesia of the entire arm and allows introduction of continuous catheters to provide prolonged postoperative pain relief. The infraclavicular approach blocks the musculocutaneous and axillary nerves more consistently because these two nerves often branch off high in the axilla and are often missed with the axillary block approach. However, multiple injections may be required for successful infraclavicular and axillary blocks.

Infraclavicular blocks are indicated for forearm, elbow, and hand surgeries. The patient is supine with the head turned

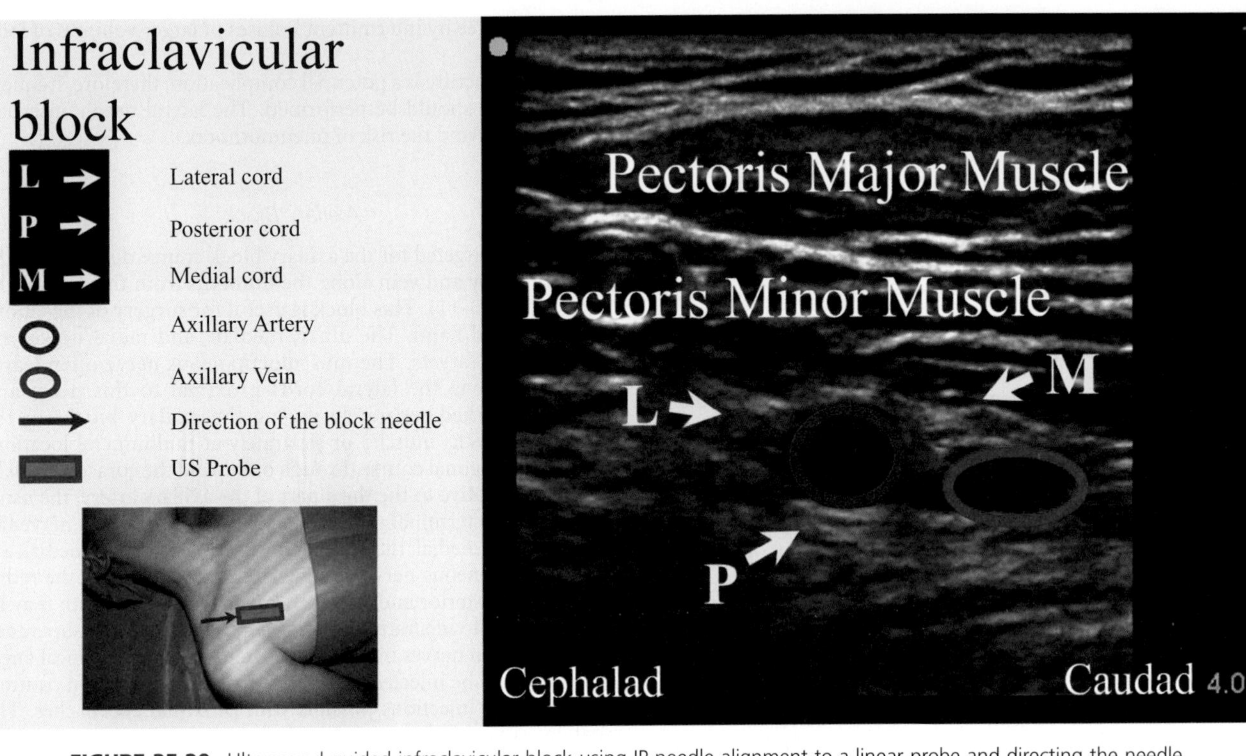

FIGURE 35-20. Ultrasound-guided infraclavicular block using IP needle alignment to a linear probe and directing the needle 15 degrees posteriorly in a cephalad-to-caudad direction. In contrast to the more proximal blocks, the nerves (cords) appear hyperechoic now due to their higher fascial content and since the surrounding tissue (muscle) is largely hypoechoic.

approximately 45 degrees to the nonoperative side, and their arm may either be at their side with hand on the abdomen or abducted with their palm placed behind their head. When preparing for this block, it is common to have the patient's elbow flexed and the hand resting on the abdomen to facilitate observation of motor responses generated with NS. Alternatively, externally rotating the arm and placing the hand behind the head stretches the cords and brings the nerves closer around the axillary artery, which may facilitate local anesthetic spread around the nerves. As always, prepare the needle insertion site and other applicable skin areas with an antiseptic solution and ensure sterility of the US probe with a standard sleeve cover or transparent dressing (not shown).

PROCEDURE USING NERVE STIMULATION TECHNIQUE

Several approaches have been described for infraclavicular block, all with various needle puncture sites and angles of insertion.[117–122] Here we describe a lateral approach,[118] which may improve plexus cord localization and reduce risk of puncture to both the pleura and axillary artery.[123,124]

- Landmarks: With the patient's arm adducted and their hand resting on their abdomen, the medial aspect of the coracoid process is palpated as one slips their finger off the clavicle.
- Needling: After skin preparation and skin wheal, a 50- to 90-mm, 18- to 22-gauge needle is inserted where the clavicle meets the medial aspect of the coracoid process, generally directed 0 to 15 degrees posterior to the horizontal plane (Fig. 35-20 illustrates this needle insertion when using US guidance). The 15-degree trajectory will likely increase the chances of contacting the more posteriorly located posterior or medial cords which may improve analgesia. A greater angle may be required to achieve adequate responses to NS, since local anesthetic injection at more than one cord may be beneficial. The cords should be approximately 4 to 6 cm deep (insertion of more than 7.5 cm may risk pleural puncture).[118] The needle puncture site may be adjusted slightly caudad to this location, as with the technique of Kapral et al.[117] If the needle is placed 2.5 cm caudad to the coracoid process, a laterally projected needle directed toward the axillary artery may be effective.[118]
- Nerve localization: The first response (elbow flexion) obtained is usually the musculocutaneous nerve arising from the lateral cord. For complete anesthesia of the hand, a separate distal response needs to be obtained from the medial (distal flexors) and posterior (distal and proximal extensors) cords.[125] A simplified approach to determining the specific cord distal responses during infraclavicular block has been described.[126] A close examination of the movements of the fifth digit (pinkie) can be useful to differentiate the cords, with lateral movement (i.e., pronation) representing the lateral cord, medial movement (i.e., flexion) representing the medial cord, and dorsal movement (i.e., extension) representing the posterior cord.[126] Some also advocate that eliciting a forearm response (pronation via the lateral cord) is essential for a complete block.[127] The artery may be punctured easily at this point, and careful aspiration is required to prevent intravascular injection.
- Injection: If a musculocutaneous nerve response is obtained, the nerve or lateral cord can be blocked by an injection of 5 to 10 mL of local anesthetic. Once responses in the hand are obtained, a further 25 mL of local anesthetic can be injected along the posterior and medial cords.

PROCEDURE USING ULTRASOUND IMAGING (FIG. 35-20)

- Scanning: Immediately medial and inferior to the coracoid process, position a linear or curved lower frequency transducer (4 to 7 MHz), depending on body habitus, in a parasagittal plane and capture the best possible short-axis view of the brachial plexus cords and axillary vessels. If the patient is quite thin or if using a more medial location (not described here) where the nerves are more superficial, a higher frequency probe may be used.

- Appearance: The pectoralis major and minor muscles are separated by a hyperechoic lining (perimysium); the pectoralis major lies superficial and lateral to the pectoralis minor. Approximately 4 to 5 cm deeper lies the axillary neurovascular bundle; the large axillary vein lies medial and caudad to the artery. The lateral cord of the plexus is often readily visualized as a hyperechoic oval structure, although the medial and posterior cords may not be readily identified because the medial cord lies between the axillary artery and vein, while the posterior cord can be hidden deep to an axillary artery acoustic shadow. In addition, the medial cord can be posterior or even slightly cephalad to the axillary artery. It is important to realize that there is a great deal of individual anatomic variation in the cord location around the artery. The nerve structures now appear hyperechoic, rather than hypoechoic as seen more proximally, presumably due to an increase in the number of fascicles and amount of (hyperechoic-appearing) connective tissue.[71]
- Needling: The skin is infiltrated with local anesthetic. For single-shot technique, a 50- to 90-mm, 18- to 22-gauge insulated needle is suitable if using NS, while a 90-mm, 17- to 20-gauge needle can be used for catheter placement. Using an IP needle alignment will be most suitable in most cases. The block needle is inserted cephalad to the probe and is then advanced caudally and posteriorly at approximately 30 degrees to the skin. The cords should be found at a depth of 4 to 6 cm, similar to blind technique.[128] It is recommended to combine US with NS for accurate nerve localization (e.g., musculocutaneous nerve or specific cord), due to the high variability of cord location.
- Local anesthetic spread: Aim to place the needle and local anesthetic posterior to the axillary artery next to the posterior cord (spread from this location is most optimal for complete block success). Performing a test dose with D5W is recommended prior to local anesthetic application to visualize spread and confirm nerve localization. Inject 20 to 25 mL of local anesthetic around the posterior cord. If local anesthetic spread is deemed inadequate to surround all cords, reposition the needle before injecting any additional local anesthetic.

COMMENTS

- In the past, numerous techniques were developed with modifications to localize nerves and avoid vessel and pleural punctures. Real-time guidance with US will address some of these issues although US-guided blocks are going through a rapid development process to determine the safest and most successful approaches.
- Techniques that incorporate multiple injections may be easier and potentially safer under combined US and NS guidance, which provides direct visualization of the anatomic structures.
- If a catheter is to be threaded, the aim should be to elicit motor responses in the hand itself. The tip of the Tuohy needle (90 mm, 17 to 20 gauge) should be directed laterally to allow the catheter to run in the direction of the nerves.
- Compared to blocks at more proximal locations, the infraclavicular block has the advantage of lower risk of blocking the phrenic nerve or stellate ganglion. However, in some cases, continuous catheters may lie along one cord and fail to provide complete anesthesia and analgesia of the entire brachial plexus with small volume infusions. This may be overcome to some degree by intermittent boluses of larger volumes of local anesthetic.
- Vessel puncture is a potential complication; therefore, frequent aspiration should be performed. The lateral needle insertion will help avoid the risk of pneumothorax.

Axillary Block

The nerves targeted for the axillary block course distally with the axillary artery and vein along the humerus from the apex of the axilla (Fig. 35-11). This block is useful for surgery of the elbow, forearm, and hand. The ulnar, median, and radial nerves are the primary targets. The musculocutaneous nerve often leaves the plexus (via the lateral cord) proximal to this point and may be blocked separately during the axillary block (in the coracobrachialis muscle) or separately at midhumeral locations (along its diagonal course through or beyond the coracobrachialis muscle). Relative to the third part of the axillary artery, the usual course of the terminal nerves is as follows: The median nerve lies anterior and medial, the ulnar nerve lies posterior and medial, the musculocutaneous nerve lies anterior and lateral, and the radial nerve lies posterior and lateral. Because the single sheath may be broken up into separate compartments by fascial septa surrounding individual nerves in the axilla, some advocate that local anesthetic should be injected at multiple sites in the axilla, in contrast to the single injections possible with proximal approaches. The patient is positioned supine with the arm abducted at 70 to 80 degrees and externally rotated, and the elbow flexed at 90 degrees.

PROCEDURE USING NERVE STIMULATION TECHNIQUE

- Landmarks: The axillary artery is marked as high in its course through the axilla as is practical. It is usually felt in the intramuscular groove between the coracobrachialis and the triceps muscles. It also passes between the insertions of the pectoralis major and the latissimus dorsi muscles on the humerus.
- Needling: A 30- to 50-mm, 22-gauge insulated needle is suitable for this block. After aseptic preparation, a skin wheal is raised over the proximal portion of the artery. The index and middle fingers of the nondominant hand straddle the artery just below this point, both localizing the pulsation and compressing the neurovascular bundle below the intended site of injection. The needle is inserted in a slight cephalad direction, followed by a two-step, four-injection process with puncture at locations just superior and inferior to the artery.
- Nerve localization: With NS technique, ideally, the nerves serving the area of proposed surgery are sought first. The median and the musculocutaneous nerves lie on the superior aspect of the artery (as viewed by the operator), whereas the ulnar and radial nerves lie below and behind the vessel. Obtaining a direct musculocutaneous nerve response (elbow flexion) indicates localization of this particular nerve, but not necessarily all nerves.
- Injection: Experience has shown that a multiple injection technique around each individual nerve is the most reliable approach (10 to 15 mL at each nerve location). Less volume may be required, but the minimum required dose/volume per nerve is not known at this time.

PROCEDURE USING ULTRASOUND IMAGING (FIG. 35-21)

- Scanning: High-frequency, linear probes are generally recommended (10 to 15 MHz) for imaging since the nerves are superficial (1 to 2 cm) below the skin. The most proximal location at the apex of the axilla may be the best for viewing all of the terminal branches of the brachial plexus. The probe is

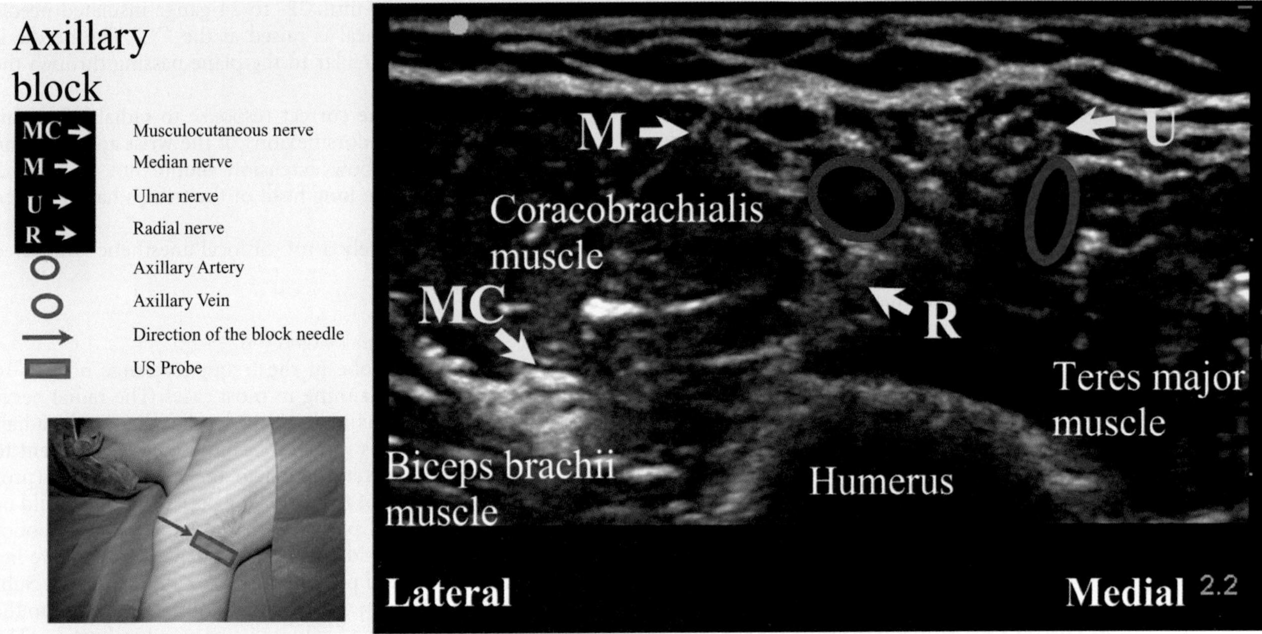

FIGURE 35-21. Ultrasound-guided axillary block using IP needle alignment to a linear high frequency probe. Typically, the block needle is advanced in sequence to reach each of the median, ulnar, and radial nerves.

positioned perpendicular to the anterior axillary fold and in cross section to the humerus at the bicipital sulcus (and at the level of the axillary pulse) to capture the transverse, or short-axis view of the neurovascular bundle.

- Appearance: In cross section:
  - The coracobrachialis and the biceps brachii muscles are seen laterally; the teres major and the triceps brachii muscles lie medially, the latter being deeper than the biceps brachii muscle
  - The anechoic and circular axillary artery lies centrally, adjacent to both the biceps brachii and coracobrachialis muscles; it is surrounded by the nerves
  - The nerves appear round-to-oval in short axis; generally they appear as hyperechoic masses due to the large amount of connective tissue (epi- and perineurium) interspersed within the hypoechoic nerve fascicles
  - The *median* nerve is often located superficial and between the artery and the biceps brachii muscle; the *ulnar* nerve is usually located medial and superficial to the artery; the *radial* nerve lies deep to the artery at the midline (clockwise: Median, ulnar, radial—but there are many variations)
  - The *musculocutaneous* nerve is commonly located in the hyperechoic plane between the biceps brachii and coracobrachialis muscles.
- Needling: A 50-mm, 22-gauge insulated needle (combined US and NS technique is recommended) is suitable. Both IP and OOP needle approaches can be used for axillary block. An OOP approach, with the needle distal to the probe and in transverse axis to the nerve, is similar to the traditional blind procedure, except that the needle will be aligned at an angle to optimize needle visibility rather than more perpendicular to the skin. An angle of 30 to 45 degrees from the skin, with the needle placed approximately 1 to 2 cm caudad to the probe, may allow optimal needle visibility (see description of the walk-down technique in the section on Common Techniques: Nerve Stimulation and Ultrasound Imaging).[37,38] The IP approach involves inserting the needle at an acute angle (20 to 30 degrees) to the skin in a lateral to medial direction (Fig. 35-21). Typically, the block needle is advanced to contact the median nerve. It is then crossed over the axillary artery to contact the ulnar nerve superficially and then finally behind the artery to the deeper radial nerve. Follow NS procedure if using this technique.
- Local anesthetic spread: Performing a test dose with D5W is recommended prior to local anesthetic application to visualize spread and confirm nerve localization. A proper injection is indicated by fluid spread completely around the nerve structure, with nerve movement away from the needle tip. Improper injection (e.g., injection outside the sheath) is indicated by a partial asymmetrical fluid expansion not immediately adjacent to the nerve structure.

COMMENTS

- Although multiple-injection NS technique has been used extensively for this and other blocks, it is important to consider that some spread of the local anesthetic solution will occur and hypesthesia can occur in an unpredictable fashion, limiting the identification of subsequent nerves. A recent evaluation of a two-injection technique—with one injection posterior to the axillary artery and the other to the musculocutaneous nerve—demonstrated that this approach may be as effective as blocking each of the ulnar, median, radial, and musculoskeletal nerves separately,[129] potentially minimizing unwanted spread to adjacent nerves.
- If forearm anesthesia is required and the musculocutaneous nerve was not localized previously, supplementary anesthesia of the musculocutaneous nerve should be attained using some reliable means of nerve localization (i.e., NS and/or US guidance) rather than blind injection into the coracobrachialis muscle. US imaging 1 to 2 cm distal to the axillary block location can clearly identify the muscle and usually the nerve.
- Intercostobrachial and medial brachial cutaneous nerve blocks can be achieved by subcutaneous injections (5 mL in total) on

the medial surface of the upper arm all the way from the biceps to triceps muscles. Both of these nerves are relatively small and can be difficult to visualize under US; however, local anesthetics can be infiltrated superficially above the median nerve toward the triceps.

- Perivascular infiltration and transarterial approaches are also traditionally performed for axillary block, although these techniques have been replaced by advanced technologies such as NS and US.
- For continuous nerve blocks, a 17- to 18-gauge Tuohy needle is required to facilitate catheter placement. Securing the catheter in the axilla may be challenging and may require a short tunnel to stabilize the catheter.
- Axillary approaches to the brachial plexus are associated with minimal complications compared to more proximal brachial plexus blocks. Neuropathy from needle puncture or intraneural injection of local anesthetic is the foremost consideration, although this may be reduced with US imaging and careful attention to injection pressures during the block. Hematoma can occur if the axillary artery is punctured, but this is a self-limiting complication.

Terminal Upper Extremity Nerve Blocks

PNB in the upper extremity are of particular value as rescue blocks to supplement incomplete surgical anesthesia and to provide long-lasting selective analgesia in the postoperative period. The peripheral nerves may be individually blocked at midhumeral, elbow, or wrist locations, depending on the specific nerve. If using US guidance, the elbow and forearm regions appear to be the most suitable block regions, and blocks at these sites may improve the accuracy of nerve localization and local anesthetic spread. The wrist is highly populated with tendons and fascial tissues (e.g., flexor and extensor retinaculae), which, on US, can be difficult to distinguish from nerves and which may also obscure visualization of nerves. With the help of color Doppler, US can be used to clearly identify the nerves at many desirable locations as they are often situated near blood vessels (Table 35-1). This chapter will focus on blocks for which NS and US imaging are most amenable but will also comment on nerve blocks at the wrist. Block
5 of the musculocutaneous nerve at the midhumeral level is discussed in the section on Axillary Block. Figures 35-11 and 35-12 illustrate the courses and cutaneous innervation of the terminal nerves of the upper extremity.

Radial Nerve

The radial nerve can be blocked at the anterosuperior aspect of the lateral epicondyle of the humerus. The radial nerve supplies the posterior compartments of the arm and forearm including skin and subcutaneous tissues. It also innervates skin on the posterior aspect of the hand laterally near the base of the thumb and the dorsal aspect of the index and the lateral half of the ring finger up to the distal interphalangeal crease. For radial nerve blocks, the patient is positioned supine with their arm slightly abducted and laterally rotated, with the elbow extended.

PROCEDURE USING NERVE STIMULATION TECHNIQUE

- Landmarks: A line is drawn on the anterior elbow between the medial and lateral epicondyles of the humerus. The radial nerve is located beneath this intercondylar line, approximately 1 to 2 cm lateral to the biceps tendon. This position should be marked with an "X."
- Needling: A 30- to 50-mm, 22- to 24-gauge insulated needle is used and a skin wheal is raised at the "X." The needle is then inserted perpendicular to the plane passing through the humeral epicondyles.
- Nerve localization: The correct response to radial NS at this location is extension (dorsiflexion) of the wrist and digits on the operative side. Elbow extension should not be elicited, since the branch to the long head of the triceps has branched off proximally.
- Injection: Approximately 5 mL of local anesthetic is injected under low pressure.

PROCEDURE USING ULTRASOUND IMAGING (FIG. 35-22)

- Scanning: A linear probe in the frequency range of 5 to 10 MHz is suitable for scanning in most cases. The radial nerve can first be located proximally at the level of the spiral (radial) groove of the humerus where it lies immediately adjacent to the humerus and posteromedial to the deep brachial (profunda brachii) artery of the arm. The patient's arm should be internally rotated and placed with the hand over the abdomen on the opposite side of the body. The spiral groove lies immediately distal and posterior to the deltoid tubercle. Subsequent tracing of the nerve from this humeral location to the anterolateral elbow may facilitate its precise localization. The probe can be rotated slowly to scan the nerve both in the longitudinal and transverse planes at the elbow for confirmation of its location.
- Appearance: At the spiral groove of the humerus, the bone is quite superficial and appears deep to the hypoechoic triceps brachii muscle as a clearly demarcated hyperechoic oval shape with dark shadowing in its interior (not shown). The nerve appears oval and predominantly hyperechoic and is located in the posterior aspect of the humerus and immediately adjacent to the small, pulsatile deep brachial (profunda brachii) artery (as verified with Doppler). At a point just proximal to the anterior compartment of the elbow, the humerus appears to have changed shape and appears smaller and almost rectangular in cross section. The hyperechoic radial nerve now lies at some distance from the humerus and is sandwiched between the brachialis and brachioradialis muscles; it remains oval in shape.
- Needling: A 30- to 50-mm, 22-gauge insulated needle is suitable if using NS. The needle can be aligned using both IP and OOP (Fig. 35-22) approaches to block the nerve at the anterosuperior aspect of the lateral epicondyle of the humerus. The nerve should be blocked slightly above the elbow since it divides into deep and superficial branches approximately 2 cm above the elbow. The block needle is advanced to approach the target nerve on its side, preferably avoiding direct needle contact with the nerve.
- Local anesthetic spread: Performing a test dose with D5W is recommended prior to local anesthetic application to visualize spread and confirm nerve localization. The aim is to inject approximately 5 mL of local anesthetic and observe spread around the nerve circumferentially.

COMMENTS

- Needle contact with the humerus indicates that the needle is too deep, while deep needle penetration without bone contact indicates that the needle is lateral to the humerus (beyond the bone).
- The radial nerve can be blocked at the wrist or even lateral distal forearm adjacent to the radial artery. At the wrist, 3 mL of solution is injected into the anatomic "snuffbox" formed

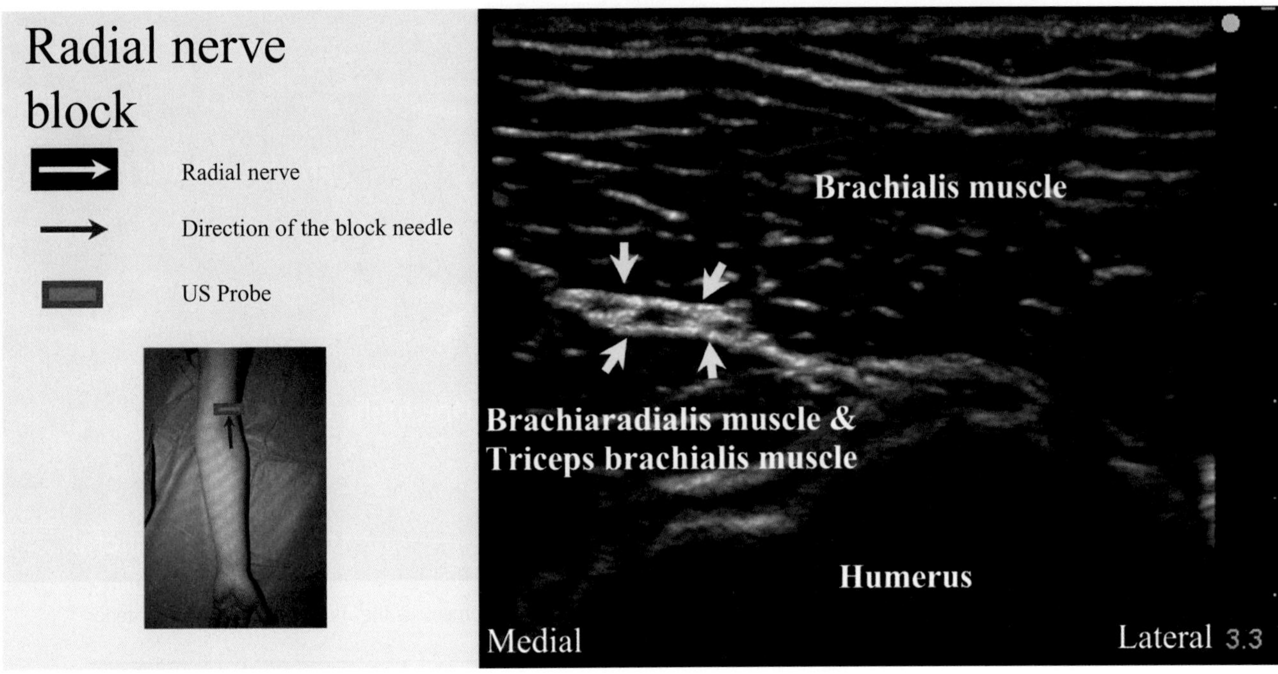

FIGURE 35-22. Ultrasound-guided radial nerve block using OOP needle alignment to a linear probe at the anterolateral elbow. The ideal placement will be a few centimeters above the elbow, where the nerve has not yet divided into superficial and deep branches.

by the tendons of the extensor pollicis longus and extensor pollicis brevis tendons. A subcutaneous wheal is then raised from this point, extending over the dorsum of the wrist 3 to 4 cm onto the back of the hand. This approach is suboptimal for most procedures since the nerve divides immediately beyond the elbow and continues as the superficial radial (sensory) and deep posterior interosseous (motor) nerves.

Median Nerve

The median nerve can be blocked at the midline of the anterior elbow or at the mid-to-distal aspect of the anterior forearm (Fig. 35-23). The nerve is located adjacent (medial) to the brachial artery at the elbow, facilitating its localization here. In the forearm, the nerve can be located at its position lateral to the ulnar nerve. The nerve supplies the skin anteriorly on the medial surface of the thumb, palm, and digits two to four, and posteriorly on the distal third of the second to fourth digits. It causes flexion at the metacarpophalangeal joints and extension at the interphalangeal joints of digits two and three. The nerve innervates muscles which produce flexion and opposition of the thumb, middle, and index fingers and pronation and flexion of the wrist. For blocks at the anterior wrist or anterior distal forearm, the patient's arm should be positioned next to the torso, with the elbow flexed slightly and the hand free to allow a wrist or thumb flexion response elicited by NS.

PROCEDURE USING NERVE STIMULATION TECHNIQUE. At the elbow:

- Landmarks: As with radial nerve block, an intercondylar line is drawn, and the nerve is located where this line crosses the pulsation of the brachial artery, usually 1 cm to the ulnar side of the biceps brachii tendon.

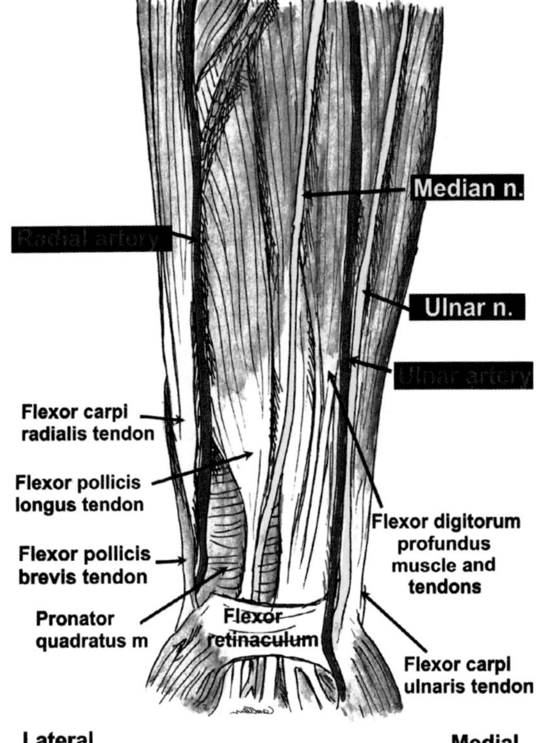

FIGURE 35-23. An illustration of the anterior forearm showing the courses of the median and ulnar nerves. The ulnar artery is a reliable landmark to localize the ulnar nerve when using ultrasound imaging.

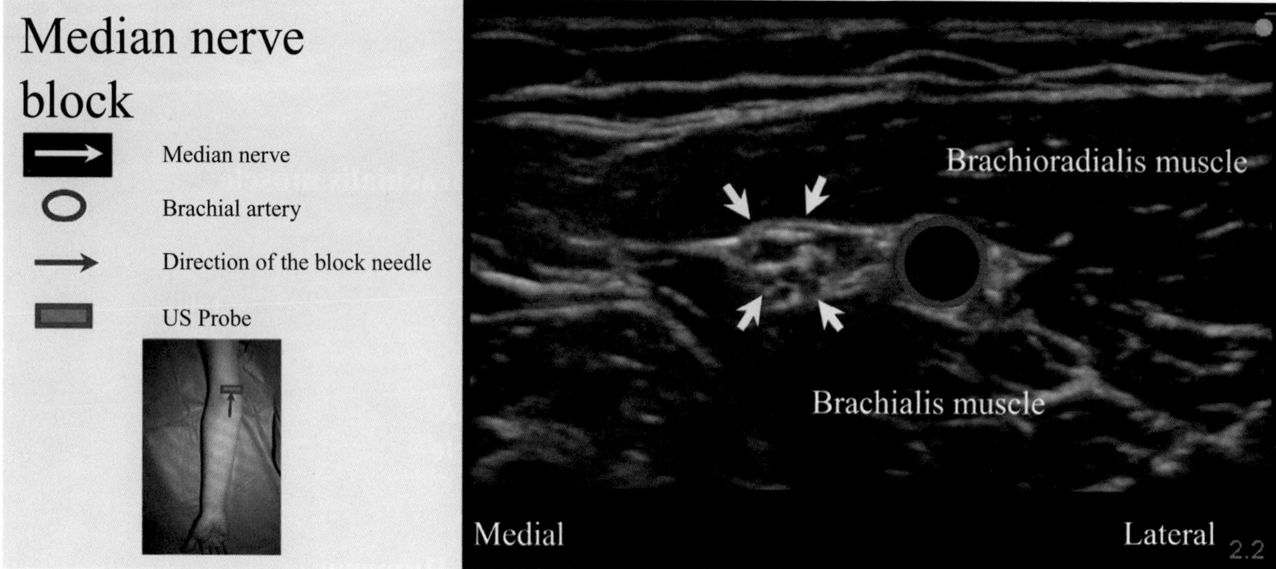

FIGURE 35-24. Ultrasound-guided median nerve block using OOP needle alignment at the medial aspect of the anterior elbow. The nerve lies medial to the large anechoic brachial artery.

- Needling: Using a 30- to 50-mm insulated needle, a skin wheal is raised at the point identified with landmarks (above), and the needle is introduced perpendicularly at this point.
- Nerve localization: Nerve responses to electrical stimulation are sought immediately adjacent to the artery. The optimal NS response for median nerve block at the elbow location is any one of the following or a combination thereof: Flexion and opposition of the thumb, middle, and index fingers; flexion of the wrist; and pronation of the forearm.
- Injection: Injection of 5 mL of local anesthetic should be sufficient to block this nerve. Care should be taken to avoid the intravascular and the intraneural injection.

In the forearm:

- It may be difficult to blindly locate this nerve in the forearm using NS, although the technique of transcutaneous electrical stimulation,[17] or similarly percutaneous electrode guidance,[18,130] can be used to locate the nerve using a probe placed on or indenting the skin's surface. Once the nerve has been localized, an insulated needle is inserted perpendicular to the plane of the forearm and NS responses are sought. A similar volume of local anesthetic should suffice.

PROCEDURE USING ULTRASOUND IMAGING (ELBOW, FIG. 35-24; FOREARM, FIG. 35-25)

- Scanning: A high-frequency (10 to 15 MHz) linear probe can be used to capture a transverse view of the nerve and localize the brachial artery, both at the elbow, where the nerve lies medial to both the artery and then the tendon of the biceps brachii muscle, and in the anterolateral forearm, where it lies lateral to the ulnar nerve and artery (localizing the ulnar nerve first will help identify the median nerve). Color Doppler may be used to confirm the location of the above named arteries.
- Appearance: At the elbow, the median nerve can be identified at approximately 1 to 2 cm in depth as a hyperechoic, yet distinctly honeycomb-like structure, lying medial to the anechoic pulsatile brachial artery. Deep to the neurovascular structures lies the musculature of the superior aspect of the elbow (pronator teres and brachialis muscles) as a hypoechoic homogeneous mass. At the forearm, the nerve appears oval-shaped and lateral to the ulnar artery.
- Needling: Both OOP and IP techniques can be used for either block location. For OOP needling at the elbow (Fig. 35-24), after adjusting the US image to have the nerve located in the middle of the screen, insert a 30- to 50-mm insulated needle perpendicular to the transversely placed probe at a 45- to 60-degree angle. NS procedure should be followed if using combined technique. IP technique, with the needle in a medial to lateral direction, may be advantageous at the elbow to allow easy tracking of the needle to ensure it avoids puncturing the brachial artery.
- Local anesthetic spread: After performing a test dose with D5W, the aim is to spread approximately 5 mL of local anesthetic around the nerve in a circular fashion, avoiding nerve contact and obtaining complete blockade.

COMMENTS

- The median nerve lies deep to the flexor retinaculum at the wrist, and there is always the potential risk of causing carpal tunnel syndrome due to elevated pressure within the tunnel from the injection solution. For this reason, the elbow or forearm locations for blocking the median nerve are the more logical choices.
- At the wrist, the median nerve lies between the tendons of the palmaris longus and the flexor carpi radialis muscles. If only the palmaris longus muscle can be felt, the nerve lies just to the radial side of its tendon. A skin wheal is raised, and a needle is inserted until it pierces the deep fascia. An injection of 3 to 5 mL of local anesthetic is sufficient to produce anesthesia.
- Blood aspirated into the tubing during elbow block indicates brachial artery puncture and the needle should be reinserted after applying pressure to the puncture site until hemostasis is achieved. Contact with the humerus indicates that the needle is too deep. Localized contraction of the arm muscles (e.g., elbow flexion and/or forearm pronation) indicates stimulation of the local muscles and also that the needle is likely too deep.

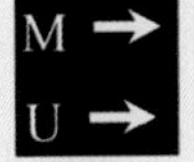

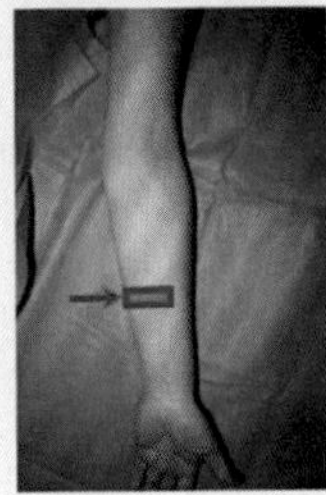

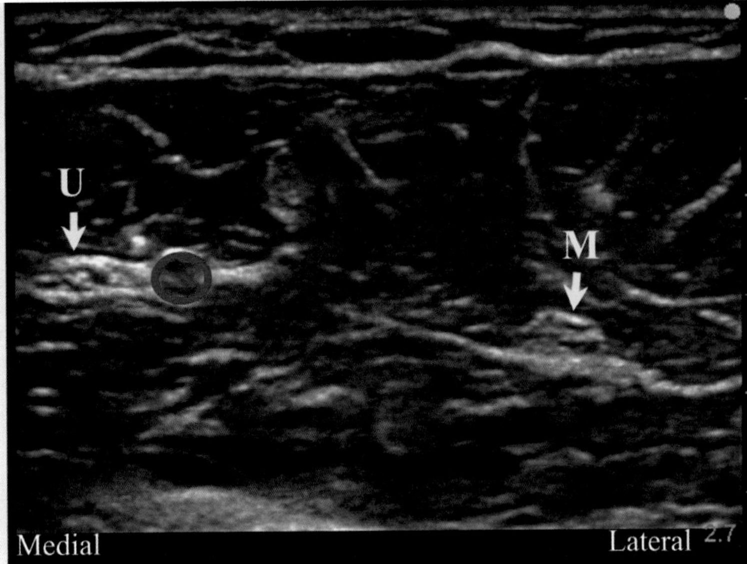

FIGURE 35-25. Ultrasound-guided ulnar nerve block in the middistal forearm using IP needle alignment to a small footprint linear ("hockey stick") probe. The ideal block location to avoid arterial puncture is where the nerve has yet to fully approach the ulnar artery.

Ulnar Nerve

In the periphery, the ulnar nerve can be blocked at the elbow, forearm, or wrist. Ulnar nerve block may be used for rescue analgesia or surgical anesthesia for surgery on the fifth digit. At the junction of the distal third and proximal two-thirds of the medial forearm, the nerve is commonly located just medial to the pulsatile ulnar artery (Fig. 35-23). US-guided technique is advised when using this block location in order to avoid the artery and localize the nerve more accurately. The ulnar nerve innervates muscles that produce flexion of the ring (fourth) and little (fifth) fingers and ulnar deviation of wrist. It supplies the skin over the medial surface (anterior and posterior) of the hand and digits four and five. Before performing the block, the patient's arm should be flexed at the elbow by 30 degrees and forearm supinated. The forearm can rest on an arm board with an additional pillow under the wrist. Prepare the needle insertion site and skin surface with an antiseptic solution. Prepare the US probe surface by applying a sterile sheath or adhesive dressing to it before needling (not shown).

PROCEDURE USING NERVE STIMULATION TECHNIQUE. At the elbow:

- Anesthetizing the ulnar nerve at the elbow may be uncomfortable for the patient. NS is not routinely used for localizing the ulnar nerve at the elbow, since the nerve is easily located (and palpated) in the cubital tunnel (ulnar groove) between the medial epicondyle of the humerus and the olecranon process of the ulna. Only a small volume (1 to 4 mL) of local anesthetic should be injected if performing the block at this location.

In the forearm:

- Similar to the median nerve, it may be difficult to blindly locate this nerve in the forearm using NS. Transcutaneous electrical stimulation[17] or percutaneous electrode guidance[18,19] can be used to locate the nerve. Once the nerve has been localized, an insulated needle attached to a nerve stimulator is inserted perpendicular to the plane of the forearm and appropriate motor responses are sought. The correct responses for ulnar nerve block at this location are flexion of the ring (fourth) and little (fifth) fingers and ulnar deviation of the wrist. Injection of 5 mL of local anesthetic is sufficient to block the nerve at the forearm. Combined US- and NS-guided technique provides good localization and accuracy with local anesthetic spread.

PROCEDURE USING ULTRASOUND IMAGING (FOREARM, FIG. 35-25)

- Scanning: A high-frequency (10 to 15 MHz) linear probe is often used for this block. The probe is placed transversely just above the midforearm level to view the ulnar nerve in short axis as it approaches the ulnar artery. The nerve is positioned above the ulna and the belly of the flexor carpi ulnaris, on the anterior surface of the arm, rather than medially to contact the bone. The operator should scan downward slowly until the pulsatile artery and nerve are viewed adjacent to each other (Doppler may be valuable here) and retract the scanhead slightly so the artery and nerve appear clearly as separate structures (Fig. 35-25).
- Appearance: The nerve in short axis is seen as a honeycomb-like, oval-shaped structure, including hypoechoic fascicular structures surrounded significantly by hyperechoic tissue. The adjacent ulnar artery appears anechoic and roughly similar in size to the nerve and lateral to it. The median nerve may be seen at the lateral edge of the image and appears similar to the ulnar nerve in size and shape.
- Needling: During IP needling, the image should be adjusted so that the nerve is toward the most lateral edge of the screen for good visibility of the needle shaft (not shown in Fig. 35-25). A short (20 to 30 mm) needle can be used in a medial-to-lateral direction to reduce the risk of vascular puncture.
- Local anesthetic spread: The aim is to spread approximately 5 mL of local anesthetic around the nerve in a circular fashion in order to avoid nerve contact but obtain a complete block. The local anesthetic injection will appear as an expansion of hypoechogenicity surrounding the nerve, which may separate the nerve from the artery.

COMMENTS

- When performing regional anesthesia in the elbow, direct injection after eliciting a paresthesia or direct injection into the groove under pressure is not advised because of the risk of damage to the nerve. Small volumes (3 to 5 mL) of local anesthetic should be used.
- During nerve block in the forearm, blood withdrawal into the tubing suggests ulnar artery puncture, and the needle should be reinserted after holding pressure. Contact with the ulna indicates that the needle is too deep.
- US imaging facilitates the unique approach of blocking the ulnar nerve in the forearm. This technique may reduce complications such as ulnar nerve neuritis or neuropraxia compared to blocks at the cubital tunnel behind the medial epicondyle.
- A linear or curved array US probe with a small footprint (26 mm; e.g., a "hockey stick" probe) may be used. This size probe is helpful for easy manipulation on the forearm and for good alignment of the needle using IP technique.
- At the wrist, the ulnar nerve lies between the ulnar artery and the tendon of the flexor carpi ulnaris muscle. A skin wheal is raised at the level of the styloid process on the palmar side of the forearm between these two landmarks, a small-gauge needle is inserted, and 3 mL of solution is injected into the area, with or without paresthesias.

Intravenous Regional Anesthesia (Bier Block)

Without using NS or US, arm anesthesia can be provided by the injection of local anesthetic into the venous system below an occluding tourniquet.

Procedure

- A small-gauge (20 or 22) intravenous catheter is inserted and taped on the dorsum of the hand in the arm to be blocked. A heparin lock or small syringe is attached, and saline is injected to maintain patency. A pneumatic tourniquet is applied over the upper arm. The tourniquet pressure should be set to 2.5 times the systolic blood pressure. The tourniquet should be inflated to confirm that the pressure is sufficient to occlude distal arterial blood flow and should be deflated before starting the block.
- The arm is elevated to promote venous drainage. An Esmarch bandage is then wrapped tightly around the limb from distal to proximal to produce further exsanguination. After exsanguination, the tourniquet is inflated to 300 mm Hg or 2.5 times the patient's systolic blood pressure and is again tested for adequate occlusion of the distal radial pulse.
- The arm is returned to the horizontal position, a 50-mL syringe with 0.5% lidocaine (without preservative) is attached to the previously inserted cannula, and the contents are injected slowly. The forearm discolors, and the patient perceives a transient "pins and needles" sensation and warmth as anesthesia ensues over the following 5 minutes. Epinephrine should not be added to the local anesthetic solution.
- For short procedures, the cannula can be removed at this point. If surgery extends beyond 1 hour, the cannula can be left in place and reinjected after 90 minutes.
- Beyond 45 minutes of surgery, many patients experience discomfort at the level of the tourniquet. Special "double-cuff" tourniquets are available for this block to alleviate this problem. The distal cuff is inflated first followed by the proximal cuff. The distal cuff is then deflated, allowing anesthesia to be induced in the area under the distal cuff. If discomfort ensues, the distal cuff is inflated over the anesthetized area of skin, and the uncomfortable proximal cuff is released. This step is critical because the major risk of this procedure is premature release of the local anesthetic solution into the circulation. If a double cuff is used, both cuffs should be tested before starting and the proper sequence for inflation and deflation meticulously followed. The potential for leakage of anesthetic into the circulation is greater with the narrower cuffs used in the double setup. Because the shifting process also increases the potential for unintentional release of anesthetic, the use of a single, wider cuff may be better for short procedures.
- If surgery is completed in less than 20 minutes, the tourniquet is left inflated for at least that total period of time. If 40 minutes has elapsed, the tourniquet can be deflated as a single maneuver. Between 20 and 40 minutes, the cuff can be deflated, reinflated immediately, and finally deflated after 1 minute to delay the sudden absorption of anesthetic into the systemic circulation, although this may not truly lower the eventual peak plasma local anesthetic levels achieved.
- Duration of anesthesia is minimal beyond the time of tourniquet release. Although bupivacaine may produce a slight prolongation of analgesia, the cardiotoxicity of systemic levels of bupivacaine makes this drug contraindicated for a Bier block.

Comments

- The simplicity of this technique is offset by the potentially significant risk of systemic local anesthetic toxicity if the tourniquet fails or is released prematurely. Complications related to systemic toxicity include seizures, cardiac arrest, and death; other noted complications include nerve damage, compartment syndrome, and thrombophlebitis.[131] Careful testing of the tourniquet and slow injection of solution into a peripheral (not antecubital) vein will reduce the chance of leakage under the tourniquet. Systemic blood levels are time-dependent, and careful attention should be paid to the sequence of tourniquet release and to patient monitoring during this period. A separate intravenous site for injection of resuscitation drugs is needed as well as ready availability of all appropriate resuscitative equipment. With careful attention to these details, this technique is one of the most effective and reliable available to the anesthesiologist.

Trunk Nerve Blocks

Anesthesia of the abdomen and chest is often obtained most simply with spinal and epidural injections of local anesthetics, but peripheral block of the spinal nerves in the paravertebral space or of the intercostal or inguinal nerves is quite suitable for many uses. This is particularly relevant when either a narrow band of anesthesia (intercostal or paravertebral) or reduced motor block is preferable. In addition, epidural injection may be hazardous because of infection or coagulopathy. Epidural anesthesia also carries concerns of systemic hypotension and epidural hematoma, which can limit its use for some patients.[132] In many clinical situations, it may be desirable to use intercostal blocks to overcome the combined anesthesia of the somatic and sympathetic fibers that occurs with neuraxial blocks; the sympathetic nerves separate from their somatic counterparts early in their course, which makes independent somatic and sympathetic blockade a practical consideration. Likewise, although paravertebral blocks may result in both somatic and sympathetic blocks, hemodynamic responses are often less than those encountered during epidural block. Sympathetic blocks are commonly performed at the major ganglia, particularly the stellate, celiac, and lumbar plexus. These blocks may require multiple injections and are technically more difficult than axial anesthesia, but they offer advantages in certain clinical situations. These blocks are not considered here, and the reader is referred to Chapter 56.

Ilioinguinal and iliohypogastric nerve blocks are used for procedures in the inguinal area including hernia repair and orchidopexy. A lumbar plexus block is not optimal in these cases, since these nerves exit the plexus more cranially (L1–L2) than those nerves targeted by the lumbar plexus block (L3–L5). Transversus abdominis plane (TAP) block[133,134] and rectus sheath blocks[135,136] can also be performed for abdominal, umbilical, or other midline surgical procedures and are often performed bilaterally. Approaches to the rectus sheath block the terminal branches of the 9th, 10th, and 11th intercostal nerves within the rectus sheath; ideally, injection is between the posterior rectus sheath and the rectus abdominis muscle. The TAP block aims to impede innervation of the abdominal wall up to the level of T8 by injecting local anesthetic between the transversus abdominis and internal oblique muscles. The initial technique of multiple injections of local anesthetic in the abdominal wall was modified to a single injection using the landmark technique by locating the "lumbar triangle of Petit."[137] With the advent of US-guided regional techniques, in which the layers of musculature can be identified, needle insertion and local anesthetic deposition between the fascial layers can be visualized in real time. Thus, the approach to the TAP block has evolved yet again and become more common.

Intercostal Nerve Block

Anesthesia of the intercostal nerves provides both motor and sensory anesthesia of the abdominal wall from the xiphoid to the pubis. Intercostal nerve blockade is used for various conditions of acute and chronic pain affecting the thorax and upper abdomen (e.g., postoperative analgesia after thoracotomies, various cardiac surgeries, and both open and laparoscopic cholecystectomies). It can be performed through several means, including continuous infusions into the subpleural space, through interpleural catheters, and by direct intercostal nerve block. The surgical site (i.e., intraoperative anatomical access) determines the available options.

These nerve blocks involve injections along the easily palpated sharp posterior angulation of the ribs, which occurs between 5 and 7 cm from the midline in the back. The blocks may be performed more laterally (8 to 10 cm from the midline)[138] or more medially (immediately beyond the transverse processes). The levels of T1–T5 may be most amenable to paravertebral block due to the overlying scapula and bulky paraspinal musculature at this region. Establishing blockade of five or six levels of intercostal nerves is a useful anesthetic procedure for providing analgesia and motor relaxation for upper abdominal procedures such as cholecystectomy and gastric surgery. Unilateral blockade of these nerves is a useful treatment for the pain of rib fracture and also serves to reduce postoperative analgesia requirements in patients with subcostal incisions. Several segments must be blocked in each of these applications because of the overlap in supply of the intercostal nerves. This technique is also useful in reducing the pain associated with the insertion of chest tubes or percutaneous biliary drainage procedures.

For intercostal blocks, the patient may be in the lateral, sitting, or prone position. For operative anesthesia, the prone position is most practical. A pillow is placed under the abdomen to provide slight flexion of the thoracic spine. The arms are draped over the edge of the stretcher or operating table so that the scapula falls away laterally from the midline. The anesthesiologist stands at the patient's side. Most anesthesiologists prefer to stand on the side that allows their dominant hand to hold the syringe at the caudad end of the patient.

Procedure Using Landmark-based Technique

LANDMARKS. The reader is referred to the Clinical Anatomy section above for descriptions of the locations of the relevant landmarks. The spinous processes in the midline from T6 to T12 are marked. The ribs are then identified along the line of their most extreme posterior angulation. The 6th and 12th ribs are marked first at their inferior borders, and a line is drawn between these two points. The rest of the ribs between them are identified, and a mark is placed on the inferior border of each rib along the angled parasagittal plane identified by the first line between the 6th and 12th ribs.

NEEDLING. After aseptic preparation, light sedation is provided for the patient, and a skin wheal is raised at each mark on the inferior border of each respective rib. Starting with the lowest rib, the index finger of the cephalad hand retracts the skin above the identifying mark in a cephalad direction. Using the other hand, the anesthesiologist inserts a needle (22 gauge, 3.75 cm) directly onto the rib, maintaining a constant 10-degree cephalad angulation. After contact is made with the rib, the cephalad traction is slowly released, the cephalad hand takes over the needle and syringe, and the needle is allowed to "walk" down to below the rib at the same angle. The needle is then advanced approximately 4 mm under the rib.

INJECTION. Once in the groove, aspiration is performed and 3 to 5 mL of a local anesthetic solution is injected. The needling and injection procedure is repeated for each segmental level and for both sides if applicable. Since the intercostal space is highly vascularized, local anesthetics are absorbed rapidly, and toxic levels of local anesthetic may be encountered when using large volumes, which can quickly lead to neurologic or cardiovascular sequelae. Maximum doses should be calculated and followed carefully for these blocks.

Procedure Using Ultrasound Imaging

The ribs can be easily visualized with the use of US. A high-frequency (5 to 15 MHz) probe can be used and is placed in a longitudinal axis. The rib will appear as a hyperechoic line casting a hypoechoic bony shadow underneath (Fig. 35-26). The pleurae can also be seen to "glitter" as they slide with respiration. The remainder of the procedure will be similar to that of blind technique. If a more medial (proximal) intercostal nerve block is desired, such as to relieve the pain of herpes zoster or of proximal rib fractures, US imaging of the costotransverse joint and ribs may be helpful. The section below on paravertebral block describes and illustrates this imaging.

Comments

- Intercostal nerve blocks can be supplemented by a number of somatic paravertebral nerve blocks or sympathetic block of the celiac plexus. Care should be taken to adjust the total dose of drug in these combined techniques so that the maximal recommended amounts are not exceeded.
- The advantages with intercostal block over sole intravenous opioid use include superior analgesia, opioid sparing, improved

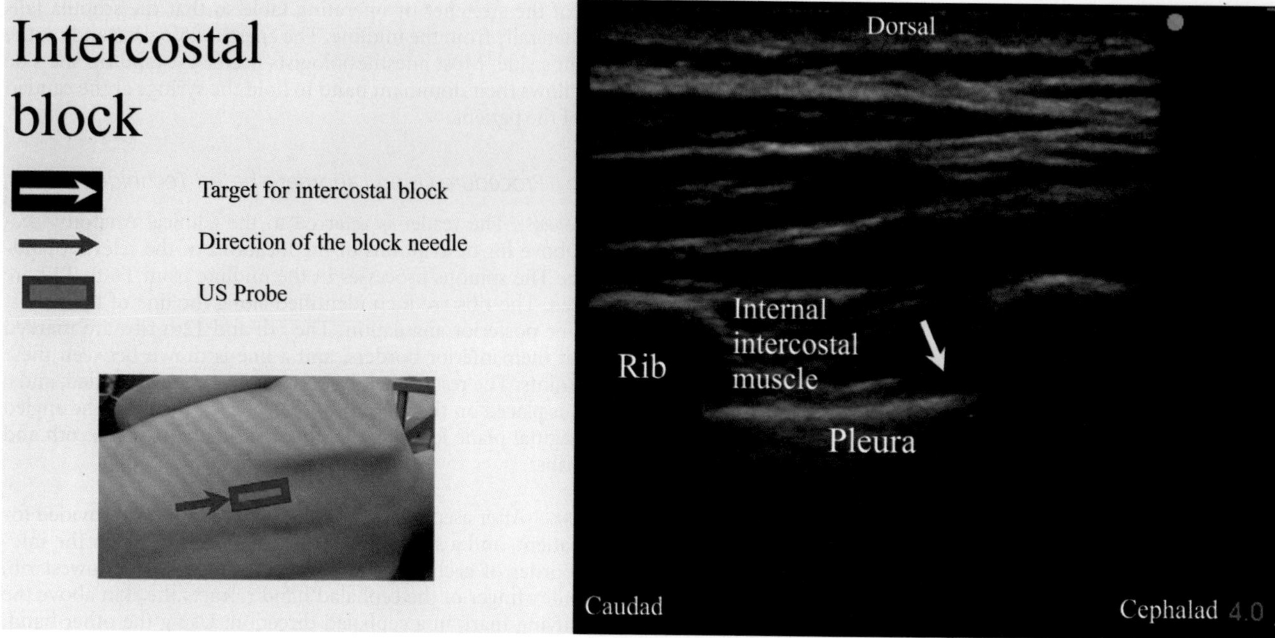

FIGURE 35-26. Ultrasound image showing the hyperechoic lines of the ribs casting a hypoechoic bony shadow. The pleura is the hyperechoic line deep to that of the ribs and has a glittery appearance, especially on respiration.

pulmonary mechanics (including earlier extubation), and reduced central nervous system depression.[138] Intercostal blocks are often used in addition to systemic analgesia (e.g., intravenous, patient-controlled analgesia).

- Despite frequent concern about the incidence of pneumothorax with intercostal blocks, this complication is rare, especially when US is used in experienced hands. This depends primarily on maintaining strict safety features of the described technique. Emphasis should be placed on absolute control of the syringe and needle at all times, particularly during injection.
- A common complication is related to the sedation required to perform this block in the prone position. Overdose can lead to airway obstruction and respiratory depression in the prone position. Attention must be paid to the patient's mental status because this block produces the highest blood levels of local anesthetics compared to any other regional anesthetic technique. When the block is performed for postoperative pain relief, the dose should be reduced to 0.25% bupivacaine or ropivacaine to minimize the chance for toxicity.
- It is possible to produce partial spinal or epidural anesthesia if the injection is made close to the midline and the anesthetic tracks along a dural sleeve to the epidural or subarachnoid space. Respiratory insufficiency can also be seen if the intercostal muscles are blocked in a patient who depends on them for ventilation. Patients with chronic obstructive disease with ineffective diaphragm motion are not good candidates for this technique.

Paravertebral Block

Techniques

This block technique is useful for segmental anesthesia, particularly of the upper thoracic segments. It is also useful if a blockade more proximal (central) than that of the intercostal nerves is needed, such as to relieve the pain of herpes zoster or of a proximal rib fracture. The thoracic paravertebral block is used for breast surgery and perioperatively for thoracic surgery. Thoracolumbar paravertebral anesthesia is commonly used for inguinal herniorrhaphy and postoperative analgesia following hip surgery. Lumbar paravertebral blockade has been used successfully for outpatient hernia operations, providing significant postoperative analgesia.

Single-injection paravertebral block used for surgical anesthesia has been shown to surpass general anesthesia with respect to postoperative pain relief, incidence of vomiting, and pain during mobility.[139] Paravertebral blocks are considered "unilateral epidurals," since they selectively block spinal nerves on the side of anesthetic application, although they also have the potential for epidural spread (i.e., they can be bilateral if desired). The anesthesia includes both somatic and sympathetic effects, with a reduced hemodynamic response (e.g., hypotension) as compared to epidural anesthesia. This nerve block requires excellent knowledge of paravertebral anatomy but can be easily performed with experience.

The upper five ribs are more difficult to palpate laterally, and blockade of their associated intercostal nerves is best performed with a paravertebral injection. This approach is technically more difficult and has slightly greater potential for complications because of the proximity of the lung and intervertebral foramina. The paravertebral block can be used at any level. At the lumbar spine, some prefer to perform lumbar plexus block to reduce the number of injections and avoid sympathetic block. The injection is made into the triangular paravertebral space where the spinal nerve has just left the intervertebral foramen. The nerve may be difficult to localize using bony landmarks in a blind fashion, and larger volumes of local anesthetic are often required. NS has been used to localize the nerve. US can be performed prior to the block to improve bony landmark identification, particularly for patients who have an obese habitus or a spinal deformity. However, real-time US guidance can be challenging and may offer limited additional value from preprocedural landmark identification, since the overriding bone tissue reflects the US beam and provides dorsal shadowing, which obscures imaging (especially of the needle) to the depth of the paravertebral space.

Paravertebral block is performed with the patient in the lateral, sitting, or prone position, the latter using a pillow placed under the patient's abdomen to produce flexion of the thoracic and lumbar spine.

Procedure Using Nerve Stimulation or Loss-of-resistance Technique

LANDMARKS. The paravertebral approach varies depending on the spinal level and the respective orientation of the vertebral spinous and transverse processes (Clinical Anatomy). Thus, paravertebral blocks in the upper thoracic region are performed at each level by identifying the spinous process of the vertebra above the level to be blocked; in the lumbar region, the spinous process of the level to be blocked is used to locate the transverse process. The appropriate spinous processes in the region to be blocked are marked and transverse lines are drawn across the cephalad border and extended laterally to overlie the transverse process (approximately 2.5 cm) (Fig. 35-27). Finally, the transverse processes are marked individually or by drawing a vertical line parallel to the spine joining the ends of the transverse lines. For a diagnostic block, a single nerve may need to be anesthetized. For pain control, several levels must be identified. The injection of at least three segments (as in intercostal blockade) is required to produce reliable segmental block because of sensory overlap from multiple nerves.

NEEDLING. After aseptic skin preparation and patient sedation, skin wheals are raised at the marked transverse processes. A 22-gauge, 70-mm insulated needle is introduced through the skin wheal in the sagittal plane and directed slightly cephalad to contact the transverse process (usually at a depth of 2 to 4 cm in the thoracic region and 5 to 8 cm in the lumbar region), or, oftentimes likely, the costotransverse ligament. Gentle cephalad or caudad exploration may be required to identify the bone. The depth of the transverse process should be carefully noted on the needle shaft. The needle is now withdrawn from the transverse process to the skin level and reinserted 10 degrees superiorly (to target the spinal nerve corresponding to the spinous process) or inferiorly (corresponding to the vertebral level below the spinous process) and 1 cm deeper than the point of bone contact. The needle should be angled slightly medially to avoid causing pneumothorax. There will be a subtle "give" at the midpoint between these landmarks (spinous and transverse processes), indicating entrance into the paravertebral space.

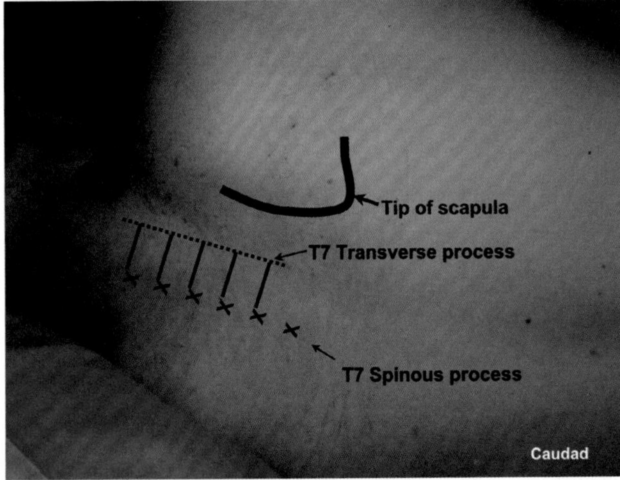

FIGURE 35-27. Landmarks for the paravertebral block at the thoracic spine. The spinous process of the level (e.g., T6) below the block (e.g., T7) is identified and a line is drawn horizontally from the cranial aspect of the spinous process to mark the transverse process. The needle is inserted at appropriate spinal levels at the lateral line marking the transverse processes.

NERVE LOCALIZATION. For NS, an initial current of 2.5 to 5 mA is used and the needle is advanced until contractions of the appropriate muscles (e.g., abdominal muscles with lumbar paravertebral block) are observed, after which the current intensity is reduced to localize the nerves at 0.5 to 0.6 mA. A test dose of local anesthetic will confirm nerve localization with abolishment of the nerve response, resulting from the current dissipation at the needle tip from the conducting solution.[26] For loss of resistance, a 22-gauge Tuohy needle is utilized. After walking off the transverse processes, a "pop" or loss-of-resistance may be felt when entering the paravertebral space.

INJECTION. When the needle has entered the paravertebral space, 3 to 7 mL of local anesthetic is injected after careful aspiration at each site, depending on the number of sites and patient size. Attention must be paid to the total milligram dose injected; the volume required to block each level limits the concentration that can be used and the total number of levels that can be blocked. If lumbar paravertebral injections are combined with intercostal blocks, the concentration and total volume for both blocks may have to be reduced.

Procedure Using Ultrasound Imaging

Imaging for these blocks is often used before block performance (i.e., "preprocedural," "supported," or "off-line" imaging) rather than during (i.e., "real-time" or "on-line" imaging) to identify the deep bony landmarks, including the articular and transverse processes. Real-time US-guided paravertebral block is an advanced block and should only be performed by experienced personnel.

SCANNING. Placing the probe transversely at the midline will provide an overview of the vertebral lamina and processes, as well as costal structures if viewing the thoracic spine (Fig. 35-28). A medial-to-lateral scan using a longitudinally placed probe can then be used to locate and mark important bony landmarks (Fig. 35-29). For this, a 5 to 7 MHz curved-array US probe (lower frequency for obese patients and higher frequency linear probes for thin adult or pediatric patients) is positioned in the sagittal plane on top of the spinous processes of the target thoracic or lumbar region. Subsequent lateral scanning will allow consecutive identification of the lamina, articular and transverse processes, and, in the thoracic spine, the ribs.

APPEARANCE. The initial transverse scan will show a hyperechoic outline of the vertebral spinous and transverse processes, the lamina, and (in the thoracic spine) the associated rib. During the lateral scan with the probe placed longitudinally to the spine, the laminae will appear first as largely overlapping linear structures. The articular processes in long axis appear as "multiple lumps," just lateral to the spinous processes and are short rectangular structures with hyperechoic lines and underlying hypoechoic bony shadowing. Moving laterally, the transverse processes

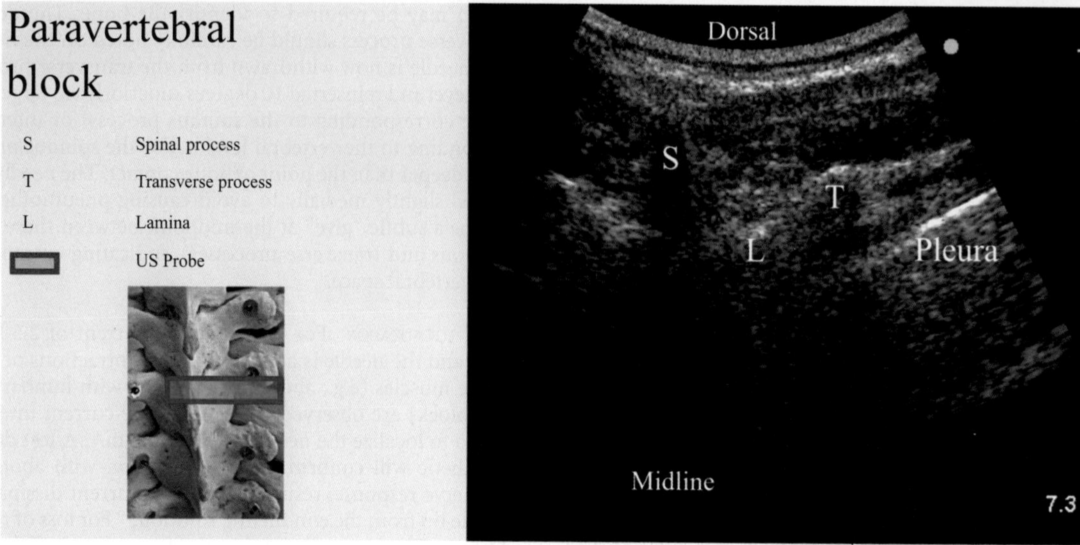

FIGURE 35-28. Probe placement and ultrasound image during paravertebral block in the thoracic spine. The probe is first placed in the midline of the spine to capture a transverse view of the vertebral and costal (if thoracic spine) elements.

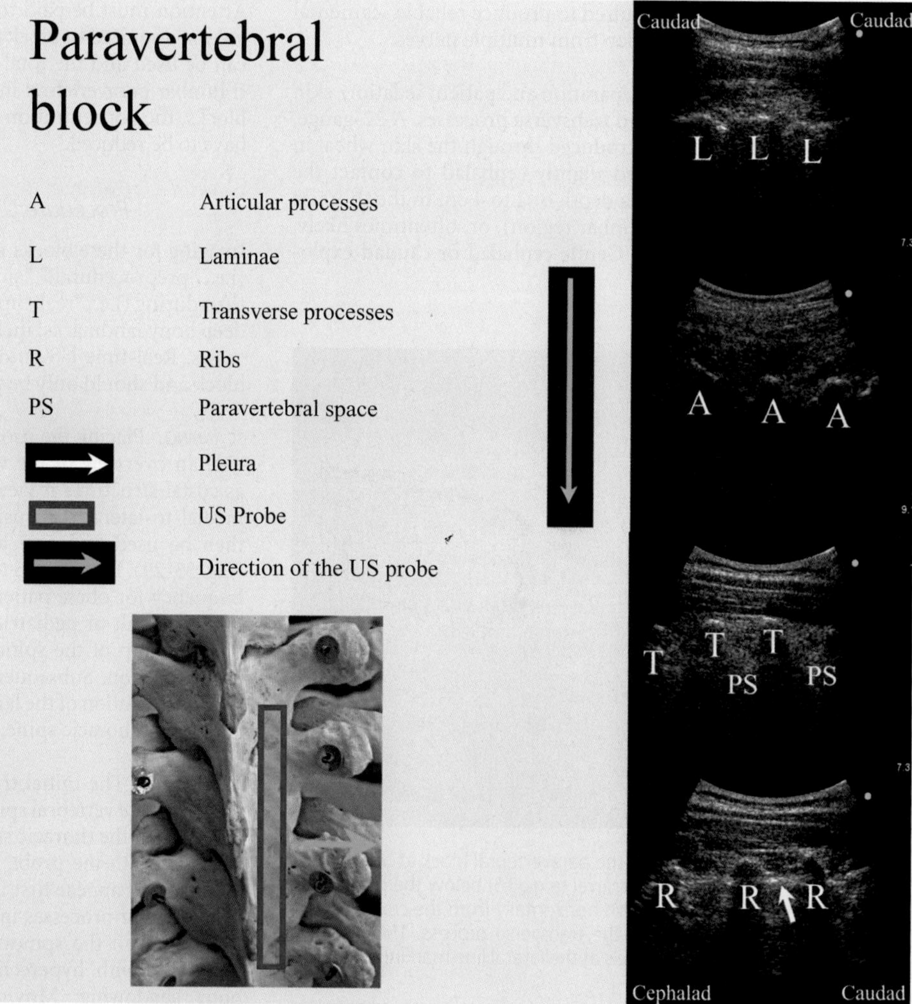

FIGURE 35-29. Ultrasound images from scanning in a medial-to-lateral direction with a curved ultrasound probe placed in the longitudinal axis.

appear and look similar to the articular processes; they will disappear from the view when the probe is moved beyond their tips, which can help distinguish them from the articular processes and mark the lateral block location. Beyond the transverse processes, the rib heads appear as long shadows within hyperechoic borders, deep to the linear hyperechoic muscle fibers of the paravertebral muscles. The paravertebral space lies deep to the transverse processes and the pleura can often be identified between and deep to the transverse process, as well as deep to the ribs.

NEEDLING. Since multiple injections are generally needed to completely cover all the dermatomes of the surgical area in clinical practice, US imaging is more suitable for a preblock assessment ("supported" US) to visualize and measure the depth of needle penetration required for the needle to contact the transverse processes. Needling will be identical to that for the blind technique, with the exception that the depth to the transverse process will be more accurately known. It is possible to perform real-time US guidance, using either IP or OOP needle alignment. The reader is referred to the Comments section for advice related to important precautions when using US guidance.

LOCAL ANESTHETIC SPREAD. Local anesthetic spread will be difficult to view if using real-time guidance during this block. The overlying bones largely reflect the US beam and obstruct visibility beyond into the paravertebral space.

Comments

- Since the paravertebral space is well vascularized, inadvertent vascular puncture will often occur, highlighting the need for frequent aspiration and injection in small aliquots.[140]
- The complication of pneumothorax is more likely with a paravertebral technique than with intercostal block. The needle should be directed medially as it passes below the transverse process and never more than 2 cm beyond the transverse process. If cough or chest pain occurs, a chest radiograph should be performed to rule out pneumothorax.
- Subarachnoid injection is also more likely in the thoracic area because of the extension of the dural sleeves to the level of the intervertebral foramina. Careful aspiration is important but may not prevent the unintentional injection of local anesthetic into the subdural space. Total spinal anesthesia can result with a 5- to 10-mL injection. Systemic toxicity is also a possibility because of the need for relatively large volumes of local anesthetic.
- If attempting real-time US guidance of paravertebral block, it is important to carefully observe the angulation of the needle, and using an IP needle alignment with respect to a longitudinal probe position may be most prudent. The needle should not be inserted with a significant medial direction as there is a risk of spinal cord injury from intraforaminal insertion and injection. Likewise, a lateral direction bears the risk of pneumothorax. If choosing to use real time US guidance during block procedure, please note: (1) with the probe placed in the sagittal/longitudinal plane, OOP needling may be more risky, as it often requires the medial or lateral angulations described above, and (2) an IP needling approach can be more risky when the probe is placed in the coronal/transverse plane.

Transversus Abdominis Plane Block

Procedure Using Landmark Technique

- The patient is positioned supine, and the "Triangle of Petit" is identified with the inferior margin being the iliac crest, the posterior margin being the latissimus dorsi muscle, and the external oblique muscle lies anteriorly.
- A blunted 22-gauge, 50- to 100-mm needle (depending on body habitus) is inserted perpendicularly, immediately posterior to the midaxillary line and above the iliac crest.
- The first and second "pops" will be felt as the needle traverses through the fascial layer of the external and internal oblique muscles, respectively. The needle should be within the plane between the internal oblique and the transversus abdominis.

Procedure Using Ultrasound Imaging

- Scanning: A high-frequency (10 to 15 MHz) linear probe is often used for this block. With the patient lying supine, the probe is placed transversely in the midline to identify the rectus muscles. The probe is then slid laterally, and the three layers of muscles—the external oblique, the internal oblique, and the transversus abdominis—can be identified (Fig. 35-30). The probe should then be positioned above the iliac crest in the anterior axillary line.
- Appearance: The intercostal nerves can be too small and scattered to be identified under US imaging; therefore, the TAP block is predominantly a muscular plane block. The three layers of the abdominal muscles can be clearly identified as they are separated by the hyperechoic fascia. Beneath the abdominal muscles is the peritoneum, which is the hyperechoic line seen on US underneath the transversus abdominis. Below this lies the peritoneal cavity, in which bowel peristalsis can be seen in real time.
- Needling: During IP needling, the image should be adjusted so that the three layers of the abdominal muscles and a small portion of the peritoneal cavity are in view. A 22-gauge, 100-mm needle can be used in a medial-to-lateral direction to reduce the risk of peritoneal puncture, and it should aim toward the muscle plane between the internal oblique and transversus abdominis muscles.
- Local anesthetic spread: The aim is to spread 20 to 30 mL of local anesthetic, without exceeding the toxic dose (e.g., 2 mg/kg of bupivacaine or 3 mg/kg of ropivacaine) on either side of the abdomen for transverse incision across the midline. The local anesthetic injection will appear as an expansion of hypoechogenicity deep to the fascial plane of the internal oblique and above that of the transversus abdominis muscle. Please refer to the accompanying video clip for a demonstration of the TAP block.

6

Comments

- It is important to ensure local anesthetic spread in the correct fascial plane, rather than injecting local anesthetic intramuscularly.
- There may be blood vessels within the abdominal muscles; therefore, color Doppler should be employed to ensure the needle trajectory is clear of blood vessels.
- For midline incisions of the abdomen, rectus sheath block can be performed by targeting the local anesthetic injection between the rectus abdominis muscle and the posterior rectus sheath, which is formed by the aponeurosis of the three layers of abdominal muscles.
- TAP blocks have been demonstrated to provide effective analgesia in the obstetrics and general surgery populations.[141–143]
- TAP blocks can be modified into transversalis fascial plane (TFP) block by targeting the local anesthetic injection into the layer between the transversus abdominis muscle

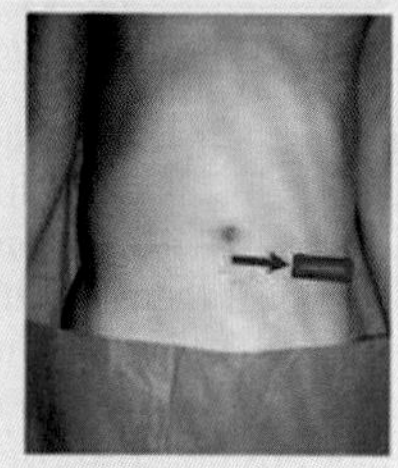

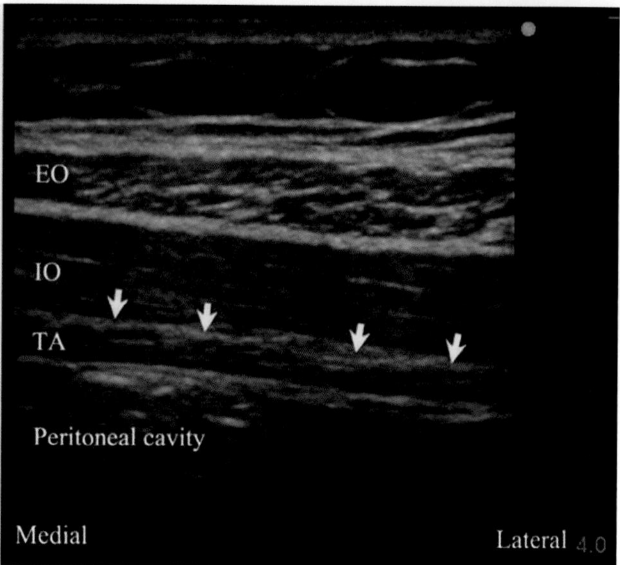

FIGURE 35-30. A high frequency linear probe placed transversely above the iliac crest in the anterior axillary line, showing the three layers of abdominal muscles, the peritoneum, and the peritoneal cavity. The needle is at an IP alignment to the probe from medial-to-lateral direction.

aponeurosis and the transversalis fascia. Local anesthetic will spread proximally over the inner surface of the quadratus lumborum muscle to anesthetize the proximal portions of the T12 and L1 nerves. The TFP block has been demonstrated to provide analgesia for anterior iliac bone graft harvesting.[144,145]

- Traditionally, paravertebral blocks and other trunk blocks are performed blindly, with either sole use of landmarks, including a loss of resistance to needle penetration of the costotransverse ligament for paravertebral block, or combined landmark and NS technique. US imaging may be beneficial for these blocks, particularly paravertebral block, in order to facilitate landmark localization. For example, preprocedural scanning can identify the tips of the transverse processes, which will help to identify correct needle insertion site. US may be particularly useful for performing blocks in obese patients (where the depth of needle insertion will be modified) or those with anatomical variation (e.g., scoliosis). This section provides a detailed description of the technique using NS guidance but will also provide illustrations in the sections on paravertebral and inguinal blocks of US imaging prior to block performance.

An overview of the anatomy of the spinal nerves is described at the beginning of the Upper Extremity section. The dermatomal innervation of the thoracic and lumbar nerves is illustrated in Figure 35-8.

Ilioinguinal and Iliohypogastric Nerve Blocks

These blocks are performed easily with blind technique, although US imaging may be used to help improve the success rate of nerve localization and deposition of local anesthetic in the correct fascial plane in close proximity to the nerves.

Procedure Using Blind Technique (Single-shot Fascial Click)

LANDMARKS. The injection site is located at about 1 to 2 cm medial and 1 to 2 cm inferior to the anterior superior iliac spine.

NEEDLING AND INJECTION. A 25-gauge, 35- to 50-mm blunted hypodermic needle can be used. The needle is inserted from the anterior abdomen (vertically) until a fascial click is detected, presumably at the junction of the internal oblique and transverse abdominis muscles. About 10- to 15-mL local anesthetic can be injected.

Procedure Using Ultrasound Imaging

SCANNING. Two different approaches have been used for US scanning of the ilioinguinal and iliohypogastric nerves.[57,146] In their clinical study, Willschke et al.[57] used a small footprint ("hockey stick"), 5 to 10 MHz probe, placed in transverse axis, just medial and superior to the anterior superior iliac spine. The cross-sectional view of the ilioinguinal nerve can be captured lying between the internal oblique and transverse abdominis muscles. In their cadaveric study, Eichenberger et al.[146] found that a 7.5 MHz probe was superior to one with a 10 MHz frequency. They used a position about 5 cm cranial and slightly posterior to the anterior superior iliac spine, where both nerves have been shown to be present between the above mentioned muscles with a 90% probability. These authors visualized both nerves as distinct entities.

APPEARANCE. The nerves appear hypoechoic with many hyperechoic dots and a distinct hyperechoic rim (Fig. 35-31). They have an oval, somewhat "boomerang" shape and appear embedded between the fascicular hypoechoic-appearing muscles. In the more cranial position, the iliac bone, with its hyperechoic border and dorsal shadowing, may be captured on the medial aspect of the screen. The thin external oblique muscle lies superficial at the cranial position, but it may not be visible more inferiorly.

NEEDLING. Both groups of authors used an OOP needling alignment, with the needle placed caudad to the probe in its center with good needle tracking. However, an IP approach is also feasible.

LOCAL ANESTHETIC SPREAD. Either one or two injections can be made, depending on the number of distinct nerves localized. The dose of local anesthetic may be lower (0.075 mL/kg has been shown

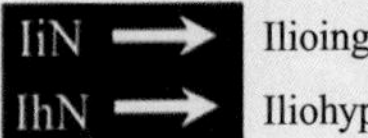

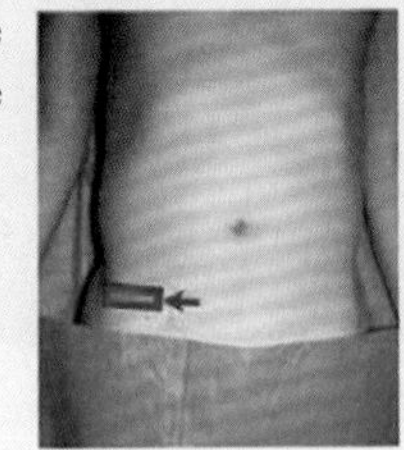

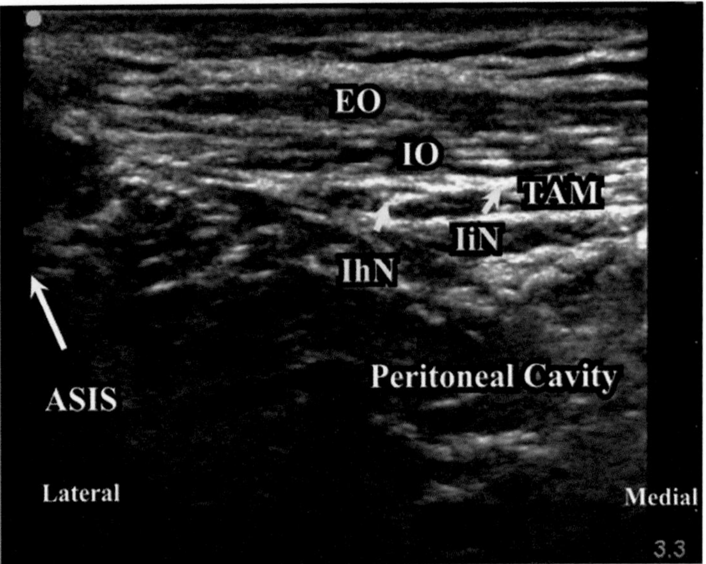

FIGURE 35-31. Ultrasound image with transverse scanning on the abdomen just medial to the anterior superior iliac spine (ASIS). Shown are the ilioinguinal and iliohypogastric nerves lying between the internal oblique and transversus abdominis muscles, just medial to the ASIS. These nerves can be blocked using an IP alignment from medial-to-lateral direction to avoid puncturing through the peritoneum.

effective for a single injection technique in children)[147] when using US imaging, since the nerves are well localized. A hypoechoic area of solution should be visualized adjacent to the nerve(s).

COMMENTS

- The ilioinguinal and iliohypogastric nerves may exist as a common trunk at the level of the anterior superior iliac spine, which further supports the use of US guidance for localizing the individual nerve.[146]
- Since there is high variability in the skin innervation from these nerves, it is impossible to confirm with clinical tests which nerve is blocked. Injecting lateral to the most laterally positioned ilioinguinal nerve, or medial to the iliohypogastric nerve, has been reported as one method to block these nerves individually.[146]
- Complications of this block are generally volume-related and include systemic toxicity and transient femoral nerve palsy. A recent assessment of the accuracy of the blind technique using US demonstrated that, even in experienced hands, needles were inserted deep to the transverses abdominis muscle over 40% of the time,[148] reinforcing the value of US in helping to prevent inaccurate needle placement or inappropriate anesthetic spread.

Penile Block

7 A penile block is used in children and adults for surgical procedures of the glans and shaft of the penis. The dorsal nerves (terminal branches of pudendal nerve; S2–S4) lie bilaterally on the outer aspect of the dorsal arteries of the penis. From the base of the penis, they divide several times and encircle the shaft of the penis before reaching the glans. This block is often performed as a circumferential infiltration of the root of the penis (ring block). Two skin wheals are raised at the dorsal base of the penis, one on each side just below and medial to the pubic spine. A 25-gauge, 37.5-mm needle is introduced on each side, and 5 mL of anesthetic (0.5 to 1 mL for infants) is injected superficially and deep along the lower border of the pubic ramus to anesthetize the dorsal nerve. For a complete ring of infiltration, an additional 5 mL (adults) is infiltrated in the subcutaneous tissue around the underside of the shaft. A larger needle or a second injection site may be needed to complete the ring. Twenty to twenty-five milliliters of 0.75% lidocaine or 0.25% bupivacaine usually suffices in adults. Epinephrine-containing solutions should not be used to avoid compromising penile circulation. US can be used to improve the efficacy of penile blocks and, in one study, was found to decrease postoperative pain and delay the administration of postoperative analgesics, although procedures using US were, on average, 10 minutes longer in duration compared to those performed blindly.[149]

Lower Extremity

Combined blocks of the lumbar and sacral plexuses provide effective surgical anesthesia to the entire lower extremity. Prior to the 1990s, an "anterior lumbar block" approach (also referred to as the "femoral three-in-one" approach), first described by Winnie et al. in 1973,[150] was commonly performed, based on the assumption that a large volume local anesthetic injection into the femoral nerve sheath would produce spread of the solution proximally to anesthetize the obturator and lateral femoral cutaneous nerves as well. Later reports of failures to obtain obturator nerve block with this approach[151,152] led to the femoral block being considered as an individual nerve block and advocated the posterior lumbar block approach for accessing the whole lumbar plexus.

PNB is indicated when spinal, caudal, or epidural techniques are contraindicated or when selective anesthesia of one leg or foot is needed. Because the anatomic landmarks identifying the fascial sheaths or compartments of the plexuses are not as clearly defined as those in the upper extremity, lower extremity blocks are often performed more distally, where the nerves have already separated into terminal branches. Thus, in addition to the fascial compartment approach (psoas block), there are peripheral approaches described at the anterior and posterior hip, knee, and ankle.

Techniques

Psoas Compartment Block

Several techniques for blocking the lumbar plexus using a posterior approach have been described; however, the one at the psoas compartment, described first by Chayen et al. in 1976,[153] remains popular. This block is performed, often with a single injection, at a point some distance lateral to the spinous process of L4, since the nerves of the lumbar plexus are in close proximity between the transverse processes of L4 and L5. Continuous psoas compartment blocks have also been shown to be effective for anesthesia (with sciatic nerve block) and perioperative analgesia in patients with hip fractures[154] and after hip arthroplasty.[155] A more cephalad approach, near L3, as described by Parkinson et al.[152] may be used, although there have been reports of renal subcapsular hematomas with blocks performed at this level.[156] This block has the advantage of blocking the entire lumbar plexus and therefore provides anesthesia/analgesia of the anterolateral and medial thigh, the knee, and the cutaneous distribution of the saphenous nerve below the knee. Although the sacral nerve roots may be anesthetized, this block will likely not provide complete anesthesia/analgesia for the entire upper leg, and sciatic nerve block will usually need to be performed as well. The patient is placed in the lateral position, with the operative side up. Adequate sedation should be provided since the plexus lies deep and the needle must penetrate several muscles. Prepare the needle insertion site and skin surface with an antiseptic solution. Prepare the US probe surface by applying a sterile sleeve or adhesive dressing to it before needling (not shown).

Procedure Using Nerve Stimulation Technique

LANDMARKS. The landmarks developed by Capdevila et al.[155] using computed tomography are illustrated here (Fig. 35-32). As compared to the depth of the lumbar plexus or transverse processes, the distance between the L4 spinous process and the lumbar plexus is not affected by body mass index. The spinous process of L4 is estimated to lie approximately 1 cm cephalad to a line between the tops of the iliac crests (intercristal line); a horizontal line is drawn laterally from the L4 spinous processes to the far side of the body. A vertical line, running parallel to the spine, is then drawn at the point of the posterior superior iliac spine to intersect the horizontal line. The lumbar plexus is then located with an "X," below a point on the horizontal line, at the junction between the lateral third and medial two-thirds between the spine and posterior superior iliac spine. The mean skin-to-lumbar plexus depth at the level of L4 is 8.4 cm in adult men and 7.1 cm in adult women based on computed tomography assessment. The distance between the posterior edges of the transverse processes of the lumbar vertebrae and the lumbar plexus is about 1.8 cm.

NEEDLING. A skin wheal is raised at the marked block site. An insulated needle (17 to 20 gauge, 110 to 150 mm long, depending on body habitus) is inserted perpendicular to all planes at the "X" until contact with the L4 transverse process is obtained (approximately 5 to 6 cm deep). After contact, the needle is withdrawn and redirected caudad below the process to a maximum depth of 2 cm deep to the transverse process.

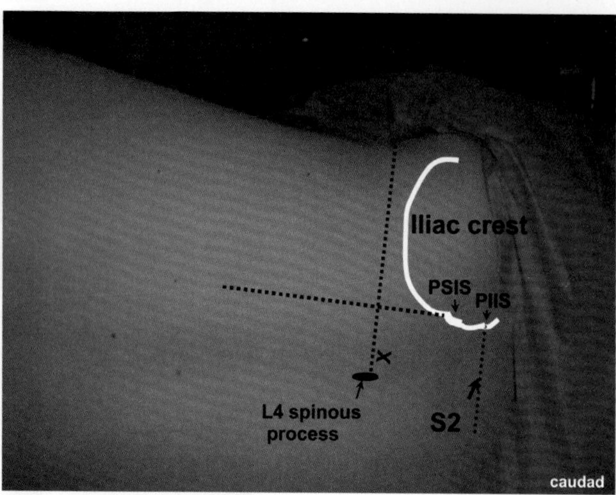

FIGURE 35-32. Surface landmarking for the psoas compartment block. The needle insertion site is one-third the distance along a horizontal line extending from the L4 transverse process to where it crosses a vertical line dissecting the posterior superior iliac spine (PSIS). PIIS, Posterior inferior iliac spine.

NERVE LOCALIZATION. With the nerve stimulator set to deliver an output current of 1 to 1.5 mA, a contraction of the quadriceps muscle (patellar twitch) is sought. The plexus is localized when the motor response is maintained at 0.3 to 0.5 mA. If a motor response is not obtained at first, cautiously moving the needle in a slight medial direction, without aiming toward the spinal cord, or in a direction 15-degree caudad or cephalad may help.

INJECTION. After the plexus is localized, 30 to 40 mL of local anesthetic is injected, using careful aspiration and administration of a test dose to rule out intravascular, epidural, or subarachnoid placement. Fifteen to twenty minutes may be required for spread of the anesthetic to all the roots of the lumbar plexus. It will take longer to produce anesthesia of the caudad branches (the lower sacral fibers that form the tibial nerve), and they may not become anesthetized at all.

Procedure Using Ultrasound Imaging

The lumbar plexus is difficult to view adequately, as the target structures are deep. Similar to paravertebral block, US imaging may be best for identifying the exact location and depth of the transverse processes prior to the block procedure. If there is desire to perform the block at L3–L4, viewing the kidneys prior to and/or during the block may help prevent renal injury and hematoma. The combined use of NS technique with US is still recommended to confirm correct needle placement.

SCANNING. A curved array probe (5 to 8 MHz) is placed in the transverse plane in the midline at the level of the L4 spinous process to provide an overview of the L4 vertebra (Fig. 35-33). The probe should be rotated to the longitudinal axis, parallel to the spine, which will allow a lateral scan to be performed to identify the tips of the transverse processes. The absence of associated ribs means that the tips of the transverse processes are fairly easily delineated.

APPEARANCE. The deep location of this block precludes clear visibility of the lumbar plexus. Indeed, the transverse processes (which are the primary landmarks) are often only vaguely delineated.

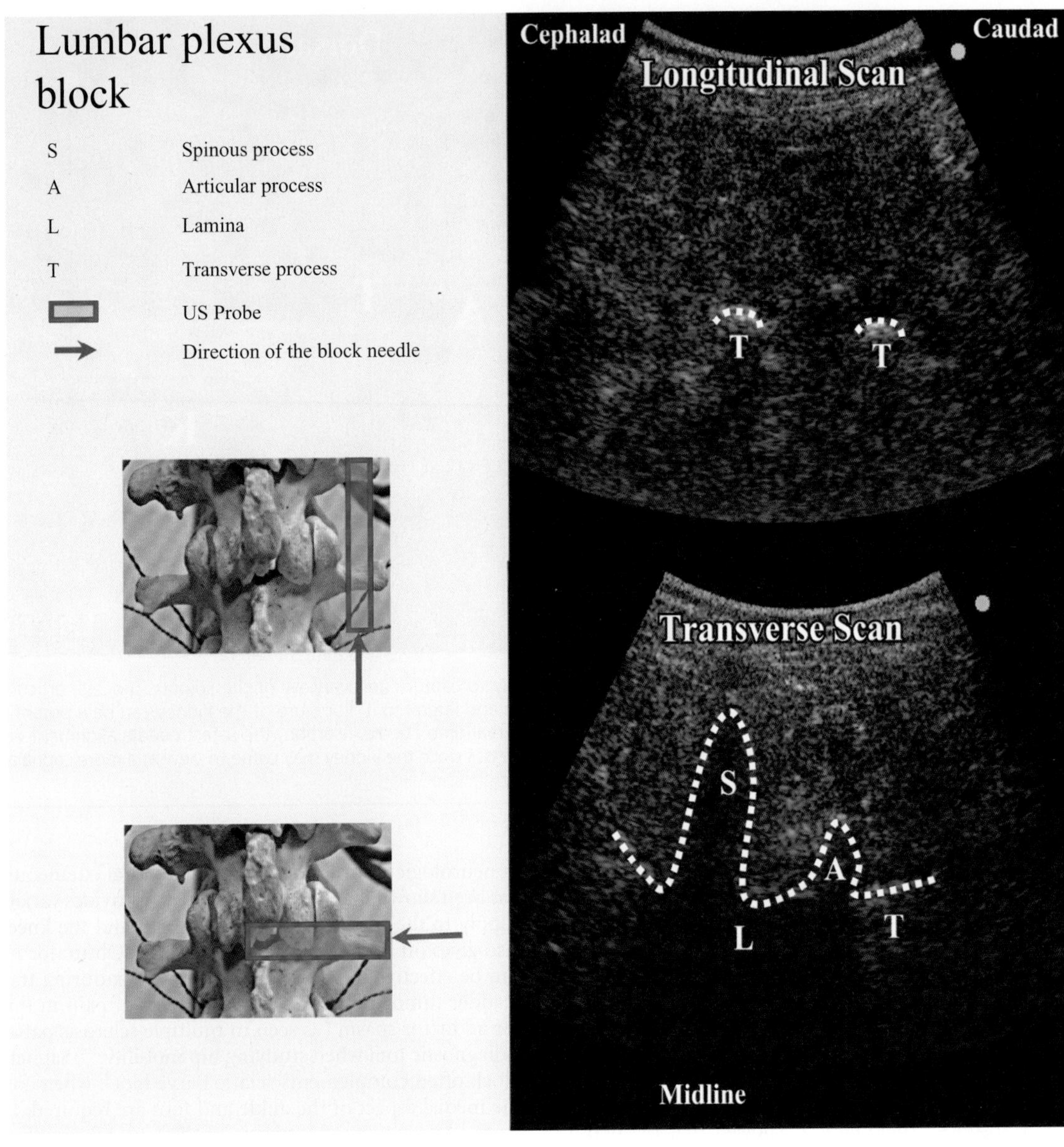

FIGURE 35-33. Ultrasound-assisted psoas compartment blockade. The curved array probe can be placed longitudinally to help mark the block location (the tips of the transverse processes; top right image). The US probe can also be positioned transversely to capture an overview of the spinal column (bottom right image). If attempting real-time needle insertion, the safest needle alignment will be IP to a longitudinally placed probe over the L3–L5 transverse processes.

Therefore, it is important to switch between transverse and longitudinal scanning between the spinous processes and the tip of the transverse processes to survey the area. In the transverse scan, the spinous processes appear hypoechoic (likely due to dorsal shadowing effect) and extend superficially, while the transverse processes are hyperechoic masses/lines at the lateral edge of the vertebra. The fascicular-appearing musculature is evident surrounding the vertebra, yet poorly delineated by most compact US machines. In the longitudinal scan, the lateral tips of the transverse processes will be identified at the most lateral point where a hyperechoic nodule is viewed.

NEEDLING. Needling will be identical to that for the blind technique, with the exception that the depth to the transverse process will be more accurately known. If choosing to perform a more cephalad approach above L4, real-time imaging may be helpful to view the kidneys (especially during inspiration when they fall toward L3–L4) (Fig. 35-34). An IP needle alignment with respect to a longitudinal probe may be most suitable to avoid excessive medial or lateral needle angulation (see Paravertebral Blockade comments).

LOCAL ANESTHETIC SPREAD. It will be difficult to view local anesthetic spread when using US guidance. If seen, a hypoechoic mass will spread within the muscle mass lateral and deep to the transverse process.

Comments

- The psoas compartment block can be beneficial for placing a catheter to provide long-lasting analgesia; the catheter is

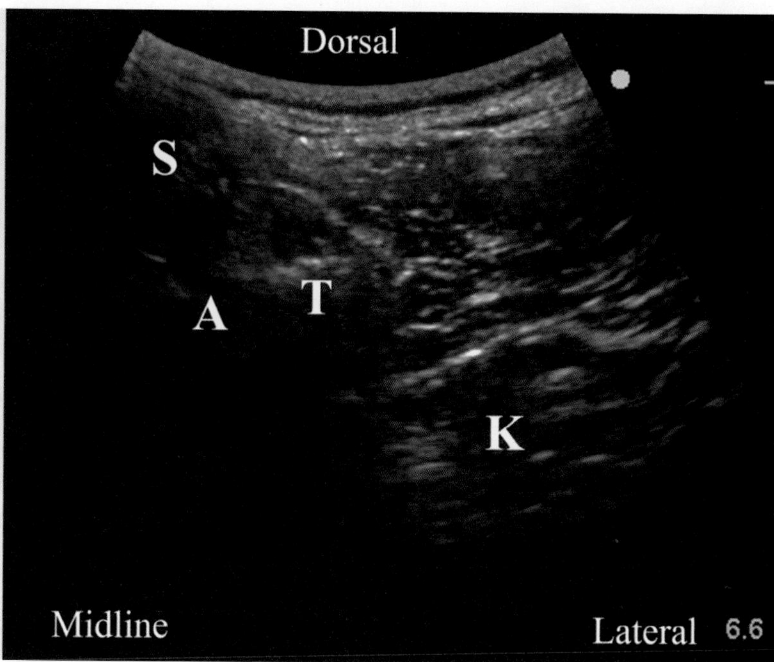

FIGURE 35-34. The curved array probe can be placed transversely to capture an overview of the spinous process, articular process, and the transverse process with the psoas muscle just deep and lateral to it. Puncture of the kidney can be a potential complication of psoas compartment block; therefore, if attempting real-time needle insertion, the safest needle alignment will be IP to a longitudinally placed probe over the L3–L5 transverse processes since the kidney may come to view at a more cephalad position.

securely fixed by the psoas muscles and kept away from any active joint region. After obtaining good localization with the stimulating needle (bevel facing caudad and lateral), a stimulating catheter is advanced 3 to 5 cm. In some cases, injecting a nonconducting solution such as D5W to expand the perineural space, while maintaining the electrical characteristics is helpful.[27] The quadriceps muscle contraction should be maintained during catheter advancement with a stimulating catheter.

- Prepuncture US may be beneficial prior to needle insertion and catheter placement. Using a higher frequency (6 to 13 MHz) linear array transducer, Ilfeld et al.[157] showed that the depth and location of each transverse process could be accurately estimated, allowing the user to minimize risks associated with needle/catheter insertion into the lumbar plexus.
- Complications of this technique include hematoma in the muscle sheath, retroperitoneal space, or kidney (hence, this block is contraindicated in patients with coagulopathy or bleeding diathesis); infection; and catheter placement within the peritoneum. Neuropathy of the nerves is possible. Unintended spread to the epidural or even subarachnoid space has also been reported.

Separate Blocks of the Terminal Nerves of the Lumbar Plexus

Anesthesia can be performed for four terminal nerves (lateral femoral cutaneous, femoral, obturator, and saphenous), although a lumbar plexus block is preferable if anesthesia of all these nerves are required. Anesthesia of the lateral femoral cutaneous nerve is occasionally used to provide sensory anesthesia for obtaining a skin graft from the lateral thigh. It can also be blocked as a diagnostic/therapeutic tool to identify cases of meralgia paresthetica (a neurologic disorder of the lateral femoral cutaneous nerve). It has been shown that the obturator nerve provides variable sensory supply to the medial aspect of the thigh and the knee joint and also gives off branches to the hip joint.[158] Obturator nerve block can be effective to prevent obturator reflex during transurethral bladder tumor resections, for treatment of pain in the hip area, for adductor spasm (as seen in multiple sclerosis patients), or as a diagnostic tool when studying hip mobility.[159] Saphenous nerve block often complements sciatic nerve block when anesthesia of the medial aspect of the ankle and foot are required. Procedures on the knee require anesthesia of the femoral and the obturator nerves, although postoperative analgesia of the knee can usually be provided by femoral nerve block alone. Single-shot femoral nerve block provides suitable postoperative analgesia after total knee arthroplasty while sparing the side effects of intrathecal morphine.[160] The use of a continuous technique can also reduce side effects as compared to continuous epidurals[161] and can facilitate rehabilitation.[162] A US-guided infrapatellar nerve block has been described for use for postoperative analgesia after outpatient arthroscopic surgery[163] but will not be included here. Since separate femoral nerve block is used extensively for analgesia, and US guidance has been described for this block, this chapter will provide a comprehensive description of this block. US guidance for obturator nerve block has been described and will be examined here. The other two nerve blocks will only be briefly discussed. The block sites for the femoral, lateral femoral cutaneous, and obturator nerves are illustrated in Figure 35-15.

Femoral Nerve/Fascia Iliacus Block

PROCEDURE USING NERVE STIMULATION

- Landmarks: The patient is placed in the supine position, with slight external rotation of the femur. A pillow can be placed under the patient's hip to facilitate palpation of the femoral pulse and accentuate other pertinent landmarks for ease of palpation. Vloka et al.[164] studied cadavers using four common needle insertion sites for femoral nerve block and found that the point where the nerve lies beneath the inguinal crease, immediately lateral to the femoral artery, was optimal for localizing the nerve. The femoral artery descends at the "midinguinal point," at the junction between the medial third and lateral two-thirds of the inguinal ligament, although it is most superficial at the femoral crease. It lies approximately 1 to 1.5 cm medial to the nerve. The inguinal crease is the skin fold located approximately 2.5 cm caudad and parallel to the inguinal ligament (Clinical Anatomy of lower extremity).

- Needling: A skin wheal is raised lateral to the area where the femoral artery pulsation is felt and a 50-mm, 22-gauge insulated needle is inserted perpendicular to the skin or using a cephalad angle of approximately 30 degrees. Aspiration is performed frequently since the femoral artery is situated closely to the nerve.
- Nerve localization: For the femoral nerve using NS, a quadriceps muscle response (patellar twitch preferably) is sought, with an endpoint of 0.5 mA used for accurate localization. Branches to the sartorius muscle arise just inferior to the inguinal ligament and leave the femoral nerve proximal to the main block location site; a response of this muscle to stimulation often indicates that the needle is too superficial and medial to the main femoral nerve. For a fascia iliacus block, loss-of-resistance technique is used instead of NS. The needle is placed vertically 5 cm lateral to the artery at the inguinal crease. Two pops are felt when the needle traverses the fascia lata and iliacus and enters the iliopsoas muscle.
- Injection: Injection of 20 mL (or less) of local anesthetic should suffice for sole femoral nerve anesthesia. Twenty to thirty milliliters of local anesthetic may be required for the fascia iliacus block. Intermittent injection with interval aspiration should be performed.

PROCEDURE USING ULTRASOUND IMAGING (FIG. 35-35)

- Scanning: A 10 MHz or higher transducer can be used for both blocks if the neurovascular structures are not located too deep (i.e., thin individuals), as this will show good distinction between the nerve and the surrounding structures (vessels and muscles). A midrange 5- to 8-MHz linear transducer is recommended if the nerve and artery are deep (>4 cm). Position the probe transverse to the nerve axis at the level of the inguinal crease. The nerve should appear approximately 1 cm deep and 1.5 cm lateral to the femoral artery, depending on body habitus (color Doppler may be used to identify the femoral artery and vein).
- Appearance: The nerve lies about 1 cm lateral and deep to the large, circular, anechoic, and pulsatile femoral artery. It often appears triangular in shape and of variable size, due to its irregular course; early branching above the inguinal ligament can increase the transverse diameter of the nerve. The fascia lata (most superficial) and iliaca (immediately adjacent to the nerve and in fact separating the nerve from the artery) may be seen superficial to the femoral nerve and often appear bright and longitudinally angled.
- Needling: Place the nerve at the medial edge of the screen, with the probe capturing a transverse view of the neurovascular structures. A 50-mm, 22-gauge needle (for single-shot) can be inserted using either IP or OOP (Fig. 35-35) needle alignment. The needle should be inserted using an acute (30 to 45 degrees) angle to maximize viewing. IP blocks may be made easier by angling the needle tip slightly away from the nerve, while accuracy of catheter placement may be improved by tilting the needle hub in a caudad direction once the needle tip is appropriately positioned.[165] Inserting the catheter

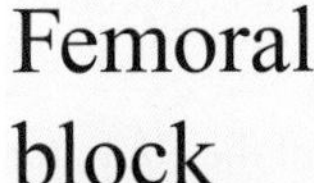

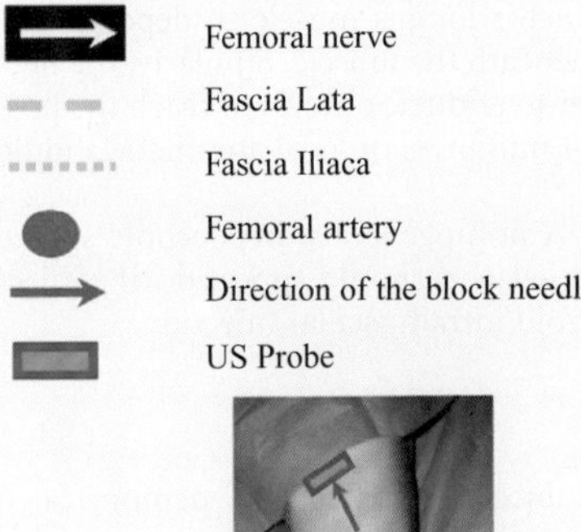

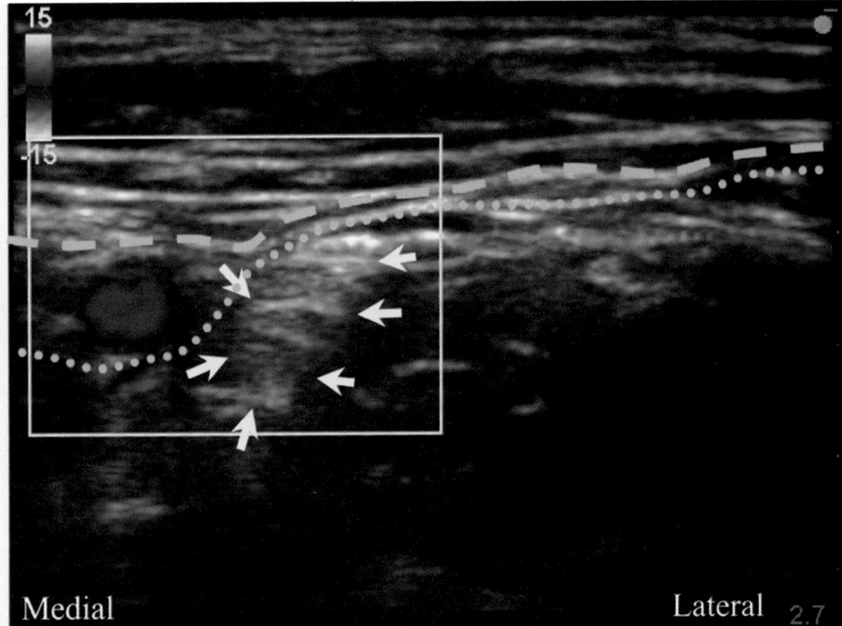

FIGURE 35-35. Ultrasound-guided femoral nerve block. The probe is placed in a slightly oblique plane (at the level of and parallel to the inguinal crease) to capture the nerve in short axis lateral to the femoral artery. The needle can be seen (not shown) as it transects the fascia lata and iliaca. The photograph illustrates an OOP approach. If IP needling is used, it should occur in a lateral-to-medial direction.

perpendicular or parallel to the nerve does not affect quality of analgesia, although the former technique may facilitate faster catheter insertion.[166] Please refer to the accompanying video clip for a demonstration of the femoral nerve block.

- For iliacus block, the needle is generally placed more laterally than with the femoral nerve block.
- Local anesthetic spread: Performing a test dose with D5W is recommended prior to local anesthetic application to visualize the spread and confirm nerve localization. Local anesthetic spread should occur within the fascial space surrounding the nerve. The solution may displace the nerve medially toward or laterally away from the artery.

COMMENTS

- When inserting a catheter, it is debatable whether a stimulating catheter improves placement,[167,168] but using a solution to expand the perineural space has been shown to be beneficial in some cases.[169,170] If a stimulating catheter is used, injection of D5W for tissue expansion will maintain motor responses to NS.[26,27]
- The lateral-to-medial needle insertion when using the IP needle alignment will ensure that the nerve is reached before reaching the femoral vessels.
- It is important to ensure that the US beam is perpendicular to the nerve's transverse axis to minimize the chance of anisotropic effects changing the echogenic properties of the structure. It has been shown that an approximate 10-degree cephalad or caudad tilt of the transducer can make the nerve isoechoic (similar-appearing) to the underlying iliopsoas muscle.[171]

Lateral Femoral Cutaneous Nerve

Using NS technique, Shannon et al.[172] found that the lateral femoral cutaneous nerve can be localized at the inguinal crease, approximately 0 to 1 cm medial to the anterior superior iliac spine (Fig. 35-15), although this mark may be highly variant[173] and should be confirmed with NS. An insulated needle (5 cm, 22 gauge is suitable) is inserted, using a perpendicular approach if the puncture is close to the anterior superior iliac spine, but in a lateral direction if it is at a distance. A "pop" may be felt as the needle penetrates the fascia lata. The primary end point for NS with this nerve is paresthesia over the lateral thigh (Fig. 35-14) with a current of approximately 0.5 to 0.6 mA. The sensory distribution may not extend proximal to the greater trochanter. Five to ten milliliters of a local anesthetic is usually sufficient to obtain a block. A recent study demonstrated that nerve targeting may not be necessary in some cases; in patients undergoing knee surgery, injection of local anesthetic immediately under the inguinal ligament provided sufficient blockade without having to inject directly around the nerve.[174]

Obturator Nerve

Since the obturator nerve branches early after its descent from the obturator foramen, blocking this nerve within the foramen near the superior pubic ramus (i.e., before it branches) is often described for blind techniques. The patient is placed supine with their hip slightly externally rotated; the hip may also be slightly flexed and abducted. If using US imaging, a straight leg has been shown to be the best position. The public tubercle is located and a mark is placed 1.5 cm both inferior and lateral to it (this mark should resemble that in Fig. 35-15). An inguinal approach is another option and may result in higher block success rates and fewer needle attempts in certain circumstances.[175]

PROCEDURE USING NERVE STIMULATION TECHNIQUE

- An insulated needle (18 to 22 gauge, 9 to 10 cm) is inserted perpendicularly until contact with the inferior pubic ramus is obtained. The needle is then redirected laterally and caudally to enter the obturator foramen and advanced 2 to 3 cm. NS using 0.5 mA for a current end point, with adductor muscle contraction, has been shown to greatly improve nerve localization.[159]

PROCEDURE USING ULTRASOUND IMAGING (FIG. 35-36). Scanning: The use of US-guided obturator block at the proximal thigh is predominantly based on the identification of three muscle layers, namely, the adductor longus, adductor brevis, and adductor magnus muscles (from superficial to deep). The anterior branch of the obturator nerve usually lies on the lateral edge between the adductor longus and brevis muscles, while the posterior branch of the obturator nerve lies between the adductor brevis and magnus muscles; however, the obturator nerve shows a considerable degree of variability at this level.[176,177] Soong et al.[178] used the Acuson Sequoia C256 machine (Siemens Medical Solutions, Malvern, PA, USA) and found that the anterior and posterior branches may be most easily visualized with the probe placed 2 cm laterally and distally to the pubic tubercle. The branches may be localized on either side of the adductor brevis muscle if the fascial planes of the muscles are highly visible (hyperechoic). The depths of the anterior and posterior branches as measured during US guidance were 15.5 and 29.3 mm, respectively; tissue compression by the probe may influence this depth. The main (common) obturator nerve may be hard to view with US imaging. An IP needling technique and color Doppler will be important to use in order to avoid adjacent blood vessels.

- Appearance: Using a high frequency probe, US visualization of the three layers of muscle—adductor longus, adductor brevis, and adductor magus—should be seen. The anterior branches of the nerve usually appear as hypoechoic circles in between a hyperechoic layer formed by the adductor longus and brevis, while the posterior branches lie between the layers of the adductor brevis and magnus muscles at this level. The nerve can also be blocked more distally at the knee.
- Needling: To anesthetize the anterior branch of the obturator nerve, a 22-gauge needle is inserted in either an IP or OOP fashion deep to the adductor longus muscle to deposit local anesthetic immediately beneath the muscle. Similarly, the needle can be inserted deeper to adductor brevis to reach the posterior branch. Five to ten milliliters of local anesthetic should suffice.
- Local anesthetic spread: A homogeneous, hypoechoic spread pattern between the muscle layers should appear during injection. It is important to avoid intramuscular injection.

COMMENTS

- Using cadavers and live subjects, Akkaya et al.[179] demonstrated that a hyperechoic triangle bordered by the superior pubic ramus, posterior edge of the pectineus muscle, and anterior aspect of the external obturator muscle is an ideal landmark to locate the obturator nerve, which lies just medial to the obturator vein.
- A recent report using US guidance suggested that a single injection of local anesthetic into the interfascial space (i.e., between the adductor longus and adductor brevis muscles) containing the anterior branch of the obturator nerve results in upward (cranial) spreading of anesthetic to block the posterior branch[180]; further spreading was encouraged by applying pressure distal to the needle insertion site.

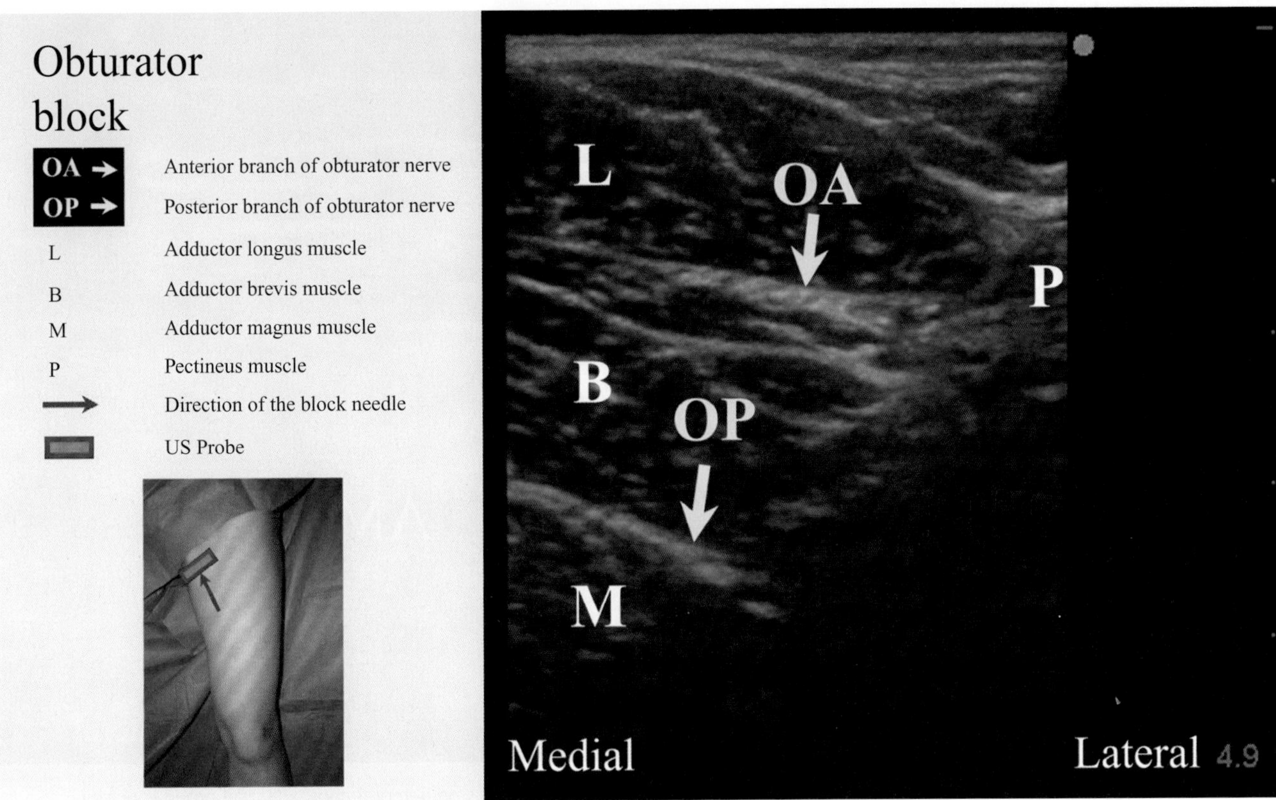

FIGURE 35-36. Ultrasound-guided obturator nerve block (anterior and posterior branches) in the proximal thigh using an OOP approach. It is important to identify the three adductor muscles—the adductor longus, adductor brevis, and adductor magnus muscles (from superficial to deep). The pectineus muscle should also be in view on the lateral side since the anterior branch of the obturator nerve is sandwiched between the adductor longus and adductor brevis deep to the pectineus muscle.

- Aspiration is essential when injecting near the unbranched obturator nerve as the obturator artery lies adjacent to the nerve, and hemorrhage involving this artery can be life-threatening.[181]

Saphenous Nerve

Many approaches to blocking the saphenous nerve have been described, with needle placement at various locations, including the midthigh, surrounding the knee, or at the ankle (as discussed in Ankle Block). A transsartorial block using a blind technique, first described by van der Wal et al.,[182] has been shown to be more effective compared to blockade at the medial femoral condyle (paracondylar block) or tibial tuberosity (below-knee field block) for producing anesthesia to the medial aspect of the foot.[183] This approach will be described here. US guidance has been used successfully with a transsartorius perifemoral,[184] subsartorial,[185] or perivenous (saphenous vein)[186,187] approach; the perifemoral approach will be discussed below. An effective approach using the sartorius and gracilis tendons as landmarks has also been described.[188] Using the more proximally located larger femoral artery (rather than the more distal saphenous branch of the descending genicular artery) as a highly visible landmark seems to help identify the sartorius muscle and nerve.

PROCEDURE USING NERVE STIMULATION TECHNIQUE (TRANSSARTORIAL)

- Landmarks: The sartorius muscle is palpated at the medial aspect of the knee joint by asking the patient to raise their extended leg 5 to 10 cm off the table. The block location is marked by the end of a 4 cm vertical line drawn from this point in a proximal direction (Benzon et al.[183] used a slightly more cephalad point 3 to 4 cm superior and 6 to 8 cm posterior to the superomedial border of the patella).
- Needling: An insulated 22-gauge needle is inserted caudally using an angle of 45 degrees with a slight posterior angle advanced from the medial aspect of the knee, in a slight posterior and caudad angle, to penetrate the sartorius muscle at a depth of approximately 2 to 3 cm.
- Nerve localization: Paresthesia at the medial malleolus should be felt with the nerve stimulator at 0.6 mA or less at a depth of 3 to 5 cm.
- Injection: Following careful aspiration, 10 mL of local anesthetic (e.g., 1.5% to 2% lidocaine) is injected.

PROCEDURE USING ULTRASOUND IMAGING (FIG. 35-37)

- Using US,[184] the sartorius muscle can be easily identified as being a superficial roof to the relatively large landmark of the femoral artery before the artery travels deep and becomes the popliteal artery via the adductor hiatus. The nerve is located between the sartorius muscle and the artery in the thigh.
- Scanning: A high-frequency linear US transducer (e.g., L38, MicroMaxx, Sonosite, Bothell, WA, USA) is placed transversely to the longitudinal axis of the extremity at the midthigh, approximately 10 to 12 cm proximal and 3 to 4 cm medial to the midpoint of the patella. The femoral artery can be identified here with certainty by power Doppler, which in turn

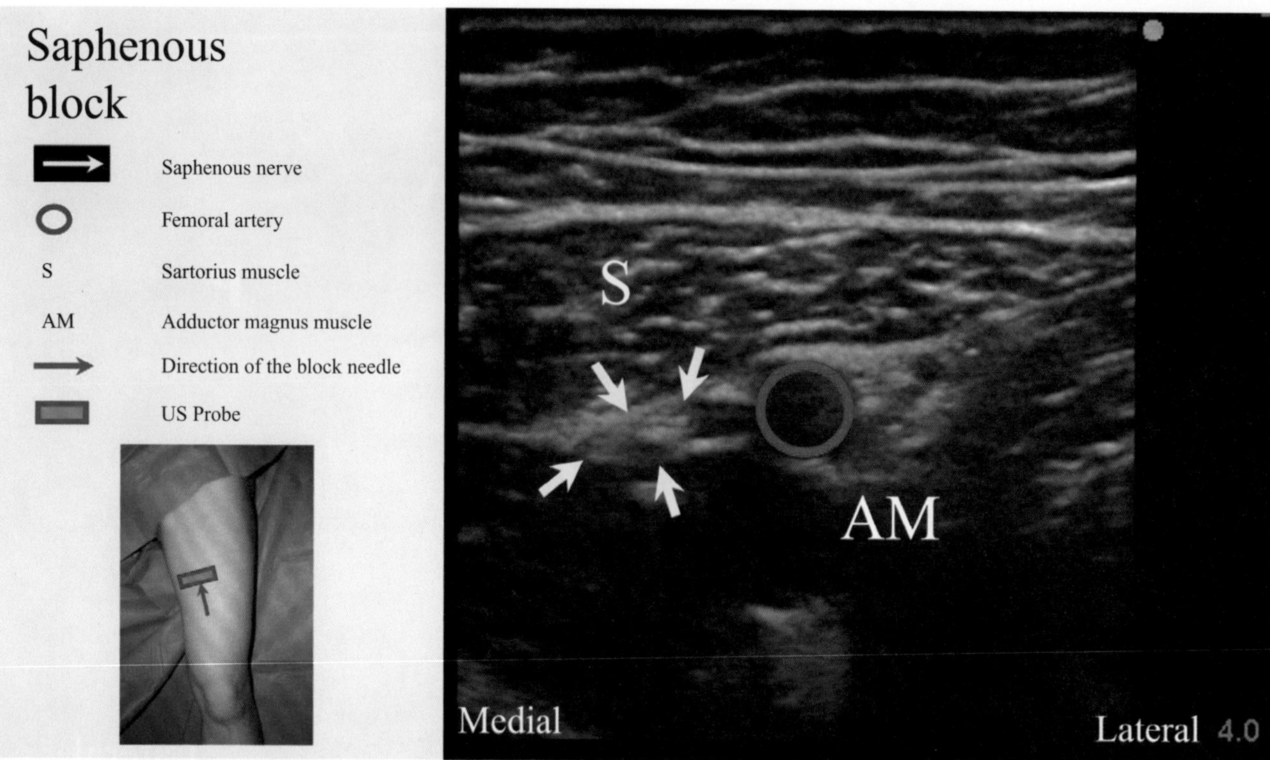

FIGURE 35-37. Ultrasound-guided saphenous nerve block using a transsartorius perifemoral approach. The probe is placed in the coronal plane at the location where the femoral nerve has yet to become the popliteal artery, approximately 10 to 12 cm proximal to and 3 to 4 cm medial to the midpoint of the patella. Using the large femoral artery as a landmark may be beneficial to more distal approaches where the nerve lies adjacent to the smaller saphenous branch of the descending genicular artery.[178] The photograph illustrates an OOP approach to the saphenous nerve block.

confirms the identity of the overlying sartorius muscle. The probe is then used to scan distally until it captures the point just prior to where the femoral artery becomes the popliteal artery. Please refer to the accompanying video clip for a demonstration of the saphenous nerve block.

9

- Appearance: Using color Doppler is important to visualize the femoral artery as a large hypoechoic (beneath the color) structure at a depth of approximately 2 to 3 cm in average-sized individuals. The sartorius muscle can then be identified as a highly delineated, lip-shaped muscle with hyperechoic borders immediately superficial to the artery. The nerve can be blocked as it lies sandwiched between the artery and the muscle at this level, or it can be blocked more distally at the knee.
- Needling: A 22-gauge needle is inserted in either an IP or OOP fashion to penetrate the sartorius muscle to deposit local anesthetic immediately beneath the muscle and medial to the artery. Five to ten milliliters of local anesthetic should suffice.
- Local anesthetic spread: A small hypoechoic mass on the medial surface of the femoral artery should appear during injection.

Sciatic Nerve Block Using Gluteal, Subgluteal, Posterior Popliteal, and Anterior Approaches

A sciatic nerve block can be used with lumbar plexus block for anesthesia of the lower extremity. Together with saphenous nerve block, the block produces adequate anesthesia of the sole of the foot and the lower leg. The large sciatic nerve is deep within the gluteal region and may be difficult to locate blindly or with US. Of benefit during US-guided blockade of the sciatic nerve and its terminal branches (tibial and common peroneal nerves) are the numerous bony and vascular landmarks that can be used for ease of identification. Knowledge of anatomy is paramount with these blocks and the block location and approach will ultimately depend on the surgical requirement. For all blocks, prepare the needle insertion site and other applicable skin areas with an antiseptic solution, and obtain sterility of the US probe with a standard sleeve cover or transparent dressing (not shown).

Posterior Sciatic Nerve Block: Classical Gluteal Approach

Position the patient semi prone (Sims' position) with the hip and knee flexed and the operative side uppermost.

PROCEDURE USING NERVE STIMULATION

- Landmarks (Fig. 35-38): An oblique line is drawn joining the posterior superior iliac spine to the midpoint of the greater trochanter (on its medial aspect). Next, a horizontal line is drawn joining the greater trochanter (at above location) to the sacral hiatus. A perpendicular line drawn at the midpoint of the oblique line and reaching the parahorizontal line is the traditional puncture site (this intersection should be approximately 5 cm caudad along the perpendicular line).
- Needling: Raise a local anesthetic skin wheal after aseptic preparation. A 100-mm, 22-gauge needle (insulated if NS is desired) is inserted perpendicular to the skin.
- Nerve localization: Nerve responses of the lower leg and foot are sought. If they are not obtained at the full depth of the

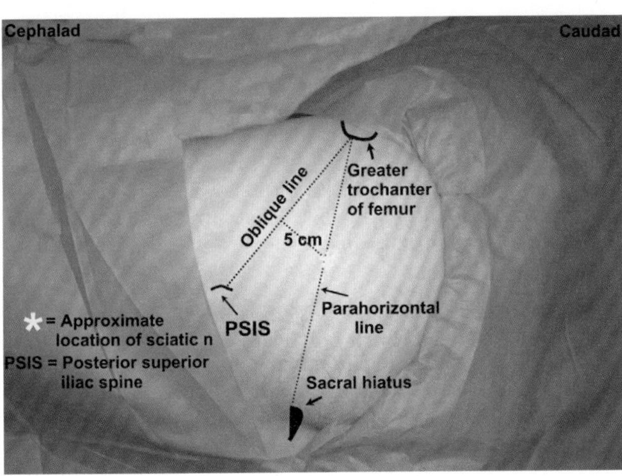

FIGURE 35-38. Landmarks for the sciatic nerve block using a posterior gluteal approach when using nerve stimulation procedure. This location will serve as a reference point when applying ultrasound imaging.

needle, the needle is withdrawn to the skin and reintroduced at a location perpendicular to the course of the nerve. Bone contact typically requires lateral needle adjustment.

- Injection: Injection of 20 to 30 mL of local anesthetic (e.g., 0.75% ropivacaine, 1% mepivacaine, 0.5% bupivacaine) is performed. If several blocks are required (i.e., lumbar plexus and/or saphenous nerve), a reduced concentration of local anesthetic may be necessary to prevent exceeding the toxic dose.

PROCEDURE USING ULTRASOUND IMAGING (FIG. 35-39)

- Scanning: A curved, lower frequency 2 to 5 MHz probe is generally used for scanning the gluteal region. Moving the probe cephalad and caudad in the gluteal region will help examine the ischial bone (a hyperechoic line with bony shadowing underneath), and the widest portion of this bone, with the ischial spine medial, should be located. The bulky gluteus maximus muscle will be seen superficial and posterior to the sciatic nerve. Vascular structures, which may be identified using color Doppler, are the internal pudendal vessels (artery and vein) that are adjacent to the ischial spine that is medial to the sciatic nerve and the inferior gluteal artery, immediately adjacent to the sciatic nerve. Alternatively, the nerve can be first located at the subgluteal region, at about the midpoint between the greater trochanter and the ischial tuberosity, and traced proximally.
- Appearance: The sciatic nerve in the gluteal region is found lateral to the ischial spine and superficial to the ischial bone. The nerve appears predominantly hyperechoic (bright) and is often wide and flat in short axis on US. Overlying the sciatic nerve is the large gluteus maximus, which is quite distinct with the usual "starry night" appearance; the inner muscle layers (superior and inferior gemellus muscles, obturator internus muscle, and quadratus femoris muscle) are often indistinct.
- Needling: Both IP and OOP approaches are appropriate for US-guided sciatic nerve block in the gluteal region. For an OOP approach, the needle is inserted inferior to the probe in a cephaloanterior direction. A fairly steep angle of insertion will be required, but placing the needle slightly inferior to the probe will reduce the angle somewhat for better visibility of the needle. With the IP approach, the needle may be moved in a lateral-to-medial direction to penetrate the gluteus maximus

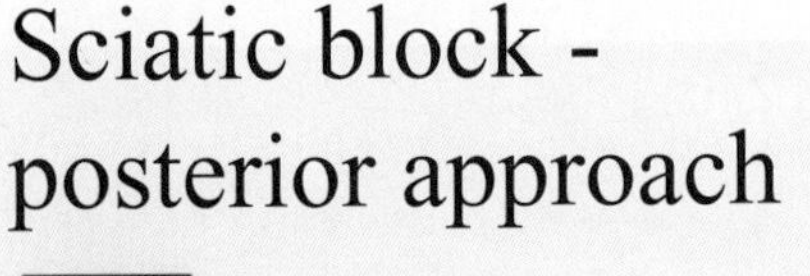

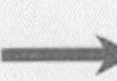

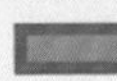

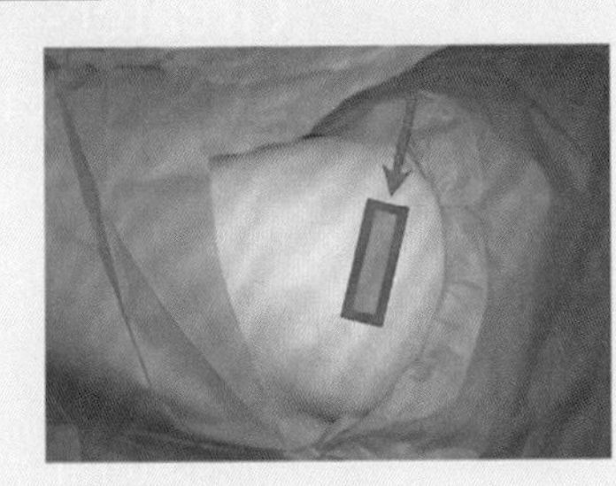

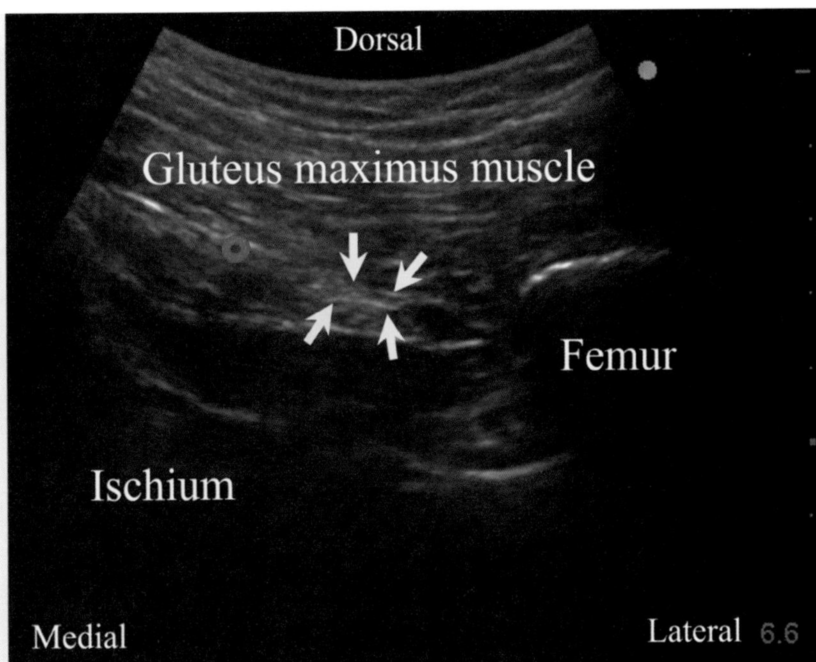

FIGURE 35-39. Ultrasound-guided sciatic nerve block using a posterior gluteal approach and an IP needle alignment to a curved low frequency probe. The lateral-to-medial needle direction may help avoid puncture of the inferior gluteal or internal pudendal vessels.

muscle before reaching the sciatic nerve above the ischial bone (Fig. 35-34).

- Local anesthetic spread: Performing a test dose with D5W is recommended prior to local anesthetic application to visualize the spread and confirm nerve localization. It is generally recommended to deposit the local anesthetic solution so that it spreads completely around the sciatic nerve.

COMMENTS

- For both IP and OOP needling approaches, scanning before needling will determine the angle, distance and depth of needle penetration.
- The OOP approach is often used for catheter insertion, and it is important to line up the site of needle insertion with the target nerve.

Posterior Sciatic Nerve Block: Subgluteal Approach

The patient is positioned semiprone (Sims' position) with the hip and knee flexed and the foot resting on the dependent knee. In some patients, the supine position with the hip flexed and knee bent is either most comfortable or necessitated due to fracture or pain at the hip. This latter position requires an assistant to support the bent leg.

PROCEDURE USING NERVE STIMULATION TECHNIQUE

- Landmarks: A horizontal line is drawn joining the medial aspect of the greater trochanter to the ischial tuberosity. The traditional puncture site is located on this line just medial to its midpoint.
- Needling: An insulated needle, 100 to 150 mm, depending on patient habitus, is used. The needle is inserted perpendicular to the skin.
- Nerve localization: Confirming sciatic nerve localization with NS is important prior to local anesthetic application. Similar responses as those for the classic gluteal approach are sought, with ankle responses preferable. It is important to distinguish the tibial (inversion or plantar flexion) and common peroneal (eversion or dorsiflexion) components of the nerve and obtain either both or, most importantly, the tibial response.
- Injection: Injection of 20 to 30 mL of local anesthetic is sufficient. If additional blocks of the lower extremity are also performed, a solution with lower concentration should be considered to prevent exceeding the toxic dose of local anesthetic.

PROCEDURE USING ULTRASOUND IMAGING (FIG. 35-40)

- Scanning: A curved, lower frequency 2 to 5 MHz probe or linear 4 to 7 MHz probe is suitable for scanning the subgluteal region. The center of the probe should be aligned with the midpoint of a line between the ischial tuberosity and the greater trochanter. If the sciatic nerve is hard to localize at the subgluteal region, it can be traced proximally from the bifurcation point at or near the apex of the popliteal fossa.
- Appearance: On the lateral side of the screen, the medial aspect of the greater trochanter appears almost pear-shaped and hypoechoic when using a curved array probe. The sciatic nerve in the subgluteal region appears predominantly hyperechoic (bright) and is often elliptical in a short-axis view using US.
- Needling: Similar to the classic gluteal approach, both IP and OOP plane needling can be performed, with the needle directed from lateral to medial for the IP technique. Using an angle of insertion of approximately 45 degrees to the skin will provide the best view of the needle and will reach the nerve, although 60 to 70 degrees may be required in certain obese individuals.
- Local anesthetic spread: The goal is to deposit local anesthetic (20 to 30 mL) next to, but not directly within, the sciatic nerve structure in the subgluteal region. A hypoechoic local anesthetic fluid collection is often seen around the hyperechoic nerve within the sheath compartment during injection.

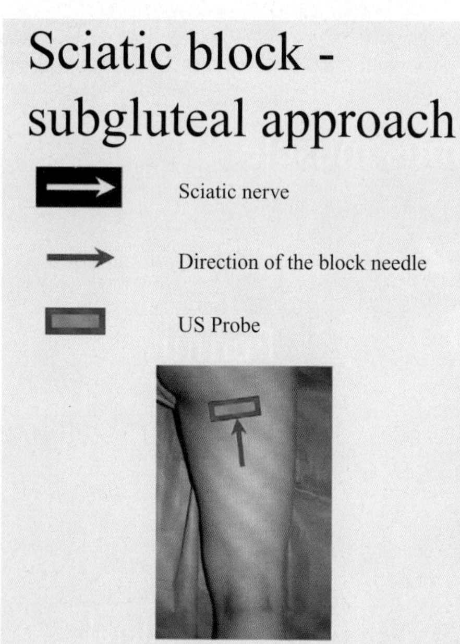

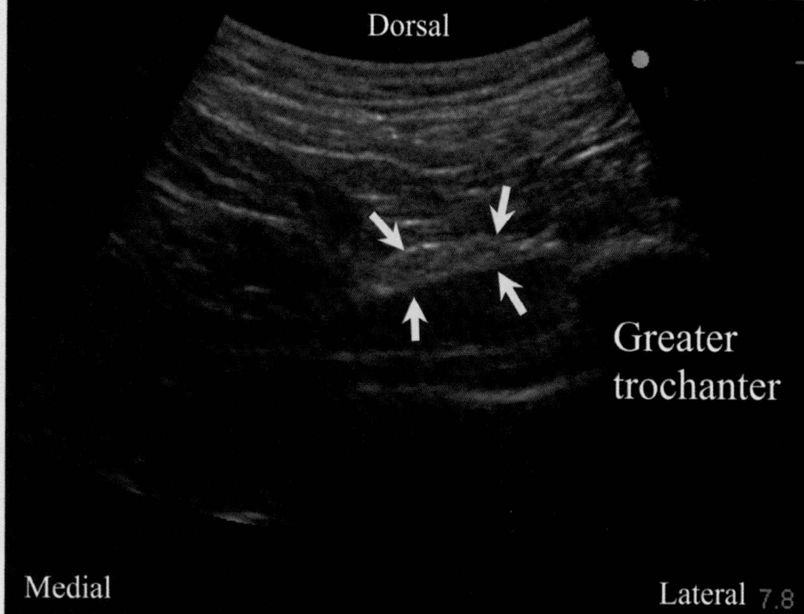

FIGURE 35-40. Ultrasound-guided sciatic nerve block with a subgluteal approach using OOP needling to a curved probe. The medially positioned ischial tuberosity is not captured in this image but will serve as a good bony landmark in most circumstances. OOP approaches will be often used since this block is often used for indwelling catheter placement, especially in children.

COMMENTS

- Since a low frequency curved array probe is necessary in many cases, the needle tip as viewed by OOP needling will be even harder to identify than when using higher resolution linear probes. Nevertheless, this approach is used often since indwelling catheters are commonly placed in the subgluteal area. It will be important to use NS in addition to US-guided technique to confirm placement of the needle and local anesthetic.

Posterior Popliteal Sciatic Block

The sciatic nerve can be blocked below the hip at the lateral midfemoral or lateral popliteal locations in addition to the posterior popliteal location,[189,190] but when using US guidance, the posterior approach allows the needle to be placed closely to the probe and thus may improve needle tracking and visibility. Furthermore, the posterior popliteal approach is most amenable to inserting indwelling catheters. The patient is positioned laterally or prone with the operative leg slightly flexed. Ideally, the ankles should be positioned beyond the end of the table so that motor responses to NS can be readily observed in the prone position. The landmarks become more visible when the knee is flexed against resistance. Please refer to the accompanying video clip for a demonstration of the sciatic nerve block from a popliteal approach.

10

PROCEDURE USING NERVE STIMULATION TECHNIQUE

- Landmarks: The puncture site is often located at the tip of a triangle formed by the popliteal crease at the base, the biceps femoris tendon laterally, and the semimembranosus tendon medially (this tendon generally lies medial to the tendon of the semitendinosus at this location). Alternatively, drawing lines 8 cm long in a cephalad direction from the insertion site of the medial and lateral tendons (above), the puncture point is at the midpoint of a line attaching the two (almost parallel) lines. It may be best to insert the needle at approximately 10 cm above the popliteal fossa in order to ensure that the sciatic nerve is blocked before its bifurcation.
- Needling: Depending on the patient, a 50-mm insulated 22-gauge needle can be inserted using an angle of 45 degrees cephalad to the skin. A fan-wise search is conducted perpendicular to this line until the nerve is contacted. If the femur is contacted by the needle, the depth is noted. The nerve should lie midway between the skin and the femur.
- Nerve localization: NS is used to localize the nerve by eliciting motor responses at the ankle or foot. The aim should be to localize the sciatic nerve before its bifurcation into its tibial and common peroneal nerve components. If only ankle inversion and/or plantarflexion (tibial nerve) or eversion and/or dorsiflexion (common peroneal) is seen, it would be appropriate to adjust the needle insertion site a few centimeters cephalad to obtain complete ankle and foot movements. Otherwise, injecting after obtaining a sole tibial nerve response has been shown to provide similar success to that after both tibial and common peroneal responses (with two injections).[191] Maintaining a motor response with currents <0.5 mA will help ensure the nerve–needle distance is appropriate for a successful block.[192]
- Injection: Twenty to thirty milliliters of local anesthetic should be deposited at the final needle location.

PROCEDURE USING ULTRASOUND GUIDANCE (FIG. 35-41)

- Scanning: A linear higher frequency 10 to 15 MHz probe is commonly used for scanning the sciatic nerve transversely in the popliteal fossa. A technique which utilizes a distal-to-proximal scan can effectively locate the sciatic nerve in the posterior popliteal fossa prior to its bifurcation (Fig. 35-41). At the popliteal crease, the transverse probe captures the tibial and common peroneal nerves, with the former being adjacent and lateral to the popliteal vessels (Doppler is very valuable here). During a proximal scan, the tibial and common peroneal nerves approach each other and join to form the sciatic nerve.
- Appearance: At the level of the popliteal crease, the tibial and common peroneal nerves lie superficial and lateral to the popliteal vessels (the common peroneal nerve is the most lateral); both nerves appear round-to-oval and hyperechoic compared to the surrounding musculature. The hyperechoic border of the femur (condyles) may be apparent. During the proximal scan, the tibial nerve moves away from the vessels and approaches the common peroneal nerve. More cephalad in the posterior thigh, the biceps femoris muscle lies superficial to the joining nerves and appears as a larger, oval-shaped structure with less internal punctate areas (hypoechoic spots) than the nerves. The sciatic nerve appears as a large, round or flat, oval hyperechoic structure. The large amount of fat and muscle may impair visualization of the nerve itself. Furthermore, the probe often needs to be tilted for optimal imaging since the nerve becomes more superficial as it descends distally.
- Needling: An OOP approach is commonly performed, especially if placing indwelling catheters. The probe is positioned directly above the sciatic nerve at or slightly cephalad to its bifurcation point and so that the nerve is in the center of the image. The needle should be inserted at the caudal surface of probe (especially if a catheter is to be inserted), with the needle tip contacting the skin approximately 3 to 4 cm caudal to the probe surface.
- Local anesthetic spread: For local anesthetic injection at the bifurcation, hypoechoic injectate will be seen to expand within the common epineural sheath. For injections above or below the bifurcation, a circumferential spread, producing a "donut" shape surrounding the hyperechoic nerve structure, is preferable. Several separate injections (medial and lateral) may be required for complete circumferential spread.

COMMENTS

- The ideal needle insertion point for sciatic nerve block using the popliteal approach remains debatable. The tibial and common peroneal branches may be blocked separately[193] or injection may occur between these nerves at the bifurcation.[194]
- Several groups have provided evidence that injection distal (caudad), rather than proximal, to the bifurcation point results in faster block onset and improved sensory block.[193–196] Recently, a randomized comparison between a single subepineural injection at the neural bifurcation and separate injections around the tibial and peroneal divisions demonstrated a higher success rate and shorter performance, onset, and total anesthesia-related times with the former approach.[197]
- US guidance, either alone or in conjunction with NS, was shown to improve the success of both single-shot and catheter-delivered local anesthetic as well as patient outcome with respect to postoperative pain, as compared to NS guidance alone.[198–200]
- The US probe may be rotated 90 degrees to show the sciatic nerve in the long axis. This is helpful to differentiate the sciatic nerve from other nonneural structures.
- During needle insertion using an OOP approach, it may be helpful to use incremental needle angulations. The needle may be best tracked within the tissue if an initial shallow angle is

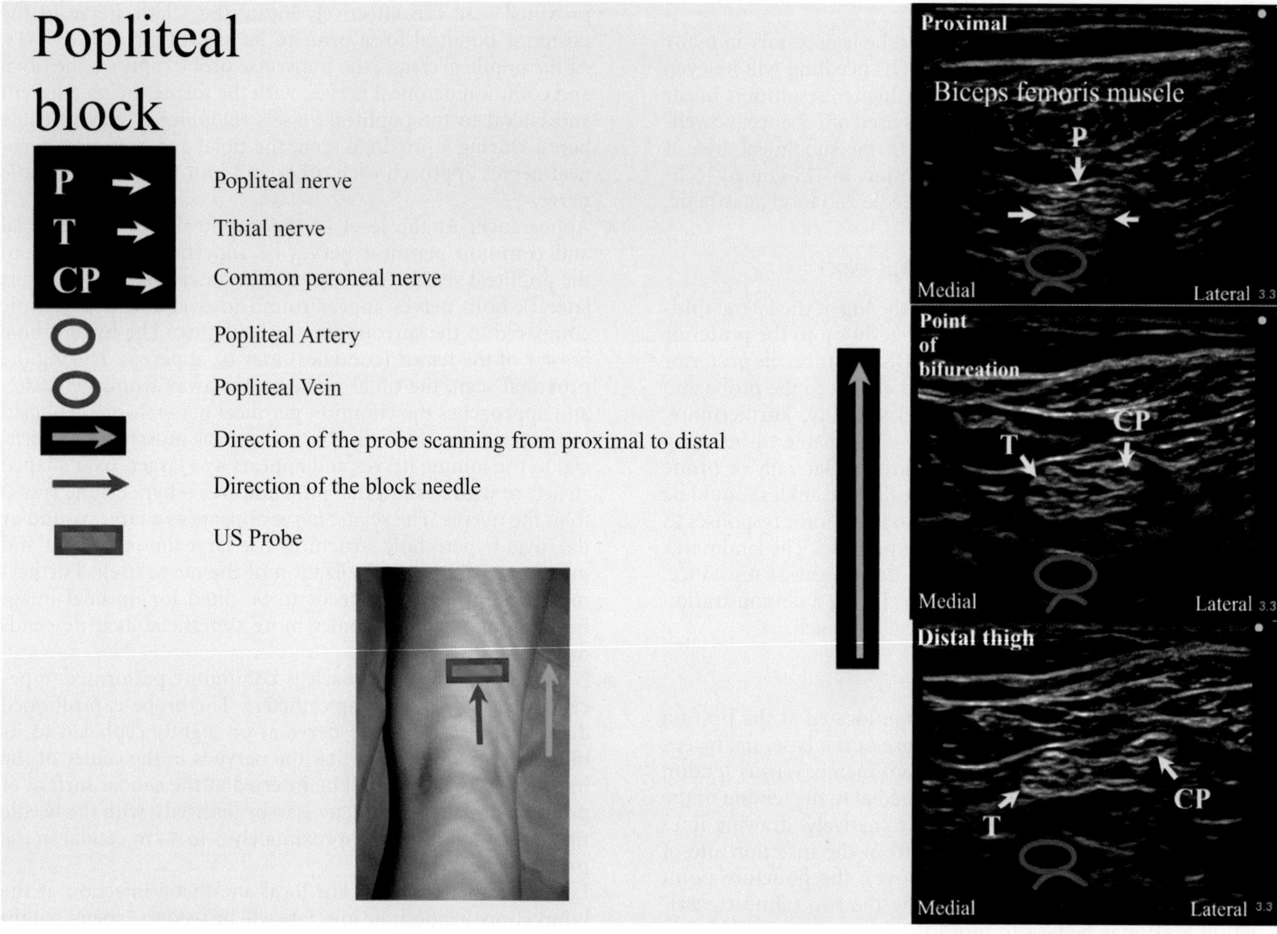

FIGURE 35-41. Ultrasound-guided popliteal nerve block. The probe is initially placed at the popliteal crease (lower image), and subsequently is used to scan proximally to capture the sciatic nerve just proximal to its bifurcation (i.e., the ideal block site), approximately 6 to 10 cm above the crease (upper).

used to clearly identify the needle tip as a hyperechoic dot, which can then be followed with subsequent steeper needle angulations (see the description of the "walk-down" technique under Practical Approaches for US guidance).[37]

Anterior Sciatic Nerve Block

This block is most suitable for patients who cannot be positioned laterally. The block is indicated for surgery below the knee, with the only sensory deficiency being the medial strip of skin supplied by the saphenous nerve. The anterior block is performed on a short portion of the sciatic nerve close to the lesser trochanter of the femur. This block may cause more discomfort since the needle traverses through more muscle layers than the other approaches of sciatic nerve block. The patient is positioned supine, with the leg to be blocked externally rotated slightly.

PROCEDURE USING NERVE STIMULATION TECHNIQUE

- Landmarks: A line is drawn connecting the anterior superior iliac spine with the pubic tubercle (inguinal ligament). A second line, parallel to the first, is drawn across the thigh from the greater trochanter. A line is then drawn downward from a point at the medial third of the upper line; the nerve is usually located at the intersection of the perpendicular line and the lower of the two parallel lines. Alternatively, the nerve is located lateral to the femoral artery pulse at the level of the inguinal crease.
- Needling: A 22-gauge, 100- to 150-mm insulated needle will be required for this deep block.
- The needle is inserted perpendicular to the skin and advanced until contact with the femur occurs. The needle is then withdrawn slightly, angulated slightly medial and cephalad, and introduced 5 cm further.
- Nerve localization: Motor responses of the ankle joint or foot are sought.
- Injection: Twenty to thirty milliliters of local anesthetic is injected after careful aspiration and administration of a test dose.

PROCEDURE USING ULTRASOUND IMAGING (FIG. 35-42)

- Scanning: It is most common to utilize a curved, lower frequency 2 to 5 MHz probe to scan the sciatic nerve in the proximal thigh. Place the probe over the proximal thigh approximately 8 cm distal to the femoral crease. A transversely placed probe is commonly used, although the nerve may be best visualized by placing the probe axis longitudinally along the course of the nerve, since capturing a longitudinal axis of the nerve may improve its identification since it has a distinctive "cable"

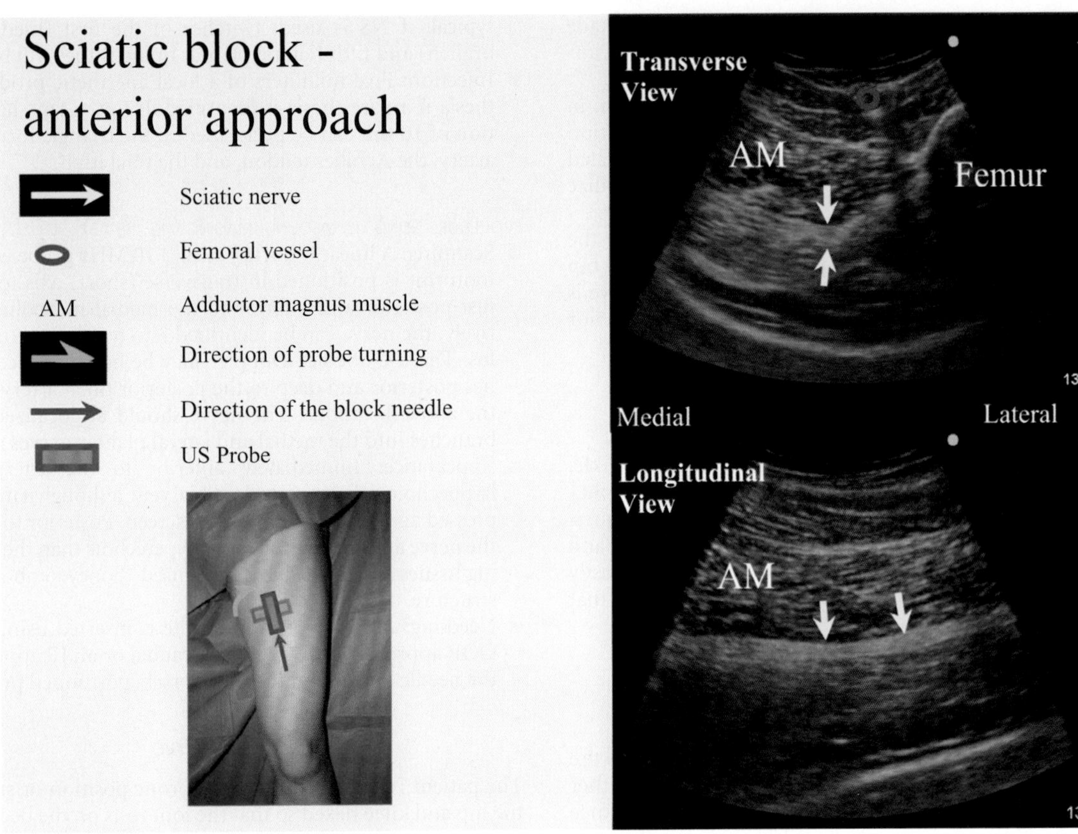

FIGURE 35-42. Ultrasound-guided sciatic block from an anterior approach. The clinical picture and upper image show probe positioning and a short-axis view of the nerve that may be used. Using a longitudinally placed probe to capture the long axis of the nerve (lower image) may be beneficial if the transverse view is difficult to capture due to bony shadowing from the lesser trochanter.

appearance. Moving in a medial-to-lateral direction may be helpful to capture an image of the nerve.

- Appearance: In transverse axis, the sciatic nerve often appears oval or round, predominantly hyperechoic, medial and posterior to the lesser trochanter, and deep to the adductor magus muscle. If using Doppler, the femoral neurovascular structures are seen superficial below the hyperechoic fascial tissue and lateral to the sciatic nerve in this projection when the leg is externally rotated. A longitudinal view captures a broad, linear, and hyperechoic cable of fibers and may allow easier identification of the nerve.[201]
- Needling: When using a probe positioned in transverse axis to the nerve, an IP approach involves advancing the needle in a medial-to-lateral and anterior to posterior direction, while an OOP approach involves inserting the needle along the midline of the probe at a location 2 to 3 cm inferior and perpendicular to the probe. If the probe is placed longitudinally, the needle direction for OOP alignment will be similar to that for the IP approach described above. Using an IP approach with the probe placed longitudinally, the needle will be placed in a cephalad-to-caudad direction, allowing it to be aimed easily toward a relatively larger target (i.e., the cable-like sciatic nerve). It is highly recommended to use combined US and NS guidance for this procedure.
- Local anesthetic spread: After careful aspiration and injection of a small amount of D5W to visualize the anesthetic spread, inject the local anesthetic while ensuring that it spreads circumferentially around the nerve.

COMMENTS

- Although depositing the local anesthetic around the nerve is desirable, it is technically challenging to reposition the needle on both sides of the nerve because of the nerve's depth within the muscle layers.
- Similar to other sciatic nerve blocks, if this block is being combined with others, the local anesthetic may need to be diluted to reduce the risk of toxicity.
- Complications are rare, but can include intravascular injection (e.g., femoral artery), infection in the injection area, hematoma formation, nerve injury, and potential CNS toxicity.

Other Approaches to Sciatic Block

- A supine approach developed by Raj et al.,[202] in which the patient's leg is maximally flexed, stretches the nerve within the space between the greater trochanter and the ischial tuberosity; needle insertion occurs at the midpoint between these two structures. In this approach, landmarks are easy to find and the position offers an alternative to patients who cannot accommodate prone or lateral positioning. This approach has recently been shown to be amenable to catheter-delivered continuous anesthesia of the sciatic nerve.[203]

- Recently, several novel approaches to sciatic nerve blockade have been described that may be useful when the patient cannot be positioned for traditional approaches:
  - Le Corroller et al.[204] have described a lateral approach, in which the patient is positioned supine and the injection occurs on the midpoint of a vertical line drawn cephalad from the greater trochanter to the anterior superior iliac spine.
  - Osaka et al.[205] have described a medial approach at the midthigh, where the patient is positioned supine, the hip and knee flexed and externally rotated. The sciatic nerve is beneath the adductor magnus muscle, 1.5 to 2 cm posterior to the femur at the upper midthigh.

Ankle Block

All five nerves of the foot can be blocked at the level of the ankle. The superficial nerves—sural, superficial peroneal, and saphenous nerves—can be blocked by simple infiltration techniques. US guidance can be useful for blocking the posterior tibial and deep peroneal (fibular) nerves, as their locations can be easily identified next to reliable landmarks (i.e., bones and vessels) that are clearly visible.

Posterior Tibial Nerve

PROCEDURE USING LANDMARK TECHNIQUE

- Landmarks: The posterior tibial nerve is the major nerve to the sole of the foot. It can be approached with the patient either in the prone position or lying supine with the hip and knee flexed so that the foot rests on the bed. The medial malleolus is identified, along with the pulsation of the posterior tibial artery behind it. The nerve is located posterior to the artery.
- Needling: A needle is introduced through the skin just behind the posterior tibial artery and directed 45 degrees anteriorly, seeking a paresthesia in the sole of the foot. Although not typical, if NS is used, twitches of the first (medial plantar branch) and fifth (lateral plantar branch) toes will be sought.
- Injection: Five milliliters of a local anesthetic produces anesthesia if a paresthesia is identified. If not, a fan-shaped injection of 10 mL can be performed in the triangle formed by the artery, the Achilles tendon, and the tibia itself.

PROCEDURE USING ULTRASOUND IMAGING (FIG. 35-43)

- Scanning: A linear ("hockey stick") 10 MHz probe with a small footprint is positioned in transverse (short) axis to the nerve just posterior and inferior to the medial malleolus. Alternatively, the nerve can be identified 3 to 5 cm above the malleolus. The use of color Doppler may be helpful, since the nerve lies posterior and deep to the posterior tibial artery at both of the above locations. The nerve should be localized before it branches into the medial and lateral plantar nerves.
- Appearance: Immediately anterior to the artery lies the hypoechoic circular posterior tibial vein, although it may be compressed and not apparent on the screen. Posterior to the artery, the nerve appears slightly more hyperechoic than the surrounding tissues and looks like a condensed "honeycomb-appearing" structure.
- Needling: A 35- to 50-mm needle is inserted using either an OOP approach with the needle caudal or an IP approach with the needle anterior to the transversely positioned probe.

Sural Nerve

The patient is placed either in the prone position or supine with the hip and knee flexed so that the foot rests on the bed. The posteriorly located sural nerve can be blocked by injection on the lateral side. The subcutaneous injection of 5 mL of local anesthetic behind the lateral malleolus, filling the groove between it and the calcaneus, produces anesthesia of the sural nerve. The effectiveness of a sural nerve block was found to be improved using a perivascular approach (i.e., identifying the lesser saphenous vein

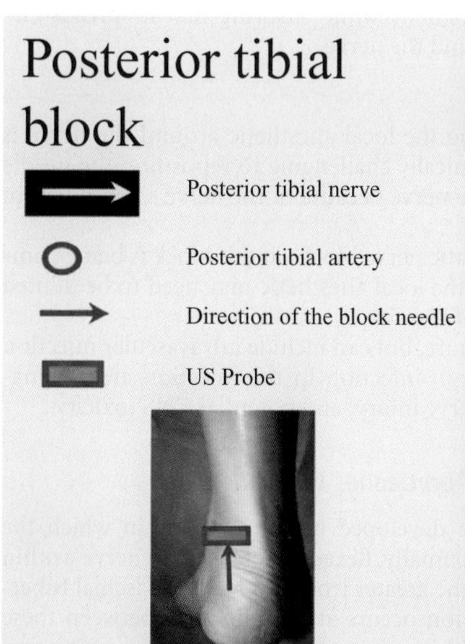

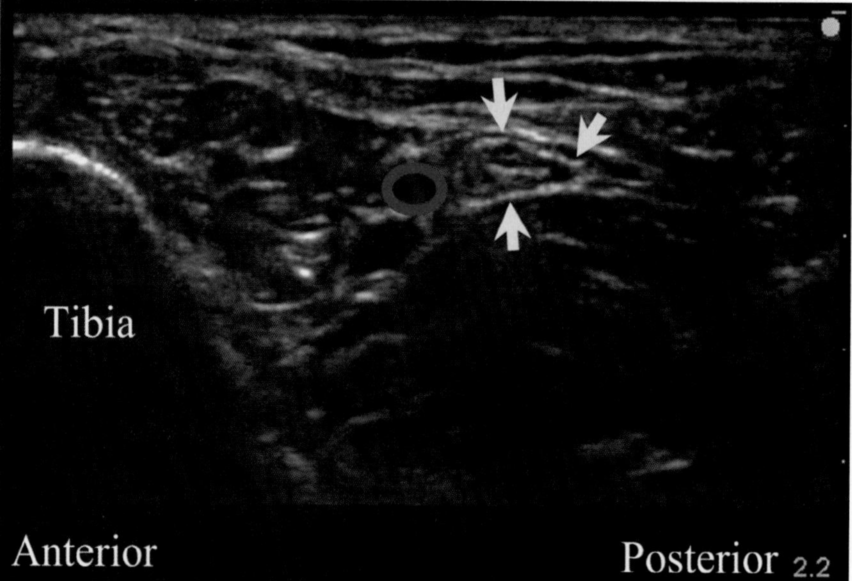

FIGURE 35-43. Ultrasound-guided posterior tibial nerve block at the ankle using an IP approach. The nerve is captured adjacent to the posterior tibial artery, prior to its division into the medial and lateral plantar nerves.

1 cm proximal to the lateral malleolus), rather than a traditional, surface landmark-based approach, under US guidance.[206]

Deep Peroneal Nerve

PROCEDURE USING LANDMARK TECHNIQUE

- Landmarks: This is the major nerve to the dorsum of the foot and lies in the deep plane of the anterior tibial artery. The patient is positioned supine, generally with the leg extended. Pulsation of the artery is sought at the level of the skin crease on the anterior midline surface of the ankle. If the artery is not palpable, the tendon of the extensor hallucis longus can be identified (the nerve lies immediately lateral to this) by asking the patient to extend the big toe.
- Needling and Injection: If the artery pulse can be felt, 5 mL of local anesthetic is injected just lateral to this. If the artery is not palpable, the tendon of the extensor hallucis longus can be identified by asking the patient to extend the big toe. If using NS, toe extension is sought for this nerve. Injection can be made into the deep planes below the fascia using either one of these landmarks.

PROCEDURE USING ULTRASOUND IMAGING (FIG. 35-44)

- Scanning: A small footprint linear ("hockey stick") 10 MHz probe is placed in transverse (short) axis to the nerve at the anterior surface of the ankle joint. Alternatively, the nerve can also be found 3 to 5 cm above the ankle joint. However, the nerve itself can be difficult to see, and only the artery can be consistently located. Color Doppler can be used at both locations to identify the anterior tibial artery lying medial to the nerve.
- Appearance: If seen, the nerve appears as a small cluster of hyperechoic fascicular appearing fibers immediately lateral to the artery, with both the nerve and the artery adjacent to the well-demarcated distal end of the tibia.
- Needling: An OOP approach will be most suitable here since the tendons lie on either side of the nerve. A 3.5- to 5-cm needle is inserted OOP and caudal to the transversely positioned small footprint probe.
- Local anesthetic spread: Injection of 4 to 5 mL of local anesthetic lateral to the nerve will help avoid the anterior tibial artery, which lies medial to the nerve. Aspiration is important to perform prior to injection.

Saphenous Nerve

The patient is placed supine with the leg extended. The saphenous nerve is anesthetized by infiltrating 5 mL of local anesthetic around the saphenous vein at the level where it passes anterior to the medial malleolus. A wall of anesthesia between the skin and the bone itself suffices to block the nerve. Alternatively, this nerve can be blocked at a more proximal site in the thigh. See the section on Separate Blocks of the Terminal Nerves of the Lumbar Plexus for blockade of this nerve more proximally in the thigh.

Superficial Peroneal Branches

A subcutaneous ridge of anesthetic solution is laid along the skin crease between the anterior tibial artery and the lateral malleolus. This subcutaneous ridge overlies the previous subfascial injection for the deep peroneal nerve. Another 5 to 10 mL of local anesthetic may be required to cover this area. The superficial peroneal nerve may be visualized using US, which may aid in more accurate injection of local anesthetic.[207]

Comments

- Anesthesia of the foot usually ensues within 15 minutes of these five injections.
- Complications of this block are rare, although neuropathy can be produced. Care should be taken not to pin any of the deep nerves against the bone at the time of injection, and intraneural injection should be avoided. Epinephrine should not be added to local anesthetics used for this block in order to avoid compromising the distal circulation.

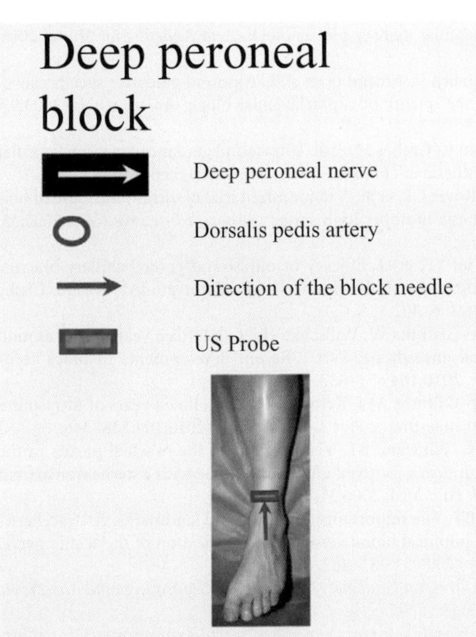

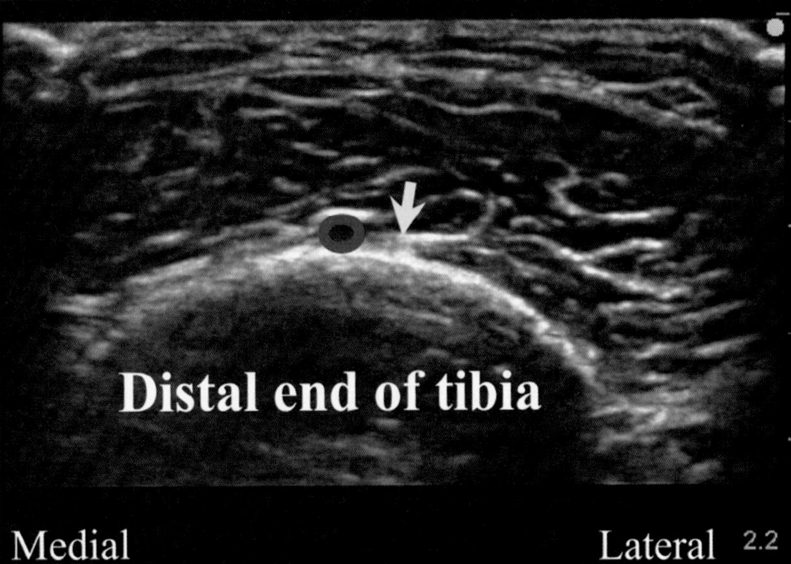

FIGURE 35-44. Ultrasound-guided deep peroneal nerve block at the anterior ankle. If possible, it is helpful to localize the medially located anterior tibial artery with Doppler in order to differentiate between the nerve and surrounding tendons.

- US imaging for the deep nerves may help avoid bone contact and avoid the multiple injections with the infiltration technique.

Continuous Catheter Technique

Continuous catheter regional anesthesia has been well documented to provide effective pain relief with reduced incidence of side effects and an improved quality of life.[208,209] Traditionally, catheters are introduced blindly once neural structures have been identified using a peripheral nerve stimulator and often after the initial local anesthetic dose has been injected via the needle. Although continuous delivery of local anesthetic has been used successfully at a number of block sites following blind catheter insertion,[210] the method is associated with at least 10% to 40% secondary block failure due to the catheters being in a suboptimal location.[211,212] This high failure rate resulted in the development of stimulating catheters to aid in their positioning close to the nerve,[213] which improved success rates. However, insertion and precise positioning of stimulating catheters requires technical expertise and can be a time-consuming process, and needle insertion with stimulating catheters remains a blind procedure since neurostimulation and anatomical landmarks are still required to locate the nerve.

In recent years, ultrasonography has been used extensively to initiate regional blocks,[214,215] and several large-scale studies have shown its efficacy in guiding the placement of perineural catheters.[216,217] However, catheter insertion for continuous regional anesthesia, whether guided by NS or US, suffers from several fundamental problems owing to the design of current needle-catheter assemblies, including dislodgement or movement of the catheter, leakage at the insertion site, and imprecise catheter placement.[210] With advancements in technology and design (e.g., catheter-over-needle),[218,219] these technical difficulties may be resolved with further research.

ACKNOWLEDGMENTS

The authors thank Drs. Derek Dillane, Vivian Ip, and Gareth Corry, and the Department of Anesthesiology and Pain Medicine, University of Alberta, for their contributions to the text and for the video clips. Many of the simplified anatomical drawings for this chapter were produced by and used with permission from Ms. Carol Chan. Most figures and material were adapted from one of the author's (B.T.) textbooks, *Atlas of Ultrasound and Nerve Stimulation-Guided Regional Anesthesia.*[37]

References

1. Tziavrangos E, Schug SA. Regional anaesthesia and perioperative outcome. *Curr Opin Anaesthesiol.* 2006;19:521–525.
2. Brown DL, Ransom DM, Hall JA, et al. Regional anesthesia and local anesthetic-induced systemic toxicity: Seizure frequency and accompanying cardiovascular changes. *Anesth Analg.* 1995;81:321–328.
3. Borgeat A, Schappi B, Biasca N, et al. Patient-controlled analgesia after major shoulder surgery: Patient-controlled interscalene analgesia versus patient-controlled analgesia. *Anesthesiology.* 1997;87:1343–1347.
4. Greengrass RA. Regional anesthesia for ambulatory surgery. *Anesthesiol Clin North America.* 2000;18:341–353, vii.
5. Singelyn FJ, Gouverneur JM. Postoperative analgesia after total hip arthroplasty: I.V. PCA with morphine, patient-controlled epidural analgesia, or continuous "3-in-1" block? A prospective evaluation by our acute pain service in more than 1,300 patients. *J Clin Anesth.* 1999;11:550–554.
6. Nielsen KC, Steele SM. Outcome after regional anaesthesia in the ambulatory setting–is it really worth it? *Best Pract Res Clin Anaesthesiol.* 2002;16:145–157.
7. Auroy Y, Narchi P, Messiah A, et al. Serious complications related to regional anesthesia: Results of a prospective survey in France. *Anesthesiology.* 1997;87:479–486.
8. Tsui B. Ultrasound-guidance and nerve stimulation: Implications for the future practice of regional anesthesia. *Can J Anaesth.* 2007;54:165–170.
9. Greenblatt GM, Denson JS. Needle nerve stimulatorlocator: Nerve blocks with a new instrument for locating nerves. *Anesth Analg.* 1962;41:599–602.
10. Sarnoff S. Functional localization of interspinal catheters. *Anesthesiology.* 1950; 11:360.
11. Boezaart AP, de Beer JF, du Toit C, et al. A new technique of continuous interscalene nerve block. *Can J Anaesth.* 1999;46:275–281.
12. Copeland SJ, Laxton MA. A new stimulating catheter for continuous peripheral nerve blocks. *Reg Anesth Pain Med.* 2001;26:589–590.
13. Perlas A, Niazi A, McCartney C, et al. The sensitivity of motor response to nerve stimulation and paresthesia for nerve localization as evaluated by ultrasound. *Reg Anesth Pain Med.* 2006;31:445–450.
14. Urmey WF, Stanton J. Inability to consistently elicit a motor response following sensory paresthesia during interscalene block administration. *Anesthesiology.* 2002;96:552–554.
15. Hadzic A, Vloka J, Hadzic N, et al. Nerve stimulators used for peripheral nerve blocks vary in their electrical characteristics. *Anesthesiology.* 2003;98:969–974.
16. Urmey WF. Using the nerve stimulator for peripheral or plexus nerve blocks. *Minerva Anestesiol.* 2006;72:467–471.
17. Ganta R, Cajee RA, Henthorn RW. Use of transcutaneous nerve stimulation to assist interscalene block. *Anesth Analg.* 1993;76:914–915.
18. Urmey WF, Grossi P. Percutaneous electrode guidance: A noninvasive technique for prelocation of peripheral nerves to facilitate peripheral plexus or nerve block. *Reg Anesth Pain Med.* 2002;27:261–267.
19. Bosenberg AT, Raw R, Boezaart AP. Surface mapping of peripheral nerves in children with a nerve stimulator. *Paediatr Anaesth.* 2002;12:398–403.
20. Tsui BC, Gupta S, Finucane B. Confirmation of epidural catheter placement using nerve stimulation. *Can J Anaesth.* 1998;45:640–644.
21. Tsui BC, Finucane B. Epidural stimulator catheter. *Tech Reg Anesth Pain Med.* 2002;6:150–154.
22. Koscielniak-Nielsen ZJ, Rassmussen H, Jepsen K. Effect of impulse duration on patients' perception of electrical stimulation and block effectiveness during axillary block in unsedated ambulatory patients. *Reg Anesth Pain Med.* 2001;26: 428–433.
23. Hadzic A, Vloka JD, Claudio RE, et al. Electrical nerve localization: Effects of cutaneous electrode placement and duration of the stimulus on motor response. *Anesthesiology.* 2004;100:1526–1530.
24. Borgeat A. Regional anesthesia, intraneural injection, and nerve injury: Beyond the epineurium. *Anesthesiology.* 2006;105:647–648.
25. Raj PP, Rosenblatt R, Montgomery SJ. Use of the nerve stimulator for peripheral blocks. *Reg Anaesth.* 1980;5:14–21.
26. Tsui BC, Wagner A, Finucane B. Electrophysiologic effect of injectates on peripheral nerve stimulation. *Reg Anesth Pain Med.* 2004;29:189–193.
27. Tsui BC, Kropelin B, Ganapathy S, et al. Dextrose 5% in water: Fluid medium for maintaining electrical stimulation of peripheral nerves during stimulating catheter placement. *Acta Anaesthesiol Scand.* 2005;49:1562–1565.
28. Sites BD, Beach ML, Spence BC, et al. Ultrasound guidance improves the success rate of a perivascular axillary plexus block. *Acta Anaesthesiol Scand.* 2006; 50:678–684.
29. Williams SR, Chouinard P, Arcand G, et al. Ultrasound guidance speeds execution and improves the quality of supraclavicular block. *Anesth Analg.* 2003;97: 1518–1523.
30. Marhofer P, Sitzwohl C, Greher M, et al. Ultrasound guidance for infraclavicular brachial plexus anesthesia in children. *Anaesthesia.* 2004;59:642–646.
31. Soeding PE, Sha S, Royse CE, et al. A randomized trial of ultrasound-guided brachial plexus anaesthesia in upper limb surgery. *Anaesth Intensive Care.* 2005;33: 719–725.
32. Liu FC, Liou JT, Tsai YF, et al. Efficacy of ultrasound-guided axillary brachial plexus block: A comparative study with nerve stimulator-guided method. *Chang Gung Med J.* 2005;28:396–402.
33. Marhofer P, Harrop-Griffiths W, Willschke H, et al. Fifteen years of ultrasound guidance in regional anaesthesia: Part 2-Recent developments in block techniques. *Br J Anaesth.* 2010;104:673–683.
34. Marhofer P, Harrop-Griffiths AW, Kettner SC, et al. Fifteen years of ultrasound guidance in regional anaesthesia: Part 1. *Br J Anaesth.* 2010;104:538–546.
35. Tsui BC, Twomey C, Finucane BT. Visualization of the brachial plexus in the supraclavicular region using a curved ultrasound probe with a sterile transparent dressing. *Reg Anesth Pain Med.* 2006;31:182–184.
36. Tsui BC, Finucane BT. The importance of ultrasound landmarks: A "traceback" approach using the popliteal blood vessels for identification of the sciatic nerve. *Reg Anesth Pain Med.* 2006;31:481–482.
37. Tsui BCH. *Atlas of Ultrasound and Nerve Stimulation-Guided Regional Anesthesia.* New York, NY: Springer; 2007.
38. Tsui BC, Dillane D. Needle puncture site and a "walkdown" approach for short-axis alignment during ultrasound-guided blocks. *Reg Anesth Pain Med.* 2006; 31:586–587.
39. Tsui BC. Facilitating needle alignment in-plane to an ultrasound beam using a portable laser unit. *Reg Anesth Pain Med.* 2007;32:84–88.

40. Selander D, Dhuner KG, Lundborg G. Peripheral nerve injury due to injection needles used for regional anesthesia. An experimental study of the acute effects of needle point trauma. *Acta Anaesthesiol Scand.* 1977;21:182–188.
41. Steele SM, Klein SM, D'Ercole FJ, et al. A new continuous catheter delivery system. *Anesth Analg.* 1998;87:228.
42. Claudio R, Hadzic A, Shih H, et al. Injection pressures by anesthesiologists during simulated peripheral nerve block. *Reg Anesth Pain Med.* 2004;29:201–205.
43. Hadzic A, Dilberovic F, Shah S, et al. Combination of intraneural injection and high injection pressure leads to fascicular injury and neurologic deficits in dogs. *Reg Anesth Pain Med.* 2004;29:417–423.
44. Selander D, Sjostrand J. Longitudinal spread of intraneurally injected local anesthetics. An experimental study of the initial neural distribution following intraneural injections. *Acta Anaesthesiol Scand.* 1978;22:622–634.
45. Tsui BC, Li LX, Pillay JJ. Compressed air injection technique to standardize block injection pressures. *Can J Anaesth.* 2006;53:1098–1102.
46. Borgeat A, Blumenthal S. Nerve injury and regional anaesthesia. *Curr Opin Anaesthesiol.* 2004;17:417–421.
47. Kaufman BR, Nystrom E, Nath S, et al. Debilitating chronic pain syndromes after presumed intraneural injections. *Pain.* 2000;85:283–286.
48. Selander D. Neurotoxicity of local anesthetics: Animal data. *Reg Anesth.* 1993;18: 461–468.
49. Ben-David B. Complications of peripheral blockade. *Anesthesiol Clin North America.* 2002;20:695–707.
50. Graf BM, Abraham I, Eberbach N, et al. Differences in cardiotoxicity of bupivacaine and ropivacaine are the result of physicochemical and stereoselective properties. *Anesthesiology.* 2002;96:1427–1434.
51. Knudsen K, Beckman SM, Blomberg S, et al. Central nervous and cardiovascular effects of i.v. infusions of ropivacaine, bupivacaine and placebo in volunteers. *Br J Anaesth.* 1997;78:507–514.
52. Muller M, Litz RJ, Huler M, et al. Grand mal convulsion and plasma concentrations after intravascular injection of ropivacaine for axillary brachial plexus blockade. *Br J Anaesth.* 2001;87:784–787.
53. Petitjeans F, Mion G, Puidupin M, et al. Tachycardia and convulsions induced by accidental intravascular ropivacaine injection during sciatic block. *Acta Anaesthesiol Scand.* 2002;46:616–617.
54. Reinikainen M, Hedman A, Pelkonen O, et al. Cardiac arrest after interscalene brachial plexus block with ropivacaine and lidocaine. *Acta Anaesthesiol Scand.* 2003;47:904–906.
55. Ruetsch YA, Fattinger KE, Borgeat A. Ropivacaine-induced convulsions and severe cardiac dysrhythmia after sciatic block. *Anesthesiology.* 1999;90: 1784–1786.
56. Marhofer P, Schrogendorfer K, Wallner T, et al. Ultrasonographic guidance reduces the amount of local anesthetic for 3-in-1 blocks. *Reg Anesth Pain Med.* 1998;23:584–588.
57. Willschke H, Marhofer P, Bosenberg A, et al. Ultrasonography for ilioinguinal/iliohypogastric nerve blocks in children. *Br J Anaesth.* 2005;95:226–230.
58. Weinberg GL, VadeBoncouer T, Ramaraju GA, et al. Pretreatment or resuscitation with a lipid infusion shifts the dose-response to bupivacaine-induced asystole in rats. *Anesthesiology.* 1998;88:1071–1075.
59. Litz RJ, Popp M, Stehr SN, et al. Successful resuscitation of a patient with ropivacaine-induced asystole after axillary plexus block using lipid infusion. *Anaesthesia.* 2006;61:800–801.
60. Rosenblatt MA, Abel M, Fischer GW, et al. Successful use of a 20% lipid emulsion to resuscitate a patient after a presumed bupivacaine-related cardiac arrest. *Anesthesiology.* 2006;105:217–218.
61. Fremling MA, Mackinnon SE. Injection injury to the median nerve. *Ann Plast Surg.* 1996;37:561–567.
62. Shah S, Hadzic A, Vloka JD, et al. Neurologic complication after anterior sciatic nerve block. *Anesth Analg.* 2005;100:1515–1517, table.
63. Selander D, Edshage S, Wolff T. Paresthesiae or no paresthesiae? Nerve lesions after axillary blocks. *Acta Anaesthesiol Scand.* 1979;23:27–33.
64. Winchell SW, Wolfe R. The incidence of neuropathy following upper extremity nerve blocks. *Reg Anesth.* 1985;10:12–15.
65. Enneking FK, Chan V, Greger J, et al. Lower-extremity peripheral nerve blockade: Essentials of our current understanding. *Reg Anesth Pain Med.* 2005;30: 4–35.
66. Gentili F, Hudson AR, Hunter D, et al. Nerve injection injury with local anesthetic agents: A light and electron microscopic, fluorescent microscopic, and horseradish peroxidase study. *Neurosurgery.* 1980;6:263–272.
67. Selander D. Peripheral nerve injury after regional anesthesia. In: Finucane BT, ed. *Complications of Regional Anesthesia.* Philadelphia, PA: Churchill Livingstone; 1999:105–115.
68. Sauter AR, Smith HJ, Stubhaug A, et al. Use of magnetic resonance imaging to define the anatomical location closest to all three cords of the infraclavicular brachial plexus. *Anesth Analg.* 2006;103:1574–1576.
69. Retzl G, Kapral S, Greher M, et al. Ultrasonographic findings of the axillary part of the brachial plexus. *Anesth Analg.* 2001;92:1271–1275.
70. Chan VWS, Perlas A, McCartney CJL, et al. Ultrasound guidance improves success rate of axillary brachial plexus block. *Can J Anaesth.* 2007;54:176–182.
71. Bonnel F. Microscopic anatomy of the adult human brachial plexus: An anatomical and histological basis for microsurgery. *Microsurgery.* 1984;5:107–118.
72. Klaastad O, Smedby O, Thompson GE, et al. Distribution of local anesthetic in axillary brachial plexus block: A clinical and magnetic resonance imaging study. *Anesthesiology.* 2002;96:1315–1324.
73. Kessler J, Gray AT. Sonography of scalene muscle anomalies for brachial plexus block. *Reg Anesth Pain Med.* 2007;32:172–173.
74. Uysal II, Seker M, Karabulut AK, et al. Brachial plexus variations in human fetuses. *Neurosurgery.* 2003;53:676–684.
75. Orebaugh SL, Pennington S. Variant location of the musculocutaneous nerve during axillary nerve block. *J Clin Anesth.* 2006;18:541–544.
76. Venieratos D, Anagnostopoulou S. Classification of communications between the musculocutaneous and median nerves. *Clin Anat.* 1998;11:327–331.
77. Amoiridis G. Median–ulnar nerve communications and anomalous innervation of the intrinsic hand muscles: An electrophysiological study. *Muscle Nerve.* 1992;15:576–579.
78. Bigeleisen PE. The bifid axillary artery. *J Clin Anesth.* 2004;16:224–225.
79. Kutiyanawala MA, Stotter A, Windle R. Anatomical variants during axillary dissection. *Br J Surg.* 1998;85:393–394.
80. Uglietta JP, Kadir S. Arteriographic study of variant arterial anatomy of the upper extremities. *Cardiovasc Intervent Radiol.* 1989;12:145–148.
81. Tsui BC. Ultrasound imaging to localize foramina for superficial trigeminal nerve block. *Can J Anesth.* 2009;56:704–706.
82. Pascal J, Charier D, Perret D, et al. Peripheral blocks of trigeminal nerve for facial soft-tissue surgery: Learning from failures. *Eur J Anaesthesiol.* 2005;22:480–482.
83. Nguyen A, Girard F, Boudreault D, et al. Scalp nerve blocks decrease the severity of pain after craniotomy. *Anesth Analg.* 2001;93:1272–1276.
84. Knize DM. A study of the supraorbital nerve. *Plast Reconstr Surg.* 1995;96:564–569.
85. Naja MZ, Al-Tannir M, Naja H, et al. Repeated nerve blocks with clonidine, fentanyl and bupivacaine for trigeminal neuralgia. *Anaesthesia.* 2006;61:70–71.
86. Haas DA. Alternative mandibular nerve block techniques: A review of the Gow-Gates and Akinosi-Vazirani closed-mouth mandibular nerve block techniques. *J Am Dent Assoc.* 2011;142:8S–12S.
87. Winnie AP, Ramamurthy S, Durrani Z, et al. Interscalene cervical plexus block: A single-injection technic. *Anesth Analg.* 1975;54:370–375.
88. Usui Y, Kobayashi T, Kakinuma H, et al. An anatomical basis for blocking of the deep cervical plexus and cervical sympathetic tract using an ultrasound-guided technique. *Anesth Analg.* 2010;110:964–968.
89. Stoneham MD, Doyle AR, Knighton JD, et al. Prospective, randomized comparison of deep or superficial cervical plexus block for carotid endarterectomy surgery. *Anesthesiology.* 1998;89:907–912.
90. de Sousa AA, Filho MA, Faglione W Jr, et al. Superficial vs combined cervical plexus block for carotid endarterectomy: A prospective, randomized study. *Surg Neurol.* 2005;63(suppl 1):S22–S25.
91. Pandit JJ, Bree S, Dillon P, et al. A comparison of superficial versus combined (superficial and deep) cervical plexus block for carotid endarterectomy: A prospective, randomized study. *Anesth Analg.* 2000;91:781–786.
92. Castresana EJ, Shaker IJ, Castresana MR. Incidence of shunting during carotid endarterectomy: Regional versus general anesthesia. *Reg Anesth.* 1997;22:23S.
93. Castresana MR, Masters RD, Castresana EJ, et al. Incidence and clinical significance of hemidiaphragmatic paresis in patients undergoing carotid endarterectomy during cervical plexus block anesthesia. *J Neurosurg Anesthesiol.* 1994;6:21–23.
94. Masters RD, Castresana EJ, Castresana MR. Superficial and deep cervical plexus block: Technical considerations. *AANA J.* 1995;63:235–243.
95. Stoneham MD, Knighton JD. Regional anaesthesia for carotid endarterectomy. *Br J Anaesth.* 1999;82:910–919.
96. Chen H, Sokoll LJ, Udelsman R. Outpatient minimally invasive parathyroidectomy: A combination of sestamibi-SPECT localization, cervical block anesthesia, and intraoperative parathyroid hormone assay. *Surgery.* 1999;126:1016–1021.
97. Miccoli P, Barellini L, Monchik JM, et al. Randomized clinical trial comparing regional and general anaesthesia in minimally invasive video-assisted parathyroidectomy. *Br J Surg.* 2005;92:814–818.
98. De Tran QH, Dugani S, Finlayson RJ. A randomized comparison between ultrasound-guided and landmark-based superficial cervical plexus block. *Reg Anesth Pain Med.* 2010;35:539–543.
99. Herring AA, Stone MB, Frenkel O, et al. The ultrasound-guided superficial cervical plexus block for anesthesia and analgesia in emergency care settings. *Am J Emerg Med.* 2012;30:1263–1267.
100. Spanknebel K, Chabot JA, DiGiorgi M, et al. Thyroidectomy using local anesthesia: A report of 1,025 cases over 16 years. *J Am Coll Surg.* 2005;201:375–385.
101. Specht MC, Romero M, Barden CB, et al. Characteristics of patients having thyroid surgery under regional anesthesia. *J Am Coll Surg.* 2001;193:367–372.
102. Tobias JD. Cervical plexus block in adolescents. *J Clin Anesth.* 1999;11:606–608.
103. Burtles R. Analgesia for 'bat ear' surgery. *Ann R Coll Surg Engl.* 1989;71:332.
104. Afridi SK, Shields KG, Bhola R, et al. Greater occipital nerve injection in primary headache syndromes–prolonged effects from a single injection. *Pain.* 2006;122: 126–129.
105. Anthony M. Cervicogenic headache: Prevalence and response to local steroid therapy. *Clin Exp Rheumatol.* 2000;18:S59–S64.
106. Winnie AP. Interscalene brachial plexus block. *Anesth Analg.* 1970;49:466.
107. Gadsden JC, Tsai T, Iwata T, et al. Low interscalene block provides reliable anesthesia for surgery at or about the elbow. *J Clin Anesth.* 2009;21:98–102.

108. Kim JH, Chen J, Bennett H, et al. A low approach to interscalene brachial plexus block results in more distal spread of sensory-motor coverage compared to the conventional approach. *Anesth Analg.* 2011;112:987–989.
109. Benumof JL. Permanent loss of cervical spinal cord function associated with interscalene block performed under general anesthesia. *Anesthesiology.* 2000; 93:1541–1544.
110. Yang WT, Chui PT, Metreweli C. Anatomy of the normal brachial plexus revealed by sonography and the role of sonographic guidance in anesthesia of the brachial plexus. *AJR Am J Roentgenol.* 1998;171:1631–1636.
111. Demondion X, Herbinet P, Boutry N, et al. Sonographic mapping of the normal brachial plexus. *AJNR Am J Neuroradiol.* 2003;24:1303–1309.
112. Sheppard DG, Iyer RB, Fenstermacher MJ. Brachial plexus: Demonstration at US. *Radiology.* 1998;208:402–406.
113. Ip VH, Tsui BC. Continuous interscalene block: The good, the bad, and the refined spread. *Acta Anaesthesiol Scand.* 2012;56:526–530.
114. Boezaart AP, Koorn R, Rosenquist RW. Paravertebral approach to the brachial plexus: An anatomic improvement in technique. *Reg Anesth Pain Med.* 2003;28:241–244.
115. Klaastad O, VadeBoncouer TR, Tillung T, et al. An evaluation of the supraclavicular plumb-bob technique for brachial plexus block by magnetic resonance imaging. *Anesth Analg.* 2003;96:862–867, table.
116. Apan A, Baydar S, Yilmaz S, et al. Surface landmarks of brachial plexus: Ultrasound and magnetic resonance imaging for supraclavicular approach with anatomical correlation. *Eur J Ultrasound.* 2001;13:191–196.
117. Kapral S, Jandrasits O, Schabernig C, et al. Lateral infraclavicular plexus block vs. axillary block for hand and forearm surgery. *Acta Anaesthesiol Scand.* 1999; 43:1047–1052.
118. Klaastad O, Smith HJ, Smedby O, et al. A novel infraclavicular brachial plexus block: The lateral and sagittal technique, developed by magnetic resonance imaging studies. *Anesth Analg.* 2004;98:252–256, table.
119. Raj PP, Montgomery SJ, Nettles D, et al. Infraclavicular brachial plexus block–a new approach. *Anesth Analg.* 1973;52:897–904.
120. Rettig HC, Gielen MJ, Boersma E, et al. A comparison of the vertical infraclavicular and axillary approaches for brachial plexus anaesthesia. *Acta Anaesthesiol Scand.* 2005;49:1501–1508.
121. Whiffler K. Coracoid block–a safe and easy technique. *Br J Anaesth.* 1981;53: 845–848.
122. Wilson JL, Brown DL, Wong GY, et al. Infraclavicular brachial plexus block: Parasagittal anatomy important to the coracoid technique. *Anesth Analg.* 1998; 87:870–873.
123. Klaastad O, Lilleas FG, Rotnes JS, et al. Magnetic resonance imaging demonstrates lack of precision in needle placement by the infraclavicular brachial plexus block described by Raj et al. *Anesth Analg.* 1999;88:593–598.
124. Koscielniak-Nielsen ZJ, Rasmussen H, Hesselbjerg L, et al. Clinical evaluation of the lateral sagittal infraclavicular block developed by MRI studies. *Reg Anesth Pain Med.* 2005;30:329–334.
125. Groen GJ, Gielen MJ, Jack NT, et al. At the cords, the pinkie towards: Interpreting infraclavicular motor responses to neurostimulation. *Reg Anesth Pain Med.* 2004;29:505–507.
126. Borene SC, Edwards JN, Boezaart AP. At the cords, the pinkie towards: Interpreting infraclavicular motor responses to neurostimulation. *Reg Anesth Pain Med.* 2004;29:125–129.
127. Borene SC, Edwards JN, Boezaart A. Response to: At the cords, the pinkie towards: Interpreting infraclavicular motor responses to neurostimulation. *Reg Anesth Pain Med.* 2004;29:505–507.
128. Brull R, McCartney CJ, Chan VW. A novel approach to infraclavicular brachial plexus block: The ultrasound experience. *Anesth Analg.* 2004;99:950–951.
129. Imasogie N, Ganapathy S, Singh S, et al. A prospective, randomized, double-blind comparison of ultrasound-guided axillary brachial plexus blocks using 2 versus 4 injections. *Anesth Analg.* 2010;110:1222–1226.
130. Urmey WF, Grossi P. Percutaneous electrode guidance and subcutaneous stimulating electrode guidance: Modifications of the original technique. *Reg Anesth Pain Med.* 2003;28:253–255.
131. Guay J. Adverse events associated with intravenous regional anesthesia (Bier block): A systematic review of complications. *J Clin Anesth.* 2009;21:585–594.
132. Horlocker TT. Peripheral nerve blocks-regional anesthesia for the new millennium. *Reg Anesth Pain Med.* 1998;23:237–240.
133. McDonnell JG, O'Donnell B, Curley G, et al. The analgesic efficacy of transversus abdominis plane block after abdominal surgery: A prospective randomized controlled trial. *Anesth Analg.* 2007;104:193–197.
134. O'Donnell BD, McDonnell JG, McShane AJ. The transversus abdominis plane (TAP) block in open retropubic prostatectomy. *Reg Anesth Pain Med.* 2006;31:91.
135. Courreges P, Poddevin F, Lecoutre D. Para-umbilical block: A new concept for regional anaesthesia in children. *Paediatr Anaesth.* 1997;7:211–214.
136. Ferguson S, Thomas V, Lewis I. The rectus sheath block in paediatric anaesthesia: New indications for an old technique? *Paediatr Anaesth.* 1996;6:463–466.
137. Rafi AN. Abdominal field block: A new approach via the lumbar triangle. *Anaesthesia.* 2001;56:1024–1026.
138. Pourseidi B, Khorram-Manesh A. Effect of intercostals neural blockade with Marcaine (bupivacaine) on postoperative pain after laparoscopic cholecystectomy. *Surg Endosc.* 2007;21:1557–1559.
139. Pusch F, Freitag H, Weinstabl C, et al. Single-injection paravertebral block compared to general anaesthesia in breast surgery. *Acta Anaesthesiol Scand.* 1999;43:770–774.
140. Naja Z, Lonnqvist PA. Somatic paravertebral nerve blockade. Incidence of failed block and complications. *Anaesthesia.* 2001;56:1184–1188.
141. Belavy D, Cowlishaw PJ, Howes M, et al. Ultrasound-guided transversus abdominis plane block for analgesia after Caesarean delivery. *Br J Anaesth.* 2009;103: 726–730.
142. El-Dawlatly AA, Turkistani A, Kettner SC, et al. Ultrasound-guided transversus abdominis plane block: Description of a new technique and comparison with conventional systemic analgesia during laparoscopic cholecystectomy. *Br J Anaesth.* 2009;102:763–767.
143. Niraj G, Searle A, Mathews M, et al. Analgesic efficacy of ultrasound-guided transversus abdominis plane block in patients undergoing open appendicectomy. *Br J Anaesth.* 2009;103:601–605.
144. Chin KJ, Chan V, Hebbard P, et al. Ultrasound-guided transversalis fascia plane block provides analgesia for anterior iliac crest bone graft harvesting. *Can J Anaesth.* 2012;59:122–123.
145. Hebbard PD. Transversalis fascia plane block, a novel ultrasound-guided abdominal wall nerve block. *Can J Anaesth.* 2009;56:618–620.
146. Eichenberger U, Greher M, Kirchmair L, et al. Ultrasound-guided blocks of the ilioinguinal and iliohypogastric nerve: Accuracy of a selective new technique confirmed by anatomical dissection. *Br J Anaesth.* 2006;97:238–243.
147. Willschke H, Bosenberg A, Marhofer P, et al. Ultrasonographic-guided ilioinguinal/iliohypogastric nerve block in pediatric anesthesia: What is the optimal volume? *Anesth Analg.* 2006;102:1680–1684.
148. Randhawa K, Soumian S, Kyi M, et al. Sonographic assessment of the conventional 'blind' ilioinguinal block. *Can J Anaesth.* 2010;57:94–95.
149. Faraoni D, Gilbeau A, Lingier P, et al. Does ultrasound guidance improve the efficacy of dorsal penile nerve block in children? *Paediatr Anaesth.* 2010;20:931–936.
150. Winnie AP, Ramamurthy S, Durrani Z. The inguinal paravascular technic of lumbar plexus anesthesia: The "3-in-1 block". *Anesth Analg.* 1973;52:989–996.
151. Marhofer P, Nasel C, Sitzwohl C, et al. Magnetic resonance imaging of the distribution of local anesthetic during the three-in-one block. *Anesth Analg.* 2000;90:119–124.
152. Parkinson SK, Mueller JB, Little WL, et al. Extent of blockade with various approaches to the lumbar plexus. *Anesth Analg.* 1989;68:243–248.
153. Chayen D, Nathan H, Chayen M. The psoas compartment block. *Anesthesiology.* 1976;45:95–99.
154. Chudinov A, Berkenstadt H, Salai M, et al. Continuous psoas compartment block for anesthesia and perioperative analgesia in patients with hip fractures. *Reg Anesth Pain Med.* 1999;24:563–568.
155. Capdevila X, Macaire P, Dadure C, et al. Continuous psoas compartment block for postoperative analgesia after total hip arthroplasty: New landmarks, technical guidelines, and clinical evaluation. *Anesth Analg.* 2002;94:1606–1613.
156. Aida S, Takahashi H, Shimoji K. Renal subcapsular hematoma after lumbar plexus block. *Anesthesiology.* 1996;84:452–455.
157. Ilfeld BM, Loland VJ, Mariano ER. Prepuncture ultrasound imaging to predict transverse process and lumbar plexus depth for psoas compartment block and perineural catheter insertion: A prospective, observational study. *Anesth Analg.* 2010;110:1725–1728.
158. Capdevila X, Coimbra C, Choquet O. Approaches to the lumbar plexus: Success, risks, and outcome. *Reg Anesth Pain Med.* 2005;30:150–162.
159. Magora F, Rozin R, Ben-Menachem Y, et al. Obturator nerve block: An evaluation of technique. *Br J Anaesth.* 1969;41:695–698.
160. Sites BD, Beach M, Gallagher JD, et al. A single injection ultrasound-assisted femoral nerve block provides side effect-sparing analgesia when compared with intrathecal morphine in patients undergoing total knee arthroplasty. *Anesth Analg.* 2004;99:1539–1543.
161. Barrington MJ, Olive D, Low K, et al. Continuous femoral nerve blockade or epidural analgesia after total knee replacement: A prospective randomized controlled trial. *Anesth Analg.* 2005;101:1824–1829.
162. Singelyn FJ, Deyaert M, Joris D, et al. Effects of intravenous patient-controlled analgesia with morphine, continuous epidural analgesia, and continuous three-in-one block on postoperative pain and knee rehabilitation after unilateral total knee arthroplasty. *Anesth Analg.* 1998;87:88–92.
163. Lundblad M, Kapral S, Marhofer P, et al. Ultrasound-guided infrapatellar nerve block in human volunteers: Description of a novel technique. *Br J Anaesth.* 2006;97:710–714.
164. Vloka JD, Hadzic A, Drobnik L, et al. Anatomical landmarks for femoral nerve block: A comparison of four needle insertion sites. *Anesth Analg.* 1999;89:1467–1470.
165. Niazi AU, Prasad A, Ramlogan R, et al. Methods to ease placement of stimulating catheters during in-plane ultrasound-guided femoral nerve block. *Reg Anesth Pain Med.* 2009;34:380–381.
166. Wang A-Z, Gu L, Zhou Q-H, et al. Ultrasound-guided continuous femoral nerve block for analgesia after total knee arthroplasty: Catheter perpendicular to the nerve versus catheter parallel to the nerve. *Reg Anesth Pain Med.* 2010;35: 127–131.
167. Hayek SM, Ritchey RM, Sessler D, et al. Continuous femoral nerve analgesia after unilateral total knee arthroplasty: Stimulating versus nonstimulating catheters. *Anesth Analg.* 2006;103:1565–1570.

168. Morin AM, Eberhart LH, Behnke HK, et al. Does femoral nerve catheter placement with stimulating catheters improve effective placement? A randomized, controlled, and observer-blinded trial. *Anesth Analg.* 2005;100:1503–1510, table.
169. Ip VH, Tsui BC. Injection of injectates is more than just for "opening the perineural space". *Reg Anesth Pain Med.* 2011;36:89–90.
170. Pham Dang C, Guilley J, Dernis L, et al. Is there any need for expanding the perineural space before catheter placement in continuous femoral nerve blocks? *Reg Anesth Pain Med.* 2006;31:393–400.
171. Soong J, Schafhalter-Zoppoth I, Gray AT. The importance of transducer angle to ultrasound visibility of the femoral nerve. *Reg Anesth Pain Med.* 2005;30:505.
172. Shannon J, Lang SA, Yip RW, et al. Lateral femoral cutaneous nerve block revisited. A nerve stimulator technique. *Reg Anesth.* 1995;20:100–104.
173. Murata Y, Takahashi K, Yamagata M, et al. The anatomy of the lateral femoral cutaneous nerve, with special reference to the harvesting of iliac bone graft. *J Bone Joint Surg Am.* 2000;82:746–747.
174. Hara K, Sakura S, Shido A. Ultrasound-guided lateral femoral cutaneous nerve block: Comparison of two techniques. *Anaesth Intensive Care.* 2011;39:69–72.
175. Jo YY, Choi E, Kil HK. Comparison of the success rate of inguinal approach with classical pubic approach for obturator nerve block in patients undergoing TURB. *Korean J Anesthesiol.* 2011;61:143–147.
176. Anagnostopoulou S, Kostopanagiotou G, Paraskeuopoulos T, et al. Obturator nerve block: From anatomy to ultrasound guidance. *Anesth Analg.* 2008;106:350–351.
177. Saranteas T, Anagnostopoulou S, Chantzi C. Obturator nerve anatomy and ultrasound imaging. *Reg Anesth Pain Med.* 2007;32:539–540.
178. Soong J, Schafhalter-Zoppoth I, Gray AT. Sonographic imaging of the obturator nerve for regional block. *Reg Anesth Pain Med.* 2007;32:146–151.
179. Akkaya T, Ozturk E, Comert A, et al. Ultrasound-guided obturator nerve block: A sonoanatomic study of a new methodologic approach. *Anesth Analg.* 2009;108:1037–1041.
180. Lee SH, Jeong CW, Lee HJ, et al. Ultrasound guided obturator nerve block: A single interfascial injection technique. *J Anesth.* 2011;25:923–926.
181. Akata T, Murakami J, Yoshinaga A. Life-threatening haemorrhage following obturator artery injury during transurethral bladder surgery: A sequel of an unsuccessful obturator nerve block. *Acta Anaesthesiol Scand.* 1999;43:784–788.
182. van der Wal M, Lang SA, Yip RW. Transsartorial approach for saphenous nerve block. *Can J Anaesth.* 1993;40:542–546.
183. Benzon HT, Sharma S, Calimaran A. Comparison of the different approaches to saphenous nerve block. *Anesthesiology.* 2005;102:633–638.
184. Tsui BC, Ozelsel T. Ultrasound-guided transsartorial perifemoral artery approach for a saphenous nerve block. *Reg Anesth Pain Med.* 2009;34:177–178.
185. Horn JL, Pitsch T, Salinas F, et al. Anatomic basis to the ultrasound-guided approach for saphenous nerve blockade. *Reg Anesth Pain Med.* 2009;34:486–489.
186. de Mey JC, Deruyck LJ, Cammu G, et al. A paravenous approach for the saphenous nerve block. *Reg Anesth Pain Med.* 2001;26:504–506.
187. Gray AT, Collins AB. Ultrasound-guided saphenous nerve block. *Reg Anesth Pain Med.* 2003;28:148.
188. Sahin L, Sahin M, Isikay N. A different approach to an ultrasound-guided saphenous nerve block. *Acta Anaesthesiol Scand.* 2011;55:1030–1031.
189. Pham DC. Midfemoral block: A new lateral approach to the sciatic nerve. *Anesth Analg.* 1999;88:1426.
190. Zetlaoui PJ, Bouaziz H. Lateral approach to the sciatic nerve in the popliteal fossa. *Anesth Analg.* 1998;87:79–82.
191. March X, Pineda O, Garcia MM, et al. The posterior approach to the sciatic nerve in the popliteal fossa: A comparison of single- versus double-injection technique. *Anesth Analg.* 2006;103:1571–1573.
192. Vloka JD, Hadzic A. The intensity of the current at which sciatic nerve stimulation is achieved is a more important factor in determining the quality of nerve block than the type of motor response obtained. *Anesthesiology.* 1998;88:1408–1411.
193. Buys MJ, Arndt CD, Vagh F, et al. Ultrasound-guided sciatic nerve block in the popliteal fossa using a lateral approach: Onset time comparing separate tibial and common peroneal nerve injections versus injecting proximal to the bifurcation. *Anesth Analg.* 2010;110:635–637.
194. Ip VH, Tsui BC. Kill 2 birds with 1 stone: Injection at the bifurcation during popliteal sciatic nerve block. *Reg Anesth Pain Med.* 2011;36:633–634.
195. Germain G, Levesque S, Dion N, et al. A comparison of an injection cephalad or caudad to the division of the sciatic nerve for ultrasound-guided popliteal block: A prospective randomized study. *Anesth Analg.* 2012;114:233–235.
196. Prasad A, Perlas A, Ramlogan R, et al. Ultrasound-guided popliteal block distal to sciatic nerve bifurcation shortens onset time: A prospective randomized double-blind study. *Reg Anesth Pain Med.* 2010;35:267–271.
197. Tran de QH, Dugani S, Pham K, et al. A randomized comparison between subepineural and conventional ultrasound-guided popliteal sciatic nerve block. *Reg Anesth Pain Med.* 2011;36:548–552.
198. Bendtsen TF, Nielsen TD, Rohde CV, et al. Ultrasound guidance improves a continuous popliteal sciatic nerve block when compared with nerve stimulation. *Reg Anesth Pain Med.* 2011;36:181–184.
199. Mariano ER, Cheng GS, Choy LP, et al. Electrical stimulation versus ultrasound guidance for popliteal-sciatic perineural catheter insertion: A randomized controlled trial. *Reg Anesth Pain Med.* 2009;34:480–485.
200. Perlas A, Brull R, Chan VWS, et al. Ultrasound guidance improves the success of sciatic nerve lock at the popliteal fossa. *Reg Anesth Pain Med.* 2008;33:259–265.
201. Tsui BC, Ozelsel T. Ultrasound-guided anterior sciatic nerve block using a longitudinal approach: "expanding the view". *Reg Anesth Pain Med.* 2008;33:275–276.
202. Raj PP, Parks RI, Watson TD, et al. A new single-position supine approach to sciatic-femoral nerve block. *Anesth Analg.* 1975;54:489–493.
203. Robards C, Wang RD, Clendenen S, et al. Sciatic nerve catheter placement: Success with using the Raj approach. *Anesth Analg.* 2009;109:972–975.
204. Le Corroller T, Wittenberg R, Pauly V, et al. A new lateral approach to the parasacral sciatic nerve block: An anatomical study. *Surg Radiol Anat.* 2011;33:91–95.
205. Osaka Y, Kashiwagi M, Nagatsuka Y, et al. Ultrasound-guided medial mid-thigh approach to sciatic nerve block with a patient in a supine position. *J Anesth.* 2011;25:621–624.
206. Redborg KE, Sites BD, Chinn CD, et al. Ultrasound improves the success rate of a sural nerve block at the ankle. *Reg Anesth Pain Med.* 2009;34:24–28.
207. Canella C, Demondion X, Guillin R, et al. Anatomic study of the superficial peroneal nerve using sonography. *AJR Am J Roentgenol.* 2009;193:174–179.
208. Capdevila X, Ponrouch M, Choquet O. Continuous peripheral nerve blocks in clinical practice. *Curr Opin Anaesthesiol.* 2008;21:619–623.
209. Chelly JE, Ghisi D, Fanelli A. Continuous peripheral nerve blocks in acute pain management. *Br J Anaesth.* 2010;105:i86–i96.
210. Ilfeld BM. Continuous peripheral nerve blocks: A review of the published evidence. *Anesth Analg.* 2011;113:904–925.
211. Ilfeld BM, Morey TE, Wright TW, et al. Continuous interscalene brachial plexus block for postoperative pain control at home: A randomized, double-blinded, placebo-controlled study. *Anesth Analg.* 2003;96:1089–1095.
212. Salinas FV. Location, location, location: Continuous peripheral nerve blocks and stimulating catheters. *Reg Anesth Pain Med.* 2003;28:79–82.
213. Kick O, Blanche E, Pham-Dang C, et al. A new stimulating stylet for immediate control of catheter tip position in continuous peripheral nerve blocks. *Anesth Analg.* 1999;89:533–534.
214. Chin KJ, Chan V. Ultrasound-guided peripheral nerve blockade. *Curr Opin Anaesthesiol.* 2008;21:624–631.
215. Marhofer P, Chan VW. Ultrasound-guided regional anesthesia: Current concepts and future trends. *Anesth Analg.* 2007;104:1265–1269.
216. Bryan NA, Swenson JD, Greis PE, et al. Indwelling interscalene catheter use in an outpatient setting for shoulder surgery: Technique, efficacy, and complications. *J Shoulder Elbow Surg.* 2007;16:388–395.
217. Davis JJ, Swenson JD, Greis PE, et al. Interscalene block for postoperative analgesia using only ultrasound guidance: The outcome in 200 patients. *J Clin Anesth.* 2009;21:272–277.
218. Tsui BC, Tsui J. Less leakage and dislodgement with a catheter-over-needle versus a catheter-through-needle approach for peripheral nerve block: an ex vivo study. *Can. J. Anesth.* 2012;59:655–661.
219. Ip V, Bouliane M, Tsui B. Potential surgical site contamination from interscalene catheter leakage with the patient in a seated position: A case report. *Can. J. Anesth.* 2012; DOI 10.1007/s12630-012-9798-1.

CHAPTER

36 Anesthesia for Neurosurgery

ARMAGAN DAGAL • ARTHUR M. LAM

Key Points

1. Anatomically, blood flow to the normal brain is supplied by the two carotid arteries and vertebral arteries. Collateral circulation is provided via the Circle of Willis.
2. Physiologically, blood flow to the brain is tightly regulated. The homeostatic mechanisms include flow–metabolism coupling, pressure autoregulation, and CO_2 reactivity.
3. These homeostatic mechanisms are affected by diseases as well as anesthetic drugs and techniques.
4. Multiple monitoring modalities are available to monitor brain function, perfusion, and oxygenation/metabolism. These include the electroencephalogram, somatosensory evoked potentials, motor evoked potentials, electromyogram, intracranial pressure, transcranial Doppler ultrasonography, brain tissue oxygenation, and jugular venous oximetry. Although most are applicable for monitoring in the neurointensive care unit, many are useful in the operating room to increase patient safety and improve outcome.
5. Definitive cerebral protective therapy remains elusive, but many techniques have been investigated and some are frequently used in the operating room on theoretical grounds. These include the use of hypothermia, control of blood glucose, and maintenance of adequate perfusion. The anemia threshold for blood transfusion remains controversial.
6. Anesthetic management of the patient with neurologic disease mandates a thorough preoperative assessment as there are often multisystem manifestations.
7. Anesthetic techniques may influence brain relaxation conditions. In general, intravenous agents cause more cerebral vasoconstriction than inhalation agents. There are no outcome studies demonstrating the superiority of any particular anesthetic agent. The use of intraoperative monitoring of evoked potentials impacts the choice of anesthetic technique.
8. Movement of water into the brain is primarily determined by the osmotic gradient, which in turn is determined by serum osmolarity. Outcome studies do not provide guidance regarding the choice of crystalloids versus colloids. In patients with brain trauma the use of albumin for resuscitation is associated with increased mortality.
9. Common neurosurgical procedures requiring special understanding and expertise include tumor excision, transsphenoidal or transcranial removal of pituitary lesions, extirpation of arteriovenous malformation, repair or clipping of aneurysms, carotid endarterectomy, and craniotomy for traumatic brain lesions including epidural and subdural hematomas.

Multimedia

1 Intracranial Compliance

2 Cerebral Blood Flow

3 Neurosurgery Tumor Excision

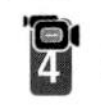
4 Mayfield Clamp

NEUROANATOMY

A basic knowledge of neuroanatomy is essential for all anesthesiologists, particularly those caring for patients with disease of the central nervous system (CNS). Components of the CNS, the brain and spinal cord, are protected by the bony structures that surround them. Yet by virtue of their protective nature, these structures are nondistensible. The intracranial volume is fixed, thereby providing little room for anything other than the brain, cerebrospinal fluid (CSF), and blood contained in the cerebral vasculature. Even the space in the spinal column, although not as restrictive as the cranium, is quickly exhausted by a space-occupying lesion such as an expanding hematoma or abscess. It is in the context of the restrictive nature of the cranium and vertebral column in which the CNS is housed that all interventions must be considered.

1 Both the brain and spinal cord have unique blood supply. The carotid artery in the neck bifurcates into the external and internal carotid arteries at the level of the third cervical vertebra, sending the internal branch through the base of the skull, giving seven branches including the ophthalmic artery, and ultimately bifurcating into the anterior and middle cerebral arteries. These vessels define the anterior cerebral circulation. The posterior circulation results from the vertebral arteries, which ascend in the posterior aspect of the neck through foramina in the cervical vertebral bodies before exiting, coursing around the brainstem, and joining the contralateral vessel to form the basilar artery. The basilar artery ascends along the brainstem before dividing into the posterior cerebral arteries. The anterior and posterior circulations anastomose through the posterior communicating arteries to provide collateral flow; collateral circulation can also occur through the anterior communicating artery connecting the bilateral anterior cerebral arteries. This system of collateralization, named the *circle of Willis* (Fig. 36-1), was described by Thomas Willis (1621–1675) with the recognition of its purpose "... that there may be a manifold way, and that more certain, for the blood about to go into divers Regions of the Brain."

The spinal column is the bony structure made up of the 7 cervical, 12 thoracic, 5 lumbar vertebrae, 5 fused sacral and 3 to 5 fused coccygeal vertebrae. It is about 70 cm long in the adult male with cervical and lumbar regions which convex forward and thoracic and sacral regions that are concave. The spinal cord exits the skull through the foramen magnum and enters the canal formed by the vertebral bodies. In the adult, the cord typically ends at the lower aspect of the first lumbar vertebral body. It is around 45 cm long in men and 43 cm long in women.

Blood supply to the cord is provided by several sources. The anterior spinal artery, which arises from the vertebral arteries, supplies the anterior two-thirds of the spinal cord. This vessel runs the length of the cord, receiving contributions from radicular arteries via intercostal vessels. The artery of Adamkiewicz is the most important radicular vessel, typically joining the anterior spinal artery in the lower thoracic region and providing blood to the thoracolumbar cord. The posterior third of the cord is supplied by two posterior spinal arteries, which arise from the vertebral arteries and also receive contributions from radicular arteries (Fig. 36-2).

NEUROPHYSIOLOGY

Cerebral metabolic rate is directly related to the number of stimulated neurons and rate of depolarization. Therefore, any activity or stimulation raises the metabolic rate. Cerebral blood flow (CBF) is tightly coupled to metabolism, on a regional as well on a global level. As an example, while visual stimulation may raise blood flow to the occipital cortex, mild hyperthermia, which raises global cerebral metabolic rate, increases flow to the entire brain.

The CSF occupies the subarachnoid space, providing a protective layer of fluid between the CNS and the tissue that surrounds it. CSF is produced by the choroid plexus in the ventricles at about 0.3 mL/min. CSF circulation follows the path from the lateral ventricles into the third ventricle via the interventricular foramina (foramina of Monro). It subsequently transits through the cerebral aqueduct of Sylvius into the fourth ventricle, and then into the space around the brain via the foramina of Magendie

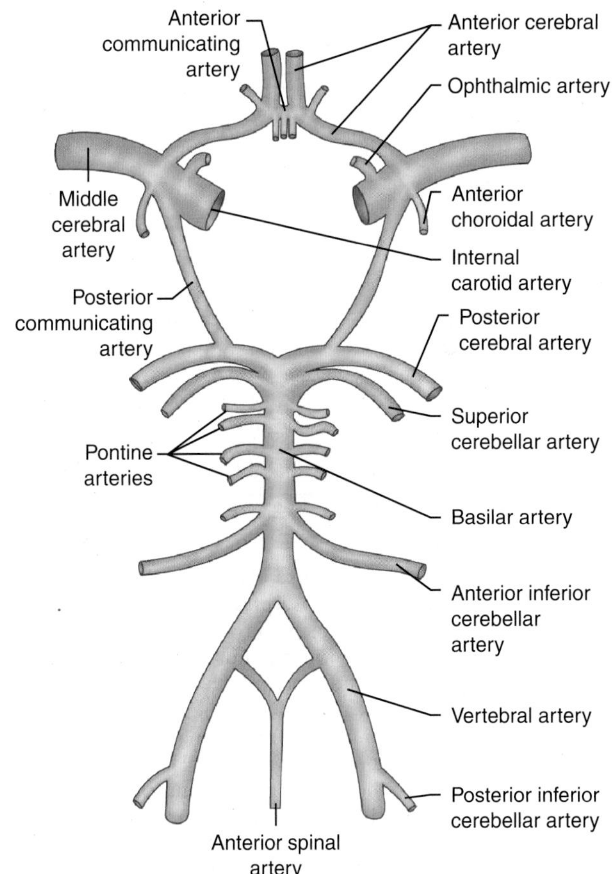

FIGURE 36-1. The circle of Willis, and other blood supply to the brain and spinal cord.

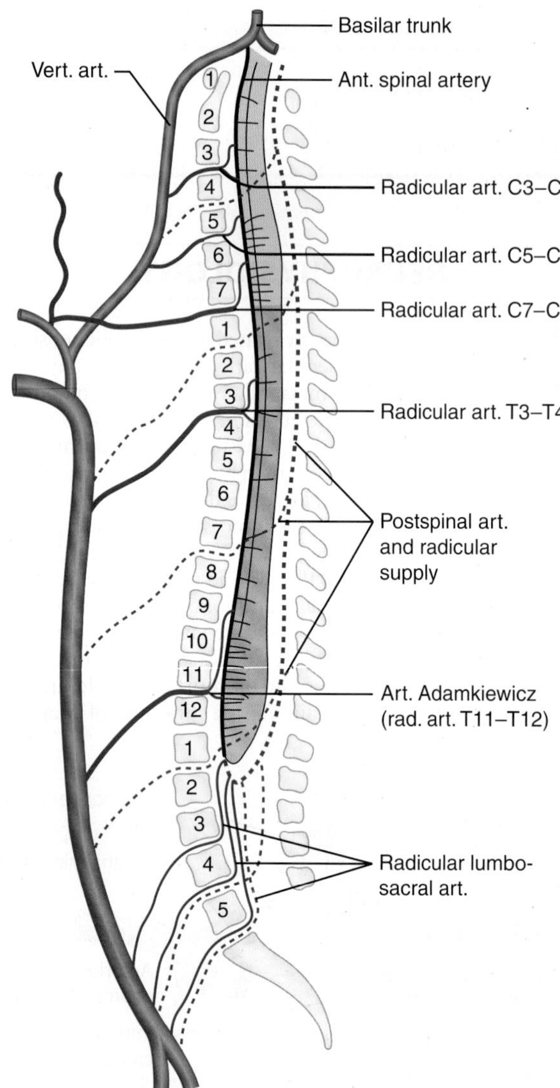

FIGURE 36-2. Blood supply to the spinal cord. Both the single anterior spinal artery and the paired posterior spinal artery arise from the vertebral arteries. The radicular arteries and particularly the artery of Adamkiewicz are important contributors. The anterior spinal artery supplies the anterior two-thirds of the spinal cord, with the posterior spinal artery supplying the rest. (vert., vertebral; art., artery; ant., anterior)

(midline posteriorly) and Luschka (laterally). It bathes both the spinal cord and the brain. Absorption into the dural venous sinuses occurs through the arachnoid granulations. Although CSF volume is approximately 150 mL, more than three times this amount is produced in a 24-hour period. This continuous flow of CSF from the source to sink allows it to participate in many functions in addition to cushioning the brain. It maintains a milieu in which the brain can function by regulating pH and electrolytes, carrying away waste products, and delivering nutrients.[1,2]

Intracranial pressure (ICP) is low except in pathologic states. The Monro–Kellie doctrine states that in the setting of a nondistensible cranial vault, the volume of blood, CSF, and brain tissue must be in equilibrium. An increase in one of these three elements, or the addition of a space-occupying lesion, can be accommodated initially through displacement of CSF into the

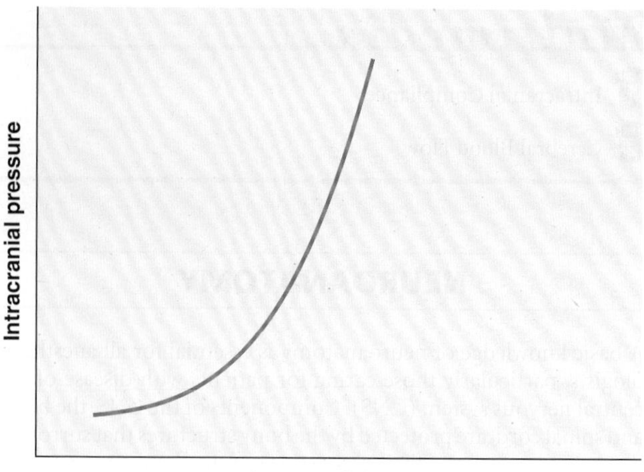

FIGURE 36-3. Intracranial compliance (elastance) curve. The brain has minimal compensatory capacity, and any increase in mass from hematoma or brain swelling will result in an inordinate increase in intracranial pressure.

thecal sac, but only to a small extent. A further increase, as with significant cerebral edema or accumulation of an extradural hematoma, will quickly lead to a marked increase in ICP due to
1 limited intracranial compliance (Fig. 36-3).

As mentioned earlier, blood flow to the brain is tightly coupled
2 to cerebral metabolism. As such, many factors affect CBF because of their effect on metabolism. Stimulation, arousal, nociception, and mild hyperthermia elevate metabolism and flow, while sedative–hypnotic agents and hypothermia decrease both metabolism
2 and flow. A number of other factors govern CBF directly without changing metabolism. A potent determinant of CBF is the arterial CO_2 tension ($Paco_2$). Within physiologic range, CBF has an approximately linear relationship with $Paco_2$. CBF changes by approximately 3% of baseline for each 1 mm Hg change in $Paco_2$ (Fig. 36-4). As CBF changes, so does cerebral blood volume (CBV), which is why hyperventilation can be used for short periods of time to relax the brain or decrease the ICP. However, this effect is thought to be short-lived. CSF pH normalizes

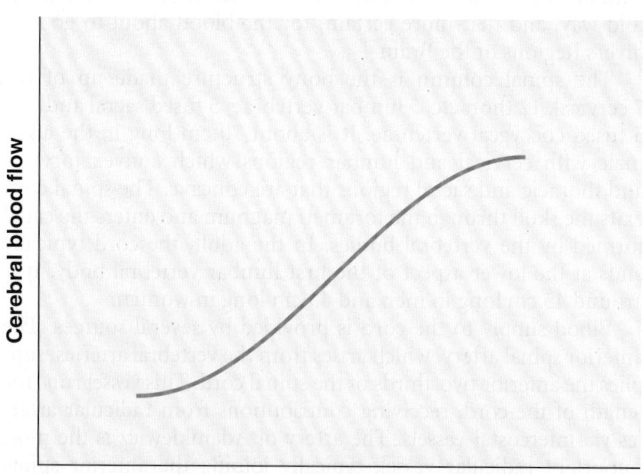

FIGURE 36-4. Cerebrovascular response to change in $Paco_2$ partial pressure. The change is linear between $Paco_2$ of 25 and 65 mm Hg.

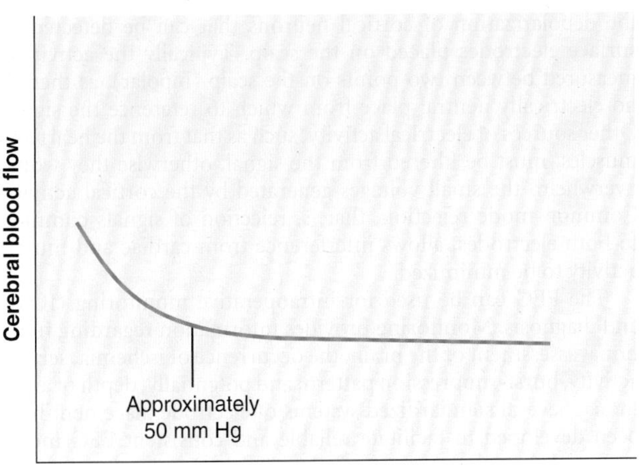

FIGURE 36-5. Cerebrovascular response to change in Pa_{O_2} partial pressure. The response of cerebral blood flow to change in Pa_{O_2} is flat until Pa_{O_2} falls below 50 mm Hg.

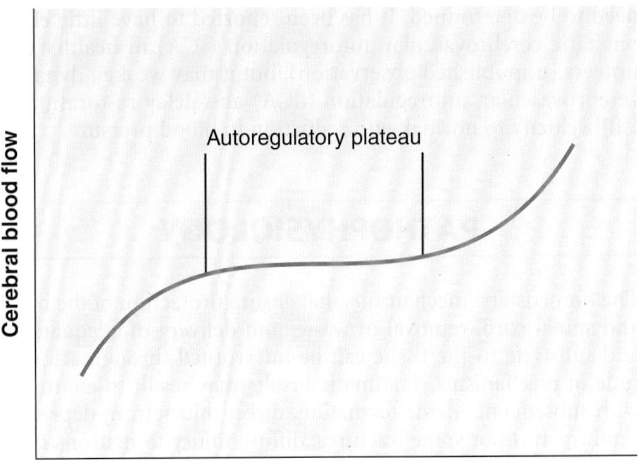

FIGURE 36-6. Cerebral autoregulation. It is generally accepted that cerebral blood flow is maintained constant between 60 and 160 mm Hg. However, these are average values, and there is considerable variation in both the lower and the upper limit of cerebral autoregulation among normal individuals.

over time, and vessel caliber returns to baseline. The exact duration of hypocapnic vasoconstriction is uncertain; a period of minutes to hours has been found in different patient populations.[3] Because the decrease in CBF occurs without a change in cerebral metabolic rate, the risk of ischemia is a theoretical concern. However, the significance of this concern is uncertain. We have no evidence of harm of moderate hyperventilation to the normal brain under general anesthesia. Early hyperventilation in traumatic brain injury (TBI) is associated with poor outcome, and the consequence of hyperventilation in TBI after the initial 24 hours is uncertain.[4–6]

In contrast to CO_2, O_2 has little effect on CBF except at abnormally low levels (Fig. 36-5). When Pa_{O_2} falls below 50 mm Hg, CBF begins to increase sharply. A teleologic explanation for this phenomenon is that CBF needs to increase only when the O_2 content of the blood begins to decrease significantly.

CBF remains approximately constant despite modest swings in arterial blood pressure. The mechanism by which CBF is maintained, originally described by Lassen,[7] is called *autoregulation* of CBF, or at times, pressure autoregulation of CBF. As cerebral perfusion pressure (CPP), defined as the difference of mean arterial pressure (MAP) and ICP, changes, cerebrovascular resistance adjusts to maintain stable flow. The resistance is varied at the arteriolar level. The range of CPP over which autoregulation is maintained is termed the *autoregulatory plateau.* Although this range is frequently quoted as a MAP range of 60 to 150 mm Hg, there is significant variability between individuals, and these numbers are only approximate. At the low end of the plateau, cerebrovascular resistance is at a minimum, and any further decrease in CPP will compromise CBF. At the high end of the plateau, cerebrovascular resistance is at a maximum, and any further increase in CPP will result in hyperemia (Fig. 36-6). Various mechanisms have been proposed to account for autoregulation, including myogenic, neurogenic, and local metabolic mediators. However, the exact mechanism remains undefined.

There is interaction between CO_2 reactivity and pressure autoregulation, although the molecular mechanism is likely different for these two homeostatic processes. When blood pressure is low, CO_2 reactivity is reduced. In contrast, under hypercapnic conditions, autoregulatory capacity is lost because of the concurrent vasodilation.

Other factors affect CBF as well. Anemia increases CBF via higher cardiac output, CPP and lower blood viscosity, as well as induced cerebral vasodilatation.[8–10] Proposed mechanisms underlying this dilatation may include upregulation of nitric oxide (NO) production, sympathetic β_2-receptor stimulation and upregulation of vascular endothelial growth factor, hypoxia-inducible factor 1α, and erythropoietin that contributes to vasodilatation and maintenance of CBF. Although it seems likely that these mediators are neuroprotective, it remains possible that they could also have harmful pathophysiologic effects.[11–13]

Anesthetic Influences

Anesthetic agents have variable influence on CBF and metabolism, CO_2 reactivity, and autoregulation.[14] Inhalation anesthetics tend to cause vasodilation in a dose-related manner, but do not per se uncouple flow and metabolism. Thus the vasodilatory influence is opposed by metabolism-mediated decrease in flow. The resultant effect is that during low doses of inhalation anesthesia, CBF is either unchanged or slightly increased. Higher doses result in dominance of the vasodilatory effect and an increase in CBF. Compared to other inhaled agents, sevoflurane in clinically relevant doses does not increase CBF, although propofol at comparable doses results in more profound cerebral vasoconstriction, and sevoflurane does not appear to impair cerebrovascular autoregulation.[15,16] Furthermore, sevoflurane anesthesia is associated with profound regional and global reduction in cerebral metabolic rate.[17] Intravenous agents including thiopental and propofol cause vasoconstriction coupled with a reduction in metabolism.[18] Ketamine, on the other hand, increases flow and metabolism.[19] CO_2 reactivity is a robust mechanism and is preserved under all anesthetic conditions.

Dexmedetomidine is a pure α_2 agonist that is increasingly utilized to provide a state of "conscious sedation" associated with minimal respiratory depression and some analgesia. It may create an ideal state to facilitate procedures such as awake craniotomy, carotid endarterectomy (CEA) under regional anesthesia, carotid angioplasty and stenting, and other neurointerventional procedures. It appears to preserve flow–metabolism coupling in healthy volunteers,[20] although its effects on the injured brain still need to be determined. It has been reported to have little effect on static cerebrovascular autoregulation (sCA) in healthy volunteers (unpublished observation), but it may weaken dynamic cerebrovascular autoregulation (dCA) and delay restoration of CBF velocity to normal with reduction in blood pressure.[21]

PATHOPHYSIOLOGY

3 The homeostatic mechanisms that ensure protection of the brain and spinal cord, removal of waste, and delivery of adequate O_2 and substrate to the tissue can be interrupted through a multitude of mechanisms. Traumatic insults may result in contusion with subsequent edema formation, direct injury from depressed skull fractures or spine fractures, diffuse injury to neurons from rapid deceleration, and disruption of the vasculature, resulting in ischemia or hemorrhage. All of these insults may ultimately compromise CNS perfusion.

Mass lesions, such as tumors, may compress adjacent structures, raise ICP, and obstruct normal flow of CSF. Hemorrhage may be spontaneous or traumatic. Depending on its location, this may cause a mass effect, impair CSF circulation, or, in the case of subarachnoid blood, breakdown of the blood may lead to further ischemic injury by causing cerebral vasospasm.

Hydrocephalus is caused by an imbalance between CSF production and removal. It frequently results in the elevation of ICP. Hydrocephalus is commonly divided into two categories: *Communicating hydrocephalus* and *obstructive hydrocephalus.* The former is characterized by a failure to absorb CSF, typically because of dysfunctional arachnoid granulations. The latter may be caused by any direct obstruction or extrinsic compression of a passageway through which CSF must pass, such as the cerebral aqueduct. This obstruction, for example, may result from a clot within the space or from a tumor adjacent to it. Depending on the circumstances, hydrocephalus can have a subtle or dramatic presentation. For example, acute hydrocephalus following an intraventricular hemorrhage may result in a rapidly progressive obtundation that improves dramatically with external ventricular drainage. In contrast, normal pressure hydrocephalus may evolve over years, resulting in barely perceptible changes in cognition and gait.

MONITORING

4 Anesthesia for neurosurgery and spine surgery requires the standard American Society of Anesthesiologists monitoring for physiologic parameters. However, the risk imposed to the CNS by these surgical procedures may warrant more extensive monitoring. For many procedures, adequate oxygenation, ventilation, and systemic blood pressure do not ensure the well being of the brain and spinal cord. Instead, the integrity of the CNS needs to be evaluated intraoperatively with monitors that specifically detect CNS function, perfusion, or metabolism. At times, the monitoring modalities can be combined to provide greater information regarding the well being of the CNS.

Central Nervous System Function

Electroencephalogram

The electroencephalogram (EEG) is the quintessential cerebral function monitor. It records the electrical activity generated by the depolarization of cortical neurons that can be detected by surface electrodes placed on the scalp. Typically the activity is measured between two points on the scalp (bipolar), as there is no electrically neutral place from which to reference the signal. Other sources of electrical activity, such as that from the heart and muscles, must be filtered from the signal, otherwise they would overwhelm the small voltages generated by the cortical activity. Common-mode rejection, that is, rejection of signals common to both electrodes, allows interference from cardiac and muscle activity to be minimized.

The EEG can be used for intraoperative monitoring (IOM) and diagnosis. Monitoring provides information regarding functional assessment of the brain, the occurrence of ischemia, seizure activity, burst-suppression pattern, and potentially, depth of anesthesia. Several standardized systems of electrode placement have been developed to facilitate reliable and consistent EEG monitoring, the most common of which is the International 10–20 System. In brief, artificial meridians are generated on the scalp running front to back and side to side, where the 10 to 20 refers to the percentage of the distance across the scalp, either from the tragus to tragus or the nasion to inion, that defines the meridian (Fig. 36-7). Electrodes can be placed at the intersection of each meridian. Each such intersection or point is given a name—either a combination of letters and a number or two letters, where the final letter is Z. The letters are F for frontal, C for central, P for parietal, T for temporal, O for occipital, A for auricular, and Fp for frontal pole. A letter followed by an odd number is a point on the left hemisphere, while a letter followed by an even number is a point on the right hemisphere. Two letters, with the second letter a Z, indicate a point along the midline.

Although sophisticated EEG monitoring for epilepsy evaluation may require recording of multiple channels, providing information on the activity between numerous points, EEG monitoring during anesthesia frequently uses a broad montage with fewer channels (two or four) to evaluate hemispheric activity. Once the signal is recorded, it can be evaluated in several ways. Viewing raw EEG may be appropriate at times, but subtle changes are difficult to detect, particularly for the infrequent user. However, the EEG can be processed to yield readily interpretable information. A common method used is *frequency domain analysis.* Using Fourier analysis, the apparent random activity of raw EEG can be broken down into a series of wave frequencies, the summation

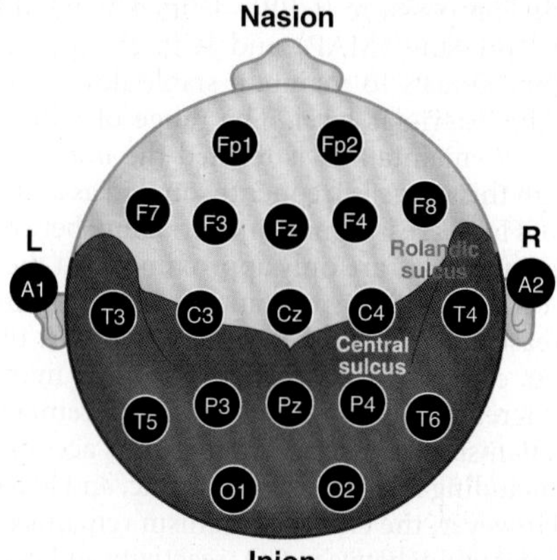

FIGURE 36-7. The international 10–20 system for electroencephalogram electrode montage. The odd numbers denote the left (*L*) hemisphere whereas the even numbers represent the right (*R*) hemisphere. See text for details.

TABLE 36-1. ELECTROENCEPHALOGRAM FREQUENCIES

Wave	Range (Hz)	Description
Delta	0–3	Low frequency, high amplitude; present in deep coma, encephalopathy, and deep anesthesia
Theta	4–7	Not prominent in adults, although may be seen in encephalopathy
Alpha	8–12	Prominent in the posterior region during relaxation with eyes closed
Beta	>12	High frequency, low amplitude; the dominant frequency during arousal

TABLE 36-2. INDICATIONS FOR ELECTROENCEPHALOGRAM MONITORING

During anesthesia	1. Carotid endarterectomy 2. Cardiopulmonary bypass procedures 3. Cerebrovascular surgery a. Aneurysm surgery involving temporary clipping b. Vascular bypass procedures 4. When burst suppression is desired for cerebral protection
In the intensive care unit	1. Barbiturate coma for patients with traumatic brain injury 2. When subclinical seizures are suspected

of which gives the overall EEG pattern. The range of frequencies seen in EEG is described in Table 36-1. The power (amplitude squared) at each frequency can then be plotted as a spectral array, whereby the effect of various influences such as anesthetic agents or an ischemic insult can be detected by how they modify the spectral analysis. A common parameter to include in the analysis of EEG is the *spectral edge frequency,* which is the frequency below which 95% of the power resides.

A progressive reduction in CBF will produce a reliable pattern change in the EEG, consisting of a loss of high-frequency activity, a loss of power, and the eventual progression to EEG silence. The monitor is therefore useful when surgical procedures jeopardize perfusion to the brain, such as when the carotid artery is cross-clamped during CEA. The EEG is particularly useful in this setting because the spectral analysis on the at-risk side can be compared in real time with the unaffected side, thus facilitating detection of ischemia by the resultant asymmetry of the spectral edge frequency.

However, the changes in the EEG spectrum seen with ischemia can occur as a result of other influences. Intravenous anesthetic agents such as propofol and thiopental, as well as inhaled agents such as isoflurane, will cause a similar decrease in the spectral edge frequency, with eventual progression to a drug-induced isoelectric EEG in a dose-related manner. During certain surgical procedures, such as extracranial-to-intracranial arterial bypass procedures, maximal suppression of cerebral metabolic rate is desirable to protect the brain during an ischemic insult. Under such circumstances, the anesthetic agent can be titrated against the EEG until the desired effect is achieved. Typically, instead of an isoelectric EEG, the goal is a state called *burst suppression.* In this state, periods of isoelectric EEG are punctuated by "bursts" of EEG activity. When burst suppression is the goal, a suppression ratio can be calculated as the percentage of an epoch in which the patient's EEG is isoelectric. The suppression ratio allows one to achieve near-complete suppression (>90%) of EEG activity, while remaining certain that regular EEG activity will return in a short while with cessation of administration of the drug. In contrast, when complete isoelectric EEG is achieved, time to arousal becomes unpredictable. Other settings in which EEG monitoring and burst suppression may be useful are listed in Table 36-2.

Using a proprietary algorithm based on probabilistic analysis, a computer-processed EEG has been used to derive a dimensionless number to monitor the degree of hypnosis or the "depth of anesthesia." The most commonly used monitor is the Bispectral index (BIS) where a number between 40 and 60 is considered optimal for the prevention of intraoperative awareness. However, a recent study failed to demonstrate the superiority of a BIS protocol over a protocol based on end-tidal anesthetic agent concentration monitoring in the prevention of intraoperative awareness.[22]

Evoked Potential Monitoring

Although EEG is a cerebral function monitor that detects spontaneous activity, evoked potential (EP) modalities detect signals that are the result of specific stimuli applied to the patient. These include somatosensory evoked potential (SSEP), brainstem auditory evoked potential (BAEP), visual evoked potential (VEP), and motor evoked potential (MEP).

The proposed benefit of EP monitoring is to identify the deterioration of neuronal function, thus enabling the opportunity to correct offending factors before becoming irreversible. Such factors include positioning of the patient (e.g., neck position, shoulder position), hypotension, hypothermia, and surgical intervention. In elective spinal surgery without EP monitoring, iatrogenic neurologic injuries have been estimated to be 0.46% for anterior cervical discectomy, 0.23% to 3.2% with scoliosis correction, and between 23.8% and 65.4% with intramedullary spinal cord tumor resection. A recent systematic review indicated that, although there is a high level of evidence that multimodal neurophysiologic monitoring is sensitive and specific for detecting intraoperative neurologic injury during spine surgery, there is very little evidence that an intraoperative response to a neuromonitoring alert reduces the rate of perioperative neurologic deterioration. Consequently there is a low level of evidence that it reduces the rate of new or worsening perioperative neurologic deficits.[23,24]

Somatosensory Evoked Potential

SSEP is a signal that is detectable on EEG and is generated in a time-locked fashion in response to a specific applied sensory input, typically a cutaneous electrical stimulation (i.e., of a peripheral sensory nerve, but also of a cranial nerve with a sensory pathway). As a result, an intact neural pathway from the periphery to the cerebral sensory cortex is essential for a signal to be generated. This monitoring modality has application in any surgical procedure that may jeopardize this pathway. Specifically, spine surgery in which the dorsal column of the spinal cord may be placed at risk is a particularly appropriate application, but it may also be used during other procedures such as craniotomy and carotid surgery where any part of the pathway may be subjected to ischemia or surgical retraction.

Because of the presence of spontaneous EEG activity, a single peripheral stimulus, which generates cortical activity of relatively low amplitude, would not be detectable amidst the background noise. Summation followed by signal averaging of repetitive stimuli is therefore necessary in order to extract meaningful signals.

Stimulation is typically done in the regions of the median nerve, ulnar nerve, and posterior tibial nerve to generate predictable and reliable signals. However, in theory, any sensory nerve could be used to generate SSEP. The SSEP is described by its polarity (the direction of the wave deflection) and its latency (the time required for a signal to be detected after the stimulus has been applied), and is quantified by both the amplitude of that signal and its latency. For example, N20 is the SSEP generated via stimulation of the median nerve that is expected to have a latency of approximately 20 ms and a negative displacement (Fig. 36-8).

Disruption of the neural pathway at any point will result in complete loss of SSEP. More commonly, ischemia, not mechanical disruption, is the intraoperative insult. As a result of ischemia, the amplitude of the signal decreases and the latency increases. A 50% decrease in signal amplitude is generally accepted as clinically significant, as is a 10% increase in latency.

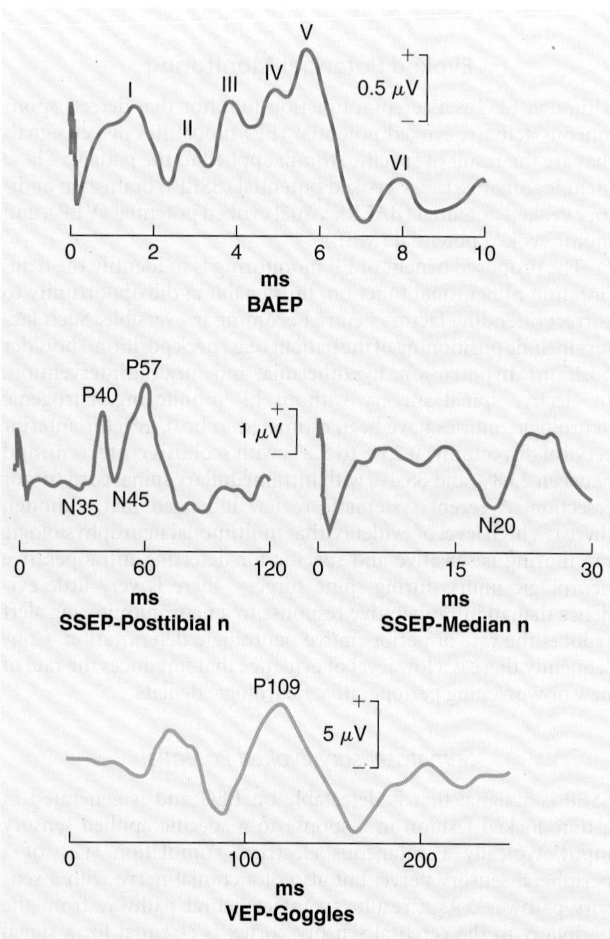

FIGURE 36-8. Representative tracings of multiple modalities of sensory evoked potential. BAEP, brainstem auditory evoked potential; ms, millisecond; n, nerve; SSEP, somatosensory evoked potential; VEP, visual evoked potential.

Brainstem Auditory Evoked Potential

BAEP is a specialized type of sensory evoked potential. Instead of an electrical stimulus applied to a somatosensory nerve, a standardized sound (click) is applied to the eighth cranial nerve via the auditory apparatus. A recognized series of peaks are generated with this technique, where the latency of each peak has significance with respect to the integrity of various parts of the auditory pathway. Although this monitoring modality is specific to cranial nerve VIII, and is particularly useful in acoustic neuroma surgery, it may be used during any surgical procedure around the brainstem to infer its integrity, although such use is associated with both low sensitivity and specificity.

Visual Evoked Potential

VEP signals are generated via light stimulation of the retina. Typically, goggles that emit LED lights are worn. Although this modality is particularly appealing to monitor the integrity of the optic nerve in settings in which visual loss is a concern, such as in prone spine surgery, the signals are not robust. They are difficult to record in a consistent fashion during anesthesia, although it appears to be more stable during propofol compared to inhalation anesthesia. Research is ongoing with respect to its intraoperative use, particularly with regard to its interpretation.

Motor Evoked Potential

MEP monitoring is different from the other evoked potential modalities described thus far. Whereas SSEP, BAEP, and VEP provide information about ascending sensory neural pathways (i.e., from the periphery to the cerebral cortex), MEP evaluates descending motor pathways (i.e., from the cerebral cortex, past the neuromuscular junction, to peripheral muscle groups). This difference allows MEP to complement SSEP, particularly in the setting of spine surgery, in which the two modalities provide information about the integrity of anatomically different areas of the spinal cord. With MEP, the stimulus is applied in a transcranial fashion over the motor cortex. The deflection, essentially an electromyographic signal, is then detected by electrodes embedded in the muscle belly. Although theoretically the stimulus can be delivered with either a magnetic or electrical source, transcranial magnetic stimulation is obliterated under anesthesia. The transcranial electrical signal is usually delivered as a rapid train of four or more stimuli, the voltage of which is adjusted to achieve adequate signals in both the upper and lower extremities. The MEP is typically detected at the thenar eminence and the abductor hallucis muscle. Transcranial electrical MEP is of substantially greater magnitude compared with SSEP, and signal averaging with repetitive stimuli is therefore not required. However, it is very sensitive to anesthetic agents, particularly inhalation anesthetics. Its amplitude can be augmented by increasing the transcranial voltage, or the number of stimuli in the train. The stimulus can cause patient movement, so MEP signals are typically obtained intermittently at points during the surgery when slight patient movements are not problematic. A bite block is mandatory to prevent injury to the tongue during transcranial stimulation.

With MEP, latency of the signal is somewhat unreliable, and not typically used to make clinical decisions. Decision making is based on amplitude alone, where a 50% decrease is considered significant (Fig. 36-9). Although MEP can be used during any spine or intracranial surgical procedure, it is becoming increasingly used during cervical spine surgery.

MEP signals are much more sensitive to volatile anesthesia than SSEP. Although there is some evidence that MEP signals are adequate during desflurane anesthesia, more research on

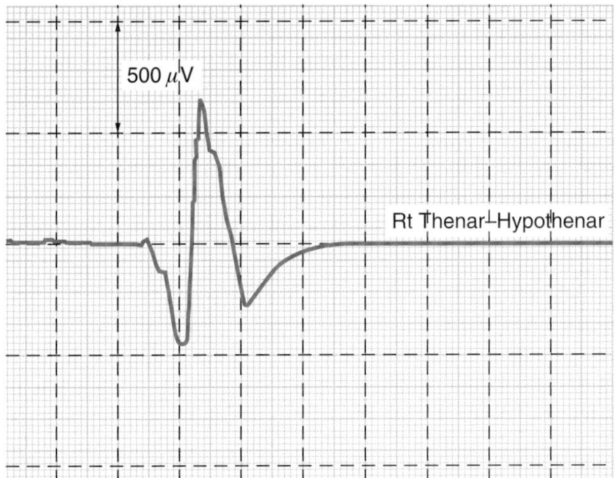

FIGURE 36-9. Representative tracing of motor evoked potential (MEP) recorded from the thenar muscles in response to transcranial electrical stimulation.

the efficacy of this technique is required, and total intravenous anesthesia is the preferred technique when MEP monitoring is required.[25] Some centers use partial neuromuscular blockade, but most centers avoid muscle relaxants altogether with MEP in order to avoid compromise of the signal.[26]

Spontaneous Electromyography

Spontaneous electromyography (EMG) is different from other evoked potentials in that a signal is not intentionally generated through stimulation at some point in a known neural pathway. Instead, it is a continuous recording of EMG activity in the muscle of regions innervated by nerve roots around which surgeons are working. Its purpose is to detect injury to those nerve roots by the surgical procedure. Impingement on a nerve root by an instrument will cause immediate motor activity that is easily detectable, which may allow the surgeon to modify his or her technique. Although spontaneous EMG is a robust signal that is tolerant of various anesthetic techniques, muscle relaxant must be avoided. Spontaneous EMG is frequently used during cervical and lumbar spine surgery where the brachial plexus and lumbosacral plexus are encountered.

Cranial Nerve Monitoring

Surgery in the posterior cranial fossa and adjacent to the brainstem places the surgeon in close proximity to cranial nerves. Although cranial nerve VIII can be monitored with BAEP as discussed earlier, several other cranial nerves can be monitored as well. Generally, only the integrity of nerves with motor components can be detected, either through spontaneous EMG or through EMG evoked by local electrical stimulation. These include cranial nerves V, VII, IX, X, XI, and XII. Cranial nerve X is usually monitored via special monitoring endotracheal tubes embedded with electrodes near the cuff.

Influence of Anesthetic Technique

As mentioned previously, anesthetic agents can have a profound influence on the amplitude and latency of evoked potentials. For instance, the quality of signals obtained with SSEP monitoring depends on the anesthetic agents used. Signals are obtainable under volatile anesthesia, but the anesthetic is typically kept at sub-MAC (minimum alveolar concentration) doses to avoid degradation in quality (increase in latency and decrease in amplitude), as amplitude of SSEP signals are depressed by volatile agents in a dose-related manner; they are recordable during low dose and obliterated with high doses. Potent volatile anesthetics should not be combined with nitrous oxide, as this technique will further compromise quality. The signals are unaffected by opioids, and opioid infusions are frequently used to facilitate low-dose volatile anesthesia. Signal quality is also excellent under intravenous anesthesia with propofol. Ketamine has been shown to enhance evoked potential monitoring. Dexmedetomidine infusion has also been used as an adjunct, allowing a reduction in propofol dose, but its effects on MEP remain controversial, with some studies reporting a lack of effect while some reports suggest a deleterious effect.[27,28]

To summarize the influence of anesthetic agents on evoked potential monitoring, general statements can be made.

1. Inhalation agents including nitrous oxide generally have more depressant effects on EP monitoring than intravenous agents.
2. Cortical EP with long latency involving multiple synapses are exquisitely sensitive to the influence of anesthetic while short latency brainstem and spinal components are resistant to anesthetic influence. Thus, BAEP can be recorded under any anesthetic technique, whereas VEP and SSEP are very sensitive.
3. Monitoring of MEP and cranial nerve EMG in general preclude the use of muscle relaxants, although the use of a short-acting neuromuscular blocking agent for the purpose of tracheal intubation is not contraindicated as its effect usually wears off before monitoring and surgery begins.
4. MEP is exquisitely sensitive to the depressant effects of inhalation anesthetics including nitrous oxide. Although it can be recorded with low-dose agents, the signals are so severely attenuated that this practice is generally not advisable. Total intravenous anesthesia without nitrous oxide is the ideal anesthetic technique for monitoring of MEP. Ketamine may enhance the amplitude of MEP, while dexmedetomidine may have either negligible or some depressant effects.
5. Opioids and benzodiazepines have negligible effects on recording of EP.
6. Propofol and thiopental attenuate the amplitude of virtually all modalities of EP but do not obliterate them. SSEP and MEP can be monitored even during burst suppression induced by these agents. BAEP can be recorded with any anesthetic technique.
7. During crucial events in which part of the central neural pathway is specifically placed at risk by surgical manipulation, as in placement of a temporary clip during aneurysm surgery, change in "anesthetic depth" should be minimized to avoid misinterpretation of the changes in EP recorded.
8. Ketamine and etomidate have been reported to enhance the quality of signals in patients with weak baseline SSEP signals, although the clinical significance and interpretation of signals obtained under these circumstances remain unclear.

Cerebral Perfusion

Although adequate CBF does not guarantee the well being of the CNS, it is one factor that is essential to its integrity. Measuring CBF is therefore an attractive method of monitoring the

CNS. Currently available techniques for quantitative measurement of CBF are not practical as an intraoperative monitor, but other methods for looking at relative changes in CBF do lend themselves to use in the operating room. Transcranial Doppler ultrasonography (TCD) and laser Doppler flowmetry are examples. Furthermore, as adequate CBF depends on an appropriate CPP, measuring ICP may be useful in certain patients to ensure conditions are adequate for sufficient CBF. Finally, numerous other modalities that evaluate CBF and that may not be practical in the operating room are used commonly in the perioperative setting.

Laser Doppler Flowmetry

Laser Doppler flowmetry is a technique that measures cortical blood flow in a small region of the brain adjacent to the placement of the device. Although it is useful for detecting relative changes in CBF, its utility is limited by several factors. First, it requires a burr hole for placement, which prevents its use in most patients. Second, it measures flow in only a small region of the brain; it could miss hypoperfusion in any area of the brain not directly monitored. Accuracy is also affected by movement and the presence of underlying major vessels. Because of these limitations, laser Doppler flowmetry has found limited applications.

Transcranial Doppler Ultrasonography

TCD is a noninvasive monitor for evaluating relative changes in flow through the large basal arteries of the brain (i.e., the circle of Willis). TCD does not measure flow directly, and therefore cannot provide information regarding absolute CBF. TCD measures flow velocity (Fig. 36-10), which is directly proportional to the flow if the diameters of these large vessels are constant. Except in well-known circumstances such as cerebral vasospasm following aneurysmal subarachnoid hemorrhage, these vessels are thought to be conductance vessels, where diameters of the basal arteries are stable.[29] Pressure autoregulation and CO_2 reactivity of CBF occurs via changes in arteriolar diameter distal to these large vessels.

Although the vessels that can be evaluated with TCD include the middle cerebral artery, internal carotid artery, anterior cerebral artery, posterior cerebral artery, ophthalmic artery, vertebral artery, and basilar artery, not all of these vessels can be monitored continuously during surgical procedures. Many of these vessels can only be evaluated with a hand-held TCD probe, which is useful for providing a brief snapshot of flow velocity in that vessel. A commercially available device for fixation of the TCD probe is essential for continuous monitoring. These devices are available either as a headband or as a rack that remains attached via fixation points on the bridge of the nose and in bilateral auditory canals. With these devices, flow velocity in the middle cerebral artery can be continuously evaluated.

In addition to the measurement of flow velocity, TCD is useful for detecting emboli. Microembolic signals can be generated by the passage of either gas or particulate matter (Fig. 36-11). The former is likely to occur as a result of venous air embolism (VAE), particularly if the patient has a patent foramen ovale, while the latter may occur during the manipulation of an atheroma in a neck vessel or as the result of thrombus formation and dislodgement on a vascular dissection.

Specific applications for intraoperative use of TCD include CEA, nonneurologic surgery in patients with TBI, and surgical procedures requiring cardiopulmonary bypass. There are also numerous indications for TCD in the perioperative setting.

Perhaps the most important use of TCD is in the neurocritical care unit, where it is used to monitor the development of vasospasm in patients who have suffered a subarachnoid hemorrhage. It has also been used for the measurement of cerebral autoregulation in patients with TBI, vasomotor reactivity in patients with occlusive vascular disease, noninvasive measurement of ICP, determination of intracranial circulatory arrest and confirmation of brain death.[30–33]

Intracranial Pressure Monitoring

Although monitoring ICP does not provide direct information about CBF, it allows the derivation of CPP, which must be in an appropriate range in order for CBF to be adequate. CPP is defined as the difference between MAP and ICP. In other words, it is the net pressure acting to move blood through the cerebral vasculature (assuming ICP is greater than right atrial pressure). CPP and CBF are not expected to be proportional, as there are other factors

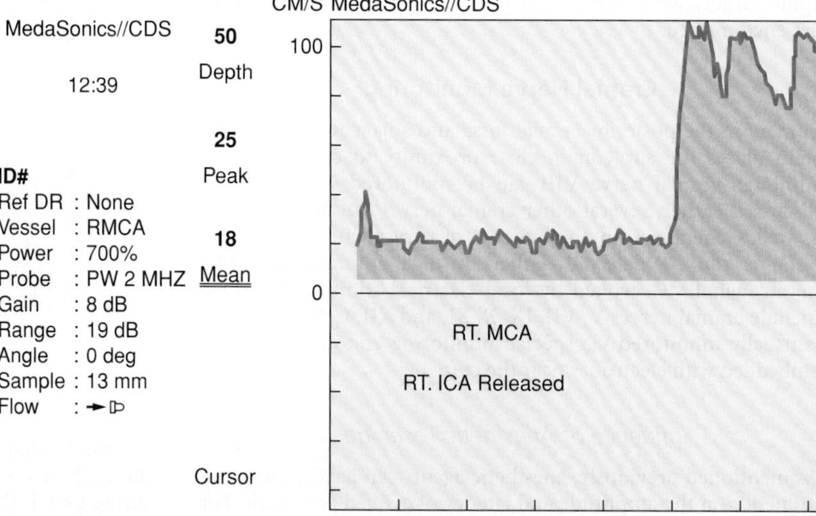

FIGURE 36-10. Transcranial Doppler tracing with release of cross-clamp during carotid endarterectomy. The resultant hyperemia is accompanied with evidence of air emboli (vertical streaks on the tracing). MCA, middle cerebral artery; ICA, internal carotid artery.

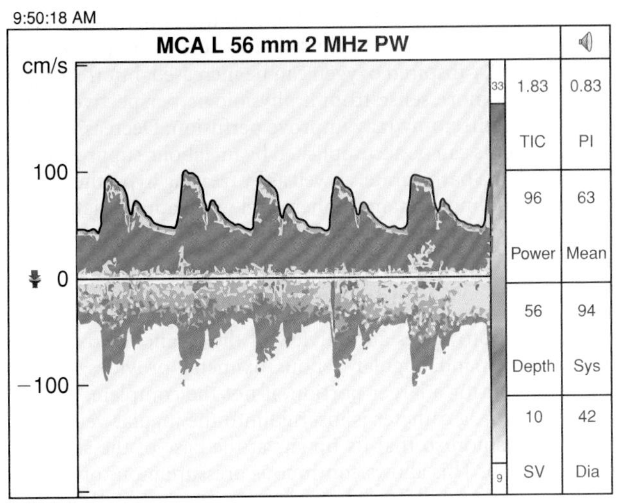

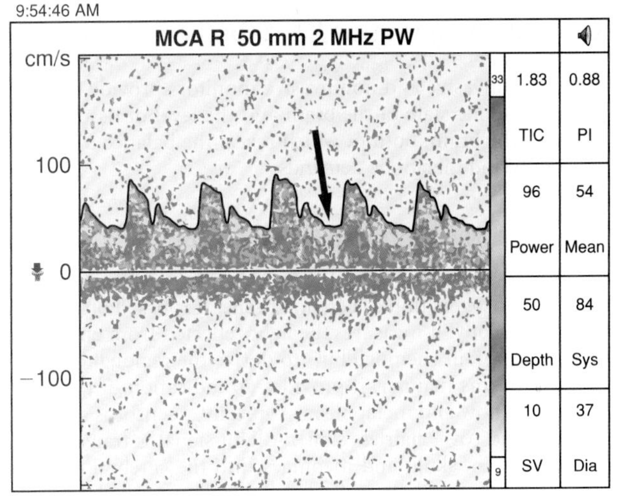

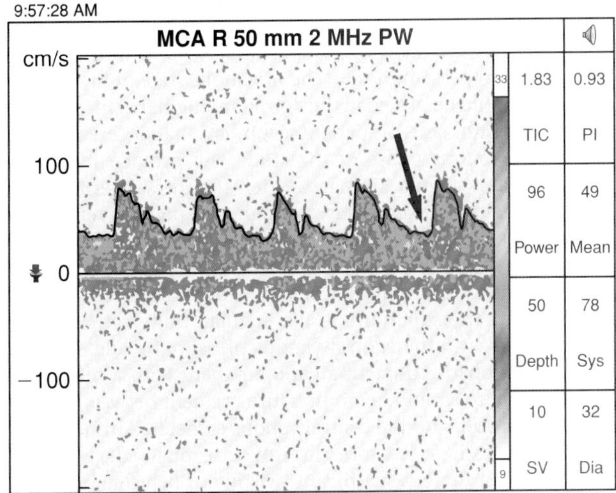

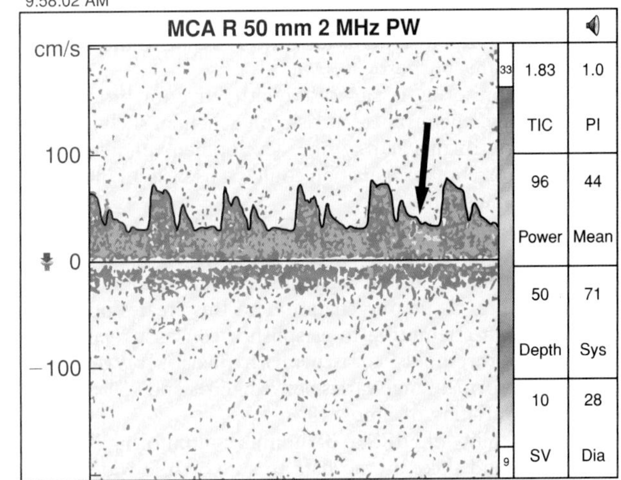

FIGURE 36-11. Particulate emboli seen on transcranial Doppler in a patient with symptoms of transient ischemic attacks consistent with right carotid artery territory embolization. The emboli are denoted by the *arrows*. MCA, middle cerebral artery; PW, pulse wave.

determining CBF (discussed elsewhere). In fact, within a physiologic range of CPP, CBF should remain approximately constant. However, a CPP that is too low will result in cerebral ischemia and CPP that is too high will cause hyperemia.

ICP monitoring is recommended in all salvageable patients with severe TBI (GCS ≤ 8) and an abnormal CT scan (hematomas, contusions, swelling, herniation, or compressed basal cistern), and in patients with severe TBI with a normal CT scan if two or more of the following features are noted at the admission: Age >40 years, unilateral or bilateral motor posturing, or SBP <90 mm Hg. However, patients who present to the operating room in the acute stage of injury will seldom have an ICP monitor in place, and the presence of elevated ICP must be inferred from the medical history, physical examination, and CT scan.

When ICP is high and CPP is low, interventions can target either ICP or MAP in order to restore a favorable balance of the two. Ideally, ICP should be maintained under 20 mm Hg. Interventions to lower ICP include suppression of cerebral metabolic activity, positional changes to decrease cerebral venous blood volume, drainage of CSF, removal of brain water with osmotic agents such as mannitol, and if absolutely essential, mild-to-moderate hyperventilation to further decrease CBV. MAP is raised via adequate intravascular resuscitation and with a vasopressor as needed. The goal CPP in TBI is >50 to 60 mm Hg.[34]

Other Modalities

Although seldom employed in the intraoperative setting, CT perfusion, single-photon emission computed tomography, positron emission tomography, and cerebral angiography all have roles, experimental or clinical, in the evaluation of CBF. However, these techniques are frequently used preoperatively and postoperatively in neurosurgical patients. On the other hand, intraoperative angiography is frequently used during neurovascular surgery to confirm placement of an aneurysm clip or to verify complete obliteration of an arteriovenous malformation (AVM). More recently, this has been superseded by indocyanine green videoangiography, as this obviates the need for radiation.[35]

Cerebral Oxygenation/Metabolism Monitors

A number of invasive and noninvasive monitors provide insight into the metabolic state of the brain and the level of tissue oxygenation of the brain, both of which reveal the balance between blood supply and metabolic demands.

Near-infrared Spectroscopy

Near-infrared spectroscopy (NIRS) is a noninvasive method of detecting the oxygenation of cerebral tissue. It is based on reflectance spectroscopy; it measures the light reflected from chromophobes in the brain (hemoglobin) to derive the regional oxygen saturation. In this manner, it provides an indication of the balance between flow and metabolism. Typically, a sensor is applied to the forehead (over hairless skin). A light signal is transmitted through the skin, skull, and meninges into the cerebral cortex. A complex analysis of the reflected light allows calculation of the oxygenation of blood in the cortex, which is a mix of venous and arterial blood. Falling saturation indicates a decline in cerebral perfusion. Exact thresholds for concern relate to the specific device used for this purpose.

Bilateral monitoring is particularly attractive for procedures that place a single hemisphere at risk for ischemia, such as CEA carotid surgery. In this setting, the development of significant asymmetry in cerebral oxygenation could be used as an indicator for the need for a shunt.

Individual variations in extracranial tissue (hence contamination), arterial to venous blood volume ratio, systemic blood pressure, $Pa{CO_2}$, hematocrit, and regional CBV are factors that can influence cerebral tissue oxygenation, and this creates potential difficulties when attempting to establish a consensus value for NIRS-derived "thresholds" for ischemia/hypoxia.[36] It is generally accepted that normal range varies between 60% and 75%, with a coefficient of variation of almost 10%.[36,37]

The applicability of NIRS in brain injury monitoring is as yet to be defined and there are no data to support the widespread application of NIRS to monitor cerebral oxygenation routinely during anesthesia and surgery. Ironically NIRS has found most acceptance in cardiac anesthesia, where access to the forehead for placement of the sensor is less of a problem than in neuroanesthesia. Nevertheless, it is a promising technology that, as advances in design are made, may find increasing application in the field of neuroanesthesia.

Brain Tissue PO_2

The brain tissue PO_2 ($Pbto_2$) monitor is an invasive probe that is inserted through a burr hole into the brain parenchyma, typically in conjunction with a fiberoptic ICP monitor. As a result, this monitor is used most commonly in patients with TBI. It measures oxygen tension in the surrounding brain. An adequate CPP in such a patient is encouraging, but it does not guarantee adequate blood supply to meet the metabolic needs of the brain. $Pbto_2$ complements ICP information in that it provides insight into oxygen delivery. A low $Pbto_2$ is indicative of inadequate oxygen delivery to that area of brain. A level of 15 mm Hg is concerning for cerebral hypoxia, and warrants intervention in TBI.[38,39] In patients with TBI, $Pbto_2$ has been shown to correlate well with the treatment effects and outcome.[40]

Its major limitation is that the information it provides reflects oxygenation at the local level—in proximity to the probe—meaning that an adequate $Pbto_2$ at that location may not guarantee adequate oxygen delivery to other regions of the brain.

Interventions to raise the $Pbto_2$ must either target oxygen delivery or oxygen consumption. In order to improve oxygen delivery, $F{IO_2}$-inspired oxygen can be increased, but treating anemia makes more sense from a physiologic perspective. Decompressive craniectomy may improve perfusion. Decreasing oxygen requirements can be accomplished by metabolic suppression with propofol or a barbiturate, as well as by treating hyperthermia with external cooling, acetaminophen, and when appropriate, nonsteroidal anti-inflammatory medications.

Jugular Venous Oximetry

Although $Pbto_2$ gives a local view of the balance of oxygen supply and demand, jugular venous oximetry provides that same information for a larger portion, if not the complete, brain. For this monitor, a catheter is inserted into the jugular vein in a retrograde fashion so that its tip sits at the base of the skull in the jugular bulb. This allows continuous pressure monitoring as well as intermittent withdrawal of a jugular venous blood sample for gas analysis. Continuous monitoring can be achieved using an oximetry catheter inserted via a conduit sheath. Confirmation of location can be made with a lateral cervical spine film.

For best representation of the metabolic state of the brain, the catheter should be placed in the dominant jugular vein, most commonly the right side. In patients who have had a cerebral angiogram, the venous phase of the study will provide information on dominant venous drainage. Often the intra-arterial contrast will drain almost exclusively through one jugular vein, regardless of the side of injection. Side dominance can also be predicted using ultrasound where the dominant vein may be larger. In the absence of this information, the right side is preferred.

Pressure transduction of the jugular bulb catheter allows comparison with the central venous pressure to rule out potential venous obstruction. In a supine patient with a neutral neck position, there should be no pressure gradient between the tip of the jugular bulb and the central venous catheter. Although rare, a significant gradient (>4 mm Hg) can occasionally develop during positioning if there is significant twisting or bending of the neck. This gradient indicates venous obstruction, potentially causing brain edema, or ischemia. The head should be repositioned until the gradient resolves.

Blood gas analysis of the sample provides several useful parameters. The saturation of jugular venous blood ($Sjvo_2$) demonstrates whether CBF is sufficient to meet the cerebral metabolic rate for oxygen ($CMRO_2$) of the brain. A normal value is in the 65% to 75% range. In TBI, $Sjvo_2$ below 50% for more than 10 minutes is undesirable and associated with poor outcome.[41] However, it has low sensitivity, and a study using PET scan indicates that a relatively large volume of tissue must be affected, approximately 13%, before $Sjvo_2$ levels decreased below 50%.[42] Intraoperative hyperventilation will lower $Sjvo_2$ as it decreases CBF. In the setting of a nontraumatized brain that is exposed to moderate hyperventilation for the duration of a neurosurgical procedure, the acceptable level for $Sjvo_2$ is unknown. In the absence of other demands, it is reasonable to guide intraoperative hyperventilation by maintaining $Sjvo_2$ >50%. It is essential that blood samples from the retrograde catheter be drawn slowly to avoid contamination from noncerebral venous blood.[43]

Measurement of simultaneous arterial and jugular venous samples allows the determination of lactate output from the brain, the presence of which indicates occurrence of anaerobic metabolism. The obvious disadvantage to jugular venous oximetry is precisely the opposite of the shortcoming for $Pbto_2$, in that it is a global monitor that could easily miss small areas of regional ischemia. The two monitors may be complementary in the setting of TBI. Intraoperatively, jugular venous oximetry is used routinely in some centers that specialize in neurosurgical procedures.

CEREBRAL PROTECTION

5 Cerebral ischemia and/or hypoxia leads to neuronal death in multiple settings. For example, ischemic stroke, TBI, and cerebral vasospasm following subarachnoid hemorrhage. Efforts to avert neurologic insult, using medications or through the manipulation of physiologic parameters, have met with meager results. In the setting of ischemic stroke, for example, thrombolysis may restore perfusion and decrease infarct size, but it may also lead to expansion of the infarct, edema, and even hemorrhage as a result of ischemia-reperfusion injury. In general, a protective strategy that is effective in experimental cerebral ischemia has not been found to be useful in the clinical setting. Of recent advances that are intriguing and controversial, none matches that generated by the concept of cerebral protection by mild or moderate hypothermia.

Persons suffering out-of-hospital cardiac arrest have been shown to have improved neurologic outcome if they are made mildly hypothermic following resuscitation.[44,45] Therefore, it would seem that mild hypothermia is protective against global ischemia/hypoxia at least in the setting of cardiac arrest.

One problem with most settings in which cerebral ischemia is encountered is that the therapeutic intervention can be applied only after the insult has occurred, that is, during the reperfusion phase. Little opportunity exists to intervene before the ischemic event. However, the operating room is a unique environment in this respect. Many ischemic insults that patients suffer in the operating room are iatrogenic and anticipated. A temporary aneurysm clip on the middle cerebral artery is an example of a focal ischemic insult that could be predicted, and a brief period of circulatory arrest induced with adenosine to facilitate clipping of a basilar artery aneurysm is an example of a global insult. The value of anticipating such events is that it allows the anesthesiologist to intervene in advance.

Despite the luxury of planning the intervention for the ischemic insult, the options anesthesiologists have for cerebral protection are few and the evidence for benefit is modest; much of this evidence has been extrapolated from animal research. Each technique will be examined in detail here.

Ischemia and Reperfusion

Ischemic insult to the brain results in energy failure. The brain depends on a continuous supply of glucose and O_2 to support aerobic metabolism, generation of adenosine triphosphate (ATP), and maintenance of cellular function. When this nutrient supply is interrupted, ATP is depleted. Cellular processes, such as those that maintain cellular membrane integrity, fail. It is reasonable then to attempt to minimize ischemic insult by lowering cerebral metabolic rate, thus decreasing the likelihood of exhausting ATP reserves during the period of ischemia. This has been the traditional paradigm for approaching the subject of intraoperative neuroprotection.

Unfortunately, further damage occurs as a result of processes that are initiated during the reperfusion stage. The reperfusion injury may be mediated via the generation of toxic oxygen species, release of excitotoxic amino acids such as glutamate, upregulation of nitric oxide synthase, and initiation of cellular apoptosis. Further therapeutic interventions would need to target these pathways as well to provide protection. A shift in the focus of neuroprotection from metabolic suppression to targeting ischemic cascades has recently been advocated.[46]

Hypothermia

It is important to distinguish mild/moderate and profound hypothermia, as they have very different practical considerations and they likely modify cerebral function in different ways.

Profound hypothermia is well known for its neuroprotective effects. Anecdotes of successful resuscitation of hypothermic drowning and avalanche victims with good neurologic recovery have been reported.[47,48] Furthermore, extensive use of deep hypothermia with circulatory arrest has been used intraoperatively for the repair of aneurysms of the thoracic aorta and for cerebral aneurysms.[49,50] When core body temperature is <20°C, and the brain is <15°C, circulatory arrest of <30 minutes appears to be well tolerated. This level of hypothermia not only decreases cerebral activity, but it also decreases the energy required for cellular housekeeping. The practical constraints against using deep hypothermia in settings in which cerebral ischemia is anticipated are numerous. Foremost is the need for cardiopulmonary bypass during the cooling and warming portion of the procedure. Hypothermia-induced coagulopathy is another concern during surgical procedures in the cold patient. Despite the drawbacks to this technique, it remains a reasonable anesthetic option to provide protection for the brain and other organs when the surgical procedure necessitates circulatory arrest.

Mild hypothermia (33° to 35°C) not only decreases cerebral metabolism, but likely modulates the immune and inflammatory response to ischemia, thus affecting the reperfusion portion of the injury as well. Animal studies have shown improved neurologic function following resuscitation from arrest.[51] This promising result in animals was later confirmed by two independent studies in humans, demonstrating that induction of hypothermia in cardiac arrest patients improved the outcome.[44,45]

Although mild hypothermia is clearly beneficial in the setting of cardiac arrest, cerebral ischemia due to an arrest is an uncommon occurrence in patients under anesthesia. In contrast, the cerebral ischemia frequently encountered by the anesthesiologist is focal in nature because of the temporary occlusion of a cerebral vessel. Although there is considerable evidence in rats that mild hypothermia is beneficial here too, there is a paucity of evidence in humans. In fact, a large multicenter study (IHAST II—Intraoperative Hypothermia for Aneurysm Surgery Trial) evaluating patients undergoing cerebral aneurysm surgery found no benefit with mild intraoperative hypothermia.[52] However, the study was not designed to study patients at the highest risk—that is, those who had undergone temporary occlusion for more than 20 minutes. Although the sample size is small, a post-hoc analysis of these at-risk patients suggest that there is a trend for either hypothermia or metabolic suppression to improve outcome.[53]

Nevertheless, hypothermia remains our most promising intervention for cerebral protection. There is a compelling physiologic rationale for its use, a clearly demonstrated effect in animals, and human data showing benefit in the setting of cardiac arrest. Unfortunately, inadequate evidence exists in humans outside cardiac arrest to recommend its routine use in the neurosurgical patient.

Despite the lack of evidence to support hypothermia in humans for cerebral protection, there is ample evidence that hyperthermia is associated with worse outcome in the setting of ischemic stroke, subarachnoid hemorrhage, cardiac arrest, and TBI.[54–57] A common extrapolation from these studies is the belief that concomitant hyperthermia and cerebral ischemia is deleterious. However, it is important to consider that these studies demonstrate an association, not a causation, of poor outcome from fever. Nevertheless, it would seem reasonable to avoid hyperthermia and treat fever aggressively in any setting in which the brain is at risk.[58]

In the operating room, during neurosurgical procedures in which the brain is at risk for ischemic insult, a goal temperature of 35° to 36°C is reasonable. Mild hypothermia (33° to 35°C) may be appropriate in many patients with a planned period of temporary focal ischemia (as in temporary occlusion for aneurysm clipping) even recognizing that there is currently a lack of solid evidence to support this therapy. Finally, deep hypothermia (<20°C) is appropriate in any situation in which a prolonged cardiac arrest is required.

Medical Therapy for Cerebral Protection

Volatile and intravenous anesthetic agents decrease cerebral metabolism, and thus seem like appropriate candidates for cerebral protection. However, evidence that the level of metabolic suppression does not correlate with the degree of protection has eroded the traditional belief in the mechanism of protection.[59] Nevertheless, numerous animal studies have found protective effects of volatile anesthetics, particularly isoflurane, in mitigating mild-to-moderate ischemic insult, although this effect may only be short-lived.[60–63] This effect may exist when applied during the insult, but also may be effective when administered prior to the insult as a preconditioning therapy.[64,65]

Barbiturates, such as thiopental, have been extensively researched in regard to cerebral protection. They have been shown to have at least short-term benefit on focal cerebral ischemia, while benefit in global ischemia remains controversial.[66–74] This effect may be mediated through a reduction in glutamate activity and intracellular calcium, an increase in γ-aminobutyric acid (GABA) activity, as well as *N*-methyl-D-aspartate (NMDA) antagonism.[75,76] Propofol likely has similar protective effects through its action on GABA receptors, as well as via free radical scavenging and limiting lipid peroxidation.[77,78] Again, the durability of this protection is unknown.

Current opinion is that anesthetic neuroprotection is primarily mediated through prevention of excitotoxic injury, not through termination of apoptotic pathways; it thus delays neuronal death and leaves a greater temporal window for intervention.[61] Without other therapeutic options to prevent eventual cell death, outcome is unlikely to be improved, save for perhaps the setting of mild ischemic insult in which apoptotic pathways are not initiated. Sufficient evidence in humans to guide clinical interventions, apart from modest hypothermia in cardiac arrest, is difficult to obtain.[45,79] Clinically, barbiturates and propofol are used intraoperatively to achieve metabolic depression as evidenced by a burst suppression EEG pattern, and although not statistically significant, results from IHAST II suggest that patients undergoing temporary occlusion for >20 minutes may benefit from metabolic suppression therapy.[53]

Glucose and Cerebral Ischemia

Although hyperglycemia has long been recognized as a frequent occurrence in critically ill patients, it was commonly viewed as benign or even beneficial.[80] Hyperglycemia could facilitate cellular uptake of glucose through noninsulin-dependent mechanisms, and thus may benefit cellular metabolism. A subsequent recognition of its association with worse outcome in many settings, including acute coronary syndrome, stroke, TBI, and critical illness, forced the medical community to reconsider the burden of hyperglycemia.[81–86] Furthermore, animal studies suggested that hyperglycemia in the setting of both cerebral and myocardial ischemia increased infarct size.[87,88]

Although considerable evidence accumulated suggesting harm associated with hyperglycemia, evidence for benefit with normalization of serum glucose using insulin has been somewhat controversial. The most influential literature is from the intensive care unit (ICU) setting, not the operating room. A prospective study in surgical ICU patients (predominantly after cardiac surgery) showed that mortality and morbidity benefit with tight glycemic control (80 to 110 mg/dL).[89] This study spurred an unfettered enthusiasm for aggressive treatment of hyperglycemia, changing practice not only in the surgical ICU but the medical ICU, and in many cases, the operating room. However, a subsequent study evaluating this therapy in a much sicker medical ICU population showed no overall mortality benefit.[90] In fact, subgroup analysis revealed increased mortality in patients who stayed in the ICU <3 days, with an improvement only in those who had a longer ICU stay. In the heterogeneous patient population who present for neurologic surgery, with operative times of several hours, not several days, it is inappropriate to extrapolate conclusions from a body of controversial ICU literature to the anesthetic environment, particularly when there is evidence for harm with short durations of therapy. Furthermore, a prospective study of intraoperative insulin therapy in cardiac surgery patients further eroded the basis for translating this ICU literature to the operating room; the insulin group had a higher incidence of death and stroke.[91]

Despite our reluctance to embrace intraoperative tight glycemic control given the current literature, it is worthwhile to consider the patient undergoing cerebrovascular surgery in particular. Given the preponderance of evidence that hyperglycemia and cerebral ischemia in combination are harmful, changing practice in these patients may be warranted. Hyperglycemia on the day of surgery for CEA is associated with worse outcome.[92] And, patients who suffer from an ischemic stroke have an improved outcome if their glucose is treated aggressively.[93] Therefore, it may be appropriate to treat neurosurgical patients who will have a period of cerebral ischemia due to temporary vascular occlusion differently from other neurosurgical patients. Better glycemic control is a reasonable goal in these patients, aiming for a range of 140 to 180 mg/dL however, we cannot state at this time that this intervention is neuroprotective.

Promising Areas of Research

Continued research in the various excitotoxic and apoptotic pathways that lead to cell death with cerebral ischemia is essential to bring promising interventions to the clinical arena. It is likely that only a multimodality approach will create durable meaningful cerebral protection.[61] Mild to moderate hypothermia continues to hold promise, given its efficacy in experimental focal ischemia. Several additional medical interventions show potential as well. Statins, which inhibit 3-hydroxy-3-methylglutaryl-coenzyme A (HMG-CoA) reductase, have nonlipid lowering effects such as improved endothelial function, as well as antithrombotic and anti-inflammatory activity, which may be neuroprotective.[94] Furthermore, the nonhematopoietic effects of erythropoietin include mitigation of lipid peroxidation and prevention of apoptosis.[95] Whether these medications will offer any benefit to neurosurgical patients remains to be determined.

A Practical Approach

In the absence of compelling evidence in humans regarding the benefit of one practice over another, it is difficult to present firm guidelines with respect to the prevention of intraoperative ischemic insult. Maintaining optimal systemic and cerebral hemodynamics, as well as oxygenation, remain the most important principles. Beyond these, for patients undergoing surgical procedures with an anticipated period of temporary focal cerebral ischemia such as cerebral aneurysm surgery or cerebrovascular bypass procedures, either volatile anesthesia or an intravenous technique can be used. It is reasonable to administer additional propofol or thiopental prior to vessel occlusion. Optimally this intervention should be guided by EEG monitoring with the goal of achieving burst suppression nearing a 50% ratio. A total intravenous anesthetic technique is preferred when maximal brain "relaxation" is desired. Euglycemia, or near euglycemia prior to vessel occlusion is desirable (140 to 180 mg/dL), but frequent glucose checks are essential throughout the anesthetic to avoid episodes of hypoglycemia if insulin is administered. Finally, hyperthermia should be avoided during this time, with the temperature kept at or below 36°C.

ANESTHETIC MANAGEMENT

Preoperative Evaluation

6 Risk stratification is indicated for neurologic or spine surgery to assess the patient's neurologic condition, as well as the inherent risk of the surgical procedure. For a smooth transition from patient referral to surgical intervention, dynamic communication between neurosurgeons, anesthesiologists, the preanesthesia clinic, neurophysiologists, and the laboratory is essential.[96,97]

Preoperative assessment allows identification of modifiable risk factors, optimization of the patient's condition, explanation of the risks and formulating the best possible anesthetic plan to improve patient safety, optimize resource utilization and increased patient satisfaction. A thorough history may be difficult to obtain from patients whose disease has resulted in a neurologic decline, such as those obtunded from TBI. Prior medical records, discussion with family physicians and family members are both helpful in this context.

Perioperative cardiac outcome is influenced by urgency, magnitude, type, duration of surgery, associate blood loss, fluid shifts, and change in body temperature. The 2007 American College of Cardiology/American Heart Association guidelines has a simplified algorithm for considering whether a patient needs preoperative cardiac testing, such as stress echocardiography, or a nuclear medicine evaluation of myocardial perfusion.[98] Spine and neurosurgical surgery fall into the intermediate-risk procedure category. The decision to perform a noninvasive cardiac test in patients with risk factors for coronary disease and poor functional status hinges on whether findings from that evaluation will affect management of the patient in the time before surgery. For neurologic patients with significant cardiac disease, current guidelines include delaying surgery for at least 2 weeks following simple balloon angioplasty, 1 month for a bare metal stent, and a full year for a drug-eluting stent. However, it is generally not feasible to delay most of the spine and neurosurgical procedures. For these patients joint consultation with cardiologists is essential. As for beta-blockers, the results of the POISE trial indicated that perioperative beta-blockade is recommended primarily in two types of patients undergoing intermediate-risk surgical procedures: Those already receiving a beta-blocker, and those who are at high risk for perioperative myocardial infarction due to documented reversible ischemia from a noninvasive study.[99,100] Furthermore, patients previously receiving a statin should continue their statin in the perioperative period.

Further considerations in the preoperative visit should include issues that will affect choice of medications and anesthetic agents. Many patients presenting for spine surgery have weakness or paralysis that may present a contraindication to the use of succinylcholine. In addition, some neurosurgical patients may have suffered from a stroke resulting in a similar contraindication. Finally, many neurosurgical patients have been exposed to antiepileptic medications, which are known to induce liver enzymes and alter drug metabolism. Previous allergies or reactions to these medications, especially phenytoin, should be elucidated.

Induction and Airway Management

With the exception of some minimally invasive spine surgery procedures and awake craniotomies, placement of an endotracheal tube is essential for most surgical procedures of the brain and spinal cord.

During induction of anesthesia, hypotension, hypertension, and prolonged apnea should be avoided. A brief period of mild hypotension is frequently encountered following induction of anesthesia. Although most patients tolerate this transient phenomenon well, it should be aggressively avoided and/or treated in patients with brain injury in which any episode of hypotension may be associated with unfavorable outcome.[101] Hypertension due to laryngoscopy, in contrast, is poorly tolerated by patients following aneurysmal subarachnoid hemorrhage, as systolic hypertension is thought to be a cause of recurrent hemorrhage from the aneurysm.[102] Finally, apnea results in a predictable increase in $Pa\text{CO}_2$, and corresponding cerebral vasodilation. Although most patients tolerate the increase in CBV, patients with poor intracranial compliance may develop severe intracranial hypertension and decompensate from apnea, as well as suffer a decrease in cerebral perfusion.

TBI patients in particular are frequently intolerant of apnea. Unfortunately, many of these patients require a rapid-sequence induction. To further complicate matters, the presence of a cervical collar for known or suspected cervical spine injury may make intubation more difficult. Careful preparation for a difficult airway is essential. Furthermore, these patients may have concomitant injuries with significant blood loss that may predispose to systemic hypotension. Vigorous resuscitation with isotonic fluid and/or blood should be administered prior to induction and continued until the patient is euvolemic. A conservative dose of thiopental, propofol, or etomidate is appropriate for induction, with succinylcholine a reasonable choice as the muscle relaxant in the setting of acute injury.

Because patients with subarachnoid hemorrhage are at risk of rebleeding from hypertension, it is reasonable to place an arterial catheter for hemodynamic monitoring prior to induction. Unacceptable increases in blood pressure during laryngoscopy should result in discontinuing the attempt, returning to mask ventilation, and deepening the anesthesia. The latter can be accomplished either with a higher concentration of inspired volatile anesthetic, or a bolus of an intravenous agent such as propofol or remifentanil. In addition, esmolol (0.5 mg/kg) can be given prior to laryngoscopy to blunt the hypertensive response.

Most intravenous anesthetic agents (propofol, thiopental, and etomidate) are indirect cerebral vasoconstrictors, reducing cerebral metabolism (CMR) leading to a corresponding reduction of CBF while preserving autoregulation and CO_2 reactivity. In contrast, ketamine has sympathomimetic properties. Its cerebral effects include an increase in CBF and ICP, but these are usually attenuated by the actions of other concurrently administered drugs.[103–105] Etomidate decreases the cerebral metabolic rate, CBF, and ICP. At the same time, because of minimal cardiovascular effects, CPP is well maintained. However, it has been reported to reduce brain tissue oxygen tension, but the mechanism is unclear. Although changes in the EEG resemble those associated with barbiturates, etomidate enhances SSEPs and causes less reduction of MEP amplitudes than thiopental or propofol.[106,107] The major limitation of etomidate is its known adrenal suppression effects. Even after a single induction dose etomidate has been shown to prolong hospital and ICU length of stay.[108–110]

The choice of muscle relaxant for use during induction deserves some consideration. Succinylcholine is contraindicated in patients with muscle denervation from stroke, myelopathy, or spinal cord injury (SCI) which results in up-regulation of acetylcholine receptor isoforms on myocyte membranes.[111] In these patients, profound hyperkalemia may result from the use of succinylcholine which has the potential to lead to a cardiac arrest.[112] However, it is generally safe to use succinylcholine in the first 24 to 72 hours after an injury, as well as, although controversial, after the spasticity is well established in about 9 months. In general a nondepolarizing muscle relaxant is appropriate for most neurosurgical patients to achieve acceptable conditions for tracheal intubation. Duration of action should be considered if MEP, spontaneous EMG, or cranial nerve monitoring is planned when adequate reversal is not possible. When used in appropriate doses, rocuronium (1.2 mg/kg) is comparable to succinylcholine (1 mg/kg) for rapid sequence induction.[113] When available, profound neuromuscular blockade from rocuronium can be reversed with sugammadex, which currently awaits approval in the United States.[114,115]

Maintenance of Anesthesia

7 The primary considerations for maintenance of anesthesia include the type of neuromonitoring planned for the procedure, optimal brain relaxation, and the balance between adequate analgesia and the ability to assess neurologic function at the end of the surgical procedure.

Most neurosurgical and spine procedures can be performed using a balanced anesthetic with volatile agents and judicious doses of opioids to reduce volatile anesthetic requirements. For both SSEP monitoring and brain relaxation, less than one MAC of volatile anesthetic is desired. When selecting an opioid, an infusion of remifentanil, fentanyl, sufentanil, or alfentanil are all reasonable options. Because of its short context half-life, remifentanil is most appropriate for neurosurgical procedures in which tracheal extubation is planned at the end of the surgery and minimal residual effect is desired to facilitate neurologic examination.[116] Other opioids with a longer duration of action are appropriate for spine surgery in which more durable analgesia following the procedure may be required. However, in most instances administration must be tapered toward the end of the procedure to avoid excessive analgesia and sedation that may interfere with prompt neurologic assessment.

Replacement of the volatile anesthetic with a continuous infusion of propofol is desirable in two settings. First, MEP monitoring virtually requires it to obtain optimal signal quality. Second, when brain relaxation is inadequate with a volatile anesthetic, propofol will provide better relaxation by further decreasing CBV.

The use of intraoperative muscle relaxant is controversial for neurosurgical procedures. It should be avoided during MEP, spontaneous EMG, or cranial nerve monitoring (except the VIIIth). However, it may be used during isolated SSEP monitoring. Some anesthesiologists are more comfortable managing a patient whose head is held in rigid fixation with muscle relaxant, but adequate anesthesia and avoidance of stimulating airway manipulations are far more important and should prevent unintended patient movement.

Dexmedetomidine, a highly selective α_2-adrenoreceptor agonist, provides sedation without causing respiratory depression, does not interfere with electrophysiologic mapping and provides hemodynamic stability. It has been found to be particularly useful for implantation of deep brain stimulators in patients with Parkinson's disease and for awake craniotomies, when sophisticated neurologic testing is required.[117,118]

Ventilation Management

Hypocapnic cerebral vasoconstriction provides the anesthesiologist with a powerful tool for manipulating CBF and CBV. Hyperventilation is routinely employed to provide brain relaxation and optimize surgical conditions. Because hyperventilation decreases CBF, it has the theoretical potential for causing or exacerbating cerebral ischemia. Clinically it has been associated with harm only in the early period of TBI, but it is still recommended to be avoided in all patients with TBI except when necessary for a brief period to manage acute increases in ICP.[119,120] In the nontrauma population, it is not clear whether there is harm in mild-to-moderate hyperventilation, particularly for the duration of a typical anesthetic. As it appears to be well tolerated, it is reasonable during neurosurgical procedures to maintain a $Paco_2$ between 30 and 35 mm Hg. Further brain relaxation should be accomplished with other modalities, such as mannitol, hypertonic saline (HTS), or intravenous anesthesia. Should hyperventilation to a $Paco_2$ below 30 mm Hg be required, it might be appropriate to guide this therapy with jugular venous oximetry when available.

The duration of effectiveness of hyperventilation is also controversial as normalization of CBF, and consequently CBV, has been reported to occur within minutes. Clinically, the effects of CBV appear to be sustained during most neurosurgical procedures of modest duration.

Fluid and Electrolytes

8 To maintain adequate cerebral perfusion, adequate intravascular volume should be maintained. With perhaps the exception of healthy patients with an AVM, the aim should always be euvolemia or slight hypervolemia. For the care of the neurosurgical patient, a large volume of hypotonic fluids including lactated Ringer's solution should not be used. Colloid has no proven advantage over crystalloid. Moreover, hetastarch can result in coagulopathy, and although low doses in healthy individuals is well tolerated, this may not be the case with patients undergoing intracranial procedures as the brain is rich in thromboplastin, the release of which may initiate coagulation abnormalities.

Both mannitol and HTS are effective in the treatment of intracranial hypertension.[121–124] Hypertonic saline (3%) administration results in less dehydration and electrolyte disturbance, and may have anti-inflammatory actions with reduction in leukocyte adhesion and endothelial cell edema.[125–127] With high-dose mannitol (2 g/kg), hyperkalemia can occur and serum potassium should be monitored.[128] Because of the presence of the blood–brain barrier, movement of water into the intracellular and interstitial compartments of the brain from the vascular compartment is primarily dependent on the osmotic pressure, and not on the oncotic pressure. Consequently, to minimize brain edema, it is important to maintain serum tonicity. The most important osmotic species in blood is sodium, so it is prudent to check the serum sodium level on a regular basis in prolonged surgical procedures during which mannitol has been given. In addition to osmotic dehydration of the brain interstitium, other proposed benefits of hypertonic solutions include a reduction in blood viscosity, increasing erythrocyte deformability, and improved cardiac output and microcirculatory flow.[129–135]

Transfusion Therapy

There has been an increasing effort to conserve the limited resource of banked blood. While anemia is associated with increased in-hospital mortality, lower hospital discharge GCS score and discharge Glasgow outcome score, paradoxically RBC transfusion to maintain a higher hemoglobin (10 gm/dL vs. 7 gm/dL) is associated with more acute lung injury, longer ICU and hospital stay, and increased mortality.[136] The lower limit of acceptable hemoglobin or hematocrit has not been well defined. The TRICC trial demonstrated that liberal transfusion targets in intensive care patients had higher mortality rates.[136] Even though this study has been criticized for various reasons, including the poor representation of neurosurgical patients, it remains the best evidence to support avoidance of transfusion down to a hematocrit of approximately 21% except in the context of ongoing hemorrhage and possibly the early phase of resuscitation for septic patients.[137] Despite the lack of evidence to support the practice, many who care for neurosurgical patients have advocated for more liberal transfusion practices to optimize oxygen delivery to the CNS.[138,139] However, there is evidence to support a similar conservative transfusion threshold in both TBI and spine patients.[140,141]

Unfortunately, most of the evidence available on transfusion thresholds relates to critically ill but euvolemic patients. In the operating room with patients undergoing neurosurgical and spine procedures, ongoing hemorrhage may necessitate transfusion well before the hemoglobin falls to 7 g/dL (or a hematocrit of 21%).

A practical approach is to consider the rate of surgical blood loss. If it is slow, then it may be appropriate simply to maintain a normal intravascular volume with isotonic crystalloid solution or with an appropriate colloid, recognizing that albumin should be avoided in patients with TBI.[142] Autologous predonation of blood, erythropoietic support, acute normovolemic hemodilution, intraoperative cell salvage, induced hypotension and the use of pharmacologic agents such as tranexamic acid, in addition to meticulous surgical hemostasis, have all been utilized with modest reductions in allogeneic blood transfusion rates during intracranial and spine surgery.[143–145] However, such practice has not been widespread, as the benefits are marginal.

Monitoring of regional and/or global cerebral oxygenation may help determine the transfusion needs, and brain tissue oxygen tension as well as NIRS have been utilized for this purpose. Currently available evidence supports a hemoglobin threshold level of 8 to 9 g/dL. In the context of ongoing bleeding, lower levels (e.g., 7 g/dL) may result in brief periods of profound anemia, which may be linked to inadequate brain perfusion.[146]

Coagulopathy of trauma in patients with severe TBI has been noted to resolve more quickly than coagulopathy in patients without severe TBI. In trauma, patients with TBI when transfused with a high PLT:RBC ratio (platelet to red blood cell) experienced improved 30-day survival.[147] A proposed mechanism may involve improved blood–brain barrier healing with activation of oligodendrocytes and repair of demyelination.[148]

Glucose Management

As discussed earlier, the combination of hyperglycemia and cerebral ischemia appears to be particularly deleterious.[149–151] Although there is a paucity of evidence addressing the topic of intraoperative glucose management, logic would dictate that glucose should be normalized prior to periods of iatrogenic ischemia.

Tight glycemic control (80 to 110 mg/dL) with intensive insulin therapy has been shown to improve morbidity and mortality in critically ill patients.[152,153] More recently, however, the findings of the NICE-SUGAR (Normoglycemia in Intensive Care Evaluation-Survival Using Glucose Algorithm Regulation) have suggested the use of intensive insulin therapy is associated with higher 90-day mortality.[154] With regard to the neurosurgical population, intensive insulin treatment may result in increased variability in blood glucose leading to cerebral osmotic shifts and higher incidences of hypoglycemia, leading to worse outcome.[155–160] Patients with neurologic injury may have poor correlation of systemic glucose with brain tissue glucose concentration. In this specific group, intensive insulin treatment may result in significantly lower brain tissue glucose concentration and the precipitation of brain energy crises. This risk is potentially greater in an anesthetized patient than an ICU patient, as the signs of hypoglycemia are masked by the anesthetic. Therefore, intraoperative glucose management with insulin requires frequent assessment of the serum glucose level. Patients who present for cerebrovascular surgery should have a preoperative glucose check. Those who are hyperglycemic should be started on an insulin infusion. Continuous closed-loop glucose control systems composed of pumps for the infusion of appropriate amounts of insulin and a glucose sensor for the detection and/or monitoring of glucose levels regulated by computerized algorithms, is an emerging method that could assist in the management of perioperative and inpatient hyperglycemia.

Intraoperative hyperglycemia is found to be common in adults undergoing urgent/emergent craniotomy for TBI and was predicted by severe TBI, the presence of subdural hematoma, preoperative hyperglycemia, and age ≥65 years.[161] A target of 140 to 180 mg/dL is adequate in most patients to achieve this goal.

Emergence

The decisions that need to be made with respect to emergence from anesthesia of neurosurgical and spine surgery patients hinge on whether the patient is an appropriate candidate for tracheal extubation. To determine this, one must evaluate what has changed over the duration of the procedure with respect to the patient's airway, oxygenation, ventilation and metabolic status. In addition, one must consider whether this patient will tolerate the hemodynamic changes that occur with extubation. Finally, postoperative plans, such as cerebral angiography, should be taken into account.

For extensive prone spine surgeries, significant dependent edema frequently occurs. Although the predictive value of a cuff leak from the endotracheal tube is poor in general, the combination of pronounced facial edema and an absent cuff leak following prone surgery should make one suspicious for upper airway edema.[162–164] Delaying extubation of the trachea under these circumstances is prudent. In addition, intraoperative administration of intravenous steroids have not been found to be useful in prevention of airway edema and delayed extubation.[165] Other factors that may delay extubation in these patients include the development of pulmonary edema and hypoxemia from fluid administration, as well as persistent hemodynamic instability.

For neurosurgical cases, usually the desire is to allow the patient to emerge from anesthesia and extubate the trachea as soon as possible after completion of the procedure. This pathway provides for an immediate neurologic examination and may obviate the need for postoperative CT scans. To facilitate emergence and extubation in the operating room, minimal use of opioids other than remifentanil is appropriate. Whether to give a longer-acting opioid, such as fentanyl or morphine, prior to emergence to treat postoperative pain is controversial. Opioids administration may delay emergence in a patient population that usually requires a relatively small amount of postoperative opioid for pain control.[166] The antitussive properties of opioids may be desirable during emergence.

Avoidance of coughing and the hemodynamic changes associated with emergence is important for all neurosurgical patients, and particularly those at high risk for postoperative hemorrhage, such as patients who have just had resection of an AVM. Coughing due to irritation of trachea can be minimized with intravenous lidocaine (1 to 1.5 mg/kg). Instillation of 4% lidocaine in the cuff of the endotracheal tube for the duration of the procedure may achieve equivalent results.[167] Labetalol, hydralazine, and nicardipine are all reasonable options for controlling hypertension on emergence.

COMMON SURGICAL PROCEDURES

Surgery for Tumors

9 The fundamental anesthetic considerations in tumor surgery are proper positioning of the patient to facilitate the surgical approach, providing adequate relaxation of the brain to optimize surgical conditions, and avoiding well-known devastating com-
3 plications, such as VAE. In addition, patients with large tumors resulting in significant intracranial hypertension are at risk of cerebral ischemia as well as herniation. Preoperative review of the level of consciousness and the CT scan should always be performed and the results taken into consideration in the anesthetic plan.

Patient positioning can be very challenging for any neurosurgical procedure, particularly for surgery in the posterior fossa. Lateral, park-bench, prone, and sitting positions are all used for surgical procedures in this region. When placing a patient in a complicated position for surgery, it is essential for the safety of the patient that all catheters and the endotracheal tube are secured particularly well. Ample help should be available at the time of positioning, particularly for obese patients. Padding adequately to avoid pressure necrosis is also essential. The head is typically
4 secured in a Mayfield apparatus. Nothing should impinge on the nose, eyes, or chin.

As the sitting position confers the greatest risk for VAE, plans should be made for treating it, should it occur. The overall incidence of VAE is about 39% in posterior fossa surgery and 11% in cervical spine procedures. A multiorifice catheter can be placed in the right atrium to evacuate air. Its location can be confirmed either with the ECG or with echocardiography. A patent foramen ovale increases the risk of paradoxical embolism. However, transpulmonary passage of air has been described and its risk may be higher with volatile than intravenous anesthesia.[168–170] Patients to be placed in the sitting position should be evaluated for a patent foramen ovale, either preoperatively or intraoperatively, and an alternate position should be considered for those who have one.

The structures in the posterior fossa, most notably the brainstem and cranial nerves, are particularly vulnerable and intolerant of surgical invasion. BAEP and cranial nerve monitoring are appropriate when the surgical procedure places the cranial nerves or brainstem at risk. SSEP and MEP monitoring can be used for any tumor resection, whether supra or infratentorial; these modalities may be particularly useful in surgeries that place specific tracts at risk.[171,172]

The brainstem is intimately involved in systemic hemodynamics, and surgery in that region may affect rapid changes in blood pressure and heart rate. Hemodynamic lability should be anticipated and treated during surgery in this region. Bradycardia can be treated with atropine, but it should also prompt communication with the surgeon, as its development may suggest a need to alter surgical technique.

Adequate brain relaxation is typically achieved with a standard anesthetic including sub-MAC volatile anesthesia, an opioid infusion, mild-to-moderate hyperventilation, and mannitol. In addition, minimizing tumor edema may be accomplished with the administration of dexamethasone.[173] Further relaxation can be achieved with discontinuation of the volatile anesthetic and initiation of a propofol infusion. HTS is a reasonable alternative to mannitol, particularly in the setting of anuric renal failure when mannitol is contraindicated. A randomized trial showed that 3% saline and mannitol have equivalent brain relaxation effects, but with the former having less electrolyte and vascular volume sequelae.[125] A brain that remains "full" may be the result of venous congestion. This problem can be mitigated with head-up tilt, but is best prevented by positioning the patient so as to minimize excessive rotation or angulation of the neck. The central venous pressure and jugular bulb venous pressure (if available) can be transduced to confirm the absence of a pressure gradient across the neck.

Vascular tumors such as meningioma may benefit from preoperative embolization. Surgical removal of large ones or ones that could not be embolized represents a high risk for significant operative blood loss. Coagulopathy can develop as a consequence of massive transfusion. It is important to perform frequent coagulation studies and administer clotting products and platelets promptly.

Pituitary Surgery

Masses in the region of the sella turcica most commonly are of pituitary origin, although other benign (meningioma, craniopharyngioma) and malignant (germ cell tumor, lymphoma) tumors may occur in this region. These tumors are typically recognized as a result of the neurologic changes they effect as they compress adjacent structures, such as visual changes with impingement of the optic chiasm, or through the systemic effects they exert via a change in hormone secretion.

Although many patients with sellar tumors may undergo surgical resection with an uncomplicated general anesthetic, there are several preoperative considerations that will affect the management of the patient. Patients should undergo a preoperative evaluation of their hormonal function to detect hypersecretion of pituitary hormones, common in pituitary adenomas, as well as panhypopituitarism. The hormones that may be secreted by pituitary tumors include prolactin, growth hormone, corticotropin, and thyroid-stimulating hormone. Patients with excess growth hormone eventually will develop acromegaly. The anesthesiologist should be prepared for a difficult airway, as well as postoperative respiratory complications in the acromegalic patient. Patients with a corticotropin-secreting adenoma will develop Cushing disease. These patients may have a typical "Cushingoid" habitus that may make airway management challenging. In addition, venous access may be difficult, and intraoperative hyperglycemia is likely. Patients with thyroid-stimulating hormone hypersecretion will exhibit signs of hyperthyroidism (e.g., tachycardia, weight loss). These patients should be managed in the preoperative period with antithyroid medications and beta-blockade. Close hemodynamic monitoring during surgery is essential.

Patients with panhypopituitarism will need hormone replacement including cortisol, levothyroxine, and possibly DDAVP (1-desamino-8-D-arginin vasopressin). These medications should be continued in the perioperative period.

Small to medium pituitary tumors can be resected from a transsphenoidal approach. Larger tumors may require a craniotomy. IOM of glucose and electrolytes is essential, particularly if the patient has pre-existing diabetes insipidus, or if the patient develops signs of diabetes insipidus during the surgery. Diabetes insipidus is a common complication of pituitary surgery due to the loss of antidiuretic hormone production. It may be temporary or permanent, and may occur either in the intraoperative or postoperative period. It is initially suspected on the basis of copious urine output, as well as rising serum sodium. A urine specific gravity of <1.005 is confirmatory. Although infusions of intravenous fluids containing free water may mitigate the electrolyte changes, replacement of antidiuretic hormone with DDAVP (0.5 to 1 μg intravenously or subcutaneously) is an effective therapy for diabetes insipidus. Volume replacement therapy may be guided with the use of central venous pressure monitoring as well as the observation of systolic variation in blood pressure.

Arteriovenous Malformations

A cerebral AVM is an abnormal vascular connection between the arterial and the venous circulation. The absence of an intervening capillary bed results in a low-resistance path for blood flow. Patients may present with hemorrhage, seizure, or focal neurologic deficit. Cerebral angiography remains the gold standard for AVM diagnosis. Although preoperative embolization of the AVM is commonly performed, either radiosurgery or an open surgical procedure is typically required subsequent to the embolization to cure the lesion. Although these lesions may be adjacent to vital structures, and an immediate postoperative neurologic examination may be desirable, emergence from anesthesia following resection of an AVM requires particular care. Because of local hemodynamic changes as a result of the AVM, the adjacent vessels must chronically vasodilate to preserve perfusion. When the low-resistance AVM has been occluded or resected, the adjacent vessels are exposed to higher pressures than to which they were previously accustomed. These vessels may not be able to autoregulate appropriately within the normal blood pressure range, and "normal perfusion pressure breakthrough" may occur. This phenomenon is defined by regional hyperemia at a normal systemic blood pressure. Normal perfusion pressure breakthrough may result in vasogenic edema and hemorrhage. It can be minimized with careful blood pressure control; preoperative embolization likely decreases its incidence as well. Following resection of large AVMs or those in the posterior fossa, taking the patient to the ICU in a ventilated and sedated state may be appropriate. Should the decision be made between the surgeon and anesthesiologist to allow emergence and tracheal extubation, aggressive management of blood pressure should be instituted, and coughing should be avoided. Intravenous labetalol and hydralazine may be adequate, but a nicardipine infusion may be most appropriate for blood pressure control. Blood pressure control needs to be conducted using an anticipated and prophylactic approach rather than a reactive one, as the delay in treating hypertension may be detrimental. Intravenous lidocaine can be used to blunt coughing.

Cerebral Aneurysm Surgery and Endovascular Treatment

Cerebral aneurysms are relatively prevalent vascular abnormalities (approximately 5% incidence at autopsy) that arise from congenital weakness of the vessel wall as well as extrinsic influences such as hypertension and cigarette smoking. They are more prevalent in women than in men. Some aneurysms become clinically significant when they rupture, resulting in arterial bleeding into the subarachnoid space. This event typically causes severe headache, and may also cause focal neurologic deficit, lethargy, and coma. For patients who survive their hemorrhage, surgical or endovascular intervention to secure the aneurysm is essential to prevent further hemorrhage. In addition, many patients are incidentally found to have cerebral aneurysms, and they may need intervention to decrease the risk of an initial subarachnoid hemorrhage. Intervention for a cerebral aneurysm may include a craniotomy and surgical clipping, or endovascular coiling.

Anesthetic considerations for cerebral aneurysm surgery are somewhat different in those patients who have experienced a subarachnoid hemorrhage as compared with those who present for elective repair. Patients with aneurysmal subarachnoid hemorrhage are at risk for numerous complications that may affect the anesthetic plan. These include cardiac dysfunction, neurogenic or cardiogenic pulmonary edema, hydrocephalus, as well as further hemorrhage from the aneurysm. This last complication is perhaps the most devastating and requires intensive treatment (see also Chapter 55).

Careful attention to hemodynamics, particularly during stimulating procedures, is essential to avoid recurrent hemorrhage. Laryngoscopy and placement of the head in the Mayfield device are two points at which transient hypertension is likely and the anesthesiologist must be particularly vigilant about maintaining an adequate depth of anesthesia.

Following subarachnoid hemorrhage, cardiac dysfunction, and pulmonary edema commonly resolve over time. The cardiac dysfunction may be severe, resulting in ECG changes, elevated troponin, and even cardiogenic shock. Echocardiography may reveal hypokinesis in a distribution not consistent with an anatomic vascular territory. Unfortunately, the need to secure the aneurysm in a timely fashion may require the anesthesiologist to provide anesthesia despite ongoing cardiac and pulmonary issues. Hemodynamic support with carefully titrated vasopressors may be necessary, recognizing the risk of elevating the blood pressure too much. Hypoxemia can often be managed with increased F_{IO_2} and positive end-expiratory pressure. With the exception of a hemodynamically unstable patient, surgical clipping of a ruptured aneurysm should rarely be postponed.

Once the aneurysm is secured with an aneurysm clip, the risk of recurrent hemorrhage from the aneurysm is removed. Although careful attention to hemodynamics as well as coughing during emergence is still important, the concern of devastating hemorrhage from the aneurysm is diminished.

The patient presenting for an elective aneurysm procedure will typically have good brain conditions, with easily achievable relaxation using mannitol (0.5 to 1 g/kg), mild-to-moderate hyperventilation, and sub-MAC volatile anesthetic in combination with an opioid infusion. Following subarachnoid hemorrhage, brain relaxation may be more difficult to achieve; intravenous anesthesia may be required. Drainage of CSF via a lumbar drain or external ventricular drain can be used at the discretion of the surgeon.

In contrast to aneurysm surgery, endovascular treatment of aneurysms is a minimally invasive procedure performed in the interventional radiology suite. The interventional neuroradiologist or neurosurgeon accesses the aneurysm via an intra-arterial catheter and typically deploys coils into the aneurysm that cause it to thrombose. This technique requires a favorably shaped aneurysm that will retain the coils once they are deployed. Increasingly sophisticated techniques, such as placing a stent in the adjacent vessel and coiling through the stent, have increased the range of aneurysms that are amenable to endovascular therapy.

Despite the less invasive nature of this procedure, it can have equally severe complications as surgery, including further hemorrhage, stroke, and vessel dissection.

Although the procedure is not particularly stimulating, the general anesthetic needs to be performed with great care. Obviously, hypertension with laryngoscopy should be avoided. Furthermore, any patient movement during the procedure can incur devastating consequences because it may result in deployment of coils in a vessel rather than the aneurysm itself. Hyperventilation should be avoided, as it will decrease CBF and make access to the aneurysm more challenging. Heparin is commonly administered during this procedure. It is meant to decrease the risk of thromboembolic complications associated with the intra-arterial catheter. Protamine must be available should arterial rupture and extravasation occur. In addition, prompt transfer to an operating room for neurosurgical intervention should also be possible.

Carotid Surgery

Carotid stenosis is a common cause of transient ischemic attack and ischemic stroke. It is amenable to surgical intervention and endovascular stenting. In older studies, CEA was found to be beneficial in reducing stroke rate in symptomatic patients (ipsilateral transient ischemic attack or nondisabling stroke) with ≥70% internal carotid artery stenosis and, to a lesser extent, in patients with 50% to 69% internal carotid artery stenosis.[174,175] In asymptomatic carotid stenosis, the benefit of surgical intervention over medical therapy appears to be somewhat smaller, and it depends on the incidence of perioperative stroke.[176,177] In addition, surgery is associated not only with a risk of stroke, but also myocardial infarction, wound infection, and cranial nerve dysfunction. At the time of the NASCET trial,[174] medical therapy consisted primarily of daily aspirin. With advances in medical therapy, including more aggressive lipid-lowering drugs as well as other effective antiplatelet agents and better antihypertensive therapy, the margin of benefit of surgery may be even less.[178] Appropriate candidate selection for surgery has therefore become extremely important. Preoperative evaluation of the asymptomatic patient depends on assessment of the risk for progression to stroke and weighing that risk against the morbidity of the procedure.

Both general and regional anesthesia may be used for CEA. Regional anesthesia is accomplished with a superficial cervical plexus block, or a combination of superficial and deep block.[179,180] This technique allows continuous neurologic assessment during the surgery, which is particularly useful at the time of carotid cross-clamp. However, some patients and surgeons may not be agreeable to this anesthetic technique. General anesthesia with an endotracheal tube is therefore a more common technique for CEA. A multicenter, randomized controlled trial, GALA, involving 3,526 patients, compared general anesthesia versus local anesthesia for carotid surgery, and did not show a significant difference between the two groups regarding quality of life, length of hospital stay, and perioperative complications of stroke, myocardial infarction, and death.[181] Both techniques are therefore similarly efficacious.

Patients undergoing carotid surgery are nevertheless at increased risk for perioperative complications, given their high prevalence of coronary artery disease, hypertension, chronic obstructive pulmonary disease, diabetes mellitus, and chronic kidney disease. Continuation of beta-blockers and statins is appropriate for patients who are receiving these medications preoperatively. Blood pressure should be maintained as close to baseline as possible throughout the surgery. Without evidence to support it, some advocate raising the blood pressure during carotid cross-clamp to improve flow through collateral vessels. This practice presupposes that collateralization is marginal and will be helped by the elevation in pressure. Collateral flow may be marginal, but it may also be absent or entirely adequate. In the latter two situations, elevation in blood pressure through the use of phenylephrine will only increase myocardial oxygen demand. However, evidence of hypoperfusion ipsilateral to the cross-clamp is reason to consider blood pressure elevation. The decision to raise blood pressure is facilitated by the concurrent use of CNS monitors.

Several CNS monitors may be used during CEA under general anesthesia. EEG allows for easy detection of a decline in spectral power on the hemisphere ipsilateral to the surgery, which would be concerning for ischemia. NIRS is also promising for its ability to demonstrate relative changes between the ipsilateral and contralateral hemispheres, but it has not come into common use as yet. TCD is particularly attractive, as it allows determination of changes in flow during carotid cross-clamp, and detection of emboli, as well as diagnosis of postoperative hyperemia. The hypoperfusion during cross-clamp can be avoided with a shunt during the surgical procedure, but at the increased risk of embolization. A decrease in flow velocity of up to 60% of baseline is generally well tolerated in the anesthetized patient during this procedure. Should a shunt be needed, the development of microembolic signals can provide feedback to the surgeon if there is a modifiable technique to the surgical procedure. At the end of the endarterectomy, during surgical closure, continued presence of a good flow velocity waveform on TCD provides confirmation of stability of the graft and lack of an intimal flap, or thrombosis. Although each monitor has attractive features, ultimately user familiarity and comfort will determine its utility.[182] Postoperatively, sustained elevation of flow velocity exceeding 100% of baseline values is highly suggestive of the development of hyperperfusion syndrome, and should prompt lowering of systemic blood pressure.

Rapid emergence and tracheal extubation at the end of the procedure is desirable because it allows immediate neurologic assessment. Hemodynamic changes can occur in the postoperative period from denervation of the carotid baroreceptor. In addition, headache, obtundation, and/or focal neurologic deficit in the postoperative period should prompt one to consider hyperemia, hemorrhage, or ischemic stroke.

Carotid artery stenting (CAS) may be used to treat carotid stenosis as well. It is an attractive procedure in that it is minimally invasive and can be performed under sedation. However, noninferiority studies have not supported stenting as compared with CEA in symptomatic patients.[183,184] Yet the SAPPHIRE trial has indicated that stenting may be a reasonable option in asymptomatic patients with tight stenosis; currently, most centers reserve stenting for patients who are poor surgical candidates.[185,186] A clinical trial in 2010, comparing CAS and CEA did not show a difference in the primary outcome of stroke, MI, or death among symptomatic and asymptomatic patients.[187] However, the patients who underwent CEA had a lower stroke rate, whereas patients who had CAS had a lower rate of myocardial infarction.

Anesthetic considerations for this procedure are important, even though it is typically performed under sedation. These patients tend to have significant medical comorbidities. Conversion to general anesthesia may incur significant risk. Furthermore, the procedure itself may induce significant hemodynamic changes, most notably bradycardia or asystole during balloon angioplasty of the internal carotid artery. Although pretreatment with atropine may prevent this complication, a brisk tachycardia is generally not desirable in these patients.

Epilepsy Surgery and Awake Craniotomy

Some intracranial neurosurgical procedures are performed on "awake" (i.e., sedated and pain free, with local anesthesia, yet able to respond to verbal or visual command) patients in order to facilitate monitoring of the region of the brain on which the surgeon is operating. These procedures require particular attention on the part of the anesthesiologist to provide patient comfort and safety. Typically these surgeries are for tumors adjacent to eloquent cortex or for resection of an epileptic focus. Frequently the decision to perform the procedure awake has been made by the neurosurgeon prior to the patient meeting the anesthesiologist. It is the role of the anesthesiologist to determine whether the patient is an appropriate candidate for an awake procedure, to coordinate with the neurosurgeon the anesthetic plan, and to support and reassure the patient through the process.

Although the patient with a difficult airway, obstructive sleep apnea, or orthopnea may present a relative contraindication to an awake craniotomy, it is the patient with severe anxiety, claustrophobia, or other psychiatric disorder who may be particularly inappropriate for this type of procedure. On the other hand, patients with neurodegenerative disorders are often elderly and may have respiratory, cardiovascular, and autonomic system compromise. Potential drug interactions and adverse effects from anti-Parkinson's medications may also occur during anesthesia.[188] Patients with dystonia or torticollis may present difficulties in airway management. Patients with psychiatric, epileptic, and chronic pain disorders will present with their own set of challenges and will need special consideration in the management of their medications perioperatively.[189–191]

Preoperative evaluation should be comprehensive and should include a thorough airway examination. Conversion to a general anesthetic remains a possibility at any point during the procedure. Extensive discussion with the patient regarding the plan is essential to prepare him or her for the experience in the operating room.

Intraoperative Management

Standard anesthesia monitors including an ECG, noninvasive arterial blood pressure, oxygen saturation, and end-tidal CO_2 are minimum requirements. Where tight control of blood pressure is required, invasive blood pressure monitoring should be employed. O_2 is provided through variable or fixed rate oxygen delivery devices with end-tidal CO_2 monitoring capability in order to verify airway patency and track respiratory rate. Attention should be given to the positioning of the patients on the operating table for maximal comfort and cooperativeness. Direct visual and verbal contacts with the patient should be maintained throughout the procedure. The environment should be made quiet, calm, and comfortable with an appropriate room temperature and humidity.

Conscious Sedation (CS) Technique

The goal of sedation is to allow the patient to have a minimally depressed level of consciousness but remain able to maintain his/her own airway and respond to verbal stimulation. Only the administration of supplemental O_2 via nasal prongs or cannula, or a facemask is required. Sedation may be given throughout the procedure or can be utilized intermittently for the surgically stimulating part of the procedure. Frequently used drugs for CS include propofol, opioids such as fentanyl or remifentanil, and dexmedetomidine.[192–194] Generally, benzodiazepines are avoided.

Propofol is one of the most frequently used drug either alone, or in combination with remifentanil. Propofol can be titrated to provide adequate sedation and a rapid, smooth recovery. However, it can decrease the incidence of seizures. At least 15 to 30 minutes is required for discontinuation of the propofol infusion prior to electrocorticographic recording. Retrospective analysis of an AAA (asleep–awake–asleep) sequence using propofol and remifentanil showed that adequate conditions are obtained in 98% of patients, with a median wake-up time of 9 minutes at the mean infusion rates of 50 μg/kg/min.[195–197]

There is growing evidence suggesting that dexmedetomidine may be the ideal sedative for awake procedures with low-dose infusion rates (0.3 to 0.6 μg/kg/hr).[119,198] Dexmedetomidine is a central-acting α_2 agonist that offers sedation and anxiolysis, helps maintain hemodynamic stability (through its central α-agonist activity) and has analgesic properties. Dexmedetomidine also causes minimal respiratory depression and has an anesthetic-sparing effect, even with infusions at the higher end of the dose range.

"Asleep Awake Asleep" (AAA) Technique

The AAA pathway is often the preferred method for epilepsy surgery and tumor resection. This anesthetic plan involves general anesthesia for the skin incision (supplemented by scalp blocks or local anesthetic infiltration), initial craniotomy, and then for the closure in the end, while the patient is allowed to emerge from anesthesia for the middle portion of the surgery in which the surgeon is working around the eloquent areas of the brain. Intraoperative mapping of cortical functions in the awake patient helps to identify the precise location of epileptic focus. During such mapping, the neurosurgeon applies electrical stimulation to the exposed brain cortex of the awake patient, which allows the neurophysiologist to report any sensory, motor, and speech effects as well as any effects on more complex cognitive functions. Such mapping can also be performed during resection of the tumor, thereby allowing for maximal tumor resection while minimizing neurologic deficits (the resection is stopped if symptoms emerge). This gives the patient better postoperative quality of life, better chance of survival.

The asleep portions of the procedure may be performed without an airway, with a laryngeal mask airway (LMA), or with an endotracheal tube in place. For suitable candidates, spontaneous ventilation with propofol anesthesia is an attractive option, as it allows straightforward emergence with minimal coughing, gagging, or straining. In addition, propofol provides a nice anesthetic for these patients because of its low incidence of nausea and vomiting during the awake period. An LMA is a suitable alternative to an endotracheal tube as it can frequently be removed with little movement of the patient as he or she emerges from anesthesia. Topical application of lidocaine to the airway prior to insertion of the LMA supplemented with lidocaine jelly on the LMA may improve patient tolerance during emergence.

An endotracheal tube provides the most secure airway, but it is also the most difficult to remove during the procedure, particularly with the patient's head secured in rigid fixation. If this pathway is chosen, several options exist to minimize coughing as the patient emerges. Prior to placement of the endotracheal tube, the larynx and trachea may be anesthetized with lidocaine. In addition, the cuff of the endotracheal tube can be filled with 4% lidocaine rather than air. Finally, allowing the patient to emerge on an infusion of low-dose remifentanil or dexmedetomidine may facilitate extubation with little movement.

During the awake portion of the procedure, all sedatives are typically withheld. For particularly stimulating events (e.g., drilling) and in coordination with the surgeon, small boluses of propofol may be given. Antiemetics may be given for nausea and small doses of fentanyl for discomfort.

Following this critical portion of the surgery, the patient may be fully anesthetized for the surgical closure. Initiating a propofol infusion and continuing with spontaneous ventilation is again a good option; otherwise, manipulation of the airway to place an LMA or endotracheal tube will be necessary while avoiding the sterile field.

General Anesthesia (GA)

Patient groups more likely to require GA includes infants and children, patients with learning difficulties, certain seizure or continuous movement disorders, severe pain, claustrophobia, and those patients who are critically ill (e.g., with high ICP).

GA may create several problem areas during surgery. For epilepsy surgery, if intraoperative localization of the epileptic focus is needed in order to provide good conditions for electrocorticography and for motor testing, the influence of anesthetic agents should be kept at a minimum, while concomitantly avoiding long periods of potential awareness on the part of the patient. Specific preoperative preparation should include informing the patients of the possibility that awareness and recall may occur at the time of electrocorticographic recording, but reassuring them that this will be brief and painless. All anesthetics will affect electrocorticography but the use of the shorter-acting anesthetic agents, either inhalation agents and/or intravenous agents will allow for faster decrease in the depth of anesthesia. During the time of recording, all or most of the anesthetic agents are discontinued. Long-term anticonvulsant therapy may lead to increased dosage requirements for opioids and neuromuscular blocking agents. Nitrous oxide should be avoided to prevent complications from a pneumocephalus. Complications that may occur during epilepsy surgery are similar to those for any craniotomy. However, severe bradycardia is a common occurrence with resection of the amygdala–hippocampus.

ANESTHESIA AND TRAUMATIC BRAIN INJURY

Overview of Traumatic Brain Injury

The presence of TBI is the primary determinant in the quality of outcome for patients suffering from trauma.[34] Anesthesiologists are involved in the care of these patients in many different settings, including the initial resuscitation in the emergency department, anesthetic management in the operating room, and ongoing care in the ICU (see also Chapter 55).

Primary injury is the result of the initial, mechanical forces on the brain tissue and skull, resulting in skull fracture, brain contusion and/or intracranial hematoma as a result of shearing and compression of neuronal, glial, and vascular tissues. The consequences of the initial TBI include physical disruption of cell membranes and infrastructure, and disturbance of ionic homeostasis secondary to increased membrane permeability. This in turn may lead to astrocytic and neuronal swelling, relative hypoperfusion, perturbation of cellular calcium homeostasis, increased free radical generation and lipid peroxidation, mitochondrial dysfunction, inflammation, apoptosis, and diffuse axonal injury. These mechanisms result in irreversible damage.[34] *Secondary injury* is the progression of the pathologic insults, such as ischemia, reperfusion and hypoxia starting immediately after the initial TBI. Systemic insults such as hypotension (systolic BP <90 mm Hg), hypoxemia (Pao_2 <60 mm Hg), hypoglycemia, hyperglycemia, hypocarbia, and hypercarbia are major contributors to secondary injury. The initial approach to patients with TBI should be similar to that of any trauma patient, as outlined in *Advanced Trauma Life Support* (ATLS) by the American College of Surgeons and followed by limitation of secondary insults. Although delayed brain ischemia appears to be the major common pathway of secondary brain damage, reperfusion hyperemia may also occur.

Airway and breathing are obviously of paramount importance in any critically ill patient but even more so in patients with head injuries, given the sensitivity of the brain to hypoxemia and hypercapnia. Prehospital tracheal intubation of the patient with TBI may be associated with worse outcomes.[199–205] If the patient arrives in the emergency department intubated, one must confirm proper placement of the endotracheal tube with a CO_2 detector and chest radiograph.[200,202–205] If the patient is not intubated, immediate attention should focus on assessing the airway and making preparations for intubation. Patients with TBI usually have several indications for intubation including: Decreased level of consciousness, increased risk of aspiration, as well as concern for hypoxemia and hypercarbia. Sometimes these patients must be intubated and sedated simply to allow further diagnostic studies. SCI occurs in up to 2% to 5% of all major trauma cases and at least 14% of these cases have the potential to have an unstable spine. Techniques to minimize cervical spine (C-spine) movement should be employed during airway management, while considerations should be given to other potential injuries.

Patients with TBI have up to a 10% incidence of an unstable cervical spine injury.[206,207] Risk factors include a motor vehicle accident and Glasgow Coma Scale (GCS) score <8. Therefore, all attempts at intubation should include in-line neck stabilization to decrease the chance of worsening a neurologic injury.[208] This maneuver may worsen the view of the glottis, making intubation more difficult.[209] Therefore, one must always have a backup plan and device in mind when performing an emergency intubation, including but not limited to LMAs and fiberoptic or videolaryngoscope technology. Patients with TBI should generally be intubated orally, as the potential presence of a basilar skull fracture could increase the risk associated with a nasal intubation. A surgical airway remains an appropriate procedure for patients with severe facial trauma and an expected difficult airway.

Minimizing the risk of aspiration of gastric contents during airway procedures is essential. The effectiveness and correct application of cricoid pressure (CP) in this setting has been questioned.[210,211] New evidence suggests that the alimentary canal at the level of cricoid ring is the postcricoid hypopharynx and not the esophagus.[212] Rice et al.[213] define the concept of "cricoid pressure unit" and discredit the logic of ineffectiveness of the CP due to previously reported displacement of the esophagus in relation to the trachea. Incorrectly applied CP may displace cervical fractures, whereas bimanual application may help to reduce this displacement.[214,215]

Another important consideration is the choice of drugs to facilitate intubation. As discussed previously, hypotension is extremely detrimental to the injured brain; therefore, the choice of drugs must be tailored to each individual patient. Sodium thiopental in a dose of 3 to 6 mg/kg is a useful drug in euvolemic hemodynamically stable patients, but is no longer available in the United States. Through its depressant effect on cerebral metabolism, thiopental decreases CBF, CBV, and ICP,[216,217] but may cause profound hypotension. Propofol and etomidate are suitable alternatives, with the latter causing less hypotension at the expense of adrenal suppression. In doses of 1.5-mg/kg lidocaine blunts the effects of laryngoscopy and intubation on ICP with minimal hemodynamic effects. Finally, although controversial, succinylcholine is not contraindicated in patients with TBI, as the effects on ICP are clinically insignificant. Succinylcholine may be the relaxant of choice when intubation needs to be established quickly.[218–220] On the other hand, rocuronium is a suitable alternative when no difficulty with the airway or intubation is anticipated. Once the trachea is intubated, the initial ventilation parameters should include 100% O_2; arterial CO_2 should be maintained in the lower normal range (35 mm Hg), and the subsequent ventilation regimen should be guided by arterial blood gas analysis.

The goal of resuscitation in any trauma patient should be to establish adequate circulation, with oxygenated blood, so that cerebral perfusion may be maintained. Blood pressure and CPP are often low after TBI. Several studies have documented worsened outcome in TBI patients who have experienced episodes of hypotension (SBP < 90 mm Hg) after TBI. Thus, continuous monitoring and optimization of blood pressure and CPP are essential. It is worth noting that there is a lack of information on what the optimal intraoperative hemodynamic goals should be. Cerebral autoregulation may be impaired after TBI. This has two possible consequences: (a) when blood pressure is low, cerebral ischemia may result, (b) in the presence of high blood pressures, cerebral hyperemia and hemorrhage may ensue. The overwhelming evidence of harm from hypotension necessitates restoration of intravascular volume.[101] Isotonic crystalloid solutions should be used to accomplish this goal; note that lactated Ringer solution is slightly hypotonic (Table 36-3). The goal is to maintain CPP in the range of 50 to 70 mm Hg, as recommended by the guidelines from the Brain Trauma Foundation in 2007.[221] Glucose-containing solution should definitely be avoided. The role of colloids is controversial. According to the Saline versus Albumin Fluid Evaluation (SAFE) study, resuscitation with albumin is associated with higher mortality rate and unfavorable outcome in TBI patients.[142] In regards to synthetic colloids, recently published studies indicate that administration of hydroxyethyl starch in patients with severe TBI may be relatively safe, but confirmation is needed.[222–224] A multicenter, clinically randomized control trial to determine whether out-of-hospital administration of hypertonic fluids would improve neurologic outcome following severe TBI has been terminated early due to futility. The investigators concluded that initial fluid resuscitation of patients with severe TBI with either HTS/dextran or HTS was not superior to 0.9% saline with respect to 6-month neurologic outcome or survival.[225]

Vasopressors and inotropes may be needed after fluid resuscitation to achieve the desired CPP, or to treat hypotension while volume restoration is ongoing. They should be used judiciously, as they are thought to increase the incidence of acute respiratory distress syndrome.[226] Currently there are no recommendations regarding the choice of vasopressors to achieve optimal CPP.

TABLE 36-3. INTRAVENOUS FLUIDS

Fluid	Osmolality (mOsm/kg)	Oncotic Pressure (mm Hg)	Na^+ (mEq/L)	Cl^- (mEq/L)	K^+ (mEq/L)	Ca^{2+}/Mg^{2+} (mEq/L)	Glucose (g/L)
Plasma	289	21	141	103	4–5	5/2	—
Crystalloid							
0.9% NS	308	0	154	154	—	—	—
0.45% NS	154	0	77	77	—	—	—
3% NS	1,030	0	515	515	—	—	—
7.5% NS	2,400	0	1,200	1,200	—	—	—
LR	273	0	130	109	4	3/0	—
D_5LR^a	527	0	130	109	4	3/0	50
D_5W^a	252	0	—	—	—	—	50
D_5 NS^a	586	0	154	154	—	—	50
$D_5$0.45% NS^a	406	0	77	77	—	—	50
Plasma-Lyte 148	294	0	140	98	5	0/3	—
Normosol-R	294	0	140	98	5	0/3	—
Mannitol (20%)	1,098	0	—	—	—	—	—
Colloid			—	—	—	—	—
Hetastarch (6%)	310	31	154	154	—	—	—
Albumin (5%)	290	19	145	145	—	—	—

^{a}In dextrose-containing solutions, it is important to distinguish between osmolality and tonicity.
NS, normal saline; LR, lactated Ringer solution; D_5W, 5% dextrose in water.

TABLE 36-4. GLASGOW COMA SCALE

Eyes	1. No eye opening
	2. Opens to painful stimulus
	3. Opens to voice
	4. Spontaneous eye opening
Verbal	1. No sounds
	2. Incomprehensible sounds
	3. Inappropriate words
	4. Confused conversation
	5. Normal speech
Motor	1. No movement
	2. Extension to painful stimulus
	3. Abnormal flexion to painful stimulus
	4. Withdrawal from painful stimulus
	5. Localization of painful stimulus
	6. Follows commands

Norepinephrine is probably the most commonly used agent to achieve these goals in adults.[227]

Patients with TBI are typically described by their localized GCS score (Table 36-4). This simple test facilitates communication between providers, and it provides prognostic information. Mild head injury is represented by a score of 13 to 15, moderate head injury by a score of 9 to 12, and severe head injury by a score of <8. The score should be determined on postresuscitation information, as hypotension may depress mental status in any patient, even those without TBI. Younger age, lower ICP on presentation, and the presence of reactive pupils were identified as the main prognostic factors in severe head injury patients. The pupil examination is particularly useful. The presence of a unilateral dilated pupil suggests uncal herniation, and is a surgical emergency, whereas the presence of bilateral fixed and dilated pupils portends a poor prognosis. Quantitative pupillary measurements have been introduced to facilitate monitoring and may help to diagnose increased ICP. Using automated pupil index, a trend was identified to indicate an inverse relationship between decreasing pupil reactivity and increasing ICP.[228]

Intracranial hypertension predisposes patients to poor outcomes, and elevated ICP refractory to therapy is associated with a worse prognosis. Some controversy exists regarding what constitutes the optimal ICP and CPP. The current accepted recommendation is to maintain CPP between 60 and 70 mm Hg, and ICP <20 to 25 mm Hg.[221] Reduction of ICP in patients with head injuries can be accomplished effectively using osmotic diuretics. Mannitol, given at 0.25 to 1 g/kg, is the most commonly used agent. The general guideline is that it can be repeatedly given, provided that serum osmolality does not exceed 320 mOsm, but there is no data to support this threshold. The mechanism of ICP reduction by mannitol may be related to its osmotic effect in shifting fluid from the brain tissue compartment to the intravascular compartment as well as its ability to improve blood rheology by decreasing blood viscosity leading to reflex vasoconstriction. In addition, mannitol, like other hypertonic fluids, decreases production of CSF. HTS (3% or 7.5%) is increasingly being used to treat elevated ICP instead of mannitol. Patients refractory to mannitol treatment may respond to HTS therapy. There is also less fluid loss from osmotic diuresis with HTS.

Hypoxia, hypercarbia, and hypocapnia should be avoided as they cause secondary injuries after TBI. Adequate oxygenation should be established to maintain Pao_2 >60 mm Hg or oxygen saturation >90%. Hyperventilation causes cerebral vasoconstriction, primarily in the small resistance arterioles in the brain; this vasoconstriction rapidly reduces the CBV and therefore the ICP. The reduction in CBV; however, is achieved at the expense of reduction in CBF and may exacerbate cerebral ischemia. The current guidelines for managing TBI indicate that prophylactic hyperventilation ($Paco_2 \leq 25$ mm Hg) is not recommended and hyperventilation should be avoided during the first 24 hours after TBI. Hyperventilation is recommended as a temporizing measure for the reduction of elevated ICP and may be utilized briefly during emergent evacuation of an expanding intracranial hematoma. When hyperventilation is required because of failure of other agents to control ICP, monitoring of $Pbto_2$, $Sjvo_2$, and the arteriovenous lactate gradient has been advocated.[230]

Induced moderate hypothermia has been considered as a therapeutic modality in head injury for many years. Several mechanisms have been proposed for the beneficial effects of hypothermia on brain protection; reduction in brain metabolic rate, attenuation of blood–brain barrier permeability, reduction of the critical threshold for oxygen delivery, calcium antagonism, blockade of excitotoxic mechanisms, preservation of protein synthesis, reduction of intracellular acidosis, modulation of the inflammatory response, a decrease in edema formation, suppression of free radicals and antioxidants and modulation of apoptotic cell death.[234–236] Furthermore, hypothermia lowers the cerebral metabolic rate by 6% to 7% for every 1°C decrease in core temperature, which consequently improves oxygen supply to the areas of ischemic brain and decreases ICP.

A 2009 Cochrane review concludes that there is no evidence that hypothermia is beneficial in the treatment of head injury.[235] A multicenter trial published in 2011, on the use of early hypothermia for TBI: The National Acute Brain Injury Study: Hypothermia II trial (NABIS:HII) was terminated early due to the lack of efficacy during an intermediate analysis.[236] Similarly, or perhaps unexpectedly, a clinical trial in pediatric head injury observed that the hypothermia group had a higher mortality rate than the normothermia group.[237] In addition, hypothermia increases the risk of pneumonia and wound infection, and may cause electrolyte and coagulation abnormalities.[238] Because of the demonstrated efficacy of hypothermia in experimental brain injury, and the perceived flaws in the clinical trials conducted thus far, the pursuit of therapeutic hypothermia for TBI remains vigorous, and there are ongoing clinical trials in both pediatric and adult TBI. (e.g., POLAR-RCT: Prophylactic Hypothermia Trial to Lessen Traumatic Brain Injury – Randomised Controlled Trial based in Australia/New Zealand, and the Eurotherm 3235 Trial based in the United Kingdom).[239,240] While the value of hypothermia remains to be established, it is important to note that hyperthermia is detrimental to the injured brain and should be prevented and/or treated.

Barbiturates may be used as an adjunct to other therapy for controlling ICP. As discussed earlier, they lower ICP via their effect on cerebral metabolism. As long as the MAP is maintained, CPP will improve. Barbiturate therapy is appropriate only in patients who are hemodynamically stable and who have been adequately resuscitated. It should not be employed if MAP and CPP cannot be maintained. Some patients with refractory elevations in ICP have sustained extensive neurologic injury, and their cerebral metabolic rate may already be low; failure to respond to barbiturates carries with it an ominous prognosis.[241] Propofol is a reasonable alternative to barbiturates for ICP management, with the added advantage of shorter duration of action. Prolonged use of high-dose propofol is not recommended as it may cause propofol infusion syndrome, which is characterized by the

TABLE 36-5. INTERVENTIONS FOR INADEQUATE CEREBRAL PERFUSION PRESSURE

Reduce brain water	1. Mannitol 2. Hypertonic saline 3. Furosemide
Remove cerebrospinal fluid	1. External ventricular drain 2. Lumbar drain 3. (Hypertonic fluid)
Decrease cerebral blood volume	1. Head-up tilt 2. Neutral neck position 3. Metabolic suppression (propofol or barbiturate) 4. Mild-to-moderate hyperventilation
Elevate mean arterial pressure	1. Adequate intravascular volume resuscitation 2. Support with vasopressor

development of lactic acidosis, cardiac failure, lipemia, and is associated with a high mortality rate.[242,243]

Both barbiturates and propofol can be used in a dose-response manner to provide ICP control, ranging from mild sedation to induced coma. If maximal metabolic suppression is desired, the infusion rate can be guided by EEG to achieve burst suppression.

Decompressive craniectomy is another management option for refractory intracranial hypertension in TBI. Although this intervention decreases ICP and improves $Pbto_2$, definitive demonstration of outcome improvement in TBI remains elusive.[244–248] The recently published Australian multicenter DECRA Trial reported on 155 adults with severe diffuse TBI and refractory ICH. According to this study, early bifrontotemporoparietal decompressive craniectomy lowers ICP and the length of stay in the ICU but leads to more unfavorable outcomes.[249] Rates of death were found to be similar in both the craniectomy group (19%) and the standard-care group (18%) at 6 months. The United Kingdom initiated (RESCUEicp) prospective multicenter randomized trial is currently ongoing (Table 36-5).

Anesthetic Management

Patients with TBI requiring surgery can be subdivided into two major groups with different perioperative concerns. These groups include those who require emergent surgery and those who require nonemergent surgery. The emergent group can also be subdivided into neurosurgical procedures and nonneurosurgical procedures. The anesthetic management of these groups will be discussed here.

Emergent Surgery

Neurosurgical

These patients commonly arrive in the operating room with an endotracheal tube in place. If their airway has not yet been secured, then the same principles that were discussed in the airway section should be applied. Often there is little time allotted for the preoperative assessment; one's approach must be concise and focused to obtain the pertinent information in a brief amount of time. These patients may have other injuries that will affect their care. The neurologic condition of the patient can be determined rapidly by obtaining the GCS score, examining the pupils, and reviewing the CT scan. The hemodynamic status of the patient is also extremely important. Patients may demonstrate the Cushing response of hypertension and bradycardia, which signifies brainstem compression from raised ICP. However, these classic findings may be masked by hypovolemia, and their absence does not rule out brainstem compression. An estimation of volume status is appropriate. Other important information includes oxygenation, which may be compromised because of pulmonary contusion; hematocrit, which may be low in the presence of additional injuries; and the extent of the evaluation obtained prior to the decision to proceed to the operating room. An incomplete evaluation, radiographic or otherwise, should leave one highly suspicious for missed injuries, such as pneumothorax or intra-abdominal hemorrhage.

Appropriate monitoring must be established rapidly so as not to delay surgical intervention. Standard monitors should be applied including ECG, pulse oximetry, capnography, and noninvasive blood pressure measurement. Two large-bore intravenous catheters are required at a minimum. Delay for placement of a central venous catheter should occur only if adequate peripheral access cannot be obtained. Consideration for a femoral venous catheter should be made, as it can be placed while preparation of the head for surgery is ongoing. An arterial catheter is desirable, but it is a secondary priority after venous access.

These patients usually do not have ICP monitors in place but one can assume the presence of intracranial hypertension in the setting of an acute space-occupying lesion. The presence of midline shift on CT scan and pupillary abnormalities on physical examination reinforce this diagnosis. Moderate hyperventilation should be used in these patients until the dura is opened, as the elevation in ICP is likely more detrimental than the short-term hyperventilation.

Blood pressure management in these patients is critical. They may arrive in the operating room in a hypertensive state. The hypertension is often a response to the stress of the injury as well as the elevated ICP. Unfortunately, this hypertension may mask an underlying volume deficit due to hemorrhage or high urine output from mannitol administered prior to arrival in the operating room. Profound hypotension may quickly follow anesthesia induction, or more likely, after the craniectomy when the intrinsic stimulus for blood pressure elevation diminishes. Risk factors for postdecompressive hypotension include low GCS score, absence of basal cisterns on CT, and bilateral dilated pupils.[250] To avoid hypotension, intravenous volume loading in the early stages of the anesthetic is essential, particularly in patients with other injuries and significant blood loss.

The choice of anesthetic agents should be based on the clinical condition of the patient. The anesthetic requirement for patients with a traumatized CNS is lower; adequate anesthesia should be administered without compromising hemodynamics. Volatile anesthesia is acceptable as it is easily titratable, whereas intravenous agents have the benefit of a greater reduction in CBV and ICP. Nitrous oxide should be avoided as it increases $CMRO_2$, CBF, and ICP in head-injured patients.[251–253] Narcotics can be used safely in these patients as long as blood pressure is not compromised and the patient is mechanically ventilated.

Nonneurosurgical

Trauma patients presenting for emergent surgical management of noncranial injuries who also have a concurrent TBI are complex to manage. The most immediately life-threatening condition

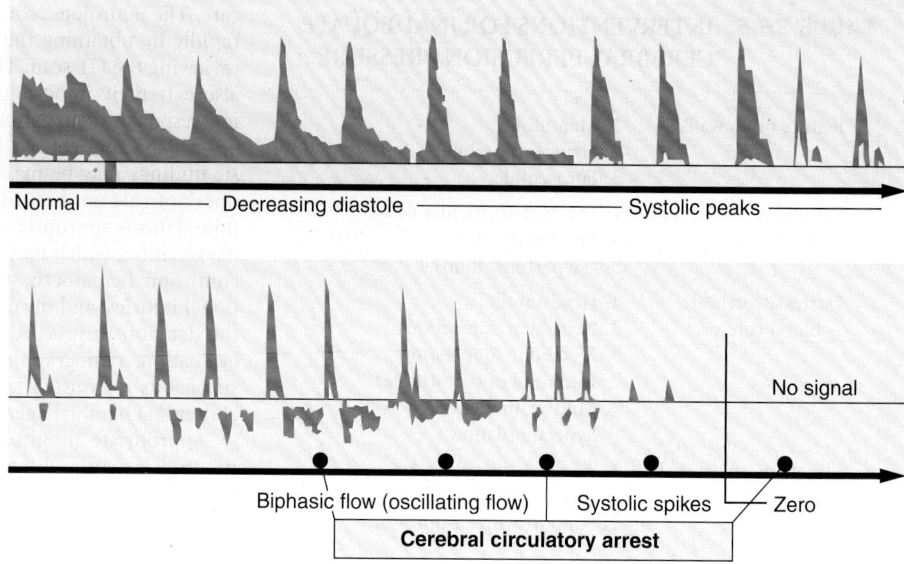

FIGURE 36-12. Transcranial Doppler tracing illustrating the characteristic changes associated with increasing intracranial pressure. The occurrence of biphasic or oscillating flow signifies the onset of intracranial circulatory arrest. Transcranial Doppler is accepted as a confirmatory test for brain death. (Reprinted from Hassler W, Steinmetz H, Gawlowski J. Transcranial Doppler ultrasonography in raised intracranial pressure and in intracranial circulatory arrest. *J Neurosurg.* 1988;68:745, with permission.)

must take priority but the presence of TBI should be considered, particularly in someone with a depressed level of consciousness or an abnormal pupil examination. If the history and examination are consistent with TBI, and a complete evaluation was not possible prior to emergent management in the operating room, obtaining an intraoperative neurosurgical consult for institution of ICP monitoring is reasonable. The presence of dilated pupils bilaterally may suggest a devastating brain injury. TCD, if available, could be used to assess for nonviable CBF patterns.[33] A well-characterized progression of TCD waveform morphology has been described for increasing ICP with a corresponding decrease in CPP (Fig. 36-12).[33,254] Increasing pulsatility of the waveform is suggestive of high ICP. Appropriate intervention should be implemented when this morphology is seen (e.g., head-up and neutral neck position, elevation of MAP, administration of mannitol, conversion to intravenous anesthesia).

Nonemergent Surgery

Patients with TBI frequently have other injuries, especially fractures requiring operative fixation. The timing of surgery in these patients remains a controversial issue.[255] One must balance the need for operative fixation of these fractures to decrease the incidence of complications related to immobility, such as atelectasis, pneumonia, and venous thromboembolism, with the risks of performing surgery in patients with head injuries. These patients have altered physiologic mechanisms, such as cerebral autoregulation, and they are at risk for secondary injury, especially that from hypotension.[256] Early fixation of major orthopedic injuries are safe and associated with fewer complications and ICU stay.[257] On the other hand, delayed fixation may allow the brain to recover in a more stable hemodynamic environment.[258] Consequently, clear definitions for resuscitation parameters are needed to better define the optimal time for surgery in patients with multiple-system trauma.[257]

In the absence of definitive evidence to guide management, we offer several conservative recommendations. In the setting of refractory elevations in ICP or very labile ICP, only emergent surgery should be performed. Because patients with TBI cannot be examined clinically during anesthesia, there should be a low threshold for placing an ICP monitor in someone who will be going to the operating room, particularly for longer surgeries and those taking place in the first 48 hours after injury. When available, advanced neuromonitoring, including TCD, jugular bulb oximetry, and brain tissue oxygenation should be used for intraoperative management.

ANESTHESIA FOR SPINE TRAUMA AND COMPLEX SPINE SURGERY

Surgery on the spinal column has become increasingly complex and lengthy, with multilevel fusions, combined anterior and posterior approaches to the spine, as well as staged procedures. The anesthetic plan for these procedures is made more complicated by the increasing age of patients requiring spine surgery and the concomitant increase in comorbid disease, as well as the need for sophisticated monitoring of the spinal cord. In addition, SCI often requires surgical intervention either for decompression of the spinal cord in patients with neurologic impairment and/or to restore the spinal column alignment and spinal stability to facilitate early patient mobilization and eventual rehabilitation. The anesthesiologist encounters many patients with disease of the spinal column, both in and out of the operating room. There are several aspects of their care, including airway management, resuscitation, and intraoperative management, that require a particular understanding of their disease. The focus of this section will be on anesthesia and SCI, but the anesthetic management will be relevant to all complex spine surgery.

Spinal Cord Injury

Primary Injury

SCI is analogous to TBI in that there is both a primary and secondary component. Initial traumatic injury typically results in damage to the bones and ligaments of the spinal column. Although SCI can occur without radiographic abnormality, which is referred to as *SCIWORA*, this phenomenon is more common in children than adults. Damage to the spinal column may occur without injury to the cord, or it can cause SCI through various insults, including compression, hemorrhage, and traumatic vasospasm, all which can result in cord ischemia and/or infarction.

The nature of the bony injury is important, as it will guide further management of the patient irrespective of the SCI. The purpose of the spinal column is to provide support to the individual while protecting the spinal cord and nerve roots. An unstable injury puts the neural elements at risk, and will necessitate some intervention to provide stability, which may be the application of a brace or surgical intervention.

Secondary Injury

Secondary injury to the spinal cord is mediated through a cascade of deleterious events similar to that seen in TBI, and begins within minutes following initial trauma. Pathologic mechanisms induce cord edema, and as a result of the rigid confines of the vertebral canal, increased pressure within that canal. This reaches its maximum between 4 and 6 days after the injury, with a consequent risk of ischemia. Pathologic consequences include induction of nitric oxide synthase, release of excitotoxic amino acids, cellular influx of calcium, oxidative stress, and lipid peroxidation.[259] Secondary injury may be exacerbated by hypotension due to hemorrhage or neurogenic shock.

Central, Anterior, Brown-Séquard, and Cauda Equina Injuries

Although a complete cord transection will result in disruption of afferent and efferent signals, many injuries damage only a portion of the spinal cord. The nature of this injury will determine its clinical manifestation. Several syndromes are well described for their classic cord lesion and corresponding signs.

Central cord syndrome is characterized by greater severity of paresis in the upper extremities than the lower, as well as bladder dysfunction and variable loss of sensation below the lesion. It is probably caused by a cervical spine lesion via hemorrhage into the cord following trauma. It is more common in elderly patients with pre-existing arthropathy.

Anterior cord syndrome is generally due to disruption of blood flow through the anterior spinal artery at the level of the injury. The anterior portion of the cord becomes ischemic, disrupting motor function below the level, with a variable effect on sensation. Pain and temperature tracts are typically interrupted as well, but two-point discrimination and proprioception remains intact.

Brown-Séquard syndrome is characterized by the interruption of a lateral half of the spinal cord, typically through penetrating trauma. Although a patient may not display all the classic findings of the Brown-Séquard syndrome, these would include loss of motor and touch sensation ipsilateral to the lesion, with pain and temperature sensation loss contralateral to the lesion.

Cauda equina syndrome is the result of injury below the level of the conus, or caudal end of the cord, typically below L2. Compression of the cauda equina results in perineal anesthesia, urinary retention, fecal incontinence, and lower extremity weakness.

American Spinal Injury Association Classification

In an effort to categorize the nature of the injury, the American Spinal Injury Association (ASIA) classification was developed in 1982 (Table 36-6). This system rates cord injuries with a letter from A through E. ASIA A is a complete cord lesion in which no motor or sensory function is preserved in the sacral segments S4–S5. ASIA B is incomplete, with only sensory spared below the lesion, including S4–S5. ASIA C indicates an injury where more than half the important muscle groups below the injury have motor scores of <3. ASIA D is an injury where more than half the muscles groups have motor scores >3. ASIA E indicates a neurologically intact individual.

TABLE 36-6. AMERICAN SPINAL INJURY ASSOCIATION (ASIA) CLASSIFICATION FOR SPINAL CORD INJURY

Classification	Description
A	Complete cord injury. No motor or sensation in sacral nerve roots S4 and S5.
B	Incomplete cord injury. Sensory preserved below the level of the injury, including S4–S5.
C	Incomplete cord injury. Motor function preserved below the level of the injury, but with strength of less than three in half the major muscle groups.
D	Incomplete cord injury. Motor function preserved below the level of the injury, with strength of three or more in at least half the major muscle groups.
E	No cord injury. Motor and sensory intact.

Comorbid Injuries

SCI occurs in up to 2% to 5% of all major trauma cases and at least 14% of these patients have the potential to have an unstable spine. Cervical spine trauma is associated with blunt cerebrovascular injury, TBI, and facial fractures.[207,260,261] Between 20% and 60% of SCI are associated with a concurrent TBI. Thoracic trauma is also associated with vascular injury; in addition, one must consider the possibility of pneumothorax, myocardial contusion, pulmonary contusion, and so forth, with trauma to the thorax.[262] Lumbar spine fractures may be associated with bowel and solid organ injury.[263]

Initial Management

Urgent Airway Management

Initial management of the patient with spine trauma follows the standard practices of care for trauma patients in general, with initial emphasis on airway, breathing, and circulation (as outlined in *ATLS*). Endotracheal intubation can be particularly difficult in the patient with SCI, especially if the lesion is in the cervical spine. In addition, intubation frequently needs to be accomplished before the presence or location of an injury can be confirmed. As a result, cervical spine injury should be presumed in all trauma patients requiring intubation prior to complete physical and radiographic evaluation. Intubation should proceed with little movement of the cervical spine. A rapid-sequence induction, with or without cricoid pressure (see discussion above), and manual in-line stabilization (MILS) of the neck is appropriate, unless a difficult airway is anticipated.

Hemodynamic Stabilization

Traumatic SCI is frequently complicated by systemic hypotension and reduced spinal cord perfusion pressure (SCPP). This in turn may contribute to secondary ischemic neurologic injury and should be avoided. SCPP is determined by the difference in MAP and cerebrospinal fluid pressure (CSFP) [SCPP = MAP – CSFP]. Spinal cord perfusion is autoregulated over a range of systemic BP in the same fashion as CBF. Systemic vasodilation from loss of sympathetic tone occurs in increasing severity with ascending levels of SCI above L2, leading to hypotension. Bradycardia complicates the picture with injuries above T6 due to compromise of the sympathetic cardiac accelerator fibers.

Restoration of intravascular volume is the first step in the treatment of hypotension in the patient with SCI. Conversely, excessive fluid administration can be associated with significant edema (including airway edema), cardiac failure, electrolyte abnormalities, coagulopathy and prolonged duration of postoperative ICU stay. The use of albumin has become debatable, similar to the concerns of increased mortality in TBI. Goal-directed treatment using cardiac output monitoring devices should be considered to help with intraoperative fluid administration.

Higher cord lesions result in greater sympathectomy, vasodilation, and thus vascular capacitance. Although volume is beneficial in this setting, a pure α-agonist such as phenylephrine is a reasonable choice to restore vascular tone. It also has the potential to induce a reflex bradycardia. Patients with higher lesions, in the upper thoracic or cervical spine, with concomitant hypotension and bradycardia should receive an agent such as dopamine or norepinephrine, which will restore cardiac inotropy and chronotropy, as well as peripheral vascular tone. Vasopressin has a vasoconstrictive and catecholamine sparing effect, that may be useful in hypotension. However, its antidiuretic effects may lead to increased water retention and hyponatremia, with potential exacerbation of intracellular edema after injury. Thus, its role in SCI is not well defined, and it should be used with some caution. Dobutamine is predominantly an inotropic agent and its use in SCI is limited because of its vasodilatory effects. Persistent bradycardia may be seen in high cervical (C1 to C5) lesions in the first 2 weeks after traumatic SCI and requires the use of anticholinergic agents or application of cardiac pacemakers.

Role for Steroids

Methylprednisolone has become a common therapy for patients with neurologic deficit resulting from SCI following large clinical studies from the 1990s, which showed important improvement in the motor function of patients with SCI.[264] However, these studies have subsequently been criticized, on the grounds that the benefits are marginal, while there is a significantly increased risk of serious side effects associated with the use of high-dose steroids, including pulmonary complications, wound infections, steroid myopathy, and gastrointestinal hemorrhage.[265,266] Current guidelines published by the American Association of Neurological Surgeons recommend the use of methylprednisolone only as a treatment option (while considering the risks and benefits associated with glucocorticoid use) and not as a standard of care.

Timing of Surgical Intervention

The purpose of surgical intervention is to decompress the neural structures and stabilize the spinal column to prevent further injury to the cord. Management of the patient with SCI frequently requires intervention for comorbid life-threatening trauma, such as intra-abdominal or pelvic hemorrhage. With the exception of patients requiring immediate surgical reduction of fractures compromising neurologic function, decompression of the spinal cord with fixation of the spinal column generally must wait until the patient is clinically appropriate for the procedure. Persistent hemodynamic instability or severe acute respiratory distress syndrome may impose a significant delay on surgical intervention. However, there is increasing interest in early fixation and mobilization. The Surgical Treatment of Acute Spinal Cord Injury Study (STASCIS) showed 24% of patients who received decompressive surgery within 24 hours of their injury experienced a 2-grade or greater improvement on the ASIA scale, compared with 4% of those in the delayed-treatment group.[267]

Intraoperative Management

Anesthetic Induction and Airway Management

Airway interventions may be required during the hospital course of the patient with known or suspected traumatic SCI. The spine should be immobilized in all trauma victims with suspected SCI until radiographically and/or clinically "cleared" with application of a cervical collar, plus immobilization with lateral head supports and straps. Increasingly CT scans have replaced radiography for clearance of cervical spine injury. Attention should be given to minimize C-spine movement during airway management. It has been clinically shown that in the normal spine, direct laryngoscopy leads to extension of the C-spine, predominantly at the atlantooccipital junction, and to a lesser extent at the C1 to C2 joint. The subaxial cervical segments (C4–C7) are minimally displaced but additional flexion occurs at the cervicothoracic junction. Instability of the occiput–atlas–axis complex may lead to anterior movement of the atlas during direct laryngoscopy, thereby reducing the space available for the spinal cord.

Several methods of tracheal intubation in this scenario exist, but no one technique has been proven superior to others. Excessive jaw thrust and chin lift should be avoided and early employment of an oral or nasal airway helps to reduce the force required for airway maintenance. Generally, a rapid sequence induction with direct or indirect laryngoscopy with MILS is the preferred practice. MILS provides better cervical stability but impairs the view of the vocal cords during conventional laryngoscopy. Nevertheless, when MILS is utilized, the incidence of neurologic impairment due to endotracheal intubation is extremely rare. Elective fixation of confirmed cervical spine or associated injuries requires careful planning for safe airway intervention. The patient may present in cervical traction or a "halo" frame, which impedes access to the airway. If the airway is potentially difficult and the patient has an existing neurologic deficit with C-spine instability, an alternative technique should be considered. Awake fiberoptic intubation has not been shown to be superior to an asleep procedure. Awake fiberoptic intubation allows a neurologic examination to be performed after intubation and positioning. However, it requires patient cooperation, and may increase stress, discomfort and disability in acutely injured patients. Provided that there is no airway patency or respiratory compromise, fiberoptic intubation in an anesthetized or deeply sedated patient provides the optimal conditions for success without causing excessive movement of the unstable spine, although some anesthesiologists might be uncomfortable with the potentially increased legal liability.

The decision whether or not to extubate the trachea at the end of the surgical procedure is influenced by many factors. These include the ease of intubation, extent and duration of surgery, surgical complications (e.g., recurrent laryngeal nerve injury), prone positioning, blood loss and subsequent fluid balance. The absence of a cuff leak in the spontaneously breathing patient has not consistently been shown to predict subsequent airway obstruction, but the presence of a cuff leak generally indicates a patent airway after extubation. When in doubt, extubating the patient's trachea with an airway exchange catheter *in situ* can facilitate emergent reintubation if necessary. Good clinical judgment is paramount, and if there is concern, it would be prudent to delay extubation.

As in most trauma situations, adequate neuromuscular blockade is required for successful intubation. Succinylcholine is the preferred agent for emergent intubation, but should be avoided between 2 days and 9 months following SCI due to the risk of induced hyperkalemia caused by denervation hypersensitivity. Rocuronium is an acceptable alternative.

Anesthetic Technique

Complex spine and trauma surgery imposes a significant risk of blood loss. An arterial catheter is essential for continuous hemodynamic monitoring and intermittent arterial blood gas and hematocrit analysis. In addition, the respiratory variation of the arterial line, or reversed pulsus paradoxus, is a useful indicator of volume responsiveness.[268]

Several large-bore peripheral intravenous catheters are appropriate for volume and blood product administration. In extensive thoracic or lumbar spine surgeries, particularly in the prone position, central venous access may be appropriate. In addition to providing more access for volume resuscitation, it enables easier access to venous circulation when arms are not accessible, helps to guide the resuscitation with mixed venous oxygen saturation determination, provides appropriate access when vasopressor drugs are used, and when advanced in to the heart may be used to aspirate air in the event of an air embolism. However, the value of the central venous pressure is controversial. It is neither a good indicator of end-diastolic volume nor a predictor of volume responsiveness in hypotension.[269] Although there is some literature suggesting a benefit to managing older patients with trauma with a pulmonary artery catheter (PAC), its use is not routinely recommended.[270] Development of less invasive and perhaps superior approach to hemodynamic monitoring has increasingly become available. Dynamic indicators of preload include respiratory variation in systolic pressure and pulse pressure, both of which can be derived from the analysis of the waveform generated by a peripherally placed arterial catheter.[271] In addition, techniques for deriving stroke volume, cardiac output, and intrathoracic blood volume have been introduced. These methods are all dependent on a quality arterial waveform without dampening. Nevertheless, when functioning properly, these techniques provide support for goal-directed fluid management and have been shown to improve outcome.

Neuromonitoring

Since the *wake up test* (in which the level of general anesthesia is transiently reduced intraoperatively to enable the patient to move an extremity in response to a verbal command) provides only a single time point of assessment of neurologic function, sophisticated neuromonitoring techniques are now used intraoperatively to continually assess the functional integrity of the spinal cord. Generally SSEP and MEP with or without nerve root monitoring are utilized, and these modalities as well as the anesthetic techniques required to allow optimal acquisition of signals had been previously discussed. When used collectively, these are referred to as multimodal IOM.

Although the use of IOM has never been validated by randomized controlled trials, it is now considered standard practice, with the primary potential benefit being identification of a deterioration of spinal cord function during the surgical procedure. Contributing factors include incorrect patient position (e.g., neck position, shoulder position), hypotension, hypothermia, and surgical retraction/injury. Identification and correction of reversible factors may help preserve spinal cord function. A recent systematic review indicated that although there is a high level of evidence that multimodal IOM is sensitive and specific for detecting intraoperative neurologic injury during spine surgery, there is a low level of evidence that IOM reduces the rate of new or worsening perioperative neurologic deficits and there is very low evidence that an intraoperative response to a neuromonitoring alert reduces the rate of perioperative neurologic deterioration.[24] Nevertheless, most spine surgeons are of the opinion that IOM allows a more aggressive surgical approach to complex spine pathology without increasing the risk of neurologic injury.[272]

Patient Positioning

The prone position provides multiple challenges to the anesthesiologist with respect to both physiologic considerations and practical considerations. The former includes hemodynamic stability that can be compromised by high intrathoracic pressure and tamponade of the heart in thin individuals. The latter includes difficulty with venous access (if the arms are tucked), and more importantly, adequate protection of pressure points. Areas at particular risk include the eyes, and face, the breasts, genitals, knees, and toes. Whether using the Mayfield device to hold the head in pins or a prone foam pillow, pressure on the eyes and nose must be avoided. Frequent confirmation that the eyes are free from contact is important, as the pillow may move over time. In addition, slight reverse Trendelenburg position may facilitate venous drainage from the head and reduce congestion and intraocular pressure.[273] Padding on the chest should not compress the neck, as this too may obstruct venous drainage. The breasts and male genitals should be checked to ensure that they are free of undue pressure. Lower extremities must be padded adequately to prevent excess weight resting on the knees and toes.

Hypothermia

Transportation, stabilization, investigation (particularly radiologic), and organization of surgery necessitates delays of minutes to hours. The ability to delay ongoing secondary injury to the spinal cord in the interim would be of great benefit in limiting ultimate neurologic dysfunction. As with the brain, there has been a wide range of reported enthusiastic research into the biochemical, histologic, and physiologic effects attributed to the application of cooling. These include a reduction in the initial rate of ATP depletion, alteration of gene expression and protein synthesis, reduction in the release of excitotoxic neurotransmitter, changes to intracellular messengers, inhibition of inflammatory responses, and a decrease in the excitatory postsynaptic potential slope in a temperature-dependent manner. Utilization of intravascular cooling catheters allows achievement of moderate systemic hypothermia more rapidly and precisely during abdominal aortic aneurysm repair and other procedures that require aortic clamping. In animal models, moderate hypothermia increases the tolerable spinal cord ischemia duration as much as 2.5 times and the effect is longer with lower temperatures in humans.[274] There is conflicting data on whether it affords any protection in circumstances of significant ongoing cord compression. Safety and efficacy of intravascular hypothermia for acute SCI have been encouraging.[275] Important determinants are cooling technique (surface or intravascular), timing, rate, duration, and degree of temperature depression, and importantly, rewarming and its associated complications such as infection.[276,277] However, a prospective randomized trial of hypothermia for acute SCI is yet to be undertaken.[278] And despite the heightened recent interest in temperature modulation for spinal function preservation and recovery, the American Association of Neurological Surgeons, and the Congress of Neurological Surgeons, published a statement in November 2007, concluding that there is insufficient scientific evidence to support or oppose systemic or local hypothermia for traumatic spine injury.[279]

Complications of Anesthesia for Spine Surgery

Autonomic Hyperreflexia

Patients with a chronic spinal cord lesion above the level of T7 may develop autonomic hyperreflexia when stimulated below the site of lesion. This is a condition characterized by intense vasoconstriction below the site of the lesion, accompanied by cutaneous vasodilation above the site, hypertension, and bradycardia. This is the result of reflex sympathetic stimulation below the lesion unmodulated by supraspinal influence from above. In severe cases, cerebral hemorrhage and myocardial ischemia can occur. To reduce the incidence of this complication, suppression of the afferent pathway by "deepening" the level of general anesthesia is necessary. Alternatively, the use of a spinal anesthetic which blocks the reflex stimulation may be the ideal anesthetic.

Postoperative Visual Loss

Postoperative visual loss (POVL) is of particular concern in prone spine surgery, although it can occur in other settings. It is estimated to occur as often as 1:1,000 following spine operations. Central retinal artery occlusion (CRAO); anterior ischemic optic neuropathy (AION); posterior ischemic optic neuropathy (PION); and cortical blindness encompass the majority of the perioperative vision losses. Though an uncommon cause of blindness in general, PION is by far the most common cause of POVL from a spine operation. Alarmed by the apparent increase in incidence, the American Society of Anesthesiology established a POVL registry to examine common factors shared by the index cases. Early reports from the POVL registry indicate that, while all of the CRAO cases were unilateral, a majority of ION cases were bilateral. These findings are consistent with the proposed etiology of CRAO resulting from direct compression of the globe when the head slipped off the headrest, and the dependent eye was left resting on the hard edge. In contrast, ION is ischemic in origin. AION results from ischemia to the anterior segment of the optic nerve, and PION from ischemia to the posterior segment of the optic nerve behind the optic disc. AION is the most common cause of blindness in the community, usually resulting from systemic hypotension secondary to gastrointestinal hemorrhage in an elderly patient. The prevalence of PION secondary to spine surgery cannot be easily explained etiologically.

Suggested risk factors for ION may include hypovolemia, hypotension, anemia, venous congestion, edema, adverse drug effects, and individual patient variation in anatomy and physiology of the optic nerve blood flow. There has been no association demonstrated with direct pressure or embolic events. A plausible mechanism is the development of venous congestion in the optic nerve secondary to the prone position and subsequent development of a compartment syndrome of the optic nerve. Both types of ION have poor potential for recovery of vision, and are indistinguishable in the later stages with both showing optic nerve atrophy.

Cortical blindness is typically associated with states of profound hypotension such as cardiac arrest or cardiac bypass procedures where emboli are common. Of the four causes of visual loss, cortical blindness has the best chance for recovery.

Currently there is no proven method to prevent perioperative blindness associated with spine surgery, nor is there a reliable method to monitor visual function during these procedures. A number of investigators have focused on monitoring of intraoperative intraocular pressure, which is unlikely to yield meaningful results. On the other hand, monitoring of VEP may provide more useful information. Careful and frequent eye checks in the prone position with documentation are recommended, but direct compression is not the cause of PION. A Mayfield headrest with pins is being used increasingly to obviate any possibility of direct compression to the globe. Hence virtually all cases of PION occur while the patient's head is in Mayfield pins. A recent case control study comparing the index cases in the POVL registry with controls suggest that the risk factors for ION include obesity, male gender, the use of Wilson frame, long surgical duration, greater estimated blood loss, and decreased percent colloid replacement of blood (as a percent of overall fluid administration).[280] Of note, there was no association with the level of blood pressure or hematocrit.

Given the increasing recognition of POVL, and the frequency of subsequent litigation, the patient should be informed preoperatively about the potential risk of blindness with complex spine surgery, and vision documented immediately upon emergence from anesthesia. Unfortunately, even with prompt diagnosis and appropriate consultation, currently there is no effective treatment once the complication occurs. Staging of a complex spine procedure to minimize the duration of the procedure, to reduce the amount of blood loss, and to decrease the quantity of fluid administered, may be the most effective means of preventing this devastating complication.

References

1. Emerich DF, Vasconcellos AV, Elliott RB, et al. The choroid plexus: Function, pathology and therapeutic potential of its transplantation. *Expert Opin Biol Ther.* [Review]. 2004;4(8):1191–1201.
2. Praetorius J. Water and solute secretion by the choroid plexus. *Pflugers Arch.* [Review]. 2007;454(1):1–18.
3. Steiner LA, Balestreri M, Johnston AJ, et al. Sustained moderate reductions in arterial CO_2 after brain trauma time-course of cerebral blood flow velocity and intracranial pressure. *Intensive Care Med.* 2004;30(12):2180–2187.
4. Diringer MN, Yundt K, Videen TO, et al. No reduction in cerebral metabolism as a result of early moderate hyperventilation following severe traumatic brain injury. *J Neurosurg.* 2000;92(1):7–13.
5. Coles JP, Minhas PS, Fryer TD, et al. Effect of hyperventilation on cerebral blood flow in traumatic head injury: Clinical relevance and monitoring correlates. *Crit Care Med.* 2002;30(9):1950–1959.
6. Warner KJ, Cuschieri J, Copass MK, et al. The impact of prehospital ventilation on outcome after severe traumatic brain injury. *J Trauma.* 2007;62(6):1330–1336.
7. Lassen NA. Cerebral blood flow and oxygen consumption in man. *Physiol Rev.* 1959;39(2):183–238.
8. Bruder N, Cohen B, Pellissier D, et al. The effect of hemodilution on cerebral blood flow velocity in anesthetized patients. *Anesth Analg.* 1998;86(2):320–324.
9. van Bommel J, Trouwborst A, Schwarte L, et al. Intestinal and cerebral oxygenation during severe isovolemic hemodilution and subsequent hyperoxic ventilation in a pig model. *Anesthesiology.* 2002;97(3):660–670.
10. Rebel A, Ulatowski JA, Kwansa H, et al. Cerebrovascular response to decreased hematocrit: Effect of cell-free hemoglobin, plasma viscosity, and CO_2. *Am J Physiol Heart Circ Physiol.* 2003;285(4):H1600–H1608.
11. Hare GM, Tsui AK, McLaren AT, et al. Anemia and cerebral outcomes: Many questions, fewer answers. *Anesth Analg.* 2008;107(4):1356–1370.

12. Hare GM, Mazer CD, Hutchison JS, et al. Severe hemodilutional anemia increases cerebral tissue injury following acute neurotrauma. *J Appl Physiol.* 2007; 103(3):1021–1029.
13. Todd MM, Farrell S, Wu B. Cerebral blood flow during hypoxemia and hemodilution in rabbits: Different roles for nitric oxide? *J Cereb Blood Flow Metab.* 1997;17(12):1319–1325.
14. Dagal A, Lam AM. Cerebral autoregulation and anesthesia. *Curr Opin Anaesthesiol.* [Review]. 2009;22(5):547–552.
15. Kaisti KK, Metsähonkala L, Teräs M, et al. Effects of surgical levels of propofol and sevoflurane anesthesia on cerebral blood flow in healthy subjects studied with positron emission tomography. *Anesthesiology.* 2002;96(6):1358–1370.
16. Summors AC, Gupta AK, Matta BF. Dynamic cerebral autoregulation during sevoflurane anesthesia: A comparison with isoflurane. *Anesth Analg.* 1999; 88(2):341–345.
17. Schlunzen L, Juul N, Hansen KV, et al. Regional cerebral glucose metabolism during sevoflurane anaesthesia in healthy subjects studied with positron emission tomography. *Acta Anaesthesiol Scand.* 2010;54:603–609.
18. Schlunzen L, Juul N, Hansen KV, et al. Regional cerebral blood flow and glucose metabolism during propofol anaesthesia in healthy subjects studied with positron emission tomography. *Acta Anaesthesiol Scand.* 2012;56:248–255.
19. Langsjo JW, Kaisti KK, Aalto S, et al. Effects of subanesthetic doses of ketamine on regional cerebral blood flow, oxygen consumption, and blood volume in humans. *Anesthesiology.* 2003;99(3):614–623.
20. Drummond JC, Dao AV, Roth DM, et al. Effect of dexmedetomidine on cerebral blood flow velocity, cerebral metabolic rate, and carbon dioxide response in normal humans. *Anesthesiology.* 2008;108(2):225–232.
21. Ogawa Y, Iwasaki K, Aoki K, et al. Dexmedetomidine weakens dynamic cerebral autoregulation as assessed by transfer function analysis and the thigh cuff method. *Anesthesiology.* 2008;109(4):642–650.
22. Avidan MS, Jacobsohn E, Glick D, et al. Prevention of intraoperative awareness in a high-risk surgical population. *N Engl J Med.* 2011;365(7):591–600.
23. Costa P, Bruno A, Bonzanino M, et al. Somatosensory- and motor-evoked potential monitoring during spine and spinal cord surgery. *Spinal Cord.* 2007;45(1):86–91.
24. Fehlings MG, Brodke DS, Norvell DC, et al. The evidence for intraoperative neurophysiological monitoring in spine surgery: Does it make a difference? *Spine (Phila Pa 1976).* 2010;35(9 suppl):S37–S46.
25. Lo YL, Chih HW, Yeh CY, et al. Intraoperative monitoring study of ipsilateral motor evoked potentials in scoliosis surgery. *Eur Spine J.* 2006;15(suppl 17):656.
26. Kakimoto M, Kawaguchi M, Yamamoto Y, et al. Tetanic stimulation of the peripheral nerve before transcranial electrical stimulation can enlarge amplitudes of myogenic motor evoked potentials during general anesthesia with neuromuscular blockade. *Anesthesiology.* 2005;102:733.
27. Bala E, Sessler DI, Nair DR, et al. Motor and somatosensory evoked potentials are well maintained in patients given dexmedetomidine during spine surgery. *Anesthesiology.* 2008;109(3):417–425.
28. Mahmoud M, Sadhasivam S, Salisbury S, et al. Susceptibility of transcranial electric motor-evoked potentials to varying targeted blood levels of dexmedetomidine during spine surgery. *Anesthesiology.* 2010;112(6):1364–1373.
29. Huber P, Handa J. Effect of contrast material, hypercapnia, hyperventilation, hypertonic glucose and papaverine on the diameter of the cerebral areteries. Angiographic determination in man. *Invest Radiol.* 1967;2:17.
30. Martin KK, Wigginton JB, Babikian VL, et al. Intraoperative cerebral high-intensity transient signals and postoperative cognitive function: A systematic review. *Am J Surg.* 2009;197(1):55–63.
31. Kincaid MS. Transcranial Doppler ultrasonography: A diagnostic tool of increasing utility. *Curr Opin Anaesthesiol.* 2008;21(5):552–559.
32. Rigamonti A, Ackery A, Baker AJ. Transcranial Doppler monitoring in subarachnoid hemorrhage: A critical tool in critical care. *Can J Anaesth.* 2008;55(2): 112–123.
33. Sharma D, Souter MJ, Moore AE, et al. Clinical experience with transcranial ultrasonography as a confirmatory test for brain death: A retrospective analysis. *Neurocrit Care.* 2011;14(3):370–376.
34. Chestnut RM. Care of central nervous system injuries. *Surg Clin North Am.* 2007;87:119.
35. Snyder LA, Spetzler RF. Current indications for indocyanine green angiography. *World Neurosurg.* 2011;76(5):405–406.
36. Highton D, Elwell C, Smith M. Noninvasive cerebral oximetry: Is there light at the end of the tunnel? *Curr Opin Anaesthesiol.* [Review]. 2010;23(5):576–581.
37. Thavasothy M, Broadhead M, Elwell C, et al. A comparison of cerebral oxygenation as measured by the NIRO 300 and the INVOS 5100 Near-Infrared Spectrophotometers. *Anaesthesia.* 2002;57(10):999–1006.
38. Valadka AB, Gopinath SP, Contant CF, et al. Relationship of brain tissue PO2 to outcome after severe head injury. *Crit Care Med.* 1998;26:1576.
39. Maloney-Wilensky E, Gracias V, Itkin A, et al. Brain tissue oxygen and outcome after severe traumatic brain injury: A systematic review. *Crit Care Med.* [Review]. 2009;37(6):2057–2063.
40. Spiotta AM, Stiefel MF, Graciaas VH, et al. Brain tissue oxygen-directed management and outcome in patients with severe traumatic brain injury. *J Neurosurg.* 2008;108:943–949.
41. Robertson CS, Gopinath SP, Goodman JC, et al. SjvO2 monitoring in head-injured patients. *J Neurotrauma.* 1995;12:891.
42. De Georgia MA, Deogaonkar A. Multimodal monitoring in the neurological intensive care unit. *Neurologist.* [Review]. 2005;11(1):45–54.
43. Matta BF, Lam AM. The rate of blood withdrawal affects the accuracy of jugular venous bulb. Oxygen saturation measurements. *Anesthesiology.* 1997;86:806.
44. Bernard SA, Gray TW, Buist MD, et al. Treatment of comatose survivors of out-of-hospital cardiac arrest with induced hypothermia. *N Engl J Med.* 2002;346:557.
45. Hypothermic after Cardiac Arrest Study Group. Mild therapeutic hypothermia to improve the neurologic outcome after cardiac arrest. *N Engl J Med.* 2002;346:549.
46. Koerner IP, Brambrink AM. Brain protection by anesthetic agents. *Curr Opin Anaesthesiol.* 2006;19:481.
47. Fritz KW, Kasperczyk W, Galaske R. [Successful resuscitation in accidental hypothermia following drowning]. *Anaesthesist.* 1988;37:331.
48. Oberhammer R, Beikircher W, Hormann C, et al. Full recovery of an avalanche victim with profound hypothermia and prolonged cardiac arrest treated by extracorporeal re-warming. *Resuscitation.* 2008;76(3):474.
49. Kunihara T, Grun T, Aicher D, et al. Hypothermic circulatory arrest is not a risk factor for neurologic morbidity in aortic surgery: A propensity score analysis. *J Thorac Cardiovasc Surg.* 2005;130:712.
50. Mack WJ, Ducruet AF, Angevine PD, et al. Deep hypothermic circulatory arrest for complex cerebral aneurysms: Lessons learned. *Neurosurgery.* 2007;60:815.
51. Leonov Y, Sterz F, Safar P, et al. Mild cerebral hypothermia during and after cardiac arrest improves neurologic outcome in dogs. *J Cereb Blood Flow Metab.* 1990;10:57.
52. Todd MM, Hindman BJ, Clark WR, et al. Intraoperative hypothermia for aneurysm surgery trial (ihast) investigators. Mild intraoperative hypothermia during surgery for intracranial aneurysm. *N Engl J Med.* 2005;352:135.
53. Hindman BJ, Bayman EO, Pfisterer WK, et al. No association between intraoperative hypothermia or supplemental protective drug and neurologic outcomes in patients undergoing temporary clipping during cerebral aneurysm surgery: Findings from the Intraoperative Hypothermia for Aneurysm Surgery Trial. *Anesthesiology.* 2010;112(1):86–101.
54. Reith J, Jorgensen HS, Pedersen PM, et al. Body temperature in acute stroke: Relation to stroke severity, infarct size, mortality, and outcome. *Lancet.* 1996;347:422.
55. Oliveira-Filho J, Ezzeddine MA, Segal AZ, et al. Fever in subarachnoid hemorrhage: Relationship to vasospasm and outcome. *Neurology.* 2001;56:1299.
56. Zeiner A, Holzer M, Sterz F, et al. Hyperthermia after cardiac arrest is associated with an unfavorable neurologic outcome. *Arch Intern Med.* 2001;161:2007.
57. Jiang JY, Macchiarelli G, Miyabayashi K, et al. Early indicators of prognosis in 846 cases of severe traumatic brain injury. *J Neurotrauma.* 2002;19:869.
58. Aiyagari V, Diringer MN. Fever control and its impact on outcomes: What is the evidence? *J Neurol Sci.* 2007;261:39.
59. Warner DS, Takaoka S, Wu B, et al. Electroencephalographic burst suppression is not required to elicit maximal neuroprotection from pentobarbital in a rat model of focal cerebral ischemia. *Anesthesiology.* 1996;84:1475.
60. Elsersy H, Sheng H, Lynch JR, et al. Effects of isoflurane versus fentanyl-nitrous oxide anesthesia on long-term outcome from severe forebrain ischemia in the rat. *Anesthesiology.* 2004;100:1160.
61. Kawaguchi M, Furuya H, Patel PM. Neuroprotective effects of anesthetic agents. *J Anesth.* 2005;19:150.
62. Kawaguchi M, Kimbro JR, Drummond JC, et al. Isoflurane delays but does not prevent cerebral infarction in rats subjected to focal ischemia. *Anesthesiology.* 2000;92:1335.
63. Soonthon-Brant V, Patel PM, Drummond JC, et al. Fentanyl does not increase brain injury after focal cerebral ischemia in rats. *Anesth Analg.* 1999;88:49.
64. Blanck TJ, Haile M, Xu F, et al. Isoflurane pretreatment ameliorates postischemic neurologic dysfunction and preserves hippocampal Ca2+/calmodulin-dependent protein kinase in a canine cardiac arrest model. *Anesthesiology.* 2000;93:1285.
65. Kapinya KJ, Lowl D, Futterer C, et al. Tolerance against ischemic neuronal injury can be induced by volatile anesthetics and is inducible NO synthase dependent. *Stroke.* 2002;33:1889.
66. Drummond JC, Cole DJ, Patel PM, et al. Focal cerebral ischemia during anesthesia with etomidate, isoflurane, or thiopental: A comparison of the extent of cerebral injury. *Neurosurgery.* 1995;37:742.
67. Michenfelder JD, Milde JH, Sundt TM Jr. Cerebral protection by barbiturate anesthesia. Use after middle cerebral artery occlusion in Java monkeys. *Arch Neurol.* 1976;33:345.
68. Selman WR, Spetzler RJ, Roski RA, et al. Barbiturate coma in focal cerebral ischemia. Relationship of protection to timing of therapy. *J Neurosurg.* 1982;56:685.
69. Smith AL, Hoff JT, Nielsen SL, et al. Barbiturate protection in acute focal cerebral ischemia. *Stroke.* 1974;5:1.
70. Bleyaert AL, Nemoto EM, Safar P, et al. Thiopental amelioration of brain damage after global ischemia in monkeys. *Anesthesiology.* 1978;49:390.
71. Gisvold SE, Safar P, Hendrickx HH, et al. Thiopental treatment after global brain ischemia in pigtailed monkeys. *Anesthesiology.* 1984;60:88.
72. Snyder BD, Ramirez-Lassepas M, Sukhum P, et al. Failure of thiopental to modify global anoxic injury. *Stroke.* 1979;10:135.
73. Steen PA, Milde JH, Michenfelder JD. No barbiturate protection in a dog model of complete cerebral ischemia. *Ann Neurol.* 1979;5:343.
74. Todd MM, Chadwick HS, Shapiro HM, et al. The neurologic effects of thiopental therapy following experimental cardiac arrest in cats. *Anesthesiology.* 1982; 57:76.

75. Zhan RZ, Fujiwara N, Endoh H, et al. Thiopental inhibits increases in [Ca2+]i induced by membrane depolarization, NMDA receptor activation, and ischemia in rat hippocampal and cortical slices. *Anesthesiology.* 1998;89:456.
76. Zhu H, Cottrell JE, Kass IS. The effect of thiopental and propofol on NMDA- and AMPA-mediated glutamate excitotoxicity. *Anesthesiology.* 1997;87(4):944.
77. Rodriguez-Lopez JM, Sanchez-Conde P, Lozano FS, et al. Laboratory investigation: Effects of propofol on the systemic inflammatory response during aortic surgery. *Can J Anaesth.* 2006;53:701.
78. Young Y, Menon DK, Tisavipat N, et al. Propofol neuroprotection in a rat model of ischaemia reperfusion injury. *Eur J Anaesthesiol.* 1997;14:320.
79. Fukuda S, Warner DS. Cerebral protection. *Br J Anaesth.* 2007;99:10.
80. Mizock BA. Alterations in carbohydrate metabolism during stress: A review of the literature. *Am J Med.* 1995;98:75.
81. Capes SE, Hunt D, Malmberg K, et al. Stress hyperglycaemia and increased risk of death after myocardial infarction in patients with and without diabetes: A systematic overview. *Lancet.* 2000;355:773.
82. Capes SE, Hunt D, Malmberg K, et al. Stress hyperglycemia and prognosis of stroke in nondiabetic and diabetic patients: A systematic overview. *Stroke.* 2001; 32:2426.
83. Gore DC, Chinkes D, Heggers J, et al. Association of hyperglycemia with increased mortality after severe burn injury. *J Trauma.* 2001;51:540.
84. Krinsley JS. Association between hyperglycemia and increased hospital mortality in a heterogeneous population of critically ill patients. *Mayo Clin Proc.* 2003;78:1471.
85. O'Neill PA, Davies I, Fullerton KJ, et al. Stress hormone and blood glucose response following acute stroke in the elderly. *Stroke.* 1991;22:842.
86. Rovlias A, Kotsou S. The influence of hyperglycemia on neurological outcome in patients with severe head injury. *Neurosurgery.* 2000;46:335.
87. Chew W, Kucharczyk J, Moseley M, et al. Hyperglycemia augments ischemic brain injury: in vivo MR imaging/spectroscopic study with nicardipine in cats with occluded middle cerebral arteries. *AJNR Am J Neuroradiol.* 1991;12:603.
88. Marfella R, D'Amico M, DiFilippo C, et al. Myocardial infarction in diabetic rats: Role of hyperglycaemia on infarct size and early expression of hypoxia-inducible factor 1. *Diabetologia.* 2002;45:1172.
89. van den Berghe G, Wouters P, Weekers F, et al. Intensive insulin therapy in the critically ill patients. *N Engl J Med.* 2001;345:1359.
90. Van den Berghe G, Wilmer A, Hermans G, et al. Intensive insulin therapy in the medical ICU. *N Engl J Med.* 2006;354:449.
91. Gandhi GY, Nuttell GA, Abel MD, et al. Intensive intraoperative insulin therapy versus conventional glucose management during cardiac surgery: A randomized trial. *Ann Intern Med.* 2007;146:233.
92. McGirt MJ, Woodworth GF, Brooke BS, et al. Hyperglycemia independently increases the risk of perioperative stroke, myocardial infarction, and death after carotid endarterectomy. *Neurosurgery.* 2006;58:1066.
93. Gentile NT, Seftchick MW, Huynh T, et al. Decreased mortality by normalizing blood glucose after acute ischemic stroke. *Acad Emerg Med.* 2006;13:174.
94. Cimino M, Gelosa P, Gianelli A, et al. Statins: Multiple mechanisms of action in the ischemic brain. *Neuroscientist.* 2007;13:208.
95. Maiese K, Li F, Chong ZZ. New avenues of exploration for erythropoietin. *JAMA.* 2005;293:90.
96. Conway JB, Goldberg J, Chung F. Preadmission anaesthesia consultation clinic. *Can J Anaesth.* 1992;39(10):1051–1057.
97. Hepner DL, Correll DJ, Beckman JA, et al. Needs analysis for the development of a preoperative clinic protocol for perioperative beta-blocker therapy. *J Clin Anesth.* 2008;20(8):580–588.
98. Fleisher LA, Beckman JA, Brown KA, et al. ACC/AHA 2007 Guidelines on Perioperative Cardiovascular Evaluation and Care for Noncardiac Surgery: Executive Summary: A Report of the American College of Cardiology/American Heart Association Task Force on Practice Guidelines (Writing Committee to Revise the 2002 Guidelines on Perioperative Cardiovascular Evaluation for Noncardiac Surgery): Developed in Collaboration With the American Society of Echocardiography, American Society of Nuclear Cardiology, Heart Rhythm Society, Society of Cardiovascular Anesthesiologists, Society for Cardiovascular Angiography and Interventions, Society for Vascular Medicine and Biology, and Society for Vascular Surgery. *Circulation.* 2007 23;116(17):1971–1996.
99. Devereaux PJ, Yang H, Guyatt GH, et al. Rationale, design, and organization of the PeriOperative ISchemic Evaluation (POISE) trial: A randomized controlled trial of metoprolol versus placebo in patients undergoing noncardiac surgery. *Am Heart J.* 2006;152(2):223–230.
100. Juul AB, Wetterslev J, Gluud C, et al. Effect of perioperative beta blockade in patients with diabetes undergoing major non-cardiac surgery: Randomised placebo controlled, blinded multicentre trial. *BMJ.* 2006;332(7556):1482.
101. Chestnut RM, Marshall LF, Klauber MR, et al. The role of secondary brain injury in determining outcome from severe head injury. *J Trauma.* 1993;34(2):216–222.
102. Fujii Y, Takeuchi S, Sasaki O, et al. Ultra-early rebleeding in spontaneous subarachnoid hemorrhage. *J Neurosurg.* 1996;84(1):35–42.
103. Kolenda H, Gremmelt A, Rading S, et al. Ketamine for analgosedative therapy in intensive care treatment of head-injured patients. *Acta Neurochir (Wien).* 1996;138(10):1193–1199.
104. Bourgoin A, Albanese J, Wereszczynski N, et al. Safety of sedation with ketamine in severe head injury patients: Comparison with sufentanil. *Crit Care Med.* 2003;31(3):711–717.
105. Schmittner MD, Vajkoczy SL, Horn P, et al. Effects of fentanyl and S(+)-ketamine on cerebral hemodynamics, gastrointestinal motility, and need of vasopressors in patients with intracranial pathologies: A pilot study. *J Neurosurg Anesthesiol.* 2007;19(4):257–262.
106. Sloan TB, Ronai AK, Toleikis JR, et al. Improvement of intraoperative somatosensory evoked potentials by etomidate. *Anesth Analg.* [Case Reports]. 1988;67(6):582–585.
107. Taniguchi M, Nadstawek J, Langenbach U, et al. Effects of four intravenous anesthetic agents on motor evoked potentials elicited by magnetic transcranial stimulation. *Neurosurgery.* 1993;33(3):407–415.
108. Hildreth AN, Mejia VA, Maxwell RA, et al. Adrenal suppression following a single dose of etomidate for rapid sequence induction: A prospective randomized study. *J Trauma.* 2008;65(3):573–579.
109. Vinclair M, Broux C, Faure P, et al. Duration of adrenal inhibition following a single dose of etomidate in critically ill patients. *Intensive Care Med.* 2008; 34(4):714–719.
110. den Brinker M, Hokken-Koelega AC, Hazelzet JA, et al. One single dose of etomidate negatively influences adrenocortical performance for at least 24h in children with meningococcal sepsis. *Intensive Care Med.* 2008;34(1):163–168.
111. Martyn JA, Richtsfeld M. Succinylcholine-induced hyperkalemia in acquired pathologic states: Etiologic factors and molecular mechanisms. *Anesthesiology.* [Review]. 2006;104(1):158–169.
112. Gronert GA, Theye RA. Pathophysiology of hyperkalemia induced by succinylcholine. *Anesthesiology.* 1975;43(1):89–99.
113. Perry JJ, Lee JS, Sillberg VA, et al. Rocuronium versus succinylcholine for rapid sequence induction intubation. *Cochrane Database Syst Rev.* 2008;(2): CD002788.
114. Magorian T, Flannery KB, Miller RD. Comparison of rocuronium, succinylcholine, and vecuronium for rapid-sequence induction of anesthesia in adult patients. *Anesthesiology.* 1993;79(5):913–918.
115. Jones RK, Caldwell JE, Brull SJ, et al. Reversal of profound rocuronium-induced blockade with sugammadex: A randomized comparison with neostigmine. *Anesthesiology.* 2008;109(5):816–824.
116. Aouad MT, Al-Alami AA, Nasr VG, et al. The effect of low-dose remifentanil on responses to the endotracheal tube during emergence from general anesthesia. *Anesth Analg.* 2009;108(4):1157–1160.
117. Mack PF, Perrine K, Kobylarz E, et al. Dexmedetomidine and neurocognitive testing in awake craniotomy. *J Neurosurg Anesthesiol.* 2004;16(1):20–25.
118. Rozet I, Muangman S, Vavilala MS, et al. Clinical experience with dexmedetomidine for implantation of deep brain stimulators in Parkinson's disease. *Anesth Analg.* 2006;103(5):1224–1228.
119. Davis DP, Dunford JV, Poste JC, et al. The impact of hypoxia and hyperventilation on outcome after paramedic rapid sequence intubation of severely head-injured patients. *J Trauma.* 2004;57(1):1–8.
120. Bratton SL, Chestnut RM, Ghajar J, et al. Guidelines for the management of severe traumatic brain injury. XIV. Hyperventilation. *J Neurotrauma.* [Practice Guideline]. 2007;24 (suppl 1):S87–S90.
121. Oddo M, Levine JM, Frangos S, et al. Effect of mannitol and hypertonic saline on cerebral oxygenation in patients with severe traumatic brain injury and refractory intracranial hypertension. *J Neurol Neurosurg Psychiatry.* 2009;80(8):916–920.
122. Vialet R, Albanese J, Thomachot L, et al. Isovolume hypertonic solutes (sodium chloride or mannitol) in the treatment of refractory posttraumatic intracranial hypertension: 2 mL/kg 7.5% saline is more effective than 2 mL/kg 20% mannitol. *Crit Care Med.* 2003;31(6):1683–1687.
123. Schwarz S, Schwab S, Bertram M, et al. Effects of hypertonic saline hydroxyethyl starch solution and mannitol in patients with increased intracranial pressure after stroke. *Stroke.* 1998;29(8):1550–1555.
124. Rozet I, Tontisirin N, Muangman S, et al. Effect of equiosmolar solutions of mannitol versus hypertonic saline on intraoperative brain relaxation and electrolyte balance. *Anesthesiology.* 2007;107(5):697–704.
125. Rizoli SB, Rhind SG, Shek PN, et al. The immunomodulatory effects of hypertonic saline resuscitation in patients sustaining traumatic hemorrhagic shock: A randomized, controlled, double-blinded trial. *Ann Surg.* 2006;243(1):47–57.
126. Pascual JL, Khwaja KA, Chaudhury P, et al. Hypertonic saline and the microcirculation. *J Trauma.* 2003;54(5 suppl):S133–S140.
127. Corso CO, Okamoto S, Leiderer R, et al. Resuscitation with hypertonic saline dextran reduces endothelial cell swelling and improves hepatic microvascular perfusion and function after hemorrhagic shock. *J Surg Res.* 1998;80(2):210–220.
128. Manninen PH, Lam AM, Gelb AW, et al. The effect of high-dose mannitol on serum and urine electrolytes and osmolality in neurosurgical patients. *Can J Anaesth.* 1987;34(5):442–446.
129. Muizelaar JP, Wei EP, Kontos HA, et al. Mannitol causes compensatory cerebral vasoconstriction and vasodilation in response to blood viscosity changes. *J Neurosurg.* 1983;59(5):822–828.
130. Burke AM, Quest DO, Chien S, et al. The effects of mannitol on blood viscosity. *J Neurosurg.* 1981;55(4):550–553.
131. Rosner MJ, Coley I. Cerebral perfusion pressure: A hemodynamic mechanism of mannitol and the postmannitol hemogram. *Neurosurgery.* 1987;21(2):147–156.
132. Mendelow AD, Teasdale GM, Russell T, et al. Effect of mannitol on cerebral blood flow and cerebral perfusion pressure in human head injury. *J Neurosurg.* 1985;63(1):43–48.

133. Kirkpatrick PJ, Smielewski P, Piechnik S, et al. Early effects of mannitol in patients with head injuries assessed using bedside multimodality monitoring. *Neurosurgery.* 1996;39(4):714–720; discussion 20–21.
134. Torre-Healy A, Marko NF, Weil RJ. Hyperosmolar therapy for intracranial hypertension. *Neurocrit Care.* 2012;17(1):117–1130.
135. Warner MA, O'Keeffe T, Bhavsar P, et al. Transfusions and long-term functional outcomes in traumatic brain injury. *J Neurosurg.* 2010;113(3):539–546.
136. Hebert PC, Wells G, Blajchman MA, et al. A multicenter, randomized, controlled clinical trial of transfusion requirements in critical care. Transfusion Requirements in Critical Care Investigators, Canadian Critical Care Trials Group. *N Engl J Med.* [Clinical Trial]. 1999;340(6):409–417.
137. Rivers E, Nguyen B, Havstad S, et al. Early goal-directed therapy in the treatment of severe sepsis and septic shock. *N Engl J Med.* 2001;345(19):1368–1377.
138. Zygun DA, Nortje J, Hutchinson PJ, et al. The effect of red blood cell transfusion on cerebral oxygenation and metabolism after severe traumatic brain injury. *Crit Care Med.* 2009;37(3):1074–1078.
139. Smith MJ, Stiefel MF, Magge S, et al. Packed red blood cell transfusion increases local cerebral oxygenation. *Crit Care Med.* 2005;33(5):1104–1108.
140. Carlson AP, Schermer CR, Lu SW. Retrospective evaluation of anemia and transfusion in traumatic brain injury. *J Trauma.* 2006;61(3):567–571.
141. Wass CT, Long TR, Faust RJ, et al. Changes in red blood cell transfusion practice during the past two decades: A retrospective analysis, with the Mayo database, of adult patients undergoing major spine surgery. *Transfusion.* 2007;47(6):1022–1027.
142. Myburgh J, Cooper DJ, Finfer S, et al. Saline or albumin for fluid resuscitation in patients with traumatic brain injury. *N Engl J Med.* 2007;357(9):874–884.
143. Holcomb JB, Wade CE, Michalek JE, et al. Increased plasma and platelet to red blood cell ratios improves outcome in 466 massively transfused civilian trauma patients. *Ann Surg.* [Multicenter Study]. 2008;248(3):447–458.
144. Karlsson M, Ternstrom L, Hyllner M, et al. Prophylactic fibrinogen infusion reduces bleeding after coronary artery bypass surgery. A prospective randomised pilot study. *Thromb Haemost.* 2009;102(1):137–144.
145. Shakur H, Roberts I, Bautista R, et al. Effects of tranexamic acid on death, vascular occlusive events, and blood transfusion in trauma patients with significant haemorrhage (CRASH-2): A randomised, placebo-controlled trial. *Lancet.* 2010;376(9734):23–32.
146. Sena MJ, Rivers RM, Muizelaar JP, et al. Transfusion practices for acute traumatic brain injury: A survey of physicians at US trauma centers. *Intensive Care Med.* 2009;35(3):480–488.
147. Brasel KJ, Vercruysse G, Spinella PC, et al. The association of blood component use ratios with the survival of massively transfused trauma patients with and without severe brain injury. *J Trauma.* 2011;71(2 suppl 3):S343–S352.
148. Rhodes KE, Raivich G, Fawcett JW. The injury response of oligodendrocyte precursor cells is induced by platelets, macrophages and inflammation-associated cytokines. *Neuroscience.* 2006;140(1):87–100.
149. Liu-DeRyke X, Collingridge DS, Orme J, et al. Clinical impact of early hyperglycemia during acute phase of traumatic brain injury. *Neurocrit Care.* 2009;11(2):151–157.
150. Jeremitsky E, Omert LA, Dunham CM, et al. The impact of hyperglycemia on patients with severe brain injury. *J Trauma.* 2005;58(1):47–50.
151. Sharma D, Jelacic J, Chennuri R, et al. Incidence and risk factors for perioperative hyperglycemia in children with traumatic brain injury. *Anesth Analg.* 2009; 108(1):81–89.
152. Mitchell I, Knight E, Gissane J, et al. A phase II randomised controlled trial of intensive insulin therapy in general intensive care patients. *Crit Care Resusc.* 2006; 8(4):289–293.
153. Thomas G, Rojas MC, Epstein SK, et al. Insulin therapy and acute kidney injury in critically ill patients a systematic review. *Nephrol Dial Transplant.* 2007; 22(10):2849–2855.
154. Finfer S, Chittock DR, Su SY, et al. Intensive versus conventional glucose control in critically ill patients. *N Engl J Med.* 2009;360(13):1283–1297.
155. Oddo M, Schmidt JM, Carrera E, et al. Impact of tight glycemic control on cerebral glucose metabolism after severe brain injury: A microdialysis study. *Crit Care Med.* 2008;36(12):3233–3238.
156. Bagshaw SM, Egi M, George C, et al. Early blood glucose control and mortality in critically ill patients in Australia. *Crit Care Med.* 2009;37(2):463–470.
157. Krinsley JS. Glycemic variability: A strong independent predictor of mortality in critically ill patients. *Crit Care Med.* 2008;36(11):3008–3013.
158. Ali NA, O'Brien JM Jr, Dungan K, et al. Glucose variability and mortality in patients with sepsis. *Crit Care Med.* 2008;36(8):2316–2321.
159. Hirshberg E, Larsen G, Van Duker H. Alterations in glucose homeostasis in the pediatric intensive care unit: Hyperglycemia and glucose variability are associated with increased mortality and morbidity. *Pediatr Crit Care Med.* 2008;9(4): 361–366.
160. Dossett LA, Cao H, Mowery NT, et al. Blood glucose variability is associated with mortality in the surgical intensive care unit. *Am Surg.* 2008;74(8):679–685; discussion 85.
161. Pecha T, Sharma D, Hoffman NG, et al. Hyperglycemia during craniotomy for adult traumatic brain injury. *Anesth Analg.* 2011;113(2):336–342.
162. De Backer D. The cuff-leak test: What are we measuring? *Crit Care.* 2005;9(1): 31–33.
163. Kriner EJ, Shafazand S, Colice GL. The endotracheal tube cuff-leak test as a predictor for postextubation stridor. *Respir Care.* 2005;50(12):1632–1638.
164. Kwon B, Yoo JU, Furey CG, et al. Risk factors for delayed extubation after single-stage, multi-level anterior cervical decompression and posterior fusion. *J Spinal Disord Tech.* 2006;19(6):389–393.
165. Emery SE, Akhavan S, Miller P, et al. Steroids and risk factors for airway compromise in multilevel cervical corpectomy patients: A prospective, randomized, double-blind study. *Spine (Phila Pa 1976).* 2009;34(3):229–232.
166. Dunbar PJ, Visco E, Lam AM. Craniotomy procedures are associated with less analgesic requirements than other surgical procedures. *Anesth Analg.* [Comparative Study]. 1999;88(2):335–340.
167. Venkatesan T, Korula G. A comparative study between the effects of 4% endotracheal tube cuff lignocaine and 1.5 mg/kg intravenous lignocaine on coughing and hemodynamics during extubation in neurosurgical patients: A randomized controlled double-blind trial. *J Neurosurg Anesthesiol.* 2006;18(4):230–234.
168. Butler BD, Hills BA. Transpulmonary passage of venous air emboli. *J Appl Physiol.* 1985;59:543.
169. Vik A, Brubakk AO, Hennessey TR, et al. Venous air embolism in swine: Transport of gas bubbles through the pulmonary circulation. *J Appl Physiol.* 1990;69:237.
170. Yahagi N, Furuya H. The effects of halothane and pentobarbital on the threshold of transpulmonary passage of venous air emboli in dogs. *Anesthesiology.* 1987; 67:905.
171. Glasker S, Pechstein U, Vongionkas VI, et al. Monitoring motor function during resection of tumours in the lower brain stem and fourth ventricle. *Childs Nerv Syst.* 2006;22:1288.
172. Neuloh G, Pechstein U, Schramm J. Motor tract monitoring during insular glioma surgery. *J Neurosurg.* 2007;106:582.
173. Kaal EC, Vecht CJ. The management of brain edema in brain tumors. *Curr Opin Oncol.* 2004;16:593.
174. Beneficial effect of carotid endarterectomy in symptomatic patients with high-grade carotid stenosis. North American Symptomatic Carotid Endarterectomy Trial Collaborators. *N Engl J Med.* 1991;325:445.
175. Chaturvedi S, Bruno A, Feasby T, et al. Carotid endarterectomy—an evidence-based review: Report of the Therapeutics and Technology Assessment Subcommittee of the American Academy of Neurology. *Neurology.* 2005;65:794.
176. Endarterectomy for asymptomatic carotid artery stenosis. Executive Committee for the Asymptomatic Carotid Atherosclerosis Study. *JAMA.* 1995;273:1421.
177. Halliday A, Mansfield A, Marro J, et al. Prevention of disabling and fatal strokes by successful carotid endarterectomy in patients without recent neurological symptoms: Randomised controlled trial. *Lancet.* 2004;363:1491.
178. Ederle J, Brown MM. The evidence for medicine versus surgery for carotid stenosis. *Eur J Radiol.* 2006;60:3.
179. de Sousa AA, Filho MA, Faglioni W Jr, et al. Superficial vs combined cervical plexus block for carotid endarterectomy: A prospective, randomized study. *Surg Neurol.* 2005;63(suppl 1):S22.
180. Pandit JJ, Bree S, Dillon P, et al. A comparison of superficial versus combined (superficial and deep) cervical plexus block for carotid endarterectomy: A prospective, randomized study. *Anesth Analg.* 2000;91:781.
181. GALA Trial Collaborative Group, Lewis SC, Warlow CP, et al. General anaesthesia versus local anaesthesia for carotid surgery (GALA): A multicentre, randomised controlled trial. *Lancet.* 2008;372(9656):2132–2142.
182. Moritz S, Kasprzak P, Arlt M, et al. Accuracy of cerebral monitoring in detecting cerebral ischemia during carotid endarterectomy: A comparison of transcranial Doppler sonography, near-infrared spectroscopy, stump pressure, and somatosensory evoked potentials. *Anesthesiology.* 2007;107:563.
183. SPACE Collaborative Group, Ringleb PA, Allenberg J, et al. 30 day results from the SPACE trial of stent-protected angioplasty versus carotid endarterectomy in symptomatic patients: A randomised non-inferiority trial. *Lancet.* 2006;368:1239.
184. Mas JL, Chatellier G, Beyssen B, et al. Endarterectomy versus stenting in patients with symptomatic severe carotid stenosis. *N Engl J Med.* 2006;355:1660.
185. Yadav JS, Wholey MH, Kuntz RT, et al. Protected carotid-artery stenting versus endarterectomy in high-risk patients. *N Engl J Med.* 2004;351:1493.
186. McClelland S 3rd. Multimodality management of carotid artery stenosis: Reviewing the class-I evidence. *J Natl Med Assoc.* 2007;99:1235.
187. Brott TG, Hobson RW 2nd, Howard G, et al. Stenting versus endarterectomy for treatment of carotid-artery stenosis. *N Engl J Med.* 2010;363(1):11–23.
188. Zanettini R, Antonini A, Gatto G, et al. Valvular heart disease and the use of dopamine agonists for Parkinson's disease. *N Engl J Med.* 2007;356(1):39–46.
189. Nicholson G, Pereira AC, Hall GM. Parkinson's disease and anaesthesia. *Br J Anaesth.* 2002;89(6):904–916.
190. Burton DA, Nicholson G, Hall GM. Anaesthesia in elderly patients with neurodegenerative disorders: Special considerations. *Drugs Aging.* 2004;21(4):229–242.
191. Krauss JK, Akeyson EW, Giam P, et al. Propofol-induced dyskinesias in Parkinson's disease. *Anesth Analg.* 1996;83(2):420–422.
192. Erickson KM, Cole DJ. Anesthetic considerations for awake craniotomy for epilepsy. *Anesthesiol Clin.* 2007;25(3):535–555, ix.
193. Skucas AP, Artru AA. Anesthetic complications of awake craniotomies for epilepsy surgery. *Anesth Analg.* 2006;102(3):882–887.
194. Manninen PH, Balki M, Lukitto K, et al. Patient satisfaction with awake craniotomy for tumor surgery: A comparison of remifentanil and fentanyl in conjunction with propofol. *Anesth Analg.* 2006;102(1):237–242.

195. Khatib R, Ebrahim Z, Rezai A, et al. Perioperative events during deep brain stimulation: The experience at cleveland clinic. *J Neurosurg Anesthesiol.* 2008;20(1):36–40.
196. Lotto M, Boulis NM. Intrathecal opioids for control of chronic low back pain during deep brain stimulation procedures. *Anesth Analg.* 2007;105(5):1410–1412.
197. Deiner S, Hagen J. Parkinson's disease and deep brain stimulator placement. *Anesthesiol Clin.* 2009;27(3):391–415.
198. Souter MJ, Rozet I, Ojemann JG, et al. Dexmedetomidine sedation during awake craniotomy for seizure resection: Effects on electrocorticography. *J Neurosurg Anesthesiol.* 2007;19(1):38–44.
199. Bulger EM, Copass MK, Sabath DR, et al. The use of neuromuscular blocking agents to facilitate prehospital intubation does not impair outcome after traumatic brain injury. *J Trauma.* 2005;58(4):718–723; discussion 23–24.
200. Winchell RJ, Hoyt DB. Endotracheal intubation in the field improves survival in patients with severe head injury. Trauma Research and Education Foundation of San Diego. *Arch Surg.* 1997;132(6):592–597.
201. Davis DP, Hoyt DB, Ochs M, et al. The effect of paramedic rapid sequence intubation on outcome in patients with severe traumatic brain injury. *J Trauma.* 2003;54(3):444–453.
202. Murray JA, Demetriades D, Berne TV, et al. Prehospital intubation in patients with severe head injury. *J Trauma.* 2000;49(6):1065–1070.
203. Davis DP, Peay J, Sise MJ, et al. The impact of prehospital endotracheal intubation on outcome in moderate to severe traumatic brain injury. *J Trauma.* 2005;58(5):933–939.
204. Davis DP. Early ventilation in traumatic brain injury. *Resuscitation.* [Review]. 2008;76(3):333–340.
205. Bochicchio GV, Ilahi O, Joshi M, et al. Endotracheal intubation in the field does not improve outcome in trauma patients who present without an acutely lethal traumatic brain injury. *J Trauma.* 2003;54(2):307–311.
206. Michael DB, Guyot DR, Darmody WR. Coincidence of head and cervical spine injury. *J Neurotrauma.* 1989;6(3):177–189.
207. Holly LT, Kelly DF, Counelis GJ, et al. Cervical spine trauma associated with moderate and severe head injury: Incidence, risk factors, and injury characteristics. *J Neurosurg.* 2002;96(3 suppl):285–291.
208. Lennarson PJ, Smith D, Todd MM, et al. Segmental cervical spine motion during orotracheal intubation of the intact and injured spine with and without external stabilization. *J Neurosurg.* 2000;92(2 suppl):201–206.
209. Hastings RH, Wood PR. Head extension and laryngeal view during laryngoscopy with cervical spine stabilization maneuvers. *Anesthesiology.* 1994;80(4):825–831.
210. Sultan P. Is cricoid pressure needed during rapid sequence induction? *Br J Hosp Med (Lond).* 2008;69(3):177.
211. Gobindram A, Clarke S. Cricoid pressure: Should we lay off the pressure? *Anaesthesia.* 2008;63(11):1258–1259.
212. Rice MJ, Mancuso AA, Gibbs C, et al. Cricoid pressure results in compression of the postcricoid hypopharynx: The esophageal position is irrelevant. *Anesth Analg.* 2009;109(5):1546–1552.
213. Rice MJ, Mancuso AA, Morey TE, et al. The anatomical correction of cricoid pressure. *Minerva Anestesiol.* 2010;76(4):304.
214. Donaldson WF 3rd, Towers JD, Doctor A, et al. A methodology to evaluate motion of the unstable spine during intubation techniques. *Spine (Phila Pa 1976).* 1993;18(14):2020–2023.
215. Butler J, Sen A. Best evidence topic report. Cricoid pressure in emergency rapid sequence induction. *Emerg Med J.* 2005;22(11):815–816.
216. Unni VK, Johnston RA, Young HS, et al. Prevention of intracranial hypertension during laryngoscopy and endotracheal intubation. Use of a second dose of thiopentone. *Br J Anaesth.* 1984;56(11):1219–1223.
217. Albrecht RF, Miletich DJ, Rosenberg R, et al. Cerebral blood flow and metabolic changes from induction to onset of anesthesia with halothane or pentobarbital. *Anesthesiology.* 1977;47(3):252–256.
218. White PF, Schlobohm RM, Pitts LH, et al. A randomized study of drugs for preventing increases in intracranial pressure during endotracheal suctioning. *Anesthesiology.* 1982;57(3):242–244.
219. Kovarik WD, Mayberg TS, Lam AM, et al. Succinylcholine does not change intracranial pressure, cerebral blood flow velocity, or the electroencephalogram in patients with neurologic injury. *Anesth Analg.* 1994;78(3):469–473.
220. Brown MM, Parr MJ, Manara AR. The effect of suxamethonium on intracranial pressure and cerebral perfusion pressure in patients with severe head injuries following blunt trauma. *Eur J Anaesthesiol.* 1996;13(5):474–477.
221. Bratton SL, Chestnut RM, Ghajar J, et al. Guidelines for the management of severe traumatic brain injury. IX. Cerebral perfusion thresholds. *J Neurotrauma.* [Practice Guideline]. 2007;24(suppl 1):S59–S64.
222. Sekhon MS, Dhingra VK, Sekhon IS, et al. The safety of synthetic colloid in critically ill patients with severe traumatic brain injuries. *J Crit Care.* 2011;26(4):357–362.
223. Huang SJ, Chen YS, Hong WC, et al. Clinical experience of hydroxyethyl starch (10% HES 200/0.5) in cerebral perfusion pressure protocol for severe head injury. *Surg Neurol.* 2006;66(suppl 2):S26–S31.
224. Neff TA, Doelberg M, Jungheinrich C, et al. Repetitive large-dose infusion of the novel hydroxyethyl starch 130/0.4 in patients with severe head injury. *Anesth Analg.* 2003;96(5):1453–1459.
225. Bulger EM, May S, Brasel KJ, et al. Out-of-hospital hypertonic resuscitation following severe traumatic brain injury: A randomized controlled trial. *JAMA.* 2010;304(13):1455–1464.
226. Contant CF, Valadka AB, Gopinath SP, et al. Adult respiratory distress syndrome: A complication of induced hypertension after severe head injury. *J Neurosurg.* 2001;95(4):560–568.
227. Steiner LA, Johnston AJ, Czosnyka M, et al. Direct comparison of cerebrovascular effects of norepinephrine and dopamine in head-injured patients. *Crit Care Med.* 2004;32(4):1049–1054.
228.
229. Chen JW, Gombart ZJ, Rogers S, et al. Pupillary reactivity as an early indicator of increased intracranial pressure: The introduction of the neurological pupil index. *Surg Neurol Int.* 2011;2:82.
230. Sheinberg M, Kanter MJ, Robertson CS, et al. Continuous monitoring of jugular venous oxygen saturation in head-injured patients. *J Neurosurg.* 1992;76(2):212–217.
231. Wang GJ, Deng HY, Maier CM, et al. Mild hypothermia reduces ICAM-1 expression, neutrophil infiltration and microglia/monocyte accumulation following experimental stroke. *Neuroscience.* 2002;114(4):1081–1090.
232. Jiang JY, Xu W, Yang PF, et al. Marked protection by selective cerebral profound hypothermia after complete cerebral ischemia in primates. *J Neurotrauma.* 2006;23(12):1847–1856.
233. Ehrlich MP, McCullough JN, Zhang N, et al. Effect of hypothermia on cerebral blood flow and metabolism in the pig. *Ann Thorac Surg.* 2002;73(1):191–197.
234. Maier CM, Sun GH, Cheng D, et al. Effects of mild hypothermia on superoxide anion production, superoxide dismutase expression, and activity following transient focal cerebral ischemia. *Neurobiol Dis.* 2002;11(1):28–42.
235. Sydenham E, Roberts I, Alderson P. Hypothermia for traumatic head injury. *Cochrane Database Syst Rev.* 2009;(2):CD001048.
236. Clifton GL, Valadka A, Zygun D, et al. Very early hypothermia induction in patients with severe brain injury (the National Acute Brain Injury Study: Hypothermia II): A randomised trial. *Lancet Neurol.* 2011;10(2):131–139.
237. Hutchison JS, Ward RE, Lacroix J, et al. Hypothermia therapy after traumatic brain injury in children. *N Engl J Med.* 2008;358(23):2447–2456.
238. Polderman KH. Application of therapeutic hypothermia in the intensive care unit. Opportunities and pitfalls of a promising treatment modality–Part 2: Practical aspects and side effects. *Intensive Care Med.* 2004;30(5):757–769.
239. http://www.anzicrc.monash.org/polar-rct.html
240. http://www.eurotherm3235trial.eu/home/index.phtml
241. Eisenberg HM, Frankowski RF, Contant CF, et al. High-dose barbiturate control of elevated intracranial pressure in patients with severe head injury. *J Neurosurg.* 1988;69:15–23.
242. Cremer OL, Moons KG, Bouman EA, et al. Long-term propofol infusion and cardiac failure in adult head-injured patients. *Lancet.* 2001;357(9250):117–118.
243. Otterspoor LC, Kalkman CJ, Cremer OL. Update on the propofol infusion syndrome in ICU management of patients with head injury. *Curr Opin Anaesthesiol.* 2008;21(5):544–551. Review.
244. Hutchinson PJ, Kirkpatrick PJ. Decompressive craniectomy in head injury. *Curr Opin Crit Care.* [Review]. 2004;10(2):101–104.
245. Sahuquillo J, Arikan F. Decompressive craniectomy for the treatment of refractory high intracranial pressure in traumatic brain injury. *Cochrane Database Syst Rev.* [Review]. 2006;(1):CD003983.
246. Jaeger M, Soehle M, Meixensberger J. Effects of decompressive craniectomy on brain tissue oxygen in patients with intracranial hypertension. *J Neurol Neurosurg Psychiatry.* [Review]. 2003;74(4):513–515.
247. Stiefel MF, Heuer GG, Smith MJ, et al. Cerebral oxygenation following decompressive hemicraniectomy for the treatment of refractory intracranial hypertension. *J Neurosurg.* 2004;101(2):241–247.
248. Aarabi B, Hesdorffer DC, Ahn ES, et al. Outcome following decompressive craniectomy for malignant swelling due to severe head injury. *J Neurosurg.* 2006;104(4):469–479.
249. Cooper DJ, Rosenfeld JV, Murray L, et al. Decompressive craniectomy in diffuse traumatic brain injury. *N Engl J Med.* 2011;364(16):1493–1502.
250. Kawaguchi M, Sakamoto T, Ohnishi H, et al. Preoperative predictors of reduction in arterial blood pressure following dural opening during surgical evacuation of acute subdural hematoma. *J Neurosurg Anesthesiol.* 1996;8(2):117–122.
251. Pelligrino DA, Miletich DJ, Hoffman WE, et al. Nitrous oxide markedly increases cerebral cortical metabolic rate and blood flow in the goat. *Anesthesiology.* 1984;60(5):405–412.
252. Matta BF, Lam AM. Nitrous oxide increases cerebral blood flow velocity during pharmacologically induced EEG silence in humans. *J Neurosurg Anesthesiol.* 1995;7(2):89–93.
253. Moss E, McDowall DG. I.c.p. increases with 50% nitrous oxide in oxygen in severe head injuries during controlled ventilation. *Br J Anaesth.* 1979;51(8):757–761.
254. Hadani M, Bruk B, Ram Z, et al. Application of transcranial Doppler ultrasonography for the diagnosis of brain death. *Intensive Care Med.* 1999;25(8):822–828.
255. Grotz MR, Giannoudis PV, Pape HC, et al. Traumatic brain injury and stabilisation of long bone fractures: An update. *Injury.* [Review]. 2004;35(11):1077–1086.
256. Pietropaoli JA, Rogers FB, Shackford SR, et al. The deleterious effects of intraoperative hypotension on outcome in patients with severe head injuries. *J Trauma.* 1992;33(3):403–407.

257. Vallier HA, Cureton BA, Ekstein C, et al. Early definitive stabilization of unstable pelvis and acetabulum fractures reduces morbidity. *J Trauma.* 2010;69(3):677–684.
258. Morshed S, Miclau T 3rd, Bembom O, et al. Delayed internal fixation of femoral shaft fracture reduces mortality among patients with multisystem trauma. *J Bone Joint Surg Am.* 2009;91(1):3–13.
259. Rothman SM, Olney JW. Glutamate and the pathophysiology of hypoxic–ischemic brain damage. *Ann Neurol.* 1986;19(2):105–111.
260. Biffl WL, Egglin T, Benedetto B, et al. Sixteen-slice computed tomographic angiography is a reliable noninvasive screening test for clinically significant blunt cerebrovascular injuries. *J Trauma.* 2006;60(4):745–751; discussion 51–52.
261. Hackl W, Hausberger K, Sailer R, et al. Prevalence of cervical spine injuries in patients with facial trauma. *Oral Surg Oral Med Oral Pathol Oral Radiol Endod.* 2001;92(4):370–376.
262. McKevitt EC, Kirkpatrick AW, Vertesi L, et al. Identifying patients at risk for intracranial and extracranial blunt carotid injuries. *Am J Surg.* 2002;183(5):566–570.
263. Rabinovici R, Ovadia P, Mathiak G, et al. Abdominal injuries associated with lumbar spine fractures in blunt trauma. *Injury.* 1999;30(7):471–474.
264. Bracken MB, Holford TR. Neurological and functional status 1 year after acute spinal cord injury: Estimates of functional recovery in National Acute Spinal Cord Injury Study II from results modeled in National Acute Spinal Cord Injury Study III. *J Neurosurg.* 2002;96(3 Suppl):259–266.
265. Hurlbert RJ. Methylprednisolone for acute spinal cord injury: An inappropriate standard of care. *J Neurosurg.* 2000;93(1 Suppl):1–7.
266. Sayer FT, Kronvall E, Nilsson OG. Methylprednisolone treatment in acute spinal cord injury: The myth challenged through a structured analysis of published literature. *Spine J.* [Review]. 2006;6(3):335–343.
267. Fehlings MG, Arvin B. The timing of surgery in patients with central spinal cord injury. *J Neurosurg Spine.* [Editorial]. 2009;10(1):1–2.
268. Michard F. Changes in arterial pressure during mechanical ventilation. *Anesthesiology.* [Review]. 2005;103(2):419–428.
269. Kumar A, Anel R, Bunnell E, et al. Pulmonary artery occlusion pressure and central venous pressure fail to predict ventricular filling volume, cardiac performance, or the response to volume infusion in normal subjects. *Crit Care Med.* 2004;32(3):691–699.
270. Friese RS, Shafi S, Gentilello LM. Pulmonary artery catheter use is associated with reduced mortality in severely injured patients: A National Trauma Data Bank analysis of 53,312 patients. *Crit Care Med.* 2006;34(6):1597–1601.
271. Montenij LJ, de Waal EE, Buhre WF. Arterial waveform analysis in anesthesia and critical care. *Curr Opin Anaesthesiol.* 2011;24(6):651–656.
272. Malhotra NR, Shaffrey CI. Intraoperative electrophysiological monitoring in spine surgery. *Spine (Phila Pa 1976).* 2010;35(25):2167–2179.
273. Ozcan MS, Praetel C, Bhatti MT, et al. The effect of body inclination during prone positioning on intraocular pressure in awake volunteers: A comparison of two operating tables. *Anesth Analg.* 2004;99(4):1152–1158.
274. Griepp RB, Griepp EB. Spinal cord perfusion and protection during descending thoracic and thoracoabdominal aortic surgery: The collateral network concept. *Ann Thorac Surg.* [Review]. 2007;83(2):S865–S869.
275. Dietrich WD 3rd. Therapeutic hypothermia for spinal cord injury. *Crit Care Med.* [Research Review]. 2009;37(7 suppl):S238–S242.
276. Levi AD, Casella G, Green BA, et al. Clinical outcomes using modest intravascular hypothermia after acute cervical spinal cord injury. *Neurosurgery.* [Research]. 2010;66(4):670–677.
277. Crock HV, Yoshizawa H, Yamagishi M, et al. Commentary on the prevention of paralysis after traumatic spinal cord injury in humans: The neglected factor–urgent restoration of spinal cord circulation. *Eur Spine J.* 2005;14(9):910–914.
278. Marion D, Bullock MR. Current and future role of therapeutic hypothermia. *J Neurotrauma.* 2009;26(3):455–467.
279. Jia X, Kowalski RG, Sciubba DM, et al. Critical care of traumatic spinal cord injury. *J Intensive Care Med.* 2011.
280. Postoperative Visual Loss Study Group. Risk factors associated with ischemic optic neuropathy after spinal fusion surgery. *Anesthesiology.* 2012;116(1):15–24.

CHAPTER

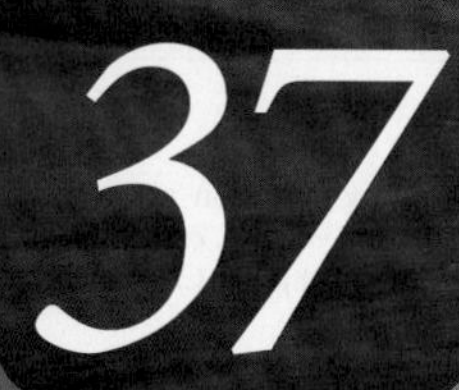

Anesthesia for Thoracic Surgery

JAMES B. EISENKRAFT • EDMOND COHEN • STEVEN M. NEUSTEIN

Key Points

1. It is important to determine prior to the onset of anesthesia and surgery whether the patient will be able to tolerate the planned lung resection.
2. Preoperative assessment of vital capacity is critical because at least three times the tidal volume (V_T) is necessary for an effective cough.
3. Smoking increases airway irritability, decreases mucociliary transport, and increases secretions. It also decreases forced vital capacity and forced expiratory flow 25% to 75%, thereby increasing the incidence of postoperative pulmonary complications.
4. The absolute indications for lung separation using a double-lumen tube have been for protection against spillage of blood, infectious material, or lavage fluid from one lung, or for ventilation in the case of bronchopleural fistula or bullae. A lobectomy or pneumonectomy is a relative indication.
5. The most important advance in checking the proper position of a double-lumen tube is the introduction of the pediatric flexible fiberoptic bronchoscope.
6. During one-lung ventilation (OLV), the dependent lung should be ventilated using a V_T that results in a plateau airway pressure <25 cm H_2O at a rate adjusted to maintain Pa_{CO_2} at 35 ± 3 mm Hg.
7. The choice of anesthetic technique for OLV must take into consideration the effects on oxygenation and therefore on hypoxic pulmonary vasoconstriction.
8. The need for OLV is much greater with video-assisted thoracoscopic surgery than with open thoracotomy because it is not possible to retract the lung during video-assisted thoracoscopic surgery as it is during an open thoracotomy.
9. The potential advantages offered by high-frequency positive-pressure ventilation during thoracic anesthesia are that lower V_T and inspiratory pressures result in a quiet lung field for the surgeon, with minimal movements of airway, lung tissue, and mediastinum.
10. Myasthenia gravis is a disorder of the neuromuscular junction, characterized by weakness and fatigability of voluntary muscles with improvement following rest. Surgical thymectomy is a commonly performed therapy.
11. In addition to a more comfortable patient, important benefits of adequate pain relief are avoidance of postoperative atelectasis and limited inspiratory thoracic cage expansion.

Multimedia

1 Position Double-lumen Tube
2 Bronchial Blocker
3 Univent
4 CPAP
5 Bronchoscopy
6 Jet Ventilation
7 Fiberoptic Intubation
8 Mediastinal Mass
9 Mediastinoscopy

Lung cancer has long been the most common cause of cancer mortality in the United States in men, and surpassed breast cancer as the leading cause of cancer deaths in women in 1987.[1] The most recent statistics from the American Cancer Society indicated that approximately 221,130 new cases of lung cancer would be diagnosed in 2011 (115,060 among men and 106,070 among women). The Society also estimated that there would be 156,940 deaths from lung cancer, which represents 27% of all cancer deaths (Fig. 37-1).[2] The increased incidence of lung cancer has led to an increase in the amount of noncardiac thoracic surgery performed in the United States.

In this chapter, the physiologic, pharmacologic, and clinical considerations for the patient undergoing pulmonary surgery are reviewed, followed by sections on anesthesia for diagnostic and therapeutic procedures, high-frequency ventilation, and special situations, including bronchopleural fistula (BPF) and tracheal reconstruction. A discussion of myasthenia gravis (MG) is included because of its relationship to the thymus gland and because thymectomy is one of the most commonly performed surgical procedures in these patients. The chapter concludes with a review of the postoperative management of the patient who has undergone noncardiac thoracic surgery.

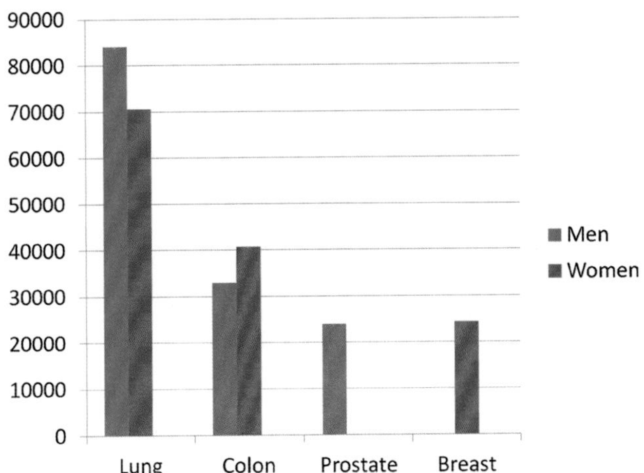

FIGURE 37-1. Estimated 2011 deaths from cancer in the United States. Lung cancer is the leading cause of cancer-related mortality. (Based on data from: The American Cancer Society, Cancer statistics, 2010. A presentation from the American Cancer Society. 2011 Estimated U.S. Cancer Deaths. Available at: http://www.cancer.org/acs/groups/content/@epidemiologysurveilance/documents/document/acspc-029997.pptx. Last accessed 11-26-2012.)

PREOPERATIVE EVALUATION

1 The preoperative evaluation of the patient for thoracic surgery should focus on the extent and severity of pulmonary disease and cardiovascular involvement (see Chapter 22). It is important to determine whether the patient will be able to tolerate the planned lung resection. To find out postoperatively that the patient cannot tolerate the resection would be catastrophic.

It is more difficult to predict postoperative pulmonary complications following elective cardiothoracic, compared with noncardiothoracic surgery.[3] Thoracic surgery is known to be associated with high risk, and patient factors that have been associated with increased risk include advanced age, poor general health status, and chronic obstructive pulmonary disease (COPD).[4]

History

Dyspnea

Dyspnea occurs when the requirement for ventilation is greater than the patient's ability to respond appropriately (see Chapter 11). Dyspnea is quantified by the degree of physical activity required to produce it, the level of activity possible (e.g., ability to walk on level ground or climb stairs), and management of daily activities. Severe exertional dyspnea usually implies a significantly diminished ventilatory reserve and a forced expiratory volume in 1 second (FEV_1) of <1,500 mL, with possible need for postoperative ventilatory support.

Cough

Recurrent productive cough for 3 months of the year for two consecutive years is necessary to make the diagnosis of chronic bronchitis. Cough indirectly increases airway irritability. If the cough is productive, the volume, consistency, and color of the sputum should be assessed. Sputum should be cultured to rule out infection and to establish whether there is a need for preoperative antibiotic therapy. Blood-stained sputum or episodes of gross hemoptysis should alert the anesthesiologist to the possibility of a tumor invading the respiratory tract (e.g., the main stem bronchus), which might interfere with endobronchial intubation.

Cigarette Smoking

Cigarette smoking increases the risk of chronic lung disease and malignancy, as well as the incidence of postoperative pulmonary complications. The number of pack-years (packs smoked per day multiplied by the number of years) is directly related to measurable changes in respiratory gas flow and closing capacity, making these patients prone to postoperative atelectasis and arterial hypoxemia.

Exercise Tolerance

Patients who can walk up three or more flights of stairs are at reduced risk, and those unable to climb two flights are generally at increased risk.[5] The best evaluation is actually the history of the patient's quality of life.[6] An otherwise healthy patient, with good exercise tolerance, generally does not require additional screening tests.

Risk Factors for Acute Lung Injury

In some cases, thoracic surgery may lead to acute lung injury (ALI) postoperatively. Perioperative risk factors that have been identified include preoperative alcohol abuse and patients undergoing pneumonectomy. Intraoperative risk factors include high ventilatory pressures and excessive amounts of fluid administration.[7]

Physical Examination

The physical examination of the patient should address the following aspects.

Respiratory Pattern

The presence of cyanosis and clubbing, the breathing pattern, and the type of breath sounds should be noted.

Cyanosis. The presence of peripheral cyanosis (in the fingers, toes, or ears) should be distinguished from causes of poor circulation (acrocyanosis). The presence of central cyanosis (in the buccal mucosa) is usually secondary to arterial hypoxemia. If cyanosis is present, the arterial hemoglobin saturation with oxygen is 80% or less (PaO_2 <50 to 52 mm Hg), which indicates a limited margin of respiratory reserve.

Clubbing. Clubbing of fingers and toes is often seen in patients with chronic lung disease, malignancies, or congenital heart disease associated with right-to-left shunt.

Respiratory Rate and Pattern. A patient's inability to complete a normal sentence without pausing for breath is an indication of severe dyspnea. Inspiratory paradox, the abdomen moving in while the chest moves out, suggests diaphragmatic fatigue and respiratory dysfunction. The patient should be assessed for paroxysmal retraction (Hoover's sign), limited diaphragmatic movement because of hyperinflation, asymmetry of chest movement secondary to phrenic nerve involvement, hemothorax, pleural effusion, and pneumothorax. The pattern and rate of breathing have important roles in distinguishing between obstructive and restrictive lung diseases. For constant minute ventilation, the work done against airflow resistance decreases when breathing is slow and deep. Work done against elastic resistance decreases when breathing is rapid and shallow (e.g., as in pulmonary infarct or pulmonary fibrosis).

Breath Sounds. Wet sounds (crackles) are usually caused by excessive fluid in the airways and indicate sputum retention or edema. Dry sounds (wheezes) are produced by high-velocity gas flow through bronchi and are a sign of airways obstruction. Distant sounds are an indication of emphysema and possibly bullae. The trachea should be in the midline. Displacement of the trachea may be secondary to a number of causes, including mediastinal mass, and should alert the anesthesiologist to a potentially difficult intubation of the trachea or airway obstruction on induction of anesthesia.

Evaluation of the Cardiovascular System

One of the most important factors in the evaluation of a patient scheduled for thoracic surgery is the presence of an increase in pulmonary vascular resistance secondary to a fixed reduction in the cross-sectional area of the pulmonary vascular bed. The pulmonary circulation is normally a low-pressure, high-compliance system capable of handling an increase in blood flow by recruitment of normally underperfused vessels. This acts as a compensatory mechanism that normally prevents an increase in pulmonary arterial pressure. In COPD, there is distention of the pulmonary capillary bed with decreased ability to tolerate an increase in blood flow (decreased compliance). Such patients demonstrate an increase in pulmonary vascular resistance when cardiac output increases because of a decreased ability to compensate for an increase in pulmonary blood flow. This results in pulmonary hypertension, signs of which include a narrowly split second heart sound, increased intensity of the pulmonary component of the second heart sound, and right ventricular and atrial hypertrophy. An increase in pulmonary vascular resistance is of significance in the management of the patient during anesthesia because several factors, such as acidosis, sepsis, hypoxia, and application of positive end-expiratory pressure (PEEP), all further increase the pulmonary vascular resistance and increase the likelihood of right ventricular failure.

In patients with ischemic or valvular heart disease, the function of the left side of the heart should also be carefully evaluated.

Electrocardiogram

A patient with COPD may present with electrocardiographic features of right atrial and ventricular hypertrophy and strain. These include a low-voltage QRS complex due to lung hyperinflation and poor R-wave progression across the precordial leads. An enlarged P wave ("P pulmonale") in standard lead II is diagnostic of right atrial hypertrophy. The electrocardiographic changes of right ventricular hypertrophy are an R/S ratio of greater than 1 in lead V_1 (i.e., R-wave voltage exceeds S-wave voltage).

Chest Radiography

Hyperinflation and increased vascular markings are usually present with COPD. Prominent lung markings often occur in bronchitis they are decreased in emphysema, particularly at the bases, where actual bullae may be present in severe cases. Hyperinflation, with an increased anteroposterior chest diameter, may be present, together with an enlarged retrosternal air space of >2 cm in diameter seen in a lateral chest radiograph.

The location of the lung lesion should be assessed by posteroanterior and lateral projections on chest radiography. In addition to tracheal or carinal shift, a mediastinal mass may indicate difficulty with ventilation, a difficult and bloody dissection, difficulty in placing a double-lumen tube (DLT; because of deviation of the main stem bronchus), or a collapsed lobe owing to bronchial obstruction with possible sepsis. Review of a computed tomography (CT) study is also useful, and often provides more information about tumor size and location than the chest radiograph.

Arterial Blood Gas Analysis

A common finding in arterial blood gas analysis of patients with COPD is hypoventilation and CO_2 retention. The "blue bloaters" (chronic bronchitis) are cyanotic, hypercarbic, hypoxemic, and usually overweight. They are in a state of chronic respiratory failure and have a decreased ventilatory response to CO_2. In these patients, the high $Paco_2$ increases cerebrospinal fluid bicarbonate concentration, the medullary chemoreceptors become reset to a higher level of CO_2, and sensitivity to CO_2 is decreased. Such patients hypoventilate when given high oxygen concentrations to breathe because of a decreased hypoxic drive.

The "pink puffers" (patients with emphysema) are typically thin, dyspneic, and pink, with essentially normal arterial blood gas values. They present with an increase in minute ventilation to maintain their normal $Paco_2$, which explains the increase in work of breathing and dyspnea. The preoperative Pao_2 correlates with the intraoperative Pao_2 during one-lung ventilation (OLV), but the intraoperative Pao_2 during two-lung ventilation correlates more closely.[8]

Pulmonary Function Testing and Evaluation for Lung Resectability

There are three goals in performing pulmonary function tests in a patient scheduled for lung resection. The first goal is to identify the patient at risk of increased postoperative morbidity and mortality. In thoracic surgery for lung cancer, the specific question is: How much lung tissue may be safely removed without making the patient a pulmonary cripple? This should be weighed against the 1-year mean survival rate of the patient with surgically untreated lung carcinoma. The second goal is to identify the patient who will need short-term or long-term postoperative ventilatory support. The third goal is to evaluate the beneficial effect and reversibility of airway obstruction with the use of bronchodilators.

Effects of Anesthesia and Surgery on Lung Volumes

Anesthesia and postoperative medications can cause changes in lung volumes and ventilatory pattern. Total lung capacity (TLC) decreases after abdominal surgery but not after surgery on an extremity. Vital capacity is decreased by 25% to 50% within 1 to 2 days after surgery and generally returns to normal after 1 to 2 weeks. Residual volume (RV) increases by 13%, whereas expiratory reserve volume decreases by 25% after lower abdominal surgery and 60% after upper abdominal and thoracic surgery. Tidal volume (V_T) decreases by 20% within 24 hours after surgery and gradually returns to normal after 2 weeks. Pulmonary compliance decreases by 33% with similar reductions in functional residual capacity (FRC) secondary to small airway closure. Most of the patients who undergo lung resection are smokers with a certain degree of COPD they are prone to postoperative complications in direct relation to the amount of lung to be resected (lobectomy or pneumonectomy) and to the severity of the preoperative lung disease.

Spirometry

2 Forced vital capacity (FVC), forced expired volume in 1 second (FEV_1), maximum voluntary ventilation (MVV), and RV/TLC correlate with outcome following thoracic surgery[9] (see Chapter 11). An abnormal preoperative vital capacity can be identified in 30% to 40% of postoperative deaths. A patient with an abnormal vital capacity has a 33% likelihood of complications and a 10% risk of postoperative mortality.

FEV_1 is a more direct indication of airway obstruction. In the past, an FEV_1 of <800 mL in a 70-kg man had been considered an absolute contraindication to lung resection. However, with the advent of thoracoscopic surgery and improved postoperative pain management, patients with smaller lung volumes are now successfully undergoing surgery. It is preferable to indicate the percentage of predicted value, rather than just using the actual results in liters. The percentage of predicted value takes into account the age and size of the patient, and the same number may have a different implication in another patient. The ratio FEV_1/FVC is useful in differentiating between restrictive and obstructive pulmonary diseases. It is normal in restrictive disease because both FEV_1 and FVC decrease, whereas in obstructive disease the ratio is usually low because the FEV_1 is markedly decreased. MVV is a nonspecific test and is an indicator of both restriction and obstruction. Although MVV has not been systematically evaluated as a predictor of morbidity, it is generally accepted that an MVV <50% of predicted value is an indication of high risk. A ratio of RV to TLC (RV/TLC) of >50% is generally indicative of a high-risk patient for pulmonary resection. By multiplying the preoperative FEV_1 by the percentage of lung tissue expected to remain following resection, a predicted postoperative FEV_1 can be calculated. Patients with a predicted postoperative FEV_1 value >40% are at reduced risk and those with predicted postoperative FEV_1 <30% are at increased risk.[10] Those patients who fall into the latter category are more likely to need postoperative ventilation.

Flow–Volume Loops

The flow–volume loop displays essentially the same information as a spirometer but is more convenient for measurement of specific flow rates (Fig. 37-2). The shape and peak airflow rates during expiration at high lung volumes are effort dependent, but indicate the patency of the larger airways. Effort-independent expiration occurs at low lung volumes and usually reflects small airway resistance, best measured by forced expiratory flow (FEF) during the middle half of the FVC ($FEF_{25-75\%}$).

In general, patients with obstructive airway disease (Fig. 37-3), such as asthma, bronchitis, and emphysema, have grossly decreased FEV_1/FVC ratios because of increased airway resistance

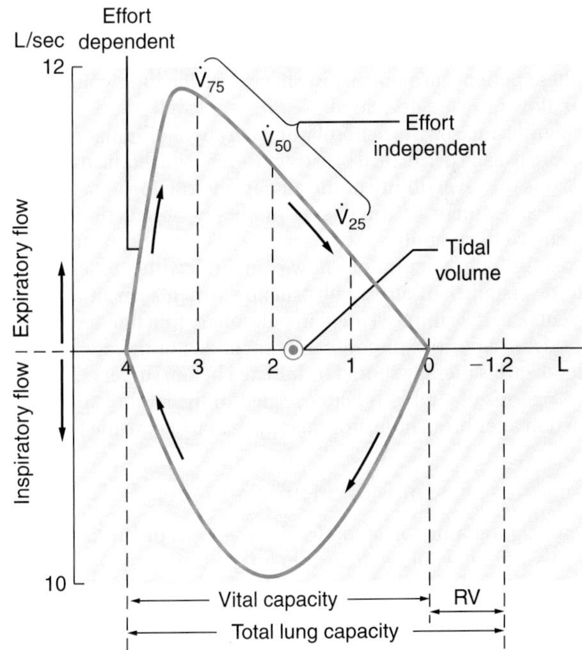

FIGURE 37-2. Flow–volume loop in a normal subject. $\dot{V}_{75}$, $\dot{V}_{50}$, and $\dot{V}_{25}$ represent flow at 75%, 50%, and 25% of vital capacity, respectively. RV, residual volume. (Reproduced from: Goudsouzian N, Karamanian A. *Physiology for the Anesthesiologist,* 2nd edition. Norwalk, CT: Appleton-Century-Crofts; 1984, with permission.)

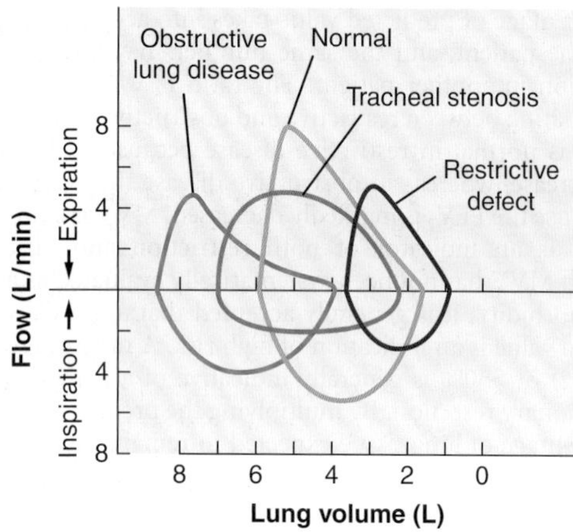

FIGURE 37-3. Flow–volume loops relative to lung volumes in a normal subject, in a patient with COPD, in a patient with fixed obstruction (tracheal stenosis), and in a patient with pulmonary fibrosis (restrictive defect). Note the concave expiratory form in the patient with COPD and the flat inspiratory curve in the patient with a fixed obstruction. (Reprinted from: Goudsouzian N, Karamanian A. *Physiology for the Anesthesiologist,* 2nd edition. Norwalk, CT: Appleton-Century-Crofts; 1984, with permission.)

and a decrease in FEV_1. Peak expiratory flow rate and MVV are usually decreased, whereas TLC increases secondary to increases in RV. In these patients, the effort-independent portion of the flow–volume curve is markedly depressed inward, with reduction of the flow rate at 25% to 75% of FVC.

In patients with restrictive disease (Fig. 37-3), such as pulmonary fibrosis and scoliosis, there is a decrease in FVC with a relatively normal FEV_1. Because the airway resistance is normal, FEV_1/FVC is also normal. TLC is markedly decreased, whereas MVV and $FEF_{25-75\%}$ are usually normal. The flow–volume curves of these patients are normal in shape, but the lung volumes and peak flow rates are decreased.

Significance of Bronchodilator Therapy. Pulmonary function tests are usually performed before and after bronchodilator therapy to assess the reversibility of the airway obstruction. This is useful in the assessment of the degree of airway obstruction and the patient's effort ability. After treatment with bronchodilators, increases in peak expiratory flow compared with a baseline indicate reversibility of airway obstruction (often seen in asthmatic patients). A 15% improvement in pulmonary function tests may be considered a positive response to bronchodilator therapy and indicates that this therapy should be initiated before surgery. The overall prognosis of COPD is better related to the level of spirometric function after bronchodilator therapy than to a baseline function.

Split-lung Function Tests

Regional lung function studies serve to predict the function of the lung tissue that would remain after lung resection. A whole (two)-lung test may fail to estimate whether the amount of postresection lung tissue will allow the patient to function at a reasonable level of activity without disabling dyspnea or cor pulmonale.

Regional Perfusion Test. This involves the intravenous injection of insoluble radioactive xenon (^{133}Xe). The peak radioactivity of each lung is proportional to the degree of perfusion of each lung.

Regional Ventilation Test. Using an inhaled, insoluble radioactive gas, the peak radioactivity over each lung is proportional to the degree of ventilation. Combining radiospirometry with whole-lung testing (FEV_1, FVC, maximal breathing capacity) has resulted in a fair degree of correlation between predicted volumes and pulmonary function tests measured after pneumonectomy.

Computed Tomography and Positron Emission Tomography Scans. Patients normally undergo CT scanning. The CT scan provides anatomic sections through the chest and can delineate the size of the tumor. It can also reveal if there is airway or cardiovascular compression.

Positron emission tomography (PET) scans use a glucose analog that is labeled with a radionuclide positron emitter. This scan can detect tumor based on the metabolic activity. Because malignant tumors are growing at such a fast rate compared with healthy tissue, the tumor cells will use up more of the sugar that has the radionuclide attached to it. There is greater uptake by malignant mediastinal lymph nodes than benign nodes. PET may be more accurate than CT for mediastinal staging.[11] Currently, PET scans can be used to further evaluate lesions that are seen on a CT scan. The PET scan can also be used to follow the results of lung cancer treatments.[12]

The CT and PET scans can be done at the same time to produce a PET–CT scan. A mass that is seen on the CT scan is more likely to be malignant if it also demonstrates enhanced glucose uptake on the PET scan.

Diffusing Capacity for Carbon Monoxide

The ability of the lung to perform gas exchange is reflected by the diffusing capacity for carbon monoxide. It is impaired in such disorders as interstitial lung disease, which affects the alveolar-capillary site. A predicted postoperative diffusing capacity for carbon monoxide <40% is associated with increased risk. Predicted postoperative diffusing capacity percent is the strongest single predictor of risk of complications and mortality after lung resection. There is little interrelationship of predicted postoperative diffusing capacity percent and predicted postoperative FEV_1, indicating that these values should be assessed independently when estimating operative risk.[13] In a recent study of 956 patients, a lower D_{LCO} ppo (diffusing capacity for carbon monoxide, predicted postoperative) and the preoperative administration of chemotherapy, were found to be predictive of postoperative complications. In that study, FEV_1 was not found to be predictive of complications.[14] In another study, the D_{LCO} ppo was the most predictive factor for postoperative morbidity and mortality.[15]

Maximal Oxygen Consumption. The maximal oxygen consumption (VO_2 max) is a predictor of postoperative complications. Patients with a VO_2 max >15 to 20 mL/kg/min are at reduced risk.[16] A VO_2 max <10 mL/kg/min indicates very high risk for lung resection.[15,17] A simpler test that can be performed is exercise oximetry—a decrease of 4% during exercise is associated with increased risk.[18] A 6-minute walk test <2,000 feet has been correlated both with a VO_2 max <15 mL/kg/min and with a decrease in oximetry reading during exercise. It has been suggested that the percentage of predicted VO_2 max may be a better indicator for risk, and a threshold of 50% to 60% could be established without an increase in surgical mortality.[19] Brunelli and Fianchini[20] had patients climb the maximum number of stairs possible. On the basis of the results of this study, these authors recommended that patients who were able to climb >14 m can safely undergo surgery, and those who were able to climb <12 m, with predicted postoperative function FEV_1 <35% not be considered for major lung resection. The inability to do a maximal stair climbing has been correlated with an increased mortality following major lung resection.[21] The preoperative evaluation of the patient for lung resection is summarized in Figure 37-4.

Whole-lung function

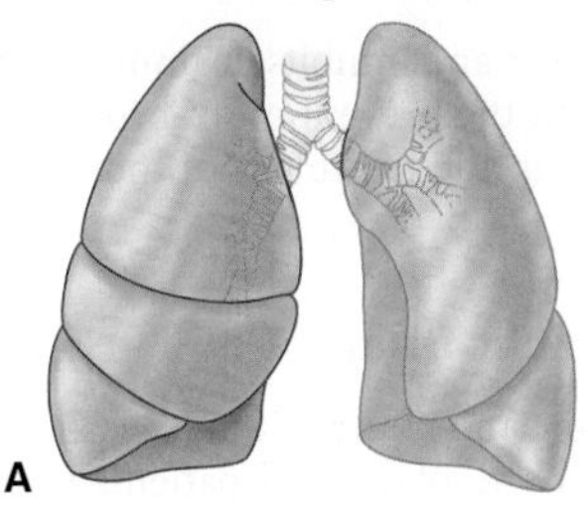

Split-lung function

1. Split-lung spirometry with DLT
2. Regional lung radiospirometry
   Regional perfusion (^{133}Xe, ^{131}I-MAA)
   Regional ventilation ^{133}Xe

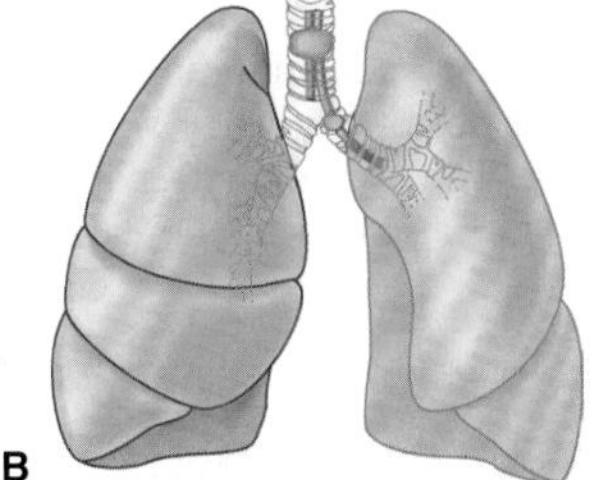

FIGURE 37-4. The order of tests to determine the cardiopulmonary status of the patient and the extent of lung resection that would be tolerated. **A:** The whole-lung function test is a basic screening test. **B:** The split-lung function tests are regional tests to determine the involvement of the diseased lung to be removed. ABG, arterial blood gas; FVC, forced vital capacity; FEV_1, forced expiratory volume in 1 second; VC, vital capacity; MVV, maximum voluntary ventilation; RV/TLC, residual volume/total lung capacity; DLT, double-lumen tube. D_LCO, diffusing capacity for carbon monoxide (Adapted from: Neustein SM, Cohen E. Preoperative evaluation of thoracic surgical patients. In: Cohen E, ed. *The Practice of Thoracic Anesthesia*. Philadelphia: JB Lippincott; 1995:187, with permission.)

PREOPERATIVE PREPARATION

The wide spectrum of physiologic changes that occur during thoracic surgery puts patients at great risk of developing postoperative complications. Morbidity and mortality increase when these changes are superimposed on an acutely or chronically compromised patient. Several conditions, including infection, dehydration, electrolyte imbalance, wheezing, obesity, cigarette smoking, cor pulmonale, and malnutrition, show particular correlations with postoperative complications. Proper, vigorous preoperative preparation can improve the patient's ability to face the surgery with a decreased risk of morbidity and mortality. It is important that conditions predisposing to postoperative complications be rigorously treated before surgery.

Smoking

There is a high prevalence of smoking among patients presenting for surgery, and there is extensive evidence that these patients are at increased risk for development of postoperative respiratory complications.[3] Approximately 33% of adult patients presenting for surgery are smokers, and there is extensive evidence that they are at increased risk for development of postoperative respiratory
3 complications.[22] Smoking increases airway irritability, decreases mucociliary transport, decreases FVC and $FEF_{25-75\%}$, and increases secretions, thereby increasing the incidence of postoperative pulmonary complications. In contrast, cessation of smoking for a period of longer than 4 to 6 weeks before surgery is associated with a decreased incidence of postoperative complications.[22] Furthermore, cessation of smoking 48 hours before surgery has been shown to decrease the percentage of carboxyhemoglobin, to shift the oxyhemoglobin dissociation curve to the right, and to increase oxygen availability. It should be emphasized, however, that most of the beneficial effects of cessation of smoking, such as improvement in ciliary function, improvement in closing volume, increase in $FEF_{25-75\%}$, and reduction in sputum production, usually occur 2 to 3 months after smoking has ceased. In one study, there was no evidence of a paradoxical increase in postoperative complications in patients who stopped smoking within 2 months before undergoing thoracic resection for lung tumor.[23] Smoking is associated with increased mortality and pulmonary complications, but these can be decreased by preoperative cessation; the risk decreases with a longer cessation.[24]

Infection

Acute or chronic infection should be vigorously treated before surgery. Broad-spectrum antibiotics are commonly used. Treatment of the acutely ill patient depends on the results of the Gram stain of the sputum and blood cultures. Unless there are other modifying circumstances such as allergic history or patients are already receiving antibiotics, cefazolin is routinely administered perioperatively. To be most effective, it needs to be given prior to skin incision.[25] In one prospective study, the incidence of mortality was lower in the group treated with prophylactic antibiotics compared with the untreated group (9% vs. 17%), and a lower incidence of postoperative pulmonary infection was also found.[26] Although not all surgeons routinely administer antibiotics prophylactically to their patients, any infection present before surgery should be vigorously treated.

Hydration and Removal of Bronchial Secretions

Correction of hypovolemia and electrolyte imbalance should be accomplished before surgery because adequate hydration decreases the viscosity of bronchial secretions and facilitates their removal from the bronchial tree. Humidification of inspired gas is extremely useful. The use of mucolytic drugs, such as acetylcysteine (Mucomyst), or oral expectorants (potassium iodide) can be beneficial to patients with viscous secretions. Commonly used methods for removing secretions from the bronchial tree include postural drainage, vigorous coughing, chest percussion, deep breathing, and the use of an incentive spirometer. These modalities often require patient cooperation and frequent verbal encouragement to maximize the benefit.

Wheezing and Bronchodilation

The presence of acute wheezing represents a medical emergency, and elective surgery should be postponed until effective treatment has been instituted. Chronic wheezing is often seen in patients with COPD and is attributable to the presence of gas flow obstruction secondary to smooth muscle contraction, accumulation of secretions, and mucosal edema. Smooth muscle contraction may occur in small airways only (detectable by changes in $FEF_{25-75\%}$) or may be widespread, with a large reduction of FEV_1 and FVC. The efficacy of bronchodilators in reversing the bronchospastic component is extremely important. A trial of bronchodilators and measurement of their effects on pulmonary function should be performed in any patient who shows evidence of air flow obstruction. Several classes of bronchodilators are available.

Sympathomimetic Drugs

Sympathomimetic drugs increase the formation of 3′,5′-cyclic adenosine monophosphate (cAMP). The balance between cAMP, which produces bronchodilation, and cyclic guanosine monophosphate, which produces bronchoconstriction, determines the state of contraction of the bronchial smooth muscle. Increasing cAMP production therefore causes relaxation of the bronchial tree. Sympathomimetic drugs, such as epinephrine, isoproterenol, isoetharine, and ephedrine, all have mixed β_1 and β_2 sympathetic agonist effects. The β_1 (cardiac effects) of these drugs are often undesirable in patients with COPD. Selective β_2 sympathomimetic drugs, such as albuterol, terbutaline, and metaproterenol, given as inhaled aerosols, are the preferred drugs for the treatment of bronchospasm, particularly in patients with cardiac disease.

Phosphodiesterase Inhibitors

Phosphodiesterase inhibitors inhibit the breakdown of cAMP by cytoplasmic phosphodiesterase. The methylxanthines, such as aminophylline, increase the level of cAMP, resulting in bronchodilation. In addition, aminophylline improves diaphragmatic contractility and increases the patient's resistance to fatigue. Therapeutic blood levels of aminophylline are 5 to 20 μg/mL and can be achieved by infusing a loading dose of 5 to 7 mg/kg over 20 minutes, followed by a continuous intravenous infusion of 0.5 to 0.7 mg/kg/hr. Aminophylline may cause ventricular dysrhythmias, and this side effect should be borne in mind when treating patients who have myocardial ischemia. Because newer medications have fewer side effects; aminophylline is now rarely used.

Steroids

Although not true bronchodilators, steroids are traditionally considered to decrease mucosal edema and may prevent the release of bronchoconstricting substances. They are of questionable benefit in acute bronchospasm. Steroids may be administered orally, parenterally, or in aerosol form, such as beclomethasone by inhaler.

Cromolyn Sodium

Cromolyn sodium stabilizes mast cells and inhibits degranulation and histamine release. It is useful in the prevention of bronchospastic attacks but is of little value in the treatment of the acute situation (see Chapter 12).

Parasympatholytic Drugs

Parasympatholytics include atropine and ipratropium (see Chapter 15). In the past, atropine has been avoided in patients with COPD and bronchitis because of the concern regarding increases in the viscosity of mucus produced by this agent. However, atropine blocks the formation of cyclic guanosine monophosphate and therefore has a bronchodilator effect.

Pulmonary Rehabilitation

Sekine et al.[26] reported that pulmonary rehabilitation led to reduced hospital stay and improved postoperative FEV_1, compared with a historical control group. The pulmonary rehabilitation included education in a variety of areas such as breathing, exercise, and nutrition.

INTRAOPERATIVE MONITORING

All patients undergoing anesthesia for thoracic surgical procedures require adherence to the Standards of Basic Anesthetic Monitoring American Society of Anesthesiologists (ASA) (see Chapter 25). In particular, these include an electrocardiogram (lead II and, if possible, V_5), chest or esophageal stethoscopes for heart and breath sound auscultation, and a temperature probe. A chest stethoscope may be placed over the dependent hemithorax to assess dependent lung ventilation. Pulse oximetry, which is a standard of care, is especially valuable during thoracic surgery because hypoxemia may occur during OLV.

Dysrhythmias occur commonly both during and after thoracic surgery, making the usual need for continuous electrocardiographic monitoring even more important. Intraoperative supraventricular tachyarrhythmias may be caused by cardiac manipulation. Dysrhythmias that occur during OLV may be a sign of inadequate oxygenation or ventilation. Postoperative dysrhythmias may be related to sympathetic nervous system stimulation from pain or to a decreased pulmonary vascular bed following lung resection. Patients who present for lung resection often have COPD due to cigarette smoking, have right-sided heart strain, and are prone to multifocal atrial tachyarrhythmias.

The axis of electrocardiogram lead II parallels that of the P wave, making this lead useful for dysrhythmia detection. The simultaneous monitoring of lead V_5 also allows for monitoring of anterolateral wall myocardial ischemia. The use of multiple leads increases the sensitivity for ischemia detection.[27] The following invasive monitors are also indicated and have led to marked improvements in patient care.

Direct Arterial Catheterization

Peripheral arterial catheterization has become an essential tool for the anesthesiologist in the management of patients undergoing major thoracic surgical procedures (see Chapter 25). It allows for continuous beat-to-beat measurement of blood pressure and frequent sampling for the determination of arterial blood gases.

Continuous blood pressure readings are critical during thoracic surgery because surgical manipulations may result in cardiac compression and there may be sudden bleeding. Immediate recognition of these changes allows time for proper identification of the etiology and the institution of appropriate treatment.

Serial arterial blood gas analyses are performed as needed in the management of patients undergoing one-lung anesthesia or during cases in which a part of the lung may be "packed away" for a period. Arterial hypoxemia may occur because of shunting of mixed venous through the collapsed lung and an inadequate hypoxic pulmonary vasoconstriction (HPV) response. Significant changes in acid–base status and hyperventilation or hypoventilation can also be identified.

A radial artery catheter (see Chapter 25) can be placed in either extremity during thoracic surgery. For a mediastinoscopic examination, one approach is to place the catheter in the right arm and to use it to monitor for possible compression of the innominate artery by the mediastinoscope. This can help avoid central nervous system complications that might result from inadequate cerebral blood flow via the right carotid artery (see "Mediastinoscopy"). The other approach would be to place the arterial catheter in the left radial artery, allowing for continuous blood pressure measurements, uninterrupted by innominate artery compression. If this is done, a pulse oximeter probe should be placed on the right upper extremity to monitor for innominate artery compression. During thoracotomy, placement of the arterial catheter in the dependent arm can be used to monitor for possible axillary artery compression, which may occur if the patient is not properly positioned. For a brief thoracoscopy case in a relatively healthy patient, it would be acceptable to proceed without an arterial catheter, as long as the pulse oximeter is functioning reliably. Such an example might be a healthy patient presenting for bilateral VAT sympathectomy for hyperhidrosis.

The patient undergoing a pulmonary resection, and especially a right pneumonectomy, is at risk for postoperative pulmonary edema. It is especially important to not fluid overload such a patient, as the likelihood of postoperative edema is greater with increased intraoperative fluid administration. Prior to its administration it would be preferable to be able to identify which patients would be likely to respond favorably to a fluid bolus. The central venous pressure (CVP) may not accurately reflect intravascular volume status, and is no longer recommended as a guide for fluid responsiveness.[28] Systolic pressure variation (SPV) and pulse pressure variation (PPV) have been reported as being able to predict fluid responsiveness.[29] In a recent paper, a PPV greater than 13% predicted fluid responsiveness, less than 9% predicted that the patient would not be responsive, and 9% to 13% reflected a gray zone.[30] Stroke volume variation has been reported to predict fluid responsiveness, specifically in patients undergoing thoracic surgery, during OLV.[31]

Central Venous Pressure Monitoring

The CVP may reflect the patient's blood volume, venous tone, and right ventricular performance; however, it is also affected by central venous obstructions and alterations of intrathoracic pressure such as PEEP (see Chapter 25). The CVP reflects right-sided heart function, not left ventricular performance. Catheters for measuring CVP may be placed for thoracotomies, and in particular, patients undergoing pneumonectomy. Uses of CVP catheters or large-bore introducers include (1) insertion of a transvenous pacemaker where necessary, (2) infusion of vasoactive drugs, and (3) insertion of a pulmonary artery (PA) catheter, which may subsequently be required during surgery or in the postoperative period. A recent study in healthy subjects indicated that, contrary to common belief, the CVP did not reflect intravascular volume status.[32]

The CVP catheter can be placed centrally from either the external or the internal jugular vein, from the subclavian veins, or from one of the arm veins. The success rate is highest using the right internal jugular vein, and a pacemaker or PA catheter can be inserted most easily from this vein. The major disadvantage of using the external jugular vein during thoracotomy is that the catheter often kinks when the patient is turned to the lateral decubitus position. The subclavian technique leads to a higher incidence of pneumothorax, which can be disastrous if it occurs in the dependent lung during OLV. If necessary and if possible, a subclavian catheter should be placed ipsilateral to the surgery. As discussed above, the CVP is no longer considered an accurate guide for fluid responsiveness. However, it is a common practice among thoracic anesthesiologists to place a CVP catheter for certain thoracic cases such as esophagectomy and pneumonectomy.

Pulmonary Artery Catheterization

The PA catheter is most reliably inserted through the right internal jugular vein using a modified Seldinger technique (see Chapter 25). Insertion of the PA catheter through either the external jugular vein or the subclavian vein often leads to obstruction of the catheter when the patient is placed in the lateral decubitus position. Misinterpretation of data from a PA catheter is a real risk in a patient with cardiac and pulmonary diseases undergoing thoracic surgery with OLV. These errors can be produced by altered ventilatory modes, the location of the PA catheter tip, ventricular compliance changes, or ventricular interdependence.[33] A major limitation of the PA catheter is the assumption that the pulmonary capillary wedge pressure (PCWP) provides a good approximation of left ventricular end-diastolic volume. The use of PCWP directly to assess preload assumes a linear relationship between ventricular end-diastolic volume and ventricular end-diastolic pressure. However, alterations in ventricular compliance affect this pressure–volume relationship during surgery. Decreases in ventricular compliance can occur with myocardial ischemia, shock, right ventricular overload, or pericardial effusion. Numerous investigators have demonstrated a poor correlation between PCWP and left ventricular end-diastolic volume in acutely ill patients.[34] This correlation is further worsened by the application of PEEP. In addition, ventricular interdependence can cause misdiagnosis when the interventricular septum encroaches on the left ventricular cavity, leading to increased values of PCWP. A PCWP associated with a decreased cardiac output can be interpreted as left ventricular failure, when in fact, left ventricular end-diastolic volume may not be increased but decreased because of compression of the left ventricle by a distended right ventricle. This situation can occur with acute respiratory failure and high levels of PEEP. Techniques such as echocardiography, which directly measure ventricular dimensions, may facilitate resolution of this complex situation.

Because most of the pulmonary blood flow is to the right lower lobe, the tip of a flow-directed PA catheter is usually located in the right lower lobe. During a left thoracotomy with OLV, the catheter tip would then be in the dependent lung and should provide accurate hemodynamic measurements. However, during a right thoracotomy with OLV, the catheter tip would most likely be in the nondependent lung, and may not be accurate. The use of intraoperative mean pulmonary artery pressure has been reported to be an indicator of safety for lung resection under thoracotomy.[35] The authors concluded that following occlusion of the main PA, upper safety limits of 33 mm Hg for right, and 35 mm Hg for left thoracotomy could be used. The authors noted that the difference between sides was minimal, and less than expected. The monitoring of $S\bar{v}o_2$ has been evaluated in patients undergoing one-lung anesthesia.[36] Changes in $S\bar{v}o_2$ were mainly dependent on changes in Sao_2. Currently, the use of the PA catheter for monitoring during thoracic surgery is generally unnecessary, and may be reserved for patients with pulmonary hypertension.

Transesophageal Echocardiography

Transesophageal echocardiography (TEE) is a useful intraoperative monitor for ventricular function, valvular function, and wall motion changes that might reflect ischemia (see Chapter 26). Its use in thoracic surgical patients has been limited, but it is widely used in patients undergoing lung transplant. The use of TEE requires special training, and may not be available at all centers. A recent review concluded that although the intraoperative use of TEE is not routinely indicated, it may be useful for diagnosing right ventricular dysfunction, in the setting of hypotension or arrhythmias following lung resection.[37] Right ventricular dysfunction may occur during OLV, clamping of the pulmonary artery for either pneumonectomy, or during lung transplantation. TEE may be used to help determine if it is necessary to utilize cardiopulmonary bypass during lung transplantation.[38]

TEE may be useful in visualizing hilar lung tumors, and evaluating possible extension into the heart. In one study, central lung tumors were seen with TEE in nine of the nine patients, peripheral lung tumors in one of the three patients, and an anterior mediastinal mass in one of one patient.[39] In this study, TEE revealed PA compression in five patients and PA infiltration in two patients. In another study investigating echocardiographic recognition of mediastinal tumors, TEE revealed that the tumors were often adjacent to the heart and identified those patients in whom there was compression of the innominate vein or PA, or infiltration of the heart.[40]

Intraoperative TEE has also revealed tumor invasion of the heart, indicating that a resection by thoracotomy without cardiopulmonary bypass was not feasible.[41] In one case report, TEE monitoring during an attempted resection of a tumor invading the left atrium showed embolization of the tumor.[42] Fragments of the tumor were seen to pass through the aortic valve. This patient subsequently died of disseminated metastases. In an exploratory thoracotomy for hemothorax, intraoperative TEE revealed the presence of a subacute aortic dissection, which was believed to be the cause of the hemothorax.[43] TEE was used intraoperatively to evaluate a large anterior mediastinal mass, providing data on right ventricular outflow compression, and ventricular contractility and filling status.[44] In another recent report, a mediastinal mass was diagnosed intraoperatively using TEE; in that case, the mass had been misdiagnosed preoperatively with transthoracic echocardiography as a pericardial effusion.[45]

Additional Noninvasive Monitoring

Although data are presently limited, it has been reported that decreased cerebral oximetry values by absolute cerebral oximetry during OLV have been correlated with postoperative complications.[46] In a subsequent study, the larger decreases in cerebral oxygen saturation occurred in patients with better preoperative lung function.[47] At this time, the data are still too limited to recommend cerebral oximetry as a routine monitor during thoracic surgery.

A recent meta-analysis of the use of noninvasive cardiac output measurements during surgery revealed poor agreement with thermodilution. Noninvasive cardiac output measurements are not commonly utilized during thoracic surgery.[48] The use of noninvasive cardiac output monitoring for thoracic surgery is not recommended at this time.

Monitoring of Oxygenation and Ventilation

Oxygenation

During the administration of all thoracic surgical anesthetics, the concentration of inspired oxygen in the breathing system must be measured using an oxygen analyzer with a low oxygen concentration limit alarm (see Chapter 24). Such analyzers vary in sophistication from fuel cells to rapidly responding paramagnetic analyzers that monitor oxygen breath-by-breath and display an oxygram (analogous to, and a mirror image of, the capnogram). Adequacy of blood oxygenation must also be ensured, and adequate illumination and exposure of the patient are helpful to assess the color of shed blood or the presence of cyanosis of the lips, nail beds, or mucous membranes. Most patients undergoing thoracic surgical or diagnostic procedures have an arterial catheter in place for continuous monitoring of blood pressure and sampling of arterial blood for blood gas analyses.

Pulse oximetry is now a standard of care for noninvasive assessment of blood oxygenation. The use of pulse oximetry is especially important during OLV, when rapid assessment of oxygenation is critical. A low Spo_2 reading provides the clinician with an indication for blood gas sampling and laboratory analysis of arterial blood. The traditional two-wavelength pulse oximeter may display spurious readings of Spo_2 in the presence of dyshemoglobins, methemoglobin and carboxyhemoglobin. Multiwavelength (8 or 12 wavelengths) pulse oximeters are now commercially available that are capable of measuring carboxyhemoglobin, methemoglobin, deoxygenated hemoglobin, and oxygenated hemoglobin ($HbO_2\%$).[49,50] In addition, continuous monitoring of total hemoglobin concentration is now available.[51]

Ventilation

All patients must be continually monitored to ensure adequacy of ventilation. Monitoring includes qualitative signs such as chest excursion (visual observation of the lungs when the chest is open) and auscultation of breath sounds. In addition, during OLV, a stethoscope can be placed on the chest wall under the ventilated dependent lung. During controlled ventilation, circuit low-pressure and high-pressure alarms with an audible signal must be used. The respiratory rate, V_T, minute volume, and inflation pressures should be observed.

Adequacy of ventilation should be confirmed by monitoring arterial blood gas analyses and $Paco_2$, in particular. This may be estimated continuously and noninvasively by using a capnograph (see Chapter 25). The end-tidal CO_2 concentration represents alveolar CO_2 ($P_{A}CO_2$), which approximates $Paco_2$. There is normally a small arterial-to-alveolar CO_2 difference (4 to 6 mm Hg), depending on alveolar dead space. The capnogram waveform is also helpful in diagnosing airway obstruction, incomplete relaxation,[52] and even malposition of the DLT.[53] During OLV, systemic hypoxemia is usually a greater problem than hypercarbia.[54] This is because CO_2 is approximately 20 times more diffusible than oxygen and $Paco_2$ is more dependent on ventilation, compared with Pao_2, which is more dependent on perfusion.

Physiology of One-lung Ventilation

Physiology of the Lateral Decubitus Position. Ventilation and blood flow in the upright position are discussed in Chapters 11

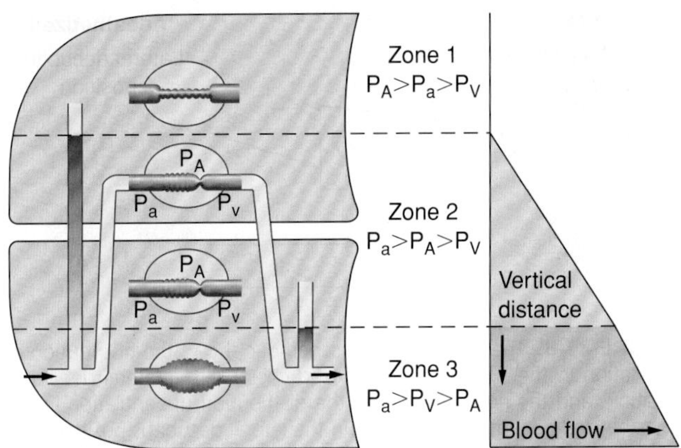

FIGURE 37-5. Schematic representation of the effects of gravity on the distribution of pulmonary blood flow in the lateral decubitus position. Vertical gradients in the lateral decubitus position are similar to those in the upright position and cause the creation of West zones 1, 2, and 3. Consequently, pulmonary blood flow increases with lung dependency, and is largest in the dependent lung and least in the nondependent lung. P_a, pulmonary artery pressure; P_A, alveolar pressure; P_v, pulmonary venous pressure. (From: Benumof JL. Physiology of the open-chest and one lung ventilation. *Thoracic Anesthesia.* New York, NY: Churchill Livingstone; 1983:288, with permission.)

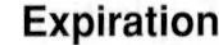

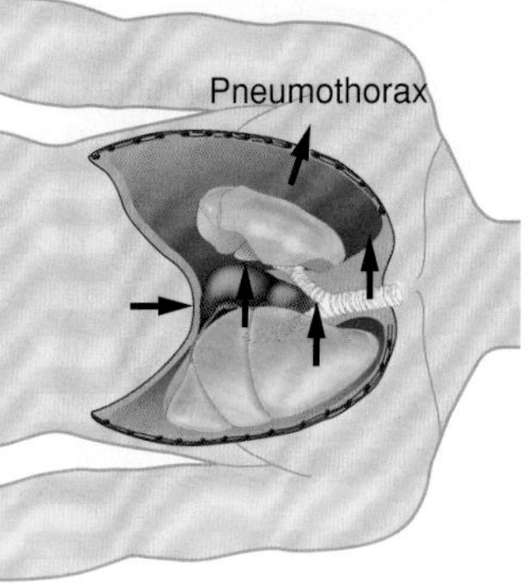

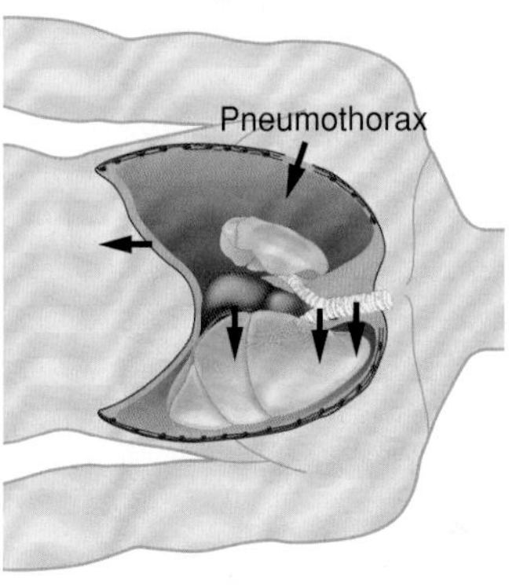

FIGURE 37-6. Schematic representation of mediastinal shift in the spontaneously breathing, open-chested patient in the lateral decubitus position. During inspiration, negative pressure in the intact hemithorax causes the mediastinum to move downward. During expiration, relative positive pressure in the intact hemithorax causes the mediastinum to move upward. (From: Tarhan S, Moffitt EA. Principles of thoracic anesthesia. *Surg Clin North Am.* 1973;53:813, with permission.)

and 28. These variables will now be considered as they pertain to the lateral decubitus position under six circumstances that are encountered during thoracic surgery.

Lateral position, awake, breathing spontaneously, chest closed. In the lateral decubitus position, the distribution of blood flow and ventilation is similar to that in the upright position, but turned by 90 degrees (Fig. 37-5). Blood flow and ventilation to the dependent lung are significantly greater than that to the nondependent lung. Good $\dot{V}/\dot{Q}$ matching at the level of the dependent lung results in adequate oxygenation in the awake patient who is breathing spontaneously. There are two important concepts in this situation. First, because perfusion is gravity-dependent, the vertical hydrostatic pressure gradient is smaller in the lateral than in the upright position; therefore, zone 1 is usually less extended. Second, in regard to ventilation, the dependent hemidiaphragm is pushed higher into the chest by the abdominal contents compared with the nondependent lung hemidiaphragm. During spontaneous ventilation, the conserved ability of the dependent diaphragm to contract results in an adequate distribution of V_T to the dependent lung. Because most of the perfusion is to the dependent lung, the $\dot{V}/\dot{Q}$ matching in this position is maintained similar to that in the upright position.

Lateral Position, Awake, Breathing Spontaneously, Chest Open. Controlled positive-pressure ventilation is the most common way to provide adequate ventilation and ensure gas exchange in an open-chest situation. Frequently, thoracoscopy is performed using intercostal blocks with the patient breathing spontaneously to allow proper lung examination. The thoracoscope provides an adequate seal of the open chest to prevent a "free" open-chest situation. Two complications can arise from the patient breathing spontaneously with an open chest. The first is mediastinal shift, usually occurring during inspiration (Fig. 37-6). The negative pressure in the intact hemithorax, compared with the less negative pressure of the open hemithorax, can cause the mediastinum to move vertically downward and push into the dependent hemithorax. The mediastinal shift can create circulatory and reflex changes that may result in a clinical picture similar to that of shock and respiratory distress. Sometimes, depending on the severity of the distress, the patient needs to be tracheally intubated immediately, with initiation of positive-pressure ventilation, and the anesthesiologist must be prepared to intubate in this position without disturbing the surgical field.

The second phenomenon is paradoxical breathing (Fig. 37-7). During inspiration, the relatively negative pressure in the intact hemithorax compared with atmospheric pressure in the open hemithorax can cause movement of air from the nondependent lung into the dependent lung. The opposite occurs during expiration. This gas movement reversal from one lung to the other represents wasted ventilation and can compromise the adequacy of gas exchange. Paradoxical breathing is increased by a large thoracotomy or by an increase in airway resistance in the dependent lung. Positive-pressure ventilation or adequate sealing of the open chest eliminates paradoxical breathing.

Lateral Position, Anesthetized, Breathing Spontaneously, Chest Closed. The induction of general anesthesia does not cause significant change in the distribution of blood flow, but it has an important impact on the distribution of ventilation. Most of the V_T enters the nondependent lung, and this results in a significant $\dot{V}/\dot{Q}$mismatch. Induction of general anesthesia causes a reduction in the volumes of both lungs secondary to a reduction in FRC. Any reduction in volume in the dependent lung is of a greater magnitude

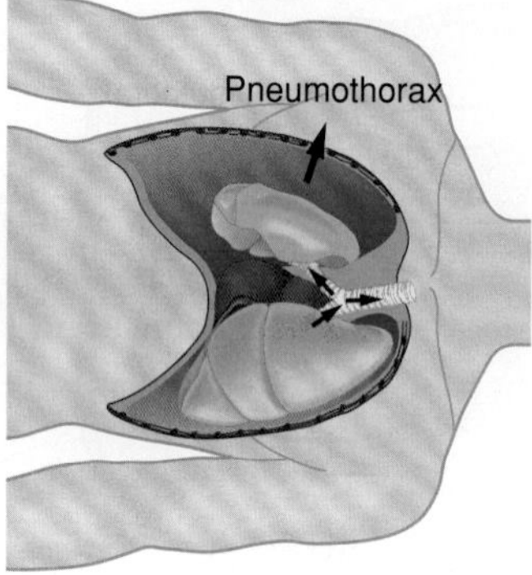

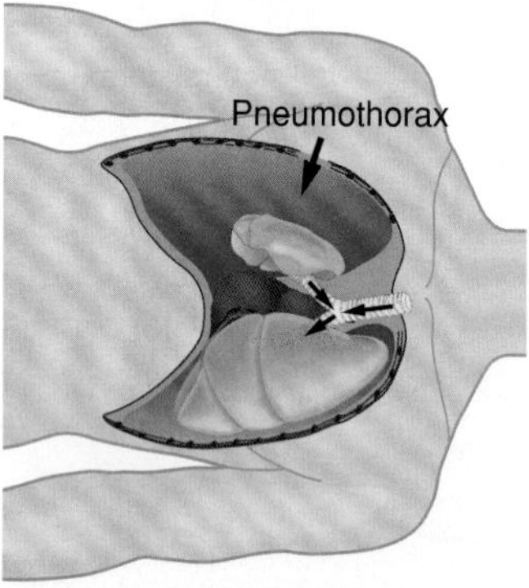

FIGURE 37-7. Schematic representation of paradoxical respiration in the spontaneously breathing, open-chested patient in the lateral decubitus position. During inspiration, movement of gas from the exposed lung into the intact lung and movement of air from the environment into the open hemithorax cause collapse of the exposed lung. During expiration, the reverse occurs, and the exposed lung expands. (From: Tarhan S, Moffitt EA. Principles of thoracic anesthesia. *Surg Clin North Am.* 1973;53:813, with permission.)

than that in the nondependent lung for several reasons. First, the cephalad displacement of the dependent diaphragm by the abdominal contents is more pronounced and is increased by paralysis. Second, the mediastinal structures pressing on the dependent lung or poor positioning of the dependent side on the operating table prevents the lung from expanding properly. The aforementioned factors will move lungs to a lower volume on the S-shaped volume–pressure curve (Fig. 37-8). The nondependent lung moves to a steeper position on the compliance curve and receives most of the V_T, whereas the dependent lung is on the flat (noncompliant) part of the curve.

Lateral Position, Anesthetized, Breathing Spontaneously, Chest Open. Opening the chest has little impact on the distribution of perfusion. However, the upper lung is now no longer restricted by the chest wall and is free to expand, resulting in a further increase in $\dot{V}/\dot{Q}$ mismatch as the nondependent lung is preferentially ventilated, owing to a now increased compliance.

Lateral position, anesthetized, paralyzed, chest open. During paralysis and positive-pressure ventilation, diaphragmatic displacement is maximal over the nondependent lung, where there is the least amount of resistance to diaphragmatic movement caused by the abdominal contents (Fig. 37-9). This further

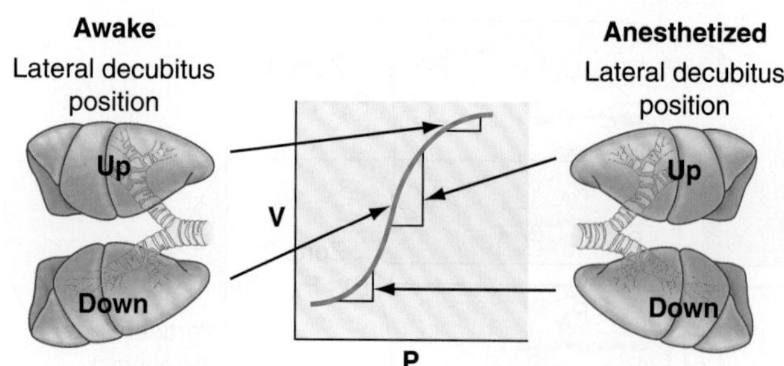

FIGURE 37-8. The left side of the schematic shows the distribution of ventilation in the awake patient (closed chest) in the lateral decubitus position, and the right side shows the distribution of ventilation in the anesthetized patient (closed chest) in the lateral decubitus position. The induction of anesthesia has caused a loss in lung volume in both lungs, with the nondependent (up) lung moving from a flat, noncompliant portion to a steep, compliant portion of the pressure–volume curve, and the dependent (down) lung moving from a steep, compliant part to a flat, noncompliant part of the pressure–volume curve. Thus, the anesthetized patient in the lateral decubitus position has most tidal ventilation in the nondependent lung (where there is the least perfusion) and less tidal ventilation in the dependent lung (where there is the most perfusion). V, volume; P, pressure. (From: Benumof JL. *Anesthesia for Thoracic Surgery.* Philadelphia, PA: WB Saunders; 1987:112, with permission.)

compromises the ventilation to the dependent lung and increases the $\dot{V}/\dot{Q}$ mismatch.

OLV, anesthetized, paralyzed, chest open. During two-lung ventilation in the lateral position, the mean blood flow to the nondependent lung is assumed to be 40% of cardiac output, whereas 60% of cardiac output goes to the dependent lung (Fig. 37-10). Normally, venous admixture (shunt) in the lateral position is 10% of cardiac output and is equally divided as 5% in each lung. Therefore, the average percentage of cardiac output participating in gas exchange is 35% in the nondependent lung and 55% in the dependent lung.

OLV creates an obligatory right-to-left transpulmonary shunt through the nonventilated, nondependent lung because the $\dot{V}/\dot{Q}$ ratio of that lung is zero. In theory, an additional 35% should be

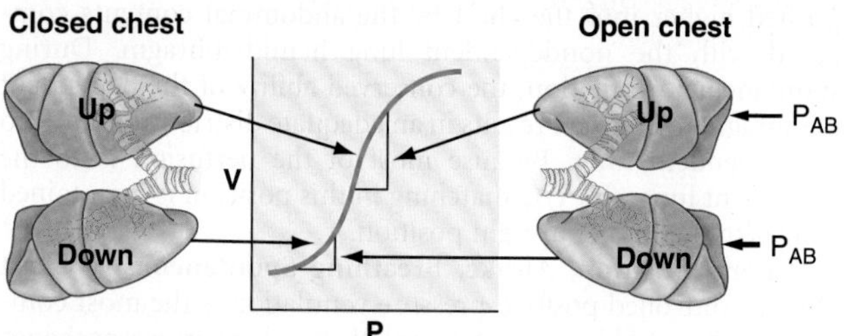

FIGURE 37-9. This schematic of a patient in the lateral decubitus position compares the closed-chested anesthetized condition with the open-chested anesthetized and paralyzed condition. Opening the chest increases nondependent lung compliance and reinforces or maintains the larger part of the tidal ventilation going to the nondependent lung. Paralysis also reinforces or maintains the larger part of tidal ventilation going to the nondependent lung because the pressure of the abdominal contents (P_{AB}) pressing against the upper diaphragm is minimal, and it is therefore easier for positive-pressure ventilation to displace this less resisting dome of the diaphragm. V, volume; P, pressure. (From: Benumof JL. *Anesthesia for Thoracic Surgery.* Philadelphia, PA: WB Saunders; 1987: 112, with permission.)

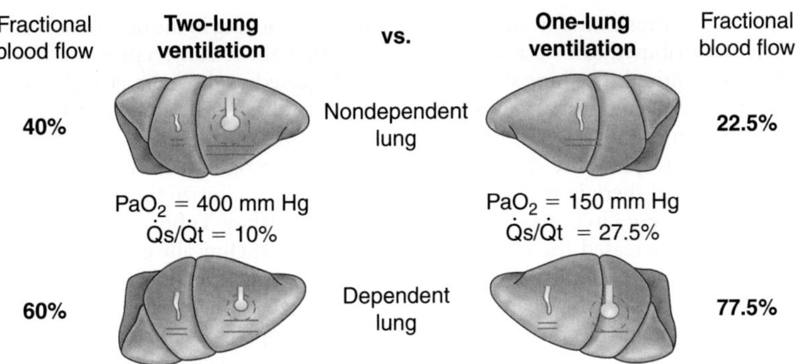

FIGURE 37-10. Schematic representation of two-lung ventilation versus one-lung ventilation (OLV). Typical values for fractional blood flow to the nondependent and dependent lungs, as well as Pa_{O_2} and $\dot{Q}s/\dot{Q}t$ for the two conditions, are shown. The $\dot{Q}s/\dot{Q}t$ during two-lung ventilation is assumed to be distributed equally between the two lungs (5% to each lung). The essential difference between two-lung ventilation and OLV is that, during OLV, the nonventilated lung has some blood flow and therefore an obligatory shunt, which is not present during two-lung ventilation. The 35% of total flow perfusing the nondependent lung, which was not shunt flow, was assumed to be able to reduce its blood flow by 50% by hypoxic pulmonary vasoconstriction. The increase in $\dot{Q}s/\dot{Q}t$ from two-lung to OLV is assumed to be due solely to the increase in blood flow through the nonventilated, nondependent lung during OLV. (From: Benumof JL. *Anesthesia for Thoracic Surgery.* Philadelphia, PA: WB Saunders; 1987:112, with permission.)

added to the total shunt during OLV. However, assuming active HPV, blood flow to the nondependent hypoxic lung will be decreased by 50% and therefore is (35/2) = 17.5%. To this, 5% must be added, which is the obligatory shunt through the nondependent lung. The shunt through the nondependent lung is therefore 22.5% (Fig. 37-10). Together with the 5% shunt in the dependent lung, total shunt during OLV is 22.5% + 5% = 27.5%. This results in a Pa_{O_2} of approximately 150 mm Hg (F_{IO_2} = 1).[55]

Because 72.5% of the perfusion is directed to the dependent lung during OLV, the matching of ventilation in this lung is important for adequate gas exchange. The dependent lung is no longer on the steep (compliant) portion of the volume–pressure curve because of reduced lung volume and FRC. There are several reasons for this reduction in FRC, including general anesthesia, paralysis, pressure from abdominal contents, compression by the weight of mediastinal structures, and suboptimal positioning on the operating table. Other considerations that impair optimal ventilation to the dependent lung include absorption atelectasis, accumulation of secretions, and the formation of a transudate in the dependent lung. All these create a low $\dot{V}/\dot{Q}$ ratio and a large $P(A{-}a)O_2$ gradient.

ONE-LUNG VENTILATION

Absolute Indications for One-lung Ventilation

Currently, a variety of thoracic surgical procedures such as lobectomy, pneumonectomy, esophagogastrectomy, pleural decortication, bullectomy, and bronchopulmonary lavage are commonly performed. Customarily the indications are classified either as
4 absolute or as relative (Table 37-1). The absolute indications include life-threatening complications, such as massive bleeding, sepsis, and pus, in which the nondiseased contralateral lung must be protected from contamination. Bronchopleural and bronchocutaneous fistulae are absolute indications because they offer a low-resistance pathway for the delivered V_T during positive-pressure ventilation. A giant unilateral bulla may rupture under positive pressure, and ventilatory exclusion is mandatory. Finally, during bronchopulmonary lavage for alveolar proteinosis or cystic fibrosis, prevention of drowning the contralateral lung is necessary.

During the last several years video-assisted thoracoscopy (VAT) was introduced to clinical practice. Unlike conventional thoracoscopy, VAT allows for an extensive variety of diagnostic and therapeutic procedures. Improvements in video-endoscopic

TABLE 37-1. INDICATIONS FOR ONE-LUNG VENTILATION

Absolute
1. Isolation of each lung to prevent contamination of a healthy lung
   a. Infection (abscess, infected cyst)
   b. Massive hemorrhage
2. Control of distribution of ventilation to only one lung
   a. Bronchopleural fistula
   b. Bronchopleural cutaneous fistula
   c. Unilateral cyst or bullae
   d. Major bronchial disruption or trauma
3. Unilateral lung lavage
4. Video-assisted thoracoscopic surgery

Relative
1. Surgical exposure—high priority
   a. Thoracic aortic aneurysm
   b. Pneumonectomy
   c. Lung volume reduction
   d. Minimally invasive cardiac surgery
   e. Upper lobectomy
2. Surgical exposure—low priority
   a. Esophageal surgery
   b. Middle and lower lobectomies
   c. Mediastinal mass resection, thymectomy
   d. Bilateral sympathectomies

Modified from: Benumof JL. Physiology of the open-chest and one lung ventilation. In: Kaplan JA, ed. *Thoracic Anesthesia.* New York, NY: Churchill Livingstone; 1983:299.

surgical equipment and a growing enthusiasm for minimally invasive surgical approaches have contributed to its use. In most cases general anesthesia with OLV is required. The lung should be well collapsed to provide the surgeon with an optimal view of the surgical field, and to facilitate palpation of the lesion in the lung parenchyma. In addition, it is difficult to place the stapler on a lung that is not completely collapsed, and there is an increase in incidence of postoperative air leak in these circumstances. The increased use of VAT has significantly increased the number of procedures that require lung separation. In some institutions, 80% to 90% of the procedures are performed using the thoracoscopic approach. In modern anesthesia practice, VAT is an absolute indication for lung separation.

Relative Indications for One-lung Ventilation

In clinical practice, a DLT is commonly used for a lobectomy or pneumonectomy; these represent relative indications for lung separation when performed through an open thoracotomy. Upper lobectomy, pneumonectomy, and thoracic aortic aneurysm repair are high-priority indications. These procedures are technically difficult, and optimal surgical exposure and a quiet operative field are highly desirable. Lower or middle lobectomy and esophageal resection are of lower priority. There are a number of additional procedures that have not been traditionally included as indications for OLV. Nevertheless, many surgeons are accustomed to operating with the lung collapsed for these cases. OLV minimizes lung trauma from retractors and manipulation, improves visualization of lung anatomy, and facilitates identification and separation of anatomic structures and lung fissures. These procedures include minimally invasive cardiac surgery, lung volume reduction, thoracic aneurysm repair, thoracic spinal procedures, mediastinal mass resection, thymectomies, and mediastinal lymph node dissection.

It is important to distinguish between the need for lung isolation versus lung separation.

Lung Isolation. Whenever the nondiseased lung is threatened with contamination by blood or pus from the diseased lung, the lungs must be isolated to prevent potentially life-threatening complications. Other indications are bronchopleural and bronchocutaneous fistulas because they offer a low-resistance pathway for the delivered V_T during positive-pressure ventilation. Finally, during bronchopulmonary lavage for alveolar proteinosis or cystic fibrosis, protection of the contralateral lung from drowning is necessary. These situations, however, are relatively uncommon and in modern anesthesia practice constitute less than 10% of all thoracic procedures.

Lung Separation. All other indications for OLV can be considered as lung separations, in which there is no risk of contamination of the dependent lung. This includes all the relative indications that are primarily for surgical exposure. VAT for diagnostic and therapeutic procedures, which requires a well-collapsed lung, should also be included in this category.[4–6] The majority of procedures where OLV is used are for lung separation; only a minority require lung isolation.[56,57]

Methods of Lung Separation

Double-lumen Endobronchial Tubes

Double-lumen endobronchial tubes are currently the most widely used means of achieving lung separation and OLV. There are several different types of DLT, but all are essentially similar in design in that two endotracheal tubes are "bonded" together. One lumen is long enough to reach a main stem bronchus, and the second lumen ends with an opening in the distal trachea. Lung separation is achieved by inflation of two cuffs: A proximal tracheal cuff and a distal bronchial cuff located in the main stem bronchus (see "Positioning Double-lumen Tubes"). The endobronchial cuff of a right-sided tube is slotted or otherwise designed to allow ventilation of the right upper lobe because the right main stem bronchus is too short to accommodate both the right lumen tip and a right bronchial cuff.

Robertshaw Tube. The Carlens tube (which had a carinal hook) was the first clinically available DLT and was used by pulmonologists for split function spirometry testing (Fig. 37-11A). Subsequently, the Robertshaw-design DLT (which lacked a carinal hook) was developed to facilitate thoracic surgery (Fig. 37-11B). This DLT is available in left-sided and right-sided forms. The absence of a carinal hook facilitates insertion. This tube design has the advantages of having D-shaped, large-diameter lumens that allow easy passage of a suction catheter, offer low resistance to gas flow, and have a fixed curvature to facilitate proper positioning and reduce the possibility of kinking. The original red rubber Robertshaw tubes were available in three sizes: Small, medium, and large. Red rubber tubes are rarely used now and have been replaced by clear, polyvinyl chloride (PVC) disposable Robertshaw-design DLTs. These are available in both right-sided and left-sided versions and in 35 French (Fr), 37 Fr, 39 Fr, and 41 Fr sizes. A 32-Fr left-sided DLT is available for small adults, and a 28 Fr for use in pediatric cases. The advantages of the disposable tubes include the relative ease of insertion and proper positioning as well as easy recognition of the blue color of the endobronchial cuff when fiberoptic bronchoscopy is used. Other advantages are the confirmation of the position on a chest radiograph using the radiopaque lines in the wall of the tube and the continuous observation of tidal gas exchange and respiratory moisture through the clear plastic. The right-sided endobronchial tube is designed to minimize occlusion of the opening of the right upper lobe bronchus. The right endobronchial cuff is doughnut-shaped and allows the right upper lobe ventilation slot to ride over the opening of the right upper lobe bronchus. The tube is also suitable for use in long-term ventilation in the intensive care unit (ICU) because it has a high-volume, low-pressure cuff. These disposable PVC tubes are generally considered the tubes of choice for achieving lung separation and OLV.[58]

A new rubber–silicone left-sided DLT, Silbronco (Silbronco DLT, Fuji Systems, Tokyo, Japan), was recently introduced into clinical practice. It has a D-shaped wire-reinforced lumen to maintain the tip at a 45-degree angle. The reinforced wall tends to prevent obstruction or kinking of the bronchial lumen, yet at the same time maintains flexibility. It is especially useful if the left main stem bronchus is angled at 90 degrees from the trachea, making it almost impossible to position a PVC DLT. This clinical scenario can be seen in patients who have previously undergone a left upper lobectomy and the expansion of the left lower lobe displaces the left main bronchus upward.[42,59]

As the left main bronchus is considerably longer than the right bronchus, there is a narrow margin of safety on the right main bronchus, with potentially a greater risk of upper lobe obstruction whenever a right-sided DLT is used. A left-sided DLT is preferred for both right- and left-sided procedures. A left-sided DLT was selected for 1,166 of the 1,170 patients in one report, and was used successfully in over 98% of those patients.[43] The authors recommended selecting the largest DLT that will safely fit the bronchus. This will provide less resistance to ventilation and is less likely to dislocate.

Some authors have suggested using the patient height as a basis for selecting a DLT. However, the correlation between airway size and height is extremely poor.[60] Tracheal and bronchial dimensions can be also directly measured from the chest radiograph

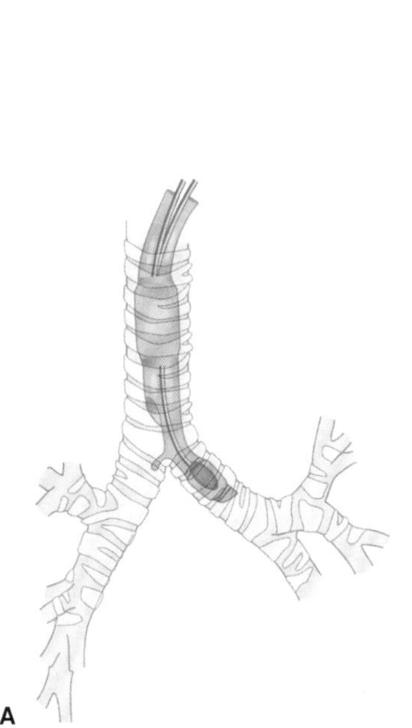
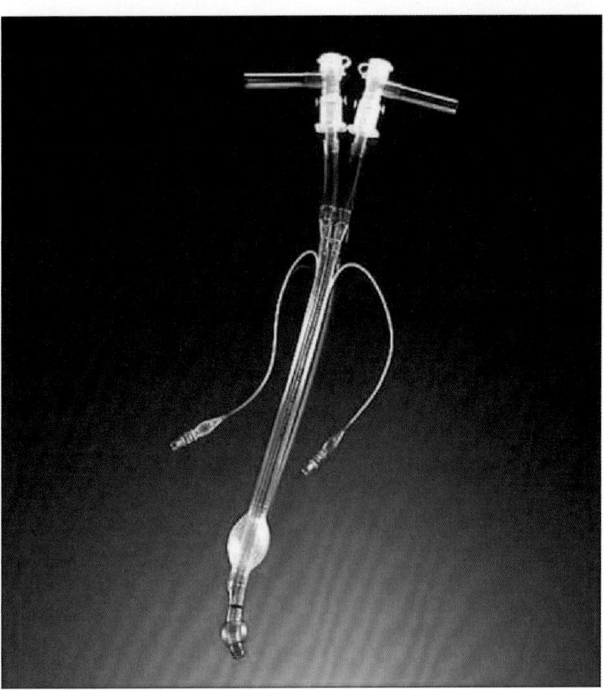

FIGURE 37-11. A: Left main stem endobronchial intubation using a Carlens tube. Note carinal "hook" used for correct positioning. (From: Hillard EK, Thompson PW. Instruments used in thoracic anaesthesia. In: Mushin WW, ed. *Thoracic Anaesthesia.* Oxford: Blackwell Scientific; 1963:315.) **B:** A left-sided Robertshaw type double-lumen tube constructed from polyvinyl chloride. (Courtesy of Nellcor Puritan Bennett, Inc., Pleasanton, California.)

or chest CT scan. It is possible to measure the diameter of the left bronchus from the chest radiograph in almost 75% of patients. In patients in whom the left main bronchus cannot be directly measured, the left bronchial diameter can be accurately estimated by measuring tracheal width. The width of the left bronchus is directly proportional to tracheal width. The left bronchial width is estimated by multiplying the tracheal width by 0.68.[61] Typically, most women will need a 37-Fr DLT and most men will be adequately managed with a 39-Fr DLT. In the past it was a more common practice to use the largest size DLT possible to avoid distal migration of the tube, and so that the pressure in the bronchial cuff could be minimized by needing less air for a seal. The common practice of fiberoptic bronchoscopy has lessened the risk of undetected distal placement or migration of the bronchial tip. A recent study demonstrated that the routine use of a 35-Fr DLT in adults regardless of height was not associated with an increase in hypoxemia or any other adverse clinical outcomes.[62]

The depth required for insertion of the DLT correlates with the height of the patient. For any adult 170- to 180-cm tall, the average depth for a left-sided DLT is 29 cm. For every 10-cm increase or decrease in height, the DLT is advanced or withdrawn 1 cm.[63]

Placement of Double-lumen Tubes. This section concentrates on the insertion of disposable Robertshaw-design DLTs because they are the most widely used. Before insertion, the DLT should be prepared and checked. The tracheal cuff (high volume, low pressure) can accommodate up to 20 mL of air, and the bronchial cuff can be checked using a 3-mL syringe. The tube should be coated liberally with water-soluble lubricant and the stylet should be withdrawn, lubricated, and gently placed back into the bronchial lumen without disturbing the tube's preformed curvature. A Macintosh blade is preferred for intubation of the trachea because it provides the largest area through which to pass the tube. The insertion of the tube is performed with the distal concave curvature facing anteriorly. After the tip of the tube is past the vocal cords, the stylet is removed and the tube is rotated through 90 degrees. A left-sided tube is rotated 90 degrees to the left, and a right-sided tube is rotated to the right. Advancement of the tube ceases when moderate resistance to further passage is encountered, indicating that the tube tip has been firmly seated in the main stem bronchus. It is important to remove the stylet before rotating and advancing the tube to avoid tracheal or bronchial laceration. Rotation and advancement of the tube should be performed gently and under continuous direct laryngoscopy to prevent hypopharyngeal structures from interfering with proper positioning. Once the tube is believed to be in the proper position, a sequence of steps should be performed to check its location.

First the tracheal cuff should be inflated, and equal ventilation of both lungs established. If breath sounds are not equal, the tube is probably too far down, and the tracheal lumen opening is in a main stem bronchus or is lying at the carina. Withdrawal of the tube by 2 to 3 cm usually restores equal breath sounds. The second step is to clamp the right side (in the case of the left-sided tube) and remove the right cap from the connector. Then the bronchial cuff is slowly inflated to prevent an air leak from the bronchial lumen around the bronchial cuff into the tracheal lumen. This ensures that excessive pressure is not applied to the bronchus and helps avoid laceration. Inflation of the bronchial cuff rarely requires >2 mL of air. The third step is to remove the clamp and check that both lungs are ventilated with both cuffs inflated. This ensures that the bronchial cuff is not obstructing the contralateral hemithorax, either totally or partially. The final step is to clamp each side selectively and watch for absence of movement and breath sounds on the ipsilateral (clamped) side; the ventilated side should have clear breath sounds, chest movement that feels compliant, respiratory gas moisture with each tidal ventilation, and no gas leak. If peak airway pressure during two-lung ventilation is 20 cm H_2O, it should not exceed 40 cm H_2O for the same V_T during OLV.

Other methods that have been used for ensuring the correct placement of a DLT include fluoroscopy, chest radiography, selective capnography, and use of an underwater seal. Determination of the presence of gas leaks when positive pressure is applied to one lumen of a DLT is easily done in the operating room (OR). If the bronchial cuff is not inflated and positive pressure is applied to the bronchial lumen of the DLT, gas leaks past the bronchial cuff and returns through the tracheal lumen. If the tracheal lumen is connected to an underwater seal system, gas will be seen to bubble up through the water. The bronchial cuff can then be gradually inflated until no gas bubbles are seen and the desired cuff seal pressure can be attained. This test is of extreme importance when absolute lung separation is needed, such as during bronchopulmonary lavage.

5 The most important advance in checking for proper position of a DLT is the introduction of the pediatric flexible fiberoptic bronchoscope (Fig. 37-12). Smith et al.[64] showed that when the disposable DLT was believed to be in correct position by auscultation and physical examination, subsequent fiberoptic bronchoscopy showed that 48% of tubes were, in fact, malpositioned. Such malpositions, however, are usually of no clinical significance.[65] When using a left-sided DLT, the bronchoscope is usually first introduced through the tracheal lumen. The carina is visualized, but no bronchial cuff herniation should be seen. The upper surface of the blue endobronchial cuff should be just below the tracheal carina. The bronchial cuff of the disposable DLT is easily visualized because of its blue color. The bronchoscope should then be passed through the bronchial lumen, and the left upper lobe

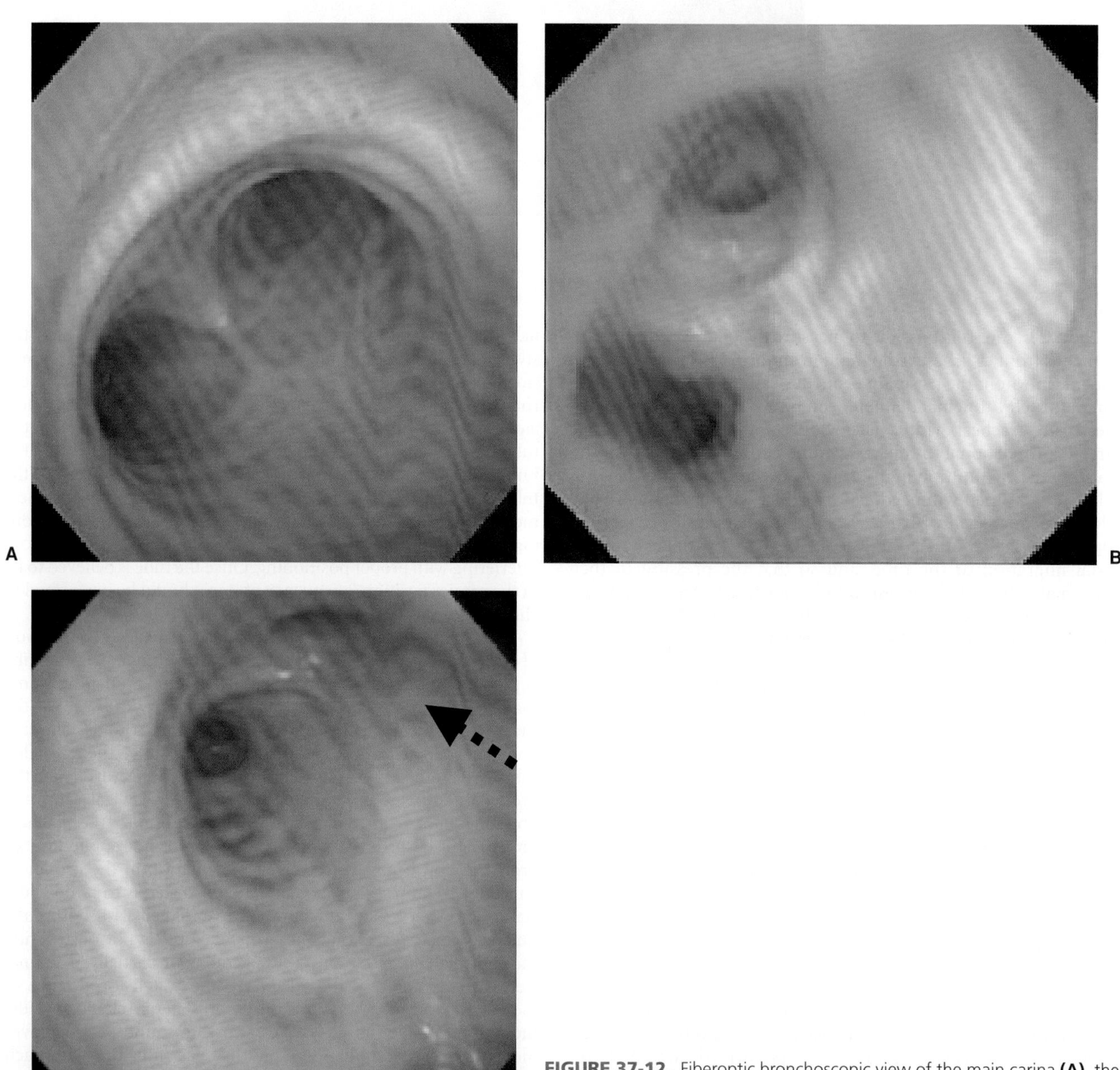

FIGURE 37-12. Fiberoptic bronchoscopic view of the main carina **(A)**, the "left bronchial carina" **(B)**, and the right bronchus **(C)**. Note the right upper lobe orifice (*arrow*).

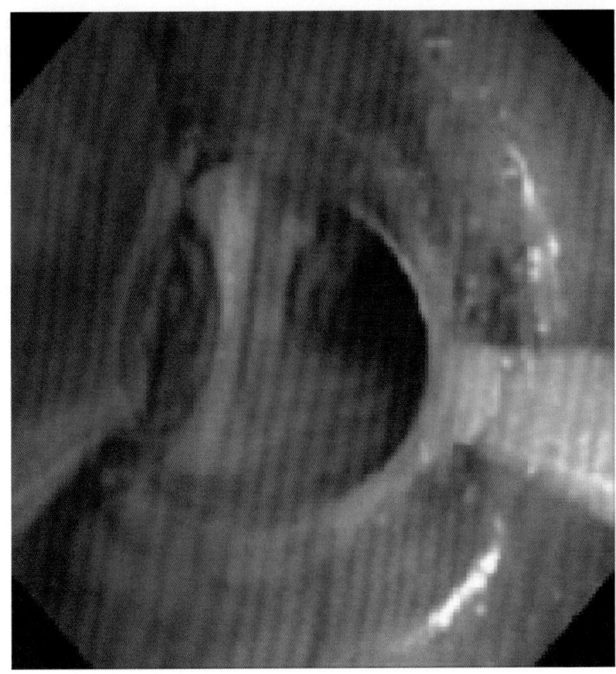

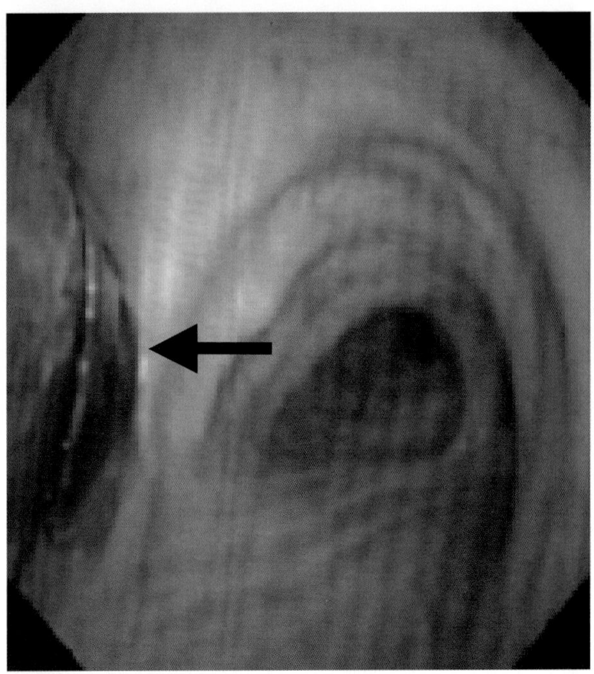

FIGURE 37-13. Malposition of the left bronchial limb of the double-lumen tube (DLT). **A:** The limb is too far into the left bronchus because the cuff is not evident. **B:** DLT is withdrawn and the balloon is now in view, indicating appropriate position of the DLT (*arrow*).

bronchial orifice should be identified. When a right-sided DLT is used, the carina should be visualized through the tracheal lumen but, more importantly, the orifice of the right upper lobe bronchus should be identified when the bronchoscope is passed through the right upper lobe ventilating slot of the DLT. Pediatric fiberoptic bronchoscopes are available in several sizes: 5.6, 4.9, and 3.6 mm in external diameter. The 4.9-mm diameter bronchoscope can be passed through DLTs of 37 Fr and larger. The 3.6-mm diameter bronchoscope is easily passed through all sizes of DLT. In general, it is recommended that the largest size that can pass through the lumen of a DLT be used because it provides better visualization and facilitates identification of the bronchial anatomy. Excellent fiberoptic images of the tracheobronchial tree can be seen by accessing the website thoracicanesthesia.com.

Problems of Malposition of the Double-lumen Tube. The use of a DLT is associated with a number of potential problems, the most important of which is malposition. There are several possibilities for tube malposition. The DLT may be accidentally directed to the side opposite the desired main stem bronchus. In this case, the lung opposite the side of the connector clamp will collapse. Inadequate separation, increased airway pressures, and instability of the DLT usually occur. In addition, because of the morphology of the DLT curvatures, tracheal or bronchial lacerations may result. If a left-sided DLT is inserted into the right main stem bronchus, it obstructs ventilation to the right upper lobe. It is therefore essential to recognize and correct such a malposition as soon as possible.

Second, the DLT may be passed too far down into either the right or the left main stem bronchus (Fig. 37-13). In this case, breath sounds are very diminished or not audible over the contralateral side. This situation is corrected when the tube is withdrawn and the opening of the tracheal lumen is above the carina.

Third, the DLT may not be inserted far enough, leaving the bronchial lumen opening above the carina. In this position, good breath sounds are heard bilaterally when ventilating through the bronchial lumen. No breath sounds are audible when ventilating through the tracheal lumen because the inflated bronchial cuff obstructs gas flow arising from the tracheal lumen. The cuff should be deflated and the DLT rotated and advanced into the desired main stem bronchus.

Fourth, a right-sided DLT may occlude the right upper lobe orifice. The mean distance from the carina to the right upper lobe orifice is 2.3 ± 0.7 cm in men and 2.1 ± 0.7 cm in women.[49] With right-sided DLTs, the ventilatory slot in the side of the bronchial catheter must overlie the right upper lobe orifice to permit ventilation of this lobe. However, the margin of safety is extremely small, and varies from 1 to 8 mm.[66] It is therefore difficult to ensure proper ventilation to the right upper lobe and avoid dislocation of the DLT during surgical manipulation. When right endobronchial intubation is required, a disposable right-sided DLT is perhaps the best choice because of the slanted doughnut shape of the bronchial cuff, which allows the ventilation slot to ride off the right upper lobe ventilation orifice and increases the margin of safety.

Fifth, the left upper lobe orifice may be obstructed by a left-sided DLT. Traditionally, it was believed that the take-off of the left upper lobe bronchus was at a safe distance from the carina and that it would not be obstructed by a left-sided DLT. However, the mean distance between the left upper lobe orifice and the carina is 5.4 ± 0.7 cm in men and 5 ± 0.7 cm in women.[67] The average distance between the openings of the right and left lumens on the left-sided disposable tubes is 6.9 cm. Therefore, an obstruction of the left upper lobe bronchus is possible while the tracheal lumen is still above the carina. There is also a 20% variation in the location of the blue endobronchial cuff on the disposable tubes because this cuff is attached to the tube at the end of the manufacturing process.

Bronchial cuff herniation may occur and obstruct the bronchial lumen if excessive volumes are used to inflate the cuff. The bronchial cuff has also been known to herniate over the tracheal

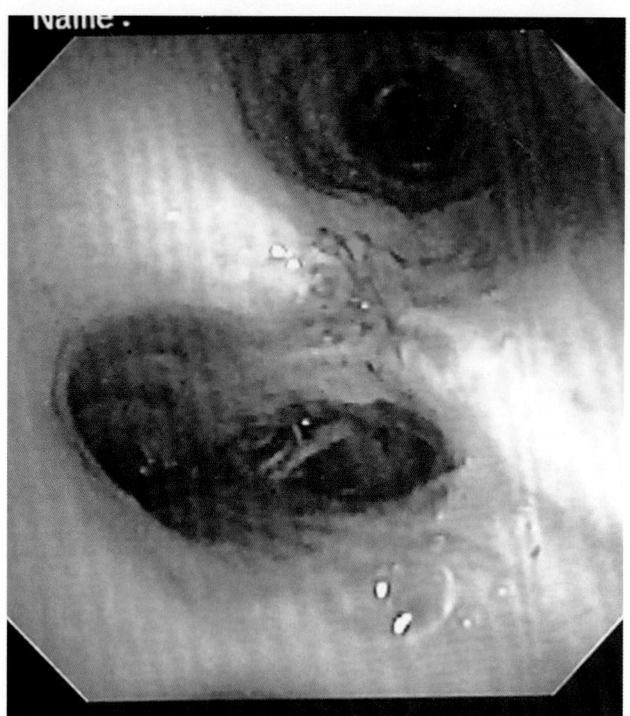

FIGURE 37-14. Bronchoscopic view showing laceration in left mainstem bronchus.

carina, and in the case of a left-sided DLT, to obstruct ventilation to the right main stem bronchus.

Another rare complication with DLTs is tracheal laceration or rupture (Fig. 37-14). Overinflation of the bronchial cuff, inappropriate positioning, and trauma owing to intraoperative dislocation that resulted in bronchial rupture have been described in association with the Robertshaw tube and the disposable DLT.[68] Therefore, the pressure in the bronchial cuff should be assessed and decreased if the cuff is found to be overinflated. If absolute separation of the lungs is not needed, the bronchial cuff should be deflated and then reinflated slowly to avoid excessive pressure on the bronchial walls. The bronchial cuff should also be deflated during any repositioning of the patient unless lung separation is absolutely required during this time.

In a recent prospective trial, 60 patients were randomly assigned to two groups. OLV was achieved with either an endobronchial blocker (blocker group) or a DLT (double-lumen group). Postoperative hoarseness and sore throat were assessed at 24, 48, and 72 hours after surgery. Bronchial injuries and vocal cord lesions were examined by bronchoscopy immediately after surgery. Postoperative hoarseness occurred significantly more frequently in the double-lumen group compared with the blocker group (44% vs. 17%, respectively). Similar findings were observed for vocal cord lesions (44% vs. 17%). The incidence of bronchial injuries was comparable between groups.[69]

Lung Separation in the Patient with a Tracheostomy

Occasionally, a patient with a permanent tracheostomy is scheduled for surgery on the lung that requires isolation. Examples of such patients include those who have undergone resection of a tumor in the floor of the mouth or on the base of the tongue, followed by extensive reconstructive surgery with the creation of a permanent tracheal stoma. Routine follow-up may reveal a lung lesion that requires a diagnostic procedure. Conventional double-lumen endobronchial tubes are designed to be inserted through the mouth, not through a tracheal stoma. The standard DLTs are usually too stiff to negotiate the curve required for insertion through a tracheal stoma and are difficult to position.[70] A separately inserted bronchial blocker may permit adequate lung separation.[71]

Saito et al.[72] described a spiral, wire-reinforced, double-lumen endobronchial tube made of silicone (Koken Medical, Tokyo, Japan) that is designed for placement through a tracheostomy. The middle section of the tube consists of two thin-walled silicone catheters with an internal diameter of 5 mm, glued together and reinforced with a stainless steel spiral wire and covered with a silicone coating with two pilot balloons. The distal section, which contains the bronchial lumen and the bronchial cuff, is made of wire-reinforced silicone to avoid excessive flexibility. The dimensions are based on the Mallinckrodt DLT (Hazelwood, MD). The bronchial cuff is located 1.2 cm from the tip, and the distance between the tip orifice and the tracheal orifice is 4.9 cm. In a clinical trial in patients with permanent tracheal stomas, the tubes functioned well in achieving lung separation, with no sign of kinking or movement, and permitted easy passage of a suction catheter.

Lung Separation in the Patient with a Difficult Airway

An airway may be recognized initially as difficult when conventional laryngoscopy reveals a grade III or IV view (see Chapter 27). When separation of the lungs is required and the patient has a clearly recognized difficult airway, then awake intubation using a flexible fiberoptic bronchoscope can be used to place a DLT, Univent tube, or single-lumen tube (SLT). The SLT may then be exchanged for a DLT or Univent tube using a tube exchanger. Furthermore, depending on the extent and duration of the surgical procedure, and the amount of fluid shift, an airway that was not initially classified as difficult may become difficult secondary to facial edema, secretions, and laryngeal trauma from the initial intubation.[73,74]

A logical approach to lung separation is shown in Figure 37-15. When lung separation is mandated and the patient has a recognized difficult airway, awake intubation using flexible fiberoptic bronchoscopy can be attempted using a DLT, Univent tube, or SLT. The same approach may be used for the patient with an unrecognized difficult airway and a failure to intubate with conventional laryngoscopy. When using a DLT over a fiberoptic bronchoscope, the anesthesiologist should keep in mind that it is a bulky tube with a large external diameter and because of the length of the DLT, only a limited part of the fiberoptic bronchoscope is available for manipulation. In addition, the mismatch between the flexibility of the fiberoptic bronchoscope and the rigidity of the DLT makes it more difficult to advance over the fiberoptic bronchoscope. The Univent tube has the same bulky external diameter and is also often difficult to pass between the vocal cords, particularly in a patient who is awake.

Single-lumen Tube can be Successfully Placed

If a failure to provide lung separation could result in a life-threatening situation, there are two possibilities to provide OLV when an SLT is already in place. First, depending on the indication for lung isolation, a tube exchanger can be used to switch to a DLT or a Univent tube. The second possibility is to direct a

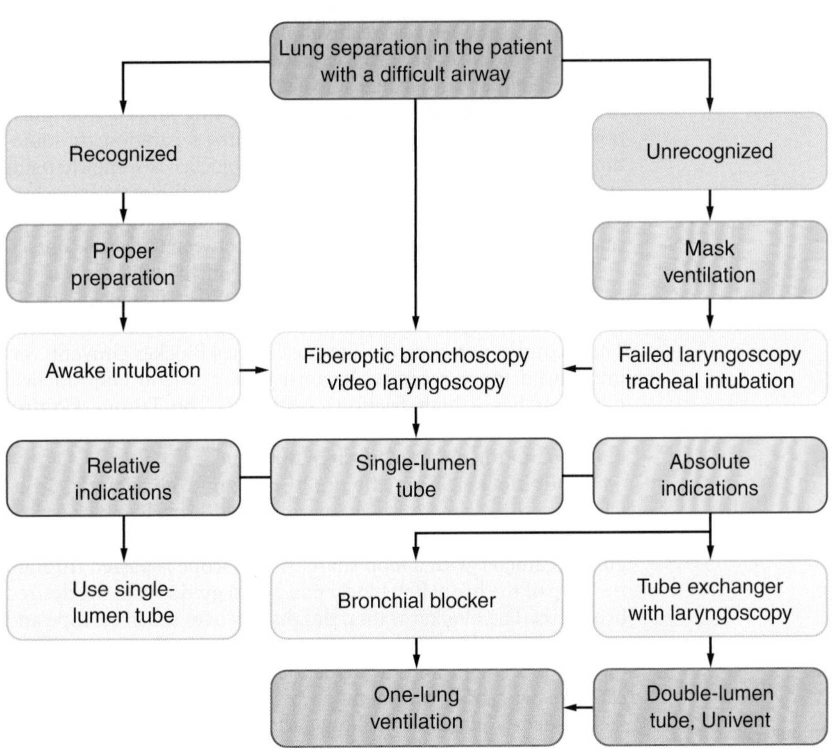

FIGURE 37-15. Lung separation in the patient with a difficult airway. (Adapted from: Cohen E, Benumof JL. Lung separation in the patient with a difficult airway. *Curr Opin Anesthesiol.* 1999;12: 29, with permission.)

bronchial blocker through the SLT into the selected main stem bronchus. These two methods, however, offer limited protection or an inadequate seal in cases such as lung lavage, pulmonary abscess, or hemoptysis, where a DLT would be the tube of choice.

Use of a Tube Exchanger

Several tube exchangers are commercially available (Cook Critical Care, Bloomington, IN; Sheridan Catheter Corporation, Argyle, NY). On these tube exchangers, the depth is marked in centimeters; they are available in a wide range of external diameters and easily adapted for either oxygen insufflation or jet ventilation. The size of the tube exchanger and the size of the tube to be inserted should be tested before use in a patient. The 11-Fr tube changer will pass through a 35- to 41-Fr DLT, whereas the 14-Fr tube exchanger does not pass through a 35 Fr. To prevent lung laceration, the tube exchanger should never be inserted against resistance. Because the first generation of tube exchangers was very stiff, there was a risk for tracheal or bronchial laceration. Recently, a new tube exchanger with a soft flexible tip was released by Cook Critical Care that is safer to use and is less likely to cause airway laceration. Finally, when passing any tube over an airway guide, a laryngoscope should be used to facilitate passage of the tube over the airway guide past supraglottic tissues.

Use of Modern Bronchial Blockers

2 **Bronchial Blocker (BB).** Lung separation can be achieved with a reusable bronchial blocker.[75] Magill described an endobronchial blocker that is placed using a bronchoscope and directed to the nonventilated lung. Inflation of the cuff at the distal end of the blocker serves to block ventilation to that lung. The lumen of the blocker permits suctioning of the airway distal to the catheter tip. Depending on the clinical circumstance, oxygen can be insufflated through the catheter lumen. A conventional tracheal tube is then placed in the trachea. This technique can be useful in achieving selective ventilation in children younger than 12 years of age. However, because the blocker balloon requires a high distending pressure, it easily slips out of the bronchus into the trachea, obstructing ventilation and losing the seal between the two lungs. This displacement can be secondary to changes in position or to surgical manipulation. The loss of lung separation can be a life-threatening situation if it was performed to prevent spillage of pus, blood, or fluid from bronchopulmonary lavage. For this reason, bronchial blockers are rarely used for these types of cases.

Indications for the use of a bronchial blocker are shown in Table 37-2. An independently passed bronchial blocker may be used with an SLT to obtain lung isolation, thereby avoiding the use of a DLT in a patient with a difficult airway. The use of a bronchial blocker also eliminates the potential risk of needing to change a DLT to an SLT at the conclusion of the procedure. The blockers are discussed later, in the chronologic order in which they were developed, and came into practice. In the past, Fogarty vascular embolectomy catheters were used for lung separation, but there is no indication for their use in the current practice of thoracic anesthesia. The balloon of the Fogarty is high pressure, low volume, and there is no lumen to allow egress of gas from the lung to facilitate deflation.

3 **Univent Tube.** The Univent (Fuji Systems Corp., Tokyo, Japan) is a single-lumen tracheal tube with a movable endobronchial blocker (Fig. 37-16). In the Univent tube, the bronchial blocker is housed in a small channel bored in the wall of the tube. The blocker contains a high-volume, low-pressure balloon, and is angled to permit external direction into the desired bronchus under direct fiberoptic bronchoscopic (FB) vision. After intubation of the trachea, the movable blocker is manipulated into the desired main stem bronchus with the aid of a fiberoptic bronchoscope. The Univent tube may be ideal for cases in which a tube change (e.g., from single to double lumen) may be difficult (e.g.,

TABLE 37-2. INDICATIONS FOR THE USE OF ENDOBRONCHIAL BLOCKERS

The Difficult Airway
Avoids the need for tube exchange (DLT to SLT)
Following laryngeal surgery
Patient with a tracheostomy
Distorted bronchial anatomy due to compression by aneurysm or tumor
Patient who requires nasotracheal intubation
Management
Makes possible segmental blockade in a patient who cannot tolerate OLV
Morbid obesity
Small size and pediatric patients
Patients from the ICU who arrive to the OR tracheally intubated
Surgical Procedures not Involving the Lung
Esophageal surgery
Spine surgery that requires a transthoracic approach
Minimally invasive cardiac surgery

ICU, Intensive care unit; OLV, one-lung ventilation; SLT, single-lumen tube; DLT, double-lumen tube; OR, operating room.

mediastinoscopy followed by thoracotomy), or in cases of bilateral lung transplantation. The Univent tube has the advantage common to all bronchial blockers: It is an SLT, and there is no need to change the tube at the end of the procedure if postoperative ventilatory support is required. This is particularly important in cases of difficult intubation, prolonged surgery with airway edema, such as thoracic aortic aneurysm surgery or extensive neurosurgical procedures on the spine with massive fluid replacement, and altered anatomy of the airway. It is also possible to suction through the blocker lumen or to apply continuous positive airway pressure (CPAP) to improve oxygenation in cases of hypoxemia.

The disadvantages of the Univent tubes are that correct positioning of the blocker may be difficult to achieve or maintain and that the external diameter is relatively large. Many anesthesiologists prefer to avoid postoperative ventilation with such a large-diameter tube, and in that case, change it to a standard tube at the conclusion of the surgery. The blocker can dislocate during surgical manipulation, and satisfactory bronchial seal and lung separation are sometimes difficult to achieve. The bronchial blocker is somewhat stiff and sometimes will not easily be directed into the main bronchus. This is particularly true for the left side. The bulky external diameter can also make it difficult to pass the tube between the vocal cords.

The first-generation Univent tube's bronchial blocker was difficult to direct into the selected main bronchus. The blocker would spin (torque) on its long axis, which made it difficult to control. The second generation, the Torque Control Blocker Univent, was introduced more recently. It consists of a silicon endotracheal tube that has a high friction coefficient. The Torque Control Blocker provides better control, which facilitates direction of the blocker into the target main stem bronchus.

Arndt Blocker. In an attempt to overcome the potential problems described previously, a snare-guided bronchial blocker has been introduced (Cook Critical Care) (Fig. 37-17A). It is a wire-guided catheter with a loop snare. A fiberscope is passed through the loop of the bronchial blocker and then guided into the desired bronchus. The blocker is then slid distally over the fiberscope and into the selected bronchus. Bronchoscopic visualization confirms blocker placement and bronchial occlusion. This balloon-tipped catheter has a hollow lumen of 1.6 mm, which allows suction to facilitate the collapse of the lung and insufflation of oxygen to the nondependent lung. The balloon is available in spherical or elliptic shape. The set contains a multiport adapter, which allows uninterrupted ventilation during the positioning of the blocker. The wire may then be removed, and a 1.6-mm lumen may be used as a suction port or for oxygen insufflations. In the first generation of this device it was not possible to reinsert the string once it had been pulled out, losing the ability to redirect the bronchial blocker if necessary. External reinforcement of the wire now allows for its reintroduction through the lumen. Finally, the external diameter necessitates a large size SLT (at least 8 mm) to be able to accommodate the bronchial blocker. The Arndt blocker is available in a 7-Fr and in a 5-Fr pediatric size. One disadvantage of the Arndt Blocker is that it is advanced blindly over the FB into the desired main bronchus. In some occasions the tip of the blocker may get caught at the main carina or at the Murphy eye of the SLT.

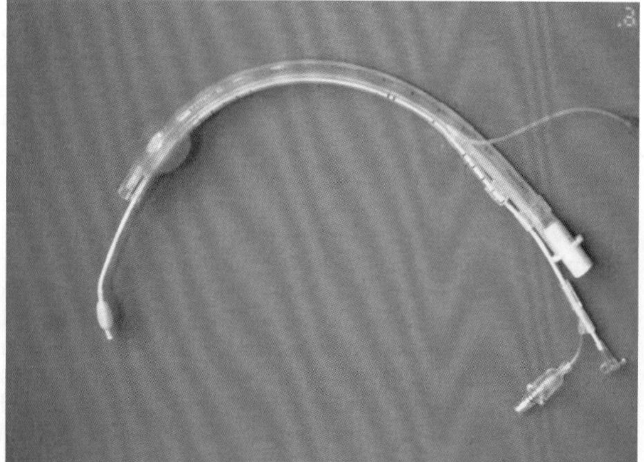
A

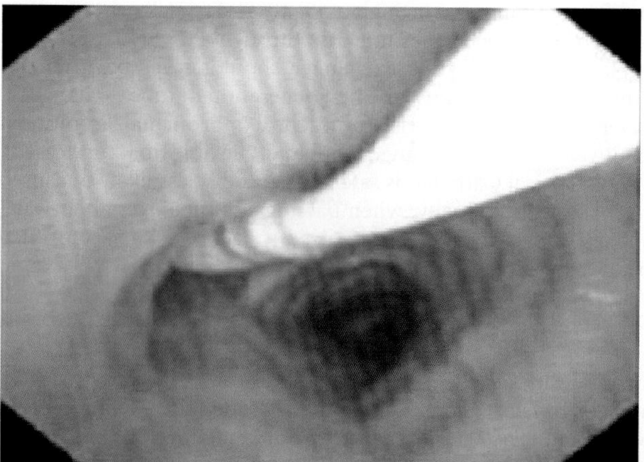
B

FIGURE 37-16. A: The Univent tube also allows lung separation using a single-lumen endotracheal tube. **B:** The Univent bronchial blocker positioned in left main stem bronchus.

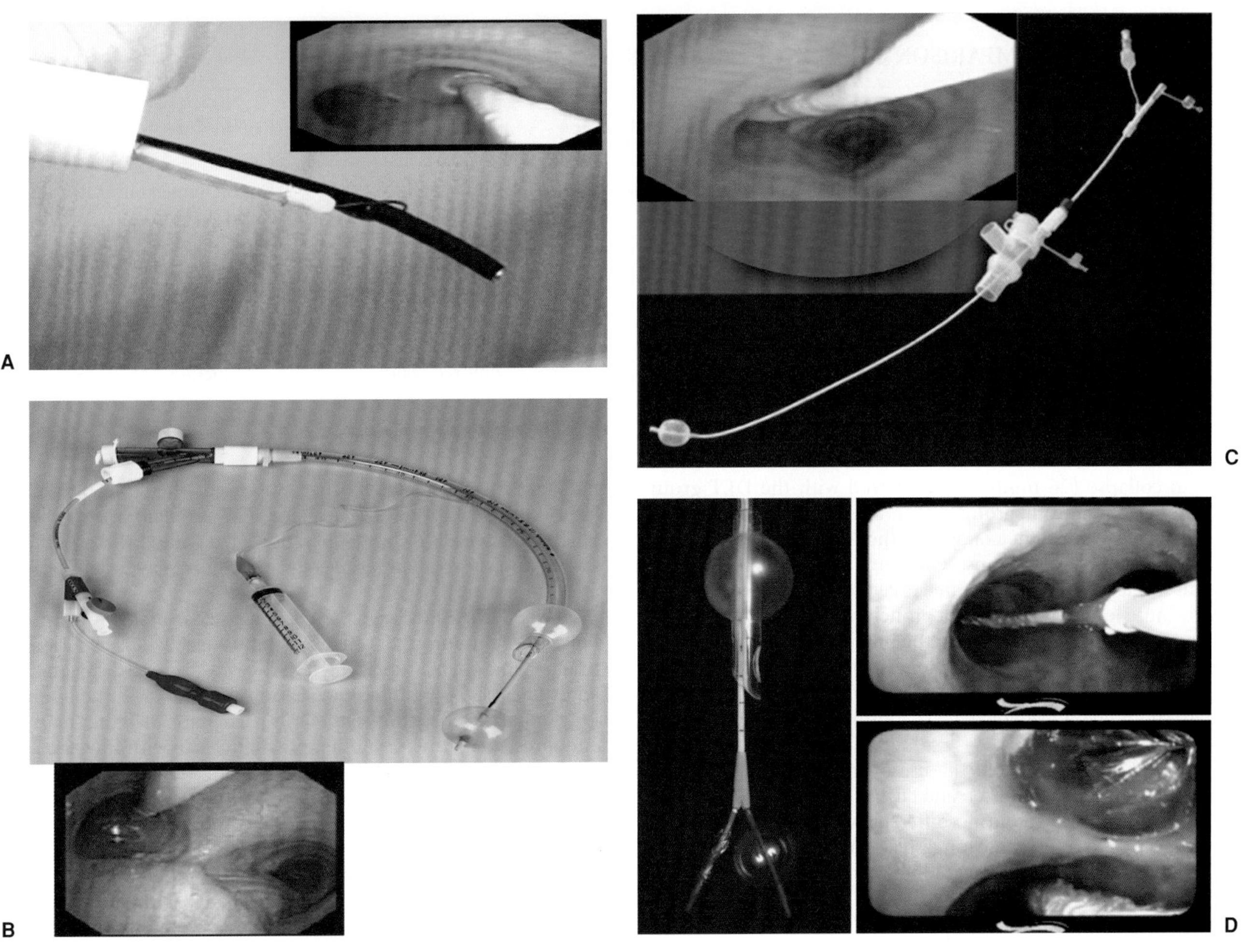

FIGURE 37-17. A: Arndt blocker; B: Cohen blocker; C: Uniblocker; D: EZ blocker.

Cohen Blocker. The Cohen Flexitip endobronchial blocker (Cook Critical Care) is designed for use as an independent bronchial blocker. It is inserted through a single-lumen endotracheal tube with the aid of a small-diameter (4-mm) fiberoptic bronchoscope[76] (Fig. 37-17B). The blocker has a rotating wheel that deflects the soft tip by more than 90 degrees and easily directs it into the desired bronchus. The blocker cuff is a high-volume, low-pressure balloon inflated via 0.4-mm lumen inside the wall of the blocker. It has a pear shape that provides adequate seal of the bronchus. Generally, it takes between 6 and 8 mL of air to seal the bronchus with the cuff. The cuff is a distinctive blue color that is easily recognizable by fiberoptic bronchoscopy. It is best to inflate the cuff under "direct vision" via the fiberoptic bronchoscope. The blocker size is 9 Fr. It has a central main lumen (1.6 mm) that allows limited suctioning of secretions and insufflations of oxygen to the collapsed lung in case of hypoxemia. This blocker and the FB do not have to pass through the tracheal tube at the same time for placement; the blocker can be passed ahead of the FB beyond the tracheal tube tip. Therefore, it can be used with a 7-mm tracheal tube.

Uniblocker. Fuji Systems introduced a new 9-Fr balloon-tipped, angled blocker with a multiple port adapter that is essentially the same design as the Univent tube blocker, but can be used as an independent blocker passed via a special connector through a standard tracheal tube (Fig. 37-17C).

EZ-Blocker. The most recent addition to the endobronchial blocker design is the EZ Blocker. (IQ Medical Ventures). This is a 7-Fr., 4 lumen, 75-cm, disposable endobronchial blocker to facilitate selective lung ventilation (Fig. 37-17D). It has a symmetric Y-shaped bifurcation and both branches have an inflatable cuff and a central lumen. The bifurcation resembles the bifurcation of the trachea. During insertion via a standard tracheal tube, each of the two distal ends is placed into a main stem bronchus. The selected lung is isolated by inflating the blocker's balloon to the least volume necessary to occlude the main stem bronchus under bronchoscopic visualization. This blocker should offer an advantage during bilateral procedures because each lung can be deflated without the need for repositioning the blocker. At the time of writing, clinical experience with the device is too limited to be able make any recommendations. The characteristics of the various bronchial blockers are summarized in Table 37-3.

The effectiveness of lung isolation among three devices—the left-sided DLT Broncho-Cath, the Torque Control Blocker Univent, and the wire-guided Arndt—has been compared in a prospective randomized trial. There was no significant difference in tube malpositions among the three groups: It took longer to position the Arndt blocker (3 minutes) compared with the left-sided DLT (2 minutes) and the Univent (2 minutes). Excluding the time for tube placement, the Arndt group also took longer for the

TABLE 37-3. COMPARISON OF BRONCHIAL BLOCKERS

	Arndt Blocker	Cohen Blocker	Uniblocker	EZ Blocker
Size	5 Fr, 7 Fr, 9 Fr	9 Fr	9 Fr	7 Fr
Guidance feature	Wire loop to snare FOB	Deflecting tip	Prefixed bend	Double-lumen bifurcated tip
Recommended tracheal tube size	9 Fr 8 mm 7 Fr 7 mm 5 Fr 4.5 mm	8 mm	8 mm	8 mm
Central lumen	1.8 mm	1.8 mm	2 mm	
Murphy eye	Present in 9 Fr	Present	None	None
Disadvantages	BB not visualized during insertion	Expensive	No steering mechanism. Prefixed bend	Lumen too small. Impossible to suction

lung to collapse (26 minutes), compared with the DLT group (17 minutes) or Univent group (19 minutes). Furthermore, unlike the other two groups, the majority of the Arndt patients required suction to achieve lung collapse. Once lung isolation was achieved, overall surgical exposure was rated excellent for the three groups. One minute longer to position a bronchial blocker or 6 minutes longer to collapse the lung with the bronchial blocker is insignificant when considering the length of the thoracic procedure. The risk benefit and the patient safety of each individual patient should be considered when choosing the methods for lung isolation.[75,77,78]

A recent study evaluated the use of the Cohen blocker, the Arndt blocker, the Uniblocker, and DLT in 4 groups of 26 patients in each group. They found no differences among the groups in the time taken to insert these lung isolation devices or in the quality of the lung collapse.[79] The grading was done by the operating surgeons who were blinded as to which device was used. The number of cuff dislocations was higher among the bronchial blocker (BB) groups. Regardless of the type of BB or DLT selected to provide OLV, the decision as to which technique to use depends on the clinical circumstances and the physician's experience and comfort with a particular device. It is important, however, that the clinician does not limit his/her practice to the use of only one device but rather be versatile and comfortable in the use of several.

Conclusion of the Surgical Procedure

Depending on the extent and the duration of the surgical procedure and the degree of fluid shift, an airway that was initially not classified as difficult may become difficult secondary to facial edema, secretions, and laryngeal trauma from the original intubation. In these cases, when planning to provide lung separation, the postoperative period should be considered and the appropriate tube placed. Many procedures that are not considered to represent absolute indications for lung separation are lengthy and complex. Complex lung resection, with or without chest wall resection, thoracoabdominal esophagogastrectomy, thoracic aortic aneurysm resection with or without total circulatory arrest, or an extensive vertebral tumor resection, may result in facial edema, secretion, and hemoptysis, requiring postoperative ventilatory support. Other indications for postoperative ventilatory support are marginal respiratory reserve, unexpected blood loss or fluid shift, hypothermia, and inadequate reversal of residual neuromuscular blockade.

If a Univent tube was used to provide OLV, the blocker may be fully retracted and the Univent tube can be used as an SLT. If an independent bronchial blocker was used, then the blocker is removed, leaving the SLT in place. The problem arises when a DLT was inserted for lung separation. In a patient with a difficult airway and subsequent facial edema, the DLT may be left in place after surgery.

If the decision to leave the DLT in place is made, it is important to keep in mind that the ICU staff is usually less experienced in managing such a tube, which may easily become dislocated. In addition, it is more difficult to suction through the lumens, and a longer, narrower suction catheter is needed to reach the tip of the endobronchial lumen. Another possibility is to withdraw the DLT to place the 19- to 20-cm mark at the teeth so that the endobronchial lumen is above the carina and both lungs can be ventilated via the bronchial lumen. Tracheal extubation from the DLT should be considered after diuresis and steroid therapy to allow reduction of the facial and airway edema.

If it is necessary to change the DLT to an SLT, a tube exchanger should be used to maintain access to the airway, as previously discussed. The tube exchanger can be passed through the bronchial limb of the DLT. Alternatively, the tube exchange may be performed under direct vision using one of several commercially available video laryngoscopes, such as the GlideScope (Verathon Medical), C-Mac (Karl Storz), or the Mc Grath (Aircraft Medical) (see Chapter 27). With these video laryngoscopes, the tube exchanger can be placed under direct vision through the vocal cords alongside the existing tube to permit passage of an SLT (Fig. 37-18). The Airtraq DL (King Systems) is a disposable video blade that is manufactured with a large channel that is large enough to accommodate a DLT.

In summary, the clinician should be able to master different methods of lung separation and make himself/herself familiar with the devices available to provide OLV. In addition, one should always plan in advance for the postoperative period when selecting the method of lung separation. Finally, in these cases, a close dialog with the surgical team is of vital importance.

MANAGEMENT OF ONE-LUNG VENTILATION

This section discusses the management of one-lung ventilation (OLV) in a paralyzed patient in the lateral decubitus position with an open chest. Inspired oxygen fraction (FIO_2), V_T and respiratory rate, dependent lung, PEEP, and nondependent lung CPAP are reviewed, and an approach to the management of OLV is presented.

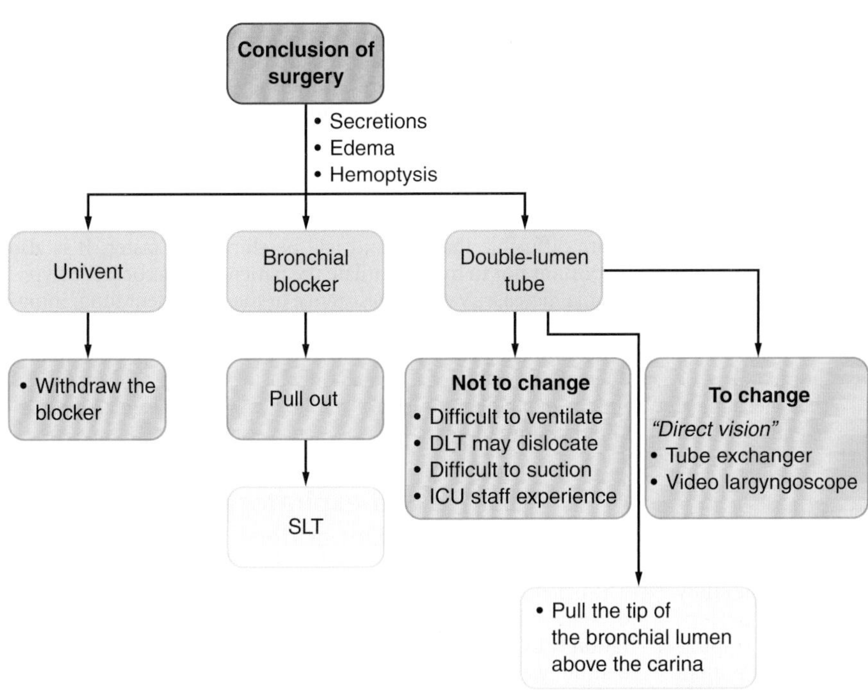

FIGURE 37-18. Conclusion of the surgical procedure. See text for discussion. SLT, single-lumen tube; DLT, double-lumen tube; ICU, intensive care unit.

Confirmation of Correct Position of DLT or Endobronchial Blocker

Following intubation with a DLT or placement of an endobronchial blocker, the correct position should be checked by clinical assessment, visualization of chest movement, auscultation, and pressure/volume flow profile. In modern anesthesia practice, a standard 4.0-mm fiberscope should be passed down the tracheal lumen to check for correct depth, or alongside the endobronchial blocker that was passed through the single lumen tracheal tube. It is a common practice to visualize the tip of the blue bronchial cuff at the level of the carina to insure that the left upper lobe orifice is not obstructed. Once the patient is turned into the lateral position, the position of the DLT should be rechecked to exclude dislocation of the tube during positioning.[80]

Inspired Oxygen Fraction

An FIO_2 of 1 is generally recommended during OLV. High oxygen concentration serves to protect against hypoxemia during the procedure and provides a higher margin of safety. A high FIO_2 may, however, cause absorption atelectasis and potentially further increase the amount of shunt because of the collapsed alveoli. The use of an FIO_2 <1 during OLV has the potential benefits of decreasing the risk of absorption atelectasis and, if N_2O is used, may allow potent inhaled anesthetics to be used in lower concentrations. Some clinicians use an O_2 80%/N_2O 20% mixture as long that the SpO_2 is maintained in a safe range. The rate of the lung collapse during OLV was addressed by Ko et al.[81] They compared the effects of three different gas mixtures (air/oxygen, FIO_2 0.4; N_2O/O_2, FIO_2 0.4; and oxygen, FIO_2 1) during OLV on lung collapse and oxygenation during subsequent OLV: They found that deflation of the nonventilated lung during thoracic surgery was delayed if air was used as part of the anesthetic gas mixture during the initial period of OLV. For thoracic procedures in which delayed collapse of the nonventilated lung will impede surgical exposure, the optimal anesthetic technique should include thorough denitrogenation of the lung by using FIO_2 of 1.

Tidal Volume and Respiratory Rate

It has been recommended that during OLV, the dependent lung be ventilated with a V_T of 10 to 12 mL/kg. Tidal volumes (V_Ts) ranging between 8 and 15 mL/kg produced no significant effect on transpulmonary shunt or PaO_2.[82] A V_T <8 mL/kg can result in a decrease in FRC and enhanced formation of atelectasis in the dependent lung. A V_T >15 mL/kg may recruit the atelectatic alveoli in the dependent lung. It will increase the pulmonary vascular resistance of the dependent lung (similar to the application of PEEP) and divert blood flow into the nondependent lung. It has been common practice during OLV to maintain the same V_T as during two-lung ventilation.

Recently, more attention has been directed toward protection of the ventilated lung with the use of smaller V_Ts to avoid ALI (see Chapter 55).[83] This concept stimulated a debate over the optimal V_T that should be used during OLV. A recent pro and con editorial argued that a (large) V_T of 12 mL/kg during OLV may cause overdistention and stretching of the lung parenchyma and therefore would increase the risk of ALI.[84] However, a (small) V_T of 6 mL/kg could lead to atelectasis in the dependent lung. Furthermore, a small V_T with PEEP may cause dynamic hyperinflation secondary to the increase in respiratory rate necessary to maintain $PaCO_2$.[85]

Mechanical ventilation practice has changed over the past few decades, with V_Ts decreasing significantly, especially in patients with ALI. The lungs of patients without ALI are still ventilated with large, and perhaps too large, V_Ts. Studies of ventilator-associated lung injury in subjects without ALI demonstrate inconsistent results. Retrospective clinical studies, however, suggest that the use of large V_T favors the development of lung injury in these patients.[86]

In a multicenter, prospective ARDS Network trial, the results unambiguously confirmed that mechanical ventilation with smaller

V_T (6 mL/kg) rather than traditional V_T (12 mL/kg) resulted in a significant increase in the number of ventilator-free days and reduction of inhospital mortality.[87]

While there is good evidence from studies in the ICU for a detrimental effect of high V_T and parenchymal overdistension, the data concerning lung injury during OLV is limited. Ventilation strategies during OLV have been compared to ARDS, because both involve ventilation of a decreased lung capacity due to unrecruited alveoli, otherwise known as the concept of "baby lung."[88] There is no evidence that these findings in patients with acute respiratory distress syndrome are applicable to patients undergoing a thoracic procedure requiring a relatively short period of controlled ventilation.

In one study, patients undergoing elective thoracotomy or laparotomy were randomly assigned to receive either mechanical ventilation with V_T of 12 or 15 mL/kg, respectively, and without PEEP, or V_T of 6 mL/kg with PEEP of 10 cm H_2O. In this study, neither time course nor concentrations of pulmonary or systemic inflammatory mediators (cytokines) differed between the two ventilatory settings within 3 hours.[89]

There are data indicating damaging effects of large V_T in patients who were ventilated for only several hours. In one study of patients undergoing pneumonectomy, 18% developed postoperative respiratory failure. The patients who developed respiratory failure had been ventilated with larger intraoperative V_T than those who did not (median, 8.3 vs. 6.7 mL/kg predicted body weight).[90] However, the authors recommended that protective lung ventilation (PV) with low V_T 6 to 7 mL/kg, PEEP to the dependent lung, frequent recruitment maneuvers, and limited administration of fluid be used during OLV.

In patients undergoing general anesthesia, lung recruitment maneuvers proved to be easy to perform and effective in reversing alveolar collapse, hypoxemia, and decreased compliance. The beneficial effect of an alveolar recruitment strategy on arterial oxygenation and respiratory compliance in anesthetized patients undergoing nonthoracic surgery in the supine position has been demonstrated.[91] Tusman et al.[91] studied 10 patients undergoing open lobectomy who received lung recruitment maneuvers. This was done by increasing peak inspiratory pressure to 40 cm H_2O, together with a PEEP of 20 cm H_2O for 10 respiratory cycles. They found that alveolar recruitment in the dependent lung augments Pao_2 values during OLV. It is important to apply the maneuvers over several minutes with a pressure of at least 20 cm H_2O and a peak of 40 cm H_2O.

Pressure-controlled ventilation (PCV) was also compared with volume-controlled ventilation (VCV) during OLV. The authors suggested that PCV may be preferred for management of OLV because the lower peak airway pressure was associated with greater perfusion of the dependent lung and smaller transpulmonary shunt.[92] A recent study investigated whether PCV results in improved arterial oxygenation compared with VCV during OLV. Fifty-eight patients with good preoperative pulmonary function scheduled for thoracic surgery were prospectively randomized into two groups. Those in group A underwent OLV initially with VCV for 30 minutes followed by PCV for a similar period of time. Those in group B underwent OLV initially with PCV for 30 minutes followed by VCV for a similar duration. Airway pressures and arterial blood gases were obtained during OLV at the end of each ventilatory mode period. The authors found no differences in arterial oxygenation during OLV between VCV (Pao_2, 206.1 ± 62.4 mm Hg) and PCV (Pao_2, 202.1 ± 56.4 mm Hg; $p = 0.534$).[93]

Cruz Pardons et al.[94] studied 110 patients scheduled for thoracic surgery requiring a minimum of 1 hour of OLV. The patients were randomized into two groups: VCV or PCV, both providing a V_T of 8 mL/kg. Measurements were taken intraoperatively and up to 24 hours postoperatively. There were no differences in the intra- or early postoperative arterial oxygenation, airway plateau pressure, and mean arterial pressure between groups, except for higher peak airway pressures in the VCV group. The respiratory rate should be adjusted to maintain a $Paco_2$ of 35 ± 3 mm Hg. Elimination of CO_2 is usually not a problem during OLV if the DLT is positioned correctly. The shunt during OLV has little influence on $Paco_2$ values because the arteriovenous PCO_2 difference is normally only 6 mm Hg. Furthermore, CO_2 is 20 times more diffusible than O_2 and will be eliminated faster. It is also important not to hyperventilate the patient's lungs because hypocapnia increases vascular resistance in the dependent lung, inhibits its nondependent lung HPV, increases shunt, and decreases Pao_2. Hypocarbia is believed to inhibit HPV secondary to a vasodilator effect. Because hypocarbia can only be achieved by hyperventilating the dependent lung, it raises the mean intra-alveolar pressure and therefore increases the vascular resistance in that lung.

Positive End-expiratory Pressure to the Dependent Lung

The beneficial effect of selective PEEP 10 cm H_2O ($PEEP_{10}$) to the dependent lung is caused by an increased lung volume at end expiration (FRC), which improves the $\dot{V}/\dot{Q}$ relationship in the dependent lung. The increase in FRC prevents airway and alveolar closure at end expiration. However, PEEP may lead to an increase in lung volume that could cause compression of the small interalveolar vessels and increase pulmonary vascular resistance. If this increase in resistance is limited to the dependent lung, blood flow can be diverted only to the nondependent (nonventilated) lung, increasing shunt fraction and further decreasing Pao_2.

The possibility that the application of PEEP can improve Pao_2 in a diseased dependent lung (low lung volume and low $\dot{V}/\dot{Q}$ ratio) with a low Pao_2 (<80 mm Hg) during OLV has been addressed by Cohen et al.[95] They found that the application of $PEEP_{10}$ during OLV in patients with a low Pao_2 may increase FRC to normal values, resulting in a lower pulmonary vascular resistance and in an improved $\dot{V}/\dot{Q}$ ratio and Pao_2. Presumably, patients with a higher Pao_2 had a dependent lung with an adequate FRC, and the application of PEEP had the negative effect of redistributing blood flow away from the dependent ventilated lung (Fig. 37-19).

In summary, in most circumstances PEEP alone would not improve arterial oxygenation, unless it could increase FRC to normal values. Since PV with low V_T is the recommended mode of ventilation during OLV, it most likely would lead to formation of atelectasis. Therefore, combining low V_T with a small amount of PEEP (5 cm H_2O) to protect from development of atlectasis is the currently recommended ventilatory strategy.

Continuous Positive Airway Pressure to the Nondependent Lung

The single most effective maneuver to increase Pao_2 during OLV is the application of CPAP to the nondependent lung.[96,97] A lower level of CPAP (5 to 10 cm H_2O) maintains the patency of the nondependent lung alveoli, allowing some oxygen uptake to occur in the distended alveoli. CPAP should be applied after delivering an inspiratory V_T to the nondependent lung to keep it slightly expanded. CPAP, applied by insufflation of oxygen under positive pressure, keeps this lung "quiet" and prevents it from collapsing completely. Insufflation of oxygen without maintaining a positive pressure failed to improve Pao_2. Intermittent reinflation of the collapsed (nondependent) lung with oxygen also resulted in a significant improvement in Pao_2.[98]

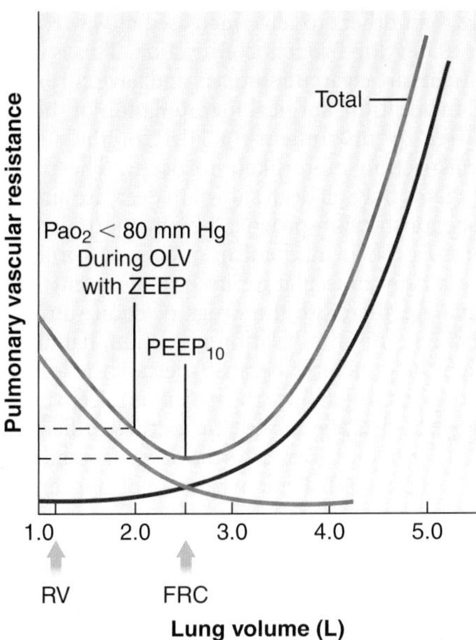

FIGURE 37-19. Effect of 10 cm H_2O positive end-expiratory pressure (PEEP) on functional residual capacity (FRC). It is postulated that, in patients having Pa_{O_2} <80 mm Hg with zero end-expiratory pressure (ZEEP), FRC is low. $PEEP_{10}$ increases FRC and thereby increases Pa_{O_2}. OLV, one-lung ventilation; $PEEP_{10}$, positive end-expiratory pressure (10 cm H_2O); RV, residual volume.

Unfortunately most thoracic procedures are initiated thoracoscopically, and the application of CPAP to the nondependent lung is generally not acceptable to most surgeons. During VAT, the lung should be well collapsed to allow the surgeon an optimal view of the surgical field and to palpate the lesion in the lung parenchyma. In addition, it is difficult to place the stapler on a lung that is not completely collapsed, and there is an increase in incidence of postoperative air leak.

The beneficial effects of CPAP 10 cm H_2O ($CPAP_{10}$) are not attributable solely to the effect of positive pressure in diverting blood flow away from the collapsed lung because (in dogs) the hyperinflation of nitrogen into the nondependent lung under 10 cm H_2O failed to improve Pa_{O_2}.

The application of high-level CPAP (15 cm H_2O) is not beneficial. At this pressure, the lung becomes overdistended, which interferes with surgical exposure. Also, this level of CPAP might have hemodynamic consequences, whereas $CPAP_{10}$ has been shown to have no significant hemodynamic effects.[99]

4 CPAP can be applied to the nondependent lung using a number of simple systems, all of which have essentially the same features: An oxygen source, tubing to connect the oxygen source to the nonventilated lung, a pressure relief valve, and a pressure gauge. The catheter to the nondependent lung is usually insufflated with 5 L/min of oxygen using a modified Ayres T-piece (pediatric) circuit, and the valve on the expiratory limb is adjusted to the desired pressure as read on the attached gauge. Instead of a pressure gauge or manometer inserted into the circuit, a weighted pop-off valve such as a ball or spring-loaded PEEP valve can be used. The amount of CPAP applied should be titrated to the clinical circumstances. In most cases, even low doses of CPAP may be sufficient to increase the Pa_{O_2} to an accepted safe level. CPAP >10 cm H_2O, is not beneficial because it creates an overdistention that interferes with surgical exposure and may have undesirable hemodynamic consequences.

High-frequency ventilation with oxygen to the nondependent lung and conventional ventilation (CV) to the dependent lung have also been used to improve Pa_{O_2} during OLV (see "High-frequency Ventilation").

Clinical Approach to Management of One-lung Ventilation

Once the patient is in the lateral position, the position of the DLT should be rechecked. Two-lung ventilation should be maintained for as long as possible, and when OLV needs to be instituted, it is generally recommended that an F_{IO_2} of 1 be used (Table 37-4).
6 The lung should be ventilated using a V_T that results in a plateau airway pressure <25 cm H_2O at a rate adjusted to maintain Pa_{CO_2} at 35 ± 3 mm Hg. This is usually monitored with the use of a capnometer or other multigas analyzer. The following measures are recommended during OLV: use of PV with low V_T 6 to 7 mL/kg, application of PEEP to the dependent lung, frequent recruitment maneuvers, and limiting the volume of fluid administered.

After initiation of OLV, depending on the lung pathology and the intensity of HPV, Pa_{O_2} can continue to decrease for up to 45 minutes. Frequent monitoring of arterial blood gases and use of a pulse oximeter continue throughout the operative period. It is also essential to work closely with the surgeon in case reinsufflation of the lung is necessary. If hypoxemia occurs during OLV, the position of the DLT should be rechecked using a fiberoptic bronchoscope. If the dependent lung is not severely diseased, a satisfactory Pa_{O_2} on two-lung ventilation should not decrease to dangerously hypoxic levels on OLV. If a left thoracotomy is being performed using a right-sided DLT, ventilation to the right upper lobe should be ensured. After the tube position has been confirmed as correct, $CPAP_{10}$ should be applied to the nondependent lung after a V_T that expands the lung. In most cases, the Pa_{O_2} increases to a safe level. During thoracoscopy, application of CPAP is usually not possible because it impedes the surgeon. This is especially so during video-assisted thoracoscopic surgery (VATS) procedures. In this case, PEEP to the ventilated lung may be tried.

TABLE 37-4. CLINICAL APPROACH TO ONE-LUNG VENTILATION (OLV) MANAGEMENT

1. Use F_{IO_2} of 1
2. Ventilate with a V_T of 6–8 mL/kg with PEEP 5 cm H_2O
3. Respiratory rate to maintain Pa_{CO_2} between 35 and 40 mm Hg
4. Check the DLT/endobronchial blocker position subsequent to the lateral decubitus positioning
5. If peak airway pressure exceeds 40 cm H_2O during OLV, DLT/endobronchial blocker malposition should be excluded
6. For hypoxemia, apply CPAP 10 cm H_2O to the nondependent lung (not during VAT)
7. If additional correction of hypoxemia is necessary add PEEP 5–10 cm H_2O to the ventilated lung
8. Frequent recruiting maneuvers
9. Avoid fluid overload
10. TIVA may be preferable to inhalation anesthetics
11. If necessary, intermittently inflate and deflate the operated lung

V_T, tidal volume; PEEP, positive end-expiratory pressure; DLT, double-lumen tube; CPAP, continuous positive airway pressure; VAT, video-assisted thoracoscopy; TIVA, total intravenous anesthetic.

ANESTHESIA FOR SURGICAL SUBSPECIALTIES

In the very rare case in which the Pa_{O_2} remains low despite these maneuvers, intermittent two-lung ventilation can be reinstituted with the surgeon's cooperation. Also, depending on the stage of surgical dissection, if a pneumonectomy is being performed, ligation of the pulmonary artery eliminates the shunt.

During OLV, the peak airway pressure, the actual V_T delivered (measured by a spirometer), the shape of the capnogram, and, if available, the pressure–volume loop, should be checked continuously. A sudden increase in peak airway pressure may be secondary to tube dislocation because of surgical manipulation, resulting in impaired ventilation. In addition, the ability to auscultate by a stethoscope over the dependent lung is extremely important.

If there is any doubt about the stability of the patient, or if the patient becomes hypotensive, dusky, or tachycardic, two-lung ventilation should be resumed until the problem has been resolved. Because of pericardial manipulation (during left thoracotomy in particular) and pulling on the great vessels, cardiac dysrhythmias and hypotension are not uncommon. Cardiotonic drugs should be prepared and kept available for use during any thoracic surgical procedure. Most thoracic surgical procedures represent only relative indications for OLV, and the benefits of OLV should always be weighed against the risks to the patient.

Attention should be directed toward the protection of the ventilated lung. PV should be used with low V_T and the lowest peak airway pressure, an I:E ratio of 1:1, with high respiratory rate or using pressure control ventilation. Patients with COPD are of particular concern because the application of PEEP may cause dynamic hyperinflation secondary to the increase in respiratory rate to maintain Pa_{CO_2}.

Frequent recruiting maneuvers should be applied to reduce the amount of atelectasis in the dependent lung. They should be applied with a sustained peak pressure of 40 cm H_2O to be effective. Fluid administration during the procedure must be limited to avoid fluid overload that could increase pulmonary capillary permeability. The risk of ALI and fluid overload increases in proportion to the amount of lung parenchyma resected.[100–102]

A balanced anesthetic technique using inhalational agents with low rates of propofol infusion alone or in combination with remifentanil is the technique of choice during OLV. It would have the least inhibitory effect on HPV and decrease the transpulmonary shunt through the nonventilated lung. A recent review by Karzai et al.[103] addressed the prediction, prevention, and treatment of hypoxemia during OLV.

A study by Yang et al.[104] compared PV with CV in two groups of 50 patients each undergoing OLV. Conventional strategy consisted of F_{IO_2} 1, VT 10 mL/kg, zero end-expiratory pressure (ZEEP), and VCV; the protective strategy consisted of F_{IO_2} 0.5, VT 6 mL/kg, PEEP 5 cm H_2O, and PCV. During OLV, although 58% of the PV group needed an increased F_{IO_2} to maintain an Sp_{O_2} >95%, peak airway pressure was significantly lower than in the CV group, whereas the mean Pa_{CO_2} values remained at 35 to 40 mm Hg in both groups. Importantly, in the PV group, the incidence of the primary end point of pulmonary dysfunction was significantly lower than in the CV group (incidence of Pa_{O_2}/F_{IO_2} <300 mm Hg, lung infiltration, or atelectasis: 4% vs. 22%).

CHOICE OF ANESTHESIA FOR THORACIC SURGERY

7 The choice of anesthesia technique for a thoracic surgical procedure must take into account the patient's cardiovascular and respiratory status and the particular effects of anesthetic drugs on these and other organ systems. Thoracic surgical patients are more likely than others to have increased airway reactivity and a propensity to develop bronchoconstriction. This is because many of these patients are cigarette smokers and have chronic bronchitis or COPD. In addition, surgical manipulation of the airways and bronchial tree by instruments, a DLT, or the surgeon makes bronchoconstriction more likely to occur. The potent inhaled anesthetic agents have all been shown to decrease airway reactivity and bronchoconstriction provoked by hypocapnia or inhaled or irritant aerosols. Their mechanism of action is probably a direct one on the airway musculature itself, and potent inhaled anesthetic agents are therefore the drugs of choice in patients with reactive airways. For an inhalation induction, halothane or sevoflurane might be preferable because they are the least pungent of the three drugs, although once the patient is asleep, isoflurane may be the preferred drug because it raises the cardiac dysrhythmia threshold and provides greater cardiovascular stability than halothane (see Chapter 17). Fentanyl does not appear to influence bronchomotor tone, but morphine may increase tone by a central vagotonic effect and by releasing histamine.

In most patients, anesthesia is safely induced with propofol or etomidate (since thiopental is no longer available in the United States). In patients with reactive airways, ketamine may be the drug of choice for induction because it has a bronchodilator effect and has been successfully used in the treatment of asthma. Shimizu et al.[105] compared the effects of isoflurane and sevoflurane on Pa_{O_2} during OLV in 20 patients undergoing thoracotomy and found no significant difference between the groups in Pa_{O_2}, concluding that both agents can be used safely. In an in vitro study, Loer et al.[106] showed that desflurane inhibits HPV, with an ED_{50} of 1.6 minimum alveolar concentration (MAC). Propofol infused in doses of 6 to 12 mg/kg/hr does not abolish HPV during OLV in humans.[107] Propofol infusion in combination with remifentanil is probably the technique of choice for producing a stable OLV with no effect on HPV. Propofol is widely used during OLV and has been investigated in terms of its effect on oxygenation. Kellow et al.[108] compared the effects of propofol and isoflurane anesthesia on right ventricular function and shunt fraction during thoracic surgery and found that isoflurane, but not propofol, was associated with an increase in shunt fraction due to HPV inhibition. However, propofol was associated with a reduction in cardiac index and right ventricular ejection fraction.

In deciding between intravenous versus potent inhaled agent for anesthesia during OLV, consideration should be given to their effects on inflammatory alterations in the deflated lung. Studies have shown that ventilation with increased V_Ts and pressures can produce a proinflammatory reaction (e.g., tumor necrosis factor, interleukins) in the nondeflated, ventilated lung.[109] De Conno et al. studied the effect on the pulmonary inflammatory response in the nonventilated lung before and after OLV in 54 adult patients undergoing thoracic surgery, and assessed if there were any immunomodulatory effects of propofol and sevoflurane. The results suggested an immunomodulatory role for sevoflurane. Compared with propofol there was a significant reduction in inflammatory mediators and a significantly better clinical outcome defined by postoperative adverse events with sevoflurane.[110] A subsequent study compared the effects of desflurane, sevoflurane, and propofol on pulmonary and systemic inflammation in 63 patients undergoing open thoracic surgery. The investigators found that OLV increases the alveolar concentrations of proinflammatory mediators in the ventilated lung and that desflurane and sevoflurane suppress the local alveolar, but not the systemic, inflammatory responses to OLV and thoracic surgery.[111]

The neuromuscular blocking drugs of choice for thoracic procedures are those that lack a histamine-releasing or vagotonic effect and that have some sympathomimetic effect (see Chapter 20). In this respect, pancuronium, vecuronium, rocuronium, and cisatracurium probably represent the drugs of choice. Succinylcholine is useful to provide rapid profound relaxation for intubation of the trachea and is not associated with an increase in airway reactivity.

Atropine or glycopyrrolate may be used to block the muscarinic effects of acetylcholine and thereby protect against cholinergically induced bronchoconstriction. It may be administered intravenously or in nebulized form (see Chapter 15).

HYPOXIC PULMONARY VASOCONSTRICTION

HPV was first described by Von Euler and Liljestrand in 1946.[112] They were studying changes in the pulmonary circulation of the cat in response to changes in inspired gas mixtures and found that 10.5% inspired O_2 (in N_2) mixtures caused an increase in pulmonary artery pressure. Breathing 100% O_2 caused a decrease in pulmonary artery pressure. They concluded that the increased pressure during hypoxia was caused by a direct effect on the pulmonary vessels. Whereas they delivered hypoxic gas mixtures to both lungs, others have studied the effects of the size of the hypoxic segment and the size of the hypoxic stimulus on perfusion pressure and on flow diversion.[113] Pulmonary perfusion pressure (in dogs) increased with the size of the hypoxic segment from zero (smallest hypoxic segment) to approximately 2.2 times baseline for the hypoxic whole lung. Flow diversion, as a percentage of flow to the test segment under normoxic conditions, decreased with increasing size of the hypoxic test segment from a maximum of 75% for very small segments to zero when the whole lung was made hypoxic. Flow diversion increased linearly as $Pa{O_2}$ was decreased over the range of 128 to 28 mm Hg. In both flow diversion and changes in perfusion pressure, the response to HPV was predictable, continuous, and maximal at a predicted $Pa{O_2}$ of 30 mm Hg (4% oxygen). Thus, HPV causes an increase in both perfusion (pulmonary artery) pressure and flow diversion.

The choice of anesthetic technique for OLV must take into consideration the effects on oxygenation and therefore on HPV. Normally, collapse of the nonventilated, nondependent lung results in activation of reflex HPV in this lung. This causes local increases in pulmonary vascular resistance and diversion of blood flow to other, better oxygenated parts of the pulmonary vascular bed (i.e., the dependent oxygenated and ventilated lung).

The relationship between $Pa{O_2}$ and the size of the hypoxic segment (Fig. 37-20) shows that, when not much of the lung is hypoxic, HPV has little effect on $Pa{O_2}$ because shunt is small in this situation. When most of the lung is hypoxic, there is no significant normoxic region to which the hypoxic region can divert flow, and then it does not matter, in terms of $Pa{O_2}$, whether the hypoxic region has active HPV. When the amount of lung made hypoxic is 30% to 70%, such as occurs during OLV, there may be a large difference between the $Pa{O_2}$ to be expected with normal HPV compared with that expected in its absence. HPV can raise $Pa{O_2}$ from potentially dangerous levels to higher and safer ones. Conversely, inhibition of HPV may cause or contribute to hypoxemia during anesthesia.

The response is believed to be accounted for by each smooth muscle cell in the pulmonary arterial wall responding to the oxygen tension in its vicinity. The mechanism of HPV has been the subject of many studies and the current status (the Redox Theory) is summarized in some excellent reviews.[114–116]

Effects of Anesthetics on Hypoxic Pulmonary Vasoconstriction

The inhalation anesthetics and many of the intravenous drugs used in anesthesia have been studied for their effects on HPV. The results have not always been consistent. Benumof[117] classified the preparations used to study these effects as in vitro, in vivo nonintact, in vivo intact, and human studies. On the basis of the results of these three types of preparation, it is generally believed that inhaled agents inhibit HPV, whereas intravenous drugs do not have this effect.[118] Studies of the effects of anesthetics and other drugs in HPV in humans are difficult since during a surgical procedure and there are many confounding variables, in particular the effects of inhaled agents on hemodynamics, for which to account.[119–121] Clinical studies therefore often fail to show a

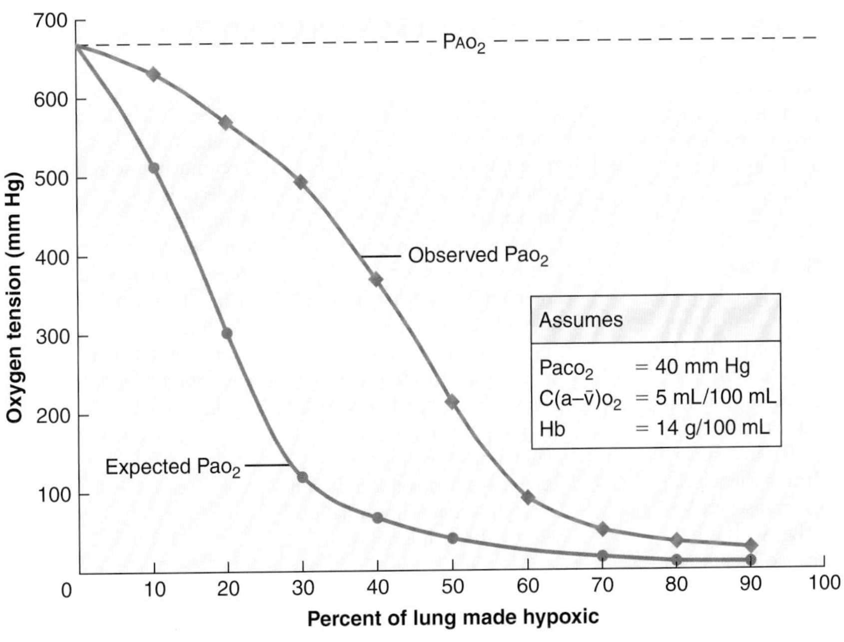

FIGURE 37-20. Role of hypoxic pulmonary vasoconstriction (HPV) in preserving $Pa{O_2}$ (in dogs). Assumptions are shown in inset. Lung is ventilated with $F{IO_2} = 1$, while increasing portions of lung are subjected to hypoxia or atelectasis. In the absence of HPV, the expected $Pa{O_2}$ would follow the blue line, whereas in the presence of an active HPV response, observed $Pa{O_2}$ is maintained close to the red line. $PA{O_2}$, alveolar $P{O_2}$; $Pa{O_2}$, arterial $P{O_2}$. (Adapted from: Marshall BE, Marshall C, Benumof JL, et al. Hypoxic pulmonary vasoconstriction in dogs: Effects of lung segment size and alveolar oxygen tension. *J Appl Physiol.* 1981;51:1543, with permission.)

difference between inhaled and intravenous agents. For example, studies have shown no clinical difference in PaO_2 and shunt between OLV patients anesthetized using propofol or sevoflurane,[122] or propofol versus isoflurane.[123] Another study[108] reported finding a larger shunt with isoflurane. A study comparing sevoflurane with propofol, both titrated to a BIS reading of 40 to 60, found no difference in effect on oxygenation.[124]

Beck et al.[122] studied 40 patients requiring OLV randomized to receive propofol (4 to 6 mg/kg/hr) or sevoflurane (1 MAC) for anesthesia maintenance. During OLV shunt fraction increased in both groups, but there was no significant difference between groups. It was concluded that inhibition of HPV by sevoflurane may only account for small increases in shunt fractions and that much of the overall shunt fraction during OLV has other causes.

Overall, the potent inhaled anesthetics are the drugs of choice during thoracic surgery. However, the technique chosen should always be dictated by the needs of the particular patient, so in the presence of cardiovascular instability or poor oxygenation when depression of HPV is a possibility, a balanced technique may be chosen.

Other Determinants of Hypoxic Pulmonary Vasoconstriction

Aside from potent inhaled agents, other drugs and maneuvers used during anesthesia may also have an inhibitory effect on regional or whole-lung HPV. Factors associated with an increase in pulmonary artery pressure antagonize the effect of increased resistance caused by HPV and result in increased flow to the hypoxic region. Such indirect inhibitors of HPV include mitral stenosis, volume overload, thromboembolism, hypothermia, vasoconstrictor drugs, and a large hypoxic lung segment. Direct inhibitors of HPV include infection, vasodilator drugs such as nitroglycerin and nitroprusside, hypocarbia, and metabolic alkalemia. All these potential inhibitors should be considered when evaluating a patient for hypoxemia during thoracic surgery.[125]

Potentiators of Hypoxic Pulmonary Vasoconstriction

Whereas in the past most research effort has been directed to studying inhibition of HPV, more recent research has investigated substances that may potentiate it. Almitrine, a respiratory stimulant drug, has been found to improve Pao_2 in patients with COPD and to have this effect in the absence of ventilatory stimulation.

Nitric Oxide and One-lung Ventilation

Nitric oxide is an endothelial-derived relaxing factor that is an important mediator for smooth muscle relaxation. HPV is inhibited by inhaled nitric oxide. Inhibition of nitric oxide synthase improved, but did not completely restore HPV in dogs suffering from sepsis.[126] Frostell et al.[127] showed that inhalation of nitric oxide selectively induced vasodilation and reversed HPV in healthy humans without causing systemic vasodilatation. It was theorized that intravenous administration of almitrine (to increase HPV) causing vasoconstriction throughout the lung, together with inhalation of nitric oxide to inhibit HPV locally and cause increased flow in the ventilated regions, would improve $\dot{V}/\dot{Q}$ matching and Pao_2 in patients with $\dot{V}/\dot{Q}$ mismatching or during OLV.[128]

Moutafis et al.[129] studied the effects of inhaled nitric oxide in combination with almitrine infusion during OLV in 40 patients undergoing thoracoscopic procedures. They found that inhaled nitric oxide alone did not affect Pao_2 during OLV, but the additional infusion of almitrine 16 mg/kg/min caused a marked increase in Pao_2. These authors suggested that this nonventilatory technique should be of value during special thoracic procedures, such as thoracoscopy, where there is a need to manipulate the pulmonary circulation to improve Pao_2 but measures such as PEEP and CPAP cannot be used. Moutafis et al.[130] also reported the use of almitrine infusion/nitric oxide inhalation to improve Pao_2 during OLV for bronchopulmonary lavage.

Although the use of almitrine appears to be attractive, this drug is not without side effects.[131] Also, the manufacturer has not made it available outside France. Phenylephrine could be a possible alternative to almitrine.[132]

ANESTHESIA FOR DIAGNOSTIC PROCEDURES

Bronchoscopy

Early bronchoscopes were of the rigid type, but in 1966 the Machida and Olympus Companies introduced the first practical bronchofiberscopes. Since then, they have been improved dramatically and have simplified many otherwise complicated bronchoscopies. The indications for bronchoscopy are shown in Table 37-5 and the instruments of choice in Table 37-6. Operator preferences and experience may play a major role in the choice of instrument.

Before bronchoscopy is performed, the patient must be evaluated for chronic lung disease, respiratory obstruction, bronchospasm, coughing, hemoptysis, and infectivity of secretions. Medications should be reviewed, and the need for a more major procedure should always be anticipated. Thus bronchoscopy may lead to

TABLE 37-5. INDICATIONS FOR BRONCHOSCOPY

Diagnostic	Therapeutic
Cough	Foreign bodies
Hemoptysis	Accumulated secretions
Wheeze	Atelectasis
Atelectasis	Aspiration
Unresolved pneumonia	Lung abscess
Diffuse lung disease	Reposition endotracheal tubes
Preoperative evaluation	
Rule out metastases	Placement of endobronchial tubes
Abnormal chest radiograph	
Assess local disease recurrence	Laser surgery of the airway
Recurrent laryngeal nerve palsy	
Diaphragm paralysis	
Acute inhalation injury	
Exclude tracheoesophageal fistula	
During mechanical ventilation	
Selective bronchography	

Adapted from: Landa JF. Indications for bronchoscopy. *Chest.* 1978;73(suppl):686, with permission.

TABLE 37-6. INSTRUMENTS OF CHOICE FOR BRONCHOSCOPY

Rigid
Foreign bodies
Massive hemoptysis
Vascular tumors
Small children
Endobronchial resections
Fiberoptic/Flexible
Mechanical problems of neck
Upper lobe and peripheral lesions
Limited hemoptysis
During mechanical ventilation
Pneumonia, for selective cultures
Positioning of double-lumen tubes
Difficult intubation
Checking position of endotracheal tube
Bronchial blockade

Adapted from: Landa JF. Indication for bronchoscopy. *Chest.* 1978;73(suppl):686, with permission.

thoracotomy or sternotomy. The planned technique for bronchoscopy should be discussed with the surgeon before the operation, and all equipment and connectors should be checked for compatibility. Monitoring during bronchoscopy should include an electrocardiogram, a blood pressure cuff, a precordial stethoscope, and a pulse oximeter. If thoracotomy is planned, an arterial cannula should also be placed, as well as other monitors (e.g., PA or CVP catheters) that may be indicated by the patient's condition. Many anesthetic techniques are useful for bronchoscopy.

Local Anesthesia

The patient should first be pretreated with a drying agent. The local anesthetics most commonly used are lidocaine and tetracaine. In all cases, the total dose of anesthetic must be considered and the potential for toxicity recognized. A nebulizer can be used to spray the oropharynx and base of the tongue, or the patient may gargle with viscous (2%) lidocaine. The tongue is then held forward, and pledgets soaked in local anesthetic are held in each piriform fossa using Krause forceps to achieve block of the internal branch of the superior laryngeal nerve (see Chapter 21). Tracheal anesthesia is achieved by a transtracheal injection of local anesthetic, or by spraying the vocal cords and trachea under direct vision using a laryngoscope or through the suction channel of the bronchofiberscope. Alternatively, a superior laryngeal nerve block can be performed by an external approach, and a glossopharyngeal block can be used to depress the gag reflex. These blocks cause depression of airway reflexes, so patients must be kept on nothing by mouth status for several hours after the examination. If fiberoptic bronchoscopy is to be performed transnasally, the nasal mucosa should be pretreated topically with 4% cocaine, or viscous lidocaine may be administered through the nares. Local anesthesia for bronchoscopy has the advantages of a patient who is awake, cooperative, and breathing spontaneously. Sedatives may be added to make the patient more comfortable. Disadvantages of local anesthesia include poor tolerance of any bleeding by the patient and the occasional lack of patient cooperation.

General Anesthesia

General anesthesia for bronchoscopy is often combined with topical laryngeal anesthesia so less general anesthesia is needed. A balanced technique uses N_2O/O_2, incremental doses of an intravenous drug such as propofol, an opioid, and a neuromuscular blocking drug. A potent inhalational anesthesia technique is also satisfactory. Alternatively, an intravenous-based technique may be used to avoid contamination of the OR atmosphere by potent inhaled agents. If desired, limited scavenging of waste gases may be achieved by placing a suction catheter in the patient's oropharynx. Unless there is some contraindication, ventilation of the lungs is usually controlled. In any patient undergoing a thoracic diagnostic procedure for a suspected malignancy, the possibility of the myasthenic syndrome with sensitivity to nondepolarizing muscle relaxants must always be considered. The doses of neuromuscular blocking drugs should be titrated to effect using a neuromuscular monitoring system.

Rigid Bronchoscopy

A modern rigid ventilating bronchoscope is essentially a hollow tube with a blunted, beveled tip. Various sizes and designs are available; however, in all of them, a side arm is provided for connection to an anesthesia source. A number of techniques have been described for maintaining ventilation and oxygenation during rigid bronchoscopic examination.

Apneic Oxygenation. After preoxygenation and induction of general anesthesia, skeletal muscle paralysis and cessation of intermittent positive-pressure ventilation, the $Paco_2$ increases. During the first minute, the increase is approximately 6 mm Hg. Subsequently, the average rate of increase is 3 mm Hg/min. Oxygen is insufflated at 10 to 15 L/min through a small catheter placed above the carina. The apneic period should be kept to the minimum necessary, particularly in high-risk patients, because the technique is limited by buildup of CO_2, respiratory acidosis, and cardiac dysrhythmias.

Apnea and Intermittent Ventilation. Oxygen and anesthesia gases are delivered to the bronchoscope via the anesthesia circuit. Ventilation is possible only when the eyepiece is in place, which limits the period for instrumentation by the surgeon. Intermittent ventilation of the lungs is achieved by squeezing the reservoir bag. In this way, assuming a good bronchoscope fit in the airway, compliance is constantly monitored, the risk of barotrauma is reduced, and V_T may be estimated. The disadvantage of this technique is that there may be a leak around the bronchoscope, which could lead to hypoventilation and hypercarbia. Packing of the oropharynx can reduce the leak, and improve ventilation in the case of such a gas leak.

Sanders Injection System. Oxygen from a high-pressure source (50 psig) is delivered, using a controllable pressure-reducing valve and toggle switch, to a 2.5- to 3.5-cm 18- or 16-gauge needle inside and parallel to the long axis of the bronchoscope. When the toggle switch is depressed, the jet of oxygen entering the bronchoscope entrains room air, and the air–oxygen mixture resulting at the distal tip of the bronchoscope emerges at a pressure to provide adequate ventilation and oxygenation. The intraluminal tracheal pressure depends on the driving pressure from the reducing valve, the size of the needle jet, the length, internal diameter, and design of the bronchoscope. Increasing the size of the needle jet increases the total gas flow for any given driving pressure. For each combination of gas-driving pressure, jet orifice, and bronchoscope diameter, only one inflation pressure can be attained, regardless of the volume or compliance of the lung. As long as the proximal end of the bronchoscope is open, the system is strictly pressure limited, and the pressure does not increase because of obstruction at the distal end. Pressure varies inversely with the cross-sectional area of the bronchoscope, so insertion of a suction catheter or biopsy forceps into the lumen causes the intratracheal pressure to increase. Provided there is not a tight fit between the bronchoscope and the airway, the risk of barotrauma is low. If the fit is tight, driving pressure should be decreased.

The advantages of the Sanders system are that because continuous ventilation is possible (because the presence of an eyepiece is not necessary for ventilation of the lungs), the duration of the bronchoscopy procedure is minimized, but the efficiency also permits extended bronchoscopy. A disadvantage is that entrainment of air by the oxygen jet results in a variable FIO_2 at the distal end of the bronchoscope, ventilation of the lungs may be inadequate if compliance is poor, and adequacy of ventilation may be difficult to assess.

Mechanical Ventilator. Ventilation of the lungs may be achieved by connecting a mechanical ventilator to an anesthesia circuit that is connected to the bronchoscope side arm. One disadvantage of this ventilation technique is the presence of a leak of anesthesia gases, and consequentially, light anesthesia.

High-frequency Positive-Pressure Ventilation. HFPPV has been used in conjunction with rigid bronchoscopy and has been compared with the Sanders injector in patients with tracheobronchial stenosis. With HFPPV of up to 150 breaths/min, blood gases were identical with both techniques. At a frequency of 500 breaths/min, oxygenation deteriorated and CO_2 was not removed effectively. HFPPV has the advantage that the tracheobronchial wall remains immobilized during ventilation.

Fiberoptic Bronchoscopy

7 New generations of fiberscopes, with their improved optics and smaller diameters, have revolutionized bronchoscopy. The flexibility has also been applied in preoperative assessment of the airway, management of difficult tracheal intubations, endotracheal tube positioning and change, bronchial toilet, correct positioning of DLTs, bronchial blockade, and evaluation of the larynx and trachea. Nasal fiberoptic bronchoscopy under topical anesthesia is well tolerated by most awake patients. The administration of an antisialagogue such as glycopyrrolate is useful in reducing secretions. Oral insertion is also possible in both awake and asleep patients and should be performed with a bite block in place to prevent damage to the bronchoscope.

Physiologic Changes Associated with Fiberoptic Bronchoscopy. In all patients, insertion of the fiberoptic bronchoscope is associated with hypoxemia. The average decline in PaO_2 is 20 mm Hg and lasts for 1 to 4 hours after the procedure. By 24 hours, the blood gas tensions are usually back to normal. It is therefore recommended that if the initial PaO_2 is 70 mm Hg ($FIO_2 = 0.21$), bronchoscopy should be performed only with the administration of supplemental oxygen. This can be provided using mouth-held nasal prongs, a special face mask with a diaphragm through which the fiberscope can be passed, or an endotracheal tube with a T-piece diaphragm adapter.

During and after fiberoptic bronchoscopy, patients experience increased airway obstruction. Thus in 35 patients, insertion of the bronchoscope was associated with an increase in FRC (17% to 30%) and decreases in PaO_2, vital capacity, FEV_1, and forced inspiratory flow.[133] All returned to baseline by 24 hours. These changes are believed to be secondary to direct mechanical activation of irritative reflexes in the airway and, possibly, to mucosal edema. They may be avoided if atropine, either intramuscular or aerosolized into the airway, is administered before the procedure. 8

The standard adult fiberoptic bronchoscope has an external diameter of 5.7 mm and a 2-mm diameter suction channel. If suction at 1 atm is applied to the fiberscope, air is removed at a rate of 14 L/min. If the fiberscope is in the airway, this causes decreases in FIO_2, PAO_2, and FRC, leading to decreased PaO_2. Suctioning should therefore be kept brief. The adult fiberscope can be passed through endotracheal tubes of 7 mm or greater internal diameter. Clearly, passage through an endotracheal tube decreases the cross-sectional area available for ventilating the patient, so if fibroscopy is planned, an endotracheal tube of the largest possible diameter should be used.

Insertion of the bronchoscope also causes a significant PEEP effect that may result in barotrauma in ventilated patients. If PEEP is already being used, it should be discontinued before passage of the fiberscope. A postendoscopy chest radiograph is advisable to exclude the presence of mediastinal emphysema or pneumothorax. In patients whose tracheas are intubated with endotracheal tubes of <8 mm internal diameter, use of pediatric fiberscopes, which have smaller diameters, would be more appropriate.

The suction channel of the adult fiberoptic bronchoscope has been used to oxygenate and ventilate the lungs of patients. By attaching a jet ventilation system (similar to that used to drive the Sanders injector for rigid bronchoscopy) to the suction connection at the head of a fiberoptic bronchoscope, successful ventilation of the lungs of patients undergoing gynecologic procedures was achieved.[134] A driving pressure of 50 psig of oxygen was used with a ventilatory rate of 18 to 20 breaths/min. This technique permitted adequate ventilation of patients with normally compliant lungs and chest walls. Ventilation of the lungs should be performed only with the tip of the instrument in the trachea because a more peripheral location may produce barotrauma.

Neodymium-yttrium-aluminum garnet (Nd-YAG) lasers are used for the resection of obstructing and endobronchial lesions (see Chapter 47). This procedure is performed under general anesthesia. The lasers may be introduced into the bronchial tree through a fiberoptic bundle passed via the suction port of the fiberoptic bronchoscope. During laser resection, FIO_2 should be kept to a minimum and titrated against oxygen saturation (as continuously monitored by pulse oximeter) to make endotracheal fire less likely (see Chapter 8). Laser therapy of bronchial tumors is also possible using a rigid bronchoscope. HFPPV through a rigid bronchoscope provides satisfactory operating conditions for laser resection of tracheal tumors and has the advantage of producing airway immobility.

Complications of Bronchoscopy

Complications of rigid bronchoscopy include mechanical trauma to the teeth, hemorrhage, bronchospasm, loss of a sponge, bronchial or tracheal perforation, subglottic edema, and barotrauma. The incidence of complications is much lower with fiberoptic bronchoscopy. Nevertheless, complications may arise owing to overdose with topical anesthetic, insertion trauma, local trauma, hemorrhage, upper airway obstruction related to passage of the instrument through an area of tracheal stenosis, hypoxemia, and bronchospasm. In most cases, it is best to intubate the trachea with an endotracheal tube after bronchoscopy under general anesthesia. This permits avoidance or treatment of some of these problems, particularly the increased airway irritability. Intubation also facilitates effective suctioning of the trachea and bronchi, and allows the patient to recover more gradually from general anesthesia.

DIAGNOSTIC PROCEDURES FOR MEDIASTINAL MASS

Patients with an anterior mediastinal mass may present a special problem for the anesthesiologist. Although such masses may cause obvious superior vena cava obstruction, they may also cause obstruction of major airways and cardiac compression, which are less obvious and may become apparent only on induction of anesthesia. Many cases of anesthetic-related airway compression from anterior mediastinal mass have been reported. In one case, total occlusion of the trachea starting 2 to 3 cm above the carina and extending to both main stem bronchi was observed, and a bronchoscope was passed through the obstruction.[135] In the second case of this report, extrinsic compression of the left main stem bronchus occurred on inspiration during recovery from anesthesia. In the third case, flow–volume studies were performed with the patient in the upright and supine positions, with marked reductions in FEV_1 and peak expiratory flow in the latter position. These findings suggested potential obstruction with onset of anesthesia; radiation therapy to the mediastinum was commenced, after which the flow–volume studies showed improved function. The planned surgical procedure was then performed under local anesthesia. In a subsequent series of 105 patients with mediastinal masses, the incidence of intraoperative cardiorespiratory complications was 38%, and the incidence of postoperative respiratory complications was 11%.[136] No cases of airway collapse were reported during anesthesia. In this series, patients were at increased risk of complications if there were preoperative cardiorespiratory signs and symptoms, obstructive and restrictive dysfunction on pulmonary function tests, and >50% tracheal compression on CT scan. In another series of patients with mediastinal mass, four patients had abnormal spirometry but underwent general anesthesia without sequelae.[137] In severe cases of airway compression, the femoral vessels should be cannulated prior to induction of anesthesia so that if the airway is lost completely cardiopulmonary bypass can be instituted immediately.[138]

The mass may be sensitive to radiation therapy, which could shrink the tumor and make an induction of general anesthesia less hazardous. However, a serious potential disadvantage of preoperative radiation therapy is that it may affect tissue histologic appearance, thereby preventing an accurate diagnosis. Furthermore, if the patient is a child, it may be difficult to obtain tissue samples under local anesthesia. No fatalities occurred in a series of 44 patients aged 18 years of age or younger with anterior mediastinal masses who underwent general anesthesia before radiation or chemotherapy. However, seven patients did have airway compromise.[139] In another report in a series of children, it was found to be safe to induce general anesthesia if the CT scan revealed that the tracheal cross-sectional area and peak expiratory flow rates were at least 50% of predicted.[140] Airway obstruction caused by an anterior mediastinal mass has been attributed to changes in lung and chest wall mechanics associated with changes in position or to onset of paralysis in muscles that previously maintained airway patency. Preoperative evaluation of a patient with an anterior mediastinal mass to avoid life-threatening total airway obstruction is shown in Figure 37-21. It is important to determine in the history if the patient has dyspnea in the supine position and to examine the CT scan to determine the extent of the tumor and its effect on surrounding structures. If such obstruction occurs, it may be relieved by passage of a rigid bronchoscope or anode tube past the obstruction, by direct laryngoscopy,[141] or by changing the position of the patient.

Airway collapse and inability to ventilate has been reported in a previously asymptomatic patient with a mediastinal mass despite spontaneous ventilation with an inhaled anesthetic and an endotracheal tube.[142] This resulted in sudden cardiopulmonary collapse. Positive-pressure ventilation was impossible, a rigid bronchoscopy was requested and the surgeons began to prepare femoral vessel access for emergent cardiopulmonary bypass. Fortunately the airway patency was re-established when the patient's spontaneous respiratory efforts improved as he awoke from general anesthesia.

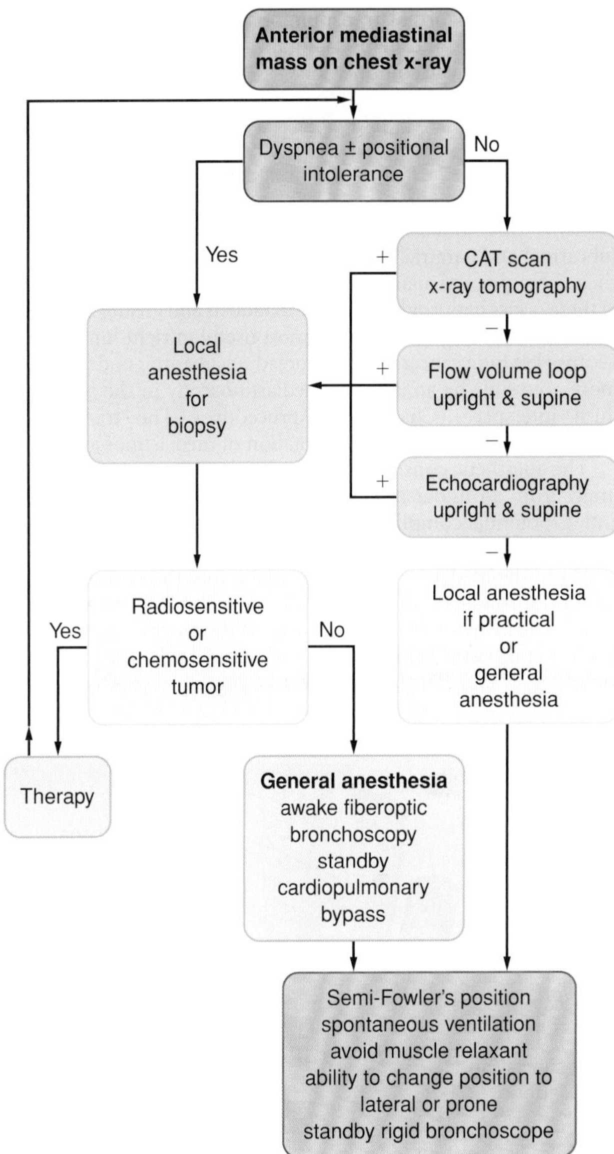

FIGURE 37-21. Flow chart describing the preoperative evaluation of the patient with an anterior mediastinal mass. + indicates positive finding; − indicates negative workup. (Reprinted from: Neuman GG, Weingarten AE, Abramowitz RM, et al. Anesthetic management of the patient with an anterior mediastinal mass. *Anesthesiology.* 1984;60:144, with permission.)

The authors emphasize the need for immediate availability of a rigid bronchoscope and that if a patient is at high risk, then serious consideration should be given to insertion of the femoral cannulas with cardiopulmonary bypass standing by before general anesthesia is induced. Cardiopulmonary bypass is not a suitable rescue modality unless the cannulae have been placed before induction because in the time required to achieve cannulation severe neurologic damage is likely to occur.[143]

In a situation in which the biopsy procedure cannot be performed under local anesthesia and there is concern that muscle paralysis may result in airway compression, fiberoptic intubation of the awake patient followed by general anesthesia with spontaneous ventilation has been described. Thus during spontaneous inspiration, the normal transpulmonary pressure gradient distends the airways and helps maintain their patency, even in the presence of extrinsic compression.

Mediastinoscopy

Mediastinoscopy was introduced as a means of assessing spread of bronchial carcinoma. The lymphatics of the lung drain first to the subcarinal and paratracheal areas, and then to the sides of the trachea, the supraclavicular areas, and the thoracic duct. Examination of these nodes has provided a tissue diagnosis and greater selectivity of patients for thoracotomy. It is most useful in right lung tumors because left lung cancers tend to spread to subaortic nodes that are more accessible by an anterior mediastinoscopy in the second or third interspace (Chamberlain procedure). The transcervical approach to the thymus is an adaptation of mediastinoscopy.

The anesthetic considerations for mediastinoscopy follow naturally from an understanding of the anatomy of this procedure and its potential complications. For cervical mediastinoscopy, the patient is placed in a reverse Trendelenburg (i.e., head-up) position, and the mediastinoscope is inserted into the superior mediastinum through a transverse incision just above the suprasternal notch. The instrument is advanced along the anterior aspect of the trachea and passes behind the innominate vessels and the aortic arch (Fig. 37-22). The left recurrent laryngeal nerve is vulnerable as it loops around the aortic arch, and any of these structures may be traumatized. Because of scarring, previous mediastinoscopy may be considered a contraindication to a repeat examination. Relative contraindications include superior vena cava obstruction, tracheal deviation, and aneurysm of the thoracic aorta.

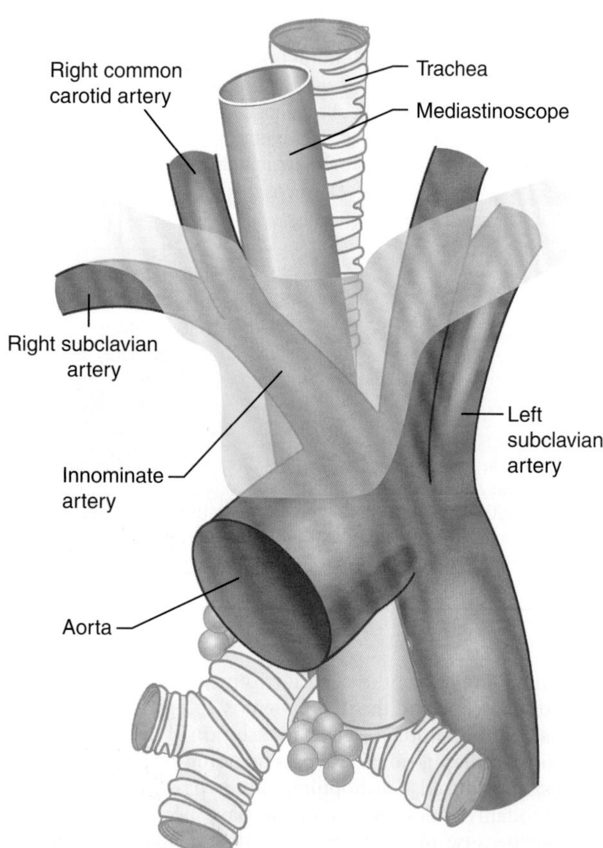

FIGURE 37-22. Anatomic relationships during mediastinoscopy. Note the position of the mediastinoscope behind the right innominate artery and aortic arch and anterior to the trachea. (From: Carlens E. Mediastinoscopy: A method for inspection and tissue biopsy in the superior mediastinum. *Dis Chest.* 1959;36:343.)

Preoperative evaluation should include a search for airway obstruction or distortion. Review of a CT scan is very helpful in this regard. Evidence of impaired cerebral circulation, history of stroke, or signs of the Eaton–Lambert syndrome resulting from oat cell carcinoma should be sought. Blood must be available for the procedure because hemorrhage is a real risk and may be life-threatening.

Most surgeons and anesthesiologists prefer general anesthesia using an endotracheal tube and continuous ventilation because this offers a more controlled situation and greater flexibility in terms of surgical manipulation. The anesthetic technique should include a muscle relaxant to prevent the patient from coughing because this may produce venous engorgement in the chest or trauma by the mediastinoscope to surrounding structures.

The incidence of morbidity with mediastinoscopy has been reported as 1.5% to 3.0%, and that of mortality as 0.09%. The most common complication is hemorrhage (0.73%) because of the proximity of major vessels and the vascularity of certain tumors. Tamponade may be the only recourse, and thoracotomy or median sternotomy may be required to achieve hemostasis. Needle aspiration of any structure is essential before any biopsy is taken. If severe bleeding occurs, induced arterial hypotension may be helpful in reducing the size of the tear in a vessel. If bleeding is venous, fluids given via an upper limb vein may enter the mediastinum, in which case a large-bore catheter should be placed in a lower limb vein. A venous laceration may also result in air embolism, particularly if the patient is breathing spontaneously. Some recommend the use of a precordial Doppler probe if the risk of air embolism is likely.

Pneumothorax is the second most common complication (0.66%). It is usually right-sided, often recognized at the time of the occurrence, and is treated according to the size. A symptomatic pneumothorax should be treated by chest tube decompression.

Recurrent laryngeal nerve injury occurred in 0.34% of cases and was permanent in 50% of these cases. The nerve may be damaged by the mediastinoscope or be involved in tumor. Such injury is not a problem unless both nerves are damaged, in which case upper airway obstruction may result. Autonomic reflexes may be initiated by manipulation of the trachea or the aorta, the latter having pressor receptors located in the arch. Vagally mediated reflexes may be blocked by atropine.

"Factitious" cardiac arrest has been reported when the right radial pulse was monitored using a plethysmograph, and the tracing suddenly disappeared in the presence of a normal electrocardiogram. A normal pulse returned after the mediastinoscope was removed, and the cause of the apparent arrest was pressure on the innominate artery by the instrument. Decreases in right arm as compared with left arm blood pressure have been reported in cases undergoing mediastinoscopy. Duration was 15 to 360 seconds. This is of particular significance if there is a history of impaired cerebral circulation or transient ischemic attacks, or if a carotid bruit is present, because transient left hemiparesis may occur after mediastinoscopy. It is therefore recommended that blood pressure be monitored in the left arm and that the right radial pulse be monitored continuously during mediastinoscopy. A decrease in the right radial pulse amplitude is an indication for repositioning the mediastinoscope, especially in a patient with a history of cerebrovascular disease.

Other reported complications include acute tracheal collapse, tension pneumomediastinum, mediastinitis, hemothorax, and chylothorax. A chest radiograph taken in the immediate postoperative period is a useful precaution in all patients after mediastinoscopy.

Thoracoscopy

Thoracoscopy (medical thoracoscopy) involves the insertion of an endoscope into the thoracic cavity and pleural space. It is used for the diagnosis of pleural disease, effusions, and infectious disease (especially in immunosuppressed patients and those with acquired immunodeficiency syndrome) and for staging procedures, chemical pleurodesis, and lung biopsy. It is usually performed by the pulmonary physician in the clinic, under local anesthesia. It is also used in therapeutic procedures such as CO_2 laser treatment of spontaneous pneumothorax or bullous emphysema[144] and Nd-YAG laser vaporization of malignant pleural tumors. A small incision is made in the lateral chest wall, and with the insertion of the instrument, fluid and biopsy specimens are easily obtained.

This procedure may be performed using local, regional, or general anesthesia; the choice depending on the expected duration of the procedure and the physical status of the patient. Pneumothorax is a potential complication of an intercostal block, but it would not have clinical sequelae during a thoracoscopy because it is created as part of the surgical procedure. The collapse of the lung provides the surgeon with a working space, and a chest tube is placed at the conclusion of the surgery. The addition of a stellate ganglion block helps suppress the cough reflex that is sometimes provoked during manipulation of the hilum of the lung.

When air enters the pleural cavity under inspection, a partial pneumothorax occurs, permitting good surgical visualization. Changes in Pa_{O_2}, Pa_{CO_2}, and cardiac rhythm are usually minimal when the procedure is performed using local or regional anesthesia.

With local anesthesia, the spontaneous pneumothorax is usually well tolerated because the skin and chest wall form a seal around the thoracoscope and limit the degree of lung collapse. Occasionally, however, the procedure is poorly tolerated, and general anesthesia must be induced. The insertion of a DLT with the patient in the lateral position may be difficult, in which case the patient may be temporarily placed in the supine position for the intubation.

If general anesthesia is required, a DLT is preferable to an SLT because positive-pressure ventilation via an SLT would interfere with endoscopic visualization. In addition, if pleurodesis is being performed, general anesthesia through a DLT allows for re-expansion of the lung and avoids the pain associated with instillation of talc for recurrent pneumothorax.

Video-assisted Thoracoscopic Surgery

VATS entails making small incisions in the chest wall, which allows the introduction of a video camera and surgical instruments into the thoracic cavity.[145] Generally, it is performed by a thoracic surgeon in the operating room under general anesthesia. Although the first thoracoscopy was performed by Jacobeus in 1910, using what was at that time a cystoscope, in more recent years the surgical techniques, instruments, and video technology have been improved to permit a wide variety of procedures to be performed using VATS. These now include diagnostic procedures for evaluation of pleural disease and effusions, staging of lung cancer, and the identification of parenchymal disease, including nodules, mediastinal tumors, and pericardial disease. They also include therapeutic procedures such as operations for pleural disease, including pleurodesis, decortication and drainage of empyema, resection of lung tissue or bullae, pericardial window or stripping, and esophageal surgery. Even lung lobectomies can now be performed by VATS.

Anesthesia Considerations

As with a traditional thoracotomy, the patient needs to be in the lateral decubitus position, and lung collapse is needed for adequate surgical exposure. This generally mandates the use of a lung-separation technique. VATS is most commonly performed
8 under general anesthesia with OLV. The need for OLV is much greater with VATS than with open thoracotomy because it is not possible to retract the lung during VATS like it is during an open thoracotomy. The operated lung should be deflated as soon as possible after tracheal intubation and positioning because it may take over 30 minutes for complete lung collapse to occur. Also, the surgeon enters the thoracic cavity much sooner during VATS than with open thoracotomy. Suction applied to the airway can help facilitate a more rapid deflation of the lung. In some cases, carbon dioxide is insufflated into the pleural cavity to facilitate visualization. Insufflation pressures should be maintained as low as possible and the CO_2 inflow rate kept <2 L/min. Higher pressures can cause mediastinal shift, hemodynamic compromise, increases in airway pressure, and increases in end-tidal CO_2. Hemodynamic compromise presents a picture similar to that because of tension pneumothorax. Significant hemodynamic changes can be produced when pressures as little as 5 mm Hg are used to insufflate CO_2 into the chest cavity.[146]

CPAP is commonly used for the treatment of hypoxemia during OLV for thoracotomy and is usually very effective. However, during VATS, CPAP interferes with the surgical exposure and is therefore best avoided. It would be preferable to use PEEP to the nonoperated (dependent lung). In addition, a lower Pa_{O_2} may have to be tolerated during VATS compared with a thoracotomy.

Postoperative Concerns

There is less pain after VATS than open thoracotomy, and an epidural catheter is usually placed before surgery only if there is a likelihood that a thoracotomy may need to be performed. A lobectomy can be performed by VAT, but an open thoracotomy may be required. The patient's respiratory function is better preserved after VATS, and their recovery is faster. However, postoperative dysrhythmias, which commonly occur after thoracotomy, have also been reported after VATS.[147] Other complications that may occur include bleeding, pulmonary edema, and pneumonia.

ANESTHESIA FOR SPECIAL SITUATIONS

Management of patients with BPF, empyema, cysts, and bullae, as well as those requiring tracheal reconstruction, is considered here. Many of these patients are appropriately managed using high-frequency ventilatory techniques; therefore, these techniques are described first (see Chapter 27).

High-frequency Ventilation

With conventional positive-pressure ventilation, V_T and rates usually exceed or approach those in the normal, spontaneously breathing patient. Gas transport to the alveoli occurs by convection in the larger airways, and then by convection and molecular diffusion in the more distal airways and alveoli. High-frequency ventilation differs from conventional positive-pressure ventilation in that smaller V_T and more rapid rates are used. Gas transport may depend more on molecular diffusion, high-velocity flow, and coaxial gas flow in the airways, with gas in the center moving distally and that in the periphery moving proximally.

There are three different types of high-frequency ventilation. HFPPV uses small V_T at rates of 60 to 120 breaths/min (1 to 2 Hz). The ventilator used has a negligible internal compliance so the V_T generated, which usually approximates the dead space volume, equals the volume set on the ventilator and represents all fresh gas. The high instantaneous gas flows generated facilitate gas exchange and movement in the conducting airways.

HFPPV may be delivered by an open or a closed system. An example of the former is the percutaneous placement of a transtracheal catheter or placement of a catheter through the nose or mouth with its distal end above the carina. Inflow is intraluminal and outflow is extraluminal. This technique has been used during bronchoscopy, tracheal resection, and reconstructive surgery. When open systems are used, the gas outflow pathway is not established mechanically and depends on natural airway patency. It is therefore subject to compromise. Also, aspiration is a potential complication with open systems.

The closed system is superior because it integrates both airway patency and outflow protection. A closed system is represented by a catheter placed in a short segment of an endotracheal tube for delivery of the HFPPV, whereas the remainder of the tube lumen represents the exit pathway for gas. A quadruple-lumen endotracheal tube (Hi-Lo Jet Tracheal Tube, Mallinckrodt, Inc.) has been designed specifically for delivery of HFPPV. One lumen is for the HFPPV delivery, one for gas outflow, one for cuff inflation, and one for measuring airway pressures at the distal end of the tube. The use of a closed system also permits application of PEEP, a situation not possible with an open arrangement.

High-frequency jet ventilation (HFJV) uses a pulse of a small jet of fresh gas introduced from a high-pressure source (50 psig) into the airway through a small catheter or additional lumen in an endotracheal tube. Rates used are usually 100 to 400 breaths/min. The fresh gas jet entrains gas from an injection cannula side-port reservoir. This system is somewhat analogous to the Sanders injector system described in the "Bronchoscopy" section, and FIO_2 is similarly variable. The jet and entrained gas flows cause forward motion of the mass of gas in the airways. HFJV can be used with an open system or with a closed arrangement, as described earlier. In the latter, PEEP may be added to enhance oxygenation. Also, with use of high fresh gas flows from an anesthesia circuit, inhaled anesthetics may be delivered as an entrained gas mixture.

High-frequency oscillation ventilation uses a mechanism that oscillates gas at rates of 400 to 2,400 breaths/min. It has not been described in association with thoracic surgical procedures. In this system, V_T is small (50 to 80 mL), and gas exchange occurs through enhanced molecular diffusion and coaxial airway flow.

9 The potential advantages offered by HFPPV during thoracic anesthesia are that lower V_T and inspiratory pressures result in a quiet lung field for the surgeon, with minimal movements of airway, lung tissue, and mediastinum. Thus, HFPPV has been used to ventilate both the nondependent and the dependent lung during thoracic surgical procedures, with adequate arterial blood gas measurements obtained throughout. At high frequencies (>6 Hz), however, CO_2 retention may become a problem.

HFJV has been used to ventilate the nondependent lung to improve Pao_2 during one-lung anesthesia, whereas the dependent lung was ventilated with conventional intermittent positive-pressure ventilation. Pao_2 increased compared with that obtained during simple collapse of the nondependent lung. A study comparing HFJV with CPAP to the nondependent lung during conventional intermittent positive-pressure ventilation to the dependent lung found that both improved Pao_2 significantly during closed and open stages of the surgery. When the chest was open, HFJV maintained satisfactory cardiac output, whereas CPAP usually decreased cardiac output; however, there were no significant differences in $Paco_2$ between HFJV and CPAP. Because similar increases in Pao_2 may be obtained using selective CPAP to the nondependent lung and much simpler equipment than that necessary to deliver high-frequency ventilation, the use of CPAP would seem preferable to high-frequency ventilation to increase Pao_2 during most one-lung anesthesia situations.

The lower pressures and V_Ts associated with high-frequency ventilation result in a small leak through BPFs, and HFJV is now generally considered the conservative treatment of choice in this condition. Another advantage of high-frequency ventilation is that the rapid-rate small V_T can be delivered through small tubes or catheters so if an airway has to be divided, the passage of a small tube across the surgical field permits ventilation of the distal airway and lung tissue. This use has been applied during sleeve resection of the lung, tracheal reconstruction, and surgery for tracheal stenosis. In all three situations, the surgeon is able to work easily around the small catheter used to provide the high-frequency ventilation.

Bronchopleural Fistula and Empyema

A BPF is an abnormal communication between the bronchial tree and the pleural cavity. Occasionally, there is an additional communication to the surface of the chest, a cutaneous BPF. BPF occurs most commonly after pulmonary resection for carcinoma. Other causes include traumatic rupture of a bronchus or bulla (sometimes caused by barotrauma or PEEP), penetrating chest wound, or spontaneous drainage into the bronchial tree of an empyema cavity or lung cyst. The incidence of BPF is higher after pneumonectomy than following other types of lung resection. The problems associated with BPF and empyema are that positive-pressure ventilation may result in contamination of healthy lung, loss of air, decreased alveolar ventilation leading to CO_2 retention, and the development of a tension pneumothorax.

If an empyema is present, it should be drained under local anesthesia before any surgery to close the BPF. Drainage is performed with the patient sitting up and leaning toward the affected side. Empyemas are often loculated, and complete drainage is not always possible. A drain to an underwater seal system is left in the cavity before administration of anesthesia for surgery of the BPF, and after drainage of an empyema, a chest radiograph should be obtained to determine the efficacy of the procedure.

The priorities in the anesthetic management of BPF are the isolation of the affected side in terms of contamination and ventilation. The ideal approach is intubation of the trachea while the patient is awake using a DLT with the patient breathing spontaneously. Supplemental oxygen should be administered, and the patient should be constantly reassured. Neuroleptanalgesia is satisfactory in providing a suitably cooperative patient, and the airway is then pretreated with topical anesthesia. The endobronchial tube selected should be such that the bronchial lumen is on the side opposite the BPF. Selection of the largest possible tube provides a close fit in the trachea, which helps stabilize the tube. Once the tube is adequately positioned in the trachea, there may be a considerable outpouring of pus from the tracheal lumen if an empyema is present; therefore, this lumen should be immediately suctioned using a large-bore suction catheter. The healthy and possibly the affected lung may then be ventilated; adequacy of oxygenation and ventilation is assessed by pulse oximetry and arterial blood gas analysis.

An alternative technique is to insert the DLT under general anesthesia, with the patient breathing spontaneously to avoid a tension pneumothorax. With either technique, the chest drainage tube must be left unclamped to avoid any bouts of coughing and to prevent the buildup of a tension pneumothorax in the event that a predisposing valvular mechanism exists. In patients who do not have an empyema, use of an SLT has been described and may be satisfactory if the BPF and air leak are small. A rapid-sequence induction with ketamine or thiopental followed by a relaxant has also been described, but is associated with considerable risk of contamination and tension pneumothorax.

BPF may also be treated conservatively using various ventilatory techniques. Thus, the bronchus of the normal lung may be intubated and ventilated, allowing the BPF to rest and heal. This approach may result in an intolerable shunt, however, and PEEP may be necessary to maintain Pao_2. Differential lung ventilation using a DLT has also been described, the healthy lung being ventilated with normal V_T, while the affected lung is exposed to a smaller V_T or to CPAP with oxygen at pressures just below the critical opening pressure of the fistula. The critical opening pressure of the BPF can be assessed by determining the lowest level of CPAP that must be applied to the bronchus on the affected side to produce continuous bubbling through the underwater seal chest drain.

For a large BPF, HFJV may be the nonsurgical treatment of choice. The use of small V_Ts results in minimal gas loss through the fistula, which may heal more quickly. In addition, hemodynamic effects are usually minimal and spontaneous efforts at ventilation are usually abolished, thereby decreasing the work of breathing and eliminating the need for relaxants or excessive sedation.

Lung Cysts and Bullae

Air-filled cysts of the lung are usually bronchogenic, postinfective, infantile, or emphysematous. They may be associated with COPD or be an isolated finding. A bulla is a thin-walled space filled with air that results from the destruction of alveolar tissue. The walls are, therefore, composed of visceral pleura, connective tissue septa, or compressed lung tissue. In general, bullae represent an area of end-stage emphysematous destruction of the lung.

Patients may be considered for surgical bullectomy when dyspnea is incapacitating, when the bullae are expanding, when there are repeated pneumothoraces owing to rupture of bullae, or if the bullae compress a large area of normal lung. Most of these patients have severe COPD and CO_2 retention, and little functional respiratory reserve. The first consideration in management is maintenance of a high FIO_2. If the bulla or cyst communicates with the bronchial tree, positive-pressure ventilation may cause it to expand or even to rupture, if it is compliant, producing a situation analogous to tension pneumothorax. If the bulla is very compliant, most of the applied V_T may be wasted in this additional dead space. Nitrous oxide should be avoided because it causes expansion of any air spaces in the body, including bullae. Once the chest is open, even more of the V_T may enter the compliant bulla, which is no longer limited by chest wall integrity, and an increase in ventilation is needed until the bulla is controlled.

The anesthetic management of these patients is challenging, particularly if the disease is bilateral. Ideally, a DLT is inserted with the patient awake or under general anesthesia but breathing spontaneously. The avoidance of positive-pressure ventilation (when possible) helps decrease the likelihood of the potential problems described previously, although oxygenation may be precarious with spontaneous ventilation. Once the endotracheal tube is in place, each lung may be controlled separately, and adequate ventilation can be applied to the healthy lung if bilateral disease is not present. Gentle positive-pressure ventilation with rapid, small V_T and pressures not to exceed 10 cm H_2O may be used during the induction and maintenance of anesthesia, especially if the bullae have been shown to have no or only poor bronchial communication by preoperative ventilation scanning. While the surgery is being performed, as each bulla is resected, the operated lung can be separately ventilated to check for air leaks and the presence of additional bullae.

If positive-pressure ventilation is to be applied before the chest is opened, the possibility of a tension pneumothorax must be kept in mind, and treatment should be readily available. The diagnosis of pneumothorax may be made by a unilateral decrease in breath sounds (this may be difficult to distinguish in a patient with bullous disease), increase in ventilatory pressure, progressive tracheal deviation, wheezing, or cardiovascular changes. Treatment of a pneumothorax involves the rapid placement of a chest tube. An added risk of chest tube placement is the creation of a cutaneous BPF, which causes problems for ventilation. Alternatively, general anesthesia is induced only after the surgeon has prepared the operative field and draped the patient. In the event of sudden deterioration in the patient's condition during induction, the surgeon may perform an immediate median sternotomy. In any event, the time from induction of anesthesia to sternotomy must be kept to a minimum.

To avoid these problems in a patient with known bullae, HFJV has been used in a patient with a large bulla undergoing coronary artery bypass graft and in another patient undergoing bilateral bullectomy. If bilateral bullectomy is to be performed, a median sternotomy is usually used. Benumof[148] described the use of sequential OLV using a DLT in the management of a patient needing bilateral bullectomy. The side with the largest bulla and least lung function, as assessed before surgery by ventilation and perfusion scans, should be operated on first. In this way, the lung with the better function should support gas exchange first. If hypoxemia develops during this one-lung situation, application of CPAP to the nonventilated lung during the deflation phase of a tidal breath should increase Pao_2.

Unlike most cases of pulmonary resection, patients after bullectomy are left with a greater amount of functional lung tissue than was previously available to them, and the mechanics of respiration are improved. At the end of the procedure, the DLT is replaced by an SLT, and the patients generally require several days to be weaned from the ventilator. During this time, the positive airway pressure used should be minimized to avoid causing a pneumothorax owing to rupture of suture or staple lines or of residual bullae.

Anesthesia for Resection of the Trachea

Tracheal resection and reconstruction are technically difficult for the surgeon and challenging for the anesthesiologist. Indications for this type of procedure include congenital lesions (agenesis, stenosis), neoplasia (primary or secondary), injuries (direct or indirect), infections, and postintubation injuries (caused by an endotracheal tube or tracheotomy). For the surgical team, the major problems are maintenance of ventilation to the lungs while the airway is being operated on and postoperative integrity of the anastomoses. In this respect, the presence of lung disease sufficiently severe to require postoperative ventilatory support is a relative contraindication to tracheal resection or reconstruction.

Monitoring of these patients should include placement of an arterial cannula in the left radial artery to permit continuous measurement of blood pressure during periods of innominate artery compression. Steroids should be administered to help reduce any tracheal edema, and a high FIO_2 should be used throughout the procedure to ensure an adequate oxygen reserve at all times in the FRC so that temporary interruptions of ventilation are less likely to produce hypoxemia.

Numerous methods have been reported to provide oxygenation and ventilation of the lungs during these procedures. A small-bore anode tube may be placed through and distal to an upper tracheal lesion so resection may occur around the tube. This technique is useful only in mild stenoses. Alternatively, an endotracheal tube may be passed through the glottis to above the stenosis, and a sterile endotracheal or bronchial tube may later be inserted into the trachea opened distal to the site of stenosis, with the sterile anesthesia tubing being led across the surgical field. After resection of the lesion, the sterile and distally placed endotracheal tube is withdrawn, and the upper tube (originally passed through the glottis) is advanced across the anastomosis. With low tracheal or bronchial lesions, resection and reconstruction may be performed around an endobronchial or DLT. During these procedures, the patient is kept in a head-down position to minimize aspiration of blood and debris into the alveoli, and ventilation must be carefully monitored throughout the procedure.

Clearly, the presence of a large-bore tube in the airway may make these resections technically difficult, and the use of high-frequency ventilation techniques may improve surgical access. Thus, a small-diameter catheter or catheters may be placed across or through the stenotic lesion or transected airway(s) and ventilation to the distal airways and lungs maintained using HFPPV or HFJV. Potential disadvantages of these high-frequency ventilation techniques are that, by necessity, the system is "open" (see "High-frequency Ventilation"), and egress of gas during exhalation may be compromised if the stenosis is tight. Also, the catheter may become occluded by blood and become displaced, and distal aspiration of debris or blood may occur. With complex resections, two anesthesia teams with two machines and anesthesia circuits or sets of ventilating equipment may be necessary to ensure adequate ventilation of the two distal airway segments. Although during carinal resections, HFPPV to the left lung alone usually provides adequate oxygenation and ventilation.

After tracheal resection or reconstructive surgery, patients should be kept with the neck and head flexed to reduce tension on the anastomotic suture lines. In some cases, this is maintained by using sutures between the chin and the anterior chest wall. Extubation of the trachea is performed as early as possible to minimize tracheal trauma due to the endotracheal tube and cuff.

Bronchopulmonary Lavage

This procedure involves irrigation of the lung and bronchial tree, and is used as a treatment for alveolar proteinosis, radioactive dust inhalation, cystic fibrosis, bronchiectasis, and asthmatic bronchitis. Lung lavage is performed under general anesthesia using a DLT so one lung may be ventilated while the other is being treated with lavage fluid.[149]

The preoperative assessment of these patients should include ventilation–perfusion scans so lavage can be performed first on the more severely affected lung (i.e., the one with the least ventilation). If involvement is equal, the left lung is generally lavaged first because gas exchange should be better through the larger, right lung. Patients are premedicated and supplied with supplemental oxygen en route to the operating room.

Anesthesia is induced with an intravenous drug and maintained with an inhaled agent in oxygen to maintain the highest possible FIO_2. Muscle relaxation facilitates placement of the DLT, and the cuff seal should be checked to maintain perfect separation at a pressure of 50 cm H_2O to prevent leakage of lavage fluid around the cuff. A fiberoptic bronchoscope is useful to check the position of the bronchial cuff of the DLT. Monitoring should include an arterial catheter, and a stethoscope should be placed over the ventilated lung to check for rales, the presence of which may indicate leakage of lavage fluid into this lung.

The patient is maintained on an FIO_2 of 1 throughout the procedure. Before lavage, this serves to denitrogenate the lungs so only oxygen and carbon dioxide remain. Instillation of fluid then allows these gases to be absorbed, resulting in greater access by the fluid to the alveolar spaces than if the more insoluble nitrogen bubbles remained.

Once the trachea is intubated, the patient is turned so the side to be lavaged is lowermost, and the DLT position and seal are checked once again. With the patient in a head-up position, warmed heparinized isotonic saline is infused by gravity from a reservoir 30 cm above the midaxillary line into the catheter to the dependent lung, while the nondependent lung is ventilated. When fluid ceases to flow in (usually after 700 to 1,000 mL in an adult), the patient is placed in a head-down position and fluid is allowed to drain out. The lavage is continued until the effluent is clear (as opposed to the milky fluid that drains initially when lavage is being performed for alveolar proteinosis), at which point the lung is suctioned and ventilation is re-established with large V_T (and pressures) because compliance is decreased owing to loss of surfactant. With each lavage, inflow and outflow volumes are monitored so the patient is not "drowned" in fluid, and there is no excessive absorption or leakage to the ventilated side. At least 90% of the saline volume should be recovered with each lavage. Two-lung ventilation is re-established and, as compliance improves, an air–oxygen mixture (addition of nitrogen) may be introduced to help maintain alveolar patency. After a further period of ventilation, in most patients, the trachea can be extubated in the operating room. In the posttreatment period, patients are encouraged to cough and engage in breathing exercises to fully re-expand the treated lung. From 3 days to 1 week after lavage of the first lung, the patient may return to the operating room for lavage of the other lung.

Problems sometimes encountered with this procedure include spillage of lavage fluid from the treated to the ventilated lung. This must be managed by stopping the lavage and ensuring functional separation of the lungs before continuing. DLT positioning is critical. Spillage may cause profound decreases in oxygenation, which may necessitate terminating the procedure and maintaining two-lung ventilation with oxygen and PEEP.

During periods when lavage fluid is being instilled into the dependent lung, oxygenation usually improves because the increased intra-alveolar pressure caused by the fluid produces diversion of the pulmonary blood flow to the nondependent, ventilated lung. Conversely, when the fluid is drained out of the dependent lung, hypoxemia may occur.[150] In some cases in which severe hypoxemia was anticipated during right lung lavage, the risk has been reduced by passing a balloon-tipped catheter into the right main pulmonary artery (checked by radiography) and inflating the balloon during periods of right lung drainage. In this way, blood flow to the dependent, right, nonventilated lung is minimized during periods of drainage. This technique is not without risk (e.g., pulmonary artery rupture) and is reserved for those patients considered to be at greatest risk for hypoxemia during lavage. If the patient has recently had a diagnostic open lung biopsy, a BPF may be present. If this is a possibility, a chest tube should be inserted on the side of the BPF, and this side should be lavaged first. The chest drain is removed several days later.

Limitations in the sizes of available DLTs preclude their use for lavage in patients weighing less than 40 kg. In such cases, cardiopulmonary bypass may be required to provide oxygenation during lavage.

Myasthenia Gravis

The thoracic anesthesiologist will most likely have to manage patients with MG for thymectomy, which is now considered the
10 treatment of choice in most cases of MG. MG is a disorder of the neuromuscular junction, the function of which is altered routinely in the modern practice of anesthesia. The incidence of MG appears to be increasing. The most accurate estimate of incidence of MG was around 30/1,000,000/year. The incidence in children and adolescents aged 0 to 19 years was found to be between 1 and 5/1,000,000/year. These rates may well be an underestimate of the true incidence rates, as mild cases will have been missed and cases in the elderly will have been misdiagnosed.[151] People of any age may be affected, but peaks of incidence occur in the third decade for women and the fifth decade for men. MG is a chronic disorder characterized by a clinical course of fluctuating painless weakness and fatigability of voluntary muscles with improvement following rest.[152,153] Onset is usually slow and insidious, any skeletal muscle or group of muscles may be affected, and the condition is associated with relapses and remissions. The most common onset is ocular; if the disease remains localized to the eyes for 2 years, the likelihood of progression to generalized MG is low. In some cases, the disease is generalized and may involve the bulbar musculature, causing problems with breathing and swallowing. Peripheral muscle involvement may cause weakness, clumsiness, and difficulty in holding up the head or in walking. The most commonly used clinical classification of MG is shown in Table 37-7.

In MG, there is a decrease in the number of postsynaptic acetylcholine receptors (AchRs) at the endplates of affected muscles. This causes a decrease in the margin of safety of neuromuscular transmission. MG is an autoimmune disorder, and about 80% of the affected patients have detectable circulating antibodies to the nicotinic AchR. These anti-AchR antibodies may cause complement-mediated lysis of the postsynaptic membrane or direct blockade of the receptors, or may modulate the receptor turnover such that the degradation rate exceeds the resynthesis rate. Studies of the endplate area show loss of synaptic folds and a widening of the synaptic cleft. A variable proportion of the patients who do not have anti-AchR antibodies have antibodies to muscle-specific tyrosine kinase (MuSK).[154]

The diagnosis of MG is suspected from the patient's history and confirmed by clinical, pharmacologic, electrophysiologic, or immunologic testing. Patients cannot sustain or repeat muscular contraction. The electrical counterpart of this is a decrement in the compound muscle action potentials evoked by repetitive stimulation of a motor nerve. This is the most specific of the nerve tests for MG but it can be performed only on certain muscles, which may not be the ones affected in an individual patient. Mechanical and electrical (electromyography) decrements improve with 2 to 10 mg of intravenous edrophonium (Tensilon test). MG patients characteristically are sensitive to nondepolarizing muscle relaxants. When the routine electromyographic results are equivocal, a regional nondepolarizing muscle relaxant test may be performed using a tourniquet to isolate the limb and limit the action of the drug. In the regional nondepolarizer muscle relaxant test, electromyograms are performed before and after the administration of 0.2 mg of curare. In equivocal cases, a positive result of a test for anti-AchR antibodies is considered diagnostic.

TABLE 37-7. CLINICAL CLASSIFICATION OF MYASTHENIA GRAVIS (MG)

Class	Description
I	Ocular myasthenia—involvement of ocular muscles only. Mild with ptosis and diplopia. Electrophysiologic testing of other musculature is negative for MG.
IA	Ocular myasthenia with peripheral muscles showing no clinical symptoms but showing a positive electromyogram for MG.
II	Generalized myasthenia
IIA	Mild—slow onset, usually ocular, spreading to skeletal and bulbar muscles. No respiratory involvement. Good response to drug therapy. Low mortality rate.
IIB	Moderate—as IIA but progressing to more severe involvement of skeletal and bulbar muscles. Dysarthria, dysphagia, difficulty chewing. No respiratory involvement. Patient's activities limited. Fair response to drug therapy.
III	Acute fulminating myasthenia—rapid onset of severe bulbar and skeletal weakness with involvement of muscles of respiration. Progression usually within 6 mos. Poor response to therapy. Patient's activities limited. Low mortality rate.
IV	Late severe myasthenia—severe MG developing at least 2 yrs after onset of group I or group II symptoms. Progression of disease may be gradual or rapid. Poor response to therapy and poor prognosis.

Adapted from: Osserman KE, Genkins G. Studies in myasthenia gravis—A review of a 20-year experience in over 1200 patients. *Mt Sinai J Med.* 1971;38:497.

Medical Therapy

Anticholinesterases are used to prolong the action of acetylcholine at the postsynaptic membrane and may also exert their own agonist effect at the AchRs. Anticholinesterases are the most commonly used medical therapy in MG (Table 37-8). Interestingly,

TABLE 37-8. ANTICHOLINESTERASE DRUGS USED TO TREAT MYASTHENIA GRAVIS

	Dose (mg)			
Drug	Oral	IV	IM	Efficacy
Pyridostigmine (Mestinon)	60	2	2–4	1
Neostigmine (Prostigmine)	15	0.5	0.7–1	1

IV, intravenous; IM, intramuscular.

no randomized controlled trial has been conducted on the use of acetylcholinesterase inhibitors in patients with MG because the response in observational studies is so obvious that a placebo group could not be justified.[155] Myasthenic patients learn to regulate their medication and titrate the dose against optimum effect. Overdosage causes the muscarinic effects of acetylcholine and may cause a cholinergic crisis. Underdosage causes weakness or a myasthenic crisis. In a patient with weakness, distinction between the two types of crisis may be made by performing a Tensilon test or by examining pupillary size, which will be large (mydriatic) in a myasthenic crisis but small (miotic) in a cholinergic crisis. Muscarinic side effects are treatable with atropine (see Chapter 15).

The immunologic basis of MG has led to the use of short- and long-term immunosuppressive drugs. Steroids are used for short-term immunosuppression, while for long-term effect azathioprine, cyclophosphamide, cyclosporine, methotrexate, mycophenolate mofetil, rituximab, and tacrolimus have been used. Steroids often produce initial deterioration before an improvement. The usual regimen is prednisone 1 mg/kg on alternate days. Rapid short-term immunomodulation has been achieved in acute exacerbations or to improve muscle strength prior to surgery. Plasma exchange or plasmapheresis may produce dramatic but transient improvements in muscle strength with decreases in anti-AchR and anti-MuSK titers, as well as other inflammatory mediators. Usually reserved for severe MG, plasma exchange has been shown to improve respiratory function in both operated and nonoperated patients with MG. Plasmapheresis causes a decrease in plasma cholinesterase levels that may prolong the effect of drugs such as succinylcholine that are normally broken down by this enzyme system.

Long-term immunomodulation is achieved by surgical thymectomy. Abnormalities are found in 75% of thymus glands removed from patients with MG (85% show hyperplasia, 15% show thymoma). After thymectomy, approximately 75% of patients either go into remission or show some improvement. Thymectomy is always indicated in those patients with thymoma, and now considered the treatment of choice in most patients with MG, except for those in Osserman class I (Table 37-7). Response to thymectomy is best if it is performed within the first 3 years following diagnosis. Clinical outcome from thymectomy is equivalent whether performed via a transsternal or video-assisted thoracoscopic approach.[156] A report describing anesthesia concerns in 17 patients who underwent robotic-assisted thoracoscopic thymectomy suggested that refinement of the surgical technique and positioning are required.[157]

Management of General Anesthesia

When possible, patients with MG should be admitted for elective surgery while in remission.[158,159] On admission, the patient's physical and emotional states should be optimized. Other diseases occasionally associated with MG should be excluded (Table 37-9). The patient's current drug therapy should be reviewed and possible drug interactions considered. Because patients are less active while in the hospital, their anticholinesterase dosage may need to be decreased. If the patient has a history of respiratory disease or bulbar involvement, preoperative evaluation should include respiratory function studies. Breathing exercises and instruction in the use of incentive spirometers may be indicated. Patients should be told of the possible need for postoperative intubation of the trachea and ventilation of the lungs. Ideally, patients with MG should be scheduled to be the first case of the day in the operating room. Patients receiving steroid therapy should receive perioperative coverage. Interactions with other immunosuppressant drugs must be considered and if the patient is in crisis preoperative plasmaphereses may be necessary.

TABLE 37-9. DISORDERS ASSOCIATED WITH MYASTHENIA GRAVIS

Thymoma
Thyroid disease
Hyperthyroidism
Hypothyroidism
Thyroiditis
Idiopathic thrombocytopenic purpura
Rheumatoid arthritis
Systemic lupus erythematosus
Anemias
Pernicious
Hemolytic
Multiple sclerosis
Ulcerative colitis
Leukemia
Lymphoma
Convulsive disorders
Extrathymic neoplasia
Sjögren syndrome
Scleroderma

Because the trachea is to be intubated and the lungs ventilated for the planned procedure in the patient with MG, traditional practice is to withhold anticholinesterase therapy on the morning of surgery so that the patient is weak on arrival at the operating room.[160] This avoids interactions with other drugs used in the operating room. Anticholinesterase therapy may be continued if the patient is physically or psychologically dependent on it. Others recommend continuing pyridostigmine, including an oral dose just before induction.[161] Premedication is satisfactorily achieved with a benzodiazepine or barbiturate. Opioids are usually avoided because of the risk of producing respiratory depression.

Monitoring should be dictated by the patient's state and planned surgical procedure, but should include an assessment of neuromuscular transmission (by means of a mechanomyogram/twitch monitor, an integrated electromyographic monitor, a kinemyograph, or an accelograph monitor)[162] if agents affecting neuromuscular transmission are to be used.

Induction of anesthesia is readily achieved with a short-acting barbiturate (if available) or propofol. In elective cases, intubation of the trachea, maintenance, and relaxation are readily achieved using potent inhaled anesthetics. Anesthesia may be deepened using a potent inhaled agent and the trachea intubated under its effect. Myasthenic patients are more sensitive than normal patients to the neuromuscular depressant effects of the potent inhaled agents. In patients with MG, isoflurane at 1.9 MAC end-tidal concentration induced a neuromuscular block of 30% to 50%, whereas halothane at 1.8 MAC induced a block of 10% to 20%. Both agents produced fade in the train-of-four ratio of 41% and 28%, respectively.[163] The less soluble inhaled agents, sevoflurane and desflurane, are even more easily administered and withdrawn; they are now the most commonly used anesthetic drugs for patients with MG. Nitahara et al.[164] studied the neuromuscular effects of sevoflurane in 16 myasthenic patients and 12 normal patients. As expected, they found a concentration-dependent decrease in T1 and T4/T1 values. The depressant effects of sevoflurane were more prominent in those myasthenic patients with baseline T4/T1 <0.90. Whichever agent is used, at the end of the procedure, the inhaled agent is discontinued and recovery of neuromuscular function begins. Experience with desflurane in MG patients undergoing video-assisted thoracoscopic thymectomy was similar.[165]

Nondepolarizing Relaxants. In some cases, patients with MG cannot tolerate the cardiovascular depressant effects of the potent inhaled anesthetics, in which case neuromuscular blocking drugs may be used, titrating dose against monitored effect. Patients with MG are sensitive (i.e., show a decrease in ED_{50} and ED_{95} when compared with non-MG patients) to the nondepolarizing neuromuscular blocking drugs.[166] All nondepolarizing relaxants have been successfully and uneventfully used with careful monitoring in patients with MG (see Chapter 20). Since the sensitivity of any individual MG patient is unknown, these drugs should be titrated in 1/10 of the usual dose. Cisatracurium may be preferred because of its short elimination half-life, small volume of distribution, lack of cumulative effect, and high clearance.[167] Sensitivity to nondepolarizing relaxants is increased during the coadministration of a potent inhaled anesthetic.[168]

Other intermediate-duration nondepolarizing agents such as vecuronium and rocuronium may be used; long-acting relaxants are best avoided in patients with MG. If necessary, the residual relaxation produced by nondepolarizers may be reversed by increments of anticholinesterase drugs, while neuromuscular transmission is carefully monitored to obtain maximum antagonism yet avoid a cholinergic crisis. All anticholinesterases have been safely used. Edrophonium may be the drug of choice because its onset of action is rapid and higher doses have a prolonged duration of action. The sensitivity of patients with MG to nondepolarizing relaxants is very variable, depending on the individual patient, the severity of MG, and the treatment. Mann et al.[169] showed that MG patients who have a T4/T1 ratio <0.9 in the preanesthetic period show increased sensitivity to atracurium. They suggest that neuromuscular monitoring using train-of-four stimulation should begin in the preinduction period following administration of adequate analgesia (fentanyl, 2 μg/kg). Itoh et al.[170] found that patients with ocular MG were less sensitive to vecuronium than were those with generalized MG. They also found that in patients with clinical MG, sensitivity to vecuronium was unrelated to the presence or absence of antibodies to the AchR. Seronegative patients were as sensitive to vecuronium as seropositive patients.[171] There are conflicting reports as to the sensitivity of patients with MG in remission. All such patients should be considered sensitive to nondepolarizers until proven otherwise.[172]

Sugammadex is a novel cyclodextrin drug that is designed to bind rocuronium with a great affinity. Before the introduction of sugammadex, anticholinesterase drugs were the only options for antagonism of residual neuromuscular blockade, and in MG patients anticholinesterases must be administered with caution so as to avoid myasthenic or cholinergic crises. Sugammadex has been reported to provide very rapid, complete, and lasting recovery from deep levels of rocuronium-induced neuromuscular blockade in normal patients.[173,174]

Sugammadex has since been reported to safely reverse deep rocuronium-induced neuromuscular blockade within 210 seconds in a patient with MG.[175] Sugammadex offers significant advantages in the management of the MG patient. At the time of writing, however, this drug is not approved for clinical use in the United States.

Succinylcholine. Myasthenic patients are resistant to the neuromuscular blocking effects of succinylcholine. The ED_{95} is 2.6 times normal in these patients.[176] Clinically, however, the use of succinylcholine has been without incident, with the usual clinical doses producing adequate relaxation for endotracheal intubation and a normal recovery time, despite the occasionally reported early onset of phase II block. Doses of 0.2 to 1 mg/kg have been used in a number of patients with MG, and most did not show fasciculation before becoming paralyzed. Fade in response to train-of-four stimulation was observed in some patients during recovery, but recovery was not delayed. Prior administration of an anticholinesterase may complicate the response to succinylcholine by delaying its metabolism.

When a rapid-sequence intubation of the trachea is required, rapid onset of muscle relaxation may be achieved with succinylcholine or with moderate doses of a nondepolarizer in the latter case, with an associated prolongation of effect. A succinylcholine (1.5 mg/kg)–vecuronium (0.01 mg/kg) sequence has been safely used in three patients with MG for thymectomy. The authors suggested that this technique may be particularly advantageous when rapid-sequence induction of anesthesia is indicated.[177] In the future, a combination technique of intubating dose rocuronium–sugammadex may replace succinylcholine for the MG patient who requires rapid-sequence induction.

Nonrelaxant Techniques. Because of concerns over the use of muscle relaxants in MG patients, there are many reports of successful use of nonrelaxant techniques. Della Rocca et al.[178] studied 68 consecutive MG patients undergoing transsternal thymectomy randomized to receive propofol/O_2/N_2O/fentanyl or sevoflurane/N_2O/O_2/fentanyl. All were tracheally extubated in the operating room, and none required intubation for postoperative respiratory depression. Madi-Jebara et al.[179] described the use of sevoflurane as the sole anesthetic combined with intrathecal sufentanil–morphine for analgesia in an adult patient who underwent transsternal thymectomy. Abe et al.[180] described propofol anesthesia combined with thoracic epidural anesthesia for thymectomy in 11 patients with MG. Chevalley et al.[181] reported use of propofol combined with epidural bupivacaine and sufentanil in 12 MG patients undergoing similar procedures. They commented that the shift away from use of muscle relaxants provided optimal operating condition and improved patient comfort. Lorimar and Hall[182] used a total intravenous anesthetic technique with propofol and remifentanil for transsternal thymectomy in an MG patient. Politis and Tobias[183] describe rapid-sequence intubation in a myasthenic patient with a full stomach using propofol, lidocaine, and remifentanil.

Baraka et al.[184] described a 19-year-old myasthenic patient with a thymoma who received remifentanil and sevoflurane anesthesia for a 2-hour thymectomy. Although the trachea was extubated 10 minutes after discontinuation of remifentanil, the patient was unresponsive to verbal stimuli and remained somnolent for 12 hours. Because the patient had been receiving pyridostigmine for the months prior to surgery, they suggest that the delayed arousal may have been the result of possible inhibition by pyridostigmine of the nonspecific esterases that normally hydrolyze remifentanil. Ingersoll-Weng et al.[185] reported use of a dexmedetomidine infusion/isoflurane technique for transsternal thymectomy in a 52-year-old woman. The patient was stable at the start of surgery but became asystolic on sternal retraction and received open cardiac massage. Resuscitation was successful, the dexmedetomidine infusion was discontinued, and surgery was completed uneventfully. Several factors may have contributed to the asystolic arrest, including a centrally mediated increase in parasympathetic activity resulting from dexmedetomidine in a patient who was also being treated with pyridostigmine, which also increases vagal tone. Thus, pyridostigmine may have interacted with dexmedetomidine in an additive or synergistic manner.

Other Drug Interactions. Medications with neuromuscular blocking properties should be used with caution in patients with MG, particularly if relaxants are being used concurrently. Such drugs include antiarrhythmics (quinidine, procainamide, calcium-channel blockers), diuretics (by causing hypokalemia), nitrogen mustards, quinine, and aminoglycoside antibiotics. Dantrolene has been used safely in a patient with MG.

Recovery from Anesthesia. Recovery from anesthesia must be carefully monitored in these patients. Extubation of the trachea should be performed when the patients are responsive and able to generate negative inspiratory pressures of greater than −20 cm H_2O. After extubation of the trachea, patients are carefully observed in the recovery area or the ICU. As soon as possible, patients should resume their usual pyridostigmine regimen. Cases of mild respiratory depression may be treatable with parenteral anticholinesterase; more severe cases may require reintubation of the trachea and mechanical ventilation of the lungs. In the immediate postoperative period, postthymectomy patients often show a marked improvement in their condition and a decreased need for anticholinesterase therapy.

Postoperative Respiratory Failure

Myasthenic patients are at increased risk for development of postoperative respiratory failure. There have been several attempts to predict before surgery which patients with MG will require prolonged postoperative ventilation of the lungs.[186] For patients who underwent transsternal thymectomy, positive predictors were a duration of MG >6 years, history of chronic respiratory disease other than that directly caused by MG, pyridostigmine dosage >750 mg/day, and a preoperative vital capacity <2.9 L. This predictive system was not found useful when applied in patients with MG undergoing transsternal thymectomy at other centers, and of no value in patients with MG undergoing other types of surgical procedures.[187] In a study of 52 MG patients following thymectomy, Mori et al.[188] concluded that those patients who received >250 mg of pyridostigmine were at greater risk for respiratory failure requiring reintubation. Each patient should therefore be treated on his or her own merits.

A study of patients undergoing transsternal thymectomy suggested that the need for postoperative mechanical ventilation correlated best with preoperative maximum static expiratory pressure. It was concluded that expiratory weakness, by reducing cough efficacy and ability to clear secretions, was the main predictive determinant. Adequate clearance of secretions is essential in these patients and may occasionally necessitate bronchoscopy.

In general, the postoperative morbidity in terms of respiratory failure is lower after transcervical rather than transsternal thymectomy.[189] Techniques described that may be useful in reducing postoperative ventilatory failure include preoperative plasma exchange and high-dose perioperative steroid therapy. If the anticipated duration of the surgical procedure is 1 to 2 hours, preoperative oral anticholinesterase therapy may be of value because the peak effect of the drug coincides with the conclusion of the surgical procedure and attempts at tracheal extubation.

Postoperative Care

In the immediate postoperative period, pain relief for patients with MG is usually provided by opioid analgesics, such as meperidine, but in reduced doses. The analgesic effect of morphine and other opioid analgesics has been reported to be increased by anticholinesterases, which has led to the recommendation that the dose of opioid analgesics be reduced by one-third in patients receiving anticholinesterase therapy. Combined regional and general anesthesia techniques have also been used to provide good surgical conditions and improved postoperative analgesia in patients with MG undergoing thymectomy. Combined epidural–general anesthesia has been reported to provide excellent intraoperative and postoperative conditions for both surgeon and patient.[190,191]

Myasthenic Syndrome (Eaton–Lambert Syndrome)

The myasthenic syndrome is a very rare immune-mediated disorder of neuromuscular transmission, associated with antibodies to the presynaptic voltage-gated calcium channel. The prevalence is estimated to be about 1/100,000.[192] It is associated with small cell carcinoma of the lung in 50% to 60% of cases. Complaints of weakness may be mistaken for MG, but in Eaton–Lambert syndrome, symptoms do not respond to administration of anticholinesterases or steroids, and activity improves strength. The defect in this condition is prejunctional, is associated with diminished release of acetylcholine from nerve terminals, and improved by agents such as 4-aminopyridine,[193] guanidine, and germine that increase repetitive firing. Affected patients are particularly sensitive to the effects of all muscle relaxants, which should be used with great caution or avoided entirely.[194] Other therapies have included immunosuppression, immune globulins, and plasmapheresis.[195]

The possibility of Eaton–Lambert syndrome should be considered in all patients with known malignant disease and those patients undergoing diagnostic procedures for suspected carcinoma of the lung. Anesthesia considerations in these patients are essentially the same as in those with MG.[196]

POSTOPERATIVE MANAGEMENT AND COMPLICATIONS

Postoperative Pain Control

After extubation of the trachea, respiratory therapy and pain management become critical components of postoperative care.
11 Adequate postoperative pain control is necessary to ensure a good respiratory effort.[197] Administration of intravenous opioids has been the standard form of pain management for years. The administration of sufficient opioid to treat pain adequately may cause sedation and respiratory depression. Patient-controlled analgesia (PCA) has been reported to decrease the amount of postoperative pain, drug use, sedation, and pulmonary complications.[198] PCA also eliminates the delays associated with personnel-administered medications and in general is very well accepted by patients.

There are other intravenous medications that can be used for pain management in addition to opioids. Low-dose ketamine infusion at 0.05 mg/kg/hr was reported to be a useful adjunct to epidural analgesia for postthoracotomy pain management.[199] Small doses of ketamine added to morphine for PCA administration have been shown to reduce the amount of morphine administered and improve respiratory parameters.[200] It reduced the incidence of oxygen desaturation below 90% during the first three postoperative nights. Gabapentin has also been successful in reducing pain following thoracic surgery, although side effects included dizziness and drowsiness.[201] Gabapentin may also reduce the incidence of postoperative delirium, and one approach could be to administer 900 mg 1 to 2 hours preoperatively.[202] Gabapentin has been reported to be not effective in reducing ipsilateral shoulder pain.[203] The injection of the periphrenic fat pad has been shown to reduce the ipsilateral shoulder pain that may occur following thoracic surgery.[204]

Intercostal nerve blocks can decrease pain and improve postoperative respiratory function. The intercostal blocks can be performed internally or externally before or after surgery using a standard technique. However, the easiest method during thoracic surgery is to have the surgeon perform the blocks under direct vision from inside the thorax while the chest is open. Bupivacaine 0.25% to 0.5%, in doses of 2 to 5 mL, can be placed in the five intercostal spaces around the incision and in intercostal spaces where chest tubes will be placed. This provides 6 to 24 hours of moderate pain relief, but patients still complain of diaphragmatic and shoulder discomfort caused by the chest tubes. Larger volumes of local anesthetics should not be used in the intercostal space because of the high absorption rate and attendant systemic toxicity that can be produced, as well as the possibility of pushing the drug centrally and producing a paravertebral sympathetic or epidural block with central sympatholysis and severe hypotension. The intraoperative placement of catheters in intercostal grooves allows for a continuous postoperative intercostal nerve block. The technique reduces pain and improves pulmonary function. Placement of a catheter in the paravertebral space allows for blockade of multiple levels of intercostal nerves. This technique has been reported to provide good analgesia, and with fewer side effects than epidural analgesia.[205] Paravertebral blocks may provide good pain relief compared with epidural after thoracotomy.[206,207]

Another approach to postoperative pain control after thoracic surgery is the use of epidural or subarachnoid opioids (see Chapter 34). Epidural morphine produces profound analgesia lasting from 16 to 24 hours after thoracotomy and does not cause a sympathetic block or sensory or motor loss. These are significant advantages over systemic opioids or infiltration of local anesthetics. Epidural opioids are most effective at alleviating pain when administered at the thoracic level. Epidural morphine has been shown to decrease pain and improve respiratory function in post-thoracotomy patients.

On the basis of a meta-analysis of 100 studies in the National Library of Medicine's PubMed database from 1966 to 2002, Block et al.[208] concluded that epidural analgesia was superior to parenteral medication; this was true regardless of agent used in the epidural catheter or the level of catheter placement. There may be a reduction in both morbidity and mortality with epidural or spinal analgesia.[209] The technique most commonly employed in academic medical centers in the United States is an infusion of bupivacaine together with a narcotic such as fentanyl administered via a thoracic epidural catheter.[210] Data in the pediatric population are limited; in one study of adolescent patients, the use of thoracic epidural analgesia provided better postoperative pain relief following minimally invasive pectus excavatum repair.[211] Acetaminophen may be a useful adjunct to thoracic epidural analgesia for treatment of ipsilateral shoulder pain following thoracotomy.[155,212] Ketorolac may be given postoperatively, but carries a risk of bleeding if given intraoperatively.

Subarachnoid (intrathecal) morphine, in a dose of 10 to 12 μg/kg, has been successfully used after thoracic surgery.[213,214] With this technique, the drug acts directly on the spinal cord, and analgesia can be produced with a smaller dose than by the epidural or intravenous routes. When morphine is given intrathecally before the induction of anesthesia, a decrease in the dose of anesthetic drugs required may occur. All patients who have received subarachnoid or epidural opioids must be closely observed for potential side effects, including delayed respiratory depression, urine retention, pruritus, nausea, and vomiting. These effects appear to be dose-related and may be reversed with naloxone. Despite over 30 years of usage, it is still not clear what dosage is optimal for this type of surgery.[215]

Noxious stimuli, including surgical incision, may lead to changes in the central nervous system that exacerbate postoperative pain. The administration of analgesic agents before surgery is termed preemptive analgesia and may prevent these neuroplastic changes, thereby decreasing postoperative pain. In an early study of preemptive analgesia, the administration of lumbar epidural fentanyl before thoracotomy incision reduced postoperative pain scores and use of PCA morphine by a small but significant amount, compared with administration of lumbar epidural fentanyl after skin incision.[216] On the basis of a meta-analysis of randomized controlled studies published between 1966 and 2004, Bong et al.[217] concluded that thoracic epidural preemptive analgesia did not provide a statistically significant reduction in postoperative pain, but was associated with a trend toward a reduction in the incidence of such pain. A subsequent study investigating the preemptive analgesic effect of infiltration of the surgical incisions with lidocaine prior to bilateral VAT incisions did help relieve pain for 24 hours, but not thereafter.[218] In that study, since there was a bilateral incision, the infiltration was only done on one side, and each patient served as his or her own control.

Interpleural analgesia is another technique for postoperative pain treatment. The injection of local anesthetic between the pleural layers can block multiple intercostal nerves and/or pain fibers traveling with the thoracic sympathetic chain. The surgeon can place the catheter under direct vision while the chest is open. The chest tubes should not be suctioned for approximately 15 minutes after injection of local anesthetic to avoid loss of the anesthetic into the drainage. The surgeon can also place in the wound a soaker catheter, through which local anesthetics can be administered postoperatively. The On-Q PainBuster (I-Flow Corporation, Lake Forrest, CA) can be used for this purpose, and is an effective adjunct in alleviating pain following thoracic surgery.[219] There may be chronic pain following thoracotomy, and also following VAT, even though the incisions are smaller with this approach.[220,221] In one report, women were more likely than men to suffer from both perioperative pain and chronic pain.[222] If it occurs, it is important to treat this chronic postoperative pain early and aggressively.[223]

In recent years, the use of VAT has become more common, and is often the initial approach for thoracic surgery. Although there can be expected to be less pain and respiratory impairment following VAT compared with thoracotomy, it is still important to have a pain management strategy as there can be a significant amount of postoperative pain. Acute postoperative pain may be either myofascial or neuropathic in origin. These can cause neuroplastic changes, which may result in chronic pain. In one study, there was a 47% incidence of chronic pain reported following VAT.[224] The incidence of chronic pain after VAT may be comparable with that following thoracotomy.[225] The pain that occurs may be related to trauma to intercostal nerves by insertion of the surgical trocars or by compression during the surgery.[226] In addition, an incision will be required to extract a lobe in the case of a lobectomy, which may exacerbate pain further.

If there is a relatively high chance of the surgeon converting the VAT to a thoracotomy, it may be preferable to place a thoracic epidural. If the preoperative lung function is poor, such that the patient may have difficulty breathing adequately postoperatively or may not tolerate systemic opioids, it also may be more prudent to place an epidural for that situation also. In contrast, for patients with good lung function who are scheduled to undergo a VAT in which a thoracotomy is unlikely, an epidural is probably unnecessary. The use of intercostal or paravertebral block combined with systemic opioids via PCA should be sufficient. In the United Kingdom, that approach has been reported to be more common for VATS lobectomy than the use of epidural analgesia.[227] In that survey, only 46% of patients undergoing VATS had a thoracic epidural placed. In contrast with an epidural, the paravertebral block is unilateral, and does not cause a sympathectomy. The administration of local anesthetic via the chest tubes is another approach which can successfully treat postoperative pain.[228] In a recent update in which the literature was reviewed regarding pain management for VAT, it was concluded that an epidural is not necessary.[229] The use of a single shot, multilevel, paravertebral block has been recommended for VATS in a recent update on the use of paravertebral blocks for thoracic surgery. The placement of a paravertebral catheter for VAT was shown to be effective for postoperative pain management in a recent prospective randomized trial.[230]

Complications Following Thoracic Surgery

Atelectasis

Patients who require thoracotomy often have pre-existing pulmonary disease that, when combined with the operative procedure, is likely to result in significant pulmonary dysfunction and possibly pneumonia. Atelectasis, the most significant cause of postoperative morbidity, has been reported to occur in up to 100% of patients undergoing thoracotomy for pulmonary resection. It occurs more commonly in the basal lobes than in the middle or upper lung regions. It may be secondary to reduction of normal respiratory effort due to splinting from pain, obesity, intrathoracic blood and fluid accumulation, and decreased compliance, all of which lead to rapid, shallow, constant V_T. Such a respiratory pattern produces small airway closure and obstruction with inspissated secretions, resulting ultimately in alveolar air resorption and terminal airway collapse. A poor cough and limited clearance of secretions add to the problem. Other sources of atelectasis include mucus plugging, which can obstruct a lobe or even an entire lung, and incomplete re-expansion of the remaining lung tissue after one-lung anesthesia.

The diagnosis of atelectasis can be made by clinical findings, chest radiography, or arterial blood gas analysis. This problem is best resolved by increasing resting lung volume or FRC. The latter can be increased by an increase in transpulmonary pressure (difference between airway pressure and interpleural pressure) or in lung compliance.

The tracheas of many patients can be extubated shortly after thoracic surgical procedures. These patients should be observed in the operating room for at least 5 minutes following extubation, and many will require a high FIO_2 by face mask. Some patients with COPD undergoing extensive thoracic surgical procedures require postoperative ventilation to avoid atelectasis and other pulmonary complications. Mechanical ventilation increases airway pressure and, to a lesser extent, interpleural pressure; therefore, transpulmonary pressure increases.

The use of incentive spirometry and CPAP has been shown to reduce postoperative complications. Additional modalities that may be helpful in preventing atelectasis include bronchodilator treatment, coughing and clearance of secretions, chest physiotherapy, mobilizing the patient, and providing adequate analgesia. Atelectasis caused by collapse of lung tissue distal to a mucus plug can be treated by positioning the patient in the lateral decubitus position with the fully expanded lung in the dependent position. This improves $\dot{V}/\dot{Q}$ matching and facilitates clearance of mucus from the nondependent obstructed lung. However, the patient should not be placed with the operative side in the dependent position after a pneumonectomy because of the risk of cardiac herniation.

The other major complications after thoracic surgery can be grouped into cardiovascular, pulmonary, and related problems.

Cardiovascular Complications

Cardiovascular complications are often the most difficult to manage in patients with associated respiratory insufficiency. The low cardiac output syndrome and postoperative cardiac dysrhythmias may be life-threatening. Invasive hemodynamic monitoring may be needed to assist in diagnosis and fluid management therapy. Other diagnostic modalities, such as echocardiography, may be required to rule out the presence of pericardial effusions or tamponade after opening the pericardium during certain types of thoracic surgical procedures. The low cardiac output syndrome must be differentiated from hypovolemia resulting from intrathoracic hemorrhage, tamponade, pulmonary emboli, or the effects of mechanical ventilation with PEEP. Postoperative fluid administration can lead to pulmonary edema resulting from the resection of lung tissue and the concomitant reduction of the pulmonary vascular bed. Re-expansion of a chronically collapsed lung may in some cases lead to re-expansion pulmonary edema (RPE); rapid re-expansion and drainage of large amounts of pleural fluid increase the risk for RPE.[231] A postoperative pulmonary embolism can originate from the remaining pulmonary artery stump. Therapeutic interventions for postoperative myocardial dysfunction include inotropic drugs, vasodilators, and combinations of these drugs, as needed, to improve ventricular function. The goal is to shift the Starling function curve up and to the left by reducing preload of either the left or right side of the heart and increasing cardiac output. Vasodilators are very effective at decreasing right ventricular afterload and improving right ventricular function because this side of the heart is especially afterload-dependent. Combinations of inotropes and vasodilators, such as dopamine and nitroglycerin, or combined drugs, such as milrinone, can be especially useful in the treatment of right-sided heart failure.

Postoperative cardiac dysrhythmias are common after thoracic surgery. Patients following pulmonary resection have postoperative supraventricular tachycardias with a frequency and severity proportional to both their age and the magnitude of the surgical procedure. Many factors contribute to these dysrhythmias, including underlying cardiac disease, degree of surgical trauma, intraoperative cardiac manipulation, stimulation of the sympathetic nervous system by pain, a reduced pulmonary vascular bed, effects of anesthetics and cardioactive drugs, and metabolic abnormalities.

In a series of 300 thoracotomies for lung resection, atrial fibrillation occurred in 20% of patients with malignant disease but in only 3% with benign disease.[232] A similar incidence of dysrhythmias is observed after pneumonectomies. Multifocal atrial tachycardia often occurs in patients with COPD and concomitant right-sided cardiac dysfunction. The right side of the heart may be further strained by the reduction in the size of the pulmonary vasculature from the lung resection, especially after right pneumonectomy. Historically, the primary antidysrhythmic drug was used to treat atrial tachycardias in thoracic surgical patients. The prophylactic use of digitalis in thoracic surgical patients is controversial, particularly in patients with signs of congestive heart failure. Arguments against its use include the potential toxic effects of the drug and the difficulty in assessing adequacy of digitalization in the absence of heart failure. A prospective, placebo-controlled, randomized study demonstrated no advantage to prophylactic digitalization of patients undergoing thoracic surgery.[233] Part of the argument for its use is the drug's efficacy in reducing the incidence of potentially fatal complications in older patients. In some studies, it has been reported to reduce the incidence of perioperative dysrhythmias. If digitalis therapy is to be instituted, normokalemia should be ensured to reduce the likelihood of digitalis toxicity.

More recently, newer drugs have replaced digitalis for dysrhythmia control. Supraventricular tachycardias can also be treated with other agents such as β-blockers or calcium-channel–blocking drugs, after ruling out underlying reversible physiologic abnormalities, such as hypoxia. Verapamil has been the standard treatment for these problems until the introduction of the ultrashort-acting β-blocker, esmolol. Esmolol has been shown to be equally effective in controlling the ventricular rate in patients with postoperative atrial fibrillation or flutter and in increasing the conversion rate to regular sinus rhythm from 8% to 34%. Owing to its short duration of action (β elimination half-life of 9 minutes) and β_1-cardioselectivity, it is the drug of choice in the postoperative period to control these dysrhythmias. Esmolol, in an intravenous loading dose of 500 μg/kg given over 1 minute followed by an infusion of 50 to 200 μg/kg/min, has been shown to be effective in the control of supraventricular tachycardias. Amiodarone has been reported to be effective in restoring and maintaining sinus rhythm.[234]

Bleeding and Respiratory Complications

Hemorrhage and pneumothorax are always major concerns after intrathoracic surgery. Because of these problems, interpleural thoracostomy tubes with an underwater seal system are routinely used after thoracic surgery. Slippage of a suture on any major vessel or airway in the chest can lead to the slow or rapid development of hypovolemic shock or a tension pneumothorax. Drainage of more than 200 mL/hr of blood is an indication for surgical re-exploration for hemorrhage. Management of the pleural drainage system is fraught with confusion. The chest bottles must be kept below the level of the chest, and the tubes should not be clamped during patient transport. These tubes can be lifesaving, but errors in technique can lead to serious complications. The creation of a pneumothorax in the nonoperative chest by central venous catheter placement is very hazardous because this lung is essential both intraoperatively during one-lung anesthesia and postoperatively after contralateral lung resection. Dehiscence of the bronchial stump may lead to the formation of a BPF, which carries a mortality rate of 20%. Surgical treatment may be needed, in which case ventilation of the patient's lungs may be difficult because of loss of V_T through the fistula. A double-lumen endobronchial tube positioned in the contralateral main stem bronchus or the use of HFJV may be required for safe management. HFJV allows ventilation with lowered peak airway pressures. However, there have been reports in which ventilation by HFJV was difficult. If a double-lumen endobronchial tube is placed, the lung with the fistula can be ventilated independently with either CPAP or HFJV.

Neurologic Complications

Central and peripheral neurologic injuries can occur during intrathoracic procedures. Such injuries often result in serious and disabling loss of function. Peripheral nerves can also be injured, either in the chest or in other parts of the body, by pressure or stretching. The nerve injury may be apparent immediately after surgery or may not become obvious until several days later. These patients often complain of a variety of unpleasant sensations, including paresthesias, cold, pain, or anesthesia in the area supplied by the affected nerves. The brachial plexus is especially vulnerable to trauma during thoracic surgery, owing to its long superficial course in the axilla between two points of fixation, the vertebrae above, and the axillary fascia below. Stretching may be the primary cause of damage to the brachial plexus, with compression playing only a secondary role. Branches of the brachial plexus may also be injured lower in the arm by compression against objects such as an ether screen or other parts of the operating table. Intrathoracic nerves can be directly injured during a surgical procedure by being transected, crushed, stretched, or cauterized. The recurrent laryngeal nerve can become involved in lymph node tissue and injured at the time of a node biopsy, especially when the biopsy is performed through a mediastinoscope. This nerve can also be injured during tracheostomy or radical pulmonary dissections. The phrenic nerve may be injured during pericardiectomy, radical pulmonary hilar dissections, division of the diaphragm during esophageal surgery, or dissection of mediastinal tumors.

Prevention is the treatment of choice for these intraoperative nerve injuries. Analgesics may be necessary to control postoperative pain in the distribution of the nerve injury and to aid in maintaining joint mobility during the healing phase. Subsequent surgical procedures may be necessary to move a swollen ulnar nerve at the elbow or to stent a partially paralyzed vocal cord.

References

1. American Lung Association. *Lung Cancer Fact Sheet.* New York, NY: American Lung Association; 2006.
2. American Cancer Society. Cancer statistics 2010. A presentation from the American Cancer Society. 2011 Estimated U.S. Cancer Deaths. Available at: http://www.cancer.org/acs/groups/content/@epidemiologysurveilance/documents/document/acspc-029997.pptx. Last accessed 12-2-2011.
3. Bapoje SR, Whitaker JF, Schulz T, et al. Preoperative evaluation of the patient with pulmonary disease. *Chest.* 2007;132:1637.
4. Smetanta GW. Preoperative pulmonary evaluation: Identifying and reducing risks for pulmonary complications. *Cleve Clin J Med.* 2006;73(suppl 1):S36.
5. Slinger PD, Johnston MR. Preoperative assessment for pulmonary resection. *J Cardiothorac Vasc Anesth.* 2000;4:202–211.
6. Reilly JJ. Evidence-based preoperative evaluation of candidates for thoracotomy. *Chest.* 1999;116:474s.
7. Licker M, Perrot M, Spiliopulos A. Risk factors for acute lung injury after thoracic surgery for lung cancer. *Anesth Analg.* 2003;97:1558.
8. Slinger PD, Sussa S, Triolet W. Predicting arterial oxygenation during one-lung anaesthesia. *Can J Anaesth.* 1992;39:1030.
9. Slinger P, Johnston M. Preoperative evaluation of the thoracic surgery patient. *Semin Anesth.* 2002;21:168.
10. Nakahara K, Ohno K, Hashimoto J, et al. Prediction of postoperative respiratory failure in patients undergoing lung resection for cancer. *Ann Thorac Surg.* 1988;46:549.
11. Vansteenkiste J, Fischer BM, Dooms C, et al. Positron-emission tomography in prognostic and therapeutic assessment of lung cancer: Systematic review. *Lancet Oncol.* 2004;5:531.
12. Gould MK, Kuschner WG, Rydzak CE, et al. Test performance of positron emission tomography and computer tomography for mediastinal staging in patients with non-small-cell lung cancer: A meta-analysis. *Ann Intern Med.* 2003; 139:879.
13. Ferguson MK, Reeder LB, Mick R. Optimizing selection of patients for major lung resection. *J Thorac Cardiovasc Surg.* 1995;109:275.
14. Amar D, Munoz D, Shi W, Zhang H, Thaler HT. A clinical prediction rule for pulmonary complications after thoracic surgery for primary lung cancer. *Anesth Analg.* 2010;110:1343–1348.
15. Ferguson MK, Vigneswaran WT. Diffusing capacity predicts morbidity after lung resection in patients without chronic obstructive pulmonary disease. *Ann Thorac Surg.* 2008;85:1158–1165.
16. Walsh GL, Morice RC, Putnam JB. Resection of lung cancer is justified in high-risk patients selected by oxygen consumption. *Ann Thorac Surg.* 1994;58:704.
17. Bollinger CT, Wyser C, Roser H, et al. Lung scanning and exercise testing for the prediction of postoperative performance in lung resection candidates at increased risk for complications. *Chest.* 1995;108:341.
18. Ninan M, Sommers KE, Landranau RJ, et al. Standardized exercise oximetry predicts post pneumonectomy outcome. *Ann Thorac Surg.* 1997;64:328.

19. Win T, Jackson A, Sharples L, et al. Cardiopulmonary exercise tests and lung cancer surgical outcome. *Chest.* 2005;127:1159.
20. Brunelli A, Fianchini A. Stair climbing test predicts cardiopulmonary complications after lung resection. *Chest.* 2002;121:1106.
21. Brunelli A, Sabbatini A, Xiume F, et al. Inability to perform maximal stair climbing test before lung resection: A propensity score analysis on early outcome. *Eur J Cardiothorac Surg.* 2005;27:367.
22. Nakagawa M, Tanaka H, Tsukuma H. Relationship between the duration of the preoperative smoke-free period and the incidence of postoperative pulmonary complications after pulmonary surgery. *Chest.* 2001;120:705.
23. Barrera R, Shi W, Amar D, et al. Smoking and cessation: Impact on pulmonary complications after thoracotomy. *Chest.* 2005;127:1927.
24. Mason DP, Subramanian S, Nowicki ER, et al. Impact of smoking cessation before resection of lung cancer: A society of thoracic surgeons general thoracic surgery database study. *Ann Thorac Surg.* 2009;88:362–371.
25. Mauermann WJ, Nemergut EC. The anesthesiologist's role in the prevention of surgical infections. *Anesthesiology.* 2006;105:413.
26. Sekine Y, Chiyo M, Iwata T, et al. Perioperative rehabilitation and physiotherapy for lung cancer patients with chronic obstructive pulmonary disease. *Jpn J Thorac Cardiovasc Surg.* 2005;53:237.
27. Landesberg G, Mosseri M, Wolf Y, et al. The probability of detecting perioperative myocardial ischemia in vascular surgery by continuous 12-lead ECG. *Anesthesiology.* 2002;96:264.
28. Marik P. Does central venous pressure predict fluid responsiveness. A systematic review of literature and tale of seven mares. *Chest.* 2008;134:172–178.
29. Marik P. Techniques for assessment of intravascular volume in critically ill patients. *J Intensive Care Med.* 2009;24:329–337.
30. Cannesson M, Le Manach YL, Hofer CK, et al. Assessing the diagnostic accuracy of pulse pressure variations for the prediction of fluid responsiveness. *Anesthesiology.* 2011;115:231–241.
31. Suehiro K, Okutani R. Stroke volume variation as a predictor of fluid responsiveness in patients undergoing one-lung ventilation. *J Cardiothorac Vasc Anesth.* 2010;24:772–775.
32. Kumar A, Anel R, Bunnell E, et al. Pulmonary artery occlusion pressure and central venous pressure fail to predict ventricular filling volume, cardiac performance, or the response to volume infusion in normal subjects. *Crit Care Med.* 2004;32:691.
33. Iberti TJ, Fischer EP, Leibowitz AB, et al. A multicenter study of physician's knowledge of the pulmonary artery catheter. *JAMA.* 1990;264:2928.
34. Raper R, Sibbald WJ. Misled by the wedge. *Chest.* 1986;89:427.
35. Koji A. Mean pulmonary artery pressure under thoracotomy as an indicator of safety for lung resection. *J Jpn Assoc Chest Surg.* 2001;15:561.
36. Thys DM, Cohen E, Eisenkraft JB. Mixed venous oxygen saturation during thoracic anesthesia. *Anesthesiology.* 1988;69:1005.
37. Pedotos A, Amar D. Right heart function in thoracic surgery: Role of echocardiography. *Curr Opin Anaesthesiol.* 2009;22:44–49.
38. Serra E, Feltracco P, Barbieri S, et al. Transesophageal echocardiography during lung transplantation. *Transplant Proc.* 2007;39:1981–1982.
39. Pothoft G, Curtius JM, Wassermann K, et al. Transesophageal echography in staging of bronchial cancers. *Pneumologie.* 1992;446:111.
40. Manguso L, Pitrolo F, Bond F, et al. Echocardiographic recognition of mediastinal masses. *Chest.* 1988;93:144.
41. Neustein SM, Cohen E, Reich DL, et al. Transesophageal echocardiography and the intraoperative diagnosis of left atrial invasion by carcinoid tumor. *Can J Anaesth.* 1993;40:664.
42. Suriani RJ, Konstadt SN, Camunas J, et al. Transesophageal echocardiographic detection of left atrial involvement in a lung tumor. *J Cardiothorac Vasc Anesth.* 1993;7:73.
43. Neustein SM, Narang J. Spontaneous hemothorax due to subacute aortic dissection. *J Cardiothorac Vasc Anesth.* 1993;7:79.
44. Redford D, Kim A, Barber B. Transesophageal echocardiography for the intraoperative evaluation of a large anterior mediastinal mass. *Anesth Analg.* 2006; 103:578.
45. Brooker RF, Zvara DA. Mediastinal mass diagnosed with intraoperative transesophageal echocardiography. *J Cardiothorac Vasc Anesth.* 2007;21:257.
46. Kazan R, Bracco D, Hemmerling TM. Reduced cerebral oxygen saturation measured by absolute cerebral oximetry during thoracic surgery correlates with postoperative complications. *Br J Anaesth.* 2009;103:811–816.
47. Suehero K, Okutai R. Cerebral desaturation during single-lung ventilation is negatively correlated with preoperative respiratory functions. *J Cardiothorac Vasc Anesth.* 2011;25:127–130.
48. Peyton P, Chong S. Minimally invasive measurement of cardiac output during surgery and critical care: A meta-analysis of accuracy and precision. *Anesthesiology.* 2010;113:1220–1235.
49. Barker SJ, Curry J, Redford D, et al. Measurement of carboxyhemoglobin and methemoglobin by pulse oximetry: A human volunteer study. *Anesthesiology.* 2006; 105:892.
50. Barker SJ, Badal JJ. The measurement of dyshemoglobins and total hemoglobin by pulse oximetry. *Curr Opin Anaesthesiol.* 2008;21:805–810.
51. Miller RD, Ward TA, Shiboski SC, et al. A comparison of three methods of hemoglobin monitoring in patients undergoing spine surgery. *Anesth Analg.* 2011;112: 858–863.
52. Eisenkraft JB. Respiratory gas monitoring. In: Reich DL, et al, eds. *Monitoring in Anesthesia and Perioperative Care.* New York, NY: Cambridge University Press; 2011.
53. Shafieha MA, Sit J, Kartha R, et al. End-tidal CO2 analyzers in proper positioning of double-lumen tubes. *Anesthesiology.* 1986;64:844.
54. Yam PCI, Innes PA, Jackson M, et al. Variation in the arterial to end-tidal Pco_2 difference during one-lung thoracic anaesthesia. *Br J Anaesth.* 1994;72:21.
55. Benumof JL. Isoflurane anesthesia and arterial oxygenation during one-lung ventilation. *Anesthesiology.* 1986;64:419.
56. Cohen E. Recommendations for airway control and difficult management in thoracic anesthesia. Are we ready for the challenge? *Minerva Anestesiol.* 2009;75: 3–5.
57. Fischer GW, Cohen E. Update of anesthesia for thoracoscopic surgery. *Curr Opin Anaesthesiol.* 2010;23:7–11.
58. Hurford WE, Alfille PH. A quality improvement study of the placement and complications of double-lumen endobronchial tubes. *J Cardiothorac Vasc Anesth.* 1993;7:517.
59. Lohser J, Brodsky J. Silibronco double-lumen tube. *J Cardiothorac Vasc Anesth.* 2006;20:129.
60. Brodsky JB, Lemmens HJM. Left double-lumen tubes: Clinical experience with 1,170 patients. *J Cardiothorac Vasc Anesth.* 2003;17:289.
61. Brodsky JB, Lemmens HJM. Tracheal width and left double-lumen tube size: A formula to estimate left-bronchial width. *J Clin Anesth.* 2005;17:267.
62. Amar D, Desiderio D, Heerdt PM, et al. Practice patterns in choice of left double-lumen tube size for thoracic surgery. *Anesth Analg.* 2008;106:379.
63. Chow MY, Go MH, Ti LK. Predicting the depth of insertion of left-sided double-lumen endobronchial tubes. *J Cardiothorac Vasc Anesth.* 2002;16:456.
64. Smith G, Hirsch N, Ehrenwerth J. Sight and sound: Can double-lumen endotracheal tubes be placed accurately without fiberoptic bronchoscopy? *Br J Anaesth.* 1987;58:1317.
65. Cohen E, Neustein SM, Goldofsky S, et al. Incidence of malposition of PVC and red rubber left-sided double lumen tubes and clinical sequelae. *J Cardiothorac Vasc Anesth.* 1995;9:122.
66. Benumof JL, Partridge BL, Salvatierra C, et al. Margin of safety in positioning modern double-lumen endotracheal tubes. *Anesthesiology.* 1987;67:729.
67. Thomas V, Neustein SM. Tracheal laceration after the use of an airway exchange catheter for double-lumen tube placement. *J Cardiothorac Vasc Anesth.* 2007;21: 718.
68. Wagner DL, Gammage GW, Wong ML. Tracheal rupture following the insertion of a disposable double-lumen endotracheal tube. *Anesthesiology.* 1985;63:698.
69. Heike Knoll H, Stephan Ziegeler S, Jan-Uwe Schreiber JU, et al. Airway injuries after one-lung ventilation: A comparison between double-lumen tube and endobronchial blocker: A randomized, prospective, controlled trial. *Anesthesiology.* 2006;105:471.
70. Andros TG, Lennon PF. One-lung ventilation in a patient with a tracheostomy and severe tracheobronchial disease. *Anesthesiology.* 1993;79:1127.
71. Bellver J, Garcia-Aguado A, Andres JD, et al. Selective bronchial intubation with the Univent system in patients with a tracheostomy. *Anesthesiology.* 1993;79: 1453.
72. Saito T, Naruke T, Carney E, et al. New double-lumen intrabronchial tube (Naruke tube) for tracheostomized patients. *Anesthesiology.* 1998;89:1038.
73. Cohen E, Benumof JL. Lung separation in the patient with a difficult airway. *Curr Opin Anesthesiol.* 1999;12:29.
74. Benumof JL. Difficult tubes and difficult airways. *J Cardiothorac Vasc Anesth.* 1998;12:131.
75. Neustein SM. The use of bronchial blockers for providing one-lung ventilation. *J Cardiothorac Vasc Anesth.* 2009;23:860–868.
76. Cohen E. The cohen flexitip endobronchial blocker: An alternative to a double lumen tube. *Anesth Analg.* 2005;101:1877.
77. Campos JH, Kernstine KH. A comparison of a left-sided Broncho-Cath with the torque control blocker Univent and the wire-guided blocker. *Anesth Analg.* 2003;96:283.
78. Campos JH. Progress in lung separation. *Thorac Surg Clin.* 2005;15:71.
79. Narayanaswamy M, McRae K, Slinger P, et al. Choosing a lung isolation device for thoracic surgery: A randomized trial of three bronchial blockers versus double-lumen tubes. *Anesth Analg.* 2009;108:1097–1101.
80. Desiderio DP, Burt M, Kolker AC, et al. The effects of endobronchial cuff inflation on double-lumen endobronchial tube movement after lateral decubitus positioning. *J Cardiothorac Vasc Anesth.* 1997;11:595–598.
81. Ko R, McRae K, Darling G, et al. The use of air in the inspired gas mixture during two-lung ventilation delays lung collapse during one-lung ventilation. *Anesth Analg.* 2009;108:1092–1096.
82. Katz JA, Larlane RG, Fairly HB, et al. Pulmonary oxygen exchange during endobronchial anesthesia: Effect of tidal volume and PEEP. *Anesthesiology.* 1982;56: 164.
83. Eichenbaum KD, Neustein SM. Acute lung injury following thoracic surgery. *J Cardiothorac Vasc Anesth.* 2010;24:681–690.
84. Slinger P. Low tidal volume is indicated during one-lung ventilation. *Anesth Analg.* 2006;103:268.
85. Gal T. Low tidal volume is not indicated during one lung ventilation. *Anesth Analg.* 2006;103:271.

86. Schultz MJ, Jack J, Haitsma JJ, et al. What tidal volumes should be used in patients without acute lung injury? *Anesthesiology.* 2007;106:1226.
87. Wrigge H, Uhlig U, Zinserling J, et al. The effects of different ventilatory settings on pulmonary and systemic inflammatory responses during major surgery. *Anesth Analg.* 2004;98:775.
88. Senturk M. New concepts of the management of one-lung ventilation. *Curr Opin Anaesthesiol.* 2006;19:1–4.
89. Wrigge H, Zinserling J, Stuber F, et al. Effects of mechanical ventilation on release of cytokines into systemic circulation in patients with normal pulmonary function. *Anesthesiology.* 2000;93:1413.
90. Fernandez-Perez ER, Keegan MT, Brown DR, et al. Intraoperative tidal volume as a risk factor for respiratory failure after pneumonectomy. *Anesthesiology.* 2006; 105:14.
91. Tusman G, Böhm SH, Vazquez da Anda G, et al. "Alveolar recruitment strategy" improves arterial oxygenation during general anaesthesia. *Br J Anaesth.* 1999; 82:8.
92. Tugrul M, Camici E, Karadeniz H, et al. Comparison of volume control with pressure control ventilation during one-lung anaesthesia. *Br J Anaesth.* 1997; 79:306.
93. Carmen MU, Casas J, Moral I, et al. Pressure-controlled versus volume-controlled ventilation during one-lung ventilation for thoracic surgery. *Anesth Analg.* 2007; 104:1029.
94. Cruz Pardons P, Garutti I, Piñeiro P, et al. Effects of ventilatory mode during one-lung ventilation on intraoperative and postoperative arterial oxygenation in thoracic surgery. *J Cardiothorac Vasc Anesth.* 2009;23:770–774.
95. Cohen E, Thys DM, Eisenkraft JB, et al. PEEP during one-lung anesthesia improves oxygenation in patients with low Pao2. *Anesth Analg.* 1985;64:200.
96. Capan LM, Turndorf H, Patel K, et al. Optimization of arterial oxygenation during one-lung anesthesia. *Anesth Analg.* 1980;59:847.
97. Hogue CW. Effectiveness of low levels of nonventilated lung continuous positive airway pressure in improving arterial oxygenation during one-lung ventilation. *Anesth Analg.* 1994;79:364.
98. Malmkvist G. Maintenance of oxygenation during one-lung ventilation. Effect of intermittent reinflation of the collapsed lung with oxygen. *Anesth Analg.* 1989; 68:763.
99. Cohen E, Eisenkraft JB, Thys DM, et al. Oxygenation and hemodynamic changes during one-lung ventilation. *J Cardiothorac Vasc Anesth.* 1988;2:34.
100. Wiedemann HP. A perspective on the fluids and catheters treatment trial (FACTT). Fluid restriction is superior in acute lung injury and ARDS. *Cleve Clin J Med.* 2008;75:42–48.
101. Wiedemann HP, Wheeler AP, Bernard GR, et al. Comparison of two fluid-management strategies in acute lung injury. *N Engl J Med.* 2006;354:2564–2575.
102. Rivers EP. Fluid-management strategies in acute lung injury–liberal, conservative, or both? *N Engl J Med.* 2006;354(24):2598–2600.
103. Karzai W, Schwarzkopf K. Hypoxemia during OLV: Prediction, prevention and treatment. *Anesthesiology.* 2009;110(6):1402–1411.
104. Yang M, Joo H, Kim K, et al. Does a protective ventilation strategy reduce the risk of pulmonary complications after lung cancer surgery? A randomized controlled trial. *Chest.* 2011;139:530–537.
105. Shimizu T, Abe K, Kinovchik K, et al. Arterial oxygenation during one-lung ventilation. *Can J Anaesth.* 1997;44:1162.
106. Loer SA, Scheeren TWL, Tarnow J. Desflurane inhibits HPV in isolated rabbit lungs. *Anesthesiology.* 1995;83:552.
107. Van Keer L, Van Aken H, Vandermeersch E, et al. Propofol does not inhibit HPV in humans. *J Clin Anesth.* 1989;1:284.
108. Kellow NH, Scott AD, White SA, et al. Comparison of the effects of propofol and isoflurane anaesthesia on right ventricular function and shunt fraction during thoracic surgery. *Br J Anesth.* 1995;75:578–582.
109. Schilling T, Kozian A, Huth C, et al. The pulmonary immune effects of mechanical ventilation in patients undergoing thoracic surgery. *Anesth Analg.* 2005;101: 957–965.
110. De Conno E, Steurer MP, Wittlinge M, et al. Anesthetic-induced improvement of the inflammatory response to one-lung ventilation. *Anesthesiology.* 2009;110: 1316–1326.
111. Schilling T, Kozian A, Senturk M, et al. Anesthetic-induced improvement of the inflammatory response to one-lung ventilation. *Anesthesiology.* 2011;115:65–74.
112. Von Euler US, Liljestrand G. Observations on the pulmonary arterial blood pressure in the cat. *Acta Physiol Scand.* 1946;12:301.
113. Marshall BE, Marshall C, Benumof JL, et al. Hypoxic pulmonary vasoconstriction in dogs: Effects of lung segment size and alveolar oxygen tensions. *J Appl Physiol.* 1981;51:1543.
114. Moudgil R, Michelakis ED, Archer SL. Hypoxic pulmonary vasoconstriction. *J Appl Physiol.* 2005;98:390.
115. Evans AM. Hypoxic pulmonary vasoconstriction. *Essays Biochem.* 2007;43:61.
116. Nagendran J, Stewart K, Hoskinson M, et al. An anesthesiologist's guide to hypoxic pulmonary vasoconstriction implications for managing single-lung anesthesia and atelectasis. *Curr Opin Anesthesiol.* 2006;19:34.
117. Benumof JL. One-lung ventilation and hypoxic pulmonary vasoconstriction: Implications for anesthetic management. *Anesth Analg.* 1985;64:821.
118. Eisenkraft JB. Effects of anesthetics on the pulmonary circulation. *Br J Anaesth.* 1990;65:63.
119. Rogers SM, Benumof JL. Halothane and isoflurane do not decrease PaO_2 during one-lung ventilation in intravenously anesthetized patients. *Anesth Analg.* 1985; 64:946.
120. Benumof JL, Augustine SD, Gibbons JA. Halothane and isoflurane only slightly impair arterial oxygenation during one-lung ventilation in patients undergoing thoracotomy. *Anesthesiology.* 1987;67:910.
121. Slinger P, Scott WAC. Arterial oxygenation during one-lung ventilation: A comparison of enflurane and isoflurane. *Anesthesiology.* 1995;82:940.
122. Beck DH, Doepfmer UR, Sinemus C, et al. Effects of sevoflurane and propofol on pulmonary shunt fraction during one-lung ventilation for thoracic surgery. *Br J Anaesth.* 2001;86:38–43.
123. Reid CW, Slinger PD, Lenis S. A comparison of the effects of propofol-alfentanil vs. isoflurane on arterial oxygenation during one lung ventilation. *J Cardiothorac Vasc Anesth.* 1996;10:860–863.
124. Pruszkowski O, Dalibon N, Moutafis M, et al. Effects of propofol vs sevoflurane on arterial oxygenation during one-lung ventilation. *Br J Anaesth.* 2007;98:539–544.
125. Ng A, Swanevelder J. Hypoxaemia associated with one-lung anaesthesia: New discoveries in ventilation and perfusion. *Br J Anaesth.* 2011;106:761–763.
126. Fischer SR, Deyo DJ, Bone HG, et al. Nitric oxide synthase inhibition restores HPV in sepsis. *Am J Respir Crit Care Med.* 1997;156:833.
127. Frostell CG, Blomqvist H, Hedenstierna G, et al. Inhaled nitric oxide selectively reverses human HPV without causing systemic vasodilation. *Anesthesiology.* 1993; 78:427.
128. Troncy E, Francoeur M, Blaise G. Inhaled nitric oxide: Clinical applications, indications and toxicology. *Can J Anaesth.* 1997;44:973.
129. Moutafis M, Liu N, Dalibon N, et al. The effects of inhaled nitric oxide and its combination with intravenous almitrine on PaO_2 during one-lung ventilation in patients undergoing thoracoscopic procedures. *Anesth Analg.* 1997;85:1130.
130. Moutafis M, Dalibon N, Colchen A, et al. Improving oxygenation during bronchopulmonary lavage using nitric oxide inhalation and almitrine infusion. *Anesth Analg.* 1999;89:32.
131. B'chir A, Mebassa A, Losserm MR, et al. Intravenous almitrine bismesylate reversibly inhibits lactic acidosis and hepatic dysfunction in patients with lung injury. *Anesthesiology.* 1998;89:823.
132. Doering EB, Hanson CW, Reily D, et al. Improvement in oxygenation by phenylephrine and nitric oxide in patients with adult respiratory distress syndrome. *Anesthesiology.* 1997;87:18.
133. Matsushima Y, Jones RL, King EG, et al. Alterations in pulmonary mechanics and gas exchange during routine fiberoptic bronchoscopy. *Chest.* 1984;86:184.
134. Satyanarayana T, Capan L, Ramanathan S, et al. Bronchofiberscopic jet ventilation. *Anesth Analg.* 1980;59:350.
135. Neuman GG, Weingarten AE, Abramowitz RM, et al. The anesthetic management of the patient with an anterior mediastinal mass. *Anesthesiology.* 1984; 60:144.
136. Bechard P, Letourneau L, Lacasse Y. Perioperative cardiorespiratory complications in adults with mediastinal mass: Incidence and risk factors. *Anesthesiology.* 2004;100:826.
137. Oley LTC, Hnatiuk MC, Corcoran MC, et al. Spirometry in surgery for anterior mediastinal masses. *Chest.* 2001;120:1152.
138. Tempe DK, Arya R, Dubey S, et al. Mediastinal mass resection: Femorofemoral cardiopulmonary bypass before induction of anesthesia in the management of airway obstruction. *J Cardiothorac Vasc Anesth.* 2001;15:233.
139. Ferrari LR, Bedford RF. General anesthesia prior to treatment of anterior mediastinal masses in pediatric cancer patients. *Anesthesiology.* 1990;72:991.
140. Shamberger RC. Preanesthetic evaluation of children with anterior mediastinal masses. *Semin Pediatr Surg.* 1999;8:61.
141. DeSoto H. Direct laryngoscopy as an aid to relieve airway obstruction in a patient with a mediastinal mass. *Anesthesiology.* 1987;67:116.
142. Gardner JC, Royster RL. Airway collapse with an anterior mediastinal mass despite spontaneous ventilation in an adult. *Anesth Analg.* 2011;113:239–242.
143. Slinger PD, Karsli C. Management of a patient with a large anterior mediastinal mass: Recurring myths. *Curr Opin Anaesthesiol.* 2007;20:1–3.
144. Barker SJ, Clarke C, Trivedi N, et al. Anesthesia for thoracoscopic laser ablation of bullous emphysema. *Anesthesiology.* 1993;78:44.
145. Brodsky JB, Cohen E. Video-assisted thoracoscopic surgery. *Curr Opin Anaesthesiol.* 2000;13:41.
146. Plummer S, Hartley M, Vaughan RS. Anaesthesia for telescopic procedures in the thorax. *Br J Anaesth.* 1998;80:223.
147. Neustein SM, Kahn P, Krellenstein DJ, et al. Incidence of arrhythmias and predisposing factors after thoracic surgery: Thoracotomy versus video-assisted thoracoscopy. *J Cardiothorac Vasc Anesth.* 1998;12:659.
148. Benumof JL. Sequential one-lung ventilation for bilateral bullectomy. *Anesthesiology.* 1987;67:268.
149. Cohen E, Eisenkraft JB. Bronchopulmonary lavage: Effects on oxygenation and hemodynamics. *J Cardiothorac Anesth.* 1990;4:119.
150. Hirsch NP. Neuromuscular junction in health and disease. *Br J Anaesth.* 2007; 99:132.
151. McGrogan A, Sneddon S, de Vries CS. The incidence of myasthenia gravis: A systematic literature review. *Neuroepidemiology.* 2010;34:171–183.
152. Drachman DB. Myasthenia gravis: Review article. *N Engl J Med.* 1994;330:1797.

153. Sathasivam S. Current and emerging treatments for the management of myasthenia gravis. *Ther Clin Risk Manag.* 2011;7:313–323.
154. McConville J, Farrugia ME, Beeson D, et al. Detection and characterization of MuSK antibodies in seronegative myasthenia gravis. *Ann Neurol.* 2004;55:580–584.
155. Mehndiratta MM, Pandey S, Kuntzer T. Acetylcholinesterase inhibitor treatment for myasthenia gravis. *Cochrane Database Syst Rev.* 2011:CD006986. Review.
156. Meyer DM, Herbert MA, Sobhani NC, et al. Comparative clinical outcomes of thymectomy for myasthenia gravis performed by extended transsternal and minimally invasive approaches. *Ann Thorac Surg.* 2009;87:385–390.
157. Pandey R, Garg R, Chandralekha, et al. Robot-assisted thoracoscopic thymectomy: Perianaesthetic concerns. *Eur J Anaesthesiol.* 2010;27:473–477.
158. Eisenkraft JB, Neustein SM. Anesthesia for esophageal and mediastinal surgery. In: Kaplan JA, ed. *Thoracic Anesthesia*, 3rd ed. New York, NY: Churchill-Livingstone; 2003:269.
159. Blichfeldt-Lauridsen L, Hansen BD. Anesthesia and myasthenia gravis. *Acta Anaesthesiol Scand.* 2012;56:17–22.
160. Tripathi M, Kaushik S, Dubey P. The effect of use of pyridostigmine and requirement for vecuronium with myasthenia gravis. *J Postgrad Med.* 2003;49:311.
161. Dillon FX. Anesthesia issues in the perioperative management of myasthenia gravis. *J Postgrad Med.* 2003;49:311.
162. Kopman AF. The datex-ohmeda M-NMT module: A potentially confusing user interface. *Anesthesiology.* 2006;104:1110–1111.
163. Nilsson E, Muller K. Neuromuscular effects of isoflurane in patients with myasthenia gravis. *Acta Anaesthesiol Scand.* 1990;34:126.
164. Nitahara K, Sugi Y, Higa K, et al. Neuromuscular effects of sevoflurane in myasthenia gravis patients. *Br J Anaesth.* 2007;98:337.
165. Gritti P, Carrara B, Khotcholava M, et al. The use of desflurane or propofol in combination with remifentanil in myasthenic patients undergoing a video-assisted thoracoscopic-extended thymectomy. *Acta Anaesthesiol Scand.* 2009;53:380–389.
166. Eisenkraft JB, Book WJ, Papatestas AE. Sensitivity to vecuronium in myasthenia gravis: A dose-response study. *Can J Anaesth.* 1990;37:301–306.
167. Baraka A, Siddik S, Kawkabani N. Cisatracurium in a myasthenic patient undergoing thymectomy. *Can J Anaesth.* 1999;46:779.
168. Baraka AS, Taha SK, Kawkabani NI. Neuromuscular interaction of sevoflurane—cisatracurium in a myasthenic patient. *Can J Anaesth.* 2000;47:562.
169. Mann R, Blobner M, Jelen-Esselborn S, et al. Preanesthetic train-of-four fade predicts the atracurium requirement of myasthenia gravis patients. *Anesthesiology.* 2000;93:346.
170. Itoh H, Shibata K, Nitta S. Difference in sensitivity to vecuronium between patients with ocular and generalized myasthenia gravis. *Br J Anaesth.* 2001;87:885.
171. Itoh H, Shibata K, Nitta S. Sensitivity to vecuronium in seropositive and seronegative patients with myasthenia gravis. *Anesth Analg.* 2003;96:1842.
172. Basaranoglu G, Erden V, Delatioglu H. Anesthesia of a patient with cured myasthenia gravis. *Anesth Analg.* 2003;96:1842.
173. Naguib M. Sugammadex: Another milestone in clinical neuromuscular pharmacology. *Anesth Analg.* 2007;104:575.
174. Kopman AF. Sugammadex: A revolutionary approach to neuromuscular antagonism. *Anesthesiology.* 2006;104:4.
175. Unterbuchner C, Fink H, Blobner M. The use of sugammadex in a patient with myasthenia gravis. *Anaesthesia.* 2010;65:302–305.
176. Eisenkraft JB, Book WJ, Papatestas AE, et al. Resistance to succinylcholine in myasthenia gravis: A dose-response study. *Anesthesiology.* 1988;69:760.
177. Baraka A, Tabboush Z. Neuromuscular response to succinylcholine-vecuronium sequence in three myasthenic patients undergoing thymectomy. *Anesth Analg.* 1991;72:827.
178. Della Rocca G, Coccia C, Diana L, et al. Propofol or sevoflurane anesthesia without muscle relaxants allow the early extubation of myasthenic patients. *Can J Anesth.* 2003;50:547.
179. Madi-Jebara S, Yazigi A, Hayek M, et al. Sevoflurane anesthesia and intrathecal sufentanil-morphine for thymectomy in myasthenia gravis. *J Clin Anesth.* 2002; 14:558.
180. Abe S, Takeuchi C, Kaneko T, et al. Propofol anesthesia combined with thoracic epidural anesthesia for thymectomy for myasthenia gravis—a report of eleven cases. *Masui.* 2001;50:1217.
181. Chevalley C, Spiliopoulos A, de Perrot M, et al. Perioperative medical management and outcome following thymectomy for myasthenia gravis. *Can J Anesth.* 2001;48:446.
182. Lorimer M, Hall R. Remifentanil and propofol total intravenous anaesthesia for thymectomy in myasthenia gravis. *Anaesth Intensive Care.* 1998;26:210.
183. Politis GD, Tobias JD. Rapid sequence intubation without a neuromuscular blocking agent in a 14 year old female patient with myasthenia gravis. *Paediatr Anaesth.* 2007;17:285.
184. Baraka AS, Haroun-Bizri ST, Georges FJ. Delayed postoperative arousal following remifentanil-based anesthesia in a myasthenic patient undergoing thymectomy. *Anesthesiology.* 2004;100:460.
185. Ingersoll-Weng E, Manecke GR, Thistlethwaite PA. Dexmedetomidine and cardiac arrest. *Anesthesiology.* 2004;100:758.
186. Eisenkraft JB, Papatestas AE, Kahn CH, et al. Predicting the need for postoperative mechanical ventilation in myasthenia gravis. *Anesthesiology.* 1986;65:79.
187. Grant RP, Jenkins LC. Prediction of the need for postoperative mechanical ventilation in myasthenia gravis: Thymectomy compared to other surgical procedures. *Can Anaesth Soc J.* 1982;29:112–116.
188. Mori T, Yoshioka M, Watanabe K, et al. Changes in respiratory condition after thymectomy for patients with myasthenia gravis. *Ann Thorac Cardiovasc Surg.* 2003;9:93.
189. Zahid I, Sharif S, Routledge T, et al. Video-assisted thoracoscopic surgery or transsternal thymectomy in the treatment of myasthenia gravis? *Interact Cardiovasc Thorac Surg.* 2011;12:40–46.
190. Burgess FW, Wilcosky B. Thoracic epidural anesthesia for transsternal thymectomy in myasthenia gravis. *Anesth Analg.* 1989;69:529.
191. Gorback MS. Analgesic management after thymectomy. *Anesthesiol Rep.* 1990;2:262–266.
192. Petty R. Lambert Eaton myasthenic syndrome. *Pract Neurol.* 2007;7:265–267.
193. Keogh M, Sedehizadeh S, Maddison P. Treatment for Lambert-Eaton myasthenic syndrome. *Cochrane Database Syst Rev.* 2011:CD003279.
194. Itoh H, Shibata K, Nitta S. Neuromuscular monitoring in myasthenic syndrome. *Anesthesia.* 2001;56:562.
195. Verschuuren JJ, Wirtz PW, Titulaer MJ, et al. Available treatment options for the management of Lambert-Eaton myasthenic syndrome. *Expert Opin Pharmacother.* 2006;7:1323–1336.
196. Telford RJ, Hollway TE. The myasthenic syndrome: Anesthesia in a patient treated with 3,4 diaminopyridine. *Br J Anaesth.* 1990;64:363.
197. Kavanagh BP, Katz J, Sandler AN. Pain control after thoracic surgery: A review of current techniques. *Anesthesiology.* 1994;81:737.
198. Whiting WG, Sandler AN, Lau LC, et al. Analgesic and respiratory effects of epidural sufentanil in post-thoracotomy patients. *Anesthesiology.* 1988;69:36.
199. Suzuki M, Haraguti S, Sugimoto K, et al. Low-dose intravenous ketamine potentiates epidural analgesia after thoracotomy. *Anesthesiology.* 2006;105:111.
200. Michelet P, Guervilly C, Helaine A. Adding ketamine to morphine for patient-controlled analgesia after thoracic surgery: Influence on morphine consumption, respiratory function, and nocturnal desaturation. *Br J Anaesth.* 2007;99:396.
201. Sihoe AD, Lee TW, Wan IY, et al. The use of gabapentin for post-operative and post-traumatic pain in thoracic surgery patients. *Eur J Cardiothorac Surg.* 2006; 29:795.
202. Kong VKF, Irwin MG. Gabapentin: A multimodal perioperative drug? *Br J Anaesth.* 2007;99:775.
203. Hout HP, Chouinard P, Girard F, et al. Gabapentin does not reduce post thoracotomy shoulder pain: A randomized, double-blind placebo controlled study. *Can J Anesth.* 2008;55:337–343.
204. Martinez-Barenys C, Busquets J, Lopez de Castro PE, et al. Randomized double-blind comparison of phrenic nerve infiltration and suprascapular nerve block for ipsilateral shoulder pain after thoracic surgery. *Eur J Cardiothorac Surg.* 2011; 40:106–112.
205. Davies RG, Myles PS, Graham JM. A comparison of the analgesic efficacy and side-effects of paravertebral vs epidural blockade for thoracotomy—a systematic review and meta-analysis of randomized controlled trials. *Br J Anesth.* 2006;96: 418.
206. Daly DJ, Myles PS. Update on the role of paravertebral blocks for thoracic surgery: Are they worth it? *Curr Opin Anaesthesiol.* 2009;22:38–32.
207. Conlon NP, Shaw AD, Grichnik KP. Postthoracotomy paravertebral analgesia: Will it replace epidural analgesia? *Anesthesiol Clin.* 2008;26:369–380.
208. Block BM, Spencer SL, Rowlingson BA, et al. Efficacy of postoperative epidural analgesia. A meta-analysis. *JAMA.* 2003;290:2455.
209. Rodgers A, Walker N, Schug S, et al. Reduction of postoperative mortality and morbidity with epidural or spinal anesthesia: Results from an overview of randomized trials. *Br Med J.* 2000;321:1.
210. Minzler B, Grimm BJ, Johnson RF, et al. The practice of thoracic epidural analgesia: A survey of academic centers in the United States. *Anesth Analg.* 2002;95:472.
211. Weber T, Matzl J, Rokitansky A, et al. Superior postoperative pain relief with thoracic epidural analgesia versus intravenous patient-controlled analgesia after minimally invasive pectus excavatum repair. *J Thorac Cardiovasc Surg.* 2007;132: 865.
212. Mac TB, Girard F, Chouinard P, et al. Acetaminophen decreases early post-thoracotomy ipsilateral shoulder pain in patients with thoracic epidural analgesia. *J Cardiothorac Vasc Anesth.* 2005;19:475.
213. Cohen E, Neustein SM. Intrathecal morphine during thoracotomy. *J Thorac Cardiovasc Anesth.* 1993;7:154.
214. Askar FZ, Kocabas S, Yucel S, et al. The efficacy of intrathecal morphine in post-thoracotomy pain management. *J Int Med Res.* 2007;35:314–322.
215. Meylan N, Elia N, Lysakowski C, et al. Benefit and risk of intrathecal morphine without local anaesthetic in patients undergoing major surgery: Meta-analysis of randomized trials. *Br J Anaesth.* 2009;102:156–162.
216. Katz J, Kavanagh BP, Sandler AN, et al. Preemptive analgesia. *Anesthesiology.* 1992;77:439.
217. Bong CL, Samuel M, Ng JM, et al. Effects of preemptive epidural analgesia on post-thoracotomy pain. *J Cardiothorac Vasc Anesth.* 2005;19:786.
218. Fiorelli A, Vicidomini G, Laperuta P, et al. Pre-emptive local analgesia in video assisted thoracic surgery sympathectomy. *Eur J Cardiothorac Surg.* 2010;37:588–593.
219. Detterbeck FC. Subpleural catheter placement for pain relief after thoracoscopic resection. *Ann Thorac Surg.* 2006;81:1552–1553.

220. Gotoda Y, Kambara N, Sakai T, et al. The morbidity, time course and predictive factors for persistent post-thoracotomy pain. *Eur J Pain.* 2001;5:89.
221. Hutter J, Miller K, Moritz E. Chronic sequels after thoracoscopic procedures for benign diseases. *Eur J Cardiothorac Surg.* 2000;17:687.
222. Ochroch EA, Gottschalk A, Troxel AB, et al. Women suffer more short and long-term pain than men after major thoracotomy. *Clin J Pain.* 2006;22:491.
223. Gottschalk A, Cohen S, Yang S, et al. Preventing and treating pain after thoracic surgery. *Anesthesiology.* 2006;104:594.
224. Steegers MA, SNik DM, Verhagen AF, et al. Only half of the chronic pain after thoracic surgery shows a neuropathic component. *J Pain.* 2008;9:955–961.
225. Wildgaard K, Ravn J, Nikolajsen L, et al. Consequences of persistent pain after lung cancer surgery: A nationwide questionnaire study. *Acta Anaesthesiol Scand.* 2011;55:60–68.
226. Wildgaard K, Ravn J, Kehlet H. Chronic post-thoracotomy pain: A critical review of pathogenic mechanisms and strategies for prevention. *Eur J Cardiothorac Surg.* 2009;36:170–180.
227. Kotemane NC, Gopinath N, Vaja R. Analgesic techniques following thoracic surgery: A survey of United Kingdom practice. *Eur J Anaesthesiol.* 2010;27:897–899.
228. Demmy TL, Nwagu C, Solan P, et al. Chest-tube delivered bupivacaine improves pain and decreases opioid use after thoracoscopy. *Ann Thorac Surg.* 2009;87:1040–1046.
229. Kaplowitz J, Papadakos PJ. Acute pain management for video-assisted thoracoscopic surgery: An update. *J Cardiothorac Vasc Anesth.* 2012;26:312–321.
230. Fibla JJ, Molins L, Mier JM, et al. The efficacy of paravertebral block using a catheter technique for postoperative analgesia in thoracoscopic surgery: A randomized trial. *Eur J Cardiothorac Surg.* 2011;40:907–911.
231. Neustein SM. Reexpansion pulmonary edema. *J Cardiothorac Vasc Anesth.* 2007; 21:887–891.
232. Beck-Nielsen J, Sorensen HR, Alstrup P. Atrial fibrillation following thoracotomy for non-cardiac cases, in particular, cancer of the lung. *Acta Med Scand.* 1973; 193:425.
233. Ritchie J, Bowe P, Gibbons JRP. Prophylactic digitalization for thoracotomy: A reassessment. *Ann Thorac Surg.* 1990;50:86.
234. Ciriaco P, Mazzone P, Canneto B, et al. Supraventricular arrhythmia following lung resection for non-small-cell lung cancer and its treatment with amiodarone. *Eur J Cardiothorac Surg.* 2000;18:12.

CHAPTER

38 Anesthesia for Cardiac Surgery

NIKOLAOS J. SKUBAS • ADAM D. LICHTMAN • AARTI SHARMA • STEPHEN J. THOMAS

Key Points

1. When treating myocardial ischemia, decreasing O_2 demand is more important than modifying O_2 supply.
2. Intraoperative ischemia is usually silent and is not usually accompanied by hemodynamic changes.
3. Slow rate, small size, and adequate perfusion are the goals in patients with coronary artery disease.
4. The pulmonary artery catheter does not always reliably detect ischemia.
5. There is no "ideal" anesthetic in cardiac surgery.
6. In aortic stenosis, a preload-dependent, hypertrophic ventricle requires adequate diastolic time and perfusion pressure.
7. In chronic aortic insufficiency, a dilated ventricle requires increased preload and decreased afterload.
8. In mitral stenosis, the left ventricle is "lazy" and "underused" and requires a slow heart rate to fill.
9. In mitral regurgitation, a preload-dependent and dilated left ventricle benefits from afterload reduction and fast heart rate.
10. Maintenance of perfusion pressure should not take precedence over ventilation during cardiac anesthesia (never forget your ABCs).
11. Fast-track anesthetic techniques depend on higher concentration of inspired volatile agents, use of vasoactive medications (β-blockers), and smaller doses of benzodiazepines and opioids.
12. The combination of systolic systemic and diastolic pulmonary pressures characterizes the performance of the left ventricle, and the combination of systolic pulmonary and central venous pressures characterizes the performance of the right ventricle.

Multimedia

1 Aortic Stenosis

2 Aortic Insufficiency

3 Mitral Stenosis

4 Mitral Regurgitation

5 Cardiopulmonary Bypass

6 Cardioplegia

7 Centrifugal and Roller Pumps

8 IABP

Anesthetizing patients who undergo cardiac surgery is exciting, intellectually challenging, and emotionally rewarding. The cardiac anesthesiologist should have a thorough understanding of normal and altered cardiac physiology; have knowledge of the pharmacology of anesthetic, vasoactive, and cardioactive drugs; and be familiar with the physiologic alterations associated with cardiopulmonary bypass (CPB) and the surgical procedures. This chapter presents a brief overview of the critical physiologic and technical considerations during cardiac surgical procedures. Some of the issues discussed are controversial because the field is continuously evolving. The authors have tried, whenever possible, not to allow their own preferences overshadow what is the consensus about the various topics presented in the chapter.

CORONARY ARTERY DISEASE

The prevention or treatment of myocardial ischemia during coronary artery bypass graft (CABG) surgery is associated with a decreased incidence of perioperative myocardial infarction. The hemodynamic management is tailored to avoid factors known to increase myocardial oxygen demand ($M\dot{V}O_2$), particularly during the vulnerable pre-CPB period. Optimizing oxygen delivery to the myocardium is equally important for the successful management of these patients because it is well recognized that most ischemic events occur with minimal or no change in $M\dot{V}O_2$.[1,2] The determinants of myocardial oxygen supply and demand are shown in Figure 38-1 and are also discussed in Chapter 10.

Myocardial Oxygen Demand

The principal determinants of $M\dot{V}O_2$ are wall tension and contractility.[3] According to Laplace's law, wall tension is directly proportional to intracavitary pressure and radius and inversely proportional to wall thickness. Therefore, myocardial oxygen demand can be reduced by interventions that (1) decrease intraventricular pressure and (2) prevent or promptly treat ventricular distention.

Demand	Supply
1. Wall stress: $\frac{PR}{2h}$ – Preload – Afterload 2. Heart rate 3. Contractility	1. Coronary blood flow: $\frac{\text{AoDP} - \text{LVEDP}}{\text{Coronary vascular resistance}}$ – Diastolic time – Collaterals, capillary density 2. Oxygen content: Hb × $SatO_2$ 3. Hb – O_2 dissociation curve 4. O_2 extraction

FIGURE 38-1. Determinants of myocardial oxygen balance. P, intracavitary pressure; R, ventricular radius; h, wall thickness; AoDP, diastolic arterial pressure; LVEDP, left ventricular end-diastolic pressure; Hb, hemoglobin; $SatO_2$, arterial oxygen saturation.

Myocardial Oxygen Supply

1 Increases in myocardial oxygen requirements can be met only by raising coronary blood flow. Arterial blood oxygen content and oxygen extraction by the myocardium are infrequent reasons for intraoperative myocardial ischemia because oxygenation and blood volume are usually well controlled during anesthesia. In addition, further oxygen extraction (blood in the coronary sinus is desaturated: Po_2 in the range of 15 to 20 mm Hg) is inadequate to meet significantly increased demand. Therefore, the principal mechanism for matching oxygen supply to alterations in $M\dot{V}O_2$ is exquisite regulation and control of coronary blood flow.

Coronary Blood Flow

The critical factors that modify coronary blood flow are the perfusion pressure and vascular tone of the coronary circulation, the time available for perfusion (determined mainly by heart rate), the severity of intraluminal obstructions, and the presence of (any) collateral circulation. The area most vulnerable to ischemia is the subendocardium of the left ventricle (LV), which is exposed to the LV intracavitary pressure and where metabolic requirements are increased because of greater systolic shortening.[4]

Perfusion of the LV subendocardium takes place almost entirely during diastole, whereas the right ventricular subendocardium is perfused in diastole and systole, assuming pulmonary hypertension is not present. This temporal disparity is explained by the different intraventricular pressures developing during systole.

The LV coronary perfusion pressure is often defined as the gradient between aortic diastolic (or mean) pressure and left ventricular diastolic pressure (LVDP; usually estimated by the pulmonary artery occlusion pressure). In the presence of intraluminal obstruction or increased vascular tone, this pressure gradient is reduced (Fig. 38-2). A low LVDP is ideal for improving perfusion (higher pressure gradient) and reducing $M\dot{V}O_2$ (decreased LV volume and wall tension). On the other hand, increasing perfusion pressure by raising the aortic pressure will increase $M\dot{V}O_2$. However, this is not as important, when one considers that tachycardia is the most important cause of intraoperative and perioperative ischemia.

Alterations in the tone of the small intramyocardial arterioles regulate diastolic vascular resistance, allowing the matching of oxygen supply with metabolic demand over a wide range of perfusion pressures.[5] The difference between autoregulated, baseline flow, and blood flow available under conditions of maximal vasodilation is termed *coronary vascular reserve* and is normally three to five times higher than basal flow. As epicardial coronary stenosis becomes more pronounced, progressive vasodilation of these resistance vessels allows preservation of basal flow, but at

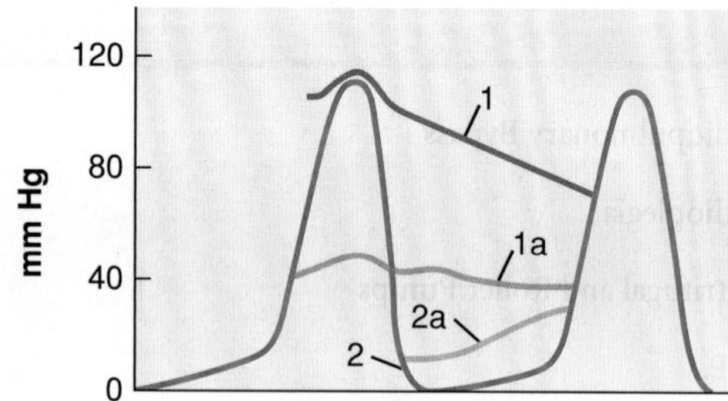

FIGURE 38-2. The pressure relationships between the aorta (*1*) and the left ventricle (*2*) determine coronary perfusion pressure. In coronary artery disease, myocardial perfusion may be compromised by decreased pressure distal to a significant stenosis (*1a*) (not quantifiable clinically) and/or by an increase in left ventricular end-diastolic pressure (*2a*). (Reprinted from Gorlin R. *Coronary Artery Disease*. Philadelphia: WB Saunders; 1976:75, with permission.)

the cost of reduced reserve. Once perfusion pressure decreases to <40 mm Hg, autoregulation of subendocardial coronary flow is lost. Whenever demand increases above available reserve, signs, symptoms, and metabolic evidence of ischemia develop.

Prinzmetal et al.[6] first described angina and myocardial infarction in patients with angiographically normal coronary vessels. Other causes of infarction include prolonged hypotension and acute coronary thrombosis. Unstable angina pectoris and/or acute coronary thrombosis are the results of plaque rupture with ensuing platelet activation and thrombus formation.[7] The presence of the potentially hyperreactive normal vessel wall adjacent to the thrombus may result in vasospasm[8] and total occlusion of the vessel lumen in the presence of a previously nonocclusive eccentric plaque or thrombus.[9] This type of acute thrombosis is believed to be the cause of most acute myocardial infarctions and associated sudden death (usually from ischemia-induced cardiac dysrhythmias).

Anesthesia is not protective against "supply" ischemia such as noted below (Fig. 38-3). It is not uncommon for an anesthetized

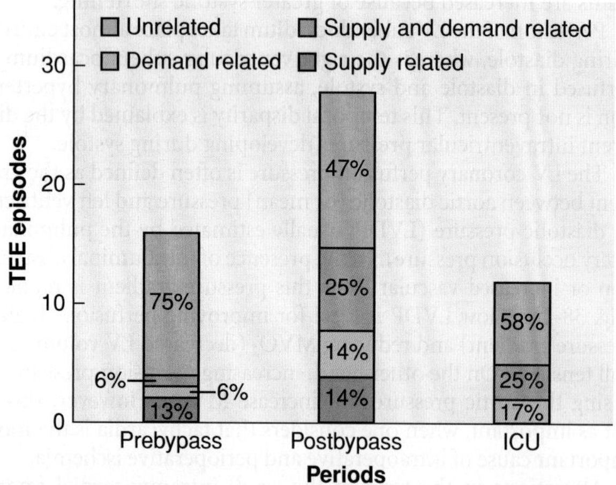

FIGURE 38-3. Association of transesophageal echocardiographic (TEE) wall motion changes with hemodynamic indices of supply and demand from continuous monitoring of 50 patients undergoing coronary artery bypass surgery. ICU, intensive care unit. (Reproduced from Leung JM, O'Kelly BV, Mangano DT, et al. Relationship of regional wall motion abnormalities to hemodynamic indices of myocardial oxygen supply and demand in patients undergoing CABG surgery. *Anesthesiology.* 1990;73:802, with permission.)

patient to show signs of ischemia without any change in heart rate,
2 blood pressure, or ventricular filling pressures. In fact, most ischemic episodes are not accompanied by hemodynamic changes. Drugs such as nitroglycerin or calcium entry blockers may be used to prevent and/or treat such episodes of coronary spasm, although prophylactic use of these agents is usually ineffective.

Hemodynamic Goals

Although the precise relationship between intraoperative ischemia and postoperative myocardial infarction remains controversial, there is consensus that the primary goal of any successful cardiac anesthetic is prevention of myocardial ischemia. Failing that, prompt identification and treatment of new ischemic episodes is essential. As is evident from the previous discussion and from the summary in Table 38-1, anesthetic decisions are designed to reduce and control those factors that increase myocardial oxygen demand (heart rate, contractility, and wall tension). At the same time, every attempt is made to optimize coronary blood flow, notably, maintaining coronary perfusion pressure and increasing
3 diastolic time. Of note, the peripheral arterial systolic pressure is different (usually higher) than the aortic root pressure, and this should be kept in mind when making decisions pertaining to coronary blood flow. The goals for patients with coronary artery disease are "slow, small, and well perfused." There is not a single "ideal" anesthetic that accomplishes all of the above. Instead, combinations of intravenous and volatile anesthetics, sedatives, muscle relaxants, and vasoactive drugs are chosen to achieve hemodynamic stability. Pharmacologic agents that may benefit coronary patients include statins[10] and angiotensin-converting enzyme inhibitors (to stabilize the atherosclerotic plaque).[11] Volatile anesthetics offer cardioprotection when applied prior to or even after the ischemic insult. A reduction in mortality and morbidity has been shown in patients undergoing CABG and aortic valve (AV) surgery. However, it is very difficult to associate these beneficial effects to pre- or postconditioning mechanisms.[12]

Monitoring for Ischemia

The ideal monitoring technique is not yet available. Analysis of the ST segment in multiple leads (most commonly leads II and

TABLE 38-1. CORONARY ARTERY DISEASE—HEMODYNAMIC GOALS

Preload	Keep the heart small: ↓ wall tension (diameter) and LVEDP; ↑ perfusion pressure gradient
Afterload	Maintain: Hypertension is better than hypotension
Contractility	Depress (if LV function is normal)
Rate	Slow
Rhythm	Sinus
$M\dot{V}O_2$	Monitor for and treat "supply"-related disturbances
CPB	Elevated filling pressures are usually not needed after CABG

↓, decrease; ↑, increase; LVEDP, left ventricular end-diastolic pressure; LV, left ventricular; $M\dot{V}O_2$, myocardial oxygen consumption; CPB, postcardiopulmonary bypass; CABG, coronary artery bypass graft.

V_4 or V_5) is currently the standard. Patients likely to develop right ventricular ischemia or those with disease of the right coronary artery might benefit from monitoring of leads V_{4R} or V_{5R}. The ST segment from various ECG leads should be continuously monitored and displayed and interactive monitors should alarm when the ST segment deviates from baseline.

Multiple attempts have been made to determine ischemic thresholds using commonly measured hemodynamic variables. Among the earliest of these was the rate–pressure product (RPP = heart rate × peak systolic arterial pressure). The RPP was considered an easily determined index of $M\dot{V}O_2$. Although RPP may correlate with oxygen demand, especially during exercise, it is not a sensitive or specific indicator of intraoperative ischemia; identical RPPs can be produced from multiple combinations of heart rate and blood pressure. Favorable conditions for oxygen balance are more likely those of lower heart rate and higher blood pressure than tachycardia and hypotension. Neither the ratio of mean arterial pressure over heart rate nor the diastolic to systolic pressure–time index is any more predictive or reliable than the RPP.[13]

Sudden elevations in pulmonary artery or capillary wedge pressure indicating LV dysfunction, large *a* waves reflecting decreased LV compliance, and *v* waves indicative of increased left atrial pressure because of ischemia-induced papillary muscle dysfunction and/or mitral regurgitation (MR) are purported signs of ischemia that may be detected with a pulmonary artery catheter (PAC). PAC-based monitoring of filling pressures, saturation of mixed venous blood in oxygen, and thermodilution cardiac output is common practice in cardiac surgery centers.[14,15] Several studies contradict this long-held
4 dogma and demonstrate that the PAC is of little value as a monitor of myocardial ischemia. Leung et al.[16] found that only 10% of all regional wall motion abnormalities were associated with an acute rise in pulmonary capillary wedge pressure in 40 patients undergoing elective CABG surgery. Haggmark et al.[17] found that neither an increase nor an abnormal pulmonary capillary wedge pressure waveform was a sensitive indicator for myocardial ischemia in 53 patients with coronary artery disease undergoing vascular surgery. A prospective study of 1,094 patients by Tuman et al.[18] showed that even high-risk cardiac surgical patients may be safely managed without routine use of a PAC, and if the need for it developed intraoperatively, delayed placement of a PAC did not influence outcome. Fontes et al.[19] assessed the limitations of PAC in the management of critically ill patients in the intensive care unit (ICU). Compared with transesophageal echocardiography (TEE), PAC predicted normal left ventricular function well, but performed poorly in judging preload and ventricular dysfunction. A more recent study showed no benefit from PACs in high-risk surgical patients.[20] Others prefer to insert a PAC in selected patients, when needed.[21] The most recent American Society of Anesthesiologists Practice Guidelines concluded that the evidence regarding the benefit that cardiac surgery patients receive from PAC is conflicting.[22] However, it is difficult to determine the value of PAC in diagnosis and treatment when the physician's ability for correct interpretation of PAC information is still in doubt.[23]

Since its introduction in the 1980s, TEE has become an invaluable diagnostic and monitoring tool during cardiac surgery. TEE permits assessment of ventricular volume, global and regional function, estimation and quantitation of valvular pathology, measurement of valve gradients and calculation of filling pressures, visualization of the thoracic aorta, and detection of intracardiac air. Practice guidelines for perioperative TEE have been recently published by the ASA.[24] Experienced cardiac anesthesiologists who are supported by continuous quality programs perform comprehensive TEE studies[25] and interpret TEE examinations at a level comparable with physicians whose primary practice is echocardiography.[26]

Multiple image planes are necessary to evaluate the three-dimensional structure of the heart. The recent introduction of real-time three-dimensional TEE introduced a real revolution in perioperative imaging, particularly of the mitral valve. The American Society of Echocardiography/Society of Cardiovascular Anesthesiologists task force for intraoperative echocardiography has published guidelines for performing a comprehensive intraoperative echocardiographic examination.[27] These recommendations describe a series of 20 standard tomographic views of the heart and great vessels that should be included in a complete intraoperative echocardiographic examination. With experience, a thorough examination can be performed in less than 10 minutes.

Selection of Anesthetic

There is no one "ideal" anesthetic for patients with coronary artery disease. The choice of anesthetic should depend primarily on the extent of pre-existing myocardial dysfunction and the pharmacologic properties of the drugs themselves. All drugs are titrated to the desired effect. The healthy patient with preserved LV function who has angina only on heavy exertion will tolerate a
5 volatile-based technique that is geared toward decreasing $M\dot{V}O_2$. Conversely, the patient with severe congestive heart failure and a previous myocardial infarction may require a less myocardial depressive regimen. Most patients with mild or even moderate dysfunction may benefit from some degree of myocardial depression, which leads to decreased oxygen demand, and may alleviate or at least reduce episodes of ischemia.

Early extubation is common practice and is achieved by multiple approaches.[28,29] The choice of anesthetic should be based on known hemodynamic, pharmacologic, and pharmacokinetic effects of each drug as they apply to the particular patient, the experience of the anesthesiologist, and the relative cost–benefit of each agent. Volatile anesthetics with low-dose narcotics or total intravenous anesthesia with short-acting drugs (e.g., midazolam, alfentanil, remifentanil, propofol) have been used to effect early extubation. The increased use of benzodiazepines and volatile agents has been associated with low incidence of awareness.[30] Intraoperative clinical variables are important factors to be considered in the timing of postoperative extubation after fast-track cardiac surgery. Inotrope use and platelet transfusion were the most significant determinants of early (<10 hours postoperatively) tracheal extubation in a Veterans Administration population.[31]

Opioids

The primary advantages of opioids are lack of myocardial depression, maintenance of a stable hemodynamic state, and reduction of heart rate. However, they cannot provide complete anesthesia. Notable side effects include (i) hypertension and tachycardia during surgical stimulation (sternotomy and aortic manipulation), especially in patients with good ventricular function; (ii) predictable hypotension when combined with benzodiazepines; (iii) lack of titratability when used in high doses; and (iv) a low incidence of intraoperative recall if used as the sole anesthetic. The current practice is to supplement the opioid with benzodiazepines and volatile agents, and many of the previous side effects may be of historical interest. A high-dose opioid-based technique may be of value only in the patient with severe myocardial dysfunction. The planned time of extubation is now one of the major factors determining the selection and dosage of opioid. Shorter-acting opioids (sufentanil and remifentanil) produce equally rapid extubation, similar ICU stay, and similar costs to fentanyl. Thus, any of these opioids can be used for fast-track cardiac surgery.[32] The beneficial cardioprotective and anti-inflammatory effects of morphine have been reconsidered recently,[33,34] bringing back into the foray the opioid that reinvigorated the practice of cardiac anesthesia.[35]

Inhalation Anesthetics

The desirable features of volatile anesthetics include dose-dependent hemodynamic changes, easy reversibility, titratable myocardial depression, amnesia, and suppression of sympathetic responses to surgical stress and CPB. Volatile anesthetics protect the myocardium from ischemia and reperfusion injury and reduce myocardial infarct size.[36] This beneficial effect has been shown when volatile anesthetics are administered before a period of prolonged ischemia ("anesthetic preconditioning") as well as during reperfusion ("anesthetic postconditioning").[37] However, it is difficult to ascertain whether these laboratory-proven benefits have contributed to improved myocardial protection in clinical practice.[38] Disadvantages include systemic hypotension (whether induced by decreased contractility or vasodilation), which may compromise the oxygen supply and lack of postoperative analgesia. Combinations of opioids and volatile anesthetics retain their advantages with minimal untoward effects. Any of the volatile agents can be used in a balanced technique.

Isoflurane is a coronary vasodilator, as are the other volatile anesthetics (although to a lesser degree). This dose-related effect is clinically insignificant in doses less than 1 MAC. Clinical studies using isoflurane to clinical rather than pharmacologic end points have not shown increased episodes of ischemia or a worsened outcome.[39]

Desflurane and sevoflurane have the fastest recovery of all volatile anesthetics. Desflurane has a rapid uptake and distribution, allowing it to be useful in cases in which hemodynamic changes mandate rapid changes in anesthetic depth. It has a cardiac profile similar to that of isoflurane. In patients undergoing noncardiac surgery, desflurane increases pulmonary artery pressure, wedge pressure, and pulmonary vascular resistance (PVR) compared with isoflurane.[40] When studying sympathetic nervous system activity, Helman et al.[41] found an increase in sympathetic activity and myocardial ischemia in patients anesthetized with desflurane as the sole anesthetic agent for coronary artery bypass surgery compared with patients anesthetized with sufentanil. Compared with isoflurane, in a technique combining fentanyl with the inhalational anesthetic, sevoflurane had an acceptable cardiovascular profile prior to CPB and similar outcome data.[42]

Intravenous Sedative Hypnotics

An alternative adjuvant anesthetic to a low-dose opioid technique is a titratable intravenous infusion of a short-acting sedative, such as midazolam,[43] propofol, or dexmedetomidine.[44] These can be continued postoperatively in the ICU and afford a predictable and fairly rapid awakening after discontinuation.[45] When compared with volatile anesthetics, propofol was associated with less favorable cardiac function, higher need for inotropic support, and elevated plasma troponins after cardiac surgery in elderly patients.[46]

Treatment of Ischemia

The use of anesthetics or vasoactive drugs that enable the heart to return to the slower-rate, smaller-size, and well-perfused state is frequently essential during anesthesia. The principal vasoactive drugs are nitrates, β-blockers, peripheral vasoconstrictors, and calcium entry blockers. Clinical scenarios for their use are given in Table 38-2. These drugs are discussed briefly here. Volatile anesthetics can also be used to control blood pressure and reduce contractility.

TABLE 38-2. TREATMENT OF INTRAOPERATIVE ISCHEMIA

Clinical Manifestation	
Increased demand	
↑ HR	Treat usual reasons, β-blocker
↑ BP	↑ anesthetic depth
↑ PCWP	Nitroglycerin
Decreased supply	
↓ HR	Atropine, pacing
↓ BP	↓ anesthetic depth, vasoconstrictor
↑ PCWP	Nitroglycerin, inotrope
No changes	Nitroglycerin, calcium channel blockers, ? heparin

↑, increase; ↓, decrease; HR, heart rate; BP, blood pressure; PCWP, pulmonary capillary wedge pressure.

Nitrates

Nitroglycerin (TNG) is the drug of choice for the treatment of acute myocardial ischemia. Its action is via systemic venodilation that decreases LV preload, wall tension, $M\dot{V}O_2$, and coronary arterial dilation, which is operative in both stenosed coronaries and collateral beds.[47] The evidence for the prophylactic use of TNG for prevention of either intraoperative ischemic episodes or postoperative cardiac complications is unconvincing.[48] At higher doses, TNG dilates arterial beds and may cause systemic hypotension. Compensatory tachycardia may increase heart $M\dot{V}O_2$. The recommended TNG dose is 0.5 to 3 μg/kg/minute and is reduced in the presence of hepatic and/or renal disease. TNG may cause methemoglobinemia especially in patients with methemoglobin reductase deficiency; this complication is more likely when large doses are administered over a prolonged time.[49] TNG is administered via special intravenous tubing that does not adsorb the drug.

Sodium Nitroprusside

Sodium nitroprusside (SNP) decreases peripheral vascular resistance by metabolic or spontaneous reduction to nitric oxide. Similar to TNG, SNP improves ventricular compliance in the ischemic myocardium. The recommended SNP dose is 0.5 to 3 μg/kg/minute and should be reduced in the presence of hepatic and/or renal disease. Adverse effects include cyanide and thiocyanate toxicity, rebound hypertension, intracranial hypertension, blood coagulation abnormalities, increased pulmonary shunting, and hypothyroidism. In vitro findings suggest that cardiac surgical patients may be at increased risk of cyanide toxicity in response to the perioperative administration of SNP.[50] Cyanide is produced when SNP is metabolized; toxic blood levels (>100 μg/dL) occur when >1.0-mg/kg SNP is administered within 2 hours or when >0.5 mg/kg/hour is administered within 24 hours. The presenting signs of cyanide toxicity include the triad of elevated mixed venous O_2 (Pv_{O_2}), requirements for increasing SNP dose (tachyphylaxis), and metabolic acidosis.[51] In addition, the patient may appear flushed. Greater risk of cyanide toxicity exists in patients who are nutritionally deficient in cobalamine (vitamin B_{12} compounds) or in dietary substances containing sulfur. Measurement of blood cyanide and pH will enable detection of abnormalities in high-risk patients for whom larger than recommended amounts of SNP have been used (8 to 10 μg/kg/minute). Treatment should consist of discontinuing infusion, administering 100% O_2, administering amyl nitrate (inhaler) or intravenous sodium nitrite and intravenous thiosulfate, except in those patients with abnormal renal function, for whom hydroxocobalamin is recommended. Circulating levels of thiocyanate increase when renal function is compromised, and central nervous system abnormalities result when thiocyanate levels reach 5 to 10 μg/dL. Lowering the SNP dose requirement or, better, replacing SNP with nicardipine, metoprolol, and esmolol reduces or eliminates the consequent buildup of cyanide. Once dissolved, SNP deteriorates in the presence of light. The container, therefore, should be wrapped in aluminum foil. An unstable SNP ion in aqueous solution reacts with various substances within 3 to 4 hours, forming colored salts. Other drugs should not be infused in the same solution as SNP.

Vasoconstrictors

Vasoconstrictors (phenylephrine, norepinephrine, vasopressin) are useful adjuncts in the prevention and treatment of ischemia because they increase systemic blood pressure, thereby improving coronary perfusion pressure, albeit at the expense of increasing afterload and perhaps $M\dot{V}O_2$. In addition, concomitant venoconstriction increases venous return and LV preload. TNG is sometimes added to counteract any increase in preload. In most situations, the increase in coronary perfusion pressure more than offsets any increase in wall tension. Peripheral vasoconstriction is indicated during episodes of systemic hypotension, especially those caused by reduced surgical stimulation or drug-induced vasodilation. No one vasoconstrictor is superior to all others. Occasionally, a combination of vasoconstrictors (e.g., norepinephrine and vasopressin) may be needed to achieve the desired blood pressure.[52]

β-blockers

β-adrenergic blockade improves myocardial oxygen balance by preventing or treating tachycardia and by decreasing contractility. Any concomitant myocardial depression is counterbalanced by the anti-ischemic effects. Indications for β-blockers include treatment of sinus tachycardia not resulting from the usual causes (e.g., light anesthesia, hypovolemia); prophylaxis of, and slowing the ventricular response to, supraventricular dysrhythmias; decreasing heart rate and contractility in hyperdynamic states; and control of ventricular dysrhythmias.[53,54] The use of β-blockers should aim at reducing the heart rate and increasing the diastolic filling time without, at the same time, decreasing the perfusion pressure and cardiac output. These therapy targets are even more important, since the POISE study revealed that death and stroke were side effects of β-blockers.[55,56] Intravenous preparations include propranolol, metoprolol, labetalol, and esmolol. Propranolol is a nonselective β-blocker with an elimination half-life of 4 to 6 hours. Metoprolol is similar to propranolol but has the purported advantage of β_1-selectivity and is less likely to trigger bronchospasm in patients with reactive airway disease. Labetalol combines β-blocking properties with those of α-blockade and is useful in treating hyperdynamic and hypertensive situations. Esmolol is a short-acting β_1-blocker that is cardioselective, with a half-life of only 9.5 minutes. It is particularly useful in treating transient increases in heart rate owing to episodic sympathetic stimulation.

Calcium Channel Blockers

Calcium channel blockers are useful in slowing the ventricular response in atrial fibrillation and flutter, as coronary vasodilators, and in the treatment of perioperative hypertension.[57,58] In vitro, all calcium entry blockers depress contractility, reduce coronary and systemic vascular tone, decrease sinoatrial node firing rate, and impede atrioventricular conduction. Unlike the β-blockers, which are similar in both structure and pharmacodynamic effect, the calcium entry blockers vary remarkably in their predominant pharmacologic action. The negative inotropic effect is greatest with verapamil and less with nifedipine, diltiazem, and nicardipine (in decreasing order). Verapamil is useful in the treatment of supraventricular tachycardia and slowing the ventricular response in atrial fibrillation and/or flutter; however, its myocardial depressant effects may limit its usefulness in some patients. In patients with reduced myocardial function, intravenous diltiazem is effective in the treatment of atrial fibrillation and flutter by slowing atrioventricular conduction with minimal myocardial depression. It is also useful in decreasing sinus rate. Calcium channel blockers have been found to have cardioprotective effects during reperfusion. Nicardipine in particular has coronary antispasmodic and vasodilatory effects more than systemic arterial vasodilatory effects.[59]

Nifedipine, amlodipine, and nicardipine are prominent peripheral vasodilators, effective in the treatment of postoperative hypertension in cardiac surgical patients, with minimal side effects.[60] The newer agent clevidipine was a better antihypertensive agent than SNP or TNG and was equivalent to nicardipine.[61] Magnesium has coronary artery vasodilating properties, reduces the size of myocardial infarction in the setting of acute ischemia, and decreases mortality associated with infarction.[62] In addition, it is an antiarrhythmic and minimizes myocardial reperfusion injury. While magnesium was found to prevent atrial fibrillation in coronary artery surgery,[63] in patients treated with β-blockers, the addition of prophylactic iv magnesium did not reduce the incidence of atrial arrhythmias.[64]

The most recent guidelines for CABG surgery have been published in 2011.[65] They recommend (i) volatile agent–based anesthetic aimed at early tracheal extubation; (ii) adequate perioperative analgesia; (iii) anesthetic care by a fellowship-trained or experienced, board-certified, TEE-trained anesthesiologist; (iv) utilization of intraoperative TEE for evaluation of acute, persistent, and life-threatening hemodynamic changes, for monitoring of ventricular function and regional wall motion abnormalities, and for concomitant valvular surgery; (v) management that augments the coronary arterial perfusion pressure to reduce the risk of perioperative myocardial ischemia and infarction; (vi) administration of β-blockers to reduce the incidence (or complications) of atrial fibrillation and cardiac mortality (particularly in patients with LVEF >30%); (vii) administration of angiotensin-converting enzyme (ACE) inhibitors or angiotensin receptor blockers perioperatively; (viii) selective use of PAC; and (ix) multimodal approach for management of perioperative bleeding and transfusion, based on use of lysine analogues, point-of-care testing, discontinuation of antiplatelet medications for at least 5 days preoperatively, among others. The reader is encouraged to consult the full document at http://circ.ahajournals.org/content/124/23/e652.

VALVULAR HEART DISEASE

Alterations in loading conditions are the initial physiologic burdens imposed by valvular heart lesions, both stenotic and regurgitant. For example, the LV is pressure overloaded in aortic stenosis (AS) and volume overloaded in aortic insufficiency and MR. In mitral stenosis, however, the LV is both volume underloaded and pressure underloaded, whereas the right ventricle (RV) faces progressively increasing left atrial and pulmonary artery pressure. Compensatory mechanisms consist of chamber enlargement, myocardial hypertrophy, and variations in vascular tone and level of sympathetic activity. These mechanisms in turn induce secondary alterations, including altered ventricular compliance, development of myocardial ischemia, chronic cardiac dysrhythmias, and progressive myocardial dysfunction.

Myocardial contractility in patients with mitral insufficiency is often transiently depressed but may progress to irreversible impairment even in the absence of clinical symptoms. Conversely, the patient with AS may complain of dyspnea, not because of impaired systolic function, but because of reduced ventricular compliance, increased left ventricular end-diastolic pressure, and pulmonary vascular congestion.

The patient presenting for valve repair or replacement often has pulmonary hypertension, severe ventricular dysfunction, and chronic rhythm disorders. Anesthetic management is predicated on understanding the altered loading conditions, preserving the compensatory mechanisms, maintaining circulatory homeostasis, and anticipating problems that may arise during and after valve surgery. In this section, we briefly describe the pathophysiology, desirable hemodynamic profile, and other pertinent anesthetic considerations for each valvular lesion.

TEE has become the standard of care in the perioperative management of patients undergoing valve surgery. TEE can further refine the preoperative diagnosis, identify valvular pathology and the mechanism of disease, and quantify the degree of stenosis and/or regurgitation. A detailed review of the perioperative role of TEE is presented in Chapter 26.

Aortic Stenosis

AS is the most common valvular disease in the United States. In a normal adult, the AV is composed of three semilunar cusps attached to the wall of the aorta. The normal AV diameter is 1.9 to 2.3 cm with an AV area of 2 to 4 cm^2. The AV cusps are suspended from symmetric outpouchings of the aortic wall that are called the *sinuses of Valsalva*. The AV cusps and the corresponding sinuses are named according to their relation to the coronary ostia: Left, right, and noncoronary (opposite the interatrial septum). On the ventricular side of the AV is the oval-shaped LV outflow tract (LVOT). Its borders are the inferior surface of the anterior leaflet of the mitral valve, the interventricular septum, and the LV free wall. The normal diameter of the LVOT is 2.2 ± 0.2 cm.

Calcific AV disease has many similar features with coronary artery disease. What in the past was thought to be "degenerative" is a disease continuum, similar to atherosclerosis. Increased mechanical stress (higher on the aortic side of AV cusps, in the flexion area) causes endothelial disruption, which leads to lipoprotein deposition, chronic inflammation, and active cusp calcification.[66] These histologic changes result in macroscopic, progressive valve thickening. Increased calcification eventually leads to leaflet immobility and outflow obstruction. Clinical factors associated with aortic sclerosis include older age, male gender, smoking, hypertension, and hyperlipidemia. Patients with bicuspid AV (increased mechanical stress) or with altered mineral metabolism (Paget disease, renal failure) have a higher prevalence of calcific AS disease. Rheumatic disease (an autoimmune disease, rarely seen in developed countries, leading to calcification and fusion along the commissures) causes mixed AS and AV regurgitation and usually coexists with mitral valve disease.

Pathophysiology

The classic symptoms of AS are angina (35%), syncope (15%), and dyspnea (50%) and are harbingers of poor outcome (death) within 5, 3 and 2 years, respectively, unless the AV is replaced. The progressive narrowing of the AV orifice results in chronic obstruction to LV ejection. Intraventricular systolic pressure increases to preserve forward flow. "Concentric" ventricular hypertrophy, in which the LV wall gradually thickens but the cavity size remains unchanged, is the compensatory response that normalizes the concomitant increase in LV wall tension. Contractility is preserved and ejection fraction is maintained at a normal range until late in the disease process (Fig. 38-4). Signs and symptoms of AS usually occur when the AV orifice is reduced to less than 0.8 to 1.0 cm^2.[67]

The costs of the concentric hypertrophy are decreased diastolic compliance and a precarious balance between myocardial oxygen supply and $M\dot{V}O_2$. Hypertrophy-induced impairment of diastolic relaxation ("stiff" LV) impedes early LV filling, and LA contraction becomes critical for maintaining adequate ventricular filling and subsequent stroke volume. In AS, the "atrial kick" may account for up to 30% to 40% of LV end-diastolic volume. The ventricular filling pressure, as reflected by pulmonary capillary wedge pressure, may vary widely with only small changes in ventricular volume (reduced compliance).

The hypertrophied muscle mass has increased basal $M\dot{V}O_2$, while demand per beat rises because of the elevated intraventricular systolic pressure. Because the capillary density is often inadequate for the hypertrophic muscle, a reduction in perfusion pressure (as when the aortic diastolic pressure is decreased and/or the ventricular filling pressure is increased) may compromise supply and total vasodilator reserve. This situation is compounded in the presence of coronary obstruction. Patients with AS often present with heart failure.

There is an inverse relationship between wall stress (afterload) and LV ejection fraction. In patients with a substantial transvalvular pressure gradient (mean >40 mm Hg), AV replacement corrects the afterload excess and improves outcome. Decreased contractility results in decreased stroke volume and a hemodynamically (and echocardiographically) decreased pressure gradient (<30 mm Hg: "Pseudo-AS" or "low-gradient AS") despite the echocardiographic presence of AS. The response to pharmacologic intervention with dobutamine or nitroprusside will clarify the diagnosis: If the calculated AV area does not change there is true AS (therefore, AV replacement is indicated), if the stroke volume increases well out of proportion to the increase in valvular gradient there is relative AS, while little or no increase in stroke volume is diagnostic of severe LV dysfunction that carries increased operative risk. However, surgical intervention has better long term than medical management alone.[68]

Anesthetic Considerations

The ideal hemodynamic environment for the patient with AS is summarized in Table 38-3. Noncardiac surgery in patients with asymptomatic severe AS may not be associated with complications (one death in 23 patients with general anesthetic, no death in 25 patients with local anesthetic), provided that their hemodynamics are invasively monitored.[69] Subsequent larger studies in these patients present conflicting results. Some show a marked increase in perioperative death and infarction rates and others do not.[70,71] The reasons for these differences are not clear, but maintenance of adequate ventricular volume and sinus rhythm is crucial.

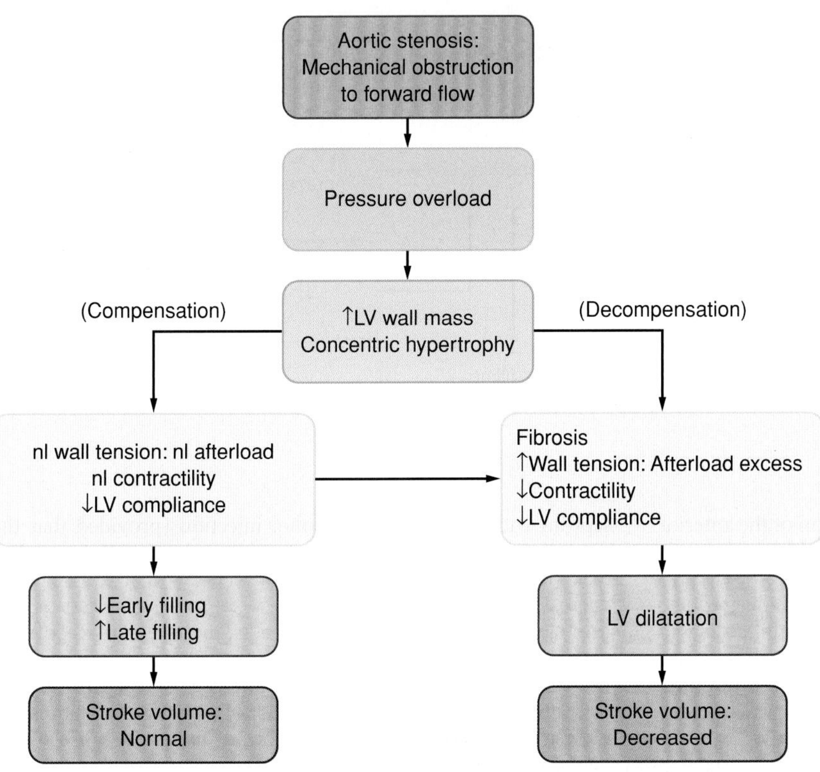

FIGURE 38-4. Pathophysiology of aortic stenosis. LV, left ventricle; nl, normal.

Hypotension must be prevented and treated promptly if it develops. Anticipation of likely hemodynamic changes is essential (e.g., expected decreases in blood pressure following spinal or epidural anesthesia); treatment should be immediate. Coronary perfusion pressure must be maintained to prevent the vicious cycle of hypotension-induced ischemia, subsequent ventricular dysfunction, and worsening hypotension. Bradycardia is a common clinical cause for hypotension in the patient with AS. Slowing the heart rate and increasing diastolic time will not increase stroke volume in the LV with concentric hypertrophy. Therefore, bradycardia will induce a fall in total cardiac output and systemic arterial pressure. This is especially pertinent in the elderly or diabetic patient, in whom sinus node disease and reduced sympathetic responses may predispose to significant bradycardia. Tachycardia must be avoided because it reduces the duration of diastolic coronary perfusion.

Ischemia may be difficult to detect because the characteristic electrocardiographic changes are often obscured by signs of LV hypertrophy and strain. Elevated LV filling pressures, although not necessarily reflecting increased volume, often require treatment to optimize coronary perfusion pressure.[68] TNG is useful in this regard, but it must be remembered that minimal reductions in ventricular volume are required. Therefore, very low doses of TNG should be used and titrated to effect. In the presence of LV dysfunction, an arterial dilator, such as nicardipine (preferred over SNP),[72] should be carefully titrated to lower afterload without affecting ventricular volume. The utility of TEE in diagnosing and grading the severity of AS is described in Chapter 26.

6

TABLE 38-3. AORTIC STENOSIS—HEMODYNAMIC GOALS

Preload	Full
Afterload	Maintain coronary perfusion gradient
Contractility	Usually not a problem, may require inotropic support if hypotension persists
Rate	Avoid bradycardia (↓ CO) and tachycardia (ischemia)
Rhythm	Sinus; may need cardioversion or β-blockers in nonsinus or fast rhythms
$M\dot{V}O_2$	Avoid tachycardia and hypotension (ischemia is an ever-present risk)
CPB	Contractility augmentation may be required secondary to myocardial stunning; blood pressure may need to be controlled later

↓, decrease; CO, cardiac output; CPB, cardiopulmonary bypass; $M\dot{V}O_2$, myocardial oxygen consumption.

Hypertrophic Cardiomyopathy

Hypertrophic cardiomyopathy is a genetically determined disease characterized by histologically abnormal myocytes and myocardial hypertrophy developing a priori, in the absence of a pressure or volume overload. The LV has a relatively small cavity relative to the wall thickness and is hyperdynamic.[73]

Pathophysiology

The physiologic consequences of hypertrophic cardiomyopathy are similar to those detailed for AS and are depicted in Figure 38-5. A subset of patients (20% to 30%) have some degree of subvalvular obstruction (hypertrophic obstructive cardiomyopathy), which may result in an LVOT gradient from a combination of anatomic

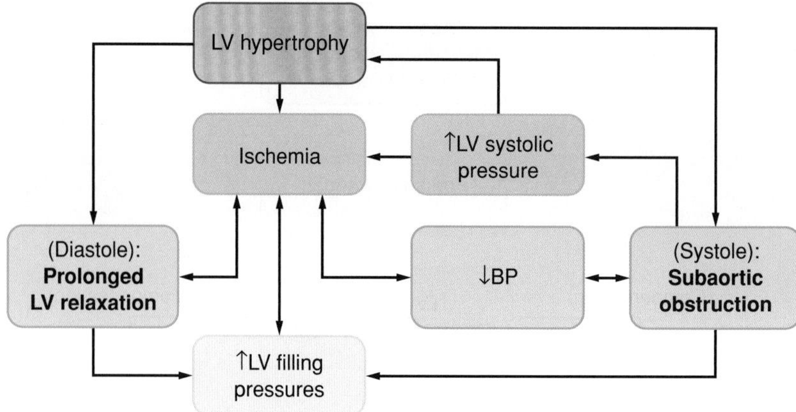

FIGURE 38-5. Pathophysiology of primary left ventricular (LV) hypertrophy in hypertrophic cardiomyopathy. BP, blood pressure.

(systolic septal bulging into the LVOT, malposition of the anterior papillary muscle) and functional (drag forces, and hyperdynamic LV contraction causing a Venturi effect) factors. The LVOT gradient is dynamic in nature, increased by any intervention that reduces the LV size (increased contractility and heart rate or decreased preload or afterload). As blood is ejected rapidly through this area, the anterior mitral valve leaflet is pulled closer to the septum (systolic anterior motion), resulting in a variable MR jet, which, in the absence of organic mitral disease, is directed posteriorly.[74]

In hypertrophic cardiomyopathy the myocardial oxygen balance is tenuous, and angina during exercise occurs even in the absence of coronary artery disease, if the coronary blood flow is unable to meet the demands of the hypertrophied myocardium.

Anesthetic Considerations

Treatment options for hypertrophic cardiomyopathy include pharmacologic "thinning" of the proximal interventricular septum with intracoronary alcohol injection (provided that the diastolic septal thickness at the site of injection is <15 mm), cardiac pacing, and surgical septal myectomy that is aimed to decrease the flow gradient (target is <30 mm Hg at rest or <50 mm Hg during exercise). The anesthetic management of patients with hypertrophic cardiomyopathy focuses on maintaining ventricular filling and avoiding the factors predisposing to outflow tract obstruction or ischemia (Table 38-4). Myocardial depression is desirable, and volatile anesthetics are useful. Because of the dependence of preload on atrial contraction, control of atrial rate and rhythm is mandatory. If junctional rhythm occurs, these patients may need atrial pacing with a transesophageal pacing probe or a PAC with pacing capability.

Although infrequent, hypertrophic cardiomyopathy occasionally coexists with valvular AS and may explain unanticipated difficulties in separating from bypass or unexpected increased pressure gradient following a seemingly uncomplicated AV replacement. A careful TEE examination of the LVOT area proximal to the newly replaced AV will resolve this dilemma. A dynamic left ventricular outflow obstruction may result following mitral valve repair, if an elongated anterior mitral leaflet is brought closer to the interventricular septum (anterior septal motion observed echocardiographically). In such cases, hypotension should be treated with volume replacement and vasoconstrictors, not inotropes.

TABLE 38-4. HYPERTROPHIC CARDIOMYOPATHY—HEMODYNAMIC GOALS

Preload	Full: Treat as in aortic stenosis
Afterload	Increase: Treat hypotension aggressively with α-adrenergic agonists
Contractility	Prefer depression
Rate	Normal range; β-blockers decrease LVOT gradient and increase LV end-diastolic pressure
Rhythm	Sinus rhythm is crucial: Atrial pacing modalities (PAC, esophageal) may be helpful
$M\dot{V}O_2$	Not a problem
CPB	Start with volume and vasoconstrictors; avoid inotropes. Check carefully for residual gradient and SAM; rule out ventricular septal defect

LVOT, left ventricular outflow tract; LV, left ventricle; PAC, pulmonary artery catheter; $M\dot{V}O_2$, myocardial oxygen consumption; CPB, cardiopulmonary bypass; SAM, systolic anterior motion.

Aortic Insufficiency

Aortic valve insufficiency (AI) is the result of annular dilatation or structural AV cusp lesions. Annular dilatation occurs with aneurysms (Marfan syndrome) or due to dissection of the ascending aorta. Calcific degeneration, rheumatic disease, bicuspid AV, endocarditis, trauma, or a jet lesion due to dynamic or fixed subvalvular stenosis results in abnormal leaflet motion and loss of coaptation and causes AI. Acute AI is caused by bacterial endocarditis, aortic dissection, or trauma.

Pathophysiology

2 In AI, blood flows into the LV from the aorta during diastole and leads to volume and pressure overload (Fig. 38-6). In chronic AI, the LV cavity increases gradually, out of proportion to the LV wall thickness (*eccentric LV hypertrophy*), sometimes to massive proportions, thus increasing the LV wall stress. The LV end-diastolic pressures are usually within the normal range, evidence of a significant increase in chamber compliance. As a result, and in

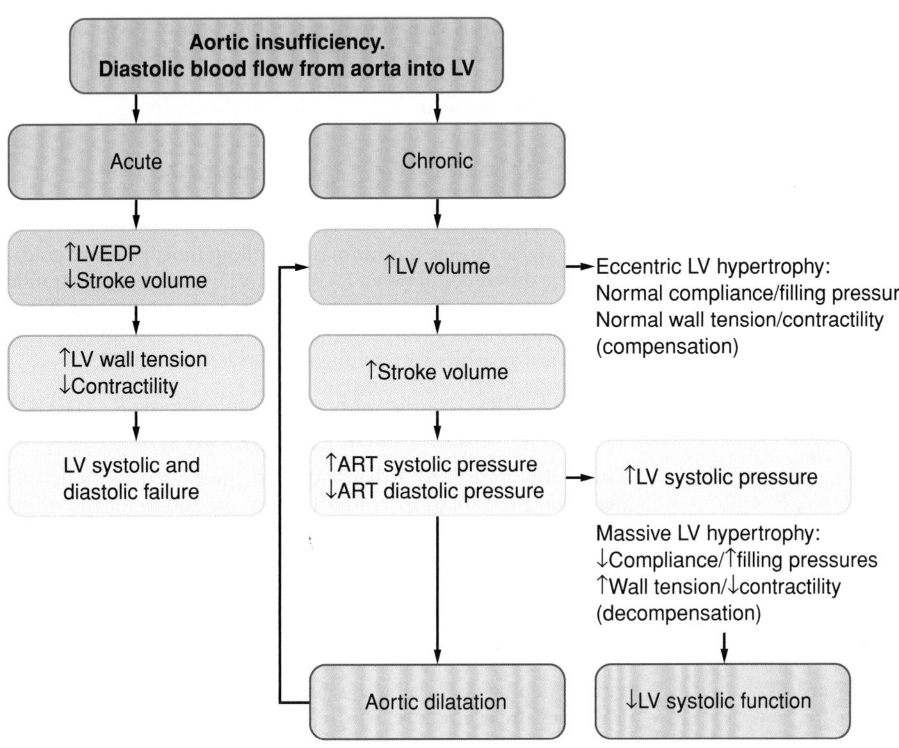

FIGURE 38-6. Pathophysiology of aortic insufficiency. LVEDP, left ventricular end-diastolic pressure; LV, left ventricle; ART, arterial.

contrast to AS, considerable alterations in LV volume can occur with only minimal changes in LV filling pressure. Although the LV may pump more than twice the normal cardiac output, $M\dot{V}O_2$ does not increase extraordinarily because the oxygen cost for muscle shortening (volume work) is low. The diastolic runoff and the moderate vasodilation reduce the LV afterload and increase the arterial pulse pressure. Thus, patients may be relatively symptom-free even when contractility is reduced. This is important in terms of planning the anesthetic, but perhaps even more so with respect to the timing of AV replacement. Ideally, the valve should be replaced just prior to the onset of irreversible myocardial damage. The outcome is better in patients with LV ejection fraction >55% or an end-diastolic LV diameter <55 mm.[75] Therefore, continued follow-up of these patients emphasizes repeated noninvasive estimations of contractility, usually after some form of afterload stress, either pharmacologic-induced or exercise-induced.

In acute AI, the previously normal in size and compliance LV is faced with a large end-diastolic volume, and the diastolic aortic to LV pressure gradient is acutely decreased.[76] As a result, the LV end-diastolic pressure rises rapidly (along the steep portion of the diastolic pressure–volume relation), the myocardial perfusion gradient is decreased, and myocardial contractility becomes impaired with severe congestive heart failure as the cardinal clinical sign. Tachycardia and peripheral vasoconstriction are the compensatory mechanisms, but they further increase the myocardial oxygen needs. In acutely ill patients, emergent AV replacement is required, whereas in less severe circumstances, mild systemic vasodilation and inotropic support may return hemodynamics toward normal.

Anesthetic Considerations

The main goal is to avoid further increases in LV wall stress. Full preload, mildly vasodilated, and modestly tachycardic describe the optimal cardiovascular state for patients with AI (Table 38-5).
7 Vasodilation (with an arterial dilator: nicardipine or SNP) promotes forward flow, although additional intravascular volume may be necessary to maintain adequate preload. The ideal heart rate is somewhat controversial. Tachycardia reduces the diastolic runoff from the aorta to the LV, and the LV volume and wall tension, and increases the diastolic blood pressure and coronary perfusion gradient, thus offsetting any increase in $M\dot{V}O_2$ secondary to increased heart rate. Bradycardia should be avoided as it results in ventricular distention, elevations in left atrial pressure, and pulmonary congestion.

TABLE 38-5. AORTIC INSUFFICIENCY—HEMODYNAMIC GOALS

Preload	Increase slightly
Afterload	Decrease: ↑ anesthetic depth or vasodilators (to decrease regurgitant fraction)
Contractility	Usually adequate
Rate	Increase: Reduces ventricular volume and raises diastolic aortic pressure
Rhythm	Usually sinus; not a problem
$M\dot{V}O_2$	Usually not a problem
CPB	Beware (and observe) for ventricular distention (pre- and post-AXC: Regurgitant flow increases if ↓ HR or nonbeating heart)

↑, increase; ↓, decrease; $M\dot{V}O_2$, myocardial oxygen consumption; CPB, cardiopulmonary bypass; AXC, aortic cross-clamp; HR, heart rate.

Ventricular distention may occur with the onset of CPB if the heart rate slows or if there is unexpected ventricular fibrillation (ineffective systolic ejection). Monitoring of heart size, rate, rhythm, and ventricular filling pressure is especially important in these patients. If LV distention occurs, insertion of an LV vent or immediate cross-clamping of the aorta should alleviate the problem. The presence of moderate-to-severe AI will affect the approach to CPB. After application of the aortic cross-clamp, cardioplegic solution is normally injected into the aortic root, delivering this solution to the coronary system, producing diastolic arrest of the heart. An incompetent AV prevents delivery of cardioplegia to the coronary system. Instead, cardioplegia will fill and distend the LV, increasing the ischemic insult incurred during CPB, and diastolic arrest of the heart becomes difficult. As a result, in the presence of AI the heart is arrested by injecting cardioplegia directly into the coronary ostia (after aortotomy) or into the coronary sinus ("retrograde").

Mitral Stenosis

Mitral valve stenosis (MS), caused by rheumatic fever, is rare in the United States. MS develops from leaflet thickening, commissural fusion, and chordal shortening and fusion due to chronic inflammation. The most frequent cause of MS is atherosclerosis-associated mitral annular calcification and endocarditis.[77]

Pathophysiology

The spectrum of physiologic disruption in patients with MS is
3 presented in Figure 38-7. Progressive decrease of the mitral valve area (MVA) impedes the blood flow from the left atrium (LA) to the LV, resulting in a pressure gradient across the mitral valve during diastole. With worsening MS, decreased LV filling will limit LV stroke volume. Although the LV myocardium may be affected by rheumatic fever and LV contractility may be impaired, LV dysfunction is caused by the combination of decreased preload and increased afterload (from reflex vasoconstriction). Proximal to the decreased MVA, the LA pressure (LAP) is elevated. According to the formula by Gorlin and Gorlin,[78]

$$\text{Valve area} = \text{flow}/(K \cdot \sqrt{\text{Pressure gradient}}) \text{ or}$$

$$\text{Pressure gradient} = [\text{flow}/(K \cdot \text{MVA})]^2$$

where flow is cardiac output/diastolic filling time; pressure gradient is the difference between LAP and LVDP; and K is a hydraulic pressure constant (this calculation assumes no regurgitant flow). At a constant MVA, rearrangement of the Gorlin formula reveals the clinical variables determining the elevated LAP in MS:

$$\text{LAP} - \text{LVDP} = [(\text{cardiac output})/(\text{diastolic time})/(K \cdot \text{MVA})]^2$$

$$\text{or LAP} = \text{LVDP} + [\text{flow}/(K \cdot \text{MVA})]^2$$

Therefore, increased cardiac output or decreased diastolic filling period results in increased LAP by the square of the original changes. This explains why tachycardia or increased forward flow, seen classically with pregnancy, thyrotoxicosis, or infection, can precipitate pulmonary edema in a patient with MS. Thus, the development of atrial fibrillation causes hemodynamic deterioration, not so much because of the loss of atrial contraction and associated decrease in preload, but because of the rapid rate, which by decreasing the diastolic filling time increases the LAP pressure even more. Upstream from the LA, the persistently elevated LAP, which eventually leads to LA dilatation (and atrial fibrillation, usually the first manifestation of MS), is reflected through the pulmonary circulation (pulmonary congestion and increased work of breathing), leading to right ventricular pressure overload with compensatory right ventricular hypertrophy. The progression and severity of pulmonary hypertension is variable; further narrowing of the valve orifice causes irreversible reactive changes in the pulmonary vasculature (rales on auscultation, hemoptysis). Once pulmonary hypertension has developed the

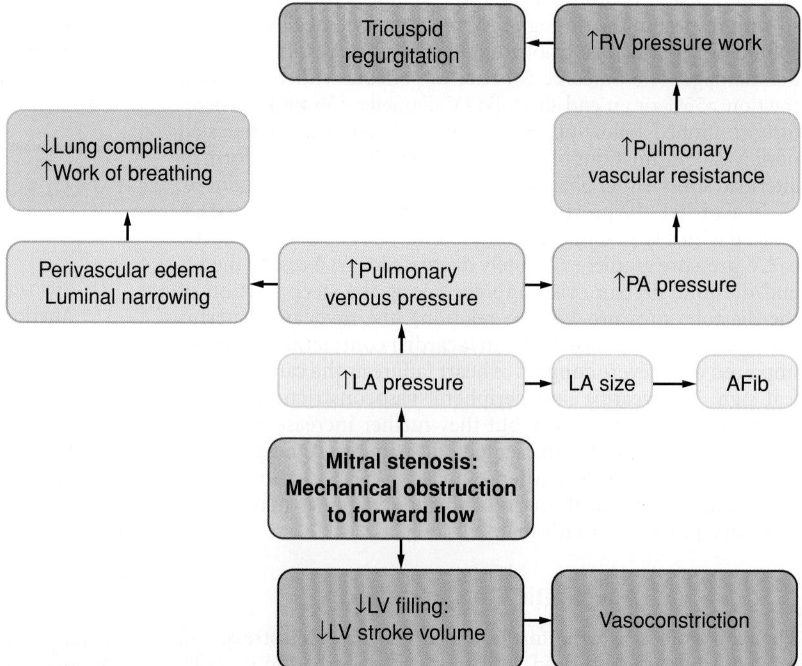

FIGURE 38-7. Pathophysiology of mitral stenosis. RV, right ventricle; PA, pulmonary artery; LA, left atrium; AFib, atrial fibrillation; LV, left ventricle.

operative risk is increased (12% vs. 3% to 8%).[79] Right ventricular dysfunction, tricuspid annular dilatation, and insufficiency (engorged neck veins) may develop as the right heart function worsens.

MS mimics left heart failure, with pulmonary congestion and decreased forward flow. The only definitive treatment is relief of obstruction with mitral valve replacement; balloon valvuloplasty and open commissurotomy are palliative maneuvers. The medical interventions should aim at decreasing the heart rate (with β- or calcium channel blockers) or treating the cause(s) responsible for the increased transmitral flow. The pulmonary capillary wedge pressure is higher than the true LVDP at least by the amount of the pressure gradient and can be used as a relative index of LV filling, even during episodes of tachycardia or increased flow.

Anesthetic Considerations

The hemodynamic goals listed in Table 38-6 are the cornerstones of prebypass anesthetic management (Table 38-6). Avoiding tachycardia precludes episodes of LA and pulmonary hypertension with potential right ventricular dysfunction, as well as inadequate LV filling with concomitant systemic hypotension. Preoperative maintenance of rate-control and β-blocking drugs, selection of anesthetics with no propensity to increase heart rate, and attainment of anesthetic levels deep enough to suppress autonomic responses are
8 methods to achieve these goals. Episodes of pulmonary hypertension and potential right-sided heart failure stemming from factors inducing pulmonary vasoconstriction must also be prevented including hypoxia, hypercarbia, and acidosis.

Treatment of hypotension in patients with MS can present a challenging dilemma. Although these patients normally take diuretics, hypovolemia is not usually the cause; hence, the response to volume administration is often disappointing. Use of a vasoconstrictor to offset mild peripheral vasodilation is acceptable, bearing in mind the effect of pulmonary vasoconstriction on right ventricular function. It is often prudent to select a drug with some inotropic effect such as ephedrine or epinephrine instead of relying on a pure vasoconstrictor, such as phenylephrine. In separating from CPB, attention is on avoiding right ventricular failure (discussed subsequently); more commonly, however, there is LV dysfunction. This may be because of intraoperative injury or sudden increase in flow to, and distention of, the chronically underloaded LV. After bypass, prominent *v* waves may be present in the pulmonary capillary wedge pressure waveform. This almost always reflects increased LV filling rather than MR provided that the cardiac output is increased when compared with preinduction values. The echocardiographic evaluation of MS is described in Chapter 26.

TABLE 38-6. MITRAL STENOSIS—HEMODYNAMIC GOALS

Preload	Maintain, avoid hypovolemia
Afterload	Prevent increase; ↑ RV afterload due to pulmonary vasoconstriction (hypoxia, hypercarbia)
	Vasopressors may be required for systemic hypotension
Contractility	LV: Usually intact; RV: May be decreased in long-standing pulmonary hypertension
Rate	Maintain at low end of normal. Avoid and treat tachycardia
Rhythm	Control ventricular response in atrial fibrillation
$M\dot{V}O_2$	Not a problem
CPB	Post-MV replacement: LV preload and filling pressures may be elevated. Cardiac function does not improve immediately

↑, increase; RV, right ventricle; $M\dot{V}O_2$, myocardial oxygen consumption; CPB, cardiopulmonary bypass; MV, mitral valve; LV, left ventricle.

Mitral Regurgitation

In MR the valve is incompetent during systole and blood regurgitates from the LV to the LA. Etiologies of MR include excessive motion of one or both leaflets, prolapse or flail due to degenerative disease or ruptured chordae tendineae following acute myocardial infarction, and restricted leaflet motion due to rheumatic heart disease or myocardial ischemia or leaflet perforation from endocarditis. In functional MR the leaflet structure is normal, but the valve is incompetent due to either decreased LV systolic pressure (ischemic cardiomyopathy) that fails to "close" the leaflets or a dilated annulus (the fiber ring from where the leaflets are suspended) that decreases the coaptation surface of the leaflets (Table 38-7).

Pathophysiology

Volume overload similar to that described with AI is the cardinal feature of MR (Fig. 38-8). The LA acts as a low-pressure outlet during LV ejection; with the onset of ventricular systole blood is ejected retrograde (there is no isovolumetric contraction period). In MR, the total LV output consists of forward (systemic, via the aorta) and retrograde (into the LA) blood volumes. The aftermaths of MR are atrial and ventricular chamber

TABLE 38-7. MECHANISMS OF MITRAL REGURGITATION

Cause	Characteristics	Location
Myxomatous degeneration	Excessive motion due to prolapse or flail	Leaflet
	Redundant tissue	
	Ruptured chordae	
Rheumatic	Thickened, calcified, restricted leaflets	Leaflet
	Commissural fusion	
Congenital	Cleft mitral valve, double orifice mitral valve	Leaflet
Miscellaneous	Drug-related (fenfluramine)	Leaflet
Endocarditis	Perforation(s)	Leaflet
	Vegetations	
Myocardial infarction	Papillary muscle rupture	Tensor apparatus
Dilated cardiomyopathy	Annular dilatation	Annulus
Ischemic heart disease	Papillary muscle dysfunction	Tensor apparatus

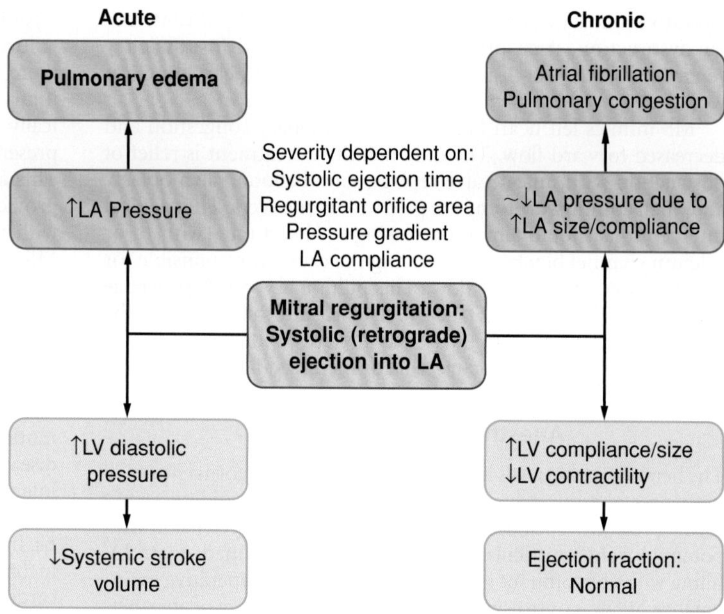

FIGURE 38-8. Pathophysiology of mitral regurgitation. LA, left atrial; LV, left ventricular.

enlargement (due to "back-and-from" blood flow), ventricular wall hypertrophy (to compensate for the increased chamber size), and increased blood volume. The LV compliance is increased so that the large LV end-diastolic volume does not cause striking increase in pressure. There is no concomitant increase in oxygen requirements because there is little pressure development. As a result, patients may have minimal symptoms as well as normal or slightly reduced ejection fraction, despite progressive myocardial dysfunction and decreased contractility The regurgitant blood volume is related to the size of the regurgitant mitral orifice, the systolic time, the pressure gradient across the valve, and the compliance of the LA. The regurgitant orifice size, in turn, depends on the valvular defect and ventricular size. Therefore, increases in heart rate, reduction of preload, and arterial dilators are effective in reducing the regurgitation of blood volume from the LV to LA.

Repairing or replacing the mitral valve increases the LV afterload and unmasks any underlying myocardial dysfunction.

TABLE 38-8. MITRAL REGURGITATION—HEMODYNAMIC GOALS

Preload	Increase slightly
Afterload	Decrease with anesthetics, arterial vasodilators
Contractility	May be depressed, titrate myocardial depressants carefully
Rate	Increase slightly; avoid bradycardia
Rhythm	If atrial fibrillation present: Control ventricular response
$M\dot{V}O_2$	Compromised if MR coexists with ischemic heart disease
CPB	Afterload is increased with competent valve, inotropic support is often needed

$M\dot{V}O_2$, myocardial oxygen consumption; MR, mitral regurgitation; CPB, cardiopulmonary bypass.

Administration of inotropes and/or vasodilators, as well as judicious increase in preload, may be necessary to successfully separate from bypass.

Acute-onset MR has a different hemodynamic picture; acute LA and LV volume overload occurs in the absence of compensatory LV enlargement. Ventricular filling pressures increase dramatically, as do pulmonary pressures. Cardiac output decreases, and pulmonary edema develops. In the setting of acute myocardial infarction, contractility may be inadequate despite pharmacologic support, and intra-aortic balloon assistance and emergency surgery may be lifesaving.

Anesthetic Considerations

Selection of anesthetics that promote vasodilation and tachycardia is ideal in the patient with MR (Table 38-8). In chronic MR, vasoactive medications are usually not necessary because of LV compensatory mechanisms. However, patients with acute MR may need aggressive pharmacologic management. In the absence of acute deterioration, pharmacologic intervention is not needed
9 usually until the postbypass period. However, vasodilators and inotropes may lead to reoccurrence or worsening of MR when, following MV repair surgery, systolic anterior motion of the anterior mitral leaflet results in obstruction of the LVOT. The pathophysiologic and clinical picture is similar to that of hypertrophic cardiomyopathy. The risk of systolic anterior motion after repair is increased when the anterior leaflet is longer than the posterior leaflet or when there is a narrow angle between the mitral and aortic annuli. If this scenario is suspected, a trial of volume expansion and vasoconstrictors is indicated. The approach to evaluation of MR severity is described in Chapter 26.

AORTIC DISEASES

Acquired (hypertension, inflammation, deceleration trauma, or iatrogenic trauma) and genetic (connective tissue disorders, bicuspid AV) conditions are the cause of aortic diseases: Aortic dissection, intramural hematoma, and aortic aneurysm. Weakening the media layers of the aorta (the term *cystic medial degeneration* denotes the disappearance of smooth muscle cells and the degeneration of elastic fibers) leads to higher wall stress, which induces dilatation and aneurysm formation, eventually resulting in intramural hemorrhage, aortic dissection, or rupture.

Aortic Dissection

Aortic dissection[80] is part of the acute aortic syndrome that includes aortic dissection, intramural hematoma, and penetrating ulcer. Aortic dissection affects mostly men (7/3 ratio) and whites (4/1 ratio), while connective tissue disorders, such as Marfan syndrome and Ehlers-Danlos syndrome affect mostly the young (age <40 years). Hypertension is the most common risk factor in older patients. Aortic dissection is caused by a tear in the aortic intima and media, which propagates proximal and distally, creating a false lumen within the aortic media. The dissection often involves aortic branches and causes poor perfusion of vital organs (brain, spinal cord, abdominal organs), cardiac tamponade, or AI. Acute aortic dissection of the ascending aorta (type A) is highly lethal, with a mortality rate of 1% to 2% per hour after onset of symptomatology and is a true surgical emergency. An aortic dissection distal to the left subclavian artery is called type B, has a 30-day mortality of 10%, and may be managed medically or with placement of a scaffold (stent). Intramural hematoma is considered a precursor to classic dissection and usually originates from ruptured vasa vasorum in the media. Intramural hematoma has the same prognosis as aortic dissection and is treated similarly.

Severe neck or chest pain (type A) or back or abdominal pain (type B) is the most common presenting complaint, although many patients have atypical symptoms mimicking stroke, myocardial infarction, vascular embolization, and abdominal pathology. Some diabetics may be totally asymptomatic. Syncope indicates development of dangerous complications (cardiac tamponade, cerebral hypoperfusion). Deficits in extremity pulses and/or differences in blood pressure are a significant finding, related to impaired blood flow to an organ or limb. It is important to diagnose correctly the type of dissection as this determines the proper treatment. A variety of diagnostic techniques (contrast-enhanced spiral computed tomography scanning or magnetic resonance imaging are slightly more sensitive and specific than TEE, which is more portable and available at bedside) are extremely accurate in the diagnosis of acute aortic dissection, but selection should consider the information required and the access to and the experience with the technique in the particular center.[81]

Patients with a high clinical suspicion of acute aortic dissection may be sent directly to the operating room for TEE-based diagnostic workup and preparation for surgery, decreasing the time period before surgical intervention.[82] Two-dimensional TEE identifies the intimal tear in 61% of the patients.[83] Apart from direct visualization of intimal tear and flaps, the site of entry and re-entry, false lumen thrombosis, coronary involvement, intramural hematoma, pericardial effusion, and AI can be diagnosed with high sensitivity and specificity.[84] However, dissections in the distal ascending aorta and proximal arch are difficult to visualize because of interposition of the left main stem bronchus between the esophagus (TEE) and aorta. Surgery is the definitive treatment for patients with type A acute aortic dissection to prevent its associated potential complications including aortic rupture, pericardial tamponade, and AI. It involves implantation of a composite graft in the ascending aorta with or without reimplantation of the coronary arteries. Type B aortic dissections can be managed medically if chronic or with implantation of a graft via an open or closed (percutaneous) approach if complicated (malperfusion symptomatology).

TABLE 38-9. ACUTE AORTIC DISSECTION—HEMODYNAMIC GOALS

Preload	May be increased if acute AI, increase further in tamponade
Afterload	Decrease with anesthetics, analgesics, arterial dilators (nitroprusside, nicardipine): Keep systolic BP <100–120 mm Hg
Contractility	May be depressed; titrate myocardial depressants carefully
Rate	Decrease to <60–80 bpm: Use β-blocker; ensure contractility is adequate
Rhythm	If atrial fibrillation present: Control ventricular response
$M\dot{V}O_2$	Compromised if aortic dissection involves coronary vessels
CPB	Alternate site of inflow (arterial) cannulation, deep hypothermic circulatory arrest possible if cerebral vessels are involved

AI, aortic insufficiency; BP, blood pressure; bpm, beats per minute; $M\dot{V}O_2$, myocardial oxygen consumption; CPB, cardiopulmonary bypass.

Anesthetic Considerations

Acute aortic dissection is a surgical emergency. Adequate intravenous access and invasive hemodynamic monitoring, including TEE, are mandatory. The hemodynamic goals are shown in Table 38-9.

Aortic Aneurysm

Thoracic aneurysms (TAs) may involve one or more aortic segments (aortic root, ascending aorta, arch, descending aorta). Most patients are asymptomatic at the time of diagnosis. Aortic root TAs may cause AI (diastolic murmur or heart failure). When large, TAs may cause local mass effect such as compression of the trachea (cough), esophagus (dysphagia), and/or recurrent laryngeal nerve (hoarseness). Detection and sizing can be done with contrast-enhanced computed tomography scanning and magnetic resonance angiography. The risk for rupture increases abruptly as TAs reach a diameter of 6 cm.[85] Surgery is indicated for ascending aorta aneurysms >5.5 cm or descending TA >6 cm.[86] Composite aortic repair (Bentall procedure) using a tube graft with a prosthetic AV sewn into one end is performed for aortic root TA associated with AI.[87] Alternatively, if AI is due to aortic root dilation, a valve-sparing procedure (preservation of the native AV cusps) is performed.[88]

The surgical replacement of aortic arch TA requires circulatory arrest during the creation of distal anastomosis and carries a risk of neurologic damage from global ischemic injury or embolization of atherosclerotic debris. Cerebral protection methods during replacement of the aortic arch include use of deep hypothermic circulatory arrest with or without arrest of cerebral circulation. Retrograde (via a superior vena cava cannula) or selective antegrade (direct cannulation of cerebral vessels) cerebral perfusion is employed to improve outcomes by providing nutrients and O_2 to the brain and flush out particulate matter from the cerebral and carotid arteries, with, so far, disputed results.[89]

Surgical replacement of the descending aorta is associated with postoperative paraplegia secondary to interruption of spinal cord blood supply (13% to 17%). A variety of methods (cerebrospinal fluid drainage, reimplantation of critical spinal arteries, maintenance of distal aortic perfusion with the use of a LA–left femoral artery bypass circuit, intraoperative epidural cooling, or use of somatosensory evoked potentials) are being used to avoid this complication, although outcome is heavily influenced by hospital and surgeon volume.[90] Alternatively, a transluminally placed endovascular stent-graft can be inserted.[91] Chapter 39 reviews recent advances in vascular stenting.

Anesthetic Considerations

The anesthetic technique is centered around two major organ systems: (1) Preservation of cardiac function (most crucial in surgery of descending TAs, where the "clamp-and-go" surgical technique imposes great fluctuations in systemic afterload and hemodynamic instability) and (2) neurologic integrity (in arch or descending TA operations). Drainage of cerebrospinal fluid will augment the spinal cord perfusion pressure. Usually, increments of 10 mL are drained at a time and the cerebrospinal fluid pressure is monitored continuously, keeping a cerebrospinal fluid pressure <15 mm Hg at all times.[92] Left heart bypass (LA to femoral artery) provides nonpulsatile retrograde aortic perfusion and supplements blood flow during aortic flow interruption, but does not perfuse the excluded aortic segment. Blood is actively removed via a cannula inserted inside the LA and advanced distal to the aortic interruption site. This technique ameliorates LV stress by reducing LV preload and afterload. The bypass flow depends on adequate preload (as assessed by the pulmonary arterial diastolic pressure or LV size via TEE) and low-normal afterload distal to the aortic cross-clamp. Too high flow of the bypass system will lead to hypotension, while increased pump flow will help decrease systemic hypertension proximal to the aortic interruption.

CARDIOPULMONARY BYPASS

Circuits

In its simplest form a CPB circuit consists of tubings (cannulae) that drain venous and return arterial blood; an oxygenator, where gas exchange occurs; and a mechanical pump that provides systemic perfusion (Fig. 38-9). The initiation of CPB involves the drainage of venous blood to the CPB machine. This is accomplished by placing a large-bore cannula(e) into the right atrium. Due to its simplicity and ease of placement, a multi-orifice "dual-stage" cannula that drains blood from the right atrium, coronary sinus, and inferior vena cava is often used. However, depending on the type of procedure (i.e., mitral valve surgery) single cannula
5 drainage may be suboptimal. Where a bloodless field is required, individual "single-stage" cannulae are placed into the superior and inferior venae cavae and then snared, thus preventing systemic venous blood from entering the heart. During CPB, the rate of venous drainage is passive and depends on several factors: Proper placement of appropriately sized cannulae, intravascular volume status, and hydrostatic pressure gradient (the difference in height between the right atrium and the venous reservoir). In the event of poor venous drainage, adjustment of the venous cannulae, raising the height of the operating table, or application of suction usually corrects the problem.

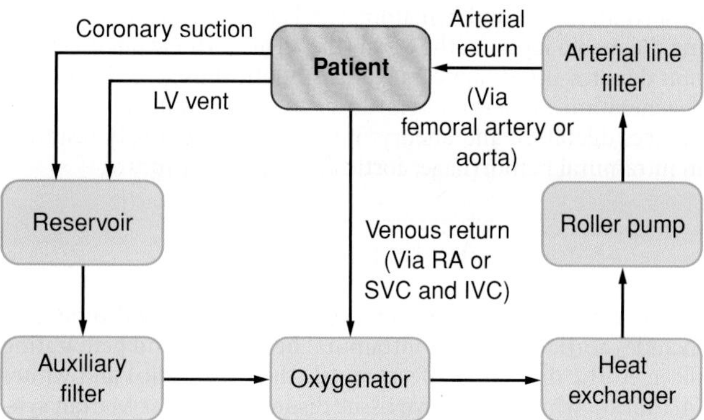

FIGURE 38-9. The basic circuit for cardiopulmonary bypass. LV, left ventricle; RA, right atrium; SVC, superior vena cava; IVC, inferior vena cava. (Reprinted from Thomson IR. Technical aspects of cardiopulmonary bypass. In: Thomas SJ, ed. *Manual of Cardiac Anesthesia.* 2nd ed. New York: Churchill Livingstone; 1993:480, with permission.)

From the venous reservoir, blood enters the oxygenator/heat exchanger unit, where it is oxygenated, carbon dioxide is removed, and the blood is warmed/cooled. The now-oxygenated blood is returned to the arterial circulation via a large "arterial" cannula. Arterial cannulae may be placed in the ascending aorta, femoral, or axillary arteries. This cycle then continues for the duration of CPB.

6 Other functions provided by the CPB machine include delivery of cardioplegia, cardiotomy suction (which scavenges shed blood from the surgical field), and vents to decompress the LV/aspirate air from the heart during de-airing procedures. Venting prevents ventricular distention that may lead to myocardial ischemia and is particularly important in patients with AI, large coronary sinus, or bronchial blood flow or when heart positioning restricts venous drainage. Common vent sites include the LV via a cannula placed in the left superior pulmonary vein (or, rarely, the LV apex) or the aortic root.

In addition to providing cardiopulmonary support, CPB circuits contain filters for the removal of bubbles and debris, in-line blood gas monitors, and volatile agent vaporizers. Warning monitors are placed in key locations of the CPB circuit. These monitors are used to detect low blood levels in the venous reservoir/oxygenator (to prevent entrainment of air to the arterial side of the circuit), high systemic line pressure (to diagnose possible arterial cannula obstruction/aortic dissection; both cause elevated line pressure), and bubbles.

Oxygenators

The use of membrane oxygenators in modern CPB machines eliminates the destructive blood–gas interface seen with older bubble oxygenators. Membrane oxygenators use bundles of hollow microporous polypropylene fibers contained in a plastic housing. Within this housing, blood flows around the fibers while fresh gas is passed though the fibers. The micropores act as channels allowing the diffusion of both oxygen and carbon dioxide. With this arrangement PO_2 on CPB is controlled by changes in FiO_2 and carbon dioxide elimination by changes in total gas flow or "sweep rate."

Pumps

7 During CPB, a mechanical pump is required to provide systemic perfusion and circulatory support. Centrifugal and roller

pumps are used in clinical practice. Roller pumps are the simplest and earliest type of pump. A length of tubing (polyvinyl chloride, silicone rubber, latex rubber) is placed in the periphery of a 210 degree rigid curved housing. At the center of this housing are two metal arms set 180 degrees apart with rollers at each end. When the arm rotates, the tubing is alternately compressed and released against the housing so that one side of the arm is compressing, while the other is releasing the tubing. Alternately compressing and releasing the tubing generates forward flow without the possibility of retrograde flow. This permits constant flow over a range of arterial resistance. It is important to note that the roller head must be nonocclusive, because when the tubing is totally compressed destruction of blood elements will result.

Roller pumps are simple and easy to use. The disadvantages include destruction of blood elements, spallation (development of plastic microemboli due to tubing compression), and complications from inflow and outflow occlusion of the pump. If pump inflow is occluded, negative pressure will develop in the roller head causing cavitation or the development of microscopic bubbles. If pump outflow becomes occluded, excessive pressure may develop proximal to the occlusion, causing the tubing connections to separate or the tubing to burst. For the most part, roller pumps have been replaced by centrifugal pumps for providing systemic support while roller pumps are most frequently used for delivering cardioplegia and providing vent/cardiotomy suction.

Centrifugal pumps use a magnetically controlled impeller housed within a rigid plastic cone. This impeller is composed of stacked smooth plastic cones that rotate to provide flow. The impeller is magnetically coupled to an electric motor located in the CPB machine. By rotating rapidly, a pressure drop across the impeller is generated, which causes blood to be sucked into the housing and then ejected. One major difference between roller head and centrifugal pumps is that flow from centrifugal pumps will vary with changes in pump preload and afterload. It is for this reason that a flowmeter must be placed on the arterial side of the bypass circuit. Advantages of centrifugal pumps include less blood trauma, lower line pressures, less cavitation, lower risk of massive air emboli, and elimination of tubing wear and spallation.

Despite the reliability of both roller and centrifugal pumps to provide systemic pressure on CPB, neither is able to deliver physiologically significant pulsatile blood flow. Pulsatile flow is the native pattern of blood flow in the human body and its lack during CPB has been cited as a cause of renal dysfunction and production of ischemic metabolic by-products. Studies show that in high-risk patients the use of pulsatile flow on CPB confers increased survival and may equate to a lower need for inotropes and mechanical support.[93] Until the controversy regarding the benefits of pulsatile flow is resolved, nonpulsatile flow will remain the most common type seen in cardiac surgery.

In the event of catastrophic CPB machine failure, a hand crank may be used to mechanically operate the biohead of a centrifugal pump to develop adequate pump flow and systemic blood pressure.

Heat Exchanger

A heat exchanger is a counter current device where either heated or cooled water is circulated around a conducting material with good thermal properties that is in contact with the patient's blood. This way blood is subsequently warmed or cooled and maintained at a desired temperature.

Prime

The fluid contained within the CPB tubing is called prime. Using crystalloid solutions, such as lactated Ringer, allows the CPB prime to achieve similar osmolarity and electrolyte composition as blood. Other solutions such as albumin (to decrease postoperative edema), mannitol (to promote diuresis), additional electrolytes (calcium to prevent hypocalcemia due to citrate in transfused blood), and heparin (to ensure a safe level of anticoagulation) are added to the prime. Many institutions use a standard volume prime for all adult patients, and others use a minimum volume based on body weight or body surface area (the average prime volume is about 1,500 mL). To prevent excessive dilutional anemia and decrease in oxygen-carrying capacity, blood may be added to the pump prime prior to initiating CPB in children, small adults, and patients with preoperative anemia. The lowest safe hematocrit on CPB is debated, but hematocrits of 17% are well tolerated.[94] Despite limited data the trend currently favors higher levels to avoid renal and neurologic consequences. Dilutional anemia on CPB is useful to the degree that it offsets changes in blood viscosity due to hypothermia. Thus, dilutional anemia may improve systemic flow. In an attempt to reduce the systemic inflammatory reaction, hemodilution, and coagulopathy associated with standard CPB circuits, miniaturized circuits have been developed. These miniaturized CPB circuits have a decreased surface area and consist of a smaller arterial venous loop/venous reservoir, pump, oxygenator, and filter. This reduction in surface area, and to a lesser extent a reduction in pump prime, has been shown to reduce blood usage.[95–97]

Anticoagulation

Contact between patient's blood and components of the CPB circuit initiates activation of the coagulation cascade. To prevent thrombosis of the CPB circuit (and the patient's death), systemic anticoagulation is required prior to insertion of cannulae and initiation of CPB. The anticoagulant of choice is heparin, a polyionic mucopolysaccharide. Following intravenous injection, the peak onset of heparin is <5 minutes with a half-life of approximately 90 minutes in normothermic patients. In hypothermic patients, there is a progressive and proportional increase in the half-life. The anticoagulant effect of heparin is derived from its ability to potentiate the activity of antithrombin III (AT). The binding of heparin to AT alters the latter's structural configuration and increases its thrombin inhibitory potency >1,000-fold. By inhibiting thrombin, AT prevents formation of fibrin clot via both the intrinsic and extrinsic pathways, in addition to inhibiting factors IX, Xa, XIa, XIIa, kallikrein, and plasmin. In patients receiving heparin preoperatively and those with congenital AT deficiencies, higher than expected doses of heparin are required to achieve adequate anticoagulation.

In the event of inadequate anticoagulation due to a relative or absolute deficiency of AT, exogenous AT can be administered in the form of a commercially available concentrate.[98] Postoperative heparin rebound and subsequent bleeding may be a concern following the administration of exogenous AT.

Partial thromboplastin time is not used in cardiac surgery to measure heparin action. This is due to the fact that modern partial thromboplastin time assays are so sensitive that heparin levels far lower than those used for safe initiation of CPB cause the sample blood to become almost unclottable within the time frame of the test. Currently, the two methods for determining adequate heparinization are measurement of the activated clotting time

(ACT) or blood-heparin concentrations. The ACT test consists of adding blood to tubes containing either diatomaceous earth (celite) or kaolin, warming and rotating the tube, and then recording the time required for clot formation. Generally, ACTs >480 seconds are considered acceptable for the initiation of CPB. Measuring heparin levels intraoperatively is an alternative method for determination of anticoagulation levels. In this method, known doses of protamine are added to a heparinized sample of blood sequentially, until the optimum dose of protamine that produces a clot in the shortest amount of time is determined. By knowing the neutralization ratio of heparin and protamine (usually 1 mg of protamine to 100 U of heparin), the heparin concentration in the sample can be determined. This method will correctly diagnose inadequate anticoagulation despite a therapeutic ACT.

Allergies to heparin are rare; more commonly, patients may present with a history of heparin-induced thrombocytopenia (HIT). There are two subtypes of HIT. The first is generally mild and consists of a transient decrease in platelet count following the administration of heparin a few days following surgery. The second type is more severe, characterized by autoimmune-mediated decrease in the platelet count due to the formation of antigenic heparin compounds (anti-PF4) that activate platelets in the face of endothelial injury. This predisposes to platelet clumping and microvascular thrombosis. This thrombosis may occur anywhere in the body and cause bowel or limb ischemia to name a few. In patients with HIT who require systemic anticoagulation, heparin alternatives should be used instead.[99] These include defibrinogenating agents (ancrod obtained from pit viper venom), hirudin, bivalirudin, and factor X inhibitors. Hirudin, which is isolated from the salivary gland of the medicinal leech (*Hirudo medicinalis*), and bivalirudin (hirulog) are both direct inhibitors of thrombin. Their action is independent of AT. The use of these agents is uncommon and the reader is advised to consult one of the several reviews on this subject.[100]

Blood Conservation in Cardiac Surgery

Blood and blood components are finite resources that are increasingly difficult to replace because of declining donation and restrictions on those that may donate. In addition, patients are increasingly demanding "bloodless" surgeries to lessen the risks of blood transfusion (infection, incompatibility reactions, transfusion error). However, because of the nature of cardiac surgery, the risk of blood and blood product transfusion is high. Bleeding as a result of reoperation, use of anticoagulants/platelet function inhibitors, and ill-defined surgical bleeding contribute to this risk. Furthermore, the inherent risk of platelet dysfunction and coagulopathy due to CPB cannot be eliminated. The use of intraoperative autologous blood donation, the scavenging and reinfusion of shed blood, and the use of antifibrinolytics (ε-aminocaproic acid, tranexamic acid) may all help to reduce the need for transfusion.[101]

Intraoperative autologous hemodilution is a well-described method of removing whole blood from a patient prior to systemic heparinization and CPB. Returning this blood following the separation from CPB returns red blood cells, active platelets, and functional coagulation factors that may mitigate surgical bleeding. Contraindications to intraoperative autologous blood donation include preoperative anemia, unstable angina/high-grade left main coronary artery disease, and AS. Blood salvage (cell saver) is another key method of intraoperative blood conservation in cardiac surgery. Following processing, units of shed blood may have hematocrits of 70%. Unfortunately, as platelets and coagulation factors are removed in the washing process, reinfusion of shed blood may worsen the CPB-associated coagulopathy by promoting a dilutional thrombocytopenia and reduction of clotting factors. Contraindications to the use of intraoperative cell salvage include infection, malignancy, and the use of topical hemostatic agents.

Antifibrinolytic use in cardiac surgery is the standard in most cardiac centers, with ε-aminocaproic acid being the primary agent used in the United States. The lysine analogues ε-aminocaproic and tranexamic acid bind to plasminogen and block its ability to bind at lysine residues of fibrinogen. This prevents the lysis of fibrin clots. Administration of these antifibrinolytics decreases bleeding after CPB and reduces the risk of blood transfusion.[102]

Aprotinin, a naturally occurring fibrinolytic, inhibits kallikrein, preserves platelet glycoprotein receptors (GIb, GIIb/IIIa), inhibits the proinflammatory cytokine release associated with CPB, as well as the inhibition of plasmin and protein C. Until recently, it was used in reoperation, aortic surgery, and whenever major bleeding was expected. However, during the course of the marketing and use of aprotinin, disturbing questions have been raised in regard to its safety. Persistent questions have lingered about renal failure and increased patient mortality.[103] This culminated, in November 2007, in response to initial patient data from the "Blood Conservation Using Antifibrinolytics: A Randomized Trial in a Cardiac Surgery Population" (BART) study,[104] in the Food and Drug Administration requesting that Bayer, the manufacturer of aprotinin, suspend its marketing until a comprehensive review of its safety is performed. Early data demonstrated that there was a higher 30-day mortality associated with the use of aprotinin as opposed to ε-aminocaproic acid or tranexamic acid. As a result, aprotinin use has ceased. A later, large retrospective study concluded that aprotinin may still be the antifibrinolytic agent of choice in extremely high-risk cases[105]; whether it returns to clinical use is to be determined.

Hemodilution due to the CPB prime is one undesired byproduct of extracorporeal circulation. One method that has been used with success to avoid excess hemodilution and reduce the need for blood transfusion is retrograde autologous priming (RAP). In RAP, the crystalloid prime contained within the CPB circuit is drained prior to the initiation of CPB and replaced by blood drained retrograde via the arterial cannula. RAP reduces hemodilution and diminishes the drop in systemic vascular resistance (SVR) associated with the initiation of CPB. When using this technique, care must be taken to avoid acute hypovolemic hypotension. Reported benefits of RAP include reduced extravascular lung water and weight gain.[106]

Ultrafiltration is another technique used in conjunction with CPB to reduce postoperative bleeding and transfusion needs. During ultrafiltration (hemoconcentration), plasma water is separated from low-molecular-weight solutes, intravascular cell components, and plasma proteins with a semipermeable membrane, using a hydrostatic pressure differential created by external suction. Conventional ultrafiltration is initiated during rewarming and is practiced more often in pediatric cardiac surgery. Advantages of hemoconcentration include a reduction in free water, increase in hemoglobin and hematocrit, preservation of hemostasis, and a decrease in levels of circulating inflammatory mediators.[107]

Myocardial Protection

The most common method of myocardial protection used today is that of intermittent hyperkalemic cold cardioplegia and moderate systemic hypothermia. Systemic hypothermia is beneficial for both myocardial and neurologic protection during cardiac surgery. The benefits of hypothermia are a reduction in metabolic rate and oxygen consumption, preservation of high-energy phosphate substrates, and a reduction in excitatory neurotransmitter release. For each degree Centigrade reduction in temperature, there is an 8% reduction in metabolic rate, so that at 28°C there is an approximate reduction in metabolic rate of 50%. Moderate systemic hypothermia can be achieved with either passive or active cooling. Using passive cooling, the patient's core temperature is allowed to equalize with the ambient temperature. This may be a slow or rapid process depending on variables such as patient's body surface area exposed and ambient temperature. Most patients undergoing cardiac surgery are actively cooled and then rewarmed using a heat exchanger.

The fundamental concept of cold cardioplegia is that a cold solution (10 to 15°C) of either blood or crystalloid with a supranormal concentration of potassium is injected into the coronary arteries or veins to induce diastolic electrical arrest. Cardioplegia may be employed via an anterograde, a retrograde, or a combination of the two routes. Anterograde cardioplegia solution is injected via the aortic root following aortic cross-clamp and into the native coronaries. The cardioplegia then follows the normal anatomic flow of blood. In patients with severe coronary disease or AI, anterograde cardioplegia may provide inadequate myocardial protection because the incompetent AV allows cardioplegia to flow inside the LV, bypassing the coronary ostia causing left ventricular distention and ischemia. In such cases, following aortic cross-clamping, an aortotomy is made and cardioplegia is delivered antegrade via handheld cannulae placed in the individual coronary ostia under direct vision. During coronary artery bypass surgery, individual grafts may be used to deliver cardioplegia once distal anastomoses have been completed. Retrograde cardioplegia is employed for myocardial protection by the placement of a catheter inside the coronary sinus. Retrograde cardioplegia is then injected via the cardiac venous system, bypassing obstructed coronaries and achieving greater myocardial protection. To maximize myocardial protection, both anterograde and retrograde are often used in combination. Depending on the time required for surgical repair, multiple injections of cardioplegia may be necessary to wash out metabolic by-products, add new high-energy and oxygen-carrying substrates, and maintain hypothermic diastolic arrest.

For the anesthesiologist monitoring a patient on CPB, the sentinel events of cardioplegic electrical arrest and resumption of electrical activity must be observed closely. LV distention and lack of rapid electrical arrest may be evidence of poor myocardial protection and the possibility of difficulty in separation from CPB. TEE is particularly helpful in diagnosing ventricular distention and its relief by venting or manual decompression of the LV.

PREOPERATIVE AND INTRAOPERATIVE MANAGEMENT

The preoperative visit should focus on the cardiovascular system but should not disregard the assessment of pulmonary, renal, hepatic, neurologic, endocrine, and hematologic functions. The anticipated events on the day of surgery, including transport to the operating room, preoperative routines (O_2 mask, vascular cannulation, anesthetic induction), and finally, the emergence in
10 the recovery room or ICU should be discussed with the patient. The importance of communicating to the anesthesiologist any symptoms such as chest pain, shortness of breath, or the need for nitroglycerin during transport or the preinduction period should be emphasized to the patient. The depth and detail of the explanation should be custom-tailored to each patient.

Data from history, physical examination, and laboratory investigations are used to define the cardiovascular anatomy and functional state. Pertinent findings suggestive of left and/or right

TABLE 38-10. PREOPERATIVE FINDINGS SUGGESTIVE OF VENTRICULAR DYSFUNCTION

History
- CAD: Previous MI, chest pain/pressure
- CHF (intermittent or chronic): Fatigue, DOE, orthopnea, PND, ankle swelling

Physical examination
- Vital signs: Hypotension, tachycardia (severe CHF)
- Engorged neck veins, apical impulse displaced laterally, S_3, S_4, rales, pitting edema, pulsatile liver, ascites

Electrocardiogram
- Ischemia/infarct, rhythm, conduction abnormalities

Chest x-ray
- Cardiomegaly, pulmonary vascular congestion/pulmonary edema, pleural effusion, Kerley B lines

Cardiovascular testing
- Catheterization data: LVEDP >18 mm Hg, EF <0.4, CI <2.0 L/min/m^2

CAD, coronary artery disease; MI, myocardial infarction; CHF, congestive heart failure; DOE, dyspnea on exertion; PND, paroxysmal nocturnal dyspnea; LVEDP, left ventricular end-diastolic pressure; EF, ejection fraction; CI, cardiac index.

ventricular dysfunction are described in Table 38-10. Increase in the severity or frequency of anginal attacks or the presence of ischemia-induced ventricular dysfunction suggests that large areas of myocardium are at risk. A history of dysrhythmias should be obtained, including the type, severity, associated symptoms, prior intervention, and successful treatment (including the presence/type/date of insertion of a rhythm management device). Integration of this information leads to appropriate selection of monitoring devices and anesthetic techniques.

Conditions commonly associated with heart disease, such as hypertension, diabetes mellitus, and cigarette smoking, must also be evaluated. The pulmonary or cardiac factors of pulmonary hypertension should be investigated. Higher systemic arterial pressures may be desirable throughout surgery in patients with a history or other evidence of carotid artery disease. Evidence for renal dysfunction must be sought since it is the most common cause of postoperative renal failure. If renal reserve is reduced, intraoperative measures such as diuretics or dopamine may be used, although there is no firm evidence to suggest that the use of any specific pharmacologic intervention is clinically beneficial.[108]

Current Drug Therapy

Almost without exception, cardiovascular drugs, including cardiac antiarrhythmics (e.g., amiodarone), β-blockers or calcium channel blockers, and nitrates as well as aspirin, antilipidemics (statins), and ACE inhibitors are continued until the time of surgery.[109] Interactions between these drugs and anesthetics are more often beneficial than harmful in maintaining hemodynamic control during periods of surgical stress and reducing morbidity and mortality.

Contrary to common belief, there is a potential long-term benefit of ACE inhibitors provided that dosing is adjusted so that hypotension is avoided.[110] On the other hand, the protracted hypotension encountered on bypass and associated with poor outcome has been associated with preoperative β-blockers or calcium channel blockers.[111] Most cardiac antidysrhythmics should also be continued to the time of surgery.

TABLE 38-11. PREOPERATIVE PHYSICAL EXAMINATION

Vital signs
Current values and range
Height, weight
For calculations of drug dosages, pump flow, cardiac index
Airway
Evaluate, identify difficulties for ventilation, intubation
Neck
Landmarks for jugular vein cannulation
Vein engorgement (CHF)
Bruits (carotid artery disease)
Heart
Murmurs: Characteristic of valve lesions, S_3 (elevated LVEDP), S_4 (decreased compliance), click (MVP prolapse)
Lateral PMI displacement (cardiomegaly)
Precordial heave, lift (hypertrophy, wall motion abnormality)
Lungs
Rales (CHF)
Rhonchi, wheezes (COPD, asthma)
Vasculature
Peripheral pulses
Sites for venous and arterial access
Abdomen
Pulsatile liver (CHF, tricuspid regurgitation)
Extremities
Peripheral edema (CHF)
Nervous system
Motor or sensory deficits

CHF, congestive heart failure; LVEDP, left ventricular end-diastolic pressure; MVP, mitral valve prolapse; PMI, point of maximal impulse; COPD, chronic obstructive pulmonary disease.

Physical Examination

Physical examination should be part of the preoperative evaluation; signs of cardiac decompensation such as an S_3 gallop, rales, jugular venous distention, or pulsatile liver should be sought. Routes for vascular access should be assessed, and the status of peripheral arteries should be evaluated. As always, the airway should be carefully evaluated with respect to ease of mask ventilation and intubation of the trachea. Other pertinent points are described in Table 38-11.

Premedication

Premedication will assist in providing a calm, anxiety-free, arousable, and hemodynamically stable patient who is prepared for surgery. Selection of drug and dosage depends on the patient's age, cardiovascular state, level of anxiety, and location. While heavy premedication is ideal for the fit person scheduled for CABG (although this patient is a rarity these days), there is inadequate time for premedication for the same-day-admit patient. Inadequate sedation may predispose to hypertension, tachycardia, or coronary vasospasm, and precipitate myocardial ischemia. These days, sedation is almost always given in the operating room after completion of regulatory paperwork.

Monitoring

We emphasize only those aspects of monitoring particularly relevant to cardiac surgery because the subject is discussed extensively in Chapters 25 and 36.

Pulse Oximeter

Vascular cannulations may be challenging and the preinduction period may be prolonged. The pulse oximeter should be the first monitor placed to detect clinically unsuspected episodes of hypoxemia and tachycardia.

Electrocardiogram

Regional ischemia may be diagnosed by appropriate lead monitoring: Lead II (and/or leads III, aVF) for the inferior myocardium (right coronary artery distribution), leads V_4 or V_5 for the anterior myocardium (left anterior descending (LAD) artery), and leads I and aVL for the lateral LV myocardial walls (circumflex artery). A strip-chart recorder or the "freeze pane" function of the hemodynamic monitor is useful for analysis and documentation of ST segment alterations and complex dysrhythmias.

Temperature

Central temperature can be measured with urinary bladder catheter or with a thermistor from a PAC.[112] Depending upon the case, nasopharyngeal or tympanic temperature probes may be used (as in cases of deep hypothermic circulatory arrest). Rectal and skin probes record peripheral temperatures, which lag behind central measurements during both cooling and rewarming periods.

Arterial Blood Pressure

Systemic arterial pressure should always be monitored invasively. The radial artery is usually cannulated,[113] although the femoral, brachial, and axillary arteries may also be used. The exact site is often a matter of personal or institutional preference. Criteria include convenience, selection of the arterial site with the "fullest" or most bounding pulse, and avoidance of the dominant hand. Occasionally, the site of surgery dictates appropriate placement; for example, the right radial artery should be used for procedures involving the descending thoracic aorta because the left subclavian artery may be included in the proximal aortic clamp. Following CPB, radial artery pressure is often misleading and may be as much as 30 mm Hg lower than central aortic pressure. The mechanism may be due to peripheral vasodilation during rewarming or marked vasoconstriction.[114] Whenever a pressure discrepancy is suspected, the central aortic pressure should be estimated (by palpation by the surgeon) or directly measured (with a needle placed directly into the aorta or via femoral artery catheterization). Timely recognition will avoid unnecessary treatment of presumed hypotension. The gradient usually disappears within 45 minutes of separation from bypass.

Central Venous Pressure and Pulmonary Artery Catheter

Access to the central circulation is mandatory for infusion of cardioactive drugs. In addition, right atrial or central venous measure reflects right ventricular filling pressure and is of critical importance whenever right ventricular dysfunction is suspected. The relationship between the transduced right atrial pressure and the LV filling is less predictable, more so in the presence of severe LV dyssynergy, pulmonary hypertension, or reduced LV compliance. In these instances, insertion of a PAC for measurement of pulmonary capillary wedge pressure provides a somewhat better index of LV filling, although TEE data are far more accurate, because they provide an estimation of actual volume. In addition, determination of cardiac output and calculation of stroke volume and PVR and SVR offer additional information to guide hemodynamic and anesthetic management.

Indications for pulmonary artery catheterization vary greatly among institutions.[22] In some, these catheters are used routinely, whereas in others they are limited to patients with severe cardiac dysfunction or pulmonary hypertension. Additional indications include combined procedures (valvular plus coronary) or prolonged intraoperative time (cardiac reoperations). Insertion of a pacing PAC can be helpful whenever exact control of rate and rhythm is desirable before access to the epicardium is possible, for example, in patients with hypertrophic cardiomyopathy or those with significant bradycardia secondary to β-blockade.

Some practitioners advocate preinduction insertion of the PAC so that the determination of baseline hemodynamics guides the anesthetic induction. However, the anxious and uncomfortable hypertensive patient is served better by a smooth anesthetic induction followed by PAC placement.

It must be remembered that the catheter often migrates toward the periphery of the lung with cardiac manipulation before and during CPB, as well as with acute preload changes. Therefore, it seems prudent to pull the catheter back a few centimeters prior to the initiation of bypass to prevent permanent wedging or possible pulmonary artery rupture.[115] Despite the controversy concerning the routine use of these catheters, there is no disagreement that the capability to estimate or measure cardiac output and ventricular filling pressures must be available in any institution performing cardiac surgery.[65] Whether this is done with a PAC or TEE is immaterial. In addition, the ability of the practitioner to interpret correctly the PAC or TEE data cannot be overemphasized.

Echocardiography

The detection of ischemia by real-time evaluation of new regional wall motion abnormalities and the assessment of valvular function (before and after intervention) and of the ascending aorta with TEE have been mentioned. It is well known that, following CPB, the LV filling pressure, irrespective of the site of measurement (LV end-diastolic pressure, LA, pulmonary capillary wedge pressure), is a poor and often misleading indicator of LV volume status.[116] Direct estimation of LV volume with TEE more appropriately directs fluid infusion and selection of vasoactive drugs in patients who are difficult to wean from CPB. In addition, residual valve lesions, intracardiac air, or new areas of ischemia or global dysfunction (due to prolonged CPB, inadequate cardioplegia or reperfusion injury) can be detected.

Central Nervous System Function and Complications

Monitoring of the brain during CPB is difficult because of lack of standardized equipment or criteria. Neurologic complications after cardiac surgery can be devastating. The 1- and 5-year survival rates after stroke are about 65% and 45%, respectively, compared with >90% and 80% to 85% for patients not having stroke.[117] Thus, many investigators have more recently focused on methods to determine the etiology and improve the detection, prevention, and treatment of postoperative neurologic complications in patients undergoing cardiac surgery.

The incidence of stroke after CABG surgery ranges from <1% (for patients <64 years) to >5% to 9% (for patients >65 years).[118] The incidence of subtle cognitive deficits that can be elicited by detailed neuropsychometric testing is much higher (60% to 70%). It is known that the neuropsychiatric deficits do improve over the initial 2 to 6 months after cardiac surgery; however, a significant percentage of patients (13% to 39%) have residual impairment. The etiology of perioperative neurologic complications is believed to be predominantly due to emboli (air, atheroma, other particulate matter) and not to hypoperfusion in susceptible patients (e.g., pre-existing cerebrovascular disease). Most overt strokes after cardiac surgery are focal and likely due to macroemboli, whereas the cognitive changes are subtle and probably result from microemboli. Risk factors for neurologic complications include advanced age (>70 years), pre-existing cerebrovascular disease (e.g., carotid artery stenosis >80%), history of prior stroke, peripheral vascular disease, ascending aortic atheroma, and diabetes. Operative factors include the duration of CPB, intracardiac procedure (e.g., valve replacement), excessive warming during and following CPB, and perhaps perfusion pressure on CPB.[119,120] Intraoperative hyperglycemia, which could theoretically result in worsened neurologic damage, has not been associated with poorer neurologic outcome.

The role of TEE in evaluating the ascending and descending aorta has been described previously. There are several management options undergoing investigation for patients with severely diseased aortas, especially those with mobile atheromas who are at increased risk of stroke. These include hypothermic fibrillatory arrest with LV vent and no aortic cross-clamp, single cross-clamp (i.e., distal and proximal grafts performed during same cross-clamp), relocation of proximal grafts to area of nondiseased aorta, no proximal grafts (internal mammary arteries only) either on CPB or using off-pump coronary artery bypass, or hypothermic circulatory arrest with resection and graft replacement of the diseased aortic segment. The technical means for cerebral protection such as the use of 20- to 40-μm arterial line filters and membrane oxygenators, newer modifications of the basic CPB apparatus, or the use of specialized equipment or procedures (including hypothermia and "tight" glucose control) have unproven benefit on neurologic outcomes.[121] Hypothermia is excellent in that it decreases cerebral metabolic rate and prolongs ischemic tolerance; however, profound hypothermia is not practical for routine cardiac surgery. Unfortunately, during routine CPB the patient is normothermic when the highest risk of embolization exists (unclamping, during rewarming, and with initial ventricular ejection). Sodium thiopental has been shown to be cerebroprotective in intracardiac procedures, but not in CABG surgery. This difference may be a result of the "reversible" neurologic impairment secondary to gas emboli, which is more likely during intracardiac procedures than CABG surgery.

Selection of Anesthetic Drugs

There are no data that document superiority of any anesthetic for either coronary or valvular surgery. The large outcome studies of Tuman et al.[122] and Slogoff et al.[123] indicated that the choice of anesthetic has no effect on the outcome in CABG patients. As was previously emphasized, the most critical factor governing anesthetic selection is the degree of ventricular dysfunction, while anticipated difficulties during tracheal intubation, the expected duration of surgery, and the anticipated time of tracheal extubation may also influence choice of anesthetics. It is desirable to be able to alter the anesthetic depth rapidly, so as to counteract the varying intensity of surgical stress. The most intense stimulation and sympathetic response is expected during tracheal intubation, incision, sternotomy, pericardiotomy, and manipulation of the aorta. The period of preparing and draping following intubation of the trachea requires minimal levels of anesthetic, as does the period of hypothermic bypass.

Volatile anesthetics are useful both as primary anesthetics and as adjuvants to prevent or treat "breakthrough" hypertension. The balance of myocardial oxygen supply and demand is usually altered favorably by reduction in contractility and afterload. Any deleterious declines in coronary perfusion pressure must be prevented or treated. Volatile agents have been used successfully in all types of valve surgery without untoward effects, although they are sometimes associated with more hemodynamic variability than is seen with opioids. Volatile anesthetics have been associated with cardioprotective effects from ischemia and reperfusion and allow for more rapid recovery of contractile function on reperfusion.[12] The ability to rapidly increase and decrease the alveolar concentration allows easy adjustment to the variable levels of surgical stimulation. Volatile anesthetics can be administered during bypass through a vaporizer mounted on the pump; they are also appropriate in the postbypass period,
11 assuming cardiac function is adequate. The use of volatile anesthetics in combination with short-acting opiates or hypnotics is more relevant nowadays, because of the relatively "fast-track" postoperative treatment.

Opioids

Opioids lack negative inotropic effects in the doses used clinically and have thus found widespread use as the primary agents for cardiac surgery. This era began in 1969, when high doses of morphine were used to anesthetize patients for AV replacement.[35] However, hypotension, histamine release, increased fluid requirements, and, often, inadequate anesthesia resulted in a decline in the use of morphine in favor of the more potent fentanyl and its analogues. Aside from bradycardia, fentanyl and its analogues are relatively devoid of cardiovascular effects and have proved to be effective anesthetics. As a primary anesthetic agent, fentanyl (50 to 100 μg/kg) or sufentanil (10 to 20 μg/kg) and oxygen provide hemodynamic stability, although they do not consistently prevent a hypertensive response to periods of increased surgical stimulation. The use of high-dose opioids prolongs the time until emergence and extubation when compared with techniques primarily based on volatile anesthetics and is no longer in fashion. In addition, although high doses of opioids produce unconsciousness and characteristic electrocardiographic slowing, recall of intraoperative events is not eliminated. Therefore, a current-era cardiac anesthetic includes adjuvant agents such as benzodiazepines to provide amnesia and volatile anesthetics or vasodilators to control hypertension. Superiority of any one opioid has not been demonstrated for either coronary or valvular surgery. Alfentanil, with an elimination half-life shorter than that of fentanyl or sufentanil, is suitable for infusion techniques and may provide optimal conditions for early extubation of the trachea. Remifentanil, an ultrashort-acting opioid, is 30 times more potent than alfentanil and undergoes hydrolysis by nonspecific esterases in minutes. Its predictable and rapid elimination is unaffected by hepatic or renal disease, making it an optimal drug for infusion techniques.

Combinations of the fentanyl-type drugs and benzodiazepines, whether given concomitantly or as premedication, result in hypotension secondary to a fall in SVR. Any opioid in high doses can produce excessive bradycardia. Vecuronium or *cis*-atracurium may magnify this problem, whereas pancuronium is often useful in preventing it. Abdominal and chest wall rigidity commonly occur with rapid injection of high doses of opioids and can be severe enough to render ventilation impossible. A low dose (priming) of nondepolarizing muscle relaxant should be given prior to opioid administration.

Nitrous Oxide

In many centers, nitrous oxide is not used during cardiac surgery. Increases in PVR associated with nitrous oxide have been demonstrated, with the greatest response in patients with pre-existing pulmonary hypertension. Nitrous oxide is also a mild myocardial depressant and elicits a compensatory, sympathetically mediated increase in SVR. These minimal changes may not be well tolerated in patients with minimal cardiovascular reserve. It is well known that nitrous oxide increases the size of any air-filled cavity. The possibility of expansion of air introduced into the circulation either before or during bypass should preclude its use immediately before, during, or after bypass.

Induction Drugs

Benzodiazepines, barbiturates, propofol, and etomidate can be used as supplements to either inhalation or opioid anesthetics and as sole induction drugs in patients with cardiac disease depending on the adequacy of ventricular function and baseline sympathetic tone. Etomidate is favored for induction in patients with limited cardiac reserve, but rarely used subsequently because of potential adrenal dysfunction associated with prolonged use. Obviously, dosage requirements must be altered to fit the clinical situation.

Neuromuscular Blocking Drugs

Muscle relaxants are components of a balanced anesthetic for cardiac surgery. Although they are not essential to surgical exposure of the heart, muscle paralysis facilitates intubation of the trachea and attenuates skeletal muscle contraction during defibrillation. Thus, they are necessary to prevent or treat opioid-induced truncal rigidity. The chief criteria for selection are the hemodynamic and pharmacokinetic properties associated with each relaxant, the patient's myocardial function, the presence of coexisting disease, current pharmacologic regimen, and anesthetic technique.[124]

Intraoperative Management

In this section we describe the anesthetic management of a patient undergoing a cardiac surgical procedure from the time of arrival in the operating room until his or her care is transferred to ICU personnel. Because the physiologic and pharmacologic rationales for anesthetic selection are previously discussed, this is rather a sequential description of what occurs and what is required during surgery. Anticipation of needs specific to each stage of the procedure and immediate availability of necessary equipment and medications prevent untoward hemodynamic aberrations and last-minute rush-in decisions.

Preparation

The operating room must be readied prior to arrival of the patient. Heparin may be drawn up prior to induction of anesthesia in the unlikely event of the need to "crash" onto CPB. Typed and cross-matched blood should be available in the operating suite. Table 38-12 provides a checklist to aid in proper preoperative preparation of the operating room.

TABLE 38-12. ANESTHETIC PREPARATION FOR CARDIAC SURGERY

Anesthesia machine
- Routine check

Airway
- Nasal cannula for O_2
- Ventilation/intubation equipment
- Suction
- Difficult airway anticipated? Special equipment
- Inspired gas humidifier

Circulatory access
- Catheters for peripheral and central venous and arterial access
- Intravenous fluids and infusion tubing and pumps
- Fluid warmer

Monitors
- Standard ASA: ECG leads, blood pressure cuff, pulse oximeter, neuromuscular blockade monitor
- Temperature: Various probes (nasal, tympanic, bladder, rectal)
- Transducers (arterial, pulmonary, and central venous pressure) zeroed
- Cardiac output computer: Proper constant inserted
  - Awareness monitor (BIS)
- Anticoagulation (ACT) monitor(s)
- Recorder

Medications
- General anesthetic: Hypnotic/induction, amnestic/benzodiazepine, volatile, opioid, muscle relaxant
- Heparin (predrawn)
- Cardioactive
  - In syringes: Nitroglycerin/nicardipine, $CaCl_2$, phenylephrine/ephedrine, epinephrine
  - Infusions: Nitroglycerin, inotrope
- Antibiotics

Miscellaneous
- Pacemaker with battery
  - Defibrillator/cardioverter with external paddles and ECG cables
  - Ultrasound system for central venous line insertion
- Compatible blood in operating room

ASA, American Society of Anesthesiologists; ECG, electrocardiogram; BIS, bispectral index; ACT, activated clotting time.

Preinduction Period

The patient's general status and level of anxiety and the effectiveness of premedication (if ordered) should be assessed prior to entry to the operating room. The patient is reminded to report chest pain, shortness of breath, or any discomfort. Supplemental oxygen via nasal cannula should be administered once the patient has been transferred to the operating table; peripheral oxygen saturation monitor, ECG leads, and noninvasive blood pressure cuff are placed, and a set of initial vital signs are recorded. Any angina should be promptly treated with oxygen, additional sedation, intravenous nitroglycerin, or, if related to anxiety-induced hypertension or tachycardia, with β-blocker and prompt induction of general anesthesia if possible.

One or two large-bore intravenous cannulae are inserted after site infiltration with local anesthetic (additional routes for infusion are desirable in patients undergoing repeat cardiac surgery). In some centers, anesthesia is then induced, and following intubation of the trachea, arterial and central venous cannulae are inserted. In other centers, however, one or both of these cannulae are inserted prior to induction of anesthesia. Preinduction or postinduction insertion of central venous or PAC has been discussed previously. Surface ultrasound is recommended for central venous access, while at all times sterile barrier technique should be adhered to.[125,126] Once they are inserted, however, initial values for all pressures and cardiac output should be recorded, and baseline determinations of arterial blood gases, hematocrit, blood glucose, and activated coagulation time should be obtained.

Throughout the preinduction period, while the intravenous and pressure monitoring catheters are inserted, the anesthesiologist must never divert his or her attention from the patient. Placing a functioning pulse oximeter with the volume loud enough to be easily heard should precede line placement. Continuous monitoring of the vital signs, careful observation of the patient, and periodic verbal contact facilitate detection of hemodynamic or ECG abnormalities, increased anxiety, or excessive response to intravenous sedation.

Induction and Intubation

The exact choice and sequence of drugs are a subtle—sometimes not so subtle—combination of art and science. The choice of specific agents (e.g., sedative, opioid, volatile drug, muscle relaxant), dose, and speed of administration depends primarily on the patient's cardiovascular reserve and desired cardiovascular profile. A smooth transition from consciousness to blissful sleep is desired without untoward airway difficulties (e.g., coughing, laryngospasm, truncal rigidity) or hemodynamic responses (e.g., hypotension from relative overdose, loss of sympathetic tone, or myocardial depression; hypertension caused by airway insertion; or jaw thrust). A "slow cardiac induction" sometimes causes, rather than alleviates, these potential problems. However, awake tracheal intubation, after proper sedation, may be appropriate in an obese patient with a wide neck if ventilation and intubation appear to be difficult. The necessity for individual approach to each patient cannot be overemphasized.

Deep planes of anesthesia, brief duration of laryngoscopy, and innumerable pharmacologic regimens have been proposed for eliminating the hypertension and tachycardia associated with intubation of the trachea. None is uniformly successful, and all drug interventions carry some degree of risk, even though they may be small. In patients with a slow heart rate prior to induction of anesthesia, the reflex response to tracheal intubation is primarily vagal, and severe bradycardia and rarely sinus arrest can occur. Identification of persistently abnormal hemodynamics or ischemia should be sought and treated.

Preincision Period

The period of time from tracheal intubation until skin incision is one of minimal stimulation as the surgical team attends to insertion of a bladder catheter, temperature probe, positioning, preparing, and draping. As a result, hypotension often develops, regardless of the anesthetic used. It may be necessary to reduce the anesthetic depth or alternatively support the systemic pressure with a vasoconstrictor. The potential risks of vasoconstriction in patients with poor left or right ventricular performance must be kept in mind. The anesthetic depth should be increased immediately prior to incision and sternotomy.

Incision to Bypass

As previously emphasized, the prebypass period is characterized by periods of intense surgical stimulation that may cause hypertension and tachycardia, or induce ischemia. Anticipating these events and deepening the anesthetic may be effective, but a vasodilator or other adjuvant is often required. Hypotension can occur during the less stressful moments before bypass, but it is more commonly associated with cardiac manipulation in preparation for, and during, atrial cannulation. This may interfere with venous return or produce episodic ectopic beats or sustained supraventricular dysrhythmias, and atrial fibrillation is not uncommon. Depending on the blood pressure and heart rate response, appropriate treatment may range from observation to vasoconstrictors, cardioversion, or rapid cannulation and institution of bypass. Maintaining adequate intravascular volume may attenuate the extent of blood pressure decrease. This is a critical period, and continual observation of the surgical field is essential.

Prebypass, ST segment analysis, and frequent TEE observation are important in identifying and localizing new ischemia. If it occurs, it should be treated appropriately and the surgeon notified. In rare cases in which a cardiac chamber is inadvertently injured and bleeding is uncontrollable, heparin is administered, the femoral vessels are cannulated, and CPB is begun using coronary suction from the field as the major means of venous return. Communication between the anesthesiologist and the surgeon is necessary to keep both apprised of the situation and to ensure the heart gets a periodic "rest during periods of manipulation."

TABLE 38-13. CHECKLIST BEFORE INITIATING CARDIOPULMONARY BYPASS

Laboratory values
- Heparinization adequate (ACT or other method)
- Hematocrit

Anesthetic
- Maintenance: Amnestics, opioids, muscle relaxants are supplemented

Monitors
- Arterial pressure: Initial hypotension and then return
- CVP: Indicates adequate venous drainage
- PCWP:
  - Elevated? LV distention (inadequate drainage, AI)
  - Pull back PAC 1–2 cm

Patient/field
- Cannulae in place:
  - No kinks or clamps or air locks
  - Arterial cannula is free of bubbles
- Face:
  - Suffusion? Inadequate SVC drainage
  - Unilateral blanching? Innominate artery cannulation
- Heart:
  - Signs of distention (AI, ischemia)

Support
- Usually not required

ACT, activated clotting time; CVP, central venous pressure; PCWP, pulmonary capillary wedge pressure; LV, left ventricle; AI, aortic insufficiency; PAC, pulmonary artery catheter; SVC, superior vena cava.

Cardiopulmonary Bypass

After heparin administration, the cannulae are inserted, and adequate levels of anticoagulation are checked to ensure the patient is ready for the institution of CPB (Table 38-13). Attention is focused on adequacy of venous drainage (no pulsatility on CVP or PA waveforms), unobstructed arterial return (appropriate systemic arterial pressure), sufficient gas exchange, and provision of necessary anesthetics and muscle relaxants. The anesthetic requirements are decreased if systemic hypothermia is used.

There is complete agreement that once full CPB is established, it is no longer necessary to ventilate the lungs.

During the initial minutes of CPB, systemic arterial pressure initially drops to 30 to 40 mm Hg as pulsatile flow ceases and the hemodilution effect of the CPB prime becomes apparent. Once adequate mixing is obtained, blood pressure increases to levels determined primarily by flow rate, and secondarily by total vascular resistance (Table 38-14). There is no consensus as to what constitutes the ideal blood pressure or flow rate for adequate vital organ perfusion, especially of the brain, during bypass.[127] Commonly, flow rates are maintained at approximately 50 to 60 mL/kg/minute, with systemic blood pressures in the 50 to 60 mm Hg range, while some believe that older patients benefit from a higher blood pressure (>70 mm Hg).

Monitoring and Management During Bypass

The common causes of blood pressure changes during CPB are listed in Table 38-14. Of primary importance is continuous observation of the surgical field and cannulae to exclude mechanical reasons. Attention can then be directed to other causes of hypotension or hypertension and their appropriate treatment. Additional areas that require periodic monitoring and occasional intervention during CPB are also described in Table 38-14. Maintenance of adequate depths of anesthesia is obviously important during bypass, although clinical signs are few. Anesthetic requirements are decreased during the period of hypothermia but return toward normal when the patient is rewarmed.

Arterial pH and mixed venous oxygen saturation, often measured online, are used to assess the adequacy of perfusion. Urine output is monitored, but it is influenced by so many variables (e.g., arterial and venous pressure, flow rate, temperature, diuretic history) that it is difficult to draw meaningful conclusions from this measurement.[128] In addition, postoperative renal failure develops from either aggravation of pre-existing renal dysfunction or persistent low cardiac output following bypass. Although many institutions administer diuretics routinely, they are just as assiduously avoided elsewhere.

Rewarming

When surgical repair is nearly complete, gradual rewarming of the patient begins. A gradient of 4 to 6°C is maintained between the patient and the perfusate to prevent formation of gas bubbles, and blood temperature should be <37°C. A slower rate of rewarming has been associated with better cognitive function 6 weeks post CABG surgery[129] Patient awareness becomes a possibility as the potentiation of anesthetic effects due to hypothermia dissipates. If adequate doses of anesthetics have not been given, administration during rewarming should be considered to prevent recall of intraoperative events. Targeting an end-tidal concentration of the inhaled agent between 0.7 and 1.3 MAC is as effective as maintaining a BIS value between 40 and 60.[130] Use of volatile anesthetics is helpful if a smooth postbypass course is anticipated and early weaning from mechanical ventilation and

TABLE 38-14. CHECKLIST DURING CARDIOPULMONARY BYPASS

Laboratory values
- Heparinization adequate (ACT or other method)
- ABGs (uncorrected): Is there acidosis?
- Hematocrit, Na^+, K^+, ionized Ca^{2+}, glucose

Anesthetic
- Discontinue ventilation

Monitors
- Arterial hypotension:
  - Inadequate venous return
    - Venous cannula: Malposition, clamp, kink, air lock
    - Bleeding, hypovolemia, IVC obstruction, table too low
  - Pump: Poor occlusion, low flow
  - Arterial cannula: Misdirected, kinked, partially clamped, aortic dissection
  - Decreased vascular tone: Anesthetics, hemodilution, idiopathic
  - Transducer/monitor malfunction: Radial artery cannula malpositioned, dampened waveform
- Arterial hypertension:
  - Pump: High flow
  - Arterial cannula: Misdirected
  - Vasoconstriction: Light anesthetic plane, response to hypothermia
  - Transducer/monitor malfunction: Radial artery cannula malpositioned/kinked
- Venous pressure:
  - Decreased? Transducer higher than atrial level?
  - Increased? True obstruction of chamber drainage? (CVP: Right, PCWP/LA: Left heart)
- EEG
- Adequate body perfusion:
  - Flow and pressure?
  - Acidosis
  - Mixed venous blood oxygen saturation
- Temperature
- Urine output

Patient/field
- Conduct of the operation
- Heart: Distention, fibrillation
- Cyanosis, venous engorgement, skin temperature
- Movement
- Signs of light anesthesia/hypercapnia: Breathing/diaphragmatic movement

Support
- Assist adequacy of pump flow:
  - Anesthetics/vasodilators for hypertension
  - Constrictors for hypotension

ACT, activated clotting time; ABGs, arterial blood gases; IVC, inferior vena cava; CVP, central venous pressure; PCWP, pulmonary capillary wedge pressure; LA, left atrium; EEG, electroencephalogram.

extubation are planned. On completion of the surgical repair, various maneuvers are performed to remove any residual air in the ventricles. The anesthesiologist is called on to vigorously inflate the lungs to remove air from the pulmonary veins and aid in filling the cardiac chambers. TEE is particularly useful in assessing the effectiveness of the de-airing process. The heart is defibrillated (if needed) and externally paced or allowed to beat (if native rhythm is present). The field is tidied up, and preparations are made to separate from CPB.

Discontinuation of Cardiopulmonary Bypass

Prior to discontinuing CPB, the patient should be normothermic, the surgical field must be dry, the appropriate laboratory values must be checked, the pulmonary compliance must be evaluated, and ventilation of the lungs must be begun (Table 38-15). If necessary, heart rate and rhythm are regulated either pharmacologically or electrically (appropriate pacing, defibrillation, cardioversion). The venous cannula(e) are then occluded incrementally and sufficient pump volume is transfused into the patient, while the bypass flow is slowly decreased (Fig. 38-10). During this time, the cardiac function is constantly evaluated from hemodynamic and TEE data and direct inspection of the heart, and the need for vasoactive or cardioactive drugs is assessed. The potential disparity, previously alluded to, between radial artery and aortic pressures must be kept in mind. Contractility, rhythm, and ventricular filling can all be estimated by careful observation of the beating heart and TEE. For example, a low blood pressure and a vigorously contracting, relatively empty ventricle suggest that volume and perhaps a vasoconstrictor are all that is needed to wean the patient from bypass, whereas adequate blood pressure in the presence of a sluggish and overdistended heart may be treated with a vasodilator and/or a small dose of an inotrope. Figure 38-11 presents a general approach to termination of CPB.

TABLE 38-15. CHECKLIST BEFORE SEPARATION FROM CARDIOPULMONARY BYPASS

Laboratory values
- Hematocrit, ABGs
- K^+: ? elevated (cardioplegia)
- Ionized Ca^{2+}

Anesthetic/machine
- Lung compliance: Evaluate (hand ventilation)
- Lungs are expanded, no atelectasis, both are ventilated (manual or mechanical)
- Vaporizers: Off
- Alarms: On

Monitors
- Normothermia (37°C nasopharyngeal, 35.5°C bladder, 35°C rectal)
- ECG: Rate, rhythm, ST
- Transducers re-zeroed and leveled
- Arterial and filling pressures
- Recorder (if available)

Patient/field
- LOOK AT THE HEART!
- De-aired: Check lead II, TEE
- Eyeball contractility, size, rhythm
- LV vent clamped/removed, caval snares released
- Bleeding: No major sites (grafts, suture lines, LV vent site)
- Vascular resistance: CPB flow $\propto$ MAP $\div$ Resistance

Support
- As needed

ABGs, arterial blood gases; ECG, electrocardiogram; TEE, transesophageal echocardiography; LV, left ventricle; CPB, cardiopulmonary bypass; MAP, mean arterial pressure.

ANESTHESIA FOR SURGICAL SUBSPECIALTIES

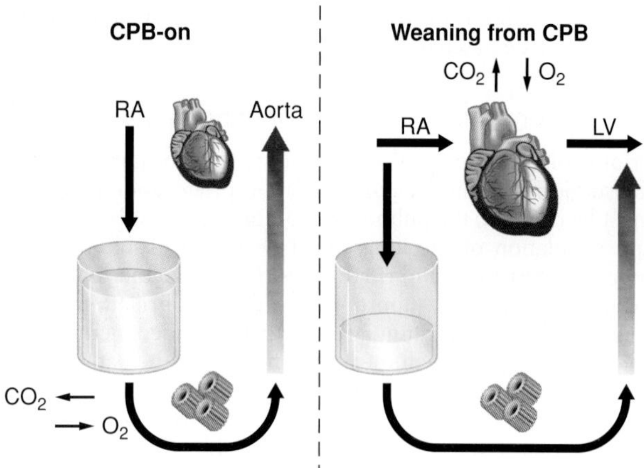

FIGURE 38-10. Weaning from cardiopulmonary bypass. While on cardiopulmonary bypass (CPB), the venous return to the heart is diverted from the right atrium (RA) to the CPB reservoir. The drainage is passive (by gravity). From the venous reservoir, the blood is "ventilated," CO_2 is removed, and O_2 is added, and then returned to the patient, usually into the aorta but occasionally via the femoral or axillary arteries. During weaning from CPB, the venous return to the CPB is reduced by gradually occluding the venous cannula, directing more of its contents to the right heart and lungs. LV, left ventricle.

TABLE 38-16. ETIOLOGY OF RIGHT OR LEFT VENTRICULAR DYSFUNCTION AFTER CARDIOPULMONARY BYPASS (CPB)

Ischemia
Inadequate myocardial protection
Intraoperative infarction
Reperfusion injury
Coronary spasm
Coronary embolism (air, thrombus, calcium)
Technical difficulties (kinked or clotted grafts)
Uncorrected structural defects
Nongraftable vessels, diffuse coronary artery disease
Residual or new valve pathology
Hypertrophic cardiomyopathy
Shunts
Pre-existing cardiac dysfunction
CPB-related factors
Excessive cardioplegia
Unrecognized cardiac distention

Inadequate cardiac performance must prompt a search for possible causes (Table 38-16); structural defects require more than mere regulation of inotropes or vasodilators. If the clinical picture is suggestive of coronary air emboli with diffuse ST segment elevation and a hypocontractile heart, continuous support on CPB with a high perfusion pressure and an empty ventricle is indicated to expel the air bubbles from the coronary circulation.

An approach to patients with inadequate cardiac output is summarized in Table 38-17. The heart rate is adjusted first. Following that, ventricular filling is optimized by transfusing blood from the CPB pump. It is important not to overdistend the heart by transfusing to an arbitrary level of filling pressure because this may result in further myocardial dysfunction. It is important to image the cardiac chambers by TEE and directly look at the heart when evaluating the response to small incremental volume infusions. The ratio of systemic to pulmonary artery pressure is also helpful[131]: Both pressures should increase in the same direction (as in Fig. 38-12A). Change in opposite directions (e.g., pulmonary pressure increases and systemic pressure decreases; Fig. 38-12C) is suggestive of LV failure.

If pharmacologic support is required, an integration of cardiac physiology (see Chapter 10) and pharmacology will lead to the rational selection of an appropriate drug or drugs. Numerous algorithms are available to guide decision making; one is presented in Figure 38-13. This algorithm uses systemic arterial and pulmonary artery pressures and cardiac output. If TEE is available, myocardial contractility and valvular function can be more readily assessed. After integrating available data, a diagnosis is made and appropriate treatment is begun. Continual reassessment of the situation is necessary to document the efficacy of treatment or to suggest new diagnoses and therapeutic approaches. If cardiac

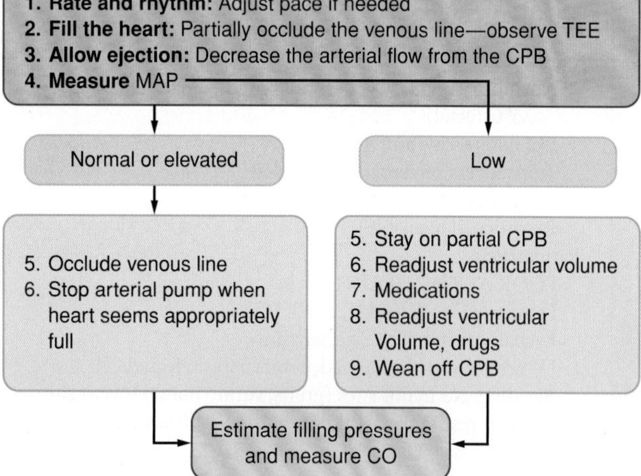

FIGURE 38-11. General approach to termination of cardiopulmonary bypass (CPB). TEE, transesophageal echocardiographic; MAP, mean arterial pressure; CO, cardiac output.

TABLE 38-17. STEPS FOR IMPROVING SYSTEMIC FLOW

1	Heart rate (A-, V-, A/V-pacing) and rhythm
2	Preload: Optimize (beware of altered compliance postbypass)
3–4	Afterload reduction if blood pressure is high and/or contractility augmentation (inotrope if low CO)
5	Preload: Recheck and adjust
6	Combine therapies
7	IABP
8	VAD

A, atrial; V, ventricular; CO, cardiac output; IABP, intra-aortic balloon pump; VAD, ventricular assist device.

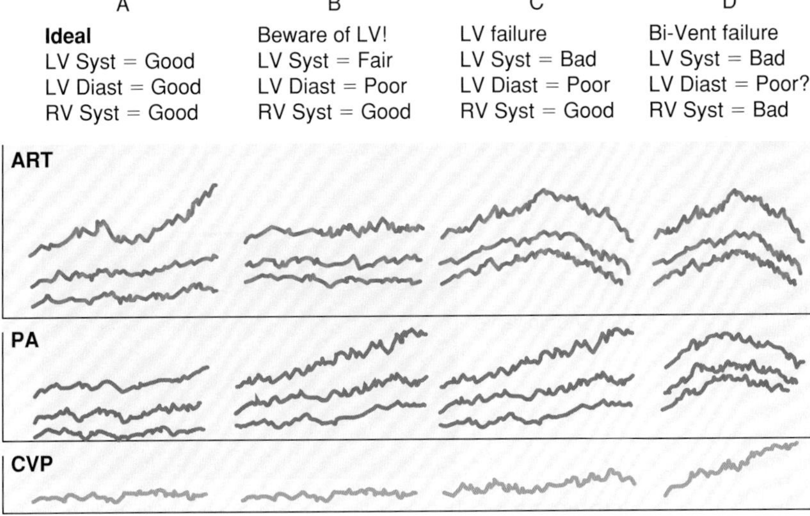

FIGURE 38-12. Hemodynamic abnormalities on termination of cardiopulmonary bypass. LV, left ventricle; syst, systolic; diast, diastolic; RV, right ventricle; ART, arterial pressure; PA, pulmonary artery; CVP, central venous pressure.

output is low and systemic pressure is adequate (Fig. 38-13A), an arteriolar dilator may improve forward flow by decreasing afterload. If systemic pressure is too low (Fig. 38-13C and D), thus prohibiting the use of vasodilators, an inotrope should be selected instead. Each inotropic drug has a distinct profile with respect to its effects on rate, contractility, SVR and PVR, and cardiac dysrhythmogenic potential (Table 38-18). If these initial therapies are
12 insufficient to promote adequate forward flow, various combinations of drugs may be tested. If systemic perfusion is still inadequate, mechanical circulatory support (MCS) is required.

A therapeutic approach to right ventricular failure (Fig. 38-13D) is outlined in Table 38-19. When pulmonary arterial pressure is normal or decreased, the cause is usually severe right ventricular ischemia secondary to intraoperative events or air. The initial response is to return to full CPB, improve perfusion, and await recovery and improvement of contractility. If this does not occur, inotropic and vasodilator therapy is established. In patients who have right ventricular failure secondary to high PVR, the mainstay of therapy is reduction of PVR with vasodilators, such as inhaled prostaglandin I_2 (PGE_2) or nitric oxide, and inotropic support. The phosphodiesterase III inhibitors, amrinone and milrinone, are particularly useful because they significantly decrease PVR and increase contractility. Overdistention of the ventricle must be assiduously avoided. Combination therapy with differential infusions refers to infusion of inotropes with vasoconstrictive properties into the left side of the circulation to maintain systemic perfusion, while avoiding an increase of the pulmonary circulation resistance. Persistent right ventricular failure precluding separation from CPB may require the insertion of a right ventricular assist device (RVAD).

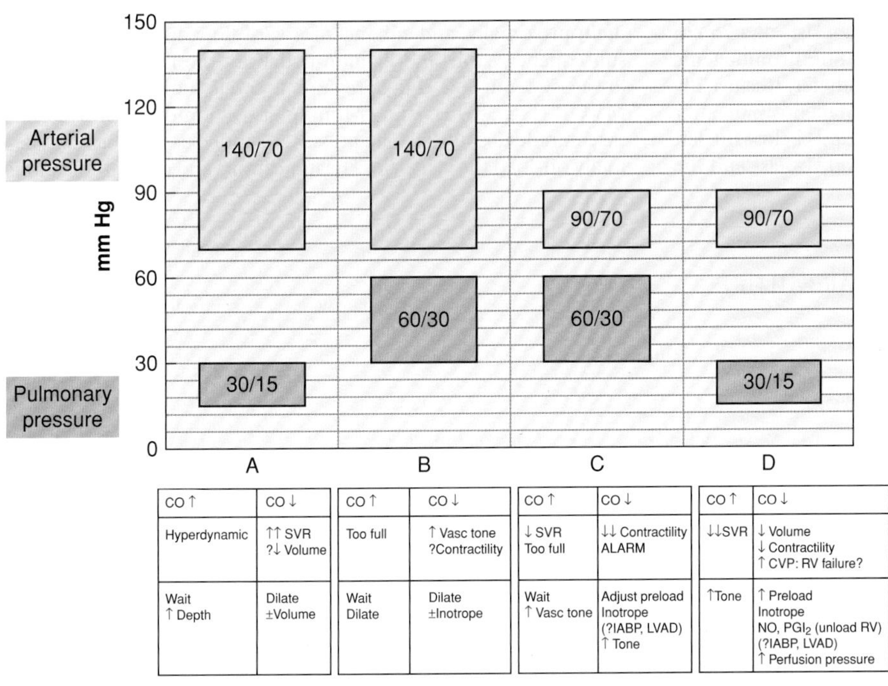

CO ↑	CO ↓	CO ↑	CO ↓	CO ↑	CO ↓	CO ↑	CO ↓
Hyperdynamic	↑↑ SVR ?↓ Volume	Too full	↑ Vasc tone ?Contractility	↓ SVR Too full	↓↓ Contractility ALARM	↓↓SVR	↓ Volume ↓ Contractility ↑ CVP: RV failure?
Wait ↑ Depth	Dilate ±Volume	Wait Dilate	Dilate ±Inotrope	Wait ↑ Vasc tone	Adjust preload Inotrope (?IABP, LVAD) ↑ Tone	↑Tone	↑ Preload Inotrope NO, PGI_2 (unload RV) (?IABP, LVAD) ↑ Perfusion pressure

FIGURE 38-13. Algorithm for the diagnosis and treatment of hemodynamic abnormalities on termination of cardiopulmonary bypass. CO, cardiac output; SVR, systemic vascular resistance; vasc, vascular; IABP, intra-aortic balloon pump; LVAD, left ventricular assist device; CVP, central venous pressure; RV, right ventricle; NO, nitric oxide; PGI_2, prostacyclin.

TABLE 38-18. MEDICATIONS GIVEN BY CONTINUOUS INFUSION

Drugs	Usual Initial Dose (μg/kg/min)	Usual Dose Range (μg/kg/min)
Amrinone[a]	2–5	2–20
Dopamine	2–5	2–20
Dobutamine	2–5	2–20
Epinephrine	0.01	0.01–0.1
Isoproterenol[b]	0.05–1	0.1–1
Lidocaine	20	20–50
Milrinone	50 μg/kg (over 3 min)	0.3–0.7
Nitroglycerin	0.5	0.5–5
Nitroprusside	0.5	0.5–5
Norepinephrine	0.1	0.1–1
Phenylephrine	1	1–3
Prostaglandin E_1	0.05–0.1	0.05–0.2
Vasopressin		0.0004

[a]Requires initial bolus of 750 μg/kg over 3 min before start of infusion.
[b]For chronotropic effect following cardiac transplantation, doses of 0.005–0.010 μg/kg/min are used.

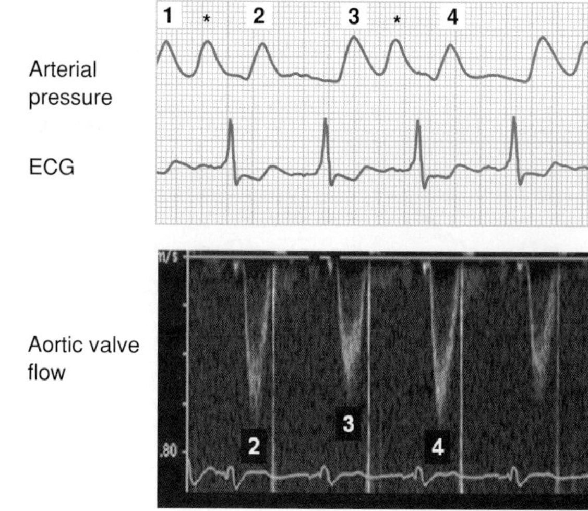

FIGURE 38-14. The physiologic effects of intra-aortic balloon pump (IABP) counterpulsation. The IABP is inflated during diastole (*asterisk*), every other beat (rate 1:2). The arterial systolic pressure is decreased after IABP augmentation (compare beats *2* and *4* with beats *1* and *3*). The diastolic arterial pressure is augmented during IABP inflation (*asterisk*). The flow through the aortic valve (approximate stroke volume) as demonstrated with pulsed wave Doppler echocardiography shows the increased forward flow after augmentation (beats *2* and *4*). ECG, electrocardiogram.

A retrospective study of 1,009 patients undergoing either CABG alone or in combination with valve surgery with CPB investigated the demographic, clinical, and echocardiographic factors associated with the use of inotropic support during separation from CPB. Wall motion score index, combined CABG and mitral valve surgery, LV ejection fraction <35%, reoperation, moderate-to-severe MR, and aortic cross-clamp time were independent predictors for use of inotropes (39% of patients).[132]

Intra-aortic Balloon Pump

The simplest and most readily available mechanical support device is the intra-aortic balloon pump.[132] It consists of a 25 cm long, sausage-shaped balloon composed of nonthrombogenic polyurethane mounted on a 90 cm vascular catheter. It is usually inserted into the femoral artery, either percutaneously or after surgical exposure, and advanced so the distal tip is below the left subclavian artery (to prevent emboli to the head vessels) and the proximal above the renal arteries.[133] Occasionally, when peripheral vascular disease prohibits passage of the balloon via the femoral artery, it is inserted via the ascending aorta.

The intra-aortic balloon pump decreases myocardial oxygen demand and increases oxygen supply to the myocardium. It uses synchronized counterpulsation to assist a beating, ejecting heart: Blood volume is moved in a direction "counter" to normal flow. The balloon is inflated during diastole and deflated during systole. The balloon inflation elevates aortic diastolic blood pressure (diastolic augmentation), thus increasing the coronary perfusion gradient proximally, and enhances forward flow distally. During the subsequent systole and balloon deflation, the LV ejects facing a lower systemic diastolic pressure (systolic unloading, reduced $\dot{M}VO_2$) (Fig. 38-14). Proper timing of balloon deflation is necessary to reduce end-diastolic pressure as much as possible to maximally off-load the ventricle. The indications and contraindications

TABLE 38-19. RIGHT VENTRICULAR FAILURE

	Pulmonary Artery Pressure			
	Increased		Normal or Decreased	
CVP	Increased	Decreased	Increased	Decreased
Diagnosis	RV and LV failure	LV failure	RV failure	
Management	Inhaled NO or PGI_2, PDE-III	Support on CPB		
	Inotropes		High perfusion pressure	
	Differential infusions		Volume (if CVP low)	
	RVAD		? CABG	

CVP, central venous pressure; RV, right ventricle; LV, left ventricle; NO, nitric oxide; PGI_2, prostaglandin I_2; PDE-III, phosphodiesterase III inhibitor; CPB, cardiopulmonary bypass; RVAD, right ventricular assist device; CABG, coronary artery bypass graft.

TABLE 38-20. INTRA-AORTIC BALLOON PUMP INDICATIONS AND CONTRAINDICATIONS

Indications

Complications of myocardial ischemia
- Hemodynamic: Cardiogenic shock
- Mechanical: Mitral regurgitation, ventricular septal defect
- Intractable dysrhythmias
- Extension of infarct: Postinfarction angina

Acute cardiac instability
- Angina: Unstable, preinfarction
- Catheterization laboratory mishap: Failed PTCA
- Bridge to transplantation
- Cardiac contusion
- ? Septic shock

Open heart surgery
- Separation from cardiopulmonary bypass
- Ventricular failure: Right or left
- Increasing inotropic requirement
- Progressive hemodynamic deterioration
- Refractory ischemia

Contraindications
- Severe aortic insufficiency
- Inability to insert
- Irreversible cardiac disease (patient is not a transplant candidate)
- Irreversible brain damage

PTCA, percutaneous transluminal coronary angioplasty.

for intra-aortic balloon pump placement are listed in Table 38-20. Myocardial function often improves with the use of the intra-aortic balloon pump, and systemic perfusion and vital organ function are preserved.[134] It is crucial to control heart rate and suppress atrial and ventricular dysrhythmias to ensure proper balloon timing. As cardiac function returns, the assist ratio is gradually weaned from every beat to every other beat and so on and, assuming no further cardiac deterioration, until it is removed.

Complications associated with the intra-aortic balloon pump are primarily related to ischemia distal to the site of balloon insertion. Direct trauma to the vessel, arterial obstruction, and thrombosis are most common, although aortic perforation and balloon rupture occur rarely. Platelet destruction and thrombocytopenia may also occur.

Ventricular Assist Device

Infrequently (1%), the heart is unable to meet systemic metabolic demands despite maximal pharmacologic therapy and insertion of the intra-aortic balloon pump. Under these circumstances, devices that actually pump blood and bypass either the LV or RV are required. MCS is increasingly an option for patients suffering from either an acute or chronic myocardial insult. In patients that are refractory to surgery (i.e., revascularization) and receiving maximal pharmacologic support, maintenance of systemic perfusion, correction of metabolic acidosis, ventricular decompression, and reduced myocardial oxygen consumption by MCS may aid in myocardial recovery. Where myocardial recovery is not possible, MCS can act as a bridge to allow for cardiac transplantation and has now become a destination therapy in its own right.

MCS can provide either short- or long-term support to a failing LV, left ventricular assist device (LVAD), RV, or RVAD, or provide biventricular support (BiVAD). The length of time needed will dictate the type of device that is used to provide MCS. For LV support, the blood is drained to the device (bypassing the failing ventricle) via a cannula placed in either the LA or the LV apex and is pumped into the systemic circulation via a cannula or graft placed in either the ascending or descending aorta. For RV support, a cannula is placed in the right atrium to divert blood from the RV, which is then pumped into the main pulmonary artery.

The types of MCS devices that are available include extracorporeal and fully implantable devices.[135] The extracorporeal devices use cannulae that divert the patient's blood to a pump or biohead that is outside the body and deliver it back to the systemic circulation. The fully implantable devices are placed in the patient's abdominal cavity with only the control lines exiting the body.

For acute short-term MCS of the LV, RV, or BiV the Thoratec® CentriMag® is often used. This device is composed of a single-use centrifugal pump, a motor, and a primary drive console. Using a bearingless magnetically levitated impeller, it provides continuous flow via a centrifugal-type rotary blood pump. The pump can rotate at speeds of 1,500 to 5,500 rpm and can provide flow rates of up to 9.9 L/minute. Other short-term devices include the Abiomed AB500™ (Abiomed, Danvers, MA) and Thoratec® PVAD™ (Thoratec Laboratories, Pleasanton, CA).[136]

Another intravascular device that may be used during high-risk coronary intervention or as a bridge to recovery is the Abiomed Impella™ (Abiomed). This device is a catheter-based intravascular microaxial blood pump. This axial flow pump is capable of delivering either 2.5 or 5 L/minute of flow (depending on the device used). It can be placed either percutaneously or via a cut down in either the femoral or axillary artery. The device is placed within the aorta with the distal/inflow portion crossing the AV and resting in the LV. LV blood is diverted to the outflow portion of the device via an impeller pump to the distal aorta providing improved systemic perfusion.[137]

Anesthetic Considerations for MCS

When considering an anesthetic plan for a patient requiring MCS one must take into account the patient's severe degree of myocardial dysfunction. This may include LV, RV, or BiV dysfunction. In addition to standard monitoring, preinduction arterial blood pressure monitoring is essential. The ablation of high sympathetic tone that heart failure patients possess may be catastrophic and cause cardiac arrest on the induction of anesthesia. As such, agents that maintain hemodynamic stability are chosen for these patients. These include the use of etomidate as an induction agent (due to its lack of vasodilatation and myocardial depression) and a careful "balanced technique." Incremental doses of midazolam and etomidate followed by a potent opioid (such as fentanyl or sufentanil) and neuromuscular blockade if titrated carefully are usually tolerated. One caveat is that, due to the slow circulation times in heart failure patients, care must be taken to allow medications time to circulate and reach the desired effect. Overzealous dosing may cause cardiovascular collapse. A good rule of thumb is that a 20% decrease in blood pressure should be treated using a direct acting agent such as phenylephrine or norepinephrine. This allows for a margin of safety and may prevent profound hypotension due to the long circulation time if the blood pressure is treated only as the patient becomes hypotensive. Volatile anesthetic agents are generally well tolerated in low doses; however, high doses of inhaled volatile agents can precipitant large changes in SVR and myocardial function. Following induction of anesthesia a PAC and TEE are routinely placed. The PAC provides important information such as central venous pressure (indication of RV function), pulmonary artery pressures, mixed venous oxygen saturation, and cardiac output. TEE is used in both the pre- and postimplant period.

Important information that needs to be determined by TEE prior to the initiation of CPB include anything that would restrict or impair LVAD filling (mitral stenosis, tricuspid regurgitation, severe RV dysfunction), the presence of aortic insufficiency (causing LV dilatation), and other anatomic issues that impact LVAD placement (PFO/ASD, intracardiac thrombus, severe atherosclerosis of the ascending aorta). Postimplant TEE is used to assess the adequacy of de-airing maneuvers, proper cannula position, and RV size and function.[138]

Considerations for VAD Patients

An in-depth discussion of the considerations for VAD patients is beyond the scope of this chapter and the reader is advised to consult one of the excellent review articles on the subject.[139]

Whether RVAD or LVAD support is required, several issues exist in common for both. In each case, maintenance of adequate preload is essential for proper device function. Once the failing ventricle is mechanically supported, the "cardiac output" of that chamber(s) is dependent upon adequate preload to fill the device and normal to low vascular resistance to promote forward flow and provide adequate systemic perfusion. Low to normal PVR is especially important in patients with an LVAD. The RV is exquisitely sensitive to changes in afterload and a failing RV will not "fill" the left side of the heart and therefore limit LVAD output. Despite extreme care, severe RV failure requiring biventricular support still occurs in approximately 30% of patients requiring an LVAD. Inotropic agents such as epinephrine, dobutamine, and milrinone as well as inhaled agents such as nitric oxide and iloprost are often used to support the RV and help maintain low PVR. Unfortunately, agents that lower PVR also tend to lower SVR. In addition, patients undergoing LVAD implantation tend to manifest profound vasodilatation following CPB. Vasopressin by virtue of not increasing PVR is preferred over norepinephrine as a vasopressor especially in patients with pulmonary hypertension.[140]

For patients on MCS that require noncardiac surgery the maintenance of adequate volume status and careful safeguarding of low to normal vascular resistance is important. The use of a PAC or TEE should be tailored to the specific patient and procedure. However, TEE is recommended in the case of patients with impaired RV function or in procedures with the potential for large volume shifts/transfusion requirements. No specific anesthetic technique is recommended in patients with MCS; however, abrupt changes in SVR due to neuraxial techniques such as spinal anesthesia make them less desirable. Patients with fully implantable devices should be considered at risk for pulmonary aspiration and treated accordingly.[141–143] Of note, in the event of cardiac arrest, chest compression is contraindicated due to the possible disruption or displacement of the VAD cannulae.

Postcardiopulmonary Bypass

The procedure is not over when the patient is safely "off pump." Continued vigilance is mandatory during decannulation, protamine administration, "drying up," and chest closure. Anesthetics are administered as clinically indicated. Atrial or junctional dysrhythmias may be caused by removal of the atrial cannulae, but often disappear once they are out. Heparin is reversed with protamine following removal of the venous cannulae; the arterial return cannula remains in place for continued transfusion of pump contents. When this is completed and bleeding is controlled, the arterial cannula is removed, and after bleeding is considered to be under control, the chest is closed. During decannulation, the possibility exists for unexpected bleeding from the atrial or aortic suture lines, and this sometimes requires rapid transfusion. Continued vigilance for new ischemia (manifested by ST segment changes, ectopy, atrial dysrhythmia, regional wall motion abnormalities by TEE) is important because it may indicate a correctable problem with the grafts. Valve patients should have the adequacy of the repair or replacement (i.e., perivalvular leak, residual stenosis) assessed by TEE.

Reversal of Anticoagulation

Protamine, a polycationic protein derived from salmon sperm, is used to neutralize heparin. The initial and total doses administered vary widely. Some use a fixed ratio of protamine to heparin, others use 1-mg protamine to 100-U heparin, and still others look to automated protamine titrations to suggest the initial dose. Regardless of the method selected, further requirements are assessed by repeated measures of the activated coagulation time or other clotting assay(s), as well as by the appearance of the surgical field.[144]

Protamine administration is associated with a broad spectrum of hemodynamic effects.[145] Idiosyncratic responses include type I anaphylactic reactions and both immediate and delayed anaphylactoid responses. True anaphylaxis, mercifully rare, is characterized by increased airway pressure, decreased SVR with systemic hypotension, and skin flushing. Increased incidence of reactions has been reported in patients sensitized to protamine from previous cardiac catheterization, hemodialysis, cardiac surgery, or exposure to neutral protamine Hagedorn insulin. Perhaps the most devastating complication associated with protamine is sudden and profound pulmonary hypertension accompanied by an elevated central venous pressure, a flaccid distended RV, and systemic hypotension. This complication, which may occur in approximately 1% of patients, is mediated by release of thromboxane and C5a anaphylatoxin. The reaction is extremely short-lived, and although reinstitution of bypass is required on rare occasions, it is usually not necessary. Whether protamine is administered via the RA, LA, or aorta, or peripherally, probably makes no difference to the occurrence of this rare reaction. Because systemic hypotension is more likely with rapid injection of protamine, slow administration into a peripheral venous site is advisable.

Postbypass Bleeding

Persistent oozing following heparin reversal is not uncommon. The usual causes include inadequate surgical hemostasis or reduced platelet count or function, and neither is identified by a prolonged activated coagulation time. Insufficient doses of protamine, dilution of coagulation factors, thrombocytopenia, and platelet dysfunction, and rarely "heparin rebound," belong in the differential diagnosis.

After adequate hemostasis is obtained, the chest is closed. This is occasionally associated with transient decreases in blood pressure, which usually respond to volume infusion. If hypotension persists, the chest should be reopened to rule out cardiac tamponade, a kinked graft, or other problems.

As the surgeon completes skin closure, the anesthesiologist prepares for an orderly transfer of the patient from the operating room to the recovery room or ICU. Medicated infusions must be maintained, as clinically indicated, with portable infusion pumps. Additional syringes with emergency cardiac medications and necessary equipment for airway management should be carried, and blood pressure(s) and ECG constantly monitored.

MINIMALLY INVASIVE CARDIAC SURGERY

Despite advantages in cardiac surgery and perfusion technology, the deleterious effects of CPB and aortic cross-clamping are well documented. The desire to avoid these complications, as well as complications associated with sternotomy, was a factor leading to the development of minimally invasive techniques not requiring CPB. As the population ages, older patients with multiple comorbid medical conditions requiring surgery are increasingly common. Avoidance of aortic manipulation and cross-clamping especially in elderly patients is associated with lower stroke rates.[146]

Newer procedures include MIDCAB (minimally invasive direct coronary artery bypass), OPCAB (off-pump coronary artery bypass), robotic surgery,[147] and more recently, percutaneous valve repair/replacement performed in the catheterization laboratory or a hybrid operating room.[148] Initially, MIDCAB was described as an alternative to angioplasty for single-vessel left anterior descending coronary (LAD) artery disease. To access the LAD and provide adequate exposure for graft anastomosis, MIDCAB was initially performed via a left thoracotomy using one-lung ventilation. MIDCAB success allowed the development of other forms of minimally invasive surgery. These include the use of parasternal and inframammary incisions, minithoracotomies, and partial sternotomy. Despite effectively decreasing complications seen from sternotomy (large scar, infection, brachial plexus palsy, and 4- to 8-week recovery period) these alternate incisions provide limited exposure and increase surgical difficulty. Another type of minimally invasive cardiac surgery uses port access technology, these days with the assistance of a robotic system. Catheters are placed percutaneously in the femoral artery and internal jugular vein to facilitate CPB. These catheters include an endovascular aortic balloon that acts as cross-clamp, a modified PAC to act as an LV vent, and a coronary sinus catheter placed for retrograde cardioplegia administration.

Following success with minimally invasive surgery, the time was right for the development of OPCAB surgery, in which exposure is via a sternotomy but CPB is not used. The first experiences with off-pump surgery were "simple" left internal mammary artery (LIMA) to LAD grafts supplemented with angioplasty. OPCAB then developed into complete multivessel coronary revascularizations. The development of retractors and stabilization devices allows the surgeon to operate on the beating heart without the need for bradycardia and without causing hypotension. Other advances include the use of intracoronary shunts and sutureless anastomotic devices.

Changes in surgical technique have forced changes in anesthetic technique.[149] High-dose narcotics were abandoned in favor of shorter-acting agents that facilitate early extubation. In addition, the lull period seen on CPB was replaced by the need to constantly monitor hemodynamics and intervene rapidly in the face of changing hemodynamics. Use of an arterial line is mandatory as changes in hemodynamics occur rapidly and may be catastrophic during cardiac manipulation. Central access is also necessary for the infusion of drugs and volume. The use of a PAC is not mandatory but does provide information about filling pressures as well as cardiac output measurements. One major problem associated with OPCAB is that exposure of the diseased coronaries and subsequent graft placement often requires positioning of the heart that is associated with hypotension and ischemia. Unfortunately, standard monitors used in cardiac surgery may not be useful in detecting this ischemia. In OPCAB surgery, positioning and retraction of the heart often results in a low-amplitude ECG with axis deviation. These changes may cause ST-T wave changes to be obscured or falsely minimized. Because the heart is obscured by laparotomy pads in the pericardial well or being lifted out of the chest, TEE may be unreliable in detecting regional wall motion changes signifying ischemia. Sudden changes in pulmonary artery pressure may be related to acute MR due to surgical positioning. In addition, displacement of the heart may cause falsely elevated central venous and pulmonary pressures despite the presence of hypovolemia. Direct observation of the heart and communication with the surgeon are critical in managing hemodynamic swings.[150,151]

As a rule, the most critical lesion is bypassed last and the least critical performed first. The coronary artery to be anastomosed must be isolated proximally and distally. This is performed using either an occluder clip or a snare. Following occlusion, there is usually a period of myocardial ischemia distal to the occlusion. Preexisting high-grade lesions might have caused formation of collateral circulation, which may ameliorate potential ischemia. Right coronary lesions will predispose to bradycardia, atrial dysrhythmias, and heart block. As a result, immediate access to cardiac pacing and cardioversion are essential. Left-sided coronary lesions may cause malignant ventricular dysrhythmias and hemodynamic collapse. Using inotropes, vasoconstrictors, and volume, sudden hemodynamic collapse may be rescued but may necessitate placement of an intra-aortic balloon pump or conversion to full CPB.

Several techniques are used to avoid rapid hemodynamic changes. These include optimizing preload prior to positioning, judicious use of inotropes and α-agonists, and placing the patient in Trendelenburg position, which allows redistribution of intravascular volume to support the heart in the vertical position.

Normothermia contributes to early extubation as well as prevention of coagulopathy. Aggressive pain control improves patient satisfaction and contributes to early extubation. Techniques for pain control in OPCAB and minimally invasive surgery include systemic opioids and nonsteroidal agents such as ketorolac (in patients without renal insufficiency), local infiltration of the surgical incision, and regional anesthesia. Regional techniques including thoracic epidurals and neuraxial narcotics are used with great success, although anticoagulation is a concern in patients with central regional anesthetics.[152] Anticoagulant protocols are controversial. Both heparin and protamine doses vary between centers. Some do not routinely reverse heparin or administer reduced doses of protamine because of the suspicion that OPCAB may cause hypercoagulability.[153]

Despite great interest in OPCAB as a way to decrease the complications associated with CPB, many remain skeptical as to the benefits. Several studies have shown the superiority of OPCAB in regard to improved neurologic outcome, while others have not.[154,155] Despite disappointing results in regard to neurocognitive and overall outcome, several short-term outcomes are improved following OPCABG. These include shorter ICU stays, decreased utilization of hospital resources, and decreased incidence of atrial fibrillation.[156]

Many have argued that the advantages of traditional CABG over CPB include a still bloodless field allowing for a better anastomosis and long-term graft patency.[157] Other studies have refuted this to prove equal long-term graft patency rates.[158] The proponents of OPCAB tend to be very familiar with the technique and perform off-pump surgery frequently. This frequency seems to make them technically facile in the peculiarities unique to OPCAB surgery. As such, this may account for varying results from center to center. Currently, there is no consensus as to the superiority of standard CABG versus OPCAB.

Relatively new to the area of minimally invasive cardiac surgery is endoscopic and robotic cardiac surgery. In these techniques, trocars are placed in the chest in anatomic locations to allow the use of long-handled surgical instruments or manipulators.

Supporters of its routine use cite decreased pain, faster healing, and greater patient satisfaction. Anesthetic considerations for endoscopic and robotic surgery are similar to those for standard minimally invasive off-pump surgery. These include one-lung ventilation, positioning issues, and normothermia.

POSTOPERATIVE CONSIDERATIONS

Bring Backs

Postoperative re-exploration is needed in 4% to 5% of cases. The indications are persistent bleeding, cardiac tamponade, and, infrequently, unexplained poor cardiac performance. Surgery is usually required within the first 24 hours but also later in cases of delayed tamponade. The possibility of cardiac tamponade must always be included in the differential diagnosis of the postoperative "dwindles" because the classic symptoms and signs are often absent.

Tamponade

In tamponade, the intracardiac pressures are deceptively elevated and do not reflect the actual volume state. Because the surrounding (intrapericardial) pressure is increased, the distending pressure (transmural pressure = intracavitary pressure – extracavitary pressure) is actually decreased. Cardiac chamber collapse is a critical feature of cardiac tamponade, and the chambers with the lowest intracardiac pressure (atria in systole and RV in diastole) are most likely to be compressed. The stroke volume is limited, and cardiac output depends on heart rate. Compensatory mechanisms include peripheral vasoconstriction to preserve venous return and systemic blood pressure, as well as tachycardia. Myocardial ischemia may occur because of the tachycardia and reduced coronary perfusion pressure.

Clinically, patients present with dyspnea, orthopnea, tachycardia, paradoxical pulse, and hypotension, but the intubated, sedated, and mechanically ventilated patient in the postanesthesia care unit following cardiac surgery may have varied clinical and hemodynamic presentations. Owing to its often atypical presentation in the cardiac surgical patient, the diagnosis of tamponade should be considered whenever hemodynamic deterioration or signs of low-output failure occur in these patients. In postoperative cardiac patients, the pericardium is no longer intact, and loculated areas of clot may compress only one chamber, causing isolated increases in filling pressure (i.e., mimicking right and/or left ventricular dysfunction). Urine output is usually diminished. Serial chest films typically show progressive mediastinal widening. The diagnosis of tamponade may be confirmed by transthoracic echocardiography (TTE) or TEE. Diastolic collapse of the RA and right ventricular and/or LV diastolic collapse are the most sensitive and specific signs of cardiac tamponade.[159] In addition, there is excessive respiratory variation of the Doppler flow velocities across the tricuspid and mitral valves. Because of the existing extracardiac compression, respiration increases the ventricular interdependence and affects the diastolic filling of the two ventricles differently. During mechanical inspiration, the increased intrathoracic pressure will impede the right ventricular and augment the LV filling. The pulsed wave Doppler echocardiographic examination of the diastolic tricuspid flow will show marked decrease as the already compromised filling gradient between the extrathoracic veins and the intrathoracic RV is further reduced. During the same time, the diastolic mitral flow will increase as the increased intrathoracic pressure is transmitted to the intrathoracic pulmonary veins, increasing the filling gradient of the LV. The opposite effects take place during mechanical exhalation when the effects of positive ventilation dissipate. The TTE approach may have important limitations: A retrosternal collection may be very difficult to be visualized in a postoperative patient, and subcostal views are rarely feasible early in the postoperative period because of the presence of chest tubes, pacemaker wires, and/or local tenderness in the subxiphoid area. Therefore, TEE is a better diagnostic tool in the immediate postoperative period.

The cure for cardiac tamponade is surgical; anesthetics can only further depress cardiac function. Therefore, drugs are selected that will preserve the compensatory mechanisms sustaining forward flow. Drugs with vasodilator (either venous or arteriolar) or myocardial depressant properties should be avoided in patients with serious hemodynamic compromise; dosages of induction agents should be appropriately reduced. Ketamine, because of its sympathomimetic effects, may be helpful in preserving heart rate and blood pressure response. It is not, however, a panacea and can induce hypotension in patients under maximal sympathetic stress. If on reopening the chest there is minimal fluid or if the patient shows little improvement, a thorough search for other causes of inadequate cardiac performance, such as clotted or kinked grafts, myocardial ischemia, or valve malfunction, is indicated.

Pain Management

Early awakening and extubation have brought the problem of postoperative pain management in cardiac surgery into focus. The standard practice has been intravenous opioids given as needed followed by conversion to oral pain medications. However, the quest is on to find an ideal postoperative pain management technique to complement the goal of early extubation and maximize patient satisfaction.[160] Several studies have shown the benefits of intrathecal administration of opioids.[161] The addition of nonsteroidal anti-inflammatory agents may play an increasing role. In cardiac patients with severe pain associated with sternal fractures due to the sternal retraction device during internal mammary harvest, epidural analgesia has been shown to be safe and effective and results in improved postoperative pulmonary function.

ANESTHESIA FOR CHILDREN WITH CONGENITAL HEART DISEASE

Because "anatomy dictates the physiology," the anesthetic management of children with congenital heart disease (CHD) requires knowledge of anatomic defects, planned surgical procedures, and comprehensive understanding of the altered physiology. The overall incidence of CHD varies between 4 and 12 per 1,000 live births. CHD can be cyanotic or acyanotic. The best way to understand the impact of a congenital defect and how anesthetic agents will interact with this defect is to envision the path blood must follow to maintain flow to the pulmonary arteries and aorta. Table 38-21 classifies various types of lesions by their physiologic impact; however, it must be remembered that there is often more than one defect present.

Preoperative Evaluation

History

In infancy, heart failure usually becomes manifest through feeding difficulties, easy fatigability, vomiting, lethargy, and labored

TABLE 38-21. PHYSIOLOGIC EFFECTS OF CONGENITAL CARDIAC LESIONS

Volume overload of the ventricle or atrium resulting in increased pulmonary blood flow
- Atrial septal defect (high flow, low pressure)
- Ventricular septal defect (high flow, high pressure)
- Patent ductus arteriosus (high flow, high pressure)
- Endocardial cushion defect (high flow, high pressure)

Cyanosis resulting from obstruction to pulmonary blood flow
- Tetralogy of Fallot
- Tricuspid atresia
- Pulmonary atresia

Pressure overload to the ventricle
- Aortic stenosis
- Coarctation of the aorta
- Pulmonary stenosis

Cyanosis due to a common mixing chamber
- Total anomalous venous return
- Truncus arteriosus
- Double outlet right ventricle
- Single ventricle

Cyanosis due to separation of the systemic and pulmonary circulation
- Transposition of the great vessels

TABLE 38-22. CLASSIFICATION OF CARDIAC MURMURS

Systolic
- Stenotic semilunar valves
- Regurgitant atrioventricular valves
- Atrial septal defect
- Ventricular septal defect
- Coarctation of the aorta
- Still murmur

Diastolic
- Regurgitant semilunar valves
- Stenotic atrioventricular valves
- Mitral flow rumble
- Tricuspid flow rumble

Continuous
- Patent ductus arteriosus
- Arteriovenous fistula
- Excessive bronchial collaterals
- Aortopulmonary window
- Venous hum
- Surgical shunt
- Severe peripheral pulmonic stenosis

breathing. In the older child, heart failure causes easy fatigability, shortness of breath, and dyspnea on exertion. Child's age and weight, presence of an upper respiratory tract infection, baseline arterial saturation, and anticipated durations of surgery and CPB must be taken into consideration.[162]

In addition, a detailed medication and surgical history should be obtained. The previous surgical procedures may be key to understanding the patient's anatomy.

Physical Examination

The physical examination of a child should seek signs and symptoms of poorly compensated congenital cardiac lesions. These children most often present with failure to thrive, which could be due to pulmonary hypertension and/or poor peripheral oxygenation and organ perfusion. The physical examination should seek to discover other signs of congestive heart failure, such as irritability, diaphoresis, tachycardia, rales, jugular venous distention, and hepatomegaly. Clinical examination of extremities should include evaluation of cyanosis, clubbing, edema, pulse volume, and blood pressure. In children with Blalock–Taussig shunts (subclavian artery to pulmonary artery), upper extremity pulses may be absent or reduced on the side of the shunt. It is important to measure blood pressure in the arms as well as in the legs in all patients in whom CHD is suspected; thus, coarctation of aorta will not be missed. Auscultation of the heart in these patients can reveal different types of murmurs depending on the lesions (Table 38-22).

The possibility of associated congenital anomalies should be considered. The overall incidence of extracardiac anomalies among children with CHD may be as high as 20%.[163]

Laboratory Evaluations

The presence of anemia in these patients may require priming of the extracorporeal circuit with red blood cells. Children with cyanotic lesions manifest with polycythemia. Polycythemia results as a consequence of bone marrow stimulation (via release of erythropoietin from the kidneys) from arterial desaturation. Increased red cell mass can lead to hyperviscosity, peripheral sludging, and reduced oxygen delivery. Sludging is augmented by dehydration from preoperative fasting and by hypothermia from low ambient operating room temperatures. In patients with hematocrit >70%, consideration should be given to preoperative electrophoresis if symptomatic hyperviscosity is present. Cyanotic children with low hematocrit may exhibit hypoxic spells more readily than if the hematocrit were normal. Polycythemia can induce a low-grade disseminated intravascular coagulation with activation of fibrinolysis, degranulation of platelets, and consumption of coagulation factors. Newborns often have inadequate liver-dependent coagulation factors because of immaturity of hepatic function. Platelet count, prothrombin time, and partial thromboplastin time should be evaluated.

Children on diuretic therapy are at risk for hypokalemia, particularly if they are receiving digitalis. Infants, particularly those with congestive heart failure, are also at risk for both hypoglycemia and hypocalcemia. Children who have undergone major cardiac procedures earlier in their lives may have been exposed to blood or blood products and are at increased risk of having abnormal serum antibodies to various blood antigens. Hence, samples of a child's blood should be sent to the blood bank for possible cross-matching.

Cardiac Evaluations

Echocardiography delineates most of the cardiac anatomy and permits noninvasive measurement of ventricular size and function, cardiac output, and severity of valve dysfunction. Cardiac catheterization is reserved for patients with poor echocardiographic windows and when there is intervening bone or air-filled lung (e.g., scoliosis or abnormalities of the peripheral pulmonary arteries). The chest radiograph of a child with CHD should be evaluated for cardiac position, size, shape, abnormal vessels, right aortic arch, scimitar syndrome (hypoplasia/aplasia of one or more lobes of right lung and hypoplasia of right pulmonary artery), aberrant pulmonary vessels, abnormal position of bronchi, vascular rings, or associated pulmonary abnormalities (e.g., pneumonia, atelectasis, or emphysema). The ECG should be reviewed for rate and rhythm abnormalities.

Premedication

The purpose of the premedication is to have a calm child without oversedation, loss of protective airway reflexes, or hemodynamic compromise. This will facilitate the separation of the child from the parents and ease the fear and anxiety associated with the perioperative period. Details on this topic are provided in Chapter 42.

Monitoring

In addition to standard monitors, additional monitors used during open heart procedures include peripheral and central temperature monitoring, invasive blood pressure monitoring, central venous pressure monitoring (which can include right atrial or left atrial pressure line placement by the surgeon intraoperatively), and TEE.

Anesthetic and Intraoperative Management

Inhalational agents hold a prominent place as induction as well as maintenance agents in pediatric cardiac anesthesia. However, patients with poor ventricular function and those with critical dependence on SVR and/or PVR will need intravenous access preinduction and avoidance or limitation of anesthetic agents that can further compromise hemodynamic function. The choice of anesthetic agents following induction is governed by ventricular function (presence or absence of congestive failure), anticipated use of CPB, and the possibility of mechanical ventilation or tracheal extubation at the end of the case. Opioids are used routinely to limit the stress response in the prebypass phase of pediatric cardiac surgery. Neonates and infants undergoing cardiac surgery and deep hypothermic CPB can generate a significant hormonal stress response. No specific relationship between opioid dose and stress response has been established. Details of dose and side effects are provided in Chapters 41 and 42. Of special note is the marked reduction in neuromuscular blocking requirements during hypothermic bypass.

The many advances in the CPB and surgical and anesthetic techniques have significantly improved the survival of children with CHD.[164] However, CPB produces marked hemostatic derangements including:

- Dilution of blood clotting factors
- Activation of the clotting cascade and consumption of clotting factors and platelets
- Reduction in coagulation enzymatic activity
- Activation of the fibrinolytic pathway.

Aminocaproic acid or tranexamic acid has been used to attenuate coagulopathy during pediatric cardiac surgery associated with CPB.

Hemodilution is a prominent problem in CPB in pediatric and neonatal populations. Modified ultrafiltration during pediatric CPB reduces total body water and serum levels of inflammatory mediators. In neonates, modified ultrafiltration results in an elevated hematocrit, improved pulmonary compliance in the immediate postbypass period, and probably improved cerebral metabolic recovery after deep hypothermic circulatory arrest, although the long-term benefit on outcome is unclear.[165] Separation from CPB will require pharmacologic and/or pacing support in some patients. In lesions in which the presence of increased PVR is known or suspected, addition of nitric oxide may be of benefit. Inhaled nitric oxide works via cGMP, causing pulmonary vasodilatation. It is truly selective for the pulmonary vascular bed and, in addition, should improve the ventilation/perfusion matching in the lungs.

Drugs that are useful in the postbypass period are given in Table 38-18.

Tracheal Extubation and Postoperative Ventilation

Children with simple lesions who have undergone CPB for procedures that do not involve ventricular incisions (atrial septal defect, ventricular septal defect without failure repaired across the tricuspid valve) can often have the endotracheal tubes removed at the conclusion of surgery or shortly thereafter in the ICU.[166,167]

Children most at risk for ventilatory failure following cardiac surgery include:

- Patients with complex surgeries requiring long bypass time and circulatory arrest time
- Patients less than a year of age and those well under their predicted weight
- Patients with Down syndrome
- Patients with pulmonary hypertension requiring preoperative ventilatory support
- Patients with postoperative cardiovascular and pulmonary complications.

In some cases, nasal continuous positive airway pressure can be employed instead of mechanical ventilation. In patients with Fontan physiology (passive pulmonary circulatory), decreasing PVR is paramount and is very much dependent on adequate ventilation, usually through mechanical means. The potentially detrimental effects of endotracheal intubation and positive pressure ventilation offset this advantage. Positive pressure ventilation is known to have a deleterious effect on pulmonary blood flow in patients with Fontan physiology. Resumption of pain-free spontaneous respiration does enhance hemodynamic performance in these patients.[166]

Regional anesthetic techniques can be used to supplement intraoperative anesthesia and provide postoperative analgesia. For example, caudal (epidural) opioids can be used in repair of coarctation of the aorta in the older child or ligation of a patent ductus arteriosus. Some physicians have used caudal or intrathecal morphine for cases involving CPB (and concomitant heparin administration), although this is not a common practice. The recommendation has been made that one allow 60 minutes to elapse between placement of a neuraxial block and administration of heparin, although there is no evidence to support this time interval.[168] Reported benefits of regional techniques include decreased stress response, improved pulmonary and gastrointestinal function, and resultant potential for cost reduction.[169] However, it is difficult to establish the superiority of a regional technique compared with intravenous analgesia.[170]

Hybrid Procedures in Pediatric Cardiac Surgery

Hybrid pediatric cardiac surgery is an emerging field that reaches across interdisciplinary lines and combines skills and techniques traditionally used by pediatric cardiac surgeons and interventional pediatric cardiologists. Advantages of hybrid procedure are real-time feedback obtained by continuous transesophageal echocardiographic monitoring, avoidance of CPB, ventricular incisions, or muscle transections.[171]

References

1. Landesberg G. The pathophysiology of perioperative myocardial infarction: Facts and perspectives. *J Cardiothorac Vasc Anesth.* 2003;17:90.
2. Biccrd BM, Rodseth RN. The pathophysiology of peri-operative myocardial infarction. *Anaesthesia.* 2010;65:733.
3. Weber KT, Janicki JS. The metabolic demand and oxygen supply of the heart: Physiologic and clinical considerations. *Am J Cardiol.* 1979;44:22.
4. Hoffman J. Transmural myocardial perfusion. *Prog Cardiovasc Dis.* 1987;29:429.
5. Bassenge E, Heusch G. Endothelial and neuro-humoral control of coronary blood flow in health and disease. *Rev Physiol Biochem Pharmacol.* 1990;116:77.
6. Prinzmetal M, Kennamer R, Merliss R. Angina pectoris: A variant form of angina pectoris. *Am J Med.* 1959;27:375.
7. Hansson GK. Mechanisms of disease. Inflammation, atherosclerosis, and coronary artery disease. *N Engl J Med.* 2005;352:1685.
8. Brown BG, Bolson EL, Dodge HT. Dynamic mechanisms in human coronary stenosis. *Circulation.* 1984;70:917.
9. Freudenberg H, Lichtlen PR. The normal wall segment in coronary stenoses – a post-mortem study. *Z Kardiol.* 1981;70:863.
10. Hindler K, Eltzschig HK, Fox AA, et al. Influence of statins on perioperative outcomes. *J Cardiothorac Vasc Anesth.* 2006;20:251.
11. Ferrari R, Guardigli G, Ceconi C. Secondary prevention of CAD with ACE inhibitors: A struggle between life and death of the endothelium. *Cardiovasc Drugs Ther.* 2010;24:331.
12. De Hert SG, Turani F, Mathur S, et al. Cardioprotection with volatile anesthetics: Mechanisms and clinical implications. *Anesth Analg.* 2005;100:1584–1593.
13. Brazier J, Cooper N, Buckberg GD. The adequacy of subendocardial oxygen delivery: The interaction of determinants of flow, arterial oxygen content and myocardial oxygen need. *Circulation.* 1974;49:968.
14. Ramsay SD, Saint S, Sullivan SD, et al. Clinical and economic effects of pulmonary artery catheterization in nonemergent coronary artery bypass graft surgery. *J Cardiothorac Vasc Anesth.* 2000;14:113.
15. London MJ, Moritz TE, Henderson WG, et al. Standard versus fiberoptic pulmonary artery catheterization for cardiac surgery in the Department of Veteran Affairs: A prospective, observational, multicenter analysis. *Anesthesiology.* 2002;96:860.
16. Leung JM, O'Kelly B, Browner WS, et al. Prognostic importance of postbypass regional wall-motion abnormalities in patients undergoing coronary artery bypass graft surgery. *Anesthesiology.* 1989;71:16.
17. Haggmark S, Hohner P, Ostman M, et al. Comparison of hemodynamic, electrocardiographic, mechanical, and metabolic indicators of intraoperative myocardial ischemia in vascular surgical patients with coronary artery disease. *Anesthesiology.* 1989;70:19.
18. Tuman KJ, McCarthy RJ, Spiess BD, et al. Effect of pulmonary artery catheterization on outcome in patients undergoing coronary artery surgery. *Anesthesiology.* 1989;70:199.
19. Fontes ML, Bellows W, Ngo L, et al. Assessment of ventricular function in critically ill patients: Limitations of pulmonary artery catheterization. *J Cardiothorac Vasc Anesth.* 1999;13:521.
20. Sandham JD, Hull RD, Brant RF, et al. A randomized, controlled trial of the use of pulmonary-artery catheters in high-risk surgical patients. *N Engl J Med.* 2003;348:5.
21. Djajani G, Karski J, Yudin M, et al. Clinical outcomes in patients undergoing elective coronary artery bypass graft surgery with and without utilization of pulmonary artery catheter-generated data. *J Cardiothorac Vasc Anesth.* 2006;20:307.
22. Practice guidelines for pulmonary artery catheterization: An updated report by the American Society of Anesthesiologists Task Force on Pulmonary Artery Catheterization. *Anesthesiology.* 2003;99:988–1014.
23. Squara P, Bennett D, Perret C. Pulmonary artery catheter: Does the problem lie in the users? *Chest.* 2002;121:2009.
24. Thys DM, Abel MD, Brooker RF, et al. Practice guidelines for perioperative transesophageal echocardiography. *Anesthesiology.* 2010;112:1084.
25. Miller JP, Lambert AS, Shapiro WA, et al. The adequacy of basic intraoperative transesophageal echocardiography performed by experienced anesthesiologists. *Anesth Analg.* 2001;92:1103.
26. Mathew JP, Fontes ML, Garwood S, et al. Transesophageal echocardiography interpretation: A comparative analysis between cardiac anesthesiologists and primary echocardiographers. *Anesth Analg.* 2002;94:302.
27. Shanewise JS, Cheung AT, Aronson S, et al. ASE/SCA guidelines for performing a comprehensive intraoperative multiplane transesophageal echocardiographic examination: Recommendations of the American Society of Echocardiography council for intraoperative echocardiography and the Society of Cardiovascular Anesthesiologists task force for certification in perioperative transesophageal echocardiography. *Anesth Analg.* 1999;89:870.
28. Cheng DC. Fast track cardiac surgery pathways: Early extubation, process of care, and cost containment. *Anesthesiology.* 1998;88:1429.
29. Myles PS, Daly DJ, Djaiani G, et al. A systematic review of the safety and effectiveness of fast-track cardiac anesthesia. *Anesthesiology.* 2003;99:982.
30. Ranta SO, Herranen P, Hynynen M. Patients' conscious recollections from cardiac anesthesia. *J Cardiothorac Vasc Anesth.* 2002;16:426.
31. London MJ, Shroyer AL, Coll JR, et al. Early extubation following cardiac surgery in a veterans population. *Anesthesiology.* 1998;88:1429.
32. Engoren M, Luther G, Fenn-Buderer N. A comparison of fentanyl, sufentanil, and remifentanil for fast-track cardiac anesthesia. *Anesth Analg.* 2001;93:859.
33. Murphy GS, Szokol JW, Marymont JH, et al. The effects of morphine and fentanyl on the inflammatory response to cardiopulmonary bypass in patients undergoing elective coronary bypass graft surgery. *Anesth Analg.* 2007;104:1334.
34. Murphy GS, Szokol JW, Marymont JH, et al. Morphine-based cardiac anesthesia provides superior early recovery compared with fentanyl in elective cardiac surgery patients. *Anesth Analg.* 2009;109:311.
35. Lowenstein E, Hallowell P, Levine FH, et al. Cardiovascular response to large doses of intravenous morphine in man. *N Engl J Med.* 1969;281:1389.
36. Jenkins DP, Pugsley WB, Alkhulaifi AM, et al. Ischemic preconditioning reduces troponin T release in patients undergoing coronary artery bypass surgery. *Heart.* 1997;77:314.
37. Tanaka K, Ludwig L, Kersten J, et al. Mechanisms of cardioprotection by volatile anesthetics. *Anesthesiology.* 2004;100:707.
38. Fraessdorf J, De Hert S, Schlack W. Anaesthesia and myocardial ischaemia/reperfusion injury. *Br J Anaesth.* 2009;103:89–98.
39. Belhomme D, Peynet J, Louzy M, et al. Evidence for preconditioning by isoflurane in coronary artery bypass graft surgery. *Circulation.* 1999;100(19 Suppl):II340.
40. Pagel S, Fu JL, Damask MC, et al. Desflurane and isoflurane produce similar alterations in systemic and pulmonary hemodynamics and arterial oxygenation in patients undergoing one-lung ventilation during thoracotomy. *Anesth Analg.* 1998;87:800.
41. Helman JD, Leung JM, Bellows WH, et al. The risk of myocardial ischemia in patients receiving desflurane versus sufentanil anesthesia for coronary artery bypass graft surgery. *Anesthesiology.* 1992;77:47.
42. Searle N, Martineau RJ, Conzen P, et al. Comparison of sevoflurane/fentanyl and isoflurane/fentanyl during elective coronary artery bypass surgery. *Can J Anaesth.* 1996;43:890.
43. Smith FJ, Bartel PR, Hugo JM, et al. Anesthetic technique (sufentanil versus ketamine plus midazolam) and quantitative electroencephalographic changes after cardiac surgery. *J Cardiothorac Vasc Anesth.* 2006;20:520.
44. Dasta JF, Jacobi J, Sesti AM, et al. Addition of dexmedetomidine to standard sedation regimens after cardiac surgery: An outcomes analysis. *Pharmacotherapy.* 2006;26:798.
45. Muellejans B, Matthey T, Scholpp J, et al. Sedation in the intensive care unit with remifentanil/propofol versus midazolam/fentanyl: A randomised, open-label, pharmacoeconomic trial. *Crit Care.* 2006;10:R91.
46. De Hert SG, Cromheecke S, ten Broecke PW, et al. Effects of propofol, desflurane and sevoflurane on recovery of myocardial function after coronary surgery in elderly high-risk patients. *Anesthesiology.* 2003;99:314.
47. Smulyan H. Nitrates, arterial function, wave reflections and coronary heart disease. *Adv Cardiol.* 2007;44:302.
48. Ali I, Buth K, Maitland A. Impact of preoperative intravenous nitroglycerin on in-hospital outcomes after coronary artery bypass grafting for unstable angina. *Am Heart J.* 2004;148:727.
49. Kaplan KJ, Taber M, Teagarden JR, et al. Association of methemoglobinemia and intravenous nitroglycerine administration. *Am J Cardiol.* 1985;55:181.
50. Cheung AT, Cruz-Shiavone GE, Meng QC, et al. Cardiopulmonary bypass, hemolysis, and nitroprusside-induced cyanide production. *Anesth Analg.* 2007;105:29.
51. Zerbe NF, Wagner BKJ. Use of vitamin B_{12} in the treatment and prevention of nitroprusside-induced cyanide toxicity. *Crit Care Med.* 1993;21:465.
52. Egi M, Bellomo R, Langenberg C, et al. Selecting a vasopressor drug for vasoplegic shock after adult cardiac surgery: A systematic literature review. *Ann Thorac Surg.* 2007;83:715.
53. Halonen J, Hakala T, Auvinen T, et al. Intravenous administration of metoprolol is more effective than oral administration in the prevention of atrial fibrillation after cardiac surgery. *Circulation.* 2006;114(1 Suppl):I1.
54. Booth JV, Ward EE, Colgan KC, et al. Metoprolol and coronary artery bypass grafting surgery: Does intraoperative metoprolol attenuate acute beta-adrenergic receptor desensitization during cardiac surgery? *Anesth Analg.* 2004;98:1224.
55. Longon MJ. Quo vadis, perioperative beta blockaed? Are you "POISE'd" on the brink? *Anesth Analg.* 2008;106:1025.

56. Warltier DC. β-Adrenergic-blocking drugs: Incredibly useful, incredibly underutilized [editorial comment]. *Anesthesiology.* 1998;88:2.
57. Opie L. Anti-ischemic properties of calcium-channel blockers: Lessons from cardiac surgery. *J Am Coll Cardiol.* 2003;41:1506.
58. Wijeysundera DN, Beattie WS, Rao V, et al. Calcium antagonists reduce cardiovascular complications after cardiac surgery: A meta-analysis. *J Am Coll Cardiol.* 2003;41:1496.
59. Apostolidou IA, Despotis GJ, Hogue CW Jr, et al. Antiischemic effects of nicardipine and nitroglycerin after coronary artery bypass grafting. *Ann Thorac Surg.* 1999;67:417.
60. Kaplan J. Clinical considerations for the use of intravenous nicardipine in the treatment of postoperative hypertension. *Am Heart J.* 1990;119:443.
61. Aronson S, Dyke CM, Stierer KA, et al. The ECLIPSE trials: Comparative studies of clevidipine to nitroglycerin, sodium nitroprusside, and nicardipine for acute hypertension treatment in cardiac surgery patients. *Anesth Analg.* 2008;107:1110.
62. Garcia LA, Dejong SC, Martin SM, et al. Magnesium reduces free radicals in an in vivo coronary occlusion-reperfusion model. *J Am Coll Cardiol.* 1998;32:536.
63. Shepherd J, Jones J, Frampton GK, et al. Intravenous magnesium sulphate and sotalol for prevention of atrial fibrillation after coronary artery bypass surgery: A systematic review and economic evaluation. *Health Technol Assess.* 2008;12:iii.
64. Cook RC, Humphries KH, Gin K, et al. Prophylactic intravenous magnesium sulphate in addition to oral β-blockade does not prevent atrial arrhythmias after coronary artery or valvular heart surgery: A randomized, controlled trial. *Circulation.* 2009;120(Suppl II):S163.
65. Hillis LD, Smith PK, Anderson JL, et al. 2011 ACCF/AHA guidelines for coronary artery bypass graft surgery: Executive summary. *Anesth Analg.* 2011;114:11.
66. Freeman RV, Otto CM. Spectrum of calcific aortic valve disease: Pathogenesis, disease progression, and treatment strategies. *Circulation.* 2005;111:3316.
67. Carabello BA. Clinical practice. Aortic stenosis. *N Engl J Med.* 2002;346:677.
68. Zile MR, Gaasch WH. Heart failure in aortic stenosis—improving diagnosis and treatment. *N Engl J Med.* 2003;348:1735.
69. O'Keefe JH Jr, Shub C, Rettke SR. Risk of noncardiac surgical procedures in patients with aortic stenosis. *Mayo Clin Proc.* 1989;64:400.
70. Kertai MD, Bountioukos M, Boersma E, et al. Aortic stenosis: An underestimated risk factor for perioperative complications in patients undergoing noncardiac surgery. *Am J Med.* 2004;116:8.
71. Zahid M, Sonel AF, Saba S, et al. Perioperative risk of noncardiac surgery associated with aortic stenosis. *Am J Cardiol.* 2005;96:436.
72. Khot UN, Novato GM, Popovi ZB, et al. Nitroprusside in critically ill patients with left ventricular dysfunction and aortic stenosis. *N Engl J Med.* 2003;348:1756.
73. Ommen SR, Nishimura RA. Hypertrophic cardiomyopathy. *Curr Probl Cardiol.* 2004;29:239.
74. Fifer MA, Vlahakes GJ. Management of symptoms in hypertrophic cardiomyopathy. *Circulation.* 2008;117:429.
75. Borer JS, Bonow RO. Contemporary approach to aortic and mitral regurgitation. *Circulation.* 2003;108:2432.
76. Bekeredjian R, Grayburn PA. Valvular heart disease. Aortic regurgitation. *Circulation.* 2005;112:125.
77. Carabello BA. Modern management of mitral stenosis. *Circulation.* 2005;112:432.
78. Gorlin R, Gorlin SG. Hydraulic formula for calculation of area of the stenotic mitral valve, other cardiac valves, and central circulatory shunts. *Am Heart J.* 1951;41:1.
79. Cardoso LF, Grinberg M, Rati MA, et al. Comparison between percutaneous balloon valvuloplasty and open commissurotomy for mitral stenosis: A prospective and randomized study. *Cardiology.* 2002;98:186.
80. Thrumurthy SG, Karthikesalingam A, Patterson BO, et al. The diagnosis and management of aortic dissection. *BMJ.* 2011;344:d8290.
81. Bosner RS, Ranasinghe AM, Loubani M, et al. Evidence, lack of evidence, controversy and debate in the provision and performance of the surgery of acute type A aortic dissection. *J Am Coll Cardiol.* 2011;58:2455.
82. Eltzschig HK, Rosenberger P, Lekowski RW Jr, et al. Role of transesophageal echocardiography in patients with suspected aortic dissection. *J Am Soc Echocardiogr.* 2005;18:1221.
83. Mohr-Kahaly S, Erbel R, Rennollet H, et al. Ambulatory follow-up of aortic dissection by transesophageal two-dimensional and color-coded Doppler echocardiography. *Circulation.* 1989;80:24.
84. Penco M, Paparoni S, Dagianti A, et al. Usefulness of transesophageal echcocardiography in the assessment of aortic dissection. *Am J Cardiol.* 2000;86:53G.
85. Davies RR, Goldstein LJ, Coady MA, et al. Yearly rupture or dissection rates for thoracic aortic aneurysms: Simple prediction based on size. *Ann Thorac Surg.* 2002;73:17.
86. Hiratzka LF, Bakris GL, Beckman JA, et al. ACCF/AHA/AATS/ACR/ASA/SCA/SCAI/SIR/STS/SVM guidelines for the diagnosis and management of patients with thoracic aortic disease: Executive summary. *Anesth Analg.* 2010;111:279.
87. Isselbacher EM. Thoracic and abdominal aortic aneurysms. *Circulation.* 2005;111:816.
88. David TE, Ivanov J, Armstrong S, et al. Aortic valve-sparing operations in patients with aneurysms of the aortic root or ascending aorta. *Ann Thorac Surg.* 2002;74:S1758.
89. Hagl C, Ergin MA, Galla JD, et al. Neurologic outcome after ascending aorta-aortic arch operations: Effect of brain protection technique in high-risk patients. *J Thorac Cardiovasc Surg.* 2001;121:1107.
90. Cowan JA Jr, Dimick JB, Henke PK, et al. Surgical treatment of intact thoracoabdominal aortic aneurysms in the United States: Hospital and surgeon volume-related outcomes. *J Vasc Surg.* 2003;37:1169.
91. Conrad MF, Cambria RP. Contemporary management of descending thoracic and thoracoabdominal aortic aneurysms: Endovascular versus open. *Circulation.* 2008;117:841.
92. Vaughn SB, LeMaire SA, Collard CD. Case scenario: Anesthetic considerations for thoracoabdominal aortic aneurysm repair. *Anesthesiology.* 2011;115:1093–1102.
93. Driessen JJ, Dhaese H, Fransen G, et al. Pulsatile compared with nonpulsatile perfusion using a centrifugal pump for cardiopulmonary bypass during coronary artery bypass grafting. Effects on systemic haemodynamics, oxygenation, and inflammatory response parameters. *Perfusion.* 1995;10:3.
94. Fang WC, Helm RE, Krieger KH, et al. Impact of minimum hematocrit during cardiopulmonary bypass on mortality in patients undergoing coronary artery surgery. *Circulation.* 1997;96(9 Suppl):II.
95. Alevizou A, Dunning J, Park JD. Can a mini-bypass circuit improve perfusion in cardiac surgery compared to conventional cardiopulmonary bypass? *Interact Cardiovasc Thorac Surg.* 2009;8:457.
96. Abdel Aal M, ElNahal N, Bakir BM, et al. Mini-cardiopulmonary bypass impact on blood conservation strategy in coronary artery bypass grafting. *Interact Cardiovasc Thorac Surg.* 2011;12:600.
97. Society of Thoracic Surgeons Blood Conservation Guideline Task Force, Ferraris VA, Brown JR, et al. 2011 update to the Society of Thoracic Surgeons and the Society of Cardiovascular Anesthesiologists blood conservation clinical practice guidelines. *Ann Thorac Surg.* 2011;91:944.
98. Avidan MS, Lefy JH, Scholz J, et al. A phase III, double-blind, placebo-controlled, multicenter study on the efficacy of recombinant human antithrombin in heparin-resistant patients scheduled to undergo cardiac surgery necessitating cardiopulmonary bypass. *Anesthesiology.* 2005;102:276.
99. Levy JH, Tanaka KA, Hursting MJ. Reducing thrombotic complications in the perioperative setting: An update on heparin-induced thrombocytopenia. *Anesth Analg.* 2007;105:570.
100. Linkins LA, Dans AL, Moores LK, et al. Treatment and prevention of heparin-induced thrombocytopenia: Antithrombotic therapy and prevention of thrombosis, 9th ed: American College of Chest Physicians evidence-based clinical practice guidelines. *Chest.* 2012;141(2 Suppl):e495S–e530S.
101. Levy JH. Pharmacologic methods to reduce perioperative bleeding. *Transfusion.* 2008;48(1 Suppl):31S.
102. Henry DA, Carless PA, Moxey AJ, et al. Anti-fibrinolytic use for minimising perioperative allogeneic blood transfusion. *Cochrane Database Syst Rev.* 2011;(3):CD001886.
103. Mangano DT, Miao Y, Vuylsteke A. Mortality associated with aprotinin during 5 years following coronary artery bypass graft surgery. *JAMA.* 2007;297:471.
104. Fergusson DA, Hervert PC, Mazer CD, et al. A comparison of aprotinin and lysine analogues in high-risk cardiac surgery. *N Engl J Med.* 2008;358:2319.
105. Karkouti K, Wijeysundera DN, Yau TM, et al. The risk-benefit profile of aprotinin versus tranexamic acid in cardiac surgery. *Anesth Analg.* 2010;110:21.
106. Severdija EE, Heijmans JH, Theunissen M, et al. Retrograde autologous priming reduces transfusion requirements in coronary artery bypass surgery. *Perfusion.* 2011;26:315.
107. Luciani GB, Menon T, Vecchi B, et al. Modified ultrafiltration reduces morbidity after adult cardiac operations: A prospective, randomized clinical trial. *Circulation.* 2001;104(12 Suppl 1):I253.
108. Zacharias M, Conion NP, Herbison GP, et al. Interventions for protecting renal function in the perioperative period. *Cochrane Database Syst Rev.* 2008;4:CD003590.
109. Filion KB, Pilote L, Rahme E, et al. Perioperative use of cardiac medical therapy among patients undergoing coronary artery bypass graft surgery: A systematic review. *Am Heart J.* 2007;154:407.
110. Lazar HL. All coronary artery bypass graft surgery patients will benefit from angiotensin-converting enzyme inhibitors. *Circulation.* 2008;117:6.
111. Levin MA, Lin HM, Castillo JG, et al. Early on-cardiopulmonary bypass hypotension and other factors associated with vasoplegic syndrome. *Circulation.* 2009;120:1664.
112. Grocott HP. Perioperative temperature and cardiac surgery. *J Extra Corpor Technol.* 2006;38:77.
113. Brzezinski M, Luisetti T, London MJ. Radial artery cannulation: A comprehensive review of recent anatomic and physiologic investigations. *Anesth Analg.* 2009;109:1763.
114. Baba T, Goto T, Yoshitake A, et al. Radial artery diameter decreases with increased femoral to radial artery pressure gradient during cardiopulmonary bypass. *Anesth Analg.* 1997;85:252–258.
115. Bussières JS. Iatrogenic pulmonary artery rupture. *Curr Opin Anaesthesiol.* 2007;20:48.
116. Hansen RM, Viquerat CE, Matthy MA, et al. Poor correlation between pulmonary arterial wedge pressure and left ventricular end-diastolic volume after coronary artery bypass graft surgery. *Anesthesiology.* 1986;64:764.
117. Puskas JD, Winston D, Wright CE, et al. Stroke after coronary artery operation. Incidence, correlates, outcome, and cost. *Ann Thorac Surg.* 2000;69:1053.
118. Ahonen J, Salmenperä M. Brain injury after adult cardiac surgery. *Acta Anaesthesiol Scand.* 2004;48:4.

119. Newman MF, Kirchner JL, Phillips-Bute B, et al. Longitudinal assessment of neurocognitive function after coronary-artery bypass surgery. *N Engl J Med.* 2001; 344:395.
120. Grocott HP, Mackensen GB, Grigore AM, et al. Postoperative hyperthermia is associated with cognitive dysfunction after coronary artery bypass graft surgery. *Stroke.* 2002;33:537.
121. Hogue CW Jr, Palin CA, Arrowsmith JE. Cardiopulmonary bypass management and neurologic outcomes: An evidence-based appraisal of current practices. *Anesth Analg.* 2006;103:21.
122. Tuman KJ, McCarthy RJ, Spiess BD, et al. Does choice of anesthetic agent significantly affect outcome after coronary artery surgery? *Anesthesiology.* 1989;70(2):189.
123. Slogoff S, Keats AS, Dear WS, et al. Steal-prone coronary anatomy and myocardial ischemia associated with four primary anesthetic agents in humans. *Anesth Analg.* 1991;72:22.
124. Murphy GS, Szokol JW, Marymont JH, et al. Recovery of neuromuscular function after cardiac surgery: Pancuronium versus rocuronium. *Anesth Analg.* 2003;96:1301.
125. Troianos CA, Hartman GS, Glas KE, et al. Guidelines for performing ultrasound guided vascular cannulation: Recommendations of the American Society of Echocardiography and the Society of Cardiovascular Anesthesiologists. *Anesth Analg.* 2012;114:46.
126. Practice guidelines for central venous access. A report by the American Society of Anesthesiologists task force on central venous access. *Anesthesiology.* 2012; 116:539.
127. Murphy GS, Hessel EA II, Groom RC. Optimal perfusion during cardiopulmonary bypass: An evidence-based approach. *Anesth Analg.* 2009;108:1394–1417.
128. Garwood S. Renal insufficiency after cardiac surgery. *Semin Cardiothorac Vasc Anesth.* 2004;8:227.
129. Grigore AM, Grocott HP, Mathew JP, et al. The rewarming rate and increased peak temperature alter neurocognitive outcome after cardiac surgery. *Anesth Analg.* 2002;94:4–10.
130. Avidan MS, Zhang L, Burnside BA, et al. Anesthesia awareness and bispectral index. *N Engl J Med.* 2008;358:1097.
131. Robitaille A, Denault AY, Couture P, et al. Importance of relative pulmonary hypertension in cardiac surgery: The mean systemic-to-pulmonary artery pressure ratio. *J Cardiothorac Vasc Anesth.* 2006;20:331.
132. McKinlay KH, Schinderle DB, Swaminathan M, et al. Predictors of inotrope use during separation from cardiopulmonary bypass. *J Cardiothorac Vasc Anesth.* 2004;18:404.
133. Klopman MA, Chen EP, Sniecinski RM. Positioning an intraaortic balloon pump using imtraoperative transesophageal echocardiographic guidance. *Anesth Analg.* 2011;113:40.
134. Field ML, Rengarajan A, Khan O, et al. Preoperative intra aortic balloon pumps in patients undergoing coronary artery bypass grafting. *Cochrane Database Syst Rev.* 2007;24:CD004472.
135. Shah KB, Tang DG, Cooke R, et al. Implantable mechanical circulatory support: Demystifying patients with ventricular assist devices and artificial hearts. *Clin Cardiol.* 2011;34(3):147–152.
136. Caccamo M, Eckman P, John R. Current state of ventricular assist devices. *Curr Heart Fail Rep.* 2011;8(2):91–98.
137. Pulido JN, Park SJ, Rihal CS. Percutaneous left ventricular assist devices: Clinical uses, future applications, and anesthetic considerations. *J Cardiothorac Vasc Anesth.* 2010;24(3):478–486.
138. Chumnanvej S, Wood MJ, MacGillivray TE, et al. Perioperative echocardiographic examination for ventricular assist device implantation. *Anesth Analg.* 2007;105(3):583–601.
139. Stone ME. Current status of mechanical circulatory assistance. *Semin Cardiothorac Vasc Anesth.* 2007;11(3):185–204.
140. Lahm T, McCaslin CA, Wozniak TC, et al. Medical and surgical treatment of acute right ventricular failure. *J Am Coll Cardiol.* 2010;56(18):1435–1446.
141. Ficke DJ, Lee J, Chaney MA, et al. Case 6–2010: Noncardiac surgery in patients with a left ventricular assist device. *J Cardiothorac Vasc Anesth.* 2010;24(6):1002–1009.
142. Riha H, Netuka I, Kotulak T, et al. Anesthesia management of a patient with a ventricular assist device for noncardiac surgery. *Semin Cardiothorac Vasc Anesth.* 2010;14(1):29–31.
143. Kartha V, Gomez W, Wu B, et al. Laparoscopic cholecystectomy in a patient with an implantable left ventricular assist device. *Br J Anaesth.* 2008;100(5):652–655.
144. Schulman S, Bijsterveld NR. Anticoagulants and their reversal. *Transfus Med Rev.* 2007;21:37.
145. Levy JH, Adkinson NF Jr. Anaphylaxis during cardiac surgery: Implications for clinicians. *Anesth Analg.* 2008;106:392.
146. Trehan N, Mishra M, Sharma OP. Further reduction in stroke after off-pump coronary artery bypass grafting: A 10-year experience. *Ann Thorac Surg.* 2001;72:S1026.
147. Leff JD, Enriquez LJ. Robotic-assisted cardiac surgery. *Int Anesthesiol Clin.* 2012; 50:78–89.
148. Billings FT, Kodali SK, Shanewise JS. Transcatheter aortic valve implantation: Anesthetic considerations. *Anesth Analg.* 2009;108:1453–1462.
149. Chassot PG, van der Linden P, Zaugg M, et al. Off-pump coronary artery bypass surgery: Physiology and anaesthetic management. *Br J Anaesth.* 2004;92:400.
150. Bainbridge D, Cheng DC. Minimally invasive direct coronary artery bypass and off-pump coronary artery bypass surgery: Anesthetic considerations. *Anesthesiol Clin.* 2008;26:437–452.
151. Huffmyer J, Raphael J. The current status of off-pump coronary bypass surgery. *Curr Opin Anaesthesiol.* 2011;24(1):64–69.
152. Fillinger MP, Yeager MP, Dodds TM, et al. Epidural anesthesia and analgesia: Effects on recovery from cardiac surgery. *J Cardiothorac Vasc Anesth.* 2002;16:15.
153. Kurlansky PA. Is there a hypercoagulable state after off-pump coronary artery bypass surgery? What do we know and what can we do? *J Thorac Cardiovasc Surg.* 2003;126:7.
154. Lev-Ran O, Ben-Gal Y, Matsa M, et al. 'No touch' techniques for porcelain ascending aorta: Comparison between cardiopulmonary bypass with femoral artery cannulation and off-pump myocardial revascularization. *J Card Surg.* 2002;17:370.
155. Sharony R, Bizekis CS, Kanchuger M, et al. Off-pump coronary artery bypass grafting reduces mortality and stroke in patients with atheromatous aortas: A case control study. *Circulation.* 2003;108(Suppl 1):II15.
156. Cheng DC, Bainbridge D, Martin JE, et al. Does off-pump coronary artery bypass reduce mortality, morbidity, and resource utilization when compared with conventional coronary artery bypass? A meta-analysis of randomized trials. *Anesthesiology.* 2005;102:188.
157. Kim KB, Lim C, Lee C, et al. Off-pump coronary artery bypass may decrease the patency of saphenous vein grafts. *Ann Thorac Surg.* 2001;72:S1033.
158. Lamy A, Devereaux PJ, Prabhakaran D, et al. Off-pump or on-pump coronary-artery bypass grafting at 30 days. *N Engl J Med.* 2012;366:1489.
159. Little WC, Freeman GL. Pericardial disease. *Circulation.* 2006;113:1622.
160. Roediger L, Larbuisson R, Lamy M. New approaches and old controversies to postoperative pain control following cardiac surgery. *Eur J Anaesthesiol.* 2006; 23:539.
161. Chaney MA. Intrathecal and epidural anesthesia and analgesia for cardiac surgery. *Anesth Analg.* 2006;102:45.
162. Malviya S, Voepel-Lewis T, Siewert M, et al. Risk factors for adverse postoperative outcomes in children presenting for cardiac surgery with upper respiratory tract infections. *Anesthesiology.* 2003;98:628.
163. Greenwood RD, Rosenthal LA, Parisi L, et al. Extracardiac abnormalities in infants with congenital heart disease. *Pediatrics.* 1975;55:485.
164. Karamlou T, Hickey E, Silliman CC, et al. Reducing risk in infant cardiopulmonary bypass: The use of a miniaturized circuit and a crystalloid prime improves cardiopulmonary function and increases cerebral blood flow. *Semin Thorac Cardiovasc Surg Pediatr Card Surg Annu.* 2005;8:3–11.
165. Raja SG, Yousufuddin S, Rasool F, et al. Impact of modified ultrafiltration on morbidity after pediatric cardiac surgery. *Asian Cardiovasc Thorac Ann.* 2006; 14:341–350. Review.
166. Alghamdi AA, Singh SK, Hamilton BC, et al. Early extubation after pediatric cardiac surgery: Systematic review, meta analysis and evidence-based recommendations. *J Card Surg.* 2010;25:586–595.
167. Mittnacht AJ, Hollinger I. Fast-tracking in pediatric cardiac surgery-the current standing. *Ann Card Anaesth.* 2010;13:92–101. Review.
168. Ip P, Chiu CS, Cheung YF. Risk factors prolonging ventilation in young children after cardiac surgery: Impact of noninfectious pulmonary complications. *Pediatr Crit Care Med.* 2002;3:269–274.
169. Lofland GK. The enhancement of hemodynamic performance in Fontan circulation using pain free spontaneous ventilation. *Eur J Cardiothorac Surg.* 2001;20: 114–119.
170. Peterson KL, DeCampli WM, Pike NA, et al. A report of two hundred twenty cases of regional anesthesia in pediatric cardiac surgery. *Anesth Analg.* 2000;90: 1014.
171. Bacha BAM, Hijazi ZM. Hybrid procedures in pediatric cardiac surgery. *Semin Thorac Cardiovasc Surg Pediatr Card Surg Annu.* 2005;78–85.

CHAPTER 39

Anesthesia for Vascular Surgery

TODD J. SMAKA • TIMOTHY E. MILLER • MICHAEL P. HUTCHENS • KATIE SCHENNING
LEE A. FLEISHER • TONG J. GAN • DAVID A. LUBARSKY

Key Points

1. The anesthesiologist may have greater influence in reducing the morbidity and costs of vascular surgery than in any other surgical procedure.
2. Atherosclerosis is a generalized inflammatory disorder of the arterial tree with associated endothelial dysfunction.
3. The absence of severe coronary stenoses can be predicted with a positive predictive value of 96% for patients without diabetes, prior angina, previous myocardial infarction (MI), or congestive heart failure (CHF).
4. The latest guidelines suggest continuing aspirin therapy in all patients with a coronary stent and discontinuing clopidogrel for as short a time interval as possible for patients with bare-metal stents <30 days or drug-eluting stents <1 year.
5. Despite the initial enthusiasm for perioperative β-blockade, newer studies have demonstrated that β-blockers may not be effective in lower-risk patients or if heart rate is not well controlled.
6. Unfortunately, despite promising bench and animal research, there is currently no clinical evidence to support the benefit of any pharmacologic intervention or protection strategy.
7. Vascular surgery patients are at high risk for postoperative nervous system disease, including delirium, stroke, and spinal cord ischemia.
8. There is some clinical evidence that elevation of blood pressure to "normal" levels during awake CEA can reverse developing neurologic deficits. Nonetheless, hypotension and hypoperfusion are not the most common cause of stroke after CEA; embolic events may be even more important, and often occur postoperatively.
9. EVAR is increasingly being considered for patients with smaller AAAs. The decision on which treatment modality is best for a large AAA usually depends on three variables: AAA size, AAA morphology, and patient perioperative risk. In general, EVAR has lower perioperative risk than OAR, but similar 2-year mortality.
10. The most common cause of emergency aortic repair is a leaking or ruptured aortic aneurysm. Ruptured aneurysms carry an associated mortality roughly 10 times greater than elective repair.

Multimedia

1 Aortic Cross Clamp for Blood Volume Redistribution

VASCULAR DISEASE: EPIDEMIOLOGIC, MEDICAL, AND SURGICAL ASPECTS

1 The anesthesiologist may have greater influence in reducing the morbidity and costs of vascular surgery than in any other surgical procedure. Since the mid-1960s, the morbidity from major vascular surgery has decreased from a 6-day mortality of >25% for major aortic repair to a 30-day mortality of <2% for endovascular abdominal aneurysm repair (EVAR). Anesthetic specialization has recently been shown to reduce early- and medium-term mortality rates for patients undergoing major vascular surgery.[1]

This chapter begins with a discussion of the pathophysiology of atherosclerotic vascular disease (AVD) and the general medical problems common in patients with peripheral vascular disease, particularly coronary artery disease (CAD). Organ protection strategies are then presented, with an emphasis on the heart and kidneys, among other organs. The specific surgical goals, anatomy, and complications for carotid, thoracic aortic, visceral, abdominal aortic, and lower extremity revascularization are placed in the context of optimal anesthetic management, including recognition of the ever-increasing use of endovascular techniques.

Pathophysiology of Atherosclerosis

2 Atherosclerosis is a generalized inflammatory disorder of the arterial tree with associated endothelial dysfunction. The commonly accepted causes of atherosclerosis are endothelial damage caused by hemodynamic shear stress, inflammation from chronic infections, hypercoagulability resulting in thrombosis, and the destructive effects of oxidized low-density lipoproteins (LDLs). Disruption of the fibrous cap over a lipid deposit can lead to plaque rupture and ulceration. Vasoactive influences can result in spasm and acute thrombosis. Platelets play a pivotal role in atherothrombosis after plaque rupture. Platelets internalize oxidized phospholipids and promote foam cell formation. In fact, platelet polymorphisms are independent risk predictors for myocardial ischemia following vascular surgery.[2]

Atherosclerosis develops as a response to injury. The primary injurious agents include lipoproteins containing apolipoprotein B, the most important of which is LDL. These lipoproteins filter into arterial intima through the endothelium. The entrapped lipoproteins then become modified into proinflammatory substances. In the subendothelial space enriched with atherogenic lipoproteins, most macrophages transform into foam cells. Foam cells aggregate to form the atheromatous core and as this process progresses, the atheromatous centers of plaques become necrotic, consisting of lipids, cholesterol crystals, and cell debris. Monocyte-derived macrophages act as scavenging and antigen-presenting cells and also produce several types of chemical mediators (e.g., cytokines, chemokines, growth regulating molecules) that are involved in inflammation. Adhesion molecules expressed by inflamed endothelium recruit leukocytes, including monocytes, which then penetrate into the intima, predisposing the vessel wall to lipid accretion and vasculitis.

The National Veterans Affairs Surgical Risk Study found that low serum albumin values and high American Society of Anesthesiologists physical classification were among the best predictors of morbidity and mortality after vascular surgery (Table 39-1).[3] Risk factors for atherosclerosis include abdominal obesity, atherogenic dyslipidemia, hypertension, insulin resistance, proinflammatory state, and prothrombotic state. Major risk factors also include cigarette smoking, elevated LDL cholesterol (LDL-C), low high-density lipoprotein, family history of premature coronary heart disease, and aging; emerging risk factors include elevated triglycerides and small LDL particles. The relative contribution of these risk factors varies (Fig. 39-1).[5]

TABLE 39-1. THE TEN MOST IMPORTANT PREOPERATIVE PREDICTORS OF POSTOPERATIVE 30-DAY MORTALITY AFTER VASCULAR SURGERY IN VETERAN'S AFFAIRS MEDICAL CENTERS[a]

Predictor	Odds Ratio
Esophageal varices	4.30
DNR status	2.96
Ventilator dependent	2.71
Emergency operation	2.40
ASA class	1.89
Creatinine >1.2 mg/dL	1.48
BUN >40 mg/dL	1.47
Operative complexity score	1.32
Age	1.03
Albumin	0.61

[a]All variables are statistically significant ($p < 0.05$) and were selected after stepwise multivariable analysis.

BUN, blood urea nitrogen; DNR, do not resuscitate.

Modified from: Khuri SF, Daley J, Henderson W, et al. Risk adjustment of the postoperative mortality rate for the comparative assessment of the quality of surgical care: Results of the National Veterans Affairs surgical risk study. *J Am Coll Surg.* 1997;185:315.

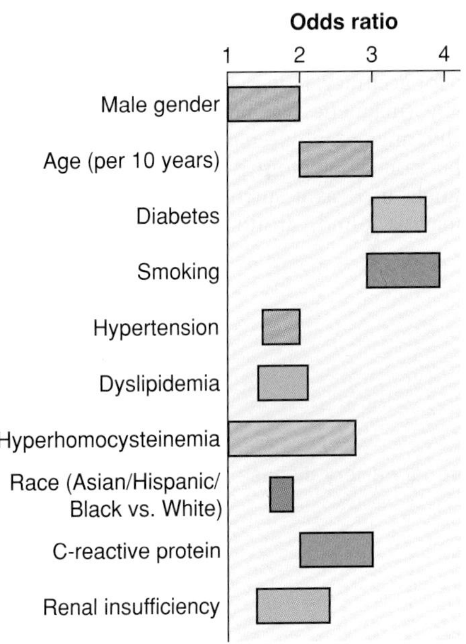

FIGURE 39-1. Approximate range of odds ratios for risk factors for symptomatic peripheral arterial disease. Some of the factors are amenable for treatment and can help in secondary prevention of complications of vascular disease. (Reprinted from: Norgren L, Hiatt WR, Dormandy JA, et al. Inter-society consensus for the management of peripheral arterial disease (TASC II). *J Vasc Surg.* 2007;45(suppl S):S5, with permission.)

Natural History of Patients with Peripheral Vascular Disease

Atherosclerosis is one of the most important and common causes of death and disability in the United States and throughout the world. More than 25 million persons in the United States have at least one clinical manifestation of atherosclerosis. Throughout the past 50 years, coronary artery atherosclerosis has been a major focus for basic and clinical investigation. However, atherosclerosis must be recognized as a systemic disease with important sequelae in many other regional circulations[5] (Fig. 39-2).

Stroke is the third leading cause of death and the principal cause of long-term disability in the United States. Six hundred thousand new or recurrent strokes occur annually. The risk of stroke is relatively uncommon (0.4% to 0.6% of patients) after noncarotid peripheral vascular surgery, but when it occurs it is associated with longer length of stay and higher mortality.[6] The principal clinical syndromes associated with aortic atherosclerosis are abdominal aortic aneurysms (AAAs), aortic dissection, peripheral atheroembolism, penetrating aortic ulcer, and intramural hematoma. Patients with peripheral arterial disease (PAD), which is atherosclerosis affecting the limb, can develop disabling symptoms of claudication or critical limb ischemia. The prevalence of claudication is 2% among older adults, but 10 times as many elderly patients have asymptomatic lower extremity atherosclerosis. PAD affecting the lower extremities can be detected by the ankle–brachial index: The ratio of the highest systolic ankle blood pressure to the highest systolic arm blood pressure. The ankle–brachial index is the single best initial screening test to perform in a patient suspected of having PAD. The index is obtained with a blood pressure cuff and a hand-held continuous-wave Doppler. A ratio <0.9 is considered abnormal and <0.4 is often associated with limb-threatening ischemia.

Catheter-based angiography is the standard method for diagnosing the PAD, against which all other imaging modalities are compared for accuracy. However, recent advances in noninvasive angiography (magnetic resonance angiography and computed tomographic angiography) enable excellent noninvasive definition of the vascular anatomy. Carotid intima-media thickness is increasingly used as a surrogate marker for atherosclerosis. A meta-analysis found carotid intima-media thickness to be a strong predictor of future vascular events,[7] though it does not significantly improve the Framingham and SCORE models for prediction of cardiovascular endpoints.[8]

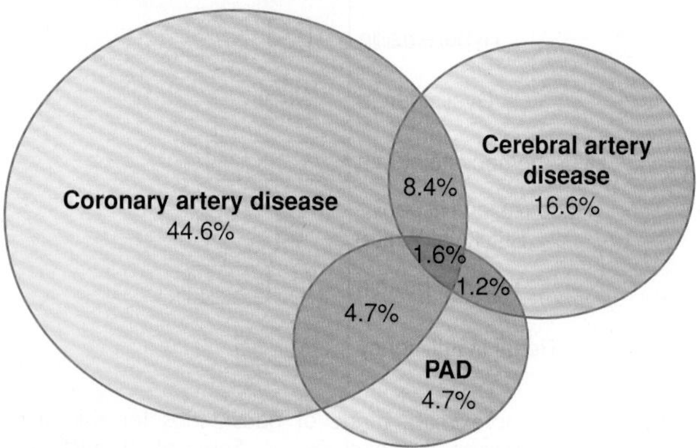

FIGURE 39-2. Typical overlap in vascular disease affecting different territories. Based on REACH data. PAD, peripheral arterial disease. (Reprinted from: Norgren L, Hiatt WR, Dormandy JA, et al. Inter-society consensus for the management of peripheral arterial disease (TASC II). *J Vasc Surg.* 2007;45(suppl S):S5, with permission.)

AAAs occur in up to 5% of men older than 65 years; most of these aneurysms are small and require only infrequent follow-up. The risk of rupture is very low for AAAs ≤4 cm in diameter but rises exponentially for AAAs >5 cm. AAAs between 4 and 5 cm in diameter should be followed every 6 to 12 months to determine whether they are increasing in size. It is interesting to note that baseline hemoglobin concentration is independently associated with AAA size and reduced long-term survival following intervention for treatment. Thus the presence or absence of anemia offers a potential refinement of existing risk stratification methods.[9]

Medical Therapy for Atherosclerosis

Continuation of chronic medical therapy, including use of antihypertensives such as β-blockers and angiotensin-converting enzyme (ACE) inhibitors, statin drugs, aspirin, and control of hyperglycemia with hypoglycemics and/or insulin, may reduce perioperative morbidity and mortality in vascular surgery. Prevention of infection, including meticulous foot care in diabetic patients, is important to avoid tissue loss. Lifestyle changes such as weight loss and exercise can forestall claudication. The use of statin drugs may reduce progression or even cause regression of atherosclerotic plaques, improve endothelial function, and reduce cardiovascular events in high-risk patients. Patients with high cardiac risk undergoing vascular surgery who received preoperative statin therapy were less likely to die.[10] Statin use is also associated with improved graft patency, limb salvage, and decreased amputation rate in patients undergoing infrainguinal bypass for AVD. Similar to β-blocker therapy, discontinuation of statin therapy for 4 days surrounding major vascular surgery is associated with an increased postoperative cardiac risk.[11] ACE inhibitors have numerous beneficial effects in patients with AVD, including plaque stabilization. Cessation of smoking may be the most effective "medical" therapy.

Chronic therapy with aspirin or other anti-inflammatory drugs may retard the progression of atherosclerosis and prevent morbid cardiovascular events. A recent meta-analysis found the time interval between discontinuation of aspirin and occurrence of vascular events to be 14.3 ± 11.3 days for acute cerebral events, 8.5 ± 3.6 days for acute coronary events, and 25.8 ± 18.1 days for acute peripheral arterial syndromes.[12] The recently reported RECO study suggested that discontinuation of aspirin for more than 5 days in patients with coronary stents is a major predictor of adverse cardiac events.[13] In patients undergoing peripheral vascular surgery, continuation of clopidogrel within 48 hours was not associated with an increased incidence of major bleeding.[14] The STRATAGEM trial randomized patients using antiplatelet agents for secondary prevention of CAD to either continuation of aspirin or placebo from 10 days before until the morning of surgery.[15] Patients with coronary stents were excluded. There was no significant difference in the composite outcome of major thrombotic and bleeding adverse events occurring within 30 days of surgery. The use in cyclooxygenase 2 (COX-2) inhibitors of patients with AVD is unclear at present, with studies suggesting increased cardiovascular events with long-term use.[16] In general, patients should continue to take aspirin until the day of surgery for carotid and lower extremity surgery, and individualize the choice for larger operations. In urgent situations when patients develop acute ischemia, systemic anticoagulation may be instituted.

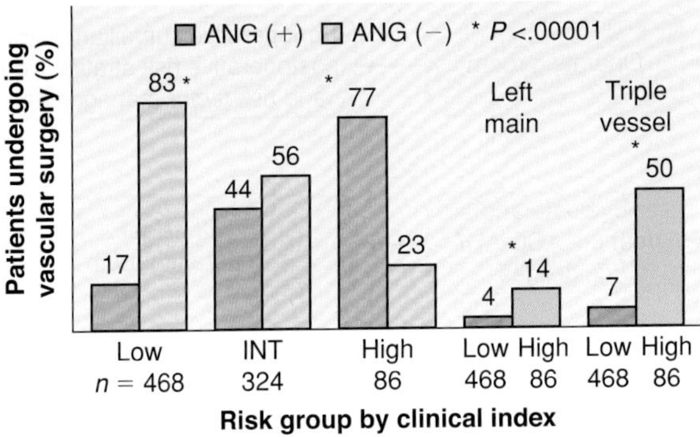

FIGURE 39-3. Clinical risk factors predict severe (left main or triple vessel) coronary artery disease. A preoperative clinical index (diabetes mellitus, prior myocardial infarction, angina, age older than 70 years, congestive heart failure) was used to stratify patients. ANG (+), angiogram positive for coronary artery disease; ANG (–), angiogram negative for coronary artery disease; INT, intermediate. (Based on data from: Paul SD, Eagle KA, Kuntz KM, et al. Concordance of preoperative clinical risk with angiographic severity of coronary artery disease in patients undergoing vascular surgery. *Circulation.* 1996;94:1561; secondary analysis of data from: Hertzer NR, Beven EG, Young JR, et al. Coronary artery disease in peripheral vascular patients: A classification of 1000 coronary angiograms and results of surgical management. *Ann Surg.* 1984;199:223.)

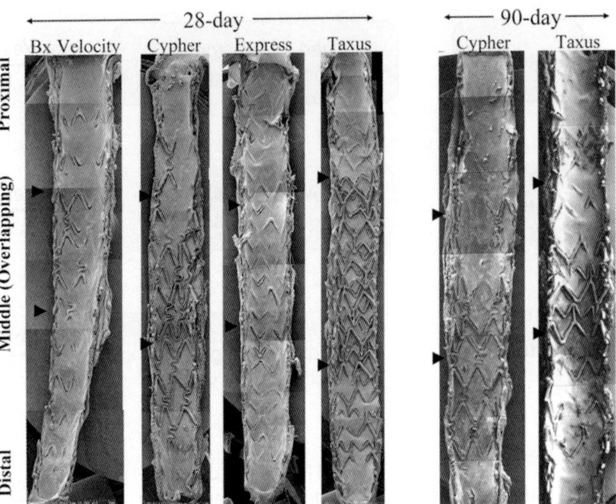

FIGURE 39-4. Scanning electron micrographs from overlapping bare metal stents (Bx) and drug-eluting stent DES implanted in the rabbit iliac artery model for 28 and 90 days. Note significantly less endothelialization in Cypher and Taxus DES as compared with Bx Velocity and Express, especially at overlapping sites at 28 days. At 90 days, the luminal surface in overlapping DES is still not fully endothelialized. *Arrows* indicate the overlapping regions. (Reprinted from: Finn AV, Nakazawa G, Joner M, et al. Vascular responses to drug eluting stents: Importance of delayed healing. *Arterioscler Thromb Vasc Biol.* 2007;27:1500, with permission.)

Chronic Medical Problems and Management in Vascular Surgery Patients

Coronary Artery Disease in Patients with Peripheral Vascular Disease

Almost two decades ago, Hertzer et al.[17] performed coronary angiography in 1,000 consecutive patients presenting for vascular surgery and identified severe correctable CAD in 25% of the entire series. The incidence of significant CAD (stenosis >70%) detected by angiography was 78% in those with clinical indications of CAD and 37% in patients without any clinical indications. However, subsequent analysis demonstrated that clinical risk factors still
3 predicted the severity of CAD (Fig. 39-3). The absence of severe coronary stenoses can be predicted with a positive predictive value of 96% for patients without diabetes, prior angina, previous myocardial infarction (MI), or congestive heart failure (CHF).

Short-term postoperative cardiac morbidity and mortality after vascular surgery is higher than after other types of noncardiac surgery. Complications after carotid endarterectomy (CEA) are generally less frequent than after other types of vascular surgery, but still produce 50% to 100% of the mortality encountered in vascular surgery patients. The presence of uncorrected CAD appears to double 5-year mortality after vascular surgery. Percutaneous coronary interventions (PCI) directed at reducing perioperative cardiac events do not appear to reduce perioperative myocardial infarction (PMI); however, PCI performed in the distant past may be protective after vascular surgery. However, in the first 6 weeks after coronary stent placement, noncardiac surgery carries considerable risks. There are two basic types of stents: Bare-metal stents and drug-eluting stents. While drug-eluting stents have a reduced incidence of restenosis, they are slow to endothelialize, and the exposed stent material remains thrombogenic far longer than bare-metal stents (Fig. 39-4).[18] Therefore, the duration of dual antiplatelet therapy (aspirin 325 mg/day and clopidogrel 75 mg/day) differs: 1 month for bare-metal stents, 12 months or more for drug-eluting stents depending upon the coronary anatomy. Aspirin is recommended for an indefinite period. Under the circumstances that prevent the use of clopidogrel for 1 year, the recommendations for duration of therapy are as follows: 3 months for sirolimus-eluting stents and 6 months for paclitaxel-eluting stents.[19] Several reports suggest that drug-eluting stents may represent an additional risk over a prolonged period (up to 12 months), particularly if antiplatelet agents are discontinued.[20] However, a case series suggests that an elevated
4 risk continues beyond 1 year.[21] The latest guidelines suggest continuing aspirin therapy in all patients with a coronary stent and discontinuing clopidogrel for as short a time interval as possible for patients with bare-metal stents <30 days or drug-eluting stents <1 year.[22] On the basis of the nonperioperative literature, there is a suggestion that holding clopidogrel for the traditional 8 days may not be necessary suggesting a shorter period of time may be optimal.[23] As noted above, there is increasing evidence to suggest that surgery can be performed with a low risk of bleeding if antiplatelet agents are continued until the day of surgery.

Recently, two distinct types of PMI: "Early" and "delayed" occurring after vascular surgery have been identified. Early PMI resembles that of acute nonsurgical MI and is probably due to acute coronary occlusion resulting from plaque rupture and thrombosis. The "delayed PMI" is associated with sustained elevation of heart rate, absence of chest pain, and prolonged premonitory episodes of ST segment depression before overt MI. The delayed PMI resembles that resulting from increase in oxygen demand in the setting of fixed coronary stenosis.[24] Myocardial oxygen supply may be diminished by anemia or hypotension, whereas oxygen demand may be increased by tachycardia and hypertension resulting from postoperative pain, withdrawal of anesthesia, or shifts in intravascular volume. Even small changes in cardiac troponin-I (cTnI) or cardiac troponin-T (cTnT) after surgery are associated with a worse perioperative and 6-month outcome, with a dose-response relationship.[25] As a result, the new definition of MI requires the rise and fall of biochemical marker

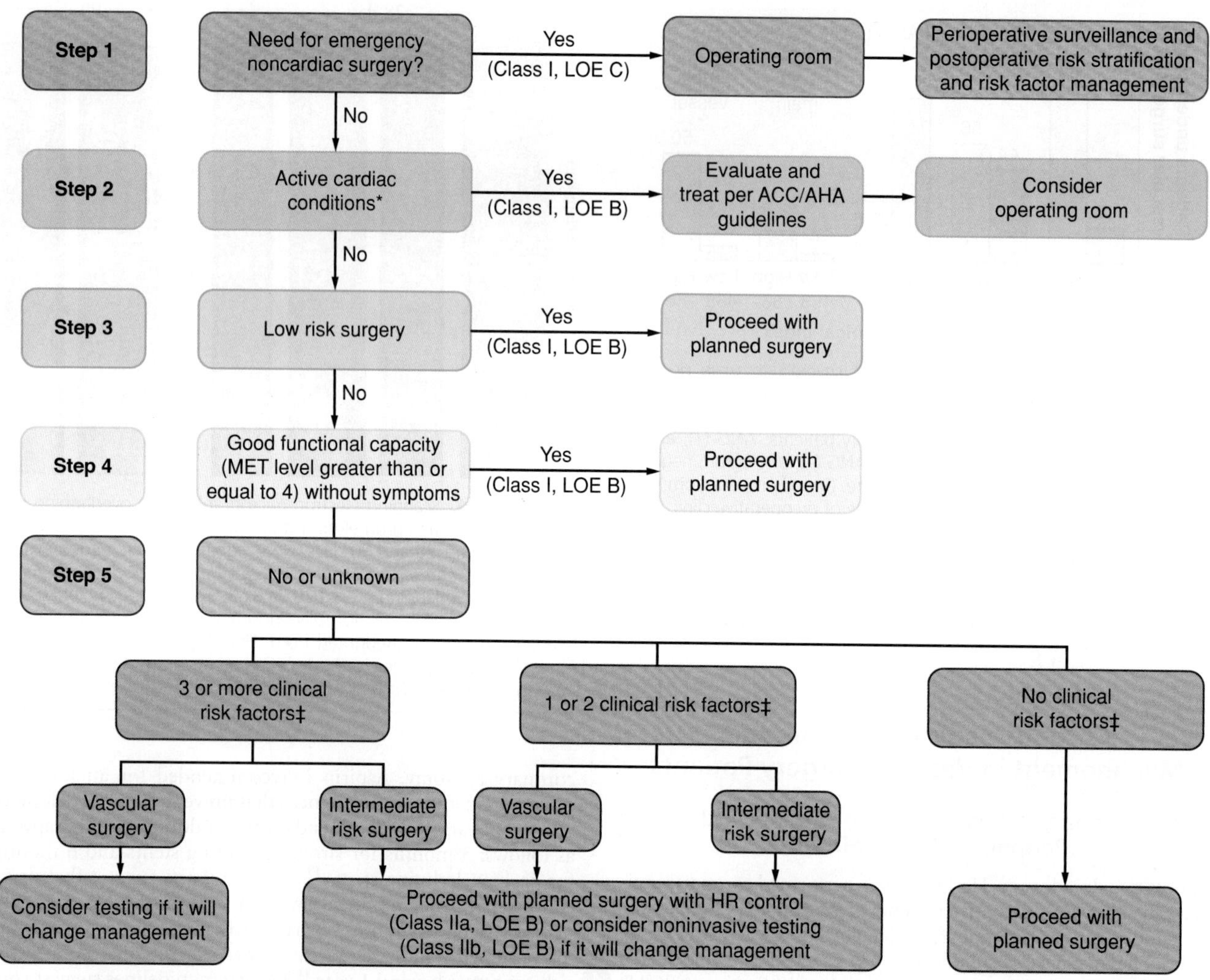

FIGURE 39-5. Cardiac evaluation and care algorithm for noncardiac surgery based on active clinical conditions, known cardiovascular disease, or cardiac risk factors for patients 50 years of age or greater. *See text for active clinical conditions. Clinical risk factors include ischemic heart disease, compensated or prior heart failure, diabetes mellitus, renal insufficiency, and cerebrovascular disease. Consider perioperative β-blockade for populations in which this has been shown to reduce cardiac morbidity/mortality: LOE, level of evidence, see following reference for details. ACC/AHA, American College of Cardiology/American Heart Association; HR, heart rate; MET, metabolic equivalent. ACC/AHA 2007 Guidelines on Perioperative Cardiovascular Evaluation and Care for Noncardiac Surgery. *Circulation* 2007;116:e418–e500.

of myocardial necrosis together with one of the following clinical or electrocardiogram (ECG) criteria: Ischemic symptoms, development of pathologic Q waves, ischemic ECG changes, or a coronary intervention.[26] Troponin screening is now recognized as an effective means of surveillance for perioperative myocardial ischemic damage.[27] In practical terms, the type of troponin that is used for surveillance, cTnI or cTnT is of little concern as both have similar diagnostic and risk stratification capabilities.

Controversy persists as to whether preoperative cardiac risk identification benefits patients. However, in 2007, the American Heart Association and American College of Cardiology (AHA/ACC) revised their guidelines and classified the clinical predictors of increased perioperative cardiovascular risk (MI, CHF, and death) as "major," "intermediate," and "minor."[28] The major predictors also defined in the guidelines as "active cardiac conditions" are acute MI (<7 days), recent MI (7 to 30 days), unstable angina, decompensated CHF, severe valvular disease, and significant dysrhythmias. Active cardiac conditions, when present, mandate intensive management, which may result in delay or cancellation of surgery unless it is emergent. "Intermediate predictors" also defined in the guidelines as "clinical risk factors" are history of ischemic heart disease (e.g., current or prior angina pectoris or prior MI), past or compensated CHF, diabetes mellitus, renal insufficiency, or cerebrovascular disease. Minor predictors (recognized markers for cardiovascular disease that have not proven to increase perioperative risk independently) are age >70 years, abnormal ECG, rhythm other than sinus, and uncontrolled systemic hypertension. The guidelines place aortic and peripheral vascular surgery in the "high-risk" surgery category with an estimated cardiac risk (MI or cardiac-related death) exceeding 5%. CEA and most endovascular procedures are regarded as the "intermediate-risk" category, with an estimated cardiac risk ranging from 1% to 5%. With these definitions, the guidelines apply a stepwise approach to the evaluation of the patient incorporating clinical risk factors, exercise capacity (defined in terms of metabolic equivalents), and urgency of surgery (Fig. 39-5).

These guidelines have shifted the paradigm toward perioperative drug therapy aimed at reducing the cardiac risk either with no noninvasive cardiac testing or only very highly selective noninvasive testing when the outcome will result in a change in the anesthetic plan. Studies in which the AHA/ACC guidelines were used to guide preoperative testing have conflicted as to whether using the guidelines can improve outcome.

Preoperative Coronary Revascularization

Myocardial revascularization may have long-term benefits in patients with triple-vessel coronary disease or poor left ventricular function. However, mortality rates associated with these techniques are consistently higher in patients with peripheral vascular disease compared with those without. Whether preoperative coronary revascularization actually protects against perioperative cardiac events is controversial. The multicenter coronary artery revascularization prophylaxis (CARP) trial randomized patients with coronary disease (except left main disease or ejection fraction <20%) before elective vascular surgery to either coronary revascularization or medical therapy. With state-of-the-art aggressive medical therapy (>80% of patients on β-blockers, >70% on aspirin, and >50% on statins in both groups), they could find no benefit to coronary revascularization.[29] A subsequent subgroup analysis of CARP trial examined the value of coronary artery bypass graft (CABG) versus percutaneous transluminal coronary angioplasty (PTCA) in those requiring coronary revascularization. Patients having a CABG had fewer MIs and tended to spend less time in the hospital after vascular surgery than patients having PTCA.[30] In patients who underwent coronary angiography in both the randomized and nonrandomized portion of the CARP trial, only the subset of patients with unprotected left main disease showed a benefit with preoperative coronary artery revascularization.[31] Thus, preoperative coronary revascularization (surgical or interventional) may be of no value in preventing cardiac events except in those patients in whom revascularization is independently indicated for acute coronary syndrome. High-risk patients should have surveillance for myocardial ischemia (typically troponin I or T) and risk-reducing strategies (including heart rate control). Should coronary revascularization be required before vascular surgery, then surgical revascularization is a suitable option compared with PCI. The safe time interval between surgical revascularization and vascular surgery is 4 to 6 weeks for surgical coronary revascularization and 2 weeks for coronary angioplasty. The safe interval for stents is much longer (see previous discussion).

The DECREASE trials evaluated the value of preoperative testing before major vascular surgery. At the time of the writing of this chapter, there is some concern regarding the validity of these trials, but no trial has been retracted. In DECREASE II, 770 patients having major vascular surgery and considered as having intermediate cardiac risk, defined as the presence of 1 or 2 cardiac risk factors, were randomized to either further risk stratification with stress imaging or proceed directly to surgery.[32] All patients received preoperative bisoprolol with a targeted heart rate (HR) of 60 to 65 initiated before, and continued after surgery. The 30-day incidence of cardiac death and nonfatal MI was similar in both groups (1.8% in the no testing group vs. 2.3% in the tested group). The conclusion of the authors was that further risk stratification in this group of patients considered at intermediate risk based on clinical history alone was unnecessary as long as perioperative β-blockers were used, and testing only delayed necessary vascular surgery. In a pilot study (DECREASE V), 101 patients with three or more risk factors and a markedly positive stress test were randomized to coronary revascularization versus medical therapy. In those patients in whom there was successful revascularization, there was significant improvement in long-term outcome.[33]

Other Medical Problems in Vascular Surgery Patients

Correcting hypertension gradually over days to weeks before surgery allows for normalization of intravascular volume and cerebral autoregulation and results in a more stable perioperative course. However, a meta-analysis of 30 observational trials of cardiovascular outcomes after surgery in hypertensive patients suggests there is a statistically but "not clinically significant" increase in cardiovascular events for hypertensive patients.[34]

Undiagnosed diabetes and abnormal glucose tolerance are common in vascular patients, and predicts perioperative myocardial ischemia.[35] Diabetic patients generally have a higher risk of MI and wound infection compared with nondiabetics undergoing AAA. Glucose management during carotid and thoracic aortic procedures may be especially important, in situations in which hyperglycemia may exacerbate neurologic injury. Intraoperative management of blood glucose concentration is an area of significant controversy, with some studies demonstrating benefit, particularly in cardiac surgery patients. However, two landmark trials of aggressive ICU glucose control have yielded opposite results, with the largest and most recent demonstrating increased mortality in patients whose capillary blood glucose concentration was kept below 110.[36]

Hypercoagulable states are more common in younger patients presenting for vascular surgery and in patients with vascular thrombi in unusual sites. Hypercoagulable responses to surgery may also predispose patients to vascular graft occlusion after surgery. Postoperative abnormalities include elevated fibrinogen levels, antithrombin III deficiency, impaired fibrinolysis, protein C deficiency, and protein S deficiency. Heparin-induced thrombocytopenia and thrombosis can occur (immunoglobulin G-mediated) after several days of exposure to heparin. Treatment includes cessation of all heparin, full anticoagulation with a direct thrombin inhibitor, and 3 weeks of warfarin therapy to prevent arterial thrombosis. Warfarin therapy alone is not recommended as it diminishes protein C and S activities and may initially promote thrombosis.

ORGAN PROTECTION IN VASCULAR SURGERY PATIENTS

Ischemia-reperfusion Injury in the Vascular Surgery Patient: Fundamental Concepts

Ischemia-reperfusion injury (IRI) is the *sine qua non* of organ failure in vascular surgery patients, and the techniques inherent to vascular surgery create a highly specific milieu that promotes multiorgan ischemia-reperfusion. It is important to recognize that IRI is an active, biphasic process (ischemia and reperfusion) in which both processes contribute to injury. Ischemia/hypoxia directly activates antiapoptotic, cell survival, and cell proliferation pathways in many cell types, including vascular endothelial cells and organ cell populations.[37] These pathways are rapid, nontranscriptional, and transcriptional—thus they change the cell and organ functions within minutes, and the altered response continues for hours to days. In addition, hypoxia, particularly if prolonged, results in mitochondrial failure and cell necrosis which present neighboring cells with cytotoxic challenges. The placement of a vascular clamp directly injures perivascular endothelium and intima, including endothelial cells. Injury and activation of endothelial cells triggers both endothelial and nonendothelial responses, including immune/coagulation activation and other potent processes. Finally, reperfusion creates shear stress as well as other changes that further activate endothelium and may induce other injurious or dysregulated processes. Overall, IRI leads to immune activation and translocation of immune/inflammatory cells such as macrophages, vascular paracrine dysregulation via secretion of vasoconstricting and vasodilating agents (endothelin-1, NOS, epoxyeicosatrienoic acids), and massive, dysregulated release of inflammatory cytokines.

Thus, IRI, particularly in vascular surgery patients, is a highly complex micro- and macrophysiologic process. This helps explain why single interventions aimed at single components of this process (e.g., increasing blood pressure to maximize flow) have proven ineffective in clinical studies. More importantly; however, this complexity is the reason why it is important to understand the rationales behind the many potential interventions.

Prevention of Myocardial Injury

Pharmacologic Approaches

Administration of β-blocking agents for primary prevention of perioperative cardiac events has been the focus of intense scrutiny. Many small trials suggest benefit, and meta-analyses of such data suggest that such strategies reduce the risk of perioperative myocardial isch-
5 emia (Table 39-2).[38] Despite the initial enthusiasm for perioperative β-blockade, newer studies have demonstrated that β-blockers may not be effective in lower-risk patients or if heart rate is not well controlled. The POISE trial enrolled 8,351 high-risk β-blocker naive patients and randomly assigned them to high-dose, extended-release metoprolol or placebo.[39] There was a significant reduction of the primary outcome of cardiovascular events, associated with a 27% reduction in MI rate, but with a significantly increased rate of 30-day all-cause mortality and stroke. Although the increased risk of stroke may have been due to hypotension associated with the large dose of metoprolol in β-blocker naive patients, the magnitude of the risk was far in excess of the magnitude of the benefit. Overall, these data suggest that administration of β-blocking agents for primary prevention of perioperative MI is both potentially beneficial and dangerous. The current ACCF/AHA guidelines on perioperative β-blockade advocate that perioperative β-blockade is a Class I indication in patients previously receiving β-blockers,[22] and β-blockers titrated to heart rate and blood pressure for patients undergoing vascular surgery who are at high cardiac risk owing to CAD or the finding of cardiac ischemia on preoperative testing (Class IIa). The recommendations discourage the routine use of higher-dose, nontitrated regimens started on the day of surgery. Flu et al.[40] demonstrated that β-blocker treatment initiated >1 week before surgery is associated with less troponin-T release and fewer strokes compared with treatment initiated <1 week before surgery.

TABLE 39-2. PHARMACOLOGIC PROPHYLAXIS AGAINST ACUTE VASCULAR EVENTS IN PATIENTS UNDERGOING VASCULAR SURGERY

Intervention	Regimen and Remarks	Recommendation[a]
Perioperative β-blockade	β-blockers should be continued in patients undergoing surgery who are receiving β-blockers for treatment of conditions with ACCF/AHA Class I guideline indications for the drugs. This represents a significant revision to 2009 guidelines based on harm from administration of extended-release metoprolol in the POISE trial (see text)	Class I
	• *Titrated to heart rate and blood pressure ("probably recommended") in vascular surgery patients who have high cardiac risk based on known coronary artery disease preoperative testing revealing cardiac ischemia.*	Class IIa
	• *Titrated to heart rate and blood pressure ("reasonable") in vascular surgery patients who have high cardiac risk based on risk factors alone.*	
α_2-agonists	Pretreatment with oral clonidine 300 μg at least 90 min before surgery and therapy continued for 72 h (oral or transdermal, 0.2 mg/d). IV clonidine 300 μg daily can also be administered for 72 h.	Class IIb
Statin therapy	Statins should be continued in patients already taking statins.	Class I
	Typical dose of atorvastatin is 20 mg once daily initiated at least 45 d prior to surgery. Withdrawal of statin therapy for >4 d after vascular surgery is associated with increased risk of cardiac complications. Administration of extended-release fluvastatin preoperatively appears ideal when prolonged postoperative ileus is expected. Statin use is also associated with improved graft patency, limb salvage, and decreased amputation rate in patients undergoing infrainguinal bypass for atherosclerotic vascular disease.	Class IIa
Calcium channel blockers	Reduced perioperative adverse cardiac events; including supraventricular tachycardia in patients undergoing various types of noncardiac surgery (primarily diltiazem). Evidence limited in patients undergoing vascular surgery.	Class IIb
Nitroglycerin	Not indicated for myocardial ischemia prophylaxis or initial treatment. May be used to treat arterial hypertension or elevated cardiac filling pressures or suspected coronary vasospasm.	Class III

[a]Class I recommendation refers to conditions for which there is evidence or general agreement that a given procedure or treatment is useful or effective; class III refers to conditions for which there is evidence and/or general agreement that the procedure/treatment is not useful/effective or in some cases may be harmful. Class II recommendations fall in between and indicate conditions for which there is conflicting evidence or a divergence of opinion about the usefulness/efficacy of a procedure/treatment. Class IIa indicates that the weight of evidence/opinion is in favor of usefulness/efficacy. Class IIb indicates that the usefulness/efficacy is less well established by evidence/opinion. In simple terms, class I recommendations are the "dos," class III recommendations are "don'ts," and class II recommendations are the "maybes." Calcium channel blockers, although not recommended as independent agents for the purpose, should be continued if a patient is receiving them.
IV, intravenous; ACE, angiotensin-converting enzyme; MI, myocardial infarction.

Commonly employed strategies for β-blocker administration in vascular surgery patients initiate oral therapy 7 to 30 days before with either atenolol 50 to 100 mg daily or metoprolol 25 to 50 mg (either extended-release once daily, or immediate-release twice daily). The intraoperative and postoperative periods are managed by intravenous administration of metoprolol titrated to heart rate and blood pressure. Alternatively, esmolol 50 to 500 μg/kg may be given intravenously over 1 minute followed by infusion of 50 to 300 μg/kg/min to achieve the target heart rate. It is important to recognize that some preparations of intravenous esmolol are dilute enough that administration of high dose infusions over 10 or more hours can result in hypervolemia and CHF, a complication that has been observed by the authors. In patients already taking β-blockers, they are continued to the day of surgery and followed by intravenous therapy to achieve the target heart rate as described previously.

α_2-adrenergic agonists (clonidine or mivazerol) have been investigated as cardioprotective agents in the perioperative environment. The data supporting these medications are intriguing but not yet supported by large randomized trials. A meta-analysis suggests beneficial effects of perioperative α_2-agonists with regard to cardiac morbidity and death in patients undergoing vascular surgery.[41] This analysis included dexmedetomidine (DEX), which was not beneficial in its own meta-analysis,[42] perhaps suggesting the effects of other α_2-agonists might be beneficial if assessed alone. The authors have evaluated transdermal clonidine (0.2 mg/day) initiated the night before surgery, and 0.3 mg oral clonidine administered 60 to 90 minutes before surgery. Clonidine reduced intraoperative myocardial ischemia and catecholamine levels as measured on the first postoperative day.[43]

ACCF/AHA guidelines and an increasing volume of data support consideration of HMG-CoA reductase inhibitors (statins) for primary prevention of perioperative MI in vascular surgery patients. Two randomized trials have demonstrated reductions in adverse cardiac outcomes with statin use (atorvastatin 20 mg daily started 30 days before surgery or fluvastatin 80 mg daily started 37 days before surgery, both continued for 2 to 4 weeks after surgery).[44,45] In addition, a meta-analysis of multiple observational trials found that preoperative statin therapy was associated with 59% reduction in relative risk of mortality after vascular surgery while no definitive conclusions could be drawn on cardiovascular morbidity.[10] Preoperative extended-release fluvastatin may be of specific benefit to patients undergoing intra-abdominal vascular surgery who often have postoperative ileus. It is unclear why statins appear to be beneficial, but pleiotropic (nonlipid lowering) effects are thought to be involved. Finally, discontinuation of statin therapy (>4 days) after major vascular surgery is associated with an increased postoperative cardiac risk, suggesting that statin therapy should be resumed early after major vascular surgery.[11] The recent ACCF/AHA guidelines advocate continuing statin therapy in patients currently taking statins as a Class I indication.[22]

ACE inhibitors also have beneficial actions with regard to acute vascular events independent of their antihypertensive action in patients with AVD. A single retrospective analysis of 3,020 patients undergoing vascular surgery at Veteran's Administration hospitals suggests that ACE inhibitor therapy, in combination with other cardiovascular agents, may reduce perioperative mortality after vascular surgery.[46] However, their use in vascular surgery is complicated by their potent perioperative hypotensive effects, and one trial of in excess of 800 patients found worsened outcomes in AAA surgical patients who received preoperative ACE inhibitors or angiotensin II receptor blockers (ARBs).[47]

A meta-analysis suggested beneficial effects of calcium channel blockers in reducing perioperative adverse cardiac events (cardiac-related death, MI, ischemia, or supraventricular tachycardia) in patients undergoing noncardiac surgery, with limited numbers of vascular surgery patients.[48] The majority of these effects were attributable to diltiazem (one of two nondihydropyridine agents). Conversely, the dihydropyridine–calcium channel blockers have been associated with increased perioperative mortality.[49] It seems clear that further evaluation of diltiazem as a cardioprotective agent is warranted, but to date no randomized trial has been conducted. On the basis of the evidence, the authors recommend that calcium channel blockers not be employed for perioperative cardioprotection.

Because it is a coronary artery dilator, nitroglycerin may seem attractive for perioperative prevention of coronary events. However, use of nitroglycerin may provoke or exacerbate hypotension with reflex tachycardia, or simply hypotension in the β-blocked patient. Several small controlled studies have shown minimal or no effect.[50–52] Therefore prophylactic nitroglycerin should not be contemplated as a cardioprotective strategy.

Choice of anesthetic technique is widely believed to influence cardiac outcomes, although data specific to vascular surgery patients is scant. High-dose narcotic anesthetics reduce the stress response after major surgery, but mandate overnight ventilation, and increase costs and the risk of ventilator-associated adverse outcomes. Volatile anesthetics promote preconditioning, reduce troponin release, hasten extubation and hospital discharge in cardiac surgery, as well as reducing death and MI compared with intravenous anesthetics.[53,54] Whether these findings are transferable to vascular surgery is unclear; however, and the best available data, a single randomized controlled trial of 88 patients, demonstrated no effect on troponin or mortality.[55]

Nonpharmacologic Approaches

Epidural analgesia may reduce perioperative myocardial ischemia because preload and afterload are reduced, the postoperative adrenergic and coagulation responses are reduced, and with thoracic administration, the coronary arteries are dilated. Although effects on cardiac outcomes in small trials have been mixed, a meta-analysis of these trials suggests that thoracic epidurals may reduce postoperative MI in high-risk patients undergoing major abdominal and vascular surgery.[56] In addition, a Cochrane review of epidural analgesia for abdominal aortic repair found a statistically significant reduction (with relative risk 0.5) in postoperative MI in the treatment group, an effect which was more pronounced in the thoracic epidural (vs. lumbar) group.[57] No randomized trial data exists to support the choice of epidural analgesia for open abdominal surgery; however, available data suggest it may be beneficial.

Anemia is an independent predictor of adverse short- and long-term cardiac outcomes in vascular surgery patients.[58,59] However, it is important to recognize that red blood cell transfusion represents far more than simple treatment of anemia—rather it is administration of a highly active biologic agent with pleiotropic effects. In general, vascular surgery patients are at high risk for myocardial ischemia and this has resulted in a more liberal transfusion strategy in this population at most centers. However, as in other surgical populations, and even after adjusting for propensity and severity of illness, transfusion worsens important outcomes including survival after vascular surgery.[60] In addition, emerging data also undermines the notion that transfusion improves outcomes in patients with myocardial ischemia and MI[61] and may support the idea that restrictive transfusion practices are safe for critically ill patients with known CAD. In contrast, Beattie et al.[62] used a propensity matched design of patients undergoing surgery from his center and found that β-blocked patients do not tolerate surgical anemia when compared with patients who are naive to β-blockers. Therefore, it may be critical to maintain adequate hemoglobin levels in β-blocked patients. It is important to recognize that all packed red cell units are not the same, and that storage time may be directly related to adverse outcomes.[63]

Postoperative management, beginning in postanesthesia care unit (PACU), may affect cardiac outcomes. Maintenance of normothermia is cardioprotective,[64] and should be pursued unless whole-body hypothermia is being employed as an organ-protective strategy (e.g., after cardiac arrest). Whether hypothermia is intended or not, its adrenergic consequences (shivering, tachycardia, hypertension) should be treated. In addition, aggressive postoperative surveillance may reduce cardiac risk as suggested by Monte Carlo simulation studies.[65]

Finally, the emergence of EVAR has prompted the hope that this procedure might reduce cardiac risk relative to open repair. Unfortunately, trials of open versus endovascular repair (OVER) have generally found no significant difference in the rate of cardiac complications. However, one randomized trial of 881 patients found a trend toward more events in the open repair group,[66] and a more recent study in patients of low to moderate risk found that EVAR was associated with a lower risk of minor, but not major cardiac complications.[67] Given the size of these studies, it is unlikely that EVAR will prove a very significant cardiac risk reduction when compared with open repair.

Prevention of Kidney Injury

Etiology and Epidemiology of Kidney Injury

Perioperative acute kidney injury (AKI) is a common complication of vascular surgery and is associated with high morbidity and mortality. The incidence of AKI is between 16% and 22% of patients undergoing aortic surgery.[68] Postoperative mortality is four- to fivefold higher in those who develop AKI when compared to those who do not and minor elevations in serum creatinine are related to increased morbidity and mortality.[69]

The pathophysiology of perioperative AKI is multifactorial, with renal IRI playing a major role. In addition to IRI, the use of nephrotoxic drugs such as ACE inhibitors, nonsteroidal anti-inflammatory drugs (NSAIDs), aminoglycosides, and diuretics in the perioperative period can contribute to AKI. Other processes contributing to perioperative AKI during vascular surgery include atheroembolization to renal arteries during surgical manipulation of the aorta and surgical injury to the renal arteries themselves. In addition, rhabdomyolysis secondary to injury or immobilization is common in vascular surgery patients.

Preoperative renal dysfunction is the most powerful predictor of postoperative renal dysfunction. Patients with pre-existing renal insufficiency have an increased risk of postoperative renal failure, as well as cardiac complications and death. If patients receive chronic dialysis treatments, they should receive dialysis on the day before or the same day as surgery. Some patients will actually be hypovolemic as a result, which can contribute to hypotension with induction of general or regional anesthesia. Interestingly, women have an increased incidence of perioperative AKI than men following cardiac and vascular surgeries. This is in contrast to the general surgical population including all age groups, in which women seem to be protected from AKI when compared to men.[70] Of note, women undergoing cardiac and vascular surgeries are older and more likely to be postmenopausal when compared to other women having surgeries, suggesting that estrogen plays a role in this protection.[71]

Several intraoperative factors including hemodynamic instability, the need for inotropic support, and the transfusion of greater than five units of packed cells or autologous blood can predict postoperative kidney injury.[72] In aortic surgery, the level of aortic clamping is correlated with postoperative kidney dysfunction, with suprarenal cross-clamping of the aorta placing the kidneys at the highest risk. With suprarenal occlusion, renal blood flow decreases by 80%. Even with infrarenal aortic clamping, renal blood flow is still reduced by 45%. These renal hemodynamic changes do not immediately revert after clamp release, and persist for at least 30 minutes beyond the systemic cardiovascular return to baseline. In addition, prolonged aortic cross-clamp time (ischemia time) is associated with elevated postoperative creatinine values.[73] Interestingly, intraoperative urine output is not predictive of postoperative renal function.[74]

In thoracic aortic repair, there are studies that suggest that an endovascular rather than open surgery may decrease the risk of perioperative AKI, especially in those patients identified as high risk.

Pharmacologic Approaches

6 Unfortunately, despite promising bench and animal research, there is currently no clinical evidence to support the benefit of any pharmacologic intervention or protection strategy. Regardless, the use of mannitol, loop diuretics, and dopamine are pervasive in clinical practice as many believe that these measures will be beneficial for renal protection. Despite the fact that the use of mannitol and other diuretics can lead to hypovolemia and thus decreased tissue perfusion. Readers are cautioned that trials of renoprotective agents as a group suffer from heterogeneity of outcome measures, definitions of renal failure, methodology, and study populations.

Mannitol is widely used in vascular surgery because it induces osmotic diuresis, decreases epithelial and endothelial cell swelling, acts as a hydroxyl free radical scavenger, and increases synthesis of prostaglandin resulting in renal vasodilation. However, there is no evidence of a renoprotective effect of mannitol in vascular surgery patients. Similarly, loop diuretics are used intraoperatively to maintain urine output, but have not been shown to improve renal outcome or patient survival. Dopamine infusion of 0.5 to 2 ug/kg body weight per minute increases renal plasma flow, sodium excretion, and glomerular filtration rate (GFR). Unfortunately, multiple randomized trials and meta-analyses have failed to show benefit with regard to the outcomes of death or prolonged dialysis.[75] Fenoldopam remains an active target of investigation and small studies have suggested benefit at the cost of increased complications (largely hypotension). Only one study has evaluated the renal effects of fenoldopam in vascular surgery, it found no renal benefit.[76]

Because of their anti-inflammatory and antioxidant effects, statins are being examined for their protective effects against perioperative AKI. A retrospective, population-based cohort study suggests that in patients older than 64 years undergoing major elective surgery, statin use decreased the rate of AKI and reduced perioperative mortality.[77] Another retrospective cohort study observed that statin use decreased the incidence of kidney dysfunction following EVAR with suprarenal endograft fixation.[78] Atrial natriuretic peptide (ANP) is also a candidate renoprotective agent which causes natriuresis, diuresis, and vasorelaxation. In a recent prospective, randomized, placebo-controlled trial, the intraoperative and postoperative infusions of ANP resulted in lower blood urea nitrogen (BUN), creatinine, and plasma B-type natriuretic peptide (BNP).[79] However, trials of ANP for renal protection have suggested a trend toward increased mortality with ANP treatment.[80]

Nonpharmacologic Approaches

Multiple nonpharmacologic strategies have been employed to prevent renal injury during aortic surgery. Selective blood perfusion of the renal arteries has been attempted to minimize the time of renal ischemia during cross-clamping. Another strategy uses cold renal artery perfusion to produce local hypothermia to decrease renal oxygen demands. A randomized trial showed that direct intra-arterial infusion of 4° C crystalloid or blood into the kidneys decreased the incidence of postoperative renal impairment.[81] Remote ischemic preconditioning is thought to prevent IRI in multiple organ systems by inducing ischemic-protection pathways. Ali et al.[82] found that intermittent cross-clamping of the internal iliacs reduced the incidence of renal insufficiency by 23%. However, repeated clamping of nonoperative arteries in patients with severe atherosclerosis likely increases the risk of surgical adverse events, and significant benefit would need to be demonstrated before adoption of such a practice.

It has been widely hoped that morbidity and mortality from EVAR would be reduced compared to open aortic aneurysm repair. The UK EVAR trials found no long-term difference in renal function between open repair and EVAR.[83] EVAR decreases kidney IRI because of the elimination of aortic cross-clamping; however, contrast-induced nephropathy is a significant cause of kidney dysfunction. As in open aortic repair (OAR), preoperative kidney function is the major predictor of postoperative renal complications. Because the renal dysfunction in EVAR is believed to stem from the use of intravenous contrast pre- and intraoperatively, prevention strategies are aimed at minimizing contrast exposure. Magnetic resonance angiography or gadolinium-based contrast studies have been proposed for patients at risk for contrast-mediated nephropathy. The use of CO_2 as contrast media and endovascular ultrasound should be used when possible to limit the use of radio-opaque dye. Allowing adequate time for renal recovery between preoperative studies and EVAR may be of benefit. Other strategies for renal protection from contrast include the use of N-acetylcysteine, sodium bicarbonate, and ensuring adequate hydration.[84]

Prevention of Pulmonary Complications

Pulmonary complications are common after major vascular surgery (10% to 30% of AAA patients) and are associated with increased mortality and length of stay.[85] Perioperative interventions clearly influence postoperative pulmonary function and likely reduce the risk of postoperative respiratory failure, prolonged mechanical ventilation, and pneumonia in surgical patients overall. Although data specific to vascular surgery are lacking, many large studies of perioperative pulmonary complications include vascular surgery patients, in particular patients undergoing aortic repair.

The American College of Physicians guidelines for reduction of perioperative pulmonary complications identify abdominal surgery, surgery lasting more than 3 hours, emergency surgery, preoperative CHF, and preoperative chronic lung disease as significant risk factors for pulmonary complications. The most effective preventive measure is postoperative lung expansion, either continuous positive airway pressure (CPAP) or incentive spirometry. Anesthetic technique is as an independent risk factor for pulmonary complications, with general anesthesia conferring an odds ratio of 1.8.[86] Although there is some heterogeneity in the overall data, the Cochrane Database analysis confirms that postoperative thoracic epidural analgesia reduces postoperative respiratory failure and duration of mechanical ventilation in patients undergoing abdominal aortic surgery.[57]

Since the initial 2,000 ARDSNET trial reported a mortality benefit of low tidal volumes (6 to 8 mL/kg)[87] in patients with acute respiratory distress syndrome, there has been interest in extension of this benefit to the perioperative population. No studies address the clinical benefit of lung-protective ventilatory strategies in vascular surgery patients. However, indirect data are intriguing. Two small clinical studies of surgical patients (in one case prolonged procedures, and in the other esophagectomy with one-lung ventilation) found reductions in systemic or bronchoalveolar lavage inflammatory markers,[88,89] and a study of cardiac surgery patients found that patients ventilated with low tidal volumes were more likely to be extubated by postoperative hour 6 and less likely to be reintubated.[90] No significant data exists to suggest that such tidal volumes are harmful.

Choice of procedure and surgical technique may influence pulmonary outcome. Aortic clamp site influences the risk of postoperative pulmonary complications (suprarenal vs. infrarenal 25% vs. 12%).[91] In randomized trials, EVAR has not demonstrated reduced risk of pulmonary complications when compared with OAR.

In short, postoperative lung expansion with CPAP or incentive spirometry and postoperative thoracic epidural analgesia reduce perioperative respiratory complications. There is some suggestion that lung protective ventilator strategies used intraoperatively may also be protective.

Protection of the Central Nervous System and Spinal Cord

7 Vascular surgery patients are at high risk for postoperative nervous system disease, including delirium, stroke, and spinal cord ischemia. All three of these complications worsen outcomes overall and can have devastating permanent consequences to the patient and their family. Importantly, anesthesiologists have access to effective preventive tools for each of these problems, and careful anesthetic management may reasonably be expected to improve surgical outcomes.

Prevention of Perioperative Delirium

Delirium (sometimes called "central nervous system failure") is a common central nervous system complication of vascular surgery. Aortic aneurysm surgery is an independent risk factor for delirium,[92] which in the past has been under-appreciated as a serious complication leading to severe adverse outcomes. Delirium is an independent risk factor for short- and long-term mortality, increased ICU and hospital stay, and skilled nursing facility discharge.[93] Unfortunately, there are no known effective perioperative interventions to reduce the incidence of delirium as a whole and few studies specifically address vascular surgery patients. However, the limited available data indicate that age, preoperative cognitive dysfunction, depression, previous amputation, alcohol abuse, and intraoperative blood transfusion are risk factors. Alcohol withdrawal remains a common cause of perioperative delirium. In patients who remain sedated postoperatively, the anesthesiologist's detailed social history may provide the only available information about preoperative substance use.

Prevention of Perioperative Stroke

Stroke is nearly twice as common in patients who have undergone AAA repairs than in the general population as long as 20 years postoperatively.[94] Open thoracoabdominal aortic aneurysm repair carries a higher risk of stroke than AAA repair, between 1.5% and 3.5%, whereas the overall risk of stroke from thoracic endovascular aortic repair (TEVAR) is 2.9%.[95] Unfortunately, there is little supporting any preventive measure for stroke in vascular surgery patients (other than those undergoing CEA), and scant data for surgical patients overall. Patients with symptomatic carotid stenosis benefit from carotid revascularization before major vascular surgery. Other potentially modifiable risk factors include atrial fibrillation and discontinuation of antiplatelet therapy, which both increase the risk of perioperative stroke.[96] However, the risks of active management of atrial fibrillation or continuation of antiplatelet therapy through surgery have not been specifically evaluated in vascular surgery patients.

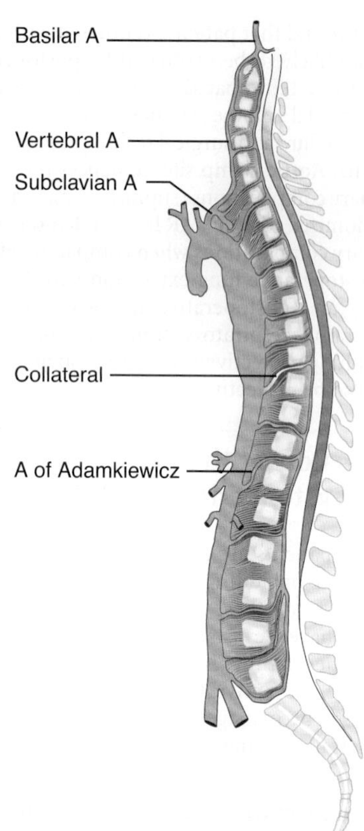

FIGURE 39-6. The artery of Adamkiewicz usually arises at the T11–T12 level and provides the blood supply to the lower spinal cord. Its variable location and the uncertainty of additional collateral blood supply explain, in part, the unpredictability of paraplegia following descending aortic surgery. (Reprinted from: Piccone W, DeLaria GA, Najafi H. Descending thoracic aneurysms. In: Bergan JJ, Yao JST, eds. *Aortic Surgery.* Philadelphia, PA: WB Saunders; 1989:249, with permission.)

TABLE 39-3. METHODS OF SPINAL CORD PROTECTION DURING DESCENDING THORACIC AORTIC SURGERY

Method
Limitation of cross-clamp duration
Distal circulatory support
Reattachment of critical intercostal arteries
CSF drainage
Hypothermia
Moderate systemic (32–34°C)
Epidural cooling
Circulatory arrest
Maintenance of proximal blood pressure
Pharmacotherapy
Systemic
Corticosteroids, barbiturates, naloxone, calcium channel antagonists, O_2 free radical scavengers, NMDA antagonists, mannitol, magnesium, vasodilators (adenosine, papaverine, prostacyclin), perfluorocarbons, colchicine
Intrathecal
Papaverine, magnesium, tetracaine, perfluorocarbons
Avoidance of postoperative hypotension
Sequential aortic clamping
Enhanced monitoring for spinal cord ischemia
Somatosensory evoked potentials
Motor evoked potentials
Hydrogen-saturated saline
Avoidance of hyperglycemia

CSF, cerebrospinal fluid; NMDA, *N*-methyl-D-aspartate.
From: Mas J-L, Chatellier G, Beyssen B, et al. Endarterectomy versus stenting in patients with symptomatic severe carotid stenosis. *N Engl J Med.* 2006;355:1660.

Prevention of Perioperative Spinal Cord Ischemia

Spinal cord ischemia occurs in 1% to 11% of operations involving a distal aortic repair. The spinal cord is supplied by two posterior arteries; together, they supply 25% of spinal cord blood flow. The anterior spinal artery (Fig. 39-6) supplies 75% of spinal cord blood flow and is the primary supply to the anterolateral cord. The anterior spinal artery is fed by a series of radicular arteries arising from the aorta, and collateralization is poor. The blood supply to the thoracolumbar cord is derived from the radicular artery of Adamkiewicz. In 75% of cases, it joins the anterior spinal artery between T8 and T12, and in 10% it joins between L1 and L2. Much of the blood flow in the anterior spinal artery depends on the artery of Adamkiewicz. Because the flow in the spinal arteries depends on collateralization and is often bidirectional, the blood supply to the spinal cord can be shunted to the rest of the body when perfusion pressures are low. Such a situation may arise when a single high aortic occlusion clamp is applied.

Standard measures to prevent spinal cord ischemia include short cross-clamping time, maintenance of normal cardiac function, and high perfusion pressures. In high aortic clamping, other methods should be considered (Table 39-3). Some surgeons place a Gott shunt, a heparinized tube that can decompress the heart and also provide distal perfusion. The Gott shunt can be placed proximally into the ascending aorta (the most common site), aortic arch, descending aorta, or left ventricle, and inserted distally into the descending aorta (most commonly), femoral artery, or abdominal aorta. Even with a Gott shunt or partial bypass, there is an obligatory time of visceral ischemia when the visceral blood supply arises from a point between the proximal and distal clamps. Placement of a shunt may result in atheroembolism, which can produce rather than prevent ischemic injury and death. Other surgeons may place a temporary ex vivo right axillofemoral bypass graft before positioning for thoracotomy. After the thoracic aortic surgery is completed, the axillofemoral graft is removed. The placement of a shunt attenuates the hemodynamic response to aortic unclamping, reduces acidosis, and could conceivably ameliorate the hormonal and metabolic changes that accompany aortic occlusion.

Other groups have chosen to use partial bypass, either from the left atrium or ascending aorta to the iliac or femoral artery to provide distal perfusion and decompress the heart. A heat exchanger may be used to induce hypothermia, which may be neuroprotective. Segmental sequential surgical repair may minimize the duration of ischemia to any given vascular bed. Intercostal artery reattachment in hopes of preserving blood flow to the anterior spinal cord may be beneficial. After reperfusion, the heat exchanger can be used to warm the patient. Other potential advantages of left atrial–left femoral artery shunt with centrifugal pump support are better operative field exposure, afterload reduction, maintenance of stable distal aortic perfusion, and reduced (but not eliminated) head and neck edema.

A markedly reduced incidence of neurologic deficits has been reported when distal aortic perfusion is combined with drainage of cerebrospinal fluid (CSF).[97] CSF drainage is used in the hope of improving the pressure gradient, allowing spinal cord blood flow as aortic occlusion lowers distal arterial pressures and increases the central venous pressure. The new endovascular techniques represent an alternative therapy when anatomy permits; lower paraplegia rates have been reported compared with open surgery.[98] However, neurologic complications still occur, and CSF drainage is commonly employed in both open and endovascular procedures for primary prevention and management.

CAROTID ENDARTERECTOMY

Carotid disease is usually a problem of embolization and less often occlusion or insufficiency. The disease may manifest itself as amaurosis fugax (transient attacks of monocular blindness) when the ophthalmic artery is embolized. Other patients may experience episodes of paresthesias, clumsiness of the extremities, or speech problems, which resolve spontaneously after a short period. These are the classic transient ischemic attacks (TIAs). However, approximately 30% of ischemic strokes are caused by obstructive carotid atherosclerosis. An isolated, cervical bruit in asymptomatic patients also seems to be associated with a higher risk of stroke, but the correlation between the location of the bruits and the type of subsequent stroke is poor.

The most common noninvasive test is carotid duplex ultrasonography, which combines B-mode anatomic imaging and pulse Doppler spectral analysis of blood flow velocity. The estimated sensitivity and specificity of the duplex scan to detect a carotid artery stenosis greater than 60% are approximately 94% and 92%, respectively, when using digital subtraction angiography as the reference standard.[99] Positive tests are usually followed by confirmatory angiography.

Management of Asymptomatic Carotid Stenosis

The optimal treatment of asymptomatic carotid stenosis is controversial.[100] For asymptomatic patients with a stenosis of >60%, the asymptomatic carotid atherosclerosis study (ACAS) detected an outcome benefit for CEA over medical therapy: Ipsilateral stroke and any perioperative stroke or death was estimated to be 11% for patients treated medically and 5.1% for surgical patients after 5 years.[101] This results in an absolute risk reduction of about 1% per year for freedom from stroke. Optimal medical therapy included recommendations to stop smoking, aspirin, blood pressure control, and statin therapy. The European asymptomatic carotid surgery trial (ACST-1) randomized 3,120 patients to CEA plus medical therapy, or medical therapy alone, and found similar results, with a stroke risk reduction of 5.9% and 6.1% at 5 years and 10 years, respectively.[102] The authors concluded that there is a benefit to CEA over medical therapy for asymptomatic stenosis only when both the perioperative risk is low, and the patient is expected to live more than 10 years.

The recent carotid revascularization endarterectomy versus stenting trial (CREST) comparing carotid angioplasty and stenting (CAS) to CEA included 1,181 asymptomatic patients, and showed no difference in the 4-year composite end point rate of any stroke, MI, or death between the two groups (CAS 3.5% vs. CEA 3.6%, hazard ratio = 1.02%, $p = 0.96$).[103] ACST-2 is now underway to compare CEA and CAS in this population.[104] However, using ACAS data, even with an operative risk for CEA/CAS of 0%, the NNT would still be above 10, with 92% of interventions being unnecessary.[105] This has led many physicians to question the role of CEA in the asymptomatic patient.

Management of Symptomatic Carotid Stenosis

The case for intervention in symptomatic patients with carotid stenosis is more clear-cut. CEA, in conjunction with aspirin therapy, has proven superior to medical therapy alone in a large trial of symptomatic patients with a stenosis >70% in the North American symptomatic carotid endarterectomy trial (NASCET).[106] The trial was stopped at 2 years due to a significant difference, with a 28% risk of stroke in the medical group compared to 13% in the CEA group. These results were confirmed by the European carotid surgery trial (ECST) of greater than 3,000 patients.[107]

There have been many trials in recent years comparing CEA with CAS for symptomatic patients. These initially reported varying results for stenting compared with CEA. The recent CREST trial randomized >2,500 patients to CAS and CEA and showed no difference of the composite endpoint of stroke, MI, or death between the two groups (7.2% vs. 6.8% for CAS and CEA respectively, hazard ratio 1.11, $p = 0.51$).[108] CAS was associated with a twofold increase in procedural death/stroke, whereas CEA is associated with a twofold increase in procedural MI. Of note, the study excluded high-risk patients, as well as those with contradictions to CAS for anatomic reasons. The recent AHA guidelines recommend CEA for high-risk patients with recent TIA and moderate (50% to 69%) or severe (79% to 99%) ipsilateral carotid artery stenosis if the perioperative morbidity and mortality risk is estimated to be <6%.[109] However, it is likely that a greater proportion of "average-risk" patients will be treated by CAS.

Preoperative Evaluation and Preparation for CEA

Most patients presenting for CEA will be taking aspirin which should be continued throughout the perioperative period. Many patients will also be taking another antiplatelet therapy. The benefit of continuing other agents at the time of CEA must be balanced against the risk of bleeding. Perioperative clopidogrel has been identified as a risk factor for post-CEA bleeding, particularly if it is continued to the day before surgery. At the authors' institution, surgeons as a rule prefer to stop clopidogrel 5 days preoperatively.

It is not advisable to delay urgent surgery that might prevent a stroke for extensive cardiac evaluation even in patients with known cardiac disease. However, the long-term risks of adverse cardiac events after CEA are related to progression of CAD. The approach to patients with both severe CAD and carotid occlusive disease is controversial. Because combined or staged operations are relatively rare (especially for symptomatic carotid disease), many case series suffer from the limitation of having been performed over many years, making generalizability to current practice difficult.

Monitoring and Preserving Neurologic Integrity

The intraoperative goals of protecting the brain and the heart often conflict. For example, increasing arterial blood pressure to augment cerebral blood flow increases the oxygen demand of the heart. The rationale behind maintaining a stable, high–normal blood pressure throughout the procedure is based on the assumption that blood vessels in ischemic or hypoperfused areas of brain 8 have lost normal autoregulation. There is some clinical evidence that elevation of blood pressure to "normal" levels during awake CEA can reverse developing neurologic deficits. Nonetheless, hypotension and hypoperfusion are not the most common cause of stroke after CEA; embolic events may be even more important, and often occur postoperatively (Fig. 39-7).[106] On balance, it is probably beneficial in the absence of neurologic monitoring to avoid hypotension during the period of cross-clamping, particularly if no shunt is used. Intravenous fluid, and vasopressors such as phenylephrine can be used to maintain blood pressure between normal and 20% above baseline. However, augmentation of blood pressure is not without risk and has been associated with an increased incidence of MI.[110] If information from the awake patient or reliable monitoring shows good cerebral blood flow, the anesthesiologist may choose to use less vasopressor and to maintain a lower blood pressure during the period of temporary carotid occlusion than would be otherwise feasible.

Hypercapnia during CEA may be detrimental if it dilates vessels in normal areas of the brain while vessels in ischemic brain areas that are already maximally dilated cannot respond. The net effect, then, is a "steal" phenomenon (i.e., a diversion of blood flow from hypoperfused brain regions to normally perfused brain regions). Conversely, hypocarbia may cause vasoconstriction and extend any area of cerebral ischemia. Most authorities therefore recommend the maintenance of normocarbia. Moderate hyperglycemia may worsen ischemic brain injury, and hyperglycemia has a documented association with worse outcome after CEA.[111]

Almost all commonly used anesthetic agents reduce cerebral metabolism, thereby decreasing the brain's requirements for oxygen. However, the notion that reduced cerebral metabolism is associated with cerebral protection has been challenged. Isoflurane, desflurane, and sevoflurane reduce cerebral oxygen requirements

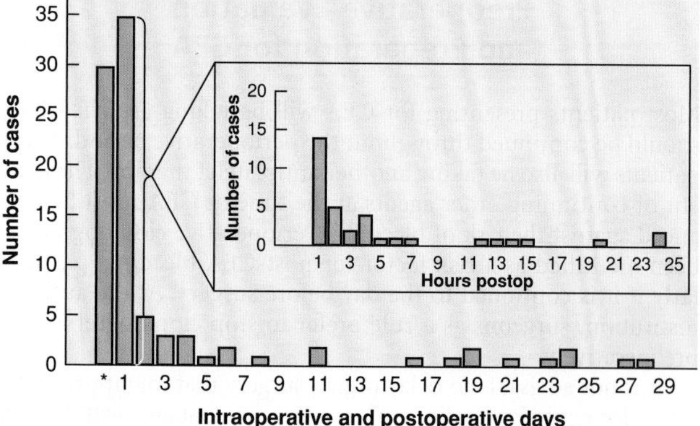

FIGURE 39-7. Data from the North American Symptomatic Carotid Trial (NASCET). Of the perioperative strokes, 35% (30/85) occurred intraoperatively, whereas 65% (55/85) occurred after the patient left the operating room (delayed events). The figure illustrates the time of onset of the 92 surgical outcome events.

comparably, but the later two agents allow for faster emergence and recovery. In addition, volatile anesthetics may provide preconditioning and neuronal protection by inducing nitric oxide synthase.

Barbiturates may offer a degree of brain protection during periods of regional ischemia. Thiopental decreases cerebral metabolic oxygen requirements to about 50% of baseline. These maximally achievable reductions in oxygen requirements correspond to a silent (i.e., isoelectric) EEG. Beyond this point, additional doses of barbiturates are neither necessary nor helpful. In cases of massive global ischemia in which basal cellular metabolism has already deteriorated, even high doses of barbiturates will not improve neurologic outcome. Therefore, some clinicians use thiopental not only for induction of anesthesia, but also for continuous infusion and/or as a 4- to 6-mg/kg bolus just before carotid occlusion. The cardiac depressant effects of the barbiturates may require inotropic support. Unfortunately, no rigorous proof is available that the use of barbiturates in the described manner can improve neurologic outcome after CEA. Excellent results have been obtained for CEA using high doses of barbiturates during carotid occlusion, without neurophysiologic monitoring or shunt placement; on average, tracheal extubation was delayed until 2 hours after surgery was completed.

Both etomidate and propofol decrease brain electrical activity and thus decrease cellular oxygen requirements. Etomidate preserves cardiovascular stability and may be beneficial in a patient population whose cardiac reserves are often limited. Propofol also allows rapid awakening of the patient and neurologic assessment at the end of surgery. Cerebral autoregulation is impaired by sevoflurane but preserved under propofol–remifentanil anesthesia.[112] Stump pressures have also been shown to be lower during sevoflurane anesthesia than with propofol: This was attributed to sevoflurane-induced vasodilation.[113] Propofol and remifentanil may be associated with a lower incidence of myocardial ischemia than a volatile-based anesthetic, but does not appear to affect overall clinical outcome.[114] Although the available evidence for the protective effects of etomidate or propofol during CEA is inconclusive, a small series in patients undergoing temporary ischemia for intracranial aneurysm clipping suggests that etomidate, propofol, or barbiturate use prolongs tolerable ischemia and reduces brain infarction.[115] Animal studies have suggested a degree of neuroprotection with both the volatile agents[116] and propofol.[117]

Hypothermia can depress neuronal activity sufficiently to decrease cellular oxygen requirements below the minimum levels normally required for continued cell viability. In theory, hypothermia represents the most effective method of cerebral protection. Even a mild decrease in temperature of about 2° to 3°C at the time of arterial hypoxemia may reduce ischemic damage to the brain. The first reported CEA was performed with the patient's head covered by ice packs. Unfortunately, this method is cumbersome, unpredictable, and rarely used. The literature provides no definitive evidence to support the hypothesis that hypothermia protects the brain sufficiently to justify the myocardial risks imposed by hypothermia and shivering. In the setting of cerebral aneurysm surgery, intraoperative hypothermia did not improve the neurologic outcome after craniotomy among good-grade patients with aneurysmal subarachnoid hemorrhage.[118]

Temporary occlusion ("cross-clamping") of the carotid artery acutely disrupts blood flow, even if flow to the ipsilateral hemisphere of the brain was already markedly diminished by severe stenosis. Continued blood supply to the brain will depend on adequate collateral blood flow through the circle of Willis if no shunt is used. If carotid stenosis has worsened gradually before CEA is performed, collaterals from the circle of Willis may have had time to develop, and the cerebral circulation may not be compromised by carotid occlusion during surgery. However, if collateral flow is compromised because of occlusive disease of the contralateral carotid artery and/or the vertebral arteries, the chances are greater that marked hypoperfusion of the brain will occur during carotid clamping. Indeed, patients with bilateral carotid disease have a higher risk of perioperative stroke after CEA than patients with unilateral disease only.

There are practice variations among surgeons in the use of shunts in carotid surgery. Surgeons who never use shunts usually rely on expedient surgery to avoid neurologic problems and do not report worse overall outcome statistics than those who do. Placement of a shunt is associated with an embolism-related stroke rate of at least 0.7% from the dislodgment and embolization of atheroma. The technical problems of shunting include air embolism, kinking of the shunt, shunt occlusion against the side of the vessel wall, and injury or disruption of the distal internal carotid artery. Patients with shunts may still develop EEG abnormalities; in these situations, shunt adjustments may be necessary. The shunt may impair surgical access to the artery, thereby increasing cross-clamp time. Most important, the use of a shunt is beneficial only if the cause of neurologic dysfunction is inadequate blood flow. However, the majority of studies suggest that as many as 65% to 95% of all neurologic deficits during CEA may be caused by thromboembolic events (Fig. 39-7). In the NASCET trial, shunting (used in 41% of patients) was not associated with a change in risk of stroke.[106]

Surgeons who use shunts selectively often use a monitoring device of cerebral perfusion to help them decide when to place the shunt. However, despite a huge body of investigative work, there is still questionable evidence that monitoring actually makes a difference.[119] Monitoring approaches include assessment of the awake patient, transcranial Doppler (TCD), somatosensory evoked potential (SSEP), EEG, cerebral oximetry, and direct xenon cerebral blood flow measurement. In each case, the goal is to avoid unnecessary shunting.

EEG monitoring is often used. EEG deterioration begins usually below a cerebral blood flow rate of about 15 mL/min/100 g brain tissue, but cellular metabolic failure does not seem to occur until blood flow falls below 10 to 12 mL/min/100 g brain tissue.[120] The most common manifestations of EEG ischemia during CEA are ipsilateral attenuation, ipsilateral slowing with attenuation, and ipsilateral slowing without attenuation. Figure 39-8 shows a processed EEG reflecting acute cerebral ischemia following left carotid artery occlusion; the placement of a shunt in this case promptly reversed the ischemic changes. However, as in all the cerebral monitoring techniques, the sensitivity in detecting perioperative stroke is limited by the fact that most strokes occur following surgery and are likely related to thromboembolic phenomena. Rapid changes in anesthetic depth may also complicate interpretation. This is particularly relevant in centers in which barbiturates or propofol infusions are used to induce EEG suppression. In the NASCET trial, 93% of patients underwent CEA with general anesthesia; 51% of patients had intraoperative cerebral monitoring (31% EEG, 14% stump pressure, 7% evoked potentials, and 3% TCD). However, the use of monitoring was not associated with reduced risk of stroke.[121] The real value of cerebral monitoring, if any, may lie in the avoidance of the placement of shunts (which can cause stroke) and blood pressure augmentation (with its detrimental effects on the heart).

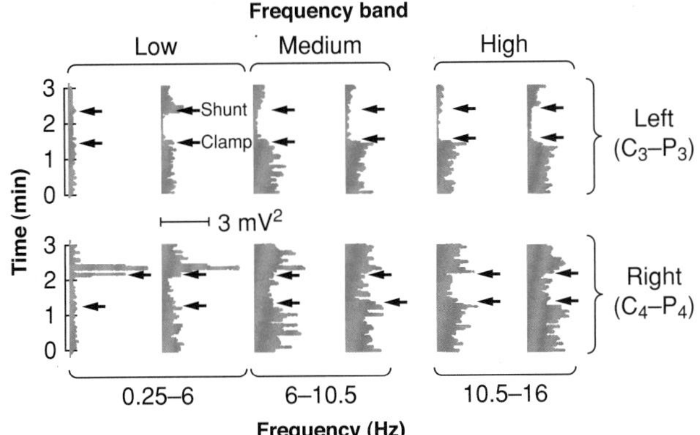

FIGURE 39-8. Acute cerebral ischemia following left carotid artery occlusion detected with processed electroencephalogram. The placement of a shunt in this case promptly reversed the ischemic changes. (Courtesy of Dr. Bruce L. Gewertz.)

EEG monitoring has other limitations. One limitation is that deep brain structures are not monitored by EEG. Also, in patients with pre-existing or fluctuating neurologic deficits the EEG may be false-negative; that is, these patients can develop perioperative strokes despite the absence of major intraoperative EEG changes. In these patients, there may be cell populations that are electrically silent or immediately adjacent to regions of infarction, and therefore not monitored by the EEG. The still-viable regions may progress to irreversible deterioration in the course of the operative procedure. Furthermore, the EEG may not be an ischemia-specific monitor because decreases in temperature and blood pressure, as well as increases in the depth of anesthesia, produce EEG changes that mimic ischemic changes. However, EEG changes secondary to anesthetics or hypothermia are more likely to be bilateral, whereas hemispheric ischemia is more likely to affect the electrical activity of only one side of the brain. Thus, the encephalographer must be made aware of adjustments to the anesthetic regimen. Bispectral index (BIS) monitoring has been shown to be a reliable indicator of ischemia is some studies, but not others. Although it primarily detects only frontal lobe activity, and is not able to detect ischemia elsewhere in the brain, a recent study found a decrease ≥14% from the basal BIS value had a high negative predictive value, with ischemia unlikely without a decrease.[122]

A retrospective series of >400 patients suggests that an "old" monitor, stump pressures (40 mm Hg cutoff) is as reliable as EEG monitoring in predicting cerebral ischemia on cross-clamp application in CEA performed under nerve block, with significant cost savings; whether these results are transferrable to general anesthesia is unclear.[123] In another study, when stump pressure and EEG were measured during CEA under regional anesthesia, both modalities had poor sensitivity as a guide to shunt placement (neurologic changes being the gold standard). Only 1.4% of patients with stump pressure >50 mm Hg required a shunt, while EEG identified cerebral ischemia in only 59.4% of patients needing shunt placement, with a false-positive rate of 1% and a false-negative rate of 40.6%. Again, whether these results are transferable to patients under general anesthesia is unclear.[124]

TCD measures middle cerebral artery blood flow velocities. TCD can also detect and quantify embolic signals, which almost always arise during dissection and/or angioplasty. A large series of 1,058 patients found the following TCD predictors of stroke after CEA: Emboli during wound closure, >90% decrease of middle cerebral artery peak systolic velocity at cross-clamping, and >100% increase of the pulsatility index of the Doppler signal at clamp release.[125] In a small case series, TCD predicted neurologic events despite a normal EEG.[126] Carotid artery clamping leads to similar changes in cerebral blood flow velocity measured by TCD in patients under regional or sevoflurane/fentanyl anesthesia. However, compared with the awake patient as a gold standard, TCD may have a low positive predictive value for neurologic deficit accompanying carotid occlusion.[127] TCD is also operator dependent, and 10% to 15% of patients do not have an adequate temporal window to make monitoring possible.

Other work has suggested that TCD is particularly useful in postoperative surveillance because most strokes occur after and not during CEA. TCD-directed dextran therapy after CEA has been shown to reduce the risk of postoperative complications. More recently, TCD-directed intravenous antiplatelet therapy has been used to reduce cerebral microembolization in patients undergoing carotid surgery.[128] TCD may also predict patients at risk of cerebral hyperperfusion syndrome following CEA or CAS.

SSEP monitoring may be particularly useful in patients with cerebral ischemia in whom EEG interpretation is more difficult.[129] SSEP monitoring is based on the detection of cortical potentials after electrical stimuli are presented to a peripheral nerve. In contrast to the EEG, which interrogates only cortical function, SSEP monitoring also evaluates deep brain structures. Any damage to these neural structures results in characteristic changes in the SSEP, usually in a decrease in amplitude and/or an increase in latency. If neural damage is severe, the cortical evoked potential is completely abolished. Severe damage occurs at about one-third of normal cerebral blood flow (i.e., at 15 mL/min/100 g brain tissue). Whereas some studies have been optimistic about the value of SSEP monitoring in the detection of cerebral ischemia, other investigators have concluded that SSEP is neither sensitive nor specific for the detection of ischemic injury during CEA. Virtually all commonly used anesthetics lead to SSEP changes that mimic changes produced by cerebral hypoxia. Therefore, a constant light plane of anesthesia needs to be maintained if increased latencies and decreased amplitudes of evoked potentials are to be ascribed to inadequate cerebral perfusion. False-negative results may also occur. On the basis of the available data, the authors conclude that this monitoring system cannot yet be considered essential in CEA.

Similarly, near infrared spectroscopy (NIRS), the most recent technology developed, has had mixed results. NIRS, or cerebral oximetry, allows continuous monitoring of cerebral oxygen saturation (rSO_2) in the frontal lobe as a marker of cerebral perfusion. Advantages are that it is easy to apply, noninvasive and can be used in all patients. Clinical reliability compared to established monitors has been inconclusive. Some studies have found a worse sensitivity and specificity compared to EEG, SSEPs, and stump pressures, whereas other authors have observed the opposite. Recently, during awake surgery cerebral oximetry using a cut off ≥19% drop in rSO_2 from baseline has been shown to have a high sensitivity and specificity when compared to the gold standard of awake testing.[130] One hundred patients were analyzed and seven developed a deterioration in conscious state following carotid cross-clamping; all had an immediate drop in rSO_2 ≥20%. There were no permanent neurologic deficits postoperatively. This suggests cerebral oximetry could be a reliable method of monitoring cerebral perfusion during CEA.

Anesthetic and Monitoring Choices for Elective Surgery

In addition to routine monitors, the authors recommend an intra-arterial catheter for blood pressure monitoring. ECG monitoring should include continuous leads II and V_5 for ST-T segment assessment. In very high-risk patients, transesophageal echocardiography (TEE) may be used as an additional monitor, especially in those with acute stroke in whom source of embolus may be an issue, or in those with left bundle branch block making ST-T segment evaluation impossible. Rarely is it necessary to use a central venous or pulmonary artery catheter (PAC), even if TEE is not available. The authors recommend restricting the use of central venous access to the rare patient with uncompensated CHF undergoing urgent CEA, and then insertion should be from the contralateral brachial or subclavian vein. The authors generally insert two peripheral intravenous catheters—one for remifentanil and vasoactive drugs and one for volume replacement. This only needs to be a medium-caliber intravenous catheter as major blood loss or significant fluid shifts during CEA are rare.

If sedatives are deemed indispensable, the smallest effective dose of midazolam is chosen for premedication to facilitate early perioperative neurologic assessment. Blood pressure and heart rate determinations from the preoperative clinic, other hospital or clinic visits, and at the time of admission are assessed to determine the range of a patient's acceptable values. The authors seek to maintain hemodynamics within this range intraoperatively. Chronic antianginal, antihypertensive, and antiplatelet medications are generally continued on the day of surgery with the exception of clopidogrel, which is stopped 1 to 5 days before surgery depending on the presence, type, and timing of coronary stenting.

Often on the day of surgery, patients present hypertensive despite having taken their morning antihypertensive and antianginal medications. These patients appear to be the most prone to hypotension after the induction of general anesthesia. Propofol or etomidate may be used for induction. Regardless of the induction agent, the clinician should be prepared to use pharmacologic blood pressure augmentation if blood pressure decreases excessively. Total fluid administration is limited in most patients to no more than 10 mL/kg of in a typical 2-hour operation because fluid overload may contribute to postoperative hypertension.

Because the respiratory depression and sedation caused by most opioids may confound the results of early neurologic assessment, long-lasting opioids are restricted whenever possible (e.g., fentanyl ≤3 μg/kg). Remifentanil provides an alternative therapy that will not produce lasting postoperative effects. The combined use of a cervical plexus block and/or surgeon-administered local anesthetic helps considerably in almost eliminating opiate requirements.

General anesthesia is maintained at a "light" level that permits EEG monitoring and results in blood pressures in the high range of normal. The trachea may be sprayed with 100 mg lidocaine to minimize stimulation by the endotracheal tube during surgery. Others have described the use of the laryngeal mask airway during CEA, which may reduce hypertensive and tachycardic episodes. The authors use remifentanil (continuous infusion 0.05 to 0.2 μg/kg/min) and light levels of desflurane or sevoflurane because of their salutary effects on the incidence of cerebral ischemia and rapid-awakening characteristics. Vasopressors are used as needed to treat hypotension or EEG changes. Because sudden onset of bradycardia and hypotension may be caused by baroreceptor reflexes with surgical irritation of the carotid sinus, some surgeons may infiltrate the carotid bifurcation with 1% lidocaine to attenuate this response. However, this practice may result in more postoperative hypertension. Relaxation is provided on the basis of the clinical need and anesthesiologist's preference. There is no proof that any one general anesthetic technique provides a superior outcome. Patients are almost always extubated at the end of the surgical procedure before or after neurologic integrity is confirmed. In patients who were easy to intubate, a deep extubation may limit the explosive hypertension that can accompany extubation. Neurologic integrity is always verified before the patient leaves the operating room. New neurologic deficits may lead to noninvasive imaging, contrast angiography, and/or surgical re-exploration.

Regional anesthesia is used by many centers for CEA. The necessary sensory blockade of the C2 to C4 dermatomes can be achieved by superficial cervical plexus block, or by subcutaneous infiltration of the surgical field. Superficial cervical plexus block may be combined with general anesthesia, and reduces postoperative opioid requirements, reduces $Paco_2$, and increases patient's satisfaction with analgesia.[131] Deep cervical plexus block does not increase the patient's comfort during the procedure compared with a simple superficial block, but increases the occurrence of complications from block placement (0.25% vs. 0%), and conversion to general anesthesia (2% vs. 0.5%).[132]

Proponents of regional anesthetic techniques claim the following advantages: Greater stability of blood pressure during surgery, inexpensive and easy cerebral monitoring, avoidance of tracheal intubation in patients with chronic obstructive lung disease, and avoidance of negative inotropic anesthetic agents in patients with limited cardiac reserves. The use of regional techniques appears to be associated with fewer episodes of EEG ischemia compared with general anesthesia.[133] In addition, overall hospital costs associated with the use of regional anesthesia may be lower. The general anesthesia versus local anesthesia for carotid surgery (GALA) trial was a multicenter trial of 3,526 patients in 95 centers for more than 8 years, and showed no definitive difference in outcomes between the two techniques.[134] There was no significant differences in the rate of stroke, MI, or mortality at 30 days.

α_2-agonists may be used for sedation during CEA. A series of >100 patients showed a low rate of need for shunting (4.3%) and no strokes when DEX was used for sedation during CEA under nerve block.[135] DEX appears to reduce hypertension/tachycardia, but increases hypotension, such that the number of hemodynamic interventions is no different from placebo; analgesia requirements in the PACU; however, are reduced with DEX.[136] Clonidine 1 μg/kg/hr suppresses the hyperadrenergic response to CEA without adverse effects on intraoperative hemodynamics or clinical neurologic monitoring.[137] The combination of superficial cervical plexus block and clonidine used to supplement general anesthesia results in an increase in hemodynamic stability after CEA and significant reductions in need for rescue antihypertensive medication postoperatively. However, preoperative clonidine (1 μg/kg) does increase the incidence of hypotension postoperatively.[138]

Disadvantages of regional anesthesia are that potential pharmacologic brain protection with anesthetics cannot be provided and that in the case of panic, sudden loss of consciousness, or onset of seizures, control of the airway may be difficult. Although emergent intubation is uncommon, it may be difficult under these circumstances and complicate surgical management. Regional anesthesia requires that the patient remains highly cooperative throughout the operation, and sedation can be provided only to a limited extent during carotid occlusion. Thus, the choice of the anesthetic technique should be determined after consultation with the patient and surgeon and must take into account the experience and expertise of the anesthesiologist.

Carotid Angioplasty and Stenting

CAS is usually performed in the vascular interventional suite by a team involving either vascular surgeons, cardiologists, or radiologists. Frequently no anesthesiologist is involved; however, anesthesiologists may be asked to provide sedation and monitoring in complex cases. The subject needs to be arousable and responsive so that serial neurologic examinations can be conducted. Adequate heparinization is crucial, with most protocols seeking to maintain activated clotting time >300 seconds. Both CEA and CAS may cause blood pressure to fall immediately after reperfusion and into the postoperative period, because of alterations in baroreceptor function. Throughout the development of CAS, concern had always been about risk and ramifications of cerebral emboli as a result of the angioplasty itself. Consequently, two main areas have been pursued to decrease the risk of embolic stroke: Proximal flow blockage and distal filters. Endovascular technology is rapidly evolving with rapid improvements in embolic protection and stent design. In addition, periprocedural antiplatelet therapy is now considered standard of care. All patients in the CAS arm of the CREST trial received aspirin 325 mg and clopidogril or ticlodipine for at least 30 days, with aspirin in all patients thereafter.[107] Results with CAS have been improving over time, and with newer embolic protection strategies, the role of CAS in both asymptomatic and symptomatic carotid disease is certain to increase.

Postoperative Management

Common problems arising after CEA or CAS include the onset of new neurologic dysfunction and hemodynamic instability; CEA may also be complicated by respiratory insufficiency. Other perioperative complications include temporary cranial nerve injuries (vagus, hypoglossal), temporary marginal mandibular nerve deficits, temporary and permanent posterior auricular nerve deficits, and mild cervical numbness, indicating injury to small sensory cervical nerves. Hematomas requiring return to surgery occur in approximately 1% of patients. Headache, wound infections, and hyperperfusion syndrome manifesting as hypertension and headache may also occur. Hyperperfusion syndrome is believed to result from blood flow to the brain that is greatly in excess of its metabolic need. It may not occur until several days after surgery, when patients present with severe ipsilateral headache and can progress to develop signs of increased cerebral excitability or frank seizures. TCD may have a role in predicting which patients will develop this syndrome. Steroids may be used in the treatment of hyperperfusion syndrome.

Blood pressure abnormalities are common after CEA; hypertension is more common than hypotension. Severe hypertension seems to occur more often in patients with poorly controlled preoperative hypertension. Both acute tachycardia and hypertension may precipitate acute myocardial ischemia and failure, and hypertension may lead to cerebral edema and/or hemorrhage. Post-CEA hypertension is significantly associated with adverse events (stroke or death), whereas postoperative hypotension and bradycardia do not appear to correlate with primary or secondary outcomes. Therefore, the authors recommend treatment of hypertension to reduce the work of the heart and in hope of decreasing neck hematoma. After excluding and/or treating other causes of hypertension such as bladder distention, pain, hypoxemia, and hypercarbia, systolic pressures of >140 mm Hg and diastolic pressures of >90 mm Hg are lowered to within the range of the patient's perioperative values, most often with labetalol in 5-mg increments. Hydralazine is a useful alternative in the setting of bradycardia or reactive airways disease. Perioperative myocardial ischemia may occur in 15% of CEA patients; angina and hypertension may be important risk factors. Usually, the hypertensive episode has its peak 2 to 3 hours after surgery, but in some individual cases it may persist for 24 hours.

Postoperative hypotension is less common, but may be caused by residual effects of anesthesia drugs, over-zealous treatment of hypertension, or baroreceptor "resetting" after the increase in flow. If the patient is asymptomatic it is usually well tolerated. Because significant hypertension and hypotension can be caused by myocardial ischemia or infarction, a 12-lead ECG should be obtained in the recovery room in hemodynamically unstable patients.

Postoperative respiratory insufficiency may be caused by recurrent laryngeal nerve or hypoglossal nerve injury, a neck hematoma, or deficient carotid body function. Wound hematomas develop in up to 2% of patients after CEA. Whereas small hematomas caused by venous oozing usually can be treated by reversing residual heparin with protamine or by applying gentle digital compression for a few minutes, an expanding hematoma must be immediately evaluated because tracheal compression and loss of the airway may ensue rapidly. In some cases, evacuation of the hematoma may not relieve the airway obstruction if lymphatic obstruction has produced massive pharyngolaryngeal edema. Indeed, four patients (0.3%) in the NASCET trial died directly because of neck hematomas.[106] Risk factors for neck hematoma may also include failure to reverse heparin and the presence of an endotracheal tube beyond the end of surgery. Hematomas are more common and delayed if a patch angioplasty has been performed. Therefore, some clinicians routinely reverse heparin with protamine in patients who have had a patch angioplasty. Some studies have suggested protamine may contribute to postoperative stroke. However, in the NASCET trial, heparin reversal using protamine (used in 40% of patients) was not associated with a change in risk of stroke.

Surgical manipulation may also damage the nerve supply to the carotid body. Although unilateral loss of carotid body function is unlikely to be significant, a bilateral loss may prevent the patient from increasing ventilation in response to a decrease in Pa_{O_2}. Therefore, supplemental oxygen should be routinely used in the recovery area. Similarly, drugs that depress respiratory drive should be avoided as much as possible in postoperative pain management. Acetaminophen constitutes effective pain relief in most patients when skin infiltration or plexus block with local anesthetic was performed in the operating room.

Routine postoperative intensive care is unusual and has been questioned. In one study, postoperative intensive care surveillance was necessary only for patients with four or more of the following risk factors: Stroke, CHF, chronic kidney failure, hypertension, dysrhythmia, and MI. Equally important, all patients requiring interventions or with adverse outcomes could be identified by the eighth postoperative hour.[139] Therefore, intensive care surveillance can be limited to high-risk patients.

Management of Emergent Carotid Surgery

The patient who awakens with a major new neurologic deficit or who develops a suspected stroke in the immediate postoperative period represents a surgical emergency. Although postoperative neurologic deficits may be due to inadequate collateral flow, carotid thrombosis may cause postoperative stroke; prompt surgical re-exploration can produce significant neurologic improvement. If a new neurologic deficit occurs in the postanesthesia recovery unit, most surgeons believe immediate re-exploration is indicated, and logic would dictate using pharmacologic methods of "cerebral protection"; however, this "logic" is controversial. Alternatively, if the deficit is deemed only focal and minor, it is most commonly because of microembolization. Consequently, noninvasive assessment of internal carotid flow and anticoagulation after exclusion of a hemorrhagic brain lesion usually constitute indicated treatment.

A patient undergoing emergency CEA may have a full stomach and thus may require protection against aspiration of gastric contents. Otherwise, an anesthetic technique similar to one for elective situations is used. For patients undergoing neck exploration for a wound hematoma following CEA, a tracheostomy or cricothyroidotomy tray should be immediately available, as well as other devices for management of the difficult airway. Esmolol is particularly useful to control hyperdynamic cardiovascular responses during awake intubation. If any difficulty is expected, the wound is opened and drained externally, and tracheal intubation is performed before general anesthesia is induced.

AORTIC RECONSTRUCTION

Aortic reconstruction may be undertaken to correct aneurysmal or occlusive disease, sometimes both coexisting. Aneurysms pose an ever-present threat to life because of their unpredictable tendency to rupture or embolize. Mortality from rupture may be as high as 85%, and even patients who receive emergent surgery have mortality rates one-half of that. Therefore, early recognition and aggressive surgical management are warranted, even in the absence of symptoms. Most centers are able to offer an endovascular approach to 60% to 70% of their patients needing repair of an infrarenal aortic aneurysm. Juxtarenal, suprarenal, and thoracoabdominal aortic aneurysms are still routinely repaired via an open approach, though some centers are trialing endovascular techniques for these aneurysms.

Epidemiology and Pathophysiology of Abdominal Aortic Aneurysm

There are approximately 200,000 new AAAs diagnosed annually, with approximately 45,000 undergoing surgical repair per year in the United States. A population-based study in Norway in 1994 to 1995 used ultrasound to measure renal and infrarenal aortic diameters; an aneurysm was present in 8.9% of men and 2.2% of women ($p < 0.001$). Risk factors for aneurysm included advanced age, smoking >40 years, hypertension, low serum high-density lipoprotein cholesterol, high level of plasma fibrinogen, and low blood platelet count. In 2005, the U.S. Preventive Services Task Force recommended that AAA screening be done in men 65 to 75 years of age who have ever smoked, citing an increased incidence in this population. They also stated that no recommendations for women can be made because there is no evidence in the literature to support a recommendation. Thoracoabdominal aortic aneurysms also occur in patients with hypertension or other risk factors for atherosclerotic disease.

AAA represents a dilatation of the abdominal aorta generally below the level of the renal arteries. The risk of rupture of the AAA is directly related to the luminal diameter of the aortic aneurysm. The aneurysm can develop an inner lining of mural thrombus, thereby decreasing the effective luminal diameter, but the size of the mural thrombus has not been shown to significantly decrease the risk of rupture. The risk of aortic rupture is related to the absolute diameter of the aortic aneurysm sac. The risk of rupture increases once the aneurysm is >4.5 to 5 cm in diameter. The size of the aneurysm is the most important predictor of subsequent rupture and mortality, but size alone does not appear to predict operative mortality. A prospective study followed 300 consecutive patients (mean age, 70 years; 70% men) who presented with AAA (average size, 4.1 cm) and were initially managed nonoperatively. The diameter of the aneurysm increased by a median of 0.3 cm per year. The 6-year cumulative incidence of rupture was 1% among patients with aneurysms <4 cm and 2% for aneurysms 4 to 4.9 cm in diameter. By comparison, the 6-year cumulative incidence of rupture was 20% among patients with aneurysms >5 cm in diameter.[140] Larger aneurysms expand even more rapidly, and aneurysms >5 cm should be considered for surgical or endovascular repair. With frequent monitoring, watchful waiting may be preferable to repair in patients with AAAs of 4 to 5.4 cm in diameter. Unfortunately, in most patients with AAA rupture (surgical mortality approaching 50%), the diagnosis of AAA was unknown beforehand. These data reinforce the importance of screening of the high-risk population to permit elective repair at the appropriate time.

Endovascular Repair versus Open Repair versus Medical Management

Before the advent of EVAR, a patient with an AAA either underwent an OAR or received medical management. OAR was reserved for patients with a large AAA (5.5 cm or larger) and who were deemed fit for surgery. In 1991, Parodi performed the first endovascular stent insertion for an infrarenal aortic aneurysm.[141] Initially, this procedure was carried out only for patients deemed unfit for OAR and who met specific aneurysm anatomic criteria. Since then, new stent technology with smaller modular designs, coupled with improved endovascular technique, has made EVAR available to a wide spectrum of patients including those who would be considered fit for OAR and who have more complex
9 aneurysm anatomy. In fact, EVAR is increasingly being considered for patients with smaller AAAs. The decision on which treatment modality is best for a large AAA usually depends on three variables: AAA size, AAA morphology, and patient perioperative risk. In general, EVAR has lower perioperative risk than OAR, but similar 2-year mortality. Also, EVAR has a higher incidence of leak, thus necessitating a lifetime of surveillance. OAR may be better suited for younger patients who do not want a lifetime of surveillance and who may have a better perioperative risk profile.

It is important to understand that an AAA is one manifestation of widespread vascular disease caused by multiple medical comorbidities; it is not a discrete disease. In a 10-year follow-up study that screened 4,734 patients older than 65 years, an infrarenal aortic diameter >2 cm was associated with increased risk of future coronary vascular disease and mortality. While the risk/benefit ratio for repair of small AAAs does not support intervention with OAR, there is emerging discussion on whether treating smaller AAAs with EVAR may be worth the benefits of intervening before additional comorbidities increase the risks of future repair.

Several studies have addressed the issue of which treatment modality is best. The EVAR-1, Dutch Randomized Endovascular Aneurysm Management (DREAM), and OVER trials all showed 30-day mortality to be significantly lower with EVAR than with OAR (1.8%, 1.2%, and 0.5% vs. 4.3%, 4.6%, and 3%, respectively).[66,142,143] The OVER trial also showed that patients receiving EVAR had a statistically significant reduction in procedure time (2.9 vs. 3.7 hours), blood loss (200 vs. 1,000 mL), transfusion requirement (0 vs. 1 units), duration of mechanical ventilation (3.6 vs. 5 hours), intensive care unit (ICU) stay (1 vs. 4 days), and hospital stay (3 vs. 7 days). On the other hand, the EVAR group was exposed to fluoroscopy for an average of 23 minutes and received an average of 132 mL of contrast, whereas the OAR group received neither. Two years after randomization, there was no significant difference in mortality, major morbidity, procedure failure, secondary therapeutic procedures, aneurysm-related hospitalizations, health-related quality of life, or erectile function.[66,144] Patients receiving OAR did experience a higher rate of wound complications and bowel obstructions.[66] Four years after randomization, both groups had similar mortality at 28%, though aneurysm-related death was lower in the EVAR group. Health-related quality of life was similar between the two groups, though the EVAR group experienced a greater number of complications (41% vs. 9% of patients, $p < 0.0001$) and reinterventions (20% vs. 6% of patients, $p < 0.0001$).[145] Six years after randomization, survival rates were similar, but the rate of secondary interventions was significantly higher for the EVAR group (29.6% vs. 18.1%, $p = 0.03$).[146] It is important to note that a meta-analysis of elective EVARs for more than 12 years demonstrated that as technical experience improved, there was a reduction in operative mortality, postoperative rupture, and incidence of leak requiring surgical intervention.[147]

Schermerhorn et al.[148] studied 22,830 matched Medicare beneficiaries who underwent AAA repair between 2001 and 2004 with follow-up through 2005 and indicated that EVAR and OAR had similar outcomes. Perioperative mortality was lower after EVAR (1.2% vs. 4.8%, $p < 0.001$), with greater benefit for those who were ≥85 years, but survival became equivalent after 3 years. Raval et al.[149] studied 7,936 patients; 2,034 of whom were ≥80 years, undergoing AAA repair between 2005 and 2008 and who were registered in the American College of Surgeons National Surgical Quality Improvement Program (ACS NSQIP) database. Older patients were more likely to experience adverse 30-day outcomes as compared with younger patients, regardless of type of AAA repair. However, older patients treated with EVAR had less overall morbidity and mortality than those treated with OAR. Those receiving EVAR had less infectious, pulmonary, cardiac, and renal complications, and had fewer requirements for blood transfusion and shorter durations of stay. Several small studies have agreed that EVAR is preferable to OAR in elderly patients.

Surprisingly, EVAR has not reduced the cost of AAA repair. The cost of the initial hospitalization for surgery should be much less expensive for EVAR than OAR because of the 3- to 5-day difference in the length of stay, but the cost of the device and the need for additional interventions, particularly radiologic follow-up of endovascular leaks, typically nullifies any cost savings.[150] A cost analysis of the DREAM trial[151] indicates that at 1 year of follow-up, EVAR is associated with a euro 4,293 (US $6,500) greater direct cost ($p = 0.01$, 95% CI 2,770 to 5,830) than OAR. The EVAR-1 investigators calculated an average aneurysm-related cost of 3,019 pound sterling (US $4,568) more for EVAR than for OAR.[142]

More than half of patients undergoing emergency AAA repair and more than a quarter of those having elective repair suffer myocardial necrosis as determined by cardiac troponin levels.[151] Myocardial injury has been shown to be less with EVAR than with OAR. There is less hemodynamic disturbance and lower Troponin T levels at 48 hours after EVAR compared to OAR.[152] In one study, aortic interruption was <1 minute for EVAR as compared with 51 minutes for OAR.[153] Patients who underwent EVAR had no significant change in heart rate, blood pressure, pulmonary capillary wedge pressure, stroke volume, or stroke work index. Thirty minutes after aortic reperfusion, 57% of patients undergoing OAR had myocardial ischemia detected by ECG or regional wall motion abnormality on transesophageal echocardiogram as compared with 33% in EVAR ($p = 0.01$). These changes were transient, and there were no differences in perioperative MI or death. EVAR has not been shown to alter the rate of cardiovascular events in patients deemed unfit for OAR.[154] Postoperative nutrition status, as determined by postoperative albumin level and nutritional risk index, is better with EVAR compared to OAR. For obese patients, defined as having a body mass index ≥30, there is a reduction in in-hospital complication rates with EVAR compared to OAR, 4% versus 26%, respectively. Obese patients undergoing EVAR also have decreased length of hospital stay, length of ICU stay, and need for ventilation. However, mortality is not different after 3 years of follow-up.[155]

Renal function deterioration does not appear to be affected by choice of surgical approach. An analysis of the 1,194 patients in the EVAR-1 and EVAR-2 trials demonstrates that renal function deteriorated slowly, but equally in fit patients randomized to either EVAR or OAR and in unfit patients randomized to either EVAR or medical management.

The EVAR-2 trial was designed to compare maximum medical therapy versus EVAR in those patients that were too unstable for OAR. The trial demonstrated that EVAR reduces aneurysm-related mortality when compared to medical therapy, but that EVAR does not improve total mortality.[156] However, this trial was limited by

TABLE 39-4. STATISTICALLY SIGNIFICANT PREDICTORS OF 30-DAY MORTALITY AFTER EVAR AAA (BASED ON THE RESULTS OF MULTIVARIABLE LOGISTIC REGRESSION MODEL, CONCORDANCE INDEX = 0.735, HOSMER–LEMESHOW GOODNESS OF FIT TEST *P* = .25)

Risk Factor	Parameter	Odds Ratio and 95% CL	*P* Value
Renal failure w/ dialysis	1.95	7.06 [5.23–9.53]	<0.0001
LE ischemia	1.27	3.55 [2.65–4.75]	<0.0001
Age ≥85 yr	1.13	3.10 [1.57–2.37]	<0.0001
Liver disease	0.93	2.52 [1.54–4.12]	0.0002
CHF	0.80	2.23 [1.89–2.64]	<0.0001
Renal failure w/o dialysis	0.65	1.91 [1.45–2.51]	<0.0001
Age 80–84 yr	0.65	1.92 [1.56–2.36]	<0.0001
Female	0.52	1.68 [1.42–1.99]	<0.0001
Neurologic	0.45	1.59 [1.29–1.94]	0.0001
Chronic pulmonary	0.45	1.57 [1.35–1.83]	<0.0001
Hospital annual volume <7	0.37	1.45 [1.18–1.80]	0.0005
Age 75–79 yr	0.34	1.40 [1.14–1.71]	0.001
Surgeon EVAR volume <3	0.26	1.30 [1.04–1.62]	0.002

CHF, Congestive heart failure; EVAR, endovascular aneurysm repair; LE, lower extremity.
Reproduced with permission. Egorova N, Giacovelli JK, Gelijns A, et al. Defining high-risk patients for endovascular aneurysm repair. *J Vasc Surg.* 2009;50(6):1271–1279.

delays in receiving the assigned treatment and a high rate of patient crossover, thus there may have been a bias against EVAR. In a more recent study, the EVAR-2 results were compared to results from 191 patients treated in a single high-volume center and who would have qualified for the EVAR-2 trial. The study suggested that EVAR is justified in these high-risk patients, though it is important to note that their patients were more likely to be on long-term antiplatelet therapy and statins than the EVAR-2 trial group.[157]

A study by Egorova et al.[158] determined there is a high-risk cohort that should not be treated with EVAR because of prohibitively high 30-day mortality, but that the cohort is small: 3.4% of patients have mortality ≥5% and 0.8% of patients have mortality >10%. Table 39-4 lists the several statistically significant predictors of 30-day mortality after EVAR, along with the associated odds ratios used to devise their scoring system for perioperative risk. Table 39-5 shows that scoring system, and it is for the cohort of patients with a total score between 10 and 12 who have ≥5% mortality, and for those with a total score of 13+ who have >10% mortality. The risk factors associated with increased 30-day mortality are, in decreasing order of significance: Renal failure with dialysis, lower extremity ischemia, age ≥85 years, liver disease, CHF, renal failure without dialysis, age 80 to 84 years, female gender, neurologic condition, chronic pulmonary condition, surgeon EVAR experience <3 cases, hospital annual volume <7 cases, and age 75 to 79 years.

Endovascular Abdominal Aneurysm Repair

A study published in 2009 by Winterborn et al.[159] of patients under surveillance for small AAA (less than 5.5 cm) demonstrated that when informed of the specific efficacy, safety, chronologic order of the care pathway, and other features of both EVAR and OAR, 84% of their patients stated they would prefer future EVAR to OAR.

Monitoring and Vascular Access

Although the incidence of perioperative conversion from EVAR to OAR is less than 1%, there still remains a real risk for the need for emergent proximal arterial control, first with an endoclamp, then with an aortic cross-clamp. In such a setting, proximal arterial access would prove indispensible, and thus it is recommended for use during EVAR. Central venous access, on the other hand, is rarely required during EVAR because hemodynamic medication infusions are seldom required and postoperative ICU stay is rare.

TABLE 39-5. RISK SCORES FOR 30-DAY MORTALITY FOR EVAR PATIENTS. A TOTAL SCORE BETWEEN 10 AND 12 PREDICTS 5% MORTALITY. A TOTAL SCORE OF 13+ PREDICTS >10% MORTALITY

Risk Factor	Score
Renal failure w/ dialysis	7
LE ischemia	5
Age ≥85 yr	4
Liver disease	3
CHF	3
Renal failure w/o dialysis	3
Age 80–84 yr	2
Female	2
Neurologic	2
Chronic pulmonary	1
Surgeon EVAR experience <3	1
Hospital annual volume <7	1
Age 75–79 yr	1

CHF, Congestive heart failure; EVAR, endovascular aneurysm repair; LE, lower extremity.
Reproduced with permission. Egorova N, Giacovelli JK, Gelijns A, et al. Defining high-risk patients for endovascular aneurysm repair. *J Vasc Surg.* 2009;50(6):1271–1279.

TABLE 39-6. SELECTED EUROSTAR REGISTRY PROCEDURE RELATED DATA COMPARING GENERAL, REGIONAL, AND LOCAL ANESTHETIC TECHNIQUES FOR PATIENTS UNDERGOING EVAR ($n = 5{,}557$ PATIENTS)

Measurements	GA ($n = 3{,}848$)	RA ($n = 1{,}399$)	LA ($n = 310$)	P (GA vs. RA)	P (GA vs. LA)	P (RA vs. LA)
Additional procedure	1,239 (32.2)	454 (32.5)	52 (16.8)	NS	<0.0001	<0.0001
Procedure duration (min)	133.3 ± 59.1 (30–660)	127.6 ± 52.8 (33–540)	115.7 ± 42.2 (25–340)	<0.0001	<0.0001	0.0009
ICU admission	619 (16.2)	116 (8.3)	6 (2)	<0.0001	<0.0001	0.0004
Hospital stay (days)	6.2 ± 8.5 (1–165)	5.1 ± 7.5 (1–106)	3.7 ± 3.1 (1–24)	<0.0001	<0.0001	0.0070
Replaced blood volume (mL)	574.4 ± 714.6 (35–6,000)	643.9 ± 672.1 (100–4,500)	357.4 ± 436.3 (10–2,000)	NS	0.0334	0.0159
Device-related complications	196 (5.1)	67 (4.8)	11 (3.6)	NS	NS	NS
Systemic complications	498 (13)	133 (9.5)	20 (6.6)	<0.0001	0.0004	NS

Values are means ± SD (ranges or %).
EVAR, Endovascular aneurysm repair; GA, general anesthesia; RA, regional anesthesia; LA, local anesthesia; NS, not significant; ICU, intensive care unit.
Adapted with permission. Ruppert V, Leurs LJ, Steckmeier B, et al. Influence of anesthesia type on outcome after endovascular aortic aneurysm repair: An analysis based on EUROSTAR data. *J Vasc Surg.* 2006;44(1):16–21.

Two large-caliber, peripheral intravenous catheters are usually sufficient. Before device insertion, systemic anticoagulation will be started with a typical heparin dose of 3,000 to 5,000 units with a goal of activated coagulation time of ≥200 seconds. At the time of device deployment, awake patients will be asked to hold their breath, and mean arterial pressure is often lowered to decrease the risk of distal migration of the stent. After device deployment, anticoagulation is reversed and activated coagulation time rechecked.

Local and Regional Anesthesia

EVAR may be carried out under almost any type of anesthesia including local, regional, neuraxial, and general techniques. The anesthetic technique selected will depend on preoperative factors such as platelet inhibitor use, low molecular weight heparin use, comorbidities limiting a patient's ability to lie flat for extended periods such as with severe chronic obstructive pulmonary disease (COPD), and on intraoperative factors such as anticipated duration, difficult arterial access, or tortuous iliac arteries. Blood loss and hemodynamic changes should be minimal when an experienced surgeon performs EVAR, but consideration must be given to the possibility for conversion to general anesthesia or for massive volume resuscitation. There are several insufficiently powered trials, large nonrandomized registries, and retrospective analyses that address local/regional anesthesia in EVAR. A literature review by Sadat et al.[160] pointed out that even though local/regional techniques tended to be used in less medically fit patients, those patients who did receive local/regional anesthesia instead of general anesthesia required less cardiovascular support during and after the surgery, had briefer ICU and hospital stays, and had lower morbidity and mortality. An analysis of 6,009 elective EVAR procedures performed between 2005 and 2008 and registered in the ACS NSQIP database showed that when compared to general anesthesia, local/regional anesthesia was associated with decreased duration of hospital stay and pulmonary morbidity.[161] An analysis of 5,557 patients in 164 centers composing the EUROSTAR registry showed that when compared to general anesthesia, local/regional anesthesia benefited patients by reducing operative time, number of ICU admissions, duration of hospital stay, and number of systemic complications.[162] Furthermore, local anesthesia was superior even to regional anesthesia for most of these parameters, though regional anesthesia was still superior to general anesthesia. Table 39-6 presents a selection of procedure related data from the EUROSTAR registry. In a study of 217 consecutive patients receiving EVAR in an approach favoring local anesthesia as the first choice for anesthetic technique, 84% of the patients were deemed appropriate for local anesthesia, and the conversion rate from local to general anesthesia was 7.6%.[163]

Conversion from EVAR to OAR

Conversion from EVAR to OAR may occur in the setting of difficult arterial access, vessel dissection at the arterial access site, poor anatomic parameters for EVAR such as with tortuous iliac arteries, stent malposition, stent migration, and aneurysm rupture. For the clinician, conversion in this setting will involve conversion to a general anesthetic and the need for adequate resuscitative equipment such as cell saver and rapid infusion devices, which must be readily available in centers performing EVARs. A primary conversion is classified as an open reoperation within 30 days following EVAR and is most commonly associated with Type I endoleak (see definition below). A secondary conversion is classified as an open reoperation after 30 days following an EVAR and is usually performed for continuing enlargement of the aneurysm sac or for a persistent endoleak. Another indication for secondary conversion is aneurysm rupture despite successful sac exclusion. The incidence of acute conversion is 1.1%, and the morbidity and mortality rates for those patients are similar to those who have elective OAR.[164]

Complications

Endoleak

Despite the minimally invasive nature of the technique, there are several complications unique to EVAR that must be anticipated. Endoleak is the most common complication, greater than 30% in some studies. An endoleak is defined as persistent blood flow outside the wall of the stent graft into the aneurysm sac. Endoleak

ANESTHESIA FOR SURGICAL SUBSPECIALTIES

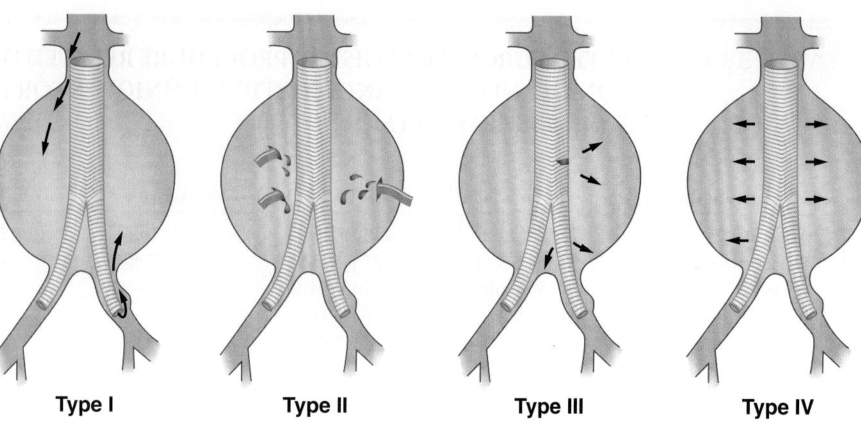

FIGURE 39-9. Categories of endoleaks. Type I: Inadequate proximal or distal seal. Type II: Backflow from collaterals, such as lumbar arterial branches or the inferior mesenteric artery. Type III: Defects in the fabric or seal failures where modular components overlap. Type IV: Porosity of graft fabrics; typically resolve after reversal of the anticoagulation employed for the endovascular abdominal aortic repair procedure. (Reprinted from: White GH, May J, Waugh RC, et al. Type III and type IV endoleak: Toward a complete definition of blood flow in the sac after endoluminal AAA repair. *J Endovasc Surg.* 1998;5:305, with permission.)

exposes the weak aneurysm wall to continued flow that may lead to rupture. White et al.[165] proposed the following classification system, with endotension being added by Gilling-Smith et al.[166] (Fig. 39-9):

- *Type I*—high flow leak adjacent to a stent that is not sealing the sac from the systemic circulation (requires immediate intervention).
- *Type II*—low flow leak due to arterial branches that have been excluded by the stent (can be treated with embolization).
- *Type III*—failure with the stent itself or at its junction with another stent (requires immediate recognition and treatment).
- *Type IV*—porosity in the stent (often resolves with reversal of anticoagulation).
- *Type V (endotension)*—persistent or recurrent pressurization of the aneurysm sac despite no detectable endoleak.

Types I and III are high-pressure leaks and generally require urgent management because of their relatively high short-term risk of sac rupture. Differentiation between types I and III is often unnecessary because both are angiographically evaluated and subsequently treated. Type II endoleak also requires correction when associated with enlarging aneurysm sac. Endoleak of all types are usually treated via the endovascular route. However, Type II endoleak without enlargement can be managed conservatively, and the rupture rate appears to be low. Like Type II endoleak, Type V endoleak (endotension) is a low flow leak and is considered less urgent, though continued endovascular evaluation may be warranted if there is impending aneurysm sac growth or patient symptoms.

Other Complications

Other problems related to EVAR include problems with arterial access; migration or malpositioning of the stent; obstruction of renal, mesenteric, or other major vascular ostia; contrast-induced nephropathy; and aneurysm rupture. Understanding surgical concerns will help prepare the clinician for potential problems. Severely atherosclerotic vessels may be difficult to cannulate and access. Percutaneous access may not be feasible in obese patients, or in patients who have had previous groin surgery, thus necessitating open groin access and arteriotomy. Aggressive attempts to negotiate less than ideal anatomy may lead to retroperitoneal hematoma and significant morbidity and mortality.

The EUROSTAR collaborators registry demonstrated a 0.21% risk of postoperative symptoms of spinal cord ischemia (6 out of 2,862 patients) in patients receiving EVAR, which is similar to the risk with OAR. Of the six patients with spinal cord ischemia, one had complete infarction of the distal cord with flaccid paraplegia and total sensory loss, two had anterior spinal artery infarction with bilateral flaccid paraplegia and loss of temperature and pain sensation, and three had bilateral nerve root or lumbar plexus damage with asymmetric motor and sensory defects. The three patients with cord infarction had no recovery, two of the three with nerve root damage had partial recovery, and one of the three with nerve root damage had complete recovery. Of the possible causes of spinal cord ischemia during AAA repair, including greater radicular artery occlusion, prolonged aortic clamping, intraoperative hypotension, atheromatous embolization, and interference with pelvic circulation, only atheromatous embolization and interference with pelvic circulation are relevant to EVAR. The EUROSTAR collaborators concluded that since all six patients with spinal cord ischemia had at least one patent hypogastric artery, thus ruling out interference with pelvic circulation as a cause of the ischemia, the ischemia was most likely caused by atheromatous embolization.[167] Interestingly, a case report by Lioupis et al.[168] details development of paraplegia 24 hours after EVAR, with resolution subsequent to immediate CSF drainage. The incidence of spinal cord ischemia is higher in patients receiving endovascular repair for a thoracic aneurysm. One study of 261 patients demonstrated an incidence of spinal cord ischemia of 10%, with half of those being reversible with CSF drainage.[169]

Postimplantation syndrome is a weakly defined yet common, transient condition characterized by fever, leukocytosis, elevated C-reactive protein level, and coagulopathy. The incidence is estimated at 35% to 60%.[170] The cause is not completely understood though endothelial activation may play a crucial role and it is not prevented by prolonged antibiotic treatment. Fever within 48 hours of EVAR is common and generally does not require microbiologic investigation, though fever beyond 48 hours of EVAR is more likely to yield positive cultures.

Open Aortic Repair

Perioperative (i.e., 30-day) mortality in elective OAR ranges from 3% to 4.6%.[66,142,143] Hypotension increases perioperative risk by 3-fold, whereas pre-existing heart disease, including CAD and CHF, increase the risk of mortality by 2.5-fold to 5-fold. Expeditious surgery with better graft materials, minimal clamp time, and blood conservation, along with better understanding of the pathophysiology of the disease, have made aortic surgery safer.

OAR was developed with the mindset of imitating normal anatomy. While it is usually easier and better to imitate normal anatomy during OAR, situations exist that require circuitous revascularization procedures, such as axillofemoral or femoral–femoral bypasses. These procedures may be required for graft infection, repeat surgery, or a hostile abdomen. A hostile abdomen includes: A postradiation state, adhesions, sepsis, and malignancy. It is emphasized these circuitous procedures have lower long-term patency rates than anatomically correct procedures.

Monitoring and Vascular Access

OAR requires continuous arterial blood pressure measurement, large-caliber venous access, and the ability to reliably and quickly administer medications. It may also be helpful to monitor certain aspects of cardiac function, to increase spinal perfusion pressure, and to minimize postoperative pain.

An arterial catheter should be placed proximal to the level of the aortic cross-clamp. Because these patients are at increased risk for future procedures involving the arteries in the nondominant arm; that is, radial artery harvest for coronary artery bypass grafting or arteriovenous fistula creation for hemodialysis access, the authors prefer to place the arterial catheter in the dominant arm. An arterial catheter may also be placed distal to the cross-clamp if there is a desire to monitor distal arterial pressure during the cross-clamp, such as with distal perfusion via a partial bypass machine.

Large-caliber venous access is best achieved with a central venous introducer because it can serve as a route for rapid administration of fluids, for central administration of medications, and for insertion of a PAC. At least one additional large-caliber venous catheter should be placed.

Intensive cardiac monitoring is usually performed with either a PAC or a TEE probe. Infrarenal OAR in the absence of cardiopulmonary disease rarely requires this intensive cardiac monitoring. The clinician will often place a PAC if the cross-clamp will be suprarenal, although large randomized trials have not demonstrated improvement in outcome with PACs.[171] Though some clinicians prefer to use TEE for intensive cardiac monitoring, it may not be advisable for higher thoracoabdominal aortic aneurysms, because the tip of the TEE probe may be very near to the aneurysm itself. This may cause mechanical injury to either the aneurysm or the esophagus because the TEE probe can push the esophagus against the aneurysm sac.

Through anterior segmental arteries that branch off the aorta, and especially through the Artery of Adamkiewicz, the aorta supplies blood to the anterior spinal cord. Ischemia of the anterior spinal cord, and the resulting paraplegia, is a serious concern during OAR. Optimizing spinal perfusion pressure may help to prevent anterior spinal cord ischemia. This is achieved with a combination of maintaining relatively higher arterial blood pressure and lower CSF pressure. CSF pressure is managed with an intrathecal drain, sometimes known as a "lumbar drain," placed at the L3–L4 or L4–L5 interspace. Some clinicians will place an intrathecal drain the night before surgery to assure sufficient clotting in the event of a traumatic tap. Allowing CSF to drain when its pressure exceeds a certain maximum, usually 5 to 10 mm Hg, will help to maintain a lower CSF pressure. It is not always possible to maintain this lower pressure, because one has to be careful not to drain the CSF too rapidly. If the CSF drains faster than 10 mL/hr, there may be a risk of intracranial herniation. Also, it is ideal if the CSF is drained at a steady rate, such as 10 mL slowly over an hour for several hours, rather than 10 mL quickly once an hour for several hours. The drain is removed after the risk of paraplegia has diminished and the coagulation status is acceptable, usually on the second or third postoperative day.

A thoracic epidural may be the best way to achieve adequate analgesia while minimizing respiratory depression, especially when the surgical exposure includes a thoracotomy, and especially if there exists concomitant pulmonary disease.[172] Epidural practice guidelines, such as those published by the American Society of Regional Anesthesia and Pain Medicine (ASRA),[33] will guide the clinician in the timing of epidural placement and removal as well as the timing of anticoagulation. At the time of this writing, heparinization may be started 1 hour after atraumatic placement of an epidural. If placement is traumatic, the guidelines state heparinization should be delayed for 24 hours. If placement reveals a "wet tap," then the catheter should not be used as an intrathecal catheter, because intrathecal local anesthetics will produce a motor block that will make it difficult to assess postoperative lower extremity neurologic function. Instead, the clinician can attempt to place the catheter at a different level. A "wet tap" does not require a delay in heparinization beyond the 1 hour required for atraumatic placement. During surgery, the epidural should be managed in such a way as to enable a postoperative lower extremity neurologic examination. A low-concentration local anesthetic, such as bupivacaine up to 0.125% or ropivacaine up to 0.2%, can be used yet still enable a postoperative examination. Some clinicians; however, will prefer to employ an opioid-only regimen to ensure there is no motor block. The epidural can be removed postoperatively once normal coagulation has been restored.

Virtually all anesthetic techniques and drugs have been used for aortic reconstructive surgery. The ability to maintain hemodynamic equilibrium and attend to detail is more crucial to outcome than is the choice of drugs. Volatile anesthetics provide a means of controlling afterload and preload but can lead to an increased need for intravascular volume. Perhaps the most important reason to routinely include volatile agents in general anesthetics is that volatile anesthetics improve preconditioning mechanisms and reduce the size of MI, should it occur.[173] In the authors' practice, a volatile anesthetic is combined with a low-dose sufentanil infusion (2 to 5 μg/kg) if an epidural is not used.

Surgical Approach

Abdominal aortic repair is performed either through a transperitoneal or a retroperitoneal exposure. In the first case, a thoracoabdominal midline incision is performed and the aorta is accessed through the peritoneum. This generous exposure is usually favored for complex aortic repair or replacement. In the retroperitoneal approach, incision is made over the lateral border of the left rectus muscle, 2 cm below the umbilicus to the 12th rib. This allows access to the aorta from the crux of the diaphragm to its bifurcation. The retroperitoneal technique allows a surgical exposure as good as the transperitoneal approach and is associated with less fluid shift, faster return of bowel function, lower pulmonary complications, shorter ICU stay, and lower overall hospital cost. The retroperitoneal approach is considered by many to be more appropriate in cases of truncal obesity, COPD, hostile abdomen, and juxtarenal aneurysm. However, the retroperitoneal approach is associated with frequent chronic wound pain, incisional hernias, and abdominal bulges. Intraoperative blood loss during OAR can be significant and depends on the size and complexity of the AAA. The postoperative course usually requires admission to the ICU for several days. The postoperative recovery period after OAR can be several months.

Aortic Cross-clamping and Unclamping

Infrarenal aortic clamping carries the lowest risk for patients; supraceliac clamping carries the highest. Clinicians should be aware that 10% to 20% of "infrarenal" aortic disease will actually involve the suprarenal portion of the aorta, necessitating suprarenal clamping. Ruptured aneurysms often must be controlled initially by

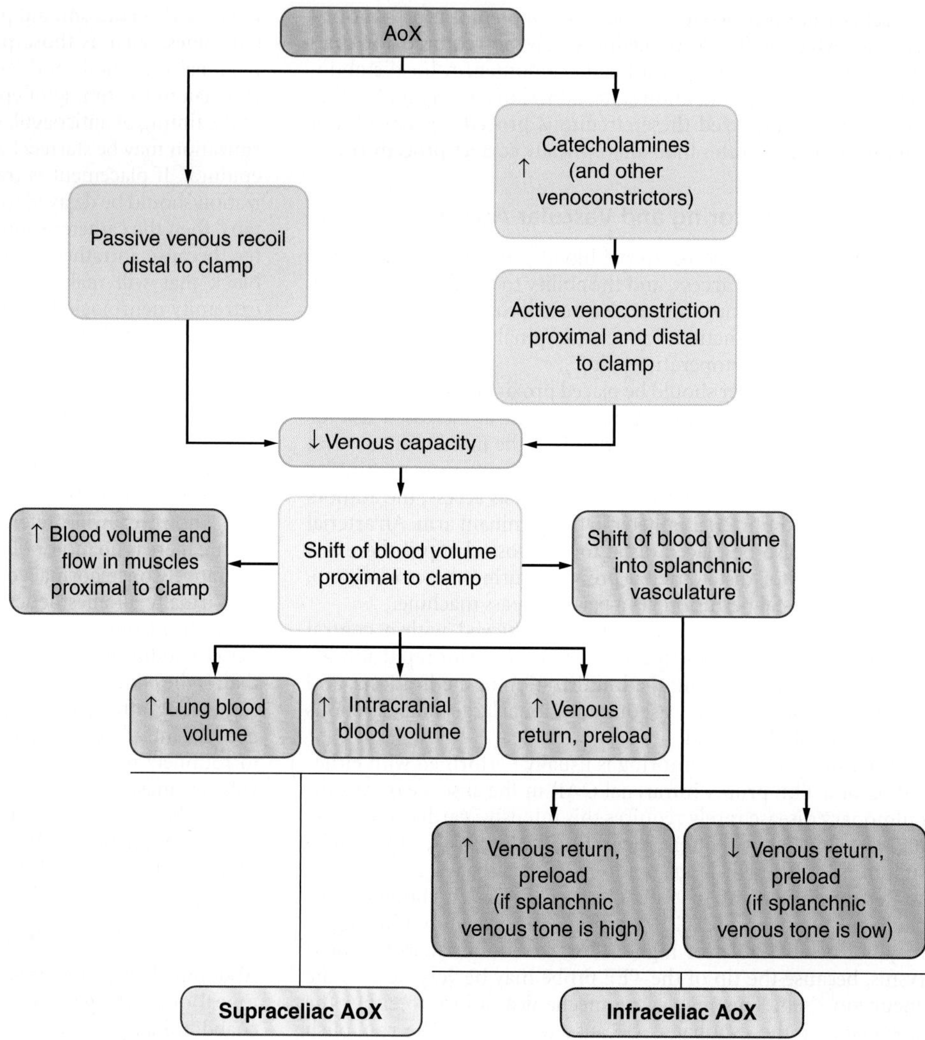

FIGURE 39-10. Blood volume redistribution during aortic cross-clamping (AoX). This schedule depicts the reason for the decrease in venous capacity, which results in blood volume redistribution from the vasculature distal-to-aortic occlusion to the vasculature proximal-to-aortic occlusion. If the aorta is occluded above the splanchnic system, the blood volume travels to the heart, increasing preload and blood volume in all organs and tissues proximal to the clamp. However, if the aorta is occluded below the splanchnic system, blood volume may shift into the splanchnic system or into the vasculature of other tissues proximal to the clamp. The distribution of this blood volume between the splanchnic and nonsplanchnic vasculature determines changes in preload. ↑ and ↓, increase and decrease, respectively. (Reprinted from: Gelman S. The pathophysiology of aortic cross-clamping and unclamping. *Anesthesiology.* 1995;82:1026, with permission.)

supraceliac clamping because of anatomic considerations. In addition to these clamp locations, there is also a lower clamp placed to eliminate retrograde bleeding from the distal anastomosis site. This lower clamp may be at the level of the iliac or femoral arteries.

The classic investigations of Gelman[174] define the pathophysiology of hemodynamic changes during aortic cross-clamping and unclamping. Aortic cross-clamping increases the mean arterial pressure and systemic vascular resistance up to 50%. This is attributed to a sudden increase in impedance to aortic flow (afterload), activation of renin, and release of catecholamines, prostaglandins, and other active vasoconstrictors. Cardiac output initially decreases in the face of high systemic vascular resistance, and that decrease may be reinforced by the decrease in oxygen consumption below the aortic cross-clamp (Figs. 39-10–39-12, Table 39-7). Some of the initial changes in hemodynamics associated with cross-clamping can be offset by boluses of a vasodilator administered immediately before placement of the clamp (e.g., nitroprusside 0.3 to 0.7 μg/kg, nicardipine 200 to 600 μg, or milrinone 50 μg/kg over 10 minutes). In this case, mechanical and pharmacologic actions cancel out each other while the body is allowed to adapt.

Preload changes are more variable than blood pressure changes. Higher central venous pressure and pulmonary artery occlusion pressures do not accompany the decrease in cardiac index in the healthy heart. However, in those with CAD, myocardial dysfunction may be associated with cross-clamping and may lead to an increase in filling pressures. Infrarenal aortic cross-clamping is well attenuated compared with suprarenal clamping; during occlusive disease repair, aortic clamping usually has limited systemic hemodynamic effect. With lower clamping, blood volume from the infrasplanchnic vasculature may shift to the compliant splanchnic vasculature limiting preload changes, and vasodilation above the level of the clamp offsets the mechanical impedance to aortic flow. Clamping an occluded artery is expected to have minimal effect. Existing collateral circulation remains intact during clamping and is responsible for maintaining lower body perfusion despite aortic cross-clamping. For higher clamps, nitrate therapy will not necessarily prevent wall motion abnormalities, and care should be exercised when using any vasodilator because of the importance of maintaining visceral and spinal perfusion pressure below the aortic cross-clamp. Furthermore, use of a thoracic epidural at the start of the case may provide enough of a sympathectomy to mollify the increase in blood pressure seen with higher clamp levels. It may be acceptable to allow a systolic blood pressure as high as 180 to 200 mm Hg as long as the surgeon has acceptable operating conditions. Even relative hypotension (<20% below resting pressure) probably should be avoided unless other means (i.e., passive shunts or

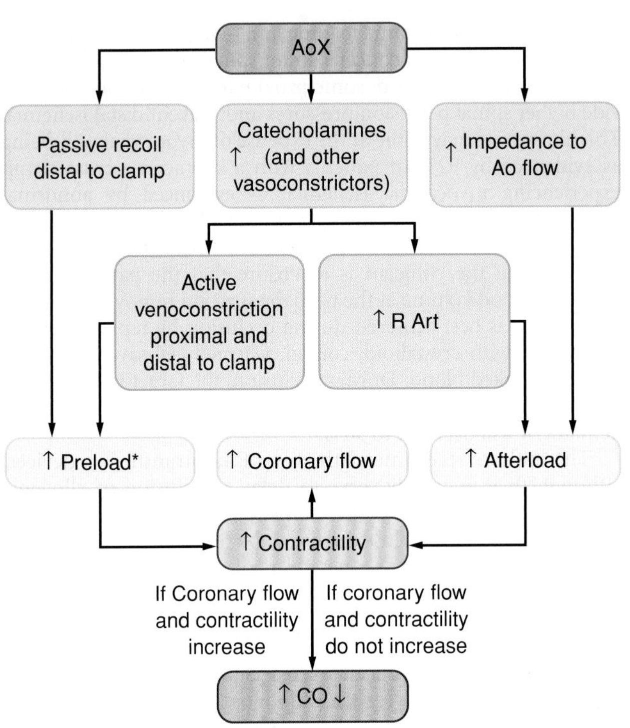

FIGURE 39-11. Systemic hemodynamic response to aortic cross-clamping (AoX). Preload does not necessarily increase. If during infrarenal aortic cross-clamping blood volume shifts into the splanchnic vasculature, preload does not increase (see Fig. 39-10). Ao, aortic; R art, arterial resistance; CO, cardiac output; ↑ and ↓, increase and decrease, respectively; *, different patterns are possible (see Fig. 42-7). (Reprinted from: Gelman S. The pathophysiology of aortic cross-clamping and unclamping. *Anesthesiology.* 1995;82:1026, with permission.)

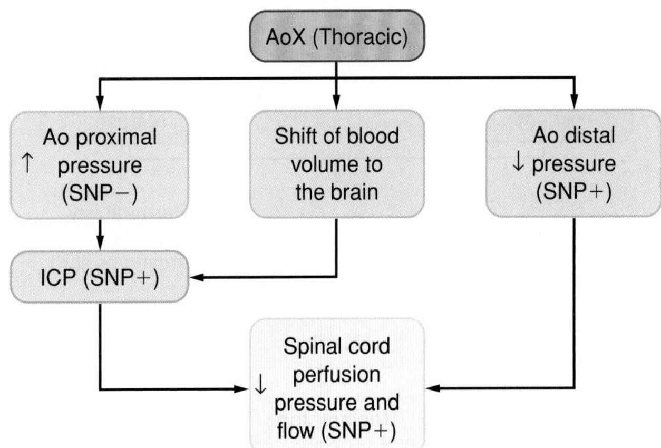

FIGURE 39-12. Spinal cord blood flow and perfusion pressure during thoracic aortic occlusion, with or without sodium nitroprusside (SNP) infusion. The changes (*arrows*) represent the response to aortic cross-clamping (AoX) per se. Ao, aortic; SNP–, SNP counteracts the effect of cross-clamping; SNP+, SNP aggravates the effect of cross-clamping; ICP, intercranial pressure; ↑ and ↓, increase and decrease, respectively. (Reprinted from: Gelman S. The pathophysiology of aortic cross-clamping and unclamping. *Anesthesiology.* 1995;82:1026, with permission.)

mechanical bypass) are used to perfuse the lower part of the body and promote visceral/spinal cord blood flow.

Reperfusion after unclamping the aorta causes systemic release of an acute load of potassium, acid, and other mediators. This can result in severe arterial hypotension unless aggressive therapy is undertaken before unclamping (Fig. 39-13). Various therapies are employed by anesthesiologists and surgeons, with no evidence to support one is superior to another. Most anesthesiologists employ some degree of fluid loading with or without vasoconstrictors (e.g., phenylephrine 100 to 200 μg, norepinephrine 8 μg, or calcium chloride 300 to 500 mg) that can offset the negative inotropic/dromotropic effects of reperfusion. Much preferable to pharmacologic manipulation is gradual unclamping, unclamping with gradual sequential release of bilateral femoral pressure, or restoring flow to one leg at a time in aortobifemoral grafts.

Management of Elective Open Aortic Repair

Hemodynamic management during OAR requires the clinician to anticipate the sudden changes in intravascular volume and systemic vascular resistance seen during clamping, unclamping, and bleeding. Prehydration may limit variations in blood pressure during surgery. The patient's vital signs should be kept within 20% of his or her normal range, as long as the heart rate does not exceed 80 to 90 beats per minute and signs of organ ischemia are absent. Increases in blood pressure or heart rate may be treated with boluses of an opioid. Left ventricular end-diastolic volume can be assessed by TEE.

ANESTHESIA FOR SURGICAL SUBSPECIALTIES

TABLE 39-7. EFFECT OF LEVEL OF AORTIC OCCLUSION ON CHANGES IN CARDIOVASCULAR VARIABLES

	% Change in Variable, by Level of Aortic Occlusion		
Cardiovascular Variable	Supraceliac	Suprarenal Infraceliac	Infrarenal
Mean arterial blood pressure	54	5[a]	2[a]
Pulmonary capillary wedge pressure	38	10[a]	0[a]
End-diastolic area	28	2[a]	9[a]
End-systolic area	69	10[a]	11[a]
Ejection fraction	−38	−10[a]	−3[a]
Abnormal motion of wall, % of patients	92	33	0
New myocardial infarctions, % of patients	8	0	0

[a]Statistically different ($P < 0.05$) from group undergoing supraceliac aortic occlusion.
Adapted with permission from Roizen MF, Ellis JE, Foss JF, et al. Intraoperative management of the patient requiring supraceliac aortic occlusion. In: Veith FJ, Hobson RW, Williams RA, Wilson SE, eds. *Vascular Surgery*, 2nd edn. New York, NY: McGraw-Hill; 1994:256.

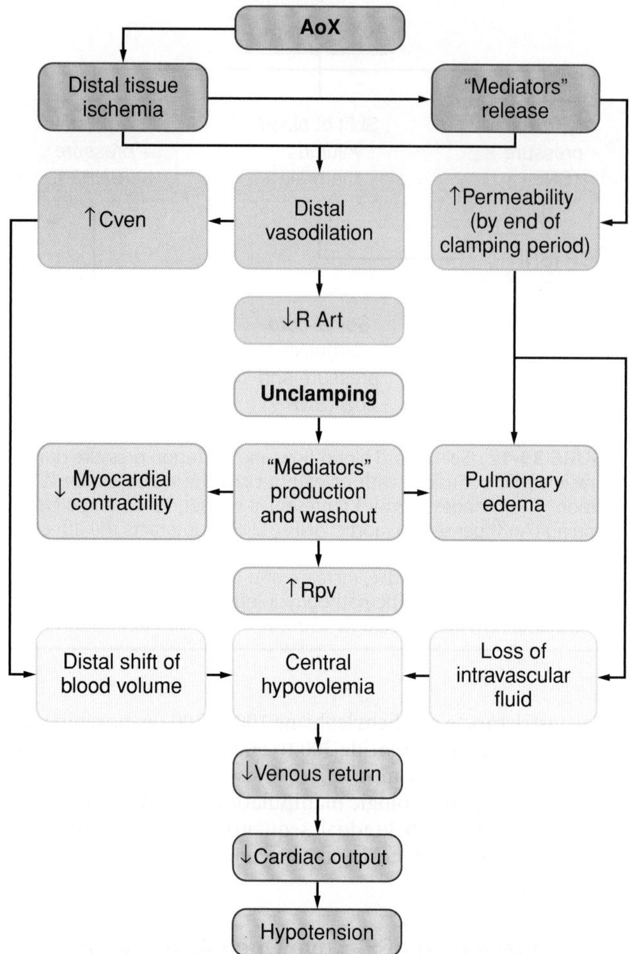

FIGURE 39-13. Systemic hemodynamic response to aortic unclamping. Preload does not necessarily increase. AoX, aortic cross-clamping; Cven, venous capacitance; R art, arterial resistance; Rpv, pulmonary vascular resistance; ↑ and ↓, increase and decrease, respectively. (Reprinted from: Gelman S. The pathophysiology of aortic cross-clamping and unclamping. *Anesthesiology.* 1995;82:1026, with permission.)

It is important to maintain temperature homeostasis, unless hypothermia is desired for potential spinal cord protection.

The application of an aortic cross-clamp causes a sudden increase in systemic vascular resistance, which in turn may cause deterioration in myocardial function. The initial deterioration improves after 10 minutes, and returns to baseline after unclamping.[175] For the half-hour immediately before cross-clamping and aortic occlusion, the patient is kept slightly hypovolemic by examining the ventricular volume by means of echocardiography or by keeping pulmonary capillary wedge pressure at 5 to 15 mm Hg. At the time of occlusion, a vasodilating drug is available for immediate use if needed. Alternatively, the concentration of volatile anesthetic may be increased or a local anesthetic may be injected into the epidural catheter; both require careful attention to avoid hypotension. If local anesthetics are used in the epidural, the resulting sympathectomy may significantly complicate the management of subsequent hypotension due to hypovolemia. One approach to reduce blood pressure in the face of aortic occlusion has been described using 15 cm H_2O positive end-expiratory pressure immediately before cross-clamp, with removal just before unclamping.[176] This approach facilitates volume loading and reduces hypotension after unclamping. If there is concern about spinal cord perfusion while the aorta is cross-clamped, some proximal hypertension may provide higher spinal perfusion pressures and prevent distal ischemia. This alternative may come at the expense of myocardial well-being as evidenced by 92% of patients with a supraceliac cross-clamp experiencing myocardial ischemia, as evidenced by abnormal motion and thickening of the left ventricle (Table 39-7). Administration of vasoconstrictors should be avoided, if possible. A primary goal of the clinician is to ensure that the patient has an adequate blood volume at the time the surgeon removes the cross-clamp. This is best achieved during occlusion by replacing blood that is lost with crystalloid, colloid, warmed cell-saver blood, or warmed banked blood. During occlusion, the target hematocrit is slightly above 30%, because after the cross-clamp is removed the hematocrit will decrease to 30%.

The authors recommend the use of autotransfusion devices, although they may only serve to delay transfusion of allogenic blood, not reduce it. The clinician should be aware that during aortic occlusion, blood loss might not be reflected in the hemodynamic monitoring because the effects of the cross-clamp on systemic vascular resistance can obscure the underlying volume status. Because a large part of the vascular tree is excluded from circulation during temporary aortic occlusion, blood loss can be considerable during supraceliac cross-clamping without the onset of hypotension or tachycardia. Blood loss into the pleural or retroperitoneal cavity may not be readily detected. Evisceration of bowel, often necessary for optimal exposure of the thoracoabdominal aorta, further depletes intravascular volume. If more blood loss is anticipated after 6 units of blood have been given, the clinician should request 10 units of platelets, and occasionally 2 units of fresh-frozen plasma.

The clinician can use filling pressures or echocardiographic estimates of volume to guide them in administering crystalloid, colloid, or blood in anticipation of the surgeon removing the cross-clamp. Vasodilators should be discontinued immediately before removal of the cross-clamp. The surgeon should remove the cross-clamp gradually to ensure that severe hypotension or bleeding does not develop. After removal of the cross-clamp, pulmonary artery pressure and central venous pressure may increase because reperfusion of ischemic tissues is associated with the release of lactic acid and other mediators that can cause pulmonary vasoconstriction. Mannitol prophylaxis may attenuate this response. Another method is to administer an infusion of human ANP starting 5 minutes after clamping. This has been shown to attenuate the increases in pulmonary artery pressure and vascular resistance, without causing severe systemic hypotension.[177]

During emergence from anesthesia, and in an effort to prevent hemodynamic variations outside the patient's normal range, the clinician can infuse nitroglycerin, esmolol, or other β-adrenergic blocking agents. If appropriate, the trachea should be extubated at the conclusion of surgery. Prophylactic β-blockade should be continued into the postoperative period if tolerated. The clinician may prefer to use a short acting agent, such as esmolol, in unstable patients and a long acting agent, such as metoprolol, in stable patients.

Thoracic and Thoracoabdominal Aneurysm Repair

Thoracic and thoracoabdominal aortic aneurysm repair are among the most challenging for clinicians. Coincident CAD and COPD are common. Lung isolation is required to facilitate surgical access to the aneurysm and to avoid an iatrogenic pulmonary contusion in the left lung. If planning to use postoperative ventilation, it may be advantageous to use a single-lumen endotracheal tube with a bronchial blocker rather than a double-lumen endotracheal tube, because edema of the head and neck frequently occurs after high cross-clamping, even with distal perfusion.

Generous exposure of the thoracic and abdominal aortas and its major branches can be obtained with a left thoracoabdominal incision and retroperitoneal dissection. The thoracoabdominal approach is favored for complex thoracoabdominal aortic replacement in the presence of stenotic or aneurysmal disease. There are two general methods of attaching the visceral branches to the aortic graft. One method is to excise the visceral branches from the parent aorta with a button of aortic wall that can later be sewn into the aortic graft. Another method is to prepare an aortic graft with attached smaller grafts that can be anastomosed to the visceral branches, sometimes with a device that allows for quick deployment and attachment. Identification of large intercostal vessels may warrant reanastomosis to the graft in order to optimize spinal cord perfusion after repair. If the patient also has mesenteric occlusive disease, endarterectomy of these branch vessels is performed before they are attached to the graft. If mesenteric revascularization is to be performed without aortic replacement, endarterectomy of the major branches of the aorta may be performed with the thoracoabdominal exposure.

Distal perfusion can be used to limit the duration of renal and mesenteric ischemia. Partial bypass, with or without an oxygenator, can be used to direct part of the patient's blood flow from either a pulmonary vein or the left atrium to the femoral artery. Perfusion to viscera below the lower aortic cross-clamp is then retrograde from the site of the femoral artery cannula. The only ischemic viscera are those between the two aortic clamps. As the visceral branches are anastamosed to the aortic graft, the clamps can be moved such that a maximum amount of viscera is being perfused either anterograde from above the upper clamp or retrograde from below the lower clamp.

Thoracic and thoracoabdominal aortic aneurysm repair has perioperative mortality as high as 20%. For this reason, TEVAR has been advocated as an alternative to OAR. The incidence of paraplegia with TEVAR seems to be reduced compared to OAR. One approach to lessen paraplegia after TEVAR has been to place a temporary stent under SSEP monitoring and deploying a permanent stent only if SSEP is unchanged. However, motor evoked potential monitoring would seem more appropriate for monitoring function of the anterior spinal column. Several authors have reported successful treatment of paraplegia by increasing spinal perfusion pressure with a combination of induced hypertension and CSF drainage. Another method described is placing an intrathecal catheter preoperatively, both for administering local anesthetic to provide anesthesia for the femoral or iliac arterial access and also for prophylactic CSF drainage.

Aortomesenteric Revascularization

Chronic mesenteric ischemia is caused by atherosclerosis or dissection, while acute mesenteric ischemia is usually caused by an acute embolic event or trauma. Surgical revascularization for chronic ischemia is indicated only in symptomatic disease, which occurs when two of the main mesenteric vessels become occluded. Elective surgery for asymptomatic occlusive disease is not justified because of the high risk of perioperative mortality, which can range from 7% to 18%. Cardiac events, hemorrhage, and bowel infarction are the most dreaded complications. In symptomatic cases of chronic ischemia, elective surgical repair with or without concomitant aortic replacement remains the best choice because percutaneous transluminal angioplasty and stenting are associated with a significant incidence of recurrence and should be reserved to specific cases. Partial cross-clamping of the aorta is preferred, if possible, and may mitigate hemodynamic changes. For acute ischemia, the presence or absence of intestinal infarction plays a major role in the patient's overall prognosis. If a single-vessel endarterectomy is performed, it may be carried out for either the celiac axis or the superior mesenteric artery.

Aortorenal Revascularization

Renal artery revascularization can be performed by endarterectomy, bypass, or ex vivo renal artery repair. Extra-anatomic renal artery bypass may be best suited for sick, debilitated patients who would not tolerate aortic clamping. Percutaneous approaches have largely replaced surgery for isolated renal artery revascularization.

Infrarenal Operations

Repair of the infrarenal aorta is performed by exposing the relevant portion of the aorta and the iliac arteries. Although it is generally recognized that distal ischemic complications are due to dislodgment of atheromatous material off the diseased aorta and that the systemic use of heparin in the absence of distal occlusive disease is unnecessary, many centers still employ heparin before aortic clamping. Aortic repair is carried out by interposition of a graft with an end-to-end anastomosis. Aortobiiliac, aortobifemoral, and aortoiliac/femoral grafts are used in most cases. Collagen-impregnated polyester fiber (Dacron) and polytetrafluoroethylene (PTFE) grafts are both used. While both graft materials have their advantages and disadvantages, the clinician should note there appears to be an association between Dacron and rare episodes of anaphylaxis, which may be related to the stabilizers used in their manufacture.

Management of Emergency Aortic Surgery

10 The most common cause of emergency aortic repair is a leaking or ruptured aortic aneurysm. Ruptured aneurysms carry an associated mortality roughly 10 times greater than elective repair. Symptoms of ruptured AAAs include pain, faintness or frank collapse, and vomiting. Pain in the back, abdomen, or both is almost always present. Therefore, many surgeons believe pain in combination with a known AAA or a pulsatile abdominal mass indicates dissection or rupture and the immediate need for surgical exploration, until proved otherwise. Ruptures most commonly occur into the retroperitoneum, a site that permits tamponade. However, retroperitoneal hemorrhage and subsequent hematoma can displace the left renal vein, inferior vena cava, and intestine, possibly leading to damage to these structures during the surgical approach. Approximately 25% of aneurysms rupture into the peritoneal cavity, often resulting in exsanguination. Other sites of rupture include structures with which the AAA may form fistulae: Inferior vena cava, iliac veins, renal veins, or bowel.

EVAR for Ruptured AAA

There have been several recent articles suggesting EVAR is superior to OAR for ruptured AAA repair.[178–180] The criticism of these conclusions is generally that the EVAR and OAR groups are not similar because the least stable patients proceed directly to the operating room for OAR, and patients with particularly challenging anatomy are deemed inappropriate for EVAR. Both of these scenarios result in the OAR group being at a disadvantage to have successful outcomes compared to EVAR. Regardless of the controversy surrounding EVAR for ruptured AAA repair, there is consensus that two keys to success are an experienced team approach and a protocol for EVAR in patients with a ruptured AAA.

Starnes et al.[179] recently reported that after implementing an algorithm favoring EVAR for ruptured AAA repair, they saw a highly significant improvement in their overall ruptured AAA 30-day mortality. During 2002 to 2007, they treated 131 patients for ruptured AAA by performing 127 OARs and 1 EVAR, with a combined 30-day mortality of 58%. For the 22 months after implementing their algorithm, they treated 56 patients by performing 24 OARs, 27 EVARs, and 5 comfort care therapies, with a combined 30-day mortality of 35% for an absolute risk reduction of 23%. Rupture time and the number of patients with hypotension (systolic blood pressure <80 mm Hg) were similar between the pre- and postalgorithm eras. The incidence of preoperative renal insufficiency was greater in the postalgorithm era. It is important to note that the 30-day mortality for those receiving OAR did not change after implementing the algorithm, therefore the reduced mortality can be attributed either to having a protocol for ruptured AAA or to performing a larger percentage of EVARs. Holt et al.[181] investigated 3,725 urgent and 4,414 ruptured AAA repairs conducted in England between 2003 and 2008. They showed that for both urgent and ruptured AAA, EVAR offered a survival advantage over OAR, and higher-volume hospitals had lower mortality for both EVAR and OAR.

At the time of this writing, the Immediate Management of the Patient with Rupture: Open Versus Endovascular repair (IMPROVE)[182] trial is being conducted. This large multicenter randomized controlled trial will help answer the question of whether EVAR is superior to OAR for ruptured AAA.

TABLE 39-8. INCIDENCE OF 30-DAY MAJOR POSTOPERATIVE OCCURRENCES IN PATIENTS UNDERGOING INFRAINGUINAL BYPASS SURGERY

Post Operative Occurrences	All Patients $n = 2,404$
Death	2.7%
Major complications	18.7%
Major complications—operative site	15.1%
Wound dehiscence	1.7%
Wound infection	3.3%
Organ space infection	0.5%
Sepsis	3.9%
Bleed	1.6%
Graft failure	7.4%
Major complications—Systemic	5.9%
Failure to wean >48 h	1.7%
Unplanned reintubation	2.3%
Pneumonia	2.1%
Acute renal failure	0.5%
Pulmonary embolism	0%
Stroke	0.5%
Coma >24 h	0
Cardiac arrest	1%
Deep venous thrombosis	1.1%

Adapted with permission. LaMuraglia GM, Conrad MF, Chung T, et al. Significant perioperative morbidity accompanies contemporary infrainguinal bypass surgery: An NSQIP report. *J Vasc Surg.* 2009;50(2):299–304.

Ruptured AAA with Shock

Shock frequently accompanies rupture. However, the absence of hypotension does not rule out the possibility of rupture, and shock may occur suddenly. The highest priority in patients in shock is rapid diagnosis with immediate laparotomy and control of the proximal aorta. A supraceliac cross-clamp will exclude the hepatic artery from circulation, which may diminish hepatic blood flow enough that metabolism of citrate is inadequate. Therefore, if hypotension related to poor myocardial contractility or coagulopathy develops, administration of calcium may be therapeutic. Vasopressin may be particularly effective in restoring blood pressure when hemorrhagic shock is resistant to catecholamines.

LOWER EXTREMITY REVASCULARIZATION

In 2009, LaMuraglia et al.[183] analyzed data from the private sector NSQIP regarding patients undergoing infrainguinal bypass surgery. They demonstrated a 30-day mortality rate of 2.7%, a 30-day major morbidity rate of 18.7%, a major systemic complication rate of 5.9%, and a major operative site-related complication rate of 15.1% (Table 39-8). Similar to aortic surgery, lower-limb revascularization has been revolutionized by the dissemination of endovascular techniques. Allaqaband et al.[184] have summarized the current landscape in epidemiology and treatment of PAD. They report that 10 million people in the United States have symptomatic PAD; 20 to 30 million have asymptomatic PAD. The prevalence of intermittent claudication increases with age, affecting >5% of patients older than 70 years. The incidence of claudication doubles or triples in patients with diabetes. Today, advances in minimally invasive percutaneous interventions have made endovascular procedures the primary modality for revascularization. Compared with open surgical procedures, endovascular interventions offer comparable or superior long-term rates of success with very low rates of morbidity and mortality.

The development of hybrid operating rooms, with a full array of imaging equipment, allows for real-time decision-making, sometimes as a combination of traditional and endovascular repair. One technique may be used for primary repair, while another for rescue. Alternatively, a percutaneous approach to superficial femoral artery occlusion may be combined with traditional surgery below the knee. Regional anesthesia may be appropriate for some patients undergoing these procedures, but the same clinical challenges remain: Managing multiple comorbidities, preservation of renal function, and radiation safety. Drug-eluting stents in the femoral artery may limit restenosis, just as in the coronary circulation. For such patients presenting for subsequent surgery, it is unclear whether stopping antiplatelet therapy perioperatively produces adverse events. Fortunately, thrombi of stented vessels are less common and less lethal in femoral arteries than in coronary arteries. Endovascular repair has also expanded to occlusive disease in the iliac arteries.

There are three clinical indications for elective surgery for chronic peripheral occlusive disease: (1) claudication, (2) ischemic rest pain or ulceration, and (3) gangrene. Patients with rest pain, ulceration, or gangrene are at variable risk for imminent limb loss and may have severe progressive ischemia. Revascularization for these patients is urgent. When a patient presents with a gangrenous (black) or pregangrenous (blue) toe, several causes other than progression of chronic arteriosclerotic occlusive disease must be considered. Emboli may originate from the heart, a proximal aneurysm, or any proximal atherosclerotic lesion. Intra-arterially administered thrombolytic agents may have been administered, precluding regional anesthesia. Local infection is particularly common in diabetic patients.

Tunneling of the graft may be more stimulating than other parts of the procedure and may cause hypertension or movement under general anesthesia. The patient is usually given heparin during the procedure. In most cases, the heparin effect is not antagonized because bleeding problems are rare and graft reocclusion is a concern. Graft patency is evaluated carefully in the recovery room. Most surgeons believe the patient's feet should be kept warm and that the patient should be well hydrated. Peripheral vasoconstriction, which may limit outflow from the new graft, is prevented. If graft thrombosis develops early in the postoperative period, the patient is promptly returned to the operating room for graft thrombectomy, as well as for evaluation and correction of the cause of the thrombosis. During graft thrombectomy significant blood loss can occur with flushing of the graft. In a study of patients undergoing traditional surgery for lower-limb revascularization, early graft failure occurred in 4.9% of patients in US Veterans Administration NSQIP database. On multivariate analysis, risks for early graft failure included younger patients (age <70 years), black race, and diabetes mellitus. Femoral-to-popliteal bypass with vein or prosthetic graft was associated with better early graft patency than any of the tibial vessel bypass procedures except for popliteal-to-tibial bypass with autogenous vein.[185] Clinicians might especially consider catheter-based regional anesthetic techniques in patients at high risk for graft failure to facilitate anesthetic management should a return trip to the operating room be necessary.

Management of Elective Lower Extremity Revascularization

The morbidity and mortality following traditional distal operations approach those following infra-aortic repair and are mainly of cardiac origin. Thus, although regional anesthesia is often used, the same management strategies and concerns previously described apply, with special attention to the postoperative period. It is during the postoperative period that most cardiac problems arise and pain relief and correction of hemodynamic and fluid disequilibria are most likely to be needed.

Similar to EVAR, regional anesthesia may be poorly tolerated by patients who are orthopneic, uncomfortable lying still for many hours, or demented and uncooperative. Regional anesthesia may offer several advantages; however, including avoidance of hyperdynamic responses to tracheal intubation and extubation, reduced incidences of postoperative respiratory and infectious complications, and reduced postoperative hypercoagulability and graft thrombosis. Other data refute any effects of regional anesthesia on thrombotic outcomes and suggest only higher costs for postoperative surveillance. In some cases, the combination of regional and general anesthesia may provide patients with the benefits of each technique.

New data on the effect of choice of anesthetic technique on outcome after lower extremity surgery comes from the NSQIP database: 14,788 patients (general anesthesia, 9,757 patients; subarachnoid block, 2,848 patients; epidural, 2,183 patients) underwent a lower extremity infrainguinal arterial bypass during the study period. Compared with subarachnoid block, the odds of graft failure were higher with general anesthesia. When compared with subarachnoid block and epidural, general anesthesia was associated with more cases of postoperative pneumonia. Compared with subarachnoid block, general anesthesia was associated with increased odds of returning to the operating room. However, there was no significant difference in 30-day mortality among the three conditions.[186]

General anesthesia for lower extremity revascularization has the advantage of obviating patient discomfort and lack of cooperation. Its use is virtually mandated in patients who are to have vein harvested from an arm. Peripheral nerve blocks ("three-in-one," femoral sciatic block) may also be useful during and after lower extremity revascularization. Compared with general anesthesia, combined sciatic and femoral nerve blocks reduced the frequency of intraoperative myocardial ischemia in a small series of patients undergoing lower extremity vascular surgery.[187]

Management of Emergency Surgery for Peripheral Vascular Insufficiency

Acute arterial occlusion resulting in severe ischemia is a surgical emergency. With acute arterial occlusion, the involved extremity suddenly becomes cold and pulseless. Patients usually complain of coldness, pain, numbness, and paresthesias, and they may lose motor and sensory functions. Abnormal sensation in the toes, feet, and legs in response to light touch and pinprick, as well as abnormal proprioception and loss of motor function in the feet and toes, are hallmarks of acute ischemia and nonviability.

The cause of the vascular insufficiency is important in planning operative treatment and anesthetic management. If the cause is an arterial embolus, Fogarty embolectomy through a groin incision under local anesthesia may suffice. However, if the cause is thrombosis of severely diseased atherosclerotic arteries, bypass repair may be required. Thus, the anesthesiologist must be prepared for a simple procedure or a complex, extended procedure. Serum potassium levels can change quickly because cell death causes release of intracellular potassium into the circulation. Myoglobin may also be released into the circulation. The development of a compartment syndrome is a possibility, therefore fasciotomies may be required. Free radical scavengers such as mannitol and *N*-acetyl cysteine may be requested to mitigate reperfusion responses; sodium bicarbonate may or may not be given at the time of reperfusion. Anticoagulants are commonly administered to patients suspected of having peripheral vascular occlusion. If a patient has received anticoagulants, the appropriateness of using regional anesthesia is controversial. However, the authors recommend that regional anesthesia should not be used when patients have received recent thrombolytic therapy.

CONCLUSION

Atherosclerosis is a systemic condition, and vascular surgery is almost always performed for but one aspect of disease. Individuals undergoing vascular repair are generally elderly patients with other major medical problems including CAD, diabetes, COPD, and renal insufficiency. Major morbidity relates to myocardial and renal well-being; therefore, the heart and kidneys should be the major foci of the anesthesiologist's attention. In carotid surgery, the goals for anesthesia management (i.e., ensuring adequate myocardial and brain perfusion and a rapidly arousable patient) may be facilitated with the use of neurophysiologic monitoring. In aortic repair, ensuring intact myocardial function is probably the best way of making certain that spinal cord, visceral, and renal perfusion will be adequate. In the case of peripheral occlusive disease, regional anesthesia plays a greater role, but the same attention to anesthetic and cardiovascular management is required.

References

1. Walsh SR, Bhutta H, Tang TY, et al. Anaesthetic specialisation leads to improved early- and medium-term survival following major vascular surgery. *Eur J Vasc Endovasc Surg.* 2010;39(6):719–725.
2. Faraday N, Martinez EA, Scharpf RB, et al. Platelet gene polymorphisms and cardiac risk assessment in vascular surgical patients. *Anesthesiology.* 2004;101(6): 1291–1297.
3. Khuri SF, Daley J, Henderson W, et al. Risk adjustment of the postoperative mortality rate for the comparative assessment of the quality of surgical care: Results of the National Veterans Affairs Surgical Risk Study. *J Am Coll Surg.* 1997;185(4):315–327.
4. Norgren L, Hiatt WR, Dormandy JA, et al. Inter-Society Consensus for the Management of Peripheral Arterial Disease (TASC II). *J Vasc Surg.* 2007;45(suppl S): S5–S67.
5. Bhatt DL, Steg PG, Ohman EM, et al. International prevalence, recognition, and treatment of cardiovascular risk factors in outpatients with atherothrombosis. *JAMA.* 2006;295(2):180–189.
6. Axelrod DA, Stanley JC, Upchurch GR, et al. Risk for stroke after elective noncarotid vascular surgery. *J Vasc Surg.* 2004;39(1):67–72.
7. Lorenz MW, Markus HS, Bots ML, et al. Prediction of clinical cardiovascular events with carotid intima-media thickness: A systematic review and meta-analysis. *Circulation.* 2007;115(4):459–467.
8. Lorenz MW, Schaefer C, Steinmetz H, et al. Is carotid intima media thickness useful for individual prediction of cardiovascular risk? Ten-year results from the Carotid Atherosclerosis Progression Study (CAPS). *Eur Heart J.* 2010;31(16):2041–2048.
9. Diehm N, Benenati JF, Becker GJ, et al. Anemia is associated with abdominal aortic aneurysm (AAA) size and decreased long-term survival after endovascular AAA repair. *J Vasc Surg.* 2007;46(4):676–681.
10. Hindler K, Shaw AD, Samuels J, et al. Improved postoperative outcomes associated with preoperative statin therapy. *Anesthesiology.* 2006;105(6):1260–1267.
11. Le Manach Y, Godet G, Coriat P, et al. The impact of postoperative discontinuation or continuation of chronic statin therapy on cardiac outcome after major vascular surgery. *Anesth Analg.* 2007;104(6):1326–1333.
12. Burger W, Chemnitius JM, Kneissl GD, et al. Low-dose aspirin for secondary cardiovascular prevention - cardiovascular risks after its perioperative withdrawal versus bleeding risks with its continuation - review and meta-analysis. *J Intern Med.* 2005;257(5):399–414.
13. Albaladejo P, Marret E, Samama CM, et al. Non-cardiac surgery in patients with coronary stents: The RECO study. *Heart.* 2011;97(19):1566–1572.
14. Stone DH, Goodney PP, Schanzer A, et al. Clopidogrel is not associated with major bleeding complications during peripheral arterial surgery. *J Vasc Surg.* 2011; 54(3):779–784.
15. Mantz J, Samama CM, Tubach F, et al. Impact of preoperative maintenance or interruption of aspirin on thrombotic and bleeding events after elective non-cardiac surgery: The multicentre, randomized, blinded, placebo-controlled, STRATAGEM trial. *Br J Anaesth.* 2011;107(6):899–910.
16. Antman EM, DeMets D, Loscalzo J. Cyclooxygenase inhibition and cardiovascular risk. *Circulation.* 2005;112(5):759–770.
17. Hertzer NR, Beven EG, Young JR, et al. Coronary artery disease in peripheral vascular patients. A classification of 1000 coronary angiograms and results of surgical management. *Ann Surg.* 1984;199(2):223–233.
18. Finn AV, Nakazawa G, Joner M, et al. Vascular responses to drug eluting stents: Importance of delayed healing. *Arterioscler Thromb Vasc Biol.* 2007;27(7):1500–1510.
19. King SB 3rd, Smith SC Jr, Hirshfeld JW Jr, et al. 2007 Focused Update of the ACC/AHA/SCAI 2005 Guideline Update for Percutaneous Coronary Intervention: A report of the American College of Cardiology/American Heart Association Task Force on Practice Guidelines: 2007 Writing Group to Review New Evidence and Update the ACC/AHA/SCAI 2005 Guideline Update for Percutaneous Coronary Intervention, Writing on Behalf of the 2005 Writing Committee. *Circulation.* 2008;117(2):261–295.
20. Schouten O, van Domburg RT, Bax JJ, et al. Noncardiac surgery after coronary stenting: Early surgery and interruption of antiplatelet therapy are associated with an increase in major adverse cardiac events. *J Am Coll Cardiol.* 2007;49(1): 122–124.
21. Rabbitts JA, Nuttall GA, Brown MJ, et al. Cardiac risk of noncardiac surgery after percutaneous coronary intervention with drug-eluting stents. *Anesthesiology.* 2008;109(4):596–604.
22. Fleisher LA, Beckman JA, Brown KA, et al. 2009 ACCF/AHA focused update on perioperative beta blockade incorporated into the ACC/AHA 2007 guidelines on perioperative cardiovascular evaluation and care for noncardiac surgery: A report of the American college of cardiology foundation/American heart association task force on practice guidelines. *Circulation.* 2009;120(21):e169–e276.
23. Metzler H, Prüller F, Münch A, et al. Premature preoperative discontinuation of antiplatelet drug therapy in cardiovascular risk patients: A preliminary study on the role of P2Y12 receptor monitoring. *Eur J Anaesthesiol.* 2010;27(2):138–145.
24. Le Manach Y, Perel A, Coriat P, et al. Early and delayed myocardial infarction after abdominal aortic surgery. *Anesthesiology.* 2005;102(5):885–891.
25. Kim LJ, Martinez EA, Faraday N, et al. Cardiac troponin I predicts short-term mortality in vascular surgery patients. *Circulation.* 2002;106(18):2366–2371.
26. Panteghini M. The new definition of myocardial infarction and the impact of troponin determination on clinical practice. *Int J Cardiol.* 2006;106(3): 298–306.
27. Mohler ER 3rd, Mantha S, Miller AB, et al. Should troponin and creatinine kinase be routinely measured after vascular surgery? *Vasc Med.* 2007;12(3):175–181.
28. Fleisher LA, Beckman JA, Brown KA, et al. ACC/AHA 2007 Guidelines on Perioperative Cardiovascular Evaluation and Care for Noncardiac Surgery: Executive Summary: A Report of the American College of Cardiology/American Heart Association Task Force on Practice Guidelines (Writing Committee to Revise the 2002 Guidelines on Perioperative Cardiovascular Evaluation for Noncardiac Surgery): Developed in Collaboration With the American Society of Echocardiography, American Society of Nuclear Cardiology, Heart Rhythm Society, Society of Cardiovascular Anesthesiologists, Society for Cardiovascular Angiography and Interventions, Society for Vascular Medicine and Biology, and Society for Vascular Surgery. *Circulation.* 2007;116(17):1971–1996.
29. McFalls EO, Ward HB, Moritz TE, et al. Coronary-artery revascularization before elective major vascular surgery. *N Engl J Med.* 2004;351(27):2795–2804.
30. Ward HB, Kelly RF, Thottapurathu L, et al. Coronary artery bypass grafting is superior to percutaneous coronary intervention in prevention of perioperative myocardial infarctions during subsequent vascular surgery. *Ann Thorac Surg.* 2006; 82(3):795–800.
31. Garcia S, Moritz TE, Ward HB, et al. Usefulness of revascularization of patients with multivessel coronary artery disease before elective vascular surgery for abdominal aortic and peripheral occlusive disease. *Am J Cardiol.* 2008;102(7):809–813.
32. Poldermans D, Bax JJ, Schouten O, et al. Should major vascular surgery be delayed because of preoperative cardiac testing in intermediate-risk patients receiving beta-blocker therapy with tight heart rate control? *J Am Coll Cardiol.* 2006;48(5):964–969.
33. Schouten O, van Kuijk JP, Flu WJ, et al. Long-term outcome of prophylactic coronary revascularization in cardiac high-risk patients undergoing major vascular surgery (from the randomized DECREASE-V Pilot Study). *Am J Cardiol.* 2009; 103(7):897–901.
34. Howell SJ, Sear JW, Foex P. Hypertension, hypertensive heart disease and perioperative cardiac risk. *Br J Anaesth.* 2004;92(4):570–583.
35. Dunkelgrun M, Schreiner F, Schockman DB, et al. Usefulness of preoperative oral glucose tolerance testing for perioperative risk stratification in patients scheduled for elective vascular surgery. *Am J Cardiol.* 2008;101(4):526–529.
36. Finfer S, Chittock DR, Su SY, et al. Intensive versus conventional glucose control in critically ill patients. *N Engl J Med.* 2009;360(13):1283–1297.
37. Semenza GL. Hypoxia. Cross talk between oxygen sensing and the cell cycle machinery. *Am J Physiol Cell Physiol.* 2011;301(3):C550–C552.
38. Wiesbauer F, Schlager O, Domanovits H, et al. Perioperative beta-blockers for preventing surgery-related mortality and morbidity: A systematic review and meta-analysis. *Anesth Analg.* 2007;104(1):27–41.
39. Devereaux PJ, Yang H, Yusuf S, et al. Effects of extended-release metoprolol succinate in patients undergoing non-cardiac surgery (POISE trial): A randomised controlled trial. *Lancet.* 2008;371(9627):1839–1847.
40. Flu WJ, van Kuijk JP, Chonchol M, et al. Timing of pre-operative beta-blocker treatment in vascular surgery patients: Influence on post-operative outcome. *J Am Coll Cardiol.* 2010;56(23):1922–1929.
41. Wijeysundera DN, Naik JS, Beattie WS. Alpha-2 adrenergic agonists to prevent perioperative cardiovascular complications: A meta-analysis. *Am J Med.* 2003; 114(9):742–752.
42. Biccard BM, Goga S, de Beurs J. Dexmedetomidine and cardiac protection for non-cardiac surgery: A meta-analysis of randomised controlled trials. *Anaesthesia.* 2008;63(1):4–14.
43. Ellis JE, Drijvers G, Pedlow S, et al. Premedication with oral and transdermal clonidine provides safe and efficacious postoperative sympatholysis. *Anesth Analg.* 1994;79(6):1133–1140.
44. Durazzo AE, Machado FS, Ikeoka DT, et al. Reduction in cardiovascular events after vascular surgery with atorvastatin: A randomized trial. *J Vasc Surg.* 2004; 39(5):967–975.
45. Schouten O, Boersma E, Hoeks SE, et al. Fluvastatin and perioperative events in patients undergoing vascular surgery. *N Engl J Med.* 2009;361(10):980–989.
46. Barrett TW, Newton K, Koudelka C, et al. Impact of combination medical therapy on mortality in vascular surgery patients. *J Hosp Med.* 2010;5(4):218–225.
47. Railton CJ, Wolpin J, Lam-McCulloch J, et al. Renin-angiotensin blockade is associated with increased mortality after vascular surgery. *Can J Anaesth.* 2010; 57(8):736–744.
48. Wijeysundera DN, Beattie WS. Calcium channel blockers for reducing cardiac morbidity after noncardiac surgery: A meta-analysis. *Anesth Analg.* 2003;97(3): 634–641.
49. Kertai MD, Westerhout CM, Varga KS, et al. Dihydropiridine calcium-channel blockers and perioperative mortality in aortic aneurysm surgery. *Br J Anaesth.* 2008;101(4):458–465.
50. Dodds TM, Stone JG, Coromilas J, et al. Prophylactic nitroglycerin infusion during noncardiac surgery does not reduce perioperative ischemia. *Anesth Analg.* 1993;76(4):705–713.

51. Coriat P, Daloz M, Bousseau D, et al. Prevention of intraoperative myocardial ischemia during noncardiac surgery with intravenous nitroglycerin. *Anesthesiology.* 1984;61(2):193–196.
52. Thomson IR, Mutch WA, Culligan JD. Failure of intravenous nitroglycerin to prevent intraoperative myocardial ischemia during fentanyl-pancuronium anesthesia. *Anesthesiology.* 1984;61(4):385–393.
53. Landoni G, Biondi-Zoccai GG, Zangrillo A, et al. Desflurane and sevoflurane in cardiac surgery: A meta-analysis of randomized clinical trials. *J Cardiothorac Vasc Anesth.* 2007;21(4):502–511.
54. Symons JA, Myles PS. Myocardial protection with volatile anaesthetic agents during coronary artery bypass surgery: A meta-analysis. *Br J Anaesth.* 2006;97(2):127–136.
55. Zangrillo A, Testa V, Aldrovandi V, et al. Volatile agents for cardiac protection in noncardiac surgery: A randomized controlled study. *J Cardiothorac Vasc Anesth.* 2011;25(6):902–907.
56. Beattie WS, Badner NH, Choi P. Epidural analgesia reduces postoperative myocardial infarction: A meta-analysis. *Anesth Analg.* 2001;93(4):853–858.
57. Nishimori M, Ballantyne JC, Low JH. Epidural pain relief versus systemic opioid-based pain relief for abdominal aortic surgery. *Cochrane Database Syst Rev.* 2006; 3:CD005059.
58. Nelson AH, Fleisher LA, Rosenbaum SH. Relationship between postoperative anemia and cardiac morbidity in high-risk vascular patients in the intensive care unit. *Crit Care Med.* 1993;21(6):860–866.
59. Dunkelgrun M, Hoeks SE, Welten GM, et al. Anemia as an independent predictor of perioperative and long-term cardiovascular outcome in patients scheduled for elective vascular surgery. *Am J Cardiol.* 2008;101(8):1196–1200.
60. Bursi F, Barbieri A, Politi L, et al. Perioperative red blood cell transfusion and outcome in stable patients after elective major vascular surgery. *Eur J Vasc Endovasc Surg.* 2009;37(3):311–318.
61. Cooper HA, Rao SV, Greenberg MD, et al. Conservative versus liberal red cell transfusion in acute myocardial infarction (the CRIT Randomized Pilot Study). *Am J Cardiol.* 2011;108(8):1108–1111.
62. Beattie WS, Wijeysundera DN, Karkouti K, et al. Acute surgical anemia influences the cardioprotective effects of beta-blockade: A single-center, propensity-matched cohort study. *Anesthesiology.* 2010;112(1):25–33.
63. Sanders J, Patel S, Cooper J, et al. Red blood cell storage is associated with length of stay and renal complications after cardiac surgery. *Transfusion.* 2011;51(11):2286–2294.
64. Frank SM, Fleisher LA, Breslow MJ, et al. Perioperative maintenance of normothermia reduces the incidence of morbid cardiac events. A randomized clinical trial. *JAMA.* 1997;277(14):1127–1134.
65. Mantha S, Foss J, Ellis JE, et al. Intense cardiac troponin surveillance for long-term benefits is cost-effective in patients undergoing open abdominal aortic surgery: A decision analysis model. *Anesth Analg.* 2007;105(5):1346–1356.
66. Lederle FA, Freischlag JA, Kyriakides TC, et al. Outcomes following endovascular vs open repair of abdominal aortic aneurysm: A randomized trial. *JAMA.* 2009; 302(14):1535–1542.
67. Becquemin JP, Pillet JC, Lescalie F, et al. A randomized controlled trial of endovascular aneurysm repair versus open surgery for abdominal aortic aneurysms in low- to moderate-risk patients. *J Vasc Surg.* 2011;53(5):1167–1173 e1.
68. Coselli JS, Bozinovski J, LeMaire SA. Open surgical repair of 2286 thoracoabdominal aortic aneurysms. *Ann Thorac Surg.* 2007;83(2):S862–S864; discussion S890–S892.
69. Ellenberger C, Schweizer A, Diaper J, et al. Incidence, risk factors and prognosis of changes in serum creatinine early after aortic abdominal surgery. *Intensive Care Med.* 2006;32(11):1808–1816.
70. Kheterpal S, Tremper KK, Heung M, et al. Development and validation of an acute kidney injury risk index for patients undergoing general surgery: Results from a national data set. *Anesthesiology.* 2009;110(3):505–515.
71. Hutchens MP, Dunlap J, Hurn PD, et al. Renal ischemia: Does sex matter? *Anesth Analg.* 2008;107(1):239–249.
72. Hiratzka LF, Bakris GL, Beckman JA, et al. 2010 ACCF/AHA/AATS/ACR/ASA/SCA/SCAI/SIR/STS/SVM guidelines for the diagnosis and management of patients with Thoracic Aortic Disease: A report of the American College of Cardiology Foundation/American Heart Association Task Force on Practice Guidelines, American Association for Thoracic Surgery, American College of Radiology, American Stroke Association, Society of Cardiovascular Anesthesiologists, Society for Cardiovascular Angiography and Interventions, Society of Interventional Radiology, Society of Thoracic Surgeons, and Society for Vascular Medicine. *Circulation.* 2010;121(13):e266–e369.
73. Georgakis P, Paraskevas KI, Bessias N, et al. Duration of aortic cross-clamping during elective open abdominal aortic aneurysm repair operations and postoperative cardiac/renal function. *Int Angiol.* 2010;29(3):244–248.
74. Knos GB, Berry AJ, Isaacson IJ, et al. Intraoperative urinary output and postoperative blood urea nitrogen and creatinine levels in patients undergoing aortic reconstructive surgery. *J Clin Anesth.* 1989;1(3):181–185.
75. Marik PE. Low-dose dopamine: A systematic review. *Intensive Care Med.* 2002; 28(7):877–883.
76. Oliver WC Jr, Nuttall GA, Cherry KJ, et al. A comparison of fenoldopam with dopamine and sodium nitroprusside in patients undergoing cross-clamping of the abdominal aorta. *Anesth Analg.* 2006;103(4):833–840.
77. Molnar AO, Coca SG, Devereaux PJ, et al. Statin use associates with a lower incidence of acute kidney injury after major elective surgery. *J Am Soc Nephrol.* 2011;22(5):939–946.
78. Moulakakis KG, Matoussevitch V, Borgonio A, et al. Evidence that statins protect renal function during endovascular repair of AAAs. *Eur J Vasc Endovasc Surg.* 2010;40(5):608–615.
79. Mitaka C, Kudo T, Jibiki M, et al. Effects of human atrial natriuretic peptide on renal function in patients undergoing abdominal aortic aneurysm repair. *Crit Care Med.* 2008;36(3):745–751.
80. Murugan R, Kellum JA. Natriuretic peptides, acute kidney injury, and clinical evidence. *Crit Care Med.* 2008;36(3):996–998.
81. Lemaire SA, Jones MM, Conklin LD, et al. Randomized comparison of cold blood and cold crystalloid renal perfusion for renal protection during thoracoabdominal aortic aneurysm repair. *J Vasc Surg.* 2009;49(1):11–19.
82. Ali ZA, Callaghan CJ, Lim E, et al. Remote ischemic preconditioning reduces myocardial and renal injury after elective abdominal aortic aneurysm repair: A randomized controlled trial. *Circulation.* 2007;116(11 suppl):I98–105.
83. Brown LC, Brown EA, Greenhalgh RM, et al. Renal function and abdominal aortic aneurysm (AAA): The impact of different management strategies on long-term renal function in the UK EndoVascular Aneurysm Repair (EVAR) Trials. *Ann Surg.* 2010;251(5):966–975.
84. Smaka TJ, Cobas M, Velazquez OC, et al. Perioperative management of endovascular abdominal aortic aneurysm repair: Update 2010. *J Cardiothorac Vasc Anesth.* 2011;25(1):166–176.
85. Kazmers A, Jacobs L, Perkins A. The impact of complications after vascular surgery in Veterans Affairs Medical Centers. *J Surg Res.* 1997;67(1):62–66.
86. Qaseem A, Snow V, Fitterman N, et al. Risk assessment for and strategies to reduce perioperative pulmonary complications for patients undergoing noncardiothoracic surgery: A guideline from the American College of Physicians. *Ann Intern Med.* 2006;144(8):575–580.
87. Ventilation with lower tidal volumes as compared with traditional tidal volumes for acute lung injury and the acute respiratory distress syndrome. The Acute Respiratory Distress Syndrome Network. *N Engl J Med.* 2000;342(18):1301–1308.
88. Michelet P, D'Journo XB, Roch A, et al. Protective ventilation influences systemic inflammation after esophagectomy: A randomized controlled study. *Anesthesiology.* 2006;105(5):911–919.
89. Wolthuis EK, Choi G, Dessing MC, et al. Mechanical ventilation with lower tidal volumes and positive end-expiratory pressure prevents pulmonary inflammation in patients without preexisting lung injury. *Anesthesiology.* 2008;108(1):46–54.
90. Sundar S, Novack V, Jervis K, et al. Influence of low tidal volume ventilation on time to extubation in cardiac surgical patients. *Anesthesiology.* 2011;114(5): 1102–1110.
91. Landry G, Lau I, Liem T, et al. Open abdominal aortic aneurysm repair in the endovascular era: Effect of clamp site on outcomes. *Arch Surg.* 2009;144(9):811–816.
92. Marcantonio ER, Goldman L, Mangione CM, et al. A clinical prediction rule for delirium after elective noncardiac surgery. *JAMA.* 1994;271(2):134–139.
93. Rudolph JL, Marcantonio ER. Review articles: Postoperative delirium: Acute change with long-term implications. *Anesth Analg.* 2011;112(5):1202–1211.
94. Eldrup N, Budtz-Lilly J, Laustsen J, et al. Long-term incidence of myocardial infarct, stroke, and mortality in patients operated on for abdominal aortic aneurysms. *J Vasc Surg.* 2012;55(2):311–317.
95. Svensson LG, Kouchoukos NT, Miller DC, et al. Expert consensus document on the treatment of descending thoracic aortic disease using endovascular stent-grafts. *Ann Thorac Surg.* 2008;85(1 suppl):S1–S41.
96. Selim M. Perioperative stroke. *N Engl J Med.* 2007;356(7):706–713.
97. Cina CS, Abouzahr L, Arena GO, et al. Cerebrospinal fluid drainage to prevent paraplegia during thoracic and thoracoabdominal aortic aneurysm surgery: A systematic review and meta-analysis. *J Vasc Surg.* 2004;40(1):36–44.
98. Glade GJ, Vahl AC, Wisselink W, et al. Mid-term survival and costs of treatment of patients with descending thoracic aortic aneurysms; endovascular vs. open repair: A case-control study. *Eur J Vasc Endovasc Surg.* 2005;29(1):28–34.
99. Jahromi AS, Cinà CS, Liu Y, et al. Sensitivity and specificity of color duplex ultrasound measurement in the estimation of internal carotid artery stenosis: A systematic review and meta-analysis. *J Vasc Surg.* 2005;41(6):962–972.
100. Schneider PA, Naylor AR. Transatlantic debate. Asymptomatic carotid artery stenosis–medical therapy alone versus medical therapy plus carotid endarterectomy or stenting. *Eur J Vasc Endovasc Surg.* 2010;40(2):274–281.
101. Endarterectomy for asymptomatic carotid artery stenosis. Executive Committee for the Asymptomatic Carotid Atherosclerosis Study. *JAMA.* 1995;273(18):1421–1428.
102. Halliday A, Harrison M, Hayter E, et al. 10-year stroke prevention after successful carotid endarterectomy for asymptomatic stenosis (ACST-1): A multicentre randomised trial. *Lancet.* 2010;376(9746):1074–1084.
103. Brott TG, Hobson RW 2nd, Howard G, et al. Stenting versus endarterectomy for treatment of carotid-artery stenosis. *N Engl J Med.* 2010;363(1):11–23.
104. Rudarakanchana N, Dialynas M, Halliday A. Asymptomatic Carotid Surgery Trial-2 (ACST-2): Rationale for a randomised clinical trial comparing carotid endarterectomy with carotid artery stenting in patients with asymptomatic carotid artery stenosis. *Eur J Vasc Endovasc Surg.* 2009;38(2):239–242.
105. Naylor AR. What is the current status of invasive treatment of extracranial carotid artery disease? *Stroke.* 2011;42(7):2080–2085.

106. Beneficial effect of carotid endarterectomy in symptomatic patients with high-grade carotid stenosis. North American Symptomatic Carotid Endarterectomy Trial Collaborators. *N Engl J Med.* 1991;325(7):445–453.
107. Randomised trial of endarterectomy for recently symptomatic carotid stenosis: Final results of the MRC European Carotid Surgery Trial (ECST). *Lancet.* 1998; 351(9113):1379–1387.
108. Mantese VA, Timaran CH, Chiu D, et al. The Carotid Revascularization Endarterectomy versus Stenting Trial (CREST): Stenting versus carotid endarterectomy for carotid disease. *Stroke.* 2010;41(10 suppl):S31–S34.
109. Furie KL, Kasner SE, Adams RJ, et al. Guidelines for the prevention of stroke in patients with stroke or transient ischemic attack: A guideline for healthcare professionals from the American Heart Association/American Stroke Association. *Stroke.* 2011;42(1):227–276.
110. Riles TS, Kopelman I, Imparato AM. Myocardial infarction following carotid endarterectomy: A review of 683 operations. *Surgery.* 1979;85(3):249–252.
111. McGirt MJ, Woodworth GF, Brooke BS, et al. Hyperglycemia independently increases the risk of perioperative stroke, myocardial infarction, and death after carotid endarterectomy. *Neurosurgery.* 2006;58(6):1066–1073.
112. Conti A, Iacopino DG, Fodale V, et al. Cerebral haemodynamic changes during propofol-remifentanil or sevoflurane anaesthesia: Transcranial Doppler study under bispectral index monitoring. *Br J Anaesth.* 2006;97(3):333–339.
113. McCulloch TJ, Thompson CL, Turner MJ. A randomized crossover comparison of the effects of propofol and sevoflurane on cerebral hemodynamics during carotid endarterectomy. *Anesthesiology.* 2007;106(1):56–64.
114. Jellish WS, Sheikh T, Baker WH, et al. Hemodynamic stability, myocardial ischemia, and perioperative outcome after carotid surgery with remifentanil/propofol or isoflurane/fentanyl anesthesia. *J Neurosurg Anesthesiol.* 2003;15(3):176–184.
115. Lavine SD, Masri LS, Levy ML, et al. Temporary occlusion of the middle cerebral artery in intracranial aneurysm surgery: Time limitation and advantage of brain protection. *J Neurosurg.* 1997;87(6):817–824.
116. Payne RS, Akca O, Roewer N, et al. Sevoflurane-induced preconditioning protects against cerebral ischemic neuronal damage in rats. *Brain Res.* 2005;1034(1–2):147–152.
117. Engelhard K, Werner C, Eberspächer E, et al. Influence of propofol on neuronal damage and apoptotic factors after incomplete cerebral ischemia and reperfusion in rats: A long-term observation. *Anesthesiology.* 2004;101(4):912–917.
118. Todd MM, Hindman BJ, Clarke WR, et al. Mild intraoperative hypothermia during surgery for intracranial aneurysm. *N Engl J Med.* 2005;352(2):135–145.
119. Pennekamp CW, Moll FL, de Borst GJ. The potential benefits and the role of cerebral monitoring in carotid endarterectomy. *Curr Opin Anaesthesiol.* 2011; 24(6):693–697.
120. Sundt TM Jr, Sharbrough FW, Piepgras DG, et al. Correlation of cerebral blood flow and electroencephalographic changes during carotid endarterectomy: With results of surgery and hemodynamics of cerebral ischemia. *Mayo Clin Proc.* 1981; 56(9):533–543.
121. Ferguson GG, Eliasziw M, Barr HW, et al. The North American Symptomatic Carotid Endarterectomy Trial : Surgical results in 1415 patients. *Stroke.* 1999; 30(9):1751–1758.
122. Estruch-Perez MJ, Ausina-Aguilar A, Barberá-Alacreu M, et al. Bispectral index changes in carotid surgery. *Ann Vasc Surg.* 2010;24(3):393–399.
123. Calligaro KD, Dougherty MJ. Correlation of carotid artery stump pressure and neurologic changes during 474 carotid endarterectomies performed in awake patients. *J Vasc Surg.* 2005;42(4):684–689.
124. Hans SS, Jareunpoon O. Prospective evaluation of electroencephalography, carotid artery stump pressure, and neurologic changes during 314 consecutive carotid endarterectomies performed in awake patients. *J Vasc Surg.* 2007;45(3):511–515.
125. Ackerstaff RG, Moons KG, van de Vlasakker CJ, et al. Association of intraoperative transcranial Doppler monitoring variables with stroke from carotid endarterectomy. *Stroke.* 2000;31(8):1817–1823.
126. Costin M, Rampersad A, Solomon RA, et al. Cerebral injury predicted by transcranial Doppler ultrasonography but not electroencephalography during carotid endarterectomy. *J Neurosurg Anesthesiol.* 2002;14(4):287–292.
127. McCarthy RJ, McCabe AE, Walker R, et al. The value of transcranial Doppler in predicting cerebral ischaemia during carotid endarterectomy. *Eur J Vasc Endovasc Surg.* 2001;21(5):408–412.
128. van Dellen D, Tiivas CA, Jarvi K, et al. Transcranial Doppler ultrasonography-directed intravenous glycoprotein IIb/IIIa receptor antagonist therapy to control transient cerebral microemboli before and after carotid endarterectomy. *Br J Surg.* 2008;95(6):709–713.
129. Manninen PH, Tan TK, Sarjeant RM. Somatosensory evoked potential monitoring during carotid endarterectomy in patients with a stroke. *Anesth Analg.* 2001; 93(1):39–44.
130. Ritter JC, Green D, Slim H, et al. The role of cerebral oximetry in combination with awake testing in patients undergoing carotid endarterectomy under local anaesthesia. *Eur J Vasc Endovasc Surg.* 2011;41(5):599–605.
131. Messner M, Albrecht S, Lang W, et al. The superficial cervical plexus block for postoperative pain therapy in carotid artery surgery. A prospective randomised controlled trial. *Eur J Vasc Endovasc Surg.* 2007;33(1):50–54.
132. Pandit JJ, Satya-Krishna R, Gration P. Superficial or deep cervical plexus block for carotid endarterectomy: A systematic review of complications. *Br J Anaesth.* 2007;99(2):159–169.
133. Illig KA, Sternbach Y, Zhang R, et al. EEG changes during awake carotid endarterectomy. *Ann Vasc Surg.* 2002;16(1):6–11.
134. Lewis SC, Warlow CP, Bodenham AR, et al. General anaesthesia versus local anaesthesia for carotid surgery (GALA): A multicentre, randomised controlled trial. *Lancet.* 2008;372(9656):2132–2142.
135. Bekker A, Gold M, Ahmed R, et al. Dexmedetomidine does not increase the incidence of intracarotid shunting in patients undergoing awake carotid endarterectomy. *Anesth Analg.* 2006;103(4):955–958.
136. McCutcheon CA, Orme RM, Scott DA, et al. A comparison of dexmedetomidine versus conventional therapy for sedation and hemodynamic control during carotid endarterectomy performed under regional anesthesia. *Anesth Analg.* 2006; 102(3):668–675.
137. Schneemilch CE, Bachmann H, Ulrich A, et al. Clonidine decreases stress response in patients undergoing carotid endarterectomy under regional anesthesia: A prospective, randomized, double-blinded, placebo-controlled study. *Anesth Analg.* 2006;103(2):297–302.
138. Pandazi A, Karamanis P, Sidiropoulou T, et al. Low-dose (1 microg/kg) clonidine premedication and hypotension after carotid artery surgery. *Vasc Endovascular Surg.* 2011;45(7):614–618.
139. Lipsett PA, Tierney S, Gordon TA, et al. Carotid endarterectomy–is intensive care unit care necessary? *J Vasc Surg.* 1994;20(3):403–409.
140. Guirguis EM, Barber GG. The natural history of abdominal aortic aneurysms. *Am J Surg.* 1991;162(5):481–483.
141. Parodi JC, Palmaz JC, Barone HD. Transfemoral intraluminal graft implantation for abdominal aortic aneurysms. *Ann Vasc Surg.* 1991;5(6):491–499.
142. Greenhalgh RM, Brown LC, Powell JT, et al. Endovascular versus open repair of abdominal aortic aneurysm. *N Engl J Med.* 2010;362(20):1863–1871.
143. Prinssen M, Verhoeven EL, Buth J, et al. A randomized trial comparing conventional and endovascular repair of abdominal aortic aneurysms. *N Engl J Med.* 2004;351(16):1607–1618.
144. Blankensteijn JD, de Jong SE, Prinssen M, et al. Two-year outcomes after conventional or endovascular repair of abdominal aortic aneurysms. *N Engl J Med.* 2005;352(23):2398–2405.
145. EVAR trial participants. Endovascular aneurysm repair versus open repair in patients with abdominal aortic aneurysm (EVAR trial 1): Randomised controlled trial. *Lancet.* 2005;365(9478):2179–2186.
146. De Bruin JL, Baas AF, Buth J, et al. Long-term outcome of open or endovascular repair of abdominal aortic aneurysm. *N Engl J Med.* 2010;362(20):1881–1889.
147. Franks SC, Sutton AJ, Bown MJ, et al. Systematic review and meta-analysis of 12 years of endovascular abdominal aortic aneurysm repair. *Eur J Vasc Endovasc Surg.* 2007;33(2):154–171.
148. Schermerhorn ML, O'Malley AJ, Jhaveri A, et al. Endovascular vs. open repair of abdominal aortic aneurysms in the Medicare population. *N Engl J Med.* 2008; 358(5):464–474.
149. Raval MV, Eskandari MK. Outcomes of elective abdominal aortic aneurysm repair among the elderly: Endovascular versus open repair. *Surgery.* 2012;151(2): 245–260.
150. Jonk YC, Kane RL, Lederle FA, et al. Cost-effectiveness of abdominal aortic aneurysm repair: A systematic review. *Int J Technol Assess Health Care.* 2007;23(2): 205–215.
151. Prinssen M, Buskens E, de Jong SE, et al. Cost-effectiveness of conventional and endovascular repair of abdominal aortic aneurysms: Results of a randomized trial. *J Vasc Surg.* 2007;46(5):883–890.
152. Barry MC, Hendriks JM, van Dijk LC, et al. A comparative study of myocardial injury during conventional and endovascular aortic aneurysm repair: Measurement of cardiac troponin T and plasma cytokine release. *Ir J Med Sci.* 2010;179(1): 35–42.
153. Cuypers PW, Gardien M, Buth J, et al. Randomized study comparing cardiac response in endovascular and open abdominal aortic aneurysm repair. *Br J Surg.* 2001;88(8):1059–1065.
154. Brown LC, Greenhalgh RM, Thompson SG, et al. Does EVAR alter the rate of cardiovascular events in patients with abdominal aortic aneurysm considered unfit for open repair? Results from the randomised EVAR trial 2. *Eur J Vasc Endovasc Surg.* 2010;39(4):396–402.
155. Jonker FH, Schlösser FJ, Dewan M, et al. Abdominal aortic aneurysm repair in obese patients: Improved outcome after endovascular treatment compared with open surgery. *Vasc Endovascular Surg.* 2010;44(2):105–109.
156. Greenhalgh RM, Brown LC, Powell JT, et al. Endovascular repair of aortic aneurysm in patients physically ineligible for open repair. *N Engl J Med.* 2010;362(20): 1872–1880.
157. Sobocinski J, Maurel B, Delsart P, et al. Should we modify our indications after the EVAR-2 trial conclusions? *Ann Vasc Surg.* 2011;25(5):590–597.
158. Egorova N, Giacovelli JK, Gelijns A, et al. Defining high-risk patients for endovascular aneurysm repair. *J Vasc Surg.* 2009;50(6):1271–1279 e1.
159. Winterborn RJ, Amin I, Lyratzopoulos G, et al. Preferences for endovascular (EVAR) or open surgical repair among patients with abdominal aortic aneurysms under surveillance. *J Vasc Surg.* 2009;49(3):576–581 e3.
160. Sadat U, Cooper DG, Gillard JH, et al. Impact of the type of anesthesia on outcome after elective endovascular aortic aneurysm repair: Literature review. *Vascular.* 2008;16(6):340–345.

161. Edwards MS, Andrews JS, Edwards AF, et al. Results of endovascular aortic aneurysm repair with general, regional, and local/monitored anesthesia care in the American College of Surgeons National Surgical Quality Improvement Program database. *J Vasc Surg.* 2011;54(5):1273–1282.
162. Ruppert V, Leurs LJ, Steckmeier B, et al. Influence of anesthesia type on outcome after endovascular aortic aneurysm repair: An analysis based on EUROSTAR data. *J Vasc Surg.* 2006;44(1):16–21.
163. Geisbusch P, Katzen BT, Machado R, et al. Local anaesthesia for endovascular repair of infrarenal aortic aneurysms. *Eur J Vasc Endovasc Surg.* 2011;42(4):467–473.
164. Newton WB 3rd, Shukla M, Andrews JS, et al. Outcomes of acute intraoperative surgical conversion during endovascular aortic aneurysm repair. *J Vasc Surg.* 2011;54(5):1244–1250.
165. White GH, May J, Waugh RC, et al. Type III and type IV endoleak: Toward a complete definition of blood flow in the sac after endoluminal AAA repair. *J Endovasc Surg.* 1998;5(4):305–309.
166. Gilling-Smith G, Brennan J, Harris P, et al. Endotension after endovascular aneurysm repair: Definition, classification, and strategies for surveillance and intervention. *J Endovasc Surg.* 1999;6(4):305–307.
167. Berg P, Kaufmann D, van Marrewijk CJ, et al. Spinal cord ischaemia after stent-graft treatment for infra-renal abdominal aortic aneurysms. Analysis of the Eurostar database. *Eur J Vasc Endovasc Surg.* 2001;22(4):342–347.
168. Lioupis C, Tyrrell M, Valenti D. A report of spinal cord ischemia following endovascular aneurysm repair of an aneurysm with a large thrombus burden and complex iliac anatomy. *Vasc Endovascular Surg.* 2010;44(1):56–60.
169. Martin DJ, Martin TD, Hess PJ, et al. Spinal cord ischemia after TEVAR in patients with abdominal aortic aneurysms. *J Vasc Surg.* 2009;49(2):302–306.
170. De La Motte L, Vogt K, Panduro Jensen L, et al. Incidence of systemic inflammatory response syndrome after endovascular aortic repair. *J Cardiovasc Surg (Torino).* 2011;52(1):73–79.
171. Sandham JD, Hull RD, Brant RF, et al. A randomized, controlled trial of the use of pulmonary-artery catheters in high-risk surgical patients. *N Engl J Med.* 2003; 348(1):5–14.
172. Panaretou V, Toufektzian L, Siafaka I, et al. Postoperative pulmonary function after open abdominal aortic aneurysm repair in patients with chronic obstructive pulmonary disease: Epidural versus intravenous analgesia. *Ann Vasc Surg.* 2012; 26(2):149–155.
173. Tanaka K, Ludwig LM, Kersten JR, et al. Mechanisms of cardioprotection by volatile anesthetics. *Anesthesiology.* 2004;100(3):707–721.
174. Gelman S. The pathophysiology of aortic cross-clamping and unclamping. *Anesthesiology.* 1995;82(4):1026–1060.
175. Matyal R, Hess PE, Asopa A, et al. Monitoring the variation in myocardial function with the Doppler-derived myocardial performance index during aortic cross-clamping. *J Cardiothorac Vasc Anesth.* 2012;26(2):204–208.
176. Johnston WE, Conroy BP, Miller GS, et al. Hemodynamic benefit of positive end-expiratory pressure during acute descending aortic occlusion. *Anesthesiology.* 2002;97(4):875–881.
177. Sumi K, Iida H, Yamaguchi S, et al. Human atrial natriuretic peptide prevents the increase in pulmonary artery pressure associated with aortic unclamping during abdominal aortic aneurysmectomy. *J Cardiothorac Vasc Anesth.* 2008;22(2): 204–209.
178. Foster J, Ghosh J, Baguneid M. In patients with ruptured abdominal aortic aneurysm does endovascular repair improve 30-day mortality? *Interact Cardiovasc Thorac Surg.* 2010;10(4):611–619.
179. Starnes BW, Quiroga E, Hutter C, et al. Management of ruptured abdominal aortic aneurysm in the endovascular era. *J Vasc Surg.* 2010;51(1):9–17.
180. Veith FJ, Lachat M, Mayer D, et al. Collected world and single center experience with endovascular treatment of ruptured abdominal aortic aneurysms. *Ann Surg.* 2009;250(5):818–824.
181. Holt PJ, Karthikesalingam A, Poloniecki JD, et al. Propensity scored analysis of outcomes after ruptured abdominal aortic aneurysm. *Br J Surg.* 2010;97(4): 496–503.
182. Powell JT, Thompson SG, Thompson MM, et al. The Immediate Management of the Patient with Rupture: Open Versus Endovascular repair (IMPROVE) aneurysm trial–ISRCTN 48334791 IMPROVE trialists. *Acta Chir Belg.* 2009;109(6):678–680.
183. LaMuraglia GM, Conrad MF, Chung T, et al. Significant perioperative morbidity accompanies contemporary infrainguinal bypass surgery: An NSQIP report. *J Vasc Surg.* 2009;50(2):299–304, 304 e1–e4.
184. Allaqaband S, Kirvaitis R, Jan F, et al. Endovascular treatment of peripheral vascular disease. *Curr Probl Cardiol.* 2006;31(11):711–760.
185. Singh N, Sidawy AN, DeZee KJ, et al. Factors associated with early failure of infrainguinal lower extremity arterial bypass. *J Vasc Surg.* 2008;47(3):556–561.
186. Singh N, Sidawy AN, Dezee K, et al. The effects of the type of anesthesia on outcomes of lower extremity infrainguinal bypass. *J Vasc Surg.* 2006;44(5): 964–968.
187. Yazigi A, Madi-Gebara S, Haddad F, et al. Intraoperative myocardial ischemia in peripheral vascular surgery: General anesthesia vs combined sciatic and femoral nerve blocks. *J Clin Anesth.* 2005;17(7):499–503.

CHAPTER

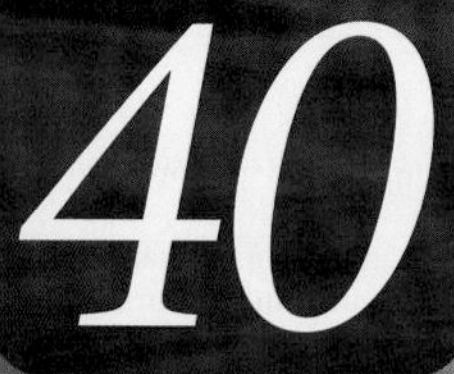

Obstetrical Anesthesia

FERNE R. BRAVEMAN • BARBARA M. SCAVONE
MARCELLE E. BLESSING • CYNTHIA A. WONG

Key Points

1. As oxygen consumption increases during pregnancy, the maternal cardiovascular system adapts to meet the metabolic demands of a growing fetus.
2. Airway edema may be particularly severe in women with preeclampsia, in patients placed in the Trendelenburg position for prolonged periods, in those who have pushed during the second stage of labor, or with concurrent use of tocolytic agents.
3. A rapid-sequence induction of anesthesia, application of cricoid pressure, and intubation with a cuffed endotracheal tube are recommended for all pregnant women receiving general anesthesia after 20 weeks' gestation.
4. The driving force for placental drug transfer is the concentration gradient of free drug between the maternal and fetal blood.
5. Labor analgesia may benefit mother and fetus and should not be withheld if requested.
6. The case-fatality rate (maternal mortality) with general anesthesia is almost 17 times greater than that with neuraxial anesthesia.
7. By virtue of age and gender as well as reduced epidural pressure after delivery, pregnant women are at a higher risk for developing postdural puncture headache.
8. Pregnancy and parturition are considered "high risk" when accompanied by conditions unfavorable to the well-being of the mother, fetus, or both.
9. Preeclampsia is classified as severe if it is associated with severe hypertension, proteinuria, or end-organ damage.
10. Antepartum hemorrhage is the leading cause of maternal mortality worldwide.
11. Heart disease during pregnancy is a leading nonobstetric cause of maternal mortality.
12. Obese parturients are more likely to have antenatal comorbidities, which may adversely affect outcome.

13 There is an increased incidence of adverse obstetric outcome, particularly after nonobstetric operations during the first trimester.

14 Any well-conducted anesthetic technique will provide safe care of the mother and fetus when the mother requires surgery during pregnancy.

Multimedia

1 Lung Volumes

2 Pudendal Nerve Block

3 C-Section Spinal

4 Fetal Heart Rate

5 Surgery Recommendations in Pregnancy

PHYSIOLOGIC CHANGES OF PREGNANCY

During pregnancy, there are major alterations in nearly every maternal organ system. These changes are initiated by hormones secreted by the corpus luteum and placenta. The mechanical effects of the enlarging uterus and compression of surrounding structures play an increasing role in the second and third trimesters. This altered physiologic state has relevant implications for the anesthesiologist caring for the pregnant patient. The most relevant changes involving hematologic, cardiovascular, ventilatory, metabolic, and gastrointestinal functions are considered in Table 40-1.

TABLE 40-1. SUMMARY OF PHYSIOLOGIC CHANGES OF PREGNANCY AT TERM

Variable	Change	Amount
Plasma volume	↑	40–50%
Total blood volume	↑	25–40%
Hemoglobin	↓	11–12 g/dL
Fibrinogen	↑	100%
Serum cholinesterase activity	↓	20–30%
Systemic vascular resistance	↓	50%
Cardiac output	↑	30–50%
Systemic blood pressure	↓	Slight
Functional residual capacity	↓	20–30%
Minute ventilation	↑	50%
Alveolar ventilation	↑	70%
Functional residual capacity	↓	20%
Oxygen consumption	↑	20%
Carbon dioxide production	↑	35%
Arterial carbon dioxide tension	↓	10 mm Hg
Arterial oxygen tension	↑	10 mm Hg
Minimum alveolar concentration	↓	32–40%

↑, increase; ↓, decrease.

Hematologic Alterations

Increased mineralocorticoid activity during pregnancy produces sodium retention and increased body water content. Thus, plasma volume and total blood volume begin to increase in early gestation, resulting in a final increase of 40% to 50% and 25% to 40%, respectively, at term. The relatively smaller increase in red blood cell volume (20%) accounts for a reduction in hemoglobin concentration (from 12 to 11 g/dL) and hematocrit (to 35%).[1] Plasma expansion and the resultant relative anemia of pregnancy plateau at approximately 32 to 34 weeks' gestation.[2] The leukocyte count ranges from 8,000 to 10,000/mm^3 throughout pregnancy. Several procoagulant factor levels increase during pregnancy, most notably fibrinogen, which doubles in mass. Anticoagulant activity decreases, as evidenced by decreased protein S concentrations and activated protein C resistance, and fibrinolysis is impaired. Increases in D-dimer and thrombin–antithrombin complexes indicate increased clotting and probable secondary fibrinolysis. Indeed, pregnancy has been referred to as a state of *chronic compensated disseminated intravascular coagulation*.[3,4] These coagulation changes peak at the time of parturition.[5] The platelet count is decreased in pregnant women, due to both dilution and increased consumption, and 6% to 15% of pregnant women at term have a platelet count $<150 \times 10^9$/L, compared with only 1% of age-matched nonpregnant controls. A further 1% of women at term have platelet counts $<100 \times 10^9$/L.[6]

Serum cholinesterase activity declines to a level of 20% below normal by term and reaches a nadir in the puerperium. However, it is doubtful that moderate succinylcholine doses lead to prolonged apnea in otherwise normal circumstances.[7] Although the total amount of protein in the circulation increases, plasma protein concentration declines to <6 g/dL at term because of dilution from increased plasma volume.[8] The albumin–globulin ratio declines because of the relatively greater reduction in albumin concentration. A decrease in serum protein concentration may be clinically significant because the free fractions of protein-bound drugs can be expected to increase.

Cardiovascular Changes

1 As oxygen consumption increases during pregnancy, the maternal cardiovascular system adapts to meet the metabolic demands of a growing fetus. Systemic vascular resistance (SVR) declines as maternal vessels lose their responsiveness to angiotensin and other pressors.[9,10] As a result, cardiac output increases by 30% to 50% above that of the nonpregnant state due primarily to a 20% to 50% increase in stroke volume and also to mild elevations in heart rate.[10]

ANESTHESIA FOR SURGICAL SUBSPECIALTIES

Arterial blood pressure decreases slightly because the decrease in peripheral resistance exceeds the increase in cardiac output. Additional increases in cardiac output occur during labor (when cardiac output may reach 12 to 14 L/min) and also in the immediate postpartum period because of added blood volume from the contracted uterus. These changes are exaggerated in multiple gestation pregnancies.[11]

Supine hypotensive syndrome, which occurs in 10% of pregnant women, occurs because the supine position leads to vena cava occlusion and thus decreased preload to the heart, resulting in lowered cardiac output and blood pressure, tachycardia, maternal mental status changes, nausea, and presyncope. Compression of the lower aorta in this position may further decrease uteroplacental perfusion and result in fetal asphyxia. From the second trimester, aortocaval compression by the enlarged uterus becomes progressively more important, reaching its maximum at 36 to 38 weeks' gestation, after which it may decrease as the fetal head descends into the pelvis.[12] Studies of cardiac output, measured with the patient in the supine position during the last weeks of pregnancy, have indicated a decrease to nonpregnant levels; however, this decrease was not observed when patients were in the lateral decubitus position.[12] Therefore, left uterine displacement by placing a wedge under the right hip or providing 15 degrees left lateral pelvic tilt should be applied routinely during the second and third trimesters of pregnancy; a minority of women may remain susceptible to vena cava and aortic compression even at this degree of tilt.[13]

Changes in the ECG may also occur. In addition to heart rate increases, left axis deviation is observed in the third trimester, possibly due to upward displacement of the heart by the gravid uterus. There is also a tendency toward premature atrial contractions, paroxysmal supraventricular tachycardia, and ventricular dysrhythmias.[14,15]

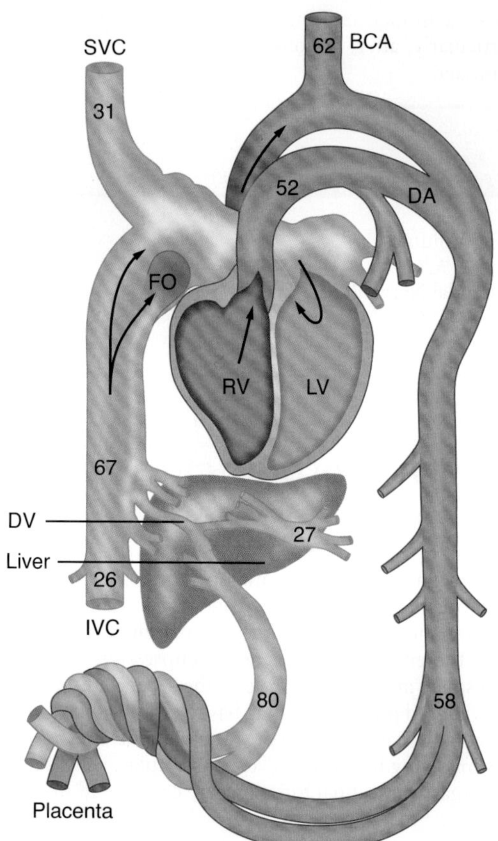

FIGURE 40-1. Diagram of the circulation in the mature fetal lamb. The numerals indicate the mean oxygen saturation (%) in the great vessels of six lambs: Right ventricle (RV), left ventricle (LV), superior vena cava (SVC), inferior vena cava (IVC), brachiocephalic artery (BCA), foramen ovale (FO), ductus arteriosus (DA), ductus venosus (DV). (Reprinted from: Born GVR, Dawes GS, Mott JC, et al. Changes in the heart and lungs at birth. *Cold Spring Harb Symp Quant Biol.* 1954;19:103, with permission.)

Respiratory Changes

Respiratory adaptations are necessary for adaptation to increasing metabolic demands, mechanical effects of the enlarging uterus, and cardiovascular changes of pregnancy.[2,16] Increased extracellular fluid and vascular engorgement and hormonal changes may lead to edema of the upper airway. Many pregnant women complain of difficulty with nasal breathing, and the friable nature of the mucous membranes during pregnancy can cause severe bleeding, especially on insertion of nasopharyngeal airways or
2 nasogastric or endotracheal tubes. Airway edema may be particularly severe in women with preeclampsia, in patients placed in the Trendelenburg position for prolonged periods, or with concurrent use of tocolytic agents. It may also be difficult to perform laryngoscopy in obese or short-necked parturients or those with enlarged breasts. Use of a short-handled laryngoscope may prove helpful. Mallampati scores increase during pregnancy and worsen further throughout labor when oropharyngeal volume also decreases.[17,18]

1 The diaphragm is displaced cephalad as the uterus increases in size. This is accompanied by an increase in the anteroposterior and transverse diameters of the thoracic cage so that total lung capacity decreases only slightly. From the fifth month, functional residual capacity (FRC) decreases by 20% to 30%, as do its subcomponents, expiratory reserve volume (ERV) (15% to 20%) and residual volume (RV) (20% to 25%) (Fig. 40-1). Concomitantly, there is an increase in inspiratory reserve volume. In most pregnant women, a decreased FRC does not cause problems, but those with pre-existing alterations in closing volume as a result of smoking, obesity, or scoliosis may experience early airway closure with advancing pregnancy, leading to hypoxemia. The Trendelenburg and supine positions also exacerbate the abnormal relationship between the closing volume and FRC. The FRC returns to normal shortly after delivery.

Airway resistance usually remains unchanged due to the competing effects of progesterone-induced relaxation of bronchiolar smooth muscle versus factors associated with increased airway resistance such as upper airway edema. Progesterone induces increases in minute ventilation, which increases from the beginning of pregnancy to a maximum of 50% above nonpregnant values at term. This is accomplished by a 30% to 50% increase in tidal volume and a small increase in respiratory rate. Alveolar dead space increases such that the dead space to tidal volume ratio remains unchanged. After delivery, as blood progesterone levels decline, ventilation returns to normal within 1 to 3 weeks.[16]

Metabolism

Basal oxygen consumption increases during early pregnancy, with an overall increase of 20% by term; CO_2 production increases. However, increased alveolar ventilation leads to a reduction in the partial pressure of carbon dioxide in arterial blood ($Paco_2$) to 32 mm Hg and an increase in the partial pressure of oxygen in arterial blood (Pa_{O_2}) to 106 mm Hg. The plasma buffer base decreases from 47 to 42 mEq/L; therefore, the pH remains practically unchanged. The maternal uptake and elimination of inhalational anesthetics are enhanced because of the increased alveolar ventilation and decreased FRC. Also, the decreased FRC and increased metabolic rate predispose the mother to development of hypoxemia during periods of apnea/hypoventilation, such as may occur during airway obstruction or prolonged attempts at tracheal intubation.[19]

Human placental lactogen and cortisol increase the tendency toward hyperglycemia and ketosis, which may exacerbate preexisting diabetes mellitus. The patient's ability to handle a glucose load is decreased, and the transplacental passage of glucose may stimulate fetal secretion of insulin, in turn leading to neonatal hypoglycemia in the immediate postpartum period.[20]

Gastrointestinal Changes

Pregnant women are at increased risk for aspiration of gastric contents compared to the general population. Aspiration pneumonitis is estimated to occur in 0.1% of cesarean deliveries performed under general anesthesia.[21] Airway difficulties present during pregnancy may contribute to this risk. In addition, gastric secretions are more acidic. Gastric emptying time is not prolonged during pregnancy, but overall gastrointestinal time is prolonged. In two recent studies of obese and nonobese, nonlaboring parturients at term, gastric emptying did not differ after ingestion of a moderate amount (300 mL) of water versus after an overnight fast.[22,23] Recent obstetric anesthesia practice guidelines by the American Society of Anesthesiologists allow for oral intake of modest amounts of clear liquids in uncomplicated laboring patients and for similar intake in patients scheduled for uncomplicated cesarean delivery up to 2 hours prior to induction of anesthesia.[24] However, the guidelines state that patients with additional risk factors for aspiration (e.g., morbid obesity, diabetes, difficult airway) or patients at increased risk for operative delivery (e.g., nonreassuring fetal heart rate [FHR] pattern) may have further restrictions of oral intake.

The lower esophageal sphincter (LES) may become distorted and incompetent and progesterone may decrease its tone. The risk of regurgitation depends, in part, on the gradient between the LES and intragastric pressures. The gravid uterus may increase intra-abdominal and intragastric pressures, decreasing the gradient. After succinylcholine administration in most patients, the gradient increases because the increase in LES pressure exceeds the increase in intragastric pressure. However, in parturients with "heartburn," the LES tone is greatly reduced.[25]

The efficacy of prophylactic nonparticulate antacids may be diminished by inadequate mixing with gastric contents, improper timing of administration, and the tendency for antacids to increase gastric volume. Administration of histamine (H_2) receptor antagonists, such as ranitidine, may be useful. A case can be made for the administration of intravenous metoclopramide before elective cesarean delivery. This dopamine antagonist hastens gastric emptying and increases resting LES tone in both nonpregnant and pregnant women.[26] The American Society of Anesthesiologists practice guidelines advise practitioners to consider the administration of nonparticulate antacids, H_2 receptor antagonists, and/or metoclopramide for aspiration prophylaxis before surgical procedures and to use neuraxial anesthesia when-
3 ever possible.[24] A rapid-sequence induction of anesthesia, application of cricoid pressure, and intubation with a cuffed endotracheal tube are recommended for pregnant women receiving general anesthesia from 20 weeks of gestation, or earlier, if symptoms of reflux are present. These recommendations also pertain to women in the immediate postpartum period because there is uncertainty as to when the risk for aspiration of gastric contents returns to normal.

Altered Drug Responses

The minimum alveolar concentration (MAC) for inhalation agents is decreased by 8 to 12 weeks' gestation and may be related to an increase in progesterone levels.[27] In addition, maximal cephalad block level after neuraxial administration of local anesthetics is higher in the second and third trimesters of pregnancy.[28] Epidural venous engorgement, which decreases intrathecal volume, may lead to increased local anesthetic spread. Pregnancy increases median nerve sensitivity to lidocaine block[29] and in vitro preparations from pregnant animals demonstrate increased susceptibility to local anesthetic blockade. This increased sensitivity may be due to progesterone or other hormonal mediators.

PLACENTAL TRANSFER AND FETAL EXPOSURE TO ANESTHETIC DRUGS

Most drugs, including many anesthetic agents, readily cross the placenta. Several factors influence the placental transfer of drugs, including physicochemical characteristics of the drug itself, maternal drug concentrations in the plasma, properties of the placenta, and hemodynamic events within the fetomaternal unit.

Drugs cross biologic membranes by simple diffusion, the rate of which is determined by the Fick principle, which states that:

$$Q/t = KA(C_m - C_f)/D$$

where Q/t is the rate of diffusion, K is the diffusion constant, A is the surface area available for exchange, C_m is the concentration of free drug in maternal blood, C_f is the concentration of free drug in fetal blood, and D is the thickness of the diffusion barrier.

The diffusion constant (K) of the drug depends on physicochemical characteristics such as molecular size, lipid solubility, and degree of ionization. Compounds with a molecular weight of <500 Da are unimpeded in crossing the placenta, whereas those with molecular weights of 500 to 1,000 Da are more restricted. Most drugs commonly used by the anesthesiologist have molecular weights that permit easy transfer.

Drugs that are highly lipid soluble cross biologic membranes more readily. The degree of ionization is important because the nonionized moiety of a drug is more lipophilic than the ionized one. Local anesthetics and opioids are weak bases, with a relatively low degree of ionization and considerable lipid solubility. In contrast, muscle relaxants are more ionized and less lipophilic, and their rate of placental transfer is therefore more limited.

The relative concentrations of drug existing in the nonionized and ionized forms can be predicted from the Henderson–Hasselbalch equation:

$$pH = pKa + \log(\text{base})/(\text{cation}).$$

The pKa is the pH at which the concentrations of free base and cation are equal. The ratio of base to cation becomes particularly important with local anesthetics because the nonionized form penetrates tissue barriers, such as the placenta. For the amide local anesthetics, the pKa values (7.7 to 8.1) are sufficiently close to physiologic pH so that changes in maternal or fetal acid–base status may significantly alter the proportion of ionized and nonionized drugs present. At equilibrium, the concentrations of nonionized drug in the fetal and maternal plasma are equal. In an acidotic fetus, local anesthetics may be relatively more ionized than in maternal blood, and "ion trapping" may occur, leading to fetal drug accumulation.[30]

The effects of maternal plasma protein binding on the rate and amount of drug transferred to the fetus are not so well understood. In sheep, the low fetomaternal ratio of bupivacaine plasma concentrations has been attributed to the difference between fetal and maternal plasma protein binding, rather than to extensive fetal tissue uptake.[31] However, if enough time is allowed for fetomaternal equilibrium to be approached, substantial accumulation of highly protein-bound drugs, such as bupivacaine, can occur in the fetus.[32]

4 As already stated, the driving force for placental drug transfer is the concentration gradient of free drug between the maternal and fetal blood. On the maternal side, the following factors interact: The dose administered, the mode and site of administration, and, in the case of local anesthetics, the use of vasoconstrictors. The rates of distribution, metabolism, and excretion of the drug, which may vary at different stages of pregnancy, are equally important. In general, higher doses result in higher maternal blood concentrations. The absorption rate varies with the site of drug injection. Compared with other forms of administration, an intravenous bolus results in the highest blood concentrations. Increased maternal blood concentrations after repeated administration of a drug greatly depend on the dose and frequency of reinjection, in addition to the kinetic characteristics of the drug. The elimination half-life of amide local anesthetic agents is relatively long, so repeated injections may lead to accumulation in the maternal plasma.[33] In contrast, 2-chloroprocaine, an ester local anesthetic, undergoes rapid enzymatic hydrolysis in the presence of pseudocholinesterase. After epidural injection, the mean half-life in the mother is approximately 3 minutes. After reinjection, 2-chloroprocaine can be detected in the maternal plasma for only 5 to 10 minutes, and no accumulation of this drug is evident.[34]

Placenta

Maturation of the placenta can affect the rate of drug transfer to the fetus, as the thickness of the trophoblastic epithelium decreases from 25 to 2 mm at term. Uptake and biotransformation of anesthetic drugs by the placenta would decrease the amount transferred to the fetus. However, placental drug uptake is limited, and there is no evidence to suggest that this organ metabolizes any of the agents commonly used in obstetric anesthesia.

Hemodynamic Factors

Any factor decreasing placental blood flow (e.g., aortocaval compression, hypotension, or hemorrhage) can decrease drug delivery to the fetus. During labor, uterine contractions intermittently reduce perfusion of the placenta. If a uterine contraction coincides with a rapid decline in plasma drug concentration after an intravenous bolus injection, by the time perfusion has returned to normal, the concentration gradient across the placenta has been greatly reduced. Thus, an intravenous injection of diazepam, administered at the onset of contraction compared to during uterine diastole, results in less drug in infants of mothers in the former group.

Several characteristics of the fetal circulation delay equilibration between the umbilical arterial and venous blood, and thus delay the depressant effects of anesthetic drugs (Fig. 40-1). The liver is the first fetal organ perfused by the umbilical venous blood, which carries drug to the fetus. Substantial uptake by this organ has been demonstrated for a variety of drugs, including thiopental, lidocaine, and halothane. During its transit to the arterial side of the fetal circulation, the drug is progressively diluted as blood in the umbilical vein becomes admixed with fetal venous blood from the gastrointestinal tract, the lower extremities, the head and upper extremities, and finally, the lungs. Because of this unique pattern of fetal circulation, continuous administration of anesthetic concentrations of nitrous oxide during elective cesarean sections caused newborn depression only if the induction-to-delivery interval exceeded 5 to 10 minutes. Rapid transfer of inhalation agents, including halothane, enflurane, and isoflurane, results in detectable umbilical arterial and venous concentrations after 1 minute.[35] Because of the rapid decline in maternal plasma drug concentrations, administration of thiopental or thiamylal as a single-bolus injection not exceeding 4 mg/kg was followed by fetal arterial concentrations of barbiturate below a level that would result in neonatal depression.[36]

Fetal regional blood flow changes can also affect the amount of drug taken up by individual organs. For example, during asphyxia and acidosis, a greater proportion of the fetal cardiac output perfuses the fetal brain, heart, and placenta. Infusion of lidocaine resulted in increased drug uptake in the heart, brain, and liver of asphyxiated baboon fetuses compared with control fetuses that were not asphyxiated.[37]

Fetus and Newborn

Any drug that reaches the fetus undergoes metabolism and excretion. In this respect, the fetus has an advantage over the newborn in that it can excrete the drug back to the mother once the concentration gradient of the free drug across the placenta has been reversed. With the use of local anesthetics, this may occur even though the total plasma drug concentration in the mother may exceed that in the fetus because there is lower protein binding in fetal plasma.[31] There is only one drug, 2-chloroprocaine, that is metabolized in the fetal blood so rapidly that even in acidosis, substantial accumulation in the fetus is avoided.[34]

In both the term and the preterm newborn, the liver contains enzymes essential for the biotransformation of amide local anesthetics. The metabolic clearance in the newborn is similar to, and renal clearance greater than, that in the adult. Elimination half-life is prolonged in the newborn due to a greater volume of distribution of the drug. Prolonged elimination half-lives in the newborn compared with the adult have been noted for other amide local anesthetics.

It is not completely understood whether the fetus and the newborn are more sensitive than the adult to the depressant and toxic effects of local anesthetics. The relative central nervous and cardiorespiratory toxicity of lidocaine has been studied in adult ewes and lambs (fetal and neonatal).[38] The doses required to produce toxicity in the fetal and neonatal lambs were greater than those required in the adult, although serum concentrations at which toxicity occurred were not different. In the fetus, this was attributed to placental clearance of drug into the mother and better maintenance of blood gas tensions during convulsions. In the newborn, a larger volume of distribution was thought to be responsible for the higher doses needed to induce toxic effects.

Bupivacaine has been implicated as a possible cause of neonatal jaundice because its high affinity for fetal erythrocyte membranes may lead to a decrease in filterability and deformability, rendering them more prone to hemolysis (see Chapter 42). However, studies failed to show increased bilirubin production in newborns whose mothers received bupivacaine for epidural anesthesia during labor and delivery.[39] Finally, observational neurobehavioral studies have revealed subtle changes in newborn neurologic and adaptive functions. In the case of most anesthetic agents, these changes are minor and transient, lasting for only 24 to 48 hours.

ANALGESIA FOR LABOR AND VAGINAL DELIVERY

Most women experience moderate-to-severe pain during parturition. In the first stage of labor, pain is caused by uterine contractions, associated with dilation of the cervix and stretching of the lower uterine segment. Pain impulses are carried in visceral afferent type C fibers accompanying the sympathetic nerves. During the first stage of labor, pain is referred to the T10 to L1 spinal cord segments. In the late first and second stages of labor, additional pain impulses from distention of the vaginal vault and perineum are carried by the pudendal nerves, composed of lower sacral fibers (S2 to S4).

Well-conducted obstetric analgesia, in addition to relieving pain and anxiety, may have other benefits. Pain may result in maternal hypertension and reduced uterine blood flow. During the first and second stages of labor, epidural analgesia blunts the increases in maternal cardiac output, heart rate, and blood pressure that occur with painful uterine contractions and "bearing-down" efforts.[40] In reducing maternal secretion of catecholamines, epidural analgesia may convert a previously dysfunctional labor pattern to normal. Maternal analgesia may also benefit the fetus by eliminating maternal hyperventilation, which often leads to reduced fetal arterial oxygen tension because of a leftward shift of the maternal oxygen–hemoglobin dissociation curve.

The most frequently chosen methods for relieving the pain of parturition are psychoprophylaxis, systemic medication, and regional analgesia. Inhalation analgesia, conventional spinal analgesia, and paracervical blockade are less commonly used. General anesthesia is rarely necessary but may be indicated for uterine relaxation in complicated deliveries. Labor varies in length and intensity, as do individual tolerance to pain and desire for pain
5 relief. Women should be supported in their choice of labor analgesia, if any, and educated about the options. Neonatal outcome appears to be similar for healthy women who deliver without pharmacologic analgesia and for women who receive analgesia. Analgesia should not be withheld if requested.[41]

Nonpharmacologic Methods of Labor Analgesia

Nonpharmacologic methods to relieve the pain of childbirth include childbirth education, emotional support, massage, aromatherapy, audiotherapy, and therapeutic use of hot and cold. More specialized techniques that require specialized training or equipment include hydrotherapy, intradermal water injections, biofeedback, transcutaneous electrical nerve stimulation, acupuncture or acupressure, and hypnosis. Conclusions regarding the efficacy of most of these techniques are not possible, as the techniques have been inadequately studied because of methodologic flaws in many study designs.[42]

Prepared Childbirth and Psychoprophylaxis

The philosophy of prepared childbirth maintains that lack of knowledge, misinformation, fear, and anxiety can heighten a patient's response to pain and consequently increase the need for analgesics. The most popular method of prepared childbirth was introduced by Lamaze. It provides an educational program on the physiology of parturition and attempts to diminish cortical pain perception by encouraging responses such as specific patterns of breathing and focused attention on a fixed object.[43] Scientific data as to whether childbirth education and psychoprophylaxis are effective in reducing childbirth pain are inconsistent and lack scientific rigor. Education, intense motivation, and cultural influences can influence the affective and behavioral responses to pain, although they probably minimally affect actual pain sensation.

Other Nonpharmacologic Methods

Continuous labor support refers to the presence during labor of nonmedical support by a trained person. Prospective, controlled trials and several systematic analyses have concluded that women who receive continuous labor support have shorter labors, fewer operative deliveries, fewer analgesic interventions, and overall satisfaction.[44] Systematic reviews of randomized controlled trials of hydrotherapy (water baths) have concluded that women experience less pain and use less analgesia, without change in the duration of labor, rate of operative delivery, or neonatal outcome.[45] Intradermal water injection consists of the injection of 0.05 to 0.1 mL of sterile water at four sites on the lower back to treat back pain during labor. Randomized controlled trials have found that the technique is effective in reducing severe back pain during labor, without any known side effects to the mother and the fetus.[46] Hypnosis requires prenatal training of the mother by a trained hypnotherapist. A meta-analysis of five randomized controlled trials concluded that women randomized to hypnosis used pharmacologic analgesia methods at a lower rate compared with women in the control groups.[42,47] The results of studies using transcutaneous electrical nerve stimulation are inconsistent, but in general, labor pain does not appear to be lessened, nor does it lower the use of other analgesic modalities.[47] In a meta-analysis including 13 trials, women who were randomized to receive acupuncture or acupressure versus control (no or "false" acupuncture) had modestly lower pain scores.[48] Similarly, relaxation techniques may also reduce pain intensity and satisfaction with pain relief compared to standard care.[49]

Systemic Medication

The advantages of systemic analgesics include ease of administration and patient acceptability. However, the drug, dose, time, and method of administration must be chosen carefully to avoid maternal or neonatal depression. Opioids are used most commonly, although tranquilizers and ketamine are used occasionally.

Opioids

Systemic opioids are commonly administered for labor analgesia, although existing data suggest that they provide little significant analgesia[50,51] (see Chapter 19). Meperidine has historically been the most commonly used systemic analgesic for the treatment of labor pain. However, in the past decade, because of concerns of the lack of efficacy and the presence of side effects, there has been a move away from its use for both labor pain and other pain conditions.[52] Meperidine can be administered by intravenous injection (effective analgesia in 5 to 10 minutes) or intramuscularly (peak effect in 40 to 50 minutes). The major side effects are a high incidence of nausea and vomiting, maternal sedation, dose-related depression of ventilation, orthostatic hypotension, and the potential for neonatal depression. Meperidine may cause transient alterations of the FHR, such as decreased beat-to-beat variability and mild tachycardia. Among other factors, the risk of neonatal depression is related to the interval from the last drug injection to delivery. The placental transfer of an active metabolite, normeperidine, which has a long elimination half-life in the neonate (62 hours), has also been implicated in contributing to neonatal depression and subtle neonatal neurobehavioral dysfunction.

Synthetic opioids such as fentanyl, alfentanil, and remifentanil are more potent than meperidine; however, their use during labor is limited by their short duration of action. These drugs offer an advantage when analgesia of rapid onset but short duration is necessary (e.g., with forceps application). For more prolonged analgesia, fentanyl or remifentanil can be administered with patient-controlled delivery devices.[53] Patient-controlled analgesia administration of opioids does carry with it the potential for drug accumulation and the risk of neonatal depression. Remifentanil has the theoretical advantage of rapid onset and offset compared with the other opioids. Bolus doses ranging from 0.2 to 1 μg/kg with lockout intervals from 1 to 5 minutes and background infusion rates from 0 to 0.1 μg/kg/min[54] have been described. However, as with other systemic opioid techniques, it is unclear whether remifentanil patient-controlled analgesia can provide satisfactory analgesia without an unacceptably high incidence of maternal, fetal, and neonatal side effects.[54]

Opioid agonists–antagonists, such as butorphanol and nalbuphine, have also been used for obstetric analgesia. These drugs have the proposed benefits of a lower incidence of nausea, vomiting, and dysphoria, as well as a "ceiling effect" on depression of ventilation. Butorphanol, 1 to 2 mg, or nalbuphine, 10 mg by intravenous or intramuscular injection, is probably the most popular. Unlike meperidine, these are biotransformed into inactive metabolites and have a ceiling effect on depression of ventilation.

Naloxone, a pure opioid antagonist, should not be administered to the mother shortly before delivery to prevent neonatal ventilatory depression because it reverses maternal analgesia at a time when it is most needed. In addition, in some instances, it has caused maternal pulmonary edema and even cardiac arrest. If necessary, the drug should be given directly to the newborn intramuscularly (0.1 mg/kg).

Ketamine

Ketamine is a potent analgesic. However, it may also induce unacceptable amnesia that may interfere with the mother's recollection of the birth. Nonetheless, ketamine is a useful adjuvant to inadequate regional analgesia during vaginal delivery or for obstetric manipulations. In low doses (0.2 to 0.4 mg/kg), ketamine provides adequate analgesia without causing neonatal depression. Constant communication is required with the patient to ensure that she is awake and able to protect her airway.

Regional Analgesia

Regional techniques provide excellent analgesia with minimal depressant effects on the mother and the fetus. The regional techniques most commonly used in obstetric anesthesia include central neuraxial blocks (spinal, epidural, and combined spinal/epidural [CSE]), paracervical and pudendal blocks, and, less frequently, lumbar sympathetic blocks (LSBs). Hypotension resulting from sympathectomy is the most frequent complication of central neuraxial blockade. Therefore, maternal blood pressure should be monitored at regular intervals, typically every 2 to 5 minutes for approximately 15 to 20 minutes after the initiation of the block and at routine intervals thereafter. The use of regional analgesia may be contraindicated in the presence of coagulopathy, acute hypovolemia, or infection at the site of needle insertion. Chorioamnionitis without frank sepsis is not a contraindication to central neuraxial blockade in obstetrics, provided antibiotics have been administered.

Because of ethical considerations and methodologic difficulties, it is difficult to design clinical studies to examine the effects of neuraxial analgesia on the progress of labor and mode of delivery. Randomized controlled trials have found no difference in the rate of cesarean delivery in women who received neuraxial compared with systemic opioid labor analgesia.[55] Meta-analyses suggests that neuraxial analgesia does not prolong the first stage of labor, although the data are heterogeneous.[55] There has been concern that early initiation of epidural analgesia during the latent phase of labor (<4 cm cervical dilation) in nulliparous women may result in a higher incidence of dystocia and cesarean delivery. Recent large randomized trials and a meta-analysis of these trials found no difference in the rate of cesarean delivery in women randomized to early neuraxial compared with systemic opioid analgesia.[56] Neuraxial analgesia is, however, associated with prolongation of the second stage of labor in nulliparous women, possibly owing to a decrease in expulsive forces or malposition of the vertex.[55] Thus, the American College of Obstetricians and Gynecologists has redefined an abnormally prolonged second stage of labor as >3 hours in nulliparous and 2 hours in multiparous women with epidural analgesia. Prolongation of the second stage may be minimized by the use of dilute local anesthetic solutions in combination with opioid.[57]

Epidural Analgesia

Epidural analgesia may be used for pain relief during labor and vaginal delivery, and if necessary, converted to anesthesia for cesarean delivery. Effective analgesia during the first stage of labor may be achieved by blocking the T10 to L1 dermatomes with low concentrations of local anesthetic, usually combined with lipid-soluble opioids. Combining drugs allows the use of lower doses of both drugs, thus minimizing side effects and complications of each. For the second stage of labor and delivery, the nerve block should be extended to include the S2 to S4 segments in order to block pain for vaginal and perineal distension and trauma.

Long-acting amides such as bupivacaine or ropivacaine are most frequently used because they produce excellent sensory analgesia while sparing motor function, particularly at low concentrations (<0.1%). Although some studies have found that ropivacaine is associated with less motor blockade than equipotent doses of bupivacaine, there was no difference in the rate of instrumental vaginal delivery among women randomized to receive epidural levobupivacaine, bupivacaine, or ropivacaine for maintenance of labor analgesia.[58]

Analgesia for the first stage of labor may be achieved with 5 to 10 mL of bupivacaine or ropivacaine (0.125%) combined with fentanyl (50 to 100 μg) or sufentanil (5 to 10 μg). There is controversy regarding the need for a test dose when using dilute solutions of local anesthetic. Because catheter aspiration is not always diagnostic, particularly when using single-orifice epidural catheters, some experts believe that a test dose should be administered to improve detection of an intrathecally or intravascularly placed catheter.[59]

Analgesia may be maintained with a continuous infusion (8 to 12 mL/hr) of bupivacaine (0.0625% to 0.1%) or ropivacaine (0.08% to 0.15%). The addition of fentanyl (1 to 2 μg/mL) or sufentanil (0.3 to 0.5 μg/mL) is often required and will allow for more dilute local anesthetic solutions to be administered. Alternatively, analgesia may be maintained with patient-controlled epidural analgesia (PCEA) with similar solutions of local anesthetic and opioid. PCEA resulted in greater patient satisfaction, a lower average hourly dose of bupivacaine (and therefore less motor block), and less need for physician intervention[60,61] compared with a continuous epidural infusion. Protocols for PCEA vary widely. Data are conflicting as to whether a background infusion improves analgesia; however, a background infusion may be helpful in selected parturients (e.g., nulliparas with long labors).[61] Common PCEA parameters include a parturient administered bolus dose of 5 to 10 mL, a lock-out interval of 10 to 20 minutes, and a background infusion of 0 to 10 mL/hr. Thirty percent to 50% of the hourly dose is often administered as a background infusion.

Women with hemodynamic stability and preserved motor function who do not require continuous fetal monitoring may ambulate with the assistance of a partner during the first stage of labor. Before ambulation, women should be observed for 30 minutes after initiation of neuraxial blockade to assess maternal and fetal well-being.

During delivery, the sacral dermatomes may be blocked with 10 mL of bupivacaine (0.25% to 0.5%), lidocaine (1.0%), or 2-chloroprocaine (2% to 3%). Many parturients have adequate analgesia for delivery without an additional bolus dose, particularly if epidural analgesia has been maintained for a long interval (hours). However, instrumental vaginal delivery may require a more dense block than that obtained with dilute local anesthetic solutions.

Spinal Analgesia

A single subarachnoid injection for labor analgesia has the advantage of fast and reliable onset of neural blockade, and it is technically easier to initiate compared with epidural analgesia. However, repeated intrathecal injections may be required for a long labor, thus increasing the risk of postdural puncture headache (PDPH). Spinal analgesia with fentanyl (15 to 25 μg) or sufentanil (2 to 5 μg) in combination with plain bupivacaine (1.25 to 2.5 mg) may be appropriate in the multiparous patient whose anticipated course of labor does not warrant a catheter technique (duration, 1.5 hours). A potential disadvantage of single-shot spinal analgesia is that the duration of labor, even in a rapidly progressing multiparous woman, may be longer than anticipated. Furthermore, if the woman requires an urgent cesarean delivery, a new anesthetic will need to be initiated. However, spinal anesthesia (a "saddle block") is a safe and effective alternative to general anesthesia or pudendal nerve block for instrumental delivery in parturients without preexisting epidural analgesia.

Combined Spinal/Epidural Analgesia

CSE analgesia is an ideal analgesic technique for use during labor. CSE combines the rapid, reliable onset of profound analgesia resulting from spinal injection with the flexibility and longer duration associated with a continuous epidural technique. After identification of the epidural space using a conventional (or specialized) epidural needle, a longer (127 mm), pencil-point spinal needle is advanced into the subarachnoid space through the epidural needle. After intrathecal injection, the spinal needle is removed and an epidural catheter is inserted. Intrathecal injection of fentanyl (10 to 25 μg) or sufentanil (2.5 to 5 μg) alone or more commonly in combination with bupivacaine (1.25 to 2.5 mg) produces profound analgesia lasting for 90 to 120 minutes with minimal motor block. Spinal opioid alone provides complete analgesia for the early latent phase of labor. However, the addition of bupivacaine is necessary for satisfactory analgesia during advanced labor. Continuous epidural analgesia or PCEA may be initiated following the spinal injection.

The most common side effects of intrathecal opioids are pruritus, nausea, vomiting, and urinary retention. The incidence of pruritus is lower if opioid is coadministered with local anesthetic.[62] Rostral spread resulting in delayed respiratory depression is rare with fentanyl and sufentanil, and usually occurs within 30 minutes of injection. Transient nonreassuring FHR patterns may occur after initiation of both epidural and spinal analgesia, with and without opioids; however, the incidence may be higher after CSE compared to epidural analgesia.[63] Presumably, uterine hypertonus and decreased uteroplacental perfusion occur as a result of rapid decrease in circulating maternal epinephrine levels after initiation of analgesia or as a result of hypotension after sympatholysis. The incidence of emergency cesarean delivery, however, is no greater after CSE than after conventional epidural analgesia.[63,64]

Mothers in early labor, or with preload-dependent medical conditions (e.g., aortic stenosis), may particularly benefit from opioid-only CSE. Spinal opioid provides complete analgesia without the need for local anesthetic in early labor, thus avoiding an acute decrease in preload, and almost always allowing motivated women to ambulate because there is no motor block. Multiparous women with advanced cervical dilation also benefit from CSE analgesia in which both intrathecal opioid and local anesthetic are injected. The onset of sacral analgesia is accomplished significantly faster with much less drug than initiation of lumbar epidural analgesia. However, because the epidural component of a CSE is not initially tested, CSE analgesia should be used with caution in women who may require urgent cesarean delivery or are at increased risk from general anesthesia (e.g., morbidly obese or anticipated difficult airway).

Paracervical Block

Bilateral paracervical block interrupts transmission of nerve impulses from the uterus and cervix during the first stage of labor. Five to 10 milliliters of dilute local anesthetic solution is injected submucosally via a needle guide in the vagina into the left and right lateral vaginal fornices. Although paracervical block effectively relieves pain during the first stage of labor, the technique has fallen out of favor during childbirth because it is associated with a high incidence of fetal asphyxia and poor neonatal outcome, particularly with the use of bupivacaine. Performing the block with dilute local anesthetic solutions, allowing 5 to 10 minutes to elapse between injections on the left and right sides, and limiting the block to women with <8 cm cervical dilation, may decrease the incidence of complications.

Paravertebral Lumbar Sympathetic Block

Paravertebral LSB is a reasonable alternative when contraindications exist to central neuraxial techniques. LSB interrupts the painful transmission of cervical and uterine impulses during the first stage of labor.[65] Although there is less risk of fetal bradycardia with LSB compared with paracervical blockade, unfamiliarity and technical difficulties associated with the performance of the block and risks of intravascular injection have decreased its use in standard practice.

Pudendal Nerve Block

The pudendal nerves, derived from the lower sacral nerve roots (S2 to S4), supply the vaginal vault, perineum, rectum, and parts of the bladder. The nerves are easily anesthetized transvaginally where they loop around the ischial spines. Ten milliliters of dilute local anesthetic solution deposited behind each sacrospinous ligament can provide adequate anesthesia for outlet forceps delivery and episiotomy repair.

Inhalation Analgesia and General Anesthesia

Inhalation labor analgesia is rare in the United States, although its use is more common in other parts of the world (see Inhaled Anesthetics, Chapter 17). Nitrous oxide, 50% by volume, is the most commonly used inhalation agent for analgesia during labor, and the mother is trained to intermittently self-administer the gas at the onset of a contraction. Studies are conflicting as to whether nitrous oxide provides benefit to the parturient[66]; however, its use appears safe for the fetus and the neonate. A major disadvantage of inhalation analgesia is the need for a waste gas scavenging system.

General anesthesia is rarely used for vaginal delivery, and precautions against gastric aspiration must always be observed (see "General Anesthesia" under "Anesthesia for Cesarean Delivery"). General anesthesia may be required when time constraints prevent induction of regional anesthesia. Potent inhalation drugs (1.5 to 2 MAC for short periods) can provide uterine relaxation for obstetric maneuvers such as second twin delivery, breech presentation, or postpartum manual removal of a retained placenta. However, in current practice, intravenous nitroglycerin (50 to 250 μg) has largely replaced the need for general anesthesia for uterine relaxation.

Although supplemental oxygen is frequently administered, there is no evidence of benefit to the mother, the fetus, or the neonate.[68,69]

Multimodal analgesia, including systemic nonsteroidal anti-inflammatory drugs and neuraxial opioids and/or local anesthetics, is optimal for postoperative analgesia. Abdominal wall nerve block techniques (transversus abdominis plane [TAP] block) have also been described after cesarean delivery.[70] Although post-cesarean delivery analgesia should take the nursing infant into account, very small amounts of drugs administered to the mother actually cross into breast milk, and even smaller amounts are absorbed from the neonatal gut. Prolonged (12 to 24 hours) postoperative pain relief in the postpartum patient can be provided by intrathecal morphine (100 to 150 μg)[71] or epidural morphine (3.5 to 4.0 mg).[72] Intrathecal morphine provides superior and longer-lasting analgesia compared to bilateral TAP block.[73] PCEA with a dilute solution of local anesthetic and lipid-soluble opioid is another option after epidural anesthesia. Side effects of neuraxial morphine include nausea, vomiting, and pruritus. Delayed respiratory depression is a rare but potentially devastating complication; therefore, the patient must be monitored carefully in the postoperative period.[74] Morbidly obese women may be at higher risk for respiratory depression.

ANESTHESIA FOR CESAREAN DELIVERY

The most common indications for cesarean delivery include arrest of dilation, nonreassuring fetal status, cephalopelvic disproportion, malpresentation, prematurity, prior cesarean delivery, and prior uterine surgery involving the corpus. The choice of anesthesia depends on the urgency of the procedure, the condition of the mother and the fetus, and the mother's wishes.

A 2001 survey of obstetric anesthesia practices in the United States revealed that most patients undergoing cesarean delivery do so under spinal or epidural anesthesia.[67] Neuraxial techniques have several advantages, such as:

- Help to avoid the necessity of airway manipulation
- Lessen the risk of gastric aspiration
- Avoid the use of depressant anesthetic drugs
- Allow the mother to remain awake during delivery
- May be associated with less operative blood loss

Compared with general anesthesia, there is less immediate neonatal depression after neuraxial compared with general anesthesia.

Neuraxial Anesthesia

Blockade to the T4 dermatome is necessary to perform cesarean delivery without maternal discomfort. The most common complication of neuraxial anesthesia is hypotension and the attendant risk of decreased uteroplacental perfusion (see "Hypotension" under "Anesthetic Complications"). Measures to decrease the incidence and severity of hypotension include left uterine displacement, intravenous fluid administration, and the liberal use of vasopressors to prevent and treat hypotension.

Most anesthesiologists administer a nonparticulate antacid before induction of anesthesia for pulmonary aspiration prophylaxis. Some practitioners also administer an H_2 receptor antagonist and metoclopramide. Sedative premedication is usually not necessary. Intraoperative monitoring mimics that for all anesthetics, although blood pressure should be measured frequently (every several minutes) for the first 20 minutes after initiation of anesthesia.

Spinal Anesthesia

Subarachnoid block is probably the most commonly administered neuraxial anesthetic for cesarean delivery because of its simplicity, speed of onset, and reliability. It is an alternative to general anesthesia for almost all but the most emergent of cesarean deliveries. Hyperbaric 0.75% bupivacaine (12.5 to 13.5 mg [1.6 to 1.8 mL]) is the most commonly used local anesthetic in the United States. It reliably provides 90 to 120 minutes of surgical anesthesia.

Despite an adequate dermatomal level for surgery, women may experience varying degrees of visceral discomfort and nausea and vomiting, particularly during exteriorization of the uterus and traction on abdominal viscera. Improved perioperative anesthesia and analgesia can be provided with the addition of fentanyl (10 to 20 μg), sufentanil (2.5 to 5 μg), or morphine (0.1 to 0.15 mg) to the local anesthetic solution. Fentanyl has a rapid onset, but is short acting and provides little additional postoperative analgesia. In contrast, morphine has a longer latency than fentanyl, but will also provide anesthesia for 12 to 18 hours after delivery.

Lumbar Epidural Anesthesia

In contrast to spinal anesthesia, epidural anesthesia is associated with a slower onset of action and a larger drug requirement to establish adequate sensory block. The major advantages of epidural compared with spinal anesthesia are the ability to titrate the extent and duration of anesthesia. To avoid inadvertent intrathecal or intravascular injection, correct placement of the epidural needle and catheter is essential. This is especially true because epidural anesthesia for cesarean delivery necessitates the administration of large doses of local anesthetic.

Aspiration of the epidural catheter for blood or cerebrospinal fluid is not reliable for detection of catheter misplacement, particularly with single-orifice catheters. Thus, most anesthesiologists administer a test dose before the initiation of surgical anesthesia. A small dose of local anesthetic (e.g., lidocaine, 45 mg, or bupivacaine, 5 mg) readily produces identifiable sensory and motor blocks if injected intrathecally. Addition of epinephrine (15 μg) with careful hemodynamic monitoring may signal intravascular injection if followed by a transient increase in heart rate and blood pressure. The use of an epinephrine test dose (15 μg) in obstetrics is controversial because false-positive results do occur

(10% increase in heart rate), especially in laboring women. In addition, epinephrine may reduce uteroplacental perfusion. Rapid injection of 1 mL of air with simultaneous precordial Doppler monitoring appears to be a reliable indicator of intravascular catheter placement.[75] Fentanyl, 100 μg, has also been used to test epidural catheter placement (significant reduction in pain).[76] A negative test, although reassuring, does not eliminate the need for incremental administration of local anesthetic.

The most commonly used agents for obstetric epidural anesthesia are 2% lidocaine with epinephrine, 5 μg/mL (1:200,000) and 3% 2-chloroprocaine. Adequate anesthesia is usually achieved with 15 to 25 mL of local anesthetic solution, administered in divided doses over 5 to 10 minutes. 2-Chloroprocaine provides rapid onset of a reliable block with minimal risk of systemic toxicity because of its extremely high rate of metabolism in maternal and fetal plasma. However, 2% lidocaine with epinephrine and sodium bicarbonate (1 mEq/10 mL lidocaine) may also be used when the rapid conversion of pre-existing epidural labor analgesia to surgical anesthesia is required for urgent cesarean delivery. Lidocaine has an onset and duration intermediate to those of 2-chloroprocaine and bupivacaine. Lidocaine should be administered with epinephrine, as lidocaine without epinephrine does not consistently provide satisfactory surgical anesthesia. Bupivacaine is no longer commonly used for obstetric epidural *anesthesia*, as it is associated with a greater risk of cardiac toxicity compared with other amide local anesthetics. Unintentional intravascular injection of bupivacaine is associated with a high incidence of maternal mortality.[77] Ropivacaine 0.5% combined with fentanyl may be used for surgical anesthesia, as the risk of toxicity is less than that of bupivacaine. The duration of motor block is shorter after ropivacaine compared with bupivacaine, but there are no differences in latency, quality of anesthesia, and duration of block.[78,79]

Combined Spinal/Epidural Anesthesia

Advantages of CSE anesthesia for cesarean delivery include the rapid onset of a dense block with a low anesthetic dose, and the ability to extend the duration of anesthesia, and perhaps to provide continuous postoperative analgesia. There is a lower incidence of breakthrough pain and intraoperative shivering, and maternal satisfaction was higher after CSE compared with epidural anesthesia for cesarean delivery.[80] Several variations of the CSE technique have been described. The standard technique uses the same spinal dose of local anesthetic as one would use for standard spinal anesthesia. In sequential CSE anesthesia, a smaller spinal dose is expected to result in inadequate anesthesia for some patients. After 15 minutes, if anesthesia is inadequate, the block is extended by injecting supplemental local anesthetic via the epidural catheter.[81] Although the incidence of hypotension is lower with this technique compared with full-dose spinal anesthesia, the induction to incision time is prolonged. A third technique is also associated with a lower incidence of hypotension without prolonging onset time. A small dose of spinal local anesthetic is followed by the routine injection of additional anesthetic through the epidural catheter approximately 5 minutes after the intrathecal dose.[82] Bupivacaine doses from 6 to 12 mg have been described for CSE anesthesia.

General Anesthesia

General anesthesia may be necessary when contraindications or relative contraindications exist to neuraxial anesthesia (e.g., coagulopathy, or moderate or severe aortic stenosis), or when the need for emergency delivery precludes central neuraxial blockade. General anesthesia should be used cautiously in women with asthma, upper respiratory tract infection, obesity, or a history of difficult tracheal intubation. Preoperative airway evaluation is particularly important in pregnant women because the inability to intubate the trachea and provide effective ventilation is the leading cause of maternal death related to anesthesia.[83] Equipment to manage the difficult airway equipment should be immediately available.[86] Mallampati classification scores worsen during labor in some parturients.[18] If airway difficulties are anticipated, a neuraxial anesthetic technique should be considered or an awake tracheal intubation performed. Pulmonary aspiration prophylaxis should be administered and the patient should be positioned with left lateral tilt to prevent aortocaval compression. Monitoring mimics that for all anesthetics.

To minimize the risk of hypoxemia during induction, denitrogenation for 3 to 5 minutes with a tight-fitting mask is essential. In an emergency, four deep breaths with 100% oxygen may suffice. A "defasciculating" dose of a nondepolarizing muscle relaxant is not necessary. Although somewhat controversial,[84] a rapid-sequence induction is usually performed. Induction with a sedative–hypnotic (e.g., propofol [2 mg/kg], ketamine [1 mg/kg], or etomidate [0.2 to 0.3 mg/kg]) is followed by succinylcholine (1 to 1.5 mg/kg) to facilitate tracheal intubation. Succinylcholine is the preferred muscle relaxant; however, when its use is contraindicated, rocuronium (0.6 mg/kg) is an acceptable alternative. A trained assistant applies cricoid pressure until the airway is properly secured with a cuffed endotracheal tube. Once correct placement of the endotracheal tube is confirmed with capnography and auscultation, the obstetrician may proceed with incision.

If there is difficulty in securing the airway, the mother should be ventilated with 100% oxygen before a subsequent attempt at tracheal intubation is made. Although some experts advise attempting to maintain cricoid pressure throughout, this practice may actually make visualization of the glottis and mask ventilation more difficult in some patients. The American Society of Anesthesiologists difficult airway algorithm[85] should be modified to include assessment of fetal status and the need for immediate delivery (Fig. 40-2). It may be safer for the mother to allow her to awaken and to reassess the method of induction and intubation, rather than to persist with traumatic efforts at tracheal intubation. However, if the fetus is in extremis, airway management with a mask or supraglottic airway device may be an acceptable alternative.[86]

In the interval between intubation and delivery, anesthesia is maintained with a 50:50 mixture of nitrous oxide in oxygen and a volatile anesthetic agent. In the past, it was common to limit the volatile agent concentration to 0.5 MAC to limit fetal exposure before delivery and to limit uterine relaxation after delivery. However, the incidence of intraoperative awareness appears to be unacceptably high with this technique.[87] Indeed, a significant number of women had bispectral index values >60 during general anesthesia with sevoflurane 1% in nitrous oxide 50%.[88] Therefore, higher concentrations of volatile agent should be used before delivery. After delivery, the nitrous oxide concentration can be increased and/or an intravenous amnestic (e.g., midazolam) and opioids can be administered.

General anesthesia for cesarean delivery is associated with lower neonatal Apgar scores at 1 minute compared with neuraxial anesthesia[89]; however, the Apgar scores at 5 minutes are comparable. Therefore, an individual trained in neonatal resuscitation should be present at delivery of the infant. After delivery, intravenous oxytocin is administered to decrease the risk of uterine atony and anesthesia is deepened with an opioid and benzodiazepine, as necessary. At the end of the procedure, the mother's trachea is extubated once she is awake and extubation criteria have been met. The usual blood loss at a cesarean delivery is 750 to 1,000 mL; transfusion is rarely necessary.

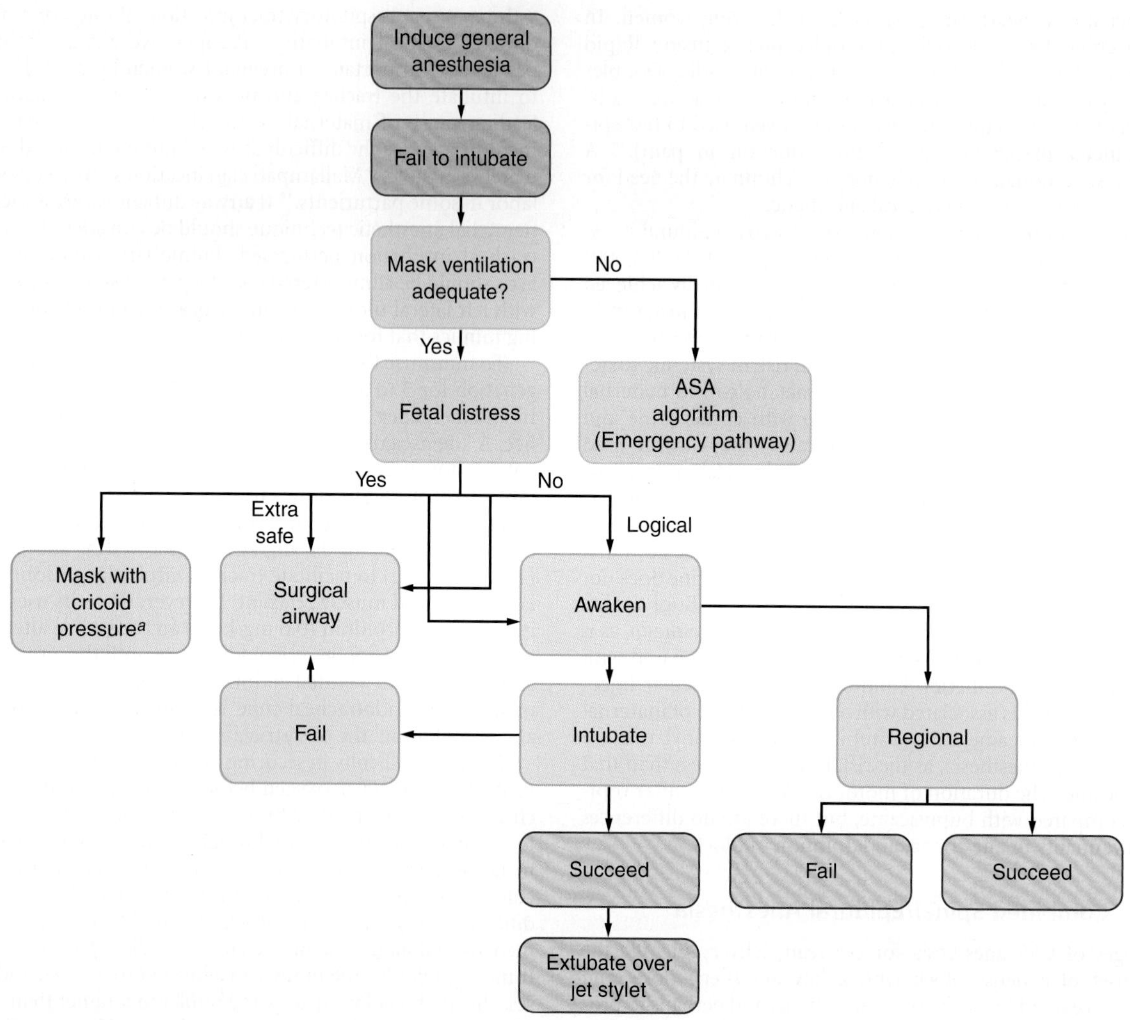

FIGURE 40-2. Management of the difficult airway in pregnancy with special reference to the presence or absence of fetal distress. When mask ventilation is not possible, the clinician is referred to the American Society of Anesthesiologists (ASA) algorithm for the emergency airway management found in Chapter 27. (Reprinted from: Kuczkowski KM, Reisner LS, Benumof JL. The difficult airway: Risk, prophylaxis, and management, Obstetric Anesthesia: Principles and Practice, 3rd ed. Chestnut DH, ed. St. Louis: Elsevier-Mosby; 2004:550, with permission.)

[a]Conventional face mask or laryngeal mask airway.

ANESTHETIC COMPLICATIONS

Maternal Mortality

A review of maternal mortality data from the US Centers for Disease Control and Prevention found that anesthesia-related maternal mortality decreased by nearly 60% from the years 1979–1990 to 1991–2002.[83] Historically, general anesthesia has been associated with a higher rate of anesthesia-related deaths than general anesthesia. During the most recent period, case-fatality rates from 6 general anesthesia fell, while those for neuraxial anesthesia rose. The risk ratio for general to neuraxial was 1.7 (95% confidence interval 0.6 to 4.6). Anesthesia-related mortality was most often associated with cesarean delivery (86%). The leading causes of death were intubation failure or induction problems (23%), respiratory failure (20%), and high spinal or epidural block (16%).[83]

Pulmonary Aspiration

The risk of inhalation of gastric contents may be increased in pregnant women, particularly if difficulty occurs with airway management. Women who have recently eaten, are laboring, received systemic opioids, or have frequent heartburn are of greatest concern.[90] Comprehensive airway evaluation, prophylactic administration of nonparticulate antacids, and use of regional anesthesia decrease the risk of aspiration. General anesthesia may be unavoidable occasionally; therefore, awake intubation may be indicated in women in whom airway difficulties are anticipated.

Hypotension

Neuraxial anesthesia is frequently associated with hypotension. Labor lowers the risk of hypotension in term pregnant women compared with nonlaboring women. Blood pressure should be monitored frequently (every 2 to 3 minutes) after the induction of neuraxial anesthesia. Techniques to reduce the incidence of hypotension during neuraxial anesthesia include left uterine displacement, intravenous fluid, and vasopressor administration. Maintaining the maternal blood pressure close to baseline reduces the incidence of maternal nausea and vomiting and is associated with higher umbilical artery pH values.[91] The administration of an intravenous bolus of crystalloid solution (1,000 to 1,500 mL) at the time of induction of neuraxial analgesia (co-load) is as effective as administration of the same volume of solution prior to the initiation of anesthesia (preload).[92] Colloid (500 mL) is superior to crystalloid solution in preventing hypotension[93] and may be considered in woman at high risk for hypotension or its consequences.

Phenylephrine is equally efficacious to ephedrine for treating maternal hypotension and results in less fetal acidosis.[94] Ephedrine crosses the placenta to a greater extent than phenylephrine and undergoes less early metabolism.[95] Stimulation of fetal β-adrenergic receptors by ephedrine increases the fetal metabolic rate; however, the clinical significance of this effect is not known. Phenylephrine may be administered as a bolus dose to treat hypotension[96] (100 to 150 μg) or continuous prophylactic infusion (starting rate, 25 to 50 μg/min).[96,97]

Total Spinal Anesthesia

High or total spinal anesthesia is a rare complication of intrathecal or epidural local anesthetic injection that occurs after excessive cephalad spread of local anesthetic in the subarachnoid or epidural space. Unintentional intrathecal administration of epidural medication as a result of dural puncture or catheter migration may also result in this complication. There is rapid ascent of sensory–motor blockade and patients may complain of dyspnea, inability to phonate, and difficulty swallowing. Profound hypotension may lead to brainstem and cerebral hypoperfusion and cause loss of conscientiousness. Immediate vasopressor administration, continued fluid administration, left uterine displacement, and leg elevation might be necessary to achieve hemodynamic stability. Reverse Trendelenburg position should not be used if hyperbaric anesthetic solution was used for spinal blockade, as there is a risk of cerebral hypoperfusion. Rapid control of the airway is essential, and endotracheal intubation may be necessary to ensure oxygenation without aspiration.

Local Anesthetic Systemic Toxicity

Local anesthetic systemic toxicity (LAST) may occur after unintended intravascular injection or drug accumulation (see Local Anesthetics). Resuscitation equipment (intravenous access, airway equipment, emergency drugs, and suction equipment) should always be available when using local anesthetics. To avoid systemic toxicity of local anesthetic agents, strict adherence to recommended dosages, methods to detect misplaced needles and catheters, and fractional administration of the induction dose are essential.

Despite these precautions, life-threatening convulsions and, rarely, cardiovascular collapse may occur. Seizure activity should be treated with an intravenous benzodiazepine, such as midazolam (1 to 5 mg), or other sedative–hypnotic. Hemodynamics, ventilation, and oxygenation must be maintained. New guidelines recommend consideration of early administration of 20% lipid emulsion (1.5 mL/kg over 1 min, followed by 0.25 mL/kg/min for at least 10 minutes after attainment of hemodynamic stability).[98] If cardiovascular collapse occurs, it should be treated according to advanced cardiac life support (ACLS) protocols. Initial small boluses of epinephrine (10 to 100 μg) are preferred; vasopressin is not recommended. Amiodarone may be used to treat ventricular dysrhythmias, particularly those due to bupivacaine. Failure to respond to lipid emulsion and vasopressor therapy should prompt consideration of cardiopulmonary bypass. A cesarean delivery may be required to relieve aortocaval compression and to ensure the efficacy of cardiac massage.[99]

Postdural Puncture Headache

7 By virtue of age and gender, pregnant women are at a higher risk for developing PDPH (see Spinal Epidural). In addition, after delivery, reduced epidural pressure may increase the risk of cerebrospinal fluid leakage through the dural opening, and estrogen withdrawal after delivery may exacerbate vascular headaches.

The incidence of PDPH is related to the diameter of the dural puncture, ranging from in excess of 70% after the use of 16-gauge needles to <1% with the smaller 25- or 26-gauge spinal needles. The incidence of cephalalgia is reduced with the use of pencil-point needles (Whitacre or Sprotte), compared with cutting bevel (Quincke) needles. Conservative treatment is indicated in the presence of mild-to-moderate discomfort, and includes bed rest, hydration, and simple analgesics. Caffeine (500 mg intravenously or 300 mg orally) has also been used in the treatment of PDPH, but the therapeutic effect is transient. Severe headache that does not respond to conservative measures for 24 hours is best treated with autologous blood patch. Using aseptic technique, approximately 20 mL of the patient's blood is injected into the epidural space close to the site of dural puncture.[100] A blood patch should not be performed for several hours after treatment with intravenous caffeine as this may precipitate a seizure. Prophylactic administration of autologous blood (after delivery, before removal of the epidural catheter) does not influence the incidence and severity of PDPH, although the duration of headache is less, compared with expectant management.[101]

Nerve Injury

Neurologic sequelae of central neuraxial blockade, although rare, have been reported. Pressure or trauma exerted by a needle or catheter on spinal nerve roots or the spinal cord produces immediate pain. Needle or catheter advancement should stop immediately on patient complaint of paresthesia or pain, and if the pain does not resolve within seconds, the needle or catheter should be withdrawn and repositioned. Anesthetics should *not* be injected when there are paresthesias. Infections such as epidural abscess or meningitis are rare and may be a manifestation of systemic sepsis or local infection. Epidural hematoma can also occur, usually in association with coagulation defects. Nerve root irritation may have a protracted recovery, lasting weeks or months. Postpartum peripheral nerve injury as a result of instrumentation, lithotomy position, or compression by the fetal head is not uncommon and may occur even in the absence of neuraxial technique.[102]

MANAGEMENT OF HIGH-RISK PARTURIENTS

8 Pregnancy and parturition are considered "high risk" when accompanied by conditions unfavorable to the well-being of the mother, the fetus, or both. Maternal problems may be related to pregnancy, such as preeclampsia–eclampsia and other hypertensive disorders

of pregnancy, or antepartum hemorrhage resulting from placenta previa or abruptio placentae. Diabetes mellitus, cardiac, chronic renal, neurologic, or sickle cell disease; and asthma, obesity, and drug abuse are not related to pregnancy but are often affected by it. Advanced maternal age (AMA) is associated with an increased risk of maternal and fetal complications. Prematurity (gestation of <37 weeks), postmaturity (≥42 weeks), intrauterine growth retardation, and multiple gestation are fetal conditions associated with risk. During labor and delivery, fetal malpresentation (breech, transverse lie), placental abruption, compression of the umbilical cord (prolapse, nuchal cord), precipitous labor, or intrauterine infection (prolonged rupture of membranes) may increase the risk to the mother or the fetus.

In general, the anesthetic management of the high-risk parturient is based on the same maternal and fetal considerations as the management of healthy mothers and fetuses. These include maintenance of maternal cardiovascular function and oxygenation, maintenance and possibly improvement of uteroplacental blood flow, and creation of optimal conditions for a painless, atraumatic delivery of an infant without significant drug effects. However, there is less physiologic reserve because many of these functions may be compromised before the induction of anesthesia. For example, significant acidosis is prone to develop in fetuses of diabetic mothers when delivered by cesarean with spinal anesthesia complicated by even brief maternal hypotension. Because the high-risk parturient may have received a variety of drugs, anesthesiologists must be familiar with potential interactions between these drugs and the anesthetic drugs they plan to administer.

Preeclampsia–Eclampsia

Hypertensive disorders, which occur in approximately 7% of all late pregnancies, are a major cause of maternal mortality. Gestational hypertension describes the development of elevated blood pressure after 20 weeks of gestation without proteinuria. Preeclampsia is defined by hypertension with proteinuria and may be associated with many other signs and symptoms. Eclampsia is present if convulsions occur. Preeclampsia–eclampsia is a disease of unknown etiology but is unique to human pregnancy. Symptoms can appear before the 20th week, with a hydatidiform mole. The condition requires the presence of a trophoblast but not a fetus.[103]

Many of the symptoms associated with preeclampsia, including placental ischemia, systemic vasoconstriction, and increased platelet aggregation, may result from an imbalance in placental production of prostacyclin and thromboxane (Figs. 40-3 and 40-4). During normal pregnancy, the placenta produces equivalent quantities of these prostaglandins, whereas in preeclamptic pregnancy, there is 7 times more thromboxane than prostacyclin.[104] An alternative etiology may be related to an inhibition of the normal trophoblastic migration of placental arterioles during the second trimester, thus preventing a low-resistance, high-flow placental circulation from developing.[105] Endothelial injury is central to the development of preeclampsia and occurs as a result of reduced placental perfusion and a production and release of substances (possibly lipid peroxidases). Abnormal endothelial function contributes to an increase in peripheral resistance and other abnormalities noted in preeclampsia through a release of fibronectin, endothelin, and other substances.

Placental ischemia results in a release of uterine renin and an increase in angiotensin (Fig. 40-3). Widespread arteriolar vasoconstriction occurs, causing hypertension, tissue hypoxia, and endothelial damage. Adherence of platelets at sites of endothelial damage results in coagulopathy. Enhanced angiotensin-mediated aldosterone secretion may lead to an increased sodium reabsorption and edema. Proteinuria may also be attributed to placental ischemia, which would lead to local tissue degeneration and a release of thromboplastin with subsequent deposition of fibrin in constricted glomerular vessels, as well as increased permeability to albumin and other plasma proteins. Furthermore, there is believed to be a decreased production of prostaglandin E, a potent vasodilator secreted in the trophoblast, which normally would balance the hypertensive effects of the renin–angiotensin system. The HELLP syndrome is a particular form of severe preeclampsia characterized by *h*emolysis, *e*levated *l*iver enzymes, and *l*ow *p*latelet count (thrombocytopenia). In contrast to preeclampsia, elevations in blood pressure and proteinuria may be mild.

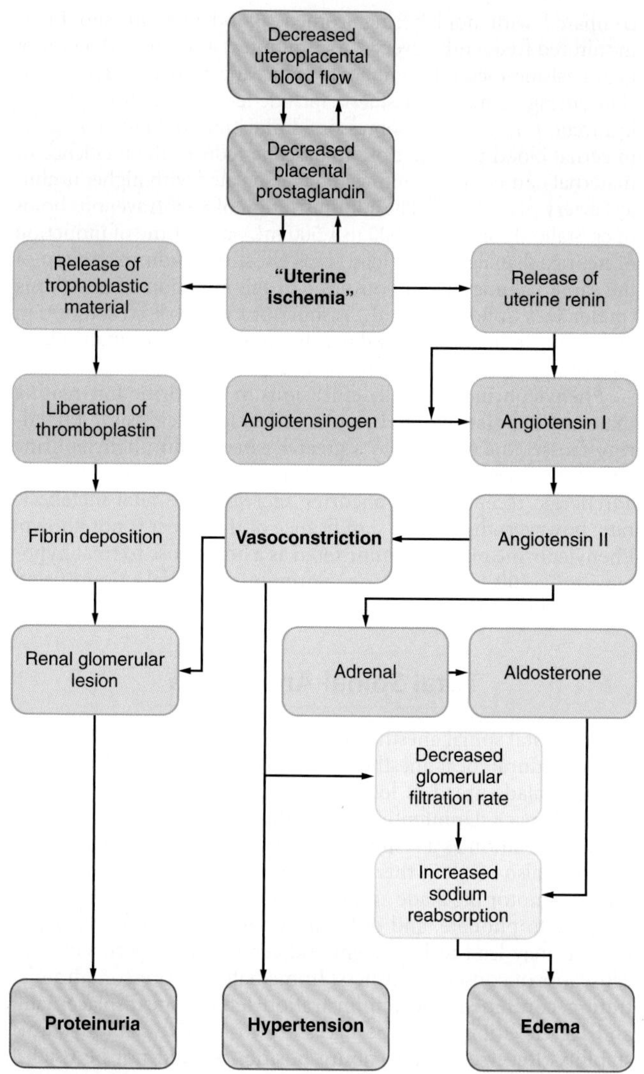

FIGURE 40-3. Proposed scheme of pathophysiologic changes in toxemia of pregnancy. (Reprinted from: Speroff L. Toxemia of pregnancy: Mechanism and therapeutic management. *Am J Cardiol.* 1973;32:582, with permission.)

9 Preeclampsia is classified as severe if it is associated with any of the following:

1. Severe hypertension
   a. Systolic blood pressure of 160 mm Hg
   b. Diastolic blood pressure of 110 mm Hg
2. Severe proteinuria of 5 g/24 hr

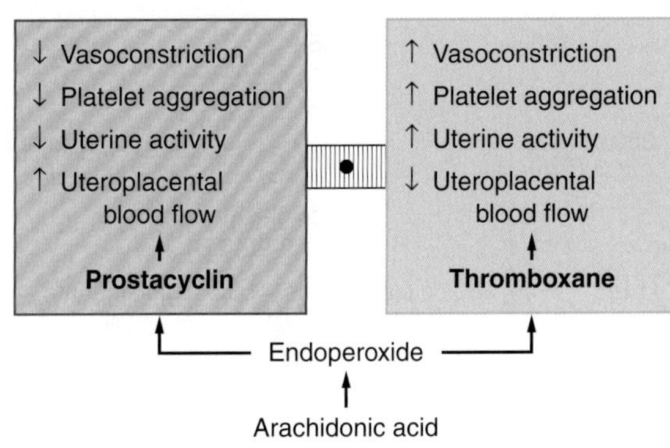

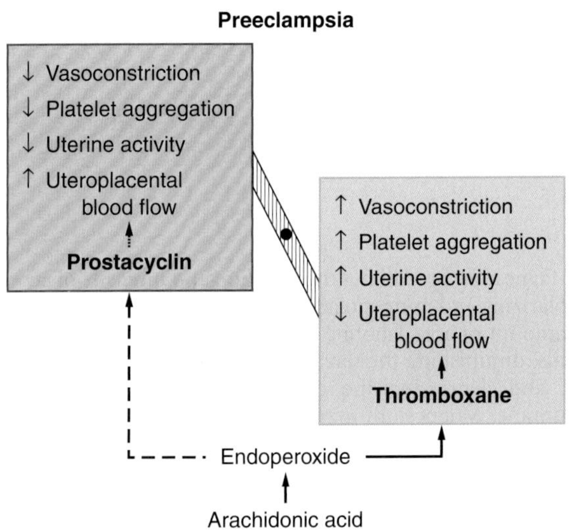

FIGURE 40-4. Comparison of the balance in the biologic actions of prostacyclin and thromboxane in normal pregnancy with the imbalance of increased thromboxane and decreased prostacyclin in preeclamptic pregnancy. (Reprinted from: Walsh SW. Preeclampsia: An imbalance in placental prostacyclin and thromboxane production. *Am J Obstet Gynecol.* 1985;152:335, with permission.)

3. Evidence of severe end-organ damage
   a. Refractory oliguria (400 mL/24 hr)
   b. Cerebral or visual disturbances
   c. Pulmonary edema or cyanosis
   d. Epigastric pain
   e. Intrauterine growth retardation
   f. Impaired liver function

Severe preeclampsia–eclampsia is a multisystem disease. Global cerebral blood flow is not diminished, but focal hypoperfusion may occur. Postmortem examination has revealed hemorrhagic necrosis in the proximity of thrombosed precapillaries, suggesting intense vasoconstriction. Cerebral edema and small foci of degeneration have been attributed to hypoxia. Petechial hemorrhages are common after the onset of convulsions. Symptoms related to these changes include headache, vertigo, cortical blindness, hyperreflexia, and convulsions. Blood pressure elevation correlates poorly with the incidence of seizures. Cerebral hemorrhage and edema account for 50% of deaths with preeclampsia–eclampsia.

Intense ocular arteriolar constriction may cause blurred vision, even temporary blindness. Heart failure may result in severe cases as a result of peripheral vasoconstriction and increased blood viscosity secondary to hemoconcentration. Left ventricular hypertrophy, subendocardial hemorrhages, cloudy swelling, and fatty and hyaline degeneration may occur.

Decreased blood supply to the liver may lead to periportal necrosis. Subcapsular hemorrhage results in epigastric pain. Rarely, there is rupture of the overstretched liver capsule and massive hemorrhage into the abdominal cavity. There may be elevated aspartate aminotransferase, lactate dehydrogenase, and alkaline phosphatase, whereas bilirubin is unaltered.

In the kidneys, there is swelling of glomerular endothelial cells and deposition of fibrin, leading to a constriction of the capillary lumina. Renal blood flow and glomerular filtration rate decrease, resulting in reduced uric acid clearance and, in severe cases, reduced clearance of urea and creatinine. Oliguria and proteinuria are characteristic symptoms of severe preeclampsia. The severity of renal involvement is reflected in the degree of proteinuria, which may reach nephrotic levels of 10 to 15 g/24 hr.

A mild pulmonary ventilation–perfusion imbalance has been reported in severe cases. It is not believed to be clinically important because the arterial oxygen tension was within normal limits. In contrast, airway edema, which may also occur in severe preeclampsia, is of great concern because it may lead to respiratory embarrassment and difficulty in tracheal intubation. Pulmonary edema occurs in approximately 2% of severe preeclamptic patients as a result of heart failure, circulatory overload, or aspiration of gastric contents during convulsions.

A reduction in intervillous blood flow may result from vasoconstriction or the development of occlusive lesions in decidual arteries, despite the elevated maternal blood pressure. Reduced placental blood flow leads to chronic fetal hypoxia and malnutrition. The risks of intrauterine growth retardation, premature birth, and perinatal death are substantially higher than in normal pregnancies and correlate with the severity of preeclampsia.

Although preeclampsia is accompanied by exaggerated retention of water and sodium, a shift of fluid and proteins from the intravascular into the extravascular compartment may result in hypovolemia, hypoproteinemia, and hemoconcentration. This phenomenon may be further affected by proteinuria. The risk of uteroplacental hypoperfusion and poor fetal outcome correlates with the degree of maternal plasma and protein depletion. The mean plasma volume in women with preeclampsia was found to be 9% less than normal, and in those with severe disease, 30% to 40% below normal.[106] The inverse relationship between the intravascular volume and the severity of hypertension was confirmed with measurements of central venous pressure (CVP) (Fig. 40-5). Volume expansion may improve maternal tissue perfusion in patients with severe preeclampsia.

Adherence of platelets at sites of endothelial damage may result in consumption coagulopathy and thrombocytopenia. It is usually mild, with the platelet count in the range of 100,000 to 150,000/mm^3. High-dose steroids (>24 mg of beta or dexamethasone in 24 hours) used to accelerate fetal lung maturity have been shown to prevent a worsening in platelet count or even increase platelet count in women with the HELLP syndrome[107] (Fig. 40-6). Elevated levels of fibrin degradation products are found less frequently, and plasma fibrinogen concentrations remain normal unless there is a placental abruption. Prolongation of prothrombin and partial thromboplastin times indicates consumption of procoagulant. Bleeding time is no longer considered a reliable test of clotting.

General Management

The definitive treatment of preeclampsia–eclampsia remains delivery of the fetus and placenta. Management is usually symptomatic until the obstetrician determines that delivery is appropriate

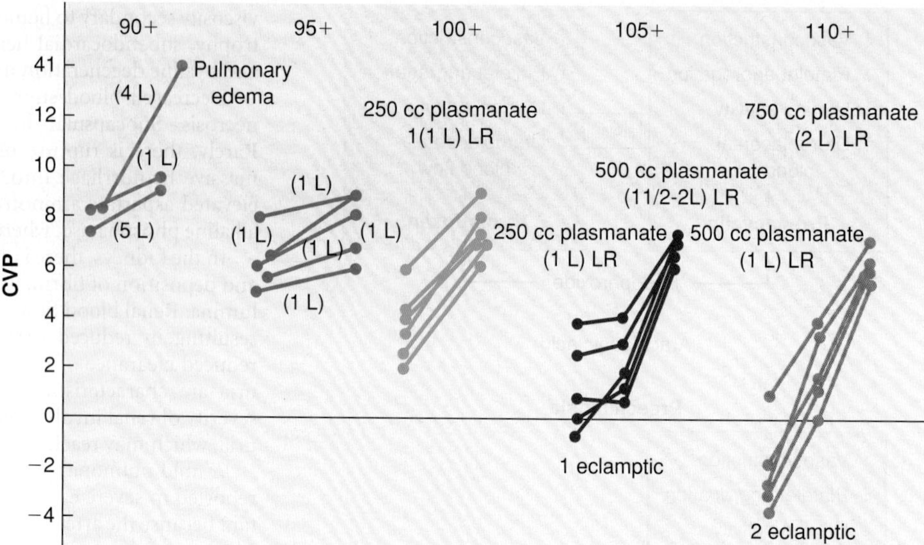

FIGURE 40-5. Initial central venous pressure measurements (three or more recordings of maternal diastolic pressure) and intravenous volume replacement required to attain the range of 6 to 8 cm H_2O in five groups of women with preeclampsia classified according to the severity of the disease (by diastolic blood pressure). LR, lactated Ringer solution. (Reprinted from: Joyce TH III, Debnath KS, Baker EA. Preeclampsia: Relationship of CVP and epidural analgesia. *Anesthesiology.* 1979;51:S297, with permission.)

for the fetus. The goals are to prevent or control convulsions, improve organ perfusion, normalize blood pressure, and correct clotting abnormalities. Mild cases may be managed expectantly with bed rest, antihypertensive medication, and fetal surveillance until the pregnancy is closer to term. Delivery is indicated in refractory cases if there is nonreassuring fetal status or if the pregnancy is already close to term. In severe cases, aggressive management should continue for at least 24 to 48 hours after delivery.

The mainstay of anticonvulsant therapy is magnesium sulfate (see Chapter 14). The patient usually receives an intravenous loading dose of 4 g in a 20% solution over 5 minutes. Therapeutic blood levels are maintained by continuous infusion of 1 to 2 g/hr. Magnesium may cause mild peripheral arterial vasodilation. Magnesium ions cross the placenta readily and may lead to fetal and neonatal hypermagnesemia. There is poor correlation between magnesium concentrations in the umbilical cord blood and the incidence of low Apgar scores and depression of ventilation at birth, which are more likely due to fetal asphyxia and prematurity. In fact, there is evidence that magnesium therapy is neuroprotective for the fetus and reduces the risk of cerebral palsy.[108]

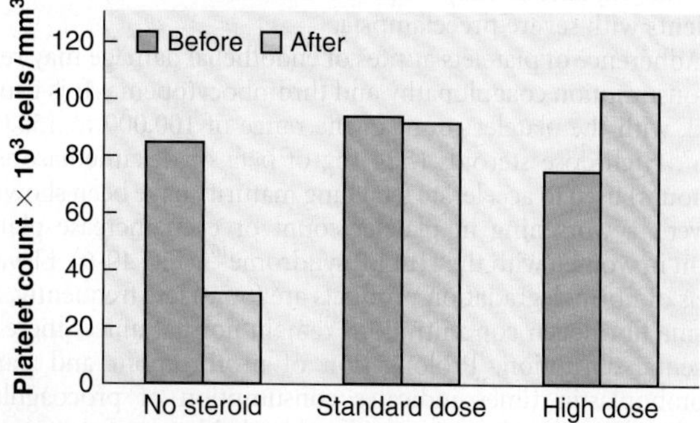

FIGURE 40-6. Mean platelet count in women with HELLP syndrome without steroids, and before and after standard steroid (<24 mg/day) and high steroid (>24 mg/day) therapy. (Adapted from: O'Brien JM, Milligan DA, Barton JR. Impact of high dose corticosteroid therapy for patients with HELLP [hemolysis, elevated liver function tests, and low platelets] syndrome. *Am J Obstet Gynecol.* 2000;183:921.)

Magnesium potentiates the duration and intensity of action of depolarizing and nondepolarizing muscle relaxants by decreasing the amount of acetylcholine liberated from the motor nerve terminals, diminishing the sensitivity of the end plate to acetylcholine, and depressing the excitability of the skeletal muscle membrane. Magnesium may also increase the severity of hypotension under regional anesthesia and make it more difficult to treat. Judicious hydration with a balanced salt solution may be required to replace intravascular volume. In all cases, careful monitoring of arterial pressure and urine output should be started as soon as possible. In severe cases, invasive central pressure monitoring may be required. A pulmonary artery catheter is safe and useful in guiding therapy for patients with pulmonary edema, renal failure, or eclampsia.[109] Monitoring should be extended to the postpartum period.

Antihypertensive therapy in preeclampsia is used to lessen the risk of cerebral hemorrhage in the mother while maintaining, even improving, tissue perfusion. Hydralazine is the most commonly used vasodilator in preeclampsia because it increases uteroplacental and renal blood flow. Nitroprusside, a potent vasodilator of resistance and capacitance vessels, with an immediate but evanescent action, is useful in preventing dangerous elevations in systemic and pulmonary artery blood pressure during laryngoscopy and intubation, and is ideal for treatment of hypertensive emergencies. Other agents used to control maternal blood pressure in preeclampsia include nitroglycerin and labetalol. Consumption coagulopathy may require infusion of fresh whole blood, platelet concentrates, fresh frozen plasma, and cryoprecipitate (see Chapter 16). Neuraxial anesthesia is contraindicated in patients with severe coagulopathy.

Anesthetic Management

Epidural, spinal, or CSE analgesia or anesthesia for labor and delivery should no longer be considered contraindicated, provided there is no severe clotting abnormality or plasma volume deficit.[110] In volume-repleted patients positioned with left uterine displacement, neuraxial analgesia does not cause an unacceptable reduction in blood pressure and leads to a significant improvement in placental perfusion.[111] With the use of radioactive xenon, it was shown that the intervillous blood flow increased by approximately

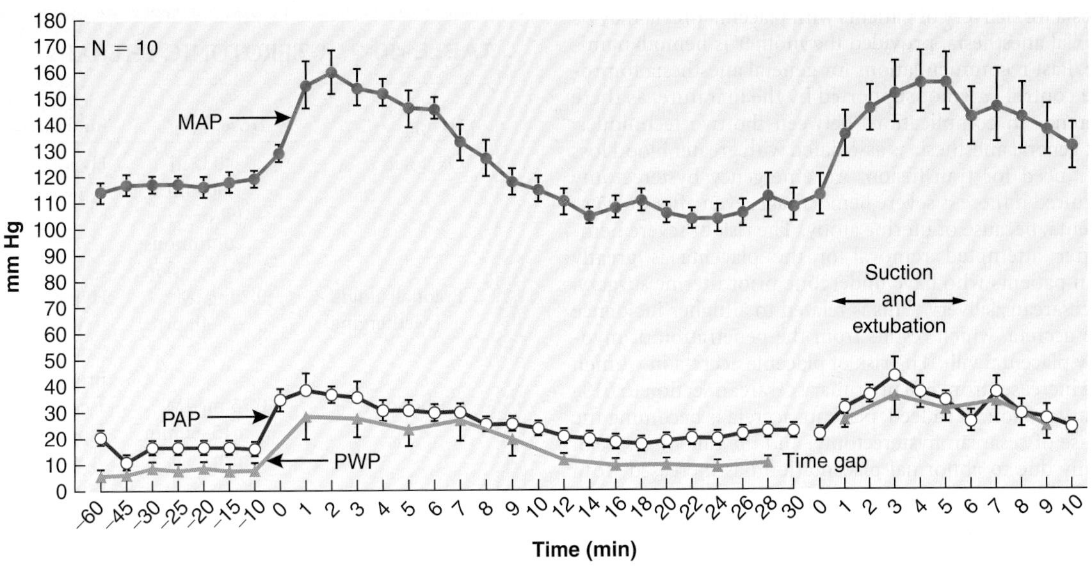

FIGURE 40-7. Mean and SE of mean arterial pressure (MAP), mean pulmonary artery pressure (PAP), and pulmonary wedge pressure (PWP) in patients with severe preeclampsia receiving thiopental and nitrous oxide (40%) with 0.5% halothane anesthesia for cesarean section. (Reprinted from: Hodgkinson R, Husain FJ, Hayashi RH. Systemic and pulmonary blood pressure during cesarean section in parturients with gestational hypertension. *Can Anaesth Soc J.* 1980;27:389, with permission.)

75% after the induction of epidural analgesia (10 mL of bupivacaine 0.25%).[112]

For cesarean delivery, the sensory level of anesthesia must extend to T3 to T4, making adequate fluid therapy and left uterine displacement even more critical. The use of spinal anesthesia in severely preeclamptic women has been discouraged in favor of the continuous epidural technique. The concern is related to the fact that severely preeclamptic women can have significant intravascular volume deficits related to widespread arteriolar vasoconstriction, which may result in catastrophic hypotension with the sudden onset of extensive sympathectomy associated with spinal anesthesia. In fact, women with severe preeclampsia appear to be at lower risk of hypotension than normotensive women having cesarean delivery.[113] Furthermore, studies to date have shown that the incidence and severity of hypotension is similar in women with severe preeclampsia having a cesarean delivery with spinal compared with epidural anesthesia.[114,115] Thus, spinal anesthesia is emerging as a suitable alternative to epidural anesthesia for cesarean delivery in severely preeclamptic women. It is important to note that severely preeclamptic women need to be adequately prepared prior to neuraxial anesthesia with judicious hydration and control of blood pressure.

General anesthesia in preeclamptic patients has its particular hazards. Rapid-sequence induction of anesthesia and intubation of the trachea are occasionally difficult because of a swollen tongue, epiglottis, or pharynx (see Chapter 27). In patients with impaired coagulation, laryngoscopy and intubation of the trachea may provoke profuse bleeding. Marked systemic and pulmonary hypertension occurring at intubation and extubation enhance the risk of cerebral hemorrhage and pulmonary edema (Fig. 40-7). However, these hemodynamic changes can be minimized with appropriate antihypertensive therapy, such as administration of labetalol or nitroprusside infusion. The use of ketamine and ergot alkaloids should be avoided. Magnesium may prolong the effects of all muscle relaxants through its actions on the myoneural junction. Therefore, relaxants should be administered with caution (using a nerve stimulator) to avoid overdosage. General anesthesia may be necessary in acute emergencies, such as abruptio placentae, and in patients who do not meet the criteria for neuraxial anesthesia.

Obstetric Hemorrhage

Worldwide, hemorrhage remains the leading cause of maternal
10 mortality, causing 25% of peripartum death. The vast majority of these deaths occur in the developing world; however, there is evidence that the rate and severity of hemorrhage are increasing in developed nations, including the United States.[116–118]

Antepartum hemorrhage occurs in association with placenta previa (abnormal implantation on the lower uterine segment and partial-to-total occlusion of the internal cervical os) and abruptio placentae. Placenta previa complicates approximately 0.4% of pregnancies, resulting in up to 0.9% incidence of maternal mortality and a 17% to 26% incidence of perinatal mortality. Risk factors for placenta previa include previous cesarean delivery, uterine surgery, or pregnancy termination. Other risk factors include smoking, AMA, multiparity, multiple gestation, and cocaine abuse. The risk for placenta previa increases in a "dose-dependent" manner with the number of previous cesarean deliveries and greater parity. The relative risk is 4.5 (95% confidence interval, 3.6 to 5.5) with one previous cesarean delivery, and it increases to 44.9 (95% confidence interval, 13.5 to 139.5) with four prior cesarean deliveries,[119,120] which should be suspected whenever a patient presents with painless, bright red vaginal bleeding, usually after the seventh month of pregnancy. Placenta previa may also be associated with an unstable or abnormal lie. The diagnosis is confirmed by ultrasonography. If bleeding is not profuse and the fetus is immature, obstetric management is conservative to prolong pregnancy. Admission to a high-risk unit is advisable if contractions or acute bleeding are present. Intravenous access and typed and cross-matched blood should be available at all times. In severe cases, or if the fetus is mature at the onset of symptoms, prompt delivery is indicated, usually by cesarean.

Anesthesia for delivery of patients with placenta previa may be with neuraxial anesthesia, provided the mother is hemodynamically stable. Past recommendations for general anesthesia to provide "more control" are not supported by the literature, as there is no difference in complications between the two techniques, except that general anesthesia is associated with greater blood loss and greater need for transfusion. An emergency hysterectomy may be required if there is severe hemorrhage, even after delivery of the placenta, because of uterine atony. The risk of severe hemorrhage after attempted removal of the placenta is greatly increased in patients who have undergone prior uterine surgery, including cesarean delivery. This is related to a higher incidence of placenta accreta, which results from the penetration of myometrium by placental villi. The risk of placenta accreta in women with previa increases from 3% in primary cesarean section to 61% in quaternary section.[121] Indeed, placenta accreta is becoming the leading cause of cesarean hysterectomy, and the rate of cesarean hysterectomy due to abnormal placentation has increased from 33/100,000 deliveries in 1994 to 1995 to 41/100,000 deliveries in 2006 to 2007.[122] The average blood loss during delivery of patients with placenta accreta is 3 to 5 L.

When placenta accreta is suspected or known, delivery is usually scheduled at 36 to 37 weeks' gestation. Under controlled, elective conditions, complications can be minimized. Some institutions may use occlusive balloon catheters placed in the internal iliac arteries prior to surgical delivery. In the face of bleeding with either placenta previa or accreta, when maintenance of fertility is desired, embolization, uterine compression sutures, and/or methotrexate therapy may be attempted to avoid hysterectomy.[123]

Abruptio placentae complicates approximately 1% of deliveries, usually in the final 10 weeks of gestation. Risk factors include smoking, trauma, cocaine abuse, multiple gestation, hypertension, preeclampsia, AMA, and preterm premature rupture of membranes. Complications include Couvelaire uterus (when extravasated blood dissects between the myometrial fibers), renal failure, disseminated intravascular coagulation, and anterior pituitary necrosis (Sheehan syndrome). The maternal mortality rate is high (1.8% to 11.0%), and the perinatal mortality rate is even higher, in excess of 50%. The diagnosis of abruptio placentae is based on the presence of uterine tenderness and hypertonus as well as vaginal bleeding of dark, clotted blood. Bleeding may be concealed if the placental margins have remained attached to the uterine wall. If the blood loss is severe (>2 L), there may be changes in the maternal blood pressure and pulse rate, indicative of hypovolemia. Fetal movement may increase during acute hypoxia or decrease if hypoxia is gradual. Fetal bradycardia and death may ensue. When placental separation is >50%, stillbirth is the likeliest outcome. Management of abruption depends on presentation, gestational age, and the degree of compromise. Management of milder cases of abruption includes artificial rupture of amniotic membranes and oxytocin augmentation of labor, if required. Distant from term, expectant management with close observation is reasonable. In the presence of nonreassuring fetal status, an emergency cesarean delivery may be performed. If fetal death has occurred, usually with severe abruption, vaginal delivery is reasonable if the mother is stable.

Postpartum hemorrhage is usually defined as blood loss >500 mL after vaginal delivery or >1,000 mL after cesarean section. The incidence of postpartum hemorrhage is increasing in the United States, mainly due to an increase in uterine atony.[116,117] Predisposing factors to atony include multiple gestations, labor induction or augmentation, cesarean delivery, polyhydramnios, chorioamnionitis, hypertensive disorders of pregnancy, retained products of conception, and antepartum hemorrhage. Treatment of postpartum hemorrhage may require

TABLE 40-2. UTEROTONIC THERAPY

Drug	Dose	Side Effects
Oxytocin	20–40 U in 1,000 mL LR by continuous IV infusion	Hypotension, tachycardia
Ergot alkaloids (Methergine)	0.2 mg IM q2–4h prn	Hypertension, vasoconstriction Coronary vasospasm Bronchospasm
Carboprost	0.25 mg IM q15–60min prn	↑ cardiac output ↑ pulmonary vascular resistance Bronchospasm Nausea
Misoprostol	800–1,000 μg PR/PV/PO q2h	Fever Nausea
Dinoprostone	20 mg PO q2h	Hypotension Nausea

LR, Lactated Ringer solution; IV, intravenous; IM, intramuscularly; prn, as needed; PR, rectally; PV, vaginally; PO, orally.

aggressive uterotonic therapy for atony or evacuation of the uterus for retained products of conception (Table 40-2). If there is a need for dilation and curettage, the anesthesiologist may be asked to provide uterine relaxation. This can be accomplished with volatile agents if the patient is under general anesthesia or with intravenous nitroglycerin if regional anesthesia or general anesthesia is used.

The anesthesiologist's role in management of obstetric hemorrhage includes both maternal resuscitation and provision of anesthesia for cesarean delivery, cesarean hysterectomy, or dilation and curettage. The choice of anesthetic technique depends on the anticipated duration of surgery, maternal condition and volume status, the potential for coagulopathy, and urgency of the procedure. General anesthesia is indicated in the presence of uncontrolled hemorrhage and/or severe coagulation abnormalities. Neuraxial anesthesia, usually continuous epidural anesthesia, has been successfully used for hysterectomy in planned, controlled situations. A saddle block is an option for anesthesia when dilation and curettage for treatment of postpartum hemorrhage is indicated and the patient is hemodynamically stable.

Maternal resuscitation in the setting of hemorrhage may require rapid securing of the airway if significant hemodynamic instability occurs, in addition to obtaining large bore intravenous, arterial, and possibly central venous access. All of these tasks may be challenging in the parturient and consideration should be given to performing them in advance of hemorrhage when hemorrhage is anticipated. Prompt transfusion of blood component therapy is crucial for replacement of blood loss, maintenance of tissue oxygenation, and correction of coagulopathy. Recently, transfusion rates for postpartum hemorrhage have increased 92% in the United States.[117,118]

Recently, there have been significant changes in transfusion practices for massive hemorrhage. The practice of transfusing packed red blood cells and fresh frozen plasma in a 1:1 ratio decreases mortality from hemorrhage in trauma patients. Early administration of platelets and cryoprecipitate has also become common in *hemostatic resuscitation protocols* for major traumatic hemorrhage, and crystalloid and colloid administration is minimized in favor of blood products (see Chapter 52). Hypothermia, metabolic acidosis, and coagulopathy commonly occur in traumatic and obstetric hemorrhage. Because of these commonalities, it has become common to extend these successful transfusion practices from the trauma literature to obstetric practice. Transfusion of cryoprecipitate should be incorporated early in obstetric hemorrhage because decreased fibrinogen levels strongly correlate with increased severity of postpartum hemorrhage.[124]

Other options are available to decrease transfusion requirements and reduce blood loss. Intraoperative cell salvage, formerly shunned because of concerns about the risk of amniotic fluid contamination of red cells, has been implemented safely during cesarean section in many centers.[125] There is also increasing interest in the use of prohemostatic agents for the treatment of obstetric hemorrhage. Many case reports and series describe the safe and effective use of activated recombinant factor VII for intractable hemorrhage.[126] Also, the antifibrinolytic drug tranexamic acid has been shown to decrease bleeding in both elective cesarean section and postpartum hemorrhage; however, further studies are needed to demonstrate its safety.[127,128]

Heart Disease

11 Heart disease during pregnancy occurs in about 1.6% of patients and is a leading nonobstetric cause of maternal morbidity and mortality, with a mortality rate ranging from 0.4% among patients in class I or II of the New York Heart Association's functional classification to 6.8% among those in classes III and IV. Medical and surgical advancements have changed the types of cardiac problems seen in pregnancy. Patients with congenital heart disease are reaching childbearing age, and the number of patients with rheumatic heart disease has declined. Older parturients (AMA) may present with aortic stenosis and insufficiency associated with a bicuspid aortic valve. AMA and obesity may be associated with coronary artery disease and myocardial ischemia. Deaths associated with congenital heart disease have decreased, but there appears to be an increase in deaths described as sudden arrhythmic death syndrome (SADS).[129] Peripartum cardiomyopathy continues to be associated with a high rate of maternal morbidity and mortality.[130,131]

Cardiac decompensation occurs most commonly at the time of maximum hemodynamic stress; in the third trimester of pregnancy, during labor and delivery, and during the immediate postpartum period. The increase in maternal blood volume, which occurs at 20 to 24 weeks' gestation, may also precipitate cardiac decompensation. During labor, cardiac output increases progressively above antepartum levels; with each uterine contraction, approximately 200 mL of blood moves into the central circulation. Consequently, stroke volume, cardiac output, and left ventricular work increase, and each contraction consistently increases cardiac output by 10% to 25% above that of uterine diastole. The greatest change occurs immediately after delivery of the placenta, when cardiac output increases to an average of 80% above prepartum values, and in some patients, it may increase by as much as 150%.

Evaluation of pre-existing heart disease is crucial and a multidisciplinary approach is necessary when managing patients with complicated cardiac disease during pregnancy and parturition. Many symptoms of pregnancy can mimic those of cardiac disease, complicating new diagnoses of cardiac disease during pregnancy. Labored breathing and venous stasis from aortocaval compression may mimic pulmonary and peripheral edema associated with congestive heart failure. Flow murmurs may be difficult to distinguish from those due to organic lesions. Finally, elevation of the diaphragm causes the heart to rotate, signs of which may be mistaken for cardiac hypertrophy. For the anesthesiologist, it is particularly important to understand how the hemodynamic consequences of different anesthetic techniques might adversely affect mothers with specific cardiac lesions. Invasive monitoring during labor and delivery is rarely indicated. Exceptions are patients with pulmonary hypertension, right-to-left shunts, or coarctation of the aorta. Because hemodynamic changes observed during labor and delivery persist into the postpartum period, if used, invasive monitoring should continue for 24 to 48 hours postpartum.

Congenital Heart Disease

Many patients with successful surgical repair of congenital heart defects are asymptomatic with minimal cardiac findings. Patients with uncorrected or partially corrected lesions may have serious cardiac decompensation with pregnancy. This includes patients with corrected tetralogy of Fallot who may have recurrence of a small ventricular septal defect or develop outflow obstruction. Neuraxial labor analgesia is recommended to minimize hemodynamic changes associated with pain. Maintenance of SVR and venous return is necessary to prevent an increase in right-to-left shunt. Phenylephrine should be used to minimize and/or treat reduction in SVR associated with sympathetic blockade.

Patients with corrected ventricular septal defects or atrial septal defects require no special care, nor do those with small asymptomatic atrial septal defects and ventricular septal defects. In symptomatic patients, neuraxial analgesia will minimize the increase in SVR associated with elevated catecholamines due to pain and may slightly decrease SVR, thus minimizing left-to-right shunting through the defect. Large ventricular septal defects or atrial septal defects are associated with pulmonary hypertension. Patients with these lesions require invasive monitoring and an analgesic technique that maintains SVR, heart rate, and pulmonary vascular resistance.

Eisenmenger's syndrome occurs when uncorrected left-to-right shunt results in pulmonary hypertension, which, when severe, reverses flow to a right-to-left shunt. Pregnancy is not well tolerated and mortality can approach 30%, most commonly from embolic phenomena. Management of these patients is challenging. Invasive monitoring of arterial and cardiac filling pressures is indicated as the right ventricle being at greater risk of dysfunction than the left ventricle. Thus, measuring the right atrial pressure is useful in this setting. Implementing labor analgesia that does not lead to deleterious hemodynamic changes is a challenge; opioid-based neuraxial techniques (e.g., CSE, continuous spinal) combined with a dilute local anesthetic may be the best option.

Cesarean delivery is most often accomplished under general anesthesia in women with Eisenmenger's syndrome. It should be recognized that arm-to-brain circulation times are rapid owing to right-to-left intracardiac shunts; drugs given intravenously have a rapid onset of action. In contrast to parenteral drugs, the rate of rise of arterial concentrations of inhaled drugs is slow because of decreased pulmonary blood flow. The myocardial depressant and vasodilating actions of volatile drugs may be hazardous in patients with Eisenmenger's syndrome, and nitrous oxide, which may increase pulmonary vascular resistance, should be avoided. Positive-pressure ventilation (PPV) of the lungs may also decrease pulmonary blood flow. Sympathetic blockade with CSE anesthesia may lead to cardiovascular decompensation. Thus, maintenance of preload using phenylephrine and fluids, guided by CVP

TABLE 40-3. HEMODYNAMIC GOALS WITH VALVULAR LESIONS

Lesion	Goal
Aortic stenosis	Sinus rhythm Maintain HR Avoid ↓ SVR Maintain venous return
Aortic insufficiency	Mild ↑ HR Avoid ↑ SVR
Mitral stenosis	Sinus rhythm ↓ HR Maintain SVR Maintain venous return
Mitral insufficiency	Sinus rhythm Mild ↑ HR Avoid ↑ SVR Avoid ↑ venous return

SVR, systemic vascular resistance; HR, heart rate.

measurements, is essential if regional anesthesia is selected. Hemodynamic monitoring for 48 hours postpartum is essential.

Valvular Heart Disease

The decrease in incidence of rheumatic heart disease in the developed world has resulted in few parturients with valvular heart disease. Aortic stenosis is now likely associated with a bicuspid valve in the patient with AMA. Table 40-3 summarizes the goals of management of patients with valvular heart disease.

Patients with prosthetic heart valves present a different challenge in pregnancy. Bioprostheses avoid the risk of thrombosis and the need for anticoagulation. There is, however, concern that pregnancy hastens the rate of valve deterioration. Mechanical valves require anticoagulation. Warfarin is associated with a lower incidence of thrombosis, than is heparin, but is associated with unacceptable fetal risk. Unfractionated heparin (UFH) and low-molecular-weight heparin (LMWH) do not cross the placenta but it is more difficult to ensure appropriate anticoagulation. The American College of Cardiology recommends any of the following options once pregnancy is confirmed[133]:

- Continue warfarin until 36 weeks, then convert to UFH or LMWH.
- Use UFH or LMWH 6 to 12 weeks, and after 36 weeks with warfarin, use 12 to 36 weeks.
- Use LMWH throughout pregnancy.

Primary Pulmonary Hypertension

Primary pulmonary hypertension (PPH) is seen predominantly in young women. Pulmonary hypertension is defined as mean pulmonary artery pressure over 25 mm Hg at rest or 30 mm Hg with exercise. The cause is unclear but is associated with endothelial dysfunction. Although uncommon in pregnancy, PPH is associated with a very high maternal mortality; pregnancy is discouraged and termination is advised should pregnancy occur.

The mode of delivery of these patients is contentious. Vaginal delivery is associated with smaller hemodynamic shifts and less risk for bleeding. However, emergency cesarean delivery for maternal or fetal deterioration may be needed. Planned cesarean delivery may offer advantage of ensuring optimal conditions and the availability of experienced staff.

Pain during labor and vaginal delivery is especially detrimental because it may further increase pulmonary vascular resistance and decrease venous return. Neuraxial analgesia is useful for preventing pain-induced increases in pulmonary vascular resistance. Dilute local anesthetic solutions with the addition of opioids will minimize the decrease in SVR. General and epidural anesthesia have been used for cesarean delivery. Spinal anesthesia may result in a sudden decrease in SVR and is thus not recommended for cesarean delivery. Risks of general anesthesia include increased pulmonary artery pressures during laryngoscopy and tracheal intubation, the adverse effects of PPV on venous return, and the negative inotropic effects of volatile anesthetics. Nitrous oxide may further increase pulmonary vascular resistance and should not be used. In addition to oxygen, the administration of isoproterenol, inhaled nitric oxide, calcium channel blockers, or sildenafil may be useful for decreasing pulmonary vascular resistance. Hemodynamic monitoring, including systemic and pulmonary arterial pressures, remains controversial in these patients, with no evidence to support the use of pulmonary artery catheters. Pulmonary artery rupture and thrombosis are risks of pulmonary artery catheters in the presence of pulmonary hypertension, but some argue that the benefits in these critically ill patients appear to offset these potential hazards. Maternal mortality is estimated between 30% and 55%, with most deaths due to right heart failure that occurs during labor and the early postpartum period.[132]

Cardiomyopathy of Pregnancy

Cardiomyopathy of pregnancy is left ventricular failure occurring late in pregnancy or in the first 6 weeks postpartum. It occurs in approximately 1 in 3,000 births and is associated with a maternal mortality of 25% to 50%. It is a diagnosis of exclusion, the etiology thought to be related to myocarditis or an abnormal immune response. Risk factors include AMA, multiparity, multiple gestation, obesity, hypertension, and preeclampsia.[131,133] Good long-term prognosis is related to recovery of left ventricular function within 6 months of delivery. A left ventricular ejection fraction of <25% at diagnosis is associated with poor long-term outcome, even with recovery after pregnancy, and these patients should be counseled against future pregnancies. If the cardiomyopathy persists, the mortality may be as high as 50%; many patients with persistent cardiomyopathy become transplant candidates. Medical management includes preload optimization, afterload reduction, and therapy to improve myocardial contractility. Patients may require thromboprophylaxis. Intrapartum anesthetic management is directed at minimizing cardiac stress and thus decompensation, and may be aided by invasive hemodynamic monitoring.

Coronary Artery Disease and Myocardial Infarction

Acute myocardial infarction during pregnancy is rare, occurring in 1 in 10,000 to 30,000 women. It is associated with a maternal mortality as high as 37% as well as a high infant mortality rate (9%). As more women with risk factors become pregnant, this complication will increase in frequency. The left anterior descending artery is most commonly affected, with 47% of infarcts associated with coronary spasm (i.e., normal angiogram) and another 16% associated with coronary artery dissection. Risk factors include smoking, obesity, AMA, diabetes, hypertension, and hyperlipidemia. Women older than 35 years are at greatest risk; the risk is 30-fold higher in women older than 40 years, compared to women younger than 20 years. The ergot alkaloids should be avoided because they can lead to coronary vasospasm, as can cocaine use.[134]

Diagnosis may be difficult as symptoms of ischemia may mimic common nonspecific complaints during pregnancy. Thus the greatest obstacle to diagnosis is a low index of suspicion. Cardiac troponin I levels are increased if cardiac muscle injury occurs. However, preeclampsia and gestational hypertension may also increase troponin levels. Therefore, electrocardiography (ECG) is an important diagnostic tool.

Delivery within 2 weeks of the infarct is associated with a high rate of reinfarction and death. Thus, delaying delivery, if possible, should be considered. Vaginal delivery is associated with lower morbidity and mortality than cesarean delivery. Intrapartum monitoring should mimic intraoperative monitoring of the nonobstetric patient with a recent myocardial infarction.

In the event of cardiac arrest in late pregnancy, left lateral displacement of the uterus should be achieved, and if cardiopulmonary resuscitation is unsuccessful, the fetus should be delivered within 5 minutes to improve maternal and infant survival.[135]

Sudden Arrhythmic Death Syndrome

SADS is defined as sudden cardiac death where all other causes are eliminated. Under this diagnosis are those cases where the heart is normal on autopsy and all stimulant drugs ruled out as cause of death. Some are identified as likely due to conduction defects by examination of relatives, the remainder are presumed to be related to arrhythmias.[129] An association between obesity and SADS has been suggested.

Diabetes Mellitus

Diabetes occurs in approximately 3% of pregnancies and 8% of gravidae of AMA. The incidence is increasing, in parallel with the increase in population obesity and type 2 diabetes.[136] Gestational diabetes mellitus is diabetes or glucose intolerance that is first diagnosed during pregnancy. Gestational diabetes mellitus is associated with increased adverse outcome, including macrosomia, neonatal hypoglycemia, hyperbilirubinemia, and intrauterine fetal demise, as well as an increased risk of obesity and diabetes in offspring later in life. Women with gestational diabetes mellitus are at increased risk for development of type 2 diabetes later in life.

Pre-existing type 1 or 2 diabetes is also associated with adverse pregnancy outcomes, including congenital malformations. Vasculopathy, nephropathy, and retinopathy may be exacerbated by pregnancy. Tight glycemic control before and during pregnancy may decrease the risk of adverse outcomes. Although a rare occurrence, normal physiologic changes of pregnancy contribute to a propensity for diabetic women, especially type 1 diabetics, to develop diabetic ketoacidosis (DKA).[137] DKA occurs at lower glucose levels in pregnancy due to enhanced lipogenesis and ketogenesis. Beta-adrenergic therapy and steroid administration may also increase the likelihood of developing DKA. Maternal mortality from DKA is unusual, fetal mortality is high.

Guidelines for the management of pregnant diabetics focus on glycemic control. A blood sugar of 60 to 120 mg/dL is desirable and insulin therapy is needed if fasting blood sugar levels are >100 mg/dL.[138] Maternal insulin requirements increase progressively during the second and third trimesters. Fetal surveillance is more intense in diabetic women. Antenatal surveillance with twice weekly nonstress tests often begins at 28 weeks. Delivery at 38 weeks' gestation may be considered if estimated fetal weight exceeds 4,500 g or fetal surveillance indicates the need for delivery.

There is no compelling evidence that one analgesic or anesthetic technique is superior to another when caring for diabetic parturients. Patients with pregestational diabetes should be assessed for comorbidities. Neuraxial labor analgesia does not appear to alter peripartum insulin and glucose requirements. Intrapartum blood glucose levels should be monitored frequently, and glucose administration and insulin therapy should be titrated to maintain maternal glucose concentration between 60 and 120 mg/dL. Insulin requirements decrease shortly after delivery.

Obesity

In the United States, more than 60% of the adult population is overweight or obese, not surprising, obesity in pregnancy mimics this
12 incidence. Obese women are more likely to have antenatal comorbidities, such as chronic hypertension, diabetes mellitus, and preeclampsia.[139] Obstetric outcome may also be affected by maternal obesity; there is a greater risk of fetal congenital cardiac anomalies, macrosomia, and shoulder dystocia. Abnormal labors and failed inductions of labor, are more likely to occur. Overall cesarean delivery rates, and specifically emergency cesarean delivery rates, increase with increasing body mass index. Preanesthetic evaluation of the obese parturient should be performed with anticipation of these complications and a multidisciplinary care plan should be generated. Careful airway evaluation is required and alternative airway equipment must be readily available, especially as the use of general anesthesia for cesarean delivery is higher in the obese parturient than in her nonobese peers. In addition, the extent of comorbidities such as hypertension and diabetes mellitus should be assessed, as these occur more frequently in obese patients.[140] Continuous neuraxial analgesia is the preferred option for pain relief during labor because it provides excellent pain relief without sedation/obtundation, prevents additional demands on the cardiorespiratory system of the obese patient. Most importantly, a well-functioning neuraxial anesthetic for labor may also be used for anesthesia for instrumental vaginal or cesarean delivery, thus avoiding airway manipulation. For cesarean delivery, the choice of anesthetic depends on maternal and fetal conditions. The panniculus must be positioned carefully to prevent cardiorespiratory embarrassment. A continuous neuraxial anesthetic technique should be considered over a "single-shot" technique because there may be unpredictable spread of local anesthetic and because a prolonged surgical duration can be anticipated. Thus, the procedure itself may outlast the effective anesthesia from the latter. Obesity is associated with an increased risk for maternal death related to increased incidence of infection, diabetes, preeclampsia, and thromboembolism. Anesthesia-related maternal mortality is also increased, primarily related to airway difficulties.

Advanced Maternal Age

In 2002, almost 14% of all births in the United States occurred in women aged 35 years or older.[141] In 2003, the percentage of primiparas 35 years and older was 10%.[142] In Canada in 2002, live births to women 30 to 34 years old accounted for 30.6% of all births; to women aged 35 to 39 years old, 14.1%; and to women 40 years and older, 2.6%. Some studies have reported higher maternal morbidity as well as perinatal morbidity and mortality in older gravidae,[143–145] suggesting that pregnancy in older women may be a "medical problem."

Both patients and health-care professionals hold the view that AMA results in poorer outcomes. Medically, this is rationalized by the higher prevalence of chronic medical conditions in older patients compared with younger ones. In one study, almost half of the pregnant women older than 45 years of age had pre-existing medical problems.[144] Cleary-Goldman et al.[145] found that 38% of 36,000 patients older than 35 years of age took medication for pre-existing conditions. In addition, many older pregnant patients have been infertile or subfertile or had a previous poor obstetric outcome. Seven percent had prior preterm delivery and 26% had a previous miscarriage.[146]

Obstetrical management should be focused on the patient's comorbidities. AMA is independently associated with gestational diabetes, preeclampsia, placental abruption, and cesarean delivery. Older gravidae are more likely to have a weight of >70 kg, hypertension, diabetes mellitus, and a bad obstetric history. These medical problems complicate the pregnancy and its management. Pregestational hypertension occurs more frequently in patients over 30 years of age.[147] Patients with chronic hypertension are more likely to develop superimposed preeclampsia (78%), deliver by cesarean (71%), and deliver before 37 weeks' gestation than the normotensive patient. Hypertensive parturients are at greater risk for placental abruption, congestive heart failure, pulmonary edema, and hypertensive encephalopathy. Further, older parturients are more likely to require prolonged hospitalization and are more likely to be admitted to the intensive care unit than younger parturients.

Cesarean delivery is performed more frequently in those with AMA. In some patients, the need for cesarean delivery is related to coexisting problems such as hypertension, preeclampsia, placental abruption, or fetal macrosomia. AMA is also independently associated with an increased likelihood for cesarean delivery. Lin et al.[148] reported that over a 5-year period, "request cesarean delivery" rates rose steadily in all patients but rose disproportionately in patients with AMA. Women over the age of 34 years were twice as likely to request cesarean delivery compared with those aged 25 years or younger. The cesarean delivery rate for mothers 30 to 34 years of age was 37%, and for mothers older than 34 years, it was 48%.[148] The complex sociodemographic explanation for the increased requests for cesarean delivery is yet to be fully ascertained and the long-term medical cost has yet to be defined.[149,150] Cesarean delivery is associated with increased maternal risk compared with uncomplicated vaginal delivery. These include short-term risks of cesarean delivery such as hemorrhage, infection, ileus, and aspiration pneumonitis. In addition, hysterectomy occurs 10 times more frequently following cesarean delivery compared with vaginal delivery. The risk of maternal death is 16 times greater. Long-term morbidity includes adhesions, bowel obstruction, bladder injury, and increased risk for placenta previa or ectopic pregnancy in subsequent pregnancies.[151]

Older women believe that their age makes their infant more vulnerable and, as such, believe a controlled cesarean delivery is safer than vaginal delivery. Other explanations for increased requests for cesarean delivery include concerns about physical stamina, protection of the pelvic floor from damage, refusal to undergo labor pain, and social convenience. Patient beliefs run counter to the many studies that show that cesarean delivery in the absence of clinical indications increases maternal mortality and perinatal morbidity.[149,150]

Perinatal complications are also significant in patients with AMA; multiple gestations,[151] both iatrogenic and naturally occurring, are more common in older gravidae. The incidence of miscarriage, congenital anomalies, preterm delivery, low birth weight, and intrauterine and neonatal death also increase with age.

PRETERM DELIVERY

Preterm labor and delivery (before 37 completed weeks of gestation) present a significant challenge to the anesthesiologist because both mother and infant may be at risk. Although preterm deliveries occur in 8% to 10% of all births, they account for approximately 80% of early neonatal deaths. In general, the mortality and morbidity rates are higher among preterm infants than among small-for-gestational-age infants of comparable weight. Severe problems that may develop in preterm infants are respiratory distress syndrome, intracranial hemorrhage, hypoglycemia, hypocalcemia, and hyperbilirubinemia. With improved neonatal intensive care, preterm infants who weigh >1,500 g often survive without severe long-term impairment. The very low-birth-weight infant (<1,500 g) is still at greater risk for significant long-term impairment.[153]

Obstetricians will try to stop preterm labor to enhance fetal lung maturity. Delaying delivery by even 24 to 48 hours may be beneficial if glucocorticoids are administered to the mother. Various agents have been used to suppress uterine activity (tocolysis), including ethanol, magnesium sulfate, prostaglandin inhibitors, β-sympathomimetics, and calcium channel blockers (Table 40-2).

It is thought that the premature infant is more vulnerable than the term newborn to the effects of drugs used in obstetric analgesia and anesthesia. However, there have been few systematic studies to determine the maternal and fetal pharmacokinetics and dynamics of drugs throughout gestation. There are several postulated causes of enhanced drug sensitivity in the preterm newborn, including:

- Less protein available for drug binding
- Higher levels of bilirubin, which may compete with the drug for protein binding
- Greater drug access to the central nervous system (CNS) because of a poorly developed blood–brain barrier
- Greater total body water and lower fat content
- A decreased ability to metabolize and excrete drugs.

However, these deficiencies of the preterm infant may not be as serious as we have been led to believe. Serum albumin and α_1-acid glycoprotein concentrations are lower in the preterm fetus; however, this would primarily affect drugs that are highly bound to these proteins. Most drugs used in anesthesia exhibit only low-to-moderate degrees of binding in the fetal serum. Approximately 50% for etidocaine and bupivacaine, 25% for lidocaine, 52% for meperidine, and 75% for thiopental.

The placenta efficiently eliminates fetal bilirubin. Thus, the hyperbilirubinemia of prematurity normally occurs in the postpartum period. With the exception of diazepam, bilirubin does not compete with anesthetic drugs because most are bound to other serum proteins (e.g., meperidine and local anesthetics bind to α_1-acid glycoproteins). It seems likely that the human blood–brain barrier develops substantially in early gestation. Thus, factors such as tissue affinity changes may account for differences between immature and mature brain uptake of highly lipid-soluble drugs.

Greater total body water in the preterm fetus results in a greater volume of distribution for drugs (see Chapter 7). Thus, to achieve equal blood concentrations, the immature fetus must receive a greater amount of drug transplacentally than the mature fetus. A study of age-related toxicity of lidocaine in sheep showed that the greater the volume of distribution, the greater the dose required to achieve toxic blood concentrations of the drug.[41] Decreased ability to metabolize or excrete drugs that is associated with prematurity is certainly not a universal phenomenon. In a study comparing the pharmacokinetics of lidocaine in preterm newborns and adults, plasma clearance was similar in both groups.[40] Neonates excreted much more unchanged lidocaine than did adults. Similarly, although meperidine metabolism is more limited in the neonate than in the adult, urinary excretion of the unchanged drug is greater in the neonate.

Gestational changes in maternal serum albumin and α_1-acid glycoprotein concentrations, which tend to decrease, may also play a role in drug availability. Serial determinations of protein binding of diazepam, phenytoin, and valproic acid in maternal serum, performed in early (8 to 16 weeks), middle (17 to 32 weeks), and late pregnancy, showed a progressive increase in the unbound fraction of these drugs.[153] This increases drug availability for placental transfer. Placental permeability itself increases as pregnancy progresses because of the increased area and decreased thickness of tissue barriers.

It therefore appears that in selection of the anesthetic drugs and techniques for delivery of a preterm infant, concerns regarding drug effects on the newborn are far less important than prevention of asphyxia and trauma to the fetus. For labor and vaginal delivery, well-conducted neuraxial anesthesia is advantageous in providing good perineal relaxation. Preterm infants with breech presentation are usually delivered by cesarean as are very low-birth-weight infants (<1,500 g). If neuraxial anesthesia is used, nitroglycerin should be available for uterine relaxation. If vaginal delivery occurs with a breech infant and there is head entrapment, general anesthesia or nitroglycerin may be needed for uterine relaxation.

HUMAN IMMUNODEFICIENCY VIRUS AND ACQUIRED IMMUNODEFICIENCY SYNDROME

Women now represent nearly half of the people worldwide living with human immunodeficiency virus (HIV) (see Chapter 13). Thus it is the rare labor and delivery unit that will not be caring for HIV-positive women. There is no evidence that pregnancy accelerates the progression of the disease. However, there is compelling interest to prevent vertical transmission of HIV from the mother to the fetus. The risk of intrauterine infection is 4.4%. Intrapartum transmission accounts for 60% of the risk of peripartum transmission and the remainder is through breastfeeding. However, when antiretroviral therapy is given to women with HIV perinatally, and to the newborn in the first weeks of life, vertical transmission is reduced by 66%.[154,155]

The choice of anesthetic technique for delivery should be based on maternal condition, obstetric considerations, and patient desires. HIV is a multiorgan disease, often with complex and changing medical management. Patients with high CD4 counts (>500 to 700/mm^3) often are not taking antiretroviral agents and have little or no end-organ damage. Patients with very low CD4 counts (<200/mm^3) are likely to be taking multiple antiretroviral and other medications. This group should have more extensive evaluation, with complete blood count, clotting studies, and liver and renal function tests. A history of cardiac or pulmonary dysfunction warrants obtaining ECG, echocardiogram, pulmonary function tests, and/or arterial blood gases in some patients.[156]

In the early years of the HIV/AIDS epidemic, concern was expressed regarding both general and neuraxial anesthesia, although there was no evidence of harm. Pulmonary disease was a concern for general anesthesia, and there were early concerns of CNS HIV infection with neuraxial anesthesia. We now have extensive experience with neuraxial anesthesia in this patient population, without reports of unique complications.[157] There has been concern that an epidural blood patch, particularly if the viral load is high, may accelerate neurologic symptoms of the disease. In a more recent case series of six patients with HIV infection and PDPH requiring epidural blood patch, there was no evidence of acceleration of HIV symptoms.[158]

SUBSTANCE ABUSE

Nearly 90% of women who abuse tobacco, drugs, or alcohol are of childbearing age. The most commonly abused substances in society as well as in pregnancy are alcohol, tobacco, cocaine, marijuana, opioids, caffeine, amphetamines, and to a lesser extent, hallucinogens and solvents. Substance abuse may significantly impact the intrapartum anesthetic management and may result in obstetric crises that require the intervention or assistance of an obstetric anesthesiologist. Diagnosis of the patient who is not under the effect of a substance at admission may be made when she, or her infant, develops withdrawal symptoms or the newborn is diagnosed with a syndrome related to in utero exposure.

Tobacco Abuse

Smoking is the most commonly abused substance in pregnancy. Smoking during pregnancy has been associated with miscarriages, intrauterine growth retardation, and increased risk of premature rupture of membrane, placental previa, abruptio placentae, preterm delivery, impaired respiratory function in newborns, and sudden infant death syndrome. The pregnant patient is at greater risk for bronchitis, pneumonia, and asthma. Nicotine causes vasoconstriction and thus may decrease placental blood flow and oxygen delivery to the fetus; of interest, smoking appears to be protective for the development of preeclampsia.

Alcohol

In a pregnant female, heavy alcohol consumption may be associated with liver disease, coagulopathy, cardiomyopathy, and esophageal varices, and can alter drug metabolism. In the fetus, alcohol has been linked to fetal alcohol syndrome. The prevalence of fetal alcohol syndrome is approximately one-third of infants of heavy maternal drinkers (>3 oz of absolute alcohol per day). Neurobehavioral deficit and IUGR have been demonstrated in infants of moderate drinkers (102 oz/day). The parturient who abuses alcohol is at further increased risk for aspiration compared with the average pregnant individual. She may have hepatic dysfunction, cardiac failure, or coagulopathy. Acute alcohol withdrawal may present within 6 to 48 hours of abstinence; thus, it may occur intrapartum or postpartum. The signs and symptoms of alcohol withdrawal include nausea and vomiting, hypertension, tachycardia, dysrhythmias, seizures, and cardiac failure. These are easily mistaken for other disease entities.

Opioids

Opioid abuse has multiple implications for both mother and fetus. The intravenous opioid abuser may have septic thrombophlebitis, HIV, endocarditis, or hepatitis. These patients are at an increased risk for developing preeclampsia and third-trimester bleeding. They will develop withdrawal symptoms should an agonist/antagonist be administered for pain relief in labor.

The anesthetic management of a chronic opioid user should include the continuation of opioids throughout labor and into the postpartum period to prevent acute opioid withdrawal. These patients are likely to have increased opioid requirements. Those patients with a history of opioid abuse who are on methadone maintenance should have a stable peripartum course. Neuraxial anesthesia is safe in these patients, but one must continue a maintenance dose of systemic opioid to prevent withdrawal symptoms, despite neuraxial labor analgesia. Neonates will have neonatal abstinence syndrome, which will require close observation and treatment.

Marijuana

Marijuana is frequently abused by women of childbearing age. Delta-9-tetrahydrocannabinol (THC) readily crosses the placenta and may directly affect the fetus. It has been associated with preterm labor and intrauterine growth retardation. The parturient who chronically uses marijuana has an increased incidence of respiratory problems, including bronchitis and emphysema, and thus may be at risk for respiratory complications related to general anesthesia. Acute marijuana use may be associated with cardiovascular stimulation at moderate doses and myocardial depression at higher doses.

Cocaine

Women acutely ingesting cocaine generally display euphoria, tachycardia, and hypertension. More serious manifestations may include seizure and coma, myocardial infarction, pulmonary edema, or subarachnoid hemorrhage. Sudden death may occur from a lethal ventricular dysrhythmia. Cocaine use in the first trimester may cause congenital anomalies. Later in pregnancy, cocaine use may be associated with premature labor, intrauterine growth retardation, and nonreassuring fetal status because of uteroplacental insufficiency or placental abruption. Therapy is supportive, primarily aimed at controlling cardiovascular and CNS consequences of cocaine use. Hypertension related to acute cocaine ingestion may be the primary etiology of cerebral hemorrhage, or cocaine may cause vasospasm and cerebral infarction. Pure β-antagonist drugs should be avoided because of the potential for worsening hypertension related to unopposed α-receptor stimulation by cocaine. The choice of anesthetic depends on maternal and fetal conditions, the planned procedure (vaginal or cesarean delivery), and urgency. General anesthesia may be associated with uncontrolled hypertension/tachycardia and life-threatening dysrhythmias in women using cocaine. Neuraxial anesthesia may also be complicated by cocaine use. Cocaine is a local anesthetic, and systemic toxicity may be additive when using amide local anesthetics for epidural anesthesia. Esters compete with cocaine for metabolism, resulting in decreased metabolism of both drugs. Chronic cocaine use may be associated with thrombocytopenia. The incidence and severity of hypotension related to neuraxial anesthesia may be greater in chronic cocaine-abusing parturients compared with controls, and hypotension may be more difficult to treat. Direct-acting agents are more effective and predictable in chronic cocaine abusers. Fetal exposure to cocaine may alter the developing brain, contributing to an increased susceptibility to addiction.[159]

Amphetamines

Amphetamines are noncatecholamine sympathomimetic drugs. They are often abused in conjunction with other CNS stimulants such as cocaine. They can be taken orally or intravenously (methamphetamine) or smoked, as crystal methamphetamine. Ecstasy is an analog of methamphetamine that has become tremendously popular in young adults. Amphetamine use leads to an increased release of norepinephrine, leading to hypertension, tachycardia, dysrhythmias, dilated pupils, hyperpyrexia, proteinuria, agitation, confusion, and seizures. These signs and symptoms closely resemble those of cocaine abuse. Methamphetamine abuse has been associated with stroke in pregnant women as well as fetal and infant deaths. Amphetamines taken early in pregnancy can result in fetal anomalies. Later in pregnancy, placental abruption may lead to fetal death. The anesthetic management of patients who abuse amphetamines is similar to that of cocaine abusers (Table 40-4).

TABLE 40-4. ANESTHETIC CONSIDERATIONS ASSOCIATED WITH COCAINE AND/OR AMPHETAMINE ABUSE

- Uncontrolled hypertension
- Cardiac dysrhythmias (ventricular tachycardia/fibrillation)
- Myocardial ischemia
- Ephedrine-resistant hypotension with neuraxial blockade (use direct-acting agent)
- Acute intake may increase MAC of volatile agents
- Chronic use may decrease dosage of anesthetic agents
- May have increased sensitivity to arrhythmogenic effects of volatile agents

MAC, minimum alveolar concentration.

FETAL MONITORING

The development of biophysical monitoring of the fetus during labor and delivery has had a tremendous impact on obstetric practice since the early 1970s. Monitoring procedures are now performed routinely, and it is important that the anesthesiologist understand the basic principles of the technology as well as the interpretation of results. With the growing sophistication of electronic devices, and specifically the science of telemetry, we can look forward to better surveillance of both mother and fetus without the loss of maternal freedom and activity that monitoring currently entails.

Electronic Fetal Monitoring

Intrapartum electronic FHR monitoring is the most common obstetric procedure performed.[160] An electronic fetal monitor is a two-channel recorder of FHR and uterine activity. In the internal system, the fetal ECG is obtained from an electrode attached to the presenting part. Intrauterine pressure is measured continuously with a transducer connected to a saline-filled catheter that is inserted transcervically. Internal monitoring is quantitative but requires rupture of the membranes and a cervical dilation of at least 1.5 cm. In addition, the presenting part must be in the true pelvis. External fetal monitoring uses data obtained indirectly from transducers secured to the mother's abdomen with adjustable straps. Ultrasound cardiography is the most commonly used method of obtaining FHR signals. Uterine activity is monitored with a tocodynamometer triggered by the changing shape of the uterus during the contraction. Indirect monitoring is mostly qualitative. Its advantage is that it can be applied without rupture of membranes, even before the onset of labor.

The following variables are considered when fetal well-being is being assessed: Uterine activity, baseline heart rate and variability, presence of accelerations, and periodic decelerations. Cervical dilation and descent of the presenting part during the first stage of labor result primarily from uterine contractions. During the active phase, contractions should occur every 2 to 3 minutes, with peak intrauterine pressures of 50 to 80 mm Hg and resting pressures of 5 to 20 mm Hg. Normally, contractions occur at a rate of five contractions in 10 minutes. When more contractions occur it is termed tachysystole.[159] Tachysystole is sometimes seen after neuraxial labor analgesia and may result from a sudden drop in serum catecholamines, which normally serve to relax the uterus.[162] Poor uterine contractility may result from overdistention (polyhydramnios, multiple gestation) or aortocaval compression. The addition of epinephrine to a local anesthetic solution may have a dose-related inhibitory effect on uterine activity.

The baseline FHR is the mean rate during a 10-minute segment and ranges between 110 and 160 beats per minute in the normal fetus.[160] Persistently elevated rates may be associated with chronic fetal distress, maternal fever, or administration of drugs such as ephedrine and atropine. Abnormally low rates may be encountered in fetuses with congenital heart block or as a late occurrence during the course of fetal hypoxia and acidosis.

Baseline FHR variability refers to fluctuations in baseline FHR that are irregular in amplitude and frequency; baseline variability is quantified as the amplitude of the peak to the trough heart rate and normally ranges between 6 and 25 beats per minute.[159] Baseline variability reflects the beat-to-beat adjustments of the parasympathetic and sympathetic nervous systems to a variety of internal and external stimuli and is mediated by the central nervous system (CNS), the peripheral nervous system, and the cardiac conduction system itself. Presence of normal variability is a reassuring sign of normal fetal acid–base status. Fetal CNS depression by asphyxia may decrease baseline variability. Therefore, a smooth FHR tracing may be an ominous finding. However, drugs that depress the CNS (sedatives, opioids, barbiturates, anesthetics) can also decrease FHR variability. Atropine may decrease variability by blocking the transmission of control impulses to the cardiac pacemaker.

An acceleration of FHR is an abrupt increase over baseline and is a reassuring sign that the fetus is not acidemic. Periodic FHR decelerations occur in association with uterine contractions (Fig. 40-8). There are three patterns observed: Early, late, and variable. Early decelerations are characterized by a symmetrical gradual decrease in FHR. The fetal heart usually begins to slow with the onset of the contraction, nadirs with the peak of the contraction, and returns to the baseline as the uterus relaxes. This type of deceleration has been attributed to fetal head compression, leading to increased vagal tone. It is not ameliorated by increasing fetal oxygenation but is blocked by atropine administration. Early decelerations are transient and well tolerated by the fetus; there is no systemic hypoxemia or acidosis.

Late decelerations are also symmetric and gradual in onset. However, they begin after the onset of uterine contraction and the low point of the deceleration occurs well after its peak. CNS or myocardial ischemia resulting from uteroplacental insufficiency and fetal hypoxemia may cause late decelerations.

Variable decelerations are the most common periodic patterns observed in the intrapartum period. They are variable in shape and

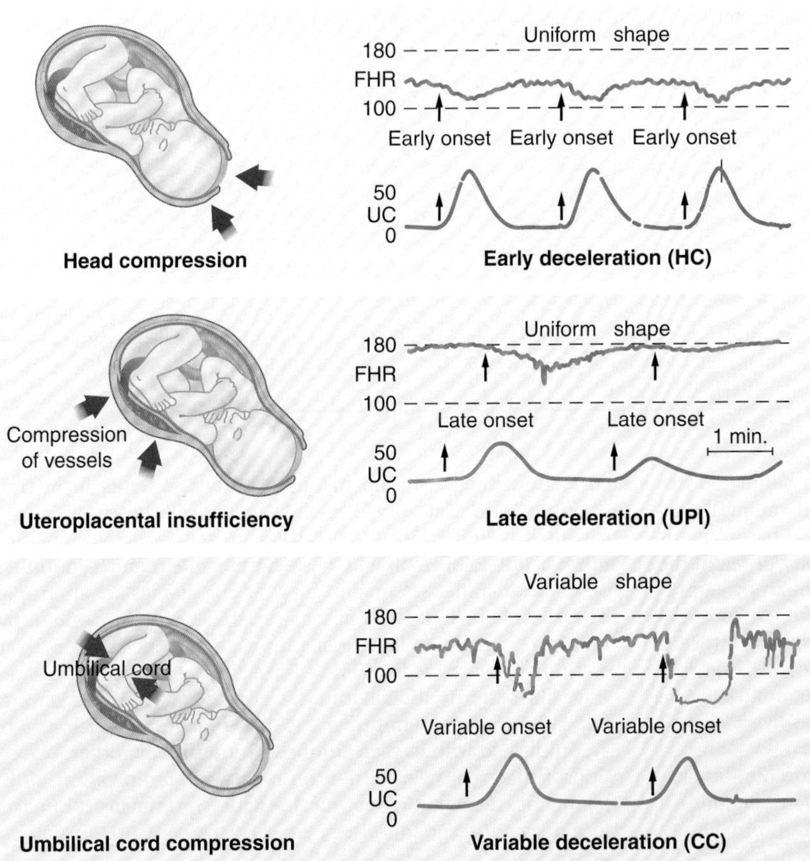

FIGURE 40-8. Classification and mechanism of fetal heart rate patterns. HC, head compression; UPI, uteroplacental insufficiency; CC, cord compression. (Reprinted from Hon EH. An introduction to fetal heart rate monitoring. New Haven, CT, Harty Press, 1969, p 29, with permission.)

Three-Tier Fetal Heart Rate Interpretation System

Category I

Category I fetal heart rate (FHR) tracings include all of the following:

- Baseline rate: 110–160 beats per minute (bpm)
- Baseline FHR variability: moderate
- Late or variable decelerations: absent
- Early decelerations: present or absent
- Accelerations: present or absent

Category II

Category II FHR tracings include all FHR tracings not categorized as Category I or Category III. Category II tracings may represent an appreciable fraction of those encountered in clinical care. Examples of Category II FHR tracings include any of the following:

Baseline rate

- Bradycardia not accompanied by absent baseline variability
- Tachycardia

Baseline FHR variability

- Minimal baseline variability
- Absent baseline variability not accompanied by recurrent decelerations
- Marked baseline variability

Accelerations

- Absence of induced accelerations after fetal stimulation

Periodic or episodic decelerations

- Recurrent variable decelerations accompanied by minimal or moderate baseline variability
- Prolonged deceleration ≥2 minutes but <10 minutes
- Recurrent late decelerations with moderate baseline variability
- Variable decelerations with other characteristics, such as slow return to baseline, "overshoots," or "shoulders"

Category III

Category III FHR tracings include either:

- Absent baseline FHR variability and any of the following:
  - Recurrent late decelerations
  - Recurrent variable decelerations
  - Bradycardia
- Sinusoidal pattern

FIGURE 40-9. Three tiered fetal heart rate interpretation system. (Reprinted from: The 2008 National Institute of Child Health and Human Development Workshop on Electronic Fetal Monitoring: Updates on Definitions, Interpretations, and Research Guidelines. *Obstet Gynec.*2008;112:661, with permission.)

abrupt in onset, with the heart rate nadir occurring within <30 seconds of the onset. Variable decelerations result from umbilical cord compression that results in activation of the carotid baroreceptor reflex. Although the initial FHR changes are of reflex origin, if the cord compressions are frequent or prolonged, fetal asphyxia may result in fetal hypoxemia and CNS insult or direct myocardial depression. If late or variable decelerations are recurrent (occur with at least one-half of contractions) or prolonged (≥15 beats per minute below baseline lasting ≥2 minutes but <10 minutes), there is a significant correlation with fetal acidosis and delivery may be undertaken.

The American College of Obstetricians and Gynecologists currently recommends a three-tiered system for the evaluation of FHR tracings.[160] Category I tracings are those with normal baseline and variability, and no late or variable decelerations. They correlate strongly with normal fetus acid–base status at the time of observation. Category II tracings include all those that are not classified as either Category I or III. They are predictive of neither normal nor abnormal acid–base status, and require continued observation and assessment. Category III tracings are abnormal. They are characterized by absent variability with any one of the following: Recurrent late decelerations, recurrent variable decelerations, or bradycardia (FHR < 100). Sinusoidal patterns (a sine-wave like pattern) also fall into Category III. Category III tracings may be corrected by improving fetal oxygenation, which may be accomplished with oxygen administration to the mother, correction of maternal hypotension or aortocaval compression, or by taking measures that reduce uterine activity. If the heart rate pattern does not respond to these conservative measures, imminent delivery may be required (Fig. 40-9).

Currently, experts agree regarding the reassuring value of a normal Category I FHR tracing. There is also consensus regarding the potentially ominous nature of Category III tracings. However, FHR patterns between these extremes present a clinical dilemma to the clinician. The high false-positive rate of FHR monitoring may lead to unnecessary cesarean deliveries.[161] A recent American College of Obstetrics and Gynecology Practice Bulletin opines not only the high false-positive rate of nonreassuring FHR tracings for predicting adverse neonatal outcomes but also the excessive inter- and intraobserver variabilities in interpretation. It also notes that the practice is associated with an increase in both instrumental vaginal and cesarean deliveries, without decreasing the incidence of cerebral palsy. The bulletin recommends continuous FHR analysis for high-risk conditions, although it allows for intermittent auscultation in an uncomplicated patient.[160]

Ancillary Tests and Fetal Pulse Oximetry

Fetal scalp pH testing has been used in the past to determine the presence of acidemia in fetuses with indeterminate FHR tracings; however, its use is decreasing, and less invasive ancillary tests such as vibroacoustic stimulation and digital scalp stimulation are more commonly employed. The elicitation of accelerations with such stimuli indicates acidemia is unlikely.

Fetal pulse oximetry is a technique in which a sensor is placed through the cervix, in contact with fetal skin that evaluates intrapartum fetal oxygenation. Fetal O_2 saturation between 30% and 70% is considered normal, and saturation readings consistently <30% for a prolonged period of time may be associated with fetal acidemia. The technique was initially touted as an adjunct to FHR monitoring in the hope that it could reduce the incidence of unnecessary cesarean delivery associated with that methodology. Unfortunately, two large studies failed to demonstrate a reduction in the incidence of cesarean delivery with the use of fetal pulse oximetry. Moreover, neonatal outcomes did not differ between subjects managed with versus without fetal pulse oximetry.[162,163] The American College of Obstetrics and Gynecology does not currently endorse the routine use of fetal pulse oximetry.[160]

NEWBORN RESUSCITATION IN THE DELIVERY ROOM

Of the approximately 3.5 million infants newly born in the United States each year, 10% require resuscitation in the delivery room.[164] The following factors may contribute to depression of the newborn: Medications used during labor and delivery, including anesthetic agents, birth trauma, and birth asphyxia (i.e., hypoxia and hypercapnia with metabolic acidosis).

Fetal Asphyxia

Fetal asphyxia, the best-studied cause of neonatal depression, usually develops as a result of interference with maternal or fetal perfusion of the placenta. As stated previously, the normal fetus is neither hypoxic nor acidotic before labor. Experimental data have revealed that transplacental gradients for pH and PCO_2 are approximately 0.05 pH units and 5 mm Hg, respectively. Although oxygen tension is low, oxygen saturation is relatively high (80% to 85%) by virtue of the leftward shift of the fetal oxyhemoglobin dissociation curve.

During labor, uterine contractions decrease or even eliminate the blood flow through the intervillous space of the placenta. On the fetal side, cord compression occurs during the final stages of approximately one-third of vaginal deliveries. Thus, mild degrees of hypoxia and acidosis occur even during normal labor and delivery, and play an important role in initiation of ventilation immediately after birth. On average, healthy, vigorous infants have an oxygen saturation of 21%, a pH of 7.24, and a PCO_2 of 56 mm Hg at birth.

Severe fetal asphyxia occasionally develops as a result of maternal or fetal complications, such as uterine hyperactivity, premature separation of the placenta, maternal hypotension, a tight nuchal cord, or a prolapsed cord. During asphyxia, changes in acid–base status are rapid. The decrease in pH results from accumulation of carbon dioxide (respiratory acidosis) and end products of anaerobic metabolism (metabolic acidosis). After oxygen stores are exhausted, the ability of fetal brain and myocardium to derive energy from anaerobic metabolism is essential for survival. However, anaerobic glycolysis is pH dependent, and its rate is greatly diminished when the pH decreases below 7. Other untoward effects of severe hypoxia and acidosis include depression of the myocardium, resulting from a decrease in its responsiveness to catecholamines; a shift to the right of the fetal oxyhemoglobin dissociation curve, resulting in reduced oxygen delivery; and an increase in pulmonary vascular resistance, which plays an important role during circulatory readjustment at birth.

Neonatal Adaptations at Birth

During birth and through the early hours and days of life, many morphologic and functional changes take place, with the cardiovascular and ventilatory systems undergoing the most dramatic alterations.[165] In the normal newborn, two events occur almost simultaneously and within seconds of delivery: The end of umbilical circulation through the placenta and expansion of the lungs. These events change the fetal circulation toward the adult type.

Survival of the neonate depends primarily on prompt establishment of effective ventilation and expansion of the lungs, which dilates the pulmonary vascular bed, resulting in decreased resistance and a significant increase in pulmonary blood flow. Pulmonary vascular resistance further decreases as oxygen tension increases and carbon dioxide levels decrease. As soon as pulmonary resistance decreases, the foramen ovale, which is a communication between the right and the left atrium, undergoes functional closure because of relative pressure changes across the valve of the foramen (Fig. 40-4). Cessation of the umbilical circulation reduces pressure in the inferior vena cava and right atrium, whereas the increase in pulmonary blood flow increases venous return and pressure in the left atrium. The ductus arteriosus does not constrict abruptly or completely after birth; functional closure may take hours, even days. Thus, shunting may still occur in the neonatal period, its direction depending on relative resistances in the pulmonary and systemic vascular beds. The smooth muscle of the ductus arteriosus constricts in response to increased oxygen tension in the newborn's blood. Catecholamines, which exist in increased concentrations in the newborn, particularly during the first 3 hours of life, also constrict the ductus arteriosus. In contrast, prostaglandins I_2 and E_2, produced by the wall of the ductus arteriosus, relax the ductal smooth muscle. Administration of prostaglandin synthesis inhibitors to fetal animals promotes closure of the ductus arteriosus.

Cardiac output and its distribution also increase; left ventricular output increases approximately 150 to 400 mL/kg/min. Cardiac output changes closely parallel the increase in oxygen consumption. The redistribution of cardiac output also leads to increases in myocardial, renal, and gastrointestinal blood flow, and decreases in cerebral, adrenal, and carotid flow.

During fetal life, respiratory gas exchange takes place through the placenta. Delivery of the infant's trunk relieves the thoracic compression that occurs as the infant passes through the birth canal, and the thorax and the lungs expand. Most infants initiate respiratory efforts a few seconds after birth. Negative pressures in excess of 40 cm H_2O bring about the initial entry of air into fluid-filled alveoli. In the mature, normal neonate, the lungs expand almost completely after the first few breaths, and the pressure–volume changes achieved with each respiration resemble those of the adult. After lung expansion, the FRC approximates 70 mL in the term newborn and changes little over the first 6 days of life. The tidal volume varies between 10 and 30 mL, the breathing frequency ranges from 30 to 60 breaths per minute, and minute ventilation exceeds 500 mL. After delivery and prompt lung expansion, reoxygenation is rapid, but it takes 2 to 3 hours to achieve a relatively normal acid–base balance, primarily by pulmonary excretion of carbon dioxide. By 24 hours, the healthy neonate has reached the same acid–base state as that of the mother before labor.

Resuscitation

The delivery room must be prepared for adequate and prompt treatment of severe neonatal depression at birth. Members of the delivery room team should be trained in resuscitation methods because both mother and infant may encounter difficulty simultaneously. One person should be designated specifically to care for the newborn during every delivery. When continued resuscitation is anticipated, a team of skilled personnel should be present. Every piece of apparatus necessary for emergency resuscitation should be checked carefully before delivery (Table 40-5). An overview of resuscitation in the delivery room is provided in Figure 40-10.

Evaluation and Treatment

The American Heart Association has released guidelines to advise the practitioner providing neonatal resuscitation.[164] Immediately after delivery, the infant should be held head-down while the cord is clamped and cut. The initial appraisal of the newborn should start from the moment of birth, with particular attention paid to determining the answer to three questions:

- Is the newborn the result of a term gestation?
- Is the newborn crying or breathing vigorously?
- Does the newborn have good muscle tone?

If the answer to all three questions is "yes," then the baby does not require further resuscitation and should be placed skin to skin with its mother if practical. If the answer to any of the above questions is "no," then further resuscitation should be provided, with the following steps taken in the order listed.

Initial Stabilization

One should place the infant supine under a radiant heat source, with the head kept low in the sniffing position, clear the airway with a bulb suction or soft catheter if necessary, dry the skin, and stimulate breathing by slapping the infant's soles lightly or rubbing its back.

Assessment of Respirations and Heart Rate

Presence of respiration versus apnea is assessed, and respiratory efforts are judged as unlabored versus gasping or labored.

An assistant should listen to the heartbeat immediately, indicating the rate by finger movement, or the rate can be detected from pulsation of the umbilical cord. Normally, the newborn's heart rate is >100 beats per minute.

Ventilation

If the newborn is apneic or gasping, or if the heart rate is <100 beats per minute after initial stabilization, then positive pressure ventilation (PPV) should begin. PPV via bag and mask should be instituted at a rate of 40 to 60 breaths per minute. The initial breath may require pressures of 30 to 40 cm H_2O. Subsequent inflation pressures should be reduced to 15 to 20 cm H_2O in an infant with normal lungs. A small plastic oropharyngeal airway may help maintain patency of the upper airway. Endotracheal intubation may be required if bag–mask ventilation is ineffective or prolonged. The administration of oxygen is controversial because studies demonstrate that both hypoxemia and excessive oxygen administration may be harmful to babies, and two recent meta-analyses suggest that room air resuscitation is associated with lower mortality than that with 100% oxygen.[165–167] Therefore, it is recommended that preductal pulse oximetry guides oxygen therapy with attention to target saturations listed in the box in Figure 40-10, and that oxygen therapy be titrated to positive heart rate response.

Chest Compressions

After adequate ventilation with oxygen for 30 seconds, if the heart rate is <60 beats per minute, then chest compressions should be initiated. It is recommended that the operator encircle the chest with both hands, supporting the back with his hands and compressing the chest with his thumbs; alternatively, one may compress with two fingers. Compressions should take place on the lower third of the sternum, to a depth that is one-third of the anterior–posterior diameter of the chest. Care must be taken not to interfere with ventilation. Recommendations call for a 3:1 compression to ventilation ratio, with 90 compressions and 30 breaths delivered per minute.

Cardiac massage and ventilation should be maintained until the heart rate exceeds 60 beats per minute.

TABLE 40-5. RESUSCITATION EQUIPMENT IN THE DELIVERY ROOM

Radiant warmer
Suction with manometer and suction trap
Suction catheters
Wall oxygen with flow meter
Resuscitation bag (≤750 mL)
Infant face masks
Infant oropharyngeal airways
Endotracheal tubes—2.5, 3, 3.5, and 4 mm
Endotracheal tube stylets
Laryngoscope(s) and blade(s)
Sterile umbilical artery catheterization tray
Needles, syringes, three-way stopcocks
Medications and solutions
1:10,000 Epinephrine
Volume expanders

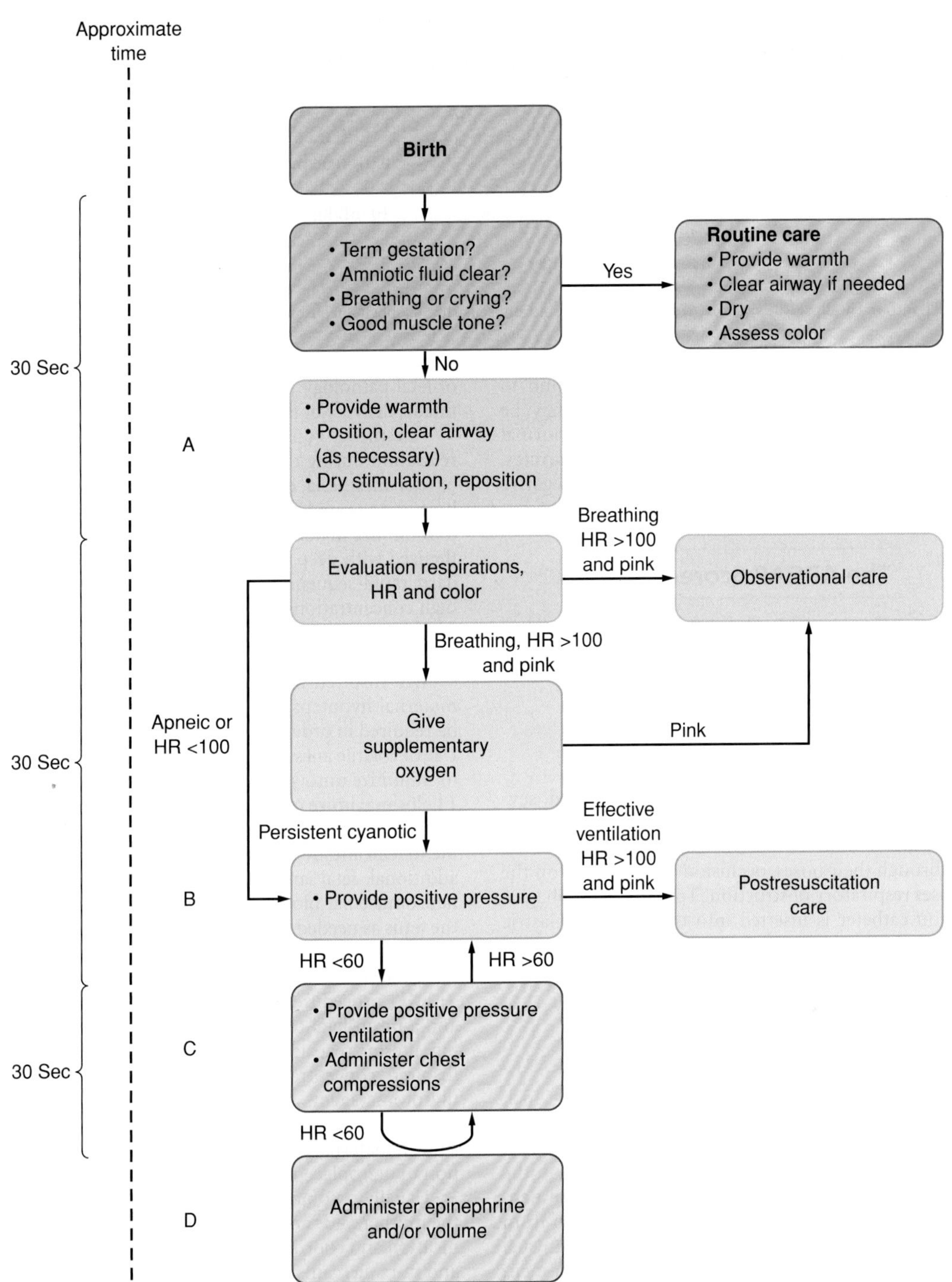

FIGURE 40-10. Algorithm for neonatal resuscitation. HR, heart rate. (Reprinted from: Kattwinkel J, Perlman JM, Aziz K, et al. Special Report—Neonatal Resuscitation; 2010. American Heart Association guidelines for cardiopulmonary resuscitation and emergency cardiovascular care. *Circulation.* 2010;122:S9, with permission.)

Medications and Volume Expansion

Persistent neonatal bradycardia is most often a result of hypoxemia, and usually responds to ventilatory efforts. If the heart rate continues at <60 beats per minute, despite adequate ventilation with 100% oxygen, then the newborn may need epinephrine, volume expansion, or both. It is recommended that epinephrine be administered intravenously as soon as access is established, at a dose of 0.01 to 0.03 mg/kg. In the absence of intravenous access, one may consider endotracheal administration of 0.05 to 0.1 mg/kg.

The use of naloxone or other medications in the delivery room is no longer recommended.

Hypovolemia frequently follows severe birth asphyxia because a greater-than-normal portion of fetal blood remains in the placenta. The infant may appear pale and have low arterial pressure,

TABLE 40-6. THERAPEUTIC GUIDELINES FOR NEONATAL RESUSCITATION

Drug or Volume Expander	Concentration	Dosage	Route/Rate
Epinephrine	1:10,000	0.01–0.03 mg/kg	IV or IT Give rapidly
Volume expanders	PRBCs Normal saline Lactated Ringer	10 mL/kg	Give over 5–10 min

IV, intravenously; IT, intratracheally; PRBCs, packed red blood cells; IM, intramuscularly; SC, subcutaneously.

tachycardia, and tachypnea. If heart rate does not respond to other measures, then acute blood volume expansion may be accomplished with the intravenous administration of normal saline or lactated Ringer solution, 10 mL/kg over 5 to 10 minutes, or, when blood loss is suspected, a similar volume of O-negative blood. Albumin is not recommended (Table 40-6).

The APGAR Score

The scoring system introduced by Apgar is a useful method of clinically evaluating the infant, particularly at 1 and 5 minutes after delivery (Table 40-7).

Diagnostic Procedures

After the neonate is successfully resuscitated and stabilized, several diagnostic procedures may be indicated. To rule out choanal atresia, each nostril should be obstructed. Because newborns must breathe through their noses, occlusion of the nostril on the patent side causes respiratory obstruction. To rule out esophageal atresia, a suction catheter is inserted into the stomach. Gastric contents are aspirated; volume in excess of 12 mL after vaginal delivery and 20 mL after cesarean delivery may result from an abnormality of the upper gastrointestinal tract.

EXIT Procedure

The EXIT (ex utero intrapartum treatment) procedure, which maintains uteroplacental support for a period of time after partial delivery of the fetus, is employed for certain fetal conditions that pose an immediate threat to neonatal life on separation from the placental circulation. The most common indications are treatment of large fetal neck masses and reversal of tracheal occlusion from clips placed for congenital diaphragmatic hernia.[168,169] The usual procedure involves partial delivery of the fetus, surgical treatment of fetal pathology (e.g., attainment of a patent fetal airway), and, finally, delivery of the fetus and clamping of the umbilical cord.

Anesthetic considerations include maintenance of uterine relaxation during the phase of fetal manipulation, administration of fetal anesthesia, ensuring adequate fetal oxygenation, fetal monitoring, and rapid reversal of uterine relaxation after cord clamping to minimize maternal blood loss.[170] Most often the mother is anesthetized with deep inhalation general anesthesia following a standard rapid-sequence induction. Maintenance of anesthesia with high concentrations of volatile anesthetic agents provides for uterine relaxation during the procedure, although a report highlighted the use of intravenous nitroglycerin for this purpose.[170] The use of high inspired inhalational anesthesia may be associated with maternal hypotension. Therefore, intravenous vasopressors may be required in order to ensure adequate uteroplacental blood flow. Use of volatile anesthetic concentrations <2 MAC is recommended to minimize untoward effects on uterine blood flow.[171] An F_{IO_2} of 1 helps maximize oxygen delivery to the placental unit.

Inhalational anesthetics rapidly cross the placenta and contribute to fetal anesthesia; intravenous opioids may be used to provide additional fetal anesthesia.[171] Intramuscular anesthetic agents, neuromuscular blocking agents, and atropine are administered to the fetus as needed after partial delivery. During the period of fetal manipulation, FHR and oxygenation can be monitored by sterile ultrasound and pulse oximetry sensors. A retrospective review of 31 EXIT procedures reported a mean FHR of 153 beats per minute and a mean fetal oxygen saturation of 71%.[168] After cord clamping, uterine relaxation must be reversed rapidly by decreasing the inspired concentration of inhalation agent and administering uterotonic agents such as oxytocin, so as to minimize maternal blood loss. The retrospective study previously referenced reported a mean maternal estimated blood loss of 848 mL and a mean duration of uteroplacental support of 30 minutes.[168]

Usually, two anesthetic teams are employed: One to tend to the mother and the other to care for the fetus/newborn. Communication and coordination between surgical, pediatric, anesthesia, and nursing teams is mandatory for successful outcomes.

TABLE 40-7. APGAR SCORES

Sign	0	1	2
Heart rate	Absent	<100 beats/min	>100 beats/min
Respiratory effort	Absent	Slow, irregular	Good, crying
Muscle tone	Limp	Some flexion of extremities	Active motion
Reflex irritability	No response	Grimace	Cough, sneeze, or cry
Color	Pale, blue	Body pink, extremities blue	Completely pink

ANESTHESIA FOR NONOBSTETRIC SURGERY IN THE PREGNANT WOMAN

In the United States, 1% to 2% undergo surgical procedures unrelated to pregnancy (approximately 80,000 anesthetics a year). The most frequent nonobstetric procedures are excision of ovarian cysts, appendectomy, breast biopsy, and surgery related to trauma. Treatment of an incompetent cervix (cervical cerclage) typically occurs early pregnancy or mid-pregnancy. Serious conditions such as intracranial aneurysms, cardiac valvular disease, and pheochromocytoma may rarely present and require surgery during pregnancy.

The objective for managing anesthesia in patients undergoing nonobstetric operative procedures is maternal safety, safe care of the fetus, and prevention of premature labor related to the surgical procedure or drugs administered during anesthesia. To achieve these goals, the effects of the patient's altered physiology must be recognized. Induction and emergence from anesthesia is more rapid than in the nonpregnant state because of increased minute ventilation, decreased FRC, and the decreased MAC of volatile agents, which may be seen as early as 8 to 10 weeks' gestation. Supine hypotensive syndrome can occur as early as the second trimester. Gastric emptying is essentially normal in the first two trimesters, but is prolonged in the third. Gastroesophageal sphincter tone is decreased after 20 weeks, thus caution regarding the unprotected airway is essential.[92] The effects of altered physiology during pregnancy are not limited to general anesthesia. There is an increased effect of local anesthetics during pregnancy; thus, the amount of local anesthetic administered should be reduced by 25% to 30% during any stage of pregnancy.

Teratogenicity may be induced at any stage of gestation. However, most of the critical organogenesis occurs in the first trimester (days 13 to 60). Although many commonly used anesthetics are teratogenic at high doses in animals, few, if any, studies support teratogenic effects of anesthetic or sedative medications in the doses used for human anesthesia care. There is some evidence for a link between maternal high-dose diazepam injection in the first trimester and cleft palate.[172] However, medicinal doses of benzodiazepine are safe when needed to treat perioperative anxiety.

Nitrous oxide has also been suggested to be teratogenic in animals when administered for prolonged periods (1 to 2 days).[173] Its effect on DNA synthesis is of concern for its use in humans. Although teratogenesis has been seen only in animals under extreme conditions, not likely to be reproduced in clinical care, some believe that nitrous oxide use is contraindicated in the first two trimesters.

Of all the information in the literature, two studies, although not new, still deserve mention. A review was taken of the entire population of the province of Manitoba, Canada, between the years 1971 and 1978.[174] State health insurance records were used to identify approximately 2,500 pregnant women who had undergone surgery during this period. Each patient was matched with a woman of similar age, living in the same area, with a pregnancy-related condition but no surgical intervention. As in earlier studies, there was no increase in the incidence of congenital anomalies in the offspring of mothers who had had surgery. However, there was an increased risk of spontaneous abortion in women who had received general anesthesia during the first or second trimesters, which was most evident after gynecologic operations. Few of the surgical group had had procedures to treat cervical incompetence, suggesting that factors other than the obstetric condition itself might be important. The results also might have been influenced by the fact that a small number of gynecologic procedures were performed with anesthesia other than general, so the effect of the surgical site alone could not be distinguished. The authors emphasized a multiplicity of factors other than the choice of the anesthetic agent (e.g., diagnostic radiologic procedures, antibiotics, analgesics, infection, decreased uterine perfusion, stress) that might have been responsible for the increased risk of abortion.

One of the largest studies regarding reproductive outcome after surgery during pregnancy is a Swedish registry review covering the years 1973 to 1981.[175] During this period, there were a total of 720,000 births, 5,405 of them after anesthesia and surgery during pregnancy. The results of this study are reassuring in that there was no increased incidence of congenital anomalies or stillbirths among infants exposed in utero to maternal surgery and anesthesia. However, in this group, there was an increased frequency of very low and low birth weights, and of deaths within 168 hours after delivery. The reasons for this are unclear and are
13 not related to any specific type of operation. The authors postulated that the maternal illness itself might have been a major contributor to adverse neonatal outcome.

Recent studies showing accelerated neuronal cell death in immature rat brain exposed to anesthetics raise concerns regarding use of general anesthetics.[176] It is premature to suggest that impairment seen in the developing rat brain with general anesthesia can be extrapolated to humans.

Intrauterine fetal asphyxia is avoided by maintaining maternal Pao_2, $Paco_2$, and uterine blood flow. $Paco_2$ can affect uterine blood flow as maternal alkalosis may cause direct vasoconstriction. Alkalosis also shifts the oxyhemoglobin dissociation curve, resulting in the release of less oxygen to the fetus at the placenta. Maternal hypotension leads to a reduction in uterine blood flow and thus fetal hypoxia. Uterine hypertension, as occurs with increased uterine irritability, will also decrease uterine blood flow.

Anesthesia and surgery may also result in preterm labor during the intra- and postoperative periods. Abdominal and pelvic procedures are associated with the greatest incidence of preterm labor. Generally, elective surgery should be delayed until the patient is no longer pregnant and she has returned to her nonpregnant physiologic state (approximately 2 to 6 weeks postpartum). Procedures that can be scheduled with some flexibility but cannot be delayed until postpartum are best scheduled in the midtrimester. This lessens the risk for teratogenicity (first-trimester medication administration) or preterm labor (greater risk in the third trimester) (Fig. 40-11).

14 If emergency surgery is required, there is no data to suggest that any well-conducted anesthetic is preferred over another, provided oxygenation and blood pressure are maintained and hyperventilation is avoided. Despite this statement, regional anesthesia should be considered as it minimizes fetal exposure to medications. Left uterine displacement should be used during the second and third trimesters, and aspiration prophylaxis should be administered to all pregnant patients after approximately 20 weeks of gestation. At a minimum, pre- and postoperative FHR and uterine activity should be assessed.[177]

Practical Suggestions

It is generally agreed that only surgical procedures that cannot be delayed for months, including emergency surgery, should be performed during pregnancy, particularly in the first trimester. The possibility of pregnancy should be considered in all female surgical patients of reproductive age. On the basis of the maternal and

fetal hazards already described, the following approach to anesthesia is suggested (Fig. 40-11):

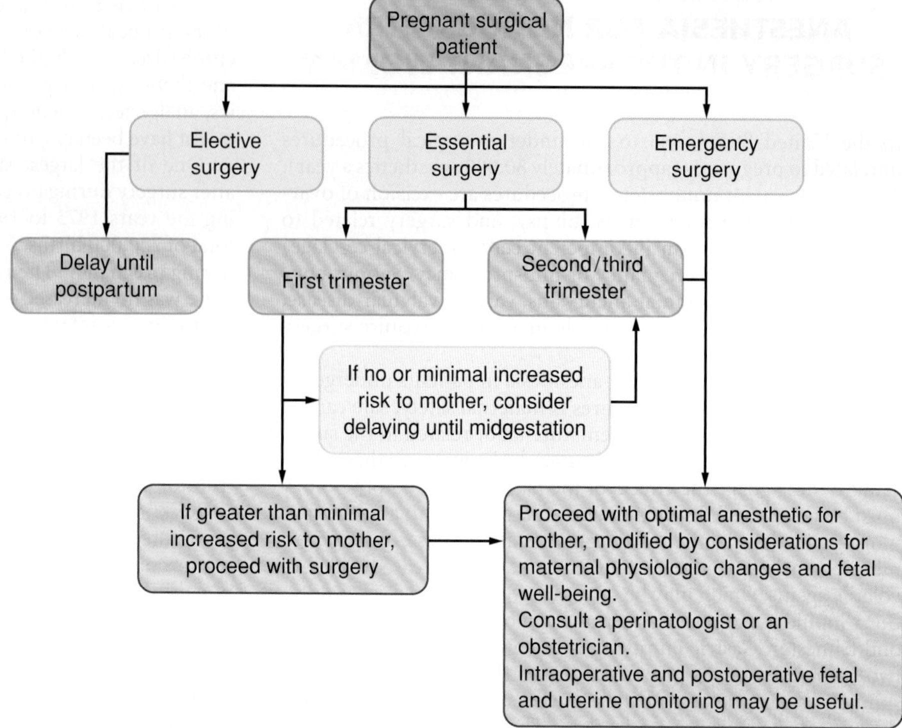

FIGURE 40-11. Recommendations for management of parturients and surgical procedures. (From: Rosen MA. Management of anesthesia for the pregnant surgical patient. *Anesthesiology.* 1999;91:1159. © 1999, Lippincott Williams & Wilkins, with permission.)

1. Anesthesiologists and surgeons should obtain consultation from an obstetrician before performing nonobstetric surgery in pregnancy.
2. The patient's apprehension should be allayed as much as possible by personal reassurance during the preanesthetic visit and by adequate sedation and premedication.
3. Pain should be relieved whenever present.
4. A nonparticulate antacid (15 to 30 mL), should be administered within half an hour before induction of anesthesia. Ranitidine and metoclopramide may be useful.
5. Beginning in the second trimester, uterine displacement must be maintained at all times.
6. Hypotension related to spinal or epidural anesthesia should be prevented as much as possible by rapid intravenous infusion of crystalloid solution during induction of anesthesia. If the mother becomes hypotensive, ephedrine or phenylephrine should be promptly administered intravenously.
7. General anesthesia should be preceded by careful denitrogenation.
8. The risk of aspiration should be minimized by application of cricoid pressure and rapid tracheal intubation with a cuffed tube.
9. To reduce fetal hazard, particularly during the first trimester, it appears preferable to choose drugs with a long history of safety. These drugs include thiopental, morphine, meperidine, muscle relaxants, and low concentrations of nitrous oxide.
10. Avoid maternal hyperventilation and monitor end-expiratory $Paco_2$ or arterial blood gases.
11. FHR may be monitored continuously or intermittently throughout surgery and anesthesia, provided that placement of the transducer does not encroach on the surgical field (this becomes technically feasible from the 16th week of pregnancy). The decision to monitor the fetus should be made in conjunction with the obstetrician based on the severity of maternal disease, the potential for fetal jeopardy, whether the fetus is viable, and whether a physician able to perform a cesarean delivery plans to be immediately available. Uterine tone may also be monitored with an external tocodynamometer if the uterus reaches the umbilicus or above.
12. Monitoring uterine activity should be continued after operation, and tocolytic agents may be required.

References

1. Taylor DJ, Lind T. Red cell mass during and after normal pregnancy. *Br J Obstet Gynaecol.* 1979;86:364.
2. Hill CC, Pickinpaugh J. Physiologic changes in pregnancy. *Surg Clin North Am.* 2008;88:391.
3. Brenner B. Haemostatic changes in pregnancy. *Thromb Res.* 2004;114:409.
4. Cerneca F, Ricci G, Simeone R, et al. Coagulation and fibrinolysis changes in normal pregnancy. Increased levels of procoagulants and reduced levels of inhibitors during pregnancy induce a hypercoagulable state, combined with a reactive fibrinolysis. *Eur J Obstet Gynecol Reprod Biol.* 1997;73:31.
5. Gerbasi FR, Bottoms S, Faraq A, et al. Changes in hemostasis activity during delivery and the immediate postpartum period. *Am J Obstet Gynecol.* 1990;162:1158.
6. Valera M, Varant O, Vayssiere C, et al. Physiologic and pathologic changes of platelets in pregnancy. *Platelets.* 2010;21:58.
7. Wildsmith JA. Serum cholinesterase, pregnancy and suxamethonium. *Anaesthesia.* 1972;27:90.
8. Coryell M, Beach E, Robinson A, et al. Metabolism of women during the reproductive cycle. XVII. Changes in electrophoretic patterns of plasma proteins through the cycle and following delivery. *J Clin Invest.* 1950;29:1559.
9. Gant NF, Daley GL, Chand S, et al. A study of angiotensin II pressor response throughout primigravid pregnancy. *J Clin Invest.* 1973;52:2682.
10. Duvekot JJ, Cheriex EC, Pieters FA, et al. Early pregnancy changes in hemodynamics and volume homeostasis are consecutive adjustments triggered by a primary fall in systemic vascular tone. *Am J Obstet Gynecol.* 1993;169:1382.
11. Kametas NA, McAuliffe F, Krampl E, et al. Maternal cardiac function in twin pregnancy. *Obstet Gynecol.* 2003;102:806.
12. Kerr MG, Scott DB, Samuel E. Studies of the inferior vena cava in late pregnancy. *Br Med J.* 1964;1:532.

13. Paech MJ. Should we take a different angle in managing pregnant women at delivery? Attempting to avoid the 'supine hypotensive syndrome.' *Anaesth Intensive Care.* 2008;36:775.
14. Carruth JE, Mivis SB, Brogan DR, et al. The electrocardiogram in normal pregnancy. *Am Heart J.* 1981;102:1075.
15. Nakagawa M, Katou S, Ichinose M, et al. Characteristics of new-onset ventricular arrhythmias in pregnancy. *J Electrocardiol.* 2004;37:47.
16. Hegewald MJ, Crapo RO. Respiratory physiology in pregnancy. *Clin Chest Med.* 2011;32:1.
17. Pilkington S, Carli F, Dakin MJ, et al. Increase in Mallampati score during pregnancy. *Br J Anaesth.* 1995;74:6.
18. Kodali B, Chandrasekhar S, Bulich LN, et al. Airway changes during labor and delivery. *Anesthesiology.* 2008;108:357–362.
19. Archer GW Jr, Marx GF. Arterial oxygen tension during apnoea in parturient women. *Br J Anaesth.* 1974;46:358.
20. Datta S, Kitzmiller JL, Naulty JS, et al. Acid-base status of diabetic mothers and their infants following spinal anesthesia for cesarean section. *Anesth Analg.* 1982;61:662.
21. McDonnell NJ, Peach MJ, Clavisi OM, et al. Difficult and failed intubation in obstetric anaesthesia: An observational study of airway management and complications associated with general anesthesia for caesarean section. *Int J Obstet Anesth.* 2009;17:292.
22. Wong CA, Loffredi M, Ganchiff JN, et al. Gastric emptying of water in term pregnancy. *Anesthesiology.* 2002;96:1395.
23. Wong CA, McCarthy RJ, Fitzgerald PC, et al. Gastric emptying of water in obese pregnant women at term. *Anesth Analg.* 2007;105:751.
24. Practice guidelines for obstetric anesthesia: An updated report by the American Society of Anesthesiologists Task Force on Obstetric Anesthesia. *Anesthesiology.* 2007;106:843.
25. Brock-Utne JG, Dow TG, Dimopoulos GE, et al. Gastric and lower oesophageal sphincter (LOS) pressures in early pregnancy. *Br J Anaesth.* 1981;53:381.
26. Wyner J, Cohen SE. Gastric volume in early pregnancy: Effect of metoclopramide. *Anesthesiology.* 1982;57:209.
27. Gin T, Chan MT. Decreased minimum alveolar concentration of isoflurane in pregnant humans. *Anesthesiology.* 1994;81:829.
28. Hirabayashi Y, Shimizu R, Saitoh K, et al. Spread of subarachnoid hyperbaric amethocaine in pregnant women. *Br J Anaesth.* 1995;74:384.
29. Butterworth JF IV, Walker FO, Lysak SZ. Pregnancy increases median nerve susceptibility of lidocaine. *Anesthesiology.* 1990;72:962.
30. Brown WU Jr, Bell GC, Alper MH. Acidosis, local anesthetics, and the newborn. *Obstet Gynecol.* 1976;48:27.
31. Kennedy RL, Miller RP, Bell JU, et al. Uptake and distribution of bupivacaine in fetal lambs. *Anesthesiology.* 1986;65:247.
32. Kuhnert PM, Kuhnert BR, Stitts JM, et al. The use of a selected ion monitoring technique to study the disposition of bupivacaine in mother, fetus, and neonate following epidural anesthesia for cesarean section. *Anesthesiology.* 1981;55:611.
33. Morishima HO, Daniel SS, Finster M, et al. Transmission of mepivacaine hydrochloride (carbocaine) across the human placenta. *Anesthesiology.* 1966;27:147.
34. Kuhnert BR, Kuhnert PM, Prochaska AL, et al. Plasma levels of 2-chloroprocaine in obstetric patients and their neonates after epidural anesthesia. *Anesthesiology.* 1980;53:21.
35. Dwyer R, Fee JP, Moore J. Uptake of halothane and isoflurane by mother and baby during caesarean section. *Br J Anaesth.* 1995;74:379.
36. Kosaka Y, Takahashi T, Mark LC. Intravenous thiobarbiturate anesthesia for cesarean section. *Anesthesiology.* 1969;31:489.
37. Morishima HO, Finster M, Pedersen H, et al. Pharmacokinetics of lidocaine in fetal and neonatal lambs and adult sheep. *Anesthesiology.* 1979;50:431.
38. Morishima HO, Pedersen H, Finster M, et al. Toxicity of lidocaine in adult, newborn, and fetal sheep. *Anesthesiology.* 1981;55:57.
39. Gale R, Ferguson JE 2nd, Stevenson DK. Effect of epidural analgesia with bupivacaine hydrochloride on neonatal bilirubin production. *Obstet Gynecol.* 1987;70:692.
40. Ueland K, Hansen JM. Maternal cardiovascular dynamics. III. Labor and delivery under local and caudal analgesia. *Am J Obstet Gynecol.* 1969;103:8.
41. Anonymous. American College of Obstetricians and Gynecologists Committee Opinion No. 339, June 2006. Analgesia and cesarean delivery rates. *Obstet Gynecol.* 2006;107:1487.
42. Smith CA, Collins CT, Cyna AM, et al. Complementary and alternative therapies for pain management in labour. *Cochrane Database Syst Rev.* 2006;CD003521.
43. Scott JR, Rose NB. Effect of psychoprophylaxis (Lamaze preparation) on labor and delivery in primiparas. *N Engl J Med.* 1976;294:1205.
44. Hodnett ED, Gates S, Hofmeyr GJ, et al. Continuous support for women during childbirth. *Cochrane Database Syst Rev.* 2011;CD003766.
45. Cluett ER, Burns E. Immersion in water in labour and birth. *Cochrane Database Syst Rev.* 2009:CD000111.
46. Fogarty V. Intradermal sterile water injections for the relief of low back pain in labour – a systematic review of the literature. *Women Birth.* 2008;21:157.
47. Dowswell T, Bedwell C, Lavender T, et al. Transcutaneous electrical nerve stimulation (TENS) for pain relief in labour. *Cochrane Database Syst Rev.* 2009;CD007214.
48. Smith CA, Collins CT, Crowther CA, et al. Acupuncture or acupressure for pain management in labour. *Cochrane Database Syst Rev.* 2011;CD009232.
49. Smith CA, Levett KM, Collins CT, et al. Relaxation techniques for pain management in labour. *Cochrane Database Syst Rev.* 2011;(12):CD009514.
50. Nelson KE, Eisenach JC. Intravenous butorphanol, meperidine, and their combination relieve pain and distress in women in labor. *Anesthesiology.* 2005;102:1008.
51. Ullman R, Smith LA, Burns E, et al. Parenteral opioids for maternal pain relief in labour. *Cochrane Database Syst Rev.* 2010;CD007396.
52. Latta KS, Ginsberg B, Barkin RL. Meperidine: A critical review. *Am J Ther.* 2002;9:53.
53. Leong WL, Sng BL, Sia AT. A comparison between remifentanil and meperidine for labor analgesia: A systematic review. *Anesth Analg.* 2011;113:818.
54. Hinova A, Fernando R. Systemic remifentanil for labor analgesia. *Anesth Analg.* 2009;109:1925.
55. Anim-Somuah M, Smyth RM, Jones L. Epidural versus non-epidural or no analgesia in labour. *Cochrane Database Syst Rev.* 2011;12:CD000331.
56. Wassen MM, Zuijlen J, Roumen FJ, et al. Early versus late epidural analgesia and risk of instrumental delivery in nulliparous women: A systematic review. *BJOG.* 2011;118:655.
57. Chestnut DH, Laszewski LJ, Pollack KL, et al. Continuous epidural infusion of 0.0625% bupivacaine-0.0002% fentanyl during the second stage of labor. *Anesthesiology.* 1990;72:613.
58. Beilin Y, Guinn NR, Bernstein HH, et al. Local anesthetics and mode of delivery: Bupivacaine versus ropivacaine versus levobupivacaine. *Anesth Analg.* 2007;105:756.
59. Birnbach DJ, Chestnut DH. The epidural test dose in obstetric patients: Has it outlived its usefulness? [editorial]. *Anesth Analg.* 1999;88:971.
60. van der Vyver M, Halpern S, Joseph G. Patient-controlled epidural analgesia versus continuous infusion for labour analgesia: A meta-analysis. *Br J Anaesth.* 2002;89:459.
61. Halpern SH, Carvalho B. Patient-controlled epidural analgesia for labor. *Anesth Analg.* 2009;108:921.
62. Asokumar B, Newman LM, McCarthy RJ, et al. Intrathecal bupivacaine reduces pruritus and prolongs duration of fentanyl analgesia during labor: A prospective, randomized controlled trial. *Anesth Analg.* 1998;87:1309.
63. Abrao KC, Francisco RP, Miyadahira S, et al. Elevation of uterine basal tone and fetal heart rate abnormalities after labor analgesia: A randomized controlled trial. *Obstet Gynecol.* 2009;113:41.
64. Albright GA, Forster RM. Does combined spinal-epidural analgesia with subarachnoid sufentanil increase the incidence of emergency cesarean delivery? *Reg Anesth.* 1997;22:400.
65. Leighton BL, Halpern SH, Wilson DB. Lumbar sympathetic blocks speed early and second stage induced labor in nulliparous women. *Anesthesiology.* 1999;90:1039.
66. Yentis S. The use of Entonox® for labour pain should be abandoned. *Int J Obstet Anesth.* 2001;10:25.
67. Bucklin BA, Hawkins JL, Anderson JR, et al. Obstetric anesthesia workforce survey: Twenty-year update. *Anesthesiology.* 2005;103:645.
68. Khaw KS, Ngan Kee WD, Lee A, et al. Supplementary oxygen for elective caesarean section under spinal anaesthesia: Useful in prolonged uterine incision-to-delivery interval? *Br J Anaesth.* 2004;92:518.
69. Backe SK, Kocarev M, Wilson RC, et al. Effect of maternal facial oxygen on neonatal behavioural scores during elective caesarean section with spinal anaesthesia. *Eur J Anaesthesiol.* 2007;24:66.
70. McDonnell JG, Curley G, Carney J, et al. The analgesic efficacy of transversus abdominis plane block after cesarean delivery: A randomized controlled trial. *Anesth Analg.* 2008;106:186.
71. Palmer CM, Emerson S, Volgoropolous D, et al. Dose-response relationship of intrathecal morphine for postcesarean analgesia. *Anesthesiology.* 1999;90:437.
72. Palmer CM, Nogami WM, Van Maren G, et al. Postcesarean epidural morphine: A dose-response study. *Anesth Analg.* 2000;90:887.
73. McMorrow RC, Ni Mhuircheartaigh RJ, Ahmed KA, et al. Comparison of transversus abdominis plane block vs spinal morphine for pain relief after caesarean section. *Br J Anaesth.* 2011;106:706.
74. Horlocker TT, Burton AW, Connis RT, et al. Practice guidelines for the prevention, detection, and management of respiratory depression associated with neuraxial opioid administration. *Anesthesiology.* 2009;110:218.
75. Leighton BL, Norris MC, DeSimone CA, et al. The air test as a clinically useful indicator of intravenously placed epidural catheters. *Anesthesiology.* 1990;73:610.
76. Morris GF, Gore-Hickman W, Lang SA, et al. Can parturients distinguish between intravenous and epidural fentanyl? *Can J Anaesth.* 1994;41:667.
77. Albright GA. Cardiac arrest following regional anesthesia with etidocaine or bupivacaine. *Anesthesiology.* 1979;51:285.
78. Crosby E, Sandler A, Finucane B, et al. Comparison of epidural anaesthesia with ropivacaine 0.5% and bupivacaine 0.5% for caesarean section. *Can J Anaesth.* 1998;45:1066.
79. Bjornestad E, Smedvig JP, Bjerkreim T, et al. Epidural ropivacaine 7.5 mg/ml for elective caesarean section: A double-blind comparison of efficacy and tolerability with bupivacaine 5 mg/ml. *Acta Anaesthesiol Scand.* 1999;43:603.
80. Choi DH, Kim JA, Chung IS. Comparison of combined spinal epidural anesthesia and epidural anesthesia for cesarean section. *Acta Anaesthesiol Scand.* 2000;44:214.

81. Thoren T, Holmstrom B, Rawal N, et al. Sequential combined spinal epidural block versus spinal block for cesarean section: Effects on maternal hypotension and neurobehavioral function of the newborn. *Anesth Analg.* 1994;78:1087.
82. Choi DH, Ahn HJ, Kim JA. Combined low-dose spinal-epidural anesthesia versus single-shot spinal anesthesia for elective cesarean delivery. *Int J Obstet Anesth.* 2006;15:13.
83. Hawkins JL, Chang J, Palmer SK, et al. Anesthesia-related maternal mortality in the United States: 1979–2002. *Obstet Gynecol.* 2011;117:69.
84. de Souza DG, Doar LH, Mehta SH, et al. Aspiration prophylaxis and rapid sequence induction for elective cesarean delivery: Time to reassess old dogma? *Anesth Analg.* 2010;110:1503.
85. Practice guidelines for management of the difficult airway: An updated report by the American Society of Anesthesiologists Task Force on Management of the Difficult Airway. *Anesthesiology.* 2003;98:1269.
86. Awan R, Nolan JP, Cook TM. Use of a ProSeal laryngeal mask airway for airway maintenance during emergency caesarean section after failed tracheal intubation. *Br J Anaesth.* 2004;92:144.
87. Robins K, Lyons G. Intraoperative awareness during general anesthesia for cesarean delivery. *Anesth Analg.* 2009;109:886.
88. Chin KJ, Yeo SW. Bispectral index values at sevoflurane concentrations of 1% and 1.5% in lower segment cesarean delivery. *Anesth Analg.* 2004;98:1140.
89. Ong BY, Cohen MM, Palahniuk RJ. Anesthesia for cesarean section–effects on neonates. *Anesth Analg.* 1989;68:270.
90. Chiloiro M, Darconza G, Piccioli E, et al. Gastric emptying and orocecal transit time in pregnancy. *J Gastroenterol.* 2001;36:538.
91. Ngan Kee WD, Khaw KS, Ng FF. Comparison of phenylephrine infusion regimens for maintaining maternal blood pressure during spinal anaesthesia for caesarean section. *Br J Anaesth.* 2004;92:469.
92. Banerjee A, Stocche RM, Angle P, et al. Preload or coload for spinal anesthesia for elective cesarean delivery: A meta-analysis. *Can J Anaesth.* 2010;57:24.
93. Morgan PJ, Halpern SH, Tarshis J. The effects of an increase of central blood volume before spinal anesthesia for cesarean delivery: A qualitative systematic review. *Anesth Analg.* 2001;92:997.
94. Lee A, Ngan Kee WD, Gin T. A quantitative, systematic review of randomized controlled trials of ephedrine versus phenylephrine for the management of hypotension during spinal anesthesia for cesarean delivery. *Anesth Analg.* 2002;94:920.
95. Ngan Kee WD, Khaw KS, Tan PE, et al. Placental transfer and fetal metabolic effects of phenylephrine and ephedrine during spinal anesthesia for cesarean delivery. *Anesthesiology.* 2009;111:506.
96. George RB, McKeen D, Columb MO, et al. Up-down determination of the 90% effective dose of phenylephrine for the treatment of spinal anesthesia-induced hypotension in parturients undergoing cesarean delivery. *Anesth Analg.* 2010; 110:154.
97. Stewart A, Fernando R, McDonald S, et al. The dose-dependent effects of phenylephrine for elective cesarean delivery under spinal anesthesia. *Anesth Analg.* 2010; 111:1230.
98. Neal JM, Bernards CM, Butterworth JF 4th, et al. ASRA practice advisory on local anesthetic systemic toxicity. *Reg Anesth Pain Med.* 2010;35:152.
99. Vanden Hoek TL, Morrison LJ, Shuster M, et al. Part 12: Cardiac arrest in special situations: 2010 American Heart Association Guidelines for Cardiopulmonary Resuscitation and Emergency Cardiovascular Care. *Circulation.* 2010;122:S829.
100. Paech MJ, Doherty DA, Christmas T, et al. The volume of blood for epidural blood patch in obstetrics: A randomized, blinded clinical trial. *Anesth Analg.* 2011; 113:126.
101. Scavone BM, Wong CA, Sullivan JT, et al. Efficacy of a prophylactic epidural blood patch in preventing post dural puncture headache in parturients after inadvertent dural puncture. *Anesthesiology.* 2004;101:1422.
102. Wong CA, Scavone BM, Dugan S, et al. Incidence of postpartum lumbosacral spine and lower extremity nerve injuries. *Obstet Gynecol.* 2003;101:279.
103. ACOG practice bulletin. Diagnosis and management of preeclampsia and eclampsia. Number 33, January 2002. American College of Obstetricians and Gynecologists. *Int J Gynaecol Obstet.* 2002;77(1):67–75.
104. Wang Y, Walsh SW, Kay HH. Placental lipid peroxides and thromboxane are increased and prostacyclin is decreased in women with preeclampsia. *Am J Obstet Gynecol.* 1992;167:946.
105. Meekins JW, Pijnenborg R, Hanssens M, et al. A study of placental bed spiral arteries and trophoblast invasion in normal and severe pre-eclamptic pregnancies. *Br J Obstet Gynaecol.* 1994;101:669.
106. Chesley LC. Plasma and red cell volumes during pregnancy. *Am J Obstet Gynecol.* 1972;112:440.
107. O'Brien JM, Milligan DA, Barton JR. Impact of high-dose corticosteroid therapy for patients with HELLP (hemolysis, elevated liver enzymes, and low platelet count) syndrome. *Am J Obstet Gynecol.* 2000;183:921.
108. Doyle LW, Crowther CA, Middleton P, et al. Magnesium sulphate for women at risk of preterm birth for neuroprotection of the fetus. *Cochrane Database Syst Rev.* 2009;CD004661.
109. Gilber WM, Towner DR, Field NT, et al. The safety and utility of pulmonary artery catheterization in severe preeclampsia and eclampsia. *Am J Obstet Gynecol.* 2000;182:1397.
110. Hogg B, Hauth JC, Caritis SN, et al. Safety of labor epidural anesthesia for women with severe hypertensive disease. National Institute of Child Health and Human Development Maternal-Fetal Medicine Units Network. *Am J Obstet Gynecol.* 1999; 181:1096.
111. Newsome LR, Bramwell RS, Curling PE. Severe preeclampsia: Hemodynamic effects of lumbar epidural anesthesia. *Anesth Analg.* 1986;65:31.
112. Jouppila P, Jouppila R, Hollmen A, et al. Lumbar epidural analgesia to improve intervillous blood flow during labor in severe preeclampsia. *Obstet Gynecol.* 1982; 59:158.
113. Aya AG, Mangin R, Vialles N, et al. Patients with severe preeclampsia experience less hypotension during spinal anesthesia for elective cesarean delivery than healthy parturients: A prospective cohort comparison. *Anesth Analg.* 2003;97:867.
114. Wallace DH, Leveno KJ, Cunningham FG, et al. Randomized comparison of general and regional anesthesia for cesarean delivery in pregnancies complicated by severe preeclampsia. *Obstet Gynecol.* 1995;86:193.
115. Hood DD, Curry R. Spinal versus epidural anesthesia for cesarean section in severely preeclamptic patients: A retrospective survey. *Anesthesiology.* 1999;90: 1276.
116. Bateman BT, Berman MF, Riley LE, et al. The epidemiology of postpartum hemorrhage in a large, nationwide sample of deliveries. *Anesth Analg.* 2010;110:1368.
117. Callaghan WM, Kuklina EV, Berg CJ. Trends in postpartum hemorrhage: United States, 1994–2006. *Am J Obstet Gynecol.* 2010;202:353.
118. Kuklina EV, Meikle SF, Jamieson DJ, et al. Severe obstetric morbidity in the United States: 1998–2005. *Obstet Gynecol.* 2009;113:293.
119. Ananth CV, Smulian JC, Vintzileos AM. The association of placenta previa with history of cesarean delivery and abortion: A meta-analysis. *Am J Obstet Gynecol.* 1997;177:1071.
120. Miller DA, Chollet JA, Goodwin TM. Clinical risk factors for placenta previa-placenta accreta. *Am J Obstet Gynecol.* 1997;177:210.
121. Silver RM, Landon MB, Rouse DJ, et al. Maternal morbidity associated with multiple repeat cesarean deliveries. *Obstet Gynecol.* 2006;107:1226.
122. Bateman BT, Mhyre JM, Callaghan WM, et al. Peripartum hysterectomy in the United States: Nationwide 14 year experience. *Am J Obstet Gynecol.* 2012;206:63.
123. ACOG Committee opinion. Number 266, January 2002: Placenta accreta. *Obstet Gynecol.* 2002;99:169–170.
124. Charbit B, Mandelbrot L, Samain E, et al. The decrease of fibrinogen is an early predictor of the severity of postpartum hemorrhage. *J Thromb Haemost.* 2007; 5:266.
125. Liumbruno GM, Liumbruno C, Rafenelli D. Intraoperative cell salvage in obstetrics: Is it a real therapeutic option? *Transfusion.* 2011;10:2244.
126. Franchini M, Franchi M, Bergamini V, et al. The use of recombinant activated FVII in postpartum hemorrhage. *Clin Obstet Gynecol.* 2010;53:219.
127. Gungorduk K, Yildirim G, Asicioglu O, et al. Efficacy of intravenous tranexamic acid in reducing blood loss after elective cesarean section: A prospective, randomized, double-blind, placebo-controlled study. *Am J Perinatol.* 2011;28:233.
128. Ducloy-Bouthors AS, Jude B, Duhamel A, et al. High dose tranexamic acid reduces blood loss in postpartum haemorrhage. *Crit Care.* 2011;15:r117.
129. Lucas S. (on behalf of the Centre for Maternal and Child Enquiries). Annex 9.1 Pathologic overview of cardiac deaths including sudden adult/arrhythmic death syndrome (SADS). *BGOG.* 2011;116:118(suppl 1).
130. Arafeh JM, Baird SM. Cardiac disease in pregnancy. *Crit Care Nurs Q.* 2006;29:32.
131. Ro A, Frishman WH. Peripartum cardiomyopathy. *Cardiol Rev.* 2006;14:35.
132. Curry R, Swan L, Steer P. Cardiac disease in pregnancy. *Curr Opin Obstet Gynecol.* 2009;21:508.
133. Palmer DG. Peripartum cardiomyopathy. *J Perinat Neonatal Nurs.* 2006;20:324.
134. Baird SM, Kennedy B. Myocardial infarction in pregnancy. *J Perinat Neonatal Nurs.* 2006;20:311; quiz 322.
135. Mallampalli A, Guy E. Cardiac arrest in pregnancy and somatic support after brain death. *Crit Care Med.* 2005;33:S325.
136. Hunt KJ, Schuller KL. The increasing prevalence of diabetes in pregnancy. *Obstet Gynecol Clin North Am.* 2007;34:173, vii.
137. Parker JA, Conway DL. Diabetic ketoacidosis in pregnancy. *Obstet Gynecol Clin North Am.* 2007;34:533, xii.
138. Mulholland C, Njoroge T, Mersereau P, et al. Comparison of guidelines available in the United States for diagnosis and management of diabetes before, during, and after pregnancy. *J Womens Health (Larchmt).* 2007;16:790.
139. Perlow JH, Morgan MA, Montgomery D, et al. Perinatal outcome in pregnancy complicated by massive obesity. *Am J Obstet Gynecol.* 1992;167:958.
140. Centre for Maternal and Child Enquires (CMACE). Improving the health of mothers, babies and children. Maternal obesity in the UK: Findings from a National Project. United Kingdom, 2010.
141. Hamilton BE, Martin JA, Sutton PD. Births: Preliminary data for 2002. *Natl Vital Stat Rep.* 2003;51:1.
142. Montan S. Increased risk in the elderly parturient. *Curr Opin Obstet Gynecol.* 2007;19:110.
143. Joseph KS, Allen AC, Dodds L, et al. The perinatal effects of delayed childbearing. *Obstet Gynecol.* 2005;105:1410.
144. Simchen MJ, Yinon Y, Moran O, et al. Pregnancy outcome after age 50. *Obstet Gynecol.* 2006;108:1084.
145. Cleary-Goldman J, Malone FD, Vidaver J, et al. Impact of maternal age on obstetric outcome. *Obstet Gynecol.* 2005;105:983.
146. Callaway LK, Lust K, McIntyre HD. Pregnancy outcomes in women of very advanced maternal age. *Aust N Z J Obstet Gynaecol.* 2005;45:12.

147. Vigil-De Gracia P, Montufar-Rueda C, Smith A. Pregnancy and severe chronic hypertension: Maternal outcome. *Hypertens Pregnancy.* 2004;23:285.
148. Lin HC, Sheen TC, Tang CH, et al. Association between maternal age and the likelihood of a cesarean section: A population-based multivariate logistic regression analysis. *Acta Obstet Gynecol Scand.* 2004;83:1178.
149. Amu O, Rajendran S, Bolaji II. Should doctors perform an elective caesarean section on request? Maternal choice alone should not determine method of delivery. *BMJ.* 1998;317:463.
150. Bell JS, Campbell DM, Graham WJ, et al. Do obstetric complications explain high caesarean section rates among women over 30? A retrospective analysis.*BMJ.* 2001;322:894.
151. Oleszczuk JJ, Keith LG, Oleszczuk AK. The paradox of old maternal age in multiple pregnancies. *Obstet Gynecol Clin North Am.* 2005;32:69, ix.
152. Holcroft CJ, Blakemore KJ, Allen M, et al. Association of prematurity and neonatal infection with neurologic morbidity in very low birth weight infants. *Obstet Gynecol.* 2003;101:1249.
153. Krauer B, Krauer F, Hytten F. *Drug Prescribing in Pregnancy.* Edinburgh: Churchill Livingstone; 1984.
154. ACOG committee opinion number 304, November 2004. Prenatal and perinatal human immunodeficiency virus testing: Expanded recommendations. *Obstet Gynecol.* 2004;104:1119.
155. Ammann AJ. Optima versus suboptimal treatment for HIV-infected pregnant women and HIV-exposed infants in clinical research studies. *J Acquir Immune Defic Syndr.* 2009;51:509.
156. Hughes SC. HIV and pregnancy: Twenty-five years into the epidemic. *Int Anesthesiol Clin.* 2007;45:29.
157. Evron S, Glezerman M, Harow E, et al. Human immunodeficiency virus: Anesthetic and obstetric considerations. *Anesth Analg.* 2004;98:503.
158. Tom DJ, Gulevich SJ, Shapiro HM, et al. Epidural blood patch in the HIV-positive patient. Review of clinical experience. San Diego HIV Neurobehavioral Research Center. *Anesthesiology.* 1992;76:943.
159. Estelles J, Rodriguez-Arias M, Maldonado C, et al. Gestational exposure to cocaine alters cocaine reward. *Behav Pharmacol.* 2006;17:509.
160. ACOG practice bulletin No. 106. Intrapartum fetal heart rate monitoring: Nomenclature, interpretation, and general management principles. *Obstet Gynecol.* 2009;114:192–202.
161. Nelson KB, Dambrosia JM, Ting TY, et al. Uncertain value of electronic fetal monitoring in predicting cerebral palsy. *N Engl J Med.* 1996;334:613.
162. Bloom SL, Spong CY, Thom E, et al. Fetal pulse oximetry and cesarean delivery. *N Engl J Med.* 2006;355:2195.
163. Garite TJ, Dildy GA, McNamara H, et al. A multicenter controlled trial of fetal pulse oximetry in the intrapartum management of nonreassuring fetal heart rate patterns. *Am J Obstet Gynecol.* 2000;183:1049.
164. Kattwinkel J, Perlman JM, Aziz K, et al. Special Report—Neonatal Resuscitation: 2010 American Heart Association guidelines for cardiopulmonary resuscitation and emergency cardiovascular care. *Circulation.* 2010;122:S9.
165. Carlton DP. Transitional changes in the newborn infant around the time of birth, Rudolph's Pediatrics. In: Bland RD, ed. New York, NY: McGraw-Hill; 2003.
166. Davis PG, Tan A, O'Donnell CPF, et al. Resuscitation of newborn infants with 100% oxygen or air: A systematic review and meta-analysis. *Lancet.* 2004;364: 1329–1333.
167. Rabi Y, Rabi D, Yee W. Room air resuscitation of the depressed newborn: A systematic review and meta-analysis. *Resuscitation.* 2007;72:353–363.
168. Bouchard S, Johnson MP, Flake AW, et al. The EXIT procedure: Experience and outcome in 31 cases. *J Pediatr Surg.* 2002;37:418.
169. MacKenzie TC, Crombleholme TM, Flake AW. The ex-utero intrapartum treatment. *Curr Opin Pediatr.* 2002;14:453.
170. Rosen MA, Andreae MH, Cameron AG. Nitroglycerin for fetal surgery: Fetoscopy and ex utero intrapartum treatment procedure with malignant hyperthermia precautions. *Anesth Analg.* 2003;96:698.
171. Gaiser RR, Cheek TG, Kurth CD. Anesthetic management of cesarean delivery complicated by ex utero intrapartum treatment of the fetus. *Anesth Analg.* 1997;84:1150.
172. Safra MJ, Oakley GP Jr. Association between cleft lip with or without cleft palate and prenatal exposure to diazepam. *Lancet.* 1975;2:478.
173. Smith BE, Gaub ML, Moya F. Teratogenic effects of anesthetic agents: Nitrous oxide. *Anesth Analg.* 1965;44:726.
174. Mazze RI, Kallen B. Reproductive outcome after anesthesia and operation during pregnancy: A registry study of 5405 cases. *Am J Obstet Gynecol.* 1989;161:1178.
175. Duncan PG, Pope WD, Cohen MM, et al. Fetal risk of anesthesia and surgery during pregnancy. *Anesthesiology.* 1986;64:790.
176. Sanchez V, Feinstein S, Lunardi N, et al. General anesthesia causes long-term impairment of mitochondrial morphogenesis and synaptic transmission in developing rat brain. *Anesthesiology.* 2011;115:992.
177. ACOG Committee opinion Number 284, August 2003: Nonobstetric surgery in pregnancy. *Obstet Gynecol.* 2003;102:431.

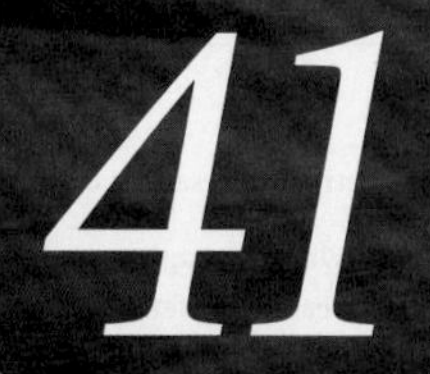

CHAPTER 41

Neonatal Anesthesia

STEVEN C. HALL • SANTHANAM SURESH

Key Points

1. Understanding the physiologic changes that occur during the transition from fetal to neonatal life is crucial to the anesthetic management of the neonate. The circulatory, pulmonary, hepatic, and renal systems are all affected in this process.
2. Important physiologic and anatomic factors account for the rapid rate of desaturation observed in neonates. These include an increase in oxygen consumption, a high closing volume, a high ratio of minute ventilation to functional residual capacity, and a pliable rib cage.
3. Persistent pulmonary hypertension of the newborn is a pathologic condition that can be primary but is often secondary to other conditions, including meconium aspiration, sepsis, congenital diaphragmatic hernia, or pneumonia. Understanding the pathophysiologic characteristics of this condition helps guide therapy.
4. Knowledge of the major anatomic differences between the infant and the adult airway helps one understand why the infant's airway is often described as "anterior" and why airway management may be challenging. These differences include a relatively large tongue, a higher glottis with anterior slanting vocal folds, a larger occiput, and a narrowing at the cricoid ring.
5. Careful attention must be given to the choice of anesthetic agents and dosing of such agents in the neonatal population. Ongoing maturational changes in the renal and hepatobiliary systems, which occur during the first 30 days of life, will affect the metabolism and elimination of many anesthetic agents.
6. Although a host of anesthetic techniques are available, including regional anesthesia, multiple factors are considered when choosing an anesthetic plan for the neonate. These include the surgical requirements, the need for postoperative ventilation, the cardiovascular stability of the neonate, and the anticipated method of postoperative pain control.
7. Special considerations must be addressed when planning an anesthetic for a neonate. Some of the controversial issues include the risk of postoperative apnea and the use of caffeine in treatment and prophylaxis, the role of oxygen concentration in the development of retinopathy of prematurity, and the neurodevelopmental effects of anesthetic agents on the fetal and neonatal brain.
8. True surgical emergencies are uncommon in the neonatal period. Knowledge of conditions with comorbidities, such as tracheoesophageal fistula, omphalocele, and congenital diaphragmatic hernia, and a thorough preoperative evaluation and stabilization of such neonates cannot be overemphasized.

Multimedia

1 Inhalation Induction

PHYSIOLOGY OF THE INFANT AND THE TRANSITION PERIOD

An infant's first year of life is characterized by an almost miraculous growth in size and maturity. The body weight alone changes by a factor of three, and there is no other period in extrauterine life when changes occur so rapidly. Before birth, fetal growth and development depend on the genetic composition of the fetus, the mother's placental function, and potential exposure to chemicals or infectious agents that can affect mother, fetus, or both. After birth, the newborn must rapidly adjust to the extrauterine environment to survive. The dramatic changes in functions of several systems will determine the viability of the neonate, as well as its ability to grow and develop properly.

The newborn period has been defined as the first 24 hours of life, and the neonatal period as the first month. There is significant change in many physiologic systems during both of
1 these periods. The first 72 hours are especially significant for the cardiovascular, pulmonary, and renal systems. The changes in these systems are interrelated; inadequate progression of change or a disease state altering one of these systems can quickly alter the maturation of one or more of the other systems. Understanding the differences in these systems from the older child, as well as the changes that occur in the neonatal period, is important in developing a comprehensive anesthetic approach.

The Cardiovascular System

Fetal Circulation

The fetal circulation is characterized by a parallel system in which both ventricles pump most of their output into the systemic circulation. Less than 10% of the combined cardiac output goes through the fetal pulmonary circulation via three main shunts; through the placenta, foramen ovale, and ductus arteriosus (Fig. 41-1A). The placenta provides oxygenated blood into the ductus venosus, the inferior vena cava, and then into the right atrium. In the right atrium, the majority of the oxygenated blood primarily flows through the foramen ovale into the left atrium,

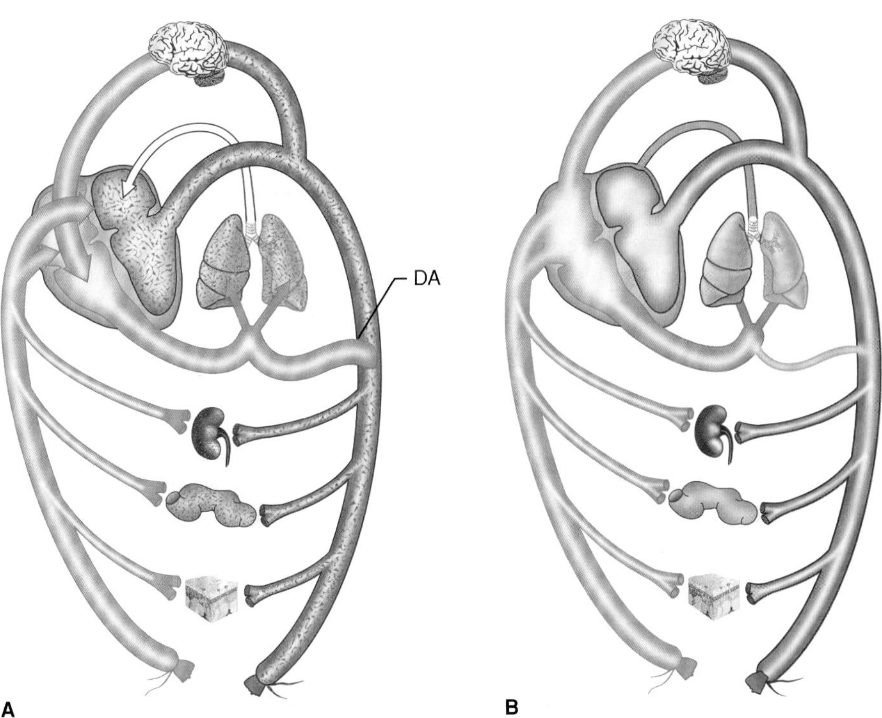

FIGURE 41-1. A: Schematic representation of the fetal circulation. Oxygenated blood leaves the placenta in the umbilical vein (*vessel without stippling*). Umbilical vein blood joins blood from the viscera (represented here by the kidney, gut, and skin) in the inferior vena cava. Approximately half of the inferior vena cava flow passes through the foramen ovale to the left atrium, where it mixes with a small amount of pulmonary venous blood, and this relatively well-oxygenated blood (*light stippling*) supplies the heart and brain by way of the ascending aorta. The other half of the inferior vena cava stream mixes with superior vena cava blood and enters the right ventricle (blood in the right atrium and ventricle has little oxygen, which is denoted by *heavy stippling*). Because the pulmonary arterioles are constricted, most of the blood in the main pulmonary artery flows through the ductus arteriosus (DA) so the descending aorta's blood has less oxygen (*heavy stippling*) than does blood in the ascending aorta (*light stippling*). **B:** Schematic representation of the circulation in the normal newborn. After expansion of the lungs and ligation of the umbilical cord, pulmonary blood flow and left atrial and systemic arterial pressures increase. When left atrial pressure exceeds right atrial pressure, the foramen ovale closes so all inferior and superior vena cava blood leaves the right atrium, enters the right ventricle, and is pumped through the pulmonary artery toward the lung. With the increase in systemic arterial pressure and decrease in pulmonary artery pressure, flow through the ductus arteriosus becomes left to right, and the ductus constricts and closes. The course of circulation is the same as in the adult. (Reprinted from: Phibbs R. Delivery room management of the newborn. In: Avery GB, ed. *Neonatology, Pathophysiology and Management of the Newborn*. Philadelphia, PA: JB Lippincott; 1981:184, with permission.)

bypassing the right ventricle and the pulmonary vascular bed. This preferential flow across the foramen occurs because of the relatively low pressure in the left atrium compared with that of the right atrium. Some blood from the right atrium does flow through the right ventricle and into the main pulmonary artery. The pulmonary vascular resistance is quite high in utero because of alveolar collapse and compression of blood vessels, inhibiting flow through the pulmonary circulation. The pulmonary vascular resistance is also high at this point because of the relatively low Pa_{O_2} and pH of the blood that does flow through the vessels. Some blood in the pulmonary artery does flow through the pulmonary circulation and then into the left atrium, but the majority of flow goes through the ductus arteriosus into the descending aorta.

CHANGES AT BIRTH. After birth, all of these shunts are eliminated or start to close quickly.[1] The placental shunt is eliminated and the ductus venosus is closed. The newborn's left ventricle is now pumping blood into the higher pressure systemic circulation exclusively. Expansion of the lungs and initiation of breathing lead to dramatic changes in both the circulatory and pulmonary systems (Fig. 41-1B). As alveoli fill with air, the compression of the pulmonary alveolar capillaries is relieved, reducing pulmonary vascular resistance and promoting flow through the pulmonary circulation. This blood is now oxygenated, raising the arterial PO_2, and further reducing pulmonary vascular resistance. Although the change in the first minutes to hours is dramatic, it usually takes 3 to 4 days for the pulmonary vascular resistance to decrease to normal levels. The foramen ovale will usually functionally close in the first hour of life as the increase in left atrial pressure from increased pulmonary circulation after the initiation of breathing exceeds right atrial pressure. The foramen is closed by a flap of tissue that covers the foramen. This foramen can reopen if there is a relative increase in right atrial pressure such as is seen with elevated pulmonary vascular resistance or fluid overload. Anatomic closure usually occurs in the first year of life, but may remain probe-patent into adulthood in 10% to 20% of patients. The ductus arteriosus starts to close in the first day of life and is usually functionally closed in the second day of life. In utero, patency of the ductus was determined by the combined relaxant effects of low oxygen tension and endogenously produced prostaglandins, especially prostaglandin E_2. In a full-term neonate, oxygen is the most important factor controlling ductal closure. When the Pa_{O_2} of blood in the ductus rises to about 50 mm Hg, the muscle in the vessel constricts. It should be noted that the ductus of a preterm infant is less responsive to increased oxygen, even though its musculature is developed.

Myocardial function is different in the neonate. The neonatal cardiac myocyte has less organized contractile elements than the child or adult.[2] Not only are there fewer myofibril elements, but they are not organized in parallel roles, as seen in the child and adult heart, making them less efficient. The neonate myocyte also has a less mature sarcoplasmic reticulum system. The underdeveloped sarcoplasmic reticulum is associated with a decrease in Ca^{2+}-adenosine triphosphatase activity, an important component of contractility. As the sarcoplasmic reticulum matures, the efficiency of calcium transport and subsequent contractility increases.[3] The neonatal myocardium cannot generate as much force as that of the older child and is relatively noncompliant. Consequently, there is limited functional reserve in the neonatal period, with afterload increases particularly poorly tolerated. After birth, there are dramatic changes in the myocardium. As the work of the ventricles increases secondary to high stroke volume and increased vascular resistance, these myocytes grow quickly in number and size. This growth is more dramatic in the left ventricle than the right ventricle because of the rise in systemic vascular resistance and fall in pulmonary vascular resistance, respectively.

Especially in the first 3 months of life, the parasympathetic nervous system influence on the heart is more mature than the sympathetic system and the myocardium does not respond to inotropic support as well as the older child or adult. There is animal evidence that there are maturational changes in β-adrenergic receptor function that explain the decreased responsiveness to inotropes in the neonate.[4] The neonatal myocardium does have increased glycogen stores and higher rates of anaerobic glycolysis, which may explain its relative resistance to hypoxia and better performance in the presence of an ischemic insult. Because the myocardium is relatively noncompliant in the newborn, preload changes can increase stroke volume and cardiac output, but not as effectively as in the older child.[5] In other words, the Frank–Starling relationship is present in the neonatal heart, but is not as effective as in the adult. The other clinical implication of a noncompliant ventricle is that, in the absence of significant increases in stroke volume, cardiac output is not well maintained in the presence of bradycardia. Lastly, neonates have immature baroreceptors. The baroreceptor is responsible for the reflex tachycardia that occurs in response to hypotension. Therefore, the immaturity of this reflex would limit the neonate's ability to compensate for hypotension. In addition, the baroresponse of the neonate is more depressed than that of the adult at the same level of anesthesia.

In summary, the neonatal heart has some significant limitations. The resting cardiac output is much higher relative to body weight than in the adult because of the higher O_2 consumption per kilogram of body weight. Stimulation of the myocardium produces a limited increase in contractility and cardiac output. The sympathetic nervous system, which usually provides the important chronotropic and inotropic support to the mature circulation during stress, is severely limited in the neonate because of lack of development. Even in the absence of stress, the neonatal heart has limited ability to increase cardiac output compared with the mature heart (Fig. 41-2). The resting cardiac output of the immature heart is close to the maximal cardiac output, so there is a limited reserve. The mature heart can increase cardiac output by 300%, whereas the immature heart can only increase cardiac output by 30% to 40%.

The Pulmonary System

The pulmonary system develops rapidly during the last trimester, with important changes in both the number of alveoli and the maturity of the pulmonary vascular system.[6] These systems have not matured enough to provide adequate gas exchange until about 24 to 26 weeks' gestation. The airways and alveoli continue to grow after birth, with alveoli increasing in number until about 8 years of age.[7] With the initiation of ventilation, the pulmonary system changes dramatically. The alveoli transition from a fluid-filled to an air-filled state and a normal ventilatory pattern with normal volumes develops in the first 5 to 10 minutes of life. In order to adequately expand the collapsed and fluid-filled alveoli, the newborn will generate an initial negative intrathoracic pressure in the range of 40 to 60 cm H_2O. By 10 to 20 minutes of life, the newborn has achieved its near-normal functional residual capacity (FRC), and the blood gases stabilize with the establishment of increased pulmonary blood flow. Table 41-1 lists the normal blood gases for the various periods of life.

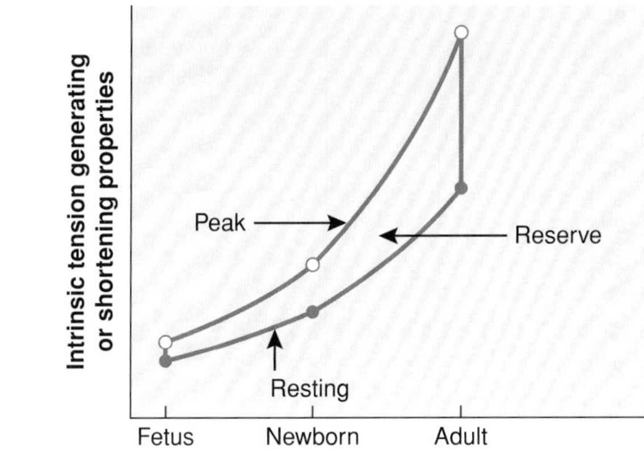

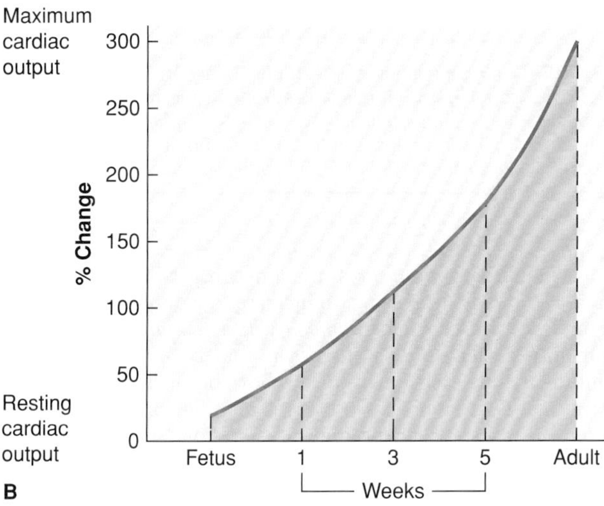

FIGURE 41-2. Schema of reduced cardiac reserve in fetal and newborn animal hearts compared with adult hearts. **A:** In the newborn infant, resting cardiac muscle performance is close to a peak of ventricular function because of limitations in diastolic, systolic, and heart rate reserve. **B:** Similarly, pump reserve early in life is limited by these factors and by much higher resting cardiac output relative to body weight, compared with that in adults. (Reprinted from: Friedman WF, George BL. Treatment of congestive heart failure by altering loading conditions of the heart. *J Pediatr.* 1985;106:700, with permission.)

The initial breaths to expand the lungs and subsequently maintain FRC are necessary components of the stabilization of the ventilatory system, as well as the circulatory system. Failure to do so will quickly lead to deterioration of both systems.

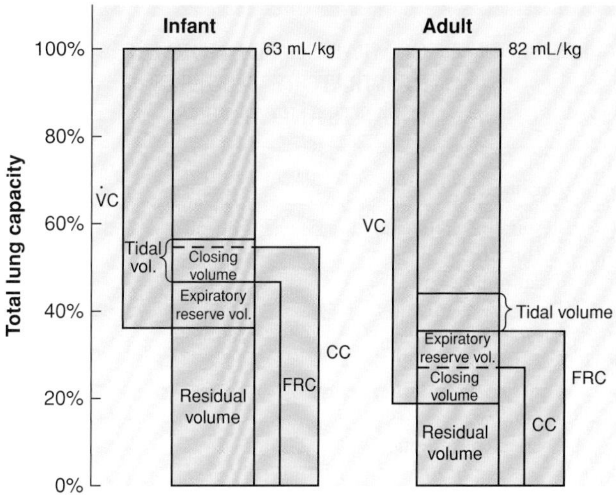

FIGURE 41-3. Static lung volumes of infants and adults. CC, closing capacity; FRC, functional residual capacity; VC, vital capacity. (Reprinted from: Smith CA, Nelson NM. *Physiology of the Newborn Infant,* 4th ed. Springfield, IL: Charles C Thomas; 1976:207, with permission.)

Tidal volume is about the same in the neonate as the child or adult on a volume/kilogram body weight measure, but the respiratory rate is increased. Closing volumes are particularly high and may be within the range of the normal tidal volume (Fig. 41-3). This increased minute ventilation mirrors the higher oxygen consumption in neonates, which is about double that seen in an adult. Because the FRC in the newborn is comparable to that of the older child or adult, but the minute ventilation is much higher, the ratio of minute ventilation to FRC is 2 to 3 times higher in the newborn. The clinical significance of this ratio is twofold. First, anesthetic induction with a volatile anesthetic agent should be faster, as should emergence. Second, the decrease in FRC relative to minute ventilation and oxygen consumption means that there is less "oxygen reserve" in the FRC compared to that
2 of older children and adults. There will be a more rapid drop in arterial oxygen levels in the newborn in the presence of apnea or hypoventilation. Table 41-2 compares normal respiratory parameters in the normal newborn and adult.

Lung compliance is relatively low, but chest wall compliance is relatively high, compared to that of older children. The pliable rib cage gives less mechanical support than in the older child, leading to significant retractions with less efficient gas exchange and functional airway closure, thus increasing the work of breathing. The intercostal muscles are poorly developed at birth, with the diaphragm providing most of the gas exchange. The diaphragm

TABLE 41-1. NORMAL BLOOD GAS VALUES IN THE NEONATE

Subject	Age	PO_2 (mm Hg)	PCO_2 (mm Hg)	pH
Fetus (term)	Before labor	25	40	7.37
Fetus (term)	End of labor	10–20	55	7.25
Newborn (term)	10 min	50	48	7.2
Newborn (term)	1 h	70	35	7.35
Newborn (term)	1 wk	75	35	7.4
Newborn (preterm, 1,500 g)	1 wk	60	38	7.37

TABLE 41-2. COMPARISON OF NORMAL RESPIRATORY VALUES IN INFANTS AND ADULTS

Parameter	Infant	Adult
Respiratory frequency (breaths/min)	30–50	12–16
Tidal volume (mL/kg)	7	7
Dead space (mL/kg)	2–2.5	2.2
Alveolar ventilation (mL/kg/min)	100–150	60
Functional residual capacity (mL/kg)	27–30	30
Oxygen consumption (mL/kg/min)	7–9	3

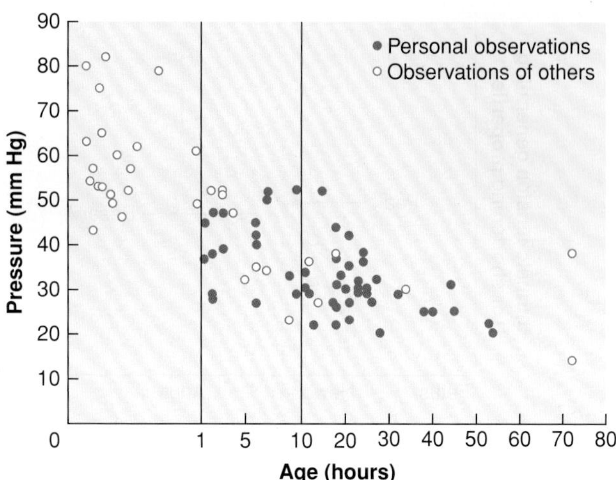

FIGURE 41-4. Correlation of mean pulmonary arterial pressure with age in 85 normal-term infants studied during the first 3 days of life. (Reprinted from: Emmanouilides GC, Moss AJ, Duffie ER, et al. Pulmonary arterial pressure changes in human newborn infants from birth to 3 days of age. *J Pediatr.* 1964;65:327, with permission.)

in the neonate has two types of fibers, the type 1, slow twitch, high-oxidative fibers that give sustained contraction with very little fatigue, and the type 2, fast twitch, low-oxidative fibers that give quick contractions, but fatigue easily. The distribution of these fibers in the newborn shows only about 25% type 1 fibers, while 55% of the fibers are type 1 in the mature diaphragm at about 2 years of age. The preterm newborn has even fewer type 1 fibers at birth, in the 10% range. This relative lack of type 1 fibers means that the newborn, especially the preterm, is at risk for diaphragmatic fatigue in the presence of significant resistance to ventilation or periods of hyperventilation.

Lastly, the continued presence of surfactant is necessary to maintain both the distensibility of the alveoli and the maintenance of an FRC at exhalation. Decreased surfactant production, due to prematurity or other conditions such as maternal diabetes, can cause respiratory distress syndrome (RDS). The decreased surfactant can cause alveolar collapse, decrease in lung compliance, hypoxia, increased work of breathing, and respiratory failure.[8] Commercially available surfactant is extraordinarily useful to both treat and prevent RDS in susceptible patients. In addition, surfactant can improve gas exchange in preterms who may not have RDS, but are stressed by sepsis, heart failure, or other systemic problems.[9] Delivered through an endotracheal tube, it can be used prophylactically in the very preterm newborn to prevent RDS, as well as treat newborns who have developed RDS.

In addition to the mechanical aspects of the pulmonary system, control of breathing has unique aspects in the neonatal period, especially in the preterm. Neonates respond less to hypercapnia than the older child. In addition, neonates respond to hypoxia with a brief period of hyperventilation, followed by hypoventilation. The initial hyperventilatory response can be prevented by hypothermia. Lastly, a periodic breathing pattern is common in neonates, especially in preterm newborns, that can persist up to a year of age.

Persistent Pulmonary Hypertension of the Newborn

The pulmonary circulation is extremely sensitive to oxygen, pH, and nitric oxide, as well as a variety of mediators such as adenosine and prostaglandins and mechanical factors such as lung inflation. Figure 41-4 illustrates the correlation of the mean pulmonary artery pressure with age during the first 3 days of life. Hypoxia and acidosis, along with inflammatory mediators, may cause pulmonary artery pressure either to persist at a high level or, after initially decreasing, to increase to pathologic levels. The result is termed *persistent pulmonary hypertension of the newborn,* 3 sometimes referred to as *persistent fetal circulation.* Persistent pulmonary hypertension of the newborn occurs in term and preterm infants, usually caused by precipitating conditions such as severe birth asphyxia, meconium aspiration, sepsis, congenital diaphragmatic hernia (CDH), and maternal use of nonsteroidal anti-inflammatory drugs with in utero constriction of the ductus arteriosus, although it is often idiopathic. Other risk factors include maternal diabetes or asthma, as well as cesarean delivery.[10] The elevated pulmonary vascular resistance causes both the ductus arteriosus and foramen ovale to remain open, with subsequent right-to-left (bypassing the pulmonary circulation) shunting. These changes result in profound hypoxia from right-to-left shunting and a normal or elevated $PaCO_2$. The hypoxemia is often noted to be out of proportion to the other presenting signs of respiratory and cardiovascular compromise. Treatment starts with correcting any predisposing disease (hypoglycemia, polycythemia) and improving poor tissue oxygenation. The response to therapy is often unpredictable. However, the goals are to achieve a Pao_2 of 50 to 70 mm Hg and a $PaCO_2$ of 50 to 55 mm Hg. In addition to standard mechanical ventilation, high-frequency ventilation, exogenous surfactant, inhaled nitric oxide, alkalinization, and extracorporeal membrane oxygenation (ECMO) have been used with varying degrees of success. Experimental therapy with other agents such as sildenafil continue to be evaluated.[11] Success in treatment and survival varies directly with the underlying cause. Significant prognostic factors are the ability of therapy to reduce pulmonary vascular resistance and associated complications such as ischemic encephalopathy.

Meconium Aspiration

Another important pulmonary issue in the newborn period is *meconium aspiration.* Interference with the normal maternal placental circulation in the third trimester may cause fetal hypoxia. Fetal hypoxia can result in an increase in the amount of muscle in the blood vessels of the distal respiratory units. Figure 41-5

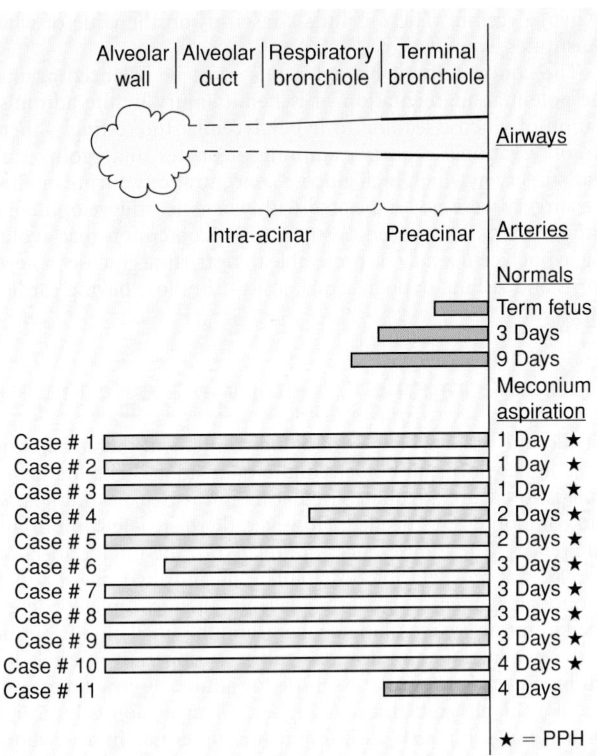

FIGURE 41-5. Diagram of muscle extension along pulmonary arterial branches (*shaded bars*). In the normal newborn, virtually no intra-acinar artery is muscular. In 9 of 10 infants with meconium aspiration and persistent pulmonary hypertension (PPH), muscle extended into the most peripheral arteries; the infant with meconium aspiration without PPH (case 11) had normal intra-acinar arteries. (Reprinted from: Murphy JD, Vawter GF, Reid LM. Pulmonary vascular disease in fetal meconium aspiration. *J Pediatr.* 1984;104:758, with permission.)

illustrates the muscle increase found in blood vessels of a series of 11 infants who died of persistent pulmonary hypertension.[12] Chronic fetal hypoxia leads to the passage of meconium in utero. The fetus breathes in utero so the meconium mixed with amniotic fluid enters the pulmonary system. Meconium aspiration can be a marker of chronic fetal hypoxia in the third trimester. This condition is different from the meconium aspiration that occurs during delivery. This meconium at birth is thick and tenacious, and mechanically obstructs the tracheobronchial system. Meconium aspiration syndrome leads to varying degrees of respiratory failure, which can be fatal in spite of all treatment modalities.

Current recommendations for intubation and suctioning for newborns at delivery with frank meconium aspiration or meconium staining (approximately 10% of newborns) emphasize a conservative approach.[13] Routine oropharyngeal suctioning of meconium is recommended immediately at the time of delivery, but tracheal intubation and suctioning should be performed selectively. If the newborn is vigorous and crying, no further suctioning is needed. If meconium is present and the newborn is depressed, the trachea should be intubated and meconium and other aspirated material suctioned from beneath the glottis. If meconium is retrieved and no bradycardia is present, reintubate and suction. If there is bradycardia, administer positive pressure ventilation and consider suctioning again later once the neonate is stabilized.

The Renal System

In utero, most of the fetal waste material is removed by the maternal placenta. In effect, the fetal kidneys are passive, receiving relatively little renal blood flow and having a low glomerular filtration rate (GFR).[14] There are four major reasons for the low renal blood flow and GFR: Low systemic arterial pressure, high renal vascular resistance, low permeability of the glomerular capillaries, and the small size and number of glomeruli. In utero, the kidneys receive only about 3% of the cardiac output, whereas they will receive about 25% of cardiac output in adulthood. At birth, this changes dramatically. The systemic arterial pressure increases and the renal vascular resistance decreases, and the kidneys now receive a progressively increased part of the cardiac output. At birth, the GFR is low, but increases significantly in the first few days, doubles in the first 2 weeks, but does not reach adult levels until about 2 years of age. The limited ability of the newborn's kidney to concentrate or dilute urine results from this low GFR and decreased tubular function. However, during the first 3 to 4 days, the circulatory changes increase renal blood flow and GFR and improve the neonate's ability to concentrate and dilute the urine. Part of the improvement in renal function is the establishment of gradients in the medullary interstitium that promotes resorption of sodium. The maturation continues, and by the time the normal full-term infant is 1 month of age, the kidneys are approximately 60% mature. Urine output is low in the first 24 hours, but then increases to an expected level of at least 1 to 2 mL/kg/hr. Diuresis after the first day of life <1 mL/kg/hr should be considered indicative of either hypovolemia or decreased renal function for another reason.

Despite the rapid maturation of renal function and the increased capacity of the neonatal kidneys, they still have limitations.[15] From an anesthetic standpoint, the half-life of medications excreted by means of glomerular filtration will be prolonged.[16] The relative inability to conserve water means that neonates, especially in the first week of life, tolerate fluid restriction poorly. In addition, the inability to excrete large amounts of water means the newborn tolerates fluid overload poorly. The newborn kidney is better able to conserve sodium than excrete sodium, making hypernatremia a risk if excess sodium is administered. However, because of the lack of tonicity in the medullary interstitium shortly after birth, there will be some obligate sodium loss in the first days of life. This improves as the countercurrent multiplier is developed in the interstitium.

Fluid and Electrolyte Therapy in the Neonate

Total body water (TBW), which is usually described in terms of percent of body weight, varies by both age and gestational status. The highest TBW is found in the fetus, but decreases to about 75% of body weight for a term infant at birth. Preterm infants have a higher TBW than term infants, often in the 80% to 85% range. TBW decreases during the first 12 months of life to about 60% to 65% of body weight and stays at this level through childhood.

TBW is distributed between two compartments, intracellular fluid (ICF) and extracellular fluid (ECF). The ECF volume is larger than the ICF volume in the fetus and newborn, usually in the 40% (ECF) and 20% (ICF) of body weight ranges. This is the opposite of the situation in infants and children. There is a significant diuresis after birth that produces a decrease in the ECF volume. In addition, ICF volume increases because of the growth of cells in the body. The ECF/ICF volumes (20% and 40% of body weight) approach adult values by about 1 year of age.

This dramatic shift is beneficial to the child, especially in increasing the mobility of reserves in the face of dehydration. Fluid can be easily mobilized from ICF volumes to replenish intravascular volume that is lost from fasting, fever, diarrhea, or other causes. This means that the nonneonate is better situated to maintain intravascular volume in these situations than the neonate.

The ECF is divided into the plasma and the interstitial fluid. The plasma water is usually about 5% of body weight and the related blood volume, assuming a hematocrit of 45%, is about 8% of body weight in infants and children. The water content is slightly higher in neonates and may approach 10% of body weight in preterms. The interstitial fluid, usually about 15% of body weight, can demonstrate large increases in disease states associated with liver failure, heart failure, renal failure, and other causes of conditions such as pleural effusions or ascites. The reason for this is the balance between oncotic and hydrostatic forces. Any condition that decreases oncotic pressure, such as loss of albumin in liver failure, promotes the loss of fluid into the interstitial fluid. On the other hand, raised hydrostatic pressures, such as seen in heart failure, can result in fluid leaving the plasma and accumulating in the interstitial space. Conditions that result in translocation of fluid from the plasma to the interstitial spaces, whether because of decreased oncotic pressure or increased oncotic pressure, are of significant consequence to the neonate. Loss of fluid from the plasma volume compromises the intravascular volume, potentially decreasing the perfusion of vital organs and systems.

The blood volume in the normal full-term newborn is approximately 85 mL/kg and approximately 90 to 100 mL/kg in the preterm, although estimates of these volumes can vary between studies. Approximately 50 mL/kg of this volume is the plasma volume. For all practical purposes, the electrolyte values in the neonatal period are the same as in the child and adult with the exception of potassium, which can be about 1 to 2 mmol/L higher than average for the first 2 days of life.[17]

Maintenance fluid requirements increase during the first days of life. They have been estimated to be 60, 80, 100, and 120 mL/kg/24 hr for the first 4 days of life, respectively. For the rest of the neonatal period, a maintenance rate of 150 mL/kg/24 hr is appropriate.

The appropriate type of maintenance fluid depends on several issues. Because of ongoing sodium loss secondary to the inability of the neonatal distal tubule to respond fully to aldosterone, intravenous fluids in the neonate must contain some sodium. Most operations on neonates involve loss of blood and ECF, which must be replaced with a fluid of similar electrolyte content (i.e., a balanced salt solution such as lactated Ringer or Plasma-Lyte). Hypotonic solutions should not be used to replace these losses because they can cause significant hyponatremia. Thus, if the neonate is already stable on a maintenance solution, it is reasonable to continue this maintenance at a constant rate, adding balanced salt solution or colloid or blood products as needed.

The other issues for fluid choice in the neonate center on appropriate glucose administration. In most cases, maintenance fluids containing 10% glucose and 0.2 normal saline with 20 mmol/L of potassium are reasonable in the first 48 hours of life. Beyond that time period, full-term infants may do well with 5% glucose instead of 10%, although preterms will often require the higher glucose load longer. Newborns of diabetic mothers, those who are small for gestational age, and those who have had continuous glucose infusions stopped have particular problems with hypoglycemia. These infants need to have their blood glucose values monitored. Neonates who are scheduled for surgery and have been receiving hyperalimentation fluids or supplementary glucose must continue to receive that fluid during surgery or must have their glucose levels monitored because of concerns of hypoglycemia. There is little consensus on the issue of what constitutes hypoglycemia.[18]

The concern about hypoglycemia must be balanced against the potential augmentation of ischemic injury by the administration of glucose leading to hyperglycemia. Interestingly, there are observational reports examining neonates undergoing cardiac surgery in which high glucose concentrations during or after the surgery were not associated with worse neurodevelopmental outcomes.[19,20] These studies support the contention that avoiding hypoglycemia may be preferable to restricting glucose in newborns and risking hypoglycemia, at least in those having cardiac surgery.

Blood Component Therapy in the Neonate

Most of the basic principles of blood component therapy are the same in newborns and older children and adults. The first principle is to ensure adequate circulating intravascular volume and add components, as needed. However, there are a few important differences. These differences are related to the interconnection of maternal and fetal blood circulations and the flow of some, but not all elements, across the placenta, the incompletely developed immune system of the neonate, and the small blood volume of the neonate. The indications in the perioperative period for red blood cells are similar to those for adults, but the target values in available guidelines are higher.[21] Transfusion is indicated for a hemoglobin <10 g/dL for major surgery or in a newborn with moderate cardiopulmonary disease, while transfusion for a hemoglobin <13 g/dL is indicated in a newborn with severe cardiopulmonary disease. It is also recommended that platelets be kept above 50,000 for invasive procedures. These recommendations are based on expert consensus, not prospective studies.

The hemoglobin in transfused blood is hemoglobin A, as opposed to the hemoglobin F in the neonate at birth. An advantage of the transfused blood is better release of oxygen at the tissue level from hemoglobin A. Fresh blood cells have the advantage of lower potassium levels, especially during rapid transfusion, than older blood, although washed or frozen cells prevent this problem. Transfusion-associated graft-versus-host disease is a rare but potentially deadly complication of red blood cell transfusion. Transfused lymphocytes in the donor blood attack the recipient bone marrow and other tissues, causing fever, pancytopenia, diarrhea, and hepatitis. To prevent this, gamma irradiation of cellular blood components is used to destroy lymphocytes and prevent transfusion-associated graft-versus-host disease. For this reason, irradiated blood is routinely used for transfusion of preterm newborns and, in many centers, for all newborns under 6 months of age. Leukoreduction by filtration is also used to reduce cytomegalic virus transmission. Lastly, because there is very weak expression of the ABO antigens at birth, ABO typing, Rh typing, and an initial antibody screen are commonly done, although cross-matching is not.

The Hepatic System

The functional capacity of the liver is immature in the newborn, especially synthetic and metabolic functions. Although most enzyme systems for both normal function and drug metabolism are present at birth, the systems have not yet been induced.[22] In utero, the maternal circulation and metabolism were responsible for the majority of elimination of drugs. As the newborn develops, the different hepatic metabolic pathways mature at different rates. Conjugation by sulfation and acetylation are relatively well developed in the newborn, with conjugation with glutathione and glucuronidation less well-developed.[23] Some of these pathways do not achieve adult levels of activity until after 1 year of age.[24,25] Because of this immaturity, some drugs that undergo hepatic biotransformation, such as morphine, have prolonged elimination half-lives in newborns.[26] Other drugs, such as lidocaine, do not undergo prolonged elimination in the newborn. In some drugs, such as caffeine, the lack of hepatic metabolism of the drug is balanced by excretion of an increased amount of unchanged drug through the kidney. Up to 85% of unmetabolized caffeine may be found in the urine in the newborn, compared with 1% in the adult.[27]

Lastly, decreased metabolism of a drug may actually increase its safety profile. Acetaminophen undergoes less biotransformation by the cytochrome P450 system in the newborn, producing less reactive metabolites that are toxic. Paradoxically, neonates can tolerate dosages of acetaminophen that would be hepatotoxic in adults.[28,29] Synthetic function of the liver is also altered in the neonatal period. Levels of albumin and other proteins necessary for binding of drugs are low in term newborns (and are even lower in preterm infants) and impacts the ability to bind drugs, producing greater levels of free drug. This phenomenon is especially true for the binding of alkaline drugs that bind to α_1—acid glycoprotein such as synthetic opioids and local anesthetics. The ability to bind to existing albumin may also be altered by hyperbilirubinemia for some medications. The need for exogenous vitamin K in the newborn is another consequence of this decrease ability. Because of decreased synthetic function, neonatal hepatic glycogen stores are low, especially in the preterm, increasing the risk of hypoglycemia in response to stress.

Anatomy of the Neonatal Airway

The anatomic and maturational factors unique to the neonatal airway are important to understand in order to effectively manage the airway (Fig. 41-6). Although previous thinking suggested that all neonates, especially preterm babies, are *obligate* nasal breathers, the majority of neonates are actually *preferential* nose breathers.[30] Anything that obstructs the nares can compromise the neonate's ability to breathe.[31] For this reason, bilateral choanal atresia of the nasopharynx can be a life-threatening surgical problem for the neonate, and the airway needs to be secured or the atresia opened to ensure adequate ventilation. The large tongue occupies relatively more space in the infant's oropharynx, promoting both soft tissue obstruction of the upper airway and increasing the difficulty of direct laryngoscopic examination and intubation of the infant's trachea. 4 In the normal adult, the glottis is at the level of C5–C6. In the full-term infant, the glottis is at the level of C4, and in the premature infant, it is at the level of C3. The combination of a large tongue and a relatively high glottis means that on laryngoscopic examination it is more difficult to establish a direct line of vision between the mouth and the larynx; there is relatively more tissue in less distance. Therefore, the infant's larynx appears to be "anterior," although the true description is cephalad. The epiglottis is omega- or tubular-shaped, with a stubby base and thick and bulky aryepiglottic folds, making it difficult to fix with laryngoscope blade. Because the tip of the epiglottis lies at C1, the close apposition with the soft palate allows the newborn to simultaneously suckle and breathe, and contributes to the preferential nasal breathing found in the neonate. The vocal cords are anterior-slanting, making visualization more difficult, but also occasionally providing some obstruction to the passage of the endotracheal tube. This phenomenon is especially true with either nasal or "blind" intubation attempts because the bevel of the blade may hang up in the anterior commissure of the angulated vocal cords instead of easily passing into the subglottic larynx.

The subglottic area is funnel-shaped, unlike the adult airway (Fig. 41-7). In adults, the narrowest aspect of the upper airway is at the vocal cords, but in the neonate there is further narrowing until the level of the cricoid ring, the first complete cartilaginous ring. Because this narrowing is susceptible to trauma from intubation or too large an endotracheal tube, uncuffed tubes have traditionally been used in the neonatal period, although cuffed tubes are increasingly popular beyond the first few months of life. The use of cuffed, small volume, high resistance endotracheal tubes have been demonstrated to provide an adequate airway with marginal changes to the diameter of the airway leading most practitioners

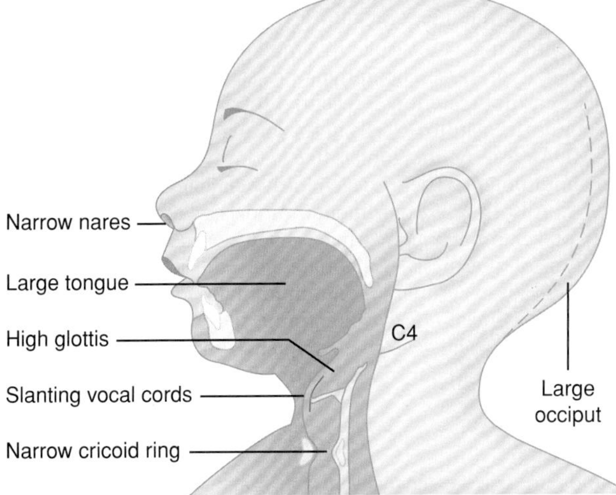

FIGURE 41-6. Complicating anatomic factors in infants. (Modified from: Smith RM. *Anesthesia for Infants and Children,* 4th ed. St Louis: Mosby; 1980:16, with permission.)

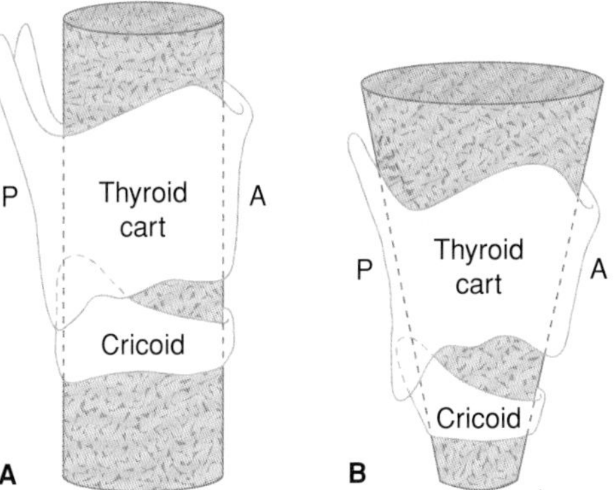

FIGURE 41-7. Configuration of the adult **(A)** versus the infant **(B)** larynx. The adult larynx has a cylindrical shape. The infant larynx is funnel-shaped because of the narrow, undeveloped cricoid cartilage. A, Anterior; P, posterior. (Reprinted from: The pediatric airway, In: Ryan JF, Coté CJ, Todres ID, eds. *A Practice of Anesthesia for Infants and Children,* 2nd ed. Orlando, FL: Grune & Stratton; 1992:61, with permission.)

to now use a cuffed tube in even neonates and young infants.[32] A narrow cricoid ring is significant because it means that the narrowest portion of the neonate's airway is not the vocal cords but the cricoid ring, this has to be kept in mind especially if an attempt to push an endotracheal tube after entrance to the glottis is considered.

Finally, the infant has a large occiput so the head flexes forward onto the chest when the infant is lying supine with his head in the midline. Further flexion of the neck can cause obstruction. Extreme extension can also obstruct the airway, so a midposition of the head with slight extension is preferred for airway maintenance. Rarely, this may require placing a small roll at the base of the neck and shoulders.

Anesthetic Drugs in Neonates

The pharmacokinetics of drugs in neonates are different than
5 in older children and adults. Factors affecting the metabolism of drugs in neonates include a larger volume of distribution, decreased protein binding, and decreased fat stores and immature renal and hepatic function. These physiologic changes alter the amount of drugs used in neonates.

- Volume of distribution. Water is predominantly in greater proportion in premature and full-term infants,[33] which increases the need for larger doses of medications that are water-soluble.
- Protein binding. Neonates have decreased protein and hence have a decrease in protein binding of most drugs. This leads to increased free drug levels, which leads to increased toxicity of drugs that are predominantly protein bound.[34]
- Fat content. Neonates have a decreased amount of fat and muscle mass, which leads to greater levels of drugs that are primarily redistributed to muscle and fat. Decreased renal and hepatic function predisposes neonates to increased blood levels from normal doses that are used for induction and maintenance of anesthesia.

Intravenous Agents

Anticholinergics

Anticholinergics such as atropine and glycopyrrolate are used frequently in neonates. They may be helpful in decreasing secretions and decreasing the response to vagal stimulation on intubation. The dose of atropine is 10 μg/kg given intravenously and 20 μg/kg if given intramuscularly. It may be desirable intramuscularly in certain situations prior to induction of anesthesia, especially in emergency surgeries. Caution should be exercised if neonates have other associated congenital abnormalities, particularly narrow angle glaucoma in which case it could increase intraocular pressure. Glycopyrrolate, a synthetic quaternary ammonium compound, has a longer duration of action than atropine and may potentially have less central effects because of decreased penetration of the blood–brain barrier.

Midazolam

This is a water-soluble benzodiazepine that can be used for premedicating infants prior to surgery. Clearance of midazolam is lower in neonates and premature infants, and hence caution has to be exercised with the amount of midazolam used. If combined with opioids, intravenous midazolam can cause severe hypotension. A common modality for midazolam administration in neonatal intensive care units is by continuous infusion. If a patient is receiving midazolam infusion, care should be taken to avoid large doses of opioids. Our recommendation is to stop midazolam during surgery, although it is recommended to resume the infusion after surgery to avoid withdrawal symptoms.

Sedative/Hypnotics

The common sedative/hypnotics used in neonates include propofol, thiopental, and ketamine.

Thiopental

Because of the large volume of distribution in neonates, it may be necessary to use large doses of thiopental for induction of anesthesia. There has been an acute shortage of thiopental for induction of anesthesia and hence is now rarely used in North America. However, because of their reduced clearance, the effect may last longer than anticipated. Thiopental can cause hypotension in neonates who are volume depleted, especially in infants who are scheduled for emergency surgery. It should be avoided in neonates with congenital heart disease because of its effect on myocardial function leading to hypotension. A dose of 2 to 4 mg/kg is usually well tolerated by most neonates for induction of anesthesia. When compared with intubation without any hypnotic, the use of intravenous thiopental demonstrated adequate maintenance of heart rate and blood pressure.[35]

Propofol

Propofol, a phenyl sedative/hypnotic, is a commonly used induction agent in infants and children. In a randomized trial comparing intravenous propofol with atropine, succinylcholine, and morphine, it was noted that propofol maintained adequate hemodynamics in neonates.[36] There is variability in elimination of propofol in neonates and preterm infants with longer elimination times.[37] Hence, while using propofol, it is important to reduce the dose to ensure early wake up and extubation. This is the most common intravenous induction agent that is used in the United States.

Ketamine

Ketamine, an *N*-methyl-D-aspartic acid (NMDA) antagonist, is used for induction of anesthesia in neonates who may have cardiovascular instability. An induction dose of 2 mg/kg intravenously with a higher dose of 4 to 5 mg/kg is used intramuscularly. Although it produces hemodynamic stability, it can cause an increase in oral secretions. Recently, there have been significant alterations in excitotoxic cells in the animal model when exposed to NMDA receptor antagonists like ketamine with resultant concern about potential neurodegenerative changes with their exposure.[38,39] All of these experimental models were using very high doses of ketamine unlike what is routinely recommended for induction of anesthesia in neonates. In addition, there are also another set of experimental data in animal studies that demonstrated a beneficial effect of ketamine in an experimental pain model.[40] Ketamine is still used frequently in neonates with congenital heart disease for induction of anesthesia.[41]

Opioids

Opioids are used extensively in the management of anesthesia in neonates. The advantage of using opioids is their ability to maintain cardiovascular stability during major surgery. The common opioids used in neonates include fentanyl, morphine, and remifentanil. Infants who are on long-term doses of opioids may develop tolerance and may have to be placed on methadone, a longer-acting opioid.[42]

Fentanyl

This synthetic opioid is commonly used for sedation in the neonate in the intensive care unit as well as in the operating room. A dose of 2 to 4 μg/kg/hr can maintain hemodynamic stability in these infants during surgery. The pharmacokinetics of fentanyl have been well studied in newborns.[43] The use of fentanyl in association with benzodiazepines may lead to hypotension and hemodynamic instability.[44] Caution must be exercised when the combination is administered during the perioperative period. Fentanyl may result in respiratory depression even with small doses. Continuous infusions may predispose to respiratory depression more frequently than bolus doses.[45] Chest wall rigidity and glottic rigidity has been described with fentanyl.[46] Small doses, as little as 1 to 2 μg/kg, can result in significant chest wall rigidity, leading to desaturation and need for mechanical ventilation. There is no significant maturational change on the brain associated with fentanyl compared with morphine. Hence, the sensitivity to fentanyl will not significantly change as the infant matures significantly. Fentanyl still continues to be the mainstay in newborns for sedation and analgesia.

Morphine

The kinetics of morphine have been studied in newborns.[47] Premature babies have been shown to have decreased clearance. Morphine clearance (range, 0.8 to 6.5 mL/min/kg) correlated significantly with gestational age ($r = 0.60$; $p < 0.01$) and birth weight ($r = 0.55$; $p < 0.01$).[48] Because of decreased clearance, dosing in neonates, especially premature infants, should be adjusted to be provided every 6 hours to allow for clearance of the drug.[47] Morphine is used frequently in the intensive care unit for postoperative pain control. Morphine infusions in the perioperative period have resulted in minor prolongation of postoperative ventilation. However, the incidence of apnea or hypotension was not observed in neonates despite prolonged morphine infusions after successful extubation.[49] A large multicenter neonatal trial (NEOPAIN) demonstrated very little neurobehavioral changes associated with preemptive analgesia with morphine in neonates in the neonatal intensive care unit.[50]

Morphine is metabolized to morphine-3-glucoronide and morphine-6-glucoronide. Morphine-6-glucoronide predisposes to respiratory depression. The sensitivity to morphine-6-glucoronide increases with increase in age because of increased maturation of the neuronal receptors.[51] A minority of infants who are scheduled for surgery may have been on ECMO. Kinetics of morphine have been carefully studied in neonates undergoing ECMO and do not show significant variability.[52]

Remifentanil

Remifentanil is an ultra short-acting opioid that is metabolized by nonspecific esterases in plasma and tissues and has a half-life of <10 minutes. The pharmacokinetics of remifentanil in neonates are similar to that of older children.[53] Remifentanil is used for maintenance of anesthesia by avoiding volatile anesthetic agents. The use of remifentanil infusion facilitated tracheal extubation in infants in a randomized trial when compared with volatile agents.[54]

Methadone

Methadone is a long-acting opioid that is used in neonates and infants in neonatal intensive care units, particularly when withdrawal from opioids is suspected. The pharmacokinetics of methadone are being studied in neonates; however, published data is not available. The "black box" warning against the use in infants with prolonged QT intervals is real and infants on long-term methadone use should be carefully monitored with serial ECGs. However, it is used frequently in managing opioid tolerance.[42]

Neuromuscular Blocking Agents

Neuromuscular blocking agents (NMBAs) are frequently used during neonatal anesthesia to facilitate tracheal intubation, assist with controlled ventilation, relax abdominal musculature, and ensure immobility. Factors that influence the choice of agent include the time of onset, duration of action, cardiovascular effects, and mechanism of clearance/elimination.

Succinylcholine

Succinylcholine, the only depolarizing muscle relaxant available, has the most rapid onset time of all the NMBAs. Neonates and infants have a larger ECF volume, leading to a larger volume of distribution and an increased dose requirement compared with children and adults. Thus, the recommended intravenous dose of succinylcholine for neonates and infants is 3 mg/kg, compared with 2 mg/kg in children, with an onset time of 30 to 45 seconds and duration of 5 to 10 minutes. The recommended intramuscular dose of succinylcholine is 4 mg/kg, with an onset time of 3 to 4 minutes and duration of approximately 20 minutes. Caution should be exercised when administering a second dose of succinylcholine because this can lead to vagally mediated bradycardia or sinus arrest. Pretreatment with atropine is recommended.[55]

The more recent succinylcholine controversy has called into question the use of succinylcholine in boys younger than 8 years.[56] The reports of hyperkalemia with cardiac arrest in such children with unrecognized muscular dystrophy have led some clinicians to take the position that succinylcholine should not be used routinely for this group of patients. The occurrence of this problem is somewhere in the range of 1 in 250,000 anesthetics, with a mortality rate of 50%. Although a concern in young children, it is not a problem in the neonatal period. Succinylcholine is still recommended in rapid-sequence situations, potential difficult airway, or if there are airway emergencies with progressive desaturation. When it is evident that a neonatal airway is obstructed by laryngospasm or other reason and no progress is made in ventilation, intramuscular or intravenous succinylcholine should be administered. Hyperkalemia can be recognized by peaked T waves. However, the clinician may not see this particular electrocardiographic change because it occurs 2 to 3 minutes after drug administration, when the anesthesiologist is attending to the airway. The hyperkalemia interferes with conduction, leading to a bradycardia and, if severe enough, cardiac arrest. The drug of first choice is intravenous calcium, 10 mg/kg. The use of sodium bicarbonate, 1 mEq/kg, to treat any metabolic acidosis that may occur with arrest is also believed to be useful because alkalosis decreases hyperkalemia. At the same time, the patient should be hyperventilated to reduce the CO_2, thereby encouraging a respiratory alkalosis. If there is refractory hypotension, an option is to administer epinephrine 5 to 10 μg/kg. One of the actions of epinephrine is to stimulate the sodium–potassium pump and cause the potassium to re-enter the cell, thereby reducing the serum level. If there is no response at this dose level, it should be increased incrementally until there is a response. Lastly, magnesium has been described as a treatment for hyperkalemia because it also antagonizes the effects of hyperkalemia, as does calcium.

Nondepolarizing Agents

The neonate's neuromuscular junction is more sensitive to nondepolarizing muscle relaxants, and the neonate has a larger volume of distribution because of a large ECF volume.[57] These two effects tend to balance each other so, roughly speaking, the dose of a nondepolarizing muscle relaxant for an infant is similar to that for a child on a milligram per kilogram basis. The ongoing organ maturation, which continues during the neonatal period, has a tremendous impact on the metabolism and clearance of the nondepolarizing agents. As a result, there is considerable variability and unpredictability in the duration of action of these agents in the neonatal period. Dosing should be titrated to effect and, when possible, guided by monitoring neuromuscular function with a nerve stimulator.

Intermediate Nondepolarizing Agents

Rocuronium

Rocuronium appears to be the drug of choice among the intermediate-acting, nondepolarizing muscle relaxants for neonates. The intubating dose of rocuronium is 0.6 mg/kg. The length of action of rocuronium in the neonate is similar to that in the older infant or child following an equipotent dose.[58] Smaller doses (0.45 mg/kg) have been demonstrated to provide adequate relaxation but predictable recovery in newborn infants. However, if a larger dose of rocuronium, 1 to 1.2 mg/kg, is administered to avoid using succinylcholine during a rapid-sequence induction, then rocuronium will be a relatively long-acting muscle relaxant. Rocuronium is metabolized by the liver; however, unlike vecuronium there are no active metabolites. Rocuronium has mild vagolytic properties and may slightly increase heart rate.

Vecuronium

Although vecuronium is considered an intermediate-acting muscle relaxant in children and adults, in infants younger than 1 year it is considered a long-acting muscle relaxant. The duration of action of vecuronium is approximately twice that observed in children because of liver immaturity.[59] Vecuronium undergoes primarily hepatic metabolism with production of active metabolites that are dependent on renal excretion. The recommended dose of vecuronium is 0.1 to 0.15 mg/kg, with an onset time of 90 seconds and duration of action of 60 to 90 minutes in the neonate. Even with increased doses, vecuronium has no effect on the cardiovascular system.

Pancuronium

Pancuronium is a long-acting NMBA with a pharmacokinetic profile similar to vecuronium. The recommended dose of 0.1 to 0.15 mg/kg has an onset time of 120 seconds and duration of 60 to 75 minutes. Unlike vecuronium, however, pancuronium primarily undergoes renal excretion.[60] Pancuronium has vagolytic and sympathomimetic actions that cause tachycardia and an increase in blood pressure.[61] In a relatively normal neonate with a normal blood pressure and normal blood volume, the use of pancuronium may result in hypertension, which has the potential to increase blood loss and increase the risk of hemorrhage in the extremely premature neonate. The risk for prolonged neuromuscular blockade in neonates, especially with altered renal function, makes pancuronium less desirable in neonates and infants undergoing minor outpatient surgical procedures.[62] The use of pancuronium for prolonged durations especially in the intensive care units can lead to muscle weakness. Prolonged use has also been associated with sensorineural hearing loss in infants.[63]

Reversal Agents

The unpredictable nature of the NMBAs in the neonatal population, as well as the inability to accurately assess neuromuscular function in many situations, necessitates reversal of all nondepolarizing NMBA in neonates. The two commonly used reversal agents are edrophonium and neostigmine. Edrophonium in a dose of 1 mg/kg achieves a 90% reversal of a neuromuscular block in 2 minutes, whereas neostigmine in a dose of 0.07 mg/kg requires 10 minutes for a 90% reversal of neuromuscular block. This difference in time to peak effect allows the anesthesiologist to decide which agent is needed. Anticholinergic drugs like atropine or glycopyrrolate is coadministered to decrease the incidence of bradycardia. Neostigmine is the most common agent used for reversal of nondepolarizing muscle relaxants in neonates. The advantages of edrophonium over neostigmine are a more rapid reversal and fewer muscarinic side effects.

Volatile Agents

Volatile agents are used for maintenance of anesthesia in the neonatal period. Although halothane was the most commonly used volatile agent for many years and had a reasonable safety profile, the introduction of sevoflurane has clearly made a difference to the use of volatile agents in neonates. Desflurane, another potent volatile agent has limited application in children. Isoflurane is used for maintenance of anesthesia for longer surgical procedures. A brief synopsis of halothane followed by a more detailed description of sevoflurane will be described in this chapter.

Halothane

Halothane is still commonly used in many parts of the world as the primary inhaled anesthetic, although it is not currently used in the United States. Its long history for induction of anesthesia and its ease of use still make it a desirable agent in children. Halothane has a weak muscle relaxant property, facilitating induction and intubation without the use of a muscle relaxant. Halothane is a potent bronchodilator and may reduce the airway reflexes associated with intubation. The use of high doses of halothane for procedures including bronchoscopic evaluation of the airway may lead to significant myocardial depression and pump failure.[64] Infants <8 weeks old and with a history of RDS with longer period of preoperative fasting are prone to hypotension. Halothane also sensitizes the myocardium to cardiac dysrhythmias. Animal experiments demonstrate the increased sensitivity to epinephrine with halothane when compared with isoflurane or sevoflurane.[65] Hence, when concurrent exogenous catecholamines are administered (including epinephrine in local anesthetic solution), careful attention to the maximum dose should be carefully monitored. With the advent of sevoflurane, the use of halothane has decreased significantly in North America.

Isoflurane

Isoflurane has become a common maintenance volatile agent in neonates and infants. Its pungent odor does not allow its use for mask induction. Isoflurane increases the heart rate and hence may predispose to cardiac dysrhythmias. It has a greater effect in potentiation of muscle relaxation and hence plays an important role as a maintenance anesthetic. It is important to remember that the dose of muscle relaxants has to be reduced when isoflurane anesthesia is used. The dose of rocuronium bromide may have to be reduced to 0.45 mg/kg compared with a normal maintenance dose of 0.6 mg/kg.[58] Isoflurane has less myocardial depression when compared with halothane in neonates.[66]

Sevoflurane

This is the newer volatile agent that offers an advantage for rapid induction and rapid awakening. It has a less pungent smell than isoflurane. Its pharmacodynamics have been studied in neonates and children with a fairly reasonable safety profile.[67] In children with congenial cardiac disease, it has been shown to produce fewer hemodynamic changes when compared with isoflurane.[68] Although it produces less myocardial depression, it has a greater effect on respiratory depression compared with halothane. Minute ventilation and respiratory frequency were significantly lower during sevoflurane than halothane anesthesia (4.5 compared with 5.4 $L/m^2/min$, and 37.5 compared with 46.7 breaths per minute, respectively, $p < 0.05$). There was also significantly less thoracoabdominal asynchrony during sevoflurane anesthesia.[69]

Desflurane

Desflurane was touted to be the best volatile agent in children because of its partition coefficient being close to that of nitrous oxide, thereby allowing a rapid uptake. However, the pungent nature of the drug has made it difficult to use it for induction of anesthesia.[70] When compared with sevoflurane, infants who were preterm were noted to wake up sooner with desflurane, although there were no reductions in postoperative respiratory events.[71]

Local Anesthetic Solutions

Local anesthetic solutions are represented by two main classes, the amino-amides (amides) and the amino-esters (esters). The main difference between the two classes is that the amides undergo enzymatic degradation by the liver and the esters are hydrolyzed by plasma cholinesterases.[72]

Amides

These are commonly used local anesthetic solutions in neonates and infants. Local anesthetics used in common clinical practice belonging to this class include lidocaine, bupivacaine, ropivacaine and, more recently, levobupivacaine. The main characteristics differentiating these drugs are their speed of onset, duration of action, and potential for cardiac toxicity. The ability of neonatal liver enzymes to metabolize and their ability to oxidize and reduce these drugs are decreased when compared with adults.[33,73] At approximately 3 months of age, the conjugation of these drugs in the liver reaches adult levels. Older children can also achieve higher levels of local anesthetic solution than adults because of alteration in pharmacokinetics of the drugs. Local anesthetic solution levels have been shown to be higher in children undergoing intercostal nerve blocks compared with adults.[74] After caudal administration of local anesthetics, peak plasma level is obtained in children and adults in approximately 30 minutes.[75] The steady-state volume of distribution (Vd_{SS}) for amides is increased in children compared with adults, although clearance (CL) is similar.[75] Elimination half-life ($t_{1/2}$) is related to the volume of distribution and clearance as follows: $t_{1/2} = (0.693 \times Vd_{SS})/CL$. This results in a larger Vd_{SS} and prolongation of the elimination half-life, especially if a continuous infusion is used. The systemic absorption of local anesthetics is often based on the site of injection. On a decreasing scale, the incidence of complications with local anesthetic solution injections decrease, with the highest concentrations seen in the intercostal area followed by the caudal space, the epidural space, and peripheral nerve blocks. With newer technique in regional anesthesia, including ultrasound guidance, the volume and dose of local anesthetic solution can be significantly reduced.[76]

Toxicity of Local Anesthetic Solutions

Local anesthetic toxicity includes cardiac toxicity, central nervous system (CNS) toxicity, local reactions, and allergic reactions. Amide local anesthetic solutions may have a greater cardiac depressing effect than ester local anesthetic solution. Common local anesthetic compounds used in the neonatal and infant period include amide local anesthetics such as lidocaine, bupivacaine, ropivacaine, and levobupivacaine, and ester local anesthetics such as chloroprocaine. A brief description of each of these agents in children is provided here.

Bupivacaine

Bupivacaine is the most commonly used local anesthetic solution in infants and children in North America. The pharmacokinetics and the pharmacodynamics have been well studied in infants and children.[77] The concentration of the local anesthetic used depends on the site, the desired density of blockade (motor and sensory), postoperative "street readiness," and the potential for cardiovascular and neurotoxicity. The concomitant use of other local anesthetics including infiltration anesthesia has to be taken into consideration before a total volume of local anesthetic solution is taken into consideration. This is especially true in neonatal surgery in which large quantities of local anesthetic solution can sometimes be injected for skin infiltration. If upper safe limits are likely to be approached, it is reasonable to avoid local anesthetic solution for infiltration and use a dilute epinephrine solution instead. The preferred concentration for peripheral nerve blockade is 0.25% bupivacaine or 0.2% ropivacaine, and the preferred concentration for single dose bolus doses is 0.25% or 0.125% solution of bupivacaine or 0.2% ropivacaine. When a continuous infusion is desired, a 0.1% or 0.125% solution of bupivacaine is preferred. In premature infants and in infants weighing under 1 kg, we prefer using 0.0625% bupivacaine, or in some cases bolus doses given every 12 hours. Although clear guidelines do not exist for local anesthetic solutions, a rough rule of thumb is to use 0.2 mg/kg/hr for continuous infusions of bupivacaine and 2 mg/kg for bolus doses.[78]

Metabolism

Bupivacaine is bound to α_1-glycoprotein. This may be altered in the newborn period.[79] It is a racemic mixture of the levo and dextro enantiomers. Although the levo enantiomer is the active form that provides the clinical effect of the local anesthetic solution, the dextro enantiomer is responsible for the adverse effects related to local anesthesia, including cardiac toxicity and neurotoxicity.

Toxicity

The major adverse effect of bupivacaine is toxicity related to the cardiovascular and the CNS. Local anesthetics have the ability to cross the blood–brain barrier and can cause alterations in the CNS functions. Continuous infusions in neonates can predispose them to CNS toxicity sooner than older infants.[80] In pediatric patients, the incidence of cardiac toxicity occurs sooner than neurotoxicity,[80] which may be partly because children may be anesthetized and devastating neurotoxicity may not be noticed until significant cardiac toxicity is seen. Manifestation of bupivacaine toxicity may also be affected by the concomitant use of volatile agents for general anesthesia.

DOSAGE. Bupivacaine can be used for most peripheral nerve blocks as well as for epidural and caudal infusions in infants and children. The maximum dosage suggested for bolus injections in the caudal space or epidural space for older children is 4 mg/kg and 2 mg/kg for neonates and infants.[78] Dosage recommendations for continuous infusions is 0.4 mg/kg/hr in older children and 0.2 mg/kg/hr in neonates and infants.[22] The concentration of the solution used for peripheral nerve blocks is usually 0.25% or 0.5%, bearing in mind the ceiling limit for maximum dosage. An example of a continuous infusion in a 4-kg neonate will be 0.2 mg/kg/hr; this will be equivalent to 0.8 mL/hr of a 0.1% solution of bupivacaine (1 mg/mL of bupivacaine).

Ropivacaine

Ropivacaine is a newer amide local anesthetic. It is a levo enantiomer with relatively less cardiovascular and CNS side effects compared with bupivacaine.[81] The pharmacokinetics of ropivacaine are such that caudal blocks with ropivacaine (2 mg/kg) in children (aged 1 to 8 years) result in plasma concentrations of ropivacaine well below toxic levels in adults.[81] This dose was also noted to produce less motor block, but provide adequate analgesia. Mean maximum plasma concentration of total ropivacaine at 2 mg/kg was 0.47 mg/L. A threshold of CNS toxicity was noted at a plasma concentration of 0.6 mg/L. Body weight-adjusted clearance was the same as in adults (5 mL/min/kg). Ropivacaine clearance depends on the unbound fraction of ropivacaine rather than the liver blood flow.

TOXICITY. Although the safety of ropivacaine has been demonstrated in animal experiments, there have been reports of CNS toxicity and cardiac toxicity associated with the use of epidural ropivacaine. It is important to understand that an overdose of ropivacaine can cause toxicity, making close attention to dosage as important with ropivacaine as with other local anesthetics. Our recommended dose is bolus dose of 2 mg/kg and an infusion rate of 0.2 mg/kg/hr.

Levobupivacaine

Levobupivacaine is a newer levo enantiomer that has fewer adverse effects than bupivacaine.[82] There are fewer pediatric trials available in literature. Because of the common use of bupivacaine in children and its low incidence of complications, levobupivacaine is not used abundantly in general pediatric anesthesiology practice. It is currently not available for use in the United States, although it is widely used in other parts of the world.

TOXICITY. Levobupivacaine, in the animal model, has been shown to have less cardiac toxicity with lower degree of myocardial depression than bupivacaine.[83]

Esters

Ester local anesthetics are metabolized by plasma cholinesterases.[84] As a result, in populations with lower pseudocholinesterases as in neonates, we see an increase in the duration of local anesthetic activity. This includes infants and neonates particularly. The duration of action of the drug is limited; hence, a continuous infusion of chloroprocaine is recommended.

Toxicity

Toxicity is based on the absence of pseudocholinesterase in the neonate.

Dosing

After a bolus dose of 1 mL/kg, a continuous infusion of chloroprocaine at 0.3 mL/kg of a 3% 2-chloroprocaine is recommended to achieve a level of T4 to T2.[85] This will be effective in producing complete surgical anesthesia for neonates undergoing hernia repair. Although the drug is not commonly used in pediatric practice, the advantage of its use is the capacity to provide complete motor block that is not prolonged.

Management of Local Anesthetic Toxicity

Lipid emulsion therapy has been demonstrated to reverse the effects of local anesthetic toxicity in experimental animal models.[86] Its effect on human models was parlayed in a case report where lipid was used as a last resort to reverse the effects of bupivacaine following a regional anesthesia technique.[87] Lipid should be readily available if local anesthesia is being used in infants. More recently an infant receiving a caudal block which resulted in cardiac toxicity was treated successfully with lipid rescue.[88]

Topical Anesthesia

Several local anesthetic preparations are now available for topical use. The most common local anesthetic preparations for topical use include lidocaine, tetracaine, benzocaine, and prilocaine. When these are applied to skin they produce effective but relatively short duration of analgesia. A topical anesthetic formulation EMLA (eutectic mixture of local anesthetic) is a mixture of lidocaine 2.5% and prilocaine 2.5%[89] and is used extensively for topical anesthesia in neonates, particularly for circumcision and venipunctures. The preparation has to be applied under an occlusive bandage for 45 to 60 minutes to obtain effective cutaneous analgesia. Although the incidence of methemoglobinemia from prilocaine is not very common in neonates, caution should be exercised when applying large doses of EMLA and caution should be exercised while applying large doses for procedures.[90]

Newer topical anesthetic solutions are now available that may offer a faster rate of onset. LMX-4, a 4% liposomal lidocaine solution can be used as topical anesthesia. There is no need for an occlusive dressing when LMX-4 is used, and it has the same efficacy as EMLA.[91,92] Liposome-encapsulated lidocaine or tetracaine has been shown to remain in the epidermis after topical application, affording a fast and lasting anesthetic effect.

ANESTHETIC MANAGEMENT OF THE NEONATE

Effective evaluation, preparation, and anesthetic management of the neonate depend on appropriate knowledge, clinical skills, and vigilance by the anesthesiologist. For safe and effective care, the anesthesiologist must take extraordinary care to understand the current status of the patient, the nature of the planned surgery, and the potential need for stabilization and preparation before surgery. After ensuring that the patient has been adequately prepared, the anesthesiologist needs to develop a detailed plan that encompasses the issues of anesthetic equipment and monitoring, airway management, drug choice, fluid management, temperature control, anticipated surgical needs, pain management, and postoperative care.

Studies have shown that morbidity and mortality related to anesthesia is higher in infants, especially neonates, compared with infants, older children, and adults.[93–96] There are probably several causes for this higher complication rate, including the emergent nature of most surgical procedures that are performed at this age, the physiologic instability of the neonate, the relative lack of experience most clinicians have with patients in this age range, and the technical challenges of monitoring and treating a very small patient. Because of the specialized nature of neonatal surgery and care, it is important that each institution that provides care to these patients have the resources of equipment, critical care facilities, nursing, laboratory, blood bank, and social work necessary to meet the needs of these patients and their families, as well as systems in place to guarantee a robust quality assurance emphasis on the provision of care. Both the American Academy of Pediatrics and the American Society of Anesthesiologists have provided guidance to many of the systems issues that should be addressed in institutions caring for these patients.[97] Physicians who agree to participate in this care need to have the preparation and ongoing experience needed to provide a consistent, high level of care.

In the distant past, concerns about physiologic instability and other challenges of caring for neonates led some practitioners to use minimal or no anesthesia for both minor and major procedures.[98–100] It is now widely recognized that neonates have stress responses similar to those of older patients, and the lack of adequate anesthetic care is as inhumane in the neonate as it is in the older child or adult.[101] Consequently, the same attention to adequate analgesia and anesthesia needs to be paid to the neonate as to other patients.

Preoperative Considerations

Preanesthetic Evaluation—History

The preanesthetic planning process starts with an evaluation of the course of intrauterine growth, followed by labor and delivery and the immediate postpartum course. The amount of history available to the anesthesiologist may vary widely. If the mother had received prepartum and postpartum care in the institution in which one is working, a significant amount of detail may be available. If the newborn is transferred from another institution, there may be limited information available. Best efforts should be made to get as much relevant information as possible, with an emphasis on maternal factors that may have affected fetal growth as well as the current status of the newborn. Additional history of the child's course since birth is important, with a particular focus on the signs that identified the surgical condition that is to be treated. Important factors include the history of feeding and hydration, need for oxygenation or ventilatory support, cardiovascular abnormalities and need for support, and any evidence of CNS problems such as seizures or intraventricular hemorrhage. Lastly, an estimation of the gestational status is made, with an emphasis on the issues of prematurity and intrauterine growth retardation with subsequent small-for-gestational age status.

The World Health Organization definition of prematurity is <37 weeks' gestation at birth. The determination of gestational age is based on the estimated date of full-term delivery, as well as physical examination of the newborn. Although these indicators are generally widely agreed on, they are subject to some degree of variation in interpretation. The greater the degree of prematurity, the more physiologic abnormalities will be expected. As one neonatologist explained, "Preterms obey no known law of physics" (Ogata E, personal communication, 2008). The implications for anesthesiologists are that the more preterm a newborn, the greater the variability of responsiveness to anesthetic agents, fluids, cardioactive drugs, and the stress of the surgical procedure.

In addition to prematurity, there is a second, related classification system. Low birth weight, defined as a birth weight of ≤2,500 g, can be due to prematurity, poor intrauterine growth, or both. Prematurity and intrauterine growth retardation are associated with increased neonatal morbidity and mortality, and it is difficult to completely separate factors associated with prematurity from those associated with intrauterine growth retardation. For discussion purposes, preterm infants are often divided into subgroups. Newborns born at 35 to 37 weeks' gestation are considered near term. These newborns have a lower incidence of major physiologic abnormalities typical of the more preterm newborn. Although they usually do not have significant pulmonary abnormalities, they may have some feeding problems or hyperbilirubinemia. This degree of prematurity does not usually have a significant impact on anesthetic management. However, infants born between 30 and 34 weeks' gestation are much more likely to show some abnormalities related to prematurity that can complicate anesthetic management.[102]

Although RDS used to be a significant source of morbidity in this population, the widespread use of exogenous surfactant has decreased the incidence dramatically, as well as the later complications of chronic lung disease. This group does have more problems with inadequate feeding, persistent patency of the ductus arteriosus, apnea in response to stress, and temperature instability. However, infants born more premature than this begin to demonstrate significant physiologic abnormalities related to prematurity. For infants with very low birth weight, defined as <1,500 g, the presence of complicating problems and morbidity and mortality are inversely related to birth weight. RDS is found in approximately 80% of infants weighing 501 to 750 g, in 65% of those 751 to 1,000 g, in 45% between 1,001 and 1,250 g, and in 25% between 1,251 and 1,500 g. In addition, symptomatic intraventricular hemorrhage is found in about 25% of infants weighing 501 to 750 g, in 12% between 751 and 1,000 g, in 8% between 1,001 and 1,250 g, and in 3% between 1,251 and 1,500 g. Other complications, such as sepsis, necrotizing enterocolitis (NEC), and bronchopulmonary dysplasia, are very high in infants with very low birth weight. Table 41-3 lists some of the most common abnormalities found in the preterm population that have implications for anesthetic evaluation, preparation, and management.

Preanesthetic Evaluation—Physical Examination

Physical examination of the newborn is focused by the condition requiring surgical intervention. Hydration is often an important issue because of both fasting and losses related to the surgical lesion. Clinical signs of dehydration include a sunken fontanelle, poor skin turgor, dry mucus membranes, sunken eyes, poor skin perfusion, delayed capillary refill, hypothermia, and a history of tachycardia or absent urine output. If there are clinical signs of dehydration, efforts should be made to correct the deficits before surgery, except in extreme, life-threatening situations. Physical examination also focuses on the respiratory and cardiovascular systems. The presence of any cardiovascular abnormalities should be noted, including poor perfusion or pulses, abnormal rhythm or rate, a murmur or gallop, hepatomegaly, or other signs of either heart failure or poor perfusion. The presence of a murmur is of concern in the neonatal period and warrants further evaluation, which is best done by a pediatric cardiologist. An electrocardiogram and echocardiogram will help define whether there is significant cardiovascular disease present that can affect the anesthetic management. Although this evaluation may take some effort and time, it is worthwhile to ensure that the anesthesiologist can plan the child's care with full knowledge of the limitations cardiovascular disease can impose.

TABLE 41-3. ABNORMALITIES ASSOCIATED WITH THE PRETERM—COMMON ANESTHETIC CONCERNS

Respiratory	Respiratory distress syndrome
	Apnea
	Pneumothorax, pneumomediastinum
	Pneumonia
	Pulmonary hemorrhage
	Bronchopulmonary dysplasia
Cardiovascular	Patent ductus arteriosus
	Hypotension
	Bradycardia
	Pulmonary hypertension
	Persistent transitional circulation
	Congenital heart disease
Central nervous system	Intraventricular hemorrhage
	Hypoxic–ischemic encephalopathy
	Seizures
	Kernicterus
	Drug withdrawal
Metabolic	Hypoglycemia
	Hyperglycemia
	Hypocalcemia
	Hypothermia
	Metabolic acidosis
Renal	Hyponatremia
	Hypernatremia
	Hyperkalemia
	Poor urine output
Gastrointestinal	Poor feeding
	Necrotizing enterocolitis
	Intestinal obstruction
Hematologic	Anemia
	Hyperbilirubinemia
	Vitamin K deficiency
Other	Retinopathy of prematurity
	Sepsis and infections

The respiratory system also must be examined in some detail. The presence of stridor or other evidence of airway obstruction, such as sternal or chest wall retractions, should be identified and investigated. Although upper airway obstruction is relatively rare in the newborn, laryngeal webs, cysts of the tongue or supraglottic region, vocal cord paralysis after a traumatic delivery, and hemangiomas of the airway can cause obstruction and need to be identified. In addition, newborns that have been previously intubated may have some degree of subglottic edema related to previous intubation. More likely are signs of lower airway disease such as tachypnea, grunting, rhonchi, retractions, and cyanosis. This may be related to the early development of RDS, but may also represent meconium aspiration, pneumonia, pneumothorax, or heart failure. The cause of any respiratory distress needs to be evaluated expeditiously prior to anesthesia to identify treatable causes and begin therapy.

Preanesthetic Evaluation—Laboratory

Most laboratory investigations are related to the underlying surgical condition such as radiologic investigations, computed tomography or magnetic resonance imaging studies, and echocardiography. However, most newborns will have, at a minimum, a blood count and glucose level drawn. The hemoglobin in a newborn is primarily fetal hemoglobin, which has a higher affinity for oxygen than adult hemoglobin. Because of this higher affinity, the hemoglobin dissociation curve is shifted to the left, releasing less oxygen to the tissues than adult hemoglobin. Newborns have a higher hemoglobin than the infant or child, often in the 15 to 18 g/dL range.[103] Rarely, a newborn will have significant polycythemia, with hemoglobin levels above 20 g/dL. If symptomatic, these patients may benefit from a lowering of the hemoglobin levels.

Glucose levels obtained close to the time of the proposed surgery are important. The stressed newborn, especially the stressed preterm or small-for-gestational age newborn, are at particular risk for hypoglycemia.[104] A glucose level between 60 and 80 mg/dL is expected in a full-term newborn, with a preterm often 10 mg/dL below that. Although there is some controversy about what actually constitutes hypoglycemia in these populations, most agree that levels <45 mg/dL warrant therapy with additional dextrose. Patients with diabetic mothers, those who have not been receiving either enteral or parenteral feeds, those who are very low birth weight, and those who have been septic are especially susceptible to hypoglycemia and require frequent monitoring and modification of parenteral fluids.

Other laboratory studies, such as electrolyte determinations and coagulation profiles, are indicated in specific patients. Hypocalcemia, in particular, can be troubling because signs of hypocalcemia are nonspecific. Unexplained hypotension, irritability, or even seizures can be presenting signs. Hypocalcemia is a problem with preterm newborns, but can also be seen in full-term newborns who have a delay in starting enteral feedings. Hyponatremia is not uncommon in newborns who have been receiving solutions with little or no salt in the first days of life, while hypernatremia may occur if there is inadequate resuscitation of the dehydrated patient when water loss is greater than salt loss. The longer a newborn has received parenteral fluids, the greater the chance of electrolyte abnormalities because of the difficulty in matching ongoing losses with replacement in the presence of an immature kidney.

Coagulation parameters are different in newborns compared with adults.[105] Although platelet counts in term newborns are usually similar to adult values, lower values are frequently seen in the preterm. Unexplained thrombocytopenia can be an early sign of sepsis, and a falling count should be an impetus to look for other signs of sepsis. Other coagulation tests are different in both the full-term and preterm newborn. The prothrombin time and partial thromboplastin time levels are about 10% longer in the newborn, but prothrombin time values approach adult levels in the first week of life and partial thromboplastin time levels within the first month of life.

Preanesthetic Plan

The anesthesiologist has a host of anesthetic techniques from which to choose and can tailor the anesthetic to the requirements of the surgery and the condition of the neonate. Major factors that should be considered in planning the anesthetic include (1) the need to have blood and blood products available before beginning the case, (2) the need for invasive monitoring, (3) the need for additional equipment for securing the airway or establishing vascular access, (4) the need to transport the child to and from the operating room, (5) the likelihood of postoperative ventilation, and (6) the plan for postoperative pain relief. Both the medical status of the patient and the planned surgical procedure will impact this planning. The anesthesiologist has the responsibility of clarifying any medical issues with the neonatologist before finalizing the plan, as well as clarifying any issues relates to the planned procedure with the surgeon. Occasionally, as planning progresses, it becomes obvious that the patient needs further medical resuscitation or evaluation before it is prudent to proceed with the procedure.

Once the anesthetic plan is clear, it should be discussed with the available parent or caregiver who has legal custody of the child. Informed consent is a process by which the anesthesiologist explains his/her understanding of the patient's status, the planned procedure, the plan for anesthetic management, alternatives to the plan, and some discussion of risks and benefits. Although there may be rare circumstances in which the legal guardian is not available to provide consent, efforts should be made in all except the most emergent of situations to have this discussion. It should be stressed that informed consent is a process, not a document. The goal of informed consent is to help the parent understand what care is being proposed, the risks and benefits involved, and reasonable alternatives. It is the discussion, in terms understandable to the parent, that is the basis of true informed consent.

Premedication

Premedication is not commonly used for neonatal anesthetics. Sedation is not usually appropriate, and analgesics are rarely indicated before taking the patient to the operating room. In the past, premedication with atropine was occasionally used, especially for older neonates, above a month of age, where an inhalation induction was considered. Because of the dominance of the parasympathetic nervous system, bradycardia on induction or in response to inhalation agents is of concern. There are some data that in the older neonate, the vagolytic activity of atropine does decrease the bradycardia and hypotension associated with volatile agents.[106,107] In older neonates, an inhalation agent may be the primary anesthetic for the case, making the addition of atropine useful. However, it is more common in neonates under a year of age to use opioids as the basis of the anesthetic, with lower doses of an inhalation agent titrated to effect. In this situation, atropine is less commonly indicated and can always be added intravenously as the anesthetic proceeds.

Intraoperative Considerations

Monitoring

Neonatal patients are at a disadvantage when it comes to perioperative monitoring because of their small size. Many of the monitoring modalities that are used in older children and adults are not available for the neonate. Examples of this include transesophageal echocardiography, pulmonary artery catheterization, and brain function monitoring. Other monitors that are used may occasionally not provide reliable information for technical reasons. Examples of this include neuromuscular blockade monitoring and automated blood pressure monitoring. Invasive monitoring such as arterial line and central venous line catheters may be technically difficult to insert, especially in the preterm. Consequently, the goal of monitoring should be to establish American Society of Anesthesiologists standard monitors of pulse oximetry, blood pressure, at the beginning of the case and add invasive monitoring, as appropriate.

Although physical observation of the patient is important in preanesthetic evaluation, it is difficult to use this monitor during a surgical procedure. Observation of the patient's color, capillary refill, warmth of skin, muscle tone, fullness of fontanelle, and chest expansion are useful monitors, but they are difficult to reliably observe once the patient is covered with surgical drapes. There is a large dependence on electronic monitors during the majority of the procedure. However, it should be remembered that heart and breath sounds heard through a precordial or esophageal stethoscope, the compliance determined during hand ventilation, the appearance of bleeding in the surgical field, and trends noted in the anesthetic record are all important observations that the anesthesiologist can use as part of the overall assessment of the patient.

Pulse oximetry is one of the most important monitors in neonatal anesthesia. Flexible probes designed for pediatric patients should be used. Placement is sometimes difficult because of the small fingers of the neonate. It may be necessary to place the probe across the web space between the thumb and the first finger, around the lateral aspect of the hand, or on the foot. Many anesthesiologists will place and check two pulse oximeter probes at the beginning of the case because of the clinical experience of having one probe malfunctioning secondary to changes in perfusion during the case. Because there may be differences in preductal and postductal saturations, probes on the left hand or either leg may give lower values than a probe on the right hand.[108] Especially in the first 2 weeks of life, there is a preponderance of fetal hemoglobin. The pulse oximeter does not compensate for the left shift of the hemoglobin desaturation curve, and pulse oximeter values read about 2% higher than arterial blood saturations.[109]

The hallmark of the pediatric anesthesiologist has been the precordial stethoscope. It has the advantages of being simple and effective in allowing continuous monitoring of heart rate, heart rhythm, strength of heart sounds, and breath sounds. A softening of heart sounds often is indicative of a drop in blood pressure. The esophageal stethoscope is more secure and less susceptible to external noise as the precordial stethoscope, while also providing the ability to measure core temperature. Although there has been recent skepticism about the usefulness of the stethoscope,[110] the stethoscope continues to be a quick, continuously available monitor that can be used to detect changes in both the circulatory and ventilatory status of the newborn.

The electrocardiograph is useful primarily to assess heart rate and rhythm. It is sometimes difficult to get the leads to adhere properly, but wiping the skin with alcohol before placement is often helpful. These leads, once applied, can bind tightly to skin, and care must be taken when removing them to avoid removal of skin, especially in the preterm. ST–T wave abnormalities may be an indicator of significant electrolyte disturbances, but abnormalities related to myocardial ischemia are not common in the perioperative period.

Blood pressure measurements are important in the management of all newborns. Noninvasive automated machines are commonly used, but it is important that a proper-sized cuff—one-half to two-thirds of the length of the upper arm—be used, and that the arterial indicator, adjacent to the exit of the hoses, be placed over the artery. The cuff should not be routinely cycled excessively, more than every 3 minutes, because of the danger of venous stasis, especially in preterms. In some cases, it is not possible to get reliable readings from an automated machine. An effective alternative is to use a manual cuff and place a Doppler probe over the brachial or radial artery. This system gives reliable systolic blood pressures over a very wide range; the Doppler probe can detect flow, even at very low blood pressures when the automated cuff may fail.

Direct arterial blood pressure monitoring offers the double advantage of accurate blood pressure readings and the ability to withdraw blood samples. A 22-gauge catheter is often used in full-term neonates and a 24-gauge catheter in preterms. A variety of sites can be used, including the radial, dorsalis pedal, and posterior tibial arteries. Less commonly, the brachial or femoral arteries are used. More recently, with the use of point of care ultrasonography, it is imperative that this measure be attempted before resorting to a cutdown using an invasive technique for access. Some patients may come to the operating room with an umbilical artery line in place. Although these can be used for monitoring, umbilical lines have both infectious and embolic risks, and may be in the way of the surgical field. All arterial lines should be flushed, either continuously or intermittently, with small amounts of heparinized saline, but caution should be used because even small amounts of flush can transmit significant pressure retrograde and cause embolic damage to the brain.

Central venous monitoring is occasionally used in neonatal surgery. Access to blood samples and central venous pressures can be especially useful in procedures, such as gastroschisis repair, in which there are anticipated large changes in both blood loss and third-space losses. Central catheters can also be used for the administration of blood, total parenteral nutrition, and cardioactive drug infusion. Insertion of these lines can be in a variety of sites, including the subclavian, internal jugular, femoral, or external jugular veins using special precautions to maintain sterile technique. The umbilical vein is not recommended as a site for central monitoring because of the risk of portal vein thrombosis. Percutaneous insertion may be assisted by ultrasound guidance. Central lines can be both challenging to insert, but also associated with significant complications related to infection, thrombosis, and emboli.[111] Meticulous technique with insertion and maintenance of the line will help minimize these complications. The use of ultrasound guidance is now routinely used in many US children's hospitals to provide a presumably safe and consistent method for gaining central venous access although a recent meta-analysis did not demonstrate any significant differences between groups.[112]

Although there may be some differential between capnography and arterial PCO_2 readings, the trend data are accurate and the shape of the waveform can give significant information about changes in ventilation, obstruction, and rebreathing. Airway pressure measurements are particularly useful in assessing changes in resistance or compliance. Although it has been traditional that hand ventilation was important in determining changes in airway and chest compliance, there is controversy about the reliability of the "feel of the hand on the bag."[113,114] Airway pressure measurements are also useful in adopting adult anesthesia ventilators for use in neonatal and pediatric patients, using peak airway pressures as a guide for setting tidal volume.[115]

Anesthetic Systems

There is a long tradition in pediatric anesthesia of using semi-open, nonrebreathing systems for general anesthesia in newborns.[116,117] Circuits such as the Jackson-Rees adaptation of the Ayre's T-piece and the Bain circuit have been the most commonly used in the United States.[118] These and related circuits have the advantage of lightweight, easy-to-open valves or lack of valves, rapid changes in anesthetic concentration, minimal work of breathing, and high circuit compliance. On the other hand, they require relatively high gas flows and require some modification for mechanical ventilation. These circuits were especially popular when spontaneous ventilation was more commonly used than it is now in neonatal patients. As the use of these circuits has diminished, familiarity with their use and application has dropped in favor of the semi-closed, rebreathing circle systems used in adult patients. There will be slower change in anesthetic concentration, less circuit compliance, and larger compression volume with these circuits, but they give the advantage of using the same circuit on patients of all ages.

Because the loss of both heat and humidity through the endotracheal tube is of concern in the neonate, the anesthetic circuit should incorporate features to minimize water and heat loss. In the past, heated vaporizers were added to the circuit for this purpose. However, there is a danger of patient absorption of water and fluid overload with their use, as well as concerns about overheating the patient or an airway burn. It is now common to use a combination of low gas flows[119] and a disposable, neonatal humidity and heat exchanger to the circuit, with warming of the gases and retention of some of the exhaled humidity.[120,121]

Lastly, the anesthesia machine used for anesthetizing neonates should have the capacity to administer medical air. There are two reasons for this. First, if nitrous oxide is contraindicated, such as in the newborn with bowel obstruction, air is mixed with oxygen to prevent the administration of only 100% oxygen. This is also used to minimize the risk of retinopathy of prematurity (ROP) by avoiding prolonged administration of 100% oxygen. Second, some patients, such as those with hypoplastic left heart syndrome, may benefit from the administration of air with additional oxygen. Without an air flowmeter in the system, this will not be possible.

Induction of Anesthesia

There is no one method of induction and maintenance of anesthesia that is best for all patients. The current medical status of the patient, the surgical condition, the presence of ongoing fluid or blood losses, the gestational age of the patient, recent fasting, and the experience of the anesthesiologist are all important considerations. Most neonates who come to the operating room will have vascular access already established; if not, the first task before induction is to establish adequate vascular access after applying monitors. Although it may rarely be appropriate to use an inhalational induction if vascular access is difficult in the older newborn, near a month of age, it is mandatory to establish access first in the newborn who is preterm, medically unstable, has a full stomach, has a potentially difficult airway, or has ongoing fluid losses.

Airway Management

Establishing the airway in the neonate requires an appreciation of the differences between the newborn and the adult airway, as discussed earlier. It is rare to administer anesthesia in the newborn period without establishing an artificial airway. Although, with meticulous technique, a mask airway can successfully be used for short periods of time, the tolerances of mask fit, adequate airway pressure, and avoidance of gastric distention are small, making this a poor choice for any but the briefest of operations. In addition, controlled ventilation is used more commonly today than spontaneous ventilation for surgical procedures, making an artificial airway necessary.

Awake intubation has been used to secure the airway without the danger of loss of airway during the procedure, but it can be a traumatic experience for both the patient and the anesthesiologist, accompanied by pain, breath holding, desaturation, and tissue trauma.[122] The desaturation associated with this technique can be ameliorated by using an oxyscope, a Miller laryngoscope blade that has a side channel to allow insufflation of oxygen during the procedure.[123,124] However, this technique is usually reserved for patients with severe hemodynamic compromise, an extraordinarily distended and tense abdomen, or a presumed

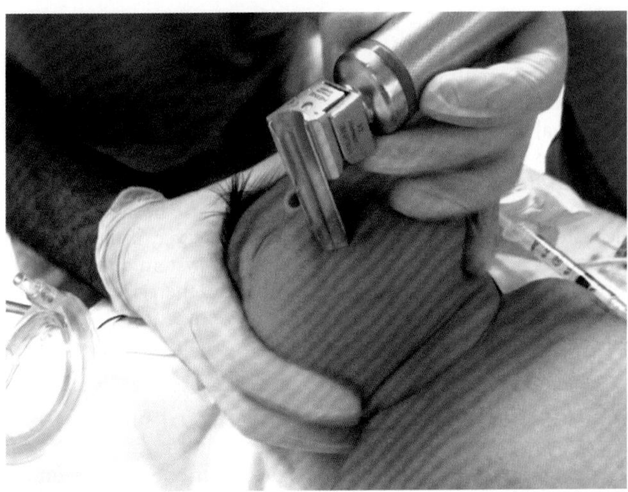

FIGURE 41-8. Insertion of Miller blade down the right side of the tongue. The blade is then turned and pressure is applied in the direction of the handle.

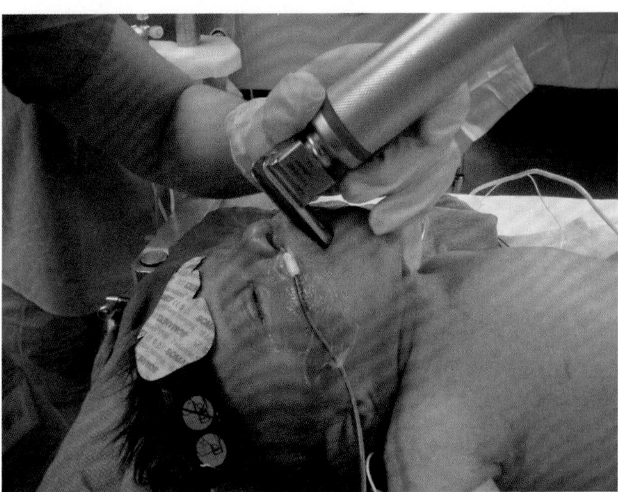

FIGURE 41-9. Cricoid pressure applied with little finger.

difficult airway, especially the newborn with micrognathia. In the latter situation, the addition of sedation with an opioid or topical application of local anesthetic can help decrease some of the trauma of the procedure. It has also been suggested that an awake intubation may be best for the anesthesiologist who is not very experienced in intubating newborns. It may be better to have a more experienced clinician, if available, attend to the airway in that situation.

Most newborns are intubated after a rapid-sequence induction. Preoxygenation is useful in adding additional safety to the procedure. Although there may be a minor concern about a period of hyperoxia in the preterm, there is no evidence that a short exposure such as preoxygenation will increase the risk of ROP. Agents for induction and muscle relaxation are discussed later. If there is concern about the difficulty of intubation, it may be prudent to induce anesthesia, ensure adequacy of mask ventilation, and then give the muscle relaxant.

Positioning for intubation is based on the known differences in the neonatal airway. Because of the large occiput of the head, the newborn already has a flexed neck. No changes in position are usually needed, although additional extension of the head may be accomplished by a shoulder roll. A Miller no. 1 blade is commonly used for the full-term newborn and a Miller no. 0 in the preterm, although there are other available blades that individual practitioners may prefer. Sliding the blade down the right side of the mouth allows the blade to be seated with minimal overlap by the tongue (Fig. 41-8). The tip of the blade is advanced to lift the epiglottis directly instead of placing it in the vallecula, as is commonly done with older patients. Every patient's anatomy is different, but if the laryngoscope is advanced in the direction parallel to the handle, one will get the best visualization. If the glottis is not easily seen, cricoid pressure can be applied with the little finger of the hand holding the handle or by an assistant, often improving the view (Fig. 41-9).

Uncuffed tubes have traditionally been used in newborns to minimize cuff pressure on the subglottic larynx, especially at the level of the cricoids. Although there has been interest in the use of cuffed tubes in newborns and infants,[125] most clinicians continue to use uncuffed tubes in newborns to maximize the internal diameter and gas flow characteristics for a given external diameter of tube. Although various formulas have been proposed for how far to advance an uncuffed tube, it is prudent to use the depth markers at the end of the tube to ensure under direct vision that the tip is advanced 2 or 3 cm past the vocal cords. A 3- or 3.5-mm internal diameter (ID) uncuffed tube is usually appropriate for a full-term newborn and a 2.5-mm ID tube is used in preterms, especially those under 1,500 g body weight. Once inserted, the presence of a positive capnograph tracing, bilateral expansion of the thorax, and bilateral breath sounds are used to ensure proper placement. Although some anesthesiologists prefer to advance the endotracheal tube past the carina and then withdraw until bilateral breath sounds are heard, there are two major disadvantages to the technique: Trauma to the airway and lack of a guarantee that the tip of the tube is not sitting right at the carina, increasing the chance of migration into a bronchus with head movement. Lastly, listen for an air leak at an airway pressure of about 20 cm H_2O to ensure that the tube is not too large for the airway, increasing the chances of subglottic edema and damage.

If intubation proves difficult, there are a variety of options. A laryngeal mask airway (LMA) can be used to provide ventilation in newborns as small as 1-kg body weight as preparations are made to use other intubating techniques.[126] It is possible to use the LMA as a guide for blind intubations in newborns with the use of a styletted tube.[127] The light wand can also be used in newborns,[128] and can be particularly useful in the newborn with micrognathia or retrognathia because of the ability to mold the wand to a "hockey stick" configuration with a sharp angle. Fiberoptic laryngoscopy, the most flexible of intubating pools routinely used in older children and adults, can also be used in the newborn. Fiberscopes are currently available that accept endotracheal tubes as small as 2.5-mm ID, although these scopes do not currently have the ability to change direction and are useful more for confirmation of tube placement. Fiberscopes that can actively change direction accept a 3.5-mm ID tube at the smallest. Insertion of the fiberscope can be done directly or through an LMA. An LMA as a conduit has been particularly useful in directly intubating newborns that could not be visualized by routine approaches.[129,130]

Lastly, an old technique that is used infrequently is digital intubation in which two fingers are advanced along the midline of the tongue and onto the epiglottis, with a styletted tube then advanced between the two fingers.[131] Once the airway is secured, ventilation is usually controlled during neonatal surgical procedures with hand ventilation or, more commonly, mechanical ventilation.[132] After establishing a baseline of acceptable ventilation, it is important to continuously monitor the peak airway pressures, chest expansion, return volume, pulse oximetry, and capnograph tracings for changes. Underlying pulmonary disease, a shift in the endotracheal tube, and surgical manipulation can be responsible for significant changes in compliance and ventilation. Initial tidal volumes of 10 mL/kg and rates of 20 to 25 breaths per minute are a reasonable starting point for most patients. With this rate and volume setting, it would be expected that peak airway pressures be approximately 20 cm H_2O. A level of positive end-expiratory pressure (PEEP) of 3 to 5 cm H_2O can be useful in preventing atelectasis. If the patient has significant pulmonary disease, he or she may require significantly higher volumes. The patient may have previously been ventilated in the neonatal intensive care unit with a ventilator modality not supported by the anesthesia ventilator. Consequently, parameters must be adjusted against physical examination and, if necessary, an arterial blood gas to ensure appropriate ventilation. If the patient has been dependent on special ventilator techniques such as high-frequency ventilation, oscillation, or nitric oxide inhalation, arrangements should be made to bring the needed equipment to the operating room and have a respiratory therapist or neonatologist who is familiar with the equipment assist in setup and, if necessary, troubleshooting.

Impact of Surgical Requirements on Anesthetic Technique

6 Every procedure has its own unique challenges. With any surgery, issues related to presurgical resuscitation, perioperative fluid and blood loss, heat loss from the surgical field, likely perioperative complications, and the likely need for postoperative intubation and ventilation should be anticipated, both on the basis of experience and communication about the unique needs of the upcoming procedure. There is a dramatic increase in the use of laparoscopic and thoracoscopic approaches to lesions, even in the smallest neonates. The considerations for these approaches are different from open procedures. There may be less blood, fluid, and heat loss, but there are additional issues related to positioning, insufflation pressures in the chest and abdomen, and prolonged surgical time. As new techniques evolve, close communication between the anesthesiologist and the surgeon is necessary to ensure adequate preparation and resolution of problems or complications.

Uptake and Distribution of Anesthetics in Neonates

Various reasons for the faster uptake of anesthetics in infants have been proposed: (1) the ratio of alveolar ventilation to FRC is 5:1 in the infant and 1.5:1 in the adult; (2) in the neonate, more of the cardiac output goes to the vessel-rich group of organs, which includes the heart and the brain; (3) the neonate has a greater cardiac output per kilogram of body mass; and (4) the infant has a lower blood gas partition coefficient for volatile anesthetics. One not well-recognized factor that may result in higher concentrations of volatile anesthetics being administered to infants has to do with the use of nonrebreathing systems such as the Bain or a Mapleson "D" circuit. When an adult circle system is used with infant tubes and bag, the clinician experienced with this equipment is used to reading the inspired, end-tidal, and dialed concentrations of the volatile anesthetic. In the circle system, the inspired concentration is a result of the combination of the end-tidal concentration that is rebreathed through the soda lime absorber and the dialed concentration. The inspired concentration is always lower than the dialed concentration, unless the flow rates are so high that a nonrebreathing system has been created. In the nonrebreathing system, the dialed concentration is the inspired concentration. Clinicians who use both systems are accustomed to these subtle differences. However, if the clinician switches back and forth between the circle system and a nonrebreathing circuit, but does so infrequently, there is a danger of not recognizing the possibility of excessive overpressure of volatile anesthetics with the nonrebreathing systems.

Anesthetic Dose Requirements of Neonates

Neonates and premature infants have lower anesthetic requirements than older infants and children.[33] The easiest way to remember the minimum alveolar concentration (MAC) values is that the MAC value in the mature state (i.e., late teenager or adult) is the same as for a full-term infant. By 6 months of age, the MAC value has increased by 50%. In the premature infant, the MAC value decreases by 20% to 30%.[34,35] The reasons for the lower MAC requirements are believed to be an immature nervous system, progesterone from the mother, and elevated blood levels of endorphins, coupled with an immature blood–brain barrier. The neonate has an immature CNS with attenuated responses to nociceptive cutaneous stimuli. These responses rapidly mature in the first several months of an infant's life, along with an increase in the MAC. Progesterone has been shown to reduce the MAC of the pregnant mother. The newborn infant has elevated progesterone levels, similar to those of the mother. Elevated levels of β-endorphin and β-lipotropin have been demonstrated in infants in the first few days of postnatal life. Endorphins do not cross the blood–brain barrier in adults; however, it is believed that the neonate's blood–brain barrier is more permeable and that endorphins might well pass into the CNS, thus elevating the pain threshold and reducing the MAC requirement.

Regional Anesthesia

There has been a tremendous increase in the use of regional anesthesia in infants and children. In general, regional techniques are combined with general anesthesia to permit early extubation and provide postoperative pain relief. Useful regional anesthesia techniques include spinal anesthesia, caudal anesthesia, epidural analgesia, penile block, and other peripheral nerve blocks (Table 41-4). Combined regional and general anesthesia is commonly provided for neonates for multiple procedures. The use of ultrasonography has revolutionized the use of regional anesthesia as vascular structures can be easily avoided while still providing a regional blockade.[133] It is important to remember that the dosage of local anesthetic solution used is limited and lipid solution is available to potentially treat any intravascular injections.[134] A dose of 1.5 mL/kg of intralipid has been suggested as a rescue dose for toxicity in children.

Spinal Anesthesia

Regional anesthesia can be provided as a sole anesthetic or in combination with general anesthesia. The use of sole regional anesthesia in neonates and infants is provided for the ex-premature infant with a potential for apnea. For patients receiving

TABLE 41-4. REGIONAL ANESTHESIA TECHNIQUES USEFUL IN NEONATES

Central neuraxial
Caudal
Epidural (lumbar, thoracic, caudal)
Spinal
Peripheral nerve blocks
Infraorbital block
Brachial plexus block (axillary, infraclavicular)
Lateral femoral cutaneous block
Penile block
Ilioinguinal block
TAP Block (transversus abdominis plane block)
Scalp blocks

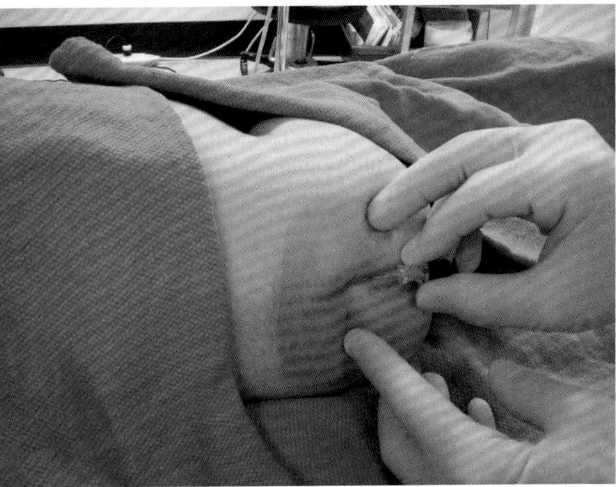

FIGURE 41-10. Caudal block. The sacral cornua are identified. A styletted needle is introduced into the caudal space through the sacral hiatus. A "pop" is felt as the sacrococcygeal ligament is accessed. After aspiration, 0.8 mL/kg of local anesthetic solution is injected. This provides analgesia for hernia repair, circumcisions, and lower abdominal surgeries.

combined general and regional anesthesia, early extubation is possible because the addition of regional anesthetic techniques eliminates the need for intraoperative narcotics in neonates, reduces or eliminates the need for muscle relaxants, and reduces the concentration of volatile agents needed for relaxation.[135] Spinal anesthesia has been reported to be effective when used as the sole anesthetic technique in premature and high-risk infants, but this technique requires excellent cooperation between the anesthesiologist and an experienced surgeon.[136] Although this is technically feasible, because of increasing advancements in general anesthesia techniques, we may be able to provide safer anesthesia with fewer complications.[137,138] Even at a dose of 0.5 to 1 mg/kg, the effects of tetracaine last only approximately 90 minutes in the neonate.

In the authors' experiences, patients have additionally benefited by providing a caudal block in addition to the spinal anesthetic and seem to have a longer duration of surgical anesthesia. Total spinal anesthesia, produced either with a primary spinal technique or secondary to an attempted epidural puncture, will present as respiratory insufficiency rather than as hypotension because of the lack of sympathetic tone in infants. The exact mechanism for the lack of cardiovascular change with spinal anesthesia in infants and young children is not clear. Consequently, the first indication of a high spinal is falling oxygen saturation rather than a falling blood pressure. Sedation can be added to regional anesthesia but may cause problems of apnea in ex-premature infants.[139]

Caudal Block

Caudal epidural block is frequently used for abdominal surgery in neonates and is probably the most commonly used regional anesthetic technique in neonates and infants. There are several different techniques described for performing a caudal block. The landmarks are the coccyx, the two sacral cornua, and the posterior superior iliac spines (Fig. 41-10). We prefer a styletted 22-gauge, short-bevel needle; the caudal space is identified both by the loss of resistance and the ease of administering the anesthetic. Once the sacrococcygeal membrane is penetrated and there is a loss of resistance, gentle aspiration is applied to the needle to determine if there is blood or cerebrospinal fluid. Injection of the anesthetic is then attempted. If there is difficulty in injecting the solution, the tip of the needle is not in the caudal space and it needs to be repositioned. If the anesthetic can be injected easily, this confirms placement in the epidural space. The needle is not advanced up the caudal canal after proper placement in the caudal epidural space has been accomplished. Other methods to identify the caudal space have been described, including stimulating technique[140] and ultrasound guidance.[141] Epinephrine is added to local anesthetic solutions for the purposes of determining if there is an intravascular injection of the anesthetic. Evidence of an intravascular injection includes (1) peaked T waves (which may be of relatively short duration, e.g., 30 seconds)[142] and (2) increase in heart rate. The other technique to minimize the potential difficulties of an intravascular injection is to fractionate the dose by dividing the dose into three aliquots and waiting approximately 20 to 30 seconds between each aliquot before continuing the injection. Caudal anesthesia is particularly effective at reducing the concentrations of volatile anesthetics needed, as well as relaxants and opioids. In addition, a single-injection caudal anesthetic can provide analgesia for 6 to 8 hours. The two local anesthetics currently in use are 0.125% bupivacaine or 0.2% ropivacaine. Epinephrine, 1:200,000, is added to local anesthetics to assist in determining if there has been an intravenous injection. Ropivacaine has been reported to be less cardiodepressant than equipotent doses of bupivacaine. Occasionally, we place a caudal catheter for providing continuous analgesia in the postoperative period. If a caudal catheter is placed, an infusion of ropivacaine or bupivacaine can be administered and provide analgesia for several days. Current recommendations for infusions in neonates and young infants are for an initial loading dose of 0.2 to 0.25 mg/kg; after 1 to 2 hours, an infusion can be begun in a dose of 0.2 mg/kg/hr.[78] The addition of clonidine, 1 to 2 μg/kg, to local anesthetic for caudal block has been used, although this has not shown to greatly increase the duration of analgesia.[143] Opioids can occasionally be used for epidural infusions. However, caution must be exercised in infants who may be prone to apnea with even moderate doses of opioids in the epidural space. Ultrasonography can be used for localization of the caudal space in infants whose anatomy may not be apparent.

Epidural Analgesia

With the introduction of newer and smaller needles and epidural catheters, we are now able to provide epidural analgesia in neonates and infants. Although most practitioners prefer using a caudal route to place catheters in the epidural space, we believe that with the introduction of ultrasound guidance, we are able to place lumbar catheters in neonates and infants easily.[144] It is imperative to limit the dose of local anesthetic solution in neonates and children to avoid toxicity.

Peripheral Nerve Blocks

Common peripheral nerve blocks in neonates include penile blocks, ilioinguinal nerve blocks, lateral femoral cutaneous blocks, transversus abdominis plane block (TAP), brachial plexus blocks, and head and neck blocks for neurosurgical procedures.

Penile Block

This is a relatively simple block that can be performed easily. The dorsal nerves of the penis are located on either side of the shaft of the penis. A ring block using a nonepinephrine-containing solution can be used to provide analgesia following circumcision.[145]

Ilioinguinal Nerve Block

The ilioinguinal and iliohypogastric nerves supply sensory innervation to the inguinal area. These nerves can be easily visualized while operating. However, we find that blockade of these nerves can provide adequate postoperative analgesia (Fig. 41-11). The anterior superior iliac spine is identified. Immediately medial to the anterior superior iliac spine, a needle is inserted toward the umbilicus and local anesthesia is fanned into the area. The advantage with the use of ultrasonography is the ability to significantly reduce the dose of local anesthesia.[76] In our practice, we routinely use ultrasonography to localize the ilioinguinal nerve, which is then blocked with minimal quantity of local anesthesia solution.

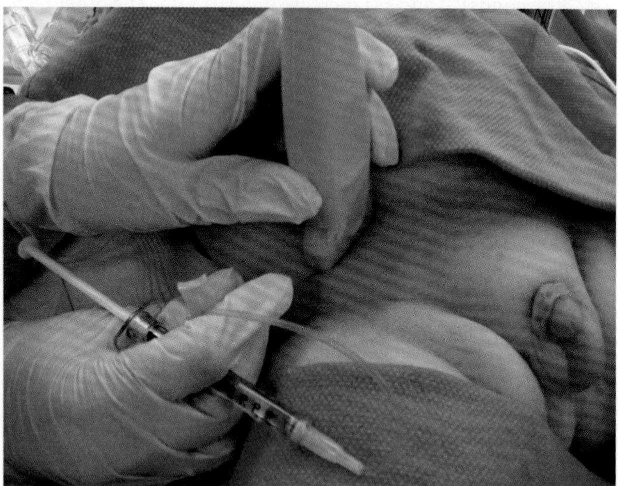

FIGURE 41-11. Ilioinguinal nerve block. Using a linear ultrasound probe, the anterior superior iliac spine is identified. The layers of the abdomen including the external oblique, transversus abdominis, and iliacus muscles are identified. The ilioinguinal and iliohypogastric nerves are located under the internal oblique muscle and in the plane between the internal oblique and the transversus abdominis muscle. A 27-gauge needle is inserted under ultrasound guidance in this plane. After aspiration, 0.1 mL/kg of local anesthetic solution is injected. This block can be used for pain relief following hernia surgery.

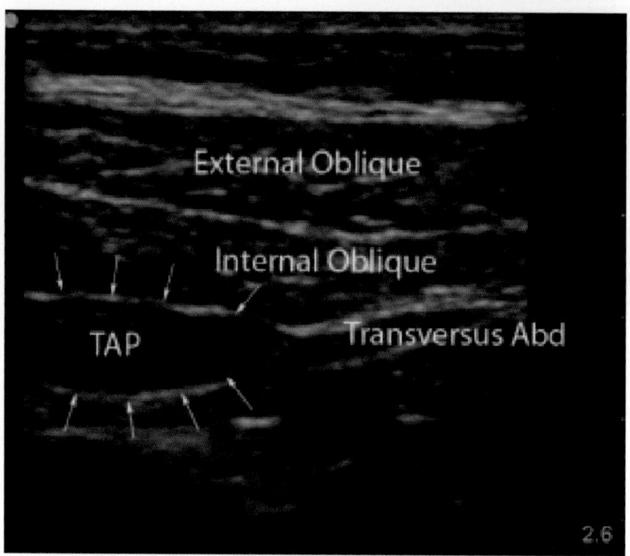

FIGURE 41-12. TAP block (Transversus abdominis plane block) Using a linear ultrasound probe with a small footprint (25 mm), the abdominal wall is scanned from medial to lateral, the three layers of the abdominal muscles are recognized, a needle is inserted into the space between the internal oblique and the transversus abdominis muscle while hydrodissecting to find the plane, 0.5 mL/kg of 0.125% bupivacaine is injected into each side to provide analgesia for the abdominal wall.

TAP Block

The TAP is a virtual space that exists between the internal oblique and the transversus abdominis muscle. This plane carries the thoraco lumbar fibers from T8 to L1 (Fig. 41-12). We have successfully used this block to provide analgesia for infants and neonates undergoing major abdominal surgery including colostomy placement.[146] This is a block we routinely use in our practice and avoid the use of opioids facilitating early extubation and return to the regular floor.

Lateral Femoral Cutaneous Blocks

The lateral femoral cutaneous nerve is a sensory branch of the lumbar plexus that supplies the lateral aspect of the thigh. This block is particularly useful in neonates who undergo muscle biopsies of the muscle of the lateral thigh.[135]

Brachial Plexus Block

This is performed for major limb surgery including major hand and arm plastic surgical procedures. The axillary approach to the brachial plexus is our preferred approach in neonates and infants. Currently, we use ultrasonography to identify each one of the branches of the brachial plexus to block them selectively,[147] thus allowing us to reduce the dose of local anesthesia needed for the block. A single shot supraclavicular approach to the brachial plexus can also be used for providing analgesia for upper extremity surgery. It is important to visualize using ultrasonography since the pleura is relatively close to the area of interest and injection. For sustained pain relief, we prefer using an infraclavicular catheter.[148]

Neurosurgical Blocks

Peripheral nerve blocks of the head and neck are useful for many surgical procedures. These may be useful in the sick neonate who requires a neurosurgical procedure. Peripheral nerve blocks of the trigeminal nerves, especially the frontal and occipital nerve branches, may be used to provide analgesia while avoiding general anesthesia.[149]

Postoperative Pain Management

The concepts of postoperative pain management are well known to most anesthesiologists. The use of intraoperative epidural anesthesia followed by postoperative epidural local anesthetics or opioids has been popular in older children and adults, and these techniques are being applied to neonates. In addition, most neonatologists are experienced with the intravenous administration of opioids for patient comfort. Each technique has its own risks and benefits.

Oral Routes

Oral routes of medications have been used for decades in neonates and children for managing pain. The commonly used oral analgesics include nonsteroidal analgesics including acetaminophen (20 mg/kg) and ibuprofen (5 mg/kg), and opioids including codeine (0.5 mg/kg) and hydrocodone (0.1 mg/kg). There may be some pharmacogenetic changes associated with the use of codeine in infants.[150]

Rectal Routes

Rectal suppositories are used frequently in neonates and infants for managing pyrexia. Rectal acetaminophen is commonly used for postoperative analgesia. A larger dose than is usually given orally is needed in infants to achieve good blood levels. A dose of 20 to 30 mg/kg is generally recommended for postoperative pain control.[151] Diclofenac, a commonly available rectal suppository in Europe, is frequently used in infants for postoperative pain control.[152]

Intravenous Analgesia

Opioids are the mainstay of analgesia in neonates and infants in the postoperative period. Morphine and fentanyl are frequently used in the neonatal intensive care unit for analgesia. However, the potential for opioid tolerance after prolonged infusion of opioids is not uncommon. To decrease the likelihood of opioid tolerance,[42] one can rotate opioids or add other medications including continuous intravenous naloxone[153] and intravenous methadone. Other intravenous nonsteroidal anti-inflammatory medications including intravenous acetaminophen has been introduced. Although not FDA approved for use in neonates, it has been gaining great interest in children for analgesia.[154] Intravenous ketorolac, a nonsteroidal anti-inflammatory drug, has been used successfully in neonates and infants for pain control.[155]

Postoperative Ventilation

The choice of an anesthetic drug should be guided by the need for postoperative management of ventilation, as well as the drug's effects on the circulation and other organs. If the surgical procedure or the neonate's condition is such that postoperative ventilation is likely, the prolonged respiratory effects of opioids or any other drug are of little concern. However, if the surgical procedure is relatively short and by itself does not require postoperative ventilation, the clinician should carefully select drugs, as well as doses of anesthetic drugs and relaxants, that will not necessitate prolonged postoperative ventilation or intubation. Postoperative ventilation places the neonate at added risk because of the problems associated with mechanical ventilation, the trauma to the subglottic area, and the potential development of postoperative subglottic stenosis or edema. However, if there is any question about the neonate's ability to maintain protective airway reflexes or normal ventilation after anesthesia, the neonate should be returned to the recovery room or newborn intensive care unit with the trachea intubated, and either ventilated or treated with a small amount of PEEP (2 to 4 cm H_2O).

SPECIAL CONSIDERATIONS

Maternal Drug Use During Pregnancy

Many drugs taken during pregnancy can affect the fetus and neonate. One area of special concern is substance abuse. During pregnancy, maternal drug use of cocaine, marijuana, and others leads to a host of problems for the neonate. Cocaine use, for instance, results in a reduced catecholamine reuptake, which may result in the accumulation of catecholamines. This has circulatory effects on the uterus, the umbilical blood vessels, and the fetal cardiovascular system. Three major problems affecting the infant are premature birth, intrauterine growth retardation, and cardiovascular abnormalities, including low cardiac output.[156] The cardiac output and stroke volume are reduced on the first day of life but return to normal by the second day. The clinical implication of this finding is that these neonates may be unstable enough in the first day of life that it may be advantageous to postpone surgery, if possible, until the second or third day of life. There is also an increase in structural cardiovascular malformations and electrocardiographic abnormalities. The most frequent lesions are peripheral pulmonic stenosis, right ventricular conduction delay, right ventricular hypertrophy, and ST segment and T-wave changes.[157] Preanesthetic history should elicit the use of drugs, including illicit use, if possible, to evaluate potential alteration of the anesthetic approach.

Temperature Control and Thermogenesis

The newborn is at risk for significant metabolic derangements caused by hypothermia. Newborns, and especially preterms, do not have the normal compensatory mechanisms that infants and children have when exposed to a cold environment. The newborn does not shiver, increase activity, or effectively vasoconstrict like older children or adults do in response to cold. In addition, the newborn has a larger body surface area-to-weight ratio that promotes heat loss, as well as low levels of subcutaneous fat for insulation. The primary mechanism the newborn has to respond to heat loss is nonshivering thermogenesis.[158] When there is a

2-degree centigrade gradient between core and skin, there is a release of norepinephrine into the bloodstream. Norepinephrine stimulates increased metabolism in a specialized tissue, brown fat, which is high in mitochondria and has abundant vascular supply. Stimulated lipolysis results in heat production, with side effects of increased oxygen consumption and production of ketone bodies and water. Ketone production causes both a metabolic acidosis and osmotic diuresis. The aerobic activity results in diversion of cardiac output to the deposits of brown fat around the kidneys, under the sternum, and between the scapulae. Because the diuresis, diversion of cardiac output away from the core circulation, and metabolic acidosis are maladaptive, every effort should be made to prevent nonshivering thermogenesis in the newborn.

Efforts to minimize nonshivering thermogenesis in the newborn are based on minimizing heat loss, both during transport to and from the neonatal intensive care unit and in the operating room. Transport should be done with the newborn in an incubator, not an open bed with overhead heaters. This will prevent heat loss from conduction and radiation. In the operating room, the room temperature is raised to its maximal level to minimize loss by conduction. Placing the patient on a forced-air warming blanket can reduce conductive heat loss dramatically,[159] as well as using plastic wrap or commercially available covers and hats to minimize heat loss from the head and all other areas not in the surgical field. The goal of all these activities is to maintain a neutral thermal environment, minimizing the stress that hypothermia can induce in the perioperative period. A complicating factor is that anesthetic agents can reduce or eliminate thermogenesis, removing any ability to compensate for cold stress.[160,161]

Respiratory Distress Syndrome

Because of the enormous technical ability of the neonatologist and the resources of neonatal intensive care units, many small infants survive and some need surgery. One of the frequent problems of preterm infants is the occurrence of the RDS secondary to a deficiency of surfactant. As discussed earlier, the use of exogenous surfactant has been widely used in premature infants of low birth weight either to prevent or to treat RDS. As a result, fewer infants now die of this entity, and the incidence of complications related to RDS has dropped. One of the long-term consequences of RDS is bronchopulmonary dysplasia. *Bronchopulmonary dysplasia* refers to a continuum of chronic disease of the lung parenchyma and airways, as well as neurodevelopment that occurs in preterms, especially under 32 weeks' gestation, who have survived RDS.[162] The theories of the cause of this condition include toxicity from oxygen administration, infection, inflammation, and barotrauma. Characteristics include airway smooth muscle hyperplasia, peribronchiolar fibrosis, enlarged alveoli, and disorganized pulmonary vasculature. Many patients improve as they age, but reactive airways, recurrent pulmonary infections, and a prolonged oxygen requirement are seen in some patients. Anesthetic concerns in these patients include evaluation of baseline oxygenation and potential presence of active bronchoconstriction. These patients often benefit from additional bronchodilator before induction. The baseline measure of oxygenation is important because these patients have less pulmonary oxygen reserve and may desaturate quickly with induction of anesthesia and hypoventilation. In patients with severe bronchopulmonary dysplasia, ventilatory management may be complicated by poor lung compliance and hyperinflation, as well as reactive airway disease. Although postanesthetic intubation is not usually required, a high index of suspicion should be used if there is significant clinical evidence of poor lung function preoperatively.

Postoperative Apnea

Apnea and bradycardia are well-recognized, major complications during and after surgery in neonates.[163] The infants at highest risk are those born prematurely, those with multiple congenital anomalies, those with a history of apnea and bradycardia, and those with chronic lung disease. The etiology of neonatal apnea is multifactorial. Decreased ventilatory control and hyporesponsiveness to hypoxia and hypercarbia may be potentiated by anesthetic agents. Respiratory muscle fatigue may also play a role because neonates have a smaller percentage of type I fibers in their diaphragm and intercostal muscles. In addition, hypothermia and anemia can also contribute to the development of postoperative apnea. The treatment of postoperative apnea or bradycardia may be as simple as tactile stimulation. However, some infants require mask ventilation or even prolonged intubation and ventilatory support. Infants with life-threatening apnea and bradycardia before surgery may be receiving CNS stimulants. Caffeine and theophylline (metabolized to caffeine) act by increasing central respiratory drive and lowering the threshold of response to hypercarbia, as well as stimulating contractility in the diaphragm. Caffeine is favored because of its wider therapeutic margin and decreased propensity for toxicity. Administering caffeine prophylactically to infants at risk of postoperative apnea to ensure adequate serum levels may prevent the need for prolonged periods of postoperative ventilatory support. The recommended loading dose is 10 mg/kg caffeine base.[164] Those infants at high risk for development of postoperative apnea may benefit from the use of a regional anesthetic as opposed to general anesthesia. Spinal anesthesia without supplemental sedation decreases the incidence of postoperative apnea and bradycardia in high-risk infants, but this advantage is lost if supplemental sedation is used.[165]

The question remains as to which infant should be admitted and monitored after outpatient surgery and for how long. The most conservative approach is to monitor all infants younger than 60 weeks' postconceptual age overnight after surgery.[166] Although the incidence of significant apnea and bradycardia is highest in the first 4 to 6 hours after surgery, it can occur up to 12 hours after surgery. In addition, the incidence of apnea directly correlates to postconceptual age. The risk of apnea goes up the younger the gestational age. An insightful approach to interpreting the various small studies is to stratify the risk of apnea, as done by Cote et al.[167] Using a meta-analysis, the study determined that the risk of apnea could be correlated with a combination of gestational age and postconceptual age. Using 95% confidence limits, the authors found that the probability of apnea in nonanemic infants free of recovery room apnea was not <5% until postconceptual age was 48 weeks with gestational age of 35 weeks. This risk was not <1%, until a postconceptual age of 56 weeks with a gestational age of 32 weeks or a postconceptual age of 54 weeks and gestational age of 35 weeks. This type of analysis allows the clinician to determine which patients should be admitted not only on the criteria of gestational and postconceptual ages, but also the amount of risk they are willing to assume.

Retinopathy of Prematurity

As the survival rate of increasingly preterm infants has grown, there is increasing concern about the development of ROP. The very preterm infant, especially those under 1,200 g of weight, are at highest risk, with an incidence of significant disease about 2%. Acute retinal changes are seen in about 45% of susceptible preterms, but there is spontaneous regression in most, permitting development of normal vision, but other infants will progress to a severe form of ROP and potential permanent blindness. Several complex factors may be responsible for the development of ROP. In the fetus, developing blood vessels grow gradually from the macula toward the edges of the developing retina. In full-term newborns, this process is complete at birth or in the first few weeks, but continues for a longer period in the preterm infant. These growing vessels are at risk for vasoconstriction and subsequent hemorrhage, followed by disorganized neovascularization or scarring. This scarring and lack of normal growth can eventually cause the retinal network to peel away resulting in retinal detachment. The spectrum or stages of disease is classified as follows:

Stage I. Mildly abnormal blood vessel growth. Many children who develop stage I improve with no treatment and eventually develop normal vision.

Stage II. Moderately abnormal blood vessel growth. Many children who develop stage II improve with no treatment and eventually develop normal vision. The disease resolves on its own without further progression.

Stage III. Severely abnormal blood vessel growth. The abnormal blood vessels grow toward the center of the eye instead of following their normal growth pattern along the surface of the retina. Some infants who develop stage III disease improve with no treatment and eventually develop normal vision. However, when infants have a certain degree of stage III and "plus disease" develops, treatment is considered. Plus disease means that the blood vessels of the retina have become enlarged and twisted, indicating a worsening of the disease. Treatment at this point provides a good chance of preventing retinal detachment.

Stage IV. Partially detached retina.

Stage V. Completely detached retina.

The most common cited cause of ROP is hyperoxia from administered oxygen, but hypoxemia, hypotension, sepsis, intraventricular hemorrhage, and other stresses have been implicated. At one time, there was concern that exposure to bright ambient light could cause ROP, but this has been disproven.[168] Although there may be spontaneous regression in early stages, there may also be progression to advanced stages and retinal detachment. The most common therapies involve using cryotherapy or laser therapy to destroy peripheral areas of the retina, slowing or reversing the abnormal growth of blood vessels. This is done to preserve the central vision from continuing distortion of the abnormal vessels in the periphery, although there is some loss of peripheral vision with this therapy.[169] In advanced stages, partial retinal detachment can be treated with a scleral buckle or vitrectomy.

The cryotherapy and laser therapies, as well as advanced procedures, are usually performed under general anesthesia in the operating room, although it is occasionally done at bedside with sedation in ventilated patients. The surgical procedures do not involve blood loss or significant surgical stress, but they do depend on a still surgical field for periods ranging from 30 to 90 minutes. The primary anesthetic challenge in these patients is related to the extreme prematurity and small size of the patients. Adequate monitoring, vascular access, and thermal stability are common challenges to management.

The risks of the development of ROP from hyperoxia have been of concern to anesthesiologists who anesthetize preterm neonates for any type of surgery. Can supplemental oxygen during an anesthetic start the development of ROP in preterm patients? We do not have an absolute direct answer to this question, but some evidence from a large collaborative study may help provide some guidance. Premature infants with confirmed early stages of ROP and a median pulse oximetry <94% saturation were randomized to a conventional oxygen arm with pulse oximetry targeted at 89% to 94% saturation or a supplemental arm with pulse oximetry targeted at 96% to 99% saturation for at least 2 weeks.[170] The patients were then re-examined for progression of disease. Use of supplemental oxygen at pulse oximetry saturations of 96% to 99% did not cause additional progression of prethreshold ROP. This study demonstrates that the use of supplemental oxygen for a prolonged period of time, not just for the short duration of a general anesthetic, was not deleterious as long as the pulse oximetry readings were kept in the 96% to 99% range. Consequently, keeping pulse oximetry readings in this range during an anesthetic should not be responsible for causing a progression of ROP in susceptible patients.

Neurodevelopmental Effects of Anesthetic Agents

There has been recent concern about the potential deleterious impact of anesthetic drugs on the developing brain. A variety of studies have shown that prolonged exposure of animal models to anesthetic agents can lead to neurodegenerative changes in the developing brain of neonatal rats.[171] However, these exposures to volatile agents and ketamine were for prolonged periods, the equivalent of several weeks of continuous exposure in the human. Nonetheless, this is an area of great concern for anesthesiologists.[172] Animal experiments have demonstrated neurocognitive changes in animals exposed to NMDA receptor antagonists like ketamine, volatile agents like isoflurane, as well as other agents including midazolam. The collective data that are currently available in literature do not support the withdrawal of these drugs from the practice of pediatric anesthesia. The data seem to be reproducible in rodents but not in other species. Future prospective trials with prospective neurocognitive testing of infants exposed to anesthesia is needed to determine if this applies to the human neonate. At the time of writing this chapter, there was no conclusive evidence to demonstrate the deleterious effect of inhaled or intravenous anesthetics on neurocognitive function in neonates and infants. Prospective studies including a current study randomizing infants to getting a spinal anesthesia versus general anesthesia should be able to provide better information on this very complex problem that may face pediatric anesthesiologists. In the meantime, several retrospective studies including data about children from a particular county in Minnesota has some data to lead to believe that there may be an association with the development of learning disability especially when exposed to multiple anesthetics before 2 years of age.[173] Although the data generated a lot of interest, it is important to understand that we need more concrete data and prospective studies to demonstrate that there are indeed neurocognitive changes associated with exposure to anesthesia in infants.

SURGICAL PROCEDURES IN NEONATES

Surgical procedures in neonates are functionally divided into two periods: Those performed in the first week and those performed in the first month. There has been a strong trend in recent years to put on emphasis of presurgical stabilization before taking the newborn to the operating room. This has reduced the emergent nature of newborn surgeries. Many procedures that used to be done on an emergent basis, even in the middle of the night, such as repair of CDH or omphalocele, are now done days later after initial therapy has been instituted. Exceptions to this include gastroschisis, which is usually attended to within 12 to 24 hours, airway lesions such as webs that are causing significant airway obstruction, and acute subdural/epidural hematomas from traumatic delivery. In most cases, however, a period of 1 to 3 days can be allowed for stabilization of the newborn or transport to an appropriate pediatric center for treatment. There is more to neonatal emergency surgery than just the immediate anesthetic and surgical procedures. Many of these infants require the support services of specialized nursing units, pediatric radiologists, pediatric intensive care physicians, specialized laboratory facilities, and they must have their complete care be the main consideration of where their surgery should be done. Many procedures are now performed using laparoscopic techniques which decreases postoperative morbidity and pain and facilitates early extubation.

Surgical Procedures in the First Week of Life

7 The most frequent major surgical procedures performed in the first week of life are for CDH, omphalocele and gastroschisis, tracheoesophageal fistula (TEF), intestinal obstruction, and meningomyelocele. Some of these conditions, such as CDH, omphalocele and gastroschisis, and meningomyelocele, are obvious at birth. It may take hours or days for a TEF or intestinal obstruction to become manifest. Because of the lack of expertise many hospitals have in the care of these patients, the transfer of these neonates to hospitals with greater expertise is often prudent after initial stabilization of the patient. Most hospitals that have expertise in these patients have a transport team that is well qualified to help with stabilization and transport. Those that do not have transport teams often have extensive protocols and procedures to work with the other institution to help ensure the safe transfer of the patient.

Two confounding factors in neonatal surgery are prematurity and associated congenital anomalies. The presence of one congenital anomaly increases the likelihood of another one. In conditions such as TEF, the mortality rate from the associated congenital heart defect is higher than that from the surgical correction of the TEF. Prematurity, particularly when associated with RDS, may adversely affect surgical outcome. The use of surfactant in the treatment of the RDS has greatly increased the number of survivors and has decreased the complexity of the issues of the infant with a combination of TEF and RDS. A neonatologist should be consulted in the case of any neonate with a congenital defect who is considered for surgery. The most serious associated congenital lesion is that of the cardiovascular system. More than 10% of infants with an isolated CDH have a cardiac anomaly,[174] with a higher incidence in newborns with associated syndromes, and approximately 15% to 25% of infants with TEF have an associated congenital cardiac anomaly.[175]

Congenital Diaphragmatic Hernia

CDH occurs with an incidence of approximately 1 in 4,000 live births. Traditionally, the mortality rate from CDH was in the range of 40% to 50%. The new strategy of permissive hypercapnia and delayed surgical repair has resulted in survival rates of >75% in some centers.[176] However, the morbidity remains high in survivors. A brief discussion of the embryologic characteristics of CDH will help the clinician understand the potentially enormous postoperative problems that may be encountered.

Embryology

Early in fetal development, the pleuroperitoneal cavity is a single compartment. The gut is herniated or extruded to the extraembryonic coelom during the ninth to tenth weeks of fetal life. During this period, the diaphragm develops to separate the thoracic and abdominal cavities (Fig. 41-13). The development of the diaphragm is usually completed by the seventh fetal week. In the ninth to tenth weeks, the developing gut returns to the peritoneal cavity. If there is delay or incomplete closure of the diaphragm, or if the gut returns early and prevents normal closure of the diaphragm, a diaphragmatic hernia will develop, producing varying degrees of herniation of the intestinal contents into the chest. The left side of the diaphragm closes later than the right side, which results in the higher incidence of left-sided diaphragmatic hernias (foramen of Bochdalek). Approximately, 90% of hernias detected in the first week of life are on the left side.

Clinical Presentation

The clinical presentation and the outcome from a diaphragmatic hernia are varied. The bowel contents may compress the lung buds and prevent development, leading to bilateral hypoplastic lungs with very little chance for survival. In most instances, however, a moderately small diaphragmatic hernia may develop later in fetal life so the lung is normal but compressed by the abdominal viscera. At the mild end of the scale, the infant might

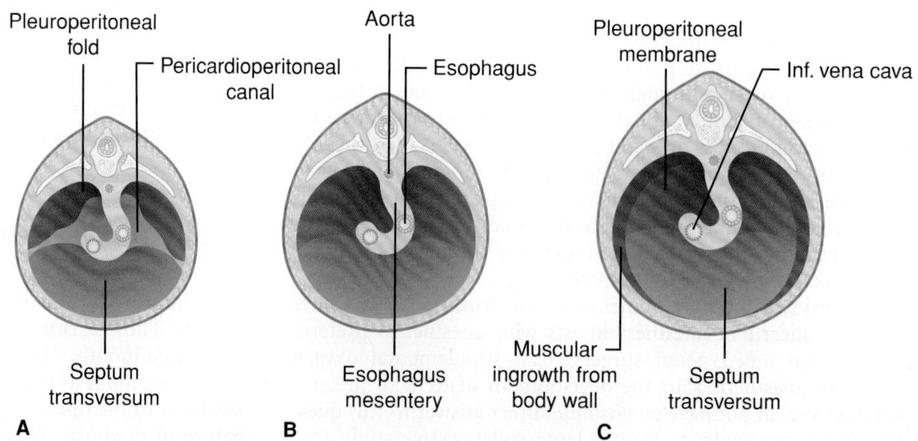

FIGURE 41-13. Schematic drawings illustrating the development of the diaphragm. **A:** The pleuroperitoneal folds appear at the beginning of the sixth week. **B:** The pleuroperitoneal folds have fused with the septum transversum and the mesentery of the esophagus in the seventh week, thus separating the thoracic cavity from the abdominal cavity. **C:** In a transverse section at the fourth month of development, an additional rim derived from the body wall forms the most peripheral part of the diaphragm. (Reprinted from: Langman J. Body cavities and serous membranes. In: Sadler TW, ed. *Langman's Medical Embryology,* 5th ed. Baltimore: Williams & Wilkins; 1985:147, with permission.)

have a relatively normal pulmonary vascular bed with varying degrees of persistent pulmonary hypertension that may rapidly revert to normal. In more severe defects, significant pulmonary hypoplasia and abnormal pulmonary vasculature lead to greater mortality.

After closure of the pleuroperitoneal membrane, muscular development of the diaphragm occurs. Incomplete muscularization of the diaphragm results in the development of a hernia sac because of intra-abdominal pressure. The condition is known as *eventration of the diaphragm,* and the diaphragm may extend well up into the thoracic cavity. The other possibility is that the innervation of the diaphragm is incomplete and the muscle is atonic. Eventration of the diaphragm is usually not symptomatic in the first week of life.

Antenatal Diagnosis

The diagnosis of CDH can be made prenatally by fetal ultrasonography or ultrafast fetal magnetic resonance imaging. Antenatal diagnosis has led to the identification of a "hidden mortality" in CDH, fetuses who did not survive gestation and neonates who died before diagnosis. Various factors have been proposed to identify predictability of survival, including early gestation diagnosis, severe mediastinal shift, polyhydramnios, a small lung-to-thorax transverse area ratio, and the herniation of liver or stomach. New techniques in fetal surgery, such as temporary endoscopic fetal tracheal occlusion, may prove beneficial to fetuses with CDH who are identified to be at risk for not surviving to term.[177] The other obvious advantage of prenatal diagnosis is that plans can be made for maternal or neonatal transport to a center with advanced neonatal critical care with availability of ECMO.

Clinical Presentation

The occurrence of symptoms depends on the degree of herniation and interference with pulmonary function. At times, the degree of interference is so great that the neonate's clinical condition begins to deteriorate immediately, whereas in other situations it may be several hours before the infant's condition is fully appreciated. In the severely involved newborn, the initial clinical findings are usually classic and readily discerned. The infant has a scaphoid abdomen secondary to the absence of intra-abdominal contents, which have herniated into the chest. Breath sounds on the affected side are reduced or absent. The diagnosis can be confirmed with a radiograph (Fig. 41-14). Immediate supportive care entails tracheal intubation and control of the airway along with decompression of the stomach. Excessive airway pressure carries a high risk for pneumothorax and worsening of a bad situation.

Preoperative Care

CDH was traditionally treated as a surgical emergency. The infants were taken immediately to surgery for decompression and repair. The thought was that removing the abdominal viscera from the thorax would allow for re-expansion of the atelectatic lung and improved oxygenation. However, as the pathophysiology of CDH was more clearly defined—pulmonary hypoplasia associated with a hyperreactive pulmonary vasculature—a strategy of preoperative stabilization with delayed surgical repair was adopted.

The stabilization of an infant with CDH may require multiple treatment modalities. The use of aggressive ventilation strategies to induce hyperventilation alkalosis has been abandoned secondary to the high incidence of iatrogenic lung injury. Conventional ventilation with permissive hypercapnia is now favored.

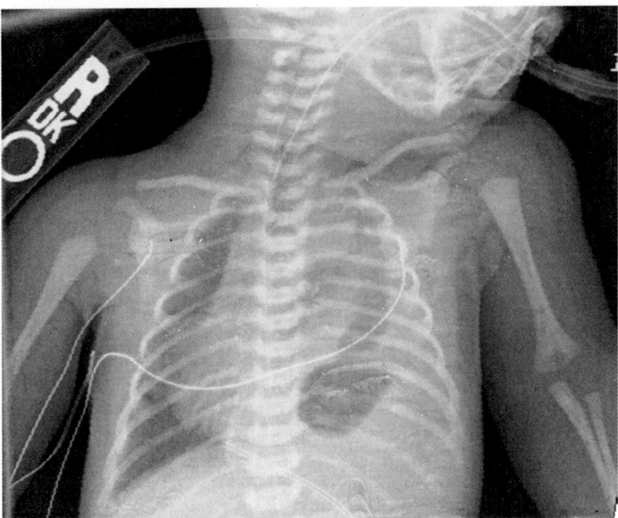

FIGURE 41-14. Infant with congenital diaphragmatic hernia. Note the loop of bowel gas in left hemithorax.

The goal is to maintain preductal arterial saturation above 85% using peak inspiratory pressures below 25 cm H_2O and allowing the PCO_2 to rise to 45 to 55 mm Hg.[176] High-frequency oscillatory ventilation, in addition to nitric oxide, has been used in place of conventional ventilation in an attempt to reduce barotraumas and has been demonstrated to be beneficial.[178] Neonates born with CDH may also have a component of surfactant deficiency, and studies have shown improvement in oxygenation in those infants given surfactant prophylactically. These have been well demonstrated in animal experiments when compared with tracheal ligation.[179]

The use of ECMO in infants with CDH was initiated in the mid-1980s. Despite extensive literature on the subject, there remains an ongoing debate as to whether ECMO improves survival in neonates with CDH. The Congenital Diaphragmatic Hernia Study Group analyzed data from the multicenter CDH Registry and determined that ECMO improves the survival rate in CDH neonates with a predicted high risk of mortality (≥80%) based on birth weight and 5-minute Apgar score. A right-sided CDH may carry a higher mortality and morbidity compared with a left-sided defect, despite the use of ECMO.[180]

Perioperative Care

Because delayed surgical repair of CDH is now the norm, neonates with CDH frequently present to the operating room already intubated and on some form of ventilatory support. Despite a period of preoperative stabilization, some infants still have a component of reactive pulmonary hypertension. The goals of ventilatory management are to ensure adequate oxygenation and avoid barotrauma. Any sudden deterioration in oxygen saturation with or without associated hypotension should raise suspicion of pneumothorax. It is important to avoid hypothermia because this increases the oxygen requirement and could precipitate pulmonary hypertension. Blood loss and fluid shifts are usually not a problem, although maintenance of intravascular volume is essential to avoid acidosis, which could also precipitate pulmonary hypertension. More recently, these patients are being operated while on ECMO and mortality of these patients can be predicted on the basis of fetal lung volumes.[181]

Anesthetic Technique

The anesthetic technique chosen depends on the size of the defect and the anticipated postoperative respiratory status. In those infants who will remain intubated after surgery, inhalation agents and narcotics may be used as tolerated. In those infants with a small defect who present to the operating room with little or no respiratory distress, it may be beneficial to avoid intraoperative narcotics and provide regional analgesia in anticipation of extubation. The use of nitrous oxide should be avoided, particularly in those situations in which abdominal closure could be difficult. Muscle relaxation is often needed to facilitate abdominal closure.

Postoperative Care

Most infants with CDH require intensive postoperative care. Recovery depends on the degree of pulmonary hypertension and pulmonary hypoplasia. It was previously believed that pulmonary hypoplasia was responsible for most deaths; however, it is now believed that potentially reversible pulmonary hypertension may be responsible for as much as 25% of reported deaths.

There is evidence to suggest that cardiac development is impaired in infants with CDH. Relative left ventricular hypoplasia with an attenuated muscle mass and cavity size have been described.

Omphalocele and Gastroschisis

Although omphalocele and gastroschisis sometimes appear similar and may be confused, they have entirely different origins and associated congenital anomalies.[182] During the fifth to tenth weeks of fetal life, the abdominal contents are extruded into the extraembryonic coelom, and the gut returns to the abdominal cavity at approximately the tenth week. Failure of part of or all the intestinal contents to return to the abdominal cavity results in an omphalocele that is covered with a membrane called the *amnion* (Fig. 41-15). The amnion protects the abdominal contents from infection and the loss of ECF. The umbilical cord is found at approximately the apex of the sac. Gastroschisis, in contrast, develops later in fetal life, after the intestinal contents have returned to the abdominal cavity. It results from interruption of the omphalomesenteric artery, which results in ischemia and atrophy of the various layers of the abdominal wall at the base of the umbilical cord. The gut then herniates through this tissue defect. The degree of herniation may be slight, or major amounts of the abdominal viscera may be found outside the peritoneal cavity. The umbilical cord is found to one side of the intestinal contents (Fig. 41-16).

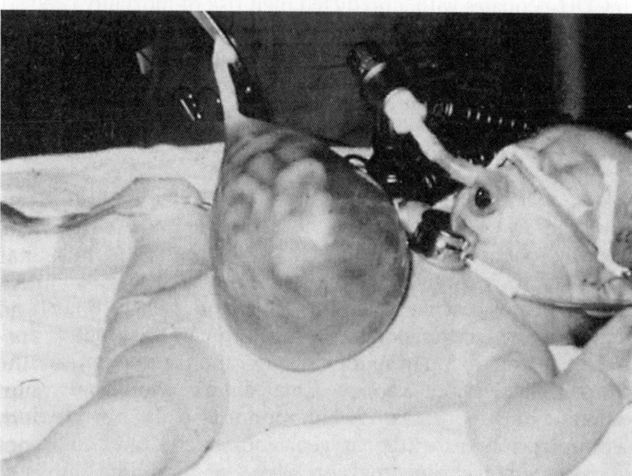

FIGURE 41-15. Omphalocele. (Reprinted from: Berry FA. Physiology and surgery of the infant. In: Berry FA, ed. *Anesthetic Management of Difficult and Routine Pediatric Patients.* New York: Churchill Livingstone; 1990:152, with permission.)

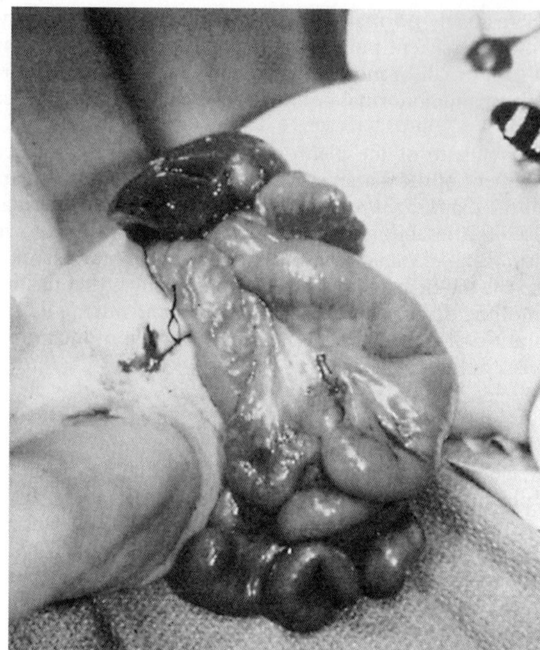

FIGURE 41-16. Gastroschisis. (Reprinted from: Berry FA. Physiology and surgery of the infant. In: Berry FA, ed. *Anesthetic Management of Difficult and Routine Pediatric Patients.* New York: Churchill Livingstone; 1990:152, with permission.)

The intestines and viscera are not covered by any membrane and therefore are highly susceptible to infection and loss of ECF. There is a very high incidence of associated congenital anomalies with omphalocele, although much lower with gastroschisis.[183] The Beckwith–Wiedemann syndrome consists of mental retardation, hypoglycemia, congenital heart disease, a large tongue, and an omphalocele. Congenital heart lesions are found in approximately 20% of infants with omphalocele. Other associated congenital defects are found with gastroschisis and omphalocele; most involve the gastrointestinal tract and consist primarily of intestinal atresia or stenosis and malrotation. Because of the uncovered gut irritating the uterine lining, premature delivery is more common in gastroschisis patients.

Antenatal Diagnosis

The overall incidence of these defects is about 1:5,000 live births. Screening for abdominal wall defects is accomplished through the use of maternal serum α-fetoprotein (AFP). AFP is a normal protein present in fetal tissues during fetal development. Closure of the abdominal wall and the neural tube (see "Meningomyelocele") prevents release of large quantities of this protein into the amniotic fluid. High levels of AFP in the amniotic fluid can cross the placenta and be detected in maternal blood. Thus, abnormal levels of maternal serum AFP in the mother raise concerns over the possibility of either an abdominal wall defect or a neural tube defect in the fetus, as do high levels of AFP in fluid obtained during amniocentesis. Levels tend to be higher when the defect is gastroschisis instead of omphalocele. The primary method of definitive fetal diagnosis of gastroschisis and omphalocele is ultrasonography. In a recent study, 88% of patients with gastroschisis and 69% with omphalocele were diagnosed prenatally with ultrasound.[184] An advantage of ultrasound is the ability to diagnosis other complicating abnormalities such as cardiac defects.

Preoperative Care

Most neonates with gastroschisis or omphalocele diagnosed prenatally are delivered by cesarean section. The advantages of this are the ability to prevent trauma to the exposed bowel and allow better coordination of the various medical specialties needed for immediate surgical management of the defect. Priorities in the delivery room care unique to an infant with gastroschisis are the need to protect the exposed bowel and minimize fluid and temperature loss. An effective way to achieve these goals involves placing the defect and lower body in a sterile, clear plastic bag to protect the defect and minimize heat and fluid loss. The bag can be filled with warm saline and a drawstring can be used to tighten the bag against the infant's body.

Preoperative stabilization of the neonate with an abdominal wall defect includes management of respiratory insufficiency, establishment of adequate intravenous access, and an assessment for associated congenital anomalies. It is expected that a significantly higher incidence in congenital anomalies will be found in omphalocele patients. Respiratory failure at birth in infants with omphalocele is a significant predictor of mortality.[185] Lung hypoplasia and abnormal thoracic development may be significant in infants with large omphaloceles. A difficult airway can be anticipated in the patient with Beckwith–Wiedemann syndrome because of the large tongue.

Surgery is not urgent in the neonate with an omphalocele and can be delayed for several days until the infant is assessed and stabilized. In those infants with severe respiratory distress or congenital heart disease who are too unstable for surgery, nonsurgical treatment with topical antiseptics and delayed closure is an option.[186] Although there has been some interest in nonoperative, bedside-staged closure of gastroschisis defects, primary operative closure continues to be the most common approach.[187]

Perioperative Care

The two major perioperative concerns are fluid loss and ventilation. The fluid volume management of the infant often entails administration of large amounts of full-strength, balanced salt solution. The adequacy of the peripheral circulation and urine output is an indicator of the adequacy of the volume resuscitation. Both conditions may present an intraoperative challenge to the anesthesiologist because with an omphalocele, after the amniotic membrane is removed, large volumes of fluid may transude or exude from the exposed abdominal viscera. The fluid that is lost is ECF, which should be replaced with full-strength, balanced salt solution. An arterial line is often used for blood pressure monitoring and frequent blood gas monitoring to assess acid–base status.

If the defect in the abdominal wall is small, a primary repair of the deficit can be accomplished. However, with a large defect, it may be difficult to return the abdominal viscera to the peritoneal cavity because the muscle and peritoneum are underdeveloped. Because of concern for the increase in the volume of gas in the intestine, nitrous oxide should not be used. Muscle relaxation is necessary to allow closure of the abdomen. With moderate size abdominal wall defects, it may not be possible to close the peritoneum, but there may be sufficient skin to close the defect. With large defects, the peritoneal cavity may be too small to contain the viscera, and attempted closure can impair circulation to the bowel, kidneys, and lower extremities, as well as compromise respiration. A pulse oximeter probe on the foot can be helpful in monitoring circulation to the lower extremities during abdominal wall closure.

Attempts have been made to find objective criteria by which to determine whether the infant will tolerate primary closure of the defect, and to avoid or minimize the circulatory and ventilatory problems. One method has been to measure intragastric pressure in infants who undergo primary closure. Intragastric pressure is measured by placing a nasogastric tube in the stomach and using a column of saline to measure the pressure.[188] Studies have used the criteria that if the intragastric pressure was ≤20 mm Hg, primary closure can proceed. Above 20 mm Hg pressures during closure, delayed closure and placement of a Dacron silo were used. With this approach, primary closure has been successful when used, with faster return to full feeds and shorter hospital length of stay compared with patients treated by delayed closure. Complications have been less with primary closure using this approach.

If primary closure is impossible, a silo is incorporated into the abdominal wall to contain and cover the abdominal viscera (Fig. 41-17). The repair is then staged from this point onward. Every 2 or 3 days, the size of the silo is reduced, in much the same fashion that a tube of toothpaste is squeezed. The infant may feel some degree of discomfort as the peritoneum and skin are stretched. Institutions vary in how they accomplish the delay closure, with some surgeons bringing the patient to the operating room for each stage and others doing this at bedside, often with the assistance of small doses of ketamine or other analgesics. Some of these patients remain on mechanical ventilation during this period, and others are extubated. In either case, both blood pressure and oxygen saturation should be closely monitored during and immediately after each stage of closure to ensure that the increase in abdominal and intrathoracic pressure does not significantly impede ventilation, oxygenation, and venous return. In some cases, further reduction must be delayed until there is more

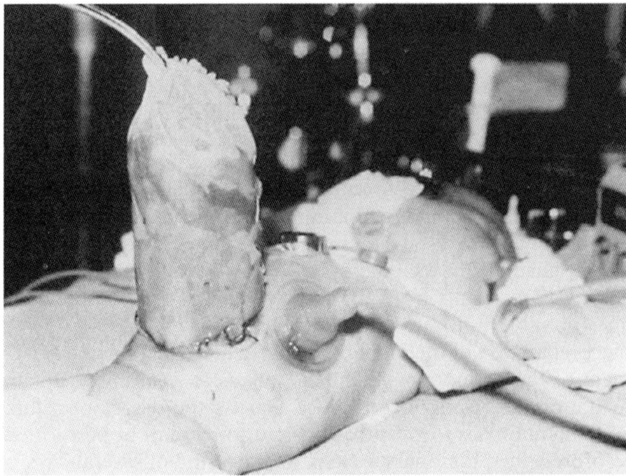

FIGURE 41-17. Dacron silo for extruded viscera. (Reprinted from: Berry FA. Physiology and surgery of the infant. In: Berry FA, ed. *Anesthetic Management of Difficult and Routine Pediatric Patients.* New York: Churchill Livingstone; 1990:154, with permission.)

abdominal growth. This is a situation that requires clinical judgment. After several stages of silo reduction, the final operation is complete closure of the abdominal wall defect under full anesthesia with complete muscle relaxation.

Postoperative Care

The postoperative care of infants with omphalocele or gastroschisis is critical. Some need tracheal intubation and assisted ventilation of the lungs for days to weeks. The ventilatory status of the patient is especially critical in omphalocele patients because up to half of these patients are born with pulmonary hypoplasia, making the balance of increased abdominal pressures and adequate ventilation and oxygenation especially challenging. Additional complications include postoperative hypertension and edema of the extremities. The increased abdominal pressure can reduce the circulation to the kidneys, which results in a release of renin. Renin activates the renin–angiotensin–aldosterone system, which is believed to cause the hypertension.

Tracheoesophageal Fistula

The treatment of esophageal atresia and TEF can be both challenging and satisfying for the anesthesiologist. Death in the perioperative period typically results from prematurity or from an associated congenital heart defect. TEF occurs in approximately 1 in 3,000 live births. Approximately 85% consist of a fistula from the distal trachea to the esophagus and a blind proximal esophageal pouch. In 10% of cases, there is a blind proximal esophageal pouch with no TEF (Fig. 41-18). The embryologic defect results from imperfect division of the foregut into the anteriorly positioned larynx and trachea and the posteriorly positioned esophagus; the division should occur between the fourth and fifth weeks of intrauterine life. Fifty percent of affected infants have associated congenital anomalies, of which approximately 15% to 25% involve the cardiovascular system.

Clinical Presentation

Atresia of the esophagus leads to inability of the fetus to swallow amniotic fluid and the subsequent development of polyhydramnios. Ultrasound may well raise the possibility of a congenital anomaly. For that reason, if polyhydramnios is present, attempts should be made to pass a nasogastric tube shortly after delivery. Passing a nasogastric tube is not routine in the delivery room; therefore, the diagnosis may not become apparent until the infant is fed. Cyanosis and choking with oral feedings should raise suspicion.

There are two major complications of esophageal atresia with a distal tracheal fistula: Aspiration pneumonia and dehydration. The presence of a distal TEF increases the likelihood of reflux of gastric juice up the esophagus and into the pulmonary system. Dehydration results from the fact that the proximal esophagus does not communicate with the stomach. Therefore, preoperative preparation of these infants is aimed at evaluation and treatment of the pulmonary system, as well as at ensuring adequate hydration and electrolyte balance. Rarely, the degree of reflux and pneumonia is so great that a gastrostomy must be performed to protect the pulmonary system, and a period of several days is needed to improve the general condition of the infant. However, if the infant is in good condition, primary repair can be performed at 24 to 48 hours. This consists of ligation of the fistula and a primary repair with approximation of the two ends of the esophagus.

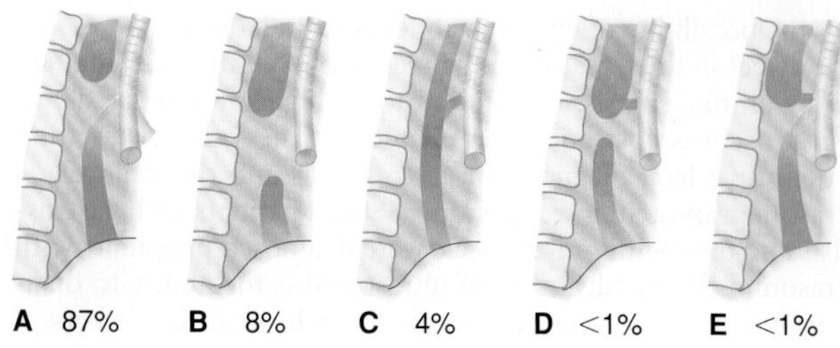

FIGURE 41-18. Diagrams of the five most commonly encountered forms of esophageal atresia and tracheoesophageal fistula, shown in order of frequency. (Reprinted from: Herbst JJ. Gastrointestinal tract. In: Behrman RE, Kleigman RM, Nelson WE, et al., eds. *Nelson Textbook of Pediatrics,* 14th ed. Philadelphia, PA: WB Saunders; 1992:942, with permission.)

Anesthetic Considerations

The repair of TEF can be done in the conventional method or by a thoracoscopic method. Both methods and the anesthetic implications for each technique will be described here. The presence of a gastrostomy reduces the potential for reflux of gastric juice during the surgical procedure. If a gastrostomy is present, the gastrostomy tube should be open to air and left at the head of the table under the anesthesiologist's observation to avoid kinking and obstruction.

CONVENTIONAL OPEN TEF CLOSURE. There are three approaches to tracheal intubation after induction of anesthesia. One is to use an inhalation induction, followed by topical spray of lidocaine and intubation while the infant is breathing spontaneously. Another technique is to use an intravenous or inhalation induction and intubate the trachea after muscle paralysis. This technique may lead to distention of the fistula and stomach with excessive positive-pressure ventilation. When controlled ventilation of the lungs is used, attempts must be made to minimize the distention of the stomach and the potential for reflux. If a gastrostomy tube is in place, the point is moot. A third technique is to intubate the neonates awake with mild sedation. This can protect the airway while reducing the chances of aspiration. Alternatively, because the fistula is usually located just above the carina on the posterior wall of the membranous trachea, the endotracheal tube can be placed just distal to the TEF. To do this, the endotracheal tube is inserted until it enters one or the other main stem bronchi. This is judged by unilateral expansion of the chest and unilateral breath sounds. The endotracheal tube is then slowly withdrawn until bilateral chest movement and breath sounds are confirmed.

The endotracheal tube might inadvertently enter the fistula when the infant is turned or during surgical manipulation. Intubation of the fistula should be suspected if there is increased difficulty in ventilation of the lungs, as well as decreased oxygen saturation and end-tidal CO_2. Because these findings may also be present when the lung is packed away to perform the surgery and because there are other explanations for these findings, intubation of the fistula should always be included in the differential diagnosis. At any time ventilation is difficult and desaturation is occurring, the surgeon must stop the procedure while the situation is clarified. The surgeon will be able to palpate the tip of the tube in the fistula if this is the problem.

The localization and isolation of H-type fistulas can be difficult. In this situation, direct laryngoscopy and bronchoscopy is performed by the surgeon, the fistula is identified, and a guidewire is fed through the fistula tract into the esophagus. The infant

TABLE 41-5. POSTOPERATIVE PAIN CONTROL FOR NEONATES AND INFANTS

Intravenous
Opioids: Morphine, fentanyl, methadone
NSAIDs: Ketorolac, intravenous acetaminophen
Oral
Acetaminophen
Ibuprofen
Hydrocodone
Codeine
Rectal
Acetaminophen
Diclofenac
Regional and local anesthesia

NSAIDs, nonsteroidal anti-inflammatory drugs.

is then intubated, with care taken not to dislodge the guidewire. Once intubated esophagoscopy is performed, the guidewire is visualized and brought out through the mouth. In this way, the surgeon can use fluoroscopy to determine the level of the fistula and decide whether a cervical or thoracic approach is necessary. During surgery, the anesthesiologist can apply traction to the wire loop to facilitate the localization of the fistula by the surgeon.

ENDOSCOPIC TEF REPAIR. The use of endoscopic methods for repair of TEF is being popularized in pediatric surgery.[189] The infant should be kept spontaneously breathing until the fistula is ligated. Maintenance of spontaneous ventilation can be challenging considering that these infants may not tolerate the use of potent inhalation agents while spontaneous ventilation is established. This approach may shorten the duration of surgical operating time while providing a minimally invasive method. The anesthetic management is still challenging.

Postoperative Care

Although there have been great advances in the treatment of TEF and esophageal atresia, postoperative care can be complicated by associated congenital heart disease, RDS, and a need for continued postoperative ventilation. The compression of the lung for several hours, along with pre-existing aspiration pneumonia in some of these infants, suggest the need, in the more difficult cases, for a short period of postoperative ventilation, or at least intubation with PEEP, as the most conservative technique for postoperative airway management. Some infants are in excellent condition at the time of surgery with no complicating factors and, therefore, should be considered for extubation immediately at the end of surgery or shortly thereafter. If extubation of the trachea is planned for the end of surgery, the anesthetic technique must be tailored accordingly. Caudal anesthesia as part of the technique is useful in these situations, reducing the concentration of maintenance volatile anesthetics, the amount of muscle relaxants, and the need for intraoperative narcotics. We prefer placing caudal epidural catheters in these children for postoperative pain control. Another option is to place a unilateral ultrasound guided paravertebral block which can again provide analgesia for the hemithorax that is the operative site. This offers good analgesia while at the same time avoiding the use of opioids, which may predispose these infants to apnea and respiratory depression.[190]

A high percentage of infants with esophageal atresia have residual difficulties of the tracheobronchial tree and esophagus for many years. These difficulties include tracheomalacia, gastroesophageal reflux, esophageal stricture, and recurrent fistulas.

Intestinal Obstruction

A useful way of classifying gastrointestinal obstruction is focus above and below the pylorus. Obstruction of the upper gastrointestinal tract is manifest by vomiting, especially after feeds, whereas obstruction of the lower gastrointestinal tract may present with abdominal distention, little or no stool passed, hematochezia, signs of pain, and vomiting.

Upper Gastrointestinal Tract Obstruction

The most common cause of upper gastrointestinal obstruction in the newborn is pyloric stenosis, but pyloric stenosis does not usually present in the first week of life. Other rare causes of obstruction, such as congenital webs, may occur. If there has been persistent vomiting, this usually means that a deficit of fluids or electrolytes will develop in the infant. The stomach contains approximately 100 to 130 mEq/L of sodium and 5 to 10 mEq/L of potassium. Persistent vomiting results in the greatest deficit of sodium. Another major concern in the infant with upper gastrointestinal tract obstruction is aspiration of gastric contents.

The anesthetic management of these patients is directed toward ensuring adequate relaxation for abdominal exploration, repair of the congenital defect, and closure of the abdomen. Nitrous oxide can be used in high intestinal obstruction because there is essentially no gas in the upper gastrointestinal tract. The next concern is whether the infant's trachea should be extubated at the end of surgery. If the infant is robust, extubation of the trachea at the end of surgery can be anticipated. The preferred technique is for general anesthesia combined with caudal epidural anesthesia. This allows light levels of volatile agent and minimal muscle relaxant use, resulting in an early extubation. Opioids may be administered, although the impact on the ability to ventilate at the end of the procedure should be considered. If the infant is moderately debilitated or if the surgical incision is extensive, a period of postoperative ventilation may well be indicated, particularly if moderate doses of opioids have been used.

Lower Gastrointestinal Tract Obstruction

Intestinal obstruction in the newborn can result from a variety of lesions. These include imperforate anus or anal atresia, duodenal atresia, jejunoileal atresia, intussusception, malrotation, volvulus, choledochal cyst, or meconium ileus. Although these are all different in etiology, their presentation is similar. The problems associated with lower gastrointestinal tract obstruction usually develop within 1 to 7 days after birth. It may take this long for the lesion to become evident because it is low in the gastrointestinal tract. An imperforate anus should be recognizable shortly after birth. However, once intestinal obstruction is diagnosed in the newborn, it becomes a surgical emergency. These patients may deteriorate rapidly. Some of these infants may have vomiting secondary to the obstruction, which poses a problem for fluid and electrolyte management. An enormous amount of fluid can be sequestered within the intestinal tract. This fluid is essentially ECF and has high sodium content. Therefore, these infants should be prepared expeditiously for surgery and have a serum sodium level of at least 130 mEq/L and a urine volume of 1 to 2 mL/kg/hr. In addition to fluid and electrolyte disturbances, delayed diagnosis or treatment of these patients can result in increased abdominal pressure, leading to respiratory embarrassment from pressure on the diaphragm and aspiration pneumonitis, as well as sepsis. Lastly, some of these conditions are associated with other congenital anomalies that complicate preanesthetic evaluation and anesthetic management.[191] Duodenal atresia, for instance, is often associated with Down syndrome, cystic fibrosis, imperforate anus, and renal abnormalities.

The preanesthetic evaluation and perioperative management is similar for all these lesions. Preanesthetic evaluation is focused on the stabilization of fluid and electrolyte status, ensuring adequate oxygenation and ventilation, hemodynamic support if the patient is septic, and identification of complicating issues such as other congenital abnormalities.

In the operating room, the need for invasive arterial and central venous monitoring is determined by the current status of the patient and the urgency of the procedure. The primary anesthetic considerations are the same as those in the preoperative period, including ongoing fluid and electrolyte resuscitation. Because these cases are usually emergent and there may be associated vomiting and abdominal distention, either an awake intubation or rapid-sequence induction is indicated. Although awake intubation may be the best approach if the patient has a probable difficult airway or has hemodynamic decompensation, a rapid-sequence induction after preoxygenation is the approach normally taken. Any induction agent can be used if judicious doses are chosen, but ketamine or etomidate are often chosen because of a concern about cardiovascular instability.

Anesthetic agents for maintenance during these cases is chosen on the basis of the patient's status and the likely surgical course. Nitrous oxide should not be used in any infant who has gaseous distention of the intestine, which is easily determined from the preoperative radiograph. Providing adequate muscle relaxation for surgery can be accomplished with various anesthetic techniques such as volatile anesthesia, muscle relaxants, and caudal or epidural block.[192] There is increasing interest in the use of remifentanil in newborns and infants because of its titratability and short duration of action, potentially increasing the options for extubation at the end of the case for some patients.[193]

The criteria for tracheal extubation at the end of surgery are the same as those described for upper gastrointestinal tract obstruction. When in doubt, it is prudent to leave the tracheal tube in place and provide a period of postoperative ventilation during which the patient's status can be re-evaluated before deciding that extubation is safe.

Meningomyelocele

Clinical Presentation

Myelomeningocele is the most common congenital primary neural tube defect. Despite the known ability of folic acid supplementation during pregnancy to largely prevent this defect, the lesion still occurs in approximately 0.5 to 1 of every 1,000 live births.[194] It results from failure of neural tube closure during the fourth week of gestation. Neural tube defects can be identified on prenatal ultrasound. Elevated maternal serum AFP detects 50% to 90% of open neural tube defects but has a false-positive rate of 5%. Amniotic fluid AFP is more reliable.

By definition, the lesion involves both the meninges and neural components, as compared with a meningocele, which does not contain neural elements. The infant is born with a cystic mass on the back comprising a neural placode, arachnoid, dura, nerve tissue and roots, and cerebrospinal fluid. The lesion most commonly occurs in the lumbosacral or sacral region, although it can extend to the thoracic region. The bony canal is also malformed, leading to multiple orthopaedic problems as the child matures. Urologic complications correlate with the level of the spinal lesion.

Newborns born with myelomeningocele have an associated anomaly of the brainstem known as the *Arnold–Chiari II (Chiari II) malformation.* The Chiari II malformation is characterized by caudal displacement of the cerebellar vermis through the foramen magnum, caudal displacement of the medulla oblongata and the cervical spine, kinking of the medulla, and obliteration of the cisterna magna.[195] The cause of Chiari II malformation rests in the small size of the skull housing the posterior fossa, forcing CNS contents out during development. Hydrocephalus requiring shunting develops in approximately 80% to 90% of infants with myelomeningocele. In contrast, only 20% of patients have symptoms of brainstem dysfunction as a result of the Chiari II malformation, but the mortality rate among those symptomatic patients is high. Complications of brainstem dysfunction include stridor, apnea and bradycardia, aspiration pneumonia, sleep-disordered breathing patterns, vocal cord paralysis, lack of coordination, and spasticity. If the symptoms are not improved by shunting, posterior fossa decompression is necessary.[196]

The infant with a myelomeningocele is usually operated on within the first 24 to 48 hours of life. This reduces the risk for development of ventriculitis or progressive neurologic deficits. Most centers close the defect and place a shunt at the same time. However, some centers may delay placement of a shunt until the infant shows symptoms of hydrocephalus. There is ongoing work to determine the benefits of intrauterine repair of myelomeningocele, hopefully with the benefits of decreased development of a Chiari II malformation, decreased hydrocephalus, and increased lower limb function. As these studies continue, the role of intrauterine repair will become clearer.[197]

Preoperative Care

The preoperative stabilization period focuses on the prevention of infection, maintenance of ECF volume, avoidance of hypothermia, and assessment for other congenital anomalies. The exposed neural placode is susceptible to trauma, leakage, and infection. The infant is usually placed in the prone position, and the placode is covered with warm saline-soaked gauze to prevent desiccation. Because of the high risk of infection, antibiotic therapy is initiated in the preoperative period. Rupture of the cyst on the back can lead to ongoing cerebrospinal fluid leakage. This fluid is replaced with full-strength, balanced salt solution. The infant is also assessed for any potentially life-threatening congenital anomalies.

Perioperative Care

The high prevalence of clinical latex allergy and latex sensitization in children with myelomeningocele has drawn much attention and led many individuals to believe that these patients have an impaired immune system that makes them more susceptible to latex allergy. The likely cause of the increased incidence of latex sensitization is repeated exposure to latex products through frequent hospitalizations and surgical procedures, as well as a program of daily bladder catheterization for those with neurogenic bladders.[198] Although it is reasonable to take special precautions to prevent latex exposure in these patients,[199] it is prudent to limit latex exposure to all patients, especially those who have repeated surgeries, bladder catheterizations, or other exposure to latex products.[200]

Positioning is critical in the infant with myelomeningocele. For induction of anesthesia, the infant may be placed supine with the defect resting in a "doughnut" to minimize trauma. Alternatively, the induction can be performed with the infant in the lateral position, although this makes intubation more challenging. The infant is turned prone for surgery. Rolls are positioned to ensure the abdomen and chest are free, avoiding pressure on the epidural venous plexus to minimize bleeding and allow adequate ventilation.

In most instances, the infant has an intravenous line placed before surgery and an intravenous induction is performed. Succinylcholine may be used to facilitate intubation without risking hyperkalemia.[201] Because increased intracranial pressure is rarely present before closure of the defect, inhalational induction is an alternative in the infant with difficult intravenous access. The anesthetic management of these newborns is rarely complicated unless there are other congenital anomalies that warrant special attention. There is no particular advantage of one technique over another because of the surgical lesion. Because these patients are usually extubated at the end of the case, a technique that allows this is usually chosen. Regional anesthesia has been reported as a safe adjunct or alternative to general anesthesia in the neonate with myelomeningocele. One small series has been published in which tetracaine spinals were used as the anesthetic for 14 infants undergoing repair of myelomeningocele.[202] In this series, there was no evidence of anesthetic-induced neurologic damage. Of note, 2 of the 14 infants had a postoperative respiratory event (1 transient apnea/bradycardia and 1 brief desaturation with bradycardia). Both of these infants had received intraoperative midazolam for sedation.

Postoperative Care

These infants must be monitored closely in the postoperative period. Respiratory complications, including stridor, apnea and bradycardia, cyanosis, and respiratory arrest, may develop after surgery in these infants with known brainstem abnormalities and potential disorders of central respiratory control. In addition, infants who were not shunted during repair may show signs of hydrocephalus, including lethargy, vomiting, seizures, apnea and bradycardia, or cardiovascular instability. These infants need to return to the operating room for insertion of a shunt. Although the majority of these patients will eventually require a shunt, a recent survey has shown that only about one-third of the patients receive one during the initial hospitalization.[203]

Hydrocephalus

Hydrocephalus in the first month of life may have several causes. It may occur after closure of a meningomyelocele because of the Chiari II malformation; it may be congenital in origin; it may be related to intraventricular hemorrhage, especially in the very preterm newborn. The incidence of hydrocephalus has been stable in recent years, with a decrease related to Chiari II malformations, but an increase secondary to hemorrhage in the preterm.[204] The cranial sutures in the neonate are open, so intracranial pressure increases are blunted or minimized. However, infants with hydrocephalus eventually have an increase in head size and sometimes in intracranial pressure, resulting in lethargy, vomiting, and cardiorespiratory problems. The anesthetic approach and the technique for tracheal intubation depend on the infant's condition. The major concern is protection of the airway and control of intracranial pressure. Awake tracheal intubation, crying, struggling, and straining can increase intracranial pressure. A rapid-sequence induction of anesthesia to control the airway and intracranial pressure is preferred. Volatile drugs, nitrous oxide, and opioids are all reasonable choices for maintenance of anesthesia, with no evidence that one technique is superior. Noninvasive intracranial pressure measurements in neurologically normal preterm neonates have shown a decrease in intracranial pressure with all drugs, including ketamine, fentanyl, and isoflurane. The failure of volatile anesthetics and ketamine to increase intracranial pressure as in adults is attributed to the compliance of the neonate's open-sutured cranium. After surgery, the trachea of these infants may remain intubated if they were experiencing periods of apnea or bradycardia before surgery because of the intracranial abnormalities. If not, the trachea can be extubated as soon as the protective reflexes have recovered.

Surgical Procedures in the First Month of Life

Surgical procedures in the first month also are considered emergent, or at least urgent, surgery. The most frequent surgical procedures in the first month are exploratory laparotomy for NEC, inguinal hernia repair, correction of pyloric stenosis, patent ductus arteriosus (PDA) ligation, a shunt procedure for hydrocephalus, and placement of a central venous catheter.

Necrotizing Enterocolitis

NEC is a disease that primarily affects premature infants who have survived the first days of life, although it can be seen in full-term newborns. One of the theories about NEC is that earlier, more rapid feeding places infants at greater risk for development of NEC. The incidence of NEC among very low birth weight infants varies between 5% and 15%.[205] The exact pathophysiology of NEC has been the source of much study and some controversy, although is likely multifactorial.[206] The condition is characterized by a cascade of pathologic events, beginning with an immature distal small and sometimes large intestine that has a decreased ability to absorb substrate, leading to stasis. The most common site is the ileocolic region, but can be seen in other areas and can be discontinuous, giving a patchy appearance. Stasis encourages bacterial proliferation, which leads to local infection. The picture is complicated by further pooling of fluid. The ischemia and infection may lead to necrosis of the intestinal mucosa, followed by perforation. The perforation leads to gangrene of the gut wall, fluid loss, peritonitis, septicemia, and disseminated intravascular coagulation. The first signs that NEC may be developing are abdominal distention, irritability, and the development of metabolic acidosis. This may be followed by radiologic evidence of pneumatosis intestinalis, portal venous air, or free abdominal air. NEC is primarily a medical disease and is treated by cessation of oral intake, administration of antibiotics, fluid and electrolyte therapy, insertion of an orogastric tube, hemodynamic support, and in some cases, the insertion of a peritoneal drain.[207] In nonresponsive cases, the infant becomes more septic with severe peritonitis, and the only solution is to perform an exploratory laparotomy to remove the gangrenous bowel and create an ileostomy.

The preoperative problems are an acute abdomen with severe peritonitis, necrosis, and gangrene of the intestine, septicemia, metabolic acidosis, and hypovolemia. These neonates may also have disseminated intravascular coagulation. Preparation of the patient is directed toward stabilization of these problems. By the time the newborn becomes a surgical candidate, the septicemia, coupled with the distended abdomen and the overall clinical deterioration of the infant, often has necessitated the use of intubation and ventilation in the neonatal intensive care unit. Appropriate laboratory investigations include an arterial blood gas, hemoglobin, glucose, electrolytes, and coagulation profile. The deteriorating status of the patient may compromise both resuscitation efforts and the desire to establish adequate vascular access and monitoring, but focused efforts should be made to provide multiple vascular access lines, an arterial line, and, if time allows, central venous line.

The anesthetic requirements are continuation of resuscitation, provision of abdominal relaxation for the surgery, and careful titration of anesthetic drugs. These infants are often so critically ill that they are very sensitive to the depressant effects of anesthesia. If the patient is not already intubated and ventilated, a rapid-sequence induction with ketamine and succinylcholine is often used. The only caution with this technique is that some patients with NEC have significant hyperkalemia secondary to dead bowel, making the use of succinylcholine problematic. High-dose rocuronium is a reasonable alternative in that situation. Maintenance of anesthesia is usually based on an opioid technique, supplemented with additional doses of ketamine or, if the patient's condition improves, low-dose inhalation agent. The use of nitrous oxide should be avoided because of the gas pockets in the abdomen.

These infants are among the most challenging cases in pediatric anesthesia. The fluid loss can be enormous, both because of surgical losses and third-space losses. Fluid management starts with full-strength, balanced salt solution for maintenance of blood pressure and urine output. Blood products are often needed during these cases. If the hematocrit is below 30% to 35%, red blood cells should be administered. On the basis of both preoperative and intraoperative laboratory work, fresh frozen plasma, platelets, and cryoprecipitate may be needed. Inotropic support may be needed in addition to these measures. The surgical technique and length of surgery is variable, depending on the findings at laparotomy. A combination of bowel resection, primary anastomoses, and enterostomies may be used. At the end of the procedure, these infants are returned intubated and ventilated to the intensive care unit, where resuscitation is continued.[208] Long-term survival is based on several factors, including the degree of prematurity, associated congenital abnormalities, the degree of surviving bowel, the total length of affected bowel, and subsequent complications. Mortality rates, especially in newborns weighing <1,500 g, are poor, with recent studies demonstrating 25% to 50% mortality before discharge.[208,209]

Inguinal Hernia Repair in the Neonate

The development of a hernia in the premature infant or neonate is a different clinical problem from the development of a hernia in an infant older than 1 year. In infants younger than 2 months who need inguinal hernia repair, there is a higher incidence of prematurity, history of RDS, history of incarceration, and congenital heart disease.[210] In preterms, the incidence of hernia may approach 20% to 30%. There is a concern about new or recurring incarceration in these patients, making hernia repair less an elective procedure than in older infants. Consequently, once identified, these patients usually are repaired within a relatively short time. If the patient is currently hospitalized, it is common to repair the hernia before discharge. Otherwise, the surgery should be scheduled within days to weeks of diagnosis.

Anesthetic Techniques for Hernia Repair

Surgical procedures below the umbilicus can be performed with either general or regional anesthesia. The choice of whether to use general or regional anesthesia depends on the preference of the surgeon and/or the anesthesiologist. However, the choice is influenced by the underlying status of the patient, previous complications, and the known risk of preterm patients to develop apnea and bradycardia during and after these procedures. As discussed earlier, there is a risk in any preterm for apnea and bradycardia after stressful procedures, but this has been most widely studied in association with inguinal hernia repair. Analysis of the many small studies have shown certain common elements.[167] Apneic events are inversely related to both gestational age and postconceptual age; the incidence is less in small-for-gestational age infants; anemia increases the incidence of apneic events; and apneic events at home are associated with a higher incidence in the perioperative period. There have been multiple studies that were recently analyzed to determine if the choice of regional or general anesthetic techniques decreased the incidence of apnea and bradycardia.[211] There is not a statistically significant difference in the studies in the incidence of apnea, bradycardia or oxygen desaturation in preterm infants, based on anesthetic technique. Consequently, the choice of anesthetic should not be based solely on the risk of preventing apneic spells. An adjunct that has some evidence in support of its use to minimize apneic spells is caffeine. The use of preservative-free caffeine in a single dose of 10 mg/kg has been suggested to decrease the incidence of apneic spells.[212]

Regional anesthesia can be used entirely for the surgery or as an adjunct to reduce general anesthetic requirements and provide postoperative analgesia. Other methods of providing intraoperative anesthesia and postoperative analgesia include the ilioinguinal–iliohypogastric nerve block or local infiltration. Ilioinguinal–iliohypogastric nerve block with 0.25% bupivacaine or 0.2% ropivacaine, with epinephrine, can be administered shortly after the induction of general anesthesia and affords excellent postoperative analgesia without the need for opioids.

Discharge after inguinal hernia repair to home is an area of some controversy. In particular, which patients can be discharged and which must be observed overnight for apnea and bradycardia? There is significant institutional variation on this issue, with the decision to admit overnight usually based on postconceptual age. There is a tendency to use 46 weeks' postconceptual age as the limit for admission, but other centers will use up to 60 weeks' postconceptual age as the limit. In our own institution, we have used a different approach. In order to make the limit easily understandable and also understanding that the basis of determining gestational age is not precise, we have all preterms admitted until they are 6 months of age. This ensures 26 weeks added to gestational age and is a compromise between the 46-week and 60-week limits, but is easy to administer. No matter what limits are used, if the infant has apneic or bradycardic spells during the perioperative period, he or she should be monitored in-house until the infant has been symptom-free for at least 12 hours.

Pyloric Stenosis

Pyloric stenosis is a relatively frequent surgical disease of the neonate and infant. It can appear as early as the second week of life. The pathologic characteristics include hypertrophy of the pyloric smooth muscle with edema of the pyloric mucosa and submucosa. This process, which develops over a period of days to weeks, leads to progressive obstruction of the pyloric valve, causing persistent vomiting. The vomiting leads to varying losses of fluids and electrolytes. The diagnosis is usually made at an early stage in the development of symptoms, especially with the help of ultrasound, so it is rare to find an infant with severe fluid and electrolyte derangements. However, an infant is occasionally seen whose problem has developed slowly over a period of weeks, resulting in severe fluid and electrolyte derangements. The stomach contents contain sodium, potassium, chloride, hydrogen ions, and water. The classic electrolyte pattern in infants with severe vomiting is hyponatremic, hypokalemic, and hypochloremic metabolic alkalosis with a compensatory respiratory acidosis. The anesthesiologist, pediatrician, and surgeon are all responsible for preparing these infants for surgery. Pyloric stenosis is a medical emergency, not a surgical emergency. The patient should not be operated on until there has been adequate fluid and electrolyte resuscitation. The infant should have normal skin turgor, and the correction of the electrolyte imbalance should produce a sodium level that is >130 mEq/L, a potassium level that is at least 3 mEq/L, a chloride level that is >85 mEq/L and increasing, and a urine output of at least 1 to 2 mL/kg/hr. These patients need a resuscitation fluid of full-strength, balanced salt solution and, after the infant begins to urinate, the addition of potassium.

Anesthetic Management

It is prudent to pass a large orogastric tube and aspirate the stomach contents because of the significant volume that may be present.[213] This procedure greatly reduces the quantity of gastric fluid. A rapid-sequence induction is advisable because of the potential for additional volume in the stomach. Although awake intubation had been popular with some clinicians in the past, it is associated with a higher incidence of complications and is traumatic to the child.[122] These patients have been fully resuscitated before coming to surgery, so there is little reason for an awake intubation. Anesthesia can be maintained by almost any technique the clinician prefers. There has been a need for muscle relaxation only for a short period during open pyloromyotomy, especially during the delivery of the pylorus at the start of the procedure and during replacement of the pylorus back into the abdomen to begin closure. However, these cases are increasingly being performed laparoscopically. Controlled ventilation reduces or eliminates the need for muscle relaxants for this surgery. At the end of the case, the patient should be wide awake before extubation. A TAP block can be provided using ultrasound guidance for postoperative pain relief with good analgesia.

Ligation of a Patent Ductus Arteriosus

As the number of small premature infants who survive has increased, so also has the number of infants who have a PDA with heart failure and respiratory failure. Prostaglandins relax the smooth muscle of the ductus so it cannot constrict. Indomethacin, a prostaglandin synthetase inhibitor, is administered to encourage closure of the ductus. However, indomethacin is often unsuccessful in the small premature infant because of the lack of muscle within the ductus. Infants with a PDA and heart failure need maximal medical management with fluid restriction, diuretics, and inotropes. These infants are at special risk because of the reduced blood volume and precarious cardiopulmonary system. If the surgery is performed in the operating room, special attention is taken to maintain normothermia, ventilation, and oxygenation during transport. If the surgery is performed at bedside in the neonatal intensive care unit, the anesthesiologist must take time before the procedure to establish where he or she will be situated, where all venous access is, and that all drugs and fluids are already prepared. An opioid-based technique with muscle relaxant is a frequent choice for anesthesia. Probably the biggest challenge during these cases is the diagnosis and management of hypotension. There can be sudden, catastrophic blood loss if the ductus tears. Consequently, syringes of balanced salt solution and blood should be immediately available. The other common cause of hypotension is compression of the lungs, heart, and great vessels by the surgeon as they are gaining exposure. This is a balance between stopping the procedure to allow the heart and blood pressure to recover versus the need to proceed with the operation. The answer comes in close communication between the anesthesiologist and the surgeon. These patients usually remain intubated after procedure, without a need to reverse the muscle relaxant. Residual opioid will provide good analgesia for the immediate postoperative period.

There are two newer techniques for closing the PDA in infants that are increasing in popularity.[214] Video-assisted thoracoscopic surgery (VATS) uses small endoscopes inserted through a series of small thoracotomy incisions to guide instruments to ligate the ductus with a thoracotomy. VATS can be done either in the operating room or, rarely, at bedside. The other approach is used by cardiologists in the cardiac catheterization to occlude the ductus with a coil. In either case, the anesthetic challenge is not so much choice of drugs, but adapting to working in an unfamiliar environment, like the catheterization suite, or understanding how the positioning, lung deflation, and need to identify the recurrent laryngeal nerve requirements of the VATS will affect their anesthetic management.

Placement of a Central Venous Catheter

The use of a central venous catheter for monitoring serum electrolytes, for hyperalimentation, and for administering medications is a well-established part of modern perioperative care. It can be placed either as part of the surgical procedure or at some other time as a separate procedure. The three major concerns in central venous catheter placement are airway management, pneumothorax, and bleeding. The airway should be secured by an endotracheal tube because of the difficulty in sharing the head, neck, and upper chest with the surgeon and as an adjunct for treating complications such as pneumothorax and bleeding. The anesthetic technique depends on the infant's condition. A pneumothorax may occur with attempts at subclavian vein puncture. The first indication of pneumothorax may be a decreasing oxygen saturation, hypotension, or difficulty with ventilation of the lungs. Because a fluoroscope is often used for central venous catheter placement, it can be used rapidly to diagnose a pneumothorax. If not, the chest should be rapidly aspirated for both diagnostic and therapeutic reasons. Bleeding is an unusual but serious complication of central venous catheter placement. It usually becomes manifest in the perioperative period as hemothorax or as hypovolemia with a decreasing hematocrit or blood pressure. The establishment of intravenous access placed before proceeding with a central line is problematic for some patients. The reason for the central line may very well be the inability to obtain peripheral access, and the clinician is left with a trade-off between prolonged attempts at starting an intravenous catheter versus proceeding directly to obtain central venous line placement. This is a clinical judgment that depends not only on the time and effort that has been spent in obtaining peripheral access, but also the underlying status of the patient. If there is a question about how to proceed, the anesthesiologist and surgeon should discuss and agree on the approach. Strict attention to skin preparation, sterile glove and drape use, and minimizing access to the central line are components important to diminish catheter-related sepsis. Subclavian approach has a higher incidence of problems than an external or internal jugular approach.

SUMMARY

8 The anesthetic management of the newborn is among the most challenging in all of anesthesiology. A strong foundation in neonatal anatomy, physiology, and pharmacology is needed, as well

as an appreciation of the disease states and surgical procedures that are unique to this population. A thorough preanesthetic evaluation and preparation, a concise plan, and meticulous technique are the basis of an effective approach. The patient's neonatologist or pediatrician and the surgeon are strong allies in providing the best care, and close communication with them is necessary. Lastly, the clinical status of a newborn can change remarkably quickly. Strict attention to detail and prospective management are the hallmarks of the anesthesiologist skilled in providing care in these difficult cases. Use of current technology including ultrasound guidance should be used for facilitating vascular access as well as regional anesthesia for pain management in these fragile infants should be vastly encouraged when available.

References

1. Friedman AH, Fahey JT. The transition from fetal to neonatal circulation: Normal responses and implications for infants with heart disease. *Semin Perinatol.* 1993;17:106.
2. Baum VC, Palmisano BW. The immature heart and anesthesia. *Anesthesiology.* 1997;87:1529.
3. Fu JD, Li J, Tweedie D, et al. Crucial role of the sarcoplasmic reticulum in the developmental regulation of Ca^{2+} transients and contraction in cardiomyocytes derived from embryonic stem cells. *Faseb J.* 2006;20:181.
4. Auman JT, Seidler FJ, Tate CA, et al. Are developing beta-adrenoceptors able to desensitize? Acute and chronic effects of beta-agonists in neonatal heart and liver. *Am J Physiol Regul Integr Comp Physiol.* 2002;283:R205.
5. Kishkurno S, Takahashi Y, Harada K, et al. Postnatal changes in left ventricular volume and contractility in healthy term infants. *Pediatr Cardiol.* 1997;18:91.
6. Hislop A. Developmental biology of the pulmonary circulation. *Paediatr Respir Rev.* 2005;6:35.
7. Mansell AL, Collins MH, Johnson E Jr, et al. Postnatal growth of lung parenchyma in the piglet: Morphometry correlated with mechanics. *Anat Rec.* 1995;241:99.
8. Merrill JD, Ballard RA. Pulmonary surfactant for neonatal respiratory disorders. *Curr Opin Pediatr.* 2003;15:149.
9. Engle WA. Surfactant-replacement therapy for respiratory distress in the preterm and term neonate. *Pediatrics.* 2008;121:419.
10. Hernandez-Diaz S, Van Marter LJ, Werler MM, et al. Risk factors for persistent pulmonary hypertension of the newborn. *Pediatrics.* 2007;120:e272.
11. Shah PS, Ohlsson A. Sildenafil for pulmonary hypertension in neonates. *Cochrane Database Syst Rev.* 2007:CD005494.
12. Murphy JD, Vawter GF, Reid LM. Pulmonary vascular disease in fatal meconium aspiration. *J Pediatr.* 1984;104:758.
13. Velaphi S, Vidyasagar D. Intrapartum and postdelivery management of infants born to mothers with meconium-stained amniotic fluid: Evidence-based recommendations. *Clin Perinatol.* 2006;33:29.
14. Drukker A, Guignard JP. Renal aspects of the term and preterm infant: A selective update. *Curr Opin Pediatr.* 2002;14:175.
15. Bartelink IH, Rademaker CM, Schobben AF, et al. Guidelines on paediatric dosing on the basis of developmental physiology and pharmacokinetic considerations. *Clin Pharmacokinet.* 2006;45:1077.
16. Alcorn J, McNamara PJ. Ontogeny of hepatic and renal systemic clearance pathways in infants: Part I. *Clin Pharmacokinet.* 2002;41:959.
17. Nash PL. Potassium and sodium homeostasis in the neonate. *Neonatal Netw.* 2007;26:125.
18. Cornblath M, Ichord R. Hypoglycemia in the neonate. *Semin Perinatol.* 2000; 24:136.
19. Ballweg JA, Wernovsky G, Ittenbach RF, et al. Hyperglycemia after infant cardiac surgery does not adversely impact neurodevelopmental outcome. *Ann Thorac Surg.* 2007;84:2052.
20. de Ferranti S, Gauvreau K, Hickey PR, et al. Intraoperative hyperglycemia during infant cardiac surgery is not associated with adverse neurodevelopmental outcomes at 1, 4, and 8 years. *Anesthesiology.* 2004;100:1345.
21. Wu Y, Stack G. Blood product replacement in the perinatal period. *Semin Perinatol.* 2007;31:262.
22. Alcorn J, McNamara PJ. Pharmacokinetics in the newborn. *Adv Drug Deliv Rev.* 2003;55:667.
23. Strassburg CP, Strassburg A, Kneip S, et al. Developmental aspects of human hepatic drug glucuronidation in young children and adults. *Gut.* 2002;50:259.
24. de Wildt SN, Kearns GL, Leeder JS, et al. Glucuronidation in humans. Pharmacogenetic and developmental aspects. *Clin Pharmacokinet.* 1999;36:439.
25. Leeder JS, Kearns GL. Pharmacogenetics in pediatrics. Implications for practice. *Pediatr Clin North Am.* 1997;44:55.
26. Lynn AM, Slattery JT. Morphine pharmacokinetics in early infancy. *Anesthesiology.* 1987;66:136.
27. Bory C, Baltassat P, Porthault M, et al. Metabolism of theophylline to caffeine in premature newborn infants. *J Pediatr.* 1979;94:988.
28. Green MD, Fischer LJ. Hepatotoxicity of acetaminophen in neonatal and young rats. II. Metabolic aspects. *Toxicol Appl Pharmacol.* 1984;74:125.
29. Green MD, Shires TK, Fischer LJ. Hepatotoxicity of acetaminophen in neonatal and young rats. I. Age-related changes in susceptibility. *Toxicol Appl Pharmacol.* 1984;74:116.
30. deAlmeida VL, Alvaro RA, Haider Z, et al. The effect of nasal occlusion on the initiation of oral breathing in preterm infants. *Pediatr Pulmonol.* 1994;18:374.
31. Miller MJ, Carlo WA, Strohl KP, et al. Effect of maturation on oral breathing in sleeping premature infants. *J Pediatr.* 1986;109:515.
32. Weiss M, Dullenkopf A, Fischer JE, et al. Prospective randomized controlled multi-centre trial of cuffed or uncuffed endotracheal tubes in small children. *Br J Anaesth.* 2009;103(6):867–873.
33. Mazoit JX. Pharmacokinetic/pharmacodynamic modeling of anesthetics in children: Therapeutic implications. *Paediatr Drugs.* 2006;8:139.
34. McNamara PJ, Alcorn J. Protein binding predictions in infants. *AAPS PharmSci.* 2002;4:E4.
35. Bhutada A, Sahni R, Rastogi S, et al. Randomised controlled trial of thiopental for intubation in neonates. *Arch Dis Child Fetal Neonatal Ed.* 2000;82:F34.
36. Ghanta S, Abdel-Latif ME, Lui K, et al. Propofol compared with the morphine, atropine, and suxamethonium regimen as induction agents for neonatal endotracheal intubation: A randomized, controlled trial. *Pediatrics.* 2007;119:e1248.
37. Allegaert K, Peeters MY, Verbesselt R, et al. Inter-individual variability in propofol pharmacokinetics in preterm and term neonates. *Br J Anaesth.* 2007;99:864.
38. Bhutta AT. Ketamine: A controversial drug for neonates. *Semin Perinatol.* 2007; 31:303.
39. Mellon RD, Simone AF, Rappaport BA. Use of anesthetic agents in neonates and young children. *Anesth Analg.* 2007;104:509.
40. Anand KJ, Garg S, Rovnaghi CR, et al. Ketamine reduces the cell death following inflammatory pain in newborn rat brain. *Pediatr Res.* 2007;62(3):283–290.
41. Radnay PA, Hollinger I, Santi A, et al. Ketamine for pediatric cardiac anesthesia. *Anaesthesist.* 1976;25:259.
42. Suresh S, Anand KJ. Opioid tolerance in neonates: A state-of-the-art review. *Paediatr Anaesth.* 2001;11:511.
43. Santeiro ML, Christie J, Stromquist C, et al. Pharmacokinetics of continuous infusion fentanyl in newborns. *J Perinatol.* 1997;17:135.
44. Burtin P, Daoud P, Jacqz-Aigrain E, et al. Hypotension with midazolam and fentanyl in the newborn. *Lancet.* 1991;337:1545.
45. Vaughn PR, Townsend SF, Thilo EH, et al. Comparison of continuous infusion of fentanyl to bolus dosing in neonates after surgery. *J Pediatr Surg.* 1996;31:1616.
46. Fahnenstich H, Steffan J, Kau N, et al. Fentanyl-induced chest wall rigidity and laryngospasm in preterm and term infants. *Crit Care Med.* 2000;28:836.
47. Bhat R, Chari G, Gulati A, et al. Pharmacokinetics of a single dose of morphine in preterm infants during the first week of life. *J Pediatr.* 1990;117:477.
48. Saarenmaa E, Neuvonen PJ, Rosenberg P, et al. Morphine clearance and effects in newborn infants in relation to gestational age. *Clin Pharmacol Ther.* 2000;68:160.
49. El Sayed MF, Taddio A, Fallah S, et al. Safety profile of morphine following surgery in neonates. *J Perinatol.* 2007;27:444.
50. Rao R, Sampers JS, Kronsberg SS, et al. Neurobehavior of preterm infants at 36 weeks postconception as a function of morphine analgesia. *Am J Perinatol.* 2007; 24:511.
51. Murphey LJ, Olsen GD. Morphine-6-beta-D-glucuronide respiratory pharmacodynamics in the neonatal guinea pig. *J Pharmacol Exp Ther.* 1994;268:110.
52. Peters JW, Anderson BJ, Simons SH, et al. Morphine metabolite pharmacokinetics during venoarterial extra corporeal membrane oxygenation in neonates. *Clin Pharmacokinet.* 2006;45:705.
53. Davis PJ, Cladis FP. The use of ultra-short-acting opioids in paediatric anaesthesia: The role of remifentanil. *Clin Pharmacokinet.* 2005;44:787.
54. Davis PJ, Galinkin J, McGowan FX, et al. A randomized multicenter study of remifentanil compared with halothane in neonates and infants undergoing pyloromyotomy. I. Emergence and recovery profiles. *Anesth Analg.* 2001;93:1380.
55. Hannallah RS, Oh TH, McGill WA, et al. Changes in heart rate and rhythm after intramuscular succinylcholine with or without atropine in anesthetized children. *Anesth Analg.* 1986;65:1329.
56. Wang JM, Stanley TH. Duchenne muscular dystrophy and malignant hyperthermia–two case reports. *Can Anaesth Soc J.* 1986;33:492.
57. Meakin GH. Muscle relaxants in paediatric day case surgery. *Eur J Anaesthesiol Suppl.* 2001;23:47.
58. Rapp HJ, Altenmueller CA, Waschke C. Neuromuscular recovery following rocuronium bromide single dose in infants. *Paediatr Anaesth.* 2004;14(4):329–335.
59. Meretoja OA, Wirtavuori K, Neuvonen PJ. Age-dependence of the dose-response curve of vecuronium in pediatric patients during balanced anesthesia. *Anesth Analg.* 1988;67:21.
60. Cook DR. Paediatric anaesthesia: Pharmacological considerations. *Drugs.* 1976; 12:212.
61. Gronert BJ, Brandom BW. Neuromuscular blocking drugs in infants and children. *Pediatr Clin North Am.* 1994;41:73.
62. Goudsouzian NG, Crone RK, Todres ID. Recovery from pancuronium blockade in the neonatal intensive care unit. *Br J Anaesth.* 1981;53:1303.

63. Cheung PY, Tyebkhan JM, Peliowski A, et al. Prolonged use of pancuronium bromide and sensorineural hearing loss in childhood survivors of congenital diaphragmatic hernia. *J Pediatr.* 1999;135:233.
64. Diaz JH. Halothane anesthesia in infancy: Identification and correlation of preoperative risk factors with intraoperative arterial hypotension and postoperative recovery. *J Pediatr Surg.* 1985;20:502.
65. Imamura S, Ikeda K. Comparison of the epinephrine-induced arrhythmogenic effect of sevoflurane with isoflurane and halothane. *J Anesth.* 1987;1:62.
66. Murray DJ, Forbes RB, Mahoney LT. Comparative hemodynamic depression of halothane versus isoflurane in neonates and infants: An echocardiographic study. *Anesth Analg.* 1992;74:329.
67. Lerman J, Sikich N, Kleinman S, et al. The pharmacology of sevoflurane in infants and children. *Anesthesiology.* 1994;80:814.
68. Russell IA, Miller Hance WC, Gregory G, et al. The safety and efficacy of sevoflurane anesthesia in infants and children with congenital heart disease. *Anesth Analg.* 2001;92:1152.
69. Brown K, Aun C, Stocks J, et al. A comparison of the respiratory effects of sevoflurane and halothane in infants and young children. *Anesthesiology.* 1998; 89:86.
70. Taylor RH, Lerman J. Induction, maintenance and recovery characteristics of desflurane in infants and children. *Can J Anaesth.* 1992;39:6.
71. Sale SM, Read JA, Stoddart PA, et al. Prospective comparison of sevoflurane and desflurane in formerly premature infants undergoing inguinal herniotomy. *Br J Anaesth.* 2006;96:774.
72. Tucker GT. Pharmacokinetics of local anaesthetics. *Br J Anaesth.* 1986;58:717.
73. Anderson BJ, Palmer GM. Recent pharmacological advances in paediatric analgesics. *Biomed Pharmacother.* 2006;60:303.
74. Rothstein P, Arthur GR, Feldman HS, et al. Bupivacaine for intercostal nerve blocks in children: Blood concentrations and pharmacokinetics. *Anesth Analg.* 1986;65:625.
75. Ecoffey C, Desparmet J, Maury M, et al. Bupivacaine in children: Pharmacokinetics following caudal anesthesia. *Anesthesiology.* 1985;63:447.
76. Willschke H, Bosenberg A, Marhofer P, et al. Ultrasonographic-guided ilioinguinal/iliohypogastric nerve block in pediatric anesthesia: What is the optimal volume? *Anesth Analg.* 2006;102:1680.
77. Beauvoir C, Rochette A, Desch G, et al. Spinal anaesthesia in newborns: Total and free bupivacaine plasma concentration. *Paediatr Anaesth.* 1996;6:195.
78. Berde CB. Convulsions associated with pediatric regional anesthesia. *Anesth Analg.* 1992;75:164.
79. Rapp HJ, Molnar V, Austin S, et al. Ropivacaine in neonates and infants: A population pharmacokinetic evaluation following single caudal block. *Paediatr Anaesth.* 2004;14:724.
80. McCloskey JJ, Haun SE, Deshpande JK. Bupivacaine toxicity secondary to continuous caudal epidural infusion in children. *Anesth Analg.* 1992;75:287.
81. Hansen TG, Ilett KF, Reid C, et al. Caudal ropivacaine in infants: Population pharmacokinetics and plasma concentrations. *Anesthesiology.* 2001;94:579.
82. Chalkiadis GA, Eyres RL, Cranswick N, et al. Pharmacokinetics of levo-bupivacaine 0.25% following caudal administration in children under 2 years of age. *Br J Anaesth.* 2004;92:218.
83. Simpson D, Curran MP, Oldfield V, et al. Ropivacaine: A review of its use in regional anaesthesia and acute pain management. *Drugs.* 2005;65:2675.
84. Tucker GT, Mather LE. Clinical pharmacokinetics of local anaesthetics. *Clin Pharmacokinet.* 1979;4:241.
85. Tobias JD, O'Dell N. Chloroprocaine for epidural anesthesia in infants and children. *Aana J.* 1995;63:131.
86. Weinberg G, Ripper R, Feinstein DL, et al. Lipid emulsion infusion rescues dogs from bupivacaine-induced cardiac toxicity. *Reg Anesth Pain Med.* 2003;28(3): 198–202.
87. Rosenblatt MA, Abel M, Fischer GW, et al. Successful use of a 20% lipid emulsion to resuscitate a patient after a presumed bupivacaine-related cardiac arrest. *Anesthesiology.* 2006;105(1):217–218.
88. Shah S, Gopalakrishnan S, Apuya J, et al. Use of Intralipid in an infant with impending cardiovascular collapse due to local anesthetic toxicity. *J Anesth.* 2009;23(3):439–441.
89. Weise KL, Nahata MC. EMLA for painful procedures in infants. *J Pediatr Health Care.* 2005;19:42; quiz 48.
90. Couper RT. Methaemoglobinaemia secondary to topical lignocaine/prilocaine in a circumcised neonate. *J Paediatr Child Health.* 2000;36:406.
91. Lillieborg S, Otterbom I, Ahlen K. Topical anaesthesia in neonates, infants and children. *Br J Anaesth.* 2004;92:450.
92. Lehr VT, Taddio A. Topical anesthesia in neonates: Clinical practices and practical considerations. *Semin Perinatol.* 2007;31:323.
93. Bhananker SM, Ramamoorthy C, Geiduschek JM, et al. Anesthesia-related cardiac arrest in children: Update from the Pediatric Perioperative Cardiac Arrest Registry. *Anesth Analg.* 2007;105:344.
94. Morray JP, Geiduschek JM, Caplan RA, et al. A comparison of pediatric and adult anesthesia closed malpractice claims. *Anesthesiology.* 1993;78:461.
95. Braz LG, Modolo NS, do Nascimento P Jr, et al. Perioperative cardiac arrest: A study of 53,718 anaesthetics over 9 yr from a Brazilian teaching hospital. *Br J Anaesth.* 2006;96:569.
96. Murat I, Constant I, Maud'huy H. Perioperative anaesthetic morbidity in children: A database of 24,165 anaesthetics over a 30-month period. *Paediatr Anaesth.* 2004;14:158.
97. Hackel A, Badgwell JM, Binding RR, et al. Guidelines for the pediatric perioperative anesthesia environment. American Academy of Pediatrics. Section on Anesthesiology. *Pediatrics.* 1999;103:512.
98. Howard CR, Howard FM, Garfunkel LC, et al. Neonatal circumcision and pain relief: Current training practices. *Pediatrics.* 1998;101:423.
99. Anand KJ, Sippell WG, Aynsley-Green A. Pain, anaesthesia, and babies. *Lancet.* 1987;2:1210.
100. Berry FA, Gregory GA. Do premature infants require anesthesia for surgery? *Anesthesiology.* 1987;67:291.
101. Anand KJ, Carr DB. The neuroanatomy, neurophysiology, and neurochemistry of pain, stress, and analgesia in newborns and children. *Pediatr Clin North Am.* 1989;36:795.
102. Tomashek KM, Shapiro-Mendoza CK, Davidoff MJ, et al. Differences in mortality between late-preterm and term singleton infants in the United States, 1995–2002. *J Pediatr.* 2007;151:450.
103. Ozyurek E, Cetintas S, Ceylan T, et al. Complete blood count parameters for healthy, small-for-gestational-age, full-term newborns. *Clin Lab Haematol.* 2006;28:97.
104. Deshpande S, Ward Platt M. The investigation and management of neonatal hypoglycaemia. *Semin Fetal Neonatal Med.* 2005;10:351.
105. Lippi G, Salvagno GL, Rugolotto S, et al. Routine coagulation tests in newborn and young infants. *J Thromb Thrombolysis.* 2007;24:153.
106. Friesen RH, Lichtor JL. Cardiovascular effects of inhalation induction with isoflurane in infants. *Anesth Analg.* 1983;62:411.
107. Murray DJ, Forbes RB, Dillman JB, et al. Haemodynamic effects of atropine during halothane or isoflurane anaesthesia in infants and small children. *Can J Anaesth.* 1989;36:295.
108. Mariani G, Dik PB, Ezquer A, et al. Pre-ductal and post-ductal O2 saturation in healthy term neonates after birth. *J Pediatr.* 2007;150:418.
109. Shiao SY. Effects of fetal hemoglobin on accurate measurements of oxygen saturation in neonates. *J Perinat Neonatal Nurs.* 2005;19:348.
110. Hubmayr RD. The times are a-changin': Should we hang up the stethoscope? *Anesthesiology.* 2004;100:1.
111. Pandit PB, Pandit FA, Govan J, et al. Complications associated with surgically placed central venous catheters in low birth weight neonates. *J Perinatol.* 1999;19:106.
112. Sigaut S, Skhiri A, Stany I, et al. Ultrasound guided internal jugular vein access in children and infant: A meta-analysis of published studies. *Paediatr Anaesth.* 2009;19(12):1199–1206.
113. Schily M, Koumoukelis H, Lerman J, et al. Can pediatric anesthesiologists detect an occluded tracheal tube in neonates? *Anesth Analg.* 2001;93:66.
114. Spears RS Jr, Yeh A, Fisher DM, et al. The "educated hand". Can anesthesiologists assess changes in neonatal pulmonary compliance manually? *Anesthesiology.* 1991;75:693.
115. Tobin MJ, Stevenson GW, Horn BJ, et al. A comparison of three modes of ventilation with the use of an adult circle system in an infant lung model. *Anesth Analg.* 1998;87:766.
116. Nakae Y, Miyabe M, Sonoda H, et al. Comparison of the Jackson-Rees circuit, the pediatric circle, and the MERA F breathing system for pediatric anesthesia. *Anesth Analg.* 1996;83:488.
117. Cote CJ. Pediatric breathing circuits and anesthesia machines. *Int Anesthesiol Clin.* 1992;30:51.
118. Spoerel WE, Bain JA. Anaesthetic breathing systems. *Br J Anaesth.* 1986;58:819.
119. Hunter T, Lerman J, Bissonnette B. The temperature and humidity of inspired gases in infants using a pediatric circle system: Effects of high and low-flow anesthesia. *Paediatr Anaesth.* 2005;15:750.
120. Luchetti M, Pigna A, Gentili A, et al. Evaluation of the efficiency of heat and moisture exchangers during paediatric anaesthesia. *Paediatr Anaesth.* 1999;9:39.
121. Monrigal JP, Granry JC. The benefit of using a heat and moisture exchanger during short operations in young children. *Paediatr Anaesth.* 1997;7:295.
122. Cook-Sather SD, Tulloch HV, Cnaan A, et al. A comparison of awake versus paralyzed tracheal intubation for infants with pyloric stenosis. *Anesth Analg.* 1998;86:945.
123. Ledbetter JL, Rasch DK, Pollard TG, et al. Reducing the risks of laryngoscopy in anaesthetised infants. *Anaesthesia.* 1988;43:151.
124. Todres ID, Crone RK. Experience with a modified laryngoscope in sick infants. *Crit Care Med.* 1981;9:544.
125. Salgo B, Schmitz A, Henze G, et al. Evaluation of a new recommendation for improved cuffed tracheal tube size selection in infants and small children. *Acta Anaesthesiol Scand.* 2006;50:557.
126. Lonnqvist PA. Successful use of laryngeal mask airway in low-weight expremature infants with bronchopulmonary dysplasia undergoing cryotherapy for retinopathy of the premature. *Anesthesiology.* 1995;83:422.
127. Hansen TG, Joensen H, Henneberg SW, et al. Laryngeal mask airway guided tracheal intubation in a neonate with the Pierre Robin syndrome. *Acta Anaesthesiol Scand.* 1995;39:129.
128. Fisher QA, Tunkel DE. Lightwand intubation of infants and children. *J Clin Anesth.* 1997;9:275.

129. Cain JM, Mason LJ, Martin RD. Airway management in two of newborns with Pierre Robin Sequence: The use of disposable vs multiple use LMA for fiberoptic intubation. *Paediatr Anaesth.* 2006;16:1274.
130. Somri M, Barna Teszler C, Tome R, et al. Flexible fiberoptic bronchoscopy through the laryngeal mask airway in a small, premature neonate. *Am J Otolaryngol.* 2005;26:268.
131. Moura JH, da Silva GA. Neonatal laryngoscope intubation and the digital method: A randomized controlled trial. *J Pediatr.* 2006;148:840.
132. Marraro G. Intraoperative ventilation. *Paediatr Anaesth.* 1998;8:373.
133. Marhofer P, Willschke H, Kettner S. Imaging techniques for regional nerve blockade and vascular cannulation in children. *Curr Opin Anaesthesiol.* 2006;19:293.
134. Weinberg GL, Ripper R, Murphy P, et al. Lipid infusion accelerates removal of bupivacaine and recovery from bupivacaine toxicity in the isolated rat heart. *Reg Anesth Pain Med.* 2006;31:296.
135. Suresh S, Wheeler M. Practical pediatric regional anesthesia. *Anesthesiol Clin North America.* 2002;20:83.
136. Williams RK, Adams DC, Aladjem EV, et al. The safety and efficacy of spinal anesthesia for surgery in infants: The Vermont Infant Spinal Registry. *Anesth Analg.* 2006;102:67.
137. Kim GS, Song JG, Gwak MS, et al. Postoperative outcome in formerly premature infants undergoing herniorrhaphy: Comparison of spinal and general anesthesia. *J Korean Med Sci.* 2003;18:691.
138. Suresh S, Hall SC. Spinal anesthesia in infants: Is the impractical practical? *Anesth Analg.* 2006;102:65.
139. Welborn LG, Rice LJ, Hannallah RS, et al. Postoperative apnea in former preterm infants: Prospective comparison of spinal and general anesthesia. *Anesthesiology.* 1990;72:838.
140. Tsui BC, Tarkkila P, Gupta S, et al. Confirmation of caudal needle placement using nerve stimulation. *Anesthesiology.* 1999;91:374.
141. Marhofer P, Bosenberg A, Sitzwohl C, et al. Pilot study of neuraxial imaging by ultrasound in infants and children. *Paediatr Anaesth.* 2005;15:671.
142. Freid EB, Bailey AG, Valley RD. Electrocardiographic and hemodynamic changes associated with unintentional intravascular injection of bupivacaine with epinephrine in infants. *Anesthesiology.* 1993;79:394.
143. Wheeler M, Patel A, Suresh S, et al. The addition of clonidine 2 microg.kg-1 does not enhance the postoperative analgesia of a caudal block using 0.125% bupivacaine and epinephrine 1:200,000 in children: A prospective, double-blind, randomized study. *Paediatr Anaesth.* 2005;15:476.
144. Willschke H, Bosenberg A, Marhofer P, et al. Epidural catheter placement in neonates: Sonoanatomy and feasibility of ultrasonographic guidance in term and preterm neonates. *Reg Anesth Pain Med.* 2007;32:34.
145. Brady-Fryer B, Wiebe N, Lander JA. Pain relief for neonatal circumcision. *Cochrane Database Syst Rev.* 2004:CD004217.
146. Bielsky A, Efrat R, Suresh S. Postoperative analgesia in neonates after major abdominal surgery: 'TAP' our way to success! *Paediatr Anaesth.* 2009;19(5): 541–542.
147. Marhofer P, Greher M, Kapral S. Ultrasound guidance in regional anaesthesia. *Br J Anaesth.* 2005;94:7.
148. Marhofer P, Sitzwohl C, Greher M, et al. Ultrasound guidance for infraclavicular brachial plexus anaesthesia in children. *Anaesthesia.* 2004;59:642.
149. Suresh S, Voronov P. Head and neck blocks in children: An anatomical and procedural review. *Paediatr Anaesth.* 2006;16:910.
150. Williams DG, Patel A, Howard RF. Pharmacogenetics of codeine metabolism in an urban population of children and its implications for analgesic reliability. *Br J Anaesth.* 2002;89:839.
151. Birmingham PK, Tobin MJ, Henthorn TK, et al. Twenty-four-hour pharmacokinetics of rectal acetaminophen in children: An old drug with new recommendations. *Anesthesiology.* 1997;87:244.
152. Moores MA, Wandless JG, Fell D. Paediatric postoperative analgesia. A comparison of rectal diclofenac with caudal bupivacaine after inguinal herniotomy. *Anaesthesia.* 1990;45:156.
153. Cheung CL, van Dijk M, Green JW, et al. Effects of low-dose naloxone on opioid therapy in pediatric patients: A retrospective case-control study. *Intensive Care Med.* 2007;33:190.
154. Bartocci M, Lundeberg S. Intravenous paracetamol: The 'Stockholm protocol' for postoperative analgesia of term and preterm neonates. *Paediatr Anaesth.* 2007;17(11):1120–1121.
155. Papacci P, De Francisci G, Iacobucci T, et al. Use of intravenous ketorolac in the neonate and premature babies. *Paediatr Anaesth.* 2004;14:487.
156. Rayburn WF. Maternal and fetal effects from substance use. *Clin Perinatol.* 2007;34:559, vi.
157. Lipshultz SE, Frassica JJ, Orav EJ. Cardiovascular abnormalities in infants prenatally exposed to cocaine. *J Pediatr.* 1991;118:44.
158. Hackman PS. Recognizing and understanding the cold-stressed term infant. *Neonatal Netw.* 2001;20:35.
159. Kongsayreepong S, Gunnaleka P, Suraseranivongse S, et al. A reusable, custom-made warming blanket prevents core hypothermia during major neonatal surgery. *Can J Anaesth.* 2002;49:605.
160. Plattner O, Semsroth M, Sessler DI, et al. Lack of nonshivering thermogenesis in infants anesthetized with fentanyl and propofol. *Anesthesiology.* 1997;86: 772.
161. Bissonnette B, Sessler DI. The thermoregulatory threshold in infants and children anesthetized with isoflurane and caudal bupivacaine. *Anesthesiology.* 1990; 73:1114.
162. Ehrenkranz RA, Walsh MC, Vohr BR, et al. Validation of the National Institutes of Health consensus definition of bronchopulmonary dysplasia. *Pediatrics.* 2005;116:1353.
163. Steward DJ. Preterm infants are more prone to complications following minor surgery than are term infants. *Anesthesiology.* 1982;56:304.
164. McNamara DG, Nixon GM, Anderson BJ. Methylxanthines for the treatment of apnea associated with bronchiolitis and anesthesia. *Paediatr Anaesth.* 2004;14:541.
165. Krane EJ, Haberkern CM, Jacobson LE. Postoperative apnea, bradycardia, and oxygen desaturation in formerly premature infants: Prospective comparison of spinal and general anesthesia. *Anesth Analg.* 1995;80:7.
166. Kurth CD, Spitzer AR, Broennle AM, et al. Postoperative apnea in preterm infants. *Anesthesiology.* 1987;66:483.
167. Cote CJ, Zaslavsky A, Downes JJ, et al. Postoperative apnea in former preterm infants after inguinal herniorrhaphy. A combined analysis. *Anesthesiology.* 1995; 82:809.
168. Kennedy KA, Fielder AR, Hardy RJ, et al. Reduced lighting does not improve medical outcomes in very low birth weight infants. *J Pediatr.* 2001;139:527.
169. Reynolds JD, Dobson V, Quinn GE, et al. Evidence-based screening criteria for retinopathy of prematurity: Natural history data from the CRYO-ROP and LIGHT-ROP studies. *Arch Ophthalmol.* 2002;120:1470.
170. Lloyd J, Askie L, Smith J, et al. Supplemental oxygen for the treatment of prethreshold retinopathy of prematurity. *Cochrane Database Syst Rev.* 2003: CD003482.
171. Fredriksson A, Ponten E, Gordh T, et al. Neonatal exposure to a combination of N-methyl-D-aspartate and gamma-aminobutyric acid type A receptor anesthetic agents potentiates apoptotic neurodegeneration and persistent behavioral deficits. *Anesthesiology.* 2007;107:427.
172. Soriano SG, Anand KJ. Anesthetics and brain toxicity. *Curr Opin Anaesthesiol.* 2005;18:293.
173. Flick RP, Katusic SK, Colligan RC, et al. Cognitive and behavioral outcomes after early exposure to anesthesia and surgery. *Pediatrics.* 2011;128(5):e1053–e1061.
174. Lin AE, Pober BR, Adatia I. Congenital diaphragmatic hernia and associated cardiovascular malformations: Type, frequency, and impact on management. *Am J Med Genet C Semin Med Genet.* 2007;145:201.
175. Greenwood RD, Rosenthal A. Cardiovascular malformations associated with tracheoesophageal fistula and esophageal atresia. *Pediatrics.* 1976;57:87.
176. Harting MT, Lally KP. Surgical management of neonates with congenital diaphragmatic hernia. *Semin Pediatr Surg.* 2007;16:109.
177. Peralta CF, Jani JC, Van Schoubroeck D, et al. Fetal lung volume after endoscopic tracheal occlusion in the prediction of postnatal outcome. *Am J Obstet Gynecol.* 2008;198:60.
178. Ng GY, Derry C, Marston L, et al. Reduction in ventilator-induced lung injury improves outcome in congenital diaphragmatic hernia? *Pediatr Surg Int.* 2008; 24:145.
179. Rodrigues CJ, Tannuri U, Tannuri AC, et al. Prenatal tracheal ligation or intra-amniotic administration of surfactant or dexamethasone prevents some structural changes in the pulmonary arteries of surgically created diaphragmatic hernia in rabbits. *Rev Hosp Clin Fac Med Sao Paulo.* 2002;57:1.
180. Fisher JC, Jefferson RA, Arkovitz MS, et al. Redefining outcomes in right congenital diaphragmatic hernia. *J Pediatr Surg.* 2008;43:373.
181. Neff KW, Kilian AK, Schaible T, et al. Prediction of mortality and need for neonatal extracorporeal membrane oxygenation in fetuses with congenital diaphragmatic hernia: Logistic regression analysis based on MRI fetal lung volume measurements. *AJR Am J Roentgenol.* 2007;189:1307.
182. Hwang PJ, Kousseff BG. Omphalocele and gastroschisis: An 18-year review study. *Genet Med.* 2004;6:232.
183. Ledbetter DJ. Gastroschisis and omphalocele. *Surg Clin North Am.* 2006;86:249.
184. Henrich K, Huemmer HP, Reingruber B, et al. Gastroschisis and omphalocele: Treatments and long-term outcomes. *Pediatr Surg Int.* 2008;24:167.
185. Tsakayannis DE, Zurakowski D, Lillehei CW. Respiratory insufficiency at birth: A predictor of mortality for infants with omphalocele. *J Pediatr Surg.* 1996;31:1088.
186. Lee SL, Beyer TD, Kim SS, et al. Initial nonoperative management and delayed closure for treatment of giant omphaloceles. *J Pediatr Surg.* 2006;41:1846.
187. Owen A, Marven S, Jackson L, et al. Experience of bedside preformed silo staged reduction and closure for gastroschisis. *J Pediatr Surg.* 2006;41:1830.
188. Olesevich M, Alexander F, Khan M, et al. Gastroschisis revisited: Role of intraoperative measurement of abdominal pressure. *J Pediatr Surg.* 2005;40:789.
189. Nguyen T, Zainabadi K, Bui T, et al. Thoracoscopic repair of esophageal atresia and tracheoesophageal fistula: Lessons learned. *J Laparoendosc Adv Surg Tech A.* 2006;16:174.
190. Hirabayashi Y, Yoshizawa Y, Inoue S, et al. Epidural analgesia for patients with tracheoesophageal fistula. *Masui.* 1988;37:370.
191. Dalla Vecchia LK, Grosfeld JL, West KW, et al. Intestinal atresia and stenosis: A 25-year experience with 277 cases. *Arch Surg.* 1998;133:490.
192. Cucchiaro G, De Lagausie P, El-Ghonemi A, et al. Single-dose caudal anesthesia for major intraabdominal operations in high-risk infants. *Anesth Analg.* 2001;92:1439.

193. Welzing L, Roth B. Experience with remifentanil in neonates and infants. *Drugs.* 2006;66:1339.
194. Shaer CM, Chescheir N, Schulkin J. Myelomeningocele: A review of the epidemiology, genetics, risk factors for conception, prenatal diagnosis, and prognosis for affected individuals. *Obstet Gynecol Surv.* 2007;62:471.
195. McLone DG, Dias MS. The Chiari II malformation: Cause and impact. *Childs Nerv Syst.* 2003;19:540.
196. McLone DG. Care of the neonate with a myelomeningocele. *Neurosurg Clin N Am.* 1998;9:111.
197. Sutton LN. Fetal surgery for neural tube defects. *Best Pract Res Clin Obstet Gynaecol.* 2008;22:175.
198. Shah S, Cawley M, Gleeson R, et al. Latex allergy and latex sensitization in children and adolescents with meningomyelocele. *J Allergy Clin Immunol.* 1998;101:741.
199. Birmingham PK, Dsida RM, Grayhack JJ, et al. Do latex precautions in children with myelodysplasia reduce intraoperative allergic reactions? *J Pediatr Orthop.* 1996;16:799.
200. Blum RH, Rockoff MA, Holzman RS, et al. Overreaction to latex allergy? *Anesth Analg.* 1997;84:467.
201. Dierdorf SF, McNiece WL, Rao CC, et al. Failure of succinylcholine to alter plasma potassium in children with myelomeningocele. *Anesthesiology.* 1986;64:272.
202. Viscomi CM, Abajian JC, Wald SL, et al. Spinal anesthesia for repair of meningomyelocele in neonates. *Anesth Analg.* 1995;81:492.
203. Sin AH, Rashidi M, Caldito G, et al. Surgical treatment of myelomeningocele: Year 2000 hospitalization, outcome, and cost analysis in the US. *Childs Nerv Syst.* 2007;23:1125.
204. Persson EK, Anderson S, Wiklund LM, et al. Hydrocephalus in children born in 1999–2002: Epidemiology, outcome and ophthalmological findings. *Childs Nerv Syst.* 2007;23:1111.
205. Lee JS, Polin RA. Treatment and prevention of necrotizing enterocolitis. *Semin Neonatol.* 2003;8:449.
206. Srinivasan PS, Brandler MD, D'Souza A. Necrotizing enterocolitis. *Clin Perinatol.* 2008;35:251.
207. Alfaleh K, Bassler D. Probiotics for prevention of necrotizing enterocolitis in preterm infants. *Cochrane Database Syst Rev.* 2008:CD005496.
208. Ehrlich PF, Sato TT, Short BL, et al. Outcome of perforated necrotizing enterocolitis in the very low-birth weight neonate may be independent of the type of surgical treatment. *Am Surg.* 2001;67:752.
209. Blakely ML, Lally KP, McDonald S, et al. Postoperative outcomes of extremely low birth-weight infants with necrotizing enterocolitis or isolated intestinal perforation: A prospective cohort study by the NICHD Neonatal Research Network. *Ann Surg.* 2005;241:984.
210. Lau ST, Lee YH, Caty MG. Current management of hernias and hydroceles. *Semin Pediatr Surg.* 2007;16:50.
211. Craven PD, Badawi N, Henderson-Smart DJ, et al. Regional (spinal, epidural, caudal) versus general anaesthesia in preterm infants undergoing inguinal herniorrhaphy in early infancy. *Cochrane Database Syst Rev.* 2003:CD003669.
212. Walther-Larsen S, Rasmussen LS. The former preterm infant and risk of postoperative apnoea: Recommendations for management. *Acta Anaesthesiol Scand.* 2006;50:888.
213. Cook-Sather SD, Tulloch HV, Liacouras CA, et al. Gastric fluid volume in infants for pyloromyotomy. *Can J Anaesth.* 1997;44:278.
214. Jacobs JP, Giroud JM, Quintessenza JA, et al. The modern approach to patent ductus arteriosus treatment: Complementary roles of video-assisted thoracoscopic surgery and interventional cardiology coil occlusion. *Ann Thorac Surg.* 2003;76:1421.

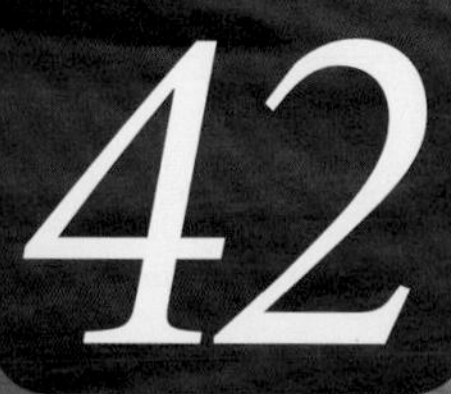

CHAPTER 42

Pediatric Anesthesia

JERROLD LERMAN

Key Points

1. The airway in neonates and infants presents unique features that require a clear understanding of the anatomy and physiology of airway structures. Laryngospasm and airway obstruction increase perioperative morbidity and mortality. Treatment of laryngospasm includes continuous positive airway pressure with 100% oxygen, jaw thrust applied at the condyles of the mandible, and early administration of atropine and propofol and/or succinylcholine to prevent serious desaturations and relax the vocal cords.
2. Laboratory evidence has raised concerns regarding the neurocognitive sequelae after general anesthetics in young animals. Recent laboratory evidence; however, suggests that exercising animals after an anesthetic mitigates the neurocognitive dysfunction. Clinical evidence in humans; however, has not directly linked anesthesia and sedation with long-term neurocognitive dysfunction. Outcome studies in humans are conflicting.
3. Drug dosing in children is complex. Several factors must be considered when choosing drug doses including developmental maturation of the cytochrome enzyme system, organ homeostasis (cardiopulmonary, renal, and hepatic functions), coexisting diseases, and obesity. Unusual drug responses or resistance may be the result of single nucleotide polymorphisms.
4. Understanding the pharmacokinetics and pharmacodynamics of inhaled anesthetics, the most commonly used anesthetics in children, helps to anticipate unexpected responses such as an anesthetic overdose during controlled ventilation or awareness after sub-MAC dosing during stimulation.
5. Upper respiratory tract infections are the most common comorbidity in children who present for surgery. Caution should be exercised when anesthetizing infants (<1 year of age) with recent colds (respiratory syncytial and other viruses may be latent) and children with colds in the preceding 2 weeks as the rate of perioperative complications is increased. Surgery should be rescheduled if any one of the following signs complicates a current infection: Fever (>38.5°C); the child has not been behaving normally (e.g., lack of appetite); purulent, green secretions; and lower respiratory tract signs (e.g., wheezing that does not clear with a deep cough).
6. Obstructive sleep apnea in children differs from adults in that large tonsils and adenoids are the primary cause of sleep apnea in the former. Perioperative respiratory complications in these

---

Portions of this chapter may appear in Lerman J, Sampathi V, Watt S. Induction, maintenance, and emergence from anesthesia. In: Andropoulos D, Gregory G, eds. *Pediatric Anesthesia.* 2012:330–360; Chapter 15. Wiley-Blackwell, Oxford, UK

children are linked to the severity of intermittent nocturnal desaturation (threshold is oxygen saturation (SaO2) <85%) as they upregulate genes responsible for opioid sensitivity. Emerging evidence suggests that sleep apnea in obese child is complicated by a systemic inflammatory response, resulting in less favorable outcomes after adenotonsillar surgery.

7 Obesity is the most rapidly growing challenge in pediatric anesthesia. Although laryngoscopy and tracheal intubation has been considered challenging, a 25-degree head-up position and exaggerated sniffing position such that the tragus lies above a horizontal line through the sternal notch facilitates tracheal intubation. Drug dosing must be adjusted to ideal or lean body weight in many instances to preclude relative drug overdoses. Perioperative respiratory complications and postoperative admission after surgery are more common in this population of children.

8 Allergies and anaphylaxis during anesthesia in children are most commonly due to latex in children. Epinephrine is the definitive treatment. Propofol allergy is extraordinarily rare in children, occurring only in those with documented egg anaphylaxis (not allergy). Although a common cause of anaphylaxis in Europe, anaphylaxis to muscle relaxants in children in North America is rare because of the absence of sensitizing agents (such as pholcodine).

9 The philosophical shift in fluid management strategy for most children ≥6 months of age in perioperative volumes has been from hypotonic glucose-containing solutions in 4–2–1 mL/kg/hr to use balanced salt solutions of 10 to 30 mL/kg. The underlying strategy is to downregulate antidiuretic hormone secretion to avoid perioperative hyponatremia. In neonates and young infants, the previous fluid strategy remains appropriate.

10 Impediments to ambulatory surgery in children include perioperative pain and vomiting. Pain should be prophylactically treated with local anesthetics and/or systemic analgesics during anesthesia to limit the need for postoperative analgesics. Continuous regional blocks are most effective in appropriate surgery. Prophylactic strategies to prevent postoperative vomiting are most effectively managed with a combination of aggressive perioperative IV fluid hydration, intravenous dexamethasone, and serotonin-receptor antagonists and avoiding forcing postoperative fluids. Ex-premature infants and full-term neonates should be monitored postoperatively in hospital until the risk of a perioperative apnea is no longer significant (up to 24 hours apnea-free).

Multimedia

Single Breath Inhalational Induction

ANATOMY AND PHYSIOLOGY

1 Airway

Understanding the anatomical differences between the infant and adult upper airways is key to managing the infant's airway safely. Table 42-1 summarizes these differences. As a result of these anatomical features, the head in the child is naturally in the "sniffing" or flexed position. The large tongue/mouth ratio presents difficulty if the mouth is closed during mask ventilation, particularly with the narrowed nares. Hence, mask ventilation requires particular skill to avoid airway obstruction. Ensuring safe mask anesthesia and a patent airway requires proper application of the "jaw thrust" as described below while avoiding pressure on the soft tissues in the submental triangle.

The most common airway problem in infants and young children is upper airway obstruction due to laryngomalacia. In this condition, the supraglottic structures converge on the glottic opening during inspiration preventing most, if not all, air entry through the glottis. The net effect is airway obstruction that is characterized by suprasternal and supraclavicular retractions, paradoxical collapse of the chest wall and/or sternum, and exaggerated diaphragmatic excursions especially if the child becomes distressed. Positive airway pressure usually resolves the acute condition. This condition resolves itself as the children grow and the oropharyngeal structures develop although in some instances surgery may be required.

A number of airway anomalies may present problems during anesthesia. Some anomalies improve with age (e.g., Pierre Robin sequence defined as micrognathia, airway distress in the first 24 hours after birth, and glossoptosis) generally becoming easy laryngoscopies around 2 years of age whereas others (such

TABLE 42-1. ANATOMICAL FEATURES OF THE UPPER AIRWAY IN INFANTS COMPARED WITH ADULTS

Head	• Larger occiput in the infant naturally positions the head in the "sniffing" position • Stabilize the head against lateral rotation • Obligate nose breathers for the first few months
Mouth	• Relative larger tongue volume in the mouth in the infant reduces the available space for instrumentation • Edentulous
Neck	• Larynx is more cephalad in the neck (C3–C4) in the infant • Epiglottis is omega shaped and longer • Vocal cords slant caudally at their insertion in the arytenoids • Narrowest part of the upper airway is the cricoid ring (a solid, conically shaped, cartilaginous structure); pseudostratified columnar epithelium covers the ring • Trachea is shorter (4–5 cm)
Tracheobronchial tree	• Acute angle of the right mainstem bronchus at the carina • Turbulent gas flow until the fifth bronchial division (resistance is related inversely to the radius to the fifth power)

as Treacher Collins syndrome, mucopolysaccharidoses) become progressively more difficult mask anesthetics and laryngoscopies with age. Several disorders present primarily with difficult mask anesthetics and ventilation while tracheal intubation is usually straightforward (e.g., Crouzon's and Apert's diseases and Down syndrome). Most airway problems in children present difficulties with tracheal intubation. It is rare to face a "cannot ventilate, cannot intubate" airway in a child. Nonetheless, it is essential to identify a child's syndrome and determine whether the airway is involved.

The cricoid ring represents the only solid cartilaginous structure in the upper airway because it is covered with pseudostratified columnar epithelium. This epithelium is subject to swelling if irritated, swelling into the lumen and reducing the radius of the airway. Because airflow in the upper airway is turbulent (Reynolds number >4,000), pressure decrease across the cricoid ring increases with changes in the radius to the fifth power. Hence, a 50% reduction in the radius of the cricoid ring increases the pressure drop by 32-fold. This increases the work of breathing, which cannot be sustained for long, resulting in respiratory failure.

The short trachea in the infant and child facilitates accidental endobronchial intubation. Careful assessment of the position of the tracheal tube in the airway is crucial to avoid this problem. Persistent hemoglobin desaturation (SaO_2 <85%) should suggest an endobronchial intubation.

The increased alveolar ventilation to functional residual capacity in the child increases the risk of hemoglobin desaturation. The increased alveolar ventilation arises from the increased oxygen consumption per kilogram required by the child compared with the adult. This fact along with the increased compliance of the rib cage (due to both anatomical and physiologic features), reduced compliance of the lungs (due to the relative lack of elastin in the infant), and reduced percent of type 1 fibers (slow-twitch, high oxidative muscle fibers) in the diaphragm predisposes the basal segments of the lungs to atelectasis under the weight of the abdomen. Together, these factors predispose the infant to rapid desaturation and respiratory failure when faced with respiratory difficulties. Additional details of the physiology of the pulmonary system may be found in Chapter 41.

Cardiovascular

Once the neonatal heart completes the transition to postnatal life, the changes in the cardiovascular system are less dramatic. In the early years, the heart has limited ability to increase stroke volume, rendering cardiac output more dependent on heart rate than in the adult. A corollary of this relationship is that hypotension in the child with a normal or increased heart rate is due to hypovolemia and should be treated with volume expansion rather than vasopressors (except in children with congenital heart disease). Systemic vascular tone is low in children up to 8 years of age, as evidenced by the lack of change in blood pressure when caudal/epidural blocks are administered.

Both heart rate and blood pressure increase with increasing age in childhood (see Table 42-2)[1] and these provide a framework from which the definitions of bradycardia and hypotension were developed.

TABLE 42-2. NORMAL RANGE OF RESTING HEART RATES AND BLOOD PRESSURE IN CHILDREN

Age	Heart Rate (beats/min)	Blood Pressure (mm Hg)
0–3 mos	100–150	65–85/45–55
3–6 mos	90–120	70–90/50–65
6–12 mos	80–120	80–100/55–65
1–3 yrs	70–110	90–105/55–70
3–6 yrs	65–110	95–110/60–75
6–12 yrs	60–95	100–120/60–75
>12 yrs	55–85	110–135/65–85

Adapted from: Bernstein D. History and physical examination. In: Kliegman RM, et al., eds. *Nelson Textbook of Pediatrics.* 19th ed. Philadelphia, PA: Saunders Elsevier; 2011:1529–1536.

Central Nervous System

Physiology

Oxygen consumption in the brain of children (5.5 mL/100 g/min) is 50% greater than that in adults (3.5 mL/100 g/min).[2] As a result, cerebral blood flow differs substantially from adults. In children 6 months to 3 years of age, the cerebral blood flow is 50% to 70% greater than in adults (50 mL/min/100 g vs. 70 to 110 mL/min/100 g). More cerebral blood flow is directed to the gray matter in children, reaching a distribution similar to that in adults by adolescence.

Apoptosis

2 That alcohol and NMDA receptor antagonists caused apoptosis (programmed cell death) in newborn rodents led investigators to discover that most general anesthetics and sedatives, which also act on NMDA and $GABA_A$ receptors, cause apoptosis in newborn rodents and nonhuman primates. Most anesthetics, with the exception of xenon, dexmedetomidine, and opioids, cause apoptosis in newborn rodents and primates after relatively prolonged exposure (>4–5 hours) and when administered in combination.[3] Brief anesthesia with ketamine (≤3 hours) or isoflurane (<2 hours) does not induce neurocognitive dysfunction.[3,4] Moreover, several drugs appear to protect or reverse the effects of anesthetics including melatonin, lithium, hypothermia, and exercise.[3]

Whether the rodent and nonhuman primate evidence of anesthetic-induced neurotoxicity is applicable to humans remains hotly debated. Since most anesthetics in young children last less than 3 hours, these data may have limited external validity, at least in terms of humans. Second, the doses of intravenous anesthetics and sedatives in rodents and primates are up to 10-fold greater than in humans[4]; such large doses may explain, in part, the neurocognitive dysfunction observed after intravenous anesthetics. Third, studies in humans who received anesthesia at a young age suggested that cognitive disability in those who received anesthesia before the age of 3 years may be more prevalent than in those who did not.[3] However, most of those studies were seriously flawed in terms of their design (retrospective), limited external validity (no pulse oximetry or capnography), different anesthetics (halothane), nonstandardized metrics (learning disability tests were not applied equally to all children), and confounding variables (complex pregnancy, drugs such as magnesium) that were not standardized. However, a large cohort of identical twins who were discordant for general anesthesia at <3 years of age in one study, when tested for intellectual aptitude 10 years later, were similar.[5] Prospective studies that are currently underway may clarify this issue. It is intriguing to know that rodents that have received a cerebral insult from ischemia, trauma or sevoflurane anesthesia have less cognitive dysfunction if they are exercised after the insult.[6,6a]

3

PHARMACOLOGY

Developmental Pharmacology

Understanding the pharmacology of medications in children is a large undertaking and a complex subject that is briefly addressed below.

For medications to be effective, they must reach their effect site. The steps involved in that process include absorption of the medication into the blood, transfer from the blood to the effect site, and termination of its action by redistribution, metabolism, and excretion.

The bioavailability of medications that are not administered intravenously depends on several factors including the route of administration, pK_a, and solubility of the drug and local perfusion. Some medications such as midazolam are poorly absorbed from the stomach at clinical doses (15% bioavailability)[7] but are well absorbed via the nares[8] whereas others such as acetaminophen are well absorbed from the stomach but are poorly and erratically absorbed from the rectum.[9] Age may have a substantial effect on the absorption of these drugs for example, gastric juice is closer to neutral pH (pH ~6) at birth and does not reach adult levels of acidity until ~3 years of age.[10] Since drugs may be administered by any of these routes, it is critical to evaluate the bioavailability of the medication via each route to determine the appropriate dose required to achieve an adequate blood concentration. The route of administration also affects whether the drug undergoes first-pass metabolism through the liver. Rectal venous drainage from the superior hemorrhoidal veins drains into the portal venous system, whereas blood from the middle and inferior hemorrhoidal veins bypasses the liver flowing directly into the iliac veins and on to the heart. Hence medications that are administered rectally may undergo first-pass hepatic metabolism if they are absorbed via the superior rectal veins.

Once in the blood, intravenous medications partition between the protein-bound fraction and the free or active fraction. Two major proteins bind medications: Albumin and α_1-acid glycoprotein. Both are synthesized in the liver. Albumin concentration is reduced in children with many diseases (cancer, nephropathy) and malnourishment. It binds acidic medications. α_1-acid glycoprotein concentration is also reduced at birth but increases slowly with increasing age as well as during periods of stress.[11] It binds basic compounds. Hence, the free fraction of medications such as lidocaine is greater in young infants than in older children because the concentration of α_1-acid glycoprotein in the former is reduced.[11] As the free fraction of medications increases, a greater dose will reach the effect site and exert physiologic or, in the case of an overdose, adverse events.

Termination of the action of most intravenous agents depends on their metabolism by the liver through phase 1 reactions (e.g., hydroxylation and oxidation) and/or phase 2 reactions (e.g., glucuronidation). The rates at which these enzyme systems mature vary widely among and within individuals depending on a host of factors. Apart from a few enzyme systems that hold importance in fetal life (e.g., CYP450 3A7),[12] the activities of the vast majority of CYP450 enzyme systems (e.g., CYP450 3A4, 2E1, and 2D6) increase with age from birth, but at divergent rates (Fig. 42-1).[12] Moreover, genetic polymorphisms of several families of enzymes (e.g., 2D6) may dramatically affect the activity of that enzyme system resulting in a wide range of activity from none to rapid and excessive (see Codeine below).[13]

Phase 1 reactions are responsible for the majority of drug metabolism in the liver acting via the cytochrome P450 enzyme system. Several enzymes are responsible for the metabolism of the vast majority of medications we administer: 3A4 (50% of medications), 2D6 (10% to 20% of medications),[13] 1A2, 2E1, and 2C9. These isozyme systems mature from birth, at which time most have limited activity (Fig. 42-1). Most of these enzyme systems mature to adult activity levels by 1 to 5 years of age. Phase 2

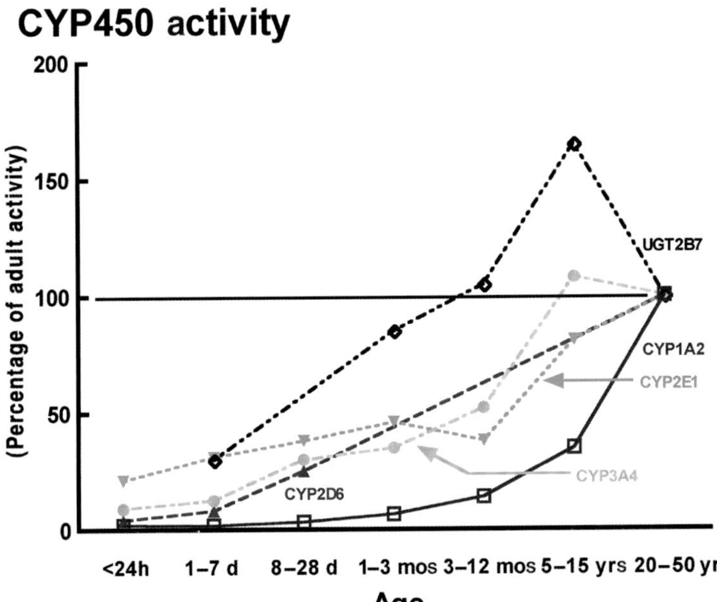

FIGURE 42-1. Developmental changes in common cytochromes of interest in pediatric anesthesia. Adapted from: Kearns GL, Abdel-Rahman SM, Alander SW, et al. Developmental pharmacology – drug disposition, action, and therapy in infants and children. *N Engl J Med.* 2003;349:1157–1167 and Alcorn J, McNamara PJ. Pharmacokinetics in the newborn. *Adv Drug Deliv Rev.* 2003;55:675.

TABLE 42-3. PHARMACOLOGY OF INHALED ANESTHETICS

	Halothane	Enflurane	Isoflurane	Sevoflurane	Desflurane
Odor	Mild, pleasant	Etheric	Etheric	Pleasant, tolerated	Etheric
Solubility					
$\lambda_{b/g}$ adults	2.4	1.9	1.4	0.66	0.42
$\lambda_{b/g}$ neonates[a]	2.14	1.78	1.19	0.66	–
$\lambda_{brain/b}$ adults[b]	1.9	1.3	1.6	1.7	1.2
$\lambda_{brain/b}$ neonates[c]	1.5	0.9	1.3	–	–
$\lambda_{fat/b}$ adults[b]	51.1	–	45	48	27
MAC					
MAC_{adults}	0.75	1.7	1.2	2.05	7
$MAC_{neonates}$	0.87	–	1.60	3.2	9.2
Metabolism					
In vivo (%)	15–20	2.4	1.4	<5	0.2

λ is the partition coefficient; b/g is blood/gas; brain/b is brain/blood; fat/b is fat/blood; MAC is the minimum alveolar concentration (%).

[a]Data from: Lerman J, Schmitt-Bantel BI, Gregory GA, et al. Effect of age on the solubility of volatile anesthetics in human tissues. *Anesthesiology.* 1986;65:307–311 and Malviya S, Lerman J. The blood/gas solubilities of sevoflurane, isoflurane, halothane, and serum constituent concentrations in neonates and adults. *Anesthesiology.* 1990;72:793–796.

[b]Data from Yasuda N, Targ AG, Eger EI II. Solubility of I-653, sevoflurane, isoflurane, and halothane in human tissues. *Anesth Analg.* 1989;69:370–373.

[c]Data from: Lerman J, Gregory GA, Willis MM, et al. Age and solubility of volatile anesthetics in blood. *Anesthesiology.* 1984;61:139–143.

systems are also immature at birth, giving rise to concerns about bilirubin toxicity. However, these systems also mature quickly with age.

Termination of the action of many medications in anesthesia depends on either redistribution of the active compound from the effect site to other vessel-rich organs (see Inhalational section) or muscle, or metabolism in the liver and excretion or direct excretion by the kidneys. Elimination of the metabolic by-products and residual active parent compounds depends on renal perfusion and elimination. The glomerular filtration rate is markedly reduced in the neonate but matures throughout childhood reaching adult rates by 5 to 15 years of age.[14]

4

Inhalational Anesthetics

The widespread appeal of the current inhalational anesthetics may be attributed to their physicochemical properties (Table 42-3), which provide a rapid onset and offset of action, cardiorespiratory homeostasis, and limited metabolism and toxicity. Halothane has all but disappeared in North American pediatric anesthetic clinical practice, having been replaced by sevoflurane as the induction agent of choice in infants and children. Enflurane has been supplanted by its optical isomer, isoflurane. Desflurane offers the most favorable pharmacokinetic and in vivo metabolic characteristics in terms of its minimal blood and tissue solubilities and resistance to metabolism, although its use as an induction agent in children is proscribed because it irritates the upper airway. Most recently, the noble gas xenon has generated much interest as an anesthetic because it is safe for the environment, lacks cardiovascular toxicity, and has no serious toxicity either in vivo or in vitro. However, xenon is very expensive, its minimum alveolar concentration (MAC) is 70%, and it causes nausea and vomiting.

All of the currently used inhalational anesthetics are methyl ethyl ether compounds except for sevoflurane, which is a methyl isopropyl ether (Table 42-3).

Pharmacokinetics

The rate of increase in alveolar to inspired anesthetic partial pressures (fraction in the alveolus (F_A) to the fraction in the inspired gas (F_I), known as the washin ratio, F_A/F_I) for inhalational anesthetics depends on six factors. The first three determine the delivery of anesthetic to the lungs and the second three determine the removal of anesthetic from the lung. The washin ratio increases from 0 toward 1 in the shape of an exponential curve for all inhalational anesthetics. The order of washin of the anesthetics is inversely related to the solubility of the anesthetics in blood; that is, the smaller the solubility in blood, the more rapid the washin.[18]

TABLE 42-4. FACTORS INCREASING THE WASHIN OF INHALATIONAL ANESTHETICS IN CHILDREN COMPARED WITH ADULTS

1. Alveolar ventilation:FRC ratio (5:1 in infants vs. 1.5:1 in adults)
2. Greater distribution of cardiac output to the vessel-rich group in infants (vessel-rich group comprises 18% of the body weight in infants compared with 8% in adults)
3. Reduced tissue solubility in infants[15]
4. Reduced blood solubility in infants[16,17]

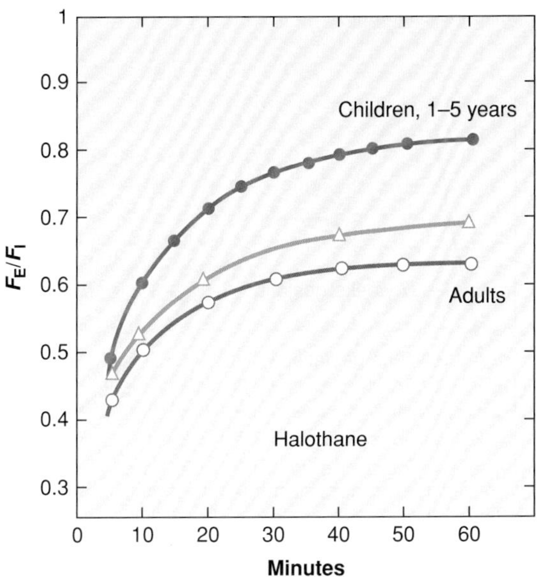

FIGURE 42-2. The more rapid washin of halothane in children compared with adults. The fractional end-tidal to inspired ratio (F_E/F_I) of halothane (*Y*-axis) over time (*X*-axis). The two *lower curves* (with *open symbols*) are from adults. Reproduced with permission from: Salanitre E, Rackow H. The pulmonary exchange of nitrous oxide and halothane in infants and children. *Anesthesiology.* 1969;30:391.

The washin curve for inhalational anesthetics is characterized by the simple exponential equation

$$F_A/F_I = 1 - e^{-kt} \tag{1}$$

where k is a constant (k = 1/time constant (τ)) and t is time in minutes. τ is the ratio of the volume of the organ to the blood flow to that organ. The smaller the time constant, the more rapidly F_A/F_I equilibrates. In children, the time constants for most organs are less than those in adults and this explains in part, the rapid equilibration of halothane in children compared with adults (Fig. 42-2).

In the case of infants and children, four factors explain the more rapid washin of halothane compared with adults. These factors are listed in order of importance from the greatest to the least in Table 42-4.

The greater alveolar ventilation: (V_A) functional residual capacity (FRC) ratio in infants and children compared with adults may be attributed to the greater metabolic rate and oxygen demand in children. Increases in alveolar ventilation speed the equilibration of inspired to alveolar anesthetic partial pressures.[19] The net effect of a greater V_A: FRC ratio is a reduction in the time constant, from 0.7 in adults to 0.2 in infants, which explains the speed of equilibration. Although a greater cardiac output should slow the rate of increase in F_A/F_I, it actually speeds the equilibration in neonates and infants. This paradoxical effect may be attributed to the greater cardiac output perfusing the vessel-rich group (VRG) (comprised of heart, brain, gastrointestinal organs, kidneys, and endocrine glands) in infants which comprises 18% of the body's weight compared with 8% in adults. Hence, the greater cardiac output in infants speeds the equilibration of F_A/F_I in the VRG, which takes up most of the anesthetic during the first couple of hours of anesthesia. The third most important factor in the rapid washin of anesthetics in infants is their reduced tissue solubility compared with that in adults.[15] The solubility of all inhalational anesthetics is reduced in tissues in infants compared with adults including the brain, muscle, and heart. Lastly, the reduced solubility of anesthetic in blood in infants speeds the washin of inhalational anesthetics in infants.[17]

To understand the relevance of differences in the tissue solubility among age groups, the τ is defined by

$$\tau = (\text{Brain volume (mL)} \times \lambda_{\text{brain/blood}}) / \text{Brain blood flow (mL/100 g/min)} \tag{2}$$

In the brain, the brain blood flow is 50 mL/100 g/min or 50 mL/100 mL/min brain. In adults, $\lambda_{\text{brain/blood}}$ is ~2, whereas in the infant it is 1. Substituting these values into Eq. 2 yields 100 × 2 (or 1)/50 or 4 minutes in adults or 2 minutes in children. Since 4τ are required to achieve 98% equilibration of F_A/F_I, the partial pressure of brain reaches alveolar pressures by 16 minutes in adults and 8 minutes in children (excluding the time to equilibrate anesthetic throughout the anesthesia workstation [AWS] and lungs). Hence, we can explain, in part, the sudden and rapid responses to inhalational anesthetic in infants and children compared with adults.

In contrast to the more soluble anesthetics of the past, the current inhalational anesthetics are less soluble in both blood and tissues. Since changes in alveolar ventilation and cardiac output affect the washin of less soluble anesthetics to a lesser extent than more soluble anesthetics, the first two factors in Table 42-4 have attenuated effects on the washin of sevoflurane and desflurane in young children. Therefore, the washin in this age group may not be substantively greater than it is in adults. Furthermore, the solubilities of these agents in blood in infants are similar to those in adults[16]; the tissue solubilities in infants compared with adults have not been reported. Hence, we expect the washin of sevoflurane and desflurane in infants to be marginally more rapid than in adults.

Estimates of the effect site equilibration half-life ($t_{1/2\text{keo}}$) for sevoflurane in adults and children have been reported using the bispectral index (BIS) to be 3.2 and 1.2 minutes, respectively.[20,21]

Two additional aspects of the pharmacokinetics of inhalational anesthetics merit consideration in infants and children. The first is the mode of ventilation. The washin of inhalational anesthetics increases rapidly during induction of anesthesia. In dogs, the washin of halothane was well tolerated during spontaneous respiration whether the inspired concentration was 0.4% or 4%.[22] The F_A/F_I plateaued in all instances at 0.6 to 0.7. As the anesthetic depth increased, ventilation was reduced, decreasing the intake of anesthetic. When the depth of anesthesia was reduced, ventilation increased and the intake and depth of anesthesia increased. This is a negative feedback control loop. However, when ventilation was controlled, 85% and 100% of the dogs that received 4% and 6% inspired halothane concentrations, respectively, did not survive.[22] Controlled ventilation is a positive feedback control loop where the delivery of inhalational anesthesia continues unabated without the negative feedback effect of respiratory depression. Ultimately, as cardiac output decreases, the uptake of anesthetic decreases and the partial pressure in the lungs increases steadily. These greater partial pressures in the lungs equilibrate with the reduced cardiac output, which circulates to the VRG to further depress them, ultimately resulting in a cardiac arrest. This study illustrates the benefits of the negative feedback control of spontaneous ventilation during inhalational anesthesia that protects against an anesthetic overdose and the risks associated with controlled ventilation. In the past, since more than one vaporizer could be used simultaneously during controlled respiration, interlocking devices were developed to prevent an inadvertent anesthetic overdose when the children could not protect themselves during controlled ventilation.

The second issue relates to shunts and their effects on the uptake and distribution of anesthetics. Left to right shunts have limited effects on the uptake and distribution of inhalational anesthetics provided the cardiac output is maintained.[23] However, right to left shunts present an entirely different and far more complex clinical problem. Whether these shunts are intrapulmonary or intracardiac or both, the washin of less soluble anesthetics are far more substantively affected in the presence of these shunts than more soluble anesthetics.[23] That is, it is much more difficult to maintain an adequate depth of anesthesia with sevoflurane in infants with significant right to left shunts. To maintain anesthesia, supplemental intravenous anesthesia is often used. Understanding this differential effect of shunts on the washin of inhalational anesthetics is beyond the scope of this chapter, but the basis may be summarized by the differential effect of ventilation on the washin of less and more soluble anesthetics.[23]

The speed of washout of inhalational anesthetics follows an exponential decay, with the speed inversely parallel to the solubility of the anesthetics in blood. That is, the washout is more rapid for anesthetics that are less soluble: Desflurane > sevoflurane > isoflurane ≥ halothane.[18] The only exception to this rule is the washout of halothane, which overlaps that of isoflurane in part, because the former is metabolized 15% to 25% in vivo (Table 42-3). Simulation demonstrated greater differences in recovery among the anesthetics after prolonged anesthesia and to >90% decrement in the anesthetic concentration.[24]

Substituting a less soluble anesthetic for a more soluble one has been proposed as a technique to accelerate the washout of anesthetics and recovery from anesthesia. However, switching from isoflurane to sevoflurane 30 minutes before the end of surgery did not speed the recovery in one report.[25] More recently, charcoal filters have been used to adsorb anesthetics and, when combined with hypercapnic hyperventilation in adults, were shown to rapidly remove anesthetics and speed recovery.[26,27]

Pharmacodynamics

The MAC is that concentration of inhalational anesthetic to which 50% of the patients move in response to a skin incision. In children, the MAC is known to depend to a great extent on age. That is, as the fetus matures and reaches term, the MAC increases peaking in infants 1 to 6 months of age for halothane[28,29] and isoflurane[30,31] and then decreases steadily thereafter with increasing age (Fig. 42-3). In the case of sevoflurane, the MAC is 3.3% in neonates and 3.2% in infants 1 to 6 months of age.[32] For children 6 months to 12 years, the MAC is constant at 2.4%.[32] In the case of desflurane, the MAC increases throughout infancy peaking in infants 6 to 12 months of age and decreases thereafter with increasing age.[33] The reason for the age-dependent differences in the MAC is unclear.

The MAC values of inhalational anesthetics in children have shown several other peculiarities. The MAC of halothane is 25% less in children with cognitive dysfunction, especially those taking antiseizure medications.[34] The MAC of desflurane in adult redheads is 20% greater than in nonredheads[35]; the same response would be expected in children of similar genetic predisposition. The MAC values for halothane and isoflurane show simple additivity with N_2O in adults and children; however, the MAC values for sevoflurane and desflurane in children are only reduced 20% to 25% in the presence of 60% N_2O.[32,36] The reason for this effect of sevoflurane and desflurane is unknown. The MAC also varies with the child's temperature. In children 4 to 10 years of age, the MAC of isoflurane decreases 5%/°C decrease in temperature.[37]

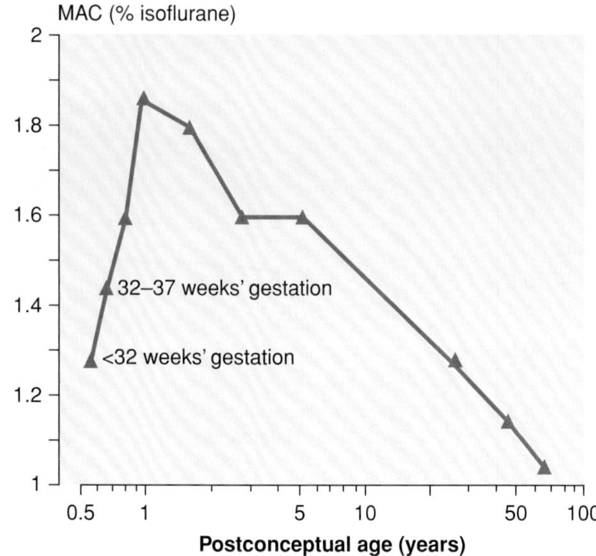

FIGURE 42-3. Age and the MAC of isoflurane from premature infants to adults. Reproduced with permission from: LeDez KM, Lerman J. The minimum alveolar concentration (MAC) of isoflurane in preterm neonates. *Anesthesiology.* 1987;67:301–307.

In addition to determining the MAC responses to skin incision, the ED_{50} to a number of other maneuvers including insertion and removal of laryngeal mask airways (LMAs), tracheal extubation, and others have been determined.[38]

Respiration

When administered in the absence of surgical stimulation, all anesthetics depress respiration and minute ventilation in a dose-dependent manner, by decreasing tidal volume and increasing respiratory rate.[39,40] Inhalational anesthetics relax intercostal muscles before the diaphragm, resulting primarily in diaphragmatic respiration. Respiratory rate increases during anesthesia, which offsets in part the reduced tidal volume. These effects are most pronounced with halothane; at concentrations ≥1.4 MAC, sevoflurane depresses respiration to a greater extent than halothane in adults,[41] although the evidence is less clear in children.[40] As the concentration of sevoflurane increases, respiratory rate also diminishes ultimately resulting in apnea. This effect is augmented in the presence of a midazolam premedication. This central effect is offset by manually assisting ventilation. In the case of desflurane, concentrations >1 MAC depress respiration in infants and children, an effect that exceeds the depression by other inhalational anesthetics.[42]

Inhalational anesthetics also depress the response to carbon dioxide and hypoxia in a dose-dependent manner.

Airway resistance increases during desflurane anesthesia,[43] and decreases during sevoflurane anesthesia.[43,44] Hence, in children with asthma, the former is best avoided and the latter is preferred. In both children and adults in the intensive care unit with refractory status asthmaticus, inhalational anesthetics have been effective.[45,46]

Upper airway responses to inhalational anesthesia (by mask) depend on both the concentration and the particular anesthetic administered. Halothane and sevoflurane do not trigger these reflex responses[39,47] whereas isoflurane and desflurane are most irritating to the airway, particularly at >1 MAC concentrations.[48,49] The package insert for desflurane cautions against using it for inhalational inductions in children. The mechanism by which inhalational anesthetics trigger upper airway reflex responses remains unclear.

When a tracheal tube is used, neither desflurane nor isoflurane triggers airway reflexes either during anesthesia or emergence.[49] When an LMA is used, extubation during deep desflurane anesthesia may increase the incidence of airway reflex responses when compared with extubation awake after desflurane or isoflurane.[50]

Cardiovascular

Inhalational anesthetics depress the heart in a dose-dependent manner. Direct effects of these anesthetics depress the heart rate, contractility, and peripheral vascular tone. Halothane depresses heart rate the most of these anesthetics, often sensitizing the myocardium to catecholamines and inducing ventricular dysrhythmias. In the past, anticholinergics were commonly used to prevent bradycardia and arrhythmias in children given halothane; however, this practice is no longer necessary with the newer ether anesthetics that infrequently cause arrhythmias. In contrast, sevoflurane and the remaining ether anesthetics exert no substantial effect on the cardiac conduction system. Sevoflurane maintains or increases heart rate during induction of anesthesia in most instances[32] likely due to withdrawal of vagal tone,[51] although on occasion nodal bradycardia has been reported during sevoflurane. Desflurane and isoflurane tend to increase the heart rate. Desflurane to a greater extent than isoflurane causes a sympathetic discharge when the inspired concentration increases rapidly and in a stepwise manner, without pretreatment with opioids[52]; similar responses in children have not been forthcoming. This effect is mediated through the right and left lungs.[53] Sevoflurane and the other inhalational anesthetics prolong the QT interval, but sevoflurane does not increase the dispersion of repolarization, making arrhythmias very rare.[54] Arrhythmias can occur in children with congenital long QT interval particularly during emergence from anesthesia.[55]

Halothane depresses myocardial contractility to the greatest extent; sevoflurane and the remaining ether anesthetics exert a much more attenuated effect in children. Hemodynamic responses to 1 × MAC of ether anesthetics suggest that they all decrease systolic blood pressure ~20% to 30% from awake values, an effect that is usually reversed with surgical stimulation.[30,32,33] Sevoflurane and halothane decrease cardiac index in children similarly, ~10% at 1 × MAC and 20% to 30% at 2 × MAC, although sevoflurane may depress cardiac index in infants less than after halothane.[56,57]

Early studies showed the dependency of cardiac output in young children on heart rate. An increase in heart rate reversed halothane-dependent decreases in cardiac output.[58] More recent evidence suggests that children can increase their stroke volume if needed to augment their cardiac output. Peripheral vascular resistance is very low in children as evidenced by the absence of a change in blood pressure when a caudal/epidural block is administered.

Sevoflurane is superior to halothane in children with congenital heart disease. It causes fewer arrhythmias and less hypotension than halothane.[59]

Most anesthetic medications prolonged the QT interval, but when the QT interval exceeds 500 milliseconds, the QT interval is considered prolonged.[60] When a prolonged QT interval occurs in the presence of a dispersion of repolarization, there is a substantial risk for the occurrence of torsades de pointes. In the presence of drugs that prolong the QT interval (e.g., most anesthetics), the risk of torsades de pointes is increased in the presence of congenital long QT interval (Romano–Ward and Jervell and Lange-Nielson syndrome), nonanesthetic medications, several medical conditions (hypomagnesemia, hypokalemia, hypocalcemia, cardiac disease, hypothyroidism), bradycardia, and the female gender.[60,61]

Central Nervous System

All inhalational anesthetics decrease cerebral vascular resistance and cerebral metabolic rate for oxygen. The decrease in vascular resistance increases cerebral blood flow in the following order: Halothane > desflurane > isoflurane > sevoflurane.[2] Sevoflurane and isoflurane decrease oxygen consumption to greater extents than halothane. Hence, the most favorable ratio of cerebral blood flow to oxygen consumption follows the reverse order: Sevoflurane > isoflurane > desflurane > halothane.

The effects of changes in blood pressure as well as carbon dioxide and oxygen tensions on cerebral blood flow during anesthesia in children have not been fully elucidated. Autoregulation of cerebral blood flow in children of all ages is similar to that in adults, although it occurs at greater blood flow rates.[2] The lower limit of autoregulation in children of all ages appears to be similar, 60 mm Hg mean arterial pressure. All inhalational anesthetics impair autoregulation, although sevoflurane does not impair autoregulation in children ≤1.5 MAC.[2] As in adults, hyperventilation restores autoregulation with isoflurane and sevoflurane. Cerebrovasodilatation to increasing carbon dioxide tension in children appears to be maintained up to ~50 mm Hg, but beyond that level maximum vasodilatation prevents any further response. Changes in cerebral blood flow in response to changes in pCO_2 during isoflurane anesthesia are greater than during sevoflurane. Hence, hyperventilation may be more effective in attenuating increased intracranial pressure during isoflurane anesthesia than during sevoflurane.

The electroencephalogram during sevoflurane is characterized by sharp, slow waves in the lower frequency range. This pattern differs substantially from that of the other anesthetics, resulting in some difficulties in interpreting BIS readings in children. That is, BIS readings are imprecise in children <5 years. They increase at sevoflurane concentrations >3%, are associated with marked variability, and are generally less than those of halothane but similar to isoflurane and desflurane at equipotent concentrations and reduced in cognitively challenged children by ~25%.[62–66] Myoclonic movement as well as EEG spike and wave activity (epileptiform) has been reported in a small number of children during inhalational inductions with sevoflurane, at concentrations 5% to 7%.[67] In patients with seizures, epileptiform EEG activity was suggested in 58% of those anesthetized with 1 to 2 MAC sevoflurane and 25% of those with 1 to 2 MAC isoflurane, with the addition of hyperventilation actually reducing the epileptiform activity.[68] With sevoflurane, these occurred not only in several patients with a history of seizures, but also in the presence of hyperventilation. Indeed, at sevoflurane concentrations approaching 8% during induction of anesthesia, ventilation should be assisted, not controlled with hyperventilation, if apnea occurs.

Renal

Inhalational anesthetics do not exert substantive effects on the kidneys in children except through their metabolism: The kidney is a site of degradation of inhalational anesthetics. Ether anesthetics, most notably methoxyflurane and to a lesser extent sevoflurane, are susceptible to CYP450 2E1 metabolism[69] releasing inorganic fluoride in similar concentrations, although only the former is known to be nephrotoxic. In part, this has been attributed to the presence of CYP450 2E1 in the kidneys and to the local release of inorganic fluoride, which is toxic to the renal tubules and in the case of methoxyflurane, caused high output renal failure and its withdrawal from the market.[70] The difference in nephrotoxicity between the two anesthetics has been attributed to two factors: The first is that the affinity of methoxyflurane for 2E1 is several folds greater than that for sevoflurane. The second is that methoxyflurane is the only anesthetic to undergo O-demethylation, which produces dichloroacetic acid, a putative cofactor in the pathogenesis of anesthetic-induced nephrotoxicity.[71]

Isoflurane and desflurane are metabolized to small extents. The risk of nephrotoxicity from inorganic fluoride from either anesthetic is remote. Indeed, very small inorganic fluoride concentrations (mean value 11 μM) have been detected after 131 MAC-hours isoflurane in children.[72]

Hepatic

There are few data regarding the effects of inhalational anesthetics on hepatic function in children. However, isolated cases of hepatic dysfunction in children have been reported after every inhalational anesthetic.[73,74] Most children who develop hepatic dysfunction recover without proceeding to liver transplantation. In the case of halothane hepatitis, serologic markers in the form of antibodies to hepatic cell membrane antigens have been detected.[75] Similar immunologic markers have been detected after isoflurane and desflurane, although none have been identified for sevoflurane to date. Although it has been suggested that repeated anesthetics with halothane cause hepatitis, this author asserts there is insufficient evidence to avoid repeated inhalational anesthetics in children.

In Vitro Metabolism

Degradation of inhalational anesthetics in the presence of carbon dioxide absorbents has been the subject of intense research and concern in both adults and children.

Sevoflurane may be degraded via the Cannizzaro reaction in carbon dioxide absorbents. The reaction is accelerated in the presence of increased temperature and Baralyme, very low fresh gas flow, high sevoflurane concentration, and used absorbent. The reaction releases five compounds, of which compound A, fluoromethyl-2,2-difluoro-1-(trifluoromethyl) vinyl ether, is the most common.[76] Nephrotoxic concentrations of compound A are believed to be >100 ppm; in children 1 MAC sevoflurane reaches 16 ppm after 5.6 MAC-hours in a circle circuit with a 2 L/min fresh gas flow.[76] To date, there have been no instances of compound A–induced nephrotoxicity in children.

Inhalational anesthetics may also be degraded in the presence of desiccated carbon dioxide absorbent yielding carbon monoxide. Desiccation occurs when a large fresh gas flows through a carbon dioxide absorber for an extended period (>48 hours) without a reservoir bag attached. When a potent inhalational anesthetic contacts the desiccated absorbent, carbon monoxide is produced. The rate of production of carbon monoxide follows the order: Desflurane ≥ enflurane > isoflurane >> halothane = sevoflurane.[77] This problem can be avoided if the AWS is turned off or the fresh gas is discontinued after each day or if the reservoir bag remains attached. Recently, carbon monoxide (≤18 ppm) was detected in the anesthesia breathing circuit in children although the source was unclear.[78]

Intravenous

Intravenous drugs are distributed first to the VRG, just as inhalational anesthetics are, and then to the muscle, vessel-poor group, and fat groups. The primary anesthetic effect occurs when the anesthetic reaches an adequate brain concentration; it is then redistributed to other tissues and metabolized to terminate its action. The pharmacokinetics of intravenous anesthetics depend on the dose and rate of drug administered, the binding of the drug in blood, the cardiac output and the distribution of cardiac output, metabolism, and excretion pathways.

Propofol

Diisopropylphenol is the most commonly used intravenous induction agent in children. This highly lipophilic drug distributes rapidly to the VRG to affect its anesthetic action. The effect site equilibration half-life ($t_{1/2keo}$) has been estimated at 0.8 or 1.2 minutes, depending on the model.[79] Its action is terminated by redistribution as well as hepatic and extrahepatic metabolism. Volume of distribution and clearance (to a lesser extent) decrease progressively during early childhood.[80] However, clearance increases throughout gestation and the neonatal period, reaching 90% of adult values by 3 months of age.[81] To maintain the 3 μg/mL blood concentration for anesthesia, a 50% greater induction and infusion dosing schedule is required in young children.[82] The net effect is a context-sensitive half-life that increases with time in children more rapidly than in adults.[82]

The ED_{50} for loss of the eyelash reflex in children varies with the child's age: 3 ± 0.2 mg/kg in infants 1 to 6 months; 1.3 to 1.6 mg/kg in children 1 to 12 years; 2.4 ± 0.1 mg/kg in children 10 to 16 years.[83] The ED_{50} and ED_{90} of propofol to insert an LMA in children is 3.5 and 5.4 mg/kg (4.7 to 6.8 mg/kg 95% CI), respectively.[84,85] The dose of propofol to facilitate tracheal intubation in children during sevoflurane anesthesia is 1 to 2 mg/kg.[86,87]

Propofol is an integral part of total intravenous anesthesia (TIVA) for maintenance of anesthesia in children undergoing medical/radiologic evaluations and surgery. For painless medical or radiologic (e.g., MRI) procedures in young children 2 to 6 years of age, an initial infusion rate of 15 mg/kg/hr (250 μg/kg/min) of propofol is recommended after either an inhalational induction or an IV induction.[82,88,89] This dose may have to be increased to stop spontaneous movement, particularly if the children have neurocognitive impairment or are younger.[90] Conversely, the infusion rate may be reduced in older children.

Based on pharmacokinetic modeling to maintain a blood concentration of 3 μg/mL, the infusion rate may be decreased during prolonged surgery to facilitate rapid emergence. The recommended stepwise reduction in the infusion rate in children 3 to 11 years of age after an intravenous induction with 2.5 mg/kg propofol is 15 mg/kg/hr (250 μg/kg/min) for 15 minutes followed by 13 mg/kg/hr (215 μg/kg/min) for 15 minutes, followed by 11 mg/kg/hr (180 μg/kg/min) for 30 minutes, followed by 10 mg/kg/hr (166 μg/kg/min) for 60 minutes, followed by 9 mg/kg/hr (150 μg/kg/min) for the next 2 hours.[82] Target-controlled infusions (TCI) in children are available in Europe, but not in North America.[91,92] These devices use preset algorithms based on the pharmacokinetics that use similar dosing algorithms with modest success.

Propofol causes pain in 70% or more of patients during intravenous induction of anesthesia[93]; the pain is greater when it is injected into a small vein (as in the hand) than in the arm.[94] This pain is most reliably prevented by administering 70% nitrous oxide before propofol or by applying a mini-Bier block with 0.5 to 1 mg/kg IV lidocaine for 60 seconds.[93–95]

Propofol has profound effects on the airway. After a rapid induction dose, a transient apnea is followed by a return of spontaneous respiration. Propofol reduces the hypopharyngeal dimensions although patency of the upper airway is preserved.[96] A jaw thrust maneuver re-establishes a patent airway, should obstruction occur.[97] An important and unique property of propofol is the ease by which an LMA can be inserted. Propofol relaxes the upper pharyngeal muscles to facilitate acceptance of the LMA. Although propofol induces apnea, atelectasis during spontaneous respiration occurs less frequently than with tracheal intubation.[98]

Propofol is the only anesthetic that has antinausea properties that may be exploited for use in children with histories of nausea and vomiting or who are undergoing emetogenic surgery.[99]

Although propofol is used for both sedation and general anesthesia, long-term sedation in infants and children is not recommended with propofol, after reports of unexpected death during propofol sedation with >4 mg/kg/hr for >48 hours.[100] In the United States, 21 children and 68 adults died in association with propofol administration over a 10-year period[101] Whether these deaths were the result of the long-chain triglycerides or propofol or both has not been clarified. At least three reports of incipient propofol infusion syndrome (PRIS) have been reported in children after only a few hours of anesthesia.[102–104] The smallest infusion rate reported to trigger PRIS was 1.9 to 2.6 mg/kg/hr.[100] Currently, long-term sedation with propofol is avoided in infants and children, especially in those with suspected inflammatory responses including sepsis.

The package insert suggests that caution should be exercised when propofol is administered to children with egg and soy allergies. See section on Allergies for a full discussion.

Ketamine

Ketamine is a phencyclidine derivative that offers enormous flexibility in the clinical care of children. This anesthetic can be used as a premedication (orally, nasally, rectally, or intramuscularly), a general anesthetic induction agent (intravenously or intramuscularly), and maintenance agent as an infusion, as a sedative (intravenously or intramuscularly), or as a neuroaxial analgesic (caudal/epidural).

Ketamine is available as a racemic mixture, in which the S enantiomer is four times more potent than the R enantiomer. Ketamine is extremely lipophilic with a rapid onset of action, within 30 seconds, and maximum effect by 1 minute; the half-time to equilibrate in the effect site (brain) is 11 seconds.[105] Effective blood concentration of ketamine for anesthesia is 3 μg/mL.[106] Clearance of ketamine is reduced in neonates, but reaches adult levels by 6 months of age.[107] Context-sensitive half-life for ketamine in a 10-kg child increases from 30 minutes after 1 hour to 55 minutes after 5 hours. Emergence after a prolonged infusion of ketamine, especially when combined with opioids and benzodiazepines, may be delayed. Ketamine is primarily metabolized via CYP450 3A4 to norketamine.

Oral ketamine may be used for premedication in a dose of 5 to 6 mg/kg.[108] It may cause nausea and vomiting postoperatively; nightmares are not common by this route. Ketamine may also be given intranasally, although the porous nature of the cribriform plate raises concern regarding the potential neurotoxicity of ketamine if it reaches the brain directly via this route. The dose of intranasal (IN) ketamine (racemic mixture) is 3 to 6 mg/kg and for S-ketamine 2 mg/kg.[109] The rectal ketamine dose for premedication is 5 to 10 mg/kg, with recovery increasing substantially in duration with larger doses of ketamine. For intramuscular use, 2 to 5 mg/kg ketamine sedates an uncooperative child in 3 to 5 minutes with a duration of action of 30 to 40 minutes.

General anesthesia may be induced with 1 to 2 mg/kg intravenously, a technique that is useful in children with cyanotic heart disease, septic shock, and conditions in which spontaneous respiration should be preserved (as in a child with an anterior mediastinal mass [AMM]). Ketamine may also be given as a continuous infusion after a single bolus loading dose of 2 mg/kg IV.[91] The regimen consists of 11 mg/kg/hr for 20 minutes followed by 7 and 5 mg/kg/hr for the same periods, then 4 mg/kg/hr for the next hour, and 3.5 mg/kg/hr thereafter. If midazolam and nitrous oxide were added, the same regimen without 20 minutes at 11 mg/kg/hr would provide adequate sedation.[91]

Ketamine is used occasionally for perioperative analgesia and has made a small resurgence for this indication in children with obstructive sleep apnea (OSA).[110] It is also used for neuroaxial analgesia. S-ketamine is the more potent and preferred enantiomer to administer. If ketamine is administered in a neuroaxial block, a preservative-free formulation should be used. *Caution: The neurotoxic risk of the racemic mixture of ketamine in the epidural space has not been established.*[111]

Side effects associated with ketamine include increased secretions, nystagmus, and nausea and vomiting. The last effect may occur in up to 33% of children. Nightmares and hallucinations have been reported after ketamine but appear to be very infrequent. Coadministration of midazolam and awakening in a dark, quiet environment may reduce the risk of nightmares postoperatively.[112]

Ketamine may be contraindicated in children with increased intracranial pressure and in those at risk for seizures (although it has been administered to many children in whom their seizures were under control).

Etomidate

This hypnotic anesthetic is infrequently used in children as its pharmacology has not been understood until recently. It is reserved for those who are hemodynamically unstable (e.g., septic shock). The dose of etomidate is 0.2 to 0.3 mg/kg intravenously in adults, with children requiring 0.3 mg/kg. The pharmacokinetics have only recently been estimated: With greater clearance and volume of distribution in young children, larger doses are required in this age group than older children.[113] Although the elimination half-life or context-sensitive half-life of etomidate has not been reported in children, repeated doses or infusions have delayed emergence which limits the use of this medication. Because etomidate causes pain at the site of injection, pretreatment with IV lidocaine and mini-Bier block is advised.

The major impediment to the use of etomidate and to its approval in many countries has been the suppression of adrenal glands, particularly in critically ill patients.[114]

Recent molecular engineering has yielded solutions to both the adrenal suppression and prolonged emergence after infusions of etomidate. Although there are no studies in humans, carbomethoxyetomidate does not substantively suppress the adrenal gland and is rapidly metabolized by tissue esterases, with an elimination half-life not unlike remifentanil.[115] If this new molecule proves safe to use in humans, this new compound may be extremely useful as an induction agent as well as a maintenance agent without suppressing the adrenal gland.

Neuromuscular Blocking Agents

With standard twitch devices readily available, every child who receives a muscle relaxant should be assessed for their twitch response before attempting to antagonize the neuromuscular blockade. The role of neuromuscular agents in children has diminished in the past decade or more with the demise in routine use of succinylcholine and the adoption of propofol as the adjunctive medication to facilitate tracheal intubation after induction of anesthesia with sevoflurane.

In Europe, the most common cause of anaphylaxis during anesthesia is muscle relaxants, with succinylcholine and rocuronium being the most common causes,[116] although in children, latex was the most common cause (42%) followed by muscle relaxants (32%) and antibiotics (9%).[116] The explanation for the frequency of anaphylaxis to relaxants in Europe remained elusive, although regional differences in the use of pholcodine, an over-the-counter cough medicine, suggested that epitopes in pholcodine (and certain cosmetics) were structurally similar to those in the aminosteroidal relaxants, which led to a cross-sensitivity and anaphylactic reactions, even upon first exposure.[117] Indeed, after pholcodine was banned in Norway, the incidence of anaphylactic reactions to muscle relaxants in that country decreased dramatically suggesting that this over-the-counter cough medicine sensitized the population to the relaxants.

Succinylcholine

As the only depolarizing muscle relaxant in clinical practice, succinylcholine remains the agent that provides the most rapid onset and offset of paralysis, without additional medications to recover the normal twitch response. Succinylcholine comprises two acetylcholine molecules fused together; it acts by depolarizing the acetylcholine receptors of the neuromuscular endplate.

The intravenous dose of succinylcholine is 3 to 4 mg/kg in neonates and infants, 2 mg/kg in children, and 1 mg/kg in adolescents.[118] The larger dose requirement with decreasing age has been attributed to the larger volume of distribution in younger infants. Paralysis usually occurs within 30 to 60 seconds and lasts approximately 5 minutes.[118] In contrast, an intramuscular dose of 4 mg/kg paralyzes 100% of children within 1 to 2 minutes, although the duration may be as great as 20 minutes.[119] Rarely is it necessary to administer succinylcholine intra- or sublingually, but this approach may be optimized with digital massage of the injection site.[120] The speed of onset of paralysis when 1.1 mg/kg is administered intralingually is intermediate between IV and IM rates, ~75 seconds.[121] It is imperative to avoid midline sublingual blood vessels to avoid a sublingual hematoma. To administer succinylcholine either IM or sublingually, a small gauge (25G) needle should be used to minimize vascular trauma. This author routinely administers atropine 20 μg/kg before succinylcholine given via any route to prevent bradycardia and asystole after a single dose in infants and children.[122]

The action of succinylcholine is terminated by pseudocholinesterase (or plasma cholinesterase) which is located on 3q26.1 and 3q26.2.[123] The residual products of metabolism have no neuromuscular activity. Pseudocholinesterase activity may be modified by a number of factors, inherited or acquired (Table 42-5). The inheritance pattern for pseudocholinesterase is autosomal recessive, which yields a host of phenotypes. Four alleles code for most of the genetic variants of pseudocholinesterase: "Usual" (U); "Atypical" (A); "Fluoride resistant" (F); and "Silent gene" (S).[123] Several minor variants (H, J, and K) have also been reported. A second gene locus that codes for pseudocholinesterase in only 10% of Caucasians has been identified. It produces a C5 band on electrophoresis that yields 30% more pseudocholinesterase enzyme than normal (Neitlich variant).[124] In addition, another gene variant with increased activity named E Cynthiana has been identified.[125]

TABLE 42-5. PSEUDOCHOLINESTERASE VARIANTS

Decreased Activity	Increased Activity
Congenital causes	Congenital causes
Gene defects	Gene defects
Usual: E^u	Cynthiana or Neitlich: C_5
Atypical: E^a	
Fluoride resistant: E^f	
Silent gene: E^s	
Rare defects	
H variant	
J variant	
K variant	
Acquired causes	Acquired causes
Hepatic insufficiency	Thyroid disease
Renal failure	Obesity
Malnutrition	Nephrotic syndrome
Severe burns	Cognitively challenged children
Chronic infections	
Pregnancy	
Neonate	
Plasmapheresis	
Drug-induced	
Organophosphates	
Cyclophosphamide	
Echothiophate iodide	
Oral contraceptives	
Metoclopramide	
Glucocorticoids	
Esmolol	
Chlorpromazine	

The genetics of pseudocholinesterase activity variant follows simple Mendelian inheritance. Individuals may be homozygous or heterozygous for the gene. The vast majority of the population has normal responses to succinylcholine; that is, homozygous usual pseudocholinesterase, U/U. About 1:30 patients are heterozygous atypical (U/A) with minimal clinical prolongation of the duration of action of succinylcholine (~15 minutes). In contrast, 1:3,000 to 1:10,000 patients are homozygous atypical (A/A) with a clinical phenotype manifesting a duration of action of 1 hour. In the case of fluoride-resistant, the frequency of homozygous F/F is 1:150,000, with a modest prolongation of succinylcholine activity of 1 to 2 hours. For the homozygous silent gene variant, S/S, the frequency is 1:10,000 patients, with a clinical duration of 6 to 8 hours. The other variants H, J, and K are associated with a 90%, 66%, and 30% reduction in pseudocholinesterase activity, respectively. The homozygous H variant yields the greatest duration of action of succinylcholine among these three 1 to 2 hours. The K variant is thought to occur in 13% of the population and the homozygous K variant occurs in 1:63, extending the duration of succinylcholine <1 hour. Interestingly, the K variant was present in 89% of A variants suggesting that more than one mutation is often present, for example, U/AK. The E Cynthiana and C5 variants destroy succinylcholine at an ultrarapid speed that may provide such a transient paralysis that the child recovers before laryngoscopy is attempted. This variant was not widely considered during the era of succinylcholine-induced masseter muscle spasm. The management of prolonged response to succinylcholine is conservative. Sedation/anesthesia and ventilation should be maintained and blood sent for identification of the gene defect.

Identification of the specific gene defect depends on the laboratory analysis of pseudocholinesterase activity and gene identification. The former involves incubating a sample of blood with dibucaine (an amide local anesthetic) that inhibits normal, but not abnormal pseudocholinesterase. When benzoylcholine is added to the blood, dibucaine suppresses the degradation of benzoylcholine by normal pseudocholinesterase by >71% (hence a dibucaine number of 71) whereas the degradation by A/A is only minimally depressed; that is, by 20%, hence the dibucaine number is 20. Intermediate inhibition is a dibucaine number of 60. A similar response occurs when fluoride is added to blood with normal pseudocholinesterase inhibited, but atypical appears resistant to it. Hence, a small dibucaine number suggests an abnormal pseudocholinesterase activity. Homozygote silent gene, S/S, conveyed no pseudocholinesterase activity, although variants of this defect also exist.[123]

SIDE EFFECTS. The salient side effects associated with succinylcholine include arrhythmias (most notably bradycardia), rhabdomyolysis (with hyperkalemia and myoglobinuria), raised intraocular pressure, fasciculations, and malignant hyperthermia (MH).

Succinylcholine causes arrhythmias by acetylcholine-associated activation of the vagal nerves. Sinus bradycardia is the most common arrhythmia, which may progress to transient asystole after a single intravenous dose of succinylcholine in a child.[126] Bradycardia can be prevented by administering an anticholinergic such as atropine (10 to 20 μg/kg) or glycopyrrolate (5 to 10 μg/kg) before succinylcholine.[122]

Rhabdomyolysis may occur when succinylcholine is administered to children with MH or a myopathy.[127,128] The muscle breakdown releases massive concentrations of hyperkalemia as well as myoglobin, both resulting in potentially fatal consequences.

Hyperkalemia may occur in response to IV succinylcholine in children with a variety of disorders: Myopathies, upper and lower motor neuron disorders, burns, severe sepsis, and chronic immobilization (e.g., drug-induced, trauma-induced) (usually for weeks).[127] There is no evidence that succinylcholine presents additional risks when administered to patients with renal failure.[129] Treatment for hyperkalemia after succinylcholine is intravenous calcium (calcium chloride 10 mg/kg) that should be repeated until the arrhythmias (ventricular wide complex) dissipate and the rhythm returns to normal sinus rhythm.

Succinylcholine increases intraocular pressure 7 to 10 mm Hg reaching a peak pressure 1 to 2 minutes after IV administration and returns to the baseline in 5 to 7 minutes.[130] This increase may be attenuated by pretreatment with anesthetics, although none provides 100% guarantee that the increase will not occur. In the presence of a lacerated globe, this increase in intraocular pressure may increase the extrusion of intraocular contents although greater increases in pressure may occur during crying and coughing.[130]

Fasciculations occur immediately after administration of IV succinylcholine. They have not been associated with any clinical sequelae. Some assert that fasciculations increase the risk of regurgitation by increasing the abdominal muscle tone. However, the crura of the diaphragm comprise skeletal muscle, which also fasciculates preventing any decrease in gastric barrier pressure. Adolescents with muscular builds are at an increased risk of developing postoperative muscle pains after succinylcholine. To prevent these pains, which can be serious, consideration should be given to avoid succinylcholine in this age group.

MH is a pharmacogenetic disorder of calcium metabolism in skeletal muscle.[128] The triggers (succinylcholine and/or inhalational anesthetics) induce an exaggerated release of intracellular calcium, which causes sustained muscle contractions. These sustained contractions generate heat and muscle breakdown with the release of intracellular potassium, myoglobin, and CPK. The earliest sign of an MH reaction is an increase in end-tidal pCO_2 that is accompanied by an increase in respiratory rate and hemoglobin desaturation. Late signs include increases in body temperature, disseminated intravascular coagulopathy, and sepsis. The definitive treatment for MH is intravenous dantrolene 2.5 mg/kg, repeated as needed until the reaction subsides.[131] (See below and Chapter 23 for further details on MH.)

Rocuronium

Rocuronium is a steroidal muscle relaxant that is an analogue of vecuronium but differs from the latter by a more rapid onset of action and reduced potency. It is eliminated almost exclusively by the liver; hence liver failure may prolong its duration of action of rocuronium.[132] In contrast, renal failure should have minimal effect on its elimination. Sevoflurane potentiates the action of rocuronium.

The potency of rocuronium is greatest in infants, least in children, and intermediate in adults. The dose should be adjusted according to the child's age: The ED_{95} in infants is 0.25 mg/kg and in children, 0.4 mg/kg.[133,134] In healthy children during sevoflurane anesthesia, 0.3 to 0.4 mg/kg rocuronium provides suitable intubating conditions in 2 to 3 minutes and permits antagonism within 20 minutes. Twice the ED_{95} or 0.6 mg/kg IV rocuronium provides relaxation in 1 to 1.5 minutes. Sevoflurane potentiates the effect of rocuronium compared with balanced anesthesia, a pharmacodynamic, not pharmacokinetic effect.[135] The time to 90% recovery of the twitch response after 0.6 mg/kg IV is 46 minutes in children. Recovery after rocuronium in infants is prolonged compared with that in children as a result of the reduced clearance and increased volume of distribution in the former.[134] At 3 to 4 × ED_{95}, 0.9 to 1.2 mg/kg IV rocuronium yields similar intubating conditions to succinylcholine within 60 seconds and may be used for rapid sequence induction (RSI), although recovery may be markedly prolonged.[136–138]

Intramuscular rocuronium (1.8 mg/kg) has been recommended for emergency situations when an IV is not available. However, this dose and route provides poor intubating conditions after 4 minutes and a duration of action of 80 minutes. The author does not recommend this route and dose of administration.

Atracurium

Atracurium is a benzylisoquinolinium muscle relaxant that undergoes spontaneous degradation in blood primarily by Hofmann elimination yielding the major metabolite, laudanosine, which is devoid of neuromuscular blocking properties.[132] It comprises 10 isomers. A typical intubating dose in infants and children is 0.5 mg/kg IV (2 to 3 × ED_{95}) with an onset of 2 minutes and a duration of action of 15 to 30 minutes. Complete recovery is usually achieved within 45 to 60 minutes. With its brief half-life, atracurium is suited for use as a continuous infusion in a dose of 6 μg/kg/min during isoflurane anesthesia and 9 μg/kg/min during a balanced intravenous anesthetic.[139] Renal and hepatic failures do not affect the duration of action of atracurium. Side effects associated with atracurium include cutaneous erythema, bronchospasm, and wheezing after a rapid large bolus administration; rarely has anaphylaxis been reported.

Cis-atracurium

Cis-atracurium is one of the 10 isomers of atracurium that has supplanted the use of atracurium. It has a potency that is threefold greater than atracurium resulting in more specificity for the receptor and fewer side effects such as histamine release.[132] It too is degraded by Hofmann elimination with a typical duration of action of 30 to 50 minutes. Suitable intubating conditions are achieved with 150 μg/kg (3 × ED_{95}) by 2 minutes after the dose.[140] Renal and hepatic failures do not affect the duration of action of *cis*-atracurium. Side effects associated with the administration of *cis*-atracurium are minimal.

Neostigmine

This author strongly recommends antagonizing all neuromuscular blocking agents in infants and children when extubation is planned,[141] provided the time interval from the last dose has not exceeded 2 hours (in most cases). The train-of-four should be ≥0.9 before the trachea is extubated.[141] Any child who appears weak, as a "fish out of water," requires antagonism or a repeat dose of antagonism of the neuromuscular blockade. In order to successfully antagonize the relaxant, vital signs including temperature must be normal.

Neostigmine is an anticholinesterase compound that antagonizes neuromuscular blockade by preventing the degradation of acetylcholine. The acetylcholine competitively displaces the muscle relaxant from the neuromuscular junction. The dose of neostigmine in infants and children is 30% to 40% less than that in adults, or 20 to 40 μg/kg, which should be administered when at least one twitch is present in the train-of-four. If the recovery of neuromuscular blockade is incomplete, repeat doses of neostigmine may be administered up to 70 μg/kg. Care must be taken to avoid exceeding 100 μg/kg as acetylcholine-associated weakness may occur.

Neostigmine should be preceded by an anticholinergic, atropine 20 μg/kg or glycopyrrolate 10 μg/kg, to minimize the effect of neostigmine on the nicotinic receptors. Atropine causes a greater increase in heart rate but has a shorter duration of action than glycopyrrolate.

Sugammadex

This γ-cyclodextrin compound is a cylindrical oligosaccharide that uniquely binds rocuronium (and to a lesser extent vecuronium) to eliminate its activity.[142] When administered in the presence of moderate to profound rocuronium-induced neuromuscular blockade, sugammadex restored the twitch response thereby providing a direct intervention for a "cannot ventilate, cannot intubate" situation. The rocuronium/sugammadex complex is excreted unchanged in the kidney. Sugammadex has been used extensively in Europe but is not approved in North America due to several episodes of hypersensitivity in preclinical trials. In children and adolescents, a single dose of ≥2 mg/kg sugammadex after partial recovery (two twitches of the train-of-four) from neuromuscular blockade with rocuronium yielded a train-of-four of 0.9 in approximately 2 minutes.[143] Dose response studies in children are required. Most recently, two reports of sugammadex reversal of rocuronium-induced anaphylaxis refractory to vasopressors suggest another important clinical role for sugammadex.[144]

Opioids

Morphine

Opioid use in infants and children has increased dramatically in the past few decades, in response to recognition that children experience pain and that pain adversely affects the speed and quality of recovery.

In children, perioperative analgesia is accomplished with intraoperative IV doses of 50 to 100 μg/kg and postoperative doses of 50 μg/kg morphine.[145] Perioperative infusions of morphine may also be administered by diluting morphine (1 mg/kg of the child's weight) in 100 mL lactated Ringer (LR) solution and infusing at 1 to 4 mL/hr. This provides analgesic blood concentrations of morphine, 10 to 40 ng/mL.[145] Morphine may also be administered via the caudal/epidural route. Doses of 25 to 50 μg/kg provide prolonged analgesia with a small incidence of side effects (vomiting, pruritus).[145] Oral morphine has also been administered, although its bioavailability is only 35% due to the first-pass effect.

Side effects after morphine include dose-dependent respiratory depression and incidence of vomiting (particularly at >100 μg/kg). Histamine release and urticaria at the site of injection are local, nonimmunologic reactions.

Fentanyl

This semi-synthetic opioid is the most widely used intraoperative analgesic in children. This very lipid soluble opioid, which is bound primarily to α_1-acid glycoprotein in blood, has a very rapid onset of action, hemodynamic stability, and brief duration of action after a single dose.[146] It may be used via the IV, IM, oral, IN, and caudal/epidural routes. It is 50 to 100 times more potent than morphine, with doses 1 to 3 μg/kg IV attenuating the sympathetic responses to minor surgical procedures, up to doses of 12 to 50 μg/kg for neonatal surgery.[147] Fentanyl is infrequently administered IM; oral fentanyl, 10 to 20 μg/kg, is used in breakthrough cancer pain. IN fentanyl (1 to 2 μg/kg) has been used as a premedication and to reduce agitation in children undergoing myringotomy and tube surgery.[109,146] Epidural fentanyl has been administered to children via the epidural space in a dose of 1 to 2 μg/mL to supplement local anesthetics. Although there is very little evidence that fentanyl augments the analgesia provided by a lumbar epidural block in a child with an effective local anesthetic concentration (e.g., 0.125% bupivacaine or 0.0625% levobupivacaine),[148] it is commonly added resulting in pruritus, nausea/vomiting, and urinary retention.

The action of clinical doses of fentanyl is terminated by redistribution and, secondarily, by clearance in the liver.[146] The initial redistribution is rapid; however, once tissue binding sites become saturated, the elimination half-life of fentanyl increases.[149] metabolized extensively by CYP450 3A4 to inactive metabolites. The context-sensitive half-life of fentanyl in adults after a brief infusion for 1 hour, 20 minutes, increases dramatically to 4 hours after an 8-hour infusion.[149] Elimination half-life may exceed 20 hours after a chronic infusion. To offset this increasing context-sensitive half-life, the dose of fentanyl must be adjusted. After a prolonged infusion of fentanyl, it is necessary to slowly taper the dose and monitor for opioid withdrawal.

Meperidine

Meperidine is no longer recommended as an analgesic because of the risk of seizures (from normeperidine) and the accumulation of normeperidine after repeated doses of meperidine. It is currently recommended only for shivering.[146] The dose of meperidine for analgesia is 1 to 2 mg/kg and for shivering 25% to 50% of that dose. The elimination half-life of meperidine in children is 3 hours.[146]

Remifentanil

Remifentanil is a unique μ-receptor opioid that undergoes spontaneous degradation in blood by tissue esterases, with an elimination half-life of approximately 5 minutes that is independent of the duration of infusion.[150] With this brief half-life, remifentanil is usually administered as a continuous infusion. The context-sensitive half-life (the time to decrease the blood concentration by 50%) of remifentanil is 3 to 8 minutes. Metabolites of remifentanil are effectively nontherapeutic.

Remifentanil is 10- to 60-fold more potent than alfentanil.[150,151] The infusion rate for remifentanil ranges from 0.05 to 0.25 μg/kg/min (although larger doses have been administered), with the dose adjusted according to the presence of concomitant medications (e.g., inhalational anesthetics). A loading dose (0.1 to 0.2 μg/kg) is usually not required as the infusion rapidly establishes an effective target organ concentration and hypotension is a real possibility.

When administered in large doses, remifentanil may cause hypotension, bradycardia, and chest wall rigidity, although the latter may be more likely vocal cord closure rather than chest rigidity.[151] Prolonged administration has resulted in tachyphylaxis. Recent evidence suggests that nitrous oxide may attenuate the risk of tachyphylaxis.[152]

Hydromorphone

Hydromorphone (or Dilaudid) is a long-acting opioid analgesic that is infrequently used in children. This μ-opioid receptor agonist is 5- to 10-fold more potent than morphine, with a recommended dose of 10 to 20 μg/kg/dose IV or IM and 1 μg/kg/hr IV or epidural continuous infusions.[146,153] Hydromorphone has an elimination half-life of 2.5 hours, similar to that of morphine. Metabolism is extensively (95%) via a single pathway to hydromorphone-3-glucuronide.

Codeine

This old, indirect acting opioid has been the mainstay of postoperative analgesia in children for decades. The analgesic effect of codeine; however, depends on its conversion to morphine (10%) and possibly to hydrocodone (11%).[154,155] Because this conversion depends on CYP450 2D6, polymorphisms of this enzyme for which more than 50 have been identified to date, may produce enormous variability in the analgesia from this drug ranging from no analgesia (e.g., no conversion to active analgesics in nonresponders) to an opioid overdose (in an ultrarapid metabolizer) which has been implicated in brain damage in one case and death in a second case postoperatively.[156,157] This popular analgesic is under increasing scrutiny currently because of these polymorphisms and the potential extreme responses to it in many jurisdictions that has resulted in its withdrarwal in some.

Codeine may be administered IM, PO, and rectal.[146,154] IV codeine is not used as it causes cardiovascular depression and seizures. The dosing range for IM, PO, and rectal routes is similar, 0.5 to 1.5 mg/kg. Oral codeine reaches a peak blood level after 1 hour and an elimination half-life of 3 hours. When administered by the IM and rectal routes, the onset of action is more rapid and the elimination half-life less.

CYP450 2D6 is a noninducible enzyme that increases in activity from birth, reaching 20% of adult activity by 1 month of age (see Figure 42-1). It is mapped onto chromosome 22. 2D6 metabolizes 25% of medications in clinical use. Polymorphisms of this enzyme are responsible for normal rates of metabolism, poor metabolizers, extensive metabolizers, and ultra-extensive metabolizers as a result of gene polymorphisms and duplication.[158,159] These vary along ethnic lines (e.g., 10% of Caucasians and 30% of Hong Kong Chinese are poor metabolizers whereas 29% of Ethiopians are ultra-extensive metabolizers) resulting in an unpredictable and varied response in children. This has prompted some to substitute alternative analgesics although few have been investigated in children. Care must be taken to prescribe the appropriate dose based on lean body weight (LBW) and whether the child's opioid receptors have been upregulated as a result of intermittent nocturnal desaturation.[160]

Acetaminophen

This nonsteroidal analgesic/antipyretic has been an effective supplement in children. Acetaminophen has no anti-inflammatory properties and is also free of platelet-inhibiting properties. Although its mechanism of action is not completely understood, it is believed to act on the peroxidase receptors of prostaglandin H_2 or via *p*-aminophenol.[161]

Oral doses of 10 to 15 mg/kg or rectal doses of 30 to 40 mg/kg yield adequate blood concentrations. Postoperative rectal dosing 20 mg/kg every 6 hours maintains blood concentrations after a rectal loading dose. Absorption after oral administration is rapid (~10 to 15 minutes) whereas after rectal administration it is slow and variable (1 to 2 hours).[162] Rectal suppositories should be lubricated to avoid mucosal tears. Repeated doses every 6 hours while maintaining the maximum 24-hour dose at <100 mg/kg confer both analgesia and antipyresis.

Two intravenous formulations of acetaminophen, paracetamol and propacetamol, are now available for use in children.[161] Propacetamol is a water-soluble prodrug that is rapidly metabolized to paracetamol once administered. The equivalent dosing of paracetamol (15 mg/kg) is one-half that of propacetamol (30 mg/kg).[163,164]

Careful attention must be paid to the dosing of IV acetaminophen as three overdoses have been reported in infants who received 10- and 20-fold overdoses of the IV formulation, with one requiring treatment with intravenous *N*-acetylcysteine.[165,166]

Ketorolac

Ketorolac is the only parenteral nonsteroidal anti-inflammatory (NSAID) medication available for use in children. It possesses anti-inflammatory and analgesic properties for mild to moderate perioperative pain,[167] and like other NSAIDs, it also inhibits platelet adhesion by reducing the synthesis of thromboxane.

Ketorolac may be administered in doses of 0.5 to 2 mg/kg, with 0.5 mg/kg being the common dose administered to children.[168,169] The elimination half-life in infants and children is quite variable, 2 to 6 hours, and varies with whether the racemate (standard preparation) or stereoisomers are administered.[168,169]

The side effects of ketorolac have raised concerns. Many surgeons avoid ketorolac during tonsillectomy and adenoidectomy because of the risk of bleeding from COX-2 inhibition of platelet aggregation. Evidence is conflicting whether ketorolac affects the incidence of bleeding after tonsillectomy.[170–172] It seems prudent to withhold administration of ketorolac until after achieving surgical hemostasis. There is evidence that ketorolac inhibits bone healing in animals; a decision regarding its use during orthopedic surgery will depend on the surgeon's view. All NSAIDs may trigger severe bronchoconstriction in asthmatics, and ketorolac is relatively contraindicated in this population, although some prescribe ketorolac in children with mild asthma.[173] Lastly idiosyncratic renal failure has been reported, which in most instances resolves spontaneously.

Diclofenac

This NSAID is also a cyclooxygenase inhibitor but with a 20-fold greater affinity for COX-2 rather than COX-1 receptors. Diclofenac may be administered IV, IM, PO, and rectally. It is a potent analgesic, almost twice as effective for acute pain than acetaminophen for the treatment of acute pain during and after surgery.[174] The intravenous dose is 0.3 mg/kg and the oral dose is 1 mg/kg.[175,176] Its bioavailability rectally is twice that orally, hence the rectal dose is half the oral dose, 0.5 mg/kg. Side effects are infrequent, 0.24% of children, with postoperative bleeding being the most frequent. Because of its limited affinity for COX-1 receptors, it is not a potent platelet inhibitor and causes far less risk of bleeding than the other NSAIDs. As with other NSAIDs, it is relatively contraindicated in children with asthma.

Sedatives

Midazolam

This benzodiazepine is the most widely used anxiolytic in children in North America. It is water soluble, with a rapid onset of action when administered orally and a brief elimination half-life.[177] Unlike diazepam, it does not cause pain upon parenteral administration. Midazolam has been administered via the oral, sublingual, nasal, IV, IM, and rectal routes.[7,177] The oral and nasal doses are discussed under "Anxiety" below. Sublingual midazolam is difficult for many children to hold without swallowing. The dose for this route is the same as for the nasal route, 0.2 to 0.3 mg/kg.[8] IV midazolam in children is warranted during TIVA or when nitrous oxide is administered to assist with amnesia. Empirical IV dosing of 0.1 to 0.2 mg/kg should be administered, with larger doses being required in adolescence. IM midazolam is infrequently used in children because of the risk of sterile abscess and pain. Rectal dose of midazolam is 0.5 mg/kg, although this route is limited to children <5 years of age.[8]

Midazolam is metabolized by CYP450 3A4 enzyme system; this enzyme reaches 30% to 40% of adult levels by 1 month and adult levels by 1 year (see Figure 42-1).[178] Approximately 50% of glucuronidated metabolite of midazolam is excreted via the kidneys.[178] Metabolism of midazolam is affected by renal and hepatic failures as well as enzyme systems that interfere with 3A4.

Dexmedetomidine

Dexmedetomidine is an α_2-agonist sedative whose relative affinity for α_2:α_1 receptors is eightfold greater than clonidine. It is available in an intravenous formulation that may be administered by the oral, nasal, IV, IM, and rectal routes.[179]

The oral dose, which requires 30 to 60 minutes to provide sedation, is 2.6 to 4 μg/kg with increasing doses being more effective but at the cost of a prolonged recovery.[179] The IN dose is 1 to 2 μg/kg with 1 μg/kg sedating ~60% of children within 1 hour.[179] IV dexmedetomidine may or may not include a loading dose: 1 μg/kg over 10 minutes, followed by an infusion of 0.3 to 0.7 μg/kg/hr, is required.[179] *This infusion rate must be carefully transcribed because unlike other medications, the infusion rate is in μg/kg/hr, not μg/kg/min.* When a loading dose is administered before the infusion, the risk of hypotension in the peri-induction period increases.

The pharmacokinetics of dexmedetomidine show a rapid early redistribution phase (half-life of 7 minutes) but a slow terminal elimination half-life, approximately 2 hours in children.[180,181] It is metabolized in the liver primarily via uridine glucuronyltransferase to inactive metabolites.

Unlike other sedative/anxiolytics, dexmedetomidine exerts its clinical effects via α_2 receptors with sedation in the locus coeruleus, hemodynamic manifestations via direct and indirect action on the sympathetic nervous system, and a host of miscellaneous side effects.[179] The unique feature of this sedative/anxiolytic is the *absence* of substantial respiratory depression.[182]

Dexmedetomidine is not a complete anesthetic. It decreases the MAC of inhalational anesthetics approximately 30% depending on the dose, provides suitable sedation for radiologic investigations (although a dose of 0.1 mg/kg IV midazolam is required to prevent movement unless large doses of dexmedetomidine are used),[88,183] facilitates awake fiberoptic intubation and awake craniotomy, provides sedation that is closest to natural sleep, provides analgesia, reduces emergence delirium (ED)[179] and facilitates motor- and sensory-evoked monitoring for spine surgery.[184]

Side effects of dexmedetomidine relate primarily to its hemodynamic effects. Bradycardia has been reported with larger dose infusions (up to 2 to 3 μg/kg/hr) and in younger age infants with an incidence as great as 16%.[183] When the bradycardia (heart rates as low as 30/min) was treated with glycopyrrolate, profound hypertension occurred.[185] This author cautions against treating bradycardia with an anticholinergic. Rapid administration of dexmedetomidine has been reported to cause transient hypertension although this is uncommon in children. However, hypotension (>20% decrease from baseline) has occurred during dexmedetomidine infusions.[180,183] The frequency of hypotension increases with an increasing dose and younger age: The greatest incidence occurs in infants, 8%. IV fluid loading may attenuate the hypotension but awaits additional studies.

PREOPERATIVE ASSESSMENT

Fasting Guidelines

The American Society of Anesthesiologists framed the fasting guidelines for infants and children in 2006.[186] The guidelines, which were based on a consensus panel and a review of the literature, concluded that the fasting intervals before elective anesthesia could be summarized as 2, 4, 6, and 8 hours as delineated in Table 42-6.[186] It is important to note that these are not age-adjusted guidelines; they apply to infants and children of all ages. Equally important is to recognize the limitations of these guidelines. Gastric emptying times after breast milk and formula have only been evaluated in infants[187]; there are no data for comparable emptying times in children (≥1 year of age).

The child who presents chewing gum requires careful consideration. First, the characteristics of gastric fluid in children who chew sugar or sugarless gum include a doubling of the gastric fluid volume, with approximately 50% showing a gastric fluid volume >0.8 mL/kg, and a trivial increase in the gastric fluid

TABLE 42-6. FASTING GUIDELINES FOR CHILDREN REQUIRING ELECTIVE ANESTHESIA[186]

Clear fluids[a]	2 h
Breast milk	4 h
Infant formula	6 h
Solids	8 h

[a]Includes clear tea. If milk is added, we recommend a 6-hour fast.

pH.[188] Hence, the gastric fluid characteristics in the child who is chewing gum are not substantially different from those in the fasted child. The child must expectorate the gum before proceeding with general anesthesia. Second, if the child swallows the gum, then the child is at risk for aspiration of gum at body temperature, which would be very difficult to extricate from the airway. Thus, anesthesia must be cancelled if the child swallows the gum. With the rarity of aspiration (~1:10,000 to 1:1,100)[189] and in the absence of coexisting medical conditions, chewing gum does not appear to increase the risk of aspiration pneumonitis in children undergoing elective surgery, provided the gum is expectorated before anesthesia.

The risk of regurgitation and aspiration is far more difficult to determine in children who present for emergency surgery after a trauma. Many factors relate to this risk including the severity and nature of the trauma, existing medical conditions, medications that were administered, and the timing and nature of the foods ingested. Very little evidence exists upon which to assess the risk of a full stomach. One study determined that the risk of regurgitation may be related to the interval between the last food ingested and the trauma or injury.[190] Since gastroparesis and intestinal stasis occur after acute pain, an inflammatory response, and opioid medications, it is likely that gastrointestinal peristalsis stops after a trauma. There is no evidence in children that administration of a prokinetic medication empties the stomach after trauma. Auscultation of bowel sounds in the abdomen does not ensure gastric emptying, although passing gas does imply peristalsis of the small and large bowels is present but does not ensure return of gastric motility. We consider children who ingested solid foods within 8 hours of a trauma to be at risk for regurgitation and aspiration and take appropriate precautions for managing the airway.

Certain medical conditions may affect gastric emptying. Although diabetes mellitus delays gastric emptying, this may require years to fully develop. Recent evidence suggests that gastroparesis may be multifactorial.[191,192] Indeed, hyperglycemia alone can delay gastric emptying in both diabetics and nondiabetics. Obesity is thought to delay gastric emptying and increase the risk of regurgitation and aspiration in children although recent evidence suggests that these children are at no greater risk for pneumonitis should aspiration occur.[193]

Laboratory Testing

Preoperative laboratory testing is infrequently ordered in healthy children without preexisting medical disease. Although preoperative hemoglobin and urinalysis were mandated in some jurisdictions in the past as screening tools for nutritional deficiencies, hemoglobinopathies, and diabetes mellitus, abnormal hemoglobin results failed to affect changes in the management of the children and hence it was discarded as a preoperative test. Children in whom a preoperative hemoglobin is indicated include those at risk for massive bleeding, those with chronic anemia in whom bleeding is highly probable, those with chronic nutritional deficiency, and those with sickle disease (see below).

A preoperative pregnancy test is required before anesthesia and sedation in most children of childbearing years in most jurisdictions. The reason for this test is the risk that some medications that are administered in the perioperative period may cause a miscarriage or, less likely, teratogenicity of an unborn fetus. The incidence of unexpected and unknown pregnancies is approximately 0.3%.[194] Evidence suggests that history alone may not reliably predict the existence of a fetus in utero. Two pregnancy tests are available: Urine and blood. The former test yields more rapid results, but both tests have a known false-positive rate. There is debate regarding the threshold age to begin pregnancy testing. Many institutions and states require preoperative pregnancy testing in females who have reached menarche; some require testing in all females who are older than a specific age, that is, 11 years. If the pregnancy test is positive and the surgery is elective, the results must be conveyed to the patient. Due consideration should be given to the risk that anesthesia and surgery might pose to the unborn fetus if surgery proceeds. If, however, the surgery is emergent, then the risk benefit ratio of proceeding must be carefully assessed.

Medical Conditions

5 Upper Respiratory Tract Infection (URTI)

Approximately 65% of children with URTIs have viruses as the cause of their infection; the remaining 34% have bacterial infections. Children who have had a recent URTI should not undergo elective anesthesia for at least 4 weeks after the infection to ensure resolution of the pathologic effects in the small airways. Because young children have 6 to 7 URTIs per year, most clinicians proceed with anesthesia 2 to 4 weeks after the original infection.[195]

When children present for elective surgery with a URTI, the author recommends canceling the anesthetic if any one of the four criteria listed in Table 42-7 is present.[196] The presence of each of these increases the risk of perioperative airway events. Additional factors that increase the risk of adverse airway events include cigarette smoking in the house, atopy, asthma, prematurity, young age, and secretions.[195,197] If an infant (<1 year of age) presents for surgery with a URTI, the chest should be examined very carefully and a low threshold maintained for cancellation as perioperative respiratory complications in these infants are substantive.[198] This age group is at risk for serious lower respiratory tract infections such as respiratory syncytial virus that may rapidly lead to pneumonia and a protracted recovery possibly involving prolonged tracheal intubation in the intensive care unit.[199]

Children who present with clear rhinorrhea, whether due to a mild URI or allergic rhinitis, should be treated with 1 to 2 drops of oxymetazoline or neosynephrine (0.25%) nose drops per nostril to dry up the nasopharyngeal secretions during anesthesia. Care must be taken to use a dilute solution of neosynephrine, as concentrated solutions may cause an unexpected hypertensive crisis. We prefer to manage these children with a face mask if at all possible, in order to minimize the risk of triggering airway reflex responses. However, if the airway must be manipulated, a supraglottic airway is less likely to trigger airway reflex responses than a tracheal tube.

TABLE 42-7. CRITERIA TO CANCEL ANESTHESIA WITH AN UPPER RESPIRATORY TRACT INFECTION[196]

1. Fever >38.5°C
2. Altered behavior (not playing as usual) and habits (not feeding as usual)
3. Purulent, productive discharge from the upper airway
4. Lower respiratory tract signs (wheezing, rhonchi) that do not clear with coughing

Asthma

Up to 20% of children have asthma or an asthmatic history, but many fewer present with severe asthma that may complicate anesthesia.[200]

Children with a history of asthma should have their pulmonary condition optimized before surgery and be stable from their chest perspective, without a recent exacerbation or recent hospitalization. In the preoperative assessment, the age of onset of asthma, number and date of the most recent hospital admissions for asthma, treatment (β_2-agonists or steroids by inhalation), and current state of asthma should be recorded. Most children with asthma have never been admitted to hospital because of their asthma. However, if they have, the asthma should be considered severe. If oral steroids have been prescribed recently for an acute exacerbation of asthma, careful preoperative examination of the chest must be performed to ensure that there is no lingering reactive airway component. On the morning of the surgery, the child's lungs should be examined to check for wheezing. If wheezing is present, the child should be instructed to cough deeply to clear any airway secretions present, and bronchodilator therapy should be initiated. Preoperative bronchodilator therapy should be administered to children with mild to moderate asthma even if they are not wheezing, as this reduces airway resistance by approximately 25% during sevoflurane anesthesia and tracheal intubation.[201] If wheezing persists, the child should be referred to their pulmonologist for reassessment and the anesthetic deferred.

Preoperative bronchodilator therapy should be administered to children who are wheezing and present for emergency or urgent nonairway surgery. If tracheal intubation can be avoided, a face mask or LMA should be used. Equipment should be prepared to administer intraoperative bronchodilator therapy should the need arise.

6 Obstructive Sleep Apnea

OSA is the most serious form of sleep-disordered breathing in children.[202] Children have obstructed airways during sleep that are associated commonly with hypercapnia and intermittent hypoxia. The gold standard for the diagnosis is a polysomnogram, although many children present for surgery with a diagnosis of OSA but without a polysomnogram. In these cases, the diagnosis is made "clinically" by the presence of loud snoring, witnessed apneas, nocturnal enuresis, attention deficit disorder and behavioral problems, and inability to concentrate in school or poor school performance. OSA occurs equally in boys and girls and in asthenic and obese children. Daytime somnolence is not a common feature in children with OSA.

Two important considerations are to assess whether the child requires admission and overnight monitoring postoperatively/160/ and whether they are at risk for increased opioid sensitivity, that is those whose minimum nocturnal SaOx is <85%.[203,204] Although children with OSA may be premedicated with very small risk, those with persistent minimum nocturnal SaO_2 <85% are at increased risk for perioperative desaturation and airway events when the usual doses of opioids are administered. Alternative analgesic strategies including local anesthetic, NSAID agents, ketamine, and α_2-agonists should be considered.[205]

Ex-premature Infants (See Chapter 41)

Infants who were born prematurely (<37 weeks gestational age) and are <60 weeks postconceptional age (defined as the sum of the gestational and postnatal ages) require 12 to 24 hours of postanesthesia monitoring for apnea and hemoglobin oxygen desaturation, irrespective of the type of surgery.[206] Factors that increase the risk of perioperative apnea in ex-premature infants include age (<60 weeks postconceptual age), anemia (<12 g% Hb), and secondary diagnoses (e.g., intraventricular hemorrhage).[206,207] Opioids are best avoided in these infants; local anesthetic blocks are preferred. Caffeine 10 mg/kg IV may be administered intraoperatively to reduce the frequency of perioperative apneas, but it will not completely eliminate the risk of apnea.[208] Once the infant has been 12 hours apnea-free, he/she may be discharged home.

In contrast to general anesthesia, regional anesthesia does not increase the risk of perioperative apnea and does not require perioperative monitoring, unless the infant also received sedation, has multisystem disease, or has a history of perioperative apneas.[209] Spinal or caudal anesthesia will provide sufficient anesthesia to perform hernia surgery, the most common surgery in ex-premature infants. If the parents have an apnea monitor at home and have been trained to manage apnea, the child may be discharged home in the parents' care.

Malignant Hyperthermia[128]

Most children who present with an MH diagnosis are offspring of a blood relative with an MH reaction or positive muscle biopsy. The first task in such a case is to verify, as best as possible, the credibility of the past MH reaction from history or records. These children should be scheduled as the first case of the day to minimize their exposure to inhaled anesthetics in both the operating room and the postanesthetic care unit (PACU). If the child is anxious, he/she should be premedicated with oral midazolam (see below) in a dose appropriate for the child's age.

To prepare the AWS for an MH-susceptible child, either a designated inhaled anesthetic-free AWS should be used or a contaminated AWS should be flushed to reduce the anesthetic concentration to <10 ppm. In the latter situation, after removing the vaporizers from the AWS, the anesthetic breathing circuit and carbon dioxide canisters should be replaced with new equipment. The fresh gas flow should be set to 10 L/min oxygen/air mixture while the ventilator ventilates an artificial lung or reservoir bag to reduce the concentration of anesthetics in the machine to ≤10 ppm, considered to be the anesthetic threshold to trigger MH reactions. The time required to achieve ≤10 ppm varies amongst the current AWSs (Table 42-8), although there is no way of verifying in any single instance that the threshold was reached. Some have proposed replacing components of the AWS to expedite and ensure the washout process while others recommend using charcoal absorbent in the inspiratory limb of the breathing circuit (for elective cases).[210] Once the breathing circuit

TABLE 42-8. WASHOUT TIMES FOR ANESTHESIA WORKSTATIONS

Ohmeda Machines (min)		Other Machines (min)	
Modulus 1	5–15	Narkomed GS	20
Excel 210	7	Drager Primus	70
AS/3	30	Drager Fabius GS	104
Aestiva (sevo)	22	Kion	>25
Aisys (sevo)	25		

Data from: Kim TW, Nemergut ME. Preparation of modern anesthesia workstations for malignant hyperthermia-susceptible patients; a review of past and present practice. *Anesthesiology.* 2011;114:205–212; data for Aestiva and Aisys from: Sabouri S, Lerman J, Heard C. Residual sevoflurane may be present after flushing the GE Anesthesia workstation for MH susceptible patients. *Anesthesiology.* 2011:A1276.

has been flushed, the fresh gas flow should NOT be reduced below the 10 L/min flow rate if a charcoal filter is not used, lest a rebound in the anesthetic concentration occurs.[211] Interestingly, MH reactions have not been reported after reducing the fresh gas flow in a flushed AWS.

A trigger-free anesthetic includes propofol, opioids, benzodiazepines, nondepolarizing muscle relaxants, nitrous oxide, and regional anesthesia.[128] Of the standard monitors, end-tidal CO_2 (the earliest indicator of an MH reaction) and temperature (preferably axillary temperature since it will reflect temperature in the largest muscle bulk in the chest) are essential. IV dantrolene should be available in sufficient quantity to treat a reaction should it occur (2.4 mg/kg IV as an initial dose, and repeated as necessary). The initial dose should maintain blood concentrations of dantrolene (>3 μg/mL) for 6 hours, after which its elimination half-life is 10 hours.[131] There is no longer any role for prophylactic preoperative dantrolene in children with MH. If dantrolene is administered, a urinary catheter should be inserted because dantrolene contains mannitol.

There is a host of additional strategies that may be utilized to stabilize the child including cooling strategies, antiarrhythmics. For further information on management of an MH reaction, please refer to Chapter 23.[128]

Children who are MH susceptible may undergo surgery as outpatients provided an MH reaction does not occur and the parents receive detailed instructions regarding how to monitor for possible MH reactions and who to call and where to go if such a reaction occurs.

Myopathies

The anesthetic for children with common myopathies, including Duchenne muscular dystrophy (DMD), Becker's muscular dystrophy, and Emery–Dreifuss syndrome, should avoid medications that are known to disrupt skeletal muscle membranes in children <8 years of age and excessive cardiac depressants in children ≥10 years with cardiomyopathy.[128] DMD is an X-linked recessive gene in which the underlying defect is the lack of dystrophin (<3% of normal) in skeletal and cardiac muscles. The onset of the disease is 2 to 6 years of age. Becker's dystrophy is a milder form of the disease with an onset in the second decade of life. Emery–Dreifuss syndrome is also a milder form of the disease often presenting with cardiac conduction defects, with syncope as the presenting finding.

The dystrophin protein complex is essential for the stability of the cytoskeleton of the muscles. Muscle contractions, whether natural or drug induced, may tear the muscle membrane and release intracellular contents including high concentrations of potassium, myoglobin, and CPK. The administration of an inhalational anesthetic (halothane >> sevoflurane ~ isoflurane) with or without succinylcholine may cause skeletal muscle contractions, releasing intracellular contents.[212] Although inhalational anesthetics have been administered to these children without untoward events, the author recommends propofol in deference to inhalational anesthesia.[128] As the children reach adolescence, the muscle wasting in DMD abates and the predominant anesthetic concern is a progressive cardiomyopathy. In the case of Emery–Dreifuss, heart block may be a complicating finding. Hence, preoperative echocardiogram and electrocardiogram are warranted before anesthetizing adolescents with DMD or Emery–Dreifuss syndrome.

Mitochondrial myopathies are a complex group of disorders that result from defects in the protein complexes of the respiratory chain in mitochondria.[128,213] The protein complexes in the chain are under bigenomic control: 85% arise from nuclear DNA and 15% from mitochondrial DNA. In children, most mitochondrial myopathies result from defects in the nuclear DNA. The distribution of defective DNA in tissues in utero determines the spectrum of the disease.[128] Children with a history of lactic acidosis during infancy should be fasted for brief periods, not receive LR solution, and receive an infusion of glucose intraoperatively. Both intravenous and inhalational anesthetics have been administered to children with mitochondrial myopathies without untoward events.[213]

Sickle Cell Disease

Sickle Cell Disease (SCD) or sickle cell anemia occurs primarily in children of sub-Sahara descent, with a frequency of sickle cell trait in African-Americans of 8% and a form of SCD of 1:600.[214] A point genetic mutation results in the replacement of the Hb AA (where A is the normal hemoglobin) with Hb SS (S is the sickle hemoglobin) in every red blood cell.[214] Thus, 100% of the cells in children with Hb SS are at risk for sickling; these children chronically have low hemoglobin concentrations (6 to 8 g%), may have had acute vasoocclusive crises, and may have received multiple red cell transfusions in the past. Vasoocclusive crises may involve a number of organs including bone, chest, and brain. Some children suffer from repeated vasoocclusive crises whereas others never experience them. These crises are not related to hypoxia, hypovolemia, or hypothermia, but rather to a systemic inflammatory response, the nature of which remains unclear. Evidence suggests that those with SCD and vasoocclusive crises have markers of a systemic inflammatory response to the disease that upregulates endogenous factors, including an adhesive factor that traps sickle red cells in arterioles and precipitates occlusive crises.[215] Whether the traditional factors of hypoxia, hypovolemia, and hypothermia exacerbate the initial process or compound the underlying inflammatory process has not been clearly established.

Two other forms of SCD, Hb SC and Hb SD, occur much less frequently than Hb SS, have an equal risk of sickling as Hb SS but have hemoglobin concentrations that are closer to normal values, approximately 10 to 11 g%. These children should be managed in a manner similar to those with Hb SS disease.[214]

Sickle cell may also present in a heterozygote form known as sickle trait, Hb AS. This disorder presents few problems during routine general and regional anesthesia and surgery provided extreme conditions, such as hypothermia and cardiopulmonary bypass, are not employed. Children with Hb AS have normal hemoglobin concentrations.

Preoperatively, a history of the frequency, severity, and precipitating triggers of sickle and vasoocclusive crises in the child should be elicited. Consultation with the treating hematologist should provide insight into the current local strategies for managing this patient. However, if the child's sickle status has not been clearly established, a sickledex test may be used to diagnose SCD in infants >6 months of age and in children. This test can be performed rapidly, inexpensively, and reliably. The sickledex test is unreliable in infants <6 months of age because Hb F interferes with the sickling process and renders the test nonconfirmatory. In fact, infants <6 months of age rarely sickle because of the presence of Hb F, which gradually wanes in concentration beyond 3 months of age. If the test is negative, the child may still have sickle trait. If the test is positive or if the child is suspected of having sickle hemoglobin from history, then a hemoglobin electrophoresis should be performed to determine the precise hemoglobinopathy present. The definitive diagnostic test for SCD is the hemoglobin electrophoresis or high-performance liquid chromatography.

To attenuate the risk of a sickle cell crisis in children with SCD in the perioperative period, many hematologists transfuse the children with packed red cells to a total hemoglobin of 10 g%.[216]

Others believe that both prophylactic blood transfusions and the need for transfusions in all children undergoing *minor* surgery are without merit.[217] The disadvantages of frequent transfusions in children who are at risk for sickle crises include sensitizing the recipient to minor antibodies (i.e., Kell and Duffy), iron overload, and transfusion reactions. It is important to consult local hematologists regarding the institutional management of children with SCD before the day of surgery to avoid surgical delays and document that discussion and management plan preoperatively with the parents and in the patient record. Optimal management of these children includes maintaining neutral thermoregulation and adequate hydration and oxygenation throughout the perioperative period.

Anterior Mediastinal Mass

Children with AMM require general anesthesia and/or sedation for a tissue (lymph node) biopsy, CT scan or MRI for diagnosis, or indwelling central line for chemotherapy.[218] Children with these tumors present a significant risk for anesthesia, since cardiac arrest has been reported in the past. Understanding the pathophysiology of the disease enables the clinician to anticipate complications and prepare the anesthetic to avoid them.

Four tissues can be found in AMMs in children: Lymphomas, teratomas, thymomas, and thyroid.[218] The most rapidly growing tumor in the anterior mediastinum is the lymphoblastic T cell lymphoma, a non-Hodgkin's lymphoma, which has a doubling time of only 12 to 24 hours. These children may present with minor findings (e.g., night sweats) that rapidly progress over 1 to 2 days to life-threatening problems (e.g., orthopnea, superior vena cava syndrome). In children, anesthesia is usually required to delimit the extent of and tumor effects on mediastinal structures in radiology as well as for tissue biopsy and chronic chemotherapy access in the operating room.

The decision to proceed with local, regional, or general anesthesia depends on the age and level of cooperation of the child, the extent of mediastinal organ compromise, and the accessibility of the node or tumor being biopsied. A multidisciplinary team that includes the surgeon, anesthesiologist, and oncologist should review all radiologic and preoperative data before embarking on the surgery.

Those children who can tolerate the surgery under local anesthesia and sedation are managed in this manner. However, the challenge is far greater in younger children, in children who cannot tolerate local anesthesia and sedation, and in those whose tumor severely compromises the airway and/or pulmonary artery. In such instances, a 12- to 24-hour course of intravenous steroids should be considered and discussed with the oncologists to shrink the tumor (usually a lymphoblastic lymphoma) to facilitate an anesthetic and reduce the risk of cardiac arrest.[219] The risks associated with 12–24 hours of steroid therapy are infrequent but include widespread tumor necrosis that may both render the diagnosis of the cell type difficult and tumor lysis syndrome.[220] Some oncologists are reluctant to treat these children with steroids because of the potential difficulty in establishing the tissue diagnosis should extensive tumor necrosis result. Establishing the tumor type is critical for determining the treatment regimen for the specific tumor type.

For most children who require a radiologic investigation, tumor biopsy, or chemotherapy access, general anesthesia with spontaneous respiration is preferred. If the child cannot lie flat, anesthesia can be induced and the trachea intubated with the child positioned in the left lateral decubitus or. less desirably, in the sitting position. The trachea should be intubated at induction of anesthesia to ensure a patent airway should it become necessary to turn the child prone because circulatory collapse occurs. Tracheal intubation is performed without muscle relaxation to preserve spontaneous respiration. Spontaneous respiration best preserves the negative intrathoracic pressure gradient to suspend the tumor above the mediastinal structures and avoid pressure on the pulmonary artery and right atrium as well as the tracheobronchial tree. It is important to remember that the capnogram may be a very useful monitor to confirm the adequacy of the pulmonary circulation (and cardiac output); the sudden loss of or reduction in the capnogram may herald compression of the pulmonary artery before systemic cardiovascular sequelae occur.

Endocarditis Prophylaxis

In 2007, the American Heart Association significantly revised the indications for bacterial endocarditis prophylaxis.[221] The new recommendations were crafted for dental procedures and adopted by the American Dental Association. The American Heart Association no longer recommends endocarditis prophylaxis for children undergoing gastrointestinal, urologic, and genitourinary surgeries, although many specialists in these areas continue to request endocarditis prophylaxis. Accordingly, it is incumbent upon the anesthesiologist to inquire of the specific specialist whether endocarditis prophylaxis should be administered.

For dental procedures, the indications for SBE prophylaxis are listed in Table 42-9.[221] The antibiotic regimen for endocarditis prophylaxis has not changed since previously published.

TABLE 42-9. SBE PROPHYLAXIS RECOMMENDATIONS BY AMERICAN HEART ASSOCIATION[221]

1. Prosthetic cardiac valve or material use to repair the cardiac valve
2. Previous infectious endocarditis
3. Congenital heart disease:
   a. Unrepaired cyanotic congenital heart disease, including palliative shunts and conduits
   b. Completely repaired congenital heart defect with prosthetic material or device, whether placed by surgery or by catheter intervention, during the first 6 mos after the procedure
   c. Repaired congenital heart disease with residual defects at the site or adjacent to the site of a prosthetic patch or prosthetic device (which inhibits endothelialization)
4. Cardiac transplantation recipients who develop cardiac valvulopathy

7 Obesity

Obesity in children is an epidemic worldwide. In children, definitions are based on growth curves, not BMI, because height and weight change with age.[222] The definitions in children are as follows: Overweight is a BMI >85%, obesity is a BMI >95%, and super (morbid) obesity is a BMI >99%. Ideal body weight (IBW) in children 1 to 18 years of age may be estimated using the child's height as Wt (kg) = Height (cm)^2 × 1.65/100. An easy, quick, and simple approach to estimate the IBW based on a child's age is

For children <8 years: Wt (kg) = 2 × Age (year) + 9

For children ≥8 years: Wt (kg) = 3 × Age (year)

Others have indicated that LBW (ideal) is 20% to 40% of total body weight (TBW), applicable also to obese children. LBW has also been estimated as IBW + 1/3(TBW – IBW).

Ninety-five percent of obesity is attributable to environmental and lifestyle factors.[222,223] Fewer than 5% of cases of obesity are attributable to diseases and genes such as Prader–Willi syndrome (Laurence–Moon–Biedl syndrome), inborn errors of metabolism, Cushing's disease, and immobility (DMD). The underlying mechanisms for these disorders include leptin mutations (receptor and prohormone convertase 1), proopiomelanocortin mutation, and MCR4 (melanocortin receptor).

Thirty percent of overweight children have restrictive pulmonary pattern results from body fat encasing the pliable chest with decreased chest wall compliance, FRC, and vital capacity.[222,223] The increased work of breathing compounds the reduced lung volumes as the closing volume approaches the tidal volume and V/Q mismatch occurs. Nocturnal hypoxemia from the above factors combined with large tonsils (see below) sets the stage for the development of pulmonary hypertension. Sleep-disordered breathing occurs in 17% (up to 33% if BMI >150%) of obese children.

Cardiovascular effects include systemic hypertension, left ventricular hypertrophy, and premature atherosclerosis. Intermittent hypoxia during sleep apnea may lead to pulmonary hypertension. Both blood volume and cardiac output are increased.

Insulin resistance and metabolic syndrome are present in 40% of moderately obese children and 50% of severely obese adolescents. Increased abdominal weight predisposes to gastroesophageal reflux, which occurs in approximately 20% of children with severe obesity. Gastric emptying rates and aspiration in obese children do not differ from those in normal children. NPO intervals are the same in obese and non-obese children. Glomerular filtration rate is increased. Fatty infiltration of the liver leads to nonalcoholic fatty liver disease, which leads to abnormal liver function tests and possibly hepatic fibrosis.

Drug dosing in obese children is complex, varying with several factors including lipid solubility, volume of distribution, and the route of elimination, hepatic or renal.[223] The drug dosing for several commonly used drugs in obese children may be estimated on the basis of their weight (Table 42-10).

These children should be positioned 25-degree head-up during preoxygenation to reduce V/Q mismatch and to facilitate tracheal intubation. The tragus should be positioned above the level of the sternal notch.[224] IV access may be difficult. Desflurane is preferred for maintenance of anesthesia as it is the least fat soluble of the inhalational anesthetics. However, if the child has asthma or lives in a home with indoor smoking, desflurane may not be preferred. Compression devices should be applied to the legs to prevent stasis and deep vein thrombosis.

Perioperative respiratory events including difficult mask ventilation, greater Mallampati airway class, bronchospasm, and rapid hemoglobin desaturation and prolonged PACU times are more common in obese children.[223]

TABLE 42-10. DRUG DOSING FOR OBESE CHILDREN

Drug	Induction Dose Based on	Maintenance Dose Based on
Thiopental[4,41]	LBW	
Propofol[46]	LBW	TBW
Synthetic opioids (fentanyl, alfentanil, and sufentanil)[4]	TBW	LBW
Morphine[47]	IBW	IBW
Remifentanil[48]	LBW	LBW
Nondepolarizing neuromuscular blockers[49]	IBW	IBW
Succinylcholine[45]	TBW	
Sugammadex[50,51]	TBW	

TBW, total body weight; LBW, lean body weight; IBW, ideal body weight.

Preoperative History

Medical, surgical, and family histories including complications should be recorded. The details of all allergies should be carefully elicited in terms of the clinical manifestations and severity. A systems approach should review each organ system including recent URTIs recorded.

Preoperative Physical Examination

The airway, respiratory, and cardiovascular systems should be examined preoperatively in every child. The airway examination should include visual inspection of the face in the anterior and profile views to detect any disproportions in facial features that might suggest a congenital facial or airway anomaly. The child should open their mouth fully, stick out their tongue, and extend their neck. Loose teeth should be identified and any removable dental appliances stored. Piercings in and around the mouth should be removed as these may become dislodged and aspirated if they are intraoral. The respiratory examination includes auscultation of the chest (front and back) with full inspiration and expiration through the mouth. If rales or rhonchi are present, the child should be instructed to cough deeply to clear them. If coughing is ineffective, then further investigations may be required including chest X-ray and a pulmonary consultation. Cardiovascular examination includes auscultation of the heart and if the child has a murmur, then further inquiry regarding cardiac symptoms (syncope, arrhythmias, tachycardia, heart failure, shortness of breath) should be solicited. If the murmur is heard during diastole, has not been diagnosed previously, or is associated with any cardiac symptomatology, then a cardiology consultation should be sought. If the child has a history of cardiac surgery, then a recent cardiology note together with an electrocardiogram and echocardiogram should be reviewed.

Anesthetic Risks; Consent/Assent

The mortality associated with anesthesia in healthy children is 1:10,000 or less.[225] Perioperative cardiac arrest rate is greater in children who are young, whose age <1 year, with congenital heart disease, and undergoing emergency surgery. This author does not give a number for the risk of cardiac arrest to parents of healthy children undergoing elective anesthesia (unless specifically requested to do so) but rather uses an analogy that the risk is greater that they would be hit by a car crossing the busy street outside the hospital than to have a serious adverse outcome during general anesthesia. Perioperative morbidity may be greater than the incidence of cardiac arrest, but depends on the child's comorbidities and the severity of the current diseases.

Specific risks discussed preoperative include the most common complications pain, nausea, and vomiting. In addition, the author reviews the small risk of unforeseen complications that may result from as yet latent diseases, dental damage, corneal abrasion, aspiration, awareness, allergic reactions, and cardiac arrest.

If asked about awareness, this author informs the parents/guardians that there is a 1% incidence of awareness reported in children,[226] which is 3- to 10-fold greater than that reported in adults. These reports, for the most part, are not consistent with those practicing pediatric anesthesia: Indeed, many of these episodes can be explained by light anesthesia during periods of stimulation.

If asked about cognitive dysfunction after anesthesia, the author informs the parents/guardians that apoptosis has been reported after almost every anesthetic in neonatal animals and some nonhuman primates.[227] Most studies in children to date have not properly investigated the risk of anesthesia on the maturing human brain precluding drawing any conclusions regarding the possible harm that anesthesia might cause. Yet, in a Dutch study of identical twins who were discordant for receiving anesthesia, neurocognitive capabilities in the twins were similar after a 10-year follow-up.[5] Accordingly, this author advises parents that there is insufficient evidence to incriminate anesthesia in causing cognitive dysfunction in young children based on the current evidence. In addition, the author suggests that when considering whether to proceed with surgery, all risks and benefits of performing anesthesia and surgery in their child must be carefully evaluated.

8 Allergies

Most allergies that are reported in hospital records are of little relevance to the conduct of anesthesia. All allergies reported to the admission nurses by patients or families are dutifully transcribed into the hospital record without censure and without regard for their relevance or authenticity. Examples of recognized side effects that do not constitute allergies include headaches after epinephrine, vomiting after opioids, and diarrhea after amoxicillin. Only true allergies that are recorded on the anesthetic record should include anaphylactic reactions and those diagnosed and confirmed by an allergist/immunologist. The remainder should be identified as hypersensitivity or idiosyncratic reactions, although the latter is not commonly practiced. Cross-sensitivity is possible, rarely, between penicillin allergy and first-generation cephalosporins; there is no cross-reactivity with second or later generation of cephalosporins.[228] If the parents report a possible penicillin allergy or sensitivity to cephalosporin that was more than 5 years ago and not confirmed by an immunologist, then this author offers to test the child using a small test dose of the intravenous antibiotic while monitoring the child and informs the parent of the outcome.

Few, if any, allergies to propofol have been reported. Although the package insert for propofol cautions against the use of propofol in children with egg allergy, evidence supports the use of propofol in children with egg allergy, provided the egg allergy was not anaphylaxis.[229] Egg lecithin, a phospholipid in propofol, is not a protein and therefore cannot induce anaphylactic reactions. However, it may bring yolk proteins with it into the formulation. AstraZeneca state that no soy protein is present in their North American formulation of propofol. Hence, children with soy allergy (usually <5 years of age) may receive propofol.

Latex allergy is an important consideration when preparing the operating room for children.[230] Numerous children with spina bifida, congenital urologic surgery, and multiple surgeries (>5 exposures) were exposed to latex products by repeated bladder catheterizations or latex gloves multiple times and developed IgE-mediated latex anaphylaxis. Since latex products both in and out of hospital have been replaced with nonlatex products, the prevalence of latex allergy in this population is decreasing. It is imperative to avoid contaminating the surgical (and anesthetic) setup with latex in order to prevent latex anaphylaxis. Children who are latex allergic and who touch toy balloons to their lips or in whose mouths dentists insert a rubber dam, will react with lip or tongue swelling, respectively. Removing all latex products from the operating room has eliminated latex anaphylactic reactions in one center.[231] If the child has latex anaphylaxis, each door entering the operating room should have signage indicating a latex-allergic patient is in the operating room; all latex products should be removed from the operating room. In otherwise healthy children with latex anaphylaxis, epinephrine is indicated in a dose of 1 to 10 μg/kg, in which 1 to 2 μg/kg reverses isolated bronchospasm up to 10 μg/kg for the very rare instance of cardiac arrest.

INDUCTION OF ANESTHESIA

Equipment

To ensure that the anesthetizing location is properly and completely prepared, it is useful to refer to a checklist. Appropriately sized equipment should be available for each child. A range of face mask sizes, oral airways, laryngoscope blades, tracheal tubes, and LMAs should be present. The author prefers cushioned clear face masks that fit the contour of the child's face and permit rapid identification of either fluid or solid material within the mask. Reliance on oral airways in establishing a patent upper airway in children has been supplanted, in part, by an appropriately applied jaw thrust maneuver.[97] The Miller and Wisconsin straight blades are preferred for tracheal intubation in infants and children because they align the axes of the mouth, pharynx, and larynx. A range of sizes of laryngoscope blades should be available in every anesthetizing location. For laryngoscopy the child should be positioned flat on the table, with the head stabilized to prevent lateral movement. The large occiput of the child puts the head in the sniffing position naturally. In infants and children with limited oxygen reserve, or when performing tracheal intubation during sedation, the Oxyscope, a straight blade fitted with a source of oxygen at the tip of the blade, may prevent oxygen desaturation. For older children and adolescents, either a Miller or Macintosh blade may be used.

The classic laryngeal mask airway (cLMA) was introduced to replace face masks in adults and has subsequently proven to be a versatile and useful airway device in children as well.[232] To fit pediatric airways, the dimensions of the adult cLMA were scaled down in size, although the mask was otherwise unmodified and made limited compensation for the difference in laryngeal anatomy. The cLMA has proven to be effective in circumstances other than elective anesthesia, including neonatal resuscitation and fiberoptic intubation. A range of sizes of the cLMA should be available.

Although effective, the cLMA does not "protect" the airway from regurgitation and laryngospasm. Since the tone of the gastroesophageal sphincter is reduced in children, compared with adults, children may be at greater risk for regurgitation in the presence of a full stomach or positive pressure ventilation. Hence, it is best to avoid LMAs in these clinical situations. Modifications of the cLMA to include a vent for regurgitant gas or liquid from the esophagus, as in the ProSeal supraglottic airway, may better protect the airway against aspiration.

Complications associated with the cLMA in children are infrequent but may include gastric inflation, aspiration, airway obstruction, and laryngospasm.[233] The frequency of complications with cLMA in infants <1 year of age is greater than that in older children and in infants managed with a face mask. Studies suggested that the epiglottis folds down into the bowl of the cLMA in a majority of children although the LMA is otherwise functioning properly; this finding may simply be moot.[233]

A range of diameters of tracheal tubes appropriate for the child's age, as well as tubes 0.5 mm ID (internal diameter in mm) smaller and larger, should always be available. The appropriate size of the uncuffed tracheal tube is based on the ID of the tube. Guidelines for uncuffed tracheal tube sizes in infants and children are as follows: Infant's weight (<1,500 g, 2.5 mm ID; 1,500 g to full-term gestation, 3 mm ID); neonate to 6 months postnatal age, 3.5 mm ID; and 0.5 to 1.5 years, 4 mm ID. For children >2 years of age, the size of uncuffed tubes may be estimated using the formula: Age (in years)/4 + 4 (or 4.5) mm ID. The size of cuffed tubes (mm ID) may be estimated using the formula: Age (in years)/4 + 3 (for children <2 years) or +3.5 (for those >2 years).

The length of a tube from the lips to midtrachea in infants <1,000 g in weight is 6 cm, 1,000 to 3,000 g is 7 to 9 cm, in term neonates 10 cm, and for infants and children, 10 + age (years) mm.

In the past, uncuffed tracheal tubes were commonly used to secure the airway of children <8 years of age. The circular shape of the tracheal tube was similar to the shape of the lumen within the cricoid ring, which allowed for a good seal without the need for a cuff on the tube. Cuffs were avoided in children out of the concern that compression of the loosely adherent pseudostratified columnar epithelium that lines the cricoid ring would swell and encroach on this narrowest portion of the upper airway and cause stridor. This increase in resistance would rapidly lead to respiratory distress, fatigue, and ultimately respiratory failure in young infants and children. To preclude this potentially serious airway complication in the perioperative period, the tracheal tube was carefully selected in children so that it either passed through the cricoid ring without resistance or did so with an audible leak at a peak inspiratory pressure 10 to 20 cm H_2O. If an audible leak was present at a peak airway pressure ≤10 cm H_2O, then the tracheal tube was changed to a half-size larger and the leak test repeated until the tube size is satisfactory. This resulted in repeat laryngoscopies and tracheal intubations and OR pollution.

Recently, there has been a shift from uncuffed to cuffed tracheal tubes in infants and children. This shift in practice has been accelerated by the introduction of the soft, high-compliance cuffed Microcuff tube (Microcuff GMbH, Weinheim, Germany).[234] These tubes have no Murphy eye, the cuff is positioned closer to the tip of the tube (than standard cuffed tubes), the cuff material is polyurethane, and the cuff shape is cylindrical (rather than spherical as in low-compliance cuffed tubes), mimicking the shape of the larynx. Several small-size studies have reported few complications when high-compliant cuffed and uncuffed tubes were used in children. Microcuff tubes confer several additional advantages over traditional uncuffed tubes, including less contamination of the OR with anesthetic gases, fewer laryngoscopies and reintubations, sealing the airway at lower pressures (~10 cm H_2O), and more consistent tidal volumes (as chest wall and abdominal compliance change during surgery).[235] However, the cost of the Microcuff tube is several folds greater than the uncuffed tube. The additional cost may be offset by savings in anesthetic gases. The cuffs on these tubes do expand when nitrous oxide is used; however, the time interval before the cuff pressure reaches 25 cm H_2O is greater with the Microcuff because they seal the airway at reduced pressures compared with other cuffed tubes for children. Overall, cuffed tracheal tubes in children substantially reduce the number of manipulations of the airway in children and operating room costs and pollution. It should be noted however, that the size of the Microcuff tubes differ from traditional tubes and no long-term outcome studies have been published in children.

Optimizing ventilation during anesthesia and surgery in infants and children has been the subject of much interest.[236] Traditional strategies held that volume-controlled pressure-limited ventilators were effective for most infants and children. However, these ventilators accounted for neither the compliance of the breathing circuit nor the variable leak around the tracheal tube. Further concerns focused on the shape of the pressure tracing during inspiration and the risk of delivering excessive peak airway pressures. In the neonatal intensive care units, pressure-controlled ventilation has been used successfully, in part because the peak inspiratory pressure is restricted and the risk of barotrauma is decreased with the constant inspiratory pressure pattern. The inspiratory pressure pattern also more evenly distributes the inspiratory gas throughout the lungs, reducing the risk of ventilation/perfusion (V/Q) mismatch. Despite the advantages of the pressure-controlled ventilators, many anesthesia ventilators were simply unable to compensate for decreases in abdominal and chest wall compliance that occurred during surgery. The new generation of anesthetic machines offers markedly improved ventilators and ventilation strategies that are hybrids of the best aspects of both volume- and pressure-regulated ventilation. These new ventilators may prove to be ideal for both preterm and term neonates. Ventilation strategies, such as the hybrid pressure-regulated volume-controlled mode, maintain a fixed tidal volume by taking into account the compressible volume of the breathing circuit.[236] This mode is used during controlled ventilation, and a pressure support mode is used once spontaneous respiration commences. For most children, the ventilation strategy will not impact on the outcome, but for those with lung disease, a poor ventilation strategy could result in a panoply of irreversible pulmonary problems. Whichever ventilation mode or strategy is planned for a particular child, it is crucial that the limits on ventilation including peak inspiratory pressure, rate, and positive end-expiratory pressure are set before the child is connected to the ventilator.

Full Stomach and Rapid Sequence Induction

The term "full stomach" refers to the presence of residual solid or liquid foods in the stomach at induction of anesthesia, a condition that places the child at risk for regurgitation and aspiration. A full stomach should be assumed in children who present for emergency surgery, in those with gastric dysmotility syndromes, and in those with diabetes. In most cases of emergency surgery, the time interval between ingestion of food and induction of general anesthesia is too brief to ensure complete evacuation of the gastric contents.[190] A full stomach may be caused by the "trauma," pain, and stress of the injury as well as by the administration of opioids, which increase gastric and intestinal paresis and further delay emptying of food from the stomach.

There are three important principles to remember in such cases: (1) there is no safe time interval after an injury that guarantees the stomach is empty of food; (2) there is no safe time interval after an injury that guarantees that there is no risk of regurgitation of gastric contents; and (3) all children (even those treated with prokinetic motility medications) are at risk for regurgitation and aspiration during induction of, maintenance of, and emergence from anesthesia.

To protect the airways of children who are at risk for regurgitation and aspiration during induction of anesthesia, an RSI of anesthesia is widely practiced. Although there is no evidence that an RSI is the best strategy, it seems reasonable to induce anesthesia as quickly as possible and to insert a tracheal tube into the larynx as quickly as possible and inflate the cuff, if a cuff is used. To perform an RSI, a tracheal tube with a stylet as well as tubes 0.5 mm ID greater or less, a functioning laryngoscope, active suction, intravenous access, and predetermined doses of anesthetic agents should be available. Induction of anesthesia may include propofol, the most common intravenous induction agent in children (2 to 4 mg/kg), or ketamine (1 to 2 mg/kg) or etomidate (0.2 to 0.3 mg/kg), the latter two favored for those who are hemodynamically unstable. We recommend succinylcholine 2 mg/kg (preceded by atropine 0.02 mg/kg) for paralysis, although rocuronium 0.8 to 1 mg/kg has also been used. (Note: *Recent concern regarding unexpected hyperkalemia and ventricular tachycardia in male children with undiagnosed muscle (wasting) diseases who received succinylcholine requires the immediate availability of intravenous calcium chloride (10 mg/kg IV, repeat as necessary) to restore normal sinus rhythm.*) If the child has a muscle wasting disorder, rocuronium should be used to secure the airway. However, if the airway appears to be difficult or precarious, then alternative strategies to secure the airway should be considered, including an inhalational anesthetic or topical local anesthetic and TIVA sedation. If an inhalational induction is performed, unexpected regurgitation may necessitate rotating the child quickly into the left lateral decubitus position and pharyngeal suctioning to prevent aspiration.

There is much debate regarding the importance and relevance of cricoid pressure in an RSI.[237] Currently, there is no evidence to support or refute the use of cricoid pressure during RSI. However, there are some concerns regarding the application of cricoid pressure in infants. In both infants and children, the cricoid ring and trachea are mobile and deformable, and as little as 5 N force can compress the infant's airway by 50%.[238] This is one-fourth to one-sixth the force recommended for cricoid pressure. Cricoid pressure may also increase the level of difficulty of tracheal intubation by distorting tracheal anatomy or compressing the cricoid ring. Very few assistants are trained properly in the location of the cricoid ring and in the magnitude of the force required to occlude the esophagus. *It remains this author's view that cricoid pressure has not been shown to reduce regurgitation in children at risk for aspiration and is not required for RSI. The practitioner should understand the advantages and disadvantages of cricoid pressure in infants and children in order to make an informed decision regarding its use.*

Emergency Drugs

Emergency drugs should always be available before inducing anesthesia. Syringes with a small gauge (23G or 25G) needle that contain weight-appropriate doses of atropine and succinylcholine should be immediately available to facilitate intramuscular or sublingual drug injection in an emergency. A syringe of propofol (1 to 2 mg/kg) should also be available to facilitate tracheal intubation or insert an LMA, as well as to break laryngospasm and increase the depth of anesthesia quickly.[239] Inotropic drugs are not routinely prepared for children undergoing elective surgery, unless the child has congenital heart disease or is critically ill. In the latter situations, preloaded syringes of phenylephrine (10 μg/mL) and epinephrine (10 μg/mL) should also be available.

Monitors

The ASA recommends basic patient monitoring during all anesthetics including electrocardiogram, arterial blood pressure, SaO_2, capnogram, and temperature, as well as additional monitors specific for the child's medical or anesthetic condition, for example, depth of anesthesia monitor. Many infants and preschool-age children fight the application of monitors while awake. Although induction of anesthesia is usually well tolerated and safe in expert hands, every effort should be made to apply at least a pulse oximeter before inducing anesthesia. The remaining monitors should be applied as soon as the child loses consciousness. Understanding the role of these monitors in pediatric anesthesia requires a basic understanding of these instruments, although three specific monitors merit mention: The capnogram, temperature, and depth of anesthesia monitoring.

Capnography

Two distinct approaches are used to analyze the end-tidal carbon dioxide tension in the breathing circuit by infrared analysis. In the first, gas is aspirated continuously from the breathing circuit and the carbon dioxide tension is detected in a remote sensor. This is known as sidestream capnography. In the second, the carbon dioxide tension is directly analyzed by a sensor interposed within the breathing circuit. The latter is known as mainstream capnography.

The accuracy of sidestream capnometry improved dramatically when circle system breathing circuits replaced t-piece circuits because there is less dilution of expiratory gas. Sidestream capnometry using gas obtained from the elbow of the circle breathing circuit provides accurate data, even in neonates who have small tidal volumes. On the other hand, mainstream capnography is infrequently used and unpopular among pediatric anesthesiologists, particularly for infants and neonates, because it increases the dead space of the breathing circuit, must be fitted at the tracheal tube/elbow and is heavy, thus increasing the risk of inadvertently bending the trachea tube and possibly kinking it.

The end-tidal pCO_2 may also be accurately monitored while the child is sedated and breathing spontaneously through a face mask or through baffled nasal prongs. This noninvasive but accurate measure of capnometry allows continuous assessment of ventilation in remote sites such as the MRI and CT scanners amongst other locations.

Temperature

Thermoregulatory homeostasis requires an understanding of the physiology of heat transfer in the child as well as the effects of anesthesia. Children have large surface areas to body weight and as such are at risk for rapid and extensive heat loss to the environment. In children, heat loss follows the order: Radiation (39%) > convection (34%) > evaporation (24%) > conduction (3%).[240] When anesthesia is induced, heat is redistributed from the central core to the periphery, from where it is lost to the environment. There is little that can be done to prevent the redistribution of heat with induction of anesthesia but there are a number of strategies that may attenuate the net loss of heat from the child.

The temperature of the operating room should be increased to about 28° C (80° F) before nonfebrile neonates and infants arrive. Since there may be a substantial (up to 1 hour) lag time between setting the operating room temperature and achieving it, the room temperature should be adjusted as the previous child leaves. The increased temperature warms the walls and the air within the room, thereby reducing both radiation and convection heat losses, respectively.[240]

Several other modalities have been used to maintain thermoneutrality in infants and children during anesthesia including water mattresses, radiant overhead heaters, and forced air warmers. Water mattresses address heat loss primarily through conductive paths and since this accounts for an insignificant fraction of the heat loss, they are unnecessary. Radiant overhead heaters are used primarily for neonates and infants. Feedback control to avoid skin burns is best served using an accurate measure of the distance of the heater from the infant's skin surface as well as continuous surface temperature monitoring on the infant's skin. However, for the majority of infants and children who require temperature control in the operating room, the most important modality is the forced air warmer. These warmers are the single most effective strategy available to minimize heat loss in children who undergo surgery lasting 1 hour or more.[241] Although it is comforting to the child to preheat the air mattress before the child enters the operating room, this practice does not affect the child's temperature at the end of anesthesia. These warmers may predispose to airborne contamination and possible surgical infection, although evidence is conflicting. It remains this author's recommendation to turn the forced air warmer off when the skin is prepped and resume heating only after the surgical drapes are in place.

A heat and moisture exchanger may be used to add humidity to the circuit although its efficiency is poor, particularly for surgery less than 1 hour and in infants.

Temperature should be monitored continuously throughout the anesthetic and in the PACU of all children who receive anesthesia or sedation. Core temperature is ideally measured in the midesophagus using an esophageal temperature probe. Although alternative sites to measure the core temperature include the rectum, nasopharynx, and axilla, each site has its limitations. Rectal temperature probes may yield inaccurate temperatures if the probe falls out of the rectum or is buried in stool. Nasopharyngeal temperature may detect brain temperature but more likely underestimates the core temperature by cooler gas passing through the breathing circuit. Axillary temperature may under- or overestimate the core temperature if it is positioned on the ipsilateral arm where the IV fluid is infusing or if the probe is either in the airspace behind the axilla being bathed by cool room air or the heat from the forced air warmer. The author prefers proper positioning of the axillary temperature probe against the axillary artery in the arm opposite to the side with the IV and with the shoulder completely adducted. In this position, an increase in temperature may be detected as an early sign of an MH reaction given the proximity of the large deltopectoral muscle group. Although some use a forehead skin temperature to track temperature, 10 MH reactions occurred in which these devices failed to reflect an increase in temperature.[242]

Temperature monitoring is important not only in MH but also to detect hypothermia. Hypothermia delays emergence from inhalational anesthesia, reduces the rate of degradation of medications. and increases infectious risks.

Depth of Anesthetic Monitoring

Recent reports of awareness in up to 1% of children who received general anesthesia for elective surgery have attracted considerable attention.[226] Careful review of the studies suggests that many of these episodes may be attributed to local practices that expose the children to concentrations of anesthesia that were insufficient for the level of stimulation. To reduce the risk of awareness, the anesthetic concentration of sevoflurane should be neither interrupted nor dramatically decreased early in anesthesia or during surgical stimulation.

The most widely studied anesthetic depth monitor in children in North America is the BIS, although other monitors such as the cerebral state index and spectral entropy monitor are available. BIS readings are affected by a number of variables that raise questions regarding their validity in children. First, the determinations vary with the anesthetic administered. For example, at equi-MAC values, the BIS measurements during halothane anesthesia are 50% greater than those during sevoflurane.[243] This likely reflects the substantial differences in the EEGs between the two anesthetics. Second, the variability in the BIS measurements during sevoflurane among children precludes precise interpretation of the BIS measurement.[64] Third, age directly affects the BIS readings, with BIS measurements in children <5 years of age are less reliable than those in children >5 years of age.[62–64] This likely stems from maturational differences in the EEG from birth to school age, which was not incorporated in the BIS algorithm. Fourth, the BIS readings decrease as the sevoflurane concentration increases but beyond 3%, BIS paradoxically increases.[63] Additional curiosities with the BIS that are not pediatric specific include its inability to accurately measure changes in the presence of nitrous oxide and ketamine, the increase in the BIS readings as muscle relaxation wears off, and lastly, the effect of position on the BIS reading with Trendelenburg position (30-degree head-down) increasing the BIS by 20%.[244]

This author's indications for the use of the BIS monitor in children include those who cannot tolerate general anesthesia because of hemodynamic instability, those in whom nitrous oxide is not used, and those who require TIVA.

PREOPERATIVE PREPARATION

Anxiolysis

It is important to reduce anxiety in children undergoing anesthesia and surgery. Anxiety is greater when preschool age and withdrawn children are separated from their parents, when anxious parents accompany their children, and when multiple personnel, bright lights, and loud noises are present at induction of anesthesia. Each of these factors should be addressed on an institutional basis to reduce the overall anxiety in young children scheduled for surgery. Goal-directed therapy for the child should primarily attenuate the child's anxiety preoperatively and anticipate more anxiety at induction of anesthesia and secondarily, address the parental anxiety.

Parental Presence at Induction of Anesthesia

Two systematic reviews established that Parental Presence at Induction of Anesthesia (PPIA) reduced the anxiety of parents but not the children.[245,246] Children 1 to 6 years of age are those for whom PPIA may be most beneficial. Parents who are most insistent on being present at induction of anesthesia are often the most disruptive, least likely to calm their child, and actually promote further noncompliant behavior in their child. Parents should never be invited to accompany their child for induction, lest both the hospital and the medical personnel find themselves responsible for any untoward sequelae that occur. The entire OR team must be like-minded regarding PPIA including detailed plans for escorting the parents out of the OR at the appropriate time. Before entering the OR, the parents must be instructed on the normal behavior of children during induction of anesthesia. If the parent is unable to cope with the OR environment or the child's loss of consciousness, he/she should not be present at their child's induction of anesthesia.

Some cognitively challenged adolescents and children may resist the transfer to the operating room. In such cases, the parents may have to be enlisted to accompany the child to the OR. Those children who resist attempts to bring them to the OR and are physically abusive despite enlisting the parent's assistance may require intramuscular ketamine (see below).

Distraction Techniques

Preoperative coloring books, stories, videos, and websites may be used to help children of all ages learn about surgery and anesthesia and the equipment that will be used for induction of anesthesia.[246] Some children's hospitals conduct operating room tours during which time the children become familiar and touch the face masks and breathing circuits. Child-life providers may help children defuse anxiety on the day of surgery by having the children play with the mask and flavor the inside using lip balm. Other distraction techniques including video games, earphones, and portable Internet devices as well as music and clowns all reduce children's anxiety. Once the child enters the operating room, the anesthesiologist should establish rapport (distract) with the child by telling a story, engaging them in conversation about a recent birthday, holiday, or vacation, or by singing as they prepare for induction of anesthesia.

Pharmacologic Sedation

For some, a premedication may be required to facilitate smooth separation from their parents. In North America, midazolam is the most widely used premedication for children because it can be given orally, nasally, rectally, intramuscularly, or intravenously to provide anxiolysis before induction of anesthesia. It should be noted that most premedications do not delay recovery and/or hospital discharge for surgeries at least 30 minutes in duration.

The dose of oral midazolam increases with decreasing age, although few bother to consider this very important factor.[247] Failure to adequately premedicate the child may lead to parents questioning the practitioner's abilities, but more importantly, may fail to provide adequate anxiolysis for separation from the parents and induction of anesthesia. The bioavailability of oral midazolam is poor, with 27% at 0.15 mg/kg and 15% at 0.45 and 1 mg/kg.[7] This author administers 0.75 to 1 mg/kg (maximum dose 15 to 20 mg) to children 18 months to 3 years of age, 0.6 to 0.75 mg/kg to children 3 to 6 years of age, 0.5 mg/kg to children 6 to 10 years of age, and 0.3 mg/kg to children >10 years to a maximum of 15 to 20 mg to ensure a 98% success rate of sedating children within 10 to 15 minutes.[248] Since oral midazolam leaves a bitter aftertaste, the current formulation is dissolved in a thick, flavored strawberry syrup. To minimize the aftertaste, the dose should be swallowed in a single bolus and then followed with a small volume of water. For children too young to swallow midazolam from a cup, it should be instilled into the lateral gutters of the mouth using a needleless syringe to prevent the child from spitting it out. Judgment should be exercised when considering oral midazolam premedication for a child who is crying continuously as few strategies, including parental presence at induction, may provide anxiolysis.

Alternative oral premedications include ketamine (5 to 6 mg/kg),[112] clonidine (2 μg/kg),[249] and dexmedetomidine (2 μg/kg).[250] Ketamine is prepared by suspending it in a thick, flavored syrup. It offers few advantages over midazolam and may cause more postoperative vomiting (POV).[112] Postoperative hallucinations and nightmares are infrequently reported after oral administration. Some have combined oral midazolam and ketamine in a 50:50 mixture with good success. Both clonidine and dexmedetomidine take 60 to 90 minutes to affect sedation and anxiolysis. They may produce bradycardia and sedation that persist beyond the duration of the anesthetic.

The IN route is effective in the crying child, although nasal administration of medications is unpleasant for most. A volume of 0.5 mL is well tolerated and covers adequate mucosal surface for rapid absorption. IN midazolam 0.1 to 0.2 mg/kg causes effective premedication, but older children complain of the bitter burning aftertaste.[251] IN sufentanil 1 to 2 μg/kg is also an effective premedication, although in one study, 23% of patients desaturated to <90% after 2 μg/kg of IN sufentanil and 45% developed chest wall rigidity after 4.5 μg/kg.[252] Succinylcholine may be required to resolve chest wall rigidity after IN sufentanil. IN dexmedetomidine (0.5 to 1 μg/kg) also provides anxiolysis and sedation,[253] although it may require up to 1 hour to affect sedation and the sedation may extend into the recovery period.

For older children and adolescents who are cognitively challenged, uncooperative, and/or behaviorally problematic despite their parents' presence, IM ketamine 2 to 5 mg/kg (concentration 100 mg/mL) administered via a small gauge, long needle (large enough to not break off if the encounter became combative) into either the deltoid muscle of an arm may be the only means to ensure safe delivery of the child to the OR.[254] These children should be seated on a gurney before administering the ketamine, as they quickly lose consciousness and motor tone, becoming difficult to lift or move onto a gurney. By this route, ketamine has an onset of action of 3 to 5 minutes and a duration of 30 to 40 minutes.

Induction Techniques

Inhalational Induction

In North America, the most common technique for inducing anesthesia in children undergoing elective surgery is an inhalational induction. Infants and children of all ages, including those who are crying and upset, can be successfully anesthetized using this approach. Distracting upset and crying children using a warm, reassuring, and calm manner often permits a successful induction of anesthesia by face mask. The notion that distraught children should be treated with "brutane" by holding children down and forcing a mask on their face with 8% sevoflurane flowing has no place in pediatric anesthesia and may psychologically scar the child for life. If the child had a poor previous experience with anesthesia, it is important to understand the nature of the past experience and design an anesthetic to minimize their anxiety.

In preschool-age children, distraction techniques and premedication are key strategies to minimize the anxiety associated with separating from their parents and undergoing induction of anesthesia. The author offers children (>3 years of age) a choice of several flavored lip balms to mark inside the mask. For younger children (<3 years of age), the author flavors the face mask for them. The smell obscures the plastic smell of the mask but more importantly it distracts the child and offers a topic for discussion. Troposmia, which means a distorted perception of an odor, is an interesting strategy in which the child is told that the flavor that was applied to the mask will transform into his/her favorite flavor as anesthesia is induced. Using this approach, 80% of children interviewed postoperatively confirmed that they smelled their favorite flavor as they were anesthetized.[255] Other distraction techniques include music, story and joke telling, magic, video and hand-held games, and clowns (see above).

With the child seated on the operating table with his/her back to the anesthesiologist's chest (or on your lap if a diaper is worn) and at least a pulse oximeter (with more monitors as tolerated), a flavored face mask is applied over the mouth and nose with 5 to 7 L/min of a mixture of 70% nitrous oxide and 30% oxygen. The adjustable pressure-limiting valve should be completely open to avoid resistance to exhalation. During this time, the child should be distracted by singing a song or telling a joke or story until the end-tidal N_2O concentration exceeds 60% or the child ceases to respond to verbal stimulation. At this point, 8% sevoflurane is delivered in one stepwise increase in concentration. If the sevoflurane concentration is increased in smaller steps or slowly, then a protracted period of excitement commonly ensues. If sevoflurane is introduced at the same time as the nitrous oxide, unpremedicated children will reject the mask because of the strong odor of sevoflurane, potentially resulting in an aversion to or fear of face masks, which almost certainly will present difficulties for future anesthetics.

As the child loses consciousness, he/she is placed in the supine position. If apneic occurs during this period (as is often the case after premedication), ventilation should be assisted manually and gently. To reduce the risk of awareness, this author recommends maintaining 8% sevoflurane and 70% nitrous oxide until intravenous access has been established. At that time, 1 to 2 mg/kg intravenous propofol is administered, the nitrous oxide may be discontinued, and an LMA or tracheal tube is inserted.[86] Bilateral air entry in the chest, the presence of a capnogram, and no air entry in the epigastrium confirm proper tracheal tube placement. After inflation of the cuff of the LMA, absence of excessive air leak at 20 cm H_2O confirms proper LMA placement. Once the airway is secured, the inspired concentration of sevoflurane may be reduced to 2% to 3% inspired and nitrous oxide may be reintroduced.

The child with mask phobia poses a real challenge for those attempting to induce anesthesia by mask.[256] Besides refusing a mask, these frightened children often steadfastly refuse needles (and therefore an intravenous induction), leaving few options for induction of anesthesia. There are many reasons why children may be fearful of face masks, including the unappealing odor of 8% sevoflurane administered to an unpremedicated child previously, a partially closed APL valve that prevented the child from exhaling, and claustrophobia. Irrespective of the reason for the mask phobia, if the mask is the focal point of the fear, it should be eliminated. In these cases, anesthesia may be induced without a face mask by inserting the elbow of the breathing circuit between two fingers and interlacing the fingers of his/her two hands (with flavor applied to the gloves) (Fig. 42-4A and B). With the hands cupped under the child's chin and 70% nitrous oxide in oxygen flowing, the hands slowly close in over the child's mouth. Since nitrous oxide is heavier than air, the cupped hands act as a reservoir for the nitrous oxide. Suction tubing may be held in close proximity to minimize spread of anesthetic to those nearby. Although this technique causes OR pollution, this author believes it is the optimal approach for managing children with mask and IV phobias. Once the hands are tight over the mouth, 8% sevoflurane may be introduced. As soon as the child stops responding, the elbow of the circuit is inserted into the mask and the mask is applied to the face.

If the child is not mask-phobic, the anesthesiologist may deliver sevoflurane from the outset of the anesthetic without the child smelling the sevoflurane by rotating the face mask 90 degrees so the balloon on the mask occludes the nares. This eliminates/decreases the smell of sevoflurane and allows anesthesia to be induced smoothly.

For older children (usually >6 years of age) who understand how to breath-hold, another induction technique is a single-breath induction of anesthesia.[257] This technique induces anesthesia within 20 seconds of the breath-hold. However, to be successful, the breathing circuit must be primed with 8%

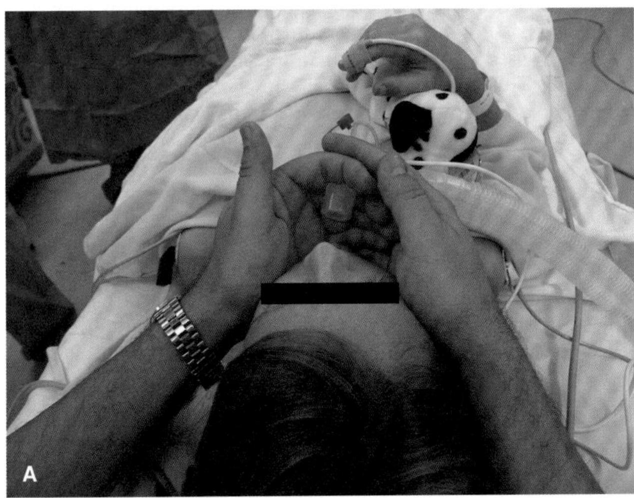

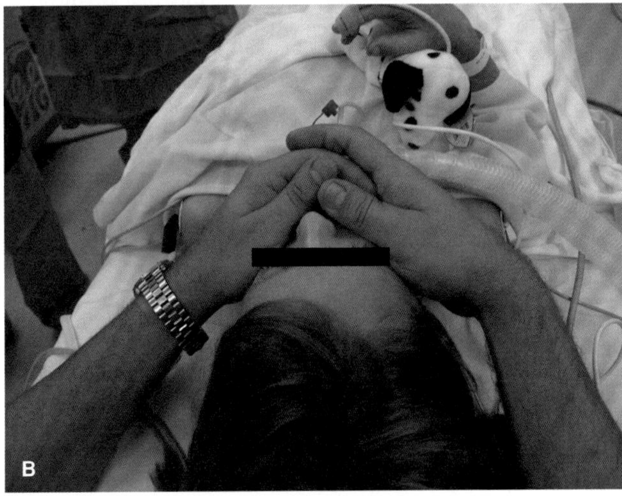

FIGURE 42-4. For the child who fears the face mask, the mask is removed and the elbow of the breathing circuit is inserted between interlaced fingers in the hand. **(A)** At this time, the fresh gas comprises 70% nitrous oxide in oxygen. The hands are gradually brought closer to the child's mouth from below the chin (nitrous oxide is heavier than air), until they completely cover the mouth. **(B)** At that point, either sevoflurane may be added to the fresh gas or a face mask applied to the face or both.

sevoflurane (with or without 70% nitrous oxide) that is verified by an agent analyzer. This is achieved by flushing the circle circuit and a 2 to 3 L reservoir bag three to four times with 8% sevoflurane in 70% nitrous oxide, exhausting the contents of the circuit through the scavenging system. A large reservoir bag is preferred in the event the child takes additional breaths. In advance of the induction, the child practices vital capacity breathing, that is, inhaling maximally through the mouth and exhaling to residual volume through the mouth (by instructing the child to exhale until there is no air left in their lungs). The child may be supine or sitting for this induction, but if the child is sitting, an assistant should be prepared to support the child's torso when he/she loses consciousness. Once the child has mastered the breathing maneuver, the child exhales to residual volume, at which point the face mask and the primed breathing circuit is applied and held tightly to the face. The child is instructed to take a single vital capacity breath through the mouth and hold it for as long as he/she can. While the child is holding his/her breath, the anesthesiologist counts aloud slowly to distract the child. In general, the child loses consciousness before the count reaches 15 seconds. As discussed above, a gradual introduction of the inhaled anesthetics may proceed smoothly in cooperative patients and one variation on that approach is demonstrated in the video.

Intravenous Induction

For children without intravenous access, there are several approaches to establishing access. First, a topical local anesthetic cream can be applied to the skin to prevent the pain of the needle puncture. Topical local anesthetic creams that are available include the eutectic mixture of local anesthetics (EMLA) cream (AstraZeneca, Wilmington, DE), which requires a 45- to 60-minute application time to produce topical anesthesia and may cause skin blanching and venoconstriction; Ametop (4% tetracaine) (Smith and New, Canada); ELA-Max (liposomal 4% lidocaine); and Synera (Zars Pharma Inc., Salt Lake City, UT). Ametop, ELA-Max, and Synera require a 30-minute application time and do not cause skin blanching or venoconstriction. A meta-analysis of EMLA and amethocaine found the latter to be more effective than the former in children.[258] The J-tip injector of powder lidocaine anesthetizes the skin, although it itself causes moderate pain in 20% of children. Investigation of the factors that predispose to painful response to IV placement include young age, more numerous previous painful procedures, greater state and trait anxiety, more active, and the presence of polymorphisms to endothelin receptor A (EDNRA rs5333) compared with those with less pain.[259] Second, 50% to 70% nitrous oxide may be administered for 1 to 2 minutes by a tight mask fit to permit IV insertion, yielding better results than with EMLA.[260] Third, IN sufentanil may be used for IV placement. These approaches may be particularly useful for children with MH and myopathies in whom a potent inhalational anesthetic must be avoided.

Once intravenous access has been established, intravenous anesthesia can be induced. Currently, propofol, ketamine, and etomidate are used for induction of anesthesia in North America; sodium thiopental is only available outside North America.

Propofol is the most widely available induction agent. It is available as Diprivan in a 1% solution that includes Intralipid (long-chain triglycerides derived from soybean oil), EDTA (ethylenediaminetetraacetic acid, a bacteriostatic agent), egg lecithin (a phospholipid membrane stabilizer), and propofol (2,6-diisopropylphenol). Since propofol is a phenol derivative, it causes pain when injected into the small peripheral veins of children. Several strategies have been used to attenuate or prevent pain, but only two techniques reliably prevent pain associated with IV propofol in small veins: 70% nitrous oxide in oxygen by inhalation or a modified Bier block using 0.5 to 1 mg/kg of 1% lidocaine injected into a vein while the arm is occluded for 45 to 60 seconds.[93,94] Propofol is a very safe induction agent for children. A bolus injection of propofol causes transient hypopnea or apnea with a minor decrease in heart rate and blood pressure.

Ketamine is also used for induction of anesthesia, although it is a second-tier induction agent because of concerns for postoperative nightmares. It is often used in the presence of circulatory instability (shock) or cyanotic heart disease.

Etomidate is only approved for children >10 years of age in the United States. A recent population pharmacokinetic study of etomidate in children concluded that the dose of etomidate should increase as age decreases because both clearance and volume of distribution increase with decreasing age.[113] However, dosing recommendations have not been forthcoming. In adults, 0.2 to 0.3 mg/kg IV etomidate is effective for induction of anesthesia. Like ketamine, it maintains blood pressure even in the presence of circulatory instability. It decreases cerebral blood flow by 20% to 30%. Minor side effects include pain on injection and myoclonic jerking. However, a far more serious side effect is suppression of adrenal function for up to 24 hours after both a single dose and a brief infusion of etomidate. Preclinical studies with a modified molecule of etomidate suggest that the anesthetic properties of etomidate may be preserved without adrenal suppression.[115] Studies in humans are pending.

Sodium thiopental has been used for almost half a century as the intravenous induction agent of choice, but in the past two decades, it was gradually supplanted by propofol as the induction agent of choice and more recently supply was cutoff to the United States out of ethical concerns regarding its use for lethal injection. Thiopental remains available in Europe and Asia. Dosing for induction of anesthesia is 3 to 5 mg/kg intravenously. It causes no serious side effects when administered as an intravenous bolus. However, because it is only metabolized at 10%/hour, emergence is delayed if it is administered as a continuous infusion.

Intramuscular Induction

The intramuscular route is infrequently used for induction of anesthesia in children because it is painful, induction is slow, and there is a risk of sterile abscess formation. The only anesthetic currently used for intramuscular injections in children is ketamine.[254] This approach is usually reserved for adolescent children who are cognitively impaired, extremely uncooperative, and large in size. For further details, see intramuscular premedication above.

Rarely do children who require emergent securing of their airways present without intravenous access. When it does occur, one of several approaches may be undertaken. Intravenous access may be established before induction of anesthesia, after anesthesia is induced with an inhalational agent, or after intramuscular injection of ketamine (3 to 5 mg/kg), atropine (0.02 mg/kg), and succinylcholine (4 mg/kg).

Rectal Induction

Rectal induction of anesthesia has been popular in young children (<5 years of age) in the past, particularly for those who were unwilling to take oral premedication or who were very frightened. Several regimens have been used for rectal induction: Methohexital 15 to 25 mg/kg, midazolam 1 mg/kg, ketamine 5 mg/kg, or thiopental 30 to 40 mg/kg.[261] A number of problems were identified with rectal anesthesia inductions, including poor bioavailability of the induction agent (due to unpredictable rectal venous absorption or evacuation of the drug from the rectum), laryngospasm (with methohexital), and delayed recovery from anesthesia. In immune-compromised patients, rectal administration of drugs may lead to sepsis. Today, rectal inductions are rarely employed. Most anesthetists prefer to involve the parents in managing the child's behavior at induction of anesthesia rather than administer a rectal medication.

PROBLEMS DURING INDUCTION OF ANESTHESIA

Oxygen Desaturation

Pulse oximetry may be the only monitor that remains functional during induction of anesthesia in the restless young child. All current oximeters include motion-artifact compensating software that provides fairly accurate measurements even when the child is moving. As the child becomes anesthetized, respiration is reduced resulting in hypoventilation. Despite the use of oxygen-enriched inspired gases, many children, particularly those with a history of a mild URI or who become deeply anesthetized, hypoventilate, or become apneic. This immediately leads to oxygen desaturation, which may be exacerbated if nitrous oxide was coadministered. The primary diagnosis at this time is segmental atelectasis and intrapulmonary shunting, providing upper airway obstruction (often referred to as mild laryngospasm) has been ruled out. To restore the SaO_2 10 to 20 cm H_2O of positive end-expiratory pressure should be applied using the adjustable pressure limit valve. The peak pressure that is delivered should be carefully adjusted to avoid inflation of the stomach. If, however, the lungs are not being ventilated, then laryngospasm should be suspected quickly and the management followed as described below.

Laryngospasm

Laryngospasm is an infrequent, but potentially life-threatening complication that occurs in children during induction and emergence from anesthesia. The frequency ranges from 0.4% to 10% among studies.[262,263] Several factors are known to increase the risk of laryngospasm in children (Table 42-11).[263]

Laryngospasm is defined as the reflex closure of the false and true vocal cords, although the precise pathogenesis of this reflex remains debatable. Complete laryngospasm is defined as the closure of the false vocal cords and apposition of the laryngeal surface of the epiglottis and interarytenoids. The net effect is complete cessation of air movement and noisy respiration, absence of movement of the reservoir bag, and an absent capnogram. In contrast, incomplete (or partial) laryngospasm is defined as incomplete apposition of the vocal cords with a residual small gap between the cords posteriorly that permits a persistent inspiratory stridor, limited movement of the reservoir bag, and progressively increasing respiratory effort. Some assert that incomplete laryngospasm is not laryngospasm at all, but for treatment purposes this is a moot point.

The clinical findings in laryngospasm begin with faint inspiratory stridor, suprasternal and supraclavicular in-drawing due to increased inspiratory effort, increased diaphragmatic excursions, and flailing of the lower ribs. As greater inspiratory effort is expended, the intensity and volume of the stridor increases, and the chest wall movement resembles that of a "rocking horse." As laryngospasm progresses, air movement through the almost closed glottis ceases and the inspiratory effort becomes completely silent. This is an ominous sign. If the progression of the laryngospasm is not interrupted, oxygen desaturation will quickly ensue. This may be followed by a decrease in heart rate. This downward spiral must be interrupted as described below.

TABLE 42-11. FACTORS ASSOCIATED WITH LARYNGOSPASM[263]

Age: greater in infants than older children and adults; the risk decreases with increasing age
Recent URTI (<2 wks)
History of reactive airway disease
Exposure to second-hand smoke
Airway anomalies
Airway surgery
Airway devices (tracheal tubes, LMA)
Stimulating the glottis during a light plane of anesthesia
Secretions in the oropharynx (e.g., blood, excess saliva, gastric juice)
Inhaled anesthesia (desflurane and isoflurane)
Inexperienced anesthesiologist

URTI, upper respiratory tract infection; LMA, laryngeal mask airway.

Management of laryngospasm requires a multifaceted and immediate response (Fig. 42-5).[262] As soon as the diagnosis is suspected, a tight-fitting face mask should be applied to the child's face and 100% oxygen delivered with continuous positive airway pressure (15 to 20 cm H_2O dialed into the adjustable pressure limiting valve). Pressures in excess of 20 cm H_2O may cause gastric inflation. Note that the reservoir bag should not be squeezed except during the child's inspiratory efforts, lest gas be driven into the stomach. If the triggering event is blood, secretions, or foreign material in the airway, these should be removed immediately. As soon as the offending agent has been expunged, the "jaw thrust" maneuver should be applied. This maneuver requires familiarity with the anatomy of the retromandibular notch, an area subtended by the condylar process of the ascending ramus of the mandible anteriorly, the mastoid process posteriorly, and the external auditory canal superiorly.[97] Bilateral digital pressure is applied to the most cephalad point on the posterior edge of the condylar process of the ascending ramus of the mandible, and the force directed toward the frontal hairline. The force should be applied for 3 to 5 seconds at a time and then released for 5 to 10 seconds, while maintaining a tight seal with the face mask against the child's face. By applying and releasing pressure on the condylar processes, the repeated painful stimuli may cause sufficient pain to induce the child to cry, which opens the vocal cords terminating the laryngospasm. In addition to causing pain, the "jaw thrust" maneuver serves to relieve upper airway obstruction in the anesthetized child by both translocating the ramus of the mandible anteriorly and rotating the temporomandibular joint so the mouth opens. Together, these maneuvers lift the tongue off the posterior pharyngeal wall establishing a patent upper airway.

The "jaw thrust" maneuver is not as effective when applied at the angle of the mandible as this region contains many fewer pain fibers and does not rotate the temporomandibular joint. Hence,

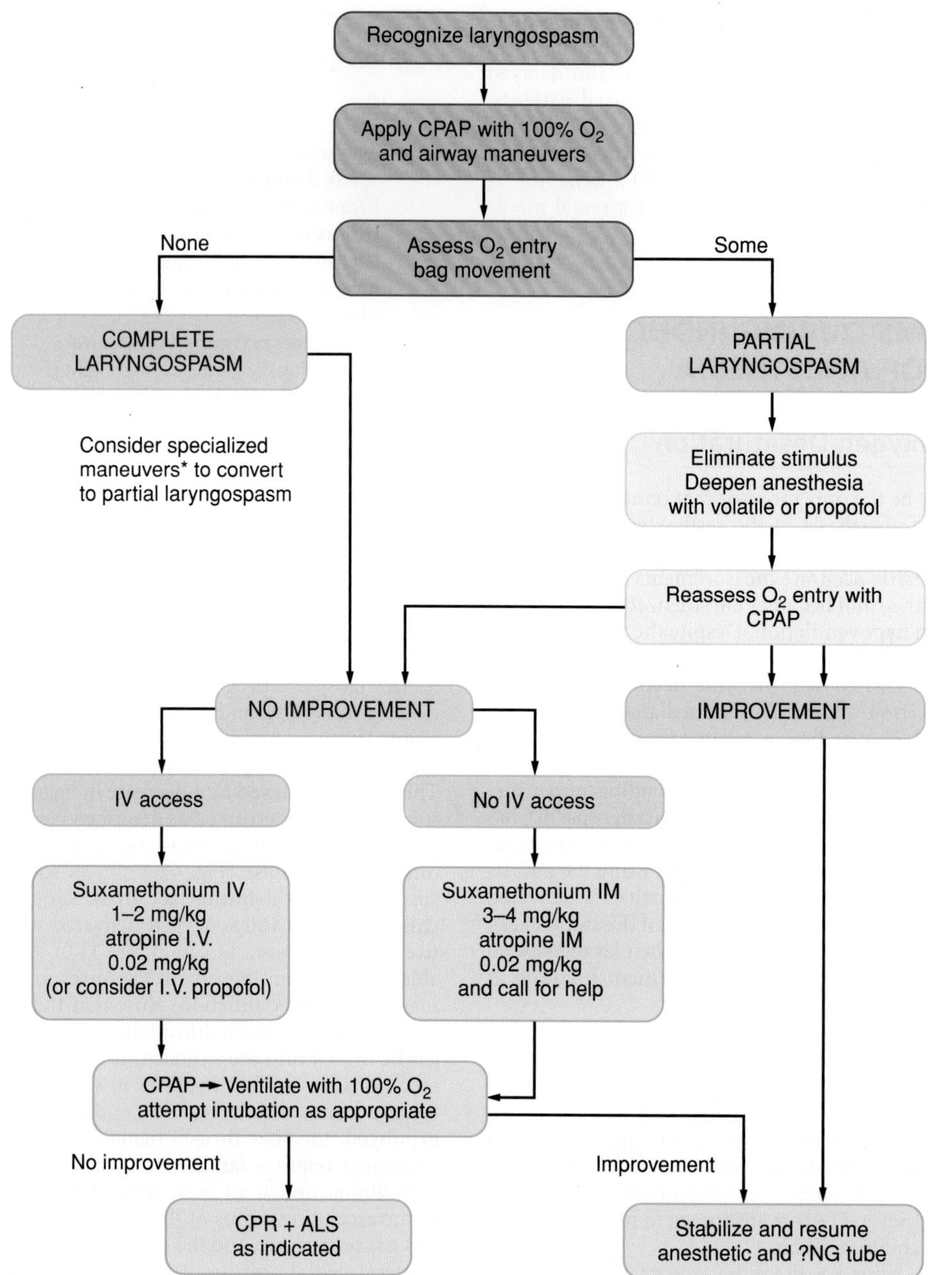

FIGURE 42-5. Algorithm to diagnose and manage laryngospasm in children. From: Hampson-Evans D, Morgan P, Farrar M. Pediatric laryngospasm. *Paediatr Anaesth.* 2008;18:303–307, with permission. *apply the jaw thrust maneuver as described on page 1243

the ability of the maneuver to establish a clear upper airway is not nearly as effective. Remember, laryngospasm cannot develop or persist if the vocal cords are moving and the child is vocalizing or crying. If positive pressure ventilation, 100% oxygen, and jaw thrust maneuver fail to break the laryngospasm, further intervention should be undertaken before desaturation and bradycardia develop. Appropriate treatment would include in the following order: IV or IM atropine (0.02 mg/kg), IV propofol (1 mg/kg), and IV or IM succinylcholine (1 to 2 mg/kg IV or 4 to 5 mg/kg IM).[264]

Some suggest that gentle chest compressions effectively break laryngospasm in children. To add chest compressions to the management of laryngospasm requires a pair of free hands. If no free hands are available, do not abandon the maneuvers described above to perform chest compressions unless there is a cardiac arrest. The risk associated with this maneuver includes sternal or rib fractures, which must be explained to the parents if they occur. Currently, the author believes there is excellent alternative treatment for laryngospasm and insufficient evidence to recommend chest compressions to relieve laryngospasm in children.

TABLE 42-12. CAUSES OF BRADYCARDIA IN INFANTS AND CHILDREN

1. Hypoxia (e.g., laryngospasm, obstructed airway, atelectasis)
2. Vagal reflex response (e.g., laryngoscopy, prolonged stretch on the extraocular muscles)
3. Increased intracranial pressure
4. Medications (e.g., clonidine, β-blockers, α-adrenergic eye drops, succinylcholine without pretreatment with atropine, sevoflurane [more common with Down syndrome], propofol infusion syndrome)
5. Electrolyte disturbance (e.g., hyperkalemia, hypocalcemia)
6. Congenital heart disease, congenital or acquired rhythm disturbance
7. Hypothermia
8. Air embolism
9. Tension pneumothorax

Bradycardia

Bradycardia is a slowing of the heart rate below age-defined limits. For infants (<1 year of age) this is 100 beats/minute (bpm); for young children 1 to 5 years of age, 80 bpm; and for children >5 years of age, 60 bpm. Since cardiac output of infants and children is heart rate dependent, a slow heart rate means a reduced cardiac output. If the heart rate decreases below these limits, corrective action should be taken to restore the heart rate, and if necessary cardiopulmonary resuscitation should be initiated. 9

Although hypoxia is the foremost cause of bradycardia in children, drug-associated causes include halothane and succinylcholine. Since sevoflurane has replaced halothane in developed countries, this cause of bradycardia has all but disappeared.[47] This is not the case in many developing countries. A single dose of succinylcholine remains a cause of bradycardia in children but is a much less common cause today because succinylcholine is not routinely used in children for tracheal intubation. The incidence of bradycardia during the first 6 minutes of sevoflurane anesthesia in children with Down syndrome is fivefold greater than that in matched controls.[265] Children who are rate dependent for cardiac output and develop bradycardia may require treatment with atropine or isoproterenol.

The causes of bradycardia in healthy children are listed in Table 42-12. To stop progressive slowing of the heart rate, the underlying cause of bradycardia should be corrected (e.g., correct hypoxia when present and administer atropine 0.02 mg/kg). Atropine is only effective when myocardial electrical activity is present and the bradycardia is of vagal origin. If asystole occurs; however, atropine cannot restore the heart rhythm, and the only definitive treatment is IV epinephrine (10 μg/kg). Secondary treatment may include isoproterenol.

MAINTENANCE OF ANESTHESIA

Techniques

Inhalational anesthetics, supplemented with intravenous analgesics and antiemetics, have been the mainstay of anesthesia although, of late, TIVA has emerged as a reasonable alternative. One key advantage that distinguishes inhalational anesthetics from intravenous anesthesia is the ability to continuously measure the end-tidal (alveolar) anesthetic concentrations of inhaled agents. This measurement provides invaluable information regarding the accuracy of our delivery system and the anesthetic partial pressures in the VRG of tissues. Currently, isoflurane, sevoflurane, and desflurane are used to maintain anesthesia in children.

TIVA has become the primary anesthetic technique for children with MH, for those undergoing spine surgery who also require motor-evoked potential monitoring, for those with a history of severe perioperative nausea and vomiting, and in some institutions, the standard anesthetic for most surgeries. Propofol and ketamine are the primary general anesthetics used with TIVA, although, unlike propofol, ketamine is emetogenic and associated with prolonged emergence when infused for prolonged periods. Propofol has been proscribed as a continuous sedative for children in ICU because of the risk of PRIS but not in anesthesia. Dosing for bolus and infusions of propofol is described above.

Supplemental analgesics are also used during both inhalational and intravenous anesthesia to prevent physiologic responses and movement to pain. Remifentanil (with a 5 minute context-sensitive half-life) 0.05 to 0.1 μg/kg/min can be administered as an infusion, whereas other opioids (fentanyl and morphine) are more often administered by intravenous boluses. Fentanyl (1 to 2 μg/kg) or morphine (0.05 to 0.1 mg/kg) can be administered intravenously; the dose is adjusted up or down depending on the child's exposure to opioids, the severity of the pain, and concomitantly administered analgesics.

Fluid Management

General Principles

Intravenous fluid administration sets should be prepared before the child arrives in the operating room. For young children, a 500-mL bag of LR solution with a graduated buretrol is appropriate; for infants (<1 year) a 250-mL bag with a buretrol is preferable. *These recommendations for the use of a buretrol and IV fluid bag are intended to limit the risk of adverse events should the entire bag inadvertently be infused in the child.* All pediatric IV sets should include a manual controller, a one-way valve (to prevent medications from passing retrograde up the IV tubing), and needleless ports and/or three-way stopcocks for medication administration. For children >8 years of age, the IV infusion set may be prepared with a macro or micro-drip without a buretrol and a 1,000-mL bag of balanced salt solution.

Intralipid infusions from total parenteral nutrition should be discontinued before transfer to the OR to reduce the risk of contaminating the Intralipid and central venous access line by repeated line accessing.

Most IV fluids administered to healthy children during elective surgery consist of a nonglucose-containing isotonic salt solution, commonly LR solution in North America. These solutions replaced glucose-containing hypotonic solutions that were associated with perioperative seizures, aspiration, and brain damage after large volumes were administered during surgery. LR solution is slightly hypotonic (280 mOm/L) and contains small concentrations of potassium and lactate. Normal saline (0.9% NaCl) is isotonic (308 mOsm/L), acidic (pH 5), and contains no ionic moieties. Normal saline is not routinely used as the primary maintenance solution since large volumes may lead to a hyperchloremic metabolic acidosis (nonanion gap type). We advocate glucose-containing solutions, such as 1% or 2.5% glucose in LR solution, as a maintenance solution in infants <6 months of age and for young children who are cachectic, chronically malnourished, tolerate fasting poorly (maple sugar disease), and suffer from debilitating disease who may be at risk for hypoglycemia.[266] These solutions should not lead to intraoperative hyperglycemia or hyponatremia. Although the shift to isotonic salt solutions dramatically decreased the incidence of perioperative hyponatremia, some specific surgeries (e.g., craniofacial surgery) may warrant perioperative monitoring of serum electrolytes.[267]

Children with specific medical conditions should have tailored intravenous solutions. For children with renal failure or renal insufficiency, normal saline has been the preferred balanced salt solution because it contains no potassium although evidence suggests it may lead to greater serum potassium concentrations than LR.[267a] Children with a mitochondrial myopathy who had lactic acidosis in infancy should be fasted for only brief periods (to avoid acidosis and hypoglycemia) and should receive only normal saline with glucose supplementation as needed.

Infants and children <2 years of age who may be hypovolemic should be assessed preoperatively to determine the magnitude of their fluid deficit: Mild, moderate, or severe. The signs of mild dehydration (5% body weight loss: Approximately 50 mL/kg deficit) include poor skin turgor and dry mouth. The signs of moderate fluid dehydration (10% of body weight loss: 100 mL/kg deficit) include sunken fontanel (if present), tachycardia, and oliguria in addition to the signs of mild dehydration. The signs of severe fluid dehydration (15% of body weight loss: 150 mL/kg deficit) include sunken eyeballs, hypotension, and anuria plus the signs of moderate dehydration.

Correction of hypovolemia requires staged infusion of isoosmolar fluid administration. Approximately 50% of the deficit should be replaced in the first hour, 25% in the second, and 25% in the third. A balanced salt solution should be used to restore euvolemia.

Elective Surgery

For elective surgery, the traditional calculation for the hourly fluid infusion rate has been based on replacing the triad of fluid deficit during fasting, on-going maintenance, and blood and third-space losses. In children, the maintenance solution calculation was predicated on the 4–2–1 mL/kg/hr rule where 4 mL/kg is for the first 10 kg, 2 mL/kg is for the second 10 kg, and 1 mL/kg is for the third 10 kg and any additional body weight thereafter.[268] In a reappraisal of their 1957 recommendation, Holliday and Segar[269] sought to address the risks associated with both administering hyponatremic solutions to children who were hypovolemic and applying their original fluid infusion rates to isotonic solutions. They reasoned that all children whether they were fasted for elective surgery, presenting with sepsis or an acute inflammatory response, or receiving specific medications such as opioids, have upregulated antidiuretic hormone that must be turned off to prevent water intoxication. To that end, they recommended establishing euvolemia as quickly as possible by infusing 10 to 40 mL/kg isotonic solution (with adjustment for those with cardiac and renal diseases) during the perioperative period. For children who require IV fluids beyond 6 hours postoperatively, a maintenance solution of isotonic fluid should be continued at half its original rate or 2–1–0.5 mL/kg/h.[269]

Blood Transfusion Therapy

Initial blood loss may be replaced with balanced salt solution at a rate of 3 mL of solution for every 1 mL of blood loss. For third-space losses, the replacement volume is based on the severity of the losses: 1 to 2 mL/kg/hr for minor surgery, 2 to 5 mL/kg/hr for moderate surgery, and 6 to 10 mL/kg/hr for major surgery and large third-space losses.

Although most pediatric surgeons are careful to minimize bleeding during surgery, it is important to remain vigilant regarding all blood loss during surgery. For procedures that are likely to result in significant tissue trauma or blood loss, appropriate size IV access must be provided for transfusion of the blood and blood products needed for volume replacement. Packed red cells cannot be rapidly infused through either 24-gauge intravenous catheters or most peripherally inserted central catheters. A 22-gauge catheter is the smallest intravenous cannula through which blood can be infused rapidly. Every effort should be expended to insert the largest intravenous catheter that the child's veins will accommodate. This replacement, together with the maintenance requirement, should be logged on the anesthetic record. As the combined volume of balanced salt solution approaches 75 to 100 mL/kg, it is important to consider the possibility of dilutional thrombocytopenia and dilution of coagulation factors; coagulation indices should be measured at this time.

The threshold for initiating packed RBC transfusions in children has undergone a renaissance in the past decade as evidence that the outcome and complications associated with a transfusion threshold of 7 g% hemoglobin is similar to that of 9 g%.[270]

The estimated blood volume in children decreases with increasing age from 95 to 100 mL/kg in premature infants to 70 mL/kg in adults.[271] Note that the estimated blood volume of obese children is reduced 10% from that of nonobese children of similar age.[271] To estimate the allowable blood loss during surgery, the following equation is used[271]:

$$\text{Maximum allowable blood loss} = \frac{(\text{starting Hct} - \text{target Hct})}{(\text{starting Hct})} \qquad (3)$$

Some modify Eq. 3 and replace the "starting Hct" in the denominator with the "average Hct." This increases the allowable blood loss before transfusion. Irrespective of which equation is used, the actual Hct should be determined before initiating blood transfusion to ensure that the Hct has actually decreased to the desired level. When initiating a blood transfusion in a child, two formulae provide rough estimates of the amount of blood required to increase the hemoglobin concentration by 1 g%: 4 mL/kg packed cells and 6 mL/kg whole blood.

10 Prophylaxis for Postoperative Vomiting

The incidence of POV in children depends on a number of factors that relate to the child (motion sickness history, age), the anesthetic (inhalational anesthetics, nitrous oxide [in specific instances], opioids), perioperative oral fluid ingestion, and the type of surgery (inguinal/orchidopexy, tonsillectomy and adenoidectomy, strabismus, and middle ear surgery). The risk of POV increases with the number of risk factors present: Age ≥3 years, duration of surgery ≥30 minutes, strabismus surgery, and a history of POV in the proband or immediate family.[272]

To reduce PONV after elective surgery, children should be fasted for brief periods and not forced to drink oral fluids postoperatively until they request them (to reduce the risk of vomiting).[273] Intraoperatively, IV fluids should be aggressively administered 20 to 30 mL/kg to reduce PONV.[274] Pain is another factor in the genesis of PONV. It can be mitigated with regional anesthesia and NSAIDs or ketamine instead of opioids. If the child is scheduled for emetogenic surgery and has a history of POV, the optimal anesthetic regimen is propofol oxygen/air and two antiemetics, although conflicting evidence exists regarding the role of substituting propofol and nitrous oxide in PONV.[275]

The optimal prophylactic antiemetic strategy to administer to children during anesthesia is dexamethasone and a 5-HT_3 receptor antagonist, such as ondansetron.[276] There is no dose–response relationship for dexamethasone: Doses between 0.0625 and 1 mg/kg are equally effective, although this author limits the maximum dose to 10 mg.[277] The dose of ondansetron for prophylaxis in children is 0.05 to 0.15 mg/kg. Although one report suggested that dexamethasone is associated with an increased incidence of postoperative tonsil bleeding,[278] those results are not consistent with the author's experience and the subsequent literature.[279,280] A single dose of glucocorticoids has been associated with several reports of tumor lysis syndrome in patients with undiagnosed acute lymphoblastic lymphoma, a very rare but potentially fatal outcome if unrecognized.[220] A single dose of dexamethasone has also been associated with a transient increase in serum glucose concentration that peaked at 2 hours postoperatively, in obese adults with poorly controlled type 2 diabetes. Data in children have not been forthcoming.

Regional Anesthesia and Pain Management

There are numerous regional blocks that may be performed to reduce nociception during and after surgery. Three common neuroaxial blocks performed in children today are caudal, epidural, and spinal blocks and these are described below. There has been a shift from neuroaxial to peripheral nerve blocks, both single-dose and continuous local anesthetic administration for perioperative pain management facilitated by the introduction of ultrasound guidance. Morbidity and mortality associated with regional anesthesia in children is exceedingly small and is not considered a substantive argument against its routine use in skilled hands.

Caudal Blockade

This block is useful for both lower abdominal and lower extremity surgeries in infants and children (<5–6 years) who are undergoing ambulatory surgery. It is usually performed under general anesthesia although in neonates, awake caudal and spinal blocks have been performed using local anesthetic infiltration and/or sedation. Single-shot caudal blocks with local anesthetic alone are commonly performed in ambulatory surgery. These blocks may last 4 to 6 hours, but if adjuvant medications are added, they may last even longer.

After induction of anesthesia and once that airway is secured, the child is turned onto the lateral decubitus (the side is determined by the anesthesiologist; left-handed anesthesiologists generally prefer the right lateral decubitus position for the child), and the key anatomical sites on the sacrum are palpated: Posterior superior iliac spines and the sacral hiatus subtended by the two sacral cornua (see also Chapter 41, section "Caudal Block"). The sacrococcygeal ligament traverses the space between the two cornua and the coccyx. The skin is then prepared with antiseptic solution and allowed to dry while local anesthetic is prepared. Once the drug has been prepared, the skin site is cut with a blunt needle (to prevent the transfer of epidermis to the caudal space) and the IV catheter (22 gauge for those ≤2 years or 20 gauge for >2 years) is passed through the subcutaneous tissue and between or just caudal to the level of the two cornua at a 45-degree angle to the skin. Once the sacrococcygeal ligament has been pierced, the cannula is laid almost flat against the skin (forming a 10-degree angle of the skin) and advanced 2 to 3 mm through the ligament. At that point, the catheter is slipped off the needle and advanced 2 to 3 mm. If any resistance is felt as the catheter is inserted, it is not within the caudal space and the entire cannula should be removed and the process repeated. If you are not certain the catheter is in the caudal canal, hold your thumb over the sacral hiatus and inject no more than 0.5 mL. If a bulge is felt desist; further injection will distort the surface anatomy and preclude a successful caudal block. If the catheter is properly positioned, then remove the needle and examine for blood or cerebrospinal fluid leaking out the catheter. Do not apply negative pressure to the catheter as veins collapse easily. Connect the syringe with local anesthetic and inject slowly 2 to 3 mL every 2 minutes, while observing the electrocardiogram. Peak T waves and an increased ST segment are sensitive indicators of an inadvertent intravascular injection during inhalational anesthesia, although blood pressure increases are more sensitive during TIVA.[281] Once the injection is complete, remove the catheter, clean the caudal skin area, and position the child for surgery.

This author prefers to administer 1 mL/kg bupivacaine 0.175% with epinephrine (1:250,000) for all surgical procedures as a single-shot caudal block. This concentration may be prepared by combining 7 mL of 0.25% bupivacaine with 3 mL of saline to give a total volume of 10 mL. This concentration permits excellent analgesic with motor blockade that resolves within 1 hour of placement. Others use ropivacaine 1 mL/kg of 0.2% or levobupivacaine 1 mL/kg of 0.15%, although a comparative study of 0.2% ropivacaine, levobupivacaine, or bupivacaine concluded that the latter two local anesthetics were more effective than the first. Adjunctive medications have been used to prolong the duration of the caudal block for several hours at best.[111,282]

If a continuous caudal block is planned for the child remaining in hospital for a period, then an 18G IV catheter should be inserted to accept a 21G epidural catheter. The catheter is inserted exactly as described above for caudal blocks and the catheter threaded to the spinal level necessary for perioperative analgesia. The catheter should be taped away from the anus or, alternately, tunneled under the skin to the side opposite the surgery. This reduces the risk of superficial infections at the catheter insertion site. Catheters that are smaller than 21 gauge may not thread to the desired dermatome level. Alternative strategies that may be used to achieve the desired level of block include the Tsui approach[283] and inserting the catheter at an intervertebral space closer to the level of surgery.

Continuous infusions of local anesthetics may be infused epidurally for up to 3 days. A recommended dosing for continuous infusions of bupivacaine to minimize the risk of toxic blood concentrations for neonates is 0.2 mg/kg/hr bupivacaine. It can be administered as 0.2 mL/kg/hr of a 0.1% solution.[284] In infants and young children, 0.2 to 0.4 mg/kg/hr should be administered using 0.3 mL/kg/hr of a 0.1% solution. In older children, 0.4 to 0.5 mg/kg/hr should be administered using 0.3 mL/kg/hr of a 0.1% or 0.125% solution. To reduce absorption of local anesthetic, epinephrine is routinely added to the local anesthetic. Fentanyl (1 to 2 μg/mL) is often added to the caudal/epidural solution, although there is little evidence that this improves the quality of the block provided the tip of the catheter is properly positioned, 0.2 to 0.3 mL/kg/hr volume of local anesthetic is administered, and at least 0.1% bupivacaine or its equivalent concentration of local anesthetic is used.[148] The addition of fentanyl to the epidural solution causes urinary retention as well as pruritus, nausea, and vomiting. In the case of levobupivacaine, a large study demonstrated no benefit from the addition of fentanyl to levobupivacaine concentrations as small as 0.0625%.[148] Ropivacaine may also be administered as a continuous epidural infusion for perioperative analgesia using a 0.2% concentration at 0.1 mL/kg/hr for infants <6 months of age and 0.2 mL/kg/hr for infants >6 months of age and children, for up to 72 hours.[285]

Careful attention must be paid to the dose of the local anesthetic (although ropivacaine and levobupivacaine are several fold less cardiotoxic than bupivacaine) in infants and children as toxic blood concentrations may cause ventricular fibrillation and cardiac arrest, which is very difficult to successfully resuscitate in the case of bupivacaine. The most effective treatment to restore normal sinus rhythm (although not FDA approved) is 1.5 mL/kg IV of 20% Intralipid,[286] repeating the bolus up to twice or until normal sinus rhythm is restored. The incidence of complications with caudal/epidural block is small, approximately 1.5:1,000.[287] Postoperatively, each child and parents/guardian should be interviewed daily for the efficacy of the block, side effects, and complications from the caudal/epidural block. Side effects of the block include nausea, vomiting, pruritus, urinary retention, and excessive motor blockade. Local infection, fluid leakage, and bleeding at the catheter site are important to recognize and treat as indicated.

Local skin infection at the catheter skin site may appear as red and swollen. These superficial infections rarely migrate internally causing epidural abscesses. If an infection is suspected, the catheter should be removed and the skin cleansed and dressed.

Epidural Block

Epidural anesthesia is performed in the same manner as in adults except that a shorter 5-cm Tuohy 18G needle is more manageable. The distances from the skin to the dura in infants and children, for example, are much smaller as are the doses.

Spinal Block

This block is useful in preterm infants and neonates who require lower abdominal superficial surgery (see Chapter 41, section "Spinal Anesthesia").

EMERGENCE AND RECOVERY FROM ANESTHESIA

As surgery concludes, a plan must be in place regarding the conditions for tracheal extubation: Will the child be awake or anesthetized? Evidence suggests that the advantages and disadvantages of the two techniques are similar, notwithstanding confounding effects by comorbidities and concomitant drugs.[288] In both scenarios, the train-of-four twitch response should be assessed and if at least one twitch is present, neuromuscular blockade should be antagonized. If there are no twitches present, antagonism should be delayed until at least one twitch appears. Equipment should be available to manage the airway (face mask, 100% oxygen) and to manage complications from extubation (e.g., active suction).

In children, the primary focus during emergence from anesthesia is the airway, the child's ability to breathe, and whether the child can protect his/her airway should bleeding or regurgitation occur during or after extubation. It is this author's practice to remove the tracheal tube or LMA when the child has fully recovered airway reflexes and is responsive. There are very few surgical or medical indications to remove the airway during a deep level of anesthesia, although opinion varies on this matter. The concern regarding a deep extubation of the trachea is that a child who is deeply anesthetized and transported with an unsecured airway depends on the expertise of the caregiver in the PACU to manage the airway until that child awakens. If the anesthesiologist must return to the operating room and if there is no physician assigned to PACU, then the caregivers may have inadequate backup should an airway emergency arise.

During an awake extubation, the practitioner can follow one of two strategies: Either the no-touch technique or direct stimulation. With the former, the child breathes 100% oxygen undisturbed and remains unstimulated until the third and final phase of emergence (as described below). The end-tidal sevoflurane concentration that is consistent with wakefulness is <0.6%. This author finds that emergence only begins when the anesthetic concentration is empirically <0.3% sevoflurane or <0.25% isoflurane, depending on the presence of concomitant medications. As the inhaled concentration decreases below these values, the child opens his/her eyes spontaneously and reaches for the tracheal tube, gags, and grimaces, all of which indicate that it is time to remove the airway. In the case of infants, they flex their hips indicating good muscle tone. In contrast, with the direct stimulating technique, the anesthetic concentration decreases toward the same concentrations (sevoflurane <0.3% and isoflurane <0.25%) at which time digital pressure may be applied to the most cephalad portion of the ascending ramus of the mandible, to the condylar process (as described in the "jaw thrust" maneuver above), for 3 to 5 seconds while directing the force toward the frontal hairline.[97] The child becomes highly aroused and gags on the tracheal tube for several seconds, but then falls back to a semiconscious state when the stimulation abates. During this quiescent period, the child may breathe shallowly or breath-hold, but if desaturation occurs, positive pressure ventilation with 100% oxygen must be instituted. When the child resumes coughing and gagging, the eyes open, respirations should be sustained and regular, the child should have purposeful movement (e.g., reaches for the tube), and then it is time to extubate. After this process, there appears to be less risk of triggering airway reflexes upon tracheal extubation. Both the no-touch and the direct stimulation strategies provide similar outcomes with safe and protected airways in children.

The timing of tracheal extubation is critical for minimizing the risk of adverse airway events during emergence from anesthesia. The optimal time to extubate the trachea in the "awake state" requires that the child has sufficiently recovered from anesthesia to support his/her own airway and that risk of adverse airway events is unlikely. During recovery from inhalational anesthesia in children, three distinct phases of emergence may be observed: Early, middle, and late phases. The early phase may last for several minutes depending on the anesthetic drugs administered, concomitant medications administered, and the age of the child. During this phase, the child coughs intermittently, gags, struggles, and moves nonpurposefully. This phase passes relatively quickly as the child emerges from anesthesia and enters the middle or quiescent phase. During the quiescent phase, the child may return to an unresponsive state, become apneic or "agitated," or breath-hold, strain, and/or desaturate, the last outcome necessitating positive pressure ventilation to restore the SaO_2 to >95%. As the child resumes quiet, spontaneous respiration, he/she enters the third and final phase of emergence, which is characterized by purposeful movement, flexing the hips and coughing and gagging on the tracheal tube, all of which increase in intensity until the child grimaces and opens the eyes spontaneously. Removing the tracheal tube during either the early or middle phase markedly increases the risk of triggering an adverse airway event (eg., laryngospasm). It is only during this third phase of emergence that the airway should be extubated making it least likely to trigger adverse airway reflex responses. The author teaches trainees that "if you think it is time to remove the tube, don't! Leave the tube in situ for another minute (or two) until the child is definitely in the late or third phase of emergence when the tracheal tube may be removed for the first and only time."

If the tube is removed prematurely, breath-holding, upper airway obstruction, and laryngospasm may ensue. The child's

TABLE 42-13. CAUSES OF DELAYED EMERGENCE FROM ANESTHESIA IN CHILDREN

Cause	Investigation/Intervention
Anesthetic-related:	
Residual drug effects: Inhalational anesthetics, opioids, propofol	• End-tidal concentration • Evaluate total drug dose
Non-anesthesia medications: Recreational drug use (cocaine, crack), herbal medicines (valerian, St. John's wort)	• History; drug toxicology screen
Depressed neuromuscular junction, residual neuromuscular blockade, or pseudocholinesterase deficiency	• Assess train-of-four
Hypothermia	• Measure the child's temperature. • Introduce heating modalities as indicated (e.g., forced air warmer, heat operating room)
Severe hypercapnia (MAC CO_2 ~200–245 mm Hg)	• Blood gas and end-tidal pCO_2
Metabolic/Other:	
Hypo or hyperglycemia; diabetic ketoacidosis	• Measure blood glucose, urinary glucose, and ketones • Arterial blood gas and electrolytes for pH and anion gap
Electrolyte and metabolic disorder	• Serum electrolytes (e.g., hyponatremia, hypomagnesemia)
Acid–base disturbance	• Blood gas analysis (anion gap or non-anion gap acidosis)
Encephalopathy	• Hepatic, renal, endocrinopathy (e.g., hypothyroidism, Addison disease), or sepsis • Blood gas analysis, electrolytes, and blood cultures if indicated
Cerebrovascular accident/hypoxia	• Check bilateral pupil size • Check responsiveness to light and pain stimulus bilaterally • Assess the presence of a gag reflex, symmetrical limb reflexes • Assess the fontanelle pressure in infants

face mask should be immediately available in order to deliver 100% oxygen through a tight fit to the face with 100% oxygen and dial 10 to 20 cm H_2O continuous positive airway pressure on the adjustable pressure limiting valve. To force the child through this "light" phase of anesthesia, pressure should be applied to the condyle of the mandible (see jaw thrust above) in 3- to 5-second intermittent applications until the child begins to breathe. If laryngospasm develops, see above for treatment.

Deep tracheal extubation requires an organized plan. In order to extubate the trachea deep, the depth of inhalational anesthesia must be 1.5 to 2 × MAC. In the case of sevoflurane, this means between 3.6% and 5% end-tidal concentration for at least 10 minutes. Some prefer to inspect the larynx at that time for foreign substances and fluids by performing laryngoscopy. Others gently stimulate the airway by moving the tube up and down. The absence of a response and the continuation of regular respirations indicate an adequate depth of anesthesia is present to remove the tube. If, however, the child coughs or breath-holds, then either a further period of anesthesia is required before a trial laryngoscopy is attempted or the deep extubation approach is abandoned and the child is awakened.

Appropriate equipment to transfer the child whose trachea is intubated must be immediately available. Either a self-inflating Laerdal bag or a t-piece should be available with a source of oxygen. The nurses who manage these children in PACU must have the skills to manage an intubated airway, emergence from anesthesia, and the airway after tracheal extubation.

The timing of removing the LMA, either awake or during deep anesthesia, in general, does not affect the incidence of upper airway adverse events. However, the presence of a URTI, specific anesthetics (e.g., desflurane, isoflurane >> halothane, sevoflurane), and specific surgeries (e.g., airway surgery) increase the risk of perioperative airway events.[195,197] When the LMA has been removed during deep anesthesia, upper airway reflex responses may only develop when the child begins to emerge from anesthesia, in the PACU. To avoid this potential problem, this author recommends that all LMAs be removed when the children are awake and only then should they be transferred to PACU.

In the vast majority of children, emergence from anesthesia progresses smoothly as described above. However, children who do not emerge from anesthesia in a timely fashion must be assessed for possible causes for delayed emergence from anesthesia (Table 42-13). The most common causes of delayed emergence include drug overdoses, increased sensitivity to drugs (e.g., OSA and opioid sensitivity), failure to taper or reduce the dose of inhalational or intravenous anesthetic, or the presence of hypothermia. Other, less frequent but potentially catastrophic events should also be considered including hypoglycemia, increased intracranial pressure, and metabolic causes including hyponatremia.

A rare but potentially fatal arrhythmia may develop during emergence in a child with an undiagnosed congenital long QT syndrome.[55] Administering medications (such as 5-HT_3 receptor antagonists) that are known to prolong the QT interval and in the presence of factors known to trigger torsades de pointes may suddenly trigger the arrhythmia.[289] Treatment with IV lidocaine (1 to 2 mg/kg), magnesium (15 to 30 mg/kg), and/or shock may be necessary to convert to sinus rhythm.

TRANSPORT TO PACU

Transferring children from the operating room to the PACU requires a stable airway, adequate oxygenation and ventilation,

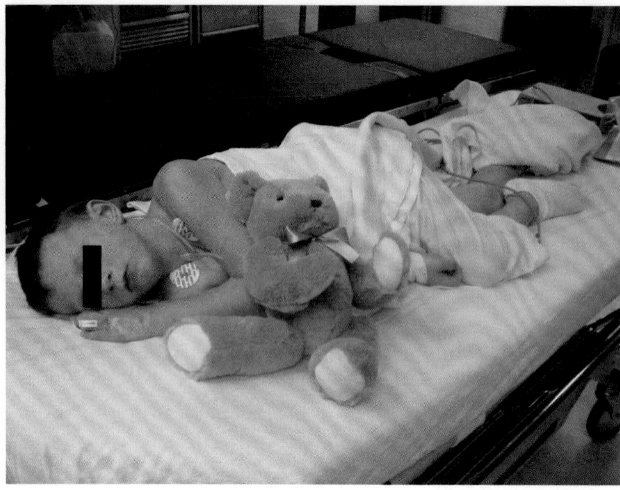

FIGURE 42-6. Position of the child after tracheal extubation in preparation for transfer to PACU and the pediatric ICU. This is known as the "recovery position" with the child lying in the lateral decubitus position, neck extended and mouth opened. In this position, oropharyngeal secretions, blood, or vomitus will drain onto the gurney rather than collect in the parapharyngeal region and trigger upper airway reflex responses.

stable heart rate and blood pressure, and adequate pain control. The child must be accompanied by an expert who has been trained to diagnose and manage postoperative problems, most notably airway obstruction.

Most children are transported to PACU without an artificial airway, breathing spontaneously. The optimal position for transfer of a child after surgery is the lateral decubitus position, known as the "recovery position."[290] In this position, the upper leg is flexed at the hip and resting on the bed in front of the lower leg. The child's upper hand should be placed under his lower cheek (Fig. 42-6). This position facilitates drainage of secretions, blood, or vomitus out of the mouth rather than onto the larynx, and the tongue falls to the lower cheek or out of the mouth rather than posteriorly onto the larynx. This position permits direct airway monitoring and intervention should the need arise.

Supplemental oxygen may be administered by nasal prongs or face mask during transport to the PACU to prevent desaturation during the transport. However, in the absence of nitrous oxide and in children whose lungs are normal, the most common reason for desaturation during transport is upper airway obstruction, an emergency that is difficult to detect by pulse oximetry when supplemental oxygen is administered. The reason for this difficulty is that the large reserve of oxygen maintains the oxygen desaturation several minutes even in the presence of complete airway obstruction or hypopnea. Therefore, this author extends the child's neck with the base of his hand (thenar and hypothenar eminences) while positioning his fingertips over the mouth/nose to feel the warm temperature in the exhaled gases to monitor respiration (and never pulls up on the chin to close the mouth) with the child in the "recovery" position.

Transporting the recovering child in the supine position predisposes to airway obstruction from posterior displacement of the tongue and facilitates the accumulation of secretions or other fluids in the supraglottic region. Furthermore, opioids depress the hypoglossal motor nuclei centrally, which relaxes the genioglossus muscle allowing the tongue to fall back and potentially obstruct the airway in the supine position.[291]

PACU COMPLICATIONS

Approximately 5% of children have complications in the PACU,[292] with 77% from vomiting, 22% from respiratory causes, and 1% or less from cardiac causes. The age distribution of the complications showed that children >8 years of age vomited more than twice as frequently as those <8 years, whereas respiratory complications in infants <1 year of age occurred twice as frequently as in those >1 year of age.

Laryngospasm, Postoperative Stridor, and Negative Pressure Pulmonary Edema

Laryngospasm, postoperative stridor, and negative pressure pulmonary edema occur both during induction of anesthesia and during or after emergence from anesthesia. Factors that increase the risk of laryngospasm are enumerated in Table 42-11.

Postextubation stridor may also occur after tracheal extubation. Stridor usually results from the epithelium within the cricoid ring swelling after the tracheal tube is removed. The swelling reduces the internal cross-sectional diameter of the cricoid ring and increases the pressure gradient (and therefore work of breathing) across the ring. Because airflow in the upper airway is turbulent, the resistance to air flow increases as the fifth power of the radius of the cricoid ring decreases. That is, if the radius of the airway within the cricoid ring decreases by 50%, the resistance to airflow increases 32-fold. In infants with increased oxygen requirements and metabolic rates, residual opioids, muscle weakness, and anesthesia may further compromise their ability to maintain an increased work of breathing during stridor, which could hasten fatigue and respiratory failure. Postextubation stridor is more common in Down syndrome and children with recent URTIs. Treatment for stridor includes humidified oxygen, sitting the child upright, reassurance, light sedation, intravenous dexamethasone (0.6 mg/kg IV), and nebulized racemic epinephrine (0.5 mL epinephrine in 2 mL saline). Heliox has been effective in reducing the work of breathing, oxygen consumption, and distress although it limits the inspired oxygen fraction. If hypoxemia or respiratory failure occurs, the trachea should be reintubated with a smaller size tube than the one originally used. To avoid further irritating the epithelium, an audible leak should be present after intubation. If a racemic epinephrine treatment is repeated more than twice, the child should be observed for rebound edema in either the PACU or a monitored unit.

Negative pressure pulmonary edema or postextubation pulmonary edema is an infrequent complication that usually occurs immediately or within several minutes after tracheal extubation in healthy, muscular adolescents and young adults, although it has been reported in infants.[293] Shortly after the trachea is extubated, the airway may become increasingly obstructed while the child appears somnolent and unresponsive. The presumptive diagnosis is laryngospasm, which may range in severity from very mild (i.e., hiccups) to severe. Ventilation by mask with 100% oxygen may be ineffective in restoring vital signs, necessitating tracheal reintubation using propofol and a muscle relaxant. As soon as the tube passes the vocal cords, pink frothy pulmonary edema fluid may appear in the tube or appear upon suctioning the tube. SaO_2 can be restored to >94% using positive pressure ventilation with positive end-expiratory pressure and 100% oxygen. Tracheal intubation and positive pressure ventilation are usually sufficient to resolve the pulmonary edema although in some instances, IV furosemide may be required. In a dose of 0.5 to 1 mg/kg, furosemide venodilates the vasculature rapidly resolving the pulmonary congestion and improving oxygenation. Although some may recover from the pulmonary edema very rapidly, others require sedation and tracheal intubation for 12 to 24 hours or more, until the pulmonary edema resolves.

Oxygen Desaturation

Failure to maintain adequate SaO_2 in the recovery room is a common problem. Unrecognized hypoxia may lead to deterioration in the child's clinical status and lead to sudden bradycardia and cardiac arrest. Continuous monitoring of the child's SaO_2 in the PACU is essential to provide an early warning sign of respiratory distress. The minimum acceptable SaO_2 in PACU is 94%. Administration of oxygen by face mask may be required to maintain the SaO_2, particularly if residual anesthesia or opioids and/or a craniofacial or muscular abnormality is present, or the child is obese or fluid overloaded. In healthy children, oxygen desaturation in PACU is generally indicative of hypoventilation and/or airway obstruction. Because there is no means of assessing ventilation in children in the PACU who do not have artificial airways, we must rely on clinical signs to quickly diagnose and treat airway obstruction and hypoventilation before complications develop.

Children should be weaned from oxygen dependency (assuming they did not require supplemental oxygen preoperatively) before they are discharged to the floor or the step-down unit. Some children remove their face masks themselves when they awaken from anesthesia; if their SaO_2 is ≥94% while breathing room air, then no additional oxygen is required. If the SaO_2 is maintained with a face mask, then the oxygen supply can be weaned to nasal prongs and then to room air provided the SaO_2 is maintained at each stage. If the child cannot maintain his/her SaO_2 despite weaning attempts, further investigation may be required (such as a chest X-ray) to rule out aspiration, pneumonia, or pneumothorax.

Emergence Agitation

The introduction of sevoflurane and desflurane anesthesia in children has caused a recrudescence of emergence agitation (also known as emergence delirium) during recovery from anesthesia. ED has a peak incidence in children (of both sexes) at 2 to 6 years of age, is more common after some anesthetics (sevoflurane ~ desflurane > isoflurane >> TIVA), lasts 10 to 15 minutes, and is terminated either spontaneously or after an IV dose of propofol, midazolam, clonidine, dexmedetomidine, ketamine, opioids, or a host of other medications.[294,295]

The diagnosis of ED in children has proven difficult for several reasons. First, the presence of pain has proved to be a significant confounding variable in establishing the diagnosis. When ED was assessed in children undergoing MRI with either sevoflurane or halothane, the incidence of ED after sevoflurane was fivefold greater than it was after halothane.[296] Second, the diagnosis of ED has been a challenge without a validated scale. To address this difficulty, we developed the pediatric anesthesia emergence delirium (PAED) score and validated it as an objective measure of ED; a score >10 or, more recently, >12 is considered strongly indicative of ED.[297]

Vomiting

The frequency of vomiting in the PACU and after hospital discharge has decreased dramatically with the introduction of prophylactic antiemetics for children at risk for PONV. Prophylaxis for PONV is recommended for surgeries with the greatest incidence of vomiting: Hernia, orchidopexy, tonsillectomy and adenoidectomy, ear surgery, strabismus surgery, and laparoscopic surgery. The incidence of vomiting increases with increasing age, peaking in females 10 to 16 years.[298] IV dexamethasone (0.0625 to 0.15 mg/kg (maximum 10 mg)) and ondansetron (0.05 to 0.15 mg/kg) reduce the perioperative incidence of PONV by up to 80% or more.[276] In fact, few children vomit in the PACU; most children who vomit, do so after ingesting their first fluids on the ward, in the car on the way home, or at home. Hence, we administer large volumes of IV fluids intraoperatively and in PACU (total 10 to 40 mL/kg) and recommend oral fluids only when the child requests to drink.[273,274] If the child continues to vomit, there is no magic solution. First, oral fluids should be withheld and intravenous access should be maintained or restarted and IV balanced salt solution administered. Second, if the child has either the ultrarapid polymorphism of CYP450 2D6 or a polymorphism of adenosine triphosphate–binding cassette subfamily B member 1 (ABCB1) non-TT type (e.g., 2677 or 3435 non-TT type) or both, then ondansetron may be ineffective.[299] Rapid assays are not available for these polymorphisms as yet. A second dose of ondansetron (0.1 mg/kg) may be given if at least 2 hours have passed since the first dose or IV metoclopramide (0.15 mg/kg) may be given.

Postoperative Pain

Management of pain in the PACU and on the ward depends on the origin of the pain, its severity, the medications already administered, and the status of the child. Regional anesthesia with neuroaxial or local blocks (penile, iliohypogastric/ilioinguinal or popliteal nerve blocks) may be used. Regional anesthesia is usually performed during general anesthesia in children (except in older adolescents) using either a direct nerve block or nerve stimulation or more recently ultrasound guidance.[300] When regional block is unsuitable, impractical, contraindicated, or refused by the parents, opioids, NSAID agents (diclofenac, tramadol, ibuprofen, and acetaminophen), and ketamine may be employed (see above).[301]

Continuous morphine infusions have been used to manage pain in children.[145] Morphine infusions may be prepared by dissolving the child's weight as milligram of morphine in 100 mL of saline and infused at 1 to 3 mL/hr. These children are ideally monitored continuously with pulse oximetry.

To tailor the morphine dose to the severity of the pain, patient-controlled analgesia (PCA) was developed for which the patient received morphine upon demand as well as a small dose continuously for background pain, if needed. PCA has been shown to be effective in children as young as 5 years, as well as by caregivers or parents who were educated regarding these devices for those <5 years of age and those who are cognitively impaired.[302] A typical morphine PCA may be programmed for a child as follows: PCA bolus 10 to 30 μg/kg; continuous rate of 10 to 40 μg/kg/hr (or in children at risk of apnea, 0 μg/kg/hr); lockout interval 6 to 10 minutes; and a 4-hour limit of 0.25 to 0.4 mg/kg.[145] Smaller doses and background infusions of PCA morphine are used in infants.[145,303] Dilaudid (hydromorphone), which is three- to five-fold more potent than morphine, may also be used. The attending nurse should routinely monitor the child's pain and if the pain is not adequately controlled, the pump settings should be reviewed and adjusted accordingly.

References

1. Bernstein D. History and physical examination. In: Kliegman RM, et al., eds. *Nelson Textbook of Pediatrics.* 19th ed. Philadelphia, PA: Saunders Elsevier; 2011:1529–1536.
2. Szabó EZ, Luginbuehl I, Bissonnette B. Impact of anesthetic agents on cerebrovascular physiology in children. *Paediatr Anaesth.* 2009;19:108–118.
3. Stratmann G. Neurotoxicity of anesthetic drugs in the developing brain. *Anesth Analg.* 2011;113:1170–1179.
4. Slikker W Jr, Zou X, Hotchkiss CE. Ketamine-induced neuronal cell death in the perinatal rhesus monkey. *Toxicol Sci.* 2007;98:145–158.
5. Bartels M, Althoff RR, Boomsma DI. Anesthesia and cognitive performance in children: No evidence for a causal relationship. *Twin Res Hum Genet.* 2009; 12:246–253.
6. Itoh T, Imano M, Nishida S, et al. Exercise inhibits neuronal apoptosis and improves cerebral function following rat traumatic brain injury. *J Neural Transm.* 2011;118:1263–1272.

6a. Shih J, May LDV, Gonzalez HE, et al. Delayed environmental enrichment reverses sevoflurane-induced memory impairment in rat. *Anesthesiology.* 2012;116: 586–602.

7. Payne K, Mattheyse FJ, Liebenberg D, et al. The pharmacokinetics of midazolam in paediatric patients. *Eur J Clin Pharmacol.* 1989;37:267–272.
8. Kogan A, Katz J, Efrat R, et al. Premedication with midazolam in young children: A comparison of four routes of administration. *Paediatr Anaesth.* 2002;12: 685–689.
9. Anderson BJ, Holford NHG, Woollard GA, et al. Perioperative pharmacodynamics of acetaminophen analgesia in children. *Anesthesiology.* 1999;90:411–421.
10. Koren G. Therapeutic drug monitoring principles in the neonate. *Clin Chem.* 1997;43:221–227.
11. Lerman J, Strong HA, LeDez KM, et al. Effects of age on the serum concentration of α1-acid glycoprotein and the binding of lidocaine in pediatric patients. *Clin Pharmacol Ther.* 1989;46:219–225.
12. Hines RN. Ontogeny of human hepatic cytochromes P450. *J Biochem Mol Toxicol.* 2007;21:169–175.
13. Ingelman-Sundberg M. Genetic polymorphisms of cytochrome *P4502D6* (CYP2D6): Clinical consequences, evolutionary aspects and functional diversity. *Pharmacogenomics J.* 2005;5:6–13.
14. Hines RN. The ontogeny of drug metabolism enzymes and implications for adverse drug events. *Pharmacol Ther.* 2008;118:250–267.
15. Lerman J, Schmitt-Bantel BI, Gregory GA, et al. Effect of age on the solubility of volatile anesthetics in human tissues. *Anesthesiology.* 1986;65:307–311.
16. Malviya S, Lerman J. The blood/gas solubilities of sevoflurane, isoflurane, halothane, and serum constituent concentrations in neonates and adults. *Anesthesiology.* 1990;72:793–796.
17. Lerman J, Gregory GA, Willis MM, et al. Age and solubility of volatile anesthetics in blood. *Anesthesiology.* 1984;61:139–143.
18. Yasuda N, Lockhart SH, Eger EI II, et al. Comparison of kinetics of sevoflurane and isoflurane in humans. *Anesth Analg.* 1991;72:316–324.
19. Eger EI II. *Anesthetic Uptake and Action.* Baltimore: Williams & Wilkins; 1974.
20. Olofsen E, Dahan A. The dynamic relationship between end-tidal sevoflurane and isoflurane concentrations and bispectral index and spectral edge frequency of the electroencephalogram. *Anesthesiology.* 1999;90:1345–1353.
21. Fuentes R, Cortínez LI, Struys MMRF, et al. The dynamic relationship between end-tidal sevoflurane concentrations, bispectral index, and cerebral state index in children. *Anesth Analg.* 2008;107:1573–1578.
22. Gibbons RT, Steffey EP, Eger EI II. The effect of spontaneous versus controlled ventilation on the rate of rise of alveolar halothane concentration in dogs. *Anesth Analg.* 1977;56:32–34.
23. Lerman J. Pharmacology of inhalational anaesthetics in infants and children. *Paediatr Anaesth.* 1992;2:191–203.
24. Eger EI II, Shafer SL. Tutorial: Context-sensitive decrement times for inhaled anesthetics. *Anesth Analg.* 2005;101:688–696.
25. Neumann MA, Weiskopf RB, Gong DH, et al. Changing from isoflurane to desflurane toward the end of anesthesia does not accelerate recovery in humans. *Anesthesiology.* 1998;88:914–921.
26. Sakata DJ, Gopalakrishnan NA, Orr JA, et al. Hypercapnic hyperventilation shorten emergence time from isoflurane anesthesia. *Anesth Analg.* 2007;104:587–591.
27. Sakata DJ, Gopalakrishnan NA, Orr JA, et al. Rapid recovery from sevoflurane and desflurane with hypercapnia and hyperventilation. *Anesth Analg.* 2007;105: 79–82.
28. Lerman J, Robinson S, Willis MM, et al. Anesthetic requirements for halothane in young children 0–1 month and 1–6 months of age. *Anesthesiology.* 1983;59:421–424.
29. Gregory GA, Eger EI II, Munson ES. The relationship between age and halothane requirements in man. *Anesthesiology.* 1969;30:488–491.
30. LeDez KM, Lerman J. The minimum alveolar concentration (MAC) of isoflurane in preterm neonates. *Anesthesiology.* 1987;67:301–307.
31. Cameron CB, Robinson S, Gregory GA. The minimum anesthetic concentration of isoflurane in children. *Anesth Analg.* 1984;63:418–420.
32. Lerman J, Sikich N, Kleinman S, et al. The pharmacology of sevoflurane in infants and children. *Anesthesiology.* 1994;80:814–824.
33. Taylor RH, Lerman J. Minimum alveolar concentration of desflurane and hemodynamic responses in neonates, infants, and children. *Anesthesiology.* 1991; 75:975–979.
34. Frei FJ, Haemmerle MH, Brunner R, et al. Minimum alveolar concentration for halothane in children with cerebral palsy and severe mental retardation. *Anaesthesia.* 1997;52:1056–1060.
35. Liem EB, Lin CM, Suleman MI, et al. Anesthetic requirement is increased in redheads. *Anesthesiology.* 2004;101:279–283.
36. Fisher DM, Zwass MS. MAC of desflurane in 60% nitrous oxide in infants and children. *Anesthesiology.* 1992;76:354–356.
37. Liu M, Hu X, Liu J. The effect of hypothermia on isoflurane MAC in children. *Anesthesiology.* 2001;94:429–432.
38. Coté CJ, Lerman J, Ward RM, et al. A practice of anesthesia for infants and children. In: Cote CJ, Lerman J, Todres ID, eds. *Pharmacokinetics and Pharmacology of Drugs Used in Children.* Philadelphia, PA: Saunders Elsevier; 2009:108; Chapter 6, Table 6-8.
39. Hatch DJ. New inhalation agents in paediatric anaesthesia. *Br J Anaesth.* 1999; 83:42–49.
40. Walpole R, Olday J, Haetzman M, et al. A comparison of the respiratory effects of high concentrations of halothane and sevoflurane. *Paediatr Anaesth.* 2001;11:157–160.
41. Doi M, Ikeda K. Respiratory effects of sevoflurane. *Anesth Analg.* 1987;66:241–244.
42. Behforouz N, Dubousset AM, Jamali S, et al. Respiratory effects of desflurane anesthesia on spontaneous ventilation in infants and children. *Anesth Analg.* 1998;87:1052–1055.
43. von Ungern-Sternberg BS, Saudan S, Petak F, et al. Desflurane but not sevoflurane impairs airway and respiratory mechanics in children with susceptible airways. *Anesthesiology.* 2008;108:216–224.
44. Dikmen Y, Eminoglu E, Salihoglu Z, et al. Pulmonary mechanics during isoflurane, sevoflurane and desflurane anaesthesia. *Anaesthesia.* 2003;58:745–748.
45. Tobias JD. Inhalational anesthesia: Basic pharmacology, end organ effects, and applications in the treatment of status asthmaticus. *J Intensive Care Med.* 2009; 24:361–371.
46. Vaschetto R, Bellotti E, Turucz E, et al. Inhalational anesthetics in acute severe asthma. *Curr Drug Targets.* 2009;10:826–832.
47. Lerman J, Davis PJ, Welborn LG, et al. Induction, recovery, and safety characteristics of sevoflurane in children undergoing ambulatory surgery: A comparison with halothane. *Anesthesiology.* 1996;84:1332–1340.
48. Lindgren L, Randell T, Saarnivaara L. Comparison of inhalation induction with isoflurane or halothane in children. *Eur J Anaesthesiol.* 1991;8:33–37.
49. Taylor RH, Lerman J. Induction, maintenance and recovery characteristics of desflurane in inhalants and children. *Can J Anaesth.* 1992;39:6–13.
50. Lerman J, Hammer GB, Verghese S, et al. Airway responses to desflurane during maintenance of anesthesia and recovery in children with laryngeal mask airways. *Paediatr Anaesth.* 2010;20:495–505.
51. Wodey E, Senhadji L, Pladys P, et al. The relationship between expired concentration of sevoflurane and sympathovagal tone in children. *Anesth Analg.* 2003; 97:377–382.
52. Ebert TJ, Muzi M. Sympathetic hyperactivity during desflurane anesthesia in healthy volunteers. A comparison with isoflurane. *Anesthesiology.* 1993;79:444–453.
53. Muzi, M, Ebert TJ, Hope WG, et al. Site(s) mediating sympathetic activation with desflurane. *Anesthesiology.* 1996;85:737–747.
54. Whyte SD, Sanatani S, Lim J, et al. A comparison of the effect on dispersion of repolarization of age-adjusted MAC values of sevoflurane in children. *Anesth Analg.* 2007;104:277–282.
55. Nathan AT, Berkowitz DH, Montenegro LM, et al. Implications of anesthesia in children with long QT syndrome. *Anesth Analg.* 2011;112:1163–1168.
56. Kawana S, Wachi J, Nakayama M, et al. Comparison of haemodynamic changes induced by sevoflurane and halothane in paediatric patients. *Can J Anaesth.* 1995;42:603–607.
57. Wodey E, Pladys P, Copin C, et al. Comparative hemodynamic depression of sevoflurane versus halothane in infants: An echocardiographic study. *Anesthesiology.* 1997;87:795–800.
58. Barash PG, Glanz S, Katz JD, et al. Ventricular function in children during halothane anesthesia: An echocardiographic evaluation. *Anesthesiology.* 1978;49:79–85.
59. Russell IA, Miller Hance WC, Gregory G, et al. The safety and efficacy of sevoflurane anesthesia in infants and children with congenital heart disease. *Anesth Analg.* 2001;92:1152–1158.
60. Cubeddu L. QT prolongation and fatal arrhythmias: A review of clinical implications and effects of drugs. *Am J Ther.* 2003;10:452–457.
61. Abriel H, Schlpafer J, Keller DI, et al. Molecular and clinical determinants of drug-induced long QT syndrome: An iatrogenic channelopathy. *Swiss Med Wkly.* 2004;134:685–694.
62. Wallenborn J, Kluba K, Olthoff D. Comparative evaluation of bispectral index and narcotrend index in children below 5 years of age. *Paediatr Anaesth.* 2007; 17:140–147.

63. Kim HS, Oh AY, Kim CS, et al. Correlation of bispectral index with end-tidal sevoflurane concentration and age in infants and children. *Br J Anaesth.* 2005; 95:362–366.
64. Tirel O, Wodey E, Harris R, et al. The impact of age on bispectral index values and EEG bispectrum during anaesthesia with desflurane and halothane in children. *Br J Anaesth.* 2006;96:480–485.
65. Davidson AJ, Huang GH, Rebmann CS, et al. Performance of entropy and bispectral index as measures of anaesthesia effect in children of different ages. *Br J Anaesth.* 2005;95:674–679.
66. Valkenburg AJ, de Leeuw TG, Tibboel D, et al. Lower bispectral index values in children who are intellectually disabled. *Anesth Analg.* 2009;109:1428–1433.
67. Wappler F, Bischoff P. Is fast induction with sevoflurane associated with an increased anesthetic risk in pediatric patients? *Anesth Analg.* 2003;96:1239–1240.
68. Iijima T, Nakamura Z, Iwao Y, et al. The epileptogenic properties of the volatile anesthetics sevoflurane and isoflurane in patients with epilepsy. *Anesth Analg.* 2000;91:989–995.
69. Kharasch ED, Thummel KE. Identification of cytochrome P450 2E1 as the predominant enzyme catalyzing human liver microsomal defluorination of sevoflurane, isoflurane, and methoxyflurane. *Anesthesiology.* 1993;79:795–807.
70. Kharasch ED, Hankins DC, Thummel KE. Human kidney methoxyflurane and sevoflurane metabolism. Intrarenal fluoride production as a possible mechanism of methoxyflurane nephrotoxicity. *Anesthesiology.* 1995;82:689–699.
71. Kharasch ED, Schroeder JL, Liggitt D, et al. New insights into the mechanism of methoxyflurane nephrotoxicity and implications for anesthetic development (part 2). *Anesthesiology.* 2006;105:737–745.
72. Arnold JH, Truog RD, Rice SA. Prolonged administration of isoflurane to pediatric patients during mechanical ventilation. *Anesth Analg.* 1993;76:520–526.
73. Jang Y, Kim AI. Severe hepatotoxicity after sevoflurane anesthesia in a child with mild renal dysfunction. *Paediatr Anaesth.* 2005;15:1140–1144.
74. Coté G, Bouchard S. Hepatotoxicity after desflurane anesthesia in a 15-month-old child with Mobius syndrome after previous exposure to isoflurane. *Anesthesiology.* 2007;107:843–845.
75. Reichle FM, Conzen PF. Halogenated inhalational anaesthetics. *Best Pract Res Clin Anaesthesiol.* 2003;17:29–46.
76. Frink EJ Jr, Green WB Jr, Brown EA, et al. Compound A concentrations during sevoflurane anesthesia in children. *Anesthesiology.* 1996;84:566–571.
77. Fang ZC, Eger EI II, Laster MJ, et al. Carbon monoxide production from degradation of desflurane, enflurane, isoflurane, halothane, and sevoflurane by sodalime and Baralyme®. *Anesth Analg.* 1995;80:1187–1193.
78. Levy RJ, Nasr VG, Rivera O, et al. Detection of carbon monoxide during routine anesthetics in infants and children. *Anesth Analg.* 2010;110:747–753.
79. Munoz HR, Cortínex LI, Ibacache ME, et al. Estimation of the plasma effect site equilibration rate constant (k_{eo}) of propofol in children using the time to peak effect. *Anesthesiology.* 2004;101:1269–1274.
80. Murat I, Billard V, Vernois J, et al. Pharmacokinetics of propofol after a single dose in children aged 1–3 years with minor burns. *Anesthesiology.* 1996;84:526–532.
81. Allegaert K, De Hoon J, Verbesselt R, et al. Maturational pharmacokinetics of single intravenous bolus of propofol. *Paediatr Anaesth.* 2007;17:1028–1034.
82. McFarlan CS, Anderson BJ, Short TG. The use of propofol infusions in paediatric anaesthesia: A practical guide. *Paediatr Anaesth.* 1999;9:209–216.
83. Westrin P. The induction dose of propofol in infants 1–6 months of age and in children 10–16 years of age. *Anesthesiology.* 1991;74:455–458.
84. Allsop E, Innes P, Jackson M, et al. Dose of propofol required to insert the laryngeal mask airway in children. *Paediatr Anaesth.* 1995;5:47–51.
85. Martlew RA, Meakin G, Wadsworth R, et al. Dose of propofol for laryngeal mask airway insertion in children: Effect premedication with midazolam. *Br J Anaesth.* 1996;76:308–309.
86. Lerman J, Houle TT, Matthews BT, et al. Propofol for tracheal intubation in children anesthetized with sevoflurane: A dose-response study. *Paediatr Anaesth.* 2009;19:218–222.
87. Kim H, Hong JY, Suk EH, et al. Optimum bolus dose of propofol for tracheal intubation during sevoflurane induction without neuromuscular blockade in children. *Anaesth Intensive Care.* 2011;39:899–903.
88. Heard C, Burrows F, Johnson K, et al. A comparison of dexmedetomidine-midazolam with propofol for maintenance of anesthesia in children undergoing magnetic resonance imaging. *Anesth Analg.* 2008;107:1832–1839.
89. Usher AG, Kearney RA, Tsui BCH. Propofol total intravenous anesthesia for MRI in children. *Paediatr Anaesth.* 2005;15:23–28.
90. Asahi Y, Kubota K, Omichi S. Dose requirements for propofol anaesthesia for dental treatment for autistic patients compared with intellectually impaired patients. *Anaesth Intensive Care.* 2009;37:70–73.
91. Mani V, Morton NS. Overview of total intravenous anesthesia in children. *Paediatr Anaesth.* 2010;20:211–222.
92. Sepúlveda P, Cortínez LI, Sáez C, et al. Performance evaluation of paediatric propofol pharmacokinetic models in healthy young children. *Br J Anaesth.* 2011;107:593–600.
93. Picard P, Tramer MR. Prevention of pain on injection with propofol: A quantitative systematic review. *Anesth Analg.* 2000;90:963–995.
94. Jalota L, Kalira V, George E, et al. Prevention of pain on injection of propofol: Systematic review and meta-analysis. *BMJ.* 2011;342:d1110.
95. Beh T, Splinter W, Kim J. In children, nitrous oxide decreases pain on injection of propofol mixed with lidocaine. *Can J Anaesth.* 2002;49:1061–1063.
96. Evans RG, Crawford MW, Noseworthy MD, et al. Effect of increasing depth of propofol anesthesia on upper airway configuration in children. *Anesthesiology.* 2003;99:596–602.
97. Larson PC Jr. Laryngospasm-the best treatment. *Anesthesiology.* 1998;89:1293–1294.
98. Lutterbey G, Wattjes MP, Doerr D, et al. Atelectasis in children undergoing either propofol infusion or positive pressure ventilation anesthesia for magnetic resonance imaging. *Paediatr Anaesth.* 2007;17:121–125.
99. Gan TJ, Meyer T, Apfel CC, et al. Consensus guidelines for managing postoperative nausea and vomiting. *Anesth Analg.* 2003;97:62–71.
100. Fodale V, La Monaca E. Propofol infusion syndrome. An overview of a perplexing disease. *Drug Saf.* 2008;31:293–303.
101. Wysowski DK, Pollock ML. Reports of death with use of propofol (Diprivan) for nonprocedural (long-term) sedation and literature review. *Anesthesiology.* 2006;105:1047–1051.
102. Koch M, De Backer D, Vincent JL. Lactic acidosis: An early marker of propofol infusion syndrome? *Intensive Care Med.* 2004;30:522.
103. Haase R, Sauer H, Eichler G. Lactic acidosis following short-term propofol infusion may be an early warning of propofol infusion syndrome. *J Neurosurg Anesthesiol.* 2005;17:122–123.
104. Westhout FD, Muhonen MG, Nwagwu CI. Early propofol infusion syndrome following cerebral angiographic embolization for giant aneurysm repair. *J Neurosurg.* 2007;106:139–142.
105. Herd DW, Anderson BJ, Keene NA, et al. Investigating the pharmacodynamics of ketamine in children. *Paediatr Anaesth.* 2008;18:36–42.
106. Dallimore D, Anderson BJ, Short TG, et al. Ketamine anesthesia in children–exploring infusion regimens. *Paediatr Anaesth.* 2008;18:708–714.
107. Anderson BJ, McKee AD, Holford NH. Size, myths and the clinical pharmacokinetics of analgesia in paediatric patients. *Clin Pharmacokinet.* 1997;33:313–327.
108. Gutstein HB, Johnson KL, Heard MB, et al. Oral ketamine preanesthetic medication in children. *Anesthesiology.* 1992;76:28–33.
109. Wolfe TR, Braude DA. Intranasal medication delivery for children: A brief review and update. *Pediatrics.* 2010;126:532–537.
110. Aspinall RL, Mayor A. A prospective randomized controlled study of the efficacy of ketamine for postoperative pain relief in children after adenotonsillectomy. *Paediatr Anaesth.* 2001;11:333–336.
111. Ansermino M, Basu R, Vandebeek C, et al. Nonopioid additives to local anaesthetics for caudal blockade in children: A systematic review. *Paediatr Anaesth.* 2003;13:561–573.
112. Funk W, Jakob W, Riedl T, et al. Oral preanesthetic medication for children: Double-blind randomized study of a combination of midazolam and ketamine vs midazolam or ketamine alone. *Br J Anaesth.* 2000;84:335–340.
113. Lin L, Zhang JW, Huang Y, et al. Population pharmacokinetics of intravenous bolus etomidate in children over 6 months of age. *Paediatr Anaesth.* 2011;22:318–326.
114. Forman SA. Clinical and molecular pharmacology of etomidate. *Anesthesiology.* 2011;114:695–707.
115. Pejo E, Cotten JF, Kelly EW, et al. In vivo and in vitro pharmacological studies of methoxycarbonyl-carboetomidate. *Anesth Analg.* 2012;115:297–304.
116. Mertes PM, Alla F, Tréchot P, et al. Anaphylaxis during anesthesia in France: An 8-year national survey. *J Allergy Clin Immunol.* 2011;128:366–373.
117. Florvaag E, Johansson SGO, Irgens A, et al. IgE-sensitization to the cough suppressant pholcodine and the effects of its withdrawal from the Norwegian market. *Allergy.* 2011;66:955–960.
118. Meakin G, Walker RW, Dearlove OR. Myotonic and neuromuscular blocking effects of increased doses of suxamethonium in infants and children. *Br J Anaesth.* 1990;65:816–818.
119. Liu LMP, DeCook TH, Goudsouzian NG, et al. Dose response to intramuscular succinylcholine in children. *Anesthesiology.* 1981;55:599–602.
120. Redden RJ, Miller M, Campbell RL. Submental administration of succinylcholine in children. *Anesth Prog.* 1990;37:296–300.
121. Mazze RI, Dunbar RW. Intralingual succinylcholine administration in children: An alternative to intravenous and intramuscular routes? *Anesth Analg.* 1968; 47:605–615.
122. Lerman J, Chinyanga HM. The heart rate response to succinylcholine in children: A comparison of atropine and glycopyrrolate. *Can Anaesth Soc J.* 1983;30:377–381.
123. Davis L, Britten JJ, Morgan M. Cholinesterase. Its significance in anaesthetic practice. *Anaesthesia.* 1997;52:244–260.
124. Neitlich HW. Increased plasma cholinesterase activity and succinylcholine resistance: A genetic variant. *J Clin Invest.* 1966;45:380–387.
125. Yoshida A, Motulsky AG. A pseudocholinesterase variant (E Cynthiana) associated with elevated plasma enzyme activity. *Am J Hum Genet.* 1969;21:486–498.
126. Leigh MD, McCoy DD, Belton MK, et al. Bradycardia following intravenous administration of succinylcholine chloride to infants and children. *Anesthesiology.* 1957;18:698–702.
127. Martyn JAJ, Richtsfeld M. Succinylcholine-induced hyperkalemia in acquired pathologic states. *Anesthesiology.* 2006;104:58–69.
128. Lerman J. Perioperative management of the paediatric patient with coexisting neuromuscular disease. *Br J Anaesth.* 2011;107(S1):i79–i89.

129. Thapa S, Brull SJ. Succinylcholine-induced hyperkalemia in patients with renal failure: An old question revisited. *Anesth Analg.* 2000;91:237–241.
130. Chidiac EJ, Rasikin AO. Succinylcholine and the open eye. *Ophthalmol Clin North Am.* 2006;19:279–285.
131. Lerman J, McLeod ME, Strong HA. Pharmacokinetics of intravenous dantrolene in children. *Anesthesiology.* 1989;70:625–629.
132. Meakin GH. Muscle relaxants in children. *Curr Opin Anaesthesiol.* 2007;20:227–231.
133. Taivainen T, Meretoja OA, Erkola O, et al. Rocuronium in infants, children and adults during a balanced anaesthesia. *Paediatr Anaesth.* 1996;6:271–275.
134. Wierda JMKH, Meretoja OA, Taivainen T, et al. Pharmacokinetics and pharmacokinetic-dynamic modelling of rocuronium in infants and children. *Br J Anaesth.* 1997;78:690–695.
135. Woloszczuk-Gebicka B, Wyska E, Grabowski T, et al. Pharmacokinetic-pharmacodynamic relationship of rocuronium under stable nitrous oxide-fentanyl or nitrous–sevoflurane anesthesia in children. *Paediatr Anaesth.* 2006;16:761–768.
136. Fuchs-Buder T, Tassonyi E. Intubating conditions and time course of rocuronium-induced neuromuscular block in children. *Br J Anaesth.* 1996;77:335–338.
137. Mazurek AJ, Rae B, Hann S, et al. Rocuronium versus succinylcholine: Are they equally effective during rapid-sequence induction of anesthesia? *Anesth Analg.* 1998;87:1259–1262.
138. Cheng CA, Aun CS, Gin T. Comparison of rocuronium and suxamethonium for rapid tracheal intubation in children. *Paediatr Anaesth.* 2002;12:140–145.
139. Brandom BW, Cook DR, Woelfel SK, et al. Atracurium infusion requirements in children during halothane, isoflurane, and narcotic anesthesia. *Anesth Analg.* 1985;64:471–476.
140. Meakin G, Meretoja OA, Perkins R, et al. Tracheal intubating conditions and pharmacodynamics following cisatracurium in infants and children undergoing halothane and thiopental-fentanyl anesthesia. *Paediatr Anaesth.* 2007;17:113–120.
141. Meretoja OA. Neuromuscular block and current treatment strategies for its reversal in children. *Paediatr Anaesth.* 2010;20:591–604.
142. Fields AM, Vadivelu N. Sugammadex: A novel neuromuscular blocker binding agent. *Curr Opin Anaesthesiol.* 2007;20:307–310.
143. Plaud B, Meretoja O, Hofmockel R, et al. Reversal of rocuronium-induced neuromuscular blockade with sugammadex in pediatric and adult surgical patients. *Anesthesiology.* 2009;110:284–294.
144. McDonnell NJ, Pavy TJG, Green LK, et al. Sugammadex in the management of rocuronium-induced anaphylaxis. *Br J Anaesth.* 2011;106:199–201.
145. Kart T, Christrup LL, Rasmussen M. Recommended use of morphine in neonates, infants and children based on a literature review: Part 2-clinical use. *Paediatr Anaesth.* 1997;7:93–101.
146. Brislin RP, Rose JB. Pediatric acute pain management. *Anesthesiol Clin North America.* 2005;23:789–814.
147. Robinson S, Gregory GA. Fentanyl-air-oxygen anesthesia for ligation of patent ductus arteriosus in preterm infants. *Anesth Analg.* 1981;60:331–334.
148. Lerman J, Nolan J, Eyres R, et al. Efficacy, safety and pharmacokinetics of levobupivacaine with and without fentanyl after continuous epidural infusion in children: A multicenter study. *Anesthesiology.* 2003;99:1166–1174.
149. Hughes MA, Glass PSA, Jacobs JR. Content-sensitive half-time in multicompartment pharmacokinetic models for intravenous anesthetic drugs. *Anesthesiology.* 1992;76:334–341.
150. Davis PJ, Cladis FP. The use of ultra-short-acting opioids in paediatric anaesthesia: The role of remifentanil. *Clin Pharmacokinet.* 2005;44:787–796.
151. Marsh DF, Hodkinson B. Remifentanil in paediatric anaesthetic practice. *Anaesthesia.* 2009;64:301–308.
152. Echevarria G, Elgueta F, Fierro C, et al. Nitrous oxide (N_2O) reduces postoperative opioid-induced hyperalgesia after remifentanil-propofol anaesthesia in humans. *Br J Anaesth.* 2011;107:959–965.
153. Berde CB, Sethna NF. Analgesics for the treatment of pain in children. *N Engl J Med.* 2002;347:1094–1103.
154. Williams DG, Hatch DJ, Howard RF. Codeine phosphate in paediatric medicine. *Br J Anaesth.* 2001;86:413–421.
155. Oyler JM, Cone EJ, Joseph RE, et al. Identification of hydrocodone in human urine following controlled codeine administration. *J Anal Toxicol.* 2000;24:530–536.
156. Voronov P, Przybylo HJ, Jagannathan N. Apnea in a child after oral codeine: A genetic variant – an ultra-rapid metabolizer. *Paediatr Anaesth.* 2007;17:684–687.
157. Ciszkowski C, Madadi P, Phillips MS, et al. Codeine, ultrarapid-metabolism genotype, and postoperative death. *N Engl J Med.* 2009;361:827–828.
158. Williams DG, Patel A, Howard RF. Pharmacogenetics of codeine metabolism in an urban population of children and its implications for analgesic reliability. *Br J Anaesth.* 2002;89:839–845.
159. Palmer SN, Giesecke NM, Body SC, et al. Pharmacokinetics of anesthetic and analgesic agents. *Anesthesiology.* 2005;102:663–671.
160. Lerman J. A disquisition on sleep-disordered breathing in children. *Paediatr Anaesth.* 2009;19(suppl 1):100–108.
161. Jahr JS, Lee VK. Intravenous acetaminophen. *Anesthesiol Clin.* 2010;28:619–645.
162. Birmingham PK, Tobin MJ, Fisher DM, et al. Initial and subsequent dosing of rectal acetaminophen in children: A 24-hour pharmacokinetic study of new dose recommendations. *Anesthesiology.* 2001;94:385–389.
163. Anderson BJ, Pons G, Autret-Leca E, et al. Pediatric intravenous paracetamol (propacetamol) pharmacokinetics: A population analysis. *Paediatr Anaesth.* 2005;15:282–292.
164. Prins SA, Van Dijk M, Van Leeuwen P, et al. Pharmacokinetics and analgesic effects of intravenous propacetamol vs rectal paracetamol in children after major craniofacial surgery. *Paediatr Anaesth.* 2008;18:582–592.
165. Nevin DG, Shung J. Intravenous paracetamol overdose in a preterm infant during anesthesia. *Paediatr Anaesth.* 2010;20:105–107.
166. Beringer RM, Thompson JP, Parry S, et al. Intravenous paracetamol overdose: Two case reports and a change to national treatment guidelines. *Arch Dis Child.* 2011;96:307–308.
167. Shende D, Das K. Comparative effect of intravenous ketorolac and pethidine on perioperative analgesia and postoperative nausea and vomiting (PONV) for paediatric strabismus surgery. *Acta Anaesthesiol Scand.* 1999;43:265–269.
168. Lynn AM, Bradford H, Kantor ED. Postoperative ketorolac tromethamine use in infants aged 6–18 months: The effect on morphine usage, safety assessment, and stereo-specific pharmacokinetics. *Anesth Analg.* 2007;104:1040–1051.
169. Cohen MN, Christians U, Henthorn T, et al. Pharmacokinetics of single-dose intravenous ketorolac in infants aged 2–11 months. *Anesth Analg.* 2011;112:655–660.
170. Gunter JB, Varughese AM, Harrington JF, et al. Recovery and complications after tonsillectomy in children: A comparison of ketorolac and morphine. *Anesth Analg.* 1995;81:1136–1141.
171. Agrawal A, Gerson CR, Selivman I, et al. Postoperative hemorrhage after tonsillectomy: Use of ketorolac tromethamine. *Otolaryngol Head Neck Surg.* 1999;120:335–339.
172. Marret E, Flahault A, Samama CM, et al. Effects of postoperative, nonsteroidal, antiinflammatory drugs on bleeding risk after tonsillectomy. Meta-analysis of randomized controlled trials. *Anesthesiology.* 2003;98:1497–1502.
173. Campobasso CP, Procacci R, Caligara M. Fatal adverse reaction to ketorolac tromethamine in asthmatic patient. *Am J Forensic Med Pathol.* 2008;29:358–363.
174. Standing JF, Savage I, Pritchard D, et al. Diclofenac for acute pain in children. *Cochrane Database Syst Rev.* 2009;4:CD005538.
175. Standing JF, Tibboel D, Korpela R, et al. Diclofenac pharmacokinetic meta-analysis and dose recommendations for surgical pain in children aged 1–12 years. *Paediatr Anaesth.* 2011;21:316–324.
176. Standing JF, Howard RF, Johnson A, et al. Population pharmacokinetics of oral diclofenac for acute pain in children. *Br J Clin Pharmacol.* 2008;66:846–853.
177. Reed MD, Rodarte A, Blumer JL, et al. The single-dose pharmacokinetics of midazolam and its primary metabolite in pediatric patients after oral and intravenous administration. *J Clin Pharmacol.* 2001;41:1359–1369.
178. Alcorn J, McNamara PJ. Ontogeny of hepatic and renal systemic clearance pathways in infants. Part I. *Clin Pharmacokinet.* 2002;41:959–998.
179. Mason KP, Lerman J. Dexmedetomidine in children: Current knowledge and future applications. *Anesth Analg.* 2011;113:1129–1142.
180. Petroz GC, Sikich N, James M, et al. A phase I, two-center study of the pharmacokinetics and pharmacodynamics of dexmedetomidine in children. *Anesthesiology.* 2006;105:1098–1110.
181. Vilo S, Rautiainen P, Kaisti K, et al. Pharmacokinetics of intravenous dexmedetomidine in children under 11 yr of age. *Br J Anaesth.* 2008;100:697–700.
182. Belleville JP, Ward DS, Bloor BC, et al. Effects of intravenous dexmedetomidine in humans. I. Sedation, ventilation and metabolic rate. *Anesthesiology.* 1992;77:1125–1133.
183. Mason DP, Zurakowski D, Zgleszewski SE, et al. High dose dexmedetomidine as the sole sedative for pediatric MRI. *Paediatr Anaesth.* 2008;18:403–411.
184. Tobias JD, Goble TJ, Bates G, et al. Effects of dexmedetomidine on intraoperative motor and somatosensory evoked potential monitoring during spinal surgery in adolescents. *Paediatr Anaesth.* 2008;18:1082–1088.
185. Mason KP, Zgleszewski S, Forman RE, et al. An exaggerated hypertensive response to glycopyrrolate therapy for bradycardia associated with high-dose dexmedetomidine. *Anesth Analg.* 2009;108:906–908.
186. Apfelbaum JL, Caplan RA, Connis RT, et al. Updated by the American Society of Anesthesiologists (ASA) Committee on standards and practice parameters. Practice guidelines for preoperative fasting and the use of pharmacologic agents to reduce the risk of pulmonary aspiration: Application to healthy patients undergoing elective procedures. *Anesthesiology.* 2011;114:495–511.
187. Cavell B. Gastric emptying in infants. *Acta Paediatr Scand.* 1971;60:370–371.
188. Schoenfelder RC, Ponnamma CM, Freyle D, et al. Residual gastric fluid volume and chewing gum before surgery. *Anesth Analg.* 2006;102:415–417.
189. Engelhardt T, Webster NR. Pulmonary aspiration of gastric contents in anaesthesia. *Br J Anaesth.* 1999;83:453–460.
190. Bricker SRW, McLuckie A, Nightingale DA. Gastric aspirates after trauma in children. *Anaesthesia.* 1989;44:721–724.
191. Samsom M, Bharucha A, Gerich JE, et al. Diabetes mellitus and gastric emptying: Questions and issues in clinical practice. *Diabetes Metab Res Rev.* 2009;25:502–514.
192. Ma J, Rayner CK, Jones KL, et al. Diabetic gastroparesis. Diagnosis and management. *Drugs.* 2009;69:971–986.
193. Cook-Sather SD, Gallagher PR, Kruge LE, et al. Overweight/obesity and gastric fluid characteristics in pediatric day surgery: Implications for fasting guidelines and pulmonary aspiration risk. *Anesth Analg.* 2009;109:727–736.
194. Manley S, de Kelaita G, Joseph NJ, et al. Preoperative pregnancy testing in ambulatory surgery. Incidence and impact of positive results. *Anesthesiology.* 1995;83:690–693.

195. von Ungern-Sternberg BS, Boda K, Chambers NA, et al. Risk assessment for respiratory complications in paediatric anaesthesia: A prospective cohort study. *Lancet.* 2010;376:773–783.
196. Tait AR, Malviya S. Anesthesia for the child with an upper respiratory tract infection: Still a dilemma? *Anesth Analg.* 2005;100:59–65.
197. Tait AR, Malviya S, Voepel-Lewis T, et al. Risk factors for perioperative adverse respiratory events in children with upper respiratory tract infections. *Anesthesiology.* 2001;95:299–306.
198. Cohen MM, Cameron CB. Should you cancel the operation when a child has an upper respiratory tract infection? *Anesth Analg.* 1991;72:282–288.
199. Pavia AT. Viral infections of the lower respiratory tract: Old viruses, new viruses, and the role of diagnosis. *Clin Infect Dis.* 2011;52(suppl 4):S284–S289.
200. Netuveli G, Hurwitz B, Levy M, et al. Ethnic variations in UK asthma frequency, morbidity, and health-service use; a systematic review and meta-analysis. *Lancet.* 2005;365(9456):312–317.
201. Scalfaro P, Sly PD, Sims C, et al. Salbutamol prevents the increase of respiratory resistance caused by tracheal intubation during sevoflurane anesthesia in asthmatic children. *Anesth Analg.* 2001;93:898–902.
202. Carroll JL. Obstructive sleep-disordered breathing in children: New controversies, new directions. *Clin Chest Med.* 2003;24:261–282.
203. Brown KA, Laferriere A, Lakheeram I, et al. Recurrent hypoxemia in children is associated with increased analgesic sensitivity to opiates. *Anesthesiology.* 2006; 105:665–669.
204. Raghavendran S, Bagry H, Detheux G, et al. An anesthetic management protocol to decrease respiratory complications after adenotonsillectomy in children with severe sleep apnea. *Anesth Analg.* 2010;110:1093–1101.
205. Aydin ON, Ugur B, Ozgun S, et al. Pain prevention with intraoperative ketamine in outpatient children undergoing tonsillectomy or tonsillectomy and adenotomy. *J Clin Anesth.* 2007;19:115–119.
206. Cote CJ, Zaslavsky A, Downes JJ, et al. Postoperative apnea in former preterm infants after inguinal herniorrhaphy: A combined analysis. *Anesthesiology.* 1995;82:809–822.
207. Murphy JJ, Swanson T, Ansermino M, et al. The frequency of apneas in premature infants after inguinal hernia repair: Do they need overnight monitoring in the intensive care unit? *J Pediatr Surg.* 2008;43:865–868.
208. Henderson-Smart DJ, Steer P. Postoperative caffeine for preventing apnea in preterm infants. *Cochrane Database Syst Rev.* 2001;4:CD000048.
209. Frawley G, Ingelmo P. Spinal anaesthesia in the neonate. *Best Pract Res Clin Anaesthesiol.* 2010;24:337–351.
210. Kim TW, Nemergut ME. Preparation of modern anesthesia workstations for malignant hyperthermia-susceptible patients; a review of past and present practice. *Anesthesiology.* 2011;114:205–212.
211. Sabouri S, Lerman J, Heard C. Residual sevoflurane may be present after flushing the GE Anesthesia workstation for MH susceptible patients. *Anesthesiology.* 2011:A1276.
212. Gurnaney H, Brown A, Litman RS. Malignant hyperthermia and muscular dystrophies. *Anesth Analg.* 2009;109:1043–1048.
213. Footitt EJ, Sinha MD, Raiman JAJ, et al. Mitochondrial disorders and general anaesthesia: A case series and review. *Br J Anaesth.* 2008;100:436–441.
214. Firth PG. Anesthesia and hemoglobinopathies. *Anesthesiol Clin.* 2009;27:321–327.
215. Firth PG. Anaesthesia for peculiar cells-a century of sickle cell disease. *Br J Anaesth.* 2005;95:287–299.
216. Vichinsky EP, Haberkern CM, Neumayr L, et al. A comparison of conservative and aggressive transfusion regimens in the perioperative management of sickle cell disease. *N Engl J Med.* 1995;333:206–213.
217. Fu T, Corrigan NJ, Quinn CT, et al. Minor elective surgical procedures using general anesthesia in children with sickle cell anemia without pre-operative blood transfusion. *Pediatr Blood Cancer.* 2005;45:43–47.
218. Lerman J. Anterior mediastinal masses in children. *Semin Anesth Perioper Med Pain.* 2007;26:133–140.
219. Borenstein SH, Gerstle T, Malkin D, et al. The effects of pre-biopsy corticosteroid treatment on the diagnosis of mediastinal lymphoma. *J Pediatr Surg.* 2000; 35:973–976.
220. McDonnell C, Barlow R, Campisi P, et al. Fatal peri-operative acute tumour lysis syndrome precipitated by dexamethasone. *Anaesthesia.* 2008;63:652–655.
221. Wilson W, Taubert KA, Gewitz M, et al. Prevention of infection endocarditis. Guidelines from the American Heart Association. A guideline from the American Heart Association Rheumatic Fever, Endocarditis, and Kawasaki Disease Committee, Council on Cardiovascular Disease in the Young, and the Council on Clinical Cardiology, Council on Cardiovascular Surgery and Anesthesia, and the Quality of Care and Outcomes Research Interdisciplinary Working Group. *Circulation.* 2007;116:1736–1754, e376–e377.
222. Brenn BR. Anesthesia for pediatric obesity. *Anesthesiol Clin North America.* 2005; 23:745–764.
223. Mortensen A, Lenz K, Abildstrom H, et al. Anesthetizing the obese child. *Paediatr Anaesth.* 2011;21:623–629.
224. Greenland KB, Edwards MJ, Hutton NJ. External auditory meatus-sternal notch relationship in adults in the sniffing position: A magnetic resonance imaging study. *Br J Anaesth.* 2010;104:268–269.
225. van der Griend BF, Lister NA, McKenzyie IM, et al. Postoperative mortality in children after 101,885 anesthetic at a tertiary pediatric hospital. *Anesth Analg.* 2011;112:1440–1447.
226. Davidson AJ, Huang GH, Czarnecki C, et al. Awareness during anesthesia in children: A prospective cohort study. *Anesth Analg.* 2005;100:653–661.
227. Hudson AE, Hemmings HC Jr. Are anaesthetics toxic to the brain? *Br J Anaesth.* 2011;107:30–37.
228. Pichichero ME. A review of evidence supporting the American Academy of Pediatrics recommendation for prescribing cephalosporin antibiotics for penicillin-allergic patients. *Pediatrics.* 2005;115:1048–1057.
229. Murphy A, Campbell DE, Baines D, et al. Allergic reactions to propofol in egg-allergic children. *Anesth Analg.* 2011;113:140–144.
230. Sampathi V, Lerman J. Perioperative latex allergy in children. *Anesth Analg.* 2011;114:673–680.
231. de Queiroz M, Combet S, Bérard J, et al. Latex allergy in children: Modalities and prevention. *Paediatr Anaesth.* 2009;19:313–319.
232. White MC, Cook TM, Stoddart PA. A critique of elective pediatric supraglottic airway devices. *Paediatr Anaesth.* 2009;19(suppl 1):55–65.
233. Park C, Bahk JH, Ahn WS, et al. The laryngeal mask airway in infants and children. *Can J Anaesth.* 2001;48:413–417.
234. Dullenkopf A, Gerber A, Weiss M. The Microcuff™ tube allows a longer time interval until unsafe cuff pressures are reached in children. *Can J Anaesth.* 2004; 51:997–1001.
235. Eschertzhuber S, Salgo B, Schmitz A, et al. Cuffed endotracheal tubes in children reduce sevoflurane and medical gas consumption and related costs. *Acta Anaesthesiol Scand.* 2010;54:855–858.
236. Habre W. Neonatal ventilation. *Best Pract Res Clin Anaesthesiol.* 2010;24:353–364.
237. Lerman J. On cricoid pressure: "May the force be with you". *Anesth Analg.* 2009; 109:1363–1366.
238. Walker RWM, Ravi R, Haylett K. Effect of cricoid force on airway calibre in children: A bronchoscopic assessment. *Br J Anaesth.* 2010;104:71–74.
239. Batra YK, Ivanova M, Ali SS, et al. The efficacy of a subhypnotic dose of propofol in preventing laryngospasm following tonsillectomy and adenoidectomy in children. *Paediatr Anaesth.* 2005;15:1094–1097.
240. Luginbuehl I, Bissonnette B. Thermal regulation. In: Coté CJ, Lerman J, Todres ID, eds. *A Practice of Anesthesia for Infants and Children.* 4th ed. Philadelphia, PA: Elsevier Inc; 2009:557–567.
241. Murat I, Berniere J, Constant I. Evaluation of the efficacy of a forced-air warmer (Bair Hugger) during spinal surgery in children. *J Clin Anesth.* 1994;6: 425–429.
242. Larach MG, Gronert GA, Allen GC, et al. Clinical presentation, treatment, and complications of malignant hyperthermia. *Anesth Analg.* 2010;110:498–507.
243. Edwards JJ, Soto RG, Bedford RF. Bispectral Index™ values are higher during halothane vs. sevoflurane anesthesia in children, but not in infants. *Acta Anaesthesiol Scand.* 2005;49:1084–1087.
244. Kaki AM, Almarakbi WA. Does patient position influence the reading of the bispectral index monitor? *Anesth Analg.* 2009;109:1843–1846.
245. Chundamala J, Wright JG, Kemp SM. An evidence-based review of parental presence during anesthesia induction and parent/child anxiety. *Can J Anaesth.* 2009; 56:57–70.
246. Yip P, Middleton P, Cyna AM, et al. Non-pharmacological interventions for assisting the induction of anaesthesia in children. *Cochrane Database Syst Rev.* 2009;8:CD006447.
247. Kain ZN, MacLaren J, McClain BC, et al. Effects of age and emotionality on the effectiveness of midazolam administered preoperatively to children. *Anesthesiology.* 2007;107:545–552.
248. Coté CJ, Cohen IT, Suresh S, et al. A comparison of three doses of a commercially prepared oral midazolam syrup in children. *Anesth Analg.* 2002;94:37–43.
249. Bergendahl H, Lonnqvist PA, Eksborg S. Clonidine in paediatric anaesthesia: Review of the literature and comparison with benzodiazepines for premedication. *Acta Anaesthesiol Scand.* 2006;50:135–143.
250. Zub D, Berkenbosch JW, Tobias JD. Preliminary experience with oral dexmedetomidine for procedural and anesthetic premedication. *Paediatr Anaesth.* 2005;15:932–938.
251. Karl HW, Rosenberger JL, Larach MG, et al. Transmucosal administration of midazolam for premedication in pediatric patients; comparison of the nasal and sublingual routes. *Anesthesiology.* 1993;78:885–891.
252. Karl HW, Keifer AT, Rosenberger JL, et al. Comparison of the safety and efficacy of intranasal midazolam or sufentanil for preinduction of anesthesia in pediatric patients. *Anesthesiology.* 1992;76:209–215.
253. Yuen VM, Hui TW, Irwin MG, et al. Optimal timing for the administration of intranasal dexmedetomidine for premedication in children. *Anaesthesia.* 2010; 65:922–929.
254. Hannallah RS, Patel RI. Low-dose intramuscular ketamine for anesthesia pre-induction in young children undergoing brief outpatient procedures. *Anesthesiology.* 1989;70:598–600.
255. Fukumoto M, Arima H, Ito S, et al. Distorted perception of smell by volatile agents facilitated inhalational induction of anesthesia. *Paediatr Anaesth.* 2005; 15:98–101.
256. Przybylo HJ, Tarbell SE, Stevenson GW. Mask fear in children presenting for anesthesia: Aversion, phobia, or both? *Paediatr Anaesth.* 2005;15:366–370.
257. Agnor R, Sikich N, Lerman J. Single-breath vital capacity rapid inhalation induction in children: 8% sevoflurane versus 5% halothane. *Anesthesiology.* 1998; 89:379–384.

258. Lander JA, Weltman BJ, So SS. EMLA and amethocaine for reduction of children's pain associated with needle insertion. *Cochrane Database Syst Rev.* 2009; 3:CD004236.
259. Kleiber C, Schutte DL, McCarthy AM, et al. Predictors of topical anesthetic effectiveness in children. *J Pain.* 2007;8:168–174.
260. Vetter T. A comparison of EMLA cream versus nitrous oxide for pediatric venous cannulation. *J Clin Anesth.* 1995;7:486–490.
261. Tanaka M, Sato M, Saito A, et al. Reevaluation of rectal ketamine premedication in children: Comparison with rectal midazolam. *Anesthesiology.* 2000;93:1217–1224.
262. Hampson-Evans D, Morgan P, Farrar M. Pediatric laryngospasm. *Paediatr Anaesth.* 2008;18:303–307.
263. Al-alami AA, Markakis Zestos M, Baraka AS. Pediatric laryngospasm: Prevention and treatment. *Curr Opin Anaesthesiol.* 2009;22:288–295.
264. Afshan G, Chohan U, Qamar-UI-Hoda M, et al. Is there a role of a small dose of propofol in the treatment of laryngeal spasm? *Paediatr Anaesth.* 2002;12:625–628.
265. Kraemer FW, Stricker PA, Gurnaney HGG, et al. Bradycardia during induction of anesthesia with sevoflurane in children with Down syndrome. *Anesth Analg.* 2010;111:1259–1263.
266. Dubois MC, Gouyet L, Murat I, et al. Lactated Ringer with 1% dextrose: An appropriate solution for peri-operative fluid therapy in children. *Paediatr Anaesth.* 1992;2:99–104.
267. Rando K, Zunini G, Negroto A. Intraoperative hyponatremia during craniofacial surgery. *Paediatr Anaesth.* 2009;19:358–363.
267a. O'Malley CMN, Frumento RJ, Hardy MA, et al. A randomized, double-blind comparison of Lactated Ringer's solution and 0.9% NaCl during renal transplantation. *Anesth Analg.* 2005;100:1518–1524.
268. Holliday MA, Segar WE. The maintenance need for water in parenteral fluid therapy. *Pediatrics.* 1957;19:823–832.
269. Holliday MA, Friedman AL, Segar WE, et al. Acute hospital-induced hyponatremia in children: A physiologic approach. *J Pediatr.* 2004;145:584–587.
270. Morley SL. Red blood cell transfusions in acute paediatrics. *Arch Dis Child Educ Pract Ed.* 2009;94:65–73.
271. Barcelona SL, Thompson AA, Coté CJ. Intraoperative pediatric blood transfusion therapy: A review of common issues. Part II: Transfusion therapy, special considerations, and reduction of allogenic blood transfusions. *Paediatr Anaesth.* 2005;15:814–830.
272. Kranke P, Eberhart LH, Toker H, et al. A prospective evaluation of the POVOC score for the prediction of postoperative vomiting in children. *Anesth Analg.* 2007;105:1592–1597.
273. Schreiner MS, Nicolson SC, Martin T, et al. Should children drink before discharge from day surgery? *Anesthesiology.* 1992;76:528–533.
274. Goodarzi M, Matar MM, Shafa M, et al. A prospective randomized blinded study of the effect of intravenous fluid therapy on postoperative nausea and vomiting in children undergoing strabismus surgery. *Paediatr Anaesth.* 2006;16:49–53.
275. Konig MW, Varughese AM, Brennen KA, et al. Quality of recovery from two types of general anesthesia for ambulatory dental surgery in children: A double-blind, randomized trial. *Paediatr Anaesth.* 2009;19:748–755.
276. Engelman E, Salengros JC, Barvais L. How much does pharmacologic prophylaxis reduce postoperative vomiting in children? Calculation of prophylaxis effectiveness and expected incidence of vomiting under treatment using Bayesian meta-analysis. *Anesthesiology.* 2008;109:1023–1035.
277. Kim MS, Coté CJ, Cristoloveanu C, et al. There is no dose-escalation response to dexamethasone (0.0625–1.0 mg/kg) in pediatric tonsillectomy or adenotonsillectomy patients for preventing vomiting, reducing pain, shortening time to first liquid intake, or the incidence of voice change. *Anesth Analg.* 2007;104:1052–1058.
278. Czarnetzki C, Elia N, Lysakowski C, et al. Dexamethasone and risk of nausea and vomiting and postoperative bleeding after tonsillectomy in children, a randomized trails. *JAMA.* 2008;300:2621–2630.
279. Brigger MT, Cunningham MJ, Hartnick CJ. Dexamethasone administration and postoperative bleeding risk in children undergoing tonsillectomy. *Arch Otolaryngol Head Neck Surg.* 2010;136:766–772.
280. Baugh RF, Archer SM, Mitchell RB, et al. Clinical practice guidelines: Tonsillectomy in children. *Otolaryngol Head Neck Surg.* 2011;144:S1–S30.
281. Polaner DM, Zuk J, Luong K, et al. Positive intravascular test dose criteria in children during total intravenous anesthesia with propofol and remifentanil are different than during inhaled anesthesia. *Anesth Analg.* 2010;110:41–44.
282. Kumar P, Rudra A, Pan AK, et al. Caudal additives in pediatrics: A comparison among midazolam, ketamine, and neostigmine coadministered with bupivacaine. *Anesth Analg.* 2005;101:69–73.
283. Tsui BC, Wagner A, Cave D, et al. Thoracic and lumbar epidural analgesia via the caudal approach using electrical stimulation guidance in pediatric patients: A review of 289 patients. *Anesthesiology.* 2004;100:683–689.
284. Berde CB. Convolutions associated with pediatric regional anesthesia. *Anesth Analg.* 1992;175:164–166.
285. Bosenberg AT, Thomas J, Cronje L, et al. Pharmacokinetics and efficacy of ropivacaine for continuous epidural infusion in neonates and infants. *Paediatr Anaesth.* 2005;15:739–749.
286. Ciechanowicz S, Patil V. Lipid emulsion for local anesthetic systemic toxicity. *Anesth Res Pract.* 2012;2012:131784.
287. Ecoffey C. Safety in pediatric regional anesthesia. *Paediatr Anaesth.* 2012;22: 25–30.
288. Pounder DR, Blackstock D, Steward DJ. Tracheal extubation in children: Halothane versus isoflurane, anesthetized versus awake. *Anesthesiology.* 1991;74:653–655.
289. Zeltser D, Justo D, Halkin A, et al. Torsade de Pointes due to noncardiac drugs: Most patient have easily identifiable risk factors. *Medicine.* 2003;82:282–290.
290. Arai YCP, Fukunaga K, Hirota S, et al. The effect of chin lift and jaw thrust while in the lateral position on stridor score in anesthetized children adenotonsillar hypertrophy. *Anesth Analg.* 2004;99:1638–1641.
291. Hajiha M, DuBord MA, Liu H, et al. Opioid receptor mechanisms at the hypoglossal motor pool and effects on tongue muscle activity in vivo. *J Physiol.* 2009; 587:2677–2692.
292. Murat I, Constant I, MaudHuy H. Perioperative anaesthetic morbidity in children: A database of 24 165 anaesthetics over a 30-month period. *Paediatr Anaesth.* 2004;14:158–166.
293. Holmes JR, Hensinger RN, Wojtys EW. Postoperative pulmonary edema in young, athletic adults. *Am J Sports Med.* 1992;19:365–371.
294. Bryan YF, Hoke LK, Taghon TA, et al. A randomized trial comparing sevoflurane and propofol in children undergoing MRI scans. *Paediatr Anaesth.* 2009;19:672–681.
295. Dahmani S, Stany I, Brasher C, et al. Pharmacological prevention of sevoflurane- and desflurane-related emergence agitation in children: A meta-analysis of published studies. *Br J Anaesth.* 2010;104:216–223.
296. Cravero J, Surgenor S, Whalen K. Emergence agitation in paediatric patients after sevoflurane anaesthesia and no surgery: A comparison with halothane. *Paediatr Anaesth.* 2000;10:419–424.
297. Sikich N, Lerman J. Develop and psychometric evaluation of the pediatric anesthesia emergence delirium scale. *Anesthesiology.* 2004;100:1138–1145.
298. Lerman J. Surgical and patient factors involved in postoperative nausea and vomiting. *Br J Anaesth.* 1992;69(suppl 1):24S–32S.
299. Ho KY, Gan TJ. Pharmacology, pharmacogenetics, and clinical efficacy of 5-hydroxytryptamine type 3 receptor antagonists for postoperative nausea and vomiting. *Curr Opin Anaesth.* 2006;19:606–611.
300. Ecoffey C. Pediatric regional anesthesia-update. *Curr Opin Anaesthesiol.* 2007; 20:232–235.
301. Anderson BJ, Palmer GM. Recent developments in the pharmacological management of pain in children. *Curr Opin Anaesthesiol.* 2006;19:285–292.
302. Birmingham PK, Suresh S, Ambrosy A, et al. Parent-assisted or nurse-assisted epidural analgesia: Is this feasible in pediatric patients? *Paediatr Anaesth.* 2009;19:1084–1089.
303. Kart T, Christrup LL, Rasmussen M. Recommended use of morphine in neonates, infants and children base on a literature review: Part 1-pharmacokinetics. *Paediatr Anaesth.* 1997;7:5–11.

CHAPTER

43 Anesthesia for Laparoscopic and Robotic Surgeries

GIRISH P. JOSHI • ANTHONY CUNNINGHAM

Key Points

1. Minimally invasive surgery reduces surgical stress and postoperative pain as well as reduces overall morbidity, thus resulting in rapid recovery, earlier ambulation, shorter hospital stay, and rapid return to daily living activities.
2. Robotic surgery offers technical advantages over laparoscopic surgery and thus should further expand the field of minimally invasive surgery.
3. Pneumoperitoneum creation and patient positioning during laparoscopic and robotic surgeries can cause significant physiologic changes, which may result in significant cardiorespiratory compromise, particularly in patients with significant cardiopulmonary dysfunctions.
4. The cardiovascular changes during pneumoperitoneum include an increase in systemic vascular resistance and mean arterial pressure, cardiac arrhythmia (bradycardia and tachycardia), while changes in cardiac filling volumes and cardiac index vary depending on the patients' status.
5. The hemodynamic changes in the morbidly obese are similar to those observed in the nonobese.
6. Pneumoperitoneum can reduce splanchnic and renal blood flows, while increasing intracranial pressures.
7. Cephalad displacement of the diaphragm caused by increased intra-abdominal pressure and patient positioning, which can lead to reduction in functional residual capacity and total lung compliance, results in basal atelectasis and increased airway pressures.
8. Carbon dioxide insufflation for creation of pneumoperitoneum increases carbon dioxide absorption, but the changes in arterial carbon dioxide concentrations remain clinically insignificant in healthy patients.
9. Balanced general anesthesia with tracheal intubation and mechanical ventilation with acceptance of higher end-tidal carbon dioxide levels remains the best practice for minimally invasive surgical procedures.
10. Aggressive multimodal analgesic as well as antiemetic prophylaxis and treatment are required to reduce these common postoperative adverse effects.
11. Should intraoperative cardiopulmonary impairment occur, it is important to confirm that the intra-abdominal pressure is <15 mm Hg as well as rule out traumatic vascular injuries, carbon dioxide embolism, subcutaneous emphysema, capnothorax, and capnomediastinum.
12. If subcutaneous emphysema extends to the chest and neck, the carbon dioxide can track to the thorax and mediastinum, thereby resulting in capnothorax or capnomediastinum.
13. Significant subcutaneous emphysema may lead to development of late hypercarbia (i.e., in the recovery room).
14. Hyperventilation and positive end-expiratory pressure should allow early resolution of capnothorax and carbon dioxide embolism.
15. If there is no improvement in the vital signs with routine management, it is imperative to release the pneumoperitoneum and place the patient in a supine (or Trendelenburg) position.

Multimedia

 Laparoscopic

INTRODUCTION

The development of "minimally invasive surgery" or "minimal access surgery" has revolutionized the field of surgery. The growth of laparoscopic surgical procedures is due to the use of smaller incisions that reduce surgical stress and postoperative pain as well as reduce overall morbidity, thus resulting in rapid recovery, earlier ambulation, shorter hospital stay, and rapid
1 return to daily living activities (Table 43-1). These benefits are achieved without compromising surgical outcomes.[1–6] In addition, a minimally invasive approach has allowed several procedures to be performed on an outpatient basis, where previously a hospital stay was necessary.[7–11] Furthermore, it has allowed the implementation of rapid rehabilitation recovery programs that have been shown to further improve perioperative outcome and reduce hospital stay.[12] Overall, there is potential for significant cost savings.

With growing surgical expertise and continuing improvements in technology, more extensive laparoscopic procedures are being performed in a wide range of patients, including morbidly obese, older, and sicker patients with significant comorbidities as well as pregnant and pediatric patients.[1] However, conventional laparoscopy has several technical limitations, such as reduced range of motion and instrument dexterity as well as a two-dimensional view of the operative field.[6] Technologic advances in computer power and robotic engineering have allowed us to address some of these limitations. Robotic surgery improves depth perception through a high-definition, magnified, and three-dimensional view of the operative field and provides intuitive instrument control that mimics natural hand and wrist movements and eliminates surgeon tremor. Overall, robotic surgery enhances surgeons' skills and thus has the potential to transform technically challenging open or laparoscopic procedures, particularly those requiring improved visualization and/or complex reconstruction necessitating extensive suturing, into technically feasible minimally invasive procedures. Robotic surgery can be applied to virtually every surgical subspecialty (e.g., general, colorectal, head and neck, gynecologic, thoracic, and cardiac surgeries). The advantages of robotic surgery are expected to broaden the appli-
2 cation of the minimally invasive surgical paradigm.

Despite the potential advantages of laparoscopic and robotic surgeries, they are associated with significant physiologic changes as well as new complications (some potentially life-threatening)
3 that are usually not seen with the traditional open approach[1] (Table 43-2). In addition, robotic procedures can have significantly prolonged operative times and require patients to be placed in extreme positions. Because the robotic system is large, it limits the access to the patient and invades the anesthesia working space. Overall, this presents significant challenges in anesthetic management. Therefore, a thorough understanding of potential physiologic changes and perioperative complications associated with laparoscopic and robotic surgeries is necessary to provide optimal patient care and improve perioperative morbidity and mortality.

This chapter discusses the anesthetic management of adult patients undergoing laparoscopic and abdominal robotic surgeries. However, endoscopic and robotic cardiac and thoracic surgeries (e.g., video-assisted thoracic surgery [VATS]) that are increasingly performed are discussed elsewhere (Chapter 37).

SURGICAL TECHNIQUES

Laparoscopic procedure entails intraperitoneal insufflation of carbon dioxide (CO_2) to create pneumoperitoneum that allows surgical exposure and manipulation. Carbon dioxide is used because it is noncombustible and more soluble in blood, which increases the safety margin and decreases the consequences of gas embolism. Unlike nitrous oxide (N_2O), CO_2 does not support combustion and, therefore, can be used safely with diathermy. Compared to helium, the high blood solubility of CO_2 and its capability for pulmonary excretion reduce the risk of adverse outcomes in the event of gas embolism. An abdominal wall lift system (i.e., a gasless laparoscopy) has been developed to achieve surgical space while avoiding the cardiopulmonary effects of CO_2 pneumoperitoneum.[13] Although this approach appears to be safe,

TABLE 43-1. ADVANTAGES OF MINIMALLY INVASIVE SURGERY

- Minimizes surgical incision and stress response
- Decreases postoperative pain and opioid requirements
- Preserves diaphragmatic function
- Improves postoperative pulmonary function
- Earlier return of bowel function
- Fewer wound-related complications
- Earlier ambulation
- Shorter hospital stays
- Early return to normal activities and work
- Reduces health costs

TABLE 43-2. POTENTIAL COMPLICATIONS DURING LAPAROSCOPY

- Creation of pneumoperitoneum (carbon dioxide insufflation and intra-abdominal pressure)
  - Hemodynamic
  - Pulmonary
  - Neurohumoral responses
- Surgical instrumentation
  - Injury: Vascular, gastrointestinal, genitourinary, nervous, thermal
  - Subcutaneous emphysema
  - Capnothorax, capnomediastinum, capnopericardium
  - Gas embolism
- Patient positioning

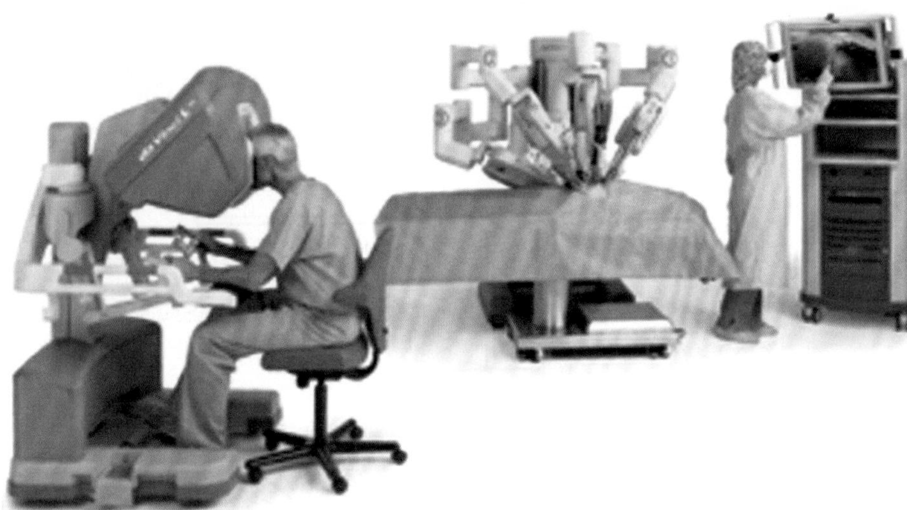

FIGURE 43-1. A control console where the surgeon is stationed and operates the robotic arms and camera. © 2012 Intuitive Surgical, Inc.

it has not been accepted in routine clinical practice because it increases operating times and surgical costs without improving clinical outcomes.[13]

The initial access necessary for CO_2 insufflation could be achieved either through a blind insertion of a Veress needle that consists of a blunt-tipped, spring-loaded inner stylet and sharp outer needle through a small subumbilical incision or a trocar inserted under direct vision. The open insertion of the trocar using a minilaparotomy approach guarantees safe creation of pneumoperitoneum and avoids the dangers of blind insertion.

Upon confirmation of appropriate placement, a variable flow electronic insufflator that automatically terminates gas flow at a preset intra-abdominal pressure (IAP) is used to achieve pneumoperitoneum. It is standard of care to maintain the IAP below 15 mm Hg, because higher pressures can have significant physiologic consequences and can increase the incidence of intraoperative complications. An access port is then inserted in place of the needle to maintain insufflation during the procedure. A video laparoscope, inserted through the port, allows visualization of the operative field. Additional access ports are inserted through a number of small skin incisions, which allow the introduction of surgical dissection and suction instruments. The secondary ports are placed under direct vision, preferably with the help of transillumination of the abdominal wall to identify superficial abdominal wall vessels.

The Da Vinci Surgical System (Intuitive Surgical Inc., Sunnyvale, California) is the most common robotic platform used currently. It consists of three components: a control console where the surgeon sits and operates the robotic arms and camera (Fig. 43-1), an equipment tower that includes an optical system, and the patient side cart that includes robotic arms.[3,4,6] Similar to a laparoscopic procedure, robotic surgery involves development of pneumoperitoneum and placement of a video camera (a high-definition three-dimensional vision system) and ports. This is followed by placement of the robotic arms, a crucial and tedious part of the procedure (Fig. 43-2). An assistant is at the patient side for suctioning, retraction, and passage of suture or sponges.

Patient position during minimally invasive surgery varies significantly based on the surgical procedure. Patients undergoing upper abdominal procedures require a reverse Trendelenburg (head-up) position, while those undergoing lower abdominal procedures require Trendelenburg (head-down) position. The head-up or head-down position can be steep. In addition, the operating tables may be rotated laterally (right or left lateral) to further facilitate surgical exposure. Also, patients undergoing pelvic surgery (e.g., radial prostatectomy and hysterectomy) may be placed in a lithotomy position. Patients undergoing urologic surgery, particularly renal procedures, may be placed in lateral or semilateral positions combined with a flexion (i.e., jackknife) position. The considerations related to patient positioning are discussed in Chapter 28.

PHYSIOLOGIC EFFECTS

The physiologic consequences of laparoscopy can be complex and depend on the interactions between the patient's pre-existing cardiopulmonary status and surgical factors such as the magnitude of IAP, degree of CO_2 absorption, alteration of patient position, and the type of surgical procedure.[2,14,15] In addition, the anesthetic technique may influence the physiologic changes; however, these effects may be minimal with modern anesthetic techniques. Of note, physiologic changes are well tolerated by most healthy patients; however, they could have adverse consequences in patients with limited cardiopulmonary reserve.

Cardiovascular Effects

The changes in the cardiovascular function during laparoscopy are due to the mechanical and neuroendocrine effects of pneumoperitoneum and the effects of absorbed CO_2 and patient positioning as well as patient factors such as cardiopulmonary status and intravascular volume (Table 43-3). The induction of pneumoperitoneum in the supine position (rather than head-down position) and limiting the IAP to 12 to 15 mm Hg minimize the alterations in cardiovascular function during laparoscopy.[2,14]

The cardiovascular changes of laparoscopy include an increase in systemic vascular resistance (SVR) and mean arterial pressure (MAP), which is caused by increased sympathetic output from
4 CO_2 absorption and a neuroendocrine response to pneumoperitoneum.[2,14,15] Pneumoperitoneum-related increased IAP results in activation of the sympathetic system with catecholamine release and the renin–angiotensin system with vasopressin release.[16] The profile of vasopressin release parallels the time course of changes

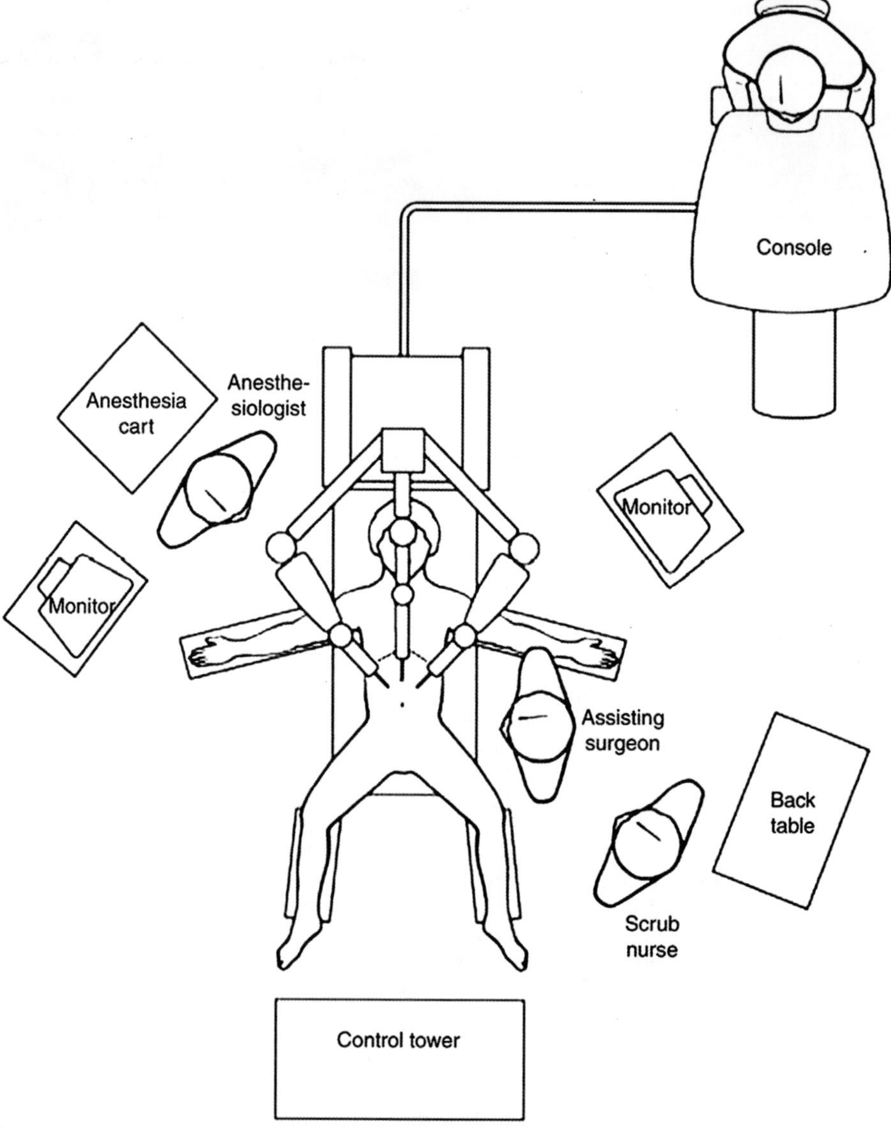

FIGURE 43-2. Layout of the operating room during robotic surgery. Reproduced from:.

TABLE 43-3. HEMODYNAMIC EFFECTS OF MINIMALLY INVASIVE SURGERY

- Increased systemic vascular resistance and mean arterial pressure
  - Causes: Hypercarbia, neuroendocrine response (e.g., increased catecholamines, vasopressin, cortisol), mechanical factors (e.g., direct compression of aorta)
- Variable change (increased or no change) in cardiac filling volumes
  - Causes: Compression of intra-abdominal organs (i.e., liver and spleen)
- Variable change (decreased or no change) in cardiac index
  - Causes: Increased afterload, decreased venous return, and cardiac filling
- Cardiac dysrhythmias (brady- or tachycardia)
  - Causes: Peritoneal stretch, hypercarbia, hypoxia, capnothorax, pulmonary embolism

in SVR. In addition, compression of the arterial vasculature from increased IAP may also lead to an increase in SVR. These neuroendocrine and mechanical responses supersede the hypercapnia-induced arteriolar dilation and decrease SVR. The increase in SVR may increase the myocardial wall tension and, thus, may increase the myocardial oxygen demand. However, myocardial ischemia, as suggested by electrocardiogram-ST–segment changes, is not observed.[17]

The changes in cardiac filling pressures and volumes during laparoscopy appear to be complex. Increased cardiac filling pressures may reflect increased intrathoracic pressures caused by pneumoperitoneum and increased sympathetic output due to hypercapnia from CO_2 absorption and surgical stress. However, cardiac filling pressures may not always reflect cardiac filling volumes. Increased IAP may compress venous capacitance vessels, causing a decrease in preload (cardiac filling volume), particularly in hypovolemic patients. In contrast, compression of the abdominal organs (e.g., liver and spleen) caused by increased IAP may increase intravascular volume, which may increase cardiac filling, particularly if the patient is placed in a head-down position.[18] Overall, the cardiac filling pressures and volumes increase, but minimally.

In healthy patients, the changes in cardiac index (CI) appear to be phasic with initial reduction after induction of pneumoperitoneum and subsequent recovery within 10 to 15 minutes. Overall, the changes in CI in healthy patients are minimal. However, in patients with severe cardiac dysfunctions, there may be a significant reduction in CI and significant hemodynamic deterioration.[19] Although reduction in CI parallels the time course of increase in SVR, the cause–effect relationship between SVR and CI is unclear. In addition, significant hypercapnia and associated respiratory acidosis may decrease myocardial contractility and lower the arrhythmia threshold. Hypercarbia can cause pulmonary vasoconstriction, which may be deleterious in patients with pulmonary hypertension or right ventricular dysfunction.

5 In the morbidly obese, the hemodynamic changes are similar to those observed in the nonobese.[20,21] Although the reasons for this observation are not clear, it is hypothesized that lack of differences in hemodynamics may be related to intrinsically higher IAP in the obese (10 mm Hg vs. 5 mm Hg in the nonobese).

In the elderly, with significant coexisting cardiopulmonary disease, pneumoperitoneum and head-down position cause several hemodynamic changes.[22] Induction of pneumoperitoneum significantly increased SVR accompanied with a significant reduction in CI and ejection fraction (EF). However, the left ventricular workload remained unchanged. Upon placement in the head-down position, the cardiac preload, as determined by the left ventricular end-diastolic area, increased and CI and EF improved.[22] Oxygenation and ventilation remained unchanged, and no patients exhibited electrocardiogram signs of myocardial ischemia. Release of pneumoperitoneum resulted in a significant decrease in SVR and increased CI and left ventricular systolic work index.

The type of surgical procedure may also influence the degree of hemodynamic derangement. Surgical disruption of the esophageal hiatus during laparoscopic fundoplication may increase mediastinal and pleural pressures, resulting in a significant reduction in CI.[23,24] Patients undergoing endoscopic radical prostatectomy in the Trendelenburg position did not experience hemodynamic changes, despite prolonged duration (average 4 hours) of pneumoperitoneum.[25]

The hemodynamic changes that occur during abdominal robotic surgery appear to be similar to those observed during laparoscopic surgery. Most of the studies evaluating such changes are performed in patients undergoing prostatectomy with steep head-down position. Peritoneal insufflation and steep (40 degrees) head-down position during robotic-assisted prostatectomy increase SVR and MAP, while other hemodynamic variables remain in acceptable limits[26,27] (Figs. 43-3 and 43-4). A recent study found that although cardiac filling pressures were increased, the cardiac performance (stroke volume, cardiac output, and mixed venous oxygen saturation as well as

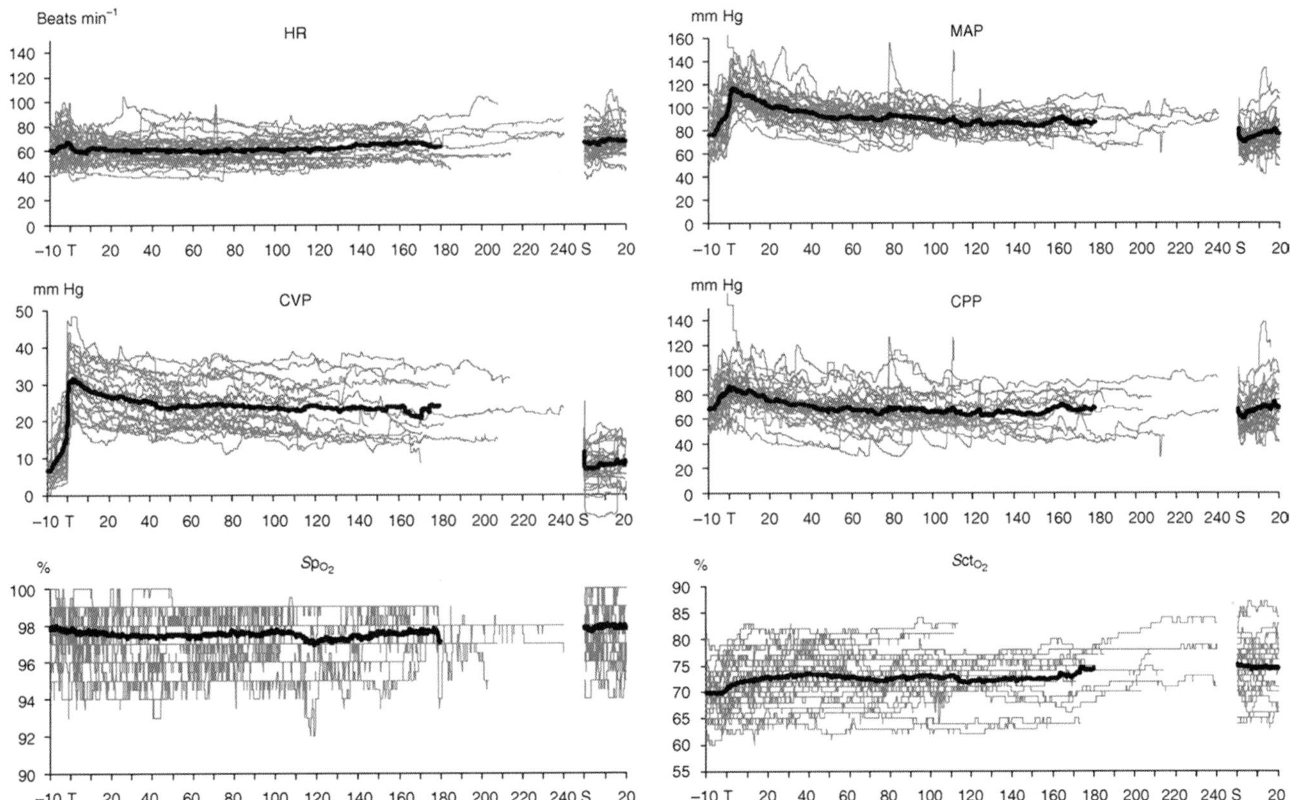

FIGURE 43-3. Hemodynamic changes (heart rate (HR), mean arterial pressures (MAPs), central venous pressures (CVPs), cerebral perfusion pressure (CPP), arterial oxygen saturation measured by pulse oximetry (SpO_2), and regional cerebral tissue oxygen saturation ($SctO_2$) in patients undergoing laparoscopic robotic prostatectomy in steep head-down position. Thin lines indicate values in individual patients and thick lines indicate mean values (From: Kalmar AF, Foubert L, Hendrickx JFA, et al. Influence of steep Trendelenburg position and CO_2 pneumoperitoneum on cardiovascular, cerebrovascular, and respiratory homeostasis during robotic prostatectomy. *Br J Anaesth.* 2012;104:433–439).

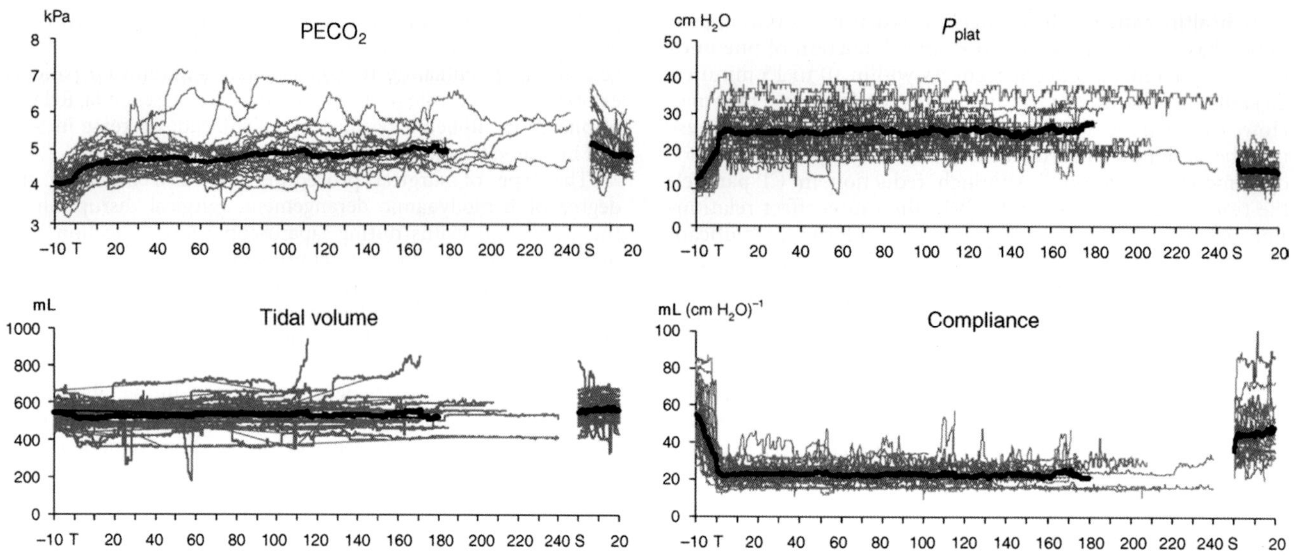

FIGURE 43-4. Changes in end-tidal CO_2 values ($PECO_2$), ventilatory plateau pressure (P_{plat}), tidal volume, and pulmonary compliance in patients undergoing laparoscopic robotic prostatectomy in steep head-down position. Thin lines indicate values in individual patients and thick lines indicate mean values (From: Kalmar AF, Foubert L, Hendrickx JFA, et al. Influence of steep Trendelenburg position and CO_2 pneumoperitoneum on cardiovascular, cerebrovascular, and respiratory homeostasis during robotic prostatectomy. *Br J Anaesth.* 2012;104:433–439).

echocardiographic cardiac dimensions) was maintained during robotic-assisted prostatectomy with patients in 45-degree head-down tilt and pneumoperitoneum with IAP 12 mm Hg[28] (Fig. 43-5). Overall, robotic surgery appears to be well tolerated in a healthy population. However, the physiologic changes in the elderly or in patients with impaired cardiopulmonary reserve undergoing robotic prostatectomy remain unknown.

Regional Perfusion (Splanchnic, Renal, Cerebral, Intraocular)

Increased IAP, systemic CO_2 absorption, and changes in patient position, along with hemodynamic changes (e.g., SVR and CI), influence splanchnic, renal, and cerebral blood flow during

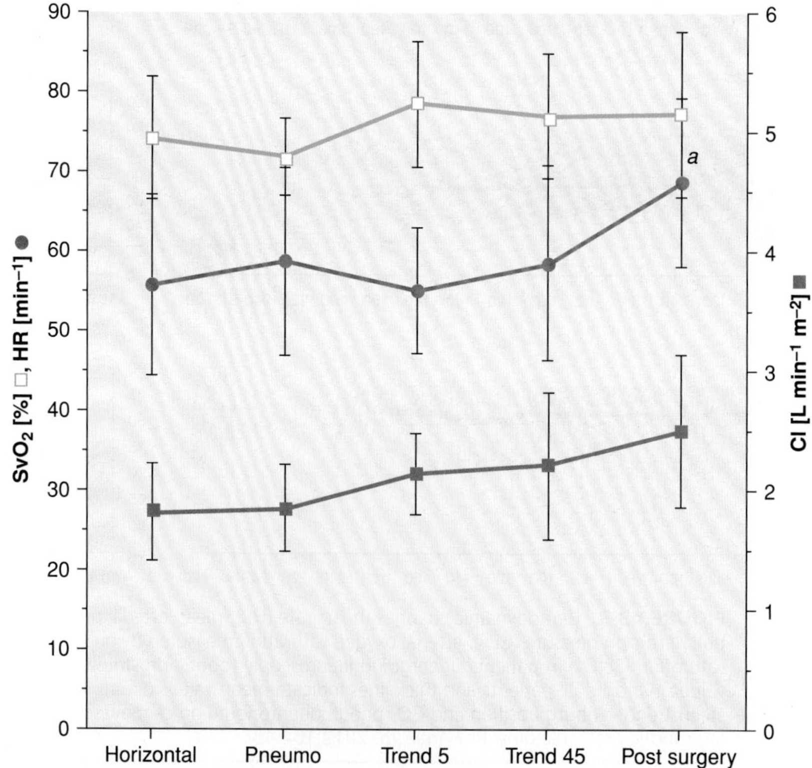

FIGURE 43-5. Changes (mean and standard deviations) in mixed venous oxygen saturation (SvO_2), heart rate (HR), and cardiac index (CI).

[a]HR significantly increased compared with horizontal, $P < .05$. (From: Lestar M, Gunnarsson L, Lagerstrand L, et al. Hemodynamic perturbations during robot-assisted laparoscopic radical prostatectomy in 45° Trendelenburg position. *Anesth Analg.* 2011;113:1069–1075).

TABLE 43-4. REGIONAL CIRCULATORY CHANGES DURING LAPAROSCOPY

- Increased cerebral perfusion and intracranial pressure
  - Caution in patient with brain tumor or ventriculoperitoneal shunt
- Decreased splanchnic blood flow
  - Variable (decreased or no change) in bowel perfusion, mechanical pneumoperitoneum compression balanced by hypercarbic vasodilatation
  - Decreased hepatic blood flow
    - Beneficial during cryoablation of liver metastasis
  - Reduced renal perfusion and urine output (reduced during pneumoperitoneum/recovery following deflation)
- Decreased femoral vein flow
  - Increased potential for deep vein thrombosis and pulmonary embolism

6 minimal access surgery (Table 43-4). However, the clinical consequences of these changes depend largely on the patient's pre-existing status.

The direct mechanical and neuroendocrine effects of pneumoperitoneum can decrease splanchnic circulation, causing reduced total hepatic blood flow and bowel circulation. However, these effects may be counterbalanced by the direct splanchnic vasodilatation caused by hypercapnia. Notwithstanding occasional reports of mesenteric ischemia following laparoscopy, the effects of pneumoperitoneum on the splanchnic circulation are not clinically significant.

The mechanical compressive and neuroendocrine effects of pneumoperitoneum may account for reduction in renal blood flow, glomerular filtration, and urine output (Table 43-5).[29,30] However, the urine output generally normalizes following pneumoperitoneum deflation with no consequent renal dysfunction. Nevertheless, there may be clinical implications in critically ill patients and those with renal dysfunction undergoing extensive laparoscopic procedures requiring prolonged pneumoperitoneum.

An increase in $PaCO_2$ during steep Trendelenburg positioning can increase cerebral blood flow and intracranial pressure with implications for patients with intracranial mass lesions. Therefore, maintenance of normocarbia is essential for preservation of cerebrovascular homeostasis.[31] However, cerebral oxygenation and cerebral perfusion remain within safe limits during combined pneumoperitoneum and Trendelenburg position.[27,32,33]

Choroidal vasodilatation and an increase in intraocular pressure may occur during CO_2 pneumoperitoneum and steep head-down position.[33] Intraocular pressure increased significantly during robotic-assisted radical prostatectomy with steep head-down position.[33] Multivariate analysis suggested that the predictors of IOP include duration of surgery and end-tidal CO_2 ($ETCO_2$).

Respiratory and Gas Exchange Effects

Changes in pulmonary function during laparoscopy include reduction in lung volume and pulmonary compliance secondary to cephalad displacement of the diaphragm caused by increased IAP and patient positioning[14,15] (Table 43-6). Reduction in functional residual capacity (FRC) and total lung compliance results in basal
7 atelectasis and increased airway pressure. In addition, the increase in minute ventilation required to avoid hypercarbia caused by systemic CO_2 absorption further increases peak airway pressures. Although these changes are well tolerated by healthy patients, significant pulmonary dysfunction may occur in patients with pre-existing pulmonary disease (see the section on complications).

The CO_2 insufflated into the peritoneal cavity is absorbed and causes hypercarbia. The absorption of gas from the peritoneal cavity depends on its diffusivity, the absorption area, and vascularity of insufflation site. Carbon dioxide absorption is greater during extraperitoneal (e.g., pelvic, hernia repair, and adrenorenal surgeries) insufflation than during intraperitoneal insufflation (e.g., cholecystectomy).[34] The CO_2 absorption reaches a plateau within 10 to 15 minutes after initiation of intraperitoneal insufflation and thus is not influenced by the duration of surgery.[35] However, it continues to increase progressively throughout extraperitoneal CO_2 insufflation.

Although laparoscopic surgery is associated with increased CO_2 absorption, the changes in arterial CO_2 ($PaCO_2$) concentra-
8 tions remain clinically insignificant in healthy patients. However, in patients with severe pulmonary disease and limited elimination of CO_2, the resulting rise in $PaCO_2$ may be significant despite aggressive hyperventilation. In addition, in this patient population, the $ETCO_2$ levels may underestimate arterial CO_2 concentrations ($PaCO_2$). Interestingly, the absorption and excretion of CO_2 in morbidly obese patients appear to be similar to that of nonobese patients.[20] However, in obese patients placed in the head-down position, arterial oxygenation and the alveolar–arterial oxygen gradient are impaired.[21]

TABLE 43-5. RENAL FUNCTION DURING LAPAROSCOPY

- Urine output reduced during laparoscopy
  - Decreased renal blood flow
  - Compression of renal parenchyma
  - Neuroendocrine
- Factors that influence urine output
  - Pre-existing renal compromise
  - Longer insufflation times
  - High intra-abdominal pressures
- Intraoperative oliguria reversible within 2 h postoperatively
- IAP <15 mm Hg safe even in patients with renal disease

TABLE 43-6. PULMONARY CHANGES DURING LAPAROSCOPY

- Diaphragm elevated
- Decreased lung volumes (e.g., functional residual capacity)
  - Increased ventilation–perfusion mismatch
  - Increased alveolar–arterial oxygen gradient
- Decreased lung compliance and increased resistance
  - Increased pleural pressures
  - Increased airway pressures
- Uneven gas distribution
- Cephalad displacement of carina
  - Endobronchial intubation

A recent study found that pH decreased during laparotomy open procedures and laparoscopic procedures with CO_2 pneumoperitoneum. However, reduced pH during the pneumoperitoneum was due to an increase in $PaCO_2$ and promptly returned to a normal value after the desufflation of the abdomen. In contrast, reduction in pH after laparotomy was from metabolic factors and persisted for approximately an hour postoperatively.[36]

A recent animal study found that the improved arterial oxygenation and gas exchange after induction of pneumoperitoneum was due to improved ventilation–perfusion matching caused by redistribution of perfusion away from the collapsed lung regions. This was probably caused by enhanced hypoxic pulmonary vasoconstriction possibly mediated via increased arterial CO_2.[37]

During robotic-assisted hysterectomy and prostatectomy performed under steep (40 degrees) head-down position, the changes in dead-space ventilation and venous admixture appear to be small.[38] Another study in patients undergoing robotic prostatectomy also found minimal changes in respiratory parameters.[27] However, the arterial end-tidal CO_2 gradient increased after 120 minutes. Therefore, $ETCO_2$ values may underestimate arterial CO_2 levels, and maintaining $ETCO_2$ between 25 and 35 mm Hg will result in $PaCO_2$ levels of 35 to 45 mm Hg. Similarly, the institution of pneumoperitoneum (IAP of 12 mm Hg) and 45-degree head-down positioning resulted in decreased lung compliance by 40%.[28] The ventilation–perfusion distribution did not differ significantly from baseline measurements, and oxygenation actually improved, probably due to optimization of intraoperative ventilation.[28]

ANESTHETIC MANAGEMENT

An optimal anesthetic technique would provide excellent intraoperative conditions while ensuring rapid recovery and low incidence of adverse effects as well as allowing early return to daily living activities.[39,40] Local and regional anesthesia (spinal and epidural) can be used for shorter laparoscopic procedures, such as diagnostic laparoscopy, which requires lower IAP and minimal head-down tilt.[40,41] Nevertheless, patient discomfort associated with creation of pneumoperitoneum and extreme position changes during the procedure can be significant. In addition, neuraxial anesthesia can cause significant sympathetic denervation, which may be associated with adverse ventilatory and circulatory responses, complicating perioperative management. Therefore, balanced general anesthesia with tracheal intubation and mechanical ventilation with acceptance of higher end-tidal carbon dioxide levels remains the best practice for minimally
9 invasive surgical procedures.

Induction of Anesthesia and Airway Management

Because of its unique recovery profile, propofol is considered the sedative–hypnotic drug of choice for induction of anesthesia. Propofol also offers an advantage over other intravenous anesthetics because of its antiemetic properties and associated euphoria on emergence. Tracheal intubation and controlled mechanical ventilation comprise the accepted anesthetic technique to reduce the increase in $PaCO_2$ and avoid ventilatory compromise from pneumoperitoneum and position changes. Although the laryngeal mask airway (LMA) has been used during short pelvic laparoscopic procedures, this evidence cannot be extrapolated to procedures requiring high IAP, steep head-down position, and upper abdominal laparoscopy as well as in patients at increased risk of regurgitation.[42,43]

Maintenance of Anesthesia

Maintenance of anesthesia with the newer inhaled anesthetics (i.e., desflurane or sevoflurane) remains the mainstay of modern anesthesia practice, probably because of the ease of titratability.[39,44] In addition, inhaled anesthetics exert some neuromuscular blocking effect. Furthermore, inhalation anesthesia may provide faster emergence as compared to total intravenous anesthesia (TIVA) with propofol. However, propofol-based TIVA is associated with a lower risk of postoperative nausea and vomiting (PONV), but its cost and apparent complexity (i.e., need for infusion and difficulty in titration) deter some practitioners.[44,45] Of note, except for patients with very high risk of PONV, the incidence of PONV with TIVA appears to be similar to that with inhalation anesthesia combined with prophylactic antiemetics.[44]

Nitrous Oxide

N_2O is widely used as part of a balanced anesthetic technique because of its amnestic and analgesic properties, as well as its ability to reduce the requirements of inhaled and intravenous anesthetic drugs and facilitate recovery.[46,47] Elimination of N_2O at the end of anesthesia produces a clinically significant acceleration in the reduction of inhaled anesthetic concentrations, further contributing to the speed of emergence.[48] However, its use during laparoscopic procedures has been controversial as a result of concerns regarding its ability to diffuse into bowel lumen, causing distension and impaired surgical access as well as increased PONV.[49] However, surgical conditions during laparoscopic procedures have been shown to be identical, regardless of whether N_2O was used.[50] In particular, surgeons were unable to distinguish between patients who had received N_2O compared to air.[50]

Although N_2O can contribute to PONV, the overall impact appears to be modest.[51] The use of propofol for induction of anesthesia and antiemetic prophylaxis, which is the current standard of care, further negates the emetic effects of N_2O.[51] A meta-analysis of randomized controlled trials found that the emetic effect of N_2O is not significant, and omitting N_2O may increase the risk of awareness.[52] Thus, there is no convincing reason to routinely avoid N_2O during laparoscopic procedures. However, omitting N_2O from the anesthesia regimen may be an option in patients at very high risk of PONV or when there are surgical difficulties.

In a laboratory experimental study, N_2O was shown to diffuse into a CO_2 pneumoperitoneum, and the levels were high enough to support combustion within 2 hours.[53] As laparoscopic surgical techniques become more complex and with the increasing use of laser and electrocautery, the chance of bowel perforation and release of highly volatile bowel gases (methane and hydrogen) into the peritoneal cavity is highly likely. However, the clinical significance of these issues remains unclear. In practice, leakage of intraperitoneal gas and replacement with fresh CO_2 are likely to wash out N_2O and reduce the risk of explosion.[54]

Intraoperative Opioids

Opioids remain an important component of a balanced general anesthetic technique and are typically titrated to achieve hemodynamic stability. However, treatment of pneumoperitoneum-induced hypertension with opioids may lead to relative opioid overdose after abdominal deflation. Therefore, it may be prudent to use an ultrashort-acting opioid (i.e., remifentanil) or sympatholytic drugs (e.g., esmolol and nicardipine) to treat pneumoperitoneum-induced hypertension. Remifentanil is a novel opioid with a short duration of action independent of the duration of infusion. Numerous studies have reported a reliable and rapid emergence from anesthesia with the use of remifentanil. Because of its short duration, transitional analgesics must be administered before emergence from anesthesia.[55]

Overall, opioids should be used sparingly because of concerns of opioid-related adverse effects such as dizziness, drowsiness, nausea, and vomiting.[55] Another concern has been raised regarding opioid-induced spasm of the sphincter of Oddi,[56] leading to misinterpretation of intraoperative cholangiographic findings during laparoscopic cholecystectomy. Many opioids, including fentanyl, have been implicated, and there are conflicting reports regarding the relative effect of individual opioids.[56] If necessary, the opioid-induced spasm of the sphincter of Oddi may be antagonized by glucagon.

Muscle Relaxants and Reversal of Residual Neuromuscular Blockade

Muscle paralysis reduces the IAP needed for the same degree of abdominal distension. However, several studies have not been able to show a correlation between the degree of muscle paralysis and the surgeon's ability.[57,58] Therefore, deep muscle paralysis may not be necessary during laparoscopic procedures. However, patient movement during robotic surgery can result in displacement of the robotic arms, which has a potential for patient harm.[59]

Recent evidence suggests that even a minor degree of residual neuromuscular blockade can increase the incidence of postoperative respiratory complications in high-risk patients such as the morbidly obese and elderly.[60–62] Unfortunately, residual neuromuscular blockade is difficult to diagnose clinically or by using train-of-four (TOF) response monitoring.[63] Recently, acceleromyography that provides a TOF ratio has been shown to reduce the incidence of residual blockade and associated unpleasant symptoms of muscle weakness in the recovery room and thus improve the overall quality of recovery.[63] Reversal with neostigmine is sometimes avoided due to concerns of higher incidence of PONV. However, the incidence of PONV and the need for antiemetics do not increase with the appropriate use of neostigmine combined with glycopyrrolate.[64,65] Therefore, reversal drugs should be used without hesitation. The dose of neostigmine should be determined by the degree of blockade at the time of reversal.[61,66]

Mechanical Ventilation

The changes in pulmonary function (e.g., reduction in lung volume, increase in peak inspiratory pressure, and decrease in pulmonary compliance) during laparoscopy may require intraoperative modification in mechanical ventilation. Typically the minute ventilation needs to be increased by 20% to 30%, which could be achieved by increasing the respiratory rate while maintaining a constant tidal volume. Lung protective ventilation strategies include the use of pressure-controlled ventilation with low tidal volumes (6 to 8 mL/kg ideal body weight) and positive end-expiratory pressure (PEEP) of 5 to 10 cm water (H_2O).[67] Use of PEEP has been shown to improve arterial oxygenation during prolonged pneumoperitoneum.[68] In addition, recruitment maneuvers are beneficial and should be applied, particularly before and after a laparoscopic procedure.[69] Unfortunately, the effects of recruitment maneuvers are short lasting and often limited by hemodynamic instability. It is important to avoid hyperventilation (and hypocapnia), as this may result in metabolic alkalosis and lead to postoperative hypoventilation. The acceptance of higher $ETCO_2$ levels may limit peak airway pressures (<50 cm H_2O) and potential barotrauma. Mild hypercapnia (i.e., $ETCO_2$ of 40 mm Hg) can improve tissue oxygenation through improved tissue perfusion, resulting from increased cardiac output and vasodilatation as well as increased oxygen off-loading from the shift of the oxyhemoglobin dissociation curve to the right.[67,70,71]

Monitoring

In addition to standard intraoperative monitoring, minimally invasive hemodynamic monitoring (e.g., arterial waveform analysis) may be appropriate in patients with significant cardiopulmonary disease to monitor the cardiovascular response to pneumoperitoneum and position changes in order to institute therapy. The arterial waveform analysis provides a relatively noninvasive means of estimating ventricular contractility and stroke volume on a beat-to-beat basis.[72,73] In addition, these monitors could guide fluid therapy by using dynamic indicators such as stroke volume variation.

Although $ETCO_2$ provides a reasonable approximation of $PaCO_2$ in healthy patients, this may not be true in patients with pre-existing cardiopulmonary disease. Therefore, monitoring of arterial blood gases may be prudent in patients with significant pulmonary disease or those with persistent refractory intraoperative hypercapnia. Also, compliance and pressure–volume loop monitoring may be helpful in diagnosing complications resulting in increased airway pressure, such as endobronchial intubation, bronchospasm, and pneumothorax. Recently, cerebral oximetry monitoring was found to provide brain oxygenation,[74–76] and could be particularly useful in high-risk patients undergoing prolonged endoscopic procedures in steep head-up or head-down procedures.[32]

Fluid Management

Maintenance of optimal intravascular volume or cardiac filling is critical in improving perioperative outcomes.[77,78] This is particularly critical during prolonged laparoscopic procedures in the high-risk patient population. However, fluid therapy remains one of the most controversial topics in perioperative management. There is continuing debate regarding the type of fluids used (i.e., crystalloids, colloids, or a type of colloid) as well as the amount of fluid administration (i.e., liberal vs. restricted or goal-directed approach).

It is increasingly becoming clear that intraoperative fluid therapy should be specific to patient characteristics and the type of surgical procedure. For mild to moderately invasive surgical procedures, crystalloid boluses (20 to 40 mL/kg) have been shown to improve outcomes, such as reduced postoperative dizziness and early ambulation.[79] For major elective surgical procedures, the use of fluid minimization and a goal-directed fluid administration approach are recommended.[77,78] In patients undergoing robotic prostatectomy, fluid minimization is recommended, as steep head-down positioning for prolonged period may result in facial, pharyngeal, and laryngeal edema. Also, large fluid volumes can lead to high urine output and interfere with the surgical procedure.

It is clear that traditional indicators used to guide fluid therapy (e.g., heart rate, arterial blood pressure, central venous pressures, and urine output) are not reliable. Urine output is reduced during laparoscopy, and its use to guide fluid therapy may lead to fluid overload. Therefore, dynamic indicators, such as stroke volume or systolic or pulse pressure variation, are preferred. Optimization of dynamic indicators can be achieved by administration of small fluid boluses.[80] Of note, deep general anesthesia and hyperventilation can influence fluid requirements and thus should be avoided.

NAUSEA AND VOMITING PREVENTION

Patients undergoing laparoscopic surgery are at a greater risk for PONV, probably due to intraperitoneal insufflation and bowel manipulation.[81] Therefore, aggressive multimodal antiemetic prophylaxis is necessary in this high-risk population. A multimodal approach to PONV prophylaxis could include use of combinations of dexamethasone, 4 to 8 mg administered after induction of anesthesia, and 5-HT_3 antagonists (e.g., ondansetron 4 mg) at the end of surgery as well as aggressive hydration, minimal opioid use, and aggressive pain control.[81–83] Other antiemetic therapy includes a scopolamine patch applied preferably prior to surgery and neurokinin-1 receptor antagonists administered preoperatively.[84,85]

PAIN PREVENTION

Compared to open surgical procedures, pain after laparoscopic procedures is considered to be less intense and of shorter duration.[86] Nevertheless, adequate pain control is critical to hasten postoperative recovery and ambulation.[55] The origin of pain after most laparoscopic and robotic procedures is predominantly visceral rather than parietal (i.e., from incision site). In addition, shoulder pain secondary to diaphragmatic irritation is also common and can limit the patient's ability to return to normal activities. The factors that could influence postoperative pain include duration of procedure, degree of IAP,[87] and the volume of residual subdiaphragmatic gas after surgery. Optimal pain therapy for patients undergoing laparoscopic and robotic surgeries includes
10 the use of multimodal analgesia techniques.[55,88] Because opioid-related adverse effects may delay recovery, nonopioid analgesics should be used when possible.

Conventional nonsteroidal anti-inflammatory drugs or cyclooxygenase-2–specific inhibitors have been shown to reduce postoperative pain and opioid requirements and thus should be considered part of analgesic therapy.[89] These analgesics could be combined with acetaminophen,[90] as the combination is superior to either drug alone.[91,92] If pain relief remains inadequate, analgesia may be supplemented with weak opioids for low- to moderate-intensity postoperative pain and with strong opioids for moderate- to high-intensity postoperative pain.[88] These drugs should be administered at the appropriate time (preoperative or intraoperative) to provide sufficient analgesia in the early recovery period as well as continued in the postoperative period. The use of these medications should depend on assessment of an individual patient's risks.

Parenteral glucocorticoids (e.g., dexamethasone) should also be considered part of a multimodal analgesia technique because they have been shown to reduce postoperative pain as well as length of hospital stay after abdominal surgery with no evidence of increased complications, including after colorectal surgery.[93,94] Although ketamine has some documented benefits,[95] its routine use remains controversial due to lack of data on optimal dose and duration.

Infiltration of the surgical wound (laparoscopy portals) with local anesthetics can provide excellent analgesia that outlasts the duration of action of the local anesthetic.[88,96,97] For hybrid or laparoscopic-assisted surgical procedures with longer incisions, continuous local anesthetic wound infusion may be used to prolong the duration of analgesia.[98] The transversus abdominis plane (TAP) block, which involves administration of local anesthetic between the layers of internal oblique and transversus abdominis muscles, may be beneficial in patients undergoing hybrid or laparoscopic-assisted procedures,[99,100] but its role in procedures with small incisions remains controversial.

Intraperitoneal instillation of long-acting local anesthetics (e.g., ropivacaine) has been shown to reduce the intensity of postlaparoscopic pain.[101,102] However, the concentration and dose of the local anesthetic as well as optimal timing of administration remain unknown. Therefore, intraperitoneal local anesthetic instillation remains controversial. Recently, intraperitoneal nebulization of ropivacaine has been shown to provide excellent postlaparoscopic pain relief, particularly shoulder pain.[103] Intravenous lidocaine infusion in the intraoperative and the postoperative periods has been reported to reduce postoperative pain and opioid requirements and improve bowel function as well as reduce the length of hospital stay.[104–106] However, the optimal dose and duration of lidocaine infusion remain unknown. No significant local anesthetic toxicity has been reported in published systematic reviews, and adverse events were not systematically evaluated. Therefore, routine use of lidocaine infusion is not recommended. Nevertheless, lidocaine infusion could be an alternative when other approaches are inadequate.

Although epidural analgesia provides excellent pain relief with improved outcomes after open major abdominal surgery, its role in laparoscopic surgery remains controversial.[86,107] Similarly, intrathecal morphine provides excellent pain relief, but it is associated with opioid-related adverse effects such as increased PONV, itching, urinary retention, and respiratory depression.[108] For most minimally invasive surgical procedures, neuraxial analgesia is not necessary because of a lack of superiority over other analgesic techniques and the potential risks of adverse effects, such as hemodynamic instability, postural hypotension, and urinary retention as well as delay of early ambulation.[109]

INTRAOPERATIVE COMPLICATIONS

Intraoperative complications during minimally invasive surgery include those related to creation of pneumoperitoneum through intraperitoneal CO_2 insufflation, patient positioning, and surgical instrumentation.[110] These include cardiopulmonary compromise, renal dysfunction, and hypothermia. Surgical complications include subcutaneous emphysema, capnothorax, capnomediastinum, capnopericardium, gas embolism, acute hemorrhage, and bowel or bladder perforation, which can occur during the laparoscopic procedure. Procedures with higher incidence of complications include upper abdominal procedures, such as fundoplication, and urologic procedures, particularly in patients with significant comorbidities.[111–115]

Cardiopulmonary Complications

Hemodynamic complications associated with laparoscopic procedures include dysrhythmias and alterations in arterial blood pressure (i.e., hypotension and hypertension). Bradyarrhythmias are attributed to increased vagal tone following peritoneal

TABLE 43-7. DIFFERENTIAL DIAGNOSIS OF CARDIOVASCULAR COLLAPSE DURING LAPAROSCOPY

- Profound vasovagal reaction
- Cardiac dysrhythmias
- Excessive intra-abdominal pressure
- Tension capno(pneumo)thorax
- Cardiac tamponade (capnomediastinum and capnopericardium)
- Significant gas embolism
- Acute blood loss
- Myocardial ischemia/infarction
- Severe respiratory acidosis (hypercapnia)
- Anesthetic drug related

stretching, especially associated with lighter levels of anesthesia; while tachyarrhythmias may be due to hypercapnia as a result of intraperitoneal CO_2 insufflation. Paroxysmal tachycardia and hypertension followed by ventricular fibrillation have been reported during laparoscopic adrenalectomy.[116] Although rare, acute cardiovascular collapse can occur (Table 43-7).

Creation of pneumoperitoneum and Trendelenburg positioning are associated with cephalad movement of the carina, which may lead to endobronchial intubation.[117,118] Pneumoperitoneum and position changes can cause significant hypoxemia (Table 43-8) and hypercarbia ($ETCO_2$ >50 mm Hg) (Table 43-9).

11 Treatment of hemodynamic dysfunction should include confirmation that the IAP has not exceeded 15 mm Hg and that vascular injuries have been ruled out, accompanied by supportive therapy including reduction in anesthetics, fluid administration, and pharmacologic interventions. In addition, hemodynamic instability in patients with a significant increase in SVR may require vasodilator therapy (Table 43-10). After cardiopulmonary stabilization, cautious slow reinsufflation may then be attempted using lower IAPs. However, with persistent signs of significant cardiopulmonary impairment, it may be necessary to convert to an open procedure.

TABLE 43-8. CAUSES OF HYPOXEMIA DURING LAPAROSCOPY

- Patient-related factors
  - Pre-existing cardiopulmonary dysfunction
  - Morbid obesity
- Low inspired oxygen concentrations
- Hypoventilation
- Ventilation–perfusion mismatch
  - Endobronchial intubation
  - Atelectasis
  - Capno(pneumo)thorax
  - Pulmonary embolization
- Reduced cardiac output
  - Inferior vena cava compression
  - Dysrhythmias
  - Myocardial depression
  - Hemorrhage
- Anemia

TABLE 43-9. DIFFERENTIAL DIAGNOSIS OF HYPERCARBIA DURING LAPAROSCOPY

- Increased carbon dioxide absorption
  - Extraperitoneal insufflation greater than intraperitoneal insufflation
  - Subcutaneous emphysema
  - Capnothorax, capnomediastinum, capnopericardium
  - Carbon dioxide embolism
- Decreased alveolar ventilation (hypoventilation, ventilation–perfusion mismatch)
  - Endobronchial intubation
  - Atelectasis (increased IAP, patient position)
  - Airway obstruction
  - Reduced cardiac output
- Increased carbon dioxide production
  - Obesity, malignant hyperthermia, fever, thyrotoxicosis
- Rebreathing of carbon dioxide
  - Defective carbon dioxide absorber
  - Malfunctioning valves

Subcutaneous Emphysema

Subcutaneous emphysema can occur from inadvertent extraperitoneal insufflation in the subcutaneous, preperitoneal, or retroperitoneal tissue or from extension of extraperitoneal insufflation.[119,120] Because there is a continuum of fascial planes, extensive subcutaneous emphysema can develop involving the abdomen, chest, neck, and groin. If the emphysema extends to the chest wall and the neck, the CO_2 can track to the thorax and mediastinum,
12 thereby resulting in capnothorax or capnomediastinum.[121] Of note, because of similar blood solubilities of CO_2 and N_2O, N_2O should not cause further expansion of a CO_2-filled space.

Predictors of subcutaneous emphysema include operative time of >200 minutes and use of six or more surgical ports.[120] Subcutaneous emphysema is indicated by the development of

TABLE 43-10. PREVENTION OF CARDIOPULMONARY CHANGES IN PATIENTS WITH SIGNIFICANT CARDIOPULMONARY DISEASE

- Induce pneumoperitoneum in supine position
- Use lower intra-abdominal pressure (10–12 mm Hg)
- Limit position change
- Early use of vasodilators and beta-blockade to control hypertension
- Monitoring
  - Arterial line for continuous blood pressure
  - Hemodynamic monitoring using pulse contour analysis
  - Transesophageal echocardiography

crepitus. Increased CO_2 absorption may cause a sudden rise in $ETCO_2$. In most cases, no specific intervention is required, and the subcutaneous emphysema resolves soon after the abdomen is deflated. However, if significant hypercarbia occurs, despite aggressive hyperventilation, it may be necessary to temporarily deflate the abdomen to allow CO_2 elimination, followed by reinsufflation with lower IAP to prevent further extravasation of
13 CO_2. Development of late hypercarbia (i.e., in the recovery room) has been reported in patients with subcutaneous emphysema.[122] Signs of hypercarbia in the postoperative period include somnolence, increased sympathetic output (i.e., increased heart rate and arterial blood pressure), and respiratory acidosis (and its consequences). If there is neck or face emphysema, a chest x-ray should be obtained in patients with cervical emphysema to rule out capnothorax or capnomediastinum.

Capnothorax, Capnomediastinum, and Capnopericardium

Capnothorax has been reported during both intraperitoneal and extraperitoneal laparoscopic procedures. Although rare, it is a potentially life-threatening complication.[110] It is most common in procedures near the diaphragm (e.g., fundoplication and adrenorenal procedures).[111,123] The suggested mechanisms include tracking of insufflated CO_2 around the aortic, caval, and esophageal hiatuses of the diaphragm into the mediastinum with subsequent rupture into the pleural space[124,125] (Table 43-11). Passage of gas through anatomic defects in the diaphragm occurring at the outer crus or through a congenital defect at the pleuroperitoneal hiatus (patent pleuroperitoneal canal) is also a likely mechanism. Accidental diaphragmatic injury and damage to the falciform ligament (e.g., during insertion of the Veress needle) and inguinal space (via retroperitoneum) can occur. Alternatively, rupture of a lung bulla or bleb could produce a tension pneumothorax independent of the pneumoperitoneum.

Capnothorax may be undetected intraoperatively or may present as an unexplained increased airway pressure, hypoxemia, hypercapnia, surgical emphysema, or, if tension capnothorax occurs, severe cardiovascular compromise with profound hypotension[125] (Table 43-12). Maintaining a high index of suspicion will facilitate early diagnosis and treatment, which can be lifesaving. Inequality in chest expansion, reduced air entry, and a bulging diaphragm (visualized by directing the videoscope toward the diaphragm) are suggestive of capnothorax.[126] In addition, subcutaneous emphysema in the head and neck may be indicative of capnothorax. A chest x-ray should confirm the diagnosis. However, a recent use of transthoracic ultrasound for the diagnosis of pneumothorax has been described.[127]

Treatment of capnothorax includes deflation of the abdomen and supportive treatment (Table 43-13). If there is minimal physiologic compromise, conservative treatment with close observation may be adequate because CO_2 is rapidly absorbed.[124,125,128] In addition to hyperventilation, use of PEEP may reduce the pressure gradient between the abdomen and the thorax during both inspiration and expiration and thus may inflate the lung and
14 resolve capnothorax. In patients with severe compromise, placement of an intercostal cannula may be necessary, followed by a chest drain if reaccumulation occurs. After stabilization, the procedure can usually be resumed at lower IAP. Conversion to an open procedure might be necessary after stabilization.

Capnomediastinum and capnopericardium, although rare, can occur during laparoscopic procedures. These complications may be associated with significant hemodynamic derangement. The diagnosis of these complications is based on chest x-ray, and their management depends on the degree of hemodynamic compromise. In most patients, deflation of the pneumoperitoneum

TABLE 43-11. CAUSES OF CAPNOTHORAX

- Inadvertent peritoneal breach
  - Dissection around the diaphragm and retroperitoneum
  - Nissen's fundoplication, gastric bypass surgery, urologic surgery
- Misdirected Veress needle (damage to the falciform ligament)
- Gas tracked through facial planes from the neck and thorax into the mediastinum and pleural space
- Passage of gas through the pleuroperitoneal hiatus (foramen of Bochdalek)
- Passage of gas through congenital defects (foramen of Morgagni)

TABLE 43-12. DIAGNOSIS OF CAPNOTHORAX

- High index of suspicion
  - Site of surgical procedures
  - Subcutaneous emphysema of the neck and thorax
- Increased end-tidal carbon dioxide and reduced end-tidal carbon dioxide with hypotension
- Decreased oxygen saturation
- Increased peak airway pressures
- Hypotension
- Unequal chest expansion and air entry
- Bulging of hemidiaphragm seen through the endoscope
- Confirmed on thoracic ultrasound and/or chest x-ray

TABLE 43-13. MANAGEMENT OF CAPNOTHORAX DURING LAPAROSCOPIC PROCEDURE

- Stop surgery and deflate the pneumoperitoneum
- Continue supportive treatment, hyperventilation, positive end-expiratory pressure
- Confirm the diagnosis of pneumothorax by clinical examination, if time permits, chest ultrasound and/or radiograph
- Treat according to the severity of cardiopulmonary compromise:
  - Minimal compromise—treat conservatively with close observation
  - Moderate to severe compromise—place intercostal cannula or temporary drain
  - Reaccumulation of capnothorax—place chest drain
- After stabilization, resume procedure with lower (10 mm Hg) intra-abdominal pressures
- If capnothorax reoccurs, it may be necessary to convert to open procedure

and close observation is adequate, while others might require supportive therapy along with hyperventilation to wash out CO_2.

Gas Embolism

Serious adverse intraoperative events attributed to gas embolism during laparoscopic procedures are widely reported. The incidence of gas embolism during laparoscopy is unclear. Studies using transesophageal echocardiography have reported a high incidence of CO_2 embolism.[129,130] Venous gas embolism detected using transesophageal echocardiography was higher in open radical retropubic prostatectomy compared with robotic-assisted laparoscopic radical prostatectomy.[131] However, the gas embolisms observed in these studies were not associated with significant cardiopulmonary effects. These studies did not observe cardiopulmonary compromise, despite a significant degree of gas embolism. Therefore, clinical relevance of these embolisms is questionable. It is possible that head-down positioning increases right atrial pressures, which may prevent cardiac entrainment of gas. In contrast, in an animal study, gas embolism occurred frequently during laparoscopic liver resection, with approximately half of the embolisms causing respiratory and/or hemodynamic disturbances, probably due to a head-up positioning during the procedure.[132]

The proposed mechanisms of gas embolism include inadvertent intravenous placement of the Veress needle or passage of CO_2 into the abdominal wall and peritoneal vessels during insufflation or into open vessels on the liver surface during gallbladder dissection. Most of the embolisms during laparoscopic hysterectomy occur during round ligament transection and broad ligament dissection.[133] During prostatectomy, most gas embolisms occur during transection of the deep dorsal venous complex.[131]

Appropriate monitoring and maintenance of a high index of suspicion should allow early detection and prevention of serious adverse sequelae from CO_2 embolism. Signs and severity of the effects of CO_2 embolism are variable and may include cardiac arrhythmia, hypoxemia, and hypotension, and an associated decrease in $ETCO_2$. The electrocardiogram might show a right strain pattern and widening of the QRS complex. Cyanosis of the head and neck resulting from inflow obstruction to the right side of the heart may also occur. Paradoxical embolism through a probe-patent foramen ovale or an atrial septal defect may result in cerebral CO_2 embolism.

If gas embolism is suspected, the abdomen should be deflated. Also, hyperventilation and rapid CO_2 washout should result in rapid absorption of the CO_2 embolus and facilitate reversal of hemodynamic impairment. In addition to aggressive cardiopulmonary resuscitation, the patient should be turned to the left lateral decubitus with a head-down position to allow the gas to rise into the apex of the right ventricle and prevent entry into the pulmonary artery. Hyperbaric oxygen and cardiopulmonary bypass have also been used to successfully treat symptomatic gas embolism.

Hypothermia

It is generally expected that the degree of hypothermia during a closed procedure, such as laparoscopy, would be less than that during an open procedure because the abdominal contents are not exposed to the atmosphere.[134,135] However, the incidence of hypothermia during laparoscopic procedures is similar to that of open abdominal operations. It is postulated that heat loss during laparoscopy occurs mainly by convection (i.e., due to flow of a fluid [liquid or gas] when it circulates through a surface at a different temperature). The potential for heat loss during laparoscopic procedures is considerable, with dry CO_2 exiting the cylinder at 21°C and being insufflated into a peritoneal cavity with a large surface area.[136]

Built-in heating elements that warm the insufflating gas have become available commercially. However, their effectiveness remains controversial[137] because heating insufflating gas without humidification may not prevent hypothermia. Therefore, heating and humidifying CO_2 to a physiologic condition has been proposed, particularly in prolonged surgical procedures.[138,139] However, larger studies are necessary to show the advantages of humidifying insufflating gas.

Complications Related to Positioning

Although complications related to positioning are discussed elsewhere (Chapter 28), this section includes complications associated with pneumoperitoneum and steep head-down positioning. In patients undergoing robotic-assisted prostatectomy, prolonged steep head-down positioning may lead to facial, pharyngeal, and laryngeal edema, which might lead to upper airway obstruction including laryngospasm. Reducing intraoperative fluid administration could minimize this edema formation. Prolonged head-down positioning and increased IAP along with large crystalloid administration could increase venous congestion in the optic canal and potentially reduce optic nerve perfusion pressure.[33,140] Acute venous congestion of the optic canal can cause ischemic optic neuropathy and lead to postoperative blindness.[141] Ocular complications, including visual loss, have been reported after robotic surgery.[142]

Prolonged caudad displacement of the shoulders can cause brachial plexus injury.[143] Therefore, careful positioning and securing the shoulders by using braces are necessary. Another potential complication reported in patients undergoing robotic surgery is corneal abrasions, which can be reduced by ocular protection using eye patches or transparent occlusive dressing over the eyes.[143]

Complications from Surgical Instrumentation

Hemorrhage may occur because of insertion of the Veress needle or trocar into major intra-abdominal vessels (i.e., aorta, common iliac vessels, or inferior vena cava) or because of injury to abdominal wall vasculature. Disruption or avulsion of the cystic or hepatic artery may cause major bleeding during laparoscopic cholecystectomy. Concealed bleeding, particularly into the retroperitoneal space, may result in delayed diagnosis of vascular injury, which may be indicated initially by unexplained hypotension and fall in hematocrit values. The anesthesiologist may therefore play a crucial role in early diagnosis of this potentially fatal complication. Uncontrollable hemorrhage requires immediate conversion to an open procedure to control bleeding and repair the vascular injury.

Other reported intra-abdominal injuries associated with trocar insertion include gastrointestinal tract perforations, hepatic and splenic tears, and mesenteric lacerations. Unrecognized gastrointestinal injuries may be associated with significant morbidity and mortality. Risk factors for gastrointestinal injuries include gastric distension and adhesions because of previous abdominal surgery. Esophageal or gastric perforation may occur during the insertion of the bougie, particularly in patients with Barrett's esophagus, ulcers, or strictures. Unrecognized bladder or ureter injury may lead to azotemia, particularly when it is associated with ascites and hyponatremia. Bladder injury may be suspected by sudden deflation of the abdomen, pneumaturia (gas bubbles in the urinary bag), and hematuria.

Placement of the Veress needle and trocars using a mini-laparotomy approach should reduce the risks of these injuries. Stomach injuries can be reduced by gastric decompression prior to surgery. Similarly, decompression of the urinary bladder by placement of a urinary catheter or asking patients to void prior to surgery should decrease the possibility of bladder trauma.

POSTOPERATIVE CONSIDERATIONS

Postoperative respiratory function is superior after laparoscopic approach as compared with open procedures. Although there have been few prospective randomized trials comparing laparoscopic and open procedures, many early studies report a lower incidence of pulmonary complications with the laparoscopic approach.

In patients with significant respiratory dysfunction and restricted CO_2 clearance, impaired postoperative ventilation from residual anesthetics and neuromuscular blockade in the immediate postoperative period may delay removal of absorbed CO_2 and cause significant hypercapnia. Of note, normalization of CO_2 concentrations may take longer after extraperitoneal insufflation than after intraperitoneal insufflation. Diaphragm dysfunction has been reported after laparoscopic procedures,[144,145] but its clinical consequence is minimal. However, postoperative respiratory failure may occur in patients with diaphragm dysfunction.[146]

Increased IAP and reverse Trendelenburg position have been reported to cause venous stasis that could increase the potential for deep vein thrombosis and pulmonary embolism.[147] Measures to reduce venous stasis, such as graduated elastic compression stockings, are indicated in the perioperative period. Minimal tissue trauma with laparoscopic techniques, facilitating early postoperative ambulation, may also reduce the risk.

AMBULATORY LAPAROSCOPIC PROCEDURES

Minimally invasive surgery has extended the range of procedures that can be performed on an outpatient basis. The safety and feasibility of laparoscopic cholecystectomy, as an outpatient surgical 15
procedure, have been well established.[7,8] Other procedures that are increasingly being performed on an outpatient basis include laparoscopic fundoplication and laparoscopic gastric band surgery. Recent systematic reviews reported that laparoscopic fundoplication could be safely performed on an ambulatory basis with an unanticipated admission rate of 7% and a readmission rate of 1%, which are similar to other ambulatory surgical procedures.[9] The most common causes for overnight admission include nausea, pain, and capnothorax. The common reasons for readmission include dysphagia and pain. The perioperative complication rate was 4% and was primarily surgery related. Another systematic review of outpatient laparoscopic adjustable gastric band surgery found that the unplanned admission rate was 0.6%, while the readmission rate was 0.55%.[10] The most common cause for failure to discharge was pain, nausea, and dysphagia and that for readmission was dysphagia. There were no mortalities reported.

A systematic review of laparoscopic gastric bypass surgery performed on a 23-hour ambulatory basis found that the unplanned admission rate after 23-hour observation was 16% and the readmission rate was 1.82%.[11] The most common reasons for readmission were related to surgery (e.g., anastomotic strictures, gastrointestinal bleeding, and internal hernia) and pulmonary embolism. Also, there was a 0.01% (2/2,201 patients) incidence of mortality. Overall, the scientific literature regarding the safety of outpatient bariatric surgery is sparse and of limited quality.[11] Therefore, the suitability of ambulatory surgery in these patients remains controversial.

It is clear from the literature that careful patient selection is critical. It should depend on the surgical procedure, the severity of comorbidities, the anesthetic technique, and the anticipated postoperative analgesic requirements, as well as patients' ability to follow postdischarge instructions. Similarly, adequate patient information and preparation as well as follow-up after surgery are necessary for the success and safety of ambulatory surgery.

SUMMARY

Minimally invasive surgery reduces postoperative pain and ileus, facilitates recovery, allows shorter hospital stays, and provides a rapid return to activities of daily living. With growing surgical expertise and improvements in technology and computer power, more extensive and prolonged procedures will be performed in a wide range of patient population. Robotic surgery offers technical advantages over laparoscopic surgery and thus should further expand the field of minimally invasive surgery.

The physiologic changes associated with pneumoperitoneum creation and patient positioning may cause significant cardiorespiratory compromise, particularly in patients with significant cardiopulmonary dysfunction. Therefore, a thorough understanding of the associated cardiopulmonary changes and the potential complications is necessary to maintain patient safety.

Balanced general anesthesia technique with mechanical ventilation remains the best practice for minimally invasive surgical procedures requiring CO_2 insufflation. Aggressive multimodal analgesia as well as antiemetic prophylaxis and treatment are required to reduce these common postoperative adverse effects.

Appropriate monitoring and maintenance of a high index of suspicion can result in early diagnosis of complications and prevent serious adverse sequelae. Should intraoperative cardiopulmonary impairment occur, it is important to confirm that the IAP is <15 mm Hg as well as rule out traumatic vascular injuries, CO_2 embolism, subcutaneous emphysema, capnothorax, and capnomediastinum. If there is no improvement in the vital signs with routine management, it is imperative to release the pneumoperitoneum and place the patient in a supine (or Trendelenburg) position. After cardiopulmonary stabilization, cautious slow reinsufflation may then be attempted. However, with persistent signs of significant cardiopulmonary impairment, it may be necessary to convert to an open procedure.

References

1. Anesthesia for minimally invasive surgery: Laparoscopy, thoracoscopy and hysteroscopy. In: Joshi GP, ed. *Anesthesiology Clinics of North America*. Philadelphia, PA: WB Saunders; 2001.
2. Joshi GP. Anesthesia for laparoscopic surgery. *Can J Anaesth*. 2002;49(6):R1–R5.
3. Mack MJ. Minimally invasive and robotic surgery. *JAMA*. 2001;285:568–572.
4. Hanly EJ, Talamini MA. Robotic abdominal surgery. *Am J Surg*. 2004;188:1 9S–26S.

5. Finkelstein J, Eckersberger E, Sadri H, et al. Open versus laparoscopic versus robot-assisted laparoscopic prostatectomy: The European and US experience. *Rev Urol.* 2010;12:35–43.
6. Weinberg L, Rao S, Escobar PE. Robotic surgery in gynecology: An updated systematic review. *Obstet Gynecol Int.* 2011;2011:852061.
7. Gurusamy KS, Junnarkar S, Farouk M, et al. Day-case versus overnight stay for laparoscopic cholecystectomy [review]. *Cochrane Database Syst Rev.* 2008(3):CD006798.
8. Gurusamy K, Junnarkar S, Farouk M, et al. Meta-analysis of randomized controlled trials on the safety and effectiveness of day-case laparoscopic cholecystectomy. *Br J Surg.* 2008;95:161–168.
9. Thomas H, Agrawal S. Systematic review of day-case laparoscopic fundoplication. *J Laparoendosc Adv Surg Tech A.* 2011;21:781–788.
10. Thomas H, Agrawal S. Systematic review of same-day laparoscopic adjustable gastric band surgery. *Obes Surg.* 2011;21:805–810.
11. Thomas H, Agrawal S. Systematic review of 23-hour (outpatient) stay laparoscopic gastric bypass surgery. *J Laparoendosc Adv Surg Tech A.* 2011;21:677–681.
12. Walter CJ, Collin J, Dumville JC, et al. Enhanced recovery in colorectal resections: A systematic review and meta-analysis. *Colorectal Dis.* 2009;11:344–353.
13. Gurusamy KS, Samraj K, Davidson BR. Abdominal lift for laparoscopic cholecystectomy. *Cochrane Database Syst Rev.* 2008;(2):CD006574.
14. O'Malley C, Cunningham AJ. Physiologic changes during laparoscopy. *Anesthesiol Clin North America.* 2001;19:1–19.
15. Gutt CN, Oniu T, Mehrabi A, et al. Circulatory and respiratory complications of carbon dioxide insufflation. *Dig Surg.* 2004;21:95–105.
16. Sammour T, Mittal A, Loveday BP, et al. Systematic review of oxidative stress associated with pneumoperitoneum. *Br J Surg.* 2009;96:836–850.
17. O'Leary E, Hubbard K, Tormey W, et al. Laparoscopic cholecystectomy: Haemodynamic and neuroendocrine responses after pneumoperitoneum and changes in position. *Br J Anaesth.* 1996;76:640–644.
18. Gannedahl P, Odelberg S, Brodin LA, et al. Effects of posture and pneumoperitoneum during anesthesia on the indices of left ventricular filling. *Acta Anaesthesiol Scand.* 1996;40:160–166.
19. Hein HAT, Joshi GP, Ramsay MAE, et al. Hemodynamic changes during laparoscopic cholecystectomy in patients with severe cardiopulmonary disease. *J Clin Anesth.* 1997;9:261–265.
20. Nguyen NT, Wolfe BM. The physiologic effects of pneumoperitoneum in the morbidly obese. *Ann Surg.* 2005;241:219–226.
21. Meininger D, Zwissler B, Byhahn C, et al. Impact of overweight and pneumoperitoneum on hemodynamics and oxygenation during prolonged laparoscopic surgery. *World J Surg.* 2006;30:520–526.
22. Harris SN, Ballantyne GH, Luther MA, et al. Alterations of cardiovascular performance during laparoscopic colectomy: A combined hemodynamic and echocardiographic analysis. *Anesth Analg.* 1996;83:482–487.
23. Talamini MA, Mendoza-Sagaon M, Gitzelmann CA, et al. Increased mediastinal pressure and decreased cardiac output during laparoscopic Nissen fundoplication. *Surgery.* 1997;122:345–352.
24. Farlo J, Thawgathurai D, Mikhail M, et al. Cardiac tamponade during laparoscopic Nissen fundoplication. *Eur J Anaesthesiol.* 1998;15:246.
25. Meininger D, Westphal K, Bremerich DH, et al. Effects of posture and prolonged pneumoperitoneum on hemodynamic parameters during laparoscopy. *World J Surg.* 2008;32:1400–1405.
26. Falabella A, Moore-Jeffries E, Sullivan M, et al. Cardiac function during steep Trendelenburg position and CO_2 pneumoperitoneum for robotic-assisted prostatectomy: A transesophageal Doppler probe study. *Int J Med Robotics Comput Assist Surg.* 2007;3:312–315.
27. Kalmar AF, Foubert L, Hendrickx JFA, et al. Influence of steep Trendelenburg position and CO_2 pneumoperitoneum on cardiovascular, cerebrovascular, and respiratory homeostasis during robotic prostatectomy. *Br J Anaesth.* 2010;104:433–439.
28. Lestar M, Gunnarsson L, Lagerstrand L, et al. Hemodynamic perturbations during robot-assisted laparoscopic radical prostatectomy in 45° Trendelenburg position. *Anesth Analg.* 2011;113:1069–1075.
29. McDougall EM, Monk TG, Wolf JS Jr, et al. The effect of prolonged pneumoperitoneum on renal function in an animal model. *J Am Coll Surg.* 1996;182:317–328.
30. Nguyen NT, Perez RV, Fleming N, et al. Effect of prolonged pneumoperitoneum on intraoperative urine output during laparoscopic gastric bypass. *J Am Coll Surg.* 2002;195:476–483.
31. Halverson A, Buchanan R, Jacobs L, et al. Evaluation of mechanism of increased intracranial pressure with insufflation. *Surg Endosc.* 1998;12:266–269.
32. Park EY, Koo BN, Min KT, et al. The effect of pneumoperitoneum in the steep Trendelenburg position on cerebral oxygenation. *Acta Anaesthesiol Scand.* 2009;53:895–899.
33. Awad H, Santilli S, Ohr M, et al. The effects of steep Trendelenburg positioning on intraocular pressure during robotic radical prostatectomy. *Anesth Analg.* 2009;109:473–478.
34. Mullet CE, Viale JP, Sagnard PE, et al. Pulmonary CO_2 elimination during surgical procedures using intra- or extraperitoneal CO_2 insufflation. *Anesth Analg.* 1993;76:622–626.
35. Kadam PG, Marda M, Shah VR. Carbon dioxide absorption during laparoscopic donor nephrectomy: A comparison between retroperitoneal and transperitoneal approaches. *Transplant Proc.* 2008;40:1119–1121.
36. Kwak HJ, Jo YY, Lee KC, et al. Acid–base alterations during laparoscopic abdominal surgery: A comparison with laparotomy. *Br J Anaesth.* 2010;105:442–447.
37. Strang CM, Freden F, Maripuu E, et al. Ventilation–perfusion distributions and gas exchange during carbon dioxide-pneumoperitoneum in a porcine model. *Br J Anaesth.* 2010;105:691–697.
38. Schrijvers D, Mottrie A, Traen K, et al. Pulmonary gas exchange is well preserved during robot assisted surgery in steep Trendelenburg position. *Acta Anaesthesiol Belg.* 2009;60:229–233.
39. Joshi GP. Fast tracking in outpatient surgery. *Curr Opin Anaesthesiol.* 2001; 14:635–639.
40. Smith I. Anesthesia for laparoscopy with emphasis on outpatient laparoscopy. *Anesthesiol Clin North America.* 2001;19:21–41.
41. Collins LM, Vaghadia H. Regional anesthesia for laparoscopy. *Anesthesiol Clin North America.* 2001;19:43–56.
42. Smith I, Joshi GP. The laryngeal mask airway for outpatient anesthesia. *J Clin Anesth.* 1993;5:22S–28S.
43. Joshi GP. The use of laryngeal mask airway devices in ambulatory anesthesia. *Semin Anesth Perioperative Med Pain.* 2001;20:257–263.
44. Joshi GP. Inhalational techniques in ambulatory anesthesia. *Anesthesiol Clin North America.* 2003;21:263–272.
45. Tonner PH, Scholz J. Total intravenous or balanced anaesthesia in ambulatory surgery? *Curr Opin Anaesthesiol.* 2000;13:631–636.
46. Smith I. Nitrous oxide in ambulatory anaesthesia: Does it have a place in day surgical anaesthesia or is it just a threat for personnel and the global environment? *Curr Opin Anaesthesiol.* 2006;19:592–596.
47. Sanders RD, Weimann J, Maze M. Biologic effects of nitrous oxide: A mechanistic and toxicologic review. *Anesthesiology.* 2008;109:707–722.
48. Peyton PJ, Chao I, Weinberg L, et al. Nitrous oxide diffusion and the second gas effect on emergence from anesthesia. *Anesthesiology.* 2011;114:596–602.
49. Leslie K, Myles PS, Chan MTV, et al. Nitrous oxide and long-term morbidity and mortality in the ENIGMA trial. *Anesth Analg.* 2010;112:387–393.
50. Taylor E, Feinstein R, White PF, et al. Anesthesia for laparoscopic cholecystectomy: Is nitrous oxide contraindicated? *Anesthesiology.* 1992;76:541–543.
51. Fernandez-Guisasola J, Gomez-Arnau JI, Cabrera Y, et al. Association between nitrous oxide and the incidence of postoperative nausea and vomiting in adults: A systematic review and meta-analysis. *Anaesthesia.* 2010;65:379–387.
52. Tramer M, Moore A, McQuay H. Omitting nitrous oxide in general anesthesia: Meta-analysis of intraoperative awareness and postoperative emesis in randomized controlled trials. *Br J Anaesth.* 1996;76:186–193.
53. Neuman GG, Sidebotham G, Negoianu E, et al. Laparoscopy explosion hazards with nitrous oxide. *Anesthesiology.* 1993;78:875–879.
54. Diemunsch PA, Van Dorsselaer T, Torp KD, et al. Calibrated pneumoperitoneal venting to prevent N_2O accumulation in the CO_2 pneumoperitoneum during laparoscopy with inhaled anesthesia: An experimental study in pigs. *Anesth Analg.* 2002;94:1014–1018.
55. Joshi GP. Multimodal analgesia techniques and postoperative rehabilitation. *Anesthesiol Clin North America.* 2005;23:185–202.
56. Jones RM, Detmer M, Hill AB, et al. Incidence of choledochoduodenal sphincter spasm during fentanyl-supplemented anesthesia. *Anesth Analg.* 1981;60:638–640.
57. Chassard D, Berrada K, Tournadre J, et al. The effects of neuromuscular block on peak airway pressure and abdominal elastance during pneumoperitoneum. *Anesth Analg.* 1996;82:525–527.
58. King M, Sujirattanawimol N, Danielson DR, et al. Requirements for muscle relaxants during radical retropubic prostatectomy. *Anesthesiology.* 2000;93: 1392–1397.
59. Gainsburg DM, Wax D, Reich DL, et al. Intraoperative management of robotic-assisted versus radical prostatectomy. *JSLS.* 2010;14:1–5.
60. Murphy GS, Brull SJ. Residual neuromuscular block: Lessons unlearned. Part I: Definitions, incidence, and adverse physiologic effects of residual neuromuscular block. *Anesth Analg.* 2010;111:120–128.
61. Brull SJ, Murphy GS. Residual neuromuscular block: Lessons unlearned. Part II: Methods to reduce the risks of residual weakness. *Anesth Analg.* 2010;111:129–140.
62. Plaud B, Debaene B, Donati F, et al. Residual paralysis after emergence from anesthesia. *Anesthesiology.* 2010;112:1013–1022.
63. Murphy GS, Szokol JW, Avram MJ, et al. Intraoperative acceleromyography monitoring reduces symptoms of muscle weakness and improves quality of recovery in the early postoperative period. *Anesthesiology.* 2011;115:946–954.
64. Tramer MR, Fuchs-Buder T. Omitting antagonism of neuromuscular block: Effect on postoperative nausea and vomiting and risk of residual paralysis. A systematic review. *Br J Anaesth.* 1999;82:379–386.
65. Cheng CR, Sessler DI, Apfel CC. Does neostigmine administration produce a clinically important increase in postoperative nausea and vomiting? *Anesth Analg.* 2005;101:1349–1355.
66. Fuchs-Buder T, Meistelman C, Alla F, et al. Antagonism of low degrees of atracurium-induced neuromuscular blockade. Dose–effect relationship for neostigmine. *Anesthesiology.* 2010;112:34–60.
67. Gertler R, Joshi GP. Modern understanding of intraoperative mechanical ventilation in normal and diseased lungs. *Adv Anesth.* 2010;28:15–33.
68. Meininger D, Byhahn C, Mierdl S, et al. Positive end-expiratory pressure improves arterial oxygenation during prolonged pneumoperitoneum. *Acta Anaesthesiol Scand.* 2005;49:778–783.

69. Futier E, Constantin JM, Pelosi P, et al. Intraoperative recruitment maneuver reverses detrimental pneumoperitoneum-induced respiratory effects in healthy weight and obese patients undergoing laparoscopy. *Anesthesiology.* 2010;113:1310–1319.
70. Hager H, Reddy D, Mandadi G, et al. Hypercapnia improves tissue oxygenation in morbidly obese surgical patients. *Anesth Analg.* 2006;103:677–681.
71. Fleischmann E, Herbst F, Kugener A, et al. Mild hypercapnia increases subcutaneous and colonic oxygen tension in patients given 80% inspired oxygen during abdominal surgery. *Anesthesiology.* 2006;104:944–949.
72. Montenij LJ, de Waal E, Buhre WF. Arterial waveform analysis in anesthesia and critical care. *Curr Opin Anesthesiol.* 2011;24:651–656.
73. Thiele RH, Durieux ME. Arterial waveform analysis for the anesthesiologist: Past, present, and future concepts. *Anesth Analg.* 2011;113:766–776.
74. Grocott HP. Avoid hypotension and hypoxia: An old anesthetic adage with renewed relevance from cerebral oximetry monitoring. *Can J Anaesth.* 2011; 58:697–702.
75. Murkin JM, Arango M. Near-infrared spectroscopy as an index of brain and tissue oxygenation. *Br J Anaesth.* 2009;103(suppl 1):i3–i13.
76. Highton D, Elwell C, Smith M. Noninvasive cerebral oximetry: Is there light at the end of the tunnel? *Curr Opin Anaesthesiol.* 2010;23:576–581.
77. Joshi GP. Intraoperative fluid restriction improves outcome after major elective gastrointestinal surgery. *Anesth Analg.* 2005;101:601–605.
78. Jacob M, Chappell D, Rehm M. Perioperative fluid administration: Another form of "work-life balance." *Anesthesiology.* 2011;114:483–484.
79. Holte K, Klarskov B, Christensen DS, et al. Liberal versus restrictive fluid administration to improve recovery after laparoscopic cholecystectomy. A randomized, double-blind study. *Ann Surg.* 2004;240:892–899.
80. Vincent JL. Let's give some fluid and see what happens *versus* the mini-fluid challenge. *Anesthesiology.* 2011;115:455–456.
81. Gan TJ, Meyer TA, Apfel CC, et al. Society for ambulatory anesthesia guidelines for the management of postoperative nausea and vomiting. *Anesth Analg.* 2007;105:1615–1628.
82. Melton MS, Klein SM, Gan TJ. Management of postdischarge nausea and vomiting after ambulatory surgery. *Curr Opin Anesthesiol.* 2011;24:612–619.
83. Le TP, Gan TJ. Update on the management of postoperative nausea and vomiting and postdischarge nausea and vomiting in ambulatory surgery. *Anesthesiol Clin.* 2010;28:225–249.
84. Diemunsch P, Joshi GP, Brichant JF. Neurokinin-1 receptor antagonists in the prevention of postoperative nausea and vomiting. *Br J Anaesth.* 2009;103:7–13.
85. George E, Hornuss C, Apfel CC. Neurokinin-1 and novel serotonin antagonists for postoperative and postdischarge nausea and vomiting. *Curr Opin Anesthesiol.* 2010;23:714–721.
86. Veldkamp R, Gholghesaei M, Bonjer HJ, et al. Laparoscopic resection of colon cancer: Consensus of the European Association of Endoscopic Surgery (EAES). *Surg Endosc.* 2004;18:1163–1185.
87. Gurusamy KS, Samraj K, Davidson BR. Low pressure versus standard pressure pneumoperitoneum in laparoscopic cholecystectomy. *Cochrane Database Syst Rev.* 2009;(2):CD006930.
88. Kehlet H, Gray AW, Bonnet F, on behalf of the PROSPECT Group. A procedure-specific systematic review and consensus recommendations for postoperative analgesia following laparoscopic cholecystectomy. *Surg Endosc.* 2005;19:1396–1415.
89. Gajraj NM, Joshi GP. Role of cyclooxygenase-2 inhibitors in postoperative pain management. *Anesthesiol Clin North America.* 2005;23:49–72.
90. McNicol ED, Tzortzopoulou A, Cepeda MS, et al. Single-dose intravenous paracetamol or propacetamol for prevention or treatment of postoperative pain: A systematic review and meta-analysis. *Br J Anaesth.* 2011;106:764–775.
91. Ong CK, Seymour RA, Lirk P, et al. Combining paracetamol (acetaminophen) with nonsteroidal antiinflammatory drugs: A qualitative systematic review of analgesic efficacy for acute postoperative pain. *Anesth Analg.* 2010;110:1170–1179.
92. Maund E, McDaid C, Rice S, et al. Paracetamol and selective and non-selective non-steroidal anti-inflammatory drugs for the reduction in morphine-related side-effects after major surgery: A systematic review. *Br J Anaesth.* 2011;106: 292–297.
93. De Oliveira GS, Almeida MD, Benzon HT, et al. Perioperative single dose systemic dexamethasone for postoperative pain: A meta-analysis of randomized controlled trials. *Anesthesiology.* 2011;115:575–588.
94. Srinivasa S, Kahokehr AA, Yu T, et al. Preoperative glucocorticoid use in major abdominal surgery: Systematic review and meta-analysis of randomized trials. *Ann Surg.* 2011;254:183–191.
95. Laskowski K, Stirling A, McKay WP, et al. A systematic review of intravenous ketamine for postoperative analgesia. *Can J Anaesth.* 2011;58:911–923.
96. Moiniche S, Jorgensen H, Wetterslev J, et al. Local anesthetic infiltration for postoperative pain relief after laparoscopy: A qualitative and quantitative systematic review of intraperitoneal, port-site infiltration and mesosalpinx block. *Anesth Analg.* 2000;90:899–912.
97. Gupta A. Local anaesthesia for pain relief after laparoscopic cholecystectomy-a systematic review. *Best Pract Res Clin Anaesthesiol.* 2005;19:275–292.
98. Thornton PC, Buggy DJ. Local anaesthetic wound infusion for acute postoperative pain: A viable option? *Br J Anaesth.* 2011;107:656–658.
99. Bonnet F, Berger J, Aveline C. Transversus abdominis block: What is its role in postoperative analgesia? *Br J Anaesth.* 2009;103:468–470.
100. Petersen PL, Mathiesen O, Torup H, et al. The transversus abdominis plane block: A valuable option for postoperative analgesia? A topical review. *Acta Anaesthesiol Scand.* 2010;54:529–535.
101. Kahokehr A, Sammour T, Soop M, et al. Intraperitoneal use of local anaesthetic in laparoscopic cholecystectomy: Systematic review and metaanalysis of randomized controlled trials. *J Hepatobiliary Pancreat Sci.* 2010;17:637–656.
102. Kahokehr A, Sammour T, Srinivasa S, et al. Systematic review and meta-analysis of intraperitoneal local anaesthetic for pain reduction after laparoscopic gastric procedures. *Br J Surg.* 2011;98:29–36.
103. Bucciero M, Ingelmo PM, Fumagalli R, et al. Intraperitoneal ropivacaine nebulization for pain management after laparoscopic cholecystetcomy: Comparison with intraperitoneal instillation. *Anesth Analg.* 2011;113:1266–1271.
104. Marret E, Rolin M, Beaussier M, et al. Meta-analysis of intravenous lidocaine and postoperative recovery after abdominal surgery. *Br J Surg.* 2008;95:1331–1338.
105. McCarthy GC, Megalla SA, Habib AS. Impact of intravenous lidocaine infusion on postoperative analgesia and recovery from surgery. A systematic review of randomized controlled trials. *Drugs.* 2010;70:1149–1163.
106. Vigneault L, Turgeon AF, Cote D, et al. Perioperative intravenous lidocaine infusion for postoperative pain control: A meta-analysis of randomized controlled trials. *Can J Anaesth.* 2011;58:22–37.
107. Levy BF, Tilney HS, Dowson HMP, et al. A systematic review of postoperative analgesia following laparoscopic colorectal surgery. *Colorectal Dis.* 2010;12:5–15.
108. Meylan N, Elia N, Lysakowski C, et al. Benefit and risk of intrathecal morphine without local anaesthetic in patients undergoing major surgery: Meta-analysis of randomized trials. *Br J Anaesth.* 2009;102:156–167.
109. Christie IW, McCabe S. Major complications of epidural analgesia after surgery: Results of six-year survey. *Anaesthesia.* 2007;62:335–342.
110. Joshi GP. Complications of laparoscopic surgery. *Anesthesiol Clin North America.* 2001;19:89–105.
111. Coelho RF, Campos ACL, Costa MAR, et al. Complications of laparoscopic fundoplication in the elderly. *Surg Laparosc Endosc Percutan Tech.* 2003;13:6–10.
112. Pareek G, Hedican SP, Gee JR, et al. Meta-analysis of the complications of laparoscopic renal surgery: Comparison of procedures and techniques. *J Urol.* 2006;175:1208–1213.
113. Fischer B, Engel N, Fehr JL, et al. Complications of robotic assisted radical prostatectomy. *World J Urol.* 2008;26:595–602.
114. Coelho RF, Palmer KJ, Rocco B, et al. Early complication rates in a single-surgeon series of 2500 robotic-assisted radical prostatectomies: Report applying a standardized grading system. *Eur Urol.* 2010;57:945–957.
115. Lasser MS, Renzulli J II, Turini GA III, et al. An unbiased prospective report of perioperative complications of robot-assisted laparoscopic radical prostatectomy. *J Urol.* 2010;75:1083–1089.
116. Cheong MA, Kim YC, Park HK, et al. Paroxysmal tachycardia and hypertension with or without ventricular fibrillation during laparoscopic adrenalectomy: Two case reports in patients with noncatecholamine-secreting adrenocortical adenomas. *J Laparoendosc Adv Surg Tech A.* 1999;9:277.
117. Lobato EB, Paige GB, Brown MM, et al. Pneumoperitoneum as a risk factor for endobronchial intubation during laparoscopic gynecologic surgery. *Anesth Analg.* 1998;86:301.
118. Rajan GRC, Foroughi V. Mainstem bronchial obstruction during laparoscopic fundoplication. *Anesth Analg.* 1999;89:252.
119. Wolf JS, Monk TG, McDougall EM, et al. The extraperitoneal approach and subcutaneous emphysema are associated with greater absorption of carbon dioxide during laparoscopic renal surgery. *J Urol.* 1995;154:959.
120. Siu W, Seifman BD, Wolf JS Jr. Subcutaneous emphysema, pneumomediastinum and bilateral pneumothoraces after laparoscopic pyeloplasty. *J Urol.* 2003;170:1936–1937.
121. Stern JA, Nadler RB. Pneumothorax masked by subcutaneous emphysema after laparoscopic nephrectomy. *J Endocrinol.* 2004;18:457–458.
122. Hall D, Goldstein A, Tynan E, et al. Profound hypercarbia late in the course of laparoscopic cholecystectomy: Detection by continuous capnometry. *Anesthesiology.* 1993;79:173.
123. Phillips S, Falk GL. Surgical tension pneumothorax during laparoscopic repair of massive hiatus hernia: A different situation requiring different management. *Anaesth Intensive Care.* 2011;39:1120–1123.
124. Joris J, Chiche JD, Lamy M. Pneumothorax during laparoscopic fundoplication: Diagnosis and treatment with positive pressure. *Anesth Analg.* 1995;81:993–1000.
125. Yee R, Hyde PR, Currie JS. Pneumothorax during laparoscopic Nissen fundoplication. *Anaesth Intensive Care.* 1996;24:93–96.
126. Hawasli A, Boutt AW. Spontaneous resolution of massive laparoscopy-associated pneumothorax: The case of the bulging diaphragm and review of the literature. *J Laparoendosc Adv Surg Tech A.* 2002;12:77–82.
127. Ueda K, Ahmed W, Ross A. Intraoperative pneumothorax identified with transthoracic ultrasound. *Anesthesiology.* 2011;115:653–655.
128. Venkatesh R, Kibel AS, Lee D, et al. Rapid resolution of carbon dioxide pneumothorax (capno-thorax) resulting from diaphragmatic injury during laparoscopic nephrectomy. *J Urol.* 2002;167:1387–1388.
129. Derouin M, Couture P, Boudreault D, et al. Detection of gas embolism by transesophageal echocardiography during laparoscopic cholecystectomy. *Anesth Analg.* 1996;82:119–124.

130. Schmandra TC, Mierdl S, Bauer H, et al. Transesophageal echocardiography shows high risk of gas embolism during laparoscopic hepatic resection under carbon dioxide pneumoperitoneum. *Br J Surg.* 2002;89:870–876.
131. Hong JY, Kim JY, Choi KH, et al. Incidence of venous gas embolism during robotic-assisted laparoscopic radical prostatectomy is lower than that during radical retropubic prostatectomy. *Br J Anaesth.* 2010;105:777–781.
132. Fors D, Eiriksson K, Arvidsson D, et al. Gas embolism during laparoscopic liver resection in a pig model: Frequency and severity. *Br J Anaesth.* 2010;105:282–288.
133. Kim CS, Kim JY, Kwon JY, et al. Venous air embolism during total laparoscopic hysterectomy: Comparison to total abdominal hysterectomy. *Anesthesiology.* 2009;111:50–54.
134. Makinen M-T. Comparison of body temperature changes during laparoscopic and open cholecystectomy. *Acta Anaesthesiol Scand.* 1997;41:736–740.
135. Stewart BT, Stitz RW, Tuch MM, et al. Hypothermia in open and laparoscopic colorectal surgery. *Dis Colon Rectum.* 1999;42:1292–1295.
136. Gray RI, Ott DE, Henderson AC, et al. Severe local hypothermia from laparoscopic gas evaporative jet cooling: A mechanism to explain clinical observations. *JSLS.* 1999;3:171–177.
137. Davis SS, Mikami DJ, Newlin M, et al. Heating and humidifying of carbon dioxide during pneumoperitoneum is not indicated: A prospective randomized trial. *Surg Endosc.* 2006;20:153–158.
138. Sammour T, Kahokehr A, Hayes J, et al. Warming and humidification of insufflation carbon dioxide in laparoscopic colonic surgery. A double-blinded randomized controlled trial. *Ann Surg.* 2010;251:1024–1033.
139. Birch DW, Manouchehri N, Shi X, et al. Heated CO(2) with or without humidification for minimally invasive abdominal surgery. *Cochrane Database Syst Rev.* 2011;(1):CD007821.
140. American Society of Anesthesiologists Task Force on Perioperative Visual Loss. Practice advisory for perioperative visual loss associated with spine surgery: An updated report by the American Society of Anesthesiologists Task Force on perioperative visual loss. *Anesthesiology.* 2012;116:274–285.
141. Newman NJ. Perioperative visual loss after nonocular surgeries. *Am J Ophthalmol.* 2008;145:604–610.
142. Weber ED, Colyer MH, Lesser RL, et al. Posterior ischemic optic neuropathy after minimally invasive prostatectomy. *J Neuroophthalmol.* 2007;27:285–287.
143. Phong SV, Koh LK. Anaesthesia for robotic-assisted radical prostatectomy: Considerations for laparoscopy in the Trendelenburg position. *Anaesth Intensive Care.* 2007;35:281–285.
144. Sharma RR, Axelsson H, Oberg A, et al. Diaphragmatic activity after laparoscopic cholecystectomy. *Anesthesiology.* 1999;91:406.
145. Erice F, Fox GS, Salib YM, et al. Diaphragmatic function before and after laparoscopic cholecystectomy. *Anesthesiology.* 1994;79:966.
146. Sadovnikoff N, Maxwell LG. Respiratory failure after laparoscopic cholecystectomy in a patient with chronic hemidiaphragm paralysis. *Anesthesiology.* 1997;87:996.
147. Beebe D, McNevin M, Belani K, et al. Evidence of venous stasis after abdominal insufflation for laparoscopic cholecystectomy. *Surg Gynecol Obstet.* 1993;176:443–447.

CHAPTER

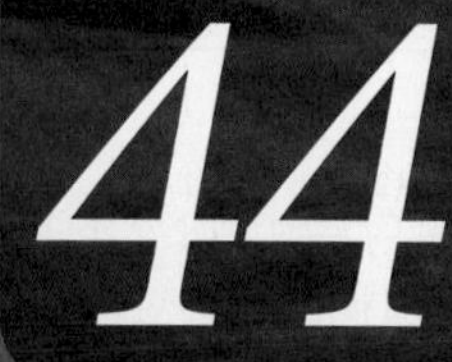

Anesthesia and Obesity

BRENDA A. BUCKLIN • ANA FERNANDEZ-BUSTAMANTE

Key Points

1. Neck circumference is the single best predictor of problematic intubation in morbidly obese patients. A larger neck circumference is associated with male sex, higher Mallampati score, grade 3 laryngoscopic views, and obstructive sleep apnea.
2. Because obese patients often have limited exercise tolerance they may appear asymptomatic even though they have significant cardiovascular disease.
3. Obstructive sleep apnea is common in obese patients and predisposes to airway management difficulties during anesthesia.
4. Elevated liver function tests (mostly elevated alanine aminotransferase) are seen in many obese patients, but no clear correlation exists between abnormalities of routine liver function tests and the capacity of the liver to metabolize drugs.
5. Forearm blood pressure is a fairly good predictor of upper arm blood pressure in most patients, but in obese patients, forearm measurements with a standard cuff may overestimate both systolic and diastolic blood pressures.
6. The head-elevated laryngoscopy position elevates the obese patient's head, upper body, and shoulders above the chest and can improve visualization for laryngoscopy and tracheal intubation.
7. Larger doses of induction agents may be required by obese patients because blood volume, muscle mass, and cardiac output increase linearly with the degree of obesity. An increased dose of succinylcholine is necessary because of an increase in pseudocholinesterase activity.
8. Positive end-expiratory pressure is the only ventilatory parameter that has consistently been shown to improve respiratory function in obese patients but it decreases venous return, cardiac output, and subsequent oxygen delivery.
9. Prompt but safe extubation reduces the likelihood that the morbidly obese patient will become ventilator-dependent, especially in patients with cardiopulmonary disease.
10. Morbid obesity is a major independent risk factor for deep venous thrombosis and sudden death from acute postoperative pulmonary embolism. Early mobilization of the morbidly obese patient is often difficult but critically important in the prevention of postoperative complications.
11. Because of the risk of perioperative hypoxemia and apnea in obese patients, postoperative pain management should include opioid-sparing multimodal analgesic techniques. Regional anesthetic techniques reduce the risk of opioid-related complications.
12. Obese patients who have received either neuraxial or parenteral opioids require careful postoperative monitoring. Delayed respiratory depression with centrally administered neuraxial opioids, when coupled with a potentially difficult airway in the obese patient, suggests that close monitoring is prudent.

Multimedia

1 Sequelae of Obesity

2 Sleep Apnea

DEFINITION AND EPIDEMIOLOGY

Introduction

The World Health Organization defines obesity as a condition with excess body fat to the extent that health and well-being are adversely affected.[1] Obesity is reaching epidemic proportions worldwide. For the first time in history, recent estimates suggest that the number of obese individuals now exceeds the number of underweight individuals. About one-third of Americans (33.8%) are currently obese.[2] The prevalence of obesity in the United States is unevenly distributed geographically, by race and ethnicity and by socioeconomic status. The overall trend is, however, to keep increasing. The prevalence of obesity is predicted to reach about 50% by 2030.[3] The Centers for Disease Control and Prevention (CDC) monitor the epidemiology of obesity and publish periodically updated data at http://www.cdc.gov/obesity/.

Obesity-related conditions including cardiovascular accidents, insulin- and noninsulin-dependent diabetes, and some types of cancer are the leading causes of death in this population.[4] Although there has been an exponential increase in the number of bariatric procedures performed, obese and morbidly obese patients undergo all types of surgical procedures. Surgery in this patient population is considered high-risk but careful planning, preoperative risk assessment, proper anesthetic management, strict venothrombotic event prevention, and effective postoperative pain control will all help to reduce the risk. With appropriate perioperative management, obese surgical patients can achieve safe and effective surgical outcomes.

The definition of obesity includes the presence of excessive body weight for the patient's age, gender, and height, and is often based on the following concepts. *Ideal body weight* (IBW) is a concept originated by life insurance companies by referencing height–weight tables. It is the weight associated with the lowest mortality rate for a given height and gender and can be estimated using Broca's index:

$$\text{IBW (kg)} = \text{height (cm)} - x,$$

where x is 100 for adult males and 105 for adult females.

Predicted body weight (PBW) is a concept similar to IBW, and is more commonly used in the medical literature. PBW is usually calculated with the following formulas in adults[5]:

$$\text{Males: PBW (kg)} = 50 + 0.91 \times (\text{height (cm)} - 152.4)$$

$$\text{Females: PBW (kg)} = 45.5 + 0.91 \times (\text{height (cm)} - 152.4)$$

Lean body weight (LBW) is the total body weight (TBW) minus the adipose tissue. It is a combination of body cell mass, extracellular water, and nonfat connective tissue. It approximates 80% and 75% of TBW for males and females, respectively, although more accurate formulas have been proposed.[6,7] In morbidly obese patients, increasing the IBW by 20% to 30% gives an estimate of LBW. In nonobese and nonmuscular individuals, TBW approximates IBW.[8]

In clinical practice it is common to utilize the *Body mass index* (BMI), also called Quetelet's index, to estimate the degree of obesity. The BMI is determined using the patient's measured weight (in kilograms) and height (in meters) and is calculated as follows:

$$\text{BMI} = \text{weight}/(\text{height})^2$$

Obesity is defined as having a BMI ≥30 kg/m^2. Obesity is further classified according to systemic disease risk (Table 44-1). *Morbid obesity,* defined as a BMI ≥40 kg/m^2, can also be further classified into super obesity (BMI ≥50 kg/m^2) and super-super obesity (BMI ≥60 kg/m^2).[9] BMI differentiates obese from nonobese adults and it estimates body fat because it adjusts for height while strongly correlating with body weight; however, it cannot distinguish between overweight and overfat, as heavily muscled individuals can be easily classified as overweight using BMI. Therefore, other factors such as age, fat content, and distribution (i.e., waist circumference and waist-to-hip ratio) should be taken into consideration, along with other health risk predictors that use the concept of BMI.[10]

The anatomic distribution of body fat has associated pathophysiologic implications.[11,12] In *android (central) obesity,* adipose tissue is located predominantly in the upper body (truncal distribution) and is associated with increased oxygen consumption and an increased incidence of cardiovascular disease. Visceral fat is particularly associated with cardiovascular disease and left ventricular dysfunction. In *gynecoid (peripheral) obesity,* adipose tissue is located predominantly in the hips, buttocks, and thighs.

ANESTHESIA FOR SURGICAL SUBSPECIALTIES

TABLE 44-1. CLASSIFICATION OF OBESITY AND SYSTEMIC DISEASE RISK ACCORDING TO WAIST CIRCUMFERENCE

BMI (kg/m^2)	Description	Risk of Systemic Disease (Small vs. Large Waist Circumference)	
		Male: <102 cm Female: <88 cm	Male: ≥102 cm Female: ≥88 cm
<18.5	Underweight		
18.5–24.9	Normal		
25–29.9	Overweight		
30–34.9	Obesity (class I)	Average	Average
35–39.9	Obesity (class II)	Increased	High
≥40	Morbid obesity (class III)	High	Very high
≥50	Super obesity	Very high	Very high
≥60	Super-super obesity	Extremely high	Extremely high

BMI, body mass index.

This fat is less metabolically active so it is less closely associated with cardiovascular disease. Body circumference indices such as waist circumference, waist-to-height ratio, and waist-to-hip ratio help to classify these patterns of obesity (e.g., android vs. gynecoid obesity) and correlate with mortality and the risk for developing obesity-related diseases. Waist circumference correlates with abdominal fat and is an independent risk predictor of disease.

Management of Obesity

Medical Therapy

The indications for pharmacologic treatment include a BMI ≥30 kg/m^2 or a BMI between 27 and 29.9 kg/m^2 in conjunction with an obesity-related medical complication. Lifestyle counseling is still the most effective tool for long-term weight loss, but it can be combined with the use of medications.[13,14] Medications used to treat obesity are formulated to reduce energy intake, increase energy utilization, or decrease absorption of nutrients. The only currently FDA-approved antiobesity medications are phentermine and orlistat.[15] Phentermine (Adipex-P) is a sympathomimetic drug that decreases appetite. Although it is only approved for 3 months use, it can induce tachycardia, palpitations, hypertension, as well as dependence, abuse, and withdrawal symptoms. It is no longer combined with fenfluramine (Phen-Fen) due to concerns of pulmonary hypertension and valvular heart disease,[16] but is being explored in combination with topiramate (Topamax).[17] This combination often causes dry mouth, paresthesias, constipation, insomnia, and dizziness. Orlistat (OTC Alli, prescribed Xenical) or tetrahydrolipstatin, blocks the absorption of dietary fat by inhibiting lipases in the gastrointestinal tract. It leads to weight loss and to improvement of blood pressure, fasting blood glucose levels, and lipid profile.[18] Fat malabsorption causes common complaints of oily spotting, liquid stools, fecal urgency, flatulence, and abdominal cramping. Chronic use of orlistat may result in fat-soluble vitamin deficiency. A prolonged prothrombin time with a normal partial thromboplastin time during orlistat treatment may reflect vitamin K deficiency and this coagulopathy should be corrected 6 to 24 hours before elective surgery.[19]

A variety of over the counter preparations, plant extracts, or herbs are often used by patients to combat obesity. Substances found in these preparations that are allegedly thought to promote fat loss include pancreatic lipase inhibitors (caffeine, green or black tea), appetite suppressants (hoodia, Korean ginseng, ephedra, sunflower oil), stimulants of energy expenditure (acai berry, caffeine), and regulators of lipid metabolism (soybean, fish oil, oolong tea, caffeine).[20] The American Society of Anesthesiologists (ASA) warns patients to tell their anesthesiologists about medications they are taking, including vitamins, herbs and other supplements, since these products may interfere with anesthesia or cause complications during surgery.[21]

Surgical Therapy (Bariatric Surgery)

Bariatric surgery is currently the most effective treatment for morbid (class III) obesity. Several guidelines exist for determining patient eligibility for bariatric surgery. Most agree that acceptable patients for surgery are those with a BMI >40 kg/m^2 or BMI >35 kg/m^2 and/or those patients with obesity-related comorbidities not controlled with medical therapy.[22] Procedures are grouped into three classifications. *Malabsorptive* procedures include jejunoileal bypass and biliopancreatic diversion, and are rarely used nowadays. *Restrictive* procedures include vertical-banded gastroplasty and adjustable gastric banding. *Combined* procedures include Roux-en-Y gastric bypass (RYGB), which combines gastric restriction with a minimal degree of malabsorption. RYGB, adjustable gastric banding, and vertical-banded gastroplasty can all be performed laparoscopically. Laparoscopic bariatric surgery is associated with less postoperative pain, lower morbidity, faster recovery, and less "third-spacing" of fluid.[23] RYGB is the most effective bariatric procedure to produce safe short- and long-term weight loss in severely obese patients. With RYGB, patients lose an average of 50% to 60% excess body weight and show a BMI decrease of approximately 10 kg/m^2 during the first 12 to 24 postoperative months. Type II diabetes resolves in a majority of patients. Laparoscopic adjustable gastric banding (LAGB) is a restrictive gastric operation that utilizes an adjustable inflatable band to alter stomach capacity for individual weight loss needs. Vertical-banded or sleeve gastroplasty also restricts food intake.

Less invasive bariatric techniques are being developed. An implantable gastric stimulator (IGS) is placed laparoscopically and emits electrical impulses to stimulate the gastric smooth muscle to stop peristalsis so that the patient feels full. The IGS can be adversely affected by defibrillation, electrocautery, lithotripsy, magnetic resonance imaging, and therapeutic radiation. Intragastric balloons and prostheses, at different experimental stages, are placed endoscopically as a temporary measure to increase satiety.[24] Adequate control of postoperative nausea and vomiting is critical to avoid possible lead and balloon dislodgement. Although apparently simple and safe as bariatric procedures, their efficacy for weight loss is still questioned.[22,25]

PATHOPHYSIOLOGY

Obesity can have an adverse effect on multiple organ systems. Table 44-2 provides a list of the most relevant organ systems with implications for clinical management. These systems will be discussed separately in this section.

Respiratory System

Fat accumulation on the thorax and abdomen decreases chest wall and lung compliance. Decreased lung compliance is partially explained by increased pulmonary blood volume related to an overall increase in blood volume. Increased elastic resistance and decreased compliance of the chest wall are further reduced while supine, leading to shallow and rapid breathing, an increased work of breathing, and limited maximum ventilatory capacity. Respiratory muscle efficiency is below normal in obese individuals. Decreased pulmonary compliance leads to decreased functional residual capacity (FRC), vital capacity, and total lung capacity. Reduction in FRC is primarily a result of reduced expiratory reserve volume (ERV), but the relationship between FRC and closing capacity, the volume at which small airways begin to close, is adversely affected (Fig. 44-1). Decreases in FRC and ERV are the most commonly reported abnormalities of pulmonary function in obese patients.[26,27] Residual volume and closing capacity are unchanged. Reduced FRC (due to decreased ERV) can result in lung volumes below closing capacity in the course of normal tidal ventilation, leading to small airway closure, ventilation–perfusion mismatch, right-to-left shunting, and arterial hypoxemia. Anesthesia and supine positioning worsen this situation such that up to a 50% reduction in FRC occurs in the obese anesthetized patient compared with 20% in the non-obese individual. Forced expiratory volume in 1 second and forced vital capacity are usually within normal limits. ERV is the most sensitive indicator of the effect of obesity on pulmonary function.

TABLE 44-2. ANESTHETIC IMPLICATIONS OF OBESITY

System	Key Concerns
Respiratory	• Increased risk of perioperative hypoxemia • Careful monitoring needed • Use supplemental oxygen • Use CPAP (if/when indicated) • Use nonsupine positioning (if possible) • Exercise extreme caution when administering respiratory depressants
Cardiovascular	• Increased blood volume, cardiac output, left ventricular thickness • Increased proinflammatory and prothrombotic mediators • Higher perioperative complications related to hypertension, thromboembolic events and left ventricular diastolic dysfunction
Gastrointestinal	• Risk of regurgitation • Higher gastric volume and lower pH increases risk of severe pneumonitis should aspiration occur • Current fasting preoperative guidelines (6 h for solids, 2 h for clear liquids) are acceptable • Preoperative assessment of liver function is recommended
Endocrine/ metabolic	• High prevalence of hyperglycemia, insulin resistance and diabetes • Close perioperative glucose monitoring • Metabolic syndrome (combination of central obesity, hypertension, dyslipidemia and impaired glucose metabolism) is frequent and doubles cardiovascular risk
Genitourinary	• Increased risk of renal disease • Higher incidence of preeclampsia and eclampsia
Neurologic	• Careful positioning with extra padding needed
Hematology	• Increased hypercoagulability and risk of perioperative thromboembolic events • Preoperative polycythemia suggests prolonged sleep apnea
Musculoskeletal	• Increased prevalence of osteoarthritis
Psychology/ psychiatry	• Depression, reduced self-esteem, social stigma

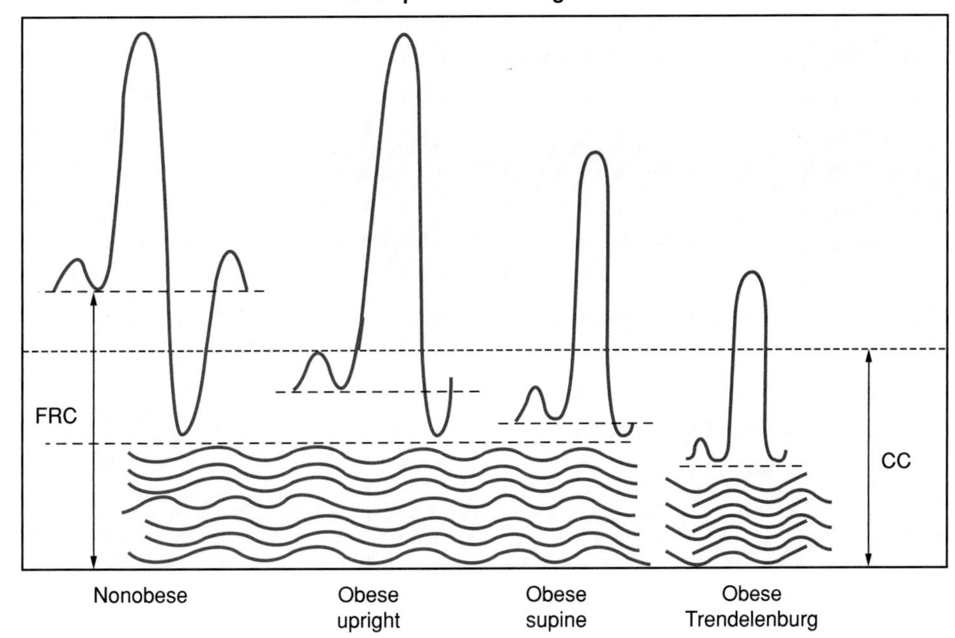

FIGURE 44-1. Effects of obesity, positioning, and anesthesia on lung volumes. FRC, functional residual capacity; CC, closing capacity; CV, closing volume; RV, residual volume. (From: Ranasinghe JS, Penning DH. Morbid Obesity. In: Suresh MS, Segal S, Preston RL, et al, eds. Shnider and Levinson's Anesthesia for Obstetrics. 5th Edition. Philadelphia: WK Health/Lippincott Williams & Wilkins, 2013:582.)

Obesity increases oxygen consumption and carbon dioxide production even at rest. This is because of the metabolic activity of excess fat and the increased workload on supportive tissues. The body attempts to meet these metabolic demands by increasing both cardiac output and alveolar ventilation. Basal metabolic activity is usually within normal limits in relationship to body surface area and normocapnia is usually maintained by an increase in minute ventilation. This requires increased oxygen consumption because most obese patients retain their normal response to hypoxemia and hypercapnia. Arterial oxygen tension in morbidly obese patients' breathing room air is lower than that predicted for similarly aged nonobese subjects in both sitting and supine positions. Chronic hypoxemia may lead to polycythemia, pulmonary hypertension and cor pulmonale.

Obese patients often suffer from OSA characterized by periodic, partial, or complete obstruction of the upper airway during sleep. In obese patients, OSA is more likely to result from airway obstruction produced by excess soft tissue. However, centrally mediated forms of sleep apnea can also occur. Physiologic abnormalities resulting from OSA include hypoxemia, hypercapnia, pulmonary hypertension, systemic vasoconstriction, and secondary polycythemia (from recurrent hypoxemia). These result in an increased risk of ischemic heart disease and cerebrovascular disease. Right ventricular failure can occur from hypoxic pulmonary vasoconstriction. Respiratory acidosis is usually limited only to periods of sleep.

The "gold standard" diagnostic test for OSA is overnight polysomnography (OPS). The inconvenience, time, and expense of OPS lead to an unknown fraction of obese patients with suspicious but no formal diagnosis of OSA.[28] Suggestive signs to look for during the preoperative visit include witnessed episodes of apnea during sleep, BMI ≥35, neck circumference ≥16 in (≥40 cm), hyperinsulinemia, and elevated glycosylated hemoglobin. Symptoms of snoring, frequent arousals during sleep and daytime sleepiness, impaired concentration, memory problems, and morning headaches are common but not predictive.[29,30] A thorough preoperative evaluation for possible OSA is recommended long enough before elective surgery to allow preparation of a perioperative management plan.[31] Preoperative initiation of continuous positive airway pressure (CPAP), especially in severe OSA cases, should be considered.[31] Patients with confirmed or suspected OSA are at high risk of presenting with a difficult airway and postoperative pulmonary complications, and should be managed accordingly.[32,33]

The *obesity hypoventilation syndrome* (OHS) *or Pickwickian syndrome* may result from long-term OSA and is seen in 5% to 10% of morbidly obese patients. The OHS is a combination of obesity and chronic hypoventilation that ultimately results in pulmonary hypertension and cor pulmonale.[34] The presence of both obesity (BMI >30 kg/m^2) and awake arterial hypercapnia ($PaCO_2$ >45 mm Hg) in the absence of known causes of hypoventilation supports the diagnosis. Prolonged OSA also alters the control of breathing, leading to CNS-mediated apneic events. This increases reliance on hypoxic drive for ventilation. The main ventilatory impairment of OHS is alveolar hypoventilation independent of intrinsic lung disease. Other characteristics of OHS include daytime hypersomnolence, hypercapnia, hypoxemia, and polycythemia. Right ventricular failure eventually ensues. These patients also have an increased sensitivity to the respiratory depressant effects of general anesthetics.

Cardiovascular and Hematologic Systems

Total blood volume is increased in the obese individual; but on a volume-to-weight basis, it is less than in nonobese individuals (50 mL/kg compared with 70 mL/kg). Most of this extra volume is distributed in the adipose tissue. Renal and splanchnic blood flows are increased. Cardiac output increases with increasing weight by as much as 20 to 30 mL/kg of excess body fat because of ventricular dilation and increases in stroke volume. The resulting increased left ventricular wall stress leads to hypertrophy, reduced compliance, and impairment of left ventricular filling (diastolic dysfunction) with elevated left ventricular diastolic pressure, and pulmonary edema.[35] When left ventricular wall thickening fails to keep pace with dilation, systolic dysfunction ("obesity cardiomyopathy") and eventual biventricular failure results (Fig. 44-2).

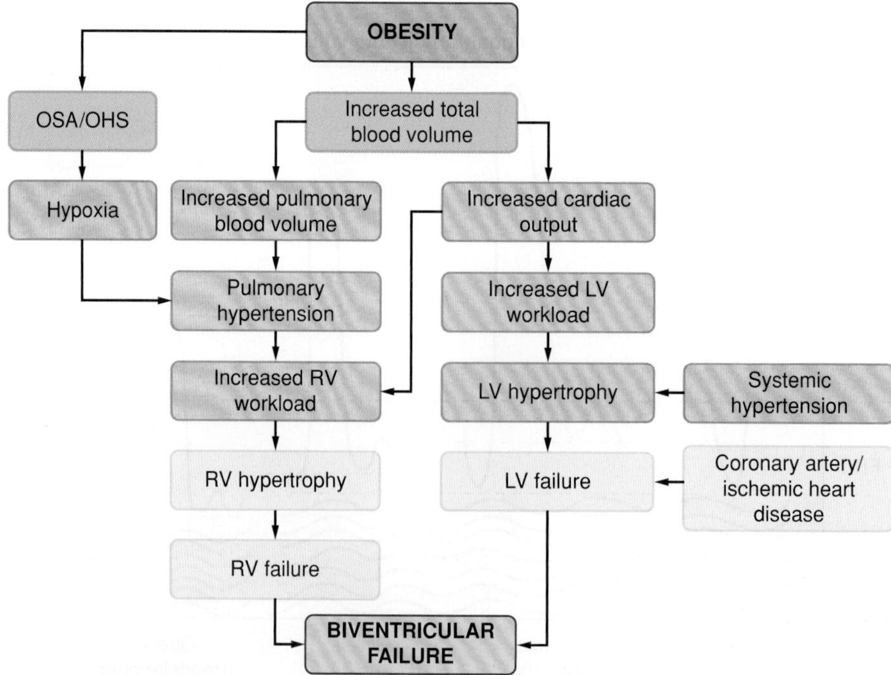

FIGURE 44-2. Interrelationship of cardiovascular and pulmonary sequelae of obesity. OSA, obstructive sleep apnea; OHS, obesity hypoventilation syndrome; LV, left ventricular; RV, right ventricular.

Obesity accelerates atherosclerosis. Symptoms such as angina or exertional dyspnea occur only occasionally because morbidly obese patients often have very limited mobility and may appear asymptomatic even when they have significant cardiovascular disease.

Blood flow to fat is 2 to 3 mL/100 g of tissue. An excess of fat requires an increase in cardiac output, to parallel an increase in oxygen consumption. This leads to a systemic arteriovenous oxygen difference that remains normal or slightly above normal. Intraoperative ventricular failure may occur from rapid intravenous fluid administration (indicating left ventricular diastolic dysfunction), the negative inotropism of anesthetic agents, or pulmonary hypertension precipitated by hypoxia or hypercapnia. Cardiac dysrhythmias may be precipitated by fatty infiltration of the conduction system, hypoxia, hypercapnia, electrolyte imbalance, coronary artery disease, increased circulating catecholamines, OSA, and myocardial hypertrophy. Frequent ECG findings seen in morbidly obese patients include low QRS voltage, multiple criteria for left ventricular hypertrophy (LVH) and left atrial enlargement, and T-wave flattening in the inferior and lateral leads.[36] In addition, there is a leftward shift of the P-wave, QRS complex, and T-wave axes, lengthening of the corrected QT interval, and prolongation of the QT interval. Substantial weight reduction reverses many of these ECG abnormalities.[37]

Cardiac output rises faster in response to exercise in the morbidly obese and is often associated with a rise in left ventricular end-diastolic pressure and pulmonary capillary wedge pressure. Similar changes occur during the perioperative period, which should prompt a low threshold for performing detailed cardiac investigations. Many obese patients have mild-to-moderate hypertension, with a 3 to 4 mm Hg increase in systolic and a 2 mm Hg increase in diastolic arterial pressure for every 10 kg of weight gained. Normotensive obese patients have reduced systemic vascular resistance, which rises with the onset of hypertension. Their expanded blood volume causes an increased cardiac output with a lower calculated systemic vascular resistance for the same level of arterial blood pressure. The renin–angiotensin system plays a major role in the hypertension of obesity by increased circulating levels of angiotensinogen, aldosterone, and angiotensin-converting enzyme. As little as 5% reduction in body weight leads to a significant reduction in renin–angiotensin activity in both plasma and adipose tissue, contributing to a reduction in blood pressure.[38]

Obese patients have a normal-to-increased level of sympathetic nervous system activity, which predisposes to insulin resistance, dyslipidemia, and hypertension.[35,39] These obesity-induced comorbidities are responsible for the increased cardiovascular risk in obese patients.[40,41] Insulin resistance enhances the pressor activity of norepinephrine and angiotensin II. Hyperinsulinemia further activates the sympathetic nervous system, causing sodium retention and contributes to obesity-induced hypertension. Hypertension causes concentric hypertrophy of the ventricle in normal-weight individuals but causes eccentric dilation in obese individuals. It is associated with increased preload and stroke work. The combination of obesity and hypertension causes left ventricular wall thickening and a larger heart volume; therefore, there is increased likelihood of cardiac failure (Fig. 44-3).

Obese individuals are also prone to cardiovascular disease because adipose tissue releases a large number of bioactive mediators. These can result in abnormal lipids, insulin resistance, inflammation, and coagulopathies.[40,41] Obese individuals have higher levels of fibrinogen (a marker for the inflammatory process of atherosclerosis), factor VII, factor VIII, von Willebrand factor, and plasminogen activator inhibitor-1 (PAI-1). Increased levels of fibrinogen, factor VII, factor VIII, and hypofibrinolysis are associated with hypercoagulability. High factor VIII levels are associated with increased cardiovascular mortality. Increased fasting triglyceride levels correlate with increased factor VII concentrations, and postprandial lipemia causes activation of factor VII. Endothelial dysfunction induced by insulin increases von Willebrand factor and factor VIII levels, predisposing to fibrin formation. Increased secretion of PAI-1 inhibits the fibrinolytic system and is associated with visceral obesity.[42]

Gastrointestinal System

Gastric volume and acidity are increased, hepatic function is altered, and drug metabolism is adversely affected by obesity. Many fasting morbidly obese patients who present for elective surgery have gastric volumes in excess of 25 mL and gastric fluid pH <2.5 (the generally accepted volume and pH indicative of high risk for pneumonitis should regurgitation and aspiration occur). Delayed gastric emptying occurs because of increased abdominal mass that causes antral distension, gastrin release, and a decrease in pH with parietal cell secretion.[43,44] Abdominal obesity increases intragastric pressure, increasing the frequency of transient lower esophageal sphincter relaxation, and/or hiatal hernia formation. An increase of >3.5 kg/m^2 in BMI is associated with a 2.7-fold increase in risk for developing new reflux symptoms.[43] An increased incidence of hiatal hernia and gastroesophageal reflux further increase aspiration risk.

Gastric emptying is faster with high-energy content intake such as fat emulsions, but because of larger gastric volume (up to 75% larger), the residual volume is increased. The combination of hiatal hernia, gastroesophageal reflux, and delayed gastric emptying, coupled with increased intra-abdominal pressure and high volume/low pH gastric content, puts the obese patient at risk for an increased incidence of severe pneumonitis should aspiration occur. Unpremedicated, nondiabetic fasting obese surgical patients who are free from significant gastroesophageal pathology are unlikely to have high volume, low pH gastric contents after routine preoperative fasting.[45] They should follow the same fasting guidelines as nonobese patients and be allowed to drink clear liquids up until 2 hours before elective surgery.[46] Weight loss significantly improves gastroesophageal reflux symptoms.[47]

Peculiar morphologic and biochemical abnormalities of the liver are associated with obesity and include fatty infiltration (high prevalence of nonalcoholic fatty liver disease or NAFLD), inflammation (nonalcoholic steatohepatitis or NASH), focal necrosis, and cirrhosis. Fatty infiltration reflects the duration rather than the degree of obesity. Histologic and liver function test abnormalities are relatively common, but clearance usually is not reduced. Abnormal liver function tests are seen in up to one-third of obese patients who have no evidence of concomitant liver disease. The most common abnormality is an increased ALT. Despite these histologic and enzymatic changes, no clear correlation exists between liver function abnormalities and the capacity of the liver to metabolize drugs.[48] Morbidly obese patients who have undergone intestinal bypass surgery have a particularly high prevalence of hepatic dysfunction and cholelithiasis. This is also common in the general obese population due to abnormal cholesterol metabolism. The high prevalence of NAFLD, NASH, and cirrhosis necessitates careful assessment for pre-existing liver disease in obese patients scheduled for surgery. Features suggestive of NASH include hepatomegaly, elevated liver enzymes, and abnormal liver histology (steatosis, steatohepatitis, fibrosis, and cirrhosis).[40]

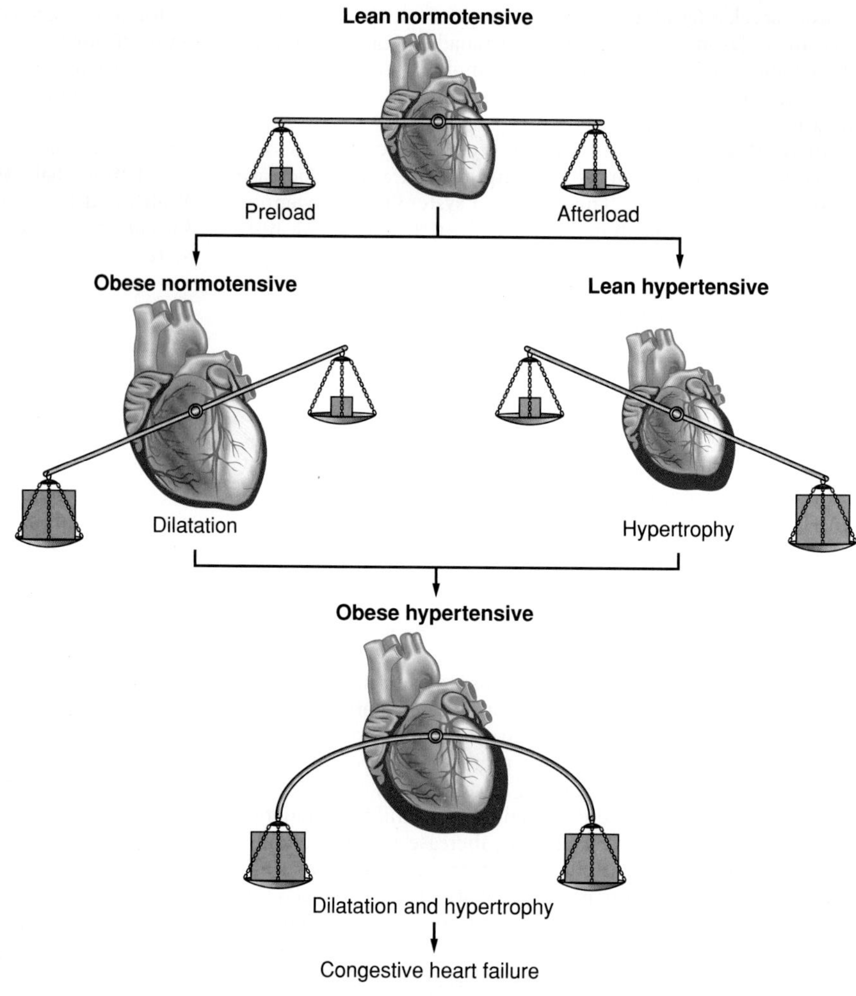

FIGURE 44-3. Adaptation of the heart to obesity and hypertension. (Reprinted from: Messerli FH. Cardiovascular effects of obesity and hypertension. *Lancet.* 1982;1:1165, with permission.)

Renal and Endocrine Systems

Impaired glucose tolerance in the morbidly obese is reflected by a high prevalence of type II diabetes mellitus as a result of resistance of peripheral adipose tissue to insulin.[35] Many obese patients have an abnormal glucose tolerance test, and the relative risk of developing diabetes increases by 25% for every 1 kg/m^2 increase in BMI above 22 kg/m^2.[35] Hyperglycemia, insulin resistance, and diabetes predispose obese patients to wound infections and an increased risk of myocardial infarction. Exogenous insulin may be required perioperatively even in obese patients with type II diabetes mellitus to oppose the catabolic response to surgery. In addition to these concerns, subclinical hypothyroidism occurs in about 25% of all morbidly obese patients. Thyroid-stimulating hormone levels are frequently elevated, suggesting the possibility that obesity leads to a state of thyroid hormone resistance in peripheral tissues. Hypothyroidism may be associated with hypoglycemia, hyponatremia, and impaired hepatic drug metabolism.

Obesity is associated with glomerular hyperfiltration as evidenced by increased renal blood flow and an increased glomerular filtration rate. Excessive weight gain increases renal tubular reabsorption and impairs natriuresis through activation of the sympathetic and renin–angiotensin systems as well as physical compression of the kidney. With prolonged obesity, there may be a loss of nephron function, with further impairment of natriuresis and further increases in arterial pressure. Obesity-related glomerular hyperfiltration decreases after weight loss, which decreases the incidence of overt glomerulopathy.[49]

Metabolic Syndrome

The metabolic syndrome, sometimes referred to as syndrome X and insulin resistance syndrome, is a cluster of metabolic abnormalities associated with an increased risk of diabetes and cardiovascular events. Individuals with this syndrome have up to a fivefold greater risk of developing type 2 diabetes mellitus (if not already present) and are also twice as likely to die from a myocardial infarction or stroke compared with those without the syndrome.[50] There are several diagnostic guidelines for metabolic syndrome.[51] The most widely used is the one delineated by the revised 2004 National Cholesterol Education Program and the American Heart Association (NCEP II/AHA),[52] which defines metabolic syndrome when three out of the following five conditions exist: (1) central obesity: Waist circumference ≥102 cm (≥40 in) in males, ≥88 cm (≥35 in) in females; (2) dyslipidemia: Triglycerides ≥150 mg/dL; (3) dyslipidemia: HDL ≤40 mg/dL in males, ≤50 mg/dL in females; (4) hypertension: ≥130/85 mm Hg or use of antihypertensives; (5) elevated fasting glucose: ≥100 mg/dL (≥5.6 mmol/L) or use of medication for hyperglycemia. Weight loss and lifestyle changes, such as following a Mediterranean diet with high intake of fruits, vegetables, and fiber, improve the metabolic syndrome features.[50,53]

PHARMACOLOGY

Pharmacologic Principles

General pharmacokinetic principles dictate, with certain exceptions, that drug dosing should take into consideration the volume of distribution (V_D) for administration of the loading dose, and the clearance for the maintenance dose.[54] A drug that is mainly distributed to lean tissues should have the loading dose calculated on the basis of LBW. If the drug is equally distributed between adipose and lean tissues, dosing should be calculated on the basis of TBW. For maintenance, a drug with similar clearance values in both obese and nonobese individuals should have the maintenance dose calculated on the basis of LBW. However, a drug whose clearance increases with obesity should have the maintenance dose calculated according to TBW.

The relative volume of the central compartment in which drugs are first distributed remains unchanged in obese patients, but absolute body water content is decreased. Lean body and adipose tissue mass are increased, affecting lipophilic and polar drug distribution (Fig. 44-4). The V_D in obese patients is affected by multiple factors including reduced total body water, increased total body fat, increased lean body mass, altered protein binding, increased blood volume, increased cardiac output, increased blood concentrations of free fatty acids, triglycerides, cholesterol, and α_1-acid glycoprotein, lipophilicity of the drug, and organomegaly.[6] Increased redistribution of a drug prolongs its elimination half-life even when clearance is unchanged or increased. Hyperlipidemia and an increased concentration of α_1-acid glycoprotein may affect protein binding, leading to a reduction in free drug concentration. Plasma albumin and total plasma protein concentrations and binding are not significantly changed by obesity, but when compared with normal-weight individuals, a relative increase in plasma protein binding may be evident. Splanchnic blood flow, blood volume, and cardiac output are all increased in obese patients. In contrast to the expected decrease in bioavailability of orally administered medications because of increased splanchnic blood flow, there is no significant difference in absorption and bioavailability when comparing obese and normal-weight subjects. Drugs that undergo phase I metabolism (oxidation, reduction, hydrolysis) are generally unaffected by changes induced by obesity, whereas phase II reactions (glucuronidation, sulfation) are enhanced.[6]

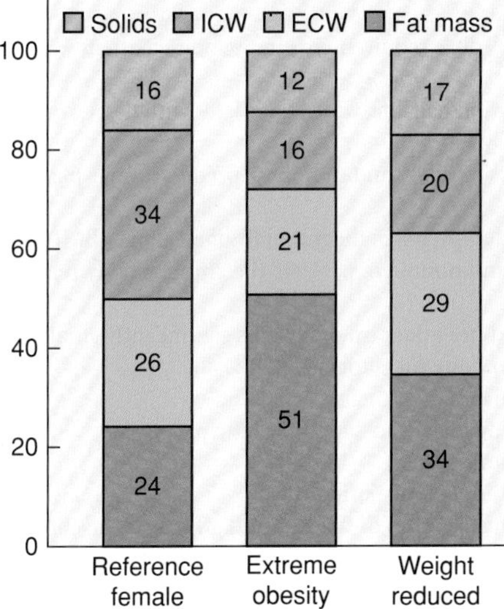

FIGURE 44-4. Body composition in extremely obese and weight-reduced states compared with reference female values. ICW, intracellular water; ECW, extracellular water. (Reprinted from: Das SK, Roberts SB, Kehayias JJ, et al. Body composition methods in extreme obesity. *Am J Physiol Endocrinol Metab.* 2003;284:E1080, with permission.)

Histologic abnormalities of the liver are common in the obese, with concomitant deranged liver function tests, but drug clearance is not usually affected. Renal clearance of drugs is increased in obesity because of increased renal blood flow and glomerular filtration rate.[49,55] As a result of the increases in glomerular filtration rate and tubular secretion, drugs such as cimetidine and aminoglycoside antibiotics that depend on renal excretion may require increased dosing. Highly lipophilic substances such as barbiturates and benzodiazepines show significant increases in V_D for obese individuals.[6] These drugs have a more selective distribution to fat stores and therefore a longer elimination half-life but with comparable clearance values to normal individuals. Less lipophilic compounds have little or no change in V_D with obesity. Exceptions to this rule include the highly lipophilic drugs digoxin, procainamide, and remifentanil.[56–58] Drugs with weak or moderate lipophilicity may be dosed on the basis of LBW. Adding 20% to the estimated IBW dose of hydrophilic medications is sufficient to include the obese patient's extra lean mass. Nondepolarizing muscle relaxants can be dosed in this manner.

Increased blood volume in the obese patient decreases plasma concentrations of rapidly injected intravenous drugs. Fat, however, has poor blood flow, and doses calculated on actual body weight could lead to excessive plasma concentrations. Calculating initial doses based on LBW with subsequent doses determined by pharmacologic response to the initial dose is a reasonable approach. Repeated injections may accumulate in fat, leading to a prolonged response because of subsequent release from this large depot.

Specific Drugs

Patients' usual medications should be continued until the time of surgery, with the possible exception of certain antihypertensives, insulin, and oral hypoglycemics. Antibiotic prophylaxis is usually indicated because of an increased incidence of wound infections in the obese.[59] Anxiolysis and prophylaxis against both aspiration pneumonitis and deep vein thrombosis (DVT) should be addressed preoperatively. Oral benzodiazepines are reliable for anxiolysis and sedation. Intravenous midazolam can also be titrated in small doses for anxiolysis during the immediate preoperative period. Dexmedetomidine, because of its minimal respiratory depressant effects, should be considered. Pharmacologic intervention with H_2-receptor antagonists, nonparticulate antacids, or proton pump inhibitors will reduce gastric volume, acidity, or both, thereby reducing the risk and severity of aspiration pneumonitis. Guidelines for dosing of common intravenous drugs utilized during anesthesia are presented in Table 44-3.

TABLE 44-3. INTRAVENOUS DRUG DOSING IN OBESITY

Drug	Dosing	Practical Anesthesia Key Points
Thiopental	Induction: LBW (somewhat increased dose)	• Increased initial dose due to increased blood volume, CO, muscle mass • Rapid distribution from plasma to periphery • Increased absolute dose • Prolonged duration of action due to high lipophilicity and increased V_D • Longer elimination half-life
Propofol	Induction: LBW (somewhat increased dose) Maintenance infusion: TBW	• Short duration of action due to rapid redistribution • Highly lipophilic • Cardiac output is major determinant of peak plasma concentration[60] • Increased V_D at steady state and increased clearance prevent increases in elimination half-life • Total clearance and V_D at steady state correlate with body weight during maintenance infusion • Negative cardiovascular effects • High affinity for fat and well-perfused organs • High hepatic extraction and conjugation relate to TBW[61]
Succinylcholine	TBW	• Pseudocholinesterase activity increases linearly with increasing weight and large extracellular fluid compartment • Dose of succinylcholine should be increased
Rocuronium	LBW	• Dosing according to LBW to prevent delayed recovery due to increased V_D • Faster onset and longer duration when dosed according to TBW[62,63] • Pharmacokinetics and pharmacodynamics not altered in obese female patients
Vecuronium	LBW	• Prolonged action when dosed according to TBW • Dosing according to LBW to prevent delayed recovery due to increased V_D and impaired hepatic clearance • Obesity does not alter distribution or elimination of the drug
Atracurium	LBW	• V_D, absolute clearance, and elimination half-life unchanged by obesity • Unchanged dose per unit body weight without prolongation of recovery because of organ function-independent elimination[64]
Cisatracurium	LBW	• Pharmacokinetics similar to atracurium but prolonged duration of action when dosed according to TBW[65]
Benzodiazepines	LBW	• Highly lipophilic drugs with larger V_D in obese patients result in longer duration of action • Midazolam has potential for prolonged sedation because larger initial doses are required to achieve adequate serum concentrations
Fentanyl	LBW	• Measured total body clearance has a nonlinear relationship to TBW and overestimates plasma concentration • Fentanyl dosing based on a derived LBW or "pharmacokinetic mass" model correlates better with clearance than TBW dosing[66,67] • Dosing based on TBW overestimates dose requirements in the obese patient
Sufentanil	LBW	• Highly lipid soluble • Increased V_D and prolonged elimination half-life, which correlates with degree of obesity • Distributes extensively in excess body fat • Similar pharmacokinetic parameters in obese and nonobese predict similar plasma concentrations • Overestimation of plasma concentration occurs in the morbidly obese range (BMI >40 kg/m^2)[67]
Remifentanil	LBW	• Pharmacokinetics similar in obese and nonobese patients (i.e., more closely related to lean body mass than LBW)[57] • Systemic clearance and V_D corrected per kilogram of TBW is significantly smaller in the obese patient. Consider age and lean body mass for dosing
Dexmedetomidine	TBW	• Highly selective α_2-adrenergic agonist • Sedative–hypnotic, anesthetic-sparing analgesic, sympatholytic properties • Lacks significant effects on respiration • Ideal analgesic adjuvant in the morbidly obese patient[68] • As part of a balanced anesthetic, infusion rates of 0.2–0.7 μg/kg/hr produce clinically effective sedation with decreased analgesic and anesthetic requirements
Neostigmine	TBW	• Prompt early reversal but delayed full recovery during neostigmine-induced reversal of vecuronium dosed according to TBW[63]
Sugammadex	N/A	• A modified γ-cyclodextrin compound that encapsulates rocuronium, (and other steroid-based neuromuscular blockers to a lesser extent) • May prove invaluable for more rapid and complete neuromuscular blockade reversal in obese patients[69]

LBW, lean body weight; VD, volume of distribution; TBW, total body weight; BMI, body mass index; N/A, not available.
Adapted from: Ogunnaike BO, Jones SB, Jones DB, et al. Anesthetic considerations for bariatric surgery. *Anesth Analg.* 2002;95:1793.

PREOPERATIVE EVALUATION

Airway

Preoperative airway assessment in obese patients is of paramount importance. In an analysis of closed malpractice claims in the United States related to airway management, obesity played a significant role in a large number of cases.[70] Anatomic changes associated with obesity that contribute to a potentially difficult airway include limited movement of the atlantoaxial joint and cervical spine by upper thoracic and low cervical fat pads; excessive tissue folds in the mouth and the pharynx; a short, thick neck; a thick submental fat pad; suprasternal, presternal, and posterior cervical fat; and large breasts in females. Excess pharyngeal tissue deposited in the lateral pharyngeal walls may not be noticed during routine airway examination. The history obtained from the patient and examination of previous records may help predict airway difficulties.

Obesity is an accepted risk factor for difficult mask ventilation and airway management. With adequate positioning and airway resources available, most obese patients can be adequately and safely managed. Overall, the magnitude of BMI by itself does not seem to have much influence on the difficulty of laryngoscopy.[71] Such difficulty, in most studies, correlates with increased age, male sex, temporomandibular joint pathology, Mallampati classes 3 and 4, OSA, and abnormal upper teeth.[72–74] The predictive role of OSA per se on difficult intubation has been recently disputed.[75] In a prospective study in bariatric patients by Neligan et al.[75] only a Mallampati score ≥3 and male gender, but not BMI, OSA or the apnea–
1 hypopnea index (AHI), predicted the risk of difficult intubation. The patient's neck circumference has been identified as the single biggest predictor of problematic intubation in morbidly obese patients.[73] The probability of a problematic intubation is approximately 5% with a 40-cm neck circumference compared with a 35% probability at 60-cm neck circumference. In this study by Brodsky et al.,[73] a larger neck circumference was associated with male gender, a higher Mallampati score, laryngoscopy grade 3 views, and OSA.

Cardiopulmonary Systems

As stated above, when evaluating the obese patient preoperatively, a review of previous anesthetic experiences, as detailed by
2 the patient, and previous anesthetic records are useful and important. Because obese patients often have limited exercise tolerance they may appear asymptomatic even though they have significant cardiovascular disease. Obese patients should be evaluated for systemic hypertension, pulmonary hypertension, signs of right and/or left ventricular failure, and ischemic heart disease. Signs of cardiac failure such as elevated jugular venous pressure, pathologic heart sounds, pulmonary crackles, hepatomegaly, and peripheral edema may all be difficult to detect because of excess adiposity. Pulmonary hypertension is fairly common in this patient population because of the chronic pulmonary impairment. The common features of pulmonary hypertension are exertional dyspnea, fatigue, and syncope (which reflect an inability to increase cardiac output during activity). Tricuspid regurgitation on echocardiography is the most useful confirmatory test of pulmonary hypertension but should be combined with clinical evaluation. An ECG may demonstrate signs of right ventricular hypertrophy such as tall precordial R waves, right axis deviation, and right ventricular strain. The higher the pulmonary artery pressure the more sensitive the ECG. Chest radiographs may show evidence of underlying lung disease and prominent pulmonary arteries.[76]

3 Evidence of sleep apnea and the obstructive hypoventilation syndrome should be obtained preoperatively not only because patients with these syndromes may present with difficult airway management issues, but also because the conditions are associated with increased perioperative pulmonary complications. A history of hypertension or a neck circumference >40 cm correlates with an increased probability of OSA. OSA is a legitimate reason to delay surgery for a proper workup.[77] OSA patients should generally be treated as inpatients; however, outpatient surgery can be considered under certain circumstances, including mild OSA, use of local or regional anesthesia with minimal sedation, availability of a 23-hour observation postanesthesia care unit, and when patients can resume oral medication at the time of discharge. OSA patients on a CPAP device at home should be instructed to bring it with them to the hospital as it may be needed postoperatively. The possibility of invasive monitoring, prolonged intubation, and postoperative mechanical ventilation should be discussed with obese patients. Arterial blood gas measurements help evaluate ventilation, as well as the need for perioperative oxygen administration and postoperative ventilation. Routine pulmonary function tests and liver function tests are not cost-effective in asymptomatic obese patients.

Metabolic Issues

Patients scheduled for repeat bariatric surgery should be screened preoperatively for long-term metabolic and nutritional abnormalities. The high prevalence of insulin resistance and diabetes in obese patients justifies the need for considering glucose checks preoperatively, and correcting abnormalities if present. Preoperative evaluation should include assessment of therapies for glycemic control, last time and dose of preoperative administration, and usual glucose values for a specific patient. Electrolytes should be checked before surgery, particularly in patients with
4 poor compliance to medications or acutely ill patients. Elevated liver function tests (mostly elevated alanine aminotransferase) are seen in many obese patients, but no clear correlation exists between abnormalities of routine liver function tests and the capacity of the liver to metabolize drugs. Other nutritional deficiencies include vitamin B12, iron, calcium, and folate. Vitamin and nutritional deficiencies can lead to a collective form of postoperative polyneuropathy, known as acute postgastric reduction surgery (APGARS) neuropathy, a polynutritional multisystem disorder characterized by protracted postoperative vomiting, hyporeflexia, and muscular weakness.[78] Differential diagnoses of this disorder include thiamine deficiency (Wernicke encephalopathy, beriberi), vitamin B12 deficiency, and Guillain–Barré syndrome. Close attention to dosing and monitoring of neuromuscular blocking agents is recommended in cases of suspected or diagnosed APGARS neuropathy. Chronic vitamin K deficiency may lead to coagulation abnormalities, requiring administration of vitamin K analog or fresh frozen plasma.

Hematologic Issues

Morbid obesity is a known risk factor for perioperative thromboembolic events, including sudden death from acute pulmonary embolism.[79] Several thromboprophylaxis protocols exist or are being developed,[80,81] but preoperative evaluation and preparation should include consideration of these plans. Guidelines from the American Society of Chest Physicians recommend, in patients undergoing bariatric surgery, the combination of intermittent pneumatic compression devices with heparin (unfractionated or low molecular weight heparin), and warn that greater doses in obese patients may be needed than in nonobese ones.[82] A prolonged postoperative thromboembolic prophylactic regimen (1 to 3 weeks) may be indicated.[80] Four risk factors for the development of DVT are particularly significant, namely venous stasis disease, BMI ≥ 60, central obesity, and OHS and/or OSA I. If present, preoperative prophylactic placement of an inferior vena cava filter should be considered.[79] A combination of short duration of surgery, lower extremity pneumatic compression, and routine early ambulation, may preclude mandatory heparin anticoagulation, except in patients with a history of previous DVT, a known hypercoagulable state, or a significant family history of DVT.[83]

INTRAOPERATIVE CONSIDERATIONS

Equipment and Monitoring

Specially designed tables or two regularly sized operating room tables may be required for safe anesthesia and surgery in obese patients. Regular operating room tables have a maximum weight limit of approximately 200 kg, but operating room tables capable of holding up to 455 kg, with a greater width, or side accessories, to accommodate the extra girth, are available. Strapping obese patients to the operating room table in combination with a malleable "bean bag" helps keep them from falling off the operating room table.

Supine positioning causes ventilatory impairment and inferior vena cava and aortic compression in obese patients. FRC and oxygenation are decreased further with supine positioning. Head-down positioning, often required during bariatric procedures, further worsens FRC and should be avoided if possible. Simply changing the obese patient from a sitting to supine position can cause a significant increase in oxygen consumption and cardiac output. The head-up position provides the longest safe apnea period during induction of anesthesia.[84] The extra time gained may help preclude hypoxemia if intubation is delayed. Both intraoperative PEEP and the head-up position significantly decrease the alveolar–arterial oxygen tension difference and increase total respiratory compliance to a similar degree, although the head-up position results in lower airway pressures. Both PEEP and the head-up position, however, decrease cardiac output significantly, which partially counteracts the beneficial effects on oxygenation.[85] Prone positioning, rarely required in the obese patient, should be correctly performed with freedom of abdominal movement to prevent detrimental effects on lung compliance, ventilation, and arterial oxygenation. Lateral decubitus positioning allows for better diaphragmatic excursion and should be favored over prone positioning whenever the surgical procedure permits. Particular care should be paid to protecting pressure areas, because pressure sores, neural injuries, and rhabdomyolysis may occur. Brachial plexus and lower extremity nerve injuries are frequent. Carpal tunnel syndrome is the most common mononeuropathy after bariatric surgery.[86,87] Other reported neurologic complications include encephalopathy (Wernicke), optic neuropathy, and myelopathy associated with vitamin B12 and copper deficiencies.[88]

Monitoring the surgical obese patient poses additional chal
5 lenges. Proper sizing of the blood pressure cuff and choice of location is important. Blood pressure measurements can be falsely elevated if a cuff is too small. Cuffs with bladders that encircle a minimum of 75% of the upper arm circumference or, preferably, the entire arm, should be used. Forearm blood pressure measurements with a standard cuff overestimate both systolic and diastolic blood pressures in obese patients.[89] Invasive arterial pressure monitoring may be indicated for the super morbidly obese patient, not only for those patients with cardiopulmonary disease but also for those patients in whom the noninvasive blood pressure cuff does not fit properly. Central venous catheterization, though not routinely needed, may be required for intravenous access in patients with inadequate peripheral access for perioperative fluid management.[90] Central venous catheters, pulmonary artery catheters and/or transesophageal echocardiography can be used selectively in patients with significant cardiopulmonary disease or in patients undergoing extensive surgery.

Airway Management

Adequate preoxygenation is vital in obese patients because rapid oxygen desaturation can occur after loss of consciousness, due to increased oxygen consumption and decreased FRC. Having the patient voluntarily take four vital capacity breaths with 100% oxygen, within 30 seconds of anesthesia induction, has been suggested as being superior to the usually recommended 3 minutes of 100% preoxygenation with normal ventilation in obese patients.[91] Use of the head-up position, or semisitting position, at approximately 25 degrees from horizontal, provides the longest period of apnea without development of hypoxia during induction of anesthesia.[84,92,93] The extra time gained may help preclude hypoxemia if intubation is delayed. Preoperative use of noninvasive positive pressure ventilation (NIPPV) or application of PEEP during induction will also combat peri-induction hypoxemia.[94,95] The head-up position may also help to prevent pulmonary aspiration of gastric contents as well as hypoxemia.

Obese patients are more likely than nonobese patients to present with difficult mask ventilation and intubation, especially if they have a short thick neck and OSA.[70–74,96,97] If a difficult intubation is anticipated, awake intubation using topical or regional anesthesia and a fiber-optic device is a prudent approach to maintain spontaneous ventilation. During awake intubation, sedative–hypnotic medications should be reduced to a minimum. Sedation with dexmedetomidine during awake intubation provides adequate anxiolysis and analgesia without respiratory depression.[98] Hypoxia and aspiration of gastric contents should be prevented at all costs during endotracheal intubation. An experienced colleague who is in the operating room or immediately available during induction and airway management can be helpful with mask ventilation or attempts at intubation. A surgeon capable of accessing the airway surgically should be readily available. The "ramped" position elevates the obese patient's upper body and
6 improves not only the laryngoscopic view compared with the standard "sniffing" position, but as mentioned previously minimizes the risk of hypoxia.[99] Towels or folded blankets under the shoulders and head can compensate for the exaggerated flexed position of posterior cervical fat (Fig. 44-5). The objective of this

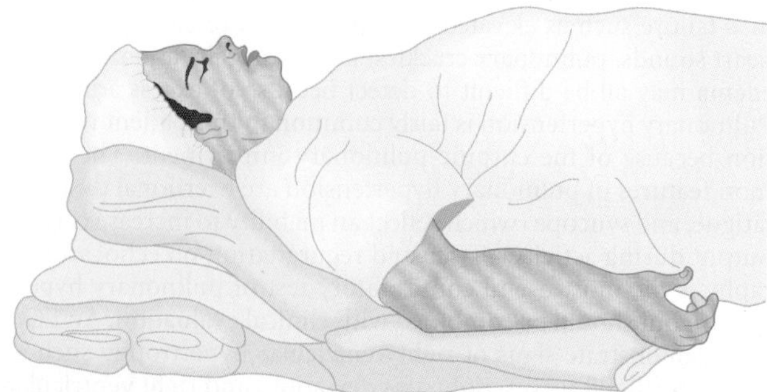

FIGURE 44-5. Ramped position with "stacking" of towels and blankets.

maneuver, known as "stacking," is to position the patient so that the tip of the chin is at a higher level than the chest to facilitate laryngoscopy and intubation.

Although direct laryngoscopy is successful in many obese patients, assuming optimal positioning has been achieved, having other intubating tools and related equipment useful during a difficult intubation is highly recommended. These tools include intubating stylets (Eschmann stylet, tube exchanger), videolaryngoscopes, laryngeal mask airways (LMA), and fiber-optic bronchoscopes. Videolaryngoscopes have proven to be efficient tools for intubating obese patients, reducing the duration of intubation and the number of attempts, with a similar or better glottic view than standard direct laryngoscopy.[100,101] Multiple laryngoscopic attempts and repeated attempts at intubation are consistent with increased airway and hemodynamic complications.[102] The ASA analysis of closed claims data also supports the recommendation to limit conventional intubation attempts to three before using other strategies.[32,70] LMA can be useful for temporarily achieving airway patency in patients with difficult mask ventilation and intubation,[103,104] or for placing a definitive endotracheal tube (intubating LMA).[32,105,106]

Induction and Maintenance

Concerns of hypoxemia, gastric regurgitation, and aspiration during induction and intubation justify the common use of rapid sequence induction (RSI) strategies. Gastroesophageal reflux disease is relatively common in obese patients, and the incidence of regurgitation and severe pneumonitis in case of aspiration is increased in this population (as discussed earlier in physiology section). Findings that nonpremedicated, nondiabetic fasting obese surgical patients with no significant gastroesophageal pathology are unlikely to have high volume, low pH gastric contents after routine preoperative fasting[45] suggest that the routine preoperative fasting guidelines (6 hours for solids, 2 hours for clear liquids) may be safe in obese patients.[107] In any case, the use of an RSI, as opposed to a standard induction technique, should be routinely and carefully evaluated in obese patients and the final decision individualized on the basis of the patient's risk of difficult mask ventilation, difficult intubation, hypoxemia, and gastric aspiration during induction.

7 No systematic analysis or comparison of anesthetic agents or techniques in obese patients is available. Larger doses of induction agents may be required because blood volume, muscle mass, and cardiac output increase linearly with the degree of obesity. Any of the commonly available intravenous induction agents may be employed after taking into consideration problems peculiar to individual patients. An increased dose of succinylcholine is necessary because of an increase in activity of pseudocholinesterase. Myalgia is not frequently seen following succinylcholine in morbidly obese patients.[108] Succinylcholine, due to its rapid onset and limited duration of action, is highly recommended for tracheal intubation especially in obese patients in which airway management is considered challenging, or for patients with a high risk of peri-induction hypoxemia or aspiration.

Continuous infusion of a short-acting intravenous agent, such as propofol, or any of the inhalation agents, or a combination, may be used to maintain anesthesia. Desflurane, sevoflurane, and isoflurane are minimally metabolized and are therefore useful agents in the obese patient, with desflurane possibly providing better hemodynamic stability and slightly faster washout.[109–111] The use of nitrous oxide (N_2O), despite its rapid elimination and analgesic properties, is limited by the high oxygen demand in this patient population. Short-acting opioids are preferred in obese patients to provide adequate analgesia but avoid postoperative respiratory depression. Remifentanil and fentanyl, carefully titrated to clinical effect, are the most common choices.[112] Dexmedetomidine, an α_2-agonist with sedative and analgesic properties, has no clinically significant adverse effects on respiration and is an attractive anesthetic adjunct in obese patients.[68] Furthermore, it reduces postoperative opioid analgesic requirements.[68,113]

Profound muscle relaxation is important during laparoscopic bariatric procedures to facilitate ventilation and to maintain an adequate working space for visualization and safe manipulation of laparoscopic instruments. It also facilitates extraction of excised tissues. Collapse of the pneumoperitoneum and tightening of the patient's musculature around port sites are early indications of inadequate muscle relaxation.[114] Vecuronium, rocuronium, and cisatracurium are useful nondepolarizing muscle blocking agents for the maintenance of muscle relaxation. Pneumoperitoneum should not be increased above a pressure of 15 mm Hg since intra-abdominal pressures of 20 mm Hg or greater can cause vena caval compression and decrease cardiac output.[112] Cephalad displacement of the diaphragm and carina from a pneumoperitoneum during laparoscopy can cause a firmly secured endotracheal tube to displace into a main stem bronchus.[115]

Anesthesia personnel may be asked to facilitate the proper placement of an intragastric balloon to help the surgeon size the gastric pouch, and also to facilitate performance of leak tests with saline or methylene blue through a nasogastric tube. Care should be taken to ensure a tight seal of the endotracheal tube cuff, otherwise aspiration of saline or methylene blue can occur. All endogastric tubes should be completely removed (not just merely pulled back into the esophagus) before gastric division to avoid unplanned stapling and transection of these devices.

Fluid Management

Excess adipose tissue may render visualization of peripheral perfusion difficult, making fluid balance difficult to assess. Blood loss is usually greater in the obese patient than in the nonobese patient for the same type of surgery, because technical difficulties of accessing the surgical site necessitate larger incisions and more extensive dissection. Therefore, fluid management is particularly challenging in the obese patient. Normovolemia should be the goal, not only to avoid hypovolemia with the associated increased hemodynamic instability and incidence of postoperative nausea and vomiting,[116] but also to avoid the hypervolemia-associated risks of decompensated congestive heart failure, peripheral tissue edema, and pulmonary complications. Rapid infusion of intravenous fluids should be avoided because pre-existing congestive cardiac failure is common in the obese patient. Recent studies, which need further confirmation, found that during laparoscopic bariatric surgery, urine output does not correlate with the rate of intraoperative fluid administration,[117] and the total volume of fluids infused does not seem to affect the incidence of postoperative rhabdomyolysis.[118]

Mechanical Ventilation

Obesity makes the selection of ventilator settings challenging, since increasing weight does not imply a proportional growth of the lung. Obese patients are more likely to be exposed to higher tidal volumes because of miscalculation of PBW or IBW,[119,120] and also to higher airway pressures due to the decreased respiratory system compliance. Although similar ventilatory parameters in nonobese patients can be used, it may be difficult to maintain plateau pressures less than 30 cm H_2O.[5] Greater inflation pressures may be tolerated in obese patients,[121] possibly because the extra adipose tissue partially attenuates lung overdistension.[122] In any case, tidal volume should be maintained at less than 13 mL/kg, since higher tidal volumes offer no added advantages during mechanical ventilation of anesthetized morbidly obese patients.[123,124] Further increasing tidal volumes only increases the peak inspiratory airway pressure, end-expiratory (plateau) airway pressure, and lung compliance without significantly improving arterial oxygen tension.[123,125,126] No specific ventilatory mode (e.g., volume vs. pressure control ventilation [PCV]) has been found significantly better for oxygenation and CO_2 clearance in obese patients, although pressure control modes have in some studies correlated with increased oxygenation.[127,128]

8 PEEP, with or without recruitment maneuvers, is the only ventilatory parameter that has consistently been shown to improve respiratory function in obese subjects.[123,129,130] Moderate PEEP (10 cm H_2O), particularly after a recruitment maneuver, has been found to be the most efficient ventilatory technique to prevent postoperative atelectasis.[131] Different methods for performing recruitment maneuvers exist. A simple one proposed by Pelosi et al.[124] is a series of 3 short (6 seconds) inflations with PCV to administer a large tidal volume by reaching an inspiratory pressure of 40 to 55 cm H_2O. These higher than usual airway pressures may be needed to compensate for the decreased chest wall compliance, achieving an adequate transpulmonary pressure to avoid alveolar collapse. The combination of recruitment maneuvers and PEEP aim at opening and maintaining patency of small airway units, therefore improving ventilation–perfusion matching and oxygenation. This practice leads to improved oxygenation, less atelectasis,[130,132] a shorter stay in the postanesthesia care unit (PACU), and decreased postoperative pulmonary complications[132] after laparoscopic bariatric surgery. Attention should be paid to avoid decreased venous return and cardiac output with PEEP or recruitment maneuvers, although they have been adequately tolerated in normovolemic morbidly obese patients.[126] Inspired oxygen fraction (FiO_2) should be titrated to the minimum levels that assures acceptable oxygenation levels but avoids reabsorption atelectasis. Some experts recommend the FiO_2 to be kept lower than 0.8 in obese patients.[124,133]

Emergence

9 Prompt but safe tracheal extubation reduces the likelihood that the morbidly obese patient will become ventilator-dependent. This is especially important in patients with underlying cardiopulmonary disease. Similar to the recommendation during induction of anesthesia, during emergence the patient should preferably be extubated in the semirecumbent position. In some institutions, policies have been developed for the mandatory presence of two anesthesia providers at emergence and extubation of morbidly obese patients.[134] Supplemental oxygen should be administrated after extubation. Some authors recommend an observation period of at least 5 minutes after extubation before transporting the patient away from the operating room.[134]

Lifting devices such as the HoverMatt (Patient handling technologies, Allentown, PA), the patient transfer device (PTD; Alimed, Dedham, MA), and gantry-style mechanical lifting devices that use slings are useful for transporting morbidly obese patients onto or off the operating room table. The PTD can be combined with the Walter Henderson maneuver (Fig. 44-6) to safely and gently transfer obese patients onto their postoperative beds.[134]

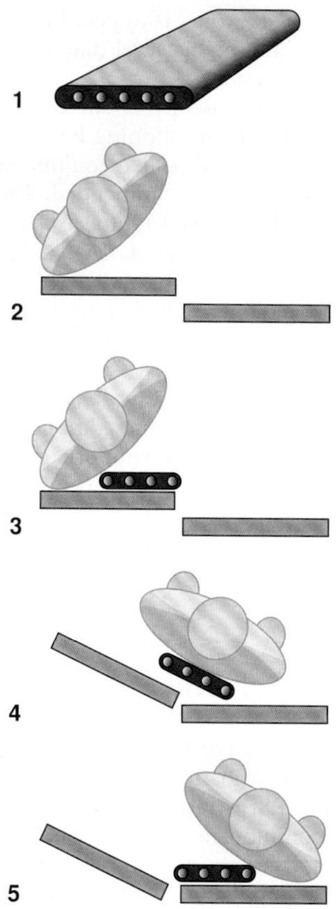

FIGURE 44-6. Illustration of the Walter Henderson maneuver. 1, patient transfer device (PTD; aka patient roller); 2, patient tilted to slip roller underneath; 3, roller slipped under patient; 4, table tilted to roll patient "downhill" onto bed; 5, patient rolled onto bed. (Reprinted from Ogunnaike BO, Whitten CW. In response to Rosenblatt MA, Reich DL, Roth R, et al. [letter]. 2004;98:1809, with permission.)

Monitored Anesthesia Care and Sedation

Monitoring of the adequacy of ventilation and oxygenation is extremely important in obese patients. Obese patients present a higher risk of sedation-induced respiratory depression, so careful titration of benzodiazepines, opioids, and propofol is mandatory to avoid hypercapnia and/or hypoxemia. Hypoxemia may require unplanned intubation, so a thorough airway examination and preparation for unintended airway management is critical even in monitored anesthesia care (MAC)/sedation cases. The prevalence of closed malpractice claims related to adverse respiratory events during monitored anesthesia cases is increasing, compared to respiratory complications or airway management complications encountered during general anesthesia.[135] In a closed claim analysis by Bhananker et al.,[136] obesity and suboptimum monitoring of pulse oximetry, end-tidal capnography or both, were significant key factors in these adverse events during MAC.

Regional Anesthesia

Neuraxial anesthetic techniques (spinal, epidural, combined spinal–epidural) and peripheral nerve blocks, used alone or in combination with general anesthesia, are being utilized more frequently as an important part of the anesthetic management of obese patients. Several studies have demonstrated the efficacy of regional techniques in reducing opioid-related complications[137,138] but there are other distinct advantages: (1) minimal or reduced manipulation of the airway, (2) administration of fewer medications with cardiopulmonary depression, (3) reduced risk of postoperative nausea and vomiting, (4) better postoperative pain control, and (5) improved postoperative outcomes.[139] When epidural anesthesia is combined with general anesthesia, time to tracheal extubation may be reduced in patients receiving a combined technique compared to general anesthesia alone.[140] However, utilization of regional anesthesia is accompanied by an increased risk of block failure in obese patients compared to those of normal weight.[141] Failure is often due to technical difficulties related to the patient's size and difficulty locating necessary anatomic landmarks. In addition, these patients also experience an increased risk of complications.[142] With proper planning, these techniques may be used successfully and should be considered in the anesthetic plan for obese patients who are candidates for regional anesthesia. However, well-functioning intravenous access should be secured prior to block placement in case complications such as a high neuraxial block or local anesthetic systemic toxicity should occur.

Neuraxial Anesthesia

Neuraxial anesthesia can produce serious cardiopulmonary alterations in obese patients undergoing surgery. Because pulmonary mechanics, lung volumes, FRC, oxygenation, and ventilation are already compromised preoperatively in these individuals, supine and Trendelenburg positioning during neuraxial anesthesia can lead to a further deterioration of lung volumes, including a reduction in FRC. FRC may fall below closing capacity promoting small airway collapse, atelectasis, ventilation–perfusion mismatch, and hypoxia, especially during supine and Trendelenburg positioning.[143] It is often helpful to measure the oxygen saturation in the sitting and supine positions to indicate the degree of pulmonary reserve before initiating neuraxial anesthesia. In addition to these pulmonary concerns, there are cardiovascular changes that warrant careful monitoring. The excess weight of the abdominal wall can compress the vena cava, causing decreased cardiac preload, reflex tachycardia, and decreased cardiac output. In a large series of obese patients undergoing nonobstetric surgery who had received spinal anesthesia, more than one-third developed hypotension.[144] Three of the patients in this series experienced cardiac arrest. There are other reports of cardiac arrest after supine positioning in morbidly obese patients.[145]

Despite these important considerations, use of neuraxial techniques can offer important advantages when compared to general anesthesia alone, particularly because it may permit utilization of fewer opioids. Parenteral opioid administration can be hazardous in these patients because of increased sensitivity, higher risk of hypoxemia, a high incidence of sleep apnea, and an increased incidence of adverse respiratory events following surgery. Administration of patient-controlled opioid analgesia has even resulted in respiratory depression in some obese patients.[146] The ASA has published guidelines for the care of patients with OSA and recommends that regional anesthetic techniques should be considered to reduce or eliminate the requirements for systemic opioids in patients with sleep apnea.[31]

Proper positioning is an important step in placement of a successful neuraxial anesthetic. Spinal or epidural placement in the sitting position will assist with identification of the midline.[147] The patient's back should be parallel to the edge of the bed to prevent lateral needle deviation away from the midline. Lateral deviation from the midline will increase the depth to the epidural or spinal spaces and can result in block failure[147] and an increased risk for intraoperative conversion to general anesthesia (in less-than-ideal circumstances). Anatomic landmarks are often obscured in these patients. If spinal processes cannot be appreciated with deep palpation, a line can be drawn from the cervical vertebral spinal process to the uppermost portion of the gluteal cleft. This line approximates the midline of the patient over the vertebral column. Ultrasound imaging can also be helpful to identify spinal processes[148] and has been shown to significantly reduce the number of needle passes and decrease the time for spinal block placement in morbidly obese patients undergoing orthopedic surgery.[149] Since the iliac crests may also be difficult to appreciate, the patient's skin folds can be used to aid in drawing a line perpendicular to the vertical line so that the intersection point can serve as a reasonable spinal or epidural needle insertion guide.

Neuraxial anesthetic placement can be particularly difficult, especially when bony landmarks are nonpalpable, there is limited back flexion,[150] and there are false losses of resistance due to fat deposition. It is often difficult to predict the depth to the epidural space but the depth to the epidural space generally correlates with BMI.[151] A recent study suggests that prepuncture ultrasonography may be useful to facilitate epidural placement in obese parturients to assist in predicting the depth to the epidural space.[152] However, ultrasound has limitations in this patient population because the image quality can be compromised due to fat overlying the epidural space and the distance to the epidural space may be inaccurate if the subcutaneous tissue is compressed. Future development of ultrasound technologies may incorporate the use of ultrasound-guided needle techniques to aid epidural placement in challenging patients.[153] In some cases, a long 25-gauge needle can be used for infiltration of local anesthetic as well as to identify spinous processes. To determine whether needle placement is midline or lateral, the patient is often helpful in directing the needle to the midline (e.g., Does it feel like I'm in the middle of your back?). A recent study demonstrated that morbidly obese parturients were significantly more helpful in identifying the midline compared to nonobese.[154] Helpfulness also varied with the patient's BMI. In most cases, standard neuraxial needles (9 to 10 cm) are usually of sufficient length if placement is midline.[155] However, longer needles (16 cm) are sometimes needed in extremely obese parturients. These needles can cause serious injury so they should only be used after careful assessment of the midline when standard needles are inadequate.

Spinal Anesthesia

Single-injection spinal anesthesia is a popular neuraxial anesthetic technique but there are concerns about technical difficulties, exaggerated spread of local anesthetic, hypotension, and an inability to prolong the block, especially in the obese patient. Spinal anesthesia is reasonable if the airway examination is reasonably normal, there is no significant cardiopulmonary disease, and the surgery is expected to be less than 90 minutes. It is often easier to insert the spinal needle when a large gauge stiff epidural needle is used as a guide for the smaller flexible spinal needle.

Decreased cerebral spinal fluid volumes have been confirmed in obese patients by magnetic resonance imaging[156] suggesting that the effective dose of spinal local anesthetic is reduced in obese patients when they receive the same anesthetic as a nonobese patient. The decreased spinal fluid volume results from displacement of the cerebral spinal fluid by soft tissue movement into the intervertebral foramen caused by an increase in abdominal pressure. This results in a direct positive correlation between the height of the block and the degree of obesity when patients receive the same volume and dose of spinal bupivacaine in the sitting position.[157] Others have demonstrated higher levels of spinal anesthesia in obese patients[158] and the need for smaller volumes of bupivacaine in obese individuals to achieve similar sensory levels.[159,160] In addition to these factors, large buttocks of obese patients may place the vertebral column in the Trendelenburg position, exaggerating the cephalad spread of spinal anesthesia. In order to avoid a high block when hyperbaric bupivacaine is used, a ramp can be placed under the patient's chest to elevate the cervical and thoracic spines to avoid the head-down position induced by large buttocks. Although there are other studies that report no clinical differences in the height of sensory block after hypobaric[161] and hyperbaric[162] spinal anesthesia in obese compared to nonobese parturients, spinal anesthesia should be performed with caution because of the consequences of extensive blockade, prolonged surgery, and the hazards of intraoperative induction of general anesthesia.

Epidural Anesthesia

Epidural anesthesia offers several advantages over single-injection spinal anesthesia including titratable dosing of local anesthetics, ability to prolong the block, decreased risk of excessive motor block, more controllable hemodynamic changes, and the option to utilize for postoperative analgesia. However, in laboring patients, a multicenter prospective observational study found that epidural anesthesia failed more often than spinal or combined spinal–epidural (CSE) anesthesia techniques.[163] Increased maternal BMI was significantly related to failure of neuraxial techniques. Hood and Dewan[164] also demonstrated an increased initial failure rate of epidural catheters in laboring patients. In the study 42% of catheters failed initially compared to 6% in the nonobese control group. In addition, Hodgkinson and Husain[165] demonstrated that the height of an epidural block for a given volume of local anesthetic is proportional to BMI and maternal weight but not height. Incremental dosing of epidural-administered local anesthetics will reduce the risk of hypotension and high block.

Catheter dislodgment is another potential problem in obese patients. Before securing the epidural catheter to the skin, the patient should move from the upright sitting position to the lateral position. In a study by Hamilton et al.,[166] the distance from the epidural space to the skin was measured as patients changed from one position to another (sitting flexed to up, up to lateral, flexed to lateral). The maximum change averaged 0.67 cm in parturients with a BMI <25, to 1.04 cm in parturients with a BMI >30. The changes in epidural catheter depth in this study were significantly increased with the BMI of patients, and the maximum observed changes in distance to skin with a change in patient position were also significantly increased with the BMI (with >4 cm change in one obese patient).[166] Because the ligamentum flavum has a mild grip on the epidural catheter, repositioning allows the epidural catheter to be pulled into the subcutaneous fat, sometimes by several centimeters. Epidural catheters should be taped in place on the skin after the patient has been repositioned, and without adjusting the catheter. This maneuver is helpful in reducing the incidence of catheter dislodgement and block failure.

In cases of inadvertent dural puncture, catheters may be threaded into the subarachnoid space for continuous spinal analgesia. Continuous spinal anesthesia may offer the benefits of a single-injection spinal anesthesia (i.e., reliability, density)[167] and reduce the risk for postdural puncture headache when an inadvertent dural puncture occurs. However, care must be used to avoid accidental administration of a large, "usual," epidural dose of local anesthetic through what is now a spinal catheter. The spinal catheters should be clearly marked so that they are not mistaken for an epidural catheter.

Combined Spinal–Epidural (CSE)

CSE anesthesia is an alternative to conventional spinal or epidural anesthesia; however, there is concern that the technique is more complicated than either spinal or epidural alone and the epidural catheter is "unproven" during the duration of spinal analgesia. Although CSE catheters fail at similar rates compared with conventional epidural catheters,[168] delayed recognition of a nonfunctional epidural catheter is a disadvantage of this technique and is particularly problematic for prolonged surgical cases. This can increase the risk of intraoperative conversion to general anesthesia. However, even if the patient does not receive a "spinal dose" during CSE placement, the return of CSF in the spinal needle is confirmation of midline needle placement. This increases the likelihood of bilateral block, improved sacral spread, and onset of analgesia in laboring parturients.[169]

Peripheral Nerve Block

Peripheral nerve blocks, with and without general anesthesia, have been increasingly utilized for obese patients undergoing surgical procedures. In obese patients, these blocks can be technically challenging and have an increased failure rate compared to techniques performed in patients of normal weight.[142,170] Although the experience and expertise of the anesthesiologist with these blocks may influence their success, a large prospective study evaluating peripheral nerve blocks determined that the risk of block failure increased proportionately with BMI.[170] Continuous supraclavicular, paravertebral, superficial cervical plexus, and continuous epidural blocks had the highest failure rates. Supplemental general anesthesia was also needed to supplement these blocks more often. Another study also evaluated success rates of supraclavicular blocks in the obese patients compared to nonobese patients and determined that success rates were also lower in the obese patients.[171] However, the rate of successful blocks in the obese patients remained high (94.3% vs. 97.3%).

Dosing of local anesthetics during regional anesthesia can be challenging in the obese patient. For instance, if a patient receives too large of a dose, they may be at risk of hypotension or systemic toxicity. Or in the case of blocks placed in the neck, the patient may experience respiratory compromise related to diaphragmatic hemiparesis in the face of pre-existing hypoventilation due to obesity. If the dose is too small, there is a risk of block failure. Although absorption of local anesthetics is dependent on the site of injection (i.e., absorption is fastest with intercostal blocks followed by epidural and spinal blocks), calculation of the local anesthetic dose is an important consideration when performing a peripheral nerve block in obese patients. The maximum safe dose of local anesthetic for a peripheral nerve block is often based on patient weight. However, the dose based on the actual weight in this patient population will increase the risk for systemic toxicity. Regardless of the route of administration (e.g., local infiltration, peripheral nerve block) local anesthetic dosing should be based on IBW rather than actual weight.

Although there are advantages to the use of peripheral nerve blocks in obese patients, placement is often difficult due to difficult positioning, obscure anatomic landmarks, and inadequate needle length. Because increased BMI is associated with an increased number of attempts at block placement and risk of block failure,[142] the use of ultrasound may be a helpful tool to increase block success[172,173] as well as safety. Unlike techniques that use nerve stimulators and/or paresthesias to identify proper needle position, ultrasound has the advantage of real-time identification of landmarks below the skin surface. Although real-time ultrasound has been shown to increase success rates,[172–174] decrease procedure time,[175] and decrease the minimum effective dose of local anesthetic solutions[176] in patients receiving peripheral nerve blocks who are of normal weight, there are few studies examining use of this technique in the obese.[172,173] Because a greater penetration depth of ultrasound is needed in the obese, the ultrasound must penetrate greater depths to reach the tissues.[177] Low-frequency transducers are needed for this degree of penetration. However, higher frequency transducers produce the best images.[177] Consequently, ultrasound images in the obese may be compromised due to an increased number of reflective surfaces and well as greater depth to the structures. Successful use of ultrasound for peripheral nerve blocks requires training and experience. Routine use of ultrasound-guided regional techniques in nonobese patients is likely to improve success rates in the obese. The American Society of Regional Anesthesia and Pain Medicine and the European Society of Regional Anesthesia have recommended education and training guidelines for ultrasound-guided regional anesthesia.[178]

POSTOPERATIVE CONSIDERATIONS

Ventilation Evaluation and Management

There is an increased incidence of atelectasis in morbidly obese patients after general anesthesia, which persists into the postoperative period.[131] Consequently, initiation of CPAP or bilevel positive airway pressure (BiPAP) has been advocated. Despite a theoretical risk, the use of noninvasive positive pressure ventilation does not seem to increase the incidence of major anastomotic leakage after gastric bypass surgery. Postoperative CPAP may improve oxygenation but does not facilitate CO_2 elimination.[179] Adequate analgesia, use of a properly fitted elastic binder for abdominal support, early ambulation, deep breathing exercises, and incentive spirometry are all useful adjuncts to avoid postoperative hypoventilation and atelectasis. Pulse oximetry and arterial blood gases should be monitored when they are indicated.

Analgesia

10 Pain management should be an important part of the postoperative care of obese patients. The goal of pain management in these individuals is not only to provide adequate analgesia but also ensure early mobilization and adequate respiratory function. Mobilization in these individuals is often difficult but critically important in the prevention of complications. Pressure ulcerations, pulmonary emboli, deep venous thrombosis, and pneumonia are some of the common complications that can be prevented by early patient mobilization. Options for pain management should include the following: (1) multimodal analgesics, (2) regional anesthesia/analgesia techniques, (3) early patient mobilization, (4) supplemental oxygen, and (5) elevation of the head of the bed. Besides delivery of a safe analgesic technique, adequate postoperative monitoring is required to ensure safety.

TABLE 44-4. SUMMARY OF PRACTICE GUIDELINES FOR THE PERIOPERATIVE MANAGEMENT OF PATIENTS WITH OBSTRUCTIVE SLEEP APNEA (OSA)

- Regional anesthetic techniques should be considered to reduce or eliminate the requirements for systemic opioids in patients with OSA.
- If neuraxial anesthesia is planned, the benefits and risks of using an opioid or opioid–local anesthetic mixture as compared to local anesthetic alone must be considered.
- If patient-controlled systemic opioids are used, continuous background infusions should be avoided or used with extreme caution.
- Nonsteroidal anti-inflammatory agents and other modalities should be considered to reduce opioid requirements.
- Supplemental oxygen should be administered continuously to all patients who are at increased perioperative risk from OSA until they are able to maintain their baseline oxygen saturation while breathing room air.
- Hospitalized patients at increased risk of respiratory compromise from OSA should be monitored with continuous pulse oximetry after discharge from the recovery room.

From: Gross JB, Bachenberg KL, Benumof JL, et al. Practice guidelines for the perioperative management of patients with obstructive sleep apnea: A report by the American Society of Anesthesiologists Task Force on Perioperative Management of patients with obstructive sleep apnea. *Anesthesiology.* 2006;104:1081–1093.

It is unclear whether OSA increases the likelihood of postoperative complications.[33,180–182] However, obesity per se increases the risk of hypoxemic events,[180] obstructive apnea, and pulmonary complications. All of these complications occur more commonly in patients with known OSA. Opioids are known to increase the
11 risk of central apnea but patients with sleep apnea are at particular risk for opioid-induced apnea.[183] Because of the risk of hypoventilation and hypoxemia in obese patients with and without sleep apnea, postoperative pain management should include opioid-sparing multimodal analgesic techniques. Regional anesthetic techniques are known to reduce the risk of opioid-related complications.[137,138] However, these techniques will be contraindicated in some patients. In those patients, the use of multimodal analgesics (e.g., local anesthetics, NSAIDs) will reduce opioid consumption and reduce the risk of respiratory depression. The ASA practice guidelines encourage the use of regional analgesic techniques instead of systemic opioids in the postoperative pain management of patients with sleep apnea. Those guidelines are summarized in Table 44-4.

Monitoring

12 Obese patients who have received either neuraxial or parenteral opioids require careful postoperative monitoring. However, in most cases, routine admission to intensive care or high acuity care units is unnecessary since admission to these units has not been shown to reduce the risk of pulmonary complications or to

change perioperative outcome.[184] Patients with a history of sleep apnea treated with noninvasive positive airway pressure should be encouraged to bring their own equipment to the hospital to reduce the risk of respiratory depression.[185] All patients receiving neuraxial opioids should be monitored for adequacy of ventilation (e.g., respiratory rate, depth of respiration [assessed without disturbing a sleeping patient]), oxygenation (e.g., pulse oximetry when appropriate), and level of consciousness.[185]

CRITICAL CARE AND RESUSCITATION

Caring for critically ill obese patients poses many of the same challenges as are seen during surgery, in terms of equipment, monitoring, and the existence of multiple comorbidities.[121] In addition, the nutritional status of the critically ill obese patient is often paradoxical and difficult to address. Hyperglycemia, whether from pre-existing diabetes or stress-induced, is common and should be corrected because hyperglycemia is associated with a higher mortality rate. Obese patients are more likely to become ventilator-dependent than nonobese patients. The combination of obesity and the commonly associated comorbidities (e.g., diabetes) found in obese patients[186] may render these patients at increased risk for the development acute lung injury (ALI) and/or acute respiratory distress syndrome (ARDS). Although an increased BMI has been associated with an increased risk of developing ALI/ARDS,[119,187] the effect on clinical outcomes is still being explored.[119,188,189]

The possible need for cardiopulmonary resuscitation should be entertained when caring for the morbidly obese critically ill patient. There are both equipment and technical concerns. Chest compressions may not be effective and mechanical compression devices may be required. The maximum 400 J of energy on regular defibrillators is sufficient for morbidly obese patients[190] because their chest wall is usually not much thicker, but the higher transthoracic impedance from the fat may obligate several attempts at defibrillation. Airway management by conventional means may be very difficult. However, tracheostomy, percutaneous cricothyrotomy, transtracheal jet ventilation, and retrograde wire intubation are time-consuming and technically difficult procedures in such emergency situations. These techniques should be reserved as final options and, when possible, should be performed by practitioners experienced in their use.[191] Direct visualization of anatomic hallmarks during emergent cricothyroidotomy can be extremely challenging in the obese patient. A novel technique has recently been proposed, in which palpation of the cricothyroid membrane can facilitate placement of an Eschmann stylet preloaded with a tracheal tube be inserted using a Seldinger-like technique.[192]

MORBIDITY AND MORTALITY

Postoperative morbidity is increased in obese patients but whether or not there is increased mortality which is controversial.[189,193,194] The most common postoperative complications are respiratory (i.e., atelectasis, pneumonia), vascular (thrombophlebitis, deep venous thrombosis) and wound (infection, dehiscence) complications. In addition, rhabdomyolysis is more common in morbidly obese patients undergoing laparoscopic procedures when compared with the open procedure, especially with prolonged procedures. The incidence of perioperative adverse events is strongly associated with pre-existing disease but not solely to BMI.[195] For example, a patient with previously diagnosed metabolic syndrome has significantly greater risk of perioperative morbidity and mortality than an obese patient with no metabolic syndrome features.[196,197] Obese patients present a higher risk of perioperative pulmonary complications, especially if preoperative respiratory conditions (e.g., OSA) are present.[112] Interestingly, the role of OSA on the incidence of postoperative hypoxemia in morbidly obese patients after laparoscopic bariatric surgery has been recently questioned.[180] Obesity increases the risk of surgical site infections (SSIs).[198,199] Some known contributing factors are hyperglycemia or diabetes,[199] longer duration of surgical procedures,[199] hypoperfusion or low tissue oxygen tension,[59,200] and low tissue antibiotic concentration. Morbid obesity significantly increases the risk of postoperative thromboembolic events, obesity, and OHS and/or OSA.[79] A combination of pneumatic compression devices, routine early ambulation, and careful perioperative anticoagulation decrease the risk of thromboembolism.[83] Because of the higher risk of postoperative complications than in nonobese patients, the practice of performing surgery on obese patients in an outpatient setting is controversial and a decision should be individualized to each patient.[112,181] Ambulatory surgery is; however, becoming more accepted and considered safe for selected patients and procedures.[112,201]

References

1. Obesity: Preventing and managing the global epidemic. Report of a WHO consultation. *World Health Organ Tech Rep Ser.* 2000;894:1–253.
2. Flegal KM, Carroll MD, Ogden CL, et al. Prevalence and trends in obesity among US adults, 1999–2008. *JAMA.* 2010;303:235–241.
3. Dietz WH. Reversing the tide of obesity. *Lancet.* 2011;378:744–746.
4. Clinical guidelines on the identification, evaluation, and treatment of overweight and obesity in adults–the evidence report. National Institutes of Health. *Obes Res.* 1998;6 (suppl 2):51S–209S.
5. Ventilation with lower tidal volumes as compared with traditional tidal volumes for acute lung injury and the acute respiratory distress syndrome. The Acute Respiratory Distress Syndrome Network. *N Engl J Med.* 2000;342:1301–1308.
6. Leykin Y, Miotto L, Pellis T. Pharmacokinetic considerations in the obese. *Best Pract Res Clin Anaesthesiol.* 2011;25:27–36.
7. Janmahasatian S, Duffull SB, Ash S, et al. Quantification of lean bodyweight. *Clin Pharmacokinet.* 2005;44:1051–1065.
8. Pai MP, Paloucek FP. The origin of the "ideal" body weight equations. *Ann Pharmacother.* 2000;34:1066–1069.
9. Leykin Y, Pellis T, Del Mestro E, et al. Anesthetic management of morbidly obese and super-morbidly obese patients undergoing bariatric operations: Hospital course and outcomes. *Obes Surg.* 2006;16:1563–1569.
10. Cefalu WT, Werbel S, Bell-Farrow AD, et al. Insulin resistance and fat patterning with aging: Relationship to metabolic risk factors for cardiovascular disease. *Metabolism.* 1998;47:401–408.
11. Menke A, Muntner P, Wildman RP, et al. Measures of adiposity and cardiovascular disease risk factors. *Obesity.* 2007;15:785–795.
12. Leitzmann MF, Moore SC, Koster A, et al. Waist circumference as compared with body-mass index in predicting mortality from specific causes. *PLoS One.* 2011; 6:e18582.
13. Wadden TA, Volger S, Sarwer DB, et al. A two-year randomized trial of obesity treatment in primary care practice. *N Engl J Med.* 2011;365:1969–1979.
14. Wadden TA, Berkowitz RI, Womble LG, et al. Randomized trial of lifestyle modification and pharmacotherapy for obesity. *N Engl J Med.* 2005;353:2111–2120.
15. Powell AG, Apovian CM, Aronne LJ. New drug targets for the treatment of obesity. *Clin Pharmacol Ther.* 2011;90:40–51.
16. Valentino MA, Lin JE, Waldman SA. Central and peripheral molecular targets for antiobesity pharmacotherapy. *Clin Pharmacol Ther.* 2010;87:652–662.
17. Gadde KM, Allison DB, Ryan DH, et al. Effects of low-dose, controlled-release, phentermine plus topiramate combination on weight and associated comorbidities in overweight and obese adults (CONQUER): A randomised, placebo-controlled, phase 3 trial. *Lancet.* 2011;377:1341–1352.
18. Bray GA, Ryan DH. Drug treatment of the overweight patient. *Gastroenterology.* 2007;132:2239–2252.
19. MacWalter RS, Fraser HW, Armstrong KM. Orlistat enhances warfarin effect. *Ann Pharmacother.* 2003;37:510–512.
20. Yun JW. Possible anti-obesity therapeutics from nature–a review. *Phytochemistry.* 2010;71:1625–1641.
21. http://www.asahq.org/For-the-Public-and-Media/Video-Press-Releases/Herbal-Medicine.aspx (Date accessed: December 29, 2011).

22. Dixon JB, Straznicky NE, Lambert EA, et al. Surgical approaches to the treatment of obesity. *Nat Rev Gastroenterol Hepatol.* 2011;8:429–437.
23. Nguyen NT. Open vs. laparoscopic procedures in bariatric surgery. *J Gastrointest Surg.* 2004;8:393–395.
24. Tsesmeli N, Coumaros D. Review of endoscopic devices for weight reduction: Old and new balloons and implantable prostheses. *Endoscopy.* 2009;41:1082–1089.
25. Shikora SA, Bergenstal R, Bessler M, et al. Implantable gastric stimulation for the treatment of clinically severe obesity: Results of the SHAPE trial. *Surg Obes Relat Dis.* 2009;5:31–37.
26. Pelosi P, Croci M, Ravagnan I, et al. The effects of body mass on lung volumes, respiratory mechanics, and gas exchange during general anesthesia. *Anesth Analg.* 1998;87:654–660.
27. Salome CM, King GG, Berend N. Physiology of obesity and effects on lung function. *J Appl Physiol.* 2010;108:206–211.
28. Kaw R, Michota F, Jaffer A, et al. Unrecognized sleep apnea in the surgical patient: Implications for the perioperative setting. *Chest.* 2006;129:198–205.
29. Yeh PS, Lee YC, Lee WJ, et al. Clinical predictors of obstructive sleep apnea in Asian bariatric patients. *Obes Surg.* 2010;20:30–35.
30. Dixon JB, Schachter LM, O'Brien PE. Predicting sleep apnea and excessive day sleepiness in the severely obese: Indicators for polysomnography. *Chest.* 2003; 123:1134–1141.
31. Gross JB, Bachenberg KL, Benumof JL, et al. Practice guidelines for the perioperative management of patients with obstructive sleep apnea: A report by the American Society of Anesthesiologists Task Force on Perioperative Management of patients with obstructive sleep apnea. *Anesthesiology.* 2006;104:1081–1093.
32. American Society of Anesthesiologists Task Force on Management of the Difficult Airway. Practice guidelines for management of the difficult airway: An updated report by the American Society of Anesthesiologists Task Force on Management of the Difficult Airway. *Anesthesiology.* 2003;98:1269–1277.
33. Memtsoudis S, Liu SS, Ma Y, et al. Perioperative pulmonary outcomes in patients with sleep apnea after noncardiac surgery. *Anesth Analg.* 2011;112:113–121.
34. Olson AL, Zwillich C. The obesity hypoventilation syndrome. *Am J Med.* 2005; 118:948–956.
35. Finer N. Medical consequences of obesity. *Medicine.* 2011;39:18–23.
36. Fraley MA, Birchem JA, Senkottaiyan N, et al. Obesity and the electrocardiogram. *Obes Rev.* 2005;6:275–281.
37. Alpert MA, Terry BE, Hamm CR, et al. Effect of weight loss on the ECG of normotensive morbidly obese patients. *Chest.* 2001;119:507–510.
38. Engeli S, Bohnke J, Gorzelniak K, et al. Weight loss and the renin-angiotensin-aldosterone system. *Hypertension.* 2005;45:356–362.
39. van Baak MA. The peripheral sympathetic nervous system in human obesity. *Obes Rev.* 2001;2:3–14.
40. Haslam DW, James WP. Obesity. *Lancet.* 2005;366:1197–1209.
41. Van Gaal LF, Mertens IL, De Block CE. Mechanisms linking obesity with cardiovascular disease. *Nature.* 2006;444:875–880.
42. Birgel M, Gottschling-Zeller H, Rohrig K, et al. Role of cytokines in the regulation of plasminogen activator inhibitor-1 expression and secretion in newly differentiated subcutaneous human adipocytes. *Arterioscler Thromb Vasc Biol.* 2000;20:1682–1687.
43. Nilsson M, Johnsen R, Ye W, et al. Obesity and estrogen as risk factors for gastroesophageal reflux symptoms. *JAMA.* 2003;290:66–72.
44. Ayazi S, Hagen JA, Chan LS, et al. Obesity and gastroesophageal reflux: Quantifying the association between body mass index, esophageal acid exposure, and lower esophageal sphincter status in a large series of patients with reflux symptoms. *J Gastrointest Surg.* 2009;13:1440–1447.
45. Harter RL, Kelly WB, Kramer MG, et al. A comparison of the volume and pH of gastric contents of obese and lean surgical patients. *Anesth Analg.* 1998;86:147–152.
46. American Society of Anesthesiologists C. Practice guidelines for preoperative fasting and the use of pharmacologic agents to reduce the risk of pulmonary aspiration: Application to healthy patients undergoing elective procedures: An updated report by the American Society of Anesthesiologists Committee on Standards and Practice Parameters. *Anesthesiology.* 2011;114:495–511.
47. Frezza EE, Ikramuddin S, Gourash W, et al. Symptomatic improvement in gastroesophageal reflux disease (GERD) following laparoscopic Roux-en-Y gastric bypass. *Surg Endosc.* 2002;16:1027–1031.
48. Cheymol G. Effects of obesity on pharmacokinetics implications for drug therapy. *Clin Pharmacokinet.* 2000;39:215–231.
49. Chagnac A, Weinstein T, Herman M, et al. The effects of weight loss on renal function in patients with severe obesity. *J Am Soc Nephrol.* 2003;14:1480–1486.
50. Kastorini CM, Milionis HJ, Esposito K, et al. The effect of Mediterranean diet on metabolic syndrome and its components: A meta-analysis of 50 studies and 534,906 individuals. *J Am Coll Cardiol.* 2011;57:1299–1313.
51. Neligan PJ. Metabolic syndrome: Anesthesia for morbid obesity. *Curr Opin Anaesthesiol.* 2010;23:375–383.
52. Grundy SM, Brewer HB Jr, Cleeman JI, et al. Definition of metabolic syndrome: Report of the National Heart, Lung, and Blood Institute/American Heart Association conference on scientific issues related to definition. *Circulation.* 2004; 109:433–438.
53. Esposito K, Marfella R, Ciotola M, et al. Effect of a Mediterranean-style diet on endothelial dysfunction and markers of vascular inflammation in the metabolic syndrome: A randomized trial. *JAMA.* 2004;292:1440–1446.
54. Casati A, Putzu M. Anesthesia in the obese patient: Pharmacokinetic considerations. *J Clin Anesth.* 2005;17:134–145.
55. Hall JE. The kidney, hypertension, and obesity. *Hypertension.* 2003;41:625–633.
56. Christoff PB, Conti DR, Naylor C, et al. Procainamide disposition in obesity. *Drug Intell Clin Pharm.* 1983;17:516–522.
57. Egan TD, Huizinga B, Gupta SK, et al. Remifentanil pharmacokinetics in obese versus lean patients. *Anesthesiology.* 1998;89:562–573.
58. Abernethy DR, Greenblatt DJ, Smith TW. Digoxin disposition in obesity: Clinical pharmacokinetic investigation. *Am Heart J.* 1981;102:740–744.
59. Kabon B, Nagele A, Reddy D, et al. Obesity decreases perioperative tissue oxygenation. *Anesthesiology.* 2004;100:274–280.
60. Upton RN, Ludbrook GL, Grant C, et al. Cardiac output is a determinant of the initial concentrations of propofol after short-infusion administration. *Anesth Analg.* 1999;89:545–552.
61. Servin F, Farinotti R, Haberer JP, et al. Propofol infusion for maintenance of anesthesia in morbidly obese patients receiving nitrous oxide. A clinical and pharmacokinetic study. *Anesthesiology.* 1993;78:657–665.
62. Leykin Y, Pellis T, Lucca M, et al. The pharmacodynamic effects of rocuronium when dosed according to real body weight or ideal body weight in morbidly obese patients. *Anesth Analg.* 2004;99:1086–1089.
63. Suzuki T, Masaki G, Ogawa S. Neostigmine-induced reversal of vecuronium in normal weight, overweight and obese female patients. *Br J Anaesth.* 2006;97: 160–163.
64. Varin F, Ducharme J, Theoret Y, et al. Influence of extreme obesity on the body disposition and neuromuscular blocking effect of atracurium. *Clin Pharmacol Ther.* 1990;48:18–25.
65. Leykin Y, Pellis T, Lucca M, et al. The effects of cisatracurium on morbidly obese women. *Anesth Analg.* 2004;99:1090–1094.
66. Shibutani K, Inchiosa MA Jr, Sawada K, et al. Accuracy of pharmacokinetic models for predicting plasma fentanyl concentrations in lean and obese surgical patients: Derivation of dosing weight ("pharmacokinetic mass"). *Anesthesiology.* 2004;101:603–613.
67. Han PY, Duffull SB, Kirkpatrick CM, et al. Dosing in obesity: A simple solution to a big problem. *Clin Pharmacol Ther.* 2007;82:505–508.
68. Feld JM, Hoffman WE, Stechert MM, et al. Fentanyl or dexmedetomidine combined with desflurane for bariatric surgery. *J Clin Anesth.* 2006;18:24–28.
69. Sacan O, White PF, Tufanogullari B, et al. Sugammadex reversal of rocuronium-induced neuromuscular blockade: A comparison with neostigmine-glycopyrrolate and edrophonium-atropine. *Anesth Analg.* 2007;104:569–574.
70. Peterson GN, Domino KB, Caplan RA, et al. Management of the difficult airway: A closed claims analysis. *Anesthesiology.* 2005;103:33–39.
71. Ezri T, Medalion B, Weisenberg M, et al. Increased body mass index per se is not a predictor of difficult laryngoscopy. *Can J Anaesth.* 2003;50:179–183.
72. El-Orbany M, Woehlck HJ. Difficult mask ventilation. *Anesth Analg.* 2009; 109:1870–1880.
73. Brodsky JB, Lemmens HJ, Brock-Utne JG, et al. Morbid obesity and tracheal intubation. *Anesth Analg.* 2002;94:732–736.
74. Juvin P, Lavaut E, Dupont H, et al. Difficult tracheal intubation is more common in obese than in lean patients. *Anesth Analg.* 2003;97:595–600.
75. Neligan PJ, Porter S, Max B, et al. Obstructive sleep apnea is not a risk factor for difficult intubation in morbidly obese patients. *Anesth Analg.* 2009;109:1182–1186.
76. McLaughlin VV, Archer SL, Badesch DB, et al. ACCF/AHA 2009 expert consensus document on pulmonary hypertension: A report of the American College of Cardiology Foundation Task Force on Expert Consensus Documents and the American Heart Association: Developed in collaboration with the American College of Chest Physicians, American Thoracic Society, Inc., and the Pulmonary Hypertension Association. *Circulation.* 2009;119:2250–2294.
77. Benumof JL. Obesity, sleep apnea, the airway and anesthesia. *Curr Opin Anaesthesiol.* 2004;17:21–30.
78. Chang CG, Adams-Huet B, Provost DA. Acute post-gastric reduction surgery (APGARS) neuropathy. *Obes Surg.* 2004;14:182–189.
79. Sapala JA, Wood MH, Schuhknecht MP, et al. Fatal pulmonary embolism after bariatric operations for morbid obesity: A 24-year retrospective analysis. *Obes Surg.* 2003;13:819–825.
80. Magee CJ, Barry J, Javed S, et al. Extended thromboprophylaxis reduces incidence of postoperative venous thromboembolism in laparoscopic bariatric surgery. *Surg Obes Relat Dis.* 2010;6:322–325.
81. Shepherd MF, Rosborough TK, Schwartz ML. Heparin thromboprophylaxis in gastric bypass surgery. *Obes Surg.* 2003;13:249–253.
82. Geerts WH, Bergqvist D, Pineo GF, et al. Prevention of venous thromboembolism: American College of Chest Physicians Evidence-Based Clinical Practice Guidelines (8th Edition). *Chest.* 2008;133:381S–453S.
83. Gonzalez QH, Tishler DS, Plata-Munoz JJ, et al. Incidence of clinically evident deep venous thrombosis after laparoscopic Roux-en-Y gastric bypass. *Surg Endosc.* 2004;18:1082–1084.
84. Boyce JR, Ness T, Castroman P, et al. A preliminary study of the optimal anesthesia positioning for the morbidly obese patient. *Obes Surg.* 2003;13:4–9.
85. Perilli V, Sollazzi L, Modesti C, et al. Comparison of positive end-expiratory pressure with reverse Trendelenburg position in morbidly obese patients undergoing bariatric surgery: Effects on hemodynamics and pulmonary gas exchange. *Obes Surg.* 2003;13:605–609.

86. Koffman BM, Greenfield LJ, Ali II, et al. Neurologic complications after surgery for obesity. *Muscle Nerve.* 2006;33:166–176.
87. Thaisetthawatkul P, Collazo-Clavell ML, Sarr MG, et al. A controlled study of peripheral neuropathy after bariatric surgery. *Neurology.* 2004;63:1462–1470.
88. Juhasz-Pocsine K, Rudnicki SA, Archer RL, et al. Neurologic complications of gastric bypass surgery for morbid obesity. *Neurology.* 2007;68:1843–1850.
89. Pierin AM, Alavarce DC, Gusmao JL, et al. Blood pressure measurement in obese patients: Comparison between upper arm and forearm measurements. *Blood Press Monit.* 2004;9:101–105.
90. Juvin P, Blarel A, Bruno F, et al. Is peripheral line placement more difficult in obese than in lean patients? *Anesth Analg.* 2003;96:1218.
91. Goldberg ME, Norris MC, Larijani GE, et al. Preoxygenation in the morbidly obese: A comparison of two techniques. *Anesth Analg.* 1989;68:520–522.
92. Dixon BJ, Dixon JB, Carden JR, et al. Preoxygenation is more effective in the 25 degrees head-up position than in the supine position in severely obese patients: A randomized controlled study. *Anesthesiology.* 2005;102:1110–1115.
93. Altermatt FR, Munoz HR, Delfino AE, et al. Pre-oxygenation in the obese patient: Effects of position on tolerance to apnoea. *Br J Anaesth.* 2005;95:706–709.
94. Delay JM, Sebbane M, Jung B, et al. The effectiveness of noninvasive positive pressure ventilation to enhance preoxygenation in morbidly obese patients: A randomized controlled study. *Anesth Analg.* 2008;107:1707–1713.
95. Gander S, Frascarolo P, Suter M, et al. Positive end-expiratory pressure during induction of general anesthesia increases duration of nonhypoxic apnea in morbidly obese patients. *Anesth Analg.* 2005;100:580–584.
96. Corso RM, Piraccini E, Calli M, et al. Obstructive sleep apnea is a risk factor for difficult endotracheal intubation. *Minerva Anestesiol.* 2011;77:99–100.
97. Siyam MA, Benhamou D. Difficult endotracheal intubation in patients with sleep apnea syndrome. *Anesth Analg.* 2002;95:1098–1102.
98. Abdelmalak B, Makary L, Hoban J, et al. Dexmedetomidine as sole sedative for awake intubation in management of the critical airway. *J Clin Anesth.* 2007; 19:370–373.
99. Collins JS, Lemmens HJ, Brodsky JB, et al. Laryngoscopy and morbid obesity: A comparison of the "sniff" and "ramped" positions. *Obes Surg.* 2004;14:1171–1175.
100. Maassen R, Lee R, Hermans B, et al. A comparison of three videolaryngoscopes: The Macintosh laryngoscope blade reduces, but does not replace, routine stylet use for intubation in morbidly obese patients. *Anesth Analg.* 2009;109: 1560–1565.
101. Marrel J, Blanc C, Frascarolo P, et al. Videolaryngoscopy improves intubation condition in morbidly obese patients. *Eur J Anaesthesiol.* 2007;24:1045–1049.
102. Mort TC. Emergency tracheal intubation: Complications associated with repeated laryngoscopic attempts. *Anesth Analg.* 2004;99:607–613.
103. Cook TM. Difficult airway in an obese patient managed with the ProSeal laryngeal mask airway. *Eur J Anaesthesiol.* 2005;22:241–243.
104. Keller C, Brimacombe J, Kleinsasser A, et al. The Laryngeal Mask Airway ProSeal(TM) as a temporary ventilatory device in grossly and morbidly obese patients before laryngoscope-guided tracheal intubation. *Anesth Analg.* 2002;94: 737–740.
105. Combes X, Sauvat S, Leroux B, et al. Intubating laryngeal mask airway in morbidly obese and lean patients: A comparative study. *Anesthesiology.* 2005;102:1106–1109.
106. Frappier J, Guenoun T, Journois D, et al. Airway management using the intubating laryngeal mask airway for the morbidly obese patient. *Anesth Analg.* 2003;96:1510–1515.
107. Maltby JR, Pytka S, Watson NC, et al. Drinking 300 mL of clear fluid two hours before surgery has no effect on gastric fluid volume and pH in fasting and non-fasting obese patients. *Can J Anaesth.* 2004;51:111–115.
108. Lemmens HJ, Brodsky JB. The dose of succinylcholine in morbid obesity. *Anesth Analg.* 2006;102:438–442.
109. De Baerdemaeker LE, Struys MM, Jacobs S, et al. Optimization of desflurane administration in morbidly obese patients: A comparison with sevoflurane using an 'inhalation bolus' technique. *Br J Anaesth.* 2003;91:638–650.
110. La Colla L, Albertin A, La Colla G, et al. Faster wash-out and recovery for desflurane vs sevoflurane in morbidly obese patients when no premedication is used. *Br J Anaesth.* 2007;99:353–358.
111. Strum EM, Szenohradszki J, Kaufman WA, et al. Emergence and recovery characteristics of desflurane versus sevoflurane in morbidly obese adult surgical patients: A prospective, randomized study. *Anesth Analg.* 2004;99:1848–1853.
112. Schumann R. Anaesthesia for bariatric surgery. *Best Pract Res Clin Anaesthesiol.* 2011;25:83–93.
113. Hofer RE, Sprung J, Sarr MG, et al. Anesthesia for a patient with morbid obesity using dexmedetomidine without narcotics. *Can J Anaesth.* 2005;52:176–180.
114. Ogunnaike BO, Jones SB, Jones DB, et al. Anesthetic considerations for bariatric surgery. *Anesth Analg.* 2002;95:1793–1805.
115. Ezri T, Hazin V, Warters D, et al. The endotracheal tube moves more often in obese patients undergoing laparoscopy compared with open abdominal surgery. *Anesth Analg.* 2003;96:278–282.
116. Schuster R, Alami RS, Curet MJ, et al. Intra-operative fluid volume influences postoperative nausea and vomiting after laparoscopic gastric bypass surgery. *Obes Surg.* 2006;16:848–851.
117. Matot I, Paskaleva R, Eid L, et al. Effect of the volume of fluids administered on intraoperative oliguria in laparoscopic bariatric surgery: A randomized controlled trial. *Arch Surg.* 2012;147(3):228–234. Epub 2011 Nov 21.
118. Wool DB, Lemmens HJ, Brodsky JB, et al. Intraoperative fluid replacement and postoperative creatine phosphokinase levels in laparoscopic bariatric patients. *Obes Surg.* 2010;20:698–701.
119. Anzueto A, Frutos-Vivar F, Esteban A, et al. Influence of body mass index on outcome of the mechanically ventilated patients. *Thorax.* 2011;66:66–73.
120. Fernandez-Bustamante A, Wood CL, Tran ZV, et al. Intraoperative ventilation: Incidence and risk factors for receiving large tidal volumes during general anesthesia. *BMC Anesthesiol.* 2011;11:22.
121. Lewandowski K, Lewandowski M. Intensive care in the obese. *Best Pract Res Clin Anaesthesiol.* 2011;25:95–108.
122. Dreyfuss D, Soler P, Basset G, et al. High inflation pressure pulmonary edema. Respective effects of high airway pressure, high tidal volume, and positive end-expiratory pressure. *Am Rev Respir Dis.* 1988;137:1159–1164.
123. Bardoczky GI, Yernault JC, Houben JJ, et al. Large tidal volume ventilation does not improve oxygenation in morbidly obese patients during anesthesia. *Anesth Analg.* 1995;81:385–388.
124. Pelosi P, Gregoretti C. Perioperative management of obese patients. *Best Pract Res Clin Anaesthesiol.* 2010;24:211–225.
125. Sprung J, Whalley DG, Falcone T, et al. The effects of tidal volume and respiratory rate on oxygenation and respiratory mechanics during laparoscopy in morbidly obese patients. *Anesth Analg.* 2003;97:268–274.
126. Bohm SH, Thamm OC, von Sandersleben A, et al. Alveolar recruitment strategy and high positive end-expiratory pressure levels do not affect hemodynamics in morbidly obese intravascular volume-loaded patients. *Anesth Analg.* 2009;109:160–163.
127. Cadi P, Guenoun T, Journois D, et al. Pressure-controlled ventilation improves oxygenation during laparoscopic obesity surgery compared with volume-controlled ventilation. *Br J Anaesth.* 2008;100:709–716.
128. Zoremba M, Kalmus G, Dette F, et al. Effect of intra-operative pressure support vs pressure controlled ventilation on oxygenation and lung function in moderately obese adults. *Anaesthesia.* 2010;65:124–129.
129. Pelosi P, Ravagnan I, Giurati G, et al. Positive end-expiratory pressure improves respiratory function in obese but not in normal subjects during anesthesia and paralysis. *Anesthesiology.* 1999;91:1221–1231.
130. Reinius H, Jonsson L, Gustafsson S, et al. Prevention of atelectasis in morbidly obese patients during general anesthesia and paralysis: A computerized tomography study. *Anesthesiology.* 2009;111:979–987.
131. Eichenberger A, Proietti S, Wicky S, et al. Morbid obesity and postoperative pulmonary atelectasis: An underestimated problem. *Anesth Analg.* 2002;95:1788–1792.
132. Talab HF, Zabani IA, Abdelrahman HS, et al. Intraoperative ventilatory strategies for prevention of pulmonary atelectasis in obese patients undergoing laparoscopic bariatric surgery. *Anesth Analg.* 2009;109:1511–1516.
133. Rothen HU, Sporre B, Engberg G, et al. Influence of gas composition on recurrence of atelectasis after a reexpansion maneuver during general anesthesia. *Anesthesiology.* 1995;82:832–842.
134. Rosenblatt MA, Reich DL, Roth R. Bariatric surgery and the prevention of postoperative respiratory complications. *Anesth Analg.* 2004;98:1810.
135. Metzner J, Posner KL, Lam MS, et al. Closed claims' analysis. *Best Pract Res Clin Anaesthesiol.* 2011;25:263–276.
136. Bhananker SM, Posner KL, Cheney FW, et al. Injury and liability associated with monitored anesthesia care: A closed claims analysis. *Anesthesiology.* 2006; 104:228–234.
137. von Ungern-Sternberg BS, Regli A, Reber A, et al. Effect of obesity and thoracic epidural analgesia on perioperative spirometry. *Br J Anaesth.* 2005;94:121–127.
138. Kehlet H, Holte K. Effect of postoperative analgesia on surgical outcome. *Br J Anaesth.* 2001;87:62–72.
139. Marret E, Remy C, Bonnet F, et al. Meta-analysis of epidural analgesia versus parenteral opioid analgesia after colorectal surgery. *Br J Surg.* 2007;94:665–673.
140. Gelman S, Laws HL, Potzick J, et al. Thoracic epidural vs balanced anesthesia in morbid obesity: An intraoperative and postoperative hemodynamic study. *Anesth Analg.* 1980;59:902–908.
141. Brodsky JB, Mariano ER. Regional anaesthesia in the obese patient: Lost landmarks and evolving ultrasound guidance. *Best Pract Res Clin Anaesthesiol.* 2011;25:61–72.
142. Nielsen KC, Guller U, Steele SM, et al. Influence of obesity on surgical regional anesthesia in the ambulatory setting: An analysis of 9,038 blocks. *Anesthesiology.* 2005;102:181–187.
143. Damia G, Mascheroni D, Croci M, et al. Perioperative changes in functional residual capacity in morbidly obese patients. *Br J Anaesth.* 1988;60:574–578.
144. Catenacci AJ, Anderson JD, Boersma D. Anesthetic hazards of obesity. *JAMA.* 1961;175:657–665.
145. Tsueda K, Debrand M, Zeok SS, et al. Obesity supine death syndrome: Reports of two morbidly obese patients. *Anesth Analg.* 1979;58:345–347.
146. VanDercar DH, Martinez AP, De Lisser EA. Sleep apnea syndromes: A potential contraindication for patient-controlled analgesia. *Anesthesiology.* 1991;74:623–624.
147. Buckley FP, Robinson NB, Simonowitz DA, et al. Anaesthesia in the morbidly obese. A comparison of anaesthetic and analgesic regimens for upper abdominal surgery. *Anaesthesia.* 1983;38:840–851.
148. Carvalho JC. Ultrasound-facilitated epidurals and spinals in obstetrics. *Anesthesiol Clin.* 2008;26:145–158.
149. Chin KJ, Perlas A, Chan V, et al. Ultrasound imaging facilitates spinal anesthesia in adults with difficult surface anatomic landmarks. *Anesthesiology.* 2011;115:94–101.

150. Ellinas EH, Eastwood DC, Patel SN, et al. The effect of obesity on neuraxial technique difficulty in pregnant patients: A prospective, observational study. *Anesth Analg.* 2009;109:1225–1231.
151. Clinkscales CP, Greenfield ML, Vanarase M, et al. An observational study of the relationship between lumbar epidural space depth and body mass index in Michigan parturients. *Int J Obstet Anesth.* 2007;16:323–327.
152. Balki M, Lee Y, Halpern S, et al. Ultrasound imaging of the lumbar spine in the transverse plane: The correlation between estimated and actual depth to the epidural space in obese parturients. *Anesth Analg.* 2009;108:1876–1881.
153. Chiang HK, Zhou Q, Mandell MS, et al. Eyes in the needle: Novel epidural needle with embedded high-frequency ultrasound transducer–epidural access in porcine model. *Anesthesiology.* 2011;114:1320–1324.
154. Marroquin BM, Fecho K, Salo-Coombs V, et al. Can parturients identify the midline during neuraxial block placement? *J Clin Anesth.* 2011;23:3–6.
155. Watts RW. The influence of obesity on the relationship between body mass index and the distance to the epidural space from the skin. *Anaesth Intensive Care.* 1993;21:309–310.
156. Hogan QH, Prost R, Kulier A, et al. Magnetic resonance imaging of cerebrospinal fluid volume and the influence of body habitus and abdominal pressure. *Anesthesiology.* 1996;84:1341–1349.
157. McCulloch WJ, Littlewood DG. Influence of obesity on spinal analgesia with isobaric 0.5% bupivacaine. *Br J Anaesth.* 1986;58:610–614.
158. Taivainen T, Tuominen M, Rosenberg PH. Influence of obesity on the spread of spinal analgesia after injection of plain 0.5% bupivacaine at the L3-4 or L4-5 interspace. *Br J Anaesth.* 1990;64:542–546.
159. Santos A, Pedersen H, Finster M, et al. Hyperbaric bupivacaine for spinal anesthesia in cesarean section. *Anesth Analg.* 1984;63:1009–1013.
160. Pitkanen MT. Body mass and spread of spinal anesthesia with bupivacaine. *Anesth Analg.* 1987;66:127–131.
161. Wong CA, Cariaso D, Johnson EC, et al. Body habitus does not influence spread of sensory blockade after the intrathecal injection of a hypobaric solution in term parturients. *Can J Anaesth.* 2003;50:689–693.
162. Norris MC. Patient variables and the subarachnoid spread of hyperbaric bupivacaine in the term parturient. *Anesthesiology.* 1990;72:478–482.
163. Bloom SL, Spong CY, Weiner SJ, et al. Complications of anesthesia for cesarean delivery. *Obstet Gynecol.* 2005;106:281–287.
164. Hood DD, Dewan DM. Anesthetic and obstetric outcome in morbidly obese parturients. *Anesthesiology.* 1993;79:1210–1218.
165. Hodgkinson R, Husain FJ. Obesity and the cephalad spread of analgesia following epidural administration of bupivacaine for Cesarean section. *Anesth Analg.* 1980;59:89–92.
166. Hamilton CL, Riley ET, Cohen SE. Changes in the position of epidural catheters associated with patient movement. *Anesthesiology.* 1997;86:778–784.
167. Milligan KR, Carp H. Continuous spinal anaesthesia for caesarean section in the morbidly obese. *Int J Obstet Anesth.* 1992;1:111–113.
168. Pan PH, Bogard TD, Owen MD. Incidence and characteristics of failures in obstetric neuraxial analgesia and anesthesia: A retrospective analysis of 19,259 deliveries. *Int J Obstet Anesth.* 2004;13:227–233.
169. Cappiello E, O'Rourke N, Segal S, et al. A randomized trial of dural puncture epidural technique compared with the standard epidural technique for labor analgesia. *Anesth Analg.* 2008;107:1646–1651.
170. Cotter JT, Nielsen KC, Guller U, et al. Increased body mass index and ASA physical status IV are risk factors for block failure in ambulatory surgery – an analysis of 9,342 blocks. *Can J Anaesth.* 2004;51:810–816.
171. Franco CD, Gloss FJ, Voronov G, et al. Supraclavicular block in the obese population: An analysis of 2020 blocks. *Anesth Analg.* 2006;102:1252–1254.
172. Chantzi C, Saranteas T, Zogogiannis J, et al. Ultrasound examination of the sciatic nerve at the anterior thigh in obese patients. *Acta Anaesthesiol Scand.* 2007;51:132.
173. Schwemmer U, Papenfuss T, Greim C, et al. Ultrasound-guided interscalene brachial plexus anaesthesia: Differences in success between patients of normal and excessive weight. *Ultraschall Med.* 2006;27:245–250.
174. Chan VW, Perlas A, McCartney CJ, et al. Ultrasound guidance improves success rate of axillary brachial plexus block. *Can J Anaesth.* 2007;54:176–182.
175. Brull R, Lupu M, Perlas A, et al. Compared with dual nerve stimulation, ultrasound guidance shortens the time for infraclavicular block performance. *Can J Anaesth.* 2009;56:812–818.
176. Casati A, Baciarello M, Di Cianni S, et al. Effects of ultrasound guidance on the minimum effective anaesthetic volume required to block the femoral nerve. *Br J Anaesth.* 2007;98:823–827.
177. Sites BD, Brull R, Chan VW, et al. Artifacts and pitfall errors associated with ultrasound-guided regional anesthesia. Part II: A pictorial approach to understanding and avoidance. *Reg Anesth Pain Med.* 2007;32:419–433.
178. Sites BD, Chan VW, Neal JM, et al. The American Society of Regional Anesthesia and Pain Medicine and the European Society Of Regional Anaesthesia and Pain Therapy Joint Committee recommendations for education and training in ultrasound-guided regional anesthesia. *Reg Anesth Pain Med.* 2009;34:40–46.
179. Gaszynski T, Tokarz A, Piotrowski D, et al. Boussignac CPAP in the postoperative period in morbidly obese patients. *Obes Surg.* 2007;17:452–456.
180. Ahmad S, Nagle A, McCarthy RJ, et al. Postoperative hypoxemia in morbidly obese patients with and without obstructive sleep apnea undergoing laparoscopic bariatric surgery. *Anesth Analg.* 2008;107:138–143.
181. Sabers C, Plevak DJ, Schroeder DR, et al. The diagnosis of obstructive sleep apnea as a risk factor for unanticipated admissions in outpatient surgery. *Anesth Analg.* 2003;96:1328–1335.
182. Gupta RM, Parvizi J, Hanssen AD, et al. Postoperative complications in patients with obstructive sleep apnea syndrome undergoing hip or knee replacement: A case-control study. *Mayo Clin Proc.* 2001;76:897–905.
183. Cullen DJ. Obstructive sleep apnea and postoperative analgesia–a potentially dangerous combination. *J Clin Anesth.* 2001;13:83–85.
184. Grover BT, Priem DM, Mathiason MA, et al. Intensive care unit stay not required for patients with obstructive sleep apnea after laparoscopic Roux-en-Y gastric bypass. *Surg Obes Relat Dis.* 2010;6:165–170.
185. American Society of Anesthesiologists Task Force on Neuraxial Opioids, Horlocker TT, Burton AW, et al. Practice guidelines for the prevention, detection, and management of respiratory depression associated with neuraxial opioid administration. *Anesthesiology.* 2009;110:218–230.
186. Honiden S, Gong MN. Diabetes, insulin, and development of acute lung injury. *Crit Care Med.* 2009;37:2455–2464.
187. Gong MN, Bajwa EK, Thompson BT, et al. Body mass index is associated with the development of acute respiratory distress syndrome. *Thorax.* 2010;65:44–50.
188. Hogue CW Jr, Stearns JD, Colantuoni E, et al. The impact of obesity on outcomes after critical illness: A meta-analysis. *Intensive Care Med.* 2009;35:1152–1170.
189. Nafiu OO, Kheterpal S, Moulding R, et al. The association of body mass index to postoperative outcomes in elderly vascular surgery patients: A reverse J-curve phenomenon. *Anesth Analg.* 2011;112:23–29.
190. DeSilva RA, Lown B. Energy requirement for defibrillation of a markedly overweight patient. *Circulation.* 1978;57:827–830.
191. Brunette DD. Resuscitation of the morbidly obese patient. *Am J Emerg Med.* 2004;22:40–47.
192. King DR. Emergent cricothyroidotomy in the morbidly obese: A safe, no-visualization technique. *J Trauma.* 2011;71:1873–1874.
193. Childers DK, Allison DB. The 'obesity paradox': A parsimonious explanation for relations among obesity, mortality rate and aging? *Int J Obes.* 2010;34:1231–1238.
194. Mullen JT, Davenport DL, Hutter MM, et al. Impact of body mass index on perioperative outcomes in patients undergoing major intra-abdominal cancer surgery. *Ann Surg Oncol.* 2008;15:2164–2172.
195. Mullen JT, Moorman DW, Davenport DL. The obesity paradox: Body mass index and outcomes in patients undergoing nonbariatric general surgery. *Ann Surg.* 2009;250:166–172.
196. Tung A. Anaesthetic considerations with the metabolic syndrome. *Br J Anaesth.* 2010;105(suppl 1):i24–i33.
197. Glance LG, Wissler R, Mukamel DB, et al. Perioperative outcomes among patients with the modified metabolic syndrome who are undergoing noncardiac surgery. *Anesthesiology.* 2010;113:859–872.
198. Anaya DA, Dellinger EP. The obese surgical patient: A susceptible host for infection. *Surg Infect.* 2006;7:473–480.
199. Cheadle WG. Risk factors for surgical site infection. *Surg Infect.* 2006;7(suppl 1):S7–S11.
200. Kabon B, Rozum R, Marschalek C, et al. Supplemental postoperative oxygen and tissue oxygen tension in morbidly obese patients. *Obes Surg.* 2010;20:885–894.
201. Thomas H, Agrawal S. Systematic review of same-day laparoscopic adjustable gastric band surgery. *Obes Surg.* 2011;21:805–810.

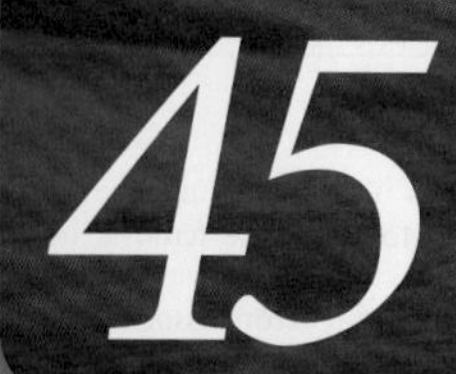

CHAPTER 45

The Liver: Surgery and Anesthesia

RANDOLPH H. STEADMAN • MICHELLE Y. BRAUNFELD

Key Points

1. The liver is the largest internal organ, accounting for 2% of the total body mass of adults. It receives 25% of the cardiac output via a dual afferent blood supply. The portal vein supplies 75% of the hepatic blood flow while the hepatic artery supplies the remainder. Because of the higher oxygen content in the hepatic artery, each vessel provides roughly 50% of the hepatic oxygen supply.
2. The liver plays a preeminent role in the intermediary metabolism of nutrients (glucose, nitrogen, and lipids) and the detoxification of chemicals, including lipophilic medications. Liver dysfunction affects the metabolism of nutrients and xenobiotics, and negatively impacts nearly every other organ system.
3. Portal hypertension, the end result of hepatic injury and fibrotic changes, results in portosystemic shunts that bypass the liver's metabolic and detoxification capabilities. When nitrogenous waste and other substances normally cleared by the liver enter the central circulation, hepatic encephalopathy ensues.
4. Additional complications of portal hypertension include variceal hemorrhage, ascites, and hepatorenal syndrome. Cardiac sequelae include hyperdynamic circulation due to decreased systemic vascular resistance, which results in an increase in cardiac output.
5. Perioperative complications encountered by cirrhotic patients include liver failure, postoperative bleeding, infection, and renal failure. Patients with a model for end-stage liver disease (MELD) score of less than 11 have a low postoperative mortality and represent an acceptable surgical risk. End-stage liver disease patients with a risk of postoperative liver failure should have elective abdominal surgery at institutions with a liver transplant program. In patients with a MELD score of 20 or higher, the high mortality risk contraindicates elective procedures until after liver transplantation.
6. Medical management undertaken to optimize cirrhotic patients undergoing surgery should be directed toward treating active infection, minimizing vasoactive infusions, optimizing central blood volume and renal status, minimizing ascites, and improving encephalopathy and coagulopathy.
7. The perioperative risk of patients with end-stage liver disease depends more on the operative site and the degree of liver impairment than the anesthetic technique.

Multimedia

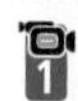
Left Liver Lobe Donation

HEPATIC FUNCTION IN HEALTH

The liver is the largest internal organ and is the body's metabolic headquarters. It weighs 1.5 kg or about 2% of the total body weight in an adult. The functional unit of the liver is the lobule, a structure roughly 1 × 2 mm that consists of plates of hepatocytes located in a radial distribution about a central vein. The afferent blood supply from the portal vein and hepatic arteriole enters at the periphery of the lobule. Bile, formed in the hepatocytes, flows into canaliculi located between the plates of hepatocytes and drains into bile ducts located at the periphery of the lobule next to portal venules and hepatic arterioles. The large pores in the endothelium lining the sinusoids allow plasma and its proteins to move readily into the tissue spaces surrounding hepatocytes, an area known as the spaces of Disse. This fluid drains into the lymphatic system. The liver generates about half of the body's lymph (Fig. 45-1).

1 The liver receives approximately 25% of the cardiac output via a dual supply. The portal venules conduct blood from the portal vein, which drains the gastrointestinal tract. The portal vein supplies 75% of the liver inflow, or about 1 L/min. The hepatic arterioles supply the remaining 25% of the hepatic blood flow. Due to the higher oxygen content of arterial blood, each vessel contributes about 50% of the hepatic oxygen supply.

The liver's high blood flow is due to low vascular resistance in the portal vein. The average portal vein pressure is 8 to 10 mm Hg while the hepatic venous pressure averages 0 mm Hg. However, when injured hepatocytes are replaced by fibrous tissue, blood flow is impeded and portal hypertension ensues. Sinusoidal pressures greater than 5 mm Hg are abnormal and define portal hypertension.[1] Sympathetic innervation from T3 to T11 controls resistance in the hepatic venules. Changes in compliance in the hepatic venous system contribute to the regulation of cardiac output and blood volume. In the presence of reduced portal venous flow, the hepatic artery can increase flow by as much as 100% to maintain hepatic oxygen delivery. The reciprocal relationship between flow in the two afferent vessels is termed the "hepatic arterial buffer response."[2]

The microcirculation of the liver lobule is divided into three zones that receive varying oxygen content.[3] Zone 1 receives oxygen-rich blood from the adjacent portal vein and hepatic artery. As blood moves through the sinusoid it passes from the intermediate zone 2 into zone 3, which surrounds the central vein. Blood entering zone 3 is oxygen poor. Pericentral hepatocytes have a greater quantity of cytochrome P450 enzymes and are the site of anaerobic metabolism. Hypoxia and reactive metabolic intermediates from biotransformation affect zone 3 more prominently than other zones.

Due to its ability to distend, the liver is capable of storing up to 1 L of blood. The liver serves as a reservoir capable of accepting blood, or releasing blood at times of low blood volume. The liver also stores vitamins, particularly vitamins B_{12} (1-year supply), D (3-month supply), and A (10-month supply). Excess body iron is transported via apoferritin to the liver for storage as ferritin, which is released when circulating iron levels are low. Thus, the liver apoferritin system serves as a blood iron buffer.

Reticuloendothelial cells called Kupffer cells line the venous sinusoids. These macrophages phagocytize bacteria that enter the sinusoids from the intestines. Less than 1% of bacteria that enter the liver pass through the systemic circulation.

2 The liver is involved in energy production and storage of nutrients absorbed from the intestines. The liver aids in blood glucose regulation through its glucose buffer function. This is accomplished by storing glucose as glycogen, converting other carbohydrates (principally fructose and galactose) to glucose, and synthesizing glucose from amino acids and triglyceride (gluconeogenesis).[4] In patients with altered liver function, blood glucose concentration can raise several fold higher than the postprandial levels found in patients with normal hepatic function.

The liver synthesizes fat, cholesterol, phospholipids, and lipoproteins. It also efficiently metabolizes fat, converting fatty acids to acetyl coenzyme A (Co A), an excellent source of energy, which can be diverted to the citric acid cycle to liberate energy for the

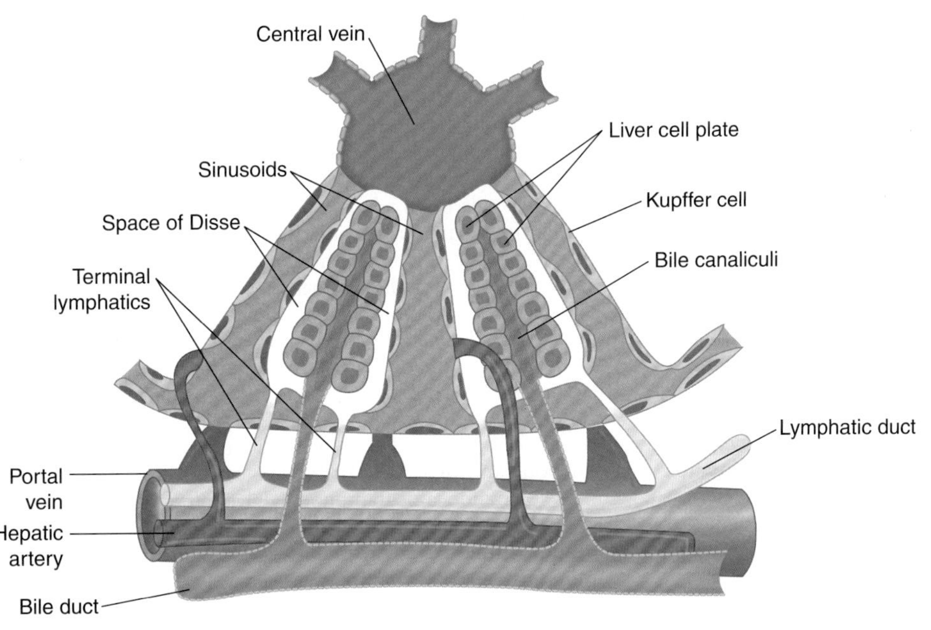

FIGURE 45-1. Basic structure of a liver lobule, showing the cellular plates, the blood vessels, the bile-collecting system, and the lymph flow system composed of the spaces of Disse and the interlobular lymphatics. (Modified from: Guyton AC, Taylor AE, Granger HJ. *Circulatory Physiology. Vol 2. Dynamics and Control of the Body Fluids.* Philadelphia, PA: WB Saunders; 1975.)

liver. The liver generates more acetyl-CoA than it consumes. The excess is packaged as acetoacetic acid for use elsewhere in the body. The majority of cholesterol synthesized in the liver is converted to bile salts and secreted in the bile. The remainder is distributed to the rest of the body where it is used to form cellular membranes and other vital structures. Fat synthesis from protein and carbohydrates occurs almost exclusively in the liver, and the liver is responsible for most fat metabolism.

The liver also plays a key role in protein metabolism. The liver synthesizes all of the plasma proteins with the exception of γ-globulins, which are formed in plasma cells. The liver is capable of forming 15 to 50 g of protein per day, an amount sufficient to replace the body's entire supply of protein in several weeks. Albumin is the major protein synthesized by the liver and is the primary determinant of plasma oncotic pressure. The liver also synthesizes the nonessential amino acids from keto acids, which are also synthesized in the liver.

The liver is capable of deamination of amino acids, which is required for energy production or the conversion of amino acids to carbohydrates or fats. Deamination produces ammonia, which is toxic. Intestinal bacteria are an additional source of ammonia. The liver removes ammonia through the formation of urea.

All of the blood clotting factors, with the exception of factors III (tissue thromboplastin), IV (calcium), and VIII (von Willebrand factor), are synthesized in the liver. Vitamin K is required for the synthesis of prothrombin (factor II) and factors VII, IX, and X.

Hepatocytes produce roughly 500 mL of bile daily. Between meals, the high pressure in the sphincter of Oddi diverts bile to the gallbladder for storage. The gallbladder holds 35 to 50 mL of bile in concentrated form. The presence of fat in the duodenum causes release of the hormone cholecystokinin from duodenal mucosa, which reaches the gallbladder via circulation and stimulates gallbladder contraction. Bile contains bile salts, bilirubin, and cholesterol. Bile salts act as a detergent, solubilizing fat into micelles, which are absorbed. Bile salts return to the liver via the portal vein, completing the enterohepatic circulation. Bile salts are needed for fat absorption, and cholestasis can result in steatorrhea and vitamin K deficiency.

The liver has the unique ability to restore itself after injury or partial hepatectomy. As much as two-thirds of the liver can be removed with regeneration of the remaining liver in a matter of weeks.[5] Hepatocyte growth factor, produced by mesenchymal cells in the liver, and other growth factors, such as epidermal growth factor (EGF), cytokines, tumor necrosis factor (TNF), and interleukin-6, are involved in stimulating regeneration. Growth factor-β, a known inhibitor of hepatocyte proliferation, is involved in halting the regenerative process, which appears to be related to the ratio of liver-to-body weight.[5,6] Inflammation, such as with a viral infection of the liver, impairs regeneration.

ASSESSMENT OF HEPATIC FUNCTION

A number of laboratory tests are available to assess the liver. Collectively termed *liver function tests* (LFTs) many, including aspartate aminotransferase (AST) and alanine aminotransferase (ALT), do not assess function but rather cellular injury. Increased serum levels of these enzymes, AST (formerly serum glutamic oxaloacetic transaminase or SGOT) and ALT (formerly serum glutamic pyruvic transaminase or SGPT), occur in many types of hepatic disease. Because AST is also found in nonhepatic tissues (including the heart, skeletal muscle, kidney, and brain), elevations are not specific for hepatic disease. ALT is primarily localized to the liver.

Fatty liver and chronic infections are associated with mild (several fold) elevations of AST and ALT. Acute hepatitis produces larger increases, but the highest concentrations, which can exceed 50 times normal, are seen with acute hepatitis necrosis. Absolute levels of these enzymes are not always helpful, as declining values may indicate recovery or conversely a lack of surviving hepatocytes. The AST/ALT ratio may be helpful in differentiating alcoholic liver disease, in which the ratio is typically >2, from viral hepatitis, which is associated with a ratio <1.

Indices of bile flow obstruction include serum levels of alkaline phosphatase (AP), 5′-nucleotidase (5′-NT), γ-glutamyl transferase (GGT), and bilirubin. AP isoenzymes are found in multiple organs including the liver, bone, kidney, intestines, placenta, and leukocytes. Normally, most circulating AP originates from liver and bone. Hepatic AP is concentrated in the microvilli of bile canaliculi and the sinusoidal surface of hepatocytes. Elevations of serum AP disproportionate to changes in AST and ALT occur with obstructions to bile flow. However, AP elevations may originate from other tissues, including the placenta during pregnancy. Although 5′-NT is also found in many tissues, elevations are highly specific for hepatobiliary obstruction. Elevations of 5′-NT may reflect the detergent action of bile salts on plasma membranes, a requirement for its release. Because 5′-NT is so specific for liver diseases, it is useful to determine whether elevated AP is of hepatic origin. Serum GGT is the most sensitive laboratory indicator of biliary tract disease but it is less specific than 5′-NT and has largely been replaced by 5′-NT.

Bilirubin originates primarily from the breakdown of hemoglobin released from senescent red blood cells. Serum bilirubin levels are determined by the van den Bergh reaction, which separates bilirubin into two fractions: A lipid-soluble, indirect-reacting form (unconjugated bilirubin) and a water-soluble, direct-reacting form (conjugated bilirubin). Elevated levels of unconjugated bilirubin indicate an excess production of bilirubin (hemolysis) or a decrease in the uptake and conjugation of bilirubin by hepatocytes. Conjugated bilirubin is elevated by impaired intrahepatic excretion or extrahepatic obstruction. Even with complete biliary tract obstruction, the bilirubin rarely exceeds 35 mg/dL because of renal excretion of conjugated bilirubin.

Tests of hepatic synthetic function focus on the measurement of serum albumin and coagulation testing. Although the liver is the primary site of albumin synthesis, excessive protein losses (enteropathy, burns, nephrotic syndrome) can also result in low albumin levels. Because of its 3-week half-life, serum albumin is not a reliable indicator of acute liver disease. In contrast, the prothrombin time (PT) and international normalized ratio (INR) are sensitive indicators of hepatic disease because of the short half-life of factor VII. The PT depends upon sufficient intake of vitamin K, which in turn depends upon adequate biliary secretion of bile salts. In patients with biliary obstruction, the PT can be prolonged despite preserved hepatic function. Other conditions that can affect the PT in the absence of liver disease include congenital coagulation factor deficiencies, consumptive coagulopathies such as disseminated intravascular coagulation (DIC), and warfarin therapy.

A number of other tests exist to assess hepatic function, though their use in the United States is limited primarily to research applications. Indocyanine green (ICG) elimination estimates hepatic blood flow and hepatocellular function due to the high extraction ratio of ICG (>70%). The MEGX test measures the conversion of lidocaine to monoethylglycinexylidide (MEGX) via hepatic demethylation. Other metabolic tests include antipyrine clearance, aminopyrine breath test, caffeine breath test, galactose elimination capacity, and urea synthesis.

Ancillary tests to confirm specific diagnoses include serologic tests for the various hepatitis viruses, autoantibodies (for the diagnosis of primary biliary cirrhosis [PBC]), ceruloplasmin (Wilson's disease), ferritin (hemochromatosis), α-1 antitrypsin (α-1 antitrypsin deficiency), and α-fetoprotein (hepatocellular carcinoma [HCC]). Serum ammonia is useful for following patients with hepatic encephalopathy (HE).

HEPATOBILIARY IMAGING

Selection of the appropriate imaging technique depends on the differential diagnosis and whether a concurrent therapeutic intervention is planned. Plain radiography has a limited role in the evaluation of liver disease. Abdominal X-rays can be useful to detect calcified or gas-containing lesions. Examples include calcified gallstones, chronic calcific pancreatitis, gas-containing liver abscesses, portal venous gas, and emphysematous cholecystitis.

Ultrasonography is the primary screening test for hepatic parenchymal disease and extrahepatic biliary disease. It is the method of choice for detecting gallstones, the presence of ascites, and portal or hepatic vein thrombosis. Its major limitations are its dependence on the operator's skill and its inability to penetrate bone or air, including bowel gas.

Radioisotope scanning has largely been replaced by computed tomography (CT) scanning. However, it is still in use in patients with suspected acute cholecystitis. Radioisotopes visualized in the gallbladder rule out obstruction of the cystic duct, while visualization of the biliary tree and common bile duct without the gallbladder indicates cystic duct obstruction and the presence of cholecystitis.

CT scanning supplements ultrasonography, providing information on the liver texture, gallbladder disease, bile duct dilatation, and mass lesions of the liver and pancreas. CT provides more resolution than ultrasonography and is less operator-dependent. Lesions can be biopsied under CT guidance. The disadvantages of CT include radiation exposure and cost.

Magnetic resonance imaging (MRI) is increasingly used for the evaluation of hepatobiliary disease. MRI is superior to CT for the assessment of malignant focal liver lesions and diffuse liver disease.[7] MRI is also useful for the evaluation of biliary disease.[8] MRI also offers the advantages of avoidance of radiation and contrast nephropathy. The primary disadvantage is the need for a 20-second breath-hold, which can require sedation or anesthesia in young and/or uncooperative patients.

Percutaneous transhepatic cholangiography (THC) is the percutaneous injection of contrast into the bile ducts under fluoroscopic guidance. It can be used to determine the site and cause of biliary obstruction and to evaluate whether cholangiocarcinoma is surgically resectable. It can also be used for balloon dilatation of biliary strictures and/or placement of an internal stent or external drain. Endoscopic retrograde cholangiopancreatography (ERCP) uses endoscopy to visualize the ampulla of Vater and selectively inject contrast material into the pancreatic and common bile ducts. ERCP has the advantage over THC of not requiring a dilated biliary tree to achieve a high probability of success. ERCP permits sphincterotomy and stone extraction, biopsy, brushings, balloon dilatation, and stent insertion.

LIVER BIOPSY

Liver biopsy continues to have a role in the evaluation of patients with liver disease. It is the method of choice to determine whether liver damage is due to necrosis, inflammation, steatosis, or fibrosis. The presence of coagulopathy or thrombocytopenia contraindicates percutaneous liver biopsy, although transjugular liver biopsy can be performed under these conditions.

HEPATIC AND HEPATOBILIARY DISEASES

Liver disease may be the result of a variety of causes, which include developmental or genetic defects, metabolic abnormalities, autoimmune diseases, infectious diseases, neoplasm, alcohol, environmental toxins, and drug toxicity. A preliminary report from the National Vital Statistics System for the year 2009 lists liver disease as the 12th leading cause of death in the United States, being responsible for over 33,000 deaths in that year. An estimated 5.5 million people in the United States have chronic liver disease (CLD) and another 20 million have biliary disease, together affecting slightly more than 8% of the population. Economic costs for care of these conditions total $8.9 billion per year.[9]

Liver disease can be divided into two main groups on the basis of the primary anatomy affected. Processes may be considered primarily hepatocellular (parenchymal) or biliary. Progressive biliary disease may eventually lead to fibrotic changes and cirrhosis, but it is characteristic of the biliary diseases that cholestasis precedes hepatocellular dysfunction. In hepatocellular diseases evidence of cholestasis and synthetic dysfunction appear synchronously (Table 45-1). The fact that hepatocellular function is preserved until late in course of cholestatic disease disadvantages patients with cholestatic liver disease awaiting liver transplantation. Priority for transplant is based on the model for end-stage liver disease (MELD) score, which is sensitive to hepatocellular dysfunction. Patients with cholestatic disease may lose transplant candidacy because of other manifestations of their disease, for example, malignancy, infection, or concurrent autoimmune disease, before they accrue enough hepatocellular damage to be offered a transplant.[10]

Liver disease may also be described as acute or chronic. The most common causes for acute liver disease are drug toxicity and infection. Acute illnesses may resolve spontaneously, segue into chronic disease, or result in acute liver failure (ALF). While the primary cause of ALF in the United States was once infectious (presumed acute hepatitis A and B), acetaminophen toxicity is currently the leading cause of this condition. Other causes of acute liver dysfunction include alcoholic hepatitis, nonacetaminophen drug toxicity, and pregnancy-related hepatic diseases. The most common causes for CLD are chronic viral hepatitis, alcoholic liver disease, and nonalcoholic fatty liver disease (NAFLD). Although the prevalence rates of chronic viral hepatitis and alcoholic liver disease have been relatively stable over the past 10 years, the prevalence of NAFLD has grown significantly and appears to be linked to the current epidemic of obesity.[11] The most important consequences of CLD are portal hypertension, cirrhosis, and malignancy.

Acute Liver Failure

ALF (previously termed fulminant hepatic failure) is defined as the appearance of encephalopathy together with coagulopathy, usually an INR ≥1.5, in a patient who has no previous history of liver disease and who has had an illness of <26 weeks' duration. Although further distinctions in duration of disease, such as hyperacute and subacute, were once used they are no longer

TABLE 45-1. BLOOD TESTS AND THE DIFFERENTIAL DIAGNOSIS OF HEPATIC DYSFUNCTION

	Bilirubin Overload (Hemolysis)	Parenchymal Dysfunction	Cholestasis
Aminotransferases	Normal	Increased (may be normal or decreased in advanced stages)	Normal (may be increased in advanced stages)
Alkaline phosphatase	Normal	Normal	Increased
Bilirubin	Increased Unconjugated	Increased Conjugated	Increased Conjugated
Serum proteins	Normal	Decreased	Normal (may be decreased in advanced stages)
Prothrombin time	Normal	Decreased (may be normal in early stages)	Normal (may be prolonged in advanced stages)
Blood urea nitrogen	Normal	Normal (may be decreased in advanced stages)	Normal
Sulfobromophthalein/ indocyanine green	Normal	Retention	Normal or retention

From: Gelman S. Anesthesia and the liver. In: Barash P, Cullen B, Stoelting R, eds. *Clinical Anesthesia.* 3rd ed. Philadelphia, PA: Lippincott-Raven; 1997:1011.

considered useful for prognosis and have been abandoned. ALF is a rare entity with an incidence of about 2,000 cases per year in the United States. Drug-related toxicity accounts for over half of the cases of ALF in the United States. Of these drug-related cases, over 80% are the result of acetaminophen ingestion. In descending order the next most common causes are idiopathic, acute viral hepatitis, autoimmune, and ischemic.[12] The natural history of adult ALF in the United States is one of spontaneous recovery in approximately 45% of patients, liver transplantation in 25%, and death without transplantation in 30%.[13] Etiology has some bearing on outcome, with the most favorable prognosis for patients with acetaminophen overdose, ischemic injury, and hepatitis A and poor prognoses for those with nonacetaminophen drug-induced liver injury (DILI), acute hepatitis B, Wilson's disease, and autoimmune hepatitis.[14]

Patients with no previous history of liver disease who present with signs or symptoms and laboratory evidence of a significant hepatitis should have an INR measured and undergo a careful mental status examination. An INR ≥1.5 and any evidence of encephalopathy should lead to admission to the hospital for ALF. History should include questions about potential infectious or toxic exposures and a detailed history of recent medications or ingestions. Questions should include details about herbal and nutritional supplements, since these have been associated with ALF as well. Except for the finding of encephalopathy, physical examination may be unrevealing. In particular, evidence of CLD should not be present, as the patient should not have had adequate time to develop the stigmata of portal hypertension and cirrhosis. Acute decompensation of CLD or "acute on chronic" liver disease is a separate condition with different etiologies, therapy, and prognostic indicators.

Standard initial labs are indicated in Table 45-2.[14] Further laboratory and investigative studies are directed by the history, for example, radiologic imaging or ultrasound for suspected hepatic vein thrombosis. Although etiologies of ALF are heterogenous, there are manifestations that are common to all patients who have massive hepatic necrosis, regardless of its provenance. The most

TABLE 45-2. INITIAL LABORATORY ANALYSIS OF SUSPECTED ACUTE LIVER FAILURE

Prothrombin time/INR
Chemistries
  Sodium, potassium, chloride, bicarbonate, calcium, magnesium, phosphate glucose
  AST, ALT, alkaline phosphatase, GGT, total bilirubin, albumin creatinine, blood urea nitrogen
Arterial blood gas
Arterial lactate
Complete blood count
Blood type and screen
Acetaminophen level
Toxicology screen
Viral hepatitis serologies
  Anti-HAV IgM, HBSAg, anti-HBc IgM, anti-HEV[a], anti-HCV[b]
Ceroloplasmin level[c]
Pregnancy test (females)
Ammonia (arterial if possible)
Autoimmune markers
  ANA, ASMA, immunoglobulin levels
HIV status[d]
Amylase and lipase

[a]If clinically indicated.
[b]Done to recognize potential underlying infection.
[c]Done only if Wilson disease is a consideration (e.g., in patients less than 40 yrs without another obvious explanation for ALF); in this case uric acid level and bilirubin to alkaline phosphatase ratio may be helpful as well.
[d]Implications for potential liver transplantation.
From: Polson J, Lee WM. AASLD position paper: The management of acute liver failure. *Hepatology.* 2005;41:1179.

TABLE 45-3. GRADES OF ENCEPHALOPATHY

I. Changes in behavior with minimal change in level of consciousness
II. Gross disorientation, drowsiness, possibly asterixis, inappropriate behavior
III. Marked confusion, incoherent speech, sleeping most of the time but arousable to vocal stimuli
IV. Comatose, unresponsive to pain, decorticate or decerebrate posturing

Note: Some patients will overlap grades; clinical judgment is required.
Adapted from: Conn HO, Leevy CM, Vhlahcevic ZR, et al. Comparison of lactulose and neomycin in the treatment of chronic portal-systemic encephalopathy. A double blind controlled trial. *Gastroenterology.* 1977;72:573.

serious, and often the proximate cause of death, is acute cerebral edema and intracranial hypertension. Effects on other organ systems include coagulopathy, circulatory dysfunction and hypotension, acute kidney injury, and metabolic derangements. Encephalopathy is a necessary finding to diagnose ALF. Encephalopathy is graded on a I to IV scale and is described in Table 45-3. The presence of cerebral edema is directly related to the depth of encephalopathy. The incidence of cerebral edema is almost negligible in stage I to stage II coma, but increases to 25% to 35% with stage III and 75% with stage IV.[15] As with the encephalopathy of cirrhosis, the underlying mechanism is not completely understood but hyperammonemia plays a significant role. Ammonia, which is toxic, is generally metabolized via the urea cycle in the liver. The brain has no cells capable of utilizing the urea cycle and thus must resort to detoxifying ammonia by synthesizing glutamine from ammonia and glutamate within astrocytes. Glutamine is osmotically active and results in osmotic astrocyte edema. Other contributors to the observed cerebral edema may include a systemic inflammatory response[16,17] and the loss of cerebral autoregulation, which leads to cerebral hyperemia.[18] Potential targets for therapy include osmotic and mechanical reduction of cerebral edema, elimination of ammonia, manipulation of cerebral blood flow and metabolism, and reduction of the inflammatory response.

General measures to reduce cerebral edema include maintaining the patient in a 30-degree head-up position and making sure the head is in neutral position so as not to impede venous return. Once a patient is intubated, muscle relaxants should be considered to minimize rises in intracranial pressure (ICP) from coughing, bucking, and shivering. Mannitol can be used to induce an osmotic diuresis, but may have limited utility in the patient with compromised renal function. Another option may be hypertonic saline, ideally targeting a serum sodium of 145 to 155 mEq/L.[19]

Although hyperventilation may acutely reduce the cerebral hyperemia associated with ALF, the response is short-lived. There is no evidence that chronic hyperventilation affords any decrease in episodes of intracranial hypertension or any survival benefit.[20] Current recommendations are to maintain normocarbia and to reserve hyperventilation for response to acute rises in ICP. Barbiturates can be used to decrease cerebral metabolism; however, their use may be limited by hypotension.

Ammonia can be eliminated by the administration of lactulose or nonabsorbable antibiotics such as rifaximin or neomycin; however, there is no evidence to support their use in the setting of ALF. Furthermore, neomycin is specifically contraindicated because of the risk of nephrotoxicity.

Corticosteroids have not been shown to be effective in ALF, but there may be a place for prophylactic antibiotics to prevent sepsis and minimize the inflammatory mediator burden. The U.S. Acute Liver Failure Study Group has recommended empiric administration of antibiotics in the following settings: (a) when surveillance cultures reveal significant isolates; (b) progression to stage III or stage IV coma; (c) refractory hypotension; or (d) when the patient exhibits elements of the systemic inflammatory response syndrome, that is, temperature >38° or <36°, heart rate >90 bpm, white blood cell count >12,000 or <4,000.[21] Other potential modalities to decrease the inflammatory response include modest hypothermia to a target temperature of 32° to 34°C and indomethacin.[22]

How to monitor the presence and progression of cerebral edema and intracranial hypertension is controversial. Serial head CTs are often obtained for patients who progress to stage III to stage IV coma, but they are not reliable for diagnosing or quantitating intracranial hypertension due to a lack of sensitivity. CT can, however, provide information on structural abnormalities such as intracranial hemorrhage.[23] Although many centers will place an ICP monitor to guide therapy in patients with stage III to stage IV coma, there are no randomized controlled studies to support this practice. Furthermore, ICP monitor placement is not a benign procedure, frequently entailing aggressive correction of coagulopathy and transport to and from the OR for a critically ill, fragile patient. Nonetheless, many believe that ICP monitors are invaluable for guiding acute therapy and for helping to determine who may no longer be a viable candidate for transplantation. In addition to measuring ICP, these monitors allow calculation of cerebral perfusion pressure (CPP = MAP – ICP), which should be kept between 50 and 80 mm Hg. In one case series, a sustained CPP <40 mm Hg for greater than 2 hours was associated with a poor neurologic outcome.[24] An effective protocol for managing intracranial hypertension in patients with stage III or stage IV encephalopathy has been described (Table 45-4) and resulted in a 95% response to treatment of episodes of ICP >20 mm Hg. Furthermore, in this prospective series, ICP was monitored in all patients, and no patients died of isolated cerebral edema. The authors used a protocol that included activated recombinant factor VII (rFVIIa) to correct coagulopathy prior to ICP placement. Significant bleeding complications from ICP monitoring were not encountered.[25]

TABLE 45-4. ICP MANAGEMENT PROTOCOL

Initiate in rapid stepwise fashion for ICP >20 mm Hg for >5 min

- Keep CPP >60 mm Hg with norepinephrine or phenylephrine infusion
- Mannitol 1 g/kg IV bolus, may repeat if serum osmolarity <320 mOsm/kg
- Hyperventilation to target PCO_2 30–35 mm Hg
- Hypothermia using cooling blanket to core temperature of 33°–34°C. Initiate neuromuscular blockade if needed with cisatracurium 0.2 mg/kg IV bolus, 3 μg/kg/min infusion—adjust to 2/4 on train of four
- Pentobarbital 5 mg/kg bolus, repeated 3–5 mg/kg boluses as necessary—titrate to ICP effect
- 3% saline: Calculate dose to achieve serum sodium in 145–155 mEq/L range

ICP, intracranial pressure; CPP, cerebral perfusion pressure; IV, intravenous.
From: Raschke RA, Curry SC, Rempe S, et al. Results of a protocol for the management of patients with fulminant hepatic failure. *Crit Care Med.* 2008;36:2244.

TABLE 45-5. KING'S COLLEGE SELECTION CRITERIA FOR LIVER TRANSPLANTATION ACCORDING TO THE ETIOLOGY OF ACUTE LIVER FAILURE

Etiology	Selection Criteria for Transplantation
Acetaminophen	Arterial pH <7.30 despite normal intravascular filling pressures (irrespective of grade of encephalopathy) OR Prothrombin time >100 s + serum creatinine >300 μmol/L in patients in grade III or IV encephalopathy
Nonacetaminophen	Prothrombin time >100 s (irrespective of grade of encephalopathy) OR Any three of the following (irrespective of grade of encephalopathy): Non-A, non-B hepatitis (cryptogenic), halothane hepatitis, or other drug toxicity Age <10 yrs or >40 yrs Jaundice to encephalopathy interval >7 d Prothrombin time >50 s Serum bilirubin >300 μmol/L

From: O'Grady JG, Alexander GJ, Hayllar KM, et al. Early indicators of prognosis in fulminant hepatic failure. *Gastroenterology.* 1989;97:439.

Equally controversial to the monitoring and significance of ICP is determining the prognosis for patients with ALF. Organs for transplantation are a scarce resource, and for some patients liver transplantation is the only life-saving option. However, this life-saving procedure comes with the requirements of major surgery and lifelong immunosuppression. Deciding which patient should receive a transplant, which may recover spontaneously, and which are unlikely to benefit from transplantation is one of the most difficult decisions encountered during the management of patients with liver disease. Unfortunately there is no ideal guideline for making these decisions. The two most widely used prognostic models are the Clichy or Paul Brousse Hospital criteria and the King's College Hospital criteria. The Clichy criteria recommend transplantation for patients in stage III or stage IV coma on the basis of age and factor V levels. The transplantation threshold is 20% factor V activity for patients <30 years or 30% factor V activity for patients >30 years.[26] There is no distinction made for the etiology of ALF, which is felt to be a weakness of these criteria. The King's College Hospital (see Table 45-5) accounted for better spontaneous outcomes of patients who had ALF on the basis of acetaminophen toxicity and divided their criteria accordingly. While the positive predictive value of King's College Hospital criteria has been shown to be clinically acceptable in ALF patients, the negative predictive value drops below 50% in nonacetaminophen patients.[27] Thus, patients who fail to fulfill these criteria include a number of patients who will die without being properly considered for transplantation. Various modifications to the King's College Hospital criteria to improve performance and other prognostic scoring models for specific etiologies have been proposed. These include the addition of blood arterial lactate, serum phosphate, and levels of Gc-globulin, a marker that could improve quantitation of hepatic necrosis.[28]

Coagulopathy is also a necessary finding for the diagnosis of ALF; however, clinically significant spontaneous bleeding is uncommon. Correction of thrombocytopenia to ≥50,000/mm³ and INR to ≤1.5 is suggested for the bleeding patient or the patient about to undergo an invasive procedure.[14,21] Specific treatment thresholds for the nonbleeding patient are difficult to define, but it is suggested that prophylactic therapy not be undertaken except for severe abnormalities, for example, platelet count ≤10,000/mm³, INR >7, and fibrinogen <100 mg/dL.[14] Occasionally, the use of rFVIIa or prothrombin complex concentrate is used to correct a resistant INR abnormality or to avoid fluid overload. It should be kept in mind that these agents carry a thrombotic risk and are contraindicated when the etiology of ALF is associated with hypercoagulability, such as pregnancy or Budd–Chiari syndrome.

Hypotension in ALF may be the result of several days of gastrointestinal losses, poor intake, or myocardial dysfunction, but likely includes a component of decreased arterial tone as liver necrosis progresses. The hypotensive ALF patient should undergo volume status and cardiac function assessment prior to consideration of inotropes or vasopressors. Vasopressors may be used either to treat systemic hypotension or to maintain an adequate CPP. On the basis of recommendations for septic patients, either norepinephrine or dopamine may be used. The use of arginine vasopressin (AVP) or its analogs cannot be recommended as there is evidence that their use is associated with increases in ICP.[29]

Acute Hepatitis

The most common causes of acute viral hepatitis are, collectively, the five identified viral hepatitidies: A (HAV), B (HBV), C (HCV), D (HDV or delta-virus), and E (HEV). HAV and HBV have been well characterized and vaccines have been developed to prevent their transmission. As a result of widespread vaccination, the incidence of new cases of HAV and HBV has decreased steadily worldwide. Unfortunately, the same cannot be said for HCV, for which there is no currently available vaccine. The number of reported new cases of HCV is decreasing but this is likely the result of better screening of transfused blood products and the adoption of universal precautions. HDV is a single-strand RNA genome that requires the helper function of HBV for virion assembly and so must occur either as a coinfection or a superinfection with HBV. HEV is a small RNA virus that has been responsible for several epidemics of hepatitis, primarily in underdeveloped countries with poor sanitation.

The diagnosis of acute hepatitis is made on the basis of classic signs and symptoms, together with laboratory studies to assess liver damage and serologic assays. Symptoms can be nonspecific, such as fatigue, poor appetite, nausea, vomiting, and abdominal pain, and many infections are subclinical. Signs may include jaundice, or a serum-sickness–type presentation with fever, arthralgia or arthritis, and rash that results from circulating hepatitis antigen–antibody complexes. Incubation periods can be several weeks to even months and patients may undergo surgery without awareness of illness. For this reason viral hepatitis should be part of the differential diagnosis when there is any evidence of postoperative liver injury.

HAV is a picornavirus that is spread primarily by the fecal–oral route or via contaminated food or water. It is highly contagious and can be spread by close personal and household contact. HAV has a mean incubation period of 4 weeks and the virus may be shed 1 to 2 weeks before and for at least 1 week after the onset of illness. HAV has a wide range of manifestation from asymptomatic disease (particularly in children) to ALF. ALF is rare (<1%) and is more likely than other causes to result in spontaneous recovery (69%) in patients without underlying liver disease.[30] There is no chronic disease state associated with HAV.

HBV is a DNA virus that is spread via parenteral, cutaneous, or mucosal exposure to infected blood or body fluids. It is an extremely hardy virus and can remain viable for days outside the body.[31] The United States has a low rate of infection and the most commonly identified risk factors are parenteral drug use and sexual contact. In highly endemic populations such as in sub-Saharan Africa, Southeast Asia, and China, infection occurs primarily during the perinatal period. Since the progression to chronic disease is approximately 90% in this age group, perpetuation of endemicity is assured. The mean incubation period is 12 weeks, but can be as long as 20 weeks. HBV surface antigen (HBsAg) is the hallmark of active HBV infection and usually appears during the incubation period, 1 to 10 weeks after exposure. ALF caused by acute HBV infection occurs in less than 1% of cases, but has only a 20% rate of spontaneous recovery. Maintenance of seropositivity for HBsAg for >6 months after recovery suggests chronic infection. Progression to chronic disease occurs in 2% to 5% of infected adults. Treatment of chronic HBV is aimed at suppressing viral replication and preventing progression of liver disease. Parameters followed are serum ALT, HBV DNA levels, positive or negative status of HBeAg (a marker of viral replication), and liver histology. There are currently six therapeutic agents approved for the treatment of chronic HBV: Adefovir dipivoxil, interferon α-2b, pegylated interferon α-2a, lamivudine, entecavir, and telbivudine.

HDV infection occurs in conjunction with HBV infection and is estimated to be present in 5% of patients with chronic HBV. Two types of HDV infection are described: Coinfection with acute HBV and superinfection on top of chronic HBV. Both types cause severe infection and may cause ALF. Suspicion should be raised for HDV infection in the patient who seems to have a fulminant course of acute HBV infection or who has had stable chronic HBV disease and acutely decompensates. The course of the patient with coinfection may be biphasic, with one peak in aminotransferases reflecting peak HBV replication and another one a few weeks later reflecting peak HDV replication. HDV superinfection can be differentiated from a flare of chronic HBV by testing for HDV RNA or IgM anti-HDV.

HCV, once referred to as non-A, non-B hepatitis until its identification in 1989, is transmitted primarily parenterally. Since the identification of HCV, the ability to serologically screen blood products for its presence has all but eliminated it as a source of posttransfusion hepatitis. Causes of transmission are often not identifiable, but the most commonly known risk factor is parenteral drug use. Incubation period averages 7 weeks, jaundice is infrequent, and there is a high rate of subclinical infection. Interestingly, patients who develop jaundice are more likely to recover completely. HCV has a high rate of progression to chronic disease (50% to 85%) and a risk of developing cirrhosis ranging from 5% to 25% over 25 to 30 years.[32] Contributing factors to the development of cirrhosis include older age, alcohol consumption, an immunosuppressed state, and obesity. HCV is currently the leading cause for liver transplantation in the United States, which is performed for cirrhosis and/or associated HCC. The optimal therapy of chronic HCV infection is the combination of pegylated interferon-α and ribavirin, with the goal of sustained viral response (SVR), defined as the absence of HCV RNA from serum by a sensitive PCR assay 24 weeks following discontinuation of therapy. Unfortunately therapy is often compromised by intolerance of drug-related constitutional or neuropsychiatric symptoms or by lab abnormalities such as neutropenia or hemolytic anemia.

Alcoholic Hepatitis

Alcoholic hepatitis is the syndrome marked by the development of jaundice and liver dysfunction in the setting of heavy alcohol use. The typical patient is a middle-aged man who has a history of excessive drinking and who has become acutely ill with the dramatic onset of jaundice. Other signs include fever, ascites, and abdominal tenderness, frequently the result of an enlarged tender liver. Encephalopathy may be present in severe alcoholic hepatitis and, if so, portends a poorer prognosis. Laboratory studies show moderate serum aminotransferase elevations (<300 IU/mL), with AST being elevated more than ALT. The AST:ALT ratio is >2 in about 70% of patients with alcoholic hepatitis.[33] The white blood count, serum bilirubin, and INR are also elevated. Elevations of serum creatinine are particularly ominous as they may indicate impeding hepatorenal syndrome (HRS). Acute kidney injury, defined as at least a 0.3 mg/dL or 50% increase in serum creatinine over baseline, is associated with a significantly increased 90-day mortality (63% vs. 7%) in patients with alcoholic hepatitis.[34]

The differential diagnosis of the patient with the clinical and laboratory findings described includes nonalcoholic steatohepatitis (NASH), viral hepatitis, DILI, fulminant autoimmune liver disease or Wilson's disease, severe ascending cholangitis, and hepatic abscess. A history of excessive alcohol use is supportive of the diagnosis of alcoholic hepatitis, but up to 20% of these patients may have a coexisting cause of liver disease.[35] While liver biopsy is not required to make the diagnosis of alcoholic hepatitis, it is important to investigate other potential causes of acute liver disease. Viral hepatitis serologies should be sent, as well as autoimmune markers and ceruloplasmin. Blood, urine, and ascitic fluid cultures should be obtained. Imaging should be done to rule out space-occupying hepatic lesions or biliary processes.

The key component of therapy for alcoholic hepatitis is abstinence. For those patients with severe alcoholic hepatitis, medical therapy should also be considered. This consists of nutritional therapy that takes into account not only protein-calorie nutrition, but vitamin and mineral deficiencies as well. The administration of a 28-day course of prednisolone is also recommended for those patients with advanced disease. In patients for whom steroids are contraindicated, consideration should be given to pentoxifylline, a phosphodiesterase inhibitor with anticytokine activity. In a randomized placebo-controlled trial the administration of pentoxifylline was associated with 40% less mortality than placebo in patients with severe alcoholic hepatitis.[36]

Drug-induced Liver Injury

Often considered as an afterthought when a patient presents with new abnormalities in liver-related laboratory studies, DILI is a significant cause of morbidity and mortality. Although the process of diagnosing DILI is not well defined and it is largely a diagnosis of exclusion, DILI should always be considered when formulating the differential diagnosis of patients presenting with liver abnormalities. Moreover DILI is a serious problem for the pharmaceutical industry, as it is the most common reason for regulatory actions such as failure of approval, removal from market, or restrictions on indications for use. Nonacetaminophen drug-induced idiosyncratic liver injury accounts for 11% to 13% of cases of ALF and, with a 20% rate of survival with supportive care, has a poorer than average rate of spontaneous recovery.[13,37]

A recent report from the international DILI Expert Working Group has defined laboratory criteria for diagnosing DILI (Table 45-6). DILI can further be characterized as hepatocellular, cholestatic, or mixed, on the basis of the relative abnormalities of laboratory values. This is done by calculating the R value, such that $R = (ALT/ULN)/(ALP/ULN)$, where ALT is the alanine aminotransferase, ALP is the alkaline phosphatase, and ULN is the upper limit of normal value. The higher the R value, the more abnormal the ALT in comparison to the ALP. Thus R values ≥5 are used to define a hepatocellular pattern of damage. R values ≤2 define a cholestatic pattern, and R values between 2 and 5 define a mixed pattern. A prognostic rule of thumb is eponymously named "Hy's law" after Hyman J. Zimmerman, a leader in DILI research. It was his observation that jaundice (defined as bilirubin >2 ULN) in patients with hepatocellular DILI carried a poor prognosis, with a mortality of >10%. This observation has been confirmed and recognized for many years by the FDA as a tool for identifying which drugs may be expected to cause significant hepatotoxicity.[38]

TABLE 45-6. CLINICAL CHEMISTRY CRITERIA FOR DRUG-INDUCED LIVER INJURY (DILI)

Any one of the following:

- More than or equal to fivefold elevation above the upper limit of normal (ULN) for alanine aminotransferase (ALT)
- More than or equal to twofold elevation above the ULN for alkaline phosphatase (ALP) (particularly with accompanying elevations in concentrations of 5′-nucleotidase or γ-glutamyl transpeptidase in the absence of known bone pathology driving the rise in ALP level)
- More than or equal to threefold elevation in ALT concentration and simultaneous elevation of bilirubin concentration exceeding 2 × ULN

Level of evidence: 2b (exploratory/retrospective cohort studies)

From: Aithal GP, Watkins PB, Andrade RJ, et al. Case definition and phenotype standardization in drug-induced liver injury. *Clin Pharmacol Ther.* 2011;89:806.

The liver is commonly involved in drug toxicity because of its central role in drug metabolism. Drugs may either be directly hepatotoxic or may propagate toxic metabolites, most often as products of phase I drug metabolism and the cytochromes P450.[39] Cell injury follows via cell stress, mitochondrial injury, or immune-mediated injury. Cell stress may result from glutathione depletion or the binding of reactive metabolites to intracellular enzymes, proteins, or lipids. Mitochondrial injury may result from the uncoupling of mitochondrial respiration with the depletion of ATP and accumulation of reactive oxygen species (ROS). Immune-mediated injury may result from the binding of reactive metabolites to cell structures, creating antigenic entities that can invoke the formation of antibodies against the cell structures themselves.

In anesthesiology perhaps the best known potentially hepatotoxic drug is halothane. Halothane was introduced to patient care in 1956 and, because of its clinical advantages of lack of flammability, potency, and patient tolerance of administration, rapidly enjoyed widespread use. However, reports of postoperative liver injury began to appear shortly thereafter, and by 1963, over 300 cases of "halothane hepatitis" had been reported.[40] The National Academy of Sciences produced a retrospective epidemiologic study on the use of halothane from these reports. The National Halothane Study reviewed cases of fatal hepatic necrosis occurring within 6 weeks of the administration of a general anesthetic, from among 34 centers in the United States. Of the 856,000 anesthetics reviewed, about 255,000 involved halothane, and 82 cases of fatal hepatic necrosis were identified. Sixty-three of these cases could be ascribed to an identifiable clinical factor, leaving 19 with otherwise unexplained hepatic necrosis. Fourteen of the nineteen had received a halothane anesthetic, but did not have consistent histologic findings. The lesions seen were similar to those seen with fatal viral hepatitis or some forms of drug-induced hepatitis.[41] Uncertainty over the direct association between halothane and the cases of fatal hepatic necrosis, together with the calculated incidence of 1 in 35,000 anesthetics even if such association did exist, led to the conclusion that halothane overall had a good safety record. The possible association with repeated exposure to halothane did not go unrecognized, and there was an editorial recommendation that halothane be avoided in patients with a history of unexplained fever and jaundice following a general anesthetic.[42]

The typical presentation of halothane hepatitis is one of nonspecific symptoms of anorexia, malaise, and fever in conjunction with a recent exposure. More specific signs include a rash and jaundice that appears 4 to 7 days after anesthetic exposure, but may be delayed for several weeks. Laboratory studies may reveal abnormalities typical of hepatocellular damage in DILI: Significant elevations in serum transaminases (500 to 2,000 IU/L), but AP elevations that are generally no more than twice the upper limit of normal.[40,43] Risk factors include female gender, obesity, age, and most important, a history of prior exposure.

It is generally agreed that halothane hepatitis is composed of two different manifestations. A relatively mild, self-limited form is characterized by elevations in liver-related lab studies without evidence of liver failure. This may occur in up to 20% of patients after halothane exposure.[44] A proposed mechanism for this hepatocellular damage is the combination of halothane degradation products and hypoxia caused by imbalance in the hepatic oxygen supply–demand relationship.[45] There is strong evidence that the severe, fulminant form of halothane hepatitis is an immune-mediated process. The association with repeated halothane exposure and the appearance of rash and eosinophilia support this hypothesis. Furthermore, circulating IgG antibodies against liver proteins, modified by the reactive trifluoroacetyl (TFA) metabolite of halothane, have been identified in the sera of patients with clinical halothane hepatitis.[46] Although other halogenated inhalational anesthetics that produce TFA metabolites such as enflurane, isoflurane, and desflurane have been associated with acute hepatic failure, the incidences of hepatitis attributed to them have been very small. Since halothane is by far the most extensively metabolized of these agents (20% halothane metabolized vs. 2% enflurane, 0.2% isoflurane, and 0.01% desflurane) the production of TFA metabolites would seem to correlate with the incidence of associated hepatitis. Indeed, an animal study examining the extent of hepatic tissue trifluoroacylation after exposure to halogenated anesthetics showed that halothane produced significantly more tissue acylation than enflurane, isoflurane, or desflurane.[47]

Pregnancy-related Liver Diseases

Abnormalities in liver studies occur in 3% to 5% of pregnancies. Although many causes reflect underlying hepatic or biliary disease, the most common causes are one of the five acute, pregnancy-related conditions: Hyperemesis gravidarum; intrahepatic cholestasis of pregnancy; preeclampsia; preeclampsia complicated by hemolysis, low platelet count, and elevated liver enzymes (HELLP syndrome); and acute fatty liver of pregnancy (AFLP; Table 45-7). Hyperemesis gravidarum is a feature of the first trimester of pregnancy and is characterized by vomiting of sufficient severity to warrant intravenous (IV) hydration. Risk factors include hyperthyroidism, molar pregnancy, and multiple pregnancies.[48] Liver enzymes may be elevated in 50% of patients, with up to 20-fold elevation, but little if any elevation of bilirubin.[49,50] It is important to distinguish hyperemesis from acute viral hepatitis or from drug toxicity with appropriate labs and a careful medication history. Therapy is primarily supportive and the condition usually resolves by the second trimester.

Intrahepatic cholestasis of pregnancy usually presents in the second to third trimester of pregnancy. The proposed etiology is interference with bile acid transport across the canalicular membrane, resulting in elevated serum bile acid elevation and pruritus. In addition to modest increases in bilirubin (usually <5 mg/dL) aminotransferases may also be elevated up to 20-fold and serum bile acids may be elevated up to 100-fold.[49] As with hyperemesis gravidarum, treatment is primarily supportive, aimed at relieving pruritus. Unlike hyperemesis, intrahepatic cholestasis of pregnancy may be associated with chronic placental insufficiency, premature labor, and sudden fetal death. Therefore, pregnancies complicated by intrahepatic cholestasis of pregnancy are considered fetal high-risk pregnancies.

The three remaining uniquely pregnancy-related conditions all present in the third trimester. Preeclampsia is diagnosed by the triad of hypertension, edema, and proteinuria. Elevation of aminotransferases is indicative of severe preeclampsia. The appearance of microangiopathic hemolytic anemia (MAHA), elevated liver enzymes, and low platelet count in the preeclamptic patient comprises the HELLP syndrome and occurs in 20% of severely preeclamptic patients. MAHA is the result of vascular endothelial injury with subsequent fibrin deposition and platelet consumption. This also leads to areas of hepatic infarction and subsequent hemorrhage, which may coalesce into large hematomas and lead

TABLE 45-7. DISTINGUISHING FEATURES OF INTRAHEPATIC CHOLESTASIS OF PREGNANCY (ICP), THE HELLP SYNDROME AND FATTY LIVER OF PREGNANCY (AFLP)

	ICP	HELLP	AFLP
% pregnancies	0.1% (United States)	0.2–0.6%	0.005–0.01%
Onset/trimester	25–32 wks	3 or postpartum	3 or postpartum
Family history	Often	No	Occasionally
Presence of preeclampsia	No	Yes	50%
Typical clinical features	Pruritus	Hemolysis	Liver failure with coagulopathy, encephalopathy hypoglycemia, DIC
	Mild jaundice	Thrombocytopenia (<50,000 often)	
	Elevated bile acids		
	Vitamin K ↓		
Aminotransferases	Mild to 10- to 20-fold elevation	Mild to 10- to 20-fold elevation	300–500 typical but variable ++
Bilirubin	<5 mg/dL	<5 mg/dL unless massive necrosis	Often <5 mg/dL, higher if severe
Hepatic imaging	Normal	Hepatic infarcts Hematomas, rupture	Fatty infiltration
Histology	Normal–mild cholestasis, no necrosis	Patchy/extensive necrosis and hemorrhage	Microvesicular fat in zone 3
Maternal mortality	0%	1–25%	7–18%
Fetal/perinatal mortality	0.4–1.4%	11%	9–23%
Recurrence in subsequent pregnancies	45–70%	4–19%	α-subunit, long-chain 3-hydroxyacyl-CoA dehydrogenase (LCHAD) defect—yes No fatty acid oxidation defect – rare

DIC, disseminated intravascular coagulation.
From: Hay JE. Liver disease in pregnancy. *Hepatology.* 2008;47:1067.

to capsular rupture and intraperitoneal bleeding. The clinical presentation is not dissimilar to severe preeclampsia, with abdominal pain, nausea, headache, hypertension, and edema. Laboratory studies show elevated aminotransferases, up to 10- to 20-fold, and modest increases in bilirubin. A peripheral smear will show the characteristic schistocytes and burr cells of MAHA. Platelet count may be used to distinguish between mild, moderate, and severe HELLP, with platelet counts of 100,000 to 150,000/mm^3, 50,000 to 100,000/mm^3, and <50,000/mm^3, respectively.

Serious maternal complications include DIC, placental abruption, eclampsia, pulmonary edema, hepatic hematoma, and hepatic capsular rupture.[51] Abdominal CT imaging is the preferred study to detect major hepatic complications of infarct, hematoma, or rupture. Contained hepatic hemorrhage can be managed conservatively with correction of volume deficit and coagulopathy. Manipulation of the abdomen or abdominal straining should be avoided. Capsular rupture or rapid extension of a hematoma is life threatening and demands more aggressive treatment for control of bleeding, usually emergency laparotomy. Rarely, there may be an indication for transplantation for the patient in whom bleeding cannot be controlled. Delivery is definitive therapy for HELLP syndrome, although up to 25% of patients may not present until the postpartum period. Therapy remains the same regardless of timing of presentation and most patients will rapidly resolve abnormalities after delivery.

AFLP is the result of rapid microvesicular fatty infiltration of the liver resulting in acute portal hypertension and encephalopathy. Although the exact mechanism of AFLP is unknown, there is an association between it and abnormalities in the enzymes involved in β-oxidation of fatty acids. Symptoms of abdominal pain, nausea, headache, and vomiting, together with laboratory findings of elevated aminotransferases, bilirubin, and thrombocytopenia, are similar to severe preeclampsia and HELLP syndrome. However, the AFLP patient may additionally have laboratory and clinical findings more unique to liver failure, such as hypoglycemia, elevated ammonia, asterixis, and encephalopathy. Although the definitive diagnosis is made histologically, there is usually reluctance to perform liver biopsy. Noninvasive studies such as ultrasound or abdominal CT are an option and may show increased echogenicity or decreased hepatic density consistent with fatty liver. However, they cannot be relied upon as they may be unremarkable in half of the patients with AFLP.[52]

Arrangements for rapid delivery should follow diagnosis of AFLP, as recovery can only follow delivery. Recovery may be prolonged in patients who are severely ill upon presentation, and there is a role for transplantation in the patient who continues to deteriorate into ALF after delivery.

CIRRHOSIS AND PORTAL HYPERTENSION

3 Cirrhosis is the end product of the long course of CLD, during which there have been either steady or recurrent episodes of parenchymal inflammation and necrosis with resultant disruption of normal hepatic architecture. Areas of fibrosis and regenerative nodules replace the normal arrangement of hepatic lobules. Blood flow through the liver is disrupted as well, with the formation of shunts between afferent (portal venous and hepatic arterial) and efferent (hepatic venous) vessels.[53] Increased resistance to blood flow through the liver leads to portal hypertension. When portal hypertension becomes severe (generally defined as a hepatic venous pressure gradient (HVPG) of >10 to 12 mm Hg), CLD becomes a systemic illness, affecting other organ systems as well.[54]

Hemostasis

Hemostasis is a dynamic process that is the product of interaction between coagulation, platelets, and fibrinolysis, resulting in the formation and revision of clot. Liver disease affects all three of these components, both quantitatively and qualitatively.

The liver is the site of synthesis for all procoagulant and anticoagulant factors, with the exception of tissue thromboplastin (III), calcium (IV), and von Willebrand factor (VIII). It is also the site for clearance of activated factors.

Cirrhotic patients are customarily considered to have a bleeding diathesis on the basis of abnormalities in conventional tests of coagulation such as PT and partial thromboplastin time (PTT). However, such tests reflect the activity of only a portion of the procoagulant factors and do not consider the concomitant decrease in anticoagulant factors, which are not customarily measured. It is the balance of procoagulant and anticoagulant forces, not the isolated measurement of either portion of the coagulation system that indicates the effective generation of thrombin. Not surprisingly, PT and PTT abnormalities correlate poorly with bleeding complications following invasive procedures, such as liver biopsy.[55–57] In fact there is evidence that, should one account for differences in the anticoagulant levels between normal and cirrhotic patients by adding thrombomodulin (an activator of the anticoagulant protein C) to the PT assay, normal and cirrhotic patients generate the same amounts of thrombin.[58] Thus, one may conclude that the decreased levels of protein C in cirrhotic patients balance the decreased levels of procoagulants, leaving thrombin generation in vivo unaltered.

Even more counterintuitive is the increasing evidence that cirrhotic patients not only have normal thrombin generation, but may actually have a procoagulant imbalance on the basis of reduced levels of anticoagulants protein C and antithrombin III, together with an increase in FVIII.[59,60] Clinically, this is supported by studies reporting not only the lack of protection of liver disease against the formation of venous thromboembolism (VTE)[61,62] but an increased risk of VTE formation associated with the presence of cirrhotic and noncirrhotic liver disease.[63]

The cholestatic diseases (e.g., PBC, sclerosing cholangitis) may eventually progress to cirrhosis, but until that happens the coagulopathy of these diseases has a different nature from that of hepatocellular dysfunction. The coagulopathy of biliary disease is characterized by functional deficiencies in the vitamin K–dependent procoagulants II, VII, IX, and X and anticoagulants protein C and protein S. Vitamin K is a fat-soluble cofactor necessary for the final step in the production of these factors: Carboxylation of the precursor produced by the liver. Bile salts are necessary for absorption of vitamin K, and impaired bile secretion in cholestasis results in vitamin K deficiency. Parenteral vitamin K can correct this deficiency and return coagulation to normal as long as the liver is still capable of manufacturing adequate amounts of factor precursors. It cannot, however, correct the coagulopathy of hepatocellular dysfunction.

Dysfibrinogenemia has been described in acute, chronic, and neoplastic liver disease and is the most common qualitative defect of coagulation factors, occurring in 70% to 80% of cirrhotics.[64] Its presence does not appear to be related to the severity of hepatic dysfunction, but instead to be associated with hepatic tissue regeneration. Excess sialic acid residues on the fibrinogen interfere with the enzymatic activity of thrombin and cause abnormal polymerization of fibrin monomers. Thus, although serum fibrinogen levels may be adequate, function is not accurately reflected.

Platelets provide primary hemostasis by interaction with the vessel wall at the site of injury and forming a physical plug. Thrombocytopenia is a well-known feature of cirrhosis. Estimates of incidence range from 30% to 64% of chronic cirrhotics, but platelet counts below 30,000/mm^3 are rare.[65] Because the liver is the primary site of thrombopoietin production, decreased levels of thrombopoietin contribute. Other factors include immunologic mechanisms, direct bone-marrow suppression, and consumptive processes such as DIC. However, the primary cause is splenic sequestration in the setting of portal hypertension. Up to 90% of the platelet population may be sequestered in the spleen. Elevated levels of von Willebrand factor are felt to compensate for decreased platelets counts, augmenting the platelet–endothelial cell interaction on vessel walls.

A second function of platelets is to promote thrombin generation. Activated platelets provide negatively charged phospholipids on their surfaces, which act as receptors for the assembly of coagulation factors and thus promote coagulation. A series of assays measuring thrombin generation concluded that platelet counts below a threshold of 100,000/mm^3 negatively correlated with thrombin production. It was further estimated that the minimum platelet count necessary to support near-normal thrombin generation was 56,000/mm^3.[58] This information provides further support to the use of platelet transfusion in the bleeding patient with platelet counts in and below that range. Platelet transfusions are not indicated in the absence of bleeding.

The fibrinolytic system limits and revises clot formation. The initial step is activation of plasmin from plasminogen by enzymes such as tissue plasminogen activator (tPA). Plasmin consumes fibrin, producing fibrin degradation products such as D-dimer. The fibrinolytic system in cirrhotic patients has many abnormalities which may account for accelerated fibrinolysis, which has a reported incidence of 30% to 46% in patients with end-stage liver disease.[66,67] The liver is the site of tPA clearance, and elevated tPA levels have been noted in patients with cirrhosis.[68] Furthermore, the liver is the site of synthesis for plasmin inhibitors, such as plasmin activator inhibitor-1 (PAI-1) and thrombin-activatable fibrinolysis inhibitor (TAFI). However, as with the process of coagulation, what matters is the balance of these factors that promote and inhibit fibrinolysis and where their net forces lie. Commonly used studies for assessing the presence and severity of accelerated fibrinolysis include the euglobulin clot lysis time (ECLT) and thromboelastography (TEG). A clot lysis index in TEG has been defined as the ratio of the clot amplitude at 60 minutes post achievement of maximum amplitude (A60) to the clot maximum amplitude (MA). A ratio of <0.85 indicates the presence of accelerated fibrinolysis and suggests the need for an antifibrinolytic agent such as epsilon aminocaproic acid or tranexamic acid in the presence of otherwise unexplained bleeding.

DIC is primarily a thrombotic diathesis, followed by widespread secondary fibrinolysis. As factors are consumed, DIC becomes a bleeding diathesis of factor and platelet deficiencies. Whether or not DIC is a feature of stable CLD is controversial. Because cirrhosis shares common lab abnormalities with DIC, standard labs cannot distinguish between consumption and decreased synthesis and so have little utility. More recent approaches to answer this question have utilized assays for substances that would be expected to be elevated as the result of excessive thrombin production, the sine qua non of DIC. These include the cleaved by-products of coagulation factor activation such as prothrombin fragment F1 + 2, fibrinopeptide A, and thrombin–antithrombin (TAT) complexes. Elevation of these would suggest that low levels of procoagulation factors are the result of consumption rather than underproduction.

It is generally agreed on the basis of examination of these special assays that overt DIC is probably not a feature of stable CLD.[69] However, an entity called "accelerated intravascular coagulation and fibrinolysis" (AICF) has been described. This may be considered a low-grade consumptive process that occurs in <30% of cirrhotics, primarily in those with severe, decompensated disease.[70] While it may not have immediate clinical consequence, patients who exhibit this phenomenon are considered at increased risk to progress to DIC in the presence of a known stimulus, such as sepsis or spontaneous bacterial peritonitis (SBP).

Cardiac Manifestations

4 The cirrhotic patient typically has a hyperdynamic circulation, characterized by a high cardiac output, low arterial blood pressure, and low systemic vascular resistance. On examination the patient is warm and appears well perfused despite systolic arterial pressures in the 80s and 90s. Although pulmonary arterial pressures may be mildly elevated, the pulmonary vascular resistance (PVR) is usually within the normal range. Consideration of the formula for calculating PVR (mean pulmonary artery pressure [mPAP] minus pulmonary capillary wedge divided by cardiac output) reveals the explanation: The cardiac output is elevated proportionally to the transpulmonary gradient (the numerator in the equation). Although these patients have an elevated intravascular volume this is not usually reflected in an elevated wedge pressure. This is due to sequestration of this volume into the massively dilated and collateralized splanchnic vascular bed. Thus, the effective circulating volume is reduced, which has consequences on other organ systems as well.

At the heart of these circulatory changes is portal hypertension. Portal hypertension causes local production of vasodilators such as natriuretic peptides, vasoactive intestinal peptide, endotoxin, glucagon, and especially nitric oxide.[71] Elevated production of nitric oxide has been observed to precede the formation of the hyperdynamic circulation in cirrhosis, and inhibition of nitric oxide formation has been shown to increase arterial pressure in cirrhotic patients. Furthermore, there is reduced circulatory responsivity to sympathetic stimulation primarily due to overproduction of vasodilators.[72]

In addition to hyperdynamic circulation the cirrhotic patient may have a combination of other cardiac functional abnormalities that are not immediately apparent in the baseline state. These abnormalities comprise four key components of a condition termed "cirrhotic cardiomyopathy." They include (1) the aforementioned increase in cardiac output and decrease in peripheral vascular resistance, (2) systolic and diastolic dysfunction, (3) cardiac resistance to β-adrenergic stimulation, and (4) electrophysiologic abnormalities.

Historically, cirrhosis has not been associated with cardiomyopathy since the hyperdynamic circulation was presumed to reflect cardiac vigor and the few patients who had overt dilated cardiomyopathy were thought to be manifesting alcoholic cardiomyopathy. However, elevated cardiac output is only a consequence of the profound decrease in afterload resulting from the dilated peripheral circulation. Systolic incompetence is revealed by physiologic or pharmacologic stress and is manifested by an inability to increase cardiac output in response to exercise and an inability to increase ejection fraction despite an increase in end-diastolic volume. Furthermore, the severity of cardiac dysfunction seems to be directly correlated with the severity of liver disease.[73]

Diastolic dysfunction has been described in cirrhotic patients as well, on the basis of diagnostic echocardiographic findings of abnormalities in transmitral flow during diastole. This consists of decrement or reversal of the E/A wave ratio and prolongation of E wave deceleration time, reflecting ventricular resistance to diastolic filling. Also supportive of the presence of diastolic dysfunction is the finding of septal and left ventricular hypertrophy on echo examination. Diastolic dysfunction renders cirrhotic patients very sensitive to changes in cardiac filling making them vulnerable to both heart failure and prerenal insufficiency.

Autonomic dysfunction is another characteristic of the altered cirrhotic cardiovascular system. Chronotropic and hemodynamic incompetence in response to various challenges such as sustained handgrip, ice water hand submersion, Valsalva maneuver, and tilt table testing has demonstrated autonomic neuropathy in 43% of cirrhotic patients. Although apparently unrelated to autonomic dysfunction, prolonged Q–Tc interval is also observed in cirrhotic patients with an incidence ranging from 30% in Child's A to 60% in Child's C patients.[74] This should be kept in mind when treating these patients with drugs known to prolong Q–T interval.

Coronary artery disease in cirrhotic patients has become an area of interest particularly as the application of liver transplantation has expanded to include older patients with comorbidities. Risk factors for coronary artery disease in cirrhotic patients are similar to those of other patient populations: Hypertension, dyslipidemia, age, gender, and obesity. However, NASH has been recognized as an increasingly important cause for transplantation and carries with it both the cardiac disease risks of its attendant maladies, obesity and diabetes, and a chronic inflammatory state. The optimal test for identifying cirrhotic patients with significant CAD is unclear. Because many of these patients cannot exercise, pharmacologic stress testing is most commonly employed. Unfortunately, studies investigating the predictive value of noninvasive functional testing, particularly dobutamine stress echocardiography, have generally shown poor sensitivity and variable quality of negative predictive value (75% to 89%).[75] Thus, among liver transplantation candidates consideration should be given to proceeding with coronary angiography if the patient is judged to have a high likelihood of CAD.[76] For less complex surgeries, however, this may not be warranted.

Renal Dysfunction

The hallmarks of renal dysfunction in cirrhosis are the seemingly inappropriate avid retention of sodium and free water, together with renal hypoperfusion and consequent decreased glomerular filtration. The extreme manifestation of this is the HRS, a prerenal functional abnormality that is the renal response to the circulatory abnormalities of advanced cirrhosis. Renal function is an important risk factor for mortality, a fact that is emphasized by its presence as one of only three variables used in calculating the MELD score, the primary predictor of 3-month mortality for patients on the liver transplantation waiting list.

Although the most dramatic and unique renal manifestation of CLD is the HRS, cirrhotic patients are also at high risk for more prosaic causes of renal dysfunction, such as parenchymal renal disease, sepsis, nephrotoxicity, and hypovolemia. It is important to remember that HRS is a diagnosis of exclusion and that other possible potentially treatable causes must be ruled out since therapies will differ.

Despite the fact that the cirrhotic patient's liver disease predominates, one should be mindful of any comorbidities that exist. Glomerulonephritis and diabetic nephropathy are not infrequent findings. NAFLD, the most common nonviral cause for adult CLD, is associated with type II diabetes. Immune complex nephropathies such as IgA nephropathy and membranous proliferative glomerulonephropathy are associated with chronic hepatitis C infection.[77] In addition, some underlying causes of liver failure are directly associated with renal dysfunction. These include such diseases as amyloidosis, systemic lupus erythematosus, autoimmune hepatitis, polycystic liver disease, and Alagille syndrome.

The cirrhotic circulatory system is characterized by marked sympathetic stimulation, and activation of the renin–angiotensin–aldosterone and vasopressin systems. These combine to save salt and water and reduce renal perfusion. Elevated levels of renal prostaglandins help to maintain renal perfusion. Thus, cirrhotic patients are very sensitive to the prostaglandin inhibition of nonsteroidal anti-inflammatory medications, although there is evidence for the safety of short-term administration of selective COX-2 inhibitor celecoxib.[78] Aminoglycosides, angiotensin-converting enzyme inhibitors, and angiotensin receptor blockers are other drug groups associated with nephrotoxicity in cirrhotic patients. Despite the expectation that contrast administration would be nephrotoxic, there is no evidence to support that concern.[79]

Cirrhotic patients are at risk for hypovolemia from a number of causes, including gastrointestinal bleeding, diuretic use, and diarrhea resulting from lactulose or rifaximin administration. Unfortunately, it can be difficult to assess intravascular volume status in patients who are total-body volume overloaded, whose measured central filling pressures may reflect transmitted elevated intra-abdominal pressures because of ascites, and whose measured serum creatinine levels are poor estimates of GFR due to decreased muscle mass.[80,81] Nonetheless, pursuit of a diagnosis by discontinuing diuretics and providing volume expansion with albumin can help differentiate hypovolemia from the other prerenal etiology of interest, HRS. Failure to improve creatinine in response to such measures is strongly suggestive of HRS as the underlying cause.

HRS is the renal manifestation of the systemic circulatory derangement of end-stage liver disease. It is considered a functional derangement, primarily on the basis of successful transplantation of kidneys from HRS patients.[82] Although it is often invoked in the differential diagnosis of acute renal dysfunction in cirrhotic patients, it accounts for only about 23% of the cases of acute kidney injury in hospitalized cirrhotic patients.[83] Nonetheless, in cirrhotic patients with ascites, the incidence of HRS is 18% at 1 year and 39% at 5 years.[84]

The initial event leading to HRS is portal hypertension. This leads to the local production of vasodilators, particularly nitric oxide, which in turn causes splanchnic vasodilation. Splanchnic vasodilation leads to a decrease in the effective circulating blood volume and a decrease in arterial blood pressure. These conditions combine to activate the sympathetic, renin–angiotensin–aldosterone and vasopressin systems. The net result is a severe reduction in renal perfusion and glomerular filtration with impaired free water excretion as the kidneys do their part to try to maintain circulatory homeostasis.

The generally agreed upon criteria for diagnosing HRS are those proposed by the International Ascites Club (Fig. 45-2).[85] Two manifestations of HRS are recognized, called type I and type II. Although they were once considered variants of the same disorder, it has become increasingly clear that they must be treated as two different entities.

Type I HRS is characterized by rapidly progressive renal failure, typically represented by at least a doubling of serum creatinine over the course of 2 weeks in close proximity to a precipitating cause such as SBP, sepsis, gastrointestinal bleeding,

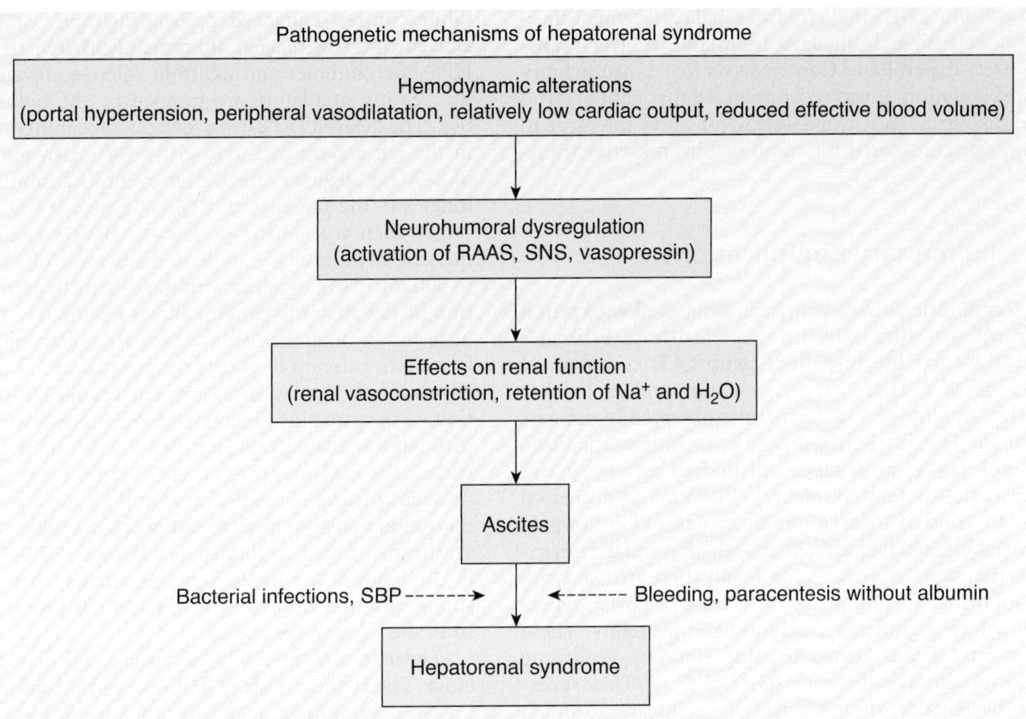

FIGURE 45-2. The pathogenetic mechanism of hepatorenal syndrome. Schematic view of the pathogenesis of hepatorenal syndrome in cirrhosis. *Dotted arrows* indicate precipitating factors that are frequently present but not necessary. RAAS, renin–angiotensin–aldosterone system; SBP, spontaneous bacterial peritonitis; SNS, sympathetic nervous system. (From: Salerno F, Gerbes A, Gines P, et al. Diagnosis, prevention and treatment of hepatorenal syndrome in cirrhosis. *Gut.* 2007;56:1312.)

or surgical stress. Patients with type I HRS have a median survival of 2 to 4 weeks without therapy.[84,86] Type I HRS is associated with failure of other organ systems, including adrenal insufficiency. Most notably; however, when type I HRS responds to medical therapy that response is usually sustained, even after withdrawal of therapy.[87]

Type II HRS is more indolent and may be considered the expected consequence of continuous and progressive activity of the circulatory homeostatic triad of the sympathetic, renin–angiotensin–aldosterone and vasopressin systems in an attempt to compensate for the progressive loss of effective circulating blood volume to the increasingly dilated splanchnic vasculature. The most compelling clinical problem in these patients is refractory ascites. Patients with type II HRS have a median survival of about 6 months.[88]

Although profound renal vasoconstriction is the proximate cause of HRS, therapy aimed at directly increasing renal perfusion by the use of prostaglandins, dopamine agonists, or endothelin antagonists has not proved successful. More effective has been therapy targeting the underlying pathology that leads to the renal vasoconstrictive response, that is, reduction of portal hypertension and/or splanchnic vasodilation.

Vasoconstrictors, such as AVP or its analogs, somatostatin or its analogs, and α-agonists such as norepinephrine and midodrine, combined with volume expansion have shown efficacy in reversing type I HRS (typically defined as a reduction in creatinine to 1.5 mg/dL).[89] AVP and its analogs are particularly attractive, since they interact with V1 receptors which mediate vasoconstriction and are particularly well represented in the splanchnic circulation. Choices among these therapies are to some extent dictated by drug availability since, for example, terlipressin is not available in the United States. Terlipressin is perhaps the most studied vasopressor for HRS and is effective in 40% to 60% of type I patients.[89,90] Predictive factors of successful treatment include a starting creatinine <5 mg/dL and a sustained rise in MAP from baseline throughout the 1- to 2-week course of treatment.[91] More importantly, when therapy is withdrawn, recurrence is uncommon and occurs in <15% of patients.[90] Although response to vasopressor plus volume expansion has been observed in type II HRS, recurrence after withdrawal of therapy is the rule.

Placement of a transjugular intrahepatic portal shunt (TIPS) lowers portal pressures and would be expected to decompress the splanchnic circulation, returning volume directly to the central circulation. Although pilot studies have shown TIPS capable of reversing both types of HRS, it has limited application primarily because of the exclusionary criteria used in these studies, for example, Child–Pugh score >12, active infection, and serum bilirubin >5 mg/dL, and risk of de novo development or worsening of HE.[92] Furthermore, even when initially successful there is a high rate of shunt stenosis and migration.

Liver transplantation is the definitive therapy for HRS. For patients with HRS who are transplant candidates, renal replacement therapy is the typical bridge to transplantation. In countries where terlipressin is available, terlipressin plus albumin volume expansion is also an option. In fact there is evidence that treatment of HRS I with terlipressin and albumin while awaiting liver transplantation may improve posttransplant outcome. Although renal recovery is anticipated, 35% of patients with pretransplant HRS will continue to require support in the immediate postoperative period, compared to 5% of patients without pretransplant HRS.[93] Gradual improvement in GFR occurs over the following 1 to 2 months, reaching 30 to 40 mL/min. There is some sense that, if allowed to continue, HRS that requires renal replacement therapy may not be reversible. In the First International Liver Transplantation Society Expert Panel Consensus on Renal Insufficiency in Liver Transplantation, it was recommended that patients who had received dialysis at least twice weekly for >6 weeks prior to transplantation be considered for combined liver–kidney transplantation.[94]

Pulmonary Complications

Pulmonary complications have long been associated with portal hypertension with or without intrinsic hepatic disease. Estimates of as high as 50% to 70% of patients with CLD complain of shortness of breath.[95] There are many commonplace mechanisms underlying pulmonary abnormalities observed in patients with liver disease. The differential diagnoses include ventilation–perfusion abnormalities associated with underlying obstructive airways disease, fluid retention, pleural effusion, and decreased lung capacities secondary to large volume ascites. α-1 antitrypsin disease is a metabolic syndrome that has both lung and liver manifestations, as may cystic fibrosis. Additionally there are two types of vascular abnormalities unique to the setting of portal hypertension, which have significant morbidity and mortality. These abnormalities have been termed hepatopulmonary syndrome (HPS) and portopulmonary hypertension (PPHTN). Their severity may even overshadow the underlying liver disease, so much so that their presence and severity influences candidacy for liver transplantation.

HPS consists of the triad of liver dysfunction, otherwise unexplained hypoxemia, and intrapulmonary vascular dilation (IPVD) that may be present in up to 20% of patients who present for liver transplantation.[96] The diagnostic criteria for HPS appear in Table 45-8.[97] These vascular lesions are of two types. Type I lesions are more common and are manifested as precapillary dilations at the alveolar level. Type II lesions are larger dilations that are more centrally located in the lungs and behave as anatomic shunts. Demonstration of IPVD may be made by agitated saline contrast-enhanced echocardiography or by technetium-labeled microaggregated albumin (TcMAA). In the absence of HPS microbubbles and albumin microaggregates injected into the venous circulation are trapped by the pulmonary capillary bed. The delayed (>3 cardiac cycles) appearance of microbubbles in the left atrium or increased (>5%) extra-pulmonary uptake of TcMAA suggests direct arteriovenous communication in the lungs and the presence of IPVDs. Type I IPVDs are functional, rather than true anatomic shunts. IPVDs result in a massive increase in pulmonary capillary diameter, from 8 to 15 μm to 50 to 500 μm. This, together with the usually hyperdynamic circulation of the cirrhotic patient, allows insufficient time for oxygen diffusion through the entire stream of capillary blood. This results in a central stream of poorly oxygenated blood that is functionally shunted. This lesion is easily correctable with the administration of oxygen, since increased FiO_2 increases oxygen diffusion through the dilated capillary. In fact, failure of 100% oxygen to correct the PaO_2 to greater than 150 mm Hg is suggestive of the presence of true anatomic or type II shunt.[98] Also of interest is the unique positional oxygenation change that occurs with this syndrome, called orthodeoxia. Because IPVDs predominate in the bases of the lungs, standing worsens hypoxemia and the supine position improves oxygenation as blood is redistributed from the bases to the apices.

The natural history of HPS is usually one of progressive hypoxemia. The pathogenesis of HPS is poorly understood, hampering the development of effective therapy. Suspected contributing factors include nitric oxide, splanchnic endotoxemia, decreased clearance of inflammatory mediators, and angiogenesis. Genetic factors are thought to contribute as well. Liver transplantation can be expected to correct hypoxemia in 85% of patients, although it may take up to a year to do so.[99] Mortality without transplantation is greater than in a matched cohort, with a median survival of 24 months and a 5-year survival of 23% versus a median survival of 87 months and a 5-year survival of 63% in transplant candidates without HPS.[100] A PaO_2 ≤50 mm Hg or a TcMAA-quantitated shunt fraction ≥20% are predictors of increased mortality regardless of whether the patient receives a transplant.

TABLE 45-8. DIAGNOSTIC CRITERIA FOR THE HEPATOPULMONARY SYNDROME

Variable	Criterion
Oxygenation defect	Partial pressure of oxygen <80 mm Hg or alveolar–arterial oxygen gradient ≥15 mm Hg while breathing ambient air
Pulmonary vascular dilatation	Positive findings on contrast-enhanced echocardiography or abnormal uptake in the brain (>6%) with radioactive lung-perfusion scanning
Liver disease	Portal hypertension (most common) with or without cirrhosis
Degree of severity	
Mild	Alveolar–arterial oxygen gradient ≥15 mm Hg, partial pressure of oxygen ≥80 mm Hg
Moderate	Alveolar–arterial oxygen gradient ≥15 mm Hg, partial pressure of oxygen ≥60 to <80 mm Hg
Severe	Alveolar–arterial oxygen gradient ≥15 mm Hg, partial pressure of oxygen ≥50 to <60 mm Hg
Very severe	Alveolar–arterial oxygen gradient ≥15 mm Hg, partial pressure of oxygen <50 mm Hg (<300 mm Hg while the patient is breathing 100% oxygen)

All criteria were determined by means of positive contrast-enhanced echocardiography (i.e., microbubble opacification of the left heart chambers three to six cycles after right atrial passage). The abbreviated formula for the alveolar–arterial gradient is as follows:

$$P_AO_2 - PaO_2 = (F_IO_2[P_{atm} - PH_2O] - [PaCO_2/0.8]) - PaO_2$$

where P_AO_2 denotes partial pressure of alveolar oxygen, PaO_2 partial pressure of arterial oxygen, F_IO_2 fraction of inspired oxygen, P_{atm} atmospheric pressure, PH_2O partial pressure of water vapor at body temperature, and $PaCO_2$ partial pressure of arterial carbon dioxide (0.8 corresponds to the standard gas-exchange respiratory ratio at rest); the normal range is 4 to 8 mm Hg (0.5 to 1.1 kPa). The normal range for the partial pressure of oxygen is 80 to 100 mm Hg (10.7 to 13.3 kPa) at sea level, while the patient is at rest and breathing ambient air. For patients older than 64 yrs of age, a value of ≤70 mm Hg (9.3 kPa) for PaO_2 or ≥20 mm Hg for the alveolar–arterial gradient is often used. Ambient air is the respired gas unless otherwise indicated. To convert millimeters of mercury to kilopascals, multiply by 0.133.

From: Rodriguez-Roisin R, Krowka MJ. Hepatopulmonary syndrome–a liver-induced lung vascular disorder. *N Engl J Med.* 2008;358:2378.

However, in the largest single-center series of liver transplantation for HPS the overall 5-year survival was 76%, an outcome comparable to transplantation in non-HPS patients.[99–101] Taken together, these findings suggest that timely transplantation in patients with HPS results in good outcomes. The transplant community has recognized this by granting MELD exception points to patients with HPS and room air PaO_2 <60 mm Hg.[102]

PPHTN is defined as pulmonary hypertension that exists in a patient who has portal hypertension with no other known cause. The specific diagnostic criteria put forth by the European Respiratory Society Task Force on Hepatopulmonary diseases[103] are

1. Clinical evidence of portal hypertension with or without hepatic disease;
2. mPAP of 25 mm Hg at rest or 30 mm Hg during exercise;
3. Mean pulmonary artery occlusion pressure (mPAOP) <15 mm Hg; and
4. PVR >240 dynes/sec/cm^5 or 3 Wood Units.

There is support for replacing the requirement that the mPAOP be <15 mm Hg with one that requires the transpulmonary gradient (TPG = mPAP – mPAOP) to be >12 mm Hg. Patients with pulmonary hypertension may be fluid overloaded as well, and such a measurement would help distinguish the contribution of volume status to an elevated mPAP. A TPG >12 mm Hg would be consistent with increased PVR, suggesting a component of pulmonary hypertension in the increased mPAP. The requirement for calculation of the PVR is a reflection of the fact that many cirrhotic patients have mildly elevated mPAP simply on the basis of an elevated cardiac output. Calculated PVR in these patients is often normal. Severity of PPHTN is graded by mPAP, with mild, moderate, and severe PPHTN defined as <35 mm Hg, 35 to 50 mm Hg, and >50 mm Hg, respectively.

The occurrence of PPHTN is 2% in a population of patients with known portal hypertension,[104] as compared to 0.13% in an unselected population.[105] Among liver transplant candidates the prevalence is 4% to 6%.[106,107] The occurrence of PPHTN is unrelated to the severity of the underlying liver disease or portal hypertension, with one epidemiologic study documenting a distribution of 51% Child's class A, 38% Child's class B, and 11% Child's class C patients among a population of patients sent to a referral center with the diagnosis of PPHTN.[108] Female patients as well as patients with underlying autoimmune hepatitis are at increased risk for PPHTN, and patients with chronic hepatitis C are at decreased risk.[106,108]

Although a theory commonly put forth for the pathophysiology of PPHTN invokes a vascular proliferative reaction to the shear stress of a chronically elevated cardiac output, the increased incidence in women and in autoimmune hepatitis suggests hormonal and immunologic processes may also contribute. Furthermore, as with other types of pulmonary hypertension increased levels of endothelin are also thought to play a role. Clinical improvement in PPHTN patients with the endothelin antagonist, bosentan, has been documented albeit in a small study.[109]

Similar to HPS patients, symptoms of PPHTN are nonspecific, commonly consisting of dyspnea, generalized weakness, and decreased exercise tolerance. Although HPS and PPHTN may coexist, such an occurrence is uncommon and PPHTN patients may have only a modest decrease in PaO_2 if at all. The single best screening study for PPHTN is the 2-D transthoracic echocardiography (TTE). TTE allows estimation of RV systolic pressure (RVSP) by the velocity of the tricuspid regurgitant jet. Assuming no pulmonary arterial or valvular lesion RSVP is a good estimate of pulmonary arterial systolic pressure. TTE also allows an estimation of central venous pressure (CVP) by caval changes in respiration and evaluation of the RV for changes suggestive of elevated right-sided pressures such as RV dilation or hypokinesis, septal flattening, or moderate to severe tricuspid regurgitation. TTE screening has a sensitivity of 97% and a specificity of 77% in diagnosing moderate to severe PPHTN in patients undergoing pretransplantation workup.[110] Right-sided cardiac catheterization is necessary, however, both to confirm elevated pressures and to measure PVR.

Therapy includes conventional measures such as diuresis, as well as some specific vasodilator therapy. Calcium channel blockers, often used in other patients with pulmonary hypertension, are contraindicated in this population because they promote mesenteric vasodilation and worsen portal hypertension. Other drugs used include prostanoids, phosphodiesterase inhibitors, and endothelin antagonists. Reported success with these modalities is on the basis of case reports or case series, and no one therapy has emerged as definitive. Liver transplantation in this population is very controversial, since pulmonary hypertension cannot be expected to resolve and may even worsen. Nonetheless, one goal of therapy is to make the patient transplant-eligible by reducing mPAP and PVR into an acceptable range.

Epoprostenol (PgI) has been shown to reduce pulmonary pressures in PPHTN and has been documented to have a survival benefit in pulmonary hypertension.[111] Epoprostenol also has an antiplatelet effect and promotes vascular remodeling. However, it must be administered as a continuous infusion via central access with little tolerance for interruption of the infusion. It has also been associated with splenomegaly and worsening thrombocytopenia, sufficient to limit its use.[112] The phosphodiesterase inhibitor sildenafil has also shown ability to reduce pulmonary pressures at 3 months, but without a sustained response at 12 months.[113] Nonetheless, it may be useful in combination therapy or it may provide a window for transplantation. Bosentan is the best studied of the endothelin antagonists. Although there are concerns for hepatic toxicity, published case reports and case series have not documented significant increases in liver enzymes with its use.[114]

The role of liver transplantation in the treatment of PPHTN is not well defined, because outcomes of transplantation are not predictable. Some patients have resolution of PPHTN with transplant, some may have no or incomplete resolution and continue to require medical therapy, and some may experience worsening of their PPHTN. Nonetheless, it is an option for a select group of patients whose pulmonary hemodynamics and cardiac function suggest they will tolerate the procedure. Evaluation of the patient for potential transplantation must include a right-heart catheterization to measure mPAP and calculate PVR. Patients with mPAP <35 mm Hg can be expected to tolerate transplant and do well postoperatively. Those with mPAP ≥35 mm Hg and elevated PVR may be considered if they respond to therapy sufficiently to reduce their mPAP below 35 mm Hg and PVR below 400 dynes/sec/cm^5.[5,115,116]

Hepatic Encephalopathy

HE is a serious, albeit reversible, neuropsychiatric complication that is a feature of both CLD and acute liver disease. The manifestations range from subtle, subclinical abnormalities that can only be discerned by formal psychometric tests (minimal HE) to clearly evident neurologic and behavioral derangements that are easily diagnosed at the bedside (overt HE). Although HE can appear as the result of portal–systemic shunting without intrinsic liver disease, the onset of HE is generally associated with advanced hepatocellular disease, and its appearance is often accompanied by other phenomena of end-stage liver disease such as ascites, hypoalbuminemia, hyperbilirubinemia, and elevations in INR. HE is an important cause of hospitalization in cirrhosis. In 2003

TABLE 45-9. WEST HAVEN CRITERIA FOR SEMIQUANTATIVE GRADING OF MENTAL STATE

Grade 1	Trivial lack of awareness
	Euphoria or anxiety
	Shortened attention span
	Impaired performance of addition
Grade 2	Lethargy or apathy
	Minimal disorientation for time or place
	Subtle personality change
	Inappropriate behavior
	Impaired performance of subtraction
Grade 3	Somnolence to semistupor, but responsive to verbal stimuli
	Confusion
	Gross disorientation
Grade 4	Coma (unresponsive to verbal or noxious stimuli)

From: Ferenci P, Lockwood A, Mullen K, et al. Hepatic encephalopathy–definition, nomenclature, diagnosis, and quantification: Final report of the working party at the 11th World Congresses of Gastroenterology, Vienna, 1998. *Hepatology.* 2002;35:716.

over 40,000 patients were hospitalized with a primary diagnosis of HE. This number increased to over 50,000 patients in 2004. Moreover, even minimal HE can affect the patient's ability to maintain employment, drive a car, perform quotidian activities, and interact with family. The fact that HE is frequently reversible emphasizes the importance of identifying and treating this condition.

The diagnosis of overt HE encompasses two sets of criteria: Neuropsychologic and neuromotor. Neuropsychologic assessment focuses on level of consciousness, attention and ability to follow commands, and affect. This is most often graded on a 0 to 4 scale using the West Haven criteria (Table 45-9).[117] Physical examination may elicit asterixis or other evidence of hyperreflexiveness such as clonus or Babinski's sign. Other focal findings can include nystagmus or decerebrate posturing. However, focal neurologic findings should prompt appropriate imaging to rule out structural neurologic lesions, since these patients are at risk for intracranial bleeding and are not immune to other neurologic pathologies such as ischemic brain disease, abscess, and tumor.

The Working Party on Hepatic Encephalopathy at the World Congress of Gastroenterology divided HE into categories according to the type of hepatic abnormality on the basis of the underlying disease process. Three types of general underlying etiology are recognized: Association with ALF, association with hepatic bypass physiology without intrinsic liver disease, and association with cirrhosis. Only HE associated with cirrhosis is further described by periodicity and quality (Table 45-10). It is generally agreed that HE is the result of the failure of the liver to adequately metabolize certain substances that when accumulated are neurotoxic, rather than failure to synthesize substances critical to normal neurotransmission. The proposed World Congress definitions support this by recognizing a type of HE that is associated with normal hepatocellular function but shunting of blood around the liver (type B). Historically, HE has been attributed to hyperammonemia resulting from inadequate hepatic metabolism of ammonia. Although ammonia continues to be considered an important contributor, severity of HE does not necessarily correlate with ammonia levels. This may be explained by recent investigations which have provided evidence for a multitude of other factors and mechanisms contributing to HE, including other gut-derived neurotoxins, γ-aminobutyric acid (GABA) and other endogenous GABA receptor agonists, oxidative stress, inflammatory mediators, hyponatremia, and abnormal serotonin and histamine neurotransmission.[118,119] Nonetheless, ammonia and its effect on astrocytes play a central role in the pathogenesis of HE. Ammonia is a by-product of nitrogen-containing compounds that is toxic and must be removed from the body. The liver is the primary site of ammonia metabolism and excretion via the urea cycle, but the brain, skeletal muscle, and possibly kidneys contribute as well. Unfortunately, neither the brain nor the skeletal muscle is capable of utilizing the urea cycle and instead use glutamine synthetase to synthesize glutamine from ammonia and glutamate. Astrocytes are major constituents of the blood–brain barrier and are the primary location for glutamine synthetase in

TABLE 45-10. PROPOSED NOMENCLATURE OF HEPATIC ENCEPHALOPATHY

HE Type	Nomenclature	Subcategory	Subdivisions
A	Encephalopathy associated with acute liver failure		
B	Encephalopathy associated with portal–systemic bypass and no intrinsic hepatocellular disease		
C	Encephalopathy associated with cirrhosis and portal hypertension/or portal–systemic shunts	Episodic HE	Precipitated
			Spontaneous[a]
			Recurrent
		Persistent HE	Mild
			Severe
			Treatment-dependent
		Minimal HE	

For definitions, see text.
[a]Without recognized precipitating factors.
From: Ferenci P, Lockwood A, Mullen K, et al. Hepatic encephalopathy–definition, nomenclature, diagnosis, and quantification: Final report of the working party at the 11th World Congresses of Gastroenterology, Vienna, 1998. *Hepatology.* 2002;35:716.

the brain. Since these are the cells capable of metabolizing ammonia, as ammonia levels rise intracellular levels of glutamine rise in concert. There are two consequences to this: (1) glutamine, which is osmotically active, pulls water intracellularly as well, causing astrocyte swelling and cerebral edema; and (2) glutamate, which is an important excitatory neurotransmitter, is first released and then consumed in producing glutamine. Experimental in vitro evidence has demonstrated glutamate release from astrocytes in response to elevated levels of ammonia.[120] It is thought that this release may be related to the neuroexcitatory signs such as agitation and seizures observed in acute HE (type A). On the other hand, a neuroinhibitory state is characteristic of the HE associated with cirrhosis (type C) and may reflect chronic adaptive changes that include downregulation of glutamate receptors and inactivation of astrocyte glutamate transporters.[120]

In addition to the decrease in glutamate activity the neuroinhibitory state observed in cirrhotic HE (type C) may also be the result of an increase in GABAergic tone. GABA is a major inhibitory neurotransmitter whose receptor complex can be activated by benzodiazepines and inhibited by flumazenil. On the basis of improvements in mental status following flumazenil administration in patients who had not received benzodiazepines, it was proposed that the production of endogenous benzodiazepine-like substances contributed to HE. Subsequent studies of plasma and CSF from HE patients were reported to demonstrate increased benzodiazepine-like substances as measured by radioreceptor assays.[121,122] Unfortunately, the benefits of flumazenil appear to be limited by its short duration of action and lack of demonstrable survival or recovery advantage.[123,124]

Inflammation and stress-induced production of ROS and reactive nitrogen species (RNOS) have also been implicated in contributing to HE. Sepsis is a well-known precipitating factor for HE. Inflammatory mediators such as TNF-α, and cytokines IL-1 and IL-6 cause cytotoxic compromise of the blood–brain barrier, leading to or worsening cerebral edema. Astrocyte swelling is a trigger for production of ROS and RNOS, which can mediate local cell membrane damage and cause further blood–brain barrier permeability.[125]

The initial step in evaluating the patient with liver disease who presents with encephalopathy is to rule out causes other than HE. The differential diagnosis includes other metabolic encephalopathies such as uremia, sepsis, glucose and electrolyte abnormalities, and endocrinopathies. Structural and vascular CNS lesions or CNS infections should also be considered. Because cirrhotic patients are exquisitely sensitive to sedative medications and have impaired hepatic (and often renal) metabolism, careful search for possible drug-related encephalopathy should be undertaken. Once other potential causes have been eliminated, the next step should be a systematic search for an underlying cause or precipitating factor (Table 45-11). Once identified, treatment or elimination should commence as soon as possible and may be sufficient for clinical improvement.

If addressing the underlying cause does not produce improvement, the next step is to employ therapy designed to either reduce the production of or increase the excretion of ammonia. Historically, the nonabsorbable disaccharide lactulose has been the mainstay of therapy and remains the first-line drug for treating HE.[126] Although the basis for its benefit is unclear there are two proposed mechanisms for its salutary effect. First, anaerobic bacteria in the colon ferment lactulose to produce weak acids and acidify the colon. This acid milieu converts ammonia into ammonium, which is poorly absorbed. Secondly, it is proposed that this acid milieu is also cathartic, and that catharsis augments reduced absorption.

Nonabsorbable antibiotics such as neomycin, metronidazole, and rifaximin are an alternative to lactulose and work by inhibiting colonic growth of ammoniagenic bacteria. Nonabsorbable antibiotics appear to be no less effective than nonabsorbable disaccharides, but concerns about toxicity associated with long-term administration limit their use. They are, however, generally better tolerated than the nonabsorbable disaccharides, which produce flatulence, frequent bowel movements, and abdominal cramping.[126–128]

TABLE 45-11. PRECIPITATING FACTORS IN HEPATIC ENCEPHALOPATHY

Constipation
Dehydration
Gastrointestinal bleeding
Bowel obstruction or ileus
Infection—esp. spontaneous bacterial peritonitis, sepsis
Excessive dietary protein
Hypokalemia
Hypoglycemia
Hypothyroidism
Hypoxia
Metabolic alkalosis
Anemia
Azotemia/uremia
Hepatic malignancy
TIPS, surgical shunt
Vascular occlusion

Although simple reduction in protein intake seems an intuitive solution, in fact protein restriction may be harmful for cirrhotic patients who tend to have little nutritional reserve due to poor intake and who have likely lost nutritional ground with every hospitalization. Practice guidelines for the treatment of HE patients recommend a normal protein intake (1 to 1.5 g/kg/day), preferably in the form of plant-based rather than animal protein because of its higher calorie to nitrogen ratio.[126]

Zinc is a cofactor in the urea cycle and may be a dietary deficiency in cirrhotic patients. Although it is unclear which patients might benefit, practice guidelines recommend consideration of chronic zinc supplementation to HE patients.

Ascites

Ascites is the most common complication of cirrhosis leading to hospitalization.[129] The occurrence of ascites marks a threshold in the nature of the underlying liver disease and is associated with a 50% mortality rate within 3 years.[130] Thus, the current recommendation is that patients who present with ascites and who are potentially candidates for liver transplantation should be referred for liver transplantation evaluation. Not all ascites is hepatic in nature; about 15% has a nonhepatic etiology. Nonhepatic causes include malignancy, cardiac failure, renal disease, pancreatitis, and tuberculosis. Perhaps the most expeditious study to define the nature of new-onset ascites is a paracentesis. Unless there is reason to suspect a particular diagnosis, routine screening studies of ascitic fluid should include a cell count and differential, and albumin and total protein levels. In particular the serum–ascites albumin gradient (SAAG) is extremely useful for delineating portal hypertensive ascites from other causes. It is calculated as the difference between simultaneously measured serum and ascites albumin levels. A SAAG $\geq$1.1 mg/dL indicates portal hypertension with 97%

accuracy.[131] Standard initial therapy for portal hypertensive ascites is salt restriction (2 g/day) and diuretics. If the underlying cause for liver disease is amenable to treatment, such as cessation of alcohol or antiviral treatment of a chronic hepatitis, such therapy should be pursued as well. Hyponatremia is common among cirrhotic patients with ascites and generally does not warrant fluid restriction unless the serum sodium level is below 120 to 125 mEq/L.[129] Rapid correction of hyponatremia is undesirable because cirrhotic patients are particularly at risk for central pontine myelinolysis, a potentially devastating neurologic complication. Observations in liver transplant recipients suggest limiting correction to ≤16 mEq/L over an 8-day period.[132]

Refractory ascites, defined as ascites that is immutable to sodium restriction, maximum doses of diuretics, and paracentesis, heralds another change in the nature of the underlying cirrhosis. It is the hallmark complication of type II HRS and indicates increased disease severity. Once patients become refractory to maximum standard medical therapy the 6-month mortality is 21%.[133] Therapeutic options for patients are limited and include serial paracentesis, liver transplantation, TIPS placement, and peritoneovenous shunt.

Although current practice is to replace albumin when ascitic fluid is drained, this practice is not well supported by randomized prospective trials. The reasons for using albumin replacement include preventing paracentesis-induced circulatory dysfunction, minimizing electrolyte disturbances, minimizing the nutritional impact of albumin loss, and preventing renal impairment. Studies have been hampered by heterogenous study populations, differences in albumin dose, and heterogeneity of end points. Nonetheless, current recommendations are that patients with drainage volumes <5 L do not need albumin replacement, and for larger volume paracentesis 6 to 8 g albumin/L may be considered.[129] TIPS placement can generally be expected to improve quality of life by obviating the need for serial paracentesis, but this must be balanced against an increase in encephalopathy and the high incidence of shunt malfunction.[134,135] Peritoneovenous shunting is an older intervention that has generally fallen into disuse because of associated complications and lack of survival benefit. However, for patients who cannot easily travel for serial paracentesis and who are not candidates for TIPS or transplantation, this may be the only option.

Infections of ascitic fluid are sufficiently common that the American Association for the Study of Liver Diseases recommends paracentesis for all hospitalized patients with ascites. SBP is diagnosed when the PMN count in ascitic fluid is ≥250 cells/mm^3 in the absence of any other identifiable intra-abdominal source. Bacterial translocation from the bowel is the most common source of SBP, although nosocomial infection from bacteremia associated with invasive procedures occurs as well. This bacterial translocation occurs via the mesenteric lymphatic system and is aided by changes in bowel flora, increased intestinal permeability, and impaired local immunity.

Because cell counts are available more quickly than culture results, the decision to treat is made empirically on that basis. Typical causative floras are *Escherichia coli, Klebsiella pneumonia*, and pneumococcus. Patients should immediately be treated with a broad-spectrum antibiotic such as cefotaxime, which covers 95% of floras.[136] In the case of nosocomial SBP or in the patient who has recently received or is currently receiving antibiotics at the time of diagnosis it is suggested that a carbapenem be considered because of the risk of multiresistant infection.[137] Sepsis may develop rapidly in these patients and SBP is a recognized precipitating factor for type I HRS. Because of this, timely administration of antibiotics in this fragile population is so important that empiric antibiotics are warranted even for patients who do not meet the diagnostic ascitic fluid PMN cell count but who exhibit signs and symptoms suggesting infection such as fever, abdominal pain, evidence of worsening hepatic or renal function, and otherwise unexplained worsening encephalopathy.[129]

Risk factors for development of SBP include a prior episode of SBP, gastrointestinal bleeding, and an ascites albumin level of <1.5 g/dL. Long-term antibiotic prophylaxis with norfloxacin or trimethoprim/sulfamethoxazole for SBP is recommended for patients who have survived an episode of SBP or who have an ascites albumin level of <1.5 g/dL and at least one of the following: Serum creatinine ≥1.2 mg/dL, blood urea nitrogen ≥25 mg/dL, serum sodium ≤130 mEq/L, or a Child–Pugh score ≥9 mg/dL with a bilirubin ≥3 mg/dL. Short-term antibiotic therapy with a third-generation cephalosporin is indicated for patients with ascites and gastrointestinal bleeding.[129]

Varices

Varices, particularly esophageal varices, are one of the end results of portal hypertension. In cirrhosis, increases in portal pressure result from distorted hepatic architecture left in the wake of inflammatory insults. Fibrosis and regenerative nodules cause impedance to splanchnic flow through the liver and lead to formation of portosystemic collaterals, particularly with the gastric and esophageal venous systems. Progression of portal hypertension leads to increased local production of nitric oxide and, eventually, massive splanchnic vasodilation. Thus portal hypertension becomes a problem not only of impedance to flow, but also of a massive increase in flow to the liver. Rupture of the high-pressure collaterals that are formed is a highly lethal and feared complication of portal hypertension.

Portal hypertension is diagnosed by measurement of the wedged hepatic venous pressure (WHVP). Although this is not a direct measure of portal pressure WHVP has been demonstrated to correlate well with it.[138] This is done by advancement of a catheter into a hepatic vein to wedge position. To correct for the contribution of increased intra-abdominal pressure from ascites, a free hepatic venous pressure or an inferior vena caval pressure should be subtracted from the measured WHVP to give the HVPG. A normal HVPG is 3 to 5 mm Hg. Patients with esophageal varices can be expected to have HVPGs of at least 10 to 12 mm Hg.[139,140]

Esophagogastroduodenoscopy is the gold-standard procedure for diagnosing varices. Presence of varices correlates with the severity of the underlying liver disease, with incidence increasing from 40% in Child's A patients to 85% in Child's C patients.[141] Varices are graded by size, with small varices being ≤5 mm and large varices being >5 mm. Also noted are the presence of red wale marks, which are whip-shaped longitudinal dilated venules. Risk for variceal bleeding correlates with the size of varices, presence of red wale marks, and variceal pressure (HVPG). Therapeutic decisions are made on the basis of these observations and measurements.

Nonselective β-blockers reduce portal pressure by two mechanisms: A decrease in cardiac output (β-1) and splanchnic vasoconstriction (β-2). There is no evidence that they prevent formation of varices; however, they are effective as primary prophylaxis for variceal bleeding in patients with large varices and those with small varices with additional risk factors such as red wale marks or Child's B or C class. For those patients who cannot tolerate β-blockers or in whom they are contraindicated, another option for primary prophylaxis of variceal bleeding is endoscopic ligation. TIPS is associated with a higher incidence of encephalopathy and higher mortality and is not indicated for primary prophylaxis.[141]

Acute variceal bleed should be managed with a combination of volume resuscitation, correction of severe coagulopathy, pharmacologic manipulation of portal pressure, and endoscopic variceal ligation. Although the temptation to vigorously volume resuscitate and completely correct all coagulation abnormalities can be overwhelming in this setting, it should be resisted. Since bleeding is, to some extent, a pressure-related phenomenon aggressive volume replacement may lead to resistant or recurrent bleeding.[142,143] The goal instead should be adequate resuscitation to maintain a hemoglobin level of 8 mg/dL and consideration of blood product transfusion to improve significant abnormalities in platelet count and INR.[141] Elective intubation for airway protection is often warranted in these patients as well. Medications to reduce portal pressure include vasopressin and its analogs and somatostatin and its analogs. Although β-blockers can reduce portal pressures, their effect on systemic pressures makes them undesirable in this setting. Early endoscopic variceal ligation in combination with pharmacotherapy is the preferred treatment for acute variceal bleed.

Resistant or early recurrent variceal bleeding occurs in about 10% to 20% of patients. A measured HVPG >20 mm Hg is a risk factor for failure of standard therapy, predicting greater length of ICU stay as well as greater transfusion requirements.[144] Balloon tamponade can be effective in this setting, but is associated with significant and potentially lethal complications such as esophageal rupture or necrosis and perforation, migration of the balloon components, and aspiration. If employed, it is recommended as a bridge to more definitive therapy such as surgical shunt or TIPS.[141]

CHRONIC CHOLESTATIC DISEASE

Biliary obstruction increases pressures in the bile ducts, leading to reflux of bile into the liver sinusoids where it may also communicate with the vascular system. Serum levels of bilirubin, bile salts, and AP (which is synthesized by the biliary epithelium) rise. If bacteria are present in bile, the patient is at risk for infectious complications such as ascending cholangitis, hepatic abscess, and sepsis as well. Cholestasis and hyperbilirubinemia are associated with an increased incidence of acute kidney injury. This may be mediated by endotoxemia, as the result of both sepsis and loss of bile salts to the vascular space. Bile salts are normally secreted into the intestine where they prevent bacterial overgrowth and bind endotoxin, thereby preventing its absorption into the portal circulation. Loss of intestinal bile salts because of biliary obstruction may cause portal and systemic endotoxemia, leading to kidney injury. Kidney injury may additionally be exacerbated by the induced diuresis, as well as impairment of myocardial contractility, resulting from elevated serum levels of bile salts.[145,146] It has also been noted that patients who come to transplant for the chronic cholestatic diseases, PBC and primary sclerosing cholangitis (PSC), have evidence of preserved or hypercoagulability on the basis of increased incidence of portal venous thrombosis, elevated levels of TAT complexes, and thromboelastographic indices consistent with hypercoagulability.[147,148]

Chronic cholestatic disease in the adult population is primarily the result of immunologic mechanisms resulting in PBC or PSC. These diseases are frequently associated with other autoimmune pathology.

PBC is a disease characterized by the progressive destruction of small intrahepatic bile ducts, together with portal inflammation that eventually leads to cirrhosis. The preponderance of PBC patients are middle-aged females, and the disease affects women and men in a 9:1 ratio. Typically, patients are asymptomatic on presentation, but may have symptoms of fatigue, right-upper quadrant abdominal pain, or pruritus. Jaundice on presentation is uncommon, and evidence of portal hypertension (i.e., progression to cirrhosis) even more so. The laboratory hallmark of PBC is the antimitochondrial antibody, which is present in 95% of patients. Liver biopsy confirms diagnosis, as well as providing histologic disease staging. The disease may follow one of three courses. The typical course is one of steady progressive loss of small bile ducts together with increasing fibrosis, leading to cirrhosis over the course of 10 to 20 years. A second form is characterized by a fluctuating course, punctuated by flares of disease resembling autoimmune hepatitis and leading to earlier liver failure. The third form, labeled the premature ductopenia variant, is marked by rapid disappearance of bile ducts with severe cholestasis and appearance of cirrhosis within 5 years. Ursodeoxycholic acid, which may have immunomodulatory effects, is the only drug demonstrated to retard progression of the disease and offer survival benefit. Liver transplantation is the most definitive therapy, but is associated with a recurrence rate of 10% to 35%.[149]

PSC is a progressive inflammatory disease of the medium and large intra and extrahepatic bile ducts. Like PBC it is often diagnosed in an asymptomatic patient who has liver biochemistries drawn for some other purpose. PSC is a disease of young men, with an M:F ratio of 7:3. Serum AP levels are elevated at presentation, and bilirubin may occasionally be elevated as well. The diagnostic studies of choice are ERCP and magnetic resonance cholangiopancreatography (MRCP), which reveal the characteristic beaded pattern of the biliary tree caused by multiple stenotic lesions. PSC has an extremely high association with inflammatory bowel disease (IBD), primarily ulcerative colitis but occasionally Crohn's disease. It is also associated with other autoimmune disease, such as insulin-dependent diabetes and psoriasis. Other contributors to the morbidity of PSC are recurrent bacterial cholangitis, cholangiocarcinoma, and, particularly in those patients with coexisting IBD, colon carcinoma. Over the average 15-year disease course of PSC, 15% to 30% of patients are likely to develop cholangiocarcinoma, which carries a very poor prognosis and may cause ineligibility for transplant.[150] Liver transplantation is the most definitive therapy for PSC, but is associated with disease recurrence.

CHRONIC HEPATOCELLULAR DISEASE

CLD is a major public health burden in the United States, with an increase in prevalence from 11.78% in the period 1988 to 1994 to 14.78% in the period 2005 to 2008. Chronic viral hepatitis, particularly hepatitis C, has historically been the most common cause of CLD, but recent data show that NAFLD has overtaken chronic hepatitis for this distinction. In the period 2005 to 2008, the prevalence of the most common causes of CLD was hepatitis B 0.34%, hepatitis C 1.68%, alcoholic liver disease 2.05%, and NAFLD 11.01%.[11] During this period the incidence of new cases of hepatitis B and C have decreased steadily, likely the result of improved blood product screening, development and wide dissemination of vaccination, and the institution of universal precautions.[151] The stable prevalence despite the decrease in new cases may reflect the survival benefit of antiviral medications and transplantation, in addition to the historically long, indolent, and frequently unrecognized course of chronic hepatitis C. Although chronic hepatitis C is still the leading cause of liver transplantation and is implicated in the increase in cases of HCC, the rise in prevalence of NAFLD together with the recognition that it can progress to cirrhosis and is a risk factor for HCC suggests that it is poised to become the next hepatic scourge.

HEPATOCELLULAR CARCINOMA

Worldwide, HCC is the third leading cause of cancer-related death. Within the United States, it is the fifth most common cancer in men and the seventh in women.[152] Risk factors include chronic viral hepatitis infection, hemochromatosis, and cirrhosis of any provenance. The prevalence of underlying cirrhosis in patients with HCC is 80% to 90%. Even if the HCC patient does not have cirrhosis, there is almost always an underlying chronic hepatitis/chronic necro-inflammatory state that seems to be key ingredient for HCC. Among patients with chronic viral hepatitis, the presence of cirrhosis or evidence of active inflammation (characterized by elevations in serum ALT) leads to increased HCC occurrence compared to patients without cirrhosis or those with persistently normal to near-normal ALT.[153] The 5-year cumulative incidence of HCC is highest for patients with chronic hepatitis C (17% in Europe and the United States, 30% in Japan) and hemochromatosis (21%). The 5-year incidence of HCC in chronic hepatitis B patients also shows geographic variation, with an incidence of 15% in areas with endemic infection and 10% in nonendemic areas.[154] This may reflect environmental influences or differences in timing and age at infection. The American Association for the Study of Liver Diseases recommends surveillance of at-risk patients. Ideally this should be in the form of liver ultrasonography every 6 months, with the use of α-fetoprotein only if ultrasound is not available.[155] α-fetoprotein lacks adequate sensitivity and specificity to be an effective screening tool, but may be valuable in diagnosis because a level >200 ng/mL in a cirrhotic patient with a hepatic mass has a high positive predictive value for HCC.[156] Diagnosis of HCC can often be made with noninvasive studies, with biopsy reserved for lesions with atypical or discordant imaging. Lesions <1 cm in diameter are followed up with repeat ultrasound. Lesions 1 to 2 cm in diameter should be studied using two different dynamic techniques, either CT, contrast ultrasonography, or MRI with contrast. Both techniques should demonstrate typical findings of the hypervascular HCC tumor, early arterial enhancement, and washout in the portal/venous phase. If they are not concordant, biopsy of the lesion is recommended. A larger lesion (>2 cm) with this typical pattern on a single dynamic study or associated with an α-fetoprotein level >200 ng/mL confirms the diagnosis of HCC.[156]

Surgical resection is the optimal treatment for HCC for those patients who have sufficient hepatic reserve. Unfortunately many patients with HCC have cirrhosis and are unable to tolerate resection. In the United States fewer than 5% of patients are candidates for resection.[152] Liver transplantation can be an option for those patients who are not resection candidates but whose disease can be expected to have transplant outcomes similar to that of other indications for transplant. The Milan criteria (one tumor <5 cm or three tumors all <3 cm) define those patients, and those patients who meet the criteria and are transplanted have 5-year survival rates of 65% to 78% compared to 5-year survival of 68% to 87% for nontumor indications.[157]

Patients who are neither surgical candidates nor transplant candidates may be managed by radiofrequency ablation or chemoembolization of their tumors. In addition, some centers use these therapies to maintain transplant eligibility for patients on the waiting list.

NONALCOHOLIC FATTY LIVER DISEASE

NAFLD describes a range of conditions characterized by excessive fat deposition in the liver. NAFLD ranges in severity from simple fat deposition (steatosis) to fat deposition together with inflammation and hepatocellular necrosis (steatohepatitis or NASH). Primary NAFLD is associated with insulin resistance and its attendant manifestations, which are components of the metabolic syndrome: Obesity, central adiposity, type II diabetes, arterial hypertension, and hypertriglyceridemia. In fact it is often referred to as the hepatic manifestation of the metabolic syndrome. The prevalence of NAFLD increases with age, is greater in males, and differs by ethnicity. In the United States, the prevalence of NAFLD is 45% in Hispanics, 33% in Caucasians, and 24% in African-Americans,[158] with an estimated overall prevalence of 30%. Unsurprisingly, NAFLD is the most common cause of elevated liver enzymes in adults.[159] NAFLD may coexist with other hepatic pathologies and exacerbates damage when it appears together with chronic hepatitis C, hemochromatosis, or alcoholic liver disease.[160] Within the disease spectrum of NAFLD, only NASH is associated with the serious consequences of HCC and cirrhosis. The gold standard for distinguishing NASH from other NAFLD is liver biopsy with the key features of macrovesicular steatosis, lobular inflammation, hepatocyte ballooning, and often perisinusoidal fibrosis. The prevalence of NASH in the United States is estimated to be 3% to 5%.[159] There is evidence, although from small studies and with different end points, that lifestyle modifications that improve insulin sensitivity such as weight loss and exercise can reduce intrahepatic lipid content in NASH.[161] Medications that may augment weight loss, such as orlistat and rimonabant, have been shown to result in histologic improvement in NASH when associated with actual weight loss. For those patients who are unable to lose weight by more conservative means, bariatric surgery has been shown to result in dramatic histologic and chemical improvement, with decreased steatosis/inflammation on biopsy and decreases in serum aminotransferases. In a meta-analysis of morbidly obese patients who underwent bariatric surgery, the pooled patient incidence of biopsy-proven NASH was 53.87%. Of these patients 81.3% showed improvement or resolution of steatohepatitis on follow-up biopsy, with 69.5% showing complete resolution.[162]

PREOPERATIVE MANAGEMENT

Hepatic Evaluation

The evaluation of hepatic function begins with a thorough history, starting with an inquiry into risk factors and the presence of symptoms attributable to CLD. Prior episodes of jaundice, particularly in relationship to surgical procedures and anesthesia, should be thoroughly investigated. Alcohol consumption, use of recreational or illicit drugs, medications (including herbal products), presence of tattoos, sexual promiscuity, consumption of raw seafood, and a history of travel to areas in which hepatitis is endemic should be sought. Symptoms of fatigue, anorexia, weight loss, nausea, vomiting, easy bruising, pruritus, dark-colored urine, biliary colic, abdominal distention, and gastrointestinal bleeding warrant further investigation for the presence of liver disease.

Physical examination findings suggestive of active liver disease include icterus, palmar erythema, spider angiomas, gynecomastia, hepatosplenomegaly, ascites, testicular atrophy, petechiae, ecchymoses, and asterixis.

In the absence of findings suggestive of liver disease, routine laboratory tests to assess hepatocellular integrity and hepatic synthetic function are not warranted. Routine laboratory testing may yield false-positive results, and true-positive results are infrequent in asymptomatic patients. Among over 19,000 Air Force trainees, 0.5% had liver-enzyme elevations; however, the cause was found in only 12 of the 99 with elevations.[163] In a study of over 7,600 surgical patients who underwent routine preoperative screening, liver-enzyme tests were abnormal in roughly 1 of 700 (0.1%) asymptomatic patients. Of the 11 patients with elevations, 3 (1 in 2,500 or 0.04%) developed jaundice.[164]

Because the normal range for laboratory test is defined as the mean plus or minus two standard deviations, 5% of normal patients can be expected to fall outside the normal range, with 2.5% following above the upper limit of normal. As a result, minor elevations of liver-enzyme results—those less than twice the normal value—may be of no clinical importance.[165] The recommended approach is to avoid testing liver enzymes in asymptomatic patients. Nonetheless, in the presence of abnormal results (in an asymptomatic patient) the safest approach is to repeat the results; and in the absence of elevations greater than twice the upper limits of normal it is reasonable to proceed with surgery.

In patients with more substantial elevations of liver enzymes, causes include alcohol abuse, medications, chronic hepatitis B and C, NASH, autoimmune hepatitis, hemochromatosis, Wilson's disease, and α-1 antitrypsin deficiency. Nonhepatic causes include celiac sprue and muscle diseases. Medications include selected antibiotics, antiepileptic drugs, lipid lowering agents, nonsteroidal anti-inflammatory agents, and sulfonylureas. Herbal medications and drugs of abuse are also associated with liver-enzyme abnormalities (Table 45-12).

TABLE 45-12. MEDICATIONS, HERBS, AND DRUGS OR SUBSTANCES OF ABUSE REPORTED TO CAUSE ELEVATIONS IN LIVER-ENZYME LEVELS

Medications
- Antibiotics
  - Synthetic penicillins
  - Ciprofloxacin
  - Nitrofurantoin
  - Ketoconazole and fluconazole
  - Isoniazid
- Antiepileptic drugs
  - Phenytoin
  - Carbamazepine
- Inhibitors of hydroxymethylglutaryl-coenzyme A reductase
  - Simvastatin
  - Pravastatin
  - Lovastatin
  - Atorvastatin
- Nonsteroidal anti-inflammatory drugs
- Sulfonylureas for hyperglycemia
  - Glipizide

Herbs and homeopathic treatments
- Chaparral
- Chinese herbs
  - jin bu huan
  - Ephedra (ma huang)
- Gentian
- Germander
- Alchemilla (lady's mantle)
- Senna
- Shark cartilage
- Scutellaria (skullcap)

Drugs and substances of abuse
- Anabolic steroids
- Cocaine
- 5-Methoxy-3,4-methylenedioxymethamphetamine (MDMA, "ecstasy")
- Phencyclidine ("angel dust")
- Glues and solvents
  - Glues containing toluene
  - Trichloroethylene, chloroform

From: Pratt DS, Kaplan MM. Primary care: Evaluation of abnormal liver-enzyme results in asymptomatic patients. *N Engl J Med.* 2000;342:1266.

Perioperative Risk Associated with Liver Disease

In patients with known liver disease, the etiology of hepatic dysfunction should be determined. Based on retrospective, small case series from the 1960s and 1970s, acute hepatitis confers a prohibitive risk for elective surgery. In a series of 36 patients with undiagnosed hepatitis who underwent laparotomy (for suspected biliary obstruction or hepatic malignancy) nearly one-third died. All patients with acute hepatitis, due to either virus or alcohol, died. The majority of patients suffered complications that included bacterial peritonitis, wound dehiscence, and hepatic failure.[166]

With improved diagnostic testing, which includes serologic testing for hepatitis C, ultrasound testing for gallstones, and improved imaging techniques for hepatic cancer, it is far more likely today that accurate diagnoses can be made preoperatively. As a result laparotomies are unlikely in patients with unsuspected hepatitis. In the absence of accumulating evidence, consensus opinion is that elective surgery should be postponed in patients with acute hepatitis.[167,168]

In patients with CLD it is not feasible to postpone surgery until recovery. A number of studies have investigated the risk of surgery in patients with cirrhosis.[169–172] Each of the studies identified various components of the Child–Turcotte–Pugh score, as well as the composite score, as important prognostic factors for perioperative mortality.

Child and Turcotte first described their classification system in 1964. They identified five factors—albumin, bilirubin, ascites, encephalopathy, and nutritional status—as important prognostic factors for patients with cirrhosis. Each of the factors was categorized according to three levels of severity and combined to generate a composite score leading to an assignment of one of three classes of severity (class A, B, or C, with C representing the most severe hepatic dysfunction). In 1972 Pugh modified the score, replacing nutritional status with PT (Table 45-13). The score was originally designed for patients undergoing portosystemic shunt procedures, but has subsequently been applied to patients with cirrhosis undergoing other surgeries. In two studies, conducted

TABLE 45-13. MODIFIED CHILD–PUGH SCORE

Presentation	Points[a] 1	2	3
Albumin (g/dL)	>3.5	2.8–3.5	<2.8
Prothrombin time			
Seconds prolonged	<4	4–6	>6
International normalized ratio	<1.7	1.7–2.3	>2.3
Bilirubin (mg/dL)[b]	<2	2–3	>3
Ascites	Absent	Slight–moderate	Tense
Encephalopathy	None	Grade I–II	Grade III–IV

[a]Class A = 5 to 6 points; B = 7 to 9 points; C = 10 to 15 points.
[b]Cholestatic diseases (e.g., primary biliary cirrhosis) produce bilirubin elevations that are disproportionate to the hepatic dysfunction. Thus, the following adjustments should be made: Assign 1 point for a bilirubin level of 4 mg/dL; 2 points for bilirubin concentrations between 4 and 10 mg/dL; and 3 points for bilirubin >10 mg/dL.
From: Kamath PS. Clinical approach to the patient with abnormal liver rest results. *Mayo Clin Proc.* 1996;71:1089, with permission.

over a decade apart, the modified Child score performed similarly in predicting perioperative mortality.[171,172] Child's class A was associated with 10%, Child's B with 30%, and Child's C with greater than 80% mortality. The 3-month mortality for hospitalized patients not undergoing surgery was 4% for class A, 14% for class B, and 51% for class C.[172]

The MELD score was originally designed to predict mortality for patients undergoing transjugular intrahepatic portocaval shunt (TIPS) procedures.[173] Subsequently it was identified as an improvement to the Child score for the allocation of organs for liver transplant candidates due to its replacement of the subjective elements of the Child score (ascites, encephalopathy) with more objective ones, INR and creatinine. The MELD score is a useful predictor of 90-day wait list mortality in liver transplant candidates.[174] The MELD score weighs the continuous variables linearly or logarithmically instead of assigning arbitrary categories, as is the case with the Child score:

$$\text{MELD score} = 9.57 \times \log_e(\text{creatinine mg/dL}) + 3.78 \times \log_e(\text{bilirubin mg/dL}) + 11.2 \times \log_e(\text{INR}) + 6.43$$

5 The MELD score appears to predict perioperative mortality of cirrhotic patients as well or better than the Child score.[175] In a single-center study of 140 surgical procedures, the *c*-statistic for the MELD score's ability to predict 30-day mortality was 0.72. A *c*-statistic of 0.5 indicates predictive ability similar to chance (a 50:50 likelihood of predicting the outcome), while a *c*-statistic of 0.7 and higher is considered useful. In the cohort of patients undergoing abdominal surgery, the *c*-statistic improved to 0.80. In this study a MELD score between 25 and 30 was associated with a 30-day mortality of 50% after abdominal surgery.[176] Each point in the MELD score up to a score of 20 equated to an additional 1% mortality; each MELD point over 20 equated to an additional 2% mortality. A larger study of 772 cirrhotics found similar results. In this study, 75% of the patients underwent abdominal surgery. A MELD score of 25 was associated with 30-day mortality of 50%. Other than the MELD score, the other important predictors of perioperative mortality in cirrhotics were age (age >70 equated to 3 MELD points) and coexisting disease (ASA physical status > IV equated to 5 MELD points).[175] The perioperative complications encountered by cirrhotic patients include liver failure, postoperative bleeding, infection, and renal failure. These authors concluded that patients with a MELD score of less than 11 have a low postoperative mortality and represent an acceptable surgical risk. However, based on the list of complications, the authors recommend that these patients should preferably have surgery at institutions with a liver transplant center. In patients with a MELD score of 20 or higher, the high mortality risk contraindicates elective procedures until after liver transplantation.[175]

Despite the fact that the MELD score is harder to calculate at the bedside, it may one day replace the Child score for predicting nontransplant surgical mortality in patients with end-stage liver disease. In one study that compared the two scoring systems, the MELD score outperformed the Child score.[175] The study authors noted that the MELD score has a wide range and stratifies risk along a continuum rather than into arbitrary categories, as the Child score does.

6 Medical management undertaken to optimize cirrhotic patients undergoing surgery should be directed toward treating active infection, minimizing vasoactive infusions, optimizing central blood volume and renal status while minimizing ascites, and improving encephalopathy and coagulopathy. However, there is little evidence to support specific goal-directed targets for preoperative care. The perioperative risk depends more on the operative site and the degree of liver impairment than the anesthetic technique. Upper abdominal surgery (cholecystectomy), when compared to hysterectomy, was associated with liver-enzyme abnormalities, while the anesthetic technique (halothane, enflurane, or fentanyl) was not.[177] In a retrospective study of 733 cirrhotic patients mortality was associated with a number of factors in addition to the Child score: Male gender, the presence of ascites, cryptogenic cirrhosis (vs. other etiologies), elevated creatinine, preoperative infection, higher ASA physical status, and surgery on the respiratory system.[178] The presence of each additional factor conferred additional risk. For instance, 1-year mortality in patients with 6 risk factors was over 80%; mortality with 2 risk factors was approximately 30%.

In addition to optimizing medical management, efforts should be made to minimize surgical risk through the consideration of less invasive surgery. Gallstones are twice as common in cirrhotic patients as in patients without cirrhosis.[169] Laparoscopic surgery appears safe in patients with Child–Pugh A and B cirrhosis. In uncontrolled retrospective studies the advantages included low mortality and shorter hospital stay.[179,180] However, Child's C patients may benefit from percutaneous drainage of the gallbladder rather than a laparoscopic approach.[180]

In a series of over 4,200 laparoscopic cholecystectomies from Taiwan, the group with cirrhosis (n = 226) had a mortality of approximately 1:100, while mortality was 1:2,000 for those without cirrhosis.[181] A meta-analysis that included 400 patients with cirrhosis showed the laparoscopic approach was associated with less blood loss, shorter operative time, and shorter hospitalization compared to an open approach.[182] Preoperative decompression of portal hypertension by TIPS may improve outcomes in patients with severe portal hypertension.[183] However, TIPS is associated with increases in pulmonary artery pressure and can worsen encephalopathy.[92,184]

INTRAOPERATIVE MANAGEMENT

Monitoring and Vascular Access

In addition to routine noninvasive monitors, the need for arterial pressure monitoring should be considered for patients with end-stage liver disease. The decision is based on the presence of preoperative systemic hypotension due to vasodilatation, anticipated blood loss, the need for intraoperative laboratory studies, coexisting disease, and age. Arterial cannulation should be considered in patients undergoing liver resection. The usefulness of CVP monitoring to predict fluid responsiveness has been questioned.[185] Some experts have abandoned CVP monitoring in the setting of liver resection.[186–188] In our practice we do not place a CVP catheter exclusively for monitoring. Pulmonary artery catheterization is used for patients with known or suspected pulmonary artery hypertension and for patients with a low cardiac ejection fraction. Transesophageal echocardiography (TEE) is a sensitive monitor for the assessment of preload, contractility, ejection fraction, regional wall motion abnormalities, and emboli. In a small series of patients with esophageal varices, TEE universally aided in diagnosis and was not associated with bleeding complications. Transgastric views were avoided to minimize esophageal manipulation.[189] TEG, if available, may be a useful guide for coagulation management.[190]

Selection of Anesthetic Technique

Neuraxial versus GA

The effect of neuraxial anesthesia on hepatic blood flow appears related to alterations of systemic blood pressure.[191,192] More recent studies support the conclusion that hepatic blood flow is reduced by epidural anesthesia, and interestingly, further reduced by an infusion of norepinephrine.[193] However, other studies suggest that vasopressors (ephedrine and dopamine) restore hepatic blood flow.[194,195] Other data conflict with this, suggesting that dopamine does not improve splanchnic blood flow.[196] Despite this confusing picture high (T-5) neuraxial blocks appear to reduce hepatic blood flow, and this effect may not be reversed when block-related hypotension is corrected with catecholamines. Thus, avoidance of high neuraxial block and hypotension seems prudent in patients with advanced liver disease.

Standard contraindications to neuraxial blockade should be considered and weighed against the procedure's benefits on a case-by-case basis. Many patients with advanced hepatic disease may not warrant consideration for neuraxial techniques due to coagulopathy and/or thrombocytopenia. Nerve blockade may be appropriate even when neuraxial blockade is contraindicated. The transversus abdominal plane (TAP) block has been used successfully for abdominal surgery, including hepatobiliary procedures.[197,198] However, the efficacy has been questioned and complications, including abdominal wall hematoma, have been reported.[199]

Volatile Anesthetics

Volatile anesthetics decrease hepatic blood flow, albeit to a variable degree.

Halothane is more likely than other inhaled anesthetics to cause cardiovascular depression and results in the greatest reduction of hepatic blood flow. Newer volatile agents, including isoflurane and sevoflurane, have less significant effects on hepatic blood flow.[200] At anesthetic concentrations of 1 MAC these agents produce very little reduction in hepatic blood flow. However, desflurane appears to more substantially decrease hepatic blood flow at 1 MAC, causing a 30% reduction at this anesthetic depth.[201] Animal studies suggest desflurane preserves total hepatic blood flow.[202] At higher anesthetic concentrations isoflurane results in a dose-dependent reduction in hepatic blood flow beyond that seen at 1 MAC. This dose-dependent reduction in hepatic blood flow does not occur with sevoflurane. In animal studies both sevoflurane and isoflurane maintain the hepatic arterial buffer response, which increases hepatic arterial blood flow in the presence of reductions of portal blood flow.[203,204]

In addition to variable effects on hepatic blood flow, concern exists regarding the production of reactive intermediates during the metabolism of volatile anesthetics. Halothane hepatitis, described elsewhere in the chapter, is largely responsible for these concerns. However, there is little evidence to suggest that other volatile anesthetics are responsible for hepatic complications. With the exception of sevoflurane, volatile anesthetics undergo metabolism that yields reactive trifluoroacetylated (TFA) intermediates. These bind to hepatic proteins and produce an immunologic reaction. However, the incidence of liver injury correlates with the extent to which inhaled anesthetics undergo oxidative metabolism. While 20% of halothane and 2.5% of enflurane are metabolized to TFA intermediates, the corresponding percentages for isoflurane and desflurane are 0.2% and 0.02%, respectively.[47]

Although there is a lack of evidence supporting a role for current volatile anesthetics in causing hepatic injury, several reports describe instances when repeated exposure to halogenated anesthetics is associated with hepatic dysfunction. Because there is no pathognomonic liver pathology, the diagnosis is based on the exclusion of other causes and a history of recent exposure. In one such case gallstones rather than isoflurane was ultimately elucidated as the cause of elevated liver enzymes.[205] A 1983 report described 24 cases of presumed enflurane-associated hepatitis, noting that the potential for toxic metabolites seems related to the degree of in vivo biotransformation of the various halogenated anesthetics.[206]

Sevoflurane undergoes more extensive metabolism than isoflurane or desflurane, rapidly producing detectable plasma concentrations of fluoride and hexafluoroisopropanol (HFIP), which are conjugated by the liver and excreted by the kidney. In distinction to the other agents, sevoflurane does not produce reactive TFA metabolites or fluoroacetylated liver proteins. This fact led to the suggestion that patients sensitized to other volatile anesthetics could be safely anesthetized with sevoflurane.[207] Indeed, despite the more extensive metabolism, there is no evidence that sevoflurane's metabolites, including compound A (produced in a reaction with carbon dioxide absorbents), produce hepatic injury.[208] In rodents there is evidence that sevoflurane protects against hepatic ischemia–reperfusion injury while isoflurane does not.[209] However, there is a single case report of ALF occurring 2 days after sevoflurane exposure for heart surgery.[210] While the cause in this case is not certain, this report suggests that patients who are sensitized to one volatile anesthetic (i.e., evidence of hepatic injury following prior exposure) should not subsequently receive any other fluorinated anesthetic.

Nitrous Oxide

Nitrous oxide administration has not been shown to cause hepatocellular injury in the absence of hepatic hypoxemia.[211] In patients with mild alcoholic hepatitis, a nitrous oxide/narcotic technique was compared to nitrous oxide/enflurane and tetracaine spinal techniques for peripheral surgery. None of the techniques were associated with biochemical worsening.[212] Due to sympathomimetic effects, nitrous oxide can lead to decreased hepatic blood flow, and inhibition of methionine synthase can occur after even brief exposures. However, the clinical significance of these effects is unclear. However, prolonged or repeated exposure could induce a vitamin B_{12} deficiency.[213]

Intravenous Anesthetics

IV anesthetics, such as propofol, etomidate and midazolam, do not appear to alter hepatic function when given for a short duration during minor procedures. The effects of IV anesthetics after prolonged infusions and in patients with advanced liver disease are not well studied. A rare syndrome of lactic acidosis, lipemia, rhabdomyolysis, hyperkalemia, myocardial failure, and death has been reported after prolonged infusions of propofol. The initial reports were in children.[214] Liver dysfunction resulting in altered lipid metabolism may predispose to the propofol infusion syndrome, as may genetic defects.[215] Patients on prolonged propofol infusions should be monitored for worsening lactic acidosis and escalating vasopressor requirements. In the event of such findings, propofol should be discontinued.

There is no evidence that opioids have an effect on hepatic function that is independent of hepatic blood flow. All opioids increase sphincter of Oddi pressure. Some authors have suggested that morphine causes spasm in the sphincter of Oddi, but a review failed to show a differential effect, concluding that morphine may be preferred over meperidine for the treatment of patients with acute pancreatitis due to less risk of seizures.[216]

Pharmacokinetic and Pharmacodynamic Alterations

The decreased functional mass of hepatocytes, coupled with lower levels of plasma proteins, and reduced hepatic blood flow due to portocaval shunts lead to reduced metabolism of drugs that rely on hepatic metabolism for clearance.

Factors that affect hepatic clearance include blood flow to the liver, the fraction of the drug unbound to plasma proteins, and intrinsic clearance. Drugs with low extraction ratios, less than 0.3, have restrictive hepatic clearance. Clearance of drugs in this class is affected by protein binding, the induction or inhibition of hepatic enzymes, age, and hepatic pathology, but clearance is not significantly affected by hepatic blood flow. Drugs with a high extraction ratio (greater than 0.7) undergo extensive first-pass metabolism, which alters their bioavailability after oral administration. Regardless of the route of administration, drugs with high extraction ratios are significantly affected by alteration in hepatic blood flow, which can occur with hemodynamic changes or hepatic inflow clamping during liver resection. High extraction ratio drugs tend to have short elimination half-lives (e.g., propranolol $t_{1/2} = 3.9$ hours).

Benzodiazepines are an example of a drug with a low extraction ratio. As is commonly the case for drugs with low extraction ratios, the elimination half-life can be prolonged (diazepam $t_{1/2} =$ 43 hours). Studies have shown conflicting effects of cirrhosis on the metabolism of midazolam, possibly due to changes in protein binding.[217,218] As hepatic protein synthesis declines with advancing liver disease, the drug fraction bound to protein decreases. Since only the unbound drug is available for metabolism by hepatic enzymes, the elimination may be unaffected despite a reduction in intrinsic hepatic clearance.[219] Bilirubin and bile acids can increase the unbound drug fracture by displacing drugs from protein binding sites. An increase in the free fraction of drug leads to enhanced effects. The volume of distribution can increase with an increase in unbound drug. However, the volume of distribution of thiopental, another drug with a low extraction ratio, is not altered in cirrhotic patients.[220] This illustrates the complex interactions that affect pharmacokinetics in patients with end-stage liver disease. However, the altered pharmacodynamic effects that occur in patients with encephalopathy frequently lead to an increased sensitivity to sedatives and analgesics.

Opioids metabolism is reduced in patients with liver disease. Dosing intervals should be increased to avoid drug accumulation. Prolonged elimination is more prominent with morphine and meperidine than the shorter duration synthetic opioids, although contradictory data exist that suggest pharmacokinetics are not significantly altered by liver disease. The clearance of the meperidine metabolite normeperidine is reduced in liver disease, which can lead to neurotoxicity.[221] The elimination of a single IV opioid bolus is less affected than a continuous infusion due to redistribution to storage sites. Remifentanil, rapidly hydrolyzed by blood and tissue esterases, is an exception among the opioids as its elimination is independent of both hepatic function and the duration of infusion. The pharmacodynamic effects of opioids are altered by liver disease, which argues for a dose reduction in patients with advanced disease because of the ability to precipitate or worsen encephalopathy.

Most induction agents, including ketamine, etomidate, propofol, and thiopental, are highly lipophilic and have high extraction ratios.[222] While elimination should be prolonged in the presence of liver disease, clearance is similar in cirrhotics to normal patients. However, the pharmacodynamic effects are more pronounced, and in some cases, as with dexmedetomidine and the benzodiazepines, the duration of action can be prolonged.[223]

The intermediate duration neuromuscular blocking agents metabolized by the liver, vecuronium and rocuronium, exhibit a prolonged duration of action in patients with liver disease.[224,225] Pancuronium's action is also prolonged. Despite this, a resistance to the initial dose of neuromuscular blocker typically occurs due to elevated γ-globulin concentrations and an increase in the volume of distribution (due to edema and/or ascites). Atracurium and cisatracurium undergo organ-independent elimination. Their durations of action are not affected by liver disease. However, their metabolite, laudanosine, is eliminated by the liver but neurotoxicity has not been reported.[226] Succinylcholine metabolism is altered due to reduced plasma cholinesterase activity in cirrhotic patients; however, the clinical impact is rarely significant.

Vasopressors

In contrast to the increased response to sedatives, patients with liver disease exhibit a reduced response to endogenous vasoconstrictors, including angiotensin II, AVP, and norepinephrine.[227]

Hyporesponsiveness to catecholamines may be modulated by the release of nitric oxide, prostacyclin, and other endothelial-derived factors in response to humoral and mechanical stimuli.[228]

Volume Resuscitation

The selection of fluid and blood products for volume resuscitation is, in general, similar in patients with and without liver disease. However, in end-stage liver disease serum albumin function is quantitatively and qualitatively decreased.[229] Albumin has three major indications in the treatment of cirrhotic patients. The first is after large volume (4 to 5 L) paracentesis.[129] The second is in the presence of SBP to prevent renal impairment, specifically in patients with bilirubin greater than 4 mg/dL or creatinine higher than 1 mg/dL.[230] The third situation is in the presence of type I HRS, where its use is beneficial in conjunction with splanchnic vasoconstrictors. In a randomized trial of terlipressin with and without concomitant albumin, a higher proportion (77%) of the group that received albumin showed a complete response (defined as a creatinine <1.5 mg/dL) compared to the terlipressin-only group (25%).[231]

Transjugular Intrahepatic Portosystemic Shunt Procedure

TIPS creates a connection between the portal and systemic circulations using a minimally invasive technique (Fig. 45-3). The indications are to decompress portal hypertension in the setting of esophageal varices and/or intractable ascites.

Sedation is commonly used to facilitate placement, though some proceduralists prefer general anesthesia, as it limits patient movement, controls diaphragmatic excursion, and reduces the risk of aspiration. In patients with recent variceal bleeding, volume resuscitation may be necessary. Due to coagulopathy, patients may require clotting factors and/or platelets before the procedure. Complications include pneumothorax or vascular injury during access to the jugular vein. Dysrhythmias can occur during catheter insertion due to stimulation of the endocardium. Providers should be prepared for the possibility of hemorrhage, which can occur in the presence of extrahepatic artery or portal vein puncture.[232]

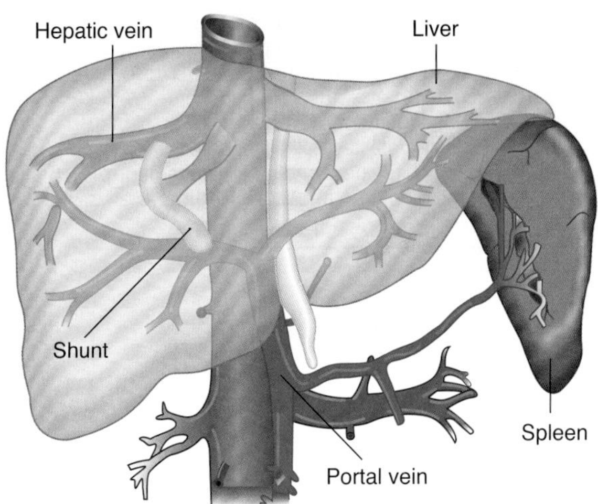

FIGURE 45-3. Transjugular intrahepatic portosystemic shunt (TIPS) procedure. A stent (or stents) is passed through the internal jugular vein over a wire into the hepatic vein. The wire and stent or stents are then advanced into the portal vein, after which blood can pass through the portal vein into the hepatic vein and bypass and decompress dilated esophageal veins. (Reproduced with permission from www.nursingcrib.com)

Hepatic Resection

In the late 1800s, the first gastrectomies and cholecystectomies were performed in Europe, but surgery on the liver was regarded as dangerous, if not impossible.[233] In 1908 Pringle described the technique of digital compression of the hepatic hilar vessels to control bleeding, which was a significant advance. Lortat-Jacob is credited with the first right hepatectomy in 1952. Another advance occurred in 1957 when segmental liver anatomy was described by Couinaud and others[234] (Figs. 45-4 and 45-5).

Despite these advances, hepatic surgery was associated with operative mortality rates of 20% or more as recently as the 1980s. Hemorrhage was a significant cause of morbidity and mortality. Persistence, along with further advances in surgery, anesthesia, and intensive care led to a reduction of mortality. Today hepatic resections are performed with mortality rates of 5% or less.

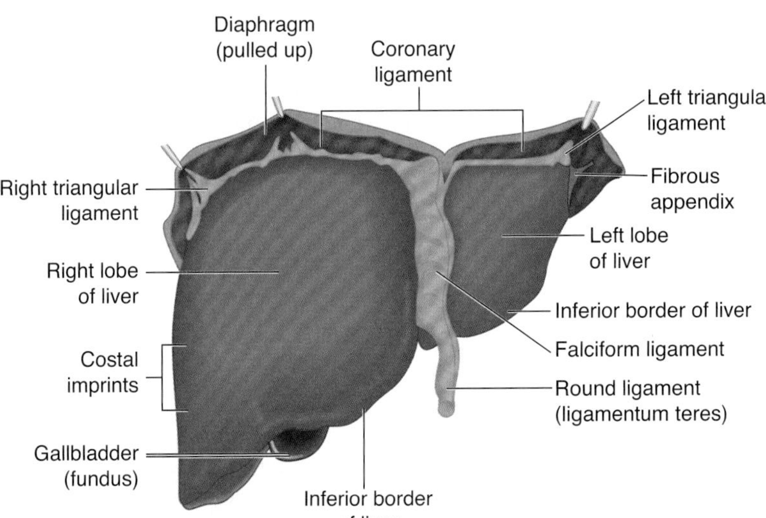

FIGURE 45-4. Superior hepatic surface: Frontal view. The anterior hepatic edge (i.e., the inferior border of the liver) delineates the superior and inferior surfaces of the liver. A sickle-shaped peritoneal fold (falciform ligament) divides the liver into two parts of unequal size, the right lobe and the left lobe. Within the free margin or base of the falciform are paraumbilical veins and the round ligament (ligamentum teres), the latter being the remnant of the obliterated umbilical vein. (From: Strunk H, Stuckmann G, Textor J, et al. Limitations and pitfalls of Couinaud's segmentation of the liver in transaxial imaging. *Eur Radiol.* 2003;13:2472–2482.)

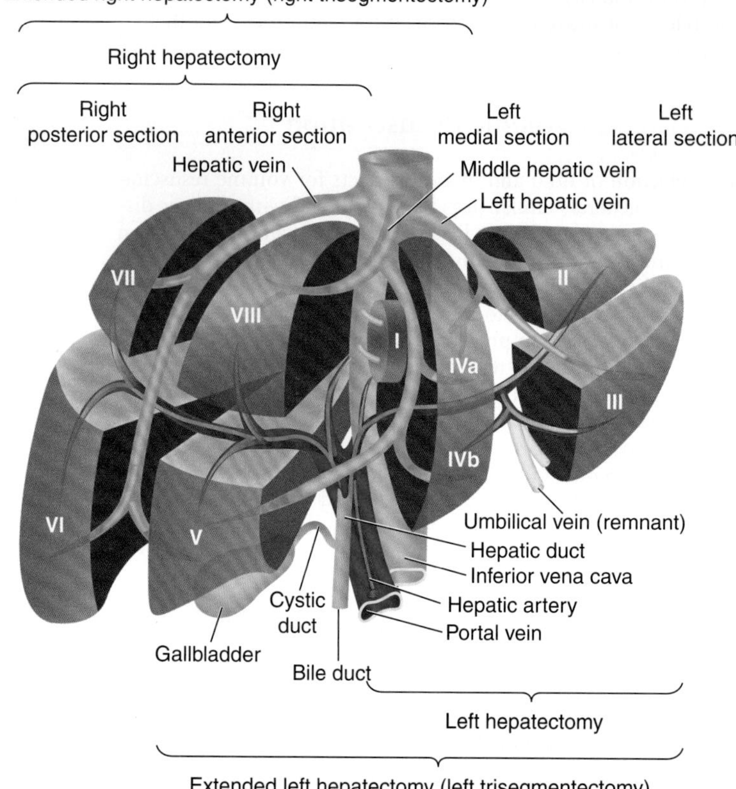

FIGURE 45-5. Schematic depiction of Couinaud segmental liver anatomy and the normal portal venous structures. *Bracketed text* shows hepatic segments resected during partial hepatectomies. (Reproduced from: Venook AP, Curley SA. Management of potentially resectable colorectal cancer liver metastases. In: Tanabe KK, Savarese DMF, eds. www.uptodate.com/contents/management-of-potentially-resectable-colorectal-cancer-liver-metastases; accessed March 2012.

Partial hepatectomy in normal, noncirrhotic livers is associated with mortality rates of 1% to 2%.[235]

Improved surgical technique with avoidance of the thoracoabdominal approach, which was associated with high morbidity, contributes to improved outcomes. Smooth fracture of liver parenchyma accompanied by bipolar coagulation made parenchymal transection possible. New transection techniques using ultrasonic dissectors, high-pressure water jets, and/or harmonic scalpels may be helpful, but they have not been proven to be superior to conventional clamp crush techniques.[236–238] Preoperative imaging techniques delineate variations in portal, arterial, and bile duct anatomy. Transfusion is necessary in less than 20% of patients.[239,240]

Yet, bleeding remains a major complication, and the hepatic veins are a significant source of blood loss. Techniques to maintain CVP at normal or even low (<5 cm H_2O) levels has been suggested as a technique to limit blood loss.[241] Whether a low CVP is deleterious to renal function is uncertain. In a single-center, uncontrolled series of nearly 500 hepatic resection patients who were managed with low CVP, no cases of renal failure were attributed to the technique.[242] Others have suggested that peripheral venous pressure is an acceptable surrogate for CVP during hepatic resection and liver transplantation.[243,244]

A number of authors question the necessity of a low CVP technique given that blood loss is less significant in the current era.[186–188,236] Others question whether CVP is a reliable monitor of fluid responsiveness.[185] Lastly, two single-center series of living liver donors came to the same conclusion that CVP is not a predictor of blood loss during hepatic resection.[245,246]

Vasopressors have a direct effect on splanchnic vessels, which reduces splanchnic pressure and decreases blood loss.[247] Portal triad clamping (of the afferent vessels) and total vascular occlusion (of the afferent vessels plus the supra- and infrahepatic vena cava) are both effective in decreasing blood loss during hepatic resection. Portal triad clamping is better tolerated and as effective as total vascular occlusions.[248] Portal triad clamping is well tolerated hemodynamically and has little effect on liver function if intermittent.[249,250] Ischemic preconditioning (10-minute inflow occlusion, followed by a 10-minute reperfusion period) followed by continuous inflow clamping for up to 75 minutes was equally effective to intermittent inflow clamping (15-minute periods followed by 5-minute reperfusion) with regard to protection against postoperative liver injury in noncirrhotic patients undergoing hepatic resection. Ischemic preconditioning plus continuous clamping resulted in less blood loss than intermittent clamping.[251]

Air embolism, a known complication of hepatic resection, can be predicted on the basis of the need for a large hepatectomy (such as a right lobectomy) or when the tumor is near the vena cava or involves portal vessels. Low CVP may increase the risk of venous air embolism, though this has not been substantiated.[252]

Techniques in use for hepatic resection continue to evolve, though indications for newer procedures are not always clearly defined. Examples include minimally invasive liver surgery, thermal ablation of hepatic tumors, and portal vein embolization to induce hypertrophy of the remnant liver.

POSTOPERATIVE LIVER DYSFUNCTION

Postoperative liver dysfunction is considered in the presence of asymptomatic elevation of hepatic transaminases, jaundice, and/or symptoms suggestive of liver failure, such as encephalopathy. Mild elevations of liver enzymes can occur after surgery, particularly upper abdominal procedures. Elevations that are less than two times the upper limit of normal are frequently transient and do not require investigation. More severe elevations suggest hepatocellular injury, which can result from a number of causes including hypoxemia, viral or bacterial insult, trauma, and chemical toxicity.

Asymptomatic, mild elevations of hepatic enzymes are not unusual within hours after surgery, but they do not usually persist for more than 2 days. Such elevations were more common after halothane than enflurane (incidence of 50% vs. 20%, respectively) but are uncommon in patients without hepatic dysfunction following currently used inhaled anesthetics.[253–257]

Jaundice, or more severe elevations of hepatic enzymes, requires investigation. Hepatic hypoxemia can result from a number of causes (Table 45-15) including cardiopulmonary etiologies (pneumonia, atelectasis, heart failure), hypoperfusion (secondary to shock), anemia, or fever. Surgery itself decreases hepatic blood flow.[258] Reabsorption of surgical or traumatic hematomas and transfusion of red blood cells are major causes of postoperative jaundice. Ten percent of transfused red cells hemolyze within 24 hours of transfusion. The bilirubin load per unit transfused is 250 mg. The liver may take time to clear the bilirubin load that results from significant hemolysis.

Unconjugated hyperbilirubinemia suggests hemolysis or an inherited disorder such as Gilbert's syndrome. Crigler–Najjar syndrome is much less common than Gilbert's. The absence or marked decrease of bilirubin glucuronyltransferase produces an unconjugated hyperbilirubinemia. Surgical and anesthetic problems are uncommon in patients with Gilbert's and Crigler–Najjar syndromes. Hemoglobinopathies (e.g., sickle cell disease), erythrocyte metabolism defects (e.g., glucose-6-phosphate dehydrogenase deficiency), transfusion reactions, and prosthetic heart valves can also cause hemolysis.

If over 50% of bilirubin is conjugated cholestasis, hepatocellular dysfunction is likely. Hypoxemia, toxic reactions, unsuspected pre-existing liver disease, trauma, and congenital disorders should be considered (Table 45-14). Some of the medicines implicated in liver disease are listed in Table 45-12. Dubin–Johnson and Rotor syndromes are congenital disorders associated with a defect in bilirubin excretion, which causes a conjugated bilirubinemia. Surgery can worsen these syndromes.

7 The nature and site of the surgical procedure is an important risk factor for postoperative liver failure.[168] Abdominal surgery appears to reduce hepatic blood flow significantly. Abdominal traction can elevate prostaglandin levels, which may be responsible.[259] Not surprisingly, hepatic resection is a risk factor for postoperative liver failure. The indication for resection in many patients is HCC, which is associated with chronic hepatitis or cirrhosis.[168] The functional reserve of the remnant hepatic parenchyma is difficult to estimate in the cirrhotic liver. In a series of 747 hepatic resections, patients with obstructive jaundice due to malignancy had a higher postoperative mortality (21%) than those with cirrhosis (8.7%), while patients with a normal liver had a postresection mortality of 1%.[260] In a series of 373 patients undergoing surgery for obstructive jaundice, those with malignancy or markedly elevated bilirubin had a 1-month mortality of >20%.[261] When renal failure accompanies hyperbilirubinemia, the mortality exceeds 50%.[262] Low intestinal levels of bile salts appear to promote the absorption of endotoxin from the gastrointestinal tract, while vasoconstrictive inflammatory mediators can precipitate renal hypoperfusion.[263]

Cardiac surgery in patients with cirrhosis is not well tolerated. Cardiopulmonary bypass exacerbates pre-existing hepatic disease by unknown mechanisms. The overall perioperative mortality in patients with cirrhosis was 31%, and 80% in patients with Child's class B cirrhosis.[264] Another series of cardiac patients reported 1-year mortality of 20%, 55%, and 84% in Child's class A, B, and C patients, respectively.[265] For comparison, the mortality in patients without cirrhosis is approximately 2%.[266] These authors concluded that cardiac surgery that involves cardiopulmonary bypass can be performed in cirrhotic patients with Child's class A cirrhosis and in selected patients with class B.

TABLE 45-14. CAUSES OF POSTOPERATIVE LIVER DYSFUNCTION

Hepatocellular	Drugs
	Anesthetics
	Ischemia
	Shock, hypotension, iatrogenic injury
	Viral hepatitis
Cholestasis	Benign postoperative cholestasis
	Sepsis
	Bile duct injury
	Drugs
	Antibiotics, antiemetics
	Choledocholithiasis or pancreatitis
	Cholecystitis
	Gilbert syndrome

TABLE 45-15. CAUSES OF HYPERBILIRUBINEMIA

Unconjugated (indirect)
Excessive bilirubin production (hemolysis)
Immaturity of enzyme systems
 Physiologic jaundice of newborn
 Jaundice of prematurity
Inherited defects
 Gilbert syndrome
 Crigler–Najjar syndrome
Drug effects

Conjugated (direct)
Hepatocellular disease (hepatitis, cirrhosis, drugs)
Intrahepatic cholestasis (drugs, pregnancy)
Benign postoperative jaundice, sepsis
Congenital conjugated hyperbilirubinemia
 Dubin–Johnson syndrome
 Rotor syndrome
Obstructive jaundice
 Extrahepatic (calculus, stricture, neoplasm)
 Intrahepatic (sclerosing cholangitis, neoplasm, primary biliary cirrhosis)

From: Friedman L, Martin P, Munoz S. Liver function tests and the objective evaluation of the patient with liver disease. In: Zakim D, Boyer T, eds. *Hepatology: A Textbook of Liver Disease.* 3rd ed. Philadelphia, PA: WB Saunders; 1996:791.

CONCLUSIONS

In patients with new-onset liver disease, elective surgery should be postponed until the course of the disease is known. In patients with pre-existing liver disease, the severity of the disease should be characterized in order to assess risk. Elective high-risk procedures (abdominal and cardiac surgery) in patients with Child's C cirrhosis should be deferred until after liver transplantation. Child's A and B patients should be medically optimized prior to surgery. While no anesthetic technique is universally contraindicated, the presence of coagulopathy may contraindicate neuraxial regional techniques. The chosen technique should be designed to maintain splanchnic, hepatic, and renal perfusion. When surgery is unavoidable in patients with advanced liver disease, transfer to a liver transplant center should be considered.

ACKNOWLEDGMENT

The authors are indebted to Brian S. Kaufman and J. David Roccaforte for their permission to use text, figures, and tables from their chapter in a prior version of *Clinical Anesthesia.*

References

1. Shah VH, Kamath PS. Portal hypertension and gastrointestinal bleeding. In: Feldman M, Friedman LS, Brandt LJ, eds. *Sleisinger and Fordtran's Gastrointestinal and Liver Disease.* 9th ed. Philadelphia, PA: Saunders Elsevier; 2010:1489.
2. Lautt WW. Mechanism and role of intrinsic regulation of hepatic arterial blood flow: Hepatic arterial buffer response. *Am J Physiol.* 1985;249:G549.
3. Robert McCuskey, Anatomy of the Liver, Chapter 1, Figure 1-11. In: Zakim and Boyer's Hepatology: A Textbook of Liver Disease. 6th ed. Philadelphia, PA: Elsevier Saunders; 2012.
4. Nordlie RC, Foster JD, Lange AJ. Regulation of glucose production by the liver. *Annu Rev Nutr.* 1999;19:379.
5. Olthoff KM. Hepatic regeneration in living donor liver transplantation. *Liver Transpl.* 2003;9:S35.
6. Viebahn CS, Yeoh GC. What fires Prometheus? The link between inflammation and regeneration following chronic liver injury. *Int J Biochem Cell Biol.* 2008;40:855.
7. Balci NC, Befeler AS, Leiva P, et al. Imaging of liver disease: Comparison between quadruple-phase multidetector computed tomography and magnetic resonance imaging. *J Gastroenterol Hepatol.* 2008;23:1520.
8. Weinreb JC, Cohen JM, Armstrong E, et al. Imaging the pediatric liver: MRI and CT. *AJR Am J Roentgenol.* 1986;147:785.
9. Kochanek KD, Xu J, Murphy SL, et al. Deaths: Preliminary data for 2009. In: Center for Disease Control and Prevention NCfHS, ed. *National Vital Statistics Reports.* Vol. 59. March 16, 2011, edn. Washington, DC: U.S. Department of Health and Human Services; 2011.
10. Goldberg DS, French B, Thomasson A, et al. Current trends in living donor liver transplantation for primary sclerosing cholangitis. *Transplantation.* 2011;91:1148.
11. Younossi ZM, Stepanova M, Afendy M, et al. Changes in the prevalence of the most common causes of chronic liver diseases in the United States from 1988 to 2008. *Clin Gastroenterol Hepatol.* 2011;9:524.
12. Lee WM. Etiologies of acute liver failure. *Semin Liver Dis.* 2008;28:142.
13. Lee WM, Squires RH Jr, Nyberg SL, et al. Acute liver failure: Summary of a workshop. *Hepatology.* 2008;47:1401.
14. Polson J, Lee WM. AASLD position paper: The management of acute liver failure. *Hepatology.* 2005;41:1179.
15. Munoz SJ. Difficult management problems in fulminant hepatic failure. *Semin Liver Dis.* 1993;13:395.
16. Blei AT. Infection, inflammation and hepatic encephalopathy, synergism redefined. *J Hepatol.* 2004;40:327.
17. Jalan R. Intracranial hypertension in acute liver failure: Pathophysiological basis of rational management. *Semin Liver Dis.* 2003;23:271.
18. Larsen FS. Cerebral circulation in liver failure: Ohm's law in force. *Semin Liver Dis.* 1996;16:281.
19. Murphy N, Auzinger G, Bernel W, et al. The effect of hypertonic sodium chloride on intracranial pressure in patients with acute liver failure. *Hepatology.* 2004;39:464.
20. Ede RJ, Gimson AE, Bihari D, et al. Controlled hyperventilation in the prevention of cerebral oedema in fulminant hepatic failure. *J Hepatol.* 1986;2:43.
21. Stravitz RT, Kramer AH, Davern T, et al. Intensive care of patients with acute liver failure: Recommendations of the U.S. Acute Liver Failure study group. *Crit Care Med.* 2007;35:2498.
22. Frontera JA, Kalb T. Neurological management of fulminant hepatic failure. *Neurocrit Care.* 2011;14:318.
23. Munoz SJ, Robinson M, Northrup B, et al. Elevated intracranial pressure and computed tomography of the brain in fulminant hepatocellular failure. *Hepatology.* 1991;13:209.
24. Lidofsky SD, Bass NM, Prager MC, et al. Intracranial pressure monitoring and liver transplantation for fulminant hepatic failure. *Hepatology.* 1992;16:1.
25. Raschke RA, Curry SC, Rempe S, et al. Results of a protocol for the management of patients with fulminant liver failure. *Crit Care Med.* 2008;36:2244.
26. Bismuth H, Samuel D, Castaing D, et al. Orthotopic liver transplantation in fulminant and subfulminant hepatitis. The Paul Brousse experience. *Ann Surg.* 1995;222:109.
27. Riordan SM, Williams R. Mechanisms of hepatocyte injury, multiorgan failure, and prognostic criteria in acute liver failure. *Semin Liver Dis.* 2003;23:203.
28. Ichai P, Samuel D. Etiology and prognosis of fulminant hepatitis in adults. *Liver Transpl.* 2008;14(suppl 2):S67.
29. Shawcross DL, Davies NA, Williams R, et al. Systemic inflammatory response exacerbates the neuropsychological effects of induced hyperammonemia in cirrhosis. *J Hepatol.* 2004;40:247.
30. Schiodt FV, Davern TJ, Shakil AO, et al. Viral hepatitis-related acute liver failure. *Am J Gastroenterol.* 2003;98:448.
31. Anonymous. Hepatitis B FAQS for health professionals. *Hepatitis B Information for Health Professionals* 2012. http://www.cdc.gov/hepatitis/HBV/HBVfaq.htm. Accessed January 27, 2012; 2012.
32. Ghany MG, Strader DB, Thomas DL, et al. Diagnosis, management, and treatment of hepatitis C: An update. *Hepatology.* 2009;49:1335.
33. Cohen JA, Kaplan MM. The SGOT/sSGPT ratio–an indicator of alcoholic liver disease. *Dig Dis Sci.* 1979;24:835.
34. Altamirano J, Fagundes C, Dominguez M, et al. Acute kidney injury is an early predictor of mortality for patients with alcoholic hepatitis. *Clin Gastroenterol Hepatol.* 2012;10:65.
35. Leevy CM, Kanagasundaram N. Alcoholic hepatitis. *Hosp Pract.* 1978;13:115.
36. Akriviadis E, Botla R, Briggs W, et al. Pentoxifylline improves short-term survival in severe acute alcoholic hepatitis: A double-blind, placebo-controlled trial. *Gastroenterology.* 2000;119:1637.
37. Ostapowicz G, Fontana RJ, Schiodt FV, et al. Results of a prospective study of acute liver failure at 17 tertiary care centers in the United States. *Ann Intern Med.* 2002;137:947.
38. Anonymous. Drug-induced liver injury premarketing clinical evaluation. http://www.fda.gov/downloads/Drugs/GuidanceComplianceRegulatoryInformation/Guidances/UCM174090.pdf. Food and Drug Administration; 2009.
39. Watkins PB, Seeff LB. Drug-induced liver injury: Summary of a single topic clinical research conference. *Hepatology.* 2006;43:618.
40. Ray DC, Drummond GB. Halothane hepatitis. *Br J Anaesth.* 1991;67:84.
41. Gall EA. Report of the pathology panel. National halothane study. *Anesthesiology.* 1968;29:233.
42. Bunker JP. Final report of the national halothane study. *Anesthesiology.* 1968;29:231.
43. Fontana RJ, Seeff LB, Andrade RJ, et al. Standardization of nomenclature and causality assessment in drug-induced liver injury: Summary of a clinical research workshop. *Hepatology.* 2010;52:730.
44. Wright R, Eade OE, Chisholm M, et al. Controlled prospective study of the effect on liver function of multiple exposures to halothane. *Lancet.* 1975;1:817.
45. Reichle FM, Conzen PF. Halogenated inhalational anaesthetics. *Best Pract Res Clin Anaesthesiol.* 2003;17:29.
46. Kenna JG, Satoh H, Christ DD, et al. Metabolic basis for a drug hypersensitivity: Antibodies in sera from patients with halothane hepatitis recognize liver neoantigens that contain the trifluoroacetyl group derived from halothane. *J Pharmacol Exp Ther.* 1988;245:1103.
47. Njoku D, Laster MJ, Gong DH, et al. Biotransformation of halothane, enflurane, isoflurane, and desflurane to trifluoroacetylated liver proteins: Association between protein acylation and hepatic injury. *Anesth Analg.* 1997;84:173.
48. Fell DB, Dodds L, Joseph KS, et al. Risk factors for hyperemesis gravidarum requiring hospital admission during pregnancy. *Obstet Gynecol.* 2006;107:277.
49. Hay JE. Liver disease in pregnancy. *Hepatology.* 2008;47:1067.
50. Bacq Y. Liver diseases unique to pregnancy: A 2010 update. *Clin Res Hepatol Gastroenterol.* 2011;35:182.
51. Baxter JK, Weinstein L. HELLP syndrome: The state of the art. *Obstet Gynecol Surv.* 2004;59:838.
52. Castro MA, Ouzounian JG, Colletti PM, et al. Radiologic studies in acute fatty liver of pregnancy. A review of the literature and 19 new cases. *J Reprod Med.* 1996;41:839.
53. Pinzani M, Rosselli M, Zuckermann M. Liver cirrhosis. *Best Pract Res Clin Gastroenterol.* 2011;25:281.
54. Ripoll C, Groszmann R, Garcia-Tsao G, et al. Hepatic venous pressure gradient predicts clinical decompensation in patients with compensated cirrhosis. *Gastroenterology.* 2007;133:481.
55. Diaz LK, Teruya J. Liver biopsy. *N Engl J Med.* 2001;344:2030.
56. Terjung B, Lemnitzer I, Dumoulin FL, et al. Bleeding complications after percutaneous liver biopsy. An analysis of risk factors. *Digestion.* 2003;67:138.
57. Segal JB, Dzik WH. Paucity of studies to support that abnormal coagulation test results predict bleeding in the setting of invasive procedures: An evidence-based review. *Transfusion.* 2005;45:1413.
58. Tripodi A, Primignani M, Chantarangkul V, et al. Thrombin generation in patients with cirrhosis: The role of platelets. *Hepatology.* 2006;44:440.
59. Lisman T, Bakhtiari K, Pereboom ITA, et al. Normal to increased thrombin generation in patients undergoing liver transplantation despite prolonged conventional coagulation tests. *J Hepatol.* 2010;52:355.
60. Tripodi A, Primignani M, Chantarangkul V, et al. An imbalance of pro- vs anticoagulation factors in plasma from patients with cirrhosis. *Gastroenterology.* 2009;137:2105.
61. Dabbagh O, Oza A, Prakash S, et al. Coagulopathy does not protect against venous thromboembolism in hospitalized patients with chronic liver disease. *Chest.* 2010;137:1145.
62. Northup PG, Mcmahon MM, Ruhl AP, et al. Coagulopathy does not fully protect hospitalized cirrhosis patients from peripheral venous thromboembolism. *Am J Gastroenterol.* 2006;101:1524.
63. Sogaard KK, Horvath-Puho E, Gronbaek H, et al. Risk of venous thromboembolism in patients with liver disease: A nationwide population-based case-control study. *Am J Gastroenterol.* 2009;104:96.

64. Francis JL, Armstrong DJ. Acquired dysfibrinogenaemia in liver disease. *J Clin Pathol.* 1982;35:667.
65. Amitrano L, Guardascione MA, Brancaccio V, et al. Coagulation disorders in liver disease. *Semin Liver Dis.* 2002;22:83.
66. Hu KQ, Yu AS, Tiyyagura L, et al. Hyperfibrinolytic activity in hospitalized cirrhotic patients in a referral liver unit. *Am J Gastroenterol.* 2001;96:1581.
67. Kujovich JL. Hemostatic defects in end stage liver disease. *Crit Care Clin.* 2005;21:563.
68. Puoti C, Bellis L, Guarisco R, et al. Quantitation of tissue polypeptide antigen (tpa) in hepatic and systemic circulation in patients with chronic liver diseases. *J Gastroenterol Hepatol.* 2009;24:1847.
69. Ben-Ari Z, Osman E, Hutton RA, et al. Disseminated intravascular coagulation in liver cirrhosis: Fact or fiction? *Am J Gastroenterol.* 1999;94:2977.
70. Joist JH. AICF and DIC in liver cirrhosis: Expressions of a hypercoagulable state. *Am J Gastroenterol.* 1999;94:2801.
71. Moller S, Henriksen JH. Cardiovascular complications of cirrhosis. *Gut.* 2008; 57:268.
72. Schepke M, Heller J, Paschke S, et al. Contractile hyporesponsiveness of hepatic arteries in humans with cirrhosis: Evidence for a receptor-specific mechanism. *Hepatology.* 2001;34:884.
73. Wong F, Girgrah N, Graba J, et al. The cardiac response to exercise in cirrhosis. *Gut.* 2001;49:268.
74. Puthumana L, Chaudhry V, Thuluvath PJ. Prolonged QTC interval and its relationship to autonomic cardiovascular reflexes in patients with cirrhosis. *J Hepatol.* 2001;35:733.
75. Raval Z, Harinstein ME, Skaro AI, et al. Cardiovascular risk assessment of the liver transplant candidate. *J Am Coll Cardiol.* 2011;58:223.
76. Ehtisham J, Altieri M, Salame E, et al. Coronary artery disease in orthotopic liver transplantation: Pretransplant assessment and management. *Liver Transpl.* 2010;16:550.
77. Mcguire BM, Julian BA, Bynon JS Jr, et al. Brief communication: Glomerulonephritis in patients with hepatitis C cirrhosis undergoing liver transplantation. *Ann Intern Med.* 2006;144:735.
78. Claria J, Kent JD, Lopez-Parra M, et al. Effects of celecoxib and naproxen on renal function in nonazotemic patients with cirrhosis and ascites. *Hepatology.* 2005;41:579.
79. Guevara M, Fernandez-Esparrach G, Alessandria C, et al. Effects of contrast media on renal function in patients with cirrhosis: A prospective study. *Hepatology.* 2004;40:646.
80. Takabatake T, Ohta H, Ishida Y, et al. Low serum creatinine levels in severe hepatic disease. *Arch Intern Med.* 1988;148:1313.
81. Papadakis MA, Arieff AI. Unpredictability of clinical evaluation of renal function in cirrhosis. Prospective study. *Am J Med.* 1987;82:945.
82. Koppel MH, Coburn JW, Mims MM, et al. Transplantation of cadaveric kidneys from patients with hepatorenal syndrome. Evidence for the functional nature of renal failure in advanced liver disease. *N Engl J Med.* 1969;280:1367.
83. Garcia-Tsao G, Parikh CR, Viola A. Acute kidney injury in cirrhosis. *Hepatology.* 2008;48:2064.
84. Gines A, Escorsell A, Gines P, et al. Incidence, predictive factors, and prognosis of the hepatorenal syndrome in cirrhosis with ascites. *Gastroenterology.* 1993;105:229.
85. Salerno F, Gerbes A, Gines P, et al. Diagnosis, prevention and treatment of hepatorenal syndrome in cirrhosis. *Gut.* 2007;56:1310.
86. Moreau R. Hepatorenal syndrome in patients with cirrhosis. *J Gastroenterol Hepatol.* 2002;17:739.
87. Arroyo V, Terra C, Gines P. Advances in the pathogenesis and treatment of type-1 and type-2 hepatorenal syndrome. *J Hepatol.* 2007;46:935.
88. Gines P, Guevara M, Arroyo V, et al. Hepatorenal syndrome. *Lancet.* 2003;362:1819.
89. Kiser TH, Maclaren R, Fish DN. Treatment of hepatorenal syndrome. *Pharmacotherapy.* 2009;29:1196.
90. Sola E, Gines P. Renal and circulatory dysfunction in cirrhosis: Current management and future perspectives. *J Hepatol.* 2010;53:1135.
91. Boyer TD, Sanyal AJ, Garcia-Tsao G, et al. Predictors of response to terlipressin plus albumin in hepatorenal syndrome (HRS) type 1: Relationship of serum creatinine to hemodynamics. *J Hepatol.* 2011;55:315.
92. Guevara M, Gines P, Bandi JC, et al. Transjugular intrahepatic portosystemic shunt in hepatorenal syndrome: Effects on renal function and vasoactive systems. *Hepatology.* 1998;28:416.
93. Gonwa TA, Morris CA, Goldstein RM, et al. Long-term survival and renal function following liver transplantation in patients with and without hepatorenal syndrome–experience in 300 patients. *Transplantation.* 1991;51:428.
94. Charlton MR, Wall WJ, Ojo AO, et al. Report of the first international liver transplantation society expert panel consensus conference on renal insufficiency in liver transplantation. *Liver Transpl.* 2009;15:S1.
95. Palma DT, Fallon MB. The hepatopulmonary syndrome. *J Hepatol.* 2006;45:617.
96. Schenk P, Fuhrmann V, Madl C, et al. Hepatopulmonary syndrome: Prevalence and predictive value of various cut offs for arterial oxygenation and their clinical consequences. *Gut.* 2002;51:853.
97. Rodriguez-Roisin R, Krowka MJ. Hepatopulmonary syndrome–a liver-induced lung vascular disorder. *N Engl J Med.* 2008;358:2378.
98. Krowka MJ. Hepatopulmonary syndrome: Recent literature (1997 to 1999) and implications for liver transplantation. *Liver Transpl.* 2000;4:S31.
99. Arguedas MR, Abrams GA, Krowka MJ, et al. Prospective evaluation of outcomes and predictors of mortality in patients with hepatopulmonary syndrome undergoing liver transplantation. *Hepatology.* 2003;37:192.
100. Swanson KL, Wiesner RH, Krowka MJ. Natural history of hepatopulmonary syndrome: Impact of liver transplantation. *Hepatology.* 2005;41:1122.
101. Gupta S, Castel H, Rao RV, et al. Improved survival after liver transplantation in patients with hepatopulmonary syndrome. *Am J Transplant.* 2010;10:354.
102. Fallon MB, Mulligan DC, Gish RG, et al. Model for end-stage liver disease (MELD) exception for hepatopulmonary syndrome. *Liver Transpl.* 2006;12:S105.
103. Rodriguez-Roisin R, Krowka MJ, Herve P, et al. Pulmonary-hepatic vascular disorders (phd). *Eur Respir J.* 2004;24:861.
104. Hadengue A, Benhayoun MK, Lebrec D, et al. Pulmonary hypertension complicating portal hypertension: Prevalence and relation to splanchnic hemodynamics. *Gastroenterology.* 1991;100:520.
105. Mcdonnell PJ, Toye PA, Hutchins GM. Primary pulmonary hypertension and cirrhosis: Are they related? *Am Rev Respir Dis.* 1983;127:437.
106. Kawut SM, Krowka MJ, Trotter JF, et al. Clinical risk factors for portopulmonary hypertension. *Hepatology.* 2008;48:196.
107. Castro M, Krowka MJ, Schroeder DR, et al. Frequency and clinical implications of increased pulmonary artery pressures in liver transplant patients. *Mayo Clin Proc.* 1996;71:543.
108. Le Pavec J, Souza R, Herve P, et al. Portopulmonary hypertension: Survival and prognostic factors. *Am J Respir Crit Care Med.* 2008;178:637.
109. Hoeper MM, Halank M, Marx C, et al. Bosentan therapy for portopulmonary hypertension. *Eur Respir J.* 2005;25:502.
110. Kim WR, Krowka MJ, Plevak DJ, et al. Accuracy of Doppler echocardiography in the assessment of pulmonary hypertension in liver transplant candidates. *Liver Transpl.* 2000;6:453.
111. Mclaughlin VV, Archer SL, Badesch DB, et al. ACCF/AHA 2009 expert consensus document on pulmonary hypertension a report of the American College of Cardiology Foundation Task Force on Expert Consensus Documents and the American Heart Association developed in collaboration with the American College of Chest Physicians; American Thoracic Society, Inc.; the Pulmonary Hypertension Association. *J Am Coll Cardiol.* 2009;53:1573.
112. Findlay JY, Plevak DJ, Krowka MJ, et al. Progressive splenomegaly after epoprostenol therapy in portopulmonary hypertension. *Liver Transpl.* 1999;5:362.
113. Reichenberger F, Voswinckel R, Steveling E, et al. Sildenafil treatment for portopulmonary hypertension. *Eur Respir J.* 2006;28:563.
114. Porres-Aguilar M, Zuckerman MJ, Figueroa-Casas JB, et al. Portopulmonary hypertension: State of the art. *Ann Hepatol.* 2008;7:321.
115. Ramsay M. Portopulmonary hypertension and right heart failure in patients with cirrhosis. *Curr Opin Anaesthesiol.* 2010;23:145.
116. Krowka MJ, Mandell MS, Ramsay MA, et al. Hepatopulmonary syndrome and portopulmonary hypertension: A report of the multicenter liver transplant database. *Liver Transpl.* 2004;10:174.
117. Ferenci P, Lockwood A, Mullen K, et al. Hepatic encephalopathy–definition, nomenclature, diagnosis, and quantification: Final report of the working party at the 11th world congresses of gastroenterology, Vienna, 1998. *Hepatology.* 2002;35:716.
118. Munoz SJ. Hepatic encephalopathy. *Med Clin North Am.* 2008;92:795.
119. Bass NM, Mullen KD, Sanyal A, et al. Rifaximin treatment in hepatic encephalopathy. *N Engl J Med.* 2010;362:1071.
120. Prakash R, Mullen KD. Mechanisms, diagnosis and management of hepatic encephalopathy. *Nat Rev Gastroenterol Hepatol.* 2010;7:515.
121. Perney P, Butterworth RF, Mousseau DD, et al. Plasma and CSF benzodiazepine receptor ligand concentrations in cirrhotic patients with hepatic encephalopathy: Relationship to severity of encephalopathy and to pharmaceutical benzodiazepine intake. *Metab Brain Dis.* 1998;13:201.
122. Mullen KD, Szauter KM, Kaminsky-Russ K. "Endogenous" benzodiazepine activity in body fluids of patients with hepatic encephalopathy. *Lancet.* 1990;336:81.
123. Lock BG, Pandit K. Evidence-based emergency medicine/systematic review abstract. Is flumazenil an effective treatment for hepatic encephalopathy? *Ann Emerg Med.* 2006;47:286.
124. Barbaro G, Di Lorenzo G, Soldini M, et al. Flumazenil for hepatic encephalopathy grade III and IVa in patients with cirrhosis: An Italian multicenter double-blind, placebo-controlled, cross-over study. *Hepatology.* 1998;28:374.
125. Haussinger D, Schliess F. Pathogenetic mechanisms of hepatic encephalopathy. *Gut.* 2008;57:1156.
126. Blei AT, Cordoba J. Hepatic encephalopathy. *Am J Gastroenterol.* 2001;96:1968.
127. Jiang Q, Jiang XH, Zheng MH, et al. Rifaximin versus nonabsorbable disaccharides in the management of hepatic encephalopathy: A meta-analysis. *Eur J Gastroenterol Hepatol.* 2008;20:1064.
128. Wright G, Chattree A, Jalan R. Management of hepatic encephalopathy. *Int J Hepatol.* 2011;2011:841407.
129. Runyon BA. Management of adult patients with ascites due to cirrhosis: An update. *Hepatology.* 2009;49:2087.
130. Arroyo V, Colmenero J. Ascites and hepatorenal syndrome in cirrhosis: Pathophysiological basis of therapy and current management. *J Hepatol.* 2003;38 (suppl 1):S69.
131. Runyon BA, Montano AA, Akriviadis EA, et al. The serum-ascites albumin gradient is superior to the exudate-transudate concept in the differential diagnosis of ascites. *Ann Intern Med.* 1992;117:215.

132. Wszolek ZK, Mccomb RD, Pfeiffer RF, et al. Pontine and extrapontine myelinolysis following liver transplantation. Relationship to serum sodium. *Transplantation.* 1989;48:1006.
133. Gines P, Cardenas A, Arroyo V, et al. Management of cirrhosis and ascites. *N Engl J Med.* 2004;350:1646.
134. Albillos A, Banares R, Gonzalez M, et al. A meta-analysis of transjugular intrahepatic portosystemic shunt versus paracentesis for refractory ascites. *J Hepatol.* 2005;43:990.
135. D'amico G, Luca A, Morabito A, et al. Uncovered transjugular intrahepatic portosystemic shunt for refractory ascites: A meta-analysis. *Gastroenterology.* 2005;129:1282.
136. Felisart J, Rimola A, Arroyo V, et al. Cefotaxime is more effective than is ampicillin-tobramycin in cirrhotics with severe infections. *Hepatology.* 1985;5:457.
137. Wiest R, Krag A, Gerbes A. Spontaneous bacterial peritonitis: Recent guidelines and beyond. *Gut.* 2012;61:297.
138. Perello A, Escorsell A, Bru C, et al. Wedged hepatic venous pressure adequately reflects portal pressure in hepatitis c virus-related cirrhosis. *Hepatology.* 1999;30:1393.
139. Garcia-Tsao G, Groszmann RJ, Fisher RL, et al. Portal pressure, presence of gastroesophageal varices and variceal bleeding. *Hepatology.* 1985;5:419.
140. Lebrec D, De Fleury P, Rueff B, et al. Portal hypertension, size of esophageal varices, and risk of gastrointestinal bleeding in alcoholic cirrhosis. *Gastroenterology.* 1980;79:1139.
141. Garcia-Tsao G, Sanyal AJ, Grace ND, et al. Prevention and management of gastroesophageal varices and variceal hemorrhage in cirrhosis. *Hepatology.* 2007;46:922.
142. Castaneda B, Morales J, Lionetti R, et al. Effects of blood volume restitution following a portal hypertensive-related bleeding in anesthetized cirrhotic rats. *Hepatology.* 2001;33:821.
143. Kravetz D, Sikuler E, Groszmann RJ. Splanchnic and systemic hemodynamics in portal hypertensive rats during hemorrhage and blood volume restitution. *Gastroenterology.* 1986;90:1232.
144. Moitinho E, Escorsell A, Bandi JC, et al. Prognostic value of early measurements of portal pressure in acute variceal bleeding. *Gastroenterology.* 1999;117:626.
145. Green J, Beyar R, Bomzon L, et al. Jaundice, the circulation and the kidney. *Nephron.* 1984;37:145.
146. Green J, Beyar R, Sideman S, et al. The "jaundiced heart": A possible explanation for postoperative shock in obstructive jaundice. *Surgery.* 1986;100:14.
147. Ben-Ari Z, Panagou M, Patch D, et al. Hypercoagulability in patients with primary biliary cirrhosis and primary sclerosing cholangitis evaluated by thromboelastography. *J Hepatol.* 1997;26:554.
148. Segal H, Cottam S, Potter D, et al. Coagulation and fibrinolysis in primary biliary cirrhosis compared with other liver disease and during orthotopic liver transplantation. *Hepatology.* 1997;25:683.
149. El-Masry M, Puig CA, Saab S. Recurrence of non-viral liver disease after orthotopic liver transplantation. *Liver Int.* 2011;31:291.
150. Mcgill JM, Kwiatkowski AP. Cholestatic liver diseases in adults. *Am J Gastroenterol.* 1998;93:684.
151. Anonymous. Viral hepatitis statistics & surveillance. 2009. http://www.cdc.gov/hepatitis/Statistics/. Accessed December 20, 2011; 2011.
152. El-Serag HB. Hepatocellular carcinoma. *N Engl J Med.* 2011;365:1118.
153. Benvegnu L, Fattovich G, Noventa F, et al. Concurrent hepatitis B and C virus infection and risk of hepatocellular carcinoma in cirrhosis. A prospective study. *Cancer.* 1994;74:2442.
154. Fattovich G, Stroffolini T, Zagni I, et al. Hepatocellular carcinoma in cirrhosis: Incidence and risk factors. *Gastroenterology.* 2004;127:S35.
155. Bruix J, Sherman M. Management of hepatocellular carcinoma: An update. *Hepatology.* 2011;53:1020.
156. Bruix J, Sherman M. Management of hepatocellular carcinoma. *Hepatology.* 2005; 42:1208.
157. Mazzaferro V, Bhoori S, Sposito C, et al. Milan criteria in liver transplantation for hepatocellular carcinoma: An evidence-based analysis of 15 years of experience. *Liver Transpl.* 2011;17(suppl 2):S44.
158. Browning JD, Szczepaniak LS, Dobbins R, et al. Prevalence of hepatic steatosis in an urban population in the United States: Impact of ethnicity. *Hepatology.* 2004;40:1387.
159. Vernon G, Baranova A, Younossi ZM. Systematic review: The epidemiology and natural history of non-alcoholic fatty liver disease and non-alcoholic steatohepatitis in adults. *Aliment Pharmacol Ther.* 2011;34:274.
160. Ratziu V, Bellentani S, Cortez-Pinto H, et al. A position statement on NAFLD/NASH based on the EASL 2009 Special Conference. *J Hepatol.* 2010;53:372.
161. Torres DM, Harrison SA. Diagnosis and therapy of nonalcoholic steatohepatitis. *Gastroenterology.* 2008;134:1682.
162. Mummadi RR, Kasturi KS, Chennareddygari S, et al. Effect of bariatric surgery on nonalcoholic fatty liver disease: Systematic review and meta-analysis. *Clin Gastroenterol Hepatol.* 2008;6:1396.
163. Kundrotas LW, Clement DJ. Serum alanine aminotransferase (alt) elevation in asymptomatic us air force basic trainee blood donors. *Dig Dis Sci.* 1993;38: 2145.
164. Schemel WH. Unexpected hepatic dysfunction found by multiple laboratory screening. *Anesth Analg.* 1976;55:810.
165. Pratt DS, Kaplan MM. Primary care: Evaluation of abnormal liver-enzyme results in asymptomatic patients. *N Engl J Med.* 2000;342:1266.
166. Powell-Jackson P, Greenway B, Williams R. Adverse effects of exploratory laparotomy in patients with unsuspected liver disease. *Br J Surg.* 1982;69:449.
167. Rizvon MK, Chou CL. Surgery in the patient with liver disease. *Med Clin North Am.* 2003;87:211.
168. Friedman LS. Surgery in the patient with liver disease. *Trans Am Clin Climatol Assoc.* 2010;121:192.
169. Aranha GV, Sontag SJ, Greenlee HB. Cholecystectomy in cirrhotic patients: A formidable operation. *Am J Surg.* 1982;143:55.
170. Doberneck RC, Sterling WA Jr, Allison DC. Morbidity and mortality after operation in nonbleeding cirrhotic patients. *Am J Surg.* 1983;146:306.
171. Garrison RN, Cryer HM, Howard DA, et al. Clarification of risk factors for abdominal operations in patients with hepatic cirrhosis. *Ann Surg.* 1984;199:648.
172. Mansour A, Watson W, Shayani V, et al. Abdominal operations in patients with cirrhosis: Still a major surgical challenge. *Surgery.* 1997;122:730.
173. Malinchoc M, Kamath PS, Gordon FD, et al. A model to predict poor survival in patients undergoing transjugular intrahepatic portosystemic shunts. *Hepatology.* 2000;31:864.
174. Freeman RB Jr, Wiesner RH, Harper A, et al. The new liver allocation system: Moving toward evidence-based transplantation policy. *Liver Transpl.* 2002;8:851.
175. Teh SH, Nagorney DM, Stevens SR, et al. Risk factors for mortality after surgery in patients with cirrhosis. *Gastroenterology.* 2007;132:1261.
176. Northup PG, Wanamaker RC, Lee VD, et al. Model for end-stage liver disease (MELD) predicts nontransplant surgical mortality in patients with cirrhosis. *Ann Surg.* 2005;242:244.
177. Viegas O, Stoelting RK. LDH5 changes after cholecystectomy or hysterectomy in patients receiving halothane, enflurane, or fentanyl. *Anesthesiology.* 1979;51:556.
178. Ziser A, Plevak DJ, Wiesner RH, et al. Morbidity and mortality in cirrhotic patients undergoing anesthesia and surgery. *Anesthesiology.* 1999;90:42.
179. Shaikh AR, Muneer A. Laparoscopic cholecystectomy in cirrhotic patients. *JSLS.* 2009;13:592.
180. Curro G, Iapichino G, Melita G, et al. Laparoscopic cholecystectomy in Child-Pugh class c cirrhotic patients. *JSLS.* 2005;9:311.
181. Yeh CN, Chen MF, Jan YY. Laparoscopic cholecystectomy in 226 cirrhotic patients. Experience of a single center in Taiwan. *Surg Endosc.* 2002;16:1583.
182. Puggioni A, Wong LL. A metaanalysis of laparoscopic cholecystectomy in patients with cirrhosis. *J Am Coll Surg.* 2003;197:921.
183. Azoulay D, Buabse F, Damiano I, et al. Neoadjuvant transjugular intrahepatic portosystemic shunt: A solution for extrahepatic abdominal operation in cirrhotic patients with severe portal hypertension. *J Am Coll Surg.* 2001;193:46.
184. Van Der Linden P, Le Moine O, Ghysels M, et al. Pulmonary hypertension after transjugular intrahepatic portosystemic shunt: Effects on right ventricular function. *Hepatology.* 1996;23:982.
185. Marik PE, Baram M, Vahid B. Does central venous pressure predict fluid responsiveness? A systematic review of the literature and the tale of seven mares. *Chest.* 2008;134:172.
186. Mansour N, Lentschener C, Ozier Y. Do we really need a low central venous pressure in elective liver resection. *Acta Anaesthesiol Scand.* 2008;52:1306.
187. Schroeder RA, Kuo PC. Pro: Low central venous pressure during liver transplantation–not too low. *J Cardiothorac Vasc Anesth.* 2008;22:311.
188. Niemann CU, Feiner J, Behrends M, et al. Central venous pressure monitoring during living right donor hepatectomy. *Liver Transpl.* 2007;13:266.
189. Spier BJ, Larue SJ, Teelin TC, et al. Review of complications in a series of patients with known gastro-esophageal varices undergoing transesophageal echocardiography. *J Am Soc Echocardiogr.* 2009;22:396.
190. Tripodi A. Tests of coagulation in liver disease. *Clin Liver Dis.* 2009;13:55.
191. Kennedy WF, Everett GB, Cobb LA, et al. Simultaneous systemic and hepatic hemodynamic measurements during high spinal anesthesia in normal man. *Anesth Analg.* 1970;49:1016.
192. Kennedy WF, Everett GB, Cobb LA, et al. Simultaneous systemic and hepatic hemodynamic measurements during high peridural anesthesia in normal man. *Anesth Analg.* 1971;50:1069.
193. Meierhenrich R, Wagner F, Schutz W, et al. The effects of thoracic epidural anesthesia on hepatic blood flow in patients under general anesthesia. *Anesth Analg.* 2009;108:1331.
194. Greitz T, Andreen M, Irestedt L. Effects of ephedrine on hemodynamics and oxygen-consumption in the dog during high epidural block with special reference to the splanchnic region. *Acta Anaesthesiol Scand.* 1984;28:557.
195. Tanaka N, Nagata N, Hamakawa T, et al. The effect of dopamine on hepatic blood flow in patients undergoing epidural anesthesia. *Anesth Analg.* 1997;85:286.
196. Hiltebrand LB, Krejci V, Sigurdsson GH. Effects of dopamine, dobutamine, and dopexamine on microcirculatory blood flow in the gastrointestinal tract during sepsis and anesthesia. *Anesthesiology.* 2004;100:1188.
197. Mcdonnell JG, O'donnell B, Curley G, et al. The analgesic efficacy of transversus abdominis plane block after abdominal surgery: A prospective randomized controlled trial. *Anesth Analg.* 2007;104:193.
198. Niraj G, Kelkar A, Jeyapalan I, et al. Comparison of analgesic efficacy of subcostal transversus abdominis plane blocks with epidural analgesia following upper abdominal surgery. *Anaesthesia.* 2011;66:465.
199. Gerges FJ, Shulman MS. Abdominal wall haematoma: An unusual complication of ultrasound guided transversus abdominis plane block. *Anaesthesia.* 2011;66:10.
200. Frink EJ Jr. The hepatic effects of sevoflurane. *Anesth Analg.* 1995;81:S46.

201. Schindler E, Muller M, Zickmann B, et al. [Blood supply to the liver in the human after 1 mac desflurane in comparison with isoflurane and halothane]. *Anasthesiol Intensivmed Notfallmed Schmerzther.* 1996;31:344.
202. Hartman JC, Pagel PS, Proctor LT, et al. Influence of desflurane, isoflurane and halothane on regional tissue perfusion in dogs. *Can J Anaesth.* 1992;39:877.
203. Matsumoto N, Koizumi M, Sugai M. Hepatolobectomy-induced depression of hepatic circulation and metabolism in the dog is counteracted by isoflurane, but not by halothane. *Acta Anaesthesiol Scand.* 1999;43:850.
204. Crawford MW, Lerman J, Saldivia V, et al. Hemodynamic and organ blood flow responses to halothane and sevoflurane anesthesia during spontaneous ventilation. *Anesth Analg.* 1992;75:1000.
205. Mclaughlin DF, Eger EI. Repeated isoflurane anesthesia in a patient with hepatic-dysfunction. *Anesth Analg.* 1984;63:775.
206. Lewis JH, Zimmerman HJ, Ishak KG, et al. Enflurane hepatotoxicity - a clinicopathologic study of 24 cases. *Ann Intern Med.* 1983;98:984.
207. Martin JL. Volatile anesthetics and liver injury: A clinical update or what every anesthesiologist should know. *Can J Anaesth.* 2005;52:125.
208. Obata R, Bito H, Ohmura M, et al. The effects of prolonged low-flow sevoflurane anesthesia on renal and hepatic function. *Anesth Analg.* 2000;91:1262.
209. Bedirli N, Ofluoglu E, Kerem M, et al. Hepatic energy metabolism and the differential protective effects of sevoflurane and isoflurane anesthesia in a rat hepatic ischemia-reperfusion injury model. *Anesth Analg.* 2008;106:830.
210. Lehmann A, Neher M, Kiessling AH, et al. Case report: Fatal hepatic failure after aortic valve replacement and sevoflurane exposure. *Can J Anaesth.* 2007;54:917.
211. Prys-Roberts C, Sear JW, Low JM, et al. Hemodynamic and hepatic effects of methohexital infusion during nitrous oxide anesthesia in humans. *Anesth Analg.* 1983;62:317.
212. Zinn SE, Fairley HB, Glenn JD. Liver function in patients with mild alcoholic hepatitis, after enflurane, nitrous oxide-narcotic, and spinal anesthesia. *Anesth Analg.* 1985;64:487.
213. Nunn JF. Clinical aspects of the interaction between nitrous oxide and vitamin B12. *Br J Anaesth.* 1987;59:3.
214. Parke TJ, Stevens JE, Rice AS, et al. Metabolic acidosis and fatal myocardial failure after propofol infusion in children: Five case reports. *BMJ.* 1992;305:613.
215. Otterspoor LC, Kalkman CJ, Cremer OL. Update on the propofol infusion syndrome in ICU management of patients with head injury. *Curr Opin Anaesthesiol.* 2008;21:544.
216. Thompson DR. Narcotic analgesic effects on the sphincter of Oddi: A review of the data and therapeutic implications in treating pancreatitis. *Am J Gastroenterol.* 2001;96:1266.
217. Trouvin JH, Farinotti R, Haberer JP, et al. Pharmacokinetics of midazolam in anesthetized cirrhotic-patients. *Br J Anaesth.* 1988;60:762.
218. Macgilchrist AJ, Birnie GG, Cook A, et al. Pharmacokinetics and pharmacodynamics of intravenous midazolam in patients with severe alcoholic cirrhosis. *Gut.* 1986;27:190.
219. Susla GM, Atkinson AJ. *Principles of Clinical Pharmacology.* 2nd ed. New York, NY: Elsevier; 2007;73–87.
220. Pandele G, Chaux F, Salvadori C, et al. Thiopental pharmacokinetics in patients with cirrhosis. *Anesthesiology.* 1983;59:123.
221. Tegeder I, Lotsch J, Geisslinger G. Pharmacokinetics of opioids in liver disease. *Clin Pharmacokinet.* 1999;37:17.
222. Servin F, Desmonts JM, Haberer JP, et al. Pharmacokinetics and protein-binding of propofol in patients with cirrhosis. *Anesthesiology.* 1988;69:887.
223. Baughman VL, Cunningham FE, Layden T, et al. Pharmacokinetic/pharmacodynamic effects of dexmedetomidine in patients with hepatic failure. *Anesth Analg.* 2000;90:U231.
224. Hunter JM, Parker CJ, Bell CF, et al. The use of different doses of vecuronium in patients with liver dysfunction. *Br J Anaesth.* 1985;57:758.
225. Magorian T, Wood P, Caldwell J, et al. The pharmacokinetics and neuromuscular effects of rocuronium bromide in patients with liver disease. *Anesth Analg.* 1995;80:754.
226. Fodale V, Santamaria LB. Laudanosine, an atracurium and cisatracurium metabolite. *Eur J Anaesthesiol.* 2002;19:466.
227. Cahill PA. Vasoconstrictor responsiveness of portal hypertensive vessels. *Clin Sci.* 1999;96:3.
228. Cahill PA, Redmond EM, Sitzmann JV. Endothelial dysfunction in cirrhosis and portal hypertension. *Pharmacol Ther.* 2001;89:273.
229. Alves De Mattos A. Current indications for the use of albumin in the treatment of cirrhosis. *Ann Hepatol.* 2011;10(suppl 1):S15.
230. Terg R, Gadano A, Cartier M, et al. Serum creatinine and bilirubin predict renal failure and mortality in patients with spontaneous bacterial peritonitis: A retrospective study. *Liver Int.* 2009;29:415.
231. Ortega R, Gines P, Uriz J, et al. Terlipressin therapy with and without albumin for patients with hepatorenal syndrome: Results of a prospective, nonrandomized study. *Hepatology.* 2002;36:941.
232. Quiroga J, Sangro B, Nunez M, et al. Transjugular intrahepatic portal-systemic shunt in the treatment of refractory ascites: Effect on clinical, renal, humoral, and hemodynamic parameters. *Hepatology.* 1995;21:986.
233. Sicklick JK, D'Angelica M, Fong Y. The Liver, pp1411–1475, In: Townsend: Sabiston Textbook of Surgery, 19th ed. Philadelphia, PA: Elsevier Saunders; 2012.
234. Fortner JG, Blumgart LH. A historic perspective of liver surgery for tumors at the end of the millennium. *J Am Coll Surg.* 2001;193:210.
235. Jarnagin WR, Gonen M, Fong Y, et al. Improvement in perioperative outcome after hepatic resection: Analysis of 1,803 consecutive cases over the past decade. *Ann Surg.* 2002;236:397.
236. Franco D. Liver surgery has become simpler. *Eur J Anaesthesiol.* 2002;19:777.
237. Lentschener C, Ozier Y. Anaesthesia for elective liver resection: Some points should be revisited. *Eur J Anaesthesiol.* 2002;19:780.
238. Clavien PA, Petrowsky H, Deoliveira ML, et al. Strategies for safer liver surgery and partial liver transplantation. *N Engl J Med.* 2007;356:1545.
239. Lentschener C, Benhamou D, Mercier FJ, et al. Aprotinin reduces blood loss in patients undergoing elective liver resection. *Anesth Analg.* 1997;84:875.
240. Jones RM, Moulton CE, Hardy KJ. Central venous pressure and its effect on blood loss during liver resection. *Br J Surg.* 1998;85:1058.
241. Wang W-D, Liang L-J, Huang X-Q, et al. Low central venous pressure reduces blood loss in hepatectomy. *World J Gastroenterol.* 2006;12:935.
242. Melendez JA, Arslan V, Fischer ME, et al. Perioperative outcomes of major hepatic resections under low central venous pressure anesthesia: Blood loss, blood transfusion, and the risk of postoperative renal dysfunction. *J Am Coll Surg.* 1998;187:620.
243. Stephan F, Rezaiguia-Delclaux S. Usefulness of a central venous catheter during hepatic surgery. *Acta Anaesthesiol Scand.* 2008;52:388.
244. Hoftman N, Braunfeld M, Hoftman G, et al. Peripheral venous pressure as a predictor of central venous pressure during orthotopic liver transplantation. *J Clin Anesth.* 2006;18:251.
245. Kim YK, Chin JH, Kang SJ, et al. Association between central venous pressure and blood loss during hepatic resection in 984 living donors. *Acta Anaesthesiol Scand.* 2009;53:601.
246. Chhibber A, Dziak J, Kolano J, et al. Anesthesia care for adult live donor hepatectomy: Our experiences with 100 cases. *Liver Transpl.* 2007;13:537.
247. Massicotte L, Perrault MA, Denault AY, et al. Effects of phlebotomy and phenylephrine infusion on portal venous pressure and systemic hemodynamics during liver transplantation. *Transplantation.* 2010;89:920.
248. Belghiti J, Noun R, Zante E, et al. Portal triad clamping or hepatic vascular exclusion for major liver resection - a controlled study. *Ann Surg.* 1996;224:155.
249. Belghiti J, Noun R, Malafosse R, et al. Continuous versus intermittent portal triad clamping for liver resection: A controlled study. *Ann Surg.* 1999;229:369.
250. Torzilli G, Makuuchi M, Inoue K. The vascular control in liver resection: Revisitation of a controversial issue. *Hepatogastroenterology.* 2002;49:28.
251. Petrowsky H, Mccormack L, Trujillo M, et al. A prospective, randomized, controlled trial comparing intermittent portal triad clamping versus ischemic preconditioning with continuous clamping for major liver resection. *Ann Surg.* 2006;244:921.
252. Giordano C, Deitte LA, Gravenstein N, et al. What is the preferred central venous pressure zero reference for hepatic resection? *Anesth Analg.* 2010;111:660.
253. Evans C, Evans M, Pollock AV. The incidence and causes of postoperative jaundice. A prospective study. *Br J Anaesth.* 1974;46:520.
254. Ebert TJ, Frink EJ Jr, Kharasch ED. Absence of biochemical evidence for renal and hepatic dysfunction after 8 hours of 1.25 minimum alveolar concentration sevoflurane anesthesia in volunteers. *Anesthesiology.* 1998;88:601.
255. Ebert TJ, Messana LD, Uhrich TD, et al. Absence of renal and hepatic toxicity after four hours of 1.25 minimum alveolar anesthetic concentration sevoflurane anesthesia in volunteers. *Anesth Analg.* 1998;86:662.
256. Bito H, Ikeda K. Renal and hepatic function in surgical patients after low-flow sevoflurane or isoflurane anesthesia. *Anesth Analg.* 1996;82:173.
257. Suttner SW, Schmidt CC, Boldt J, et al. Low-flow desflurane and sevoflurane anesthesia minimally affect hepatic integrity and function in elderly patients. *Anesth Analg.* 2000;91:206.
258. Gelman SI. Disturbances in hepatic blood flow during anesthesia and surgery. *Arch Surg.* 1976;111:881.
259. Seltzer JL, Goldberg ME, Larijani GE, et al. Prostacyclin mediation of vasodilation following mesenteric traction. *Anesthesiology.* 1988;68:514.
260. Belghiti J, Hiramatsu K, Benoist S, et al. Seven hundred forty-seven hepatectomies in the 1990s: An update to evaluate the actual risk of liver resection. *J Am Coll Surg.* 2000;191:38.
261. Dixon JM, Armstrong CP, Duffy SW, et al. Factors affecting morbidity and mortality after surgery for obstructive jaundice: A review of 373 patients. *Gut.* 1983;24:845.
262. Wait RB, Kahng KU. Renal failure complicating obstructive jaundice. *Am J Surg.* 1989;157:256.
263. Kramer HJ. Impaired renal function in obstructive jaundice: Roles of the thromboxane and endothelin systems. *Nephron.* 1997;77:1.
264. Klemperer JD, Ko W, Krieger KH, et al. Cardiac operations in patients with cirrhosis. *Ann Thorac Surg.* 1998;65:85.
265. Filsoufi F, Salzberg SP, Rahmanian PB, et al. Early and late outcome of cardiac surgery in patients with liver cirrhosis. *Liver Transpl.* 2007;13:990.
266. Abramov D, Tamariz MG, Fremes SE, et al. Trends in coronary artery bypass surgery results: A recent, 9-year study. *Ann Thorac Surg.* 2000;70:84.

CHAPTER

46 Endocrine Function

JEFFREY J. SCHWARTZ • SHAMSUDDIN AKHTAR • STANLEY H. ROSENBAUM

Key Points

1. The major risk of anesthesia in the poorly controlled thyrotoxic patient is thyroid storm, which must be aggressively treated with β-blockers, iodide, and antithyroid drugs.
2. Asymptomatic or mild hypothyroidism does not appear to significantly increase anesthetic risk and is not a contraindication to surgery. Moderate to severe hypothyroidism should be corrected before surgery to prevent multisystem complications.
3. Patients who have received corticosteroids for >1 week in the past year may have adrenal suppression and should receive supplemental steroids in the perioperative period.
4. Preoperative preparation of the pheochromocytoma patient with α-blockers decreases intraoperative hemodynamic instability.
5. Pheochromocytoma manipulation is associated with severe hypertension that should be treated aggressively with nitroprusside, phentolamine, or other rapidly acting vasodilators.
6. The major perioperative risks to the diabetic patient come from coexisting disease, especially coronary artery disease. Coexisting disease must be aggressively sought and optimized.
7. Very tight control of perioperative blood glucose levels appears to increase the risk of hypoglycemic complications without clearly reducing the risk of hyperglycemic complications.
8. Endotracheal intubation may be unpredictably difficult in patients with acromegaly.

Multimedia

1. NIM Thyroid
2. Vitamin D Metabolism
3. Catecholamines
4. Metabolism of Endogenous Catecholamines

THYROID GLAND

The thyroid gland secretes thyroid hormones, thyroxine (T_4), and 3,3′,5-triiodothyronine (T_3), which are the major regulators of cellular metabolic activity. Thyroid hormones exert a variety of actions by regulating the synthesis and activity of various proteins. They are necessary for proper cardiac, pulmonary, and neurologic function during both health and illness.

Thyroid Metabolism and Function

The production of thyroid hormone is initiated by the active uptake and concentration of iodide in the thyroid gland (Fig. 46-1). Dietary iodine is reduced to iodide in the gastrointestinal (GI) tract. Circulating iodide is taken up by the thyroid gland, where it is then bound to tyrosine residues to form various iodotyrosines. After organification, monoiodotyrosine or diiodotyrosine is coupled enzymatically by thyroid peroxidase to form either T_3 or T_4. These hormones are attached to the thyroglobulin protein and stored as colloid in the gland. The release of T_3 and T_4 from the gland is accomplished through proteolysis from the thyroglobulin and diffusion into the circulation. Thyrotropin (thyroid-stimulating hormone [TSH]) is produced in the anterior pituitary gland, and its secretion is regulated by thyrotropin-releasing hormone produced in the hypothalamus. TSH is responsible for maintaining the uptake of iodide and proteolytic release of thyroid hormone. Excess iodide inhibits the synthesis and secretion of thyroid hormone. Circulating thyroid hormone inhibits thyroid-releasing hormone and TSH secretion in a negative-feedback loop. The thyroid gland is solely responsible for the daily secretion of T_4 (80 to 100 μg/day). The half-life of T_4 in the circulation is 6 to 7 days.

Approximately 80% of T_3 is produced by the extrathyroidal deiodination of T_4 and 20% is produced by direct thyroid secretion. The half-life of T_3 is 24 to 30 hours. Most of the effects of thyroid hormones are mediated by the more potent and less protein-bound T_3. The degree to which these hormones are protein bound in the circulation is the major factor influencing their activity and degradation. T_4 is metabolized by monodeiodination to either T_3 or reverse T_3 (rT_3). T_3 is biologically active, whereas rT_3 is inactive. The major fraction of circulating hormone is bound to thyroxine-binding globulin (TBG), with a smaller fraction bound to albumin and transthyretin. Less than 0.1% is present as free, unbound hormone. Changes in serum-binding protein concentrations have a major effect on total T_3 and T_4 serum concentrations. The plasma normally contains 5 to 12 μg/dL of T_4 and 60 to 180 ng/dL of T_3. Many drugs can affect thyroid function, including amiodarone and dopamine.[1]

Although the thyroid hormone is important to many aspects of growth and function, the anesthesiologist is most often concerned with the cardiovascular manifestations of thyroid disease.[2] Thyroid hormones affect tissue responses to sympathetic stimuli and increase the intrinsic contractile state of cardiac muscle.

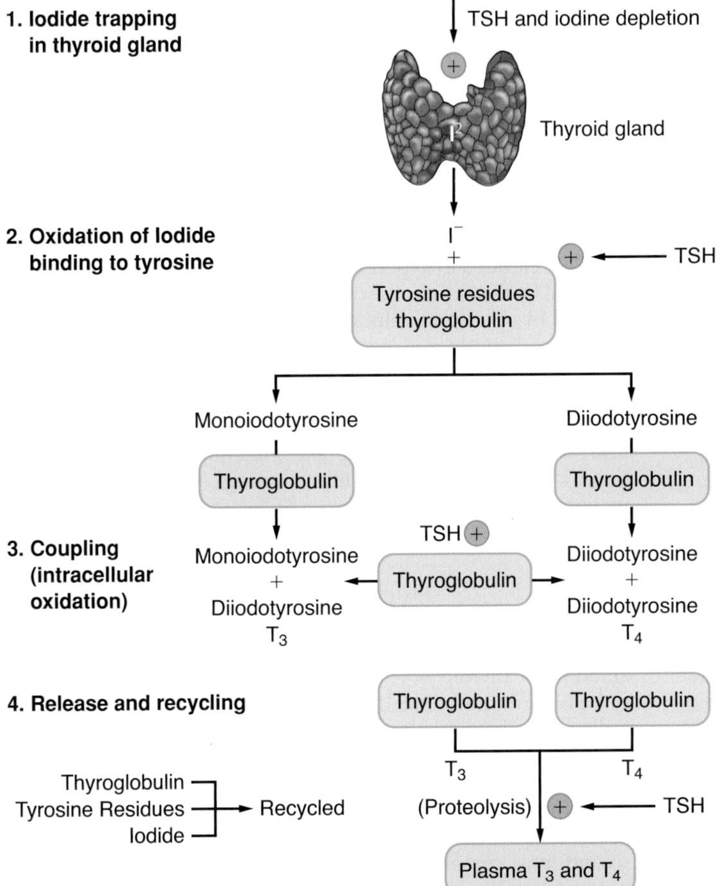

FIGURE 46-1. Thyroid hormone biosynthesis consists of four stages: (1) organification, (2) binding, (3) coupling, and (4) release. TSH, thyroid-stimulating hormone; T_3, triiodothyronine; T_4, thyroxine.

TABLE 46-1. TESTS OF THYROID GLAND FUNCTION

	T_4	T_3	THBR	TSH
Hyperthyroidism	Elevated	Elevated	Elevated	Normal or low
Primary hypothyroidism	Low	Low or normal	Low	Elevated
Secondary hypothyroidism	Low	Low	Low	Low
Sick euthyroidism (decreased peripheral conversion of T_4 to T_3)	Normal	Low	Normal	Normal
Pregnancy	Elevated	Normal	Low	Normal

T_4, total serum thyroxine; T_3, serum triiodothyronine; THBR, thyroid hormone binding rate; TSH, thyroid-stimulating hormone.

β-adrenergic receptors are increased in number, and cardiac α-adrenergic receptors are decreased by thyroid hormone.[3]

Tests of Thyroid Function

Serum Thyroxine

The serum T_4 assay is a standard test for evaluation of thyroid gland function (Table 46-1). The total T_4 is elevated in approximately 90% of patients with hyperthyroidism, and it is low in 85% of those who are hypothyroid. The concentration of T_4 is measured by radioimmunoassay (RIA). The serum T_4 concentration is influenced by thyroid hormone protein–binding capacity. An increase or decrease in TBG levels or in protein binding may therefore alter the total T_4 but not the concentration of the free T_4. Because of the effect of TBG on circulating total T_4, the T_4 levels should never be used alone to evaluate thyroid disease. Elevations in the TBG concentration are the most common cause of hyperthyroxinemia in euthyroid patients. Increases in TBG due to acute liver disease, pregnancy, or drugs (oral contraceptives, exogenous estrogens, clofibrate, opioids) may be the causative factor. Because a total T_4 can be misleadingly high in euthyroidism or normal in hypothyroidism, some measure of free thyroid hormone activity (free T_4) must also be used.

Serum Triiodothyronine

The serum T_3 is also measured by RIA. Serum T_3 levels are often determined to detect disease in patients with clinical evidence of hyperthyroidism in the absence of elevations of T_4. T_3 may be the only thyroid hormone produced in excess. T_3 concentrations may be depressed by factors that impair the peripheral conversion of T_4 to T_3 (sick euthyroid syndrome). In 50% of hypothyroid patients, the serum T_3 concentration is low; in the remaining 50%, it is normal.

Tests for Assessing Thyroid Hormone Binding

Because conventional assays measure total hormone levels, which can be affected by protein binding without affecting free hormone levels, it is necessary to find some measure of thyroid-binding proteins to correctly interpret total thyroxine levels. A direct measurement of unbound T_3 and T_4 can be performed by equilibrium dialysis or by unbound immunoassays. Indirect measurement of free hormone levels can be calculated by multiplying the total hormone level by the thyroid hormone binding ratio, which can be calculated from the T_3-resin uptake. This product is the free T_3 or T_4 index. The T_3 uptake test measures the ability of the patient's serum to bind exogenously introduced T_3 and reflects the amount of TBG and the extent of T_3 saturation on TBG. The T_3 uptake is inversely related to the degree of unsaturation of TBG.

Thyroid-Stimulating Hormone

The radioimmunoassay for this hormone is sensitive and specific enough to become the first test in evaluating suspected thyroid dysfunction. It is often higher than 20 μIU/mL in primary hypothyroidism (normal 0.4 to 4.5 μIU/mL). Hyperthyroidism can be suspected from depressed TSH levels. A condition characterized by elevated TSH and normal T_4 may represent subclinical hypothyroidism. A low TSH level in a clinically hypothyroid patient indicates disease at the pituitary or hypothalamic level. The goal of thyroid replacement therapy is to normalize TSH levels.[3] Starvation, fever, stress, corticosteroids, and T_3 or T_4 can all depress TSH levels.

Radioactive Iodine Uptake

The thyroid gland has the ability to concentrate large amounts of inorganic iodide. The oral administration of radioactive iodine (^{131}I) can be used to indicate thyroid gland activity. Thyroid uptake is elevated in hyperthyroidism unless the hyperthyroidism is caused by thyroiditis, in which case the uptake is low or absent. Because of overlap in values, it is difficult to distinguish euthyroid from hypothyroid people. Radioactive iodide uptake may be increased by a variety of factors, including dietary iodine deficiency, renal failure, and congestive heart failure. Because uptake is under TSH control, elevated free T_4 levels and corticosteroids decrease radioactive iodide uptake. Functioning ("hot") thyroid tissue is rarely malignant. Nonfunctioning ("cold") tissue may be malignant or benign.

Hyperthyroidism

Hyperthyroidism results from the exposure of tissues to excessive amounts of thyroid hormone (Table 46-2). The most common cause is the multinodular diffuse goiter of Graves disease. This typically occurs between the ages of 20 and 40 years and is predominant in women. Most patients with this condition demonstrate a syndrome characterized by diffuse glandular enlargement, ophthalmopathy, dermopathy, and clubbing of the fingers. A thyroid-stimulating autoantibody may be present. Thyroid adenoma is the second most common cause. Another cause of increased thyroid hormone synthesis is thyroiditis. Subacute thyroiditis frequently

TABLE 46-2. CAUSES OF HYPERTHYROIDISM

Intrinsic thyroid disease
Hyperfunctioning thyroid adenoma
Toxic multinodular goiter
Abnormal TSH stimulator
Graves disease
Trophoblastic tumor
Disorders of hormone storage or release
Thyroiditis
Excess production of TSH
Pituitary thyrotropin (rare)
Extrathyroidal source of hormone
Struma ovarii
Functioning follicular carcinoma
Exogenous thyroid
Iatrogenic
Iodine induced

TSH, thyroid-stimulating hormone.

follows a respiratory illness and is characterized by a viral-like illness with a firm, painful gland. This type of thyroiditis is frequently treated with anti-inflammatory agents alone. Rarely, subacute thyroiditis may occur in a patient with a normal-sized painless gland. Hashimoto thyroiditis is a chronic autoimmune disease that usually produces hypothyroidism but may occasionally produce hyperthyroidism. Hyperthyroidism may also be associated with pregnancy, ^{131}I therapy, thyroid carcinoma, trophoblastic tumors, or TSH-secreting pituitary adenomas. Iatrogenic hyperthyroidism may follow thyroid hormone replacement or may occur after iodide exposure (angiographic contrast media) in patients with chronically low iodide intake (Jod-Basedow phenomenon). The antiarrhythmic agent amiodarone is iodine rich and is another cause of iodine-induced thyrotoxicosis.[4]

The major manifestations of hyperthyroidism are weight loss, diarrhea, skeletal muscle weakness and stiffness, warm and moist skin, heat intolerance, and nervousness. Cardiovascular manifestations include increased left ventricular contractility and ejection fraction, tachycardia, elevated systolic blood pressure, and decreased diastolic blood pressure. Hypercalcemia, thrombocytopenia, and a mild anemia may be present. Elderly patients may present with heart failure, atrial fibrillation, or other cardiac dysrhythmias. They may also present with apathetic hyperthyroidism characterized by depression and withdrawal, without the usual systemic signs or symptoms.

Treatment and Anesthetic Considerations

The most important goal in managing the hyperthyroid patient is to make the patient euthyroid before any surgery, if possible. The drugs propylthiouracil and methimazole are thiourea derivatives that inhibit organification of iodide and the synthesis of thyroid hormone.[5] Propylthiouracil also decreases the peripheral conversion of T_4 to T_3. Normal thyroid glands usually contain a store of hormone that is large enough to maintain a euthyroid state for several months, even if synthesis is abolished. Therefore, hyperthyroid patients are unlikely to be regulated to a euthyroid state with antithyroid drugs alone in <6 to 8 weeks. Toxic reactions from these drugs are uncommon but include skin rash, nausea, fever, agranulocytosis, hepatitis, and arthralgias.

Inorganic iodide inhibits iodide organification and thyroid hormone release—the Wolff-Chaikoff effect. Iodide is also effective in reducing the size of the hyperplastic gland and has a role in the preparation of the patient for emergency thyroid surgery. Antithyroid drugs should be started before iodide treatment because of the possibility of worsening the thyrotoxicosis.

β-adrenergic antagonists are effective in attenuating the manifestations of excessive sympathetic activity and should be used in all hyperthyroid patients unless contraindicated. β-adrenergic blockade alone does not inhibit hormone synthesis, but specifically propranolol does impair the peripheral conversion of T_4 to T_3 over 1 to 2 weeks. Propranolol given over 12 to 24 hours decreases tachycardia, heat intolerance, anxiety, and tremor. Any β-blocker may be used, and long-acting agents may be more convenient. The combination of propranolol (in doses titrated to effect) plus potassium iodide (2 to 5 drops every 8 hours) is frequently used before surgery to ameliorate cardiovascular symptoms and reduce circulating concentrations of T_4 and T_3. Preoperative preparation usually requires 7 to 14 days.

Heart failure secondary to poorly controlled paroxysmal atrial fibrillation may improve with slowing of the ventricular rate, but abnormalities of left ventricular function secondary to hyperthyroidism may not be corrected with the use of β-antagonists. If a hyperthyroid patient with clinically apparent disease requires emergency surgery, β-adrenergic blockade should be administered to achieve a heart rate <90 beats per minute. β-blockers do not prevent thyroid storm. Glucocorticoids such as dexamethasone (8 to 12 mg/day) are used in the management of severe thyrotoxicosis because they reduce thyroid hormone secretion and the peripheral conversion of T_4 to T_3.

Iopanoic acid, a radiographic contrast agent that decreases peripheral conversion of T_4 and releases iodine that inhibits synthesis, is useful for emergency preparation.

Radioactive iodine therapy is an effective treatment for some patients with thyrotoxicosis.[6] However, it should not be administered to patients who are pregnant because it crosses the placenta and may destroy the fetal thyroid. A side effect of radioiodine therapy is hypothyroidism; 10% to 60% of cases occur in the first year of therapy and an additional 2% occur per year thereafter.

A variety of anesthetic techniques and drugs have been used for hyperthyroid patients undergoing surgery. All antithyroid medications are continued through the morning of surgery. The goal of intraoperative management in the hyperthyroid patient is to achieve a depth of anesthesia that prevents an exaggerated sympathetic response to surgical stimulation while avoiding the administration of medication that stimulates the sympathetic nervous system. Pancuronium should be avoided. It is best to avoid using ketamine, even when a patient is clinically euthyroid. Hypotension that occurs during surgery is best treated with direct-acting vasopressors rather than a medication that provokes the release of catecholamines. The incidence of myasthenia gravis is increased in hyperthyroid patients; thus, the initial dose of muscle relaxant should be reduced and a twitch monitor should be used to titrate subsequent doses. Regional anesthesia is an excellent alternative when appropriate; however, epinephrine-containing solutions should be avoided.

1 Thyroid storm is a life-threatening exacerbation of hyperthyroidism that most commonly develops in the undiagnosed or untreated hyperthyroid patient because of the stress of surgery or nonthyroid illness.[7] Operating on an acutely hyperthyroid gland may provoke thyroid storm, although this is probably not due to mechanical release of hormone.[8] Its manifestations include hyperthermia, tachycardia, dysrhythmias, myocardial ischemia, congestive heart failure, agitation, and confusion. It must be distinguished from, or considered with, pheochromocytoma,

TABLE 46-3. MANAGEMENT OF THYROID STORM

Administer IV fluids
Administer sodium iodide, 250 mg PO or IV q6h
Administer propylthiouracil, 200–400 mg PO or via NGT q6h
Administer hydrocortisone, 50–100 mg IV q6h
Administer propranolol, 10–40 mg PO q4–6h, or esmolol infusion to treat hyperadrenergic signs
Cooling blankets and acetaminophen and meperidine (25–50 mg) IV q4–6h may be used to prevent shivering
Use digoxin for heart failure especially in the presence of atrial fibrillation with rapid ventricular response

IV, intravenous(ly); PO, oral(ly); NGT, nasogastric tube.

malignant hyperthermia, and light anesthesia. Although free T_4 levels are often markedly elevated, no laboratory test is diagnostic. Treatment involves large doses of propylthiouracil and supportive measures to control fever and restore intravascular volume. Hemodynamic monitoring (pulmonary artery catheter, arterial catheter) is especially useful in guiding the treatment of patients with significant left ventricular dysfunction (Table 46-3). Again, it is essential to remove or treat the precipitating event.

Anesthesia for Thyroid Surgery

Thyroidectomy as an alternative to prolonged medical therapy is used less frequently now than in the past. Indications include failed medical therapy, underlying cancer, and symptomatic goiter. It is usually performed under general endotracheal anesthesia, although the use of the laryngeal mask airway is increasing.[9] Use of a laryngeal mask airway allows real-time visualization of vocal cord function because the patient is allowed to breathe spontaneously. Limited thyroidectomy may also be performed under bilateral superficial cervical plexus block. The anesthesiologist must be prepared to manage an unexpected difficult intubation because the incidence of difficult intubation during goiter surgery is 5% to 8%.[10] Thyroid cancer increases the risk, but the size of the goiter is not predictive. Large goiters, especially if associated with evidence of significant airway obstruction or tracheal deviation, may warrant securing the airway while the patient is awake. Large substernal goiters can behave as anterior mediastinal masses and cause intrathoracic airway obstruction after induction of general anesthesia. Computed tomography (CT) or magnetic resonance imaging (MRI) should be reviewed. The complications after thyroidectomy include recurrent laryngeal nerve (RLN) damage, tracheal compression secondary to hematoma or tracheomalacia, and hypoparathyroidism. Hypoparathyroidism secondary to the inadvertent surgical removal of parathyroid glands is most frequently seen after total thyroidectomy. The symptoms of hypocalcemia develop within 24 to 96 hours after surgery[11] (see Chapter 14). Laryngeal stridor progressing to laryngospasm may be one of the first indications of hypocalcemic tetany. Intravenous administration of calcium chloride or calcium gluconate is warranted in this situation. Magnesium levels should also be monitored and corrected if low. Bilateral RLN injury is an extremely rare injury and necessitates reintubation. Unilateral nerve injury is more common and is often transient.[12] Unilateral damage to the RLN is characterized by hoarseness and a paralyzed vocal cord, whereas bilateral injury causes aphonia (see Chapter 27). It is wise to evaluate vocal cord function before and after surgery by laryngoscopy or by asking the patient to phonate by saying the sound for "E." Routine postoperative visualization of the vocal cords is not warranted. Some surgeons elect to monitor RLN function intraoperatively. A nerve stimulator may be used by the surgeon to stimulate suspicious structures and contraction of the laryngeal muscles noted. Alternatively, the NIM (Nerve Integrity Monitor; Medtronic Xomed) endotracheal tube can be used. This endotracheal tube has two pairs of electrodes embedded in the shaft of the endotracheal tube just above the cuff. When properly positioned, the electrodes will be in contact with the vocal cords and an electromyographic signal can be monitored. Muscle relaxants and topical laryngeal anesthesia must be avoided to obtain appropriate signals. Postoperative extubation of the trachea should be performed under optimal conditions. Intraoperative laryngeal nerve injury or collapse of the tracheal rings from previous weakening may mandate emergency reintubation.

Hypothyroidism

Hypothyroidism is a relatively common disease (0.3% to 5% of the adult population) that results from inadequate circulating levels of T_4 or T_3 or both.[13] The development of hypothyroidism is often slow and progressive, making the clinical diagnosis difficult, especially in more subtle cases. Hypofunctioning of the thyroid gland has many causes (Table 46-4). Primary failure of the thyroid gland refers to decreased production of thyroid hormone, despite adequate TSH production, and accounts for 95% of all cases of thyroid dysfunction. The remainder of the cases are caused by either hypothalamic or pituitary disease (secondary hypothyroidism) and are associated with other pituitary deficiencies.

A lack of thyroid hormone produces a variety of signs and symptoms. These early findings are often nonspecific and difficult to recognize. A history of radioiodine therapy, external neck irradiation, or the presence of a goiter is helpful in diagnosis. There is a generalized reduction in metabolic activity, resulting in lethargy, slow mental functioning, cold intolerance, and slow movements. The cardiovascular manifestations of hypothyroidism reflect the importance of thyroid hormone for myocardial contractility and catecholamine function. These patients exhibit bradycardia, decreased cardiac output, and increased peripheral resistance.[14] The accumulation of a cholesterol-rich pericardial fluid produces

TABLE 46-4. CAUSES OF HYPOTHYROIDISM

Primary hypothyroidism
Autoimmune
Irradiation to the neck
Previous ^{131}I therapy
Surgical removal
Thyroiditis (Hashimoto disease)
Severe iodine depletion
Medications (iodines, propylthiouracil, methimazole)
Hereditary defects in biosynthesis
Congenital defects in gland development
Secondary or tertiary hypothyroidism
Pituitary
Hypothalamic

Reproduced from Petersdorf RG, ed. *Harrison's principles of internal medicine.* 10th ed. New York: McGraw-Hill; 1983, with permission.

low voltage on the electrocardiogram (ECG). Heart failure only rarely occurs in the absence of coexisting heart disease. Angina pectoris itself is unusual in hypothyroidism but can appear when thyroid hormone treatment is initiated. Ventilatory responsiveness to hypoxia and hypercapnia is depressed in hypothyroid patients. This depression is potentiated by sedatives, opioids, and general anesthesia. Postoperative ventilatory failure requiring prolonged ventilation is rarely seen in hypothyroid patients in the absence of coexisting lung disease, obesity, or myxedema coma. Other abnormalities found in hypothyroidism include anemia, coagulopathy, hypothermia, sleep apnea, and impaired renal free water clearance with hyponatremia. Decreased GI motility can compound the effect of postoperative ileus. In long-standing or severe disease, the stress response may be blunted and adrenal depression may occur.

Treatment and Anesthetic Considerations

Treatment of symptomatic hypothyroidism is with hormone replacement therapy.[15] Controversy remains regarding the preoperative anesthetic management of the hypothyroid patient. Although it seems logical, given the multisystem effects of thyroid hormone, to recommend that all hypothyroid surgical candidates be restored to a euthyroid state before surgery, such a recommendation is, in general, based on individual case reports. There have been few controlled studies to support the position that most hypothyroid patients are unusually sensitive to anesthetic drugs, have prolonged recovery times, or have a higher incidence of cardiovascular instability or collapse.

No increase in serious complications in patients with mild or moderate hypothyroidism undergoing general anesthesia has been noted.[16] One study noted a higher incidence of intraoperative hypotension and postoperative GI and neuropsychiatric complications in mild and moderately hypothyroid patients undergoing noncardiac surgery, but still noted there were no compelling clinical reasons to postpone surgery in these patients.[17] Surgery in severely hypothyroid patients should be postponed when possible until these patients are at least partially treated.

The management of hypothyroid patients with symptomatic coronary artery disease has been a subject of particular controversy.[18] The need for thyroid hormone replacement therapy must be weighed against the risk of precipitating myocardial ischemia. Several studies and a literature review found no differences in the frequency of intraoperative or postoperative complications when mild or moderately hypothyroid patients underwent cardiac surgery. In symptomatic patients or unstable patients with cardiac ischemia, thyroid replacement should probably be delayed until after coronary revascularization.

2 There appears to be little reason to postpone elective surgery in patients who have mild or moderate hypothyroidism. However, thyroid replacement therapy is indicated for patients with severe hypothyroidism or myxedema coma and for pregnant patients who are hypothyroid. Untreated hypothyroidism in pregnant patients is associated with an increased incidence of spontaneous abortion and mental and physical abnormalities in the offspring.

A number of anesthetic medications have been used without difficulty in hypothyroid patients. Although ketamine has been proposed as the ideal induction agents, all intravenous induction agents have been used in the hypothyroid patient. The maintenance of anesthesia may be safely achieved with either intravenous or inhaled anesthetics. There appears to be little, if any, decrease in the minimum alveolar concentration for volatile agents. Regional anesthesia is a good choice in the hypothyroid patient, provided the intravascular volume is well maintained. Monitoring is directed toward the early recognition of hypotension, congestive heart failure, and hypothermia. Scrupulous attention should be paid to maintaining normal body temperature.

TABLE 46-5. MANAGEMENT OF MYXEDEMA

Tracheal intubation and controlled ventilation as needed
Levothyroxine, 200–300 μg IV over 5–10 min initially, and 100 μg IV q24h
Hydrocortisone, 100 mg IV, then 25 mg IV q6h
Fluid and electrolyte therapy as indicated by serum electrolytes
Cover to conserve body heat; no warming blankets

IV, intravenous(ly).

Myxedema coma represents a severe form of hypothyroidism characterized by stupor or coma, hypoventilation, hypothermia, hypotension, and hyponatremia. This is a medical emergency with a high mortality rate (25% to 50%) and, as such, requires aggressive therapy (Table 46-5). Only lifesaving surgery should proceed in the face of myxedema coma. Intravenous thyroid replacement is initiated as soon as the clinical diagnosis is made. An intravenous loading dose of T_4 (sodium levothyroxine, 200 to 300 μg) is given initially and followed by a maintenance dose of T_4, 50 to 200 μg/day intravenously.[19] Alternatively, T_3 may be used because it has a more rapid onset. Improvements in heart rate, blood pressure, and body temperature may occur within 24 hours. However, replacement therapy with either form of thyroid hormone may precipitate myocardial ischemia. There is also an increased likelihood of acute primary adrenal insufficiency in these patients, and they should receive stress doses of hydrocortisone. Steroid replacement continues until normal adrenal function can be confirmed.

PARATHYROID GLANDS

Calcium Physiology

The normal adult body contains approximately 1 to 2 kg of calcium (Ca^{2+}), of which 99% is in the skeleton.[20] Plasma calcium is present in three forms: (a) a protein-bound fraction (50%), (b) an ionized fraction (45%), and (c) a diffusible but nonionized fraction (5%) that is complexed with phosphate, bicarbonate, and citrate (see Chapter 14). This division is interesting because it is the ionized fraction that is physiologically active and homeostatically regulated. The normal total serum calcium concentration is 8.8 to 10.4 mg/dL. Albumin binds approximately 90% of the protein-bound fraction of calcium, and total serum Ca^{2+} consequently depends on albumin levels. In general, an increase or decrease in albumin of 1 g/dL is associated with a parallel change in total serum Ca^{2+} of 0.8 mg/dL. The serum ionized Ca^{2+} concentration is affected by temperature and blood pH through alterations in Ca^{2+} protein binding to albumin. Acidosis decreases protein binding (increases ionized Ca^{2+}), and alkalosis increases protein binding (decreases ionized Ca^{2+}). The concentration of free Ca^{2+} ion is of critical importance in regulating skeletal muscle contraction, coagulation, neurotransmitter release, endocrine secretion, and a variety of other cellular functions. As a consequence, the maintenance of serum Ca^{2+} concentration is subject

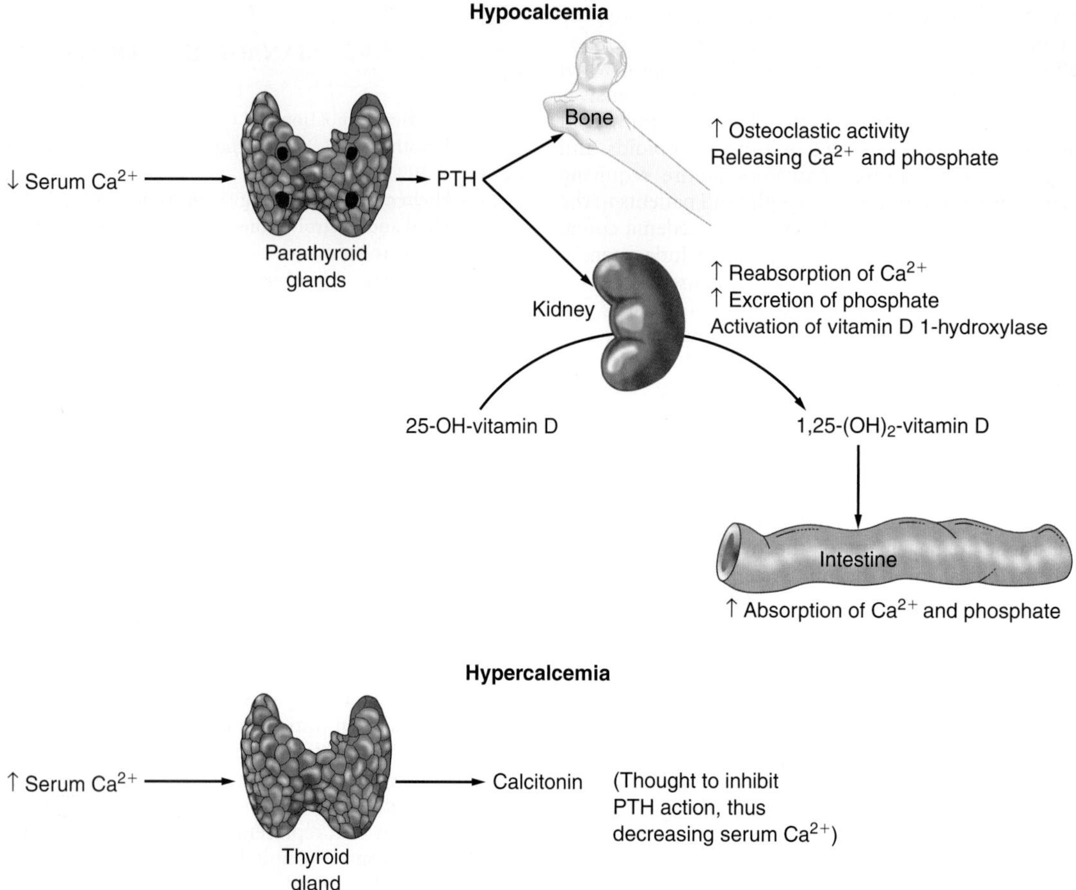

FIGURE 46-2. Parathyroid hormone (PTH) and vitamin D metabolism and action. 25-OH, 25-hydroxycholecalciferol; 1,25-$(OH)_2$, 1,25-dihydroxycholecalciferol. (From McClatchey KD. *Clinical laboratory medicine*. 2nd ed. Philadelphia, PA: Lippincott Williams & Wilkins; 2002.)

to tight hormonal control by parathyroid hormone (PTH) and vitamin D (Fig. 46-2).

PTH acts to maintain the extracellular fluid Ca^{2+} concentration through direct effects on bone resorption and renal Ca^{2+} resorption at the distal tubule and indirectly through its effects on the synthesis of 1,25-dihydroxyvitamin D. The renal effects of PTH include phosphaturia and bicarbonaturia, in addition to enhanced Ca^{2+} and magnesium resorption. Most evidence suggests that rapid changes in blood Ca^{2+} levels are primarily the result of hormonal effects on bone and, to a lesser extent, to renal Ca^{2+} clearance, whereas maintenance of overall Ca^{2+} balance depends more on the indirect effects of the hormone on intestinal calcium absorption.

PTH secretion is primarily regulated by the serum ionized Ca^{2+} concentration. This negative-feedback mechanism is exquisitely sensitive in maintaining calcium levels in a normal range. Release of PTH is also influenced by phosphate, magnesium, and catecholamine levels. Acute hypomagnesemia directly stimulates PTH release, whereas chronic magnesium depletion appears to inhibit proper functioning of the parathyroid gland. The plasma phosphate concentration has an indirect influence on PTH secretion by causing reciprocal changes in the serum ionized Ca^{2+} concentration.

Vitamin D is absorbed from the GI tract and can be produced enzymatically by ultraviolet irradiation of the skin. Vitamin D (cholecalciferol) is made from cholesterol metabolites and is inactive. Calciferol is hydroxylated in the liver to 25-hydroxycholecalciferol (25-OHD) and in the kidney is further hydroxylated to 1,25-dihydroxycholecalciferol [1,25$(OH)_2$D] or 24,25-dihydroxycholecalciferol [24,25$(OH)_2$D]. 25-OHD is the major circulating form of vitamin D. The synthesis of this hormone is not regulated by a hormone or by Ca^{2+} or phosphate levels. 1,25$(OH)_2$D and 24,25$(OH)_2$D are the major active metabolites of vitamin D, and their production is reciprocally regulated at the kidney. Hypocalcemia and hypophosphatemia cause an increased production of 1,25$(OH)_2$D and a decreased production of 24,25$(OH)_2$D. 1,25$(OH)_2$D stimulates bone, kidney, and intestinal absorption of calcium and phosphate. Vitamin D deficiency can lead to decreased intestinal absorption of Ca^{2+} and secondary hyperparathyroidism.

Hyperparathyroidism

Primary hyperparathyroidism is most commonly due to a benign parathyroid adenoma (90% of cases) or hyperplasia (9%) and very rarely to a parathyroid carcinoma.[21] Primary hyperparathyroidism may also exist as part of a multiple endocrine neoplastic (MEN) syndrome. Hyperplasia usually involves all four glands. Although most patients with primary hyperparathyroidism are hypercalcemic, most are asymptomatic at the time of diagnosis. When symptoms occur, they usually result from the hypercalcemia that accompanies the disease. Primary hyperparathyroidism occurring during pregnancy is associated with a high maternal and fetal morbidity rate (50%). The placenta allows the fetus to concentrate calcium, promoting fetal hypercalcemia and leading to hypoparathyroidism in the newborn. Pregnant women with primary hyperparathyroidism should generally be treated with surgery.

Hypercalcemia is responsible for a broad spectrum of signs and symptoms. Nephrolithiasis is the most common manifestation, occurring in 60% to 70% of patients. Polyuria and polydipsia are also common complaints. An increase in bone turnover may lead to generalized demineralization and subperiosteal bone resorption; however, only a small group of patients (10% to 15%) have clinically significant bone disease. Patients may experience generalized skeletal muscle weakness and fatigability, epigastric discomfort, peptic ulceration, and constipation. Psychiatric manifestations include depression, memory loss, confusion, or psychosis. Between 20% and 50% of patients are hypertensive, but this usually resolves with successful treatment of the disease. Cardiac function is enhanced in the early stages of hypercalcemia. Calcium flux into the cells is reflected in the plateau phase of the action potential (phase 2). As extracellular calcium increases, the inward flux is more rapid, and phase 2 is shortened (see Chapter 10). The corresponding ECG change is a shorter QT interval. Cardiac contractility may increase until a level between 15 and 20 mg/dL is reached. At this point, there is a prolongation of the PR segment and QRS complex that can result in heart block or bundle-branch block. Bradycardia also occurs.

An elevated serum Ca^{2+} concentration is a valuable diagnostic indicator of primary hyperparathyroidism. The serum phosphate concentration is nonspecific, with many patients having normal or near-normal levels. The reported incidence of hyperchloremic acidosis varies widely in primary hyperparathyroidism, but most patients usually have a serum chloride concentration in excess of 102 mEq/L. Rarely does a patient with hypercalcemia secondary to ectopic PTH production (malignancy) present with hyperchloremic acidosis. The definitive diagnosis of primary hyperparathyroidism is made by RIA demonstration of an elevation in PTH levels in the presence of hypercalcemia. An elevated nephrogenous cyclic adenosine monophosphate is noted in >90% of patients with primary hyperparathyroidism.

Hypercalcemia may also result from the ectopic production of PTH or PTH-like substances from lung, genitourinary, breast, GI, and lymphoproliferative malignancies. Tumors may also produce hypercalcemia through direct bone resorption or the production of osteoclast-activating factor. In the absence of a clinically obvious neoplasm, there may be difficulty in differentiating between PTH-producing malignancies and primary hyperparathyroidism. PTH fragments from malignant tissue differ from native PTH, so precise clinical identification may aid in distinguishing between ectopic PTH production and primary hyperparathyroidism.

Secondary hyperparathyroidism represents an increase in parathyroid function as a result of conditions that produce hypocalcemia or hyperphosphatemia. Chronic renal disease is a common cause of hyperphosphatemia (due to decreased phosphate excretion) and decreased vitamin D metabolism. The hypocalcemia that results leads to an increased production of PTH. GI disorders accompanied by malabsorption may also lead to a secondary increase in parathyroid activity. Tertiary hyperparathyroidism refers to the development of hypercalcemia in a patient who has had prolonged secondary hyperparathyroidism that has caused adenomatous changes in the parathyroid gland and unregulated PTH.

Treatment and Anesthetic Considerations

Surgery is the treatment of choice for the patient with symptomatic disease. However, there is considerable controversy surrounding the choice of treatment in the asymptomatic patient. It is not clear whether mild primary hyperparathyroidism decreases longevity. Surgery is often chosen over medical therapy because it offers definitive treatment and is generally safe.

Preoperative preparation focuses on the correction of intravascular volume and electrolyte irregularities. It is particularly important to evaluate the patient with chronic hypercalcemia for abnormalities of the renal, cardiac, or central nervous systems. Emergency treatment of hypercalcemia is undertaken before surgery when the serum Ca^{2+} concentration exceeds 15 mg/dL (7.5 mEq/L). Lowering of the serum Ca^{2+} concentration is initially accomplished by expanding the intravascular volume and establishing a sodium diuresis. This is achieved with the intravenous administration of normal saline and furosemide. Rehydration alone is capable of lowering the serum Ca^{2+} level by ≥2 mg/dL. Hydration dilutes the serum Ca^{2+}, and sodium diuresis promotes Ca^{2+} excretion through an inhibition of sodium and Ca^{2+} resorption in the proximal tubule. Hypokalemia and hypomagnesemia may result.

Another element in the treatment of hypercalcemia is the correction of hypophosphatemia. Hypophosphatemia increases GI absorption of Ca^{2+}, stimulates the breakdown of bone, and impairs the uptake of Ca^{2+} by bone. Low serum phosphate levels impair cardiac contractility and may contribute to congestive heart failure. Hypophosphatemia also causes skeletal muscle weakness, hemolysis, and platelet dysfunction.

Other medications that have a role in lowering the serum Ca^{2+} include bisphosphonates, mithramycin, calcitonin, and glucocorticoids. Bisphosphonates are pyrophosphate analogs that inhibit osteoclast action. They are the drugs of choice for severe hypercalcemia. Toxic effects include fever and hypophosphatemia. Mithramycin, a cytotoxic agent, inhibits PTH-induced osteoclast activity and can lower the serum Ca^{2+} levels by ≥2 mg/dL in 24 to 48 hours. Toxic effects include azotemia, hepatotoxicity, and thrombocytopenia. Calcitonin is useful in transiently lowering the serum Ca^{2+} level 2 to 4 mg/dL through direct inhibition of osteoclastic bone resorption. The advantages of calcitonin are the mild side effects (urticaria, nausea) and the rapid onset of activity. Calcitonin resistance usually develops within 24 to 48 hours. Glucocorticoids are effective in lowering the serum Ca^{2+} concentration in several conditions (sarcoidosis, some malignancies, hyperthyroidism, vitamin D intoxication) through their actions on osteoclast bone resorption, GI absorption of calcium, and the urinary excretion of calcium. Glucocorticoids are usually of no benefit in the treatment of primary hypercalcemia. Finally, hemodialysis or peritoneal dialysis can be used to lower the serum Ca^{2+} level when alternative regimens are ineffective or contraindicated.

There is no evidence that a specific anesthetic drug or technique has advantages over another. A thorough knowledge of the clinical manifestations attributable to hypercalcemia is of the greatest value in choosing an anesthetic technique. Special monitoring is usually not required. Because of the unpredictable response to neuromuscular blocking drugs in the hypercalcemic patient, a conservative approach to muscle paralysis makes sense. There is an increased requirement for vecuronium, and probably all nondepolarizing muscle relaxants, during onset of neuromuscular blockade.[22] Careful positioning of the osteopenic patient is necessary to avoid pathologic bone fractures.

Anesthesia for Parathyroid Surgery

General anesthesia is most commonly used for parathyroid surgery. Minimally invasive parathyroidectomy is superior to conventional bilateral cervical exploration in patients with sporadic primary hyperparathyroidism[23] and can usually be performed under bilateral cervical plexus block.[24] Some centers use an intraoperative rapid PTH assay to help determine when a hyperfunctioning gland has been removed. There is in vitro, but no clinical,[25] evidence that propofol can interfere with the assay, so many surgeons prefer that propofol not be used within 15 minutes of an assay. Postoperative complications include RLN injury, bleeding, and transient or complete hypoparathyroidism. Unilateral RLN is characterized by hoarseness and usually requires no intervention. Bilateral RLN injury is a rare complication, producing aphonia and requiring immediate tracheal intubation.

After successful parathyroidectomy, a decrease in the serum Ca^{2+} level should be observed within 24 hours. Patients with significant preoperative bone disease may have hypocalcemia after removal of the PTH-secreting glands. This "hungry bone" syndrome comes as a result of the rapid remineralization of bone. Thus, serum Ca^{2+}, magnesium, and phosphorus levels should be closely monitored until stable. The serum Ca^{2+} nadir usually occurs within 3 to 7 days.

Hypoparathyroidism

An underproduction of PTH or resistance of the end-organ tissues to PTH results in hypocalcemia (<8 mg/dL).[26] The normal physiologic response to hypocalcemia is an increase in PTH secretion and $1,25(OH)_2D$ synthesis, with an increase in Ca^{2+} mobilization from bone, GI absorption, and renal tubule reclamation. The most common cause of acquired PTH deficiency is inadvertent removal of the parathyroid glands during thyroid or parathyroid surgery. Other causes of acquired hypoparathyroidism include ^{131}I therapy for thyroid disease, neck trauma, granulomatous disease, or an infiltrating process (malignancy or amyloidosis). Severe hypomagnesemia (<0.8 mEq/L) from any cause can produce hypocalcemia by suppressing PTH secretion and interfering with PTH action. Renal insufficiency leads to phosphorus retention and impaired $1,25(OH)_2D$ synthesis, which results in hypocalcemia. These patients are commonly treated with vitamin D, which increases intestinal calcium absorption and suppresses secondary increases in PTH secretion. Hypocalcemia due to pancreatitis and burns results from the suppression of PTH and from the sequestration of calcium.

Clinical Features and Treatment

The clinical features of hypoparathyroidism are a manifestation of hypocalcemia. Neuronal irritability and skeletal muscle spasms, tetany, or seizures reflect a reduced threshold of excitation. Latent tetany may be demonstrated by eliciting the Chvostek or Trousseau sign. Chvostek sign is a contracture of the facial muscle produced by tapping the facial nerve as it passes through the parotid gland. Trousseau sign is contraction of the fingers and wrist after application of a blood pressure cuff inflated above the systolic blood pressure for approximately 3 minutes. Other common complaints of hypocalcemia include fatigue, depression, paresthesias, and skeletal muscle cramps. The acute onset of hypocalcemia after thyroid or parathyroid surgery may manifest as stridor and apnea. Cardiovascular manifestations of hypocalcemia include congestive heart failure, hypotension, and a relative insensitivity to the effects of β-adrenergic agonists (see Chapter 10). Delayed ventricular repolarization results in a prolonged QT interval on the ECG. Although prolongation of the QT interval may be a reliable sign of hypocalcemia in an individual patient, the ECG is relatively insensitive for the detection of hypocalcemia.

The treatment of hypoparathyroidism consists of electrolyte replacement. The objective is to have the patient's clinical symptoms under control before anesthesia and surgery. Hypocalcemia caused by magnesium depletion is treated by correcting the magnesium deficit. Serum phosphate excess is corrected by the removal of phosphate from the diet and the oral administration of phosphate-binding resins (aluminum hydroxide). The urinary excretion of phosphate can be increased with a saline volume infusion. Ca^{2+} deficiencies are corrected with Ca^{2+} supplements or vitamin D analogs. Patients with severe symptomatic hypocalcemia are treated with intravenous calcium gluconate (10 to 20 mL of 10% solution) given over several minutes and followed by a continuous infusion (1 to 2 mg/kg/hour) of elemental Ca^{2+}. The correction of serum Ca^{2+} levels should be monitored by measuring serum Ca^{2+} concentrations and following clinical symptoms. When oral or intravenous calcium is inadequate to maintain a normal serum–ionized calcium level, vitamin D is added to the regimen.

ADRENAL CORTEX

The adrenal cortex functions to synthesize and secrete three types of hormones. Endogenous and dietary cholesterol is used in the adrenal biosynthesis of glucocorticoids (cortisol), mineralocorticoids (aldosterone and 11-deoxycorticosterone), and androgens (dehydroepiandrosterone). Cortisol and aldosterone are the two essential hormones, whereas adrenal androgens are of relatively minor physiologic significance in adults. The major biologic effects of adrenal cortical hyperfunction or hypofunction occur as a result of cortisol or aldosterone excess or deficiency. Abnormal function of the adrenal cortex may render a patient unable to respond appropriately during a period of surgical stress or critical illness.

Glucocorticoid Physiology

Cortisol (hydrocortisone) is the most potent endogenous glucocorticoid and is produced by the inner portions of the adrenal cortex. Cortisone is a glucocorticoid produced in small amounts. Cortisol is produced under the control of adrenocorticotropic hormone (ACTH; corticotropin), a polypeptide synthesized and released by the anterior pituitary gland. Glucocorticoids exert their biologic effects by diffusing into the cytoplasm of target cells and combining with specific high-affinity receptor proteins.

The daily production of endogenous cortisol is approximately 20 mg. The maximal output is 150 to 300 mg. Most of the circulating hormone is bound to the α-globulin cortisol-binding globulin. It is the relatively small amount of free hormone that exerts the biologic effects. Endogenous glucocorticoids are inactivated primarily by the liver and are excreted in the urine as 17-hydroxycorticosteroids. Cortisol is also filtered at the glomerulus and may be excreted unchanged in the urine. Although the rate of cortisol secretion is decreased by approximately 30% in the elderly patient, plasma cortisol levels remain in a normal range because of a corresponding decrease in hepatic and renal clearance.

Cortisol secretion is directly controlled by ACTH, which in turn is regulated by the corticotropin-releasing factor from the hypothalamus. ACTH is synthesized in the pituitary gland from a precursor molecule that also produces β-lipotropin and β-endorphin. The secretion of ACTH and corticotropin-releasing factor is governed chiefly by glucocorticoids, the sleep–wake cycle, and stress. Cortisol is the most potent regulator of ACTH secretion, acting by a negative-feedback mechanism to maintain cortisol levels in a physiologic range. ACTH release follows a diurnal pattern, with maximal activity occurring soon after awakening. This diurnal pattern of activity occurs in normal subjects and in those with adrenal insufficiency. Psychological or physical stress (trauma, surgery, intense exercise) also promotes ACTH release, regardless of the level of circulating cortisol or the time of day.

Cortisol has multiple effects on intermediate carbohydrate, protein, and fatty acid metabolism, as well as maintenance and regulation of immune and circulatory function. Glucocorticoids enhance gluconeogenesis, elevate blood glucose, and promote hepatic glycogen synthesis. The catabolic effect of glucocorticoids is partially blocked by insulin. The net effect on protein metabolism is enhanced degradation of muscle tissue and negative nitrogen balance. In supraphysiologic amounts, glucocorticoids suppress growth hormone secretion and impair somatic growth. The anti-inflammatory actions of cortisol relate to its effect in stabilizing lysosomes and promoting capillary integrity. Cortisol also antagonizes leukocyte migration inhibition factor, thus reducing white cell adherence to vascular endothelium and diminishing leukocyte response to local inflammation. Phagocytic activity does not decrease, although the killing potential of macrophages and monocytes is diminished. Other diverse actions include the facilitation of free water clearance, maintenance of blood pressure, a weak mineralocorticoid effect, promotion of appetite, stimulation of hematopoiesis, and induction of liver enzymes.

Mineralocorticoid Physiology

Aldosterone is the most potent mineralocorticoid produced by the adrenal gland. This hormone binds to receptors in sweat glands, the alimentary tract, and the distal convoluted tubule of the kidney. Aldosterone is a major regulator of extracellular volume and potassium homeostasis through the resorption of sodium and the secretion of potassium by these tissues. The major regulators of aldosterone release are the renin–angiotensin system and serum potassium (Fig. 46-3). The juxtaglomerular apparatus that surrounds the renal afferent arterioles produces renin in response to decreased perfusion pressures and sympathetic stimulation. Renin splits the hepatic precursor angiotensinogen to form the decapeptide, angiotensin I, which is then altered enzymatically by converting enzyme (primarily in the lung) to form the octapeptide angiotensin II. Angiotensin II is the most potent vasopressor produced in the body. It directly stimulates the adrenal cortex to produce aldosterone. The renin–angiotensin system is the body's most important protector of volume status. Other stimuli that increase the production of aldosterone include hyperkalemia and, to a limited degree, hyponatremia, prostaglandin E, and ACTH.

Glucocorticoid Excess (Cushing Syndrome)

Cushing syndrome, caused by either overproduction of cortisol by the adrenal cortex or exogenous glucocorticoid therapy, results in a syndrome characterized by truncal obesity, hypertension, hyperglycemia, increased intravascular fluid volume, hypokalemia, fatigability, abdominal striae, osteoporosis, and muscle weakness. Most cases of Cushing syndrome that occur spontaneously are due to bilateral adrenal hyperplasia secondary to ACTH produced by an anterior pituitary microadenoma or nonendocrine tumor (e.g., of the lung, kidney, or pancreas) (see Chapter 36). The primary overproduction of cortisol and other adrenal steroids is caused by an adrenal neoplasm in approximately 20% to 25% of patients with Cushing syndrome. These tumors are usually unilateral, and approximately half are malignant. When Cushing syndrome occurs in patients older than 60 years of age, the most likely cause is an adrenal carcinoma or ectopic ACTH produced from a nonendocrine tumor. Finally, an increasingly common cause of Cushing syndrome is the prolonged administration of exogenous glucocorticoids to treat a variety of illnesses.

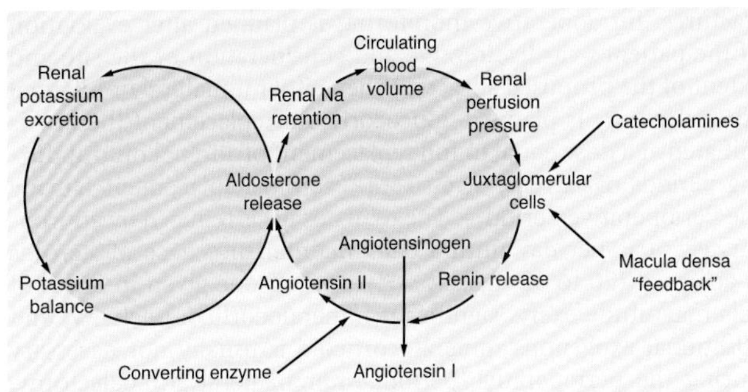

FIGURE 46-3. Interrelationship of the volume and potassium feedback loops on aldosterone secretion. (Reprinted from Petersdorf RG, ed. *Harrison's principles of internal medicine*. 10th ed. New York: McGraw-Hill; 1983, with permission.)

The signs and symptoms of Cushing syndrome follow from the known actions of glucocorticoids. Truncal obesity and thin extremities reflect increased muscle wasting and a redistribution of fat in facial, cervical, and truncal areas. Impaired calcium absorption and a decrease in bone formation may result in osteopenia. Sixty percent of patients have hyperglycemia, but overt diabetes mellitus (DM) occurs in <20%. Hypertension and fluid retention are seen in most patients. Profound emotional changes, ranging from emotional lability to frank psychosis, may be present. An increased susceptibility to infection reflects the immunosuppressive effects of corticosteroids. Hypokalemic alkalosis without distinctive physical findings is common when adrenal hyperplasia is caused by ectopic ACTH production from a nonendocrine tumor.

The laboratory diagnosis of hyperadrenocorticism is based on a variable elevation in plasma and urinary cortisol levels, urinary 17-hydroxycorticosteroids, and plasma ACTH. Once the diagnosis is established, simultaneous measurement of plasma ACTH and cortisol levels can determine whether the Cushing syndrome is due to primary pituitary or adrenal disease.[27]

Alternatively, a dexamethasone suppression test can be used. Patients with pituitary adenomas frequently show depression in cortisol and 17-hydroxycorticosteroid levels when a high dose of dexamethasone is administered because the tumor retains some negative-feedback control, while adrenal tumors do not.

Anesthetic Management

General considerations for the preoperative preparation of the patient include treating hypertension and diabetes and normalizing intravascular fluid volume and electrolyte concentrations. Diuresis with the aldosterone antagonist spironolactone helps mobilize fluid and normalize potassium concentration. Careful positioning of the osteopenic patient is important to avoid fractures. Intraoperative monitoring is planned after evaluation of the patient's cardiac reserve and consideration of the site and extent of the proposed surgery. When either unilateral or bilateral adrenalectomy is planned, glucocorticoid replacement therapy is initiated at a dose equal to full replacement of adrenal output during periods of extreme stress (see "Steroid Replacement During the Perioperative Period"). The total dosage is reduced by approximately 50% per day until a daily maintenance dose of steroids is achieved (20 to 30 mg/day). Hydrocortisone given in doses of this magnitude exerts significant mineralocorticoid activity, and additional exogenous mineralocorticoid is usually not necessary during the perioperative period. After bilateral adrenalectomy, most patients require 0.05 to 0.1 mg/day of fludrocortisone (9-α-fluorohydrocortisone) starting around day 5 to provide mineralocorticoid activity. Slightly higher doses may be needed if prednisone is used for glucocorticoid maintenance because it has little intrinsic mineralocorticoid activity. The fludrocortisone dose is reduced if congestive heart failure, hypokalemia, or hypertension develops. For the patient with a solitary adrenal adenoma, unilateral adrenalectomy may be followed by normalization of function in the contralateral gland over time. Treatment plans should therefore be individualized, and adjustments in dosage may be necessary. The production of glucocorticoids or ACTH by a neoplasm may not be eliminated if the tumor is unresectable. These patients often need continuous medical therapy with steroid inhibitors such as metyrapone to control their symptoms.

There are no specific recommendations regarding the use of a particular anesthetic technique or medication in patients with hyperadrenocorticism. When significant skeletal muscle weakness is present, a conservative approach to the use of muscle relaxants is warranted. Etomidate has been used for temporizing medical treatment of severe Cushing syndrome because of its inhibition of steroid synthesis.

Mineralocorticoid Excess

Hypersecretion of the major adrenal mineralocorticoid aldosterone increases the renal tubular exchange of sodium for potassium and hydrogen ions. This leads to hypertension, hypokalemic alkalosis, skeletal muscle weakness, and fatigue. Possibly as many as 1% of unselected hypertensive patients have primary hyperaldosteronism. The increase in renal sodium reabsorption and extracellular volume expansion is partly responsible for the high incidence of diastolic hypertension in these patients. Patients with primary hyperaldosteronism (Conn syndrome) characteristically do not have edema. Secondary aldosteronism results from an elevation in renin production. The diagnosis of primary or secondary hyperaldosteronism should be entertained in the nonedematous hypertensive patient with persistent hypokalemia who is not receiving potassium-wasting diuretics. Hyposecretion of renin that fails to increase appropriately during volume depletion or salt restriction is an important finding in primary aldosteronism. The measurement of plasma renin levels is useful in distinguishing primary from secondary hyperaldosteronism. It is of limited value in differentiating patients with primary aldosteronism from those with other causes of hypertension because renin activity is also suppressed in approximately 25% of patients with essential hypertension.

Anesthetic Considerations

Preoperative preparation for the patient with primary aldosteronism is directed toward restoring the intravascular volume and the electrolyte concentrations to normal. Hypertension and hypokalemia may be controlled by restricting sodium intake and administration of the aldosterone antagonist spironolactone. This diuretic works slowly to produce an increase in potassium levels, with dosages in the range of 25 to 100 mg every 8 hours. Total-body potassium deficits are difficult to estimate and may be in excess of 300 mEq. Whenever possible, potassium should be replaced slowly to allow equilibration between intracellular and extracellular potassium stores. The usual complications of chronic hypertension need to be assessed.

Adrenal Insufficiency (Addison Disease)

The undersecretion of adrenal steroid hormones may develop as the result of a primary inability of the adrenal gland to elaborate sufficient quantities of hormone or as the result of a deficiency in the production of ACTH.

Clinically, primary adrenal insufficiency is usually not apparent until at least 90% of the adrenal cortex has been destroyed. The predominant cause of primary adrenal insufficiency used to be tuberculosis; however, today, the most frequent cause of Addison disease is idiopathic adrenal insufficiency secondary to autoimmune destruction of the gland. Autoimmune destruction of the adrenal cortex causes both a glucocorticoid and a mineralocorticoid deficiency. A variety of other conditions presumed to have an autoimmune pathogenesis may also occur concomitantly with idiopathic Addison disease. Hashimoto thyroiditis in association with autoimmune adrenal insufficiency is termed Schmidt syndrome. Other possible causes of adrenal gland destruction include certain bacterial, fungal, and advanced human immunodeficiency virus infections; metastatic cancer; sepsis; and hemorrhage. Secondary adrenal insufficiency occurs when the anterior pituitary fails to secrete sufficient quantities of ACTH. Pituitary failure may result from tumor, infection, surgical ablation, or radiation therapy. Pituitary surgery may cause transient adrenal insufficiency requiring supplemental glucocorticoids.[28]

Patients receiving chronic corticosteroid therapy will not generally have frank adrenal insufficiency, but may have hypothalamic-pituitary-adrenal (HPA) suppression and may develop acute adrenal insufficiency during the stress of the perioperative period. Relative adrenal insufficiency is a common finding in critically ill surgical patients with hypotension requiring vasopressors.[29]

Clinical Presentation

The cardinal symptoms of idiopathic Addison disease include chronic fatigue, muscle weakness, anorexia, weight loss, nausea, vomiting, and diarrhea. Hypotension is almost always encountered in the disease process. Female patients may exhibit decreased axillary and pubic hair growth because of the loss of adrenal androgen secretion. An acute crisis can present as abdominal pain, severe vomiting and diarrhea, hypotension, decreased consciousness, and shock. Diffuse hyperpigmentation occurs in most patients with primary adrenal insufficiency and is secondary to the compensatory increase in ACTH and β-lipotropin. These hormones stimulate an increase in melanocyte production. Mineralocorticoid deficiency is characteristically present in primary adrenal disease; as a result, there is a reduction in urine sodium conservation. Hyperkalemia may be a cause of life-threatening cardiac dysrhythmias. Adrenal insufficiency secondary to pituitary disease is not associated with cutaneous hyperpigmentation or mineralocorticoid deficiency. Salt and water balance is usually maintained unless severe fluid and electrolyte losses overwhelm the subnormal aldosterone secretory capacity. Organic lesions of pituitary origin require a diligent search for coexisting hormone deficiencies. Acute adrenal insufficiency from inadequate replacement of steroids on chronic steroid therapy is rare and can present as refractory, distributive shock. In critically ill patients, adrenal insufficiency may not present with classic symptoms. The clinical picture may resemble that of sepsis without a source of infection.[30] A high degree of suspicion must be maintained if the patient has cardiovascular instability without a defined cause.[31,32]

Diagnosis

The patient's pituitary–adrenal responsiveness should be determined when the diagnosis of primary or secondary adrenal insufficiency is first suspected. Biochemical evidence of impaired adrenal or pituitary secretory reserve unequivocally confirms the diagnosis. Patients who are clinically stable may undergo testing before treatment is initiated. Those believed to have acute adrenal insufficiency should receive immediate therapy.

Plasma cortisol levels are measured before and 30 and 60 minutes after the intravenous administration of 250 μg of synthetic ACTH. There are multiple determinants for adequate adrenal reserve; usually the plasma cortisol rises at least 500 nmol/L 60 minutes after the injection of the synthetic ACTH.[33] Patients with adrenal insufficiency usually demonstrate little or no adrenal response.

Treatment and Anesthetic Considerations

Normal adults secrete about 20 mg of cortisol (hydrocortisone) and 0.1 mg of aldosterone per day. Glucocorticoid therapy is usually given twice daily in sufficient dosage to meet physiologic requirements. A typical regimen in the unstressed patient may consist of prednisone, 5 mg in the morning and 2.5 mg in the evening, or hydrocortisone, 20 mg in the morning and 10 mg in the evening. The daily glucocorticoid dosage is typically 50% higher than basal adrenal output to cover the patient for mild stress. Replacement dosages are adjusted in response to the patient's clinical symptoms or the occurrence of intercurrent illnesses. Mineralocorticoid replacement is also administered on a daily basis; most patients require 0.05 to 0.1 mg/day of fludrocortisone. The mineralocorticoid dose may be reduced if severe hypokalemia, hypertension, or congestive heart failure develops, or it may be increased if postural hypotension is demonstrated.

Secondary adrenal insufficiency often occurs in the presence of multiple hormone deficiencies. A decrease in ACTH production results in the decreased secretion of cortisol and adrenal androgens, but aldosterone control by more dominant mechanisms remains intact. A liberal salt diet is encouraged. Glucocorticoid substitution follows the same guidelines previously outlined for primary adrenal insufficiency.

Immediate therapy of acute adrenal insufficiency is mandatory, regardless of the etiology, and consists of electrolyte resuscitation and steroid replacement (Table 46-6). Initial therapy begins with the rapid intravenous administration of an isotonic crystalloid solution. A dose of 100 mg of hydrocortisone is administered as an intravenous bolus over several minutes. Steroid replacement is continued during the first 24 hours with 100 mg of intravenous hydrocortisone given every 8 hours. If the patient is stable, the steroid dose is reduced starting on the second day. After adequate fluid resuscitation, if the patient continues to be hemodynamically unstable, inotropic support may be necessary. Invasive monitoring is extremely valuable as a guide to both diagnosis and therapy.

Steroid Replacement During the Perioperative Period

Perioperatively, patients with adrenal insufficiency and those with HPA suppression from chronic steroid use require additional corticosteroids to mimic the increased output of the normal adrenal gland during stress. The normal adrenal gland can secrete up to 100 mg/m^2 of cortisol per day or more during the perioperative period.[34] The pituitary–adrenal axis is usually considered to be intact if a plasma cortisol level of >19 μg/dL is measured during acute stress, but there is no precise threshold. The degree of adrenal responsiveness has been correlated with the duration of surgery and the extent of surgical trauma. The mean maximal plasma cortisol level measured during major surgery (colectomy, hip osteotomy) was 47 μg/dL. Minor surgical procedures (herniorrhaphy) resulted in mean maximal plasma cortisol levels of 28 μg/dL. Adrenal activity may also be affected by the anesthetic technique used. Regional anesthesia is effective in postponing the elevation in cortisol levels during surgery of the lower abdomen and extremities.[35] Deep general anesthesia may also suppress the elevation of stress hormones such as ACTH and cortisol during the surgical procedure.

Although symptoms indicative of clinically significant adrenal insufficiency have been reported during the perioperative period, these clinical findings have rarely been documented in direct association with glucocorticoid deficiency.[36] There is evidence in adrenally suppressed primates that subphysiologic steroid replacement causes perioperative hemodynamic instability and increased mortality.

3 Identifying which patients require steroid supplementation can be difficult. Provocative testing with ACTH stimulation is too costly to justify compared with the risk of brief steroid supplementation. HPA suppression can occur after 5 daily doses of prednisone ≥20 mg. Recovery of HPA function occurs gradually and can take up to 9 to 12 months. HPA suppression can occur with topical, regional, and inhaled steroids. Alternate-day therapy decreases the risk of HPA suppression.

The clinical problem is how much steroid to give. There is no proven optimal regimen for perioperative steroid replacement (Table 46-7). A low-dose cortisol replacement program using an intravenous infusion of 25 mg of cortisol before the induction

TABLE 46-6. MANAGEMENT OF ACUTE ADRENAL INSUFFICIENCY

Hydrocortisone, 100 mg IV bolus, followed by hydrocortisone, 100 mg q6h for 24 h
Fluid and electrolyte replacement as indicated by vital signs, serum electrolytes, and serum glucose

IV, intravenous(ly).

TABLE 46-7. MANAGEMENT OPTIONS FOR STEROID REPLACEMENT IN THE PERIOPERATIVE PERIOD

Hydrocortisone, 25 mg IV, at the time of induction followed by hydrocortisone infusion, 100 mg over 24 hours
Hydrocortisone, 100 mg IV, before, during, and after surgery

IV, intravenous(ly).

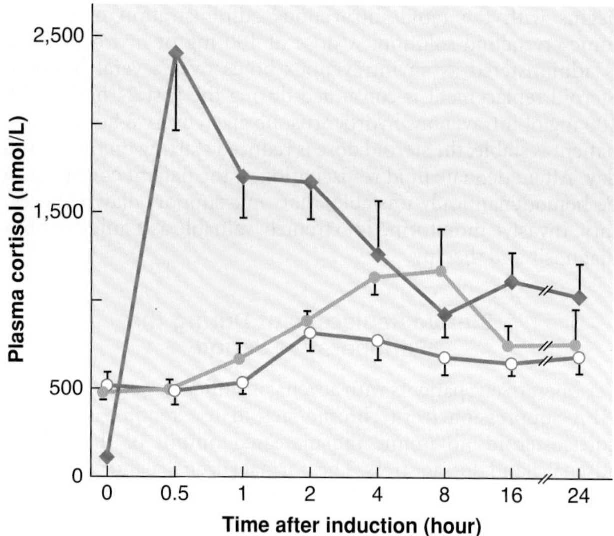

FIGURE 46-4. Plasma cortisol concentrations (mean ± SEM) were measured in three groups of patients undergoing elective surgery. Group I control patients, $n = 8$ (*closed circles*), had never received corticosteroids. Group II patients, $n = 8$ (*open circles*), received preoperative corticosteroids with a normal response to preoperative adrenocorticotropic hormone (ACTH; corticotropin) stimulation testing. These patients and control patients received no corticosteroid substitution during the perioperative period. Group III, $n = 6$ (*closed diamonds*), consisted of patients receiving long-term corticosteroid therapy with an abnormal response to ACTH stimulation testing during the perioperative period. These patients (group III) received intravenous (IV) cortisol, 25 mg, after the induction of anesthesia plus a continuous IV infusion of cortisol, 100 mg, during the next 24 hours. Plasma cortisol levels in group III were significantly lower than in the other two groups before the induction of anesthesia. After IV administration of cortisol to group III patients, plasma concentrations were significantly higher than in groups I and II for the next 2 hours ($p < .01$). Thereafter, the mean plasma concentrations were similar for all groups. There were no clinical signs of circulatory insufficiency in any group. (Reprinted from Symreng T, Karlberg BE, Kagedol B, et al. Physiological cortisol substitution of long-term steroid-treated patients undergoing major surgery. *Br J Anaesth.* 1981;53:949, with permission.)

of anesthesia, followed by a continuous infusion of cortisol (100 mg) in the next 24 hours, has been advocated[37] (Fig. 46-4). This low-dose cortisol replacement program was used in patients with proven adrenal insufficiency and resulted in plasma cortisol levels as high as those seen in healthy control subjects subjected to a similar operative stress. One study with a limited number of patients found no problems with cardiovascular instability if patients received their usual dose of steroids.[38] An extensive review concluded that the best evidence was that patients should receive their usual daily dose but no supplementation.[39] Although the low-dose approach appears logical, many clinicians are unwilling to adopt this regimen until further trials have been undertaken in patients receiving physiologic steroid replacement. A popular regimen calls for the administration of 200 to 300 mg of hydrocortisone per 70 kg body weight in divided doses on the day of surgery. The lower dose is adjusted upward for longer and more extensive surgical procedures. Patients who are using steroids at the time of surgery receive their usual dose on the morning of surgery and are supplemented at a level that is at least equivalent to the usual daily replacement. Glucocorticoid coverage is rapidly tapered to the patient's normal maintenance dosage during the postoperative period. Although no conclusive evidence supports an increased incidence of infection or abnormal wound healing when supraphysiologic doses of supplemental steroids are used acutely, the goal of therapy is to use the minimal drug dosage necessary to adequately protect the patient.

Exogenous Glucocorticoid Therapy

The therapeutic use of supraphysiologic doses of glucocorticoids has expanded, and the anesthesiologist should be familiar with the various preparations (Table 46-8). Dexamethasone, methylprednisolone, and prednisone have less mineralocorticoid effect than cortisone or hydrocortisone. Prednisone and methylprednisolone are precursors that must be metabolized by the liver before anti-inflammatory activity can occur and should be used cautiously in the presence of liver disease.

Mineralocorticoid Insufficiency

Isolated mineralocorticoid insufficiency has been reported as a congenital biosynthetic defect, after unilateral adrenalectomy for removal of an aldosterone-secreting adenoma, during protracted

TABLE 46-8. GLUCOCORTICOID PREPARATIONS

Generic Name	Anti-inflammatory	Mineralocorticoid	Approximate Equivalent Dose (mg)
Short acting			
Hydrocortisone	1.0	1.0	20.0
Cortisone	0.8	0.8	25.0
Prednisone	4.0	0.25	5.0
Prednisolone	4.0	0.25	5.0
Methylprednisolone	5.0	–	4.0
Intermediate acting			
Triamcinolone	5.0	–	4.0
Long acting			
Dexamethasone	30.0	–	0.75

Relative milligram comparisons with cortisol. The glucocorticoid and mineralocorticoid properties of cortisol are set as 1.0.

heparin therapy, and in patients with a deficiency in renin production. This syndrome is commonly seen in patients with mild renal failure and long-standing DM. A feature common to all patients with hypoaldosteronism is a failure to increase aldosterone production in response to salt restriction or volume contraction.

Most patients present with hypotension, hyperkalemia that may be life-threatening, and a metabolic acidosis that is out of proportion to the degree of coexisting renal impairment. Patients with low renin secretion, hypoaldosteronism, and renal dysfunction respond to ACTH stimulation. Nonsteroidal anti-inflammatory drugs, which inhibit prostaglandin synthesis, may further inhibit renin release and exacerbate the condition. Patients with isolated hypoaldosteronism are given fludrocortisone orally in a dose of 0.05 to 0.1 mg/day. Patients with low renin secretion usually require higher doses to correct the electrolyte abnormalities. Caution should be observed in patients with hypertension or congestive heart failure. An alternative approach in these patients is the administration of furosemide alone or in combination with mineralocorticoid.

ADRENAL MEDULLA

3 The adrenal medulla is derived embryologically from neuroectodermal cells. As a specialized part of the sympathetic nervous system, the adrenal medulla synthesizes and secretes the catecholamines epinephrine (80%) and norepinephrine (20%). Preganglionic fibers of the sympathetic nervous system bypass the paravertebral ganglia and pass directly from the spinal cord to the adrenal medulla. The adrenal medulla is analogous to a postganglionic neuron, although the catecholamines secreted by the medulla function as hormones, not as neurotransmitters.

4 The synthesis of norepinephrine begins with hydroxylation of tyrosine to dopa (Fig. 46-5). This rate-limiting step in catecholamine biosynthesis is regulated so synthesis is coupled to release. In the adrenal medulla and in those rare central neurons using epinephrine as a neurotransmitter, most of the norepinephrine is converted to epinephrine by the enzyme phenylethanolamine-*N*-methyltransferase. It is likely that the capacity of the adrenal medulla to synthesize epinephrine is influenced by the flow of glucocorticoid-rich blood from the adrenal cortex through the intra-adrenal portal system because it is known that high concentrations of glucocorticoid are able to induce the enzyme phenylethanolamine-*N*-methyltransferase.

In the adrenal medulla, catecholamines are stored in chromaffin granules complexed with adenosine triphosphate and Ca^{2+}. The normal adrenal releases epinephrine and norepinephrine by exocytosis in response to stimulation by preganglionic sympathetic neurons. The circulatory half-life (10 to 30 seconds) of these catechols is considerably longer than the brief receptor activity of norepinephrine released as a neurotransmitter from postganglionic sympathetic nerve endings. Biotransformation of circulating norepinephrine and epinephrine is accomplished chiefly by the enzyme catechol-*O*-methyltransferase, located in the liver and kidney. Monoamine oxidase is of less importance in the metabolism of circulating catechols. Metanephrine and vanillylmandelic acid are the major end products of catecholamine metabolism. These metabolites and a small amount of unchanged catecholamine (1%) appear in the urine.

The outflow of postganglionic sympathetic neurotransmitters and circulating catecholamine from the adrenal medulla is coordinated by higher cortical centers connected to the brainstem. The intrinsic activity of the brainstem sympathetic areas is modulated by higher cortical functions, emotional reactions (anger, fear), and various physiologic stimuli, including changes in the physical and chemical properties of the extracellular fluid (hypoglycemia, hypotension). The adrenal medulla and sympathetic nervous system are often stimulated together in a generalized fashion, although many physiologic conditions exist in which they act independently.

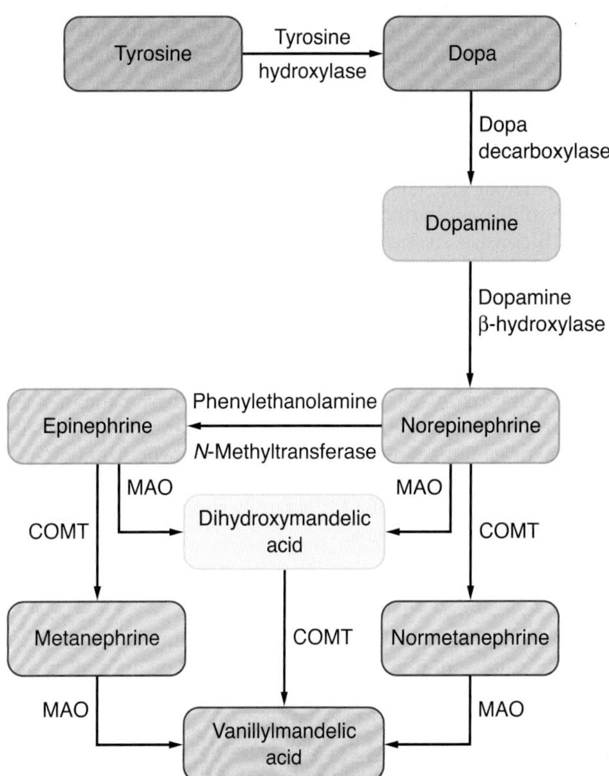

FIGURE 46-5. Synthesis and metabolism of endogenous catecholamines. COMT, catechol-*O*-methyltransferase; MAO, monoamine oxidase. (Reprinted from Stoelting RK, Dierdorf SF, eds. *Anesthesia and co-existing disease*. New York: Churchill-Livingstone; 1983, with permission.)

Pheochromocytoma

The only important disease process associated with the adrenal medulla is pheochromocytoma. These tumors produce, store, and secrete catecholamines. Most pheochromocytomas secrete both epinephrine and norepinephrine, with the percentage of secreted norepinephrine being greater than that secreted by the normal gland. Although pheochromocytomas occur in <0.2% of hypertensive patients, it is important to aggressively evaluate the patient with clinically suspect symptoms because surgical extirpation is curative in >90% of patients and complications are often lethal in undiagnosed cases.[40] Postmortem series have reported high perioperative mortality rates in undiagnosed patients undergoing relatively minor surgical procedures. Most deaths are from cardiovascular causes. Perioperative morbidity is related to tumor size and the degree of catecholamine secretion.[41]

Most (85% to 90%) pheochromocytomas are solitary tumors localized to a single adrenal gland, usually the right. Approximately 10% of adults and 25% of children have bilateral tumors. The tumor may originate in extra-adrenal sites (10%), anywhere along the paravertebral sympathetic chain; however, 95% of the tumors are located in the abdomen, and a small percentage are located in the thorax, urinary bladder, or neck. Malignant spread of these highly vascular tumors occurs in approximately 10% of cases.

In approximately 5% of cases, this tumor is inherited as a familial autosomal dominant trait. It may be part of the polyglandular syndrome referred to as multiple endocrine neoplasia (MEN) IIA or IIB. Type IIA includes medullary carcinoma of the thyroid, parathyroid hyperplasia, and pheochromocytoma; type IIB consists of medullary carcinoma of the thyroid, pheochromocytoma, and neuromas of the oral mucosa. Pheochromocytomas may also arise in association with von Recklinghausen neurofibromatosis or von Hippel-Lindau disease (retinal and cerebellar angiomatosis). The pheochromocytoma of the familial syndromes is rarely extra-adrenal or malignant. Bilateral tumors occur in approximately 75% of cases. When these patients present with a single adrenal pheochromocytoma, the chances of subsequent development of a second adrenal pheochromocytoma are sufficiently high that bilateral adrenalectomy should be considered. Every member of a MEN family should be considered at risk for pheochromocytoma.

Clinical Presentation

Pheochromocytoma may occur at any age, but it is most common in young to middle adult life. The clinical manifestations are mainly due to the pharmacologic effects of the catecholamines released from the tumor. These tumors are not innervated, and catecholamine release is independent of neurogenic control. Most patients have sustained hypertension, although occasionally it is paroxysmal.[42] When true paroxysms occur, the blood pressure may rise to alarmingly high levels, placing the patient at risk for cerebrovascular hemorrhage, heart failure, dysrhythmias, or myocardial infarction. Headache, palpitations, tremor, profuse sweating, and either pallor or flushing may accompany an attack. Pheochromocytoma can masquerade as malignant hyperthermia. Physical examination of the patient with pheochromocytoma may be unrevealing during the period between attacks, unless the patient presents with symptoms and signs of sequelae related to long-standing hypertension. A catecholamine-induced cardiomyopathy may be accompanied by heart failure and cardiac dysrhythmias. Paroxysms are commonly not associated with clearly defined events, but may be precipitated by displacement of the abdominal contents or, in the case of a bladder tumor, by micturition.

Diagnosis

Biochemical determination of free catecholamine concentration and catecholamine metabolites in the urine is the most common screening test used to establish the diagnosis of pheochromocytoma.[43] Urinary vanillylmandelic acid and unconjugated norepinephrine and epinephrine levels are measured in a 24-hour urine collection and are expressed as a function of the creatinine clearance (Fig. 46-6). Excess production of catecholamines is diagnostic for pheochromocytoma. Free catecholamines represent <1% of the originally released hormone, and urinary levels are not always elevated to a significant degree. Hence, differentiation from normal subjects may be difficult. A change in the ratio of unconjugated epinephrine to norepinephrine may be the only biochemical finding. Certain drugs interfere with urinary assays, and some patients with paroxysmal hypertension have normal values between attacks.

Although routine laboratory data are unlikely to provide specific diagnostic insight, ECG, chest radiograph, and complete

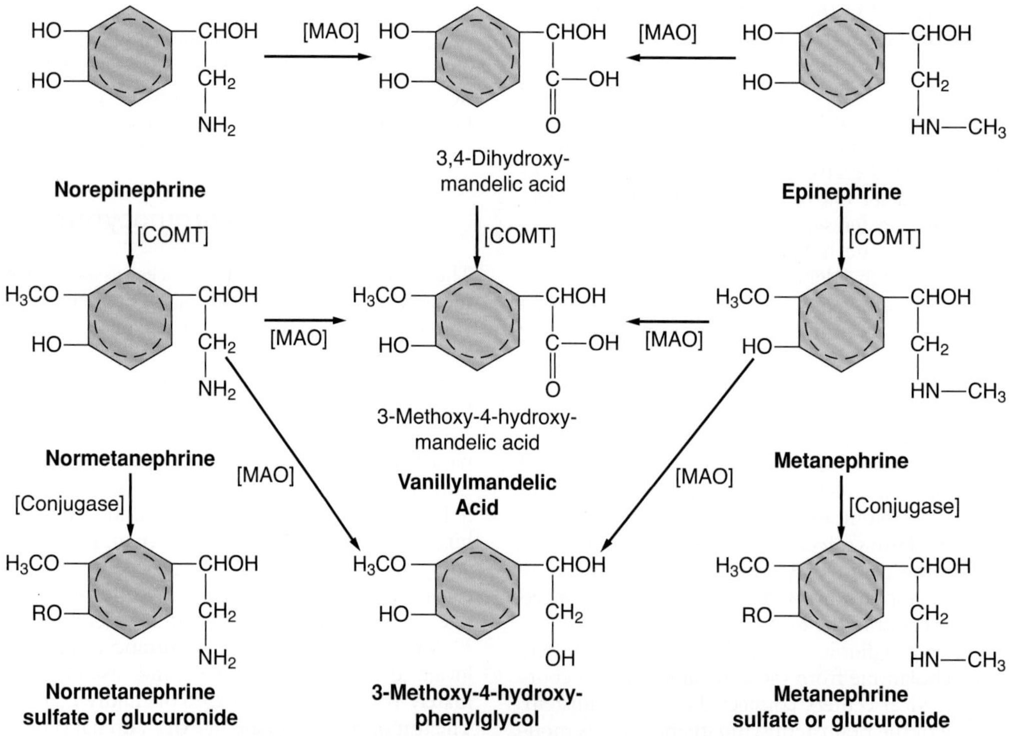

FIGURE 46-6. Catabolism of norepinephrine and epinephrine.

blood cell count can provide valuable information to the clinician who entertains the diagnosis. Left ventricular hypertrophy and nonspecific T-wave changes are two of the more common ECG findings. Evidence of acute myocardial infarction or tachyarrhythmia has also been reported. The chest radiograph may reveal cardiomegaly, and the blood count often shows an elevated hematocrit consistent with a reduced intravascular volume and hemoconcentration. Standardized imaging methods such as CT and MRI are used in the noninvasive localization of these tumors.[44] Improvements in imaging may obviate the need for abdominal exploration or venous sampling to localize the tumor in selected patients.[45] Ultrasound and MRI are especially useful in pregnant patients. ^{131}I-Metaiodobenzylguanidine scintigraphy is also effective in localizing recurrent or extra-adrenal masses.

Anesthetic Considerations

Preoperative Preparation

4 The reduction in perioperative mortality rates from a high of 45% to between 0% and 3%, from excision of pheochromocytoma followed by the introduction of α-antagonists for preoperative therapy. Perioperative blood pressure fluctuations, myocardial infarction, congestive heart failure, cardiac dysrhythmias, and cerebral hemorrhage all appear to be reduced in frequency when the patient has been treated before surgery with α-blockers and the intravascular fluid compartment has been re-expanded. Extended treatment with α-antagonists is also effective in treating the clinical manifestations of catecholamine myocarditis. However, α-blocker therapy has never been studied in a controlled way, and there are some groups that question its necessity in light of the availability of potent titratable vasodilators for intraoperative use.[46] A list of drugs frequently used in the management of pheochromocytoma is given in Table 46-9.

α-adrenergic blockade is initiated once the diagnosis of pheochromocytoma is established (see Chapter 15). Phenoxybenzamine, a long-acting (24 to 48 hours), noncompetitive presynaptic (α_2) and postsynaptic (α_1) blocker, has traditionally been used at doses of 10 mg every 8 hours. Increments are added until the blood pressure is controlled and paroxysms disappear. Most patients need between 80 and 200 mg/day. The absorption after oral administration is variable, and side effects are common. Certain cardiovascular reflexes such as the baroreceptor reflex are blunted, and postural hypotension is common. Selective competitive α_1-blockers, such as doxazosin, terazosin, and prazosin, have also been used effectively. Because postural hypotension can be pronounced with the commencement of therapy, the initial 1-mg dose is given at bedtime. Postural changes are also seen with maintenance therapy. A comparison of patients with pheochromocytoma receiving phenoxybenzamine or prazosin has shown both drugs to be equally effective in controlling blood pressure. Although the optimal period of preoperative treatment has not been established, most clinicians recommend beginning α-blockade therapy at least 10 to 14 days before the proposed surgery; however, periods as short as 3 to 5 days have been used.[47] During this time, the contracted intravascular volume and hematocrit return toward normal and the blood pressure is stabilized. Despite the real possibility of hypotension after vascular isolation of the tumor, most clinicians continue α-blockers until the morning of surgery.

β-adrenergic blockade is occasionally added after α-blockade has been established. This addition is considered in patients with persistent tachycardia or cardiac dysrhythmias that may be caused by nonselective α-blockade or epinephrine-secreting tumors. β-blockers should not be given until adequate α-blockade is ensured to avoid the possibility of unopposed α-mediated vasoconstriction. There is no clear preoperative advantage of one β-antagonist over another, although the short half-life of esmolol may allow better control of heart rate and arrhythmias in the perioperative setting. Labetalol, a β-adrenergic antagonist with α-blocking activity, is effective as a second-line medication, but can increase blood pressure when this drug is used alone.

α-methyltyrosine is an agent that inhibits the enzyme tyrosine hydroxylase, the rate-limiting step in catecholamine biosynthesis. This medication is currently reserved for patients with metastatic disease or for situations in which surgery is contraindicated and long-term medical therapy is required. When α-methyltyrosine is used in combination with α-adrenergic–blocking agents, there is a significant reduction in catecholamine biosynthesis.

Unrecognized pheochromocytoma during pregnancy may be life-threatening to the mother and fetus. Although the safety of adrenergic-blocking agents during pregnancy has not been established, these agents probably improve fetal survival in pregnant patients with pheochromocytoma. The trend is to perform surgery during the first trimester or at the time of cesarean delivery. There is no reason to terminate an early pregnancy, but the patient should be aware of the risk of spontaneous abortion resulting from abdominal surgery to remove the tumor.[48]

Perioperative Anesthetic Management

Symptomatic patients continue to receive medical therapy until tachycardia, cardiac dysrhythmias, and paroxysmal elevations in blood pressure are well controlled. If it is not possible to initiate α-blocking therapy before surgery or if the patient has received <48 hours of intensive treatment, it may be necessary to infuse nitroprusside during the induction of anesthesia. A low-dose infusion is often initiated in anticipation of the marked blood pressure elevations that can occur with laryngoscopy and surgical stimulation.

Improvements in imaging now allow most patients with solitary tumors without evidence of metastases or local invasion to undergo a laparoscopic retroperitoneal approach. If the surgeon needs to assess for bilateral disease or the dissection is too difficult, then the procedure can be converted to an open one. During laparoscopic surgery, creation of the pneumoperitoneum may cause release of catecholamines and large changes in hemodynamics that can be controlled with a vasodilator.[49]

Although there is no clear advantage to one anesthetic technique over another, drugs that are known to liberate histamine are avoided. Because of the potential for ventricular irritability, halothane is not administered. A potent sedative hypnotic, in combination with an opioid analgesic, is used for induction. It is extremely important to achieve an adequate depth of anesthesia before proceeding with laryngoscopy to minimize the sympathetic nervous system response to this maneuver. Maintenance is provided with an opioid analgesic and a potent inhalation agent.
5 Manipulation of the tumor may produce a marked elevation in blood pressure. Acute hypertensive crises are treated with intravenous infusions of nitroprusside or phentolamine or any vasodilator mentioned later. Phentolamine is a short-acting α-adrenergic antagonist that may be given as an intravenous bolus (2 to 5 mg) or by continuous infusion. Tachydysrhythmia is controlled with intravenous boluses of propranolol (1-mg increments) or by a continuous infusion of the ultrashort-acting selective β_1-adrenergic antagonist esmolol. The disadvantage of long-acting β-blockers may be persistence of bradycardia and hypotension after the tumor is removed. Even esmolol may be problematic because there are cases of cardiac arrest after clamping of the venous drainage in patients receiving large doses of esmolol.

TABLE 46-9. DRUGS USED IN THE MANAGEMENT OF PHEOCHROMOCYTOMA

Drug	Action	Preoperative Blood Pressure Control	Pressor Crisis	Comment
Phentolamine	Nonselective α-antagonist	–	1–5 mg IV; 0.5–1 mg/minute IV	Short duration of action ~5 minute
Phenoxybenzamine	Nonselective α-antagonist	20 mg/day PO up to 160 mg/day in divided doses	–	Long half-life; may accumulate
Doxazosin (terazosin dosing similar)	Selective α_1-antagonist	1 mg/day PO up to 8 mg/day PO	–	First-dose phenomena; may cause syncope
Propranolol	Nonselective β-antagonist	40 mg/day PO up to 480 mg/day in divided doses to control tachycardia	1–2 mg IV bolus	Should never be given without first creating α-blockade
Atenolol	Selective β_1-antagonist	50–100 mg/day PO	–	Long-acting drug eliminated unchanged by kidney
Esmolol	Selective β_1-antagonist	–	250–500 μg/kg/minute IV loading followed by maintenance infusion 25–250 μg/kg/minute	Short acting; elimination half-life ~9 minute
Labetalol	α-antagonist and β-antagonist	200 mg/day PO in divided doses up to 800 mg/day	10 mg IV bolus	A much weaker α-blocker than β-blocker; may cause hypertensive response
Nitroprusside	Direct vasodilator	–	0.5–1.5 μg/kg/minute initially, increased to maximum of 8 μg/kg/minute; titrate to effect	Powerful vasodilator; short acting
Magnesium sulfate	Direct vasodilator and membrane stabilizer	–	2–4 g IV bolus followed by 1–2 g/hour and additional 1–2 g boluses as needed	May potentiate neuromuscular blockade
Nicardipine	Calcium channel antagonist	–	1–2 μg/kg/min increased to 7.5 μg/kg/minute; titrate to effect	–
α-methyltyrosine	Inhibitor of biosynthesis of catecholamine	1–4 g/day PO in divided doses	–	Suitable for patients not amenable to surgery; may be nephrotoxic

IV, intravenous(ly); PO, oral(ly).

Almost every vasodilator has been tried and recommended as an adjuvant to control hypertension. Magnesium sulfate given as an infusion with intermittent boluses has successfully controlled blood pressure.[50] Nicardipine, clevidipine,[51] nitroglycerin, diltiazem, fenoldopam, and prostaglandin E_1 have all been used anecdotally. The reduction in blood pressure that may occur after ligation of the tumor's venous supply can be dangerously abrupt and should be anticipated through close communication with the surgical team. Restitution of any intravascular fluid deficit is the initial therapy in this situation. After replenishment of the intravascular volume, if the patient remains hypotensive, phenylephrine is administered. Norepinephrine or vasopressin may also be needed.[51] After surgery, catecholamine levels return to normal over several days. Approximately 75% of patients become normotensive within 10 days. Hypoglycemia must be watched for as insulin levels rise from loss of catecholamine-induced β-cell suppression.

DIABETES MELLITUS

A fasting glucose level below 100 mg/dL is considered normal. Individuals with documented fasting glucose levels above 126 mg/dL are considered diabetics, while those with levels between 100 and 125 mg/dL are considered prediabetics.[52] An estimated 20.8 million Americans (7% of the U.S. population) have DM and about 40 million Americans have prediabetes. DM is the most commonly occurring endocrine disease found in surgical patients, and 25% to 50% of diabetics will require surgery at some point in their lives. Although the most serious complications of DM are related to its character as a chronic disease, it can cause difficulties in the short-term management of acute illness. DM can remain clinically inapparent until exacerbated by the stress of trauma or surgery.[53] Some observational studies report that hyperglycemia is present in 32% to 38% of patients in community hospitals, 41% of critically ill patients with acute coronary syndromes, and 80% of patients after cardiac surgery.[54] In these reports, approximately one-third of non-intensive care unit (ICU) patients and approximately 80% of ICU patients had no history of diabetes before admission.[54]

The principles of the treatment of DM will be easier to understand if one reviews the physiology of glucose metabolism and the stress response and then considers some of the specific pathologic entities that comprise the clinical picture of DM.

Classification

DM primarily manifests as a disease of glucose metabolism; however, it significantly affects lipid and protein metabolism and has an impact on a wide range of endocrinologic functions. Despite a variety of etiologic factors, its hallmark is a deficiency, either absolute or relative, in the amount of insulin effect to the tissues.

DM is classified into four broad types: type 1 diabetes, type 2 diabetes, gestational DM, and diabetes due to other causes.[52]

Type 1 accounts for 5% to 10% of all DM cases and is distinguished from type 2, which accounts for the remaining 90% to 95% of all DM cases. The patient with type 1 DM typically experiences the onset of disease early in life. Consequently, this form was also referred to as juvenile-onset diabetes. In general, the patient with type 1 DM is not obese, has an abrupt onset of the disease, and has very low levels of circulating insulin. Disease in these patients cannot be controlled with diet or oral hypoglycemic agents; rather, it mandates treatment with insulin as there is an absolute deficiency of insulin due to destruction of β cells. It is difficult to maintain an optimal glucose level in patients with type 1 DM. They are more likely to become ketotic and sustain progressive end-organ complications of diabetes.[52]

Patients with type 2 DM, also called adult-onset diabetes, typically experience a gradual onset of the disease later in life. However, the milder type 2 form can occur in young people, and many older adults can acquire a severe and brittle form of type 1. Because of the obesity epidemic, many adolescent and teenagers are presenting more frequently with this disorder.[52] Patients with type 2 DM are often obese, have resistance to the effects of insulin (commonly referred to as insulin resistance), and, hence, may have normal or even elevated levels of insulin. In milder forms, this version of diabetes can often be treated with diet, lifestyle modifications, and oral hypoglycemic agents. Because these patients are relatively resistant to ketosis, their disease may not be clinically apparent until exacerbated by the stress of surgery or intercurrent illness.

Other types of DM can be a result of a disease that damages the pancreas and thus impairs insulin secretion. Pancreatic surgery, chronic pancreatitis, cystic fibrosis, and hemochromatosis can damage the pancreas and impair insulin secretion sufficiently to produce clinical DM. DM can also result from one of the endocrine diseases that produces a hormone that opposes the action of insulin. Hence, a patient with a glucagonoma, pheochromocytoma, or acromegaly may be diabetic. An increased effect of glucocorticoids, either from Cushing disease or steroid therapy, may also oppose the effect of insulin enough to elicit clinical diabetes and would certainly complicate the management of pre-existing diabetes. Treatment of human immunodeficiency virus/acquired immunodeficiency syndrome, genetic defects in β-cell function, and genetic defects in insulin action can also induce diabetes.[52] Gestational diabetes is a common medical problem of pregnancy and may presage future type 2 DM. Different diagnostic criteria are used to diagnose gestational diabetes.[52]

Physiology

Insulin has multiple and complex interactions with lipid, protein, and glucose metabolism. It also has many nonmetabolic functions.[55] For our purposes, it is easiest to regard the effects of insulin on glucose metabolism as primary and to view its effects on other metabolic functions only as they relate to glucose.

Insulin is a small protein produced by the β cells of the islets of Langerhans in the pancreas. The basal rate of insulin secretion is about 1 U/hour, which can increase by 5- to 10-fold after ingestion of food. Normal production in the adult human is approximately 40 to 50 U/day. Insulin acts through its specific receptor on cells. The half-life of insulin in the circulation is 5 minutes. However, it may clinically appear to have a longer duration of action, due to delays in binding and release from the cellular receptors.[56] These facts lead us to the important principle that once a high level of insulin saturates all the binding sites, insulin will not have a more potent effect, just a more long-lasting effect.

Insulin is metabolized in the liver and kidneys. In patients with hepatic dysfunction, the loss of gluconeogenesis and a prolongation of insulin effect increase the risk of hypoglycemia. Similarly, in patients with renal disease, the action of insulin is prolonged. They are more prone to hypoglycemia, and exogenous insulin should be administered judiciously in diabetic patients with renal disease.

Insulin release is related to a number of events. First is the direct effect of glucose and amino acids to stimulate insulin release. The mechanism involves interaction with hormones from the GI tract released during enteral feeding. The autonomic nervous system, also through vagal stimulation, increases insulin release, as does β-adrenergic stimulation and α-adrenergic blockade. Nitric oxide stimulates insulin secretion, and potassium depletion decreases insulin secretion.

The most fundamental action of insulin is to stimulate increased cellular uptake of glucose in skeletal muscle cells, adipose tissue, and cardiac cells. This is particularly important in skeletal muscle cells, where muscle activity also increases glucose uptake and is an important variable in the management of the physically active diabetic patient. The brain, liver, and immune cells are exceptions, where insulin does not affect glucose transport. Hence, the diabetic patient has hyperglycemia because of inadequate cellular uptake of glucose. Along with glucose, potassium enters the cells under the influence of insulin, so the diabetic patient is also likely to have an imbalance of potassium concentrations across cell membranes.

Other important metabolic functions of insulin include the stimulation of glycogen formation, as well as the suppression of gluconeogenesis and lipolysis. The patient with insulin deficiency has low glycogen stores and active gluconeogenesis. This implies that in the diabetic patient, because of an absence of glycogen, protein must be broken down to make glucose. Insulin also increases the uptake of amino acids into muscle cells. Hence, an insulin deficiency leads to catabolism and negative nitrogen balance.

Fat metabolism is also abnormal in the diabetic state, with acceleration of lipid catabolism and increased formation of ketone bodies. A deficiency of insulin leads to increased fatty acid liberation from adipose tissue. These fatty acids have multiple metabolic effects, including interference with carbohydrate phosphorylation in muscle, which leads to further hyperglycemia. Low concentrations of insulin, which may be inadequate to prevent hyperglycemia, are often sufficient to block lipolysis. This effect explains the common clinical situation in which a patient is hyperglycemic without being ketotic.

Glucagon is a polypeptide released from the α cells of the pancreas and acts both to stimulate the release of insulin and to oppose some of the effects of insulin. It has both a direct and an indirect ability to increase circulating glucose levels. In some patients, after total pancreatic resection, glucose balance is not as poor as might be expected because of the concomitant absence of glucagon. Glucagon release is stimulated by hypoglycemia, epinephrine, and cortisol and is suppressed by glucose ingestion.

The metabolic effects of stress are intricately involved with the same pathways as those involved in DM. During stress, elevations in the circulating levels of cortisol, glucagon, catecholamines, and growth hormone all act to cause hyperglycemia. In addition, glucagon and adrenergic stimulation exert a suppressive effect on insulin release. Furthermore, inflammatory mediators released during stress enhance the release of the counter-regulatory hormones and directly affect the intracellular signaling pathways of insulin, culminating in significant insulin resistance.[57,58] Hence, mild hyperglycemia may occur in the stressed patient who does not have DM. In the diabetic patient, stress makes the hyperglycemia more difficult to control. In a patient with minimal or subclinical DM before the stressful episode, the hyperglycemia may become difficult to manage during the stress-related event.

Diagnosis

For decades, the diagnosis of diabetes was based on plasma glucose criteria, either the fasting plasma glucose (FPG) or the 2-hour value in the 75-g oral glucose tolerance test (OGTT). Starting in 2009, the criteria to diagnose DM was amended and now includes hemoglobin A1C (HbA1C) >6.5%.[52] Correlation of HbA1C with average glucose levels is presented in Table 46-10. Other criteria for diagnosing DM are listed in Table 46-11. As with most diagnostic tests, a test result diagnostic of diabetes should be repeated to rule out laboratory error, unless the diagnosis is clear on clinical grounds.[59]

TABLE 46-10. CORRELATION OF HEMOGLOBIN A1C WITH AVERAGE GLUCOSE

	Mean Plasma Glucose	
A1C (%)	mg/dL	mmol/dL
6	126	7.0
7	154	8.6
8	183	10.2
9	212	11.8
10	240	13.4
11	269	14.9
12	298	16.5

These estimates are based on ADAG data of 2,700 glucose measurements over 3 months per A1C measurement in 507 adults with type 1, type 2, and no diabetes. The correlation between A1C and average glucose was 0.92. (From Nathan DM, Kuenen J, Borg R, et al. A1c-derived average glucose study group. Translating the A1C assay into estimated average glucose values. *Diabetes Care.* 2008;31:1473–1478.)

TABLE 46-11. CRITERIA FOR THE DIAGNOSIS OF DIABETES

1. A1C ≥6.5%. The test should be performed in a laboratory using a method that is certified and standardized.[a]
2. Fasting plasma glucose ≥126 mg/dL (7 mmol/L). Fasting is defined as no caloric intake for at least 8 hours.[a]
3. Two-hour plasma glucose ≥200 mg/dL (11.1 mmol/L) during an oral glucose tolerance test (OGTT). The test should be performed as described by the World Health Organization, using a glucose load containing the equivalent of 75 g anhydrous glucose dissolved in water.[a]
4. In a patient with classic symptoms of hyperglycemia or hyperglycemic crisis, a random plasma glucose ≥200 mg/dL (11.1 mmol/L).

[a]In the absence of unequivocal hyperglycemia, result should be confirmed by repeat testing. (Adapted from Surks MI, Sievert R. Drugs and thyroid function. *N Engl J Med.* 1995;333:1688–1694.)

Treatment

Patients with type 1 DM require insulin to survive. Further, the risk of microvascular complications can be decreased if glycemic control is maintained near normal levels of blood glucose (HbA1C <7%).[52] Patients may be on a range of doses of short-acting and long-acting insulin, with doses given 3 to 4 times per day, depending on the desire for tight control. In some clinical situations, an insulin pump may be used to administer a constant level of insulin.

Patients with type 2 DM may initially be treated with diet control, exercise, and metformin therapy.[60] Metformin is a biguanide that decreases hepatic glucose output and enhances the sensitivity of both hepatic and peripheral tissues to insulin.[61] If this fails to control glucose levels or the diabetes worsens, therapy with insulin and additional oral agents are indicated.[52] The goal is to decrease HbA1C levels below 7% safely, without causing hypoglycemia. Each new class of noninsulin agents added to initial therapy is expected to reduce HbA1C by 0.9% to 1.1%.[62] Selected properties of noninsulin glucose-lowering drugs are noted in Table 46-12. Sulfonylureas (glyburide, glipizide, glimepiride) and glinides (repaglinide, nateglinide) enhance β-cell insulin secretion. Rosiglitazone (Avandia) and pioglitazone (Actos) are thiazolidinediones that increase insulin sensitivity. α-glucosidase inhibitors (acarbose, miglitol) decrease postprandial glucose absorption. Amylin analogs (pramlinide [Symlin]) suppress glucagon secretion and slow gastric emptying. Incretin mimetics (exenatide [Byetta]), as the name implies, immulate natural incretin hormones (glucagon-like peptide-1 [GLP-1], glucose-dependent insulinotropic polypeptide [GIP]) and increase insulin production, inhibit glucagon secretion, and decrease glucose absorption. Dipeptidyl-peptidase-4 inhibitors (sitagliptin [Januvia]) also slow degradation of incretin hormones and improve postprandial hyperglycemia. Bariatric surgery may be considered for adults with a body mass index >35 kg/m^2 and type 2 diabetes, especially if the diabetes or associated comorbidities are difficult to control with lifestyle and pharmacologic therapy.[52]

TABLE 46-12. **PROPERTIES OF SELECTED GLUCOSE-LOWERING DRUGS**

Class	Compounds	Mechanism	Actions
Biguanides	Metformin	Activate AMP-kinase	Decrease hepatic glucose production Decrease intestinal glucose absorption Increase insulin action
Sulfonylureas (second generation)	Glibenclamide/Glyburide Glipizide Gliclazide Glimepiride	Close KATP channels on β-cell plasma membranes	Increase insulin secretion
Meglitinides	Repaglinide Nateglinide	Close KATP channels on β-cell plasma membranes	Increase insulin secretion
Thiazolidinediones (Glitazones)	Pioglitazone Rosiglitazone	Activate the nuclear transcription factor PPAR-γ	Increase peripheral insulin sensitivity
α-glucosidase inhibitors	Acarbose Miglitol	Inhibit intestinal α-glucosidase	Intestinal carbohydrate digestion (and consequently, absorption is slowed)
GLP-1 receptor agonists (incretin mimetics)	Exenatide Liraglutide	Activate GLP-1 receptors (β-cells/ endocrine pancreas; brain/ autonomous nervous system)	Increase insulin secretion (glucose dependent) Decrease glucagon secretion (glucose dependent) Slow gastric emptying Increase satiety
DPP-4 inhibitors (incretin enhancers)	Sitagliptin Vildagliptin Saxagliptin Linagliptin	Inhibit DPP-4 activity, prolong survival of endogenously released incretin hormones	Increase active GLP-1 concentration Increase active GIP concentration Increase insulin secretion Decrease glucagon secretion
Bile acid sequestrants	Colesevelam	Bind bile acids/cholesterol	Unknown
Dopamine-2 agonists	Bromocriptine	Activate dopaminergic receptors	Alter hypothalamic regulation of metabolism Increase insulin sensitivity

Adapted from Standards of medical care in diabetes–2012. *Diabetes Care.* 2012;35(Suppl 1):S11–S63.

Anesthetic Management

Successful management of diabetic patients is as, or more dependent upon chronic complication management than acute glycemia.

Preoperative

Preoperative evaluation and management has three important goals: One is determining end-organ complications of DM. This requires a thorough history and physical, a recent ECG, blood urea nitrogen, potassium, creatinine, glucose, and urinalysis. Second is determining the patient's glucose-lowering regimen. Patients may be on different types of insulin regimens and oral hypoglycemic agents. Preoperative counseling has to be specific to the patient's glucose-lowering regimen. The third goal is to determine patient glycemic control and the need for preoperative intervention to control glucose.

End-Organ Complications of Diabetes

6 Atherosclerosis develops earlier and is more widespread in diabetic patients compared with nondiabetics. Manifestations include coronary artery disease, peripheral vascular disease, cerebrovascular disease, and renovascular disease. The incidence of postoperative myocardial infarction is increased in diabetic patients, and the complication rate is higher. Coronary artery disease can manifest at a young age or atypically in type 1 diabetics. Silent myocardial ischemia and infarction occur more commonly in diabetic patients, perhaps because of sensory neuropathy of the visceral afferents to the heart. DM may be associated with a cardiomyopathy in the face of angiographically normal coronary arteries, possibly with diffuse disease in arteries too small to be visualized. The American College of Cardiology (ACC)/American Heart Association guidelines recognize DM as an intermediate risk factor when evaluating patients for noncardiac surgery.[63] Preoperative hyperglycemia, as documented by increased HbA1C, has consistently been associated with poor perioperative outcomes in a variety of clinical situations.[56,64]

Diabetic nephropathy occurs in 20% to 40% of patients with diabetes and is the leading cause of end-stage renal disease (ESRD). Albuminuria usually precedes a steady decline in renal function. Microalbuminuria (30 to 299 mg/24 hours) has been shown to be the earliest stage of diabetic nephropathy in type 1 diabetes and a marker for development of nephropathy in type 2 diabetes.[52,65]

Patients with diabetes can develop heterogeneous types of neuropathies with diverse clinical manifestations. Most common among the neuropathies are chronic sensorimotor distal symmetric polyneuropathy and autonomic neuropathy.[66] Cardiovascular autonomic neuropathy is clinically the most important. It presents as resting tachycardia, exercise intolerance, and orthostatic hypotension. Autonomic function may be tested by measuring the beat-to-beat variation in heart rate during breathing, heart rate response to a Valsalva maneuver, and orthostatic changes in diastolic blood pressure and heart rate. Diabetic patients with autonomic neuropathy are at increased risk for intraoperative hypotension, requiring vasopressor support, and perioperative cardiorespiratory arrest.[67–69] There may be an exaggerated pressor response to tracheal intubation.[70] Autonomic neuropathy predisposes to intraoperative hypothermia.[71]

Diabetic patients may also have GI neuropathies (e.g., esophageal enteropathy, gastroparesis, constipation, diarrhea, fecal incontinence). They may have delayed gastric emptying, and therefore they may be at increased risk of pulmonary aspiration of gastric contents. Autonomic function tests can predict the presence of solid food particles in gastric contents, but not increased gastric volume or acidity. Metoclopramide or erythromycin may be useful in emptying the stomach of solid food.[52]

In up to 40% of juvenile patients with DM presenting for renal transplantation, laryngoscopy can be difficult.[72] This may be due to diabetic stiff joint syndrome, a frequent complication of type 1 DM, leading to decreased mobility of the atlanto-occipital joint. The "prayer sign," an inability to approximate the palmar surfaces of the interphalangeal joints, is associated with stiff joint syndrome and may predict difficult laryngoscopy. Diabetic patients are at an increased risk of cognitive decline, dementia, fractures, cancer, obstructive sleep apnea, and hearing disorders.[52]

Determining Glucose-Lowering Regimen and Preoperative Counseling

Though specific protocols vary from institution to institution, a typical protocol followed at our institution is as follows.[73] Patients who are on oral antihyperglycemic medications are advised to discontinue their medications the night before surgery. No oral hypoglycemic medications are administered or advised on the morning of surgery. Medications are reinstituted after the patient has resumed a normal diet. Patients who are on sulfonylureas are particularly at risk for developing hypoglycemia. Metformin should be discontinued preoperatively because it has been associated with severe lactic acidosis during episodes of hypotension, poor perfusion, or hypoxia. However, similar perioperative outcomes have been reported in patients who have undergone surgery without discontinuing metformin.[74]

For patients who are taking short- or long-acting insulin preparations, adjustment of the insulin should take into account the timing of their insulin regimen. Patients who take both evening and morning doses of insulin should take their usual dose of evening short-acting insulin, but reduce their intermediate- or long-acting insulin dose by 20% the night before surgery. On the morning of surgery, they should omit their morning short-acting insulin and reduce the intermediate- or long-acting dose by 50% (and take this only if the fasting glucose is >120 mg/dL). If patients are using a premixed insulin, they are instructed to reduce their evening dose prior to surgery by 20% and hold insulin completely on the morning of the procedure.[73] Patients with type 1 diabetes need some basal insulin at all times.

Preoperative Glycemic Control

It is axiomatic that the patient should attain the best possible preoperative metabolic control; however, no randomized control study has documented that achieving a certain glycemic range preoperatively for a certain period of time will improve perioperative outcome.[75] Currently, no evidence-based guidelines exist regarding when to cancel a surgical procedure due to hyperglycemia. Given the multitude of patient factors involved as well as the variety of surgical procedures and procedure urgency, it is unlikely that recommendations based on outcomes will be forthcoming. Providers need to weigh several issues when considering this question. First, the urgency of surgery should be considered. Second, hyperglycemia could represent an unstable metabolic state, such as diabetic ketoacidosis, which should be rapidly assessed in the preoperative area. Elective surgery in an unstable metabolic state is not recommended (see "Emergencies"). Furthermore, the chronic glycemic state of the patient should be considered. If the patient has chronically elevated glucose values, this represents poor glucose control, as opposed to a new illness. In this situation, there are opportunities for providers to identify and address the problem prior to the patient arriving in the preoperative area. The value of canceling elective surgery in this situation is unclear. Another consideration is that the hyperglycemia may be caused by the illness for which the patient presented for surgery (e.g., osteomyelitis), which would not be expected to improve until the patient undergoes surgery. Providers must therefore assess the patient for stability, the need for the procedure, the risks of the procedure, and the ability of the patient to achieve glucose control if the surgery is postponed. Some institutions have used a cutoff value of 300 mg/dL as a trigger in the preoperative area for evaluation for ketoacidosis via either urine ketone dipstick or whole blood chemistry. In other institutions it is left to the discretion of the physician.[73] However, it is recommended to postpone nonurgent or elective surgery if there is an acute rise in glucose to >400 mg/dL.[73]

Intraoperative

The details of the anesthetic plan depend intimately on the end-organ complications. Invasive monitoring may be indicated for the patient with heart disease, awake intubation may be necessary if a difficult intubation is predicted, fluid management and drug choices may depend on renal function, and aspiration must be considered if there is gastroparesis.

Blood glucose levels should be measured before and after surgery. The need for additional measurements is determined by the duration and magnitude of surgery, as well as the brittleness of the diabetes. Hourly measurements are reasonable in high-risk patients, especially those receiving continuous insulin through either an insulin pump or infusion.

The standard glucose dosage for an adult patient is 5 to 10 g/hour (100 to 200 mL of 5% dextrose solution hourly). Intraoperative administration of glucose should be guided by the patient's glucose level with the goal of preventing hypoglycemia or hyperglycemia. Routine administration of glucose-containing intravenous fluids is not recommended. It is best to separately record dextrose administration and fluids given.

Monitoring of the patient who arrives in the operating room with significant metabolic impairment, such as diabetic ketoacidosis, is similar to management in the medical ICU, including hourly determinations of blood glucose, arterial pH, electrolytes, and fluid balance. Frequent reassessments with medical consultation as necessary guide the use of fluids, electrolytes, especially potassium, insulin, phosphate, and glucose.

Another area of monitoring that is extremely important in the diabetic patient is positioning on the operating table. Injuries to the limbs or nerves are more likely in the patient who arrives in the operating room already compromised by diabetic peripheral vascular disease or neuropathy. The peripheral nerves may already be partly ischemic and therefore particularly vulnerable to pressure or stretch injuries.[76]

Hyperglycemia and Perioperative Outcomes

Prior to the past decade, little attention was paid to the control of hyperglycemia in the perioperative period or in the acute phase of critical illness managed in the ICU. Permissive or stress-induced hyperglycemia was generally accepted as the norm. Stress-induced hyperglycemia is defined as a transient response to the stress of an acute injury or illness.[54] Observational studies have reported significant prevalence of hyperglycemia in hospitalized patients. Seventy percent of diabetic patients with acute coronary syndrome and 80% of cardiac surgery patients in the perioperative period may develop hyperglycemia.[60] Hyperglycemia in a hospital setting is defined as any blood glucose >140 mg/dL.[77] Hyperglycemia significantly impairs chemotaxis, phagocytosis, generation of reactive oxygen species, and intracellular killing of bacteria.[78] Vascular reactivity is also decreased by hyperglycemia and is proposed to be related to decreased nitric oxide production. Acute hyperglycemia has also been shown to lead to poor outcomes in the setting of myocardial infarction and stroke.[78] There is evidence that hyperglycemia in hospitalized patients leads directly to adverse consequences.[78]

In surgical patients, *post*operative hyperglycemia is associated with an increased risk of infection, renal and pulmonary complications, and also mortality (Fig. 46-7).[56,79–83] Many studies have addressed the effects of hyperglycemia *peri*operatively and confirmed similar associations.[75,84–86] One study demonstrated that for every 20 mg/dL increase in the mean intraoperative glucose, the risk of an adverse outcome increased by more than 30%.[84]

Two other glycemic factors are also associated with poor perioperative outcomes. Hypoglycemia is a rare occurrence compared to hyperglycemia, but it is the principal factor limiting optimization of glycemic control and is associated with increased mortality.[87,88] Finally, glucose variability (changes in the measured level of blood glucose) is an independent predictor of mortality.[89] This indicates that measures of glycemia, other than glucose concentration, may be important in the pathophysiology of hyperglycemia. Three different methods of expression of glucose variability are utilized: standard deviation (SD) of glucose, the mean amplitude of glycemic excursions (MAGE), and the glycemic lability index (GLI). MAGE is the mean of absolute values of any Δglucose (consecutive values) that are >1 SD of the entire set of glucose values. GLI is the squared difference between consecutive glucose measures per unit of actual time between those samples. Of these three methods, the GLI may be the best discriminator for mortality.[90] However, no prospective trials have determined whether decreased glucose variability with insulin results improved perioperative outcomes.

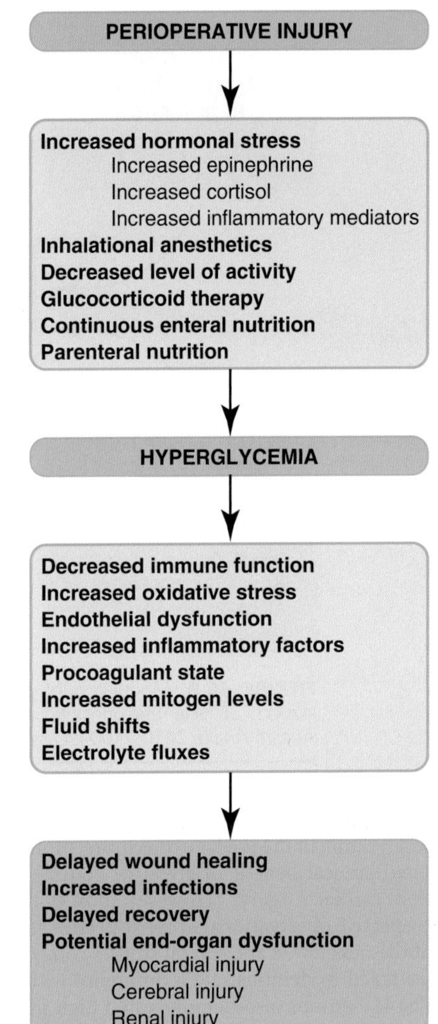

FIGURE 46-7. Relation among perioperative injury, hyperglycemia, and outcomes. (Reproduced from Akhtar S, Barash PG, Inzucchi SE. Scientific principles and clinical implications of perioperative glucose regulation and control. *Anesth Analg*. 2010;110(2):478–497, with permission.)

Perioperative Glycemic Control

Many factors influence the glucose levels in the perioperative period (Fig. 46-8). Endogenous insulin secretions, exogenous insulin administration, insulin resistance, endogenous glucose production, exogenous glucose administration, and overall glucose consumption are some of the key factors that determine glucose levels in a patient.

Insulin secretion can be decreased because of the direct effects of anesthetics, while significant insulin resistance develops postoperatively. Degree of insulin resistance is directly related to surgical trauma (Fig. 46-9). Insulin resistance can not only be modified by the stress of surgery and the inflammatory state but it may also be affected by nutritional intake and level of activity. Postoperative ambulation and physical activity can alter glucose consumption acutely. Intraoperative and postoperative hyperglycemia are predicable in patients who present for cardiac and high-risk noncardiac surgery and/or have poor glycemic control preoperatively (e.g., diabetics, or patients who have an ongoing metabolic insult secondary to trauma or sepsis).[56]

Glycemic Goals

In 2001, van den Berghe et al. published a landmark paper[91] that demonstrated a mortality benefit of tight glucose control in critically ill patients in the surgical ICU. From this study originated the concept of intensive insulin therapy (IIT) as a means of normalizing elevated glucose levels in critically ill patients. IIT was defined by a target glucose range of 80 to 110 mg/dL, and standard care implied a target glucose range of 180 to 200 mg/dL.[91] Although the study van den Berghe et al. was a single-center, nonblinded trial, other retrospective studies also supported their

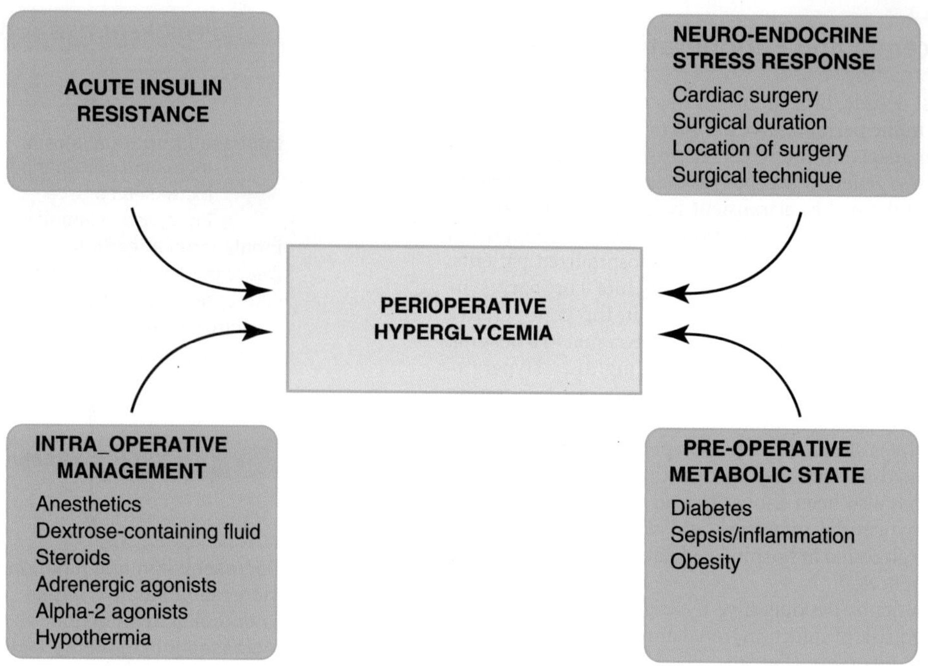

FIGURE 46-8. Modulators of perioperative hyperglycemia. (Reproduced from Akhtar S, Barash PG, Inzucchi SE. Scientific principles and clinical implications of perioperative glucose regulation and control. *Anesth Analg*. 2010;110(2):478–497, with permission.)

findings and many centers adopted IIT protocols for management of hyperglycemia in the ICU. Furthermore, numerous studies documented clinical benefit of glycemic control in patients who underwent cardiac surgery.[56] However, most of the evidence was from prospective observational or retrospective studies. Over the course of the next few years, several studies comparing IIT to standard care failed to demonstrate a difference with respect to mortality. The IIT groups also demonstrated high incidences of hypoglycemia (8% to 28%), which was 6 times higher than the control group.[92–95]

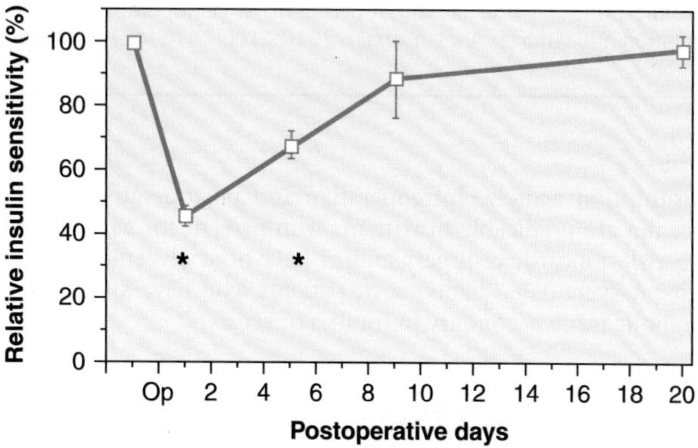

FIGURE 46-9. Time course for postoperative insulin resistance in patients undergoing open cholecystectomy. Relative insulin sensitivity represented as a percentage that is calculated as postoperative insulin sensitivity/perioperative insulin sensitivity × 100. Insulin sensitivity was determined within 5 days preoperatively and at days 1 (n = 9), 5, 9, and 20 (n = 5) postoperatively. *Statistically significant difference. Op, day of the operation. (Reproduced from Thorell A, Efendic S, Gutnaik M, et al. Insulin resistance after abdominal surgery. *Br J Surg*. 1994;81: 59–63, with permission.)

7 The largest study to date, the NICE-SUGAR study, a multicenter, multinational randomized controlled trial, compared the effect of intensive glycemic control (target 81 to 108 mg/dL, mean blood glucose attained 115 mg/dL) to standard glycemic control (target 144 to 180 mg/dL, mean blood glucose attained 144 mg/dL) on outcomes among 6,104 critically ill participants, almost all of whom required mechanical ventilation.[96] Surprisingly, 90-day mortality was significantly higher in the intensive versus the conventional group in both surgical and medical patients, as was mortality from cardiovascular causes. Severe hypoglycemia was also more common in the intensively treated group (6.8% vs. 0.5%). The results of this study were in stark contrast to the van den Berghe et al. study, which reported a 42% relative reduction in ICU mortality in critically ill surgical patients treated to a target blood glucose of 80 to 110 mg/dL.

One situation where tight glucose control with insulin may be beneficial is in patients who are administered exogenous glucose via total parenteral nutrition.[97] This was the case in van den Berghe et al. study where patients received significant exogenous glucose early in the ICU. Furthermore, the control group in NICE-SUGAR trial had reasonably good blood glucose management and was maintained at a mean glucose of 144 mg/dL, only 29 mg/dL above the intensively managed patients. Accordingly, this study's findings do not negate the concept that glycemic control in the ICU is important. However, they do strongly suggest that it may not be necessary to target blood glucose values to a highly stringent target of <110 mg/dL, and that it may actually be dangerous to control glucose too tightly.

Several studies published subsequent to the NICE-SUGAR trial underscored the findings of that investigation. Annane et al.[98] found no reduction in mortality and increased hypoglycemia in a randomized controlled trial of IIT with glucocorticoids in the treatment of septic shock. The control group was given standard insulin therapy plus glucocorticoids. Three recent meta-analyses of randomized trials investigating IIT demonstrated no overall effect on mortality and increased hypoglycemia rates in the IIT groups compared with controls.[97,99,100] An observational cohort study published prior to the NICE-SUGAR trial compared outcomes before and after institution of an IIT policy. Hypoglycemia was increased and no survival benefit was noted with the institution of IIT.[101]

In summary, association between perioperative hyperglycemia and poor outcomes is strong. Though hyperglycemia develops frequently in patients who undergo cardiac or high-risk noncardiac surgery, the value of controlling glucose levels tightly *intraoperatively* has not been proven conclusively. Poor glycemic control is probably a marker of significant metabolic perturbation, which is beyond the regulatory capacity of the body. Given that in the NICE-SUGAR trial the standard insulin therapy control group (140 to 180 mg/dL range) had similar outcomes (if not better) than the IIT group, the 140 to 180 mg/dL range is now generally accepted as the new goal. In 2009, the American Association of Clinical Endocrinologists and the American Diabetes Association (AACE/ADA) released formal recommendations for the management of hyperglycemia in the ICU.[102] The recommended threshold to initiate an insulin infusion is no higher than 180 mg/dL. Once insulin therapy has been initiated, the 140 to 180 mg/dL goal range is targeted.

In addition to the AACE/ADA, various other professional organizations have published guidelines for the management of glucose levels in the ICU. The Surviving Sepsis Campaign targets a blood glucose level of 150 mg/dL while maintaining glucose levels <180 mg/dL; the Institute for Healthcare Improvement target is <180 mg/dL; the 2009 European Society of Cardiology guidelines for perioperative cardiac management in noncardiac surgery patients do take into account the results of the NICE-SUGAR study and recommend maintaining glucose levels <180 mg/dL in postsurgery patients.[103] The ACC/American Heart Association targets 110 to 180 mg/dL in patients undergoing noncardiac surgery[53]; however, this predates the NICE-SUGAR trial. The Society of Thoracic Surgeons (for cardiac surgery) targets 150 to 180 mg/dL, while the most recent guidelines from the American College of Physicians recommend keeping glucose <180 mg/dL in critically ill patients[104] (Table 46-13).

In noncritically ill hospitalized patients, the goal is to keep the fasting premeal glucose <140 mg/dL and random glucose <180 mg/dL. This should ideally be achieved by basal plus bolus insulin dosing rather than sliding-scale insulin. Practitioners should also keep in mind that target glucose levels for terminally ill, elderly, frail, and nursing home patients have not been established. There is general consensus that in these populations, the risk of hypoglycemia outweighs the risk of hyperglycemia and less stringent targets may be more appropriate.[52,105]

Management of Perioperative Hyperglycemia

In view of the complex nature of glycemic control in the perioperative period, maintaining glucose levels within a specific range can be demanding. The narrower the desired glycemic range, the more resource intensive the protocol will be.

There are multiple insulin preparations, with varying duration of actions, that can be administered in many different ways.[106] The simplest way is to administer short-acting insulin subcutaneously. Only a few studies have adopted this route and have not been very successful in maintaining glucose in the desired range (40% to 60% of the time) and achieving it in a timely manner. In the perioperative setting, the state of peripheral perfusion is extremely variable and vasoconstriction is very common, often secondary to hypovolemia or hypothermia. Hence, absorption of any drug administered subcutaneously can be erratic and unreliable. Similarly, sliding-scale protocols have also been disappointing. Most study protocols that have demonstrated desirable glycemic control in the acute care setting have used continuous intravenous insulin infusion combined with intravenous bolus injections. Targeted glucose levels are achieved successfully and timely using these dynamic scale protocols combined with frequent blood glucose determinations. Once a certain requirement of insulin in a 24-hour period is known, the patient can be transitioned to basal–bolus insulin protocol. This requires giving a certain amount of long-acting insulin (which provides a fraction of basal insulin requirement), supplemented by 3 to 4 doses of short-acting insulin bolus based on blood glucose measurements.[54]

Blood glucose can be determined by central laboratory, blood–gas analysis machines, or various point-of-care testing devices that use capillary blood (fingerstick). Point-of-care devices are most commonly used in many acute care areas for glucose monitoring and management. Practitioners should keep in mind that the accuracy of these handheld meters can vary by 20%.[107] Glucose meter analysis (arterial and capillary blood) may provide higher glucose values, whereas blood–gas meter analysis of arterial blood may yield lower glucose values compared with central laboratory values. The hemodynamic state of the patient may also affect the accuracy of the blood glucose measurement by the point-of-care devices. Furthermore, whole blood glucose

TABLE 46-13. CURRENT RECOMMENDATIONS FOR GLYCEMIC CONTROL IN CRITICALLY ILL PATIENTS

Organization	Year	Patient Population	Treatment Threshold (mg/dL)	Target Glucose Level (mg/dL)
American Heart Association	2009	Patients undergoing noncardiac surgery	180	110–180
American Heart Association	2009	Patients with acute coronary syndrome	180	<140
Society of Thoracic Surgeons	2009	Cardiac surgery in ICU	150	150–180
European Society of Cardiology	2009	Patients after major noncardiac surgery	180	140–180
Surviving Sepsis Campaign	2009	ICU patients	180	<150
Institute for Healthcare Improvement	2009	ICU patients	180	<180
American Diabetes Association	2011	ICU patients	180	140–180
American College of Physicians	2011	ICU patients	180	140–180

values and plasma glucose values are different, and the same is true for arterial and venous blood. Therefore, a real possibility exists of overdosing or underdosing a patient with insulin. Hence, aberrant glucose values should be verified by central laboratory measurements, and practitioners should be aware of the performance of the point-of-care devices used in their institutions.[108]

Type 1 Diabetes

Type 1 diabetics require insulin or they will rapidly develop ketoacidosis and its complications. This can be given by administering one-half to two-thirds of the patient's usual intermediate-acting insulin subcutaneously on the morning of surgery. In addition to this basal insulin, a regular insulin sliding scale (RISS) can be added and titrated to blood glucose measurement.[109] Alternatively, an insulin infusion of 0.5 to 2 U/hour (100 U regular insulin in 1,000 mL normal saline at 5 to 20 mL/hour) can meet basal metabolic needs and be adjusted to maintain blood glucose at the desired level.[106] With either method, a slow glucose infusion (5% dextrose in water at 75 to 125 mL/hour) will prevent hypoglycemia while the patient is fasting.

Type 2 Diabetes

Patients who are on oral antihyperglycemic medications are advised to discontinue their medications the night before surgery. No oral hypoglycemic medications are administered or advised on the morning of surgery. Patients on chronic insulin are treated based on their insulin regimen. Perioperative glucose control can be achieved by insulin infusion titrated to blood glucose (typically in the ICUs) or basal long-acting insulin supplemented by a RISS. The use of a RISS as the sole method of control is to be discouraged, because it can predispose to wide glucose variations.[54]

Postoperatively, as the patient resumes oral intake, therapy can be transitioned to the patient's chronic regimen. Type 2 diabetics who have had a gastric bypass procedure can have rapid resolution of their glucose intolerance and will often need their oral agents and insulin reduced or even discontinued in the postoperative period. This effect appears to be due to changes in the incretin hormones such as GIP and GLP-1, rather than weight loss.[110]

Emergencies

Patients may present with metabolic instability, or it may develop perioperatively. Stress, trauma, and infection may all lead to increased insulin requirements and insulin resistance.[111]

Hyperosmolar Nonketotic Coma

An occasional elderly patient with minimal or mild DM may present with remarkably high blood glucose levels (>600 mg/dL) and profound dehydration. Such patients usually have enough endogenous insulin activity to prevent ketosis; even with blood sugar concentrations of 1,000 mg/dL, they are not in ketoacidosis. Presumably, it is the combination of an impaired thirst response and mild renal insufficiency that allows the hyperglycemia to develop. The marked hyperosmolarity may lead to coma and seizures, with the increased plasma viscosity producing a tendency to intravascular thrombosis. It is characteristic of this syndrome that the metabolic disturbance responds quickly to rehydration and small doses of insulin. If there are no cardiovascular contraindications, 1 to 2 L of normal saline, or equivalent, should be infused over 1 to 2 hours. Insulin, by bolus or infusion, should be administered. With rapid correction of the hyperosmolarity, cerebral edema is a risk, and recovery of mental acuity may be delayed after the blood glucose level and circulating volume have been normalized.

Diabetic Ketoacidosis

Diabetic ketoacidosis is defined by the biochemical triad of ketonemia, hyperglycemia, and acidemia.[112] If the diabetic patient has insufficient insulin effect to block the mobilization and metabolism of free fatty acids, the metabolic by-products acetoacetate and β-hydroxybutyrate accumulate. These ketone bodies are organic acids and cause a metabolic acidosis with an increased unmeasured anion gap. Clinically, the patient often presents because of intercurrent illness, trauma, or the untoward cessation of insulin therapy. Although hyperglycemia is almost always present, the degree of hyperglycemia does not correlate with the severity of acidosis. Blood sugar levels are often in the 250 to 500 mg/dL range. The patient is always dehydrated because of the combination of the hyperglycemia-induced osmotic diuresis and the nausea and vomiting typical of this syndrome. Because leukocytosis, abdominal pain, GI ileus, and mildly elevated amylase levels are all common in ketoacidosis, an occasional patient is misdiagnosed as having an intra-abdominal surgical problem.

Diagnostic criteria for diabetic ketoacidosis include (a) ketonemia or significant ketonuria; (b) blood glucose >250 mg/dL or known DM; and (c) serum bicarbonate below 18 mmol/L and/or arterial pH <7.3.[113] Treatment of diabetic ketoacidosis includes insulin administration and fluid and electrolyte replacement (Table 46-14). Route of administration of insulin is determined by the severity of diabetic ketoacidosis. Mild to moderate diabetic ketoacidosis can be treated with subcutaneously administered insulin analogs. However, severe diabetic ketoacidosis requires intravenous insulin administration. Typically a continuous infusion is started at 0.14 U/kg/hour. If the blood glucose does not fall by 10% in the first hour, a bolus of 0.14 U/kg is administered. Another alternative is to administer 0.1 U/kg as a bolus followed by an infusion at 0.1 U/kg/hour. When blood glucose levels decrease below 250 mg/dL, glucose should be added to the intravenous fluid while insulin therapy continues. Fluid requirements can be marked; 1 to 2 L of normal saline, or equivalent, should be given over 1 to 2 hours. After the first hour, they may need to be continued at 500 mL/hour. Further deficits can be replaced more gradually. Potassium replacement is a key concern

TABLE 46-14. MANAGEMENT OF DIABETIC KETOACIDOSIS

- Regular insulin, 10 U IV bolus, followed by an insulin infusion nominally at (blood glucose/150) U/h
- Isotonic IV fluids as guided by vital signs and urine output; anticipate 4–10 L deficit
- When urine output is >0.5 mL/kg/hour, give potassium chloride, 10–40 mEq/hour (with continuous ECG monitoring when the rate is >10 mEq/hour)
- When serum glucose is decreased to 250 mg/dL, add dextrose 5% at 100 mL/hour
- Consider sodium bicarbonate to correct pH <6.9

IV, intravenous(ly); ECG, electrocardiogram.

in patients with diabetic ketoacidosis. Because of the diuresis, the total-body potassium stores are reduced. However, acidosis by itself causes a shift of potassium ions out of the cell. Thus, the serum potassium concentration may be normal or even slightly elevated while the patient is acidotic. As soon as the metabolic acidosis is corrected, the potassium ions shift back into the cells. Consequently, the serum potassium concentration can decline acutely. Therefore, early and vigorous potassium replacement is required in these patients, with the exception of those patients in renal failure. Hypophosphatemia also occurs with the correction of the acidosis and, if severe, may cause impairment of ventilation, resulting from skeletal muscle weakness in the vulnerable patient. Instead of diabetic ketoacidosis, the diabetic patient with a metabolic acidosis may have lactic acidosis, which results from poor tissue perfusion or sepsis. It is diagnosed by the presence of an increased serum lactate concentration without an elevated ketone concentration.

Diabetic ketoacidosis must also be distinguished from the syndrome of alcoholic ketoacidosis. This typically occurs in the poorly nourished alcoholic patient after acute intoxication. Except for the presence of chemical ketoacidosis, alcoholic ketoacidosis is not clinically related in any way to DM. The alcoholic patient may be hypoglycemic or mildly hyperglycemic. The predominant ketone in this syndrome is β-hydroxybutyrate, which tends to react less sensitively in the standard laboratory nitroprusside reaction measurement of ketones. Hence, the diagnosis may be obscured. Administration of dextrose and parenteral fluids is the specific treatment for alcoholic ketoacidosis; insulin is not indicated (except in the rare circumstance in which the patient also has clear-cut DM).

Hypoglycemia

Hypoglycemia is the clinical occurrence most feared in the management of diabetic patients. The precise level at which symptomatic hypoglycemia occurs is variable. The normal, fasted patient may have blood sugar levels ≤50 mg/dL without symptoms. However, the diabetic patient who has a chronically elevated blood sugar level may be symptomatic at levels significantly above this glucose concentration. Hypoglycemia is almost impossible to diagnose clinically in the unconscious patient.

Clinically significant hypoglycemia is defined by Whipple's triad: (a) symptoms of neuroglycopenia, (b) simultaneous blood glucose concentration <40 mg/dL, and (c) relief of symptoms with glucose administration. Although a subclinical stress response may be initiated at glucose levels <70 mg/dL, a blood glucose level of approximately 55 mg/dL results in activation of the sympathetic nervous system and autonomic symptoms, which include sweating, palpitations, tremor, and hunger. Neuroglycopenic symptoms occur with blood glucose levels of approximately 45 mg/dL, and include behavioral and cognitive impairment, drowsiness, speech difficulty, blurred vision, seizures, coma, and death. Many of the autonomic as well as the early neurologic symptoms are notably absent in the intubated, sedated, critically ill, or anesthetized patient. In the anesthetized patient, these signs of sympathetic hyperactivity can easily be misinterpreted as inadequate or "light" anesthesia. In the anesthetized, sedated, or seriously ill patient, the mental changes of hypoglycemia are also unrecognizable. Furthermore, in patients being treated with β-adrenergic–blocking agents or in patients with advanced diabetic autonomic neuropathy, the sympathetic hyperactivity of hypoglycemia may be obscured. Thus, the clinical diagnosis of hypoglycemia in the surgical patient may be difficult to make, and only a high degree of suspicion and frequent blood glucose checks can prevent this complication. Treatment is with 25 g of intravenous dextrose (50 mL of dextrose 50% in water) or 1 mg of intramuscular glucagon if the patient is not alert, and 8 oz of juice if the patient is alert. The goal is to achieve a blood glucose level >100 mg/dL.

Hypoglycemia is more likely to occur in the diabetic surgical patient if insulin or sulfonylureas are given without supplemental glucose. With renal insufficiency, the action of insulin and oral hypoglycemic agents is prolonged.

PITUITARY GLAND

The pituitary gland is located below the base of the brain in a bony structure called the sella turcica. The pituitary gland and the hypothalamus together form a central unit that regulates the release of various hormones. The pituitary gland is divided into two components. The *anterior pituitary* (adenohypophysis) secretes prolactin, growth hormone, gonadotropins (luteinizing hormone and follicle-stimulating hormone), TSH, and ACTH. The *posterior pituitary* (neurohypophysis) secretes the hormones vasopressin and oxytocin. Hormone release from the anterior and posterior pituitary is regulated by the hypothalamus. Regulatory peptides or preformed hormones from the hypothalamus are transported to the pituitary gland through vascular or tissue connections.

Anterior Pituitary

Hyposecretion of anterior pituitary hormones is usually due to compression of the gland by tumor. This may begin as an isolated deficiency, but it usually develops into multiglandular dysfunction. Male impotence or secondary amenorrhea in the woman is an early manifestation of panhypopituitarism. Panhypopituitarism after postpartum hemorrhagic shock (Sheehan syndrome) is due to necrosis of the anterior pituitary gland. Radiation therapy delivered to the sella turcica or nearby structures and surgical hypophysectomy are other causes of panhypopituitarism. Panhypopituitarism is treated with specific hormone replacement therapy, which should be continued in the perioperative period. Stress doses of corticosteroids are necessary for patients receiving steroid replacement because of inadequate ACTH.

The hypersecretion of various anterior pituitary hormones is usually caused by an adenoma. Excess prolactin secretion with galactorrhea is a common hormonal abnormality associated with pituitary adenoma. Cushing disease may occur secondary to excess ACTH production, and gigantism or acromegaly may occur as a consequence of excess growth hormone production in the child or adult, respectively. Excessive secretion of TSH is rare.

Acromegaly in the adult patient may pose several problems for the anesthesiologist.[114] Hypertrophy occurs in skeletal, connec-
8 tive, and soft tissues.[115] The tongue and epiglottis are enlarged, making the patient susceptible to upper airway obstruction. The incidence of difficult intubation is 20% to 30% and may be clinically unpredictable.[116] Hoarseness may reflect thickening of the vocal cords or paralysis of an RLN due to stretching. Dyspnea or stridor is associated with subglottic narrowing. Peripheral nerve or artery entrapment, hypertension, and DM are other common findings. The anesthetic management of these patients is complicated by distortion of the facial anatomy and upper airway. Induction of general anesthesia may put the patient at increased risk if mask fit is improper or vocal cord visualization is impaired.

When the preoperative history suggests upper airway or vocal cord involvement, it is prudent to consider intubation of the trachea while the patient is awake.

Posterior Pituitary

The posterior pituitary, or neurohypophysis, is composed of terminal nerve endings that extend from the ventral hypothalamus. Vasopressin (antidiuretic hormone [ADH]) and oxytocin are the two principal hormones secreted by the posterior pituitary. Both hormones are synthesized in the supraoptic and paraventricular nuclei of the hypothalamus. They are bound to inactive carrier proteins, neurophysins, and transported by axons to membrane-bound storage vesicles located in the posterior pituitary. ADH is a nonapeptide that circulates as a free peptide after its release. The primary functions of ADH are maintenance of extracellular fluid volume and regulation of plasma osmolality. Oxytocin elicits contraction of the uterus and promotes milk secretion and ejection by the mammary glands.

Vasopressin

ADH promotes resorption of solute-free water by increasing cell membrane permeability to water alone. The target sites for ADH are the collecting tubules of the kidneys. A decrease in free water clearance causes a decrease in serum osmolality and a corresponding increase in circulating blood volume. Under normal conditions, the primary stimulus for the release of ADH is an increase in serum osmolality.

Osmoreceptors located in the hypothalamus are sensitive to changes in the normal serum osmolality of as little as 1% (normal osmolality is approximately 285 mOsm/L). Stretch receptors in the left atrium and perhaps pulmonary veins, which are sensitive to moderate reductions in the blood volume, are also capable of stimulating ADH secretion. The need to restore plasma volume may at times override osmotic inhibition of ADH release. Various physiologic and pharmacologic stimuli also influence the secretion of ADH. Positive-pressure ventilation of the lungs, stress, anxiety, hyperthermia, β-adrenergic stimulation, and any histamine-releasing stimulus can promote the release of ADH.

ADH also has other actions. It can increase blood pressure by constricting vascular smooth muscle (see Chapter 38). This activity is most significant in the splanchnic, renal, and coronary vascular beds, and provides the rationale for administering exogenous vasopressin in the management of hemorrhage due to esophageal varices. Caution must be taken when this drug is used in patients with coronary artery disease. ADH (even in small doses) can precipitate myocardial ischemia through vasoconstriction of the coronary arteries. It is unclear whether selective arterial infusion is safer than systemic administration with regard to cardiac and vascular side effects. ADH is also often used in vasodilatory shock as an adjuvant to other pressor agents.

ADH also promotes hemostasis through an increase in the level of circulating von Willebrand factor and factor VIII. Desmopressin (DDAVP), an analog of ADH, is commonly used to treat some types of von Willebrand disease (see Chapter 16). DDAVP is also frequently used to reverse the coagulopathy of renal failure.

Diabetes Insipidus

Diabetes insipidus results from inadequate secretion of ADH or resistance on the part of the renal tubules to ADH (nephrogenic diabetes insipidus). Failure to secrete adequate amounts of ADH results in polydipsia, hypernatremia, and a high output of poorly concentrated urine. Hypovolemia and hypernatremia may become so severe as to be life-threatening. This disorder usually occurs after destruction of the pituitary gland by intracranial trauma, infiltrating lesions, or surgery[117] (see Chapter 36). Patients in whom diabetes insipidus develops secondary to severe head trauma or subarachnoid hemorrhage often have impending brain death. Treatment of diabetes insipidus depends on the extent of the hormonal deficiency. During surgery, the patient with complete diabetes insipidus receives an intravenous infusion of aqueous ADH (100 to 200 mU/hour), combined with administration of an isotonic crystalloid solution. The serum sodium and plasma osmolality are measured on a regular basis and therapeutic changes are made accordingly. ADH may also be given intramuscularly (as vasopressin tannate in oil). DDAVP administered intranasally has prolonged antidiuretic activity (12 to 24 hours) and is associated with a low incidence of pressor effects. As a consequence of the large outpouring of ADH in response to surgical stress, patients with a residually functioning gland usually do not need parenteral ADH during the perioperative period unless the plasma osmolality rises above 290 mOsm/L. Nonhormonal agents that have efficacy in the treatment of incomplete diabetes insipidus include the oral hypoglycemic chlorpropamide (200 to 500 mg/day). This drug stimulates the release of ADH and sensitizes the renal tubules to the hormone. Hypoglycemia is a serious side effect that limits the usefulness of the drug. Clofibrate, a hypolipidemic agent, is also capable of stimulating ADH release and has been used in the outpatient setting. None of these medications are effective in the patient with nephrogenic diabetes insipidus. Paradoxically, the thiazide diuretics exert an antidiuretic action in patients with this disorder.

Inappropriate Secretion of Antidiuretic Hormone

Inappropriate and excessive secretion of ADH may occur in association with a number of diverse pathologic processes, including head injuries, intracranial tumors, pulmonary infections, small cell carcinoma of the lung, and hypothyroidism (see Chapter 36). The clinical manifestations occur as a result of a dilutional hyponatremia, decreased serum osmolality, and a reduced urine output with a high osmolality. Weight gain, skeletal muscle weakness, and mental confusion or convulsions are presenting symptoms. Peripheral edema and hypertension are rare. The diagnosis of the syndrome of inappropriate ADH secretion is one of exclusion, and other causes of hyponatremia must be ruled out first. The prognosis is related to the underlying cause of the syndrome.

The treatment for patients with mild or moderate water intoxication is restriction of fluid intake to 800 mL/day. Patients with severe water intoxication associated with hyponatremia and mental confusion may require more aggressive therapy, with the intravenous administration of a hypertonic saline solution. This may be administered in conjunction with furosemide. Caution must be observed in patients with poor left ventricular function. Isotonic saline is substituted for hypertonic solutions once the serum sodium is brought into a safe range. Too-rapid correction of hyponatremia may induce central pontine myelinolysis and cause permanent brain damage. Serum sodium should not be raised by more than 12 mEq/L in 24 hours. Other drugs that may be used in the patient with syndrome of inappropriate ADH are demeclocycline and lithium. Demeclocycline interferes with the ability of the renal tubules to concentrate urine and is frequently used in outpatients. Lithium is usually not used because of the high incidence of toxicity.

ENDOCRINE RESPONSE TO SURGICAL STRESS

Anesthesia, surgery, and trauma elicit a generalized endocrine metabolic response characterized by an increase in the plasma levels of cortisol, ADH, renin, catecholamines, and endorphins and by metabolic changes such as hyperglycemia and a negative nitrogen balance.[118,119] Various neural and humoral factors (e.g., pain, anxiety, acidosis, local tissue factors, hypoxia) play a role in activating this stress response. There is an acute response to critical illness that is characterized by normal pituitary function, but targets organ insensitivity. During the chronic phase of critical illness, there is generalized endocrine hypofunction probably of a hypothalamic origin.[120]

The induction of anesthesia increases the levels of circulating catecholamines and is a form of metabolic stress. Regional anesthesia may block part of the metabolic stress response during surgery, probably by blockade of the neural communication from the surgical area. It is theorized that the persistently high levels of circulating catecholamines in trauma and critical illness lead to stress hyperglycemia through a direct inhibition of insulin release. Bypass of the gut hormonal actions in patients receiving intravenous glucose feedings, especially if given in large amounts, contributes to the impairment of insulin release during illness and can create a particularly difficult management problem for diabetic patients.

Endorphins are a group of endogenous peptides with opioid activity that have been isolated from the central nervous system. It is well documented that β-endorphin is released from the anterior pituitary, where it is contained as part of β-lipoprotein, a 91-chain amino acid, which is a cleavage product of the precursor peptide for ACTH. Large increases in the central nervous system and plasma concentrations of endorphins in response to emotional or surgical stimuli suggest that these substances play a role in the body's response to stress. These substances modulate painful stimuli by binding to opiate receptors located throughout the brain and spinal cord.

Numerous experiments have focused on the stress response and its relation to the depth of anesthesia. Regional anesthesia and general anesthesia appear to blunt the release of various stress hormones during the period of surgical stimulation in a dose-dependent fashion. Historically, anesthesiologists have relied on the indirect measurement of hemodynamic variables such as blood pressure and heart rate to evaluate the level of autonomic activity in response to anesthesia and surgery. It is assumed that the physiologic manifestations of stress are potentially harmful, especially in patients with limited functional reserve. As such, anesthetic techniques and pain management strategies are designed to limit this neurohormonal response in the hope of providing the patient with some benefit. Further investigations are needed to assess the impact of these efforts on perioperative morbidity and mortality.

References

1. Surks MI, Sievert R. Drugs and thyroid function. *N Engl J Med.* 1995;333:1688–1694.
2. Deegan RJ, Furman WR. Cardiovascular manifestations of endocrine dysfunction. *J Cardiothorac Vasc Anesth.* 2011;25:705–720.
3. Klein I, Danzi S. Thyroid disease and the heart. *Circulation.* 2007;116:1725–1735.
4. Mulligan DC, McHenry CR, Kinney W, et al. Amiodarone-induced thyrotoxicosis: Clinical presentation and expanded indications for thyroidectomy. *Surgery.* 1993;114:1114–1119.
5. Cooper DS. Antithyroid drugs. *N Engl J Med.* 2005;352:905–917.
6. Franklyn JA. The management of hyperthyroidism. *N Engl J Med.* 1994;330:1731–1738.
7. Smallridge RC. Metabolic and anatomic thyroid emergencies: A review. *Crit Care Med.* 1992;20:276–291.
8. Hermann M, Richter B, Roka R, et al. Thyroid surgery in untreated severe hyperthyroidism: Perioperative kinetics of free thyroid hormones in the glandular venous effluent and peripheral blood. *Surgery.* 1994;115:240–245.
9. Farling PA. Thyroid disease. *Br J Anaesth.* 2000;85:15–28.
10. Bouaggad A, Nejmi SE, Bouderka MA, et al. Prediction of difficult tracheal intubation in thyroid surgery. *Anesth Analg.* 2004;99:603–606.
11. Szubin L, Kacker A, Kakani R, et al. The management of post-thyroidectomy hypocalcemia. *Ear Nose Throat J.* 1996;75:612–614, 616.
12. Wagner HE, Seiler C. Recurrent laryngeal nerve palsy after thyroid gland surgery. *Br J Surg.* 1994;81:226–228.
13. Lindsay RS, Toft AD. Hypothyroidism. *Lancet.* 1997;349:413–417.
14. Stathatos N, Wartofsky L. Perioperative management of patients with hypothyroidism. *Endocrinol Metab Clin North Am.* 2003;32:503–518.
15. Toft AD. Thyroxine therapy. *N Engl J Med.* 1994;331:174–180.
16. Bennett-Guerrero E, Kramer DC, Schwinn DA. Effect of chronic and acute thyroid hormone reduction on perioperative outcome. *Anesth Analg.* 1997;85: 30–36.
17. Ladenson PW, Levin AA, Ridgway EC, et al. Complications of surgery in hypothyroid patients. *Am J Med.* 1984;77:261–266.
18. Whitten CW, Latson TW, Klein KW, et al. Anesthetic management of a hypothyroid cardiac surgical patient. *J Cardiothorac Vasc Anesth.* 1991;5:156–159.
19. Weinberg AD, Ehrenwerth J. Anesthetic considerations and perioperative management of patients with hypothyroidism. *Adv Anesth.* 1987;4:185–212.
20. Mihai R, Farndon JR. Parathyroid disease and calcium metabolism. *Br J Anaesth.* 2000;85:29–43.
21. Fraser WD. Hyperparathyroidism. *Lancet.* 2009;374:145–158.
22. Roland EJ, Wierda JM, Eurin BG, et al. Pharmacodynamic behaviour of vecuronium in primary hyperparathyroidism. *Can J Anaesth.* 1994;41:694–698.
23. Udelsman R, Lin Z, Donovan P. The superiority of minimally invasive parathyroidectomy based on 1650 consecutive patients with primary hyperparathyroidism. *Ann Surg.* 2011;253:585–591.
24. Shindo ML, Rosenthal JM, Lee T. Minimally invasive parathyroidectomy using local anesthesia with intravenous sedation and targeted approaches. *Otolaryngol Head Neck Surg.* 2008;138:381–387.
25. Kivela JE, Sprung J, Richards ML, et al. Effects of propofol on intraoperative parathyroid hormone monitoring in patients with primary hyperparathyroidism undergoing parathyroidectomy: A randomized control trial. *Can J Anaesth.* 2011;58:525–531.
26. Shoback D. Hypoparathyroidism. *N Engl J Med.* 2008;359:391–403.
27. Vaughan ED Jr. Diseases of the adrenal gland. *Med Clin North Am.* 2004;88: 443–466.
28. Inder WJ, Hunt PJ. Glucocorticoid replacement in pituitary surgery: Guidelines for perioperative assessment and management. *J Clin Endocrinol Metab.* 2002;87: 2745–2750.
29. Rivers EP, Gaspari M, Abi Saad G, et al. Adrenal insufficiency in high-risk surgical ICU patients. *Chest.* 2001;119:889–896.
30. Lamberts SWJ, Bruining HA, DeJong FH. Corticosteroid therapy in severe illness. *N Engl J Med.* 1997;337:1285–1292.
31. Axelrod L. Perioperative management of patients treated with glucocorticoids. *Endocrinol Metab Clin North Am.* 2003;32:367–383.
32. Sutherland FWH, Naik SK. Acute adrenal insufficiency after coronary artery bypass grafting. *Ann Thorac Surg.* 1996;62:1516–1517.
33. Dorin RI, Qualls CR, Crapo LM. Diagnosis of adrenal insufficiency. *Ann Intern Med.* 2003;139:194–204.
34. Coursin DB, Wood KE. Corticosteroid supplementation for adrenal insufficiency. *JAMA.* 2002;287:236–240.
35. Engquist A, Brandt MR, Fernandes A, et al. The blocking effect of epidural analgesia on the adrenocortical and hyperglycemic responses to surgery. *Acta Anaesthesiol Scand.* 1977;21:330–335.
36. Salem M, Tainsh RE Jr, Bromberg J, et al. Perioperative glucocorticoid coverage: A reassessment 41 years after emergence of a problem. *Ann Surg.* 1994;219:416–425.
37. Symreng T, Karlberg BE, Kagedal B, et al. Physiological cortisol substitution of long-term steroid-treated patients undergoing major surgery. *Br J Anaesth.* 1981; 53:949–954.
38. Glowniak JV, Loriaux DL. A double-blind study of perioperative steroid requirements in secondary adrenal insufficiency. *Surgery.* 1997;121:123–129.
39. Marik PE, Varon J. Requirement of perioperative stress doses of corticosteroids. *Arch Surg.* 2008;143(12):1222–1226.
40. Prys-Roberts C. Phaeochromocytoma: Recent progress in its management. *Br J Anaesth.* 2000;85:44–57.
41. Kinney MAO, Warner ME, van Heerden JA, et al. Perianesthetic risks and outcomes of pheochromocytoma and paraganglioma resection. *Anesth Analg.* 2000;91:1118–1123.
42. Kinney MAO, Narr BJ, Warner MA. Perioperative management of pheochromocytoma. *J Cardiothorac Vasc Anesth.* 2002;16:359–369.
43. Chen H, Sippel RS, O'Dorisio MS, et al. The North American Neuroendocrine Tumor Society consensus guideline for the diagnosis and management of neuroendocrine tumors. *Pancreas.* 2010;39:775–783.

44. Witteles RM, Kaplan EL, Roizen MF. Sensitivity of diagnostic and localization tests for pheochromocytoma in clinical practice. *Arch Intern Med.* 2000;160:2521–2524.
45. Geoghegan JG, Emberton M, Bloom R, et al. Changing trends in the management of phaeochromocytoma. *Br J Surg.* 1998;85:117–120.
46. Ulchaker JC, Goldfarb DA, Bravo EL, et al. Successful outcomes in pheochromocytoma surgery in the modern era. *J Urol.* 1999;161:764–767.
47. Pacak K. Preoperative management of the pheochromocytoma patient. *J Clin Endocrinol Metab.* 2007;92:4069–4079.
48. Hamilton A, Sirrs S, Schmidt N, et al. Anaesthesia for phaeochromocytoma in pregnancy. *Can J Anaesth.* 1997;44:654–657.
49. Joris JL, Hamoir EE, Hartstein GM, et al. Hemodynamic changes and catecholamine release during laparoscopic adrenalectomy for pheochromocytoma. *Anesth Analg.* 1999;88:16–21.
50. James MF, Cronje L. Pheochromocytoma crisis: The use of magnesium sulfate. *Anesth Analg.* 2004;99:680–686.
51. Lord MS, Augoustides JGT. Perioperative management of pheochromocytoma: Focus on magnesium, clevidipine, and vasopressin. *J Cardiothorac Vasc Anesth.* 2012;26:526–631.
52. Standards of medical care in diabetes–2012. *Diabetes Care.* 2012;35(Suppl 1): S11–S63.
53. Corathers SD, Falciglia M. The role of hyperglycemia in acute illness: Supporting evidence and its limitations. *Nutrition.* 2011;27(3):276–281.
54. Smiley D, Umpierrez GE. Management of hyperglycemia in hospitalized patients. *Ann N Y Acad Sci.* 2010;1212:1–11.
55. Kim JA, Montagnani M, Koh KK, et al. Reciprocal relationships between insulin resistance and endothelial dysfunction: Molecular and pathophysiological mechanisms. *Circulation.* 2006;113(15):1888–1904.
56. Akhtar S, Barash PG, Inzucchi SE. Scientific principles and clinical implications of perioperative glucose regulation and control. *Anesth Analg.* 2010;110(2):478–497.
57. Bagry HS, Raghavendran S, Carli F. Metabolic syndrome and insulin resistance: Perioperative considerations. *Anesthesiology.* 2008;108(3):506–523.
58. Biddinger SB, Kahn CR. From mice to men: Insights into the insulin resistance syndromes. *Annu Rev Physiol.* 2006;68:123–158.
59. Sacks DB, Arnold M, Bakris GL, et al. Guidelines and recommendations for laboratory analysis in the diagnosis and management of diabetes mellitus. *Clin Chem.* 2011;57(6):e1–e47.
60. Qaseem A, Humphrey LL, Sweet DE, et al. Oral pharmacologic treatment of type 2 diabetes mellitus: A clinical practice guideline from the American college of physicians. *Ann Intern Med.* 2012;156(3):218–231.
61. Bailey CJ, Turner RC. Metformin. *N Engl J Med.* 1996;334(9):574–579.
62. Bennett WL, Maruthur NM, Singh S, et al. Comparative effectiveness and safety of medications for type 2 diabetes: An update including new drugs and 2-drug combinations. *Ann Intern Med.* 2011;154(9):602–613.
63. Fleisher LA, Beckman JA, Brown KA, et al. 2009 ACCF/AHA focused update on perioperative beta blockade incorporated into the ACC/AHA 2007 guidelines on perioperative cardiovascular evaluation and care for noncardiac surgery: A report of the American College of Cardiology Foundation/American Heart Association Task Force on practice guidelines. *Circulation.* 2009;120(21):e169–e276.
64. Pichardo-Lowden A, Gabbay RA. Management of hyperglycemia during the perioperative period. *Curr Diab Rep.* 2012;12(1):108–118.
65. Garg JP, Bakris GL. Microalbuminuria: Marker of vascular dysfunction, risk factor for cardiovascular disease. *Vasc Med.* 2002;7(1):35–43.
66. Freeman R. Not all neuropathy in diabetes is of diabetic etiology: Differential diagnosis of diabetic neuropathy. *Curr Diab Rep.* 2009;9(6):423–431.
67. Charlson ME, MacKenzie CR, Gold JP. Preoperative autonomic function abnormalities in patients with diabetes mellitus and patients with hypertension. *J Am Coll Surg.* 1994;179(1):1–10.
68. Latson TW, Ashmore TH, Reinhart DJ, et al. Autonomic reflex dysfunction in patients presenting for elective surgery is associated with hypotension after anesthesia induction. *Anesthesiology.* 1994;80(2):326–337.
69. Page MM, Watkins PJ. Cardiorespiratory arrest and diabetic autonomic neuropathy. *Lancet.* 1978;1(8054):14–16.
70. Vohra A, Kumar S, Charlton AJ, et al. Effect of diabetes mellitus on the cardiovascular responses to induction of anaesthesia and tracheal intubation. *Br J Anaesth.* 1993;71(2):258–261.
71. Kitamura A, Hoshino T, Kon T, et al. Patients with diabetic neuropathy are at risk of a greater intraoperative reduction in core temperature. *Anesthesiology.* 2000;92(5):1311–1318.
72. Hogan K, Rusy D, Springman SR. Difficult laryngoscopy and diabetes mellitus. *Anesth Analg.* 1988;67(12):1162–1165.
73. Alexanian SM, McDonnell ME, Akhtar S. Creating a perioperative glycemic control program. *Anesthesiol Res Pract.* 2011;2011:465974.
74. Duncan AI, Koch CG, Xu M, et al. Recent metformin ingestion does not increase in-hospital morbidity or mortality after cardiac surgery. *Anesth Analg.* 2007;104(1):42–50.
75. King JT, Goulet JL, Perkal MF, et al. Glycemic control and infections in patients with diabetes undergoing noncardiac surgery. *Ann Surg.* 2011;253(1):158–165.
76. Harati Y. Diabetic peripheral neuropathies. *Ann Intern Med.* 1987;107(4):546–559.
77. Umpierrez GE, Hellman R, Korytkowski MT, et al. Management of hyperglycemia in hospitalized patients in non-critical care setting: An endocrine society clinical practice guideline. *J Clin Endocrinol Metab.* 2012;97(1):16–38.
78. Inzucchi SE. Clinical practice. Management of hyperglycemia in the hospital setting. *N Engl J Med.* 2006;355(18):1903–1911.
79. Vriesendorp T, Morelis Q, Devries J, et al. Early post-operative glucose levels are an independent risk factor for infection after peripheral vascular surgery. A retrospective study. *Eur J Vasc Endovasc Surg.* 2004;28(5):520–525.
80. Pomposelli JJ, Baxter JK 3rd, Babineau TJ, et al. Early postoperative glucose control predicts nosocomial infection rate in diabetic patients. *JPEN J Parenter Enteral Nutr.* 1998;22(2):77–81.
81. Swenne CL, Lindholm C, Borowiec J, et al. Peri-operative glucose control and development of surgical wound infections in patients undergoing coronary artery bypass graft. *J Hosp Infect.* 2005;61(3):201–212.
82. Noordzij PG, Boersma E, Schreiner F, et al. Increased preoperative glucose levels are associated with perioperative mortality in patients undergoing noncardiac, nonvascular surgery. *Eur J Endocrinol.* 2007;156(1):137–142.
83. Schmeltz LR, DeSantis AJ, Thiyagarajan V, et al. Reduction of surgical mortality and morbidity in diabetic patients undergoing cardiac surgery with a combined intravenous and subcutaneous insulin glucose management strategy. *Diabetes Care.* 2007;30(4):823–828.
84. Gandhi GY, Nuttall GA, Abel MD, et al. Intraoperative hyperglycemia and perioperative outcomes in cardiac surgery patients. *Mayo Clin Proc.* 2005;80(7):862–866.
85. Frisch A, Chandra P, Smiley D, et al. Prevalence and clinical outcome of hyperglycemia in the perioperative period in noncardiac surgery. *Diabetes Care.* 2010; 33(8):1783–1788.
86. Polito A, Thiagarajan RR, Laussen PC, et al. Association between intraoperative and early postoperative glucose levels and adverse outcomes after complex congenital heart surgery. *Circulation.* 2008;118(22):2235–2242.
87. Krinsley J, Preiser JC. Intensive insulin therapy to control hyperglycemia in the critically ill: A look back at the evidence shapes the challenges ahead. *Crit Care.* 2010;14(6):330.
88. Zoungas S, Patel A, Chalmers J, et al. Severe hypoglycemia and risks of vascular events and death. *N Engl J Med.* 2010;363(15):1410–1418.
89. Krinsley JS. Glycemic variability: A strong independent predictor of mortality in critically ill patients. *Crit Care Med.* 2008;36(11):3008–3013.
90. Mackenzie IM, Whitehouse T, Nightingale PG. The metrics of glycaemic control in critical care. *Intensive Care Med.* 2011;37(3):435–443.
91. van den Berghe G, Wouters P, Weekers F, et al. Intensive insulin therapy in critically ill patients. *N Engl J Med.* 2001;345(19):1359–1367.
92. Van den Berghe G, Wilmer A, Hermans G, et al. Intensive insulin therapy in the medical ICU. *N Engl J Med.* 2006;354(5):449–461.
93. Arabi YM, Dabbagh OC, Tamim HM, et al. Intensive versus conventional insulin therapy: A randomized controlled trial in medical and surgical critically ill patients. *Crit Care Med.* 2008;36(12):3190–3197.
94. Brunkhorst FM, Engel C, Bloos F, et al. Intensive insulin therapy and pentastarch resuscitation in severe sepsis. *N Engl J Med.* 2008;358(2):125–139.
95. Preiser JC, Devos P, Ruiz-Santana S, et al. A prospective randomised multi-centre controlled trial on tight glucose control by intensive insulin therapy in adult intensive care units: The Glucontrol study. *Intensive Care Med.* 2009;35(10): 1738–1748.
96. Finfer S, Chittock DR, Su SY, et al. Intensive versus conventional glucose control in critically ill patients. *N Engl J Med.* 2009;360(13):1283–1297.
97. Marik PE, Preiser JC. Toward understanding tight glycemic control in the ICU: A systematic review and metaanalysis. *Chest.* 2010;137(3):544–551.
98. Annane D, Cariou A, Maxime V, et al. Corticosteroid treatment and intensive insulin therapy for septic shock in adults: A randomized controlled trial. *JAMA.* 2010;303(4):341–348.
99. Griesdale DE, de Souza RJ, van Dam RM, et al. Intensive insulin therapy and mortality among critically ill patients: A meta-analysis including NICE-SUGAR study data. *CMAJ.* 2009;180(8):821–827.
100. Kansagara D, Fu R, Freeman M, et al. Intensive insulin therapy in hospitalized patients: A systematic review. *Ann Intern Med.* 2011;154(4):268–282.
101. Treggiari MM, Karir V, Yanez ND, et al. Intensive insulin therapy and mortality in critically ill patients. *Crit Care.* 2008;12(1):R29.
102. Moghissi ES, Korytkowski MT, DiNardo M, et al. American Association of Clinical Endocrinologists and American Diabetes Association consensus statement on inpatient glycemic control. *Endocr Pract.* 2009;15(4):353–369.
103. Poldermans D, Bax JJ, Boersma E, et al. Guidelines for pre-operative cardiac risk assessment and perioperative cardiac management in non-cardiac surgery. *Eur Heart J.* 2009;30(22):2769–2812.
104. Qaseem A, Humphrey LL, Chou R, et al. Use of intensive insulin therapy for the management of glycemic control in hospitalized patients: A clinical practice guideline from the American College of Physicians. *Ann Intern Med.* 2011;154(4):260–267.
105. Sinclair AJ, Paolisso G, Castro M, et al. European Diabetes Working Party for Older People 2011 clinical guidelines for type 2 diabetes mellitus. Executive summary. *Diabetes Metab.* 2011;37(Suppl 3):S27–S38.
106. Inzucchi SE. The Yale Diabetes Center Diabetes Facts and Guidelines 2011–2012. http://endocrinology.yale.edu/patient/50135_Yale%20National%20F.pdf. Accessed January 4, 2012.
107. Rice MJ, Pitkin AD, Coursin DB. Review article: Glucose measurement in the operating room: More complicated than it seems. *Anesth Analg.* 2010; 110(4):1056–1065.

108. Maerz LL, Akhtar S. Perioperative glycemic management in 2011: Paradigm shifts. *Curr Opin Crit Care.* 2011;17(4):370–375.
109. Coursin DB, Connery LE, Ketzler JT. Perioperative diabetic and hyperglycemic management issues. *Crit Care Med.* 2004;32(4 Suppl):S116–S125.
110. Cummings DE, Overduin J, Foster-Schubert KE. Gastric bypass for obesity: Mechanisms of weight loss and diabetes resolution. *J Clin Endocrinol Metab.* 2004;89(6):2608–2615.
111. Nyenwe EA, Kitabchi AE. Evidence-based management of hyperglycemic emergencies in diabetes mellitus. *Diabetes Res Clin Pract.* 2011;94(3):340–351.
112. Savage MW, Dhatariya KK, Kilvert A, et al. Joint British Diabetes Societies guideline for the management of diabetic ketoacidosis. *Diabet Med.* 2011;28(5):508–515.
113. Peterson C, Fox JA, Devallis P, et al. Starvation in the midst of cardiopulmonary bypass: Diabetic ketoacidosis during cardiac surgery. *J Cardiothorac Vasc Anesth.* 2012;26:910–916.
114. Melmed S. Acromegaly. *N Engl J Med.* 2006;355:2558–2573.
115. Smith M, Hirsch NP. Pituitary disease and anaesthesia. *Br J Anaesth.* 2000;85:3–14.
116. Schmitt H, Buchfelder M, Radespiel-Troger M, et al. Difficult intubation in acromegalic patients: Incidence and predictability. *Anesthesiology.* 2000;93:110–114.
117. Nemergut EC, Dumont AS, Barry UT, et al. Perioperative management of patients undergoing transsphenoidal pituitary surgery. *Anesth Analg.* 2005;101:1170–1181.
118. Weissman C. The metabolic response to stress: An overview and update. *Anesthesiology.* 1990;73:308–327.
119. Desborough JP. The stress response to trauma and surgery. *Br J Anaesth.* 2000;85:109–117.
120. Langouche L, Van Den Berghe G. The dynamic neuroendocrine response to critical illness. *Endocrinol Metab Clin North Am.* 2006;35:777–791.

CHAPTER

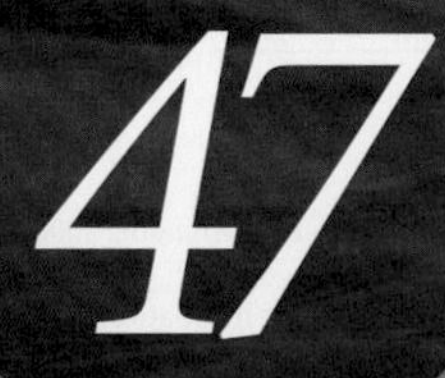

Anesthesia for Otolaryngologic Surgery

LYNNE R. FERRARI • CHARLES NARGOZIAN

Key Points

1. The restricted spaces in the airway require an understanding and cooperative relationship between surgeon and anesthesiologist, and the use of specially adapted equipment suitable to these cramped areas.
2. Despite only mild-to-moderate tonsillar enlargement on physical examination, children with obstructive sleep apnea have upper airway obstruction while awake and apnea during sleep. The clinician should not underestimate the severity of the problem based on tonsillar size alone.
3. Post-tonsillectomy hemorrhage may result in unappreciated large volumes of swallowed blood originating from the tonsillar fossa. These patients must be considered to have a full stomach, and anesthetic precautions addressing this situation must be taken.
4. The middle ear and sinuses are air-filled, nondistensible cavities. During procedures in which the eardrum is replaced or perforation is patched, nitrous oxide should be discontinued or, if this is not possible, limited to a maximum of 50% during the application of the tympanic membrane graft to avoid pressure-related displacement.
5. Systemic absorption of vasoconstrictive agents during FESS surgical procedures may cause hypertension, bradycardia, tachycardia, and arrhythmias. Preoperative evaluation should include a thorough investigation of the patient's cardiovascular status. Rapid response by the anesthesiologist to these effects is necessary in preventing complications.
6. Prior radiation therapy may lead to fibrosis and ankylosis in the temporomandibular joint, rendering orotracheal intubation difficult.
7. Prior to extubation after temporomandibular arthroscopy, the oral cavity and neck must be examined carefully to rule out the presence of extracapsular extravasation of irrigation fluid. Extravasation can lead to airway closure.
8. After extensive facial trauma or resection of tumors of the upper airway, it is prudent to keep the patient's trachea intubated until edema has subsided. Extraoral facial edema should lead the physician to suspect intraoral edema and possible airway compromise.

Multimedia

1. Airway Abscess
2. Facial Nerve
3. Jet Ventilation
4. Epiglottis
5. Laser ENT
6. Tracheostomy

EVALUATING THE AIRWAY

Air flows through the upper respiratory passages, into the trachea, bronchi, bronchioles, and into alveoli in the healthy human. Air flow occurs seemingly without either thought or effort, and the actual work of respiration in the unobstructed airway is minimal. However, airway obstruction due to malformation, tumor, infection, or trauma may significantly alter the clinical presentation and make gas exchange a laborious, energy-consuming process. The increased work of breathing can leave the patient exhausted, incapable of maintaining adequate gas exchange, and finally succumbing to ventilatory failure. Significant obstruction and anatomic distortion may be present in a patient with minimal evidence of disease because clinically evident upper airway obstruction is a late sign. It is a most unwelcome experience for the anesthesiologist to unexpectedly discover an obstructed upper airway at the time of attempted tracheal intubation.

In the presence of tumor, other mass lesions, or infection in the airway, it may be useful to obtain radiologic evaluation of the airway with plain films of the tracheal and laryngeal air columns or computed tomography and MRI studies of the airway. Significant anatomic distortion is usually evident and may help the anesthesiologist determine the most appropriate technique for securing the airway.

ANESTHESIA FOR PEDIATRIC EAR, NOSE, AND THROAT SURGERY

1 The safe management of the pediatric patient undergoing surgery of the ear, nose, and throat is particularly challenging to the anesthesiologist. The restricted spaces in the airway of the child require an understanding and cooperative relationship between surgeon and anesthesiologist, and the use of specially adapted equipment suitable to these cramped areas.

Tonsillectomy and Adenoidectomy

Untreated adenoidal hyperplasia may lead to nasopharyngeal obstruction, causing failure to thrive, speech disorders, obligate mouth breathing, sleep disturbances, orofacial abnormalities with a narrowing of the upper airway, and dental abnormalities. Surgical removal of the adenoids is usually accompanied by tonsillectomy; however, purulent adenoiditis, despite adequate medical therapy, and recurrent otitis media with effusion secondary to adenoidal hyperplasia are improved with adenoidectomy alone.

Tonsillectomy is one of the more commonly performed pediatric surgical procedures.[1] Chronic or recurrent acute tonsillitis, peritonsillar abscess, tonsillar hyperplasia, and obstructive sleep apnea syndrome are the major indications for surgery.[2–4] In addition, patients with cardiac valvular disease are at risk for endocarditis from recurrent streptococcal bacteremia secondary to infected tonsils. Tonsillar hyperplasia may lead to chronic airway obstruction resulting in sleep apnea, carbon dioxide (CO_2) retention, cor pulmonale, failure to thrive, swallowing disorders, and speech abnormalities. These risks are eliminated with removal of the tonsils.

Obstruction of the oropharyngeal airway by hypertrophied tonsils leading to apnea during sleep is an important clinical entity referred to as *obstructive sleep apnea syndrome.* Despite only mild-to-moderate tonsillar enlargement on physical examination, these patients have upper airway obstruction while awake and apnea during sleep. The goals of treatment are to relieve airway obstruction and increase the cross-sectional area of the pharynx, which is successful in two-thirds of pediatric cases.[5] Some patients require the use of nasal continuous positive airway pressure during sleep, whereas others may require a tracheostomy to bypass the chronic upper airway obstruction that is present. The two most frequent levels of obstruction during sleep are at the soft palate and the base of the tongue.[6] Most children have tremendous improvement in their symptoms after tonsillectomy.

In children with long-standing hypoxemia and hypercarbia, increased airway resistance can lead to cor pulmonale (Fig. 47-1). Patients have electrocardiographic evidence of right ventricular hypertrophy, with one-third of them having chest radiographs consistent with cardiomegaly. Each apneic episode causes progressively increasing pulmonary artery pressure with significant systemic and pulmonary artery hypertension, leading to ventricular dysfunction and cardiac dysrhythmias.[7] These patients often have dysfunction in the medulla or hypothalamic areas of the central nervous system causing persistently elevated CO_2, despite relief of airway obstruction. This group of patients has a hyperreactive pulmonary vascular bed, and the increased pulmonary vascular resistance and myocardial depression in response to hypoxia, hypercarbia, and acidosis are far greater than what is expected for that degree of physiologic alteration in the normal population. Cardiac enlargement is frequently reversible with digitalization and surgical removal of the tonsils and adenoids.

Preoperative Evaluation

A thorough history is the basis for the preoperative evaluation. Because patients requiring tonsillectomy and adenoidectomy have frequent infections, the parent should be questioned for current use of antibiotics, antihistamines, or other medicines. A history of sleep apnea should be sought. The physical examination should begin with observation of the patient. The presence of audible respirations, mouth breathing, nasal quality of the speech, and chest retractions should be noted. Mouth breathing may be the result of chronic nasopharyngeal obstruction. An elongated face, retrognathic mandible, and a high-arched palate may be present.[8] The oropharynx should be inspected for evaluation of tonsillar size to determine the ease of mask ventilation and tracheal intubation (Fig. 47-2). The presence of wheezing or rales on auscultation of the chest may be a lower respiratory manifestation of pharyngitis or tonsillitis. The presence of inspiratory stridor or prolonged expiration may indicate partial airway obstruction from hypertrophied tonsils or adenoids.

Measurement of hematocrit and coagulation parameters is suggested. Many nonprescription cold medications and

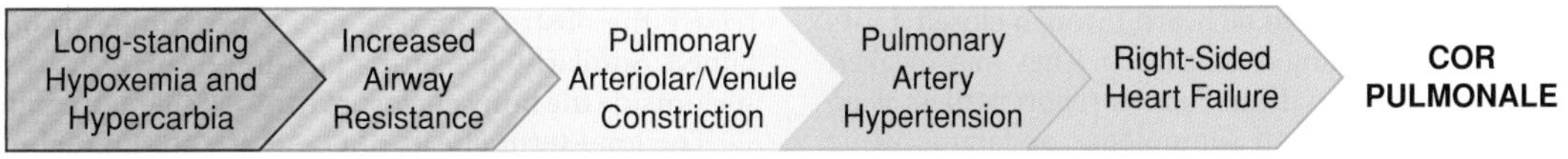

FIGURE 47-1. Events leading to cor pulmonale.

ANESTHESIA FOR SURGICAL SUBSPECIALTIES

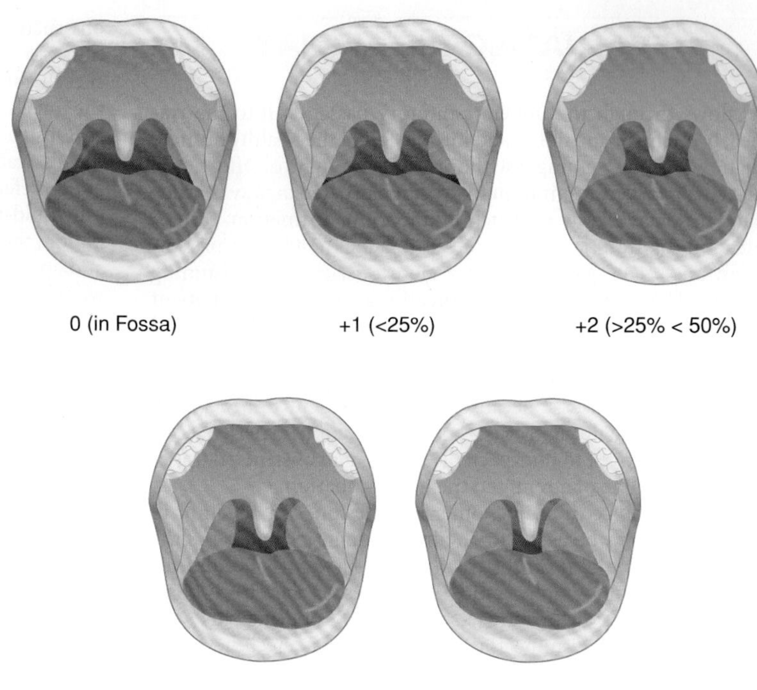

FIGURE 47-2. Classification of tonsil size, including percentage of oropharyngeal area occupied by hypertrophied tonsils.

antihistamines contain aspirin, which may affect platelet function, and this potential anticoagulation should be taken into consideration. Chest radiographs and electrocardiograms (ECGs) are not required unless specific abnormalities are elicited during the history, such as recent pneumonia, bronchitis, upper respiratory infection (URI), or history consistent with cor pulmonale, which is seen in children with obstructive sleep apnea syndrome. In those children with a history of cardiac abnormalities, an echocardiogram may be indicated.

Sleep Disordered Breathing and Obstructive Sleep Apnea

Sleep disordered breathing (SDB) is a spectrum of disorders ranging from primary snoring to obstructive sleep apnea syndrome (OSAS). SDB affects 10% of the population but only 1% to 4% will progress to OSAS. OSAS is characterized by periodic, partial, or complete obstruction of the upper airway during sleep.[9–11] Proper screening and diagnosis of obstructive sleep apnea prior to surgery for both children and adults is essential in reducing the associated risks. The STOP questionnaire has been developed as a tool to screen adult patients for obstructive sleep apnea and includes information on **S**noring, daytime somnolence and **T**iredness, **O**bservation of apnea during sleep and elevations in blood **P**ressure. Predicting risk in children, however, is far more complicated.[12,13]

Repetitive arousal from sleep to restore airway patency is a common feature as are episodic sleep-associated oxygen desaturation, hypercarbia, and cardiac dysfunction as a result of airway obstruction. Individuals who experience obstruction during sleep may have snoring loud enough to be heard through closed doors or observed pauses in breathing during sleep. They may awaken from sleep with a choking sensation. Parents report restless sleep in affected children and frequent somnolence or fatigue while awake despite adequate sleep hours. These children fall asleep easily in nonstimulating environments and are difficult to arouse at usual awakening time. Type 1 OSAS is characterized by lymphoid hyperplasia without obesity whereas type 2 OSAS patients are obese with minimal lymphoid hyperplasia. Approximately 10% of OSAS is present in preschool and school-aged children and is thought to decline after 9 years of age.

Obesity changes craniofacial anthropometric characteristics. Therefore, a body mass index of 95% for age or greater is a predisposing physical characteristic that increases the risk of developing OSAS.[14] Children with craniofacial abnormalities including a
2 small maxilla and mandible, a large tongue for a given mandibular size, and a thick neck have a similar increased risk. Many of these children have syndromes which are associated with additional comorbidities. Anatomic nasal obstruction and Class 4 touching tonsils reduce oropharyngeal cross-sectional area which constitutes an additional risk. Pharyngeal size is determined by the soft-tissue volume inside the bony enclosure of the mandible; an anatomic imbalance between the upper airway soft-tissue volume and craniofacial size will result in obstruction. The magnitude of pharyngeal muscle contraction is controlled by neural mechanisms and the interaction between the anatomical balance and neural mechanisms determines pharyngeal airway size. Increased neural mechanisms can compensate the anatomical imbalance in obstructive sleep apnea patients during wakefulness. When these neural mechanisms are suppressed during sleep or anesthesia, pharyngeal dilator muscles do not contract maximally and therefore the pharyngeal airway severely narrows because of the anatomical imbalance. Increasing bony enclosure size will provide relief of airway obstruction. This is only accomplished surgically by mandibular advancement. Increasing the distance between the mentum and the cervical column by positioning will transiently relieve the obstruction as long as the sniffing position is maintained. Similarly, the sitting position displaces excessive soft tissue outside the bony enclosure through the submandibular space.

The long-term effects of OSAS are not limited to the airway. These children have other systemic comorbidities. Increased body mass index and obesity may lead to increased cognitive vulnerability as illustrated by the increased frequency of hyperactivity and increased levels of C-reactive protein. The duration of OSA has no relation to reversibility of neurobehavioral impairment since many believe that episodic hypoxia alters the neurochemical substrate of the prefrontal cortex causing neuronal cell loss. Metabolic syndrome consists of insulin resistance, dyslipidemia, and hypertension. It is felt that OSAS is a risk factor for metabolic syndrome in obese children but not in nonobese patients. Cardiovascular and hemodynamic comorbidities are more common in OSAS patients. These consist of altered regulation of blood pressure as well as alterations in sympathetic activity and reactivity. Also present are endothelial dysfunction and initiation and propagation of inflammatory response facilitated by increases in levels of C-reactive protein. Systemic inflammation using interleukins as a marker is a component of OSAS in both obese and nonobese children and is reversed after tonsillectomy. Systemic hypertension, changes in left ventricular geometry, and intermittent hypoxia leading to pulmonary artery hypertension are well-described comorbidities present in patients with OSAS.

The mainstay of the management is surgical removal of tonsils and adenoids which carries an 85% success rate in resolving OSAS. Recurrence may occur in children with craniofacial abnormalities and in others. If surgical intervention does not resolve the problem, nocturnal CPAP is the next treatment modality. However, many of these children may present for imaging studies or require sedation prior to removal of the tonsils or adenoids.

Anesthetic Management

The goals of the anesthetic management for tonsillectomy and adenoidectomy are to render the child unconscious in the most atraumatic manner possible, to provide the surgeon with optimal operating conditions, to establish intravenous access to provide a route for volume expansion and medications when necessary, and to provide rapid emergence so that the patient is awake and able to protect the recently instrumented airway. Premedication may be used as determined by the anesthesiologist during the preanesthetic visit. Sedative premedication should be avoided in children with obstructive sleep apnea, intermittent obstruction, or very large tonsils. Administration of opiates to patients with obstructive sleep apnea is associated with an increased risk of oxygen desaturation secondary to chronic hypoxemia and alterations in respiratory control.[15] Use of an antisialagogue will minimize secretions in the operative field.

Anesthesia is commonly induced with a volatile anesthetic agent, oxygen, and nitrous oxide (N_2O) by mask. Parental presence in the operating room (OR) during mask induction may be helpful in the anxious unpremedicated child. Tracheal intubation is best accomplished under deep inhalation anesthesia or aided by a short-acting nondepolarizing muscle relaxant. Many clinicians may choose to eliminate the neuromuscular blocking agent in favor of enhancing the depth of anesthesia with the use of propofol. The addition of 0.5 to 1 μg/kg of dexmedetomidine infused during the procedure may help to attenuate emergence delirium in toddlers at the conclusion of the anesthetic.[16] Blood in the pharynx may enter the trachea during the surgical procedure. For this reason, the supraglottic area may be packed with petroleum gauze, or a cuffed endotracheal tube may be used. If a cuffed endotracheal tube is selected, careful attention to the inflation pressure of the cuff is essential if postextubation croup is to be avoided. Monitoring consists of precordial stethoscope, ECG, automated blood pressure, pulse oximetry, and end-tidal capnography.

Emergence from anesthesia should be rapid, and the child should be alert before transfer to the recovery area. The child should be awake and able to clear blood or secretions from the oropharynx as efficiently as possible before removal of the endotracheal tube. Maintenance of airway and pharyngeal reflexes is essential in the prevention of aspiration, laryngospasm, and airway obstruction. There is no difference in the incidence of airway complications on emergence between patients who are extubated awake or deeply anesthetized.[17]

The use of the laryngeal mask airway (LMA) for adenotonsillectomy was described in 1990; however, it was not until the widespread availability of a streamlined flexible model that it was routinely used for this purpose.[18,19] There is an emerging trend to use the flexible LMA for tonsillectomy, which protects the vocal cords from blood or secretions that may be present in the oropharynx.[20] The wide, rigid tube of the standard LMA model does not fit under the mouth gag and is easily compressed or dislodged during full mouth opening. The flexible model has a soft, reinforced shaft that easily fits under the mouth gag without becoming dislodged or compressed. Adequate surgical access can be achieved, and the lower airway is protected from exposure to blood during the procedure.[21,22] Since the cuff is larger and occupies a greater percentage of the posterior hypopharynx, there is a greater risk of airway fire if the electrocautery touches the LMA. Insertion is possible after either the intravenous administration of 3 mg/kg of propofol or when sufficient depth of anesthesia is achieved using a volatile agent administered by face mask. The same depth of anesthesia should be obtained during insertion of the LMA as would be required for performing laryngoscopy and endotracheal intubation. Positive-pressure ventilation should be avoided when the LMA is used during tonsillectomy, although gentle assisted ventilation is both safe and effective if peak inspiratory pressure is kept below 20 cm H_2O.

Tonsillar enlargement can make LMA insertion difficult; care in placement is essential.[23] Maneuvers to overcome this difficulty include increased head extension, lateral insertion of the mask, anterior displacement of the tongue, pressure on the tip of the LMA using the index finger as it negotiates the pharyngeal curve, or use of the laryngoscope if all else fails. Dislodgment of the device does not occur during extreme head extension, assuming good position and ventilation were obtained before changes in head position.[24]

Advantages of the LMA over traditional endotracheal intubation are a decrease in the incidence of postoperative stridor and laryngospasm and an increase in immediate postoperative oxygen saturation. If the child is breathing spontaneously at a regular rate and depth, the LMA may be removed before emergence from anesthesia. The oropharynx should be gently suctioned with a soft, flexible catheter, the LMA deflated and removed, an oral airway inserted, and the respirations assisted with 100% oxygen delivered by face mask. It is often distressing for young children to awaken with the LMA still in place. Although the device is an appropriate substitute for an oral airway in the adult population, this is not so in children. If the practitioner wants to remove the LMA when the child has emerged from anesthesia, it should be deflated and removed as soon as possible after the return to consciousness. In addition, because it is not possible to pass a nasogastric tube beyond the LMA cuff even when deflated, the stomach cannot be emptied at the conclusion of surgery.

Complications

The incidence of emesis after tonsillectomy ranges from 30% to 65%.[25] Whether emesis is due to irritant blood in the stomach or stimulation of the gag reflex by inflammation and edema at the surgical site remains unclear. Central nervous system stimulation from the gastrointestinal tract, as may be seen with gastric distention from the introduction of swallowed or insufflated air, may trigger the emetic center. Decompressing the stomach with an orogastric tube may be helpful in preventing this response. Treatment with ondansetron, 0.10 to 0.15 mg/kg, either with or without dexamethasone, 0.5 mg/kg, has been shown to be very effective in reducing post-tonsillectomy nausea and vomiting.[26–28] Postoperative administration of meperidine increases the probability of emesis, and alternative analgesic agents should be administered. Dehydration secondary to poor oral intake as a result of nausea, vomiting, or pain can occur after tonsillectomy in 1% of cases. Vigorous intravenous hydration during surgery can offset the physiologic effects of lower postoperative fluid intake.

3 The most serious complication of tonsillectomy is postoperative hemorrhage, which occurs at a frequency of 0.1% to 8.1%. The recent utilization of coblation tonsillectomy may result in an incidence of post-tonsillectomy hemorrhage up to 11.1%.[4,29,30] Approximately 75% of postoperative tonsillar hemorrhage occurs within 6 hours of surgery. Most of the remaining 25% occurs within the first 24 hours of surgery, although bleeding may be noted until the sixth postoperative day.[31,32] Sixty-seven percent of postoperative bleeding originates from the tonsillar fossa, 26% in the nasopharynx, and 7% in both. Initial attempts to control bleeding may be made using pharyngeal packs and cautery. If this fails, patients must return to the OR for exploration and surgical hemostasis.

Unappreciated large volumes of blood originating from the tonsillar bed may be swallowed. These patients must be considered to have a full stomach, and anesthetic precautions addressing this situation must be taken. A rapid-sequence induction accompanied by cricoid pressure and a styletted endotracheal tube is controversial but may be of benefit in some circumstances. Because the amount of blood swallowed can be considerable, blood pressure must be checked in both the erect and supine positions to exclude orthostatic changes resulting from decreases in vascular volume. Intravenous access and hydration must be established before the induction of anesthesia. A variety of laryngoscope blades and endotracheal tubes, as well as functioning suction apparatus, should be prepared in duplicate because blood in the airway may impair visualization of the vocal cords and cause plugging of the endotracheal tube.

Pain after adenoidectomy is usually minimal, but pain after tonsillectomy is severe. This contributes to poor fluid intake and overall discomfort of patients. An increase in postoperative pain medication requirements has been noted in patients having laser or electrocautery as part of the operative tonsillectomy compared with those who have had sharp surgical dissection and ligation of blood vessels to achieve hemostasis.[7,33] Intraoperative administration of corticosteroids may decrease edema formation and subsequent patient discomfort. Although infiltration of the peritonsillar space with local anesthetic and epinephrine has been shown to be effective in reducing intraoperative blood loss, it does not decrease postoperative pain.

Peritonsillar abscess, or quinsy tonsil, is a condition that may require immediate surgical intervention to relieve potential or existing airway obstruction. An acutely infected tonsil may undergo abscess formation, producing a large mass in the lateral pharynx that can interfere with swallowing and breathing (Figs. 47-3–47-5). Fever, pain, and trismus are frequent symptoms. Treatment consists of surgical drainage of the abscess, either with or without tonsillectomy, and intravenous antibiotic therapy. Although the airway seems compromised, the peritonsillar abscess is usually in a fixed location in the lateral pharynx and does not interfere with ventilation of the patient by face mask after induction of general anesthesia. Visualization of the vocal cords should not be impaired because the pathologic process is supraglottic and

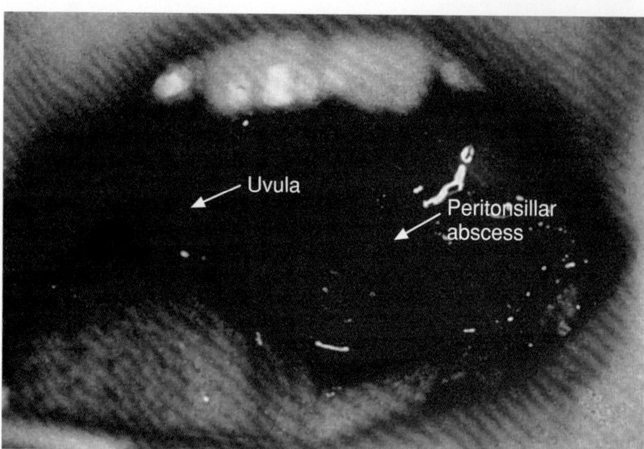

FIGURE 47-3. Patient with a peritonsillar abscess on the left side. Note the displacement of the uvula. (Courtesy of Michael Cunningham, MD, Boston, MA.)

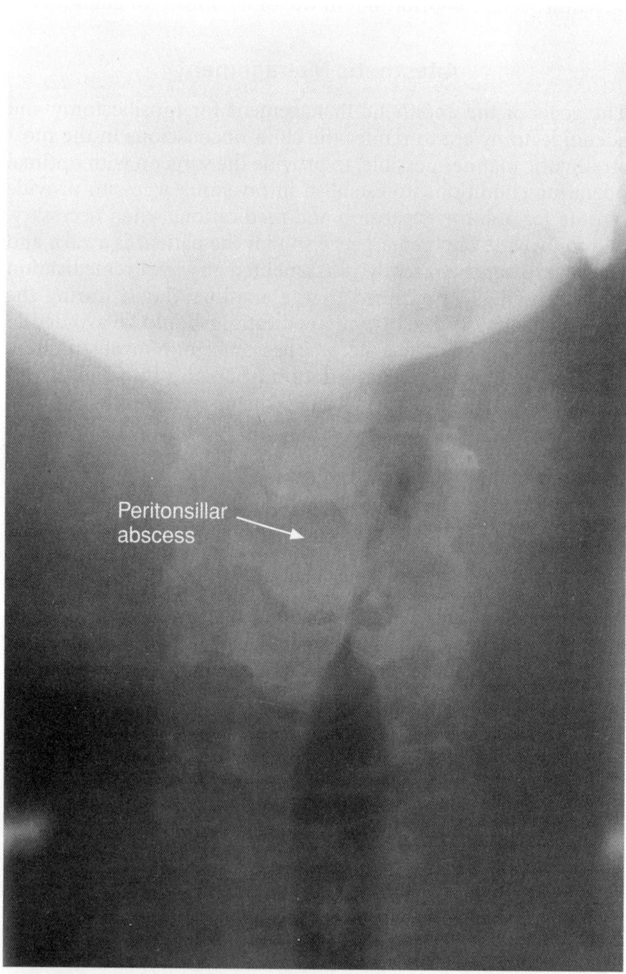

FIGURE 47-4. Neck radiograph of a patient with a peritonsillar abscess (*arrow*).

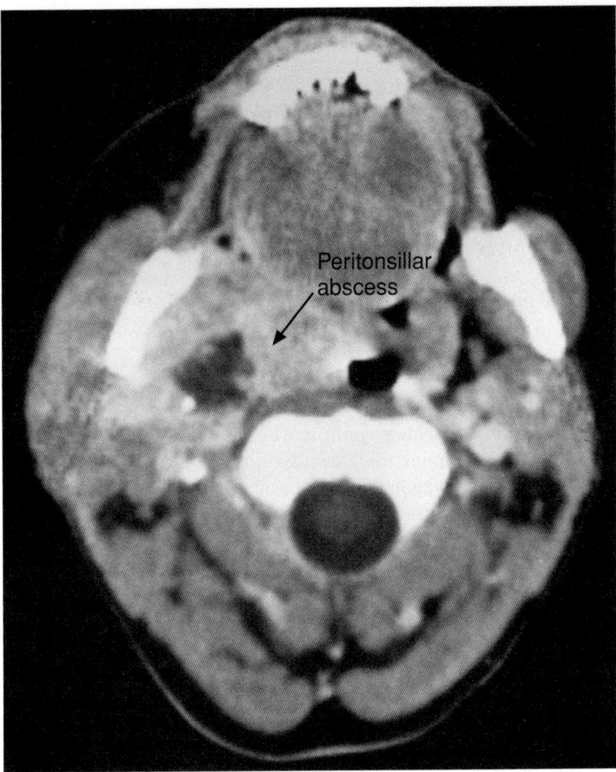

FIGURE 47-5. Computed tomography scan of a patient with a peritonsillar abscess (*arrow*).

well above the laryngeal inlet. Laryngoscopy must be carefully performed, avoiding manipulation of the larynx and surrounding structures. Intubation should be gentle because the tonsillar area is tense and friable and inadvertent rupture of the abscess can occur, leading to spillage of purulent material into the trachea.

Acute postoperative pulmonary edema is an infrequent but potentially life-threatening complication encountered when airway obstruction is suddenly relieved. One proposed mechanism is that during inspiration before adenotonsillectomy, the negative intrapleural pressure that is generated causes an increase in venous return, enhancing pulmonary blood volume. In the healthy child without airway obstruction, pleural pressure ranges from −2.5 cm to −10 cm H_2O during inspiration. Intrapleural pressure generated in the child with airway obstruction can be as much as −30 cm H_2O, which causes disruption of the capillary walls of the pulmonary microvasculature when transmitted to the interstitial peribronchial and perivascular spaces. Concurrent with a negative transpulmonary gradient is an increase in venous return to the right side of the heart, thus increasing preload, which in the setting of "leaky capillaries" facilitates transudation of fluid into the alveolar space. To counterbalance this negative gradient, positive intrapleural and alveolar pressures are generated during exhalation, which decreases pulmonary venous return and blood volume. This phenomenon is similar to an expiratory "grunt" mechanism in which the transpleural pressures generated are similar to those present during a Valsalva maneuver.

The rapid relief of airway obstruction results in decreased airway pressure, an increase in venous return, an increase in pulmonary hydrostatic pressure, hyperemia, and finally pulmonary edema. The all-important counterbalance of the expiratory grunt in limiting pulmonary venous return is lost when the obstruction is relieved. Contributing factors are the increased volume load on both ventricles as well as the inability of the pulmonary lymphatic system to remove acutely large amounts of fluid. The anesthesiologist may attempt to prevent this situation during induction of anesthesia by applying moderate amounts of continuous positive pressure to the airway, thus allowing time for circulatory adaptation to take place. This physiologic sequence is similar to that seen in patients with severe acute airway obstruction secondary to epiglottitis or laryngospasm.

Negative-pressure pulmonary edema is signaled by the appearance of frothy pink fluid in the endotracheal tube of an intubated patient or the presence of a decreased oxygen saturation, wheezing, dyspnea, and increased respiratory rate in the immediate postoperative period in a previously extubated patient. Mild cases may present with minimal symptoms. The differential diagnosis of negative-pressure pulmonary edema includes aspiration of gastric contents, adult respiratory distress syndrome, congestive heart failure, volume overload, and anaphylaxis. A chest radiograph illustrating diffuse, usually bilateral interstitial pulmonary infiltrates combined with an appropriate clinical history will confirm the diagnosis.[7,34,35]

Treatment is usually supportive, with maintenance of a patent airway, oxygen administration, and diuretic therapy in some cases. Endotracheal intubation and mechanical ventilation with positive end-expiratory pressure may be necessary in severe cases. Resolution is usually rapid and may occur within hours of inception. Most cases resolve within 24 hours without treatment. There is currently no reliable method for predicting which children will experience this clinical syndrome after their airway obstruction has been resolved.

Adenoidectomy patients may be safely discharged on the same day after recovering from anesthesia. Although most tonsillectomy patients previously required postoperative admission to the hospital for observation, administration of analgesics, and hydration, many centers are discharging tonsillectomy patients on the day of surgery without adverse outcomes, and this trend will likely continue.[35,36] Patients should be observed for early hemorrhage for a minimum of 4 to 6 hours and be free from significant nausea, vomiting, and pain prior to discharge. The ability to take fluid by mouth is not a requirement for discharge home. However, intravenous hydration must be adequate to prevent dehydration. Excessive somnolence and severe vomiting are indications for hospital admission. There are patients for whom early discharge is not advised, and those patients should be admitted to the hospital after tonsillectomy. The characteristics of such patients are listed in Table 47-1. Admission to an ICU is controversial and reserved for those children with very severe OSA, comorbidities that cannot be managed on the floor, and children who have demonstrated significant airway obstruction and desaturation in the initial postoperative period that required intervention beyond repositioning and oxygen supplementation.[37]

Ear Surgery

The ear and its associated structures are target organs for many pathologic conditions. General anesthesia for surgery of the ear has its own set of unique considerations that must be addressed.

Myringotomy and Tube Insertion

Chronic serous otitis in children can lead to hearing loss. Drainage of accumulated fluid in the middle ear is an effective treatment for this condition. Myringotomy, which creates an opening in the tympanic membrane for fluid drainage, may be performed

TABLE 47-1. TONSILLECTOMY AND ADENOIDECTOMY INPATIENT GUIDELINES: RECOMMENDATION OF THE AMERICAN ACADEMY OF OTOLARYNGOLOGY—HEAD AND NECK SURGERY

Admit patients to the hospital after adenotonsillectomy if they meet any of the following criteria:

- Age ≤3 yrs
- Severe OSA with an apnea–hypopnea index of 10 or more obstructive events/hour, oxygen saturation nadir <80% or both
- Abnormal coagulation values with or without an identified bleeding disorder in the patient or family
- Systemic disorders that put the patient at increased preoperative cardiopulmonary, metabolic, or general medical risk
- Child with craniofacial or other airway abnormalities including, but not limited to, syndromic disorders such as Treacher Collins syndrome, Crouzon syndrome, Goldenhar syndrome, Pierre Robin anomalad, CHARGE syndrome, achondroplasia, and, most prominently, Down syndrome, as well as isolated airway abnormalities such as choanal atresia and laryngotracheal stenosis
- When extended travel time, weather conditions, and home social conditions are not consistent with close observation, cooperation, and ability to return to the hospital quickly at the discretion of the attending physician

CHARGE, *c*oloboma of the eye, *h*eart defects, *a*tresia of the choanae, *r*etardation of growth and/or development, *g*enital and/or urinary abnormalities, and *e*ar abnormalities.

alone. During healing, the drainage path may become occluded; therefore, ventilation tube placement is usually included. The insertion of a small plastic tube in the tympanic membrane serves as a vent for the ostium and allows for continued drainage of the middle ear until the tubes are naturally extruded in 6 months to 1 year, or surgically removed at an appropriate time (Fig. 47-6).

Myringotomy and tube insertion is a relatively short procedure, and anesthesia may be effectively accomplished with a potent inhalation agent, oxygen, and N_2O administered by face mask. Premedication is not recommended because most sedative drugs used for premedication will far outlast the duration of the surgical procedure. Patients with chronic otitis frequently have accompanying recurrent URI. It is often the eradication of middle ear fluid that resolves the concomitant URI. Because tracheal intubation is not required for routine patients, the criteria for cancellation of surgery and anesthesia may be different for this procedure. Insertion of myringotomy tubes may be undertaken in most children with a concomitant URI provided that this can be completed with facemask anesthesia and endotracheal intubation is avoided. No significant difference in perioperative morbidity between asymptomatic patients and those fulfilling URI criteria has been demonstrated.[38,39] It is recommended that patients with URI symptoms receive supplemental postoperative oxygen.

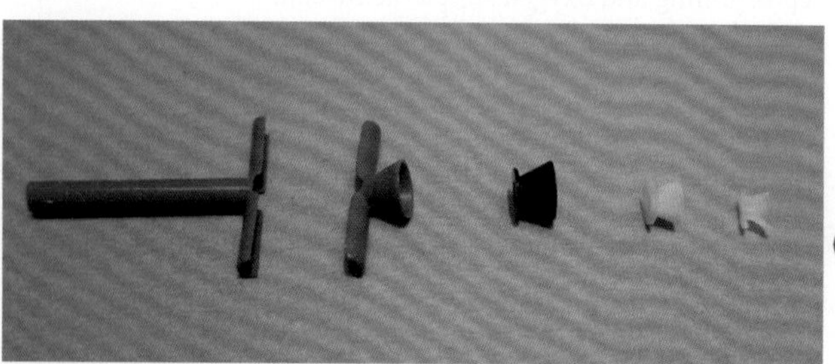

FIGURE 47-6. Two types of myringotomy tubes. Both the ventilating T-tube and the beveled-button ventilating tube are shown in full and cross-sectional views.

Middle Ear and Mastoid

Tympanoplasty and mastoidectomy are two of the most common procedures performed on the middle ear and accessory structures. To gain access to the surgical site, the head is positioned on a headrest, which may be lower than the operative table, and extreme degrees of lateral rotation may be required. Extreme tension on the heads of the sternocleidomastoid muscles must be avoided. The laxity of the ligaments of the cervical spine and the immaturity of odontoid process in children make them especially prone to C1 to C2 subluxation.

2 Ear surgery often involves surgical identification and preservation of the facial nerve, which requires isolation of the nerve by the surgeon and verification of its function by means of electrical stimulation (Fig. 47-7). This is accomplished by brainstem auditory-evoked potential and electrocochleogram monitoring, which requires that complete muscle relaxation be avoided.[40] If an opioid-relaxant technique is chosen, however, at least 30% of the muscle response, as determined by a twitch monitor, should be preserved. This fact suggests that it is not mandatory to avoid skeletal muscle relaxants in the anesthetic management of patients undergoing surgical procedures when monitoring of facial nerve function is necessary.

Bleeding must be kept to a minimum during surgery of the small structures of the middle ear. Relative hypotension, keeping the mean arterial pressure 25% below baseline, is effective. Concentrated epinephrine solution, often 1:1,000, can be injected in the area of the tympanic vessels to produce vasoconstriction. Close attention should be paid to the volume of injected epinephrine so that dysrhythmias and wide swings in blood pressure may be avoided.

4 The middle ear and sinuses are air-filled, nondistensible cavities. An increase in the volume of gas in these structures results in an increase in pressure. N_2O diffuses along a concentration gradient into the air-filled middle ear spaces more rapidly than nitrogen moves out. Passive venting occurs at 20 to 30 cm H_2O pressure, and it has been shown that the use of N_2O results in pressures that exceed the ability of the eustachian tube to vent the middle ear within 5 minutes, leading to pressure buildup.[41]

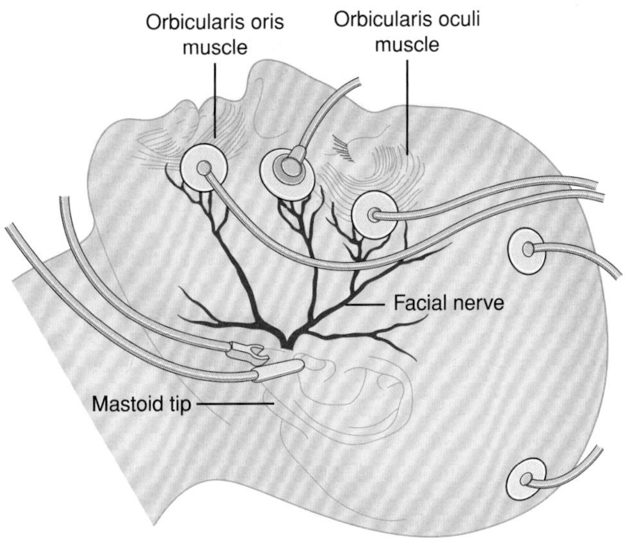

FIGURE 47-7. Illustration of facial nerve and monitoring electrodes. (Courtesy of Steve Ronner, PhD, Boston, MA.)

TABLE 47-2. CAUSES OF STRIDOR

Supraglottic Airway	Larynx	Subglottic Airway
Laryngomalacia	Laryngocele	Tracheomalacia
Vocal cord paralysis	Infection (tonsillitis, peritonsillar abscess)	Vascular ring
Subglottic stenosis	Foreign body	Foreign body
Hemangiomas	Choanal atresia	Infection (croup, epiglottitis)
Cysts	Cyst	
	Mass	
	Large tonsils	
	Large adenoids	
	Craniofacial abnormalities	

During procedures in which the eardrum is replaced or a perforation is patched, N_2O should be discontinued or, if this is not possible, limited to a maximum of 50% during the application of the tympanic membrane graft to avoid pressure-related displacement.

After N_2O is discontinued, it is quickly reabsorbed, creating a void in the middle ear with resulting negative pressure. This negative pressure may result in serous otitis, disarticulation of the ossicles in the middle ear (especially the stapes), and hearing impairment, which may last up to 6 weeks after surgery. The use of N_2O is related to a high incidence of postoperative nausea and vomiting, which is a direct result of negative middle ear pressure during recovery. The vestibular system is stimulated by traction placed on the round window by the negative pressure that is created. Although all patients have the potential for nausea and vomiting after surgery, children younger than 8 years of age seem to be most affected. If the use of N_2O cannot be avoided, vigorous use of antiemetics is warranted.

Airway Surgery

Stridor

Noisy breathing due to obstructed airflow is known as *stridor.* Inspiratory stridor results from upper airway obstruction; expiratory stridor results from lower airway obstruction; and biphasic stridor is present with midtracheal lesions. The evaluation of a patient with stridor begins with a thorough history. The age of onset suggests a cause: Laryngotracheomalacia and vocal cord paralysis are usually present at or shortly after birth, whereas cysts or mass lesions develop later in life (Table 47-2). Information indicating positions that make the stridor better or worse should be obtained, and placing a patient in a position that allows gravity to aid in reducing obstruction can be of benefit during anesthetic induction.

Physical examination reveals the general condition of a patient and the degree of the airway compromise. Laboratory examination may include assessment of hemoglobin, a chest radiograph, and barium swallow, which can aid in identifying lesions that may be compressing the trachea. Other radiologic examinations such as MRI and computed tomography scan may be indicated in isolated instances but are not routinely ordered. Specific note of the signs and symptoms listed in Table 47-3 should be made.

Laryngomalacia is the most common cause of stridor in infants. It is most often due to a long epiglottis that prolapses posteriorly and prominent arytenoid cartilages with redundant aryepiglottic folds that obstruct the glottic opening during inspiration.[42] The definitive diagnosis is obtained by direct laryngoscopy and rigid or flexible bronchoscopy. Preliminary examination is usually carried out in the surgeon's office. A small, flexible fiberoptic bronchoscope is inserted through the nares into the oropharynx, and the movement of the vocal cords is observed. Alternatively, it may be accomplished in the OR before anesthetic induction in an awake patient or in a lightly anesthetized patient during spontaneous respiration. Patients must be breathing spontaneously so that the vocal cords can move freely. After deepening anesthesia and topicalization of the vocal cords is performed using 1% to 2% lidocaine, a rigid bronchoscope is inserted through the vocal cords and the subglottic area is inspected; the lower trachea and bronchi are evaluated with a rigid or flexible fiberoptic bronchoscope.

Bronchoscopy

Small infants may be brought into the OR unpremedicated. Older children and adults may experience respiratory depression

TABLE 47-3. CLINICAL COMPONENT OF THE EVALUATION OF PATIENTS WITH STRIDOR

Respiratory rate	Chest retractions
Heart rate	Nasal flaring
Wheezing	Level of consciousness
Cyanosis	

and worsening of airway obstruction if heavy premedication is administered, so only light sedation is suggested. The airway must be protected from aspiration of gastric contents during prolonged airway manipulation; therefore, premedication with the full regimen of acid aspiration prophylaxis may be indicated.

The goals of the anesthetic are analgesia, an unconscious patient, and a "quiet" surgical field.[43] Coughing, bucking, or straining during instrumentation with the rigid bronchoscope may cause difficulty for the surgeon and result in damage to the patient's airway. At the conclusion of the procedure, patients should be returned to consciousness quickly, with airway reflexes intact. For most patients, a pulse oximeter, blood pressure cuff, ECG, and precordial stethoscope are applied before induction of anesthesia. Inhalation induction by mask is accompanied by oxygen and a volatile agent administered in increasing concentrations in children and intravenous drugs in adults. Patients should be placed in the position that produces the least adverse effect on airway symptoms (often the sitting position). An intravenously administered antisialagogue may help decrease secretions that might compromise the view through the bronchoscope.

The size of a bronchoscope refers to the internal diameter. Because the external diameter may be significantly greater than in an endotracheal tube of similar size (Table 47-4), care must be taken to select a bronchoscope of proper external diameter to avoid damage to the laryngeal structures. A rigid bronchoscope can be used for ventilation of the lungs during examination of the airway. It is inserted through the vocal cords, and ventilation is accomplished through a side port, which can be attached to the anesthesia circuit. During ventilation with the viewing telescope in place, high resistance may be encountered as a result of partial occlusion of the lumen. High fresh gas flow rates, large tidal volumes, and high inspired volatile anesthetic concentrations are often necessary to compensate for leaks around the ventilating bronchoscope and the high resistance encountered when the viewing telescope is in place. Manual ventilation at higher-than-normal rates is most effective in achieving adequate ventilation. Adequate time for exhalation must be provided for passive recoil of the chest.[44]

3 An alternative method of ventilation is the jet ventilation technique, which involves intermittent bursts of oxygen delivered under pressure through a 16-gauge catheter attached to a rigid bronchoscope.[45] Intermittent flow is accomplished by depressing the lever of an on–off valve. The use of jet ventilation techniques is associated with the additional risks of pneumothorax or pneumomediastinum due to rupture of alveolar blebs or a bronchus.[46] Because ventilation may be intermittent and at times suboptimal, oxygen should be used as the carrier gas during bronchoscopic examination. Intravenous drugs that cause excessive respiratory depression should be avoided. It is wise to ask the surgeon if movement of the vocal cords will be required at the conclusion of the procedure or if tracheal or bronchial dynamics will be evaluated during the procedure so that the anesthetic may be planned accordingly (i.e., spontaneous respirations preserved during light levels of anesthesia vs. no respiratory efforts and the use of short-acting muscle relaxants).

Maintenance of anesthesia is usually accomplished with a volatile anesthetic augmented by propofol infusion (100 to 200 μg/kg/min). Intravenous anesthetics combined with muscle relaxation best maintain a constant level of anesthesia because the delivery of volatile anesthetics through the bronchoscope may be interrupted, and anesthetic depth can vary. At the conclusion of rigid bronchoscopy, an endotracheal tube is usually placed in the trachea to control the airway during recovery of anesthesia. Securing the airway is particularly important if muscle relaxants have been used since passive regurgitation of gastric contents may be more likely to occur in paralyzed patients. An additional advantage of placing an endotracheal tube is that if the surgeon should want to examine the distal airways, a small, flexible fiberoptic bronchoscope can be passed through the endotracheal tube.

TABLE 47-4. COMPARISON OF EXTERNAL DIAMETER OF STANDARD ENDOTRACHEAL TUBES VERSUS RIGID BRONCHOSCOPE

Endotracheal Tube	Rigid Bronchoscope	
Internal Diameter (mm)	External Diameter (mm)	External Diameter (mm)
2.5	3.5	4.2
3	4.3	5
3.5	4.9	5.7
4	5.5	6.7
5	6.8	7.8
6	8.2	8.2

Pediatric Airway Emergencies

Upper airway emergencies may be life-threatening and demand immediate treatment. Rapid respiratory failure can occur in patients with croup, epiglottitis, or foreign body aspiration, and few clinical situations are more challenging to the anesthesiologist.

Epiglottitis

4 Acute epiglottitis is one of the most feared infectious diseases in children and adults, and is the result of *Haemophilus influenzae* type B. A conservative estimate of the incidence of epiglottitis is 10 to 40 cases per million people in the United States. Since 1985, with the widespread vaccination against *H. influenzae* type B (Hib), which was the most common organism related to epiglottitis, the overall incidence of the disease among children has dropped dramatically. It can progress with extreme rapidity from sore throat to airway obstruction to respiratory failure and ultimately to death if proper diagnosis and intervention are not rapidly implemented. Patients are usually between 2 and 7 years of age, although epiglottitis has been reported in younger children and in adults. Epiglottitis in the very young (younger than 1 year) is unusual and occurs in only about 4% of cases and in adults, it peaks between ages 20 to 40 years. Vaccination against *H. influenzae* type B polysaccharide is now recommended before 2 years of age to provide immunity before the greatest period of vulnerability in pediatric patients.

Characteristic signs and symptoms of acute epiglottitis include sudden onset of fever, dysphagia, drooling, thick muffled voice, and preference for the sitting position with the head extended and leaning forward. Retractions, labored breathing, and cyanosis may be observed in cases in which respiratory obstruction is present. However, in the early stages, the patient may be pale and toxic without respiratory distress. *Supraglottitis* may be a more appropriate designation because it is the tissues of the supraglottic structures—from the vallecula to the arytenoids—that are involved in the infectious process. At no time, especially in the emergency department or radiography suite, should direct visualization of the epiglottis be attempted in the unanesthetized patient. The differential resulting from negative pressure inside and atmospheric pressure outside the extrathoracic airway results in slight narrowing during normal inspiration. The pressure differential on inspiration is exaggerated in the patient with airway obstruction. This dynamic collapse of the airway may become life-threatening in the struggling, agitated patient, and every attempt should be made to keep the patient calm. Blood drawing, intravenous catheter insertion, and excessive manipulation of the patient, as well as sedation, should be avoided before securing the airway to avoid the possibility of total obstruction.

If the clinical situation allows, oxygen should be administered by mask, and lateral radiographs of the soft tissues in the neck may be obtained. Thickening of the aryepiglottic folds and swelling of the epiglottis may be noted (the "thumbprint" sign). Radiologic examination should be carried out only if skilled personnel and adequate equipment accompany the patient at all times. The patient with severe airway compromise should proceed from the emergency department directly to the operating suite accompanied by both the anesthesiologist and surgeon. Parental presence in this situation may calm an anxious and frightened child.

In all cases of epiglottitis, an artificial airway is established by means of tracheal intubation. In some centers in which personnel experienced in the management of the compromised airway are not available, tracheostomy is a less-favored alternative. In the OR, the child is kept in the sitting position while monitors are placed. A pulse oximeter and precordial stethoscope are essential. If it is believed to be helpful, one parent may accompany the child and remain in the OR during the induction of general anesthesia. The OR must be prepared with equipment and personnel for laryngoscopy, rigid bronchoscopy, and tracheostomy. Anesthetic induction is accomplished by inhalation of oxygen and increasing concentrations of sevoflurane. After loss of consciousness occurs, intravenous access should be secured and the child lowered into the supine position. Laryngoscopy followed by oral tracheal intubation is then accomplished without the use of muscle relaxants. The endotracheal tube chosen should be at least one size (0.5 mm) smaller than would normally be chosen, and a stylette is often useful. Once the surgeon has examined the larynx, noting the appearance of the epiglottis, aryepiglottic folds, and surrounding tissues, the endotracheal tube may be changed to a nasotracheal tube and secured. Tissue and blood cultures are taken, and antibiotic therapy is initiated. The child is then transferred to the ICU for continued observation and radiographic confirmation of tube placement. Sedation is appropriate at this time. Tracheal extubation is usually attempted 48 to 72 hours later in the OR, when a significant leak around the nasotracheal tube is present and visual inspection of the larynx by flexible fiberoptic bronchoscopy confirms reduction in swelling of the epiglottis and surrounding tissues.

Laryngotracheobronchitis

Laryngotracheobronchitis (LTB), or croup, occurs in children from 6 months to 6 years of age, but is primarily seen in children younger than 3 years of age. It is usually viral in etiology, and its onset is more insidious than that of epiglottitis. The child presents with low-grade fever, inspiratory stridor, and a "barking" cough. Radiologic examination confirms the diagnosis, and subglottic narrowing of the airway column secondary to circumferential soft-tissue edema produces the "steeple" sign characteristic of LTB. Approximately 6% of patients with LTB require admission to the hospital. Treatment includes cool, humidified mist and oxygen therapy, usually administered in a tent for mild-to-moderate cases. More severe cases of LTB are accompanied by tachypnea, tachycardia, and cyanosis. Racemic epinephrine administered by nebulizer is beneficial. The use of steroids has been surrounded by a great deal of controversy, but current opinion is that a short course of steroids may be beneficial. In rare circumstances, thick secretions are present in the airway, and the child requires intubation to allow pulmonary toilet and suctioning to be performed. Management in the ICU and extubation are carried out in the same fashion as for epiglottitis.

Foreign Body Aspiration

A major cause of morbidity and mortality in children and adults is aspiration of a foreign body. Any history of coughing, choking, or cyanosis while eating should suggest the possibility of foreign body aspiration. Peanuts, popcorn, jelly beans, and hot dogs are some of the ingested items most commonly associated with pulmonary aspiration. Any patient who presents to the emergency department with refractory wheezing should be suspected of this diagnosis. Physical findings include decreased breath sounds, tachypnea, stridor, wheezing, and fever. These signs indicate an obstructive process with inflammation present in the airway. Some foreign bodies are identifiable on radiologic examination; however, 90% are radiolucent, and air trapping, infiltrate, and atelectasis are all that are noted.

The most common site of foreign body aspiration is the main stem bronchus, the right being more frequent than the left (Fig. 47-8). Food particles comprise the majority of aspirated items; however, beads, pins, and small toys are not unusual. Each

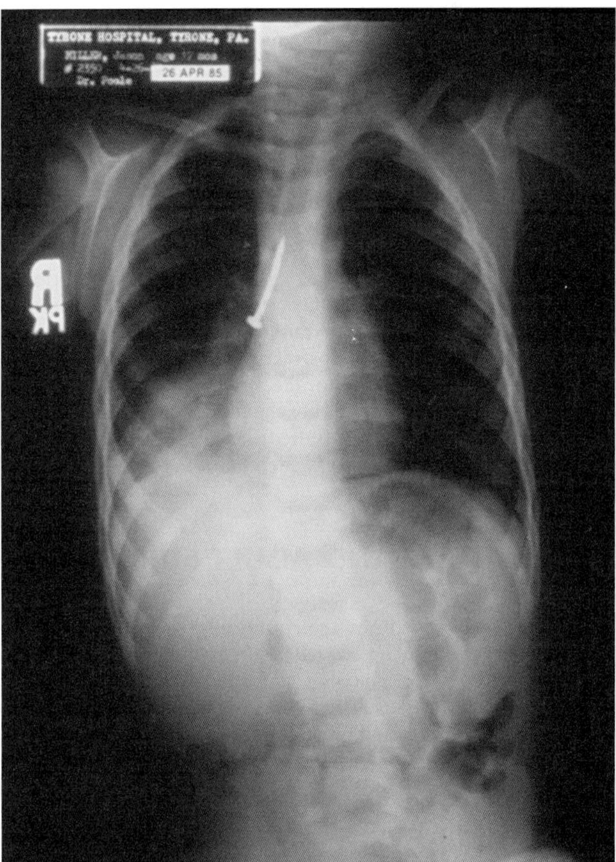

FIGURE 47-8. Aspirated foreign body in the right mainstem bronchus.

type of aspirated item has potential complications associated with it. Vegetable items expand with moisture encountered in the respiratory tract and can fragment into multiple pieces, thus creating a situation in which the original foreign body is in one bronchus and, with coughing, a fragment is dislodged and transported to the other bronchus. Oil-containing objects, such as peanuts, cause a chemical inflammation, and sharp objects cause bleeding in addition to the obstruction.

All aspirated foreign bodies in the airway should be removed in the OR and considered to be emergency situations. No sedation should be administered to patients before removal of the foreign body. If the patient has recently eaten, full-stomach precautions must be taken and anesthesia should be induced intravenously (topical anesthetic cream may be applied to the skin before intravenous catheter insertion in small children) by rapid sequence, and gentle cricoid pressure maintained during intubation of the trachea. If the child has not eaten recently, anesthesia may be induced by inhalation of sevoflurane in oxygen by mask. Inhalation induction can be prolonged secondary to obstruction of the airway, and N_2O should be avoided to prevent air trapping distal to the obstruction. After evacuation of the stomach by orogastric tube, the airway may be given over to the surgeon, who introduces a rigid bronchoscope and removes the aspirated object.

Spontaneous ventilation should be preserved until the location and nature of the foreign body have been determined. Ventilation via the bronchoscope requires careful attention. Hypoxia and hypercarbia may occur because of inadequate ventilation caused by an excessively large leak around the bronchoscope or, more commonly, inability to provide adequate gas exchange through a narrow-lumen bronchoscope fitted with an internal telescope. These conditions are remedied by frequent removal of the telescope and withdrawal of the bronchoscope to the midtrachea, allowing effective ventilation. Bronchospasm may occur during examination of the respiratory tract and should be treated with increasing depths of anesthesia, nebulized albuterol, or intravenous bronchodilators. Although rare, pneumothorax should be suspected if acute deterioration occurs during the procedure.

Once the foreign body has been removed, examination of the entire tracheobronchial tree is carried out to detect any additional objects or fragments. Often, vigorous irrigation and suctioning distal to the obstruction are required to remove secretions and prevent the possibility of postobstructive pneumonia. Steroids are administered if inflammation of the airway mucosa is observed. Close postoperative observation of the patient is required so that early intervention may be instituted in the event of respiratory compromise secondary to airway edema or infection.

PEDIATRIC AND ADULT SURGERY

Certain surgical procedures are commonly performed in both adults and children, including nasal surgery and laser surgery of the airway. Surgery for maxillofacial trauma and upper airway tumors or infection, as well as temporomandibular joint (TMJ) arthroscopy, are conducted more commonly in adults.

Laser Surgery of the Airway

5 One of the greatest advances in airway surgery has been the use of the laser (*l*ight *a*mplification by *s*timulated *e*mission of *r*adiation). For use in the airway, the laser provides precision in targeting lesions, minimal bleeding and edema, preservation of surrounding structures, and rapid healing. The laser consists of a tube with reflective mirrors at either end and an amplifying medium between them to generate electron activity, resulting in the production of light.[47] The CO_2 laser is the most widely used in medical practice, having particular application in the treatment of laryngeal or vocal cord papillomas, laryngeal webs, resection of redundant subglottic tissue, and coagulation of hemangiomas. The laser is an especially useful modality for the surgeon because the invisible beam of light affords an unobstructed view of the lesion during resection. The energy emitted by a CO_2 laser is absorbed by water contained in blood and tissues. Human tissue is approximately 80% water, and laser energy absorbed by tissue water rapidly increases the temperature, denaturing protein and vaporizing the target tissue. The thermal energy of the laser beam cauterizes capillaries as it vaporizes tissues; thus, bleeding and postoperative edema are minimized.

The properties that give the laser a high degree of specificity also supply the route by which a misdirected laser beam may cause injury to a patient or to unprotected OR personnel.[48] The eyes are especially vulnerable, and all OR personnel should wear laser-specific eye goggles with side protectors to prevent injury. Because of the limited penetration (0.01 mm) of the CO_2 laser, it may cause injury only to the cornea. Other lasers such as the neodymium–yttrium-aluminum-garnet (Nd:YAG) have deeper penetration, and may cause retinal injury and scarring. The eyes of a patient undergoing laser treatment must be protected by taping them shut, followed by the application of wet gauze pads and a metal shield. Any stray laser beam is absorbed by the wet gauze, preventing penetration of the eyes. Laser radiation increases the temperature of the absorbent material, and flammable objects such as surgical drapes must be kept away from the path of the laser beam. To avoid cutaneous burns from deflected beams, wet towels should be applied to exposed skin of the face and neck when the laser is being used in the airway. Laser smoke plumes may cause damage to the lungs; interstitial pneumonia has been reported with long-term exposure. In addition, it has been postulated that cancer cells and virus particles, including human immunodeficiency virus, are vaporized during laser application, and the resultant smoke plume, if inhaled, may be a vehicle for spread. The use of specially designed surgical masks for filtering laser smoke is recommended.

Most anesthetic techniques are suitable for laser surgery, provided that patients are immobile and the laser beam can be directed at a target that is entirely still and in full view. Both N_2O and oxygen support combustion; therefore, the primary gas for anesthetic maintenance should consist of blended air and oxygen or helium and oxygen. A pulse oximeter should be used at all times to ensure adequate oxygenation at the lowest possible inspired concentration of oxygen.

Anesthesia during laser surgery may be administered with or without an endotracheal tube. The choice of endotracheal tube used during laser surgery can affect the safety of the technique. All standard polyvinyl chloride (PVC) endotracheal tubes are flammable and can ignite and vaporize producing hydrochloric acid when in contact with the laser beam. Red rubber endotracheal tubes wrapped with reflective metallic tape do not vaporize but deflect the laser beam instead; however, the introduction of commercially available laser-specific endotracheal tubes has essentially replaced the use of these endotracheal tubes. Cuffed endotracheal tubes should be inflated with sterile saline to which methylene blue has been added so that a cuff rupture from a misdirected laser spark is readily detected by the blue dye and extinguished by the saline.[49] Endotracheal tubes have been manufactured specifically for use during laser surgery. Some have a double cuff to

TABLE 47-5. COMPARISON OF STANDARD PLASTIC VERSUS METAL ENDOTRACHEAL TUBES

	External Diameter (mm)	
Internal Diameter (mm)	Plastic	Metal
3 (uncuffed)	4.3	5.2
3.5 (uncuffed)	4.9	5.7
4 (uncuffed)	5.5	6.1
4.5 (cuffed)	6.2	7
5 (cuffed)	6.8	7.5
5.5 (cuffed)	7.5	7.9
6 (cuffed)	8.2	8.5

ensure protection of the airway in the event of a cuff rupture, and some have a special matte finish that effectively prevents reflected laser beam scattering; some have both. Nonreflective flexible metal endotracheal tubes are also specifically manufactured for use during laser surgery. The outer diameter of each size of metal laser tube is considerably greater than the PVC counterpart, especially in the small sizes used for pediatric anesthesia (Table 47-5). 5

An apneic technique is preferred by some surgeons, especially when working on the airway of small infants and children. The advantage of this technique is an unobstructed surgical field to the absence of an endotracheal tube, which may obscure the surgical field. In this circumstance, a child is anesthetized and rendered immobile by the use of a muscle relaxant or deep inhalation of a volatile anesthetic. The patient's trachea is not intubated, and the airway is given over to the surgeon, who uses the laser for brief periods. Between laser applications, the patient's lungs are ventilated by mask. Because apnea is a component of this technique, it is prudent to ventilate the lungs with oxygen. Although this technique has been widely used with safety, there is a greater potential for debris and resected material to enter the trachea as well as the potential for airway trauma as a result of repeated endotracheal intubation.

The use of a jet ventilator is a modification of the apneic technique that does not require tracheal intubation but does provide for oxygenation; ventilation during laser surgery uses a jet ventilator. The operating laryngoscope is fitted with a catheter through which oxygen is delivered under pressure through a variable reducing valve. Additional room air is entrained, and the patient's lungs are ventilated with this combination of gases. This technique produces a quiet surgical field because large chest excursions of the diaphragm are eliminated and ventilation is uninterrupted. In morbidly obese patients and those with severe small airway disease, effective ventilation is difficult to impossible with this technique, and an alternate technique should be used.

The final technique that may be used is spontaneous ventilation without the aid of an endotracheal tube (Figs. 47-9 and 47-10). In this technique, a surgical laryngoscope fitted with an oxygen insufflation port is inserted into the larynx. Anesthesia may be induced with a volatile agent by mask but is maintained with total intravenous agents without muscle relaxant in the spontaneously breathing patient. Propofol may be infused with or without a short-acting narcotic, and the vocal cords may be sprayed with 4% lidocaine to decrease reactivity. This technique is advantageous in that longer periods of uninterrupted laser application may be provided. Disadvantages include the absence of complete control of the airway, limited protection from laryngospasm, limited protection from debris entering the airway, vocal cords' motion, and difficult scavenging.

Nasal Surgery

Close communication between the anesthesiologist and the otorhinolaryngologist during nasal surgery is essential for a successful outcome and avoidance of major complications. Functional endoscopic sinus surgery (FESS) is the most common procedure performed in the nasal area. Historically, nasal procedures were completed under topical or local anesthesia with sedation so that the patient could signal the surgeon if problems arose.[50] As endoscopic nasal surgery grew larger in scope and duration, general anesthesia became preferred and local anesthesia with sedation was reserved for the simpler cases.

To achieve optimal visualization of the surgical field, bleeding must be kept to a minimum. Current anesthetic practice includes the use of vasoconstrictors, elevation of the head, and modest hypotension. Preoperative evaluation of the patient includes a focused cardiovascular history to determine coronary artery disease, peripheral artery disease, and cardiac arrhythmias. Positive findings may alter the degree of head elevation, use of topical constrictors, or the anesthetic technique and the degree of induced hypotension.

Intranasal vasoconstriction has been accomplished by the use of local anesthetics combined with cocaine, epinephrine, and phenylephrine. Systemic absorption of these agents can cause hypotension, hypertension, bradycardia, tachycardia, and arrhythmias.[51,52] For patients on beta-blocker or calcium channel–blocker therapy, alpha-agonist–induced hypertension may lead to pulmonary edema and cardiac failure. Prompt treatment is needed to prevent serious complications.

The patient is positioned with the head elevated 15 degrees to facilitate venous drainage. This position may give some modest hypotension; however, there is the potential for venous pooling in the lower extremities. General anesthesia is maintained with either inhalation based or total intravenous anesthesia (TIVA). Many surgeons now prefer TIVA since it has been shown to reduce blood loss and improve visualization of the surgical field. Comparing isoflurane and fentanyl anesthesia to remifentanyl and propofol resulted in better visualization and less blood loss for the TIVA group at equal reduction in blood pressure.[53,54] TIVA may also have the added benefit of reducing both coughing on emergence and postoperative nausea and vomiting.

Skull Base Surgery

Skull base surgery may be considered the logical extension of nasal surgery involving otorhinolaryngology, neurosurgery, and anesthesia. The majority of adult patients undergoing skull base surgery have malignant tumors with a smaller group of patients having benign tumors, congenital malformations, or other abnormalities. These patients often require radiologic procedures to determine the location and extent of the lesion prior to surgery. Noninvasive tests include CAT scans and MRIs to ascertain the extent of bony and soft-tissue abnormalities, whereas more invasive angiography may be needed to determine tumor location and blood supply. These studies may then be used to program intraoperative localizing systems to help guide the surgical dissection.[55] Finally, embolization of lesions may be performed a day or two prior to surgery to shrink the lesion and decrease blood loss during the operative procedure.[56]

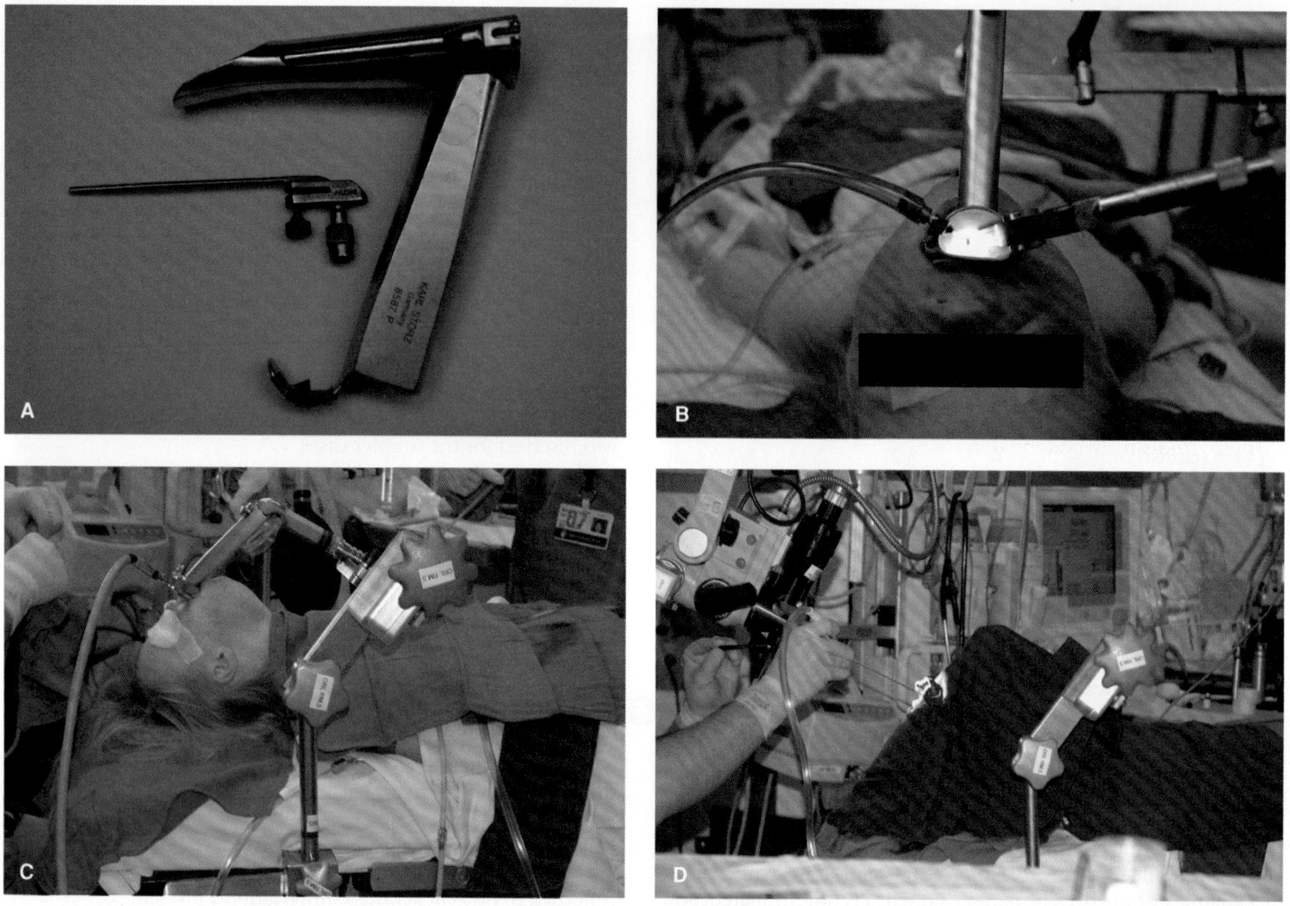

FIGURE 47-9. **A:** The surgical laryngoscope and the jet ventilator needle. **B:** The surgical view of the laryngoscope positioned in the patient's pharynx and connected to a continuous flow of oxygen through the jet ventilator needle. **C:** View of the anesthetized, spontaneously breathing patient. **D:** Laser-aided resection of vocal cord lesion.

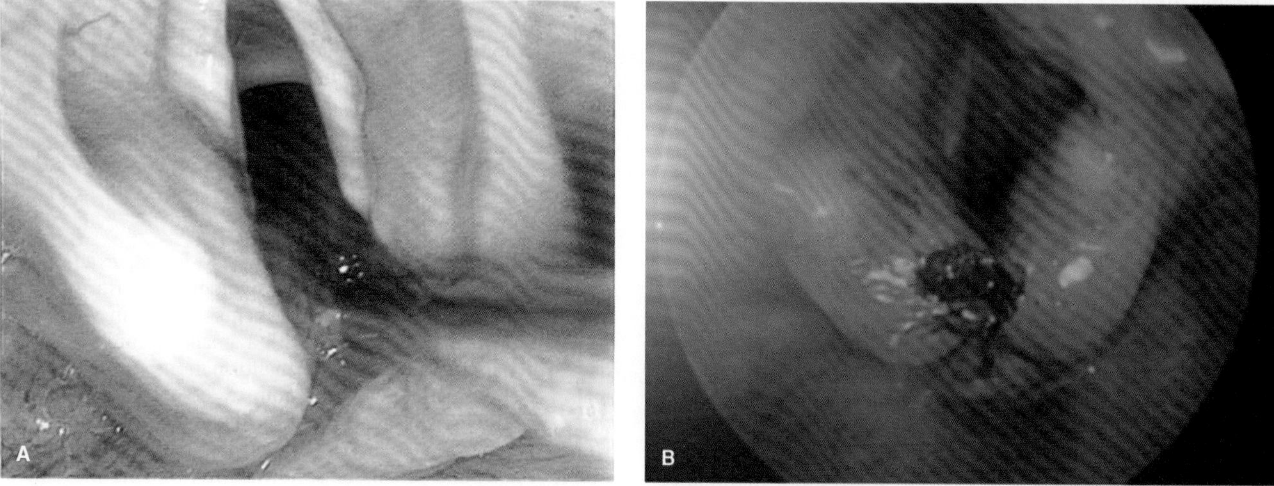

FIGURE 47-10. **A:** Unrepaired posterior laryngeal cleft. **B:** Laryngeal cleft post surgical repair.

Special attention during the preoperative assessment should be given to prior surgical procedures which may affect the airway, chemotherapy, and radiation treatment. Prior surgical
6 procedures may alter a previously easy airway which subsequently may require advanced airway management techniques to intubate the trachea. Prior chemotherapy can have anesthetic implications depending on the agents used. Adriamycin and other cardiotoxic agents whose effects are dose dependent may require a cardiac evaluation including an echocardiogram. Decreased cardiac function may impact the type of anesthetic agents used and require the use of pulmonary catheter for monitoring. Neurotoxic agents may lessen the dose of muscle relaxants or cause their duration of action to be prolonged requiring neuromuscular monitoring. Prior radiation therapy usually does not cause systemic problems unless the pituitary gland is damaged which can give rise to the problems of panhypopituitarism leading to hypothyroidism, hypoadrenocorticism, and diabetes insipidus. However, prior radiation therapy may lead to fibrosis and ankylosis in the temporomandibular joint, rendering orotracheal intubation difficult. Previous radiation to the operative site may also increase blood loss and results in poor wound healing. Secondary radiation fibrosis may also make the surgical dissection more difficult and time consuming. It may also necessitate the use of free or vascularized grafts to close the surgical site. The location of the donor site and potential anastomotic sites must also be considered when positioning the patient.

Close attention must be paid to the evaluation of the head and neck is during the physical examination. Usually these patients do not have a difficult airway or require special techniques for intubation. Although intubation may not be difficult, the route and fixation of the endotracheal tube must be given consideration. For lesions requiring a midline surgical approach, oral intubation is the preferred route. If the lesion does not cross the midline, an oral or nasal approach may be used. Nasal endotracheal tubes may be secured by use of a heavy suture through the nasal septum and around the tube. Oral endotracheal tubes may be secured by either wiring the endotracheal tube to the teeth, suturing it to the gingival periosteum, or by using a circummandibular wire.

There are two noteworthy points for anesthetic consideration: The use of muscle relaxation and deliberate hypotension.[57] Similar to other procedures in which the facial nerve is at risk for injury or transection during dissection, it is necessary to avoid paralysis so that the facial nerve may be periodically stimulated to verify its integrity. Muscle relaxants may be given if nerve stimulation is no longer required. Minimizing blood loss and a plan for replacement with blood products must be considered. Deliberate hypotension or hemodilution can be used to minimize blood loss during the procedure. Their use together is contraindicated since tissue oxygen delivery may be inadequate. Recently, antithrombolytic therapy has been used with success in craniofacial procedures and may be of benefit in these cases.[58,59] Directed donor or autologous blood donation have been used to minimize or decrease the exposure to allogenic blood products. Blood salvage techniques, such as cell saver, are usually not appropriate given that most surgical sites are not reached through sterile approaches.

Upper Airway Infections

Infectious processes of the upper airway can occur in the adult and present the same problems of airway compression, distortion, and compromise. Inflammation of the upper airway caused mainly by gram-negative bacteria, may present with the same symptoms as epiglottitis in the pediatric age group. While these patients present with fever, chills, drooling, and difficulty speaking and swallowing, they do not usually appear with critical airways from swelling. These same symptoms may occur with Ludwig's angina which is a generalized cellulitis of the submandibular region.[60] The infection is often the result of dental abscesses and extends into the submandibular, submental, and sublingual areas. Involvement of the sublingual spaces pushes the tongue upward and backward compromising the airway.[61] Associated swelling of the soft tissue in the supraglottic region can lead to obstruction of the airway and asphyxiation making this a surgical emergency to drain the abscess and relieve the airway compromise.

Airway management can be very difficult in these cases.[62] Awake tracheostomy with local anesthesia has been considered the safest in these patients. Alternative techniques of intubation include fiberoptic nasal intubation and direct laryngoscopy after inhalational anesthesia. These patients require care in an ICU
6 whether they have a tracheotomy or an endotracheal tube once the abscess has been drained as increased swelling may develop. The trachea should not be extubated until there is some resolution of the swelling.

Temporomandibular Joint Arthroscopy

Arthroscopic surgery of the TMJ as an outpatient procedure has been made possible by the development of small gauge arthroscopes and lasers. Indications for arthroscopic surgery include dislocation of cartilage causing clicking or lock jaw, immobility secondary to fibrosis, osteoarthritis, synovitis, or simply arthralgia.[63,64]

Immobility caused by pain is often relieved by general anesthesia allowing for easy intubation. When immobility is caused by
7 fibrosis resulting from long-standing immobility, nasal fiberoptic intubation may be required for tracheal intubation. Complications are rare but include temporary or total deficits of cranial nerves V, VII, and VIII along with hearing loss. Of particular importance to the anesthesiologist is partial or complete closure of the airway due to extravasation of the fluid used to irrigate the joint during arthroscopy.[65] The patient's airway should be examined for evidence of swelling indicating significant extravasation of fluid to avert a potential disaster.

Maxillofacial Trauma

Traumatic disruption of the bony, cartilaginous, and soft-tissue components of the face and upper airway challenges the anesthesiologist to recognize the nature and extent of the injury and consequent anatomic alteration, create a plan for securing the airway safely, implement the plan without doing further damage, maintain the airway during the administration of an anesthetic, and determine when and how to extubate the patient's trachea. Also necessary is the creation of a comfortable environment for both surgeon and anesthesiologist in a limited work space.

It is conventional to divide the facial skeleton into thirds. The lower third consists of the mandible, with its subdivisions of midline symphysis, body, angle, ramus, condyle, and coronoid process. The middle third contains the zygomatic arch of the temporal bone, blending into the zygomaticomaxillary complex, the maxillae, nasal bones, and orbits. The superior third consists of the frontal bone. This combination of bony buttresses and arches creates a normal vector of force dispersion and distribution to absorb the normal forces of mastication as well as external trauma. Thus, a blow to the mandible may be of sufficient magnitude to fracture the mandible at the point of impact or elsewhere, but does not extend the fracture line into the base of the skull. However, the force from a blow to the midface, especially from in front and above, does not follow a normal vector of force dispersion and redistribution. Rather, it tends to create an abnormal shearing force, which may tear the facial skeleton from the cranial skeleton and extend the fracture into the base of the skull. In any patient with severe midfacial trauma, a fracture of the base of the skull must be considered.

The mandible is a tubular bone and, as such, derives its strength from the cortices and is least vulnerable to fracture where the cortex is thickest at the anteroinferior margin. Moving posteriorly, the cortex thins, and a greater incidence of fractures is found at the angle of the mandible, the ramus, and the condyle.[66,67] Another common point of fracture is in the body of the mandible at the level of the first or second molar. Clinical experience indicates that this distribution occurs after high-velocity, high-impact trauma, such as occurs in an automobile accident. After trauma inflicted by a fist, a blunt weapon, or a fall, there is a greater tendency for a fracture of the symphysis, parasymphysis, and body to occur. This difference may result not only from lesser versus greater energy impact and redistribution, but also from the person's tendency to turn the head away from an impending blow and thus take the force of impact on the side of the face and the body of the mandible rather than on the symphysis.[68]

The mandible has a unique, horseshoe shape that causes forces to gather at points of vulnerability, often distant from the point of impact. If this phenomenon is unrecognized, it can create serious problems in diagnosis. It may be known, for example, that the patient was struck on the symphysis, but it must also be recognized that he or she may have a fracture of the condyle, perhaps with involvement of the TMJ and limitation of jaw mobility.

In 1901, Rene LeFort of Lille, France, published the results of a series of rather bizarre experiments.[69] He attempted to determine if there is a reliable means of detecting facial fractures by examining facial soft-tissue injuries and by using the nature and extent of these injuries as indicators of bony disruption. He concluded that extensive soft-tissue injury does not necessarily indicate bony trauma, and conversely, serious fractures may exist with relatively little soft-tissue disruption. In the course of his studies, LeFort determined the common lines of midface fracture, which are thus eponymous and called LeFort I, LeFort II, and LeFort III fractures.

The LeFort I fracture is a horizontal fracture of the maxilla, passing above the floor of the nose but involving the lower third of the septum, mobilizing the palate, maxillary alveolar process, and the lower third of the pterygoid plates and parts of the palatine bones. The fracture segment may be displaced posteriorly or laterally or rotated about a vertical axis.

The LeFort II fracture is pyramidal, beginning at the junction of the thick upper part of the nasal bone, with the thinner portion forming the upper margin of the anterior nasal aperture. The fracture crosses the medial wall of the orbit, including the lacrimal bone beneath the zygomaticomaxillary suture; crosses the lateral wall of the antrum; and passes posteriorly through the pterygoid plates. The fracture segment may be displaced posteriorly or rotated about an axis.

In a LeFort III fracture, the line of fracture parallels the base of the skull, separating the midfacial skeleton from the base of the cranium. The line of fracture passes through the base of the nose and the ethmoid bone in its depth, and through the orbital plates. The cribriform plate of the ethmoid may or may not be fractured. The fracture line crosses the lesser wing of the sphenoid, then downward to the pterygomaxillary fissure and sphenopalatine fossa. From the base of the inferior orbital fissure, the fracture extends laterally and upward to the frontozygomatic suture and downward and backward to the root of the pterygoid plates. A LeFort III fracture results from massive force applied to the midface. The zygomata are displaced, applying rotational force to the zygomatic arches. The arches are usually fractured as a result.

With a LeFort III fracture, the midface is mobilized and often distracted posteriorly. The normal convexity of the face becomes concave, giving rise to the characteristic "dish face deformity" of a LeFort III fracture. Even if this facial concavity is not clinically evident, the presence of a LeFort III fracture should be suspected if the incisive edges of the maxillary and mandibular teeth are apposed, instead of the normal position in which the maxillary incisors shingle over the mandibular incisors. This apposition serves as a subtle clue to minimal posterior displacement of the midface.

The patient who has sustained facial trauma may present with an obvious pathologic process that can distract the physician from completing a total evaluation of the patient. In the patient with facial trauma, other injuries may not be as apparent but may represent a greater threat to the patient's well-being. One study revealed that in patients with maxillofacial injury due to low-velocity, low-impact blows, 4% had additional major life-threatening injuries and 10% had additional minor injuries. With high-velocity, high-impact accidents, 32% had major additional injuries and 31% had minor additional injuries.[70] Of great importance, cervical spine fractures occurred in 1.2% of high-velocity injuries. Another study has reported a 5.5% incidence of cervical spine injury in patients with facial skeletal trauma.[71] Any level of the cervical spine may be involved, but injuries at C2 (31%) and C6 to C7 (50%) predominate. Cranial fractures and intracranial injury also are not uncommon.

Once an understanding of the facial trauma that was sustained and the consideration of concomitant injuries assessed, the patient can be examined and a plan for safe tracheal intubation devised. While tracheal intubation can usually be accomplished without difficulty, there are some situations which require further explanation.

Patients who do not open their mouth during the preoperative evaluation require further thought. One must ascertain if the limit mouth opening is the result of pain, trismus, or mechanical problem or some combination of the three. Simple fractures of the mandible can be very painful on movement of the jaw. Once the patient is anesthetized, the mouth can be opened and tracheal intubation can proceed without difficulty. Occasionally, there may be mechanical interference with opening from injury to the temporomandibular area either directly or indirectly. Direct trauma to the mandibular condyle or zygomatic arch may cause fractures that interfere with normal function of the TM joint. Indirect trauma is caused by transmittal of force up the body and ramus to the condyles. Compression fractures of condyles in the glenoid fossa and greenstick fractures of the condyles may result impeding opening.

Trismus, spasm of the muscles of mastication, can result from trauma or infection and interfere with mouth opening. It too is usually overcome by general anesthesia and muscle relaxation. The caveat here is that should the trismus be of long standing some degree of joint immobility will occur. If the trismus is caused by a facial infection, the affected muscles may become edematous and swell causing a mechanical interference with opening.

Lastly, the issue of nasotracheal intubation should be addressed for the patient with facial trauma. It is indicated in situations where oral intubation is impossible, for the patient without protective airway reflexes or in situations where prolonged intubation is anticipated. The major contraindication to nasotracheal intubation is the LeFort III fracture where the cribriform plate of the ethmoid bone may be involved. Foreign material from the nasopharynx may result in causing meningitis or even more devastating, the endotracheal tube can enter the cranial cavity. Even positive-pressure bag and mask ventilation can force foreign material or air into the skull.[72] Radiographic studies should be done prior to nasotracheal intubation whenever trauma to the is suspected.

Nasal fiberoptic intubation can be accomplished either with the patient awake, sedated, or after the induction of general anesthesia. A recent development in the management of the traumatized airway when awake fiberoptic intubation is the preferred method of securing the airway is the use of dexmedetomidine. Dexmedetomidine is an α_2-agonist that results in a moderate level of sedation without causing respiratory distress or hemodynamic instability during fiberoptic intubation.[73] Patients at risk for cervical spinal cord compression had excellent cooperation for postintubation neurologic examination when treated with a loading dose of 1 μg/kg bolus over 10 minutes followed by an infusion of 0.2 to 0.7 μg/kg/hr.[74] Side effects of hypertension, hypotension, and bradycardia may occur.

Extubation

8 Extubating the trachea at the end of a procedure is often straightforward and uneventful. Some clinicians will position the patient on their side to allow any pooled secretions or blood from the nasopharynx from irritating the vocal cords. This helps prevent coughing and laryngospasm making emergence that much smoother.

After trauma, infection, or extensive oral resection for tumor, the endotracheal tube must not be removed until there is clearly subsidence of any edema that might compromise the unprotected airway. Particular attention must be given to the submandibular area, where extensive edema forces the tongue upward and posteriorly compromising the airway. An edematous tongue protruding beyond the incisors is a warning sign of edema. If substantial edema is present, a waiting period of 24 to 36 hours is usually indicated. Serious infection may require a longer period of time to resolve.

Extubation in these patients should not be attempted until there is clear evidence of an air leak around the endotracheal tube once the cuff is deflated. As a safety precaution, the endotracheal tube can be removed over a tube changer.[75] The tube changer can be left in place until it is certain that the spontaneously breathing patient is able to maintain adequate gas exchange. Supplemental oxygen can also be delivered through the tube changer if needed remembering that barotrauma may occur if there is not adequate egress of air leading to pneumomediastinum, pneumothorax, and possible death.[76] Another useful technique is to place a fiberoptic bronchoscope through the tube and into the airway and to remove the tube over the bronchoscope so that it can be replaced immediately if necessary.

When tracheostomy has been incorporated into the anesthetic and the surgical plan, it is maintained at the termination of the procedure. These patients need to be in the ICU whether breathing spontaneously or needing mechanical ventilation. Care must be taken to ensure that the tracheostomy tube not get dislodged or removed which may result in a catastrophic outcome.

ACKNOWLEDGMENTS

The authors would like to acknowledge Ms. Jessie Barnes Hurley for her tireless assistance in the preparation of this manuscript.

The authors would also like to acknowledge the prior contributions of Dr. Alexander Gotta to this chapter in previous editions and thank him for his many years of clinical leadership in this area.

References

1. Brodsky L. Modern assessment of tonsils and adenoids. *Pediatr Clin North Am.* 1989;36:1551–1569.
2. Berkowitz RG, Zalzal GH. Tonsillectomy in children under 3 years of age. *Arch Otolaryngol Head Neck Surg.* 1990;116:685–686.
3. Ferrari L. Anesthesia for Pediatric ENT Procedures. *Progr Anesthesiol, Danamiller Memorial Education Foundation.* 2001;15:15–27.
4. Deutsch ES. Tonsillectomy and adenoidectomy. Changing indications. *Pediatr Clin North Am.* 1996;43(6):1319–1338.
5. Section on Pediatric Pulmonology, Subcommittee on Obstructive Sleep Apnea Syndrome. American Academy of Pediatrics. Clinical practice guideline: diagnosis and management of childhood obstructive sleep apnea syndrome. *Pediatrics.* 2002;109(4):704–712.
6. Chaban R, Cole P, Hoffstein V. Site of upper airway obstruction in patients with idiopathic obstructive sleep apnea. *Laryngoscope.* 1988;98(6 pt 1):641–647.
7. Blum RH, McGowan FX Jr. Chronic upper airway obstruction and cardiac dysfunction: anatomy, pathophysiology and anesthetic implications. *Paediatr Anaesth.* 2004;14(1):75–83.
8. Smith RM, Gonzalez C. The relationship between nasal obstruction and craniofacial growth. *Pediatr Clin North Am.* 1989;36:1423–1434.
9. Lerman J. Unraveling the mysteries of sleep-disordered breathing in children. *Anesthesiology.* 2006;105(4):645–647.
10. Gross JB, Bachenberg KL, Benumof JL, et al. Practice guidelines for the perioperative management of patients with obstructive sleep apnea: a report by the American Society of Anesthesiologists Task Force on Perioperative Management of patients with obstructive sleep apnea. *Anesthesiology.* 2006;104(5): 1081–1093.
11. Brown KA. Outcome, risk, and error and the child with obstructive sleep apnea. *Paediatr Anaesth.* 2011;21(7):771–780.
12. Chung F, Yegneswaran B, Liao P, et al. STOP questionnaire: a tool to screen patients for obstructive sleep apnea. *Anesthesiology.* 2008;108(5):812–821.
13. Chung SA, Yuan H, Chung F. A systemic review of obstructive sleep apnea and its implications for anesthesiologists. *Anesth Analg.* 2008;107(5):1543–1563.
14. Tsuiki S, Isono S, Ishikawa T, et al. Anatomical balance of the upper airway and obstructive sleep apnea. *Anesthesiology.* 2008;108(6):1009–1015.
15. Brown KA, Laferriere A, Lakheeram I, et al. Recurrent hypoxemia in children is associated with increased analgesic sensitivity to opiates. *Anesthesiology.* 2006;105 (4):665–669.
16. Pestieau S, Quezado Z, Johnson Y, et al. High-dose dexmedetomidine increases the opioid-free interval and decreases opioid requirement after tonsillectomy in children. *Can J Anaesth.* 2011;58(6):540–550.
17. Patel RI, Hannallah RS, Norden J, et al. Emergence airway complications in children: a comparison of tracheal extubation in awake and deeply anesthetized patients. *Anesth Analg.* 1991;73:266–270.
18. Alexander CA. A modified intavent laryngeal mask for ENT and dental anaesthesia. *Anaesthesia.* 1990;45:892–893.
19. Haynes SR, Morton NS. The laryngeal mask airway: A review of its use in paediatric anaesthesia. *Paediatr Anaesth.* 1993;3:65.
20. Johr M. Anaesthesia for tonsillectomy. *Curr Opin Anaesthesiol.* 2006;19:260–261.
21. Williams PJ, Bailey PM. Comparison of the reinforced laryngeal mask airway and tracheal intubation for adenotonsillectomy. *Br J Anaesth.* 1993;70(1):30–33.
22. Nair I, Bailey PM. Review of uses of the laryngeal mask in ENT anaesthesia. *Anaesthesia.* 1995;50(10):898–900.
23. Mason DG, Bingham RM. The laryngeal mask airway in children. *Anaesthesia.* 1990;45(9):760–763.
24. Goudsouzian N, Cleveland R. Stability of the laryngeal mask airway during marked extension of the head. *Paediatr Anaesth.* 1993;3:117–119.
25. Gunter JB, McAuliffe JJ, Beckman EC, et al. A factorial study of ondansetron, metoclopramide, and dexamethasone for emesis prophylaxis after adenotonsillectomy in children. *Paediatr Anaesth.* 2006;16(11):1153–1165.
26. Sukhani R, Pappas AL, Lurie J, et al. Ondansetron and dolasetron provide equivalent postoperative vomiting control after ambulatory tonsillectomy in dexamethasone-pretreated children. *Anesth Analg.* 2002;95(5):1230–1235, table of contents.
27. Randall DA, Hoffer ME. Complications of tonsillectomy and adenoidectomy. *Otolaryngol Head Neck Surg.* 1998;118(1):61–68.
28. Czarnetzki C, Elia N, Lysakowski C, et al. Dexamethasone and risk of nausea and vomiting and postoperative bleeding after tonsillectomy in children: a randomized trial. *JAMA.* 2008;300(22):2621–2630.
29. Windfuhr JP, Deck JC, Remmert S. Hemorrhage following coblation tonsillectomy. *Ann Otol Rhinol Laryngol.* 2005;114(10):749–756.
30. Windfuhr JP, Chen YS, Remmert S. Hemorrhage following tonsillectomy and adenoidectomy in 15,218 patients. *Otolaryngol Head Neck Surg.* 2005;132(2):281–286.
31. Crysdale W, Russell D. Complications of tonsillectomy and adenoidectomy in 9409 children observed overnight. *Can Med Assoc J.* 1986;135:1139.
32. Linden BE, Gross CW, Long TE, et al. Morbidity in pediatric tonsillectomy. *Laryngoscope.* 1990;100:120–124.
33. Broadman LM, Patel RI, Feldman BA, et al. The effects of peritonsillar infiltration on the reduction of intraoperative blood loss and post-tonsillectomy pain in children. *Laryngoscope.* 1989;99(6 pt 1):578–581.

34. Mehta VM, Har-El G, Goldstein NA. Postobstructive pulmonary edema after laryngospasm in the otolaryngology patient. *Laryngoscope.* 2006;116(9):1693–1696.
35. Brigger MT, Brietzke SE. Outpatient tonsillectomy in children: a systematic review. *Otolaryngol Head Neck Surg.* 2006;135(1):1–7.
36. Pizzuto M, Volk M, Kingston L. Common Topics in Otolaryngology. *Pediatr Clin North Am.* 1998;45(4).
37. Statham MM, Elluru RG, Buncher R, et al. Adenotonsillectomy for obstructive sleep apnea syndrome in young children: prevalence of pulmonary complications. *Arch Otolaryngol Head Neck Surg.* 2006;132(5):476–480.
38. Tait A, Malviya S, Voepel-Lewis T, et al. Risk Factors for Perioperative Adverse Respiratory Events in Children with Upper Respiratory Tract Infections. *Anesthesiology.* 2001;95(2):299–306.
39. Tait AR, Malviya S. Anesthesia for the child with an upper respiratory tract infection: still a dilemma? *Anesth Analg.* 2005;100(1):59–65.
40. Levine RA, Ronner SF, Ojemann RG. Auditory evoked potential and other neurophysiologic monitoring techniques during tumor surgery in the cerebellopontine angle. In: Loftus C, Traynelis V, eds. *Intraoperative Monitoring Techniques in Neurosurgery.* New York, NY: McGraw Hill, Inc.; 1994:175–176.
41. Casey WF, Drake-Lee AB. Nitrous oxide and middle ear pressure: A study of induction methods in children. *Anaesthesia.* 1982;37:896–900.
42. Zalzal GH. Stridor and airway compromise. *Pediatr Clin North Am.* 1989;36:1389–1402.
43. Ferrari LR, Vasallo S. Anesthesia for otorhinolaryngology procedures. In: Cote C, Ryan J, Todres I, Goudsouzian N, eds. *A Practice of Anesthesia for Infants and Children.* Philadelphia, PA: W.B. Saunders; 1992:318–320.
44. Soriano SG, Kim C, Jones DT. Surgical airway, rigid bronchoscopy and transtracheal jet ventilation in the pediatric patient. *Anesthesiol Clin North Am.* 1998;16:827.
45. Sanders RD. Two ventilating attachments for bronchoscopes. *Del Med J.* 1967:170–192.
46. Steward DJ. Percutaneous transtracheal ventilation for laser endoscopic procedures in infants and small children. *Can J Anaesth.* 1987;34:429–430.
47. Hermens JM, Bennett MJ, Hirshman CA. Anesthesia for laser surgery. *Anesth Analg.* 1983;62:218–229.
48. McLesky CH. Anesthetic management of patients undergoing endoscopic laser surgery. *IARS Review Course Lectures.* Cleveland: International Anesthesia Research Society (IARS); 1988:135.
49. Sosis MB, Dillon FX. Saline-filled cuffs help prevent laser-induced polyvinylchloride endotracheal tube fires. *Anesth Analg.* 1991;72:187–189.
50. Lee WC, Kapur TR, Ramsden WN. Local and regional anesthesia for functional endoscopic sinus surgery. *Ann Otol Rhinol Laryngol.* 1997;106(9):767–769.
51. John G, Low JM, Tan PE, et al. Plasma catecholamine levels during functional endoscopic sinus surgery. *Clin Otolaryngol Allied Sci.* 1995;20(3):213–215.
52. Groudine SB, Hollinger I, Jones J, et al. New York State guidelines on the topical use of phenylephrine in the operating room. The Phenylephrine Advisory Committee. *Anesthesiology.* 2000;92(3):859–864.
53. Tirelli G, Bigarini S, Russolo M, et al. Total intravenous anaesthesia in endoscopic sinus-nasal surgery. *Acta Otorhinolaryngol Ital.* 2004;24(3):137–144.
54. Wormald PJ, van Renen G, Perks J, et al. The effect of the total intravenous anesthesia compared with inhalational anesthesia on the surgical field during endoscopic sinus surgery. *Am J Rhinol.* 2005;19(5):514–520.
55. Cartellieri M, Vorbeck F, Kremser J. Comparison of six three-dimensional navigation systems during sinus surgery. *Acta Otolaryngol.* 2001;121(4):500–504.
56. Gruber A, Bavinzski G, Killer M, et al. Preoperative embolization of hypervascular skull base tumors. *Minim Invasive Neurosurg.* 2000;43(2):62–71.
57. Jellish WS, Murdoch J, Leonetti JP. Perioperative management of complex skull base surgery: the anesthesiologist's point of view. *Neurosurg Focus.* 2002;12(5):e5.
58. Goobie SM, Meier PM, Pereira LM, et al. Efficacy of tranexamic acid in pediatric craniosynostosis surgery: a double-blind, placebo-controlled trial. *Anesthesiology.* 2011;114(4):862–871.
59. Henry DA, Carless PA, Moxey AJ, et al. Anti-fibrinolytic use for minimising perioperative allogeneic blood transfusion. *Cochrane Database Syst Rev.* 2011;(3):CD001886.
60. Greenberg SL, Huang J, Chang RS, et al. Surgical management of Ludwig's angina. *ANZ J Surg.* 2007;77(7):540–543.
61. Kulkarni AH, Pai SD, Bhattarai B, et al. Ludwig's angina and airway considerations: a case report. *Cases J.* 2008;1(1):19.
62. Ovassapian A, Tuncbilek M, Weitzel EK, et al. Airway management in adult patients with deep neck infections: a case series and review of the literature. *Anesth Analg.* 2005;100(2):585–589.
63. Annandale T. On displacement of the inter-articular cartilage of the lower jaw, and its treatment by operation. *Lancet.* 1887;1:411.
64. Sanders B. Arthroscopic surgery of the temporomandibular joint: treatment of internal derangement with persistent closed lock. *Oral Surg Oral Med Oral Pathol.* 1986;62(4):361–372.
65. Hendler BH, Levin LM. Postobstructive pulmonary edema as a sequela of temporomandibular joint arthroscopy: a case report. *J Oral Maxillofac Surg.* 1993;51(3):315–317.
66. Huelke DF, Patrick LM. Mechanics in the Production of Mandibular Fractures: Strain-Gauge Measurements of Impacts to the Chin. *J Dent Res.* 1964;43:437–446.
67. Nahum AM. The biomechanics of facial bone fracture. *Laryngoscope.* 1975;85(1):140–156.
68. Olson RA, Fonseca RJ, Zeitler DL, et al. Fractures of the mandible: a review of 580 cases. *J Oral Maxillofac Surg.* 1982;40(1):23–28.
69. LeFort R. Etude experimentale sur les fractures de la machoire superieure. *Rev Chir.* 1901;23:208.
70. Luce EA, Tubb TD, Moore AM. Review of 1,000 major facial fractures and associated injuries. *Plast Reconstr Surg.* 1979;63(1):26–30.
71. Davidson JS, Birdsell DC. Cervical spine injury in patients with facial skeletal trauma. *J Trauma.* 1989;29(9):1276–1278.
72. Dacosta A, Billard JL, Gery P, et al. Posttraumatic intracerebral pneumatocele after ventilation with a mask: case report. *J Trauma.* 1994;36(2):255–257.
73. Bergese SD, Khabiri B, Roberts WD, et al. Dexmedetomidine for conscious sedation in difficult awake fiberoptic intubation cases. *J Clin Anesth.* 2007;19(2):141–144.
74. Avitsian R, Lin J, Lotto M, et al. Dexmedetomidine and awake fiberoptic intubation for possible cervical spine myelopathy: a clinical series. *J Neurosurg Anesthesiol.* 2005;17(2):97–99.
75. Loudermilk EP, Hartmannsgruber M, Stoltzfus DP, et al. A prospective study of the safety of tracheal extubation using a pediatric airway exchange catheter for patients with a known difficult airway. *Chest.* 1997;111(6):1660–1665.
76. Duggan LV, Law JA, Murphy MF. Brief review: Supplementing oxygen through an airway exchange catheter: efficacy, complications, and recommendations. *Can J Anaesth.* 2011;58(6):560–568.

CHAPTER

48 Anesthesia for Ophthalmologic Surgery

KATHRYN E. MCGOLDRICK • STEVEN I. GAYER

ANESTHESIA FOR SURGICAL SUBSPECIALTIES

Key Points

1. Although apprehension is predictable in potentially blind patients awaiting surgery, this problem is often exacerbated in the elderly, whose coping mechanisms may be diminished by depression or dementia.
2. With intraocular procedures, profound akinesia and meticulous control of IOP are requisite. However, with extraocular surgery, the significance of IOP fades, whereas concern about elicitation of the oculocardiac reflex assumes prominence.
3. Inhalation anesthetics cause dose-related reductions in intraocular pressure (IOP). The exact mechanisms are unknown, but postulated causes include depression of a control center in the diencephalon, reduction of aqueous humor production, enhancement of aqueous outflow, or relaxation of the extraocular muscles.
4. The oculocardiac reflex is triggered by pressure on the globe and by traction on the extraocular muscles, as well as on the conjunctiva or on the orbital structures. This reflex, the afferent limb of which is trigeminal and the efferent limb is vagal, may also be elicited by performance of a retrobulbar block, by ocular trauma, and by direct pressure on tissue remaining in the orbital apex after enucleation.
5. Ophthalmic drugs may significantly alter the patient's reaction to anesthesia. Similarly, anesthetic drugs and maneuvers may dramatically influence intraocular dynamics.
6. Several anesthetic options are available for many types of ocular procedures, including general anesthesia, retrobulbar block, peribulbar anesthesia, sub-Tenon (episcleral) block, topical analgesia, and intracameral injection.
7. The complications of ophthalmic anesthesia can be both vision- and life-threatening.

Multimedia

Open Eye Injury

Anesthesia for ophthalmic surgery presents many unique challenges (Table 48-1). In addition to possessing technical expertise, the anesthesiologist must have detailed knowledge of ocular anatomy, physiology, and pharmacology. It is essential to appreciate that ophthalmic drugs may significantly alter the reaction to anesthesia and that, concomitantly, anesthetic drugs and maneuvers may dramatically influence intraocular dynamics. Patients undergoing ophthalmic surgery may represent extremes of age and notable coexisting medical diseases (e.g., diabetes mellitus, coronary artery disease, essential hypertension, chronic lung disease), but they are likely to be in the elderly age group. Indeed, the elderly constitute the most rapidly growing subset of the US population, with the 2009 Census reporting 37.8 million Americans age 65 years or older, an increase of 30% since 1990. Impressively, almost 19 million Americans were 75 years or older in 2009, an increase of 46% from 1990. Moreover, the elderly are a uniquely vulnerable group with reduced functional reserve and a myriad of age-related diseases. The economic implication of these age-related diseases is staggering. For example, age-related macular degeneration is the leading cause of blindness in individuals older than 65 years in the United States, affecting more than 1.75 million people. Because of the rapid aging of our population, this number will increase to almost 3 million by 2020.[1] More recent prevalence studies suggest that the number of persons with Alzheimer disease in the United States is approximately 5 million. Given that the percentage of individuals with Alzheimer disease increases by a factor of 2 with approximately every 5 years of age, 1% of persons who are 60 years old and about 30% of those who are 85 years old have the disease. Without advances in therapy, the number of symptomatic cases in the United States is predicted to increase to 13.2 million by 2050.[2] Current annual expenditures on care for patients with Alzheimer disease exceed $84 billion,[3]
1 a statistic that underscores the urgency of seeking more effective therapeutic and prophylactic interventions. Moreover, although apprehension is predictable in blind or potentially blind patients awaiting surgery, this problem is often exacerbated in the elderly, whose coping mechanisms may be diminished by depression or dementia.

It is mandatory to be knowledgeable about the numerous surgical procedures that are unique to the specialty of ophthalmology. Although the list of ocular surgical interventions is lengthy, these procedures may, in general, be classified as *extraocular* or *intraocular.* This distinction is critical because anesthetic considerations are different for these two major surgical categories. For example, with intraocular procedures, profound akinesia (relax-
2 ation of recti muscles) and meticulous control of intraocular pressure (IOP) are requisite. However, with extraocular surgery, the significance of IOP fades, whereas concern about elicitation of the oculocardiac reflex assumes prominence.

TABLE 48-1. REQUIREMENTS OF OPHTHALMIC SURGERY

- Safety
- Akinesia
- Analgesia
- Minimal bleeding
- Avoidance or obtundation of oculocardiac reflex
- Control of intraocular pressure
- Awareness of drug interactions
- Smooth emergence

OCULAR ANATOMY

The anesthesiologist should be knowledgeable about ocular anatomy to enhance his or her understanding of surgical procedures and to aid the surgeon in the performance of regional blocks when needed[4] (Fig. 48-1). Salient subdivisions of ocular anatomy include the orbit, the eye itself, the extraocular muscles, the eyelids, and the lacrimal system.

The orbit is a bony box, or pyramidal cavity, housing the eyeball and its associated structures in the skull. The walls of the orbit are composed of the following bones: Frontal, zygomatic, greater wing of the sphenoid, maxilla, palatine, lacrimal, and ethmoid. A familiarity with the surface relationships of the orbital rim is mandatory for the skilled performance of regional blocks.

The optic foramen, located at the orbital apex, transmits the optic nerve and the ophthalmic artery, as well as the sympathetic nerves from the carotid plexus. The superior orbital fissure transmits the superior and inferior branches of the oculomotor nerve; the lacrimal, frontal, and nasociliary branches of the trigeminal nerve; the trochlear and abducens nerves; and the superior and inferior ophthalmic veins. The inferior orbital or sphenomaxillary fissure contains the infraorbital and zygomatic nerves and communication between the inferior ophthalmic vein and the pterygoid plexus. The infraorbital foramen, located about 4 mm below the orbital rim in the maxilla, transmits the infraorbital nerve, artery, and vein. The lacrimal fossa contains the lacrimal gland in the superior temporal orbit. The supraorbital notch, located at the junction of the medial one-third and temporal two-thirds of the superior orbital rim, transmits the supraorbital nerve, artery, and vein. The supraorbital notch, the infraorbital foramen, and the lacrimal fossa are clinically palpable and function as major landmarks for administration of regional anesthesia.

The eye itself is actually one large sphere with part of a smaller sphere incorporated in the anterior surface, constituting a structure with two different radii of curvature. The coat of the eye

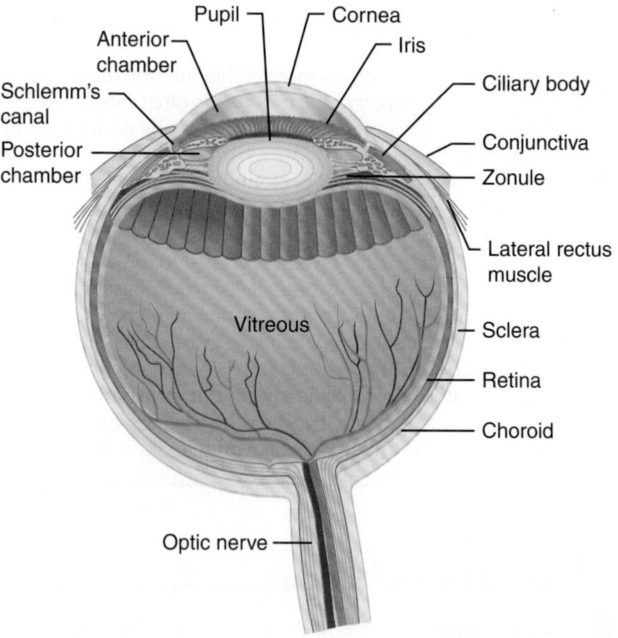

FIGURE 48-1. Diagram of ocular anatomy.

is composed of three layers: Sclera, uveal tract, and retina. The fibrous outer layer, or *sclera*, is protective, providing sufficient rigidity to maintain the shape of the eye. The anterior portion of the sclera, the cornea, is transparent, permitting light to pass into the internal ocular structures. The double-spherical shape of the eye exists because the corneal arc of curvature is steeper than the scleral arc of curvature. The focusing of rays of light to form a retinal image commences at the cornea.

The *uveal tract*, or middle layer of the globe, is vascular and in direct apposition to the sclera. A potential space, known as the *suprachoroidal space*, separates the sclera from the uveal tract. This potential space, however, may become filled with blood during an expulsive or suprachoroidal hemorrhage, often associated with surgical disaster. The iris, ciliary body, and choroid compose the uveal tract. The iris includes the pupil, which controls the amount of light entering the eye by contractions of three sets of muscles. The iris dilator is sympathetically innervated; the iris sphincter and the ciliary muscle have parasympathetic innervation. Posterior to the iris lays the ciliary body, which produces aqueous humor (see "Formation and Drainage of Aqueous Humor"). The ciliary muscles, situated in the ciliary body, adjust the shape of the lens to accommodate focusing at various distances. Large vessels and a network of small vessels and capillaries known as the *choriocapillaris* constitute the choroid, which supplies nutrition to the outer part of the retina.

The *retina* is a neurosensory membrane composed of ten layers that convert light impulses into neural impulses. These neural impulses are then carried through the optic nerve to the brain. Located in the center of the globe is the vitreous cavity, filled with a gelatinous substance known as *vitreous humor*. This material is adherent to the most anterior 3 mm of the retina, as well as to large blood vessels and the optic nerve. The vitreous humor may pull on the retina, causing retinal tears and retinal detachment.

The crystalline lens, located posterior to the pupil, refracts rays of light passing through the cornea and pupil to focus images on the retina. The ciliary muscle, whose contractile state causes tautness or relaxation of the lens zonules, regulates the thickness of the lens.

In addition, six extraocular muscles move the eye within the orbit to various positions. The bilobed lacrimal gland provides most of the tear film, which serves to maintain a moist anterior surface on the globe. The lacrimal drainage system—composed of the puncta, canaliculi, lacrimal sac, and lacrimal duct—drains into the nose below the inferior turbinate. Blockage of this system occurs frequently, necessitating procedures ranging from lacrimal duct probing to dacryocystorhinostomy, which involves anastomosis of the lacrimal sac to the nasal mucosa.

Covering the surface of the globe and lining the eyelids is a mucous membrane called the *conjunctiva*. Because drugs are absorbed across the membrane, it is a popular site for administration of ophthalmic drugs.

The eyelids consist of four layers: (1) the conjunctiva, (2) the cartilaginous tarsal plate, (3) a muscle layer composed mainly of the orbicularis and the levator palpebrae, and (4) the skin. The eyelids protect the eye from foreign objects; through blinking, the tear film produced by the lacrimal gland is spread across the surface of the eye, keeping the cornea moist.

Blood supply to the eye and orbit is by means of branches of both the internal and external carotid arteries. Venous drainage of the orbit is accomplished through the multiple anastomoses of the superior and inferior ophthalmic veins. Venous drainage of the eye is achieved mainly through the central retinal vein. All these veins empty directly into the cavernous sinus.

The sensory and motor innervations of the eye and its adnexa are very complex, with multiple cranial nerves supplying branches to various ocular structures. A branch of the oculomotor nerve supplies a motor root to the ciliary ganglion, which in turn supplies the sphincter of the pupil and the ciliary muscle. The trochlear nerve supplies the superior oblique muscle. The abducens nerve supplies the lateral rectus muscle. The trigeminal nerve constitutes the most complex ocular and adnexal innervation. In addition, the zygomatic branch of the facial nerve eventually divides into an upper branch, supplying the frontalis and the upper lid orbicularis, whereas the lower branch supplies the orbicularis of the lower lid.

OCULAR PHYSIOLOGY

Despite its relatively diminutive size, the eye is a complex organ, concerned with many intricate physiologic processes. The formation and drainage of aqueous humor and their influence on IOP in both normal and glaucomatous eyes are among the most important functions, especially from the anesthesiologist's perspective. An appreciation of the effects of various anesthetic manipulations on IOP requires an understanding of the fundamental principles of ocular physiology.

Formation and Drainage of Aqueous Humor

Two-thirds of the aqueous humor is formed in the posterior chamber by the ciliary body in an active secretory process involving both the carbonic anhydrase and the cytochrome oxidase systems (Fig. 48-2). The remaining third is formed by passive filtration of aqueous humor from the vessels on the anterior surface of the iris.

At the ciliary epithelium, sodium is actively transported into the aqueous humor in the posterior chamber. Bicarbonate and chloride ions passively follow the sodium ions. This active mechanism results in the osmotic pressure of the aqueous humor being many times greater than that of plasma. It is this disparity in osmotic pressure that leads to an average rate of aqueous humor production of 2 μL/min.

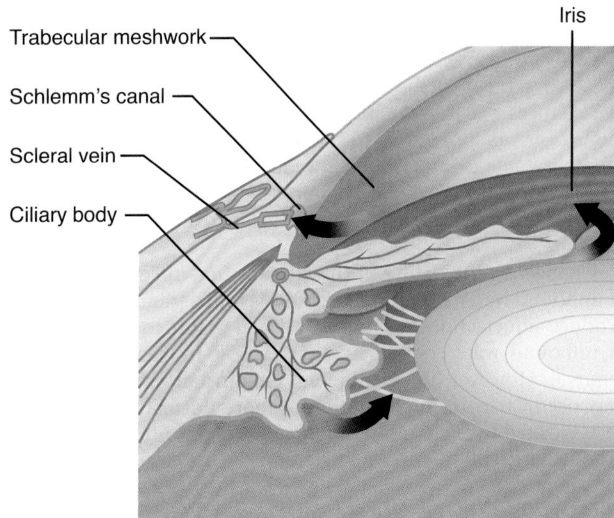

FIGURE 48-2. Ocular anatomy concerned with control of intraocular pressure.

Aqueous humor flows from the posterior chamber through the pupillary aperture and into the anterior chamber, where it mixes with the aqueous formed by the iris. During its journey into the anterior chamber, the aqueous humor bathes the avascular lens and, once in the anterior chamber, it also bathes the corneal endothelium. Then the aqueous humor flows into the peripheral segment of the anterior chamber and exits the eye through the trabecular network, Schlemm's canal, and episcleral venous system. A network of connecting venous channels eventually leads to the superior vena cava and the right atrium. Thus, obstruction of venous return at any point from the eye to the right side of the heart impedes aqueous drainage, elevating IOP accordingly.

Maintenance of Intraocular Pressure

IOP normally varies between 10 and 21.7 mm Hg and is considered abnormal above 22 mm Hg. This level varies 1 to 2 mm Hg with each cardiac contraction. Also, a diurnal variation of 2 to 5 mm Hg is observed, with a higher value noted on awakening. This higher awakening pressure has been ascribed to vascular congestion, pressure on the globe from closed lids, and mydriasis—all of which occur during sleep. If IOP is too high, it may produce opacities by interfering with normal corneal metabolism.

During anesthesia, a rise in IOP can produce permanent visual loss. If the IOP is already elevated, a further increase can trigger acute glaucoma. If penetration of the globe occurs when the IOP is excessively high, rupture of a blood vessel with subsequent hemorrhage may transpire. IOP becomes atmospheric once the eye cavity has been entered, and any sudden rise in pressure may lead to prolapse of the iris and lens, and loss of vitreous. Thus, proper control of IOP is critical.

Three main factors influence IOP: (1) External pressure on the eye by the contraction of the orbicularis oculi muscle and the tone of the extraocular muscles, venous congestion of orbital veins (as may occur with vomiting and coughing), and conditions such as orbital tumor; (2) scleral rigidity; and (3) changes in intraocular contents that are semisolid (lens, vitreous, or intraocular tumor) or fluid (blood and aqueous humor). Although these factors affect IOP, the major control of intraocular tension is exerted by the fluid content, especially the aqueous humor.

Sclerosis of the sclera, not uncommonly seen in the elderly, may be associated with decreased scleral compliance and increased IOP. Other degenerative changes of the eye linked with aging can also influence IOP, the most significant being a hardening and enlargement of the crystalline lens. When these degenerative changes occur, they may lead to anterior displacement of the lens–iris diaphragm. A resultant shallowness of the anterior chamber angle may then occur, reducing access of the trabecular meshwork to aqueous. This process is usually gradual, but, if rapid lens engorgement occurs, angle-closure glaucoma may transpire.

Changes in the nature of the vitreous that affect the amount of unbound water also influence IOP. Myopia, trauma, and aging produce liquefaction of vitreous gel and a subsequent increase in unbound water, which may lower IOP by facilitating fluid removal. However, under different circumstances, the opposite may occur; that is, the hydration of more normal vitreous may be associated with elevation of IOP. Hence, it is often prudent to produce a slightly dehydrated state in the surgical patient with glaucoma.

Intraocular blood volume, determined primarily by vessel dilation or contraction in the spongy layers of the choroid, contributes importantly to IOP. Although changes in arterial or venous pressure may secondarily affect IOP, excursions in arterial pressure have much less importance than do venous fluctuations. In chronic arterial hypertension, ocular pressure returns to normal levels after a period of adaptation brought about by compression of vessels in the choroid as a result of increased IOP. Thus, a feedback mechanism reduces the total volume of blood, keeping IOP relatively constant in patients with systemic hypertension.

However, if venous return from the eye is disturbed at any point from Schlemm's canal to the right atrium, IOP increases substantially. Trendelenburg position, cervical collar, and even a tight necktie can produce increased intraocular blood volume and distention of orbital vessels, as well as attenuated aqueous drainage.[5] Straining, vomiting, or coughing greatly increase venous pressure and raise IOP as much as 40 mm Hg or more. The deleterious implications of these activities cannot be overemphasized. Laryngoscopy and tracheal intubation may also elevate IOP, even without any visible reaction to intubation, but especially when the patient coughs. Topical anesthesia of the larynx may attenuate the systemic hypertensive response to laryngoscopy but does not reliably prevent associated increases in IOP.[6] Ordinarily, the pressure elevation from such increases in blood volume or venous pressure dissipates rapidly. However, if the coughing or straining occurs during ocular surgery when the eye is open, as in penetrating keratoplasty, the result may be a disastrous expulsive hemorrhage, at worst, or a disconcerting loss of vitreous, at best.

Despite the notable role of venous pressure, scleral rigidity, and vitreous composition, maintenance of IOP is determined primarily by the rate of aqueous formation and the rate of aqueous humor outflow. The most important influence on formation of aqueous humor is the difference in osmotic pressure between aqueous humor and plasma. This fact is illustrated by the equation:

$$\text{IOP} = K[(\text{OPaq} - \text{OPpl}) + \text{CP}] \quad (48\text{-}1)$$

where K is the coefficient of outflow, OPaq is the osmotic pressure of aqueous humor, OPpl is the osmotic pressure of plasma, and CP is the capillary pressure. Hypertonic solutions such as mannitol are used to lower IOP because a small change in the solute concentration of plasma can markedly influence the formation of aqueous humor and hence IOP.

Fluctuations in aqueous humor outflow may also produce a dramatic alteration in IOP. The most significant factor controlling aqueous humor outflow is the diameter of Fontana spaces, as illustrated by the equation:

$$A = \frac{r^4(\text{Piop} - \text{Pv})}{8\eta L} \quad (48\text{-}2)$$

where A is the volume of aqueous outflow per unit of time, r is the radius of Fontana spaces, Piop is the IOP, Pv is the venous pressure, η is the viscosity, and L is the length of Fontana spaces. When the pupil dilates, Fontana spaces narrow, resistance to outflow is increased, and IOP rises. Because mydriasis is undesirable in both closed-angle glaucoma and open-angle glaucoma, miotics are applied conjunctivally in patients with glaucoma.

Glaucoma

Glaucoma is a condition characterized by elevated IOP, resulting in impairment of capillary blood flow to the optic nerve with eventual loss of optic nerve tissue and function. Two different anatomic types of glaucoma exist: Open-angle or chronic simple glaucoma and closed-angle or acute glaucoma. (Other variations of these processes occur but are not especially germane to anesthetic management.)

With open-angle glaucoma, the elevated IOP exists with an anatomically open anterior chamber angle. It is believed that sclerosis of trabecular tissue results in impaired aqueous humor filtration and drainage. Treatment consists of medication to produce miosis and trabecular stretching. Commonly used eye drops are epinephrine, timolol, dipivefrin, and betaxolol. Closed-angle glaucoma is characterized by the peripheral iris moving into direct contact with the posterior corneal surface, mechanically obstructing aqueous humor outflow. People who have a narrow angle between the iris and the posterior cornea are predisposed to this condition. In these patients, mydriasis can produce such increased thickening of the peripheral iris that corneal touch occurs and the angle is closed. Another mechanism producing acute, closed-angle glaucoma is swelling of the crystalline lens. In this case, pupillary block occurs, with the edematous lens blocking the flow of aqueous humor from the posterior to the anterior chamber. This situation can also develop if the lens is traumatically dislocated anteriorly, thus physically blocking the anterior chamber.

It was previously believed by some clinicians that patients with glaucoma should not be given atropine. However, this claim is untenable. Atropine in the dose range used clinically has no effect on IOP in either open-angle or closed-angle glaucoma. When 0.4 mg of atropine is given parenterally to a 70-kg person, approximately 0.0001 mg is absorbed by the eye.[7] Garde et al.[8] reported, however, that scopolamine has a greater mydriatic effect than atropine and recommended not using scopolamine in patients with known or suspected closed-angle glaucoma.

Equation 48-2, describing the volume of aqueous outflow per unit of time, clearly demonstrates that outflow is exquisitely sensitive to fluctuations in venous pressure. Because a rise in venous pressure produces an increased volume of ocular blood and decreased aqueous outflow, it is obvious that considerable elevation of IOP occurs with any maneuver that increases venous pressure. Hence, in addition to preoperative instillation of miotics, other anesthetic goals for the patient with glaucoma include perioperative avoidance of venous congestion and overhydration. Furthermore, hypotensive episodes are to be avoided because these patients are allegedly vulnerable to retinal vascular thrombosis.

Primary congenital glaucoma is classified according to age of onset, with the infantile type presenting any time after birth until 3 years of age. The juvenile type presents between the ages of 37 months and 30 years. Moreover, childhood glaucoma may also occur in conjunction with various eye diseases or developmental anomalies such as aniridia, mesodermal dysgenesis syndrome, and retinopathy of prematurity.

Successful management of infantile glaucoma critically depends on early diagnosis. Presenting symptoms include epiphora, photophobia, blepharospasm, and irritability. Ocular enlargement, termed *buphthalmos,* or "ox eye," and corneal haziness secondary to edema are common. Buphthalmos is rare, however, if glaucoma develops after 3 years of age because by then the eye is much less elastic.

Because infantile glaucoma is frequently associated with obstructed aqueous humor outflow, management of it often requires surgical creation, by goniotomy or trabeculotomy, of a route for aqueous humor to flow into the canal of Schlemm. However, advanced disease may be unresponsive to even multiple goniotomies, and the more radical trabeculectomy or some other variety of filtering procedure may be necessary.

The juvenile form of glaucoma, in which the cornea and eye size are normal, is commonly associated with a family history of open-angle glaucoma and is treated similarly to primary open-angle glaucoma.

In cases of pediatric secondary glaucoma, goniotomy and filtering may be unsuccessful, whereas cyclocryotherapy may effect a reduction in IOP, pain, and corneal edema. The ciliary body is destroyed with a cryoprobe cooled to –70°C, thus dramatically decreasing aqueous formation.

It is essential to appreciate that the high IOP frequently encountered in infantile glaucoma can be reduced by >15 mm Hg when a surgical plane of general anesthesia is achieved. However, one study demonstrated minimal effect of halothane on IOP when the concentration ranged narrowly between 0.5% and 1%.[9] Some clinicians maintain that ketamine is a useful drug to use for examination under anesthesia when infantile glaucoma is part of the differential diagnosis because ketamine does not appear to reduce IOP, giving a spuriously low reading. Moreover, even normal infants sporadically have pressures in the mid-20s. Hence, diagnosis is not based exclusively on the numerical pressure recorded under anesthesia. Other factors such as corneal edema and increased corneal diameter, tears in Descemet membrane, and cupping of the optic nerve are considered in making the diagnosis. If these aberrations are noted, surgical intervention may be mandatory, even in the setting of a reputedly normal IOP.

EFFECTS OF ANESTHESIA AND ADJUVANT DRUGS ON INTRAOCULAR PRESSURE

Central Nervous System Depressants

3 Inhalation anesthetics purportedly cause dose-related decreases in IOP. The exact mechanisms are unknown, but postulated causes include depression of a central nervous system (CNS) control center in the diencephalon, reduction of aqueous humor production, enhancement of aqueous humor outflow, or relaxation of the extraocular muscles.[7] Moreover, virtually all CNS depressants—including barbiturates, neuroleptics, opioids, tranquilizers,[7] and hypnotics, such as etomidate and propofol—lower IOP in both normal and glaucomatous eyes. Etomidate, despite its proclivity to produce pain on intravenous injection and skeletal muscle movement, is associated with a significant reduction in IOP.[10] However, etomidate-induced myoclonus may be hazardous in the setting of a ruptured globe.

Controversy surrounds the issue of ketamine's effect on IOP. Administered intravenously or intramuscularly, ketamine initially was believed to increase IOP significantly, as measured by indentation tonometry.[11] Corssen and Hoy[12] also reported a slight but statistically significant increase in IOP that appeared unrelated to changes in blood pressure or depth of anesthesia. However, nystagmus made proper positioning of the tonometer difficult and may have resulted in less-than-accurate measurements.

Conflicting results arose from a study in which 2 mg/kg of ketamine given intravenously to adults failed to have a significant effect on IOP.[13] Furthermore, a pediatric study reported no increase in IOP after an intramuscular ketamine dose of 8 mg/kg. Indeed, values obtained were similar to those reported with halothane and isoflurane.[14,15]

Some of the confusion may arise from differences in premedication practices and from the use of different instruments to measure IOP. More recent studies have used applanation tonometry rather than indentation tonometry. However, even if future studies should confirm that ketamine has minimal or no effect on IOP, ketamine's proclivity to cause nystagmus and blepharospasm makes it a less-than-optimal agent for many types of ophthalmic surgery.

Ventilation and Temperature

Hyperventilation decreases IOP, whereas asphyxia, administration of carbon dioxide, and hypoventilation have been shown to elevate IOP.[16]

Hypothermia lowers IOP. On initial consideration, hypothermia might be expected to raise IOP because of the associated increase in viscosity of aqueous humor. However, hypothermia is linked with decreased formation of aqueous humor and with vasoconstriction; hence, the net result is a reduction in IOP.

Adjuvant Drugs

Ganglionic Blockers, Hypertonic Solutions, and Acetazolamide

Ganglionic blockers such as tetraethylammonium and pentamethonium cause a dramatic decrease in IOP. Trimethaphan also substantially lowers IOP in normal subjects, despite mydriasis.

Intravenous administration of hypertonic solutions such as dextran, urea, mannitol, and sorbitol elevates plasma osmotic pressure, thereby decreasing aqueous humor formation and reducing IOP. As effective as urea is in reducing IOP, intravenous mannitol has the advantage of fewer side effects. Mannitol's onset, peak (30 to 45 minutes), and duration of action (5 to 6 hours) are similar to those of urea. Moreover, both drugs may produce acute intravascular volume overload. Sudden expansion of plasma volume secondary to efflux of intracellular water into the vascular compartment places a heavy workload on the kidneys and heart, often resulting in hypertension and dilution of plasma sodium. Furthermore, mannitol-associated diuresis, if protracted, may trigger hypotension in volume-depleted patients.

Intravenous administration of acetazolamide inactivates carbonic anhydrase and interferes with the sodium pump. The resultant decrease in aqueous humor formation lowers IOP. However, the action of acetazolamide is not limited to the eye, and systemic effects include loss of sodium, potassium, and water secondary to the drug's renal tubular effects. Such electrolyte imbalances may then be linked to cardiac dysrhythmias during general anesthesia.

An advantage of acetazolamide is its relative ease of administration. Whereas large volumes of hypertonic solutions must be infused to reduce IOP, acetazolamide is easily given as a typical adult dose of 500 mg dissolved in 10 mL of sterile water. Acetazolamide may also be given orally, and topical carbonic anhydrase inhibitors are commercially available.

Neuromuscular Blocking Drugs

Neuromuscular blocking drugs have both direct and indirect actions on IOP.

Equipotent paralyzing doses of all the nondepolarizing drugs, including pancuronium,[17] directly lower IOP by relaxing the extraocular muscles (Fig. 48-3). However, if paralysis of the respiratory muscles is accompanied by alveolar hypoventilation, the latter secondary effect may supervene to increase IOP.

In contrast to nondepolarizing drugs, the depolarizing drug succinylcholine elevates IOP. Lincoff et al.[18] reported extrusion of vitreous after succinylcholine administration to a patient with a surgically open eye. An average peak IOP increase of about 8 mm Hg is produced within 1 to 4 minutes of an intravenous

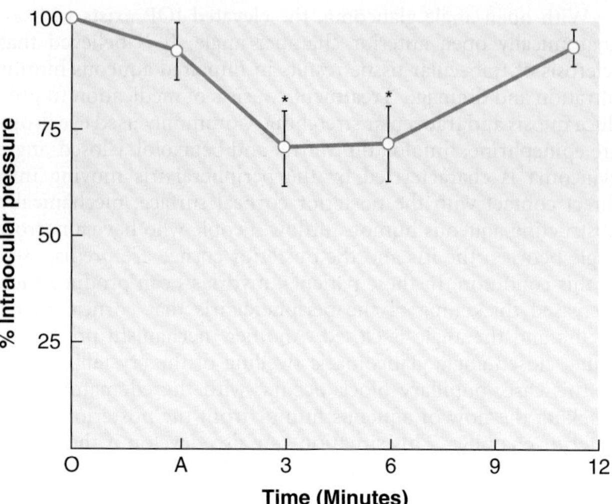

FIGURE 48-3. Mean intraocular pressure after administration of thiopental, 3 to 4 mg/kg, and pancuronium, 0.08 mg/kg at 0. *A* = loss of lid reflex; * = $p < 0.05$. (Reprinted from: Litwiller RW, DiFazio CA, Rushia EF. Pancuronium and intraocular pressure. *Anesthesiology.* 1975;42:750, with permission.)

dose. Within 7 minutes, return to baseline usually transpires.[19] The ocular hypertensive effect of succinylcholine has been attributed to several mechanisms, including tonic contraction of extraocular muscles,[7] choroidal vascular dilation, and relaxation of orbital smooth muscle. One study speculates that the succinylcholine-induced increase in IOP is multifactorial but primarily the result of the cycloplegic action of succinylcholine, producing a deepening of the anterior chamber and increased outflow resistance.[20] Because they studied eyes with the extraocular muscles detached and still observed an elevation in IOP, these investigators proposed that changes in extraocular muscle tone do not contribute substantially to the increase in IOP observed after succinylcholine administration.

A variety of methods have been advocated to prevent succinylcholine-induced elevations in IOP. However, although some attenuation of the increase results, none of these techniques consistently and completely block the ocular hypertensive response. Prior administration of such drugs as acetazolamide, narcotics, β-blockers, and nondepolarizing neuromuscular blocking drugs has been suggested. The efficacy of pretreatment with nondepolarizing drugs is controversial.

In 1968, using indentation tonometry, Miller et al.[21] reported that pretreatment with small amounts of gallamine or *d*-tubocurarine prevented succinylcholine-associated increases in IOP. However, in 1978, using the more sensitive applanation tonometer, Meyers et al.[22] were unable to consistently circumvent the ocular hypertensive response after similar pretreatment therapy (Table 48-2). In addition, Verma[23] claimed that a "self-taming" technique in which a small dose of succinylcholine is administered prior to induction was protective, but in a controlled study using applanation tonometry, Meyers et al.[24] challenged this claim. Although intravenous pretreatment with lidocaine, 1 to 2 mg/kg, may blunt the hemodynamic response to laryngoscopy,[6,25] such therapy does not reliably prevent the ocular hypertensive response associated with succinylcholine and intubation.[26] However, Grover et al.[27] claimed that pretreatment with lidocaine, 1.5 mg/kg intravenously, 1 minute before induction with thiopental and succinylcholine offered protection from IOP increases

TABLE 48-2. EFFECTS OF SUCCINYLCHOLINE ON INTRAOCULAR PRESSURE: DOUBLE-BLIND *d*-TUBOCURARINE OR GALLAMINE PRETREATMENT

		Intraocular Pressure (mm Hg, MEAN ± SE)		
Pretreatment[a]	Mean Age (yr)	Baseline	3 min After Pretreatment	1 min After Succinylcholine[b]
d-Tubocurarine	13.4	13 ± 1	12.3 ± 1.2	24 ± 1.3
Gallamine	8.7	10.9 ± 1.1	10.6 ± 1	23.4 ± 2.3

[a]*d*-Tubocurarine, 0.09 mg/kg, or gallamine, 0.3 mg/kg.
[b]1 to 1.5 mg/kg intravenously.
Reprinted from: Meyers EF, Krupin T, Johnson M, et al. Failure of nondepolarizing neuromuscular blockers to inhibit succinylcholine-induced increased intraocular pressure: A controlled study. *Anesthesiology*. 1978;48:149, with permission.

because of succinylcholine and may therefore be of value in rapid-sequence induction for open eye injuries.

Certainly, succinylcholine—if unaccompanied by pretreatment with a nondepolarizing neuromuscular blocking drug—is not the ideal agent for patients with penetrating ocular wounds and careful consideration should be used before giving it after the eye has been opened. Nonetheless, it is no longer valid to recommend that succinylcholine be used only with extreme reluctance in ocular surgery. Clearly, any succinylcholine-induced increment in IOP is usually dissipated before surgery is started.

The forced duction test (FDT) is an intraoperative maneuver that helps the ophthalmologist to determine whether strabismus is due to muscle paresis versus a restrictive force. It is discussed in detail in the strabismus section of this chapter. Of concern, Jampolsky[28] warned that succinylcholine should be avoided in patients undergoing repeat strabismus surgery because the FDT does not return to baseline for approximately 30 minutes after administration of the drug. More recent and quantitatively sophisticated studies by Dell and Williams[29] supported this caveat, although the latter investigators suggest waiting only 20 minutes after administration of succinylcholine before performing the FDT. However, in light of the black box warning issued by the Food and Drug Administration stating that use of succinylcholine in children may rarely be associated with hyperkalemia and cardiac arrest, it should be reserved for emergency intubation or when immediate airway control is needed, so the drug is typically avoided in pediatric strabismus surgery.

OCULOCARDIAC REFLEX

Bernard Aschner and Giuseppe Dagnini first described the oculocardiac reflex in 1908. This reflex is triggered by pressure on the globe and by traction on the extraocular muscles, as well as on the conjunctiva or the orbital structures. Moreover, the reflex may also be elicited by performance of a retrobulbar block,[30] by ocular trauma, and by direct pressure on tissue remaining in the orbital
4 apex after enucleation. The afferent limb is trigeminal and the efferent limb is vagal. Although the most common manifestation of the oculocardiac reflex is sinus bradycardia, a wide spectrum of cardiac dysrhythmias may occur, including junctional rhythm, ectopic atrial rhythm, atrioventricular blockade, ventricular bigeminy, multifocal premature ventricular contractions, wandering pacemaker, idioventricular rhythm, asystole, and ventricular tachycardia.[31] This reflex may appear during either local or general anesthesia; however, hypercarbia and hypoxemia are believed to augment the incidence and severity of the problem, as may inappropriate anesthetic depth.

Reports on the alleged incidence of the oculocardiac reflex are remarkable in their striking variability. Berler[30] reported an incidence of 50%, but other sources quote rates ranging from 16% to 82%. Commonly, those articles disclosing a higher incidence included children in the study population, and children tend to have more vagal tone.

A variety of maneuvers to abolish or obtund the oculocardiac reflex have been promulgated. None of these methods have been consistently effective, safe, and reliable. Inclusion of intramuscular anticholinergic drugs such as atropine or glycopyrrolate in the usual premedication regimen for oculocardiac reflex prophylaxis is ineffective.[32]

Atropine given intravenously within 30 minutes of surgery is believed to reduce incidence of the reflex. However, reports differ concerning dosage and timing. Moreover, some anesthesiologists claim that prior intravenous administration of atropine may yield more serious and refractory cardiac dysrhythmias than the reflex itself. Clearly, atropine may be considered a potential myocardial irritant. A variety of cardiac dysrhythmias[33] and several conduction abnormalities,[34] including ventricular fibrillation, ventricular tachycardia, and left bundle-branch block, have been attributed to intravenous atropine.

Although administration of retrobulbar anesthesia may provide some cardiac antidysrhythmic value by blocking the afferent limb of the reflex arc, such a regional technique is not devoid of potential complications, which include, but are not limited to, optic nerve damage, retrobulbar hemorrhage, and stimulation of the oculocardiac reflex arc by the retrobulbar block itself.

It is generally believed that the aforementioned prophylactic measures, fraught with inherent hazards, are usually not indicated in adults. If a cardiac dysrhythmia appears, initially the surgeon should be asked to cease operative manipulation. Next, the patient's anesthetic depth and ventilatory status are evaluated. Commonly, heart rate and rhythm return to baseline within 20 seconds after institution of these measures. Moreover, Moonie et al.[35] noted that, with repeated manipulation, bradycardia is less likely to recur, probably secondary to fatigue of the reflex arc at the level of the cardioinhibitory center. However, if the initial cardiac dysrhythmia is especially serious or if the reflex tenaciously recurs, atropine should be administered intravenously, but only after the surgeon stops ocular manipulation.

For pediatric strabismus surgery; however, some anesthesiologists administer intravenous atropine, 0.02 mg/kg, before commencing surgery.[36] Alternatively, glycopyrrolate,

0.01 mg/kg administered intravenously, may be associated with less tachycardia than atropine in this setting.

ANESTHETIC RAMIFICATIONS OF OPHTHALMIC DRUGS

There is considerable potential for drug interactions during
5 administration of anesthesia for ocular surgery. Topical ophthalmic drugs may produce undesirable systemic effects or may have deleterious anesthetic implications. Systemic absorption of topical ophthalmic drugs may occur from either the conjunctiva or the nasal mucosa after the drainage through the nasolacrimal duct. In addition, from spillover, some percutaneous absorption through the immature epidermis of the premature infant may transpire.[37] Occluding the nasolacrimal duct by pressing on the inner canthus of the eye for a few minutes after each instillation greatly decreases systemic absorption. Some of the potentially worrisome topical ocular drugs include anticholinesterases, cocaine, cyclopentolate, epinephrine, phenylephrine, and timolol. In addition, intraocular sulfur hexafluoride and other intraocular gases have important anesthetic ramifications. Furthermore, certain ophthalmic drugs given systemically may produce untoward sequelae germane to anesthetic management. Drugs in this category include glycerol, mannitol, and acetazolamide.

Anticholinesterase Agents

Echothiophate, also known as *phospholine iodide*, is a long-acting anticholinesterase miotic that lowers IOP by decreasing resistance to the outflow of aqueous humor. It is used to treat glaucoma that is refractory to other therapies and also to treat some children with accommodative esotropia. It is absorbed into the systemic circulation after instillation in the conjunctival sac. Any of the long-acting anticholinesterases may prolong the action of succinylcholine because, after ≥1 month of therapy, plasma pseudocholinesterase activity may be <5% of normal. It is said, moreover, that normal enzyme activity does not return until 4 to 6 weeks after discontinuation of the drug.[38] Hence, the anesthesiologist should anticipate prolonged apnea after a usual dose of succinylcholine. In addition, a delay in metabolism of ester local anesthetics should be expected.

Cocaine

Cocaine, introduced to ophthalmology in 1884 by Koller, has limited topical ocular use because it can cause corneal pits and erosion. However, as the only local anesthetic that inherently produces vasoconstriction and shrinkage of mucous membranes, cocaine has been used in nasal packs during dacryocystorhinostomy. The drug is so well absorbed from mucosal surfaces that plasma concentrations are achieved that are comparable to those after direct intravenous injection. Because cocaine interferes with catecholamine uptake, it has a sympathetic nervous system potentiating effect.

The usual maximal dose of cocaine used in clinical practice is 200 mg for a 70-kg adult, or 3 mg/kg. Although 1 g is considered to be the usual lethal dose for an adult, considerable variation occurs. Furthermore, systemic reactions may appear with as little as 20 mg.

Meyers[39] described two cases of cocaine toxicity during dacryocystorhinostomy, underscoring that cocaine is contraindicated in hypertensive patients or in patients receiving drugs such as tricyclic antidepressants or monoamine oxidase inhibitors. In addition, sympathomimetics, such as epinephrine or phenylephrine, should not be given with cocaine.

Obviously, before administering cocaine or another potent vasoconstrictor for dacryocystorhinostomy, the physician should carefully search out possible contraindications. To avoid toxic levels, doses of dilute solutions should be meticulously calculated and carefully administered. If serious cardiovascular effects occur, labetalol should be used to counteract them.[40] Beta blocking agents should not be administered in this situation owing to the potential to exacerbate hypertension as a result of unopposed α-adrenergic stimulation. Labetalol offers the advantages of combined α-blockade and β-blockade. In addition, labetalol is preferable to esmolol because of its longer duration of action. It is important to appreciate, however, that labetalol has not been shown to reverse coronary artery vasoconstriction in humans. In the setting of cocaine-associated chest pain and/or myocardial infarction, β-blockers should not be administered acutely. Rather, nitroglycerin should be given.

Cyclopentolate

Despite the popularity of cyclopentolate as a mydriatic, it is not without side effects, which include CNS toxicity. Manifestations include dysarthria, disorientation, and frank psychotic reactions. Purportedly, CNS dysfunction is more likely to follow use of the 2% solution as opposed to the 1% solution. Furthermore, cases of convulsions in children after ocular instillation of cyclopentolate have been reported. Hence, for pediatric use, 0.5% to 1% solutions are recommended. At higher concentrations, cyclopentolate also causes cycloplegia.

Epinephrine

Although topical epinephrine has proved useful in some patients with open-angle glaucoma, the 2% solution has been associated with such systemic effects as nervousness, hypertension, angina pectoris, tachycardia, and other dysrhythmias.[41] Consequently, dipivefrin hydrochloride, a prodrug of epinephrine formed by the diesterification of epinephrine and pivalic acid, is often used instead. The addition of pivaloyl groups to the epinephrine molecule enhances its lipophilic character, greatly facilitating its penetration into the anterior chamber where it reduces aqueous production and augments outflow. The prodrug delivery system is a more efficient way of delivering the therapeutic benefits of epinephrine, with less drug and with fewer side effects than conventional epinephrine therapy. Dipivefrin 0.1% is less irritating than 1% or 2% epinephrine, and, unlike cholinergic agents used to treat glaucoma, it does not produce miosis or accommodative spasm. Dipivefrin should not be used, however, in patients with narrow angles because any dilation of the pupil may trigger an attack of angle-closure glaucoma.

Phenylephrine

Pupillary dilation and capillary decongestion are reliably produced by topical phenylephrine. Although systemic effects secondary to topical application of prudent doses are rare,[42] severe hypertension, headache, tachycardia, and tremulousness have been reported.

In patients with coronary artery disease, severe myocardial ischemia, cardiac dysrhythmias, and even myocardial infarction may develop after topical 10% eye drops. Those with cerebral aneurysms may be susceptible to cerebral hemorrhage after phenylephrine in this concentration. In general, a safe systemic level follows absorption from either the conjunctiva or the nasal mucosa after drainage by the tear ducts. However, phenylephrine should not be given in the eye after surgery has begun and venous channels are patent.

Children are especially vulnerable to overdose and may respond in a dramatic and adverse fashion to phenylephrine drops. Hence, the use of only 2.5%, rather than 10%, phenylephrine is recommended in infants and the elderly, and the frequency of application should be strictly limited in these patient populations.

Timolol and Betaxolol

Timolol, a nonselective β-adrenergic blocking drug, historically has been a popular antiglaucoma drug. Because significant conjunctival absorption may occur, timolol should be administered with caution to patients with known obstructive airway disease, congestive heart failure, or greater than first-degree heart block. Life-threatening asthmatic crises have been reported after the administration of timolol drops to some patients with chronic, stable asthma.[43] The development of severe sinus bradycardia in a patient with cardiac conduction defects (left anterior hemiblock, first-degree atrioventricular block, and incomplete right bundle branch block) has been reported after timolol.[44] Moreover, timolol has been implicated in the exacerbation of myasthenia gravis[45] and in the production of postoperative apnea in neonates and young infants.[46]

In contrast to timolol, a newer antiglaucoma drug, betaxolol, a β_1-blocker, is said to be more oculospecific and have minimal systemic effects.[47] However, patients receiving an oral β-blocker and betaxolol should be observed for potential additive effect on known systemic effects of β-blockade. Caution should be exercised in patients receiving catecholamine-depleting drugs. Although betaxolol has produced only minimal effects in patients with obstructive airway disease, caution should be exercised in the treatment of patients with excessive restriction of pulmonary function. Moreover, betaxolol is contraindicated in patients with sinus bradycardia, congestive heart failure, greater than first-degree heart block, cardiogenic shock, and overt myocardial failure.

Intraocular Sulfur Hexafluoride

For a patient with a retinal detachment, intraocular sulfur hexafluoride or other gases, such as certain perfluorocarbons, may be injected into the vitreous to facilitate reattachment mechanically. The recommendations that follow do not apply to open-eye procedures, during which volume and pressure changes are readily compensated for by fluid and gas leak.

Stinson and Donlon[48] suggested terminating nitrous oxide 15 minutes before gas injection to prevent significant changes in the size of the intravitreous gas bubble. The patient is then given virtually 100% oxygen, or a combination of oxygen and air (admixed with a small percentage of volatile agent), for the balance of the operation without adversely affecting intravitreous gas dynamics. Furthermore, if a patient requires reoperation and general anesthesia after intravitreous gas injection, nitrous oxide should be avoided for 5 days subsequent to air injection and for 10 days after sulfur hexafluoride injection[49] (Table 48-3).

Perfluoropropane and octafluorocyclobutane may also be used in vitreoretinal surgery to support the retina. Like sulfur hexafluoride, these gases are relatively insoluble and require discontinuance of nitrous oxide at least 15 minutes before injection. By varying the concentration, volume, and type of gas used, bubbles can be produced that will last up to 70 days before being completely absorbed. If the patient requires reoperation, it must be remembered that perfluoropropane lingers in the eye for a protracted period.[50] A Medic-Alert bracelet might be helpful in these circumstances to warn against administration of nitrous oxide during the window of vulnerability. If nitrous oxide is administered during this interval, the bubble will rapidly expand, risking retinal and optic nerve ischemia secondary to central retinal artery occlusion.

TABLE 48-3. DIFFERENTIAL SOLUBILITIES OF GASES

	Blood: Gas Partition Coefficients
Sulfur hexafluoride	0.004
Nitrogen	0.015
Nitrous oxide	0.468

Systemic Ophthalmic Drugs

In addition to topical and intraocular therapies, various ophthalmic drugs given systemically may result in complications of concern to the anesthesiologist. These systemic drugs include glycerol, mannitol, and acetazolamide. For example, oral glycerol may be associated with nausea, vomiting, and risk of aspiration. Hyperglycemia or glycosuria, disorientation, and seizure activity may also occur after oral glycerol.

The recommended intravenous dose of mannitol is 1.5 g/kg given over a 30- to 60-minute interval. However, serious systemic problems may result from rapid infusion of large doses of mannitol. These complications include renal failure, congestive heart failure, pulmonary congestion, electrolyte imbalance, hypotension or hypertension, myocardial ischemia, and, rarely, allergic reactions. Clearly, the patient's renal and cardiovascular status must be thoroughly evaluated before mannitol therapy.

Acetazolamide, a carbonic anhydrase inhibitor with renal tubular effects, should be considered contraindicated in patients with marked hepatic or renal dysfunction or in those with low sodium levels or abnormal potassium values. As is well known, severe electrolyte imbalances can trigger serious cardiac dysrhythmias during general anesthesia. Furthermore, people with chronic lung disease may be vulnerable to the development of severe acidosis with long-term acetazolamide therapy. Topically active carbonic anhydrase inhibitors have been developed, are now commercially available, and appear to be relatively free of clinically important systemic effects.

PREOPERATIVE EVALUATION

Establishing Rapport and Assessing Medical Condition

Preoperative preparation and evaluation of the patient begin with the establishment of rapport and communication among the anesthesiologist, the surgeon, and the patient. Most patients realize that surgery and anesthesia entail inherent risks, and they appreciate a candid explanation of potential complications, balanced with information concerning probability or frequency of permanent adverse sequelae. Such an approach also fulfills the medicolegal responsibilities of the physician to obtain informed consent.

A thorough history of the patient and physical examination are the foundation of safe patient care. Questionnaires, in lieu of medical evaluation, lack sensitivity to detect pertinent medical issues.[51] A complete list of medications that the patient is currently taking, both systemic and topical, must be obtained so potential drug interactions can be anticipated and essential medication will be administered during the hospital stay. Naturally, a history of any allergies to medicines, foods, or tape should be documented. Clearly, knowledge of any personal or family history of adverse reactions to anesthesia is mandatory. The requisite laboratory data vary, depending on the medical history and physical status of the patient, as well as the nature of the surgical procedure. Indeed, the American Society of Anesthesiologists (ASA) task force on preoperative evaluation concluded that routine preoperative tests are commonly not useful in assessing and managing patients' perioperative experience. In a more recent multicenter study of cataract patients, for example, Schein et al.[52] demonstrated that "routine" testing does not improve patient safety or outcome. Some physicians and laypersons misinterpreted the results and conclusions of this investigation, believing that patients having cataract surgery need no preoperative evaluation. It is vital to note that all patients in this trial received regular medical care and were evaluated by a physician preoperatively. Patients whose medical status indicated a need for preoperative laboratory tests were excluded from the study. Clearly, testing should be based on the results of the history and physical examination. Because "routine" testing for the >1.5 million cataract operations in the United States is estimated to cost $150 million annually, the favorable economic impact of this "targeted" approach is obvious.

Many elderly adult candidates for ophthalmic surgery are on antiplatelet or anticoagulant therapy because of a history of coronary or vascular pathology. Such patients are at higher risk for perioperative hemorrhagic events, including retrobulbar hemorrhage, circumorbital hematoma, intravitreous bleeding, and hyphema. Traditionally, antiplatelet and anticoagulant medications were withheld for an "appropriate" length of time before eye surgery. However, this strategy may increase the risk of such adverse events as myocardial ischemia or infarction, cerebrovascular accident, and deep venous thrombosis. Several studies exploring this controversial issue suggest that cataract and other ophthalmic procedures can be safely performed under regional anesthesia without discontinuing anticoagulants,[53,54] especially if the prothrombin time is approximately 1.5 times control.[55] A multicenter study of almost 20,000 cataract patients older than 50 years attempted to establish the risks and benefits of continuing aspirin or warfarin therapy.[56] Despite the large population studied, the rate of complications was so low that absolute differences in risk were minimal. Patients who continued therapy did not have more ocular hemorrhage; those who discontinued treatment did not have a greater incidence of medical events. A recent meta-analysis of 11 studies revealed that continuing warfarin therapy for cataract patients was associated with an increased risk of bleeding, but almost all were self-limiting and not clinically relevant. No patient had bleeding-related compromise of visual acuity.[57] Nonetheless, it is critical to appreciate that these investigations focused specifically on cataract operations. Oculoplastic or retinal surgery may be another matter.

Another area of potential concern involves patients whose coronary artery disease is being managed with drug-eluting stents. Although bare-metal stents are susceptible to in-stent restenosis, drug-eluting stents are more vulnerable to stent thrombosis, a complication with a high mortality rate. Thus, patients with drug-eluting stents are typically on dual antiplatelet therapy with aspirin and clopidogrel for extended periods of time. Although prospective trials are clearly needed, a conclusion that is emerging is that the risk of thrombotic complications in patients with drug-eluting stents appears to heavily outweigh the risk of bleeding complications. Therefore, given current information, a convincing case can be made for continuing dual antiplatelet therapy in the perioperative period and for delaying elective surgery for at least 4 to 6 weeks after placement of a bare metal stent and for at least 12 months after drug-eluting stent placement.[57,58]

Eye surgery patients are often at the extremes of age, ranging from premature babies with retinopathy of prematurity to nonagenarians. Hence, special age-related considerations such as altered pharmacokinetics and pharmacodynamics apply. In addition, elderly patients frequently have multiple comorbidities that include thyroid dysfunction, cardiopulmonary, and renal diseases. Hypertension is encountered in the majority of geriatric patients. Those with poorly controlled blood pressure should not receive dilating eye drops, such as phenylephrine, without consulting an anesthesiologist. Systemic absorption of high concentrations (e.g., >2.5% phenylephrine) or improperly instilled mydriatics can precipitate a hypertensive crisis with potentially devastating consequences.

As our society becomes increasingly geriatric, the number of ophthalmic surgery patients presenting with implanted cardiac defibrillators (ICDs) and pacemakers grows. The theoretical possibility of eye injury from patient movement in the event of ICD discharge during surgery exists. Although there is a broad spectrum of ophthalmic surgical procedures, the majority of cases use minimal bipolar cautery. For some, such as clear-corneal cataract surgery, no cautery is used. Thus, there is low risk of electromagnetic interference precipitating device discharge. Despite millions of procedures performed each year, there have not been any case reports of ICD activation during ophthalmic surgery and none of the device manufacturers have documented such an incident.[59,60] A retrospective survey of ophthalmic-anesthesia providers found that >80% did not use a magnet to reprogram or inactivate an ICD before surgery.[60]

Perioperative movement is a possible cause of patient eye injury and potential anesthesiologist liability. An analysis of ophthalmic monitored anesthesia care (MAC) closed claims cases that resulted in blindness or poor visual outcome found that >80% were associated with inadequate anesthesia and/or patient movement either during the block or intraoperatively.[61] Cough, orthopnea, and restlessness are the most common precipitators of excessive motion. Intraoperative movement during general anesthesia may also induce dire visual consequences. Because most ophthalmic surgical procedures are elective, should an enhanced risk of perioperative movement be noted during the preoperative assessment, the prudent course may be to postpone surgery until the patient is in optimal condition to remain relatively still,[62] or to perform the procedure under general anesthesia. Deliberate patient selection is requisite in order to prescribe the optimal anesthesia care plan.

The anesthesiologist must be aware of the anesthetic implications of congenital and metabolic diseases with ocular manifestations. Diabetic patients often present with ocular complications, and the anesthesiologist must be knowledgeable about the systemic disturbances of physiology that affect these patients. Indeed, the list of congenital and metabolic diseases associated with ocular pathologic effects that have important anesthetic implications is lengthy. A partial summary includes syndromes such as Crouzon, Apert, Goldenhar (oculoauriculovertebral dysplasia), Sturge–Weber, Marfan, Lowe (oculocerebrorenal syndrome), Down (trisomy 21), Wagner–Stickler, and Riley–Day (familial dysautonomia). Other diseases in this category are homocystinuria, myotonia dystrophica, and sickle cell disease.[63]

Anesthesia Options

The requirements of ophthalmic surgery include safety, akinesia, analgesia, minimal bleeding, avoidance or obtundation of the oculocardiac reflex, prevention of intraocular hypertension, awareness of drug interactions, and a smooth emergence devoid of vomiting, coughing, or retching (Table 48-1). Moreover, the exigencies of ophthalmic anesthesia mandate that the anesthesiologist be positioned remote from the patient's airway, sometimes creating certain logistic problems.

6 A number of anesthetic options exist, including general anesthesia, retrobulbar block, peribulbar anesthesia, sub-Tenon (episcleral) block, topical anesthesia, and intracameral injection. General anesthesia is administered for most children. Some adolescent and most adult patients can be cared for with regional or topical anesthesia and MAC, with or without sedation. The choice of anesthesia technique should be individualized on the basis of the patient's needs and preferences, the nature and duration of the procedure, and the preferences and skills of the anesthesiologist and the surgeon.

Traditionally, the most commonly selected regional anesthetic technique for cataract surgery had been the retrobulbar block. Since the mid-1990s, peribulbar injection has surpassed retrobulbar block in popularity because of a relatively superior safety profile. Recently, however, topical analgesia has become more commonly used for cataract surgery in the United States (59% vs. 41% for block techniques),[64] and sub-Tenon blocks have surged in popularity in the United Kingdom and New Zealand.[65] Anesthesia for adult patients undergoing retina surgery is still accomplished primarily with peribulbar or retrobulbar block,[66] although some surgeons prefer general anesthesia for certain patients. More recently, anesthesiologists have had increasing interest in administering ocular anesthesia, and workshops in ophthalmic regional anesthesia are often conducted at major regional and national meetings. Many ophthalmologists and administrators encourage anesthesiologists to administer the blocks to facilitate operating room efficiency.

When a regional anesthetic of the orbit is administered, either by the anesthesiologist or the ophthalmologist, it is the responsibility of the anesthesiologist to monitor the patient's vital signs, electrocardiogram (ECG), and oxygen saturation. Sedation may be administered before performance of the block and/or initiation of surgery. The anesthesiologist must be vigilant for the oculocardiac reflex, signs of brainstem anesthesia, and the need for airway support or other interventions.

Side of Anesthesia and Surgery

In an attempt to ensure proper patient, side, site, and procedure selection, The Joint Commission (formerly known as the Joint Commission on Accreditation of Healthcare Organizations) held a "Wrong Site Summit" in May 2003 in which they developed a "Universal Protocol for Preventing Wrong Site, Wrong Procedure, Wrong Person Surgery." The policy is tripartite, involving preoperative verification, marking of the intended site, and a "time-out" immediately before the start of surgery.[67] Patient involvement and effective communication are key components.

Ophthalmologic surgery and regional anesthesia confer greater risk than many other surgical procedures owing to the potential for laterality errors. Patients (and medical staff) may be confused as to the side, site, or actual procedure. Sedatives or anesthetic agents may enhance the likelihood of error. Some patients, such as children and infants, may lack the competence to intervene. Similarity of names can be conducive to mistakes. Procedural factors may be contributory; a wrong side may be draped or prepared, a patient's cap may obscure a clearly marked surgical site. Human factors play a key role in the problem. Failure to cross-check consent forms, patient charts, and patients, tragically, occasionally still occurs. Our distraction-rich environment, coupled with dysfunctional oral/written communication, and lack of proper adherence to safety protocols also play a role.

Anesthesia Techniques

More than 40 years ago, it was common for ophthalmic procedures to involve large ocular incisions. General endotracheal anesthesia, with deep and sustained neuromuscular paralysis and placement of sandbags to surround the patient's head, were typical strategies to ensure perioperative immobility. In more recent years, general anesthesia typically has been reserved for children and adults who are unable to communicate, cooperate, or remain suitably stationary. Although endotracheal anesthesia is necessary for patients at risk of aspiration, the laryngeal mask airway (LMA) has been increasingly accepted as a means to secure the airway in patients with no risk factors for aspiration who are having eye surgery with general anesthesia.[68] The LMA is not only safe and effective in this setting, but it also offers the advantage of less increase in IOP on insertion and removal than is encountered with an endotracheal tube.[69] Similarly, less bucking and coughing on emergence and during the recovery phase have been noted.[70] Vigilance must be maintained, however, to detect initial misplacement or intraoperative displacement of the LMA. In addition, intraoperative laryngospasm in infants and neonates is not uncommon with an LMA.

Retrobulbar and Peribulbar Blocks

Needle-based ophthalmic regional anesthesia was first described by Knapp[71] in 1884. Then, in the early 20th century, Atkinson[72] introduced the retrobulbar block. Retrobulbar block is a practical means to achieve analgesia and profound akinesia of the globe. The peribulbar block is a more recently introduced needle-based technique that varies from the retrobulbar block in terms of the depth and angulation of needle placement within the orbit. Traditionally, the four rectus muscles, along with connective tissue septae, were believed to create a defined compartment known as the *orbital cone.* This so-called cone extends from the rectus muscle origins around the optic foramen at the apex of the orbit to the attachment of the muscles to the globe anteriorly. Retrobulbar blocks are accomplished by directing a needle toward the orbital apex with sufficient depth and angulation such that the cone is penetrated (Figs. 48-4 and 48-5).[73] Local anesthetic is then instilled in the cone, behind the eye. Cadaveric dissections, however, have shown the fallacy of the classic concept of the cone. There is no complete intermuscular septum encircling the rectus muscles, linking them together to form an impermeable compartment behind the globe akin to the brachial plexus sheath in the axilla.[74]

Ripart et al.[75] clearly demonstrated that extraconal injections of dye into cadaveric specimens diffused into the intraconal space, and solutions placed within the cone distributed to the extraconal

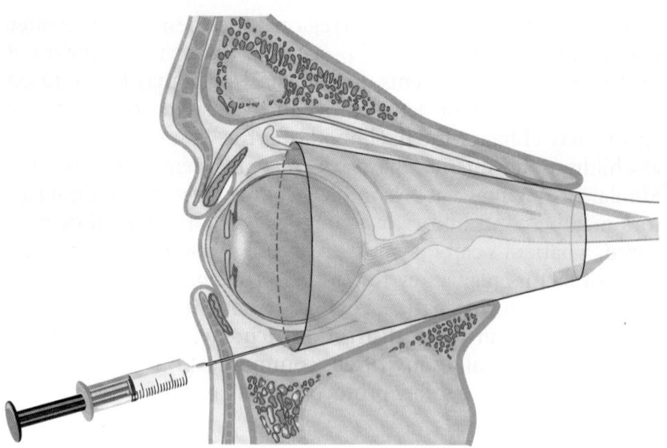

FIGURE 48-4. Retrobulbar (intraconal) block and schematic representation of the intraorbital muscle cone.

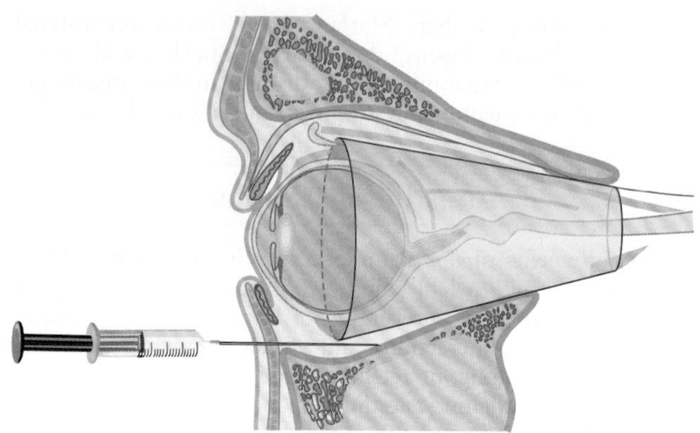

FIGURE 48-6. Peribulbar (extraconal) block and schematic representation of the intraorbital muscle cone.

space. Thus, the peribulbar block is executed by directing a needle to less depth and with minimal angulation, parallel to the globe, toward the greater wing of the sphenoid bone (Figs. 48-6 and 48-7). Local anesthetic instilled in this extraconal space will eventually penetrate toward the optic nerve and other structures, establishing conduction anesthesia. The peribulbar block is theoretically safer because the needle tip is kept at a greater distance from vital intraorbital structures and brain.

A retrobulbar, or the so-called intraconal block, positions local anesthetics deep within the orbit proximate to the nerves and muscle origins. Thus, it requires low volume, has rapid onset, and yields intense depth of anesthesia. The peribulbar, or extraconal block, placed further from the optic and other orbital nerves, requires larger volumes of local anesthetic and has longer latency of onset. The needle entry point for both blocks is at the same inferotemporal location. The junction of the lateral third and medial two-thirds of the inferior orbital rim in line with the lateral limbal margin has been the conventional access point. However, locating the needle entry point more laterally may serve to decrease the likelihood of injecting local anesthetics into the delicate inferior rectus muscle. This is important because intramuscular injection of anesthetics has been postulated as a potential cause of postoperative strabismus.[76] Medial approaches at the caruncle have also been popularized more recently.[77] Supplementation of anesthesia with an injection above the globe may not be prudent because the preponderance of vessels lie in the superior orbit. In addition, the belly of the superior oblique muscle and the trochlear muscle can be encountered superonasally.

Katsev et al.[78] demonstrated that the tips of commonly used 1.5-inch (38-mm) needles can reach critical structures in the densely packed apex of the orbit in almost 20% of retrobulbar blocks. Consequently, 1.25-inch (31-mm) needles are appropriate. Controversy exists over the advantages of sharp versus dull needles. Dull needles may require more force to penetrate the globe. However, sharp needles are less painful to insert and may cause less damage in the face of inadvertent globe puncture.[79] In the past, patients were asked to gaze superonasally while a block was conducted. Unsold et al.[80] found that this maneuver caused the optic nerve to stretch directly in the path of the incoming needle during retrobulbar injection, exposing it to risk of needle trauma. Patients should be instructed to maintain gaze in the neutral position, leaving the optic nerve lax within the orbit in the course of needle insertion.[81] Elevations in IOP after a retrobulbar block can be minimized by application of gentle noncontinuous digital pressure or use of an ocular decompression device.[82]

Akinesia of the eyelids is obtained by blocking the branches of the facial nerve supplying the orbicularis muscle. Lid akinesia is often a direct consequence of the larger volume of local anesthetic

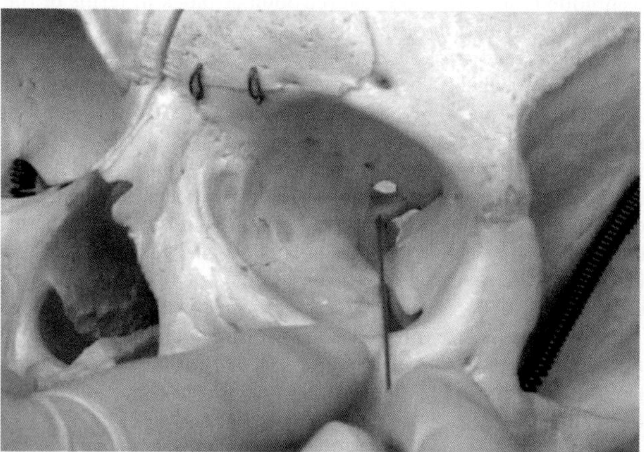

FIGURE 48-5. Needle placement for retrobulbar block.

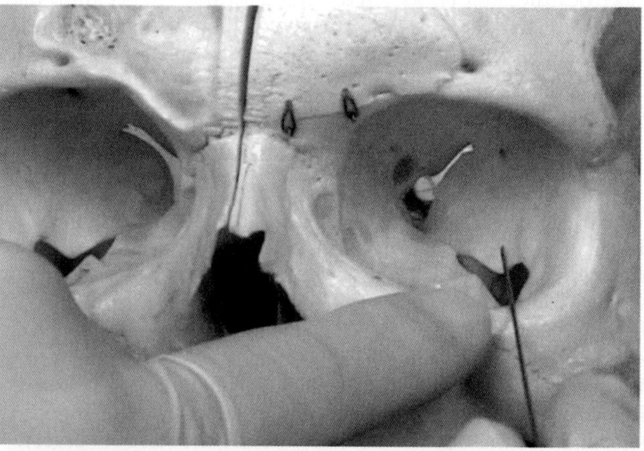

FIGURE 48-7. Needle placement for peribulbar block.

used for peribulbar blocks. Retrobulbar blocks, in contrast, often leave the orbicularis oculi fully functional. Thus, a facial nerve block is performed in conjunction with retrobulbar block to prevent squeezing of the eyelid that could result in extrusion of intraocular contents during corneal transplantation, for example. Since facial nerve block was first used for ophthalmic surgery by Van Lint in 1914, numerous methods of facial nerve blockade have been described. These techniques block the facial nerve after its exit point from the skull in the stylomastoid foramen. Moving distally to proximally to the foramen, the techniques include the Van Lint, Atkinson, O'Brien, and Nadbath–Rehman methods. Although each has advantages and disadvantages, the Nadbath–Rehman approach can potentially produce the most serious systemic consequences. With this approach, a 27-gauge, 12-mm needle is inserted between the mastoid process and the posterior border of the mandibular ramus. Because of the proximity of the jugular foramen (10 mm medial to the stylomastoid foramen) to the injection site, ipsilateral paralysis of cranial nerves IX, X, and XI can occur, producing hoarseness, dysphagia, pooling of secretions, agitation, respiratory distress, or laryngospasm. Moreover, because the Nadbath–Rehman block produces complete hemifacial akinesia that interferes with oral intake, this approach is not recommended for outpatients.

7 Complications associated with needle-based ophthalmic anesthetics may be local or systemic, and may result in blindness or even death (Table 48-4). Bleeding may be superficial or deep, arterial or venous. Superficial hemorrhage may produce an unsightly circumorbital hematoma. Retrobulbar hemorrhage, when arterially based, may produce precipitous bleeding and a palpable, dramatic increase in IOP, as well as globe proptosis and entrapment of the upper lid. With the globe's vascular supply in jeopardy, the patient's long-term ultimate visual acuity may be quickly compromised. Consultation with an ophthalmologist should be immediately sought, and fundoscopic examination, tonometric measurement of IOP, ultrasound to assess presence/location of blood, and even a lateral canthotomy may be warranted. Continuous ECG monitoring is indicated because the oculocardiac reflex may occur as blood extravasates from the muscle cone. The decision to proceed with surgery in the presence of a mild or moderate hemorrhage depends on numerous factors, including the degree of bleeding, the nature of the planned ophthalmologic surgery, and the patient's condition.

Penetration of the sclera is a distinct, although rare, possibility with needle-based anesthesia techniques. Mechanical trauma, with potential retinal detachment, and chemical injury to delicate retina tissue caused by local anesthetics can occur. Blindness or very poor vision may be the result. Globe puncture is defined as a single entry into the eye, whereas perforation is caused by two full-thickness wounds—an entry and a subsequent exit. The globe's posterior pole is the most commonly penetrated area. Risk factors for posterior pole needle injury include presence of an elongated globe, recessed orb, and/or atypical-shaped eye. The anteroposterior distance of an eye may be long because of myopia or presence of globe-enveloping intraorbital hardware such as a scleral buckle. Some patients have an abnormal outpouching of the eye, termed *staphyloma.* Most staphyloma are located at the posterior of the globe, surrounding the juncture of the eye with the optic nerve. By definition, a retrobulbar anesthetic is conducted by purposefully angling the needle steeply and deeply within the orbit behind the globe. If the globe is longer than one assumes, it is at greater risk of penetration or puncture by the retrobulbar needle. In one study, ultrasound detection determined that the tip of the needle, placed in retrobulbar fashion, can be much closer to the posterior pole of the globe than presupposed by physicians.[83] Peribulbar anesthesia entails shallower placement of the needle without directing the needle inward toward the orbital apex; thus, it is associated with a lower incidence of globe-needle injury. Be aware, however, that it is still possible to engage the needle with sclera laterally.

The risk of penetrating the sclera with a needle is also inversely proportional to the anesthesiologist's education and experience. This notion is affirmed by several reports of globe injuries rendered by inadequately educated or trained personnel in the early 1990s.[84] In a survey of 284 directors of anesthesiology and ophthalmology programs, no formal training or education in ophthalmic regional anesthesia techniques was provided to anesthesia residents in most academic programs.[85] This survey concluded that anesthesiologists who perform needle-based ophthalmic blocks should have knowledge of orbital anatomy and the ocular risk factors that were noted previously. Thus, appropriate preanesthesia history-taking includes direct interrogation concerning myopia or previous scleral buckle surgery, as both imply increased globe length. Bayes et al.[86] showed that a history of correction for myopia as a child or young adult was both highly sensitive and specific for having an elongated axial length. Physical examination of surface anatomy should note the position of the globe within the orbit and whether enophthalmos is present. A recessed eye is at greater risk of needle-tip misadventure. The most important laboratory examination is the preoperative ultrasound. For patients undergoing cataract surgery, an ultrasound is *always* performed to calculate the appropriate intraocular lens to insert intraoperatively. In addition, it reveals the length and shape of the eye. An axial length >26 mm confers greater risk of penetration or perforation. In the event that the ultrasound report is not found in the patient's chart, the anesthesiologist should inquire about the results before embarking on a needle-based block.

In the future, portable real-time ultrasonography may have a role in reducing the risk of penetrating injury (Fig. 48-8). The eye is easily accessible, its geometry and surrounding elements are relatively straightforward, and the tissue contents of the orbit lack gas-filled or osseous structures, making this an ideal area for ultrasonic imaging. Suitable transducers need to be developed and machines need to be more readily available.[87]

TABLE 48-4. COMPLICATIONS OF NEEDLE-BASED OPHTHALMIC ANESTHESIA

Stimulation of oculocardiac reflex arc
Superficial hemorrhage → circumorbital hematoma
Retrobulbar hemorrhage ± retinal perfusion compromise → loss of vision
Globe penetration ± intraocular injection → retinal detachment, loss of vision
Trauma to optic nerve or orbital cranial nerves → loss of vision
Optic nerve sheath injection → orbital epidural anesthesia
Extraocular muscle injury, leading to postoperative strabismus, diplopia
Intra-arterial injection, producing immediate convulsions
Central retinal artery occlusion
Inadvertent brainstem anesthesia → contralateral amaurosis, mydriasis, muscle paresis. Neurocardiopulmonary compromise

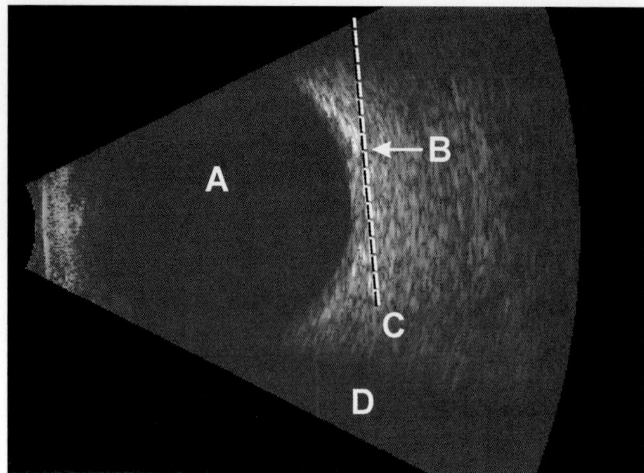

FIGURE 48-8. Ultrasound-guided block with overlay. **(A)** Globe. **(B)** Needleshaft. **(C)** Needle tip. **(D)** Optic nerve.

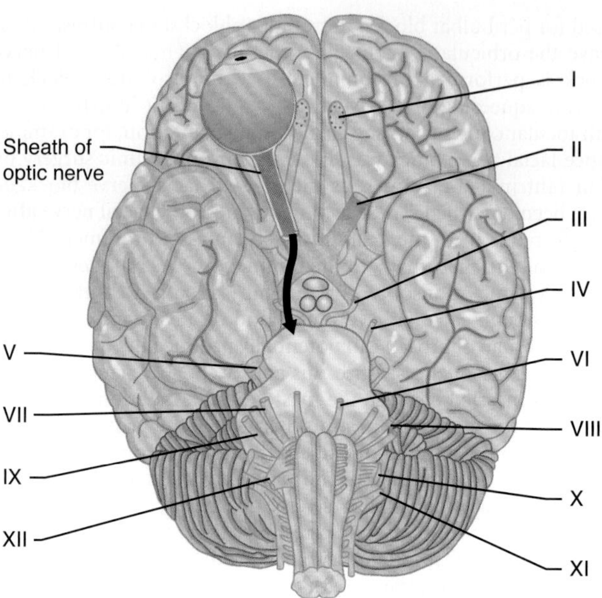

FIGURE 48-9. Base of the brain and the path that local anesthetic agents might follow if inadvertently injected into the subarachnoid space. This route includes the cranial nerves, pons, and midbrain. (Reprinted from: Javitt JC, Addiego R, Friedberg HL, et al. Brain stem anesthesia after retrobulbar block. *Ophthalmology*. 1987;94:718, with permission.)

Brainstem anesthesia and inadvertent intravascular injection of local anesthetics are two additional potentially devastating consequences of needle-based ocular anesthesia. In the course of accidental intravascular arterial injection, local anesthetics flow from the needle via a branch of the ophthalmic artery in retrograde fashion to the internal carotid artery and then to the Circle of Willis. Rapid redistribution of local anesthetic to the brain results in immediate onset of convulsions. Cardiopulmonary instability may also occur.

Although the incidence of brainstem anesthesia is rare, it is even less common with peribulbar versus retrobulbar blocks. Brainstem anesthesia is a consequence of the direct spread of local anesthetic agents to the brain along the meningeal sheath surrounding the optic nerve. In contradistinction to intra-arterial injection, symptoms are typically not immediate. There is a continuum of sequelae dependent on the concentration and volume of drug that gains access centrally, as well as the specific areas into which the anesthetic spreads (Fig. 48-9). One case report described the insidious onset of unconsciousness and apnea over 7 minutes, without concomitant seizures or cardiovascular collapse.[88] Nicoll et al.[89] reported 16 cases of apparently central spread of anesthetics in a series of 6,000 retrobulbar blocks. Eight patients developed respiratory arrest. Examination of the conscious patient's contralateral, nonblocked eye for amaurosis, mydriasis, and extraocular muscle paresis may confirm the diagnosis of brainstem anesthesia. The abducens and oculomotor nerves are more commonly affected than the superior oblique muscle's trochlear nerve. Other protean CNS signs may include violent shivering; eventual loss of consciousness; apnea; and hemiplegia, paraplegia, quadriplegia, or hyperreflexia. Blockade of cranial nerves VIII to XII results in deafness, vertigo, vagolysis, dysphagia, aphasia, and loss of neck muscle power. It is axiomatic that personnel skilled in airway maintenance and ventilatory and circulatory support should be immediately available whenever retrobulbar or other needle-based anesthetic blocks are administered.

Cannula-based Techniques

Cannula-based ophthalmic regional anesthesia was first described by Swan[90] in 1956. The sub-Tenon block was rediscovered and popularized in the 1990s as another practical means to achieve analgesia and akinesia of the globe, while offering potential advantages in certain circumstances over needle-based blocks.[91] Imaging studies have shown that local anesthetics instilled beneath Tenon capsule spread into the posterior orbit.[92] The block is accomplished by inserting a blunt cannula through a small incision in the conjunctiva and Tenon capsule, also known as the *episcleral membrane*, with subsequent infusion of local anesthetics (Fig. 48-10). Onset of analgesia is rapid. The ultimate extent of globe akinesia is proportional to the volume of local anesthetic injected. One large prospective study by Guise[65] of 6,000 such blocks found this technique to be highly effective. Advantages, particularly for very myopic patients who have elongated axial lengths, include decreased

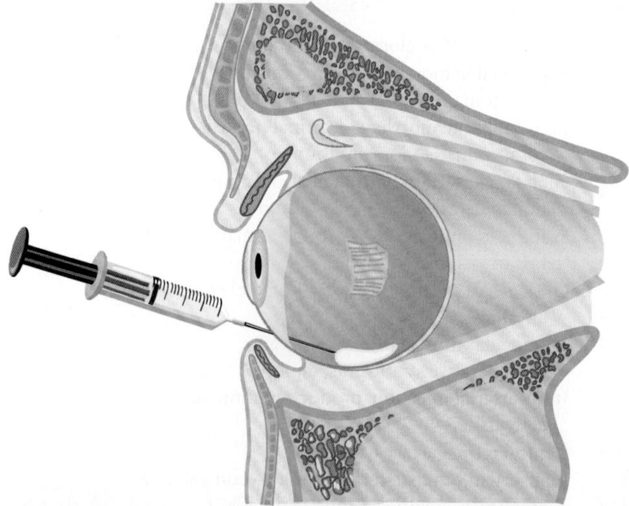

FIGURE 48-10. Sub-Tenon (episcleral) block with blunt cannula.

risk of posterior pole penetration or perforation because needles are not placed into the posterior orbit.

After application of topical anesthetic, the episcleral space can be accessed from all quadrants with blunt-tipped scissors; however, the incision is most commonly made in the inferonasal quadrant. The cannula is guided through the opening with the aid of a toothless forceps. It is common for local anesthetics to leak retrograde out of the incision site. Conjunctival bleeding, chemosis, and ballooning up of the conjunctiva are also common. Fortunately, these are cosmetic issues that rarely affect outcome. Guise[65] estimated the incidence of minor hemorrhage to be <10% and had to abandon only one case because of a large subconjunctival hemorrhage that was not sight-threatening. Thus, the sub-Tenon block may be a prudent ocular anesthesia technique for the anticoagulated patient at risk for retrobulbar hemorrhage.

Major complications of sub-Tenon anesthesia include globe perforation,[93] hemorrhage, rectus muscle trauma, postoperative strabismus, orbital cellulitis, and brainstem anesthesia.[94] More complications are reported with longer (18 to 25 mm), rigid, metallic cannulae. Shorter (12 mm), more flexible, plastic cannulae may be preferable; however, they are associated with a higher incidence of conjunctival hemorrhage and chemosis. Variations of sub-Tenon blocks include ultrashort cannulae (6 mm) and needle-based episcleral block techniques[95] A new technique of an incisionless sub-Tenon's block has been pioneered by Allman et al.[96] There has been a report of a death associated with a sub-Tenon block, potentially secondary to central spread of local anesthetic.[97] However, the definitive pathogenesis remains an enigma.[98]

Topical Analgesia

Ophthalmologists have also been returning to a technique that was popularized during the early 1900s—the use of topical anesthetic agents, particularly when the surgical incision is being made through clear cornea. Indeed, surface analgesia was the technique of choice for cataract surgery until the evolution of effective needle-based methods of regional anesthesia and improved safety of general anesthesia in the 1930s. Multiple advances in cataract surgery that have enabled faster operations, with greater control and less trauma, have allowed ophthalmologists to re-examine the use of topical anesthesia for this procedure. Phacoemulsification, with its small incisions, is clearly the procedure of choice in using topical anesthesia; however, planned extracapsular procedures can also be performed under topical anesthesia, thereby circumventing potential complications of peribulbar or retrobulbar block.

Fully anticoagulated patients may be excellent candidates for topical analgesia, as are monocular patients who are spared the trauma of prolonged local anesthetic–induced postoperative amaurosis. Potential disadvantages of topical anesthesia include eye movement during surgery, patient anxiety or discomfort, and, rarely, allergic reactions. Patient selection is critical and should be restricted to individuals who are alert and able to follow instructions, and who can control their eye movements. Patients who are demented or photophobic, or who cannot communicate, are inappropriate candidates, as are those with an inflamed eye. Similarly, patients with dense cataracts or with small pupils who may require significant iris manipulation or those who need large scleral incisions may be contraindicated for topical anesthesia.

Topical analgesia can be achieved with local anesthetic drops or gels. Anesthetic gels produce greater levels of drug in the anterior chamber than equal doses of drops and may afford superior surface analgesia.[99] Intracameral injection of 0.1 to 0.2 mL of 1% preservative-free lidocaine into the anterior chamber supplements the analgesic effects but may be deleterious to corneal endothelium.[100] Concerns about increased potential for postoperative endophthalmitis with gel-based topical analgesia exist because gels might theoretically form a barrier to bactericidal agents. Therefore, if administered, gels should be applied after antiseptic solutions, taking care to apply anesthetic drops before the use of caustic bactericidal preps.

Choice of Local Anesthetics, Block Adjuvants, and Adjuncts

Anesthetics for ocular surgery are selected on the basis of onset and duration needed. Fast-onset, brief-duration local anesthetics are optimal for procedures such as cataract surgery or pterygium excision. Longer-acting agents are indicated for lengthier operations such as vitreoretinal surgery. Bupivacaine 0.75% concentration has been shown to have potential to cause extraocular muscle toxicity. Lower concentrations do not have such a propensity.[101] A tradition of mixing different local anesthetics to produce a block with shorter latency of onset, yet longer duration of effect, has been a paradigm of ophthalmic anesthesia. Vasoconstrictors may improve the quality of the block by delaying washout of drug from the orbit. There is concern, however, that epinephrine, the most common vasoconstrictor additive, may compromise retinal perfusion[102]; it is best avoided in patients with glaucomatous optic nerve damage. The addition of clonidine 0.5 μg/kg to the local anesthetics in a retrobulbar block for vitreoretinal surgery prolongs the duration of analgesia and reduces the frequency of postoperative pain severe enough to require pharmacologic intervention.[103]

Sodium bicarbonate, morphine sulfate, and even vecuronium have been used as local anesthetic adjuvants in ophthalmic surgery. Without question, however, hyaluronidase has been the most popular ancillary agent used to modify ocular local anesthetic actions since it was introduced by Atkinson in 1949. It acts by hydrolyzing hyaluronic acid, a natural substance that binds cells together, keeping them cohesive. Thus, hyaluronidase increases tissue permeability, serves to promote dispersion of local anesthetics through tissues within the orbit, reduces the increase in orbital pressure associated with the volume of injected anesthetics, and enhances the quality of orbital blockade. Furthermore, hyaluronidase may reduce the risk of local anesthetic–induced extraocular muscle injury because clustered increases of postoperative diplopia were reported after national shortages of the drug in 1998 and 2000.[104] Studies since that time have supported these findings.[105] However, it is possible that many who were administering orbital blocks may have modified their technique in response to the absence of hyaluronidase by placing needles deeper, using more injections, or depositing larger volumes of local anesthetics.

Intravenous osmotic agents, such as mannitol and glycerin, as well as carbonic anhydrase inhibitors can be given to reduce vitreous volume and decrease IOP after they are artificially increased by local anesthetics. Digital pressure to soften the globe was described more than 50 years ago.[106] Mechanical devices that apply pressure to the globe were developed shortly thereafter; and a number of these devices are commercially available. Essentially, they are all variations on a ball, balloon, or bag theme. The Super Pinky ball and the Honan IOP Reducer (The Lebanon Corporation, Lebanon, Indiana) are examples.[82] Immediately after administration of regional orbital anesthesia, the compression device may be positioned on the eye for 5 to 20 minutes. Reduction of IOP to below baseline levels is not uncommon. However, excessive pressure on the globe by these devices may impede blood flow, causing ischemic optic neuropathy or central retinal artery occlusion, possibly leading to blindness.[107] The Honan device addresses this potentially catastrophic complication with a pneumatic bellows that maintains even compression of the globe coupled to a manometric gauge that indicates a numeric value of applied pressure. A safety valve limits the amount of inflation of the bellows. With the increasing popularity of smaller incisions, lower-profile prosthetic lenses, and topical analgesia for cataract surgery, there is less need for IOP-reducing devices.

General Principles of Monitored Anesthesia Care

Many advocate the intravenous administration of an appropriate agent immediately prior to ocular regional anesthesia to provide comfort and amnesia. Polypharmacy and deep sedation in the form of high doses of opioids, benzodiazepines, and hypnotics may be unwise because of the pharmacologic vagaries in the geriatric population and the attendant risks of respiratory depression, airway obstruction, hypotension, CNS aberrations, and prolonged recovery time. This undesirable technique has all the disadvantages of a general anesthetic in the absence of an endotracheal tube or LMA without the advantage of controllability that general anesthesia offers. After the block has been performed, the patient should be relaxed but sufficiently responsive to avoid head movement associated with snoring or sudden abrupt movement on awakening. Perioperative patient movement is a leading cause of patient eye injury and anesthesiologist liability.[61] Clearly, patients under conscious sedation must be capable of remaining relatively still, responding rationally to commands, and maintaining airway patency. Undersedation should likewise be avoided because tachycardia and hypertension may have deleterious effects, especially in patients with coronary artery disease. Moreover, patients with orthopedic deformities or arthritis must be meticulously positioned and given comfortable padding on the operating table. Adequate ventilation about the face is essential to avoid carbon dioxide accumulation, particularly as supplemental oxygen can delay signs of desaturation.[108] Use of exogenous oxygen can also contribute to surgical fire, particularly during oculoplastic surgery performed with electrocautery. Consider air or mixed air/oxygen instead of oxygen for these procedures. Tightly occluded drapes may also promote accumulation of oxygen. In fact, burn injuries during facial surgery with supplemental oxygen account for nearly 20% of MAC closed claims cases.[61] Patients must be comfortably warm as the hazards of shivering in patients having delicate eye surgery are well known. Further, shivering causes a risk for patients with coronary artery disease. Continuous ECG monitoring is vital, lest performance of the retrobulbar block, pressure on the orbit, or tugging on the extraocular muscles stimulates the oculocardiac reflex arc and produces dangerous cardiac dysrhythmias. Likewise, pulse oximetry is essential. The adequacy of the sedated patient's ventilation should be assessed by clinical signs as well as exhaled carbon dioxide. Unequivocally, MAC should reflect "maximum anesthesia caution, not minimal anesthesiology care."[109]

Studies have confirmed that most cataract operations performed in the United States are conducted with the patient under some form of local anesthesia (either retrobulbar, peribulbar, sub-Tenon, or topical analgesia), with monitoring equipment used in 97% of cases and an anesthesiologist present in 78% of cases.[110] An international survey of ophthalmologists reported routine use of anesthesia-trained personnel in 96% and 97% of cases in the United States and Australia, respectively.[111] On the other side of the spectrum, ophthalmologists from Malaysia and Thailand had anesthesia monitoring 31% and 18% of the time, respectively. Indeed, many anesthesiologists fear that the Centers for Medicare and Medicaid Services will decide not to reimburse for MAC for "routine" cataract cases.

An important study by Rosenfeld et al.[112] assessed the need for MAC in cataract surgery. These investigators prospectively studied the incidence and nature of interventions required by anesthesia personnel in 1,006 consecutive cataract operations (both phacoemulsification and extracapsular techniques were included) performed under peribulbar block. They also analyzed germane information, including patient demographic data, medical history, and preoperative laboratory tests, for ability to predict those patients at greatest risk for intervention. They found that 37% of patients required some type of intervention and that, in general, the majority of those interventions could not have been predicted before surgery. Patients younger than 60 years required intervention in >60% of cases. The interventions ranged from minor forms, such as verbal reassurance and hand holding, to administering such intravenous medications as supplemental sedation or antihypertensive, pressor, or antiarrhythmic agents, or to providing respiratory assistance. Although hypertension, lung disease, renal disease, and a diagnosis of cancer were related to interventions, these four conditions combined accounted for only a small portion of the needed interventions. Moreover, although many of the interventions were relatively minor, several were more serious, and 30% of the interventions were considered (by the involved anesthesia personnel) to be critical to the success of the operation. The investigators concluded that MAC by qualified anesthesia personnel is reasonable and justified and contributes to the quality of patient care when cataract surgery is performed with local anesthesia. Fung et al.[113] examined satisfaction scores for community-based cataract surgery via topical anesthesia and discovered that patients' value and regard for the anesthesiologist's role actually increased from the preoperative to the postoperative interview. In view of the fact that topical anesthesia produces analgesia that is less profound and provides operating conditions that are less ideal than regional or general anesthesia, it seems likely that anesthesia care is equally appropriate to provide comfort, support, and indicated drugs for these patients as well. For both ethical and surgical reasons, the ophthalmologist's attention must not be distracted from the microsurgical field.

ANESTHETIC MANAGEMENT IN SPECIFIC SITUATIONS

General Concepts and Objectives

Most patients undergoing eye surgery are either younger than 10 years or older than 55 years. In children, operations on the ocular adnexa, including lid surgery, repair of lacrimal apparatus, and adjustment of extraocular muscles, are common. However, surgery on the anterior segment, such as cataract removal, glaucoma procedures, and trauma repair, is not limited to the adult population. Nor are posterior segment operations such as scleral buckling and vitrectomy the exclusive domain of geriatrics.

Most ocular procedures demand profound analgesia but minimal skeletal muscle relaxation. The airway must be protected from obstruction, and the anesthesiologist must work at a distance—along with anesthetic apparatus—from the surgical field. The anesthesiologist and surgeon should agree on the selection of local or general anesthesia. Additional preparation must include identification of underlying diseases, such as asthma, diabetes mellitus, or nephropathy. The patient should also be prepared emotionally for the recovery period, when he or she may awaken with one or both eyes closed by bandages. This preparation is important not only to spare the patient fear and anxiety but to prevent much of the thrashing about that fright might produce, to the detriment of the eye.

Preoperative sedation is chosen carefully and is usually administered intravenously immediately before surgery because most ophthalmic procedures are performed on an ambulatory basis. Except for strabismus correction, retinal detachment surgery, and cryosurgery, ophthalmic procedures are usually associated with little pain. Thus, the routine use of opioid premedication, replete with emetic potential, is ill-advised. Rather, premedication should be prescribed with a view toward amnesia, sedation, and antiemesis.

Analgesia and akinesia are then secured through either local or general anesthesia, with careful attention paid to proper control of IOP and to the possible appearance of the oculocardiac reflex. The anesthesiologist strives to provide a smooth intraoperative course and to prevent coughing, retching, and vomiting, lest harmful increases in IOP transpire that could hinder successful surgery. If general anesthesia is elected, extubation of the trachea should be accomplished before there is a tendency to cough. The administration of intravenous lidocaine, 1.5 to 2 mg/kg, before extubation of the trachea is helpful in attenuating coughing. If the patient is deemed to be at extremely high risk for postoperative nausea and vomiting, prophylactic multimodal antiemetic therapy may be selected in conjunction with total intravenous anesthesia with propofol.

"Open-Eye, Full-Stomach" Encounters

The anesthesiologist involved in caring for a patient with a penetrating eye injury and a full stomach confronts special challenges. He or she must weigh the risk of aspiration against the risk of blindness in the injured eye that could result from elevated IOP and extrusion of ocular contents.

As in all cases of trauma, attention should be given to the exclusion of other injuries, such as skull and orbital fractures, intracranial trauma associated with subdural hematoma formation, and the possibility of thoracic or abdominal bleeding.

Although regional anesthesia is often a valuable alternative for the management of trauma patients who have recently eaten, this option had traditionally been considered contraindicated in patients with penetrating eye injuries because of the potential to extrude intraocular contents via pressure generated by injection of local anesthetics. Nonetheless, some anecdotal case reports of successful use of ophthalmic blocks in this setting have been published.[114] Recognizing that there are several distinct permutations of eye injuries, Scott et al.[115] developed techniques to safely block patients with *select* open-globe injuries. In a 4-year period, 220 disrupted eyes were repaired via regional anesthesia at Bascom Palmer Eye Institute. A significant number of injuries were caused by intraocular foreign bodies and dehiscence of cataract or corneal transplant incisions. Blocked eyes tended to have more anterior, smaller wounds than those repaired via general anesthesia. There was no outcome difference—that is, change of visual acuity from initial evaluation until final examination—between the eyes repaired via regional versus general anesthesia. Moreover, combined topical anesthesia and sedation for *selected* patients with open-globe injuries has also been reported.[116]

Nonetheless, it is not always possible to determine the extent of disruption preoperatively, and general anesthesia is typically considered prudent in this setting. Preoperative prophylaxis against aspiration may involve administering H_2 receptor antagonists to elevate gastric fluid pH and to reduce gastric acid production. Metoclopramide may be given to induce peristalsis and enhance gastric emptying.

Traditionally, an induction agent and nondepolarizing neuromuscular blocking drug technique was described as the method of choice for the emergency repair of an open eye injury; the nondepolarizing drug pancuronium in a dose of 0.15 mg/kg has been shown to lower IOP. However, this method has its disadvantages, including risk of aspiration and death during the relatively lengthy period—ranging from 75 to 150 seconds—during which the airway is unprotected. Performance of the Sellick maneuver during this interval may afford some protection. Furthermore, a premature attempt at intubation of the trachea produces coughing, straining, and a dramatic rise in IOP, emphasizing the need to confirm the onset of drug effect with a peripheral nerve stimulator while appreciating, nonetheless, that muscle groups vary in their response to muscle relaxants. Moreover, the cardiovascular side effects of tachycardia and hypertension may prove worrisome in patients with coronary artery disease. Also, the long duration of action of intubating doses of pancuronium may mandate postoperative mechanical ventilation of the lungs. Intermediate-acting nondepolarizing drugs such as vecuronium have briefer durations of action, and less dramatic, if any, circulatory effects, but nevertheless have an onset of action similar to that of pancuronium.

Several studies have explored the use of extremely large doses of nondepolarizing muscle relaxants to accelerate the onset of adequate relaxation for endotracheal intubation. Using vecuronium doses of 0.2 and 0.4 mg/kg, Casson and Jones[117] found mean onset times of 95 and 87 seconds, respectively. Ginsberg et al.[118] found that by increasing the vecuronium dose from 100 to 400 μg/kg the corresponding times to endotracheal intubation decreased from 183 to 96 seconds.

Succinylcholine offers the distinct advantages of swift onset, superb intubating conditions, and brief duration of action. If administered after careful pretreatment with a nondepolarizing drug and an induction dose of thiopental (4 to 6 mg/kg), succinylcholine produces only small increases in IOP.[119] Although the advisability of this technique has been debated vociferously, there are no published reports of loss of intraocular contents from a pretreatment barbiturate–succinylcholine sequence when used in this setting.[120] Moreover, in 1993, McGoldrick[121] pointed out that the 1957 watershed article of Lincoff et al.[18] states: "Various communications have been received from ophthalmologists who have used succinylcholine in surgery. This includes several reports of cases in which succinylcholine was given to forestall impending vitreous prolapse only to have a prompt expulsion of vitreous occur." Under such desperate circumstances, it is extremely difficult to attribute the expulsion of vitreous directly to succinylcholine.[121]

Rocuronium, with its purportedly rapid onset, may prove to be a useful drug in these circumstances, provided adequate doses (1.2 mg/kg intravenously) are administered. Unfortunately, it has an intermediate duration of action that could be disadvantageous, compared with succinylcholine, in a patient with an unrecognized difficult airway. Sugammadex may provide a solution. It is an oligosaccharide chelating agent that rapidly reverses the effects of aminosteroid neuromuscular blocking agents, particularly rocuronium. Recovery of >90% train-of-four responses may be accomplished in <120 seconds.[122] Thus, in the future, a new paradigm for the "open-globe, full-stomach" scenario may entail rapid-sequence induction with high-dose rocuronium to achieve swift onset of superb intubating conditions, followed by quick termination of neuromuscular blocking effect by sugammadex if the situation is encountered in which one cannot intubate or cannot ventilate.[123] As of this writing, however, sugammadex has not been approved for use in the United States.

It was hoped that rapacuronium, with its swift onset, would emerge as a viable alternative to succinylcholine. However, rapacuronium is no longer available in the United States because of its role in triggering intractable bronchospasm in some patients. New ultrashort-acting nondepolarizing alternatives to succinylcholine are currently undergoing clinical investigation in human volunteers. One approach to the management of open-eye, full-stomach situations is summarized by Baumgarten and Reynolds,[124] who wrote in 1985:

> It may be possible to devise a combination of intravenous anesthetics and nondepolarizing relaxants that totally prevents coughing after rapid intubation. Until this combination is devised and confirmed in a large, controlled double-blind series, clinicians should not apply the priming principle to the open eye-full stomach patient. Use of a blockade monitor to predict intubating conditions may be unreliable, since muscle groups vary in their response to nondepolarizing relaxants. At this time, succinylcholine with precurarization probably remains the most tenable compromise in the open eye-full stomach challenge.

Patients with open-globe injuries requiring general anesthesia whose airway assessment is reassuring may occasionally have a contraindication to succinylcholine, such as malignant hyperthermia susceptibility, Duchenne muscular dystrophy, or certain types of myotonia. These patients may be managed using appropriately large doses of a nondepolarizing neuromuscular blocker to enable accelerated onset of paralysis and satisfactory intubating conditions. Maintenance could then be accomplished with a total intravenous anesthetic technique.

When confronted with a patient whose airway anatomy or anesthetic history suggests potential difficulties, the anesthesiologist should consult with the ophthalmologist concerning the probability of saving the injured eye. In selected instances, general anesthesia may be avoided by using topical or regional anesthesia. If this approach is not feasible, awake fiberoptic laryngoscopy and intubation may be the safest option, realizing that substantial increases in IOP may occur if the patient gags or coughs. These risks, which can be minimized by thorough topical anesthesia of the airway, assume relative unimportance when balanced against the risk of being unable to ventilate and oxygenate the patient.

Strabismus Surgery

Approximately 3% of the population has malalignment of the visual axes, which may be accompanied by diplopia, amblyopia, and loss of stereopsis (Table 48-5). Indeed, strabismus surgery is the most common pediatric ocular operation performed in the United States, and it entails a variety of techniques to weaken an extraocular muscle by moving its insertion on the globe (recession) or to strengthen an extraocular muscle by eliminating a short strip of the tendon or muscle (resection).

Infantile strabismus occurs within the first 6 months of life and is often observed in the neonatal period. Although most patients with strabismus are healthy, normal children, the incidence of strabismus is increased in those with CNS dysfunction such as cerebral palsy and meningomyelocele with hydrocephalus. Moreover, strabismus may be acquired secondary to oculomotor nerve trauma or sensory abnormalities such as cataracts or refractive aberrations.

In addition to the well-known propensity of strabismus surgery to trigger the oculocardiac reflex (previously discussed), there is also an increased incidence of malignant hyperthermia in patients with conditions such as strabismus or ptosis. This observation is consistent with the impression that people susceptible to malignant hyperthermia often have localized areas of skeletal muscle weakness or other musculoskeletal abnormalities. Other aspects of strabismus surgery of interest to anesthesiologists include succinylcholine-induced interference with the FDT and an increased incidence of postoperative nausea and vomiting.

In formulating a surgical treatment plan for incomitant strabismus, ophthalmologists often find the FDT to be exquisitely helpful in differentiating between a paretic muscle and a restrictive force preventing ocular motion. To perform the FDT, the surgeon grasps the sclera of the anesthetized eye with a forceps near the corneal limbus and moves the eye into each field of gaze, concomitantly assessing tissue and elastic properties. This simple test provides valuable clues to the presence and site of mechanical restrictions of the extraocular muscles and is most valuable in patients who have previously undergone strabismus surgery, in those who may have paralysis of one of the extraocular muscles, and in those who have sustained orbital trauma.

France et al.[125] quantitated the magnitude and duration of change of the FDT after succinylcholine administration. They demonstrated that quantification of the force necessary to rotate the globe remained notably increased over control for 15 minutes, even though the rise in IOP and the skeletal muscle paralysis lasted <5 minutes. Because succinylcholine interferes with FDT, its use is contraindicated <20 minutes before testing. Hence, France et al.[125] suggested performing the FDT on the anesthetized patient either while mask inhalation anesthesia is being administered, before intubation of the trachea; after intubation, facilitated by nondepolarizing neuromuscular blocking drugs; or after intubation under moderately deep inhalation anesthesia, unaided by succinylcholine. (As previously discussed, succinylcholine is widely avoided in elective pediatric surgical cases as a result of the FDA warning of rare reports of acute rhabdomyolysis, subsequent hyperkalemia, dysrhythmia, and potential cardiac arrest.)

Eye movement under general anesthesia is well documented, and in nonaligned eyes this tendency is augmented such that divergent squints diverge more and convergent squints converge less. Another recent report discloses that surgeons at a regional eye teaching hospital in the United Kingdom who specialize in strabismus surgery are increasingly requesting that, if the FDT is being used, nondepolarizing neuromuscular blockade be incorporated into the anesthetic management so muscle tone is minimal or absent during testing.[29]

Once intubation of the trachea has been accomplished, anesthesia is commonly maintained with desflurane, sevoflurane or isoflurane, nitrous oxide, and oxygen. The patient is carefully monitored with a precordial stethoscope, ECG, blood pressure device, pulse oximeter, end-tidal carbon dioxide measurement, and temperature probe. If bradycardia occurs, the surgeon is asked to discontinue ocular manipulation, and the patient's ventilatory status and anesthetic depth are quickly assessed. If additional intravenous atropine is indicated, it is not given while the oculocardiac reflex is active in case even more dangerous cardiac dysrhythmias are triggered.

The LMA is gaining popularity for strabismus surgery in the United States, provided the patient is not at risk for aspiration. The laryngeal mask can be inserted without the use of muscle relaxants, causes less hemodynamic perturbation, and is associated with less straining and coughing on removal.

Vomiting after eye muscle surgery is common, giving credibility to the existence of the oculogastric reflex. The administration of droperidol, 0.075 mg/kg at induction of anesthesia before manipulation of the eye, has been shown to reduce the incidence of vomiting after strabismus surgery to a clinically acceptable level of approximately 10% without prolonging recovery time.[126] Moreover, a lower dose of droperidol, 0.02 mg/kg intravenously, administered immediately after anesthetic induction in patients with strabismus may decrease both the incidence and severity of nausea and vomiting.[127] Many physicians have stopped using droperidol owing to the FDA "black box" warning. However, the droperidol doses used for postoperative nausea and vomiting are extremely low and unlikely to be associated with notable cardiovascular events. Indeed, considerable concern has been expressed about the quality and quantity of evidence and the validity of the FDA conclusion.[128]

Prophylactic intravenous administration of a serotonin receptor antagonist such as ondansetron, dolasetron, or granisetron also appears to be efficacious. Combination therapy consisting of one or two antiemetics, each with a different mechanism of action, plus a glucocorticoid such as dexamethasone, has been shown to be efficacious and safe in patients at high risk for postoperative nausea and vomiting.[128] Moreover, a total intravenous technique with propofol has also been associated with a low incidence of emesis after strabismus surgery.[129] In addition, avoiding narcotics may be helpful, although a recent paper found no difference in postoperative nausea or vomiting in children who received a remifentanil–sevoflurane mixture versus sevoflurane sans the narcotic.[130] One study demonstrates that the nonopioid analgesic ketorolac, in a dose of 0.75 mg/kg intravenously, provides analgesia comparable with that of morphine in pediatric patients with strabismus, but with a much lower incidence of nausea and vomiting in the first 24 hours.[131]

Intraocular Surgery

Advances in both anesthesia and in technology now permit a level of controlled intraocular manipulation that was not possible one-quarter century ago (Table 48-5).

Proper control of IOP is crucial for such intraocular procedures as glaucoma drainage surgery, open sky vitrectomy, penetrating keratoplasty (corneal transplantation), and traditional intracapsular cataract extraction. Before scleral incision (when IOP becomes equal to atmospheric pressure), a low-normal IOP is essential because abrupt decompression of a hypertensive eye could result in iris or lens prolapse, vitreous loss, or expulsive choroidal hemorrhage. Available data have not demonstrated a major difference in the rate of complications such as vitreous loss and iris prolapse between local anesthesia and general anesthesia.

Many anesthetic techniques may be safely used for elective intraocular surgery. If general anesthesia is selected, virtually any of the inhalation drugs may be given after intravenous induction of anesthesia with a barbiturate or propofol, neuromuscular blocking drug, and topical laryngeal lidocaine. Because complete akinesia is essential for delicate intraocular surgery, nondepolarizing drugs are administered, followed by neuromuscular function monitoring to ensure a 90% to 95% twitch suppression level during surgery. Because proper control of IOP is critical, controlled ventilation of the lungs is used, along with end-tidal carbon dioxide monitoring to ensure avoidance of hypercarbia.

Maximal pupillary dilation is important for many types of intraocular surgery and can be induced by continuous infusion of epinephrine 1:200,000 in a balanced salt solution, delivered through a small-gauge needle placed in the anterior chamber. Almost simultaneous with its administration, the drug is removed by aspirating it from the anterior chamber. The iris usually dilates immediately on contact with the epinephrine infusion, and drug uptake is presumably limited by the associated intense vasoconstriction of the iris and ciliary body. However, epinephrine may also be potentially absorbed by drainage through the canal of Schlemm into the venous system or by spillover of the infusion into the conjunctival vessels or drainage to the nasal mucosa.

At the completion of surgery, any residual neuromuscular blockade is reversed. On resumption of spontaneous ventilation, the patient's trachea is extubated (often in the lateral position) with the patient still deeply anesthetized and after intravenous administration of lidocaine to prevent coughing. Atropine and neostigmine may be safely used to reverse neuromuscular blockade, even in patients with glaucoma because this combination of drugs, in conventional doses, has minimal effects on pupil size and IOP.

Retinal Detachment Surgery

Surgery to repair retinal detachments involves procedures affecting intraocular volume, frequently using a synthetic silicone band or sponge to produce a localized or encircling scleral indentation (Table 48-5). Furthermore, internal tamponade of the retinal break may be accomplished by injecting an expandable gas such as sulfur hexafluoride into the vitreous. Because of blood gas partition coefficient differences, the administration of nitrous oxide may enhance the internal tamponade effect of sulfur hexafluoride intraoperatively, only to be followed by a dramatic drop in IOP and volume on discontinuation of nitrous oxide. The injected sulfur hexafluoride bubble, in the presence of concomitant administration of nitrous oxide, can cause a rapid and dramatic rise in IOP, reaching a peak within 20 minutes[48,49] (see "Intraocular Sulfur Hexafluoride"). Because the resultant rise in IOP may compromise retinal circulation, Stinson and Donlon[48] recommended cessation of nitrous oxide administration 15 minutes before gas injection to prevent significant changes in the volume of the intravitreous gas bubble. Furthermore, Wolf et al.[49] stated that if a patient requires anesthesia after intravitreous gas injection, nitrous oxide should be omitted for 5 days after an air injection and for 10 days after sulfur hexafluoride injection. In cases in which perfluoropropane has been injected, the nitrous oxide proscription should be in effect for longer than 70 days. Alternatively, silicone oil, a vitreous substitute, may be injected to achieve internal tamponade of a retinal break. Moreover, it should be pointed out that cervicofacial subcutaneous emphysema and

TABLE 48-5. CONCERNS WITH VARIOUS OCULAR PROCEDURES

Procedure	Concerns
Strabismus repair	Forced duction testing Oculocardiac reflex Oculogastric reflex Malignant hyperthermia
Intraocular surgery	Proper control of IOP Akinesia Drug interactions Associated systemic disease
Retinal detachment surgery	Oculocardiac reflex Proper control of IOP Nitrous oxide interaction with air, sulfur hexafluoride, or perfluorocarbons

IOP, intraocular pressure.

ANESTHESIA FOR SURGICAL SUBSPECIALTIES

pneumomediastinum have been reported after the injection of pressurized gas during retinal detachment surgery.[132] Although the precise mechanism of injury remains speculative, it was hypothesized that the pressure indicator for the perfluorocarbon gas injection may have malfunctioned.

It should be emphasized that resorption time is not always uniform or predictable. For example, reports have appeared where a 19-year-old woman with type 1 diabetes injected with sulfur hexafluoride 25 days before subsequent surgery and a 37-year-old man with insulin-dependent diabetes injected with perfluoropropane gas 41 days before subsequent surgery were given nitrous oxide and developed central retinal artery occlusion and permanent blindness in the affected eye.[133] Because the pressure in the retinal arterial vessels is lower in patients with diabetes, the elderly, and those with atherosclerosis, these patients are likely at higher risk for this devastating complication.[134,135] The international distributors of medical-grade gases, in cooperation with the American distributors and the FDA, have begun to provide hospital band-type warning bracelets for patients who receive intraocular gas injection to alert health professionals to the presence of the bubble and the need to avoid nitrous oxide administration.

Retinal detachment operations are basically extraocular but may briefly become intraocular if the surgeon elects to perforate and drain subretinal fluid. Furthermore, rotation of the globe with traction on the extraocular muscles may elicit the oculocardiac reflex, so the anesthesiologist must be vigilant about potential cardiac dysrhythmias. In addition, because it is desirable to have a soft eye while the sclera is being buckled, intravenous administration of acetazolamide or mannitol is common during retinal surgery to lower IOP.

These patients are usually managed in the same manner as those having intraocular surgery, except that maintenance of intraoperative skeletal muscle paralysis is not as critical as during intraocular surgery. Hence, inhalational anesthetics need not be accompanied during surgery by nondepolarizing neuromuscular blocking drugs.

Principles of Laser Therapy

In 1957, in a laboratory at Columbia University, the first design for the laser was born. The invention has revolutionized industry, refined scientific measurements, provided therapy for countless medical and surgical conditions, and inspired 13 Nobel Prizes. The principle is based on the consequences of a photon meeting an electron in an excited state. Sometimes the collision produces a second photon that has the same color and direction as the original. When repeated on a large scale, this process creates an orderly beam of light. The term *laser* was coined to describe this photon-cloning effect, and the acronym signifies *l*ight *a*mplified by *s*timulated *e*mission of *r*adiation.

Laser radiation has many notable properties. Because it is monochromatic, all the photons have the same wavelength, energy, and frequency. It is coherent, with all the photons in phase. Moreover, laser radiation is collimated, so its beam is nondivergent. These properties allow the precision that is associated with laser surgery. The amount of radiant energy (joules) absorbed by tissues is the product of power (watts) multiplied by duration (seconds). Surgical lasers typically are used in either a continuous or a pulsed mode.

The effect that a particular laser beam exerts on tissue depends predominantly on its wavelength and power density. A specific laser's wavelength depends on its lasing medium, which also gives the laser its name. In general, the longer the wavelength, the more strongly absorbed the light. The converse is true; the shorter the wavelength, the more scattered the light. The power of the laser beam is converted to heat at a shallow depth. Coherent light of high-power density excels in cutting or vaporizing tissue. Lower-power densities are used to photocoagulate tissue and promote hemostasis. Of course, another variable that can be manipulated to produce a given effect is the duration of contact between laser beam and tissue. Additional uses of lasers of low-power density include the photoactivation of systemically administered dyes to precisely treat localized disease sites, such as with age-related macular degeneration.

Lasers are used to treat a wide spectrum of eye conditions, including three of the most common causes of visual loss in the United States: Diabetic retinopathy, glaucoma, and age-related macular degeneration. Recently, the use of lasers expanded to include the rapidly growing field of refractive surgery. Argon, krypton, diode, dye-tuned, neodymium: Yttrium-aluminum-garnet (Nd:YAG), and excimer lasers are among those commonly used for ophthalmic surgery. Owing to concern that indirect exposure to laser energy could cause ocular damage to operating room personnel, staff working with or near the laser wear protective goggles designed to block the particular wavelength of light emitted by the laser in use.

The argon laser emits blue-green light with a wavelength of approximately 488 to 515 nm (approximately 0.5 μm). This laser has low maximum power and is easily transmitted by fiberoptic bundles. Light from the argon laser is strongly absorbed by hemoglobin, melanin, and other pigments, rendering it useful in retinal detachment surgery to photocoagulate or cauterize pigment epithelium and the adjacent neurosensory retina, thus creating an adhesion between the retina and the "wall of the eye" to keep the retina attached. This photocoagulative property of the argon and similar lasers achieves its therapeutic effect in the treatment of diabetic retinopathy by focal and controlled necrosis of a limited amount of ischemic retina. The argon laser is also used with some efficacy to treat the late complications that can develop in the natural history of retinal vein occlusion. Because emissions of the argon laser can penetrate the cornea and lens, causing severe retinal damage, personnel in the vicinity of the argon laser should wear orange protective goggles.

The Nd:YAG, commonly called the *YAG laser,* emits light in the infrared range (wavelength, 1,064 nm [1.06 μm]) and is useful in posterior lens-capsule surgery. The Nd:YAG laser has high-power density and is efficacious in creating an opening in opacified posterior capsule membranes that develop in approximately one-third of cases after phacoemulsification or other extracapsular cataract surgery. Personnel working in the vicinity of this laser should wear green goggles and realize that their ability to detect cyanosis will be impaired.

An excimer laser (sometimes, and more correctly, called an *exciplex laser*) is a form of high-power, ultraviolet chemical laser frequently used in delicate refractive surgery (LASIK), commonly referred to as *laser corrective surgery.* The term *excimer* is short for "excited dimer," and *exciplex* is short for "excited complex." An excimer laser generally uses a combination of inert gas (argon, krypton, or xenon) and a reactive gas (fluorine or chlorine). Under appropriate conditions of electrical stimulation, a pseudomolecule called a *dimer* is generated, which can exist only in an energized state and gives rise to laser light in the ultraviolet range, typically with wavelengths of 125 to 200 nm. The ultraviolet light from an excimer laser is well absorbed by biologic matter and organic compounds. Instead of burning or cutting material, the excimer laser supplies enough energy to disrupt the molecular bonds of surface tissue through ablation. This property allows removal of exceptionally fine layers of surface material with almost no heating or change to neighboring tissue. These lasers are usually operated with a pulse rate of around 100 Hz and a pulse duration of 10 ns, although some may operate as high as 8 kHz and 30 ns.

Age-related macular degeneration is the most common cause of blindness in the elderly and has become alarmingly prevalent. The treatment of the generally more severe wet form of age-related macular degeneration has interestingly progressed over the years from the initial photocoagulation of the neovascular membrane that develops in the central retina or macula. Cauterization obliterates this membrane, but can also damage the adjacent healthy macular tissue. The next modality used to treat age-related macular degeneration was the cold laser to photoactivate an intravenously injected drug, verteporfin, which chemically changed on light exposure of 693 nm in the presence of oxygen. By precisely applying the cold laser light to the area of the neovascular membrane, the photoactivated verteporfin produced highly reactive oxygen radicals and "selectively" necrosed the diseased tissue. Because of ill effects on nearby healthy tissue, this approach has been superseded by a more effective, nonlaser treatment with intravitreous injection of monoclonal antibody drugs such as ranibizumab (FDA-approved) or bevacizumab (off-label).

POSTOPERATIVE OCULAR COMPLICATIONS

The incidence of eye injuries associated with nonocular surgery is low. In a study by Roth et al.[136] of 60,965 patients undergoing nonocular surgery from 1988 to 1992, the incidence of eye injury was 0.056% (34 patients). Twenty-one of these 34 patients sustained corneal abrasion, although other injuries included conjunctivitis, blurry vision, red eye, chemical injury, direct ocular trauma, and blindness. Independent risk factors for greater relative risk of ocular injury were protracted surgical procedures, lateral intraoperative positioning, head or neck surgery, general anesthesia, and (for some unknown reason) surgery on a Monday. A specific mechanism of injury could be identified in only 21% of cases. In the ASA Closed Claims Study published in 1992 (which analyzed only cases involving litigation), eye injuries represented merely 3% of all claims, but the serious nature of some of the injuries was reflected in large financial awards.[137] Similar to the findings of Roth et al., in the Closed Claims Study the specific mechanism of injury could be ascertained in only a minority of cases. Another Closed Claims Study published in 2004 and examining injuries associated with regional anesthesia reported that the proportion of regional anesthesia claims linked to eye blocks increased from 2% in the 1980s to 7% in the 1990s.[138] These injuries were typically permanent and related to the anesthesiologist's block technique or patient movement. More than half of the claims resulted in blindness. As sub-Tenon's and topical anesthesia for cataract removal became more common, it was thought that a reduction in claims would occur. This has not, in fact, been the case.[139]

Although infrequent and often transient, eye injuries occasionally can result in blindness or more limited, but nonetheless permanent, visual impairment. Postoperative complications after nonocular surgery include corneal abrasion and minor visual disturbances, chemical injuries, thermal or photic injury, and serious visual disturbances, including blindness. Serious injury may result from such diverse conditions as acute corneal epithelial edema, glycine toxicity and other visual disturbances associated with transurethral resection of the prostate, retinal ischemia, ischemic optic neuropathy, cortical blindness, and acute glaucoma. It appears that certain types of surgery, including complex spinal surgery in the prone position; operations involving extracorporeal circulation; and neck, nasal, or sinus surgery may increase the risk of serious postoperative visual complications.

Corneal Abrasion

Although the most common ocular complication of general anesthesia is corneal abrasion,[140] the incidence varies widely, depending on the perioperative circumstances. In a prospective study, Cucchiara and Black[141] found a 0.17% incidence of corneal abrasion in 4,652 neurosurgical patients whose eyes were protected, whereas Batra and Bali[140] one decade earlier reported a 44% incidence of corneal abrasion when eyes were left unprotected and partly open. A more recent study of over 100,000 nonophthalmologic procedures found an incidence of 0.15% which decreased to 0.079% following a teaching initiative.[142] A variety of mechanisms can result in corneal abrasion, including damage caused by the anesthetic mask, surgical drapes, and spillage of solutions. During intubation of the trachea, moreover, the end of plastic watch bands or hospital identification cards clipped to the laryngoscopist's vest pocket can injure the cornea. Ocular injury may also occur from loss of pain sensation, obtundation of protective corneal reflexes, and decreased tear production during anesthesia. Therefore, it may be prudent to tape the eyelids closed immediately after induction, and during mask ventilation and laryngoscopy. In addition to taping the eyelids closed, applying protective goggles and instilling petroleum-based ointments into the conjunctival sac may provide protection. Disadvantages of ointments include occasional allergic reactions; flammability, which may make their use undesirable during surgery around the face and contraindicated during laser surgery; and blurred vision in the early postoperative period. The blurring and foreign-body sensation associated with ointments may actually increase the incidence of postoperative corneal abrasions if they trigger excessive rubbing of the eyes while the patient is still emerging from anesthesia. Even water-based (methylcellulose) ointments may be irritating and cause scleral erythema. It would seem prudent, therefore, to close the eyelids with tape during general anesthesia for procedures away from the head and neck. For certain procedures on the face, ocular occluders or tarsorrhaphy may be indicated. Special attention should also be devoted to frequent checking of the eyes during procedures on a prone patient.

Patients with corneal abrasion usually complain of a foreign-body sensation, pain, tearing, and photophobia. The pain is typically exacerbated by blinking and ocular movement. It is wise to have an ophthalmologic consultation immediately. Treatment typically consists of the prophylactic application of antibiotic ointment and patching the injured eye shut. Although permanent sequelae are possible, healing usually occurs within 24 hours.

Chemical Injury

Spillage of solutions during skin preparation may result in chemical damage to the eye. The FDA has reported serious corneal damage from eye contact with Hibiclens, a 4% chlorhexidine gluconate solution formulated with a detergent. Again, with meticulous attention to detail, this misadventure is preventable. Treatment consists of liberal bathing of the eye with balanced salt solution to remove the offending agent. After surgery, it may be desirable to have an ophthalmologist examine the eye to document any residual injury or lack thereof.

Photic Injury

Direct or reflected light beams may permanently damage the eye. For patients undergoing nonocular laser surgery, the potential for serious injury to the cornea or retina from certain laser beams requires that the patient's eyes be protected with moist gauze pads and metal shields, and that operating room personnel wear protective glasses. These goggles must be appropriately tinted for the specific wavelength they are intended to block. Clear goggles may be worn when working with the carbon dioxide laser, whereas for work with the argon, Nd:YAG, or Nd:YAG-KTP (potassium titanyl phosphate) laser, the goggles must be tinted orange, green, and orange-red, respectively.

Mild Visual Symptoms

After anesthesia, transient, mild visual disturbances such as photophobia or diplopia are common. Blurred vision in the early postoperative period may reflect residual effects of petroleum-based ophthalmic ointments or ocular effects of anticholinergic drugs administered in the perioperative period (see "Corneal Abrasion").

In contrast, the complaint of postoperative visual loss is rare and is cause for alarm. Several of the following conditions may be associated with visual loss after anesthesia and surgery, and should be included in the differential diagnosis: Hemorrhagic retinopathy, retinal ischemia, retinal artery occlusion, ischemic optic neuropathy, cortical blindness, and acute glaucoma.

Hemorrhagic Retinopathy

Retinal hemorrhages that occur in otherwise healthy people secondary to hemodynamic changes associated with turbulent emergence from anesthesia or protracted vomiting are termed *Valsalva retinopathy*. Fortunately, these venous hemorrhages are usually self-limiting and resolve completely in a few days to a few months.

Because no visual changes occur unless the macula is involved, most cases are asymptomatic. However, if bleeding into the optic nerve occurs, resulting in optic atrophy, or if the hemorrhage is massive, permanent visual impairment may ensue. In some instances of massive hemorrhage, vitrectomy may offer some improvement.

Retinal venous hemorrhage has also been described after injections of local anesthetics, steroids, or saline into the lumbar epidural space, and these cases have been summarized by Purdy and Ajimal.[143] The patients all received large injections (≥40 mL) into the epidural space, and they subsequently developed blurry vision or headaches. On funduscopic examination, retinal hemorrhage was consistently observed. Eight of the nine patients described had complete recovery. It is believed that the hemorrhage is produced by rapid epidural injection, which causes a sudden increase in intracranial pressure. This increase in cerebrospinal fluid pressure causes an increase of retinal venous pressure, which may cause retinal hemorrhages. It is possible that obesity, hypertension, coagulopathies, pre-existing elevated cerebrospinal fluid pressure (as seen in pseudotumor cerebri), and such retinal vascular diseases as diabetic retinopathy may be risk factors. Caution is recommended when injecting drugs or fluid into the epidural space; a slow injection rate and using the minimal volume necessary to accomplish the desired objective are strongly recommended.

Retinal bleeding may also originate from the arterial circulation. This bleeding may be associated with extraocular trauma. Funduscopic examination shows cotton–wool exudates, and this condition is known as *Purtscher retinopathy*. Purtscher retinopathy should be ruled out when a trauma patient complains of postanesthetic visual loss. This condition is associated with a poor prognosis, and most patients sustain permanent visual impairment.

Retinal Ischemia

Retinal ischemia or infarction may also result from direct ocular trauma secondary to external pressure exerted by an ill-fitting anesthetic mask, especially in a hypotensive setting, and from embolism during cardiac surgery, or from the intraocular injection of a large volume of sulfur hexafluoride or other gases in the presence of high concentrations of nitrous oxide. It may also result from increased ocular venous pressure associated with impaired venous drainage or elevated IOP.

The importance of carefully positioning patients and scrupulously monitoring external pressure on the eye cannot be overemphasized, especially when the patient is in the prone or jack-knife position. When the head is dependently positioned, venous pressure may be elevated. If external pressure is applied to the globe from improper head support, perfusion pressure to the eye is likely to be reduced. An episode of systemic hypotension in this setting could further decrease perfusion pressure and thereby decrease intraocular blood flow, resulting in possible retinal ischemia.

It is imperative that a padded or foam headrest be used for procedures done with patients in the prone position. The patient's eyes must be in the opening of this headrest and they must be checked at frequent intervals for pressure. Alternatively, Mayfield tongs can be used. During some spine procedures, a steep head-down position may be used to decrease venous bleeding and enhance surgical exposure. This position, in combination with deliberate hypotension and infusion of large quantities of crystalloid, may increase the risk of compromising the ocular circulation. It seems prudent to avoid combining these three risk factors to any significant degree.

Central retinal arterial occlusion and branch retinal arterial occlusion are important, and frequently preventable, causes of postoperative visual loss. Most case reports follow spinal, nasal, sinus, or neck surgery, as well as after coronary artery bypass graft (CABG) surgery. In addition to external pressure on the eye, causes can include emboli from carotid plaques or other sources, as well as vasospasm or thrombosis after radical neck surgery complicated by hemorrhage and hypotension, and after intranasal injection of α-adrenergic agonists. Several cases have followed intra-arterial injections of corticosteroids or local anesthetics in branches of the external carotid artery, with possible retrograde embolization to the ocular blood supply.[144] Mabry[145] suggested that the mechanism of injury involves positioning the needle intra-arterially to produce retrograde flow into the branches of the ophthalmic artery, and the perfusion pressure that must be overcome during the injection. Therefore, when injecting in the nasal and sinus areas, topical vasoconstrictors should be applied to decrease the size of the vascular bed, and a small (25-gauge) needle on a low-volume syringe should be used to minimize injection pressure. Moreover, because some cases have followed injections of corticosteroids combined with other drugs, it is believed that this practice may predispose to formation of drug crystals and therefore should be discouraged.

In cases of central retinal arterial occlusion, signs of eye injury including proptosis, chemosis, hyphema, corneal abrasion, and lid bruising are apparent. Pathognomonic findings on funduscopic examination reveal a pale, edematous retina and a cherry-red spot. Platelet-fibrin, cholesterol, calcific, or crystalloid emboli may be found in narrowed retinal arterioles. Embolic or arteritic causes may be discovered via echocardiogram, carotid ultrasound, and temporal artery biopsy. Computed tomography (CT) and magnetic resonance imaging (MRI) studies are negative.

Prevention is much more successful than treatment. It may be possible to apply ocular massage (contraindicated if glaucoma is a possibility) to dislodge an embolus to more peripheral sites, and intravenous acetazolamide and 5% carbon dioxide inhalation have been used to increase retinal blood flow. The prognosis, however, typically is poor, and approximately 50% of patients with central retinal arterial occlusion eventually have optic atrophy.

Ischemic Optic Neuropathy

Ischemic optic neuropathy in the nonsurgical setting is the most common cause of *sudden* visual loss in patients older than 50 years, and it may be either arteritic or nonarteritic. Our discussion is limited to postoperative ischemic optic neuropathy and contrasts the similarities and differences between anterior ischemic optic neuropathy and posterior ischemic optic neuropathy. Because of a perceived increase in the incidence of postoperative visual loss since the mid-1990s, the Committee on Professional Liability of the ASA established the Postoperative Visual Loss Database on July 1, 1999, to better identify associated risk factors so these tragic complications might be prevented in the future.[146] Because the incidence of postoperative vision loss after spine surgery in the prone position is estimated to range from 0.017% to 0.1%, and the condition can occur in healthy individuals of all ages, it would seem prudent to discuss this potential complication preoperatively with the patient during the informed consent process.

Anterior Ischemic Optic Neuropathy

Although the multifactorial pathophysiology of anterior ischemic optic neuropathy has not been completely established, it is believed to involve temporary hypoperfusion or nonperfusion of the vessels supplying the anterior portion of the optic nerve, although intra-axonal edema and disturbed autoregulation to the optic nerve head may also play a role.[144] Coexisting systemic disease, especially involving the cardiovascular system and (to a lesser extent) the endocrine system, is common in patients in whom anterior ischemic optic neuropathy develops. Male gender also strongly predominates. Other risk factors for postoperative anterior ischemic optic neuropathy include CABG and other thoracovascular operations, as well as spinal surgery. Although massive bleeding, anemia, and hypotension are commonly described intraoperative risk factors, a retrospective survey of surgeons who perform spinal fusion surgery disclosed that hypotension and anemia were equally prevalent in patients in whom ischemic optic neuropathy developed and in those in whom it did not.[147] Other possible risk factors are increased IOP or orbital venous pressure. Although emboli may also play a role, anterior ischemic optic neuropathy is not usually caused by emboli because emboli preferentially lodge in the central retinal artery rather than in the short posterior ciliary arteries that supply the anterior optic nerve.

Increased IOP caused by extrinsic compression of the eye decreases retinal blood flow that can produce both retinal and optic nerve injuries. Moreover, increased IOP can result from large infusions of crystalloid when the head is steeply dependent, as during many spinal operations.[148] Increased orbital venous pressure results in a decreased perfusion pressure gradient to the optic nerve head. Interestingly, one patient who had ischemic optic neuropathy despite perioperative normotension had marked facial edema after surgery of protracted duration.[148] Similarly, a study in cardiac surgery patients revealed that increases in IOP correlated with the degree of hemodilution and the use of crystalloid priming solution.[149] Patients with anterior ischemic optic neuropathy were more likely to have significant weight gain within 24 hours of open heart surgery, again suggesting the role of elevated ocular venous pressure in impeding blood flow to the optic nerve.

According to Roth and Gillesberg,[144] a complex interaction of factors such as ocular venous pressure, hemodilution, hypotension, release of endogenous vasoconstrictors, and individual risk factors such as atherosclerosis and aberrant optic nerve circulation may be implicated in the development of anterior ischemic optic neuropathy. Therefore, specific recommendations for preventative strategies are elusive. Clearly, however, external pressure on the eyes must be meticulously avoided. It also seems prudent to minimize time in the prone position when the head is notably dependent. In patients with pre-existing cardiovascular disease, significant hypertension, or glaucoma, it seems advisable to maintain systemic blood pressure as close to baseline as possible.[144]

Patients with anterior ischemic optic neuropathy typically have painless visual loss that may not be noted until the first postoperative day (or possibly later), an afferent pupillary defect, altitudinal field defects, and optic disc edema or pallor. MRI or CT initially shows enlargement of the optic nerve. However, optic atrophy is detected by MRI later.

The prognosis for anterior ischemic optic neuropathy varies but is often grim. Although there is no recognized treatment for anterior ischemic optic neuropathy, Williams et al.[150] reviewed the various therapies that may be instituted. These include intravenous acetazolamide, furosemide, mannitol, and steroids. Maintaining the head-up position could be helpful if increased ocular venous pressure is operative. Surgical optic nerve sheath fenestration or decompression is not only ineffective, but may actually be harmful.[151]

Posterior Ischemic Optic Neuropathy

The posterior optic nerve has a less luxuriant blood supply than the anterior optic nerve. Most perioperative ION cases associated with spine surgery occur in the posterior optic nerve where there is poor collateral flow, rendering the nerve vulnerable to prolonged pathophysiologic changes in blood flow. In contrast to anterior ischemic optic neuropathy, relatively few cases have been reported after CABG, and posterior ischemic optic neuropathy appears to be less related to coexisting cardiovascular disease. As with anterior ischemic optic neuropathy, male patients outnumber female patients substantially. Many cases have been associated with surgery involving the neck, nose, sinuses, or spine. In approximately one third of cases reported, facial edema has been noted.[144] Approximately 11% of cases were associated with cardiopulmonary bypass procedures.

Posterior ischemic optic neuropathy is produced by reduced oxygen delivery to the retrolaminar part of the optic nerve. Compression of the pial vessels (supplied by small collaterals from the ophthalmic artery) or embolic phenomena have been postulated to produce ischemia.[144]

A hypoxic insult in this region results in a slower development of ischemic damage so a symptom-free period often precedes the loss of vision. In some patients, the onset of symptoms may be delayed several days. Typical findings include an afferent pupillary defect or nonreactive pupil. Disc edema is not a feature of posterior ischemic optic neuropathy because of its retro-orbital position. CT scan in the early postoperative period may reveal enlargement of the intraorbital portion of the optic nerve. Bilateral blindness is more common with posterior ischemic optic neuropathy than with anterior ischemic optic neuropathy, possibly indicating involvement of the optic chiasm. Concomitant disease of the eye or ocular blood supply may be related to posterior ischemic optic neuropathy.[144] Some cases may show partial improvement spontaneously, but often no improvement is noted. Steroids may be considered for treatment. Preventive strategies are as outlined for anterior ischemic optic neuropathy.

A review of the first 6 years of cases submitted to the ASA Postoperative Visual Loss Registry found that spinal surgery patients at greatest risk for ischemic optic neuropathy and visual compromise include those with predisposing patient-specific factors, surgery exceeding 6 hours' duration, and blood loss of more than a liter.[152] In the 83 reported cases, there was no causative evidence of traumatic eye injury from edema or direct pressure on the globe. Mean blood pressures and hematocrits varied widely among those who developed postoperative blindness. However, 34% of cases had the lowest mean arterial blood pressure or systolic blood pressure ≥40% below baseline, and in only 6% of cases were the mean arterial or the systolic pressures <20% below baseline. The ASA practice advisory for perioperative visual loss associated with spine surgery concludes that there is no established "transfusion threshold" and that deliberate intraoperative hypotension during surgery has not been proven as contributory to postoperative loss of vision.[153] The consultants and specialty society members, however, expressed concern about the use of deliberate hypotension in high-risk patients and recommended that the use of this technique be determined on a case-by-case basis. Further, they recommended that high-risk patients should be positioned so that their heads are level with or higher than the heart, if possible. Patients' heads should be maintained in a neutral forward position, avoiding neck flexion, extension, lateral flexion, or rotation, if at all possible. Finally, consideration should be given to using *staged* spine procedures, in order to avoid excessively protracted periods in the prone position, for high-risk patients.

In 2012, the first multicenter study to identify risk factors for ION patients compared with patients without ION after prone spinal fusion surgery using detailed perioperative data was published.[154] Cases with anterior and posterior ION were combined. After multivariate analysis, risk factors for ION after spinal fusion surgery included male sex, obesity, Wilson frame use, prolonged anesthesia duration, greater estimated blood loss, and lower percent colloid administration. No statistically significant independent effect on ION of older age, hypertension, atherosclerosis, smoking, or diabetes was identified. These recent findings suggest that the etiology of ION may be more heavily influenced by intraoperative factors than by any known preexisting comorbidities or vasculopathy. Fully half of the risk factors strongly support the speculation that acute venous congestion of the optic canal is a potential contributor to ION in this setting.[155] Perhaps over time, investigators will be able to determine what role, if any, an inflammatory response, either locally or systemically, plays in the genesis of ION.[155]

Cortical Blindness

Brain injury rostral to the optic nerve may cause cortical blindness. The impairment is produced by damage to the visual path beyond the lateral geniculate nucleus or the visual cortex in the occipital lobe. Similar to anterior ischemic optic neuropathy, cortical blindness is a significant concern in patients undergoing CABG, and systemic disease is often present. Emboli and sustained, profound hypotension are common causes. Other events implicated in the pathophysiology include cardiac arrest, hypoxemia, intracranial hypertension, exsanguinating hemorrhage, vascular occlusion, thrombosis, and vasospasm.

Differential diagnostic features include a normal optic disc on fundoscopy and normal pupillary responses. There is, however, loss of optokinetic nystagmus with normal eye motility. CT and MRI are helpful in delineating the extent of brain infarction associated with cortical blindness. Occipital lesions are frequently bilateral and CT findings typically indicate posterior cerebral artery thrombosis, basilar artery occlusion, posterior cerebral artery branch occlusion, or watershed infarction. Lesions after CABG often include the parieto-occipital area.

Whereas most cases of ischemic optic neuropathy do not improve significantly or completely, visual recovery from cortical blindness in previously healthy patients may be considerable but prolonged. Preventive strategies include maintenance of adequate systemic perfusion pressure and, in cardiac surgery, minimizing manipulation of the aorta, meticulous removal of air and particulate matter during valvular procedures, and use of an arterial line filter in selected patients during bypass.

Acute Glaucoma

Although topical application of such mydriatic drugs as atropine and scopolamine is contraindicated in patients with known, chronic glaucoma, the systemic use of anticholinergics in usual premedicating doses is safe for glaucomatous eyes. The use of an atropine–neostigmine combination for reversal of neuromuscular blockade is also safe in patients with glaucoma. Topical ophthalmic medications that are being administered to control glaucoma should be continued through the perioperative period.

Acute angle-closure glaucoma typically occurs spontaneously but has been reported, albeit rarely, after both spinal and general anesthesia. Acute angle-closure glaucoma caused by pupillary block is a serious, multifactorial disease. Risk factors include genetic predisposition, shallow anterior chamber depth, increased lens thickness, small corneal diameter, female gender, and advanced age. One study[156] explored possible precipitating events in at-risk patients and found no evidence that the type of anesthetic agent, the duration of surgery, the volume of parenteral fluids, or the intraoperative blood pressure were related to the development of acute angle-closure glaucoma.

Despite its seriousness, acute angle-closure glaucoma may be difficult to recognize.[157] However, physicians should be knowledgeable about this potential complication because diagnostic delay may detrimentally affect visual outcome and cause permanent optic nerve damage. Fazio et al.[158] recommended that the preoperative evaluation include a thorough ocular history and a penlight examination to detect a shallow anterior chamber. Those patients considered at risk should then undergo a preoperative ophthalmic evaluation and perioperative miotic therapy. After surgery, these patients should be scrupulously watched for red eye or a fixed dilated pupil, as well as for complaints of pain and blurred vision. Acute glaucoma is a true emergency, and ophthalmologic consultation should be secured immediately to acutely decrease IOP with systemic and topical therapy. The intense periorbital pain typically described by these patients is an important aid in differential diagnosis.

Postcataract Ptosis

Ptosis after cataract surgery is not uncommon, and multiple factors have been implicated in its etiology.[159,160] These include the presence of a pre-existing ptosis, injection of anesthetic solution into the upper lid when performing facial nerve block, retrobulbar injection, injection of peribulbar anesthesia through the upper eyelid at the 12-o'clock position, ocular compression or massage, the eyelid speculum, placement of a superior rectus bridle suture with traction on the superior rectus–levator complex, creation of a large conjunctival flap, prolonged or tight patching in the postoperative period, and postoperative eyelid edema. Feibel et al.[159] believed that the development of postcataract ptosis is multifactorial and that no single aspect of cataract surgery is the sole contributor. More recently, Taylor et al.[160] used MRI immediately after diagnosis of diplopia in four patients who received peribulbar block. They found peribulbar edema consistent with direct local anesthetic–induced myotoxicity after presumed inadvertent intramuscular injection. Although local anesthetics are clearly myotoxic, the local anesthetic injection cannot be isolated as the primary factor because postsurgical ptosis is also seen in patients undergoing surgery with general anesthesia.

References

1. Eye Diseases Prevalence Research Group. Prevalence of age-related macular degeneration in the United States. *Arch Ophthalmol.* 2004;122:564.
2. Hebert LE, Scherr PA, Bienias JL, et al. Alzheimer disease in the US population: Prevalence estimates using the 2000 Census. *Arch Neurol.* 2003;60:119.
3. Wimo A, Winblad B. Health economical aspects of Alzheimer disease and its treatment. *Psychogeriatrics.* 2001;1:189.
4. Bruce RA. *Ocular Anatomy, Anesthesia for Ophthalmology.* In: Bruce RA, McGoldrick KE, Oppenheimer P. eds. Birmingham: Aesculapius; 1982:3.
5. Teng C, Gurses-Ozden R, Liebmann JM, et al. Effect of a tight necktie on intraocular pressure. *Br J Ophthalmol.* 2003;87:946.
6. Stoelting RK. Circulatory changes during direct laryngoscopy and tracheal intubation: Influence of duration of laryngoscopy with or without prior lidocaine. *Anesthesiology.* 1977;47:381.
7. Duncalf D, Foldes FF. Effect of anesthetic drugs and muscle relaxants on intraocular pressure. In: Smith RB. eds. *Anesthesia in Ophthalmology.* Boston, MA: Little Brown; 1973:21.
8. Garde JF, Aston R, Endler GC, et al. Racial mydriatic response to belladonna preparations. *Anesth Analg.* 1978;57:572.
9. Watcha MF, Chu FC, Stevens JL, et al. Effects of halothane on intraocular pressure in anesthetized children. *Anesth Analg.* 1990;71:181.
10. Thompson MF, Brock-Utne JG, Bean P, et al. Anaesthesia and intraocular pressure: A comparison of total intravenous anaesthesia using etomidate with conventional inhalational anaesthesia. *Anaesthesia.* 1982;37:758.
11. Yoshikawa K, Murai Y. Effect of ketamine on intraocular pressure in children. *Anesth Analg.* 1971;50:199.
12. Corssen G, Hoy JE. A new parenteral anesthetic—CI581: Its effect on intraocular pressure. *J Pediatr Ophthalmol.* 1967;4:20.
13. Peuler M, Glass DD, Arens JF. Ketamine and intraocular pressure. *Anesthesiology.* 1975;43:575.
14. Ausinsch B, Rayburn RL, Munson ES, et al. Ketamine and intraocular pressure in children. *Anesth Analg.* 1976;55:773.
15. Ausinsch B, Graves SA, Munson ES, et al. Intraocular pressure in children during isoflurane and halothane anesthesia. *Anesthesiology.* 1975;42:167.
16. Duncalf D, Weitzner SW. Ventilation and hypercapnia on intraocular pressure in children. *Anesth Analg.* 1963;43:232.
17. Litwiller RW, Difazio CA, Rushia EL. Pancuronium and intraocular pressure. *Anesthesiology.* 1975;42:750.
18. Lincoff HA, Breinin GM, DeVoe AG, et al. Effect of succinylcholine on the extraocular muscles. *Am J Ophthalmol.* 1957;44:440.
19. Pandey K, Badolas RP, Kumar S. Time course of intraocular hypertension produced by suxamethonium. *Br J Anaesth.* 1972;44:191.
20. Kelly RE, Dinner M, Turner LS, et al. Succinylcholine increases intraocular pressure in the human eye with the extraocular muscles detached. *Anesthesiology.* 1993;79:948.
21. Miller RD, Way WL, Hickey RF. Inhibition of succinylcholine-induced increased intraocular pressure by nondepolarizing muscle relaxants. *Anesthesiology.* 1968; 29:123.
22. Meyers EF, Krupin T, Johnson M, et al. Failure of nondepolarizing neuromuscular blockers to inhibit succinylcholine-induced increased intraocular pressure: A controlled study. *Anesthesiology.* 1978;48:149.
23. Verma RS. "Self-taming" of succinylcholine-induced fasciculations and intraocular pressure. *Anesthesiology.* 1979;50:245.
24. Meyers EF, Singer P, Otto A. A controlled study of the effect of succinylcholine self-taming on IOP. *Anesthesiology.* 1980;53:72.
25. Stoelting RK. Blood pressure and heart rate changes during short duration laryngoscopy for tracheal intubation: Influences of viscous or intravenous lidocaine. *Anesth Analg.* 1978;57:197.
26. Smith RB, Babinski M, Leano N. Effect of lidocaine on succinylcholine-induced rise in IOP. *Can Anaesth Soc J.* 1979;26:482.
27. Grover VK, Lata K, Sharma S, et al. Efficacy of lignocaine in the suppression of the intraocular pressure response to suxamethonium and tracheal intubation. *Anaesthesia.* 1989;44:22.
28. Jampolsky A. Strabismus: Surgical overcorrections. *Highlights Ophthalmol.* 1965; 8:78.
29. Dell R, Williams B. Anaesthesia for strabismus surgery: A regional survey. *Br J Anaesth.* 1999;82:761.
30. Berler DK. Oculocardiac reflex. *Am J Ophthalmol.* 1963;12(56):954.
31. Alexander JP. Reflex disturbances of cardiac rhythm during ophthalmic surgery. *Br J Ophthalmol.* 1975;59:518.
32. Mirakur RK, Clarke RSJ, Dundee JW, et al. Anticholinergic drugs in anaesthesia: A survey of their present position. *Anaesthesia.* 1978;33:133.
33. Massumi RA, Mason DT, Amsterdam EA, et al. Ventricular fibrillation and tachycardia after intravenous atropine for treatment of bradycardias. *N Engl J Med.* 1972;287:336.
34. McGoldrick KE. Transient left bundle branch block during local anesthesia. *Anesthesiol Rev.* 1981;8(6):36.
35. Moonie GT, Rees DI, Elton D. Oculocardiac reflex during strabismus surgery. *Can Anaesth Soc J.* 1964;11:621.
36. Steward DJ. Anticholinergic premedication for infants and children. *Can Anaesth Soc J.* 1983;30:325.
37. Nachman RL, Esterly NB. Increased skin permeability in preterm infants. *J Pediatr.* 1971;79:628.
38. Ellis EP, Esterdahl M. Echothiophate iodide therapy in children: Effect upon blood cholinesterase levels. *Arch Ophthalmol.* 1967;77:598.
39. Meyers EF. Cocaine toxicity during dacryocystorhinostomy. *Arch Ophthalmol.* 1980;98:842.
40. Gay GR, Loper KA. Control of cocaine-induced hypertension with labetalol (letter). *Anesth Analg.* 1988;67:92.
41. Lansche RK. Systemic effects of topical epinephrine and phenylephrine. *Am J Ophthalmol.* 1966;49:95.
42. Brown MM, Brown GC, Spaeth GL. Lack of side effects from topically administered 10% phenylephrine eye drops: A controlled study. *Arch Ophthalmol.* 1980;98:487.
43. Jones FL, Eckberg NL. Exacerbation of asthma by timolol. *N Engl J Med.* 1979; 301:170.
44. Kim JW, Smith PH. Timolol-induced bradycardia. *Anesth Analg.* 1980;59:301.
45. Shavitz SA. Timolol and myasthenia gravis. *JAMA.* 1979;242:1612.
46. Bailey PL. Timolol and postoperative apnea in neonates and young infants. *Anesthesiology.* 1984;61:622.
47. Vinker S, Kaiserman I, Waitman DA, et al. Prescription of ocular beta-blockers in patients with obstructive pulmonary disease: Does a central electronic medical record make a difference? *Clin Drug Investig.* 2006;26:495.
48. Stinson TW, Donlon JV. Interaction of SF6 and air with nitrous oxide. *Anesthesiology.* 1979;51:S16.
49. Wolf GL, Capriano C, Hartung J. Effects of nitrous oxide on gas bubble volume in the anterior chamber. *Arch Ophthalmol.* 1985;103:418.
50. Lee EJK. Use of nitrous oxide causing severe visual loss 37 days after retinal surgery. *Br J Anaesth.* 2004;93:464.
51. Marcus EN, Gayer S, Anderson DR. Medical evaluation of patients before ocular surgery (editorial). *Am J Ophthalmol.* 2003;136:338.
52. Schein OD, Katz J, Bass EB, et al. The value of routine preoperative medical testing before cataract surgery. *N Engl J Med.* 2000;342:168.
53. Charles S, Rosenfeld PJ, Gayer S. Medical consequences of stopping anticoagulants prior to intraocular surgery or intravitreal injections. *Retina.* 2007;27(7):813.
54. Feitl ME, Krupin T. Retrobulbar anesthesia. *Ophthalmol Clin North Am.* 1990; 3:83.
55. Katz J, Feldman MA, Bass EB, et al. Risks and benefits of anticoagulant and antiplatelet medication use before cataract surgery. *Ophthalmology.* 2003;110: 1784.
56. Jamula E, Anderson J, Douketis JD. Safety of continuing warfaran therapy during cataract surgery: a systematic review and meta-analysis. *Thromb Res.* 2009; 124:292–299.
57. Douketis JD, Berger PB, Dunn AS, et al. The perioperative management of antithrombotic therapy: American College of Chest Physicians Evidence-Based Clinical Practice Guidelines (8th ed). *Chest.* 2008;133(6 suppl):299S.
58. American Society of Anesthesiologists Committee on Standards and Practice Parameters. Practice alert for the perioperative management of patients with coronary artery stents: a report by the American Society of Anesthesiologists Committee on Standards and Practice Parameters. *Anesthesiology.* 2009;110:22.
59. Bayes J. A survey of ophthalmic anesthetists on managing pacemakers and implanted cardiac defibrillators. *Anesth Analg.* 2006;103:1615.
60. Stoller GL. Ophthalmic surgery and the implantable cardioverter defibrillator. *Arch Ophthalmol.* 2006;124:123.
61. Bhananker SM, Posner KL, Cheney FW, et al. Injury and liability associated with monitored anesthesia care: A closed claims analysis. *Anesthesiology.* 2006;104:228.

62. Gayer S. Key components of risk associated with ophthalmic anesthesia. *Anesthesiology.* 2006;105:859.
63. McGoldrick KE. Ocular pathology and systemic diseases. In: McGoldrick KE, ed. *Anesthetic Implications, Anesthesia for Ophthalmic and Otolaryngologic Surgery.* Philadelphia, PA: WB Saunders; 1992:210.
64. Leaming DV. Practice styles and preferences of ASCRS members: 2002 survey. *J Cataract Refract Surg.* 2003;29:1421.
65. Guise PA. Sub-Tenon anesthesia: A prospective study of 6000 blocks. *Anesthesiology.* 2003;98:964.
66. Gayer S, Flynn HW Jr. Sub-Tenon's injection for local anesthesia in posterior segment surgery (discussion). *Ophthalmology.* 2000;107:46.
67. The Joint Commission on Accreditation of Healthcare Organizations. Universal protocol for preventing wrong site, wrong procedure, wrong person surgery. Accessed October 19th, 2007. http://www.jointcommission.org/PatientSafety/UniversalProtocol.
68. Wainwright AC. Positive pressure ventilation and the laryngeal mask airway in ophthalmic anaesthesia. *Br J Anaesth.* 1995;75:249.
69. Lamb K, James MFM, Janicki PK. The laryngeal mask airway for intraocular surgery: Effects on intraocular pressure and stress responses. *Br J Anaesth.* 1992; 69:143.
70. Thomson KD. The effect of the laryngeal mask airway on coughing after eye surgery under general anesthesia. *Ophthalmic Surg.* 1992;23:630.
71. Knapp H. On cocaine and its use in ophthalmic and general surgery. *Arch Ophthalmol.* 1884;13:402.
72. Atkinson WS. Retrobulbar injection of anesthetic within the muscular cone. *Arch Ophthalmol.* 1936;16:494.
73. Gayer S. Ophthalmic anesthesia: More than meets the eye. In: Schwartz AJ, ed. *American Society of Anesthesiologists Refresher Courses in Anesthesiology.* Philadelphia, PA: Lippincott Williams & Wilkins; 2006:55.
74. Korneef L. The architecture of the musculofibrous apparatus in the human orbit. *Acta Morphol Neerl Scand.* 1977;15:35.
75. Ripart J, Lefrant J, de la Coussaye J, et al. Peribulbar versus retrobulbar anesthesia for ophthalmic surgery. *Anesthesiology.* 2001;94:56.
76. Capó H, Roth E, Johnson T, et al. Vertical strabismus after cataract surgery. *Ophthalmology.* 1996;103:918.
77. Ripart J, Lefrant J, Lalourcey L, et al. Medial canthus (caruncle) single injection periocular anesthesia. *Anesth Analg.* 1996;83:1234.
78. Katsev DA, Drews RC, Rose BT. An anatomic study of retrobulbar needle path length. *Ophthalmology.* 1989;96:1221.
79. Waller SG, Taboada J, O'Connor P. Retrobulbar anesthesia risk: Do sharp needles really perforate the eye more easily than blunt needles? *Ophthalmology.* 1993;100:506.
80. Unsold R, Stanley JA, DeGroot J. The CT topography of retrobulbar anesthesia. *Graefes Arch Clin Exp Ophthalmol.* 1981;217:125.
81. Liu C, Youl B, Moseley I. Magnetic resonance imaging of the optic nerve in extremes of gaze. Implications for the positioning of the globe for retrobulbar anesthesia. *Br J Ophthalmol.* 1992;76:728.
82. Gayer S, Denham D, Alarakhia K, et al. Ocular decompression devices: Liquid mercury balloon versus the tungsten powder balloon. *Am J Ophthalmol.* 2006; 142:500.
83. Birch A, Evans M, Redembo E. The ultrasonic localization of retrobulbar needles during retrobulbar block. *Ophthalmology.* 1995;102:824.
84. Grizzard WS, Kirk NM, Pavan PR, et al. Perforating ocular injuries caused by anesthesia personnel. *Ophthalmology.* 1991;98:1011.
85. Miller-Meeks MJ, Bergstrom T, Karp KO. Prevalent attitudes regarding residency training in ocular anesthesia. *Ophthalmology.* 1994;101:1353.
86. Bayes J, Zheng H, Rosow CE. Early use of eyeglasses for myopia predicts long axial length of the eye. *Anesth Analg.* 2010;110:119.
87. Gayer S. Ocular ultrasound guided anesthesia. In: Singh AD, Hayden BC, eds. *Ophthalmic Ultrasonography.* Philadelphia, PA: Elsevier; 2012:195–200.
88. Chang J-L, Gonzalez-Abola E, Larson CE. Brain stem anesthesia following retrobulbar block. *Anesthesiology.* 1984;61:789.
89. Nicoll JMV, Acharya PA, Ahlen K, et al. Central nervous system complications after 6000 retrobulbar blocks. *Anesth Analg.* 1987;66:1298.
90. Swan KC. New drugs and techniques for ocular anesthesia. *Trans Am Acad Ophthalmol Otolaryngol.* 1956;60:368.
91. Gayer S, Cass GD. Sub-Tenon techniques should be one option among many. *Anesthesiology.* 2004;100:196.
92. Niemi-Murola L, Krootila K, Kivisaari R, et al. Localization of local anesthetic solution by magnetic resonance imaging. *Ophthalmology.* 2004;111:342.
93. Frieman BJ, Friedberg MA. Globe perforation associated with sub-Tenon's anesthesia. *J Ophthalmol.* 2001;131:520.
94. Ruschen H, Bremner FD, Carr C. Complications after sub-Tenon's eye block. *Anesth Analg.* 2003;96:273.
95. Ripart J, Metge L, Prat-Pradal D, et al. Medial canthus single-injection episcleral (sub-Tenon) anesthesia: Computed tomography imaging. *Anesth Analg.* 1998;87:42.
96. Allman KG, Theron AD, Byles DB. A new technique of incisionless, minimally invasive sub-Tenon's anaesthesia. *Anaesthesia.* 2008;63(7):782.
97. Quantock C, Goswami T. Death potentially secondary to sub-Tenon's block. *Anaesthesia.* 2007;62:175.
98. Palte H, Gayer S. Death after a sub-Tenon's block. *Anaesthesia.* 2007;62:531.
99. Bardocci A, Lofoco G, Perdicaro S, et al. Lidocaine 2% gel versus lidocaine 4% unpreserved drops for topical anesthesia in cataract surgery: A randomized controlled trial. *Ophthalmology.* 2003;110:144.
100. Eggeling P, Pleyer U, Hartman C, et al. Corneal endothelial toxicity of different lidocaine concentrations. *J Cataract Refract Surg.* 2000;26:1403.
101. Zhang C, Phamonvaechavan R, Rajan A, et al. Concentration-dependent bupivacaine myotoxicity in rabbit extraocular muscle. *J AAPOS.* 2010;14:323.
102. Netland PA, Harris A. Color Doppler ultrasound measurements after topical and retrobulbar epinephrine in primate eyes. *Invest Ophthalmol Vis Sci.* 1997;38:2655.
103. Yazbeck-Karam VG, Siddik-Sayyid SM, Abi Nader EL, et al. Supplementation of retrobulbar block with clonidine in vitreoretinal surgery: Effect on postoperative pain. *J Clin Anesth.* 2011;23:393.
104. Brown SM, Coats DK, Collins MLZ, et al. Second cluster of strabismus cases after periocular anesthesia without hyaluronidase. *J Cataract Refract Surg.* 2001; 27:1876.
105. Hamada S, Devys JM, Xuan TH, et al. Role of hyaluronidase in diplopia after peribulbar anesthesia for cataract surgery. *Ophthalmology.* 2005;112(5):879.
106. Kirsch RE. Further studies on the use of digital pressure in cataract surgery. Optimal length of time for application of digital pressure. *Arch Ophthalmol.* 1957; 58:641.
107. Jay WM, Aziz MZ, Green K. Effect of intraocular pressure reducer on ocular and optic nerve blood flow in phakic rabbit eyes. *Acta Ophthalmologica.* 1986;64:52.
108. Downs JB. Has oxygen administration delayed appropriate respiratory care? Fallacies regarding oxygen therapy. *Respir Care.* 2003;48:611.
109. Hug CC. MAC should stand for maximum anesthesia caution, not minimal anesthesiology care (editorial). *Anesthesiology.* 2006;104:221.
110. Norregaard JC, Schein OD, Bellan L, et al. International variation in anesthesia care during cataract surgery: Results from the International Cataract Surgery Outcomes Study. *Arch Ophthalmol.* 1997;115:1304.
111. Eichel R, Goldberg I. Anaesthesia techniques for cataract surgery: A survey of delegates to the Congress of the International Council of Ophthalmology, 2002. *Clin Experiment Ophthalmol.* 2005;33:469.
112. Rosenfeld SI, Litinsky SM, Snyder DA, et al. Effectiveness of monitored anesthesia care in cataract surgery. *Ophthalmology.* 1999;106:1256.
113. Fung D, Cohen MM, Stewart S, et al. What determines patient satisfaction with cataract care under topical local anesthesia and monitored sedation in a community hospital setting? *Anesth Analg.* 2005;100:1644.
114. Gayer S. Rethinking anesthesia strategies for patients with traumatic eye injuries: Alternatives to general anesthesia. *Curr Anesth Crit Care.* 2006;17:191.
115. Scott IU, McCabe CM, Flynn HW Jr, et al. Local anesthesia with intravenous sedation for surgical repair of selected open globe injuries. *Am J Ophthalmol.* 2002; 134:707.
116. Boscia F, La Tegola MG, Columbo G, et al. Combined topical anesthesia and sedation for open-globe injuries in selected patients. *Ophthalmology.* 2003; 110:1555.
117. Casson WR, Jones RM. Vecuronium induced neuromuscular blockade. *Anaesthesia.* 1986;41:354.
118. Ginsberg B, Glass PS, Quill T, et al. Onset and duration of neuromuscular blockade following high-dose vecuronium administration. *Anesthesiology.* 1989; 71:201.
119. Konchiergeri HN, Lee YE, Venugopal K. Effect of pancuronium on intraocular pressure changes induced by succinylcholine. *Can Anaesth Soc J.* 1979;26:479.
120. Libonati MM, Leahy JJ, Ellison N. The use of succinylcholine in open eye surgery. *Anesthesiology.* 1985;62:637.
121. McGoldrick KE. The open globe: Is an alternative to succinylcholine necessary? (editorial). *J Clin Anesth.* 1993;5:1.
122. de Boer H, Driessen JJ, Marcus MA, et al. Reversal of rocuronium-induced (1.2 mg/kg) neuromuscular block by sugammadex: A multicenter dose-finding and safety study. *Anesthesiology.* 2007;107:239.
123. Kopman AF. Sugammadex: A revolutionary approach to neuromuscular antagonism (editorial). *Anesthesiology.* 2006;104:631.
124. Baumgarten RK, Reynolds WJ. Priming principle and the open eye-full stomach. *Anesthesiology.* 1985;63:561.
125. France NK, France TD, Wordburn JD Jr, et al. Succinylcholine alteration of the forced duction test. *Ophthalmology.* 1980;87:1282.
126. Lerman MD, Eustis S, Smith DR. Effect of droperidol pretreatment on post-anesthetic vomiting in children undergoing strabismus surgery. *Anesthesiology.* 1986;65:322.
127. Brown RE, James DG, Weaver RG, et al. Low-dose droperidol versus standard-dose droperidol for prevention of postoperative vomiting after pediatric strabismus surgery. *J Clin Anesth.* 1991;3:306.
128. Gan TJ, Meyer TA, Apfel CC, et al. Society of Ambulatory Anesthesia guidelines for the management of postoperative nausea and vomiting. *Anesth Analg.* 2007;105:1615.
129. Watcha MF, Simeon RM, White PF, et al. Effect of propofol on the incidence of postoperative vomiting after strabismus surgery in pediatric outpatients. *Anesthesiology.* 1991;75:204.
130. Oh AY, Kim JH, Hwang JW, et al. Incidence of postoperative nausea and vomiting after pediatric strabismus surgery with sevoflurane or remifentanil–sevoflurane. *Br J Anaesth.* 2010;104:756.

131. Munro HM, Riegger LQ, Reynolds PI, et al. Comparison of the analgesic and emetic properties of ketorolac and morphine for paediatric outpatient strabismus surgery. *Br J Anaesth.* 1994;72:624.
132. Colson JD. Cervicofacial subcutaneous emphysema and pneumomediastinum after retinal detachment surgery: Just another monitored anesthesia eye case. *J Clin Anesth.* 2011;23:410.
133. Seaberg RR, Freeman WR, Goldbaum MH, et al. Permanent postoperative vision loss associated with expansion of intraocular gas in the presence of a nitrous oxide-containing anesthetic. *Anesthesiology.* 2002;97:1309.
134. Dallinger S, Findl O, Strenn K, et al. Age dependence of choroidal blood flow. *J Am Geriatr Soc.* 1998;46:484.
135. Recchia FM, Brown GC. Systemic disorders associated with retinal vascular occlusion. *Curr Opin Ophthalmol.* 2000;11:462.
136. Roth S, Thisted RA, Erickson JP, et al. Eye injuries after nonocular surgery: A study of 60,965 anesthetics from 1988–1992. *Anesthesiology.* 1996;85:1020.
137. Gild WA, Posner KL, Caplan RA, et al. Eye injuries associated with anesthesia. *Anesthesiology.* 1992;76:204.
138. Lee LA, Posner KL, Domino KB, et al. Injuries associated with regional anesthesia in the 1980s and 1990s: A closed claims analysis. *Anesthesiology.* 2004;101:143.
139. Szypula K, Ashpole KJ, Bogod D, et al. Litigation related to regional anesthesia: an analysis of claims against the NHS in England 1995–2007. *Anaesthesia.* 2010; 65:443.
140. Batra YK, Bali M. Corneal abrasions during general anesthesia. *Anesth Analg.* 1977;56:363.
141. Cucchiara R, Black S. Corneal abrasion during anesthesia and surgery. *Anesthesiology.* 1988;69:978.
142. Martin DP, Weingarten TN, Gunn PW, et al. Performance improvement system and perioperative corneal injuries. *Anesthesiology.* 2009;111:320.
143. Purdy EP, Ajimal GS. Vision loss after lumbar epidural steroid injection. *Anesth Analg.* 1988;86:119.
144. Roth S, Gillesberg I. Injuries to the visual system and other sense organs. In: Benumof JL, Saidman LJ, eds. *Anesthesia and Perioperative Complications.* 2nd ed. St. Louis: Mosby; 1999:377.
145. Mabry RL. Visual loss after intranasal corticosteroid injection. *Arch Otolaryngol.* 1981;107:484.
146. Lee LA. Postoperative visual loss data gathered and analyzed. *ASA Newsl.* 2000; 64:25.
147. Myers MA, Hamilton SR, Bogosian AJ, et al. Visual loss as a complication of spinal surgery. *Spine.* 1997;22:1325.
148. Dilger JA, Tetzlaff JE, Bell GR, et al. Ischemic optic neuropathy after spinal fusion. *Can J Anaesth.* 1998;45:63.
149. Shapira OM, Kimmel WA, Lindsey PS, et al. Anterior ischemic optic neuropathy after open heart operations. *Ann Thorac Surg.* 1996;61:660.
150. Williams EL, Hart WM, Tempelhoff R. Postoperative ischemic optic neuropathy. *Anesth Analg.* 1995;80:1018.
151. The Ischemic Optic Neuropathy Decompression Trial Research Group. Optic nerve decompression surgery is not effective and may be harmful. *JAMA.* 1995; 273:625.
152. Lee LA, Roth S, Posner KL, et al. The American Society of Anesthesiologists Postoperative Visual Loss Registry: Analysis of 93 spine surgery cases with postoperative visual loss. *Anesthesiology.* 2006;105:652.
153. American Society of Anesthesiologists Task Force on Perioperative Blindness. Practice advisory for perioperative visual loss associated with spine surgery: A report by the American Society of Anesthesiologists Task Force on Perioperative Blindness. *Anesthesiology.* 2006;104:1319.
154. The Postoperative Visual Loss Study Group. Risk factors associated with ischemic optic neuropathy after spinal fusion surgery. *Anesthesiology.* 2012;116:15.
155. Warner M. Cracking open the door on perioperative visual loss (editorial). *Anesthesiology.* 2012;116:1.
156. Drance SM. Angle-closure glaucoma among Canadian Eskimos. *Can J Ophthalmol.* 1973;8:252.
157. Gayer S. Prone to blindness: Answers to postoperative visual loss. *Anesth Analg.* 2010;112:11–12.
158. Fazio DT, Bateman JB, Christensen RE. Acute angle-closure glaucoma associated with surgical anesthesia. *Arch Ophthalmol.* 1985;103:360.
159. Feibel RM, Custer PL, Gordon MO. Postcataract ptosis: A randomized, double-masked comparison of peribulbar and retrobulbar anesthesia. *Ophthalmology.* 1993;100:660.
160. Taylor G, Devys JM, Heran F, et al. Early exploration of diplopia with magnetic resonance imaging after peribulbar anaesthesia. *Br J Anaesth.* 2004;92:899.

CHAPTER

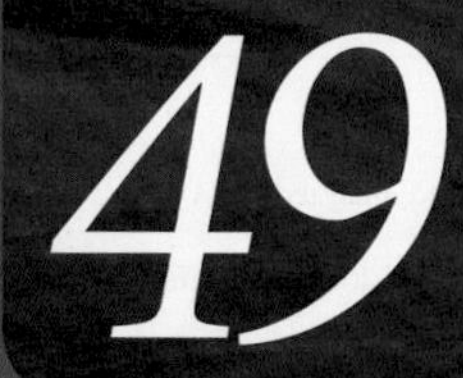

The Renal System and Anesthesia for Urologic Surgery

MARK STAFFORD-SMITH • ANDREW SHAW • AARON SANDLER • CATHERINE KUHN

Key Points

1. Renal filtration and reabsorption are susceptible to alterations by surgical illness and anesthesia. Autoregulation of renal blood flow (RBF) is effective over a wide range of mean arterial pressures (50 to 150 mm Hg). Autoregulation of urine flow does not occur, but a linear relationship between mean arterial pressure above 50 mm Hg and urine output is observed.
2. Renal medullary blood flow is low (2% of total RBF) but central to the kidneys' ability to concentrate urine. During periods of reduced renal perfusion, the metabolically active medullary thick ascending limb may be especially vulnerable to ischemic injury.
3. The physiologic response to surgical stress invokes intrinsic mechanisms for sodium and water conservation. Renal cortical vasoconstriction causes a shift in perfusion toward juxtamedullary nephrons, a decrease in glomerular filtration rate, and retention of salt and water result.
4. The stress response may induce a decrease in RBF and glomerular filtration rate, causing afferent arteriolar vasoconstriction. If this situation is not reversed, ischemic damage to the kidney may result in acute renal failure (ARF).
5. Anesthetic-induced reductions in RBF have been described for many agents but are usually clinically insignificant and reversible. Likewise, anesthetic agents have not been shown to interfere with the renal response to physiologic stress.
6. Isolated ARF carries a mortality of up to 60% in surgical patients, with acute tubular necrosis being the cause of ARF in most of these patients.
7. Overall, there are no conclusive comparative studies demonstrating superior renal protection or improved renal outcome with general versus regional anesthesia.
8. Surgical patients with nondialysis-dependent chronic kidney disease are at higher risk of developing end-stage renal disease. The single most reliable predictor of new postoperative need for dialysis is preoperative renal insufficiency.
9. Maintaining adequate intravascular volume and hemodynamic stability with aggressive management of kidney hypoperfusion is a basic principle of anesthetic care to prevent acute kidney injury.
10. Urologic patients are often elderly, have numerous comorbidities, and require critical evaluation prior to any urologic procedure.

11 Combining epidural with general anesthetic techniques for some major surgeries may offer advantages for accelerated recovery, improved analgesia, and even better outcomes, but these techniques must be conducted with respect for other perioperative issues, including thromboprophylaxis for prevention of deep venous thrombosis.

12 Watchful waiting, minimally invasive principles, and technologic innovation (e.g., laparoscopy, robotics) have changed the favored approach to many kidney, bladder, and prostate disorders, in some cases reducing the number of high-risk surgeries, in others creating other safer less morbid alternate treatments.

13 Absorption of irrigating solution related most often to transurethral prostate or bladder tumor resections can cause "TUR syndrome," a condition that, while becoming less common, has the potential to be serious and even life-threatening during several hours following surgery. Knowledge of specific concerns relevant to the different irrigating solutions, and vigilance of the anesthesiologist to factors that minimize absorption, recognition of signs and symptoms, and appropriate treatment are key to favorable outcomes with this condition.

Multimedia

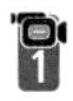
1 Laparoscopic

2 Robotic Prostatectomy

INTRODUCTION AND CONTEXT

The kidney plays a central role in implementing and controlling a variety of homeostatic functions, including excreting metabolic waste products in the urine, while keeping extracellular fluid volume and composition constant. Acute kidney injury (AKI) can occur as a direct result of surgical or medical disease, prolonged reduction in renal oxygen delivery, nephrotoxin insult, or a combination of these three factors. The first part of this chapter reviews renal physiology and pathophysiologic states as they relate to anesthetic practice, and then addresses strategies for recognizing and managing patients at risk for AKI and renal failure. The second part describes current urologic procedures and their attendant anesthetic management issues.

RENAL ANATOMY AND PHYSIOLOGY

Gross Anatomy

The two normal *kidneys* are reddish-brown organs and are ovoid in outline, but the medial margin is deeply indented and concave at its middle (Fig. 49-1) where a wide, vertical cleft (the hilus) transmits structures entering and leaving the kidney. The *hilus* lies at approximately the level of the first lumbar vertebra. The kidneys lie in the paravertebral gutters, behind the peritoneum, with the right kidney lying slightly lower than the left one because of the presence of the liver. At its upper end, the ureter has dilated to give rise to the *renal pelvis,* which passes through the hilus into the kidney proper. There it is continuous with several short funnel-like tubes (calyces) that unite it with the renal parenchyma. The renal blood vessels lie anterior to the pelvis of the kidney, but some branches may pass posteriorly. Renal pain sensation is conveyed back to spinal cord segments T10 through L1 by sympathetic fibers. Sympathetic innervation is supplied by preganglionic fibers from T8 to L1. The vagus nerve provides parasympathetic innervation to the kidney, and the S2 to S4 spinal segments supply the ureters.

The kidneys are enclosed by a thick, fibrous capsule, itself surrounded by a fatty capsule that fills the space inside the loosely applied renal (Gerota's) fascia. The developing kidney is first formed in the pelvis and then ascends to its final position on the posterior abdominal wall. During its ascent, the kidney receives blood supply from several successive sources, such that an accessory renal artery from the aorta may be found entering the lower pole of the kidney. When first formed, the rudimentary kidneys are close together and may fuse to give rise to a horseshoe kidney. This organ is unable to ascend, "held in place" by the inferior mesenteric artery, and thus when present it remains forever a pelvic organ.

The *bladder* is located in the retropubic space and receives its innervation from sympathetic nerves originating from T11 to L2, which conduct pain, touch, and temperature sensations, whereas bladder stretch sensation is transmitted via parasympathetic fibers from segments S2 to S4. Parasympathetics also provide the bladder with most of its motor innervation.

The *prostate, penile urethra,* and *penis* also receive sympathetic and parasympathetic fibers from the T11 to L2 and S2 to S4 segments, respectively. The pudendal nerve provides pain sensation to the penis via the dorsal nerve of the penis. Sensory innervation of the *scrotum* is via cutaneous nerves, which project to lumbosacral segments, whereas testicular sensation is conducted to lower thoracic and upper lumbar segments.

Ultrastructure

Inspection of the cut surface of the kidney reveals the paler *cortex,* adjacent to the capsule, and the darker, conical pyramids of the renal *medulla* (Fig. 49-1). The pyramids are radially striated and are covered with cortex, extending into the kidney as the renal columns. *Collecting tubules* from each lobe of the kidney (pyramid and its covering of cortex) discharge urine into the calyceal system via renal papillae at the entrance of each pyramid into the calyx proper. These collecting tubules originate deep within the radial striations (medullary rays) of the kidney and convey urine formed in the structural units of the kidneys, the *nephrons.* The parenchyma of each kidney contains approximately 1×10^6 tightly packed nephrons, each one consisting of a tuft of capillaries (the *glomerulus*) invaginated into the blind, expanded end (glomerular corpuscle) of a long tubule that leaves the renal corpuscle to form the proximal convoluted tubule in the cortex. This leads into the straight tubule, which loops down into the medullary pyramid (*loop of Henle*) and hence back to the cortex to become continuous with the distal convoluted tubule. This then opens into a collecting duct that is common to a number of nephrons and passes through the pyramid to enter the lesser calyx at the papilla. It is in

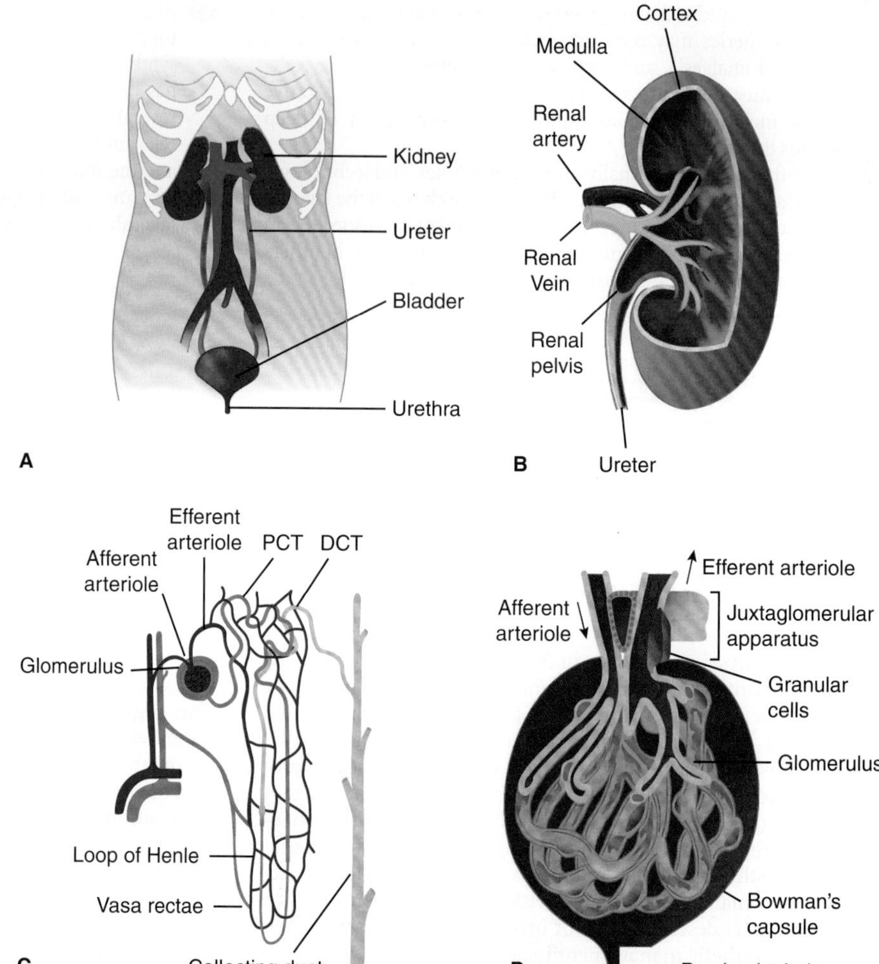

FIGURE 49-1. The gross anatomy **(A)** and internal structure of the genitourinary system and kidney. Internal organization of the kidney includes cortex and medulla regions and the vasculature **(B)**. The nephron is the functional unit of the kidney **(C)**. Plasma filtration occurs in the glomerulus **(D)**; 20% of plasma that enters the glomerulus passes through the specialized capillary wall into the Bowman capsule and enters the tubule to be processed and generate urine. PCT, proximal convoluted tubule, DCT, distal convoluted tubule. (From: http://www.incontinenceaid.com/files/images/Urinary_system_components.jpg **[A]**; **B**; http://www.pathology.vcu.edu/education/PathLab/pages/renalpath/rpsrhome.htm from Lecture 1 (modified with permission) **[C]**.)

these parts of the nephron (proximal tubule, loop of Henle, distal tubule, and collecting duct) that urine is formed, concentrated, and conveyed to the ureters. The distal convoluted tubule comes into very close contact with the afferent glomerular arteriole, and the cells of each are there modified to form the *juxtaglomerular apparatus,* a complex physiologic feedback control mechanism contributing in part to the precise control of intra- and extrarenal hemodynamics that is a hallmark feature of the normally functioning kidney.

As is the case for the renal tubules, the vasculature of the kidney is highly organized. The renal artery enters the kidney at the hilum and then divides many times before producing the arcuate arteries that run along the boundary between cortex and outer medulla. Interlobular arteries branch from arcuate arteries toward the outer kidney surface, giving rise as they pass through the cortex to numerous afferent arterioles, each leading to a single glomerular capillary tuft. The barrier where filtration from the vascular to tubular space within the glomerulus occurs is highly specialized and includes fenestrated negatively charged capillary endothelial cells and tubular epithelial cells (podocytes) separated by a basement membrane. Normally, selective permeability permits approximately 25% of the plasma elements to pass into the Bowman capsule; only cells and proteins >60 to 70 kDa cannot cross. However, abnormalities of this barrier can occur with diseases that may permit filtration of much larger proteins and even red blood cells; these changes manifest as the *nephrotic syndrome* (proteinuria >3.5 g/24 hr) or *glomerulonephritis* (hematuria and proteinuria). The glomerular capillaries exit the Bowman capsule and merge to form the efferent arteriole and peritubular capillaries that nourish the tubules. The renal vasculature is unusual in having this arrangement of two capillary beds joined in series by arterioles. Blood supply to the entire tubular system comes from the glomerular efferent arteriole, which branches into an extensive capillary network. Some of these peritubular capillaries, the *vasa recta,* descend deep into the medulla to parallel the loops of Henle. The vasa recta then return in a cortical direction with the loops, join other peritubular capillaries, and empty into the cortical veins.

Correlation of Structure and Function

Because renal tissue makes up only 0.4% of body weight but receives 25% of cardiac output, the kidneys are by far the most highly perfused major organs in the body, and this facilitates plasma filtration at rates as high as 125 to 140 mL/min in adults. The functions of the kidney are many and varied, including waste filtration, endocrine and exocrine activities, immune and metabolic functions, and maintenance of physiologic homeostasis. As well as tight regulation of extracellular solutes such as sodium, potassium, hydrogen, bicarbonate, and glucose, the kidney also generates ammonia and glucose and eliminates nitrogenous and other metabolic wastes including urea, creatinine, and bilirubin. Finally, circulating hormones secreted by the kidney influences red blood cell generation, calcium homeostasis, and systemic blood pressure.

The kidney fulfills its dual roles of waste excretion and body fluid management by filtering large amounts of fluid and solutes from the blood and secreting waste products into the tubular fluid. Filtration and reabsorption are affected by comorbid disease, surgery, and anesthesia and are the focus of the next section.

Glomerular Filtration

Production of urine begins with water and solute filtration from plasma flowing into the glomerulus via the afferent arteriole. The *glomerular filtration rate* (GFR) is a measure of glomerular function expressed as milliliters of plasma filtered per minute. The *ultrafiltration constant* (Kf) is directly related to glomerular capillary permeability and glomerular surface area. The two major determinants of filtration pressure are glomerular capillary pressure (P_{GC}) and glomerular oncotic pressure (π_{GC}). P_{GC} is directly related to renal artery pressure and is heavily influenced by arteriolar tone at points upstream (afferent) and downstream (efferent) from the glomerulus. An increase in afferent arteriolar tone, as occurs with intense sympathetic or angiotensin II stimulation, causes filtration pressure and GFR to fall. Milder degrees of sympathetic or angiotensin activity cause a selective increase in efferent arteriolar tone, which tends to increase filtration pressure and GFR. The π_{GC} is directly dependent on plasma oncotic pressure. Afferent arteriolar dilatation enhances GFR by increasing glomerular flow, which in turn elevates glomerular capillary pressure.

Autoregulation of Renal Blood Flow and Glomerular Filtration Rate

Renal blood flow (RBF) *autoregulation* maintains relatively constant rates of RBF and glomerular filtration over a wide range of arterial blood pressure. Renal autoregulation of blood flow and filtration is accomplished primarily by local feedback signals that modulate glomerular arteriolar tone to protect the glomeruli
1 from excessive perfusion pressure (Fig. 49-2).

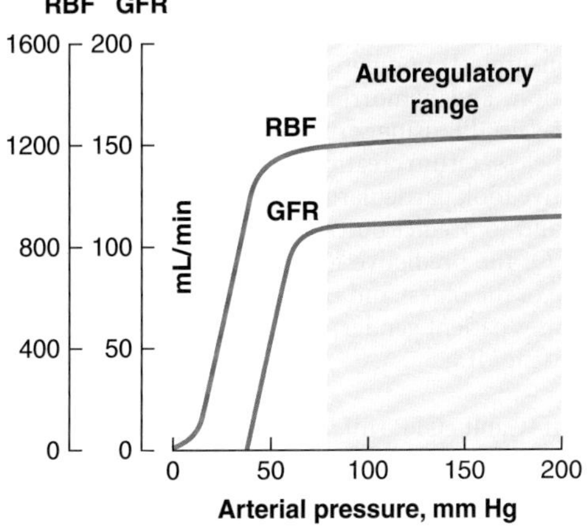

FIGURE 49-2. Renal blood flow (RBF) autoregulation maintains RBF and glomerular filtration rate (GFR) relatively constant with changes in systolic blood pressure from about 80 to 200 mm Hg. (From: http://www2.kumc.edu/ki/physiology/course/two/2_8.htm, with permission.)

In health, autoregulation of RBF is effective over a wide range of systemic arterial pressures. Several mechanisms for regulating blood flow to the glomerulus have been described, and all involve modulation of afferent glomerular arteriolar tone. The *myogenic reflex theory* holds that an increase in arterial pressure causes the afferent arteriolar wall to stretch and then constrict (by reflex); likewise, a decrease in arterial pressure causes reflex afferent arteriolar dilatation. The other proposed mechanism of RBF autoregulation is a phenomenon called *tubuloglomerular feedback,* which is also responsible for autoregulation of GFR.

Tubuloglomerular feedback allows the composition of distal tubular fluid to influence glomerular function through actions involving the juxtaglomerular apparatus. When RBF falls, the concomitant decrease in GFR results in less chloride delivery to the juxtaglomerular apparatus, which causes the afferent arteriole to dilate. Glomerular flow and pressure then increase, and GFR returns to previous levels. Chloride also acts as the feedback signal for control of efferent arteriolar tone. When GFR falls, declining chloride delivery to the juxtaglomerular apparatus triggers release of *renin,* which ultimately causes the formation of *angiotensin II.* In response to angiotensin, efferent arteriolar constriction increases glomerular pressure, which increases glomerular filtration. It is important to realize that autoregulation of urine flow does not occur, and that above a mean arterial pressure of 50 mm Hg there is a linear relationship between mean arterial pressure and urine output.

Tubular Reabsorption of Sodium and Water

Active, energy-dependent reabsorption of sodium begins almost immediately as the glomerular filtrate enters the proximal tubule. Here, an adenosine triphosphatase pump drives the sodium into tubular cells while chloride ions passively follow. Glucose, amino acid, and other organic compound reabsorption are strongly coupled to sodium in the proximal tubule. Normally, the proximal tubule reabsorbs two-thirds of the filtered sodium, but no active sodium transport occurs in the loop of Henle until the medul-
2 lary thick ascending limb is reached. Cells of the medullary thick ascending limb are metabolically active in their role of reabsorbing sodium and chloride and have a high oxygen consumption compared with the thin portions of the descending and ascending limbs.

Reabsorption of water is a passive, osmotically driven process tied to the reabsorption of sodium and other solutes. Water reabsorption also depends on peritubular capillary pressure; high capillary pressure opposes water reabsorption and tends to increase urine output. The proximal tubule reabsorbs approximately 65% of filtered water in an isosmotic fashion with sodium and chloride. The descending limb of the loop of Henle allows water to follow osmotic gradients into the renal interstitium. However, the thin ascending limb and medullary thick ascending limb are relatively impermeable to water and play a key role in the production of concentrated urine. Only 15% of filtered water is reabsorbed by the loop of Henle; the remaining filtrate volume flows into the distal tubule. There, and in the collecting duct, water reabsorption is controlled entirely by *antidiuretic hormone* (ADH) secreted by the pituitary gland. Conservation of water and excretion of excess solute by the kidneys would be impossible without the ability to produce concentrated urine. This is accomplished by establishing a hyperosmotic medullary interstitium and regulation of water permeability of the distal tubule and collecting duct via the action of ADH.

ADH increases the water permeability of the collecting ducts and allows for passive diffusion of water (under considerable osmotic pressure) back into the circulation. The posterior pituitary

gland releases ADH in response to an increase in either extracellular sodium concentration or extracellular osmolality. In addition, ADH release can be triggered by an absolute or relative reduction in
3 intravascular fluid volume. The arterial baroreceptors are activated when hypovolemia leads to a decrease in blood pressure, whereas atrial receptors are stimulated by a decline in atrial filling pressure. Both of these circulatory reflex systems stimulate release of ADH from the pituitary and cause retention of water by the kidney in an effort to return the intravascular volume toward normal. ADH also causes renal cortical vasoconstriction when it is released in large amounts, such as during the physiologic stress response to trauma, surgery, or other critical illness. This induces a shift of RBF to the hypoxia-prone renal medulla.

The Renin–Angiotensin–Aldosterone System

Renin release by the afferent arteriole may be triggered by hypotension, increased tubular chloride concentration, or by sympathetic stimulation. Renin enhances *angiotensin II* production, which in turn induces renal efferent arteriolar vasoconstriction. Angiotensin II also promotes ADH release from the posterior pituitary, sodium reabsorption by the proximal tubule, and aldosterone release by the adrenal medulla. *Aldosterone* stimulates the distal tubule and collecting duct to reabsorb sodium (and water), resulting in intravascular volume expansion. Sympathetic nervous system stimulation may also directly cause release of aldosterone. This leads to renal cortical vasoconstriction, a decrease in GFR, and salt and water retention.

Renal Vasodilator Mechanisms

Opposing the saline retention and vasoconstriction observed in stress states are the actions of *atrial natriuretic peptide* (ANP), *nitric oxide*, and the renal *prostaglandin* system. ANP is released by the cardiac atria in response to increased stretch under conditions of volume expansion. Both natriuresis and aquaresis increase as ANP blocks reabsorption of sodium in the distal tubule and collecting duct. ANP also increases GFR, causes systemic vasodilatation, inhibits the release of renin, opposes production and action of angiotensin II, and decreases aldosterone secretion.[1,2] Likewise, nitric oxide produced in the kidney opposes the renal vasoconstrictor effects of angiotensin II and the adrenergic nervous system, promotes sodium and water excretion, and participates in tubuloglomerular feedback.[3]

Prostaglandins are produced by the kidney as part of a complex system that modulates RBF and opposes the actions of ADH and the renin–angiotensin–aldosterone system.[4] Stress states, renal ischemia, and hypotension stimulate the production of renal prostaglandins through the enzymes phospholipase A_2 and cyclooxygenase. Prostaglandins produced by cyclooxygenase activity cause dilatation of renal arterioles (antiangiotensin II), whereas their distal tubular effects result in an increase in sodium and water excre-
4 tion (anti-ADH and aldosterone). The renal prostaglandin system is important in maintaining RBF and sodium and water excretion during times of high physiologic stress and poor renal perfusion.[4]

CLINICAL ASSESSMENT OF THE KIDNEY

Most agree that measures such as urine output correlate poorly with perioperative renal function[5]; however, much about the kidneys can be learned from knowing how effectively they clear circulating substances and inspection of the urine (i.e., urinalysis).

Renal Function Tests

Filtration is a useful method to clinically assess kidney function. As a key indicator of disease, knowledge of limited filtration capacity is important to guide drug dosing for agents cleared by the kidneys and helps with preoperative risk stratification. Also, acute declines in filtration capacity indicate kidney injury and predict a more complicated clinical course.[2] *GFR*, as previously mentioned, refers to the plasma volume filtered per unit time by the kidneys, and normal values range from 90 to 140 mL/min. Normal GFRs relate to the patient age, size, and gender. In general, GFR declines 10% per decade after age 30 and is approximately 10 mL/min higher in men than women. A GFR below 60 mL/min meets criteria for chronic kidney disease (CKD) and is considered impaired, while values lower than 15 mL/min are often associated with uremic symptoms and may require dialysis.

An "ideal" substance to assess GFR through its clearance from the circulation must have specific properties, including a steady supply, free filtration, and no tubular reabsorption or excretion; ideally, it is also cheap and easy to measure. Unfortunately, the perfect ideal substance is yet to be identified. The "gold standard" GFR tools involve expensive and cumbersome measurements (e.g., inulin, ^{51}Cr-EDTA or ^{99}Tc-DTPA clearance), while the most practical and inexpensive test involves an imperfect "ideal" substance, *creatinine*. However, despite creatinine's limitations, its relatively steady supply from muscle metabolism, modest tubular secretion, and proven usefulness in numerous clinical settings make it the most used renal filtration marker currently available. Although more ideal substances and other "early biomarkers" of AKI are being evaluated as clinical tools, current candidates (e.g., cystatin C) have yet to replace creatinine.

Estimates of GFR (eGFR) can be made by determining *creatinine clearance* (CrCl) from urine and blood creatinine tests. In stable, critically ill patients, 2-hour urine collections are sufficient to calculate CrCl,[6] using the following formula:

$$\text{CrCl (mL/min)} = U_{Cr}\ \text{(mg/dL)} \times V\ \text{(mL)}/P_{Cr}\ \text{(mg/dL)} \times \text{time (min)}$$

where U_{Cr} = urine creatinine, V = total volume of urine collected, P_{Cr} = plasma creatinine, time = collection time.

However, if patient characteristics are known, GFR can also be estimated from a single steady-state serum creatinine value. Notably, predictive formulas are developed using data from stable (nonsurgical) populations, and factors such as fluid shifts, hemodilution, and hemorrhage may add an "unsteadiness" to perioperative eGFR using serum creatinine.

Nonetheless, serum creatinine remains, so far, an unsurpassed perioperative tool, particularly to reflect *trends* of change in renal filtration and to predict outcome, even during the perioperative period.[7–9] Of the predictive formulas, the Cockroft–Gault equation is one of the oldest and most durable.[10] The Cockroft–Gault equation uses patient gender, age (years), weight (kg), and serum creatinine (mg/dL):

$$\text{Cockroft–Gault eGFR (mL/min)} = (140 - \text{age}) \times \text{weight (kg)}/(\text{Cr} \times 72)(\times 0.85 \text{ for female patients})$$

More recently, a method developed from the Modification of Diet in Renal Disease (MDRD) study that adds other factors including ethnicity (black vs. nonblack) to Cockroft–Gault equation has gained popularity.[11]

An abbreviated MDRD formula is available that can estimate GFR measured in milliliters per minute per 1.73 m^2:

$$\text{GFR} = 186 \times (\text{serum creatinine} - \text{mg/dL})^{-1.154} \times (\text{age})^{-0.203}$$
$$(\times 0.742 \text{ for female patients})$$
$$(\times 1.210 \text{ for black patients})$$

However, even a detailed MDRD eGFR under ideal conditions sometimes correlates poorly with a gold standard-determined GFR, with more than a 30% error in 10% of patients, and 2% deviating more than 50%.[11]

Some consensus definitions for significant perioperative renal dysfunction exist. For example, the Society of Thoracic Surgeons defines postoperative AKI as either a new requirement for dialysis or a rise in serum creatinine to >2 mg/dL involving at least a 50% increase in serum creatinine above baseline.[12] Another definition requires a creatinine rise of >25% or 0.5 mg/dL (44 μmol/L) within 48 hours.[13] The Acute Dialysis Quality Initiative (ADQI) Group definition for critically ill patients grades AKI by an acute creatinine rise of 50% as *r*isk, 100% as *i*njury, or 200% as *f*ailure (the RIFLE criteria).[14] The Acute Kidney Injury Network (AKIN) definition, a 1.5-fold or 0.3 mg/dL (≥26.4 μmol/L) creatinine rise within a 48-hour period or more than 6 hours of oliguria (>0.5 mL/kg/hr), is a modification of its RIFLE predecessor.[14,15] Notably, serum creatinine does not usually rise significantly until GFR rates fall below 50 mL/min, so preoperative serum creatinine may be normal in patients even with some degree of renal dysfunction (Fig. 49-3).

Blood urea nitrogen (BUN) is sometimes used to assess renal function but possesses few of the characteristics of an ideal substance. Tubular urea transport changes with some conditions (e.g., dehydration), and urea generation can be highly variable, particularly during the postoperative period (i.e., catabolic state). In addition, hemodilution (e.g., cardiopulmonary bypass [CPB]) may affect circulating BUN levels.

Urinalysis and Urine Characteristics

Urine inspection can reveal abnormal cloudiness, color, and unexpected odors. Detailed descriptions of urine examination are available[16]; therefore, only a summary is provided here. Cloudy urine is due to suspended elements such as white or red blood cells and/or crystals. Lightly centrifuged urine sediment will normally contain 80 ± 20 mg of protein per day and up to two red blood cells per high-power field (400×); higher levels of red blood cells or protein reflect abnormal kidney function. Urine protein electrophoresis can differentiate proteinuria from a glomerular (filtering), tubular (reuptake), overflow (supply that saturates the reuptake system), or tissue (e.g., kidney inflammation) abnormality.[17] In contrast, color changes reflect dissolved substances; this occurs most commonly with dehydration, but other causes include food colorings, drugs, and liver disease (e.g., bilirubin). Unusual odors are less common but can also be diagnostic (e.g., maple syrup urine disease). Chromogenic "dipstick" chemical tests can determine urine pH and provide a semiquantitative analysis of protein, blood, nitrites, leukocyte esterase, glucose, ketones, urobilinogen, and bilirubin. In addition, microscopy can identify crystals, cells, tubular casts, and bacteria.

Urine *specific gravity* (the weight of urine relative to distilled water) normally ranges between 1.001 and 1.035, and can be used as a surrogate for osmolarity (normal 50 to 1,000 mOsm/kg), with 1.010 reflecting a specific gravity similar to that of plasma. High specific gravity (>1.018) implies preserved renal concentrating ability, unless high levels of glucose, protein, or contrast dye injection have raised specific gravity without significantly changing osmolarity.

Although poor urine output (e.g., <400 mL urine/24 hr) may reflect hypovolemia or impending *prerenal* renal failure, a majority of perioperative AKI episodes develop in the absence of oliguria.[1] The normal response to hypovolemia is renal solute retention; fluid and electrolyte retention produces a concentrated urine with a low sodium content (<20 mEq/L). In contrast, impaired

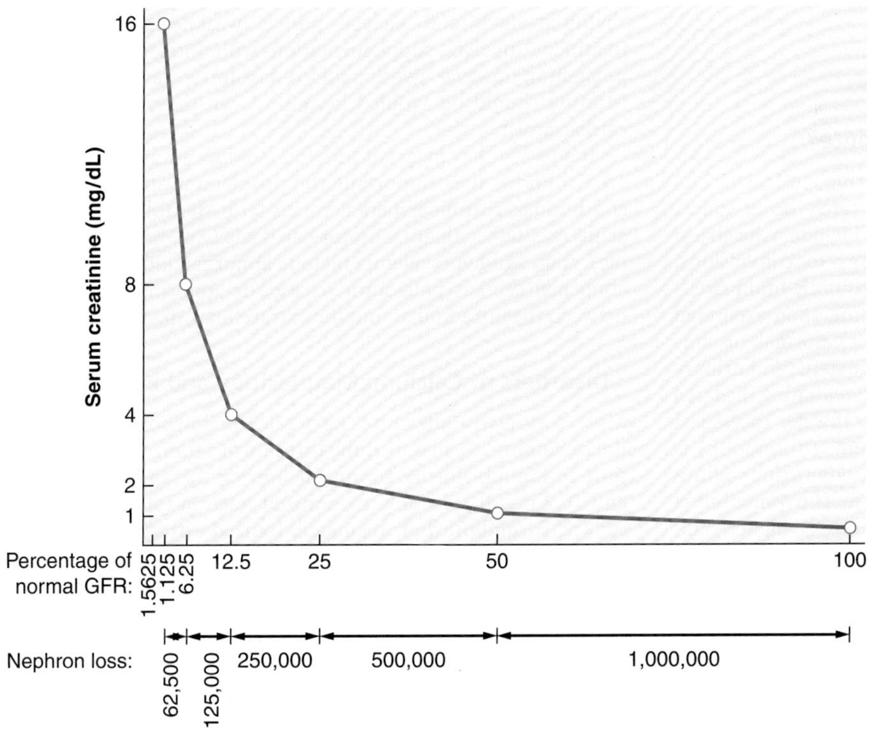

FIGURE 49-3. The nonlinear relationship between changes in renal filtration and serum creatinine level means that a large reduction (e.g., 75%, 120 to 30 mL/min) in glomerular filtration rate (GFR) may be associated with a modest rise in serum creatinine. Proportional reductions in GFR and (approximate) nephron loss (x axis) have an inverse logarithmic relationship with serum creatinine concentration (y axis). (Modified from: Faber MD, Kupin WL, Krishna G, et al. In: Lazarus JM, Brenner BM, eds. *Acute Renal Failure: The differential diagnosis of ARF.* 3rd ed. New York, NY: Churchill Livingstone, 1993, 133, with permission.)

concentrating ability due to AKI causes urine to approach plasma osmolarity (isosthenuria) with a higher sodium content (>40 mEq/L). The kidneys' ability to retain electrolytes is also reflected in the *fractional excretion of sodium* (FE_{Na}), a test that uses a spot sample of urine and blood to compare sodium and creatinine excretion; this test can be useful to distinguish hypovolemia and renal injury:

$$FE_{Na} = U_{Na}/P_{Na} \times P_{Cr}/U_{Cr} \times 100$$

where U_{Na} = urine sodium, P_{Na} = plasma sodium, U_{Cr} = urine creatinine, and P_{Cr} = plasma creatinine.

FE_{Na} <1% implies that sodium is being normally conserved while values above 1% are consistent with acute tubular necrosis (ATN).

PERIOPERATIVE NEPHROLOGY

Pathophysiology

Altered renal function can be thought of as a clinical continuum ranging from the normal compensatory changes seen during stress to frank renal failure. Clinically, there is considerable overlap between compensated and decompensated renal dysfunctional states. The kidney under stress reacts in a predictable manner to help restore intravascular volume and maintain blood pressure. The sympathetic nervous system reacts to trauma, shock, or pain by releasing norepinephrine, which acts much like angiotensin II on the renal arterioles. Norepinephrine also activates the renin–angiotensin–aldosterone system and causes ADH release. The net
5 result of modest activity of the stress response system is a shift of blood flow from the renal cortex to the medulla, avid sodium and water reabsorption, and decreased urine output. A more intense stress response may induce a decrease in RBF and GFR by causing afferent arteriolar constriction. If this extreme situation is not reversed, ischemic damage to the kidney may result, and AKI may become clinically manifest.

Electrolyte Disorders

Disorders of Sodium Balance

Hyponatremia is the most commonly occurring electrolyte disorder[18,19] (see also Chapter 14). Symptoms rarely occur unless sodium values are <125 mmol/L, and these include a spectrum ranging from anorexia, nausea, and lethargy to convulsions, dysrhythmias, coma, and even death due to osmotic brain swelling.[20–22] Hyponatremia may occur in the setting of an expanded (e.g., transurethral resection [TUR] syndrome), normal, or contracted extracellular fluid volume, and volemic status and urinary sodium concentration are key markers in differentiating the large number of potential causes of hyponatremia. If water excess is a reason for hyponatremia, dilute urine (sodium >20 mmol/L) is expected. Conversely, avid renal sodium retention (urine sodium <20 mmol/L) suggests sodium loss as a cause. If hyponatremia is acute, the risk of neurologic complications is higher, and cautious treatment is indicated to prevent cerebral edema and seizures. This should be accomplished with intravenous hypertonic saline and furosemide to enhance water excretion and prevent sodium overload (see transurethral resection syndrome section).

Hypernatremia (serum sodium >145 mmol/L) is generally the result of sodium gain or water loss, most commonly the latter. Dehydration of brain tissue can cause symptoms ranging from confusion to convulsions and coma. In cases of hypernatremia, laboratory studies often show evidence of hemoconcentration (increased hematocrit and serum protein concentrations). In addition, urine output is usually low (<500 mL/day) and hyperosmolar (>1,000 mOsm), with very low urinary sodium concentration and evidence of prerenal failure (elevations of BUN and serum creatinine). Occasionally, the urine is not maximally concentrated, suggesting an osmotic diuresis or an intrinsic renal disorder such as diabetes insipidus. The primary goal of treatment is restoration of serum tonicity, which can be achieved with isotonic or hypotonic parenteral fluids and/or diuretics unless irreversible renal injury is present, in which situation dialysis may be necessary.

Disorders of Potassium Balance

Even minor variations in serum potassium concentration can lead to symptoms such as skeletal muscle weakness, gastrointestinal ileus, myocardial depression, malignant ventricular dysrhythmias, and asystole. Nearly 98% of total body potassium is intracellular. Circulating potassium levels are tightly controlled via renal and gastrointestinal excretion and reabsorption, but potassium also moves between the intra- and extracellular compartments under the influence of insulin and β_2-adrenoceptors. In the kidney, 70% of potassium reabsorption occurs in the proximal tubule and another 15% to 20% in the loop of Henle. The collecting duct is responsible for potassium excretion under the influence of aldosterone.

Hypokalemia may be due to a net potassium deficiency or transfer of extracellular potassium to the intracellular space. Notably, total body depletion may exist even with normal extracellular potassium levels (e.g., diabetic ketoacidosis). Causes of hypokalemia include extrarenal loss (e.g., vomiting, diarrhea), renal loss (impaired processing due to drugs, hormones, or inherited renal abnormalities), potassium shifts between the extra- and intracellular spaces (e.g., insulin therapy), and, occasionally, inadequate intake. Clinical manifestations of hypokalemia include ECG changes (flattened T waves—"no pot, no T", U waves, prodysrhythmic state) and skeletal muscle weakness. Hypokalemia treatment involves supplementation with intravenous or oral potassium; however, overly rapid potassium intravenous administration should be avoided because it can cause hyperkalemic cardiac arrest.

If a patient has *hyperkalemia* (elevated serum potassium level >5.5 mEq/L), it is important to consider the duration of the condition as chronic hyperkalemia is far better tolerated than an acute rise. Other than laboratory artifacts (e.g., hemolyzed sample), causes of hyperkalemia include abnormal kidney excretion, abnormal cellular potassium release, or abnormal distribution between the intracellular and the extracellular space.

Disorders of Calcium, Magnesium, and Phosphorus

Most of a grown adult's 1 to 2 kg of calcium is in bone (98%), with the remaining 2% in one of the three forms: Ionized, chelated, or protein-bound. Normal serum calcium values range between 8.5 and 10.2 mg/dL, but only the ionized fraction (50%) is biologically active and precisely regulated. Ionized extracellular calcium concentration (iCa^{++}) is controlled by the combined actions of parathyroid hormone (PTH), calcitonin, and vitamin D and further modulated by dietary and environmental factors. Hypocalcemia due to reduced serum protein levels is physiologically unimportant. Extracellular magnesium represents only 0.3% of total (mainly intracellular) stores, making normal serum levels (1.6 to 2.2 mg/dL) a poor reflection of total body magnesium.

Phosphorus is a major intracellular anion that plays a role in regulation of glycolysis, ammoniagenesis, and calcium homeostasis and is an essential component of adenosine triphosphate and red blood cell 2,3-diphosphoglyceric acid synthesis.

The clinical manifestations of *hypocalcemia* include cramping, digital numbness, laryngospasm, carpopedal spasm, bronchospasm, seizures, and respiratory arrest. A positive Chvostek sign (facial muscle twitching in response to tapping the facial nerve) or Trousseau sign (carpal spasm induced by brachial artery occlusion) are the classic hallmarks of hypocalcemia but in practice are often absent. Mental status changes, including irritability, depression, and impaired cognition, may also occur. Cardiac manifestations include QT interval shortening and dysrhythmias.

Hypocalcemia may be due to several mechanisms, including a decrease in PTH secretion or action, reduced vitamin D synthesis or action, resistance of bone to PTH or vitamin D effects, or calcium sequestration. Citrate used for regional anticoagulation with dialysis can also cause hypocalcemia and may also lead to hypomagnesemia from decreased PTH secretion. Parathyroidectomy during neck surgery reduces PTH levels and is a common cause of acquired hypoparathyroidism.

Clinical symptoms of *hypercalcemia* correlate with its acuity and include constipation, nausea and vomiting, drowsiness, lethargy, weakness, stupor, and coma. Cardiovascular manifestations may include hypertension, shortened QT interval, heart block, and other dysrhythmias. The most frequent causes of hypercalcemia are primary hyperparathyroidism and malignancy. Other causes include thiazide (increased renal calcium reabsorption) or lithium (inhibits PTH release) therapy and rarer medical conditions including granulomatous disease, thyrotoxicosis, and multiple endocrine neoplasia (MEN) types I and II.

Hypomagnesemia (<1.6 mg/dL) may sometimes be asymptomatic, but clinically important problems can and do manifest, including neuromuscular, cardiac, neurologic, and related electrolytic (hypokalemia and hypocalcemia) abnormalities. Causes of hypomagnesemia can be divided in four broad categories: Decreased intake, gastrointestinal loss, renal loss, and redistribution. Nutritional hypomagnesemia can result from malabsorption syndromes in patients receiving parenteral nutrition, and it is also present in 25% of alcoholics. Redistribution occurs with acute pancreatitis, administration of catecholamines, and in "hungry bone syndrome" after parathyroidectomy.[10] Magnesium can be supplemented orally or via the parenteral route.

Clinical manifestations of *hypermagnesemia* (>4 to 6 mg/dL) are serious and potentially fatal. Minor symptoms include hypotension, nausea, vomiting, facial flushing, urinary retention, and ileus. In more extreme cases, flaccid skeletal muscular paralysis, hyporeflexia, bradycardia, bradydysrhythmias, respiratory depression, coma, and cardiac arrest may occur. Hypermagnesemia generally occurs in two clinical settings: Compromised renal function (GFR <20 mL/min) and excessive magnesium intake (e.g., excessive intravenous therapy in preeclampsia). Although mild hypermagnesemia in the setting of normal renal function can be treated with supportive care and withdrawal of the cause, in some cases dialysis is necessary.

Hypophosphatemia is clinically more important than hyperphosphatemia and can result in symptoms including muscle weakness, respiratory failure, and difficulty in weaning critically ill patients from mechanical ventilation when serum levels are <0.32 mmol/L. In addition, low phosphate levels may diminish oxygen delivery to tissues and rarely cause hemolysis. Hypophosphatemia can result from intracellular redistribution (from catecholamine therapy), from inadequate intake or absorption secondary to alcoholism or malnutrition, or from increased renal or gastrointestinal losses.[12] Intravenous and oral supplementation can be used to treat hypophosphatemia.

Hyperphosphatemia (>5 mg/dL) is generally related to accompanying hypocalcemia although increased phosphate levels may also lead to calcium precipitation and decreased intestinal calcium absorption.[13,14] Significantly elevated serum phosphate levels are most commonly due to reduced excretion from renal insufficiency but can also result from excess intake or redistribution of intracellular phosphorus. Treatment of chronic hyperphosphatemia includes dietary phosphate restriction and oral phosphate binders.

Acid–Base Disorders

The primary determinant of serum pH is the balance between plasma bicarbonate (HCO_3^-) concentration and the PCO_2 in the extracellular space. Acid–base homeostasis involves tight regulation of HCO_3^- and $PaCO_2$. Primary extracellular pH derangements due to abnormal bicarbonate reabsorption and proton (H^+) elimination by the kidney lead to metabolic acidosis or alkalosis, while factors that abnormally affect respiratory drive influence $PaCO_2$, leading to respiratory acidosis or alkalosis. Because combined problems are often seen in perioperative critically ill patients, an approach to both "pure" and "mixed" acid–base disorders is presented here.

Metabolic Acidosis

The *anion gap* (AG) represents the total serum concentration of unmeasured anions and can be calculated as $AG = (Na^+ + K^+) - (HCO_3^- + Cl^-)$. It allows differentiation of the causes of metabolic acidosis into normal AG (8 ± 4) and increased AG (>16 mmol/L) varieties. Conditions that cause an increase in negatively charged ions other than bicarbonate and chloride (e.g., lactate, salicylate) increase the AG. In contrast, non-AG metabolic acidosis results from renal or gastrointestinal HCO_3^- loss and is associated with high chloride levels (hyperchloremic metabolic acidosis). The usual compensatory response to all types of metabolic acidoses is hyperventilation, which leads to a partial pH correction toward normal. Winter's formula predicts expected $PaCO_2$ for a metabolic acidosis as follows: $PaCO_2 = (1.5 \times HCO_3^-) + 8$.

Metabolic Alkalosis

Metabolic alkalosis is a common primary acid–base disturbance associated with increased plasma HCO_3^-. Increased extracellular HCO_3^- is due to a net loss of H^+ and/or addition of HCO_3^-. The most common cause of metabolic alkalosis is gastrointestinal acid loss due to vomiting or nasogastric suctioning; the resulting hypovolemia leads to secretion of renin and aldosterone and enhanced absorption of HCO_3^-. Thiazides and loop diuretics both induce a net loss of chloride and free water and can cause a volume "contraction" alkalosis.

Respiratory Acidosis

If the lungs fail to eliminate CO_2, hypercapnia and respiratory acidosis result, characterized by increased $PaCO_2$ and decreased blood pH. Acute and chronic causes can be differentiated by examining arterial pH, $PaCO_2$, and HCO_3^- values. In the early phase of respiratory acidosis, increased $PaCO_2$ stimulates renal generation and secretion of H^+. The kidneys continue to adapt to the increased pH through greater titratable acid excretion (e.g., ammonium) and HCO_3^- generation. Therefore, acute respiratory acidosis is characterized by an elevated $PaCO_2$, acidemia, and a relatively normal HCO_3^-. In contrast, chronic respiratory acidosis is associated with an elevated HCO_3^- (often accompanied by a relatively normal pH) due to renal compensation.

Respiratory Alkalosis

Increased minute ventilation is the primary cause of respiratory alkalosis, characterized by decreased $PaCO_2$ and increased pH. Patients with acute, uncompensated respiratory alkalosis have normal plasma HCO_3^-. In chronic respiratory alkalosis, renal compensation leads to decreased plasma HCO_3^-. The causes of respiratory alkalosis relate to abnormal respiratory drive from stimulants or toxins (e.g., salicylate, caffeine, nicotine, progesterone), central nervous system abnormalities (e.g., anxiety, stroke, increased intracranial pressure), pulmonary abnormalities (e.g., pulmonary embolism, pneumonia), mechanical hyperventilation, or systemic conditions such as liver failure and sepsis.

Mixed Acid–Base Disorders

It is not uncommon for a metabolic derangement to coexist with a respiratory derangement, particularly in intensive care patients. A general approach to the diagnosis of mixed acid–base disorders requires a step-wise approach that begins with a focused history and physical examination. An arterial blood gas and a concurrent serum chemistry panel (including Na^+, K^+, Cl^-, and total CO_2 concentrations) should also be obtained, and the use of an acid–base map may help differentiate simple from mixed disorders (Fig. 49-4).

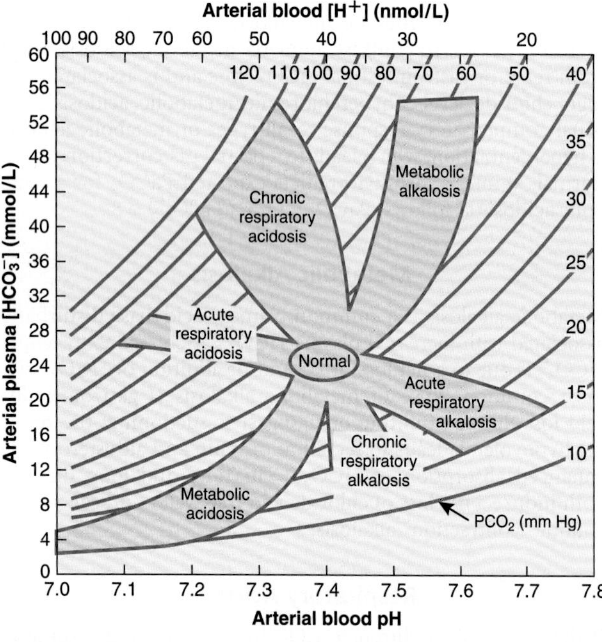

FIGURE 49-4. Acid–base map. Plotting the PCO_2 and H^+ (from the arterial blood gas) against plasma HCO_3^- (from the serum chemistry panel) for a patient can identify simple acid–base disorders. When mixed disorders exist, values may fall outside the shaded areas. (From: DuBose TD Jr. In: Brenner BM, ed. *Acid-Base Disorders, Brenner & Rector's The Kidney.* 7th ed. Philadelphia, PA: WB Saunders; 2004:938, with permission.)

Acute Kidney Conditions

Acute Kidney Injury

Acute kidney injury (AKI) is now the preferred term for an acute deterioration in renal function. It is associated with a decline in glomerular filtration and results in inability of the kidneys to excrete nitrogenous and other wastes. This manifests as an accumulation of creatinine and urea in the blood (uremia) and is often accompanied by reduced urine production, although nonoliguric forms of postoperative AKI are common.[16] Isolated AKI carries a mortality of <10%.[17] In surgical patients, ATN is the most common cause of AKI. AKI frequently occurs in the setting of critical illness with multiple organ failure when the mortality is
6 alarmingly high (up to 90%).[18] Notably, extracorporeal renal support appears to have little impact in altering the generally poor outcome associated with AKI in critically ill surgical patients.[19,20] Even studies that advocate the use of extracorporeal technology report mortality of between 50% and 70%.[21–24]

AKI can be caused by *prerenal* factors causing renal hypoperfusion, *intrinsic* renal causes, or *postrenal* causes (obstructive uropathy). There are many pathophysiologic similarities between the various causes of kidney injury.

Prerenal Azotemia

Prerenal azotemia is the increase in BUN associated with renal hypoperfusion or ischemia that has not yet caused renal parenchymal damage. The metabolically active cells of the medullary thick ascending limb of the loop of Henle are especially vulnerable to hypoxic damage because of their relatively high oxygen consumption.[25] AKI ensues when necrosis of tubular cells releases debris into the tubules, causing flow obstruction, increased tubular back pressure, and leak of tubular fluid. Often, prerenal AKI is precipitated in patients with pre-existing renal vasoconstriction (e.g., volume depletion, heart failure, or sepsis) by nephrotoxin exposure or further reductions in cardiac output.[26]

Intrinsic Acute Kidney Injury

The term *intrinsic* not only implies a primary renal cause of AKI but also includes AKI due to ischemia, nephrotoxins, and renal parenchymal diseases. ATN remains the most common ischemic lesion and represents an extension of prerenal azotemia, whereas cortical necrosis may follow a massive renovascular insult such as prolonged suprarenal aortic clamping or renal artery embolism. Nephrotoxins often act in concert with hypoperfusion or underlying renal vasoconstrictive states to damage renal tubules or the microvasculature. Several common nephrotoxins, some of which are difficult to avoid in a hospitalized patient population, are listed in Table 49-1.

Postrenal Acute Kidney Injury (Obstructive Uropathy)

Downstream obstruction of the urinary collecting system is the least common pathway to established AKI, accounting for <5% of cases.[27] Because it can generally be corrected, it is extremely important to exclude with a renal ultrasound examination as a source of AKI. The obstructing lesion may occur at any level of the collecting system, from the renal pelvis to the distal urethra. Intraluminal pressure rises and is eventually transmitted back to the glomerulus, thereby reducing glomerular filtration pressure and rate.

TABLE 49-1. NEPHROTOXINS COMMONLY FOUND IN THE HOSPITAL SETTING

Exogenous	Endogenous
Antibiotics (aminoglycosides, cephalosporins, amphotericin B, sulfonamide, tetracyclines, vancomycin)	Calcium (hypercalcemia)
Anesthetic agents (methoxyflurane, enflurane)	Uric acid (hyperuricemia and hyperuricosuria)
Nonsteroidal anti-inflammatory drugs	Myoglobin (rhabdomyolysis)
(Aspirin, ibuprofen, naproxen, indomethacin, ketorolac)	Hemoglobin (hemolysis)
Chemotherapeutic–immunosuppressive agents	Bilirubin (obstructive jaundice)
(Cisplatinum, cyclosporin A, methotrexate, mitomycin, nitrosoureas, tacrolimus)	Oxalate crystals
Contrast media	Paraproteins

Nephrotoxins and Perioperative Acute Kidney Injury

Nephrotoxin exposure is a common occurrence in hospitalized patients and frequently plays a role in the cause of AKI in this population. Nephrotoxins may take the form of drugs, nontherapeutic chemicals, heavy metals, poisons, and endogenous compounds (Table 49-1). The nephrotoxins most likely to contribute to renal dysfunction/failure in the perioperative period are certain antimicrobial and chemotherapeutic–immunosuppressive agents, radiocontrast media, nonsteroidal anti-inflammatory drugs (NSAIDs), and the endogenous heme pigments myoglobin and hemoglobin. These diverse groups of renal toxins share a common pathophysiologic characteristic: They disturb either renal oxygen delivery or oxygen utilization and thereby promote renal ischemia.

Antimicrobial and chemotherapeutic–immunosuppressive agents are effective because they are cellular toxins. When these drugs are filtered, reabsorbed, secreted, and eventually excreted by the kidney, toxic concentrations in renal cells can be reached. The aminoglycoside antibiotics and amphotericin B are particularly difficult to avoid because they are effective antimicrobials, with few available alternatives. Their effect can be additive with other nephrotoxic factors causing impairment of kidney function. Hypovolemia, fever, renal vasoconstriction, and concomitant therapy with other nephrotoxic agents should be avoided wherever possible. Electrolyte disorders such as hypercalcemia, hypomagnesemia, hypokalemia, and metabolic acidosis can further enhance nephrotoxic damage to the kidney.

Cyclosporin A and tacrolimus are indispensable components of many immunosuppressive drug regimens, but in combination with other nephrotoxins and clinical factors, they can cause acute and exacerbate chronic kidney injuries in transplant recipients.[23]

Radiocontrast media poses a threat to the renal function of patients with diabetic nephropathy, pre-existing renal vasoconstriction (heart failure, hypovolemia), or renal insufficiency.[24] Radiocontrast dye has effects on renal function that develop 24 to 48 hours after exposure and peak at 3 to 5 days. Measures that may prevent AKI or lessen the severity of renal damage include prehydration, smaller contrast doses, and judicious withholding of other nephrotoxins, such as NSAIDs. Elective surgery should be postponed until the effects of the dye have resolved. The idea that pretreatment with *N*-acetylcysteine can prevent radiocontrast nephropathy in patients with renal insufficiency[25] has now largely been abandoned.

NSAIDs produce reversible inhibition of prostaglandin synthesis and are well-known nephrotoxins.[26] Except in cases of massive overdose, NSAIDs produce renal dysfunction only in patients with coexisting renal hypoperfusion or vasoconstriction. Advanced age, hypovolemia, end-stage hepatic disease, heart failure, sepsis, chronic renal insufficiency, and major surgery are risk factors for development of NSAID-induced AKI.[27]

Myoglobin and hemoglobin are both capable of causing AKI in critically ill surgical patients. Myoglobin seems to be a more potent nephrotoxin than hemoglobin because it is more readily filtered at the glomerulus and can be reabsorbed by the renal tubules, where it chelates nitric oxide and thus induces medullary vasoconstriction and ischemia.[28] Hypovolemia and acidemia potentiate the toxicity of both pigments. Reduced intravascular volume causes a decrease in RBF and GFR, which results in a smaller volume of tubular fluid with a relatively higher concentration of pigment. There is also evidence suggesting that pigment precipitation inside the tubular lumen is enhanced under acidotic conditions and that tubular obstruction plays a role in the pathogenesis of AKI.[28,29]

Preventive treatment of pigment-induced AKI is directed at increasing RBF and tubular (urine) flow while correcting any existing acidosis. These goals may be accomplished by expanding the intravascular fluid volume with crystalloid infusion, stimulating an osmotic diuresis with mannitol, and increasing the urine pH with intravenous bicarbonate therapy.[30] Adequate systemic resuscitation from shock is a prerequisite if AKI is to be avoided, especially in massive crush injuries and electrical burns. Forced mannitol-alkali diuresis is indicated as the second step in the preventive treatment of myoglobinuria, with urine flow rates of up to 300 mL/hr and a urine pH of >6.5 advocated for patients with massive crush injuries.[30]

The nephrotoxicity of volatile agents remains controversial. Inhalation anesthetics such as enflurane, isoflurane, and sevoflurane can generate free fluoride ions during their metabolism, which (when levels are >50 μM/L) may cause polyuric AKI by interfering with tubular concentrating ability. However, peak fluoride levels during administration of these agents seldom reach toxic levels, and there are few reports describing volatile agent–induced nephrotoxicity.[31] The potential of sevoflurane-induced nephrotoxicity has been related to the production of compound A during prolonged, low fresh gas flow, sevoflurane anesthesia.[32] Although there
7 are insufficient data to conclude that sevoflurane-induced kidney injury occurs in the human population, even during low gas flow anesthesia, it is probably prudent to maintain a fresh gas flow of at least 2 L/min formation during sevoflurane anesthesia.[33]

Chronic Kidney Disease

Patients with nondialysis-dependent CKD are at increased risk of developing *end-stage renal disease* (ESRD). ESRD is the term used to describe a clinical syndrome characterized by renal dysfunction that would prove fatal without renal replacement therapy. These patients have GFRs <25% of normal. Lesser degrees of renal dysfunction may be categorized as chronic renal insufficiency (25% to 40% of normal GFR) or decreased renal reserve (60% to 75% of normal GFR). Patients with decreased renal reserve are often asymptomatic and frequently do not have elevated blood
8 levels of creatinine or urea. Established renal insufficiency results in patently abnormal serum creatinine and BUN values, but nocturia (due to reduced concentrating ability) may be the only symptom.

The *uremic syndrome* represents an extreme form of chronic renal failure, which occurs as the surviving nephron population and GFR decreases below 10% of normal. It results in inability of the kidney to perform its two major functions: Regulation of the volume and composition of the extracellular fluid and excretion of waste products. Water balance in ESRD becomes difficult to manage because the number of functioning nephrons is too small either to concentrate or to fully dilute the urine. This results in failure both to conserve water and to excrete excess water. Patients with uremic syndrome often require frequent or continuous dialysis.

Life-threatening hyperkalemia may occur in CKD because of slower-than-normal potassium clearance. Situations predisposing patients with renal failure to hyperkalemia are presented in Table 49-2. Derangements in calcium, magnesium, and phosphorus metabolism are also commonly seen in CKD (Table 49-3).

TABLE 49-2. FACTORS CONTRIBUTING TO HYPERKALEMIA IN CHRONIC RENAL FAILURE

Potassium Intake
Increased dietary intake
Exogenous IV supplementation
Potassium salts of drugs
Sodium substitutes
Blood transfusion
Gastrointestinal hemorrhage
Potassium Release from Intracellular Stores
Increased catabolism, sepsis
Metabolic acidosis
β-Adrenergic blocking agents
Digitalis intoxication (Na–K-ATPase inhibition)
Insulin deficiency
Succinylcholine
Potassium Excretion
Acute decrease in GFR
Constipation
Potassium-sparing diuretics
Angiotensin-converting enzyme inhibitors (decreased aldosterone secretion)
Heparin (decreased aldosterone effect)

IV, intravenous; Na–K-ATPase, Na–K-adenosine triphosphatase; GFR, glomerular filtration rate.

TABLE 49-3. THE UREMIC SYNDROME

Water Homeostasis
Extracellular fluid expansion
Electrolyte and Acid–base
Hyponatremia
Hyperkalemia
Hypercalcemia or hypocalcemia
Hyperphosphatemia
Hypermagnesemia
Metabolic acidosis
Cardiovascular
Heart failure
Hypertension
Pericarditis
Myocardial dysfunction
Dysrhythmias
Respiratory
Pulmonary edema
Central hyperventilation
Hematologic
Anemia
Platelet hemostatic defect
Immunologic
Cell-mediated and humoral immunity defects
Gastrointestinal
Delayed gastric emptying, anorexia, nausea, vomiting, hiccups, upper gastrointestinal tract inflammation/hemorrhage
Neuromuscular
Encephalopathy, seizures, tremors, myoclonus
Sensory and motor polyneuropathy
Autonomic dysfunction, decreased baroreceptor responsiveness, dialysis-associated hypotension
Endocrine Metabolism
Renal osteodystrophy
$\downarrow$ Glucose intolerance
Hypertriglyceridemia, $\uparrow$ atherosclerosis

Metabolic acidosis occurs in two forms in ESRD: A hyperchloremic, normal AG acidosis and a high AG acidosis from inability to excrete titratable acids. Both render patients susceptible to an endogenous acid load such as may occur in shock states, hypovolemia, or with an increase in catabolism.

Cardiovascular complications of the uremic syndrome are primarily due to volume overload, high renin–angiotensin activity, autonomic nervous system hyperactivity, acidosis, and electrolyte disturbances. Hypertension due to extracellular fluid volume expansion, autonomic factors, and hyperreninemia is an almost universal finding in ESRD. Together with volume overload, acidemia, anemia, and possibly the presence of high-flow arteriovenous fistulae created for dialysis access, hypertension may contribute to the development of myocardial dysfunction and heart failure. Pericarditis may occur secondary to uremia or dialysis, with pericardial tamponade developing in 20% of the latter group.[34] Pulmonary problems associated with CKD are limited to changes in lung water and control of ventilation. Pulmonary edema and restrictive pulmonary dysfunction are commonly seen in patients with renal failure and are usually responsive to dialysis. Hypervolemia, heart failure, reduced serum oncotic pressure, and increased pulmonary capillary permeability are relevant factors in the development of pulmonary edema. Chronic metabolic acidosis may also be responsible for the hyperventilation seen in patients with ESRD, but increased lung water and poor pulmonary compliance can also stimulate hyperventilation.

The anemia of CKD occurs as a result of reduced levels of erythropoietin, red cell damage, ongoing gastrointestinal blood loss, and iron or vitamin deficiencies. Platelet dysfunction may aggravate blood loss, but it is responsive to dialysis, cryoprecipitate administration, and desmopressin acetate (or 1-deamino-8-D-arginine vasopressin [DDAVP]). Acquired defects in both cellular and humoral immunity probably account for the high prevalence of serious infections (60%) and high mortality from sepsis in CKD (30%).

Drug Prescribing in Renal Failure

If a drug depends solely on the kidney for clearance, then a simple approach to prescribing might involve a calculated percentage reduction in drug dosage that matches the reduction in GFR. Although GFR can be accurately measured, an estimated clearance derived from serum creatinine is usually adequate for these purposes. Unfortunately, clearance of most medications involves a more complex combination of both hepatic and renal functions, and drug level measurement or algorithms for specific drugs are often recommended.

AKI may affect absorption of a drug. For example, a reduced first-pass effect through the gastrointestinal tract and liver is associated with increased serum levels of oral β-blockers and opioids in patients with AKI. Also, an increase in the volume of distribution is seen in most patients with CKD due to increased plasma volume and decreased plasma protein binding. However, plasma protein binding is highly variable, with acidic drugs having reduced binding and basic agents (e.g., amide local anesthetics) having increased binding. Importantly, for drugs with less binding, "normal" drug levels may reflect dangerously high active (unbound) drug levels. For example, therapeutic phenytoin levels are typically reported as being in the range of 10 to 20 mg/mL normally but 4 to 10 mg/mL in cases of renal failure. Finally, hepatic metabolism of drugs is difficult to predict in the setting of renal failure because some hepatic enzymes are inhibited whereas others are induced, and accompanying liver disorders may alter the relationship of drug clearance with GFR.

Anesthetic Agents in Renal Failure

With the exception of methoxyflurane and possibly enflurane, anesthetic agents do not directly cause renal dysfunction or interfere with the normal compensatory mechanisms activated by the stress response. The nephrotoxicity of methoxyflurane appears to be due to its metabolism, which results in release of the fluoride ions believed responsible for the renal injury.[35] It has been suggested that renal, not hepatic, metabolism of methoxyflurane may be responsible for generating fluoride ions locally that contribute to nephrotoxicity.[36] Enflurane nephrotoxicity may also occur[37] but is of minor clinical importance, even in patients with preexisting renal dysfunction. Although direct anesthetic effects on the kidney are usually not harmful, indirect effects may combine with hypovolemia, shock, nephrotoxin exposure, or other renal vasoconstrictive states to produce renal dysfunction. If the chosen anesthetic technique causes a protracted reduction in cardiac output or sustained hypotension that coincides with a period of intense renal vasoconstriction, renal dysfunction or failure could result. This is true for either general or regional anesthesia. There are no comparative studies demonstrating superior renal protection or improved renal outcome with general versus regional anesthesia.

Significant renal impairment may affect the disposition, metabolism, and excretion of the commonly used anesthetic agents. Inhalation anesthetics are, of course, an exception to the rule that drugs with central nervous system activity (which generally are lipid soluble) must be converted to more hydrophilic compounds by the liver before being excreted by the kidney. The water-soluble metabolites of agents that are not inhaled may accumulate in renal failure and display prolonged pharmacodynamic effects if they possess even a small percentage of the pharmacologic activity of the parent drug. Drugs that are eliminated unchanged by the kidneys (e.g., certain nondepolarizing muscle relaxants, the cholinesterase inhibitors, many antibiotics, digoxin) have a prolonged elimination half-life when given to patients with kidney failure. Many drugs used in anesthesia are highly protein-bound and may demonstrate exaggerated clinical effects when protein binding is reduced by uremia.

Induction Agents and Sedatives

Although now rarely used, sodium thiopental serves as a good illustrative example of how reduced protein binding in CKD may affect the clinical use of an anesthetic agent. Burch and Stanski[38] showed that the free fraction of an induction dose of thiopental is almost doubled in patients with renal failure. This accounts for the exaggerated clinical effects seen with thiopental in CKD patients and the substantial reduction in the necessary induction dose of this agent in uremic patients when compared with patients with normal renal function.

Ketamine is less extensively protein-bound than thiopental, and renal failure appears to have less influence on its free fraction. Redistribution and hepatic metabolism are largely responsible for termination of the anesthetic effects, with <3% of the drug excreted unchanged in the urine. Norketamine, the major metabolite, has one-third the pharmacologic activity of the parent drug and is further metabolized before it is excreted by the kidney.[39]

Etomidate, although only 75% protein-bound in normal patients, has a larger free fraction in patients with ESRD.[40] The decrease in protein binding does not seem to alter the clinical effects of an etomidate anesthetic induction in patients with renal failure.

Propofol undergoes extensive, rapid hepatic biotransformation to inactive metabolites that are renally excreted. Its pharmacokinetics appear to be unchanged in patients with renal failure,[41] and there are no reports of prolongation of its effects in ESRD.

The benzodiazepines, as a group, are extensively protein-bound. CKD increases the free fraction of benzodiazepines in the plasma, and this potentiates their clinical effect. Certain benzodiazepine metabolites are pharmacologically active and have the potential to accumulate with repeated administration of the parent drug to anephric patients. For example, 60% to 80% of midazolam is excreted as its (active) α-hydroxy metabolite,[42] which accumulates during long-term infusions in patients with renal failure.[42] AKI appears to slow the plasma clearance of midazolam, whereas repeated diazepam or lorazepam administration in CKD may carry a risk of active metabolite-induced sedation. Alprazolam is one of the few drugs related to anesthesia practice that has undergone pharmacodynamic studies in patients with CKD. Schmith et al.[43] found that when decreased protein binding and increased free fraction of alprazolam are taken into account, patients with CKD are actually more sensitive to its sedative effects than healthy persons.

Dexmedetomidine is primarily metabolized in the liver. Volunteers with renal impairment receiving dexmedetomidine experienced a long-lasting sedative effect than subjects with normal kidney function. The most likely explanation is that less protein binding of dexmedetomidine occurs in subjects with renal dysfunction.[44]

Opioids

Single-dose studies of the pharmacokinetics of morphine in renal failure demonstrate no alteration in its disposition. However, chronic administration results in accumulation of its 6-glucuronide metabolite, which has potent analgesic and sedative effects.[45] There is also a decrease in protein binding of morphine in ESRD, which mandates a reduction in its initial dose. Meperidine is remarkable for its neurotoxic, renally excreted metabolite (normeperidine) and is not recommended for use in patients with poor renal function. Hydromorphone is metabolized to hydromorphone-3-glucuronide, which is excreted by the kidneys. This active metabolite accumulates in patients with renal failure and may cause cognitive dysfunction and myoclonus.[46] Codeine also has the potential for causing prolonged narcosis in patients with renal failure and cannot be recommended for long-term use.[45]

Fentanyl appears to be a better choice of opioid for use in ESRD because of its lack of active metabolites, unchanged free fraction, and short redistribution phase.[47] Small-to-moderate doses, titrated to effect, are well tolerated by uremic patients.

Alfentanil has been shown to have reduced protein binding but no change in its elimination half-life or clearance in ESRD and is extensively metabolized to inactive compounds.[48] Therefore, caution should be exercised in administering a loading dose, but the total dose and infusion dose should be similar to those for patients with normal renal function. The free fraction of sufentanil is unchanged in ESRD; however, its pharmacokinetics are variable, and it has been reported to cause prolonged narcosis.[49]

Remifentanil is rapidly metabolized by blood and tissue esterases to a weakly active (about 4,600 times less potent) μ-opioid agonist and renally excreted metabolite, remifentanil acid. Renal failure has no effect on the clearance of remifentanil, but elimination of the principal metabolite, remifentanil acid, is markedly reduced. However, the clinical implications of this metabolite are likely limited.[50]

Muscle Relaxants

Muscle relaxants are the most likely group of drugs used in anesthetic practice to produce prolonged effects in ESRD because of their dependence on renal excretion (Table 49-4). Only succinylcholine, atracurium, *cis*-atracurium, and mivacurium appear to have minimal renal excretion of the unchanged parent compound. Most nondepolarizing muscle relaxants must be either hepatically excreted or metabolized to inactive forms in order to terminate their activity. Some muscle relaxants have renally excreted, active metabolites that may contribute to their prolonged duration of action in patients with ESRD. Although the following discussion focuses on the pharmacology of individual muscle relaxants, coexisting acidosis and electrolyte disturbances, as well as drug therapy (e.g., aminoglycosides, diuretics, immunosuppressants, magnesium-containing antacids), may alter the pharmacodynamics of muscle relaxants in patients with renal failure.[51]

Succinylcholine has a long history of use in CKD that has been somewhat confused by conflicting reports of plasma cholinesterase activity in renal failure.[52,53] Provided the serum potassium concentration is not dangerously elevated, its use can be justified as part of a rapid-sequence induction technique because its duration of action in ESRD is not significantly prolonged. Use of a continuous infusion of succinylcholine, however, is more problematic because the major metabolite, succinylmonocholine, is weakly active and excreted by the kidney. Concern about the increase in serum potassium levels after succinylcholine administration (0.5 mEq/L in normal subjects) implies that the serum potassium should be normalized to the extent possible in patients with renal failure, but clinical experience has shown that the acute small increase in potassium following administration of succinylcholine is generally well tolerated in patients with *chronically* elevated serum potassium levels. Use of the long-acting muscle relaxants doxacurium, pancuronium, and pipecuronium might also be questioned in patients with known renal insufficiency. In a single-dose study of doxacurium, Cook et al.[54] demonstrated an increased elimination half-life, reduced plasma clearance, and prolonged duration of effect in patients with renal failure. Similar findings have been reported for the pharmacokinetics of pipecuronium.

TABLE 49-4. NONDEPOLARIZING MUSCLE RELAXANTS IN RENAL FAILURE

Drug	% Renal Excretion	Half-life (hr) Normal/ESRD	Renally Excreted Active Metabolite	Use in ESRD
d-Tubocurarine	60	1.4–2.2	–	Avoid
Metocurine	45–60	6/11.4	–	Avoid
Pancuronium	30	2.3/4–8	+	Avoid
Gallamine	>85	2.5/6–20	–	Avoid
Pipecuronium	37	1.8–2.3/4.4	+	Avoid
Doxacurium	30	1.7/3.7	–	Avoid
Vecuronium	30	0.9/1.4	+	Avoid infusion
Rocuronium	30	1.2–1.6/1.6–1.7	–	Variable duration
Atracurium/ *cis*-atracurium	<5	0.3/0.4	–	Normal
Mivacurium	<7	2 min/2 min	–	Duration 1.5 × normal
Rapacuronium	<12	0.5/0.5	++	Normal single dose

ESRD, end-stage renal disease.

Intermediate-acting muscle relaxants (atracurium, *cis*-atracurium, vecuronium, and rocuronium) have a distinct advantage in ESRD because of their shorter duration. The risk of a clinically significant, prolonged block is much reduced. Atracurium and its derivative, *cis*-atracurium, undergo enzymatic ester hydrolysis and spontaneous nonenzymatic (Hoffman) degradation with minimal renal excretion of the parent compound. Their elimination half-life, clearance, and duration of action are not affected by renal failure,[55] nor have they been reported to cause prolonged clinical effects in ESRD. These characteristics strongly support their use in patients with renal disease. One potential concern is that an atracurium metabolite, laudanosine, may cause seizures in experimental animals and may accumulate with repeated dosing or continuous infusion.[56] However, this has not been realized in intensive care patients with renal failure receiving prolonged infusions of atracurium. Consistent with its greater potency and lower dosing requirements, *cis*-atracurium metabolism results in lower laudanosine blood levels than does atracurium in ESRD patients.

The pharmacokinetics of vecuronium were initially reported as unchanged in renal failure, but it was later demonstrated that its duration of action was prolonged as a result of reduced plasma clearance and increased elimination half-life.[55] In addition, the active metabolite, 3-desmethylvecuronium, was shown to accumulate in anephric patients receiving a continuous vecuronium infusion who subsequently had prolonged neuromuscular blockade. An intubating dose would be expected to last approximately 50% longer in patients with ESRD.[57]

Rocuronium, a rapid-onset muscle relaxant, has a pharmacokinetic profile in normal subjects similar to that of vecuronium.[58] Single-dose pharmacokinetic studies in patients with renal failure have reported conflicting results. Szenohradszky et al.[59] reported that renal failure increased the volume of distribution and elimination half-life of rocuronium but had no effect on its clearance. Cooper et al.[60] found that its clearance was reduced, and the duration of block was widely variable in patients with renal failure, although the mean duration of relaxation and spontaneous recovery was not statistically different from that in control subjects.

The short-acting muscle relaxant mivacurium is enzymatically eliminated by plasma pseudocholinesterase at a somewhat slower rate than succinylcholine. Low pseudocholinesterase activity correlates with slower recovery from a bolus dose of mivacurium in anephric patients.[53] The maintenance infusion dose has been reported to be both lower[61] and similar[62] to that in normal control subjects.

The pharmacokinetics of the clinically available anticholinesterases are affected by renal failure.[63] They have a prolonged duration of action in ESRD because of their heavy reliance on renal excretion. The anticholinergic agents atropine and glycopyrrolate, used in conjunction with the anticholinesterases, are similarly excreted by the kidney. Therefore, no dosage alteration of the anticholinesterases is required when antagonizing neuromuscular blockade in patients with reduced renal function.

Diuretic Drugs: Effects and Mechanisms

Fluid overload occurs when salt or water intake exceeds renal and extrarenal losses and is characterized by increased total body water and usually sodium. Fluid overload may be evenly distributed among the body compartments (e.g., congestive heart failure), or the interstitial space may be increased while the circulating blood volume may be normal or even decreased (e.g., posttraumatic or postoperative fluid shifts). Edema results when Starling forces favor passage of fluid into the interstitial space. A variety of chronic medical conditions (congestive heart failure, renal failure, or hepatic cirrhosis) can lead to fluid overload and edema that may even require surgery to be delayed for treatment to reduce operative risk. The first line of therapy for fluid overload that includes all body compartments involves restriction of salt and water ingestion; however, diuretic therapy is often indicated.

The Physiologic Basis of Diuretic Action

Diuretics are typically grouped according to their site and mechanism of action (Fig. 49-5). Under normal conditions, kidney function assures that <1% of the filtered Na^+ load enters the urine (i.e., the fractional excretion of Na^+ (FENa) is <1%). The Na^+/K^+-ATPase pump on the basolateral surface (blood side) of renal tubular cells is primarily responsible for active pumping of Na^+ out of cells into blood in exchange for K^+. This pump causes a net movement of positive charge out of the cell (2 K^+ in, for every 3 Na^+ out) creating an electrochemical gradient that also causes Na^+ to enter the luminal (urine) side of the cell. Renal tubular cells in different portions of the nephron have different luminal "systems" to allow this Na^+ influx. These systems are the sites of action where the different diuretics work.

Proximal Tubule Diuretics

In the proximal tubule, a specialized luminal transporter exchanges protons (H^+) for sodium ions; the result is sodium reabsorption and acidification of the urine. The excreted H^+ combines with bicarbonate (HCO_3^-) in the tubule to form carbonic acid: $H^+ + HCO_3^- \rightarrow H_2CO_3$. Carbonic acid converts to water (H_2O) and carbon dioxide (CO_2) in a reaction catalyzed by carbonic anhydrase: $H_2CO_3 \rightarrow H_2O + CO_2$. The same enzyme, carbonic anhydrase, allows this reaction to occur in reverse within tubular cells, converting H_2CO_3 to HCO_3^- and H^+, generating more H^+ for countertransport with Na^+, and releasing bicarbonate that passes into the circulation. Carbonic anhydrase inhibitors are drugs that inhibit this enzyme; the net effect of these agents is that sodium and bicarbonate, that would otherwise have been reabsorbed, remain in the urine and result in an alkaline diuresis.

Although patients may develop a metabolic acidosis when taking these agents, compensatory processes in the tubules accommodate the effects of carbonic anhydrase inhibitors so that their long-term use rarely causes this problem. However, these agents can be useful, for example, with contraction alkalosis from aggressive diuresis with loop diuretics (see later discussion); administration of these drugs can reduce $PaCO_2$ and improve PaO_2 for patients with little accompanying change in blood pH. Specific uses for carbonic anhydrase inhibitors include the treatment of mountain sickness, open-angle glaucoma, and to increase respiratory drive in patients with central sleep apnea.[64,65]

Osmotic Diuretics

Substances such as mannitol that are freely filtered at the glomerulus but poorly reabsorbed by the renal tubule will cause an osmotic diuresis. In the water-permeable segments of the proximal tubule and loop of Henle, fluid reabsorption occurs, and filtered mannitol is concentrated. Eventually oncotic pressure in the tubular fluid resists further fluid reabsorption. Mannitol also draws water from cells into the plasma and effectively increases RBF.

Mannitol has been widely used, especially for the prophylaxis of specific types of acute renal failures (ARFs) and in the treatment of increased intracranial pressure (see Chapter 36). In select patient populations, such as cadaveric kidney transplant recipients, it has been found to be effective.[66] However, in a controlled trial of mannitol prophylaxis in patients with mild chronic renal failure, it was less effective than hydration alone for prevention of contrast-associated nephropathy.[67] Although animal studies

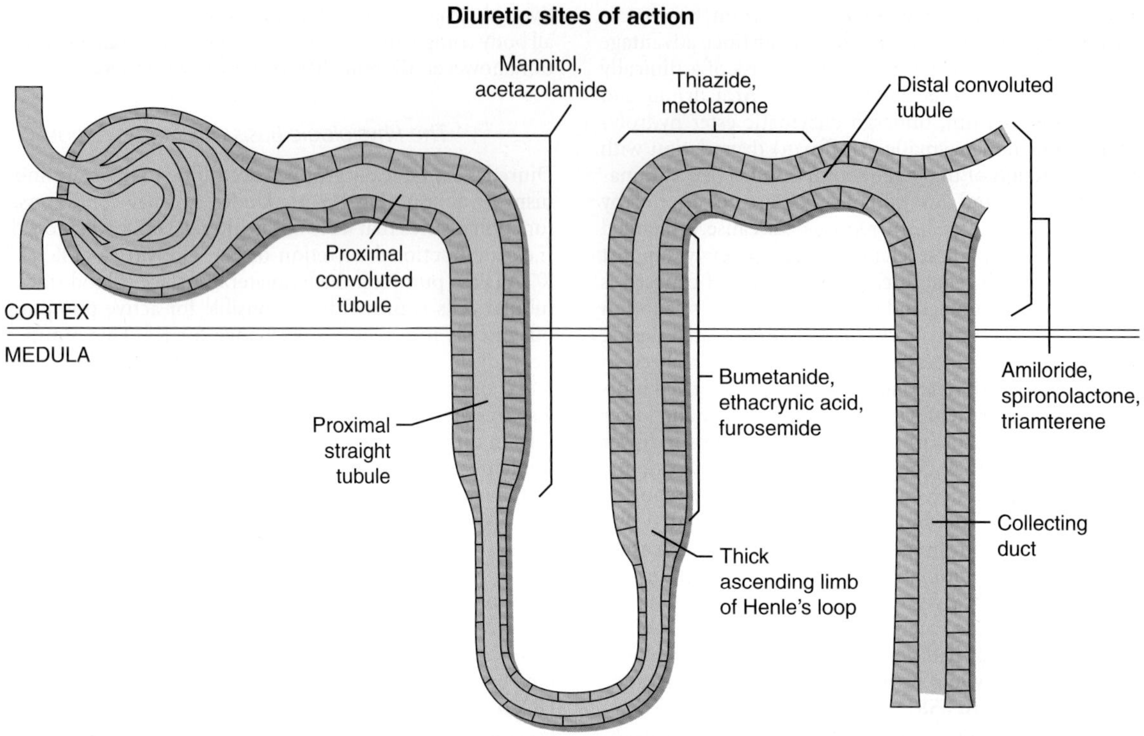

Diuretic sites of action

CORTEX
MEDULA
Mannitol, acetazolamide
Thiazide, metolazone
Distal convoluted tubule
Proximal convoluted tubule
Proximal straight tubule
Bumetanide, ethacrynic acid, furosemide
Amiloride, spironolactone, triamterene
Collecting duct
Thick ascending limb of Henle's loop

FIGURE 49-5. Site of action of commonly available diuretics. (From: Mende CW: Current issues in diuretic therapy. *Hosp Pract.* 1990;25(suppl 1):15, with permission.)

showed initial promise, apart from AKI prophylaxis in kidney transplantation, there is no clear evidence that mannitol is effective either for the prevention or treatment of AKI.[68] As mannitol shifts water between fluid compartments, there can be effects on plasma and intracellular electrolyte concentrations, including hyponatremia and hypochloremia and intracellular increases in K^+ and H^+. Patients with normal renal function quickly correct these changes, but patients with renal impairment may develop significant circulatory overload with hemodilution and pulmonary edema, hyperkalemic metabolic acidosis, central nervous system depression, and even severe hyponatremia requiring urgent hemodialysis.[69]

Loop Diuretics

The electrochemical gradient established by the Na^+/K^+-ATPase in the loop of Henle drives the transport of one Na^+, one K^+, and two Cl^- ions into the tubule cells from the tubular fluid. Because the thick ascending limb segment of the loop of Henle is water-impermeable, reabsorption of solute concentrates the interstitium and dilutes the tubular fluid. Loop diuretics, such as furosemide, bumetanide, and torsemide, directly inhibit the electroneutral transporter, preventing salt reabsorption from occurring. Because 25% of filtered NaCl is normally reabsorbed in the loop of Henle, loop diuretics cause a large salt load to pass to the distal convoluted tubule that is beyond the extra reserve of this tubular segment to reabsorb; consequently, large volumes of dilute urine ensue.

Loop diuretics are a first-line therapeutic modality for treatment of acute decompensated congestive heart failure. Although loop diuretics have no proven mortality benefit, they reduce left ventricular filling pressures and very effectively relieve the symptoms of congestion, pulmonary edema, extremity swelling, and hepatic congestion. Adverse effects of loop diuretics include hypokalemia, hyponatremia, and also AKI. Heart failure patients with atrial fibrillation may also be prescribed digitalis, which in combination with furosemide, can lead to hypokalemia-induced dysrhythmias. Loop diuretics, especially furosemide, may cause ototoxicity particularly in patients with renal insufficiency.[70]

Distal Convoluted Tubule Diuretics

Distal convoluted tubule diuretics, such as thiazides (e.g., hydrochlorothiazide) and metolazone, act in the early part of this segment to block the NaCl cotransport mechanism across apical plasma membranes. Because the distal tubule is relatively water-impermeable, net NaCl absorption causes urinary dilution. Clinically, distal convoluted tubule diuretics are used for the treatment of hypertension (often as sole therapy), volume overload disorders, and to relieve the symptoms of edema in pregnancy.

Adverse reactions associated with distal tubule diuretics include electrolyte disturbances and volume depletion. Hydrochlorothiazide specifically has been associated with a number of other side effects including pancreatitis, jaundice, diarrhea, and aplastic anemia.

Distal (Collecting Duct) Acting Diuretics

Unlike in the more proximal nephron segments, NaCl absorption in the collecting duct cells is not electroneutral. That is, a net electrical gradient is maintained both by the Na^+/K^+-ATPase Na^+ ion channels and in the luminal membranes. As a result, the tubule lumen is negatively charged with respect to the blood. This normally causes K^+ secretion into the tubular lumen through K^+-specific ion channels. Distal K^+-sparing diuretics (e.g., amiloride and triamterene) directly inhibit luminal Na^+ entry, blocking this mechanism, and resulting in a K^+-"sparing" effect. In addition, H^+ secretion is inhibited.

A second class of distal-acting, potassium-sparing diuretics is the competitive aldosterone antagonists (e.g., spironolactone and eplerenone). Ordinarily, the mineralocorticoid hormone aldosterone is released by the body in response to angiotensin II or hyperkalemia. Aldosterone normally stimulates Na^+ reabsorption and K^+ excretion by the collecting duct. Inhibition of the aldosterone effect by these drugs causes a mild natriuresis and K^+ retention. Distal K^+-sparing agents are used primarily for K^+-sparing diuresis (e.g., in patients with volume overload receiving digitalis or with hypokalemic alkalosis). In addition, these drugs are especially useful in treating disorders involving secondary hyperaldosteronism, such as cirrhosis with ascites. Spironolactone treatment has been shown to improve survival with volume overload and left ventricular dysfunction or heart failure.[71] Hyperkalemia and hyperkalemic, hyperchloremic metabolic acidoses are significant complications of the injudicious use of spironolactone, triamterene, or amiloride.

Dopaminergic Agonists

Intravenous infusion of low-dose dopamine (1 to 3 μg/kg/min) is natriuretic owing primarily to a modest increase in the GFR and reduction in proximal Na^+ reabsorption mediated by dopamine type 1 (DA_1) receptors.[72] Fenoldopam is a selective DA_1 receptor agonist with little cardiac stimulation. At higher doses, the pressor response to dopamine is beneficial in patients with hypotension, but it has little or no renal effect in critically ill or septic patients.[72,73] The so-called "renal-dose" dopamine for the treatment of AKI, although widely used, has not been demonstrated to have significant renoprotective properties in numerous studies[74–76] and can cause worsened splanchnic oxygenation, impaired gastrointestinal function, impaired endocrine and immunologic system function, blunting of ventilatory drive, and increased risk of postcardiac surgery atrial fibrillation.[77–79]

High-risk Surgical Procedures

Cardiac Surgery

Cardiac operations requiring CPB can be expected to result in AKI or failure in up to 7% of patients.[80,81] There are numerous risk factors associated with the development of postoperative AKI in this population (Fig. 49-6).[82] Interestingly, patients with preoperative CKD appear to tolerate surgery and CPB remarkably well.[83] Renal ischemia-reperfusion, inflammatory mediators, and toxin exposure are considered to be primary pathogenetic mechanisms involved in AKI. Renal risk factors contributing through these mechanisms include preoperative left ventricular dysfunction, duration of CPB, pulse pressure hypertension,[84] and aprotinin therapy.[85]

Although some retrospective studies suggest "beating heart" off pump coronary artery bypass grafting lowers renal risk compared with the traditional CPB techniques,[86] randomized studies

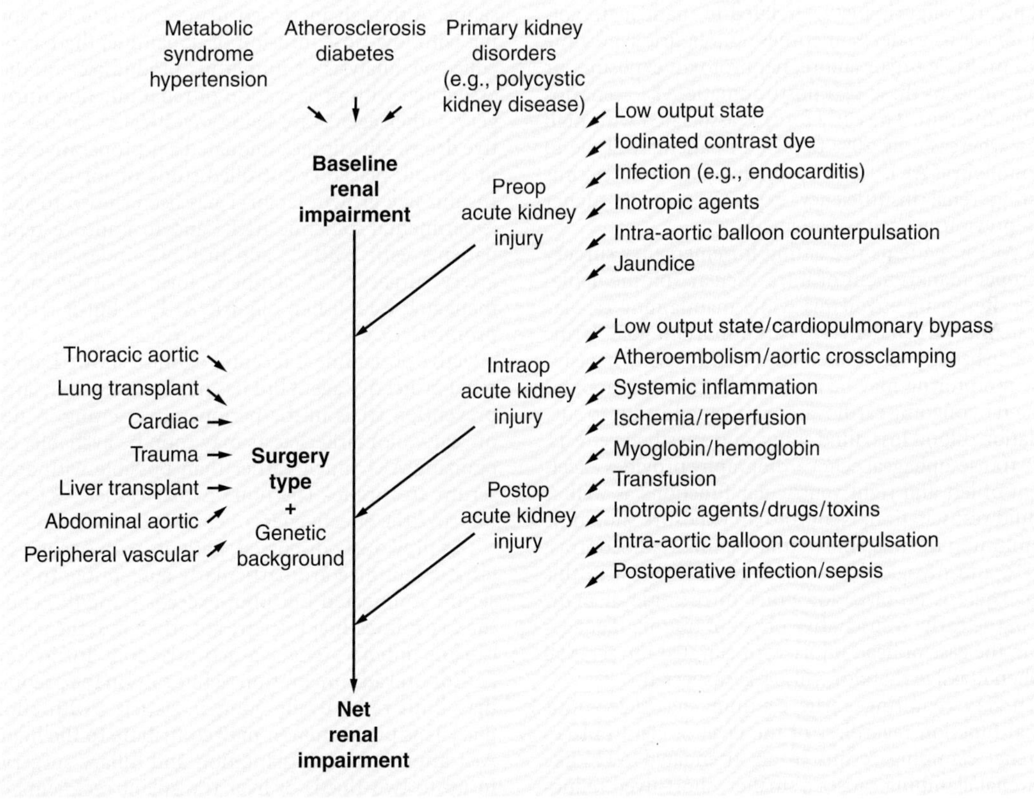

FIGURE 49-6. Clinical risk factors that predict perioperative acute kidney injury and renal dysfunction. Preop, preoperative; Intraop, intraoperative; Postop, postoperative. (From: Stafford-Smith M, Patel UD, Phillips-Bute BG, et al. Acute kidney injury and chronic kidney disease after cardiac surgery. *Adv Chronic Kidney Dis.* 2008;15:257–277, with permission.)

have been inconclusive. However, despite the fact that pulsatile CPB suppresses plasma renin activity, postoperative renal function in patients with normal kidneys undergoing pulsatile or nonpulsatile CPB is equivalent.

Numerous agents have been used intraoperatively without success in attempts to protect the kidney during cardiac surgery. Mannitol use during CPB is partly aimed at avoiding hemoglobin-induced AKI, by promoting urine flow and reducing renal cell swelling. Dopamine is infused at low doses (<5 μg/kg/min) as a renal vasodilator without benefit. Costa et al.[87] administered low-dose dopamine during CPB to patients with preoperative renal dysfunction and were able to induce a saluresis without affecting GFR or protecting the kidney from ischemic injury. Dopexamine improved CrCl and systemic oxygen delivery in one cardiac surgery study,[88] but a systemic review of 21 randomized, controlled trials failed to confirm benefit.[89] Other studies examining the renal protective effects of fenoldopam, ANP, and insulin-like growth factor-1 in this population have not shown a consistently protective effect.

Noncardiac Surgery

Several common noncardiac surgical procedures can compromise previously normal renal function. Emergency surgery has been reported as a risk factor for AKI, with trauma surgery figuring as a prominent subgroup of emergency procedures.[90] ATN is the typical renal lesion associated with trauma, and it may be produced by a number of ischemic mechanisms. Most often, hypovolemic shock, pigmenturia, multiple organ failure, or exogenous nephrotoxins are responsible for sequential or simultaneous insults to the kidney. AKI that develops in the trauma patient may be characterized by an early oliguric picture related to inadequate volume resuscitation, or by a later, sometimes nonoliguric syndrome associated with multiple organ failure, nephrotoxin exposure, or sepsis. The outcomes of these two posttraumatic AKI scenarios are dramatically different. The early form is associated with high mortality rates, whereas only 20% to 30% of patients will die in
9 the case of nonoliguric AKI.[91] Not surprisingly, trauma victims with pre-existing renal insufficiency experience much higher mortality than previously healthy patients.[92]

Preventing AKI in patients presenting for emergency surgery begins with proper management of intravascular volume depletion and shock. Restoring euvolemia while maintaining cardiac output and systemic oxygen delivery is an important goal. Urine flow, once established, is maintained at ≥0.5 mL/kg/hr. Invasive hemodynamic monitoring may be required to guide intraoperative management of ongoing cardiovascular instability due to surgical manipulation, blood loss, fluid shifts, and anesthetic effects. Intraoperative transesophageal echocardiography provides excellent assessment of left and right ventricular functions as well as guidance of fluid resuscitation. Nephrotoxin exposure should be kept to a minimum in the unstable trauma victim. Radiocontrast media, NSAIDs, and myoglobin pose the greatest threat in this patient group. There is no place for either furosemide or mannitol therapy in the early, resuscitative phase of trauma management, except in the case of head injury with elevated intracranial pressure or when massive rhabdomyolysis is suspected.

Vascular surgery requiring aortic clamping has deleterious effects on renal function regardless of the level of clamp placement. Suprarenal clamping results in an attenuated ATN-like lesion.[93] Infrarenal clamping causes a smaller, short-lived reduction in GFR and is associated with a lower risk of AKI, whereas surgery involving the thoracic aorta has a 25% incidence of AKI.[94] Two major predictors of AKI following aortic surgery are pre-existing renal dysfunction and perioperative hemodynamic instability.[95] Olsen et al.[96] reported in a large series of patients undergoing abdominal aortic aneurysm repair that the overall incidence of AKI was 12%. Patients who had emergency surgery for ruptured aneurysm had a very high incidence of hemodynamic instability, and AKI developed in 26%; in contrast, elective aortic surgery was associated with good hemodynamic control and a 4% incidence of renal failure. Atheromatous renal artery emboli and prolonged aortic clamp time may contribute to ischemic renal injury in these patients.

The endovascular approach (endostent) to major aortic surgery has gained popularity.[97] The etiology of AKI after endovascular and open repair of aortic aneurysm is multifactorial (renal ischemia, atheroembolism, hemodynamic instability). Although hemodynamic changes during endovascular procedures on the aorta may be less dramatic than those accompanying open repair, the prevalence of renal complications appears to be similar. During endovascular procedures, patients may be exposed to substantial amounts of radiocontrast dye, which can exacerbate postoperative renal dysfunction, especially in those with pre-existing renal insufficiency. The long-term incidence of renal insufficiency/failure (followed up to 24 months postoperatively) is similar after endovascular and open repair of aortic aneurysm. It is thus important that before endovascular procedures, patients are adequately hydrated, and the total dose of radiocontrast dye is limited.

Most efforts to preserve renal function in aortic surgery have centered on diuretic and renal vasodilator therapies, although a large body of evidence no longer supports the use of either intravenous mannitol or dopamine to prevent AKI in this setting. Indeed, a clinical study of infrarenal aortic clamping found that combined mannitol and low-dose dopamine treatment was no more effective in preventing AKI than volume expansion with saline. Although increased urine flow rate is a consistent finding with low-dose infusion of dopamine, there is no evidence in collective analysis of numerous randomized studies that this is associated with preservation of renal function during aortic surgery. Other agents are being investigated for use as renoprotective drugs. Nifedipine attenuated a postoperative decrease in GFR in a small, placebo-controlled study of aortic surgery patients.[98] Insulin-like growth factor-1 has been shown to speed healing in experimental ischemic AKI[99] and to improve renal function in patients with ESRD[100] and in those undergoing aortic or renal artery surgery.[101] A synthetic form of ANP may be useful in managing established oliguric ARF,[102] but it has not been used prophylactically in high-risk surgical patients. Fenoldopam, a selective dopamine-1 receptor agonist, showed some promise as a renal protective agent but has not been tested in large multicenter prevention trials in the perioperative setting. A new generation of "early biomarker" tests may soon be available, capable of recognizing AKI much earlier than possible with accumulation of serum creatinine. The hope is that earlier AKI recognition will improve the effectiveness of current interventions.

As previously discussed, patients with hepatic failure or cholestatic jaundice are particularly susceptible to AKI. When the serum conjugated bilirubin exceeds 8 mg/dL, endotoxins from the gastrointestinal tract are absorbed into the portal circulation, causing intense renal vasoconstriction. Intravenous mannitol and/or oral administration of bile salts in the preoperative period may limit renal dysfunction in patients with cholestatic jaundice. This phenomenon may contribute to the high incidence of AKI after liver transplantation and biliary surgery. AKI occurs in up to two-thirds of liver transplant recipients.[103] Many liver transplant candidates have overt hepatorenal syndrome, renal dysfunction, and presumably underlying renal vasoconstriction. When such patients are exposed to intraoperative hemodynamic instability, massive transfusion, and nephrotoxins, AKI frequently follows.[104]

NEPHRECTOMY

A review of urologic surgical procedures is outlined below, including sections on nephrectomy, cystectomy, prostatectomy, TUR procedures, and therapies for urolithiasis. For each section, general disease principles and treatment rationales are briefly discussed, perioperative management and potential complications reviewed, and then important aspects related to specific procedures within the section highlighted (e.g., simple vs. radical nephrectomy). 10 Selected additional topics are outlined at the end of the section. Notably, a deliberate approach has been taken to minimize repetition by referring the reader to other chapter sections whenever appropriate.

Nephrectomy procedures involve partial, radical, or simple resection of the kidney. Each year in the United States, there are approximately 46,000 nephrectomies for benign or malignant disease, and an additional 5,500 donor surgeries for renal transplant. While radical nephrectomy is the standard for resectable kidney cancer, simple nephrectomy is typical for benign disease. Some kidney tumors invade the renal vein extending as far as the inferior vena cava or right atrium; these tumors require additional procedures to safely retrieve their intravascular component. Kidney transplant donor nephrectomy involves simple nephrectomy with measures to avoid organ trauma and optimize graft function. The so-called "nephron sparing" or partial nephrectomy is indicated for limited benign disease but increasingly is being considered for wider indications including selected cancerous lesions.

The approach and incision for nephrectomy are based on surgical priorities and surgeon preference. Retroperitoneal approaches require a flank incision and lateral decubitus positioning with flank extension (Fig. 49-7), allowing access to the kidney with avoidance of the peritoneal cavity. This approach has obvious advantages for treatment of infection but also simplifies procedures with prior abdominal surgery or obesity. Difficulties with the retroperitoneal approach include access to the vena cava, risk of unintentional pneumothorax, and the adverse effects of

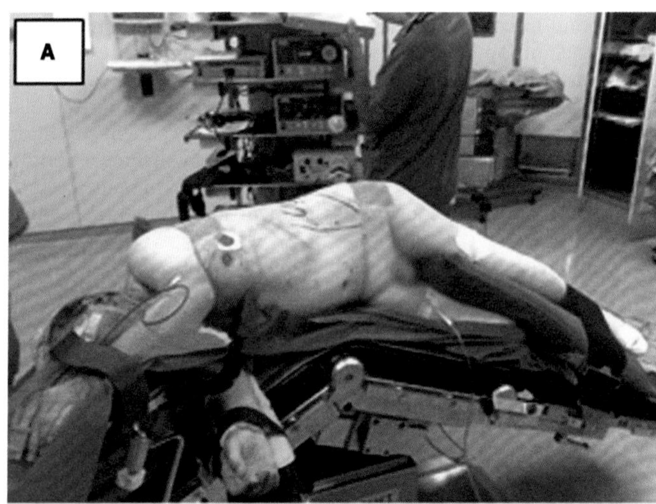

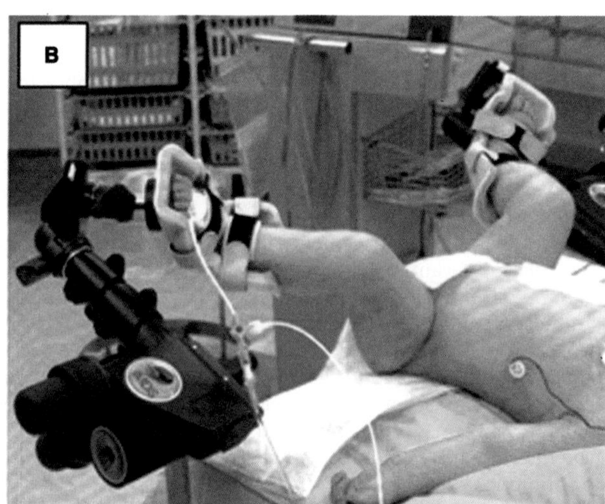

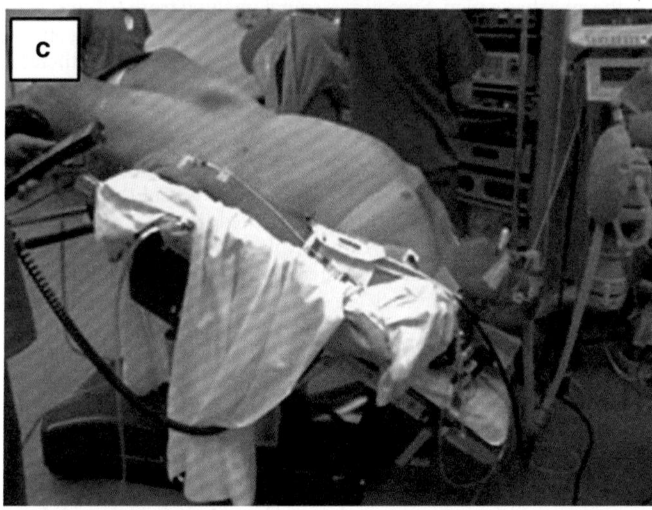

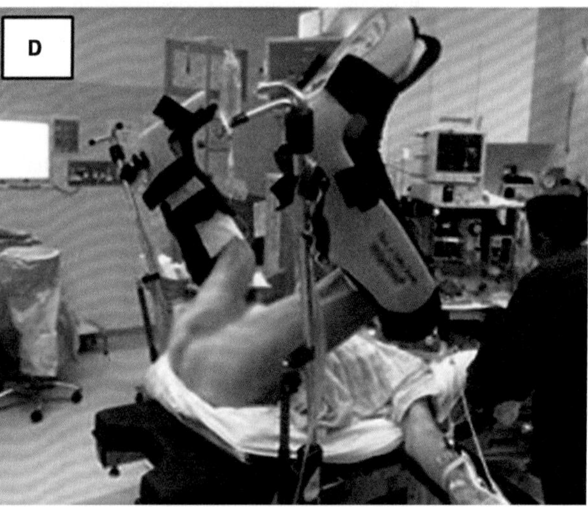

FIGURE 49-7. Common positioning options for urologic surgery include right lateral decubitus with waist extension **(A)**, lithotomy **(B)**, supine with steep (30 to 45 degrees) Trendelenberg **(C)**, and exaggerated lithotomy **(D)**. (From: http://www.opitek.dk/en/products/pedistirrup, with permission **[A]**; http://www.virtualmedicalcentre.com/treatment/radical-perineal-prostatectomy-rpp/163, with permission **[D]**.)

lateral decubitus position and flank extension on respiratory vital capacity, which can be reduced up to 20% (see Chapter 28).

Anterior approaches to nephrectomy involve supine positioning and breach of the peritoneal cavity through midline, subcostal, or thoraco-abdominal incisions that provide direct access to both the kidney and major vascular structures. Although transperitoneal approaches add the risk of visceral injury and peritonitis, they improve access to the renal pedicle (e.g., trauma, hemorrhage) with best access to both kidneys being through midline incisions (e.g., bilateral nephrectomy for end-stage polycystic kidney disease). The thoraco-abdominal approach enters both the peritoneal and pleural spaces and rarely may require single-lung ventilation.

In recent years, *laparoscopic* retro- and transperitoneal approaches to nephrectomy have surpassed their open equivalents in popularity, particularly for simple and donor procedures, but these techniques are even being used for "nephron-sparing" partial nephrectomy. Other recent innovations include robotic-assisted, single port laparoscopic, and even transvaginal minimally invasive nephrectomies.

Preoperative Considerations

Recruits for donor nephrectomy surgery are typically healthy individuals; however, perioperative risk for other nephrectomy procedures often relates to the indication for surgery. Although smoking and obesity are the most important risk factors for renal cancer, many other cardiovascular risk factors are also strongly associated with renal cancer risk including advanced age, male gender, chronic or ESRD, and hypertension. Hence, protocols for assessment and management of perioperative cardiac risk are particularly relevant to nephrectomy surgery.[105]

Simple nephrectomy for infectious indications is uncommon but most often involves diabetic patients and can be grouped into two categories. Elective procedures involve irreversible kidney damage due to chronic pyelonephritis (e.g., xanthogranulomatous).[106] In contrast, emergent procedures are associated with very high mortality rates (up to 43%) and generally involve critically ill patients with acute emphysematous pyelonephritis unresponsive to antibiotics.

Several hereditary conditions that are associated with kidney cancer also have attributes that must be considered in anesthetic planning[107]; for example, individuals with Birt–Hogg–Dubé syndrome have pulmonary cysts that increase the risk of intraoperative spontaneous pneumothorax, while patients with von Hippel–Lindau syndrome, the commonest of these disorders, have high rates of pheochromocytoma and neuroendocrine tumors.

Ten to forty percent of patients presenting with renal cancer have associated paraneoplastic syndromes.[108] Beyond fever, cachexia, and weight loss, these subdivide into endocrine and nonendocrine categories. Tumor-related endocrine effects include hypercalcemia (PTH-like effects), hypertension (renin), anemia/polycythemia (erythropoietin), nonmetastatic hepatic dysfunction (Stauffer syndrome), galactorrhea, Cushing's syndrome, and ectopic insulin and glucagon production, while nonendocrine effects include amyloidosis, neuromyopathies, vasculopathy, nephropathy, coagulopathy, and elevated prostaglandin levels. Of renal cancers presenting with hypercalcemia, 50% are paraneoplastic in origin. Renal tumors may also be associated with a hypercoagulable state; sudden intraoperative clot formation has been reported.[109]

As for most major urologic surgeries, other investigations for nephrectomy surgery include routine ECG, chest X ray, complete blood cell count, electrolyte profile with serum BUN and creatinine, liver function tests, serum calcium assessment, bleeding profile, and urine analysis. Although normal serum creatinine level and evidence of contralateral function by intravenous pyelogram are sometimes considered sufficient assessment to predict adequate postoperative renal function, a noninvasive differential renal scan (iodine-131 or technetium-99m computerized isotope renograph) is often performed for more precise prediction of postoperative GFR.

Urologic surgery patients often present with additional disease workup that can provide a wealth of information beyond routine studies and assessment of their urinary tract. Abdominal CT scans detail tumor size, location, and invasion of the renal collecting system or perirenal fat, while MRI is most valuable to assess for vena caval and/or cardiac chamber involvement.

Standard recommended preoperative management of chronic drug therapies is all that is necessary for most nephrectomy procedures, although dose adjustment may be considered if significant changes in renal function are anticipated.

Intraoperative Considerations

Preparation for even the most "straightforward" nephrectomy surgery demands sufficient monitoring and vascular access to respond to complications, most notably significant hemorrhage, an uncommon but ever-present risk in such procedures. Beyond standard monitoring (e.g., ASA guidelines) and two large bore peripheral intravenous catheters, requirements for intravascular access and additional monitoring are dictated by patient condition and complexity of the procedure but generally include a peripheral intra-arterial catheter for continuous blood pressure recording and repeated blood gas assessment and sometimes central venous access.

While central venous line placement is not essential for most nephrectomy surgeries, patient and procedural factors such as comorbidities (e.g., cardiac history) and bleeding risk (e.g., tumor extension into venous structures) may warrant such monitoring. If placement of a central venous catheter is deemed necessary, selection of the side *ipsilateral* to the nephrectomy surgery for subclavian or internal jugular central venous puncture should be considered to minimize the risk of bilateral pneumothorax.

Assessment of infection, bony metastases, and bleeding risk may influence the decision to include neuraxial procedures in the anesthesia plan. Sometimes spinal imaging from CT and MRI scans can provide added detail useful when contemplating epidural catheter placement. If a lumbar or thoracic epidural catheter is placed, this is usually done prior to anesthesia induction to allow for a meaningful test dose sequence and to facilitate pre-incision administration of epidural opiates. Varied opinions regarding intraoperative local anesthetic dosing of the epidural catheter involve concerns over hemodynamic stability and the likelihood of significant blood loss during the procedure.

Neuraxial injection or catheter placement prior to anesthesia induction (e.g., epidural catheter insertion) can be followed by placement of intra-arterial and central venous access after anesthesia
11 induction in most cases. Bladder catheter placement is essential for all nephrectomy procedures; urinary output monitoring provides information on intravascular volume status in the absence of central venous pressure monitoring, avoids the possibility of urinary retention, and also provides valuable information postoperatively regarding renal function, bleeding sources, and the possibility of clot-related urinary tract obstruction. Noninvasive cardiac output monitoring (e.g., esophageal Doppler, LidCO, NiCO) techniques may be useful for cardiac monitoring in selected patients.

Standard pre-anesthesia induction considerations include postoperative planning (e.g., PACU vs. stepdown vs. ICU disposition) and administration of intravenous antibiotic prophylaxis within 1 hour prior to surgical incision. Plans for postoperative analgesia strategy may dictate disposition particularly to involve a care team capable of recognizing and treating potential complications of the various analgesia strategies.

Anesthesia induction agent selection to achieve hypnosis, paralysis, and blunting of the hemodynamic intubation response should be matched to any use of regional anesthesia, the anticipated duration of the procedure, and the patient's renal function. Intraoperative and postoperative pain management can be accomplished by intravenous or other opioid therapies such as patient-controlled analgesia or neuraxial analgesia. Continuous epidural analgesia attenuates the neuroendocrine response but may also improve postoperative ventilatory mechanics and resolve ileus sooner and has been associated with improved survival in intermediate-to-high-risk noncardiac surgery.[110]

Potential intraoperative complications include injury to major blood vessels (e.g., inferior vena cava, aorta), gastrointestinal organs (e.g., spleen, liver, pancreas), and unrecognized entry into the pleural space with resultant pneumothorax. Complications associated with hemorrhage during nephrectomy are uncommon but mandate preparatory steps beyond monitoring and generous intravenous access. Confirmation that blood products are present or readily available should occur immediately prior to surgery. Routine fluid and patient warming technology, availability of colloid volume expanders, and even a rapid transfusion device for selected cases should also be considered. Since unexplained changes in pulmonary mechanics or hypotension during a nephrectomy procedure may reflect diaphragmatic injury and pneumothorax, such changes should be discussed with the surgeon to facilitate prompt intervention. This may require direct repair of a rent in the diaphragm as well as needle decompression of a pneumothorax and chest tube insertion.

Particularly in the setting of limited renal reserve, in addition to consideration of transfusion "triggers" and strict avoidance of unjustifiable blood product administration, a note of caution is warranted regarding the potential for resuscitation "overshoot" in response to acute hemorrhage. Strict attention to appropriate monitors during fluid resuscitation, assisted by good communication with the surgeon, will help avoid the risk of pulmonary edema from fluid overload.

Postoperative Considerations

Up to 20% of patients undergoing nephrectomy develop postoperative complications, and operative mortality rates following radical nephrectomy are as high as 2%. Added to standard concerns, such as hemorrhage and unrecognized visceral injury, are atelectasis, ileus, superficial and deep wound infections, temporary or permanent renal failure, and incisional hernia. The most common radical nephrectomy complications are adjacent organ (4% bowel, spleen, liver, diaphragm, or pancreas) and vascular injury (2%). Overall complication rates are similar whether an open or laparoscopic approach is used.[111–113] Bleeding requiring transfusion occurs in up to 5.7% of all cases.[114–116] Other less common major complications include myocardial infarction, congestive heart failure, pulmonary embolism, cerebrovascular accident, pneumonia, and thrombophlebitis.

A logical expectation of nephrectomy surgery would be the need to adjust postoperative dosing of drug therapies to accommodate the anticipated decrease in GFR associated with an approximate 50% loss of kidney tissue. Although a drop in GFR can be anticipated, interestingly, adaptation of the remaining kidney usually results in a modest 25% decline postoperatively.

The pain of nephrectomy, laparoscopic or open, is significant. Analgesia can be achieved with epidural or spinal analgesia strategies, systemic opioids, and nonopioid adjuncts including intravenous acetominophen. Recent findings of improved recovery using epidural analgesia for major abdominal surgeries[117] have not been assessed specifically for nephrectomy surgery.

Specific Procedures

Simple and Donor Nephrectomies

Simple nephrectomy is sufficient intervention for irreversible nonmalignant disease such as untreatable infection, unsalvageable kidney trauma, or a nonfunctioning kidney due to calculi or hypertensive disease. Up to 86% of patients with hypertension that is presumed to be renovascular in origin with noncorrectable unilateral renal artery disease have improved hypertension control after simple nephrectomy.

During donor procedures, several steps are added to simple nephrectomy, including administration of drugs intravenously just prior to explantation to achieve low-level anticoagulation (e.g., 3,000 USP heparin units) and forced diuresis (e.g., mannitol 12.5 g, furosemide 40 mg), extension of (laparoscopic) incisions to assure atraumatic organ extraction, and postharvest protamine administration. Procured organs are infused with cold preservative (e.g., University of Wisconsin or histidine–tryptophan–ketoglutarate solutions) and stored on ice and/or cold machine perfused. Just over one-third of renal transplants in the United States are from living donors and, compared to cadavers, living kidney donation is associated with improved short- and long-term outcomes (i.e., recipient and graft survival).

Radical Nephrectomy

Renal cell carcinoma is the main indication for radical nephrectomy and accounts for 90% to 95% of kidney neoplasms and 3% of all malignancies in adults. With the exception of hereditary syndromes with high tumor rates (see above), a positive family history incurs a two- to three-fold increased risk of kidney cancer, but such individuals constitute only 2% of radical nephrectomies. Hematuria, a palpable mass and flank pain, is the classic triad at presentation, but nowadays renal tumors are more often (approximately 72%) diagnosed incidentally during workup for other nonurologic problems. Occasionally, tumors declare due to signs or symptoms of vena caval involvement such as dilated abdominal veins, (left) varicocele, lower extremity edema, or pulmonary embolism. Symptomatic tumors usually reflect more advanced disease and are more often associated with metastasis and a poor prognosis. Transitional cell cancers of the upper urothelial tract (ureters, renal pelvis) are also treated by radical nephrectomy with resection of the associated ureter including a cuff of bladder tissue. Up to one-third of kidney cancer patients have metastases at diagnosis, but many are still candidates for surgery.

Radical nephrectomy involves renal artery and vein ligation with subsequent removal *en bloc* of the kidney, perinephric fat, Gerota's fascia, proximal ureter, and often the adjacent adrenal gland. Lymph node dissection is then performed from the diaphragm to the aortic bifurcation. Most renal cancers stay within Gerota's fascia and can be completely removed, but a disappointing 20% to 30% of patients with successful surgery still have their disease return. Although radical nephrectomy is standard for central and large tumors, the value of nephron-sparing partial nephrectomy for early stage and small renal cell cancers is being evaluated. While nonsurgical therapies are available, renal cell cancers are resistant to radiation and chemotherapy. Blood loss during radical nephrectomy is highly dependent on the location and extent of the tumor. Laparoscopic innovations have reduced bleeding for all types of nephrectomy surgeries.

Radical Nephrectomy with Inferior Vena Cava Tumor Thrombus

Between 4% and 10% of patients with renal cell carcinoma have the so-called "tumor thrombus" extension beyond the kidney either limited to the renal vein or extending into the inferior vena cava. Although often restricted to the vessel lumen, the thrombus may become adherent to the vessel wall,[118] and right atrial involvement is present in 1% of cases. Radical nephrectomy procedures involving resection of tumor thrombus are particularly challenging due to their risk of sudden major bleeding and potential for acute hemodynamic instability (e.g., inferior vena cava clamping or tumor pulmonary embolism).

Renal tumors with IVC thrombus are classified by the extent of tumor thrombus within the IVC and right atrium (levels I–IV; Fig. 49-8) and require different procedures in addition to radical nephrectomy.[119] In general, thrombus extraction can occur with simple proximal and distal caval control alone for tumors that go no further than the infrahepatic IVC. As thrombus extends into the intrahepatic IVC or higher, isolating the vessel to extract the thrombus becomes more challenging and ultimately can only be achieved safely using CPB with or without aortic crossclamping and cardiac arrest. In addition to sternotomy incision, such procedures require standard heparin anticoagulation and employ an added circuit venous line filter to trap tumor fragments (Fig. 49-8). Other interventions used at some institutions in the treatment of renal tumor caval thrombus include venovenous bypass, inferior vena cava filter insertion, and even deep hypothermic circulatory arrest.

Appropriate considerations when monitoring these complex procedures include radial arterial catheterization, central venous and pulmonary artery catheter placement, and intraoperative transesophageal echocardiography (Fig. 49-8). In cases where supradiaphragmatic tumor thrombus is present, placement of a pulmonary artery catheter prior to thrombus resection is contraindicated due to risk of embolization of tumor fragments. If the thrombus extends into the suprahepatic IVC, hepatic mobilization with Pringle maneuver (clamping of the hepatoduodenal ligament to interrupt blood flow through the hepatic artery and portal vein) may be required, generally for less than 30 minutes.[120] Additional preparation includes all steps standard for procedures involving CPB (see Chapter 38), including large bore peripheral intravenous access, vasoactive infusions, fluid, and blood products. Preoperative therapeutic embolization of the tumor is sometimes also used in cases of arterial thrombus, extensive parasitic vessel formation, or with anticipated difficulty in isolating

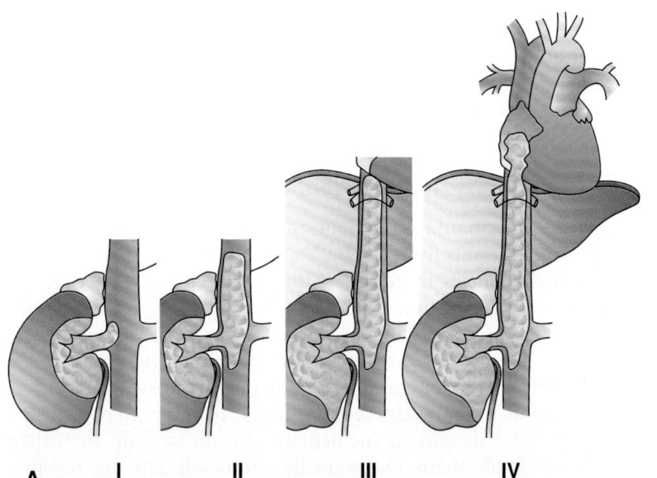

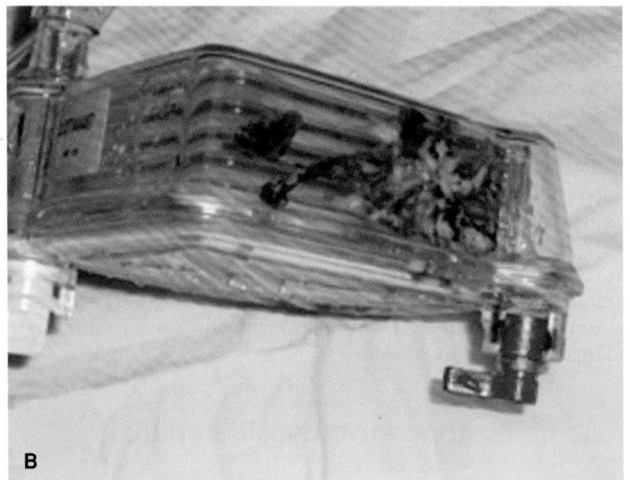

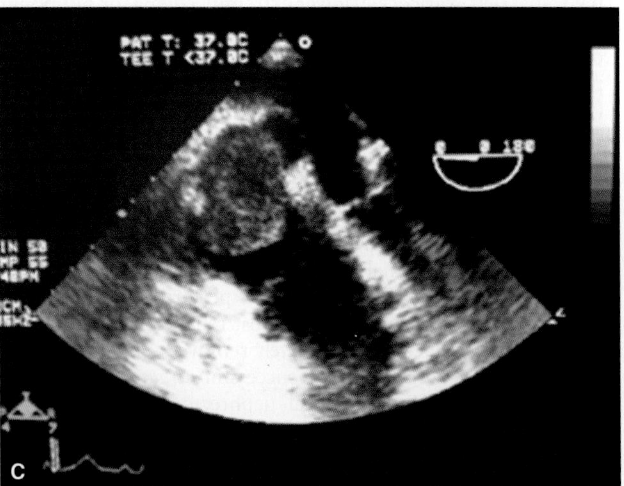

FIGURE 49-8. Radical nephrectomy with inferior vena cava thrombus removal for renal cell carcinoma is a major operative procedure. Surgical complexity is predicted by the extent of intravascular tumor thrombus, as classified by the most proximal level of tumor extension (levels I–IV; **A**). Evidence of thrombus emboli in the venous filter following cardiopulmonary bypass **(B)** highlights the friability of intravascular renal cell carcinoma thrombus. Intraoperative transesophageal echocardiography demonstrates right atrial extension of a renal cell tumor **(C)**. (From: Nesbitt JC, Soltero ER, Dinney CP, et al. Surgical management of renal cell carcinoma with inferior vena cava tumor thrombus. Ann thorac surg. 1997;63:1592–1600, with permission **[A]**.)

the renal artery. Despite the potential for significant blood loss, cell saver technology use is discouraged due to the potential for returning tumor cells to the circulation.

"Nephron-sparing" Partial Nephrectomy

Minimizing unnecessary loss of healthy tissue is a logical part of surgical planning for any kidney resection. Partial nephrectomy is often sufficient for benign tumors, but this procedure is also becoming an alternate to radical nephrectomy for some cancerous renal cell tumors, particularly when renal parenchyma must be preserved; examples include bilateral tumors, CKD, tumors in a single remaining kidney, or where the contralateral kidney is at risk for future disease or tumor. Even when the contralateral kidney is normal, studies are now demonstrating comparable long-term results with nephron-sparing partial nephrectomy procedures as with radical nephrectomy for patients with a single, localized small tumor (<4 cm) and even medium-sized (<7 cm) peripherally located tumors. Limitations of partial nephrectomy include a higher perioperative risk of bleeding and urine leak, and a local tumor recurrence rate of 1% to 6%.

Laparoscopic and Robotic Nephrectomies

Laparoscopic and robotic techniques can be applied to retroperitoneal and transperitoneal approaches and all types of nephrectomies (i.e., radical, simple, or partial). Compared to open approaches, these minimally invasive strategies employ access through small airtight "ports." Insufflation of carbon dioxide into the peritoneal cavity or retroperitoneal space is used to separate structures and enhance visibility. In recent years, laparoscopic techniques have surpassed open nephrectomies in popularity, particularly for simple and radical procedures. Laparoscopic approaches to radical nephrectomy are even being successfully employed in the treatment of locally invasive kidney cancer. Laparoscopic partial nephrectomy is technically more demanding than its open counterpart and currently involves temporary clamping of the renal hilum to optimize visibility during excision and minimize blood loss. The warm ischemic time related to clamping can cause AKI, particularly if the duration exceeds 30 minutes.[121,122]

Some studies have reported comparisons of equivalent open and laparoscopic procedures. Laparoscopic radical nephrectomy for cancer involves smaller incisions, less blood loss, decreased postoperative analgesic requirement, shorter hospital stay and convalescent period, and similar long-term outcomes when compared with open radical nephrectomy.[123,124] Likewise, laparoscopic "nephron-sparing" partial nephrectomy results in less bleeding and a shorter hospital stay, and for selected tumors has 5- and 10-year outcomes similar to those of open partial nephrectomy.[125,126] Laparoscopic donor nephrectomy has no adverse effects on the success of kidney transplant but is associated with less pain and analgesic requirement, faster hospital discharge, and better quality of life compared with open donor nephrectomy.[127] Institutional experience with laparoscopic and robotic assistance with nephrectomy procedures may influence anesthetic planning and the perceived need for invasive procedures (e.g., central venous pressure monitoring).

Traditional open nephrectomy is associated with a significant incidence of chronic pain ranging from 5% to 26%.[128,129] The hope is that laparoscopic approaches will reduce the incidence of chronic pain syndromes. The perceived differences between laparoscopic and open nephrectomy procedures have influenced clinical practice including anesthesia planning for postoperative pain management. Compared to open nephrectomy, the reduced pain and shorter recovery times have meant that epidural anesthesia is less likely to be selected for laparoscopic approaches, with postoperative pain control for these procedures provided by a multimodal strategy involving opiates and appropriate non-opioid adjuncts. NSAIDs are rarely used to avoid their potential nephrotoxic effects. Recent small studies have reported good success with continuous local anesthetic infusions via catheters placed in the rectus and retroperitoneal sheaths intraoperatively (across the intercostal, ilioinguinal, and ileohypogastric nerves). Benefits include reduced pain levels, opioid requirements, nausea, time to recovery and discharge, and cost.[130,131]

Robotic approaches to nephrectomy surgery are beginning to be employed but have very similar considerations to laparoscopic nephrectomy in terms of issues such as pneumoperitoneum. Notably, robotic nephrectomy has specific positioning requirements due to the robotic equipment, and care must be taken to assure that the robotic arms do not cause pressure injury to the patient. Depending on the experience of the surgical team, robotic procedures may also take more time. Notably, the role of robot assistance is also being similarly explored and developed for several other major urologic surgeries (e.g., partial nephrectomy, radical cystectomy, pyeloplasty, and radical cystectomy).[132]

Physiology of Pneumoperitoneum

Despite potential surgical advantages of laparoscopic surgery, the consequences of pneumoperitoneum, most notably systemic CO_2 absorption and obstruction of venous return from the lower body, are important particularly for patients with cardiopulmonary disease (Table 49-5)[133] (see Chapter 33). These include an

TABLE 49-5. PHYSIOLOGY OF CO_2 PNEUMOPERITONEUM IN THE TRENDELENBURG POSITION

Organ System	Effect
Cardiovascular	↑ Systemic vascular resistance ↑ Mean arterial pressure ↑ Myocardial oxygen consumption ↓ Renal, portal, and sphlanchnic flow
Respiratory	↑ Ventilation–perfusion mismatch ↓ Functional residual capacity ↓ Vital capacity ↓ Compliance ↑ Peak airway pressure Pulmonary congestion and edema Hypercarbia, respiratory acidosis
Central nervous system	↑ Intracranial pressure ↑ Cerebral blood flow ↑ Intraocular pressure Catecholamine release
Endocrine	Activation of renin–angiotensin system
Others	Gastroesophageal regurgitation Venous air embolism Neuropraxia, especially brachial Tracheal tube displacement Facial and airway edema

From: Irvine M, Patil V. Anaesthesia for robot-assisted laparoscopic surgery. *Continuing Education in Anaesthesia, Critical Care & Pain.* 2009;9:125–129, with permission.

average 30% decrease in cardiac output with the institution of pneumoperitoneum which, due to an associated increase in systemic vascular resistance (afterload), is often accompanied by little change or even an increase (up to 16%) in mean arterial blood pressure. Systemic vascular resistance and cardiac output usually return to near normal values over the 10 minutes following institution of pneumoperitoneum. Preoperative fluid loading, with additional pre-induction colloid boluses before institution of pneumoperitoneum, result in higher stroke volume and urine output compared to standard intraoperative fluid regimens, but studies are lacking regarding any evidence of improved outcome using this strategy.[134]

A strategy involving hydration and limiting insufflation pressures to below 12 mm Hg is advocated. Presumably related to derangements of renal perfusion, pneumoperitoneum insufflation pressures of >15 mm Hg have been associated with postoperative AKI. Following laparoscopic donor nephrectomy, some donors develop oliguria despite hemodynamic stability and liberal fluid management strategies. The etiology of this is unclear, but it is usually self-limited. Urine output of >2 mL/kg/hr is also encouraged, although there is no clear evidence that the diuretic effects of furosemide, mannitol, "renal dose" dopamine, fenoldopam, or ANP analogs are of any value in protecting the kidney.[135]

Other effects of pneumoperitoneum include restricted diaphragmatic excursion, acid–base abnormalities due to systemic absorption of CO_2, neurohumoral responses, and the potential for venous gas embolism. Reductions in pulmonary compliance and functional residual capacity, combined with CO_2 absorption, often cause respiratory acidosis. Cephalad displacement of the abdominal contents, particularly in obese patients, can also add atelectasis and ventilation–perfusion mismatch. Cardiac valvular dysfunction has been reported during laparoscopic nephrectomy,[136] and cardiac ischemia can develop in "at-risk" patients with coronary artery disease. There is also an immediate increase in intracranial pressure with the institution of the pneumoperitoneum.

Hemodynamic instability or hypoxia that occurs with CO_2 insufflation due to the above-mentioned perturbations must be addressed, and a small number of patients will require conversion to an open surgical approach. However, despite the numerous disturbances, a majority of patients can be safely managed through episodes of pneumoperitoneum with appropriate circulatory support, thoughtful ventilator management, and good communication between surgeon and anesthesiologist that includes a willingness to adjust CO_2 insufflation pressures. Notably, adequate neuromuscular blockade plays a role in keeping insufflation pressures at the lowest level required to achieve optimal surgical exposure.

Offsetting advantages of laparoscopic approaches are risks also seen in settings other than nephrectomy including trauma during trocar placement (approx. 0.5%) and increased rates of postoperative deep venous thrombosis.

CYSTECTOMY AND OTHER MAJOR BLADDER SURGERIES

Cystectomy surgery involves removal of all or part of the urinary bladder. While radical cystectomy is standard for most muscle-invasive malignant disease, simple cystectomy is primarily for benign bladder disease. Of the 69,250 cases of bladder cancer expected in 2011 in the United States, approximately 90% will undergo a surgical procedure for their disease. Radical cystectomy combines bladder removal with resection of other pelvic organs and lymph nodes. Partial or simple cystectomy and transurethral resection of bladder tumor (TURBT) (see transurethral resection procedures section) are other procedures used in the treatment of benign and malignant bladder diseases.

In removing the entire bladder, simple and radical cystectomy procedures oblige a companion surgery to allow for future urine collection. The so-called "diversion procedures" involve redirecting the ureters, most commonly to a pouch fashioned from ileum (ileal conduit), that passively drains urine into a bag through a stoma on the patient's abdominal wall. Alternate options include the so-called "continent" diversion reconstructive procedures which are becoming more popular. Since diversion surgeries can make future diagnosis of appendicitis difficult, some surgeons routinely also perform an appendectomy as part of urinary diversion procedures.

Supine or modified lithotomy positioning (Fig. 49-7) and midline incision with avoidance of the umbilicus are standard for open cystectomy surgery; however, a transverse abdominal incision is occasionally used. Much like nephrectomy surgery, both retroperitoneal and transperitoneal approaches are feasible for cystectomy, and laparoscopic and robotic-assisted techniques are becoming popular both for cystectomy and diversion procedures.

Preoperative Considerations

The most common patients presenting for cystectomy are those with bladder cancer. Approximately 90% have transitional cell tumors, and approximately 90% of these have already invaded muscle at diagnosis. Bladder tumors occasionally present with urinary retention but are generally diagnosed by hematuria (microscopic or macroscopic) with or without voiding symptoms such as urgency, frequency, and dysuria. Prior to cystectomy, patients have usually undergone one or several cystoscopies for tumor biopsy or resection, and many have already received radiation and chemotherapy.

Risk factors for bladder cancer and atherosclerosis overlap, and perioperative protocols for cardiac risk assessment and management are relevant to cystectomy surgery.[105] Smoking history is most important, doubling the risk of bladder cancer, while occupational exposures in the leather, dye, and rubber industry and drinking water with high arsenic levels also contribute. A smoking history also raises the risk for respiratory disease. Men are about four times more likely than women to be diagnosed with bladder cancer with white men twice as likely as African-American men. The average patient presenting with bladder cancer is 65 years old. Paraneoplastic syndromes similar to those seen with kidney cancer have been reported with bladder cancer but are relatively rare.

Intraoperative Considerations

Anesthetic management for cystectomy is similar to that for nephrectomy surgery (see above), including preparation for the potential for major bleeding. Although patients strictly could undergo cystectomy surgery with epidural anesthesia alone, this is rarely chosen due to the extended duration of surgery. Particular attention should be paid to the approach to assessment of intravascular volume during cystectomy surgery given the considerable potential for bleeding and hypovolemia and the absence of meaningful urine output data. Combining intraoperative epidural analgesia with a general anesthetic for cystectomy may reduce bleeding and improve postoperative analgesia without otherwise affecting complication rates.[137]

Postoperative Considerations

Simple cystectomy with diversion procedure involves a more limited dissection of pelvic structures relative to radical cystectomy and is generally associated with considerably less blood loss and lower complication rates.[138] Following radical cystectomy with diversion, some patients will require admission to an intensive care unit. Average blood loss ranges between 560 and 3,000 mL, and transfusion is common. Hospital lengths of stay can be long but vary considerably among centers. The mortality rate for radical cystectomy with diversion procedure is approximately 1%, and perioperative complications are common (27.3%).[139] Early problems include acute pyelonephritis following ureteral catheter removal, ileus, injury to local structures such as the obturator nerve (adductor palsy and gait disturbance), and impaired lymph drainage (lymphocele, leg edema).

Specific Procedures

Partial Cystectomy

Nonmalignant indications for partial bladder resection include bladder endometriosis and benign tumors (e.g., lymphangioma). Wherever partial cystectomy will suffice, the effects of added surgery and poorer quality of life associated with a urinary diversion procedure can be eliminated. Hence, the current interest in methods to identify bladder cancer patients for whom partial cystectomy with pelvic lymph node dissection may be as good a treatment as radical cystectomy. Selective "bladder-sparing" protocols that use responsiveness of a tumor to chemotherapy and radiation therapy as a guide to surgical decision making appear to successfully identify about one-third of the patients whose long-term outcome with partial cystectomy are equivalent to radical cystectomy, without the need for a diversion procedure.[132]

Simple and Radical Cystectomy

Simple cystectomy is indicated for benign disease such as neurogenic bladder, refractory bladder pain syndrome (interstitial cystitis), bladder damage from radiation, and refractory incontinence.

Radical cystectomy involves resection of the bladder but also related pelvic structures including pelvic lymphadenectomy of obturator and iliac nodes. In the male, the bladder en bloc with pelvic peritoneum, prostate and seminal vesicles, ureteric remnants, and a small piece of membranous urethra, and in the female, the uterus, ovaries, fallopian tubes, vaginal vault, and urethra. Alternate terminology to radical cystectomy for these major procedures include the following: In the male, "radical cystoprostatectomy" and, in the female, "radical cystectomy with pelvic exenteration."

Ileal Conduit and Other Diversion Procedures

The concept of ileal conduit surgery is relatively straightforward, involving creation of an ileal pouch that is attached to both ureters and the abdominal wall as a stoma. In contrast, continent diversion procedures are numerous and diverse in their approaches to urine collection and drainage. Continent urinary diversions can be categorized into (1) ureterosigmoidostomy, (2) continent cutaneous diversions, and (3) "neobladder" diversions to the native urethra.[140] Ureterosigmoidostomy is only occasionally used and involves tunneling the ureters to the sigmoid colon, with urine storage and elimination being through the rectum. Continent cutaneous reservoirs resemble ileal conduit surgery, but the stomal attachment to the abdominal wall is modified to produce a valve mechanism, with urine drainage achieved by intermittent catheter drainage. Many continent cutaneous variants exist that involve the use of different bowel segments as the source for the reservoir (e.g., ileum, ileocecum, ascending colon, sigmoid colon, or transverse colon). Finally, continent orthotopic diversions involve "neobladder" construction from terminal ileum, cecum, or sigmoid colon, which is attached to proximal urethra and its intact rhabdosphincter mechanism. Notably, all urinary diversion procedures involve extensive dissection and are considerably more challenging if the patient has received preoperative radiation therapy. Complications of urinary diversion surgery include bowel obstruction, urinary tract infection, deep venous thrombosis and pulmonary embolism, pneumonia, upper urinary tract damage, and skin breakdown around the stoma.

After recovery, patients with urinary diversions are vulnerable to conditions that require subsequent surgeries; these include problems at the stoma site (e.g., stricture, hernia, prolapse, retraction 5% to 10%), fistulae between urinary tract and bowel (3%), bowel obstruction, reservoir or other genitourinary stone diseases (5%), impotence, primary tumor recurrence, and even bowel cancer in the bladder pouch. In addition, postradical cystectomy bladder cancer victims are subjected to frequent surveillance procedures due to their high risk for future upper urinary tract urothelial malignancies (3%) and may require radical nephroureterectomy.

Anesthetic considerations for patients who present with existing diversion procedures include metabolic and electrolyte abnormalities such as hyperchloremic metabolic acidosis (common), hypokalemia, hypocalcemia and hypomagnesemia, and high rates of urinary tract infection and pyelonephritis. In addition, these individuals frequently suffer from chronic diarrhea and may have problems related to malabsorption (e.g., vitamin B_{12} deficiency).

PROSTATECTOMY

Almost all procedures involving complete resection of the prostate (i.e., prostatectomy) are for adenocarcinoma of the prostate, since nonmalignant surgical disease of the prostate is typically so amenable to TUR (see the next section). Despite prostate cancer being a disease limited to men, it is the second most common cancer in most countries with an incidence that increases significantly with age and is approximately 50% more common in African-American men than in Caucasian men (Fig. 49-9).[141]

Current evidence-based opinion on the optimal management of prostate cancer is rapidly evolving, including the relative value of intervention (i.e., hormonal, cryo-, chemo-, internal and external radiation therapy, highly focused ultrasound ablation, and surgery) compared to an expanded role for "watchful waiting" in low-risk groups, as identified by measures such as tumor aggressiveness (e.g., Gleason score) and biomarkers (e.g., prostate-specific antigen levels). A second related concept is also emerging—that prostate cancer may exist in clinically significant (approximately 15%) and "insignificant" forms.[142] In general, surgical approaches are likely in younger men, while elderly patients who may die from disorders other than their prostate cancer are being more frequently advised to pursue nonsurgical therapy.

Prostatectomy can be performed using retropubic or perineal approaches and is amenable to endoscopic techniques with or without robotic assistance. The retropubic approach requires the

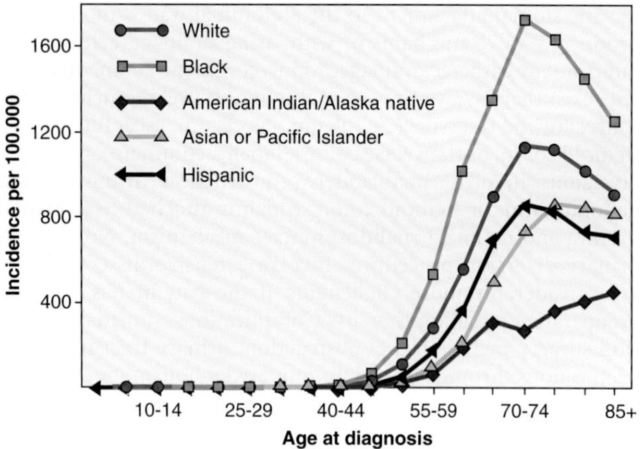

FIGURE 49-9. Crude incidence rates for prostate cancer, by race/ethnicity. (From: www.seer.cancer.gov [accessed March 2012]).

patient to be supine with the bed extended and in Trendelenberg position (Fig. 49-7) and allows access to the prostate gland and related lymph nodes from behind the pubic symphysis (and the best chance of sparing the neurovascular bundle), using either a vertical midline or Pfannensteil (horizontal low suprapubic) incision. In contrast, the perineal approach requires the patient be in exaggerated lithotomy and steep Trendelenberg position (Fig. 49-7), with an incision between the scrotum and the anal sphincter that provides adequate access to the prostate (but not lymph nodes).

Preoperative Considerations

Beyond advanced age, relatively few factors predict likelihood of contracting prostate cancer. Family history more than doubles the chances of the disease, while African-American descent increases the risk by approximately 50% (Fig. 49-9). Otherwise, factors such as smoking, obesity, diet, history of vasectomy, prostatitis, or sexually transmitted diseases have little or no effect on prostate cancer risk. Due to the advanced age of the population presenting for prostatectomy, an emphasis on comorbid disease in preoperative evaluation is particularly relevant. Paraneoplastic syndromes similar to those seen with kidney cancer are occasionally evident in prostate cancer patients.

Intraoperative Considerations

Anesthetic management for open prostatectomy is similar to that for cystectomy surgery (see above), including attentiveness to the potential for major bleeding. Epidural catheter placement is usually in the low thoracic spinal region, guided in part by the chosen option for anesthesia, including spinal/epidural alone, general alone, or combined spinal/epidural and general anesthesia. A surgical block to at least the T10 level is required for procedures performed using neuraxial block alone. In one study, patients experienced 33% less pain when preemptive epidural dosing occurred prior to incision.[143] Radical prostatectomy may take longer than the duration of a single-dose spinal anesthetic, so epidural or combined spinal–epidural is recommended. Notably, a neuraxial alone strategy for perineal prostatectomy is likely to be poorly tolerated due to the uncomfortable exaggerated lithotomy and head-down positioning requirements. Exaggerated lithotomy position for prostatectomy has also been associated in some studies with higher rates of neurologic injury (21% with transient sensory or motor deficit); patients appearing to be at greater risk when surgery lasts longer than 180 minutes.[144,145] In addition, even with general anesthesia, some patients tolerate the exaggerated lithotomy–head-down position for perineal prostatectomy poorly due to elevated ventilation pressures and impaired oxygenation.

As with cystectomy surgery, the approach to intravascular volume assessment during prostatectomy must consider the potential for bleeding and hypovolemia and limited meaningful urine output data; the need for arterial and/or pressure central venous monitoring should be guided by patient comorbidities. Neuraxial anesthesia for prostatectomy has been associated with decreased blood loss in some studies.[146] However, any blood-sparing benefits of neuraxial anesthesia appear to be lost when it is combined with mechanical ventilation (and general anesthesia), possibly due to the effect of increased intrathoracic pressure on prostatic venous pressures.[147] Notably, breaching of the rich prostatic venous plexuses also creates the potential for acute hemodynamic instability from major venous air embolism, which has been reported during both retropubic and perineal prostatectomy approaches; suspicion of this complication warrants immediate steps to flood the surgical field and alter patient positioning to raise venous pressures above atmospheric, in addition to other standard resuscitation measures.[148]

Postoperative Considerations

Simple prostatectomy requires a limited dissection relative to radical prostatectomy and is generally associated with less blood loss and lower complication rates. Nonetheless, most radical prostatectomy patients are not admitted to an intensive care unit. Average blood loss for radical prostatectomy surgery is between 500 and 1500 mL,[149] and approximately 10% of patients will require a perioperative blood transfusion.[150] In addition to vascular injury, the commonest serious intraoperative complications are bowel or ureteral injury. The mortality rate for radical prostatectomy is less than 1%. Impaired lymph drainage (lymphocele, leg edema) is associated in some studies with increased rates of postoperative deep venous thrombosis and pulmonary embolism.[150]

Transversus abdominis plane local anesthetic blocks are used at some institutions for pain management to facilitate retropubic prostatectomy fast tracking recovery protocols[151]; ultrasound guidance for these procedures can minimize procedure-related risk of adjacent structure injury (e.g., bowel).

Specific Procedures

Simple Prostatectomy

Simple open prostatectomy is occasionally required for resection of very large prostate glands affected by benign prostatic hypertrophy (BPH),[152] but, in the era of medical therapies such as α-1 selective adrenergic receptor blockers and 5-α reductase inhibitors, this is an infrequent procedure. Currently, retropubic prostatectomy is the most common approach in the United States.

Radical Prostatectomy

Radical prostatectomy involves removal of the entire prostate gland, seminal vesicles, and generally the surrounding nerves and veins. The part of the urethra within the prostate gland's transition zone is also removed. Preservation of one or both cavernous nerves (part of the neurovascular bundle on each side of the prostate) can improve postsurgery quality of life (i.e., reduced urinary incontinence and erectile dysfunction) but limits the extent of possible resection. Notably, the incidence of positive margins with tumor resection during radical prostatectomy is significant (~30%). The value of more aggressive resection with sural nerve grafting to address erectile dysfunction remains unclear.[153] Controversial early data on the association of epidural anesthesia and analgesia with lower rates of cancer recurrence[154] have not been substantiated in more recent reports.

Laparoscopic and Robotic Prostatectomy

Minimally invasive laparoscopic and robotic-assisted approaches to prostatectomy are gaining popularity (see Chapter 43). While these techniques are characterized by less pain, shorter hospital stays, faster recovery, and improved patient satisfaction,[155] they also present added challenge for the anesthesiologist, including prolonged procedure duration, the risk of hypothermia, occult blood loss, and the physiologic stresses of pneumoperitoneum added to exaggerated Trendelenburg with or without lithotomy positioning.

Laparoscopic and robotic prostatectomy procedures require general anesthesia with endotracheal intubation. Standard monitoring and adequate intravenous access must be established prior to patient positioning since access after positioning is very difficult (Fig. 49-10). Pulse oximeter probe placement should avoid the ear lobe to anticipate the potential for inaccurate readings in this location, presumably related to the venous engorgement with head-down positioning and pneumoperitoneum.[156] Intra-arterial and central venous monitoring are not routine but may be indicated based on patient comorbidities. Anesthetic planning must take into account that, due to the fixed position of the robot arms, movements such as coughing can cause injury internally or at port sites. Exaggerated Trendelenburg positioning is required for the procedure, and some practitioners deliberately refrain from dosing epidural catheters to avoid cephalad spread of epidural drugs during the procedure.

Steep Trendelenburg (30 to 45 degrees head-down) to facilitate pelvic access during laparoscopic and robotic prostatectomy procedures increases the risk of several important complications (Fig. 49-7). To prevent sliding, patients must be well situated on the operating table (e.g., within a vacuum bean bag) then firmly secured (e.g., tape, safety belt). Arms should be placed on angled armboards *prior* to lowering the end table section during lithotomy positioning to minimize the risk of pinched or crushed fingers. The patient's arms are generally tucked at the side, and pressure points carefully padded. Additional padding should distribute localized pressure from shoulder braces, which sometimes support a significant fraction of the patient's body weight (Fig. 49-10). Beyond brachial plexus protection with shoulder padding, attention should be paid to radial (at the humerus), ulnar (at the elbow), and lateral femoral cutaneous (by the lithotomy leg holders) nerves to minimize axonal injuries. Finally, since oral ulceration and even conjunctival burns have been attributed to lithotomy-related reflux of gastric contents, steps such as preoperative antacid therapy, stomach drainage by orogastric tube, and waterproof eye taping should all be considered.[157]

Lack of easy access to the patient is a concern during robotic prostatectomy, primarily caused by the sheer size of current robot arms (Fig. 49-10). Hence, positioning preparation must be thorough and completed prior to robot docking. A Mayo instrument standing directly above the patient's head reliably prevents robotic arms from causing pressure-related facial injuries and/or endotracheal tube displacement (Fig. 49-10).[158] Operating room staff must also be trained for robot emergencies, particularly timely removal of the device. Notably, while cardioversion and defibrillation are possible with the robot docked, cardiopulmonary resuscitation with chest compressions is nearly impossible.

The physiology of steep Trendelenburg positioning is well tolerated by healthy patients,[159] but this cannot be assumed for those with serious comorbidities. Adding to the stresses of head-down positioning during laparoscopic prostatectomy are the effects of CO_2 pneumoperitoneum (see nephrectomy section; Table 49-5). Although no formal guidelines exist, additional monitoring for patients with cardiac disease (e.g., compensated congestive heart failure) may be justified to assess responses to position-related intravascular volume shifts. Respiratory effects of robotic prostatectomy are numerous and often require considerable adjustments to mechanical ventilation parameters. Endotracheal tube cuff location should be just beyond the vocal cords, to minimize the potential for developing a mainstem intubation with the cephalad shift of the diaphragm and mediastinum from the combination of head-down and pneumoperitoneum.[156] The related encroachment of abdominal contents on the diaphragm also has significant effects on pulmonary function, particularly in obese patients, including reductions in functional residual capacity, vital capacity, and overall lung compliance that translate into the need for higher peak airway pressures for equivalent tidal volumes. In addition, obese patients experience greater ventilation; perfusion mismatching. One study reported an average 8% lower tidal volumes, 22% higher respiratory rates, and a 38% higher peak inspiratory pressures to maintain similar end-tidal carbon dioxide levels but lower oxygen saturation levels, during robotic compared to open retropubic radical prostatectomy.[160] Interestingly, CO_2 insufflation for retroperitoneal laparoscopic procedures requires greater increases in minute ventilation to compensate for absorbed CO_2 than equivalent transperitoneal procedures.[157] Tolerance of mildly elevated CO_2 levels (permissive hypercarbia) during some phases of the surgery may be a good strategy in some patients but is potentially ill-advised for patients with CKD where even mild respiratory acidosis can be associated with significant hyperkalemia.[161] Transcranial Doppler[162] and cerebral oximetry[159] to monitor intracranial perfusion have been suggested for patients with cerebrovascular disease. Potential adverse effects on intraocular pressure of head-down positioning in at-risk patients (e.g., poorly controlled glaucoma) have not been rigorously studied. Despite all these physiologic perturbations, the need to convert from laparoscopic/robotic assisted to open techniques for major urologic procedures is remarkably infrequent.[157]

During robotic prostatectomy, one of the major surgical steps involves re-anastomosis of the severed urethral ends after prostate gland resection, this is often made more complicated by urine from the bladder neck spilling directly into the operative field, obscuring the surgeon's view and impeding progress. Anticipation of this problem by the anesthesiologist can assist the surgeon through cautious fluid restriction, particularly prior to urethral anastomosis. A generally restrictive approach to fluid administration may also attenuate the development of mild facial, periorbital, and even occasionally laryngeal edema associated with prolonged steep lithotomy position.[156,157] However, edema accumulation is rarely sufficient to threaten airway patency after tracheal extubation.

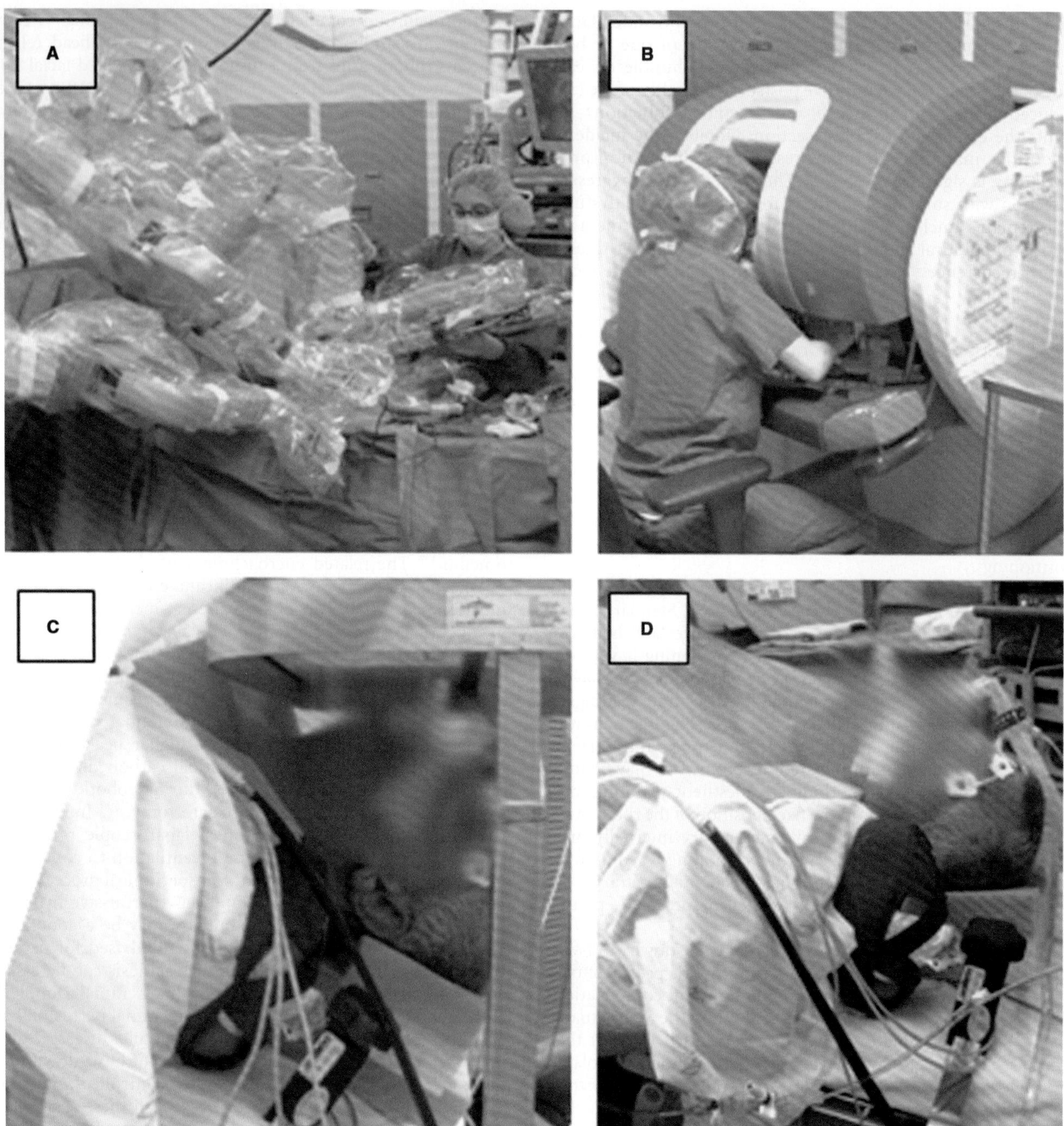

FIGURE 49-10. Images from a robotic radical prostatectomy procedure highlights the significant difficulty in accessing patients after the robot is docked **(A)**, the remote location of the surgeon **(B)**, the utility of a carefully placed Mayo stand to protect the patient's face and endotracheal tube **(C)**, and the value of shoulder support padding to avoid pressure injuries **(D)**.

TRANSURETHRAL SURVEILLANCE AND RESECTION PROCEDURES

Transurethral endoscopy is commonly used, relatively noninvasive surgical tool in the armamentarium of the urologist, that can play an important role in the management and treatment of urothelial cancers (e.g., cystoscopy/ureteroscopy surveillance, TURBT), urolithiasis (e.g., ureteroscopic stent placement, basket stone retrieval), and BPH (e.g., transurethral resection of the prostate [TURP]). Despite the benign and noninvasive appearance of transurethral tissue resection surgeries (TURBT, TURP), these procedures are occasionally associated with significant morbidity and even mortality.

Cystoscopy and TURBT procedures are used in the surveilance, staging, and management of transitional cell bladder cancers (see cystectomy section). For patients with superficial cancers that do not invade the bladder muscle, bladder biopsy and subsequent TURBT may be curative, but such patients require ongoing cystoscopy surveillance and often receive biologic therapies (e.g., Bacillus Calmette-Guerin [BCG]S vaccine) that reduce the recurrence rate of bladder cancer, presumably by boosting the immune response. Nonetheless, about 50% of patients with a resected bladder cancer will develop another bladder or ureteral cancer in the future.

TURP is a mainstay, and even "gold standard" therapy to alleviate urine obstructive symptoms related to BPH. BPH describes
12 the smooth muscle and epithelial cell proliferation within the transition zone of the prostate that histologically characterizes this disorder. The symptoms of BPH reflect the combination of bladder outlet obstruction (static) and increased smooth muscle tone (dynamic). While TURP surgery with electrocautery has been for many decades central to the treatment of BPH, a proliferation of other options explains the steady decrease in the use of TURP for BPH treatment, partly due to the significant side effects that can occur with this procedure (e.g., incontinence, impotence). Medical therapy for BPH is common, directed at both static and dynamic components of the disease (α-1 adrenergic antagonists and α-1A reductase inhibitors), and is part of the current more conservative watchful waiting approach to surgical treatment of BPH. Numerous alternate procedures to TURP are now being used for BPH; in 2005, TURP represented 39% of BPH procedures compared to 81% in 1999. Description of these alternate procedures is beyond the scope of this text, but some of these include transurethral needle ablation (TUNA), transurethral microwave thermal therapy (TUMT), transurethral ablation prostatectomy (TURAPY), holmium laser ablation of the prostate (HoLAP), interstitial laser coagulation (ILC), ultrasound/high intensity focused ultrasound (HIFU), and water intensity hyperthermia (WIT).

Positioning concerns for cystoscopy, TURBT, and TURP are the same as for other procedures in lithotomy position (Fig. 49-10) and in particular relate to adequate padding of pressure points and avoidance of peroneal nerve compression.

Preoperative Considerations

Patients presenting for TURP are likely to be elderly and may have other serious comorbidities. Cardiovascular and pulmonary status should be carefully assessed to evaluate the patient's ability to tolerate the intravascular volume changes associated with the procedure. Patients on anticoagulant therapy may not be candidates for spinal anesthesia, depending on the indication for anticoagulation. The risk of stopping the anticoagulant perioperatively may or may not be worth the advantages of spinal anesthesia for a particular patient. Decisions about this should be made in conjunction with the surgeon, as the risk of postoperative bleeding following TURP will likely dictate an interval of normal coagulation or bridging treatment with short-acting anticoagulants such as heparin.

Intraoperative Considerations

Choice of anesthetic technique for cystoscopy, TURBT, and TURP procedures should be tailored to the individual and can be performed safely with either general or regional anesthesia.[163] Neuraxial block allows the patient to remain awake and may hasten the diagnosis of bladder or prostatic capsule perforation and the TUR syndrome and may also decrease blood loss compared with general anesthesia.[164,165] For ambulatory surgery patients, care must be taken in the selection of spinal anesthetic medications so as to avoid prolonged anesthetic duration and delayed discharge from the facility. Combined spinal–epidural techniques or general anesthesia may have advantages if the length of surgery is unpredictable. Notably, the lower central venous pressure associated with regional anesthesia may actually increase the likelihood of significant irrigation fluid absorption.[166]

Hypothermia can complicate TURP procedures: Body temperature decreases approximately 1° C/hr of surgery, and shivering occurs in 16% of patients who receive room-temperature irrigation fluids. Hypothermia does not develop if irrigation solutions are warmed to body temperature.[167]

Approximately 2.5% of patients require transfusion during TURP surgery. Average blood loss is 2 to 4 mL/min,[168] but individual bleeding rates can be difficult to assess due to mixing with irrigating fluid. The patient's vital signs may be useful to guide transfusion,[169] but, with prolonged resections, serial assessments of hemoglobin level are advisable.

Surgical perforation of the prostatic capsule occurs in 2% of TURP procedures, usually resulting in extraperitoneal fluid extravasation. Awake patients with a neuraxial anesthetic may complain during surgery of new onset pain localized to the lower abdomen and back.[169,170] Bladder perforation during TURBT more commonly results in extravasation of fluid intraperitoneally and may produce abdominal distension and complaints of abdominal and shoulder pain in awake patients.[171] Notably, evidence of perforation often only becomes clear postoperatively.

Postoperative Considerations

Although abnormal bleeding after TURP occurs in fewer than 1% of resections,[168] 2% to 3% of patients will require transfusion perioperatively.[172,173] Blood loss following TURBT is usually less than 100 mL, although postoperative hemorrhage can rarely occur. Thromboplastin, a thrombogenic stimulant found in high concentrations in prostate cancer cells, can rarely trigger disseminated intravascular coagulation.[169] Another cause of post-TURP bleeding is release of prostatic tissue plasminogen activators. These factors convert plasminogen to plasmin, causing fibrinolysis. Treatment of these conditions is supportive and may include transfusion of coagulation factors and platelets.[174]

As outlined above, bladder, prostatic capsule, or urethral perforation are uncommon but serious complications that may manifest postoperatively with or without symptoms of TUR syndrome (see later). Fever related to TURP procedures may indicate bacteremia secondary to spread of bacteria through open prostatic venous sinuses, particularly with a history of infectious prostatitis.

The most common complications following TURP surgery are the need for urinary recatheterization (4%), prostatic capsule perforation (2%), and postoperative hemorrhage requiring transfusion (1%).[175] The 30-day mortality following TURP is 0.2%[176–180] and most commonly relates to serious cardiac and respiratory complications.[181]

Specific Procedures

Cystoscopy and Ureteroscopy

While surveillance cystoscopy is often performed under local anesthesia outside the operating room with minimal monitoring or sedation and without the involvement of anesthesia personnel, some cystoscopy and most ureteroscopy procedures, particularly for those patients with comorbidities, occur in the operating room setting. Cystoscopy and ureteroscopy are rarely associated with significant complications, and perioperative considerations should generally parallel those for the disease being screened for or managed (see related sections).

Transurethral Bladder Tumor Resection

During any simple cystoscopy or ureteroscopy procedure, abnormal tissue may require one or more planned or unanticipated diagnostic biopsies or biopsy/resections. As outlined above (see cystectomy section), risk factors for bladder cancer and atherosclerosis overlap and cardiac risk assessment is relevant to TURBT surgery.[182] A serious intraoperative complication of TURBT is bladder perforation by the rigid cystoscope during tissue resection, which occasionally occurs due to unexpected patient movement. For this reason, muscle relaxation is preferred during general anesthesia, particularly in lateral wall resections where the obturator nerve may be stimulated by electrocautery, producing a violent contraction of the ipsilateral thigh muscles. Neuraxial anesthesia to the T9 to T10 dermatomal level also provides adequate anesthesia for the procedure and prevents the obturator reflex. Regional anesthesia may also facilitate detection of bladder perforation. Postoperative pain is usually minimal and responds well to nonopiate and opiate medications.

Transurethral Prostate Resection (TURP)

Standard procedure during TURP surgery involves inserting a "resectoscope," a specialized endoscopy instrument with an electrode capable of both coagulating and cutting tissue, into the urethra then bladder, and the tissue protruding into the prostatic urethra is then resected.[183] There has been much recent interest in the use of lasers rather than electrocautery to resect excess prostate tissue. A variety of different lasers have been utilized. Laser techniques have advantages over traditional electrocautery approaches particularly related to traditional irrigation fluid restrictions: Laser resection has no requirement for a nonconductive fluid, so 0.9% saline may be used, avoiding complications of absorption related to hypo-osmolarity and solute toxicity (see TUR syndrome below). Furthermore, the potential for systemic absorption may be reduced due to the lower irrigation infusion rates and pressures necessary for laser procedures.[184,185] Lasers also have coagulative properties, resulting in less blood loss and lower rates of transfusion.

Irrigating Solutions and Transurethral Resection Syndrome

Key to a surgeon's endoscopic view during transurethral procedures is a crystal clear irrigating solution, infused with a pump or via gravity (and drained away) to flush out blood and resected tissue and keep space between structures. Safety characteristics of the irrigating solution are important since, with tissue resection or urinary tract injury, significant amounts of the fluid may inadvertently enter the circulation; for example, during TURP through openings in the venous plexus or retroperitoneal rents in the prostatic capsule or consequent to perforation of the urinary bladder into the peritoneal space during TURBT. Other procedures where inadvertent perforation can cause the TUR syndrome include cystoscopy, ureteroscopy (URS), percutaneous nephrolithotomy (PNL), and laser vaporization of the prostate.

13 The spectrum of morbidities associated with irrigating solution absorption are termed the TUR syndrome. A variety of nonconductive *nonelectrolytic* solutions are in common use. The crystalloids have current-dispersing properties due to their ionic characteristics that make them unsuitable for use with unipolar electrocautery. When absorbed in significant amounts, nonelectrolytic irrigation solutions combine electrolyte disturbances with hypervolemia. Notably, newer transurethral *bipolar* electrocautery and laser techniques now allow irrigation with isotonic crystalloid solutions (e.g., 0.9% saline), but until these technologies totally replace unipolar electrocautery, nonconducting osmotically active irrigating solutions will continue to be used, each variant having its own concerns (Table 49-6).[186]

It is, therefore, important that the anesthesiologist be aware of solutions used for transurethral procedures at their own institution, since TUR syndrome for each irrigating solution has its own profile (Table 49-6). Nonetheless, *TUR syndrome* historically describes a common cluster of symptoms related to hypervolemic water intoxication; the principal components are (a) excessive volume expansion (respiratory distress, congestive heart failure,

TABLE 49-6. PROPERTIES OF COMMONLY USED IRRIGATING SOLUTIONS FOR TRANSURETHRAL RESECTION PROCEDURES

Solution	Osmolality (mOsm/L)	Advantages	Disadvantages
Distilled water	0	Improved visibility	Hemolysis Hemoglobinemia Hemoglobinuria Hyponatremia
Glycine (1.5%)	200	Less likelihood of TUR syndrome	Transient postoperative visual syndrome Hyperammonemia Hyperoxaluria
Sorbitol (3.3%)	165	Same as glycine	Hyperglycemia, possible lactic acidosis Osmotic diuresis
Mannitol (5%)	275	Isosmolar solution Not metabolized	Osmotic diuresis Possibility of acute intravascular volume expansion

TURP, transurethral resection of the prostate.
Adapted from: Krongrad A, Droller MJ. Complications of transurethral resection of the prostate. In: Marshall FF, ed. *Urologic Complications: Medical and Surgical, Adult and Pediatric.* 2nd ed. St. Louis: Mosby-Year Book, 1990, 05, with permission.

TABLE 49-7. SIGNS AND SYMPTOMS OF ACUTE HYPONATREMIA

Serum Na^+ (mEq/L)	CNS Changes	ECG Changes
120	Confusion	Possible widening of QRS complex
	Restlessness	
115	Somnolence	Widened QRS complex
	Nausea	Elevated ST segment
110	Seizures	Ventricular tachycardia or fibrillation
	Coma	

CNS, central nervous system; ECG, electrocardiogram.
Adapted from: Jensen V. The TURP syndrome. *Can J Anaesth.* 1991;38:90, with permission.

pulmonary edema, hypertension, bradycardia, hypotension, etc.), (b) hyponatremia (mental confusion, nausea, etc.; Table 49-7), and (c) other problems specific to each of the irrigating solutions.[187–189] Notably, any future trend toward limiting irrigation to physiologic solutions (e.g., 0.9% saline), should eliminate all but the hypervolemic component of the TUR syndrome.

Of available irrigating solutions, distilled water is rarely utilized due to its hypotonicity. Water intoxication with distilled water rapidly causes severe hyponatremia, leading to hemolysis, hemoglobinemia, and renal failure. Sorbitol and glucose solutions cause hyperglycemia when they are absorbed. Glycine, an amino acid normally metabolized to ammonia, may cause a depressed mental status and even coma (due to hyperammonemia) that can last 24 to 48 hours postoperatively.[190,191] Also reported with glycine are blurred vision, minimally or nonreactive pupils, and transient blindness.[192,193] Since glycine has structural similarities to aminobutyric acid, these visual disturbances are thought to reflect neurotransmitter-mediated brainstem or cranial nerve inhibition rather than cerebral edema.[193]

Absorption of very large amounts of irrigant (>2 L) is usually required to manifest the TUR syndrome. The incidence of symptomatic TUR syndrome is highest during TURP procedures where it may be as high as 1.4%.[172] Typically, intraoperative irrigation infusion rates of 300 mL/min are used during TURP procedures for optimal surgical visualization.[181] Some intravascular absorption is to be expected; rates of 20 mL/min are typical, but these can reach as high as 200 mL/min.[194] Factors that predict increased irrigation fluid absorption during a TURP procedure include the number and size of open venous sinuses (i.e., greater blood loss implies greater potential for irrigation absorption), surgical disruption of the prostatic capsule, longer duration of resection, higher hydrostatic pressure of the irrigating fluid, and lower venous pressure at the irrigant–blood interface.[168]

To minimize fluid absorption, procedural guidelines include limiting resection time to <1 hour and suspending the irrigating fluid bag no more than 30 cm above the operating table at the beginning and 15 cm in the final stages of resection.[168,195] In addition, avoidance of hypotonic intravenous fluids and treatment of regional anesthesia-induced hypotension with judicious use of intravenous vasopressor agents rather than intravenous fluids should be considered.

Symptomatic TUR syndrome is much less common following TURBT (and usually related to symptoms of bladder perforation), but it is important to be aware of the possibility of its occurrence since it may present somewhat differently due to the slower rate of fluid absorption.[171] Most notably, the time course of symptoms following bladder perforation during TURBT reflects the slower absorption from the abdominal cavity, compared to direct prostatic venous plexus entry with TURP. For example, nadir serum sodium values are generally reached between 1 and 6 hours following TURP, whereas TUR syndrome following TURBT occurs between 2 and 9 hours postoperatively.[171]

Clinical manifestations of the TUR syndrome range from mild (restlessness, nausea, shortness of breath, dizziness) to severe (seizures, coma, hypertension, bradycardia, cardiovascular collapse). In the awake patient with a regional block, a classic triad of symptoms has been described that consists of an increase in both systolic and diastolic pressures associated with an increase in pulse pressure, bradycardia, and mental status changes.[169,187]

Early symptoms associated with TUR syndrome are mostly related to acute intravascular volume expansion, independent of changes in serum osmolality and sodium.[189] Initial hypertension and bradycardia from acute volume overload may evolve into left heart failure, pulmonary edema, and even cardiovascular collapse.[196] With the continued absorption of hypotonic irrigation fluid, cerebral edema as a consequence of dilutional hyponatremia may develop. Rapid change, as opposed to a specific low threshold serum sodium concentration, is responsible for most of the signs and symptoms of TUR syndrome (Table 49-7).[187]

When neurologic or cardiovascular complications of TURP procedures are recognized intraoperatively, prompt intervention is necessary (Table 49-8). First, the surgeon should be informed of the patient's status change so that the procedure can be completed or terminated as quickly as possible. The hallmark of patient treatment is to restore extracellular tonicity. Although the traditional recommended rate of serum sodium correction is 0.5 mEq/L/hr, this is for chronic hyponatremia, and no established rate for correction of acute hyponatremia exists. Symptomatic patients with serum sodium concentrations <120 mEq/L should have their extracellular tonicity corrected with hypertonic saline. Sodium chloride in a 3% solution should be infused at a rate no greater than 100 mL/hr. Serum electrolytes should be followed closely, and the hypertonic saline discontinued when the patient is asymptomatic or serum sodium concentration exceeds

TABLE 49-8. TREATMENT OF THE TRANSURETHRAL RESECTION SYNDROME

- Ensure oxygenation and circulatory support
- Notify surgeon and terminate procedure as soon as possible
- Consider insertion of invasive monitors if cardiovascular instability occurs
- Send blood to laboratory for evaluation of electrolytes, creatinine, glucose, and arterial blood gases
- Obtain 12-lead electrocardiogram
- Treat mild symptoms (with serum Na^+ concentration >120 mEq/L) with fluid restriction and loop diuretic (furosemide)
- Treat severe symptoms (if serum Na^+ <120 mEq/L) with 3% sodium chloride IV at a rate <100 mL/h
- Discontinue 3% sodium chloride when serum Na^+ >120 mEq/L

120 mEq/L. Treatment with hypertonic saline has been associated with development of demyelinating central nervous system lesions (central pontine myelinolysis) due to rapid increases in plasma osmolality, and this approach should be reserved for patients with severe, life-threatening symptoms.[197] The demyelination is the result of excessive shrinkage of brain cells after rapid hydration with hyperosmolar solution as the brain cells have extruded important osmoles to compensate for the chronic hypotonicity. Notably, reports of demyelination after correction of acute symptomatic hyponatremia are rare, and there are no reports of demyelination after treatment of acute TUR syndrome.[189]

THERAPIES FOR UROLITHIASIS

Stone disease of the urinary tract, urolithiasis, can be subdivided on the basis of the location of the stone into nephrolithiasis (kidney), ureterolithiasis (ureter), or cystolithiasis (bladder). Nephrolithiasis is a common clinical problem, with an increasing incidence. The lifetime prevalence of nephrolithiasis is 10% in men and 5% in women. Up to 50% of patients with an initial stone episode will have a recurrence within 5 years.[198]

The composition of kidney stones varies (Table 49-9). The most common type of stones contain calcium and are radio-opaque. Stones form when the concentration of stone-forming salts in the urine is elevated, (e.g., oxalate) or when the level of stone inhibitors in the urine is low (e.g., citrate). This results in supersaturation of the urine with salts, allowing crystals to form and grow, particularly in situations where urine volume is low. This pathophysiology explains the principles of the medical management of kidney stones: Increasing urine volume and maneuvers to restore urinary salt balance, through dietary and medical treatment.[199,200]

The preferred diagnostic modality for urolithiasis is helical noncontrast CT scan which can identify radio-opaque and radiolucent stones in the entire urinary system and determine whether hydronephrosis is present. Ultrasound imaging is also informative for stones in the kidney and proximal ureter but cannot image the distal ureter and may miss smaller stones. Compared to helical CT and ultrasonography, plain radiographs (Kidney–Ureter–Bladder, KUB) provide no additional information about obstruction or hydronephrosis and can miss stones in the kidney or ureter. Intravenous pyelography is rarely used since it offers no added information compared to other diagnostic modalities and exposes the patient to radiation and contrast-related renal injury.[200]

TABLE 49-9. SPECTRUM OF KIDNEY STONES TYPES: COMPOSITION, FREQUENCY, AND CAUSES

Stone Composition	Frequency	Mechanism
Calcium oxalate or Calcium phosphate	70–80%	Hypercalciuria • High sodium and protein diet • Hypercalcemia, e.g., hyperparathyroidism • Chronic metabolic acidosis Low urine output • Chronic dehydration Hyperuricosuria • High purine, high protein intake • Gout Hyperoxaluria • Low dietary calcium • High oxalate diet • Genetic Low urine citrate • Chronic metabolic acidosis • Renal tubular acidosis • Inflammatory bowel disease
Uric Acid	10–15%	Low urine pH Chronic metabolic acidosis Hyperuricosuria Obesity Lesch–Nyhan syndrome
Magnesium ammonium phosphate (struvite)	10–15%	Urinary infections (urea-splitting bacteria), e.g., Proteus, Klebsiella, Staphylococcus, Pseudomonas, Providentia, and Corynebacterium urealyticum
Cystine	<1%	Cystinuria—autosomal recessive
Others: Indinavir	<1%	Antiretroviral drug for HIV
Triamterene		Potassium-sparing diuretic
Xanthine		Xanthine oxidase inhibitor therapy, e.g., allopurinol

Modified from: Hall PM. Nephrolithiasis: Treatment, causes, and prevention. *Cleve Clin J Med.* 2009;76:583–591 with permission; Brown P. Management of urinary tract infections associated with nephrolithiasis. *Curr Infect Dis Rep.* 2010;12:450–454, with permission.

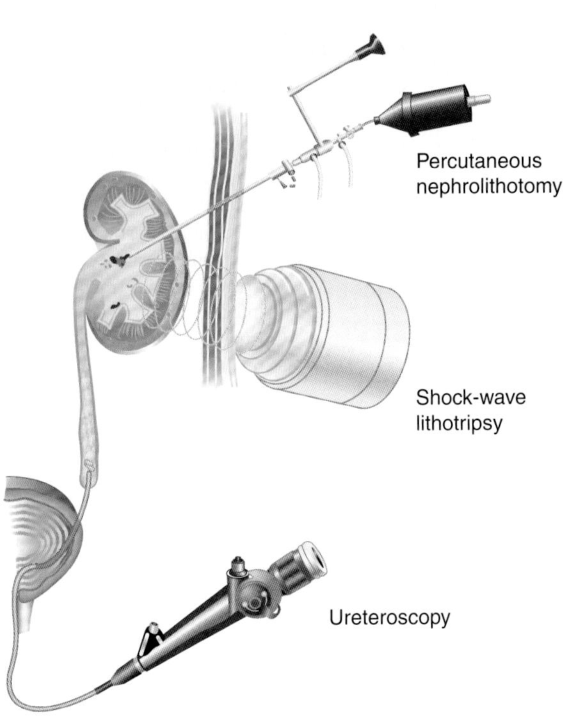

FIGURE 49-11. Urinary tract stones: Intervention choices. From: Samplaski MK, Irwin BH, Desai M. Less-invasive ways to remove stones from the kidneys and ureters. *Cleve Clin J Med.* 2009;76:592–598, with permission.

Patients with kidney stones typically present with intermittent or continuous moderate to severe colicky pain in the ipsilateral flank and upper abdomen. Testicular or labial pain is more typical with distal ureteric stones. Occasionally, patients present with painless urinary infection or hematuria. Conservative nonsurgical therapy for smaller stones consists of analgesics (e.g., nonsteroidal anti-inflammatory drugs and/or opiates) and aggressive fluid administration to promote urine flow and passage of the stone. The so-called "medical expulsive therapy" (MET) to promote ureter relaxation and the spontaneous passage of small ureteral stones involves treatment with calcium-channel blockers (e.g., nifedipine), α-blockers (e.g., tamsulosin), and sometimes, corticosteroids[200,201] The likelihood of stone passage without surgery relates to the size of the stone, its location, and the presence or absence of urinary system anatomic abnormalities such as strictures. If stones do not pass spontaneously or respond to MET, various surgical options can be considered, as discussed above (Fig. 49-11).

Preoperative Considerations

Anesthetic planning for urolithiasis surgery should include standard considerations. Typical calcium salt stone disease presents in the third to fifth decades of life[200] and is commonly associated with comorbidities such as obesity, hypertension, and hyperparathyroidism. Patients with renal failure or CKD should be assessed for the sequelae of these conditions, including platelet dysfunction, anemia, and electrolyte abnormalities. Bladder stones are often diagnosed in patients with poor voiding capacity, for example, paraplegic patients, and the associated perioperative concerns for these patients should be addressed. Although paraplegic patients with sensory deficits below T6 lack pain perception for cystoscopy procedures, they are at risk for *autonomic hyperreflexia* and require anesthesia to block the afferent stimulation that can provoke this reaction (e.g., bladder distension). This can be achieved with deeper levels of general anesthesia or regional anesthesia.[202] Patients with idiopathic hypercalciuria are often treated with thiazide diuretics, and serum potassium should be assessed preoperatively.[200]

Perioperative opioid analgesic dosing for urolithiasis procedures can be challenging. Patients with recurrent nephrolithiasis may be receiving chronic opioid therapy and demonstrate tolerance intra- and postoperatively. In contrast, when severe colic is alleviated by surgery for an opioid naive patient already treated with opiates, postoperative somnolence is quite common. Renal colic is often associated with nausea and vomiting, and preoperative aspiration prophylaxis should be considered.

Unless open surgery is planned, there is rarely a need for blood transfusion for stone surgery. Selection of appropriate monitors should be dictated by patient comorbidities, as significant blood loss or fluid shifts are unusual with these procedures. However, if patient difficulty achieving vascular access during a procedure is anticipated (e.g., percutaneous nephrolithotripsy), there should be a low threshold for establishing invasive monitoring prior to the procedure. Antibiotic prophylaxis is important, particularly with infected stones or pyelonephritis. When lasers are required, appropriate eye protection should be provided for the perioperative team and patient.

Intraoperative Considerations

Compared with other more invasive urologic procedures, stone surgeries generally do not involve large amounts of blood loss or fluid shifts, with the possible exception of percutaneous nephrolithotripsy (see later). Information about anesthetic choice and potential intraoperative issues is discussed in the individual sections below and in the sections on nephrectomy and transurethral surgery elsewhere in this chapter. Monitoring decisions and anesthetic choices should be made on the basis of patient comorbidity, and intraoperative care should focus on those as well.

Postoperative Considerations

Postoperative concerns for urolithiasis procedures are generally minor. Interestingly, patients with severe renal colic prior to less-invasive surgeries (e.g., URS) may have less or no pain postoperatively with relief of their urinary obstruction and stone retrieval. However, immediately following urinary tract instrumentation, many patients experience rather uncomfortable bladder and ureteral spasms. Occasionally, open surgery is required for upper urinary tract stone removal, with postoperative concerns comparable to nephrectomy patients having similar incisions; these include pain, which may be sufficient to require epidural analgesia, and monitoring requirements to ensure that adequate resuscitation related to any blood loss has occurred. This pain is typically responsive to NSAIDs, oxybutynin, and belladonna and opium suppositories.

Monitoring the adequacy of urine output and maintaining any urinary irrigation or drainage system (e.g., stents, three-way Foley catheters) to promote clearance of blood in the urinary system is important, as clots or stone fragments can cause acute urinary obstruction.

After extraction or lithotripsy of stones, particularly struvite stones or in the setting of pyelonephritis, patients may develop a pattern of rigors, hypotension, and fever, which can lead to shock. Urine culture results can be misleading in predicting which patients will develop sepsis since urine below the level of a stone may be clean, yet urine upstream of the stony obstruction may be infected. A sepsis picture can be noted during the procedure but is more likely to occur postoperatively. Indications of intravascular bacterial seeding from infected urine needs prompt attention with blood cultures, fluids and resuscitation, and institution of appropriate antibiotic therapy to prevent more serious sequelae of a sepsis syndrome. The potential acuity of this situation should not be underestimated, as even healthy ASA 1 to 2 patients can develop systemic inflammatory response syndrome (SIRS) and require aggressive resuscitation and intensive care.[203]

Specific Procedures

Shock Wave Lithotripsy

Shock wave lithotripsy (SWL) is best suited for intranephric stones that are small to moderate in size but can be used for proximal ureteral stones as well. The principle of SWL is to use focused sound waves to break the stone into pieces small enough to pass through the ureters, bladder, and urethra during normal urination. This requires transmission of the sound wave beam via an interface with the patient's body. Early SWL was conducted via immersion in a water bath, which created this interface. In addition to the significant positioning maneuvers associated with this procedure, patients are prone to hypothermia during the procedure. Dysrhythmias can be a special problem as the transmission of the ultrasonic pulse is timed and triggered by the ECG. Significant respiratory and hemodynamic changes are associated with immersion and emergence from the water bath, which can be problematic particularly for patients with cardiopulmonary disease.[204] Modern "dry" SWL uses a smaller water-filled coupling device to provide an interface with the patient, which simplifies the procedure considerably. Newer SWL machines also have a more tightly focused sound beam and can deliver the required energy at pressures in each acoustic pulse that are less painful for the patient. These advances allow most procedures to be conducted in an outpatient setting, with topical local anesthesia and analgesia/sedation provided with combinations of nonsteroidal anti-inflammatory medications and opiates. General anesthesia and/or deep sedation are rarely required.

Several factors affect the likelihood of success of SWL. Since increased distance from beam to stone reduces the effectiveness of SWL, this procedure is less successful in obese patients.

Extremely hard stones (such as cysteine and calcium oxalate) are more resistant to lithotripsy and may best be addressed with other treatment modalities.[205] Patients may require more than one treatment for complete stone comminution. As pulse counts increase, so does the risk of kidney injury and even subcapsular hematoma.[199] SWL is the least-invasive and most commonly performed procedure for the management of stone disease, however, even for this approach several relative and absolute contraindications exist (Table 49-10).

TABLE 49-10. CONTRAINDICATIONS TO SHOCK WAVE LITHOTRIPSY

Absolute contraindications	Bleeding disorder or anticoagulation Pregnancy
Relative contraindications	Large calcified aortic or renal artery aneurysms Untreated urinary tract infection Obstruction distal to the renal calculi Pacemaker, ICD, or neurostimulation implant Morbid obesity

ICD, implantable cardioverter-defibrillator.

Percutaneous Nephrolithotomy

PNL is useful for the management of larger intranephric stones, especially those resistant to SWL, staghorn calculi, and some proximal ureteral stones. PNL requires initial placement of a ureteral stent via cystoureteroscopy performed in the lithotomy position. This stent will prevent ureteral obstruction as fragments of stone pass through the ureter following PNL. Following stent placement, the patient is repositioned to an oblique prone position for percutaneous puncture of the renal pelvis under fluoroscopic guidance, which is followed by placement of a nephrostomy tube to facilitate placement of a nephroscope for stone extraction with forceps or other instruments. Large stones may require use of an ultrasound or laser probe, also placed via the nephrostomy, to fragment them to facilitate removal. The combination of fluoroscopy and direct vision of the renal pelvis and ureters with nephro- and ureteroscopy is used to ensure that complete removal of the stone(s) has been achieved. Large volumes of irrigation are used to cool the ultrasound probe and wash away the debris, making TUR syndrome an occasional complication of PNL. Because of the large irrigant volume, blood loss can be underappreciated, and unexplained hemodynamic instability during these procedures is often a manifestation of blood loss. Published rates of transfusion during or after PNL range from 5% to 14%.[206] Pneumothorax, though rare, is a possible complication of the procedure depending on the approach used for insertion of the nephroscope.

General anesthesia with endotracheal intubation allows for a secure airway for positioning into the prone position and is most commonly used in many centers; however, spinal anesthesia can also be used.[207] For certain patients, local infiltration with sedation may even suffice.[208]

Ureteroscopy for Removal of Stones

Ureteroscopy for removal of stones (URS) is the procedure of choice for mid-ureteral and distal ureteral stones that have failed conservative management. It is also indicated for treatment of bilateral ureteral stones and can be considered in patients for whom cessation of anticoagulation is not advisable. Morbidly obese patients for whom SWL is not advised are also candidates for this procedure.[199] Although more invasive than SWL, URS generally achieves a higher stone-free rate and can be used to remove stones in all portions of the ureter. Newer technology has allowed smaller, more flexible ureteroscopes, and lasers are now incorporated to facilitate stone disintegration. Various "basket" and other retrieval devices can be inserted through the ureteroscope. The postoperative complications from ureterosopic stone retrieval include perforation of the ureter (5%) and stricture formation (<2%) and rarely TUR syndrome.[209] The procedure can be performed using urethral local anesthesia with intravenous sedation and monitored anesthesia care, spinal, or general anesthesia. The previous section addresses anesthetic concerns related to cystoscopy and ureteroscopy.

Open and Laparoscopic Pyelolithotomy or Nephrectomy

With the advent of the previously discussed modalities for the treatment of urolithiasis, the use of laparoscopic or open surgery for removal of stones has declined considerably, and they should not be considered first-line treatment for stone disease. Patients who have failed SWL or PNL or who require open surgery for other indications are candidates for open treatment of stone disease. This can be accomplished laparoscopically (retroperitoneal or transperitoneal) or open, depending on the capabilities of the surgeon. Compared with less-invasive approaches, both laparoscopic and open procedures result in more postoperative pain, longer hospital stays and recovery and are associated with higher complication rates.

UROGYNECOLOGY AND PREGNANCY-RELATED UROLOGIC PROCEDURES

A variety of urogynecologic procedures that treat pelvic floor prolapse are directed at symptomatic improvement of stress incontinence. These procedures are relatively noninvasive, often accomplished using a transvaginal approach with the patient in the lithotomy position, and frequently performed as outpatient procedures with same-day discharge home. Anesthesia can be accomplished with local infiltration accompanied by heavy sedation and monitored anesthetic care, neuraxial anesthesia using spinal or combined spinal/epidural local anesthetic injection, or general anesthesia. Local preferences may dictate anesthetic choice, as suggested by reports from some centers regarding the selection of spinal anesthesia that describe on the one hand improved patient and surgeon satisfaction,[210] and on the other a four-fold higher urinary retention rate[211] and 1 hour longer postanesthesia care unit stay.

Renal colic is the most common nonobstetric cause of abdominal pain requiring hospitalization in pregnant women.[199] Medical management of these patients must consider the fetal gestational age regarding decisions about appropriate analgesics (e.g., nonsteroidal anti-inflammatory drugs in the third trimester may cause premature closure of the fetal ductus arteriosus and adverse renal effects). Diagnostic tests preferably avoid ionizing radiation and favor the use of ultrasound whenever possible. Interventions in pregnant patients with symptomatic nephrolithiasis have traditionally been limited to ureteral stents to relieve pain and prevent obstruction, with definitive therapy delayed postpartum; however, the need for repeated stent exchanges is common. More recent data supports the safety and efficacy of URS for stone removal during pregnancy. SWL is contraindicated in pregnancy.[212,213]

Surgical urologic issues related to the obstetrical patient are uncommon, with the exception of inadvertent injury to the ureter or bladder during cesarean section which, if recognized, should be repaired intraoperatively.[214] Ureteral stenting is also occasionally required to enable ureter identification during a cesarean/hysterectomy procedure for placenta accreta or percreta.[215]

Impotence Surgery and Medication

The impotence drugs sildenafil (Viagra), tadalafil (Cialis), and vardenafil (Levitra) all inhibit cyclic GMP (cGMP)-specific phosphodiesterase type 5 (PDE 5) in vascular smooth muscle (Fig. 49-12). Blocking PDE 5 impairs cGMP breakdown, the mediator of nitric oxide effects that produce erectile responses to sexual stimulation through penile arterial vasodilation and corpus cavernosum smooth muscle relaxation. These agents have effects on other vessels and can be a useful treatment for pulmonary artery hypertension (trade names; sildenafil—Revatio, tadalfil—Adcirca).

Rational perioperative management of PDE 5 inhibitor agents is important. Notably, while impotence therapies should be discontinued before surgery to minimize the risk of hypotension, pulmonary hypertension therapies must continue throughout the perioperative period. Although inhaled nitric oxide therapy can safely be used with PDE 5 inhibitors since its effects are limited to the pulmonary vasculature, whenever these agents are combined with systemic nitric oxide donors such as nitroglycerin or sodium nitroprusside, exaggerated hypotensive responses are likely due to their dramatic potentiation of the peripheral vasodilator effects of nitric oxide.

Erectile dysfunction refractory to medical therapies can be treated by penile prosthesis implantation. Most prostheses are inflatable, with a secondary fluid reservoir and/or pump either behind the abdominal wall or inside the scrotum. Semirigid prostheses that do not involve pumps or reservoirs are also available, but these are less commonly used. Although penile implant procedures are relatively noninvasive, many recipients are elderly with multiple comorbidities, including vascular disease and diabetes. Traditionally, implantation has been performed under general or neuraxial anesthesia, but regional block (combined proximal dorsal nerve block and crural block) with sedation and monitored anesthesia care is also suitable if an abdominal incision is not required.[216]

Pediatric Surgical Urologic Disorders

The anesthesiologist caring for a pediatric patient undergoing a urologic procedure must first and foremost have a strong grasp of concepts of pediatric anesthesiology. General anesthesia is typical for these procedures, although a caudal block may provide good postoperative pain control (see Chapter 42).

Nephrectomy and Adrenalectomy

Many adult urologic procedures are also performed in children, although frequently for different indications. Nephrectomy, for example, is used to treat Wilms' tumor and nonfunctioning kidney due to obstructive uropathy, stone disease, vesicoureteral reflux, or multicystic dysplastic kidney. Pediatric nephrectomy is amenable to open or laparoscopic approaches with general anesthesia.[217]

Adrenalectomy for neuroblastoma (28%), pheochromocytoma (21%), or adenoma (14%) can most often be achieved laparoscopically, although conversion to an open procedure, most often necessary due to tumor adherence to surrounding organs, is more common than in adults (10%).[218]

As for adults, the preoperative workup and preparation of patients with pheochromocytoma should be thorough. Since inherited syndromes such as neurofibromatosis, von Hippel–Lindau disease, tuberous sclerosis, Sturge–Weber syndrome, and MEN are commonly associated with pediatric pheochromocytoma, other related characteristics of these conditions should also be considered in preoperative preparation.[219] As for adult pheochromocytoma, preoperative therapy with α-1 adrenergic blocking agents (e.g., phenoxybenzamine) is recommended (see Chapter 46).[220]

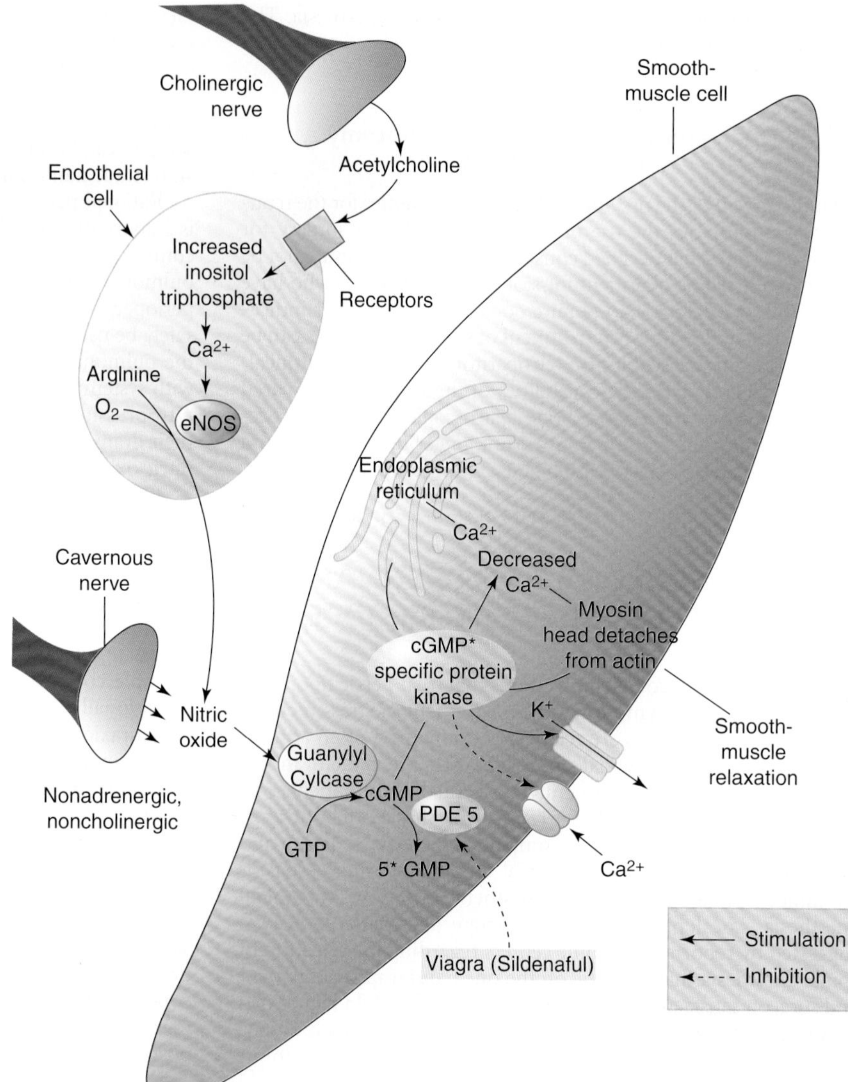

FIGURE 49-12. Nitric oxide–mediated vascular smooth muscle relaxation, including the inhibiting effects of sildenafil on cyclic GMP-specific phosphodiesterase type 5 (PDE 5). (Accessed at www.wiley.com/college/boyer/0470003790/cutting_edge/viagra/viagra.htm. This material is reproduced with permission of John Wiley & Sons, Inc.)

Reconstructive Urologic Procedures

A number of urologic procedures related to congenital urologic deformities are performed almost exclusively on children. Many of these procedures are reconstructive in nature, intended to functionally repair a defect present at birth.

Bladder exstrophy, where part of the urinary bladder remains outside the body through a defect in the abdominal wall, occurs in 1 per 10,000 to 50,000 live births with a 2:1 male:female ratio.[221] Associated abnormalities are frequently present in the pelvic bones and external genitalia. Repair requires one or more of the following three procedures in a staged fashion, with primary closure of the abdominal wall and osteotomy usually occurring before 4 months of age, epispadias repair between 8 and 24 months of age, and bladder neck reconstruction at 40 to 60 months.[222]

Repair of ureteropelvic junction obstruction (UPJO) and ureterovesical reimplantation to treat vesicoureteral reflux requires general anesthesia and may be performed open or laparoscopically. Reconstruction of the lower urinary tract is more frequently achieved using an open approach, although laparoscopy is beginning to gain favor.

Posterior urethral valves (PUVs) are persistent embryonic membranes that cause bladder outlet obstruction and can lead to incomplete emptying, bladder hypertrophy, and even renal insufficiency or failure. PUVs occur exclusively in males, with an incidence of 1 to 2 per 10,000 male births and may be diagnosed before or after birth by ultrasound. While temporary treatment involves catheterization and antibiotics to prevent infection, definitive surgical repair is required, usually in the early postnatal period. Nonetheless, approximately one-third of the patients with PUV develop end-stage renal disease and require dialysis and/or renal transplantation.[223]

Undescended testis (cryptorchidism) affects 2% to 4% of male newborns. Cryptorchidism that persists at 1 year of age (1%) requires surgical repair (orchiopexy) normally as an outpatient procedure under general anesthesia.[224]

Hypospadius, an abnormal location of the urethral meatus on the ventral aspect of the penis resulting from incomplete embryologic development, occurs in 0.3% to 0.8% of male infants. Surgical repair is most commonly performed around 6 months of age as an outpatient procedure under general anesthesia, often supplemented with caudal analgesia. More complex repairs may require a second staged procedure around 12 months.

Circumcision of newborns is usually accomplished under ring block or local anesthetic infiltration without the presence of an anesthesiologist, although in older children general anesthesia with or without neuraxial anesthesia may be more appropriate.

UROLOGIC SURGICAL EMERGENCIES

Urologic emergencies are relatively rare, but three urologic emergency surgeries are worthy of mention. *Testicular torsion* requires emergency attention due to the high risk, if otherwise untreated, for infarction or gangrene which would require orchiectomy. In contrast, patients with *Fournier Gangrene* and *sepsis* associated with nephrolithiasis are noteworthy since emergent definitive surgical therapy is the most effective way to reverse their infectious process and improve their prognosis. These latter patients are generally very seriously ill, and often the anesthesiologist provides ongoing resuscitation and applies critical care principles while delivering anesthetic care.

Testicular Torsion

Testicular torsion has a bimodal incidence, in the neonatal period and during early pubertal to teenage years. Testicular torsion affects approximately 1 in 4,000 young men, and 65% of cases occur in teenagers. When the spermatic cord twists, venous outflow from a testicle is obstructed, and eventually this compromises arterial flow, leading to ischemia and infarction.[225] Patients with testicular torsion present with acute scrotal pain and tenderness, most cases not involving a history of trauma. A predisposing anatomic "bell-clapper deformity," which allows the testes to rotate freely in the tunica vaginalis, is the most common cause of this problem. Other risk factors include testicular tumors, a history of cryptorchidism, and an increase in testicular volume (e.g., puberty). Common misdiagnoses include epididymitis/orchitis, incarcerated hernia, and varicocele.[225] Absence of the cremasteric reflex is usually present on physical examination, and Doppler ultrasonography demonstrates decreased or absent blood flow. Equivocal physical examination findings dictate surgical exploration.

Apart from the considerable pain that torsion causes, the most important priority is the viability of the testicle. Testicular torsion requires immediate intervention, as viability decreases significantly with the duration of testicular ischemia. Success in saving the testicle relates to the timing from symptom onset to de-torsion, with success rates of 90%, 50%, and 10% with delays of 6, 12, and greater than 24 hours, respectively.[226]

Anesthesia for testicular torsion surgery must respect its emergent nature, including the likelihood that the patient has not fasted. Regional or general anesthesia is appropriate, but spinal anesthesia is relatively contraindicated due to the high risk of postdural puncture headache in the young population where the problem is most often manifested.

Fournier Gangrene

Fournier gangrene is a form of necrotizing fasciitis affecting the genitalia. It presents most commonly in older men, and frequently associated comorbidities include diabetes mellitus, morbid obesity, and immune suppression.[227] Minor genital trauma is often the inciting event, but rapid widespread inflammation, infection, and ultimately polymicrobial sepsis characterize the condition. Fournier gangrene patients often present with already established septic shock warranting the emergent status for surgery, but fluid resuscitation and institution of broad-spectrum antibiotic therapy (commonly staphylococci, streptococci, enterobacteriaceae, and anaerobes) are also priorities.[228] Surgical management consists of incision, drainage, and debridement of affected tissue. Hyperbaric oxygen therapy is also employed at some centers[229,230] but does not replace emergent surgical debridement. Morbidity and mortality are significant, with advanced age and presence of septic shock at presentation portending the highest risk.[231]

Anesthetic planning must incorporate assessment of the degree of sepsis and hemodynamic status of the patient. General anesthesia with endotracheal intubation and positive pressure ventilation is standard. Intra-arterial and central venous access are often indicated to facilitate resuscitation of the patient. Transfusion may be necessary since the extensive tissue resection can involve significant blood loss. Patients often require postoperative intensive care admission to manage the sequelae of sepsis and often undergo repeated procedures for additional debridement, wound care, and eventually wound closure.[228]

Emergency Treatment of Nephrolithiasis

Most patients who require surgical or interventional treatment of nephrolithiasis can be managed electively, but patients with infection associated with urinary tract obstruction, AKI, bilateral obstructing stones, intractable pain or vomiting, or obstruction in a solitary (native or transplanted) kidney should be managed urgently to avoid sepsis and preserve renal function.[205] Procedures indicated for these conditions to alleviate obstruction include cystoscopy with stent insertion, percutaneous nephrostomy, and very rarely, open pyelolithotomy or nephrectomy for definitive treatment related to stones unsuccessfully treated by less-invasive interventions. Identification of patients who have infected urine and obstruction is important as they are at high risk of developing sepsis, which can manifest preoperatively, intraoperatively, or postoperatively. As with any infection, the principles of drainage and institution of appropriate antibiotic therapy are paramount, and in the presence of complete urinary obstruction, antibiotic therapy alone is insufficient treatment. If the urinary tract can be decompressed with a stent or nephrostomy, definitive management can be postponed until the patient has responded to antibiotic therapy.[199] Patients with nephrolithiasis complicated by urinary tract infection are at higher risk for infection with antibiotic-resistant pathogens, which requires targeted antibiotic therapy.[232]

Another category of patients requiring urgent surgery are patients with declining renal function in the setting of urinary obstruction, (e.g., ureteral obstruction from renal papillary necrosis, blood clots, or urethral obstruction due to blood clots or stricture).[198] Other situations (e.g., obstructed solitary or transplanted kidney, hemorrhage, and blood clots) may dictate urgent, rather than elective, surgery to relieve the urinary obstruction and preserve renal function, though in the absence of infection this group of patients may not be as acutely ill.

Anesthetic considerations for emergent nephrolithiasis surgery are similar to those for equivalent elective procedures (see above). Additional considerations include the potential need for more invasive monitoring, for example, direct arterial blood pressure monitoring in the setting of sepsis. Similarly, hemodynamically unstable septic patients often have ongoing needs for fluid resuscitation, pharmacologic support of the circulation, and in the setting of deteriorating renal function may require alterations from standard anesthetic agent selections. Since evidence of sepsis may not manifest until the postoperative period, raised awareness for such concerns should continue through into the postanesthetic recovery period.

References

1. Alpert RA, Roizen MF, Hamilton WK, et al. Intraoperative urinary output does not predict postoperative renal function in patients undergoing abdominal aortic revascularization. *Surgery.* 1984;95:707–711.
2. Conlon PJ, Stafford-Smith M, White WD, et al. Acute renal failure following cardiac surgery. *Nephrol Dial Transplant.* 1999;14:1158–1162.
3. Levin A. Cystatin C, serum creatinine, and estimates of kidney function: Searching for better measures of kidney function and cardiovascular risk. *Ann Intern Med.* 2005;142:586–588.
4. Grubb A, Bjork J, Lindstrom V, et al. A cystatin C-based formula without anthropometric variables estimates glomerular filtration rate better than creatinine clearance using the Cockcroft-Gault formula. *Scand J Clin Lab Invest.* 2005; 65:153–162.
5. Alpert MA, Govindarajan G, Del Rosario ML, et al. The role of the renin-angiotensin system in the pathophysiology, prevention, and treatment of renal impairment in patients with the cardiometabolic syndrome or its components. *J Cardiometab Syndr.* 2009;4:57–62.
6. Sladen RN, Endo E, Harrison T. Two-hour versus 22-hour creatinine clearance in critically ill patients. *Anesthesiology.* 1987;67:1013–1016.
7. Bloor GK, Welsh KR, Goodall S, et al. Comparison of predicted with measured creatinine clearance in cardiac surgical patients. *J Cardiothorac Vasc Anesth.* 1996; 10:899–902.
8. Gowans EM, Fraser CG. Biological variation of serum and urine creatinine and creatinine clearance: ramifications for interpretation of results and patient care. *Ann Clin Biochem.* 1988;25:259–263.
9. Morgan DB, Dillon S, Payne RB. The assessment of glomerular function: creatinine clearance or plasma creatinine? *Postgrad Med J.* 1978;54:302–310.
10. Cockcroft DW, Gault MH. Prediction of creatinine clearance from serum creatinine. *Nephron.* 1976;16:31–41.
11. Levey AS, Bosch JP, Lewis JB, et al. A more accurate method to estimate glomerular filtration rate from serum creatinine: a new prediction equation. Modification of Diet in Renal Disease Study Group. *Ann Intern Med.* 1999;130:461–470.
12. Ferguson TB Jr, Dziuban SW Jr, Edwards FH, et al. The STS National Database: Current changes and challenges for the new millennium. Committee to Establish a National Database in Cardiothoracic Surgery, The Society of Thoracic Surgeons. *Ann Thorac Surg.* 2000;69:680–691.
13. Barrett BJ, Parfrey PS. Prevention of nephrotoxicity induced by radiocontrast agents. *N Engl J Med.* 1994;331:1449–1450.
14. Bellomo R, Ronco C, Kellum JA, et al. Acute renal failure – definition, outcome measures, animal models, fluid therapy and information technology needs: The Second International Consensus Conference of the Acute Dialysis Quality Initiative (ADQI) Group. *Crit Care.* 2004;8:R204–R212.
15. Mehta RL, Kellum JA, Shah SV, et al. Acute Kidney Injury Network: Report of an initiative to improve outcomes in acute kidney injury. *Crit Care.* 2007;11:R31.
16. Greenberg A, ed. *Primer on Kidney Diseases.* 4th ed. Philadelphia, PA: Elsevier Saunders; 2005.
17. Stafford-Smith M. Antifibrinolytic agents make alpha1- and beta2-microglobulinuria poor markers of postcardiac surgery renal dysfunction. *Anesthesiology.* 1999;90:928–929.
18. Anderson RJ, Chung HM, Kluge R, et al. Hyponatremia: A prospective analysis of its epidemiology and the pathogenetic role of vasopressin. *Ann Intern Med.* 1985;102:164–168.
19. Verbalis JG. Hyponatremia: Epidemiology, pathophysiology, and therapy. *Curr Opin Nephrol Hypertens.* 1993;2:636–652.
20. Arieff AI. Hyponatremia, convulsions, respiratory arrest, and permanent brain damage after elective surgery in healthy women. *N Engl J Med.* 1986;314:1529–1535.
21. Arieff AI, Ayus JC, Fraser CL. Hyponatraemia and death or permanent brain damage in healthy children. *Br Med J.* 1992;304:1218–1222.
22. Ayus JC, Wheeler JM, Arieff AI. Postoperative hyponatremic encephalopathy in menstruant women. *Ann Intern Med.* 1992;117:891–897.
23. Wilkinson A, Cohen D. Renal failure in the recipients of nonrenal solid organ transplants. *J Am Soc Nephrol.* 1999;10:1136–1144.
24. Rudnick M, Feldman H. Contrast-induced nephropathy: What are the true clinical consequences? *Clin J Am Soc Nephrol.* 2008;3:263–272.
25. Alonso A, Lau J, Jaber B, et al. Prevention of radiocontrast nephropathy with N-acetylcysteine in patients with chronic kidney disease: a meta-analysis of randomized, controlled trials. *Am J Kidney Dis.* 2004;43:1–9.
26. Taber SS, Mueller BA. Drug-associated renal dysfunction. *Crit Care Clin.* 2006;22: 357–374, viii.
27. Huerta C, Castellsague J, Varas-Lorenzo C, et al. Nonsteroidal anti-inflammatory drugs and risk of ARF in the general population. *Am J Kidney Dis.* 2005;45:531–539.
28. Oh KJ, Lee HH, Lee JS, et al. Reversible renal vasoconstriction in a patient with acute renal failure after exercise. *Clin Nephrol.* 2006;66:297–301.
29. Melli G, Chaudhry V, Cornblath DR. Rhabdomyolysis: An evaluation of 475 hospitalized patients. *Medicine (Baltimore).* 2005;84:377–385.
30. Singh D, Chander V, Chopra K. Rhabdomyolysis. *Methods Find Exp Clin Pharmacol.* 2005;27:39–48.
31. Eichhorn JH, Hedley-Whyte J, Steinman TI, et al. Renal failure following enflurane anesthesia. *Anesthesiology.* 1976;45:557–560.
32. Eger EI, Gong D, Koblin DD, et al. Dose-related biochemical markers of renal injury after sevoflurane versus desflurane anesthesia in volunteers. *Anesth Analg.* 1997;85:1154–1163.
33. Conzen PF, Kharasch ED, Czerner SF, et al. Low-flow sevoflurane compared with low-flow isoflurane anesthesia in patients with stable renal insufficiency. *Anesthesiology.* 2002;97:578–584.
34. Gunukula SR, Spodick DH. Pericardial disease in renal patients. *Semin Nephrol.* 2001;21:52–56.
35. Crandell WB, Pappas SG, Macdonald A. Nephrotoxicity associated with methoxyflurane anesthesia. *Anesthesiology.* 1966;27:591–607.
36. Kharasch ED, Hankins DC, Thummel KE. Human kidney methoxyflurane and sevoflurane metabolism. Intrarenal fluoride production as a possible mechanism of methoxyflurane nephrotoxicity. *Anesthesiology.* 1995;82:689–699.
37. Mazze RI, Calverley RK, Smith NT. Inorganic fluoride nephrotoxicity: Prolonged enflurane and halothane anesthesia in volunteers. *Anesthesiology.* 1977;46: 265–271.
38. Burch PG, Stanski DR. Decreased protein binding and thiopental kinetics. *Clin Pharmacol Ther.* 1982;32:212–217.
39. Gan TJ. Pharmacokinetic and pharmacodynamic characteristics of medications used for moderate sedation. *Clin Pharmacokinet.* 2006;45:855–869.
40. Carlos R, Calvo R, Erill S. Plasma protein binding of etomidate in patients with renal failure or hepatic cirrhosis. *Clin Pharmacokinet.* 1979;4:144–148.
41. Kirvela M, Olkkola KT, Rosenberg PH, et al. Pharmacokinetics of propofol and haemodynamic changes during induction of anaesthesia in uraemic patients. *Br J Anaesth.* 1992;68:178–182.
42. Vinik HR, Reves JG, Greenblatt DJ, et al. The pharmacokinetics of midazolam in chronic renal failure patients. *Anesthesiology.* 1983;59:390–394.
43. Schmith VD, Piraino B, Smith RB, et al. Alprazolam in end-stage renal disease. II. Pharmacodynamics. *Clin Pharmacol Ther.* 1992;51:533–540.
44. De Wolf AM, Fragen RJ, Avram MJ, et al. The pharmacokinetics of dexmedetomidine in volunteers with severe renal impairment. *Anesth Analg.* 2001;93:1205–1209.
45. Chan GL, Matzke GR. Effects of renal insufficiency on the pharmacokinetics and pharmacodynamics of opioid analgesics. *Drug Intell Clin Pharm.* 1987;21:773–783.
46. Babul N, Darke AC, Hagen N. Hydromorphone metabolite accumulation in renal failure. *J Pain Symptom Manage.* 1995;10:184–186.
47. Murphy EJ. Acute pain management pharmacology for the patient with concurrent renal or hepatic disease. *Anaesth Intensive Care.* 2005;33:311–322.
48. Davis PJ, Stiller RL, Cook DR, et al. Effects of cholestatic hepatic disease and chronic renal failure on alfentanil pharmacokinetics in children. *Anesth Analg.* 1989;68:579–583.
49. Wiggum DC, Cork RC, Weldon ST, et al. Postoperative respiratory depression and elevated sufentanil levels in a patient with chronic renal failure. *Anesthesiology.* 1985;63:708–710.
50. Pitsiu M, Wilmer A, Bodenham A, et al. Pharmacokinetics of remifentanil and its major metabolite, remifentanil acid, in ICU patients with renal impairment. *Br J Anaesth.* 2004;92:493–503.
51. Szenohradszky J, Caldwell JE, Wright PM, et al. Influence of renal failure on the pharmacokinetics and neuromuscular effects of a single dose of rapacuronium bromide. *Anesthesiology.* 1999;90:24–35.
52. Ryan DW. Preoperative serum cholinesterase concentration in chronic renal failure. Clinical experience of suxamethonium in 81 patients undergoing renal transplant. *Br J Anaesth.* 1977;49:945–949.
53. Cook DR, Freeman JA, Lai AA, et al. Pharmacokinetics of mivacurium in normal patients and in those with hepatic or renal failure. *Br J Anaesth.* 1992;69:580–585.
54. Cook DR, Freeman JA, Lai AA, et al. Pharmacokinetics and pharmacodynamics of doxacurium in normal patients and in those with hepatic or renal failure. *Anesth Analg.* 1991;72:145–150.
55. Della Rocca G, Pompei L, Coccia C, et al. Atracurium, cisatracurium, vecuronium and rocuronium in patients with renal failure. *Minerva Anestesiol.* 2003;69: 605–611, 12, 5.
56. Fahey MR, Rupp SM, Canfell C, et al. Effect of renal failure on laudanosine excretion in man. *Br J Anaesth.* 1985;57:1049–1051.
57. Lynam DP, Cronnelly R, Castagnoli KP, et al. The pharmacodynamics and pharmacokinetics of vecuronium in patients anesthetized with isoflurane with normal renal function or with renal failure. *Anesthesiology.* 1988;69:227–231.
58. Robertson EN, Driessen JJ, Booij LH. Pharmacokinetics and pharmacodynamics of rocuronium in patients with and without renal failure. *Eur J Anaesthesiol.* 2005;22:4–10.
59. Szenohradszky J, Fisher DM, Segredo V, et al. Pharmacokinetics of rocuronium bromide (ORG 9426) in patients with normal renal function or patients undergoing cadaver renal transplantation. *Anesthesiology.* 1992;77:899–904.
60. Cooper RA, Maddineni VR, Mirakhur RK, et al. Time course of neuromuscular effects and pharmacokinetics of rocuronium bromide (Org 9426) during

isoflurane anaesthesia in patients with and without renal failure. *Br J Anaesth.* 1993;71:222–226.
61. Phillips BJ, Hunter JM. Use of mivacurium chloride by constant infusion in the anephric patient. *Br J Anaesth.* 1992;68:492–498.
62. Blobner M, Jelen-Esselborn S, Schneider G, et al. Effect of renal function on neuromuscular block induced by continuous infusion of mivacurium. *Br J Anaesth.* 1995;74:452–454.
63. Morris RB, Cronnelly R, Miller RD, et al. Pharmacokinetics of edrophonium in anephric and renal transplant patients. *Br J Anaesth.* 1981;53:1311–1314.
64. Larson EB, Roach RC, Schoene RB, et al. Acute mountain sickness and acetazolamide. Clinical efficacy and effect on ventilation. *JAMA.* 1982;248:328–332.
65. White DP, Zwillich CW, Pickett CK, et al. Central sleep apnea. Improvement with acetazolamide therapy. *Arch Intern Med.* 1982;142:1816–1819.
66. Better OS, Rubinstein I, Winaver JM, et al. Mannitol therapy revisited (1940–1997). *Kidney Int.* 1997;52:886–894.
67. Solomon R, Werner C, Mann D, et al. Effects of saline, mannitol, and furosemide to prevent acute decreases in renal function induced by radiocontrast agents. *N Engl J Med.* 1994;331(21):1416–1420.
68. Conger JD. Interventions in clinical acute renal failure: what are the data? *Am J Kidney Dis.* 1995;26:565–576.
69. Borges HF, Hocks J, Kjellstrand CM. Mannitol intoxication in patients with renal failure. *Arch Intern Med.* 1982;142:63–66.
70. Gallagher KL, Jones JK. Furosemide-induced ototoxicity. *Ann Intern Med.* 1979; 91:744–745.
71. Pitt B, Zannad F, Remme WJ, et al. The effect of spironolactone on morbidity and mortality in patients with severe heart failure. Randomized Aldactone Evaluation Study Investigators. *N Engl J Med.* 1999;341:709–717.
72. Jose PA, Felder RA. What we can learn from the selective manipulation of dopaminergic receptors about the pathogenesis and treatment of hypertension? *Curr Opin Nephrol Hypertens.* 1996;5:447–451.
73. Bellomo R, Cole L, Ronco C. Hemodynamic support and the role of dopamine. *Kidney Int Suppl.* 1998;66:S71–S74.
74. Marik PE. Low-dose dopamine: A systematic review. *Intensive Care Med.* 2002; 28:877–883.
75. Kellum JA, Decker JM. Use of dopamine in acute renal failure: A meta-analysis. *Crit Care Med.* 2001;29:1526–1531.
76. Prins I, Plotz FB, Uiterwaal CS, et al. Low-dose dopamine in neonatal and pediatric intensive care: A systematic review. *Intensive Care Med.* 2001;27:206–210.
77. Holmes CL, Walley KR. Bad medicine: Low-dose dopamine in the ICU. *Chest.* 2003;123:1266–1275.
78. Argalious M, Motta P, Khandwala F, et al. "Renal dose" dopamine is associated with the risk of new-onset atrial fibrillation after cardiac surgery. *Crit Care Med.* 2005;33:1327–1332.
79. Denton MD, Chertow GM, Brady HR. "Renal-dose" dopamine for the treatment of acute renal failure: Scientific rationale, experimental studies and clinical trials. *Kidney Int.* 1996;50:4–14.
80. Abel RM, Buckley MJ, Austen WG, et al. Etiology, incidence, and prognosis of renal failure following cardiac operations. Results of a prospective analysis of 500 consecutive patients. *J Thorac Cardiovasc Surg.* 1976;71:323–333.
81. Swaminathan M, Shaw A, Phillips-Bute B, et al. Trends in acute renal failure associated with coronary artery bypass graft surgery in the United States. *Crit Care Med.* 2007;35:2286–2291.
82. Filsoufi F, Rahmanian PB, Castillo JG, et al. Early and late outcomes of cardiac surgery in patients with moderate to severe preoperative renal dysfunction without dialysis. *Interact Cardiovasc Thorac Surg.* 2008;7:90–95.
83. Bechtel JF, Detter C, Fischlein T, et al. Cardiac surgery in patients on dialysis: Decreased 30-day mortality, unchanged overall survival. *Ann Thorac Surg.* 2008; 85:147–153.
84. Aronson S, Fontes ML, Miao Y, et al. Risk index for perioperative renal dysfunction/failure: critical dependence on pulse pressure hypertension. *Circulation.* 2007; 115:733–742.
85. Mangano DT, Tudor IC, Dietzel C. The risk associated with aprotinin in cardiac surgery. *N Engl J Med.* 2006;354:353–365.
86. Hix JK, Thakar CV, Katz EM, et al. Effect of off-pump coronary artery bypass graft surgery on postoperative acute kidney injury and mortality. *Crit Care Med.* 2006;34:2979–2983.
87. Costa P, Ottino GM, Matani A, et al. Low-dose dopamine during cardiopulmonary bypass in patients with renal dysfunction. *J Cardiothorac Anesth.* 1990;4:469–473.
88. Berendes E, Mollhoff T, Van Aken H, et al. Effects of dopexamine on creatinine clearance, systemic inflammation, and splanchnic oxygenation in patients undergoing coronary artery bypass grafting. *Anesth Analg.* 1997;84:950–957.
89. Renton MC, Snowden CP. Dopexamine and its role in the protection of hepatosplanchnic and renal perfusion in high-risk surgical and critically ill patients. *Br J Anaesth.* 2005;94:459–467.
90. Novis BK, Roizen MF, Aronson S, et al. Association of preoperative risk factors with postoperative acute renal failure. *Anesth Analg.* 1994;78:143–149.
91. Stene JK. Renal failure in the trauma patient. *Crit Care Clin.* 1990;6:111–119.
92. Cachecho R, Millham FH, Wedel SK. Management of the trauma patient with pre-existing renal disease. *Crit Care Clin.* 1994;10:523–536.
93. Myers BD, Miller DC, Mehigan JT, et al. Nature of the renal injury following total renal ischemia in man. *J Clin Invest.* 1984;73:329–341.
94. Godet G, Fleron MH, Vicaut E, et al. Risk factors for acute postoperative renal failure in thoracic or thoracoabdominal aortic surgery: A prospective study. *Anesth Analg.* 1997;85:1227–1232.
95. Svensson LG, Coselli JS, Safi HJ, et al. Appraisal of adjuncts to prevent acute renal failure after surgery on the thoracic or thoracoabdominal aorta. *J Vasc Surg.* 1989;10:230–239.
96. Olsen PS, Schroeder T, Perko M, et al. Renal failure after operation for abdominal aortic aneurysm. *Ann Vasc Surg.* 1990;4:580–583.
97. Svensson LG, Kouchoukos NT, Miller DC, et al. Expert consensus document on the treatment of descending thoracic aortic disease using endovascular stent-grafts. *Ann Thorac Surg.* 2008;85:S1–S41.
98. Antonucci F, Calo L, Rizzolo M, et al. Nifedipine can preserve renal function in patients undergoing aortic surgery with infrarenal crossclamping. *Nephron.* 1996;74:668–673.
99. Ding H, Kopple JD, Cohen A, et al. Recombinant human insulin-like growth factor-I accelerates recovery and reduces catabolism in rats with ischemic acute renal failure. *J Clin Invest.* 1993;91:2281–2287.
100. Vijayan A, Franklin SC, Behrend T, et al. Insulin-like growth factor I improves renal function in patients with end-stage chronic renal failure. *Am J Physiol.* 1999;276:R929–R934.
101. Franklin SC, Moulton M, Sicard GA, et al. Insulin-like growth factor I preserves renal function postoperatively. *Am J Physiol.* 1997;272:F257–F259.
102. Allgren RL, Marbury TC, Rahman SN, et al. Anaritide in acute tubular necrosis. Auriculin Anaritide Acute Renal Failure Study Group. *N Engl J Med.* 1997;336: 828–834.
103. Yalavarthy R, Edelstein CL, Teitelbaum I. Acute renal failure and chronic kidney disease following liver transplantation. *Hemodial Int.* 2007;11 suppl 3:S7–S12.
104. Lopez Lago AM, Fernandez Villanueva J, Garcia Acuna JM, et al. Evolution of hepatorenal syndrome after orthotopic liver transplantation: Comparative analysis with patients who developed acute renal failure in the early postoperative period of liver transplantation. *Transplant Proc.* 2007;39:2318–2319.
105. Fleisher LA, Beckman JA, Brown KA, et al. ACC/AHA 2007 Guidelines on Perioperative Cardiovascular Evaluation and Care for Noncardiac Surgery: Executive Summary: A Report of the American College of Cardiology/American Heart Association Task Force on Practice Guidelines (Writing Committee to Revise the 2002 Guidelines on Perioperative Cardiovascular Evaluation for Noncardiac Surgery): Developed in Collaboration With the American Society of Echocardiography, American Society of Nuclear Cardiology, Heart Rhythm Society, Society of Cardiovascular Anesthesiologists, Society for Cardiovascular Angiography and Interventions, Society for Vascular Medicine and Biology, and Society for Vascular Surgery. *Circulation.* 2007;116:1971–1996.
106. Khaira HS, Shah RB, Wolf JS Jr. Laparoscopic and open surgical nephrectomy for xanthogranulomatous pyelonephritis. *J Endourol.* 2005;19:813–817.
107. Richard S, Lidereau R, Giraud S. The growing family of hereditary renal cell carcinoma. *Nephrol Dial Transplant.* 2004;19:2954–2958.
108. Palapattu GS, Kristo B, Rajfer J. Paraneoplastic syndromes in urologic malignancy: The many faces of renal cell carcinoma. *Rev Urol.* 2002;4:163–170.
109. Galvez JA, Clebone A, Garwood S, et al. Fatal intraoperative cardiac thrombosis in a patient with renal cell carcinoma. *Anesthesiology.* 2011;114:1212.
110. Wijeysundera DN, Beattie WS, Austin PC, et al. Epidural anaesthesia and survival after intermediate-to-high risk non-cardiac surgery: A population-based cohort study. *Lancet.* 2008;372:562–569.
111. Dunn MD, Portis AJ, Shalhav AL, et al. Laparoscopic versus open radical nephrectomy: A 9-year experience. *J Urol.* 2000;164:1153–1159.
112. Permpongkosol S, Link RE, Su LM, et al. Complications of 2,775 urological laparoscopic procedures: 1993 to 2005. *J Urol.* 2007;177:580–585.
113. Pareek G, Hedican SP, Gee JR, et al. Meta-analysis of the complications of laparoscopic renal surgery: Comparison of procedures and techniques. *J Urol.* 2006; 175:1208–1213.
114. Gill IS, Matin SF, Desai MM, et al. Comparative analysis of laparoscopic versus open partial nephrectomy for renal tumors in 200 patients. *J Urol.* 2003;170: 64–68.
115. Simmons MN, Gill IS. Decreased complications of contemporary laparoscopic partial nephrectomy: Use of a standardized reporting system. *J Urol.* 2007; 177:2067–2073; discussion 73.
116. Turna B, Frota R, Kamoi K, et al. Risk factor analysis of postoperative complications in laparoscopic partial nephrectomy. *J Urol.* 2008;179:1289–1294; discussion 94–95.
117. Lassen K, Soop M, Nygren J, et al. Consensus review of optimal perioperative care in colorectal surgery: Enhanced Recovery After Surgery (ERAS) Group recommendations. *Arch Surg.* 2009;144:961–969.
118. Schefft P, Novick AC, Straffon RA, et al. Surgery for renal cell carcinoma extending into the inferior vena cava. *J Urol.* 1978;120:28–31.
119. Neves RJ, Zincke H. Surgical treatment of renal cancer with vena cava extension. *Br J Urol.* 1987;59:390–395.
120. Nesbitt JC, Soltero ER, Dinney CP, et al. Surgical management of renal cell carcinoma with inferior vena cava tumor thrombus. *Ann Thorac Surg.* 1997;63:1592–1600.
121. Porpiglia F, Renard J, Billia M, et al. Is renal warm ischemia over 30 minutes during laparoscopic partial nephrectomy possible? One-year results of a prospective study. *Eur Urol.* 2007;52:1170–1178.

122. Desai MM, Gill IS, Ramani AP, et al. The impact of warm ischaemia on renal function after laparoscopic partial nephrectomy. *BJU Int.* 2005;95:377–383.
123. Eskicorapci SY, Teber D, Schulze M, et al. Laparoscopic radical nephrectomy: The new gold standard surgical treatment for localized renal cell carcinoma. *ScientificWorldJournal.* 2007;7:825–836.
124. Permpongkosol S, Chan DY, Link RE, et al. Long-term survival analysis after laparoscopic radical nephrectomy. *J Urol.* 2005;174:1222–1225.
125. Russo P. Is laparoscopic partial nephrectomy as effective as open partial nephrectomy in patients with renal cell carcinoma? *Nat Clin Pract Urol.* 2008;5:12–13.
126. Gill IS, Kavoussi LR, Lane BR, et al. Comparison of 1,800 laparoscopic and open partial nephrectomies for single renal tumors. *J Urol.* 2007;178:41–46.
127. Nicholson ML, Elwell R, Kaushik M, et al. Health-related quality of life after living donor nephrectomy: A randomized controlled trial of laparoscopic versus open nephrectomy. *Transplantation.* 2011;91:457–461.
128. Waller JR, Hiley AL, Mullin EJ, et al. Living kidney donation: A comparison of laparoscopic and conventional open operations. *Postgrad Med J.* 2002;78:153–157.
129. Owen M, Lorgelly P, Serpell M. Chronic pain following donor nephrectomy–a study of the incidence, nature and impact of chronic post-nephrectomy pain. *Eur J Pain.* 2010;14:732–734.
130. Biglarnia AR, Tufveson G, Lorant T, et al. Efficacy and safety of continuous local infusion of ropivacaine after retroperitoneoscopic live donor nephrectomy. *Am J Transplant.* 2011;11:93–100.
131. Panaro F, Gheza F, Piardi T, et al. Continuous infusion of local anesthesia after living donor nephrectomy: A comparative analysis. *Transplant Proc.* 2011;43:985–987.
132. Yates DR, Vaessen C, Roupret M. From Leonardo to da Vinci: The history of robot-assisted surgery in urology. *BJU Int.* 2011;108:1708–1713; discussion 14.
133. Branche PE, Duperret SL, Sagnard PE, et al. Left ventricular loading modifications induced by pneumoperitoneum: A time course echocardiographic study. *Anesth Analg.* 1998;86:482–487.
134. Mertens zur Borg IR, Di Biase M, Verbrugge S, et al. Comparison of three perioperative fluid regimes for laparoscopic donor nephrectomy: A prospective randomized dose-finding study. *Surg Endosc.* 2008;22:146–150.
135. Feltracco P, Ori C. Anesthetic management of living transplantation. *Minerva Anestesiol.* 2010;76:525–533.
136. Fahy BG, Barnas GM, Nagle SE, et al. Changes in lung and chest wall properties with abdominal insufflation of carbon dioxide are immediately reversible. *Anesth Analg.* 1996;82:501–505.
137. Ozyuvaci E, Altan A, Karadeniz T, et al. General anesthesia versus epidural and general anesthesia in radical cystectomy. *Urol Int.* 2005;74:62–67.
138. Rowley MW, Clemens JQ, Latini JM, et al. Simple cystectomy: Outcomes of a new operative technique. *Urology.* 2011;78:942–945.
139. Novotny V, Hakenberg OW, Wiessner D, et al. Perioperative complications of radical cystectomy in a contemporary series. *Eur Urol.* 2007;51:397–401; discussion 401–402.
140. Mullen R, Scollay JM, Hecht G, et al. Death within 48 h–adverse events after general surgical procedures. *Surgeon.* 2012;10:1–5.
141. http://seer.cancer.gov/ (Accessed 6 April 2012)
142. Ploussard G, Epstein JI, Montironi R, et al. The contemporary concept of significant versus insignificant prostate cancer. *Eur Urol.* 2011;60:291–303.
143. Gottschalk A, Smith DS, Jobes DR, et al. Preemptive epidural analgesia and recovery from radical prostatectomy: A randomized controlled trial. *JAMA.* 1998; 279:1076–1082.
144. Price DT, Vieweg J, Roland F, et al. Transient lower extremity neurapraxia associated with radical perineal prostatectomy: A complication of the exaggerated lithotomy position. *J Urol.* 1998;160:1376–1378.
145. Keller H. Re: Transient lower extremity neurapraxia associated with radical perineal prostatectomy: A complication of the exaggerated lithotomy position. *J Urol.* 1999;162:171.
146. Salonia A, Crescenti A, Suardi N, et al. General versus spinal anesthesia in patients undergoing radical retropubic prostatectomy: Results of a prospective, randomized study. *Urology.* 2004;64:95–100.
147. Malhotra V. Anesthesia considerations radical prostatectomy. *Revista Mexicana de Anestesiologia.* 2006;29:89–92.
148. Memtsoudis SG, Malhotra V. Catastrophic venous air embolus during prostatectomy in the Trendelenburg position. *Can J Anaesth.* 2003;50:1084–1085.
149. Whalley DG, Berrigan MJ. Anesthesia for radical prostatectomy, cystectomy, nephrectomy, pheochromocytoma, and laparoscopic procedures. *Anesthesiol Clin North America.* 2000;18:899–917, x.
150. Klevecka V, Burmester L, Musch M, et al. Intraoperative and early postoperative complications of radical retropubic prostatectomy. *Urol Int.* 2007;79:217–225.
151. Dudderidge T, Doyle P, Mayer E, et al. Evolution of care pathway for laparoscopic radical prostatectomy. *J Endourol.* 2011;26(6):660–665.
152. Sutherland DE, Perez DS, Weeks DC. Robot-assisted simple prostatectomy for severe benign prostatic hyperplasia. *J Endourol.* 2011;25:641–644.
153. White WM, Kim ED. Interposition nerve grafting during radical prostatectomy: Cumulative review and critical appraisal of literature. *Urology.* 2009;74:245–250.
154. Biki B, Mascha E, Moriarty DC, et al. Anesthetic technique for radical prostatectomy surgery affects cancer recurrence: A retrospective analysis. *Anesthesiology.* 2008;109:180–187.
155. Fuchs KH. Minimally invasive surgery. *Endoscopy.* 2002;34:154–159.
156. Irvine M, Patil V. Anaesthesia for robot-assisted laparoscopic surgery. *Continuing Education in Anaesthesia, Critical Care & Pain.* 2009;9:125–129.
157. Conacher ID, Soomro NA, Rix D. Anaesthesia for laparoscopic urological surgery. *Br J Anaesth.* 2004;93:859–864.
158. Pathan H, Gulati S. A case of airway occlusion in robotic surgery. *J Robotic Surg.* 2007;1:169–170.
159. Kalmar AF, Foubert L, Hendrickx JF, et al. Influence of steep Trendelenburg position and CO(2) pneumoperitoneum on cardiovascular, cerebrovascular, and respiratory homeostasis during robotic prostatectomy. *Br J Anaesth.* 2010;104: 433–439.
160. Gainsburg DM, Wax D, Reich DL, et al. Intraoperative management of robotic-assisted versus open radical prostatectomy. *JSLS.* 2010;14:1–5.
161. Sladen RN. Anesthetic considerations for the patient with renal failure. *Anesthesiol Clin North America.* 2000;18:863–882, x.
162. Colomina MJ, Godet C, Pellise F, et al. Transcranial Doppler monitoring during laparoscopic anterior lumbar interbody fusion. *Anesth Analg.* 2003;97:1675–1679.
163. Reeves MD, Myles PS. Does anaesthetic technique affect the outcome after transurethral resection of the prostate? *BJU Int.* 1999;84:982–986.
164. Mackenzie AR. Influence of anaesthesia on blood loss in transurethral prostatectomy. *Scott Med J.* 1990;35:14–16.
165. McGowan SW, Smith GF. Anaesthesia for transurethral prostatectomy. A comparison of spinal intradural analgesia with two methods of general anaesthesia. *Anaesthesia.* 1980;35:847–853.
166. Gehring H, Nahm W, Baerwald J, et al. Irrigation fluid absorption during transurethral resection of the prostate: Spinal vs. general anaesthesia. *Acta Anaesthesiol Scand.* 1999;43:458–463.
167. Allen TD. Body temperature changes during prostatic resection as related to the temperature of the irrigating solution. *J Urol.* 1973;110:433–435.
168. Hatch PD. Surgical and anaesthetic considerations in transurethral resection of the prostate. *Anaesth Intensive Care.* 1987;15:203–211.
169. Krongrad A, Droller M. Complications of transurethral resection of the prostate. In: Marshall F, ed. *Urologic Complications: Medical and Surgical, Adult and Pediatric.* 2nd ed. St. Louis: Mosby-Year Book; 1990:305.
170. Mebust WK, Holtgrewe HL, Cockett AT, et al. Transurethral prostatectomy: Immediate and postoperative complications. a cooperative study of 13 participating institutions evaluating 3,885 patients. 1989. *J Urol.* 2002;167:999–1003.
171. Dorotta I, Basali A, Ritchey M, et al. Transurethral resection syndrome after bladder perforation. *Anesth Analg.* 2003;97:1536–1538.
172. Reich O, Gratzke C, Bachmann A, et al. Morbidity, mortality and early outcome of transurethral resection of the prostate: A prospective multicenter evaluation of 10,654 patients. *J Urol.* 2008;180:246–249.
173. Ahyai SA, Gilling P, Kaplan SA, et al. Meta-analysis of functional outcomes and complications following transurethral procedures for lower urinary tract symptoms resulting from benign prostatic enlargement. *Eur Urol.* 2010;58:384–397.
174. Ansell J. Acquired bleeding disorders. In: Rippe J, Irwin R, Alpert J, Dalen J, eds. *Intensive Care Medicine.* 2nd ed. Boston: Little, Brown; 1991:1013.
175. Wasson JH, Reda DJ, Bruskewitz RC, et al. A comparison of transurethral surgery with watchful waiting for moderate symptoms of benign prostatic hyperplasia. The Veterans Affairs Cooperative Study Group on Transurethral Resection of the Prostate. *N Engl J Med.* 1995;332:75–79.
176. Mebust WK, Holtgrewe HL, Cockett AT, et al. Transurethral prostatectomy: immediate and postoperative complications. A cooperative study of 13 participating institutions evaluating 3,885 patients. *J Urol.* 1989;141:243–247.
177. Melchior J, Valk WL, Foret JD, et al. Transurethral prostatectomy: Computerized analysis of 2,223 consecutive cases. *J Urol.* 1974;112:634–642.
178. Perrin P, Barnes R, Hadley H, et al. Forty years of transurethral prostatic resections. *J Urol.* 1976;116:757–758.
179. Fuglsig S, Aagaard J, Jonler M, et al. Survival after transurethral resection of the prostate: A 10-year followup. *J Urol.* 1994;151:637–639.
180. Matani Y, Mottrie AM, Stockle M, et al. Transurethral prostatectomy: A long-term follow-up study of 166 patients over 80 years of age. *Eur Urol.* 1996;30: 414–417.
181. Fitzpatrick JM. Minimally invasive and endoscopic management of benign prostatic hyperplasia. In: Wein A, Kavoussi L, Novick A, Partin A, Peters C, eds. *Campbell-Walsh Urology.* 9th ed. Philadelphia, PA: Saunders Elsevier; 2007:2803.
182. Gettman M, Segura J. *Indications and Outcomes of Ureteroscopy for Urinary Stones.* Totowa, NJ: Humana Press; 2004.
183. Freiha F, Deem S, Pearl RG. Urology: Transurethral resection of the protate (TURP). In: Jaffe RA, Samuels SI, eds. *Anesthesiologist's Manual of Surgical Procedures.* New York, NY: Raven Press; 1994:553.
184. Shah HN, Kausik V, Hegde S, et al. Evaluation of fluid absorption during holmium laser enucleation of prostate by breath ethanol technique. *J Urol.* 2006; 175:537–540.
185. Akata T, Yoshimura H, Matsumae Y, et al. [Changes in serum Na+ and blood hemoglobin levels during three types of transurethral procedures for the treatment of benign prostatic hypertrophy]. *Masui.* 2004;53:638–644.
186. Rocco B, Albo G, Ferreira RC, et al. Recent advances in the surgical treatment of benign prostatic hyperplasia. *Ther Adv Urol.* 2011;3:263–272.
187. Jensen V. The TURP syndrome. *Can J Anaesth.* 1991;38:90–96.
188. Agin C. Anesthesia for transurethral prostate surgery. In: Lebowitz P, ed. *Anesthesia for Urologic Surgery.* Boston: Brown; 1993:25.

189. Gravenstein D. Transurethral resection of the prostate (TURP) syndrome: A review of the pathophysiology and management. *Anesth Analg.* 1997;84:438–446.
190. Roesch RP, Stoelting RK, Lingeman JE, et al. Ammonia toxicity resulting from glycine absorption during a transurethral resection of the prostate. *Anesthesiology.* 1983;58:577–579.
191. Hoekstra PT, Kahnoski R, McCamish MA, et al. Transurethral prostatic resection syndrome–a new perspective: encephalopathy with associated hyperammonemia. *J Urol.* 1983;130:704–707.
192. Ovassapian A, Joshi CW, Brunner EA. Visual disturbances: An unusual symptom of transurethral prostatic resection reaction. *Anesthesiology.* 1982;57:332–334.
193. Barletta JP, Fanous MM, Hamed LM. Temporary blindness in the TUR syndrome. *J Neuroophthalmol.* 1994;14:6–8.
194. Hahn RG, Ekengren JC. Patterns of irrigating fluid absorption during transurethral resection of the prostate as indicated by ethanol. *J Urol.* 1993;149:502–506.
195. Rippa A. Transurethral resection of the prostate: Aids and accessories. In: Smith A, ed. *Smith's Textbook of Endourology.* St. Louis: Quality Medical; 1996:1190.
196. Hahn RG, Stalberg HP, Ekengren J, et al. Effects of 1.5% glycine solution with and without 1% ethanol on the fluid balance in elderly men. *Acta Anaesthesiol Scand.* 1991;35:725–730.
197. Black R. Disorders of plasma sodium and plasma potassium. In: Rippe J, Irwin R, Alpert J, Dalen J, eds. *Intensive Care Medicine.* 2nd ed. Boston: Little, Brown; 1991:794.
198. Hall PM. Nephrolithiasis: Treatment, causes, and prevention. *Cleve Clin J Med.* 2009;76:583–591.
199. Preminger GM, Tiselius HG, Assimos DG, et al. 2007 guideline for the management of ureteral calculi. *Eur Urol.* 2007;52:1610–1631.
200. Hollingsworth JM, Rogers MA, Kaufman SR, et al. Medical therapy to facilitate urinary stone passage: A meta-analysis. *Lancet.* 2006;368:1171–1179.
201. Auge BK, Preminger GM. Update on shock wave lithotripsy technology. *Curr Opin Urol.* 2002;12:287–290.
202. Lambert DH, Deane RS, Mazuzan JE Jr. Anesthesia and the control of blood pressure in patients with spinal cord injury. *Anesth Analg.* 1982;61:344–348.
203. Mariappan P, Tolley DA. Endoscopic stone surgery: Minimizing the risk of postoperative sepsis. *Curr Opin Urol.* 2005;15:101–105.
204. Abbott MA, Samuel JR, Webb DR. Anaesthesia for extracorporeal shock wave lithotripsy. *Anaesthesia.* 1985;40:1065–1072.
205. Samplaski MK, Irwin BH, Desai M. Less-invasive ways to remove stones from the kidneys and ureters. *Cleve Clin J Med.* 2009;76:592–598.
206. Stoller ML, Lee KL, Schwartz BF, et al. Autologous blood use in percutaneous nephrolithotomy. *Urology.* 1999;54:444–449.
207. Mehrabi S, Karimzadeh Shirazi K. Results and complications of spinal anesthesia in percutaneous nephrolithotomy. *Urol J.* 2010;7:22–25.
208. Aravantinos E, Karatzas A, Gravas S, et al. Feasibility of percutaneous nephrolithotomy under assisted local anaesthesia: A prospective study on selected patients with upper urinary tract obstruction. *Eur Urol.* 2007;51:224–227; discussion 8.
209. Johnson DB, Pearle MS. Complications of ureteroscopy. *Urol Clin North Am.* 2004;31:157–171.
210. Foon R, Toozs-Hobson P, Cooper G. Anaesthesia for incontinence surgery: Spinal anaesthesia or sedation? *J Obstet Gynaecol.* 2010;30:605–608.
211. Wohlrab KJ, Erekson EA, Korbly NB, et al. The association between regional anesthesia and acute postoperative urinary retention in women undergoing outpatient midurethral sling procdures. *Am J Obstet Gynecol.* 2009:571.e1–571.e5.
212. Lifshitz DA, Lingeman JE. Ureteroscopy as a first-line intervention for ureteral calculi in pregnancy. *J Endourol.* 2002;16:19–22.
213. Ulvik NM, Bakke A, Hoisaeter PA. Ureteroscopy in pregnancy. *J Urol.* 1995;154: 1660–1663.
214. Yossepowitch O, Baniel J, Livne PM. Urological injuries during cesarean section: Intraoperative diagnosis and management. *J Urol.* 2004;172:196–199.
215. Belfort MA. Placenta accreta. *Am J Obstet Gynecol.* 2010;203:430–439.
216. Hsu GL, Hsieh CH, Chen HS, et al. The advancement of pure local anesthesia for penile surgeries: Can an outpatient basis be sustainable? *J Androl.* 2007;28:200–205.
217. Casale P, Kojima Y. Robotic-assisted laparoscopic surgery in pediatric urology: An update. *Scand J Surg.* 2009;98:110–119.
218. St Peter SD, Valusek PA, Hill S, et al. Laparoscopic adrenalectomy in children: A multicenter experience. *J Laparoendosc Adv Surg Tech A.* 2011;21:647–649.
219. Waguespack SG, Rich T, Grubbs E, et al. A current review of the etiology, diagnosis, and treatment of pediatric pheochromocytoma and paraganglioma. *J Clin Endocrinol Metab.* 2010;95:2023–2037.
220. Ein SH, Pullerits J, Creighton R, et al. Pediatric pheochromocytoma. A 36-year review. *Pediatr Surg Int.* 1997;12:595–598.
221. Meinhardt H. Computational modelling of epithelial patterning. *Curr Opin Genet Dev.* 2007;17:272–280.
222. Baird AD, Nelson CP, Gearhart JP. Modern staged repair of bladder exstrophy: A contemporary series. *J Pediatr Urol.* 2007;3:311–315.
223. Nasir AA, Ameh EA, Abdur-Rahman LO, et al. Posterior urethral valve. *World J Pediatr.* 2011;7:205–216.
224. Barthold JS, Gonzalez R. The epidemiology of congenital cryptorchidism, testicular ascent and orchiopexy. *J Urol.* 2003;170:2396–2401.
225. Ringdahl E, Teague L. Testicular torsion. *Am Fam Physician.* 2006;74:1739–1743.
226. Davenport M. ABC of general surgery in children. Acute problems of the scrotum. *BMJ.* 1996;312:435–437.
227. Paty R, Smith AD. Gangrene and Fournier's gangrene. *Urol Clin North Am.* 1992; 19:149–162.
228. Norton KS, Johnson LW, Perry T, et al. Management of Fournier's gangrene: An eleven year retrospective analysis of early recognition, diagnosis, and treatment. *Am Surg.* 2002;68:709–713.
229. Korhonen K, Hirn M, Niinikoski J. Hyperbaric oxygen in the treatment of Fournier's gangrene. *Eur J Surg.* 1998;164:251–255.
230. Mindrup SR, Kealey GP, Fallon B. Hyperbaric oxygen for the treatment of fournier's gangrene. *J Urol.* 2005;173:1975–1977.
231. Corcoran AT, Smaldone MC, Gibbons EP, et al. Validation of the Fournier's gangrene severity index in a large contemporary series. *J Urol.* 2008;180:944–948.
232. Brown P. Management of urinary tract infections associated with nephrolithiasis. *Curr Infect Dis Rep.* 2010;12:450–454.

CHAPTER

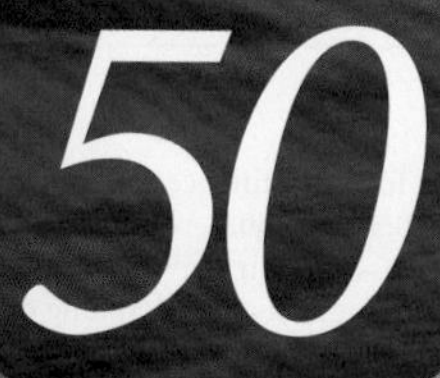

Anesthesia for Orthopedic Surgery

TERESE T. HORLOCKER • DENISE J. WEDEL

Key Points

1. Orthopedic surgery is well suited to neuraxial and peripheral regional anesthetic techniques. Improved surgical outcomes have increased their popularity.
2. The frequency of neurologic injuries following scoliosis correction is approximately 1%, with half of these resulting in partial or complete paraplegia. Neurophysiologic monitoring and the wake-up test are often used to monitor spinal cord integrity.
3. Orthopedic procedures are frequently associated with significant blood loss. The anesthesiologist must be proficient at blood salvage techniques, induced hypotension, and normovolemic hemodilution to decrease blood loss and transfusion requirements.
4. Visual changes, including blindness, may occur following major spine surgery.
5. Multimodal analgesia protocols are effective in decreasing opioid consumption and opioid-related side effects following orthopedic surgical procedures.
6. Proper positioning for orthopedic procedures is paramount to providing optimal surgical conditions, as well as avoiding potential stretch and compression injuries.
7. Neuraxial and peripheral continuous blockades improve surgical outcome, including increased joint range of motion and decreased hospital stay, following total joint replacement.
8. Orthopedic patients are at high risk for thromboembolic complications, with the highest risk reported among hip fracture patients.
9. Regional anesthetic techniques reduce the risk of thromboembolism. However, they do not replace the need for pharmacologic prophylaxis.
10. Thromboprophylaxis may result in neuraxial or perineural bleeding in patients who have undergone regional blockade.

Multimedia

1. Scoliosis
2. Brachial Plexus Injury
3. Prone Position
4. Prone Position Facial
5. Interscalene Block
6. Ankle Block

Perioperative management of the patient undergoing orthopedic surgery involves knowledge of the specific orthopedic surgical techniques, including duration, extent, predicted blood loss, and associated complications (including nerve injury). Regional anesthetic techniques allow both intraoperative surgical anesthesia and postoperative analgesia, creating a further subspecialty within orthopedic anesthesia. Another vitally important part of orthopedic anesthesia is patient positioning. Experience and knowledge in positioning the patient are required to produce optimal surgical conditions and avoid potential injuries. Likewise, because orthopedic procedures are frequently associated with major blood loss, the orthopedic anesthesiologist must be experienced in techniques that decrease these risks, able to use intraoperative hypotension and blood salvage techniques, and able to manage transfusion-related complications.

Orthopedic surgical patients usually require early mobilization and rehabilitation, both of which can be expedited by appropriate selection of anesthetic techniques and management of postoperative analgesia. A multimodal approach, often utilizing continuous neuraxial or peripheral neural infusions, is associated with enhanced recovery and improved functional outcome. However, patients undergoing major orthopedic surgery are at risk for venous thromboembolism. Knowledge of the current pharmacologic and mechanical methods of thromboprophylaxis is required to prevent the occurrence of these thromboembolic complications, while potential interactions between anticoagulants and anesthetic drugs or regional anesthetic techniques must be thoroughly understood to reduce the risk of perioperative bleeding and neurologic injury for expanding hematomas.

PREOPERATIVE ASSESSMENT

The anesthesiologist's preoperative assessment is crucial to the formulation and execution of the anesthetic plan. The patient must be evaluated for pre-existing medical problems, previous anesthetic complications, potential airway difficulties, and considerations relating to intraoperative positioning.

Progression of cardiac symptoms and exercise tolerance in patients with a history of *coronary artery disease* may be difficult to assess because of the limitations in mobility induced by the underlying orthopedic condition. As a result, pharmacologic functional cardiovascular testing may be warranted. Overall, patients undergoing orthopedic procedures are considered at intermediate risk for cardiac complications perioperatively. Perioperative cardiac morbidity may be decreased by the initiation of β-blockade in selected patients.[1]

Many patients undergoing orthopedic surgery have *rheumatoid arthritis*. Systemic manifestations of this disease include pulmonary, cardiac, and musculoskeletal involvement. Particularly significant to the anesthesiologist is involvement of the cervical spine, temporomandibular joint, and larynx. Rheumatoid involvement of the cervical spine may result in limited neck range of motion, which interferes with airway management. Atlantoaxial instability, with subluxation of the odontoid process, can lead to spinal cord injury during neck extension. Patients with rheumatoid arthritis are often receiving chronic steroid therapy and may require perioperative steroid replacement.

The patient's medications should be reviewed and the patient instructed which medications to continue until the time of surgery. Specifically, antihypertensive medications and chronic opioid therapy should *not* be discontinued. Patients taking opioids for a period of greater than 4 weeks often develop tolerance and opioid-induced hyperanalgesia, although there can be significant patient variability.[2] The patient should also be queried regarding the use of hemostasis-altering drugs; many patients are instructed by their surgeon to begin thromboprophylaxis with aspirin or warfarin preoperatively. Likewise, patients with cardiac-stents may require maintenance of their antiplatelet medications.[3]

Preoperative evaluation should include a focused *physical examination.* Patients should be assessed for limitation in mouth opening or neck extension, adequacy of thyromental distance, and state of dentition. The heart and lungs should be auscultated. In addition, the proposed site of needle placement for regional anesthesia should be assessed for evidence of infection and anatomic abnormalities or limitations. A brief neurologic examination, with documentation of any pre-existing deficits, is crucial. At this time, the patient should also be evaluated for any potential positioning difficulties related to arthritic involvement of other joints or body habitus.

Hemoglobin and creatinine values are determined for all patients undergoing major procedures; other laboratory and imaging studies are performed as indicated by preoperative medical conditions. Ideally, the patient should undergo a preoperative educational session in which the surgical procedure, anesthetic/analgesic options, and the postoperative rehabilitative plan are described.

SELECTION OF ANESTHETIC TECHNIQUE

Many orthopedic surgical procedures, because of their localized peripheral site, lend themselves to regional anesthetic techniques. Neural structures may be blocked at the peripheral nerve, plexus,
1 or neuraxial level. Regional anesthetics offer several advantages over general anesthetics among these patients, including enhanced rehabilitation, more rapid hospital dismissal, improved postoperative analgesia, decreased incidence of nausea and vomiting, less respiratory and cardiac depression, improved perfusion via sympathetic block, reduced blood loss, and decreased risk of thromboembolism. It is important to explain these benefits and encourage regional anesthesia when appropriate. The specific regional technique and local anesthetic solution used depend on a variety of factors, including duration of surgery, duration of postoperative analgesia, degree of sensory/motor block required to allow rehabilitation/ambulation, and indication for postoperative sympathectomy. Likewise, any patient who has an absolute contraindication to regional anesthesia (patient refusal, infection at the site of needle placement, systemic coagulopathy) is a candidate for general anesthesia. Importantly, a contraindication may often exist for neuraxial blockade, but more distal peripheral techniques remain appropriate. For example, a femoral nerve catheter may be maintained in the setting of thromboprophylaxis with low–molecular-weight heparin (LMWH), while an epidural catheter should be removed prior to initiation of LMWH therapy.[4] The relative risks and benefits of regional and general anesthesia are discussed in the following sections.

SURGERY TO THE SPINE

Spinal Cord Injuries

Spinal injury occurs at a rate of 11,000 cases per year (see also Chapter 36). Approximately half of these are at the cervical level. The examination of a person with a suspected spinal cord injury begins with a prompt neurologic examination and a rapid assessment for possible injury to other systems. Cervical injuries are frequently associated with head injury, thoracic fractures with pulmonary and cardiovascular injury, and lumbar fractures with abdominal and long-bone injuries. The patient should be examined immediately for signs of respiratory insufficiency, airway obstruction, rib fractures, and chest wall or facial trauma.

Serial neurologic examination is necessary to assess the function of the spinal cord above the level of the fracture. The fifth cervical segment is perhaps the most important in providing clinical evidence of cervical spinal injury. This segment controls motor function of the deltoid, biceps, brachialis, and brachioradialis muscles. If these muscles are flaccid, the fifth cervical nerve is involved, and there will be partial diaphragmatic paralysis. A complete lesion at the fourth cervical segment is not compatible with survival unless artificial respiration is initiated. Spinal shock occurs acutely and results in complete cessation of spinal cord functions below the level of the lesion. This results in flaccid paralysis, loss of visceral and somatic sensation, and paralytic ileus. Vasopressor reflexes are also lost. Spinal shock may persist from a few days to 3 months.

Surgical treatment of spinal cord injuries is based on the presence or absence of neurologic function and the radiographic evaluation of vertebral displacement and instability. Patients with unstable spines who are not quadriplegic or paraplegic may become so during transport or positioning for surgery.

Tracheal Intubation

Airway management is critical in patients with cervical spinal cord injury. The most common cause of death with acute cervical spinal cord injury is respiratory failure. All patients with severe trauma or head injuries should be assumed to have an unstable cervical fracture until proven otherwise radiographically. During transport, the patient should be moved on a rigid board with the neck immobilized to prevent further injury. Awake fiberoptic-assisted intubation may be necessary, with general anesthesia induced only after voluntary upper and lower extremity movement is confirmed. Blind nasotracheal intubation may be used if there is no evidence of facial or basal skull fractures. In a truly emergent situation, oral intubation with direct laryngoscopy is the usual approach. The trachea should be intubated with minimum flexion or extension of the neck.

Respiratory Considerations

Ventilatory impairment increases with higher levels of spinal injury. A high cervical lesion that includes the diaphragmatic segments (C4 to C5) results in respiratory failure, and death occurs unless artificial pulmonary ventilation is used. Lesions between C5 and T7 cause significant alterations in respiratory function, owing to the loss of abdominal and intercostal support. The indrawing of flaccid thoracic muscles during inspiration produces paradoxical respirations, resulting in a vital capacity reduction of 60%. Inability to cough and effectively clear secretions results in atelectasis and infection.

Cardiovascular Considerations

During spinal shock, there is loss of sympathetic vascular tone below the injury. If the cardioaccelerator fibers (T1 through T4) are damaged, bradycardia results. Therefore, hemorrhagic shock may not produce a compensatory tachycardia in these patients; the rate may remain at 40 to 60 beats per minute. Monitoring of central venous or pulmonary artery pressures may be necessary for fluid management in a patient with a high cervical lesion. Autonomic instability should be treated with vasoconstrictors, vasodilators, and positive chronotropic drugs as needed.

Succinylcholine-induced Hyperkalemia

Hyperkalemia may develop after administration of succinylcholine to a patient with spinal cord injury. The amount of potassium released depends on the extent of the patient's motor deficit. It is considered safe to administer succinylcholine for the first 48 hours. After that time, there is a proliferation of acetylcholine receptors in the muscle, and they become supersensitive to depolarizing muscle relaxants.[5] The increases in serum potassium are maximal between 4 weeks and 5 months after spinal injury. Serum potassium levels may increase from normal to as high as 14 mEq/L, causing ventricular fibrillation or cardiac arrest. Therefore, succinylcholine should be avoided in all spinal cord–injured patients after 48 hours. There are no contraindications to the nondepolarizing agents.

Temperature Control

Disruption of the sympathetic pathways carrying temperature sensation, and subsequent loss of vasoconstriction below the level of injury, causes spinal cord–injured patients to be poikilothermic. Maintenance of normal temperature can be achieved by applying exogenous heat to the skin, increasing ambient air temperature, warming intravenous fluids, and humidifying gases.

Maintaining Spinal Cord Integrity

All patients with spinal cord trauma should be considered to have compromised spinal cords, and an important component of anesthetic management is the preservation of spinal cord blood flow. Blood pressure and intravascular volume should be maintained within normal levels to ensure adequate spinal cord perfusion pressure. Sustained hypotension may worsen neurologic deficits. Hyperventilation should be avoided because hypocarbia decreases spinal cord blood flow. These considerations, as well as spinal cord monitoring, are discussed in detail later in this chapter.

Autonomic Hyperreflexia

After recovery from spinal shock, 85% of patients exhibit autonomic hyperreflexia when there has been complete cord transection above T5. The syndrome, which can also occur with injuries at lower levels, is characterized by severe paroxysmal hypertension with bradycardia (baroreceptor reflex), dysrhythmias, and cutaneous vasoconstriction below, and vasodilation above, the level of the injury. The episode is typically precipitated by distention of the bladder or rectum, but can be induced by any noxious stimulus. Many patients with spinal injuries and autonomic hyperreflexia will report characteristic headaches with bladder distention. The lack of supraspinal inhibition allows the sympathetic outflow below the lesion to react to the stimulus unopposed. If autonomic hyperreflexia occurs, it should be treated by removal of the stimulus, deepening anesthesia, and administration of direct-acting vasodilators. Untreated, the hypertensive crisis may progress to seizures, intracranial hemorrhage, or myocardial infarction.

Scoliosis

Scoliosis is a deformity of the spine resulting in lateral curvature and rotation of the vertebrae, as well as deformity of the rib cage (Fig. 50-1). The incidence of scoliosis predominantly reflects the incidence of idiopathic scoliosis, which represents 75% to 90%

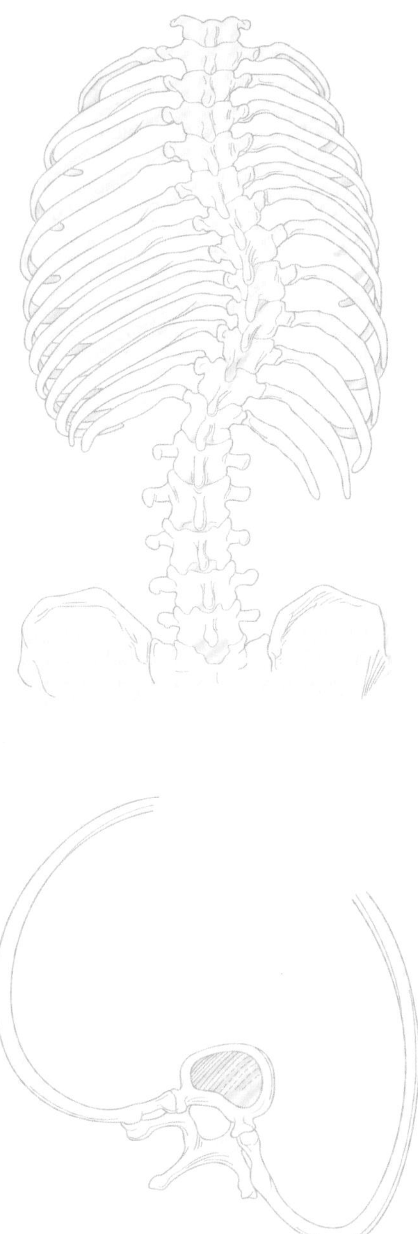

FIGURE 50-1. Deformity of the vertebrae and rib cage in scoliosis. Primary curvature occurs most frequently in the thoracic and lumbar regions. The vertebral bodies are wedge-shaped, and the posterior angles of the ribs are shallow on the side of concavity. On the convex side, the rib angles are more acute. (Reprinted from: Horlocker TT, Cucchiara RF, Ebersold MJ. Vertebral column and spinal cord surgery. In: Cucchiara RF, Michenfelder JD, eds. *Clinical Neuroanesthesia*. New York, NY: Churchill Livingstone; 1990:325, with permission.)

of cases. The remaining 10% to 25% of cases are associated with neuromuscular diseases and congenital abnormalities, including congenital heart disease, trauma, and mesenchymal disorders. The severity of scoliosis is defined by the angle of scoliosis or *Cobb angle*. Surgical correction is performed for Cobb angles >50 degrees, with the intent of *halting*, not reversing, progression of respiratory and cardiac dysfunction. Likewise, quality of life is improved, but only modestly.

Pulmonary Considerations

1 Scoliosis has profound effects on the respiratory and cardiovascular systems (Fig. 50-2). In patients with untreated scoliosis, respiratory failure and death usually occur by 45 years of age. Vital capacity appears to be a reliable prognostic indicator of perioperative respiratory reserve. Postoperative ventilation will most likely be required for patients with a vital capacity <40% of predicted. Although the long-term effect of scoliosis repair is to halt the decline in respiratory function, pulmonary function acutely deteriorates for 7 to 10 days after surgery.

The primary abnormality in gas exchange is ventilation–perfusion maldistribution, which contributes to hypoxemia. However, hypercapnia develops with increasing age as compensatory mechanisms fail. Prolonged hypoxia, hypercapnia, and pulmonary vascular constriction may result in irreversible pulmonary vascular changes and pulmonary hypertension. In general, the prognosis of scoliosis associated with neuromuscular disease is worse than that of idiopathic scoliosis. These patients frequently need postoperative ventilatory support.

Cardiovascular Considerations

Cardiovascular function is also affected in patients with scoliosis. At autopsy, these patients exhibit right ventricular hypertrophy and hypertensive pulmonary vascular changes. Prolonged alveolar hypoxia due to hypoventilation and ventilation–perfusion mismatch eventually causes irreversible vasoconstriction and pulmonary hypertension. Scoliosis is also associated with congenital heart conditions, including mitral valve prolapse, coarctation of the aorta, and cyanotic heart disease, suggesting a common embryonic insult or collagen defect.

Surgical Approach and Positioning

The prone position is used for the posterior approach to the spine (see also Chapter 28). Pressure points should be carefully padded. An orthopedic frame, such as the Jackson table or Wilson frame, can be used to free the chest and abdomen. In correct prone positioning for thoracolumbar spine surgery, the head is turned, the neck is slightly flexed, and the arms are anteriorly flexed and abducted to reduce tension on the brachial plexus (Fig. 50-3). Alternatively, the head may remain in the neutral position, supported by a foam headrest or a skull holder with pins. If only one arm is
2 abducted, the head should be laterally rotated toward the ipsilateral arm to prevent stretch injury to the brachial plexus. Because rotation of the neck in patients with cervical spondylosis may alter carotid or vertebral circulation and compromise the spinal cord, patients should be evaluated for neck pain or neurologic symptoms with neck rotation before surgery. The chest and iliac crest are supported by chest rolls or other supports to leave the abdomen free. Breasts should be positioned medially to avoid traumatic injury. The dependent ear and eye should be checked frequently during surgery to avoid injury and ischemia. Necrosis of the dependent ear cartilage may occur if the pinna is doubled back on itself. Eyes should be taped closed to avoid corneal abrasion, which occurs in the dependent eye with a frequency of 0.17%.[6]

The anterior approach to the thoracolumbar spine is achieved with the patient in the lateral position, usually with the convexity of the curve uppermost. Removal of one or more ribs may be necessary for adequate surgical exposure. Likewise, placement of a double-lumen endotracheal tube, with collapse of the lung on the operative side, may be required for surgery above T8. Thus, the thoracolumbar approach for anterior spinal fusion may be associated with more postoperative respiratory insufficiency than posterior fusion because of lung and diaphragmatic manipulation.

FIGURE 50-2. The factors in idiopathic scoliosis that contribute to respiratory function abnormalities and failure. V_D, dead space volume; V_T, tidal volume; $AaDO_2$, alveolar to arterial oxygen gradient. (Reprinted from: Kafer ER. Respiratory and cardiovascular functions in scoliosis. *Bull Eur Physiopathol Respir.* 1977;13:299, with permission.)

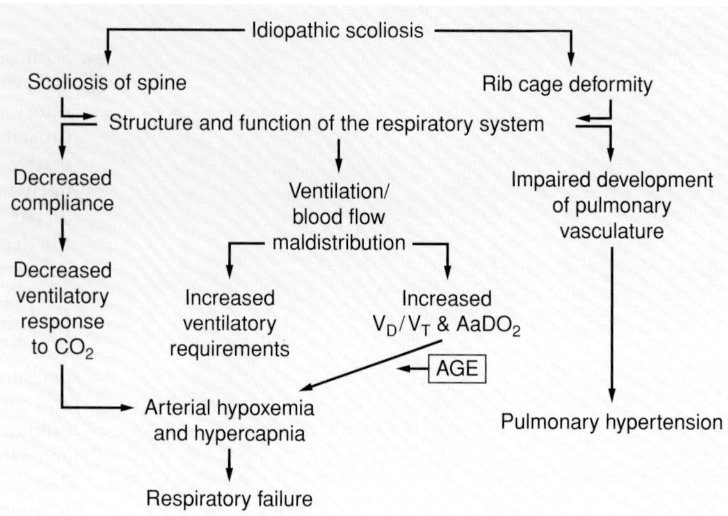

Combined anterior and posterior spinal procedures yield higher union rates and greater correction in patients undergoing scoliosis correction. It remains unclear whether these two major procedures should be performed on the same day or whether the posterior fusion should be delayed to allow the patient to recover from the anterior (first) procedure. Furthermore, the actual timing of the second procedure remains controversial. Although the degree of correction and the arthrodesis rates are similar for one- or two-stage procedures, the morbidity and number of complications, such as increased blood loss and transfusion requirements, decreased nutritional parameters, and longer hospital stays, may be increased for staged procedures.[7] However, these results are not consistent.[8] Because the risk of significant complications is present with either same-day or staged anterior–posterior fusion, prospective studies are needed to clarify this issue.

Anesthetic Management

The primary aim of preoperative evaluation of patients with scoliosis is to detect the presence and extent of cardiac or pulmonary compromise. Respiratory reserve is assessed by exercise tolerance, vital capacity, and arterial blood gases. Cardiac studies are performed as indicated to optimize preoperative cardiovascular status. A brief neurologic examination will document pre-existing neurologic deficits. Finally, cervical mobility and upper airway anatomy are assessed to discover any potential airway or positioning difficulties.

Anesthetic considerations for surgical correction of scoliosis by *spinal fusion and instrumentation* include management of a patient in the prone position, hypothermia secondary to a long procedure with an extensive exposed area, and replacement of blood and fluid losses, which may be extensive.[9] More recently, attention has been focused on the maintenance of spinal cord integrity, prevention and treatment of venous air embolism (VAE), and reduction of blood loss through hypotensive anesthetic techniques.

Adequate hemodynamic monitoring and venous access are essential in the management of patients undergoing spinal fusion and instrumentation. The radial artery is cannulated for direct blood pressure measurement and assessment of blood gases. A central venous catheter is helpful in evaluating blood and fluid management and can be used to aspirate air if VAE occurs. Patients with evidence of pulmonary hypertension, or severe coexistent cardiovascular or pulmonary disease, may require a pulmonary artery catheter.

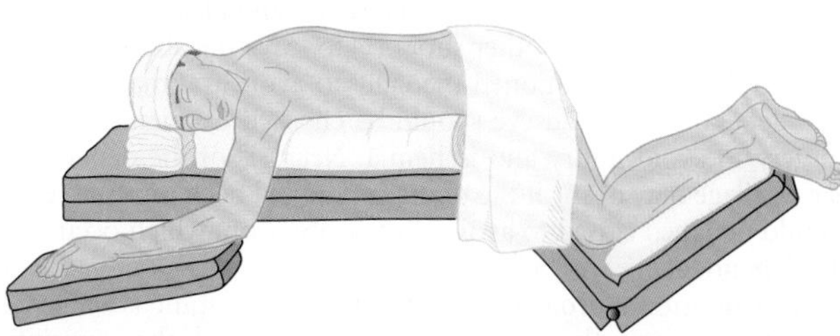

FIGURE 50-3. Prone position. The head is turned with the dependent ear and eye being protected from pressure. Chest rolls are in place, the arms are brought forward without hyperextension, and the knees are flexed. (Reprinted from: Horlocker TT, Cucchiara RF, Ebersold MJ. Vertebral column and spinal cord surgery. In: Cucchiara RF, Michenfelder JD, eds. *Clinical Neuroanesthesia*. New York, NY: Churchill Livingstone; 1990:325, with permission.)

Degenerative Vertebral Column Disease

Spinal stenosis, spondylosis, and spondylolisthesis are all forms of degenerative vertebral column disease. It is not unusual for more than one of these degenerative changes in the spine to occur concomitantly, leading to a more rapid progression of neurologic symptoms and the need for surgical intervention.

Surgical Approach and Positioning

3 Cervical laminectomy is performed in the prone, lateral, or sitting position, whereas thoracolumbar laminectomy is usually
4 performed prone. Considerations for positioning a prone patient have been previously discussed (see also Chapter 28). Patients undergoing cervical laminectomy should be assessed before surgery for cervical range of motion and the presence of neurologic symptoms during flexion, extension, or rotation. With the anterior approach, the surgical incision approximates the anterior border of the sternocleidomastoid muscle and is therefore

near critical anatomic structures. Lateral retraction of the carotid artery may endanger blood flow to the brain, particularly in the elderly patient. Retraction of the esophagus and trachea medially may cause pharyngeal laceration, laryngeal edema, and recurrent laryngeal nerve paralysis. Cerebrospinal fluid leaks and trauma to the vertebral artery have also been reported.

In the sitting position for cervical laminectomy, blood flows away from the site of operation, producing a clear operative field and better surgical exposure. In this position, the patient sits with head, arms, and chest supported. The patient must be carefully positioned and the dependent areas must be padded to prevent compression injuries to nerves and skin. Extreme cervical flexion may obstruct the airway. Hypotension can be minimized by gradual attainment of the sitting position. A disadvantage of the sitting position is the increased occurrence of VAE. Although the incidence of VAE in sitting posterior fossa cases is 40%, the incidence is only 5% to 25% in sitting cervical spine procedures.[10]

Recently, surgical advances have made it possible to perform minimally invasive surgery (MIS) procedures with smaller incisions and decreased soft tissue trauma. MIS techniques can be classified as endoscopic or nonendoscopic (mini-open). Although endoscopic approaches decrease some approach morbidities, they are associated with high instrumentation cost, steep learning curves, and new complication profiles.[11,12] Furthermore, the high costs have not been shown to be justified by superior clinical benefits. Nonendoscopic MIS approaches use direct visualization and standard operative techniques and report lower complication rates, reduced length of stay, and faster recovery time. Although certain MIS procedures may produce early cost benefits, longer follow-up, better outcome, and cost data are needed to determine if MIS techniques are cost effective compared to open or nonsurgical interventions.[11]

Anesthetic Management

Either general or neuraxial anesthesia may be safely administered for relatively uncomplicated lower thoracic and lumbar spine surgery; a randomized trial in 2009 concluded that general anesthesia was associated with higher surgeon satisfaction and less nausea and vomiting.[13] General anesthesia is preferred for essentially all thoracic and cervical procedures because of the high spinal level that would be required with a regional technique. General anesthesia ensures airway access, is associated with greater patient acceptance, and can be used for prolonged operations. Succinylcholine should be avoided if there are progressive neurologic deficits.

Spinal Cord Monitoring

2 Paraplegia is one of the most feared complications of major spine surgery (see also Chapter 36). The incidence of neurologic injuries associated with scoliosis correction is 1.2%, with partial or complete paraplegia occurring in half the cases. When patients awaken paraplegic, neurologic recovery is unlikely, although immediate removal of instrumentation improves the prognosis. It is therefore essential that any intraoperative compromise of spinal cord function be detected as early as possible and reversed immediately. The two methods developed to accomplish this are the wake-up test and neurophysiologic monitoring.

The *wake-up test*, first described by Vauzelle et al.,[14] consists of the intraoperative awakening of patients after completion of spinal instrumentation. Surgical anesthesia is typically provided with a balanced technique of nitrous oxide, a volatile drug, and opioids, although use of opioids with a short-acting volatile anesthetic (e.g., sevoflurane), or an infusion of propofol, is also possible. The opioids are important to provide analgesia while the patient is awake and to permit the patient to tolerate the endotracheal tube. During the 30 to 45 minutes before intraoperative wake-up, the volatile anesthetic, or propofol, and muscle relaxants are discontinued and the patient is allowed to awaken gradually. The patient is addressed by name and asked to move both hands, and after a positive response, both feet. Patients usually respond within 5 minutes. If there is satisfactory movement of the hands, but not the feet, the distraction on the rod is released one notch, and the wake-up test repeated. Although recall of the event occurs in only 0% to 20% of patients and is rarely viewed as unpleasant,[15] it is important to describe to the patient before surgery what will transpire so that anxiety will be minimized should the patient be fully aware during the wake-up. It is extremely rare for a patient who was neurologically intact when awakened during surgery to have a neurologic deficit on completion of the procedure. However, certain hazards of the wake-up test do exist and include recall, pain, air embolism, dislocation of spinal instrumentation, and accidental tracheal extubation or removal of intravenous and arterial lines.

An adjunct or alternative to the wake-up test is neurophysiologic monitoring. Somatosensory stimulation follows the dorsal column pathways of proprioception and vibration: Pathways supplied by the posterior spinal artery. Accordingly, the motor pathway, which is supplied by the anterior spinal artery, is not addressed by monitoring somatosensory evoked potentials (SSEP). High concentrations of inhaled agents cannot be used when monitoring SSEP. Motor evoked potentials (MEP), in contrast, monitor motor pathways but are technically more difficult to use. Muscle relaxants cannot be used in patients having MEP monitoring. If both SSEP and MEP are to be monitored during spine surgery, one might consider providing anesthesia with an ultrashort-acting opioid infusion with a low-dose inhaled anesthetic and monitoring of the electroencephalogram or bispectral index to minimize the potential for intraoperative awareness. It is of critical importance to note that postoperative paraplegia has occurred despite preservation of intraoperative SSEPs. Combined use of MEPs and SSEPs may increase the early detection of spinal cord ischemia.[9,16]

Acute alterations in SSEP amplitude or latency signify spinal cord compromise and may be the result of direct trauma, ischemia, compression, or hematoma. If changes occur, it is recommended that surgery be discontinued, blood pressure returned to normal or 20% above normal, and volatile agents decreased or discontinued. Arterial blood gases may be drawn to rule out a metabolic derangement. If the waveform does not return to normal, the surgeon should release distraction on the cord. A wake-up test is often performed at this time to definitely exclude neurologic deficits. In addition to neural injury, SSEPs are altered by volatile anesthetics, hypercarbia, hypoxia, hypotension, and hypothermia.[17,18]

Blood Loss

The rate of transfusion in adult spine surgery ranges from 50% to 81%.[19] Most of the blood loss in spinal instrumentation and fusion occurs with decortication and is proportional to the number
3 of vertebral levels decorticated.[20] Measures to decrease blood loss and transfusion requirements during major spine surgery have traditionally included preoperative autologous donation, proper positioning and the use of intraoperative blood salvage, induced hypotension, intraoperative normovolemic hemodilution, and the administration of antifibrinolytics (aprotinin and tranexamic acid), although reported results are inconsistent.[21–23] Recent systematic reviews have concluded that good evidence

exists consistently for positioning and use of tranexamic acid.[19,24] However, the safety of antifibrinolytics is not fully known. While tranexamic acid is currently recommended in the adult population, optimal dosing has yet to be determined in pediatric patients.[25] Importantly, the FDA has suspended aprotinin use on the basis of safety data in the cardiac literature.[19,24]

Patients undergoing major spine surgery may acquire a perioperative coagulopathy from dilution of coagulation factors and/or platelets or fibrinolysis. The mechanisms of coagulopathy and the role of coagulation testing during these procedures are poorly defined. However, it appears that a significant deviation from normal values of either the prothrombin time or the activated partial thromboplastin time is predictive of bleeding and may be used to guide transfusion therapy.[26] Another rare cause of bleeding during spine surgery is trauma to the aorta, vena cava, or iliac vessels. Unexplained hypotension or signs of hypovolemia without obvious blood loss should alert the anesthesiologist to this possibility.

Visual Loss after Spine Surgery

4 In the 1990s, cases of unilateral and bilateral blindness were reported after spine surgery.[27–29] The diagnoses included optic neuropathy, retinal artery occlusion, and cerebral ischemia. Most cases were associated with complex instrumented fusions[28]; many cases were associated with significant (prolonged) intraoperative hypotension, anemia, large intraoperative blood loss, and prolonged surgery.[29] However, these conditions are present during many major spine procedures without visual sequelae.

Ischemic optic neuropathy was the most common cause of visual loss after spine surgery and accounted for 83 of 93 spine surgery cases.[30] Using a case control design with multivariate analysis, the American Society of Anesthesiologists Visual Loss Study Group's risk factors for ischemic optic neuropathy after spinal surgery included male sex, obesity, Wilson frame use, anesthetic duration, increased blood loss, and the use of non-colloid for fluid replacement.[31] Using this model, the only preoperative factor that is modifiable is surgical frame selection. In addition, anesthesiologists may use these results to guide fluid administration. It is also recommended that the risk of visual loss should be considered in the preoperative discussion for patients undergoing lengthy spine surgery in the prone position.

Venous Air Embolus

VAE is a catastrophic event that may occur during spine surgery. The large amount of exposed bone and the elevated location of the surgical incision relative to the heart predispose to VAE. Capnography, mass spectrometry, and precordial Doppler are noninvasive, yet effective, in detecting VAE. VAE can occur in all positions associated with laminectomies because the wound is above the cardiac level. Incidences of VAE (defined by aspiration of air through a central venous catheter) in patients undergoing neurosurgical procedures in the sitting, supine, prone, and lateral positions are 25%, 18%, 10%, and 8%, respectively.[10] The actual incidence of VAE in spine surgery is unknown; however, poor neurologic recovery is often reported.[32] The presenting sign is often unexplained hypotension and an increase in the end-tidal nitrogen concentration, or a precipitous fall in the end-tidal CO_2 concentration. The anesthesiologist, therefore, should be aware of the possibilities of VAE because prompt diagnosis and treatment increase patient survival. If VAE is suspected, the wound should be irrigated with saline, nitrous oxide discontinued, and vasopressors administered. Massive embolism may necessitate turning the patient supine and initiating cardiopulmonary resuscitation.

Postoperative Care

Most patients undergoing surgery to the spine can be extubated immediately after the operation if the procedure was relatively uneventful and preoperative vital capacity values were acceptable. Residual opioid or muscle relaxant may lead to hypoventilation or apnea, especially in patients with an associated neuromuscular disease. Some patients who have experienced considerable blood loss and who have received large amounts of intravenous fluids, particularly if they were prone, may have severe facial edema that renders immediate tracheal extubation unwise. Aggressive postoperative pulmonary care, including incentive spirometry, is necessary to avoid atelectasis and pneumonia. Continued hemorrhage in the postoperative period is another concern. Careful monitoring of systemic and central venous pressures, urine output, and wound drainage is essential. Neurologic status must also be monitored closely for deterioration.

5 Traditionally, postoperative analgesia is typically provided by systemic opioids. However, wound instillation with local anesthetic or injection of intrathecal morphine is associated with improved pain scores and decreased side effects in the early postoperative period.[33] Multimodal analgesia, a multidisciplinary approach to pain management with the aim of maximizing the positive aspects of the treatment while limiting the associated side effects, has become the gold standard for postoperative pain relief. Because many of the negative side effects of analgesic therapy are opioid-related (and dose-dependent), limiting perioperative opioid use is a major principle of multimodal analgesia. Anti-inflammatory medications and acetaminophen are valuable adjuvants to systemic opioids. The addition of nonopioid analgesics reduces opioid use, improves analgesia, and decreases opioid-related side effects. Recently a perioperative oral multimodal approach, including scheduled extended release oxycodone, gabapentin, acetaminophen, and "as needed" short-acting oxycodone for breath-through pain, has been described. Compared to intravenous opioids, the oral regimen was associated with less opioid consumption, decreased pain, less nausea, and less drowsiness.[34]

Epidural and Spinal Anesthesia after Major Spine Surgery

Previous spine surgery has been considered to represent a relative contraindication to the use of regional anesthesia. The presence of postoperative spinal stenosis or other degenerative changes in the spine or pre-existing neurologic symptoms may preclude the use of regional anesthesia in these patients. Likewise, many of these patients experience chronic back pain and are reluctant to undergo epidural or spinal anesthesia, fearing exacerbation of their pre-existing back complaints. Finally, postoperative anatomic changes make needle or catheter placement more difficult and complicated after major spine surgery; needle insertion can be accomplished only at nonfused segments.

Spread of epidural local anesthetic following spine surgery may be affected by adhesions, producing an incomplete or "patchy" block. Obliteration of the epidural space may increase the incidence of dural puncture and make subsequent epidural blood patch placement impossible. Several retrospective studies have demonstrated that epidural anesthesia may be successfully performed in patients with previous spine surgery; however, successful catheter placement was possible on the first attempt in only 50% of patients, even with an experienced anesthesiologist. In addition, although adequate epidural anesthesia was eventually produced in 40% to 95% of patients, there appeared to be a higher incidence of traumatic needle placement, inadvertent dural puncture, and unsuccessful epidural needle or catheter placement, especially if spinal fusion extended to L5 through S1.[35–37]

Spinal anesthesia may produce a more reliable block and cause less trauma than epidural anesthesia. Although needle placement may be more difficult or traumatic in these patients, the spread of local anesthetic in the subarachnoid space and quality of block would not be affected. A spinal anesthetic may be more desirable after spine surgery because the technique does not depend on a subjective loss of resistance, but instead has a definite end point—the presence of cerebrospinal fluid.

The overall success and neurologic complication rates was examined in 937 patients with spinal stenosis or lumbar disc disease undergoing neuraxial block, 207 (22%) of whom had previously undergone spine surgery, although the majority were simple laminectomies or discectomies. Success rates did not differ between patients who had previous surgery and those who had undergone a spine procedure. Ten patients experienced new or progressive neurologic deficits when compared with preoperative findings; the neuraxial technique was the primary cause in four patients. The authors concluded that patients with pre-existing spinal canal pathology have a higher incidence of neurologic complications after neuraxial blockade than that previously reported for patients without such underlying pathology.[38] These findings validate those of Moen et al.[39,40] who reported a higher frequency of (undiagnosed) spinal stenosis in patients who developed paraplegia following uneventful neuraxial block.

SURGERY TO THE UPPER EXTREMITIES

Orthopedic surgical procedures to the upper extremity are well suited to regional anesthetic techniques. In addition to intraoperative anesthesia, brachial plexus and peripheral nerve blocks may be used in the treatment and prevention of reflex sympathetic dystrophy (complex regional pain syndrome). Continuous catheter techniques provide postoperative analgesia and allow early limb mobilization. Conversely, although the benefits of regional anesthesia in this patient population are well established, orthopedic surgical procedures often involve peripheral nerves with pre-existing deficits, such as ulnar nerve transposition and carpal tunnel release. In addition, the operative site may be adjacent to neural structures, as with total shoulder arthroplasty or fractures of the proximal humerus. The decision to perform regional anesthesia in a patient with pre-existing neurologic deficits or who is at risk for perioperative neurapraxia should be made on an individual basis after discussion with the patient and surgeon. Meticulous regional anesthetic technique with appropriate use of local anesthetic solutions and vasoconstrictors, careful patient positioning, and serial postoperative neurologic examinations may reduce the incidence of neurologic dysfunction.

Local anesthetic selection is based on the duration and degree of sensory or motor block required. Although prolonged blockade of the lower extremities interferes with ambulation and therefore delays outpatient discharge, persistent upper extremity block is not a contraindication to hospital dismissal. However, the patient should be informed of the anticipated duration of analgesia during the postoperative visit and instructed to protect the blocked extremity until block resolution.

Surgery to the Shoulder and Upper Arm

Reconstructive shoulder surgery, including total shoulder arthroplasty and rotator cuff repair, presents unique management and positioning considerations to the anesthesiologist. For example, 4% of patients undergoing total shoulder arthroplasty have a documented postoperative neurologic deficit, including 3% of patients with injury to the brachial plexus. The level of injury is at the level of the nerve trunks, which is the level at which an interscalene block is performed, making it impossible to determine
5 the etiology of the nerve injury (surgical vs. anesthetic). Most of these nerve injuries represent a neurapraxia; 90% resolve in 3 to 4 months.[41] In addition, nerve injury often occurs in association with upper extremity trauma. Radial nerve palsy is identified in up to 18% of patients with humeral shaft fractures, whereas injury to the axillary nerve and brachial plexus is associated with proximal humerus fractures. However, the significant incidence of neurologic deficits demonstrates the importance of clinical examination before regional anesthetic techniques in these patients.

Surgical Approach and Positioning

Surgical procedures to the upper arm and shoulder are typically performed with the patient in the "beach chair" position (see Chapter 28). The patient's head, neck, and hips must be secured to prevent additional lateral movement. The head and neck must remain firmly supported by the operating table and secured in a neutral position; excessive rotation or flexion of the head away from the operative side results in stretch injury to the brachial
6 plexus. Care must also be taken to avoid pressure on the eyes and ears. All airway connections should be tightened and possibly reinforced with tape because after surgical draping, access to the patient's face and airway is limited. Case reports of stroke after general anesthesia in the sitting position have been reported, particularly in the setting of induced hypotension. It has been suggested that, during induced hypotension, the systolic blood pressure should not be decreased by more than 20% to 30% from baseline (to 80 to 90 mm Hg in normal patients).[42] Although there were no strokes in a series of 4,169 sedated, blocked, and spontaneously breathing patients who underwent induced hypotension during shoulder surgery in the sitting position, the absolute risk remains undetermined.[43]

A tourniquet cannot be used during proximal upper extremity surgical procedures, and significant blood loss may occur. Therefore, arterial cannulation may be helpful for direct blood pressure measurement and monitoring of intraoperative hemoglobin concentrations during total shoulder arthroplasty and reduction of humeral fractures. In theory, VAE may occur during surgical procedures to the shoulder because the operative site is higher than the heart, but the incidence is low.

Anesthetic Management

Surgery to the shoulder and humerus may be performed under regional or general anesthesia. With careful positioning and appropriate sedation, interscalene or supraclavicular blockade alone can provide excellent surgical anesthesia (Table 50-1). However, general anesthesia or a combination of regional and general anesthesia is often chosen because of limited access to the patient's airway during these surgical procedures. Interscalene brachial plexus block may be performed before surgical incision or after postoperative upper extremity neurologic function has been determined. Severe hypotension and bradycardia

TABLE 50-1. REGIONAL ANESTHETIC TECHNIQUES FOR UPPER EXTREMITY SURGERY

Brachial Plexus Technique	Level of Blockade	Peripheral Nerves Blocked	Surgical Applications	Comments
Axillary	Peripheral nerve	Radial, ulnar, median; musculocutaneous unreliably blocked	Surgery to forearm and hand, less utilized for procedures about the elbow	Unsuitable for proximal humerus or shoulder surgery; patient must be able to abduct the arm to perform
Infraclavicular	Cords	Radial, ulnar, median, musculocutaneous, axillary	Surgery to elbow, forearm, and hand	Catheter site (near coracoid process) easy to maintain; no risk of hemothorax, pneumothorax
Supraclavicular	Distal trunk–proximal cord	Radial, ulnar, median, musculocutaneous, axillary	Surgery to mid humerus, elbow, forearm, and hand	Risk of pneumothorax—unsuitable for outpatient procedures; phrenic nerve paresis in 30% of cases
Interscalene	Upper and middle trunks	Entire brachial plexus, although inferior trunk (ulnar nerve) not blocked in 15–20% of cases	Surgery to shoulder, proximal/midhumerus	Phrenic nerve paresis in 100% of patients for block duration—unsuitable for patients unable to tolerate 25% reduction in pulmonary function

Duration of block performed with long-acting local anesthetic (bupivacaine or ropivacaine) is 12–20 h; intermediate-acting agents (lidocaine or mepivacaine) will resolve after 4–6 h.

(e.g., Bezold–Jarisch reflex) have been reported in awake, sitting patients undergoing shoulder surgery under an interscalene block. The cause is presumed to be stimulation of intracardiac mechanoreceptors by decreased venous return, producing an abrupt withdrawal of sympathetic tone and enhanced parasympathetic output. This effect results in bradycardia, hypotension, and syncope. The frequency is decreased when prophylactic β-blockers are administered.[44]

Interscalene block should be performed with caution in patients with a pre-existing brachial plexopathy because of the risk of perioperative exacerbation of neurologic deficits. The ipsilateral diaphragmatic paresis and 25% loss of pulmonary function produced by interscalene block also contraindicates this block in patients with severe pulmonary disease.[45] The reduction in pulmonary function is present for the duration of the interscalene block.

Surgery to the Elbow

Although use of general anesthesia is appropriate, surgical procedures to the distal humerus, elbow, and forearm are commonly performed using regional anesthetic techniques. Infraclavicular and supraclavicular approaches to the brachial plexus are the most reliable and provide consistent anesthesia to the four major nerves of the brachial plexus: Median, ulnar, radial, and musculocutaneous. However, the small but definite risk of pneumothorax associated with supraclavicular and infraclavicular blocks usually makes this approach unsuitable for outpatient procedures. Typically, the pneumothorax occurs 6 to 12 hours after hospital discharge; therefore, a postoperative chest radiograph is not helpful. Although chest tube placement is advised for pneumothorax >20% of lung volume, the lung may also be re-expanded with a small Teflon catheter under fluoroscopic guidance, eliminating the need for hospital admission. The axillary approach to the brachial plexus eliminates the risk of pneumothorax and reliably provides adequate anesthesia for surgery near the elbow.[46]

Surgery to the Wrist and Hand

Surgery to the distal forearm, wrist, and hand may be performed under general or regional anesthesia. Brachial plexus block provides comprehensive and consistent regional anesthesia for the distal upper extremity and can be used for outpatients.[47,48] Although the brachial plexus may be successfully blocked at several sites, the interscalene approach is seldom used for wrist and hand procedures because incomplete anesthesia of the ulnar nerve is noted in 15% to 30% of patients. In addition, although the supraclavicular approach results in blockade of all four major nerves, the risk of pneumothorax reduces its suitability for outpatient procedures. Therefore, the axillary approach is most commonly used for surgical procedures to the forearm, wrist, and hand.

Minor hand procedures such as carpal tunnel release, reduction of phalanx fractures, and superficial wound debridements may require only local infiltration or peripheral blockade at the midhumeral, elbow, or wrist level. Inflation of an upper arm tourniquet in these patients causes significant discomfort in 45 to 60 minutes and limits the duration of the surgical procedure. Intravenous regional anesthesia (Bier block) using a double tourniquet permits more extensive surgery and longer tourniquet times than distal peripheral block, but does not provide postoperative analgesia.

Continuous Brachial Plexus Anesthesia

Overall, there are early, but no long-term, benefits with a single-injection regional anesthetic technique compared with a general anesthetic. However, placement of an indwelling perineural catheter results in more substantial and lasting benefits, including avoidance of hospital admission/readmission, decreased opioid-related side effects and sleep disturbance, and improved rehabilitation.[49,50] Thus, anesthetic management of patients undergoing elbow surgery is focused on *postoperative* analgesia, rather than *intraoperative* anesthesia to improve perioperative outcomes. Brachial plexus catheters may be inserted using interscalene, infraclavicular, and axillary approaches. After surgery, the catheters may be left indwelling for 4 to 7 days without adverse effects. A continuous infusion of dilute local anesthetic solution, such as bupivacaine 0.125%, prevents vasospasm and increases circulation after limb replantation or vascular repair. More concentrated solutions result in complete sensory block and allow early joint mobilization after painful surgical procedures to the elbow. Ambulatory (at-home) applications provide superior analgesia with fewer side effects than conventional systemic analgesic therapy.[49]

SURGERY TO THE LOWER EXTREMITIES

Although orthopedic procedures to the lower extremity may be performed under both general and regional anesthesia, the ability to provide superior postoperative analgesia, rapid postoperative rehabilitation, and reduced cost of medical care may result from thoughtfully implemented regional anesthetic and analgesic techniques.[51–53]

Multiple studies demonstrate significantly reduced intraoperative blood loss during total hip arthroplasty completed under central neuraxial blockade compared with general anesthesia.[54] Likewise, postoperative pulmonary thromboembolism (PTE) from deep venous thrombosis (DVT) is an important cause of morbidity and mortality in orthopedic surgical patients. Historical investigations reported a decreased incidence of DVT and PTE in patients whose surgery was conducted under regional anesthesia.[55,56] However, these patients did not receive pharmacologic thromboprophylaxis. The potential benefit of regional anesthesia in reducing thromboembolic complications is discussed later in this chapter.

Surgery to the Hip

More than 200,000 total hip replacements are performed annually in North America. Patients undergoing surgical procedures to the hip for arthritic conditions typically are elderly and often have pre-existing medical conditions that may affect perioperative outcome. In addition, because hospital costs appear to be directly related to the length of hospital stay, anesthetic techniques associated with improved recovery and reduced complications may decrease the total hospital costs among these patients.[51–53]

Surgical Approach and Positioning

The lateral decubitus position is frequently used to facilitate surgical exposure for total hip arthroplasty, whereas the fracture table is often used for repair of femur fractures. In transferring the patient from the supine to lateral decubitus position, care must be taken to maintain the head and shoulders in a neutral position. The patient is supported while the position is secured with hip rests or other mechanical devices. The dependent arm is abducted and placed on a padded arm rest; a rolled towel or wrapped intravenous fluid bag is placed in the axilla to avoid compression of the brachial plexus and vascular structures. The upper arm is placed on a padded overarm board.

Positioning on the fracture table (Fig. 50-4) also requires adequate personnel to move the patient, with one person assigned to apply traction to the fractured limb. The fracture table affords two advantages: Maintenance of traction on the fractured extremity, allowing manipulation for closed reduction and fixation, and access to the fracture site for radiography in several planes. The patient must be carefully monitored for hemodynamic changes during positioning, whether under regional or general anesthesia. Care must be taken to pad the perineal post before positioning the patient's pelvis. Usually, the arm ipsilateral to the fractured hip is placed on an arm board or in a sling to keep it from obstructing the fluoroscopic view.

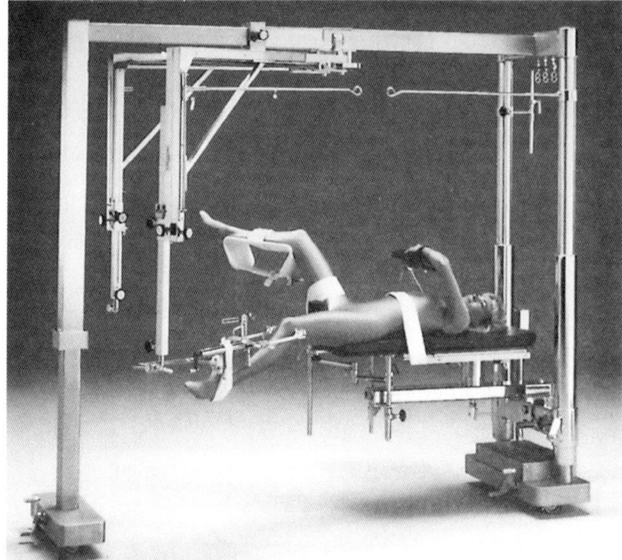

FIGURE 50-4. The fracture table. The patient must be moved carefully with continuous traction on the fractured limb. The ipsilateral arm is positioned on an arm board or sling without stretching the brachial plexus. (Courtesy of Midmark Corporation, Versailles, OH.)

Anesthetic Technique

Regional techniques may be used to provide intraoperative anesthesia as well as postoperative analgesia. Both hypobaric and isobaric spinal anesthetic solutions are effective. Adequate intravenous hydration before placing the neuraxial block protects against a precipitous drop in blood pressure that can occur secondary to sympathetic blockade and peripheral vasodilation. Placement of an epidural catheter allows prolonged anesthesia as well as postoperative analgesia. More recently, both single-dose and continuous lumbar plexus techniques have been performed to provide postoperative analgesia in patients undergoing major hip surgery. Single-injection techniques are associated with short-term improvements in analgesia (approximately 6 hours) and a modest decrease in blood loss.[57] However, prolonged analgesia with continuous psoas compartment block was associated with decreased postoperative pain, fewer episodes of cognitive dysfunction, and decreased ileus and facilitated hospital discharge.[52,53] The lumbar plexus block also contributes to the intraoperative anesthetic,
7 allowing decreased dosing of volatile agents, opioids, and/or spinal anesthetic solutions (Table 50-2).

Blood Loss

Regional anesthetic techniques reduce blood loss in patients undergoing hip surgery.[58] Deliberate hypotension can also be used with general anesthesia as a means of reducing surgical blood loss and has been recommended when the benefits can be

TABLE 50-2. LUMBOSACRAL TECHNIQUES FOR MAJOR LOWER EXTREMITY SURGERY

Peripheral Technique	Area of Blockade	Duration of Blockade[a]	Perioperative Outcomes[b]
Lumbar plexus		12–18 h	
Femoral	Femoral, partial lateral femoral cutaneous, and obturator		Improved analgesia and joint range of motion, decreased hospital stay compared to PCA; fewer technical problems, less urinary retention and hypotension than epidural analgesia (TKA)
Fascia iliaca	Femoral, partial lateral femoral cutaneous, obturator, and sciatic (S1)		Improved analgesia and joint range of motion compared to PCA (TKA)
Psoas compartment	Complete lumbar plexus; occasional spread to sacral plexus or neuraxis		Reduced morphine consumption, pain at rest compared to PCA (TKA, THA); reduced blood loss (THA); analgesia equivalent to continuous femoral block (TKA)
Sciatic	Posterior thigh and leg (except saphenous area)	18–30 h	Supplemental sciatic required (TKA); proximal approaches allow block of posterior femoral cutaneous nerve (TKA)

[a]Duration of block performed with long-acting local anesthetic (bupivacaine or ropivacaine); intermediate-acting agents (lidocaine or mepivacaine) will resolve after 4–6 h.
[b]Outcomes most marked in patients who receive a continuous lumbar plexus catheter with infusion of 0.1–0.2% bupivacaine or ropivacaine at 6–12 mL/h for 48–72 h.
PCA, patient-controlled analgesia; TKA, total knee arthroplasty; THA, total hip arthroplasty.
From: Horlocker TT. Anesthesia and pain management. In: Berry DJ, Trousdale RT, Dennis D, et al., eds. *Revision Hip and Knee Arthroplasty.* Philadelphia, PA: Lippincott Williams and Wilkins; in press, with permission.

expected to outweigh the risks.[59] Diltiazem, nitroprusside with and without captopril, β-blockers, and nitroglycerin have also been used to induce hypotension.

Total Knee Arthroplasty

More than 300,000 total knee arthroplasties are performed annually in North America. These procedures are often associated with significant postoperative pain, particularly when continuous-motion machines are applied to the affected joint. Failure to provide adequate analgesia impedes aggressive physical therapy and rehabilitation, which is critical to maintaining joint range of motion and potentially delays hospital dismissal. Thus, the anesthesiologist must devise a plan for not only intraoperative anesthesia, but also postoperative analgesia.

Anesthetic Technique and Positioning

Regional anesthetic techniques that can be used for surgical procedures about the knee include neuraxial and peripheral leg blocks. Surgical anesthesia for operative procedures on the knee in which a tourniquet will be used requires blockade of all four nerves (femoral, lateral femoral cutaneous, obturator, and sciatic nerves) innervating the leg. Spinal anesthesia can be accomplished with hyperbaric or isobaric solutions, although the latter are favored by most orthopedic anesthesiologists. Injection of hyperbaric solutions often results in a higher level of sensory and motor blockades than needed for the surgical procedure, with subsequent earlier offset of anesthesia. Epidural blockade offers the advantage of a continuous catheter technique that can be continued into the postoperative period.

Although it is possible to perform major knee surgery under peripheral nerve blocks, more often a femoral three-in-one or lumbar plexus (psoas) block is combined with a spinal or general anesthetic. This is less difficult technically, reduces the amount of local anesthetic (and associated systemic toxicity), and provides postoperative analgesia for 12 to 24 hours. Continuous lumbar plexus techniques, with or without supplemental sciatic block, allow for prolonged postoperative analgesia. The routine performance of a sciatic block remains controversial. From investigations that did not include a sciatic block, it is apparent that blockade of the sacral plexus is crucial to some, but not all, patients undergoing major knee surgery.[60–62]

The supine position optimizes surgical exposure during knee arthroscopy or arthroplasty, lower extremity amputations, and procedures to the tibia and fibula. Care must be taken to cushion the extremities and bony prominences.

Postoperative Analgesia after Major Joint Replacement

Pain after total joint replacement, particularly total knee arthroplasty, is severe. Traditionally, postoperative analgesia following total joint replacement was provided by either intravenous patient-controlled analgesia or epidural analgesia. However, each technique has distinct advantages and disadvantages. For example, opioids do not consistently provide adequate pain relief and often cause sedation, constipation, nausea and vomiting, and pruritus. Epidural infusions containing local anesthetics (with or without an opioid) provide superior analgesia but are associated with hypotension, urinary retention, motor block limiting ambulation, and spinal hematoma secondary to anticoagulation.[63]

Numerous reports have documented that single-dose and continuous peripheral nerve techniques that block the lumbar plexus (fascia iliaca, femoral, psoas compartment blocks), with or without sciatic nerve blockade, can be used with success for patients having total joint replacement.[52,53,60,62–72]

Several studies have also demonstrated that unilateral peripheral block provides a quality of analgesia and surgical outcomes similar to that of continuous epidural analgesia, but with fewer side effects.[64,66,70] These reports suggest that continuous peripheral techniques may be the optimal analgesic method following total joint arthroplasty. Appreciation of the indications, benefits, and side effects associated with both conventional and novel analgesic approaches is paramount to maximizing rehabilitative efforts and improving patient satisfaction. The use of peripheral or neuraxial regional anesthetic techniques and a combination of opioid and nonopioid analgesic agents for breakthrough pain (multimodal analgesia) results in superior pain control, attenuation of the stress response, and decreased opioid requirements.

In recent years, there has been increased interest in high-volume local wound infiltration/infusion techniques in these operations with a combined administration of local anesthetics, NSAIDs, and epinephrine [local infiltration analgesia (LIA)]. However, positive results have been inconsistently repeated. LIA likely has a place for intraoperative use in TKA, but most probably not in THA. The placement of a postoperative wound or intra-articular catheter with a local anesthetic infusion supplements the initial infiltration.[73,74] The simplicity and low risk of this technique have increased its application. However, overall the LIA technique must be evaluated against the efficacy, safety, and cost of other evidence-based analgesic techniques.[74]

Knee Arthroscopy and Anterior Cruciate Ligament Repair

Outpatient knee surgery may be performed under a variety of anesthetic techniques. The complexity/duration of the surgical procedure will determine the usefulness of peripheral blocks compared with neuraxial or general anesthesia. Because diagnostic knee arthroscopy is a relatively minor procedure that may be performed under local anesthesia with sedation, the performance of a single-dose or continuous lower extremity block is probably not warranted in the majority of patients. The optimal anesthetic technique would allow rapid operating suite turnover and patient recovery, excellent operating conditions, and minimal side effects. Unfortunately, each approach is associated with advantages and disadvantages. For example, concerns over transient neurologic symptoms propelled a search for an alternative to intrathecal lidocaine; to date, its reliable sensory and motor blocks (of limited duration) have not been duplicated. Bupivacaine has a low incidence of transient neurologic symptoms. However, the time to hospital discharge following administration of low-dose bupivacaine (5 to 7.5 mg) with fentanyl (10 μg) may be as long as 3 hours. Conversely, general anesthesia is associated with nausea and vomiting, side effects prevalent in the patient population undergoing knee arthroscopy. Evidence has failed to demonstrate a clinically significant difference in patient outcome with respect to anesthetic technique.[75] Patient preference may also have a significant impact on selection of anesthetic technique.

Repair of the anterior cruciate ligament (ACL) is also performed as an outpatient procedure. However, the surgery is more extensive than knee arthroscopy, and postoperative pain may be significant. The anesthetic considerations are similar to those of diagnostic knee arthroscopy, with the additional need to provide substantial analgesia. In a comprehensive evaluation of analgesia following ACL, Williams et al.[76] reported that femoral catheters reliably maintain pain scores below the moderate-to-severe pain threshold for the first 4 days after ACL reconstruction. Selected patients may be discharged home with an indwelling femoral catheter to provide sustained pain relief for 48 hours.[77] Hospital discharge criteria generally include successful oral intake, ambulation, and voiding by the patient. Thus, patients who have undergone a neuraxial technique will not be discharged until complete block resolution (although the requirement to void is somewhat controversial).

Intra-articular Injection

Intra-articular injections of local anesthetics, opioids, or combinations have become routine for perioperative pain management after arthroscopic knee surgery. A number of reports enthusiastically recommend the use of this technique; however, the results remain conflicting.[78,79] Comparison of reports is difficult because of variability in underlying anesthetic techniques, different dosages and concentrations of local anesthetic, and lack of control groups. The safety of injecting large volumes of intra-articular bupivacaine has been ascertained, and side effects are rare after intra-articular doses of morphine. Because these techniques are simple, are low risk and seem to afford pain relief under some conditions, they will likely be continued.

Surgery to the Ankle and Foot

Innervation of the foot is provided by the femoral nerve (via the saphenous nerve) and by the sciatic nerve (via the posterior tibial, sural, and deep and superficial peroneal nerves).[61] Therefore, central neuraxial blockade and peripheral nerve blocks at the upper leg, knee, or ankle are appropriate regional anesthetic techniques for foot surgery. The selection of the regional technique is based on the surgical site, use of a calf or thigh tourniquet, degree of weight bearing/ambulation, and the need for postoperative analgesia. For example, inflation of a thigh tourniquet for longer than 15 to 20 minutes necessitates a general or neuraxial anesthetic, regardless of the surgical site. Common surgical procedures and considerations regarding the choice of regional technique are discussed in Table 50-3.[80]

The distal surgical site and the ability to block the pain pathways at multiple sites give regional anesthesia an advantage over general anesthesia for surgery to the ankle and foot. Peripheral blockade avoids the cardiovascular and respiratory side effects, as well as the urinary retention associated with neuraxial and general anesthesia. Often, patients undergoing lower extremity peripheral techniques may be discharged directly from the operating room to the outpatient nursing station, reducing recovery time and charges. The use of long-acting local anesthetics and the addition of epinephrine or clonidine allow prolongation of postoperative analgesia. Mepivacaine and lidocaine may be more appropriate in the ambulatory setting, where fast-onset and reliable surgical anesthesia is essential. Placement of an indwelling catheter is the standard for major foot and ankle surgery and allows for superior and prolonged analgesia with minimal opioid-related side effects.[81]

Prolonged peripheral or plexus blockade provides excellent pain relief; however, the risk of accidental nerve trauma in an anesthetized extremity is theoretically higher outside the hospital environment. The patient should be informed of the risks and instructed in appropriate care of the extremity. Patients who are unable or unwilling to comply with recommended medical care may not be good candidates for regional anesthesia techniques and/or should be fully recovered before discharge. In all cases, a follow-up telephone call on the first postoperative day should include questions concerning residual areas of neural blockade or altered neural function, such as paresthesias. Any patient concerns regarding the anesthetic or surgery should also be discussed. Patients with indwelling plexus or peripheral catheters should be

TABLE 50-3. ANESTHETIC TECHNIQUES FOR COMMON FOOT AND ANKLE OPERATIONS

	Surgical Procedure	Regional Technique	Comments
Forefoot[a]	Hallux valgus	Metatarsal, ankle, popliteal blockade	Sural nerve block not necessary for surgery
	Amputations	Ankle, popliteal blockade	Popliteal blockade is the technique of choice in the presence of infection or swelling
Midfoot[a]	Transmetatarsal amputations	Popliteal, ankle blockade	
Hindfoot[a]	Ankle arthroscopy	Spinal, epidural, or general anesthesia	Operation typically requires good muscle relaxation for manipulation; thigh tourniquet
	Achilles tendon repair	Spinal, epidural, or popliteal blockade	Spinal or epidural anesthesia whenever thigh tourniquet is required
	Triple arthrodesis	Spinal or epidural	Neuraxial technique preferred for bone graft harvesting; popliteal blockade for postoperative analgesia

[a]Femoral or saphenous block required if the incision extends to the medial aspect of the foot or ankle.
From: Hadzic A, Vloka JD. Anesthesia for ankle and foot surgery. *Tech Reg Anesth Pain Manage.* 1990;3:113–119, with permission.

queried regarding the presence of residual block, signs of local anesthetic toxicity, and catheter migration.[81]

MICROVASCULAR SURGERY

Microvascular surgery includes both *replantation,* the reattachment of a completely severed body part, and *revascularization,* the re-establishment of blood flow through a severed body part. Most replantation surgery involves the upper extremity. Anesthetic management in microvascular surgery includes maintenance of blood flow through microvascular anastomoses, positioning considerations associated with a long surgical procedure during which the patient must lie completely still, and replacement of blood and fluid losses, which may be extensive.

Maintenance of blood flow through microvascular anastomoses is paramount to limb or graft viability. Blood flow may be improved by increasing the perfusion pressure, preventing hypothermia, and using vasodilators and sympathetic blockade. Microvascular perfusion pressure depends on both adequate intravascular volume and oncotic pressure. Blood loss during microvascular surgery is typically continual and insidious. Unrecognized bleeding and migration of intravascular fluid into the third space reduce microvascular perfusion pressure and must be corrected. However, overzealous use of crystalloid results in generalized edema, including the replanted body part, whereas excessive transfusion of blood products increases blood viscosity and therefore decreases flow. Evidence suggests that use of phenylephrine to support blood pressure does not jeopardize blood flow to the tissue being replanted.[82] Rheologically, the oxygen-carrying capacity of blood is optimized with a hematocrit of 30%. Arterial cannulation allows frequent assessment of hemoglobin levels and acid–base status, as well as direct blood pressure measurement.

Body temperature is also a determinant of blood flow. Hypothermia not only results in peripheral vasoconstriction, but causes sympathetic activation, shivering, increased oxygen demand, a leftward shift of the oxygen–hemoglobin dissociation curve, and altered coagulation. Therefore, hypothermia must be prevented in microvascular surgical patients. The operating room temperature should be increased to 21°C, intravenous solutions should be warmed, and the patient should be covered with a forced-air warming blanket.

The use of vasodilators has also been studied in the treatment of perioperative vasospasm. Local anesthetics and papaverine, applied topically, may be used to provide relaxation of vascular smooth muscle in the intraoperative setting. All the volatile anesthetics are potent vasodilators and can increase tissue blood flow 200% to 300%, even at typical expired anesthetic concentrations. Direct-acting vasodilating agents, such as sodium nitroprusside, trimethaphan, and hydralazine, produce vasodilation but do not prevent vasospasm because of direct surgical stimulation. Nitroprusside has been shown to reduce perfusion in a microvascular free flap.[82] In addition, the volatile anesthetics and intravenous agents may also result in hypotension and decreased microvascular perfusion pressure. Regional anesthetic techniques provide sympathectomy and vasodilation to the proximal (innervated) segment of an extremity, but have no effect on vasospasm in the replanted (denervated) tissue. Antithrombotics (heparin), fibrinolytics (streptokinase, urokinase, low-molecular-weight dextran), and smooth muscle relaxants (papaverine, local anesthetics) are also used to preserve blood flow in microvascular anastomoses.

Microvascular surgery may be performed under regional or general anesthesia or both. The type of anesthesia does not affect graft survival.[83] Regional anesthesia has several advantages over general anesthesia. The sympathectomy associated with local anesthetic blockade results in vasodilation and increased blood flow. A single-injection regional anesthetic technique may be of insufficient duration for many microvascular procedures. However, placement of an indwelling catheter (epidural, plexus, or peripheral) provides extended intraoperative anesthesia and continuous postoperative analgesia. General anesthesia ensures airway access and reduces the possibility of patient movement during critical surgical events. A combination of general and continuous regional anesthesia allows prolonged intraoperative anesthesia and postoperative analgesia, reduces the amount of inhalation agent, and increases the patient's acceptance of lengthy surgical procedures. However, regardless of anesthetic technique, conditions that stimulate vasospasm or vasoconstriction, such as pain, hypotension, and hypovolemia, must be avoided. Whether administration of a vasopressor with vasoconstrictive qualities or addition of epinephrine to local anesthetic solutions may decrease anastomotic blood flow is controversial.[82]

PEDIATRIC ORTHOPEDIC SURGERY

Pediatric patients present with a variety of orthopedic conditions, including congenital deformities, traumatic injuries, infections, and malignancies (see also Chapter 42). Anesthetic management of the pediatric orthopedic patient involves not only the usual pediatric patient considerations, such as airway management, fluid replacement, and maintenance of body temperature, but also the unique concerns associated with orthopedic surgery. Coexisting neuromuscular conditions, such as arthrogryposis or myelomeningocele, may predispose pediatric orthopedic patients to latex allergy and malignant hyperthermia.

Orthopedic procedures may be performed with children anesthetized with regional, general, or a combination of anesthetic techniques. The patient's age, operative site and positioning, and surgical duration are important factors in the selection of an anesthetic. Children older than 7 years of age may tolerate a primary regional anesthetic technique, whereas younger children may benefit from a general or combination regional/general anesthesia. Neural blockade may be initiated after induction of general anesthesia and before surgical incision to provide possible preemptive analgesia, or, on completion of the surgical procedure, to extend the duration of postoperative analgesia. Often, regional anesthetic procedures are technically easier to perform on children because the relative lack of subcutaneous tissue facilitates identification of bony and vascular landmarks as well as spread of local anesthetic solutions. The advantages of regional anesthesia in children are similar to those in adults and include earlier ambulation and hospital discharge, decreased incidence of nausea and vomiting, and prolonged postoperative analgesia.

Surgical procedures to the lower extremity may be safely and successfully performed under caudal, epidural, and spinal anesthesia.[84,85] However, the anatomic differences between the pediatric and adult spine and spinal cord must be appreciated.[84–86] In addition, femoral, lateral femoral cutaneous, and sciatic nerve blocks allow prolonged anesthesia and analgesia to the blocked extremity, but often require additional intraoperative supplementation with intravenous or inhalation agents.[87]

Upper extremity procedures may be performed with any of the anesthetic techniques previously described for adults.[85] The superficial location of the brachial plexus, decreased neural diameter, and rapid diffusion of local anesthetics contribute to the high success rate, which approaches 100%.[88] Blockade of the brachial plexus is usually accomplished with perivascular, sheath, nerve stimulator, or ultrasound techniques in children younger than 7 years of age because elicitation of paresthesias is regarded as uncomfortable (and therefore unacceptable) by the younger pediatric patients. Intravenous regional (Bier) block is particularly useful in the pediatric population for limited procedures such as closed reduction of forearm fractures.

OTHER CONSIDERATIONS

Tourniquets

Tourniquets are often used to minimize blood loss and provide a bloodless operating field. Appropriate selection of tourniquet cuff size and inflation pressure is paramount in reducing the risk of neuromuscular injury related to tourniquet ischemia. The cuff should be large enough to comfortably circle the limb to ensure circumferentially uniform pressure. The point of overlap should be placed 180 degrees from the neurovascular bundle because there is some area of decreased compression at the overlap point. The width of the inflated cuff should be more than half the limb diameter.

Opinions differ as to the pressure required in tourniquets to prevent bleeding. In general, a cuff pressure 100 mm Hg above a patient's measured systolic pressure is adequate for the thigh, and 50 mm Hg above systolic pressure is adequate for the arm, with the understanding that if hypertensive episodes occur, the cuff pressure should be increased. Bleeding from the surgical site after cuff inflation may rarely be due to inadequate occlusion of the major arterial inflow, which is corrected by cuff reapplication and use of the proper degree of inflation. Bleeding during tourniquet inflation is more commonly due to intramedullary blood flow in the long bones, particularly in the skeletally immature patient, and to small arterial vessels between the two bones of distal extremities. Overinflation of the tourniquet does *not* resolve these problems. Likewise, the duration of safe tourniquet inflation is generally considered to be 2 hours. Five minutes of intermittent perfusion between 1- and 2-hour inflations, followed by repeated exsanguination through elevation and compression, *may* allow more extended use, although this remains controversial.[89,90]

Damage to underlying vessels, nerves, and skeletal muscles has been reported following tourniquet inflation.[91] Injury is a function of both inflation pressure and duration of inflation. Direct pressure from the cuff is more damaging than the ischemia distally. Arterial spasm, venous thrombosis, and nerve injury are all demonstrable after several hours. Clinical examination, electromyography, and effluent blood analysis all show completely reversible changes for inflations of 1 to 2 hours, which is the basis for the recommendation of this period as the safe duration for tourniquet use; longer inflation times are associated with prolonged or irreversible changes in neurologic and/or muscular function.[89,91]

Transient systemic metabolic acidosis and increased arterial carbon dioxide levels have been demonstrated after tourniquet deflation and do not cause deleterious effects in healthy patients.[92] Measurable changes include a 10% to 15% increase in heart rate, a 5% to 10% increase in serum potassium, and a rise of 1 to 8 mm Hg in carbon dioxide tension in blood. Prolonged inflation or the simultaneous release of two tourniquets is not recommended. It may produce clinically significant acidosis, particularly in patients with an underlying acidosis from other causes. Tourniquet release has also been associated with cerebral embolic phenomena.[93]

When a pneumatic tourniquet is used with regional anesthetic techniques, some patients complain of dull, aching pain or become restless, even though seemingly adequate analgesia exists for the operation itself. Patient discomfort usually appears approximately 45 minutes after the tourniquet is inflated and becomes more intense with time. No satisfactory explanation for its genesis has been found. Current explanations involve pain transmission through both A delta and C fibers and its modulation in the dorsal horn synapses. The C (slow pain) fibers recover faster as the block wanes. Analogous phenomena may be observed at the same time point during general anesthesia. Evidence of lightening anesthesia (increase in blood pressure and pulse rate) may appear even though the same concentrations of anesthetic are being delivered.[94,95] The definitive treatment for tourniquet pain is release of the tourniquet. Relief of pain is prompt and

TABLE 50-4. CRITERIA FOR DIAGNOSIS OF FAT EMBOLUS SYNDROME

Major
Axillary/subconjunctival petechiae
Hypoxemia (Pao_2 <60 mm Hg; Fio_2 <0.4)
Central nervous system depression (disproportionate to hypoxemia)
Pulmonary edema
Minor
Tachycardia (>110 beats/min)
Hyperthermia
Retinal fat emboli
Urinary fat globules
Decreased platelets/hematocrit (unexplained)
Increased erythrocyte sedimentation rate
Fat globules in sputum

Diagnosis of fat embolus syndrome requires at least one sign from the major and four signs from the minor criteria categories.
From: Gurd AR. Fat embolism: An aid to diagnosis. *J Bone Joint Surg Br.* 1970; 52:732, with permission.

complete. During surgery, however, opioids and hypnotics are usually effective.

Fat Embolus Syndrome

Fat embolus syndrome (FES) is associated with multiple traumatic injuries and surgery involving long-bone fractures.[96] Risk factors include male gender, age (20 to 30 years), hypovolemic shock, intramedullary instrumentation, rheumatoid arthritis, total hip arthroplasty using the technique of cementing femoral stems designed for press-fit application, and bilateral total knee surgery. The incidence of FES in isolated long-bone fractures is 3% to 4%, and the mortality rate associated with this condition is significant, ranging from 10% to 20%.

Clinical and laboratory signs of FES have been classified by Gurd[97] as major or minor (Table 50-4), with a diagnosis requiring at least one major and four minor criteria, as well as the exclusion of other posttraumatic causes of hypoxemia. Major signs of the syndrome include the presence of axillary or subconjunctival petechiae, significant hypoxemia, central nervous system depression in excess of that expected because of the level of hypoxemia, and pulmonary edema. Classified as minor signs are tachycardia, hyperthermia, retinal fat emboli on funduscopic examination, urinary fat globules, an unexplained decrease in hematocrit or platelets, an increased erythrocyte sedimentation rate, and fat globules in the sputum. Symptoms usually occur 12 to 40 hours after the injury and can range from mild dyspnea to frank coma. Decreased arterial oxygen tension is the most consistent abnormal laboratory value. Fulminant episodes can occur within hours of the traumatic injury, causing severe hypoxemia, respiratory failure, and severe neurologic impairment. Disseminated intravascular coagulation can also occur in conjunction with FES.

Appropriate treatment of FES requires early recognition of the syndrome, reversal of possible aggravating factors such as hypovolemia, early surgical stabilization of fracture sites, and aggressive respiratory support. Corticosteroid therapy is controversial but may be beneficial. Other pharmacologic interventions, including heparin and dextran, have not been shown to be effective in treating FES.[96]

Methyl Methacrylate

Methyl methacrylate is an acrylic bone cement used during arthroplastic procedures. Insertion of this cement is associated with sudden onset of hypotension in some patients. This hypotension has been attributed to absorption of the volatile monomer of methyl methacrylate, embolization of air and bone marrow during femoral reaming, lysis of blood cells and marrow induced by the exothermic reaction, and conversion of methyl methacrylate to methacrylate acid. Adequate hydration and maximizing inspired oxygen concentration minimize the hypotension and hypoxemia that can accompany cementing of the prosthesis. Because air can be entrained during this procedure, nitrous oxide should be discontinued several minutes before this point.

Venous Thromboembolism

8 Venous thromboembolism is a major cause of death after surgery or trauma to the lower extremities. Without prophylaxis, venous thrombosis develops in 40% to 80% of orthopedic patients, and 1% to 28% show clinical or laboratory evidence of pulmonary embolism. Fatal pulmonary embolism occurs in

TABLE 50-5. VENOUS THROMBOEMBOLISM PREVALENCE AFTER MAJOR ORTHOPEDIC SURGERY

	Deep Venous Thrombosis[a]		Pulmonary Embolism	
Procedure	Total (%)	Proximal (%)	Total (%)	Fatal (%)
Total hip replacement	42–57	18–36	0.9–28	0.14–2
Total knee replacement	41–85	5–22	1.5–10	0.1–1.7
Hip fracture surgery	46–60	23–30	3–11	2.5–7.5

[a]Total or proximal deep venous thrombosis prevalence based on the use of mandatory venography in prospective randomized clinical trials in which patients received either prophylaxis or a placebo.
From: Geerts WH, Bergqvist D, Pineo GF, et al. Prevention of venous thromboembolism: American College of Chest Physicians evidence-based clinical practice guidelines (8th edition). *Chest.* 2008;133:381S–453S, with permission.

TABLE 50-6. ANTITHROMBOTIC REGIMENS TO PREVENT THROMBOEMBOLISM IN ORTHOPEDIC SURGICAL PATIENTS

Hip and Knee Arthroplasty and Hip Fracture Surgery

- LMWH[a] started 12 h before surgery or 12–24 h after surgery, or 4–6 h after surgery at half the usual dose and then increasing to the usual high-risk dose the following day
- Fondaparinux[a] (2.5 mg started 6–8 h after surgery)
- Adjusted-dose warfarin started preoperatively or the evening after surgery (INR target, 2.5; INR range, 2–3)
- Intermittent pneumatic compression is an alternative option to anticoagulant prophylaxis in patients who have a high risk of bleeding
- Rivaroxaban[a] (10 mg started 6–10 h after surgery)
- Dabigatran[a] (110 mg 1–4 h after surgery; followed by 220 mg on subsequent days)[b]

Spinal Cord Injury

- LMWH once primary hemostasis is evident
- Intermittent pneumatic compression is an alternative option when anticoagulation is contraindicated early after the injury
- During the rehabilitation phase, conversion to adjusted-dose warfarin (INR target, 2.5; INR range, 2–3)

Elective Spine Surgery

- Routine use of thromboprophylaxis, apart from early and persistent mobilization, not routinely recommended for patients without additional risk factors

Knee Arthroscopy

- Routine use of thromboprophylaxis, apart from early and persistent mobilization, not routinely recommended

[a]Use with caution in patients receiving neuraxial anesthesia/analgesia.
[b]Dabigatran is approved for thromboprophylaxis in Europe and non-valvular atrial fibrillation in the United States.
LMWH, low-molecular-weight heparin; INR, international normalized ratio.
From: Geerts WH, Bergqvist D, Pineo GF, et al. Prevention of venous thromboembolism: American College of Chest Physicians evidence-based clinical practice guidelines (8th edition). *Chest.* 2008;133:381S-453S, with permission.

0.1% to 8% of patients[98] (Table 50-5). The incidence of fatal pulmonary embolism is highest in patients who have undergone surgery for hip fracture. Although fatal pulmonary embolism may be the most common preventable cause of hospital death, many physicians fail to use prophylaxis appropriately because of concern about bleeding complications from anticoagulation. Effective thromboprophylaxis requires knowledge of clinical risk factors in individual patients, such as advanced age, prolonged immobility or bed rest, prior history of thromboembolism, cancer, pre-existing hypercoagulable state, and major surgery. In many patients, multiple risk factors may be present, and the risks are cumulative. After identification of the risk of thromboembolism, an assessment may be made regarding the risks and benefits of physical or pharmacologic techniques used to prevent thromboembolism.

Antithrombotic Prophylaxis

Thromboprophylaxis is based on identification of risk factors. Guidelines for antithrombotic therapy, including selection of pharmacologic agent, degree of anticoagulation desired, and duration of therapy, continue to evolve.[98] Recommendations from the Eighth American College of Chest Physicians in 2008 are based on prospective randomized studies that assess the efficacy of therapy, using contrast venography or fibrinogen leg scanning to diagnose asymptomatic thrombi (Table 50-6). For patients undergoing major joint replacement, administration of LMWH, warfarin, fondaparinux, or rivaroxaban is recommended. Similar recommendations are made for patients with acute spinal cord injury. Conversely, other orthopedic patients are considered low risk, and no pharmacologic prophylaxis is warranted.

Neuraxial Anesthesia and Analgesia in the Patient Receiving Antithrombotic Therapy

Several studies show a decrease in the incidence of both DVT and PTE in (non-pharmacologically thromboprophylaxed) patients undergoing hip surgery under epidural[54–56] and spinal[99–101] anesthesia. Similar findings have been reported for knee surgery performed under epidural anesthesia.[102,103] Proposed mechanisms for this effect include (1) rheologic changes resulting in hyperkinetic lower extremity blood flow, reducing venous stasis and preventing thrombus formation; (2) beneficial circulatory effects from epinephrine added to the local anesthetic solutions; (3) altered coagulation and fibrinolytic responses to surgery under central neural blockade, resulting in a decreased tendency for blood to clot and better fibrinolytic function; (4) the absence of positive-pressure ventilation and its concomitant effects on circulation; and (5) direct local anesthetic effects such as decreased
9 platelet aggregation. It is important to note that most of the studies examining the value of epidural and spinal anesthesia in preventing DVT and PTE involved patients who were not receiving currently recommended pharmacologic prophylaxis. In addition, despite the reduction in thromboembolism in the presence of a neuraxial block, the risk of thromboembolism remains significant, and pharmacologic thromboprophylaxis is required.

The more recent introduction of more efficacious anticoagulants and antiplatelet agents has further increased the complexity of patient management (Table 50-7). Anesthesiologists must balance the risk of thromboembolic and hemorrhagic complications. Spinal hematoma was considered a rare complication of neuraxial blockade until the introduction of LMWH as a thromboprophylactic agent in the 1990s. The calculated incidence (approximately 1 in 3,000 epidural anesthetics), along with the catastrophic nature of spinal bleeding (only 30% of patients had good neurologic recovery),[40,104] warranted an alternate approach to analgesic management following total hip and knee replace-
10 ment. Although psoas compartment and femoral catheters are suitable (if not superior) alternatives to neuraxial infusions, there are no investigations that examine the frequency and severity of hemorrhagic complications following plexus or peripheral blockade in anticoagulated patients. Cases of major bleeding (significant decreases in hemoglobin and/or blood pressure) associated with nonneuraxial techniques occurred after deep plexus or deep peripheral block (i.e., psoas compartment, lumbar sympathetic, sciatic blockade) and have involved heparin, LMWH, warfarin, and thienopyridine derivatives. These cases suggest that significant blood loss, rather than neural deficits, may be the most serious complication of nonneuraxial regional techniques in the anticoagulated patient. Current recommendations are to apply the neuraxial guidelines to deep plexus and deep peripheral blocks (Table 50-8).[4]

TABLE 50-7. PHARMACOLOGIC ACTIVITIES OF ANTICOAGULANTS, ANTIPLATELET AGENTS, AND THROMBOLYTICS

Agent	Effect on Coagulation Variables: PT	Effect on Coagulation Variables: APTT	Time to Peak Effect	Time to Normal Hemostasis after Discontinuation
Intravenous heparin	↑	↑↑↑	Minutes	4–6 h
Subcutaneous heparin	–	↑	40–50 min	4–6 h
Low-molecular-weight heparin	–	–	3–5 h	12–24 h
Warfarin	↑↑↑	↑	4–6 days (less with loading dose)	4–6 days
Dabigatran	↑	↑↑	2 h	4–7 days
Rivaroxaban	↑↑	↑↑	3 h	1–2 days
Antiplatelet agents				
Aspirin	–	–	Hours	5–8 days
Other NSAIDs			Hours	1–3 days
Ticlopidine, clopidogrel, prasugrel			Hours	5–14 days
Platelet glycoprotein IIb/IIIa receptor inhibitors			Minutes	8–48 h
Fibrinolytics	↑	↑↑	Minutes	24–36 h

PT, prothrombin time; aPTT, activated partial thromboplastin time; ↑, clinically insignificant increase; ↑↑, possibly clinically significant increase; ↑↑↑, clinically significant increase; NSAID, nonsteroidal anti-inflammatory drug.
Adapted from: Horlocker TT, Wedel DJ. Anticoagulation and neuraxial block: Historical perspective, anesthetic implications, and risk management. *Reg Anesth Pain Med.* 1998;23:129–134, with permission.

TABLE 50-8. RECOMMENDATIONS FOR MANAGEMENT OF PATIENTS RECEIVING NEURAXIAL BLOCKADE AND ANTICOAGULANT DRUGS

Warfarin	Discontinue chronic warfarin therapy 4–5 days before spinal procedure and evaluate INR. INR should be within the normal range at the time of procedure to ensure adequate levels of all vitamin K–dependent factors. Postoperatively, daily INR assessment with catheter removal occurring with INR <1.5
Antiplatelet medications	No contraindications with aspirin or other NSAIDs. Thienopyridine derivatives (clopidogrel and prasugrel) should be discontinued 5–7 days and ticlopidine 14 days prior to procedure. GP IIb/IIIa inhibitors should be discontinued to allow recovery of platelet function prior to procedure (8 h for tirofiban and eptifibatide, 24–48 h for abciximab)
Thrombolytics/fibrinolytics	There are no available data to suggest a safe interval between procedure and initiation or discontinuation of these medications. Follow fibrinogen level and observe for signs of neural compression
LMWH	Delay procedure at least 12 h from the last dose of thromboprophylaxis LMWH dose. For "treatment" dosing of LMWH, at least 24 h should elapse prior to procedure. LMWH should not be administered within 24 h after the procedure. Indwelling epidural catheters should be maintained only with once-daily dosing of LMWH and strict avoidance of additional hemostasis-altering medications, including NSAIDs
Unfractionated SQ heparin	There are no contraindications to a neuraxial procedure if total daily dose is less than 10,000 U. For higher dosing regimens, increase neurologic monitoring and cautiously coadminister antiplatelet medications
Unfractionated IV heparin	Delay needle/catheter placement 2–4 h after last dose; document normal aPTT. Heparin may be restarted 1 h following procedure. Sustained heparinization with an indwelling neuraxial catheter associated with increased risk; monitor neurologic status aggressively
Dabigatran	Discontinue 5–7 days prior to procedure; for shorter time periods, document normal TT. First postoperative dose 24 h after needle placement and 6 h post catheter removal (whichever is later)
Rivaroxaban	According to European guidelines, 22–26 h should elapse between discontinuation of rivaroxaban and neuraxial block in patients with normal renal function.[105] Longer intervals are required in patients with renal insufficiency. Indwelling neuraxial catheters are contraindicated due to the "boxed warning." Four to six hours is recommended between spinal block and initiation of rivaroxaban therapy postoperatively[105]

INR, international normalized ratio; NSAIDs, nonsteroidal anti-inflammatory drugs; GP IIb/IIIa, platelet glycoprotein receptor IIb/IIIa inhibitors; LMWH, low-molecular-weight heparin; SQ, subcutaneous; aPTT, activated partial thromboplastin time; TT, thrombin time.
Unless otherwise specified, recommendations from Horlocker TT, Wedel DJ, Benzon H, et al. Regional anesthesia in the anticoagulated patient: Defining the risks (the second ASRA Consensus Conference on Neuraxial Anesthesia and Anticoagulation). *Reg Anesth Pain Med.* 2003;28:172–197.

References

1. Almanaseer Y, Mukherjee D, Kline-Rogers EM, et al. Implementation of the ACC/AHA guidelines for preoperative cardiac risk assessment in a general medicine preoperative clinic: Improving efficiency and preserving outcomes. *Cardiology.* 2005;103:24–29.
2. Buvanendran A, Thillainathan V. Preoperative and postoperative anesthetic and analgesic techniques for minimally invasive surgery of the spine. *Spine (Phila Pa 1976).* 2010;35:S274–S280.
3. American Society of Anesthesiologists Committee on Standards and Practice Parameters. Practice alert for the perioperative management of patients with coronary artery stents: A report by the American Society of Anesthesiologists Committee on Standards and Practice Parameters. *Anesthesiology.* 2009;110: 22–23.
4. Horlocker TT, Wedel DJ, Rowlingson JC, et al. Regional anesthesia in the patient receiving antithrombotic or thrombolytic therapy: American Society of Regional Anesthesia and Pain Medicine Evidence-Based Guidelines (Third Edition). *Reg Anesth Pain Med.* 2010;35:64–101.
5. Martyn JA, White DA, Gronert GA, et al. Up-and-down regulation of skeletal muscle acetylcholine receptors. Effects on neuromuscular blockers. *Anesthesiology.* 1992;76:822–843.
6. Cucchiara RF, Black S. Corneal abrasion during anesthesia and surgery. *Anesthesiology.* 1988;69:978–979.
7. Ferguson RL, Hansen MM, Nicholas DA, et al. Same-day versus staged anterior-posterior spinal surgery in a neuromuscular scoliosis population: The evaluation of medical complications. *J Pediatr Orthop.* 1996;16:293–303.
8. McDonnell MF, Glassman SD, Dimar JR 2nd, et al. Perioperative complications of anterior procedures on the spine. *J Bone Joint Surg Am.* 1996;78:839–847.
9. Fehlings MG, Brodke DS, Norvell DC, et al. The evidence for intraoperative neurophysiological monitoring in spine surgery: Does it make a difference? *Spine (Phila Pa 1976).* 2010;35(9 suppl):S37–S46.
10. Albin MS, Chang JL, Babinski M, et al. Intracardiac catheters in neurosurgical anesthesia. *Anesthesiology.* 1979;50:67–68.
11. Allen RT, Garfin SR. The economics of minimally invasive spine surgery: The value perspective. *Spine (Phila Pa 1976).* 2010;35:S375–S382.
12. Cardoso MJ, Rosner MK. Does the Wilson frame assist with optimizing surgical exposure for minimally invasive lumbar fusions? *Neurosurg Focus.* 2010;28: E20.
13. Sadrolsadat SH, Mahdavi AR, Moharari RS, et al. A prospective randomized trial comparing the technique of spinal and general anesthesia for lumbar disk surgery: A study of 100 cases. *Surg Neurol.* 2009;71:60–65; discussion 65.
14. Vauzelle C, Stagnara P, Jouvinroux P. Functional monitoring of spinal cord activity during spinal surgery. *Clin Orthop Relat Res.* 1973;93:173–178.
15. Pathak KS, Brown RH, Nash CL Jr, et al. Continuous opioid infusion for scoliosis fusion surgery. *Anesth Analg.* 1983;62:841–845.
16. Schwartz DM, Auerbach JD, Dormans JP, et al. Neurophysiological detection of impending spinal cord injury during scoliosis surgery. *J Bone Joint Surg Am.* 2007;89:2440–2449.
17. Burke D, Hicks RG. Surgical monitoring of motor pathways. *J Clin Neurophysiol.* 1998;15:194–205.
18. Pathak KS, Ammadio M, Kalamchi A, et al. Effects of halothane, enflurane, and isoflurane on somatosensory evoked potentials during nitrous oxide anesthesia. *Anesthesiology.* 1987;66:753–757.
19. Elgafy H, Bransford RJ, McGuire RA, et al. Blood loss in major spine surgery: Are there effective measures to decrease massive hemorrhage in major spine fusion surgery? *Spine (Phila Pa 1976).* 2010;35:S47–S56.
20. Nuttall GA, Horlocker TT, Santrach PJ, et al. The predictors of blood transfusions in spinal instrumentation and fusion surgery. *Spine (Phila Pa 1976).* 2000;25:596–601.
21. Copley LA, Richards BS, Safavi FZ, et al. Hemodilution as a method to reduce transfusion requirements in adolescent spine fusion surgery. *Spine (Phila Pa 1976).* 1999;24:219–222; discussion 223–214.
22. Murray DJ, Forbes RB, Titone MB, et al. Transfusion management in pediatric and adolescent scoliosis surgery. Efficacy of autologous blood. *Spine (Phila Pa 1976).* 1997;22:2735–2740.
23. Brodsky JW, Dickson JH, Erwin WD, et al. Hypotensive anesthesia for scoliosis surgery in Jehovah's Witnesses. *Spine (Phila Pa 1976).* 1991;16:304–306.
24. Tse EY, Cheung WY, Ng KF, et al. Reducing perioperative blood loss and allogeneic blood transfusion in patients undergoing major spine surgery. *J Bone Joint Surg Am.* 2011;93:1268–1277.
25. Grant JA, Howard J, Luntley J, et al. Perioperative blood transfusion requirements in pediatric scoliosis surgery: The efficacy of tranexamic acid. *J Pediatr Orthop.* 2009;29:300–304.
26. Horlocker TT, Nuttall GA, Dekutoski MB, et al. Accuracy of coagulation tests during spinal fusion and instrumentation. *Anesth Analg.* 2001;93:33–38.
27. Dilger JA, Tetzlaff JE, Bell GR, et al. Ischaemic optic neuropathy after spinal fusion. *Can J Anaesth.* 1998;45:63–66.
28. Myers MA, Hamilton SR, Bogosian AJ, et al. Visual loss as a complication of spine surgery. A review of 37 cases. *Spine (Phila Pa 1976).* 1997;22:1325–1329.
29. Warner ME, Warner MA, Garrity JA, et al. The frequency of perioperative vision loss. *Anesth Analg.* 2001;93:1417–1421; table of contents.
30. Lee LA, Roth S, Posner KL, et al. The American Society of Anesthesiologists Postoperative Visual Loss Registry: Analysis of 93 spine surgery cases with postoperative visual loss. *Anesthesiology.* 2006;105:652–659; quiz 867–658.
31. Postoperative Visual Loss Study Group. Risk factors associated with ischemic optic neuropathy after spinal fusion surgery. *Anesthesiology.* 2012;116:15–24.
32. Horlocker TT, Wedel DJ, Cucchiara RF. Venous air embolism during spinal instrumentation and fusion in the prone position. *Anesth Analg.* 1992;75:152.
33. Bianconi M, Ferraro L, Ricci R, et al. The pharmacokinetics and efficacy of ropivacaine continuous wound instillation after spine fusion surgery. *Anesth Analg.* 2004;98:166–172.
34. Rajpal S, Gordon DB, Pellino TA, et al. Comparison of perioperative oral multimodal analgesia versus IV PCA for spine surgery. *J Spinal Disord Tech.* 2010; 23:139–145.
35. Crosby ET, Halpern SH. Obstetric epidural anaesthesia in patients with Harrington instrumentation. *Can J Anaesth.* 1989;36:693–696.
36. Daley MD, Rolbin SH, Hew EM, et al. Epidural anesthesia for obstetrics after spinal surgery. *Reg Anesth.* 1990;15:280–284.
37. Hubbert CH. Epidural anesthesia in patients with spinal fusion. *Anesth Analg.* 1985;64:843.
38. Hebl JR, Horlocker TT, Kopp SL, et al. Neuraxial blockade in patients with preexisting spinal stenosis, lumbar disk disease, or prior spine surgery: Efficacy and neurologic complications. *Anesth Analg.* 2010;111:1511–1519.
39. Hebl JR, Kopp SL, Schroeder DR, et al. Neurologic complications after neuraxial anesthesia or analgesia in patients with preexisting peripheral sensorimotor neuropathy or diabetic polyneuropathy. *Anesth Analg.* 2006;103:1294–1299.
40. Moen V, Dahlgren N, Irestedt L. Severe neurological complications after central neuraxial blockades in Sweden 1990–1999. *Anesthesiology.* 2004;101:950–959.
41. Lynch NM, Cofield RH, Silbert PL, et al. Neurologic complications after total shoulder arthroplasty. *J Shoulder Elbow Surg.* 1996;5:53–61.
42. Dutton RP. Controlled hypotension for spinal surgery. *Eur Spine J.* 2004;13(suppl 1): S66–S71.
43. Yadeau JT, Casciano M, Liu SS, et al. Stroke, regional anesthesia in the sitting position, and hypotension: A review of 4169 ambulatory surgery patients. *Reg Anesth Pain Med.* 2011;36:430–435.
44. Liguori GA, Kahn RL, Gordon J, et al. The use of metoprolol and glycopyrrolate to prevent hypotensive/bradycardic events during shoulder arthroscopy in the sitting position under interscalene block. *Anesth Analg.* 1998;87:1320–1325.
45. Urmey WF, Talts KH, Sharrock NE. One hundred percent incidence of hemidiaphragmatic paresis associated with interscalene brachial plexus anesthesia as diagnosed by ultrasonography. *Anesth Analg.* 1991;72:498–503.
46. Schroeder LE, Horlocker TT, Schroeder DR. The efficacy of axillary block for surgical procedures about the elbow. *Anesth Analg.* 1996;83:747–751.
47. Chan VW, Peng PW, Kaszas Z, et al. A comparative study of general anesthesia, intravenous regional anesthesia, and axillary block for outpatient hand surgery: Clinical outcome and cost analysis. *Anesth Analg.* 2001;93:1181–1184.
48. McCartney CJ, Brull R, Chan VW, et al. Early but no long-term benefit of regional compared with general anesthesia for ambulatory hand surgery. *Anesthesiology.* 2004;101:461–467.
49. Ilfeld BM, Morey TE, Wright TW, et al. Interscalene perineural ropivacaine infusion: A comparison of two dosing regimens for postoperative analgesia. *Reg Anesth Pain Med.* 2004;29:9–16.
50. Ilfeld BM, Wright TW, Enneking FK, et al. Total elbow arthroplasty as an outpatient procedure using a continuous infraclavicular nerve block at home: A prospective case report. *Reg Anesth Pain Med.* 2006;31:172–176.
51. Duncan CM, Hall Long K, Warner DO, et al. The economic implications of a multimodal analgesic regimen for patients undergoing major orthopedic surgery: A comparative study of direct costs. *Reg Anesth Pain Med.* 2009;34:301–307.
52. Horlocker TT, Kopp SL, Pagnano MW, et al. Analgesia for total hip and knee arthroplasty: A multimodal pathway featuring peripheral nerve block. *J Am Acad Orthop Surg.* 2006;14:126–135.
53. Hebl JR, Kopp SL, Ali MH, et al. A comprehensive anesthesia protocol that emphasizes peripheral nerve blockade for total knee and total hip arthroplasty. *J Bone Joint Surg Am.* 2005;87(suppl 2):63–70.
54. Sculco TP. Global blood management in orthopaedic surgery. *Clin Orthop Relat Res.* 1998;357:43–49.
55. Modig J, Borg T, Bagge L, et al. Role of extradural and of general anaesthesia in fibrinolysis and coagulation after total hip replacement. *Br J Anaesth.* 1983; 55:625–629.
56. Modig J, Borg T, Karlstrom G, et al. Thromboembolism after total hip replacement: Role of epidural and general anesthesia. *Anesth Analg.* 1983;62:174–180.
57. Stevens RD, Van Gessel E, Flory N, et al. Lumbar plexus block reduces pain and blood loss associated with total hip arthroplasty. *Anesthesiology.* 2000;93: 115–121.
58. Sharrock NE, Salvati EA. Hypotensive epidural anesthesia for total hip arthroplasty: A review. *Acta Orthop Scand.* 1996;67:91–107.
59. Rosberg B, Fredin H, Gustafson C. Anesthetic techniques and surgical blood loss in total hip arthroplasty. *Acta Anaesthesiol Scand.* 1982;26:189–193.
60. Ben-David B, Schmalenberger K, Chelly JE. Analgesia after total knee arthroplasty: Is continuous sciatic blockade needed in addition to continuous femoral blockade? *Anesth Analg.* 2004;98:747–749.

61. Enneking FK, Chan V, Greger J, et al. Lower-extremity peripheral nerve blockade: Essentials of our current understanding. *Reg Anesth Pain Med.* 2005;30:4–35.
62. Pham Dang C, Gautheron E, Guilley J, et al. The value of adding sciatic block to continuous femoral block for analgesia after total knee replacement. *Reg Anesth Pain Med.* 2005;30:128–133.
63. Choi PT, Bhandari M, Scott J, et al. Epidural analgesia for pain relief following hip or knee replacement. *Cochrane Database Syst Rev.* 2003. http://onlinelibrary.wiley.com/doi/10.1002/14651858.CD003071/abstract;jsessionid=246CD83293B4CE925DA525E38B8A6F80.d03t01
64. Capdevila X, Barthelet Y, Biboulet P, et al. Effects of perioperative analgesic technique on the surgical outcome and duration of rehabilitation after major knee surgery. *Anesthesiology.* 1999;91:8–15.
65. Chelly JE, Greger J, Gebhard R, et al. Continuous femoral blocks improve recovery and outcome of patients undergoing total knee arthroplasty. *J Arthroplasty.* 2001;16:436–445.
66. Singelyn FJ, Gouverneur JM. Postoperative analgesia after total hip arthroplasty: I.v. PCA with morphine, patient-controlled epidural analgesia, or continuous "3-in-1" block?: A prospective evaluation by our acute pain service in more than 1,300 patients. *J Clin Anesth.* 1999;11:550–554.
67. Singelyn FJ, Gouverneur JM. Extended "three-in-one" block after total knee arthroplasty: Continuous versus patient-controlled techniques. *Anesth Analg.* 2000; 91:176–180.
68. Allen HW, Liu SS, Ware PD, et al. Peripheral nerve blocks improve analgesia after total knee replacement surgery. *Anesth Analg.* 1998;87:93–97.
69. Kaloul I, Guay J, Cote C, et al. The posterior lumbar plexus (psoas compartment) block and the three-in-one femoral nerve block provide similar postoperative analgesia after total knee replacement. [Erratum appears in *Can J Anaesth.* 2005;52(1):119]. *Can J Anaesth.* 2004;51:45–51.
70. Singelyn FJ, Deyaert M, Joris D, et al. Effects of intravenous patient-controlled analgesia with morphine, continuous epidural analgesia, and continuous three-in-one block on postoperative pain and knee rehabilitation after unilateral total knee arthroplasty. *Anesth Analg.* 1998;87:88–92.
71. Capdevila X, Macaire P, Dadure C, et al. Continuous psoas compartment block for postoperative analgesia after total hip arthroplasty: New landmarks, technical guidelines, and clinical evaluation. *Anesth Analg.* 2002;94:1606–1613.
72. Ganapathy S, Wasserman RA, Watson JT, et al. Modified continuous femoral three-in-one block for postoperative pain after total knee arthroplasty. *Anesth Analg.* 1999;89:1197–1202.
73. White PF, Kehlet H. Improving postoperative pain management: What are the unresolved issues? *Anesthesiology.* 2010;112:220–225.
74. Kehlet H, Andersen LO. Local infiltration analgesia in joint replacement: The evidence and recommendations for clinical practice. *Acta Anaesthesiol Scand.* 2011;55:778–784.
75. Horlocker TT, Hebl JR. Evidence based report: Outpatient knee arthroscopy–is there an optimal anesthetic technique? *Reg Anesth Pain Med.* 2003;28:58–63.
76. Williams BA, Kentor ML, Vogt MT, et al. Reduction of verbal pain scores after anterior cruciate ligament reconstruction with 2-day continuous femoral nerve block: A randomized clinical trial. *Anesthesiology.* 2006;104:315–327.
77. Klein SM, Greengrass RA, Gleason DH, et al. Major ambulatory surgery with continuous regional anesthesia and a disposable infusion pump. *Anesthesiology.* 1999;91:563–565.
78. Stein C, Comisel K, Haimerl E, et al. Analgesic effect of intraarticular morphine after arthroscopic knee surgery. *N Engl J Med.* 1991;325:1123–1126.
79. Ng HP, Nordstrom U, Axelsson K, et al. Efficacy of intra-articular bupivacaine, ropivacaine, or a combination of ropivacaine, morphine, and ketorolac on postoperative pain relief after ambulatory arthroscopic knee surgery: A randomized double-blind study. *Reg Anesth Pain Med.* 2006;31:26–33.
80. Hadic A, Vloka JD. Anesthesia for ankle and foot surgery. *Tech Reg Anesth Pain Manage.* 1999;3:113–119.
81. Ilfeld BM, Morey TE, Wang RD, et al. Continuous popliteal sciatic nerve block for postoperative pain control at home: A randomized, double-blinded, placebo-controlled study. *Anesthesiology.* 2002;97:959–965.
82. Banic A, Krejci V, Erni D, et al. Effects of sodium nitroprusside and phenylephrine on blood flow in free musculocutaneous flaps during general anesthesia. *Anesthesiology.* 1999;90:147–155.
83. Li J, Guo Z, Zhu Q, et al. Fingertip replantation: Determinants of survival. *Plast Reconstr Surg.* 2008;122:833–839.
84. Yaster M, Maxwell LG. Pediatric regional anesthesia. *Anesthesiology.* 1989;70: 324–338.
85. Cousins MJ, Carr DB, Horlocker TT, et al. *Neural Blockade in Clinical Anesthesia and Pain Medicine.* Philadelphia, PA: Wolters Kluwer; Lippincott Williams and Wilkins; 2009:1306.
86. Dalens B. Regional anesthesia in children. *Anesth Analg.* 1989;68:654–672.
87. Maccani RM, Wedel DJ, Melton A, et al. Femoral and lateral femoral cutaneous nerve block for muscle biopsies in children. *Paediatr Anaesth.* 1995;5: 223–227.
88. Wedel DJ, Krohn JS, Hall JA. Brachial plexus anesthesia in pediatric patients. *Mayo Clin Proc.* 1991;66:583–588.
89. Horlocker TT, Hebl JR, Gali B, et al. Anesthetic, patient, and surgical risk factors for neurologic complications after prolonged total tourniquet time during total knee arthroplasty. *Anesth Analg.* 2006;102:950–955.
90. Sapega AA, Heppenstall RB, Chance B, et al. Optimizing tourniquet application and release times in extremity surgery. A biochemical and ultrastructural study. *J Bone Joint Surg Am.* 1985;67:303–314.
91. Pedowitz RA. Tourniquet-induced neuromuscular injury. A recent review of rabbit and clinical experiments. *Acta Orthop Scand Suppl.* 1991;245:1–33.
92. Kadoi Y, Ide M, Saito S, et al. Hyperventilation after tourniquet deflation prevents an increase in cerebral blood flow velocity. *Can J Anaesth.* 1999;46: 259–264.
93. Della Valle CJ, Jazrawi LM, Di Cesare PE, et al. Paradoxical cerebral embolism complicating a major orthopaedic operation. A report of two cases. *J Bone Joint Surg Am.* 1999;81:108–110.
94. Valli H, Rosenberg PH. Effects of three anaesthesia methods on haemodynamic responses connected with the use of thigh tourniquet in orthopaedic patients. *Acta Anaesthesiol Scand.* 1985;29:142–147.
95. Hagenouw RR, Bridenbaugh PO, van Egmond J, et al. Tourniquet pain: A volunteer study. *Anesth Analg.* 1986;65:1175–1180.
96. Akhtar S. Fat embolism. *Anesthesiol Clin.* 2009;27:533–550.
97. Gurd AR. Fat embolism: An aid to diagnosis. *J Bone Joint Surg Am.* 1970;52: 732–737.
98. Geerts WH, Bergqvist D, Pineo GF, et al. Prevention of venous thromboembolism: American College of Chest Physicians Evidence-Based Clinical Practice Guidelines (8th Edition). *Chest.* 2008;133:381S–453S.
99. Davis FM, Laurenson VG, Gillespie WJ, et al. Deep vein thrombosis after total hip replacement. A comparison between spinal and general anaesthesia. *J Bone Joint Surg Am.* 1989;71:181–185.
100. Donadoni R, Baele G, Devulder J, et al. Coagulation and fibrinolytic parameters in patients undergoing total hip replacement: Influence of the anaesthesia technique. *Acta Anaesthesiol Scand.* 1989;33:588–592.
101. Thorburn J, Louden JR, Vallance R. Spinal and general anaesthesia in total hip replacement: Frequency of deep vein thrombosis. *Br J Anaesth.* 1980;52: 1117–1121.
102. Nielsen PT, Jorgensen LN, Albrecht-Beste E, et al. Lower thrombosis risk with epidural blockade in knee arthroplasty. *Acta Orthop Scand.* 1990;61:29–31.
103. Sharrock NE, Haas SB, Hargett MJ, et al. Effects of epidural anesthesia on the incidence of deep-vein thrombosis after total knee arthroplasty. [Erratum appears in *J Bone Joint Surg Am.* 1991;73(6):952]. *J Bone Joint Surg Am.* 1991;73: 502–506.
104. Horlocker TT, Wedel DJ. Neuraxial block and low-molecular-weight heparin: Balancing perioperative analgesia and thromboprophylaxis. *Reg Anesth Pain Med.* 1998;23:164–177.
105. Gogarten W, Vandermeulen E, Van Aken H, et al. Regional anaesthesia and antithrombotic agents: Recommendations of the European Society of Anaesthesiology. *Eur J Anaesthesiol.* 2010;27:999–1015.

CHAPTER

51 Transplant Anesthesia

MARIE CSETE • DALIA BANKS • GERARD MANECKE • KATHRYN GLAS

Key Points

1. Brain death is declared when the clinical picture is consistent with irreversible cessation of all brain functions.
2. The mainstay of donor management is maintenance of euvolemia, oxygenation, perfusion, and normothermia, as well as communication with multiple surgical teams.
3. Donation after cardiac death organs now account for over 10% of organ transplants in the United States.
4. Living kidney and liver donors must be healthy and without significant cardiopulmonary, neurologic, or psychiatric disease, diabetes, obesity, or hypertension.
5. Immune suppression is associated with severe infections, increased risk of malignancy, and progressive vascular disease.
6. Renal transplant recipients are often anemic, with hyperdynamic cardiac indices.
7. For renal transplantation, the major anesthetic consideration is maintenance of renal blood flow. Typical hemodynamic goals during transplant are systolic pressure >90 mm Hg, mean systemic pressure >60 mm Hg, and central venous pressure >10 mm Hg.
8. Patients with end-stage liver disease (ESLD) have multiorgan dysfunction with secondary cardiac, pulmonary, and renal complications of ESLD.
9. Liver transplantation is traditionally described in three phases: dissection, anhepatic, and neohepatic, with reperfusion marking the neohepatic phase.
10. Intraoperative management of lung transplant patients should focus on fluid and ventilatory strategies designed to minimize acute lung injury and primary graft dysfunction.
11. Left ventricular assist devices are increasingly common in patients presenting for heart transplantation.
12. Nonischemic cardiomyopathy has replaced ischemic cardiomyopathy as the most common indication for heart transplantation.
13. For all transplant recipients, antibiotic, antiviral, antifungal, immunosuppression, and disease-specific drug regimens should be disrupted minimally in the perioperative period.

Multimedia

1 Left Liver Lobe Donation

Transplantation is the standard of care for many end-stage diseases. About 113,000 patients are on solid-organ transplant waiting lists in the United States. Organ donation has not kept pace with demand, resulting in many practice changes to increase the donor pool, including more use of living-related organ donation, donor organs once considered marginal (extended criteria donors [ECDs]), grafts from "donation after cardiac death" (DCD) donors, as well as paired kidney donations (kidney swaps). All of these changes impact anesthetic management of organ recipients.

The United Network of Organ Sharing (UNOS; www.unos.org) was created by the 1984 National Organ Transplant Act to manage the organ procurement and transplant network for efficient and equitable distribution of donated organs. The system for organ placement received a technology upgrade in 2006 with the launch of DonorNet, an electronic resource for matching and distribution of organs around the United States. Speed of placement is important, as brain-dead donors are unstable, and ECD grafts are particularly important to transplant with minimal cold ischemic times. In general, maximum cold ischemic times are 4 to 6 hours for heart or lung grafts, 12 to 24 hours for livers, and up to 72 hours for kidneys. The UNOS website data contain center- and region-specific transplant databases, regularly updated.

The Scientific Registry of Transplant Recipients (www.ustransplant.org) is a source of transplant data important to clinicians, patients, and researchers. US centers performed 27,527 transplants in 2009, and almost 200,000 Americans are living with transplanted organs. Data on death rates while on transplant waiting lists are sobering, pointing to the complexity of illness in these patients and the need for more organ donation. In 2008, the rate of death on the waiting list for hearts was 17%, for kidneys 6.3%, and for livers 11.4%. In 2010, in the United States (including Washington, D.C., and Puerto Rico), 28,663 transplants were performed: 16,899 kidneys, 350 pancreata, 828 kidneys/pancreata, 6,291 livers, 2,333 hearts, 1,770 lungs, 41 hearts/lungs, and 151 intestinal transplants. In major transplant centers, specialist anesthesiology teams participate in the preoperative assessment and optimization of patients for major organ transplant procedures. Directors of liver transplant anesthesiology teams are now required to complete transplant continuing medical education. Solid-organ transplantation is also a critical component of many anesthesia training programs.

ANESTHETIC MANAGEMENT OF ORGAN DONORS

Brain-dead Donors

Brain-dead, heart-beating donors present many challenging management issues because collected experience in a single center is usually small, and research in brain-dead human subjects is
1 sparse. Brain death is declared when the clinical picture is consistent with irreversible cessation of all brain function.[1] Legal and medical brain death criteria differ from state to state, but all require cessation of both cerebral and brainstem functions. Brain-dead donors are unresponsive to sensory stimuli and have no brainstem reflexes, including ventilatory drive with apnea testing. Physicians involved in the transplant recipient process should not be involved in declaration of brain death of a donor. Potentially reversible causes of coma must be ruled out (hypothermia, hypotension, drugs, toxins) before declaration of brain death. Flat electroencephalogram is consistent with brain death. Transcranial Doppler and traditional or isotope angiography are used to confirm the clinical examination and lack of circulation to the brain.[2] Brain-dead patients may have intact spinal reflexes, so they may require neuromuscular blockade during organ procurement.

Brain death is associated with hemodynamic instability, wide swings in hormone levels, systemic inflammation, and oxidant stress, all of which negatively impact donor organ function.[3] Just after brain death, adrenergic surges can cause ischemia and ischemia–reperfusion injuries. Studies of head trauma patients suggest that the onset of brain death is associated with a transient period of hypotension with increased cardiac index and tissue perfusion. During this period, vasoactive drugs administered to increase blood pressure can cause rapid circulatory deterioration.[4] This period precedes the autonomic storm associated with herniation of the brain and emphasizes the wide dynamic swings in blood chemistries and hemodynamics after brain death. The timing of therapies to support hemodynamics is difficult as catecholamine storm is often followed quickly by pituitary failure. Once pituitary failure ensues, hormone therapy may help stabilize donors hemodynamically and thereby extend the donor pool.[5–8] However, with the inherent difficulty of controlling studies in brain-dead patients, proof that routine donor hormone therapy is beneficial is difficult to obtain. A standard hormone therapy regimen is triiodothyronine (4-μg intravenous [IV] bolus, then 3 μg/hr); methylprednisolone, 15 mg/kg intravenously every 24 hours; desmopressin, 1 U then 0.5 to 4 U/hr to maintain systemic vascular resistance (SVR) at 800 to 1,200 dyne/s/cm^5 (and reduce the polyuria of diabetes insipidus). Insulin infusion to maintain blood glucose 120 to 180 mg/dL is also recommended, and recent studies support glucose control for maintaining donor kidney graft quality.[9] Evidence that desmopressin is better than norepinephrine for maintaining donor heart quality is solid, evidence for triiodothyronine is not strong.[10] Other medications that should be available for the donor operation are broad-spectrum antibiotics, mannitol and loop diuretics, and heparin.

Because donor yield for hearts is only 42%, consensus conferences have been used to improve evaluation and utilization of cardiac donor organs.[11] Donor heart history is very important, and electrocardiography and echocardiography are mandatory. The ideal heart donor is <50 years old and is hemodynamically stable. Presence of major chest trauma, cardiac disease, active infection, prolonged cardiac arrest, malignancy, human immunodeficiency virus or hepatitis, or intracardiac injections moves the donor from ideal to marginal status. Overall health status of the donor prior to determination of brain death can facilitate a directed laboratory evaluation. Cardiac catheterization is often requested for male donors >45 years old, for females >50 years old, or for young donors with significant personal or family history of coronary artery disease. For recipients with pulmonary hypertension, younger donors, short ischemic time, low donor inotrope requirement, and oversized organs are preferred. Human leukocyte antigen (HLA) typing and ABO blood group compatibility are performed. The donor heart size should be within 20% to 30% of the recipient's heart size.

Anesthetic management during organ harvest is guided by the needs of the procurement teams, who may come from several centers and have discrepant requests, depending on the organs procured. UNOS has created a resource for managing organ donors in an effort to improve donor care and, therefore, the function of donated organs.[a] Transport of ventilated donors to the operating room (OR) often requires positive end-expiratory pressure (PEEP) valves attached to the Ambu bag to maintain

[a]See the Critical Pathway for the Adult or Pediatric Organ Donor at http://store.unos.org/category.php?category=CAT1013.

oxygenation. Recently, in a rare prospective trial, a lung-sparing ventilation strategy was shown to increase the lung donor pool. Patients ventilated with tidal volumes of 6 to 8 mL/kg body weight and 8 to 10 cm water (H_2O) PEEP were more likely to be lung donors than patients managed with tidal volumes 10 to 15 mL/kg and 3 to 5 cm PEEP.[12]

2 The mainstay of donor management is maintenance of euvolemia; therefore, central venous pressure (CVP) monitoring is standard. CVP is maintained at 6 to 12 mm Hg, and when pulmonary artery (PA) catheters are used to assess cardiac function, pulmonary capillary wedge pressure is maintained at <12 mm Hg. The type of fluid used for resuscitation can make a difference. In a study of 64 brain-dead donors, high molecular weight hydroxyethyl starch (HES, 200/0.6) had a negative impact on long-term renal function in recipients of these donor grafts compared with low molecular weight (130/0.4) HES.[13] The goals of volume and hormonal therapies are to minimize the use of vasopressors as the use of high-dose dopamine is associated with renal graft failure.[7] Efforts should be made to maintain serum sodium levels below 155 mmol/L; higher levels are associated with poor liver graft function.[14] A large European trial showed that brain-dead donors treated with 4 μg/kg/min dopamine generated better functioning kidney grafts than untreated controls.[15]

Generally, packed cells are used to maintain hematocrit of 30%, and fresh-frozen plasma (FFP) is used to maintain the international normalized ratio (INR) <1.5, although these practices are not evidence based. Surgeons procuring the lungs will want to keep the CVP low, and diuretics may be requested just prior to collection of the lungs. Surgeons procuring kidneys usually want high filling pressures. Donor oxygenation, perfusion, and normothermia are all important anesthetic goals, and the precise end points of therapy require coordination and communication with the various surgical teams. Generally, arterial PCO_2 is maintained at 30 to 35 mm Hg.

Prior to lung removal, surgeons will perform bronchoscopy. An adapter, such as the Portex fiberoptic bronchoscopic swivel adapter (SIMS Portex, Inc., Keene, New Hampshire), facilitates ventilation during the procedure. Glucocorticoids may be requested, and on occasion, prostaglandin E_1 is requested to improve circulation of the lung preservation solution. Surgical techniques have been developed to allow three recipients from one thoracic donor: two single-lung transplants and a heart transplant.[16] The heart is removed first, leaving a small cuff of left atrium attached to the lungs. The harvesting team will ask for systemic heparinization just prior to exsanguination and excision. Cardioplegia is administered, the heart stops ejecting, and the heart is removed. The trachea is transected and the lungs are removed en bloc for later separation.

Donor lungs are more susceptible to injury in brain-dead patients before procurement than are other organs, likely from contusion, aspiration, or edema with fluid resuscitation. Consequently, many multiorgan donors do not meet the current strict criteria for lung donors. These criteria are listed in Table 51-1. The Pulmonary Council of the International Society for Heart and Lung Transplantation reviews evidence (or lack thereof) for these criteria.[17] Lungs once considered marginal are being used increasingly because of this severe shortage of donor lungs. Exclusion of donors based on arterial blood gas or chest roentgenogram (CXR) (Table 51-1) is based on relatively small trials.[18] With experience, lung transplantation using donors outside these boundaries does not negatively impact the recipient, and most centers rely on bronchoscopy to determine lung suitability for transplantation.[19] Sputum Gram stains and cultures are routinely obtained on all lung donors. A positive Gram stain does not seem to impact outcome; however, organisms on bronchoalveolar lavage are associated with decreased survival.[20] One study suggested that evidence of aspiration seen on bronchoscopy, bilateral pulmonary infiltrates, or persistent purulent secretions is a criterion for donor exclusion.[21] Advanced donor age (>55 years) together with long ischemic time (>6 hours) are associated with poor transplant outcomes. In addition to the usual hematologic criteria, donor–recipient compatibility is based on height and/or total lung capacity.

TABLE 51-1. IDEAL DECEASED LUNG DONOR

Age <55 years
ABO compatibility
Clear chest radiograph
PaO_2 >300 on FiO_2 1, PEEP 5 cm H_2O
Tobacco history <20 pack-years
Absence of chest trauma
No evidence of aspiration or sepsis
Negative sputum Gram stain
Absence of purulent secretions at bronchoscopy

PEEP, positive end-expiratory pressure.

For heart retrieval, the surgeons perform a pericardiotomy, and the aortic root is cannulated for infusion of cardioplegia solutions. Following ligation of the great veins, the heart is compressed and exsanguinated, cardioplegia is given to induce cardiac arrest, and the aorta is cross-clamped. After cardiectomy the donor heart is preserved in cold ice slush. For donors who provide both lungs and the heart to a single recipient, a combined cardiopulmonary surgical extraction is performed.

A shortage of available donors has led to increased use of marginal donors and separate alternate transplant lists of recipients who consent to accept marginal donors. Increased risk of primary graft dysfunction is the main reason to avoid marginal donors. Marginal donors are typically used for patients who do not meet the standard recipient criteria, with advanced age a common reason for alternative listing. Common donor factors that lead to marginal status are abnormal hepatitis screening tests, left ventricular dysfunction or coronary artery disease, advanced age, and DCD.

Donation After Cardiac Death

In 2007 hospitals were mandated by the Joint Commission, in collaboration with local Organ Procurement Organizations, to develop DCD policies and protocols in response to organ donor
3 shortages. Since that time, DCD grafts have increased in the United States, accounting for 10.6% of all organ transplants,[22] while a few European countries have not adopted the practice at all. The criteria for death of DCD donors (previously called non–heart-beating donors) are distinct from those of brain-dead donors. DCD donors typically have severe whole-brain dysfunction but have electrical activity in the brain. Death is defined by cessation of circulation (arterial monitoring showing pulse pressure is zero, or Doppler monitoring showing no flow) and respiration. Life support measures are used to control the timing of death and organ procurement and to maximize the function of organs from these donors. Based in part on a study by the Institute of Medicine,[23] the American Society of Anesthesiologists (ASA) developed a reference document for management of DCD patients,[b] but every hospital must

[b]http://www.asahq.org/clinical/OrganDonationsamplepolicy.pdf.

develop its own protocols reflecting local constraints. Optimally, end-of-life care, including analgesia, is provided by the same medical team responsible for the care of the patient in the intensive care unit (ICU). Anesthesiologists do not necessarily have to be involved in DCD donor management, even when withdrawal of care occurs in the OR.[24] The main principles for institutional guidelines are outlined in the ASA report and include the following: The decision to withdraw care must be made prior to and independent of any discussion about organ donation. Suitable DCD donors are those in whom death is anticipated within 1 to 2 hours of withdrawal of life support. With experience, DCD donors with longer time to cardiorespiratory arrest can be used successfully for kidney transplantation.[25]

Detailed protocols for interactions with family members of the donor, transplant teams, organ procurement organizations (OPOs), and OR personnel must be established as part of DCD planning. Informed consent is required for organ donation and for any preorgan recovery procedures, such as drug administration or vascular cannulation. A plan for the donor's care should be in place if the patient does not die within the anticipated time frame, and ideally care should be transferred back to the team that knows the patient and family. Once the family decision to consent to DCD is made, the OPO can help guide management of the patient while the allocation of organs is being arranged. Uncontrolled, unanticipated crises that force the conversation about consent under extreme circumstances are obviously more difficult and may mean that the OPO cannot be involved in donor management because of time constraints. Nonetheless, uncontrolled DCD donors can be used for transplantation.[26,27]

Circulation and respiration must be absent for a minimum of 2 minutes before the start of organ recovery. Organ recovery started >5 minutes after respiratory and circulatory arrest may compromise donor organ quality, but this limit has now been extended with reasonable transplant outcomes. Predicting which patients will expire in 1 to 2 hours cannot be done with certainty. The most experienced program with DCD, University of Wisconsin, developed an evaluation tool to help predict which patients would die within 1 to 2 hours of withdrawal of support (Table 51-2).[28]

DCD donors provided 1,306 transplanted kidneys in 2008 (an increase of 12% over 2007), but 20.9% of DCD kidneys were discarded. DCD donors provided 276 livers (down from 2007), but 32.3% of the livers had to be discarded. Over half the pancreata of DCD donors had to be discarded, and 32 pancreata transplants from DCD donors were performed. These numbers point to the need to optimize DCD protocols, including matching to appropriate recipients. DCD lungs are used efficiently, and only 5.6% were discarded. Pediatric DCD donors also provide quality organs for transplantation.[29] Although DCD donors extend the donor pool, they are associated with increased recipient complications, decreased graft survival, and increased cost of transplantation.[30] DCD livers, for example, have consistently poorer outcomes than brain-dead donors' livers, but careful selection of both donors and recipients for these marginal grafts can still help expand the donor pool.[31]

TABLE 51-2. UNIVERSITY OF WISCONSIN SCORING TOOL TO PREDICT BREATHING AFTER WITHDRAWAL OF CARE IN POTENTIAL DONOR AFTER CARDIAC DEATH

Criteria	Points
Spontaneous Respiration (after 10 min)	
RR >12/min	1
RR <12/min	3
TV >200 cc	1
TV <200 cc	3
NIF >20 cm H_2O	1
NIF <20 cm H_2O	3
No spontaneous respiration	9
BMI	
<25	1
25–29	2
>30	3
Vasopressors	
None	1
One	2
Multiple	3
Age (yr)	
<30	1
31–50	2
≥51	3
Intubation	
Endotracheal tube	3
Tracheostomy	1
Oxygenation (after 10 min)	
O_2 Sat >90%	1
O_2 Sat 80%–89%	2
O_2 Sat <79%	3
Scoring	
<12 High risk for continuing to breathe after extubation	
13–18 Moderate risk for continuing to breathe after extubation	
19–24 Low risk for continued breathing after extubation	
RR, TV, NIF, BMI, body mass index; Sat, saturation.	

Adapted from: the University of Wisconsin website; Lewis J, Peltier J, Nelson H, et al. Development of the University of Wisconsin donation after cardiac death evaluation tool. *Prog Transplant.* 2003;13:265.

Living Kidney Donors

Safety and comfort are the primary considerations in the care of
4 living donors. Living donors must be healthy and without significant cardiopulmonary, neurologic, or psychiatric disease, diabetes, obesity, or hypertension. Renal function must be normal, with no history of renal stones or proteinuria. Open nephrectomy has been largely replaced by laparoscopic donor nephrectomy, which is associated with significantly less pain than the open procedure and shorter hospital length of stay and time to full recovery, but otherwise similar complication rates to the open procedure.[32] With experience, laparoscopic donor nephrectomies have been performed in more complex patients, with a low incidence of conversion to open nephrectomy and transfusion only rarely required.[33] Both anesthetics and insufflation of the peritoneum with carbon dioxide (CO_2) necessary for the laparoscopic procedure decrease renal blood flow. Nonetheless, as laparoscopic nephrectomies have become shorter (limiting the period of reduced renal perfusion), early graft function is similar to that of grafts obtained with the open procedure.[34] Patients undergoing the laparoscopic procedure often receive more fluids than open

nephrectomy donors, probably reflecting attempts to maintain renal perfusion during the period of compromise. Fluid loading overnight before surgery (vs. fluid administration starting with surgery) is associated with better creatinine clearance during the procedure, but this advantage is lost by postoperative day 2,[35] likely because donors have good renal function at baseline and the period of renal perfusion compromise is generally short. A reasonable fluid protocol is to administer crystalloid at 10 mL/kg/hr above calculated losses and to maintain urine output at about 100 mL/hr[36] or to titrate fluids to a CVP end point, although CVP may not accurately reflect volume status with the patient in lateral decubitus and with pneumoperitoneum.[37] Nitrous oxide is contraindicated for laparoscopic donor nephrectomy because distended bowel can get in the way of the surgeons.[38] For patient comfort, central venous lines (if used) are generally placed after induction of anesthesia.

Donor nephrectomy should be an uncomplicated procedure and donor tracheas can be extubated in the OR. Deep venous thrombosis prophylaxis is warranted.[39] For open nephrectomy, the patient is positioned in the lateral decubitus position with the bed flexed to expose and arch the flank. Donors are generally managed with general anesthesia, but epidural and combined epidural–spinal techniques (supplemented with intravenous propofol)[40] as well as general–epidural combined techniques are used. Postoperative pain following donor nephrectomy can be severe, and patient-controlled analgesia is often used. But the pain can still be severe enough to limit respiratory effort and mobilization of the patient. Furthermore, a survey of 123 donors showed that one-third of them had chronic pain after the open procedure,[41] suggesting postoperative pain management is often not optimal. Early complications include pulmonary (atelectasis, pneumothorax, pneumonia), urinary tract infections, and wound problems; long-term complications include reduced renal function, hypertension, albuminuria, and psychiatric issues (anxiety, depression).[39] Some centers admit donors to a step-down or medical ICU for a day after surgery, but the total hospital stay is usually only 2 to 4 days. Bladder catheters are removed on postoperative day 1. Patients should be advised that full recovery (i.e., feeling normal) takes 4 to 6 weeks, especially after the open procedure. Fortunately, perioperative mortality is rare but cannot be denied as a possible outcome during preoperative patient discussions.

Living Liver Donors

Left lobe liver donation (segments II and III) is usually done in the context of parent-to-child donation with recipients <15 kg. Although left lateral segmentectomy is a big operation, it is generally well tolerated (Fig. 51-1). Nonetheless, living left lobe donors must be healthy and without a history or risk for thromboembolic disease. By comparison, donor right hepatectomy needed for adult-to-adult liver transplantation is a major procedure (Fig. 51-2) and carries significant risk. The residual liver volume of the donor must be >35% of original volume to prevent "small for size" syndrome in the donor. Because risk for this syndrome is increased in older donors or in patients with cholestatic or hepatocellular disease, including steatosis,[42] adult-to-adult living donors should have no liver disease. Mortality of right liver resection for donation is estimated at 0.2% to 0.5%.[42] Complication rates are high for right liver donors (up to 30% of donors), including air embolism, atelectasis, pneumonia,[43] and biliary tract damage. An estimated 3.2% of donors in experienced centers suffer major complications.[44] Most centers do not perform adult-to-adult liver transplants in very ill recipients.

Large liver resections may require virtually complete hepatic venous exclusion (cross-clamping of the hepatic pedicle usually without cava clamping). Not unexpectedly, venous return falls significantly. Without the collaterals developed by patients with chronic liver disease, normal donors may experience significant hypotension when the hepatic pedicle is cross-clamped. Blood pressure is maintained largely through reflex increases in endogenous vasopressin and norepinephrine levels.[45] For these reasons, volume loading is reasonable prior to clamping, but some centers try to reduce blood loss by maintaining low CVP, while CVP monitoring is not routine in other centers. Sufficiently powered studies to prove that the benefits of low CVP (reduced transfusion requirements) outweigh the risks (renal compromise, air embolism) are unlikely to be performed, and institutional practices vary widely. If vasopressors are needed, vasopressin and norepinephrine are reasonable choices to enhance normal endogenous reflexes. Isovolemic hemodilution has been reported to reduce allogeneic red cell requirements in major hepatic resections.[46] At experienced centers, blood loss is usually <1 L, and 20% to 40% of patients require transfusion.[47–49] Blood salvage is useful, and some centers offer autologous donation programs for donors. Both can reduce the need for allogeneic blood transfusions.[50] Transesophageal echocardiography (TEE), if expertise is available, is ideal and may obviate central line placement. Most donor tracheas can be extubated safely in the OR. Hypothermia is a preventable reason for not extubating in the OR. A wide variety of general anesthetics are used for liver donors, although one small single-center trial suggested that desflurane resulted in better hepatic and renal functions after right liver donation than propofol–remifentanil anesthesia.[51]

Postoperative pain management in these patients is a matter of controversy because of perioperative coagulopathy (see Chapter 57). Some institutions use epidural catheters, providing excellent analgesia without complications. However, with large liver resection, INR rises significantly after surgery, peaking at 1 day[52] or within a few days after surgery, at a time when the catheter is usually removed. (Platelet counts also fall after large liver resections but usually remain in normal ranges.) For this reason, many centers will not place epidural catheters in right liver donors and rely on IV patient-controlled analgesia to manage postoperative pain. Laparoscopic resection of left lobe liver (segments II and III)[53] and right lobe[54] is available in some centers.

Hypophosphatemia (with excessive loss of phosphate in the urine) is common after hepatectomy,[55] and should be treated with sodium phosphate infusions to maintain phosphate levels 3.5 to 5.4 mg/dL, unless patients have significant renal compromise (creatinine clearance <50 mL/hr). Liver function tests other than INR are also abnormal in the postoperative period after liver resection and usually return to baseline levels within 3 months, although small changes in liver function tests can persist for up to a year after hepatectomy. Some living liver donors can experience chronic low platelet counts after hepatectomy.[56]

Living Lung Donors

Living lung donation is not a common procedure. Selection criteria for living lung donors are listed in Table 51-3.[57] Reported morbidity is low,[58] but follow-up of these donors is not well reported. If two donors are used for one recipient, scheduling difficulties are considerable. The surgical procedure is performed in three ORs simultaneously, one for each donor and the recipient. Donors are generally managed with combined general anesthesia and epidural analgesia.

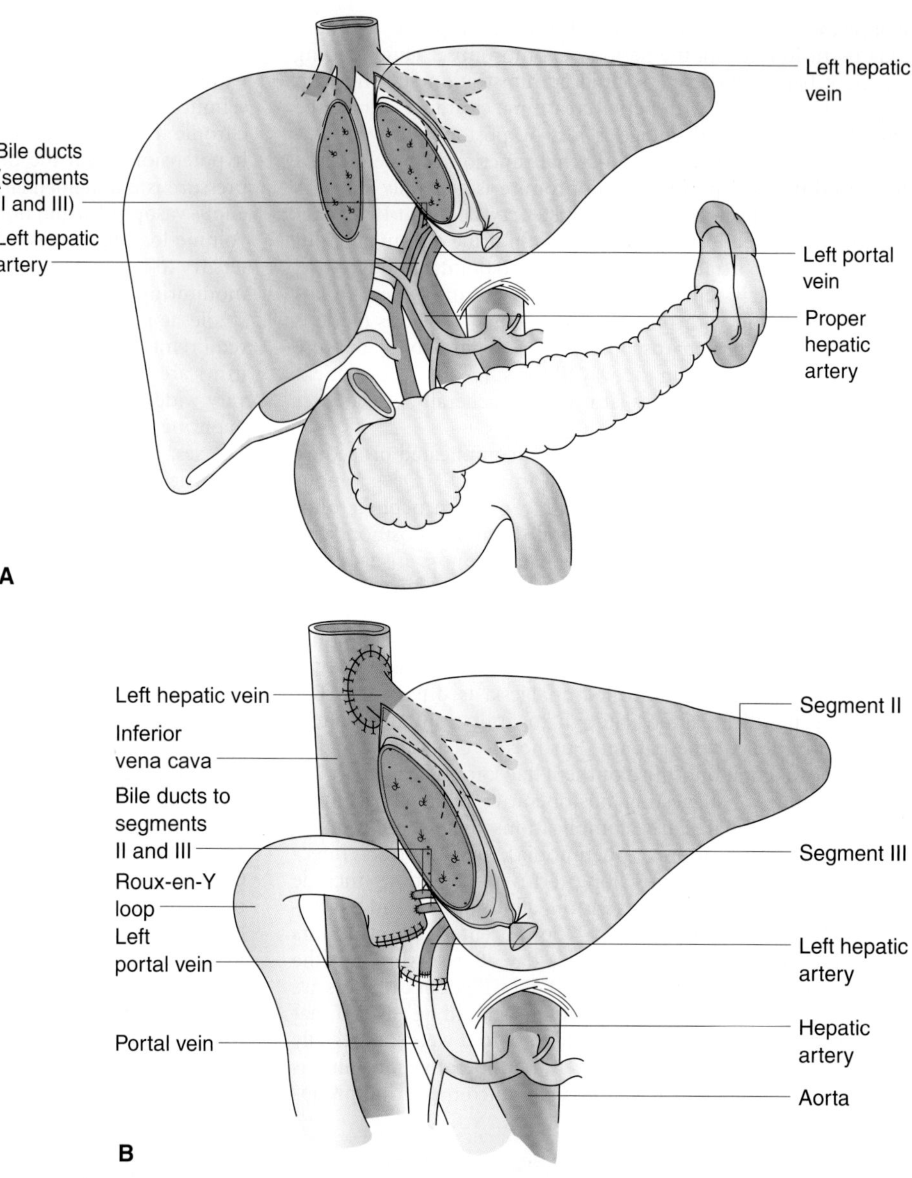

FIGURE 51-1. Left lateral segment (segments II and III) living donor transplantation. **A:** Donor operation. **B:** Recipient operation complete.

TABLE 51-3. LIVING LUNG DONOR CRITERIA

Member of recipient's extended family
Age 18–55 years
No prior thoracic surgery on donor side
Good general health
Taller than recipient preferred
ABO compatible
FVC and FEV_1 >85% predicted
PO_2 >80 mm Hg on room air
No chronic viral diseases
Normal electrocardiogram and echocardiogram
Normal stress test in donors older than 40 years old

FVC, forced vital capacity; FEV_1, forced expiratory volume in 1 second.
Adapted from: www.unos.org.

IMMUNOSUPPRESSIVE AGENTS

Pharmacologic suppression of the immune response to allografts is associated with major side effects. Considerable variability in intestinal absorption, genetic and induced differences in metabolism of these drugs, changing dosage requirements with aging, and idiosyncratic complications all mandate individualization of immunosuppressive regimens. Immunosuppressed patients who are undertreated risk rejection; overimmunosuppression can be
5 toxic, especially to the kidneys. All immunosuppression regimens carry major risks, such as infection, malignancy, and progressive vascular disease. Immunosuppression regimens differ considerably from center to center, and anesthesiologists must communicate with the transplant team to obtain the schedule and dose of immunosuppressive agents for each patient. It is particularly important to review drug regimens with transplant coordinators when posttransplant patients are scheduled for surgery because

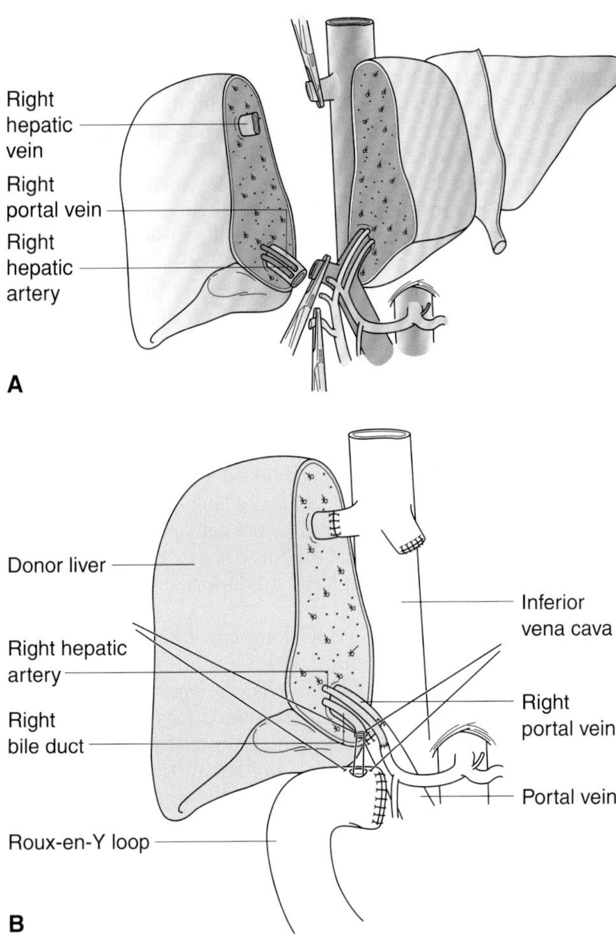

FIGURE 51-2. Right lobe (segments V to VIII) living donor transplantation. **A:** Donor operation. **B:** Recipient operation completed.

the transplant team needs information about peak and trough drug levels that may not be accessible on the hospital record.

Immunosuppressed patients coming to the OR deserve special attention to sterile technique and maintenance of antibiotic, antifungal, and antiviral regimens during the perioperative period. Complications of chronic immunosuppression are summarized in Table 51-4.

TABLE 51-4. COMPLICATIONS OF CHRONIC IMMUNE SUPPRESSION

System	Complication
Central nervous system	Lowered seizure threshold
Cardiovascular	Diabetes
	Hypertension
	Hyperlipidemia
	Atherosclerosis
Renal/electrolyte	Decreased glomerular filtration rate
	Hyperkalemia
	Hypomagnesemia
Hematologic/immune	Increased risk of infections
	Increased risk of malignancy
	Pancytopenia
Endocrine/other	Osteoporosis
	Poor wound healing

Calcineurin Inhibitors

The modern transplant era began with the introduction of the calcineurin inhibitor (CNI) cyclosporine into clinical practice. CNIs are still a mainstay of immunosuppression for solid-organ transplant recipients. Tacrolimus (FK-506) is also widely used. Inhibition of calcineurin, among other effects, modifies NFAT (nuclear factor of activated T cells) and frees nuclear factor-κB to translocate to the nucleus, where it enhances transcription of T-cell interleukin-2 (IL-2). Via these signal transduction pathways, CNI inhibits T-lymphocyte activation, differentiation, and cytokine production.[59] Calcineurin is involved in diverse cellular processes, so its inhibition can cause many significant side effects. These include hypertension (often requiring therapy), hyperlipidemia, ischemic vascular disease (including in heart recipients), diabetes, and nephrotoxicity. Cyclosporine causes acute nephropathy, which is usually reversible with drug cessation. But chronic renal damage from cyclosporine is a more refractory problem. A variety of other drugs are used with CNI to reduce the amount of CNI required. Ischemic cardiac disease is the leading cause of death of kidney transplant recipients, in part because of underlying disease that preceded transplantation. But CNI can exacerbate risk factors for coronary artery disease. It is important to note that end-stage liver disease (ESLD) does not confer protection from coronary artery disease, and liver transplant patients are also at risk for progression of ischemic cardiac disease after transplantation. Neurologic side effects also complicate CNI therapy, including tacrolimus-induced polyneuropathy[60] and encephalopathy.[61] When immunosuppression is interrupted by surgery or when multiple potentially interacting drugs are used, tacrolimus trough levels should be reassessed.

Tacrolimus is metabolized by cytochrome P450 3A4 and causes its up-regulation. Cyclosporine may rarely prolong the action of pancuronium.[62,63] To switch from oral to intravenous dosing of cyclosporine, usually about one-third the oral dose is used. Usual doses of tacrolimus are 0.15 to 0.3 mg/kg/day given in two doses. To switch from oral to intravenous tacrolimus, a starting dose of about one-tenth the oral dose can be used.

Corticosteroids

Corticosteroids disrupt expression of many cytokines in T cells, antigen-presenting cells, and macrophages. These drugs are used both for maintenance immunosuppression and in pulse dosing for acute rejection. Especially for growing children, corticosteroid-sparing regimens are increasingly popular. The well-known side effects are hypertension, diabetes, hyperlipidemia, weight gain (including Cushingoid features), and gastrointestinal ulceration (see Chapter 49). Communication with the transplant service is important in determining timing and dose of steroid administration perioperatively in patients who are taking the drug chronically. Corticosteroids are generally withheld during liver transplantation in recipients with hepatitis C because of concern that they contribute to hepatitis C recurrence.[64] Nonetheless, a recent multicenter study showed little advantage to a steroid-free immunosuppression regimen in patients with hepatitis C followed for 2 years after their transplants.[65]

Polyclonal and Monoclonal Antibodies

Antithymocyte globulin (ATG) is purified rabbit immunoglobulin-G (IgG) taken from animals immunized with human thymocytes, so that previous exposure to rabbits is a risk factor for serum sickness with ATG exposure. Polyclonal ATG suppresses the immune system by depleting immune cells, mostly T cells, but it interacts with a wide variety of cell surface molecules involved in adhesion and cell trafficking and ischemia–reperfusion injury. It has a long history of use in treating acute rejection and induction of immunosuppression, particularly in sensitized transplant recipients and in steroid- and calcineurin-sparing regimens.[66] Anesthesiologists should be aware that acute and severe serum sickness is a rare side effect of ATG administration,[67] presenting as jaw pain, and is treated by stopping the drug, plasmapheresis, and corticosteroids.[68]

OKT3 antibody is directed against a component of the T-cell receptor complex and affects immunosuppression by blocking T-cell function. Acute administration of OKT3 in awake patients (especially first administration) may result in generalized weakness, fever, chills, and some hypotension. More severe hypotension, bronchospasm, and pulmonary edema have been reported. Formulations of OKT3 may require syringe filtering before administration.

"Humanized" antibodies are antibodies engineered to contain human constant regions in the immunoglobulin protein, so that patients do not develop an antimouse immunologic response. Muromonab-CD3 is a humanized form of OKT3, usually used for acute rejection.[69]

IL-2 receptor (CD25) antagonists, such as basiliximab and daclizumab, are newer humanized antibodies directed against a portion of the IL-2 receptor expressed on activated T cells. About half of the heart transplant centers now use IL-2 receptor antagonists in their initial immunosuppression regimen to reduce the dose and cardiovascular side effects of calcineurin inhibitors. Gastrointestinal upset is the most commonly cited side effect of these drugs. However, basiliximab has been implicated in causing pulmonary edema in young renal transplant patients.[70]

Belatacept is directed against the CD80/CD86 ligands on antigen-presenting cells that activate T cells through the CD28 (costimulatory) pathway. It is approved for maintenance immunosuppression for kidney transplant recipients. Infusion reactions can include hypotension, but acute reactions are usually mild.[71] New targets for immunosuppressive drugs include complement and B cells as well as drugs directed at molecules that exacerbate ischemia–reperfusion.[72] Coagulopathy has been reported as a side effect of alemtuzumab (Campath),[73] which recognizes CD52 on B cells. Rituximab is another anti–B-cell antibody that acts at CD20 and is used for humoral rejection.

Tolerance of organ grafts without pharmacologic immunosuppression is possible using combined bone marrow and solid-organ transplants, with marrow and the solid organ derived from the same donor.[74]

Other Immunosuppressive Drugs

Mammalian target of rapamycin (mTOR) inhibitors are often used in combination with CNI to decrease the complications of dose-related side effects (calcineurin-sparing regimens) such as nephrotoxicity. TOR is involved in complex signaling processes that promote synthesis of proteins, including several that regulate cellular proliferation. Thus, mTOR inhibitors such as sirolimus (Rapamycin) are antiproliferative, used both in immunosuppression and increasingly in cancer therapies. Similar to cyclosporine and tacrolimus, sirolimus is metabolized in liver via P450 CYP3A isoenzymes, but coadministration of sirolimus and a calcineurin inhibitor does not increase calcineurin inhibitor drug requirements. In fact, the combination may be synergistic.[75] Diltiazem raises the plasma concentration of sirolimus.[76]

Azathioprine is hydrolyzed in blood to 6-mercaptopurine, a purine analog and metabolite with the ability to incorporate into DNA during the S phase of the cell cycle. Because DNA synthesis is a necessary prerequisite to mitosis, azathioprine exerts an antiproliferative effect. Antiproliferative drugs rely on the fact that immune activation implies explosive proliferation of lymphocytes. Side effects occur because other proliferating cells (gastrointestinal tract, bone marrow) are also affected. Repression of bone marrow cell cycling can cause pancytopenia. Cardiac arrest and severe upper airway edema are rare complications.[77] The intravenous dose is about half the oral dose.

Mycophenolate mofetil is metabolized into a molecule that inhibits purine synthesis. It too can cause leukopenia and thrombocytopenia as side effects, as well as red cell aplasia[78]; additionally it is teratogenic.[79] The usual oral dose is 1 to 1.5 g twice a day. Mycophenolate has largely replaced azathioprine in combination regimens.[80]

Mesenchymal stem cells (MSCs) are anti-inflammatory stem cells, currently in multiple clinical trials for solid-organ transplantation. MSCs are multipotent cells that are easily derived from marrow, fat, or other organs and expanded ex vivo. Their first use in the context of organ transplantation was for the treatment of grade IV graft versus host disease in marrow transplant recipients.[81] MSCs have pleiotropic effects on the immune response, including antiproliferative T-cell function. The goal of MSC trials for solid-organ transplantation is to reduce the amount of pharmacologic immunosuppression needed. Although these are allogeneic cells, they do not elicit a classical immune response, so third-party MSCs can be used in any patient without the need for donor-specific MSC. No adverse acute reactions to MSC infusion or injection have been reported after thousands of treatments.

CORNEAL TRANSPLANTATION

Corneas are the most common organs transplanted in the United States, with >40,000 transplants per year. Corneal transplants can be performed under local anesthesia (often with IV sedation) or general anesthesia. Recipients of cornea grafts are often elderly. A major anesthetic goal is maintaining low intraocular pressure (see Chapter 48 – EYE). For particularly complex procedures, diuretics and intravenous fluid restriction may be warranted to prevent edema.[82] Patient positioning (head-up angle of the bed) on transfer from the OR should be directed by the surgeon. Rejection of corneal allografts is the most common cause of graft loss in the first year after transplantation.

RENAL TRANSPLANTATION

Preoperative Considerations

The prevalence of end-stage renal disease (ESRD) is about 0.17% in the United States, where 16,899 kidney transplants were performed in 2010, representing no change in transplant volume in 5 years despite growing need. The most common recipient age group was 50 to 64 years (6,684 patients), and 2,813 recipients

TABLE 51-5. DIAGNOSES OF PATIENTS ON ADULT RENAL TRANSPLANT WAITING LIST

Diagnosis	Patients on List (%)
Type 2 diabetes	30.0
Hypertensive nephrosclerosis	21.5
Glomerular disease	19.7
Polycystic kidney disease	6.6
Tubular/interstitial disease	5.0
Renovascular/other vascular	3.6
Congenital or metabolic disease	3.1
Neoplasm	0.3
Other	0.5

Adapted from: unos.org.

were over 65 years. Thirty-seven percent overall received living donor grafts. Mortality on the waiting list in 2009 was 6.3%.[c]

Diseases treated with renal transplants are shown in Table 51-5, calculated from the 2008 waiting list data. Many of these underlying diagnoses are also risk factors for coronary artery disease, so preoperative evaluation is focused on cardiovascular function, but a comprehensive medical workup is essential.

About half the mortality of patients on dialysis is due to heart failure. Cardiovascular complication is a leading cause of death after renal transplantation. Therefore, cardiovascular risk factor modification is imperative before and after transplantation,[83] includ-
6 ing hypertension and hyperlipidemia. Renal transplant recipients are often anemic, with hyperdynamic cardiac indices. Patients >50 years (with or without risk factors for coronary disease) are generally screened with dobutamine stress tests or myocardial scintigraphy. The interval at which these studies are repeated in patients listed for transplantation varies from center to center. Peripheral vascular disease should also be assessed. Pulmonary function tests (PFTs) should be reviewed by anesthesiologists prior to transplantation (see Chapter 11). PFTs are particularly important in type 1 diabetics who often present with reduced lung volumes and diffusing capacity. The precise cause of abnormal PFTs in these patients is not known, but clinical studies suggest that long-term normoglycemia after kidney or pancreas transplantation is associated with improved pulmonary function.[84] Hypercoagulable states are common in patients with renal disease and deserve detailed evaluation so that they can be managed perioperatively.[85]

All solid-organ transplant patients are screened for tumors (mammography, Papanicolaou [Pap] test, colonoscopy, prostate-specific antigen) and infection (dental evaluation, viral serologies). Patients should have good control of their diabetes before transplantation and have an evaluation for psychiatric stability and social support. Severe heart, lung, or liver disease, most malignancies, and active or untreatable infections such as tuberculosis are exclusion criteria for renal transplantation.

Dialysis-dependent patients should be dialyzed before surgery. Cadaveric grafts can be safely transplanted after 24 hours of cold ischemia time, and potentially after 36 hours, allowing scheduling of preoperative dialysis. With preoperative dialysis, severe hyperkalemia during surgery is unusual.

[c]ustransplant.org.

ECDs are often used for kidney transplantation. Factors used in designation of ECD kidneys are age, creatinine, stroke as cause of death, and hypertension. Healthy older living donor kidneys have outcomes similar to standard criteria donor kidneys.[86] For example, donors over 50 years old are considered ECD if they have a history of hypertension, creatinine >1.5 mg/dL, or cause of death was cerebrovascular accident.[87] DCD donors are also an ECD category. ECDs affect the scheduling of transplantation as minimization of cold ischemia times is essential and delayed graft function may complicate the intraoperative course of DCD graft recipients.[88] Some centers report increased rates of primary nonfunction in DCD kidney grafts, contributing to early graft loss.[89]

Kidney allocation is a bit more complex than liver allocation. Blood type O kidneys are allocated to type O recipients, and blood type B kidneys are transplanted only in B recipients, except in the case of zero antigen mismatched candidates. Zero mismatched kidneys have the same HLA A, B, and DR antigens, and there is mandatory sharing of these kidneys through UNet with a complicated set of rules governing priority for these donors (see http://optn.transplant.hrsa.gov/PoliciesandBylaws2/policies/pdfs/policy_7.pdf).

Intraoperative Protocols

Renal transplantation is generally done under general anesthesia. Small studies have suggested good outcomes with epidural anesthesia[90] or combined epidural–spinal anesthesia. But concerns over uremic platelet dysfunction and residual heparin from preoperative dialysis have limited the use of regional anesthesia for kidney transplantation. Rapid-sequence induction is indicated in diabetic patients with gastroparesis (preceded by oral sodium bicitrate). Anemic, hyperdynamic patients may have higher dose requirements for induction agents such as propofol.[91] Rocuronium is useful for patients in whom rapid-sequence induction is indicated, but the duration of block is variable in patients with ESRD.[92] Similarly, plasma clearance of rapacuronium is reduced with renal failure, but titration of dose to neuromuscular blockade monitoring end points prevents delayed recovery.[93] Generally, the long-acting nondepolarizing muscle relaxants are avoided and shorter-acting agents such as cisatracurium are used. Before incision, antibiotics are given. A central venous catheter (usually triple lumen) is placed for CVP monitoring and drug administration in most centers, and a bladder catheter is placed.

Incision is usually in the lower right abdomen to facilitate placement of the graft in the iliac fossa. The recipient iliac artery and vein are used for graft vascularization, followed by connection of the ureter to the recipient bladder. If the kidney is too large for the iliac fossa, it can be positioned in the retroperitoneal space. Iliac vessels may be used for anastomoses, or the aorta and inferior vena cava may be required.

7 The major anesthetic consideration is maintenance of renal blood flow. No data are available to determine whether inhaled versus balanced intravenous techniques are better at preserving (graft) renal flow. Similarly, the choice of inhaled gas has not been shown to significantly impact posttransplant renal function. Isoflurane, sevoflurane, and desflurane are all used to manage renal transplant patients. Morphine effect is prolonged in the setting of ESRD, and high doses of meperidine can cause accumulation of its metabolite, normeperidine, in these patients. Similarly remifentanil metabolite accumulation occurs in ESRD, whereas fentanyl, alfentanil, and sufentanil pharmacokinetics are clinically normal.[94]

Hypertensive renal transplant patients often require antihypertensive drugs perioperatively. Calcium channel blockers have been best studied for renal protection of cyclosporine-treated hypertensive transplant patients. But after surgery, angiotensin-converting enzyme inhibitors and α-blockers may be as effective as calcium channel blockers.[95] Typical hemodynamic goals during transplant are systolic pressure >90 mm Hg, mean systemic pressure >60 mm Hg, and CVP >10 mm Hg. These goals are usually achievable without vasopressors, using isotonic fluids and adjustment of anesthetic doses. Hemodynamic management varies widely from center to center, so close communication between surgeon and anesthesiologist is imperative. Plasma-Lyte is the crystalloid of choice for kidney transplantation, and it preserves acid–base balance and electrolytes when compared with Ringer's lactate or normal saline.[96]

Once the first anastomosis is started, diuresis is initiated (both mannitol and furosemide are often given). Heparin and verapamil should also be available in the OR. In some centers, anesthesiologists are asked to administer the first doses of immunosuppression. A kidney graft is defective in concentrating urine and reabsorbing sodium, so attention to electrolytes is important.

Glucose control is also important for patients undergoing transplantation. A small, single-center prospective study of living kidney donor recipients identified glucose >160 mg/dL as a risk factor for acute perioperative renal dysfunction, likely associated with more severe ischemia–reperfusion injury.[97] Tight glucose control after kidney transplant is associated with less rejection, and diabetics with poorly controlled glucose levels after transplantation have increased mortality.[98] For these reasons, tight blood glucose control (80 to 110 mg/dL) is a reasonable anesthetic management goal during renal transplantation. Dopamine does not reliably improve renal function in this setting. The selective DA1 agonist fenoldopam is used to preserve renal function during kidney transplantation in some centers and is a superior renal protectant,[99] although not extensively studied.

Transfusion is rarely required in the OR, although renal transplant patients are often anemic coming to surgery (and may be receiving erythropoietin). Because of immunosuppression, if cytomegalovirus (CMV)-negative patients receiving a CMV-negative organ are transfused, CMV-negative blood is preferred. Leukocyte filters are also effective in preventing CMV transmission but are probably inferior to CMV-negative blood.[100] The entire surgery should take about 3 hours.

Most surgical complications of renal transplantation are not recognized in the OR. The common postoperative complications are ureteral obstruction and fistulae, vascular thromboses, lymphoceles, wound complications,[101] and bleeding.

Patient-controlled analgesia is a good choice for postoperative pain management, and despite prolonged action, morphine can be used safely if patients are monitored intensively. Nonsteroidal anti-inflammatory agents and cyclooxygenase-2 inhibitors are contraindicated. Pain can be severe, prompting some centers to explore combination blocks (ilioinguinal–iliohypogastric and intercostal nerve blocks)[102] or transversus abdominis plane blocks[103] for posttransplant patients. Chronic pain after kidney transplantation is common,[104] suggesting that more attention should be given to early postoperative pain management. Kidney transplant recipients are generally discharged from the hospital within a week of surgery.

In children, the most common causes of ESRD requiring transplantation are congenital (largely anatomic developmental) anomalies. Only 15% of pediatric transplants are performed for children <2 years of age.[105] Kidney size mismatch can complicate the surgery in small children. Adult donor kidneys may have to be placed in the retroperitoneum of small children. Although chronic peritoneal dialysis may help expand the abdominal volume,[106] attention to peak inspiratory pressures at closure is important, and increased pressures should be reported to the surgical team. Pediatric renal transplantation is associated with somewhat lower rates of success than adult transplantation, with vascular thromboses of the grafts more common in younger children.

LIVER TRANSPLANTATION

Preoperative Considerations

Liver transplant programs vary considerably in the numbers of transplants performed, with only 20 centers reporting transplant volumes >100 patients in either 2009 or 2010. However, the number of transplants performed in a given center is only a small percentage of patients evaluated for liver transplantation. The anesthesiologist's input into the workup of liver transplant recipients is essential for decisions regarding candidacy and optimal
8 preparation of patients for transplantation. Patients with ESLD have multiorgan dysfunction with cardiac, pulmonary, and renal compromise because of their liver disease (Table 51-6). Furthermore, 58% of patients transplanted in 2010 were age 50 to 64 years, and 11.3% were >65 years old. Common liver diagnoses leading to liver transplantation are shown in Table 51-7.

Adult liver transplant recipients are prioritized for transplantation by severity of illness, using the MELD (model for ESLD) score, which was originally developed to predict survival of patients with liver disease independent of liver transplantation[107]:

$$\begin{aligned}\text{MELD Score} = {} & 0.957 \times \text{Log}_e \text{ (creatinine in mg/dL)} \\ & + 0.378 \times \text{Log}_e \text{ (total bilirubin in mg/dL)} \\ & + 1.12 \times \text{Log}_e \text{ (INR)} \\ & + 0.643\end{aligned}$$

Pediatric patients are prioritized for transplant using the pediatric ESLD score (PELD):

$$\begin{aligned}\text{PELD Score} = {} & (0.463\ [\text{age}^d]) - 0.687 \\ & \times \text{Log}_e \text{ (albumin g/dL)} \\ & + 0.480 \times \text{Log}_e \text{ (total bilirubin mg/dL)} \\ & + 1.857 \times \text{Log}_e \text{ (INR)} \\ & + 0.667 \text{ (growth failure}^e) \times 10\end{aligned}$$

Patients with acute liver failure are given priority for donor livers, then the patients with the highest MELD score and compatible blood group are next.

All liver transplant patients are screened for infectious diseases including human immunodeficiency virus (HIV), CMV, and Epstein-Barr virus. As for other solid-organ transplants, major infection and malignancy may exclude patients from consideration for transplantation. Several centers have had good experience transplanting patients who have HIV, and HIV-infected patients who require liver transplants should be referred to these centers.[108]

Renal dysfunction is common in patients undergoing liver transplantation. Serum creatinine levels are not extremely useful in capturing renal function in patients with liver disease. Even a small increase in serum creatinine in these patients suggests significant renal dysfunction; hence, the reason that creatinine is emphasized in MELD scoring. Ongoing evaluation of MELD/PELD scores of

[d] <1 year old = 1; >1 year old = 0.

[e] >2 standard deviations (SD) below mean for age = 1; ≤2 SD below median for age = 0.

TABLE 51-6. MULTISYSTEM COMPLICATIONS OF END-STAGE LIVER DISEASE

System	Consequence
Central Nervous System	Fatigue
Encephalopathy (confusion to coma)	Blood–brain barrier disruption and intracranial hypertension (acute liver failure)
Pulmonary	
Respiratory alkalosis	Hypoxemia/hepatopulmonary syndrome
Pulmonary hypertension	Reduced right heart function
Cardiovascular	
Reduced systemic vascular resistance	Hyperdynamic circulation
Diastolic dysfunction	
Prolonged QT interval	
Blunted responses to inotropes	
Blunted responses to vasopressors	
Diabetes	
Gastrointestinal	
Gastrointestinal bleeding from varices	
Ascites	
Delayed gastric emptying	
Hematologic	
Decreased synthesis of clotting factors	Risk of massive surgical bleeding
Hypersplenism (pancytopenia)	
Impaired fibrinolytic mechanisms	
Renal	
Hepatorenal syndrome	Impaired renal excretion of drugs
Hyponatremia	
Endocrine	
Glucose intolerance	
Osteoporosis	Fracture susceptibility
Nutritional/metabolic	Muscle wasting and weakness
Other	
Poor skin integrity; pruritus	
Increased volume of distribution for drugs	
Decreased citrate metabolism	Calcium requirement with rapid fresh-frozen plasma infusion

wait-listed patients is mandated, with the sickest patients requiring the most frequent laboratory studies to update scores.

Difficult decisions about patient candidacy are common in evaluating liver transplant candidates. Several are discussed here to highlight the need for regular involvement of a transplant anesthesiologist in the candidacy evaluation process. Patients with ESLD generally have very low SVR, high cardiac index, and increased mixed venous oxygen saturation. Liver disease is not protective against coronary artery disease. Most patients are screened for cardiac disease using dobutamine stress echocardiography or myocardial stress scintigraphy, although the effectiveness of diagnosing coronary artery disease in these patients is not well established.[109] Patients with evidence of significant coronary lesions usually require cardiac catheterization to identify stenoses amenable to angioplasty preoperatively. These studies can be done safely even in patients with significant renal dysfunction.[110] Patients with severe coronary artery disease are generally not candidates for liver transplantation. Functional assessment of patients in addition to laboratory and imaging studies is important, and one study found that a distance of <250 m on a 6-minute walk test is an independent predictor of death on the transplant waiting list.[111] A recent, small retrospective studies suggests that troponin I levels >0.07 ng/mL may predict liver transplant patients at risk for cardiovascular complications.[112]

Significant aortic stenosis also presents a difficult dilemma pretransplant. Because cardiac surgery is considered risky in a patient with ESLD, patients with aortic stenosis can be treated with valvuloplasty before liver transplantation. Then, after the liver graft is stable, aortic valve replacement can be considered. Similarly, patients with hypertrophic obstructive cardiomyopathy (HOCM) and left ventricular outflow tract obstruction can be treated with alcohol ablation of the septum before surgery to improve cardiac function during transplantation.[113] These HOCM patients can benefit particularly from TEE monitoring because PA capillary wedge pressure does not accurately reflect left ventricular (LV) volume in this population. Patients with patent foramen ovales may be at risk for intraoperative stroke, and some centers work with cardiologists to close larger shunts noninvasively before surgery.

TABLE 51-7. DIAGNOSES LEADING TO LIVER TRANSPLANTATION IN ADULTS

Pathology	Diagnoses
Hepatocellular disease	Hepatitis C
	Laennec cirrhosis (alcoholic)
	Combined HCV/Laennec cirrhosis
	Autoimmune hepatitis
	Cryptogenic (idiopathic) cirrhosis
	Hepatitis B
	Small hepatocellular carcinoma (usually with other hepatocellular diseases)
	Nonalcoholic steatohepatitis
Cholestatic disease	Primary biliary cirrhosis
	Primary sclerosing cholangitis
Acute liver failure	Viral (unknown)
	Acute hepatitis viruses (A, B, C)
	Drug-induced liver failure
	Wilson disease

HCV, hepatitis C virus.

Portopulmonary hypertension (PPH) patients coming to transplant are particularly challenging. Diagnosis of PPH is made in the (a) setting of liver disease (b) mean positive airway pressure ≥25 mm Hg, pulmonary vascular resistance (PVR) >240 dyne/s/cm^5, and PA occlusion pressure ≤12 mm Hg.[114] Echocardiography is also used to screen patients for portopulmonary hypertension and intracardiac shunts. Systolic PA pressure estimates are made by capturing the maximum velocity of regurgitant flow across the tricuspid valve, and this velocity is used in the Bernoulli equation for the pressure gradient between the right ventricle and the right atrium ($\Delta P = 4V^4$). If moderate to severe pulmonary hypertension (estimated systolic PA pressure >50 mm Hg) is suggested, right heart catheterization is needed for direct pressure measurements. Multiple case reports and small retrospective reviews demonstrate that patients with portopulmonary hypertension are at substantial risk of perioperative death. There is general agreement that a mean PA pressure >50 mm Hg is an absolute contraindication to liver transplantation. Patients with PA pressures between 35 and 50 mm Hg and pulmonary vascular resistance >250 dyne/s/cm^{-5} are also likely at increased risk. Efforts to lower PA pressure before transplantation pay off and considerably reduce the risk of transplantation.[115] Epoprostenol is the usual first-line therapy for portopulmonary hypertension and is effective in lowering PA pressures significantly in many patients, but it requires home IV delivery. Inhaled iloprost has been used in Europe for PPH patients with good results.[116] Sildenafil is also useful for treatment of portopulmonary hypertension[117] and can be given via nasogastric tube during surgery. Controlling PA pressures is critical in patients with the most severe PPH, and a few patients have been successfully managed with the mixed endothelin antagonist bosentan[118] or the selective endothelin-A receptor antagonist ambrisentan (Cartin-Ceba) or imatinib.[119] Right heart dysfunction that does not reverse after treatment of primary pulmonary hypertension is considered a contraindication to liver transplantation.[120] Inhaled nitric oxide is extremely useful for managing PA pressures during liver transplantation.

PFTs are often abnormal in ESLD, with most patients showing reduced diffusion capacity for carbon monoxide. Hepatopulmonary syndrome (HPS, a widened alveolar–arterial gradient in room air due to liver disease), can lead to severe hypoxemia. Contrast echocardiography is used to diagnose intrapulmonary vasodilation using agitated saline. The microbubbles act as a contrast, and if intracardiac shunts are present, they appear within three heart beats after injection in the left ventricle. The later appearance of bubbles suggests intrapulmonary shunting. Once a contraindication to transplantation, HPS is now an indication for transplantation as it is the only therapy that can reverse the underlying physiology.[121] If HPS is severe and completely unresponsive to oxygen, transplantation is risky because the immediate perioperative period may be complicated by frank graft hypoxia and failure. Fortunately, most patients with HPS have some element of physiologic ventilation–perfusion mismatch, are oxygen responsive, and, with this "room to move," can be safely transplanted.

Some patients with refractory ascites and normal renal function can have relief from ascites with terlipressin treatment,[122] but this is unfortunately not available in the United States.

Recently, a large number of new drugs for the treatment of hepatitis C have entered clinical trials and the market,[123] including protease inhibitors, viral polymerase inhibitors, viral replication complex inhibitors, new interferon formulations, and new ribavirin formulations. Because clinical experience with these agents is small, the anesthetic implications and potential for drug interactions with anesthetics are not known.

Intraoperative Procedures

Uncomplicated liver transplants can take as few as 3 hours, and tracheas can be extubated at the end of the case, but predicting which patients will be straightforward is not always easy. Consequently, intensive preparation for surgery is important. Rapid-sequence induction of general anesthesia is indicated because patients with ESLD often have gastroparesis[124] in addition to increased intra-abdominal pressure from ascites. The authors place invasive lines and monitors after induction of general anesthesia: Two arterial catheters, one in the left radial and one in the right femoral artery (left femoral if a kidney transplant is planned). PA catheters and continuous echocardiography are used for monitoring volume status, and TEE is particularly useful for patients with cardiac lesions undergoing transplantation[125] (see Chapter 28). At least two large-bore (9 Fr) catheters are placed for rapid intravenous infusions. In many centers, anesthesiologists also place percutaneous lines specifically for use in venovenous bypass (VVB) if necessary, but many centers only rarely use VVB. Bladder catheters and nasogastric tubes are placed in all patients. A rapid infusion system with the ability to deliver at least 500 mL/min of warmed blood is primed and is in the room. Before surgical incision, blood product availability is confirmed, and some blood products are in the room and checked (routinely 10 U red cells and 10 U FFP). Normothermia, essential for optimal hemostasis, is maintained with fluid warmers and convective air blankets over the legs and over the upper body.

9 Liver transplantation is traditionally described in three phases: Dissection, anhepatic, and neohepatic, with reperfusion of the graft marking the start of the neohepatic phase. During the dissection phase of surgery, blood loss may be high. The major anesthetic goals of this phase are correction of coagulopathies and maintenance of intravascular volume for renal protection. Some centers advocate low CVP management of liver transplant patients to reduce blood loss,[126] but this technique may be harmful in patients with higher MELD scores[127] and marginal renal function.

Coagulation Management

Although standard laboratory coagulation studies do not predict bleeding well, they are still the best tests available in real time in the OR. For this reason, FFP is used to maintain INR ≤1.5 in patients with anticipated or ongoing bleeding. Point of care INR is extremely useful in patients with massive blood loss, providing information in seconds. In the authors' experience, point of care INR and clinical laboratory INR values may be different, but once the offset is known, the two INR values track well. Rapid infusion of FFP can quickly lead to ionized hypocalcemia because of the citrate load that is not metabolized by a diseased liver. Infusion of calcium chloride ($CaCl_2$), adjusted to ionized Ca^{2+} levels, is better at maintaining constant calcium (Ca^{2+}) levels than are intermittent boluses. Platelet transfusion has traditionally been used to maintain platelet counts >50,000/mm^3; however, recent data suggest that platelet transfusion is detrimental to graft and patient survival.[128] Importantly, we find that maintaining fibrinogen >150 mg/dL with cryoprecipitate is critical for hemostasis. Cell-saver blood may also be used to limit allogeneic transfusions, although it is generally not used in patients with hepatocellular carcinoma.

Many other factors contribute to poor hemostasis in liver transplant patients besides poor clotting factor synthesis, including renal failure, infection, endothelial dysfunction, and high portal pressures.[129] This complexity in the etiology of underlying bleeding problems is likely a factor in the unpredictability of bleeding during liver transplant patients.

In addition to complex coagulopathies of ESLD, many patients with liver disease have a superimposed hypercoagulable state (see Chapter 16). For example, patients with autoimmune liver diseases may have antiphospholipid antibodies. In general, prohemostatic factors are also elevated in patients with liver disease, including von Willebrand factor and factor VIII, and low values of ADAMTS-13, antithrombin, protein C, and plasminogen disrupt the normal balance of hemostatic agents.[129] So, in addition to monitoring discrete parts of the coagulation profile to guide transfusion therapies, it is important to look at a measure of whole-blood clotting to assess thrombotic potential. Most centers use thromboelastography (TEG) to help sort out complex coagulation disturbances and their evolution during liver transplantation, to help with interpretation of standard laboratory tests of coagulation, and to get a picture of overall clotting and fibrinolysis status. Using TEG, normal or hypernormal whole clotting in the presence of high INR and low fibrinogen and platelets (and usually elevated D-dimers) should be taken as a caution that the patient may have a clinically significant hypercoagulable state. Under these circumstances, the authors' approach is to maintain transfusion therapies, as noted previously, and to avoid pharmacologic procoagulant drugs. For the majority of patients with synthetic dysfunction, thrombocytopenia, and hypofibrinogenemia, whole-blood clotting is delayed. In these patients, many centers supplement transfusion therapy with antifibrinolytic agents. Considerable center-dependent variation in use and dosing of antifibrinolytics makes generalizations difficult. In the authors' experience, ε-aminocaproic acid (EACA; 5 g load and 1 g/hr infusion) to support hemostasis during surgery is useful in most coagulopathic patients during liver transplantation, provided there is no evidence or history of hypercoagulability. Other centers use considerably less drug, less often. Fibrinolysis acutely worsens immediately after reperfusion to varying degrees, depending largely on the amount of tissue plasminogen activator released from the graft.[130] A (re)bolus of EACA (again, doses are highly variable) is helpful to maintain hemostasis once this postreperfusion exacerbation of fibrinolysis is documented. Some centers use transexamic acid instead of EACA, which is also a plasminogen inhibitor but has a longer half-life than EACA.

Activated factor VII can be used safely during liver transplantation,[131] but is usually reserved for rescue of refractory critical bleeding unresponsive to more standard management because of its expense and because the risk of thrombosis in liver disease patients is not known. When this drug is given, INR rapidly normalizes,[132] although the amount of circulating clotting factors does not change, complicating laboratory coagulation studies. NovoSeven administration is also useful for surgical hemostasis for placement of intracranial pressure (ICP) monitors in patients with acute liver failure and for selected patients undergoing liver transplantation with difficult red cell crossmatches or in patients who refuse transfusion on religious grounds.

Pulmonary embolism is an unusual complication of liver transplantation, reflecting the complex coagulation imbalance of ESLD and liver transplantation. If diagnosed promptly, low-dose tissue plasminogen activator (0.5 to 4 mg) into the CVP port of a pulmonary artery catheter (PAC) can lyse the clot quickly.[133]

Perioperative renal dysfunction is a major challenge that is common in liver transplantation and can be exacerbated by hypovolemia and anesthetic-induced impairment of renal blood flow. Creatinine levels can significantly underestimate the degree of renal dysfunction, especially in ESLD patients with significant muscle wasting.[134] Hepatorenal syndrome (HRS) is a functional renal disorder associated with liver disease, categorized as type 1 (acute severe decompensation, creatinine >2.5 mg/dL), which is usually fatal, and type 2 (chronic, moderate renal failure with creatinine >1.5 and glomerular filtration rate <40 mL/min). HRS in general is the diagnosis of renal failure if the patient has ascites, is not in shock, has not been exposed to nephrotoxic drugs, has no parenchymal renal disease, has a creatinine level >1.5 mg/dL, and does not improve after 2 days of diuretic withdrawal and albumin therapy (1 g/kg/day up to 100 g/day).[135] Albumin may play a role in preventing and treating HRS in the setting of spontaneous bacterial peritonitis.[136] In addition, large-volume (>5 L) drainage of ascites with incision is a paracentesis and should be accompanied by albumin therapy to prevent renal decompensation, with recommended albumin doses of 6 to 8 g/L of ascites drained. Terlipressin (in Europe) and norepinephrine[137] may be useful for HRS because they relieve splanchnic vasodilatation. The α_1-agonist midodrine is useful for improving renal function in some patients.[138] No prospective trials have been done to support use of one vasopressor over another during transplantation, and intraoperative pharmacologic renal support is largely guided by the hepatology literature. Dopamine is not useful for preserving renal function during liver transplantation. The most important consideration for patients with HRS is to ensure adequate volume replacement before instituting diuresis in the OR.

The *anhepatic phase* begins when the liver is functionally excluded from the circulation. Historically, the vena cava is clamped above (suprahepatic anastomosis) and below (infrahepatic anastomosis) the liver, and the portal vein and hepatic artery are clamped. With complete cava cross-clamp, venous return falls by 50% to 60%, often resulting in hypotension. VVB may be used to increase venous return and, therefore, blood pressure, to increase renal and gut perfusion pressures, and to decompress portal pressures for a better surgical field. VVB is rarely used in the authors' center because surgeons use cava-sparing techniques, and hemodynamics during the anhepatic period can be managed with volume loading and vasopressors as needed. VVB carries potential complications, including arm lymphedema, air embolism, and vascular injury, and its benefit is limited when anhepatic times are short. Surgical techniques that preserve caval flow (piggyback technique)[139] are standard in most US centers and make intraoperative management significantly easier.

Reperfusion of the graft is the most treacherous time of the liver transplant. Communication between the surgical and anesthesia teams is essential in precise preparation for reperfusion. Caval clamps are removed first, and the integrity of the caval anastomoses are ensured. Caval reperfusion is usually hemodynamically well tolerated. However, portal vein reperfusion often results in hemodynamic instability. The original descriptions of reperfusion syndrome emphasized (often severe) hypotension and bradycardia with portal reperfusion.[140] Now, with flushing techniques that precede reperfusion and changes in preservation solution, bradycardia is less common. Typically, reperfusion is associated with hypotension (further drop of already low SVR and increase in carbon monoxide [CO]), which may or may not require treatment.

The authors' preparation for reperfusion is to give sodium bicarbonate just before unclamping (25 to 50 mEq) to meet the acid load from the graft. For particularly prolonged acidosis tris(hydroxymethyl)aminomethane (THAM) infusion is useful.[141] Importantly, the authors administer 500 to 1,000 mg of $CaCl_2$ precisely at the time of portal reperfusion to counteract the effects of potassium on the heart. If, despite these preparations, T waves on electrocardiogram (ECG) become elevated, the same treatment is repeated. Some anesthesiologists prefer to treat ECG changes only after they are diagnosed. Lidocaine, atropine, and norepinephrine are available at the time of reperfusion in case of ventricular dysrhythmias, bradyarrhythmias, and severe hypotension. Hepatic artery unclamping is usually hemodynamically uncomplicated.

One small study suggested that methylene blue (1 to 1.5 mg/kg bolus) reduces hemodynamic instability after reperfusion,[142] but was not supported in a follow-up retrospective review from another center.[143] Methylene blue is thought to mediate its effects by scavenging reactive oxygen species and nitric oxide. On the other hand, a study in which inhaled nitric oxide (iNO) was given during the entire transplant suggested significant acute benefits (decreased hepatocyte apoptosis) and earlier graft recovery, including faster coagulation factor synthesis.[144]

Neohepatic Period

Calcium is not required after reperfusion so that one early indication of graft metabolic function is the lack of a calcium requirement, even when FFP is infused rapidly. Usually within 30 minutes, the base deficit improves with graft metabolism of citrate and lactate. Within the first hour, the CO decreases (after an acute increase after portal reperfusion) as SVR increases with graft metabolism of vasoactive substances unleashed at reperfusion. In addition, the graft appearance should be noted. It should have a smooth edge and no evidence of engorgement. Bile is made in the first half-hour after reperfusion in a good-functioning graft. Often, renal function improves after reperfusion, probably because of graft metabolism of renal vasoconstrictors. Similar to kidney transplantation, ECD grafts are increasingly used to reduce wait-list mortality. The major classes of ECD liver donors are advanced age, steatosis, DCD, and split grafts,[145] as well as donors with extended hospital stays.[146] These grafts are often slow to function metabolically in the OR. For these and other classes of ECD livers, cold ischemia times should be limited, which can significantly impact the OR schedule.

During the neohepatic period, biliary anastomoses are completed and sources of surgical bleeding are corrected. Drains are placed and the abdomen is closed. Fast-tracking protocols for liver transplant patients are common in experienced centers.[147]

Pediatric Liver Transplantation

Indications for pediatric liver transplantation differ considerably from that of adults, with biliary atresia the most common indication (43%). Inherited metabolic diseases are the indication for 13% of pediatric liver transplants.[148] Portopulmonary hypertension is rare in children, but biliary atresia is associated with atrial septal defects and situs inversus.[149] Children <1 year of age with inherited liver disease are often very small for age. In small children, a radial artery catheter and at least one large (18-g) peripheral intravenous line are placed after induction of anesthesia. Surgeons may place tunneled central lines before incision, useful for intraoperative transfusions, postoperative administration of drugs, as well as CVP monitoring. Children with previous Kasai operations for biliary atresia may have massive bleeding during dissection because of adhesions. Small children receiving large grafts may have respiratory compromise with abdominal closure. Because hepatic artery thrombosis (HAT) is a more common complication in children than adults, some centers choose to have the INR at the end of surgery in the 1.8 to 2 range; postoperative aspirin and alprostadil are often used to prevent HAT. If flow is inadequate (by poor Doppler signals) in the artery after anastomosis, intraoperative reanastomosis or a new anastomosis may be required acutely. Aortic cross-clamping may be required for these anastomoses. Biliary complications are also common in pediatric transplant recipients, especially those receiving adult left lateral segment grafts, with hepatic artery thrombosis a significant contributor to biliary complications. Some centers report longer surgical procedures and higher transfusion requirements in pediatric patients who receive a living donor graft versus a deceased donor graft.[150] Use of split livers (one liver for two patients) puts a strain on transplant teams, but is an effective way to extend the donor pool.

Acute Liver Failure

Anesthetic considerations for both adults and children with acute liver failure (ALF) are focused on protection of the brain and treating cerebral edema[151] (see Chapter 39). Patients with a diagnosis of ALF should be managed in the ICU, because they can have a rapidly progressive course of elevated ICP, leading to herniation and death. In the authors' center, because these patients are relatively rare, the care of ALF patients follows a protocol developed by a multidisciplinary team, including anesthesiology. ICP monitoring is useful in managing these patients but risks intracranial bleeding; nonetheless its use is advocated by the US Acute Liver Failure Study Group.[152] Some centers have gained expertise in transcranial Doppler monitoring in place of invasive ICP monitoring[153,154] thereby avoiding the risk of ICP monitoring in coagulopathic patients. In the authors' experience, bispectral index monitoring, especially in patients without ICP monitors, can help detect acute changes in cerebral blood flow, such as with vascular clamping in the OR. Anesthetic management of these patients starts in the ICU, with intubation as needed for airway protection in the setting of encephalopathy or for initiation of therapeutic hypothermia. Mild hypothermia (core temperature 34° to 35°C)[155] is used in most centers for ALF, rather than colder hypothermic treatments used for head trauma. The head is positioned midline and the head of the bed raised. Hyperventilation is also commonly used to manage ICP but is best used as a rescue therapy. Mannitol is used for osmotherapy to an end point of 310 mOsm/L. Hypertonic saline is also useful for lowering ICP in some patients, although there are limited data to support its use.[156] Liver-assist devices can help bridge patients with ALF to transplantation. In the United States, the molecular adsorbent recirculating system has been in use for more than a decade. These devices may also contribute to a rapid enough recovery that some ALF patients can be spared from transplantation.[157]

Vasodilating anesthetics, including all inhaled agents, should be avoided, especially without ICP monitoring. In the authors' experience, pentothal infusion is a good maintenance anesthetic, and acute rises in ICP can be managed with etomidate. Patients may come to the OR on *N*-acetylcysteine, a glutathione donor. When antihypertensive therapy is required, labetalol does not cause significant cerebral vasodilation in these patients.[158] Acute cerebral vasodilatation often accompanies reperfusion. Management of intracranial hypertension and cerebral edema is based on very small studies of patients with acute liver failure and on adaptations of studies directed at control of intracranial hypertension in other settings (see Chapter 39).

PANCREAS AND ISLET TRANSPLANTATION

The majority of pancreas transplants (about 75%) are done as simultaneous pancreas and kidney transplants from a single deceased donor. Pancreata grafted in these procedures have historically had better long-term survival than grafts done after kidney transplantation or independent pancreas grafts. Independent pancreas grafts are usually performed for patients with type 1 diabetes who have frequent metabolic complications (hypoglycemia) but preserved renal function. With proper donor selection and aggressive attention to targeted antibiotic coverage, better graft survival rates after isolated pancreas transplant outcomes have recently been reported.[159]

The preoperative assessment of pancreas transplant recipients focuses on the end-organ complications of type 1 diabetes (reviewed in Chapter 44). Monitoring will depend on cardiac status, but generally patients do not require PA catheters and have been evaluated for cardiac disease as part of the transplant workup. Nonetheless, cardiovascular disease is present in many patients undergoing pancreas transplantation, although they tend to be younger than liver transplant recipients.

The major difference between pancreas transplantation and other procedures is that strict attention to control of blood glucose is indicated to protect newly transplanted β cells from hyperglycemic damage. No formula for controlling blood glucose has emerged as a standard of intraoperative management. In general, if adult patients arrive with glucose >250 mg/dL, 10 U of insulin can be given intravenously, followed by an infusion of insulin. The infusion starting rate varies, depending on the initial blood glucose level. Once blood glucose levels are controlled (<150 mg/dL), intravenous 5% dextrose (about 100 mL/hr) should also be infused as the insulin infusion is continued. The most important issue is to check the response to insulin frequently and adjust infusions as necessary. No literature exists for a patient with an implanted insulin pump, but it seems reasonable to continue to use the pump at basal rates in these patients as long as its operation is reviewed[160] and blood glucoses are monitored regularly during surgery.

Islet transplants were revived by the Edmonton protocol, published in 2000.[161] The major changes introduced included a glucocorticoid-free immunosuppression regimen and immediate transplantation of islets after isolation. Since that time, islets have been cultured after isolation in many centers, which makes surgical scheduling easier. Islets are generally infused into the portal circulation; acute portal hypertension may result from the infusion. This surgery should not be complicated by significant blood loss.

SMALL BOWEL AND MULTIVISCERAL TRANSPLANTATION

In 2003, the American Gastroenterological Association published a medical position statement on indications for intestinal transplantation.[f] Indications for intestinal transplantation include impending liver failure in patients with intestinal failure (or short-gut syndromes requiring total parenteral nutrition [TPN]), frequent severe dehydration in patients with intestinal failure, and severe complications of central lines for TPN (sepsis, thrombosis of central veins). Patients who develop liver failure from TPN for intestinal failure are candidates for combined liver-intestine transplantation. In these cases, liver failure should be irreversible, and biopsy findings are often required for this conclusion in patients without overt ESLD.[162] In general, intestinal transplantation is usually performed only in patients with life-threatening complications of the intestinal failure, mostly in children, but increasingly in adult recipients.

For anesthesiologists, a major hurdle for these transplants is line placement adequate for transfusion of blood products and fluids, which may be substantial during these long cases. Anesthesiologists should review angiographic studies to determine venous patency before attempting central line placement. Ultrasound devices are helpful in identifying the known patent vessels for cannulation, but surgical cut-downs for venous access may be necessary, including transhepatic or intraoperative renal vein catheterization[163] (see Chapter 41). Superior vena cava or inferior vena cava obstruction may require preoperative intervention (surgical and/or lytic) for adequate vascular access for surgery.[164] Antibiotic regimens should be continued during the surgery. Nitrous oxide, as in liver transplantation, is avoided.

Common complications of intestinal failure include dehydration and electrolyte abnormalities, gastric acid hypersecretion, pancreatic insufficiency, bone disease, and TPN-induced liver failure.[165] Because electrolyte abnormalities are common, they should be monitored continuously during surgery and appropriate replacement instituted. Because enteral feeding will not be possible until weeks after surgery, TPN should be continued in the perioperative period.

Like reperfusion of liver grafts, intestinal graft reperfusion is associated with an acute release of acid and potassium from the graft. Anticipatory bicarbonate and $CaCl_2$ administration are used to counteract the effects of acid and potassium on the heart. After reperfusion, coagulopathy may worsen, and is usually managed by reassessment of INR, fibrinogen and platelet counts, and correction with blood products.

LUNG TRANSPLANTATION

Lung transplantation is accepted therapy for end-stage pulmonary and pulmonary vascular disease, based on documented improvement in longevity and quality of life.[166,167] The Department of Health and Human Services Organ Procurement and Transplantation Network reports >22,000 lung transplant procedures in the United States since 1988, and the 2011 Registry of the International Society for Heart and Lung Transplantation reports over 38,000 lung transplants worldwide since 1989.[166] With median

[f]http://www.guideline.gov/summary/summary.aspx?ss=15&_id=3795&nbr=3021#s23.

waiting time ranging between 500 and 1,000 days, however, many patients die awaiting transplant because of the shortage of suitable organs. The past 16 years have seen a slow but steady improvement in overall outcomes in lung transplantation. Data compiled during that period reveal a median posttransplant survival of 5.5 years and a 53% survival rate at 5 years. The most common indications for lung transplantation are chronic obstructive pulmonary disease (35%), idiopathic pulmonary fibrosis (23%), cystic fibrosis (CF, 17%), and α_1-antitrypsin deficiency (6%).[166]

Surgical options for lung transplantation are single-lung transplant, en bloc double, sequential double, and heart–lung transplantation. The International Society for Heart and Lung Transplantation registry for 2011 indicates a continued increase in double-lung transplants over the past 14 years, with a relatively stable number of single-lung transplants,[166] a trend likely related to reports of improved 1-year survival after double-lung transplantation. There has been a recent trend toward avoiding the use of cardiopulmonary bypass (CPB) in single and sequential double-lung transplantation, although CPB is always made available as a backup and often used for patients with pulmonary hypertension. Double-lung transplantation is most commonly used in patients with pulmonary vascular disease and CF, although its use is increasing in chronic obstructive pulmonary disease and idiopathic pulmonary fibrosis. Single-lung transplantation for emphysema has favor because of good short-term outcomes, with the added advantage of availing another donor lung to another recipient. Lung transplant centers vary in applying single- or double-lung transplant to different diagnoses as well as the application of CPB, and the procedure indications are still debated.[167] Double-lung transplantation, however, is indicated if a single-lung transplantation would allow a continuing pathologic process to place either the native or transplanted lung in jeopardy. For example, in CF patients, infection in the native lung can easily spread to the transplanted lung. In pulmonary hypertension, remaining pulmonary vascular disease in the native lung would result in progressive pulmonary hypertension and thus hypertensive vasculopathy in the transplanted lung. Finally, a severely emphysematous lung, with its high compliance, would be at risk for air trapping and barotrauma when coexisting with a transplanted lung with normal compliance.[168]

Recipient Selection

The International Guidelines for the Selection of Lung Transplant Candidates were updated in 2006 by consensus agreement of several thoracic societies (summarized in Table 51-8).[166] In general, patients should be considered for lung transplantation if they exhibit poor pulmonary function despite maximal medical therapy. Contraindications to lung transplantation are based on their impact on long-term survival (see Table 51-8). Patients with significant cardiac disease can be considered for heart–lung

TABLE 51-8. LUNG RECIPIENT SELECTION GUIDELINES

General Indications	
End-stage lung disease	
Failed maximal medical treatment of lung disease	
Age within limits for planned transplant	
Life expectancy <2–3 yrs	
Ability to walk and undergo rehabilitation	
Sound nutritional status (70%–130% of ideal body weight)	
Stable psychosocial profile	
No significant comorbid disease	
Disease-Specific Indications	
COPD	FEV_1 <25% of predicted value after bronchodilators and/ or $PaCO_2$ = 55 mm Hg and/or pulmonary hypertension (especially with cor pulmonale)
	Chronic O_2 therapy
Cystic fibrosis	FEV_1 <30% predicted
	Hypoxemia, hypercapnia, or rapidly declining lung function
	Weight loss and hemoptysis
	Frequent exacerbations, especially young females
	Absence of antibiotic-resistant organisms
Idiopathic pulmonary fibrosis	Vital capacity <60%–65% of predicted
	Resting hypoxemia
	Progression of disease despite therapy (steroids)
Pulmonary hypertension	NYHA functional status class III or IV, despite prostacyclin therapy
	Mean right atrial pressure <15 mm Hg
	Mean pulmonary artery pressure <55 mm Hg
	Cardiac index <2 L/min/m^2
Eisenmenger syndrome	NYHA class III or IV, despite optimal therapy
Pediatric	NYHA class III or IV
	Disease unresponsive to maximal therapy
	Cor pulmonale, cyanosis, low cardiac output

COPD, chronic obstructive pulmonary disease; FEV_1, forced expiratory volume in 1 second; NYHA, New York Heart Association.

transplantation but are not candidates for isolated lung transplant. A new lung allocation system has been in use since May 2005.[166] Candidates are now given a lung allocation score to determine their wait-list status, instead of the historical scoring system, which relied heavily on time on the transplant waiting list. The new system weighs net benefit of transplant and clinical urgency.

As for other transplant recipients, patients are screened for malignancy (mammography, Pap test, and colonoscopy). PFT, left and right heart catheterization, and transthoracic echocardiography are used to evaluate candidate recipients. Lung transplantation is not advocated for acute disease processes, such as acute respiratory distress syndrome. Specific age limits were recommended in the past; however, current guidelines list age >65 years as only a relative contraindication to transplantation. CF is associated with complex pulmonary infections and colonization with microbial flora that can negatively impact transplant outcomes.[167,168] However, with the exception of patients colonized with *Burkholderia cepacia,* most CF patients can be successfully transplanted despite chronic bacterial infections.[169]

Preanesthetic Considerations

Medical evaluation prior to listing a patient for transplantation requires the expertise of many medical specialties. If the patient has been on the waiting list for an extended period, it is important to review recent laboratory and functional data because disease progression may have resulted in a change in status since the original workup. It is critical to confirm ABO compatibility of donor and recipient prior to surgery. Lung transplant candidates have poor pulmonary status and are frequently receiving multiple therapies, including oxygen, inhaled bronchodilators, steroids, and pulmonary vasodilators. These medications should be continued in the perioperative period. Because short ischemic times are necessary for optimal organ function, the procedure must be done as soon as a lung becomes available. Because these procedures are done on an urgent or emergent basis, the patient often presents with a full stomach.

Although lung transplant patients are understandably anxious, they also have minimal pulmonary reserve, and sedation must be given carefully under monitored conditions. After determining oxygen saturation, slow, incremental dosing of a short-acting benzodiazepine (0.25 to 1 mg midazolam) may be used for anxiolysis. Premedication with narcotics such as fentanyl must be administered with extreme caution, if at all, because of the ventilatory depressant effect. Use of metoclopramide, histamine-2 antagonists, and a nonparticulate antacid are usually warranted because of full-stomach considerations. Many patients are unable to rest supine or in Trendelenburg position for central venous catheterization. Placement of large-bore peripheral IV and arterial access is usually adequate for initiation of the anesthetic, with central access achieved after induction. Placement of a PAC is usually warranted for monitoring cardiac output and pulmonary vascular resistance, with a catheter capable of continuous cardiac output and mixed venous oxygenation (MvO_2) saturation preferable. Thoracic epidural catheters are placed preoperatively at some centers, especially in patients who are believed unlikely to require CPB with its associated anticoagulation. The American Society for Regional Anesthesia consensus statement on regional anesthesia in the anticoagulated patient[170] states that there is currently insufficient evidence to determine the risk of neuraxial hematoma in patients receiving neuraxial anesthesia and full systemic anticoagulation. Another option is to place the epidural in the early postoperative period, after coagulopathies are corrected. The epidural can be placed using light sedation during weaning from mechanical ventilation, allowing better neurologic monitoring and pain control prior to tracheal extubation.

Intraoperative Management

Single-lung Transplantation

Lung transplant recipients are often chronically intravascularly volume depleted and also tend to suffer chronic pulmonary hypertension. These factors predispose these patients to hypotension and decreased cardiac output upon anesthetic induction. Restriction of anesthetic doses because of this concern increases the risk of awareness in this patient population. Monitoring with processed electroencephalogram may thus be useful. Anesthetic management guided by bispectral index monitoring has been associated with a reduction of the incidence of intraoperative awareness in this population.[171] Because fluid restriction is beneficial for postoperative management, small fluid boluses, particularly with colloid, and judicious induction with etomidate, benzodiazepine, and narcotics are prudent. These patients often remain intubated for hours to days postoperatively, so a fast-track anesthetic technique is usually unnecessary. Communication with the surgical team about this issue is advised, however, because some patients, particularly those with chronic obstructive pulmonary disease undergoing single-lung transplant, may be extubated early. A balanced technique combining narcotic and inhalation anesthetics or benzodiazepines is usually an effective approach to maintenance of the anesthetic state. Muscle relaxation is maintained with nondepolarizers, such as rocuronium or vecuronium, without impacting hemodynamics. Nitrous oxide is rarely used because it may exacerbate bullous emphysematous disease, pulmonary hypertension, or intraoperative hypoxemia.

Lung isolation, preferably with a double-lumen endobronchial tube, is necessary for single-lung and bilateral sequential lung transplantation. The double-lumen tube, compared with bronchial blockade techniques, allows better suctioning of secretions, improved deflation of the operative lung during dissection, and application of continuous positive airway pressure to the operative lung if indicated. A bronchial blocker is more easily dislodged with surgical manipulation, may not provide isolation of the right upper lobe, and requires repositioning midsurgery in the case of a bilateral sequential procedure. A left-sided endobronchial tube is preferred, because a right-sided tube may be difficult to position relative to the right upper lobe bronchus.

10 Fluid restriction and lung ventilation strategies designed to protect the lung allograft are indicated as these patients are at risk for acute lung injury and pulmonary edema. This implies use of small tidal volumes (6 mL/kg) and oxygenation techniques, using PEEP and the lowest acceptable fraction of inspired oxygen (FiO_2) settings.[172] Fluid restriction recommendations are based on data showing that elevated CVP is associated with increased mortality after lung transplantation.[173] Intermittent fluid boluses to maintain CVP <7 cm H_2O and use of vasoactive drugs to maintain hemodynamic parameters are recommended. Cardiac output monitoring using PAC, or minimally invasive techniques such as esophageal Doppler or pulse contour analysis are useful for guiding fluid restriction while ensuring adequate cardiac output. Lung recipients are susceptible to pulmonary hypertension and right ventricular (RV) dysfunction or failure during single-lung ventilation. Optimizing oxygenation and ventilation does not always improve RV function, and vasodilator or inotropic support may be required. Inhaled nitric oxide is an option for improving respiratory and RV status.

During single-lung ventilation, hypoxemia is common. Strategies to improve oxygenation and ventilation are discussed in Chapter 56. Newer anesthesia machines with pressure-controlled ventilation and other advanced options have diminished the need for ICU ventilators during the operative procedure. CPB is indicated during lung transplantation if adequate oxygenation cannot be maintained despite ventilatory and pharmacologic maneuvers and PA clamping by the surgeon. Inability to ventilate, oxygenate, or maintain adequate RV function is an indication for CPB.

Single-lung transplantation can be performed via lateral thoracotomy. If the surgeon is concerned about a need for CPB, then the patient must be positioned to allow rapid access to either the aorta and right atrium or to the femoral artery and vein. Access can be accomplished via either anterior thoracotomy with partial sternotomy or lateral thoracotomy with decreased angulation of the hips to allow access to the femoral vessels. Determination of operative side is based on preoperative ventilation–perfusion studies and prior thoracic surgeries. The lung with poorer function is typically the one replaced.

After pneumonectomy, the surgeon will size the donor vascular tissue to the recipient vessels and sequentially anastomose the atrial/pulmonary vein patch, bronchus, and pulmonary artery. The lung is kept cold with ice in the surgical field until reperfusion. Circulation is restored to the donor lung, suture lines are checked for hemostasis, and then ventilation is begun. Systemic hypotension can occur during reperfusion but is usually not as significant as that with liver graft reperfusion. The anesthesiologist is often asked to assess the bronchial anastomosis using fiberoptic bronchoscopy and to perform bronchopulmonary toilet on the transplanted lung if necessary (removal of blood, secretions). TEE is useful to assess pulmonary venous drainage of the transplanted lung (*vide infra*). Perfadex (Vitralife, Goteborg, Sweden), a low-molecular-weight dextran solution, improves early graft function and is now used widely for preservation during procurement.[174] There can, nonetheless, be reperfusion injury to the lung presenting as pulmonary edema. PEEP and lung protective strategies are particularly useful in this scenario.

Intraoperative TEE is a valuable tool in the assessment of lung transplant patients. A comprehensive TEE examination should be performed after induction of anesthesia with attention focused on biventricular function, presence of valvular regurgitation, patent foramen ovale or atrial septal defect, and pulse wave Doppler flow patterns in the pulmonary veins. Significant RV dysfunction, valvular regurgitation, or intra-atrial shunt may lead the surgeon to utilize CPB. TEE can be helpful in monitoring RV function during initial clamping of the PA. Acute deterioration of RV function is an indication for the institution of CPB. After reperfusion, another TEE examination should be performed. Pulmonary vein anastomotic obstruction can be diagnosed with careful Doppler examination of the pulmonary venous inflow (see Chapter 28). Because this condition leads to acute graft failure, rapid diagnosis and treatment in the OR are important.

At the completion of the procedure, the patient should be evaluated for exchange of the double-lumen tube to a large (8-mm internal diameter or larger) single-lumen endotracheal tube. Significant oropharyngeal edema, high PEEP requirement, or need for differential lung ventilation justify leaving the double-lumen tube in place postoperatively to allow improvement in clinical status prior to endotracheal tube exchange.

Double-lung Transplantation

Bilateral lung transplant is performed in the supine position via the clamshell incision (Fig. 51-3). The arms can be suspended on a padded bar above the patient or tucked at the sides. If the arms are suspended, care must be taken to avoid stretching the brachial plexi. These cases can also be performed via midline sternotomy. En bloc double-lung transplant requires CPB, and a single-lumen endotracheal tube is sufficient. Bilateral sequential transplantation requires lung isolation, preferably via a double-lumen endotracheal tube. Bilateral sequential transplant is now the preferred procedure because a tracheal anastomosis is unnecessary and there is less surgical bleeding. Most centers electively institute CPB for this procedure in the presence of preoperative pulmonary hypertension and urgent CPB for indications previously discussed. Serial implantation implies longer ischemic time for the second lung, but this has not been shown to adversely affect outcome. In some institutions, sequential bilateral transplantation with CPB is performed using a double-lumen endobronchial tube, allowing immediate ventilation and oxygenation of the first transplanted lung while the second is being transplanted. In most institutions the bronchial circulation is not re-established, so a transplanted lung on CPB does not receive oxygenated bronchial blood flow. Thus, ventilation of a newly transplanted lung with 50% oxygen, even during CPB, may be advisable. The clamshell incision is extensive and can cause significant postoperative pain. Thoracic epidurals are often used to provide pain relief.

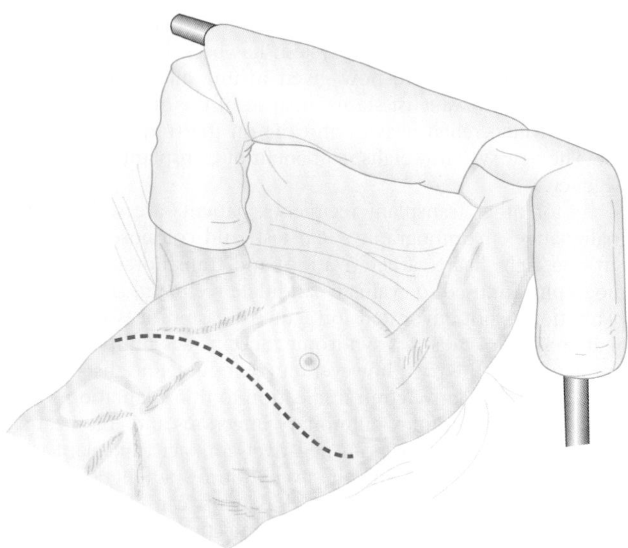

FIGURE 51-3. Clamshell–Manecke responsible.

Pediatric Lung Transplantation

The Registry of the International Society for Heart and Lung Transplantation Pediatric Report was last published in 2011.[175] Pediatric lung transplantation has increased over the past decade, with adolescents accounting for the majority of the procedures: 127 pediatric lung transplants were reported worldwide in 2009, compared with only 73 in 1999. The most common diagnoses are CF, congenital heart disease, and primary pulmonary hypertension. Congenital heart disease is the most common indication in infants. Overall survival is similar for pediatric and adult populations. Infants have better survival than adolescents after lung transplantation, but overall, survival of pediatric recipients is still improving. An evaluation of patients with CF listed and receiving lung transplantation showed that only 1% of the patients showed a survival benefit from surgery, a remarkably poor result.[176] However, quality of life still appears improved by lung transplantation in patients with CF. Efforts to quantify quality of life are ongoing. The role of lung transplantation for treatment of CF deserves further study to determine optimal age, pretransplant diagnosis, status, and firm indicators. Most pediatric patients receive double-lung transplantation with CPB, with a single-lumen endotracheal tube. The clamshell incision is used. Central and arterial access is necessary for perioperative monitoring.

Primary Graft Dysfunction

The most common causes of acute graft lung failure are acute rejection, inadequate pulmonary venous drainage, and an entity called primary graft dysfunction (PGD). The etiology of PGD, a major cause of posttransplant morbidity and mortality, is multifactorial.[177,178] PGD, defined as allograft dysfunction occurring within 72 hours of transplantation, is graded on a scale of 0 to 3. Grade 3 is defined as PaO_2/FiO_2 <200 with radiographic infiltrates consistent with pulmonary edema. Grade 3 PGD is associated with statistically increased 30-day mortality.[177] Grades 1 and 2 are also associated with infiltrates, although less severe, with PaO_2/FiO_2 ratios >300 and between 200 and 300, respectively. Grade 0 means no PGD, the PaO_2/FiO_2 ratio is >300, and no pulmonary infiltrates are present. Possible factors contributing to PGD include prolonged organ ischemia time with ischemia–reperfusion injury, advanced donor age, pulmonary hypertension in the recipient, and the use of CPB. Anesthetic management has not emerged as a risk factor for PGD. To date there are no specific data to support a link between transfusion and PGD, although an association is suspected.[177] However, data are limited on transfusion during lung transplantation, in contradistinction to the large amounts of data on transfusion requirements during kidney or liver transplantation. Wang et al.[179] and Oto et al.[180] found that patients undergoing double-lung transplants, procedures with CPB, or those with Eisenmenger syndrome or CF had increased transfusion requirements during lung transplantation. Further study is needed to determine whether and how transfusion negatively impacts lung transplant outcomes. The transplant literature does not show a correlation between fluid management in the OR and outcome, although management of pulmonary transplant patients as if they have acute lung injury with a protective strategy, as described above, is recommended. Severe, life-threatening PGD has been successfully managed with extracorporeal membrane oxygenation (ECMO).[180]

Inhaled Nitric Oxide

Inhaled nitric oxide (iNO) therapy may be used to decrease pulmonary vascular resistance and improve oxygenation (see Chapter 56). NO has an extremely short duration of action in vivo, rapidly inactivated by reacting with heme to produce methemoglobin. Because iNO is preferentially delivered to ventilated areas, vascular relaxation in these areas leads to improved blood flow and hence, improvements in ventilation–perfusion matching and oxygenation. Rapid inactivation of iNO in the pulmonary vasculature prevents its systemic distribution and systemic vasodilatation and hypotension.

Some anesthesiologists use iNO routinely for lung transplantation,[181] while others believe its potential adverse side effects should lead to restriction of its use.[182] Proponents argue that use of iNO in the recipient, and possibly even the donor, takes advantage of immunomodulatory and antimicrobial activities of NO that reduce recipient lung injury.[183] Opponents argue that iNO use should be limited to the population at risk for needing CPB during lung transplantation and to patients with reperfusion injury. They cite risks of methemoglobinemia, NO-metabolite–related lung injury, and decreased sensitivity of exhaled NO monitoring as a diagnostic tool for acute lung rejection. Although small studies have suggested benefit of prophylactic iNO, a randomized clinical trial of 30 patients undergoing double-lung transplant at an institution with high usage of CPB showed no benefit of prophylactic iNO in prevention of pulmonary edema.[184]

NO may mediate other clinically beneficial effects. NO activates guanylate cyclase in platelets to attenuate platelet aggregation and adhesion.[185] iNO can decrease pulmonary vascular resistance, improve oxygenation, decrease inflammatory response to surgery or trauma, impede microbial growth, and have a vasodilatory effect limited only to the pulmonary system. Its use in successful management of lung transplant patients is well documented.[186,187]

Heart–lung Transplant (Adult and Pediatric)

Heart–lung transplantation is the least common intrathoracic transplant procedure, with only 72 reported for 2005 to 2006.[188] Bilateral sequential lung transplant has largely replaced heart–lung transplantation and improved pharmacologic management of pulmonary hypertension. RV failure obviates the need for the heart–lung procedure. As indications for lung transplantation have evolved to replace heart–lung transplant for diagnoses such as primary pulmonary hypertension and CF, congenital heart disease and acquired heart disease are increasingly common indications for heart–lung transplantation.[189] Most pediatric heart–lung transplants are currently performed for children aged 11 to 17 years. The use of this procedure for CF is rapidly diminishing, leaving pulmonary vascular disease and congenital heart disease as the main indications for pediatric heart–lung transplantation.[189] Anesthetic management of these patients is similar to that of isolated heart or lung transplant patients. Because a tracheal anastomosis is performed, a single-lumen endotracheal tube is sufficient. The endotracheal tube is either removed or withdrawn above the suture line during CPB to facilitate the tracheal anastomosis. Inotropes may be needed for RV dysfunction immediately after bypass. Pulmonary reperfusion injury can also occur, requiring management of acute lung injury as described for lung transplantation.

HEART TRANSPLANTATION

The South African pioneer of heart transplant (HT) surgery, Christiaan Barnard, performed the first human HT on December 3, 1967,[190] marking a momentous breakthrough in modern medicine and technology. Subsequently, Norman Shumway, the father of HT in the United States, was the first to successfully carry out the procedure in 1968.[191] This accomplishment was the result of many years of early groundbreaking experimental work by Alexis Carrel, who invented the first perfusion pump, opening the way to organ transplantation, as well as Frank Mann, Richard Lower, and many more. Recent HT history has been marked by tremendous insights and advances in all aspects, including donor allocation and selection criteria, surgical technique, as well as immunosuppression, which have improved survival significantly.[80]

As of June 30, 2010, the total number of heart transplants reported to the International Society for Heart and Lung Transplantation Registry was 100,210.[192] Currently, the number of patients on the wait list reported by UNOS is 3,171. With improving techniques and addition of immunosuppression for HT, 1-year survival is approaching 90% and 7-year survival 75%.[193] In the past 5 years, the disease processes for which cardiac transplantation is

TABLE 51-9. STAGES IN THE DEVELOPMENT OF HEART FAILURE WITH RECOMMENDED THERAPY BY STAGE

Stage	Risk Classification	Therapeutic Intervention
A	High risk for developing HF (hypertension, DM or lipid disorders)	Lifestyle modification and appropriate drug therapy such as angiotensin blockers and statins.
B	Asymptomatic patients with structural heart disease (Previous MI, LV dysfunction, valvular heart disease)	Lifestyle modification, disease-modifying drug therapy, and possibly an implantable defibrillator.
C	Symptomatic patients with structural heart disease (dyspnea and fatigue, impaired exercise tolerance)	Routine drug therapy (diuretics), selective drug therapy (aldosterone antagonists, hydralazine, and nitrates) and biventricular pacemakers and implantable defibrillators.
D	Refractory HF despite maximal medical or resynchronization therapy.	Therapeutic options in this high-risk cohort include end-of-life care, chronic intravenous inotropic support, permanent mechanical support, SVR, and HT.

HF, heart failure; LV, left ventricle; MI, myocardial infarction; DM, diabetes mellitus; SVR, surgical ventricular restoration; HT, heart transplantation.

Adapted from: Jessup M, Abraham WT, Casey DE, et al. 2009 focused update: ACCF/AHA Guidelines for the Diagnosis and Management of Heart Failure in Adults: A report of the American College of Cardiology Foundation/American Heart Association Task Force on Practice Guidelines: Developed in collaboration with the International Society for Heart and Lung Transplantation. *Circulation.* 2009;119:1977.

indicated have changed significantly and can currently be divided into the following categories: nonischemic cardiomyopathy 53.3%, ischemic cardiomyopathy 37.7%, congenital heart disease 2.9%, valvular cardiomyopathy 2.7%, retransplantation 2.6%, miscellaneous 0.8%.[194]

Nontransplant Therapies for Heart Failure

Changes in clinical management of heart failure (HF) in the past decade, along with insights into outcomes after HT after decades of the procedure, have resulted in a new management strategy for patients with HF. The American College of Cardiology (ACC) and American Heart Association (AHA) collaborated to develop a staging system for HF and therapy, and therapies are based on this stage of disease severity (Table 51-9).[195]

Nonsurgical treatment options to improve ventricular function in patients with HF include neurohormonal inhibition with angiotensin-converting enzyme inhibitors, β-blockers, as well as cardiac resynchronization therapy. New drugs in the commercialization process target other molecular pathways, including relaxin and tumor necrosis factor–like weak (TWEAK) inducer of apoptosis, a multifunctional cytokine. Relaxin, an endogenous peptide, mediates systemic vasodilatation and improved renal function in the setting of HF through production of nitric oxide, inhibition of endothelin, and inhibition of angiotensin II.[196] An early clinical trial of relaxin in HF patients demonstrated decreases in pulmonary wedge pressure and improvements in cardiac index.[197] TWEAK, a member of the TNF superfamily of cytokines,[198] acts at the receptor fibroblast growth factor–inducible molecule 14 (Fn14). Fn14, a highly inducible cell-surface receptor, normally regulates various physiologic processes. In particular, it seems to play an important beneficial role in tissue repair following acute injury.[199,200] Another regimen that has proven helpful for increasing cardiac function in HF patients is the combination of phosphodiesterase-3 inhibitor, enoximone, and β-blockade, which retained myocardial inotropy.[201,202]

Cardiac resynchronization therapy (CRT) has developed a larger role in the most recent ACC/AHA guidelines for medical treatment of patients with late stages of HF. In support of the guidelines, the Comparison of Medical Therapy, Pacing and Defibrillation in Heart Failure trial demonstrated a significantly reduced hospitalization and death rate in advanced, chronic HF patients treated with CRT.[203,204] Although CRT and new pharmacologic agents have improved the quality of life in HF patients, surgical procedures or ventricular-assist devices are still required for a subset of HF patients.

Surgical ventricular restoration is a procedure designed to remodel LV function through restoration of ventricular geometry in patients with a dilated LV. It has emerged as an alternative to HT for selected patients. The procedure requires identification of areas of left ventricular scarring, the boundary between damaged and healthy myocardium, and knowledge of the volume and size of the left ventricle.[205] A purse-string suture is placed to encircle the scar, and the healthy portions of the ventricular wall are approximated and joined together with or without a patch. Finally, the scarred ventricular wall is sutured over the patch for mechanical reinforcement. With this technique the mechanical consequences of a scarred myocardium are reduced, LV volume is reduced, and the LV is reshaped for a more functional geometry.[205]

Ventricular Assist Devices

The American Heart Association Statistics Committee and Stroke Statistics Subcommittee reported that there are >100,000 patients in the United States with end-stage HF, with an associated 5-year mortality as high as 50%.[206] Ventricular assist device (VAD) implantation, used as a bridge to transplantation, for clinical recovery or as a destination therapy (DT) has revolutionized treatment

TABLE 51-10. INTERMACS PATIENT PROFILES AND TIMING OF INTERVENTION

Patient Profile	Intervention
I. Critical cardiogenic shock despite maximal medical support	VAD intervention within hours
II. Progressive clinical decline despite inotropic support	VAD intervention within days
III. HF requiring mild to moderate inotropic dependence	Elective VAD implantation within weeks
IV. Recurrent HF that can be stabilized with medical intervention	Elective VAD intervention within months
V. Comfortable at rest and able to perform daily activities but exertion intolerant	Variable; depends on nutrition, organ function, and activity
VI. Exertion limited; able to perform mild activity, but fatigue results within a few minutes	Variable; depends on nutrition, organ function, and activity
VII. Advanced NYHA functional class III	Mechanical circulatory support is not indicated at this time

HF, heart failure; VAD, ventricular assist device; NYHA, New York Heart Association.
Adapted from: Stevenson et al.

for patients who cannot be weaned from inotropic therapy or restored to New York Heart Association class III despite medical therapy optimization or for those who are not transplant candi-
11 dates.[207] The utilization of these devices has seen rapid growth in recent years, with DT especially becoming more frequent.

In 2005 a VAD registry, the Interagency Registry for Mechanical Assisted Circulatory Support (INTERMACS), was established to manage, track, and refine VAD placements nationwide and has since been updated.[208] INTERMACS recently provided seven clinical profiles to identify severity of HF and provide a platform for the assessment of VAD implantation risk (Table 51-10).[209–211]

VADs have three main clinical applications: bridge to transplant (BTT), bridge to recovery (BTR), and DT.[207] Because of the shortage of organ donors for heart transplants, BTT application is not common. BTR is also limited and depends on the extent of myocardial injury and the etiology of disease. However, with improved technology, the greatest potential for VAD therapy is DT for the refractory HF population who are ineligible for cardiac transplant and can benefit from long-term support.

The landmark Randomized Evaluation of Mechanical Assistance for the Treatment of Congestive Heart Failure (REMATCH) clinical trial reported an 81% improvement in survival and improved quality of life of terminally ill HF patients with implanted heart pumps versus optimal medical management.[212] A DT study following the REMATCH trial demonstrated an additional 17% improvement in 1-year survival of patients receiving the HeartMate XVE (Thoratec Corp., Pleasanton California).[213] The HeartMate II Left Ventricular Assist System has been extensively studied as BTT and DT for advanced heart failure. Results of the DT trial[214] showed 1-year survival of 68% and 2-year survival of 58% for treated patients, with significant improvements in quality of life and functional status.

Based on these findings, it is likely that anesthesiologists will see more patients for initial device placement, perioperative management of left ventricular assist devices (LVADs) and patients with VAD DT undergoing general surgical procedures. Criteria for VAD implantation are essentially the same as the definition of cardiogenic shock: Cardiac index <2 L/min, SVR >2,100 dyne/s/cm^5, pulmonary capillary wedge >20 mm Hg, systemic hypotension <80 mm Hg, or urine output <20 mL/hr with metabolic acidosis. The usual contraindications for device implantation include irreversible end-organ failure, advanced pulmonary disease unrelated to cardiac function, sepsis, and metastatic cancer.

Three generation of VADs are available. Some are Food and Drug Administration–approved for therapy, but others can only be used in the context of a regulated clinical trial. The first generation generally consists of pumps such as the Thoratec VAD (Thoratec, Pleasanton, California) or HeartMate (Thoratec, Pleasanton, California), which provide pulsatile flow. Second-generation VADs are smaller devices making use of electromechanical impellers to drive blood forward (e.g., HeartMate II, Jarvik 2000 [Jarvik Heart, New York]). The newest, third-generation devices are an upgrade of the previous instruments and utilize new technologies, including bearingless, magnetically, and/or hydrodynamically suspended impellers that minimize heat generation and improve durability. VADs vary in significant ways according to location of device (intra-, extra- or paracorporeal), the source of driving power (pneumatic or electric), the level of anticoagulation required (none, aspirin, warfarin), flow range, filling pattern (fill-to-empty or various other modes), and power source (battery or alternating current). A number of reviews are available for further information on the different devices and management issues.[215,216]

A brief summary of key considerations for VADs is included here. VADs are usually positioned in parallel with the circulation. LVADs are positioned with the inflow cannula in either the left atrium or left ventricle and drains to the pump (Fig. 51-4). The outflow cannula returns blood to the patient via an anastomosis with the ascending aorta. Right VADs (RVADs) are similar, however, the inflow cannula is placed in the right atrium or right ventricle with drainage to the pump. The outflow cannula returns blood to the patient via an anastomosis with the main PA. In nonpulsatile axial flow pumps (e.g., HeartMate II), the operation is based on a rotating impeller pump, which drives blood to the systemic circulation at a fixed rate depending on pump speed and the inflow–outflow pressure gradient. The advantages of these systems are that they are smaller, more durable, and they typically

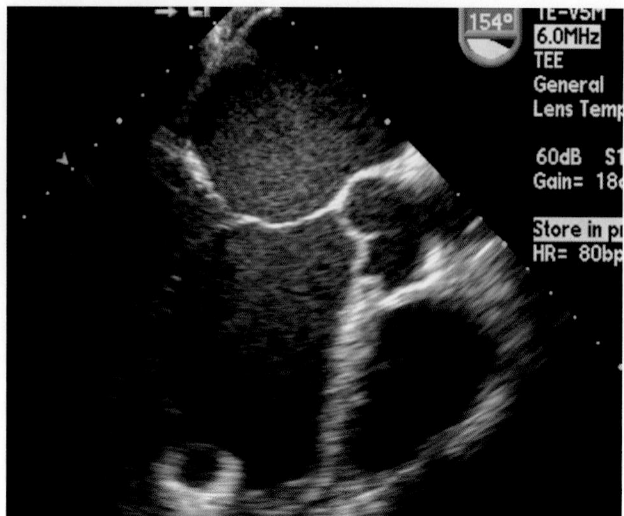

FIGURE 51-4. Echo 1: Midesophageal long axis view showing the left ventricular assist device inflow cannula in the left ventricle apex.

generate higher flows at lower pressures. The systems require low-dose anticoagulation and are suitable for patients with a body surface area of <1.2 m^2.[217–219]

LVAD pump flow is directly affected by intravascular volume and afterload. Failure to correct hypovolemia and increased afterload will result in decreased LVAD flow and hypotension because of low functional cardiac output. Often a perfusionist or a dedicated VAD nurse is available for device management and troubleshooting in the OR. Patients presenting for VAD implantation have myriad medical problems in various stages of decompensated HF. There is frequently an associated elevation in PVR and impaired RV function as well as impaired hepatic function or coagulopathy, renal insufficiency, and reduced response to catecholamines.

Intraoperative management of LVAD patients requires a protocol including availability of blood products (packed red blood cells, FFP, and platelets). Invasive monitoring is required, often inclusive of an arterial line, large-bore introducer with PAC, or a second central venous catheter in the setting of difficult venous access.

TEE plays a central role in VAD implantation both pre-CPB and post-CPB. The pre-CPB examination includes an evaluation for any intracardiac shunts. An unrecognized, untreated intracardiac shunt can lead to significant hypoxemia in the post-CPB period. Evaluation of aortic valve competency is important, as aortic insufficiency will cause recirculation through an LVAD and poor systemic perfusion. Therefore, an incompetent aortic valve should be oversewn or replaced. Lastly, right ventricular function should be assessed as well as evaluation for cardiac thrombus and aortic atheroma.

Post-CPB TEE examination should focus on adequate deairing, evaluation of inflow cannula position, and a recheck for patent foramen ovale. Confirmation of proper LVAD function includes evaluating LV decompression, aortic valve closure during LVAD systole, and outlet cannula presence in the aorta with appropriate flow. Epinephrine, norepinephrine, and other resuscitation drugs should be available. NO should be available in the event of right heart failure (Fig. 51-5).[216,220] Anesthesiologists and intensivists should be aware of recent studies showing that, with the increasing use of an axial flow LVAD as a DT, patients can develop an acquired von Willebrand factor deficiency.[221,222] Cerebral hyperperfusion and consequent neurologic dysfunction are also risks after LVAD implantation.[223]

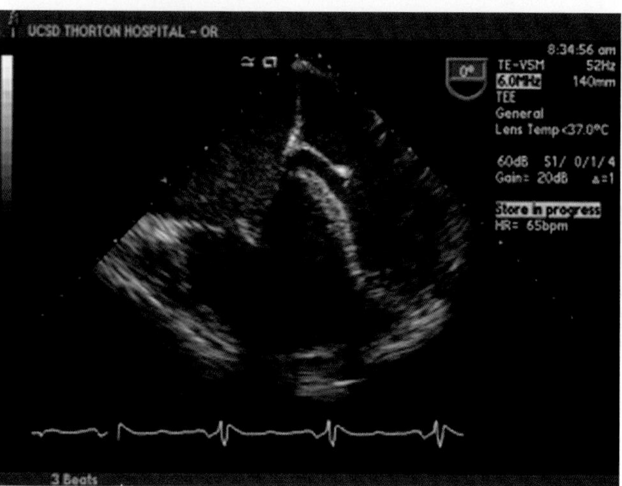

FIGURE 51-5. Echo 2: Massive right ventricle dilation, paradoxical septum motion with or without an empty left ventricle.

The Tandem Heart (Cardiac Assist Inc., Pittsburgh, Pennsylvania) is a percutaneous ventricular assist device usually placed in a cardiac catheterization laboratory or in the OR. The indications are short-term hemodynamic support (from a few hours up to 14 days), giving the heart time to recover and potentially regain native function. The left-sided inflow cannula is advanced from the femoral vein into the left atrium by puncturing the interatrial septum. The outflow cannula is placed in the femoral artery. With this device, the activated clotting time is usually maintained at 200 sec.[224]

The Total Artificial Heart (SynCardia Systems, Inc., Tucson, Arizona) is used as a bridge to transplantation in patients with irreversible biventricular failure[225] in a few specialized centers across the United States (Fig. 51-6).

Heart Transplant Recipient Selection

Medical therapy of CHF, together with the evolving field of mechanical circulatory support, has yielded dramatically improved nontransplant options for patients and consequently
12 changed the selection criteria and considerations for HT. According to guidelines released in 2011 by the Registry of the International Society for Heart and Lung Transplantation, nonischemic

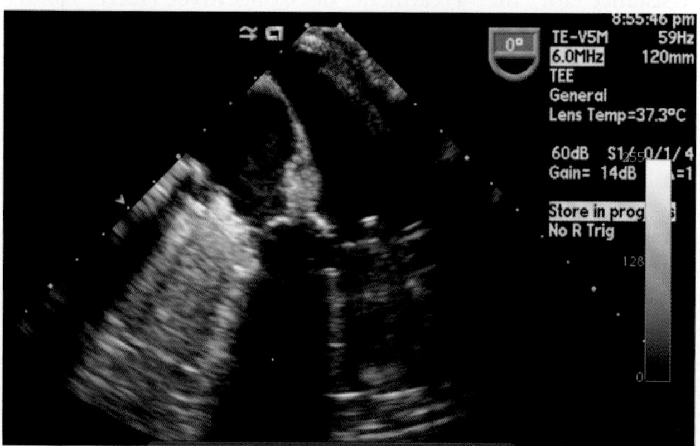

FIGURE 51-6. Echo 3: Total artificial heart.

cardiomyopathy was the most common indication for HT from January 2005 to June 2010, a shift from the previous registry report that documented ischemic cardiomyopathy as the most common diagnosis.[194] Although the median age for transplant recipients has not changed significantly, the past decade has seen a considerable increase in the number of patients in their 60s and 70s undergoing HT. Between January 2002 and June 2010, 19% of the recipients received an LVAD preoperatively; this number increased dramatically to 30% in 2009.[194] With the advances made in cardiac surgery, an increasing number of congenital heart disease patient survive into adulthood. As a result, a higher percentage of these patients are receiving an HT. Donor demographics have changed in other ways. In 2009, 14% of donors were aged 50 to 60 years, compared with 4% of donors in this age group in 1990. In summary, the profile of the typical recent heart allograft recipient has changed dramatically so that anesthesiologists are likely to see patients on LVADs, more patients with congenital lesions, as well as a large subset of elderly transplant patients.

Donor heart placement is not done at the national level. Currently, the limited ischemic time of approximately 4 to 5 hours excludes a national sharing of donor hearts or matching donor hearts according to HLA compatibility.[226] The first step in donor placement is to rule out any contraindication to heart donation, including malignancies. The second step is to match a specific donor to a suitable transplant candidate.[226]

Size matching is especially important for recipients with pulmonary hypertension. Pulmonary hypertension is associated with increased perioperative mortality, so that severe, irreversible pulmonary hypertension (PVR >6 Wood units/m^2 and high transpulmonary gradient >15 mm Hg) is a contraindication to HT. Right heart catheterization is often utilized during recipient evaluation to determine the transpulmonary gradient. Severe recipient hepatic, renal, or pulmonary disease or any other major debilitating comorbid condition is a contraindication because of the effects of immunosuppressive agents on these organs. UNOS indications for cardiac transplant are patients requiring continuous mechanical or inotropic support, peak O_2 uptake <14 mL/kg/min, LVEF <20%, inoperable congenital heart disease, intractable malignant arrhythmias, and pulmonary vascular resistance <2 Wood units.

Surgical Technique in Heart Transplantation

The four main anastomosis of the HT procedure are the right and left atrial anastomoses and the end-to-end aortic and pulmonary anastomoses. There are two accepted surgical techniques for HT, the original biatrial technique first described by Lower and Shumway.[191,227] in 1960, which preserves portions of recipient's native atria to create two atrial anastomoses (Fig. 51-7). Sievers et al.[228] introduced the bicaval technique in 1991 in which the donor right atrium is attached directly to the inferior and superior vena cava and the left atrial anastomosis is done as a cuff (Fig. 51-8).[80] This technique better preserves atrial geometry, tricuspid annulus shape, and right ventricular function, with less tricuspid and mitral regurgitation and less conduction disturbances. Supported by several studies,[229,230] the latter technique has quickly gained popularity.

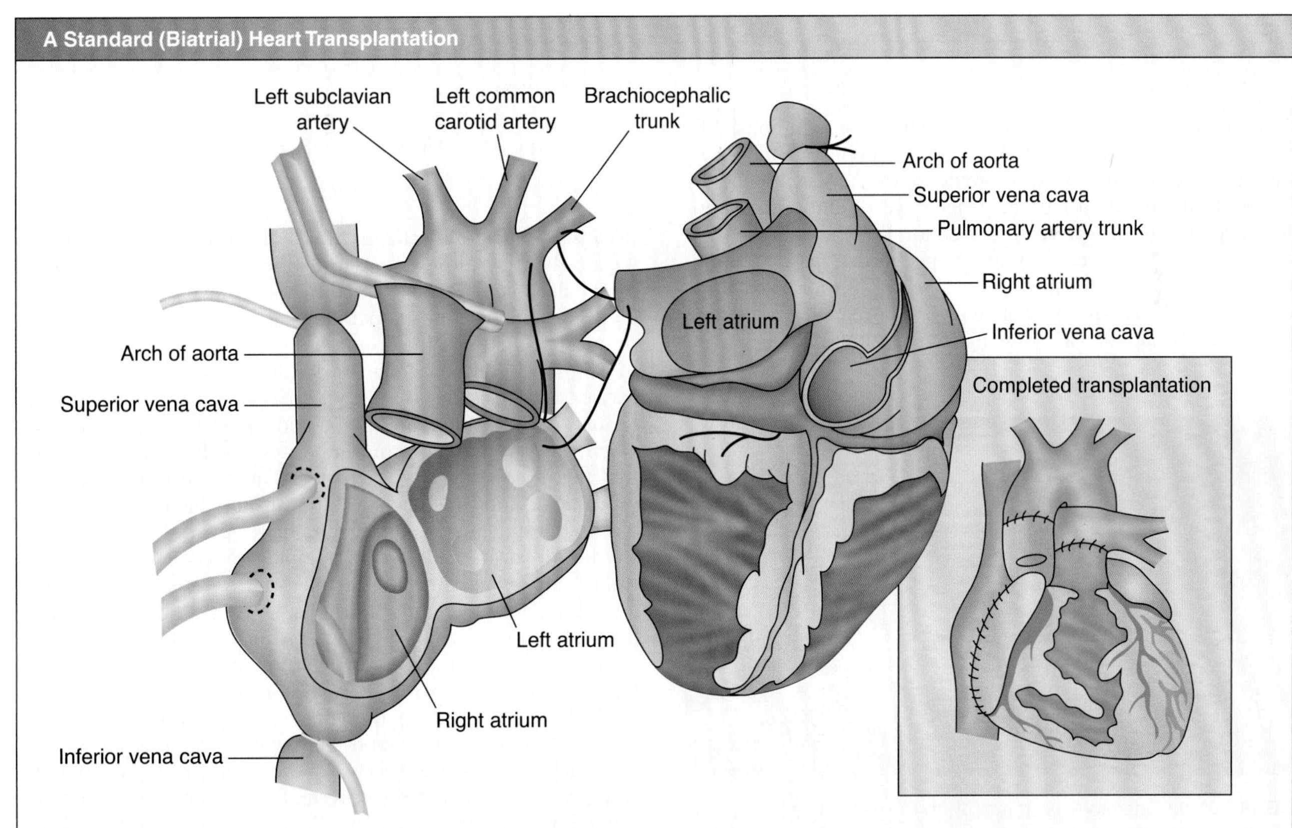

FIGURE 51-7. Biatrial technique. Reprinted with permission from *N Engl J Med.* 2006;355:3.

ANESTHESIA FOR SURGICAL SUBSPECIALTIES

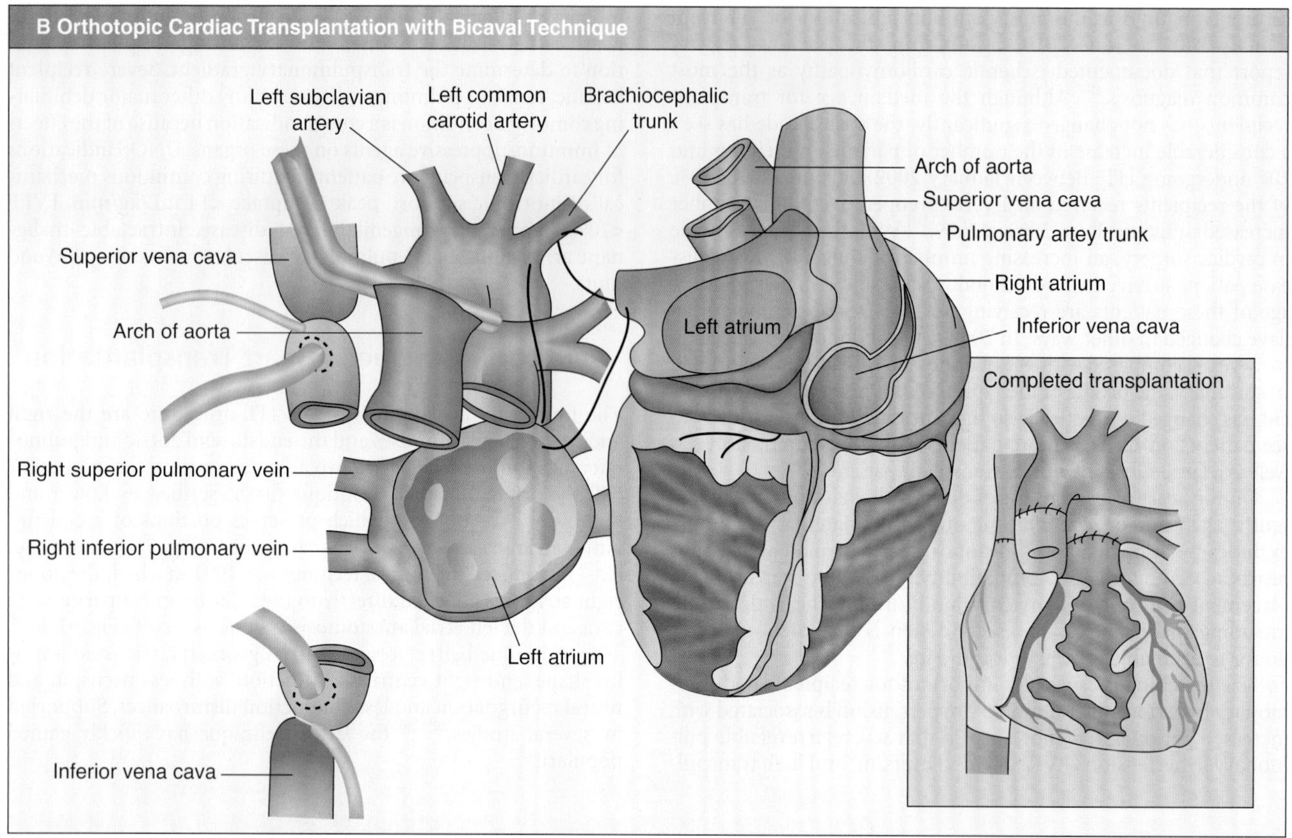

FIGURE 51-8. Bicaval technique. Reprinted with permission from *N Engl J Med.* 2006;355:3.

There are two approaches for HT. The most common is the orthotopic approach, in which the donor heart is placed in the normal anatomic location. The heterotopic approach is an infrequently utilized technique, indicated in patients with significant pulmonary hypertension to preserve the donor RV and in significant size mismatch, which can complicate pediatric transplantation.[80] The donor heart is implanted in the lower right thorax, resulting in two parallel circulations. Native RV supports right circulation, and donor RV supports left (systemic) circulation (Fig. 51-9).[231,232]

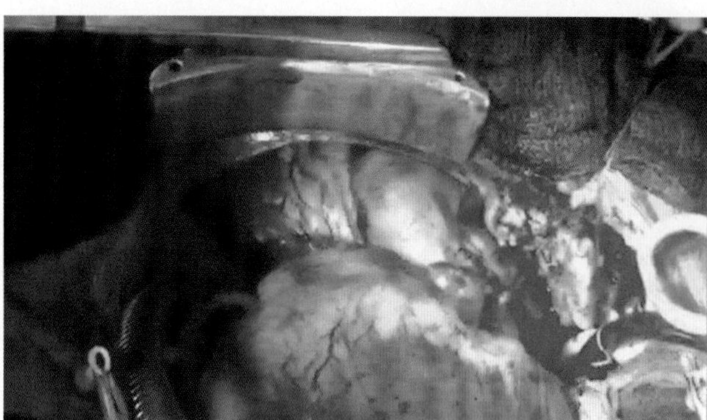

FIGURE 51-9. Heterotopic heart transplant. The transplanted heart is the one in the right chest, under the retractor. It sits in the right pleural cavity, the original native heart is the one in the normal anatomical position.

Anesthetic Management for Heart Transplantation

Because donor cold ischemia times of more than 4 to 5 hours negatively affect donor heart function, heart transplantation is essentially an emergency procedure requiring expeditious preoperative evaluation and preparation of the recipient. Close communication between the donor and recipient teams is important to minimize graft ischemia times. Ideally, the recipient heart is excised as soon as the donor heart arrives at the recipient hospital. Induction of recipient anesthesia and surgical incision are made when the donor team communicates the final determination that the donor organ is acceptable. Timing decisions are based on distance and time necessary to transport the donor organ, as well as the time it takes to prepare the recipient. History of prior sternotomy or difficult airway can increase recipient preparation time. When evaluating the recipient, a few issues need special attention: Nothing by mouth status, level of cardiovascular support (inotropic infusions, chronic medications for heart failure, presence of LVAD), and presence of hemodynamic monitoring lines or antiarrhythmic devices, such as pacemaker, CRT device, or defibrillator. Antiarrhythmic devices need to be interrogated and reprogrammed to a mode that will not be affected by electrocautery interference. Because of the emergency nature of these cases, patients frequently have recently eaten, and rapid-sequence induction may be necessary. Patients are frequently taking angiotensin-converting enzyme inhibitors, which could increase the risk of intraoperative hypotension, or anticoagulants, which can increase the risk of bleeding. Vasopressin or methylene blue infusions can be beneficial for treatment of angiotensin-converting enzyme inhibitor–induced vasoplegia, and FFP should be ordered if the INR is elevated.

Many anesthetic management issues related to the heart transplant patient are similar to those for open-heart surgeries (see Chapter 38). The notable differences are strictest attention to sterility and immunosuppression during HT and issues related to early donor heart function and denervation. The right or the left internal jugular venous (IJV) approach for a central line placement is appropriate; however, some surgeons prefer to leave the right IJV for future endomyocardial biopsies. PACs capable of monitoring continuous cardiac out and mixed venous oxygen saturation are preferable for intraoperative use as well as postoperative monitoring.

Antibiotics and immunosuppressive medications are usually given prior to incision. Large-bore intravenous access is necessary for administration of resuscitation medications if no central line is present for induction. Inotropes should be readily available prior to induction. Dobutamine, epinephrine, milrinone, norepinephrine, dopamine, vasopressin, and phenylephrine have all been used effectively in the perioperative management of HT patients. Presence of an LVAD or prior sternotomy increases the length and the risks associated with the procedure. Aminocaproic acid or tranexamic acid is used for antifibrinolytic effects to minimize bleeding and transfusions, especially in LVAD patients.

Intraoperative Management

The induction sequence is of critical importance, as patients presenting for HT are dependent on their endogenous sympathetic drive, so extreme caution with induction should be exercised.[233] High-dose narcotic techniques have been used for induction and management of cardiac transplant patients for many years with good results.[234] Balanced anesthetic techniques, using lower doses of narcotics, with etomidate and inhalation anesthetics, can be used as well.[235] Hypotension may not respond to standard vasopressors, and inotrope use should be rapidly instituted or increased if response to phenylephrine, for example, is inadequate.

A comprehensive TEE examination should be performed after induction of anesthesia and after weaning from CPB. The native heart can be monitored prior to CPB for changes in ventricular function or an increase in valvular regurgitation. Early diagnosis of deterioration can facilitate rapid therapy and hemodynamic stability. Manipulation of the heart is minimized prior to aortic cross-clamping if thrombus is noted.

Heparin dosing is similar to that for other CPB procedures. Cannulation of the aorta is performed high along the ascending aorta, near the aortic arch. The superior and inferior vena cavae are cannulated individually. By encircling the cavae with tourniquets, all blood flow is directed through the cannula into the bypass circuit, and the surgical field is bloodless. Prior to resection of the native heart, the PA catheter should be withdrawn from the surgical field. The catheter can be readvanced after removal of the superior caval cannula. Maintenance of CPB and weaning from CPB are associated with the same issues as for other cardiac surgical procedures. Ischemic time for the donor heart starts with aortic cross-clamp during the harvest and ends with removal of the cross-clamp from the recipient aorta. TEE is very useful for deairing and evaluation of ventricular, valvular, and intracardiac shunts prior to weaning from CPB. Because the donor heart is denervated, normal physiologic feedback loops controlling inotropy and chronotropy are lost. Isoproterenol is used frequently for its direct effects on cardiac β-receptors to increase graft heart rate. Temporary epicardial pacing is sometimes useful until isoproterenol has had adequate time to reach maximal effect. (Vasoactive drug effects in denervated hearts are reviewed in Table 51-11.) Residual native atrial tissue may continue to have electrical activity, seen clinically as two P waves on ECG. The native P wave has no physiologic effects on the donor heart. Inotrope selection for weaning from CPB is similar to other cardiac surgical procedures (see Chapter 38). Right ventricular failure is the most common complication encountered during weaning of CPB, indicated by high mean PA pressures exceeding 30 mm Hg. The risk of donor right heart failure is increased in these cases, as the donor right heart is not accustomed to high pulmonary resistance and may fail acutely. Therapy of right heart failure should be prompt and aggressive, and measures should be taken to reduce pulmonary vascular resistance and improve RV contractility.[236]

TABLE 51-11. EFFECT OF DENERVATION ON CARDIAC PHARMACOLOGY

	Effect On	
Substance	**Recipient**	**Mechanism**
Digitalis	Normal increase of contractility, minimal effect on atrioventricular node	Direct myocardial effect, denervation
Atropine	None	Denervation
Adrenaline	Increased contractility Increased chronotropy	Denervation hypersensitivity
Noradrenaline	Increased contractility Increased chronotropy	Denervation No neuronal uptake
Isoproterenol	Normal increase in contractility, normal increase in chronotropy	
Quinidine	No vagolytic effect	Denervation
Verapamil	Atrioventricular block	Direct effect
Nifedipine	No reflex tachycardia	Denervation
Hydralazine	No reflex tachycardia	Denervation
β-blocker	Increased antagonist effect	Denervation

Reprinted with permission from: Deng MC. Cardiac transplantation. *Heart.* 2002;287:177.

Adequate oxygenation and ventilation, avoidance of hypercarbia and acidosis, and maintenance of adequate perfusion pressure to the right ventricle are all fundamental.

If IV agents do not facilitate weaning from CPB, iNO and inhaled prostacyclin (iloprost) have been shown to be beneficial in this setting.[237–239] Failure to respond to these measures may indicate the need for mechanical right heart support.[240,241]

Pediatric Heart Transplantation

Heart transplant is now an accepted procedure in infants and children with a 5-year survival rate of ~70%. The latest International Registry for Heart and Lung Transplantation revealed 350 to 400 pediatric HT procedures are performed worldwide each year, representing about 10% of the total number of heart transplants.[189] The pretransplant diagnosis was congenital heart disease or idiopathic/viral cardiomyopathy in 75% of these patients. In the United States, retransplantation is an increasing indication. ECMO is used as a bridge to transplant at some centers, although it is acknowledged to be only a short-term option.[189] Although ECMO is the therapeutic choice for circulatory support in most pediatric cardiac patients, some pediatric patients (mostly adolescents) benefit from placement of a ventricular assist device.[242] Preoperative evaluation focuses on cardiopulmonary status and the particulars of the cardiac physiology in congenital heart disease patients (see Chapter 41) Palliative procedures may have been performed prior to transplant, and reoperation increases surgical risk. Central venous catheters and intra-arterial catheters are placed routinely, although frequently after induction. After an inhalation induction, anesthetic management frequently involves high-dose narcotics and intermittent benzodiazepines. Marginal donors are, not surprisingly, also being used for pediatric heart grafts, including size mismatches of over 3 times recipient body weight, high donor inotrope requirement, prolonged ischemic time, and ABO mismatch.[243–246] Hyperacute rejection does not occur because of the immaturity of the immune system and absence of preformed antibodies to various antigens, including blood group antigens. For ABO mismatched grafts, recipient isohemagglutinin titers are obtained pretransplantation, then plasma exchange is performed during CPB. Four-year follow-up data show similar morbidity and mortality compared with ABO-compatible recipients. Furthermore, waiting-list survival is improved because of expansion of the donor pool.

COMPOSITE TISSUE TRANSPLANTATION

Upper extremity or face transplantations are exceedingly complex procedures performed only in a few centers. To date, 26 upper extremity transplants have been performed. Anesthesiologists should be involved in perioperative protocol development for these new procedures from the initial planning stages of a program, especially because well-planned regional nerve blocks can be very useful for upper extremity transplants and other anesthesia-specific concerns can be addressed in advance.[247] Limb transplants recipients may be heparinized.[247] Bilateral limb allografts expose the recipient to two reperfusion events. The common feature of these grafts is that they contain multiple organs (blood vessels, nerves, muscle, skin). Multiple anastomoses imply a very long surgical procedure. Composite tissue recipients require intense immunosuppression, in part because the skin is highly antigenic, and some immunosuppressants that are unfamiliar to anesthesiologists may be administered intraoperatively. In addition to complex triple-drug immunosuppression, at least one center uses donor marrow infusions in an effort to induce tolerance to the allograft. Another common feature of composite tissue transplants generally is the potential for massive blood loss.

For face donors, surgeons prefer to procure the face first, before other organs are procured. The graft recovery is complex, with isolation of motor and sensory nerves, as well as venous and arterial vessels. Multiple surgeons are involved in both graft recovery and implantation. Recipient nose and mouth deformities will certainly require individualized airway care. Protocols for these patients are just being developed, but the choice of anesthetic and fluid management is directed at preventing microvasculature constriction and postoperative edema. A recent report of three successful face transplants highlights the immunologic complexity of this procedure. In addition to usual ABO matching, T- and B-cell matching was performed and an induction regimen of mycophenolate mofetil, ATG, and methylprednisolone was used.[249]

Management of the Transplant Patient for Nontransplant Surgery

As the population of transplant recipients increases, the incidence of elective or emergent nontransplant surgery in this group will also increase. These patients cannot always return to the transplant center for surgery, so anesthesiologists outside transplant centers will encounter these patients.

For solid-organ recipients, evaluation of patients is centered on the function of the grafted organ. In renal and liver transplant patients, the level of renal dysfunction will often determine the choice of drugs, particularly neuromuscular blockers, and dose modification of drugs is dependent on renal excretion, such as antibiotics. Table 51-12 lists medications that can cause renal dysfunction when administered to a patient receiving immunosuppressive agents. A major consideration for renal transplant recipients is maintenance of renal perfusion with adequate volume replacement. Thus, CVP monitoring is useful for preventing prerenal damage to transplanted kidneys, but CVP lines must be placed using strict aseptic technique. It is important to note that signs of infection may be masked in transplant patients. Failing, rejecting, or reinfected liver grafts are often accompanied by deterioration of renal function. Protection of the kidneys is a central part of anesthesia

TABLE 51-12. DRUGS THAT MAY CAUSE RENAL DYSFUNCTION WHEN COADMINISTERED WITH CALCINEURIN INHIBITORS

Amphotericin	Cotrimoxazole
Cimetidine	Vancomycin
Ranitidine	Tobramycin
Melphalan	Gentamicin
Nonsteroidal anti-inflammatory drugs	

Adapted with permission from: Kostopanagiotou G, Smyrniotis V, Arkadopoulos N, et al. Anesthetic and perioperative management of adult transplant recipients in non-transplant surgery. *Anesth Analg.* 1999;89:613.

TABLE 51-13. DRUGS AFFECTING CYCLOSPORINE OR TACROLIMUS BLOOD LEVELS

Increase Blood Levels	Decrease Blood Levels
Bromocriptine	Carbamazepine
Chloroquine[a]	Octreotide[a]
Cimetidine[b]	Phenobarbital
Clarithromycin	Phenytoin
Cotrimoxazole	Rifampin
Danazol	Ticlopidine
Erythromycin	
Fluconazole	
Itraconazole	
Ketoconazole	
Metoclopramide	
Nicardipine	
Verapamil	

[a]Reported with cyclosporine; may not interact with tacrolimus.
[b]May not interact with cyclosporine.

plans, and CVP or TEE is useful to guide fluid replacement, especially in cases where large fluid shifts are anticipated.

13 For all transplant recipients, antibiotic, antiviral, antifungal, and immune suppression regimens should be disrupted as little as possible in the perioperative period. The types of infection to which transplant recipients are susceptible change over time, with donor-derived and hospital-acquired infections predominating in the first posttransplant month.[249] Infections acquired by transplant patients in months 2 to 6 versus later after transplantation are also distinct, and these patterns should guide surgical prophylaxis and perioperative diagnostic procedures. Infectious disease specialists are important consults in preoperative transplant patients. A study of solid-organ transplant patients who developed appendicitis highlights the risks of infection in this population: Transplant recipients are likely to have more complications and longer hospital stays.[250] Complications of immune suppression are reviewed in Table 51-4, and important drug interactions with calcineurin inhibitors in Table 51-13. Significant intraoperative fluid shifts can cause an acute decrease in cyclosporine or tacrolimus blood levels. In these cases, consideration should be given to repeat testing of drug levels during the day of surgery. Nonsteroidal anti-inflammatory medications should be avoided for a number of reasons. First, many patients have underlying renal dysfunction related to immunosuppressive agents. Second, the risk of gastrointestinal hemorrhage is increased in patients already at risk for gastritis from chronic steroids.

Patients who present for surgery with signs of acute rejection or infection may benefit from delay of surgery to optimize their status. Both rejection and infection in the face of surgery are associated with increased risk of morbidity and mortality. Regional and general anesthetic techniques have been used successfully in posttransplant patients. In addition to the standard ASA monitors, invasive monitors should be used if warranted based on surgical procedure and general health status of the patient. Invasive monitoring is not indicated solely on the basis of prior transplantation. Nasal intubation should be avoided because of the potential risk for infection presented by nasal flora.

Virtually all liver diseases can recur in grafted livers, including autoimmune diseases, fatty liver, and especially hepatitis C. The degree of liver dysfunction from recurrent disease should be evaluated with hepatologists and by using standard laboratory tests.

For lung transplant recipients with a tracheal anastomosis, denervation has occurred below the level of the suture line, and the cough reflex is diminished or absent. These patients are at increased risk of retained secretions and pneumonia and have an increased airway hyperreactivity and bronchospasm. Because most lung transplants are now being done with bronchial instead of tracheal anastomoses, the risk of tracheal suture line stenosis or disruption with manipulation is markedly diminished. Advantages of regional anesthetic techniques in lung transplant patients include minimization of airway manipulation and decreased infectious risk.

Comparison of preoperative PFT, arterial blood gas, and CXR results with prior studies can help diagnose acute infection or rejection. Significant decreases in forced expiratory volume in 1 second, vital capacity and total lung capacity, and an obstructive pattern may indicate acute rejection. Arterial blood gas in the presence of rejection will show an increased A–a (Alveolar–arterial) gradient from stable baseline gases, along with perihilar infiltration on CXR. However, rejection and infection can be difficult to distinguish clinically. If the patient is suspected of having an active pulmonary process, consultation with pulmonary medicine for a possible diagnostic bronchoscopy should be considered prior to surgery.

Transplanted hearts are denervated, impacting perioperative management significantly. The transplanted heart cannot respond to indirect acting agents, such as ephedrine and even dopamine, or to peripheral attempts to induce hemodynamic changes, such as carotid massage, Valsalva maneuver, or laryngoscopy. β-effects of epinephrine and norepinephrine are exaggerated in heart transplant recipients (vs. α-effects). Isoproterenol is the mainstay of chronotropic therapy in these patients. ECG analysis may show two P waves, one from the native atrium and one from the implanted atrium. The native P wave will not conduct to the implanted heart, and these nonconducted P waves should not be confused with complete heart block. Isoproterenol should be available as an inotrope and chronotrope. Dobutamine can also be helpful; norepinephrine and epinephrine should be reserved for refractory cardiogenic shock. Because the denervated heart does not reflexively compensate for hemodynamic changes induced by regional anesthetics, general anesthesia is usually preferred.

Preoperative evaluation of heart transplant recipients should focus on cardiac functional status. Significant rejection will present with symptoms of heart failure. All heart transplant patients should be evaluated with ECG and transthoracic echocardiography prior to surgery. New findings should be discussed with the cardiology consultant to determine the need for stress testing or myocardial biopsy. Invasive monitors should be placed only when warranted by the clinical status and surgical procedure. CVP or, increasingly, TEE monitoring is helpful in managing fluid resuscitation and inotropic support.

References

1. A definition of irreversible coma. Report of the Ad Hoc Committee of the Harvard Medical School to Examine the Definition of Brain Death. *JAMA*. 1985;205:337.
2. Hevesi Z, Lopukhin SY, Giuditta A, et al. Supportive care after brain death for the donor candidate. *Int Anesthesiol Clin*. 2006;4:21.
3. Nijboer WN, Schuurs TA, van der Hoeven JAB, et al. Effect of brain death and donor treatment on organ inflammatory response and donor organ viability. *Curr Opin Organ Transpl*. 2004;9:110.
4. Belzberg H, Shoemaker WC, Wo CCJ, et al. Hemodynamic and oxygen transport patterns after head trauma and brain death: Implications for management of the organ donor. *J Trauma*. 2007;63:1032.
5. Novitzky D, Cooper DK, Rosendale JD, et al. Hormonal therapy of the brain-dead organ donor: Experimental and clinical studies. *Transplantation*. 2006;82:1396.

6. Rosendale JD, Kauffman HM, McBride MA, et al. Aggressive pharmacologic donor management results in more transplanted organs. *Transplantation.* 2003;75:482.
7. Salim A, Vassiliu P, Velmahos GC, et al. The role of thyroid hormone administration in potential organ donors. *Arch Surg.* 2001;136:1377.
8. Kutsogiannis DJ, Pagliarello G, Doig C, et al. Medical management to optimize donor organ potential: review of the literature. *Can J Anesth.* 2006;53:820.
9. Blasi-Ibanez A, Hirose R, Feiner J, et al. Predictors associated with terminal renal function in deceased organ donors in the intensive care unit. *Anesthesiology.* 2009; 110:333.
10. Ranasinghe AM, Bonser RS. Endocrine changes in brain death and transplantation. *Best Pract Res Clin Endocrinol Metab.* 2011;25:799.
11. Zaroff JG, Rosengard BR, Armstrong WF, et al. Maximizing use of organs recovered from the cadaveric donor: Cardiac recommendations. Consensus Conference Report, Crystal City, VA, March 28–29, 2001. *Circulation.* 2002;106:836.
12. Mascia L, Pasero D, Slutsky AS, et al. Effect of a lung protective strategy for organ donors on eligibility and availability of lungs for transplantation: A randomized controlled trial. *JAMA.* 2010;304:2620.
13. Blasco V, Leone M, Antonini F, et al. Comparison of the novel hydroxyethylstartch 130/0.4 and hydroxyethylstarch 200/0.6 in brain-dead donor resuscitation on renal function after transplantation. *Br J Anaesth.* 2008;100:504.
14. Figueras J, Busquets J, Grande L, et al. The deleterious effect of donor high plasma sodium and extended preservation in liver transplantation: A multivariate analysis. *Transplantation.* 1993;61:410.
15. Schnulle P, Gottmann U, Hoeger S, et al. Effects of donor pretreatment with dopamine on graft function after kidney transplantation: A randomized controlled trial. *JAMA.* 2009;302:1067.
16. Todd TR, Goldberg M, Koshal A, et al. Separate extraction of cardiac and pulmonary grafts from a single donor. *Ann Thorac Surg.* 1988;46:356.
17. Orens JB, Boehler A, Perrot M, et al. A review of lung transplant donor criteria. *J Heart Lung Transplant.* 2003;22:1183.
18. Harjula A, Baldwin JC, Starnes VA, et al. Proper donor selection for heart-lung transplantation. The Stanford experience. *J Thorac Cardiovasc Surg.* 1987;94: 874.
19. Bhorade SM, Vigneswaran W, McCabe MA, et al. Liberalization of donor criteria may expand the donor pool without adverse consequence in lung transplantation. *J Heart Lung Transplant.* 2000;19:1200.
20. Studer SM, Orens JB. Cadaveric donor selection and management. *Semin Respir Crit Care Med.* 2006;27:492.
21. Sekine Y, Waddell TK, Matte-Martyn A, et al. Risk quantification of early outcome after lung transplantation: Donor, recipient, operative, and post-transplant parameters. *J Heart Lung Transplant.* 2004;23:96.
22. Klein AS, Messersmith EE, Ratner LE, et al. Organ donation and utilization in the United States, 1999–2008. *Am J Transplant.* 2010;10(pt2):973.
23. Committee on Non-Heart-Beating Transplantation II. *The Scientific and Ethical Basis for Practice and Protocols, Division of Health Care Services, Institute of Medicine: Non-heart-beating organ transplantation: Practice and protocols.* Washington, DC: National Academy Press; 2000.
24. Van Norman GA. Another matter of life and death: What every anesthesiologist should know about the ethical, legal, and policy implications of the non-heart-beating cadaver organ donor. *Anesthesiology.* 2003;98:763.
25. Reid AW, Harper S, Jackson CH, et al. Expansion of the kidney donor pool by using cardiac death donors with prolonged time to cardiorespiratory arrest. *Am J Transplant.* 2011;11:995.
26. Gagandeep S, Matsuoka L, Mateo R, et al. Expanding the donor kidney pool: Utility of renal allografts procured in a setting of uncontrolled cardiac death. *Am J Transplant.* 2006;6:1682.
27. Nunez JR, Varela A, del Rio F, et al. Bipulmonary transplants with lungs obtained from two non-heart-beating donors who died out of hospital. *J Thorac Cardiovasc Surg.* 2004;127:297.
28. Lewis J, Peltier J, Nelson H, et al. Development of the University of Wisconsin donation after cardiac death evaluation tool. *Prog Transplant.* 2003;13:265.
29. Abt P, Kashyap R, Orloff M, et al. Pediatric liver and kidney transplantation with allografts from DCD donors: A review of UNOS data. *Transplantation.* 2006; 82:1708.
30. Saidi RF, Elias N, Kawai T, et al. Outcome of kidney transplantation using expanded criteria donors and donation after cardiac death. *Am J Transplant.* 2007; 7:2769.
31. Scaro AI, Wang E, Lyuksemburg V, et al. Donation after cardiac death liver transplantation: Time for policy to catch up with practice. *Liver Transpl.* 2012;18:5.
32. Wilson CH, Sanni A, Rix DA, et al. Laparoscopic versus open nephrectomy for live kidney donors. *Cochrane Database Syst Rev.* 2011;11:CD006124.
33. Ahearn AJ, Posselt AM, Kang SM, et al. Experience with laparoscopic donor nephrectomy among more than 1000 cases: Low complication rates, despite more challenging cases. *Arch Surg.* 2011;146:859.
34. Brook NR, Gibbons N, Nicol DL, et al. Open and laparoscopic donor nephrectomy: Activity and outcomes from all Australasian transplant centers. *Transplantation.* 2010;89:1482.
35. Mertens zur Borg IR, Di Biase M, Verbrugge S, et al. Comparison of three perioperative fluid regimes for laparoscopic donor nephrectomy: A prospective randomized dose-finding study. *Surg Endosc.* 2008;22:146.
36. Biancofiore G, Amorese G, Lugli D, et al. Laparoscopic live donor nephrectomy: The anaesthesiologist's perspective. *Eur J Anaesthesiol.* 2004;21:74.
37. Feldman LS, Anidiar M, Metrakos P, et al. Optimization of cardiac preload during laparoscopic donor nephrectomy: A preliminary study of central venous pressure versus esophageal Doppler monitoring. *Surg Endosc.* 2004;18:412.
38. El-Galley R, Hammontree L, Urban D, et al. Anesthesia for laparoscopic donor nephrectomy: Is nitrous oxide contraindicated? *J Urol.* 2007;178:225.
39. Feltracco P, Ori C. Anesthetic management of living transplantation. *Minerva Anestesiol.* 2010;76:525.
40. Haberal M, Emirolu R, Arslan G, et al. Living-donor nephrectomy under combined spinal-epidural anesthesia. *Transplantation.* 2002;34:2448.
41. Owen M, Lorgelly P, Serpell M. Chronic pain following donor nephrectomy—a study of the incidence, nature and impact of chronic post-nephrectomy pain. *Eur J Pain.* 2010;14:732.
42. Clavien PA, Petrowski H, DeOliveira ML, et al. Strategies for safer liver surgery and partial liver transplantation. *N Engl J Med.* 2007;356:1545.
43. Ayanoglu HO, Ulukaya S, Yuzer Y, et al. Anesthetic management and complications in living donor hepatectomy. *Transplant Proc.* 2003;35:2970.
44. Hwang S, Lee S-G, Lee Y-J, et al. Lessons learned from 1,000 living donor liver transplantations in a single center: How to make living donation safe. *Liver Transpl.* 2006;12:920.
45. Eyraud D, Richard O, Borie DC, et al. Hemodynamic and hormonal responses to the sudden interruption of caval flow: Insights from a prospective study of hepatic vascular exclusion during major liver resections. *Anesth Analg.* 2002;95:1173.
46. Rhim CH, Johnson LB, Kitisin K, et al. Intra-operative isovolemic hemodilution is safe and effective in eliminating allogeneic blood transfusion during right hepatic lobectomy: Comparison of living donor versus non-donors. *HPB (Oxford).* 2005;7:201.
47. Niemann CU, Roberts JP, Ascher NL, et al. Intraoperative hemodynamics and liver function in adult-to-adult living donor livers. *Liver Transpl.* 2002;8:1126.
48. Cammu G, Troisi R, Cuomo O, et al. Anaesthetic management and outcome in right-lobe living liver-donor surgery. *Eur J Anaesthesiol.* 2002;19:93.
49. Lentschener C, Ozier Y. Anaesthesia for elective liver resection: Some points should be revisited. *Eur J Anaesthesiol.* 2002;19:788.
50. Lutz JT, Valentin-Gamazo C, Gorlinger K, et al. Blood transfusion requirements and blood salvage in donors undergoing right hepatectomy for living related liver transplantation. *Anesth Analg.* 2003;96:351.
51. Ko JS, Gwak MS, Choi SJ, et al. The effects of desflurane and propofol-remifentanil on postoperative hepatic and renal functions after right hepatectomy in liver donors. *Liver Transpl.* 2008;14:1150.
52. Gouvea G, Diaz R, Auler L, et al. Perioperative coagulation profile in living liver donors as assessed by rotational thromboelastography. *Liver Transpl.* 2010;16:387.
53. Soubrane O, Cherqui D, Scatton O, et al. Laparoscopic left lateral sectionectomy in living donors:safety and reproducibility of the technique in a single center. *Ann Surg.* 2006;244:815.
54. Koffron AJ, Kung R, Baker T, et al. Laparoscopic-assisted right lobe donor hepatectomy. *Am J Transplant.* 2006;6:2522.
55. Nafidi O, Lepage R, Lapointe RW, et al. Hepatic resection-related hypophosphatemia is of renal origin as manifested by isolated hyperphosphaturia. *Ann Surg.* 2007;245:1000.
56. Trotter JF, Gillespie BW, Terrault NA, et al. Adult-to-Adult Living Donor Transplantation Cohort Study Group: Laboratory test results after living liver donation in the adult-to-adult living donor liver transplantation cohort study. *Liver Transpl.* 2011;17:409.
57. Barr ML, Belghiti J, Villamil FG, et al. A report of the Vancouver Forum on the care of the live organ donor: Lung, liver, pancreas, and intestine data and medical guidelines. *Transplantation.* 2006;81:1373.
58. Nishioka M, Yokoyama C, Iwasaki M, et al. Donor quality of life in living-donor lobar lung transplantation. *J Heart Lung Transplant.* 2011;30:1348.
59. Panther F, Strasen J, Czolbe M, et al. Inhibition of nuclear translocation of calcineurin suppresses T-cell activation and prevents acute rejection of donor hearts. *Transplantation.* 2011;91:597.
60. De Weerdt A, Claeys KG, De Jonghe P, et al. Tacrolimus-related polyneuropathy: Case report and review of the literature. *Clin Neurol Neurosurg.* 2008;110(3):291–294.
61. Wu Q, Marescaux C, Wolff V, et al. Tacrolimus-associated posterior reversible encephalopathy syndrome after solid organ transplantation. *Eur Neurol.* 2010; 64:169.
62. Sidi A, Kaplan RF, Davis RF. Prolonged neuromuscular blockade and ventilatory failure after renal transplantation and cyclosporine. *Can J Anaesth.* 1990;37:543.
63. Crosby E, Robblee JA. Cyclosporine-pancuronium interaction in a patient with a renal allograft. *Can J Anaesth.* 1998;35:300.
64. Kato T, Gaynor JJ, Yoshida H, et al. Randomization trial of steroid-free induction versus corticosteroid maintenance among orthotopic liver transplant recipients with hepatitis C virus: Impact on hepatic fibrosis progression at one year. *Transplantation.* 2007;84:829.
65. Klintmalm GB, Davis GL, Teperman L, et al. A randomized, multicenter study comparing steroid free immunosuppression and standard immunosuppression for liver transplant recipients with chronic hepatitis C. *Liver Transpl.* 2011;17: 1394.

66. Gaber AO, Monaco AP, Russell JA, et al. Rabbit antithymocyte globulin (Thymoglobulin[R]). *Drugs.* 2010;70:691.
67. Busani S, Rinaldi L, Begliomini B, et al. Thymoglobulin-induced severe cardiovascular reaction and acute renal failure in a patient scheduled for orthotopic liver transplantation. *Minerva Anestesiol.* 2006;72:243.
68. Boothpur R, Hardinger KL, Skelton RM, et al. Serum sickness after treatment with rabbit anti-thymocyte globulin in kidney transplant recipients with previous rabbit exposure. *Am J Kidney Dis.* 2010;55:141.
69. Wilde MI, Goa KL. Muromonab CD3: A reappraisal of its pharmacology and use as prophylaxis of solid organ transplant rejection. *Drugs.* 1996;51:865.
70. Bamgbola FO, Del Rio M, Kaskel FJ, et al. Non-cardiogenic pulmonary edema during basiliximab induction in three adolescent renal transplant patients. *Pediatr Transplant.* 2003;7:31.
71. Martin ST, Tichy EM, Gabardi S. Belatacept: A novel biologic for maintenance immunosuppression after renal transplantation. *Pharmacotherapy.* 2011;31:394.
72. Klipa D, Mahmud N, Ahsan N. Antibody immunosuppressive therapy in solid organ transplant: Part II. *MAbs.* 2010;2:607.
73. Farid SG, Barwick J, Goldsmith PJ. Alemtuzumab (Campath-1H)-induced coagulopathy in renal transplantation. *Transplantation.* 2009;87:1751.
74. Scandling JD, Busque S, Dejbakhsh-Jones S, et al. Tolerance and chimerism after renal and hematopoietic cell transplantation. *N Engl J Med.* 2008;358:362.
75. Barten MJ, Streit F, Boeger M, et al. Synergistic effects of sirolimus with cyclosporine and tacrolimus: Analysis of immunosuppression on lymphocyte proliferation and activation in rat whole blood. *Transplantation.* 2004;77:1154.
76. Tsunoda SM, Aweeka FT. Drug concentration monitoring of immunosuppressive agents: Focus on tacrolimus, mycophenolate mofetil and sirolimus. *BioDrugs.* 2000;14:355.
77. Jungling AS, Shangraw RE. Massive airway edema after azathioprine. *Anesthesiology.* 2000;92:888.
78. Engelen W, Verpooten GA, Van der Planken M, et al. Four cases of red blood cell aplasia in association with the use of mycophenolate mofetil in renal transplant patients. *Clin Nephrol.* 2003;60:119.
79. Perez-Aytes A, Ledo A, Boso V, et al. In utero exposure to mycophenolate mofetil: A characteristic phenotype? *Am J Med Genet A.* 2008;146:1.
80. Hunt SA, Haddad F. The changing face of heart transplantation. *J Am Coll Cardiol.* 2008;52:587.
81. Le Blanc K, Frassoni F, Ball L, et al. Mesenchymal stem cells for treatment of steroid-resistant, severe, acute graft-versus-host disease: A phase II study. *Lancet.* 2008;371:1579.
82. Skelton VA, Henderson K, Liu C. Anaesthetic implications of osteo-odontokeratoprosthesis surgery. *Eur J Anaesthesiol.* 2000;17:390.
83. Hunter K. Anesthesiology in renal and pancreas transplantation. *Curr Opin Organ Transpl.* 2003;8:243.
84. Dieterle CD, Schmauss S, Arbogast H, et al. Pulmonary function in patients with type 1 diabetes before and after simultaneous pancreas and kidney transplantation. *Transplantation.* 2007;83:566.
85. Bunnapradist S, Danovitch GM. Evaluation of adult kidney transplant candidates. *Am J Transplant.* 2007;7:2333.
86. Young A, Kim SJ, Speechley MR, et al; Donor Nephrectomy Outcomes Research (DONOR) Network. Accepting kidneys from older living donors: Impact on transplant recipient outcomes. *Am J Transplant.* 2011;11:743.
87. Ojo AO. Expanded criteria donors: process and outcomes. *Semin Dial.* 2005;18:463.
88. Bellingham JM, Santhanakrishnan C, Neidlinger N, et al. Donation after cardiac death: A 29-year experience. *Surgery.* 2011;150:692.
89. Snoeijs MG, Winkens B, Heemskerk MB, et al. Kidney transplantation from donors after cardiac death: A 25-year experience. *Transplantation.* 2010;90:1106.
90. Akpek EA, Kayhan Z, Donmez A, et al. Early postoperative renal function following renal transplantation surgery: Effect of anesthetic technique. *J Anesth.* 2002;16:114.
91. Goyal P, Puri GD, Pandey CK, et al. Evaluation of induction doses of propofol: Comparison between end stage renal disease and normal renal function patients. *Anaesth Intensive Care.* 2002;30:584.
92. Robertson EN, Driessen JJ, Vogt M, et al. Pharmacodynamics of rocuronium 0.3 mg kg (−1) in adult patients with and without renal failure. *Eur J Anaesthesiol.* 2005;22:929.
93. Fisher DM, Dempsey GA, Atherton DP, et al. Effect of renal failure and cirrhosis on the pharmacokinetics and neuromuscular effects of rapacuronium administered by bolus followed by infusion. *Anesthesiology.* 2000;93:1384.
94. SarinKapoor H, Kaur R, Kaur H. Anaesthesia for renal transplant surgery. *Acta Anaesthesiol Scand.* 2007;51:1354.
95. Olyaei AJ, deMattos AM, Bennett WM. A practical guide to the management of hypertension in renal transplant recipients. *Drugs.* 1999;58:1011.
96. Hadimioglu N, Saadawy I, Saglam T, et al. The effect of different crystalloid solutions on acid-base balance and early kidney function after kidney transplantation. *Anesth Analg.* 2008;107:264.
97. Parekh J, Niemann CU, Dang K, et al. Intraoperative hyperglycemia augments ischemia reperfusion injury in renal transplantation: A prospective study. *J Transplant.* 2011;2011:652458.
98. Wiesbauer F, Heinze G, Regele H, et al. Glucose control is associated with patient survival in diabetic patients after renal transplantation. *Transplantation.* 2010;89:612.
99. Sorbello M, Morello G, Paratore A, et al. Fenoldopam vs dopamine as a nephroprotective strategy during living donor kidney transplantation: Preliminary data. *Transplant Proc.* 2007;39:1794.
100. Nichols WG, Price TH, Gooley T, et al. Transfusion-transmitted cytomegalovirus infection after receipt of leukoreduced blood products. *Blood.* 2003;101:4195.
101. Parada B, Figueiredo A, Mota Am Furtado A. Surgical complications in 1000 renal transplants. *Transplant Proc.* 2003;35:1085.
102. Shoeibi G, Babakhani B, Mohammadi SS. The efficacy of ilioinguinal-iliohypogastric and intercostals nerve co-blockage for postoperative pain relief in kidney recipients. *Anesth Analg.* 2009;108:330.
103. Mukhtar K, Khattak I. Transversus abdominis plane block for renal transplant recipients. *Br J Anaesth.* 2010;104:663.
104. Masaitis-Zagaiewska A, Pietrasik P, Krawczyk J, et al. Similar prevalence but different characteristics of pain in kidney transplant recipients and chronic hemodialysis patients. *Clin Transplant.* 2011;25:E14.
105. Giessing M, Muller D, Winkelmann B, et al. Kidney transplantation in children and adolescents. *Transplant Proc.* 2007;39:2197.
106. Healey PJ, McDonald R, Waldhausen JH, et al. Transplantation of adult living donor kidneys into infants and small children. *Arch Surg.* 2000;135:1035.
107. Freeman RB Jr, Wiesner RH, Harper A, et al. UNOS/OPTN Liver Disease Severity Score, UNOS/OPTN Liver and Intestine, and UNOS/OPTN Pediatric Transplantation Committees: The new liver allocation system: Moving toward evidence-based transplantation policy. *Liver Transpl.* 2002;8:851.
108. Kemmer NM, Sherman KE. Liver transplantation trends in the HIV population. *Dig Dis Sci.* 2011;56:3393.
109. Diaz G, O'Connor M. Cardiovascular and renal complications in patients receiving a solid-organ transplant. *Curr Opin Crit Care.* 2011;17:382.
110. Kumar N, Dahri L, Brown W, et al. Effect of elective coronary angiography on glomerular filtration rate in patients with advanced chronic kidney disease. *Clin J Am Soc Nephrol.* 2009;4:1907.
111. Carey EJ, Steidley DE, Aqel BA, et al. Six-minute walk distance predicts mortality in liver transplant candidates. *Liver Transpl.* 2010;16:1373.
112. Coss E, Watt KDS, Pedersen R, et al. Predictors of cardiovascular events after liver transplantation: A role for pretransplant troponin levels. *Liver Transpl.* 2011;17:23.
113. Paramesh AS, Fairchild RB, Quinn TM, et al. Amelioration of hypertrophic cardiomyopathy using nonsurgical septal ablation in a cirrhotic patient prior to liver transplantation. *Liver Transpl.* 2005;11:236.
114. Rodriguez-Roisin R, Krowka MJ, Herve P, et al; ERS Task Force Pulmonary-Hepatic Vascular Disorders (PHD) Scientific Committee. Pulmonary-hepatic vascular disorders (PHD). *Eur Respir J.* 2004;24:861.
115. Ashfaq M, Chinnakotla S, Rogers L, et al. The impact of treatment of portopulmonary hypertension on survival following liver transplantation. *Am J Transplant.* 2007;7:1258.
116. Melgosa MT, Ricci GL, Garcia-Pagan JC, et al. Acute and long-term effects of inhaled iloprost in portopulmonary hypertension. *Liver Transpl.* 2010;16:348.
117. Makisalo H, Koivusalo A, Vakkuri A, et al. Sildenafil for portopulmonary hypertension in a patient undergoing liver transplantation. *Liver Transpl.* 2004;10:945.
118. Hoeper MM, Halank M, Marx C, et al. Bosentan therapy for portopulmonary hypertension. *Eur Respir J.* 2005;25:502.
119. Tapper EB, Knowles D, Heffron T, et al. Portopulmonary hypertension: Imatinib as a novel treatment and the Emory experience with this condition. *Transplant Proc.* 2009;41:1969.
120. Ramsay MA. Portopulmonary hypertension and hepatopulmonary syndrome, and liver transplantation. *Int Anesthesiol Clin.* 2006;44:69.
121. Pastor CM, Schiffer E. Therapy insight: Hepatopulmonary syndrome and orthotopic liver transplantation. *Nat Clin Pract Gastroenterol Hepatol.* 2007;4:614.
122. Fimiani B, Della Guardia D, Puoti C, et al. The use of terlipressin in cirrhotic patients with refractory ascites and normal renal function: A multicentric study. *Eur J Intern Med.* 2011;22:587.
123. Soriano V, Vispo E, Poveda E, et al. Directly acting antivirals against hepatitis C virus. *J Antimicrob Chemother.* 2011;66:1673.
124. Verne GN, Soldevia-Pico C, Robinson ME, et al. Autonomic dysfunction and gastroparesis in cirrhosis. *J Clin Gastroenterol.* 2004;38:72.
125. Aniskevich S, Shine TS, Feinglass NG, et al. Dynamic left ventricular outflow tract obstruction during liver transplantation: The role of transesophageal echocardiography. *J Cardiothorac Vasc Anesth.* 2007;21:577.
126. Massicotte L, Lenis S, Thibeault L, et al. Effect of low central venous pressure and phlebotomy on blood product transfusion requirements during liver transplantations. *Liver Transpl.* 2006;12:117.
127. Schroeder RA, Collins BH, Tuttle-Newhall E, et al. Intraoperative fluid management during orthotopic liver transplantation. *J Cardiothorac Vasc Anesth.* 2004;18:438.
128. de Boer MT, Christensen MC, Asmussen M, et al. Impact of intraoperative transfusion of platelet and red blood cells on survival after liver transplantation. *Anesth Analg.* 2008;106:32.
129. Tripoli A, Mannucci PM. The coagulopathy of chronic liver disease. *N Engl J Med.* 2011;365:147.

130. Porte RJ, Bontempo FA, Knot EA, et al. Systemic effects of tissue plasminogen activator-associated fibrinolysis and its relation to thrombin generation in orthotopic liver transplantation. *Transplantation.* 1989;47:978.
131. Meijer K, Hendriks HG, De Wolf JT, et al. Recombinant factor VIIa in orthotopic liver transplantation: Influence on parameters of coagulation and fibrinolysis. *Blood Coagul Fibrinolysis.* 2003;14:169.
132. Surudo T, Wojcicki M, Milkiewicz P, et al. Rapid correction of prothrombin time after low-dose recombinant factor VIIA in patients undergoing orthotopic liver transplantation. *Transplant Proc.* 2003;35:2323.
133. Boone JD, Sherwani SS, Herborn JC, et al. The successful use of low-dose recombinant tissue plasminogen activator for treatment of intracardiac/pulmonary thrombosis during liver transplantation. *Anesth Analg.* 2011;112:319.
134. Sherman DS, Fish DN, Teitelbaum I. Assessing renal function in cirrhotic patients: Problems and pitfalls. *Am J Kidney Dis.* 2003;41:269.
135. Guevara M, Arroyo V. Hepatorenal syndrome. *Expert Opin Pharmacother.* 2011;12:1405.
136. Sort P, Navasa M, Arroyo V, et al. Effect of intravenous albumin on renal impairment and mortality in patients with cirrhosis and spontaneous bacterial peritonitis. *N Engl J Med.* 1999;341:403.
137. Duvoux C, Zandirenas D, Hezode C, et al. Effects of noradrenalin and albumin in patients with type 1 hepatorenal syndrome: A pilot study. *Hepatology.* 2002; 36:374.
138. Moreau R, Lebrec D. The use of vasoconstrictors in patients with cirrhosis: Type I HRS and beyond. *Hepatology.* 2006;43:385.
139. Steib A, Saada A, Clever B. Orthotopic liver transplantation with preservation of portocaval flow compared with venovenous bypass. *Liver Transpl Surg.* 1997;3:518.
140. Aggarwal S, Kang Y, Freeman JA, et al. Postreperfusion syndrome: Hypotension after reperfusion of the transplanted liver. *J Crit Care.* 1993;8:154.
141. Nahas GG, Sutin KM, Fermon C, et al. Guidelines for the treatment of acidaemia with THAM. *Drugs.* 1998;55:191.
142. Koelzow H, Gedney JA, Baumann J, et al. The effect of methylene blue on the hemodynamic changes during ischemia reperfusion injury in orthotopic liver transplantation. *Anesth Analg.* 2002;94:824.
143. Fukuzawa K, Pretto EA. The effect of methylene blue during orthotopic liver transplantation on post reperfusion syndrome and postoperative graft function. *J Hepatobiliary Pancreat Sci.* 2011;18:406.
144. Lang JD Jr, Teng X, Chumley P, et al. Inhaled NO accelerates restoration of liver function in adults following orthotopic liver transplantation. *J Clin Invest.* 2007;117:2583.
145. Foster R, Zimmerman M, Trotter JF. Expanding donor options: Marginal, living, and split donors. *Clin Liver Dis.* 2007;11:417.
146. Cameron AM, Ghobrial RM, Yersiz H, et al. Optimal utilization of donor grafts with extended criteria. *Ann Surg.* 2006;243:748.
147. Taner CB, Willingham DL, Bulatao IG, et al. Is mandatory ICU stay needed after liver transplantation? Feasibility of fast tracking to the surgical ward after liver transplantation. *Liver Transpl.* 2012;18:361.
148. Bennett J, Bromley P. Perioperative issues in pediatric liver transplantation. *Int Anesthesiol Clin.* 2006;44:125.
149. McDiarmid SV. Current status of liver transplantation in children. *Pediatr Clin North Am.* 2003;50:1335.
150. Alper I, Ulukaya S. Anesthetic management in pediatric liver transplantation: A comparison of deceased or live donor liver transplantations. *J Anesth.* 2010;24:399.
151. Blei AT. Brain edema in acute liver failure. *Crit Care Clin.* 2008;24:99.
152. Stravitz RT, Kramer AH, Davern T, et al. Intensive care unit care of patients with acute liver failure: Recommendations of the U.S. Acute Liver Failure Study Group. *Crit Care Med.* 2007;35:2498.
153. Aggarwal S, Kang Y, De Wolf A, et al. Transcranial Doppler monitoring of cerebral blood flow velocity during liver transplantation. *Transplant Proc.* 1993; 25:1799.
154. Bindi ML, Biancofiore G, Esposito M, et al. Transcranial Doppler sonography is useful for the decision-making at the point of care in patients with acute hepatic failure: A single center's experience. *J Clin Monit Comput.* 2008;22:449.
155. Jalan R, Olde Damink SW, Deutz NE, et al. Moderate hypothermia in patients with acute liver failure and uncontrolled intracranial hypertension. *Gastroenterology.* 2004;127:1338.
156. Sundaram V, Shaikh OS. Acute liver failure: Current practice and recent advances. *Gastroenterol Clin North Am.* 2011;40:523.
157. Camus C, Lavoue S, Gacouin A, et al. Liver transplantation avoided in patients with fulminant hepatic failure who received albumin dialysis with the molecular adsorbent recirculating system while on the waiting list: Impact of the duration of therapy. *Ther Apher Dial.* 2009;13:549.
158. Lidofsky SD, Bass NM, Prager MC, et al. Intracranial pressure monitoring and liver transplantation for fulminant hepatic failure. *Hepatology.* 1992;16:1.
159. Schnickel GT, Busuttil RW, Lipshutz GS. Improvement in short-term pancreas transplant outcome by targeted antimicrobial therapy and refined donor selection. *Am Surg.* 2011;77:1407.
160. Mokshagundam SPL. Perioperative management of diabetes mellitus. *Crit Care Nurs Q.* 2004;27:135.
161. Shapiro AM, Lakey JR, Ryan EA, et al. Islet transplantation in seven patients with type 1 diabetes mellitus using a glucocorticoid-free immunosuppressive regimen. *N Engl J Med.* 2000;343:230.
162. Langnas AN. Advances in small-intestine transplantation. *Transplantation.* 2004; 77:S75.
163. Goldman LJ, Santamaria ML, Gamez M. Anaesthetic management of a patient with microvillus inclusion disease for intestinal transplantation. *Paediatr Anaesth.* 2002;12:278.
164. Mims TT, Fishbein TM, Feierman DE. Management of a small bowel transplant with complicated central venous access in a patient with asymptomatic superior and inferior vena cava obstruction. *Transplant Proc.* 2004;36:388.
165. Goulet O, Ruemmele F, Lacaille F, et al. Irreversible intestinal failure. *J Pediatr Gastroenterol Nutr.* 2004;38:250.
166. Christie JD, Edwards LB, Kucheryavaya AY, et al. The Registry of the International Society for Heart and Lung Transplantation: Twenty-eighth Adult Lung and Heart-Lung Transplantation Report—2011. *J Heart Lung Transplant.* 2011; 30:1104.
167. Orens JB, Garrity ER Jr. General overview of lung transplantation and review of organ allocation. *Proc Am Thorac Soc.* 2009;6:13.
168. Weill D, Keshavjee S. Lung transplantation for emphysema: Two lungs or one. *J Heart Lung Transplant.* 2001;20:739.
169. Hadjiliadis D, Steele MP, Chapparo C, et al. Survival of lung transplant patients with cystic fibrosis harboring panresistant bacteria other than *Burkholderia cepacia*, compared with patients harboring sensitive bacteria. *J Heart Lung Transplant.* 2007;26:834.
170. Horlocker TT, Wedel DJ, Benzon H, et al. Regional anesthesia in the anticoagulated patient: Defining the risks (the second ASRA consensus conference on neuraxial anesthesia and anticoagulation). *Reg Anesth Pain Med.* 2003;28:172.
171. Myles PS, Leslie K, Forbes A, et al. Bispectral index monitoring to prevent awareness during anaesthesia: The B-Aware randomised controlled trial. *Lancet.* 2004;363:1757.
172. Wiedemann HP, Wheeler AP, Bernard GR, et al. Comparison of two fluid-management strategies in acute lung injury. *N Engl J Med.* 2006;354:2564.
173. Pilcher DV, Scheinkestel CD, Snell GI, et al. A high central venous pressure is associated with prolonged mechanical ventilation and increased mortality following lung transplantation. *J Thorac Cardiovasc Surg.* 2005;129:912.
174. Oto T, Griffiths AP, Rosenfeldt F, et al. Preservation solutions in lung transplantation: Outcomes from Perfadex, Papworth, and Euro-Collins Solutions. *Ann Thorac Surg.* 2006;82:1842.
175. Benden C, Aurora P, Edwards LB, et al. Registry of the International Society for Heart and Lung Transplantation: Fourteenth Pediatric Lung and Heart-Lung Transplantation Report—2011. *J Heart Lung Transplant.* 2011;30:1123–1132.
176. Liou TG, Adler FR, Cox DR, et al. Lung transplantation and survival in children with cystic fibrosis. *N Engl J Med.* 2007;357:2143.
177. Barr ML, Kawut SM, Whelan TP, et al. Report of the ISHLT Working Group on Primary Lung Graft Dysfunction Part IV: Recipient-related risk factors and markers. *J Heart Lung Transplant.* 2005;24:1468.
178. Christie JD, Carby M, Bag R, et al. Report of the ISHLT Working Group on Primary Lung Graft Dysfunction Part II: Definition. A consensus statement of the International Society for Heart and Lung Transplantation. *J Heart Lung Transplant.* 2005;24:1454.
179. Wang YW, Kurichi JE, Blumenthal NP, et al. Multiple variables affecting blood usage in lung transplantation. *J Heart Lung Transplant.* 2006;25:533.
180. Oto T, Rosenfeldt F, Rowland M, et al. Extracorporeal membrane oxygenation after lung transplantation: Evolving techniques improves outcomes. *Ann Thorac Surg.* 2004;78:1230.
181. Lang JD, Lell W. Pro: Inhaled nitric oxide should be used routinely in patients undergoing lung transplantation. *J Cardiothorac Vasc Anesth.* 2001;15:785.
182. McQuitty CK. Con: Inhaled nitric oxide should not be used routinely in patients undergoing lung transplantation. *J Cardiothorac Vasc Anesth.* 2001;15:790.
183. Meyer KC, Love RB, Zimmerman JJ. The therapeutic potential of nitric oxide in lung transplantation. *Chest.* 1998;113:1360.
184. Perrin G, Roch A, Michelet P, et al. Inhaled nitric oxide does not prevent pulmonary edema after lung transplantation measured by lung water content. *Chest.* 2006;129:1024.
185. Beghetti M, Sparling C, Cox PN, et al. Inhaled NO inhibits platelet aggregation and elevates plasma but not intraplatelet cGMP in healthy human volunteers. *Am J Physiol Heart Circ Physiol.* 2003;285:H637.
186. Cornfield DN, Milla CE, Haddad IY, et al. Safety of inhaled nitric oxide after lung transplantation. *J Heart Lung Transplant.* 2003;22:903.
187. Hoehn T, Huebner J, Paboura E, et al. Effect of therapeutic concentrations of nitric oxide on bacterial growth in vitro. *Crit Care Med.* 1998;26:1857.
188. Trulock EP, Christie JD, Edwards LB, et al. Registry of the International Society for Heart and Lung Transplantation: Twenty-fourth Official Adult Lung and Heart-Lung Transplantation Report—2007. *J Heart Lung Transplant.* 2007; 26:782.
189. Aurora P, Boucek MM, Christie J, et al. Registry of the International Society for Heart and Lung Transplantation: Tenth Official Pediatric Lung and Heart/Lung Transplantation Report—2007. *J Heart Lung Transplant.* 2007;26:1223.
190. Barnard CN. The operation. A human cardiac transplant: An interim report of a successful operation performed at Groote Schuur Hospital, Cape Town. *S Afr Med J.* 1967;41:1271.
191. Lower RR, Shumway NE. Studies on orthotopic homotransplantations of the canine heart. *Surg Forum.* 1960;11:18.

192. Hertz MI, Aurora P, Benden C, et al. Scientific Registry of the International Society for Heart and Lung Transplantation: Introduction to the 2011 annual reports. *J Heart Lung Transplant.* 2011;30:1123.
193. Taylor DO, Brown RN, Jessup ML, et al. Progress in heart transplantation: Riskier patients yet better outcomes: A 15 year multi-institutional study. *J Heart Lung Transplant.* 2007;26:S61.
194. Stehlik J, Edwards LB, Kucheryavaya AY, et al. The Registry of the International Society for Heart and Lung Transplantation: Twenty-eighth Adult Heart Transplant Report—2011. *J Heart Lung Transplant.* 2011;30:1078.
195. Jessup M, Abraham WT, Casey DE, et al. 2009 focused update: ACCF/AHA Guidelines for the Diagnosis and Management of Heart Failure in Adults: A report of the American College of Cardiology Foundation/American Heart Association Task Force on Practice Guidelines: Developed in collaboration with the International Society for Heart and Lung Transplantation. *Circulation.* 2009;119:1977.
196. Teichman SL, Unemori E, Dschietzig T. Relaxin, a pleiotropic vasodilator for the treatment of heart failure. *Heart Fail Rev.* 2009;14:321.
197. Dschietzig T, Teichman SL, Unemori E, et al. Intravenous recombinant human relaxin in compensated heart failure: A safety, tolerability and pharmacodynamic trial. *J Card Fail.* 2009;15:182.
198. Burkly LC, Michaelson JS, Hahm K, et al. TWEAKing tissue remodeling by a multifunctional cytokine: Role of TWEAK/Fn14 pathway in health and disease. *Cytokine.* 2007;40:1.
199. Winkles JA. The TWEAK-Fn 14 cytokine-receptor axis: Discovery, biology, and therapeutic targeting. *Nat Rev Drug Discov.* 2008;7:411.
200. Jain M, Jakubowski A, Cui L, et al. A novel role for tumor necrosis factor like weak inducer of apoptosis (TWEAK) in the development of cardiac dysfunction and failure. *Circulation.* 2009;119:2058.
201. POISE Study Group. Effects of extended-release metoprolol succinate in patients undergoing non-cardiac surgery (POISE trial): A randomized controlled trial. *Lancet.* 2008;371:183.
202. London MJ, Zaugg M, Schaub MC, et al. Perioperative beta-adrenergic receptor blockade: Physiologic foundations and clinical controversies. *Anesthesiology.* 2004;100:170.
203. Bristow MR, Saxon LA, Boehmer J, et al. Cardiac-resynchronization therapy with or without an implantable defibrillator in advanced chronic heart failure. *N Engl J Med.* 2004;350:2140.
204. Anand IS, Carson P, Galle E, et al. Cardiac resynchronization therapy reduces the risk of hospitalizations in patients with advanced heart failure: Results from the comparison of medical therapy, pacing and defibrillation in heart failure (COMPANION) trial. *Circulation.* 2009;119:969.
205. Eisen HJ. Surgical ventricular reconstruction for heart failure. *N Engl J Med.* 2009;360:1781.
206. Rosamond W, Flegal K, Furie K, et al. Heart disease and stroke statistics: 2008 update: A report from the American Heart Association Statistics Committee and the Stroke Statistics Subcommittee. *Circulation.* 2008;117:e25.
207. Rose EA, Gelijns AC, Moskowitz AJ, et al. Long-term use of a left ventricular device for end-stage heart failure. *N Engl J Med.* 2001;345:1435.
208. Kirklin JK, Naftel DC, Kormos RL, et al. Third INTERMACS Annual Report: The evolution of destination therapy in the United States. *J Heart Lung Transplant.* 2011;30:115.
209. Wilson SR, Mudge GH, Stewart GC, et al. Evaluation for a ventricular assist device: Selecting the appropriate candidate. *Circulation.* 2009;119:2225.
210. Stevenson LW, Couper G. On the fledgling field of mechanical circulatory support. *J Am Coll Cardiol.* 2007;50:748.
211. Stevenson L. When is heart failure a surgical disease? In: Rose EA, Stevenson L, eds. *Management of End-Stage Heart Disease.* Philadelphia, PA, and New York, NY: Lippincott-Raven; 1998:129–146.
212. Rose EA, Moskowitz AJ, Packer M, et al. The REMATCH trial: Rationale, design, and end points. Randomized evaluation of mechanical assistance for the treatment of congestive heart failure. *Ann Thorac Surg.* 1999;67:723.
213. Lietz K, Long JW, Kfoury AG, et al. Outcomes of left ventricular assist device implantation as destination therapy in the post-REMATCH era: Implications for patient selection. *Circulation.* 2007;116:497.
214. Slaughter MS, Rogers JG, Milano CA, et al. Advanced heart failure treated with continuous-flow left ventricular assist device. *N Engl J Med.* 2009;361:2241.
215. Thunberg CA, Gaitan BD, Arabia FA, et al. Ventricular assist devices today and tomorrow. *J Cardiothorac Vasc Anesth.* 2010;24:656.
216. Chumnanvej S, Wood MJ, MacGillivray TE, et al. Perioperaive echocardiographic examination for ventricular assist device implantation. *Anesth Analg.* 2007;105:583.
217. CardiacAssist: TandemHeart pVAD product information. Available at: http://www.cardiacassist.com.
218. Thoratec: HeartMate II clinical outcomes. Available at: http:// www.thoratec.com/vad-trials-outcomes/clinical-outcomes/heartmatell-lvad.aspx.
219. Thoratec: HeartMate II LVAS operating manual. Available at: http://www.thoratec.com/medical-professionals/resource-library/ifusmanuals/download/81.
220. Nicolosi A, Pagel PS. Perioperative considerations in the patient with a left ventricular assist device. *Anesthesiology.* 2003;98:56.
221. Crow S, Chen D, Milano C, et al. Acquired von Willebrand syndrome in continuous-flow ventricular assist device recipients. *Ann Thorac Surg.* 2010;90:1263.
222. Meyer AL, Malehsa D, Bara C, et al. Acquired von Willebrand syndrome in patients with an axial flow left ventricular assist device. *Circ Heart Fail.* 2010;3:67.
223. Lietz K, Brown K, Ali SS, et al. The role of cerebral hyperperfusion in postoperative neurologic dysfunction after left ventricular assist device implantation for end-stage heart failure. *J Thorac Cardiovasc Surg.* 2009;137:10.
224. Kar B, Adkins LE, Civitello AB, et al. Clinical experience with the TandemHeart® percutaneous ventricular assist device. *Tex Heart Inst J.* 2006;33:111.
225. Copeland JC, Smith RG, Arabia FA, et al. Cardiac replacement with a total artificial heart as a bridge to transplantation. *N Engl J Med.* 2004;351:859.
226. McCarthy PM, Quader MA, Hoercher KJ. Evolving strategies for surgical management of patients with severe left ventricular dysfunction. *Heart Lung Circ.* 2003;12:31.
227. Rodeheffer RJ, Naftel DC, Stevenson LW, et al. Secular trends in cardiac transplant recipient and donor management in the United States, 1990 to 1994. A multi-institutional study. Cardiac Transplant Research Database Group. *Circulation.* 1996;94:2883.
228. Sievers HH, Weyand M, Kraatz EG, et al. An alternative technique for orthotopic cardiac transplantation, with preservation of the normal anatomy of the right atrium. *Thorac Cardiovasc Surg.* 1991;39:70.
229. Schnoor M, Schafer T, Luhman D, et al. Bicaval versus standard technique in orthotopic heart transplantation: A systematic review and meta-analysis. *J Thorac Cardiovasc Surg.* 2007;134:1322.
230. Jacob S, Sellke F. Is bicaval orthotopic heart transplantation superior to the biatrial technique? *Interact Cardiovasc Thorac Surg.* 2009;9:333.
231. Newcomb AE, Esmore D, Rosenfeldt FL, et al. Heterotopic heart transplantation: an expanding role in the twenty-first century? *Ann Thorac Surg.* 2004;78:1345.
232. Copeland H, Kalra N, Gustafson M, et al. A case of heterotopic heart transplant as a "Biologic Left Ventricular Assist" in restrictive cardiomyopathy. *World J Pediatr Congen Heart Surg.* 2011;2:637.
233. Waterman PM, Bjerke R. Rapid-sequence induction technique in patients with severe ventricular dysfunction. *J Cardiothorac Anesth.* 1988;2:602.
234. Demas K, Wyner J, Mihm FG, et al. Anaesthesia for heart transplantation. A retrospective study and review. *Br J Anaesth.* 1986;58:1357.
235. Hensley FA, Martin DE, Larach DR. Anesthetic management for cardiac transplantation in North America—1986 survey. *J Cardiothorac Anesth.* 1987;1:429.
236. Woods J, Monteiro P, Rhodes A. Right ventricular dysfunction. *Curr Opin Crit Care.* 2007;13:532.
237. Ardehali A, Hughes K, Sadeghi A, et al. Inhaled nitric oxide for pulmonary hypertension after heart transplantation. *Transplantation.* 2001;72:638.
238. Mosquera I, Crespo-Leiro MG, Tabuyo T, et al. Pulmonary hypertension and right ventricular failure after heart transplantation: Usefulness of nitric oxide. *Transplant Proc.* 2002;34:166.
239. Rajek A, Pernerstorfer T, Kastner J, et al. Inhaled nitric oxide reduces pulmonary vascular resistance more than prostaglandin E(1) during heart transplantation. *Anesth Analg.* 2000;90:523.
240. Fonger JD, Borkon AM, Baumgartner WA, et al. Acute right ventricular failure following heart transplantation: Improvement with prostaglandin E1 and right ventricular assist. *J Heart Transplant.* 1986;5:327.
241. Augoustides JG, Ochroch EA. Novel pulmonary vasodilators. *Int Anesthesiol Clin.* 2005;43:101.
242. Fynn-Thompson F, Almond C. Pediatric ventricular assist devices. *Pediatr Cardiol.* 2007;28:149.
243. Boucek MM, Mathis CM, Kanakriyeh MS, et al. Donor shortage: use of the dysfunctional donor heart. *J Heart Lung Transplant.* 1993;12(6, Pt 2):S186.
244. Morgan JA, John R, Park YK, et al. Successful outcome with extended allograft ischemic time in pediatric heart transplantation. *J Heart Lung Transplant.* 2005; 1:58.
245. West LJ, Pollock-Barziv SM, Dipchand AI, et al. ABO-incompatible heart transplantation in infants. *N Engl J Med.* 2001;344:793.
246. Rao JN, Hasan A, Hamilton JRL, et al. ABO-incompatible heart transplantation in infants: The Freeman Hospital experience. *Transplantation.* 2004;77:1389.
247. Edrich T, Pomahac B, Lu JT, et al. Perioperative management of partial face transplantation involving a heparin antibody-positive donor. *J Clin Anesth.* 2011; 23:318.
248. Pomahac B, Pribaz J, Eriksson E, et al. Three patients with full facial transplantation. *N Engl J Med.* 2012;366:715.
249. Kostopanagiotou G, Smyrniotis V, Arkadopoulos N, et al. Anesthetic and perioperative management of adult transplant recipients in nontransplant surgery. *Anesth Analg.* 1999;89:613.
250. Fishman JA. Infection in solid-organ transplant recipients. *N Engl J Med.* 2007; 357:2601.
251. Savar A, Hiatt JR, Busuttil RW. Acute appendicitis after solid organ transplantation. *Clin Transplant.* 2006;20:78.

CHAPTER

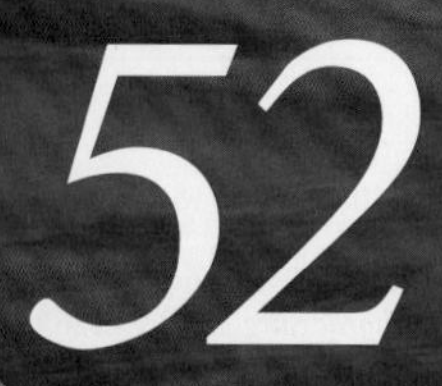

52 Trauma and Burns

LEVON M. CAPAN • SANFORD M. MILLER • KEVIN J. GINGRICH

Key Points

1. Airway management is tailored to the type of injury, the nature and degree of airway compromise, and the patient's hemodynamic and oxygenation status.
2. Fast computed tomography technology with the capability of sagittal image reconstruction is replacing conventional multiple view plain radiographic evaluation of cervical spine injury. Further, magnetic resonance imaging is replacing flexion/extension plain radiographic evaluation of the relatively infrequent ligamentous injuries of the cervical spine.
3. Penetrating neck injuries usually present with obvious clinical manifestations, whereas blunt cervical trauma may be more subtle.
4. Morbidity and mortality of flail chest is primarily related to underlying pulmonary contusion that develops over a period of a few hours after injury. A liberal indication for tracheal intubation of these patients may be associated with increased morbidity and mortality.
5. Head injury and hemorrhagic shock are the most common causes of traumatic death.
6. Lethal triad or bloody vicious cycle refers to the development of acidosis, hypothermia, and coagulopathy, which, if untreated, may lead to death.
7. Approximately 10% of patients with hemorrhagic shock may have severe coagulopathy at the time of admission and the early operative phase, requiring hemostatic resuscitation with plasma, platelets, and coagulation factors.
8. The most important therapeutic maneuvers in head injured patients are normalization of intracranial pressure, cerebral perfusion pressure, and oxygen delivery.
9. Brain ischemia is the most threatening consequence of head injury. By causing cerebral vasoconstriction, hyperventilation further aggravates ischemia.
10. The term blunt cardiac injury has replaced myocardial contusion and encompasses varying degrees of myocardial damage, coronary artery injury, and rupture of the cardiac free wall, the septum, or a valve.
11. Transesophageal echocardiography is very useful in the trauma setting, providing information about right and left ventricular volume, ejection fraction, wall motion abnormalities, pulmonary hypertension, cardiac output, acute ischemia, blunt cardiac injury, cardiac septal or valvular damage, coronary artery injury, pericardial tamponade, and aortic injury.
12. In the trauma patient persistent hypotension is usually a result of bleeding, tension pneumothorax, neurogenic shock, and/or cardiac injury such as pericardial tamponade or myocardial contusion.
13. Inspired by military experience, many studies of civilian trauma have demonstrated the benefit of hemostatic resuscitation involving high ratios of fresh frozen plasma or platelets to packed red blood cell transfusion. However, many of these studies have been found to have survivor bias, necessitating further work in this area.
14. Monitoring of blood coagulation status with thromboelastography is useful in bleeding patients receiving massive transfusion.
15. Prothrombin complex concentrates containing factors II, VII, IX, and X are available in the United States and are used primarily to reverse the effects of warfarin in acute trauma patients.

Multimedia

1 Management of the Major Trauma Patient

2 Nail Trachea Case

3 Pneumothorax

Injury is responsible for 9% of the total annual mortality (5 million people) in the world.[1] Traffic accidents alone killed 3,500 people every day in 2009; almost half of the victims were pedestrians, cyclists, and motorcyclists.[2] Violence, encompassing homicides, suicides, and war-related injuries, is also estimated to kill about 1.5 million people every year in the world of whom the vast majority reside in low- and middle-income countries.[3]

In the United States, according to data from the National Safety Council intentional injuries (suicide, homicide, and assault) claimed 55,000 lives in 2008, while in 2010, unintentional (motor vehicle, falls, drowning, poisoning, etc.) mortality claimed 126,000 lives. Trauma, with an estimated 181,000 deaths per year, was the third leading cause of death after heart disease and cancer. Unintentional injuries were the fifth, suicides the tenth, and assault the fifteenth leading causes of death overall. For the age range between 15 and 31, accidents, suicide, and homicide were the three leading causes of death. Morbidity caused by injuries is far in excess of mortality; in 2010, a total of 37.9 million emergency room visits were related to unintentional injuries. The estimated cost of unintentional injuries alone that year was $731 billion, including the costs of fatal and nonfatal injuries, employer costs, vehicle damage, and fire losses.[4]

Approximately 75% of the hospital deaths from high-energy trauma such as motor vehicle accidents, falls, and gunshot or stab wounds occur within 48 hours after admission, most commonly from central nervous system (CNS), thoracic, abdominal, retroperitoneal, or vascular injuries.[5] CNS injury and hemorrhage are the most common causes of early trauma mortality.[6] Nearly one-third of these patients die within the first 4 hours after admission, representing the majority of operating room (OR) trauma deaths. Of the hospital deaths, 5% to 10% occur between the third and seventh day of admission, usually from CNS injuries, and the rest in subsequent weeks, most commonly as a result of multiorgan failure.[5] Pulmonary thromboembolism and infectious complications may also contribute to mortality during this phase.[5] Interestingly, injuries caused by low energy impacts, mainly from falls usually in the elderly, also produce significant mortality from head injury and complications of skeletal injuries. Of these deaths, 20% occur within 48 hours, 32% after 3 to 7 days, and 48% after 7 days. Pre-existing conditions such as congestive heart failure, cirrhosis, warfarin, and/or β-blocker usage increase the mortality rate in trauma patients.[7]

INITIAL EVALUATION AND RESUSCITATION

The strategy of initial management can be defined as a continuous, priority-driven process of patient assessment, resuscitation, and reassessment. The general approach to evaluation of the acute trauma victim has three sequential components: rapid overview, primary survey, and secondary survey (Fig. 52-1). Resuscitation is initiated, if needed, at any time during this continuum. *Rapid overview* takes only a few seconds and is used to determine whether the patient is stable, unstable, dying, or dead. The *primary survey* involves rapid evaluation of functions that are crucial to survival. The ABCs of airway patency, breathing, and circulation are assessed. Then a brief neurologic examination is performed, and the patient is examined for any external injuries that might have been overlooked.

The *secondary survey* involves a more elaborate systematic examination of the entire body to identify additional injuries. Radiographic and other diagnostic procedures may also be performed if the stability of the patient permits. Within this general framework the anesthesiologist, aside from managing the airway, contributes as part of the team for evaluation and resuscitation, while gathering information needed for possible future anesthetic management.

Injuries may be missed during initial evaluation and even during emergency surgery, resulting in significant pain, complications, residual disability, delay of treatment, or death.[8] Reported missed diagnoses include cervical spine, thoracoabdominal, pelvic, nerve, and external soft tissue injuries, and extremity fractures. Some of these injuries may present during administration of anesthesia, such as spinal cord damage in a patient with unrecognized cervical spine injury, massive intraoperative bleeding from an unrecognized thoracoabdominal injury during extremity surgery, or sudden intraoperative hypoxemia in a patient with unrecognized pneumothorax.

A *tertiary survey* within the first 24 hours after admission (which may include a period of anesthesia) can potentially diagnose the majority of clinically significant injuries missed during initial evaluation by repeating the primary and secondary examinations and reviewing the results of radiologic and laboratory testing.[8]

Airway Evaluation and Intervention

Airway evaluation involves the diagnosis of any trauma to the airway or surrounding tissues, recognition and anticipation of the respiratory consequences of these injuries, and prediction of the potential for exacerbation of these or other injuries by any contemplated airway management maneuvers (see Chapter 27). Although nontraumatic causes of airway difficulty, such as preexisting factors may be present, only the management of trauma-related problems is discussed in this section. Generally, the American Society of Anesthesiologists's (ASA) difficult airway algorithm can be applied with certain modifications to various trauma airway management scenarios. For instance, cancellation of airway management when difficulty arises may not be an option. Likewise awake rather than asleep intubation or a surgical airway from the outset may be the preferred technique in some situations. The ASA's difficult airway algorithm as modified for various trauma conditions is available.[9] Airway management is tailored to the type of injury, the nature and degree of airway compromise, and the patient's hemodynamic and oxygenation status.

Airway Obstruction

Airway obstruction is probably the most frequent cause of asphyxia and may result from posteriorly displaced or lacerated pharyngeal soft tissues; cervical or mediastinal hematoma; bleeding, secretions, or foreign bodies within the airway; and/or

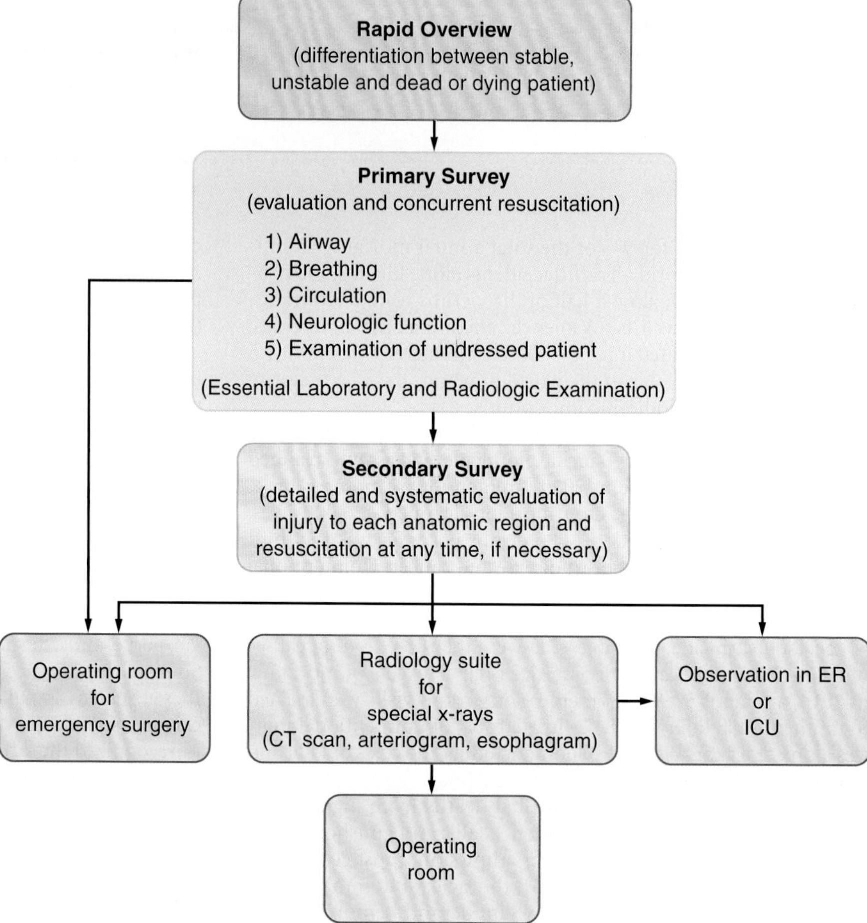

FIGURE 52-1. Clinical sequence for initial management of the major trauma patient. CT, computed tomography; ER, emergency room; ICU, intensive care unit.

displaced bone or cartilage fragments. Bleeding into the cervical region may produce airway obstruction not only because of compression by the hematoma, but also from venous congestion and upper airway edema as a result of compression of neck veins. Signs of upper and lower airway obstruction include dyspnea, cyanosis, hoarseness, stridor, dysphonia, subcutaneous emphysema, and hemoptysis. Cervical deformity, edema, crepitation, tracheal tug and/or deviation, or jugular venous distention may be present before these symptoms appear and may help indicate that specialized techniques are required to secure the airway.

The initial steps in airway management are chin lift, jaw thrust, clearing of the oropharynx, placement of an oropharyngeal or nasopharyngeal airway, and, in inadequately breathing patients, ventilation with a self-inflating bag. Immobilization of the cervical spine and administration of oxygen should be applied simultaneously. Blind passage of a nasopharyngeal airway or a nasogastric or nasotracheal tube should be avoided if a basilar skull fracture is suspected because it may enter the anterior cranial fossa. A cuffed oropharyngeal airway (Combitube or King's airway) or a laryngeal mask airway (LMA) may permit ventilation with a self-inflating bag, although neither provides protection against aspiration of gastric contents. They may be used as temporary measures and can serve as a bridge for a brief period to re-establish the airway patency or to facilitate intubation aided by a flexible fiberoptic bronchoscope (FOB). If they do not provide adequate ventilation, the trachea must be intubated immediately using either direct laryngoscopy or a cricothyroidotomy, depending on the results of airway assessment.

Maxillofacial, neck, and chest injuries, as well as cervicofacial burns, are the most common trauma-related causes of difficult tracheal intubation. Airway assessment should include a rapid examination of the anterior neck for feasibility of access to the cricothyroid membrane. Tracheostomy is not desirable during initial management because it takes longer to perform than a cricothyroidotomy and requires neck extension, which may cause or exacerbate cord trauma in patients with cervical spine injuries. Conversion to a tracheostomy should be considered later to prevent laryngeal damage if a cricothyroidotomy will be in place for more than 2 to 3 days. Possible contraindications to cricothyroidotomy include age younger than 12 years and suspected laryngeal trauma. Permanent laryngeal damage may result in the former, and uncorrectable airway obstruction may occur in the latter situation.

Full Stomach

A full stomach is a background condition in acute trauma: the urgency of securing the airway often does not permit adequate time for pharmacologic measures to reduce gastric volume and acidity. Thus, rather than relying on these agents, the emphasis should be placed on selection of a safe technique for securing the airway when necessary: rapid-sequence induction with cricoid pressure for those patients without serious airway problems, and awake intubation with sedation and topical anesthesia, if possible, for those with anticipated serious airway difficulties.

In agitated and uncooperative patients, topical anesthesia of the airway may be impossible, whereas administration of sedative agents may result in apnea or airway obstruction, with an increased risk of aspiration of gastric contents and inadequate conditions for tracheal intubation. After locating the cricothyroid membrane and denitrogenating the lungs, a rapid-sequence induction may be used to allow securing of the airway with direct laryngoscopy or, if necessary, immediate cricothyroidotomy. Personnel and material necessary to perform translaryngeal ventilation or cricothyroidotomy must be in place before induction of general anesthesia.

Head, Open Eye, and Contained Major Vessel Injuries

The principles of tracheal intubation are similar for these injuries. Apart from the need to ensure adequate oxygenation and ventilation, these patients require deep anesthesia and profound muscle relaxation before airway manipulation. This helps prevent hypertension, coughing, and bucking, and thereby minimizes intracranial, intraocular, or intravascular pressure elevation, which can result in herniation of the brain, extrusion of eye contents, or dislodgment of a hemostatic clot from an injured vessel, respectively. The preferred anesthetic sequence to achieve this goal in patients who are not hemodynamically compromised includes preoxygenation and opioid loading, followed by relatively large doses of an intravenous anesthetic and muscle relaxant. Hemodynamic responses to this sequence should be carefully monitored and promptly corrected. Systemic hypotension, intracranial pressure (ICP) elevation, and decreased cerebral perfusion pressure (CPP; CPP equals mean arterial pressure minus ICP) may occur whether cerebral autoregulation is present or absent in patients with head injuries, and if untreated it can produce secondary ischemic insults. Ketamine is probably contraindicated in patients with head and vascular injuries because it may increase both intracranial and systemic vascular pressures. However, no significant increase in intraocular pressure (IOP) has been documented. Any muscle relaxant, including succinylcholine, may be used as long as the fasciculation produced by this agent is inhibited by prior administration of an adequate dose of a nondepolarizing muscle relaxant. Alternatively, rocuronium can provide intubating conditions within 60 seconds with a dose of 1.2 to 1.5 mg/kg; neuromuscular blockade produced by this dose lasts approximately 2 hours. Of course, neither muscle relaxants nor intravenous anesthetics are indicated when initial assessment suggests a difficult airway. As in any other trauma patient, hypotension dictates either reduced or no intravenous anesthetic administration.

Cervical Spine Injury

Overall, 2% to 4% of blunt trauma patients have cervical spine (C-spine) injuries, of which 7% to 15% are unstable.[10] The most common causes include high-speed motor vehicle accidents, falls, diving accidents, and gunshot wounds. Head injuries, especially those with low Glasgow coma scores (GCS) and focal neurologic deficits, are likely to be associated with C-spine injuries. Approximately 2% to 10% of head trauma victims have C-spine injuries, while 25% to 50% of patients with C-spine injuries have an associated head injury.[10] The incidence of assault-related injuries depends on the mechanism, being highest after gunshot wounds (1.35%), lowest after stab wounds (0.12%), and intermediate after blunt trauma (0.4%) to the cervicothoracic region.

Initial Evaluation

Accurate and timely evaluation is important because 2% to 10% of blunt trauma induced C-spine injury patients develop new or worsening neurologic deficits after admission, partly attributable to delayed diagnosis and improper C-spine protection and/or manipulation.[10] Often there is no time to evaluate the injury, and emergency airway management may have to be performed without ruling out C-spine injury while the patients are in a rigid collar and neck stabilizing devices. Clearance of the neck at the earliest possible time after airway management should be performed to minimize the complications associated with the collar, such as pressure ulceration, ICP elevation in head injured patients, compromised central venous access, and airway management challenges if reintubation is needed.

In the conscious patient with a suspected injury, diagnosis is relatively easy. According to the American National Emergency X-Radiography Utilization Study (NEXUS), a clinical evaluation revealing no posterior midline tenderness in the neck and no focal neurologic deficit in an injured patient with a normal level of alertness, no evidence of intoxication, and absence of painful distracting injury indicates a low probability of a C-spine injury, and there is thus no need for radiographic evaluation.[11] Recently, however, it has been shown that a significant number of major trauma patients cleared by these criteria had clinically important unstable C-spine injuries requiring treatment. Therefore, routine computerized tomography (CT) in addition to clinical evaluation is recommended to rule out C-spine injury in major trauma victims.[12] Probably the reason for the lower reliability of the NEXUS criteria is difficulty in evaluating distracting injuries.

The Canadian C-spine rule for radiography after trauma is another tool designed to identify low-risk patients.[10] With this diagnostic tool, proper answers to the following three questions eliminate the possibility of injury and the need for radiographic studies: (a) Is there any high-risk factor mandating radiography? (b) Are there low-risk factors that permit safe evaluation of the range of motion of the neck? (c) Can the patient rotate the neck laterally for 45 degrees in each direction without pain? (Fig. 52-2).

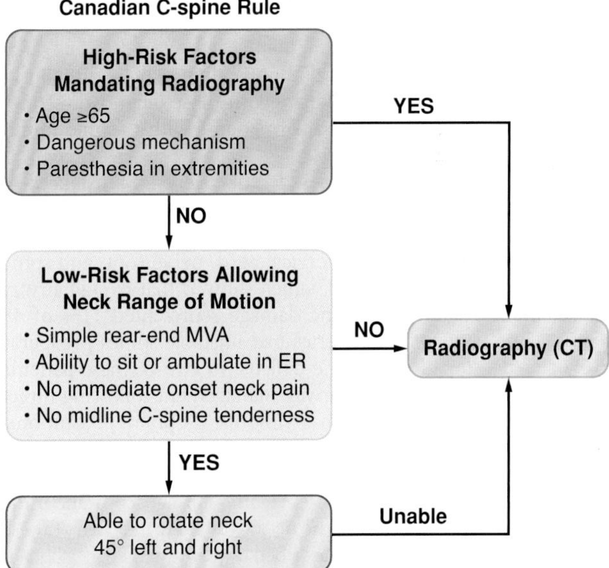

FIGURE 52-2. Canadian cervical spine rule designed to diagnose cervical spine injury and identify patients who require further radiographic (computed tomography) evaluation. (Adapted with permission from Stiell IG, Clement CM, McKnight RD, et al. The Canadian C-spine rule versus the NEXUS low-risk criteria in patients with trauma. *N Engl J Med.* 2003;349:2510.)

ANESTHESIA FOR SURGICAL SUBSPECIALTIES

Comparison of these two sets of criteria showed that the Canadian rule is more reliable than those for NEXUS in diagnosing C-spine injury in responsive patients.[13]

2 For those patients who cannot be cleared clinically and thus require radiographic evaluation, it is now clear that the diagnostic capability of three-view plain films is inferior to that provided by modern multidetector CT scans. Currently in modern trauma centers radiographic evaluation of the C-spine is performed using thin cut CT images with sagittal and coronal reconstruction. There is, however, a subset of patients with a normal CT scan who are either comatose, obtunded or are awake but have neck pain. Given the fact that CT is not sensitive in picking up soft tissue and ligamentous injury, ruling out ligamentous C-spine injury in these patients is difficult and the diagnostic strategy is somewhat controversial. Dynamic fluoroscopy to obtain flexion/extension series has limited value because it is extremely low yield, relatively dangerous, and cost ineffective.[14] It requires repeat examinations, it is difficult to identify specific ligamentous injury, and often the lower cervical spine cannot be visualized. In many trauma centers it is no longer performed.

Magnetic resonance imaging (MRI) is a reliable tool; a normal examination can conclusively exclude C-spine injury.[15] It is thus the gold standard for ruling out C-spine injury. However, it is so sensitive that it can detect subtle injuries that are clinically insignificant. It cannot be performed in multiple trauma patients who have metallic skeletal fixators. It is expensive and requires patient transport. Finally, it cannot be performed in the first few days after injury, the period when airway management is most commonly performed. A more recently proposed approach, which is practiced in many countries and in many, but not all, trauma centers in the United States, is to rely on the CT study performed using multidetector devices with <3-mm cuts. The diagnostic capability of this method is excellent, with the possibility of missing 1 unstable C-spine injury in about 5,000 patients not cleared by clinical examination.[16]

There are certain situations that theoretically could be missed with CT examination. Acute rupture of a transverse atlantal ligament produces significant instability despite the absence of a neurologic deficit and normal alignment while the patient is supine on a CT scanner. Likewise, in a head-injured patient, a mild to moderate central cord syndrome, which is referred to as spinal cord injury without radiological abnormality, may be difficult to discern with a CT scan. Familiarity with these diagnostic strategies may help in the assessment of patients with C-spine injury before airway management.

Interestingly, published series describe very few instances of neurologic deficits related to airway management in C-spine–injured patients. Recently, Hindman et al.[17] reviewed the closed claims data for perioperative cervical cord, nerve root, and spine injury between 1970 and 2007, which showed that overall airway management–related neurologic damage represented 11% of 48 claims. Nine patients in the series had unstable spines preoperatively and developed neurologic deficits. In two of these patients the injury was attributed to airway management following direct laryngoscopy and intubation without C-spine precautions. McLeod and Calder[18] reviewed nine allegedly intubation-related cervical spinal cord injuries. Of these, three patients in two reports developed increased neurologic deficit after laryngoscopy and intubation without stabilization of the neck. It is likely that two of these patients are the same patients described by Hindman et al.[17] Thus it is possible that airway management–related cervical cord injury in C-spine injured patients can occur, but if it does, it is rare.

Airway Management

Almost all airway maneuvers, including jaw thrust, chin lift, head tilt, and oral airway placement, result in some degree of C-spine movement.[10] To secure the airway with direct laryngoscopy, manual in-line stabilization (MILS) of the neck is the standard care of these patients in the acute stage. A hard cervical collar alone, which is routinely placed, does not provide absolute protection, especially for rotational movements of the neck. MILS is best accomplished by having two operators in addition to the physician who is actually managing the airway. The first operator stabilizes and aligns the head in neutral position without applying cephalad traction. The second operator stabilizes both shoulders by holding them against the table or stretcher. The anterior portion of the hard collar, which limits mouth opening, may be removed after immobilization.

In the presence of MILS, the glottic view may be suboptimal in 10% to 15% of patients during direct laryngoscopy because of limitation of neck extension. Airway management may be further compromised in some patients because of enlargement of the prevertebral space by a hematoma from the vertebral fracture. Consequently, greater anterior pressure needs to be applied to the tongue by the laryngoscope blade to visualize the larynx. This increased anterior pressure is transmitted to the spine and can increase the movement of the unstable vertebral segment. Thus, the more the restriction of the glottic view during direct laryngoscopy, the greater the pressure on the tongue, the spine, and the unstable segment with potential displacement of the unstable fragment. Santoni et al.[19] demonstrated that during various phases of direct laryngoscopy and intubation, the pressures exerted on the tongue and indirectly to the spine were greater with MILS than without MILS (Fig. 52-3). This finding confirmed the results of a videofluoroscopic study by Lennarson et al.[20] who demonstrated significant anteroposterior displacement when MILS was applied to cadavers with destabilized C-spines.

Although convincing, these data should not eliminate the current standard practice of applying MILS during airway management of these patients. Currently, there is no scientifically rigorous clinical trial to show conclusively that airway management without MILS is associated with a favorable spinal cord outcome. Based on the available data, it is, however, reasonable to allow some relaxation of the MILS to improve the glottic view when visualization of the larynx is restricted.

Other measures and techniques, including the McCoy laryngoscope, rigid fiberoptic video laryngoscopes (Glidescope, Verathon, Bothell, Washington; Airtraq, Airtraq LLC, Fenton, Missouri; McGrath, LMA North America, San Diego, California), FOB, lightwand, translaryngeal (retrograde) intubation, and cricothyroidotomy, can be used to secure the airway in the acute phase in patients requiring cervical spine immobilization. So far the existing data suggest that neck motion with modern video laryngoscopes is similar to that produced by the Macintosh blade, although they provide better glottic views. A gum elastic bougie passed through the endotracheal tube, or a satin-sheathed stylet placed through its Murphy aperture, may also be helpful. They can be inserted through the larynx more easily than the tube itself because their small diameter does not block the view of the glottis during direct laryngoscopy. Cricoid pressure may optimize the view, but it should be applied with great care as it may produce undue motion of the unstable spine if excessive force is used. Supraglottic intubating airways with or without the aid of FOB can be used, but neck movement with these devices appears to be comparable to that produced by conventional laryngoscopes. Flexible fiberoptic laryngoscopy, lightwand, and possibly translaryngeal-guided intubation (see "Maxillofacial Injuries" section) cause almost no neck movement, but blood or secretions in the airway, a long preparation time, and difficulty in their use in comatose, uncooperative, or anesthetized patients reduce their utility during initial management. Nasotracheal intubation carries the risks of epistaxis, failure

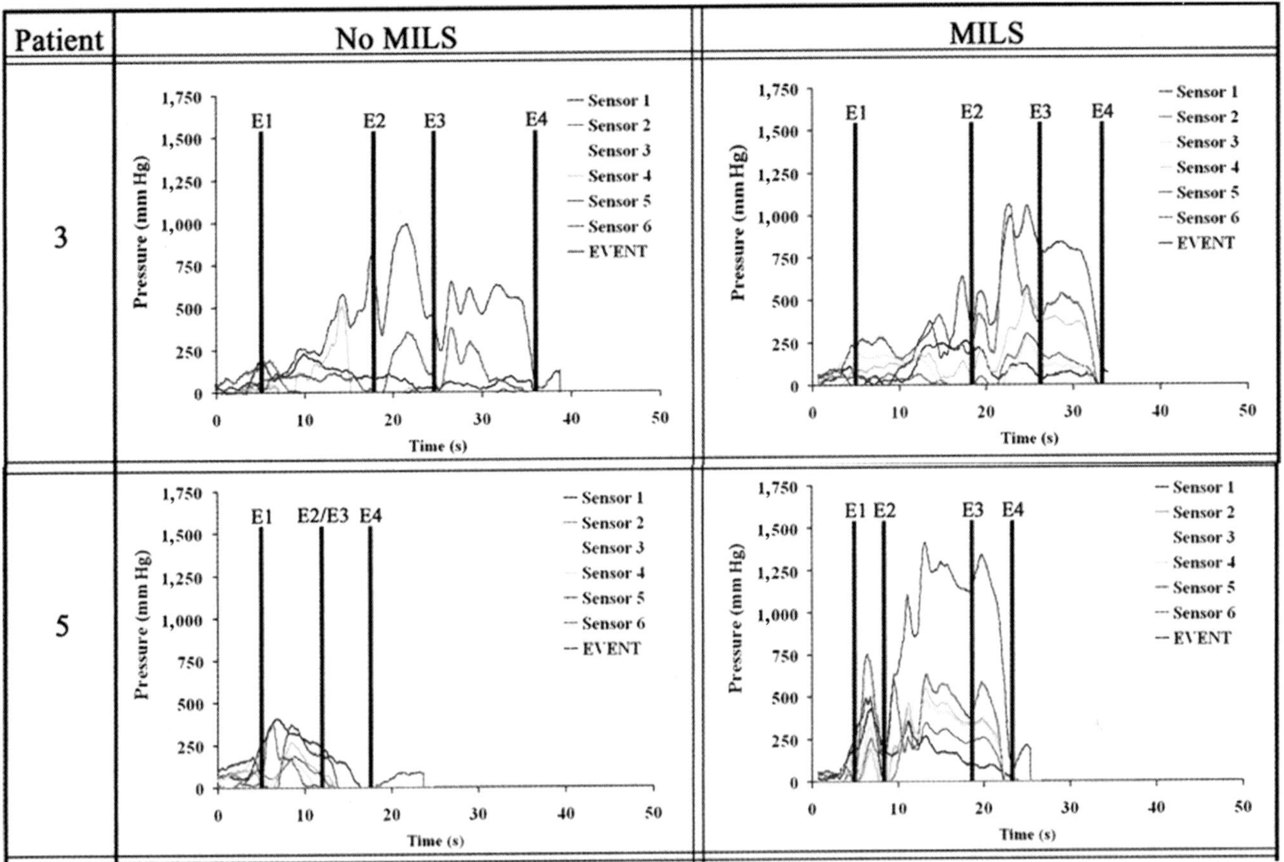

FIGURE 52-3. Pressures applied by the MacIntosh laryngoscope blade on the tongue and indirectly on the cervical spine during various phases of direct laryngoscopy and intubation in two patients. Note that applied pressure is greatest from the time of final position of the blade to the completion of intubation, especially with application of manual in line stabilization of the head and neck. (Reproduced with permission from Santoni BG, Hindman BJ, Puttlitz CM, et al. Manual in line stabilization increases pressures applied by the laryngoscope blade during direct laryngoscopy and orotracheal intubation. *Anesthesiology.* 2009;110:24.)

of intubation, and the possibility of entry of the endotracheal tube into the cranial vault or the orbit if there is damage to the cranial base or the maxillofacial complex. Absence of the usual signs of cranial base fracture (battle sign, raccoon eyes, or bleeding from the ear or the nose) cannot be relied on to exclude the possibility of its occurrence because with rapid prehospital transport, these signs may not be immediately apparent.

In the subacute phase of C-spine injury when time constraints, full stomach, and patient cooperation issues do not exist, the use of FOB in the awake, sedated patient with appropriate topical anesthesia is preferred. Advantages of this technique are minimal movement of the neck, positioning of the patient awake, maintenance of protective reflexes, and the ability to assess the neurologic status after intubation.

Direct Airway Injuries

Direct airway damage can occur anywhere between the nasopharynx and the bronchi. Sometimes more than one site may be involved, resulting in persistent airway dysfunction after one of the problems is corrected.[21] Head, face, and neck injuries are more common in military personnel in combat than in the civilian population; effective torso protection by body armor used in combat leaves these regions unprotected.[22]

Maxillofacial Injuries

In addition to soft tissue edema of the pharynx and peripharyngeal hematoma, blood or debris in the oropharynx may be responsible for partial or complete airway obstruction in the acute stage of these injuries. Occasionally, teeth or foreign bodies in the pharynx may be aspirated into the airway causing some degree of obstruction, which may occur or be recognized only during attempts at tracheal intubation. Another problem is the dynamic nature of soft tissue injuries in this region. A hematoma or edema in the face, tongue, or neck may expand during the first several hours after injury and ultimately occlude the airway. Serious airway compromise may develop within a few hours in up to

50% of patients with major penetrating facial injuries or multiple trauma, caused by progressive inflammation or edema resulting from liberal administration of fluids.

The face, head, and neck are vulnerable to missile and explosion 3 injuries.[22] Although rare, massive hemorrhage, most frequently from the internal maxillary artery or its branches, and less frequently from the facial, external carotid, or sphenopalatine arteries and other small branches, may be life threatening, requiring anterior, posterior, or anteroposterior packing, intermaxillary fixation, and, when these measures are ineffective, angioembolization.[23,24] Tracheal intubation or a surgical airway is necessary as an initial measure to avert airway compromise in these circumstances.

Fracture-induced encroachment on the airway or limitation of mandibular movement, pain, and trismus may limit mouth opening. Fentanyl in titrated doses of up to 2 to 4 μg/kg over a period of 10 to 20 minutes may produce an improvement in the patient's ability to open the mouth if mechanical limitation is not present.

The selection of an airway management technique in the presence of a maxillofacial fracture is based on the patient's presenting condition. Most patients with isolated facial injuries do not require emergency tracheal intubation. Surgery may be delayed for as long as a week with no adverse effect on the repair. Patients who present with airway compromise may be intubated using direct laryngoscopy; the decision about the use of anesthetics and muscle relaxants is based on the results of airway evaluation. When there is bleeding into the oropharynx, a flexible fiberoptic laryngoscope may be useless because of obstruction of the view. A retrograde technique, using a wire or epidural catheter passed through a 14-gauge catheter introduced into the trachea through the cricothyroid membrane, may be used if the patient can open his or her mouth. A surgical airway is indicated when there is airway compromise, when direct laryngoscopy has failed or is considered impossible, when the jaws will be wired, or when a tracheostomy will be performed anyway after definitive repair of the fracture.[25] Tracheostomy may be indicated as an emergency procedure in the emergency room within a few minutes of arrival, as a delayed procedure in the OR for airway control within 12 hours of arrival, or as an elective procedure during definitive surgery in the OR more than 12 hours following admission to the hospital.[22] Comminuted mandibular, midfacial bilateral LeFort III, and panfacial fractures are likely to be managed with tracheostomy for definitive surgery.[25] To avoid the possible complications of tracheostomy, submental or submandibular intubation, which involves externalizing the proximal end of an orotracheal flexible armored tube through a small submental incision has been performed. Thus, the trachea remains surgically intact.[26] Nasogastric or nasotracheal intubation should be avoided when a basilar skull or maxillary fracture is suspected because of the possibility that the tube may enter the cranium or the orbit. Hemorrhagic shock and life-threatening cranial, laryngotracheal, thoracic, and cervical spine injuries may accompany major facial fractures, and airway management must be tailored accordingly. The likelihood of cranial injury increases in midface fractures involving the frontal sinus, as well as the orbitozygomatic and orbitoethmoid complexes.

Cervical Airway Injuries

Injury to the cervical air passages can result from blunt or penetrating trauma. The incidence of blunt and penetrating laryngotracheal injuries admitted to major trauma centers is 0.34% and 4%, respectively.[27] Similarly to maxillofacial injuries, wartime laryngotracheal injuries are more severe and occur more frequently (5% to 6%) than peacetime injuries (0.91%).[28] Although the pharynx and esophagus are close to the cervical air passages, their involvement in peacetime trauma is less likely than airway injuries (0.08% after blunt and 0.9% after penetrating trauma).[27] Clinical signs such as air escape, hemoptysis, and coughing are present in almost all patients with penetrating injuries, facilitating the diagnosis. In contrast, major blunt laryngotracheal damage may be missed, either because the patient is asymptomatic or unresponsive, or because suggestive signs and symptoms are missed in the initial evaluation. The typical presentation includes hoarseness, muffled voice, dyspnea, stridor, dysphagia, odynophagia, cervical pain and tenderness, ecchymosis, subcutaneous emphysema, and flattening of the thyroid cartilage protuberance (Adam's apple). Whether the trauma is blunt or penetrating, attempts at blind tracheal intubation may produce further trauma to the larynx and complete airway obstruction if the endotracheal tube enters a false passage or disrupts the continuity of an already tenuous airway.[29] Thus, whenever possible, intubation of the trachea should be performed using an FOB, or the airway should be secured surgically. A CT scan of the neck provides valuable information and should be performed before any airway intervention in all stable patients without respiratory and hemodynamic compromise. Originally, the severity of laryngeal injury was classified based on endoscopic findings. With modern CT equipment, information similar to that provided by FOB can be obtained with CT scanning. A classification of laryngeal injuries is depicted in Table 52-1.[30,31]

The strategy for tracheal intubation depends on the clinical presentation.[29] The tracheas of some patients with penetrating airway injuries, especially stab wounds, may be intubated through the airway defect without the need for anesthetics or optical equipment. The presence of cartilaginous fractures or mucosal abnormalities necessitates awake intubation with an FOB or awake tracheostomy.[21] Laryngeal damage precludes cricothyroidotomy. Tracheostomy should be performed with extreme caution because up to 70% of patients with blunt laryngeal injuries may have an associated cervical spine injury.[29] Uncooperative or confused patients may not tolerate awake airway manipulation. It may be best to transport these patients to the OR, induce anesthesia with inhalational agents, and intubate the trachea without muscle relaxants.[29] Episodes of airway obstruction during spontaneous breathing under an inhalational anesthetic can be managed by positioning the patient upright in addition to the usual maneuvers.

TABLE 52-1. CLASSIFICATION OF LARYNGEAL INJURIES

Grade	Laryngeal Findings	Airway
1	No fractures Minor lacerations Minimal edema	Minimal airway symptoms
2	Undisplaced fractures Mucosal damage without cartilage exposure	Mild airway compromise
3	Displaced fractures Vocal fold immobility	Significant airway compromise
4	Multiple fractures with instability	Significant airway compromise
5	Laryngotracheal separation	Catastrophic airway obstruction

Adapted from Schaefer SD. Primary management of laryngeal trauma. *Ann Otol RhinolLaryngol.* 1982; 91:399 and Fuhrman GM, Stieg FH 3rd, Buerk CA, et al. Blunt laryngeal trauma: Classification and management protocol. *J Trauma* 1990;30:87.

Complete transection of the trachea is rare but when it occurs it is life threatening. The distal segment of the trachea retracts into the chest, causing airway obstruction either spontaneously or during airway manipulation. Surgery involves pulling up the distal end and performing an end-to-end anastomosis to the proximal segment or suturing it to the skin as a permanent tracheostomy. In extreme situations, such as complete or near-complete transection of the larynx and trachea, femorofemoral bypass or percutaneous cardiopulmonary support may be considered if time permits.[32]

Thoracic Airway Injuries

Whereas penetrating trauma can cause damage to any segment of the intrathoracic airway, blunt injury usually involves the posterior membranous portion of the trachea and the mainstem bronchi, usually within approximately 3 cm of the carina. A significant number of these injuries result from iatrogenic causes such as tracheal intubation.[33] Pneumothorax, pneumomediastinum, pneumopericardium, subcutaneous emphysema, and a continuous air leak from the chest tube are the usual signs of this injury. They occur frequently but are not specific for thoracic airway damage. In patients intubated without the suspicion of a tracheal injury, difficulty in obtaining a seal around the endotracheal tube or the presence on a chest radiograph of a large radiolucent area in the trachea corresponding to the cuff suggests a perforated airway. Other radiographic findings include a radiolucent line along the prevertebral fascia due to air tracking up from the mediastinum, peribronchial air or sudden obstruction along an air-filled bronchus, and the "dropped lung" sign when complete intrapleural bronchial transection causes the apex of the collapsed lung to descend to the level of the hilum. Occasionally, simultaneous esophageal injury with a tracheoesophageal fistula may be present.[34]

Airway management is similar to that of cervical airway injury. Anesthetics, and especially muscle relaxants, may produce irreversible obstruction, presumably because of relaxation of structures that maintain airway patency in the awake patient. However, airway loss may also occur during attempts at awake intubation, often as a result of further distortion of the airway by the endotracheal tube, patient agitation, or rebleeding into the airway. After intubation of the trachea, the adequacy of airway intervention is evaluated mainly by auscultation and capnography. Pulmonary contusion, atelectasis, diaphragmatic rupture with thoracic migration of the abdominal contents, and pneumothorax may complicate the interpretation of chest auscultation. Likewise, carbon dioxide (CO_2) elimination may be decreased or absent in shock and cardiac arrest.

The outcome after surgical repair of these injuries is often suboptimal and complicated by stump leak and empyema, suture line stenosis, or the need for tracheostomy or pneumonectomy. The recent trend is selective conservative management with an endotracheal tube placed using bronchoscopic guidance distal to the tracheal injury.[35] Patients with lesions >4 cm, cartilaginous rather than membranous injuries, concomitant esophageal trauma, progressive subcutaneous emphysema, severe dyspnea requiring intubation and ventilation, difficulty with mechanical ventilation, pneumothorax with an air leak through the chest drains, and mediastinitis are still managed surgically. Those without these problems may be treated nonoperatively with a reasonable outcome.[33,35]

Management of Breathing Abnormalities

Of the several causes that may alter respiration after trauma, tension pneumothorax, flail chest, and open pneumothorax are immediate threats to the patient's life and therefore require rapid diagnosis and treatment. Hemothorax, closed pneumothorax, pulmonary contusion, diaphragmatic rupture with herniation of abdominal contents into the thorax, and atelectasis from a mucous plug, aspiration, or chest wall splinting can also interfere with breathing and pulmonary gas exchange and deteriorate into life-threatening complications.

Although cyanosis, tachypnea, hypotension, neck vein distention, tracheal deviation, and diminished breath sounds on the affected side are the classic signs of tension pneumothorax, neck vein distention may be absent in hypovolemic patients and tracheal deviation may be difficult to appreciate. Diagnosis with an ultrasound probe placed on the second intercostal space on the suspected side to search for lung sliding and comet tail signs has the potential to provide rapid diagnosis; absence of these signs suggests the presence of pneumothorax.[36] Inability to position most trauma patients upright and the likelihood of inadequate imaging decrease the diagnostic value of chest radiographs.[37] In the supine position the "deep sulcus sign," which results from the tendency of pleural air to track in the lateral and caudal regions, is usually the diagnostic chest radiographic sign of tension pneumothorax.[37] The definitive diagnosis is made by CT scanning.[36] However, in hypoxemic and hypotensive patients, immediate insertion of a 14-gauge angiocatheter through the fourth intercostal space in the midaxillary line or, at times, through the second intercostal space at the midclavicular line, is essential. There is no time for radiologic confirmation in this setting.

4 A flail chest results from fractures of more than two sites of at least three adjacent ribs or rib fractures with associated costochondral separation or sternal fracture. An underlying pulmonary contusion with increased elastic recoil of the lung and work of breathing is the main cause of respiratory insufficiency or failure and resulting hypoxemia.[38] It often develops over a 3- to 6-hour period, causing gradual deterioration of the chest radiograph and arterial blood gases (ABGs).[38] Coexisting hemopneumothorax, paradoxical chest wall movement, and/or pain-induced splinting may contribute to the gas exchange abnormalities. Repeat evaluation by physical examination, chest radiograph, and ABG determinations is essential for early recognition of these complications. Preliminary bedside ultrasound examination showing replacement of the normal A lines with pathologic B lines also suggests pulmonary contusion.[39] The fraction of lung volume contused, as determined by chest radiograph or CT scan, may be predictive of the subsequent development of acute respiratory distress syndrome (ARDS). The likelihood increases abruptly once the contusion volume exceeds 20% of total lung volume.[40] Without significant gas exchange abnormalities, chest wall instability alone is not an indication for respiratory support. There is evidence that liberal use of tracheal intubation and mechanical ventilation in the presence of a flail chest or pulmonary contusion increases the rate of pulmonary complications and mortality and prolongs the hospital stay.[38,41] Effective pain relief by itself can improve respiratory function and often prevents the need for mechanical ventilation. For this purpose, continuous epidural analgesia with local anesthetics and opioids, preferably directed to thoracic segments, provides better pain relief and ventilatory function than parenteral opioids, reducing morbidity and mortality in elderly patients with chest wall trauma.[38] Other therapeutic measures include supplemental oxygen, continuous positive airway pressure (CPAP) of 10 to 15 cm water (H_2O) by facemask, airway humidification, chest physiotherapy, incentive spirometry, bronchodilators, airway suctioning (using FOB, if necessary), and nutritional support.[38] Overzealous infusion of fluids and transfusion of blood products may result in deterioration of oxygenation by worsening the underlying pulmonary injury.[38]

Pulmonary contusion, respiratory insufficiency or failure despite adequate analgesia, clinical evidence of severe shock, associated severe head injury or injury requiring surgery, airway obstruction, and significant pre-existing chronic pulmonary disease are indications for tracheal intubation and mechanical ventilation. Outcome in these patients may be dependent on the pattern of ventilation. In head injury patients, unless the clinical evidence suggests imminent cerebral herniation, hyperventilation must be avoided because it increases cerebral vasoconstriction, thus decreasing perfusion with accumulation of cerebral lactic acid immediately after its institution.[42] In hypovolemic patients, hyperventilation may interfere with venous return and cardiac output, leading to hypotension, further decrease in organ perfusion, and even cardiac arrest. Ventilation with low tidal volumes (6 to 8 mL/kg) and moderate positive end-expiratory pressure (PEEP), producing low inspiratory alveolar or plateau pressures, appears to be the best pattern to prevent deterioration of hemodynamics and decrease the likelihood of ARDS.[43] In intubated, spontaneously breathing patients, airway pressure release ventilation, in which spontaneous breathing is superimposed on mechanical ventilation by intermittent sudden, brief decrease of CPAP, provides improved ventilation/perfusion ($\dot{V}/\dot{Q}$) matching and systemic blood pressure, lower sedation requirements, greater oxygen (O_2) delivery, shorter periods of intubation, and a decreased incidence of ventilator-associated pneumonia, which occurs in up to 30% of ventilated patients with pulmonary contusion.[41,44,45] Severe unilateral pulmonary contusion unresponsive to these measures may be treated by differential lung ventilation via a double-lumen endobronchial tube. In bilateral severe contusions with life-threatening hypoxemia, high-frequency jet ventilation may enhance oxygenation and cardiac function, which may be compromised by concomitant myocardial contusion or ischemia.[46]

Systemic air embolism occurs mainly after penetrating lung trauma and blast injuries, or less frequently after blunt thoracic trauma that produces lacerations of both distal air passages and pulmonary veins.[47] Positive-pressure ventilation after tracheal intubation may then result in entrainment of air into the systemic circulation. Hemoptysis, circulatory instability, and CNS dysfunction immediately after starting artificial ventilation, as well as detection of air in blood from the radial artery, establishes the diagnosis. Air bubbles may also be seen in the coronary arteries during thoracotomy. Surgical management involves immediate thoracotomy and clamping of the hilum of the lacerated lung. Respiratory maneuvers that minimize or prevent air entry into the systemic circulation include isolating and collapsing the lacerated lung by means of a double-lumen tube or ventilation with the lowest possible tidal volumes via a single-lumen tube.[47] Transesophageal echocardiography (TEE) of the left side of the heart may permits visualization of air bubbles and their disappearance with therapeutic maneuvers.

Management of Shock

5 Hemorrhage is the most common cause of traumatic hypotension and shock and is, after head injury, the second most common cause of mortality after trauma. Other causes are abnormal pump function (myocardial contusion, pericardial tamponade, pre-existing cardiac disease, or coronary artery or cardiac valve injury), pneumothorax or hemothorax, spinal cord injury, and rarely, anaphylaxis or sepsis (Table 52-2).

In bleeding patients the primary goal is the urgent surgical control of the source of bleeding. Certain types of bleeding sources, however, may be temporarily controlled with nonsurgical measures, such as finger compression of open neck injuries and tourniquet control of external bleeding from extremities. Tourniquets should be removed as soon as urgent surgical control is achieved to avoid pressure-induced nerve damage, skin necrosis, or limb ischemia.

Evaluation of the severity of hemorrhagic shock in the initial phase is based on the mechanism and anatomical pattern of injury, hemodynamic data, and the response to fluid resuscitation. Free falls from heights >6 m, high-energy deceleration impact, and high velocity gunshot wounds are very likely to produce major damage and bleeding. Thoracoabdominal and pelvic injuries also are likely to be associated with major bleeding. Immediate evaluation of these anatomical sites with radiographs of the chest and pelvis, focused abdominal sonography for trauma (FAST), CT, or rarely, diagnostic peritoneal lavage (DPL), is necessary. Patients with significant intra-abdominal fluid recognized with these tests and hemodynamic instability require immediate surgical intervention. Those who are suspected to have occult abdominal bleeding based on a high-risk mechanism of injury but who are hemodynamically stable must undergo further evaluation with CT. The modern multislice CT devices available in most trauma centers can provide early whole-body scanning with or without contrast within a few minutes.[48] By using contrast, a delayed-phase CT can also demonstrate the active bleeding site.

Clinical assessment using hemodynamic data is based on a few relatively insensitive and nonspecific clinical signs. For example, tachycardia, which is traditionally used as an index of hypovolemia, may be absent in up to 30% of hypotensive trauma patients because of increased vagal tone, chronic cocaine use, or other reasons.[49] Inability of the patient to elevate the heart rate in the face of hypoperfusion is considered a predictor of increased mortality independent of severity of injury, systemic blood pressure, or the presence of a head injury.[49] In contrast, by increasing catecholamine output, tissue injury and associated pain may maintain tachycardia and normal systemic blood pressure in the presence or absence of hypovolemia without necessarily increasing the cardiac index or tissue oxygen delivery. In fact, in this situation an increase in intestinal vascular resistance and a decrease in splanchnic blood flow may occur, and if prolonged, may allow entry of intestinal micro-organisms into the circulation and increase the likelihood of subsequent sepsis and organ failure.[50–52] Thus, equating a normal heart rate and systemic blood pressure with normovolemia during initial resuscitation may lead to loss of valuable time for treating underlying occult hypovolemia or hypoperfusion. This is especially true in the elderly trauma population (age >65) in whom significant tissue hypoperfusion in the presence of normal blood pressure is more likely than in younger patients.[53] Traditionally, the normal systolic blood pressure (SBP) is defined as 90 mm Hg. Recent findings suggest that trauma patients with this level or lower emergency department (ED) SBP have a higher mortality, higher blood lactate levels, and greater base deficits than civilian trauma patients with a SBP of 110 mm Hg and injured soldiers with a SBP of 100 mm Hg[54,55] (Fig. 52-4). Thus, the optimal SBP in the trauma patient appears to be 100 to 110 mm Hg. Although traditional vital signs are relatively unreliable for recognizing life-threatening shock, heart rate, systemic blood pressure, pulse pressure, respiratory rate, urine output, and mental status are still used as early clinical indicators of the severity of hemorrhagic shock. (Table 52-3).[50,56] Shock index (SI), a value derived by dividing the heart rate by the SBP, appears to be a more accurate indicator of early hemorrhagic shock and a predictor of mortality than the individual vital signs. In normal individuals, SI varies between 0.58 and 0.64 (mean 0.61) increasing from 0.70 to 0.80 (mean 0.75) after a moderate degree of blood loss. In the elderly, it has been demonstrated that age times SI identifies early shock and predicts mortality better than SI itself.[57]

TABLE 52-2. GUIDELINES FOR MANAGEMENT OF TRAUMATIC SHOCK

	Etiology					
	Hemorrhage or Extensive Tissue Injury	Cardiac Tamponade	Myocardial Contusion	Pneumothorax or Hemothorax	Spinal Cord Injury	Sepsis
Primary mechanisms	Hypovolemia	Ventricular inflow restriction	Diminished ventricular performance and elevated pulmonary vascular resistance	Lung collapse Mediastinal shift, causing inflow and outflow obstruction of the heart	Vasodilatation and relative hypovolemia caused by loss of sympathetic tone	Intestinal perforation causing peritoneal contamination
Typical signs and symptoms	Tachycardia Narrow pulse pressure Cold, clammy skin from vasoconstriction	Tachycardia Hypotension Dilated and engorged neck veins Muffled heart sounds Diminished BP response to fluid challenge	Dysrhythmia Tachycardia Hypotension	Tachycardia Hypotension Dilated and engorged neck veins Absent breath sounds Hyperresonance to percussion Tracheal shift Dyspnea Subcutaneous emphysema	Hypotension without tachycardia, cutaneous vasoconstriction, or narrow pulse pressure	Develops mainly a few hours after colon injury In hypovolemic patients, signs and symptoms indistinguishable from hypovolemic shock In normovolemic patients, fever, modest tachycardia, warm, pink skin, near normal BP, wide pulse pressure Hypotension may develop
Treatment continuum, from least to most intense	Crystalloids initially Transfusion if 2,000 mL of crystalloid in 15 min does not restore BP	Pericardiocentesis Pericardial window Emergency room thoracotomy	Fluids Fluids and vasodilators Fluids and inotropes	Release of air with 14-gauge catheter Chest tube	Fluids Fluids and vasopressors Fluids, vasopressors, and inotropes, if myocardial damage is present	Fluids and antibiotics Fluids, antibiotics, and inotropes for hypotension

BP, blood pressure.
Reproduced with permission from American College of Surgeons, Committee on Trauma. Shock, *Advanced Trauma Life Support Student Course Manual.* 8th ed. Chicago: American College of Surgeons; 2008:55–71.

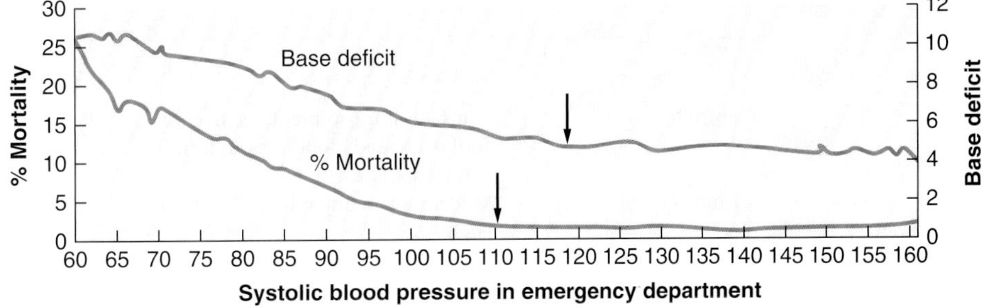

FIGURE 52-4. Relationship between emergency department systolic blood pressure, base deficit, and overall mortality rate of trauma patients; head injury patients are not included. Note that mortality and base deficit decrease as systolic blood pressure increases, stabilizing at 110 mm Hg rather than at the generally accepted 90 mm Hg. BP, blood pressure. (Adapted with permission from Eastridge BJ, Salinas J, Wade CE, et al. Hypotension begins at 110 mm Hg: Redefining "hypotension" with data. *J Trauma.* 2007;63:291.)

TABLE 52-3. ADVANCED TRAUMA LIFE SUPPORT CLASSIFICATION OF HEMORRHAGIC SHOCK[a]

	Class I	Class II	Class III	Class IV
Blood loss (mL)	≤750	750–1,500	1,500–2,000	≥2,000
Blood loss (% blood volume)	≤15	15–30	30–40	≥40
Pulse rate (per min)	<100	>100	>120	≥140
Blood pressure	Normal	Normal	Decreased	Decreased
Pulse pressure	Normal or increased	Decreased	Decreased	Decreased
Respiratory rate (breaths/min)	14–20	20–30	30–40	>35
Urine output (mL/hr)	≥30	20–30	5–15	Negligible
Mental status	Slightly anxious	Mildly anxious	Anxious and confused	Confused, lethargic
Fluid replacement (3:1 rule)	Crystalloid[b]	Crystalloid	Crystalloid + blood	Crystalloid + blood

[a]For a 70-kg male patient, based on initial presentation.
[b]The 3:1 rule is based on empiric observation that most patients require 300 mL balanced electrolyte solution for each 100 mL blood loss. Without other clinical and monitoring parameters, this guideline may result in excessive or inadequate fluid resuscitation.
Adapted with permission from American College of Surgeons, Committee on Trauma. *Shock, Advanced Trauma Life Support Student Course Manual.* 8th ed. Chicago: American College of Surgeons; 2008:55–71.

Finally, the response to initial fluid resuscitation in the form of lactated Ringer's or normal saline solution of about 2 L, or 20 mL/kg in children, over a period of 15 to 30 minutes may allow estimation of the severity of hemorrhage (Table 52-4).[45] The goal of therapy is to re-establish organ perfusion. Overinfusing fluids in patients who have normalized their SBP may lead to further bleeding by increasing arterial and venous pressures, diluting clotting factors and platelets, reducing body temperature, and decreasing blood viscosity.[58,59] Bickell et al.[60] showed that delaying fluid resuscitation until surgical control of bleeding in victims of penetrating trauma improved survival to hospital discharge and decreased the length of hospital stay. Although many experimental studies have confirmed the findings of Bickell et al.,[60] it has also become clear that withholding fluids completely can result in as much harm as vigorous resuscitation.[61] In contrast, slow infusion of isotonic or hypertonic crystalloids and preferably of packed red blood cells (PRBCs), titrated to slightly lower than normal systemic pressure, had beneficial effects on animal survival without tissue injury or organ failure. A clinical study conducted subsequent to Bickell et al.[60] on hypotensive resuscitation demonstrated better outcome in penetrating, but not in blunt trauma.[62] Nevertheless, while this practice is contraindicated in traumatic brain and spinal cord injuries and in elderly patients with chronic systemic hypertension where adequate perfusion is crucial,[59] it emphasizes the useful fact that fluid administration in excess of that needed to achieve normovolemia prior to control of hemorrhage may be deleterious.[58] Early use of vasopressors to maintain hemodynamic stability has also been shown to be associated with deleterious effects.[63] However, judicious use of these drugs along with carefully titrated fluids may offer some advantages.

Crystalloids are used in the vast majority of trauma centers for initial resuscitation.[59] Hypertonic saline (250 mL 7.5% with 6% dextran-70) is safe and may be associated with lower intracranial pressure than normal saline in brain-injured patients[59] and may improve hemodynamics in hypotensive penetrating trauma patients.[64] Although colloid solutions are associated with an increased risk of organ failure and death in trauma victims, a meta-analysis showed no difference in mortality between colloids and crystalloids.[65] If used, hydroxyethyl starch solutions (maximum 20 mL/kg) should probably be given priority over albumin solutions because the possible deleterious effects of colloids have mostly been associated with albumin.

Some of the proven markers of organ perfusion can be used during early management to set the goals of resuscitation. Of

TABLE 52-4. RESPONSE TO INITIAL FLUID RESUSCITATION[a]

	Rapid Response	Transient Response	Minimal or No Response
Vital signs	Return to normal	Transient improvement, recurrence of decreased blood pressure, and increased heart rate	Remain abnormal
Estimated blood loss	Minimal (10%–20%)	Moderate and ongoing (20%–40%)	Severe (>40%)
Need for more crystalloid	Low	High	High
Need for blood	Low	Moderate to high	Immediate
Blood preparation	Type and crossmatch	Type specific	Emergency blood release
Need for operative intervention	Possible	Likely	Highly likely
Early presence of surgeon	Yes	Yes	Yes

[a]2,000 mL of isotonic solution in adults; 20 mL/kg bolus of Ringer's lactate in children.
Adapted with permission from American College of Surgeons, Committee on Trauma. *Shock, Advanced Trauma Life Support Student Course Manual.* 8th ed. Chicago: American College of Surgeons; 2008:55–71.

these, the base deficit and blood lactate level are the most useful and practical tools during all phases of shock, including the earliest. The base deficit reflects the severity of shock, the oxygen debt, changes in O_2 delivery, the adequacy of fluid resuscitation, and the likelihood of multiple organ failure and survival with reasonable accuracy in *previously healthy* adult and pediatric trauma patients.[59] Base deficit is considered a better prognostic marker than the arterial pH. A base deficit between –2 and –5 mmol/L suggests mild shock, between –6 and –9 mmol/L indicates moderate shock, whereas ≤–10 mmol/L is a sign of severe shock.[59] An admission base deficit below –5 to –8 mmol/L correlates with increased mortality. Thus, normalization of the base deficit is one of the end points of resuscitation. Elevation of the blood lactate level is less specific than base deficit as a marker of tissue hypoxia because it can be generated in well-oxygenated tissues by increased epinephrine-induced skeletal muscle glycolysis, accelerated pyruvate oxidation, decreased hepatic clearance of lactate, and early mitochondrial dysfunction. All these conditions may be present in the trauma patient. Thus, blood lactate and base deficit may not closely correlate with each other. Nevertheless, in most trauma victims an elevated lactate level correlates with other signs of hypoperfusion, rendering it an important marker of dysoxia and an end point of resuscitation. The normal plasma lactate concentration is 0.5 to 1.5 mmol/L; levels >5 mmol/L indicate significant lactic acidosis. The half-life of lactate is approximately 3 hours; thus, the level decreases rather gradually after correction of the cause. Failure to clear lactate within 24 hours after reversal of circulatory shock is a predictor of increased mortality.[59]

Measurement of hemoglobin (Hgb) or hematocrit (Hct) helps in managing the bleeding trauma patient. However, decision making based on a single Hct value may lead to erroneous management decisions. Trauma patients, if not treated with adequate crystalloids or colloids or those receiving PRBC transfusion, can maintain a normal Hct despite ongoing bleeding and delay in surgical control. On the other hand, serial Hct measurements and consideration of the type and amount of fluid received may be useful in deciding the timing and amount of transfusion.[66] The usefulness of Hgb or Hct as a PRBC transfusion threshold remains unclear, although the recommended target Hgb concentration in all phases of management is 7 to 9 g/dL, including brain-injured patients in whom tissue oxygenation is most relevant.[59] In brain-injured patients, although several studies demonstrated that increasing the Hgb level to 9 or 10 g/dL from lower levels with PRBCs of <19 days storage increased brain oxygenation in 75% of patients,[67,68] data from other sources showed either increased morbidity and mortality with PRBC transfusion[69] or improved neurological outcome when the Hct value was kept <30 (Hgb <10 g/dL) for longer periods.[70] Transfusion of PRBC has been shown to be an independent risk factor for mortality, lung injury, increased infection rate, renal failure, and intensive care unit (ICU) and hospital length of stay in trauma patients, especially when the transfused red cells are older than 14 days; this finding was true independent of the severity of shock.[71,72] Nevertheless, this concern should not preclude timely and adequate administration of blood products.

Normally, type-specific crossmatched blood can be available in most centers in about 30 minutes, including transport time. Type-specific uncrossmatched blood can be available in even less time for patients with severe hemorrhage. However, if the situation dictates immediate transfusion, type O, Rh-positive, AB-negative fresh frozen plasma (FFP) is satisfactory in most situations. Controversy exists about the use of uncrossmatched type O PRBC because of concern about the development of alloantibodies and allergic reactions. Dutton et al.,[73] reviewing their experience in 161 patients receiving 581 units of universal donor blood, demonstrated that only 1 of the 10 Rh-negative males receiving O, Rh-positive blood developed alloantibodies. All four females in the series received type O, Rh-negative blood without apparent problem.

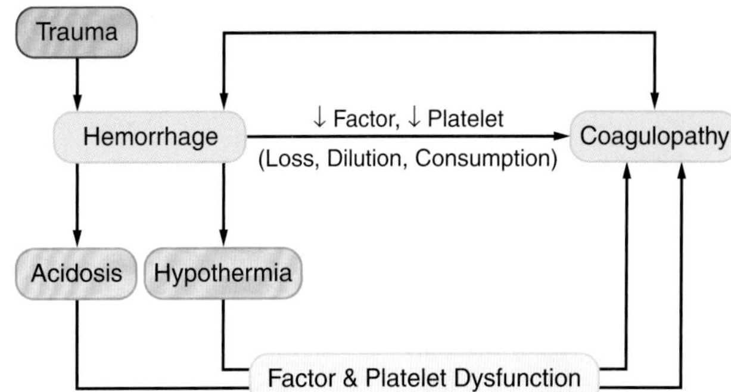

FIGURE 52-5. Schematic representation of bloody vicious cycle or lethal triad. Trauma-induced hemorrhage causes acidosis, hypothermia, and coagulopathy. Acidosis and hypothermia produce factor and platelet dysfunction, enhancing coagulopathy, which in turn causes increased bleeding. The cycle continues until death ensues, unless effective treatment by timely control of bleeding and correction of acidosis, hypothermia, and coagulopathy is instituted.

6 One of the principal goals during early management of the hemorrhaging trauma victim is to avoid the development of the so-called vicious cycle or lethal triad, consisting of acidosis, hypothermia, and coagulopathy (Fig. 52-5). Both acidosis and hypothermia are major factors in the induction of coagulopathy. Resuscitation with fluids and PRBCs, which have no hemostatic activity, further adds to this effect by diluting platelets, already reduced in number and dysfunctional, and coagulation factors. Bleeding and intravascular coagulation further augments coagulopathy via loss or consumption of damaged or depleted platelets and coagulation factors. Augmented coagulopathy further increases the blood loss, necessitating additional fluid replacement and thus maintaining the vicious cycle.

The practice of administering large volumes of crystalloids, colloids, and PRBCs with no hemostatic components for initial resuscitation is considered to be the major factor in the development of often lethal coagulopathy. Most trauma patients are hypercoagulable when admitted to the ER and do not develop coagulopathy
7 when administration of hemostatic agents is delayed. However, in the estimated 10% of patients with severe trauma and shock who enter the hospital in a hypocoagulable state[74] or rapidly develop hypocoagulation, resuscitative fluids and PRBCs may further worsen the coagulopathy and facilitate the vicious cycle. A computer simulation study by Hirshberg et al.[75] clearly demonstrated that with current fluid resuscitation techniques, most major trauma patients are coagulopathic at the time they arrive to the OR. In their study, the prothrombin time (PT) would increase to below hemostatic levels after replacement of one blood volume, fibrinogen function would become inadequate at replacement of 1.25 blood volumes, and finally, platelets with replacement of 1.75 blood volumes. Experience gained from the Iraq and Afghanistan wars attests to the accuracy of the findings of Hirshberg et al.[75] Holcomb et al.[76] strongly recommend starting liquid plasma replacement along with fluids and PRBCs as soon as the patient arrives in the ER and continuing it throughout surgery.

Liquid plasma differs from FFP in that it is frozen at –180°C within 8 to 24 hours, whereas FFP is frozen within 8 hours. It contains all of the stable proteins found in FFP, although in slightly lower concentrations. The major difference is a 25% reduction of factor VIII. One unit of FFP contains approximately 7% of the

TABLE 52-5. MASSIVE TRANSFUSION PROTOCOL USED IN GRADY MEMORIAL HOSPITAL IN ATLANTA

Package	PRBCs	Plasma	Platelets	Cryoprecipitate
Initiation	**6 U (UD/TS)**	**6 U (UD)**		
1 (0.5 hr)	6 U (UD/TS)	6 U (UD)	1 apheresis[a]	
2 (1 hr)	6 U (UD/TS)	6 U (TS)		10 U
3 (1.5 hr)	6 U (UD/TS)	6 U (TS)	1 apheresis[a]	
4 (2 hr)	6 U (UD/TS)	6 U (TS)		10 U
5 (2.5 hr)	6 U (UD/TS)	6 U (TS)	1 apheresis[a]	
6 (3 hr)	6 U (UD/TS)	6 U (TS)		10 U

UD, universal donor; TS, type specific.
[a]One apheresis unit of platelet is equal to 8–10 standard units.
Reproduced with permission from Dente CJ, Shaz BH, Nicholas JM, et al. Early predictors of massive transfusion in patients sustaining torso gunshot wounds in a civilian level 1 trauma center. *J Trauma.* 2010;68:298.

coagulation factor activity of a 70-kg man. Thawing of FFP or liquid plasma takes about 30 minutes. The recommended ratio of FFP and platelets to PRBCs varies widely, ranging from 1:10 to 2:3 for FFP to PRBCs and from 6:10 to 12:10 for platelets to PRBCs.[77] Nevertheless, military data demonstrate that the death rate was 65% when the plasma to PRBC ratio was 1:8, 34% when it was 1:2.5, and 19% for 1:1.4.[78]

Currently many trauma centers use hemostatic resuscitation (massive transfusion) protocols during initial resuscitation of major traumatic hemorrhage in the ED and OR. These involve administering a relatively limited quantity of crystalloid solutions and volume replacement with liquid plasma or FFP and PRBCs. In addition, platelets and cryoprecipitate are given regularly. One such protocol, used in Grady Memorial Hospital in Atlanta, Georgia, is shown in Table 52-5.[79]

Timely initiation of massive transfusion or hemostatic resuscitation protocol is associated with improved survival and reduced transfusion.[80,81] However, identification of these patients early enough is difficult. Much effort has been directed recently at specifying criteria to identify these patients. Cotton et al.[82] recently validated previously proposed simple criteria as an early massive transfusion trigger. The ABC score is calculated by assigning a value of 0 or 1 to each of four parameters: penetrating mechanism, positive FAST, arrival SBP <90 mm Hg, and heart rate >120 beats per minute. A score of ≥2 was associated with an increased likelihood of massive transfusion. Larson et al.[81] demonstrated that the presence of any two of the of four admission findings (heart rate >110 beats per minute, SBP <110 mm Hg, base deficit <–6, and Hgb <11) predicted massive transfusion with high likelihood. Finally Callcut et al.[83] demonstrated that each of the five massive transfusion trigger variables proposed by the military did not have the same predictive ability. Of SBP <90 mm Hg, Hgb <11 g/dL, body temperature <35.5°C, International Normalized Ratio (INR) >1.5, and base deficit <–6, INR was the most predictive of massive transfusion. However, generally the presence of three or more of these five triggers suggests a greater likelihood for the need of massive transfusion. Finally, rapid thromboelastography (r-TEG) can be useful to decide on early (<1 hour) administration of FFP and platelets.[84]

Rapid establishment of venous access with large-bore cannulae placed in peripheral veins that drain both above and below the diaphragm is essential for adequate fluid resuscitation in the patient who is severely injured. When vascular collapse and extremity injury impair access to arm or leg vessels, percutaneous cannulation of the internal jugular, subclavian, or femoral veins can be performed. Ultrasound guidance may facilitate cannulation of the internal jugular vein and prevent needle entry and infusion of fluids into the pleural space in patients with a large hemothorax. Ultrasound may also be used for infraclavicular access to the axillary vein, the cephalic or basilic veins at the midarm level, or to the femoral vein. If necessary, a cutdown to a saphenous or arm vein can be rapidly performed in older children and adults. In children <5 years of age, intraosseous cannulation has a high success rate and a low incidence of complications. Infusion rates comparable with those obtained with intravenous lines are possible in small children, although a pressure infusion device may be necessary to achieve adequate flow.

Patients who arrive in the ED in cardiac arrest require advanced cardiac life support. However, the success rate of external cardiac massage in hypovolemic trauma victims is likely to be low.[85] ED thoracotomy not only permits performance of open cardiac massage, but also aids resuscitation efforts by allowing drainage of pericardial blood, control of cardiac and great vessel bleeding, application of a cross-clamp to the aorta, and rapid administration of fluids through a small Foley catheter introduced into the right atrium, or in desperate situations, through a large-bore catheter or introducer in the descending aorta. This procedure is not indicated in blunt torso trauma. The mortality rate is similar regardless of whether it is attempted or not.[86] In penetrating injuries, depending on the presenting condition of the patient, the initial success rate may be as high as 70%, but the neurologically intact hospital discharge rate is only 10% to 15%.[86,87]

EARLY MANAGEMENT OF SPECIFIC INJURIES

Head Injury

Approximately 40% of deaths from trauma are caused by head injury, and indeed, even a moderate brain injury may increase the mortality rate of patients with other injuries. In nonsurvivors, progression of the damaged area beyond the directly injured region (secondary brain injury) can be demonstrated at autopsy.[88] The major factor in secondary injury is tissue hypoxia, which results in lactic acidosis, free radical generation, prostaglandin synthesis and release of excitatory amino acids (primarily glutamate), lipid peroxidation and breakdown of cell membranes, entry of large

TABLE 52-6. EFFECTS ON OUTCOME OF SECONDARY INSULTS OCCURRING FROM TIME OF INJURY THROUGH RESUSCITATION[a]

Secondary Insults	No. of Patients	Total Patients (%)	6-Month Outcome (%) Good/ Moderate	Severe/ Vegetative	Dead
Total cases	717	100	43.0	20.2	36.8
Neither	308	43.0	63.9	10.2	26.9
Hypoxia	161	22.4	50.3	21.7	28.0
Hypotension	62	11.4	32.9	17.1	50.0
Both	166	23.2	20.5	22.3	57.2

[a]Data from hospital emergency departments enrolled in Traumatic Coma Data Bank.
Reprinted with permission from Prough DS, Lang J. Therapy of patients with head injuries: Key parameters for management. *J Trauma.* 1997;42(Suppl):10S.

quantities of sodium, calcium, and water into the cells, and leakage of fluid from the blood vessels into the extracellular space.[89,90] This process results in brain edema and both regional and global disturbances of the cerebral circulation. Thus, of all the possible secondary insults to the injured brain, decreased oxygen delivery as a result of hypotension and hypoxia has the greatest detrimental impact (Table 52-6).[91,92]

Brain injury by itself does not cause hypotension in adults except as a preterminal event. However, more than half of the patients with severe head trauma have other injuries that render approximately 15% of them hypotensive. Approximately 30% are hypoxic on admission as a result of central respiratory depression or associated chest injuries. Furthermore, exposure to these insults is likely to occur during any phase of the continuum of hospital care: in the radiology unit, the OR, the postanesthesia care unit, the ICU, or elsewhere. The most common early complications of head trauma are intracranial hypertension, brain herniation, seizures, neurogenic pulmonary edema, cardiac dysrhythmias, bradycardia, systemic hypertension, and coagulopathy.

Diagnosis

Mental impairment after trauma may have any of several etiologies. However, the possibility of hypoxia and shock must always be considered first. If consciousness remains depressed despite ventilation and fluid replacement, a head injury is assumed to be present and the patient is managed accordingly. As noted, hypotension is the most important cause of death in the head-injured patient. Chesnut[92] demonstrated that a single episode of SBP <90 mm Hg is associated with a 50% increase in mortality, and subsequent episodes or lower pressures increase mortality even further.[93] Therefore, every effort should be made to support the blood pressure with fluids and vasopressors (preferably phenylephrine, which does not constrict cerebral vessels) and ensure adequate oxygenation *before* the unconscious patient is evaluated. A baseline neurologic examination should be performed after initial resuscitation but before any sedative or muscle relaxant agents are administered, and this should be repeated at frequent intervals because the patient's condition may change rapidly. Anesthetic and adjunct drugs may render an adequate neurologic examination impossible; thus, long-acting muscle relaxants, opioids, sedatives, or hypnotics should be given selectively.[91,94]

Consciousness can be initially assessed within a few seconds using the AVPU system (*a*lert; responds to *v*erbal stimuli; responds to *p*ain; *u*nresponsive) (Table 52-7). More precise information is provided by the GCS (Table 52-7), which provides a standard means of evaluating the patient's neurologic status. In this test, the sum of the scores obtained for eye opening, verbal response, and

TABLE 52-7. TWO-LEVEL INITIAL EVALUATION OF CONSCIOUSNESS

Level 1. AVPU System	
A = Alert	
V = Responds to verbal stimuli	
P = Responds to painful stimuli	
U = Unresponsive	
Level 2. Glasgow Coma Scale (GCS)	
Eye opening (E)	
Spontaneous, already open and blinking	4
To speech	3
To pain	2
None	1
Verbal response (V)	
Oriented	5
Answers but confused	4
Inappropriate but recognizable words	3
Incomprehensible sounds	2
None	1
Best motor response (M)	
Obeys verbal commands	6
Localizes painful stimulus	5
Withdraws from painful stimulus	4
Decorticate posturing (upper extremity flexion)	3
Decerebrate posturing (upper extremity extension)	2
No movement	1
GCS ≤8 = deep coma, severe head trauma, poor outcome	
GCS 9–12 = conscious patient with moderate injury	
GCS >12 = mild injury	

motor activity correlates with the state of consciousness, the severity of the head injury, and the prognosis.[94] Assessment of motor function should be performed on the extremity that responds best. The limb affected by neurologic injury is examined, but the result is not considered in the GCS.

Dilatation and sluggish response of the pupil is a sign of compression of the oculomotor nerve by the medial portion of the temporal lobe (uncus). A maximally dilated and unresponsive "blown" pupil suggests uncal herniation under the falx cerebri. The presence of similar findings in ocular injuries makes interpretation of pupillary findings difficult when eye and head injuries coexist. However, the pupillary reaction to light is usually more sluggish in the head-injured patient.

CT scanning is used for the diagnosis of most acute head injuries. Positive CT findings after acute head injury include midline shift, distortion of the ventricles and cisterns, effacement of the sulci in the uninjured hemisphere, and the presence of a hematoma at any location in the cranial vault. Subdural hematomas usually have a concave border, whereas epidural hematomas present with a convex outline classically termed a *lenticular* configuration. Patients in severe coma (GCS <8) have a 40% likelihood of an intracranial hematoma. Those with higher GCS scores are less likely to have had intracranial bleeding although it is evident that the significant incidence of this complication even in these patients necessitates a CT study, preferably with contrast enhancement. Other benefits of CT scanning include detection of intracranial air and depressed skull fractures.

Management

The primary objective of the early management of brain trauma is to prevent or alleviate the secondary injury process that may follow any complication that decreases the oxygen supply to the brain, including systemic hypotension, hypoxemia, anemia, raised ICP, acidosis, and possibly hyperglycemia (serum glucose >200 mg/dL). These insults cause exacerbation of trauma-induced cerebral ischemia and metabolic derangements, worsen-
8 ing the outcome.[95,96] *The most important therapeutic maneuvers in these patients are aimed at normalizing ICP, CPP, and oxygen delivery.* The Brain Trauma Foundation and the American Association of Neurological Surgeons have published evidence-based guidelines for the treatment of head-injured patients.[91] Primary therapy includes normalization of the systemic blood pressure (mean blood pressure >80 mm Hg) and maintaining the PaO_2 >95, the ICP <20 to 25 mm Hg, and the CPP 50 to 70 mm Hg. Maintaining the CPP at levels above 70 mm Hg, the former standard, is no longer advised because it may be associated with an increased incidence of ARDS.[91] The patient is kept at 30-degree head elevation, sedation and paralysis are given as necessary, and cerebrospinal fluid is drained through a ventriculostomy catheter if available. Rapid and adequate restoration of the intravascular volume with isotonic crystalloid and, if necessary, with colloid solutions should be aimed at maintaining the CPP between 50 and 70 mm Hg while attempting to minimize further brain swelling. Lactated Ringer's (LR) solution, which is slightly hypotonic (Na^+ = 130 mEq/L, osmolality ~255 mOsm/L), may promote swelling in uninjured areas of the brain if it is given in large quantities. Edema tends to occur in injured brain regions regardless of the type of solution administered because of increased permeability of the blood–brain barrier. To minimize edema formation, it is wise to monitor serum osmolality and to replace LR solution with isotonic normal saline. If serum osmolality cannot be measured, this change can be made empirically after 3 L of LR solution.

Much of the focus has been on in-hospital management of patients with brain trauma, but there is increasing interest in the impact of prehospital care on the outcome in these patients. Multiple studies have demonstrated an association between prehospital endotracheal intubation and mortality of patients with severe brain trauma.[97,98] In a large multicenter retrospective study, Davis et al.[99] found that patients with GCS ≤8, in whom endotracheal intubation was attempted at the accident site, had a higher mortality than those who were not intubated until arrival at the emer-
9 gency room (adjusted odds ratio of 2.91; *P* <.01). The authors speculated that this may result from physiological insults during intubation (elevated ICP, oxygen desaturation, or inadvertent postintubation hyperventilation and cerebral hypoperfusion with ischemia) and concluded that there may be no benefit to prehospital endotracheal intubation.

Normalization of the ICP has been shown to reduce mortality.[100] Effective reduction in ICP can be provided, or at least aided, by administration of mannitol, an important part of the management of severe head injury. It is administered in boluses of 0.25 to 0.5 g/kg and repeated every 4 to 6 hours as needed to control the ICP.[91] Higher doses, up to 2 g/kg, are recommended by some authors.[101] In addition to its osmotic diuretic effect, this agent may improve cerebral blood flow (CBF) and O_2 delivery by reducing the hematocrit and thus the blood viscosity, improving CBF and oxygen delivery.[91] There is a risk of hypovolemia and resultant hypotension when therapeutic doses of mannitol are used. If the ICP elevation persists, additional doses of mannitol should be given cautiously. Acute mannitol toxicity, manifested by hyponatremia, high serum osmolality, and a gap between calculated and measured serum osmolality >10 mOsm/L, may result when the drug is given in large doses (2 to 3 g/kg) or to patients with renal failure. Mannitol should be used with great care in the presence of hypotension, sepsis, nephrotoxic drugs, or preexisting renal disease, because these may also precipitate renal failure.[91] Further, the effects of mannitol result from its activity in regions of the brain where the blood–brain barrier is intact. It may exacerbate edema in injured areas in which it may easily enter the tissues.

The addition of relatively small volumes of hypertonic saline in concentrations between 3% (6 to 8 mL/kg) and 7.5% (4 mL/kg) followed by infusion of LR may be beneficial in multiple trauma patients with head injury.[102] In addition, hypertonic saline (15% solution), in bolus doses of 0.42 mL/kg, is as efficacious as mannitol for initial therapy of elevated ICP in this patient population.[101] Like mannitol, hypertonic saline draws fluid from the intracellular space and, thus, in addition to restoring the blood volume, it reduces brain edema and prevents elevation of the ICP.[103] On the other hand, hypertonic saline may, also like mannitol, increase edema in the injured region of the brain.[104] The intravascular volume expansion produced by hypertonic saline is transient. It can be prolonged by addition of 6% dextran-70 or hetastarch to the solution. However, administration of hypertonic saline cannot be maintained for long periods. It may cause hypernatremia, hyperosmolality, or hyperchloremic acidosis, probably from renal bicarbonate loss secondary to increased levels of chloride (Cl^-). Serum concentrations of sodium (Na^+) and Cl^- and the patient's acid–base status should be followed, and the administration of hypertonic saline should be discontinued if plasma Na^+ reaches 160 mEq/L. Because of these considerations, and the fact that there has been no standardization of the concentration, the dose, or the duration of treatment, the use of hypertonic saline should still be considered experimental therapy.[91,105] Resuscitation with colloid solutions (hetastarch, pentastarch, pentafraction, human albumin 5% and

25%, or dextran) provides a sustained improvement in vital signs, but the increase in colloid osmotic pressure produced by these solutions may not have an important role in reducing brain edema.

Hyponatremia in these patients results from intravascular volume expansion rather than sodium loss; thus treatment with saline solutions is not appropriate. Because of a synergistic action between mannitol and loop diuretics in improving the ICP, addition of furosemide may be a safer and more effective treatment than increasing the dose of mannitol when intracranial hypertension persists. Until about 1995, hyperventilation to a $PaCO_2$ of 25 to 30 mm Hg was a mainstay of the therapy of head injury. However, brain ischemia, which is probably the most threatening consequence of head injury, is likely to occur during the first 6 hours after trauma even when the CPP is maintained above the generally recommended 50 to 70 mm Hg.[106] This hypoperfusion seems to be caused largely by increased cerebral vascular resistance, which may be enhanced by hyperventilation. However, some degree of hyperventilation may be necessary for short periods of time in patients who have severe injuries and elevated ICP that does not respond to normal ventilation and diuretics, although this should not be used during the first 24 hours following injury.[91] Its use after the initial phase should be based on monitoring of the ICP and, if available, the jugular venous oxygen saturation ($SjvO_2$) and arteriojugular venous difference of oxygen ($AVDO_2$). It should be noted that hyperventilation in the severely brain-injured patient may also be associated with acute lung injury.[107]

Measurement of the $SjvO_2$ is used in some centers as a guide to therapy of the head-injured patient.[108] A catheter is passed retrograde into the jugular bulb under fluoroscopic control. The O_2 saturation may be measured with a co-oximeter or continuously by means of a fiberoptic sensor.[108] An $SjvO_2$ of <50% is considered critical desaturation. The $AVDO_2$ is a standard measure of the brain's oxygen supply to demand ratio. It is equal to $1.34 \times \text{Hgb} \times (SaO_2 - SjvO_2)$ (the saturations are expressed as decimal values), and normally is approximately 6. An increase in this value is a sign of insufficient blood flow, whereas a subnormal level indicates hyperemia. A reduction in ICP with elevation of CPP during treatment is reflected by a rise in $SjvO_2$ and a narrowing of the $AVDO_2$, presumably reflecting an improvement in the circulation to the brain. Unfortunately, several shortcomings of the technique have hindered its universal acceptance. Because all of the cerebral veins drain into the cavernous sinus and from there into the jugular bulbs, $AVDO_2$ measures only global O_2 consumption, which may well be very different from the situation in the injured region. Indeed, Coles[106] has demonstrated by positron emission tomography (PET) scanning that a significant increase in the region of critical hypoperfusion resulting from hyperventilation was not necessarily associated with a correspondingly abnormal $SjvO_2$ or $AVDO_2$ (Fig. 52-6). Patient or catheter movement may also alter the measured jugular bulb venous oxygen tension. Thus, there may be a high proportion of inaccurate values—as high as nearly two-thirds—although recent advances in the technique have probably reduced these errors. Cruz[109] has suggested that jugular venous monitoring should be used only in sedated, paralyzed patients.

If the ICP remains elevated despite all of these measures, pentobarbital (3 to 10 mg/kg given over 0.5 to 2.5 hours, followed by a maintenance infusion of 0.5 to 3.0 mg/kg/hr, aimed at a serum concentration between 2.5 and 4.0 mg/dL) may be required. High-dose barbiturates are of no value in the routine therapy of head injury and should be used only for refractory ICP elevation. Of course, immediate surgical decompression, especially of epidural hematomas, is an important factor in reducing morbidity and mortality.

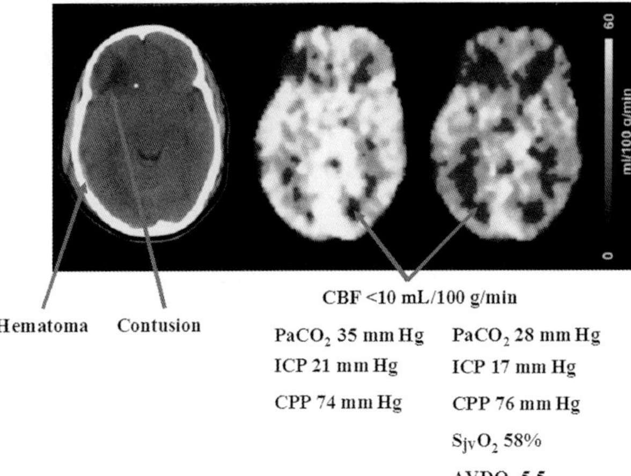

FIGURE 52-6. Effects of hyperventilation on cerebral blood flow (CBF). The left image is a computed tomography scan of the patient whose positron emission tomography scans are shown in the other two images. Note that there is a significant decrease in the CBF and an increase in the areas of hypoperfusion despite improvement in the intracranial pressure (ICP), and normal $SjvO_2$ (jugular venous oxygen saturation), and $AVDO_2$ (arteriojugular venous difference of oxygen). CPP, cerebral perfusion pressure. (Adapted with permission from Coles JP. Regional ischemia after head injury. *Curr Opin Crit Care.* 2004;10:120.)

Over the past decade there has been much debate regarding optimal blood glucose in critically ill patients. Brain-injured patients are unique members of this group because brain metabolism is altered by the injury and is heavily dependent on glucose. Hypoglycemia (<40 gm/dL), which may cause metabolic crisis, and hyperglycemia (>200 gm/dL) can cause detrimental effects through excitotoxicity, oxidative stress, and inflammatory cytokine release. Tight insulin control therapy (80 to 110 mg/dL) has been associated with episodes of hypoglycemia. As a result, the current recommendations are to maintain glucose levels of 110 to 180 mg/dL.[110]

Nearly 75% of severely brain-injured patients expire within the first 3 days from the initial trauma. Many of the survivors will later succumb to non-neurologic organ dysfunction involving pulmonary failure and cardiac impairment, which may be related to sympathetic hyperactivity. β-blocker therapy has been proposed as a treatment that may be beneficial in these patients.[111] The optimal agent, the dose level, the timing, and the duration of treatment, however, remain to be determined.

If the patient is hemodynamically stable, a CT scan is performed. The strictest attention should be paid to ensure adequate oxygenation, ventilation, blood pressure, and ICP control during the procedure. If the patient is hemodynamically unstable or requires emergency surgery for associated injuries and has a history suggesting a head injury, even though a significant intracranial hematoma is unlikely on clinical grounds, intraoperative ICP monitoring is indicated to permit rapid detection of ICP elevation. Both intracranial hematomas and hemorrhage in other regions have a high surgical priority. In the multiple trauma victim, prioritization between the two is based on the severity of each injury. Because there is no time to obtain a CT scan of the head in patients with both profuse hemorrhage and brain herniation, the patient is brought directly to the OR for simultaneous control of the bleeding site and evacuation of the intracranial hematoma.

TABLE 52-8. SIX-MONTH OUTCOMES FOR PATIENTS WITH BRAIN INJURY IN VARIOUS STUDIES

Name of Study	No. of Patients	Year Published	6-Month Outcome (%) Good/ Moderate	Severe/ Vegetative	Dead	Comments
Three-country (Jennett et al.[a])	700	1977	38	11	51	Various treatments, some untreated
Miller et al.[b]	158	1981	47	12	40	Vent, surgery, ICP monitoring, hyperventilation, and Rx
Traumatic Coma Data Bank (TCDB)[c]	717	1997	43	20	37	Total patients, standard therapy
TCDB[c]	308	1997	54	19	27	Patients without hypotension or hypoxia
Palmer et al.[115]	56	2000	70	14	16	1995 BTF Guidelines
Rudehill et al.[112]	1,508	2002	69	11	20	Standard protocol, early management
Patel et al.[117]	129	2002	63	13	20	NCCU Protocol

ICP, intracranial pressure; BTF, Brain Trauma Foundation; Rx, other treatment; NCCU, neurosurgical critical care unit.
Results of various treatment protocols for brain injuries. The three-country study surveyed patients who had received a wide variety of treatment; some were untreated. Miller et al. relied on hyperventilation and, when necessary, barbiturates. The TCBD patients were treated similarly; note the difference in outcome of the patients who did not experience hypotension or hypoxia (see Table 52-6). The final three studies are described in the text.
[a]Jennett B, Teasdale G, Galbraith S. Severe head injuries in three countries. *J Neurol Neurosurg Psychiatry.* 1977;40:291.
[b]Miller JD, Butterworth JF, Gudeman SK, et al. Further experience in the management of severe head injury. *J Neurosurg.* 1981;54:289.
[c]Prough DS, Lang J. Therapy of patients with head injuries: Key parameters for management. *J Trauma.* 1997;42(Suppl):10S.

The site of the craniotomy can be determined by a ventriculogram or an ultrasound examination with a pencil-tip probe; both tests may be performed under local anesthesia through a frontal burr hole.

It may be possible to improve the outlook for brain-injured patients:

1. The earlier definitive treatment is initiated, the better the outcome is likely to be. Rudehill et al.[112] have demonstrated improvement in outcomes in a large series of patients when care was initiated by anesthesiologists at the accident scene.
2. Meanwhile, the wide variety of types and severities of injury and of responses to treatment—both among different patients and in the same patient at different times—imply that therapeutic interventions must be individualized.[113,114] These aims may be met, at least partly, by carefully structured intensive care.[115,116] Therapeutic goals should be set explicitly and reviewed, and altered if necessary, at every change of shift.

Indeed, early intervention and controlled management may explain much of the improvement in outcomes that has been obtained over the past 15 years, including the results obtained by Patel et al.[117] and by Palmer et al.[115] using strict protocol driven therapies (in the latter case, the 1995 Brain Trauma Foundation Guidelines) (Table 52-8).

Spine and Spinal Cord Injury

Initial Evaluation

The objective in the evaluation of spinal trauma is to diagnose instability of the spine and the extent of neurologic involvement. Not stabilizing the spine in the first hours after a major accident until a definitive diagnosis is established carries the risk of converting a neurologically intact patient into a para- or quadriplegic. During transport to the hospital, the patient should be immobilized with a hard collar, a spine board, and tape. After admission, patients should not be left on a rigid spine board for longer than 1 hour, especially when they are paralyzed, because of the risk of decubitus ulcers.

In the conscious patient, the diagnosis is relatively easy: a history of a motor vehicle, industrial, or athletic accident, an act of violence, or a fall; penetrating trauma resulting in a neurologic deficit below a specific spinal level; or pain and tenderness over the involved vertebrae strongly suggest a spine injury. It should be noted, however, that spinal pain is not always localized to the level of injury.[118] Obviously, these symptoms are difficult to elicit in the comatose patient. In these circumstances, flaccid areflexia, loss of rectal sphincter tone, paradoxical respiration, and bradycardia in a hypovolemic patient suggest the diagnosis. In cervical spine trauma, an ability to flex but not to extend the elbow and response to painful stimuli above but not below the clavicle also indicate neurologic injury. Current guidelines consider absence of neck pain or paresthesia and a negative physical examination—lack of tenderness with palpation and during voluntary flexion and extension of the neck—in a neurologically intact, conscious patient as adequate indications for ruling out a cervical spine injury without further radiologic studies. Alcohol intoxication and distracting associated injuries do not seem to alter these criteria as long as the patient is alert, conscious, and able to concentrate. A large meta-analysis of obtunded trauma patients demonstrated that modern multislice helical CT imaging is sufficient to detect unstable cervical spine injuries. However, this approach may still miss some patients at risk for subsequent cervical cord insult.[119]

Depending on the degree of deficit, spinal cord injuries are categorized as *complete* or *incomplete.* Intact sensory perception over the sacral distribution and voluntary contraction of the anus (sacral sparing) are present in incomplete, but not in complete, injuries. There is practically no possibility of significant neurologic recovery in complete injury, whereas functional restoration may occur in up to 50% of patients after incomplete injuries. In some patients the development of *spinal shock,* which is manifested by absolute flaccidity and loss of reflexes, precludes distinguishing between complete and incomplete injuries during the initial phase of treatment. Therefore, even in the absence of sacral sparing, the possibility of neurologic recovery dictates that all possible efforts be made at this time to prevent further damage and to preserve cord function. A similar principle applies to the evaluation of the level of injury. After the first few days, spinal cord edema subsides and the final level is commonly a few segments lower than on initial presentation. Thus, early therapeutic efforts should not be abandoned even in the patient with a high-level injury, which carries a grim functional prognosis.

Spinal shock is probably caused by direct trauma to the spinal cord and usually subsides within days to weeks. The term is frequently used as a misnomer for *neurogenic shock,* which is defined as hypotension and bradycardia caused by the loss of vasomotor tone and sympathetic innervation of the heart as a result of functional depression of the descending sympathetic pathways of the spinal cord. It is usually present after high thoracic and cervical spine injuries and improves within 3 to 5 days.

Initial Management

The spinal cord, a microcosm of the brain, is also vulnerable to a secondary injury process that may be a product of hypotension, hypoxia, and probably other physiologic complications.[120] Prompt recognition and aggressive treatment of these insults, which may also result from associated trauma, may minimize exacerbation of spinal cord lesions and improve the long-term outlook of these patients.[95,121]

Immobilization and Intubation

Maintenance of immobilization of the injured spine is of paramount importance. If a cervical spine fracture is suspected, immobilization or manual inline stabilization of the neck is necessary before the patient is moved. If the patient has a thoracic or lumbar injury, a careful log-rolling maneuver should be used.[120,122]

About one-third of paraplegic patients require airway management, mostly within the first 24 hours after injury. Signs of respiratory distress or fatigue, or a rising respiratory rate or $PaCO_2$, are major indications for ventilatory assistance. Severe bradycardia or dysrhythmias may result from unopposed vagal activity during tracheal intubation or suctioning: the patient must be preoxygenated and atropine (0.4 to 0.6 mg) should be given before any instrumentation. If bradycardia develops during airway management, treatment includes additional atropine, glycopyrrolate, isoproterenol, or, if necessary, cardiac pacing.

The techniques of intubation in spine-injured patients are discussed in the "Airway Management" section.

Steroids

Since the early 1990s, high-dose methylprednisolone has been used in many centers in an attempt to improve the outcome from spinal cord injuries. The drug is given as a bolus of 30 mg/kg within 8 hours of injury, followed in 1 hour by an infusion of 5.4 mg $\times$ kg^{-1} $\times$ hr^{-1} for the next 23 to 47 hours. The National Acute Spinal Cord Injury Studies[123,124] indicated some improvement in motor function in treated patients who had partial sensory and motor loss. However, the findings of these studies have not been duplicated in any other prospective or retrospective trials[125] and have been criticized because of multiple major deficiencies in the analysis of the data.

Furthermore, steroid therapy is associated with an increased rate of sepsis, pneumonia, and days of intensive care and positive pressure ventilation[126] and is also associated with increased mortality in the 36% to 74% of patients with spine injuries who also have head injuries.[127] Because of these findings, most centers have abandoned the use of steroids in spinal cord–injured patients.

Systemic hypothermia, minocycline, riluzole, and magnesium are possibly effective therapies that are currently or will soon be in clinical trials.[128]

Respiratory Complications

Respiratory complications are common in all phases of the care of spinal cord–injured patients and are the most frequent cause of death in the acute stage.[129,130] In the initial period, these problems may be augmented by associated brain, neck, chest, or abdominal injury, alcohol intoxication, or the effects of self-administered or iatrogenic drugs. Injuries at C5 or lower are usually associated with normal tidal volumes because the function of the diaphragm is intact, whereas patients with injuries at C4 or above may require permanent ventilatory assistance. Nevertheless, accessory respiratory muscle paresis may cause a significant loss of expiratory reserve even when the injury involves the lower spinal segments.[131,132] Pulmonary edema is another significant cause of respiratory dysfunction. A severe catecholamine surge follows acute trauma to the spinal cord.[133] Although the resultant severe hypertension lasts for only a few minutes, its effects persist. It may produce both pulmonary capillary damage, as a result of shifting of a large portion of the blood volume into the pulmonary circulation, and left ventricular dysfunction. Overzealous fluid therapy to treat the patient's initial hypotension may lead to acute pulmonary edema when the sympathetic activity returns approximately 3 to 5 days after the injury.

Paradoxical respiration in the quadriplegic patient results from partial chest wall collapse during inspiration. It may produce limitation of the tidal volume and an increased risk of hypoventilation.[132] The situation is aggravated when the patient is in an upright position. The diaphragm cannot maintain its normal domed shape, the only way it can contract efficiently, because the weight of the thoracic contents is not opposed by the normal tone of the abdominal muscles. Thus, in contrast to other diseases that produce respiratory insufficiency, the supine position improves respiration in persons with quadriplegia (Fig. 52-7).[132]

Other causes of inadequate respiration in the early phase of spinal cord injury are aspiration of gastric contents, atelectasis, pneumonia, and bronchoconstriction. Management includes careful observation of the patient's breathing and preparation to ventilate the lungs and intubate the trachea at the first sign of respiratory depression.[132]

Hemodynamic Management

Hemodynamic management of quadriplegic patients includes a complete assessment, with a pulmonary artery catheter if necessary, as early as possible after injury. In as many as 25% of patients with cervical spinal cord injuries, left ventricular dysfunction may contribute to the hypotension.[134] There is evidence to support the maintenance of mean arterial pressure >85 mm Hg.[135] Decreased preload can be treated with fluid infusion using cardiac function

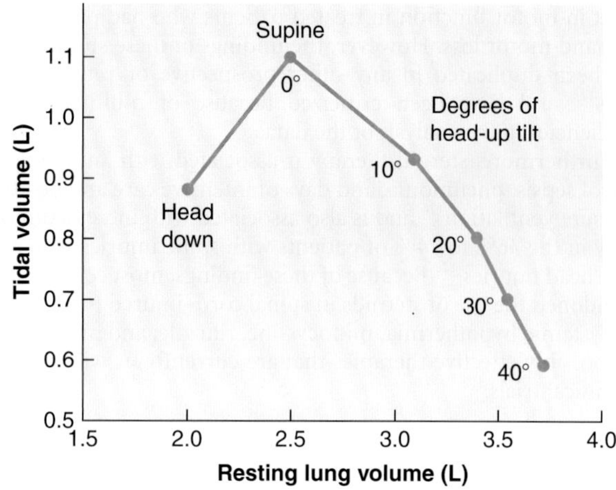

FIGURE 52-7. Effect of semi-Fowler's position on ventilation in quadriplegic patients. (Reprinted with permission from Winslow C, Bode RK, Felton D, et al. Impact of respiratory complications on length of stay and hospital costs in acute cervical spine injury. *Chest.* 2002;121:1548.)

curves as a guide. In general, volume may be safely replaced to a central venous or pulmonary capillary wedge pressure (PCWP) of 18 mm Hg.[134] This avoids, or at least limits, the severity of the pulmonary edema described previously. Hypotension, despite adequate fluid infusion, acidosis, or low mixed venous PO_2, requires treatment with inotropes such as dopamine.

A recent review by Christie et al.[136] indicates that these patients frequently experience deep vein thrombosis, which may adversely affect both hemodynamic and pulmonary function. The authors recommend the initiation of low-molecular weight heparin therapy within 72 hours of the injury, which should be held on the day of any surgical procedure.

Anesthetic Considerations

Any anesthetic technique compatible with the patient's general condition is satisfactory for the spinal cord–injured patient. Hypotension is very common during anesthesia in quadriplegics. Placement of a TEE or a central venous or pulmonary artery catheter may facilitate management of the patient's volume and blood pressure status.

Succinylcholine may produce a sudden, severe increase in serum K^+ in spine-injured patients. Levels as high as 14 mEq $\times$ L^{-1} may be reached: the result may be irreversible ventricular dysrhythmias and cardiac arrest. Although succinylcholine is probably safe during the 4 to 7 days after injury, it is probably best to avoid it altogether in the paraplegic patient and to use rapid-onset nondepolarizing agents such as rocuronium when a rapid-sequence induction is required.

Neck Injury

Both penetrating and blunt trauma may injure the major structures in the neck, vessels, respiratory and digestive tracts, and nervous system. Hemorrhage, asphyxia, mediastinitis, paralysis, stroke, or death may result if these injuries are not promptly recognized and treated.

Penetrating neck injuries usually present with obvious clinical manifestations; blunt cervical trauma may be more subtle. Airway compromise or obstruction, brisk bleeding from the wound site, an expanding pulsatile hematoma, and shock with or without external bleeding are obvious signs of cervical vascular injury and dictate immediate airway management and vascular control. Decreased or absent upper-extremity or distal carotid pulses, as well as carotid bruit or thrill, are pathognomonic for cervical arterial injury. Hemothorax, pneumothorax, and signs of air embolism are also suggestive. Respiratory distress, cyanosis, or stridor are obvious signs of airway injury and require immediate tracheal intubation. Other signs that strongly suggest airway injury are dysphonia, hoarseness, cough, hemoptysis, air bubbling from the wound, subcutaneous crepitus, and laryngeal tenderness. Because of their dynamic nature, cervical airway injuries may rapidly progress to obstruction. The patient, therefore, should be observed carefully and the trachea intubated at the first sign of problems.

Esophageal injuries, whether in the neck or the chest, are insidious and difficult to diagnose. Dysphagia, odynophagia, hematemesis, subcutaneous crepitus, prevertebral air on a lateral cervical radiograph, and major concomitant injuries to other cervical structures suggest an esophageal injury and call for confirmation with an esophagram.

The neurologic manifestations of a penetrating neck injury vary depending on the injured structure. Partial spinal cord transection produces Brown-Sequard syndrome with ipsilateral motor and contralateral sensory deficit below the injury. Complete spinal cord transection, depending on the level of injury, produces paraplegia or quadriplegia, usually with neurogenic shock. Occasionally, luminal occlusion of the carotid and vertebral arteries may lead to a hemispheric cerebrovascular accident; associated hypotension increases the likelihood of this event.

Patients with severe active bleeding, persistent hypotension, and air bubbling through the wound require immediate surgery without further diagnostic studies.[137] Controversy exists over the indications for surgical management of stable penetrating neck injuries. Mandatory exploration is associated with negative findings in approximately 70% of patients.[137] Thus, in many centers, patients are evaluated with noninvasive diagnostic tests and undergo surgery only when there are positive findings.[137] A prospective multicenter study showed that clinical signs and symptoms often reliably indicate the cervical structures injured and prevent unnecessary imaging, and if imaging is needed, multidetector CT is a highly sensitive and specific screening tool.[138]

Blunt cervical vascular injuries usually present with a hematoma that may compress the cervical veins, displace the airway, and produce pharyngeal and laryngeal congestion. Injury to an artery may produce an intimal tear, pseudoaneurysm, fistula, or thrombosis. If a carotid or vertebral artery is involved, cerebral ischemia may occur. Often thrombosis develops gradually over minutes to a few hours, thus the appearance of neurologic symptoms is delayed in approximately 40% of patients. Symptomatic patients may present with a cervical bruit, altered mental status, or lateralizing neurologic deficits, including hemiparesis, transient ischemic attacks, amaurosis fugax, or Horner syndrome. The mortality rate associated with blunt carotid injury varies between 15% and 28%, and 15% to 50% of survivors have neurologic deficits.[139] Identification of a blunt or penetrating carotid injury in an asymptomatic patient using ultrasound, CT, or CT angiography not only allows early institution of antiplatelet therapy, systemic anticoagulation, endovascular intervention, or surgical repair,[139,140] but also occasionally prevents the neurologic deficits that may follow surgery for associated injuries in an unprotected patient.

Airway injuries after blunt trauma are rare but carry an overall mortality rate of 2%.[137] Their severity varies from a simple mucosal tear or hematoma to a comminuted laryngeal cartilage fracture or complete cricotracheal separation (see Table 52-1). They frequently require primary laryngeal repair or tracheostomy. Anesthetic management is not only complicated by relatively complex airway management problems[29,32] (discussed in the "Airway Evaluation and Intervention" section), but also with associated skull base, intracranial, open neck, cervical spine, esophageal, or pharyngeal injuries.[137,141]

Chest Injury

Although a high percentage of thoracic injuries can be treated conservatively, patients who need surgery may have major intraoperative physiologic disturbances.

Chest Wall Injury

Rib, scapula, and sternal fractures, in addition to interfering with adequate respiration, may be associated with severe underlying thoracic, abdominal, cranial, and skeletal injuries. The management principles for these injuries are similar to those previously described for flail chest, although the need for mechanical ventilation is less likely in single rib fractures treated with systemic analgesics than in a flail chest. Effective pain relief, preferably with continuous thoracic epidural anesthesia or paravertebral or intercostal block, is central to management.[141]

Pleural Injury

Closed pneumothorax is easy to miss in major trauma. The presence of subcutaneous emphysema, pulmonary contusion, and rib fractures should draw suspicion of coexisting pneumothorax.[142] Tension pneumothorax involving >50% of a hemithorax presents with dyspnea, tachycardia, cyanosis, agitation, diaphoresis, neck vein distention, tracheal deviation, and displacement of the maximal cardiac impulse to the contralateral side.

Although an upright plain chest radiograph provides the best opportunity for detection of pneumothorax, this position may be impossible or contraindicated in patients who are experiencing major hemorrhage or those with suspected spine injury. Air in the pleural space tends to accumulate in the anteromedial sulcus first, and then in lateral and caudal regions, often producing hemodynamic alterations and the "deep sulcus sign" on the anteroposterior chest radiogram in supine or semirecumbent patients. Transthoracic ultrasound may be used for the emergency diagnosis of pneumothorax. Normally, movement of the lung beneath the chest wall produces "comet tail" artifacts from echo-dense areas on the lung surface. In the presence of pneumothorax, neither lung motion, nor sliding, nor comet tails can be seen. In one study of blunt and penetrating trauma victims, ultrasound was more sensitive than a supine chest film but did not detect all pneumothoraces. Further, ultrasound detection of rib and sternal fractures also appeared to be more accurate than the chest radiograph. It was recommended that a chest film and the ultrasound can complement each other, but that chest CT be used as the definitive test.[36] Ultrasound examination may also be helpful in detecting residual pleural air after placement of thoracostomy tube, pulmonary embolism, pneumonia, and hemothorax.[143] It has been suggested that a small closed pneumothorax can be safely managed by observation alone without a chest tube even in those patients who require positive-pressure ventilation as long as continuing vigilance is maintained.[144,145] Based on the most recent Advanced Trauma Life Support recommendation[145] and our own experience, we strongly believe that once diagnosed, a traumatic pneumothorax, no matter how small, should be treated with thoracostomy drainage before tracheal intubation and positive-pressure ventilation.

Bleeding intercostal vessels are responsible for most hemothoraces. Severe airway deviation may be produced by a hemothorax, although it is not as common as it is after a pneumothorax. Treatment consists of drainage with a 30 to 40F catheter chest tube (26 to 32F catheter is used for pneumothorax). Initial drainage of 1,000 mL of blood or collection of >200 mL/hr for several hours is an indication for thoracotomy. Retained clotted blood after tube thoracostomy may be treated conservatively with intrapleural fibrinolytic agents.[146] Additional indications for thoracotomy are a "white lung" appearance on the anteroposterior chest radiograph or a continuous major air leak from the chest tube, which may result from a direct airway injury or major lung laceration. Hemodynamically stable patients with persistent bleeding of <150 mL/hr are often managed with video-assisted thoracoscopic surgery (VATS) to control bleeding, which requires collapse of the lung on the involved side using a double-lumen tube or a bronchial blocker. VATS can also be useful in diagnosis of suspected diaphragmatic or mediastinal injuries, evaluation of some bronchopleural fistulas, and evacuation of clotted blood or an empyema that does not drain with a chest tube or respond to intrapleural fibrinolytic therapy.[146] Use of VATS decreases the need for open thoracotomy and the number of negative explorations in stable trauma patients.[147]

Pulmonary Contusion

Pulmonary contusion often accompanies chest wall injury, but may also develop in isolation. Its management is discussed in the "Management of Breathing Abnormalities" section.

Penetrating Cardiac Injury

Pericardial tamponade, cardiac chamber perforation, and fistula formation between the cardiac chambers and the great vessels are the consequences of a penetrating cardiac trauma. Any penetrating wound of the chest, especially one within the "cardiac window" (midclavicular lines laterally, clavicles superiorly, and costal margins inferiorly), can cause this injury. These injuries are often fatal at the scene, especially if they are gunshot rather than stab wounds and involve the right rather than the thicker walled left ventricle. Because of the dynamic nature of cardiac injuries and the risk of sudden hemodynamic deterioration, these patients must be transported directly to the OR and immediate sternotomy or left thoracotomy must be performed as soon as the injury is suspected. Emergency cardiopulmonary bypass may be needed. Pneumopericardium visible on a plain chest radiograph after penetrating chest trauma should increase the suspicion, although it is not seen in all patients. Transthoracic echocardiography can be used for screening stable patients, but it may be inconclusive in obese patients and in those with pneumothorax. TEE provides an accurate diagnosis in these patients, but it is impractical during the initial evaluation phase of trauma.[148] Of the alternative diagnostic measures, the central venous pressure (CVP) is not always accurate, and a subxiphoid pericardial window is invasive, must be performed in the OR under general anesthesia, takes longer, and cannot detect an intracardiac shunt.

Pericardial Tamponade

Both penetrating and blunt trauma can cause hemopericardium. The classic findings of pericardial tamponade—tachycardia, hypotension, distant heart sounds, distended neck veins, pulsus paradoxus, or pulsus alternans—are difficult to appreciate or may be absent in a hypovolemic trauma patient. A chest radiograph may reveal a globular heart, although this sign is often not appreciated. Transthoracic echocardiography with placement of the probe in the subxiphoid region, which is part of FAST, or intraoperative TEE can demonstrate blood in the pericardial sac and the presence of ventricular diastolic collapse, which indicates at least a 20% reduction in cardiac output.

Initial management consists of evacuation of the pericardial blood by ultrasound-guided pericardiocentesis or surgery as soon as possible. Even a small amount of blood drainage improves hemodynamics. Intracardiac volumes should be optimized with intravenous fluids. If anesthesia is contemplated for surgery, ketamine or etomidate, which produce relatively little myocardial depression, is preferred. Administration of anesthesia should be delayed until draping and preparation are completed. Patients *in extremis* with penetrating trauma-related pericardial tamponade may be candidates for ED thoracotomy. Rarely, laceration of the pericardium may permit complete or partial herniation of the heart through the defect with catastrophic consequences. Immediate thoracotomy and reduction of the heart is indicated.

Blunt Cardiac Injury

10 The term blunt cardiac injury has replaced myocardial contusion and encompasses varying degrees of myocardial damage, coronary artery injury, and rupture of the cardiac free wall, septum, or a valve following blunt trauma.[149] Myocardial injury consists of myofibrillar disintegration, edema, bleeding, or necrosis that, depending on its severity, presents as minor electrocardiogram (ECG) or enzyme abnormalities, complex arrhythmias, or cardiac failure caused by direct mechanical impact or indirectly by coronary occlusion. Arrhythmias last no more than a few days. Ventricular wall motion abnormalities may persist for up to 1 year, but any increased risk of perioperative cardiac complications appears to last for no more than 1 month.

The prominent clinical findings are angina, sometimes responding to nitroglycerin, dyspnea, chest wall ecchymosis and/or fractures; dysrhythmias of any type; and right-sided or left-sided congestive heart failure. Orliaguet et al.[149] proposed an algorithm for the diagnosis and treatment of several clinical scenarios caused by this injury (Fig. 52-8). The diagnosis is based on the 12-lead ECG, troponin I level, and echocardiography. The ECG is very sensitive, although not specific. A normal trace cannot rule out the diagnosis, but it is the best screening test. Common ECG abnormalities include almost any type of arrhythmia, ST- or T-wave changes, and conduction delays. Patients with a normal ECG undergoing minor surgery do not require any further testing. Patients with severe injuries need measurement of troponin I and TEE to diagnose any abnormalities caused by the cardiac injury (Fig. 52-8). Echocardiography can demonstrate wall motion abnormalities, valve malfunction, hemopericardium, intracardiac thrombi, venous or systemic embolism, and end-diastolic and fractional ventricular wall area changes. It thus aids not only in the diagnosis of blunt cardiac injury, but also in hemodynamic management. Treatment options depend on the diagnosis (Fig. 52-8). They include antiarrhythmic agents, inotropes, fluid loading, high-frequency jet ventilation to optimize cardiac function, and surgery for hemopericardium, valvular or septal lesions, or coronary artery injury or disease.

Valvular injuries present as insufficiency of the aortic, mitral, or tricuspid valves. Acute traumatic insufficiency of the aortic and mitral valves is poorly tolerated, increasing the ventricular wall stress and rapidly progressing to pulmonary edema. Ventricular septal defects can be recognized by increased pulmonary vascularity with a normal heart size on the chest radiograph. An atrial septal defect is usually missed in clinical examination but may be recognized by echocardiography.

Commotio cordis (agitated heart) is an entity characterized by the development of sudden ventricular tachyarrhythmias, cardiac arrest, and often death following a blow to the chest in young

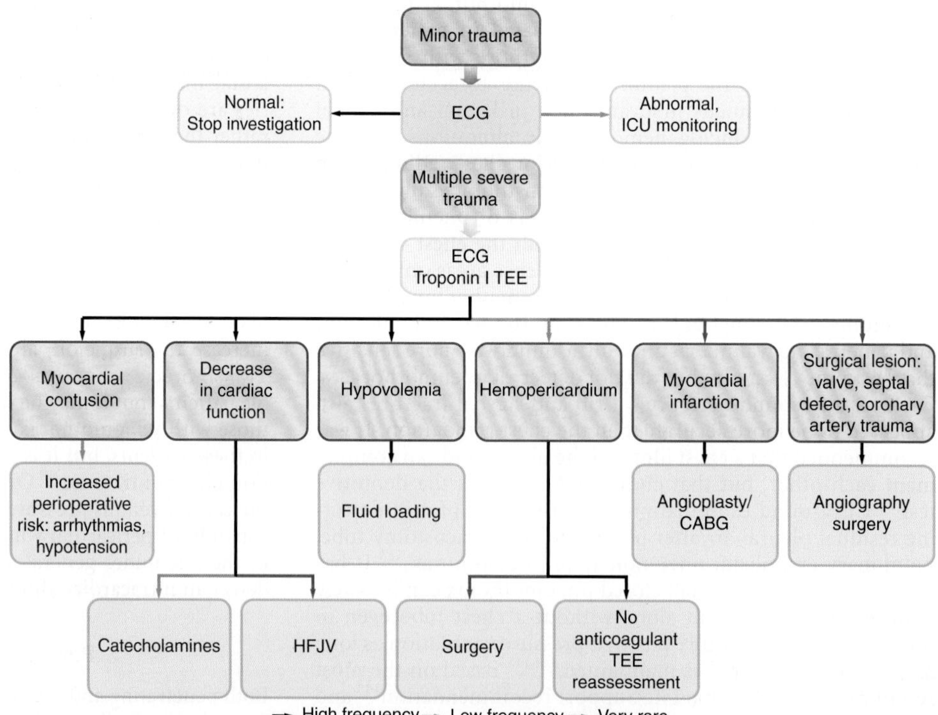

FIGURE 52-8. Algorithm for management of various clinical scenarios produced by severe blunt cardiac injury (BCI). Evaluation of severe multiple trauma-induced BCI uses electrocardiogram (ECG), troponin I, and transesophageal echocardiography (TEE). *Arrows* represent the frequency of occurrence of each scenario and the frequency of management measures. *Thick arrows* represent high frequency, *thin arrows* low frequency, and *dotted arrows* very rare occurrences. CABG, coronary artery bypass graft; HFJV, high-frequency jet ventilation. (Adapted with permission from Orliaguet G, Ferjani M, Riou B. The heart in blunt trauma. *Anesthesiology.* 2001;95:544.)

TABLE 52-9. COMMON CLINICAL, RADIOGRAPHIC, AND ULTRASOUND FEATURES OF THORACIC AORTIC INJURIES

Clinical	Radiographic	Spiral Computed Tomography	Ultrasound
Increased arterial pressure and pulse amplitude in upper extremities Decreased arterial pressure and pulse amplitude in lower extremities Absent or weak left radial artery pulse Osler's sign: discrepancy between left and right arm blood pressure Retrosternal or interscapular pain Hoarseness Systolic flow murmur over the precordium or medial to the left scapula Neurologic deficits in the lower extremities	Widened mediastinum Blurring of the aortic contours Widened paraspinal interfaces Left apical cap Opacified aortopulmonary window Broadened paratracheal stripe Displacement of the left mainstem bronchus Displaced superior vena cava Rightward deviation of the esophagus and trachea Nasogastric tube shift Left hemothorax Sternal and/or upper rib fractures Lung contusion Pneumothorax	Mediastinal hematoma Aortic wall irregularity Intimal flap False aneurysm Pseudocoarctation Intramural hematoma Intraluminal clot or medial flap	Intimal flap Turbulent flow Dilated aortic isthmus Acute false aneurysm Intraluminal medial flap Hemothorax Hemomediastinum

people, most often during competitive or recreational sports. The blow would have occurred during the 10- to 20-millisecond period of the T-wave upstroke. *Commotio cordis* differs from myocardial contusion because of the absence of any structural cardiac injury. Treatment involves immediate defibrillation.[150]

Thoracic Aortic Injury

Penetrating trauma can injure any part of the thoracic aorta, including its branches, to any extent. Blunt trauma, on the other hand, most commonly causes damage at the isthmus, the junction between the free and fixed portions of the descending aorta, which is just distal to the origin of the left subclavian artery. The *ligamentum arteriosum* and left mainstem bronchus anchor the isthmus, fixing it in relation to the proximal aorta and making it vulnerable to traction forces and tearing. The presenting symptoms, signs, and radiographic and ultrasound findings are shown in Table 52-9, although there may be no clinical findings or a constellation of symptoms or signs in the ED. Only 20% to 30% of patients with mediastinal widening actually have this injury. Measuring the left mediastinal width (≥6 cm) and its fraction of the total mediastinal width (≥0.6) may increase the specificity and positive predictive value of the plain film.[151]

Contrast-enhanced spiral CT with volume-rendered image reconstruction techniques permits a reliable noninvasive diagnosis and eliminates the need for biplanar aortography. Transesophageal echocardiography is equally capable of diagnosing subadventitial aortic injuries that require intervention.[152] Lesions of the intima and media and concomitant blunt cardiac injuries are also more likely to be detectable by TEE than CT.[152] However, CT, especially those obtained with multidetector devices, is generally preferred for diagnosis because it provides an accurate diagnosis, and introducing a TEE probe under these circumstances is impractical and probably fraught with the danger of aortic rupture. Furthermore, many of these patients have suspected craniofacial or esophageal injuries, preventing introduction of the probe. TEE is especially useful for the anesthesiologist intraoperatively when associated injuries require immediate surgery without time for CT scanning of the chest.

Traumatic aortic injury can be classified into three categories: grade 1 injury consists of an intramural hematoma, limited intimal flap and/or mural thrombus; grade 2 injury consists of subadventitial rupture, injury to the media, altered aortic geometry, and/or small hemomediastinum; grade 3 injury consists of transsection with massive blood extravasation and intraluminal obstruction, causing pseudocoarctation and ischemia (Fig. 52-9).[153]

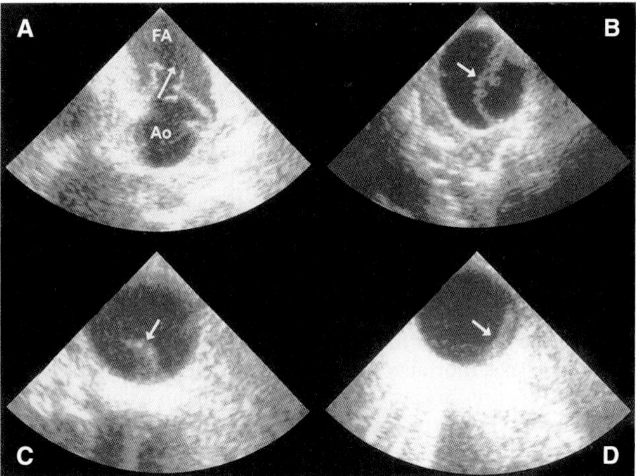

FIGURE 52-9. Typical transesophageal echocardiographic appearances of three grades of traumatic aortic injury. **(A)** Grade 3 injury. Adventitia of the aortic wall is damaged and a false aneurysm (FA) is communicating (*arrow*) with the aortic lumen (Ao). **(B)** Grade 2 injury. Large medial flap moves back and forth during each cardiac cycle. Adventitia is intact **(C, D)** Grade 1 injury. Intimal flap **(C)** and intramural hematoma **(D)** (shown with *arrows*) without hemomediastinum or alteration of aortic geometry. (Reprinted with permission from Goarin J-P, Cluzel P, Gosgnach M, et al. Evaluation of transesophageal echocardiography for diagnosis of traumatic aortic injury. *Anesthesiology.* 2000;93:1373.)

TABLE 52-10. CHANGE IN THE MANAGEMENT OF BLUNT THORACIC AORTIC INJURIES FROM 1997 TO 2007

	$AAST_1$ N = 253	$AAST_2$ N = 193
Diagnosis		
Aortogram	220 (87%)	16 (8%)
CT scan	88 (35%)	180 (93%)
TEE	30 (12%)	2 (1%)
REPAIR		
Open	207 (100%)	68 (35%)
Endovascular	—	125 (65%)
Outcomes		
Mortality	53/241 (22%)	25/193 (13%)
Paraplegia		
All patients	18 (9%)	2 (2%)
Open repair	18 (9%)	2 (3%)
Endovascular	0	1/125 (1%)
Renal failure	18 (9%)	17 (9%)
Repair site complication	1/207 (1%)	25/125 (20%)

$AAST_1$, American Association for the Surgery of Trauma 1997 Study; $AAST_2$, American Association for the Surgery of Trauma 2007 Study; TEE, transesophageal echocardiogram; CT, computed tomography.

Reproduced with permission from Demetriades D, Velmahos GC, Scalea TM, et al. Diagnosis and treatment of blunt thoracic aortic injuries: Changing perspectives. *J Trauma.* 2008;64:1415.

Management strategies in the diagnosis and treatment of blunt aortic injuries have gone through major changes during the past 10 years with substantially improved early outcomes (Table 52-10). In the area of diagnosis, contrast-enhanced CT angiography has practically replaced aortography and TEE, whereas endovascular thoracic aortic repair has replaced open surgery as the primary surgical treatment.[154] Intraoperatively, patients undergoing endovascular repair with a stent are monitored with contrast aortography and intravascular ultrasound. Thus, aortography has not been completely eliminated.

Although currently the majority of blunt thoracic aortic injuries are managed using endovascular stents, repairs via the traditional open left thoracotomy are still occasionally performed. This technique requires lung isolation with a double-lumen tube or a bronchial blocker, partial heparinization, and, at times, partial left heart bypass to decompress the left heart and perfuse the distal aorta during a "clamp and sew" technique. A clamp is placed just distal to the take off of the left subclavian artery. Although bleeding is excessive, mortality and morbidity, especially paraplegia or renal dysfunction, are also very common with this technique.[154,155]

Endovascular aortic repair is minimally invasive and is associated with many fewer early complications such as paraplegia, stroke, bleeding, or death than are encountered after open thoracotomy (see Table 52-10). An endoleak between the graft and the vascular wall is one of the early recognized complications. A radial artery cannula should be placed on the right side as sometimes the left subclavian artery is covered by the stent. A central venous catheter is placed for administration of vasoactive drugs. Embolization of aortic atheromas to the brain is one of the complications of this procedure. TEE may help to image the atheroma prior to stent deployment. During aortography and stent placement, ventilation may have to be stopped and the systemic blood pressure may have to be lowered to a mean of 60 mm Hg.

The incidence of long-term graft complications is not known, but it appears that the survival curves between open thoracotomy and endovascular techniques converge at 2 years, and the rates of aneurysm-related mortality converge at 6 years.[155]

Surgical prioritization when multiple injuries are present depends on the hemodynamic and neurologic status of the patient. Although the aorta should be repaired as early as possible, control of active hemorrhage from other sites and surgery for intracranial hematomas have a higher surgical priority, unless the aorta is leaking. In most instances, a blood clot between the aorta and the mediastinal pleura occludes the vessel. Any disturbance of the tamponaded region may reinitiate bleeding. A rapid flow of blood in a large artery tends to pull its endothelium with it and thus may rupture an injured vessel that is sealed with a clot or a hematoma. Such an increase in the aortic blood flow is usually caused by increased myocardial contractility. Every effort should be made to prevent increased cardiac contractility and hypertension.

Diaphragmatic Injury

Injury to the diaphragm may permit migration of abdominal contents into the chest where they may compress the lung, producing abnormalities of gas exchange, or the heart, resulting in dysrhythmias and/or hypotension. Because the defect produced by blunt injury is larger than that resulting from a penetrating injury, migration of abdominal contents, which requires a defect of at least 6 cm in diameter, is also more common after blunt trauma. The liver protects the right side of the diaphragm, thus traumatic herniation is more common on the left side, but right-sided diaphragmatic injuries are more frequently missed.[156]

Diagnosis of a diaphragmatic hernia can be made by laparoscopy, or in selected cases, VATS. Nevertheless, noting that the end of a nasogastric tube is above the diaphragm on the chest radiograph is a certain sign that the stomach is displaced into the chest. A chest radiograph that shows intestinal markings and lung compression or a contrast-enhanced abdominal CT scan that includes the lower third of the thorax can provide important information. Failure to retrieve the instilled fluid during DPL or drainage of DPL fluid from a thoracostomy tube also indicates this injury.

Abdominal and Pelvic Injuries

Table 52-11 summarizes the strengths and weaknesses of the currently available diagnostic tools used for abdominal injuries.[157] Because of the unpredictable course of bullets in the body, exploratory laparotomy or, in selected cases, laparoscopy is required in most patients after a gunshot wound to the abdomen. Occasionally, in hemodynamically stable patients, abdominal and flank gunshot wounds may be evaluated with an initial CT scan. Stab wounds may be managed with tractotomy to determine whether the peritoneum is involved. Laparoscopy, laparotomy, or DPL may be indicated after a positive tractotomy.

Patients with blunt abdominal trauma are evaluated by CT scan unless they are hemodynamically unstable and there are overt abdominal signs such as tenderness, guarding, and gross distension, in which case surgery without CT scan may be indicated. Absence of abdominal distention, however, does not rule out intra-abdominal bleeding. At least 1 L of blood can accumulate before the smallest change in girth is apparent, and the diaphragm can also move cephalad, allowing further significant blood loss without any change in abdominal circumference.

The diagnostic ability of the FAST is inferior to CT scan evaluation, which has recently undergone significant technologic improvements. The FAST is operator dependent, has good

TABLE 52-11. DIAGNOSTIC TOOLS IN ABDOMINAL TRAUMA: STRENGTHS AND WEAKNESSES

Diagnostic Tool	Strength	Weakness
Physical examination	Expeditious, safe, and inexpensive; potential for serial examination	Diagnosis of specific injury (e.g., diaphragm)
Diagnostic peritoneal lavage	Expeditious, safe, and inexpensive	Diagnosis of diaphragmatic injury, hollow viscus injury, retroperitoneal injury; can be oversensitive and nonspecific
Computed tomography	Evaluation of peritoneum and retroperitoneum	Diagnosis of diaphragmatic injury, hollow viscus injury
	Staging of solid organ injury	Expensive; controversial need for contrast
Ultrasonography	Expeditious, safe, and inexpensive; accurate for free peritoneal fluid	Diagnosis of diaphragmatic injury, hollow viscus injury, penetrating injury, good specificity, but moderate sensitivity
	Potential for serial examinations	Less accurate in the presence of large retroperitoneal hematomas
Laparoscopy	Diagnosis of peritoneal penetration, diaphragmatic injury	Diagnosis of hollow viscus injury, retroperitoneal injury
	Evaluation of bleeding or solid organ injury	Expensive
	Potential for therapy	
Video-assisted thoracoscopic surgery	Evaluation of lung, diaphragm, mediastinum, chest wall, and pericardium; potential for treatment	Requires operating room; expensive Diagnosis of abdominal injuries

Reprinted with permission from Villavicencio RT, Aucar JA. Analysis of laparoscopy in trauma. *J Am Coll Surg.* 1999;189:11.

specificity but only moderate sensitivity, can diagnose injuries associated with intraperitoneal fluid but not those without it, but cannot determine the severity of organ injury.[158]

The FAST is most needed in hemodynamically unstable patients who may not be safe to transport to CT unit shortly after admission to the ED. Its sensitivity in those patients is found to be low, preventing the development of an ultrasound-based clinical pathway to diagnose blunt abdominal injury and to decide between conservative and operative management.[158] Performing serial FAST examinations may decrease the false-negative results, but in the unstable patient there is often limited time for decision making. Known clinical conditions that decrease the sensitivity of the FAST include pelvic and spine injuries, subcutaneous emphysema, and obesity. On the other hand, the FAST requires one-third of the time is less expensive to perform than CT, and is without the hazard of radiation.

Screening with abdominal ultrasonography is performed by placing a 3.0 to 5.0 MHz probe on four distinct areas of the abdomen: subxiphoid, to detect pericardial blood; right upper quadrant, for blood in the hepatorenal pouch; left upper quadrant, to detect perisplenic blood; and just above the pubic symphysis, for blood in the rectovesical pouch.

Laparoscopy is an excellent screening tool in abdominal trauma patients. An analysis showed that it avoided laparotomy in 63% of patients and missed only 1% of the injuries.[157] It is also possible to repair diaphragmatic, bladder, and solid organ injuries with this technique. The complication rate of laparoscopy in trauma is approximately 1%, including pneumothorax, small bowel injury, intra-abdominal vascular injury, extraperitoneal CO_2 insufflation, and CO_2 embolization.[157]

Fractures of the Pelvis

Pelvic fractures occur in widely varied anatomic forms and physiologic severity. Major hemorrhage, which is one of the major causes of mortality, occurs in about 25% of patients; exsanguination occurs in 1% of injuries. Other major causes of mortality include associated injuries, such as chest, brain, intra-abdominal, and long bone injuries, and postoperative complications, such as sepsis, pulmonary embolism, and renal failure. In most of these fractures, bleeding results from venous disruption by fragments of bone. Retroperitoneal pelvic bleeding is self-limited in most patients with venous injuries because of the tamponading effect, except in those with open fractures. Approximately 18% to 20% of patients have arterial bleeding which does not stop. The retroperitoneal space in these patients may serve as a distensible container, which expands superiorly and anteriorly and may totally obliterate the lower part of the abdominal cavity. Component therapy with blood products is important in these patients until the bleeding is controlled.[159] Large retroperitoneal hematomas may also cause respiratory difficulty because of pressure on the diaphragm.

Early detection and intervention to control bleeding are important. Pelvic ring disruption, arterial extravasation (CT blush), and elevated bladder pressure secondary to compression by hematoma volumes >500 mL are important signs that can be detected on CT examination, making it a key diagnostic measure. In addition, continuing hemodynamic instability after adequate fracture stabilization is suggestive of pelvic hemorrhage. Following external pelvic ring stabilization using external fixators, pelvic binder, or a C-clamp to decrease the mobility of the bone fragments and help control blood loss, angiography can indicate the type and location of bleeding. Arterial bleeding, which is present in 15% to 20% of patients, is treated with embolization. The angiography suite should be prepared in advance not only for anesthesia, but also for invasive monitoring and resuscitation. In hemodynamically unstable patients, deciding whether to transport the patient to the OR to control bleeding from associated injuries or to proceed to interventional radiology for angiography and possible embolization is difficult, although surgery of abdominal, thoracic, and head injuries are given priority. In most centers, it takes at least

45 minutes to begin angiography, during which time a considerable amount of blood may be lost. Recent data suggest that after external stabilization of the pelvis, extraperitoneal (preperitoneal) packing in the OR under general anesthesia followed by angiography, and if arterial bleeding is noticed, embolization, may be more beneficial than only external fixation and angiography.[160] In this manner, pelvic venous bleeding is managed expeditiously. Packing involves a 6- to 7-cm midline vertical incision starting from the pubic symphysis, accessing the hematoma, and introducing two or three abdominal lap pads deep into the pelvis. The incision for packing is not continuous with the abdominal incision. Although this concept contrasts with the traditional understanding that opening a retroperitoneal hematoma caused by a pelvic fracture must be avoided to prevent excessive bleeding, with the present approach hematoma is entered extraperitoneally, instead of intraperitoneally, which indeed increases the bleeding. Laparotomy may be indicated, although it should be based on solid indications. Nontherapeutic laparotomy may worsen the outcome.[161] Pelvic fractures may also injure the bladder and the urethra. Thus, a urethrogram should be performed before insertion of a urinary catheter.

Extremity Injuries

Surgical repair of extremity fractures, whether open or closed, should be performed as soon as possible. Delayed fracture repair is associated with an increased risk of deep vein thrombosis (DVT), pneumonia, sepsis, and the pulmonary and cerebral complications of fat embolism. In open fractures, an additional important concern is infection. Wounds left unrepaired for more than 6 hours are likely to become septic.

Associated vascular trauma must be recognized early. Most vascular injuries exhibit at least some part of the classic syndrome of *pain, pulselessness, pallor, paresthesias,* and *paresis.* The definitive diagnosis is made with arteriography. In selected patients, a duplex ultrasound study may be used as a screening test. Patients with vascular trauma should be operated on expeditiously, often without preoperative angiography. These patients may bleed slowly but substantially both pre- and intraoperatively; thus, delayed surgery and prolonged skeletal repair may lead to unrecognized hemorrhagic shock, which may at times become irreversible. Damage control, that is, controlling bleeding and external fixation of the fractures, may be the management of choice.

Compartment syndrome, which is characterized by severe pain in the affected extremity, should be recognized early so that emergency fasciotomy can be effective in preventing irreversible muscle and nerve damage. In unconscious patients, swelling and tenseness of the extremity indicate the presence of this complication. The definitive diagnosis is made by measuring compartment pressures using a transducer attached to a fluid-filled extension tube and a needle inserted into the various compartments of the extremity. A pressure exceeding 40 cm H_2O is an indication for immediate surgery. Caution must be exercised when using epidural or nerve block analgesia for perioperative pain relief in the presence of extremity fractures. Absence of pain can delay the diagnosis of compartment syndrome.

Burns

Determination of the size and depth of a burn sets the guidelines for resuscitation, as well as the indications for surgical intervention.[162] A partial-thickness burn is red, blanches to touch, and is sensitive to painful stimuli and heat. Superficial partial-thickness (first-degree) burns involve the epidermis and upper dermis and heal spontaneously. Deep partial-thickness (second-degree) burns involve the deep dermis and require excision and grafting to ensure rapid return of function. A full-thickness (third-degree) burn does not blanch, even with deep pressure, and is insensate. Complete destruction of the dermis requires wound excision and grafting to prevent wound infection that may lead to local sepsis and systemic inflammation. Fourth-degree burns involve muscle, fascia, and bone, necessitating complete excision and leaving the patient with limited function. Laser Doppler imaging can be used as an aid to judge burn wound depth.[163] The size of the burned area as a fraction of the total body surface area (TBSA) is estimated by the "rule of nines." In an adult, the head contributes to 9%; the upper extremities, 18%; the trunk, 36%; and the lower extremities, 36% of the TBSA. These proportions are somewhat different in children, depending on the age and size. To estimate the size of a burn, the palmar surface of a child (excluding the digits) represents about 0.5% of the TBSA over a wide range of ages. Accuracy of the rule of nines has been challenged and it has been found to overestimate the TBSA of the head and arms. Further, it has been demonstrated that TBSA varies according to body mass index. A proposed rule for normal weight and obese patients is summarized in Table 52-12.[164]

TABLE 52-12. NEW PROPOSED RULE TO ESTIMATE BODY SURFACE AREAS OF NORMAL AND OBESE PATIENTS

	Normal Overweight (% BSA)	Obese (% BSA)	Morbidity Obese (% BSA)
Head	5	5	5
Arms	15	15	15
Trunk	35	40	45
Legs	45	40	35

Adapted from Neaman KC, Andres A, McClure AM, et al. A new method for estimation of involved BSAs for obese and normal-weight patients with burn injury. *J Burn Care Res.* 2011;32:421.

Information about the mechanism of injury facilitates the diagnosis of associated clinical abnormalities. For example, thermal trauma caused by flames in a closed space is likely to be associated with airway damage. Burns resulting from motor vehicle, airplane, or industrial accidents may be complicated by other traumatic injuries. Finally, burns caused by electrocution may show little external evidence but may be associated with severe fractures, hematomas, visceral injury, and skeletal and cardiac muscle injury resulting in pain, myoglobinuria, and dysrhythmias, or other ECG abnormalities.

Full-thickness burns involving >10% of the TBSA; partial-thickness burns covering >25% of TBSA in adults or over 20% at the extremes of age; burns involving the face, hands, feet, or perineum; inhalation, chemical, and electrical burns; and burns in patients with severe pre-existing medical disorders are considered major burns.[162] A severe burn is a systemic disease that stimulates the release of mediators such as interleukins, tumor necrosis factor, and neopterins, locally (producing wound edema) and into the circulation, resulting in immune suppression, hypermetabolism, protein catabolism, insulin resistance, sepsis, and multisystem organ failure. Patients with burns >40% TBSA consistently develop catabolism and weight loss, which may last up to 1 year. Prevention of sepsis, maintenance of normal body temperature, and pain management may decrease the extent of catabolism. Pharmacologically, recombinant human growth hormone, insulin-like growth factor-1, low-dose insulin infusion, β-blockade, and the synthetic testosterone analog oxandrolone can decrease protein catabolism or improve anabolism.[165,166]

Airway Complications

Respiratory distress in the initial phase of a burn is usually caused by airway injury involving the pharynx or the trachea. Singed facial hair, facial burns, dysphonia or hoarseness, cough, soot in the mouth or nose, and swallowing difficulties in patients with or without respiratory distress should increase the suspicion of upper (frequent) and lower (occasional) airway injury. In the upper airway, glottic and periglottic edema and copious, thick secretions may produce respiratory obstruction. This may be aggravated by fluid resuscitation even in the absence of significant inhalation injury.[167] In lower airway burns, decreased surfactant and mucociliary function, mucosal necrosis and ulceration, edema, tissue sloughing, and secretions produce bronchial obstruction, air trapping, and bronchopneumonia. The development of parenchymal lung injury takes approximately 1 to 5 days and presents with the clinical picture of ARDS. Pneumonia and pulmonary embolism (PE) are late complications that occur 5 or more days after burns. The presence of a lung injury markedly increases the mortality rate from thermal injuries.[168] Administration of the highest possible concentration of O_2 by facemask is the first priority in moderately to severely burned patients with a patent airway. In patients with massive burns, stridor, respiratory distress, hypoxemia, hypercarbia, loss of consciousness, or altered mentation, immediate tracheal intubation is indicated. The intubation technique selected depends on the operator's experience, the age of the patient, and the extent of airway compromise. In adults, awake fiberoptic intubation under adequate topical anesthesia is probably the safest approach, but other techniques (Air-Traq[R], Air Traq LCC, Fenton, Missouri; King View, King Systems, Nobelsville, Indiana; Glidescope, Verathon, Washington; Intubating LMA, LMA North America, San Diego, California) or retrograde intubation may be used. In most pediatric patients, awake intubation is not possible. An inhalation induction with O_2 and sevoflurane, followed by intubation using a fiberoptic bronchoscope or conventional laryngoscope, is appropriate.[162] A surgical airway entails a significant risk of pulmonary sepsis and late upper airway sequelae, and it should be reserved for those whose airway management cannot be handled in any other way.[162] Immediately after securing the airway, ventilation with low levels of PEEP will prevent the pulmonary edema that may develop secondary to loss of laryngeal auto-PEEP in patients with significant airway obstruction before intubation. Airway humidification, bronchial toilet, and bronchodilators if needed for bronchospasm are also indicated.

The pediatric airway is particularly challenging because it may be occluded by minimal amounts of swelling due to its small diameter. Prophylactic intubation may therefore be required in children who are suspected of having an inhalation injury, even though they are not yet in respiratory distress. Prophylactic tracheal intubation may also be indicated in adults when the resources for careful follow-up are insufficient. Information obtained from radiologic, ABG, and endoscopic examinations and pulmonary function testing may be useful to predict which patient will need tracheal intubation and possibly decrease the risks of airway manipulation.

Serial fiberoptic laryngoscopy is easy to perform and can provide direct information about the glottic and periglottic structures. It may avoid tracheal intubation in patients who would otherwise be considered candidates for this procedure. Fiberoptic bronchoscopy has the additional advantage of providing information about the lower airway, although it is more uncomfortable for the patient and requires topical anesthesia of the tracheobronchial tree.

The chest radiograph, ABGs, and pulmonary function tests are usually normal in the immediate postburn period, even in patients with pulmonary complications. However, these tests should be performed at this time for later comparison. The treatment of smoke inhalation in burns involves ventilatory management, intensive care, and treatment of carbon monoxide (CO) and cyanide (CN^-) toxicity.

Ventilation and Intensive Care

Hypoxemia may persist despite tracheal intubation, ventilation with PEEP, bronchodilators, and suction of airway secretions. In the first 36 hours, this is caused by acute pulmonary edema. From day 2 to 5, hypoxia may result from atelectasis, bronchopneumonia, and airway edema following mucosal necrosis and sloughing, viscous secretions, and distal airway obstruction. Later there may be nosocomial pneumonia, hypermetabolism-induced respiratory failure, and ARDS. Treatment of these complications is individualized, using ventilatory maneuvers such as low tidal volume (5 to 6 mL) with titrated PEEP, bronchoscopic lavage, antibiotics, chest physiotherapy, and other supportive measures. Lack of response to therapy because of severe ventilation–perfusion mismatching or shunt may be an indication for the use of nitric oxide, a potent, short-acting vasodilator, via the airway.[169] Patients with ARDS may benefit from high-frequency oscillatory ventilation, both intraoperatively and in the ICU.[170] Prophylactic measures against DVT, gastric ulcers, and hypothermia should be used routinely. Burns with TBSA ≥40% and those necessitating ICU admission carry the risk of venous thromboembolism requiring prophylaxis.[171] Further, pulmonary procoagulant activity with inhibited fibrinolysis in mechanically ventilated patients with burn and inhalation injuries results in alveolar fibrin depositions and pulmonary inflammation, which may decrease with anticoagulants.[172]

Carbon Monoxide Toxicity

In burn victims, CO inhalation is almost always associated with smoke inhalation, which increases morbidity and mortality compared with CO toxicity alone. CO produces tissue hypoxia primarily by its 200-fold greater affinity for hemoglobin than oxygen and by its ability to shift the hemoglobin dissociation curve to the left, impairing O_2 unloading to the tissues. It also interferes with mitochondrial function, uncoupling oxidative phosphorylation, and reducing adenosine triphosphate production, thus causing metabolic acidosis. Probably because of this effect on the mitochondria, CO can be a direct myocardial toxin preventing survival in patients who suffer cardiac arrest even though they have been resuscitated and treated with hyperbaric oxygen.

A normal oxygen saturation on a pulse oximeter does not exclude the possibility of CO toxicity, although low arterial O_2 saturation measured by a co-oximeter should raise the suspicion.[173] Portable devices such as the Masimo Rad-5 (Masimo Corp., Irvine, California) are capable of measuring carboxyhemoglobin and methemoglobin levels noninvasively via a finger sensor along with pulse oximetry, alerting the clinician about spuriously high O_2 saturation values. If CO toxicity is not accompanied by a lung injury and thus by decreased PaO_2, tachypnea is absent. The carotid bodies are sensitive to the arterial O_2 tension and not to the O_2 content. The classic cherry-red color of the blood is also absent in most patients because it occurs only at carboxyhemoglobin

TABLE 52-13. SYMPTOMS OF CARBON MONOXIDE TOXICITY AS A FUNCTION OF THE BLOOD COHB LEVEL

Blood COHb Level (%)	Symptoms
<15–20	Headache, dizziness, and occasional confusion
20–40	Nausea, vomiting, disorientation, and visual impairment
40–60	Agitation, combativeness, hallucinations, coma, and shock
>60	Death

COHb, carboxyhemoglobin.

(COHb) concentrations above 40%, and it may also be obscured by coexistent hypoxia and cyanosis.

The patient's inspired oxygen should be maintained at the highest possible concentration, even when there is no evidence of significant smoke-induced lung injury, until CO toxicity is ruled out by measurement of blood COHb. A high fraction of inspired oxygen (FiO_2) not only improves oxygenation, but also promotes elimination of CO; an FiO_2 of 1.0 decreases the blood half-life of COHb from the 4 hours seen in room air to about 60 to 90 minutes, and to 20 to 30 minutes at 3 atm in a hyperbaric chamber.[162] The greater the blood concentrations of COHb, the more severe the presenting symptoms (Table 52-13). Delayed neuropsychiatric disorders have been described in patients exposed to toxic levels of CO, and there is evidence to suggest that early hyperbaric O_2 treatment may prevent these symptoms.[162] The decision to institute this treatment should be based on comparing the risks of transport, decreased patient access, and delay in emergency treatment against the possible neurologic sequelae. Currently, hyperbaric O_2 is recommended for patients with COHb >30% at admission if the treatment of life-threatening problems—shock, neurologic injury, metabolic acidosis, myocardial ischemia, infarction, or arrhythmias—will not be compromised.

Cyanide Toxicity

Another cause of tissue hypoxia in burned patients is CN^- toxicity. Cyanide or hydrocyanic acid is produced by incomplete combustion of synthetic materials and may be inhaled or absorbed through mucous membranes. As in CO toxicity, the usual clinical presentation is unexplained metabolic acidosis. Nonspecific neurologic symptoms such as agitation, confusion, or coma are also common findings. Elevated plasma lactate levels in severe burns may result from hypovolemia or CO or CN^- toxicity. However, lactic acidosis after smoke inhalation in a patient without a major burn suggests CN^- toxicity.[174] The definitive diagnosis can be made only by determination of the blood cyanide level, which is toxic above 0.2 mg/L and lethal at levels beyond 1 mg/L. A spectrophotometric assay using methemoglobin as a colorimetric indicator provides a timely and reliable determination of blood CN^-.[175] The pulse oximetry reading will be accurate in the absence of CO toxicity and nitrate therapy–induced methemoglobinemia.

Increased CN^- in the blood can cause generalized cardiovascular depression and cardiac rhythm disturbances, especially in patients with lactic acidosis. Fortunately, the half-life of CN^- is short (approximately 1 hour),[174] and rapid improvement of hemodynamics should be expected after rescue of the victim from the toxic environment. Immediate administration of O_2, which is required for all burn victims, may be lifesaving for this complication. Although there are specific therapies for CN^- toxicity (e.g., amyl nitrate, sodium nitrite, thiosulfate), given the short half-life of the ion, it is not clear whether these measures offer significant help to the patient whose blood CN^- usually decreases to low levels during transport from the field to the hospital.[176] Of course, if circumstances permit, hyperbaric O_2 treatment can be used for all the complications of thermal injury: CO and CN^- poisoning, smoke-induced lung damage, and cutaneous burns.

Fluid Replacement

Immediately after a serious burn microvascular permeability increases, causing the loss of a substantial amount of protein-rich fluid into the interstitial space. A major burn, a delay in initiation of resuscitation, or an inhalation injury increases the size of the leak.[162] Further, there seems to be a correlation between inhalation injury and cutaneous burns in the production of edema: pulmonary edema increases cutaneous edema and vice versa.[177] If resuscitation is successful, edema formation stops within 18 to 24 hours.[177] This fluid flux is enhanced by increased intravascular hydrostatic and interstitial osmotic pressures and decreased interstitial hydrostatic pressure. In addition, cardiac contractility may decrease because of circulating mediators, a diminished response to catecholamines, decreased coronary blood flow, and increased systemic vascular resistance.[162,178] This may result in shock, whose origin is primarily hypovolemic and, to a much smaller extent, cardiogenic.[178] If the hypotension is treated appropriately with fluids, the hemodynamic picture is replaced within 24 to 48 hours by one resembling sepsis or septic shock, with increased heart rate, cardiac output, and rate pressure product, and diminished systemic vascular resistance caused by the release of inflammatory mediators.[178]

Fluid resuscitation is essential in the early care of the burned patient with an injury >15% TBSA. Smaller burns can be managed with replacement at 150% of the calculated maintenance rate and careful monitoring of fluid status. Intravascular volume should be restored with utmost care to prevent excessive edema formation in both damaged and intact tissues resulting from the generalized increase in capillary permeability caused by the injury. Edema from overaggressive resuscitation has many deleterious and potentially life-threatening effects. Mention has already been made of the facilitation of upper airway edema after rapid fluid infusion in large cutaneous burns with or without smoke inhalation.[167] Likewise, chest wall edema may develop after administration of large quantities of fluid to patients with burns in this area, causing respiratory difficulties and necessitating excision of burned tissue from the anterior axillary line to improve breathing. Abdominal edema may also occur, and when resuscitation volume exceeds 300 mL/kg/24 hr, increased intra-abdominal pressure may produce *abdominal compartment syndrome* with impedance of venous return.[179,180] Edema formation may also increase the tissue pressure in the burned area, resulting in reduction of blood flow to distal sites. This, together with decreased tissue oxygen tension, may produce necrosis of damaged but viable cells, increasing the extent of injury and the risk of infection.

Crystalloid solutions are preferred for resuscitation during the first day following a burn injury; leakage of colloids during this phase may increase edema.[181] Nevertheless, crystalloid resuscitation, especially in children, may cause a rapid decline in plasma protein concentration and necessitate administration of 5% albumin in LR solution after the first day following a burn >30% TBSA and/or significant inhalation injury when the capillary leak stops.[182] It is believed that this will moderate the tendency to edema formation associated with the administration of large amounts of isotonic (0.9% saline or LR) solutions. Some centers use plasma with crystalloid routinely and partly attribute the good outcomes of their patients to this practice.[183] Administration of fluids in excess of the amount recommended by the Parkland formula appears to be relatively frequent in modern burn management and is termed *fluid creep.* Avoidance of early overresuscitation, routine use of colloids, and adherence to protocols are recommended to prevent this problem.[184] Plasma exchange therapy may also remove inflammatory mediators and decrease capillary permeability, lowering fluid requirements and improving base deficit and lactate in these patients.[185] Alternatively, hypertonic saline solutions draw intracellular water into the bloodstream and thus decrease the fluid volume needed to maintain perfusion and extracellular volume and limit the severity of edema in patients with burns occupying >50% TBSA, circumferential extremity burns, or inhalational injury.[162] Unfortunately, hypertonic solutions may cause hypernatremia and intracellular water depletion. Patients and experimental animals receiving these fluids for burn therapy often did not show an overall fluid-sparing effect and had an unacceptably high incidence of renal failure and death compared with those receiving LR solution.[181,186,187]

Of the many resuscitation formulas available, the Parkland (Baxter) and modified Brooke formulas are tailored to the clinical condition of the patient and are accepted in most centers (Table 52-14).[182] The addition of glucose is not necessary except in children, especially those weighing <20 kg. Albumin 5% may be administered after the first day following injury at a rate of 0.3, 0.4, or 0.5 mL/kg of the percentage burned per 24 hours for burns of 30% to 50%, 50% to 70%, or 70% to 100% TBSA, respectively. These formulas are guidelines only, and none can be expected to provide adequate restoration of intravascular volume in all burn victims, especially small children and patients with inhalation injuries. Therefore, administration of fluids during the initial phase should be titrated to the specific goals described in Table 52-14, and, if a pulmonary artery catheter is placed, acceptable cardiac output, filling pressures, and a mixed venous oxygen tension (PvO_2) of 35 to 40 mm Hg. Careful monitoring of the Hct may also guide fluid management. An increase in Hct during the first day suggests inadequate fluid resuscitation because hemolysis and sequestration are actually expected to cause a decrease in this parameter. Acute anemia, as may occur during excision and grafting of burns, is usually well tolerated. Blood replacement is usually not initiated until the Hct is below 20% in healthy patients requiring limited operations, approximately 25% in those who are healthy but need extensive procedures, and 30% or more when there is a history of pre-existing cardiovascular disease.

Standard clinical end points of resuscitation such as urine output and vital signs are used routinely to guide fluid therapy. The pulmonary artery catheter is associated with the risk of infectious complications and is used less frequently than in the past. A transpulmonary thermodilution technique using Pulsiocath thermistor-tipped catheter (Pulsion Medical Systems, Munich, Germany) is less invasive and may be employed to measure cardiac index, intrathoracic blood volume index, extrathoracic lung water index, extravascular lung volume index, and systemic vascular resistance. This technique requires placement of central venous and arterial catheters without cardiac or pulmonary cannulation.[188]

When in rare instances fluid resuscitation fails, despite administration of crystalloids in excess of 6 mL/kg per percentage TBSA, and invasive or semi-invasive monitoring suggests adequate intravascular volume, vasopressor and/or inotropic agents may be indicated. Dopamine in small doses (5 μg/kg/min) and/or β-adrenergic agents may improve urine output without further need for fluids.[182] Electrolyte abnormalities may occur after the first day for several reasons but are primarily a result of topical agents applied to control pain, decrease vapor loss, prevent desiccation, and slow bacterial growth.[182] Nonaqueous topicals (silver sulfadiazine), if administered without providing free water such as 5% dextrose, may result in hypernatremia and its CNS consequences including intracranial bleeding. In contrast, aqueous topical agents such as 5% silver nitrate solution may cause hyponatremia and its consequences of cerebral edema and seizure secondary to electrolyte leaching. Central pontine demyelination may occur if the hyponatremia is corrected rapidly with salt solutions. Serum ionized calcium and magnesium should also be monitored.

TABLE 52-14. GUIDELINES FOR INITIAL FLUID RESUSCITATION AFTER THERMAL INJURY

Adults and Children >20 kg
Parkland formula[a]
4.0 mL crystalloid/kg/% burn/first 24 hr
Modified Brooke Formula[a]
2.0 mL lactated Ringer's/kg per % burn per first 24 hr
Children <20 kg
Crystalloid 2–3 mL/kg per % burn per 24 hr[a]
Crystalloid with 5% dextrose at maintenance rate
100 mL/kg for the first 10 kg and 50 mL/kg for the next 10 kg for 24 hr
Clinical End Points of Burn Resuscitation
Urine output: 0.5–1 mL
Pulse: 80–140 per min (age dependent)
Systolic BP: 60 mm Hg (infants); children 70–90 plus 2x age in years mm Hg; adults MAP > 60 mm Hg
Base deficit: <2

BP, blood pressure; MAP, mean arterial pressure.
[a]50% of calculated volume is given during the first 8 hr, 25% is given during the second 8 hr, and the remaining 25% is given during the third 8 hr.

OPERATIVE MANAGEMENT

Overall, nearly 25% of trauma patients present with pre-existing conditions such as cirrhosis; cardiovascular, pulmonary, and renal diseases; coagulation disorders; diabetes; and alcohol or drug abuse that may increase trauma-related morbidity and mortality and require additional care.[7,189] Premedication is rarely indicated, especially in those who are hypovolemic, head injured, or intoxicated. If needed, small doses of opioid (morphine, 1 to 2 mg; fentanyl, 25 to 50 μg) or sedative (midazolam, 0.5 to 1.0 mg) may be administered with close monitoring of vital signs. Regional analgesia may be provided for stable patients with skeletal injuries awaiting surgery. Femoral nerve block, for example, provides excellent analgesia for femoral shaft fractures. Evaluation of the multiple trauma patient emergently transported to the OR involves reviewing pre-existing conditions, vital signs, oxygenation, and preoperative fluid replacement and confirmation of correct position and patency of a previously inserted endotracheal tube.

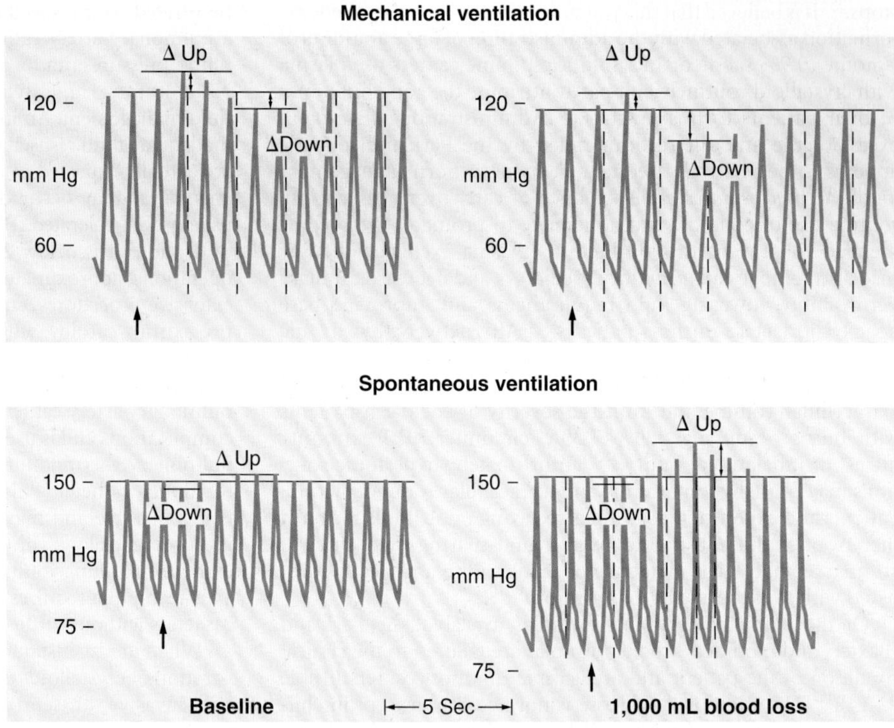

FIGURE 52-10. Arterial pressure records of a mechanically ventilated patient before (*left*) and after (*right*) 1,000 mL blood loss. Note the increase in systolic pressure variation and δ-down component following hemorrhage. Decrease in blood pressure occurs during exhalation with mechanical ventilation and inspiration in spontaneously breathing subjects (*upgoing arrow* defines inhalation). δ-Up is the difference between the end-expiratory systolic pressure and the maximum systolic pressure over a respiratory cycle. See text for definition of systolic pressure variation and δ-down component. (Reprinted with permission from Rooke GA, Schwid HA, Shapira Y. The effect of graded hemorrhage and intravascular volume replacement on systolic pressure variation in humans during mechanical and spontaneous ventilation. *Anesth Analg.* 1995;80:925.)

Monitoring

Hemodynamic Monitoring

Direct intra-arterial pressure monitoring, which permits beat-to-beat data acquisition and sampling for measurement of blood gases, should be in place before surgery. An ultrasound-guided technique or a surgical cut-down may be necessary to facilitate access. The radial artery is the vessel of choice in abdominal or chest trauma in which the aorta may be cross-clamped, making a femoral or dorsalis pedis cannula nonfunctional. The right radial artery is preferred in cases of chest trauma in which cross-clamping of the descending aorta might result in occlusion of the left subclavian artery. In mechanically ventilated patients, the magnitude of systolic pressure variation (the difference between the maximum and minimum systolic pressure over the respiratory cycle) and its Δ-down component (the difference between systolic pressure at end expiration and the lowest value during the respiratory cycle) can provide reliable information about the intravascular volume status and predict responsiveness to fluid loading (Fig. 52-10). A systolic pressure variation >5 mm Hg and a Δ-down >2 mm Hg suggest hypovolemia.[190]

The ability to predict fluid responsiveness is of crucial importance in preventing over- or underinfusion of fluids and their consequences. Interest has been centered in *automatically* obtaining systolic blood pressure variation (SPV), pulse pressure variation (PPV), and stroke volume variation (SVV) during the mechanical ventilation cycle to predict fluid responsiveness. Indeed several such devices, such as the PICCO (Pulsion Medical Systems, Munich, Germany), LIDCO (Lidco Ltd., United Kingdom), and FloTrac CO Monitor (Edwards Laboratories, USA) are able to display SPV, PPV, and SVV, which appear to predict responsiveness to fluid administration with greater accuracy than static markers of preload such as central venous pressure, pulmonary artery occlusion pressure, and even global end diastolic volume or left ventricular end diastolic area.[191] Threshold values to discriminate responders from nonresponders to fluid infusion have been determined (PPV or SVV >12% for responders). These dynamic indices of preload can be obtained with an arterial line without central venous or pulmonary artery catheters. Limitations of this technology include their ability to work only in intubated and mechanically ventilated patients with tidal volumes >7 to 8 mL/kg, closed chest, and normal cardiac rhythm; their doubtful reliability in patients with stiff lungs or those receiving PEEP; and most importantly, lack of information about their accuracy in acutely injured patients.[192]

Delaying emergent surgery to place a central venous line is rarely indicated unless a large-bore catheter is needed for volume resuscitation. However, if the patient is elderly, if there is a likelihood of myocardial damage, or if there is multiple organ damage with a requirement for prolonged surgery and massive fluid replacement, early placement of a CVP or pulmonary artery catheter may be indicated before the development of coagulopathy renders it hazardous. If a pulmonary artery catheter is placed, mixed venous O_2 may convey information about organ perfusion.

11 The TEE provides valuable diagnostic information in blunt cardiac injury, cardiac septal or valvular damage, coronary artery injury, pericardial tamponade, and aortic rupture.[193] It also permits assessment of cardiac function, including right and left ventricular volume, ejection fraction, wall motion abnormalities, pulmonary hypertension, and cardiac output and detects acute ischemia more accurately than either ECG or pulmonary artery pressure monitoring. Monitoring left ventricular volume alone can provide information about the adequacy of the intravascular volume. This technique also allows visualization of fat and air entry into the right heart or the left heart through a patent foramen ovale during internal fixation of lower extremity fractures.[194] It is possible that the TEE probe may be introduced into an unrecognized esophageal tear because the insidious nature of esophageal injury makes diagnosis difficult during the first 24 hours after trauma.

Urine Output

Urine output is routinely monitored as an indicator of organ perfusion, hemolysis, skeletal muscle destruction, and urinary tract integrity after trauma. Its reliability for monitoring perfusion is decreased by prolonged shock prior to surgery and osmotic diuresis caused by administration of mannitol or radiopaque dye. Dark, cola-colored urine in the trauma patient suggests either hemoglobinuria resulting from incompatible blood transfusion or myoglobinuria caused by massive skeletal muscle destruction after blunt or electrical trauma. Although the definitive diagnosis is made by serum electrophoresis, rapid differential diagnosis can be made by centrifugation of a blood specimen. Pink-stained serum suggests hemoglobinuria whereas unstained serum indicates myoglobinuria. Both of these conditions may result in acute renal failure. Prevention involves inducing diuresis with fluids and mannitol and, in myoglobinuria, although controversial, additional alkalinization of the urine with sodium bicarbonate to pH >5.6. Red-colored urine usually is caused by hematuria, which, in the traumatized patient, suggests urinary tract injury.

Oxygenation

Frequently trauma patients develop hypoxemia (O_2 saturation <90%), hypothermia, hypotension, and/or decreased peripheral perfusion. Although modern pulse oximeters are designed to be unaffected by these conditions, inaccurate measurement of O_2 saturation (SpO_2) is still observed. Of the available devices, finger or earlobe pulse oximeters are more affected by decreased perfusion than forehead oximeters probably because the latter senses the pulsation of the supraorbital artery, a branch of the carotid artery, which is presumably less affected by shock or hypothermia. However, SpO_2 results with this monitor may be affected by venous pulsation, especially in patients receiving positive pressure ventilation or in any situation that distends the tributaries of the superior vena cava.[195] It has been suggested that using these sensors with a head band that exerts 10 to 20 mm Hg pressure may minimize the inaccuracy.[195]

With recent advances in technology, multiwavelength pulse co-oximeters are also capable of providing other physiologic data including pulse rate, SpO_2, perfusion index, carboxyhemoglobin, and methemoglobin. These monitors can also measure noninvasive continuous hemoglobin concentration with reasonable accuracy. The ability of these monitors (Masimo Rad-7 and Rad-57 Pulse CO-oximeter, Irvine, California) to measure methemoglobin and carboxyhemoglobin concentration noninvasively renders them useful in acute burn injury management. Although these monitors provide more accurate information than conventional pulse oximeters, to the best of the authors' knowledge they have not yet been tested in major trauma victims.

Organ Perfusion and Oxygen Utilization

As discussed previously, unrecognized hypoperfusion may lead to splanchnic ischemia with resulting acidosis in the intestinal wall, permitting the passage of luminal micro-organisms into the circulation and release of inflammatory mediators, causing sepsis and multiorgan failure.[50–52] Base deficit and blood lactate level, which have already been discussed in the section "Management of Shock," are considered acceptable markers of organ hypoperfusion in the *apparently* resuscitated patient and may be used intraoperatively to set the optimal end points of resuscitation.[52] Another parameter that may provide information intraoperatively about the global perfusion of the body is the arterial–end tidal CO_2 difference. Values >10 mm Hg after resuscitation predict mortality.[196] It may be useful in the decision about when to perform damage control surgery, and intraoperatively, in guiding resuscitation with fluids, inotropes, and vasopressors. A large gap is usually due to decreased lung perfusion resulting in high $PaCO_2$ and low end-tidal CO_2. Severe chest trauma, hypotension, or metabolic acidosis also increases the likelihood of discordance between arterial and end tidal CO_2.[197]

Oxygen transport variables, once routinely monitored as markers of organ perfusion, especially in the ICU setting, are used less frequently and in a limited number of centers primarily because they require pulmonary artery catheterization. They consist of oxygen delivery (DO_2), O_2 consumption ($\dot{V}O_2$), and O_2 extraction ratio. The DO_2 index (DO_2I) is a particularly useful end point because it integrates three important variables: hemoglobin concentration, arterial oxygen saturation, and cardiac output. The minimum acceptable value for this marker is 500 mL/min/m^2,[198] performing as effectively as the previously recommended DO_2I of ≥600 mL/min/m^2. A computerized ICU decision protocol developed to standardize shock resuscitation in some centers uses DO_2I >500 mL/min/m^2 as a goal.[198] The oxygen consumption index ($\dot{V}O_2I$) is also an important variable. Subsequent organ failure may occur if it decreases below a value of 170 mL/min/m^2, indicating a flow-dependent phase of O_2 utilization.[52] Increasing DO_2I until $\dot{V}O_2I$ attains flow independence may prevent organ failure; however, this approach is not practical clinically, mainly because there are also DI_2I-independent regulators of $\dot{V}O_2$.[198]

Finally, a global O_2 extraction ratio <0.25 to 0.3 suggests absence of dysoxia. However, it is possible that dysoxia may be present in an individual organ in the presence of a normal overall O_2 extraction ratio. Monitoring of O_2 transport variables, the most useful of which is DO_2I, is usually done in the ICU when invasive monitoring permits measurement of cardiac output and mixed venous O_2. These values can also be monitored in the OR whenever arterial and pulmonary artery lines are present.

It has recently been demonstrated that central venous, instead of pulmonary artery, monitoring with CVP >10 mm Hg, mean systemic blood pressure of 65 mm Hg, and Hgb >10 g/dL as threshold values also suggest adequate organ perfusion.[199] It should be emphasized that various pre-existing and trauma-related conditions may affect the interpretations of these perfusion markers. For example, the base deficit may reflect a nongap acidosis, elevated lactate may be secondary to impaired clearance due to hepatic dysfunction, and arterial to end-tidal CO_2 gradient may be caused by chronic obstructive lung disease. Thus, management decisions must be individualized, taking into account the patient's general condition.

Coagulation

Conventional blood coagulation monitoring includes a baseline and subsequent serial measurements of PT, INR, activated partial thromboplastin time (aPTT), platelet count, blood fibrinogen level, and fibrin degradation products (FDP). Although trauma center laboratories cannot provide results of the standard coagulation tests rapidly, at least INR can be monitored with a point of care device and provide some information. Thromboelastography (TEG; (Haemonetics, Boston, Massachusetts) and rotation TEM (ROTEM; Pentapharm, Munich, Germany) are point of care devices that provide a relatively rapid, comprehensive, and quantitative graphic evaluation of clotting function.[200,201] The TEG determines the time necessary for initial fibrin formation, the rapidity of fibrin deposition, the clot consistency, the rate of clot formation, and the times required for clot retraction and lysis[200] (Fig. 52-11). Basically, the R and K values are indices of formation, buildup, and crosslinking of fibrin and depend on the function of coagulation factors. The maximum amplitude is the

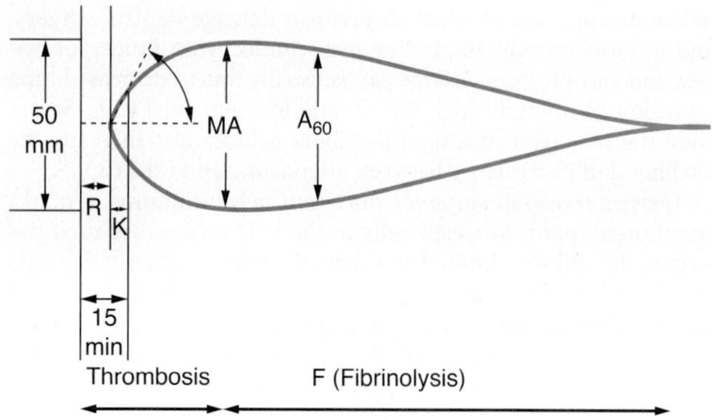

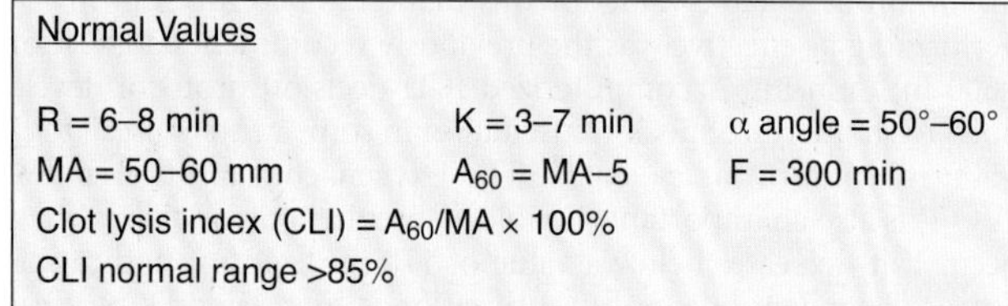
Normal Values

R = 6–8 min | K = 3–7 min | α angle = 50°–60°
MA = 50–60 mm | A_{60} = MA–5 | F = 300 min
Clot lysis index (CLI) = A_{60}/MA × 100%
CLI normal range >85%

FIGURE 52-11. Thrombelastogram. R is the interval from blood deposition in the cuvette to an amplitude of 1 mm on the thrombelastogram; K is the time between the end of R and a point with an amplitude of 20 mm on the thrombelastogram; MA is the maximum amplitude of thrombelastogram; α angle is the slope of the external divergence of the tracing from the R value point; A_{60} is the amplitude of thromboelastogram 60 minutes after maximum amplitude; F is the time from MA to return to 0 amplitude (normal >300 minutes).

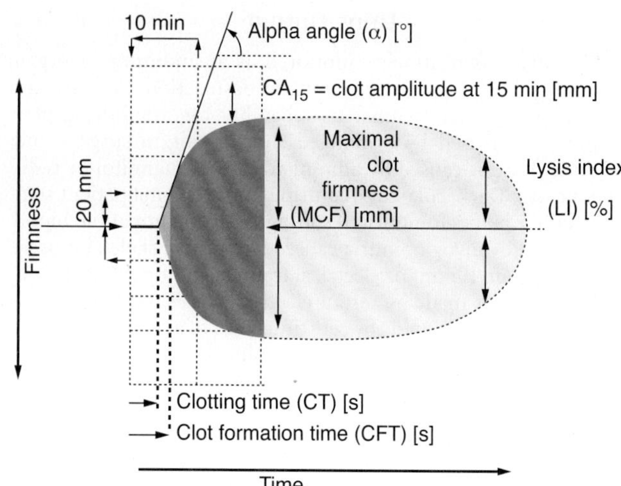

FIGURE 52-12. Rotation thromboelastometry graph depicting each clotting parameter. (Reproduced by permission from Rugeri L, Levrat A, David JS, et al. Diagnosis of early coagulation abnormalities in trauma patients by rotation thromboelastography. *J Thromb Haemostas.* 2007;5:289.)

widest portion of the curve and indicates the absolute strength of the fibrin clot. It represents platelet function. The *a*-angle is the slope of the external divergence of the tracing from the R-value point, indicating the speed of clot formation and fibrin crosslinking. The value of this parameter is determined by both coagulation factors and platelets. Hypothermia can cause coagulopathy by interfering with both platelets and coagulation factors.[202] When the blood of a cold and coagulopathic patient is placed in the TEG cuvette, which is normally heated to 37°C, a near-normal trace may be obtained. Newer TEG devices are temperature adjustable. Thus, the temperature in the cuvette can be adjusted to that of the patient. Likewise, by using activators, rapid TEG (r-TEG) can be performed to obtain timely results.[84] ROTEM is a modified TEM that uses a ball-bearing system for power transduction and is less susceptible to movements or vibration that may affect the TEG.[201] It measures clot formation and fibrinolysis. Results of coagulation parameters are obtained within 10 to 15 minutes because of activation with specific materials for each of clotting, platelet, and fibrinogen function. Figure 52-12 shows a typical TEM graph in which clotting time (CT), clot formation time (CFT), maximum clot firmness (MCF), and the amplitude of clot at 10 minutes (CA_{10}) and 15 minutes (CA_{15}) can be determined.[201] After 30 to 60 minutes, the clot lysis index at 30 and 60 minutes (CLI_{30}-CLI_{60}), which is the ratio between the amplitudes at 30 and 60 minutes, and amplitude of the graph at the point of CT may be obtained. As in TEG, each parameter represents the status of a specific function.

Anesthetic and Adjunct Drugs

Apart from regional anesthesia techniques, which are used in patients with minor extremity injuries and stable hemodynamics, anesthetic and adjunct drugs for general anesthesia need to be tailored to five major clinical conditions: airway compromise, hypovolemia, head or open eye injuries, cardiac injury, and burns. The varying contribution of these conditions to the clinical picture of a given patient necessitates priority-oriented planning.

Airway Compromise

Anesthetics and muscle relaxants should be avoided before the airway is secured if there is significant airway obstruction or if there is doubt as to whether the patient's trachea can be intubated because of anatomic limitations. If time permits, lateral neck radiographs, CT scanning, and endoscopy can be used to define better the problems. Topical anesthesia with mild sedation can be used to secure the airway with a conventional blade, video laryngoscope, or FOB. If a rapid sequence induction is contemplated, ketamine and etomidate may confer advantages over thiopental and propofol. In equipotent doses in normovolemic patients, they produce less cardiovascular depression. Although succinylcholine, with its short onset time and duration, is still the muscle relaxant of choice for rapid-sequence induction, rocuronium (1.2 to 1.5 mg/kg) has almost the same onset time and does not have the undesirable side effects associated with succinylcholine (e.g., increased intragastric, intraocular, and intracranial pressures and potassium release in patients with burns and neurologic diseases). Its longer duration of action may be disadvantageous and may lead to hypoxia if both ventilation and intubation prove to be impossible. Under these circumstances, one of the available video laryngoscopes or other aids can be employed to overcome the problem. Surgical standby for cricothyroidotomy should be considered if failure of these techniques is anticipated. Bradycardia, dysrhythmias, and cardiac arrest may occur after succinylcholine in the presence of hypoxia and hypercarbia. Some of these complications may also follow an apparently uneventful intubation performed without succinylcholine.

Hypovolemia

In the absence of controlled human studies of anesthetic drug effect in hemorrhage and hemorrhagic shock, our current knowledge in this area is based on the results of experimental work, mostly in swine. Anesthetic agents not only have direct cardiovascular depressant effects, but also inhibit compensatory hemodynamic mechanisms such as central catecholamine output and baroreflex (neuroregulatory) mechanisms, which maintain systemic pressure in hypovolemia. Hemorrhage and hypovolemia lead to a higher than normal blood concentration following a given dose of intravenous agents, increased sensitivity of the brain to anesthetics, preferential distribution of the cardiac output to the brain and the heart, cerebral hypoxia, dilutional hypoproteinemia producing a larger free fraction of intravenous drugs, and acidosis, all of which increase the effects of drugs on the brain and the heart.

The pharmacokinetic and pharmacodynamic responses of intravenous agents to experimental hemorrhagic shock vary depending on the severity of the hemorrhage, the specific agent, and whether the effect analyzed is hypnosis or immobility to noxious stimuli. For example, in swine with compensated hemorrhage, when administered as a continuous infusion, blood propofol concentration increased by <20%, while during uncompensated shock (i.e., in hypotensive animals), it increased by almost 4 times.[203] On the other hand, under the same experimental conditions, plasma remifentanil concentration doubled during compensated shock, but increased almost 27 times in uncompensated shock.[203] Remifentanil degradation relies on tissue and blood esterases. It is possible that hydrolysis by tissue esterases is more intense than by their blood counterparts because the decreased tissue blood flow in uncompensated shock is able to produce such a major reduction in remifentanil metabolism. Another example is that hemorrhage has a similar potentiating effect on the production of hypnosis and immobility by propofol.[204] In contrast, the potentiating effect of hemorrhagic shock on isoflurane induced hypnosis is much smaller than on its immobilizing effect.[204]

Because of the decrease in size of the central compartment and in systemic clearance, plasma concentrations of fentanyl and remifentanil are increased.[203,205] A decreased volume of distribution also increases the blood level of etomidate by 20% in shock,[206] and for propofol this effect is even greater. There is also variation in the extent of brain sensitivity to these agents. Although etomidate pharmacodynamics are unchanged,[207] a significant increase in the sensitivity of the brain and heart to propofol is noted in animals, even after fluid resuscitation.[206] Based on these experimental findings, Shafer[208] calculated that in patients with shock, the dose of propofol should be only 10% to 20% of that given to a healthy patient. Although he calculated that etomidate dose should not require adjustment for shock, the authors decrease the dose by at least 25% to 50% when we suspect hypovolemia. As to the opioids, the calculated dose for fentanyl and remifentanil is approximately one-half that for healthy patients (Fig. 52-13).[208] Of the remaining intravenous agents, thiopental and midazolam are also known to have significant cardiovascular depressant activity, whereas ketamine has stimulatory effects when the autonomic nervous system is intact.

There are also differences among anesthetics in the direction and extent of their effects on compensatory mechanisms. For example, the baroreceptor depression produced by intravenous agents is usually milder than that of inhalational agents. Opioid agents have little direct cardiovascular or baroreflex depressant effect; however, these agents can cause hypotension by inhibiting central sympathetic activity, especially in the hypovolemic trauma patient whose apparent hemodynamic stability is maintained by hyperactive sympathetic tone.

Two important principles in the use of anesthetic agents are accurate estimation of the degree of hypovolemia and reduction of doses accordingly. The presence of hypotension suggests uncompensated hypovolemia in which case anesthetics almost invariably produce further deterioration of systemic blood pressure and sometimes cardiac standstill. Intravascular volume, to

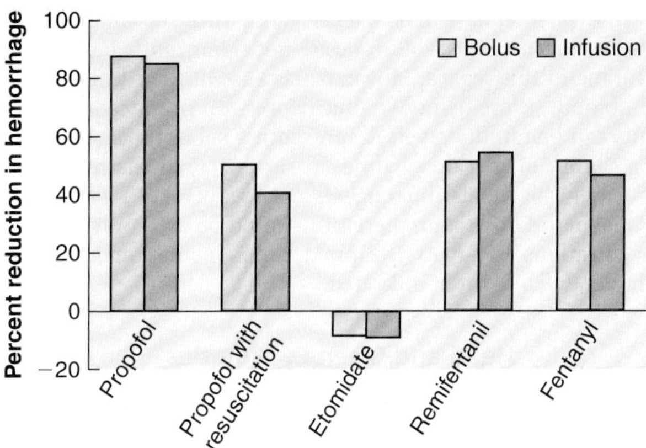

FIGURE 52-13. Calculated dose reduction of various anesthetics administered as bolus or infusion in moderate hemorrhagic shock. Calculation is based on pharmacokinetic and pharmacodynamic studies performed in experimental hemorrhagic shock. (Reprinted with permission from Shafer SL. Shock values. *Anesthesiology.* 2004;101:567.)

the extent possible, must be restored before their use. When time constraints or continuing hemorrhage prevent restoration of blood volume, the airway must be secured without the benefit of anesthesia (perhaps using only rapidly acting muscle relaxants and small doses of opioids, etomidate, or ketamine), even though this approach may result in recall of induction and intraoperative events in up to 40% of patients.[209] Hypothermia, alcohol intoxication, drug use before anesthesia, and metabolic disturbances in the acute trauma patient cannot reliably prevent recall. However, scopolamine, (0.6 mg), and midazolam, if the patient can tolerate it, given before airway management may decrease the likelihood of this complication. Intraoperative use of the bispectral index monitor and, whenever possible, titrating anesthetics to bispectral index levels <60 may prevent recall in trauma patients.

In normotensive but hypovolemic patients, restoration of volume and selection of an agent with the least cardiovascular depressant effect appears logical. Ketamine and etomidate are the preferred induction agents,[207] although at low doses other intravenous anesthetics are also unlikely to produce hypotension. Therefore, the use of any of these drugs in reduced doses is probably more important than the particular agent chosen.

Maintenance of anesthesia in the hypovolemic trauma patient raises concerns similar to those pertaining to induction. Experimental data have shown that depending on its severity, hemorrhagic shock decreases minimum alveolar concentration (MAC) by approximately 25%. Restoration of intravascular volume did not, but administration of naloxone did normalize MAC in these animals, suggesting that shock-induced release of endorphins is primarily responsible for this effect.[210]

Although nitrous oxide's (N_2O) myocardial depressant effect is normally somewhat counterbalanced by its ability to increase sympathetic outflow, in acute hemorrhage there is already a dramatic increase in sympathetic activity and stimulation of baroreceptors. Under these circumstances, patients are unlikely to respond to the sympathetic effect of N_2O, and the cardiovascular depressant properties of the gas are unmasked. These may be similar to those of other inhalation agents. In addition, by reducing FiO_2, use of N_2O incurs a risk of hypoxemia in patients with reduced cardiac output or pulmonary compromise. Despite causing little impairment of reflex tachycardia and having a vasodilatory action that preserves organ blood flow in normovolemic patients, isoflurane can impair cardiac output and organ blood flow in hypovolemia—that is, it can cause cardiovascular depression. Desflurane and sevoflurane are not significantly better than isoflurane in this regard. However, because of their low solubility in blood, severe hemodynamic depression produced by these agents can be rapidly reversed, preventing suboptimal perfusion for a significant period of time. In summary, in the hypovolemic patient all inhalational agents may reduce both global and regional blood flows and, therefore, should be used only in small concentrations (<1 MAC). Opioid supplementation is usually well tolerated and often indicated.

Head and Open Eye Injuries

The importance of deep anesthesia and adequate muscle relaxation during airway management of patients with head or open eye injuries has already been discussed. Anesthetic agents selected for management of brain injury should produce the least increase in ICP, the least decrease in mean arterial pressure, and the greatest reduction in cerebral metabolic rate ($CMRO_2$). As demonstrated by intraoperative $SjvO_2$ measurements in patients with acute head injury, the most important factor in causing cerebral ischemia is increased ICP from intracranial hematoma. Prompt decompression is the most crucial means of ensuring cerebral well-being. Hypotension caused by anesthetics or other factors contributes to the development or progression of cerebral ischemia. Utmost attention should be paid during anesthesia to avoidance of hypotension (mean arterial pressure <60 mm Hg or SBP <90 mm Hg). With the possible exception of ketamine, all intravenous anesthetics cause comparable degrees of cerebrovascular constriction. Again, with the exception of ketamine, $CMRO_2$ is also reduced by all the available intravenous anesthetics. An important drawback to these agents is that their cardiovascular depressant effects may reduce CPP. This problem can be ameliorated by administering pretreatment doses of opioids (fentanyl, 2 to 3 μg/kg), which permit reduction of the anesthetic dose. This may also prevent the myoclonic movements associated with etomidate and occasionally with propofol, and thus reduce the risks of ICP and IOP increase. Nevertheless, myoclonus is best prevented by careful timing of the dose of muscle relaxants. Another measure to preserve CPP during anesthesia is to administer vasopressors, being aware that hypovolemia may be masked by their use.

Ordinarily, administration of succinylcholine should follow pretreatment doses of nondepolarizing agents to prevent fasciculation-induced elevation of ICP and IOP.[211] Avoiding succinylcholine usually does not alleviate the problem because laryngoscopy and tracheal intubation produce a greater and longer-lasting increase in these pressures. Rocuronium, 1.2 to 1.5 mg/kg, has an onset time comparable with that of succinylcholine. None of the nondepolarizing muscle relaxants causes an elevation of ICP or IOP in the absence of associated tracheal intubation.

All inhalation anesthetics may increase CBF and cerebral blood volume (CBV), and thus the ICP. Cerebral autoregulation, CO_2 responsiveness, and $CMRO_2$ are reduced. Unlike thiopental, which decreases both CBF and $CMRO_2$ in parallel, inhalational anesthetics decrease $CMRO_2$ while increasing the CBF. The extent of this uncoupling varies with the agent and the dose. Isoflurane has the least vasodilatory effect and thus is the most widely used inhalation anesthetic, although desflurane and sevoflurane have comparable effects on the cerebral circulation. In hyperventilated patients with cerebral tumors or mild edema, isoflurane does not raise the ICP if it is administered at an inspired concentration of <1 MAC. In the presence of severe head injury, when cerebral autoregulation and CO_2 responsiveness are impaired, isoflurane has the potential to increase CBF and ICP even at levels <1 MAC and with hyperventilation. Therefore, it may be prudent not to use this agent in the presence of elevated ICP, at least until the skull is opened and the ICP is controlled. In these patients, anesthesia can be maintained initially with opioids plus thiopental, propofol, midazolam, or etomidate.

Nitrous oxide may increase CBF, CBV, and ICP when administered with inhalation anesthetics if the $PaCO_2$ is normal or increased. This effect may be eliminated when this agent is administered with adequate doses of barbiturates or hyperventilation. The effect on $CMRO_2$ is variable: both an increase and a decrease have been observed. Thus, N_2O probably is not deleterious in patients with head injury with minimal ICP elevation if it is used after a bolus dose or during infusion of intravenous anesthetics.

In a spontaneously breathing patient, opioids may produce hypoventilation with an associated increase in CBF and ICP. Therefore, they should be used in small doses in head trauma, preferably with the patient mechanically ventilated. Some reports suggest that opioids and, to a smaller extent, opiates may interfere with CPP by increasing ICP, decreasing mean arterial pressure, or both.[212,213] Fentanyl and sufentanil are most implicated, and it appears that this phenomenon occurs with severe head injury.[63] Although the clinical significance of these findings is not yet clear, it is prudent to administer fentanyl or its analogs slowly, when the arterial pressure is normal or slightly elevated, ensuring preservation of systemic blood pressure with vasoactive agents, if necessary.

A recent survey by Grathwohl et al.[214] compared the results of total intravenous anesthesia using ketamine with volatile agent anesthesia in a series of combat-related head injuries from Iraq. Although there are unavoidable shortcomings to the study, it nevertheless indicates that the specific anesthetic agents chosen probably do not affect the neurologic outcome as long as the vital signs are maintained.

Cardiac Injury

If there is pericardial tamponade, preload and myocardial contractility must be maintained. Any decrease in these parameters may exacerbate an already existing right ventricle (RV) inflow occlusion. A decrease in heart rate should also be treated promptly to maintain adequate cardiac output. Because all of the available anesthetics can depress myocardial contractility and cause vasodilation, it is preferable to administer these agents after evacuation of the pericardial blood under local anesthesia. If general anesthesia is required to relieve the tamponade, induction should be delayed until the patient is prepared and draped. Both anesthetics and controlled ventilation, particularly with PEEP, impair cardiac output. Deep anesthesia and high airway pressures should be avoided before evacuation of the hemopericardium. In chronic pericardial effusion, ketamine supports the cardiac index better than other intravenous agents. In acute pericardial tamponade, even minor insults can bring cardiac activity to a halt. Ketamine thus remains the agent of choice. It should be given in small doses after adequate fluid infusion. Similar principles apply to the use of maintenance agents, which should be given in the smallest possible doses until the heart is decompressed. TEE monitoring may aid management between induction and pericardiotomy.

In blunt myocardial injury, the objective is not only to maintain cardiac contractility, but also to lower the elevated pulmonary vascular resistance that may result from concomitant pulmonary contusion, atelectasis, or aspiration. All anesthetics should preferably be administered after restoration of intravascular volume and titrated to maintain adequate systemic blood pressure and cardiac output. If necessary, inotropes, preferably amrinone or milrinone, which produce some pulmonary vasodilation, may be used. Anesthetic maintenance by intravenous anesthetics and opioids to avoid the myocardial depression produced by inhalational agents should also be considered.

Burns

A hypermetabolic state characterized by tachycardia, tachypnea, catecholamine surge, increased O_2 consumption, and augmented catabolism follows the initial few hours of a burn and continues into the convalescent phase, necessitating increased oxygen, ventilation, and nutrition.[162,166,178,215] Early extensive and repeated escharotomies with coverage by skin grafts attenuate the postburn hypermetabolic response, decrease insulin resistance, decrease fluid loss, and improve survival.[216] They are usually performed between the second day and the second week, often necessitating massive transfusion, temperature control, and management of fluid, electrolyte, and coagulation abnormalities. Usually, an autograft harvested from either the patient, a cadaver, or both is used. An artificial skin substitute, Integra-ting (Integra Life Sciences, Plainsboro, New Jersey), consisting of a dermal inner layer made of bovine collagen and chondroitin-6-sulfate and a neoepidermal outer layer made of polysiloxane polymer may also be used with more favorable reduction of resting energy expenditure and elevation of serum proteins compared with that of cadaver skin.[188]

Anesthetic management of escharotomies presents several difficulties. Burned tissue may prevent access for ECG, pulse oximeter, neuromuscular function, and noninvasive blood pressure monitoring. Needle electrodes or surgical staples, a reflectance pulse oximeter, and an arterial catheter may be necessary. Large-bore intravenous catheters are essential. Hyperthermia occurs, but hypothermia is more likely in the OR and is to be avoided. Exposure and evaporative fluid loss necessitate maintenance of the OR temperature between 28°C and 32°C, use of countercurrent fluid and blood warming devices, surface heating with forced dry, warm air, and humidified inspired gases. Blood loss can be controlled by restricting the escharotomy to 15% to 20% TBSA, using extremity tourniquets, administering topical thrombin and fibrin sealants on the excised area, applying dilute epinephrine solution topically (1:10,000) or by injection (0.5 mg per 1,000 mL), and using compression bandages.[217] Epinephrine doses of up to 6.7 mg topically or 0.8 mg by injection into the surgical area are well tolerated. The affinity of β-adrenergic receptors to ligands is decreased after burns. The administration of a large amount of blood and blood products subjects the patient to complications of transfusion, such as coagulopathy, requiring monitoring of coagulation status and administration of adequate replacement therapy.

Shock, hyperdynamic circulation, decreased serum albumin concentration, increased α1-acid glycoprotein concentration, and altered receptor sensitivity change the response to various drugs during the resuscitative and convalescent phases.[162] The doses of intravenous anesthetics should be reduced during the resuscitation phase to prevent excessive hemodynamic depression. Burn patients have excruciating pain and exceedingly high opioid requirements. A proven anesthetic regimen for excision and grafting of burns is isoflurane plus large doses of opioid. The response to depolarizing and nondepolarizing muscle relaxants remains unaltered during the first 24 hours after burn injury. However, after the first day, succinylcholine should be avoided for at least 1 year because it can result in a potentially lethal increase of serum K^+ when the burn size exceeds 10% of TBSA. The mechanism of this response is related to up-regulation (increase) of acetylcholine receptors, which ultimately occupy the entire muscle membrane, the additional expression of two newly described isoforms of acetylcholine receptor, and nicotinic (neural) α-7 acetylcholine receptors. The latter can be depolarized not only by acetylcholine and succinylcholine, but also by choline, which thus plays an important role in the development of hyperkalemia.[218] Resistance develops to all nondepolarizing muscle relaxants in patients with burns of >30% TBSA starting at approximately 1 week and peaking 5 to 6 weeks after injury, probably from pharmacodynamic causes.[162,163] Increasing the dose can partly overcome this resistance. For instance, rocuronium, which is important for rapid-sequence induction and treatment of laryngospasm when succinylcholine is contraindicated, has an onset time delayed by about 50 seconds (30% longer than patients without burn) when a 0.9 mg/kg dose is used. Increasing the dose to 1.2 mg/kg decreases the delay by 30 seconds, but the onset time remains about 25 to 30 seconds longer than that observed in patients without burns. Intubating conditions also improve by increasing the dose. Recovery time from the block is shorter in burned patients than in normal individuals.[219]

For serial wound debridement, ketamine in intermittent doses, neuraxial or peripheral nerve blocks via an indwelling catheter, or sedation with opioids and intravenous agents may be employed. In a preliminary study, patients receiving fentanyl experienced higher body temperatures than those who received morphine. This was attributed to the well-established anti-inflammatory properties of morphine.[220]

Management of Intraoperative Complications

Persistent Hypotension

12 Persistent hypotension following trauma is usually the result of one of four mechanisms: bleeding, tension pneumothorax, neurogenic shock, or cardiac injury. Although many other causes, such as citrate intoxication (hypocalcemia), hypothermia, coronary artery disease, allergic reactions, or incompatible transfusion may be responsible for this complication, they occur infrequently.

Hypotension is most likely due to bleeding. The source may be obvious, such as external bleeding from the skull or an open vessel in the extremities, or hidden. The thoracic and abdominal cavities and the pelvic retroperitoneal space are the most common sites of occult hemorrhage that results in hypotension. Management includes early diagnosis and control of the bleeding site plus effective fluid resuscitation. The latter can best be accomplished using an infusion system with large-diameter tubing (5 mm) and a countercurrent heat exchanger. The system should be connected to a 14-gauge or larger cannula, preferably inserted into veins both above and below the diaphragm. The Rapid Infuser system (Belmont Instrument Corp, Bellerica, Massachusetts), which consists of a reservoir, countercurrent heating system, and roller pump, is capable of delivering up to 1,600 mL/min of warm fluids once the rate of infusion is programmed.

Of the isotonic crystalloid solutions, LR is preferred over normal saline. Experimental evidence shows that resuscitation with normal saline during uncontrolled hemorrhage is associated with greater urine output and thus greater fluid requirement compared with LR, resulting in hyperchloremic acidosis and dilutional coagulopathy.[221] Acidosis does not occur with LR, but tissue edema may result from its slight hypotonicity (~255 mOsm/L), and neutralization of the citrate anticoagulant in PRBCs may occur because of its Ca^{2+} content.

Human serum albumin (5% and 25%) and hydroxyethyl starch are the most commonly used colloids. Hetastarch, a high molecular weight (670 kDa) polymeric glucose compound, is the most commonly used hydroxyethyl starch in the United States. Because of its molecular weight, it remains within the blood vessels and can restore the blood volume. However, it also has an adverse effect on coagulation, especially on platelets, factor VIII, and von Willebrand factor if it is given in doses exceeding 20 mL/kg. Its intravascular retention and adverse effects on coagulation are related not only to its molecular weight but also to molar substitution, which is defined as the number of hydroxyethyl groups per glucose subunit; the higher the molar substitution, the higher the intravascular retention and thus the more severe the coagulopathy. Efforts to reduce molecular weight and molar substitution in order to maintain intravascular retention and yet minimize coagulopathy recently resulted in the development of a new compound, hydroxyethyl starch 130/0.4 (Voluven[R], Fresenius Kabi Norge AS, Halden, Norway), with a molecular weight of 130 kDa and molar substitution of 0.4. It appears to provide adequate vascular volume expansion with less coagulation abnormality in major orthopedic surgery patients. Theoretically, the combined use of fluids and moderate doses of vasopressor may rapidly restore blood pressure to normal levels, limit the fluid volume infused, and improve short-term survival.

Neurogenic shock from spinal cord injury may be missed during initial evaluation, especially in unconscious patients. However, differentiation of neurogenic shock from hemorrhagic shock is important. Patients with spinal cord injury are often bradycardic and readily respond to catecholamine administration. Mistaking neurogenic shock for hemorrhagic shock may lead to excessive fluid infusion and pulmonary edema in the spinal cord–injured patient. The reverse error may also occur: depriving patients with hemorrhagic shock of fluids because of misdiagnosis of neurogenic shock. Invasive central hemodynamic monitoring may be indicated in such patients.[134] In some patients, of course, hemorrhagic shock and neurogenic shock may coexist.

Cardiac causes of persistent hypotension include blunt cardiac injury and pericardial tamponade. Intraoperative TEE can be useful in the differential diagnosis. The RV is most commonly involved in blunt cardiac injury. If there is a concomitant increase in pulmonary vascular resistance (e.g., from an associated pulmonary contusion), the RV pressure increases while its output decreases, resulting in an increased CVP. The raised RV pressure causes the interventricular septum to shift toward the left, decreasing left ventricular compliance, increasing its diastolic pressure, and decreasing cardiac output. These alterations in cardiac anatomy and ventricular dynamics can be displayed by TEE, information that can be useful during interpretation of elevated cardiac filling pressures.

In the absence of TEE, a pulmonary artery catheter may be helpful. Equalization of pressures across the cardiac chambers during diastole suggests pericardial tamponade. A similar picture may also be seen in severe blunt cardiac injury, causing difficulty in differential diagnosis. This effect, however, is rare and is usually associated with critical hemodynamic instability. Differential diagnosis in these instances can be established by pericardiocentesis. Septal encroachment into the left ventricle from RV contusion results in an increase in pulmonary artery wedge pressure. Decreasing the rate of fluid infusion in these patients results in a further decrease in cardiac output. Treatment includes fluid infusion, pulmonary vasodilators if the systemic blood pressure is normal, and inotropic support if the systemic blood pressure is low. Absence of response to this treatment is an indication for placement of an intra-aortic balloon pump. Pulmonary artery catheterization may also help detect an oxygen step-up from a septal injury. During thoracotomy, a distended RV should also raise the suspicion of a septal defect.

Hypothermia

Shock, alcohol intoxication, exposure to cold, fluid resuscitation, and abnormalities in thermoregulatory mechanisms render the major trauma patient hypothermic during the initial phase of injury. A core body temperature below 35°C is often associated with acidosis, hypotension, and coagulopathy, which in turn may lead to an increased risk of severe bleeding, need for transfusion, and mortality.[59] Admission hypothermia, which is present in approximately 50% of patients, is an independent risk factor after major trauma,[222] and the mortality rate increases with decreasing temperature. Severe hypothermia, which in the trauma patient is defined as core temperature below 32°C,[223] was associated with a 100% mortality rate in one study,[224] although survival of a few patients with admission temperatures even lower than 32°C has been reported.[225] The intraoperative risk of hypothermia is also higher for trauma victims than for electively operated patients. Increased heat loss is seen most commonly in patients with spinal cord, extensive soft tissue, and burn injuries and in patients who consumed ethanol preoperatively or those undergoing body cavity surgery.

Other deleterious effects of hypothermia are cardiac depression, myocardial ischemia, arrhythmias, peripheral vasoconstriction, impaired tissue oxygen delivery, elevated oxygen consumption during rewarming, blunted response to catecholamines, increased blood viscosity, metabolic acidosis, abnormalities of K^+ and Ca^{2+} homeostasis, reduced drug clearance, and increased risk of infection.[222–226] Rewarming after hypothermia, especially at a rapid rate, may release accumulated metabolic products into the central circulation, causing further myocardial depression, hypotension, and increased acidosis.

Prevention of hypothermia and correction of body temperature to normal appear to decrease mortality rate, blood loss, fluid requirement, organ failure, and length of ICU stay.[227] Convective warming with forced dry air at 43°C can prevent a temperature drop in most trauma victims but cannot effectively treat severe hypothermia because the low specific heat of air has little heat content to give to the cold trauma patient, and often, due to the nature of the surgical procedure, only a limited body surface area is exposed to warming.[227] Circulating-water warmers that cover a relatively smaller body surface area than forced air warmers may produce faster rewarming (Fig. 52-14).[228] Airway warming can reduce the heat loss caused by the latent heat of vaporization, but

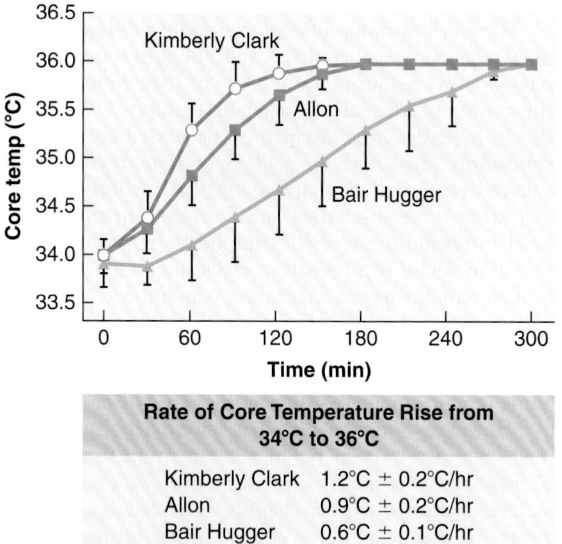

FIGURE 52-14. The rate of rise in core temperature with circulating water and forced air devices used in healthy anesthetized volunteers. Circulating water devices warm the body faster than forced air devices. (Reproduced with permission from Wadhwa A, Komatsu R, Orhan-Sungur M, et al. New circulating water devices warm more quickly than forced-air in volunteers. *Anesth Analg.* 2007;105:1681.)

this technique also transfers very little heat.[227] Administration of warm intravenous fluids is the most effective way to prevent and treat hypothermia in the trauma patient, provided they are administered at a relatively rapid rate. For each liter of fluid given at 40°C to a patient with a body temperature of 33°C, 29.33 kJ of heat energy are gained (the specific heat of water is 4.19 kJ/L/°C). Countercurrent heat exchange systems (Belmont Rapid Infuser, Belmont Instrument Corp., Bellerica, Massachusetts) warm the fluid to 40°C, and the delivered fluid temperature is little affected by the rate of administration.

Deliberate therapeutic hypothermia in hemorrhaging patients, and selectively in brain-injured patients with GCS between 4 and 7, may have some salutary effects on outcome.[59] However, in view of contradictory reports about beneficial and deleterious effects such as hypotension, hypovolemia, electrolyte disorders, insulin resistance, reduced insulin secretion, and increased risk of infection, it is prudent to evaluate the results of future studies before introducing this measure into clinical practice.[229,230]

Coagulation Abnormalities

Multiple factors may be responsible for coagulopathy in trauma: dilution of coagulation factors and platelets; tissue hypoperfusion; disturbance of fibrinogen/fibrin polymerization and platelet activity caused by decreased serum ionized (active) Ca^{++} with infusion of colloids or by binding to citrate in PRBC, FFP, and platelet units;[231] hypoxia, hypothermia and acidosis; disseminated intravascular coagulation (DIC); and primary fibrinolysis.[232,233] DIC results from acute release of thromboplastin from injured brain, fat, amniotic fluid or other sources, or subacutely from endothelial inflammation or failure interfering with clearance of activated coagulation factors, causing microthrombi and consumption coagulopathy.[234] It has also been suggested that early coagulopathy, before fluid administration, is caused by tissue hypoperfusion, which increases thrombomodulin and diverts thrombin from fibrin generation to activation of protein C.[235] More recently Johansson et al.[236] demonstrated elevated admission circulating syndecan-1 levels, a marker of degradation of the subendothelial glycocalyx, in trauma patients, suggesting that the precipitating event is vascular damage resulting from catecholamine release and increasing permeability, inflammation, and coagulopathy, probably implying that the interplay among these mechanisms is the pathogenesis of trauma-induced coagulopathy.[237]

Hypothermia affects platelet morphology, function, and sequestration; retards enzyme activity; and decreases coagulation factor function by about 10% for each 1°C drop in temperature, slowing the initiation and propagation of platelet plugs and fibrin clot as well as enhancing fibrinolytic activity.[74,77,232,238] The mechanism of hypothermia-induced coagulopathy is complex and depends on the extent of temperature decrease. Down to 33°C, there is little alteration in coagulation enzyme activity, explaining the practically unchanged values reported for aPTT.[239] Within this temperature range, coagulopathy results from altered platelet aggregation or adhesion.[239] Thus, the aPTT at temperatures from 33°C to 37°C does not provide any meaningful information about coagulation status, even when the test is performed at the hypothermic patient's temperature, because it does not measure platelet adhesion. In contrast, thromboelastography at the patient's temperature may be reflective of the degree of coagulopathy.[231] Both enzymatic activity and platelet aggregation are abnormal below 33°C.[239] Metabolic acidosis is probably a stronger coagulation enzyme inhibitor than hypothermia. It interferes with the generation of thrombin, a factor essential in activating cofactors, platelets, and enzymes, in addition to converting fibrinogen to fibrin. This effect of acidosis is potentiated by hypothermia (Fig. 52-15).[240]

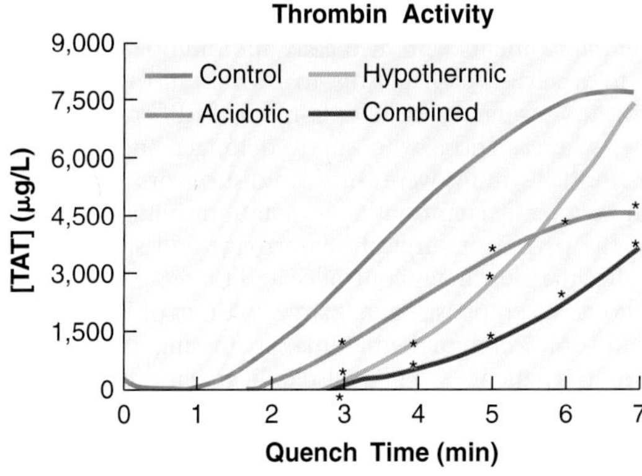

FIGURE 52-15. Thrombin generation rate in normal, acidotic, hypothermic, and acidotic and hypothermic swine. Thrombin generation was determined by measuring thrombin-antithrombin III concentration in blood samples obtained at 1-minute intervals in each condition. Note that acidosis and hypothermia decrease thrombin generation rate. (Reproduced with permission from Martini WZ, Pusateri AE, Uscilowicz JM, et al. Independent contributions of hypothermia and acidosis to coagulopathy in swine. *J Trauma.* 2005;58:1002, discussion 1009.)

Diagnosis

The perioperative diagnosis of coagulopathy is often made by observing bleeding from wounds or puncture sites, rather than by interpretation of laboratory tests. However, the differential diagnosis between consumptive and dilutional coagulopathy requires laboratory testing. The availability of point of care coagulation testing (INR, thromboelastography, and thromboelastometry) reduces the delay in obtaining the results of these tests (Cotton, 2011). In general, the inability to determine the type of coagulopathy does not present a problem because the initial treatment is similar for both conditions. Nevertheless, the diagnosis of DIC has prognostic significance because its treatment involves elimination of its cause(s). The presence of elevated circulating FDP, especially when >40 mg/mL, is suggestive of DIC, but the result of this study will reach the clinician long after the completion of initial resuscitation. A fibrinogen level <100 mg/dL is also suggestive of DIC, but reduction to this value often takes a long time, decreasing the diagnostic value of the test, although serial measurements may be useful. A diagnostic scoring system consisting of platelet count, prothrombin time, fibrinogen level, and FDP measurements has been suggested to rule DIC in or out.[241]

Treatment

Fresh Frozen Plasma

As discussed above, newer guidelines recommend administration of thawed FFP immediately after the arrival of severely traumatized, bleeding, coagulopathic patients.[59,242] The recommended dose is 10 to 15 mL/kg; but additional doses may be needed.[59,242] Following initial administration, FFP is indicated when the transfusion exceeds 10 U of PRBC within a 6-hour period and when the PT and/or partial thromboplastin time values exceed 1.5 times normal.[59,242] Inspired by the experience gained during recent wars, many trauma centers have changed their transfusion protocols and modified the PRBC to FFP ratio from 4:1 to 1:1 or 2:1. Many civilian studies indeed showed the benefit of early treatment with high FFP to PRBC ratios administered to bleeding trauma patients,[58,243,244] although others did not and suggested 2:1 or even
13 3:1 as a more optimal ratio.[242,245] Many studies that demonstrated

a benefit of high plasma to PRBC ratio have been found to have *survivor bias.* Patients who died early and did not have the opportunity to receive a high plasma to PRBC ratio were considered to be deaths secondary to low plasma to PRBC ratio component therapy, whereas those who survived longer and received high plasma to PRBC ratios were considered survivors due to the component therapy.[246] Hemostatic resuscitation should be most active during the period of surgical hemorrhage and should be terminated after the bleeding is controlled and there is no coagulopathy.

It should be emphasized that large volumes of FFP may worsen traumatic intracerebral hematoma, increasing the mortality of head-injured patients.[247] FFP is also indicated for reversal of coagulopathy in patients receiving vitamin K antagonist oral anticoagulants if prothrombin complex concentrates or factor IX concentrates are not available.[59] The risks associated with FFP include circulatory overload, ABO incompatibility, transmission of infectious diseases, mild allergic reactions, and transfusion-related acute lung injury, in which platelet concentrates are also implicated.[59]

TABLE 52-15. CONDITIONS REQUIRED TO JUSTIFY THE USE OF RECOMBINANT FACTOR VIIa (rFVIIa) IN COAGULOPATHIC TRAUMA PATIENTS

- Surgical bleeding is controlled
- PRBC, platelet, FFP, and cryoprecipitate or fibrinogen administration results in Hct >24% and platelets >50 × 10^9/L, fibrinogen >1.5 to 2.0 g/L
- Severe acidosis (<7.25) is corrected
- Antifibrinolytics are used
- Severe hypothermia and hypocalcemia are corrected

PRBC, packed red blood cells; FFP, frozen fresh plasma; Hct, hematocrit.

Platelets

Platelet transfusion is indicated when the platelet count falls below 50 × 10^9/L. It is possible that in patients with DIC or hyperfibrinolysis and in those with head injury and massive bleeding, higher levels (75 or 100 × 10^9/L) may be beneficial. High platelet to PRBC ratios (1:1 or 1:2) appear to decrease mortality in trauma patients.[243] Platelets can be administered either as pooled concentrates or single-donor apheresis units. From each unit of whole blood, platelet concentrates of 7.5 × 10^{10}/L can be prepared, which increase platelet count by 5 to 10 × 10^9/L; 4 to 8 U are usually sufficient. Apheresis platelet units contain 3 to 6 × 10^{11}/L platelets, and a single unit is usually sufficient to provide hemostasis.[59]

Fibrinogen

In the trauma patient, a plasma fibrinogen level below 1.5 g/L (normal 2 g/L) in the presence of nonsurgical bleeding indicates replacement with 3 to 4 g of fibrinogen concentrate or cryoprecipitate 50 mg/kg (15 to 20 U).[59] Obtaining a fibrinogen level from the laboratory not only may take about an hour and also may be erroneous; for example in patients receiving colloids, the fibrinogen
14 level may be overestimated.[59] Repeated use of point of care devices, TEG or thromboelastometry, allows titration of fibrinogen or cryoprecipitate and other blood products (see Fig. 52-12). For example, in normal individuals a maximum clot firmness of 7 mm measured with thromboelastometry corresponds to a plasma fibrinogen concentration of 2 g/L; maximum clot firmness values <7 mm require administration of fibrinogen or cryoprecipitate.[201]

Antifibrinolytic Agents

The synthetic lysin analog antifibrinolytic agents, tranexamic acid and ε-aminocaproic acid, competitive inhibitors of plasmin and plasminogen, are effective in reducing bleeding in cardiac and elective surgery, even when a significant hyperfibrinolysis is absent.[59] The recently reported Clinical Randomization of Antifibrinolytic in Significant Hemorrhage study of 20,000 patients from 274 sites demonstrated that tranexamic acid given within 3 hours of injury (1 g in a 10-minute bolus and then 1 g infused over the next 8 hours) decreased mortality from hemorrhage; this reduction was 37% if the drug was given within 1 hour after injury. On the other hand, tranexamic acid given beyond 3 hours of injury increased bleeding-related mortality.[248]

It is unlikely that antifibrinolytics will be used in major trauma centers because the FFP used in the massive transfusion protocol contains all of the endogenous antifibrinolytic elements and the protocol is routinely activated in severe trauma patients.[249] Nevertheless, they should be considered in patients who demonstrate fibrinolysis during serial thromboelastographic or thromboelastometric monitoring. The usual dose of tranexamic acid is 10 to 15 mg/kg followed by 1 to 5 mg/kg/hr. The dose of ε-aminocaproic acid is 100 to 150 mg/kg followed by 15 mg/kg/hr.[59]

Factor VIIa

By activating factor X, factor VIIa produces a thrombin burst, which in turn converts fibrinogen to fibrin. This thrombin release is augmented by platelet activation. Severe acidosis, hypothermia, and hemodilution block the effects of factor VIIa. Thus to obtain benefit, it should be administered after platelet and fibrinogen levels are adequate and pH and hypothermia are corrected to at least 7.25 and 33°C, respectively. The dose of recombinant factor VIIa is controversial.[59] The originally recommended dose is 200 μg/kg followed by 100 μg/kg 2 more times from 1 to 3 hours later.[250] More recently, an initial dose of 100 to 140 g/kg, with a similar dose repeated 1 and 3 hours later, if needed, has been shown to provide adequate hemostatic plasma levels.[251] Recombinant factor VIIa may be indicated for off-label use if major bleeding persists after standard measures of hemostasis are used and conditions listed in Table 52-15 are reached.[59] A clear explanation should be given to the patient's family about its potential for arterial and venous thromboembolism (5.6% vs. 3% with placebo).[252]

15 Prothrombin complex concentrate (PCC, factor IX complex) contains factors II, VII, IX, and X. In the trauma setting, it is used for rapid reversal of vitamin K antagonist oral anticoagulants (warfarin), especially in patients with intracranial bleeding.[253] A similar effect can be obtained by administering FFP, but at a much slower rate and a larger infused volume; however, there is a smaller risk of viral transmission.[254] PCC is not effective for reversing direct thrombin inhibitor anticoagulants (dabigatran [Pradaxa]), which have been recently used to prevent stroke in patients with atrial fibrillation. Whether PCC is effective in bleeding trauma patients who are not on warfarin is not clear. As with recombinant factor VIIa, thrombotic complications are increased with PCC.[254]

Electrolyte and Acid-Base Disturbances

Intraoperative hyperkalemia may develop as a result of three mechanisms. First, in patients with irreversible shock, cell membrane permeability is altered, thus massive K^+ efflux results in severe hyperkalemia; in this situation, survival is unlikely. Second, after repair of a major vessel, subsequent reperfusion of the ischemic tissues results in a sudden release of K^+ into the general circulation. Third, transfusion at a rate faster than 1 U every 4 minutes in an acidotic and hypovolemic patient may cause an increase in plasma K^+ levels. Frequent monitoring of serum K^+, gradual and intermittent unclamping of vascular shunts, and avoiding transfusion at higher rates than needed help reduce the rate of K^+ increase. If a rise in K^+ is detected, treatment with regular insulin, 10 U intravenously, with 50% dextrose, 50 mL, and sodium bicarbonate, 8.4%, 50 mL is indicated. If there is a dysrhythmia, $CaCl_2$, 500 mg, should also be administered. Insulin and dextrose can be repeated 2 or 3 times at 30- to 45-minute intervals, if necessary. Hemodialysis may be indicated in desperate situations.

Metabolic acidosis is caused by shock in most trauma patients. Other rare causes of acidosis in this population are alcoholic lactic acidosis, alcoholic ketoacidosis, diabetic ketoacidosis, and CO or CN^- poisoning after inhalation injuries. The differential diagnosis between hypovolemic, diabetic, and alcoholic acidosis, all of which have anion gaps, requires measurement of blood lactate, urinary ketone bodies, and blood sugar and assessment of intravascular volume. Alcoholic ketoacidosis is treated with intravenous dextrose, whereas diabetic ketoacidosis is managed with insulin. No specific treatment except intravenous normal saline exists for alcoholic lactic acidosis.

Treatment of metabolic acidosis involves correction of the underlying cause: management of hypoxemia, restoration of intravascular volume, optimization of cardiac function, or treatment of CO or CN^- toxicity. Symptomatic treatment with sodium bicarbonate has serious disadvantages, including leftward shift of the oxyhemoglobin dissociation curve causing decreased O_2 unloading, a hyperosmolar state secondary to the excessive sodium load, hypokalemia, further hemodynamic depression, overshoot alkalosis a few hours after giving the drug, and intracellular acidosis if adequate ventilation or pulmonary blood flow cannot be provided. Nevertheless, because of the possibility that severe acidosis can cause dysrhythmias, myocardial depression, hypotension, and resistance to exogenous catecholamines, some clinicians administer bicarbonate to buy time if the pH is <7.2.

Intraoperative Death

Death is a much greater threat during emergency trauma surgery than it is in any other operative procedure. Approximately 0.7% of patients admitted for acute trauma die in the OR, accounting for approximately 8% of postinjury deaths.[255] Uncontrollable bleeding is the cause of approximately 80% of intraoperative mortality; brain herniation and air embolism are the most common causes of death in the remaining patients.[255] A multicenter, retrospective study has defined certain features that increase the likelihood of OR death (Table 52-16).[255] Rapid transport to the OR, rapidly stabilizing life-threatening injuries while deferring definitive surgery (damage control), simultaneous thoracotomy and laparotomy for thoracoabdominal injuries, appropriate management of retroperitoneal hematoma, and early correction of hypothermia and shock may reduce intraoperative mortality rates.[255]

Of these measures, the damage control principle has reduced not only the intraoperative, but also the overall mortality from

TABLE 52-16. CLINICAL FEATURES ASSOCIATED WITH INTRAOPERATIVE MORTALITY

Category	Clinical Features
Mechanism of injury	Gunshot wound
	Pedestrian injuries
Injury severity	Mean injury severity score >41
	Mean revised trauma score >3.0
Preoperative physiologic profile	Mean BP in the field <50 mm Hg
	Mean BP on arrival to ED <60 mm Hg
	Best systolic BP in the ED <90 mm Hg
	Circulatory shock time >10 min
	Best mean pH <7.18
	Mean preoperative crystalloid resuscitation >3,850 mL; mean red cell transfusion >834 mL
Type of injury	Significant head, chest, abdominal, and pelvic injuries individually or in combination after blunt trauma
	Significant chest and abdominal injuries individually or in combination after penetrating trauma
Organ injury	Brain
	Liver
	Aorta or other major vascular injury
	Cardiac injury
Operating room resuscitation and physiologic status	Systolic BP <90 mm Hg during first hour
	Systolic BP <90 mm Hg for >30 min
	Deterioration of mean pH from 7.19 to 7.01
	Mean intraoperative blood loss 5,172 mL; mean blood replacement 4,541 mL
	Mean platelet transfusion 784 mL
	Mean fresh frozen plasma 1,418 mL
	Mean intraoperative temperature 32.2°C
	Intraoperative cardiac arrest

BP, blood pressure; ED, emergency department.
Data from Hoyt DB, Bulger EM, Knudson MM, et al. Death in the operating room: An analysis of a multi-center experience. *J Trauma.* 1994;37:426.

trauma surgery, although morbidity from sepsis, abscess formation, and gastrointestinal fistulas may increase.[256] Originally described in three stages, the current suggestion is that it should be managed in four phases. In the first phase, attention is directed in the ED to recognition of the pattern of injury, control of bleeding if possible, and rapid transport to the OR, as well as the decision to initiate damage control resuscitation by limiting crystalloid infusion, allowing permissive hypotension, activating rewarming, and initiating blood component replacement with early administration of FFP and platelets at high ratios with PRBC.[257]

The second phase occurs in the OR where, in addition to efforts to maintain the patient's intravascular volume, temperature, acid-base status, and coagulation at near normal levels with damage control resuscitation, the surgeons rapidly control bleeding and leave the abdominal cavity open without fascial closure, but temporarily covered by a Vac-Pac dressing, which allows an enlarged space for edematous organs and controlled egress of fluid.

The third phase takes place in the ICU where intravascular volume, hypothermia, acidosis, and coagulation abnormalities are corrected. In the fourth phase, the stabilized patient is returned to the OR for definitive surgery and abdominal closure. The fourth phase involves multiple returns to the OR at 24- to 48-hour intervals for organ repair, abdominal washout, and debridement before the final closure of the abdomen. The damage control principle, originally proposed for abdominal trauma, is now applied to injuries at other anatomical sites, including the chest, pelvis, extremities, and soft tissues.[258]

EARLY POSTOPERATIVE CONSIDERATIONS

The concerns in the early postoperative period are similar to those of the intraoperative phase. Re-evaluation and optimization of the circulation, oxygenation, temperature, CNS function, coagulation, electrolyte and acid-base status, and renal function are the hallmarks of postoperative management. Pain control in this group of patients may have more than a humanitarian purpose; it can improve pulmonary function, ventilation, and oxygenation in patients with chest injury or a long abdominal incision. For sedation in mechanically ventilated patients, both propofol (25 to 75 μg/kg/min) and midazolam (0.1 to 20 μg/kg/min) infusions alone or in combination are equally effective and safe, although wake-up time in patients receiving midazolam is longer (660 ± 400 minutes) than in those receiving propofol alone (110 ± 50 minutes) or in both agents combined (190 ± 200 minutes).[259] Morphine 0.02 to 0.04 mg/kg/hr or fentanyl 1 to 3 μg/kg/hr may be added for analgesia. Small boluses of midazolam (3 to 5 mg), propofol (50 mg), morphine (2 to 3 mg), or fentanyl (25 to 50 μg) may also be given as required.[259]

Acute Renal Failure

Acute renal failure is a possibility if prolonged shock or crush syndrome occurs during early management. In a study aimed at finding the predictors of acute renal failure, trauma was one of the seven independent predictors of this complication.[260] Following an episode of shock in patients who have not received an osmotic load (radiopaque material, mannitol) or diuretic, determination of 2- or 6-hour creatinine and free water clearances may help predict the development of posttraumatic renal dysfunction.[261] Creatinine clearance <25 mL/min and free water clearance ≥–15 mL/hr suggest the likelihood of acute renal failure. Decreased urine flow rate is not a good predictor, and the blood urea nitrogen does not rise until at least 24 hours after surgery or trauma.[261]

The cause of renal failure in crush syndrome is probably rhabdomyolysis-induced myoglobin release into the circulation. Serum creatinine kinase levels increase in these patients; levels >5,000 U/L are associated with renal failure.[262] The differentiation of myoglobinuria from hemoglobinuria was described in the "Urine Output" section. A clear supernatant suggests myoglobin, whereas a rose color indicates hemoglobin. The traditional prophylaxis for renal failure after rhabdomyolysis includes fluids, mannitol, and bicarbonate. However, more recent data suggest that bicarbonate and mannitol are ineffective.[262]

Abdominal Compartment Syndrome

Abdominal compartment syndrome results from intra-abdominal hypertension with organ dysfunction after major abdominal trauma and surgery (primary syndrome), although other patients

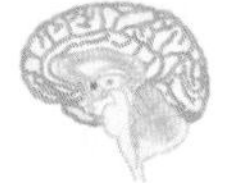

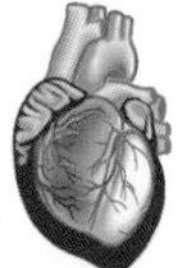

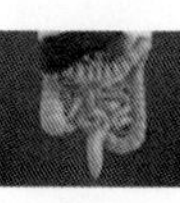

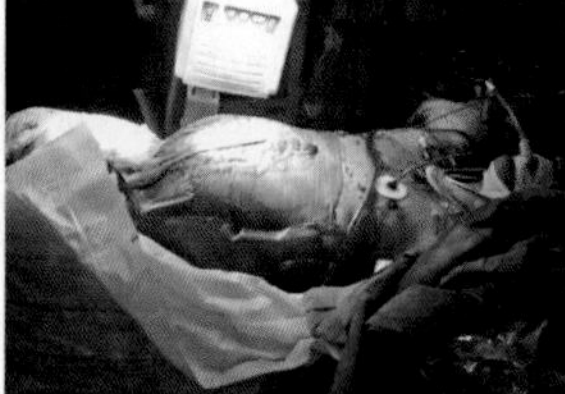

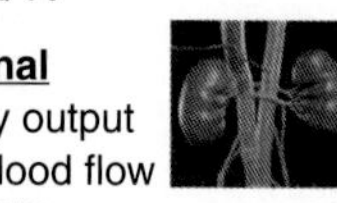

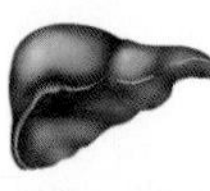

FIGURE 52-16. Physiologic effects of abdominal compartment syndrome. Image in the center is a patient whose abdomen was left open but covered with nonadhesive dressing. C_{dyn}, dynamic pulmonary compliance; CO, cardiac output; CPP, cerebral perfusion pressure; CVP, central venous pressure; GFR, glomerular filtration rate; ICP, intracranial pressure; PAOP, pulmonary artery occlusion pressure; P_{aw}, mean airway pressure; pHi, intramucosal pH; PIP, peak inspiratory pressure; Qsp/Qt, intrapulmonary shunt; SMA, superior mesenteric artery; SVR, systemic vascular resistance; Vd/Vt, dead space ventilation. (Adapted with permission from Cheatham ML. Intra-abdominal hypertension and abdominal compartment syndrome. *N Horizons*. 1999;7:96.)

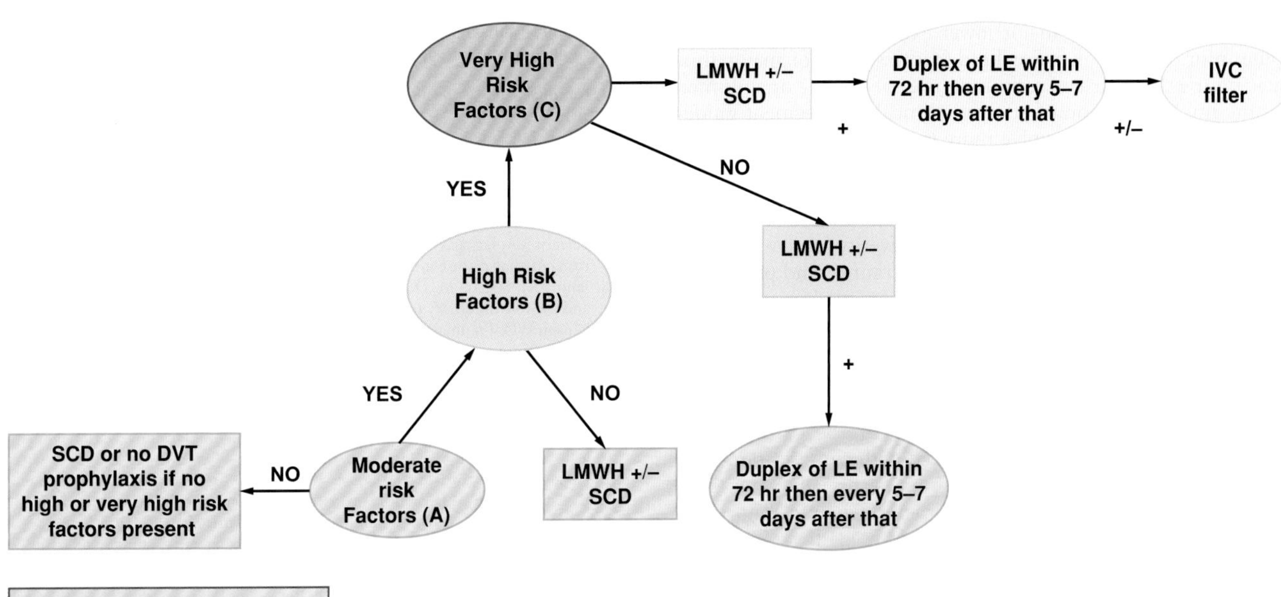

A. Moderate risk factor
- Age >40[a]
- ISS>9[a]
- Surgical procedure within 72 hr[a]
- Immobilization[a]
- Pregnancy[a]
- Estrogen therapy[a]
- History of DVT or PE[a]
- Malignancy[a]
- Hypercoagulability[a]
- Extensive soft tissue trauma[a]
- CHF[a]

B. High risk factors
- Age>50[a]
- ISS>16[a]
- Femoral line placed in bay[a]
- GCS<9[a]
- Venous injury[a]
- **Major lower extremity injury[b]**

C. Very High/ "refractory" risk factors
- Spinal cord injury[a,b]
- AIS (head and neck>/=3)-long bone fracture[a]
- Multiple >/3 long bone fractures[a]
- **Severe pelvic fracture[a,b]**
- **Mechanical ventilation longer than 3 days[b]**
- **Severe LE fracture + ISS >16[b]**
- Cannot be anticoagulated High or very high risk factors[a]

FIGURE 52-17. Prophylaxis model based on combination of Eastern Association for Surgery of Trauma (EAST) recommendations and the data from Baldwin et al. in blunt trauma patients. Venous thromboembolism risks are classified as moderate, high, and very high. Risk criteria in each of these groups are marked with a superscript of "a" (meaning based on EAST guidelines) and "b" (meaning based on Baldwin et al. data). Low molecular weight heparin is used unless contraindicated. AIS, abbreviated injury score; CHF, congestive heart failure; DVT, deep vein thrombosis; GCS, Glasgow coma score; IVC, inferior vena cava; ISS, injury severity score; LE, lower extremity; PE, pulmonary embolism; SCD, sequential compression device. (Reproduced by permission from Baldwin K, Namdari S, Esterhai SL, et al. Venous thromboembolism in patients with blunt trauma: Are comprehensive guidelines the answer? *Am J Orthop.* 2011;40:E83.)

may develop the syndrome without surgery, for example, during massive fluid resuscitation following major trauma or burns (secondary syndrome).[263–266] The syndrome results from massive edema of abdominal organs produced by shock-induced inflammatory mediators, excessive fluid resuscitation, surgical manipulation, and closure of the abdominal fascia. The significant cardiac, pulmonary, renal, gastrointestinal, hepatic, and CNS dysfunction caused by this syndrome result in a high mortality rate (Fig. 52-16).

Clinically, a tense, severely distended abdomen, raised peak airway pressure, CO_2 retention, and oliguria should direct the clinician to measure the intravesical pressure via a Foley catheter, which reflects the intra-abdominal pressure. Values >20 to 25 mm Hg may indicate inadequate organ perfusion and necessitate abdominal decompression, which, if delayed, may result in progression to multiorgan failure and death.[263,266] Almost all of these patients require mechanical ventilation. If a pulmonary artery catheter is in place, attributing a relatively high PCWP to the ventilator and continuing high-volume fluid infusion may further increase intra-abdominal edema and increase mortality.[267] Interestingly, patients who will develop abdominal compartment syndrome often do not respond to fluid administration with elevated cardiac output, despite an increasing PCWP.[267]

It should be emphasized that recent advances in the management of acute trauma and critical care, such as limiting crystalloid infusion, hemostatic resuscitation, damage control, and open abdomen strategies have substantially decreased the incidence of postinjury abdominal compartment syndrome.[268] Postinjury intra-abdominal hypertension still occurs commonly in severely injured high-risk patients, but it is not associated with multiorgan failure in most instances. In other words, unlike in the past, intra-abdominal hypertension is seldom a harbinger of abdominal compartment syndrome or multiorgan failure. It is believed that limiting crystalloid infusion is the most important factor in this salutary evolution.[268]

Thromboembolism

The overall incidence of venous thromboembolism (VTE) involving DVT and PE is 3.2% in blunt trauma patients.[269] However,

DVT occurs in 30% of major lower-extremity injuries, 30% of spine injuries, 46% of major head injuries, 33% of major thoracic injuries, and 15% of serious injuries of the face or abdomen despite implementation of effective clinical management guidelines.[269] When injuries involve more than one of these high-risk regions, the likelihood of DVT is even higher.[269] Fortunately, only a relatively small fraction (0.3%) of severely injured patients have PE.[269] Statistically significant risk factors for VTE are mechanical ventilation for longer than 3 days, injury severity score >15, spinal cord injury, major lower extremity bony trauma, and pelvic ring injury.[269] In most instances, DVT is asymptomatic, and in many of those in whom leg swelling develops, concurrent lower-extremity injuries may be implicated. The diagnosis of proximal DVT in symptomatic patients can be made by duplex ultrasonography, but this method has low sensitivity in the absence of symptoms.[270] Venography, which is the gold standard, can be performed in equivocal cases, although it is associated with complications and inherent logistical problems. Hypoxemia, especially when sudden and associated with dyspnea and hemodynamic abnormalities, even very early after injury, is highly suggestive of PE. The definitive diagnosis is established by spiral CT and pulmonary angiography. In hemodynamically unstable patients, resuscitation takes precedence over radiologic diagnosis. Management is symptomatic and includes tracheal intubation, positive pressure ventilation with FiO_2 of 1.0, administration of fluids and inotropes (amrinone or milrinone), and continuous arterial and CVP monitoring. TEE is helpful because it may demonstrate RV performance, tricuspid regurgitation, or, in some cases, the thrombus within the pulmonary artery, the right heart chambers, or in transit through a patent foramen ovale to the left atrium.

Baldwin et al.[269] reviewed their experience of VTE in more than 10,000 blunt trauma patients over a period of 10 years. These patients were managed using the clinical management guidelines recommended by the Eastern Association for the Surgery of Trauma (EAST).[271] Based on their experience, they proposed the management pathway shown in Figure 52-17, which combined the EAST-defined risks with their own for moderate, high, and higher risk factors; their modified pathway is based on this. Currently, prophylaxis involves application of sequential compression devices, even if one of the lower extremities is free of trauma, and low molecular weight heparin if bleeding is unlikely to exacerbate the injury. Low-dose unfractionated heparin appears to be ineffective in trauma patients.[272] Mechanical devices such as sequential compression boots should be applied as early as possible after injury. Late (>4 days) initiation of prophylaxis, whether because of massive transfusion, low anticipated risk due to absence of comorbidity, or because of fear of intracranial bleeding after a severe head injury, has been shown to triple the risk of venous thromboembolism.[273] Consideration should be given to placement of a vena cava filter if the risk of bleeding is unacceptably high. Removable vena cava filters are now available and are likely to be used prophylactically in high-risk patients more often than permanent filters, which are associated with long-term complications. In patients with severe hemodynamic depression or cardiac arrest unresponsive to resuscitative measures, thrombolytic agents may be considered, despite the risk of hemorrhage.

References

1. World Health Organization: Injuries. Health topics: Injuries. 2008. http://www.who.int/topics/injuries/en/. Accessed November 5, 2012.
2. World Health Organization. World Report on Road Traffic Injury Prevention. 2004. http://whqlibdoc.who.int/publications/2004/9241562609.pdf. Accessed November 5, 2012.
3. World Health Organization. World Report on Violence and Health. 2002. http://whqlibdoc.who.int/publications/2002/9241545615_eng.pdf. Accessed November 5, 2012.
4. National Safety Council. *Injury Facts*. 2012 ed. Chicago: National Safety Council; 2012.
5. Acosta JA, Yang JC, Winchell RJ, et al. Lethal injuries and time of death in a level 1 trauma center. *J Am Coll Surg*. 1998;186:528–531.
6. Sakellaridis N, Pavlou E, Karatzas S, et al. Comparison of mannitol and hypertonic saline in the treatment of severe brain injuries. *J Neurosurg*. 2011;114:545–548.
7. Ferraris VA, Ferraris SP, Saha SP. The relationship between mortality and preexisting cardiac disease in 5,971 trauma patients. *J Trauma*. 2010;69:645–652.
8. Janjua KJ, Sugrue M, Deane SA. Prospective evaluation of early missed injuries and the role of tertiary trauma survey. *J Trauma*. 1998;44:1000–1005.
9. Wilson WC. Trauma: airway management. ASA difficult airway algorithm modified for trauma and five common intubation scenarios. *ASA Newsl*. 2005;69:9.
10. Crosby ET. Airway management in adults after cervical spine trauma. *Anesthesiology*. 2006;104:1293–1318.
11. Hoffman JR, Mower WR, Wolfson AB, et al. Validity of a set of clinical criteria to rule out injury to the cervical spine in patients with blunt trauma. National Emergency X-Radiography Utilization Study Group. *N Engl J Med*. 2000;343:94–99.
12. Duane TM, Mayglothling J, Wilson SP, et al. National Emergency X-Radiography Utilization Study criteria is inadequate to rule out fracture after significant blunt trauma compared with computed tomography. *J Trauma*. 2011;70:829–831.
13. Stiell IG, Clement CM, McKnight RD, et al. The Canadian C-spine rule versus the NEXUS low-risk criteria in patients with trauma. *N Engl J Med*. 2003;349:2510–2518.
14. Anglen J, Metzler M, Bunn P, et al. Flexion and extension views are not cost-effective in a cervical spine clearance protocol for obtunded trauma patients. *J Trauma*. 2002;52:54–59.
15. Muchow RD, Resnick DK, Abdel MP, et al. Magnetic resonance imaging (MRI) in the clearance of the cervical spine in blunt trauma: a meta-analysis. *J Trauma*. 2008;64:179–189.
16. Panczykowski DM, Tomycz ND, Okonkwo DO. Comparative effectiveness of using computed tomography alone to exclude cervical spine injuries in obtunded or intubated patients: meta-analysis of 14,327 patients with blunt trauma. *J Neurosurg*. 2011;115:541–549.
17. Hindman BJ, Palecek JP, Posner KL, et al. Cervical spinal cord, root, and bony spine injuries: a closed claims analysis. *Anesthesiology*. 2011;114:782–795.
18. McLeod AD, Calder I. Spinal cord injury and direct laryngoscopy–the legend lives on. *Br J Anaesthesia*. 2000;84:705–709.
19. Santoni BG, Hindman BJ, Puttlitz CM, et al. Manual in-line stabilization increases pressures applied by the laryngoscope blade during direct laryngoscopy and orotracheal intubation. *Anesthesiology*. 2009;110:24–31.
20. Lennarson PJ, Smith DW, Sawin PD, et al. Cervical spinal motion during intubation: efficacy of stabilization maneuvers in the setting of complete segmental instability. *J Neurosurg*. 2001;94:265–270.
21. Verschueren DS, Bell RB, Bagheri SC, et al. Management of laryngo-tracheal injuries associated with craniomaxillofacial trauma. *J Oral Maxillofac Surg*. 2006;64:203–214.
22. Brennan J, Gibbons MD, Lopez M, et al. Traumatic airway management in Operation Iraqi Freedom. *Otolaryngol Head Neck Surg*. 2011;144:376–380.
23. Cogbill TH, Cothren CC, Ahearn MK, et al. Management of maxillofacial injuries with severe oronasal hemorrhage: A multicenter perspective. *J Trauma*. 2008;65:994–999.
24. Chen YF, Tzeng IH, Li YH, et al. Transcatheter arterial embolization in the treatment of maxillofacial trauma induced life-threatening hemorrhages. *J Trauma*. 2009;66:1425–1430.
25. Holmgren EP, Bagheri S, Bell RB, et al. Utilization of tracheostomy in craniomaxillofacial trauma at a level-1 trauma center. *J Oral Maxillofac Surg*. 2007;65:2005–2010.
26. Gadre KS, Waknis PP. Transmylohyoid/Submental intubation: review, analysis, and refinements. *J Craniofac Surg*. 2010;21:516–519.
27. Demetriades D, Velmahos GG, Asensio JA. Cervical pharyngoesophageal and laryngotracheal injuries. *World J Surg*. 2001;25:1044–1048.
28. Danic D, Prgomet D, Sekelj A, et al. External laryngotracheal trauma. *Eur Arch Otorhinolaryngol*. 2006;263:228–232.
29. O'Connor PJ, Russell JD, Moriarty DC. Anesthetic implications of laryngeal trauma. *Anesth Analg*. 1998;87:1283–1284.
30. Schaefer SD. Primary management of laryngeal trauma. *Ann Otol Rhinol Laryngol*. 1982;91:399–402.
31. Fuhrman GM, Stieg FH 3rd, Buerk CA. Blunt laryngeal trauma: Classification and management protocol. *J Trauma*. 1990;30:87–92.
32. Yamazaki M, Sasaki R, Masuda A, et al. Anesthetic management of complete tracheal disruption using percutaneous cardiopulmonary support system. *Anesth Analg*. 1998;86:998–1000.
33. Gomez-Caro A, Ausin P, Moradiellos FJ, et al. Role of conservative medical management of tracheobronchial injuries. *J Trauma*. 2006;61:1426–1434; discussion 1434–1435.
34. Martel G, Al-Sabti H, Mulder DS, et al. Acute tracheoesophageal burst injury after blunt chest trauma: Case report and review of the literature. *J Trauma*. 2007;62:236–242.

35. Beiderlinden M, Adamzik M, Peters J. Conservative treatment of tracheal injuries. *Anesth Analg.* 2005;100:210–214.
36. Kirkpatrick AW, Sirois M, Laupland KB, et al. Hand-held thoracic sonography for detecting post-traumatic pneumothoraces: The extended focused assessment with sonography for trauma (EFAST). *J Trauma.* 2004;57:288–295.
37. Ball CG, Kirkpatrick AW, Fox DL, et al. Are occult pneumothoraces truly occult or simply missed? *J Trauma.* 2006;60:294–298 discussion 298–299.
38. Cohn SM, Dubose JJ. Pulmonary contusion: an update on recent advances in clinical management. *World J Surg.* 2010;34:1959–1970.
39. Stone MB, Secko MA. Bedside ultrasound diagnosis of pulmonary contusion. *Pediatr Emerg Care.* 2009;25:854–855.
40. Hamrick MC, Duhn RD, Ochsner MG. Critical evaluation of pulmonary contusion in the early post-traumatic period: risk of assisted ventilation. *Am Surg.* 2009; 75:1054–1058.
41. Schweiger JW. The pathophysiology, diagnosis, and management strategies for flail chest injury and pulmonary contusion. *Anesth Analg.* 2001;92(Suppl., IARS Review Course Lectures):86–93.
42. Caulfield EV, Dutton RP, Floccare DJ, et al. Prehospital hypocapnia and poor outcome after severe traumatic brain injury. *J Trauma.* 2009;66:1577–1582; discussion 1583.
43. Wolthuis EK, Choi G, Dessing MC, et al. Mechanical ventilation with lower tidal volumes and positive end-expiratory pressure prevents pulmonary inflammation in patients without preexisting lung injury. *Anesthesiology.* 2008;108:46–54.
44. Walkey AJ, Nair S, Papadopoulos S, et al. Use of airway pressure release ventilation is associated with a reduced incidence of ventilator-associated pneumonia in patients with pulmonary contusion. *J Trauma.* 2011;70:E42–E47.
45. McCunn M, Habashi NM. Airway pressure release ventilation in the acute respiratory distress syndrome following traumatic injury. *Int Anesthesiol Clin.* 2002;40:89–102.
46. Riou B, Zaier K, Kalfon P, et al. High-frequency jet ventilation in life-threatening bilateral pulmonary contusion. *Anesthesiology.* 2001;94:927–930.
47. Ho AM, Ling E. Systemic air embolism after lung trauma. *Anesthesiology.* 1999; 90:564–575.
48. Huber-Wagner S, Lefering R, Qvick LM, et al. Effect of whole-body CT during trauma resuscitation on survival: A retrospective, multicentre study. *Lancet.* 2009;373:1455–1461.
49. Mizushima Y, Ueno M, Watanabe H, et al. Discrepancy between heart rate and makers of hypoperfusion is a predictor of mortality in trauma patients. *J Trauma.* 2011;71:789–792.
50. American College of Surgeons Committee on Trauma: Shock. *Advanced Trauma Life Support Student Course Manual.* 8th ed. Chicago: American College of Surgeons; 2008:55–71.
51. Mackway-Jones K, Foex BA, Kirkman E, et al. Modification of the cardiovascular response to hemorrhage by somatic afferent nerve stimulation with special reference to gut and skeletal muscle blood flow. *J Trauma.* 1999;47:481–485.
52. Porter JM, Ivatury RR. In search of the optimal end points of resuscitation in trauma patients. A review. *J Trauma.* 1998;44:908–914.
53. Oyetunji TA, Chang DC, Crompton JG, et al. Redefining hypotension in the elderly: Normotension is not reassuring. *Arch Surg.* 2011;146:865–869.
54. Eastridge BJ, Salinas J, McManus JG, et al. Hypotension begins at 110 mm Hg: Redefining "hypotension" with data. *J Trauma.* 2007;63:291–297; discussion 297–299.
55. Eastridge BJ, Salinas J, Wade CE, et al. Hypotension is 100 mm Hg on the battlefield. *Am J Surg.* 2011;202:404–408.
56. Garrioch MA. The body's response to blood loss. *Vox Sang.* 2004;87(Suppl):74–76.
57. Zarzaur BL, Croce MA, Magnotti LJ, et al. Identifying life-threatening shock in the older injured patient: An analysis of the National Trauma Data Bank. *J Trauma.* 2010;68:1134–1138.
58. Maegele M, Lefering R, Yucel N, et al. Early coagulopathy in multiple injury: An analysis from the German Trauma Registry on 8724 patients. *Injury.* 2007; 38:298–304.
59. Rossaint R, Bouillon B, Cerny V, et al. Management of bleeding following major trauma: An updated European guideline. *Crit Care.* 2010;14:R52.
60. Bickell WH, Wall MJ, Pepe PE, et al. Immediate versus delayed fluid resuscitation for hypotensive patients with penetrating torso injuries. *N Engl J Med.* 1994; 331:1105–1113.
61. Stern SA. Low-volume fluid resuscitation for presumed hemorrhagic shock: Helpful or harmful? *Curr Opin Crit Care.* 2001;7:422–430.
62. Dutton RP, Mackenzie CF, Scalea TM. Hypotensive resuscitation during active hemorrhage: Impact on in-hospital mortality. *J Trauma.* 2002;52:1141–1146.
63. Sperry RJ, Bailey PL, Reichman MV, et al. Fentanyl and sufentanil increase intracranial pressure in head trauma patients. *Anesthesiology.* 1992;77:416–420.
64. Wade AL, Dye JL, Mohrle CR, et al. Head, face, and neck injuries during Operation Iraqi Freedom II: Results from the US Navy-Marine Corps Combat Trauma Registry. *J Trauma.* 2007;63:836–840.
65. Roberts I, Alderson P, Bunn F, et al. Colloids versus crystalloids for fluid resuscitation in critically ill patients. *Cochrane Database Syst Rev.* 2004;(4):CD000567.
66. Zehtabchi S, Sinert R, Goldman M, et al. Diagnostic performance of serial haematocrit measurements in identifying major injury in adult trauma patients. *Injury.* 2006;37:46–52.
67. Smith MJ, Stiefel MF, Magge S, et al. Packed red blood cell transfusion increases local cerebral oxygenation. *Crit Care Med.* 2005;33:1104–1108.
68. Leal-Noval SR, Munoz-Gomez M, Arellano-Orden V, et al. Impact of age of transfused blood on cerebral oxygenation in male patients with severe traumatic brain injury. *Crit Care Med.* 2008;36:1290–1296.
69. Salim A, Hadjizacharia P, DuBose J, et al. Role of anemia in traumatic brain injury. *J Am Coll Surg.* 2008;207:398–406.
70. Carlson AP, Schermer CR, Lu SW. Retrospective evaluation of anemia and transfusion in traumatic brain injury. *J Trauma.* 2006;61:567–571.
71. Malone DL, Dunne J, Tracy JK, et al. Blood transfusion, independent of shock severity, is associated with worse outcome in trauma. *J Trauma.* 2003;54:898–905; discussion 905–907.
72. Weinberg JA, McGwin G Jr, Marques MB, et al. Does the age of transfused blood affect outcomes? *J Trauma.* 2008;65:794–798.
73. Dutton RP, Shih D, Edelman BB, et al. Safety of uncrossmatched type-O red cells for resuscitation from hemorrhagic shock. *J Trauma.* 2005;59:1445–1449.
74. Tieu BH, Holcomb JB, Schreiber MA. Coagulopathy: Its pathophysiology and treatment in the injured patient. *World J Surg.* 2007;31:1055–1064.
75. Hirshberg A, Dugas M, Banez EI, et al. Minimizing dilutional coagulopathy in exsanguinating hemorrhage: A computer simulation. *J Trauma.* 2003;54:454–463.
76. Holcomb JB, Jenkins D, Rhee P, et al. Damage control resuscitation: Directly addressing the early coagulopathy of trauma. *J Trauma.* 2007;62:307–310.
77. Spahn DR, Rossaint R. Coagulopathy and blood component transfusion in trauma. *Br J Anaesth.* 2005;95:130–139.
78. Borgman MA, Spinella PC, Perkins JG, et al. The ratio of blood products transfused affects mortality in patients receiving massive transfusions at a combat support hospital. *J Trauma.* 2007;63:805–813.
79. Dente CJ, Shaz BH, Nicholas JM, et al. Early predictors of massive transfusion in patients sustaining torso gunshot wounds in a civilian level I trauma center. *J Trauma.* 2010;68:298–304.
80. Cotton BA, Au BK, Nunez TC, et al. Predefined massive transfusion protocols are associated with a reduction in organ failure and postinjury complications. *J Trauma.* 2009;66:41–48; discussion 48–49.
81. Larson CR, White CE, Spinella PC, et al. Association of shock, coagulopathy, and initial vital signs with massive transfusion in combat casualties. *J Trauma.* 2010;69(Suppl 1):S26–S32.
82. Cotton BA, Dossett LA, Haut ER, et al. Multicenter validation of a simplified score to predict massive transfusion in trauma. *J Trauma.* 2010;69(Suppl 1):S33–S39.
83. Callcut RA, Johannigman JA, Kadon KS, et al. All massive transfusion criteria are not created equal: Defining the predictive value of individual transfusion triggers to better determine who benefits from blood. *J Trauma.* 2011;70:794–801.
84. Cotton BA, Faz G, Hatch QM, et al. Rapid thrombelastography delivers real-time results that predict transfusion within 1 hour of admission. *J Trauma.* 2011; 71:407–414; discussion 414–417.
85. Luna GK, Pavlin EG, Kirkman T, et al. Hemodynamic effects of external cardiac massage in trauma shock. *J Trauma.* 1989;29:1430–1433.
86. Durham LA, Richardson RJ, Wall MJ, et al. Emergency center thoracotomy: Impact of prehospital resuscitation. *J Trauma.* 1992;32:775–779.
87. Millham FH, Gridlinger GA. Survival determinants in patients undergoing emergency room thoracotomy for penetrating chest injury. *J Trauma.* 1993;34:332–336.
88. Shackford SR, Mackersie RC, Davis JW, et al. Epidemiology and pathology of traumatic deaths occurring at a level I trauma center in a regionalized system; the importance of secondary brain injury. *J Trauma.* 1989;29:1392–1397.
89. Verweij BH, Amelink GJ, Muizelaar JP. Current concepts of cerebral oxygen transport and energy metabolism after severe traumatic brain injury. *Prog Brain Res.* 2007;161:111–124.
90. Werner C, Engelhard K. Pathophysiology of traumatic brain injury. *Br J Anaesth.* 2007;99:4–9.
91. Brain Trauma Foundation American Academy of Neurosurgeons. Guidelines for the management of severe traumatic brain injury. *J Neurotrauma.* 2007;24 (Suppl 1):S1–S106.
92. Chesnut RM. Avoidance of hypotension: Conditio sine qua non of successful head injury management. *J Trauma.* 1997;42(Supp):4S–9S.
93. McHugh GS, Engel DC, Butcher I, et al. Prognostic value of secondary insults in traumatic brain injury: Results from the IMPACT study. *J Neurotrauma.* 2007;24:287–293.
94. American College of Surgeons Committee on Trauma. *Head Trauma, Advanced Trauma Life Support Student Course Manual.* 8th ed. Chicago: American College of Surgeons; 2008:131–150.
95. Chesnut RM. Management of brain and spine injuries. *Crit Care Clin.* 2004; 20:25–55.
96. Duncan T, Krost WS, Mistovich JJ, et al. Beyond the basics: Brain injuries. *Emerg Med Serv.* 2007;36:65–69; quiz 70–71.
97. Davis DP, Peay J, Sise MJ, et al. The impact of prehospital endotracheal intubation on outcome in moderate to severe traumatic brain injury. *J Trauma.* 2005;58:933–939.
98. Wang HE, Peitzman AB, Cassidy LD, et al. Out-of-hospital endotracheal intubation and outcome after traumatic brain injury. *Ann Emerg Med.* 2004;44:439–450.
99. Davis DP, Koprowicz KM, Newgard CD, et al. The relationship between out-of-hospital airway management and outcome among trauma patients with Glasgow Coma Scale Scores of 8 or less. *Prehosp Emerg Care.* 2011;15:184–192.
100. Farahvar A, Gerber LM, Chiu YL, et al. Response to intracranial hypertension treatment as a predictor of death in patients with severe traumatic brain injury. *J Neurosurg.* 2011;114:1471–1478.

101. Latorre JG, Greer DM. Management of acute intracranial hypertension: A review. *Neurologist.* 2009;15:193–207.
102. White H, Cook D, Venkatesh B. The use of hypertonic saline for treating intracranial hypertension after traumatic brain injury. *Anesth Analg.* 2006;102:1836–1846.
103. Freshman SP, Battistella FD, Mateucci M, et al. Hypertonic saline (7.5%) versus mannitol: A comparison for treatment of acute head injuries. *J Trauma.* 1993;35:344–348.
104. Lescot T, Degos V, Zouaoui A. Opposed effects of hypertonic saline on contusions and noncontused brain tissue in patients with severe traumatic brain injury. *Crit Care Med.* 2006;34:3029–3033.
105. Doyle JA, Davis DP, Hoyt DB. The use of hypertonic saline in the treatment of traumatic brain injury. *J Trauma.* 2001;50:367–383.
106. Coles JP. Regional ischemia after head injury. *Curr Opin Crit Care.* 2004;10: 120–125.
107. Mascia L, Zavala E, Bosma K, et al. High tidal volume is associated with the development of acute lung injury after severe brain injury: An international observational study. *Crit Care Med.* 2007;35:1815–1820.
108. Chan KH, Dearden NM, Miller JD, et al. Multimodality monitoring as a guide to treatment of intracranial hypertension after severe brain injury. *Neurosurgery.* 1993;32:547–552.
109. Cruz J. Jugular venous oxygen saturation monitoring. *J Neurosurg.* 1992;77:162–163.
110. Jeremitsky E, Omert LA, Dunham CM, et al. The impact of hyperglycemia on patients with severe brain injury. *J Trauma.* 2005;58:47–50.
111. Heffernan DS, Inaba K, Arbabi S, et al. Sympathetic hyperactivity after traumatic brain injury and the role of beta-blocker therapy. *J Trauma.* 2010;69:1602–1609.
112. Rudehill A, Bellander B, Weitzberg E, et al. Outcome of traumatic brain injuries in 1,508 patients: impact of prehospital care. *J Neurotrauma.* 2002;19:855–868.
113. Elf K, Nilsson P, Enblad P. Outcome after traumatic brain injury improved by an organized secondary insult program and standardized neurointensive care. *Crit Care Med.* 2002;30:2129–2134.
114. Warner DS, Borel CO. Treatment of traumatic brain injury: One size does not fit all. *Anesth Analg.* 2004;99:1208–1210.
115. Palmer S, Bader MK, Qureshi A, et al. The impact on outcomes in a community hospital setting of using the AANS traumatic brain injury guidelines. Americans Associations for Neurologic Surgeons. *J Trauma.* 2001;50:657–664.
116. Watts DD, Hanfling D, Waller MA, et al. An evaluation of the use of guidelines in prehospital management of brain injury. *Prehosp Emerg Care.* 2004;8:254–261.
117. Patel HC, Menon DK, Tebbs S, et al. Specialist neurocritical care and outcome from head injury. *Intensive Care Med.* 2002;28:547–553.
118. Domeier RM, Evans RW, Swor RA, et al. Prehospital clinical findings associated with spinal injury. *Prehosp Emerg Care.* 1997;1:11–15.
119. Traynelis VC, Kasliwal MK. Cervical clearance. *J Neurosurg.* 2011;115:536–539; discussion 539–540.
120. Stevens RD, Bhardwaj A, Kirsch JR, et al. Critical care and perioperative management in traumatic spinal cord injury. *J Neurosurg Anesthesiol.* 2003;15:215–229.
121. Vale FL, Burns J, Jackson AB, et al. Combined medical and surgical treatment after acute spinal cord injury: Results of a pilot study to assess the merits of aggressive medical resuscitation and blood pressure management. *J Neurosurg.* 1997;87:239–246.
122. Bernhard M, Gries A, Kremer P, et al. Spinal cord injury (SCI)—prehospital management. *Resuscitation.* 2005;66:127–139.
123. Bracken MB, Shepard MJ, Collins WF Jr, et al. Methylprednisolone or naloxone treatment after acute spinal cord injury. Results of the Second National Acute Spinal Cord Injury Study. *J Neurosurg.* 1992;76:23–31.
124. Bracken MB, Shepard MJ, Holford TR, et al. Methylprednisolone or tirilazad mesylate after acute spinal cord injury: Results of the third National Acute Spinal Cord Injury randomized controlled trial. *J Neurosurg.* 1998;89:699–706.
125. Sayer FT, Kronvall E, Nilsson OG. Methylprednisolone treatment in acute spinal cord injury: the myth challenged through a structured analysis of published literature. *Spine J.* 2006;6:335–343.
126. Gerndt SJ, Rodriguez JL, Pawlik JW, et al. Consequences of high-dose steroid therapy for acute spinal cord injury. *J Trauma.* 1997;42:279–284.
127. Tolonen A, Turkka J, Salonen O, et al. Traumatic brain injury is under-diagnosed in patients with spinal cord injury. *J Rehabil Med.* 2007;39:622–626.
128. Kwon BK, Okon E, Hillyer J, et al. A systematic review of non-invasive pharmacologic neuroprotective treatments for acute spinal cord injury. *J Neurotrauma.* 2011;28:1545–1588.
129. Berlly M, Shem K. Respiratory management during the first five days after spinal cord injury. *J Spinal Cord Med.* 2007;30:309–318.
130. Brown R, DiMarco AF, Hoit JD, et al. Respiratory dysfunction and management in spinal cord injury. *Respir Care.* 2006;51:853–868;discussion 869–870.
131. Alexander MS, Biering-Sorensen F, Bodner D, et al. International standards to document remaining autonomic function after spinal cord injury. *Spinal Cord.* 2009;47:36–43.
132. Winslow C, Rozovsky J. Effect of spinal cord injury on the respiratory system. *Am J Phys Med Rehabil.* 2003;82:803–814.
133. Theodore J, Robin ED. Pathogenesis of neurogenic pulmonary edema. *Lancet.* 1975;2:749–751.
134. Mackenzie CF, Shin B, Krishnaprasad D, et al. Assessment of cardiac and respiratory function during surgery on patients with acute quadriplegia. *J Neurosurg.* 1985;62:843–849.
135. Casha S, Christie S. A systematic review of intensive cardiopulmonary management after spinal cord injury. *J Neurotrauma.* 2011;28:1479–1495.
136. Christie S, Thibault-Halman G, Casha S. Acute pharmacological DVT prophylaxis after spinal cord injury. *J Neurotrauma.* 2011;28:1509–1514.
137. Demetriades D, Salim A, Brown C. Neck injuries. *Curr Probl Surg.* 2007;44:13–85.
138. Inaba K, Branco BC, Menaker J, et al. Evaluation of multidetector computed tomography for penetrating neck injury: A prospective multicenter study. *J Trauma.* 2012;72:577.
139. Biffl WL, Moore EE, Ryu RK, et al. The unrecognized epidemic of blunt carotid arterial injuries. Early diagnosis improves neurologic outcome. *Ann Surg.* 1998; 228:462–469.
140. Jewett BS, Shockley WW, Rutledge R. External laryngeal trauma: analysis of 392 patients. *Arch Otolaryngol Head Neck Surg.* 1999;125:877–880.
141. Ho AM, Karmakar MK, Critchley LA. Acute pain management of patients with multiple fractured ribs: A focus on regional techniques. *Curr Opin Crit Care.* 2011;17:323–327.
142. Ball CG, Kirkpatrick AW, Laupland KB, et al. Incidence, risk factors, and outcomes for occult pneumothoraces in victims of major trauma. *J Trauma.* 2005;59:917–924; discussion 924–925.
143. Reissig A, Copetti R, Kroegel C. Current role of emergency ultrasound of the chest. *Crit Care Med.* 2011;39:839–845.
144. Yadav K, Jalili M, Zehtabchi S. Management of traumatic occult pneumothorax. *Resuscitation.* 2010;81:1063–1068.
145. American College of Surgeons Committee on Trauama. *Thoracic Trauma, Advanced Trauma Life Support Student Course Manual.* 8th ed. Chicago: American College of Surgeons; 2008:85.
146. Boersma WG, Stigt JA, Smit HJ. Treatment of haemothorax. *Respir Med.* 2010; 104:1583–1587.
147. Mineo TC, Ambrogi V, Cristino B, et al. Changing indications for thoracotomy in blunt chest trauma after the advent of videothoracoscopy. *J Trauma.* 1999;47:1088–1091.
148. Porembka DT, Johnson DJ, Hoyt BD, et al. Penetrating cardiac trauma: a perioperative role for transesophageal echocardiography. *Anesth Analg.* 1993;77:1275–1277.
149. Orliaguet G, Ferjani M, Riou B. The heart in blunt trauma. *Anesthesiology.* 2001;95:544–548.
150. Maron BJ, Estes NA 3rd. Commotio cordis. *N Engl J Med.* 2010;362:917–927.
151. Wong YC, Ng CJ, Wang LJ, et al. Left mediastinal width and mediastinal width ratio are better radiographic criteria than general mediastinal width for predicting blunt aortic injury. *J Trauma.* 2004;57:88–94.
152. Vignon P, Boncoeur MP, Francois B. Comparison of multiplane transesophageal echocardiography and contrast-enhanced helical CT in the diagnosis of blunt traumatic cardiovascular injuries. *Anesthesiology.* 2001;94:615–622; discussion 5A.
153. Goarin JP, Cluzel P, Gosgnach M, et al. Evaluation of transesophageal echocardiography for diagnosis of traumatic aortic injury. *Anesthesiology.* 2000;93:1373–1377.
154. Demetriades D, Velmahos GC, Scalea TM, et al. Diagnosis and treatment of blunt thoracic aortic injuries: Changing perspectives. *J Trauma.* 2008;64:1415–1418; discussion 1418–1419.
155. Singh KE, Baum VC. The anesthetic management of cardiovascular trauma. *Curr Opin Anaesthesiol.* 2011;24:98–103.
156. Morgan BS, Watcyn-Jones T, Garner JP. Traumatic diaphragmatic injury. *J R Army Med Corps.* 2010;156:139–144.
157. Villavicencio RT, Aucar JA. Analysis of laparoscopy in trauma. *J Am Coll Surg.* 1999;189:11–20.
158. Gaarder C, Kroepelien CF, Loekke R, et al. Ultrasound performed by radiologists-confirming the truth about FAST in trauma. *J Trauma.* 2009;67:323–327; discussion 328–329.
159. White CE, Hsu JR, Holcomb JB. Haemodynamically unstable pelvic fractures. *Injury.* 2009;40:1023–1030.
160. Cothren CC, Osborn PM, Moore EE, et al. Preperitonal pelvic packing for hemodynamically unstable pelvic fractures: A paradigm shift. *J Trauma.* 2007;62:834–839; discussion 839–842.
161. Verbeek D, Sugrue M, Balogh Z. Acute management of hemodynamically unstable pelvic trauma patients: time for a change? Multicenter review of recent practice. *World J Surg.* 2008;32:1874–1882.
162. MacLennan N, Heimbach DM, Cullen BF. Anesthesia for major thermal injury. *Anesthesiology.* 1998;89:749–770.
163. Hemington-Gorse SJ. A comparison of laser Doppler imaging with other measurement techniques to assess burn depth. *J Wound Care.* 2005;14:151–153.
164. Neaman KC, Andres LA, McClure AM, et al. A new method for estimation of involved BSAs for obese and normal-weight patients with burn injury. *J Burn Care Res.* 2011;32:421–428.
165. Pereira CT, Herndon DN. The pharmacologic modulation of the hypermetabolic response to burns. *Adv Surg.* 2005;39:245–261.
166. Williams FN, Branski LK, Jeschke MG, et al. What, how, and how much should patients with burns be fed? *Surg Clin North Am.* 2011;91:609–629.
167. Haponik EF, Meyers DA, Munster AM, et al. Acute upper airway injury in burn patients: serial changes of flow-volume curves and nasopharyngoscopy. *Am Rev Respir Dis.* 1987;135:360–366.
168. Smith DL, Cairns BA, Ramadan F, et al. Effect of inhalation injury, burn size and age on mortality: A study of 1447 consecutive burn patients. *J Trauma.* 1994; 37:655–659.

169. Sheridan RL, Hurford WE, Kacmarek RM, et al. Inhaled nitric oxide in burn patients with respiratory failure. *J Trauma.* 1997;42:629–634.
170. Walia G, Jada G, Cartotto R. Anesthesia and intraoperative high-frequency oscillatory ventilation during burn surgery. *J Burn Care Res.* 2011;32:118–123.
171. Pannucci CJ, Osborne NH, Wahl WL. Venous thromboembolism in thermally injured patients: Analysis of the National Burn Repository. *J Burn Care Res.* 2011;32:6–12.
172. Hofstra JJ, Vlaar AP, Knape P, et al. Pulmonary activation of coagulation and inhibition of fibrinolysis after burn injuries and inhalation trauma. *J Trauma.* 2011;70:1389–1397.
173. Vegfors M, Lennmarken C. Carboxyhemoglobinaemia and pulse oximetry. *Br J Anaesth.* 1991;66:625–626.
174. Baud FJ, Barriot P, Toffis V, et al. Elevated blood cyanide concentrations in victims of smoke inhalation. *N Engl J Med.* 1991;325:1761–1766.
175. Tung A, Lynch J, McDade WA. A new biological assay for measuring cyanide in blood. *Anesth Analg.* 1997;85:1045–1051.
176. Breen PH, Isserles SA, Westley J, et al. Combined carbon monoxide and cyanide poisoning: A place for treatment? *Anesth Analg.* 1995;80:671–677.
177. Miller K, Chang A. Acute inhalation injury. *Emerg Med Clin North Am.* 2003;21:533–557.
178. Williams FN, Herndon DN, Suman OE, et al. Changes in cardiac physiology after severe burn injury. *J Burn Care Res.* 2011;32:269–274.
179. Namias N. Advances in burn care. *Curr Opin Crit Care.* 2007;13:405–410.
180. Ivy ME, Atweh NA, Palmer J, et al. Intra-abdominal hypertension and abdominal compartment syndrome in burn patients. *J Trauma.* 2000;49:387–391.
181. Edgar DW, Fish JS, Gomez M, et al. Local and systemic treatments for acute edema after burn injury: A systematic review of the literature. *J Burn Care Res.* 2011;32:334–347.
182. Sheridan RL. Burns. *Crit Care Med.* 2002;30:S500–S514.
183. Fodor L, Fodor A, Ramon Y, et al. Controversies in fluid resuscitation for burn management: Literature review and our experience. *Injury.* 2006;37:374–379.
184. Saffle JI. The phenomenon of "fluid creep" in acute burn resuscitation. *J Burn Care Res.* 2007;28:382–395.
185. Klein MB, Edwards JA, Kramer CB, et al. The beneficial effects of plasma exchange after severe burn injury. *J Burn Care Res.* 2009;30:243–248.
186. Huang PP, Stucky FS, Dimick AR, et al. Hypertonic sodium resuscitation is associated with renal failure and death. *Ann Surg.* 1995;221:543–554.
187. Elgjo GI, Poli de Figueiredo LF, Schenarts PJ, et al. Hypertonic saline dextran produces early (8–12 hrs) fluid sparing in burn resuscitation: A 24-hr prospective, double-blind study in sheep. *Crit Care Med.* 2000;28:163–171.
188. Branski LK, Herndon DN, Pereira C, et al. Longitudinal assessment of Integra in primary burn management: a randomized pediatric clinical trial. *Crit Care Med.* 2007;35:2615–2623.
189. Morris JR, MacKenzie EJ, Edelstein SL. The effect of preexisting conditions on mortality in trauma patients. *JAMA.* 1990;263:1942–1946.
190. Rooke GA, Schwid HA, Shapira Y. The effect of graded hemorrhage and intravascular volume replacement on systolic pressure variation in humans during mechanical and spontaneous ventilation. *Anesth Analg.* 1995;80:925–932.
191. Marik PE, Dellinger RP. Is the cortrosyn test necessary in high basal corticoid patients with septic shock? *Crit Care Med.* 2009;37:386–387.
192. Michard F. Stroke volume variation: From applied physiology to improved outcomes. *Crit Care Med.* 2011;39:402–403.
193. Porembka DT. Importance of transesophageal echocardiography in the critically ill and injured patient. *Crit Care Med.* 2007;35:S414–S430.
194. Capan LM, Miller SM, Patel KP. Fat embolism. *Anesth Clin North Am.* 1993; 11:25–53.
195. Agashe GS, Coakley J, Mannheimer PD. Forehead pulse oximetry: Headband use helps alleviate false low readings likely related to venous pulsation artifact. *Anesthesiology.* 2006;105:1111–1116.
196. Tyburski JG, Carlin AM, Harvey EH. End-tidal CO2-arterial CO2 differences: A useful intraoperative mortality marker in trauma surgery. *J Trauma.* 2003;55: 892–896; discussion 896–897.
197. Lee SW, Hong YS, Han C. Concordance of end-tidal carbon dioxide and arterial carbon dioxide in severe traumatic brain injury. *J Trauma.* 2009;67:526–530.
198. McKinley BA, Kozar RA, Cocanour CS, et al. Normal versus supranormal oxygen delivery goals in shock resuscitation: The response is the same. *J Trauma.* 2002;53:825–832.
199. McKinley BA, Sucher JF, Todd SR, et al. Central venous pressure versus pulmonary artery catheter-directed shock resuscitation. *Shock.* 2009;32:463–470.
200. Mallett SV, Cox JA. Thromboelastography. *Br J Anaesth.* 1992;69:307–313.
201. Rugeri L, Levrat A, David JS, et al. Diagnosis of early coagulation abnormalities in trauma patients by rotation thrombelastography. *J Thromb Haemost.* 2007;5:289–295.
202. Johnston TD, Chen Y, Reed RL. Functional equivalence of hypothermia to specific clotting factor deficiencies. *J Trauma.* 1994;37:413–417.
203. Kurita T, Uraoka M, Morita K, et al. Influence of haemorrhage on the pseudo-steady-state remifentanil concentration in a swine model: A comparison with propofol and the effect of haemorrhagic shock stage. *Br J Anaesth.* 2011;107:719–725.
204. Kurita T, Takata K, Morita K, et al. The influence of hemorrhagic shock on the electroencephalographic and immobilizing effects of propofol in a swine model. *Anesth Analg.* 2009;109:398–404.
205. Egar TD, Kuramkote S, Gong G, et al. Fentanyl pharmacokinetics in hemorrhagic shock. A porcine model. *Anesthesiology.* 1999;91:156–166.
206. Johnson KB, Egan TD, Kern SE, et al. The influence of hemorrhagic shock on propofol: A pharmacokinetic and pharmacodynamic analysis. *Anesthesiology.* 2003;99:409–420.
207. Johnson KB, Egan TD, Layman J, et al. The influence of hemorrhagic shock on etomidate: A pharmacokinetic and pharmacodynamic analysis. *Anesth Analg.* 2003;96:1360–1368.
208. Shafer SL. Shock values. *Anesthesiology.* 2004;101:567–568.
209. Weiskopf RB, Bogetz MS, Roizen MF, et al. Cardiovascular and metabolic sequelae of inducing anesthesia with ketamine or thiopental in hypovolemic swine. *Anesthesiology.* 1984;60:214–221.
210. Kurita T, Takata K, Uraoka M, et al. The influence of hemorrhagic shock on the minimum alveolar anesthetic concentration of isoflurane in a swine model. *Anesth Analg.* 2007;105:1639–1643.
211. Libonati MM, Leahy MJ, Ellison N. The use of succinylcholine in open eye surgery. *Anesthesiology.* 1985;62:637–640.
212. de Nadal M, Munar F, Poca MA, et al. Cerebral hemodynamic effects of morphine and fentanyl in patients with severe head injury. Absence of correlation to cerebral autoregulation. *Anesthesiology.* 2000;92:11–18.
213. Moss E. Alfentanil increases intracranial pressure when intracranial compliance is low. *Anaesthesia.* 1992;47:134–136.
214. Grathwohl KW, Black IH, Spinella PC, et al. Total intravenous anesthesia including ketamine versus volatile gas anesthesia for combat-related operative traumatic brain injury. *Anesthesiology.* 2008;109:44–53.
215. Branski LK, Herndon DN, Byrd JF, et al. Transpulmonary thermodilution for hemodynamic measurements in severely burned children. *Critical Care.* 2011;15:R118.
216. Chen XL, Xia ZF, Wei HF. Escharectomy and allografting during shock stage reduces insulin resistance induced by major burn. *J Burn Care Res.* 2011;32:e59–e66.
217. Sterling JP, Heimbach DM. Hemostasis in burn surgery—a review. *Burns.* 2011; 37:559–565.
218. Martyn JAJ, Fukushima Y, Chon Y, et al. Muscle relaxants in burns, trauma and critical illness. *Int Anesthesiol Clin.* 2006;44:123.
219. Han T, Kim H, Bae J, et al. Neuromuscular pharmacodynamics of rocuronium in patients with major burns. *Anesth Analg.* 2004;99:386–392.
220. Kahn SA, Beers RJ, Lentz CW. Do fentanyl and morphine influence body temperature after severe burn injury? *J Burn Care Res.* 2011;32:309–316.
221. Todd SR, Malinoski D, Muller PJ, et al. Lactated Ringer's is superior to normal saline in the resuscitation of uncontrolled hemorrhagic shock. *J Trauma.* 2007;62:636–639.
222. Wang HE, Callaway CW, Peitzman AB, et al. Admission hypothermia and outcome after major trauma. *Crit Care Med.* 2005;33:1296–1301.
223. Tsuei BJ, Kearney PA. Hypothermia in the trauma patient. *Injury.* 2004;35:7–15.
224. Jurkovich GJ, Greiser WB, Luterman A, et al. Hypothermia in trauma victims: An ominous predictor of survival. *J Trauma.* 1987;27:1019–1025.
225. Ireland S, Endacott R, Cameron P, et al. The incidence and significance of accidental hypothermia in major trauma—a prospective observational study. *Resuscitation.* 2011;82:300–306.
226. Smith C, Soreide E. Hypothermia in trauma victims. *ASA Newsletter.* 2005;69:17.
227. Gentilello LM. Advances in the management of hypothermia. *Surg Clin North Am.* 1995;75:243–256.
228. Wadhwa A, Komatsu R, Orhan-Sungur M, et al. New circulating-water devices warm more quickly than forced-air in volunteers. *Anesth Analg.* 2007;105:1681–1687.
229. Peterson K, Carson S, Carney N. Hypothermia treatment for traumatic brain injury: A systematic review and meta-analysis. *J Neurotrauma.* 2008;25:62–71.
230. Sydenham E, Roberts I, Alderson P. Hypothermia for traumatic head injury. *Cochrane Database Syst Rev.* 2009;(2):CD001048.
231. Mittermayr M, Streif W, Haas T, et al. Hemostatic changes after crystalloid or colloid fluid administration during major orthopedic surgery: The role of fibrinogen administration. *Anesth Analg.* 2007;105:905–917.
232. Kashuk JL, Moore EE, Sawyer M, et al. A: Primary fibrinolysis is integral in the pathogenesis of the acute coagulopathy of trauma. *Ann Surg.* 2010;252:434–442; discussion 443–444.
233. Bolliger D, Gorlinger K, Tanaka KA. Pathophysiology and treatment of coagulopathy in massive hemorrhage and hemodilution. *Anesthesiology.* 2010;113:1205–1219.
234. Hess JR, Lawson JH. The coagulopathy of trauma versus disseminated intravascular coagulation. *J Trauma.* 2006;60:S12–S19.
235. Brohi K, Cohen MJ, Ganter MT, et al. Acute traumatic coagulopathy: initiated by hypoperfusion: modulated through the protein C pathway? *Ann Surg.* 2007; 245:812–818.
236. Johansson PI, Stensballe J, Rasmussen LS, et al. A high admission syndecan-1 level, a marker of endothelial glycocalyx degradation, is associated with inflammation, protein C depletion, fibrinolysis, and increased mortality in trauma patients. *Ann Surg.* 2011;254:194–200.
237. Holcomb JB. A novel and potentially unifying mechanism for shock induced early coagulopathy. *Ann Surg.* 2011;254:201–202.
238. DeLoughery TG. Coagulation defects in trauma patients: etiology, recognition, and therapy. *Crit Care Clin.* 2004;20:13–24.
239. Wolberg AS, Meng ZH, Monroe DM 3rd, et al. A systematic evaluation of the effect of temperature on coagulation enzyme activity and platelet function. *J Trauma.* 2004;56:1221–1228.

240. Martini WZ, Pusateri AE, Uscilowicz JM, et al. Independent contributions of hypothermia and acidosis to coagulopathy in swine. *J Trauma.* 2005;58:1002–1009.
241. Levi M. Disseminated intravascular coagulation. *Crit Care Med.* 2007;35:2191–2195.
242. Kashuk JL, Moore EE, Sawyer M, et al. Postinjury coagulopathy management: goal directed resuscitation via POC thrombelastography. *Ann Surg.* 2010;251: 604–614.
243. Gunter OL Jr, Au BK, Isbell JM, et al. Optimizing outcomes in damage control resuscitation: Identifying blood product ratios associated with improved survival. *J Trauma.* 2008;65:527–534.
244. Duchesne JC, Hunt JP, Wahl G, et al. Review of current blood transfusions strategies in a mature level I trauma center: Were we wrong for the last 60 years? *J Trauma.* 2008;65:272–276; discussion 276–278.
245. Snyder CW, Weinberg JA, McGwin G Jr, et al. The relationship of blood product ratio to mortality: survival benefit or survival bias? *J Trauma.* 2009;66:358–362; discussion 362–364.
246. Ho AM, Dion PW, Yeung JH, et al. Prevalence of survivor bias in observational studies on fresh frozen plasma: Erythrocyte ratios in trauma requiring massive transfusion. *Anesthesiology* 2012;116:716–728.
247. Etemadrezaie H, Baharvahdat H, Shariati Z, et al. The effect of fresh frozen plasma in severe closed head injury. *Clin Neurol Neurosurg.* 2007;109:166–171.
248. Collaborators C-T. Effects of tranexamic acid on death, vascular occlusive events, and blood transfusion in trauma patients with significant haemorrhage (CRASH-2): A randomised, placebo-controlled trial. *Lancet.* 2010;376:23–32.
249. Gruen RL, Mitra B. Tranexamic acid for trauma. *Lancet.* 2011;377:1052–1054.
250. Boffard KD, Riou B, Warren B, et al. Recombinant factor VIIa as adjunctive therapy for bleeding control in severely injured trauma patients: Two parallel randomized, placebo-controlled, double-blind clinical trials. *J Trauma.* 2005;59:8–15; discussion 15–18.
251. Martinowitz U, Michaelson M. Guidelines for the use of recombinant activated factor VII (rFVIIa) in uncontrolled bleeding: A report by the Israeli Multidisciplinary rFVIIa Task Force. *J Thromb Haemost.* 2005;3:640–648.
252. European Medicines Agency. NovoSeven (eptacog alfa). http://www.ema.europa.eu/ema/index.jsp?curl=pages/medicines/human/medicines/000074/human_med_000936.jsp&mid=WC0b01ac058001d124 (Accessed Dec. 11, 2012).
253. Imberti D, Barillari G, Biasioli C, et al. Emergency reversal of anticoagulation with a three-factor prothrombin complex concentrate in patients with intracranial haemorrhage. *Blood Transfus.* 2011;9:148–155.
254. Sorensen B, Spahn DR, Innerhofer P, et al. Clinical review: Prothrombin complex concentrates—evaluation of safety and thrombogenicity. *Critical Care.* 2011;15:201.
255. Hoyt DB, Bulger EM, Knudson MM, et al. Death in the operating room: an analysis of a multi-center experience. *J Trauma.* 1994;37:426–432.
256. Nicholas JM, Rix EP, Easley KA, et al. Changing patterns in the management of penetrating abdominal trauma: the more things change, the more they stay the same. *J Trauma.* 2003;55:1095–1108; discussion 1108–1110.
257. Duchesne JC, Kimonis K, Marr AB, et al. Damage control resuscitation in combination with damage control laparotomy: A survival advantage. *J Trauma.* 2010;69:46–52.
258. Morshed S, Corrales LA, Lin K, et al. Femoral nailing during serum bicarbonate-defined hypo-perfusion predicts pulmonary organ dysfunction in multi-system trauma patients. *Injury.* 2011;42:643–649.
259. Sanchez-Izquierdo-Riera JA, Caballero-Cubedo RE, Perez-Vela JL, et al. Propofol versus midazolam: Safety and efficacy for sedating the severe trauma patient. *Anesth Analg.* 1998;86:1219–1224.
260. Kheterpal S, Tremper KK, Englesbe MJ, et al. Predictors of postoperative acute renal failure after noncardiac surgery in patients with previously normal renal function. *Anesthesiology.* 2007;107:892–902.
261. Shin B, Mackenzie CF, Helrich M. Creatinine clearance for early detection of posttraumatic renal dysfunction. *Anesthesiology.* 1986;64:605–609.
262. Brown CV, Rhee P, Chan L, et al. Preventing renal failure in patients with rhabdomyolysis: Do bicarbonate and mannitol make a difference? *J Trauma.* 2004; 56:1191–1196.
263. Balogh Z, McKinley BA, Cocanour CS, et al. Secondary abdominal compartment syndrome is an elusive early complication of traumatic shock resuscitation. *Am J Surg.* 2002;184:538–543; discussion 543–544.
264. Cheatham ML. Intra-abdominal hypertension and abdominal compartment syndrome. *N Horizons.* 1999;7:96–115.
265. Maxwell RA, Fabian TC, Croce MA, et al. Secondary abdominal compartment syndrome: An underappreciated manifestation of severe hemorrhagic shock. *J Trauma.* 1999;47:995–999.
266. Balogh Z, McKinley BA, Holcomb JB, et al. Both primary and secondary abdominal compartment syndrome can be predicted early and are harbingers of multiple organ failure. *J Trauma.* 2003;54:848–859; discussion 859–861.
267. Balogh Z, McKinley BA, Cocanour CS, et al. Patients with impending abdominal compartment syndrome do not respond to early volume loading. *Am J Surg.* 2003;186:602–607; discussion 607–608.
268. Balogh ZJ, Martin A, van Wessem KP, et al. Mission to eliminate postinjury abdominal compartment syndrome. *Arch Surg.* 2011;146:938–943.
269. Baldwin K, Namdari S, Esterhai JL, et al. Venous thromboembolism in patients with blunt trauma: Are comprehensive guidelines the answer? *Am J Orthop.* 2011; 40:E83–E87.
270. Jongbloets LM, Lensing AW, Koopman MM, et al. Limitations of compression ultrasound for the detection of symptomless postoperative deep vein thrombosis. *Lancet.* 1994;343:1142–1144.
271. Frankel HL, FitzPatrick MK, Gaskell S, et al. Strategies to improve compliance with evidence-based clinical management guidelines. *J Am Coll Surg.* 1999; 189:533–538.
272. Geerts WH, Jay RM, Code KI, et al. A comparison of low-dose heparin with low-molecular-weight heparin as prophylaxis against venous thromboembolism after major trauma. *N Engl J Med.* 1996;335:701–707.
273. Nathens AB, McMurray MK, Cuschieri J, et al. The practice of venous thromboembolism prophylaxis in the major trauma patient. *J Trauma.* 2007;62:557–562; discussion 562–563.

CHAPTER

53 Emergency Preparedness for and Disaster Management of Casualties from Natural Disasters and Chemical, Biologic, Radiologic, Nuclear, and High-Yield Explosive (CBRNE) Events

MICHAEL J. MURRAY

ANESTHESIA FOR SURGICAL SUBSPECIALTIES

Key Points

1. There are certain principles that are common to all such events, independent of their etiology, and as a group anesthesiologists are as well prepared if not better prepared to assist their communities in planning for and in caring for patients from a disaster.
2. Any time a situation arises in which medical capability is significantly below standards to which we are accustomed in the United States the anesthesiologist is indeed practicing in an austere environment.
3. If one has a pet, family or friends living with them, or has legal responsibility for a loved one (elderly parents, disabled person) one must have a plan for these individuals that provides care for them.
4. Despite the best effort of law enforcement, fire and rescue teams, and emergency medical agencies, hospitals will continue to play a vital role in helping communities respond to catastrophic events.
5. Anesthesiologists' basic understanding of physiology and pharmacology, their airway skills, their fluid resuscitation expertise, their ability to manage ventilators and to provide anesthesia in the field environment, in the emergency department, in the operating room, and in intensive care units (ICUs) will be invaluable.
6. If assigned to triage patients, the anesthesiologist will be expected to classify patients into four groups—those requiring immediate care, delayed care, first aid, and expectant.
7. Anesthesiologists should position themselves at the head of the bed and assume responsibility for the airway and venous access. For the former it would be ideal to have two or three assistants (one providing in-line C-spine stabilization, another individual applying cricoid pressure, and a third individual administering medications).
8. The toxicity of the nerve agents depends on the compound delivered, the dose that is delivered (LC), and the time (t) that an individual is exposed to that dose.
9. There are three categories of biologic weapons (Table 53-1). Category A are those weapons which are highly contagious and fit all the characteristics of a relatively ideal biologic agent.

Multimedia

1 Disaster Preparedness

INTRODUCTION

Preparing to manage, to deal with the sequelae of, and to mitigate future disasters originating from natural events, industrial accidents or, of more interest recently, caused intentionally by terrorists using chemical, biologic, radiologic, nuclear, or high-yield explosive (CBRNE) agents is a high priority for the majority of governments the world over. Even large multinational corporations recognize the need for planning to assist during disasters and to decrease future risk of disasters. Two thousand such corporations, each with $5 billion or more in assets, participate in the World Economic Forum, a private not-for-profit foundation established in Switzerland. Through its Global Agenda Council on Humanitarian Assistance, partnering with the United Nations, humanitarian aid is provided throughout the world following natural disasters wherever there is a need. The resulting public–private collaboration has a distinguished track record; however, the Council recognizes the need to do more with respect to disaster risk reduction and disaster (www.weforum.org/issues/disaster-management). Money may also play a role—natural disasters that occurred in 2011 caused more than 350 billion dollars in losses (www.weforum.org/content/global-agenda-council-catastrophic-risks-2012). Whatever the reason, though, the aid provided is the only mechanism to mitigate the effects of disasters in many areas of the world where economic resources are inadequate. The United States also is cognizant of the benefits to its foreign policy by assisting in humanitarian missions. The U.S. Agency for International Development (USAID) spends a significant portion of its budget each year to provide humanitarian assistance in the wake of natural disasters such as floods, volcanic eruptions, and earthquakes but spends just as much to mitigate the effects of future catastrophes. The American Society of Anesthesiologists has recognized the importance of such activities and in the past decade has established a Committee on Emergency Preparedness and Trauma (COTEP) and a Global Health Initiative. While no one can doubt the altruistic motives for these actions, as a member-driven organization it has been driven in these endeavors from requests from members during this same time frame: After 9-11 strike, after Hurricanes Katrina and Ike, after the tornados that struck the central and southeast part of the country over the last couple years, and most recently after the earthquake that struck Haiti in 2010. ASA members who have been involved in relief efforts, members who have either been in the military or are in the military, and international members who have experienced terrorism on a more frequent basis have created a cacophony of voices calling for more education and training on how to prepare for a disaster and how to manage the victims of such disasters. Most residency program directors would agree that anesthesiologists are well prepared to manage individual patients but are lacking when it comes to education in managing the numbers of patients that might arise from a mass casualty event. Books have been written on such topics and governments have created large bureaucracies to address such events, so it would be naïve to think that a chapter in a book could adequately prepare one to cope with all contin-
1 gencies. However, there are certain principles that are common to all such events, independent of their etiology, and as a group anesthesiologists are as well prepared if not better prepared to assist their communities in planning for and in caring for patients from a disaster. We must expend the energy to be better educated as the initial response to any disaster always occurs at the local level; therefore, as anesthesiologists we must be prepared to provide assistance during such emergencies. Other physicians, hospital administrators, and nongovernment organizations (NGOs) all place anesthesia providers at the top of the list of healthcare workers who are needed to manage the sequelae of natural disasters and mass casualty events. We are in such demand that the NGO, Doctors Without Borders (*Medicins san Frontiers*), waives its policy that clinicians commit for 9- to 18-month rotations; there is an option for anesthesia providers of 1- to 3-month assignments (www.doctorswithoutboarders.org/work/field/recruitment.cfn). Whether it is providing anesthesia so that an extremity can be amputated allowing someone trapped in the rubble of a building following an earthquake can be extracted, starting an intravenous infusion in a child or adult debilitated by diarrhea, treating the effects of a chemical agent, managing a ventilator in someone with anthrax, or providing anesthesia to a casualty from an explosion, anesthesia providers have the requisite skills to assist in all these scenarios—these are services we provide on a daily basis.

However, disasters and mass casualty events are not something in which we participate on a daily basis so therefore education and training for these situations is critically important, beginning with preparation to respond to the most likely disasters to occur in our respective geographic location, for example, hurricanes on the Atlantic Seaboard and Gulf of Mexico, earthquakes on the West Coast of North America or tornadoes in the Midwest and Southeast of the United States. Even though natural and industrial disasters have occurred for millennia, the use of CBRNE agents and devices by terrorists in recent decades has emphasized the need for increased preparedness.

However, time and time again history shows that enthusiasm for education is high after an event and then tapers off; maintaining that enthusiasm is difficult,[1] and therefore most if not all healthcare facilities[2] are not prepared to deal with mass casualty incidents the exception being those facilities staffed by physicians with prior military training.[3] In dealing with acts of terrorism geography is not helpful in anticipating what might occur, but that is not to say that one cannot anticipate what to expect. One can learn from experience; terrorists have been successful in their minds' eyes with improvised explosive devices (IEDs), and even in those situations in which IEDs were not used, terrorists have chosen to use certain weapons of mass destruction (WMD) more often than others. For example, if they were to choose a chemical agent, a nerve agent is most likely and amongst those sarin has been the agent of choice. Similarly amongst biologic agents, anthrax, which was used in 2001, or smallpox would be the most likely choice because of the high lethality and infectivity associated with those two agents.[4,5] Twice in the past 20 years "dirty" bombs have either been planned or planted (and fortunately not used) so such devices would be the most likely source of radiation used by terrorists. However, to underscore what was stated above based on past experience a natural or industrial event would be most likely (Table 53-1).

To prepare for the kinds of scenarios described above, there are certain terms with which one must be familiar. A mass casualty *incident* is one that results in a number of patients that a community healthcare system has the resources to treat,

TABLE 53-1. EXAMPLES OF CBRNE EVENTS

	Natural	Industrial	Terrorist
Chemical	—	Accidental release of methyl isocyanate in Bhopal, India, 1984	Release of sarin by Aum Shinrikyo Tokyo Subway, 1995
Biologic	Spanish Flu Pandemic, 1918		US Anthrax Attacks, 2001
Radiologic	Tsunami affecting Fukushima nuclear power plant in Okuma, Japan, 2011	Three Mile Island, 1979 Chernobyl, 1986	Dirty Bomb—Chechen Rebels, 1995
Nuclear	Solar Flairs	—	—
Explosive	Mount St. Helens volcanic eruption, 1980	Fire at petroleum plant in Abule-Egba, Lagos, Nigeria in 2006	Suicide bombers

despite turmoil and confusion. A mass casualty *event* is one that overwhelms the hospital or the community's healthcare system. One also must be cognizant of the fact that though she or he might never plan to participate in a humanitarian mission overseas and therefore think that there is no need to train to work in an austere environment, depending on the circumstances of the disaster in which one finds one's self the environment may be
2 very austere indeed. Any time a situation arises in which medical capability is significantly below standards to which we are accustomed in the United States the anesthesiologist is indeed practicing in an austere environment. This austerity might occur in a:

- Mass casualty event in which the number of cases overwhelms capacity
- Natural disaster in which the hospital is damaged or loses electricity or water
- Disaster (natural/industrial/terrorist) in which care is provided on site

As described above, graduates of anesthesia training programs in North America can cope well in such situations, provided that they understand the basic requisites of disaster management, the focus of this chapter.

PREPARATION—PERSONAL PREPAREDNESS

Family Plan

In order to manage the numbers of casualties that would be expected during a mass casualty one must be prepared.[6,7] Often overlooked during emergency preparedness and disaster management training is the development of a family plan and a personal preparedness plan. The former is important whether one is single or lives alone. Whether or not one has a pet, family, or friends living with them, or has legal responsibility for a loved one (elderly
3 parents, disabled person) one must have a plan for these individuals that provides care for and information to loved ones. There are a number of websites that guide one through the creation of such a plan (Appendix I). During hurricane Katrina ~35% of policemen and firemen did not show up for work—this should not come as a surprise to anyone.[8] These individuals may have had to evacuate a parent in an assisted living facility or children in a day care center. Just as the military requires service members to have a family care plan (and a Will and Last Testament!), as a critically important healthcare provider we must have family care plans as well. However, if you know that you will be unavailable during a disaster then you have a responsibility to inform your employer or group of your personal situation. Even evacuation requires a plan. All family plans should include periodic family drills and updates. Plans might include situations such as what to do if there is a fire, what to do if parents do not make it home, the location of second copies of all important documents, where to meet if the house or neighborhood is destroyed or not accessible. Many assume that they will be able to communicate with loved ones during a disaster but often cell phone towers are damaged or so many people are trying to use the system that the network is overwhelmed. Plan in advance so that you are prepared for these contingencies.

And just as service members have a duffel bag or sea bag packed with toiletries, bedding, change of clothes, money, flash lights, and battery operated radio, those with such important roles as ours ideally should have a packed duffel bag as well. In a hurricane, earthquake, flood, tornado, or huge solar flair, loss of electric power is very likely. ATMs, gas pumps, toll booths and so on do not function without electricity—hence the need for some cash, flash lights, battery controlled radio (to stay abreast of the news)—and a vehicle that has a fuel tank that is not on empty!

Government Plan

In September 2011, the United States Department of Homeland Security published its first edition of a 111-page document National Preparedness Goal.[9] Figure 53-1 lists the multiple issues for which FEMA must prepare, and with which agencies it must coordinate—with the United States Departments of Justice, of Health and Human Services, of Agriculture, of Commerce, and of Defense. Of note is that within the "Response" section, medical response is one of eleven for which the government has planned—a response which is under the auspices of the Department of Health and Human Services (DHHS). DHHS created and maintains a National Disaster Medical System (NDMS). Unfortunately, the system has not been adequately established and maintains. As

Prevention	Protection	Mitigation	Response	Recovery
Planning				
Public information and warning				
Operational coordination				
Forensics and attribution Intelligence and information sharing Interdiction and disruption Screening, search, and detection	Access control and identity verification Cybersecurity Intelligence and information sharing Interdiction and disruption Physical protective measures Risk management for protection programs and activities Screening, search, and detection Supply chain integrity and security	Community resilience Long-term vulnerability reduction Risk and disaster resilience assessment Threats and hazard identification	Critical transportation Environmental response/health and safety Fatality management services Infrastructure systems Mass care services Mass search and rescue operations On-scene security and protection Operational communications Public and private services and resources Public health and medical services Situational assessment	Economic recovery Health and social services Housing Infrastructure systems Natural and cultural resources

FIGURE 53-1. Lists the multiple issues for which FEMA must prepare, and with which agencies it must coordinate.

highlighted by the US response to the earthquake in Haiti in 2010 the DHHS maintains only three International Medical Surgical Response Teams (IMSuRT), teams that were established with the idea that they would provide care to US citizens injured in areas of conflict. Unfortunately only one is funded and equipped and prior to Haiti, it had only been activated and used once—for the earthquake that occurred in 2003 in Bam, Iran.

Other teams that DHHS maintains in its NDMS in addition to the IMSuRTs are as follows:

Disaster Medical Assistance Team (DMAT)—a team that supposedly can rapidly mobilize and whose goal is to set up and staff with physicians, nurses and other support personnel emergency facilities and pharmaceutical dispensaries geographically as close as possible to a disaster. The teams are supposed to be self-sustaining for at least 72 hours before they require outside logistics. Just as the reserve military forces do, a DMAT is supposed to train 1 week-end a month. Not many surgeons and not many anesthesiologists have joined a DMAT as the team does not have the capacity to perform surgical procedures! Disaster Mortuary Team (DMORT) as the name implies is a team that would manage large numbers of dead following a mass casualty event with capacity to conduct forensic examinations. National Veterinary Response Team (NVRT) is a team established to provide veterinary services as well as zoonotic disease surveillance.

Most recently, the DHHS through its NDMS is planning and creating 15 Medical Specialty Enhancement Teams (MSETs). MSETsare going to consist of a group of precredentialed anesthesiologists and surgeons (30 of each), along with a few pediatricians. The concept is that there would be a pool of specialists who would be activated during a crisis, whether domestic or international, and would have sufficient logistic support that the team could deploy to either a fixed facility or a field site. Once activated MSET members would be federal employees during their deployments for a minimum of 2 weeks and would be protected by workers' compensation laws, the federal tort claims act, and the Uniformed Services Employment and Reemployment Rights Act (USERRA). DHHS knows that many anesthesia providers do not have time for monthly drills or frequent call ups that the DMATs have. Although MSET members would be encouraged to train with DMATs, participation in an MSET will require far less of an investment in time. However, if activated, members of the teams would be expected to deploy or risk being dropped from the team and program. MSETs are a work in progress and many of the details of logistics and training are unanswered. It is hoped that once successfully established the size and number of teams could be expanded and the teams better developed to respond to future disasters, whether they be acts of nature or of terrorists. Please note however that as mentioned above, the initial response is local—such teams might take 2 or 3 days or longer to mobilize and deploy.

NGOs' Plans

Ever since the anthrax attacks of 2000 and 2001, the destruction of the World Trade Center Towers on September 11, 2001, the SARS epidemic of 2004, and the continued devastation caused by nature (hurricanes, earthquakes, tornadoes, floods, and fires), The Joint Commission (TJC), the American Hospital Association, and state and county health departments have more closely monitored and evaluated hospitals' and communities' emergency preparedness. In 2003, TJC published its "Health Care at the Crossroads: Strategies for Creating and Maintaining Community-Wide Emergency Preparedness Systems".[10] The white paper has not been updated but emergency preparedness is one of the "standards" TJC uses to certify hospitals. Since 2003 it has hosted annual conferences, the most recent addressing how the two hospitals and their employees responded to the tornado that struck Joplin on May 20, 2011.[11]

TJC recognizes that there has been a change in healthcare delivery in the United States over the last several years and decades, reflective of similar problems faced worldwide, that has left the healthcare system under-funded with limited resources and ever
4 increasing demand. Despite the best effort of law enforcement, fire and rescue teams, and emergency medical agencies, hospitals will continue to play a vital role in helping communities respond to catastrophic events, whether natural, unintentional, or terrorist-initiated. TJC was proactive in recognizing that, "It is no longer sufficient to develop disaster plans and dust them off if a threat appears imminent. Rather a system of preparedness across communities must be in place everyday".[10] The TJC acknowledged the need, despite decreasing healthcare resources, for what it describes as "surge capacity" within healthcare systems to handle the potentially hundreds, if not thousands or more, of patients who might be victims of catastrophic events. By planning and drilling, TJC hopes to reduce the appeal to terrorists of using WMD as an effective means of terrorism, and to help communities better respond to natural disasters. The white paper TJC published focused on three major areas:

I. Enlisting the community to develop the local response.
II. Focusing on the key aspects of the system that prepares the community to mobilize to care for patients, protect its staff, and serve the public.
III. Establishing the accountabilities, oversight, leadership, and sustainment of a community-preparedness system.

While the guidelines are just that—guidelines that are not mandatory nor required by law, all hospitals aspire to have TJC accreditation and from that perspective, the white paper was important in that hospitals do have biannual drills of their emergency preparedness and disaster management plans, sometimes coordinating with local law enforcement agencies and health departments and emergency medical response teams to create as realistic scenarios as possible. Unfortunately, the participation of anesthesia departments in these drills is often minimal. Drills are usually held on week days during working hours—because anesthesia departments are fully staffed and completely operational during those hours hospital administrators certify that they can handle the number of casualties coming through their ED; for financial reasons, the drills are not very realistic—surgical procedures are never canceled and the system is never tested at night or on weekends. At night when there is minimal telecommunications personnel in place how would a hospital mobilize its staff? Many have telephone "trees" but again because they are not tested many anesthesia providers have long since misplaced their contact information. Even if tested, how operational would the plan be during a major disaster when communication systems are overwhelmed? Short text communication would be the best way for departments to alert personnel to the disaster. Other advantages to having anesthesia departments actually participate in drills would be the establishment of trust with liaisons in the emergency response community and with local law enforcement agencies. How much better the outcome would have been if that had been the case in Moscow during the 2002 Nord-Ost siege when the Spetsnaz forces most likely used carfentanil against Chechen rebels without informing emergency response or hospital personnel resulting in 170 deaths.[12]

Impediments to the establishment of effective response plans are not only financial but also based on a lack of awareness of what occurs during a disaster. As Israelis know from their years of dealing with suicide bombers, and as the Japanese found out during the release of sarin by Aum Shinrikyo terrorist group in the Tokyo subway system in 1996, victims do NOT go to level I trauma centers, nor do they wait to be transported by emergency medical teams—they fan out in all directions to whatever healthcare facility they can find and they do so on foot, by private vehicles, by whatever means available.[13] St. Luke's hospital in Tokyo found itself inundated with close to 900 patients after the subway sarin attacks—its ED, lobby entrance—almost the entire first floor of the hospital was crammed with patients—none of whom had been decontaminated, and all of whom created a chaotic situation that was difficult to manage, and which delayed treatment for those who needed it most. The affected patients required treatment best understood by anesthesiologists who use cholinesterase inhibitors daily and best administered by intravenous lines inserted by these same providers. Furthermore, because of the size of most anesthesia departments, assuming 70% of providers will actually respond to a mass casualty event or disaster, there will be sufficient personnel for the providers to cover all the healthcare facilities operating suites (including obstetrical suites—a disaster has yet to occur that prevents pregnant women from going into labor and delivering). Other places anesthesia providers can assist in management of healthcare delivery during a disaster include:

- to assist in triage outside the hospital (who better to manage the pain or labored respiration of the expectant patient?),
- to assist in decontamination (who better to evaluate for the presence of anticholinesterase (nerve) agents or cyanide toxicity),
- to assist with vascular access or airway management (made more difficult if wearing a HAZMAT suit and even more difficult if one has never worn such a suit), or
- to assist in ventilator management in the ICU or in overflow areas of the hospital such as the PACU of patients with respiratory failure caused by a nerve agent or biologic agent.

ROLE OF ANESTHESIOLOGIST IN MANAGING MASS CASUALTIES

It is difficult to anticipate every situation in which anesthesiologists could be asked to assist in managing mass casualty situations. For example, on October 26, 2002, terrorists held 750 hostages at the Nord-Ost Theater in Moscow. Many believe that the authorities instilled nebulized or volatile carfentanil into the air ducts of the opera house, thereby immobilizing the terrorists.[12] Unfortunately, because of the incapacitating effect of carfentanil, the hostages became victims too. Patients were transported from the theater to hospitals without any treatment prior to arrival. Ideally, anesthesiologists or other healthcare providers with an opioid antagonist such as naloxone should have been readily available and present at the site to manage both hostages and the terrorists. Unfortunately, this was not the case.

Anesthesiologists' basic understanding of physiology and pharmacology, their airway skills, their fluid resuscitation exper-
5 tise, their ability to manage ventilators and to provide anesthesia in the field environment, in the emergency department, in the operating room, and in intensive care units (ICUs) will be invaluable. In these mass casualty situations, many patients suffer burns, fractures, lacerations, soft tissue trauma, and amputations that will require triage, stabilization in the emergency room or in some other facility near the emergency room, and either more definitive treatment in the operating room or in the ICU.

During a mass casualty incident an anesthesiologist may well be asked to provide anesthetic services in an area other than the operating room or ICU. One will not know where one will be working until reporting to the hospital and the command and control center established to manage the incident.[14] The site of the command and control center is pre-established and outlined in the hospital's emergency preparedness plan, but typically within the hospital's emergency department or in close proximity. Other entrances to the hospital are typically closed during a mass casualty incident for the purposes of maintaining control of the numbers of patients that might present and to allow for decontamination of patients if necessary avoiding exposure of hospital personnel to contagious agents or transferrable substances such as nerve agents. The lack of such control and decontamination of the Tokyo subway sarin attack victims in 1995 resulted in a number of healthcare workers becoming ill by absorbing sarin from patients who had not been properly decontaminated.[13] Not only were they unable to work but they became patients themselves, increasing the number of patients requiring care and consuming resources.

Triage

6 If assigned to triage patients, the anesthesiologist will be expected to classify patients into four groups—those requiring immediate care, delayed care, first aid, and expectant. The latter group includes those expected not to survive, or, because of the number of patients arriving, those for whom there are not adequate personnel or resources to adequately resuscitate without jeopardizing the lives of many more patients who would not receive the care they require and for whom the prognosis is more favorable. Experience has taught that initially triage officers are "conservative"—they try to save as many as possible, but over days, if not hours they gain experience and become better at identifying patients for whom resources exist to improve outcome. In the future, biotechnology may play a role[15] but at present hospitals must rely on physicians' experience and again because of their knowledge of the hospitals resources—in the OR and ICU they may well be the ideal triage officer. He or she will have to assess and decide if patients fall into one of the four groups. "Expectant" patients are usually transported to an area separate from the ED where they can be provided comfort care, such a site must be situated such that newly arriving patients are not exposed to the sight of dying patients. Anesthesiologists may well be assigned to provide such care because of expertise in managing airways, in establishing intravenous access for the administration of medications, and

our familiarity with the available anxiolytic and analgesic medications. As emotionally difficult as the process might be of identifying or managing patients not expected to survive is the assessment of patients who may have been injured or been affected during a disaster but do not appear to require treatment, but who might require delayed care. Depending on the agent, diagnosis of those requiring therapy:

- Chemical (nerve) agents: If only headache, meiosis, rhinorrhea, and lacrimation after exposure, patients can be decontaminated (see later) and dismissed. Patients with dyspnea, bronchospasm, or arrhythmias will require treatment with atropine.
- Biologic agents: Fever, rash, dyspnea, cough
- Radiation/nuclear: Nausea within 6 hours of exposure; because of the prevalence for those with this symptom, check leukocyte count, dismiss, and have the patient return in 48 hours for repeat check—if no change in count, no therapy is indicated.
- Explosive: If tympanic membranes are intact and SpO_2 is within normal limits, other injuries are unlikely.

Decontamination

In most situations, people in contact with chemical agents or radioactive materials are decontaminated by those with proper training—the decontamination is normally performed first and then patients are evaluated and triaged. The process is usually fairly straightforward; clothes are removed and individuals are washed with copious amounts of water (the contaminated water and apparel can present quite a challenge!); if individuals have been exposed to a chemical agent, a dilute solution of sodium hypochlorite 0.5% (household bleach) can be used.

However, if the patient presents with life-threatening injury, the patient is treated first and decontaminated afterward. Patients with severe chemical agent poisoning may present with acute respiratory failure requiring emergency tracheal intubation. In this scenario, an anesthesiologist would be assigned to the decontamination station. For obvious reasons the intubation would have to be performed with the anesthesiologist wearing a hazard material (HAZMAT) or a biohazard suit with multiple-layered gloves and a gas mask. The suits are not insulated and if the decontamination is performed outside the hospital the extremes of temperature can significantly hinder performance, as does the decreased manual dexterity because of the gloves and the impairment in vision from the face hoods. Ideally individuals with prior training would manage the airway intubation but depending on circumstances that may not happen. As many have learned from the past experience, it is best to anticipate the unexpected, and to be flexible if the maximum numbers of patients are to be saved. Preparation of equipment and drugs before the arrival of contaminated patients decreases the difficulties with manual dexterity that are encountered while wearing the multiple-layered or rubber gloves. Consider securing the airway with a laryngeal mask airway, when indicated, rather than with a tracheal tube.

Emergency Department

Another place where an anesthesiologist might be assigned is the emergency department. While some level I trauma centers have an anesthesia team assigned to support the emergency department, this is not the norm. Depending on the types of casualties, but especially for casualties from a violent explosion, anesthesiologists might be assigned to manage the airway and secure
7 central venous access. Anesthesiologists should position themselves at the head of the bed and assume responsibility for the airway and venous access. For the former, it would be ideal to have two or three assistants (one providing in-line C-spine stabilization, another individual applying cricoid pressure, and a third individual administering medications.) Sometimes it is necessary to remind emergency room physicians and trauma surgeons that "A" (airway) and "B" (breathing) come before "C" (circulation); certainly, the primary and secondary surveys can be conducted during this critical time point but ventilation and oxygenation must be assured.

In previous industrial accidents and fires, appropriate management of the airway has been critical. Patients with large-area burns will require establishment of intravenous access for provision of intravascular volume resuscitation. Depending on the event (burn vs. a crush injury—protocols for fluid resuscitation vary), in patients with extensive soft tissue and skeletal muscle damage, alkalinization of the urine with volume resuscitation and diuresis may be organ-and life-saving. If chemical weapons are also used, again depending on the severity of the injury, not only may tracheal intubation be required, but ventilator management may be necessary.

The remainder of this chapter review the four major types of agents available to terrorists, recognizing that similar injuries can be caused by industrial catastrophes (thousands of deaths and injuries from methyl isocyanate in Bhopal, India, December 1984) or natural disasters (radiation exposure as a result of the tsunami that hit Japan in 2011).

CHEMICAL

Nerve Agents

Prior to the last century, it was unthinkable that rogue states or terrorists would use chemical agents. During the first World War, more than one million soldiers and civilians were exposed to chemical gas injuries with over 100,000 of them dying. In 1935, Italy invaded Abyssinia (Ethiopia) and during that invasion, sprayed mustard gas from aircrafts. When Japan invaded China in 1937, mustard gas, phosgene, and hydrogen cyanide were used. In that same year, German chemical laboratories produced the first nerve agent, tabun. During 1963 to 1967, Egypt used phosgene and mustard agents in support of South Yemen during the civil war in that country. When Iraq attacked Iran in the 1980s, mustard gas and nerve agents were used. In all these examples, chemical agents were used by the military during armed conflict. The governments mentioned above have all signed in the Chemical Weapons Convention. January 2012 marked the end of an era as the United States, in compliance with the Chemical Weapons Convention ratified by the Senate in 1997, the U.S. Army Chemical Materials Agency completed destruction of 27,000 tons of chemical weapons that it had manufactured and stored over the years.[16]

However, as one era ended another one had already begun. In 1994 and 1995, the use of the nerve agent, sarin, by the Japanese cult Aum Shinrikyo was a major turning point for it was the first time that a terrorist group had used a nerve agent in a terrorist attack. More than 5,000 persons were evaluated at hospitals of whom approximately 1,000 had been exposed to the nerve agent and 18 died. There is no doubt in anyone's mind that chemical agents will be used again in the future. The nerve agents are so named because of their mechanism of action (Table 53-2).

Similar to organophosphate insecticides and to the anticholinesterase drugs anesthesiologists use daily, nerve agents inhibit acetylcholinesterase. This inhibition results in excessive amounts of acetylcholine (the reason a cholinergic agent such as atropine

TABLE 53-2. TOXICITY OF NERVE AGENTS

Series	G[a]	V	Novichok[b]
	GA (tabun)	VE	
	GB (sarin)	VG	
	GD (soman)	VM	
	GF	VR	
		VX	

[a]Developed by but never used by Germany during 1930s.
[b]Manufactured by the USSR in 1980s and 1990s. G series agents are known as Nonpersistent whereas the V agents are persistent (in the environment) and 10× more toxic than the G agents. VX is the only agent ever fielded by the United States.

or glycopyrrolate is administered any time we inject an anticholinesterase such as neostigmine) at preganglionic muscarinic and postganglionic muscarinic and nicotinic receptors, leading to copious secretions, meiosis, arrhythmias, bronchospasm, tonic muscle contractions, respiratory paralysis, seizures, and death. Similar to managing the side effects of neostigmine, a cholinergic agent and competitive muscarinic blocker (i.e., atropine or glycopyrrolate) is administered to attenuate and block the muscarinic side effects of the agents.

When anticipating a nerve agent attack, US military personnel pretreat themselves with low-dose pyridostigmine and don personal protective equipment; the latter prevents the agent from contacting and wetting skin from which it is readily absorbed, and low-dose pyridostigmine binds to acetylcholinesterase preventing any nerve agent that is absorbed from binding to the enzyme. Pyridostigmine is a reversible drug that will be metabolized over time whereas the nerve agents bind irreversibly.

US military personnel carry syringes of atropine and of pralidoxime chloride (2-PAM-CL), an oxime that reactivates acetylcholinesterase by removing the nerve agent from its binding site on the enzyme. Spontaneous reactivation of enzyme complex is variable, which partly accounts for differences in acute toxicity between the nerve agents. 2-PAM-CL is administered to reactivate the dialkylphosphonyl acetylcholinesterase enzyme more quickly,[17] thus making the complex resistant to spontaneous hydrolysis and more likely to reactivation by oximes. The most optimistic estimates are that after exposure 30 minutes will elapse before casualties are transported to EDs, the diagnosis of nerve agent attack is made and the oxime can be administered. Thirty minutes is equally optimistic as there have been deaths at chemical weapon manufacturing facilities within 2 minutes of accidental exposure. Toxicity of the nerve agents is not just related to which agent, but also to the dose of agent to which one is exposed, and also the duration of exposure. However, if numbers of casualties arrive at a triage site outside a hospital ED, the sooner one administers an oxime such as 2-PAM-CL the better. Most of the nerve agents can be reversed with the exception of soman. With soman, aging of AChE occurs so fast that no clinically relevant spontaneous reactivation of AChE can occur. The oxime must be administered before all the enzyme become aged. Even though aging occurs more slowly and reactivation occurs relatively rapidly in the case of nerve agents other than soman, early oxime administration is still clinically important in patients poisoned with these agents. Experimental studies on the treatment of nerve agent poisoning have to be interpreted with caution. Some studies have used prophylactic protocols, whereas the drugs concerned (atropine, oxime) would only be given to a civilian population after exposure. The experimental use of pyridostigmine before nerve agent exposure, although rational, is not of relevance in the civilian context. With the possible exception of the treatment of cyclosarin (GF) and soman poisoning, a review of available experimental evidence suggests that there are no clinically important differences between the different oximes in the treatment of nerve agent poisoning, if studies employing pretreatment with pyridostigmine are excluded.[17]

Diagnosis

Patients exposed to a nerve agent, either ingested, inhaled, or via the transdermal route present with evidence of muscarinic site stimulation: Airway, pupillary, and GI tract constriction; bradycardia; and activation of the glands within the eyes, nose, mouth, and sweat glands manifested by intense lacrimation, rhinorrhea, salivation, and sweating. The degree of exposure correlates with the amount of secretions produced. Nicotinic stimulation at preganglionic sites leads to tachycardia and hypertension, and at the nicotinic acetylcholine receptor on the neuromuscular junction, fasciculations, twitching, fatigue, and flaccid paralysis. The excessive parasympathetic activity leads to miosis and loss of accommodation so that patients complain of blurred vision. Within the respiratory system, the increased parasympathetic activity leads to bronchorrhea and bronchoconstriction which together with the respiratory muscle fatigue initially manifests as coughing, wheezing, and shortness of breath. The agent on the skin will produce localized sweating and fasciculations obvious to the naked eye. Within the cardiovascular system, activity within the muscarinic system leads to bradycardia, but depending on the degree of nicotinic activity in the preganglionic nodes, a patient's heart rate may be low, normal, or high. Within the GI tract, the increased parasympathetic activity leads to nausea, vomiting, diarrhea, and incontinence. This overall unopposed parasympathetic activity leads to a pneumonic of "DUMBELS" (D—diarrhea, U—urination, M—miosis, B—bronchorrhea and bronchoconstriction, E—emesis, L—lacrimation, and S—salivation).

Treatment

8 The toxicity of the nerve agents depends on the compound delivered, the dose that is delivered (LC), and the time (t) that an individual is exposed to that dose. For example, a patient exposed to 10 mg/m^3 of an agent for 10 minutes would have an LCt of 100 mg/min/m^3. The same could be achieved by being exposed to a concentration of 100 mg/m^3 for only 1 minute. The treatment for nerve agent poisoning is one with which every anesthesiologist is familiar. Atropine is a competitive muscarinic blocker. Pralidoxime chloride is the better long-term treatment as it reactivates acetylcholinesterase by removing the organophosphate compound. Atropine is administered at a dose of 2 to 6 mg or more and repeated every 5 to 10 minutes until secretions begin to decrease (the patient is no longer salivating) and ventilation is improved. In severe casualties, 15 to 20 mg would not be unusual and some casualties have required gram amounts of atropine. The US military travels with automatic injectors containing 2 mg of atropine and 600 mg of 2-PAM-CL.

Depending on the extent of exposure, treatment is different. For minimal exposure, often seen with brief exposure to nerve agent vapor, patients may complain of headache and tightness in the chest and manifest meiosis, rhinorrhea, and salivation. Individuals must be removed from further exposure, clothing removed, topical atropine to the eye if pain is significant, and wet decontamination if there was any liquid exposure. With moderate exposure, the same signs are present, but now the patient demonstrates more severe rhinorrhea, complains of dyspnea, and on examination, there is evidence of bronchospasm and muscle fasciculation. Patients with moderate (and severe) poisoning require treatment with atropine and 2-PAM-CL intramuscularly. Casualties again must have their clothing removed and if they were exposed to liquid nerve agent, they need to go through a wet decontamination process. With severe exposure, the same symptoms as mentioned above are present, but now the patient manifests severe respiratory compromise, flaccid paralysis, incontinence, arrhythmias, and convulsions. After decontamination the patient will require repetitive doses of intravenous atropine, along with intramuscular 2-PAM-CL, IV benzodiazepines to treat the seizures (caused by the muscarinic effects of the nerve agents within the CNS[18]), and intubation and mechanical ventilation depending on the degree of respiratory compromise.

With nerve injury casualties, decontamination is critical. It needs to be done as quickly as possible, first by leaving the area of exposure. As commented at the beginning of this chapter, healthcare and emergency workers in Japan became victims themselves by standing unprotected in the subway cars in which there was liquid sarin with some vapor.[13] Patients are decontaminated by removing their clothing and washing with copious amounts of water and 0.5% hypochlorite (dilute household bleach). The bleach is not as critical as washing with copious amounts of water. Depending on the number of casualties, emergency departments have plans in place to set up fire trucks side-by-side with a "chamber" established between the two trucks in which individuals would disrobe as they came into the chamber and be exposed to water sprays as they walked through the chamber to the other side. From there, depending upon the severity of the symptoms, they would receive atropine, 2-PAM-CL, and further treatment.

Pulmonary Agents

The so-called pulmonary agents are by nature gases at room temperature, and almost any gas could be considered a pulmonary agent if released in sufficient quantity in a closed environment to displace O_2 with the exposed subjects dying by asphyxiation. Chlorine and phosgene are considered the classical pulmonary agents and the two most likely to be used by terrorists. If quantities are released that are sufficient to displace O_2, then death results from asphyxia. In addition, these two gases are extremely toxic to the lungs; individuals who survive the acute exposure if they have inhaled even small amounts often develop acute lung injury or acute respiratory distress syndrome (ARDS). However, the treatment is no different from what a critical care anesthesiologist would do in managing a patient with silo filler's disease or farmer's lung, which develops after exposure to nitrogen dioxide when a farm worker opens or enters a silo that has inadequate ventilation. The treatment of the resulting noncardiogenic pulmonary edema from NO_2 or the pulmonary agents is supportive: Mechanical ventilation using small tidal volumes (6 to 8 mL/kg), peak airway pressures <30 cm H_2O), positive end expiratory pressure, and inspired oxygen concentrations of 50% to 60% or less.

Blood Agents

The third and final class of chemical toxins includes the blood agents—hydrogen cyanide and cyanogen chloride. Because of the instability of the latter, hydrogen cyanide is more likely to be used by terrorists in a closed environment as an aerosol. Again, anesthesiologists are familiar with this class of substances because of our clinical use of sodium nitroprusside as an intravascular vasodilator, which we know, has cyanide as a metabolite. Cyanide inhibits cellular respiration by interrupting the oxidative electron transfer process in mitochondria. The treatment for cyanide toxicity is similar to what we anesthesiologists would do for someone who had an accidental overdose of sodium nitroprusside: Intravenous thiosulfate and supportive care including tracheal intubation, ventilation with 100% oxygen, and inotropes and vasopressors to stabilize the cardiovascular system.

BIOLOGIC

History

This section considers the naturally occurring infectious agents as well as those most likely to be used by terrorists. Many of the latter caused plagues in the past or were used as weapons. Infectious organisms have been used as biologic weapons since the dawn of history. Ghengis Khan is reported to have used cats infected with fleas bearing the plague to destroy towns in his conquest of Asia. British forces distributed blankets that harbored small pox virus (the blankets had been used by patients who had smallpox) to American Indians killing more than 50% of the infected tribes.[19] In World War II, Unit 731, a Japanese military unit is reported to have dropped plague-infected fleas over populated areas of China causing outbreaks of plague and killing several hundred thousand people.[19]

The ideal biologic agent is one that has the greatest potential for adverse public health consequences, generating mass casualties, and with potential for easy large-scale dissemination that could cause mass hysteria and civil disruption. Such a weapon should be relatively easy to produce, inexpensive, highly infectious, and contagious, resulting in widespread morbidity and mortality. In order to be effective, there should be little or no natural immunity, which is currently the case with diseases such as smallpox for which we no longer routinely vaccinate individuals except in the military and in high-risk public health areas. There
9 are three categories of biologic weapons (Table 53-3). Category A are those agents which are highly contagious and fit all the characteristics of a relatively ideal biologic agent.

Smallpox

The last case of naturally occurring smallpox in the world was reported in 1977 in Somalia.[20] In 1978, two laboratory workers in the United Kingdom were infected with smallpox.[20] In 1980, the World Health Organization (WHO) announced that the world was free of this scourge. Terrorists might consider using small pox as weapon because an increasing number of peoples no longer carry immunity; routine vaccination for smallpox is no longer carried out, except in the military and for some public healthcare workers considered at high risk of contracting the disease (individuals who the government would rely on to staff vaccination stations if there were a break-out).[20] Forty percent to eighty percent of patients exposed to the smallpox virus will come down with the disease. Smallpox is highly infective, requiring only 10 to 100 organisms to infect an individual. The mortality rate is approximately 30% in unvaccinated patients and as high as 50% if smallpox occurs in communities that have no native immunity against smallpox. The protective effect of the smallpox vaccine decreases with time, but even at 20 years, the vaccine would provide some protection.

When an unvaccinated person is initially infected, she or he develops a prodrome of malaise, headache, and backache with the onset of fever to as high as 40°C. The fever decreases over the next 3 or 4 days at which time a rash develops. This progression is in contradistinction to chicken pox in which the rash develops

TABLE 53-3. BIOLOGIC AGENTS USED FOR WARFARE

Category A	Category B	Category C
B. anthracis (anthrax)	*Coxiella burnetti* (Q fever)	Various equine encephalitic viruses
Variola major (smallpox)	*Vibrio cholerae* (cholera)	
Y. pestis (plague)	*Burkholderii mallei* (glanders)	
Clostridium botulinum (botulism)	Enteric pathogens (*E. coli* 0157: H7, salmonella, shigella)	
F. tularenis (tularemia)	Cholera, cryptosporidium	
Viral hemorrhagic fever (Ebola, Lassa, Marburg, Argentine)	Various encephalitic viruses	
	Various biologic toxins	

Category A are those agents which are highly contagious and fit all the characteristics of a relatively ideal biologic agent.
Category B agents are relatively easy to disseminate but have low mortality rates.
Category C agents are emerging pathogens that might be engineered for biologic warfare.

at the same time as the fever. Unlike chicken pox, smallpox has a predilection for the distal extremities and face, though no part of the body is spared. Also, all lesions in a patient with smallpox are at the same stage, whereas with chicken pox, lesions are at multiple different stages including papules, vesicles, pustules, and scabs. Most cases of smallpox are transmitted through aerosolized droplets that are inhaled, but clothes and blankets that have come in contact with pustules, until the scab falls off, are infectious; the organism can be transmitted in these linens.

Smallpox has probably been present in humans since 10,000 BC. It is transmitted human to human, and if used as a bioterrorism agent, would likely be dispersed by aerosols in the environment with the hope that multiple humans would be infected and would transmit it to other humans. There is evidence that the former Soviet Union has developed transgenic smallpox viruses that are very infectious and for which the US vaccine may not be completely protective. The time of onset after exposure to such a virus might be very short. Currently there are only two WHO-approved depositories of smallpox, at the CDC in Atlanta, Georgia, and at the Institute of Virus Preparations in Russia. With the collapse of the Soviet Union, there was a concern that some stores of smallpox made it into rogue countries that may have developed their own biologic weapons. A look at how the WHO eradicated smallpox might be helpful in understanding how the Unite States has prepared to respond to smallpox as a biologic weapon. In the 18th century, 400,000 Europeans a year were dying from smallpox. Though only 1% of patients who survive smallpox become blind, it accounted for one-third of all cases of blindness in Europe. The WHO eradicated smallpox by identifying patients with smallpox and placing them in strict quarantine. Such patients are readily identified because of the presence of smallpox lesions on the face. Patients were quarantined and all their contacts were vaccinated as there was a 3- to 7-day window with the naturally occurring virus before the patient developed symptoms and signs of smallpox.[21]

Vaccination against smallpox is controversial. The vaccine is made from a live vaccinia virus developed in calf lymph, but is not an attenuated smallpox virus itself. Smallpox is a member of the Orthopox genus of the pox varidae family of double-stranded deoxyribonucleic acid (DNA) viruses that also contain cowpox, monkeypox, and vaccinia. In the event of a documented case of smallpox, the CDC plans to quarantine the patient and immediate patient contacts within a certain geographic radius would be vaccinated. There are stockpiles of vaccines placed strategically throughout the United States just for such an event. A bifurcated needle is dipped into the reconstituted vaccine and then 10 to 15 jabs are made into the dermis of the upper deltoid. Because of the side effects of smallpox vaccinations, people with immunologic disorders, eczema (active or with a history of severe eczema), and pregnant or nursing women should not receive the vaccine. The CDC monitors for adverse side effects of vaccination; most are not serious, such as fever, rash, malaise, although two cases of cardiomyopathy[22] have been reported. There is no plan to vaccinate the US population. Many obstacles have been overcome to develop second and third generation small pox vaccines. Before 2001, the vaccine that was used, Dryvax, similar to what Jenner used in the 18th century, contained live attenuated virus and was the reason that immunocompromised individuals developed adverse events when vaccinated. From 2001 to the present vaccine, ACAM (Acambis Modified Vaccinia Ankara) has been used to vaccinate against smallpox. Dryvax and ACAM are fairly similar though the latter may be a little safer to use than Dryvax but not so much safer than immunocompromised individuals are offered the vaccine. To avoid the dangers of a live vaccine, an inactive vaccine (modified vaccinia Ankara (MVA) [Imvamune]) was developed[23]; the United States has a contract to purchase 20 million doses. The available evidence is that even immunocompromised individuals such as those with HIV infection might tolerate immunization.

The CDC and the state departments of health will implement their quarantine and vaccination plans should an index case or cluster cases occur.

Anthrax

Bacillus anthracis (anthrax) was probably used as a biologic weapon in the middle ages when troops laying siege to a town would catapult infected animal carcasses over the ramparts into the inhabited areas. For reasons discussed later, this method was not a particularly effective way of infecting the native population. During the 20th century, several countries including the United States, Great Britain, Russia, and Iraq studied ways to weaponize anthrax. Anthrax has appeal as a bioterrorism agent because if it can be "weaponized" (normally if anthrax spores are inhaled, they clump in the nasal pharynx). *B. anthracis* must be finely ground so that it readily aerosolizes and can get to and deposit in the terminal bronchioles and alveoli.[24] Inhalation anthrax, which was relatively uncommon in the past, has an 80% fatality rate. One of the letters that was mailed in the anthrax attacks of 2001 contained 2 g of weapons-grade anthrax. With an LD50 of 1,000 spores, under optimum conditions, this was enough material to infect 50 million individuals. In a terrorist attack, for maximum "effect" anthrax could be aerosolized and sprayed from airplanes or delivered through a dispersion device mounted on top of a missile. The attacks on North America in 2001 and the accidental release of spores at a biologic facility in the city of Sverdlovsk in the former Soviet Union in 1979 are illustrative of the potential of anthrax as a weapon. In the United States, 5 of 11 cases died (50% mortality rate); in the former Soviet Union, 66 of 77 died (86% mortality rate).[25] The Aun Shinrikyo also released anthrax spores in Tokyo in 1993. Fortunately, they used a nonpathogenic strain of anthrax and so there were no casualties.[24] As demonstrated in 2001 in the United States, terrorists are sophisticated enough that they might be successful in obtaining and releasing weapons-grade anthrax. Such attacks, even if detected early[26] would create mass hysteria and greatly affect the entire country and world.[27]

Anthrax is a gram-positive, spore-forming bacillus that is transmitted to humans from contaminated animals, their byproducts, or carcasses. Spores may persist in soil for years. The disease is all but gone from North America, but is still prevalent in many developing countries, and herbivores, especially cattle, usually die within 24 to 48 hours of contracting the disease. They have such a huge number of organisms that humans, who are relatively resistant to infection, can be exposed and contract the disease.[28]

There are three primary types of anthrax infection: Cutaneous, inhalation, and GI. Ninety-five percent of cases are cutaneous. From a public health perspective, we are worried most about inhalation anthrax, which worldwide usually affects 2,000 to 20,000 people per annum. People can be exposed through contact with animals in an agricultural setting or in an industrial setting, for example, a rendering plant or tanning facility, or as mentioned previously, in the production of biologic weapons.[29]

Anthrax has additional appeal to bioterrorists because inhalation anthrax is hard to detect. It manifests as an influenza-like disease with fever, myalgias, malaise, and a nonproductive cough with or without chest pain.[30] After a few days, the patient appears to get better, but then a couple days later the patient becomes much sicker with dyspnea, cyanosis, hemoptysis, stridor, and chest pain. The most notable finding on physical examination and laboratory testing is a widened mediastinum. Usually when a patient develops profound dyspnea, death ensues within 1 to 2 days. In the past, penicillin G was the treatment of choice, but since weaponized anthrax has been engineered to be resistant to penicillin G, ciprofloxacin or doxacycline is more commonly used. In the outbreaks in Florida, Washington, D.C. and New Jersey contacts of infected patients or people exposed to the spores were treated with ciprofloxacin or doxacycline. A recent study concluded 8 years later that this drug regimen is the best strategy for managing a small-scale attack as occurred in 2001.[31]

Plague

The oldest cases of *Yersinia pestis* (bubonic plague) were documented in China in the third century. *Y. pestis* has been thought to be the etiologic agent in multiple epidemics and three pandemics, the first of which was during the Roman emperor Justinian's reign, the second pandemic was during the 14th century—the Black Death—that killed one-third of the population of Europe, and the last at the end of the 19th century killed millions in China and India.[32] The first documented use of plague as a biologic weapon was in 1346 when the Tartars in their siege of the fortress at Kaffa catapulted infected corpses into the city.[19] The plague was used by Unit 731 to infect large areas of China, and as many as 200,000 Chinese may have died. More recently, the United States and Russia have studied *Y. pestis* as a bioagent, examining ways to aerosolize and ways to distribute the bacillus. Surprisingly, the organism is only viable for approximately 60 minutes after being distributed; if dispersed by an airplane, its viability would limit its infectivity for only 10 km from the dispersion site.

Y. pestis is a nonmotile, gram-positive bacillus. Rodents and fleas are its natural hosts, and they reinfect each other by fleas biting infected rodents. Soil can be contaminated and therefore rodents can acquire the disease simply by digging in an infected area. Humans are an accidental host, and they acquire the disease usually from a fleabite, though rarely there can be direct inoculation of infected material into a person. Direct person-to-person transmission occurs with pneumonic plague.

There are two types of plague: Bubonic and pneumonic. With bubonic plague, after a fleabite, there is a 2- to 6-day incubation period at which time there is the sudden onset of fever, chills, weakness, and headache. Intense painful swelling occurs in the lymph nodes, usually in the groin, axilla, or neck. This swelling or buboes are typically oval in nature, 1 to 10 cm in diameter and extremely tender. Up to 25% of patients will have pustules, papules, or skin lesions near these buboes. Without treatment, patients become septic, develop septic shock with cyanosis and gangrene in peripheral tissues, leading to the "black death" descriptor that was used during the epidemics in Europe. As mentioned, material from these buboes is infective only if inoculated into human tissue. However, patients who have bubonic plague can seed their lungs in which case they develop pneumonic plague. During coughing, they aerosolize *Y. pestis* which is highly contagious. Mortality for either form of the disease is over 50%. Diagnosis is made with a Gram stain or culture of organisms from blood, sputum, or buboes.

The treatment of choice is streptomycin, but chloramphenicol and tetracycline are acceptable alternatives. These patients with pneumonic plague should be managed as one would manage a patient with drug resistance to tuberculosis as the respiratory secretions are highly infectious. There is currently no vaccine against *Y. pestis.*

Tularemia

Francisella tularenis (tularemia) has some similarities to anthrax and plague, but is not nearly as dangerous. It was studied as a biologic weapon in the 20th century because it is highly infectious, requiring an innoculum of perhaps as small as only ten organisms.[33] During World War II, tularemia developed in soldiers along the German-Russian front that was thought secondary to the use of *F. tularenis* as a biologic weapon. The fact that both armies were infected underscores one of the dangers of using infectious agents as biologic weapons. Often these are dispersed with aerosols, and despite the best predictions of air currents, they are notoriously unpredictable; with the shifting air currents, one's own troops could become infected. Unit 731 of the Japanese army also studied the use of *F. tularenis* as a biologic weapon, and the United States and Russia were known to have grown large quantities of *F. tularenis* and stored it.

F. tularenis is a gram-negative, pleomorphic rod. There are several animal hosts, with the cotton-tailed rabbit being one of the most susceptible. Normally, humans acquire *tularenis* with direct contact of an infected animal or from the bite of an infected tick or deerfly.[33] Occasionally, the ingestion of infected food or inhalation of a small amount of aerosol will initiate the disease. There are two strains of *F. tularenis,* Jellison A and B, with the B strain being relatively innocuous, and in North America the A strain is quite virulent. Normally, a patient will develop a cutaneous ulcer at the site of entry after contact with an animal. As few as 10 or

50 organisms can invade the body either through hair follicles or miniabrasions. The incubation period is 2 to 6 days, at which time there is swelling and ulceration at the site of entry. As the swelling continues, the skin eventually breaks creating an ulcer, which develops a necrotic base that becomes black as it scars.

It is most likely that *F. tularenis* would be delivered from an aerosol from an airplane, in which case following inhalation, there is a 3- to 5-day incubation period, and then the onset of disease is marked with fever, pharyngitis, bronchitis, pneumonia, pleuritis, and hilar lymphadenopathy. Mortality rate for pneumonic tularemia is 5% to 15%.

The treatment of choice for tularemia is streptomycin, though gentamicin, tetracycline, and chloramphenicol have been used. There is a concern that the former Soviet Union, perhaps the United States, and perhaps terrorists have engineered *F. tularenis* to be resistant to a number of agents. Prophylaxis with streptomycin, ciprofloxacin, or doxycycline has been recommended in the past for individuals exposed to the organism. There was a vaccine available that comprised of an attenuated whole organism strain, but it is not available.

Botulism

The first known work with *Clostridium botulinum* (botulism) as a biologic weapon was in World War II. Both the Germans and Japanese military and scientific communities experimented with *C. botulinum*. Unit 731 fed pure cultures of *C. botulinum* to Chinese captives with devastating effects. Both the United States and former Soviet Union are known to have produced large quantities of *C. botulinum* toxin as has Iraq, Iran, Syria, and North Korea. In fact, after the first Gulf War, Iraq admitted to having over 19,000 L of concentrated botulism toxin of which almost half were loaded on military weapons.[34] Nineteen thousand liters of botulinum toxin is enough to kill the world's population three times over! More recently, Aum Shinrikyo, the cult in Japan, dispersed aerosols of botulinum toxin on three different occasions in Japan. Fortunately, their dispersal methods and the agent were associated with multiple problems and no one was injured. Of concern is that a terrorist organization working with a rogue state acquired and used botulinum as a bioterrorist weapon.

Botulinism manifests as neuroparalysis caused by the toxin from *C. botulinum*. Unlike all the other biologic mentioned previously, it is not caused by a live organism and is, therefore, not contagious. The organism from which botulinum toxin is derived is a gram-positive spore, which is an obligatory anaerobe, widely distributed in soil and in marine and agricultural products. Humans ingest *C. botulinum* without apparent effects until the organism begins to release toxins of which there are several. Toxins are distributed from the gastrointestinal (GI) tract, or from the lungs if inhaled, in the blood stream to cholinergic nerve endings where they block the release of acetylcholine at muscarinic and nicotinic receptors by inhibiting the intracellular fusion of the vesicles containing acetylcholine to nerve-terminal membrane for release into the synaptic cleft. This mechanism is the exact opposite of the chemical nerve agents such as sarin that result in an increase in the amount of acetylcholine at the cholinergic receptors but the end result is the same. Patients develop a progressive weakness and a flaccid paralysis that begin in the extremities, and progress until the respiratory muscles cease to contract. Of note, *C. botulinum* toxin is the most potent poison known to humans; the LD100 dose is only 1 pg.[35]

Shortly after ingestion or inhalation of the toxin, the incubation period is between 2 hours and 8 days, but most commonly between 12 and 36 hours.[36] As muscles become weak patients develop diplopia, dysphonia, dysarthria, dysphagia, and eventually dyspnea and finally paralysis. Along with the effects noted within the skeletal muscle system caused by the lack of acetylcholine at the nicotinic receptor, muscarinic blockade results in decreased salivation, ileus, and urinary retention, again the opposite of what is seen with nerve agent poisoning.

Toxins can be removed through gastric lavage, use of cathartics, and with enemas. The treatment of patients includes the use of a trivalent antitoxin. Patients with profound respiratory embarrassment should have their airways protected and mechanical ventilation initiated. Without the use of antitoxin, it takes the patient 2 to 8 weeks to recover. The mortality rate is quoted as 5% to 10%.

Hemorrhagic Fevers

There are a number of viral hemorrhagic fevers that are listed as category A agents including the arena viruses (lassa fever and others), bunya viruses (hanta), flaviruses (Dengue), and filoviruses (ebola and marburg). There are at least 18 viruses that cause human hemorrhagic fevers, which form a special group of viruses characterized by viral replication in lymphoid cells, after which patients develop fever and myalgia with an incubation of anywhere from 2 to 18 days, depending on the agent itself and the amount that is inhaled or inoculated across the dermis.[35] They encompass syndromes that vary from febrile hemorrhagic fever with edema to septic shock, which rapidly leads to death. Both the United States and the former Soviet Union have experimented and have weaponized several of these viruses. Studies in nonhuman primates suggest that the agents are highly infectious, requiring only a few virions to produce illness.[36] The Aum Shrinrikyo cult in Japan went to Africa in the 1990s to try to obtain an ebola virus which they planned to weaponize. There is no known incident where these agents have been used as a biologic weapon, but there is clear interest and potential for this use, so much so that the US government has recently initiated discussions on how to increase research into diagnostic tests and treatment with antivirals of the filoviruses (ebola viruses and marburg viruses).[37]

The viruses are single-stranded, ribonucleic acid (RNA) viruses which have a rodent or insect reservoir and are communicated to humans by inhalation of an aerosol, through contact with an infected animal, or the bite of an infected insect. Humans are not a reservoir for the virus. The hemorrhagic fevers are contagious, and person-to-person transmission in Africa has occurred. The incubation period is within several days of contact or inhalation of the agent, at which time patients present with fever, myalgia, and evidence of a capillary leak (systemic leak or pulmonary edema), thrombocytopenia and disseminated intravascular coagulation (DIC). The fatality rate, depending on the specific virus used is anywhere from 2% to 60%. There are no specific antiviral therapies for this class of viruses. Ribavirin, interferon-alpha, and hyperimmune globulin are often administered, with ribavirin being more protective against some of the viruses than others, but unfortunately one does not initially know what the etiologic agent is when the patient first presents. There is a live attenuated virus vaccine for yellow fever, but there are none for any of the other agents, though there is extensive, ongoing testing with the development of vaccines for several of these most dangerous viruses.

RADIATION—NUCLEAR

The greatest likelihood of dealing with patients who are exposed to ionizing radiation would come from a nuclear power plant or reactor accident, and in decreasing order of likelihood from a terrorist action and lastly from a detonation of a nuclear bomb. With respect to nuclear power plants, the US Nuclear Regulatory Commission has not found that people living in adjacent counties have increased rates of cancers but continues to study the issue.[38] Unfortunately, that is not the case when there is release of radioactive material as has occurred in the past at Chernobyl, and most recently at the Fukushima Daiichi nuclear power plant in Japan following the earthquake and tsunami on 11 March 2011. As the details of the disaster in Japan are still not completely clear, this discussion will focus on Chernobyl as it is claimed that the meltdown that occurred in Japan released only 10% as much radiation as occurred at Chernobyl.[39]

On April 26, 1986, workers at the Chernobyl nuclear power plant did not recognize or respond to evidence of one of the reactors malfunctioning, with loss of cooling capacity and an explosion of the nuclear reactor.[40] Two workers died as a direct effect of the explosion, while those who remained in shielded areas survived unless they went to fight the fire in which case they eventually died of radiation injury. Short-term gamma and beta emissions from the explosion and subsequent gamma and beta radiation from the reactor core debris killed many more with long-term health effects to the entire community. Because of a lack of protective clothing and respirators, the radioactive material that exploded into the atmosphere rained down for several days affecting many more workers and thousands of civilians. Primary sources of radiation were iodine-131, strontium-90, and cesium-137. During the subsequent 24 hours, 140,000 people were evacuated and potassium iodide tablets were distributed to as many people in the area as possible. Two hundred and thirty patients were subsequently hospitalized with many patients succumbing to infections because of bone marrow suppression, and in those patients in whom bone marrow transplantation was attempted, 17 of 19 died because of associated radiation burns. All told, radiation burns caused 21 deaths. Oropharyngeal burns occurred in 28 patients. Over the next several years, the average radiation exposure around Chernobyl was four times normal due to residual ground contamination. Almost two decades later, the effects of Chernobyl continue to be felt in the immediate vicinity and in the area down-wind from the reactor site.[40] The experience from Chernobyl should indicate the kind of injuries and results that anesthesiologists can anticipate from nuclear accidents including radiation burns, bone marrow suppression, the destruction of the lining of the GI tract, GI bleeding with translocation of bacteria, infection, sepsis, septic shock, and death. As evidenced by the experiences in Chernobyl, potassium iodide is indicated to protect the thyroid gland from taking up iodine-131, and other drugs are being considered such as 5-androstenediol.

There have been other situations from which we can learn during which people have been exposed to ionizing radiation. On March 28, 1979, at the Three Mile Island nuclear power plant, the number 2 nuclear reactor overheated, and because the pressure relief valve failed to close, radioactive coolant was released into the containment facility.[41] As is often the case, there were numerous communication missteps, which resulted in the release of inconsistent information, generating genuine fear among individuals living nearby the nuclear power plant. There were no biologic effects of the event, but severe psychological sequelae did result.

On September 13, 1987, in Goiania, Brazil, a lead canister containing between 1,400 and 1,600 curies of cesium-137 contaminated 250 people; four of whom died, but multiple individuals had short- and long-term health sequelae.[42] Mitigation efforts required the removal of 6,000 tons of clothing, furniture, dirt, trees, and other materials. The cesium had been left in a building in a lead canister when it was abandoned by its occupants; the canister was taken, opened by looters, and children played with the material.

Potential Sources of Ionizing Radiation Exposure

We are exposed to radiation on an annual basis from cosmic radiation, radon, medical devices, and in multiple stores and factories. In essence, half of our exposure comes from natural sources with most of the remaining exposure originating from medical imaging and devices.[38] A chest radiograph leads to 5 to 10 mrem of exposure, whereas a computerized tomographic scan can lead up to 5,000 mrem of exposure.

Obviously the greatest concern is the exposure to ionizing radiation that is unintentional as occurred at the Chernobyl nuclear power plants. Intentional exposure threats are the result of military conflict or terrorism. With respect to the former, the two situations in which this occurred were in Hiroshima and Nagasaki in 1945.

In Hiroshima, the bomb ("little boy") was only a 12.5-kiloton bomb, which killed an estimated 66,000 people and injured 69,000 more. The bomb that fell at Nagasaki ("fat boy") was a 22-kiloton plutonium implosion bomb, which killed between 39,000 and 74,000 people with 75,000 people sustaining severe injuries. We learned from that experience that the majority of casualties are from the initial blast, from fire, and from the collapse of buildings. Radiation exposure subsequently killed many more. With any nuclear explosion, many individuals will be injured or die from the tertiary effect of the blast. Patients could have burn, crush, or radiation injury or any combination thereof.

More recently, we recognize that exposure to ionizing radiation may be as a result of terrorism. The most likely event will be the use of a dispersion device such as a conventional weapon, that is, a bomb, surrounded with radionuclides such as cesium or strontium. In fact, in 1987, Iraq tested a 1-ton "dirty" bomb, and in 1996, Islamic terrorists in Chechnya placed a bomb packed with cesium-137 in a Moscow park that did not explode. While a radiation dispersion device remains the most likely event, terrorists could also target a nuclear power plant using commercial jet, munitions, or internal sabotage.

While a blast, crush, or thermal injury is readily apparent, the effects of ionizing radiation are usually not apparent. Individuals should be familiar with types of ionizing radiation, which include alpha particles, beta particles, gamma rays, x-rays, and neutrons. One also needs to understand how radiation is measured (Table 53-4). There are several methods which take into account not only the decay rate of a radioactive isotope (becquerel [Bq] or a curie [Ci]) or the dose absorbed usually quantified as the amount absorbed by any type of tissue or material. The radiation-absorbed dose (rad) = 0.01 Gray (Gy) which is the international system of units (SI) for denoting the amount of energy deposited in joules per kilogram. One Gy equals 100 rad. A sievert is the SI unit for measurement of *human* exposure to radiation in joules per kilogram, with 1 sievert = 100 rem (roentgen equivalent for man).

In a nuclear accident or catastrophe, patients could have several types of radiation exposure such as external radiation from an x-ray–emitting device or from gamma rays or beta particles, they can be contaminated with debris emitting ionized radiation or they can inhale or ingest gaseous radioactive material,[43] and some of this material can become incorporated into tissue such as with radioactive iodine isotopes. In order to protect individuals, the distance from the source or explosion is important, the amount of shielding, the time one is exposed, and the amount of

TABLE 53-4. RADIATION EXPOSURE TERMS

- ***Becquerel (Bq):*** The International System of units (SI) measurement of radioactivity, defined as decay events per second. 1 Bq = 1 disintegration per second.
- ***Curie (Ci):*** The traditional measure of radioactivity, as measured by radioactive decay. 1 Ci = 2.7×10^{10} disintegrations per second.
- ***Radiation-absorbed dose (rad):*** The energy deposited by any type of radiation to any type of tissue or material. 1 rad = 0.01 Gy.
- ***Gray (Gy):*** The SI unit for the energy deposited by any type of radiation, in joules per kilogram. 1 Gy = 100 rad.
- ***Roentgen equivalent man (rem):*** The unit of human exposure to radiation. 1 rem = 0.01 Sv.
- ***Sievert (Sv):*** The SI unit for measurement of human exposure to radiation, in joules per kilogram. 1 Sv = 100 rem.

radioactive material to which one is exposed. Human tissue will block alpha particles (though if inhaled, alpha particles can penetrate up to 50 microns into the pulmonary epithelium material leading to the development of lung cancer), but will not stop beta particles or gamma rays. Beta particles are stopped by aluminum shields, but gamma rays can penetrate even concrete walls and lead is required to shield for both gamma and x-rays.

The most likely injury from ionizing radiation is to those tissues that have the greatest turnover rate, *that is,* the sensitivity of tissues to radiation from greatest to least is for lymphoid, GI, reproductive, dermal, bone marrow, and nervous system tissue. In reality, the response of lymphoid and bone marrow to ionizing radiation cause the greatest problems. The thrombocytopenia, granulocytopenia, and the GI injury lead to bleeding and bacterial translocation across the GI epithelium, the net result of which is sepsis, bleeding—the hallmarks of acute radiation syndrome, which lead to death.

Because ionizing radiation is invisible, individuals may appear normal. Patients who present with nausea, vomiting, diarrhea, and fever are likely to have severe acute radiation syndrome. Hypotension, erythemia, and CNS dysfunction will manifest later. "Short-term" effects such as these, however, may not appear until days to weeks after the exposure, depending on the amount of exposure (as little as 0.75 to 1 Gy), whereas hematopoetic syndrome (severe lymphoid and bone marrow suppression) results from exposure to 3 to 6 Gy and may lead to death within 8 to 50 days. Long-term effects include thyroid cancer and psychological injury as has been documented many times in the past.

Management

Should a radiation disaster occur, it would be followed by a huge coordinated local, state, and federal response which at the federal level would include the US Department of Homeland Security, the Department of Energy, the Department of Justice, FEMA, the Environmental Protection Agency, and the Nuclear Regulatory Commission. Of most importance, depending on the type of catastrophe, would be the immediate evacuation of the area. If evacuation is impossible, a safe place should be sought within the home or building. The principle of disaster management always involves containment (avoid bringing patients with material emitting ionizing radiation to the hospital). Therefore, as part of the containment process, to the extent possible patients should be decontaminated at the site. Removal of clothing is critically important. Beta and gamma rays and neutrons will be gone unless there is still material emitting this radiation on a person's clothing. Rather than guess, it is best to disrobe. In previous mass casualty situation, maintenance of casualties' privacy has been a concern, but not one with an easy solution. Afterward, patients' skin should be washed with warm soapy water. Depending on the number of casualties, and especially because individuals will arrive by private vehicles or on foot, decontamination areas may have to be set up outside of hospitals with care taken to isolate belongings, with the same consideration given to biologic fluids as for clothing including saliva, blood, urine, stool, as they may be contaminated with radioisotopes and may require special handling precautions.

Potassium iodide can attenuate most of the radiation-induced thyroid effects, and but must be given as quickly as possible because after 24 hours, there is little protective effect. Treatment is largely supportive as these patients will develop acute radiation syndrome manifested by bleeding and sepsis. Treatment guidelines for management of post-irradiation sepsis have been developed and advocated by the military.[44] The use of granulocyte-colony–stimulating factor may be of benefit. Other treatments would include oral and GI decontamination using nasopharyngeal lavage, oral lavage and brushing, early stomach lavage, or administration of emetic and osmotic laxatives. Blocking agents include potassium iodide and strontium lactate. Mobilizing agents include ammonium chloride, calcium gluconate, and diuretics, which may enhance renal excretion. Chelation therapy that has been recommended includes calcium diethylenetriamine pentaacetic acid (DTPA) as an initial dose and then zinc DTPA.[45] Granulocyte macrophage colony–stimulating factor and thrombopoietin or interleukin-11, though postulated, have not been proven to be of benefit. For individuals with a contaminated GI tract, selective decontamination may be helpful, though again has not been demonstrated to be of benefit in this situation.[46]

Unfortunately, because of the possibility of blast, thermal, and crush injuries, along with the radiation injury, the care of the injured may require the care of patients who have multiple combined injuries. The initial response should be as per the advanced trauma life support (ATLS) guidelines, which include an assessment of the airway, breathing, and circulation, and extent of trauma and then decontamination of the patient after which the patient is stabilized and further evaluated. Wounds must be considered contaminated. "Dirty wounds" should not be closed, but cleaned and debrided, excised, and observed. Unfortunately, in this situation, there is also the possibility that there may be the combined effects of a radiation-releasing event and either the use of chemical or biologic weapons.[46] Because of the kinds of terrorism, some of it reportedly government sponsored, communities and the US government have had to plan for the unthinkable, that is, detonation of a nuclear device on US soil.[47,48]

EXPLOSIVE

Management of traumatic injury is covered in Chapter 52 (Anesthesia for Trauma and Burn Injury), but a chapter on disaster management would not be complete without mentioning the use of explosive devices by terrorists. As the media reports daily, particularly in Afghanistan, the use of improvised explosive device (IED) is the terrorist's favorite weapon. Patients have burns, fractures, lacerations, multiple shrapnel injuries, soft tissue trauma, and traumatic amputations. As the weapons have become more sophisticated and powerful, the extent of injuries has increased significantly. In 2012, US military personnel are experiencing more multiple than single traumatic extremity amputations.[49]

Patients with any evidence of burns to the face or airway will require appropriate airway management. Patients should be intubated, awake if possible, as a significant number of these patients will have mild to moderate glottic edema at the time of intubation. Those patients with burns must be managed aggressively with respect to fluid resuscitation. With isolated total body surface injury, fluid resuscitation is aggressive. With polytrauma, and no third degree burns then "damage control resuscitation/surgery" is the norm.[50] Patient's body temperature is maintained (operating rooms maintained at >100 °F) and surgery is performed as soon as possible to stop the bleeding, thereby decreasing the need for blood products and the chances of developing a dilutional coagulopathy. Patients who do develop a coagulopathy appear to benefit from a ratio of pRBCs to fresh frozen plasma to platelets of 1:1:1.[51] One study has demonstrated that tranexamic acid decreases the need for additional blood products. In patients with crush injury and markedly elevated creatine phosphokinase, alkalinization of the urine may attenuate renal failure from myoglobinuria.

CONCLUSION

While it could occur it is unlikely that an anesthesiologist would be at the initial site of a natural or intentional disaster, but it could happen. Most likely they will become involved if the hospital at which they work provides care for a number of these patients. As in the previous situations, anesthesiologists could find themselves being involved in triage, in the emergency room, operating room, or ICU.[52] As suggested for several of these situations, airway management and ventilator management may be critical, as would the establishment of intravascular access and volume resuscitation.

Obviously, it is critical to have a high index of suspicion if you are managing the index case or two or more patients with presenting signs and symptoms that are suggestive of the use of a biologic weapon. The individual who is the point of contact for the index case should notify the hospital infectious disease specialist and the local and state health departments. Factors that might indicate the intentional release of a biologic agent would include unusual temporal or geographic clustering of cases, an uncommon age distribution, or a significant number of cases (more than one) of acute flaccid paralysis that might suggest use of botulinum toxin.

If called to the hospital to be involved in managing such a catastrophe, the anesthesiologist must review basic decontamination and isolation techniques and as commented previously, must follow those guidelines scrupulously.

What is clear is that the anesthesiologists have the requisite training and experience to be of vital importance in managing such casualties. However, based on their training, they may not be emotionally prepared to manage these patients. They must remember that unlike their normal practice, they may have to triage patients, accept the fact that the standard of care may be changed, and focus their efforts on interventions which will carry the greatest benefit for the greatest number of casualties.

This process begins when the anesthesiologist gets the call at home or in the hospital of an impending mass casualty. She or he must first report to the command and control center and, though most likely they may work in the operating room, they could also be used in the triage area in the emergency department or in the ICU. Of utmost importance is familiarity with the hospital's disaster plan. One must also develop one's own family care plan in anticipation of absence from the home for extended periods of time. Ensuring one's own safety through the appropriate use of protective devices to serve as barriers against radiologic, biologic, and chemical weapons is also of vital importance.

References

1. Dara SI, Ashton RW, Farmer JC. Engendering enthusiasm for sustainable disaster critical care response: Why this is of consequence to critical care professionals? *Crit Care.* 2005;9(2):125–127.
2. Gomez D, Haas B, Ahmed N, et al. Disaster preparedness of Canadian trauma centres: The perspective of medical directors of trauma. *Can J Surg.* 2011;54(1):9–16.
3. Ciraulo DL, Frykberg ER, Feliciano DV, et al. A survey assessment of the level of preparedness for domestic terrorism and mass casualty incidents among eastern association for the surgery of trauma members. *J Trauma.* 2004;56(5):1033–1039; discussion 1039–1041.
4. Moore ZS, Seward JF, Lane JM. Smallpox. *Lancet.* 2006;367(9508):425–435.
5. Tepper M, Whitehead J. Clinical predictors of bioterrorism-related inhalational anthrax. *Lancet.* 2005;365(9455):214; author reply 215.
6. Lynch DK. Plan ahead. *Anesth Analg.* 2010;110(3):653–654.
7. Merchant RM, Leigh JE, Lurie N. Health care volunteers and disaster response–first, be prepared. *N Engl J Med.* 2010;362(10):872–873.
8. Masterson L, Steffen C, Brin M, et al. Willingness to respond: Of emergency department personnel and their predicted participation in mass casualty terrorist events. *J Emerg Med.* 2009;36(1):43–49.
9. Homeland Security, FEMA. *National Preparedness Goal.* 2011; 1–111. http://www.fema.gov/pdf/prepared/npg.pdf
10. The Joint Commission on Accreditation of Healthcare Organizations. Health care at the crossroads. Strategies for creating and sustaining community-wide emergency preparedness systems. 2003; 1–44. http://www.jointcommission.org/assets/1/18/health_care_at_the_crossroads.pdf
11. Peter Shin FJ. An HIT solution for clinical care and disaster planning: How one health center in Joplin, MO survived a tornado and avoided a Health Information disaster. *Online Journal of Public Health Informatics.* 2012;4(1):1–7.
12. Martin Enserink RS. Questions swirl over knockout gas used in hostage crisis. *Science.* 2002;298:1150–1151.
13. Okumura T, Takasu N, Ishimatsu S, et al. Report on 640 victims of the Tokyo subway sarin attack. *Ann Emerg Med.* 1996;28(2):129–135.
14. Zane RD, Prestipino AL. Implementing the hospital emergency incident command system: An integrated delivery system's experience. *Prehosp Disaster Med.* 2004;19(4):311–317.
15. Goransson Nyberg A, Stricklin D, Sellstrom A. Mass casualties and health care following the release of toxic chemicals or radioactive material–contribution of modern biotechnology. *Int J Environ Res Public Health.* 2011;8(12):4521–4549.
16. Chemical, Biological, Radiological and Nuclear Defense Information Analysis Center (CBRNIAC). U.S. Army Chemical Materials agency creates a safer tomorrow. *CBRNIAC Newsletter.* 2012;13(2):4–7.
17. Kassa J, Karasova JZ, Musilek K, et al. A comparison of the neuroprotective efficacy of newly developed oximes (K117, K127) and currently available oxime (obidoxime) in tabun-poisoned rats. *Toxicol Mech Methods* 2009;19(3):232–238.
18. Aroniadou-Anderjaska V, Figueiredo TH, Apland JP, et al. Primary brain targets of nerve agents: the role of the amygdala in comparison to the hippocampus. *Neurotoxicol.* 2009;30(5):772–776.
19. Beeching NJ, Dance DA, Miller AR, et al. Biological warfare and bioterrorism. *BMJ.* 2002;324(7333):336–339.
20. Breman JG, Henderson DA. Diagnosis and management of smallpox. *N Engl J Med.* 2002;346(17):1300–1308.
21. *The World Health Organization Smallpox Eradication Programme.* 2012; Course. Available from: http://choo.fis.utoronto.ca/fis/courses/lis2102/KO.WHO.case.html.
22. From the Centers for Disease Control and Prevention. Smallpox vaccine adverse events among civilians–United States, March 4-10, 2003. *JAMA.* 2003;289(15):1921–1922.
23. Frey SE, Newman FK, Kennedy JS, et al. Clinical and immunologic responses to multiple doses of IMVAMUNE (Modified Vaccinia Ankara) followed by Dryvax challenge. *Vaccine.* 2007;25(51):8562–8573.
24. Inglesby TV, Henderson DA, Bartlett JG, et al. Anthrax as a biological weapon: Medical and public health management. Working Group on Civilian Biodefense. *JAMA.* 1999;281(18):1735–1745.
25. Kalamas AG. Anthrax. *Anesthesiol Clin North America.* 2004;22(3):533–540, vii.
26. Janse I, Hamidjaja RA, Bok JM, et al. Reliable detection of Bacillus anthracis, Francisella tularensis and Yersinia pestis by using multiplex qPCR including internal controls for nucleic acid extraction and amplification. *BMC Microbiol.* 2010;10:314.
27. Martin G. Anthrax: Lessons learned from the U.S. Capitol experience. *Mil Med.* 2003;168(9 suppl):9–14.
28. Swartz MN. Recognition and management of anthrax–an update. *N Engl J Med.* 2001;345(22):1621–1626.

29. Dixon TC, Meselson M, Guillemin J, et al. Anthrax. *N Engl J Med.* 1999;341(11): 815–826.
30. Shafazand S, Doyle R, Ruoss S, et al. Inhalational anthrax: Epidemiology, diagnosis, and management. *Chest.* 1999;116(5):1369–1376.
31. Schmitt B, Dobrez D, Parada JP, et al. Responding to a small-scale bioterrorist anthrax attack: Cost-effectiveness analysis comparing preattack vaccination with postattack antibiotic treatment and vaccination. *Arch Intern Med* 2007;167(7): 655–662.
32. Prentice MB, Rahalison L. Plague. *Lancet.* 2007;369(9568):1196–1207.
33. Zietz BP, Dunkelberg H. The history of the plague and the research on the causative agent Yersinia pestis. *Int J Hyg Environ Health.* 2004;207(2):165–178.
34. Josko D. Botulin toxin: A weapon in terrorism. *Clin Lab Sci.* 2004;17(1):30–34.
35. Franz DR, Jahrling PB, McClain DJ, et al. Clinical recognition and management of patients exposed to biological warfare agents. *Clin Lab Med.* 2001;21(3):435–473.
36. Bhalla DK, Warheit DB. Biological agents with potential for misuse: A historical perspective and defensive measures. *Toxicol Appl Pharmacol.* 2004;199(1):71–84.
37. Kuhn JH, Dodd LE, Wahl-Jensen V, et al. Evaluation of perceived threat differences posed by filovirus variants. *Biosecur Bioterror.* 2011;9(4):361–371.
38. Fact Sheet on Biological Effects of Radiation, U.S.N.R. Commission, Editor, 2011.
39. Masamichi Chino Hn, Haruyasu Nagai, Hiroaki Terada, et al. Preliminary estimation of release amounts of 131I and 137Cs Accidentally Discharged from the fukushima daiichi nuclear power plant into the atmosphere. *J Nucl Sci Tech.* 2011; 48(7):1129–1134.
40. Shibata Y, Yamashita S, Masyakin VB, et al. 15 years after Chernobyl: New evidence of thyroid cancer. *Lancet.* 2001;358(9297):1965–1966.
41. Collins DL. Human responses to the threat of or exposure to ionizing radiation at Three Mile Island, Pennsylvania, and Goiania, Brazil. *Mil Med.* 2002;167 (2 suppl):137–138.
42. Collins DL, de Carvalho AB. Chronic stress from the Goiania 137Cs radiation accident. *Behav Med.* 1993;18(4):149–157.
43. Ibrahim SA, Simon SL, Bouville A, et al. Alimentary tract absorption (f1 values) for radionuclides in local and regional fallout from nuclear tests. *Health Phys.* 2010;99(2):233–251.
44. Brook I, Elliott TB, Ledney GD, et al. Management of postirradiation sepsis. *Mil Med.* 2002;167(2 suppl):105–106.
45. Knudson GB, Elliott TB, Brook I, et al. Nuclear, biological, and chemical combined injuries and countermeasures on the battlefield. *Mil Med.* 2002;167(2 suppl): 95–97.
46. Shi C, Lu S. Radiation injuries. *Int J Low Extrem Wounds.* 2011;10(3):120–121.
47. Sternberg S. Experts plan for how to deal with nuclear terror strike. USA Today March 15, 2011. http://www.usatoday.com/news/nation/2011-03-15-nukemed14_ST_N.htm
48. National Security Staff Interagency Policy Coordination Subcommittee for Preparedness and Response to Radiological and Nuclear Threats. *Planning Guidance for Response to a Nuclear Detonation.* 2nd Ed. 2010.
49. Zoroya G. IEDs contribute to increase in multiple amputations. USA Today June 4, 2012. http://www.usatoday.com/news/military/story/2012-06-04/IED-amputations-military-Afghanistan/55385376/1
50. Holcomb JB, Jenkins D, Rhee P, et al. Damage control resuscitation: Directly addressing the early coagulopathy of trauma. *J Trauma.* 2007;62(2): 307–310.
51. Borgman MA, Spinella PC, Perkins JG, et al. The ratio of blood products transfused affects mortality in patients receiving massive transfusions at a combat support hospital. *J Trauma.* 2007;63(4):805–813.
52. Baker DJ. Management of casualties from terrorist chemical and biological attack: A key role for the anaesthetist. *Br J Anaesth.* 2002;89(2):211–214.

Family Emergency Plan

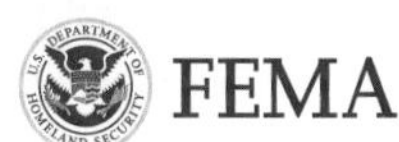

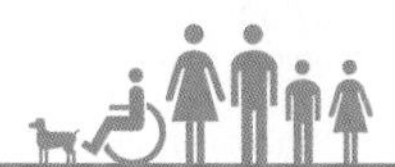

Make sure your family has a plan in case of an emergency. Before an emergency happens, sit down together and decide how you will get in contact with each other, where you will go and what you will do in an emergency. Keep a copy of this plan in your emergency supply kit or another safe place where you can access it in the event of a disaster.

Out-of-Town Contact Name: ____________________ Telephone Number: ____________________

Email: ____________________

Neighborhood Meeting Place: ____________________ Telephone Number: ____________________

Regional Meeting Place: ____________________ Telephone Number: ____________________

Evacuation Location: ____________________ Telephone Number: ____________________

Fill out the following information for each family member and keep it up to date.

Name: ____________________ Social Security Number: ____________________
Date of Birth: ____________________ Important Medical Information: ____________________

Name: ____________________ Social Security Number: ____________________
Date of Birth: ____________________ Important Medical Information: ____________________

Name: ____________________ Social Security Number: ____________________
Date of Birth: ____________________ Important Medical Information: ____________________

Name: ____________________ Social Security Number: ____________________
Date of Birth: ____________________ Important Medical Information: ____________________

Name: ____________________ Social Security Number: ____________________
Date of Birth: ____________________ Important Medical Information: ____________________

Name: ____________________ Social Security Number: ____________________
Date of Birth: ____________________ Important Medical Information: ____________________

Write down where your family spends the most time: work, school and other places you frequent. Schools, daycare providers, workplaces and apartment buildings should all have site-specific emergency plans that you and your family need to know about.

Work Location One
Address:
Phone Number:
Evacuation Location:

Work Location Two
Address:
Phone Number:
Evacuation Location:

Work Location Three
Address:
Phone Number:
Evacuation Location:

Other place you frequent
Address:
Phone Number:
Evacuation Location:

School Location One
Address:
Phone Number:
Evacuation Location:

School Location Two
Address:
Phone Number:
Evacuation Location:

School Location Three
Address:
Phone Number:
Evacuation Location:

Other place you frequent
Address:
Phone Number:
Evacuation Location:

Important Information	Name	Telephone Number	Policy Number
Doctor(s):			
Other:			
Pharmacist:			
Medical Insurance:			
Homeowners/Rental Insurance:			
Veterinarian/Kennel (for pets):			

Dial 911 for Emergencies

Family Emergency Plan

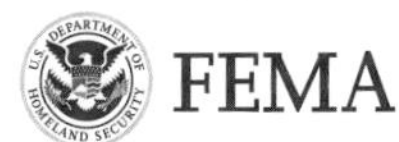

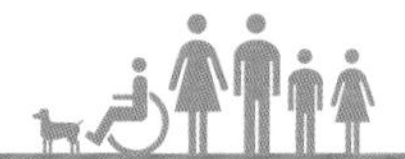

Make sure your family has a plan in case of an emergency. Fill out these cards and give one to each member of your family to make sure they know who to call and where to meet in case of an emergency.

ADDITIONAL IMPORTANT PHONE NUMBERS & INFORMATION:

< FOLD HERE >

Family Emergency Plan

EMERGENCY CONTACT NAME:
TELEPHONE:

OUT-OF-TOWN CONTACT NAME:
TELEPHONE:

NEIGHBORHOOD MEETING PLACE:
TELEPHONE:

OTHER IMPORTANT INFORMATION:

Ready ®

DIAL 911 FOR EMERGENCIES

ADDITIONAL IMPORTANT PHONE NUMBERS & INFORMATION:

Family Emergency Plan

EMERGENCY CONTACT NAME:
TELEPHONE:

OUT-OF-TOWN CONTACT NAME:
TELEPHONE:

NEIGHBORHOOD MEETING PLACE:
TELEPHONE:

OTHER IMPORTANT INFORMATION:

Ready ®

DIAL 911 FOR EMERGENCIES

ADDITIONAL IMPORTANT PHONE NUMBERS & INFORMATION:

< FOLD HERE >

Family Emergency Plan

EMERGENCY CONTACT NAME:
TELEPHONE:

OUT-OF-TOWN CONTACT NAME:
TELEPHONE:

NEIGHBORHOOD MEETING PLACE:
TELEPHONE:

OTHER IMPORTANT INFORMATION:

Ready ®

DIAL 911 FOR EMERGENCIES

ADDITIONAL IMPORTANT PHONE NUMBERS & INFORMATION:

Family Emergency Plan

EMERGENCY CONTACT NAME:
TELEPHONE:

OUT-OF-TOWN CONTACT NAME:
TELEPHONE:

NEIGHBORHOOD MEETING PLACE:
TELEPHONE:

OTHER IMPORTANT INFORMATION:

Ready ®

DIAL 911 FOR EMERGENCIES

SECTION VIII

Perioperative and Consultative Services

CHAPTER

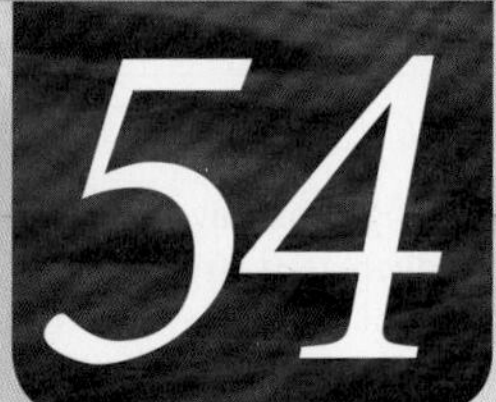

Postanesthesia Recovery

MICHAEL A. FOWLER • BRUCE D. SPIESS

Key Points

1. The postoperative planning begins with the preoperative evaluation and formation of an intraoperative anesthetic plan. The type of anesthetic (i.e., inhalation technique, total intravenous anesthetic, sedation, local, regional) influences the type and length of postanesthesia care unit (PACU) recovery.
2. The level of PACU care depends on the type/approach of surgery, type of anesthetic, intraoperative course of events, as well as patient pre-existing and evolving comorbidities. Typical recovery settings include inpatient recovery, ambulatory recovery (phase 1 for more intensive needs and phase 2 for less intensive needs), short stay (23-hour admit), and recovery from specific procedures (i.e., computed tomography, magnetic resonance imaging, invasive radiology, cardiac, pediatric, and radiation procedures).
3. The transfer of care to a PACU nurse includes assuring that the patient has had appropriate monitoring applied, admission vital signs were taken, a direct and thorough report received that allows for rapid evaluation should complications arise, as well as a nurse capable of handling the acuity of the patient's medical/surgical problems.
4. Relative hypovolemia should be evaluated and managed in PACU based on the patient's comorbidities, preoperative status (i.e., bowel preparation, postdialysis), type and duration of surgery, blood loss, and urine output.
5. Postoperative analgesia should be individualized to requirements and expectations. A multimodal approach includes the appropriate use of nonsteroidal anti-inflammatory drugs, narcotics, adjuncts, regional and local anesthetics, as well as anxiety relief and appropriate emotional support.
6. Discharge criteria should be tailored to the individual patient's underlying disease, recovery course, and postdischarge level of care.
7. The cardiac risks during the postoperative stay include myocardial ischemia, which may be minimized with continued use of β-blockers, analgesia, nitrates, supplemental oxygen, adequate circulating volume, oxygen-carrying capacity, heart rate control, and an understanding of hypercoagulable states.
8. The respiratory risks of a patient must take into account the preoperative respiratory disease status. Residual anesthetics, opioids, and sedatives all impair responsiveness to increasing CO_2 and decreasing O_2 levels. Pain itself can decrease respiration/minute

ventilation, leading to CO_2 retention and hypoxia. Supplemental O_2 application alone does not guarantee hypoxemia will not occur.

9 The evaluation of a patient's ability to void may be affected by the type of surgery (i.e., genitourinary surgery, hernia repairs) or the type of anesthetic (i.e., regional, neuraxial, or opioids).

10 Glycemic monitoring and control should persist as a continuum from intraoperative management. Good glycemic control may help with fighting infection, improve wound healing, which can result in better surgical outcomes. Hypoglycemia occurs because of nothing by mouth status, intraoperative administration of insulin, as well as the patient using programmable insulin pumps.

11 Hypothermia can lead to an increased length of stay in PACU, lethargy, decreased minute ventilation, decreased strength, and increased cardiac demand. It is important to assure that the patient is dry and insulated. The use of air warming blankets, warming mats, and intravenous fluid warmers all minimize hypothermia.

12 Many elderly patients experience a varied degree of postoperative confusion, delirium, or cognitive dysfunction in the PACU. Many pediatric patients also experience postemergence delirium leading to increased length of stay in the PACU.

13 Postoperative nausea and vomiting is a major cause of patient discomfort and dissatisfaction, as well as an aspiration risk and causes prolonged PACU stay.

Multimedia

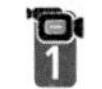 Tracheostomy

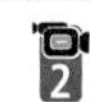 Aspiration

POSTANESTHESIA RECOVERY

1 Each patient recovering from an anesthetic has circumstances that require an individualized problem-oriented approach. Postoperative planning begins with the preoperative evaluation and formation of an intraoperative anesthetic plan. Postanesthesia recovery must continue to adapt to meet the needs of the changing perioperative landscape, advances in technology, changing surgical techniques; and to respond to improved evidence-based research. Dissemination of anesthesia services beyond the perisurgical arena has brought changes and greater demands on recovery units.

Standards for Postanesthesia Care

The ASA House of Delegates approved Standards for Postanesthesia Care on October 12, 1988. These standards were last amended on October 27, 2004.[1]

VALUE AND ECONOMICS OF POSTANESTHESIA CARE UNIT

The quality of postanesthesia care is composed of many variables such as tracking of complications, time per patient spent in recovery, overall clinical outcomes, and patient satisfaction. The value of postanesthesia care is a measure of the quality of care provided compared with the amount of resources spent per patient outcome. The postanesthesia care unit (PACU) helps to use resources efficiently by having trained staff that routinely care for postsurgical patients, thereby recognizing/preventing complications, and by having physicians instituting appropriate and timely therapies.

The actual cost of PACU care incorporates costs of staffing, space, and hardware (resource utilization). Triage and discharge policies affect both how many admissions occur and what resources each admission consumes. Nurse staffing continues to be the largest direct cost in the PACU. The mix of nursing staff, experience of nurses, staffing ratios, and the complexity and duration of PACU stay affect the overall personnel cost per admission. The level of monitoring provided affects the capital expenditure for equipment, and disposable items account for operating expenditures. The patient acuity mix also determines needs for staffing and equipment such as ventilators, additional monitors, intravenous pumps, and patient-controlled analgesia pumps. The type of physician coverage—such as dedicated coverage versus on-demand coverage—can affect response time, efficiency of care, costs, and patient outcomes. The use of routine postoperative diagnostic testing and therapies without evidence-based need can lead to unnecessary treatments, increasing cost per patient and possible worse patient outcomes.

Cost comparisons between institutions are difficult because charges and cost factors vary widely across institutions, in different regions of the United States, and between countries. They constantly change over time. Regulatory requirements, standards of care, medical–legal climates, and institutional requirements vary greatly between regions and even between facilities in the same locale. It is difficult to establish cost-effectiveness goals of a single PACU because of the differing requirements of individual patients having the same procedures. This difference can be the result of levels of patient comorbidities, level of procedure complexity, surgeon, type of anesthetic, as well as patient perception and expectations. These are just some of the factors that can determine the type of care needed postoperatively. Continued pressures from many fronts to contain costs and maximize cost-effectiveness force each surgical facility to continually evaluate the value of its PACU care to each individual patient.

PACU directors are challenged to optimize clinical results while minimizing expenditures. Innovative PACU practices should guarantee safe care, minimize cost, and fulfill regulatory and institutional requirements. Medical professionals (physicians, nursing, and support staff) must work in concert to identify practices that are wasteful versus those that have proven yield/benefit. The impact of many PACU-proposed interventions on clinical outcomes are not easily substantiated by controlled scientific analysis. Useless testing, unnecessary or unjustifiable therapy, and inappropriate PACU admissions should be eliminated. However, using a more expensive therapy may generate real savings by decreasing additional therapies, testing, admissions, or length of stay. Another important element essential for patient safety and efficiency in the PACU is communication with the intraoperative anesthesiology service. Communication is perhaps the least expensive tool in medicine and the one most universally proven to be involved in human error events. Utilization of PACU resources is directly related to anesthetic duration and technique. In one study, 22.1% of 37,000 patients had a minor anesthesia-related event or complication that prolonged PACU stays and consumed PACU resources.[2] Another study showed how postoperative adverse events increase the amount of nursing resources needed in the PACU.[3] Close coordination between the PACU and the anesthesiology service should reduce the frequency and impact of such events.

Improvements in surgical and anesthetic techniques might create an opportunity to shorten the length of stay in the PACU, but realized change is frequently reduced by transportation delays, persistence of pain or nausea, waiting for space, or surgeon discharge delays.[4] Cost-saving measures in other areas may also increase the cost of PACU care; for example, fast-tracking to discharge to home rather than to a hospital bed. The cost savings of not occupying a hospital bed is offset by an increase in PACU stay and therefore greater consumption of PACU resources.[5] The savings may be cost savings for the patient and beneficial for the facility as a whole but at a greater expense to the PACU. True savings are only realized when operational changes yield a decrease in expenditures for staff, supplies, or equipment. For example, patients who are able to bypass the PACU creates a savings opportunity only if paid nursing hours are reduced or if more surgical cases are covered with the same hours. With the use of less-invasive surgical techniques combined with innovative anesthetic techniques, such as regional anesthetics, shorter PACU stays can result in real savings opportunities. However, the areas of scheduling, clerical, or maintenance tasks must not consume excess staffing hours, without savings realized. Finally, trimming costs could entail an increase in unwanted risk to patients. Differentiating between cost-effective postanesthesia care and unsafe practice remains a matter of constant professional judgment and debate daily in most PACUs.

LEVELS OF POSTOPERATIVE/ POSTANESTHESIA CARE

With continued demand to increase overall healthcare efficiency, caution must be taken to provide the most appropriate care for each patient. As anesthesia services expand to cover a variety of patient types in ever-increasing areas outside the operating room, selecting the correct type of recovery is essential. For the many differing anesthesia areas ranging from inpatient surgery, ambulatory surgery, to off-site procedures, the level of postoperative care that a patient requires is determined by the degree of underlying illness, comorbidities, and the duration as well as the type of anesthesia and surgery. These factors are used to assess the risk of postoperative complications. Less-invasive surgeries or procedures combined with shorter-duration anesthetic regimens facilitate high levels of arousal and minimal cardiovascular or respiratory depression at the end of surgery.

Using a less intensive postanesthesia setting for selected patients can reduce costs for a surgical procedure and allow the facility to divert scarce PACU resources to patients with greater needs. Alert patients are more satisfied when spared the unnecessary assessments in interventions of PACU care. Amenities such as recliners, reading material, television, music, and food improve perceptions (emotional satisfaction) without affecting quality or safety. Earlier reunion with family or visitors in the low-intensity setting is desirable assuming that postoperative care is safe and appropriate.

Creation of separate PACUs for inpatients, ambulatory, or off-site patients is one possible way to streamline PACU care for appropriately triaged patients. Phase I recovery would be reserved for more intense recovery and would require more one-on-one care for staff. Phase II recovery should be less intensive and is appropriate for patients after less-invasive procedures requiring less attention from nursing while recovering. If separation of different phases of care is not possible, then providing the appropriate level of monitoring and coverage to the degree of postoperative impairment achieves similar results in a single PACU
2 area. However, care equal to a full-intensity PACU must always be available, given the incidence of complications after anesthesia and surgery.[6] As the aging population generates an increase in the complexity of surgical care in the face of tighter control of resources, maintaining appropriate PACU capacity and safety by observing applicable PACU guidelines and standards will be increasingly important.[7,8]

POSTANESTHETIC TRIAGE

Patients must be carefully evaluated to determine which level of care is appropriate. Triage should be based on clinical condition, length/type of procedure and anesthetic, and the potential for complications that require intervention. Alternatives to PACU care must be used in a nondiscriminatory fashion. Arbitrary criteria based on age, American Society of Anesthesiologists (ASA) classification, ambulatory versus inpatient versus off-site procedure status, or type of insurance should not be used for determining the level of recovery care. An individual patient undergoing a specific procedure or anesthetic should receive the same appropriate level of postoperative care whether the procedure is performed in a hospital operating room, an ambulatory surgical center, an endoscopy room, an invasive radiology suite, or an outpatient office. If doubt exists about a patient's safety in a lower-intensity setting, the patient should be admitted to a higher level of care for recovery. Patient safety should always be favored regardless of the cost.

After superficial procedures using local infiltration, minor blocks, or sedation, patients can almost always recover with less intensive monitoring and coverage. Healthy patients undergoing more extensive procedures (e.g., hernia repairs, arthroscopic procedures, minor orthopedic procedures) under local, plexus, or peripheral nerve blockade might also bypass phase I recovery and go directly to phase II. The increasing use of continuous peripheral nerve catheters for surgery has shortened PACU time and can eliminate many hospital admissions.[9] Innovative anesthetic techniques, advanced surgical techniques, and use of bispectral index monitoring help facilitate fast-track postoperative care.[10]

For more intensive procedures and patients with greater acuity, bypassing the PACU and direct admission to intensive care units (ICUs) can reduce demands on the PACU as well as reduce errors with decreased number of hand offs. This still requires proper postoperative reporting to the accepting unit including how to communicate with the surgical service and anesthesiologist. These ICUs must be trained and prepared to receive immediate postoperative patients as well as meet the standards of the PACU.

SAFETY IN THE POSTANESTHESIA CARE UNIT

The PACU medical director (every PACU should have medical oversight) must ensure that the PACU environment is as safe as possible for both patients and staff. Beyond usual safety policies, maintain staffing and training to ensure appropriate coverage and skill mix are available to deal with unforeseen crises. Incidence of adverse events in the PACU correlates with nursing workload and staff availability.[3] Ideally, all staff should have PACU certification, and staffing ratios should never fall below acceptable standards.[8] Less skilled or training staff must be appropriately supervised, and a sufficient number of certified personnel must always be available to handle worst-case scenarios.

The PACU staff protects patients who are temporarily incompetent and preserves patients' rights to observance of advanced directives and to informed consent for additional procedures. The staff is obligated to optimize each patient's privacy, dignity, and to minimize the psychological impact of unpleasant or frightening events. Observance of procedures for hand-washing, sterility, and infection control should be strictly enforced.[11] Medical directors must safeguard against potential for personal assault of patients during recovery such as unwarranted restraints and procedures without consent. Access to the PACU should be strictly controlled. With increasing acceptance of reuniting patients with family/friends, safety and privacy need to be continually addressed.

The PACU environment must also be safe for professionals. Air handling should guarantee that personnel are not exposed to unacceptable levels of trace anesthetic gases, although trace gas monitoring is not necessary. Ensure that staff members receive appropriate vaccinations, including that for hepatitis B. Practitioners must adhere to policies for radiation safety, infection control, disposal of sharps, universal precautions for blood-borne diseases, and safeguarding against exposure to pathogens such as methicillin-resistant *Staphylococcus*, vancomycin-resistant *Enterococcus, Clostridium difficile*, or tuberculosis. Always keep masks, gloves, gowns, eye protection, and appropriate particulate respiratory equipment easily accessible. Following current infection control policies and guidelines are essential for patient and staff safety. Ensure that sufficient help is available to avoid injury while lifting and positioning patients or while dealing with emergence situations. Precise documentation and clear delineation of responsibility is essential for proper care of patients and can protect staff against unnecessary medicolegal exposure.

ADMISSION TO THE POSTANESTHESIA CARE UNIT

Every patient admitted to a PACU should have heart rate, rhythm, systemic blood pressure, airway patency, peripheral oxygen saturation, ventilatory rate/character, and level of pain recorded and periodically monitored.[7] Assessment with periodic recording every 5 minutes for the first 15 minutes and every 15 minutes thereafter is a minimum. Document temperature, level of consciousness, mental status, neuromuscular function, hydration status, degree of nausea on admission/discharge, and more frequently if appropriate, are also minimum standards of care. Every patient should be continuously monitored with a pulse oximeter and at least a single-lead electrocardiogram (ECG). Extra leads, particularly precordial V3 to V6, are appropriate if left ventricular ischemia is likely. Capnography is necessary for patients receiving mechanical ventilation or those at risk for compromised ventilatory function. Transduction and recorded output from invasive monitors such as central venous, systemic, or pulmonary arterial catheters must be accomplished. Diagnostic (laboratory) testing should be ordered only for specific indications.

Anesthesiology personnel should manage the patient until a PACU nurse secures admission vital signs, attaches appropriate monitors, and care is transferred with a complete report to the nursing staff. A succinct but thorough report that includes sufficient information to allow rapid evaluation and intervention for postoperative complications must be legibly recorded using a standardized format printed on the PACU record (Table 54-1). This report should be similar to the OR timeout, providing patient identification, procedure performed, anesthetic type and
3 continuing therapies. Documentation of the time and amount of all neuromuscular relaxants, respiratory depressant medications, and reversal agents should be standard. Outlined orders, specific therapeutic end points, and, most importantly, how to contact the responsible anesthesiologist all must be transmitted. The anesthesiologist should never transfer responsibility to PACU personnel until the patient's airway status, ventilation, and hemodynamics are appropriate for the caregivers to whom he or she entrusts the patient's care. Leaving a patient in the hands of someone unfamiliar or incapable of adequately handling the acuity of the medical situation in a rush to perform "the next case" may constitute abandonment of care. Check the function of indwelling cannulae, intravenous catheters, monitors and verify medication type and rates of any intravenous infusions before leaving.

POSTOPERATIVE PAIN MANAGEMENT

Relief of surgical pain with minimal side effects is a major goal during PACU care and a top priority for patients.[7,12–14] Periodically assess and document level of pain throughout recovery. The Joint Commission for Accreditation of Health Organizations has mandated that a numerical pain scale be used with periodic recording and an acceptable score for discharge. Inadequate postoperative analgesia is a major source of preoperative fear/dissatisfaction for surgical patients. In addition to improving comfort, analgesia reduces sympathetic nervous system response, thereby avoiding hypertension, tachycardia, and dysrhythmias. In hypo-
4 volemic patients, the sympathetic nervous system activity may well mask relative hypovolemia. Administration of analgesics can precipitate hypotension in an apparently stable patient, especially if direct or histamine-induced vasodilation occurs. It is important to assess a tachycardic patient with low or normal blood pressure who complains of pain carefully before giving analgesics that might precipitate or accentuate hypotension.

The actual degree of postoperative pain can be difficult to establish. Severity of pain varies among surgical procedures and anesthetic techniques. Staff members are relatively ineffective at quantifying level of discomfort. Patients are able to communicate despite having received sedative hypnotic drugs. Furthermore, patients may be impaired in their communication abilities coming into the hospital or may be affected by the entire medical experience, and thereby may be afraid to express their needs. Inexperienced nurses overestimate a patient's pain, whereas more experienced nurses tend to underestimate the pain.[15] Either error can lead to inappropriate treatment. Use of a numeric pain scale yields more reliable results but requires that a patient be willing to communicate. A wide divergence can exist between a patient's cognitive perception of pain and sympathetic nervous system response, related to psychological, cultural, and cardiovascular differences among individuals. Some patients perceive severe pain with minimal sympathetic nervous system activity, whereas others exhibit hypertension and tachycardia with minimal complaint of discomfort. The best measure of analgesia is the patient's perception. Heart rate, respiratory rate and depth, sweating, nausea, and vomiting all may be signs of pain but their

TABLE 54-1. COMPONENTS OF A POSTANESTHESIA CARE UNIT ADMISSION REPORT

Preoperative History/Procedures
- Medication allergies or reactions
- Pertinent earlier surgical procedures
- Underlying medical illness
- Chronic medications
- Acute problems (e.g., ischemia, acid–base status, dehydration)
- Premedications (e.g., antibiotics and time given, β-adrenergic blockers, antiemetics)
- Preoperative pain control (e.g., nerve blocks, adjunct medications, narcotics)
- Preoperative pain assessment (chronic and acute pain scores)
- NPO status

Intraoperative Factors
- Surgical procedure
- Type of anesthetic
- Type and difficulty of airway management
- Relaxant/reversal status
- Time and amount of opioids administered
- Type and amount of intravenous fluids administered
- Estimated blood loss
- Urine output
- Unexpected surgical or anesthetic events
- Intraoperative vital sign ranges
- Intraoperative laboratory findings
- Drugs given (e.g., steroids, diuretics, antibiotics, vasoactive medications, antiemetics)

Assessment and Report of Current Status
- Airway patency
- Ventilatory adequacy
- Level of consciousness
- Level of pain
- Heart rate and heart rhythm
- Endotracheal tube position
- Systemic pressure
- Intravascular volume status
- Function of invasive monitors
- Size and location of intravenous catheters
- Anesthetic equipment (e.g., epidural catheters, peripheral nerve catheters)
- Overall impression

Postoperative Instructions
- Expected airway and ventilatory status
- Acceptable vital sign ranges
- Acceptable urine output and blood loss
- Surgical instructions (e.g., positioning, wound care)
- Anticipated cardiovascular problems
- Orders for therapeutic interventions
- Diagnostic tests to be secured
- Therapeutic goals and end points before discharge
- Location of responsible physician

NPO, nothing by mouth.

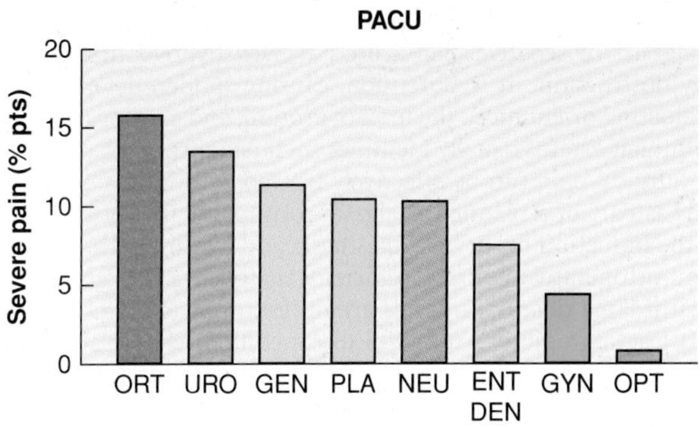

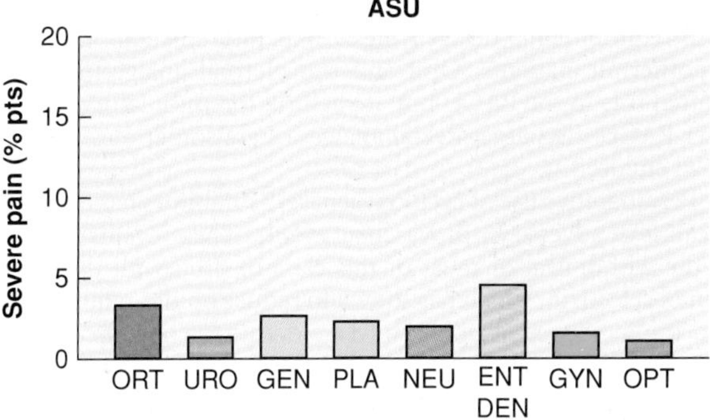

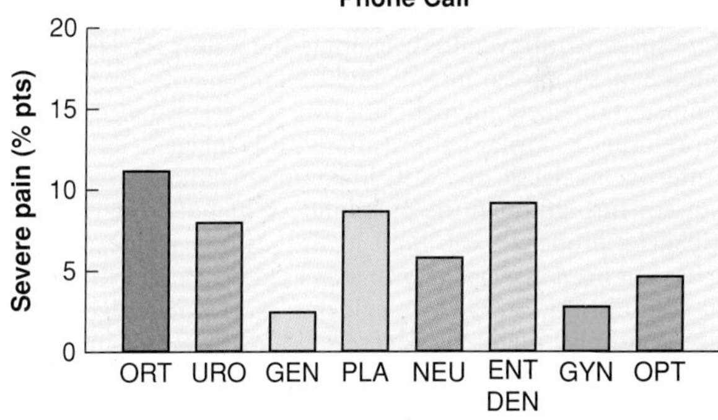

FIGURE 54-1. Percentage of patients experiencing severe pain in the postanesthesia care unit (PACU), the ambulatory surgery unit (ASU), and during phone call follow-up at 24 hours. ORT, orthopedics; URO, urology; GEN, general; PLA, plastics; NEU, neurology; ENT, ear, nose, throat; DEN, dental; GYN, gynecology; OPT, ophthalmology. (Reprinted from: Chung F, Ritchie E, Su J. Postoperative pain in ambulatory surgery. *Anesth Analg.* 1997;85:808, with permission.)

absence or presence is not in itself reliable as a measure of the presence of pain.

5 Careful identification of patient subgroups, assessment of individual analgesic requirements, and implementation of a planned, multimodal approach will provide seamless pain control through and beyond the PACU interval.[16] In a study of postoperative pain in 10,008 ambulatory patients, only 5.3% related severe pain in the PACU and 1.7% in the discharge area (Fig. 54-1). However, a much higher percentage of patients relate that moderate-to-severe pain recurs after discharge.[17,18] To avoid masking signs of an unrelated condition or a surgical complication, ascertain that the nature and intensity of pain are appropriate for the surgical procedure. The central nervous system (CNS) signs of hypoxemia, acidemia, or cerebral hypoperfusion often mimic those of

pain, especially during emergence. Administration of parenteral analgesics or sedatives can acutely worsen hypoventilation, airway obstruction, or hypotension, causing sudden deterioration. Evaluating orientation, the level of arousal, and cardiovascular or pulmonary status usually identifies such patients.

Surgical pain can be effectively treated with intravenous opioids as part of a planned analgesic continuum that begins prior to the induction of surgical anesthesia and continues throughout the postoperative course. Sufficient analgesia is the end point, even if large doses of opioids are necessary in tolerant patients. Short-acting opioids are useful to expedite discharge and minimize nausea in ambulatory settings,[19] although duration of analgesia can be a problem. During intravenous titration of opioids, assess for incremental respiratory or cardiovascular depression. Disadvantages of intramuscular administration include larger dose requirements, delayed onset, and unpredictable uptake in hypothermic patients. Oral and transdermal analgesics have a limited role in the PACU but are helpful for ambulatory patients after PACU discharge. Rectal analgesics are sometimes useful in small children.

Perioperative use of cyclooxygenase-2 inhibitors has decreased because of adverse cardiovascular events. These events have led to the withdrawal of most of this class of drug with the exception of celecoxib, which has shown to reduce opioid requirements and the incidence of opioid adverse events.[20] The concerns surrounding the negative cardiac side effects have made the overall appropriateness of this therapy more complicated. Nonselective nonsteroidal anti-inflammatory drugs such as ibuprofen or acetaminophen are also effective, especially when administered orally before surgery. Intravenous acetaminophen, now available in the United States can also lower opioid requirements. Preoperative administration likely augments the overall level of analgesia rather than offering a substantial preemptive advantage.[21] Ketorolac is an effective analgesic and anti-inflammatory that lowers opioid requirements, although the possibility of hemorrhage due to its antiplatelet properties can limit its use. Although intraoperative use has not been associated with increased bleeding, preoperative oral administration has some evidence of postoperative hemorrhage. Ketorolac might also decrease ischemic events in patients with coronary artery disease through analgesic and antiplatelet actions. Use of clonidine to supplement analgesia is effective but can cause hypotension. Agonist–antagonist analgesics offer little advantage. Interventions such as repositioning, reassurance, or extubation also help minimize discomfort.

Other analgesic modalities provide pain relief in and beyond the PACU.[22] Intravenous opioid loading in the PACU is important for smooth transition to intravenous patient-controlled analgesia. Injection of opioids into the epidural or subarachnoid space during anesthesia or in the PACU yields prolonged postoperative analgesia in selected patients.[23,24] Nausea and pruritus are troubling side effects, and immediate or delayed ventilatory depression can occur related to vascular uptake and cephalad spread in cerebrospinal fluid. Nausea should resolve with antiemetics, whereas pruritus and ventilatory depression often respond to naloxone infusion. Addition of local anesthetic or clonidine enhances analgesia and decreases the risk of side effects from epidural opioids, although local anesthetics add risk of hypotension or motor blockade. Epidural analgesia is effective after thoracic and upper abdominal procedures and helps wean obese patients or those with chronic obstructive pulmonary disease (COPD) from mechanical ventilation. Whether epidural analgesia improves surgical outcomes remains debatable.

Continuous flow catheters with pressure delivery systems of local anesthetics have been used intrawound to reduce pain and opioid requirements, increase patient satisfaction, and reduce length of hospital stay.[25] These same delivery systems have been safely used with continuous peripheral nerve catheters for in-hospital as well as outpatient use.[26,27] With the use of ultrasound-guided techniques for catheter placement, appropriately selected outpatients can safely receive the pain control benefits of regional anesthesia.[9] However, extensive written and oral postoperative instructions must be provided, with systems in place for 24-hour access by patients for catheter-related complications.

Placement of long-acting regional analgesic blocks reduces pain, controls sympathetic nervous system activity, and often improves ventilation.[22] After shoulder procedures, interscalene block yields almost complete pain relief with only moderate inconvenience from motor impairment. Paralysis of the ipsilateral diaphragm can impair postoperative ventilation in patients with marginal reserve, although the impact is small in most patients.[28] Suprascapular nerve block might be an alternative to avoid this potentially serious side effect. Percutaneous intercostal or paravertebral blocks reduce analgesic requirements after thoracic, breast, or high abdominal incision, although beneficial effects on postoperative pulmonary function are questionable. Transversus abdominis plane (TAP) blocks are effective for lower abdominal surgeries as well as those innervated by the ilioinguinal and iliohypogastric nerves. Caudal analgesia or paravertebral blocks can also be effective in children after inguinal or genital procedures, whereas infiltration of local anesthetic into joints, soft tissues, or incisions decreases the intensity of pain. Other modalities, such as guided imagery, hypnosis, transcutaneous nerve stimulation, music, massage, or acupuncture, have limited utility for surgical pain but may provide a positive patient experience.

Use of patient-controlled analgesia, spinal opioids, or neural blockade mandates anticipation of risk beyond the PACU. The plan for extended postoperative analgesia should be prepared before induction of surgical anesthesia, and then orient the anesthetic and PACU care toward that plan. These plans should be in agreement with the patient, surgeon, and anesthesiologist. If one analgesic modality proves inadequate, take particular care when implementing a second technique.

Fear, anxiety, and confusion often accentuate postoperative pain during recovery, especially after general anesthesia. Titration of an intravenous sedative such as midazolam attenuates this psychogenic component, although analgesic requirements may increase slightly because benzodiazepines interact with γ-aminobutyric acid receptors. It is important to distinguish between requirements for analgesia and for anxiolysis. Opioids are poor sedatives and anxiolytics, whereas benzodiazepines are poor analgesics. However, when opioid dose appears larger than what might be anticipated as what the patient should require, one should consider the possibility that anxiety is playing a large role in the dysphoric event in the PACU.

DISCHARGE CRITERIA

When possible before discharge from postoperative care, each patient should be sufficiently oriented to assess his or her physical condition and be able to summon assistance. Airway reflexes and motor function must be adequate to maintain patency and prevent aspiration. One should ensure that ventilation and oxygenation are acceptable, with sufficient reserve to cover minor deterioration in unmonitored settings. Blood pressure, heart rate, and indices of peripheral perfusion should be relatively constant for at least 15 minutes and appropriately near baseline. Achieving normal body temperature is not an absolute requirement, but there should be resolution of shivering. Acceptable analgesia

TABLE 54-2. TWO MOST COMMONLY USED POSTANESTHESIA CARE UNIT DISCHARGE CRITERIA SYSTEMS

Modified Aldrete Scoring System	Postanesthetic Discharge Scoring System
Respiration	**Vital signs**
2 = Able to take deep breath and cough	2 = BP + pulse within 20% preop baseline
1 = Dyspnea/shallow breathing	1 = BP + pulse within 20–40% preop baseline
0 = Apnea	0 = BP + pulse >40% preop baseline
O_2 saturation	**Activity**
2 = Maintains Spo_2 >92% on room air	2 = Steady gait, no dizziness or meets preop level
1 = Needs O_2 inhalation to maintain O_2 saturation >90%	1 = Requires assistance
0 = O_2 saturation <90% even with supplemental oxygen	0 = Unable to ambulate
Consciousness	**Nausea and Vomiting**
2 = Fully awake	2 = Minimal/treated with PO medication
1 = Arousable on calling	1 = Moderate/treated with parenteral medication
0 = Not responding	0 = Severe/continues despite treatment
Circulation	**Pain**
2 = BP ± 20 mm Hg preop	Controlled with oral analgesics and acceptable to patient:
1 = BP ± 20–50 mm Hg preop	2 = Yes
0 = BP ± 50 mm Hg preop	1 = No
Activity	**Surgical Bleeding**
2 = Able to move four extremities voluntary or on command	2 = Minimal/no dressing changes
1 = Able to move two extremities	1 = Moderate/up to two dressing changes required
0 = Unable to move extremities	0 = Severe/more than three dressing changes required
Score ≥9 for discharge	Score ≥9 for discharge

BP, blood pressure; PO, oral.

must be achieved and vomiting appropriately controlled. Patients should be observed for at least 15 minutes after the last intravenous opioid or sedative is administered to assess peak effects and side effects. If regional anesthetics have been administered, longer observation could be appropriate. One should monitor oxygen saturation for 15 minutes after discontinuation of supplemental oxygen to detect hypoxemia and then assess likely complications of surgery (e.g., bleeding, vascular compromise, pneumothorax) or of underlying conditions (e.g., hypertension, myocardial ischemia, hyperglycemia, bronchospasm). One should also document a brief neurologic assessment of orientation, eye signs, facial symmetry, and extremity movement and review results of diagnostic tests. If these generic criteria cannot be met, postponement of discharge or transfer to a specialized unit is advisable. There is no demonstrable benefit from a mandatory minimum duration of PACU care.

Scoring systems such as the Modified Aldrete Score or Postanesthesia Discharge Scoring System (Table 54-2) are two commonly used systems for patient assessment and attempt to simplify and standardize patient discharge criteria. Fixed PACU discharge criteria must be used with caution because variability among patients is tremendous. Scoring systems that quantify physical status or establish thresholds for vital signs are useful for
6 assessment but cannot replace individual evaluation.[29,30] Ideally, each patient should be evaluated for discharge by an anesthesiologist using a consistent set of criteria, considering the severity of underlying disease, the anesthetic and recovery course, and the level of care at the destination (Table 54-2). A plan for the continued management of likely postdischarge symptoms such as pain, nausea, headache, dizziness, drowsiness, and fatigue must be made prior to discharge.[18]

POSTOPERATIVE EVALUATION

The Centers for Medicare and Medicaid Services (CMS) have instituted compliance policies for those entities that participate in the Medicare and Medicaid programs. The policy for postanesthesia follow-up requires a written documentation that is performed by an individual that is qualified to administer anesthesia no later than 48 hours postprocedure. The time frame starts as soon as the patient arrives to the recovery area or ICU. The evaluation should be performed only after the patient has sufficiently recovered from anesthesia to be able to participate such as answer questions or perform simple tasks. The postanesthesia evaluation must contain the following elements:

- Respiratory function, including respiratory rate, airway patency, and oxygen saturation
- Cardiovascular function, including pulse rate and blood pressure
- Mental status
- Temperature
- Pain
- Nausea and vomiting
- Postoperative hydration.

CARDIOVASCULAR COMPLICATIONS

The purpose of this section is not to entirely review all the possible cardiovascular events that might beset a patient in the PACU, rather it is to help the reader decide what events might be 7 unique to the PACU. The cardiac risks during the postoperative stay include myocardial ischemia, which may be minimized with continued use of β-blockers, analgesia, nitrates, supplemental oxygen, adequate circulating volume, oxygen-carrying capacity, heart rate control, and an understanding of hypercoagulable states. In the PACU, some reflexes previously blunted by general anesthetics, sedatives, and opioids return toward baseline revealing an unexpected cardiovascular compromise. Perhaps the two most common types of patients to encounter troubles will be the patient with coronary artery disease and the patient with congestive heart failure. In the PACU it is a rare event for a patient to complain, *de novo,* of anginal type chest pain. The patients have significant blood opioid levels, and endorphins may be high because of the operation. The anesthetic makes the sensorium dulled and dysfunctional. The first sign of myocardial ischemia may well be hypotension, and the use of newer sedation techniques using drugs like dexmedetomidine can lead to hypotension postoperatively which can cloud the picture of a patient's cardiac disease. The most common sign of myocardial ischemia is tachycardia. Tachycardia is very often a reaction to, not the cause of, myocardial ischemia. That does not mean that all tachycardia heralds myocardial ischemia, but in a patient who seems at risk for coronary artery disease, new-onset tachycardia that is not caused by pain should be taken seriously. The ECG may show classic ST–T wave elevation or depression depending on lead placement and area of ischemia. But the lack of ST–T wave elevation does not rule out coronary artery disease. Transmural myocardial infarctions outside the PACU show no ECG diagnostic changes 10% to 30% of the time. So the clinician must be especially suspicious of a series of hemodynamic changes in a person at risk for coronary artery disease. Early intervention with nitrates, opioids, β-blockers, and even anticoagulants may save a life. Cardiology should be involved to gain immediate and timely access to the cardiac catheterization laboratory or for angiolytic drug therapy. Involvement and communication with the surgical service must be immediate and decisions especially as to anticoagulation and lytic therapy should be made among several services in consultation. Thus, cardiac ischemia in the PACU may manifest subtly! With increasing use of bare metal and drug-eluting stents (DES), recognition of those patients who have stopped antiplatelet therapy and are in postoperative hypercoagulable states can quickly occlude these stents. This situation requires quick recognition and response for intervention in the cath lab.

Congestive heart failure is epidemic in our ever-aging population. The outpatient cardiology services have an expanding armamentarium of new inotropic/vasodilator therapy, devices, and interventions that allow patients to compensate for their congestive heart failure. One should know not only the ejection fraction but the activities of daily living, exercise tolerance, and other risk indices. The ejection fraction is only an estimate of the fractional shortening of the myocardial actin and myosin fibrils. Although it is a useful estimate of severity of impairment, one is struck by how stable some patients may be with a large dilated heart contracting at a 15% ejection fraction. They are compensated but have little reserve. The potential problems of bleeding, volume shifts, and respiratory compromise in the PACU could quickly cause decompensation. There are also no absolute numbers with regard to fluid restriction. The usage of transesophageal echocardiography revolutionized cardiac anesthesia. It, along with transthoracic echo, may be of great use in the PACU. Within a very few minutes a puzzling hypotensive situation might be explained by an echocardiogram. In the fast-paced dynamic environment of the PACU, placing a pulmonary artery (PA) catheter may give useful information, but may also take valuable time away from patient triage and treatment. The echocardiogram allows rapid viewing of myocardial contractility, regional wall motion, volume status, and valvular dysfunction.

The PACU has in the recent history taken on a new role in some hospitals. Cardiac surgical care is pushing toward "early extubation" or "fast-tracking." In years past, especially when a "cardiac anesthetic" involved very large dosages of semisynthetic opioids that obligated patients to ≥24 hours of ventilation, the ICU was the standard place for all postoperative heart patients. Today, there is no such entity as a cardiac anesthetic. Balanced anesthetic techniques are used most often. Those who write about early extubation have pushed the limits from 24 hours all the way to extubation of patients on the operating table. Series are available with few if any reintubation catastrophes or events when this technique is practiced with good teams. The natural extension is to establish some highly specialized PACUs that function as step-down or short-term ICUs. In a study of 85 prospective patients[31] undergoing "off-pump" coronary artery bypass graft procedures, the patients were extubated in 12 ± 2 minutes after the chest was closed. They were then taken to a special part of the PACU where they were monitored for a number of hours (up to 480 minutes in some situations). Patients were then either discharged to the cardiac floors or sent to an ICU. Of the 85 patients in this study, only 4 failed the PACU stay and had to be admitted to an ICU. Bradycardia was the cause for failure in three cases and one there was one case of myocardial infarction. Two patients later returned to the ICU from the cardiac ward; there was one case of atrial fibrillation and another case of myocardial infarction. During the same time 304 patients who were not undergoing off-pump coronary artery bypass graft surgery were admitted to the cardiac ICU. The cost for PACU stay was $5,140.00 less than for an ICU-admitted patient. Although this study seems quite favorable, the two groups of patients were not comparable.

Studies from the mid-to-late 1990s looking at high-risk vascular and thoracic surgery patients showed that they could each be adequately cared for in an adequately staffed and prepared PACU.[32] The conclusion was that a hospital could well improve its patient throughput by putting more resources into expanded PACU care and not so much into ICU services. Several nursing reviews are available to give input as to how to structure such new units.[33,34]

Anesthesiology services are in increased demand throughout most hospitals. The PACU will likely need to prepare to care for those patients or to staff "ectopic" sites. In the evoked potential laboratories, for example, ablation procedures for dysrhythmias and the newer "mini-Maze" procedures may require care in the PACU. Automated implantable defibrillators are placed in hybrid suites, operating rooms, or catheterization laboratories. Now there is the possibility of percutaneous valve replacements as well as some hybrid and percutaneous coronary revascularization procedures. If these patients require deep sedation or general anesthesia, the patient will also require PACU care.

The cardiac patient is the common patient today. The new procedures and pressure to ever streamline operating room care is pressuring the PACU to become more and more a cardiac mini-ICU. The smart PACU medical director and hospital administrator will see that with targeted resources, patients may well be safely cared for in a more cost-effective manner with quicker throughput by using a PACU approach.

POSTOPERATIVE PULMONARY DYSFUNCTION

Mechanical, hemodynamic, and pharmacologic factors related to surgery and anesthesia impair ventilation, oxygenation, and airway maintenance.[35] Heavy smoking, obesity, sleep apnea, severe asthma, and COPD increase the risk of postoperative ventilatory events.[36] Preoperative pulmonary function testing has limited predictive value for postoperative complications,[37] perhaps with the exception of postoperative bronchospasm in smokers.[38]

Inadequate Postoperative Ventilation

In PACU patients, mild respiratory acidemia due to atelectasis and decreased minute ventilation is expected; thus, elevated $Paco_2$ does not necessarily indicate inadequate postoperative ventilation. Inadequate ventilation should be suspected when (1) respiratory acidemia occurs coincident with tachypnea, anxiety, dyspnea, labored ventilation, or increased sympathetic nervous system activity; (2) hypercarbia reduces the arterial pH below 7.30; or (3) $Paco_2$ progressively increases with a progressive decrease in arterial pH.

Inadequate Respiratory Drive

During early recovery from anesthesia, residual effects of intravenous and inhalation anesthetics blunt the ventilatory responses to both hypercarbia and hypoxemia. Sedatives augment depression from opioids or anesthetics and reduce the conscious desire to ventilate (a significant component of ventilatory drive).

Hypoventilation and hypercarbia can evolve insidiously during transfer and admission to the PACU. Although effects of intraoperative medications are usually waning, the peak depressant effect of an intravenous opioid given just before transfer occurs in the PACU. Coincident depression of medullary centers that regulate the sympathetic nervous system can blunt signs of acidemia or hypoxemia such as hypertension, tachycardia, and agitation, concealing hypoventilation. Patients might communicate lucidly and even complain of pain while experiencing significant opioid-induced hypoventilation. A balance must be struck between an acceptable level of postoperative ventilatory depression and a tolerable level of pain or agitation. Patients with abnormal CO_2/pH responses from morbid obesity, chronic airway obstruction, or sleep apnea are more sensitive to respiratory depressants.[39] Risk for apnea after anesthesia in preterm infants depends on type of anesthetic, postconceptual age, and preoperative hematocrit. Preterm infants should be monitored for at least 12 hours (see Chapter 41). Children with active or recent upper respiratory infection are more prone to breath-holding, severe cough, and arterial desaturations below 90% during recovery, especially if they have a history of reactive airway disease or secondhand smoke exposure or have undergone intubation and/or airway surgery.[40] If hypoventilation from opioids is excessive, forced arousal and careful titration (20 to 40 μg at a time) of intravenous naloxone reverses respiratory depression without affecting analgesia. Flumazenil (0.1 mg titrated to effect up to 1.5 mg) directly reverses depressant effects of benzodiazepines on ventilatory drive but is usually unnecessary.

The abrupt diminution of a noxious stimulus (e.g., tracheal extubation, placement of a postoperative block) may promote hypoventilation or airway obstruction by altering the balance between arousal from discomfort and depression from medication. Intracranial hemorrhage or edema sometimes presents with hypoventilation, especially after posterior fossa craniotomy. Bilateral carotid body injury after endarterectomy can ablate peripheral hypoxic drive. Chronic respiratory acidemia from COPD alters CNS sensitivity to pH and makes hypoxic drive dominant, but hypoventilation from supplemental oxygen rarely occurs.

Increased Airway Resistance

High resistance to gas flow through airways increases work of breathing and CO_2 production. If inspiratory muscles cannot generate sufficient pressure gradients to overcome resistance, alveolar ventilation fails to match CO_2 production and progressive respiratory acidemia occurs.

In postoperative patients, increased upper airway resistance is caused by obstruction in the pharynx (posterior tongue displacement, change in anteroposterior and lateral dimensions from soft-tissue collapse), in the larynx (laryngospasm, laryngeal edema), or in the large airways (extrinsic compression from hematoma, tumor, or tracheal stenosis). Weakness from residual neuromuscular relaxation,[41] myasthenia gravis or myasthenic syndromes can contribute, but it is seldom the primary cause of airway compromise. If the airway is clear of vomitus or foreign bodies, simple maneuvers such as improving the level of consciousness, lateral positioning, chin lift, mandible elevation, or placement of an oropharyngeal or nasopharyngeal airway usually relieve obstruction. A nasopharyngeal airway is better tolerated when the patient has functional gag reflexes. Acute extrinsic upper airway compression (e.g., an expanding neck hematoma) must be relieved.

During emergence, stimulation of the pharynx or vocal cords by secretions, blood, foreign matter, or extubation can generate laryngospasm.[42] Laryngeal constrictor muscles occlude the tracheal inlet and reduce gas flow. Patients who smoke or are chronically exposed to smoke have irritable airway conditions, have copious secretions, or have undergone upper airway surgery are at higher risk.[35,40] Laryngospasm can usually be overcome by providing gentle positive pressure (10 to 20 mm Hg continuous) in the oropharynx by mask with 100% O_2. Prolonged laryngospasm is relieved with a small dose of succinylcholine (e.g., 0.1 mg/kg) or deepening sedation with propofol. An intubating dosage of succinylcholine should not be used to break postoperative laryngospasm, especially if the alveolar partial pressure of oxygen (PAO_2) is decreased by hypoventilation. As little as 5 to 10 mg of succinylcholine can break the laryngospasm. Unless assisted ventilation is provided, declining PAO_2 causes serious hypoxemia before spontaneous ventilation resumes[43] (Fig. 54-2). If the functional residual capacity (FRC) is abnormally reduced, the decreased volume of O_2 available in the lungs accelerates the development of hypoxemia. Severe laryngeal obstruction can occur secondarily because of hypocalcemia after parathyroid excision.

Soft-tissue edema worsens airway obstruction, especially in children and adults recovering from procedures on the neck. Nebulized vasoconstrictors like epinepherine help somewhat, but steroids have little effect acutely. Patients with C1 esterase inhibitor deficiency can develop severe angioneurotic edema after even slight trauma to the airway. Pathologic airway obstruction (e.g., severe edema, epiglottitis, retropharyngeal abscess, encroaching tumors) might require emergency tracheal intubation, but airway manipulation is dangerous because minor trauma from intubation attempts can convert a marginal airway into a total obstruction. Judgment by the individual anesthesiologist regarding timing, patient status, available equipment along with airway management skills all play a part of the decision as to where, when, and how to intubate. Sedatives or muscle relaxants used

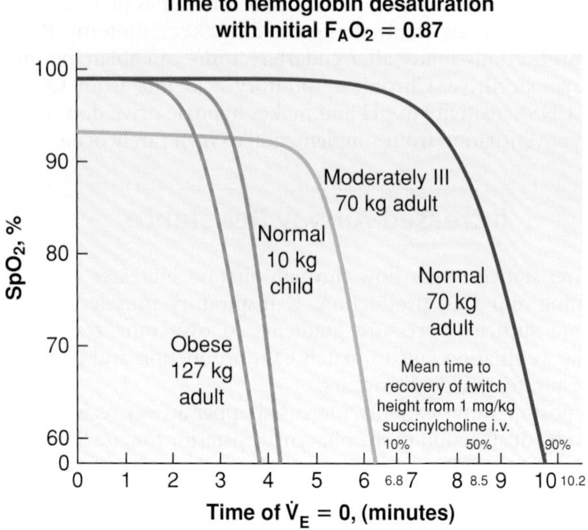

FIGURE 54-2. Rate of Spo_2 decline after onset of apnea. (Reprinted from: Benumof JL, Dagg R, Benumof R. Critical hemoglobin desaturation will occur before return to an unparalyzed state following 1 mg/kg intravenous succinylcholine. *Anesthesiology.* 1997;87:979, with permission.)

to facilitate intubation can worsen obstruction by compromising the patient's volitional efforts to maintain the airway and by eliminating spontaneous ventilation. Equipment and personnel necessary for emergency cricothyroidotomy or tracheostomy should be available. Needle cricothyroidotomy using a 14-gauge intravenous catheter or a commercially available kit permits oxygenation and marginal ventilation until the airway is secured, especially if jet ventilation with 100% oxygen is used.

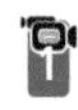

Reduction of cross-sectional area in small airways increases overall airway resistance because resistance varies inversely with the fourth power of radius during laminar flow and with the fifth power during turbulent flow. Pharyngeal or tracheal stimulation from secretions, suctioning, aspiration, or a tracheal tube can trigger a reflex constriction of bronchial smooth muscle in emerging patients with reactive airways. Histamine release precipitated by medication or allergic reactions also increases airway smooth muscle tone. Decreased radial traction on small airways reduces cross-sectional area in patients with COPD or with decreased lung volume secondary to obesity, surgical manipulation, excessive lung water, or splinting. Preoperative spirometric evidence of increased airway resistance predicts an increased risk of postoperative bronchospasm.[38] Smokers and patients with bronchospastic conditions are at highest risk.[44] If ventilatory requirements are increased by warming, hyperthermia, or work of breathing, high flow rates convert laminar flow to higher-resistance turbulent flow. Prolonged expiratory time or audible turbulent air flow (wheezing) during forced vital capacity expiration often unmasks subclinical airway resistance. (Resistance is higher during expiration because intermediate-diameter airways are compressed by positive intrathoracic pressure.) High airway resistance does not always cause wheezing because flow might be so impeded that no sound is produced. Signs of increased resistance mimic those of decreased pulmonary compliance. Spontaneously breathing patients exhibit accessory muscle recruitment, labored ventilation, and increased work of breathing with either condition. Mechanically ventilated patients exhibit high peak inspiratory pressures.

The treatment of small airway resistance is directed at an underlying etiology. One must eliminate laryngeal or airway stimulation. Patients often respond to their pre-existing regimen of albuterol, pirbuterol, or salmeterol inhalers. Levalbuterol or metaproterenol nebulized in oxygen resolves postoperative bronchospasm with minimal tachycardia. Nebulized racemic epinephrine effectively relaxes smooth muscle, but side effects of tachycardia and flushing can be seen. Isoproterenol has also been nebulized with good results. Intramuscular or sublingual terbutaline can be added. Administration of steroid therapy offers little acute improvement, but may prevent later recurrence. Bronchospasm that is resistant to β_2-sympathomimetic medication may improve with an anticholinergic medication such as atropine or ipratropium. If bronchospasm is life-threatening, an intravenous epinephrine infusion yields profound bronchodilation. Increased small airway resistance caused by mechanical factors (e.g., loss of lung volume, retained secretions, pulmonary edema) usually does not resolve with bronchodilators. Restoration of lung volume with incentive spirometry or deep tidal ventilation increases radial traction on small airways. Reducing left ventricular filling pressures might relieve airway resistance caused by increased lung water, although interstitial fluid accumulation can persist. Also, extended contraction of airway smooth muscle obstructs venous and lymphatic flow, leading to airway wall edema that resolves slowly.

Decreased Compliance

Reduced pulmonary compliance accentuates the work of breathing. In the extreme, low compliance causes progressive respiratory muscle fatigue, hypoventilation, and respiratory acidemia. Parenchymal changes also affect compliance. Reduction of FRC leads to small airway closure and distal lung collapse, requiring greater energy expenditure to re-expand the lung. Pulmonary edema increases the lung's weight and inertia and elevates surface tension by interfering with surfactant activity, making expansion more difficult. Pulmonary contusion or hemorrhage interferes with lung expansion, as do restrictive lung diseases, skeletal abnormalities, intrathoracic lesions, hemothorax, pneumothorax, or cardiomegaly. Obesity affects pulmonary compliance, especially when adipose tissue compresses the thoracic cage or increases intra-abdominal pressure in supine or lateral positions. Extrathoracic factors such as tight muscles of the chest or abdominal dressings and gas in the stomach or bowel reduce compliance. Most notably after intra-abdominal laparoscopic procedures, retained CO_2 may impair diaphragm movement. The CO_2 has the capability to dissecting into the thorax creating either a pneumothorax or pneumomediastinum, which is usually a self-limited event as the CO_2 is relatively rapidly absorbed. There is usually no need for chest tube intervention. An intra-abdominal tumor, hemorrhage, ascites, bowel obstruction, or pregnancy impairs diaphragmatic excursion and reduces compliance.

Work of breathing is improved by resolving problems that reduce compliance. Allowing patients to recover in a semisitting (semi-Fowler) position reduces work of breathing. Incentive spirometry and chest physiotherapy help restore lung volume, as does positive end-expiratory pressure (PEEP) or continuous positive airway pressure (CPAP). In patients with COPD and highly compliant lungs, positive airway pressure might force the rib cage and diaphragms toward their excursion limits, accentuating inspiratory muscular effort.

Neuromuscular and Skeletal Problems

Postoperative airway obstruction and hypoventilation are accentuated by incomplete reversal of neuromuscular relaxation. Residual paralysis compromises airway patency, ability to overcome airway resistance, airway protection, and ability to clear secretions.[45] In the extreme, paralysis precludes effective spontaneous ventilation. Intraoperative use of shorter-acting relaxants might decrease the incidence of residual paralysis but does not eliminate the problem. Marginal reversal can be more dangerous than near-total paralysis because a weak, agitated patient exhibiting uncoordinated movements and airway obstruction is more easily identified. A somnolent patient exhibiting mild stridor and shallow ventilation from marginal neuromuscular function might be overlooked, allowing insidious hypoventilation and respiratory acidemia or regurgitation with aspiration to occur. PACU staff should be aware of patients who have received nondepolarizing muscle relaxants but no reversal agents because they often exhibit low levels of residual paralysis.[46] Safety of techniques designed to avoid reversal of short- and intermediate-duration relaxants has not been substantiated, and reversal of nondepolarizing relaxants is recommended.[7] The selective relaxant binding agent used widely in Europe but currently unavailable in the United States, γ-cyclodextrins (i.e., Sugammadex), is a promising reversal drug that can avoid the side effects of other anticholinesterases and anticholinergics.[47] Patients with neuromuscular abnormalities such as myasthenia gravis, Eaton–Lambert syndrome, periodic paralysis, or muscular dystrophies exhibit exaggerated or prolonged responses to muscle relaxants. Even without relaxant administration, these patients can exhibit postoperative ventilatory insufficiency. Medications potentiate neuromuscular relaxation (e.g., antibiotics, furosemide, propranolol, phenytoin), as does hypocalcemia or hypermagnesemia.

Diaphragmatic contraction is compromised in some postoperative patients, forcing more reliance on intercostal muscles and reducing the ability to overcome decreased compliance or increased ventilatory demands. Impairment of phrenic nerve function from interscalene block, trauma, or thoracic and neck operations can "paralyze" one or rarely both diaphragms.[28] Adequate ventilation will normally be maintained with only one diaphragm, and marginal ventilation by external intercostal muscles alone. However, with high work of breathing, muscle weakness, or increased ventilatory demands, a nonfunctional diaphragm impairs minute ventilation. Thoracic spinal or epidural blockade interferes with intercostal muscle function and reduces ventilatory reserve, especially in patients with COPD. Abnormal motor neuron function (e.g., Guillain–Barré syndrome, cervical spinal cord trauma), flail chest, or severe kyphosis or scoliosis can cause postoperative ventilatory insufficiency.

Simple tests help assess mechanical ability to ventilate. The ability to sustain head elevation in a supine position, a forced vital capacity of 10 to 12 mL/kg, an inspiratory pressure more negative than −25 cm H_2O, and tactile train-of-four assessment imply that strength of ventilatory muscles is adequate to sustain ventilation and to take a large enough breath to cough. However, none of these clinical end points reliably predicts recovery of airway protective reflexes,[46] and failure on these tests does not necessarily indicate the need for assisted ventilation.

The use of noninvasive mechanical ventilation techniques such as continuous positive airway pressure or bilevel ventilation can help safely extubate some patients earlier or prevent reintubating others. By using these noninvasive airway techniques, patients can often overcome some of the above discussed issues interfering with normal respiration. Thus reducing the risk of remaining intubated or reintubation. Units other than ICUs are able to manage these patients therefore offloading the burden on the ICU.

Occasionally, a clinical picture suggests ventilatory insufficiency when ventilation is adequate. Voluntary limitation of chest expansion to avoid pain (splinting) causes labored, rapid, shallow breathing characteristic of inadequate ventilation. Splinting seldom causes actual hypoventilation and usually improves with analgesia and repositioning. Ventilation with small tidal volumes due to thoracic restriction or reduced compliance seems to generate afferent input from pulmonary stretch receptors, leading to dyspnea, labored breathing, and accessory muscle recruitment in spite of appropriate minute ventilation. Occasional large, "satisfying" lung expansions often relieve these symptoms. Finally, spontaneous hyperventilation to compensate for a metabolic acidemia might generate tachypnea or labored breathing, which is mistaken for ventilatory insufficiency.

Increased Dead Space

Ventilation of unperfused dead space or of poorly perfused alveoli with high ventilation/perfusion ($\dot{V}/\dot{Q}$) ratios is less effective in removing CO_2. Expansion of dead space volume or reduction of tidal volume increases the fraction of each breath wasted in dead space $\dot{V}_D/\dot{V}_T$ and the amount of CO_2 from the previous exhalation that is rebreathed. A proportionally larger increase in total minute ventilation is required to meet any increase in CO_2 production. Patients with high $\dot{V}_D/\dot{V}_T$ are at greater risk for postoperative ventilatory failure.

Occasionally, an acute increase in dead space contributes to respiratory acidemia in postoperative patients. Although upper airway dead space is reduced after tracheal intubation and tracheostomy, excessive tubing volume or valve reversal in breathing circuits promotes rebreathing of CO_2. PEEP or CPAP elevates physiologic dead space, especially in patients with high pulmonary compliance. Pulmonary embolization with air, thrombus, or cellular debris increases physiologic dead space, although impact on CO_2 excretion is often compensated by accelerated minute ventilation from hypercarbic and hypoxic drives or reflex responses. Decreased cardiac output can transiently increase $\dot{V}_D/\dot{V}_T$ by decreasing perfusion to well-ventilated, nondependent lung. Irreversible increases in dead space occur if adult respiratory distress syndrome (ARDS) related to sepsis, transfusion-related acute lung injury (TRALI), or hypoxia destroys pulmonary microvasculature. Dead space may appear high if an inhalation interrupts the previous exhalation and the spent alveolar gas is retained. This "gas trapping" occurs when high airway resistance lengthens the time required to exhale completely, or if improper inspiration/expiration ratios or high ventilatory rates are used during mechanical ventilation.

Increased Carbon Dioxide Production

Carbon dioxide production varies directly with metabolic rate, body temperature, and substrate availability. During anesthesia, CO_2 production falls to approximately 60% of the normal 2 to 3 mL/kg/min as hypothermia lowers metabolic activity and neuromuscular relaxation reduces tonic muscle contraction. Therefore, during recovery, metabolic rate and CO_2 production can increase by 40%. Shivering, high work of breathing, infection, sympathetic nervous system activity, or rapid carbohydrate metabolism during intravenous hyperalimentation accelerates CO_2 production. Malignant hyperthermia generates CO_2 production many times greater than normal, which rapidly exceeds ventilatory reserve and causes severe respiratory and metabolic acidemia. Even mild increases of CO_2 production can precipitate respiratory acidemia if low compliance, airway resistance, or neuromuscular paralysis interferes with ventilation. With the exception of adjusting hyperalimentation, improving work of breathing, reducing shivering, or treating hyperthermia, there is little yield from addressing CO_2 production in PACU patients.

Inadequate Postoperative Oxygenation

Systemic arterial partial pressure of oxygen ($Pa{O_2}$) is the best indicator of pulmonary oxygen transfer from alveolar gas to pulmonary capillary blood. Arterial hemoglobin saturation monitored by pulse oximetry yields less information on alveolar–arterial gradients and is not helpful in assessing impact of hemoglobin dissociation curve shifts or carboxyhemoglobin.[48] Evaluation of metabolic acidemia or mixed venous oxygen content yields insight into peripheral oxygen delivery and utilization. Adequate arterial oxygenation does not mean that cardiac output, arterial perfusion pressure, or distribution of blood flow will maintain tissue oxygenation. Sepsis, hypotension, anemia, or hemoglobin dissociation abnormalities can generate tissue ischemia despite adequate oxygenation.

In postoperative patients, the acceptable lower limit for $Pa{O_2}$ varies with individual patient characteristics. A $Pa{O_2}$ below 65 to 70 mm Hg causes significant hemoglobin desaturation, although tissue oxygen delivery might be maintained at lower levels. Maintaining $Pa{O_2}$ between 80 and 100 mm Hg (saturation: 93% to 97%) ensures adequate oxygen availability. Little benefit is derived from elevating $Pa{O_2}$ above 110 mm Hg because hemoglobin is saturated and the amount of additional oxygen dissolved in plasma is negligible. During mechanical ventilation, a $Pa{O_2}$ above 80 mm Hg with 0.4 $F{I}{O_2}$ and 5 cm H_2O PEEP,[48] CPAP or spontaneous breathing trial usually predicts sustained adequate oxygenation after tracheal extubation.

Distribution of Ventilation

Loss of dependent lung volume commonly causes $\dot{V}/\dot{Q}$ mismatching and hypoxemia. A reduction in FRC decreases radial traction on small airways, leading to collapse and distal atelectasis that can worsen for 36 hours after surgery.[49] Reduced ventilation in dependent lung is particularly damaging because gravity directs pulmonary blood flow to dependent areas. Obese patients sustain large decreases in FRC during surgery. Older patients normally exhibit some airway closure at end expiration, and those with COPD have more severe closure that is exacerbated by small reductions in FRC. Retraction, packing, manipulation, or peritoneal insufflation during upper abdominal surgery reduces FRC, as does compression from leaning surgical assistants.[50] Prone, lithotomy, or Trendelenburg positions are disadvantageous, especially in obese patients. Right upper lobe collapse secondary to partial right main stem intubation is a frequently overlooked cause. During one-lung anesthesia, the weight of unsupported mediastinal contents, pressure from abdominal contents on the dependent diaphragm, and lung compression all reduce dependent lung volume. Gravity and lymphatic obstruction promote interstitial fluid accumulation and further $\dot{V}/\dot{Q}$ mismatching. This "down lung syndrome" may appear as unilateral pulmonary edema on the chest film.

Postoperatively, acute pulmonary edema from overhydration, ventricular dysfunction, airway obstruction, or increased capillary permeability (e.g., including transfusion-related acute lung injury, drug reactions) leads to hypoxemia by interfering with both $\dot{V}/\dot{Q}$ matching and diffusion of oxygen. Strong inspiratory efforts against an obstructed airway decrease FRC and promote negative-pressure pulmonary edema. Small airway occlusion from compression, retained secretions, or aspiration leads to distal hypoventilation and hypoxemia, as does main stem intubation. Pneumothorax or hemothorax also reduce lung volume.

Conservative measures that restore lung volume often improve oxygenation. If possible, patients should recover in a semisitting or reverse Trendelenberg position to reduce abdominal pressure on the diaphragms. Pain with ventilation encourages shallow breathing, so analgesia helps maintain FRC, especially with upper abdominal or chest wall incisions. Deep ventilation, cough, chest physiotherapy, and incentive spirometry seem to help expand FRC, mobilize secretions, and accustom a patient to incisional discomfort, but actual efficacy is debated.[51,52] For serious postoperative reduction of FRC, positive pressure is effective. CPAP (5 to 7 cm H_2O) or bilevel can be delivered by face mask for several hours until factors promoting loss of lung volume resolve. If hypoxemia is severe or patient acceptance of CPAP or the often more tolerable bilevel mask is poor, tracheal intubation is usually required. Intubation for delivery of noninvasive ventilation does not mandate positive-pressure ventilation. Ventilatory requirements should be assessed independently, considering $Pa{CO_2}$, arterial pH, and work of breathing. Usually, 5 to 10 cm H_2O of CPAP or PEEP improves $Pa{O_2}$ without risking hypotension, increased intracranial pressure, or barotrauma. If $Pa{O_2}$ does not improve, one must re-evaluate the etiology. An occasional patient with ARDS or pulmonary contusion might require expiratory pressures in excess of 10 cm H_2O for improved oxygenation.

Tracheal intubation eliminates normal expiratory resistance and the "physiologic PEEP" (2 to 5 cm H_2O) that helps maintain lung volume during spontaneous ventilation. Exposing an intubated trachea to ambient pressure may cause a gradual reduction in FRC. Healthy, slender patients will often tolerate short periods of intubation without positive pressure, but generally it is prudent to use 5 cm H_2O CPAP for intubated postoperative patients.

Distribution of Perfusion

Poor distribution of pulmonary blood flow also interferes with $\dot{V}/\dot{Q}$ matching and oxygenation. Flow distribution is primarily determined by hydrodynamic factors (PA and venous pressures, vascular resistance), which are affected by gravity, airway pressure, lung volume, and cardiac dynamics. Flow distribution is modulated by hypoxic pulmonary vasoconstriction (HPV), which diverts flow from air spaces that exhibit low $Pa{O_2}$. In postoperative patients, position affects oxygenation if gravity forces blood flow to areas with reduced ventilation. For example, placing a poorly ventilated lung in a dependent position can reduce $Pa{O_2}$. Postoperative changes in PA pressure, airway pressure, and lung volume also have complex effects on blood flow distribution that can adversely affect $\dot{V}/\dot{Q}$ matching. Residual inhalation anesthetics, vasodilators, and sympathomimetics directly affect vascular tone and HPV, partially explaining larger alveolar–arterial oxygen gradients after general anesthesia. (Changes in distribution of ventilation also contribute.) Patients with liver cirrhosis exhibit poor $\dot{V}/\dot{Q}$ matching caused by small arteriovenous shunts that form throughout their lungs. Circulating endotoxin impairs HPV, contributing to hypoxemia in septic patients.

In the PACU, few interventions are useful to improve $\dot{V}/\dot{Q}$ matching by changing the distributions pulmonary blood flow. Maintain PA and airway pressures within an acceptable range. When possible, avoid placing an atelectatic or diseased lung in a dependent position. Placing poorly ventilated parenchyma in a nondependent position could improve $\dot{V}/\dot{Q}$ matching, but positioning a diseased lung in an "up" position may promote drainage of purulent material into the unaffected lung. Avoiding vasodilatory medications may improve $Pa{O_2}$ but benefits from the medication usually outweigh drawbacks of impaired HPV.

Inadequate Alveolar P_{AO_2}

Postoperative hypoxemia is occasionally caused by a global reduction of P_{AO_2}, usually from inadequate ventilation, and marked increase in P_{ACO_2} (see the alveolar gas equation in Chapter 11). Hypoventilation must be severe to cause hypoxemia based on the alveolar gas equation. Complete apnea or airway obstruction by a foreign body, soft-tissue edema, or laryngospasm as well as very high small airway resistance all lead to rapid depletion of alveolar oxygen, and precludes effective ventilation. If cessation of ventilation does occur, the rate of P_{AO_2} decline varies with age, body habitus, degree of underlying illness, and initial P_{AO_2}[43] (Fig. 54-3).
8 Hypoxemia might also occur if opioids or residual anesthetic levels severely depress ventilatory drives. Partial airway obstruction does not usually reduce P_{AO_2}, especially when patients are receiving supplemental oxygen. Increasing the oxygen content of the FRC with supplemental oxygen safeguards against hypoxemia from hypoventilation or airway obstruction, and eliminates the use of the pulse oximeter as a monitor of hypoventilation. Rarely, excessive concentrations of other gases reduce P_{AO_2}. After general anesthesia, rapid outpouring of nitrous oxide displaces alveolar gas and can lower P_{AO_2} if a patient is hypoventilating or breathing ambient air, but this "diffusion hypoxia" would usually occur before PACU admission. Volume displacement of oxygen could also occur during severe hypercarbia in a patient breathing ambient air, although acidemia is often a greater problem.

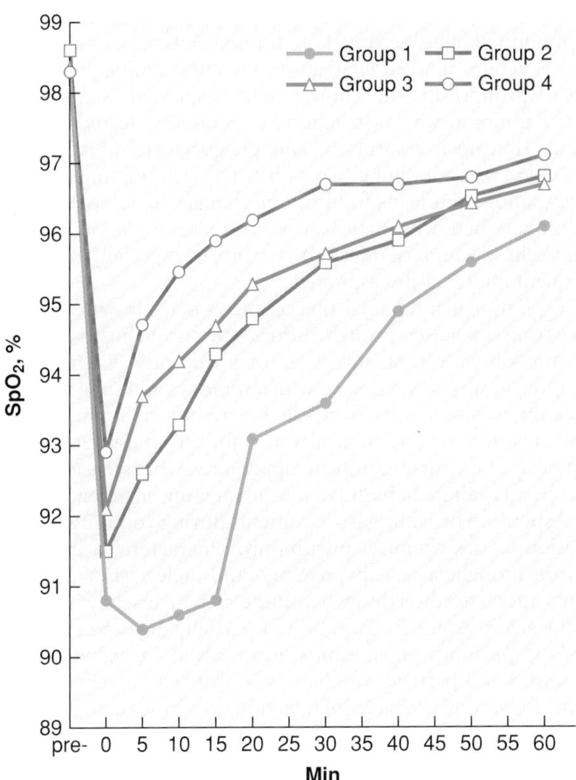

FIGURE 54-3. Sp_{O_2} versus postanesthesia care unit time in patients spontaneously breathing room air after general anesthesia (group 1, 0 to 1 year of age; group 2, 1 to 3 years; group 3, 3 to 14 years; group 4, 14 to 58 years). (Reprinted from: Xue FS, Huang YG, Tong SY, et al. A comparative study of early postoperative hypoxemia in infants, children, and adults undergoing elective plastic surgery. *Anesth Analg.* 1996;83:709, with permission.)

Reduced Mixed Venous P_{O_2}

Mixed venous partial pressure of oxygen ($P\bar{v}_{O_2}$) is affected by arterial oxygen content, cardiac output, distribution of peripheral blood flow, and tissue oxygen extraction. If arterial oxygen content decreases or tissue extraction increases, $P\bar{v}_{O_2}$ falls. The lower the $Pv\text{-}o_2$ in blood that is shunted or flows through low $\dot{V}/\dot{Q}$ units, the greater the reduction of Pa_{O_2}. Blood with a low $P\bar{v}_{O_2}$ also extracts larger volumes of oxygen from alveolar gas, amplifying the effect of hypoventilation or airway obstruction on P_{AO_2}. Very low $P\bar{v}_{O_2}$ increases the risk of resorption atelectasis in poorly ventilated alveoli. In postoperative patients, shivering, infection, and hypermetabolism lower $P\bar{v}_{O_2}$ by increasing peripheral oxygen extraction. Low cardiac output and hypotension also lower $P\bar{v}_{O_2}$ by decreasing tissue oxygen delivery. Supplemental oxygen reduces the impact of low $P\bar{v}_{O_2}$ on alveolar oxygen extraction and on arterial oxygenation.

Obstructive Sleep Apnea

Obstructive sleep apnea (OSA) is a syndrome in which patients exhibit a period of partial or complete obstruction of the upper airway. This obstruction in turn interrupts sleep patterns, resulting in daytime hypersomnolence, decreased ability to concentrate, increased irritability, as well as aggressive and distractible behavior in children. The airway obstruction may cause episodic oxygen desaturation, hypercarbia, and possibly lead to cardiac dysfunction. It is estimated that 9% of women and 24% of men in the United States show disordered breathing while asleep, and 2% of women and 4% of men show overt symptoms of OSA.[53] These numbers are likely to increase as the population ages and become increasingly obese. In May 2003, the ASA Task Force on Perioperative Management of Patients with Obstructive Sleep Apnea issued guidelines based on the ASA scoring system for OSA and classifying patients as having mild, moderate, or severe OSA based on the apnea–hypopnea index.[54]

The perioperative management of the OSA patient must start preoperatively with a well-planned anesthetic taking into account the type, location, and recovery of surgery. Postoperative management concerns include analgesia, oxygenation, patient positioning, and monitoring. Regional anesthesia with minimal sedation is best for recovery versus increased use of opioids. Supplemental oxygen should be used immediately postoperatively. Patients who use CPAP or noninvasive positive-pressure ventilation should continue to use these therapies. Positioning should be used to minimize the patients' ability to obstruct the airway, which can be limited based on the type of surgery. Adult OSA patients show improvement in apnea–hypopnea index scores while in lateral, prone, and sitting positions compared with supine. With regard to monitoring, there is agreement among the consultants on the task force that pulse oximetry should be used until the patients' oxygen saturation remains above 90% on room air while sleeping. The use of telemetry for monitoring pulse oximetry, ECG, or ventilation can be beneficial in reducing adverse postoperative events and should be used on a patient need basis. With increasing studies in the area of OSA, the increased standardization of information regarding this patient population will lead to greater evidence-based treatment and supported clinical care.

Anemia

Preoperative hematocrit and intraoperative hemorrhage determine a patient's red cell mass and oxygen-carrying capacity after surgery. Reduction of hematocrit caused by dilution has less impact. The hematocrit at which oxygen delivery becomes insufficient to match tissue needs varies with cardiac reserve, oxygen consumption, hemoglobin dissociation, PaO_2, and blood flow distribution. The actual level at which shock, lack of tissue oxygen delivery, occurs is known as the *critical* DO_2 level. For animals and humans who have normal myocardial function and are euvolemic, critical DO_2 requires at least 3 to 3.5 g/dL hemoglobin concentration. Of course, a hemoglobin concentration this low may not be an appropriate transfusion trigger. However, it does illustrate the large excess of hemoglobin available to meet metabolic O_2 demands. Each patient has a minimum hematocrit below which tissues use inefficient anaerobic metabolism, generating a lactic acidemia. Patients with vascular disease are at increased risk of vital organ ischemia as hematocrit falls. Work from the ASA and the cardiac anesthesia/surgery societies (Society of Thoracic Surgeons and Society of Cardiovascular Anesthesiologists) have published guidelines for transfusion and blood management. It is well accepted now that patients who are stable, not bleeding, and euvolemic can tolerate a hemoglobin of 6 g/dL. Transfusion may be of some benefit between 6 and 8 g/dL and it is rarely of use above 10 g/dL. Furthermore, transfusion of red cells to assist in weaning a patient from the ventilator has been shown to make the weaning process prolonged and/or make it far more difficult to remove the patient from the ventilator.

Supplemental Oxygen

The incidence of hypoxemia in postoperative patients is high. In PACU patients placed on room air, 30% of patients younger than 1 year of age, 20% aged 1 to 3 years, 14% aged 3 to 14 years, and 7.8% of adults had hemoglobin saturations fall below 90%, with many falling below 85%[55] (Fig. 54-3). Clinical observation and assessment of cognitive function do not accurately screen for hypoxemia, so monitoring with oximetry is essential throughout the PACU admission.[56] One cannot predict which patients will become hypoxemic or when hypoxemia will occur. Patients with lung disease or obesity, those recovering from thoracic or upper abdominal procedures, and those with preoperative hypoxemia are at increased risk.[57] Postoperative hypoxemia occurs in children, especially those with respiratory infections or chronic adenotonsillar hypertrophy. Hypoxemia occurs frequently after regional anesthesia.[24]

Supplemental oxygen should be administered only to patients at high risk of hypoxemia or with low SpO_2 readings (Table 54-3). However, some recommend supplemental oxygen be administered in the PACU during initial recovery and perhaps during transport to the PACU.[7] Supplemental oxygen does not address underlying causes of hypoxemia in postoperative patients, its use does not guarantee that hypoxemia will not occur, and it is likely to mask hypoventilation.[58] Although oxygen might cause minor mucosal drying, routine humidification is of little benefit unless intubation bypasses natural humidification. Oxygen apparatus can increase the risk of corneal abrasion during emergence.

TABLE 54-3. COMMON OXYGEN DELIVERY SYSTEMS WITH CORRELATING O_2 FLOW RATES TO DELIVERED FIO_2 RANGES

System	O_2 Flow Rate (L/min)	FIO_2
Nasal cannula	1	0.21–0.24
	2	0.23–0.28
	3	0.27–0.32
	4	0.31–0.36
	5	0.35–0.40
	6	0.39–0.44
Simple mask	5	0.30–0.40
	8	0.40–0.60
Partial rebreathing mask	10	0.50–0.65
Nonrebreathing mask	10–15	0.60–near 1

Perioperative Aspiration

During anesthesia, depression of airway reflexes places patients at risk for intraoperative pulmonary aspiration that may manifest in the PACU, or for aspiration during recovery. Pulmonary morbidity from perioperative aspiration varies with the type and volume of the aspirate. Although aspiration of gastric contents is most widely feared, surgical patients also experience other aspiration syndromes.

Aspiration of clear oral secretions during induction, facemask ventilation, or emergence is common and usually insignificant. Cough, mild tracheal irritation, or transient laryngospasm are immediate sequelae, although large-volume aspiration predisposes to infection, small airway obstruction, or pulmonary edema. Aspiration of blood secondary to trauma, epistaxis, or airway surgery generates marked changes on the chest radiograph that are out of proportion with clinical signs. Aspirated "sterile" blood causes minor airway obstruction but is rapidly cleared by mucociliary transport, resorption, and phagocytosis. Massive blood aspiration or aspiration of clots obstructs airways, interferes with oxygenation, and leads to fibrinous changes in air spaces and to pulmonary hemochromatosis from iron accumulation in phagocytic cells. Secondary infection is a threat, especially if tissue or purulent matter is also aspirated.

Aspiration of food, small objects, pieces of teeth, or dental appliances causes persistent cough, diffuse reflex bronchospasm, airway obstruction with distal atelectasis, or pneumonia. Complications are often localized and treated with antibiotics and supportive care once the foreign matter is expelled or removed. Secondary thermal, chemical, or traumatic airway injury from aspirated objects can occur. Of course, complete upper airway or tracheal obstruction by an aspirated object is a life-threatening emergency.

Aspiration of acidic gastric contents during vomiting or regurgitation causes chemical pneumonitis characterized initially by diffuse bronchospasm, hypoxemia, and atelectasis.[59] The morbidity increases directly with volume and inversely with the pH of the acidic aspirate. Aspiration of partially digested food worsens and prolongs pneumonitis, especially if vegetable matter is present. Food particles mechanically obstruct airways and are a nidus for secondary bacterial infection. In serious cases, epithelial degeneration, interstitial and alveolar edema, and hemorrhage into air spaces rapidly progress to ARDS with high-permeability pulmonary edema. Destruction of pneumocytes, decreased surfactant activity, hyaline membrane formation, and emphysematous changes can follow, leading to $\dot{V}/\dot{Q}$ mismatching and reduced compliance. Destruction of microvasculature increases pulmonary vascular resistance and dead space ventilation.

The incidence of serious aspiration is relatively low in PACU patients, but the risk is still significant. Frequency of postoperative vomiting remains high, especially if gas has accumulated in the stomach. Protective airway reflexes such as cough, swallowing, and laryngospasm are suppressed by depressant medications such as inhalation anesthetics, barbiturates, and opiates, so observe carefully patients with decreased levels of consciousness. Persisting effects of laryngeal nerve blocks or topical local anesthetics used to reduce airway irritability decrease postoperative airway protection, as does residual sedation. Reflexes are also impaired by residual neuromuscular paralysis.[46,60] Patients can sustain airway patency and spontaneous ventilation, pass a head lift test, have a tactile train-of-four T4/T1 ratio >0.7, and still have impaired airway reflexes from residual paralysis. The T4/T1 ratio should exceed 0.9 before reflexes are completely competent.[60] Risk of aspiration also increases if reversal is omitted. Hypotension, hypoxemia, or acidemia cause both emesis and obtundation, increasing aspiration risk.

Preventing aspiration is critical because effective therapy is limited.[61] For patients at high risk, preoperative administration of nonparticulate antacids such as sodium citrate increases the pH of gastric fluid without excessively increasing volume. Avoid particulate antacids. Histamine type 2 receptor blockers such as famotidine or ranitidine reduce the volume and increase the pH of gastric secretions. Metoclopramide increases gastroesophageal sphincter tone and accelerates gastric emptying. Inserting a nasogastric tube is often ineffective to remove particulate matter and interferes with gastroesophageal sphincter integrity.

In the PACU, vigilance against aspiration is important. Trendelenburg position might promote regurgitation but aids in airway clearance if regurgitation or vomiting occurs. Head elevation in unconscious patients should be avoided because it creates a gravitational gradient from pharynx to lung. High-risk patients should not have the trachea extubated until airway reflexes are restored. That being said, even though a patient is awake and able to follow commands he or she may well still have depressed gag reflex for some considerable number of hours after surgery/anesthesia. The introduction of opioids and other sedatives may well turn a situation of relatively good airway protection into one of potential aspiration. Aspiration of acidic fluid can still occur around an inflated tracheal tube cuff, so frequently monitor the upper airway for secretions or vomitus. One should avoid cuff deflation until extubation because the rigid tube impairs laryngospasm, swallowing, and other protective reflexes. The pharynx should use suction completely and the trachea extubated at end inspiration with positive airway pressure to promote expulsion of material trapped below the cords but above the inflated cuff. Observation is essential after extubation because airway reflexes might be temporarily impaired. Anatomic distortion in the airway from soft-tissue trauma or surgical intervention interferes with airway protection. Mandibular fixation makes expulsion of vomitus, blood, or secretions difficult, so have equipment for release of mandibular fixation available and ensure that patients demonstrate cognitive and physical ability to clear the airway before the trachea is extubated.

Discovery of gastric secretions in the pharynx mandates immediate lateral head positioning (assuming cervical spine integrity) and suction of the airway. If airway reflexes are compromised, tracheal intubation is often appropriate. After intubation, the trachea is suctioned through the tracheal tube before positive-pressure ventilation; this avoids widely disseminating aspirated material into distal airways. Instillation of saline or alkalotic solutions is not recommended. Assessing the pH of tracheal aspirate is useless because buffering is immediate. Checking pharyngeal aspirate pH is more accurate but of little practical value. Suspicion that aspiration has occurred mandates 24 to 48 hours of monitoring for development of aspiration pneumonitis. If the likelihood of aspiration is small in an ambulatory patient, outpatient follow-up can be done, assuming hypoxemia, cough, wheezing, or radiographic abnormalities do not appear within 4 to 6 hours. The patient should receive explicit instructions to contact a medical facility at the first appearance of malaise, fever, cough, chest pain, or other symptoms of pneumonitis. If likelihood of aspiration is high, the patient should be admitted to the hospital. Observation includes serial temperature checks, white blood cell counts with differential, chest radiograph, and blood gas determination. Chest physiotherapy, incentive spirometry, and restarting medications for pre-existing pulmonary conditions minimize the loss of lung volume, $\dot{V}/\dot{Q}$ mismatching, and infection. Fluffy infiltrates may appear on the chest radiograph any time within 24 hours. Hypoxemia might develop quickly or evolve insidiously as injury progresses, so frequent pulse oximetry monitoring is important.

If hypoxemia, increased airway resistance, consolidation, or pulmonary edema evolves, the patient should be supported with supplemental oxygen, PEEP, or CPAP. Mechanical ventilation may be necessary. Steroids yield no improvement and may increase the risk of bacterial super infection. Bacterial infection does not always follow aspiration, so prophylactic antibiotics merely promote colonization by resistant organisms. If bacterial infection is apparent, institute antibiotic therapy based on culture results. If cultures are equivocal, use broad-spectrum antibiotics with coverage for gram-negative rods and anaerobes, including *Bacteroides fragilis.* Overall therapy is similar to that for ARDS. Pulmonary edema from increased capillary permeability should not be treated with diuretics unless high filling pressures or hypervolemia exist.

POSTOPERATIVE RENAL COMPLICATIONS

Ability to Void

9 The ability to void should be assessed because opioids and autonomic side effects of regional anesthesia interfere with sphincter relaxation and promote urine retention. Urinary retention is common after urologic, inguinal, and genital surgery, and retention frequently delays discharge.[4] Observation after these surgeries is needed to determine if inability to urinate is a possible surgical complication. Neither the patient nor staff can accurately estimate bladder volume through sensation or palpation. An ultrasonic bladder scan helps assess bladder volume before discharge and avoid the archaic practice of routine "straight catheterization." It is reasonable to discharge selected ambulatory patients from the facility and inpatients to a floor before they void.[7,62,63] When inpatients are transferred prior to voiding, ensure that urination can be monitored to avoid complications from urinary retention. Give ambulatory patients who are discharged without voiding a specific time interval in which to void (i.e., 10 to 12 hours after discharge). If retention persists, the patient must contact a healthcare facility. High return rates after urologic procedures are related to urinary retention.[64]

Renal Tubular Function

Analysis of urine yields information about postoperative renal tubular function. Urine color is not useful for assessing concentrating ability, but it does assist recognition of hematuria, hemoglobinuria, or pyuria. Urine osmolarity (reflecting the number of particles in solution) is a more reliable index of tubular function than specific gravity, which is affected by molecular weight of solutes. An osmolarity >450 mOsm/L indicates intact tubular concentrating ability. A urine sodium concentration far below or a potassium concentration above serum concentrations also indicates tubular viability, as does acidification or alkalinization of urine. Osmolarity, electrolyte, and pH values close to those in serum may indicate poor tubular function or acute tubular necrosis.

Inorganic fluoride released during metabolism of certain inhalation anesthetics can cause a transient reduction of tubular concentrating ability after long anesthetics. Higher fluoride levels cause renal tubular necrosis. Interaction of sevoflurane with dry carbon dioxide absorbents (often found in first cases or peripheral locations) generates compound A, vinyl ether that degrades to release inorganic fluoride. Although transient impairment of protein retention and concentrating ability may occur, use of sevoflurane does not seriously affect renal function.

Oliguria

Oliguria (≤0.5 mL/kg/hr) occurs frequently during recovery and usually reflects an appropriate renal response to hypovolemia. The stress response of surgery also increases antidiuretic hormone (ADH), which can lead to decreased urine output. However, decreased urine output might indicate abnormal renal function. The acceptable degree and duration of oliguria vary with baseline renal status, the surgical procedure, and the anticipated postoperative course. In patients without catheters, one should assess interval since last voiding, and bladder volume to help differentiate oliguria from inability to void. One should check indwelling urinary catheters for kinking, for obstruction by blood clots or debris, and for the catheter tip being positioned above the urinary level in the bladder, and aggressively evaluate oliguria if intraoperative events could jeopardize renal function (e.g., aortic cross-clamping, severe hypotension, possible ureteral ligature, massive transfusion). Systemic blood pressure must be adequate for renal perfusion, based on preoperative pressures. Administration of desmopressin for hematologic purposes seldom affects postoperative urinary output. After urine is sent for electrolyte and osmolarity determinations, a 300 to 500 mL intravenous crystalloid bolus helps assess whether oliguria represents a renal response to hypovolemia. If output does not improve, consider a larger bolus or a diagnostic trial of furosemide, 5 mg intravenously. Furosemide increases urine output if oliguria reflects tubular resorption of fluid. Patients receiving chronic diuretic therapy might require a diuretic effect to maintain postoperative urine output.

Persistence of oliguria despite hydration, adequate perfusion pressure, and a furosemide challenge increases the likelihood of acute tubular necrosis, ureteral obstruction, renal artery or vein occlusion, or inappropriate ADH secretion. Cystoscopy, intravenous pyelography, angiography, or radionuclide scanning may help clarify renal status. Osmotic or loop diuretics may be useful to attenuate renal damage. The use of low-dose dopamine or dobutamine has not proven to improve renal function. Fenoldopam used perioperatively has shown to reduce the risk of acute kidney injury for select high-risk cardiac surgical patients.[65] Consultation with a nephrologist is prudent.

Polyuria

Relying on high postoperative urinary output to gauge intravascular volume status or renal viability can be misleading. Profuse urine output often reflects generous intraoperative fluid administration, but osmotic diuresis caused by hyperglycemia and glycosuria is another common cause, particularly if glucose-containing crystalloid solutions are infusing. Polyuria might also reflect intraoperative diuretic administration. However, sustained polyuria (4 to 5 mL/kg/hr) can indicate abnormal regulation of water clearance or high-output renal failure, especially if urinary losses compromise intravascular volume and systemic blood pressure. Diabetes insipidus occurs secondary to intracranial surgery, pituitary ablation, head trauma, or increased intracranial pressure. A urine specific gravity of ≤1.005 and a urine osmolality <200 mOsm/kg are the hallmark of diabetes insipidus. A random plasma osmolality is generally >285 mOsm/kg. Diagnostic or therapeutic administration of vasopressin is useful.

METABOLIC COMPLICATIONS

Postoperative Acid–Base Disorders

Categorization of postoperative acid–base abnormalities into primary and compensatory disorders is difficult because rapidly changing pathophysiology can often generate multiple primary disorders.

Respiratory Acidemia

Respiratory acidemia is frequently encountered in PACU patients because anesthetics, opioids, and sedatives promote hypoventilation by depressing CNS sensitivity to pH and $Paco_2$. In awake, spontaneously breathing patients with adequate analgesia, hypercarbia and acidemia are usually mild ($Paco_2$ 45 to 50 mm Hg, pH 7.36 to 7.32). Deeply sedated patients exhibit more profound acidemia unless supplemental ventilation is administered. Patients with residual neuromuscular paralysis, increased airway resistance, or decreased pulmonary compliance might not sustain adequate ventilation despite an intact CNS drive, especially if CO_2 production is elevated by fever, shivering, or hyperalimentation. The kidneys require hours to generate a compensatory metabolic alkalosis, so compensation for acute postoperative respiratory acidemia is limited.

Symptoms of respiratory acidemia include agitation, confusion, ventilatory dissatisfaction, and tachypnea. Sympathetic nervous system response to low pH causes hypertension, tachycardia, and dysrhythmias. Respiratory acidemia caused by CNS depression often produces less intense signs of sympathetic nervous system activity. In patients with head injury, intracranial tumors, or cerebral edema, respiratory acidemia increases cerebral blood flow and intracranial pressure. At very low pH, catecholamines cannot interact with adrenergic receptors, so heart rate and blood pressure decrease precipitously. Treatment consists of correcting the imbalance between CO_2 production and alveolar ventilation. Raising the level of consciousness by the judicious reversal of opioids or benzodiazepines improves ventilatory drive. It is important to ensure that the patient does not have increased airway resistance or residual neuromuscular blockade. If spontaneous ventilation cannot maintain CO_2 excretion, tracheal intubation and mechanical ventilation are necessary. Reducing CO_2 production by controlling fever or shivering may be helpful.

Metabolic Acidemia

Evaluation of acute postoperative metabolic acidemia is relatively straightforward (Table 54-4). Occasionally, ketoacidosis occurs in diabetic patients. During ketoacidosis, serum glucose levels are elevated and ketones are detectable in blood or urine. Patients

TABLE 54-4. CAUSES OF ACIDEMIA

Normal anion gap acidosis
GI loss of bicarbonate
Diarrhea
Urinary diversion
GI fistulas or drains
Renal loss of bicarbonate
Renal tubular acidosis
Renal insufficiency
Recovery phase of ketoacidosis
Increased anion gap acidosis
Ketoacidosis (diabetic, alcoholic, severe cachexia)
Lactic acidosis (seizures, neuroleptic malignant syndrome, MH, severe asthma, pheochromocytoma, cardiogenic shock, hypovolemia, severe anemia, regional ischemia, sepsis, hypoglycemia)
Respiratory acidosis

GI, gastrointestinal; MH, malignant hyperthermia.

with renal failure or renal tubular acidosis usually exhibit a preoperative metabolic acidemia. Large volumes of saline infusions during surgery can generate a mild hyperchloremic, metabolic acidemia, but use of lactated Ringer solution avoids this problem.[66] Rarely, a patient manifests acidemia from toxic ingestion of aspirin or methanol. Once these unusual causes are excluded, postoperative metabolic acidemia almost always represents lactic acidemia secondary to insufficient delivery or utilization of oxygen in peripheral tissues. Peripheral hypoperfusion is often caused by low cardiac output (hypovolemia, cardiac failure, dysrhythmia) or peripheral vasodilation (sepsis, catecholamine depletion, sympathectomy). Arteriolar constriction from hypothermia or pressor administration reduces tissue perfusion and induces abnormal blood flow distribution. Hypoxemia, severe anemia, impaired hemoglobin dissociation, CO poisoning, and inability to use oxygen in the mitochondria (cyanide or arsenic poisoning) also generate lactic acidemia.

A spontaneously breathing patient will increase minute ventilation in response to metabolic acidemia and quickly generate a respiratory alkalosis to compensate for metabolic acidemia. However, general anesthetics and analgesics suppress this ventilatory response. The sympathetic response to acute postoperative metabolic acidemia is often milder than the response to respiratory acidemia because hydrogen and bicarbonate ions cross the blood–brain barrier with more difficulty than CO_2. Treatment consists of resolving the condition causing accumulation of metabolic acid. For example, ketoacidosis is treated with intravenous potassium, insulin, and glucose. Improving cardiac output or systemic blood pressure will reduce lactic acid production, as will rewarming. If conditions causing lactate accumulation are improved and acidemia is mild, renal excretion of hydrogen ions will restore normal pH. For severe or progressive acidemia, intravenous bicarbonate or calcium gluconate helps restore pH.

Respiratory Alkalemia

Pain or anxiety during emergence causes hyperventilation and acute respiratory alkalemia. Excessive mechanical ventilation also generates respiratory alkalemia, especially if hypothermia or paralysis has decreased CO_2 production. Pathologic causes of "central" hyperventilation include sepsis, cerebrovascular accident, or paradoxic CNS acidosis (an imbalance of bicarbonate concentration across the blood–brain barrier caused by prolonged hyperventilation). Acute respiratory alkalemia can generate confusion, dizziness, atrial dysrhythmias, and abnormal cardiac conduction. Alkalemia decreases cerebral blood flow, causing hypoperfusion and even stroke in patients with cerebrovascular disease. If the alkalemia is severe, reduced serum ionized calcium concentration precipitates muscle fasciculation or hypocalcemic tetany. Very high pH depresses cardiovascular, CNS, and catecholamine receptor functions. Metabolic compensation for acute respiratory alkalemia is limited because time constants for bicarbonate excretion are large. Treatment necessitates reducing alveolar ventilation, usually by administering analgesics and sedatives for pain and anxiety. Rebreathing of CO_2 has little application in the PACU.

Metabolic Alkalemia

Metabolic alkalemia is rare in PACU patients unless vomiting, gastric suctioning, dehydration, alkaline ingestion, or potassium-wasting diuretics caused an alkalemia that existed before surgery. Excessive intraoperative bicarbonate administration causes postoperative metabolic alkalemia, but alkalemia from metabolism of lactate or citrate usually does not appear within the first 24 hours. Respiratory compensation through retention of CO_2 is rapid but limited because hypoventilation eventually causes hypoxemia. Hydration and correction of hypochloremia and hypokalemia allow the kidney to excrete excess bicarbonate.

Glucose Disorders and Control

10 Adequate glucose control has been recommended to reduce morbidity in a variety of postsurgical patients. The control of glucose in diabetic and nondiabetic patients has shown to reduce complications and hospital length of stay and improve patient outcomes. However, the potential for hypoglycemia and coma should not be discounted. Insulin therapy should be based on serum glucose levels and requires careful and timely monitoring of blood glucose levels to avoid hypoglycemia. This plan includes clear and concise hand off of information when patients care is transferred. Urine glucose measurements should be reserved to assess osmotic diuresis and estimate renal transport thresholds by comparison with serum levels.

Hyperglycemia

Glucose infusions and stress responses commonly elevate serum glucose levels after surgery. For most patients during anesthesia, glucose should not be included in maintenance intravenous solutions. Moderate postoperative hyperglycemia (150 to 250 mg/dL) resolves spontaneously and has little adverse effect in the nondiabetic patient. Higher glucose levels cause glycosuria with osmotic diuresis and interfere with serum electrolyte determinations. Severe hyperglycemia increases serum osmolality to a point that cerebral disequilibrium and hyperosmolar coma occur. Type I diabetic patients are at risk for ketoacidosis. Potassium replacement and serial blood glucose determinations are essential.

Hypoglycemia

Hypoglycemia in the PACU can be caused by endogenous insulin secretion or by excessive or inadvertent insulin administration. Serious postoperative hypoglycemia is rare and easily treated with intravenous 50% dextrose followed by glucose infusion. Either sedation or excessive sympathetic nervous system activity masks signs and symptoms of hypoglycemia after anesthesia. Diabetic patients and especially patients who have received insulin therapy intraoperatively must have serum glucose levels measured to avoid the serious problems related to hypoglycemia. Extreme care with documenting and reporting the use of insulin is paramount to provide safe and appropriate care.

Electrolyte Disorders

Hyponatremia

Postoperative hyponatremia occurs if free water is infused intravenously during surgery or if sodium-free irrigating solution is absorbed during transurethral prostatic resection or hysteroscopy. Accumulation of serum glycine or its metabolite, ammonia, might exacerbate symptoms. Free water retention is also caused by inappropriate ADH secretion, prolonged labor induction with oxytocin, or respiratory uptake of nebulized droplets. Theoretically, excessive infusion of isotonic saline leads to excretion of hypertonic urine, desalination, and iatrogenic hyponatremia. Symptoms of moderate hyponatremia include agitation, disorientation, visual disturbances, and nausea, whereas severe hyponatremia causes unconsciousness, impaired airway reflexes, and CNS irritability that progress to grand mal seizures. Therapy includes intravenous normal saline and intravenous furosemide to promote free water excretion. Infusion of hypertonic saline may be useful for severe hyponatremia, in which diligence not to increase serum sodium by 0.5 mEq/hr is needed to avoid CNS lesions or pulmonary edema. Monitor serum sodium concentration and osmolarity.

Hypokalemia

Postoperative hypokalemia is often inconsequential but might generate serious dysrhythmias, especially in patients taking digoxin. A potassium deficit caused by chronic diuretic therapy, nasogastric suctioning, or vomiting often underlies hypokalemia. Urinary and hemorrhagic losses, dilution, and insulin therapy generate acute hypokalemia that worsens during respiratory alkalemia. Excess sympathetic nervous system activity, infusion of calcium, or β-mimetic medications exacerbates effects of hypokalemia. Adding potassium to peripheral intravenous fluids often restores serum concentration, but concentrated solutions infused through a central catheter may be necessary. So often practitioners think 10 to 30 mEq of potassium will bring the patient back to normal. Potassium is an intracellular ion and a plasma potassium deficit is indicative of a far greater intracellular deficit. It is the intracellular-to-extracellular ratio that may well be important, and rapid changes can contribute to as many dysrhythmias as can mild hypokalemia alone.

Hyperkalemia

A high serum potassium level raises the suspicion of spurious hyperkalemia from a hemolyzed specimen or from sampling near an intravenous catheter containing potassium or banked blood. Postoperative hyperkalemia occurs after excessive potassium infusion or in patients with renal failure or malignant hyperthermia. Acute acidemia exacerbates hyperkalemia. Treatment with intravenous insulin and glucose acutely lowers potassium, whereas intravenous calcium counters myocardial effects. Hemodialysis may be necessary for very high potassium levels or symptomatic patients.

Calcium and Magnesium

Although underlying parathyroid disease or massive fluid replacement reduces total body and ionized calcium, symptomatic hypocalcemia seldom occurs in the PACU. A rare patient might exhibit upper airway obstruction from hypocalcemia after parathyroid excision. Reduction of the ionized fraction by acute alkalemia may cause myocardial conduction and contractility abnormalities, decreased vascular tone, or tetany. Transfusion of blood containing chelating agents (e.g., citrate) rarely causes symptomatic hypocalcemia. Administration of calcium chloride or calcium gluconate to hypocalcemic patients improves cardiovascular dynamics.

Magnesium plays a key role in restoration of neuromuscular function after surgery and in maintenance of cardiac rhythm and conduction. Hypermagnesemia is rare because the kidneys are effective at excreting excessive magnesium. Obstetric patients who have been receiving magnesium for tocolysis or control of severe pregnancy-induced hypertension can present postoperatively hyporeflexive, and at higher serum levels show prolonged atrioventricular conduction or complete heart block. Treatment entails intravenous calcium and diuretics.

MISCELLANEOUS COMPLICATIONS

Incidental Trauma

Each patient admitted to the PACU should be carefully evaluated for traumatic complications. Discovery of a complication necessitates careful documentation, notification of physicians responsible for extended care, consultation with specialists, and follow-up.

Ocular Injuries and Visual Changes

Corneal abrasion caused by drying or inadvertent eye contact during facemask ventilation or intubation is a common intraoperative eye injury. The incidence of this type of injury in a nonophthalmic patient is estimated to be between 0.034% and 0.17%, with the higher incidence related to prone or lateral positioning.[67] Corneal injury can occur during emergence in the PACU from patients rubbing their eyes, if a rigid oxygen face mask rides up on the eye, or if the eye is rubbed with a pulse oximeter probe and from eye make-up (particularly mascara) being rubbed in the eyes. Abrasions cause tearing, decreased visual acuity, pain, and photophobia. Fluorescein staining aids diagnosis. Abrasions usually heal spontaneously within 72 hours without scarring, but severe injury can cause cataract formation and impair vision. There is no standard treatment for corneal abrasions, but symptomatic treatment includes artificial tears, topical antibiotics, topical analgesics, and eye closure.

Visual acuity is often impaired after anesthesia. Autonomic side effects of medications impair accommodation, and residual ocular lubricant clouds vision. Impairment of retinal perfusion by ocular compression generates postoperative visual disturbances ranging from loss of acuity to permanent blindness.[68,69] Ischemic optic atrophy can also occur in the absence of external compression.[70] Risk of blindness is higher after long procedures in the prone position, as well as in patients with vascular disease, pre-existing hypertension, diabetes, and sickle cell anemia. A significant percentage of postoperative patients suffer deficits in acuity unrelated to ocular trauma, some of whom require permanent refractive adjustment.[71] Anesthesiologists should be alert for visual impairment and check acuity when assessing patients at higher risk for ischemic optic atrophy.

Hearing Impairment

Hearing impairment after anesthesia and surgery is relatively common.[72] Although impairment is often subclinical, patients sometimes experience decreased auditory acuity, tinnitus, or roaring. Incidence of detectable hearing impairment is particularly high after dural puncture for spinal anesthesia (8% to 16%), and varies with needle size, needle type, and patient age. Impairment can be unilateral or bilateral and usually resolves spontaneously. Hearing loss also occurs after general anesthesia for both noncardiac and cardiac surgeries, and is often related to disruption of the round window or tympanic membrane rupture. Eustachian tube inflammation and otitis secondary to endotracheal intubation can also impact hearing.

Oral, Pharyngeal, and Laryngeal Injuries

Laryngoscope blades, surgical instruments, rigid oral airways, and dentition can all cause trauma of oral soft tissues. Lip, tongue, or gum abrasions are treated with an ice pack and analgesia. Penetrating injuries caused by tissue entrapment between teeth and rigid devices may require topical antibiotics. After a traumatic tracheal intubation, hematoma or edema might cause partial upper airway obstruction. Nebulized racemic epinephrine often improves stridor more quickly than steroids. Dental damage can occur during airway manipulations or during emergence if a patient bites on a rigid oral airway or forcefully clenches his or her teeth. Document tooth or dental appliance damage, obtain a dental consultation, and observe for signs of foreign body aspiration.[73]

Sore throat and hoarseness after tracheal intubation occur in 20% to 50% of patients, depending on the degree of trauma during laryngoscopy and oropharyngeal suctioning, the duration of intubation, and the type of endotracheal tube. Mucosal irritation also presents as an unquenchable dryness in mouth and throat. The use of local anesthetic ointments to lubricate endotracheal tubes may cause additional mucosal irritation. Topical viscous lidocaine attenuates irritation from nasogastric tubes but may increase risk of aspiration during recovery. In children, the severity of postextubation laryngeal edema or tracheitis varies with age, intubation duration, and degree of trauma or tube movement. Most recover with cool mist therapy, but nebulized racemic epinephrine and dexamethasone may be needed in more severe cases. Laryngoscopy and intubation can also cause hypoglossal, lingual, or recurrent laryngeal nerve damage, vocal cord evulsion, desquamation of laryngeal or tracheal mucosa, edema or ulceration, and tracheal perforation. Postoperative sore throat and dysphagia also occurs without intubation, related to the use of laryngeal mask airways,[74] oral airways, trauma from suctioning, or drying from unhumidified gases. Neck and jaw soreness is commonly seen after facemask anesthetics.

Nerve Injuries

Nerve injuries caused by improper positioning during anesthesia generate serious long-term complications (see Chapter 28).[75] Spinal cord injury can be caused by positioning for intubation or by hematoma accumulation after placement of neuraxial anesthetics. Peripheral nerve compression during general or regional anesthesia sometimes causes permanent sensory and motor deficits, as do stretch injuries from hyperextension of an extremity.[76] Any bruising or skin breakdown noted postoperatively should prompt evaluation for underlying nerve damage. Many postoperative neuropathies have no identifiable cause. This remark is particularly true for ulnar neuropathy, which may be related to subtle positioning problems, pre-existing impairment, or sensitivity of the nerve to ischemia.[77] Every complaint of nonsurgical pain, numbness, or weakness from a postoperative patient should be carefully evaluated. In the event of neuropathic weakness, electromyographic studies may determine the location of the lesion and possible reversibility of the nerve deficit. Sensory neuropathies rarely last longer than 5 days and should be referred to a neurologist if the deficit exceeds this time or if it progresses.[78]

Postdural puncture headache may first occur in the PACU, although most appear within 24 to 48 hours. Headache is more frequent after difficult subarachnoid anesthetics with multiple attempts and after dural puncture during attempted epidural placement. Subarachnoid air bubbles from loss-of-resistance testing may contribute. In the PACU, treatment is supportive with hydration, analgesics, and positioning. In severe cases, early intervention with the definitive treatment of epidural blood patch might be considered. Nerve injury secondary to needle contact or intraneuronal injection during placement of regional anesthesia is rare but does occur.[76,79] In one study, 6.3% of 4,767 patients experienced paresthesia during placement of spinal anesthesia, but only 0.126% had persisting symptoms.[80] In the PACU, patients often complain of pain, focal numbness, residual paresthesia, or dysesthesia. Symptoms are usually transient. Administer analgesia, reassure the patient, document findings, and follow for the possibility of an evolving neurologic deficit.

During recovery from spinal anesthesia, some patients exhibit lower extremity discomfort, buttock pain, and other signs of sacral or lumbar neurologic irritation. This problem is more common in obese patients, after procedures in lithotomy position, and after spinal anesthesia with 5% lidocaine.[79] Symptoms are transient and treated supportively. Rarely, a patient exhibits headache and meningeal signs caused by chemical meningitis after injection of a spinal drug that is contaminated or outside the acceptable pH range.

Soft-tissue and Joint Injuries

If pressure points are improperly padded, soft-tissue ischemia and necrosis occur, especially with lateral or prone positioning. Prolonged scalp pressure causes localized alopecia, whereas entrapment of ears, breasts, genitalia, or skin folds causes inflammation or necrosis. Regional ischemia from major arterial compression is rare. Thermal, electrical, or chemical burns from cautery equipment, preparatory solutions, or adhesives also occur. Extravasation of intravenous medications or fluids can cause sloughing, localized chemical neuropathy, or compartment syndromes. Excessive joint or muscle extension leads to postoperative backache, joint pain, stiffness, and even joint instability. After regional anesthesia, extremities must be properly secured and padded to prevent nerve injury.

Skeletal Muscle Pain

Postoperative muscle pain is caused by many intraoperative factors. Prolonged lack of motion or unusual muscle stretch during positioning often contributes to muscle stiffness and aching. Postoperative myalgia has been reported to range between 5% and 83% of patients after the use of succinylcholine,[81] while the pathogenesis of this myalgia remains unclear.[79,82] Acute myalgia also occurs after administration of other relaxants and in patients receiving no relaxant. Delayed onset muscle fatigue can appear days after surgery and resolves spontaneously.

Hypothermia and Shivering

Although intraoperative temperature maintenance is a goal, patients still exhibit postoperative hypothermia. During anesthesia, heat is redistributed and also is lost by evaporation during skin preparation, by humidification of dry gases in the airway, and by radiation and convection from the skin and wound. Temperature reduction is accelerated by cold intravenous fluids and low ambient temperatures. The thermoregulatory threshold, below which humans actively regulate body temperature, is decreased during general anesthesia and is less effective under anesthesia. Ability to maintain body temperature is also compromised because paralysis and anesthesia impair shivering and thermoregulatory vasoconstriction, and because nonshivering thermogenesis is ineffective in adults. Rate of heat loss is similar during general or regional anesthesia, but rewarming is slower after regional anesthesia because residual vasodilation and paralysis impede heat generation and retention. Cachectic, traumatized, or burned patients experience greater temperature reduction, as do infants because of a low ratio of body mass-to-surface area.

11 Hypothermia complicates and prolongs care in the PACU.[83] Average PACU stay is increased by 40 to 90 minutes for hypothermic patients.[84] Postoperative hypothermia increases sympathetic nervous system activity with increased epinephrine and norepinephrine levels,[85] elevates peripheral vascular resistance, and decreases venous capacitance. Risk of myocardial ischemia[86] and dysrhythmia from mechanical myocardial stimulation is increased. Vasoconstriction interferes with the reliability of pulse oximetry and intra-arterial pressure monitoring. Hypoperfusion jeopardizes marginal tissue grafts and promotes tissue hypoxia and metabolic acidemia. The higher affinity of hemoglobin compromises oxygen unloading to hypothermic tissues. Platelet sequestration, decreased platelet function, and reduced clotting factor function contribute to coagulopathy. Moderate hyperglycemia occurs, cellular immune responses are compromised, and postoperative infection rates increase.[87] A decrease in the minimal alveolar concentration of inhalation anesthetics (5% to 7% per 1°C cooling) accentuates residual sedation. Low perfusion and impaired biotransformation might increase the duration of neuromuscular relaxants and sedatives. Moderate hypothermia (28° to 32°C) is associated with cardiac dysrhythmias. Severe hypothermia (≤28°C) interferes with cardiac rhythm generation and impulse conduction. On ECG, the PR, QRS, or QT intervals lengthen, and J waves appear. Spontaneous ventricular fibrillation occurs at temperature <28°C.

During emergence, hypothalamic regulation generates shivering to increase endogenous heat production.[88] Shivering increases the risk of incidental trauma, disrupts medical devices, and interferes with ECG and pulse oximetry monitoring. Oxygen consumption and CO_2 production can increase 200%. Associated increases in minute ventilation and cardiac output might precipitate ventilatory failure in patients with limited reserve or myocardial ischemia in those with coronary artery disease.[86] Shivering is accentuated by tremors related to emergence from inhalation anesthesia. Tremors exhibit clonic and tonic components, and likely reflect decreased cortical influence on spinal cord reflexes.

Restoration of normothermia is an important goal during recovery. Supplemental oxygen should be instituted and forced-air warming devices are most useful for treating hypothermia. Intravenous fluids and blood should be warmed. For most patients, shivering from mild-to-moderate hypothermia is uncomfortable but self-limited, and needs no treatment other than rewarming and reassurance. Many medications have been recommended to suppress shivering, but meperidine is most efficacious in conjunction rewarming.[7] Fentanyl has also been used with patients in whom meperidine is contraindicated. Withholding reversal of relaxants in ventilated, sedated patients attenuates shivering but increases rewarming time. If temperature is near normal (>96° to 97°F) and shivering is resolved, transfer from PACU to an inpatient floor or a discharge area is acceptable.

The Surgical Care Improvement Project sponsored by CMS, The Joint Commission (TJC) and other national partners, is a program that uses several quality measures to help improve the safety and outcomes of surgical patients. One of those measures important to anesthesiologists is maintaining patient's temperature above 36°C. While this measure really begins with care in the operating room, the PACU has a 15-minute window beginning with PACU admission during which patient temperature of at least 36°C should be recorded. Maintaining adequate temperature has shown to reduce wound infections in surgical patients, produce better outcomes and reduce length of stay.

Hyperthermia

Hyperthermia is relatively uncommon in the PACU. Occasionally, a patient exhibits short-lived hyperthermia from close draping or aggressive intraoperative heat preservation. Postoperative fever sometimes reflects a pre-existing infection (e.g., sinusitis, upper respiratory or urinary tract infection) or an infection exacerbated by the surgical procedure (e.g., resection of infected tonsils or appendix, abscess drainage, urinary tract manipulation). Elevated temperature might indicate a drug or transfusion reaction. Muscarinic blocking agents such as atropine interfere with cooling and might contribute to fever, but they are seldom the cause in adults. Other hypermetabolic states such as thyroid storm must be considered. High fever occurs with malignant hyperthermia, but signs such as tachycardia, muscle rigidity, dysrhythmia, hyperventilation, and acidemia establish the diagnosis first.

Ambient cooling, chest physiotherapy, incentive spirometry, and antipyretics are usually sufficient to treat postoperative fever. One should withhold offending medications or blood products if a drug or transfusion reaction is suspected and notify the physician responsible for extended care to ensure postdischarge evaluation. Therapy for thyroid storm or malignant hyperthermia is well described elsewhere.

Persistent Sedation

Approximately 90% of patients regain consciousness within 15 minutes of admission to the PACU; unconsciousness persisting for a greater period is considered prolonged.[89] Even a highly susceptible patient should respond to a stimulus within 30 to 45 minutes after a reasonably conducted anesthetic. In a patient with prolonged sedation, research the level of preoperative responsiveness to uncover intoxication with drugs and alcohol or pre-existing mental dysfunction. One should note the time and amount of preoperative and intraoperative sedative medications, and review any unusual intraoperative events. The rate and character of spontaneous ventilation helps judge residual opioid effect. Physical assessment should include a tactile stimulus such as a light skin pinch, which elicits greater arousal than verbal stimulation, perhaps because sensory input is amplified through the reticular activating system. Diagnostic value of pupillary response is low.

Residual sedation from inhalation anesthetics might cause prolonged unconsciousness, especially after long procedures, in obese patients, or when high concentrations are continued through the end of surgery. Prolonged sedation is less likely after anesthesia with low solubility agents such as sevoflurane or desflurane. Premedications that have sedative effects (e.g., diphenhydramine, hydroxyzine, promethazine, droperidol, lorazepam, midazolam, meclizine, and scopolamine) contribute to postoperative somnolence. Sedation from intraoperative opioid or sedative administration is dose related. Opioids are the only drugs that cause bradypnea; thus, regardless of what other drug effects, if the respiratory rate is <14 to 16, then opioids are clearly affecting the patient's level of consciousness. To assess sedation from opioids, one can administer low-dose intravenous naloxone (0.04-mg increments every 2 minutes, up to 0.2 mg). With careful titration, respiratory depression and sedation can be reversed without dangerous reversal of analgesia. If unconsciousness is related to residual opioid effects, ventilatory rate and arousal will increase with ≤0.2 mg of intravenous naloxone, unless a patient has received a massive opioid overdose.

Flumazenil (0.2 mg intravenously per minute to a total of 1 mg), a competitive benzodiazepine antagonist, differentiates sedation from midazolam and diazepam, although duration of action is short. Risk of inducing seizures must be considered in reversing chronic benzodiazepine users. Neither naloxone nor flumazenil should be used as a routine element of postoperative care.[7] Pharmaceutic reversal should be reserved for specific indications in individual patients. Administration of intravenous physostigmine (0.5 to 1 mg) counteracts but does not reverse sedation caused by inhalation anesthetics, other sedatives, and anticholinergics. If administration of naloxone, flumazenil, or physostigmine does not improve the level of consciousness, unconsciousness is most likely not related to reversible residual anesthetic medications. However, it is still possible that an unrecognized, preoperative overdose with depressant oral drugs (i.e., anticholinergic and antihistamines) is responsible.

The increasing use of dexmedetomidine for sedation cases can lead to persistent sedation in the PACU. These patients are usually easy to arouse and follow commands readily. Patients sedated with dexmedetomidine tend to less respiratory depression unless other respiratory depressant medications have also been given. The minimal effect on respiratory drive by dexmedetomidine allows safe discharge from the PACU as long as the destination of the patient is sufficient to care for the mild sedation.

Profound residual neuromuscular paralysis rarely might mimic unconsciousness by precluding any motor response to stimuli. This phenomenon could occur after gross overdosage, if reversal agents are omitted, in patients with unrecognized neuromuscular disease, or with phase II blockade from succinylcholine use in a patient with pseudocholinesterase deficiency. Observation of purposeful motion, spontaneous ventilation, or reflex muscular movement eliminates residual paralysis as an explanation. CNS depression secondary to intravenous local anesthetic toxicity or inadvertent subarachnoid injection can mimic postoperative coma. Children who were exhausted before surgery are often difficult to arouse after anesthesia, especially if sleep patterns are disrupted by emergency surgery at night. Hypothermia below 33°C impairs consciousness and increases the depressant effect of medications. Core temperatures below 30°C can cause fixed pupillary dilation, areflexia, and coma. A serum glucose level will eliminate severe hypoglycemia or hyperglycemic hyperosmolar coma as causes. Suspicion that unresponsiveness is caused by hypoglycemia indicates an immediate empiric trial of intravenous 50% dextrose. Hyposmolar states (<260 mOsm/L) such as acute hyponatremia (Na <125 mEq/L) are ruled out by checking serum electrolyte and osmolarity. Arterial blood gas analysis reveals CO_2 narcosis ($Paco_2$ >200 to 250 mm Hg) as well as carboxyhemoglobin levels for carbon monoxide poisoning. A patient may also be feigning unresponsiveness or having a hysterical reaction that presents as unconsciousness.

If a diagnosis remains elusive, consult a neurologist for a thorough neurologic evaluation. Occasionally, unresponsiveness reflects subclinical grand mal seizures secondary to delirium tremens or an underlying seizure disorder. Cerebral anoxia from hypoperfusion or prolonged profound hypoxemia must be considered. In injured patients or those recovering from intracranial surgery, evaluate for unrecognized head trauma, intracerebral hemorrhage, or increased intracranial pressure. Patients sometimes awaken very slowly after long intracranial procedures.[90] Cerebral thromboembolism is another possibility in patients who have undergone internal jugular or subclavian cannulation. Patients with atrial fibrillation, carotid bruits, or hypercoagulable states are also at increased risk of thromboembolism. Paradoxic air or fat embolism through a right-to-left intracardiac shunt should be considered. After cardiac, proximal major vascular, or invasive neck surgery, risk of postoperative stroke ranges from 2.2% to 5.2%.[91] Postoperative cerebrovascular accidents in other patients are rare, showing a 0.03% to 0.08% incidence in the fourth decade but increasing to 3% to 4% by the eighth decade, and usually become evident after the PACU interval.[92]

Altered Mental Status

Recovering patients sometimes exhibit inappropriate mental reactions, ranging from lethargy and confusion to physical combativeness and extreme disorientation.

Emergence Reactions

Aside from the disturbance to staff and other patients, a stormy emergence reaction has significant medical consequences. The risk of incidental trauma increases, including contusion or fracture, corneal abrasion, and sprains from struggling. Thrashing jeopardizes suture lines, orthopedic fixations, vascular grafts, drains, tracheal tubes, and vascular catheters. Agitated patients manifest high levels of sympathetic nervous system tone, tachycardia, and hypertension. Less appreciated is the risk of injury to PACU staff struggling to protect a combative patient.

For a short period after regaining consciousness, some patients appear unable to appropriately process sensory input. Most exhibit somnolence, slight disorientation, and sluggish mental reactions that rapidly clear. Others experience wide emotional swings such as weeping or escalating resistance to positioning and restraint. Predicting which patients will have adverse psychologi-
12 cal reactions is difficult. Emergence delirium, which is prevalent in children and young adults, is difficult to predict preoperatively and does not appear to be related to specific types of anesthesia.[93] In young children, anxiety is heightened by parental separation. Heightened anxiety seems to be the one consistent factor in predicting emergence delirium.[94] Many therapies have been tried to prevent or stop emergence delirium in pediatric patients without much success; however, the use of dexmedetomidine has shown promise in reducing this phenomenon without increasing time to extubate or time to discharge.[95] Ketamine and propofol have also been used with some success.[96] Very young children may react inappropriately to sound when hearing acutely improves after myringotomies. Patients with mental retardation, psychiatric disorders, organic brain dysfunction, or hostile preoperative interactions manifest those problems after surgery. Inability to speak secondary to oral fixation or tracheal intubation generates frustration or fear that exaggerates emergence reactions. Ethnic, cultural, and psychological characteristics play some role. A language barrier or a new postoperative hearing impairment accentuates an emergence reaction because input from PACU

staff might not be understood. The incidence of stormy emergence is probably higher after procedures with high emotional significance. Recall of intraoperative events can generate severe panic and anxiety during emergence.[97] In patients who abuse alcohol, opioids, cocaine, or other illicit drugs, intoxication or withdrawal can elicit bizarre emergence behavior. Disorientation, paranoia, and combativeness occur after use of scopolamine as a premedication or antiemetic, which can be treated with intravenous physostigmine. Ketamine or droperidol can cause dysphoria and hallucination, although acute reactions are rare. Etomidate contributes to restlessness.

Pain amplifies agitation, confusion, and aggressive behavior during emergence[98]; therefore, it is helpful to ensure adequate postoperative analgesia early in the PACU course. Urinary urgency or gastric distention from trapped gas generates discomfort and agitation, as do tight dressings, painful phlebotomy, and poor positioning. Endotracheal or nasogastric tubes and urinary catheters are also uncomfortable. Check for unusual pain sources such as corneal abrasion, entrapment of body parts, infiltrated vascular catheters, or small devices left beneath a patient. Nausea, dizziness, and pruritus are distressing during emergence. Some patients struggle to move from a supine into a more comfortable semisitting or lateral position, especially those with gastroesophageal reflux, pulmonary congestion, or obesity. Emerging patients often resist physical restraint. Residual paralysis elicits agitation or uncoordinated motions that make a patient appear disoriented and combative. Observation of weakness or a peculiar flapping nature of voluntary motion helps in the diagnosis. However, patients can appear fully recovered by head lift and train-of-four monitoring but still perceive impaired swallowing, visual acuity, and sense of strength.[99]

Combativeness, confusion, or disorientation might reflect respiratory dysfunction. Moderate hypoxemia often presents with clouded mentation, disorientation, and agitation resembling that caused by pain. Respiratory acidemia elicits profound agitation, although acidemia caused by ventilatory center depression generates less agitation because higher CNS functions are also depressed. Hypercarbia is more likely to cause lethargy or somnolence. Limitation of inspiratory volume by chest dressings, gastric distention, or splinting causes a vague dissatisfaction with lung inflation similar to air hunger. This also occurs during mechanical ventilation with low delivered volumes and is probably mediated by stretch receptors in the lung. Inability to generate a forceful cough or clear secretions causes distress, as well as high work of breathing. Interstitial pulmonary edema elicits symptoms of air hunger before airway flooding occurs. Agitation can be profound, even with adequate ventilation and oxygenation.

Metabolic abnormalities interfere with lucidity. Lactic acidemia causes anxiety and mild disorientation; acute hyponatremia clouds the sensorium; and hypoglycemia causes first agitation and then diminished responsiveness. Seizure activity might mimic agitation and combativeness. Seizures should be higher in the differential diagnosis in patients with epilepsy, head trauma, and chronic alcohol or cocaine abuse. Cerebral hypoperfusion can produce disorientation, agitation, and combativeness, which can be seen after head trauma or space-occupying lesions. Action such as increasing the mean arterial pressure might be required to assure cerebral perfusion pressure.

There are few interventions that prevent "stormy" emergence reactions.[94] Altered mental status is treated supportively because most emergence reactions disappear within 10 to 15 minutes. Verbal reassurances that surgery is completed and that the patient is doing well are invaluable. One should use the patient's name frequently with reassurance of well-being, and stress the time and location. When practical, one should allow patients to choose their own position and provide adequate analgesia. In selected cases, parenteral sedation relieves fear or anxiety and smoothes emergence. Identifying whether a patient is reacting to pain or to anxiety is important. Benzodiazepines and barbiturates are ineffective analgesics, whereas opioids are poor sedatives. One should not administer sedative or analgesic medications if altered mental status might reflect a physiologic abnormality such as hypoxemia, hypoglycemia, hypotension, or acidemia, and use restraints only if a patient's or staff's safety is jeopardized.

Delirium and Cognitive Decline

12 A high percentage of elderly patients (5% to 50%) experience some degree of postoperative confusion, delirium, or cognitive decline.[100,101] Patients exhibit fluctuations in level of consciousness and orientation, or deterioration of memory, mental functions, and acquisition of new information. The problem may be related to exacerbation of central cholinergic insufficiency by narcotics, sedatives, or anticholinergics. However, stress of surgery, fever, pain, emesis, sleep deprivation, and loss of routine undoubtedly contribute. Presence of pre-existing dementia, cognitive abnormalities, organic brain syndrome, or hearing and visual impairment predicts postoperative delirium, as does evidence of physical infirmity such as high ASA physical status or lack of stress response to surgery. Cognitive dysfunction also occurs at lower incidence (15% greater than control) in younger patients, more frequently resolves within 3 months, and may be related to inactivity during recuperation.[102] Although signs often appear on the first to third postoperative day, onset is sometimes evident in the PACU.

Overall, recovery of cognitive function is slower in the elderly.[103] Because older patients are often skilled at concealing declining capabilities, careful assessment of preoperative capabilities helps identify deficits that affect postoperative status. Postoperative lethargy, clouded sensorium, or delirium sometimes reflects an acute physiologic change. Hyperosmolarity from hyperglycemia or hypernatremia as well as hyponatremia can alter consciousness. Cerebral fluid shifts with decreased mentation occur in patients on dialysis and after rapid correction of severe dehydration. Patients receiving atropine premedication or chronic meperidine therapy might exhibit anticholinergic-induced delirium. Disorientation or clouded sensorium can reflect chronic use of psychogenic drugs, premedication with long-acting sedatives, or unrecognized intoxication. Life-threatening conditions such as seizures, hypoxemia, hypoglycemia, hypotension, acidemia, or cerebrovascular accident sometimes present with confusion, disorientation, inability to vocalize, or reduced level of consciousness, especially if earlier premonitory signs and symptoms are misinterpreted.

Postoperative Nausea and Vomiting

13 Postoperative nausea and vomiting (PONV) continues to be a significant challenge to be avoided after many types of anesthetics. Not only is PONV considered by many patients the most unpleasant aspect following an anesthetic, many describe this as their greatest fear of subsequent anesthetics.[104] Patients are often more concerned about PONV than pain or other risks associated with anesthesia and surgery. In addition to patients' dissatisfaction with nausea and vomiting, there exist medical risks (increased abdominal pressure, increased central venous pressure, aspiration of gastric contents, sympathetic nervous system response with increasing blood pressure and heart rate as well as parasympathetic responses producing bradycardia and hypotension). PONV represents a significant burden to be avoided due to

patient satisfaction and safety as well as the economic impact of prolonged PACU stays and unanticipated admissions.

The incidence of PONV varies with many potential causes. Patients often experience nausea and emesis after discharge from the PACU which may coincide with increased oral intake or waning effect of antiemetics. Surgeries associated with a higher risk of PONV are eye procedures, peritoneal or intestinal irritation, ear–nose–throat procedures especially with middle ear manipulation, dental and cosmetic procedures. Patient groups at increased are those with a previous history of PONV or motion sickness, menstruating females, children over the age of 2, obesity, and nonsmokers.[105] Perioperative factors that may increase the incidence include no PO intake (starvation, dehydration), autonomic imbalance, pain, and the effects of anesthetics on the chemotactic center.

Incidence of PONV is lower following regional rather than general anesthesia especially with a decreased use of opioids.[106] The use of nonopioid analgesics may reduce the frequency of emesis while providing adequate pain control. Induction agents such as propofol and barbiturates are associated with reduced incidence compared to etomidate and ketamine. A total intravenous anesthetic (TIVA) technique with propofol greatly reduces PONV incidence compared to a pure inhalation anesthetic. There is little significant difference among inhalation agents, although sevoflurane and desflurane might generate slightly higher rates of nausea. The choice of anticholinergic reversal agents may be a contributing factor but remains unclear to what degree.

Several interventions have been evaluated and can be implemented to reduce the incidence of PONV. The use of meclizine 25 mg preoperatively for patients predisposed to motion sickness can be effective. Prophylaxis with 5-HT3 receptor antagonists (i.e., ondansetron) prior to emergence significantly reduces incidence and is cost effective. Dexamethasone also has antiemetic effects and can be used effectively with other prophylactic agents. Hydration is effective, easy and cost effective. The use of droperidol prophylaxis has decreased due to a 2001 FDA black box warning with prolonged QT on EKG, but still remains an effective rescue method in select patients with EKG monitoring. The FDA letter regarding the use of droperidol did not address the usual prophylaxis dose of 0.625 mg, but recommended EKG monitoring for 2 to 3 hours after administration. In September of 2011, the FDA published a similar safety announcement regarding prolonged QT with the use of ondansetron, which was first documented in 2005. There were no recommendations regarding routine EKG monitoring with the use of ondansetron but caution and monitoring should be used with those patients with known prolonged QT syndromes.[107] Rescue with nonselective antihistamines (i.e., promethazine) is effective but caution is advised in patients where increased sedation can be problematic such as children and OSA. Acupuncture and acupressure can provide relief but due to provider proficiency, patient acceptance and proven efficacy compared to antiemetic medications, these methods are less frequently used.[108] More serious causes of nausea and vomiting such as hypotension, hypoxia, hypoglycemia, increased intracranial pressure, or gastric bleeding should be considered prior to treatment.

References

1. Standards for Postanesthesia Care (Approved by House of Delegates on October 12, 1988 and last amended on October 27, 2004). Available at: www.asahq.org/publicationsAndServices/standards/36.pdf.
2. Bothner U, Georgieff M, Schwilk B. The impact of minor perioperative anesthesia-related incidents, events, and complications on postanesthesia care unit utilization. *Anesth Analg.* 1999;89:506.
3. Cohen MM, O'Brien-Pallas LL, Copplestone C, et al. Nursing workload associated with adverse events in the postanesthesia care unit. *Anesthesiology.* 1999;91:1882.
4. Pavlin DJ, Rapp SE, Polissar NL, et al. Factors affecting discharge time in adult outpatients. *Anesth Analg.* 1998;87:816.
5. Song D, Chung F, Ronayne M, et al. Fast-tracking (bypassing the PACU) does not reduce nursing workload after ambulatory surgery. *Br J Anaesth.* 2004;93:768.
6. Hines R, Barash PG, Watrous G, et al. Complications occurring in the postanesthesia care unit: A survey. *Anesth Analg.* 1992;74:503.
7. American Society of Anesthesiologists Task Force on Postanesthetic Care. Practice guidelines for postanesthetic care: A report by the American Society of Anesthesiologists Task Force on Postanesthetic Care. *Anesthesiology.* 2002;96:742.
8. Sullivan EE. Standards of perianesthesia nursing practice 2002. *J Perianesth Nurs.* 2002;17:275.
9. Swenson JD, Bay N, Loose E, et al. Outpatient management of continuous peripheral nerve catheters placed using ultrasound guidance: An experience in 620 patients. *Anesth Analg.* 2006;103:1436.
10. Apfelbaum JL, Walawander CA, Grasela TH, et al. Eliminating intensive postoperative care in same-day surgery patients using short-acting anesthetics. *Anesthesiology.* 2002;97:66.
11. Pittet D, Stephan F, Hugonnet S, et al. Hand-cleansing during postanesthesia care. *Anesthesiology.* 2003;99:530.
12. Macario A, Weinger M, Carney S, et al. Which clinical anesthesia outcomes are important to avoid? The perspective of patients. *Anesth Analg.* 1999;89:652.
13. Strassels SA, Chen C, Carr DB. Postoperative analgesia: Economics, resource use, and patient satisfaction in an urban teaching hospital. *Anesth Analg.* 2002;94:130.
14. Apfelbaum JL, Chen C, Mehta SS, et al. Postoperative pain experience: Results from a national survey suggest postoperative pain continues to be undermanaged. *Anesth Analg.* 2003;97:534.
15. Rundshagen I, Schnabel K, Standl T, et al. Patients' vs nurses' assessments of postoperative pain and anxiety during patient- or nurse-controlled analgesia. *Br J Anaesth.* 1999;82:374.
16. American Society of Anesthesiologists Task Force on Acute Pain Management. Practice guidelines for acute pain management in the perioperative setting: An updated report by the American Society of Anesthesiologists Task Force on Acute Pain Management. *Anesthesiology.* 2004;100:1573.
17. Chung F, Ritchie E, Su J. Postoperative pain in ambulatory surgery. *Anesth Analg.* 1997;85:808.
18. Wu CL, Berenholtz SM, Pronovost PJ, et al. Systematic review and analysis of postdischarge symptoms after outpatient surgery. *Anesthesiology.* 2002;96:994.
19. Peng PW, Sandler AN. A review of the use of fentanyl analgesia in the management of acute pain in adults. *Anesthesiology.* 1999;90:576.
20. Ekman EF, Wahba M, Ancona F. Analgesic efficacy of perioperative celecoxib in ambulatory arthroscopic knee surgery: A double-blind, placebo-controlled study. *Arthroscopy.* 2006;22:635.
21. Moiniche S, Kehlet H, Dahl JB. A qualitative and quantitative systematic review of preemptive analgesia for postoperative pain relief: The role of timing of analgesia. *Anesthesiology.* 2002;96:725.
22. White PF. The role of non-opioid analgesic techniques in the management of pain after ambulatory surgery. *Anesth Analg.* 2002;94:577.
23. Gwirtz KH, Young JV, Byers RS, et al. The safety and efficacy of intrathecal opioid analgesia for acute postoperative pain: Seven years' experience with 5,969 surgical patients at Indiana University Hospital. *Anesth Analg.* 1999;88:599.
24. de Leon-Casasola OA, Lema MJ. Postoperative epidural opioid analgesia: What are the choices? *Anesth Analg.* 1996;83:867.
25. Baig MK, Zmora O, Derdemezi J, et al. Use of the ON-Q pain management system is associated with decreased postoperative analgesic requirement: Double blind randomized placebo pilot study. *J Am Coll Surg.* 2006;202:297.
26. Capdevila X, Pirat P, Bringuier S, et al. Continuous peripheral nerve blocks in hospital wards after orthopedic surgery: A multicenter prospective analysis of the quality of postoperative analgesia and complications in 1,416 patients. *Anesthesiology.* 2005;103:1035.
27. Ilfeld BM, Enneking FK. Continuous peripheral nerve blocks at home: A review. *Anesth Analg.* 2005;100:1822.
28. Casati A, Fanelli G, Cedrati V, et al. Pulmonary function changes after interscalene brachial plexus anesthesia with 0.5% and 0.75% ropivacaine: A double-blinded comparison with 2% mepivacaine. *Anesth Analg.* 1999;88:587.
29. Aldrete JA. The post-anesthesia recovery score revisited. *J Clin Anesth.* 1995;7:89.
30. White PF, Song D. New criteria for fast-tracking after outpatient anesthesia: A comparison with the modified Aldrete's scoring system. *Anesth Analg.* 1999; 88:1069.
31. Noiseux N, Bracco D, Prieto I, et al. Do patients after off-pump coronary artery bypass grafting need the intensive care unit? A prospective audit of 85 patients. *Interact Cardiovasc Thorac Surg.* 2008;7:32.
32. Schweizer A, Khatchatourian G, Hohn L, et al. Opening of a new postanesthesia care unit: Impact on critical care utilization and complications following major vascular and thoracic surgery. *J Clin Anesth.* 2002;14:486.
33. Heland M, Retsas A. Establishing a cardiac surgery recovery unit within the post anaesthesia care unit. *Collegian.* 1999;6:10.
34. Baltimore JJ. Perianesthesia care of cardiac surgery patients: A CPAN review. *J Perianesth Nurs.* 2001;16:246.
35. Rose DK, Cohen MM, Wigglesworth DF, et al. Critical respiratory events in the postanesthesia care unit, patient, surgical, and anesthetic factors. *Anesthesiology.* 1994;81:410.

36. Schwilk B, Bothner U, Schraag S, et al. Perioperative respiratory events in smokers and nonsmokers undergoing general anaesthesia. *Acta Anaesthesiol Scand.* 1997;41:348.
37. Ballantyne JC, Carr DB, deFerranti S, et al. The comparative effects of postoperative analgesic therapies on pulmonary outcome: Cumulative meta-analyses of randomized, controlled trials. *Anesth Analg.* 1998;86:598.
38. Warner DO, Warner MA, Offord KP, et al. Airway obstruction and perioperative complications in smokers undergoing abdominal surgery. *Anesthesiology.* 1999; 90:372.
39. Strauss SG, Lynn AM, Bratton SL, et al. Ventilatory response to CO_2 in children with obstructive sleep apnea from adenotonsillar hypertrophy. *Anesth Analg.* 1999; 89:328.
40. Tait AR, Malviya S, Voepel-Lewis T, et al. Risk factors for perioperative adverse respiratory events in children with upper respiratory tract infections. *Anesthesiology.* 2001;95:299.
41. D'Honneur G, Lofaso F, Drummond GB, et al. Susceptibility to upper airway obstruction during partial neuromuscular block. *Anesthesiology.* 1998;88:371.
42. Asai T, Koga K, Vaughan RS. Respiratory complications associated with tracheal intubation and extubation. *Br J Anaesth.* 1998;80:767.
43. Benumof JL, Dagg R, Benumof R. Critical hemoglobin desaturation will occur before return to an unparalyzed state following 1 mg/kg intravenous succinylcholine. *Anesthesiology.* 1997;87:979.
44. Warner DO, Warner MA, Barnes RD, et al. Perioperative respiratory complications in patients with asthma. *Anesthesiology.* 1996;85:460.
45. Berg H, Roed J, Viby-Mogensen J, et al. Residual neuromuscular block is a risk factor for postoperative pulmonary complications. A prospective, randomised, and blinded study of postoperative pulmonary complications after atracurium, vecuronium and pancuronium. *Acta Anaesthesiol Scand.* 1997;41: 1095.
46. Debaene B, Plaud B, Dilly MP, et al. Residual paralysis in the PACU after a single intubating dose of nondepolarizing muscle relaxant with an intermediate duration of action. *Anesthesiology.* 2003;98:1042.
47. de Boer HD, Driessen JJ, Marcus MA, et al. Reversal of rocuronium-induced (1.2 mg/kg) profound neuromuscular block by sugammadex: A multicenter, dose-finding and safety study. *Anesthesiology.* 2007;107:239.
48. Stoller JK, Kester L. Respiratory care protocols in postanesthesia care. *J Perianesth Nurs.* 1998;13:349.
49. Rothen HU, Sporre B, Engberg G, et al. Airway closure, atelectasis and gas exchange during general anaesthesia. *Br J Anaesth.* 1998;81:681.
50. Karayiannakis AJ, Makri GG, Mantzioka A, et al. Postoperative pulmonary function after laparoscopic and open cholecystectomy. *Br J Anaesth.* 1996;77:448.
51. Thomas JA, McIntosh JM. Are incentive spirometry, intermittent positive pressure breathing, and deep breathing exercises effective in the prevention of postoperative pulmonary complications after upper abdominal surgery? A systematic overview and meta-analysis. *Phys Ther.* 1994;74:3.
52. Overend TJ, Anderson CM, Lucy SD, et al. The effect of incentive spirometry on postoperative pulmonary complications: A systematic review. *Chest.* 2001; 120:971.
53. Young T, Palta M, Dempsey J, et al. The occurrence of sleep-disordered breathing among middle-aged adults. *N Engl J Med.* 1993;328:1230.
54. Gross JB, Bachenberg KL, Benumof JL, et al. Practice guidelines for the perioperative management of patients with obstructive sleep apnea: A report by the American Society of Anesthesiologists Task Force on perioperative management of patients with obstructive sleep apnea. *Anesthesiology.* 2006;104:1081.
55. Xue FS, Huang YG, Tong SY, et al. A comparative study of early postoperative hypoxemia in infants, children, and adults undergoing elective plastic surgery. *Anesth Analg.* 1996;83:709.
56. Moller JT, Johannessen NW, Espersen K, et al. Randomized evaluation of pulse oximetry in 20,802 patients: II. perioperative events and postoperative complications. *Anesthesiology.* 1993;78:445.
57. Xue FS, Li BW, Zhang GS, et al. The influence of surgical sites on early postoperative hypoxemia in adults undergoing elective surgery. *Anesth Analg.* 1999;88:213.
58. Moller JT, Wittrup M, Johansen SH. Hypoxemia in the postanesthesia care unit: An observer study. *Anesthesiology.* 1990;73:890.
59. Ng A, Smith G. Gastroesophageal reflux and aspiration of gastric contents in anesthetic practice. *Anesth Analg.* 2001;93:494.
60. Eriksson LI, Sundman E, Olsson R, et al. Functional assessment of the pharynx at rest and during swallowing in partially paralyzed humans: Simultaneous videomanometry and mechanomyography of awake human volunteers. *Anesthesiology.* 1997;87:1035.
61. Practice guidelines for preoperative fasting and the use of pharmacologic agents to reduce the risk of pulmonary aspiration. Application to healthy patients undergoing elective procedures: A report by the American Society of Anesthesiologist Task Force on preoperative fasting. *Anesthesiology.* 1999;90:896.
62. Mulroy MF, Salinas FV, Larkin KL, et al. Ambulatory surgery patients may be discharged before voiding after short-acting spinal and epidural anesthesia. *Anesthesiology.* 2002;97:315.
63. Marshall SI, Chung F. Discharge criteria and complications after ambulatory surgery. *Anesth Analg.* 1999;88:508.
64. Twersky R, Fishman D, Homel P. What happens after discharge? Return hospital visits after ambulatory surgery. *Anesth Analg.* 1997;84:319.
65. Cogliati AA, Vellutini R, Nardini A, et al. Fenoldopam infusion for renal protection in high-risk cardiac surgery patients: A randomized clinical study. *J Cardiothorac Vasc Anesth.* 2007;21:847.
66. Waters JH, Gottlieb A, Schoenwald P, et al. Normal saline versus lactated Ringer's solution for intraoperative fluid management in patients undergoing abdominal aortic aneurysm repair: An outcome study. *Anesth Analg.* 2001;93:817.
67. Moos DD, Lind DM. Detection and treatment of perioperative corneal abrasions. *J Perianesth Nurs.* 2006;21:332.
68. Myers MA, Hamilton SR, Bogosian AJ, et al. Visual loss as a complication of spine surgery. A review of 37 cases. *Spine.* 1997;22:1325.
69. Warner ME, Warner MA, Garrity JA, et al. The frequency of perioperative vision loss. *Anesth Analg.* 2001;93:1417.
70. Williams EL, Hart WM Jr, Tempelhoff R. Postoperative ischemic optic neuropathy. *Anesth Analg.* 1995;80:1018.
71. Warner ME, Fronapfel PJ, Hebl JR, et al. Perioperative visual changes. *Anesthesiology.* 2002;96:855.
72. Sprung J, Bourke DL, Contreras MG, et al. Perioperative hearing impairment. *Anesthesiology.* 2003;98:241.
73. Warner ME, Benenfeld SM, Warner MA, et al. Perianesthetic dental injuries: Frequency, outcomes, and risk factors. *Anesthesiology.* 1999;90:1302.
74. Brimacombe J, Holyoake L, Keller C, et al. Pharyngolaryngeal, neck, and jaw discomfort after anesthesia with the face mask and laryngeal mask airway at high and low cuff volumes in males and females. *Anesthesiology.* 2000;93:26.
75. Practice advisory for the prevention of perioperative peripheral neuropathies. A report by the American Society of Anesthesiologists Task Force on prevention of perioperative peripheral neuropathies. *Anesthesiology.* 2000;92:1168.
76. Cheney FW, Domino KB, Caplan RA, et al. Nerve injury associated with anesthesia: A closed claims analysis. *Anesthesiology.* 1999;90:1062.
77. Warner MA, Warner DO, Matsumoto JY, et al. Ulnar neuropathy in surgical patients. *Anesthesiology.* 1999;90:54.
78. Warner MA. Perioperative neuropathies. *Mayo Clin Proc.* 1998;73:567.
79. Auroy Y, Benhamou D, Bargues L, et al. Major complications of regional anesthesia in France: The SOS regional anesthesia hotline service. *Anesthesiology.* 2002; 97:1274.
80. Horlocker TT, McGregor DG, Matsushige DK, et al. A retrospective review of 4,767 consecutive spinal anesthetics: Central nervous system complications. perioperative outcomes group. *Anesth Analg.* 1997;84:578.
81. Schreiber JU, Mencke T, Biedler A, et al. Postoperative myalgia after succinylcholine: No evidence for an inflammatory origin. *Anesth Analg.* 2003;96:1640.
82. Bettelli G. Which muscle relaxants should be used in day surgery and when. *Curr Opin Anaesthesiol.* 2006;19:600.
83. Sessler DI. Complications and treatment of mild hypothermia. *Anesthesiology.* 2001;95:531.
84. Lenhardt R, Marker E, Goll V, et al. Mild intraoperative hypothermia prolongs postanesthetic recovery. *Anesthesiology.* 1997;87:1318.
85. Sun LS, Adams DC, Delphin E, et al. Sympathetic response during cardiopulmonary bypass: Mild versus moderate hypothermia. *Crit Care Med.* 1997;25: 1990.
86. Frank SM, Fleisher LA, Breslow MJ, et al. Perioperative maintenance of normothermia reduces the incidence of morbid cardiac events. A randomized clinical trial. *JAMA.* 1997;277:1127.
87. Ammori JB, Sigakis M, Englesbe MJ, et al. Effect of intraoperative hyperglycemia during liver transplantation. *J Surg Res.* 2007;140:227.
88. De Witte J, Sessler DI. Perioperative shivering: Physiology and pharmacology. *Anesthesiology.* 2002;96:467.
89. Zelcer J, Wells DG. Anaesthetic-related recovery room complications. *Anaesth Intensive Care.* 1987;15:168.
90. Schubert A, Mascha EJ, Bloomfield EL, et al. Effect of cranial surgery and brain tumor size on emergence from anesthesia. *Anesthesiology.* 1996;85:513.
91. Wong GY, Warner DO, Schroeder DR, et al. Risk of surgery and anesthesia for ischemic stroke. *Anesthesiology.* 2000;92:425.
92. Kim J, Gelb AW. Predicting perioperative stroke. *J Neurosurg Anesthesiol.* 1995; 7:211.
93. Vlajkovic GP, Sindjelic RP. Emergence delirium in children: Many questions, few answers. *Anesth Analg.* 2007;104:84.
94. Voepel-Lewis T, Malviya S, Tait AR. A prospective cohort study of emergence agitation in the pediatric postanesthesia care unit. *Anesth Analg.* 2003;96:1625.
95. Isik B, Arslan M, Tunga AD, et al. Dexmedetomidine decreases emergence agitation in pediatric patients after sevoflurane anesthesia without surgery. *Paediatr Anaesth.* 2006;16:748.
96. Abu-Shahwan I, Chowdary K. Ketamine is effective in decreasing the incidence of emergence agitation in children undergoing dental repair under sevoflurane general anesthesia. *Paediatr Anaesth.* 2007;17:846.
97. Schwender D, Kunze-Kronawitter H, Dietrich P, et al. Conscious awareness during general anaesthesia: Patients' perceptions, emotions, cognition and reactions. *Br J Anaesth.* 1998;80:133.
98. Lynch EP, Lazor MA, Gellis JE, et al. The impact of postoperative pain on the development of postoperative delirium. *Anesth Analg.* 1998;86:781.
99. Kopman AF, Yee PS, Neuman GG. Relationship of the train-of-four fade ratio to clinical signs and symptoms of residual paralysis in awake volunteers. *Anesthesiology.* 1997;86:765.

100. Cook DJ, Rooke GA. Priorities in perioperative geriatrics. *Anesth Analg.* 2003;96:1823.
101. Zakriya KJ, Christmas C, Wenz JFS, et al. Preoperative factors associated with postoperative change in confusion assessment method score in hip fracture patients. *Anesth Analg.* 2002;94:1628.
102. Johnson T, Monk T, Rasmussen LS, et al. Postoperative cognitive dysfunction in middle-aged patients. *Anesthesiology.* 2002;96:1351.
103. Dodds C, Allison J. Postoperative cognitive deficit in the elderly surgical patient. *Br J Anaesth.* 1998;81:449.
104. Kerger H, Turan A, Kredel M, et al. Patients' willingness to pay for anti-emetic treatment. *Acta Anaesthesiol Scand.* 2007;51:38.
105. Sinclair DR, Chung F, Mezei G. Can postoperative nausea and vomiting be predicted? *Anesthesiology.* 1999;91:109.
106. Williams BA, Kentor ML, Vogt MT, et al. Economics of nerve block pain management after anterior cruciate ligament reconstruction: Potential hospital cost savings via associated postanesthesia care unit bypass and same-day discharge. *Anesthesiology.* 2004;100:697.
107. Charbit B, Albaladejo P, Funck-Brentano C, et al. Prolongation of QTc interval after postoperative nausea and vomiting treatment by droperidol or ondansetron. *Anesthesiology.* 2005;102(6):1094–1100.
108. Lee A, Done ML. The use of nonpharmacologic techniques to prevent postoperative nausea and vomiting: A meta-analysis. *Anesth Analg.* 1999;88:1362.

CHAPTER

Critical Care Medicine

MATTHEW R. HALLMAN • MIRIAM M. TREGGIARI • STEVEN DEEM

Key Points

1. Simple and inexpensive interventions in the ICU, such as the utilization of checklists and strict attention to aseptic technique during central venous catheterization, can result in substantial improvements in patient outcomes.
2. Administration of high-dose corticosteroids to patients presenting with traumatic brain injury is associated with 20% increase in the relative risk of death.
3. Administration of thrombolytic therapy (rt-PA) to patients presenting within 4.5 hours of onset of acute ischemic stroke results in improved neurologic outcome.
4. Patients who are resuscitated from cardiac arrest due to ventricular fibrillation have improved neurologic outcome and possibly reduced mortality when treated with mild therapeutic hypothermia (32° to 34°C) for 12 to 24 hours after hospital admission.
5. In patients with severe sepsis or septic shock, early and aggressive use of fluid resuscitation, appropriate antibiotics, infectious source control, and vasopressors/inotropes as needed improves survival.
6. Separation from mechanical ventilation in patients who are recovering from respiratory failure is accelerated by respiratory therapy–driven protocols and daily trials of spontaneous breathing.
7. Ventilation with low tidal volume (6 mL/kg) in patients with acute lung injury and acute respiratory distress syndrome reduces mortality, compared to traditional tidal volumes (12 mL/kg).
8. Red blood cell transfusion in the ICU should be restricted (transfusion threshold hemoglobin <7 g/dL) with the possible exception of patients with a diagnosis of active bleeding, early septic shock, acute myocardial infarction, or unstable angina, or with primarily neurologic or neurosurgical problems.
9. Nurse-driven sedation protocols and reduction of sedation reduce the duration of mechanical ventilation and ICU length of stay.
10. The incidence of ventilator-associated pneumonia (VAP) can be reduced with strict hand washing during patient care and semirecumbent positioning of the patient. Antibiotic therapy of VAP should utilize a "de-escalating" strategy, and can be limited to an 8-day course in uncomplicated cases.

Multimedia

1. Cerebral Blood Flow
2. Swan Pressure Tracing
3. Swan Real Life
4. A-line Insertion
5. Mechanical Ventilation Pressure
6. A-line Infection

INTRODUCTION: ANESTHESIOLOGISTS AND CRITICAL CARE MEDICINE

Historically, Critical Care Medicine evolved as a specialty nearly simultaneously in Europe and North America, but has followed strikingly different models in regards to the involvement of anesthesiologists. The first intensive care unit (ICU) in Europe may have been located in Denmark in the 1950s, and concurrently the first critical care physician, or "intensivist," may well have been an anesthesiologist.[1] Anesthesiologists continued to play a defining role in the development of Critical Care Medicine in most of Europe, Australia, New Zealand, Japan, and elsewhere and comprise the majority of intensivists in many countries around the world today. In North America, anesthesiologists were also integral to the development of Critical Care Medicine as a specialty. However, in contrast to other countries, in the United States anesthesiologists have played an ever-diminishing role in the specialty, and today comprise a small minority of the intensivist workforce.[2]

Although it has been suggested that the first ICU in North America was established at Johns Hopkins in 1923 to care for postoperative neurosurgical patients, it was not until the late 1950s and early 1960s that true multidisciplinary ICUs began to appear. The driving forces behind ICU development included advances in surgical techniques, polio epidemics which resulted in widespread respiratory failure, and later the recognition of the acute respiratory distress syndrome (ARDS). Anesthesiologists played a natural role in the evolution of ICUs, given their familiarity with surgical resuscitation and mechanical ventilation. Early on, however, the concept of "intensivists" did not exist, and patients were often managed by their primary physician (be it a surgeon or an internist) and nurses, with formal or informal consultation given by specialists, including anesthesiologists.

In the early 1960s, the first Critical Care Medicine training program was established at the University of Pittsburgh under the direction of an anesthesiologist, Peter Safar. At this point, the concept of "intensivist" was born; as defined by Dr. Safar, the qualities and qualifications of such an individual should include inquisitiveness, thoughtfulness, a high level of motivation, action orientation, diplomacy, and scientific training. In the late 1960s, a group including Dr. Safar and another anesthesiologist, Ake Grenvik, were instrumental in inaugurating the Society of Critical Care Medicine (SCCM). Anesthesiologists working through SCCM were instrumental in developing the board certification process for Critical Care Medicine, and in 1986 the first Critical Care Medicine Certification examination was administered by the American Board of Anesthesiology.[3] From the 1960s until the present, numerous anesthesiologists made important contributions to the development of the specialty, to critical care–related research, and to improvements in the care of critically ill patients. However, as of 2010 only about 1,300 anesthesiologists had completed the certification process in Critical Care Medicine in the United States, and anesthesiologists comprised only 8% of adult intensivists certified in the past 10 years.[4]

Anesthesiology and Critical Care Medicine: The Future

Although it seems certain that anesthesiologists will continue to play an important role in Critical Care Medicine worldwide, in the United States anesthesiology is currently at a crossroads in regards to its continued involvement in Critical Care Medicine. There are several forces that will shape the evolution of the specialty of Critical Care Medicine as a whole and the contribution that anesthesiologists will make to this evolution: (1) Increasing evidence that intensivists increase the quality of care and improve outcomes; (2) business/economic factors, whereby employers, insurers, and hospitals recognize the cost savings associated with intensivists in the ICU, as exemplified by the Leapfrog Initiative (further discussed in the following section); and (3) the aging population and increasing demand for critical care services, which will result in a shortage of intensivists starting in 2007 that will grow to a greater than 20% deficit by the year 2020, given current training levels[2] (Table 55-1). This prediction does not take into account any additional demands placed on the healthcare system, if any, by the Leapfrog Initiative and thus is likely an underestimate of the true future need for intensivists.

Given the above observations, it is clear that opportunities for careers in Critical Care Medicine will be amply available in the coming years. Anesthesiology as a specialty would seem ideally suited to help satisfy the increasing demand for intensivists. Anesthesiologists are hospital based; have sound fundamental training in physiology, pharmacology, invasive procedures, and monitoring; and have excellent historical and concurrent role models for the anesthesiologist as intensivist. However, economic and lifestyle incentives have recently dissuaded anesthesiology trainees from pursuing further training and careers in Critical Care Medicine.

TABLE 55-1. LEAPFROG ICU PHYSICIAN STAFFING (IPS) STANDARD

Hospitals fulfilling the IPS standard will operate adult and/or pediatric ICUs that are managed or comanaged by intensivists who

1. Are present during daytime hours and provide clinical care exclusively in the ICU
2. At other times can, at least 95% of the time,
   i. return ICU pages within 5 min and
   ii. arrange for an FCCS-certified[a] nonphysician effector to reach ICU patients within 5 min.

[a]Fundamental Critical Care Support (course training to prepare nonintensivists to manage the first 24 h of critical illness, sponsored by the Society of Critical Care Medicine).

From: http://www.leapfroggroup.org/for_hospitals/leapfrog_hospital_survey_copy/leapfrog_safety_practices/icu_physician_staffing

Critical care services are currently not reimbursed at rates commensurate with surgical anesthesia, and critical care practice is accurately perceived as more time-consuming and the workload more unpredictable than an operating room–based practice. However, these factors may change in the coming years, as reimbursement for surgical anesthesia and critical care services equalize and the lifestyle constraints associated with critical care are moderated by creative organizational strategies, including the use of physician extenders and other mechanisms for reducing the "24–7" workload. Lastly, the increase in the anesthesiology residency training requirement to include 4 months of intensive care may imbue trainees with a greater interest in Critical Care Medicine as a career choice. As stated above, anesthesiology in the United States is at a crossroads; with proper imagination, emphasis, support, and training the specialty can reassert itself as a leader in the field of Critical Care Medicine.

Critical Care Medicine: A Systems and Evidence-based Approach

Critical care encompasses all disciplines of medicine. It is clearly beyond the scope of a single chapter to provide detailed coverage of all aspects of critical illness, including physiology, pathophysiology, and management of disease. In addition, many critical care issues are commonly encountered by anesthesiologists that practice solely in the operating room and are covered in detail elsewhere in this text. Thus, this chapter will focus on topics that are relatively unique to the ICU, on therapeutic approaches, and upon practices for which strong evidence exists, particularly when supported by randomized controlled trials (RCTs).

Grading of levels of evidence and practice guidelines in an effort to improve clinician confidence in recommendations has become standard practice. Several different grading systems exist, with no clear evidence that one is superior to another; furthermore, given uncertainty about the methodology of grading systems and their effects on patient outcomes,[5] we have chosen not to include "grades" or levels of evidence in this chapter.

PROCESS OF CARE IN THE ICU

The method by which care is delivered may affect outcomes as much or more than the specific interventions employed. For example, care delivery models that reduce errors and encourage utilization of evidence-based practices may have a profound effect on outcomes, in addition to reducing costs. A single adverse event in the ICU may cost as much as $4,000 and increase length of stay by 1 day.[6] Additional data suggest that implementation of evidence-based practices in the ICU is not consistent and that more uniform implementation could save up to approximately 200,000 lives per year in the United States.[7]

As advances in medical and surgical therapeutics have increased the complexity of care for an aging and increasingly ill population of patients, it has become increasingly clear that the involvement of intensivists in the management of the critically ill is desirable. Several studies have suggested that mortality and other intermediate end points such as ICU length of stay can be reduced when "high-intensity" physician staffing models that mandate management or comanagement by intensivists are used.[8] These studies, as summarized in a meta-analysis by Pronovost et al. and further supported by two subsequent cohort studies,[8–10] have provoked a reconsideration of the ideal staffing model for ICUs in the United States, particularly amongst the business community.

The Business Roundtable, a national association of CEOs of Fortune 500 companies, formed the Leapfrog Group in 1999. The Leapfrog Group is a coalition of over 150 purchasers and providers of healthcare benefits, including large companies such as General Motors, Motorola, and Merck and insurers such as Aetna. The stated goal of the Leapfrog Group is to improve health care, in particular by reducing deaths due to medical error. To accomplish this mission, the group formulated the Leapfrog Initiative, which includes a series of "safety standards" that healthcare providers (largely hospitals) should strive for if they are to provide care for Leapfrog Group employees. Prompted by the data associating intensivists with improved outcomes, the Leapfrog Initiative included an ICU Physician Staffing (IPS) standard that promotes the continuous involvement of intensivists in the care of critically ill patients (Table 55-1).[11] Less than 10% of hospitals met this standard prior to its publication, and a recent survey suggests that there has been little improvement in compliance since then.[12,13] Reported barriers to implementation of the Leapfrog Initiative include lack of ICU directors, cost, loss of control and continuity in patient care, and loss of income.[13] However, considerable cost savings as a result of Leapfrog Initiative implementation have been estimated which continues to provide additional impetus for widespread adoption of these practices.[14]

1 In addition to improved ICU staffing, other simple interventions in the process of care have been shown to improve outcomes. These include efforts to reduce errors of omission by utilizing checklists during procedures and patient rounds,[15] and by explicitly outlining the daily goals of care during rounds.[16] Such efforts incur little or no cost, may incur substantial benefits, but are severely underutilized in the United States at present.

NEUROLOGIC AND NEUROSURGICAL CRITICAL CARE

Neuromonitoring

Several neuromonitoring devices used in the ICU setting may help in assessing pathophysiologic processes and adjusting therapy. The following section will discuss some commonly used neuromonitoring devices, including transcranial Doppler (TCD) ultrasonography, brain tissue oxygenation ($PbrO_2$), and microdialysis. Intracranial pressure (ICP) monitoring and jugular venous oximetry are discussed in chapters on Standard Monitoring Techniques, Anesthesia for Neurosurgery, and Burns and Trauma, and will not be discussed in detail here.

Transcranial Doppler Ultrasonography

TCD measures blood flow velocities and can indirectly estimate cerebral blood flow, ICP, cerebral autoregulation, and intracranial compliance. In patients with subarachnoid hemorrhage (SAH) or traumatic brain injury (TBI) TCD can be used as a tool to identify vasospasm as flow velocities through a given blood vessel tend to increase during spasm. In patients with TBI, flow velocities are depressed, and impaired autoregulation and vascular reactivity are common. In these patients, monitoring of TCD and jugular venous oxygen saturation (SjO_2) (see later) may be used to define the optimum cerebral perfusion pressure (CPP).[17] In addition, TCD indices may predict neurologic outcome in patients with TBI.[18] While anatomic variations preclude obtaining TCDs in all patients, the major barrier to more widespread adoption of this modality is the expertise required to obtain and interpret the data accurately.

Brain Tissue Oxygenation

Brain tissue oxygen pressure ($PbrO_2$) measurements are performed by introducing a small, oxygen-sensitive catheter into the brain tissue. The device monitors a very local area of the brain tissue, and this technique is increasingly used for evaluation of cerebral oxygenation (normal $PbrO_2$ values: 25 to 30 mm Hg).[19] Monitoring may be performed in relatively undamaged parts of the brain or, preferably, in the penumbra region of an intracerebral lesion.[20] Various studies have shown that an increase in ICP and a decrease in CPP or arterial oxygenation, and hyperventilation may result in decreased $PbrO_2$. This monitoring modality has been shown to be helpful in detecting intraoperative brain hypoxia during episodes of hyperventilation.[21] In patients with TBI, ischemic episodes defined as $PbrO_2$ <10 mm Hg for longer than 15 minutes in the first week after the injury were found to be associated with unfavorable neurologic outcome, and values of 0 (not responding to an oxygen challenge) are compatible with brain death.[22] A $PbrO_2$ of 15 mm Hg or less has been recommended as a threshold to initiate treatment.[23] Improvement in $PbrO_2$ in response to increased CPP, blood transfusion,[24] initiation of barbiturate coma,[25] and after decompressive hemicraniectomy have all been observed.[26] However, only retrospective observational studies have examined the effects of $PbrO_2$ monitoring on outcomes after neurologic injury, with variable results reported.[27,28] This may in part be due to the fact that $PbrO_2$ monitors are very focused in their sampling territory, and data obtained from a monitor placed in a nonrepresentative area of the cortex may not be generalizable to the rest of the brain. A phase II, multicenter trial of $PbrO_2$-guided therapy of patients with TBI (BOOST-2) is currently enrolling since 2011 and will hopefully provide more information about the influence of this monitoring modality on patient outcomes.

Microdialysis

Microdialysis uses a probe as an interface to the brain to continuously monitor the chemistry of a small focal volume of the cerebral extracellular space. This method uses internally perfused semipermeable membrane probes, which allow neurochemical water-soluble substances to be collected outside the brain for further analysis. Like $PbrO_2$ monitors, the catheter is typically placed in a cerebral territory deemed to be at risk for further damage. In patients with SAH this is the vascular territory associated with the hemorrhage, in nonfocal TBI it is commonly the right frontal lobe, and in focal TBI and ischemic stroke it is commonly the penumbra region.[29] The catheter allows measurement of energy-related metabolites, neurotransmitters, inflammatory markers, and exogenous substances such as drugs. The most commonly measured substances in clinical practice are lactate, pyruvate, glucose, and glutamate.[29] This monitoring modality thus provides insight into the bioenergetic status of the brain. Increased lactate, decreased glucose, and an elevated lactate/pyruvate ratio indicate accelerated anaerobic metabolism. This metabolic pattern commonly occurs with cerebral ischemia or hypoxia, and increased glycolysis in this setting is associated with a poor outcome. Extracellular excitatory amino acids such as glutamate may provide a marker for secondary brain insults, as indicated by elevation during periods of hypoxia and intracranial hypertension. Like $PbrO_2$ monitors, microdialysis catheters must be correctly positioned for the information they produce to be useful. Further, metabolism can be altered without changes of cerebral oxygenation and may not correlate with high ICP or low CPP, and correlation between microdialysis values and outcome is lacking.[30]

Diagnosis and Clinical Management of the Most Common Types of Neurologic Failure

Traumatic Brain Injury

TBI is the leading cause of death from blunt trauma, with an incidence of approximately 10/100,000 per year. With a proportion of 20% of deaths occurring in patients between the age of 5 and 45 years, TBI represents the leading cause of death in this age group. The most powerful predictors of poor outcome from injury through resuscitation are age >55 years, poor pupillary reactivity, postresuscitation Glasgow Coma Scale (GCS), hypotension, hypoxia, and an unfavorable intracranial diagnosis as established by radiologic features (e.g., CT scan). In addition, early hyperglycemia (>200 mg/dL) is a reliable independent predictor of poor outcome.

The GCS (see the chapter on Burns and Trauma) is the most widely used clinical measure of injury severity in patients with TBI. The advantages of this scale are that it provides an objective method of measuring consciousness, it has high intra- and interrater reliability across observers with a wide variety of experience, and it has an excellent correlation with outcome. However, the GCS is unmeasurable in up to 25% to 45% of the patients at admission and is inaccurate when only the partial score is used, such as in patients with tracheal intubation whose verbal response cannot be assessed. TBI qualifies as severe when the GCS is 8 or less. The predictive value of the GCS at admission is about 69% for good neurologic outcome and 76% for unfavorable outcome. After 7 days these figures approximate 80% for both favorable and unfavorable outcomes.[31]

Pupillary dilatation and light reactivity are also useful predictors of neurologic outcome. When both pupils are dilated and unreactive, the likelihood of poor neurologic outcome or death is as high as 90% to 95%. When both pupils are reactive, the likelihood of poor neurologic outcome is approximately 30% to 40%, while the probability of good outcome is 50% to 70%.

Hypotension is a strong predictor of poor outcome in TBI. Chesnut et al.[32] reported that there was a 15-fold increased risk of mortality in patients with early hypotension and an 11-fold increase in mortality in patients with late hypotension.

Radiologic imaging is important in the diagnosis and in assessing the prognosis of patients with TBI. A number of computerized tomography (CT scan)–based scoring systems have been developed and correlated with outcome, but the amount of midline shift appears to be the single most predictive feature of outcome. Subarachnoid blood, intraventricular blood, and diffuse axonal injury patterns portend worse outcomes, while epidural hematomas generally have better outcomes.[33] In addition, it should be noted that about one-third to one-half of the patients present no lesion at admission and develop new lesions secondarily, which is associated with substantially worse neurologic outcome.

The goal of resuscitation in TBI and other types of brain injury is to prevent continuing cerebral insult after a primary injury has already occurred. The extent of the primary cerebral injury is usually determined by the mechanism of the trauma, the cause, and the duration of cerebral ischemia. A primary insult is often associated with intracranial hypertension and systemic hypotension, leading to decreased cerebral perfusion and brain ischemia. Concomitant hypoxemia aggravates brain hypoxia, especially in the presence of hyperthermia, which increases brain metabolic demand. The combined effect of these factors leads to secondary brain injury characterized by excitotoxicity, oxidative stress, and inflammation. The resulting cerebral ischemia may be the single most important secondary event affecting outcome following a cerebral insult. Prevention of secondary injury is the main goal of resuscitative efforts.

TABLE 55-2. ICU MANAGEMENT OF PATIENTS WITH SEVERE TRAUMATIC BRAIN INJURY

Basic principles applied to all patients, assuming initial surgical management	• Head elevation 30–45 degrees[a]
	• CPP 50–70 Torr
	  • Euvolemia, vasopressors as needed
	• ICP <20 Torr
	  • Mannitol, hypertonic saline
	  • CSF drainage
	• SaO_2 ≥95%; $PaCO_2$ 35–40 Torr
	• Temperature ≤37°C
	• Glucose <180 mg/dL
	• Sedation and analgesia
	• Early enteral nutrition
	• Seizure, stress ulcer, and DVT prophylaxis

Refractory intracranial hypertension Consider one or all of these interventions, depending on individual circumstances	• Optimized hyperventilation with SjO_2 and/or $PbrO_2$ monitoring • Barbiturate coma • Mild therapeutic hypothermia (33°–35°C) • Decompressive craniectomy

[a]Unless contraindicated by spine injury, hemodynamic instability, or otherwise.
CPP, cerebral perfusion pressure; ICP, intracranial pressure; CSF, cerebrospinal fluid; SaO_2, arterial oxygen saturation; $PaCO_2$, arterial carbon dioxide tension; DVT, deep venous thrombosis; SjO_2, jugular venous oxygen saturation; $PbrO_2$, brain tissue oxygen tension.

Traumatized areas of the brain manifest impaired autoregulation and disruption of the blood–brain barrier. If space-occupying lesions or edema are present, these will contribute to reduced brain compliance, leading to increased ICP and a consequent deleterious effect on cerebral blood flow. The rationale for attempting to optimize CPP arises from the fact that cerebral regions surrounding the primary lesion may be close to the ischemic threshold. Therefore, the goals of neuroresuscitation are oriented at restoration of cerebral blood flow by maintenance of adequate CPP, reduction of ICP, evacuation of space-occupying lesions, initiation of therapies for cerebral protection, and avoidance of hypoxia.

Unfortunately, the ICU treatment of TBI is hindered by a lack of rigorous RCTs to prove benefit, or lack thereof, for many of the management strategies utilized today. The Brain Trauma Foundation has published Guidelines for the Management of Severe Traumatic Brain Injury and revised them as recently as 2007.[23] However, only one recommendation in 15 subject areas reaches "Level I," meaning based on high-quality, randomized trials. Thus, treatment is based largely on pathophysiologic principles and uncontrolled trials. A general guideline for management of patients with severe TBI appears in Table 55-2. Basic principles of management of acute TBI, including osmotherapy, are discussed further in the chapter on Trauma and Burns; sedation, hyperventilation, hypothermia, corticosteroids, and antiseizure prophylaxis are discussed in further detail below.

Sedation of neurologically impaired patients should typically be achieved with short-acting sedatives to allow for frequent assessment of neurologic examination.[34] Although no studies have investigated the effect of sedation on outcome in patients with neurologic disorders, a common practice is to provide sedation with propofol, benzodiazepines, or dexmedetomidine in patients following TBI. These agents have favorable effects on cerebral oxygen balance, although propofol is more potent in this regard. Undesirable effects of sedatives are those leading to a reduction in CPP due to hemodynamic depression or to an increase in CBF accompanied by a simultaneous increase in ICP, a condition potentially occurring, for example, with the use of ketamine.

Propofol rapidly penetrates the central nervous system and has rapid elimination kinetics. Despite the induction of systemic hypotension, propofol decreases cerebral metabolism resulting in a coupled decline in cerebral blood flow, with consequent decrease in ICP. Propofol's favorable pharmacologic and neurophysiologic profile has led to its widespread use in neurointensive care, and high-dose propofol has been advocated as a substitute for barbiturate therapy in patients with refractory intracranial hypertension. However, prolonged (>24 hours), high-dose (>80 μg/kg/min) propofol administration has been associated with lactic acidosis, cardiac failure, and death ("propofol infusion syndrome") in children and adults with TBI.[35] Thus, the use of high-dose propofol to control refractory intracranial hypertension is not recommended, and barbiturates should be considered if ICP is not controlled by moderate doses of propofol.

The mechanisms by which barbiturates exert their cerebral protective effect appear to be mediated by a reduction in ICP via alteration in vascular tone, reduction of cerebral metabolic rate, and inhibition of free radical peroxidation. Although barbiturates are effective in reducing ICP, their routine use in TBI does not appear beneficial and may in fact result in excess mortality in patients with diffuse brain injury.[36,37] This effect may in part relate to the profound cardiovascular depressant effects of barbiturates. Based on one small randomized trial, barbiturates do appear to reduce mortality in patients with refractory high ICP.[38] Thus, high-dose barbiturate therapy may be considered in hemodynamically stable severe TBI patients with intracranial hypertension refractory to maximal medical and surgical ICP-lowering therapy. In some patients pentobarbital may induce cerebral hypoxia by reducing CBF in excess of metabolism, and therefore SjO_2 monitoring may be considered during barbiturate therapy.

The centrally acting α-2 agonist dexmedetomidine has both sedative and analgesic effects. Its most desirable property is that it can allow for a more interactive and awake patient than other sedatives (see section on sedation later). While it has not been studied specifically in brain-injured patients, Drummond et al.[39] have shown that cerebral blood flow–cerebral metabolic rate of oxygen ($CMRO_2$) coupling remains intact in healthy volunteers during dexmedetomidine infusion.

Although neuromuscular blockade may result in a fall in ICP, the routine use of neuromuscular blockade is discouraged since its use has been associated with longer ICU course, a higher incidence of pneumonia, and a trend toward more frequent sepsis without any improvement in outcome.

Hyperventilation effectively reduces ICP by reducing CBF. However, the role that hyperventilation should play in routine management of TBI is not clear. Primarily, this is related to concerns that hyperventilation may lead to critically low CBF, resulting in worsening cerebral ischemia.[40] In small randomized trials, prophylactic hyperventilation has not proven to be beneficial in TBI.[41] In contrast, it has been proposed that "optimized hyperventilation" in the presence of "luxury perfusion" (excess CBF) may increase global cerebral oxygen metabolism and help normalize global cerebral glucose extraction. Cruz[42] reported that an optimized hyperventilation strategy resulted in a reduction in mortality compared to CPP management in concurrent matched control patients, although this was not a randomized trial. On the basis of the available evidence, prolonged or prophylactic hyperventilation should be avoided after severe TBI, especially in the first 24 hours after the injury. Hyperventilation may be necessary for brief periods to reduce intracranial hypertension refractory to sedation, osmotic therapy, and CSF drainage and should be guided by SjO_2 and/or $PbrO_2$.[23] A marked fall in either of these values suggests a harmful effect of hyperventilation and that it should be reduced or discontinued.

Experimentally, hypothermia causes a reduction in cerebral metabolism by decreasing all cell functions, both related to neuronal electric activity and those responsible for cellular integrity. In addition, mild hypothermia has been shown to decrease the release of substrates associated with tissue injury such as glutamate and aspartate. A meta-analysis of eight randomized trials of the use of mild hypothermia (33° to 35°C) in patients with TBI, and including 748 patients, indicated that despite a marginal improvement in poor neurologic outcome, there was no mortality advantage and there was an increased risk of pneumonia.[43] An additional randomized trial of very early hypothermia published subsequently again found no outcome benefit to hypothermia.[44] Therefore, mild hypothermia should not be routinely induced in patients with TBI, although it may be useful for rescue therapy of patients with refractory intracranial hypertension. On the other hand, immediate rewarming of TBI patients with spontaneous hypothermia may further worsen outcome and should be done with caution.[45]

2 Corticosteroids to reduce posttraumatic inflammatory injury in TBI were advocated for 30 years or more, but without convincing evidence of benefit. The CRASH study, published in 2004, prospectively randomized over 10,000 patients presenting with acute TBI to receive high-dose methylprednisolone or placebo for 48 hours after hospital admission. Methylprednisolone administration was associated with an approximately 20% increase in the relative risk of death at 2 weeks in the entire cohort, and detriment was evident across subgroups divided by severity and type of injury.[46] Thus, high-dose corticosteroids should not be administered as therapy for acute TBI.[23] Likewise, intravenous magnesium administration did not improve outcomes in patients with TBI and might even have a negative effect in the treatment of significant brain injury.[47]

Anticonvulsants are effective at preventing early posttraumatic seizures within 7 days following head trauma. However, the evidence does not indicate that prevention of early seizures improves outcome following TBI.[48] Seizures should therefore be treated on an as-needed basis.

Finally, it should be noted that use of albumin as fluid replacement therapy in patients with TBI has been associated with increased mortality in a subgroup analysis of an RCT comparing saline and albumin.[49] Routine albumin administration to patients with TBI should be avoided (Table 55-2).

Subarachnoid Hemorrhage

The incidence of SAH in the United States varies from 7.5 to 12.1 cases per 100,000 population. SAH is most commonly caused by the rupture of an intracranial aneurysm. Other causes of SAH include trauma, vertebral and carotid artery dissection, dural and spinal arteriovenous malformations, mycotic aneurysms, sickle cell disease, cocaine abuse, coagulation disorders, and pituitary apoplexy. Aneurysmal SAH is associated with considerable morbidity and mortality, with only one-third of the patients suffering from SAH being functional survivors. The leading causes of death and disability are the direct effect of the initial bleed, cerebral vasospasm, and rebleeding. The Report of the Cooperative Study of Intracranial Aneurysms and SAH estimated that 33% of the patients would die before receiving medical attention.[50,51] Although the number of early deaths may not have changed substantially, the overall case fatality rate of aneurysmal SAH has fallen over time, and although there is geographic variation mortality is reported in the 40% to 50% range in most studies.[52] Approximately 40% to 50% of patients survive with good neurologic outcome after SAH (independence as measured by the modified Rankin scale).[52] Severity of the initial bleed is the most important determinant of SAH outcome.

At the time of aneurysm rupture, there is a critical reduction in CBF due to increase in ICP toward arterial diastolic values. The persistence of a no-flow pattern is associated with acute vasospasm and swelling of perivascular astrocytes, neuronal cells, and capillary endothelium. After SAH, injury to the posterior hypothalamus may stimulate release of norepinephrine (NE) from the adrenal medulla and sympathetic cardiac efferent nerves. The release of NE has been associated with ischemic changes in the subendocardium (neurogenic stunned myocardium), cardiac dysrhythmias, and pulmonary edema.

In survivors of the initial bleed, emphasis has been placed on early aneurysm control with either surgery or interventional neuroradiology (coiling). Approximately 10% to 23% of unsecured aneurysms will rebleed in the first 2 weeks, most within the first 6 to 12 hours after the initial hemorrhage, and rebleeding is associated with mortality approximating 80%. Early aneurysm occlusion substantially reduces the risk of this complication. With the improvement of the operative management, delayed complications have become increasingly important causes of death and disability.

Cerebral vasospasm after SAH is identified by angiography in up to 60% of patients and is correlated with the amount and location of subarachnoid blood. A reduction in cerebral blood flow associated with vessel narrowing is ultimately responsible for the appearance of delayed ischemic neurologic deficits (DINDS). DINDS occur in approximately one-third of patients suffering from SAH. In a systematic review of the literature, Dorsch[53] found an overall death rate of 31% (vs. 17% in patients without vasospasm), permanent deficits in 35%, and good outcome in 34% of the patients who developed symptomatic vasospasm. DINDS typically present as alteration in consciousness and/or transient focal neurologic deficits that rarely occur within the first 3 days after aneurysm rupture, typically peak in 7 to 10 days, and resolve over 10 to 14 days. If severe, vasospasm can result in cerebral infarction and persistent neurologic deficits, which contribute to considerable long-term morbidity.

TCD has been used to identify and quantify cerebral vasospasm on the basis that blood flow velocity increases as the diameter of the vessel decreases. Changes in measured velocities over time may be more reliable than absolute values in predicting symptomatic vasospasm. Velocities greater than 200 cm/s have been associated with a high risk of infarction but there is a poor correlation between the TCD velocities and angiographic findings, especially for the posterior circulation.

Oral nimodipine (60 mg every 4 hours for 21 days) as prophylaxis for cerebral vasospasm is recognized as an effective treatment in improving neurologic outcome (reduction of cerebral infarction and poor functional outcome) and mortality from cerebral vasospasm in patients suffering from SAH.[54] Because angiographic studies did not demonstrate a difference in the frequency of vasospasm compared with a placebo-treated group, the benefits of nimodipine have been attributed to a cytoprotective effect related to the reduced availability of intracellular calcium and improved microvascular collateral flow. No other pharmacologic therapies to prevent or treat cerebral vasospasm have demonstrated effective results in clinical trials with the exception of statins. Tseng et al. conducted a meta-analysis of available studies examining the effect of statin therapy on outcomes in SAH and found a reduction in the risk of DINDS in those patients receiving a statin. Further, statin therapy appeared safe and may reduce the incidence of vasospasm although the quality of evidence was insufficient to conclude this definitively.[55]

Hypervolemic, hypertensive, and hemodilution ("triple-H") therapy is one of the mainstays of prevention and treatment of cerebral ischemia associated with SAH-induced vasospasm despite the lack of evidence for its effectiveness, especially for prophylactic use.[56] The rationale for hypervolemia is derived from the observation that hypovolemia is associated with poor outcomes after SAH and is often present because of blood loss and/or hypothalamic dysfunction and secretion of natriuretic peptides. Volume expansion is therefore considered beneficial to optimize the hemodynamic profile. The rationale for hypertension derives from the concept that a loss of cerebral autoregulation associated with vasospasm results in pressure-dependent cerebral blood flow. Finally, hemodilution is a consequence of hypervolemic therapy and is thought to optimize the rheologic properties of the blood and thereby to improve microcirculatory flow. There is no consensus with regard to the goals of the therapy and it is unclear which component of this therapy is necessary or sufficient to treat vasospasm.[57] Common complications of treatment are pulmonary edema and myocardial ischemia. Since the blood–brain barrier may be disrupted, aggravation of vasogenic edema or hemorrhagic infarction has also been described.[58]

Interventional neuroradiology with the use of balloon angioplasty can reverse or improve vasospasm-induced neurologic deficits if initiated early after the development of ischemic symptoms. Although observational data suggest a beneficial effect of angioplasty on long-term outcomes, these findings have not been confirmed in RCTs, and the risks of angioplasty include intimal dissection, vessel rupture, ischemia, and infarction.

Hydrocephalus is another cause of neurologic dysfunction after SAH, occurring in 25% of patients surviving the hemorrhage. The presence of blood in the ventricular system obstructs ventricular drainage and CSF absorption sites (subarachnoid villi). Ventricular drainage is usually successful in improving neurologic symptoms due to hydrocephalus. A minority of patients will require a permanent ventriculo-peritoneal shunt. Seizures also occur in 13% of patients with SAH and are more common in patients with a neurologic deficit; thus, prophylactic anticonvulsant therapy should be considered, but consensus for its use is generally lacking.[59]

A relatively common complication after SAH (10% to 34%) is hyponatremia. Hyponatremia usually develops several days after the hemorrhage and is attributed to two main causes: (1) A syndrome of inappropriate antidiuretic hormone (SIADH), which is associated with euvolemia or mild hypervolemia and an excess of free water, and (2) cerebral "salt wasting," which is marked by depletion of sodium and water. The differentiation of these two entities can be difficult but is theoretically important, in that SIADH is treated by free water restriction, and cerebral salt wasting with volume repletion and sodium administration. Thus, assessment of intravascular volume status is a key component when deciding on the treatment regimen for hyponatremia associated with SAH. Other medical complications are relatively common after SAH and include pneumonia, neurogenic pulmonary edema and acute lung injury (ALI), sepsis, gastrointestinal (GI) bleeding, deep venous thrombosis (DVT), and pulmonary embolism (PE).

Acute Ischemic Stroke

Although evidence indicates that the incidence of stroke has declined over the past 30 years, stroke remains one of the leading causes of disability and death in the United States. Nearly 90% of strokes can be attributed to an ischemic mechanism such as atherosclerosis, thrombosis, cardio-embolism, or hypotension. Other major causes of stroke are intracerebral hemorrhage and SAH.[60] Unusual causes of stroke such as carotid artery dissection, hypercoagulation syndromes, or infective endocarditis should be considered in younger patients without apparent risk factors. Transient ischemic attacks may precede stroke and thus should be considered as a warning sign. The prognosis after stroke varies depending on the size and location of the lesion. In patients with acute ischemic stroke, the duration of coma appears to be the most important predictor of outcome and successful therapy.

Rapid clot lysis and restoration of circulation have been proposed as measures to limit the extent of brain injury and improve outcome after stroke. In accordance with the American Heart Association guidelines, systemic thrombolysis using IV alteplase (rt-PA) should be administered to patients presenting with acute ischemic stroke within 3 hours of symptom onset so long as no
3 contraindications exist.[61] A recent meta-analysis of trials including almost 3,700 patients found that the treatment window may be extended to 4.5 hours. In this analysis neurologic outcomes at 90 days in those patients treated with rt-PA within 4.5 hours of symptom onset were better than those treated with placebo, but no mortality benefit was found.[62] After 4.5 hours the risk of hemorrhage (5% to 7% overall) appears to outweigh the benefits of treatment. It is clear that earlier treatment leads to improved outcomes and that treatment should be initiated as soon as possible.

There is no evidence that intra-arterial thrombolysis or mechanical thrombectomy is superior or inferior to intravenous administration of rt-PA, but they may be considered in patients with large MCA territory ischemic strokes and in situations where systemic rt-PA is contraindicated. Intravenous streptokinase, aspirin, heparin, warfarin, ticlopidine, or other antithrombotic or antiplatelet aggregating drugs are generally not recommended within 24 hours of treatment with either systemic or arterial rt-PA.

Unfractionated heparin (UFH) and low-molecular-weight heparin (LMWH) have not been shown to prevent stroke progression or reduce the rate of stroke recurrence when administered within 48 hours of the acute event, and therefore their use is not recommended. In general, heparin is only recommended for early secondary prophylaxis in patients with suspected cardiac embolism. Aspirin 325 mg has been shown to reduce the risk of early recurrent ischemic stroke and is recommended within 24 to 48 hours of stroke onset in most patients, but increases the risk of hemorrhagic stroke. The frequency of DVT in acute stroke is reduced by anticoagulants, especially LMWH, but not by antiplatelet agents. However, it is unclear if the frequency of PE is also reduced.

The majority of patients with acute ischemic stroke present with severe arterial hypertension. If intracerebral hemorrhage is excluded, treatment of hypertension should be delayed since reduction of the perfusion pressure could compromise the viable brain surrounding the ischemia (ischemic penumbra). However, severe hypertension (systolic blood pressure >220 mm Hg, or mean arterial blood pressure of >130 mm Hg, or diastolic >120 mm Hg) should be controlled because of increased risk of hemorrhagic transformation in anticoagulated patients or after thrombolysis. Although there is no evidence for an optimal level of blood pressure, there is general consensus that the systolic pressure should not be lowered below 150 to 160 mm Hg. If the event is accompanied by raised ICP due to cerebral edema, the principles of treatment of raised ICP discussed above with regard to TBI similarly apply. Cytotoxic brain edema usually occurs 24 to 96 hours after acute ischemic stroke, and osmotherapy constitutes the basis of ICP reduction. Steroids are of no value in the treatment of ischemic stroke. Because hyperglycemia is associated with poor outcome in ischemic stroke, tight glucose control has been recommended by some. However, a randomized trial of glucose–potassium and insulin infusion that targeted normoglycemia in patients with acute stroke failed to demonstrate a mortality benefit at 90 days.[63]

Space-occupying middle cerebral artery infarctions (malignant MCA syndrome) and cerebellar infarctions have a high mortality rate and, in selected cases where signs of intractable intracranial hypertension are present, hemicraniectomy or decompressive
surgery of the posterior fossa, respectively, could be life saving 2
and improve outcome.[64] Surgery seems to be less beneficial in
patients presenting with aphasia, in patients older than 50 years, 3
and in patients undergoing delayed surgery (greater than 24 hours after presentation).

Anoxic Brain Injury

Anoxic brain injury most commonly occurs as a result of cardiac arrest, either in or out of the hospital. Of patients who survive their initial cardiac arrest, in-hospital mortality ranges from approximately 50% to 90%, and a high percentage of survivors suffer brain injury with significant long-term disability. The pathophysiology of anoxic brain injury is multifactorial and includes excitatory neurotransmitter release, accumulation of intracellular calcium, and oxygen free radical generation. Unfortunately, pharmacologic therapies aimed at several of these pathways, including barbiturates, benzodiazepines, corticosteroids, calcium channel antagonists, and free radical scavengers, have failed to improve the outcome of anoxic brain injury.

4 Mounting evidence supports a role for mild therapeutic hypothermia in anoxic brain injury. A Cochrane review in 2009 found that available evidence supports the induction of mild hypothermia (temperature 32° to 34°C) in survivors of out-of-hospital ventricular fibrillation/ventricular tachycardia arrest.[65] Hypothermia was associated with a relative increase in patients with a favorable neurologic outcome (moderate disability or less) of 40% to 50%, and in one study it was also associated with relative 6-month mortality reduction by approximately 25%.[66] Thus, mild therapeutic hypothermia should be routinely applied to comatose survivors of out-of-hospital cardiac arrest due to ventricular fibrillation; it should also be considered in other scenarios, including in-hospital cardiac arrest and cardiac arrest due to asystole and pulseless electrical activity.

CARDIOVASCULAR AND HEMODYNAMIC ASPECTS OF CRITICAL CARE

Principles of Monitoring and Resuscitation

Shock states are associated with impairment of adequate oxygen delivery resulting in decreased tissue perfusion and tissue hypoxia. It is important to emphasize that global hemodynamic monitoring may not reflect regional perfusion or the peripheral tissue energy status. Occasionally, despite increased cardiac output (CO) and oxygen delivery peripheral tissues suffer from hypoxia due to blood flow maldistribution and uncoupling between oxygen delivery and oxygen utilization from mitochondrial dysfunction and energetic failure (cytopathic hypoxia).

Invasive monitoring in shock states provides insight into the circulatory status, organ perfusion, tissue microcirculation, and cellular metabolic status of the critically ill patient. Hemodynamic monitoring ranges from the simple monitoring of ECG and pulse oximetry, to continuous arterial pressure measurement via an arterial catheter, the monitoring of cardiac filling pressures with central venous or pulmonary artery catheters (PACs), to cardiac echocardiography. Several experimental monitoring devices detecting microenvironmental conditions at the tissue level are under continuous investigation.

Functional Hemodynamic Monitoring

Pulmonary Artery Catheter

The PAC measures hemodynamic indices including central venous pressure (CVP), pulmonary artery pressure and occlusion pressure (PaOP), CO (thermodilution method), systemic vascular resistance (SVR) and pulmonary vascular resistance, and mixed venous oxygen saturation (SvO_2) and provides data for deriving oxygenation variables (oxygen delivery [DO_2], consumption [VO_2], and extraction [O_2ER]). The information provided by the PAC may assist in the differentiation of cardiogenic and noncardiogenic circulatory and respiratory failure and help guide fluid, inotropic, and vasopressor therapy. The technical and physiologic principles of the PAC are discussed in detail in other chapters.

Despite the theoretical benefits of pulmonary artery catheterization, there are few data to support a positive effect of PAC utilization on mortality or other substantive outcome variables. Patient populations including those with ARDS, congestive heart failure, and septic shock and high-risk surgical patients have all been the subject of investigations targeting the effect of PAC use on outcome.[67,68] These trials have all failed to show benefit. As a consequence of these studies questioning the benefits of the PAC, the frequency of its use has substantially decreased in both medical and surgical patients.[69]

There is reason to believe that some or all of the following factors may be responsible for the observed lack of benefit associated with PAC use: (1) Device or procedure-related complications; (2) inaccurate data; (3) fundamentally incorrect assumptions about the meaning of the measured data; (4) inappropriate decisions resulting from misinterpretation of the data; and (5) harmful effects of well-intended therapies. As an example of factor number 3, there is increasing evidence that CVP and PA pressure do not predict the hemodynamic response to intravenous fluid administration in normal subjects or patients with shock.[70,71] As an example of factor number 5, the ability to increase DO_2 with fluid resuscitation and inotropic therapy in patients with septic shock identifies a better prognosis. This observation led to a therapeutic strategy known as "supraphysiologic resuscitation" to defined end points (cardiac index >4.5 L/min, DO_2 >600 mL/m^2/min, and VO_2 >170 mL/m^2/min) in patients with septic and surgical/trauma-related shock. However, a large, randomized, prospective study found that this approach was associated with increased mortality in patients with septic shock, and this approach is no longer favored.[72]

As with all interventions, the decision to insert a PAC must weigh the risks of monitoring against the potential benefits in terms of adaptation of treatment to the information obtained from the monitoring. While there are likely specific patient populations and disease states that may benefit from this monitoring modality, further research is necessary to define these groups.

A somewhat less invasive and less costly alternative to placing a PAC for the measurement of SvO_2 is to measure central venous oxygen saturation ($ScvO_2$) via a fiberoptic central venous catheter. $ScvO_2$ is approximately 5 mm Hg higher than SvO_2 in critically ill patients, but appears to correlate well with SvO_2 during changes in hemodynamic status.[73] Targeting an $ScvO_2$ >70% as a component of early goal–directed therapy in patients with septic shock has been associated with a reduction in mortality.[74]

Arterial Pressure Waveform Analysis

4 In addition to static pressure measurements such as CVP and PaOP, dynamic indicators of preload include respiratory variation in systolic pressure and pulse pressure, both of which can be derived from the analysis of the waveform generated by a peripherally placed arterial catheter. In addition, techniques for deriving stroke volume, CO, and intrathoracic blood volume are available. These techniques present a less invasive approach to hemodynamic monitoring of critically ill patients.

The variation in systolic blood pressure and pulse pressure during positive pressure ventilation (PPV) is highly predictive of the response to intravascular fluid administration in both normal subjects and critically ill patients. During PPV there is an inspiratory reduction in right ventricular stroke volume due to decreased venous return and a subsequent reduction in left ventricular end-diastolic volume appearing during the expiratory phase of the respiratory cycle. Therefore, the left ventricular stroke volume varies cyclically with ventilation and is paralleled by a similar variation in systolic blood pressure and pulse pressure; these effects are exaggerated during absolute and relative hypovolemia. Systolic and pulse pressure variations are superior predictors of fluid responsiveness (compared to static measures such as CVP and PaOP) in patients with a variety of critical illnesses, including septic shock, ALI, and following cardiac surgery.[75]

Analysis of the systemic arterial pulse contour allows derivation of CO after initial calibration using an indicator-dilution technique. Two commercially available devices utilize either lithium (injected through a peripheral IV; LiDCO) or thermal dilution (injected through a central venous catheter; PiCCO) for initial calibration. CO derived using pulse contour analysis correlates well with thermodilution CO in a variety of conditions and has the advantage of providing continuous measurement without necessitating the placement of a PAC. The PiCCO device also allows for measurement of intrathoracic blood volume using transpulmonary thermodilution; the latter may be a more accurate reflection of preload than static central pressure measurements. Although further validation of these techniques in critically ill patients is necessary, the use of pulse contour analysis may potentially obviate the need for pulmonary artery catheterization to measure CO, particularly if combined with the measurement of $ScvO_2$ as an indicator of the balance between oxygen delivery and consumption.

Transesophageal Doppler sonography using a small probe in a large nasogastric tube (6 mm) monitors descending aortic flow velocity continuously. When combined with the cross-sectional area of the aorta it allows for less invasive monitoring of CO compared to the PAC. The disadvantages of this technique are that it is inaccurate if not positioned correctly, it is easily dislodged, and that it does not measure the supra-aortic output or the aortic cross-sectional area directly. Instead, aortic cross-sectional area is determined using a nomogram and assumed to remain constant throughout systole.[76] Two cases of intrabronchial displacement of the probe have been reported.

Echocardiography

Echocardiography is an even less invasive hemodynamic monitoring tool, see Chapter 26. Both transthoracic echocardiography (TTE), and transesophageal echocardiography (TEE) provide accurate diagnostic information with regard to dynamic ventricular function, valvular anatomy, pericardial anatomy and intracardiac pressures. While TEE has long been used in the ICU, especially in cardiac surgical patients, TTE use is becoming more widespread as the size and cost of the equipment are coming down. The major limitation of echocardiography is that it does not provide continuous monitoring and requires a high standard of training and experience. However, a number of studies have now shown that with very limited training practitioners can accurately and rapidly perform focused cardiac examinations. Melamed et al. provided intensivists with 2 hours of formal didactic training followed by 4 hours of hands-on training in focused point-of-care echocardiography. Using formal TTEs obtained by professional sonographers and interpreted by attending cardiologists as a gold standard, the intensivists were able to correctly identify ventricular (dys)function more than 80% of the time.[77] Ultrasound has the additional benefit of being easily adapted to other uses in addition to cardiac assessment such as to guide placement of vascular catheters, assessment of lung pleura and parenchyma, and venous thrombosis detection. Although the role of echocardiography in routine critical care management remains undefined, it has been suggested that this technique can replace pulmonary arterial catheterization in the ICU without adversely affecting outcomes.[78] However, it should be kept in mind that data on outcomes with the use of focused echocardiography are lacking.

Definition and Types of Circulatory Failure

The common denominator of shock is circulatory instability characterized by severe hypotension and inadequate tissue perfusion. Shock states are classified according to the primary cause of circulatory failure. *Distributive* or *vasodilatory* shock results from a reduction in SVR, often associated with an increased CO, whereas *cardiogenic* (left or right cardiac failure) and *hypovolemic* shock are low CO states usually characterized by increased peripheral resistance. *Obstructive* shock, as the name suggests, is characterized by an obstruction to CO such as may happen with a tension pneumothorax or pericardial tamponade. The most common forms of shock encountered in the ICU are cardiogenic, septic (a form of distributive shock), and hypovolemic shock. Despite extensive research and aggressive management, the mortality from shock remains staggeringly high; approximately 35% to 40% of patients die within 28 days of the onset of septic shock, and the mortality rate is 70% to 80% for patients with cardiogenic shock. The mortality from hypovolemic shock is highly variable and depends upon the etiology and the rapidity of recognition and treatment. Cardiogenic and septic shock are discussed in more detail in the following section; the causes and treatment of traumatic shock, including hypovolemic and obstructive shock, are discussed in the chapter on Trauma and Burns.

Cardiogenic Shock

The initiating event in cardiogenic shock is a primary pump failure. Heart failure may result from extensive myocardial infarction (MI), cardiomyopathy, dysrhythmias, mechanical complications (mitral regurgitation, ventricular septal defect), tamponade, and so on. The pathophysiologic characteristics include a reduction in contractility, usually accompanied by dilatation of cardiac cavities and venous congestion. Determining the etiology of cardiogenic shock is of utmost importance as the treatment varies considerably based on the underlying mechanism; β-blockers are contraindicated in nonischemic ventricular failure exacerbations and diuresis is frequently indicated, whereas in acute ischemic ST elevation MI (STEMI) β-blockers are a mainstay of treatment and there is little role for acute diuresis. A 12-lead ECG, serum troponin measurements, B-type natriuretic peptide levels, and TTE should be obtained in all patients presenting with heart failure as this information is helpful in differentiating between the various causes of heart failure.[79] Absence of pulmonary congestion at initial clinical evaluation does not exclude a diagnosis of cardiogenic shock due to predominant left ventricular failure and is not associated with a better prognosis. The onset of pump failure is associated with two compensatory mechanisms: A reflex vasoconstriction in systemic vessels causing an increase in left ventricular workload and myocardial oxygen demand, and a redistribution of blood volume toward the heart and the lungs. However, cardiogenic shock developing within 36 hours of an acute MI has been associated with variably decreased SVRs, possibly mediated by the presence of a systemic inflammatory response.

Several studies have demonstrated that the incidence and severity of left ventricular failure complicating acute MI were directly related to the extent of ventricular mass necrosis. Consequently, therapy should minimize myocardial oxygen demand and raise oxygen delivery to the ischemic area; this goal is complicated by the fact that many resuscitative approaches to correct hypotension (preload augmentation, inotropes, and vasopressors; see later) increase myocardial oxygen consumption. In patients without hypotension, pharmacologic vasodilatation using nitrates or sodium nitroprusside may reduce myocardial oxygen consumption and improve ventricular ejection by reducing left ventricular afterload and possibly produce a shift of blood from the lungs to the periphery by reducing venous tone. B-type natriuretic peptide (nesiritide) and fenoldopam have similar effects, but have not shown any benefit in large randomized trials and are not recommended.[80] When pharmacologic interventions are not sufficient to restore hemodynamic stability, the use of mechanical support with the insertion of intra-aortic balloon pump counterpulsation and ventricular assist devices can help unload the ventricles.

In patients with MI, coronary reperfusion can be achieved with systemic thrombolysis or, preferably, primary percutaneous coronary intervention (PCI). The American Heart Association/American College of Cardiology guidelines recommend treatment of STEMI by PCI within 90 minutes of presentation or, if not available, by thrombolytic therapy within 30 minutes of presentation.[81] A randomized trial comparing emergency revascularization with primary PCI or coronary artery bypass surgery to a regimen of thrombolysis did not demonstrate a mortality difference at 30 days. However, at 6 months and 1 year, there was a significant mortality reduction with emergency revascularization in patients under age of 75 years.[82] The addition of intra-aortic balloon counterpulsation to PCI in acute STEMI did not reduce infarct size or otherwise improve outcomes.[83]

Septic Shock

Septic shock is a form of distributive shock associated with the activation of the systemic inflammatory response and is usually characterized by a high CO, low SVR, hypotension, and regional blood flow redistribution, resulting in tissue hypoperfusion. Other causes of distributive shock include acute spinal cord injury, pancreatitis, burns, fulminant hepatic failure, multiple traumatic injuries, toxic shock syndrome, anaphylaxis and anaphylactoid reactions, and drug or toxin reactions, including insect bites, transfusion reactions, and heavy metal poisoning. In patients with systemic infections, the physiologic response can be staged on a continuum from a systemic inflammatory response syndrome (SIRS), to sepsis, severe sepsis, and septic shock (Table 55-3). The hemodynamic profile of septic shock is influenced by several sepsis-induced physiologic changes including hypovolemia and vasodilatation, in addition to cardiac depression. Sepsis is associated with a global decrease in cardiac contractility, and echocardiographic measurements of the left ventricle size demonstrate an inability of the ventricle to dilate in septic patients.[84]

In endotoxemia and sepsis, metabolic needs are increased and the ability of the tissues to extract and utilize oxygen may be impaired. Thus, a metabolic acidosis may be present despite normal levels of oxygen transport. A decrease in cellular O_2 extraction capacity may result from factors other than hypoperfusion, such as direct cellular damage by toxins and/or mediators or maldistribution of blood flow (cytopathic hypoxia). The impact of impaired perfusion on organ function depends on individual susceptibility to hypoxia. The peculiar anatomy and the microcirculatory structure of intestinal villi with their countercurrent flow mechanism render the superficial layers of the mucosa particularly vulnerable to ischemia. The GI tract has been implicated as the "motor" of *multiple organ dysfunction syndrome* (MODS) and "splanchnic resuscitation" has been advocated as a central objective in patients with septic shock. Intramucosal pH and PCO_2 monitoring has been proposed as a technique to assess the splanchnic metabolic state.

Though hypoperfusion is the dominant cause of lactic acidosis in sepsis, various degrees of intermediary metabolic alterations may contribute to the increased lactate production independent of perfusion. Normally, lactate is cleared by the liver metabolic activity via the Cori cycle. Subsequently, with the development of liver perfusion impairment this organ may turn to a net lactate producer. Furthermore, the increase in the rate of glucose metabolism may also occur due to inhibition of the step-limiting enzyme, pyruvate dehydrogenase, for pyruvate to enter the Krebs cycle. An increase in the relative proportion of inactive to active enzyme results in pyruvate accumulation and lactate production.

MODS refers to the presence of altered organ function in an acutely ill patient such that homeostasis cannot be maintained without intervention.[85] The exact pathophysiology of MODS is not yet fully understood, although alterations in systemic hemodynamics, organ perfusion, and tissue microcirculation resulting in tissue hypoxia play a role in initiating and maintaining the syndrome. MODS accounts for most deaths in the ICU.

While organ failure only qualifies a dichotomous event that is either present or absent, organ dysfunction represents a continuum of physiologic derangements. Different severity scores have been proposed to quantify the range of severity of MODS. A commonly used score that correlates with a higher mortality in

TABLE 55-3. DEFINITIONS OF SEPSIS AND ORGAN FAILURE

Clinical Evidence of Infection:
Infection: Microbial phenomenon characterized by an inflammatory response to the presence of microorganisms or the invasion of normally sterile tissue by those organisms.
Bacteremia: The presence of viable bacteria in the blood.

Systemic Inflammatory Response Syndrome (SIRS): Systemic inflammatory response to a variety of severe clinical insults. The response is manifested by two or more of the following conditions:
Core temperature <36°C or >38°C.
Tachycardia >90 beats/min.
Tachypnea >20 breaths/min while breathing spontaneously, or $PaCO_2$ <4.3 kPa.
White blood count >12,000 cells/mm^3, <4,000 cells/mm^3, or >10% immature forms

Sepsis: The systemic response to infection. This systemic response is manifested by three or more of the conditions described above (SIRS) and presented clinical or microbiologic evidence of infection.

Severe Sepsis: Sepsis associated with organ dysfunction, hypoperfusion, or hypotension. Hypoperfusion and perfusion abnormalities may include, but are not limited to, lactic acidosis, oliguria, or an acute alteration in mental status.

Septic Shock: Sepsis with hypotension, despite adequate fluid resuscitation, along with the presence of perfusion abnormalities that may include, but are not limited to, lactic acidosis, oliguria, or an acute alteration in mental status. Patients who are on inotropic or vasopressor agents may not be hypotensive at the time that perfusion abnormalities are measured.

Sepsis-induced Hypotension: A systolic BP of <90 mm Hg or a reduction of >40 mm Hg from baseline in the absence of other causes for hypotension.

Multiple Organ Dysfunction Syndrome: Presence of several altered organ function in an acutely ill patient such that homeostasis cannot be maintained without intervention.

From American College of Chest Physicians/Society of Critical Care Medicine Consensus Conference: Definitions for sepsis and organ failure and guidelines for the use of innovative therapies in sepsis. *Crit Care Med* 1992;20:864, with permission.

the ICU was developed by Marshall et al.[86] This scoring system assigns increasingly high values based on markers of increasing respiratory, renal, cardiovascular, hepatic, hematologic, and central nervous system dysfunction.

Based on the etiology, MODS can be classified as either primary or secondary. *Primary* MODS is the result of a well-defined insult in which a primary organ dysfunction occurs early and can be directly attributable to the insult itself (e.g., ARDS due to pulmonary contusion). *Secondary* MODS represents an abnormal host response (e.g., ARDS in patients with sepsis) and is the result of a systemic inflammatory response initiated by a primary insult involving another organ system.

Clinical Management of Shock/Circulatory Failure Based on Hemodynamic Parameters

The mainstay of treatment of hemodynamic instability is correction of hypotension and restoration of regional blood flow with intravascular volume expansion and vasopressors and/or inotropes. Adequacy of regional perfusion is usually assessed by evaluating indices of organ function, including myocardial ischemia, renal dysfunction (urine output and renal function tests), arterial lactate levels as an indicator of anaerobic metabolism, central nervous system dysfunction as indicated by abnormal sensorium, and hepatic parenchymal injury as determined by liver function tests. However, these functional assessments of satisfactory organ perfusion may not allow rapid adjustments in therapy compared to more direct continuous monitoring of global and/or regional perfusion. Therefore, additional end points of treatment consist of mean arterial pressure and DO_2, or some surrogate of the latter (SvO_2 or $ScvO_2$).

5 Recommendations from the Surviving Sepsis Campaign, an international initiative aiming at improving outcomes in patients with severe sepsis, propose a number of interventions (bundles) to guide management of patients with septic shock (Table 55-4).[87]

Management of Hypotension with Fluid Replacement Therapy

Intravascular volume expansion is the first line of therapy in most forms of shock. Appropriate clinical indicators of the response to a fluid challenge (intravenous bolus of 250 to 1,000 mL crystalloids over 5 to 15 minutes) are heart rate (HR), blood pressure, and urine output as well as invasively acquired measures including CVP, PaOP, systolic and pulse pressure variations, and CO. An increase in CO following volume expansion unmasks an absolute or relative hypovolemic state (preload dependency). Lack of change or a decrease in CO following volume expansion suggests a euvolemic status, volume overload, or cardiac failure.

The choice of crystalloids versus colloids for volume expansion has been debated for decades, without clear resolution. Two meta-analyses examined how the choice of crystalloid or colloid solutions affects survival in critically ill patients. Results from these analyses were conflicting, demonstrating either noninferiority or increased mortality with the use of albumin-containing fluids.[88,89] A multicenter, randomized, double-blind trial compared the effect of fluid resuscitation with 4% albumin or saline on mortality in ICU patients.[90] Outcomes were similar in both groups at 28 days. Another trial in 537 patients with severe sepsis compared volume resuscitation with hetastarch to Ringer's lactate; although there was no difference in mortality between groups, patients randomized to receive hetastarch had a higher risk of renal failure and the need for renal replacement therapy (RRT).[91] Additional evidence

TABLE 55-4. MANAGEMENT OF SEVERE SEPSIS AND SEPTIC SHOCK

- Initiation of early goal–directed resuscitation during the first 6 h after onset of sepsis
- Blood cultures to identity causative organisms before starting antibiotic therapy, and prompt imaging studies performed identify potential source of infection
- Administration of empiric broad-spectrum antibiotics within 1 h of diagnosis, and reassessment of appropriate therapy upon availability of microbiology results
- Control of source of infection
- Administration of either crystalloid or colloids as choice for fluid resuscitation
- Fluid challenge to achieve adequate filling pressures, and reduction of rate of fluids with rising filling pressure and no improvement in tissue perfusion
- Use of norepinephrine or dopamine as first-line vasopressors for a target mean arterial pressure ≥65 mm Hg
- Use of vasopressin at fixed rate as an adjunct to catecholamines
- Use of low dopamine for renal protection not recommended
- Consideration for dobutamine in low cardiac output states despite fluid resuscitation
- Targeting supranormal values of oxygen delivery is not recommended
- Stress-dose steroid therapy for septic shock if blood pressure is poorly responsive to fluid and vasopressors
- Targeting a hemoglobin of 7–9 g/dL in the absence of tissue hypoperfusion, coronary artery disease, or acute hemorrhage
- Appropriate use of fresh frozen plasma and platelets
- Use of low tidal volume, limitation of inspiratory plateau pressure, and application of at least a minimal amount of positive end-expiratory pressure for ALI patients
- Elevation of the head of the bed to a semirecumbent position unless contraindicated
- Avoidance of routine use of pulmonary artery catheter in patients with ALI
- Use a conservative fluid strategy for patients with acute lung injury who are not in shock
- Use of protocols for ventilation weaning and sedation/analgesia, with daily sedation interruption if using continuous infusion sedation
- Avoidance of neuromuscular blockade
- Equivalence of continuous venovenous hemofiltration and intermittent hemodialysis
- Use of bicarbonate to correct arterial pH above 7.15 is not recommended
- Use of deep vein thrombosis and stress ulcer prophylaxis with H_2 blockers or proton pump inhibitors is recommended
- Consideration of limitation of life support when appropriate

ALI, acute lung injury.
Adapted from: Dellinger RP, Levy MM, Carlet JM, et al. Surviving Sepsis Campaign: International guidelines for management of severe sepsis and septic shock: 2008. *Crit Care Med.* 2008;36:296–327.

continues to accumulate linking hetastarch administration to an increased rate of renal failure.[92] Thus, crystalloid appears at least as good as colloid for fluid resuscitation in the majority of critically ill patients and may be safer overall.

Management of Shock with Vasopressors/Inotropes

If patients remain persistently hypotensive despite volume expansion and markers of adequate preload, the use of vasopressors and/or inotropic drugs is indicated. Pharmacologic agents include adrenergic agonists with inotropic and vasoconstrictor effects (NE, dopamine, dobutamine, epinephrine, phenylephrine); other vasoconstrictors are vasopressin and nitric oxide synthase inhibitors. Select agents will be discussed below.

Norepinephrine

NE increases systemic arterial pressure by increasing SVR, with variable effects on CO and HR. These effects are mainly mediated by α- and β-adrenergic receptor agonism. Older studies comparing the hemodynamic and splanchnic effects of NE to dopamine in patients with sepsis suggest that NE may improve the oxygen supply–demand ratio in the splanchnic bed whereas dopamine may have a deleterious effect on this relationship. However, it should be noted that the hemodynamic parameters targeted in this study were outside the range of what is currently recommended.[93]

A more recent review of clinical trials comparing NE to dopamine in over 2,000 patients with shock of all kinds found a 28-day mortality benefit in patients treated with NE. While the majority of patients had septic shock, when the septic shock subgroup was analyzed the mortality benefit was no longer statistically significant. Dopamine was associated with more than twice the risk of developing a cardiac dysrhythmia.[94] A Cochrane meta-analysis found similar results with a nonsignificant trend toward improved mortality in patients treated with NE compared to dopamine and an increased risk of dysrhythmias in the dopamine group.[95]

A concern that NE may compromise renal perfusion has led to some hesitancy to use this drug; however, the majority of available evidence suggests that NE improves renal function in volume-resuscitated, hypotensive patients with septic shock. It is worth noting that the combination of excessively high doses of any vasopressor with inadequate effective plasma volume expansion may reduce organ perfusion and should be avoided.

Dopamine

Dopamine raises mean arterial pressure primarily by increasing cardiac index and less so by increasing SVR. These effects are mediated by dopaminergic receptor agonism as well as by α- and β-adrenergic receptor agonism. Dopamine does not have consistent selective dopaminergic effects on renal blood flow, but rather improves urine output by either improving overall hemodynamics, a direct diuretic effect, or decreasing the release of antidiuretic hormone via baroreceptor responses.[96] While some have advocated for the use of "renal dose" dopamine, a large randomized trial and a meta-analysis comparing low-dose dopamine to placebo in critically ill patients found no differences in either renal function tests or survival, and the use of low-dose dopamine is therefore not recommended.[97] In addition to the above concerns regarding mortality, splanchnic perfusion, and dysrhythmias with dopamine, there is evidence that dopamine may also have pro-inflammatory actions and may suppress the innate immune response.[98]

Dobutamine

Dobutamine is a β-1 and β-2 receptor agonist that demonstrates potent inotropic and chronotropic effects and mild peripheral vasodilatation, with the ultimate effect of increasing oxygen delivery and consumption. Dobutamine is the drug of choice in patients with circulatory failure primarily due to cardiac pump failure (cardiogenic shock). However, dobutamine should not be used as first-line single therapy when hypotension is present and is frequently combined with other agents such as NE. In patients with septic shock dobutamine may be useful in the presence of impaired cardiac contractility with resulting inadequate CO and oxygen delivery. Several studies show that dobutamine alone or added to standard vasopressor regimens increases both oxygen delivery and consumption in septic and elderly septic patients.[99] In patients with septic shock, the combination of NE plus dobutamine resulted in increased gastric mucosal perfusion compared to NE alone.[100] Other studies comparing the effects of NE plus dobutamine versus epinephrine or dopamine alone suggested an improved balance between oxygen delivery and consumption with the combination therapy.

Despite these physiologic benefits of dobutamine in septic shock, detrimental effects have been observed when therapy is oriented to supranormal CO, DO_2, and VO_2 in critically ill patients, as discussed previously.[72] Based on this and other studies, the use of aggressive strategies such as high-dose dobutamine to drive cardiac index above a predefined "supraphysiologic" level is not recommended as routine therapy in the critically ill. In contrast, a clinical trial of early goal–directed therapy during the first 6 hours of septic shock to maintain central venous oxyhemoglobin saturation ($ScvO_2$) of 70% or greater with volume resuscitation, packed red blood cell (RBC) transfusion to a hematocrit of 30% and, if not sufficient, with dobutamine up to 20 μg/kg/min demonstrated a 16% absolute reduction in 28-day mortality compared to standard therapy.[74] It is not clear whether the observed benefits of early goal–directed therapy were due to the early initiation of treatment, achievement of the goal end points, or specific elements of treatment (e.g., blood transfusion or dobutamine). However, this early approach of increasing oxygen delivery in septic shock patients by targeting an indicator of supply/demand relationship is substantially different from the supraphysiologic resuscitation in general ICU populations previously described.

In summary, dobutamine treatment is the first line of treatment in patients with shock and decreased cardiac contractility and performance. In patients with septic shock, dobutamine may be useful as second-line agent, after adequate fluid resuscitation and if introduction of vasopressors has not restored sufficient levels of oxygen delivery, reflected by an $ScvO_2$ of >70% (which approximates a mixed venous oxygen saturation, SvO_2, of >65%) and increased lactate clearance. However, further corroborating data are necessary to determine the true benefits of early optimization of oxygen delivery. Targeting supranormal levels of oxygen delivery and consumption is not recommended.

Epinephrine

Epinephrine is a β-1, β-2, α-adrenergic receptor agonist that exhibits a dose-related response. It increases arterial blood pressure by increasing cardiac index through both inotropic and chronotropic effects. It also increases SVR, DO_2, and VO_2. The increased VO_2 is via activation of metabolic pathways.

In patients with septic shock, epinephrine may reduce splanchnic perfusion despite an increase in global hemodynamic and oxygen transport. Compared with a combination of dobutamine and NE, epinephrine resulted in similar hemodynamic profiles in patients with cardiogenic shock, but was associated with a transient elevation in serum lactate levels compared to the NE and dobutamine group.[101] It was also associated with an increase in HR and greater incidence of dysrhythmias. There were similar findings of equivalency when dobutamine combined with NE was compared to epinephrine in patients with septic shock.[102]

Lactate elevation with epinephrine therapy is observed consistently, but whether this reflects a reduction in vital organ perfusion with resulting anaerobic metabolism, increased production consequent to a thermogenic effect in skeletal muscle, or reduced clearance remains to be defined. However, epinephrine treatment at best brings no additional benefit to other catecholamine therapy in the management of patients with septic shock and may increase dysrhythmias and lactate production.

Vasopressin

Vasopressin is a potent vasoconstrictor when administered in low doses to patients in shock, particularly those with distributive shock due to sepsis or hepatic failure, or with circulatory failure following cardiopulmonary bypass.[103] This may in part be related to a relative deficiency of vasopressin in these settings. Vasopressin may also be useful in resuscitation from cardiac arrest, particularly if due to asystole, and is offered as an option in the current ACLS algorithm for treatment of ventricular fibrillation.[104]

Vasopressin administration during shock typically results in dramatically increased systemic blood pressure, with either no effect or a mild decrease in CO, little change in HR, and no effect on pulmonary vascular resistance. Although vasopressin has the potential to reduce mesenteric and renal blood flow, it does not appear to do so when administered at low dose during vasodilatory shock.[105,106] In addition, vasopressin and its analogs have been shown to improve urine output in the hepatorenal syndrome, supporting a positive effect of vasopressin on renal blood flow in vasodilatory states. Clinical trials of vasopressin or vasopressin analogues (terlipressin) have consistently demonstrated a catecholamine sparing effect of vasopressin in patients with severe burns or septic shock, but a mortality benefit has not been demonstrated.[107–109] The largest of these trials conducted by the Vasopressin and Septic Shock Trials Group (VASST) compared vasopressin to NE in over 700 patients.[109] There was no overall difference in 28- or 90-day mortality, but patients with less severe septic shock (defined as baseline NE requirement of <15 μg/min) did better with vasopressin. Based on these data, the Surviving Sepsis Campaign suggests that vasopressin at the dose of 0.03 U/min may be added to NE with the expectation that the effect on blood pressure be similar to that produced by NE. The experts also propose that epinephrine should be the first choice alternative agent in septic shock that is poorly responsive to NE or dopamine.

Additional Treatment Considerations for Critically Ill Patients with Septic Shock

Activated Protein C

Clinical or subclinical manifestations of intravascular disseminated coagulation and consumption coagulopathy are present in essentially all patients with septic shock. The activation of protein C is thought to be an important mechanism for modulating sepsis-induced consumption coagulopathy. The rationale for replacing activated protein C relates to its anticoagulant and profibrinolytic properties, which interrupt the consumption coagulopathy and are particularly effective at preventing microvascular thrombosis. Drotrecogin-alfa, a human recombinant activated protein C, was approved by the Food and Drug Administration (FDA) for treatment of patients with severe sepsis as defined by an APACHE II score >25 based on results from a single RCT. However, subsequent clinical trials and a meta-analysis failed to show any mortality benefit. Based on these findings Drotrecogin-alfa was removed from the market in October 2011.[110]

Corticosteroids

Although high-dose corticosteroids for the treatment of septic shock are of no benefit, lower doses, on the order of hydrocortisone 200 to 300 mg/day, can reduce dependency on vasopressors and expedite the resolution of shock, but they do not confer a mortality benefit.[111,112] Adrenal function testing prior to initiation of steroid therapy is not considered necessary to identify patients with relative adrenal insufficiency, as the effects of corticosteroids are similar irrespective of the test results. This issue is discussed in depth in the endocrinology section of this chapter.

Treatment of Infection

Identifying the source of the infection, source control, and early initiation of appropriate antibiotic therapy are critical priorities in addition to hemodynamic support. Appropriate cultures should always be obtained before antimicrobial therapy is initiated. At least two blood cultures (one drawn percutaneously and one drawn from a vascular access device) as well as urine, respiratory, cerebralspinal fluid, wound, and other fluid collection cultures should be obtained. Diagnostic studies should be performed promptly to assist the identification of the source of infection and the causative organism, especially for foci amenable to source control measures (e.g., abscess drainage). Empiric antibiotic therapy should be started as soon as possible, within 1 hour of recognition of sepsis, after appropriate culture collection. A retrospective review by Kumar et al.[113] calculated that mortality may increase as much as 7.6% for each hour if antibiotic treatment is delayed after identification of sepsis. Initial empiric therapy should be broad enough and include one or more drugs that have activity against the likely pathogens and which penetrate into the presumed site of infection. After antibiotic susceptibility testing is available, restriction of the number of antibiotics and narrowing the spectrum of antimicrobial treatment is appropriate. For a more detailed discussion and specific sites of infection, please refer to the section on nosocomial infection.

ACUTE RESPIRATORY FAILURE

Acute respiratory failure is characterized by a derangement in pulmonary gas exchange or an imbalance between the work of breathing and respiratory muscle capacity and is usually accompanied by hypoxemia and/or hypercapnia. Indeed, in some cases respiratory failure may be caused by "nonrespiratory" issues, for example, coma that results in the inability to protect the airway. Acute respiratory failure is a relatively common phenomenon; depending on the type of ICU, the majority of patients may be mechanically ventilated at any given time, and virtually all critically ill patients are mechanically ventilated for some portion of their ICU stay. Suffice it to say that the treatment of acute respiratory failure is primarily supportive and typically necessitates supplemental oxygen and often mechanical ventilation with or without airway intubation. Acute respiratory failure typically resolves when the initiating condition is adequately treated. The following sections will discuss the basic principles of mechanical ventilation, some of the more challenging types of respiratory failure, and potential therapeutic approaches to respiratory failure.

Principles of Mechanical Ventilation

Mechanical ventilation in the ICU is provided through the application of positive pressure to the airway; at its simplest, a preset tidal volume (volume control) or inspiratory pressure (pressure control) and rate provide a minimal minute ventilation. Any breathing that the patient does above this set minute ventilation is either supported (continuous mandatory ventilation [CMV]) or not (intermittent mandatory ventilation [IMV]). However, ICU ventilators have become increasingly powerful and complex, capable of delivering high inspiratory flows and utilizing microprocessors that simultaneously monitor and respond to multiple characteristics of the respiratory circuit. Thus, ventilatory modes used today include pressure support ventilation, pressure control ventilation, volume control ventilation, pressure-regulated volume control, high-frequency ventilation, proportional assist ventilation, airway pressure release ventilation, synchronous IMV, and others. In reality, despite strong regional, local, and individual biases, there is little evidence to suggest that the mode of mechanical ventilation contributes significantly to any major outcome measure, and the choice of mode is at this point largely one of clinician preference. Thus, this discussion will not dwell on specific modes of ventilation.

Mechanical PPV has been traditionally considered supportive therapy that is applied until the initiating cause of respiratory failure improves sufficiently such that the patient can breathe without assistance. However, evidence suggests that mechanical ventilation may be injurious in certain settings. Traditionally, tidal volumes of 10 to 15 mL/kg were routinely used to ventilate patients in the ICU. The use of such "supraphysiologic" tidal volumes (normal resting tidal volumes are 5 to 7 mL/kg) evolved from the observation that the use of smaller-sized volumes was associated with the development of atelectasis and hypoxemia in anesthetized patients in the operating room. However, large tidal volumes can result in cardiovascular compromise, barotrauma, ventilator-induced (or ventilator-associated) lung injury (VILI or VALI) and excess mortality, as discussed below.

PPV results in increased intrathoracic pressure, which reduces venous return, and in turn results in reduced CO and blood pressure. In addition, PPV can result in alveolar over-distention and alveolar rupture, which manifests as pneumothorax, pneumomediastinum, and subcutaneous emphysema (barotrauma). Both of these effects are amplified in patients with obstructive lung disease (asthma and chronic obstructive pulmonary disease; COPD). In these patients, limitation of expiratory flow leads to air trapping and the development of intrinsic positive end-expiratory pressure (PEEP) or auto-PEEP. Air trapping results in alveolar overdistention and increases the risk of barotrauma, and auto-PEEP can contribute substantially to increased intrathoracic pressure and cardiovascular depression. Auto-PEEP cannot be detected without holding exhalation for a prolonged interval (expiratory pause) with both inspiratory and expiratory ventilator valves closed; thus, auto-PEEP may not be appreciated unless specifically investigated.

The development of air trapping and auto-PEEP leads to significant morbidity and mortality in patients with obstructive lung disease. Thus, the ventilatory strategy in these patients should focus on prolongation of expiratory time by limiting minute ventilation through use of low tidal volumes (6 to 8 mL/kg or less) and a low rate (8 to 12 breaths per minute) and by reducing the inspiratory time of the respiratory cycle. Low minute ventilation is often associated with hypercapnia and respiratory acidosis ("permissive hypercapnia"); however, this does not appear to be harmful, and the benefits of reduced air trapping and auto-PEEP far outweigh any possible detriment. In order to decrease inspiratory time, the inspiratory flow rate must increase, and this results in increased peak airway pressure. However, most of the peak pressure is dissipated in the endotracheal tube and large airways, and more importantly, end-expiratory, static or plateau, and mean airway pressures will fall with increased expiratory time. In order to accomplish the above goals, deep sedation is often required. Rarely is neuromuscular blockade required. The adoption of this type of ventilatory strategy in the 1980s and 1990s was associated with a dramatic reduction in mortality due to acute, severe asthma and respiratory failure, from as high as 23% to less than 5%.[114]

In contrast to barotrauma, VILI or VALI refers to microscopic injury to the lung due to over-distention (volutrauma) and cyclic reopening of alveoli (atelectrauma). VALI has been well demonstrated in numerous experimental models and is histologically similar to the features seen in ALI of other causes, with diffuse alveolar damage (DAD) and increased microvascular permeability.[115] In addition, VALI is associated with the systemic release of inflammatory mediators that may contribute to multiple organ failure. Clinically, patients felt to be at risk for VALI are those with abnormally low recruitable lung volumes, in particular those with ALI and ARDS. Thus, a "lung-protective" ventilatory strategy utilizing low tidal volume ventilation has been proven to save lives when applied to patients with ALI/ARDS (see later). In addition, accumulating evidence suggests that the use of low tidal volume ventilation may reduce of risk of developing ALI/ARDS in critically ill patients.[116,117]

In summary, although tidal volumes of 10 to 12 mL/kg may still be indicated for some patients, in most cases an initial tidal volume of 8 mL/kg is probably appropriate, and volumes as low as 4 mL/kg may be appropriate in some cases. In addition, since lung volumes correlate with height rather than weight, tidal volume selection should be based on predicted or ideal body weight, rather than actual weight to avoid lung over-distention. Predicted body weight (PBW) can be calculated from the formula: PBW = 50 + 2.3 (height [inches] − 60) (males) or 45.5 + 2.3 (height [inches] − 60) (females).

Although mechanical ventilation generally implies airway intubation, either translaryngeal or via tracheotomy, noninvasive positive pressure ventilation (NPPV) or continuous positive airway pressure (CPAP) can be delivered via a tight sealing nasal or full-face mask. NPPV is applied using either standard ICU ventilators (typically set to pressure support or pressure control modes, with or without PEEP) or specially designed ventilators that deliver CPAP or bi-level positive airway pressure (Bi-PAP). These dedicated noninvasive ventilators generate high gas flow, can cycle between a high inspiratory pressure and a lower expiratory pressure, and can sense and respond to patient inspiratory effort. Originally developed for home ventilation in patients with obstructive sleep apnea and chronic respiratory failure, newer models are targeted for use in the ICU and incorporate monitoring packages that allow assessment of delivered tidal volumes and respiratory patterns. However, there is no evidence that the type of ventilator used for NPPV affects patient outcome, and the choice of equipment is typically based on availability and familiarity.

NPPV compared to standard therapy has been associated with improved outcomes in a variety of causes of respiratory failure, including cardiogenic pulmonary edema, chronic obstructive pulmonary disease (COPD), and ALI in immunosuppressed patients.[118,119] Improved outcomes include the avoidance of endotracheal intubation, a reduction in complications associated with intubation including ventilator-associated pneumonia (VAP), and reduced mortality. However, NPPV is not without risk and has been associated with increased complications in some studies, including a higher rate of MI in patients with cardiogenic pulmonary edema, and increased mortality in patients with respiratory failure after extubation.[120,121] Therefore, NPPV is best and most safely utilized when patient characteristics are ideal, including an awake, cooperative patient (with the exception of rapidly reversible obtundation due to high PCO_2), a low risk for regurgitation and aspiration of gastric contents, and a high likelihood that the process resulting in respiratory failure is rapidly reversible. Further research including larger, randomized trials of NPPV is necessary to better define the particular subgroups of patients who will benefit from this approach.

"Weaning" from mechanical ventilation is better termed "liberation" or "separation" from ventilation, as weaning implies that ventilation must be gradually withdrawn in order to allow respiratory muscle and patient adaptation to the process. In reality, separation from mechanical ventilation is more a function of the resolution of the cause of respiratory failure, rather than the technique used to withdraw ventilatory support. This is supported by a study showing that daily trials of unassisted ventilation ("T-piece trials") resulted in more rapid separation from ventilation than other more gradual approaches, in particular IMV "weaning."[122] In addition, the so-called "weaning parameters" are inadequate
6 predictors of the success or failure of withdrawal of ventilatory support and add little to routine management. Thus, the process of separation from mechanical ventilation is expedited when respiratory therapy–driven protocols are used that focus on daily assessment of the ability to breathe without assistance, assuming improvement of the inciting process, adequate oxygenation, and hemodynamic stability.[123] Once the patient can breathe comfortably for 30 to 120 minutes without support, the trachea can be extubated, assuming that there are no other precluding factors such as airway abnormalities and coma.

Acute Lung Injury and Acute Respiratory Distress Syndrome

ALI and ARDS are syndromes of acute, hypoxemic respiratory failure marked pathologically by DAD, with resulting increased lung permeability and diffuse alveolar edema.[124] ARDS can occur as a result of direct injury to the lung (e.g., aspiration or pneumonia) or in association with extrapulmonary infection (sepsis) or injury (e.g., multiple trauma). ARDS/DAD is associated with an inflammatory cell infiltration of the lung, increased systemic markers of inflammation, and progression through exudative, fibroproliferative, and fibrotic phases of injury over days to weeks.

TABLE 55-5. THE BERLIN DEFINITION OF THE ACUTE RESPIRATORY DISTRESS SYNDROME

Timing	Within 1 week of a known clinical insult or new or worsening respiratory symptoms
Chest imaging[a]	Bilateral opacities—not fully explained by effusions, lobar/lung collapse, or nodules
Origin of edema	Not fully explained by cardiac failure or fluid overload. Need objective assessment (e.g., echocardiography) if no risk factor present
Oxygenation	
Mild	200 mm Hg $<PaO_2/FIO_2 \leq 300$ mm Hg; PEEP or CPAP ≥ 5 cm H_2O
Moderate	100 mm Hg $<PaO_2/FIO_2 \leq 200$ mm Hg; PEEP ≥ 5 cm H_2O
Severe	$PaO_2/FIO_2 \leq 100$ mm Hg with PEEP ≥ 5 cm H_2O

[a]Chest radiography or computed tomography scan.
Adapted from Ranieri VM, Rubenfeld GD, Thompson BT, et al. Acute respiratory distress syndrome: the Berlin Definition. *JAMA*. 2012;307:2526–2533.

In order to better standardize the definition of ARDS for epidemiologic and research purposes, in 1994 a joint American–European Conference proposed criteria for characterizing ARDS according to the severity of gas exchange abnormality.[125] Despite some controversy, these criteria were generally accepted and used to guide research study design and enrollment for nearly two decades.[125] However, in 2012 a new consensus conference proposed the "Berlin Definition," which eliminates the distinction between "acute lung injury" and ARDS, and rather categorizes ARDS by severity based on the degree of hypoxemia (mild, moderate, severe; Table 55.5).[126] The three categories are associated with increasing mortality. In contrast to the previous American-European Conference definition, the Berlin Definition of ARDS was empirically evaluated using patient-level meta-analysis, and is thus better validated as a research and descriptive tool.

ALI/ARDS is highly prevalent in the ICU population and accounts for 10% to 15% of all ICU admissions.[126] Of predisposing factors, sepsis carries the highest risk (approximately 30%) and is the most common cause of ALI/ARDS. Mortality associated with ARDS appears to have fallen over the past 20 years, although this observation is mainly confined to RCTs versus observational studies.[126,127] Moreover, ARDS mortality varies greatly with the population of patients studied; for example, ARDS mortality in trauma patients is in the 10% to 15% range, whereas mortality in medical ICU patients is as high as 60%. Patients with ARDS continue to die primarily as a result of associated conditions (sepsis, multiple organ failure, etc.) and uncommonly die of hypoxemia per se.

Clinically, ARDS and ALI are characterized by reduced static thoracic (lung and chest wall) compliance and severe impairment of gas exchange, including high intrapulmonary shunt and dead space fraction. These mechanics and gas exchange abnormalities create a challenge in terms of optimizing mechanical ventilation, as maintenance of adequate oxygenation and CO_2 elimination are both problematic. In addition, although the *P*/*F* ratio does not appear to predict mortality, high dead space fraction does and may reflect the extent of pulmonary vascular injury.[128] Pulmonary hypertension often develops as the syndrome progresses and can complicate hemodynamic management.

Although ALI/ARDS appears to be a diffuse process by chest X-ray, lung opacification is surprisingly heterogeneous when the lung is imaged by CT. Areas of dense opacification are frequently confined to the posterior, dependent portion of the lung, leaving a small, relatively normal, recruitable volume available for ventilation. This low recruitable lung volume has been termed the "baby lung" and has important implications for ventilatory management in ARDS, as discussed below.[115]

The treatment of ALI/ARDS is largely supportive and includes aggressive treatment of inciting events, avoidance of complications, and mechanical ventilation. In regard to the latter, it is critical that tidal volumes and static ventilatory pressures are mini-
7 mized in order to avoid further injury to the remaining relatively uninjured lung. A large, randomized, prospective trial found that a strategy that used tidal volumes of 6 mL/kg or less and maintained static (plateau) airway pressure at ≤ 30 cm H_2O resulted in a relative mortality reduction of 22% when compared to a control group ventilated with tidal volumes of 12 mL/kg.[129] This approach was corroborated in a similar, smaller trial.[130] This is the only intervention that has been unequivocally proven to reduce mortality in patients with ARDS.

Since ARDS is marked by high intrapulmonary shunt, hypoxemia is relatively unresponsive to oxygen therapy. Thus, strategies to recruit collapsed lung are necessary. This is most commonly achieved by using PEEP. The optimal balance between PEEP and FIO_2 has long been debated, but at this point there is no strong evidence to favor either a "high PEEP, low FIO_2" or a "minimal PEEP, high FIO_2" strategy.[131] Other maneuvers to promote recruitment of lung include the use of esophageal manometry to titrate PEEP and tidal volume, recruitment maneuvers or sigh breaths, pressure-controlled ventilation, inverse ratio ventilation (prolonged inspiratory time), prone positioning, and high-frequency ventilation. Of these techniques, prone positioning has been the most rigorously studied, and a meta-analysis of seven RCTs of patients with ARDS and ALI found a mortality benefit to prone positioning in patients with a *P*/*F* ratio <100. Because prone positioning is associated with an increased risk of endotracheal tube dislodgement and pressure ulcers it is a therapy that should be reserved for "rescue" situations when conventional strategies have failed.[132]

Inhaled nitric oxide (iNO) also variably and transiently improves oxygenation in ALI/ARDS by improving blood flow to ventilated alveoli. However, several randomized, prospective trials have failed to show any relevant long-term outcome benefits associated with iNO administration to patients with ALI/ARDS.[133,134] iNO may still be useful as "rescue" therapy in selected patients with severe, refractory hypoxemia, although its benefits in this setting have not been rigorously tested.

Given that ALI/ARDS is marked by high-permeability pulmonary edema, it is intuitive that administration of excessive fluids be avoided. Results from an RCT found that a conservative fluid management strategy that emphasized diuresis resulted in improved oxygenation and more ventilator-free days and days not in the ICU, but no significant difference in mortality compared to liberal fluid management.[135] Another intervention to facilitate reduction of lung water in ALI and ARDS is coadministration of albumin with furosemide.[136] Although a small study suggested that administration of inhaled β-agonists might enhance lung water clearance in patients with ALI and ARDS, a subsequent large RCT failed to show benefit to this therapy.[137]

Multiple therapies have been tested in an effort to halt the inflammatory and proliferative phases of injury, with mixed success. Corticosteroid administration to patients with ALI and ARDS has been associated with reduced mortality in two small randomized trial and smaller case series and cohort studies.[138,139] A large RCT sponsored by the ARDS Network randomized patients between days 7 and 28 of ARDS onset to methylprednisolone versus placebo.[140] Although there was no difference in 28-day mortality in the intention-to-treat analysis, patients receiving steroids between 7 and 14 days after ARDS onset appeared to benefit, while those starting treatment more than 14 days after ARDS onset appeared to suffer harm. Furthermore, the group receiving methylprednisolone had more ventilator-free days and shock-free days at day 28, in addition to improved oxygenation and respiratory system compliance. Thus, it appears that patients with ARDS may benefit from corticosteroid treatment within a narrow window of time, but further study is necessary before strong conclusions can be drawn.

Additional areas of controversy in the management of patients with ALI and ARDS include the use of neuromuscular blockade and extracorporeal membrane oxygenation (ECMO). Although the use of neuromuscular blockade to facilitate mechanical ventilation of patients with ALI and ARDS has generally been on the decline due to fears of increased risk of critical illness myopathy, a French, multicenter trial that randomized patients with severe ARDS (*P*/*F* ratio <150) to early treatment with cisatracurium versus placebo raises some doubt about these fears.[141] The cisatracurium-treated group had a reduction in the hazard ratio for death, after adjustment, compared to the placebo group, and there was no increase in ICU-acquired paresis. Reservations about this approach remain, however, and further research is necessary before routine neuromuscular blockade for severe ARDS can be recommended.

The use of ECMO to support patients with severe ARDS had a resurgence during the influenza pandemic of 2009, with some observational data suggesting a survival benefit to ECMO.[142] In addition, a UK-based multicenter trial randomized patients with severe ARDS to consideration for ECMO at a specialized referral center versus conventional treatment at their originating hospital. Patients randomized to ECMO consideration had an increased likelihood of disability-free survival at 6 months.[143] Skepticism remains regarding the widespread use of ECMO for management of severe ARDS given the invasive nature of this approach, cost considerations, and need for transfer to specialized centers.

ACUTE RENAL FAILURE

Acute renal failure (ARF) is reported to occur in up to 66% of critically ill patients. Unfortunately, the true incidence is difficult to pinpoint due to variability in patient populations and the use of multiple diagnostic criteria. In 2004, a consensus group proposed standard criteria for classifying the severity of renal injury and the associated outcomes. The criteria, known as the RIFLE criteria, have been subsequently validated in several studies.[144,145] These criteria are expected to improve the ability to identify, study, and treat renal failure in the ICU.[145] (Table 55-6).

Despite these caveats regarding the diagnosis of ARF, the incidence appears to be fairly stable over the past 20 years.[146] Moreover, the hospital mortality associated with ARF requiring dialysis has remained approximately 60% for nearly five decades.[146,147] This is discouraging when one considers reductions in mortality in association with other organ failures over the same time interval. The reasons for the lack of improvement in outcome are unclear, but likely include insensitive means for identifying patients with incipient renal failure and lack of effective preventive and therapeutic measures.

In the ICU, ARF occurs due to prerenal causes and tubular injury (acute tubular necrosis [ATN]) in the vast majority of cases.[146] Other potential causes of ARF in the ICU include glomerulonephritis, vasculitis, interstitial nephritis, macro and microvascular disease (e.g., thrombotic thrombocytopenic purpura), toxins (nonsteroidal anti-inflammatory drugs, cisplatin, aminoglycosides, radiologic contrast, myoglobin, and hemoglobin), and urinary tract obstruction. The initial evaluation of ARF should focus on identifying easily correctable causes; thus, urine sodium concentration and fractional excretion of sodium can help identify prerenal azotemia, urinalysis can identify possible glomerulonephritis or interstitial nephritis, and ultrasonography can rule out postrenal or obstructive sources of ARF. In azotemic patients who have received diuretics, the fractional excretion of urea may be more sensitive than the fractional excretion of sodium in detecting a prerenal cause.[148]

In incipient and established ARF, supportive care is the rule, with the focus on maintenance of euvolemia, avoidance of renal toxins, adjustment of medication doses, and monitoring of electrolytes and acid–base status. Pharmacologic approaches to the prevention and treatment of ARF have been uniformly disappointing; these include low-dose dopamine,[97] aniritide (recombinant atrial natriuretic peptide), and diuretics.[149] The evidence supporting diuretic use has been conflicting, but a meta-analysis showed no effect on outcomes.[149] Nonetheless, diuretics should be administered with caution in early ARF and in response to defined physiologic problems such as hypervolemia or hyperkalemia until higher level evidence showing

TABLE 55-6. RIFLE CLASSIFICATION OF ACUTE KIDNEY INJURY

	Serum Creatinine	Urine Output	In-hospital Mortality Odds Ratio
Risk[a]	↑ Serum Cr ≥1.5× baseline	<0.5 mL/kg/h for 6 h	2.5
Injury	↑ Serum Cr ≥2× baseline	<0.5 mL/kg/h for 12 h	5.4
Failure[b]	↑ Serum Cr ≥3× baseline or ↑ ≥0.5 mg/dL if baseline ≥4 mg/dL	<0.3 mL/kg/h for 24 h or anuria × 24 h	10.1
Loss	Complete loss of renal function for >4 weeks		
End stage	End-stage renal disease		

[a]Some authors consider any increase in serum creatinine ≥0.3 mg/dL to qualify as meeting the risk criteria.
[b]Some authors consider any patient requiring renal replacement therapy, even if the serum creatinine is normal, to meet the failure criteria.
Adapted from: Bellomo R, Ronco C, Kellum J, et al. Acute renal failure-definition, outcome measures, animal models, fluid therapy, and information technology needs: The Second International Consensus Conference of the Acute Dialysis Quality Initiative (ADQI) Group. *Crit Care.* 2004;8:R204–R212; Uchino S, Kellum JA, Bellomo R, et al. Acute renal failure in critically ill patients: A multinational, multicenter study. *JAMA.* 2005;294:813–818.

benefit and safety is available. In the specific setting of contrast-induced nephropathy, intravascular volume expansion with saline or sodium bicarbonate prior to contrast administration appears to be of benefit in preventing nephropathy and improving other outcomes.[150,151] However, prophylactic administration of *N*-acetyl cysteine does not appear to reduce the risk of contrast-induced nephropathy.[152]

Although hemodialysis (RRT) is typically considered a supportive measure in ARF, recent interest has focused on the potential for RRT to improve renal recovery and reduce mortality. Research on RRT in the ICU has focused on the type and intensity or dose of dialysis; the timing of initiation of RRT is also of interest, but has not been rigorously studied in this setting.

The intensity of RRT is determined by both the frequency of treatment and the degree of solute clearance per time. Although increased intensity of dialysis improves outcome in patients with chronic end-stage renal disease, these benefits have not been reproduced in patients with ARF in two large, randomized clinical trials.[153,154] It appears that RRT three times per week is as effective as daily RRT so long as the prescribed RRT dose is delivered.

Continuous renal replacement therapy (CRRT) (including continuous venovenous hemofiltration and hemodialysis) has long been known as a useful technique when hemodynamic instability is present; in contrast to intermittent hemodialysis, effective solute removal is possible with CRRT in the presence of arterial hypotension. Despite this theoretical advantage to CRRT, several studies, including a relatively large, multicenter RCT, found no survival benefit to CRRT compared to intermittent hemodialysis.[155] The two techniques are considered equivalent.

ENDOCRINE ASPECTS OF CRITICAL CARE MEDICINE

Glucose Management in Critical Illness

Hyperglycemia is commonly encountered in critically ill patients and occurs in both diabetics and nondiabetics. Hyperglycemia results primarily because of increased glucose production and insulin resistance caused by inflammatory and hormonal mediators that are released in response to injury. Hyperglycemia may also be aggravated by various therapeutic and supportive interventions, including the use of corticosteroids and total parenteral nutrition (PN). Although the risks of hyperglycemia for patients with diabetes who are ketosis-prone have long been appreciated, mounting evidence suggests that hyperglycemia is detrimental to critically ill patients in a broader sense. Hyperglycemia is associated with increased risk of postoperative infection (wound and otherwise) and poor outcome in patients with stroke or TBI.[156] In addition, the blood glucose level is a risk factor for mortality in diabetic patients admitted with acute MI.[157]

Given the above considerations, strict glycemic control in critically ill patients has been advocated as leading to multiple outcome benefits. A single RCT of surgical patients published in 2001 found that intensive insulin therapy (goal glucose <110 mg/dL) reduced ICU mortality by approximately 50% compared to more conventional therapy (goal glucose <215).[158] Based largely on the results of this one trial there was widespread adoption of protocols to target blood glucose between 80 and 110 mg/dL. Unfortunately, the benefits of the initial trial were not reproduced in multiple subsequent trials, and in fact an increased risk of hypoglycemia and associated harm have been observed.[159] After an additional large, multicenter, multinational RCT of intensive insulin therapy (NICE-SUGAR study) showed increased mortality in the tight glucose control group, the practice of maintaining blood glucose between 80 and 110 mg/dL was widely abandoned.[160] Current serum glucose targets are somewhat variable, but most agree that 140 to 180 mg/dL is acceptable in most patients.

Adrenal Function in Critical Illness

The stress response to injury includes an increase in serum cortisol levels in most critically ill patients.[161] However, adrenal insufficiency may also occur in critically ill patients for several reasons, including inhibition of adrenal stimulation or corticosteroid synthesis by drugs or cytokines and direct injury to or infection of the pituitary or adrenal glands.[162] Thus, adrenal insufficiency has been reported to occur with increased frequency in critically ill patients with trauma, burns, sepsis, and other conditions in comparison with the general population.

The diagnosis of adrenal insufficiency in critical illness is complicated by limitations of commonly used tests of adrenal function. Cortisol is highly protein bound, and serum proteins, including albumin, are commonly depressed in critically ill patients. Although total serum cortisol levels are low in critically ill patients with hypoproteinemia, free cortisol levels are elevated.[163] This suggests that earlier reports that utilized total serum cortisol levels in critically ill patients may have overestimated the incidence of adrenal insufficiency. However, until free cortisol assays are more widely available, the diagnosis of adrenal insufficiency in critical illness must be based on clinical suspicion and total cortisol levels.

In addition to absolute adrenal insufficiency (low baseline cortisol and poor response to ACTH administration/stimulation) a condition of relative adrenal insufficiency (defined as an increase in serum cortisol of ≤ 9 μg/dL in response to ACTH administration, independent of the baseline cortisol level) has been described in patients in septic shock and with other illnesses. Low-normal baseline cortisol levels, high baseline cortisol levels, and a poor response to ACTH are all predictors of increased mortality in critical illness.[164,165]

Although high-dose corticosteroids for the treatment of septic shock are of no benefit, evidence suggests that lower doses, on the order of hydrocortisone 200 to 300 mg/day, can reduce dependency on vasopressors and shorten the duration of shock. Evidence for a mortality benefit is less clear with some trials showing improved mortality and others showing lack of efficacy.[111,112] A meta-analysis of randomized and quasi-randomized trials through 2008 and dating back to the 1950s suggests that low-dose hydrocortisone (200 to 300 mg/day or equivalent) given for a period of at least 4 days should be considered only in patients with vasopressor-dependent septic shock as this was the only subgroup showing any mortality benefit.[166] There does not appear to be an increased risk of gastric ulceration, superinfection, or neuromuscular weakness according to this analysis, but hypernatremia and hyperglycemia are more common in patients receiving steroids.

Thyroid Function in Critical Illness

Measures of thyroid function, including levels of thyrotropin (TSH), T_3, and T_4, are deranged in the majority of critically ill patients. Depression of T_3 occurs within hours of injury or illness and can persist for weeks. TSH levels may be normal initially, but fall to inappropriately low levels as illness progresses. T_4 levels are also often low, but can be normal or high. Low hormone levels may occur for a variety of reasons, including altered binding and metabolism early in the course of illness, and depressed neuroendocrine function with more prolonged courses. In addition, certain drugs, in particular the vasopressor dopamine, can depress thyroid function through central mechanisms.[167] Low thyroid hormone levels, particularly for T_3, correlate with the severity of illness and are associated with an increased risk of death.[161]

It is controversial as to whether the observed abnormalities in thyroid hormones represent an appropriate response to illness or true hypothyroidism; thus, the terms "euthyroid sick syndrome" and "nonthyroidal illness" have been coined to describe thyroid function abnormalities in critical illness.[168] Furthermore, it is not clear whether replacement of thyroid hormones is indicated or beneficial in critical illness. T_3 administration to brain-dead organ donors appears to improve hemodynamic stability, although randomized trials found minimal or no benefit to T_3 or T_4 administration in patients undergoing cardiopulmonary bypass and cardiac surgery.[169] In addition, several small studies have found no benefit to T_3 or T_4 administration to patients with a variety of critical illnesses. Larger, randomized prospective trials are necessary to define the role of routine thyroid hormone supplementation in nonthyroidal illness.

Importantly, true hypothyroidism may be present in the critically ill, particularly in the geriatric population, and should be considered in the face of refractory shock, adrenal insufficiency, unexplained coma, and prolonged, unexplained respiratory failure. True hypothyroidism is marked by an elevation of TSH (usually >25 mU/L) in the face of a low T_4 level.

Somatotropic Function in Critical Illness

Growth hormone (GH) levels are low in prolonged critical illness, and it has been conjectured that deficiencies of GH and insulin-like growth factor-1 (IGF-1) contribute to the muscle wasting seen in acute illness.[161] However, although small trials have found that GH administration can attenuate muscle catabolism in critical illness, a large, randomized prospective trial found that administration of large doses of GH to critically ill patients resulted in increased mortality.[170] Thus, GH administration during critical illness cannot be advocated at this time, although further exploration of the benefits of smaller doses of GH may be warranted.

ANEMIA AND TRANSFUSION THERAPY IN CRITICAL ILLNESS

Anemia is a frequent if not obligate accompaniment of critical illness. The vast majority of patients admitted to the ICU are anemic at some point in their hospital stay, and more than one-third of them will receive transfused blood.[171,172] Importantly, both anemia (Hb < 9 g/dL) and the amount of transfused blood are independently associated with mortality.[171,172] However, this association does not denote cause and effect, particularly for anemia, which may just be a marker of the severity of illness.

The cause of anemia in critical illness is multifactorial and related to blood loss from the primary injury or illness, iatrogenic blood loss due to daily blood sampling, nutritional deficiencies and marrow suppression.[173] Given that approximately 13% of ICU patients may have iron, folate, or vitamin B_{12} deficiencies, these parameters should be checked prior to blood transfusion.

Treatment of anemia in critical illness is the source of considerable debate. In unstressed subjects, severe anemia (Hb ≤ 5 g/dL) is amazingly well tolerated due to physiologic compensations that maintain oxygen delivery and extraction. However, it has long been assumed that critically ill patients have less efficient compensatory mechanisms and reduced physiologic reserve and thereby require a higher Hb concentration than unstressed individuals. Historically, this was translated to a transfusion threshold at an Hb concentration of approximately 10 g/dL.[174] However, transfusion of RBCs is not without risks including infection, transfusion-related acute lung injury (TRALI), transfusion-associated circulatory overload (TACO), transfusion-related immunomodulation (TRIM), microchimerism, and more (see the chapter on Hemostasis and Transfusion Medicine for a more complete discussion of transfusion risks).[175] These negative effects of transfusion may help explain why a large RCT of transfusion requirements in critical illness (the "TRICC" study) found that 30-day mortality was not affected when a restrictive transfusion threshold (Hb <7 g/dL) was used, compared to a more conventional threshold of <10 g/dL.[176] Furthermore, a trend in mortality reduction favored the restrictive group, and various subgroups of patients (less than 55 years of age and less severely ill by APACHE scoring) had a significantly lower mortality when they were transfused using the restrictive strategy. A similar trial in pediatric patients found no mortality difference between restrictive and liberal transfusion strategies, suggesting that a restrictive strategy is safe in critically
8 ill children.[177] These data strongly suggest that routine transfusion of critically ill patients is not necessary and may be harmful unless the Hb concentration is below 7 g/dL and are supported by observational studies that associate transfusion with increased morbidity and mortality in critical illness.[75] Unfortunately, data collected from ICUs at multiple centers in the United States since the publication of the TRICC study suggest that the transfusion threshold remains substantially higher, at a mean Hb of 8.6 g/dL.[171] More recent data from Canada reveal considerable heterogeneity in transfusion thresholds across centers.[178]

There are multiple possible reasons for the persistence of a high transfusion threshold in the ICU. Although the TRICC study included a broad spectrum of critically ill patients, some groups were excluded (active bleeding) or underrepresented (neurologic or neurosurgical injury). Furthermore, although a retrospective analysis of the TRICC data suggested that patients with coronary artery disease did not benefit from more liberal transfusion unless they had unstable angina or acute MI, concern remains about the tolerance for anemia in this group of patients. Lastly, Hb is an important determinant of oxygen delivery (DO_2), and transfusion is an integral component of goal-directed therapeutic strategies that aim to optimize DO_2 in early shock states.[74] In the absence of these possible exclusions (active bleeding, acute neurologic injury, active myocardial ischemia, or the early resuscitation of septic shock) restriction of blood transfusion to a threshold of <7.0 g/dL should be considered the standard of care and potentially life saving.

Alternatives to the transfusion of red cells for treatment of anemia are not currently available for widespread use. Several hemoglobin-based oxygen carriers (HBOCs) have been studied in clinical trials involving trauma and surgery, but results have been mixed, and none are currently FDA approved for use. Compassionate use of HBOCs in patients who have refused blood transfusion for religious reasons has been reported.

Prevention of anemia in critical illness is an appealing alternative to transfusion. One simple and potentially cost-saving approach is to reduce the volume and frequency of blood draws in the ICU. As noted earlier, iatrogenic blood loss is a major factor in the development of anemia of critical illness. Another potential approach is the administration of recombinant erythropoietin and iron. A large RCT found that administration of recombinant erythropoietin to critically ill patients on day 3 of an ICU stay and every week thereafter reduced transfusion requirements significantly, without affecting mortality or other outcome variables.[179] However, a subsequent RCT with a lower recommended transfusion threshold found no reduction in blood transfusion in association with erythropoietin administration.[180] Interestingly, there was a reduction in mortality in trauma patients who received erythropoietin compared to placebo. This may reflect nonerythropoietic effects of this agent given the lack of effect on blood transfusion. Given the current high cost of erythropoietin, it is not a cost-effective alternative at this time for general use in critically ill patients, although further investigation of its utility in trauma patients is warranted.

NUTRITION IN THE CRITICALLY ILL PATIENT

Critical illness can lead to hypermetabolic states and if nutritional support is inadequate or delayed, patients are at immediate risk of malnutrition. Poor nutritional status is associated with increased mortality and morbidity among critically ill patients. Therefore, appropriate nutrition is an important aspect of critical care and adequate nutritional support should be considered a standard of care. While over 200 formulas have been promoted for predicting daily calorie requirements of the critically ill patient, the American Society for Parenteral and Enteral Nutrition (ASPEN) and SCCM guidelines do not specify any specific formula.[181] It is acceptable to use a simple formula based on the patient's ideal body weight (25 to 30 kcal/kg/day), of which 15% to 20% should be represented by proteins (1.2 to 2 g/kg/day). In the obese patient (BMI > 30), permissive underfeeding at a level 60% to 70% of ideal body weight–predicted needs is acceptable.

Patient metabolic requirements should be established early after ICU admission and enteral feeding tolerance evaluated without delay (within 24 hours of admission). Evidence suggests that early enteral nutrition (EN) initiated within 4.4 hours after ICU admission results in less organ dysfunction than delayed feeding (36.5 hours after ICU admission).[182] Feeding intolerance due to high gastric residual volume can be improved by the administration of gastric prokinetic agents and positioning an enteric tube postpyloric. However, a systematic review comparing gastric versus postpyloric feeding did not suggest a clinical benefit from postpyloric tube feeding with regard to pneumonia, ICU length of stay, and mortality.[183] There is some suggestion that intermittent enteral feeding, as opposed to a continuous feeding regimen, is more likely to allow earlier attainment of the enteral calorie goal.[184]

Most of the trials evaluating PN do not demonstrate any favorable impact on outcome. In fact, EN is associated with lower infection risk and PN is associated with increased rates of complications and death. Therefore, EN is preferred over PN whenever possible because of its lower cost and less frequent complications.[185] Although not rigorously investigated, in patients unable to tolerate enteral feedings, PN may be considered. There has been considerable debate regarding the timing of initiation of PN, with Canadian and American guidelines generally recommending delayed initiation, while European guidelines have recommended early initiation.[181,186] A recent prospective randomized trial comparing initiation of PN at or before ICU day 2 with PN initiation at ICU day 8 showed the delayed initiation group had a decrease in infections, shorter duration of mechanical ventilation, less need for RRT, and a cost savings.[187] However, it is unclear how long of a delay in initiating PN is acceptable, assuming that EN is contraindicated or not tolerated despite vigorous attempts. Overall, strategies to optimize delivery of EN (starting at the target rate, use of a feeding protocol with a higher threshold of gastric residuals volumes, use of motility agents, and use of small bowel feeding) and minimize the risks of EN (elevation of the head of the bed) should be considered. There are no studies that demonstrate a benefit from the use of supplemental PN in patients unable to tolerate adequate EN.[185] Strategies that maximize the benefit and minimize the risks of PN (hypocaloric dose, withholding lipids) should be considered.

Complications associated with enteral feedings include aspiration of gastric feeding, diarrhea, and fluid and electrolyte imbalance. To prevent aspiration with gastric feeding, the head of the patient's bed should be raised 30 to 45 degrees during feeding; jejunal access can be considered in patients with recurrent tube feeding aspiration. Diarrhea is a common complication during enteral feeding associated with many potential causes, including medications (antibiotics or sorbitol-containing products), altered bacterial flora (*Clostridium difficile*), formula composition (including osmolality), infusion rate, hypoalbuminemia, bacterial contamination of the enteral fluid, and the patient's related conditions. To prevent or reduce diarrhea all potential etiologies should be considered and corrected. Exchanging a polymeric formula with fiber with a more expensive elemental amino acid diet may improve feeding tolerance. However, animal studies demonstrated that elemental diets promote bacterial overgrowth and may result in greater bacterial translocation.

Among special formulations, immunonutrition has been hypothesized to influence infectious morbidity and mortality in critically ill patients via a beneficial effect on GI immunologic function. This effect appears to be much greater in surgical patients, such as those with burns and in trauma. Specific enteral formulations, particularly those with high concentrations of glutamine, nucleotides, omega-3 fatty acids, and antioxidants, have the strongest data to support their use. The beneficial effects in medical ICU patients are less well established, and two recent RCTs found no benefit to nutritional supplementation with immunomodulatory agents in patients with ALI.[188,189] Two meta-analyses suggest that the administration of supplemental antioxidant micronutrients (selenium, zinc, and vitamins A, C, and E) may be associated with increased survival, although the overall quality of trials included in the meta-analyses is poor.[190,191]

SEDATION OF THE CRITICALLY ILL PATIENT

Critically ill patients are often deeply sedated, in part due to concerns for patient comfort, but also because of potential benefits afforded by a reduction in the sympathoadrenal response to injury. In addition, complications associated with under-sedation include ventilator dyssynchrony, patient injury, agitation, anxiety, stress disorders, and, possibly, unplanned tracheal extubation. That said, the bulk of available evidence from observational and randomized trials suggests that practices that favor light sedation, bolus administration versus continuous infusion of sedatives, and that promote daily trials of awakening in ICU patients result in a variety of benefits, including a shortened duration of mechanical ventilation and decreased time in the ICU.[192–197] Beyond lengthening the duration of mechanical ventilation, other complications associated with over-sedation include excessive cardiovascular and respiratory depression and infectious complications.[198]

The depth of sedation may also play a role in long-term outcomes after discharge from the ICU and hospital. Increasing evidence suggests that patients admitted to the ICU are at risk of developing symptoms of posttraumatic stress disorders, and of experiencing delusional memories. Approximately two-thirds of ICU patients have amnesia for the entire ICU course, and high-dose sedative administration is associated with both lack of recall and development of PTSD.[199,200] Furthermore, follow-up of patients enrolled in RCTs have found that sedation regimens that promote light sedation or daily awakening are not associated with increased long-term cognitive, psychological, or functional problems.[197,201,202]

Several factors such as interindividual variability, changes over time, severity of disease, intensity of painful stimuli, drug interactions, and organ dysfunction influence the analgesic and sedative needs of ICU patients. Therefore, it is important to titrate medications according to established therapeutic goals and revaluate sedation requirements frequently. Several scales are available to assess sedation levels over time. The most commonly used are the Ramsay sedation scale, the sedation–agitation scale and the Richmond agitation–sedation scale. Features common to all of these scales are the grading of sedation over different depths and allowance for indicators of agitation. There is no evidence that one scale is superior to another at this time, although the Richmond agitation–sedation scale has been more rigorously prospectively validated for reliability and validity.[203]

Confusion and agitation are common in ICU patients and may have unfavorable consequences on patient outcome. Patients experiencing agitation have been reported to have a higher incidence of major complications, higher admission to rehabilitation centers, and increased duration of hospital stay. Agitation is also a predictive factor for mortality. Agitation needs to be distinguished from delirium, which is very common in ICU patients and equally associated with increased length of stay, morbidity, and mortality.[204] Delirium can be difficult to diagnose in ICU patients since features of delirium, such as altered status of consciousness, are shared with several disorders typical of ICU patients. The distinguishing characteristics of delirium include acute onset and fluctuating course, inattention, disorganized thinking, and altered level of consciousness. Structured screening instruments are available and recommended for the diagnosis of delirium in the ICU.[205,206]

Nonpharmacologic and pharmacologic means can be used to provide comfort and safety to ICU patients. The former include verbal and written communication, frequent reorientation, maintenance of a day–night cycle, noise reduction, and ensuring ventilation synchrony. A randomized trial comparing continuous sedation to no sedation combined with nonpharmacologic techniques including those described above found an increase in ventilator-free days and a trend toward reduced ICU mortality in the no-sedation group.[196]

Pharmacologic agents include hypnotics–anxiolytics, opioids, and antipsychotics. Hypnotics most commonly used are propofol, midazolam, and lorazepam; each of these drugs has its own particular advantages, but there are insufficient data at this time to suggest a difference in relevant patient outcomes among them. A prospective, randomized, nonblinded trial compared a continuous infusion of lorazepam, midazolam, and propofol in trauma patients.[207] Midazolam appeared to be the most titratable drug, with the lowest incidence of over- and under-sedation. Lorazepam was the most cost-effective choice for sedation despite the observation that over-sedation occurred twice as often with lorazepam when compared to propofol or midazolam. A meta-analysis including 27 randomized trials comparing propofol versus midazolam suggested that tracheal extubation occurred earlier with the use of propofol for patients who were ventilated for a duration shorter than 36 hours.[208] However, no differences were found with regard to the ICU length of stay or mortality. Greater levels of hypotension and elevated triglyceride levels were observed with the use of propofol. Since then, an open label randomized trial found that continuous infusion of propofol was associated with shorter length of mechanical ventilation and ICU stay compared to intermittent lorazepam administration.[209]

Adverse effects unique to hypnotic–anxiolytic drugs include a hyperosmolar acidosis due to the diluent mixed with lorazepam (propylene glycol) and the potentially lethal "propofol infusion syndrome."[35] Both of these complications can be avoided by minimizing the administered dose of the respective agent.

Dexmedetomidine is a unique sedative agent for several reasons: (1) Mechanistically, it is an α-2 adrenergic receptor agonist, similar to clonidine, (2) it provides sedation without inducing unresponsiveness or coma, (3) it has some analgesic effect, and (4) it has little effect on respiratory drive. Dexmedetomidine has been effectively used as a single agent or in combination with other drugs in postsurgical and medical ICU patients. Two RCTs comparing dexmedetomidine to lorazepam and midazolam infusions, respectively, suggest that dexmedetomidine administration may be associated with a lower risk of delirium development.[210,211] However, the acquisition costs of dexmedetomidine are high, it is currently FDA approved for use for only up to 24 hours, and there is insufficient evidence to recommend its routine use at the current time.[212]

Morphine and fentanyl are the most commonly used opioids to provide analgesia in the ICU. Morphine should be avoided in patients with renal failure due to active metabolites that accumulate in the presence of impaired renal elimination.

Delirium in the ICU is commonly treated with antipsychotic agents such as haloperidol, and, more recently, newer antipsychotics such as olanzapine, quetiapine, risperidone, and ziprazadone. However, a small feasibility study found that scheduled haloperidol or ziprazadone was not superior to placebo in reducing delirium in mechanically ventilated ICU patients.[213] On the other hand, another small pilot study found that quetiapine administration (50 mg enterally twice daily) was superior to placebo plus as-needed haloperidol in reducing delirium in critically ill patients.[214] Larger studies are necessary to determine the true benefits of antipsychotic agents in the prevention and treatment of delirium in critically ill patients.

Neuromuscular blockade may be occasionally indicated in ICU patients with severe TBI or respiratory failure (see previous discussion under ALI/ARDS section), but routine use is discouraged because of concerns that this practice may predispose to critical illness polyneuropathy and myopathy (see section on acquired neuromuscular disorders in critical illness) and because of an increased risk of nosocomial pneumonia in patients receiving these agents.

9 In summary, sedation and analgesia should be provided in the ICU population to ensure patient comfort and safety. In establishing treatment algorithms, analgesia should be prioritized over sedation. Titration and assessment of analgesia and sedation should be an integral part of ICU monitoring so that over- and under-sedation can be avoided. The establishment of nurse-guided sedation protocols and daily interruption of sedation have been shown to be effective in reducing the length of mechanical ventilation and ICU stay.

COMPLICATIONS IN THE ICU: DETECTION, PREVENTION, AND THERAPY

Nosocomial Infections

Nosocomial infections are a major source of morbidity and mortality in the critically ill. At some level, nosocomial infections are unavoidable and occur because of the nature of intensive care: Patients are critically ill with altered host defenses, they require invasive devices (endotracheal tubes, intravascular catheters, etc.)

for support, monitoring, and therapy that provide portals of entry for infectious organisms, and they receive therapies that increase the risk of infection (glucocorticoids, PN). On the other hand, many nosocomial infections are preventable with relatively simple interventions.[215] This became more financially relevant in the United States in 2008, when the Center for Medicare and Medicaid Services (CMS) ceased reimbursing hospitals for preventable complications, one of which includes catheter-related urinary tract infection (UTI).

Several types and sources of infections are relatively unique to ICU care and should be included in the differential diagnosis when signs suggestive of infection arise. These infections include sinusitis, VAP, intravascular catheter-associated bacteremia, catheter-associated UTI, and invasive fungal infection. The diagnosis, prevention, and treatment of these will be discussed in the following section.

Sinusitis

Radiographic sinusitis is common in critically ill patients with indwelling oral and nasal tubes. Nasal intubation confers a greater risk than oral intubation of radiographic sinusitis, occurring in approximately 95% and 25% of patients with nasal and oral tubes after 1 week of intubation, respectively.[216] Several reports suggest that approximately 10% of radiographically diagnosed sinusitis is infected as determined by quantitative cultures, although the incidence may be much higher. van Zanten et al.[217] reported that bacterial sinusitis was responsible for 16% of fevers of unknown origin in a surgical ICU. The organisms cultured from sinuses represent those that are responsible for other nosocomial infections, particularly VAP (staphylococcal species, enteric gram-negative bacteria, and non-lactose–fermenting gram-negative rods such as *Pseudomonas* and *Acinetobacter*). Bacterial sinusitis may predispose to the development of VAP, possibly because of micro-aspiration of infected secretions.

Prevention of sinusitis should focus on efforts to improve sinus drainage, including semirecumbent positioning and avoidance of nasal tubes. Bacterial sinusitis should be considered in patients with unexplained fever and leukocytosis in the ICU. If radiographic sinusitis is documented, any nasal tubes should be removed, and nasal irrigation and short-term administration of nasal decongestants should be considered. If the patient is severely ill, broad-spectrum antibiotic coverage should be considered. If these maneuvers do not result in resolution of signs and symptoms of infection in 2 to 3 days, and in the absence of infection elsewhere, otolaryngologic consultation and consideration of sinus drainage procedures should be undertaken.

Ventilator-associated Pneumonia

Endotracheal intubation and mechanical ventilation increase the risk of nosocomial pneumonia, thus the term ventilator-associated pneumonia or VAP. The likelihood of developing VAP increases with the duration of mechanical ventilation, although the incremental risk may fall over time from a high of 3% per day in the first week of intubation/ventilation to 1% per day after 15 days in the ICU.[218] The quoted incidence of VAP is dependent on the criteria used to diagnose pneumonia (clinical vs. invasive technique); as discussed below, traditional clinical criteria are likely both insensitive and nonspecific and may lead to a falsely high or low incidence of VAP. For example, in a study comparing an invasive diagnostic technique to traditional clinical criteria in patients suspected of having VAP, only 50% of the patients in the invasive group met criteria for VAP compared to the clinical diagnostic group.[219] Given this caveat, studies that solely or primarily relied on invasive techniques to diagnose VAP suggest an incidence greater than 15% at 1 week of ICU stay and greater than 20% at 2 weeks.[218]

Although the mortality in patients with VAP ranges between 30% and 70%, the attributable mortality (the number of patients who die because of VAP rather than with VAP) is more difficult to pinpoint. This may be due to differences in the type of ICU, patient factors, diagnostic techniques across studies, or differences in the virulence of the causative pathogens. Thus, although earlier work suggested an attributable mortality of VAP greater than 40%,[220] more recent and rigorously conducted work suggests that the effect of VAP on mortality is minimal.[221]

VAP can be categorized as "early-onset," occurring within the first 48 to 72 hours of intubation/ventilation, or "late-onset," occurring thereafter. Early-onset VAP is generally caused by organisms such as *Haemophilus influenzae, Streptococcus pneumoniae,* methicillin-sensitive *Staphylococcus aureus,* and other relatively antibiotic-sensitive oral flora that enter the trachea around the time of intubation. Late-onset VAP is associated with more virulent and antibiotic-resistant organisms such as methicillin-resistant *S. aureus, Pseudomonas aeruginosa,* and *Acinetobacter.* In general, early-onset organisms are associated with zero or low attributable mortality, whereas late-onset organisms, particularly *Pseudomonas* and *Acinetobacter* species, are associated with higher mortality.[220]

10 There are a number of interventions that can reduce the incidence of VAP, some of which are relatively simple and inexpensive and others which are more costly and/or associated with some risk. The simplest and least expensive and yet very effective interventions are strict hand washing between patients and semirecumbent positioning of the patient (head height at 30 degrees or greater from horizontal). These practices should be rigorously applied in all ICUs (granted that semirecumbent positioning is not possible in all patients).

A somewhat more controversial subject involves the use of prophylaxis to prevent GI bleeding. As mentioned earlier, acid-suppression therapies have been associated with an increased risk of VAP because they allow bacterial overgrowth in the stomach. Further, the risk of significant GI bleeding is very low in the ICU, even in high-risk patients (those with coagulopathy or on mechanical ventilation). Thus, GI prophylactic therapy should be reserved for only these high-risk patients, and sucralfate should be considered as an alternative agent to acid-suppressive regimens despite its potentially reduced effectiveness.

Somewhat more expensive interventions to reduce VAP that may be useful in certain patients include subglottic suctioning and oscillating beds.[222] Intermittent subglottic suctioning using specially designed tracheal tubes has been shown to reduce the incidence of VAP in several small studies and may reduce the duration of mechanical ventilation and length of ICU stay.[223] However, these tubes are more expensive than conventional tracheal tubes, and their cost-effectiveness has not been established, particularly if their use is instituted in all intubated patients. Oscillating beds have been shown to reduce the incidence of VAP in surgical populations and patients with neurologic injury. However, these beds are very costly and cannot be recommended for routine use.[222] In patients who do not tolerate semirecumbent positioning because of fractures, hemodynamic instability, or otherwise, the use of oscillating beds should be considered.

Given that gastric and oropharyngeal colonization with resistant organisms appears to be a risk factor for the development of VAP, intervention to "decontaminate" these sites has been investigated. Selective digestive decontamination (SDD) typically involves the application of a mix of nonabsorbable antimicrobial agents, such as polymyxin, amphotericin, and aminoglycoside, in paste form to coat the oropharynx and as an elixir applied orally and via a nasogastric tube to decontaminate the GI tract, with or without the concomitant administration of systemic antibiotics. SDD does reduce the incidence of VAP and has been associated with variable mortality reduction in some studies. SDD is also associated with the development of antibiotic resistance, and concerns regarding the long-term impact of resistance have limited the widespread adoption of SDD.[222] However, more limited oral decontamination with chlorhexidine appears to reduce VAP rates without leading to excess antibiotic resistance.[224]

An additional and important approach to reduce the overall mortality from VAP involves refinement of the diagnostic process and limitation of antibiotic therapy to avoid the development of antibiotic resistance. As mentioned earlier, an invasive diagnostic strategy is likely more accurate than traditional clinical criteria to diagnose VAP. Invasive strategies typically involve collection of bronchial–alveolar specimens using lavage or protected brushes and then quantitating bacterial growth in the laboratory. Thus, VAP is diagnosed only when bacteria are seen within bronchoalveolar cells microscopically or when bacterial growth exceeds specific thresholds ($\geq 10^4$ colony-forming units/mL for bronchoalveolar lavage and $\geq 10^3$ colony-forming units/mL for protected brush specimens). Specimens have typically been obtained bronchoscopically, although data suggest that specimens obtained by direct aspiration through the tracheal tube are comparable to bronchoscopic specimens, suggesting it is quantitation of bacterial growth rather than the "invasiveness" of the technique that is important.[225] The important adjunct to this diagnostic approach is that although antibiotics may be started at the time clinical criteria for pneumonia are met and quantitative cultures are sent, they are stopped if the threshold values for VAP are not reached.

A moderately sized RCT of invasive versus noninvasive strategies to diagnose and treat VAP found that the invasive approach resulted in a mortality reduction at 14 days and a trend toward mortality reduction at 28 days.[219] In addition, the invasive strategy was associated with less multiple organ failure and reduced antibiotic use. Surprisingly, the invasive strategy did not result in a reduced incidence of emergence of resistant bacteria, although the incidence of *Candida* growth was reduced. A more recent RCT sponsored by the Canadian Critical Care Trials Group did not confirm the benefits found in the previous RCT; however, several methodologic weaknesses reduce the generalizability of this study.[226] Thus, the data favor the use of an invasive strategy to diagnose VAP when and if possible.

It is clear that delay in treatment of nosocomial infections including VAP is associated with increased mortality. Thus, treatment should not be delayed pending diagnostic evaluation; rather treatment should be started after culture specimens are sent if the clinical suspicion of VAP is high. Antibiotics can then be narrowed in spectrum or discontinued depending on the results from quantitative cultures after 48 to 72 hours. This approach is known as "de-escalating therapy" and is designed to ensure adequate antibiotic treatment up front, but avoid overuse of antibiotics in the long run.[220] Antibiotic selection should be predicated on hospital bacterial growth and resistance patterns. In general, for patients with early-onset VAP, antibiotics can be relatively narrow in spectrum and limited to a single agent; for late-onset VAP, broader spectrum antibiotics should be initiated and include agents from two different classes directed toward resistant gram-negative organisms and in many cases an agent directed against methicillin-resistant *S. aureus* (Table 55-7).

The optimal duration of antibiotic therapy for VAP is not well defined. A recent meta-analysis found that 8 days of antibiotic therapy was effective for treatment of VAP in terms of mortality and recurrent infections and resulted in more antibiotic-free days.[227] However, patients who had VAP caused by non-lactose–fermenting gram-negative rods (including *Pseudomonas*) had a higher infection recurrence rate if they received an initial 8-day course of therapy. It is unclear whether intermediate courses of therapy would have avoided infection recurrence. Thus, it is reasonable to choose an 8-day course of therapy for many patients with VAP; however, if there is an inadequate early clinical response or infection with non-lactose–fermenting gram-negative rods a longer course should be considered.

TABLE 55-7. EMPIRIC THERAPY OF VENTILATOR-ASSOCIATED PNEUMONIA

Common Organisms	Antibiotics
Early-onset VAP	
Enteric gram-negative rods • *Escherichia coli* • *Enterobacter* species • *Proteus* species • *Klebsiella* species • *Haemophilus influenzae* • Methicillin-sensitive *Staphylococcus aureus* • *Streptococcus pneumoniae*	*β*-lactam/*β*-lactamase inhibitor combination, *or* second-generation cephalosporin, *or* fluoroquinolone
Late-onset or Severe Early-onset VAP	
Above, *plus:* • *Pseudomonas aeruginosa* • *Acinetobacter* species • Methicillin-resistant *Staphylococcus aureus* (MRSA)	*β*-lactam/*β*-lactamase inhibitor combination, *or* third- or fourth-generation cephalosporin, *or* fluoroquinolone *plus* aminoglycoside, *or* second, structurally unrelated agent with antipseudomonal activity *plus* vancomycin or linezolid[a]

[a]If likelihood of MRSA is high.

Catheter-related Blood Stream Infections

6

Catheter-related blood stream infection (CRBSI) as strictly defined by the Center for Disease Control (CDC) includes the following criteria: (1) Clinical suspicion of catheter-related infection (including low likelihood of infection elsewhere) plus (2) positive culture of blood drawn from the catheter or of a segment of catheter plus (3) matching positive blood culture drawn from another site, preferably by direct venotomy or arterial puncture. Given this strict definition, the incidence of CRBSI is less than 5% in most studies. However, the incidence of bacteremia is affected by several factors, including the conditions and technique of insertion, type and location of catheter, and the duration of catheterization and can vary widely from study to study. The attributable mortality of CRBSI is approximately 11%, which is much lower than that for primary bacteremia or bacteremia associated with another site of infection.[228] The cost associated with a CRBSI is quite high and has been estimated between $22,000 and $54,000.[229]

Catheter infection is more likely when placement occurs under emergency conditions and is reduced by the use of strict aseptic technique with full barrier precautions. This includes pre-insertion hand washing, full gown and gloves, and the use of a large barrier drape.[230] In addition, skin cleansing with chlorhexidine is more effective than other agents at reducing catheter-related infection. Attention to these practices can dramatically reduce catheter-related infection.[229,231,232] These simple interventions should be considered as standards of care and are recommended by the CDC.

Catheter-related infection and bacteremia increase with the duration of catheterization, particularly for durations of greater than 2 days. However, routine catheter replacement at 3 or 7 days does not reduce the incidence of infection and results in increased mechanical complications. Thus, routine guide wire exchange of catheters is not recommended.

Catheters coated with either antiseptics (chlorhexidine and silver sulfadiazine) or antibiotics (rifampin and minocycline) reduce bacterial colonization of catheters as well as bacteremia. This effect becomes manifest only after days 5 to 6 of the catheter being in place; thus the CDC recommends the use of antimicrobial-coated catheters in patients with an expected duration of catheterization of greater than 5 days, particularly if the local rate of catheter-related infection is high.[233] Ultimately, a key component of strategies to reduce catheter-related infection is to limit the duration of insertion, and the need for continued central venous catheterization should be reviewed every day.[229,231] Catheter-related infection is insertion site dependent, increasing in frequency from subclavian to internal jugular to femoral vein sites. In addition, infection appears to be less likely for arterial than venous catheters.

Catheter-related venous thrombosis occurs commonly, and is associated with an increased risk of infection. Routine flushing of catheter ports with heparin reduces both the incidence of thrombosis and infection. However, heparin solutions contain antimicrobial preservatives and it is unclear if the heparin or the preservative is responsible for the beneficial effect. In addition, heparin may induce thrombocytopenia. Therefore, the CDC does not recommend the routine use of heparin flushing.[233]

Organisms commonly responsible for catheter-related bacteremia include *S. epidermidis* and *S. aureus,* enteric gram-negative bacteria, *P. aeruginosa* and *Acinetobacter,* and occasionally *Enterococcal* species. Note that although coagulase-negative staphylococci are commonly isolated from blood cultures in the ICU, they are likely responsible for true infection in a minority of cases.[234] When catheter-related bacteremia is confirmed, the offending catheter should be removed and appropriate antibiotics continued for a minimum of 7 days; longer courses should be considered for *S. aureus* bacteremia given the predilection for this organism to cause endocarditis. Suspected catheter-related infections can be addressed by sending screening cultures drawn through the catheter and from a peripheral site; guide wire exchange of the catheter with culture of the intracutaneous segment and tip can also be considered in this situation, but should a catheter-associated infection be confirmed, the catheter should be removed, not exchanged. Depending on the patient's severity of illness, a strong suspicion of catheter-related bacteremia should trigger the institution of broad-spectrum antibiotic coverage, including coverage for methicillin-resistant staphylococcal species and non-lactose–fermenting gram-negative rods, until culture results return, with subsequent de-escalation of therapy. Similar to VAP, early appropriate antibiotic coverage of catheter-related bacteremia will likely reduce mortality, although this has not been systematically studied.

Urinary Tract Infection

The urinary tract is the second most common source of infection in the ICU, with infections occurring in up to one-third of patients. The incidence of UTI increases with the duration of bladder catheterization.[215,235] The responsible organisms are similar to those causing other nosocomial infections and include staphylococcal species, *Enterococcus,* enteric gram-negative bacteria, and non-lactose–fermenting gram-negative bacteria such as *Pseudomonas.* Bacteriuria is associated with bacteremia about 5% of the time. Similar to other ICU-acquired infections, UTIs are associated with increased mortality, although the attributable mortality is not clear.

Prevention of ICU-acquired UTIs includes using careful hand washing and aseptic technique during catheter insertion and minimization of catheterization duration. The use of silver alloy and antibiotic-coated catheters may also reduce the incidence of UTI, although the evidence is insufficient at this point to recommend general use of coated catheters.[236]

Invasive Fungal Infections

Invasive fungal infection in nonneutropenic patients is caused by *Candida* species in the vast majority of cases, is increasingly common in the ICU population, and accounts for 5% to 10% of all blood stream infections in the ICU.[228,237] In addition, although fungal infection is not usually associated with pneumonia in a general ICU population, recent studies suggest that *Aspergillus* may be a common cause of VAP in patients with varying degrees of immunosuppression.[238] Other than neutropenia, risk factors for *Candida* blood stream infection include the presence of central venous catheters, uremia and dialysis-dependent renal failure, and administration of PN, multiple broad-spectrum antibiotics, and steroids. In addition, colonization of multiple sites by *Candida* is a risk factor for the development of fungemia.[239] The attributable mortality due to *Candida* blood stream infection is high, approaching 40%, and mortality appears to be much higher in medical versus surgical ICU patients. Invasive *Candida* infection is also associated with increased duration of mechanical ventilation, and ICU and hospital length of stay.

In addition to simple blood stream infection, *Candida* species are associated with UTI, postoperative peritonitis, and disseminated blood-borne infection. *Candida* is frequently cultured from the urine of catheterized patients, and candiduria is associated with the development of blood stream infection. True Candida peritonitis is also difficult to separate from contamination of culture specimens, but given that the mortality associated with Candida peritonitis is approximately 50%, treatment is warranted if clinical signs suggest infection. Disseminated blood-borne infection can result in endophthalmitis, endocarditis, and hepatic and pulmonary abscesses, is likely to occur when initial treatment of candidemia is delayed, and is associated with a high mortality. Lastly, although *Candida* is frequently grown from sputum cultures, true Candida pneumonia is unlikely. However, sputum colonization is a risk factor for blood stream infection.

Candida albicans is responsible for approximately 50% of invasive *Candida* infections in critically ill patients. *Candida tropicalis, Candida paraisopolis, Candida glabrata,* and *Candida krusei* account for the remainder, in descending order of frequency. Speciation is important as *C. glabrata* and, particularly, *C. krusei* are resistant to treatment with the most commonly used therapeutic agent fluconazole.

Prevention of invasive *Candida* infection involves avoidance of risk factors, including limitation of intravascular catheterization, PN, and antibiotic administration. Prophylactic therapy with fluconazole is effective at reducing the risk of invasive *Candida* infection in high-risk patients, but this strategy has been studied most extensively in the neutropenic population. Prophylactic fluconazole appears to increase the incidence of invasive infection with more resistant species, such as *C. glabrata* and *C. krusei;* thus, prophylactic therapy should be reserved for only the high-risk patient.[240]

Candida grows slowly in blood culture medium, and invasive infection can be indolent, making diagnosis of invasive candidiasis difficult. Serologic and molecular tests can be directed at detection of cell wall components. Other *Candida* antigens and antibodies against these components are available but lack sensitivity and are not widely clinically available. Thus, a high level of suspicion for invasive *Candida* infection in critically ill patients is necessary, particularly in patients with multiple risk factors, including multiple site colonization. "Preemptive" therapy should be considered in patients with a high likelihood of invasive *Candida* infection while awaiting blood culture results, as delay in treatment is associated with increased mortality. Unfortunately, many cases of invasive candidiasis are identified only at autopsy.[237]

Documented *Candida* blood stream infection should be treated aggressively, with therapy started promptly (or preemptively, as described above), and continued for at least 2 weeks after the last positive blood culture. An ophthalmologic examination is warranted in patients with documented or suspected blood stream infection, as patients with endophthalmitis may require longer courses of therapy. Intravascular catheters that are potential sources of blood stream infection should be removed.

It is not clear that routine treatment of candiduria is warranted, as candiduria often clears without treatment or with discontinuation of the bladder catheter; in addition, candiduria often recurs after initially successful antifungal therapy.[241] However, if candiduria is associated with signs of systemic infection, antifungal treatment should be considered; a similar approach can be taken when *Candida* is cultured from the peritoneal space.

Organisms sensitive to the azole derivative fluconazole cause the majority of invasive *Candida* infections in the ICU, and fluconazole is the first-line treatment given its reasonable efficacy and limited toxicity. Infections caused by resistant organisms such as *C. glabrata* and *C. krusei* may respond to newer-generation azoles such as voriconazole, and this is a reasonable therapeutic approach in the hemodynamically stable patient. Echinocandins such as caspofungin, micafungin, and anidulafungin are another class of antifungal agents with broad-spectrum activity and seemingly limited toxicity that are the treatment of choice in the unstable patient. Amphotericin B is generally reserved for refractory, life-threatening infections due to its toxicity. The reader is directed elsewhere for a more detailed discussion of antifungal agents.[240]

Stress Ulceration and Gastrointestinal Hemorrhage

Gastric mucosal breakdown with resulting gastritis and ulceration ("stress ulceration") can lead to GI bleeding in the ICU. Clinically significant GI bleeding is that which results in hemodynamic instability and/or a sudden fall in hematocrit that results in blood transfusion. The incidence of clinically significant stress-related GI bleeding was once felt to be quite high (20% or greater), but more recent studies suggest that the incidence is much lower and is less than 5% in high-risk patients and less than 1% for low-risk patients.[242] The major risk factors for stress-related GI bleeding are mechanical ventilation and coagulopathy; secondary risk factors amongst mechanically ventilated patients include renal failure, thermal injury, and possibly head injury, although the latter two factors have not been recently evaluated.[242–244] EN may protect against significant GI bleeding.[244]

Agents used to prevent stress ulceration and GI bleeding include methods to suppress acid production such as H_2 receptor antagonists (H_2RAs) and proton pump inhibitors (PPIs) and cytoprotective agents such as sucralfate. However, the agent of choice (and whether any prophylaxis is beneficial or indicated) is somewhat controversial for the following reasons: (1) Although ranitidine was shown to be more effective than sucralfate in preventing clinically significant GI bleeding in high-risk patients in a large, randomized prospective trial, the incidence of bleeding with both agents was quite low (1.7% vs. 3.8%).[245] Furthermore, a meta-analysis suggested that neither ranitidine nor sucralfate is superior to placebo in reducing clinically important bleeding.[246] (2) Acid suppression may favor gastric colonization with enteric flora, which may in turn increase the risk of nosocomial pneumonia. Multiple small, randomized trials suggested a higher incidence of VAP when ranitidine was compared to sucralfate, and in the above-quoted large trial there was a trend toward increased VAP in the ranitidine group. An increase in the incidence of *C. difficile* colitis in patients treated with PPIs has also been reported. (3) It appears that stress ulcer prophylaxis is more widely used than necessary, is often administered to low-risk patients, and results in an overall cost that may be higher than the benefit. Thus, although stress ulcer prophylaxis, predominantly with H_2RAs, is commonly used in critically ill patients, the utility of this intervention is unclear.

PPIs are very effective at suppressing gastric acid production and have been shown to be as effective as ranitidine and cimetidine at reducing stress ulcer–related bleeding in the ICU. In addition, PPIs may be more effective than ranitidine in preventing rebleeding due to stress ulceration.[247] However, PPIs cannot be recommended for routine use as prophylactic agents due to insufficient data and cost considerations. In addition, PPIs also have the potential to increase the risk of VAP, given their effective suppression of gastric acid secretion.

Venous Thromboembolism

Venous thromboembolism (VTE) occurs frequently in critically ill patients, with incidences of DVT of 10% to 30% and PE of 1.5% to 5%. However, the reported incidence varies widely depending on the study design, tests used to detect DVT, and the patient population studied. Virtually all critically ill patients have one or more risk factors for VTE; risk factors can be grouped according to their importance as described by Anderson and Spencer.[248] Determination of VTE risk is important in that it will help in choosing prophylactic therapy and in determining the level of suspicion for VTE in individual patients (Table 55-8).

In addition to classic lower extremity DVT, upper extremity DVT occurs with increased frequency in the ICU population. This is directly associated with the use of central venous catheters in the subclavian and internal jugular sites. Upper extremity DVT can result in pulmonary embolism in up to two-thirds of cases, with occasional fatalities. Catheter-related thrombosis is also associated with increased risk of catheter-associated infection and bacteremia. Finally, upper extremity DVT is associated with considerable long-term morbidity, particularly related to postthrombotic syndrome.[249]

The literature supporting prophylactic measures to prevent VTE in the ICU population is relatively poor and marked by small, heterogeneous studies. In addition, studies supporting VTE prophylaxis in the ICU generally show differences only in intermediate end points, such as asymptomatic DVT, with no differences in the incidence of PE or death. This is particularly true for VTE prophylaxis in patients with traumatic injury and makes evidence-based recommendations for prophylaxis difficult. Finally, the risks of VTE prophylaxis, including heparin-induced thrombocytopenia and bleeding, must be weighed when considering prophylaxis

TABLE 55-8. RISK FACTORS FOR VENOUS THROMBOEMBOLISM

Strong risk factors (odds ratio >10)
- Fracture (hip or leg)
- Hip or knee replacement
- Major trauma
- Spinal cord injury

Moderate risk factors (odds ratio 2–9)
- Arthroscopic knee surgery
- Central venous lines
- Chemotherapy
- Congestive heart or respiratory failure
- Hormone replacement therapy
- Malignancy
- Oral contraceptive therapy
- Paralytic stroke
- Pregnancy/postpartum
- Previous venous thromboembolism
- Thrombophilia

Weak risk factors (odds ratio <2)
- Bed rest >3 days
- Immobility due to sitting (e.g., prolonged car or air travel)
- Increasing age
- Laparoscopic surgery (e.g., cholecystectomy)
- Obesity
- Pregnancy/antepartum
- Varicose veins

From: Anderson FA Jr, Spencer FA. Risk factors for venous thromboembolism. *Circulation*. 2003;107:I9–16, with permission.

in the ICU population. Nonetheless, it is generally agreed that high-risk patients without contraindications should receive prophylaxis with LMWH, and that patients with low-to-moderate risk should receive low-dose UFH. Patients with contraindications to LMWH or UFH should probably receive prophylaxis with mechanical devices (serial compression devices), although there is no compelling evidence to suggest that they are effective in the ICU population.[250] In patients at high risk for DVT and contraindications to anticoagulation the preventative placement of a vena cava filter may be considered, although there are little data to support this practice. To reduce central venous catheter–associated thrombosis and infection, catheter tips should be positioned in the superior vena cava and catheters may be flushed with a dilute heparin solution. Heparin bonding of catheters may also reduce local thrombosis. Importantly, it should be recognized that the incidence of VTE in patients receiving pharmacologic prophylaxis remains substantial, ranging between 5% and 30% depending on the therapy and population studied.

Given the high incidence of asymptomatic DVT in critically ill patients, a high index of suspicion for VTE must be maintained in the ICU. However, despite the high incidence of DVT, routine screening studies for DVT do not appear to improve clinical outcomes in the ICU. Thus, VTE should be considered in critically ill patients in the face of relatively nonspecific findings, such as unexplained tachycardia, tachypnea, fever, asymmetric extremity edema, and gas exchange abnormalities, including high dead space ventilation. Compression Doppler ultrasonography is the most commonly utilized test for diagnosis of DVT and has good positive and negative predictive value compared to contrast venography[251]; helical computerized tomography of the chest (CT) has supplanted radionuclide ventilation–perfusion scanning as the primary test for the diagnosis of PE.[252,253] CT scanning can also be extended to include the extremities to diagnose DVT. However, ventilation–perfusion scanning and/or pulmonary angiography may have utility in specific circumstances, including in the presence of renal insufficiency (concerns about contrast-induced nephrotoxicity) or equivocal results on CT scan. In addition, pulmonary angiography may be the test of choice when the likelihood of PE is high and anticoagulation is contraindicated, necessitating immediate placement of a vena cava filter. Although low D-dimer levels have a high negative predictive value in ruling out VTE in outpatients, this test appears to have less utility in the ICU setting due to the frequent occurrence of high levels in critically ill patients.[254]

The mainstay of treatment for VTE is heparin, which should be started prior to confirmatory studies if clinical suspicion is high. LMWH may be superior to UFH in efficacy with comparable rates of bleeding for the treatment of VTE; the choice of drug should be based on clinical circumstances and availability. The advantages of UFH in the ICU population are its titratability and rapid reversibility, which may be desirable in patients at high risk for bleeding. In patients with PE and hemodynamic instability, thrombolytic therapy should be considered if not contraindicated. Although the data supporting thrombolytic therapy for treatment of PE are limited, patients with massive PE and/or shock are likely to benefit from thrombolysis; patients with more subtle signs of instability, including right ventricular dilation, may also benefit.[255]

For patients who have contraindications to anticoagulation or who have recurrent PE despite anticoagulation, vena cava filters can be placed in the SVC or IVC, depending on DVT location. Ultimately, given the long-term thrombotic complications associated with these devices, patients with vena cava filters should be anticoagulated when no longer contraindicated, and the devices should be removed when they are no longer required.

Acquired Neuromuscular Disorders in Critical Illness

Neuromuscular abnormalities developing as a consequence of critical illness can be found in the majority of patients hospitalized in the ICU for a week or more. The spectrum of illness ranges from isolated nerve entrapment with focal pain or weakness, to disuse muscle atrophy with mild weakness, to severe myopathy and/or neuropathy with associated severe, prolonged weakness. Although various studies have attempted to distinguish neuropathic from myopathic syndromes, resulting in a bewildering list of associated acronyms, it is likely that there is considerable overlap between the two in terms of risk factors, presentation, and prognosis.[256]

Prospective studies have shown that 25% to 36% of patients receiving intensive care are weak by clinical evaluation; electrodiagnostic studies (nerve conduction and electromyography) suggest that neuromuscular abnormalities are present in 42% to 47% of patients in the ICU for 7 days or more and in 68% to 100% of patients with sepsis or the SIRS. In addition to sepsis, factors strongly associated with the development of ICU-acquired neuromuscular abnormalities include duration of illness and hyperglycemia. Although corticosteroid and neuromuscular blocking drug administration have also been associated with ICU-acquired neuromuscular abnormalities, these agents do not consistently appear as risk factors, and their ultimate role in the pathogenesis of this problem is as yet undefined.[257]

ICU-acquired neuromuscular abnormalities can result in severe weakness with flaccid quadriplegia that lasts for weeks or months and likely prolong the duration of mechanical ventilation and ICU stay and hospitalization and provide a significant impediment to long-term functional recovery from critical illness.[258,259] In addition, acquired weakness in the ICU may be a significant contributor to ICU and hospital mortality.

Prevention of acquired neuromuscular disorders in the ICU centers on avoidance or minimization of contributory risk factors, including high-dose steroids, prolonged neuromuscular blockade, and hyperglycemia. In regards to the latter, the only prospectively proven intervention for prevention of polyneuropathy as defined by electrophysiologic testing is tight glycemic control utilizing intensive insulin therapy (goal glucose <110 mg/dL).[158,260] In addition, efforts to reduce the risk of infection and ICU length of stay including rigorous hand washing and infection control procedures, semirecumbent positioning, careful aseptic technique and barrier protection for central venous catheter placement, and lung-protective ventilation will likely result in a reduction in the incidence and ramifications of ICU-acquired neuromuscular abnormalities.

The diagnosis of ICU-acquired neuromuscular abnormalities should be entertained in all critically ill patients with unexplained weakness; electrodiagnostic studies can help confirm the diagnosis and rule out other, potentially treatable causes of weakness such as Gullain–Barré syndrome. Muscle biopsy is confirmatory in cases of myopathy, but given its invasive nature, biopsy is not warranted outside of research settings. Unfortunately, no treatment for ICU-acquired neuromuscular abnormalities has been identified; avoidance of potentially contributing agents and aggressive physical therapy are warranted. Discharge planning should include the potential need for long-term nursing and rehabilitative care.

References

1. Berthelsen PG, Cronqvist M. The first intensive care unit in the world: Copenhagen 1953. *Acta Anaesthesiol Scand.* 2003;47:1190–1195.
2. Angus DC, Kelley MA, Schmitz RJ, et al. Caring for the critically ill patient. Current and projected workforce requirements for care of the critically ill and patients with pulmonary disease: Can we meet the requirements of an aging population? *JAMA.* 2000;284:2762–2770.
3. Spielman FJ. Critical care medicine: Anesthesiology steps forward. *Bull Anesth Hist.* 2003;21:12–13.
4. *ABMS 2010 Certificate Statistics.* Chicago, IL: American Board of Medical Specialties; 2010.
5. Kavanagh BP. The GRADE system for rating clinical guidelines. *PLoS Med.* 2009; 6:e1000094. http://www.plosmedicine.org/article/info%3Adoi%2F10.1371%2Fjournal.pmed.1000094
6. Kaushal R, Bates DW, Franz C, et al. Costs of adverse events in intensive care units. *Crit Care Med.* 2007;35:2479–2483.
7. Pronovost PJ, Rinke ML, Emery K, et al. Interventions to reduce mortality among patients treated in intensive care units. *J Crit Care.* 2004;19:158–164.
8. Pronovost PJ, Angus DC, Dorman T, et al. Physician staffing patterns and clinical outcomes in critically ill patients: A systematic review. *JAMA.* 2002;288:2151–2162.
9. Treggiari MM, Martin DP, Yanez ND, et al. Effect of intensive care unit organizational model and structure on outcomes in patients with acute lung injury. *Am J Respir Crit Care Med.* 2007;176:685–690.
10. Nathens AB, Rivara FP, MacKenzie EJ, et al. The impact of an intensivist-model ICU on trauma-related mortality. *Ann Surg.* 2006;244:545–554.
11. ICU Physician Staffing Fact Sheet. The Leapfrog Group for Patient Safety. http://www.leapfroggroup.org/for_hospitals/leapfrog_hospital_survey_copy/leapfrog_safety_practices/icu_physician_staffing; accessed January 16, 2012.
12. Angus DC, Shorr AF, White A, et al. Critical care delivery in the United States: Distribution of services and compliance with Leapfrog recommendations. *Crit Care Med.* 2006;34:1016–1024.
13. Kahn JM, Matthews FA, Angus DC, et al. Barriers to implementing the Leapfrog Group recommendations for intensivist physician staffing: A survey of intensive care unit directors. *J Crit Care.* 2007;22:97–103.
14. Pronovost PJ, Needham DM, Waters H, et al. Intensive care unit physician staffing: Financial modeling of the Leapfrog standard. *Crit Care Med.* 2006;34:S18–S24.
15. Hales BM, Pronovost PJ. The checklist–a tool for error management and performance improvement. *J Crit Care.* 2006;21:231–235.
16. Pronovost P, Berenholtz S, Dorman T, et al. Improving communication in the ICU using daily goals. *J Crit Care.* 2003;18:71–75.
17. Chan KH, Miller JD, Dearden NM, et al. The effect of changes in cerebral perfusion pressure upon middle cerebral artery blood flow velocity and jugular bulb venous oxygen saturation after severe brain injury. *J Neurosurg.* 1992;77:55–61.
18. Budohoski KP, Reinhard M, Aries MJ, et al. Monitoring cerebral autoregulation after head injury. Which component of transcranial Doppler flow velocity is optimal? *Neurocrit Care.* 2011;17(2):211–218.
19. Haitsma IK, Maas AI. Advanced monitoring in the intensive care unit: Brain tissue oxygen tension. *Curr Opin Crit Care.* 2002;8:115–120.
20. Longhi L, Pagan F, Valeriani V, et al. Monitoring brain tissue oxygen tension in brain-injured patients reveals hypoxic episodes in normal-appearing and in perifocal tissue. *Intensive Care Med.* 2007;33:2136–2142.
21. Ibanez J, Vilalta A, Mena MP, et al. [Intraoperative detection of ischemic brain hypoxia using oxygen tissue pressure microprobes]. *Neurocirugia (Asturias, Spain).* 2003;14:483–489, discussion 90.
22. Smith ML, Counelis GJ, Maloney-Wilensky E, et al. Brain tissue oxygen tension in clinical brain death: A case series. *Neurol Res.* 2007;29(7):755–759.
23. Guidelines for the management of severe traumatic brain injury. *J Neurotrauma.* 2007;24(suppl 1):S1–S106.
24. Smith MJ, Stiefel MF, Magge S, et al. Packed red blood cell transfusion increases local cerebral oxygenation. *Crit Care Med.* 2005;33:1104–1108.
25. Thorat JD, Wang EC, Lee KK, et al. Barbiturate therapy for patients with refractory intracranial hypertension following severe traumatic brain injury: Its effects on tissue oxygenation, brain temperature and autoregulation. *J Clin Neurosci.* 2008;15:143–148.
26. Stiefel MF, Heuer GG, Smith MJ, et al. Cerebral oxygenation following decompressive hemicraniectomy for the treatment of refractory intracranial hypertension. *J Neurosurg.* 2004;101:241–247.
27. Martini RP, Deem S, Yanez ND, et al. Management guided by brain tissue oxygen monitoring and outcome following severe traumatic brain injury. *J Neurosurg.* 2009;111:644–649.
28. Narotam PK, Morrison JF, Nathoo N. Brain tissue oxygen monitoring in traumatic brain injury and major trauma: Outcome analysis of a brain tissue oxygen-directed therapy. *J Neurosurg.* 2009;111:672–682.
29. Bhatia A, Gupta AK. Neuromonitoring in the intensive care unit. II. Cerebral oxygenation monitoring and microdialysis. *Intensive Care Med.* 2007;33:1322–1328.
30. Nelson DW, Thornquist B, MacCallum RM, et al. Analyses of cerebral microdialysis in patients with traumatic brain injury: Relations to intracranial pressure, cerebral perfusion pressure and catheter placement. *BMC Med.* 2011;9:21.
31. Thatcher RW, Cantor DS, McAlaster R, et al. Comprehensive predictions of outcome in closed head-injured patients. The development of prognostic equations. *Ann N Y Acad Sci.* 1991;620:82–101.
32. Chesnut RM, Marshall SB, Piek J, et al. Early and late systemic hypotension as a frequent and fundamental source of cerebral ischemia following severe brain injury in the Traumatic Coma Data Bank. *Acta Neurochir Suppl (Wien).* 1993;59:121–125.
33. Nelson DW, Nystrom H, MacCallum RM, et al. Extended analysis of early computed tomography scans of traumatic brain injured patients and relations to outcome. *J Neurotrauma.* 2010;27:51–64.
34. Mirski MA, Muffelman B, Ulatowski JA, et al. Sedation for the critically ill neurologic patient. *Crit Care Med.* 1995;23:2038–2053.
35. Cremer OL, Moons KG, Bouman EA, et al. Long-term propofol infusion and cardiac failure in adult head-injured patients. *Lancet.* 2001;357:117–118.
36. Schwartz ML, Tator CH, Rowed DW, et al. The University of Toronto head injury treatment study: A prospective, randomized comparison of pentobarbital and mannitol. *Can J Neurol Sci.* 1984;11:434–440.
37. Ward JD, Becker DP, Miller JD, et al. Failure of prophylactic barbiturate coma in the treatment of severe head injury. *J Neurosurg.* 1985;62:383–388.
38. Eisenberg HM, Frankowski RF, Contant CF, et al. High-dose barbiturate control of elevated intracranial pressure in patients with severe head injury. *J Neurosurg.* 1988;69:15–23.
39. Drummond JC, Dao AV, Roth DM, et al. Effect of dexmedetomidine on cerebral blood flow velocity, cerebral metabolic rate, and carbon dioxide response in normal humans. *Anesthesiology.* 2008;108:225–232.
40. Robertson CS, Valadka AB, Hannay HJ, et al. Prevention of secondary ischemic insults after severe head injury. *Crit Care Med.* 1999;27:2086–2095.
41. Muizelaar JP, Marmarou A, Ward JD, et al. Adverse effects of prolonged hyperventilation in patients with severe head injury: A randomized clinical trial. *J Neurosurg.* 1991;75:731–739.
42. Cruz J. The first decade of continuous monitoring of jugular bulb oxyhemoglobin saturation: Management strategies and clinical outcome. *Crit Care Med.* 1998;26:344–351.
43. Henderson WR, Dhingra VK, Chittock DR, et al. Hypothermia in the management of traumatic brain injury. A systematic review and meta-analysis.*Intensive Care Med.* 2003;29:1637–1644.
44. Clifton GL, Drever P, Valadka A, et al. Multicenter trial of early hypothermia in severe brain injury. *J Neurotrauma.* 2009;26:393–397.
45. Clifton GL, Miller ER, Choi SC, et al. Hypothermia on admission in patients with severe brain injury. *J Neurotrauma.* 2002;19:293–301.

46. Roberts I, Yates D, Sandercock P, et al. Effect of intravenous corticosteroids on death within 14 days in 10008 adults with clinically significant head injury (MRC CRASH trial): Randomised placebo-controlled trial. *Lancet.* 2004;364:1321–1328.
47. Temkin NR, Anderson GD, Winn HR, et al. Magnesium sulfate for neuroprotection after traumatic brain injury: A randomised controlled trial. *Lancet Neurol.* 2007;6:29–38.
48. Temkin NR, Dikmen SS, Wilensky AJ, et al. A randomized, double-blind study of phenytoin for the prevention of post-traumatic seizures. *N Engl J Med.* 1990; 323:497–502.
49. Myburgh J, Cooper J, Finfer S, et al. Saline or albumin for fluid resuscitation in patients with traumatic brain injury. *N Engl J Med.* 2007;357:874–884.
50. Kassell NF, Torner JC, Jane JA, et al. The International Cooperative Study on the Timing of Aneurysm Surgery. Part 2: Surgical results. *J Neurosurg.* 1990;73:37–47.
51. Kassell NF, Torner JC, Haley EC Jr, et al. The International Cooperative Study on the Timing of Aneurysm Surgery. Part 1: Overall management results. *J Neurosurg.* 1990;73:18–36.
52. Nieuwkamp DJ, Setz LE, Algra A, et al. Changes in case fatality of aneurysmal subarachnoid haemorrhage over time, according to age, sex, and region: A meta-analysis. *Lancet Neurol.* 2009;8:635–642.
53. Dorsch NW. Cerebral arterial spasm–a clinical review. *Br J Neurosurg.* 1995; 9:403–412.
54. Barker FG 2nd, Ogilvy CS. Efficacy of prophylactic nimodipine for delayed ischemic deficit after subarachnoid hemorrhage: A metaanalysis. *J Neurosurg.* 1996; 84:405–414.
55. Tseng MY. Summary of evidence on immediate statins therapy following aneurysmal subarachnoid hemorrhage. *Neurocrit Care.* 2011;15:298–301.
56. Treggiari MM, Walder B, Suter PM, et al. Systematic review of the prevention of delayed ischemic neurological deficits with hypertension, hypervolemia, and hemodilution therapy following subarachnoid hemorrhage. *J Neurosurg.* 2003;98:978–984.
57. Diringer MN, Bleck TP, Claude Hemphill J 3rd, et al. Critical care management of patients following aneurysmal subarachnoid hemorrhage: Recommendations from the Neurocritical Care Society's Multidisciplinary Consensus Conference. *Neurocrit Care.* 2011;15:211–240.
58. Shimoda M, Oda S, Tsugane R, et al. Intracranial complications of hypervolemic therapy in patients with a delayed ischemic deficit attributed to vasospasm. *J Neurosurg.* 1993;78:423–429.
59. Lanzino G, D'Urso PI, Suarez J. Seizures and anticonvulsants after aneurysmal subarachnoid hemorrhage. *Neurocrit Care.* 2011;15:247–256.
60. Roger VL, Go AS, Lloyd-Jones DM, et al. Heart disease and stroke statistics– 2011 update: A report from the American Heart Association. *Circulation.* 2011; 123:e18–e209.
61. Adams HP Jr, del Zoppo G, Alberts MJ, et al. Guidelines for the early management of adults with ischemic stroke: A guideline from the American Heart Association/ American Stroke Association Stroke Council, Clinical Cardiology Council, Cardiovascular Radiology and Intervention Council, and the Atherosclerotic Peripheral Vascular Disease and Quality of Care Outcomes in Research Interdisciplinary Working Groups: The American Academy of Neurology affirms the value of this guideline as an educational tool for neurologists. *Stroke.* 2007;38:1655–1711.
62. Lees KR, Bluhmki E, von Kummer R, et al. Time to treatment with intravenous alteplase and outcome in stroke: An updated pooled analysis of ECASS, ATLANTIS, NINDS, and EPITHET trials. *Lancet.* 2010;375:1695–1703.
63. Gray CS, Hildreth AJ, Sandercock PA, et al. Glucose-potassium-insulin infusions in the management of post-stroke hyperglycaemia: The UK Glucose Insulin in Stroke Trial (GIST-UK). *Lancet Neurol.* 2007;6:397–406.
64. Vahedi K, Hofmeijer J, Juettler E, et al. Early decompressive surgery in malignant infarction of the middle cerebral artery: A pooled analysis of three randomised controlled trials. *Lancet Neurol.* 2007;6:215–222.
65. Arrich J, Holzer M, Herkner H, et al. Hypothermia for neuroprotection in adults after cardiopulmonary resuscitation. *Cochrane Database Syst Rev.* 2009: CD004128.
66. The Hypothermia after Cardiac Arrest Study Group. Mild therapeutic hypothermia to improve the neurologic outcome after cardiac arrest. *N Engl J Med.* 2002;346:549–556.
67. Richard C, Warszawski J, Anguel N, et al. Early use of the pulmonary artery catheter and outcomes in patients with shock and acute respiratory distress syndrome: A randomized controlled trial. *JAMA.* 2003;290:2713–2720.
68. Sandham JD, Hull RD, Brant RF, et al. A randomized, controlled trial of the use of pulmonary-artery catheters in high-risk surgical patients. *N Engl J Med.* 2003;348:5–14.
69. Koo KK, Sun JC, Zhou Q, et al. Pulmonary artery catheters: Evolving rates and reasons for use. *Crit Care Med.* 2011;39:1613–1618.
70. Kumar A, Anel R, Bunnell E, et al. Pulmonary artery occlusion pressure and central venous pressure fail to predict ventricular filling volume, cardiac performance, or the response to volume infusion in normal subjects. *Crit Care Med.* 2004;32:691–699.
71. Michard F, Boussat S, Chemla D, et al. Relation between respiratory changes in arterial pulse pressure and fluid responsiveness in septic patients with acute circulatory failure. *Am J Respir Crit Care Med.* 2000;162:134–138.
72. Hayes MA, Timmins AC, Yau EH, et al. Elevation of systemic oxygen delivery in the treatment of critically ill patients. *N Engl J Med.* 1994;330:1717–1722.
73. Reinhart K, Kuhn HJ, Hartog C, et al. Continuous central venous and pulmonary artery oxygen saturation monitoring in the critically ill. *Intensive Care Med.* 2004;30:1572–1578.
74. Rivers E, Nguyen B, Havstad S, et al. Early goal-directed therapy in the treatment of severe sepsis and septic shock. *N Engl J Med.* 2001;345:1368–1377.
75. Marik PE, Corwin HL. Efficacy of red blood cell transfusion in the critically ill: A systematic review of the literature. *Crit Care Med.* 2008;36:2667–2674.
76. Baillard C, Cohen Y, Fosse JP, et al. Haemodynamic measurements (continuous cardiac output and systemic vascular resistance) in critically ill patients: Transoesophageal Doppler versus continuous thermodilution. *Anaesth Intensive Care.* 1999;27:33–37.
77. Melamed R, Sprenkle MD, Ulstad VK, et al. Assessment of left ventricular function by intensivists using hand-held echocardiography. *Chest.* 2009;135:1416–1420.
78. Vieillard-Baron A, Prin S, Chergui K, et al. Hemodynamic instability in sepsis: Bedside assessment by Doppler echocardiography. *Am J Respir Crit Care Med.* 2003;168:1270–1276.
79. Jessup M, Abraham WT, Casey DE, et al. 2009 focused update: ACCF/AHA Guidelines for the Diagnosis and Management of Heart Failure in Adults: A report of the American College of Cardiology Foundation/American Heart Association Task Force on Practice Guidelines: Developed in collaboration with the International Society for Heart and Lung Transplantation. *Circulation.* 2009;119:1977–2016.
80. O'Connor CM, Starling RC, Hernandez AF, et al. Effect of nesiritide in patients with acute decompensated heart failure. *N Engl J Med.* 2011;365:32–43.
81. Antman EM, Hand M, Armstrong PW, et al. 2007 focused update of the ACC/ AHA 2004 guidelines for the management of patients with ST-elevation myocardial infarction: A report of the American College of Cardiology/American Heart Association Task Force on Practice Guidelines. *J Am Coll Cardiol.* 2008;51:210–247.
82. Hochman JS, Sleeper LA, Webb JG, et al. Early revascularization in acute myocardial infarction complicated by cardiogenic shock. SHOCK Investigators. Should we emergently revascularize occluded coronaries for cardiogenic shock. *N Engl J Med.* 1999;341:625–634.
83. Patel MR, Smalling RW, Thiele H, et al. Intra-aortic balloon counterpulsation and infarct size in patients with acute anterior myocardial infarction without shock: The CRISP AMI randomized trial. *JAMA.* 2011;306:1329–1337.
84. Vieillard Baron A, Schmitt JM, Beauchet A, et al. Early preload adaptation in septic shock? A transesophageal echocardiographic study. *Anesthesiology.* 2001;94: 400–406.
85. American College of Chest Physicians/Society of Critical Care Medicine Consensus Conference: Definitions for sepsis and organ failure and guidelines for the use of innovative therapies in sepsis. *Crit Care Med.* 1992;20:864–874.
86. Marshall JC, Cook DJ, Christou NV, et al. Multiple organ dysfunction score: A reliable descriptor of a complex clinical outcome. *Crit Care Med.* 1995;23:1638–1652.
87. Dellinger RP, Levy MM, Carlet JM, et al. Surviving Sepsis Campaign: International guidelines for management of severe sepsis and septic shock: 2008. *Crit Care Med.* 2008;36:296–327.
88. Wilkes MM, Navickis RJ. Patient survival after human albumin administration. A meta-analysis of randomized, controlled trials. *Ann Intern Med.* 2001;135:149–164.
89. Cochrane Injuries Group Albumin Reviewers. Human albumin administration in critically ill patients: Systematic review of randomised controlled trials. *BMJ.* 1998;317:235–240.
90. Finfer S, Bellomo R, Boyce N, et al. A comparison of albumin and saline for fluid resuscitation in the intensive care unit. *N Engl J Med.* 2004;350:2247–2256.
91. Brunkhorst FM, Engel C, Bloos F, et al. Intensive insulin therapy and pentastarch resuscitation in severe sepsis. *N Engl J Med.* 2008;358:125–139.
92. Bayer O, Reinhart K, Sakr Y, et al. Renal effects of synthetic colloids and crystalloids in patients with severe sepsis: A prospective sequential comparison. *Crit Care Med.* 2011;39:1335–1342.
93. Martin C, Viviand X, Leone M, et al. Effect of norepinephrine on the outcome of septic shock. *Crit Care Med.* 2000;28:2758–2765.
94. Vasu TS, Cavallazzi R, Hirani A, et al. Norepinephrine or dopamine for septic shock: A systematic review of randomized clinical trials. *J Intensive Care Med.* 2012;27(3):172–178.
95. Havel C, Arrich J, Losert H, et al. Vasopressors for hypotensive shock. *Cochrane Database Syst Rev.* 2011:CD003709.
96. Martin C, Papazian L, Perrin G, et al. Norepinephrine or dopamine for the treatment of hyperdynamic septic shock? *Chest.* 1993;103:1826–1831.
97. Bellomo R, Chapman M, Finfer S, et al. Low-dose dopamine in patients with early renal dysfunction: A placebo-controlled randomised trial. Australian and New Zealand Intensive Care Society (ANZICS) Clinical Trials Group. *Lancet.* 2000;356:2139–2143.
98. Hartemink KJ, Groeneveld AB. Vasopressors and inotropes in the treatment of human septic shock: Effect on innate immunity? *Inflammation.* 2012;35(1):206–213.
99. Shoemaker WC, Appel PL, Kram HB. Hemodynamic and oxygen transport effects of dobutamine in critically ill general surgical patients. *Crit Care Med.* 1986;14:1032–1037.
100. Duranteau J, Sitbon P, Teboul JL, et al. Effects of epinephrine, norepinephrine, or the combination of norepinephrine and dobutamine on gastric mucosa in septic shock. *Crit Care Med.* 1999;27:893–900.
101. Levy B, Perez P, Perny J, et al. Comparison of norepinephrine-dobutamine to epinephrine for hemodynamics, lactate metabolism, and organ function

variables in cardiogenic shock. A prospective, randomized pilot study. *Crit Care Med.* 2011;39:450–455.
102. Annane D, Vignon P, Renault A, et al. Norepinephrine plus dobutamine versus epinephrine alone for management of septic shock: A randomised trial. *Lancet.* 2007;370:676–684.
103. Holmes CL, Patel BM, Russell JA, et al. Physiology of vasopressin relevant to management of septic shock. *Chest.* 2001;120:989–1002.
104. Wenzel V, Krismer AC, Arntz HR, et al. A comparison of vasopressin and epinephrine for out-of-hospital cardiopulmonary resuscitation. *N Engl J Med.* 2004;350:105–113.
105. Patel BM, Chittock DR, Russell JA, et al. Beneficial effects of short-term vasopressin infusion during severe septic shock. *Anesthesiology.* 2002;96:576–582.
106. Dunser MW, Mayr AJ, Ulmer H, et al. Arginine vasopressin in advanced vasodilatory shock: A prospective, randomized, controlled study. *Circulation.* 2003;107:2313–2319.
107. Albanese J, Leone M, Delmas A, et al. Terlipressin or norepinephrine in hyperdynamic septic shock: A prospective, randomized study. *Crit Care Med.* 2005;33:1897–1902.
108. Cartotto R, McGibney K, Smith T, et al. Vasopressin for the septic burn patient. *Burns.* 2007;33:441–451.
109. Russell JA, Walley KR, Singer J, et al. Vasopressin versus norepinephrine infusion in patients with septic shock. *N Engl J Med.* 2008;358:877–887.
110. Marti-Carvajal AJ, Sola I, Lathyris D, et al. Human recombinant activated protein C for severe sepsis. *Cochrane Database Syst Rev.* 2011:CD004388.
111. Annane D, Sebille V, Charpentier C, et al. Effect of treatment with low doses of hydrocortisone and fludrocortisone on mortality in patients with septic shock. *JAMA.* 2002;288:862–871.
112. Sprung CL, Annane D, Didier K, et al. Hydrocortisone therapy for patients with septic shock. *N Engl J Med.* 2008;358:111–124.
113. Kumar A, Roberts D, Wood KE, et al. Duration of hypotension before initiation of effective antimicrobial therapy is the critical determinant of survival in human septic shock. *Crit Care Med.* 2006;34:1589–1596.
114. Feihl F, Perret C. Permissive hypercapnia. How permissive should we be? *Am J Respir Crit Care Med.* 1994;150:1722–1737.
115. Moloney ED, Griffiths MJ. Protective ventilation of patients with acute respiratory distress syndrome. *Br J Anaesth.* 2004;92:261–270.
116. Determann RM, Royakkers A, Wolthuis EK, et al. Ventilation with lower tidal volumes as compared with conventional tidal volumes for patients without acute lung injury: A preventive randomized controlled trial. *Crit Care.* 2010;14:R1.
117. Gajic O, Frutos-Vivar F, Esteban A, et al. Ventilator settings as a risk factor for acute respiratory distress syndrome in mechanically ventilated patients. *Intensive Care Med.* 2005;31:922–926.
118. Nava S, Carbone G, DiBattista N, et al. Noninvasive ventilation in cardiogenic pulmonary edema: A multicenter randomized trial. *Am J Respir Crit Care Med.* 2003;168:1432–1437.
119. International Consensus Conferences in Intensive Care Medicine: Noninvasive positive pressure ventilation in acute Respiratory failure. *Am J Respir Crit Care Med.* 2001;163:283–291.
120. Esteban A, Frutos-Vivar F, Ferguson ND, et al. Noninvasive positive-pressure ventilation for respiratory failure after extubation. *N Engl J Med.* 2004;350:2452–2460.
121. Mehta S, Jay GD, Woolard RH, et al. Randomized, prospective trial of bilevel versus continuous positive airway pressure in acute pulmonary edema. *Crit Care Med.* 1997;25:620–628.
122. Esteban A, Frutos F, Tobin MJ, et al. A comparison of four methods of weaning patients from mechanical ventilation. Spanish Lung Failure Collaborative Group. *N Engl J Med.* 1995;332:345–350.
123. MacIntyre NR, Cook DJ, Ely EW Jr, et al. Evidence-based guidelines for weaning and discontinuing ventilatory support: A collective task force facilitated by the American College of Chest Physicians; the American Association for Respiratory Care; and the American College of Critical Care Medicine. *Chest.* 2001;120:375S–395S.
124. Schuster DP. What is acute lung injury? What is ARDS? *Chest.* 1995;107:1721–1726.
125. Bernard GR, Artigas A, Brigham KL, et al. Report of the American-European consensus conference on ARDS: Definitions, mechanisms, relevant outcomes and clinical trial coordination. The Consensus Committee. *Intensive Care Med.* 1994;20:225–232.
126. Ranieri VM, Rubenfeld GD, Thompson BT, et al. Acute respiratory distress syndrome: the Berlin Definition. *JAMA.* 2012;307:2526–2533.
127. Phua J, Badia JR, Adhikari NK, et al. Has mortality from acute respiratory distress syndrome decreased over time? A systematic review. *Am J Respir Crit Care Med.* 2009;179:220–227.
128. Nuckton TJ, Alonso JA, Kallet RH, et al. Pulmonary dead-space fraction as a risk factor for death in the acute respiratory distress syndrome. *N Engl J Med.* 2002;346:1281–1286.
129. The Acute Respiratory Distress Syndrome Network. Ventilation with lower tidal volumes as compared with traditional tidal volumes for acute lung injury and the acute respiratory distress syndrome. *N Engl J Med.* 2000;342:1301–1308.
130. Villar J, Kacmarek RM, Perez-Mendez L, et al. A high positive end-expiratory pressure, low tidal volume ventilatory strategy improves outcome in persistent acute respiratory distress syndrome: A randomized, controlled trial. *Crit Care Med.* 2006;34:1311–1318.
131. Briel M, Meade M, Mercat A, et al. Higher vs lower positive end-expiratory pressure in patients with acute lung injury and acute respiratory distress syndrome: Systematic review and meta-analysis. *JAMA.* 2010;303:865–873.
132. Sud S, Friedrich JO, Taccone P, et al. Prone ventilation reduces mortality in patients with acute respiratory failure and severe hypoxemia: Systematic review and meta-analysis. *Intensive Care Med.* 2010;36:585–599.
133. Taylor RW, Zimmerman JL, Dellinger RP, et al. Low-dose inhaled nitric oxide in patients with acute lung injury: A randomized controlled trial. *JAMA.* 2004;291:1603–1609.
134. Sokol J, Jacobs SE, Bohn D. Inhaled nitric oxide for acute hypoxic respiratory failure in children and adults: A meta-analysis. *Anesth Analg.* 2003;97:989–998.
135. Wiedemann HP, Wheeler AP, Bernard GR, et al. Comparison of two fluid-management strategies in acute lung injury. *N Engl J Med.* 2006;354:2564–2575.
136. Martin GS, Moss M, Wheeler AP, et al. A randomized, controlled trial of furosemide with or without albumin in hypoproteinemic patients with acute lung injury. *Crit Care Med.* 2005;33:1681–1687.
137. Matthay MA, Brower RG, Carson S, et al. Randomized, placebo-controlled clinical trial of an aerosolized beta-agonist for treatment of acute lung injury. *Am J Respir Crit Care Med.* 2011;184:561–568.
138. Meduri GU, Headley AS, Golden E, et al. Effect of prolonged methylprednisolone therapy in unresolving acute respiratory distress syndrome: A randomized controlled trial. *JAMA.* 1998;280:159–165.
139. Meduri GU, Golden E, Freire AX, et al. Methylprednisolone infusion in early severe ARDS: Results of a randomized controlled trial. *Chest.* 2007;131:954–963.
140. Steinberg KP, Hudson LD, Goodman RB, et al. Efficacy and safety of corticosteroids for persistent acute respiratory distress syndrome. *N Engl J Med.* 2006;354:1671–1684.
141. Papazian L, Forel JM, Gacouin A, et al. Neuromuscular blockers in early acute respiratory distress syndrome. *N Engl J Med.* 2010;363:1107–1116.
142. Noah MA, Peek GJ, Finney SJ, et al. Referral to an extracorporeal membrane oxygenation center and mortality among patients with severe 2009 influenza A(H1N1). *JAMA.* 2011;306:1659–1668.
143. Peek GJ, Elbourne D, Mugford M, et al. Randomised controlled trial and parallel economic evaluation of conventional ventilatory support versus extracorporeal membrane oxygenation for severe adult respiratory failure (CESAR). *Health Technol Assess.* 2010;14:1–46.
144. Bellomo R, Kellum JA, Ronco C. Defining and classifying acute renal failure: From advocacy to consensus and validation of the RIFLE criteria. *Intensive Care Med.* 2007;33:409–413.
145. Bellomo R, Ronco C, Kellum J, et al. Acute renal failure-definition, outcome measures, animal models, fluid therapy, and information technology needs: The Second International Consensus Conference of the Acute Dialysis Quality Initiative (ADQI) Group. *Crit Care.* 2004;8:R204–R212.
146. Singri N, Ahya SN, Levin ML. Acute renal failure. *JAMA.* 2003;289:747–751.
147. Uchino S, Kellum JA, Bellomo R, et al. Acute renal failure in critically ill patients: A multinational, multicenter study. *JAMA.* 2005;294:813–818.
148. Carvounis CP, Nisar S, Guro-Razuman S. Significance of the fractional excretion of urea in the differential diagnosis of acute renal failure. *Kidney Int.* 2002;62:2223–2229.
149. Ho KM, Sheridan DJ. Meta-analysis of frusemide to prevent or treat acute renal failure. *BMJ.* 2006;333:420.
150. Briguori C, Airoldi F, D'Andrea D, et al. Renal Insufficiency Following Contrast Media Administration Trial (REMEDIAL): A randomized comparison of 3 preventive strategies. *Circulation.* 2007;115:1211–1217.
151. Marenzi G, Assanelli E, Marana I, et al. N-acetylcysteine and contrast-induced nephropathy in primary angioplasty. *N Engl J Med.* 2006;354:2773–2782.
152. ACT investigators. Acetylcysteine for prevention of renal outcomes in patients undergoing coronary and peripheral vascular angiography: Main results from the randomized Acetylcysteine for Contrast-induced nephropathy Trial (ACT). *Circulation.* 2011;124:1250–1259.
153. Bellomo R, Cass A, Cole L, et al. Intensity of continuous renal-replacement therapy in critically ill patients. *N Engl J Med.* 2009;361:1627–1638.
154. Palevsky PM, Zhang JH, O'Connor TZ, et al. Intensity of renal support in critically ill patients with acute kidney injury. *N Engl J Med.* 2008;359:7–20.
155. Vinsonneau C, Camus C, Combes A, et al. Continuous venovenous haemodiafiltration versus intermittent haemodialysis for acute renal failure in patients with multiple-organ dysfunction syndrome: A multicentre randomised trial. *Lancet.* 2006;368:379–385.
156. McCowen KC, Malhotra A, Bistrian BR. Stress-induced hyperglycemia. *Crit Care Clin.* 2001;17:107–124.
157. Malmberg K, Norhammar A, Wedel H, et al. Glycometabolic state at admission: Important risk marker of mortality in conventionally treated patients with diabetes mellitus and acute myocardial infarction: Long-term results from the Diabetes and Insulin-Glucose Infusion in Acute Myocardial Infarction (DIGAMI) study. *Circulation.* 1999;99:2626–2632.
158. van den Berghe G, Wouters P, Weekers F, et al. Intensive insulin therapy in the critically ill patients. *N Engl J Med.* 2001;345:1359–1367.
159. Wiener RS, Wiener DC, Larson RJ. Benefits and risks of tight glucose control in critically ill adults: A meta-analysis. *JAMA.* 2008;300:933–944.

160. Finfer S, Chittock DR, Su SY, et al. Intensive versus conventional glucose control in critically ill patients. *N Engl J Med.* 2009;360:1283–1297.
161. Van den Berghe G, de Zegher F, Bouillon R. Clinical review 95: Acute and prolonged critical illness as different neuroendocrine paradigms. *J Clin Endocrinol Metab.* 1998;83:1827–1834.
162. Cooper MS, Stewart PM. Corticosteroid insufficiency in acutely ill patients. *N Engl J Med.* 2003;348:727–734.
163. Hamrahian AH, Oseni TS, Arafah BM. Measurements of serum free cortisol in critically ill patients. *N Engl J Med.* 2004;350:1629–1638.
164. Annane D, Sebille V, Troche G, et al. A 3-level prognostic classification in septic shock based on cortisol levels and cortisol response to corticotropin. *JAMA.* 2000;283:1038–1045.
165. Lipiner-Friedman D, Sprung CL, Laterre PF, et al. Adrenal function in sepsis: The retrospective Corticus cohort study. *Crit Care Med.* 2007;35:1012–1018.
166. Annane D, Cariou A, Maxime V, et al. Corticosteroid treatment and intensive insulin therapy for septic shock in adults: A randomized controlled trial. *JAMA.* 2010;303:341–348.
167. Van den Berghe G, de Zegher F, Lauwers P. Dopamine and the sick euthyroid syndrome in critical illness. *Clin Endocrinol (Oxf).* 1994;41:731–737.
168. De Groot LJ. Dangerous dogmas in medicine: The nonthyroidal illness syndrome. *J Clin Endocrinol Metab.* 1999;84:151–164.
169. Bennett-Guerrero E, Jimenez JL, White WD, et al. Cardiovascular effects of intravenous triiodothyronine in patients undergoing coronary artery bypass graft surgery. A randomized, double-blind, placebo-controlled trial. Duke T3 study group. *JAMA.* 1996;275:687–692.
170. Takala J, Ruokonen E, Webster NR, et al. Increased mortality associated with growth hormone treatment in critically ill adults. *N Engl J Med.* 1999;341:785–792.
171. Corwin HL, Gettinger A, Pearl RG, et al. The CRIT Study: Anemia and blood transfusion in the critically ill–current clinical practice in the United States. *Crit Care Med.* 2004;32:39–52.
172. Vincent JL, Baron JF, Reinhart K, et al. Anemia and blood transfusion in critically ill patients. *JAMA.* 2002;288:1499–1507.
173. Rodriguez RM, Corwin HL, Gettinger A, et al. Nutritional deficiencies and blunted erythropoietin response as causes of the anemia of critical illness. *J Crit Care.* 2001;16:36–41.
174. Adams RC, Lundy JS. Anesthesia in cases of poor surgical risk: Some suggestions for decreasing the risk. *Surg Gynecol Obstet.* 1942;64:1011–1019.
175. Hendrickson JE, Hillyer CD. Noninfectious serious hazards of transfusion. *Anesth Analg.* 2009;108:759–769.
176. Hebert PC, Wells G, Blajchman MA, et al. A multicenter, randomized, controlled clinical trial of transfusion requirements in critical care. Transfusion Requirements in Critical Care Investigators, Canadian Critical Care Trials Group. *N Engl J Med.* 1999;340:409–417.
177. Lacroix J, Hebert PC, Hutchison JS, et al. Transfusion strategies for patients in pediatric intensive care units. *N Engl J Med.* 2007;356:1609–1619.
178. Hutton B, Fergusson D, Tinmouth A, et al. Transfusion rates vary significantly amongst Canadian medical centres. *Can J Anaesth.* 2005;52:581–590.
179. Corwin HL, Gettinger A, Pearl RG, et al. Efficacy of recombinant human erythropoietin in critically ill patients: A randomized controlled trial. *JAMA.* 2002; 288:2827–2835.
180. Corwin HL, Gettinger A, Fabian TC, et al. Efficacy and safety of epoetin alfa in critically ill patients. *N Engl J Med.* 2007;357:965–976.
181. McClave SA, Martindale RG, Vanek VW, et al. Guidelines for the provision and assessment of nutrition support therapy in the adult critically ill patient: Society of Critical Care Medicine (SCCM) and American Society for Parenteral and Enteral Nutrition (A.S.P.E.N.). *JPEN J Parenter Enteral Nutr.* 2009;33:277–316.
182. Kompan L, Kremzar B, Gadzijev E, et al. Effects of early enteral nutrition on intestinal permeability and the development of multiple organ failure after multiple injury. *Intensive Care Med.* 1999;25:157–161.
183. Marik PE, Zaloga GP. Gastric versus post-pyloric feeding: A systematic review. *Crit Care.* 2003;7:R46–R51.
184. MacLeod JB, Lefton J, Houghton D, et al. Prospective randomized control trial of intermittent versus continuous gastric feeds for critically ill trauma patients. *J Trauma.* 2007;63:57–61.
185. Zaloga GP. Parenteral nutrition in adult inpatients with functioning gastrointestinal tracts: Assessment of outcomes. *Lancet.* 2006;367:1101–1111.
186. Singer P, Berger MM, Van den Berghe G, et al. ESPEN guidelines on parenteral nutrition: Intensive care. *Clin Nutr.* 2009;28:387–400.
187. Casaer MP, Mesotten D, Hermans G, et al. Early versus late parenteral nutrition in critically ill adults. *N Engl J Med.* 2011;365:506–517.
188. Rice TW, Wheeler AP, Thompson BT, et al. Enteral omega-3 fatty acid, gamma-linolenic acid, and antioxidant supplementation in acute lung injury. *JAMA.* 2011;306:1574–1581.
189. Stapleton RD, Martin TR, Weiss NS, et al. A phase II randomized placebo-controlled trial of omega-3 fatty acids for the treatment of acute lung injury. *Crit Care Med.* 2011;39:1655–1662.
190. Visser J, Labadarios D, Blaauw R. Micronutrient supplementation for critically ill adults: A systematic review and meta-analysis. *Nutrition.* 2011;27:745–758.
191. Heyland DK, Dhaliwal R, Suchner U, et al. Antioxidant nutrients: A systematic review of trace elements and vitamins in the critically ill patient. *Intensive Care Med.* 2005;31:327–337.
192. Kollef MH, Levy NT, Ahrens TS, et al. The use of continuous i.v. sedation is associated with prolongation of mechanical ventilation. *Chest.* 1998;114:541–548.
193. Brook AD, Ahrens TS, Schaiff R, et al. Effect of a nursing-implemented sedation protocol on the duration of mechanical ventilation. *Crit Care Med.* 1999;27:2609–2615.
194. Kress JP, Pohlman AS, O'Connor MF, et al. Daily interruption of sedative infusions in critically ill patients undergoing mechanical ventilation. *N Engl J Med.* 2000;342:1471–1477.
195. Girard TD, Kress JP, Fuchs BD, et al. Efficacy and safety of a paired sedation and ventilator weaning protocol for mechanically ventilated patients in intensive care (Awakening and Breathing Controlled trial): A randomised controlled trial. *Lancet.* 2008;371:126–134.
196. Strom T, Martinussen T, Toft P. A protocol of no sedation for critically ill patients receiving mechanical ventilation: A randomised trial. *Lancet.* 2010;375:475–480.
197. Treggiari MM, Romand JA, Yanez ND, et al. Randomized trial of light versus deep sedation on mental health after critical illness. *Crit Care Med.* 2009;37:2527–2534.
198. Schweickert WD, Gehlbach BK, Pohlman AS, et al. Daily interruption of sedative infusions and complications of critical illness in mechanically ventilated patients. *Crit Care Med.* 2004;32:1272–1276.
199. Samuelson K, Lundberg D, Fridlund B. Memory in relation to depth of sedation in adult mechanically ventilated intensive care patients. *Intensive Care Med.* 2006;32:660–667.
200. Girard TD, Shintani AK, Jackson JC, et al. Risk factors for post-traumatic stress disorder symptoms following critical illness requiring mechanical ventilation: A prospective cohort study. *Crit Care.* 2007;11:R28.
201. Kress JP, Gehlbach B, Lacy M, et al. The long-term psychological effects of daily sedative interruption on critically ill patients. *Am J Respir Crit Care Med.* 2003;168:1457–1461.
202. Jackson JC, Girard TD, Gordon SM, et al. Long-term cognitive and psychological outcomes in the awakening and breathing controlled trial. *Am J Respir Crit Care Med.* 2010;182:183–191.
203. Ely EW, Truman B, Shintani A, et al. Monitoring sedation status over time in ICU patients: Reliability and validity of the Richmond Agitation-Sedation Scale (RASS). *JAMA.* 2003;289:2983–2991.
204. Ely EW, Shintani A, Truman B, et al. Delirium as a predictor of mortality in mechanically ventilated patients in the intensive care unit. *JAMA.* 2004;291:1753–1762.
205. Ely EW, Inouye SK, Bernard GR, et al. Delirium in mechanically ventilated patients: Validity and reliability of the confusion assessment method for the intensive care unit (CAM-ICU). *JAMA.* 2001;286:2703–2710.
206. Bergeron N, Dubois MJ, Dumont M, et al. Intensive Care Delirium Screening Checklist: Evaluation of a new screening tool. *Intensive Care Med.* 2001;27: 859–864.
207. McCollam JS, O'Neil MG, Norcross ED, et al. Continuous infusions of lorazepam, midazolam, and propofol for sedation of the critically ill surgery trauma patient: A prospective, randomized comparison. *Crit Care Med.* 1999;27:2454–2458.
208. Walder B, Elia N, Henzi I, et al. A lack of evidence of superiority of propofol versus midazolam for sedation in mechanically ventilated critically ill patients: A qualitative and quantitative systematic review. *Anesth Analg.* 2001;92:975–983.
209. Carson SS, Kress JP, Rodgers JE, et al. A randomized trial of intermittent lorazepam versus propofol with daily interruption in mechanically ventilated patients. *Crit Care Med.* 2006;34:1326–1332.
210. Pandharipande PP, Pun BT, Herr DL, et al. Effect of sedation with dexmedetomidine vs lorazepam on acute brain dysfunction in mechanically ventilated patients: The MENDS randomized controlled trial. *JAMA.* 2007;298:2644–2653.
211. Riker RR, Shehabi Y, Bokesch PM, et al. Dexmedetomidine vs midazolam for sedation of critically ill patients: A randomized trial. *JAMA.* 2009;301:489–499.
212. Coursin DB, Maccioli GA. Dexmedetomidine. *Curr Opin Crit Care.* 2001;7: 221–226.
213. Girard TD, Pandharipande PP, Carson SS, et al. Feasibility, efficacy, and safety of antipsychotics for intensive care unit delirium: The MIND randomized, placebo-controlled trial. *Crit Care Med.* 2010;38:428–437.
214. Devlin JW, Roberts RJ, Fong JJ, et al. Efficacy and safety of quetiapine in critically ill patients with delirium: A prospective, multicenter, randomized, double-blind, placebo-controlled pilot study. *Crit Care Med.* 2010;38:419–427.
215. Vincent JL. Nosocomial infections in adult intensive-care units. *Lancet.* 2003; 361:2068–2077.
216. Rouby JJ, Laurent P, Gosnach M, et al. Risk factors and clinical relevance of nosocomial maxillary sinusitis in the critically ill. *Am J Respir Crit Care Med.* 1994; 150:776–783.
217. van Zanten AR, Dixon JM, Nipshagen MD, et al. Hospital-acquired sinusitis is a common cause of fever of unknown origin in orotracheally intubated critically ill patients. *Crit Care.* 2005;9:R583–R590.
218. Cook DJ, Walter SD, Cook RJ, et al. Incidence of and risk factors for ventilator-associated pneumonia in critically ill patients. *Ann Intern Med.* 1998;129: 433–440.
219. Fagon JY, Chastre J, Wolff M, et al. Invasive and noninvasive strategies for management of suspected ventilator-associated pneumonia. A randomized trial. *Ann Intern Med.* 2000;132:621–630.

220. Hoffken G, Niederman MS. Nosocomial pneumonia: The importance of a de-escalating strategy for antibiotic treatment of pneumonia in the ICU. *Chest.* 2002;122:2183–2196.
221. Bekaert M, Timsit JF, Vansteelandt S, et al. Attributable mortality of ventilator-associated pneumonia: A reappraisal using causal analysis. *Am J Respir Crit Care Med.* 2011;184:1133–1139.
222. Collard HR, Saint S, Matthay MA. Prevention of ventilator-associated pneumonia: An evidence-based systematic review. *Ann Intern Med.* 2003;138:494–501.
223. Muscedere J, Rewa O, McKechnie K, et al. Subglottic secretion drainage for the prevention of ventilator-associated pneumonia: A systematic review and meta-analysis. *Crit Care Med.* 2011;39:1985–1991.
224. Chlebicki MP, Safdar N. Topical chlorhexidine for prevention of ventilator-associated pneumonia: A meta-analysis. *Crit Care Med.* 2007;35:595–602.
225. Wood AY, Davit AJ 2nd, Ciraulo DL, et al. A prospective assessment of diagnostic efficacy of blind protective bronchial brushings compared to bronchoscope-assisted lavage, bronchoscope-directed brushings, and blind endotracheal aspirates in ventilator-associated pneumonia. *J Trauma.* 2003;55:825–834.
226. The Canadian Critical Care Trials Group. A randomized trial of diagnostic techniques for ventilator-associated pneumonia. *N Engl J Med.* 2006;355:2619–2630.
227. Pugh R, Grant C, Cooke RP, et al. Short-course versus prolonged-course antibiotic therapy for hospital-acquired pneumonia in critically ill adults. *Cochrane Database Syst Rev.* 2011:CD007577.
228. Renaud B, Brun-Buisson C. Outcomes of primary and catheter-related bacteremia. A cohort and case-control study in critically ill patients. *Am J Respir Crit Care Med.* 2001;163:1584–1590.
229. Pronovost P, Needham D, Berenholtz S, et al. An intervention to decrease catheter-related bloodstream infections in the ICU. *N Engl J Med.* 2006;355:2725–2732.
230. Polderman KH, Girbes AR. Central venous catheter use. Part 2: Infectious complications. *Intensive Care Med.* 2002;28:18–28.
231. Berenholtz SM, Pronovost PJ, Lipsett PA, et al. Eliminating catheter-related bloodstream infections in the intensive care unit. *Crit Care Med.* 2004;32: 2014–2020.
232. Kim JS, Holtom P, Vigen C. Reduction of catheter-related bloodstream infections through the use of a central venous line bundle: Epidemiologic and economic consequences. *Am J Infect Control.* 2011;39:640–646.
233. O'Grady NP, Alexander M, Burns LA, et al. Guidelines for the prevention of intravascular catheter-related infections. *Clin Infect Dis.* 2011;52:e162–e193.
234. Ringberg H, Thoren A, Bredberg A. Evaluation of coagulase-negative staphylococci in blood cultures. A prospective clinical and microbiological study. *Scand J Infect Dis.* 1991;23:315–323.
235. Di Filippo A, De Gaudio AR. Device-related infections in critically ill patients. Part II: Prevention of ventilator-associated pneumonia and urinary tract infections. *J Chemother.* 2003;15:536–542.
236. Johnson JR, Kuskowski MA, Wilt TJ. Systematic review: Antimicrobial urinary catheters to prevent catheter-associated urinary tract infection in hospitalized patients. *Ann Intern Med.* 2006;144:116–126.
237. Eggimann P, Garbino J, Pittet D. Epidemiology of Candida species infections in critically ill non-immunosuppressed patients. *Lancet Infect Dis.* 2003;3:685–702.
238. Meersseman W, Lagrou K, Maertens J, et al. Galactomannan in bronchoalveolar lavage fluid: A tool for diagnosing aspergillosis in intensive care unit patients. *Am J Respir Crit Care Med.* 2008;177:27–34.
239. Verduyn Lunel FM, Meis JF, Voss A. Nosocomial fungal infections: Candidemia. *Diagn Microbiol Infect Dis.* 1999;34:213–220.
240. Echeverria PM, Kett DH, Azoulay E. Candida prophylaxis and therapy in the ICU. *Semin Respir Crit Care Med.* 2011;32:159–173.
241. Eggimann P, Garbino J, Pittet D. Management of Candida species infections in critically ill patients. *Lancet Infect Dis.* 2003;3:772–785.
242. Cook DJ, Fuller HD, Guyatt GH, et al. Risk factors for gastrointestinal bleeding in critically ill patients. Canadian Critical Care Trials Group. *N Engl J Med.* 1994;330:377–381.
243. Metz CA, Livingston DH, Smith JS, et al. Impact of multiple risk factors and ranitidine prophylaxis on the development of stress-related upper gastrointestinal bleeding: A prospective, multicenter, double-blind, randomized trial. The Ranitidine Head Injury Study Group. *Crit Care Med.* 1993;21:1844–1849.
244. Cook D, Heyland D, Griffith L, et al. Risk factors for clinically important upper gastrointestinal bleeding in patients requiring mechanical ventilation. Canadian Critical Care Trials Group. *Crit Care Med.* 1999;27:2812–2817.
245. Cook D, Guyatt G, Marshall J, et al. A comparison of sucralfate and ranitidine for the prevention of upper gastrointestinal bleeding in patients requiring mechanical ventilation. Canadian Critical Care Trials Group. *N Engl J Med.* 1998;338:791–797.
246. Messori A, Trippoli S, Vaiani M, et al. Bleeding and pneumonia in intensive care patients given ranitidine and sucralfate for prevention of stress ulcer: Meta-analysis of randomised controlled trials. *BMJ.* 2000;321:1103–1106.
247. Morgan D. Intravenous proton pump inhibitors in the critical care setting. *Crit Care Med.* 2002;30:S369–S372.
248. Anderson FA Jr, Spencer FA. Risk factors for venous thromboembolism. *Circulation.* 2003;107:I9–I16.
249. Joffe HV, Goldhaber SZ. Upper-extremity deep vein thrombosis. *Circulation.* 2002;106:1874–1880.
250. Geerts W, Selby R. Prevention of venous thromboembolism in the ICU. *Chest.* 2003;124:357S–363S.
251. Kearon C, Ginsberg JS, Hirsh J. The role of venous ultrasonography in the diagnosis of suspected deep venous thrombosis and pulmonary embolism. *Ann Intern Med.* 1998;129:1044–1049.
252. Goldhaber SZ, Elliott CG. Acute pulmonary embolism: Part I: Epidemiology, pathophysiology, and diagnosis. *Circulation.* 2003;108:2726–2729.
253. Anderson DR, Kahn SR, Rodger MA, et al. Computed tomographic pulmonary angiography vs ventilation-perfusion lung scanning in patients with suspected pulmonary embolism: A randomized controlled trial. *JAMA.* 2007;298:2743–2753.
254. Kollef MH, Zahid M, Eisenberg PR. Predictive value of a rapid semiquantitative D-dimer assay in critically ill patients with suspected venous thromboembolic disease. *Crit Care Med.* 2000;28:414–420.
255. Goldhaber SZ, Elliott CG. Acute pulmonary embolism: Part II: Risk stratification, treatment, and prevention. *Circulation.* 2003;108:2834–2838.
256. Deem S. Intensive-care-unit-acquired muscle weakness. *Respir Care.* 2006; 51:1042–1052, discussion 52–53.
257. Stevens RD, Dowdy DW, Michaels RK, et al. Neuromuscular dysfunction acquired in critical illness: A systematic review. *Intensive Care Med.* 2007;33:1876–1891.
258. Herridge MS, Cheung AM, Tansey CM, et al. One-year outcomes in survivors of the acute respiratory distress syndrome. *N Engl J Med.* 2003;348:683–693.
259. Deem S, Lee CM, Curtis JR. Acquired neuromuscular disorders in the intensive care unit. *Am J Respir Crit Care Med.* 2003;168:735–739.
260. Hermans G, Wilmer A, Meersseman W, et al. Impact of intensive insulin therapy on neuromuscular complications and ventilator dependency in the medical intensive care unit. *Am J Respir Crit Care Med.* 2007;175:480–489.

CHAPTER

Acute Pain Management

STEPHEN M. MACRES • PETER G. MOORE • SCOTT M. FISHMAN

Key Points

1. The inadequate relief of postoperative pain has adverse physiologic effects that can contribute to significant morbidity and mortality, resulting in the delay of patient recovery and return to daily activities.
2. The pain pathway is not "hardwired" and nociceptive input is not passively transmitted from the periphery to the brain. Tissue injury tends to fuel neuroplastic changes within the nervous system, which results in both peripheral and central sensitization.
3. In order for preventive analgesia to be successful, three critical principles must be adhered to: (1) The depth of analgesia must be adequate enough to block all nociceptive input during surgery, (2) the analgesic technique must be extensive enough to include the entire surgical field, and (3) the duration of analgesia must include both the surgical and postsurgical periods.
4. The various opioid analgesics available today have distinct pharmacologic differences that we can credit to their intricate interaction with the three main opioid receptors mu, delta, and kappa. The opioid receptors are members of a G protein–coupled (guanosine triphosphate regulatory proteins) receptor family, which signals via a second messenger such as cyclic adenosine monophosphate or an ion channel.
5. The therapeutic benefit of nonsteroidal anti-inflammatory drugs is believed to be mediated through the inhibition of cyclooxygenase enzymes, types 1 and 2, which convert arachidonic acid to prostaglandins.
6. Short-term use of parecoxib and valdecoxib in patients following coronary artery bypass surgery is associated with an increased risk of thromboembolic events. The authors, therefore, do not recommend prescribing a cyclooxygenase 2 inhibitor for patients with a known history of coronary artery disease or cerebrovascular disease.
7. The five variables associated with all modes of patient-controlled analgesia include (1) bolus dose, (2) incremental (demand) dose, (3) lockout interval, (4) background infusion rate, and (5) 1- and 4-hour limits. A typical patient-controlled analgesia regimen in an otherwise healthy adult would be an incremental dose of 1 to 2 mg of morphine with an 8- to 10-minute lockout. The authors do not recommend a background infusion of opioid in the opioid-naive patient.
8. *Epidural analgesia* is a critical component of multimodal perioperative pain management and improved patient outcome. Meta-analyses investigating the efficacy of epidural analgesia found epidural analgesia to be superior to systemically administered opioids.
9. Continuous peripheral nerve block has proven to be an effective technique for postoperative pain management, which is superior to opioid analgesia with fewer opioid-related side effects and rare neurologic and infectious complications.
10. Should a perioperative nerve injury occur, it is incumbent on the physician to determine which combination of anesthetic, surgical, and patient risk factors are involved in any nerve injury and to not assume a priori that the regional anesthetic is the culprit.
11. The opioid-dependent patient is often identified just moments prior to surgery and the anesthesia team needs to be innovative. The anesthesiologist needs to be flexible enough to tailor an individual anesthetic that incorporates a multimodal approach, combining regional anesthesia with general anesthesia and nonopioid coanalgesics with opioid analgesics. Opioids remain the mainstay of perioperative pain management, and an adequate dose of opioid needs to be maintained to avoid precipitating withdrawal symptoms.

12 The key components to establishing a successful perioperative pain management service begins with an institutional commitment to support the service. The team must be built around a physician leader with training and experience in pain medicine. There must be other anesthesiologists available to support the service.

Multimedia

1 Nociceptive Pathways
2 Pain Sensitization
3 Pain Processing
4 Universal Pain Assessment Tool
5 Brachial Plexus
6 Interscalene Block
7 Supraclavicular Block
8 Femoral Nerve Block
9 Ultrasound Guided Saphenous Nerve Block
10 Ultrasound Guided Poplietal Nerve Block
11 TAP Block

INTRODUCTION

There are approximately 75 million surgical procedures performed each year in the United States and more than half are performed in the inpatient setting. Appropriate management of acute perioperative pain using multimodal or balanced analgesia is therefore crucial. In 1992 clinical practice guidelines were promulgated by the Agency for Health Care Policy and Research, which provided guidelines for physicians for the treatment of acute pain.[1] Soon thereafter the American Society of Anesthesiologists developed treatment guidelines for acute postoperative pain, which have been updated and amended as of 2012.[2] Despite significant advances in our knowledge and treatment of acute pain and dissemination of these guidelines, significant deficits continue to persist and the management of acute postoperative pain is still less than optimal.

1 The inadequate relief of postoperative pain has adverse physiologic effects that can contribute to significant morbidity and mortality, resulting in the delay of patient recovery and return to daily activities.[3] In addition, poor postoperative pain control contributes to patient dissatisfaction with the surgical experience and may have adverse psychological consequences.[4] Poorly managed postoperative pain can also increase the incidence of persistent postoperative pain conditions. Because aggressive treatment of acute postoperative pain is considered to be so beneficial, the Joint Commission on Accreditation of Healthcare Organizations has declared that "pain is the fifth vital sign" and all institutions seeking accreditation from this group must develop pain management programs.

ACUTE PAIN DEFINED

Acute pain has been defined as "the normal, predicted, physiologic response to an adverse chemical, thermal, or mechanical stimulus."[5] Generally, acute pain resolves within 1 month. However, poorly managed acute pain that might occur following surgery can produce pathophysiologic processes in both the peripheral and central nervous systems that have the potential to produce chronicity.[4] Acute pain-induced change in the central nervous system is known as *neuronal plasticity.* This can result in sensitization of the nervous system resulting in allodynia and hyperalgesia. Surgical procedures that can be associated with chronic painful conditions include amputation of a limb, lateral thoracotomy, inguinal herniorrhaphy, abdominal hysterectomy, saphenous vein stripping, open cholecystectomy, nephrectomy, and mastectomy.[4]

ANATOMY OF ACUTE PAIN

1 The nociceptive pathway is an afferent (Fig. 56-1) three-neuron dual ascending (e.g., anterolateral and dorsal column medial lemniscal pathways) system, with descending modulation (Fig. 56-2) from the cortex, thalamus, and brainstem.[6] Nociceptors are free nerve endings located in skin, muscle, bone, and connective tissue

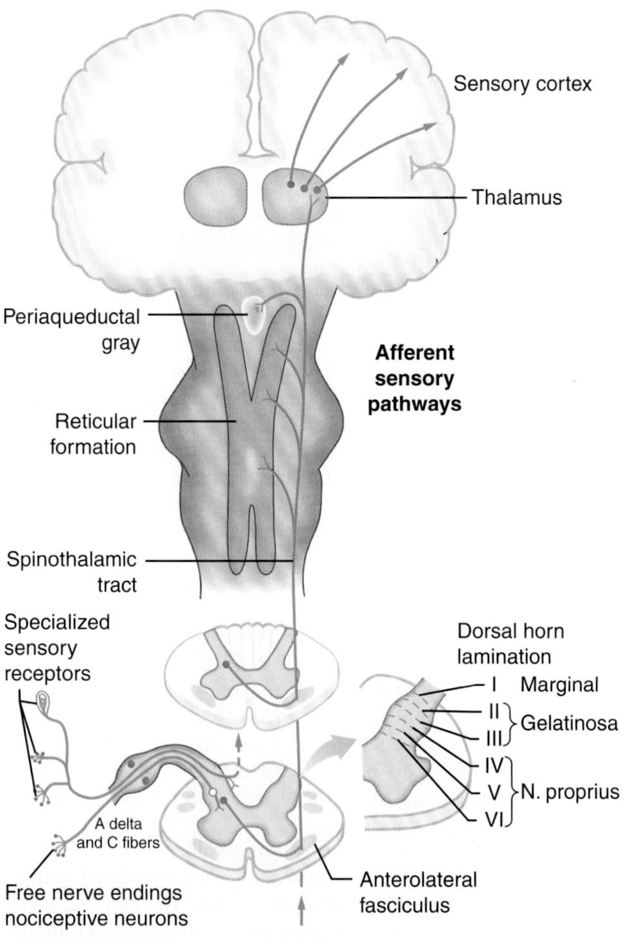

FIGURE 56-1. Afferent nociceptive pathway.

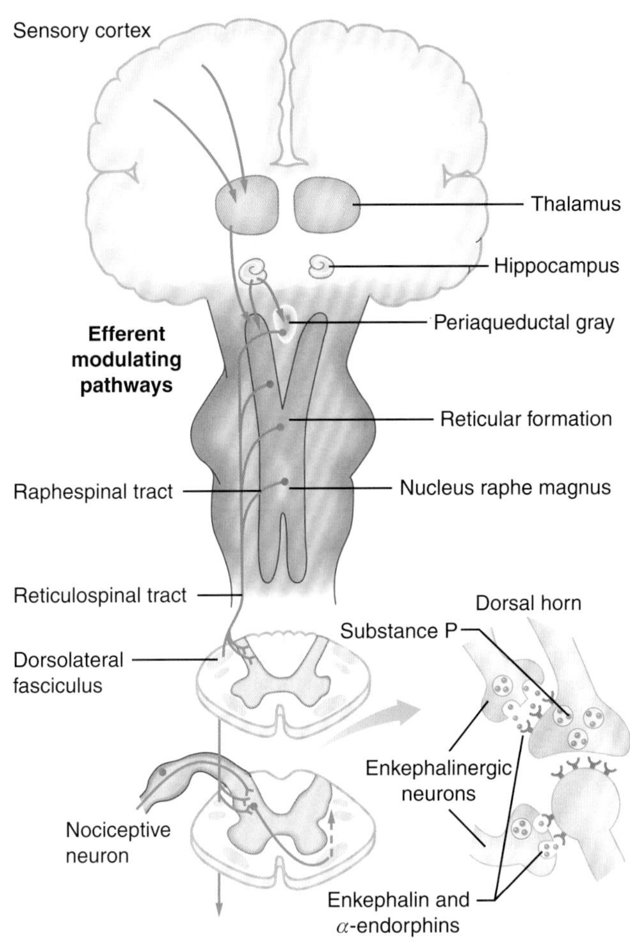

FIGURE 56-2. Efferent pathways involved in nociceptive regulation.

TABLE 56-1. PRIMARY AFFERENT NERVES

Fiber Class[a]	Velocity	Effective Stimuli
Aβ (myelinated) (12–20 μ dia)	Group II (>40–50 m/s)	Low-threshold mechanoreceptors Specialized nerve endings (pacinian corpuscles)
Aδ (myelinated) (1–4 μ dia)	Group III (10 < × < 40 m/s)	Low-threshold mechanical or thermal High-threshold mechanical or thermal Specialized nerve endings
C (unmyelinated) (0.5–1.5 μ dia)	Group IV (<2 m/s)	High-threshold thermal, mechanical, and chemical Free nerve endings

[a]Aβ/Aδ/C is the Erlanger–Gasser classification and refers to axon size; II/III/IV is the Lloyd–Hunt classification and is defined on conduction velocity in muscle afferents. Because of the relationship between size and state of myelination with conduction velocity, these designations are often used interchangeably.
From: Warfield CA, Bajwa ZH, eds. *Principles and Practice of Pain Medicine.* 2nd ed. New York, NY: McGraw Hill; 2004, p14.

with cell bodies located in the dorsal root ganglia. The first-order neurons that make up the dual ascending system have their origins in the periphery as A delta and polymodal C fibers (Table 56-1). A delta fibers transmit "first pain," which is described as sharp or stinging in nature and is well localized. Polymodal C fibers transmit "second pain," which is more diffuse in nature and is associated with the affective and motivational aspects of pain. First-order neurons synapse on second-order neurons in the dorsal horn primarily within laminas I, II, and V, where they release excitatory amino acids and neuropeptides (Figs. 56-3 and 56-4). Some fibers can ascend or descend in Lissauer's tract prior to terminating on neurons that project to higher centers. Second-order neurons consist of nociceptive-specific and wide dynamic-range (WDR) neurons. Nociceptive-specific neurons are located primarily in lamina I, respond only to noxious stimuli, and are thought to be involved in the sensory-discriminative aspects of pain. WDR neurons are predominately located in laminae IV, V, and VI, respond to both nonnoxious and noxious input, and are involved with the affective–motivational component of pain. Axons of both nociceptive-specific and WDR neurons ascend the spinal cord via the dorsal column-medial lemniscus and the anterior lateral spinothalamic tract to synapse on third-order neurons in the contralateral thalamus, which then project to the somatosensory cortex where nociceptive input is perceived as pain (Fig. 56-1).

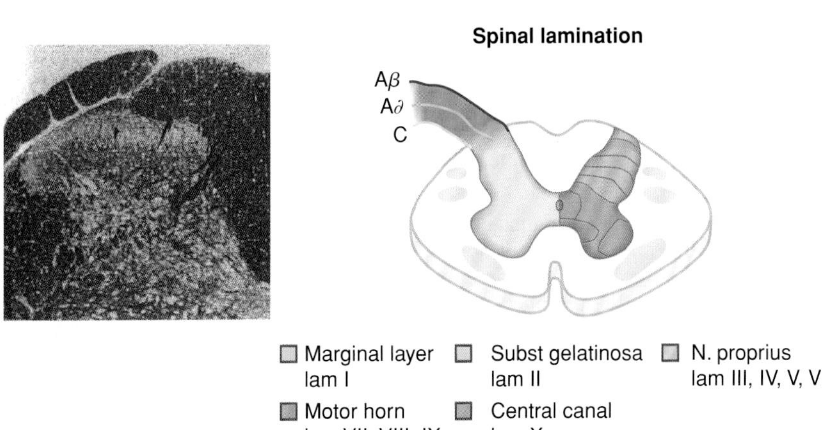

FIGURE 56-3. Schematic on the right showing the Rexed lamination and the approximate organization of the approach of the afferent to the spinal cord as they enter at the dorsal root entry zone and then penetrate into the dorsal horn to terminate in laminae I and II (A/C) or penetrate more deeply to loop upward to terminate as high as the dorsum of lamina III (Aβ). Inset on the left shows histologic appearance of the left dorsal quadrant, and large, myelinated axons. (From: Warfield CA, Bajwa ZH, eds. *Principles and Practice of Pain Medicine.* 2nd ed. New York, NY: McGraw Hill Medical Publishing Division; 2004.)

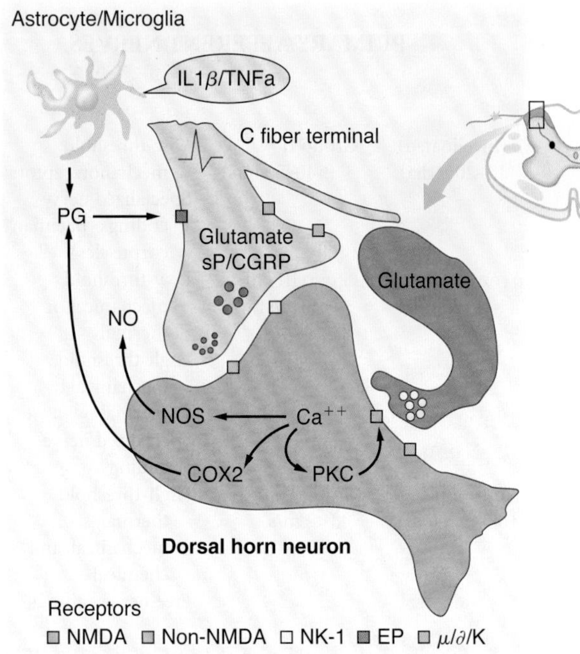

FIGURE 56-4. Schematic summarizing the organization of dorsal horn systems that contribute to the processing of nociceptive information. (1) Primary afferent C fibers release peptide (e.g., substance P [sP], calcitonin gene–related peptide [CGRP], and so on) and excitatory amino acid (glutamate) products. Small dorsal root ganglion (DRG) cells, as well as some postsynaptic elements contain nitric oxide synthase (NOS) and are able, upon depolarization, to release NO (nitric oxide). (2) Peptides and excitatory amino acids evoke excitation in second-order neurons. For glutamate, direct monosynaptic excitation is mediated by non-*N*-methyl-D-aspartate (NMDA) receptors (i.e., acute primary afferent excitation of WDR neurons is not mediated by the NMDA or neurokinin 1 (NK-1) receptor). (3) Interneurons excited by afferent barrage induce excitation in second-order neurons via an NMDA receptor. This leads to a marked increase in intracellular Ca^{2+} and the activation of kinases and phosphorylating enzymes. Prostaglandins (PGs) generated by cyclooxygenase-2 (COX-2) and NO by NOS are formed and released. These agents diffuse extracellulary and facilitate transmitter release (retrograde transmission) from primary and nonprimary afferent terminals, either by a direct cellular action (e.g., NO) or by an interaction with a specific class of receptors (e.g., EP receptors for prostanoids). (4) Nonneuronal sources of prostaglandins may include activated astrocytes and microglia that are stimulated by circulating cytokines, which are released secondary to peripheral nerve injury and inflammation. Terminal excitability can be altered by activation of a variety of receptors located on the sensory terminal, including those for, μ, δ, and κ opioids. (From: Warfield CA, Bajwa ZH, eds. *Principles and Practice of Pain Medicine*. 2nd ed. New York, NY: McGraw Hill Medical Publishing Division; 2004.)

Pain Processing

A key development in our understanding of pain processing is
2 that the pain pathway is not "hardwired" and nociceptive input is not passively transmitted from the periphery to the brain.[7] Tissue injury tends to fuel neuroplastic changes within the nervous system, which results in both peripheral and central sensitization.
2 Clinically this can manifest as *hyperalgesia,* which is defined as an exaggerated pain response to a normally painful stimulus, and *allodynia,* which is defined as a painful response to a typically nonpainful stimulus[7] (Fig. 56-5).

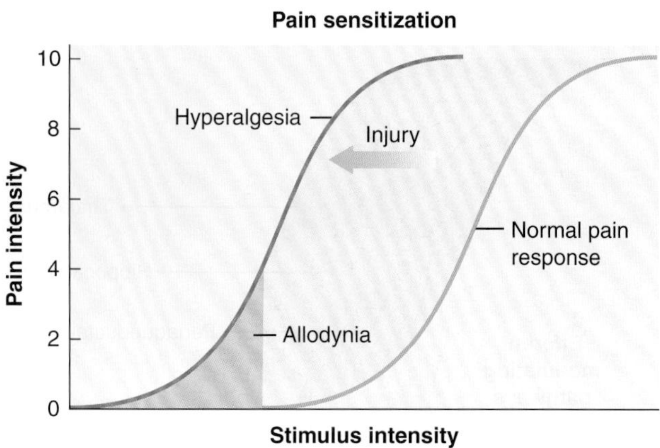

FIGURE 56-5. Pain sensitization. (Obtained with permission from: Dave Klemm, http:www.georgetown.edu/dml/facs/graphics/index.htm.)

3 The four elements of pain processing include (1) transduction, (2) transmission, (3) modulation, and (4) perception (Fig. 56-6). *Transduction* is the event whereby noxious thermal, chemical, or mechanical stimuli are converted into an action potential. *Transmission* occurs when the action potential is conducted through the nervous system via the first-, second-, and third-order neurons, which have cell bodies located in the dorsal root ganglion, dorsal horn, and thalamus, respectively. *Modulation* of pain transmission involves altering afferent neural transmission along the pain pathway. The dorsal horn of the spinal cord is the most common site for modulation of the pain pathway, and modulation can involve either *inhibition* or *augmentation* of the pain signals.[6] Examples of *inhibitory* spinal modulation include (1) release of inhibitory neurotransmitters such as γ-amino butyric acid (GABA) and glycine by intrinsic spinal neurons, and (2) activation of descending efferent neuronal pathways from the motor cortex, hypothalamus, periaqueductal gray matter, and the nucleus raphe magnus, which results in the release of norepinephrine, serotonin, and endorphins in the dorsal horn. Spinal modulation, which results in *augmentation* of pain pathways, is manifested as central sensitization, which is a consequence of neuronal plasticity. The phenomenon of "wind-up" is a specific example of central plasticity that results from repetitive C-fiber stimulation of WDR neurons in the dorsal horn. *Perception* of pain is the final common pathway, which results from the integration of painful input into the somatosensory and limbic cortices. Generally speaking, traditional analgesic therapies have only targeted pain *perception.* A *multimodal approach* to pain therapy should target all four elements of the pain processing pathway.

CHEMICAL MEDIATORS OF TRANSDUCTION AND TRANSMISSION

Tissue damage following surgical procedures leads to the activation of small nociceptive nerve endings and local inflammatory cells (e.g., macrophages, mast cells, lymphocytes, and platelets) in the periphery. Antidromic release of substance P and glutamate from small nociceptive afferents results in vasodilation, extravasation of plasma proteins, and stimulation of inflammatory cells to release numerous algogenic substances (Table 56-2 and Fig. 56-7). This chemical milieu will both directly produce pain transduction via nociceptor stimulation as well as facilitate pain transduction

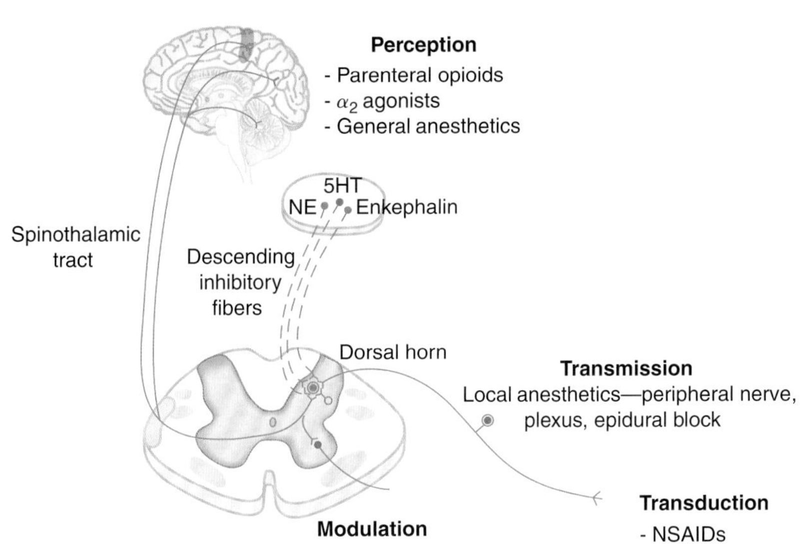

FIGURE 56-6. The four elements of pain processing: Transduction, transmission, modulation, and perception. 5HT, serotonin; NE, norepinephrine; NMDA, *N*-methyl-D-asparate; NSAIDs, nonsteroidal anti-inflammatory drugs; CCK, cholecystokin; NO, nitric oxide.

by increasing the excitability of nociceptors. *Peripheral sensitization* of polymodal C fibers and high-threshold mechanoreceptors by these chemicals leads to *primary hyperalgesia*, which by definition is an exaggerated response to pain at the site of injury.

As is the case in the periphery, the dorsal horn of the spinal cord contains numerous transmitters and receptors involved in pain processing. Three classes of transmitter compounds integral to pain transmission include (1) the excitatory amino acids glutamate and aspartate, (2) the excitatory neuropeptides substance P and neurokinin A, and (3) the inhibitory amino acids glycine and GABA. The various pain receptors include (1) the NMDA (*N*-methyl-D-aspartate), (2) the AMPA (α-amino-3-hydroxy-5-methylisoxazole-4-proprionic acid), (3) the kainate, and (4) the metabotropic (Fig. 56-8).

TABLE 56-2. **ALGOGENIC SUBSTANCES**

Substance	Source	Effect
Bradykinin	Macrophages and plasma kininogen	Activates nociceptors
Serotonin	Platelets	Activates nociceptors
Histamine	Platelets and mast cells	Produces vasodilation, edema and pruritus Potentiates the response of nociceptors to bradykinin
Prostaglandin	Tissue injury and cyclooxygenase pathway	Sensitize nociceptors
Leukotriene	Tissue injury and lipooxygenase pathway	Sensitize nociceptors
Excess H^+ ions	Tissue injury and ischemia	Increases pain and hyperalgesia associated with inflammation
Cytokines (e.g., interleukins and tissue necrosis factor)	Macrophages	Excite and sensitize nociceptors
Adenosine	Tissue injury	Pain and hyperalgesia
Neurotransmitters (e.g., glutamate and substance P)	Antidromic release by peripheral nerve terminals following tissue injury	Substance P activates macrophages and Mast cells Glutamate activates nociceptors
Nerve growth factor	Macrophages	Stimulates mast cells to release histamine and serotonin Induces heat hyperalgesia Sensitizes nociceptors

Data derived from: Dougherty PM, Raja SN. Neurochemistry of somatosensory and pain processing. In: Benzon HT, Raja SN, Molloy RE, et al., eds. *Essentials of Pain Medicine and Regional Anesthesia.* Elsevier, Churchill Livingstone; 2005:7.

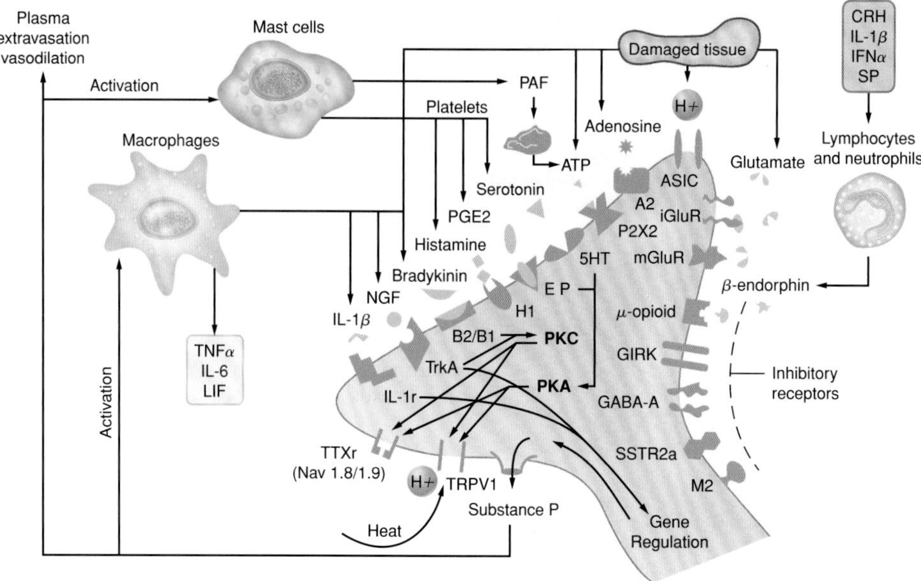

FIGURE 56-7. Schematic of the neurochemistry of somatosensory processing at peripheral sensory nerve endings. (From: Benzon HT, Raja SN, Molloy RE, et al., eds. *Essentials of Pain Medicine and Regional Anesthesia.* 2nd ed. Elsevier, Churchill Livingstone; 2005:8.)

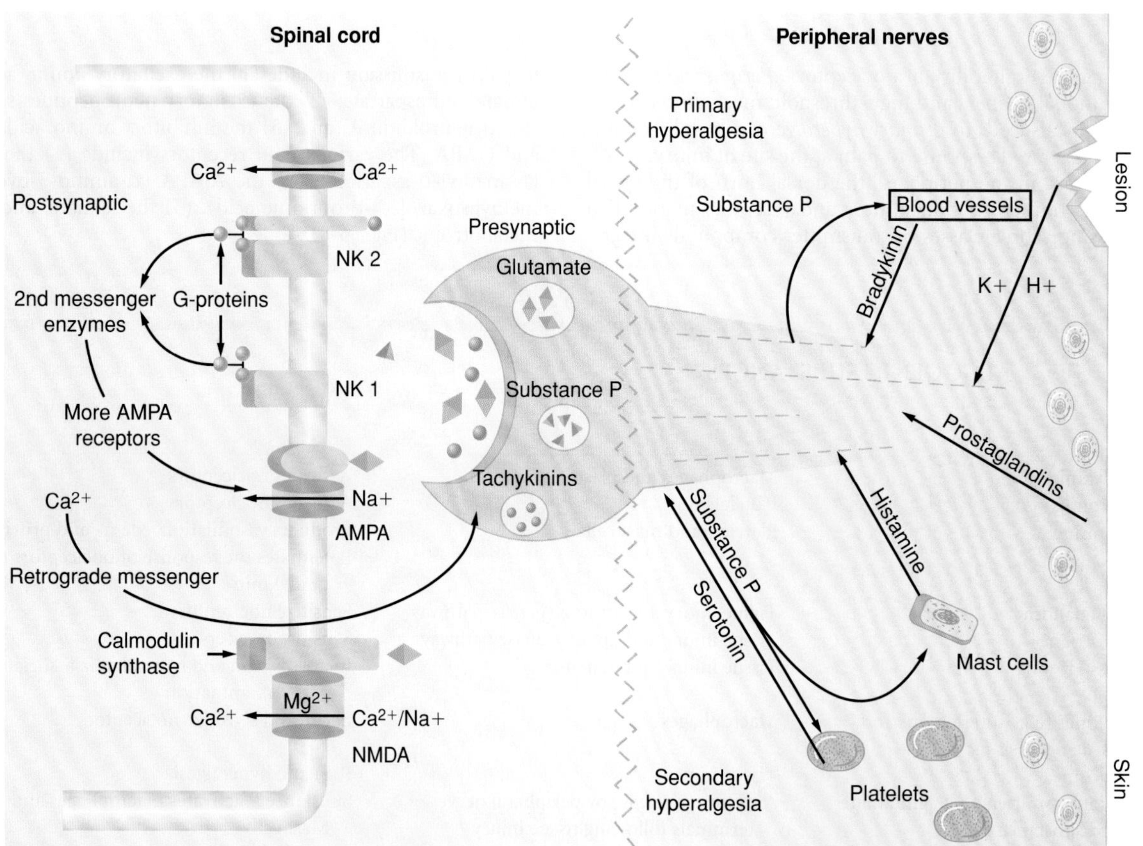

FIGURE 56-8. Schematic representation of peripheral and spinal mechanism involved in neuroplasticity. Primary hyperalgesia results from tissue release of toxic substances. These toxic substances spread to adjacent tissues, prolonging the hyperalgesic state (secondary hyperalgesia). As C fiber terminals increase in frequency of release of neurotransmitters, such as glutamate, substance P, tachykinins, brain-derived neurotrophic factor, and calcitonin gene–related peptide, the effects of these neurotransmitters are summated, resulting in prolonged depolarizations of second-order neurons ("wind-up"). Function changes at the second-order neuron occur as a result of neurotransmitter binding to postsynaptic receptors, which results in activity-dependent plasticity of the spinal cord. AMPA, α-amino-3-hydroxy-5-methyl-4-isoxazole propionic acid; NK, neurokinin; NMDA, *N*-methyl-D-asparate.

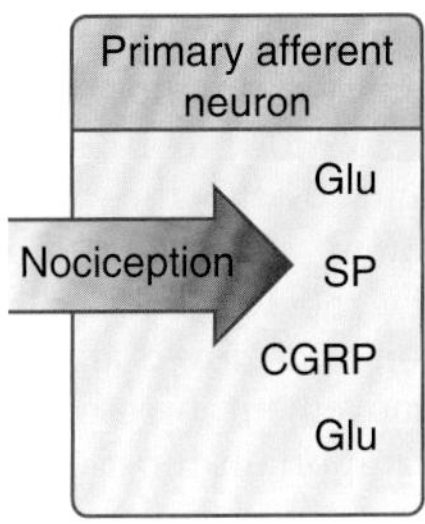

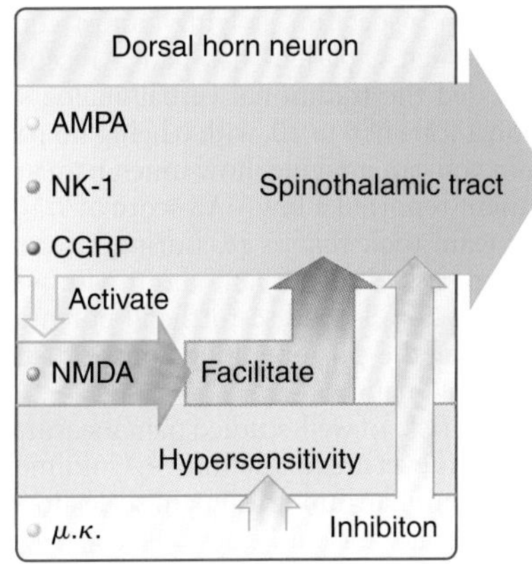

FIGURE 56-9. Primary nociceptive transmission in the spinal cord. Primary afferent nociceptive input is transmitted via α-amino-3-hydroxy-5-methyl-4-isoxazole propionic acid (AMPA), neurokinin-1 (NK1), and calcitonin gene–related peptide (CGRP) synapses, whose signals work their way to the thalamus. Glutaminergic (*N*-methyl-D-asparate [NMDA]) synapses do not participate significantly in primary nociceptive transmission, but instead play a crucial role in spinal sensitization. Accordingly, even after complete NMDA blockade in the spinal cord, primary afferent nociceptive information is transmitted to the thalamus. NMDA antagonists thus have an antihyperalgesic rather than an analgesic effect in the spinal cord. Glu, glutamate; SP, substance P. (Reprinted from: International Association for the Study of Pain: Pain Control Updates. *IASP Newletter* 2005;13(2):3, with permission.)

The AMPA and kainate receptors, which are sodium channel dependent, are essential for fast synaptic afferent input. On the other hand, the NMDA receptor, which is calcium channel dependent, is only activated following prolonged depolarization of the cell membrane. Release of substance P into the spinal cord will remove the magnesium block on the channel of the NMDA receptor giving glutamate free access to the NMDA receptor. Repetitive C-fiber stimulation of WDR neurons in the dorsal horn at intervals of 0.5 to 1 Hz can precipitate the occurrence of wind-up and *central sensitization* (Fig. 56-9). This leads to *secondary hyperalgesia,* which, by definition, is an increased pain response evoked by stimuli outside the area of injury.

THE SURGICAL STRESS RESPONSE

Although similar, postoperative pain and the surgical stress response are not the same. Surgical stress causes release of cytokines (e.g., interleukin-1, interleukin-6, and tumor necrosis factor-α) and precipitates adverse neuroendocrine and sympathoadrenal responses, resulting in detrimental physiologic responses, particularly in high-risk patients.[4]

The increased secretion of the catabolic hormones such as cortisol, glucagon, growth hormone, and catecholamines and the decreased secretion of the anabolic hormones such as insulin and testosterone, characterize the neuroendocrine response. The end result of this is hyperglycemia and a negative nitrogen balance, the consequences of which include poor wound healing, muscle wasting, fatigue, and impaired immunocompetency.

The sympathoadrenal response has detrimental effects on numerous organ systems; these are listed in Table 56-3.[8]

TABLE 56-3. CONSEQUENCES OF POORLY MANAGED ACUTE PAIN

Cardiovascular	Tachycardia, hypertension, and increase in cardiac work load
Pulmonary	Respiratory muscle spasm (splinting), decrease in vital capacity, atelectasis, hypoxia, and increased risk of pulmonary infection
Gastrointestinal	Postoperative ileus
Renal	Increased risk of oliguria and urinary retention
Coagulation	Increased risk of thromboemboli
Immunologic	Impaired immune function
Muscular	Muscle weakness and fatigue. Limited mobility can increase the risk of thromboembolism
Psychological	Anxiety, fear, and frustration results in poor patient satisfaction

Data derived from: Joshi GP, Ogunnaike BO. Consequences of inadequate postoperative pain relief and chronic persistent postoperative pain. *Anesthesiol Clin North America.* 2005;23:21; Rowlingson JC. Update on acute pain management. International Anesthesia Research Society Review Course Lectures. 2006:95; Kehlet H. Multimodal approach to control postoperative pathophysiology and rehabilitation. *Br J Anaesth.* 1997;78:606.

PREVENTIVE ANALGESIA

Preventive analgesia includes any antinociceptive regimen delivered at any time during the perioperative period that will attenuate pain-induced sensitization. The term "preventive analgesia" replaces the older terminology "preemptive analgesia", which is defined as an analgesic regimen that is administered prior to surgical incision and is more effective at pain relief than the same regimen administered after surgery. Although use of the term preemptive analgesia has been popular in the past, evidence of its clinical benefit in humans has been mixed and the term should be considered obsolete. The goal of preventive analgesia is to block the development of sustained pain. Theoretically, this occurs by preventing NMDA receptor activation in the dorsal horn that is associated with wind-up, facilitation, central sensitization expansion of receptive fields, and long-term potentiation, all of which can lead to a chronic pain
3 state.[7] In order for preventive analgesia to be successful, three critical principles must be adhered to: (1) The depth of analgesia must be adequate enough to block all nociceptive input during surgery, (2) the analgesic technique must be extensive enough to include the entire surgical field, and (3) the duration of analgesia must include both the surgical and postsurgical periods. Patients with pre-existing chronic pain may not respond as well to these techniques because of pre-existing sensitization of the nervous system.

STRATEGIES FOR ACUTE PAIN MANAGEMENT

The majority of postoperative pain is nociceptive in character, but there are a small percentage of patients who can experience neuropathic pain postoperatively. It is critical to recognize this fact because patients with neuropathic pain are at increased risk of progressing to a chronic pain state. Neuropathic pain is a result of accidental nerve injury secondary to cutting, traction compression, or entrapment.[4] Clinical features may include continuous burning, paroxysmal shooting, or electric pain with associated allodynia, hyperalgesia, and dysesthesias. There can be a delay in the onset of the pain, and it can follow a nondermatomal distribution. Surgical procedures that are a relatively high risk for neuropathic pain include limb amputations, breast surgery, gallbladder surgery, thoracic surgery, and inguinal hernia repair.[4] Nociceptive pain responds best to opioids, nonsteroidal anti-inflammatory drugs (NSAIDs), para-aminophenol agents, and regional anesthesia techniques.[10] Neuropathic pain, on the other hand, may benefit from the addition of the nonopioid analgesic adjuvants such as the NMDA receptor antagonists, α_2-agonists, and the α_2–δ subunit calcium channel ligands, which will be discussed in detail.

Strategies for acute pain management should also consider the sex of the patient as sex differences appear to exist for pain perception as well as response to opioid analgesics. Evidence suggests that women experience more pain following surgery than men, and therefore require more morphine to achieve a similar level of pain relief.[11]

ASSESSMENT OF ACUTE PAIN

The need for assessment of the patient in pain is illustrated by the postoperative patient who is said to be relatively pain-free, but who, on inspection, is lying almost completely still in bed. Too often, such a patient has had a recent cursory evaluation that included the traditional verbal analog score (VAS) 0 to 10 scale ("on a scale of 0 to 10, with 0 being no pain and 10 being the worst pain you can imagine, how much pain are you in" from which the patient reported a low VAS score of 1/10) (Fig. 56-10). The treating team took that as reassuring information and moved along. No one asked the patient about pain with movement, breathing, moving bowels, and so forth, all potentially important functional goals for the postoperative course that may be undermined by untreated pain.

A variety of well-studied pain measurement scales exist that can be helpful yet are not definitive. Unidimensional instruments such as the familiar numerical pain scale already mentioned, the visual analog scale, and the "faces" (Fig. 56-10) pain rating scale can provide some degree of guidance about a patient's experience of pain, but all of these are completely subjective and are open to wide variation between subjects and within subjects at different times.

Multidimensional instruments, such as the McGill Pain Questionnaire or the Brief Pain Inventory provide a broader picture of a patient's experience, but are usually more cumbersome to administer and, in the end, suffer the same limitations as all other attempts to measure pain. A number of tools to assess cancer-related and noncancer chronic pain have been advanced and validated.[12] Most of these focus on persistent background pain and do not help identify intermittent or breakthrough pain. Several assessment scales specifically address breakthrough or episodic pain. The Breakthrough Pain Questionnaire was introduced by Portenoy and Hagen to assess breakthrough pain in cancer

FIGURE 56-10. Linear verbal analog score and faces pain assessment tool.

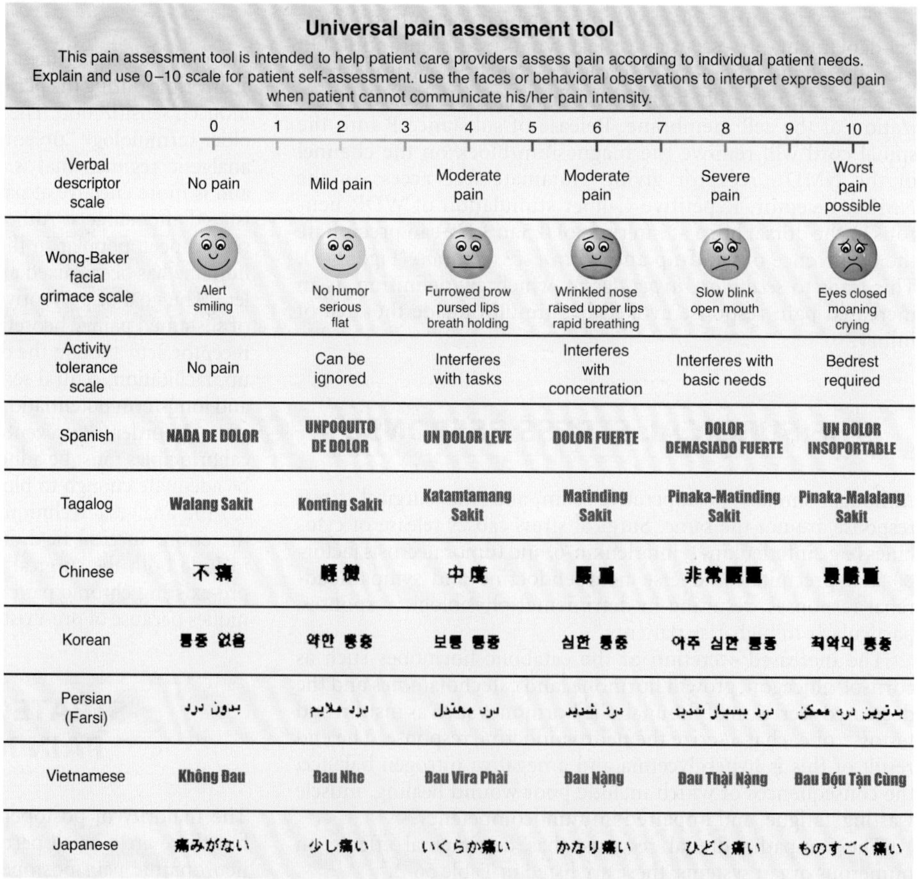

Universal pain assessment tool

This pain assessment tool is intended to help patient care providers assess pain according to individual patient needs. Explain and use 0–10 scale for patient self-assessment. use the faces or behavioral observations to interpret expressed pain when patient cannot communicate his/her pain intensity.

	0	1	2	3	4	5	6	7	8	9	10
Verbal descriptor scale	No pain		Mild pain		Moderate pain		Moderate pain		Severe pain		Worst pain possible
Wong-Baker facial grimace scale	Alert smiling		No humor serious flat		Furrowed brow pursed lips breath holding		Wrinkled nose raised upper lips rapid breathing		Slow blink open mouth		Eyes closed moaning crying
Activity tolerance scale	No pain		Can be ignored		Interferes with tasks		Interferes with concentration		Interferes with basic needs		Bedrest required
Spanish	**NADA DE DOLOR**		**UNPOQUITO DE DOLOR**		**UN DOLOR LEVE**		**DOLOR FUERTE**		**DOLOR DEMASIADO FUERTE**		**UN DOLOR INSOPORTABLE**
Tagalog	**Walang Sakit**		**Konting Sakit**		**Katamtamang Sakit**		**Matinding Sakit**		**Pinaka-Matinding Sakit**		**Pinaka-Malalang Sakit**
Chinese	不痛		輕微		中度		嚴重		非常嚴重		最嚴重
Korean	통증 없음		약한 통증		보통 통증		심한 통증		아주 심한 통증		최악의 통증
Persian (Farsi)	بدون درد		درد ملایم		درد معتدل		درد شدید		درد بسیار شدید		بدترین درد ممکن
Vietnamese	**Không Đau**		**Đau Nhe**		**Đau Vira Phài**		**Đau Nặng**		**Đau Thậi Nặng**		**Đau Độu Tận Cùng**
Japanese	痛みがない		少し痛い		いくらか痛い		かなり痛い		ひどく痛い		ものすごく痛い

TABLE 56-4. THREE CLASSES OF ACUTE PAIN

1. Breakthrough: Pain that escalates above a persistent background pain.
2. Transitory and Intermittant: Pain that is episodic in the absence of background pain.
3. Background: Pain that is persistent but may vary over time.

patients, and has also been studied in patients with acute noncancer pain, for which it can offer a picture of both breakthrough and background pain states.[13]

Ultimately, we are left with a maxim first attributed to Dr. John Bonica, the father of pain medicine: "Pain is what a patient says it is." The best way to begin assessing a patient's pain is to *ask* about it and *listen* to the answers. Attempts to reduce the experience to finite details may lead to failure to ask the right questions, distance us from our patients, focus us away from the whole person, and potentially miss golden diagnostic clues that could lead to effective interventions.

Effective treatment of acute pain requires assessment as well as vigilant reassessment to determine if the primary goals are met, adversity has occurred, or changes are necessary. Acute pain may be viewed as breakthrough, intermittent, or background in nature (Table 56-4). The assessment process for each of these is relatively similar and will help to resolve the related condition into broad pathophysiologic groups such as cancer versus noncancer, and nociceptive versus neuropathic, or mixed pain states. Such an approach supports a rational process for developing a useful differential diagnosis and approaches. Table 56-5 lists the common features of pain that are usually reviewed during the assessment for acute pain. A thorough physical examination must also be performed with particular attention to the neurologic examination, which may offer clues to aberrant neural processing. Such neurologic findings may indicate nerve injury, alerting the astute clinician to a neuropathic rather than a nociceptive pain state that requires a different analgesic approach.[14] A provocative physical examination may include examination of the affected areas with maneuvers that may provoke pain such as range of motion testing, walking, and cough. The benefits of provocative testing must outweigh the associated suffering incurred by the patient. Medical imaging is also a common part of the acute pain workup. Overemphasis on imaging data should, however, be avoided as this can potentially lead to misinterpretation of the patient's underlying pain syndrome.

TABLE 56-5. FEATURES OF PAIN COMMONLY ADDRESSED DURING ASSESSMENT

Onset of pain
Temporal pattern of pain
Site of pain
Radiation of pain
Quality (character) of pain
Intensity (severity) of pain
Exacerbating factors (what makes the pain start or get worse?)
Relieving factors (what prevents the pain or makes it better?)
Response to analgesics (including attitudes and concerns about opioids)
Response to other interventions
Associated physical symptoms
Associated psychological symptoms
Interference with activities of daily living

OPIOID ANALGESICS

Opioids are the mainstay for the treatment of acute postoperative pain, and morphine is the "gold-standard." The various opioid
4 analgesics available today have distinct pharmacologic differences that we can credit to their intricate interaction with the three main opioid receptors: mu, delta, and kappa. The opioid receptors are members of a G protein–coupled (guanosine triphosphate regulatory proteins) receptor family, which signals via a second messenger such as cyclic adenosine monophosphate or an ion channel. In the ascending pain pathway opioid receptors are located in three areas that include (1) the periphery, following inflammation; (2) the spinal cord dorsal horn; and (3) supraspinally in the brainstem, thalamus, and cortex. Mu opioid receptors are also found in the periaqueductal grey, the nucleus raphe magnus, and the rostral ventral medulla, which constitutes the descending inhibitory pain pathway. The three primary mechanisms of action for opioid analgesia at the level of the spinal cord, include (1) inhibition of calcium influx presynaptically, which results in depolarization of the cell membrane and decreased release of neurotransmitters and neuropeptides into the synaptic cleft; (2) enhancing potassium efflux from the cell postsynaptically, which results in hyperpolarization of the cell and a decrease in pain transmission, and (3) activation of a descending inhibitory pain circuit via inhibition of GABAergic transmission in the brainstem. Peripheral opioid receptors, which mediate analgesia, are located on primary afferent neurons. Activation of these receptors inhibits the release of pronociceptive and proinflammatory substances like substance P, which accounts for the analgesic and anti-inflammatory effects. The "broad-spectrum" opioid, methadone, has NMDA receptor antagonist properties and inhibits the reuptake of serotonin and norepinephrine, which may make it useful in the treatment of neuropathic pain.

There is great diversity in the available routes of administration of opioid analgesics. Table 56-6 is a list of relevant pharmacokinetic data. Table 56-7 offers equianalgesic dosing guidelines for the various opioids. The reader is referred to the section "Perioperative Pain Management of the Opioid-dependent Patient" for a complete discussion of incomplete cross-tolerance between the different opioids and dosing considerations.

Common opioid-induced side effects include sedation, nausea and vomiting, respiratory depression, and constipation. Less common side effects include confusion, urinary retention, dizziness, and myoclonus. Tolerance rarely develops to the constipating effects of the opioids. Alvimopan, a peripherally acting mu receptor antagonist that has negligible systemic absorption, attenuates opioid-induced constipation and shortens postoperative ileus and length of hospital stay.[15] Opioid-induced hyperalgesia (OIH) is a relatively rare phenomenon whereby patients who are receiving opioids suddenly and paradoxically become more sensitive to pain despite continued treatment with opioids. Evidence suggests that OIH is more likely to develop following high doses of phenanthrene opioids such as morphine.[16] Changing the opioid to a phenyl piperidine derivative such as fentanyl may thwart OIH. There is also evidence that coadministration of an NMDA receptor

TABLE 56-6. OPIOID ANALGESIC PHARMACOKINETICS

Drug	Onset of Effect	Peak Effect	Duration of Effect	Elimination t½	VD (L/kg)	Protein Binding (%)	Metabolism Pathway	Active Metabolites	Major Excretion Pathway
Alfentanil	Immediate	1.5–2 min	<10 min	1.5–1.85 h	0.4–1	92%	Liver	—	Urine
Codeine	Oral: 10–30 min, IV: 15 min	0.5–1 h	Oral: 4–6 h, IV: 5 h	2.5–3 h	—	—	Liver	Morphine	Urine
Fentanyl injection	IV: immediate, IM: 7–8 min	—	IV: 0.5–1 h, IM: 1–2 h	3.65 h	4	Alters with increasing ionization	Liver	—	Urine
Fentanyl transdermal	—	24–72 h	72 h	≈17 h	6	Decreases with increasing ionization	Liver: CYP3A4	—	Urine
Fentanyl transmucosal	—	—	—	7 h	4	80–85%	Liver: CYP3A4	—	Urine
Hydromorphone	IM/Subcutaneous: 15 min Oral: 30 min	0.5–1 h	IR: 4–5 h, ER: 24 h, IM/Subcutaneous: 4–5 h	IR: 2.3 h, ER: 18.6 h IM/Subcutaneous: 2.6 h	≈4	8–20%	Liver: Glucuronidation	—	Urine
Levorphanol	IM: 15–30 min	Oral: 1 h	—	IV: 11–16 h	IV: 10–13	40%	—	—	—
Meperidine	—	—	2–4 h	3–6 (parent), <20 h (normeperidine)		60–80%	Liver	Normeperidine	—
Methadone	Parenteral: 10–20 min Oral: 30–60 min	—	4 h	8–59 h	2–6	85–90%	Liver primarily CYP3A4 and to lesser extent CYP2D6	—	Urine and fecal
Morphine sulfate	IM/Subcutaneous: 10–30 min	Epidural: 10–15 min, Oral: 1 h	Subcutaneous/ IM: 4–5 h	1.5–2 h	1–6	20–35%	Liver: glucuronidation	Morphine 6 glucuronide	Urine
Oxycodone	Within 60 min	—	IR: 3–4 h CR[a]: 12 h	IR: 3.2 h, CR: 4.5 h	2.6	45%	Liver: Somewhat involves CYP2D6	Noroxycodone and oxymorphone	Urine
Oxymorphone	Parenteral: 5–10 min	—	Parenteral: 3–6 h	1.3 h	≈3	—	Liver	—	Urine
Propoxyphene*	—	2–2.5 h	—	6–12 h (parent), 30–36 h (norpropoxyphene)	—	80%	Liver	Norpropoxyphene	Urine
Remifentanil	Rapid	—	—	10–20 min	0.35	70%	Hydrolysis by esterases	—	Urine
Sufentanil	IV: immediate, Epidural: 10 min[b]	—	Epidural: 1.7 h	2.7 h	—	91–93%, 79% in neonates	Liver and small intestine	—	—
Tramadol	—	—	2 h (tramadol), 3 h (M1, active metabolite)	6.3 h (tramadol), 7.4 h (M1, active metabolite)	2.6–2.9	20%	Liver: CYP2D6 and CYP3A4	O-desmethyl-tramadol (M1) via CYP2D6	Urine

Removed from the US market in November 2010 secondary to increased risk of cardiogenic death.
IV, intravenous; CT, cytochrome; IR, immediate release; ER, extended release; IM, intramuscularly.
Adapted with permission from: Drug Facts and Comparisons, Wolter Kluwer Health.

TABLE 56-7. OPIOID EQUIANALGESIC DOSING

Drug	IV/IM/SQ	Oral (mg)
Morphine (MS Contin)	10 mg	30
Hydromorphone (Dilaudid)	1.5–2 mg	6–8
Hydrocodone (Vicodin)	NA	30–45
Oxymorphone (Opana IR and ER)	1 mg	10
Oxycodone (Percocet, Oxycontin)	10–15 mg	20
Levorphanol (Levo-Dromoran)	2 mg	4
Fentanyl	100 μg	NA
Meperidine (Demerol)	100 mg	300
Codeine	100 mg	200
Methadone	The conversion ratio for methadone is variable. Please see Table 56-8.	

IV, intravenous; IM, intramuscular; SQ, subcutaneous; IR, immediate release; ER, extended release.
Data derived from: Carroll IR, Angst MS, Clark JD. Management of perioperative pain in patients chronically consuming opioids. *Reg Anesth Pain Med.* 2004;29:576; Toombs JD, Kral LA. Methadone treatment for pain states. *Am Fam Phys.* 2005;71:1353; Hadi I, Morley-Forster PK, Dain S, et al. Brief review: Perioperative management of the patient with chronic non-cancer pain. *Can J Anaesth.* 2006;53:1190.

antagonist can abolish opioid-induced tolerance and OIH.[16] Finally, opioid analgesics have profound immunomodulatory effects, which include inhibition of cellular and humoral immune functions, depressed natural killer cell activity, promotion of angiogenesis and inhibition of apoptosis. Such effects can be beneficial or deleterious depending upon the clinical situation.[17,18]

Morphine is the prototype opioid and is the "gold standard" to which all other analgesics are compared. Although the plasma half-life of the drug is approximately 2 hours its analgesic duration of action is closer to 4 to 5 hours. Morphine undergoes hepatic glucuronidation to morphine-6-glucuronide and morphine-3-glucuronide, both of which are cleared by the kidney. Morphine-6-glucuronide is an active metabolite of morphine and is thought to be responsible for most of the analgesia associated with chronic dosing of the drug. Morphine-3-glucuronide, on the other hand, is considered to be devoid of analgesic activity. With chronic dosing these metabolites can accumulate and can be particularly problematic in patients with renal failure. Dosing adjustment is therefore necessary and monitoring of side effects is important. Morphine-6-glucuronide contributes to side effects such as drowsiness, nausea and vomiting, coma, and respiratory depression. Morphine-3-glucuronide, on the other hand, is thought to cause agitation, myoclonus, delirium, and hyperalgesia.

Hydromorphone is a semisynthetic opioid that has 4 to 6 times the potency of morphine. It is available for oral, rectal, parenteral, and neuraxial administration. Whereas the oral bioavailability of the drug is reported to be 20% to 50%, its bioavailability via the subcutaneous route is 78%, making it the ideal drug for long-term subcutaneous administration in the opioid-tolerant patient. Like morphine, hydromorphone is biotransformed in the liver. The active metabolites are dihydromorphine and dihydroisomorphine and the inactive metabolite is hydromorphone-3-glucuronide. Although hydromorphone has traditionally been the preferred opioid for patients with acute pain and impaired kidney function, evidence suggests that hydromorphone-3-glucuronide can accumulate in those with renal failure and may contribute to side effects such as neuroexcitation and cognitive impairment. Opioid-related side effects such as nausea, vomiting, sedation, cognitive impairment, and pruritus are reported to be less intense with hydromorphone vis-à-vis morphine. In fact, the incidence of pruritus following neuraxial administration of hydromorphone is reported to be approximately 5% versus the 11% to 77% range reported for neuraxial morphine.[19]

Fentanyl, a synthetic opioid chemically related to the phenylpiperidines, is a relatively selective mu receptor agonist, which is considered to be 80 times the potency of morphine following intravenous administration. It is extensively metabolized in the liver to norfentanyl and other inactive metabolites, which are excreted in the urine and bile. Fentanyl is therefore suitable for patients in renal failure. The drug is available for intravenous, subcutaneous, transdermal, transmucosal, and neuraxial administration. The transdermal administration of fentanyl using iontophoresis (Ionsys, Janssen-Cilag LTD) is a novel on-demand drug delivery system that does not require venous access.

Sufentanil, alfentanil, and *remifentanil* are analogs of fentanyl that have analgesic effects similar to those of morphine and the other mu receptor agonists. *Sufentanil* is approximately 1,000 times the potency of morphine and is primarily used in the operating room either intravenously or neuraxially.[20] Like fentanyl, sufentanil is very lipophilic, and although their pharmacokinetic and pharmacodynamic profiles are similar, sufentanil has a smaller volume of distribution and shorter elimination half-life.[20] The high intrinsic potency of sufentanil makes it an excellent choice for epidural analgesia in the opioid-dependent patient.[21] *Alfentanil* is approximately 10 times the potency of morphine and, like sufentanil, is used primarily in the operating room either intravenously or neuraxially. *Remifentanil* is an ultra–short-acting synthetic opioid. The potency of the drug is approximately equal to that of fentanyl. Remifentanil is rapidly degraded by tissue and plasma esterases, which accounts for its incredibly short terminal elimination half-life of 10 to 20 minutes.[20] Rapid clearance and lack of accumulation make this a very desirable opioid in the operative setting. One disadvantage, however, is that discontinuation of a remifentanil infusion results in rapid loss of analgesia. There is also evidence to suggest that remifentanil infusions may be associated with the development of opioid-induced hyperalgesia. Further studies are clearly needed to better define this phenomenon.

Meperidine, a phenylpiperidine, is a synthetic mu opioid receptor agonist with a short half-life. The drug is recommended for the short-term management of acute pain only and has absolutely no role in the management of chronic pain. The drug is biotransformed by the liver to normeperidine, a potentially neurotoxic metabolite, which has a 12- to 16-hour half-life. Repetitive dosing of meperidine can cause accumulation of normeperidine, which may precipitate tremulousness, myoclonus, and seizures. It is therefore recommended that the total daily intravenous dose in an otherwise healthy adult without renal or central nervous system disease should not exceed 600 mg/day and should not be administered for longer than 48 hours.[22] We do not recommend administration of meperidine as an intravenous patient–controlled analgesia (PCA). The drug is contraindicated in patients receiving monoamine oxidase inhibitors as this may precipitate a syndrome characterized by muscle rigidity, hyperpyrexia, and seizures.

Methadone is a relatively inexpensive synthetic opioid considered to be a broad-spectrum opioid because it is a (1) mu receptor agonist, (2) NMDA antagonist, and (3) inhibitor of monoamine transmitter reuptake, making it potentially useful for the treatment

TABLE 56-8. CONVERSION RATIOS FROM MORPHINE TO METHADONE

Daily Chronic Oral Morphine Dose[a]		Conversion Ratio Oral Morphine: Oral Methadone	
<100 mg	(e.g., 90 mg PO morphine)	3:1	(e.g., 30 mg PO methadone)
100–300 mg	(e.g., 300 mg PO morphine)	5:1	(e.g., 60 mg PO methadone)
300–600 mg	(e.g., 600 mg PO morphine)	10:1	(e.g., 60 mg PO methadone)
600–800 mg	(e.g., 720 mg PO morphine)	12:1	(e.g., 60 mg PO methadone)
800–1,000 mg	(e.g., 900 mg PO morphine)	15:1	(e.g., 60 mg PO methadone)
>1,000 mg	(e.g., 1,200 mg PO morphine)	20:1	(e.g., 60 mg PO methadone)

PO, by mouth.
[a]When converting from morphine to methadone use the table with caution. There is considerable variation from one individual to another. It is recommended that a clinician well versed in chronic pain therapy perform this task.
Data derived from: Toombs JD, Kral LA. Methadone treatment for pain states. *Am Fam Phys.* 2005;71:1353; Drug, Facts and Comparisons. St. Louis, MO: Wolters Kluwer Health, 2008; Ayonrinde OT, Bridge DT. The rediscovery of methadone for cancer pain management. *Med J Austr.* 2000;173:536.

of neuropathic pain. The drug is well absorbed from the gastrointestinal tract with a reported bioavailability of approximating 80%. The drug is extensively metabolized in the liver by the cytochrome P450 (CYP450) system to inactive metabolites, which are cleared in the bile and urine; unlike morphine, it is generally not necessary to adjust the dosage of methadone in patients with renal insufficiency. Methadone has an elimination half-life of 22 hours, and following a single dose the duration of analgesia is approximately 3 to 6 hours. With repetitive dosing, however, methadone can accumulate and slow tissue release into the blood stream can result in a long elimination half-life of up to 128 hours and duration of analgesia of 8 to 12 hours. This long half-life explains the potential risk for cumulative toxicity, and therefore the importance of monitoring for side effects such as excessive sedation and confusion following the initiation of an around-the-clock dosing regimen.

Finally, opioid rotation is a very useful technique to restore analgesic sensitivity in the highly tolerant patient, and methadone is a common choice for opioid rotation. Because cross-tolerance is incomplete, the calculated equianalgesic dose of any new opioid is always lower than expected. One must be particularly cautious, however, when converting from morphine to methadone as the morphine/methadone equianalgesic ratio appears to be curvilinear; whereas the morphine-to-methadone conversion ratio is 3:1 at morphine doses of <100 mg/day, the ratio is 20:1 at morphine doses of >1,001 mg/day (Table 56-8). Methadone is principally metabolized by the CYP3A4 subtype enzyme of the cytochrome P450 system and to a lesser extent by the CYP1A2 and CYP2D6 subtypes. Consequently, there is the potential for numerous drug interactions with methadone, as shown in Table 56-9. Whereas inhibition of methadone metabolism will theoretically provoke

TABLE 56-9. METHADONE DRUG INTERACTIONS

Clinical Significance	Increase Methadone Concentration/Effects	Decrease Methadone Concentration/Effects
Documented clinical effects	Ciprofloxacin (Cipro), diazepam (Valium), ethanol (acute use), fluconazole (Diflucan), urinary alkalinizers	Amprenavir (Agenerase), efavirenz (Sustiva), nelfinavir (Viracept), nevirapine (Viramune), phenobarbital, phenytoin (Dilantin), rifampin (Rifadin), ritonavir (Norvir), urinary acidifiers
Documented enzyme effects	Cimetidine (Tagamet), fluoxetine (Prozac)	Carbamazepine (Tegretol)
Clinical effects uncertain	Omeprazole (Prilosec), quinidine, paroxetine (Paxil)	
Predicted interaction	Delavirdine (Rescriptor), grapefruit juice or fruit	Ethanol (chronic use)
No current clinical evidence	Ketoconazole (Nizoral), macrolide antibiotics (erythromycin, clarithromycin [Biaxin], troleandomycin [TAO]), tricyclic antidepressants, verapamil (Calan)	

Information derived from: Raja SN, Dougherty PM. Anatomy and physiology of somatosensory and pain processing, *Essentials of Pain Medicine and Regional Anesthesia,* 2nd ed. In: Benzon HT, Raja SN, Molloy RE, Liu S, Fishman SM, eds. Philadelphia, PA: Elsevier, Churchill Livingstone, 2005, 1; Rowlingson JC. Update on acute pain management. International Anesthesia Research Society Review Course Lectures. 2006:95; Power I. Recent advances in postoperative pain therapy. *Br J Anaesth.* 2005;95:43; Weinbroum AA. A single small dose of postoperative ketamine provides rapid and sustained improvement in morphine analgesia in the presence of morphine-resistant pain. *Anesth Analg.* 2003;96:789; Sveticic G, Gentilini A, Eichenberger U, et al. Combinations of morphine with ketamine for patient-controlled analgesia: A new optimization method. *Anesthesiology.* 2003;98:1195.

toxicity, induction of methadone metabolism could potentially precipitate inadequate analgesia or even withdrawal symptoms. Frequent adjustments of the methadone dosage may therefore be required if medications are added to or eliminated from a patient's drug regimen. A rare side effect associated with methadone is a pause-dependent dysrhythmia associated with bradycardia, QT prolongation, and Torsades de point.

Buprenorphine is a potent semisynthetic opioid that is derived from thebaine. The drug is classified as a mixed agonist–antagonist and partial mu receptor agonist with an analgesic potency 25 to 50 times greater than that of morphine. Buprenorphine is a lipophilic opioid with moderate intrinsic activity and a high affinity for the mu opioid receptor, with a half-life for dissociation from the receptor of 166 minutes compared with 7 minutes for fentanyl. The drug is metabolized by the gut and the liver and has a half-life of about 3 hours, but this bears little connection to the rate of disappearance of its clinical effects because of its avid binding to the mu receptor, as previously noted. The drug can be delivered by various routes of administration include intravenous, intramuscular, neuraxial, subcutaneous, sublingual, and transdermal. Buprenorphine is also an excellent alternative for the treatment of acute pain in the patient who cannot tolerate morphine secondary to allergy or other sensitivity. In humans, buprenorphine is reported to have a ceiling effect for respiratory depression but not for analgesia. Buprenorphine is reported to have anti-inflammatory effects and therefore may be efficacious when administered intra-articularly. Investigators have demonstrated that buprenorphine will significantly prolong the analgesic effects of a peripheral nerve block when 0.3 mg of the drug is combined with 40 mL of a local anesthetic mixture consisting of 1% mepivacaine, 0.2% tetracaine, and epinephrine 1:200,000.[23]

NONOPIOID ANALGESIC ADJUNCTS

5 The *NSAIDs* are among the most commonly used drugs in the world because of their anti-inflammatory, analgesic, and antipyretic effects (Table 56-10). The therapeutic benefit of NSAIDs is believed to be mediated through the inhibition of cyclooxygenase (COX) enzymes (prostaglandin H_2 synthetases), types 1 and 2, which convert arachidonic acid to prostaglandin H_2 (PGH_2). The COX enzyme consists of two active sites: (1) The cyclooxygenase site and (2) the peroxidase site. NSAIDs mediate their effects by binding to the cyclooxygenase site (Fig. 56-11)

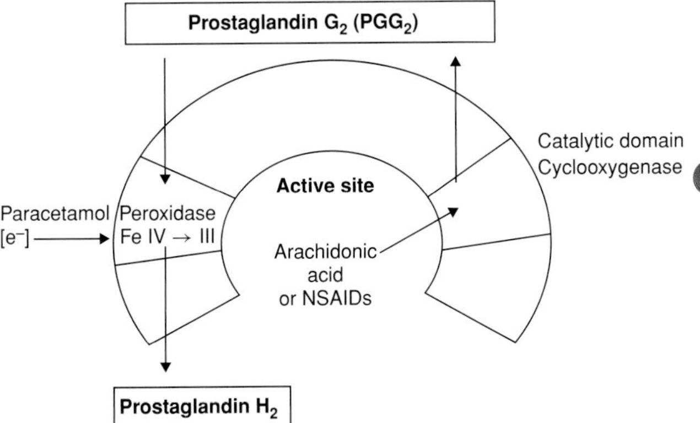

FIGURE 56-11. From Kam, P.C.A., COX-3: Uncertainties and controversies, *Curr Anaesth Crit Care.* 2009; (20) 50.

COX-1 is the constitutive enzyme that produces prostaglandins, which are important for general "house-keeping" functions such as gastric protection and hemostasis. COX-2, on the other hand, is the inducible form of the enzyme that produces prostaglandins that mediate pain, inflammation, fever, and carcinogenesis. Prostaglandin E_2 is the key mediator of both peripheral and central pain sensitization. Peripherally, prostaglandins do not directly mediate pain; rather, they contribute to hyperalgesia by sensitizing nociceptors to other mediators of pain sensation such as histamine and bradykinin.[24] Centrally, prostaglandins enhance pain transmission at the level of the dorsal horn by (1) increasing the release of substance P and glutamate from first-order pain neurons, (2) increasing the sensitivity of second-order pain neurons, and (3) inhibiting the release of neurotransmitters from the descending pain-modulating pathways.

NSAIDs have proved effective in the treatment of postoperative pain. In addition, they are opioid-sparing and can significantly decrease the incidence of opioid-related side effects such as postoperative nausea and vomiting and sedation.[25] Unlike the opioids, NSAIDs exhibit a "ceiling effect" with respect to maximum analgesic effects. Parenteral NSAIDs such as ketorolac are commonly employed as part of a multimodal approach for acute perioperative pain management. The optimal dose of ketorolac for postoperative pain control is 15 to 30 mg intravenously every 6 to 8 hours not to exceed 5 days. The dose should be decreased in patients with renal failure.

Despite the benefits of NSAIDs in the perioperative period they are not without some significant side effects. Platelet dysfunction, gastrointestinal ulceration, and an increased risk of nephrotoxicity are several reasons why the nonselective NSAIDs may be avoided in the perioperative period. The risk of nephrotoxicity is increased in patients with hypovolemia, congestive heart failure, and chronic renal insufficiency.[24] The COX-2–selective inhibitors were developed in an attempt to minimizing their side effects. The COX-2–specific inhibitor celecoxib (Celebrex) is available in the United States. Rofecoxib (Vioxx) and valdecoxib (Bextra) also released in the same period were recalled by the manufacturers because of concerns about adverse cardiovascular risks. Celecoxib is the only COX-2–specific inhibitor currently available in the United States for acute postoperative pain. The recommended oral loading dose is a 400 mg followed by 200 mg orally every 12 hours for several days. Parecoxib (Dynastat) is an injectable COX-2–specific inhibitor that is available only in Europe for the treatment of moderate-to-severe postoperative pain. The recommended dose of the drug in Europe is 40 mg intravenously or intramuscularly initially followed by 20 to 40 mg every 4 to 6 hours not to exceed 80 mg/day. Unlike the nonselective NSAIDs, however, COX-2–specific inhibitors offer the potential advantages of a reduced incidence of gastrointestinal ulceration and they do not inhibit platelet function. Because prostaglandins play a crucial role in renal function through their effect on blood flow, natriuresis and glomerular filtration, traditional NSAIDs, and the COX-2 inhibitors can cause fluid retention and hypertension.

6 Short-term use of parecoxib and valdecoxib in patients following coronary artery bypass surgery is associated with an increased risk of thromboembolic events.[26]

The authors, therefore, do not recommend prescribing a COX-2 inhibitor for patients with a known history of coronary artery disease or cerebrovascular disease. Both COX-1 and COX-2 play significant roles in bone fusion following fracture, and the use of the traditional NSAIDs has been found to inhibit the healing process, particularly following lumbar spinal fusion surgery. The effect of COX-2 inhibitors on bone fusion following orthopedic procedures continues to be controversial, and no recommendations can be made at this time. NSAIDs and

TABLE 56-10. NONOPIOID ANALGESICS (ADULT DOSING GUIDELINES)

Drug	Route	Half-Life (h)	Dose (mg)	Comments
Para-aminophenols				
Acetaminophen	PO and IV	2	500–1,000 mg q4–6h. Maximum daily dose (MDD) in the healthy adult is 4,000 mg. Intravenous dosing guidelines: Adult >50kg: 1 g q4–6h not to exceed 4 g/day Adult <50kg: 15mg/kg q4–6h not to exceed 3 g/day. Pedi >33 kg: 15 mg/kg q4–6h not to exceed 3 g/day. Pedi 10–33 kg: 15mg/kg q4–6h not to exceed 2 g/day.	Hepatotoxicity can occur in chronic alcoholics receiving therapeutic doses. Administer intravenous formulation over 15 minutes.
Salicylates				
Acetylsalicylic acid	PO	0.25	500–1,000 mg q4–6h MDD is 4,000 mg in the healthy adult.	Salicylic acid has a $T_{1/2}$ 2–3 h at low doses and >20 h at higher doses. Because of the risk of Reyes syndrome avoid the use of aspirin in children <12 years old.
Diflunisal	PO	8–12	500 mg q8–12h	Decrease the dose in the elderly to 500–1,000 mg/day
Choline magnesium trisalicylate	PO	9–17	Loading dose (LD) = 1,000 mg 1,000–1,500 mg q12h	Unlike aspirin does not increase bleeding time. MDD = 2,000–3,000 mg
NSAIDs Propionic acids				
Ibuprofen Intravenous formulation (Caldolor) available in the United States in 2009.	PO and IV	2	400 mg q4–6h	Intravenous ibuprofen: Infuse over 30 minutes to avoid phlebitis Limit adult dose to 3,200 mg/day.
Naproxen	PO	12–15	250 mg q6–8h	LD = 500 mg. MDD = 1,500 mg
Ketoprofen	PO	2.1	25–50 mg q6–8h	MDD = 300 mg
Oxaprozin	PO	42–50	600 mg q12–24h	MDD = 1,200 mg
Indolacetic acids				
Indomethacin	PO	2	25 mg q8–12h	MDD = 200 mg
Sulindac	PO	7.8	150 mg q12h	MDD = 400 mg. Active metabolite has a half-life of 16 h
Etodolac	PO	7.3	300–400 mg q8–12h	MDD = 1,000 mg
Pyrrolacetic acids				
Ketorolac	IV	6	30 mg initially followed by 15–30 mg q6–8h not to exceed 5 days.	MDD = 120 mg. Hypovolemia should be corrected prior to administration. Decrease the dose in the elderly (>65 years of age) and in renal failure.
Phenylacetic acids				
Diclofenac potassium	PO	2	50 mg q8h	MDD = 150 mg
Enolic acids (Oxicams)				
Meloxicam	PO	15–20	7.5–15 mg q24h	COX-2 selectivity similar to celecoxib
Piroxicam	PO	50	20–40 mg q24h	
Naphthylalkanone				
Nabumetone	PO	22.5	500–750 mg q8–12h	LD = 1,000 mg. MDD = 2,000 mg. Active metabolite has half-life = 22.5 h
COX-2 inhibitor				
Celecoxib	PO	11	100–200 mg q12h	LD = 400 mg. MDD = 400 mg. Avoid this drug in patients allergic to sulfonamides.

PO, by month; COX-2, cyclooxygenase.

Data derived from: *Principles of Analgesic Use in the Treatment of Acute Pain and Cancer Pain.* 5th ed. Glenview, IL: American Pain Society, 2003; Drug, Facts and Comparisons. St. Louis, MO: Wolters Kluwer Health, 2008.

COX-2–selective inhibitors should not be administered to patients with known hypersensitivity to the drugs or to patients with Samters triad (aka aspirin triad), which is a medical condition consisting of asthma, aspirin insensitivity, and nasal polyposis. Finally, avoid celecoxib and valdecoxib in patients with allergic-type reactions to sulfonamides.

The *para-aminophenol* derivative acetaminophen (aka paracetamol) has both analgesic and antipyretic properties, similar to aspirin, but is devoid of any anti-inflammatory effects. The drug is primarily a centrally acting inhibitor of the cyclooxygenase enzyme with minimal peripheral effects. Acetaminophen neither enters the active site of the COX enzyme nor binds to the cyclooxygenase site, but instead it prevents COX activation by reducing heme at the peroxidase site of the enzyme (Fig. 56-11). In addition, there may be modulation of descending inhibitory serotoninergic pathways and the drug may act on the opioid, cannabinoid, and NMDA receptors.[27] Acetaminophen is devoid of many of the side effects generally associated with the NSAIDs, such as gastrointestinal ulceration, impaired platelet function, adverse cardiorenal effects, and impairment of bone fusion following orthopedic procedures. Acetaminophen is opioid-sparing and can be used in conjunction with an NSAID as part of a multimodal analgesic program. In adults, 2 g of oral acetaminophen is equivalent to 200 mg of celecoxib.

Propacetamol is the intravenous prodrug formulation of paracetamol and is a popular adjuvant for perioperative pain control in Europe. The drug has the disadvantage that it must be reconstituted prior to administration. Two grams of propacetamol is equivalent to 1 g of paracetamol. Fortunately, a ready-to-use intravenous formulation of paracetamol (Perfalgan) has been released in Europe. Intravenous acetaminophen (Ofirmev) was released in the United States in November of 2010. The drug is available as a 1 g (1,000 mg/100 mL) infusion that does not require reconstitution and can be infused through a peripheral IV over 15 minutes. See Table 56-10 for dosing guidelines.

The *NMDA receptor antagonists* such as ketamine and dextromethorphan may be useful analgesic adjuncts. Excitatory neurotransmitter stimulation of the NMDA receptor is believed to be involved in the development and maintenance of several phenomena including (1) persistent postoperative pain, (2) hypersensitivity, wind-up, and allodynia, (3) opioid-induced tolerance, and (4) OIH. Low-dose ketamine (0.25- to 0.5-mg intravenous bolus followed by an infusion of 2 to 4 μg/kg/min) can provide significant analgesia and is opioid-sparing. The mechanism of action of ketamine is NMDA receptor blockade, but in addition the drug interacts with opioidergic, cholinergic, and monoaminergic receptors and blocks sodium channels.[28]

NMDA receptor antagonists may act synergistically when combined with an opioid. The ideal intravenous PCA morphine–ketamine combination ratio is 1:1 with an 8-minute lockout.[29] A double-blind study, however, demonstrates that the combination of ketamine (1 mg/mL) with morphine (1 mg/mL) administered as an intravenous PCA to patients following major abdominal surgery does not significantly improve pain relief.[30] In patients with morphine-resistant pain, however, the combination of 250 μg/kg of ketamine plus 15 μg/kg of morphine has been reported to provide significant analgesia.[28] Results are promising, but more studies will certainly be required to clearly define the role of ketamine for postoperative analgesia.

Dextromethorphan, the d-isomer of the codeine analog levorphanol, is a noncompetitive NMDA receptor antagonist that has been used for many years as an antitussive. Dextromethorphan does not have a direct analgesic effect; rather, analgesia is likely mediated by its NMDA receptor antagonism. The drug can be administered orally, intravenously, and intramuscularly. There is a sustained-release suspension available that contains dextromethorphan, 30 mg/5 mL, and is marketed as Delsym (Adams Respiratory Therapeutics). Following oral administration the drug is metabolized to dextrorphan, which is the metabolite that accounts for most of the side effects, the most common of which is nausea and vomiting. Because the intravenous administration of large doses can lead to hypotension and tachycardia, the intramuscular route may be the preferred route of delivery. Dextromethorphan has been shown to both inhibit secondary hyperalgesia following peripheral burn injury and cause a reduction in temporal summation of pain. The preoperative administration of 150 mg of oral dextromethorphan can reduce the PCA morphine requirements of patients undergoing abdominal hysterectomy, and the preincisional administration of 120 mg of intramuscular dextromethorphan provides preemptive analgesia in patients undergoing elective upper abdominal surgery. Finally, a randomized double-blind placebo-controlled study has demonstrated that dextromethorphan dosed 200 mg orally every 8 hours (e.g., 2 hours prior to surgery, then 8 hours and 16 hours thereafter) can provide a modest reduction in morphine consumption following knee surgery.[31]

The *α_2-adrenergic agonists* clonidine (half-life, 9 to 12 hours) and dexmedetomidine (half-life, 2 hours) may be administered perioperatively to provide analgesia, sedation, and anxiolysis. The presynaptic activation of α_2-receptors that results in the decreased release of norepinephrine is believed to mediate analgesia. Whereas clonidine is a selective partial agonist for the α_2-adrenoreceptor, dexmedetomidine is super selective for the receptor. Their respective α_2/α_1 binding ratios are 220:1 for clonidine versus 1,620:1 for dexmedetomidine. Analgesia is mediated supraspinally (locus coeruleus), spinally (substantia gelatinosa), and peripherally. Dexmedetomidine is reported to have greater affinity for the 2A subtype of the receptor, which may account for the drug's superior analgesic properties vis-à-vis clonidine. Clonidine can be administered orally, transdermally, intravenously, perineurally, and neuraxially for perioperative pain management. Premedication with 5 μg/kg of oral clonidine in patients undergoing knee surgery can decrease the use of PCA morphine and decrease the incidence of postoperative nausea and vomiting. In addition, the combination of oral clonidine, 3 to 5 μg/kg with 0.2 mg/24 hours of transdermal clonidine can decrease postoperative PCA morphine requirement by 50% following prostatectomy surgery. In a double-blind placebo-controlled study, investigators demonstrated that addition of 25 μg of intrathecal clonidine to a bupivacaine (15 mg) morphine (250 μg) spinal anesthetic cocktail, for total knee arthroplasty (TKA), could reduce postoperative morphine use and improve VAS pain scores at 24 hours.[32] Clonidine in doses of 0.5 to 1 μg/kg may enhance the efficacy and increase the duration of local anesthetics in peripheral nerve blockade. In addition, the intra-articular use of clonidine can be beneficial. Side effects include sedation, hypotension, and bradycardia if the dose exceeds 150 μg as part of a peripheral nerve block.

Dexmedetomidine is the D-enantiomer of medetomidine. It is a highly selective α_2-agonist that does not interact with the GABA-mimetic system and therefore does not depress the respiratory drive.[33] Other advantages include analgesia, titratable sedation (e.g., "cooperative sedation"), and anxiolysis. In addition, the centrally mediated reduction in sympathetic tone is reported to have a cardioprotective effect, particularly in high-risk patients undergoing vascular surgery. There is a low incidence of bradycardia and hypotension, which can be treated with atropine, ephedrine, or volume infusion.[33] Dexmedetomidine is a useful adjunct to both opioid and nonopioid analgesics as part of a multimodal analgesic protocol. Combining the drug with ketamine and opioids can obviate the respiratory depressant effects of the latter and the psychomimetic effects of the former.[34] The recommended dose of dexmedetomidine is a loading dose of 1 μg/kg intravenously over 10 minutes followed by an infusion of 0.2 to 0.7 μg/kg/hr,[33] A dexmedetomidine infusion (0.2 to 0.7 μg/kg/hr) combined with peripheral nerve blockade can provide superb analgesia, anxiolysis, and sedation during prolonged procedures.

The gabapentinoids (*α_2–δ subunit calcium channel ligands*), gabapentin (Neurontin) and pregabalin (Lyrica), are indicated for the treatment of partial onset seizures, neuropathic pain (e.g., postherpetic neuralgia), and other chronic pain states (e.g., fibromyalgia) but have been commonly prescribed for off-label use for acute perioperative pain relief. Numerous meta-analysis indicates that the perioperative administration of gabapentinoids improves postoperative pain (both at rest and with movement) and decreases postoperative opioid requirement. In addition, there is a decreased incidence of postoperative vomiting, pruritus and urinary retention probably secondary to the opioid-sparing effects of the drugs.[35]

Compared to traditional analgesics, which decrease afferent input from the site of tissue injury, the gabapentinoids decrease the hyperexcitability of dorsal horn neurons caused by tissue damage.[36] Although structurally similar to GABA (gamma-aminobutyric acid) these drugs are not GABAergic and do not bind $GABA_A$ $GABA_b$ $GABA_c$ radioligand sites or allosteric GABA receptor sites. The analgesic mechanism of action of the gabapentinoids may involve 3 distinct processes: (1) Decreased release of neurotransmitter via presynaptic binding of the calcium receptor (Ca_v α_2 δ), (2) redistribution of the calcium channel away from its functional membrane bound site to its nonfunctional cytosolic site, and (3) inhibition of activation of the transcription factor nuclear factor κB (NF- κB), which reduces gene transcription of COX-2 and interleukin-6 (IL-6).[37]

Gabapentin prevents the development of central excitability and is antihyperalgesic. Meta-analysis of the analgesic effects of gabapentin suggests that it should be part of any multimodal analgesic regimen for perioperative pain management.[38] In a double-blinded, randomized, placebo-controlled study, gabapentin was administered as a 1,200-mg oral dose 1 to 2 hours prior to surgery in patients scheduled to undergo elective arthroscopic anterior cruciate ligament (ACL) repair.[39] Advantages of this regimen included a 50% reduction in postoperative morphine consumption and improved early knee flexion following surgery. In another double-blind placebo-controlled study,[40] patients undergoing abdominal hysterectomy reported superior postoperative analgesia following the administration of gabapentin 1 to 2 hours preoperatively. The recommended adult dose of gabapentin as part of a multimodal pain regimen for postoperative pain management is 900 mg orally 1 to 2 hours prior to surgery.[40] The gastrointestinal absorption of gabapentin occurs through a saturable transport system resulting in bioavailability that decreases with increasing doses. Therefore, increased doses of the drug result in incrementally smaller increases in plasma drug concentration (e.g., nonlinear pharmacokinetics).[41] Common side effects include dizziness, drowsiness, and ataxia.

Pregabalin is a newer gabapentinoid with greater potency than gabapentin that may be useful for the treatment of acute perioperative pain. A recent meta-analysis suggests that pregabalin has significant opioid-sparing effects in the first 24 hours following surgery and postoperative vomiting is reduced.[36] There is also strong evidence suggesting that the perioperative use of pregabalin can reduce the incidence of chronic neuropathic pain following TKA and can reduce the time necessary to achieve effective joint range of motion.[42] Compared to gabapentin, pregabalin has a linear pharmacokinetic profile (dose-independent absorbtion), increased potency, and fewer side effects. Further investigation will be required to better define useful drug combinations and dosing regimens for gabapentin and pregabalin.

The *local anesthetic* lidocaine has been shown to be analgesic, antihyperalgesic, and anti-inflammatory following intravenous administration.[43] The perioperative infusion of lidocaine has been shown to not only improve postoperative analgesia in patients recovering from laparoscopic colectomy, but it also can decrease postoperative opioid requirements, attenuate postoperative ileus, and accelerate time to discharge from the hospital.[43] Further studies are certainly warranted to establish both the safety and efficacy of this novel approach.

The *glucocorticoids* are well known for their analgesic, anti-inflammatory, and antiemetic effects. Inhibition of cytosolic phospholipase A_2 upstream from the lipoxygenase and COX enzymes in the prostaglandin cascade most certainly accounts for both their anti-inflammatory and analgesic effects by inhibiting leukotriene and prostaglandin production. The mechanism of the antiemetic effect of the corticosteroids is less clearly understood but appears to be centrally mediated.[44] Although corticosteroids are well recognized as effective analgesics following oral surgery, the analgesic benefits following general surgery, orthopedic surgery, and back surgery have had mixed reviews. Results from a recent study suggest that the combination of dexamethasone (8 mg intravenously) and gabapentin (800 mg orally) administered 1 hour prior to varicocele surgery improves postoperative analgesia and decreases the incidence of postoperative nausea and vomiting.[44] Side effects associated with the use of corticosteroids include gastrointestinal upset, impairment of the immune system, and delayed wound healing; however, because of the small doses used perioperatively, corticosteroids are considered to be relatively safe. Future studies will better define the role of corticosteroids in perioperative pain management.

METHODS OF ANALGESIA

Patient-controlled Analgesia

PCA is any technique of pain management that allows the patients to administer their own analgesia on demand. We will highlight some important aspects of PCA as a complete review of PCA is beyond the scope of this chapter; we refer the reader to the comprehensive review by Macintyre on this topic.[45] In the United States, the most commonly used drugs are morphine, hydromorphone, and fentanyl. Hydromorphone is recommended as an alternative in renal failure; however, fentanyl might be a better choice as it has no active metabolites. Meperidine is not recommended for use in an intravenous PCA secondary to accumulation of its potentially toxic metabolite normeperidine.

7 The five variables associated with all modes of PCA include (1) bolus dose, (2) incremental (demand) dose, (3) lockout interval, (4) background infusion rate, and (5) 1- and 4-hour limits. A typical PCA regimen in an otherwise healthy adult would be an incremental dose of 1 to 2 mg of morphine with an 8- to 10-minute lockout (Table 56-11). The authors do not recommend a background infusion of opioid in the opioid-naive patient. A background infusion should be reserved for the patient with chronic malignant or nonmalignant pain who is opioid-tolerant or in patients with persistent pain who have failed a trial of incremental PCA dosing. In the elderly, the dose of the PCA should be decreased. The relative risk factors for use of an opioid PCA are listed in Table 56-12. If more than two risk factors exist, you may want to avoid using a PCA in the standard dosing regimen and administer opioids only as needed.

TABLE 56-11. USUAL INTRAVENOUS OPIOID PATIENT–CONTROLLED ANALGESIA REGIMENS IN THE OPIOID-NAIVE ADULT PATIENT

Opioid	Demand Dose	Lockout (min)	Basal Infusion
Morphine	1–2 mg	6–10	0–2 mg/h
Hydromorphone	0.2–0.4 mg	6–10	0–0.4 mg/h
Fentanyl	20–50 μg	5–10	0–60 μg/h
Sufentanil	4–6 μg	5–10	0–8 μg/h
Tramadol	10–20 mg	6–10	0–20 mg/h

Data derived from: Macintyre PE. Safety and efficacy of patient-controlled analgesia. *Br J Anaesth.* 2001;87:36; Grass JA: Patient-controlled analgesia. *Anesth Analg.* 2005;101(suppl):S44.

Opioid-related side effects include nausea and vomiting, pruritus, sedation, and confusion. Consensus guidelines for the treatment of nausea and vomiting include prescribing various combinations of dopamine antagonists, serotonin antagonists, and glucocorticoids.[46] Pruritus can be ameliorated with the use of diphenhydramine, hydroxyzine, or a low dose of an opioid antagonist (e.g., naloxone) or mixed agonist–antagonist (e.g., nalbuphine). Excessive sedation may respond to a change in the opioid; however, use of a multimodal analgesic technique, which incorporates the use of a regional anesthetic (e.g., epidural or peripheral nerve blockade), an NSAID, acetaminophen, or other nonopioid analgesics such as an NMDA receptor antagonist or an α_2–δ subunit calcium channel ligand, will have an opioid-sparing effect, which should attenuate opioid-induced sedation.

Neuraxial Analgesia

Although opioid analgesics have been prescribed to patients for many centuries, the exact mechanism of action was not completely understood until 1971 when the opioid receptor was discovered. Within 5 years time, Yaksh reported that morphine could produce spinally mediated analgesia in a rat model. Soon thereafter in 1979 and 1981, respectfully, Wang and then Onofrio reported significant pain relief following the neuraxial administration of morphine in patients with severe cancer-related pain. Since these discoveries, the intrathecal administration of opioids and the epidural administration of opioids plus a local anesthetic has produced significant comfort for our patients.

TABLE 56-12. RELATIVE RISK FACTORS ASSOCIATED WITH THE USE OF PATIENT-CONTROLLED ANALGESIA

Pulmonary disease
Obstructive sleep apnea
Renal or hepatic dysfunction
Congestive heart failure
Closed head injury
Altered mental status
Lactating mothers

8 *Epidural analgesia* is a critical component of multimodal perioperative pain management and improved patient outcome. Meta-analysis investigating the efficacy of epidural analgesia found epidural analgesia to be superior to systemically administered opioids.[47] The efficacy of an epidural technique is determined by numerous factors that can include (1) catheter incision site congruency, (2) choice of analgesic drugs, (3) rates of infusion, (4) duration of epidural analgesia, and (5) type of pain assessment (rest vs. dynamic). Ideally, the epidural catheter is positioned congruent with the surgical incision (Fig. 56-12). Thoracic epidural catheter placement is recommended for both thoracic and upper abdominal surgical procedures because of the observed improvement in coronary artery blood flow, attenuation of pulmonary complications, and the reduction in the duration of postoperative ileus. Combining a local anesthetic plus an opioid in the epidural space is believed to have a synergistic effect.[47] The optimal duration of epidural analgesia has not been determined, but recommendations are that the infusion be continued for at least 2 to 4 days. Other than analgesia, epidural infusions lasting <24 hours do not appear to offer any clear cardiovascular advantages.

Epidurally administered opioids have the distinct advantage of producing analgesia without causing significant sympatholytic effect or motor blockade. Analgesia occurs by way of a *spinal mechanism* and through a *supraspinal mechanism* following systemic adsorption. The spinal mechanism occurs following diffusion of the drug into the spinal fluid, and is determined by meningeal permeability. Opioids with intermediate lipophilicity (e.g., hydromorphone, alfentanil, meperidine) have the ability to easily move between the aqueous and lipid regions of the arachnoid membrane and therefore have high meningeal permeability, which potentially confers higher bioavailability in the spinal cord. However, in a comprehensive review of the topic Bernards et al.[48] concluded that morphine has greater bioavailability in the spinal cord than alfentanil, fentanyl, and sufentanil.

In general, the epidural administration of hydrophilic opioids tends to have a slow onset, long duration, and a mechanism of action that is primarily spinal in nature. The epidural administration of lipophilic opioids, on the other hand, have a quick onset, short duration, and a mechanism of action that is primarily supraspinal, secondary to rapid systemic uptake. However, the data are controversial and the site of action of lipophilic opioids such as fentanyl may primarily be determined by the mode of administration. Bolus administration of fentanyl appears to have a segmental analgesic effect whereas epidural infusion of fentanyl appears to have a nonsegmental (systemic) effect. There are some data, however, that suggest that there can be significant spinal mechanisms of action of the lipophilic opioids, particularly with the thoracic epidural infusion of fentanyl. In the opioid-tolerant patient

FIGURE 56-12. Dermatome guide for placement of epidural catheters.

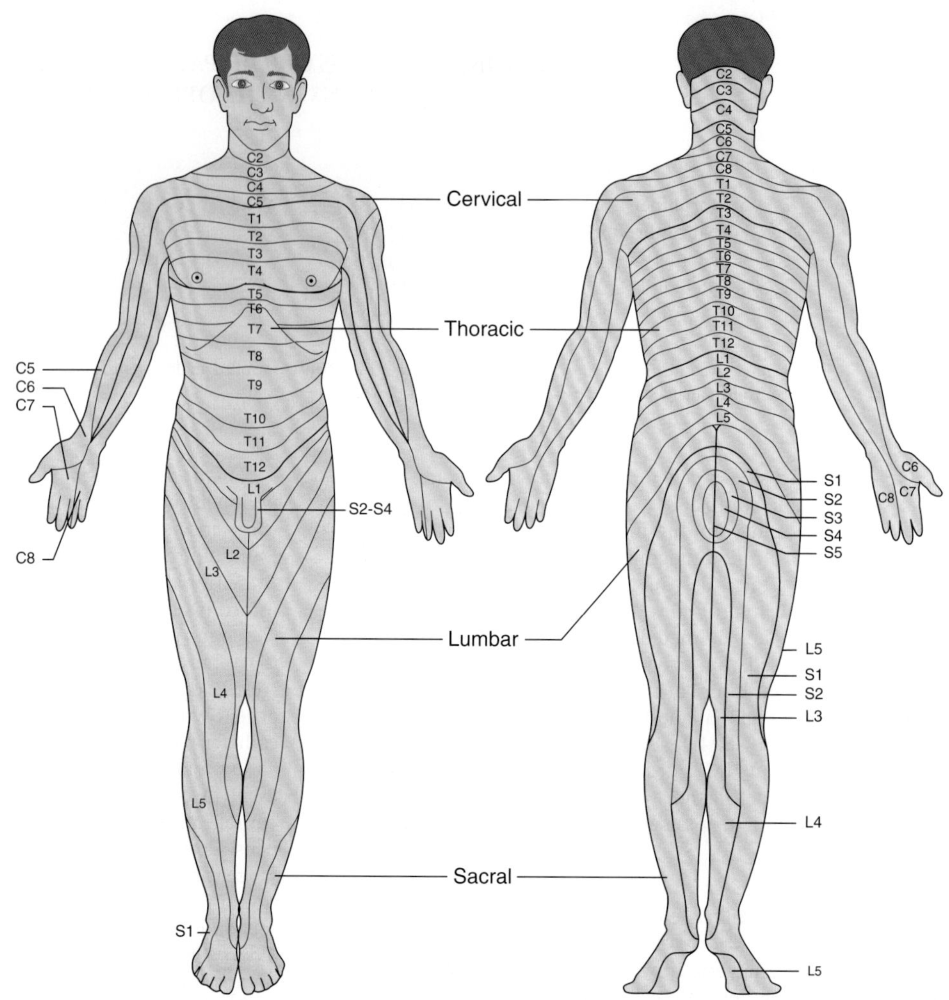

taking >250 mg/day of oral morphine, sufentanil may be considered to be the epidural opioid of choice because of its high intrinsic activity.

As previously mentioned, local anesthetic–opioid combinations are the most common form of epidural infusion because the combination is considered to be synergistic. Local anesthetics have the unique ability to block the stress response by blocking afferent input to the spinal cord. Although bupivacaine plus fentanyl may be the most common combination, bupivacaine plus morphine makes more sense from a bioavailability point of view. Hydromorphone plus bupivacaine also makes very good sense as this combination has all the advantages of a hydrophilic opioid with excellent meningeal permeability but less risk of pruritus. Remember, epidural infusions may consist of just a hydrophilic opioid if the patient cannot tolerate side effects from the local anesthetic or if the epidural is incongruent with the surgical incision. Likewise, an epidural infusion may consist simply of a local anesthetic if the patient cannot tolerate opioid-related side effects, provided that the epidural is correctly placed and is congruent with the surgical incision. Table 56-13 contains epidural dosing guidelines.

Adjuvant medications, which may enhance analgesia, include clonidine and ketamine. Clonidine (2 μg/mL) can be combined with an opioid and a local anesthetic and is usually infused at a rate of 5 to 20 μg/hr. Side effects that limit its clinical usefulness include hypotension, bradycardia, and sedation. An epidural infusion consisting of ropivacaine 0.2%, fentanyl 5 μg/mL, and clonidine 2 μg/mL infused at a rate of 3 to 7 mL/hr following a TKA has been reported to cause no significant sedation in this dosage range.[49] The safety of epidurally administered ketamine has not been determined, and routine use cannot be recommended at this time.

A novel approach to postoperative pain control is extended-release epidural morphine (Depodur). The system consists of morphine encapsulated within a liposome delivery system, which provides controlled release of morphine for up to 48 hours. Double-blinded studies indicate that the epidural administration of liposomal morphine has proven to be efficacious in the treatment of postoperative pain associated with total hip arthroplasty (THA), TKA, and cesarean section. Depodur is only approved for lumbar epidural administration.

Intrathecal analgesia with a variety of drugs is a widely accepted practice for the treatment of both acute and chronic pain. Rathmell et al.[50] have thoroughly reviewed the role of intrathecal analgesia for acute pain. Opioid analgesics are the most commonly administered drugs for this purpose, including morphine, hydromorphone, meperidine, methadone, fentanyl, and sufentanil. Their distribution within the intrathecal space following administration

TABLE 56-13. GUIDELINES FOR ADULT EPIDURAL CATHETER DOSING REGIMEN[a]

Catheter Placement	Surgical Dermatome		
	Lumbar (e.g., total knee arthroplasty or lower extremity bypass surgery)	Low thoracic (e.g., exploratory laparotomy, xiphopubic incision)	Mid-to-high thoracic (e.g., thoracotomy, sternotomy)
Lumbar T_{12}–caudal	Catheter congruent with incision! Bupivacaine 0.05–0.1% or Ropivacaine 0.1–0.2% with Fentanyl 2–5 μg/mL or morphine 0.1 mg/mL or hydromorphone 0.02 mg/mL	Catheter/incision incongruency! [c]May consider Bupivacaine or Ropivacaine with a hydrophilic opioid. *This is not ideal!* [d]Hydrophilic opioids are required! Morphine 0.1 mg/mL or Hydromorphone 0.02 mg/mL	Not Applicable
Low thoracic T_8–T_{12}	Not applicable	Catheter congruent with incision! Bupivacaine 0.05–0.1% or Ropivacaine 0.1–0.2% with Fentanyl 2–5 μg/mL or morphine 0.1 mg/mL or hydromorphone 0.02 mg/mL	Catheter/incision incongruency! May consider Bupivacaine or Ropivacaine with an opioid but *this is not ideal!* Lipophilic Fentanyl 2–5 μg/mL. *This is not the ideal opioid!* [d]Hydrophilic opioids are a better choice! 1. Morphine 0.1 mg/mL or 2. Hydromorphone 0.02 mg/mL
Mid-to-high thoracic T_4–T_8	Not applicable	Not applicable	Catheter Congruent with incision! Bupivacaine 0.05–0.1% or Ropivacaine 0.1–0.2% with Fentanyl 2–5 μg/mL or morphine 0.1 mg/mL or hydromorphone 0.02 mg/mL

[a]Rate of infusion, 2–10 mL/h. Recommended adult dose for epidural bupivacaine. Do not exceed 400 mg/24 h!
[b]May consider Clonidine 1–2 μg/mL in the epidural. Remember hypotension, bradycardia, and sedation are common at doses greater than 14 μg/h.
[c]Local anesthetic efficacy is diminished with catheter/incision incongruency!
[d]Hydrophilic opioids provide a broad band of analgesia! Morphine is the gold-standard. Epidural hydromorphone may cause less pruritus.

is complex. Hydrophilic opioids (e.g., morphine) penetrate the spinal cord and bind to specific pre- and postsynaptic receptors within the dorsal horn. They traverse the dura slowly, bind to epidural fat poorly, and slowly enter the plasma. They tend to have a slow onset of action, long duration, and provide a broad band of analgesia. Delayed respiratory depression is more common with hydrophilic opioids secondary to rostral spread.[50] Lipophilic opioids (e.g., fentanyl), on the other hand, tend to bind to nonspecific receptors in the white matter. They rapidly cross the dura and are quickly sequestered into epidural fat and swiftly enter the systemic circulation. As a general rule lipophilic opioids tend to have a rapid onset of action, short duration, and a narrow band of analgesia. Delayed respiratory depression is less of a problem with the lipophilic opioids. Other side effects associated with intrathecal opioids include nausea and vomiting, urinary retention, and pruritus. The incidence of pruritus with intrathecal hydromorphone is reported to be significantly less than with morphine (refer to Table 56-14 for dosing guidelines).

Other useful analgesic additives include the α_2-agonists, NSAIDs, NMDA receptor antagonists, acetylcholinesterase inhibitors, adenosine, epinephrine, and benzodiazepines. The α_2-agonists alter pain transmission by binding to pre- and postsynaptic receptors within the dorsal horn of the spinal cord. Evidence suggests that intrathecal clonidine is synergistic with spinal local anesthetics, prolongs sensory and motor blockades, and causes less urinary retention than intrathecal morphine.[50] Intrathecal clonidine does not cause respiratory depression or pruritus. Intrathecal doses of 150 μg, however, are reported to increase the incidence of hypotension, bradycardia, and nausea[50] (refer to Table 56-15 for additional dosing recommendations). Anecdotal reports suggest that the neuraxial administration of an NSAID, either accidentally or intentionally, is both safe and effective. Further investigation for the treatment of postoperative pain is required of the role of intrathecal NSAIDs as well as the acetylcholinesterase inhibitors, NMDA receptor antagonists, adenosine, and benzodiazepines.

Peripheral Nerve Blockade

Single-injection peripheral nerve blockade has been shown to provide pain control that is superior to opioids with fewer side effects.[51] Single-injection techniques are limited in duration but continuous peripheral nerve block (CPNB) techniques can extend the benefits of peripheral nerve blockade well into the
9 postoperative period. CPNB has proven to be an effective technique for postoperative pain management; it is superior to opioid analgesia with fewer opioid-related side effects and rare neurologic and infectious complications.[52,53] The benefits of CPNB in

TABLE 56-14. INTRATHECAL ANALGESIA DOSING GUIDELINES[a]

Surgical Procedure	Intrathecal Drug Dose
Labor analgesia	Sufentanil 2.5–5 μg
Cesarean section (C-section)	Morphine 100 μg. The addition of clonidine 60 μg is synergistic and can increase the duration of spinal analgesia after C-section but also increases intraoperative sedation.
Outpatient knee arthroscopy	Fentanyl 10–25 μg will improve intraoperative analgesia without prolonging postoperative motor blockade.
Total knee arthroscopy	Morphine 200–300 μg
Total hip arthroplasty	Morphine 100–200 μg
Thoracotomy and major abdominal surgery	Morphine 500 μg. The incidence of side effects such as nausea and vomiting, urinary retention, and pruritus increase significantly with doses >300 μg.

[a]50–100 μg of intrathecal hydromorphone approximates 100–200 μg of intrathecal morphine.

Data derived from: *Principles of Analgesic Use in the Treatment of Acute Pain and Cancer Pain.* 5th ed. Glenview, IL, American Pain Society, 2003; Rathmell JP, Lair TR, Nauman B. The role of intrathecal drugs in the treatment of acute pain. *Anesth Analg.* 2005;101(5 suppl):S30.

the ambulatory setting include prolonged postoperative analgesia, facilitated discharge from the hospital, fewer opioid-related side effects, and greater patient satisfaction.[54] Finally, CPNB has proven to be an extraordinarily useful technique in the austere and remote environment of the battlefield by providing site-specific and opioid-sparing analgesia for the wounded soldier. Tables 56-16 and 56-17 present indications and contraindications for specific peripheral nerve blocks. Table 56-18 has recommended dosing regimen of CPNB.

The Brachial Plexus

Above the Clavicle

The *interscalene block* is the ideal peripheral nerve block for painful orthopedic and vascular procedures performed on the shoulder and upper arm, but is a poor choice for forearm and hand surgery as the ulnar nerve is commonly spared. It is the most cephalad approach to the brachial plexus and was originally described by Winnie[55] in 1970. In his now-classic description, the plexus is approached at the C6 level (cricoid cartilage) where the roots of the brachial plexus (C5 to T1) pass between the anterior and middle scalene muscles in the interscalene groove. The direction of the needle is medial, dorsal, and caudad with the needle entry approximately 60 degrees from the sagittal plane. A motor response to the biceps, deltoid, or pectoralis major muscle has been shown to be an acceptable end point when performing an interscalene block with a neurostimulation. An important caveat is that if you produce a diaphragmatic or trapezius muscle contraction while performing the block, your block needle is either too anterior (phrenic nerve stimulation) or too posterior (spinal accessory nerve stimulation) to the interscalene groove.

This block is easily performed using ultrasound guidance with a posterior in-plane approach and the transducer positioned in an axial oblique plane. The needle tip can be advanced under real time and positioned near the nerve roots between the middle and anterior scalene muscles. A recent study has confirmed that regardless of motor response, as long as the needle tip is positioned between the two most lateral nerve structures you will achieve a successful blockade of the plexus.[56] Your end point for injection of local anesthetic has now become real-time observation of hydrodissection and not motor stimulation.

Single-injection interscalene blockade for shoulder surgery reduces postoperative VAS pain scores, total opioid consumption, postoperative nausea and vomiting, time for request of first dose of analgesic, time to discharge, and unplanned hospital admissions.[57] Interscalene blockade provides postoperative analgesia, which is superior to subacromial bursae blockade, suprascapular nerve blockade, infusion of intra-articular local anesthetic, and parenteral opioids. To extend the period of postoperative analgesia, continuous catheter techniques have been successfully

TABLE 56-15. INTRATHECAL ANALGESIA OTHER DOSING GUIDELINES

Intrathecal Drug	Dosing	Comments
Clonidine	15–45 μg improves the quality of spinal blockade in outpatient surgery.	Side effects increase significantly at intrathecal doses >150 μg.
Epinephrine	0.1–0.6 mg Dose-related increase 1. Return of motor function 2. Return of micturition	Not recommended for outpatient surgery
Neostigmine	6.25–50 μg Dose-related increase: 1. Motor blockade 2. Time for resolution of the block 3. Nausea and vomiting	Further studies of the appropriate intrathecal dose that optimizes analgesia while minimizing side effects are warranted.

Data derived from: Rathmell JP, Lair TR, Nauman B. The role of intrathecal drugs in the treatment of acute pain. *Anesth Analg.* 2005;101(5 suppl):S30; Liu SS, McDonald SB. Current issues in spinal anesthesia. *Anesthesiology.* 2001;94:888.

TABLE 56-16. **BRACHIAL PLEXUS BLOCKADE**

Peripheral Nerve Block	Indications	Contraindications	Comments
Interscalene	Total shoulder arthroplasty and hemiarthroplasty Open rotator cuff repair Open anterior reconstruction Open reduction, internal fixation (ORIF) and joint fusion.	Refusal by the patient, infection, or hematoma in the vicinity of the block, allergy to local anesthetics, and progressive neuropathy or lesion of unknown etiology. In the anticoagulated patient follow the recommendations set forth for neuraxial blockade until practice guidelines for peripheral nerve blocks are promulgated.	Catheter techniques are useful for painful surgeries such as shoulder arthroplasty. Ultrasound-guided regional anesthesia (UGRA) can shorten the onset time of the block and decrease the dose of local anesthetic required. Low-volume UGRA of the brachial plexus can decrease the risk of hemidiaphragmatic paresis (HDP). Pneumothorax (PTX) is a risk with the classic approach. Winnie's *perivascular approach* and the *plumb bob approach* can minimize but not totally eliminate the risk of PTX. Ultrasound guidance has the potential of significantly decreasing the risk of PTX. Low-volume UGRA can almost eliminate the risk of HDP.
Supraclavicular	Provides anesthesia to the entire upper extremity with a single injection of local anesthetic.	See above	Catheter techniques are beneficial and relatively easy to perform.
Infraclavicular	This approach is ideally suited for surgery on the distal upper arm, the entire forearm, wrist, and hand.	See above Also chest deformities and healed but dislocated fractures of the clavicle.	Ultrasound guidance can significantly improve the safety and effectiveness of this block.
Axillary	Surgery distal to the elbow: Arteriovenous fistula, Colles fracture, Dupytrens contracture release, wrist fusion and ORIF.	See above	Separate blockade of the musculocutaneous and intercostobrachial nerves are usually necessary. Catheter techniques can be useful. Consider ultrasound guidance.
Midhumeral	Surgery on the: forearm, wrist and hand	See above	When you need adequate blockade of the radial nerve (e.g., wrist surgery) consider this block over the axillary approach.

employed in both the inpatient and outpatient settings. In a randomized placebo-controlled study of patients undergoing total shoulder arthroplasty, investigators concluded that continuous nerve blockade with 0.2% ropivacaine provided potent analgesia that improved postoperative shoulder mobility and shortened the time to discharge.[58]

The *supraclavicular approach* to the brachial plexus provides anesthesia to the entire upper extremity with a single injection of local anesthetic. The supraclavicular approach is carried out at a point where the plexus is reduced to its fewest component parts, the superior, middle, and inferior trunks, as they pass under the clavicle and over the first rib. An important landmark is the subclavian artery, which is often palpable in the supraclavicular fossa. The nerves of the brachial plexus lie in a cephaloposterior relationship to the artery at this level. When performing the block with a peripheral nerve stimulator, stimulation of the middle trunk (hand twitch) is reported to be associated with the highest success rates.

In the now "classic" Kulenkampff description,[59] needle insertion is 1 cm above the midpoint of the clavicle in a plane that is parallel to the patient's head and neck. This approach requires the elicitation of multiple paresthesias and multiple injections. The incidence of pneumothorax has been reported to be as high as 0.5% to 5% with this technique. With the introduction of ultrasound-guided supraclavicular blockade, however, the safety of this approach has improved dramatically. Real-time imaging of the needle tip in order to optimize its position not only decreases the risk of pneumothorax but increases the quality and shortens the onset time of the block.[60] The optimal position of the needle tip when performing this block with ultrasound guidance is reported to be in the corner bordered by the subclavian artery medially, the first rib inferiorly, and the divisions of the

TABLE 56-17. LUMBAR AND SACRAL PLEXUS BLOCKADE

Peripheral Nerve Block	Indications	Contraindications	Comments
Lumbar plexus	Total knee reconstruction and joint replacement surgery. Anterior and posterior cruciate ligament repair. Patellar tendon or fracture repair. May be combined with sciatic nerve block for hip surgery.	Refusal by the patient, infection, or hematoma in the vicinity of the block, allergy to local anesthetics, and progressive neuropathy or lesion of unknown etiology.	Catheter techniques may be useful for painful surgical procedures such as cruciate ligament grafting or joint replacement surgery.
		In the anticoagulated patient follow the recommendations set forth for neuraxial blockade until practice guidelines for peripheral nerve blocks are promulgated.	Excellent blockade of femoral, obturator, and lateral femoral cutaneous nerves. A true 3-in-1 block. Avoid this technique in the anticoagulated patient.
Femoral nerve	Total knee arthroplasty (TKA) Antereior cruciate ligament repair, femoral neck fractures, and saphenous vein stripping. Muscle biopsies involving the ventral, medial, or lateral thigh.	See above	Good choice for TKA. May be combined with a sciatic nerve block for TKA. Catheter techniques are useful. Ultrasound guidance confirms placement of the needle tip between the fascia iliaca and the iliopsoas muscle.
Sciatic nerve	Above-the-knee amputation. Combine with a lumbar plexus block. Ankle joint replacement. Ankle arthrodesis. Calcaneal osteotomy. Achilles tendon repair.	See above	Numerous approaches have been described. The *parasacral approach* is the most cephalad. The *infragluteal parabiceps approach* is useful. Catheter techniques are useful for prolonged analgesia. Ultrasound guidance can confirm needle placement in the subgluteal space.
Popliteal fossa	Below-the-knee amputation. Combine with a saphenous nerve block. *Ankle surgery:* Triple arthrodesis, arthroscopy, and Achilles tendon repair. *Foot surgery:* Bunion surgery and transmetatarsal amputation.	See above	Lateral and posterior approaches have been described. Catheter insertion following ambulatory foot surgery can provide prolonged analgesia. Ultrasound guidance is very useful. Use the "seesaw" sign to confirm identification of the common peroneal and tibial nerves.

TABLE 56-18. RECOMMENDED DOSING REGIMEN OF LOCAL ANESTHETICS FOR CONTINUOUS PERIPHERAL NERVE BLOCKADE

Catheter	Agent	Rate of Infusion	PCA Bolus (mL)	Lockout (min)
Interscalene Infraclavicular	Ropivacaine 0.2% or bupivacaine 0.15–0.2%	5–8 mL/h	2–4	15–20
Femoral	Ropivacaine 0.2% or	5–10 mL/h	—	—
Popliteal	bupivacaine 0.15–0.2%	—	5–10	30–60
		5–8 mL/h	2	15–20
Paravertebral	Ropivacaine 0.2%	0.1–0.2 mL/kg/h	—	—
	Bupivacaine 0.25% with 0.1 mL/kg/h 1:400,000 epinephrine	—	—	

PCA, patient-controlled analgesia.

Data derived from: Karmakar MK, Chui PT, Joynt GM, et al. Thoracic paravertebral block for management of pain associated with multiple fractured ribs in patients with concomitant lumbar spinal trauma. *Reg Anesth Pain Med.* 2001;26:169; Liu S: Update in use of continuous perineural catheters for postoperative analgesia. IARS 2006 Review Course Lectures. *Anesth Analg suppl.* 2006: 64.

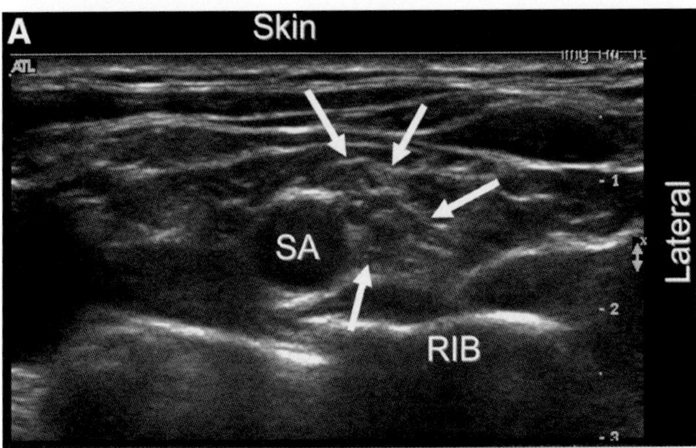

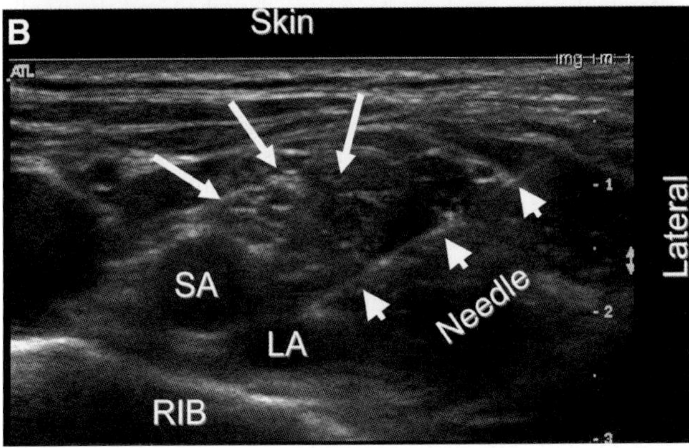

FIGURE 56-13. Ultrasound-guided supraclavicular nerve block. SA, subclavian artery; LA, local anesthetic. (Reprinted from: Soares LG, Brull R, Lai J, et al. Eight ball, corner pocket: The optimal needle position for ultrasound-guided supraclavicular block. *Reg Anesth Pain Med.* 2007; 32:2, with permission.)

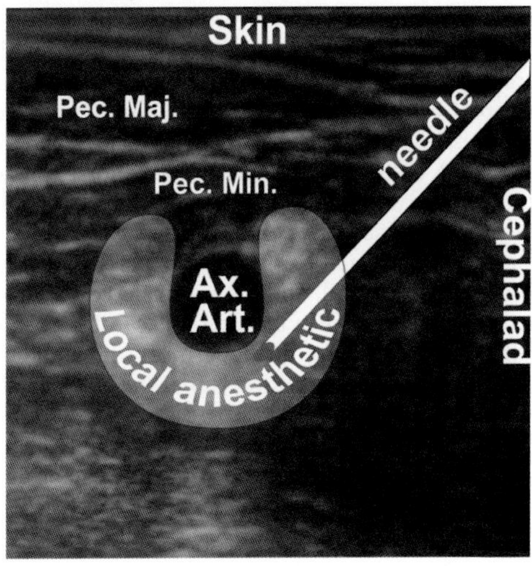

FIGURE 56-14. Ultrasound-guided infraclavicular nerve block. Ultrasonic anatomy, initial needle position, and desired U-shaped anesthetic distribution. Pec. Maj., pectoralis major muscle; Pec. Min., pectoralis minor muscle; Ax. Art., axillary artery. (Reused with permission from: Dingemans E, Williams SR, Arcand G et al. Neurostimulation in ultrasound guided infraclavicular block. *Anesth Analg.* 2007;104:1274.)

brachial plexus superiorly and laterally.[61] Administration of local anesthetic at this location allows the brachial plexus to be displaced superiorly (Fig. 56-13) and a dense block sets up within minutes.[61] Although the supraclavicular approach is amenable to continuous catheter techniques, the literature on this subject is meager.

Below the Clavicle

The *infraclavicular block* is ideally suited for surgical procedures below the midhumerus such as the hand, wrist, forearm, or elbow.[62] The block targets the brachial plexus at the level of the cords where it is in close proximity to the axillary artery.[63] The popularity of this approach has been less than enthusiastic because of unreliable surface landmarks and the potential risks of pneumothorax and vascular puncture. Ultrasound guidance has dramatically improved both the safety and efficacy of the infraclavicular approach and success rates are reported to be in the 90% to 100% range.[64] Ideal positioning is reported to be with the arm abducted to 110 degrees, externally rotated, and the elbow flexed 90 degrees. With this positioning, the plexus lies closer to the surface, facilitating ultrasound visualization, and the block is performed with relative ease. The needle puncture is made at the apex of the deltopectoral groove in the sagittal plane. Because this is a deep block, visualization of individual cords may be challenging so that the axillary artery becomes an important landmark. The optimal injection site is craniposterior and adjacent to the axillary artery.[65] This area is closest to all three cords and potentially optimizes local anesthetic spread. A prospective randomized trial comparing ultrasound-guided infraclavicular blockade, with and without neurostimulation, has confirmed that the "U-shaped" distribution of local anesthetic around the posterior, medial, and lateral aspects of the axillary artery will reliably produce complete blockade of the brachial plexus (Fig. 56-14).[63] The authors conclude that infraclavicular blockade is more rapidly performed and a block of better quality is achieved when you use local anesthetic spread as your end point for injection as opposed to neurostimulation.

A recent large-scale study documented the analgesic benefit and favorable safety profile of single-injection infraclavicular nerve blockade.[66] Placement of continuous infraclavicular nerve catheters has the advantage of providing prolonged analgesia for several days following surgery. Benefits include improved pain scores, decreased opioid requirements, less sedation, and less sleep disturbance with continuous infraclavicular nerve blockade.[67] The block can be performed with the arm *abducted* or *adducted* position. This flexibility in positioning can be advantageous particularly in the trauma patient who has significant pain and limited mobility. Placement of continuous infraclavicular catheters provides the advantage of a secure point of insertion that will not dislodge easily with patient movement. It is also relatively easy to keep clean and sterile particularly if the patient is to be discharged home with the catheter in situ to be removed at a latter date.

The Lumbar Plexus

Posterior Approach (Psoas Compartment Block)

The lumbar plexus is formed from the ventral rami of the L1 to L4 spinal nerve roots, with a small contribution from T12 in some patients. The plexus lies within the substance of the psoas muscle in between the anterior and posterior masses and gives rise to the femoral (saphenous), obturator, lateral femoral cutaneous, ilioinguinal, iliohypogastric, and genitofemoral nerves. The nerves provide sensory innervation to the abdomen and groin, the anterior, lateral, and medial aspects of the thigh, the knee joint, and the medial part of the calf. Motor innervation is supplied to the abdominal muscles, the hip flexors, thigh adductors, and the quadriceps muscles. Numerous posterior and anterior approaches for lumbar plexus blockade (LPB) have been described[68] and the block is indicated for major surgeries of the hip and knee.

The posterior approach to the lumbar plexus reliably blocks the femoral, lateral femoral, and obturator nerves.[69] The block is performed with the patient in the lateral decubitus position usually with the operative side in the uppermost (independent) position. The advantage of this position is that the block can be combined with a sciatic nerve block. The disadvantage, however, is the increased risk of epidural spread. When combined with sciatic nerve blockade, virtually any surgical procedure can be performed on the lower extremity. Although ultrasound-guided LPB has been described in the literature, it has not been studied extensively. The depth of the plexus in adults may make ultrasound guidance both difficult and unreliable and preclude its use; however, in children ultrasound-guided LPB may prove to be efficacious.[70]

LPB alone and combined with sciatic nerve blockade has been safely and effectively used in the outpatient setting for knee arthroscopy. For more painful and invasive procedures such as TKA, THA, and ACL repair, however, the benefit of LBP for postoperative pain management becomes even more evident. When compared with epidural analgesia there is a reduced requirement for urinary catheter insertion, and the risk of epidural hematoma formation secondary to postoperative anticoagulation is nearly eliminated. Continuous LPB with a catheter technique is reported to provide optimal analgesia both at rest and during physiotherapy following THA and may provide opioid-free analgesia following both TKA and THA.[71]

Complications are associated with the placement of sciatic and psoas compartment blocks. Therefore, extreme care should be exercised if you choose to place these blocks. The incidence of sciatic nerve injury following TKA, unrelated to regional anesthesia technique, is reported to be in the range of 0.2% to 2.4%.[72] Risk factors include valgus deformity (≥10 degrees), tourniquet time ≥120 minutes, pre-existing neuropathy, and postoperative bleeding.[73] Sciatic nerve blockade can mask these complications. Intermittent bolusing of the sciatic catheter (e.g., discontinuous catheter technique) allows neurologic examination between boluses. Complications associated with the placement of a psoas compartment block includes epidural spread, spinal anesthesia, systemic toxicity, unilateral sympathectomy, renal subscapular hematoma, and neurologic injury.[73] Psoas compartment blockade should be avoided in the anticoagulated patient.

Anterior Approach (Femoral Nerve Block)

The femoral nerve is formed from the posterior divisions of the ventral rami of L2 to L4 and is the largest terminal branch of the lumbar plexus. The nerve emerges from the lower lateral border of the psoas muscle and passes beneath the inguinal ligament in the groove between the iliacus and psoas muscles. In the inguinal region the nerve is covered by two fascial layers, the fascia lata and fascia iliaca, and whereas the fascia lata separates the subcutaneous tissue from the muscle and vessels, the fascia iliaca completely envelopes both the iliopsoas muscle and the femoral nerve, physically separating the nerve from the femoral artery and vein.[74] Although the nerve can be visualized with ultrasound, both above and below the inguinal ligament it is ideally visualized at the level of the inguinal crease, and at this level, the nerve is positioned approximately 0.5 cm lateral to the femoral artery. The nerve provides motor innervation to the quadriceps femoris, sartorius, and pectineus muscles as well as sensory innervation to the anterior thigh, knee and the medial aspect of the lower extremity terminating as the saphenous nerve. Recent ultrasound-guided evidence indicates that the topographic relationship of the femoral nerve at the inguinal crease is *medial and lateral* to each other rather than *anterior and posterior* and both divisions are in close proximity to each other under the fascia iliaca.[75]

In 1973, Winnie and colleagues[76] described a paravascular approach to femoral nerve blockade as a "3-in-1" technique suggesting that the fascial sheath that surrounds the femoral nerve acts as a conduit to reliably anesthetize the femoral, obturator, and lateral femoral cutaneous nerves. In reality, the obturator nerve is commonly spared.

Since the original description several anterior approaches to femoral nerve blockade have been described and the needle insertion site varies considerably. Needle insertion at the inguinal (femoral) crease (2 to 4 cm below the inguinal ligament) immediately lateral to the femoral pulse results in a 100% success rate for surgical anesthesia when using a peripheral nerve stimulator technique. With the patient in the supine position, a 2-inch (50-mm) insulated short bevel needle is advanced at a 60-degree angle in posterior and cephalad directions. Although a quadriceps "twitch" has been described as the appropriate muscle stimulation using a peripheral nerve stimulation technique, recent evidence supports either a quadriceps or sartorius evoked muscle twitch as an acceptable stimulation end point associated with equivalent degrees of femoral nerve blockade.[77] Eliciting a motor response at 0.3 to 0.5 mA confirms the ideal needle position, and local anesthetic can be incrementally injected with periodic aspiration to avoid intravascular injection.

Another very successful approach to femoral nerve blockade is the fascia iliaca compartment block. The injection site is distant from any neurovascular structures and therefore does not require neurostimulation to be successful.[73] The block has been described in both children and adults and is reported to be more successful than the 3-in-1 block. Continuous peripheral nerve catheter placement is reported to be faster with the fascia iliaca approach.[73]

Femoral nerve blockade is tremendously effective for postoperative pain control following arthroscopic reconstruction of the ACL with *patellar tendon autograft*. Single-injection femoral nerve blockade improves postoperative pain control, delays the time to first request for an analgesic, and provides analgesia superior to intra-articular ropivacaine. Femoral nerve blockade alone is an inadequate block for ACL reconstruction with *hamstring autograft* because of postoperative pain in the sciatic nerve distribution. A combination of femoral nerve blockade and sciatic nerve blockade is necessary in this case. In addition, continuous catheter techniques can prolong analgesia well into the postoperative period. Femoral nerve blockade alone or in combination with sciatic nerve blockade provides superior pain control and a reduction in unanticipated hospital admissions when used for more invasive and complex outpatient knee surgeries such as high osteotomy, multiple ligament reconstruction, and meniscal reconstruction. A meta-analysis concludes that femoral nerve blockade is as effective as epidural analgesia following TKA.[78] Femoral nerve blockade provides site-specific analgesia and is an integral part of any multimodal analgesic regimen following major knee or hip surgery.[79]

Ultrasound-guided femoral nerve blockade has also been described.[74] Care must be taken to place the tip of the needle within the space between the fascia iliaca and the iliopsoas muscle lateral to the femoral artery (Fig. 56-15). Local anesthetic can then be injected under real time and hydrodissection can be directly observed near the medial and lateral divisions of the femoral nerve. Placement of a continuous femoral nerve block catheter is

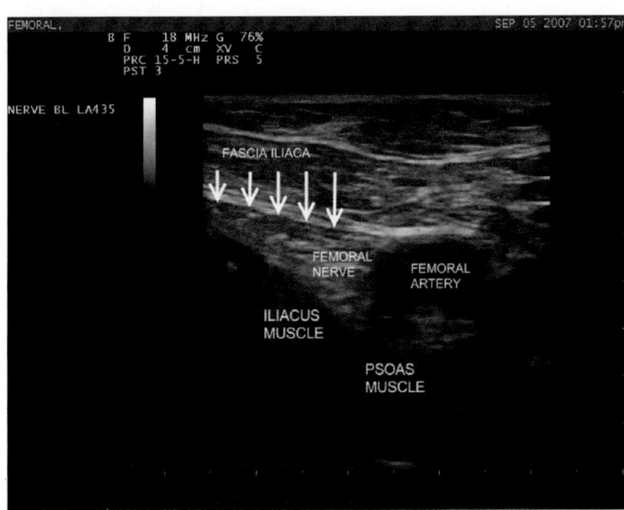

FIGURE 56-15. Ultrasound-guided femoral nerve blockade: Short axis ultrasound image of the infrainguinal structures. Femoral nerve blockade can be performed with a needle approach that is either in-plane or out-of-plane. The needle tip must be positioned within the space between the fascia iliaca and the iliopsoas muscle before local anesthetic is injected in order to achieve a successful block of the femoral nerve.

highly recommended as part of a multimodal analgesic regimen for both TKA and THA. Ultrasound-guided placement of the catheter perpendicular to or parallel to the femoral nerve has been described and as long as the tip of the catheter is in close proximity to the femoral nerve both techniques are equally effective.[80] In combination with ultrasound guidance, the fascia iliaca approach has also been successfully used for the placement of continuous peripheral nerve catheters in the outpatient setting.[54] Advantages of ultrasound guidance for femoral nerve blockade versus guidance by peripheral nerve stimulation include (1) decreased time for onset of complete sensory blockade, (2) reduction in local anesthetic volume, and (3) an increased success of sensory block.

Saphenous nerve blockade is frequently combined with a lateral popliteal block or sciatic block for procedures involving the lower leg. The saphenous nerve is the only branch of the lumbar plexus below the knee and is the largest sensory terminal branch of the femoral nerve. The nerve provides sensory innervation to the medial, anteromedial, and posteromedial parts of the knee, leg, and medial malleolus and, in some people, the medial aspect of the large toe. Several approaches have been described at the level of the patella and medial malleolus. The paravenous approach is based on the close relationship of the saphenous vein and nerve at the level of the tibial tuberosity. Ultrasound-guided saphenous nerve blockade deep to the sartorius muscle near the adductor canal has also been described in the literature and this may prove to be a useful approach.[81]

Sacral Plexus

The sciatic nerve originates from the sacral plexus and is derived from the ventral rami of the fourth lumbar to the third sacral nerve roots. The three major components of the sciatic nerve include the tibial and common peroneal nerves and the posterior femoral cutaneous nerve to the thigh. The sciatic nerve provides sensory, motor, and some sympathetic innervation to the lower extremity and, its blockade in combination with an LPB, can provide complete anesthesia and postoperative analgesia for lower extremity surgery. Numerous proximal and distal techniques, using anterior, posterior, and lateral approaches to the sciatic nerve with the patient in the supine, prone lateral, and lithotomy positions, have been described. Patient comfort is a key factor in determining the preferred approach. *Proximal* sciatic nerve blockade is often combined with a psoas compartment block or a femoral nerve block for procedures on the lower extremity including THA, TKA, and ACL repair, as previously discussed. In addition, the combination of a femoral and a sciatic nerve block is also indicated for complex outpatient knee surgeries, above- and below-the-knee amputations, and ankle and foot surgery.

Following foot and ankle surgery, sciatic nerve blockade provides safe, effective, and long-lasting postoperative analgesia. The infragluteal parabiceps approach offers distinct advantages over the more traditional approaches as the approach relies on easily palpable soft-tissue landmarks. Inversion of the foot following nerve stimulation at <0.4 mA is the preferred evoked motor response because inversion is found to be associated with a more rapid onset and complete blockade. Unfortunately, single-shot proximal sciatic nerve blockade with a long-acting local anesthetic can only provide analgesia for 10 to 20 hours. Continuous proximal sciatic nerve blockade has been successfully applied for foot and ankle surgery and below-the-knee amputation. Continuous parasacral sciatic nerve blockade has been described in patients undergoing complex lower extremity surgery including TKA, osteotomy, above-the-knee amputation, osteosarcoma resection, and other procedures on the leg. The advantage of this approach is complete anesthesia of all three branches of the sciatic nerve.

Ultrasound guidance provides real-time visualization and high-quality images of the sciatic nerve. Using a curved 2- to 5-MHz (megahertz) transducer, very good quality images of the sciatic nerve have been described in the gluteal, infragluteal, and proximal thigh locations[82] (Figs. 56-16 and 56-17). Successful ultrasound-guided blockade of the sciatic nerve within the subgluteal has also been described with the hyperechoic nerve being easily imaged with a 2- to 5-MHz transducer at the level of the greater trochanter and ischial tuberosity.[83] Ultrasound-guided subgluteal blockade with a stimulating catheter has also been

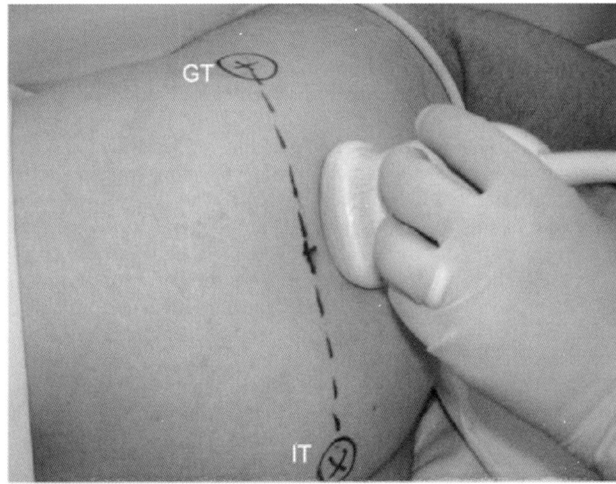

FIGURE 56-16. Ultrasound-guided sciatic nerve blockade. Ultrasound transducer positioned transverse in the infragluteal region. GT, greater trochanter; IT, ischial tuberosity. (Reprinted from: Chan VW, Nova H, Abbas S, et al. Ultrasound examination and localization of the sciatic nerve. *Anesthesiology*. 2006;104:310, with permission.)

PERIOPERATIVE AND CONSULTATIVE SERVICES

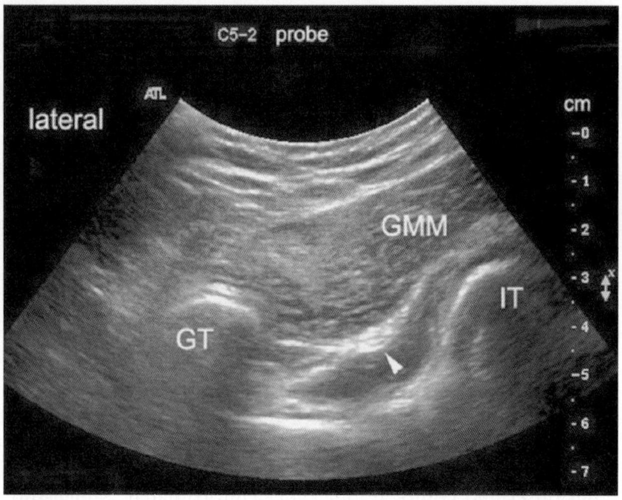

FIGURE 56-17. Ultrasound image of the sciatic nerve. The *arrow* points to the sciatic nerve. GT, greater trochanter; GMM, gluteus maximus muscle; IT, ischial tuberosity. (Reprinted from: Chan VW, Nova H, Abbas S, et al. Ultrasound examination and localization of the sciatic nerve. *Anesthesiology.* 2006;104:311, with permission.)

described in children undergoing various lower extremity surgical procedures.[84] The authors describe excellent postoperative analgesia and patient satisfaction.

Distal sciatic nerve blockade is typically performed in the popliteal fossa using a lateral or posterior approach. In the adult patient, the block is preferably performed at least 100 mm superior to the popliteal crease cephalad to the bifurcation of the sciatic nerve into the tibial and common peroneal nerves. When using neurostimulation as the end point for injection of local anesthetic, inversion of the foot is the ideal motor response that best predicts complete sensory blockade. The popliteal approach to sciatic nerve blockade typically spares the posterior cutaneous nerve to the thigh, thus preserving hamstring function. This approach therefore has the added benefit of being less restrictive on ambulation, which is useful following ambulatory surgery. The block provides superior analgesia for foot and ankle surgery and is often paired with a saphenous nerve block for surgeries involving the medial aspect of the leg and foot. Compared with subcutaneous local anesthetic infiltration and ankle blockade, popliteal sciatic nerve blockade provides significantly longer postoperative analgesia and has a high degree of patient satisfaction. Ultrasound guidance significantly improves the accuracy of needle placement through real-time imaging of the nerve and potentially improves efficacy.[85] The image of the sciatic nerve in the popliteal space will vary depending on the type of transducer used, but the linear 5- to 12-MHz transducer provides the highest resolution image.[85] With the posterior approach and a short-axis (transverse cross-sectional) view, active or passive dorsiflexion of the foot can produce external rotation of the sciatic nerve, which facilitates its identification. Real-time visualization of circumferential spread of local anesthetic around the nerve with ultrasound guidance will not only decrease the failure rate but it will expedite block onset compared with conventional techniques, reduce complications, and provide greater patient satisfaction.[85]

Continuous popliteal sciatic nerve blockade can significantly extend the duration of superb postoperative analgesia and has been successfully implemented in both the inpatient and outpatient settings. Pain-related sleep disruption is less, and hospital length of stay is shorter, which can potentially lead to a reduction in healthcare costs.[86] Risks associated with at-home perineural infusions of local anesthetic include catheter site infection, nerve injury, and catheter migration with subsequent local anesthetic toxicity. Complications are relatively rare.[54,87]

Paravertebral blockade (PVB) can provide segmental analgesia for numerous surgical procedures including thoracotomy, mastectomy, nephrectomy, cholecystectomy and rib fractures, spinal surgery, and video-assisted thorascopic surgery, as well as inguinal and abdominal procedures. The paravertebral space (PVS) does not actually exist but is considered to be a potential space created by fluid distention of the tissues.[88] The PVS is defined anteriorly by the parietal pleura, posteriorly by the costotransverse ligament, superiorly by the occiput, inferiorly by the alar of the sacrum, and medially by the vertebral body, intervertebral disc, and the intervertebral foramen. Laterally, the PVS is contiguous with the intercostal space.[88] The PVS contains the anterior and posterior ramus of the spinal nerve root and the white and grey rami communicantes. Injection of local anesthetic into this potential space will therefore produce a dense sensory and sympathetic block resulting in unilateral segmental analgesia.[2] Generally speaking, PVB is performed at the thoracic level. When performed in the lumbar region it is better known as a *psoas compartment block* and when performed at the cervical level it is referred to as a *deep cervical plexus block.*[88]

Blind percutaneous PVB can be performed with the patient in the seated, prone, or lateral decubitus position. The block is administered with either a spinal needle or a Tuohy needle and multiple- and single-injection and catheter techniques have been described. Needle insertion is 2.5 cm lateral to the superior aspect of the spinous process (paramedial line) and advanced perpendicular to the skin in all planes until it contacts the transverse process, which is at a depth of about 2 to 5 cm in the adult. The needle is "walked" off the transverse process superiorly or inferiorly and advanced no more than 1 to 1.5 cm into the PVS. Loss of resistance to air or saline may be used but it has an indistinct end point. However, nerve stimulation and ultrasound both have the potential to facilitate needle placement. Although single-level (T4) and multilevel (C7 to T6) blocks can be performed, four injections can provide a more reliable loss of sensation than a single injection.[89] The recommended bolus dose of bupivacaine, to be distributed over single or multiple levels, is 1.5 mg/kg (0.3 mL/kg of 0.5% bupivacaine) not to exceed 150 mg total dose. The addition of epinephrine 1:400,000 to 1:200,000 can prolong the blockade and serves to facilitate detection of intravascular injection. Ropivacaine 0.5% may be a safer alternative to bupivacaine, and besides it has been shown to have a more rapid onset, a broader initial spread, and a longer duration of action. The recommended dose for an infusion is 0.1 mL/kg/hr of 0.25% bupivacaine or 0.1 to 0.2 mL/kg/hr of 0.2% ropivacaine.[90] Complications include hypotension, vascular puncture, pleural puncture, pneumothorax, and epidural or intrathecal trespass. The risk of pleural puncture can be decreased with the assistance of sonographic guidance to identify the transverse process. Likewise, the risk of pleural puncture can be decreased when the paravertebral catheter is placed percutaneously under direct visualization of the parietal pleura by the surgeon or the anesthesiologist prior to closure of a thoracotomy incision.

The advantages of PVB include lower postoperative VAS pain scores, a reduction in postoperative opioid consumption, and, therefore, less opioid-induced postoperative nausea and vomiting, less pain with movement, and shorter hospital stays. Continuous PVB compares favorably with thoracic epidurals for post-thoracotomy analgesia. Continuous PVB provides analgesia that is equivalent to thoracic epidural blockade but without the side effects of hypotension, postoperative nausea and vomiting, and urinary retention[91] and may therefore be a reasonable alternative to a thoracic epidural catheter for postoperative analgesia.

Miscellaneous Regional Anesthesia Techniques

The *rectus sheath block* (RSB) is a regional anesthetic technique for use in adults to provide relaxation of the anterior abdominal wall during laparotomy. The RSB has been described in both adults and children and can provide effective postoperative analgesia for both umbilical and midline surgical incisions. The block is performed by depositing local anesthetic in the potential space between the rectus abdominis muscle and the posterior rectus sheath. Traditionally, the RSB has relied on a "blind" technique using a short bevel needle with an end point for injection defined as a loss of resistance or an audible "pop." Complications associated with the block include intraperitoneal injection of local anesthetic, perforation of the bowel, and puncture of a mesenteric vessel. Ultrasound-guided RSB has been described in both the pediatric and adult populations and real-time imaging of the optimal needle position will eliminate or at least minimize the uncertainty and potential complications associated with the "blind" technique.

The *transversus abdominis plane* block is very similar to the RSB in that it anesthetizes neural afferents that supply the anterior abdominal wall. This block can provide adequate postoperative analgesia in patients undergoing major abdominal surgery. It is performed by injecting local anesthetic into the transversus abdominis plane via the triangle of Petit, which is defined by the latissimus dorsi muscle posteriorly, the external oblique muscle anteriorly, and the iliac crest caudally. This is a blind approach that uses a "double-pop" technique to advance the needle into the appropriate fascial plane. Fortunately, the transversus abdominis plane block can be performed using ultrasound guidance[92] and, as is the case with the RSB, potentially increasing the success rate of the block while decreasing complications.

Placement of a *continuous wound catheter* is a relatively simple and sometimes effective technique in which the surgeon places a catheter into the wound at the end of surgery and a local anesthetic infusion is begun. Appropriate placement of the catheter in the preperitoneal space, rather than the subcutaneous space, is required for adequate analgesia. Local anesthetics may inhibit the first and second stages of wound healing, so routine use may not be recommended.[93] Further study of this promising modality is recommended.

Recently, there has been an interest in continuous *intra-articular* and *periarticular* infiltration of local anesthetic with or without opioid for TKA. The advantage of the approach is that quadriceps strength can be maintained thus facilitating ambulation and possibly earlier discharge from the hospital. A major disadvantange of this approach relates to reports of chondrolysis that may limit its usage. Other major disadvantages include the potential for large wound effusions and an increased risk for infection with a catheter in place, The *periarticular soft-tissue injection* of local anesthetic combined with an NSAID (e.g., ropivacaine and ketorolac) combined with an intra-articular catheter for 24 hours has been described.[94] This technique appears to be safe and effective, and the risk of infection is minimized by removing the catheter on postoperative day 1. A single-injection technique referred to as *local infiltration analgesia* (LIA), following TKA, has also been described in the literature. Although injection of local anesthetic in the soft tissue around the knee joint is of proven efficacy, there are concerns about local anesthetic systemic toxicity. Likewise, there are reports of major complications including deep infection and wound dehiscence in the LIA groups.[95]

Continuous Peripheral Nerve Blockade Caveats

Interest in CPNB increased following the Food and Drug Administration warning in 1997 on the risk of spinal hematoma in patients who received epidural placement and low-molecular-weight heparin concurrently.[96] Although bleeding complications can be associated with the placement of CPNB catheters, the actual risks related to this technique are not well defined. Hemorrhagic complications, rather than neurologic deficits, appear to be the predominant risk associated with the performance of peripheral nerve blockade in the anticoagulated patient.[97] Major hemorrhage can occur following performance of psoas compartment blockade (e.g., LPB) and lumbar sympathetic blockade.[97] Special risk seems likely in any patient who may be anticoagulated perioperatively.

Practice-based guidelines for the performance of *neuraxial techniques* in the anticoagulated patient are available online at the American Society of Regional Anesthesia (ASRA) Web site at http://www.asra.com/consensus-statements and are based on the recommendations set forth in the consensus statement by Horlocker et al.[97] At the time of this publication, however, no consensus statement has been promulgated by the society outlining practice guidelines for the performance of *peripheral nerve blocks* in anticoagulated patients. Until guidelines are developed for the performance of peripheral nerve blockade in the anticoagulated patient, Horlocker et al.[97] recommend a conservative approach by adapting the guidelines set forth by ASRA for the performance of neuraxial blockade, which they acknowledge may be overly restrictive.

Despite the fact that a sustained-release morphine is currently available for epidural use, the routine application of timed-release formulations of local anesthetic and opioids for both neuraxial and peripheral analgesia is remote. The argument for their use is simplicity and prolonged analgesia; however, once administered, there is no turning back and the dose cannot be titrated to effect nor can it be turned off so a neurovascular check of the patient can be performed. Continuous catheter systems may be cumbersome and potentially more expensive but they are titratable and they can be turned on and off as appropriate and they can be intermittently bolused when indicated.

COMPLICATIONS FROM REGIONAL ANESTHESIA

The opinion of some that regional anesthesia is safer than general anesthesia may be based on the fact that regional anesthesia has been associated with reduced postoperative mortality secondary to thromboembolic phenomenon and myocardial infarction.[98,99] Nonetheless, data from the American Society of Anesthesiologists Closed Claims Project database suggests that the comparative safety of regional anesthesia in comparison to general anesthesia cannot be accurately determined. In a review of Closed Claims data, however, death is more common with claims involving general anesthesia and permanent-disabling and nondisabling temporary injuries are more often associated with regional anesthesia.[100] Serious complications associated with regional anesthesia include cardiac arrest, radiculopathy, cauda equina syndrome, and paraplegia. Fortunately, the incidence of severe anesthesia-related complications are rare (<0.1%); however, the incidence of cardiac arrest and neurologic complications are higher following spinal anesthesia than after all other types of regional procedures. The incidence of cardiac arrest following spinal anesthesia is $6.4 \pm 1.2/10{,}000$ versus $1.0 \pm 0.4/10{,}000$ for other forms of regional anesthesia. The incidence of neurologic injury after spinal anesthesia ($6 \pm 1/10{,}000$ cases) is greater than all other regional techniques (e.g., epidural, peripheral nerve block and intravenous regional anesthesia) combined ($1.6 \pm 0.5/10{,}000$ cases).

TABLE 56-19. RISK FACTORS FOR NERVE INJURY DURING THE PERFORMANCE OF REGIONAL ANESTHESIA

Variables	Risk Factors
Patient	Body habitus Pre-existing neurologic disorder (e.g., diabetes mellitus or patients who have received chemotherapy in the recent past) Male gender Advanced age
Surgical	Direct surgical trauma or stretch Prolonged tourniquet time Hematoma Infection Tightly applied casts or surgical dressings Patient positioning
Regional anesthesia	Mechanical injury from the needle or catheter Chemical neurotoxicity from the local anesthetic Ischemic injury to the nerve

Data derived from: Neal JM, Hebl JR, Gerancher JC, et al. Brachial plexus anesthesia: Essentials of our current understanding. *Reg Anesth Pain Med.* 2002;27:402; Horlocker TT: Complications of regional anesthesia. IARS 2004 Review Course Lectures. *Anesth Analg Suppl.* 2004:56; Ben-David B. Complications of peripheral blockade. *Anesthesiol Clin North America.* 2002;20:457; Hebl JR, Horlocker TT, Pritchard DJ. Diffuse brachial plexopathy after interscalene blockade in a patient receiving cisplatin chemotherapy: The pharmacologic double crush syndrome. *Anesth Analg.* 2001;92:249.

10 Should a perioperative nerve injury occur, it is incumbent on the physician to determine which combination of anesthetic, surgical, and patient risk factors are involved in any nerve injury and not assume a priori that the regional anesthetic is the culprit. The risk factors for nerve injury are listed in Table 56-19. *Patient risk factors* for perioperative nerve injury may include any pre-existing systemic neuropathy (e.g., diabetes mellitus) or drug-induced neuropathy (e.g., vincristine or *cis*-platin). Risk factors for ulnar nerve injury include male sex, prolonged hospitalization, increasing age, extremes of body habitus, and diabetes. Diabetics, for example, have a decreased requirement for local anesthetic yet an increased risk for local anesthetic-induced nerve injury. This phenomenon has been described as the "double-crush" syndrome and proposes that axons injured at one site have an increased susceptibility to injury distally. Interestingly enough, in spite of this risk, regional anesthesia has been safely performed on patients with pre-existing ulnar neuropathy who underwent ulnar nerve transposition.[101]

TABLE 56-20. ADVANTAGES OF ULTRASOUND-GUIDED REGIONAL ANESTHESIA

1. Hastenened block performance.
2. Fewer needle passes resulting in less patient discomfort and potentially a decreased risk of vascular puncture and hematoma formation in the anticoagulated patient.
3. Faster initial onset of the block.
4. Decreased dose of local anesthetic.
5. Preprocedural scanning can reveal anticipated as well as unanticipated structures such as hemodialysis catheters, ventriculoperitoneal shunts, vascular and neurologic anomalies.

Liu SS, Ngeow JE, YaDeau JT. Ultrasound-guided regional anesthesia and analgesia: A qualitative review, *Reg Anesth Pain Med.* 2009;34(1):47–59.

TABLE 56-21. ULTRASOUND-GUIDED REGIONAL ANESTHESIA (UGRA) AND PATIENT SAFETY

1. Peripheral nerve injury
   The incidence of peripheral nerve injury with UGRA is similar to reports of nerve injury following the use of peripheral nerve stimulation (PNS).
2. Local anesthetic systemic toxicity (LAST)
   Compared to PNS, UGRA decreases the risk of unintended vascular puncture but does not necessarily decrease the risk of local anesthetic toxicity.
3. Hemidiaphragmatic paresis (HDP)
   Low-volume UGRA of the brachial plexus can decrease the risk of HDP following an interscalene approach and almost eliminate it following a supraclavicular approach.
4. Pneumothorax (PTX)
   Since UGRA allows the anesthesiologist to directly visualize the pleura this should decrease the risk of PTX; however, PTX has been reported following the performance of UGRA.

Neal, JM. Ultrasound-guided regional anesthesia and patient safety: An evidence-based analysis. *Reg Anesth Pain Med.* 2010;35(2 suppl):S59–67.

Ultrasound guidance technology for the performance of peripheral nerve blockde has become very popular over the past decade. Direct visualization of the needle and the associated anatomic structures and real-time hydrodissection of local anesthetic around target nerves should theoretically increase the safety and decrease complications associated with peripheral nerve blockade. However, ultrasound-guided regional anesthesia (UGRA) does not completely eliminate all the risks associated with the performance of peripheral nerve blockade. Advantages associated with the use of UGRA are listed in Table 56-20. Relevant patient safety issues are listed in Table 56-21. See Chapters 21 (Local Anesthetics), 34 (Epidural and Spinal Anesthesia), and 35 (Peripheral Nerve Blockade) for additional details on the reported complications of regional anesthesia.

PERIOPERATIVE PAIN MANAGEMENT OF THE OPIOID-DEPENDENT PATIENT

Although this discussion focuses on the patient with chronic pain syndromes, these strategies for perioperative pain management are easily adaptable to other opioid-dependent populations. Chronic pain is defined as "pain without apparent biologic value that has persisted beyond the normal tissue healing time usually taken to be three months" (International Association for the Study of Pain) and "pain of a duration or intensity that adversely affects the function or well-being of the patient" (American Society of Anesthesiologists). Chronic pain is often associated with anxiety and depression, which may require treatment with various anxiolytics, antidepressants, anticonvulsants, antiarrhythmics, and skeletal muscle relaxants in addition to opioids. Symptoms unique to chronic pain include tight musculature, limited range of motion, and lack of energy, sleep disturbance, irritability, and social withdrawal. Associated psychiatric diagnoses may include hypochondriasis and psychosis.

Over the past decade, the percentage of patients with chronic pain for whom chronic opioids have been prescribed has increased dramatically. Although the goal of opioid therapy for chronic pain is improvement of pain, function, and quality of life, unacceptable opioid side effects and concerns about adverse hormonal effects and immune modulation from long-term exposure can cause patients to abandon therapy. In addition, long-term opioid use results in physical dependence, the potential for withdrawal symptoms on abrupt discontinuation of the opioid, and the development of tolerance and OIH.

Physical dependence is a "physiologic state of adaptation to a specific psychoactive substance characterized by the emergence of a *withdrawal syndrome* during abstinence, which may be relieved in total or in part by readministration of the substance." Opioid *withdrawal* is characterized by an increased sympathetic and parasympathetic response that results in hypertension, tachycardia, diaphoresis, abdominal cramping, and diarrhea. Clinical experience suggests that patients are considered to be *physically dependent* on an opioid if they have been receiving the equivalent of 30 mg of intravenous morphine daily for a period of at least 2 to 4 weeks, and therefore failure to provide adequate amounts of opioids perioperatively will precipitate withdrawal symptoms. *Tolerance* is a rightward shift of the dose–response curve and by definition is "a state in which an increased dosage of a psychoactive substance is needed to produce a desired effect." Escalating doses of opioid may also be explained by an underlying progression of the disease state or by the development of OIH. Tolerance can be innate or acquired. Innate tolerance is a genetically predetermined sensitivity to a drug, whereas acquired tolerance can have a pharmacokinetic, learned, or pharmacodynamic basis. Pharmacokinetic tolerance involves a diminution in the effects of a drug because of changes in distribution and metabolism usually secondary to enzyme induction of the cytochrome 450 system, which results in accelerated metabolism. Learned tolerance refers to compensatory behavior that masks intoxication. Pharmacodynamic tolerance refers to neuroadaptive changes that occur following chronic exposure to opioids, which may involve receptor desensitization secondary to receptor down-regulation, internalization, and uncoupling of opioid receptors from G proteins. Opioids exhibit *cross-tolerance* to each other but the degree of cross-tolerance varies widely and is often incomplete.[102] Clinicians use incomplete cross-tolerance to their advantage to restore analgesic sensitivity in highly tolerant patients through opioid rotation.[102] Because cross-tolerance is incomplete, analgesia is restored with the new opioid at >50% below the predicted equianalgesic dose.[102] It must be stressed that the development of tolerance or physical dependence in no way implies that the patient is addicted to an opioid. *Addiction* is a biopsychosocial disease characterized by dysfunctional behavior that involves craving, compulsive use, loss of control, and the continued use of a drug in spite of adverse consequences. Finally, addiction should not be confused with *pseudoaddiction*, which, by definition, describes the patient who has behavioral features of addiction secondary to undertreatment of the pain syndrome. Pseudoaddiction is usually diagnosed retrospectively because once the dose of opioid is increased, pain resolves and aberrant behavior abates.

TABLE 56-22. SUGGESTED GUIDELINES FOR PERIOPERATIVE PAIN MANAGEMENT IN THE OPIOID-TOLERANT PATIENT

Preoperative

1. Evaluation: Evaluation should include early recognition and high index of suspicion.
2. Identification: Identify factors such as total opioid dose requirement and previous surgery/trauma resulting in undermedication, inadequate analgesia, or relapse episodes.
3. Consultation: Meet with addiction specialists and pain specialists with regard to perioperative planning.
4. Reassurance: Discuss patient concerns related to pain control, anxiety, and risk of relapse.
5. Medication: Calculate opioid dose requirement and modes of administration; provide anxiolytics or other medications as clinically indicated.

Intraoperative

1. Maintain baseline opioids (oral, transdermal, intravenous).
2. Increase intraoperative and postoperative opioid dose to compensate for tolerance.
3. Provide peripheral neural or plexus blockade; consider neuraxial analgesic techniques when clinically indicated.
4. Use nonopioids as analgesic adjuncts.

Postoperative

1. Plan preoperatively for postoperative analgesia; formulate primary strategy as well as suitable alternatives.
2. Maintain baseline opioids.
3. Use multimodal analgesic techniques.
4. Patient-controlled analgesia: Use as primary therapy or as supplementation for epidural or regional techniques.
5. Continue neuraxial opioids: Intrathecal or epidural analgesia.
6. Continue continuous neural blockade.

After Discharge

7. If surgery provides complete pain relief, opioids should be slowly tapered, rather than abruptly discontinued.
8. Develop a pain management plan before hospital discharge. Provide adequate doses of opioid and nonopioid analgesics.
9. Arrange for a timely outpatient pain clinic follow-up or a visit with the patient's addictionologist.

Data derived from: Mitra S, Sinatra RS. Perioperative management of acute pain in the opioid-dependent patient. *Anesthesiology.* 2004;101:212.

11 The onus for the identification of the opioid-dependent patient rests with the patient's surgical team, preoperative evaluation staff, and the anesthesia team.[103] Ideally the patient and the healthcare teams will formulate a perioperative pain management plan prior to surgery, and the chronic pain service, if available, should be consulted. Often, however, the opioid-dependent patient is identified just moments prior to surgery and the anesthesia team needs to be innovative. The anesthesiologist needs to be flexible enough to tailor an individual anesthetic that incorporates a multimodal approach, combining regional anesthesia with general anesthesia and nonopioid coanalgesics with opioid analgesics. Opioids remain the mainstay of perioperative pain management, and an adequate dose of opioid needs to be maintained to avoid precipitating withdrawal symptoms (Table 56-22).

Preoperative management of the patient involves determining the patients "baseline" opioid requirement, and on the day of surgery the patient should be instructed to take the normal opioid dose. If for some reason the patient neglects to take the opioid on the day of surgery, the anesthesiologist can administer an equivalent dose preoperatively. During the preinduction period the dose of fentanyl, morphine, or hydromorphone administered for sedation can be 25% to 50% higher than the dose used in the opioid-naive patient. Patients prescribed transdermal fentanyl patches are usually instructed to maintain their fentanyl patch into the operating room and this can serve as their baseline opioid requirement. Occasionally, however, in the case of major surgery, in which the risk of major blood loss or sepsis is significant, patients may be instructed to discontinue their transdermal patch, and an intravenous fentanyl infusion can be initiated to maintain adequate plasma concentrations. Patients maintained on methadone should continue their baseline dose throughout the perioperative period. In the United States, methadone is available for both oral and intravenous administration. The reader is reminded that patients receiving >200 mg of methadone per day can develop a prolonged QT interval, which places them at risk for Torsades de pointe. It is therefore recommended that a baseline electrocardiogram be obtained for comparison. Patients who are maintained on the partial opioid agonist buprenorphine may continue to receive the drug for postoperative pain control, and either morphine or methadone may be administered to supplement analgesia if required. Full antagonists (e.g., naloxone and naltrexone) and the partial agonists–antagonists (e.g., nalbuphine, pentazocine, and butorphanol) should be avoided because they will precipitate withdrawal symptoms in opioid-dependent patients.

Intraoperative management of the opioid-dependent patient requires the prudent use of fentanyl, morphine, or hydromorphone in order to provide effective intraoperative anesthesia, postoperative analgesia, and to prevent opioid withdrawal. This requires the administration of the patients' baseline opioid requirement plus their intraoperative requirements secondary to surgical stimulation. Exact opioid dosing guidelines do not exist but because of receptor down-regulation secondary to chronic opioid administration, opioid doses may need to be increased 30% to 100% vis-à-vis the opioid-naive patient. Because of receptor down-regulation an alternative opioid may be useful in this setting. Opioid rotation takes advantage of the fact that the new opioid will bind a different opioid receptor subtype and be metabolized differently. Following the cancer pain model, the dose of the new opioid is <50% of the calculated equianalgesic dose because of incomplete cross-tolerance.[102] Although the alternative opioid may be administered for several days postoperatively, prudence dictates that a physician or pharmacist well versed in pain management convert the patient to the appropriate oral opioid regimen for discharge from the hospital.

The optimal intraoperative dose of opioid varies considerably from patient to patient; therefore, monitoring intraoperative vital signs such as heart rate, pupil size, and respiratory rate can be useful and allows the clinician to avoid the negative consequences of overdosing or underdosing the patient with opioid. Reversing neuromuscular blockade toward the end of a general anesthetic and allowing the patient to breathe spontaneously can be a prudent technique. Patients with a respiratory rate >20 breaths per minute and significantly dilated pupils require additional opioid. Titrating fentanyl, morphine, or hydromorphone to a respiratory rate of 12 to 14 breaths per minute and a moderately miotic pupil is recommended. It is also recommend that patients who are receiving chronic methadone therapy may receive an additional intraoperative dose of 0.1 mg/kg intravenously, which can be titrated to hemodynamic effect and pupillary response.

Postoperative management of the opioid-dependent patient can be very challenging. Ideally, the optimal amount of opioid has been administered to the patient during the intraoperative period, allowing them to emerge from anesthesia comfortably sedated and pain-free. On arrival to the recovery room, intravenous opioids may be administered on an "as-needed" basis; however, initiation of an intravenous PCA opioid with both a basal and an incremental (bolus) dose will minimize the risk of breakthrough pain. The recommended basal infusion should equate to the patient's hourly preoperative oral opioid dose requirement as this will avoid precipitating withdrawal symptoms, and the bolus dose, as calculated from the background infusion, is the 1-hour dose of the background infusion. For example, a patient taking 90 mg of oral morphine per day equates to 30 mg of intravenous morphine per day, which can be administered as a basal morphine infusion of 1.25 mg/hr. The bolus dose would be equivalent to 1.25 mg with a lockout interval of 6 to 10 minutes. Basal infusions are not required for patients who are maintained on their transdermal fentanyl patches as these provide adequate basal analgesia. Therefore, a fentanyl PCA with a bolus dose and an appropriate lockout interval is all that is required. Patients recovering from same-day surgery will be initially treated with intravenous doses of opioids in the recovery room; however, they can be quickly transitioned to an oral regimen consisting of their baseline opioid requirement plus an appropriate amount of short-acting opioid for breakthrough pain consistent with the invasiveness of the surgery.

Nonopioid coanalgesics are opioid-sparing and should be part and parcel of any multimodal perioperative pain management regimen in the opioid-dependent patient. Low-dose ketamine is highly recommended. A bolus dose of 0.25 to 0.5 mg/kg followed by an infusion of 2 to 4 μg/kg/min is reported to enhance analgesia in this population of patients. The preoperative administration of acetaminophen, a COX-2 inhibitor, an α_2–δ subunit calcium channel ligand (e.g., gababentin), and α_2-agonists (e.g., clonidine) may also be particularly beneficial in the perioperative pain management of these patients.

Regional anesthesia is highly recommended in this patient population. Peripheral nerve blockade as a single-injection technique or as a continuous catheter can be very useful. Likewise, if indicated epidural analgesia should be part and parcel of the multimodal pain regimen for these patients. During the perioperative period, however, the epidural and systemic requirements for morphine have been reported to increase three- to fourfold. Epidural infusions that have been recommended include a combination of either fentanyl (2 to 5 μg/mL), morphine (0.1 to 0.2 mg/mL), or hydromorphone (0.02 to 0.04 mg/mL) combined with a local anesthetic such as bupivacaine (0.05% to 0.2%) or ropivacaine (0.1% to 0.2%). Switching to an opioid with high intrinsic efficacy may be useful. A combination of sufentanil (2 μg/mL) with 0.1% bupivacaine has been shown to be quite efficacious in an opioid-tolerant patient refractory to the analgesic effects of epidural morphine. The neuraxial administration of opioid is usually a very small fraction of the patient's baseline opioid requirement. Notwithstanding the fact that patients obtain excellent analgesia from the epidural, opioid serum levels and supraspinal receptor binding may not be totally adequate at preventing opioid withdrawal symptoms. It may therefore be necessary for the patient to receive at least part of their baseline opioid dose either orally or intravenously (PCA) to prevent opioid withdrawal symptoms. A physician well versed in chronic pain management and comfortable in the equianalgesic dosing of opioids via different routes of administration should ideally be involved in the care of the patient. Careful monitoring of the patient for excessive sedation or respiratory depression is mandatory, and caregivers in the recovery room and on the postsurgical units should be alerted to the potential risk for respiratory depression when parenteral and neuraxial opioids are combined.

ORGANIZATION OF PERIOPERATIVE PAIN MANAGEMENT SERVICES

There is a growing recognition in the healthcare industry that the undertreatment of pain is a widespread problem that cuts across all phases of patient care. The effective management of pain is a crucial component of good perioperative care and recovery from surgery. Unrelieved pain and inadequate pain relief have detrimental physiologic and psychological effects on patients by slowing recovery and creating burdens for patients and their families, and by increasing costs to the healthcare system. Although the acute postoperative pain service plays an integral role in the pain management of the surgical patients, there are considerable barriers that challenge the establishment and/or effectiveness of acute pain teams in managing patients across the continuum of care. There is good evidence that the overall incidence of moderate-to-severe pain in surgical patients is about 25% to 40% despite the availability of pain treatment.[104] A major obstacle to the establishment of postoperative pain services is its cost in a privatized health system wherein limited reimbursement for postoperative care discourages the establishment of a service. The value of an acute pain service apart from its benefit for patient care also comes from the added value of reducing hospital costs by improving surgical outcome and by facilitating patient recovery and early discharge.[105] While providing direct patient care along previous lines such as the management of continuous epidural and regional catheter infusions and other modalities, the perioperative pain management service must also play a leading role in patient education and the education of other physicians, nurses, and caregivers to ensure their competence in effectively assessing, managing, and meeting a patient's needs. The success of a perioperative pain management team can be established not only in the context of the direct patient care that the team provides, but also through its role in educating other healthcare professionals and service as physician leaders responsible for setting clinical standards and practice guidelines in the healthcare system.

12 The key components to establishing a successful perioperative pain management service begins with an institutional commitment to support the service. The team must be built around a physician leader with training and experience in pain medicine. There must be other anesthesiologists available to support the service. The institutional must support the service, which may be manifest through support of a nurse coordinator or the availability of a pharmacist to consult on the many pharmaceutical issues that arise in patients on preoperative medications that may conflict with the perioperative pain management plan. The perioperative pain management chief is responsible for the development and implementation of clinical pathways and protocols that are effective across the continuum. These protocols must include pain assessment tools that are adopted across the continuum of care by all caregivers.

Although it is convenient to regard postoperative pain primarily as acute pain caused by tissue injury associated with surgery, this may exclude other important factors that contribute to a patient's suffering following surgery. Acute postsurgical pain can also be caused by prolonged patient positioning or pressure effects from prolonged immobility. Many patients presenting for elective surgery may also suffer chronic pain from underlying illness or injury (e.g., degenerative diseases or malignancy) that may contribute significantly to the intensity of the postoperative pain experienced by the patient. Postoperative pain remains a substantial problem that is often masked by a patient's acceptance of pain as a natural consequence of surgery. Other common patient barriers include cultural and language barriers, stoicism and/or opiophobia, and personal experience or the experiences of friends and relatives. For these reasons, postoperative pain management begins preoperatively with patient education to alleviate the attendant anxiety, apprehension, and fear of surgery, to understand the patient's fears and concerns, and to come to an agreement with the patient that pain control is an expected goal of care. Education is also the key to changing attitudes of other caregivers to more effectively treat their patient's pain. In developing a perioperative pain service it is important to bear in mind that the importance of effective perioperative pain management extends well beyond the mere establishment of dedicated personnel but must also encompass a leadership role in transforming the institutional culture to elevate the relief of pain and suffering to its place as a primary goal of patient care.[106]

SPECIAL CONSIDERATIONS IN THE PERIOPERATIVE PAIN MANAGEMENT OF CHILDREN

Acute pain management in children undergoing surgery or invasive procedures offers several specific and unique challenges for the anesthesiologist. The challenges include the importance of the child's parents and siblings support, preoperative fear and anxiety in the child, developmental and communication issues, difficulties in evaluating pain and the effectiveness of treatment, and the child's reaction to pain, surgery, and the environment including crying and resistance to care. These problems all summate to emphasize the importance of a holistic approach to pain management that focuses on family-centered care wherein significant efforts are made to reduce preoperative stress and anxiety and to engage the parents in gaining the cooperation of the child.[107] There is also good evidence that the level of preoperative anxiety and stress adversely impacts postoperative pain and recovery from surgery. A number of methods can be used to reduce preoperative anxiety in children. They include preoperative parental education and counseling about the operative experience,[108] distraction techniques including videos and music, hand-held video games, game-playing with the support of the family and/or child life specialists, and parental presence coupled with oral midazolam (0.5 mg/kg) administration to ease anxiety associated with the transition to the induction of anesthesia. As parental behavior and attitudes can be major determinants of a child's behavior during the inhalational induction of anesthesia, the anesthesiologist is obliged to counsel and inform parents as to the importance of modulating their fear and anxiety should they want to be present during anesthetic induction.

Effective pain management in the postoperative period depends on effective assessment and the precision of the evaluation tools used to measure pain intensity.[109] A child's responses to pain may be variable and unpredictable because of their age and development, verbal communication skills, fear and anxiety, withdrawal, prior experiences, parental presence or absence, and the parent's reactions to the care.[110] A comprehensive approach to assessment that employs multiple assessment tools including behavioral responses offers the best option for success. The use of visual analog "faces" pain scales referenced to the appropriate cultural identity of the patient can be useful in assessing postoperative pain severity. There is some question as to the value of parental or practitioner evaluation of a child's pain intensity relative to the visual analog scale, but parents can play a key role in the assessment and management of their child's pain in the postoperative period, particularly when their child is reluctant to communicate or suffers from a cognitive disorder.[111]

Nonparenteral Analgesics

Nonopioid Analgesics

The use of nonopioid analgesics administered orally or by rectal suppository are important adjuvant analgesic therapies under a wide variety of circumstances. The release of intravenous acetaminophen (Ofirmev) in November 2011 has progressively replaced nonparenteral administration of acetaminophen in pediatric perioperative practice. See Table 56-10 for dosing guidelines in children. Intravenous acetaminophen can be used across a wide spectrum of surgical procedures and may be sufficient for outpatient procedures. Nonparenteral administration of acetaminophen either by oral administration (10 to 20 mg/kg) or by rectal suppository (20 to 40 mg/kg) after induction of anesthesia remains an acceptable alternative to parenteral administration. Although the short-term use of the NSAIDs (e.g., ibuprofen and ketorolac) are equipotent with acetaminophen and can be used with safety, the overall convenience and fewer side effects of acetaminophen have favored its use in children. Oral clonidine (4 μg/kg) given as a preoperative medication has also been used with good effect for sedation and postoperative pain management in children undergoing adenotonsillectomy. The greater degree of postoperative sedation with clonidine relative to other analgesics may limit its universal acceptance.

Opioid Analgesics

Codeine in combination with acetaminophen is commonly used with good effect for the management of moderate postoperative pain in the ambulatory patient.[112] The atypical opioid tramadol (3 mg/kg) has also been used as an oral preparation, usually in combination with midazolam (0.5 mg/kg) prior to the induction of anesthesia in children undergoing adenotonsillectomy. Oral tramadol can also be used for postoperative analgesia in children undergoing oral or dental procedures.[113] Intranasal sufentanil (0.2 μg/k) can also be used to manage preoperative anxiety and postoperative analgesia in children and may be more effective than oral tramadol.[113]

Patient-controlled Analgesia

PCA is established as an important postoperative pain management tool in adults and is increasingly used in older children to good effect.[114,115] There are safety concerns with the use of PCA in children that mandate a high level of surveillance with respect to the functioning of the equipment and careful patient monitoring that may be a limitation to its use in infants. PCA by proxy is a safety risk as there is no complete assurance that parents will be competent in assessing the intensity of their child's pain or be able to regulate the bolus dosages in order to avoid opioid overdosage.[116]

Epidural Neuraxial Analgesia

The use of epidural neuraxial analgesia either as a single-shot technique or a continuous catheter technique has become a key component of the perioperative pain management plan for infants and young children undergoing abdominal, urologic, or orthopedic procedures.[117] The use of a single-shot "kiddy" caudal using a local anesthetic with morphine is effective in relieving pain associated with minor procedures in the outpatient setting. Although the overall morbidity is low, there is serious risk associated with epidural analgesia in children related to the systemic toxicity of the local anesthetic and the need to place the epidural under general anesthesia. The risk of irreversible cardiac toxicity, although primarily associated with the use of bupivacaine, can also occur with the ropivacaine and levobupivacaine at an incidence of about 30% to 50% relative to bupivacaine. The risks are increased in children with hepatic dysfunction or when large volumes of local anesthetic are injected into the epidural space through a small, sharp, immobile needle. In the rare event that cardiac toxicity occurs, the anesthesiologist must be prepared to initiate chest compressions and lung ventilation to minimize the risk of anoxic injury and immediately start an intravenous bolus infusion of 20% intralipid (1 to 2 mL/kg) followed by a continuous infusion (0.25 to 0.5 mL/kg/min) until normal cardiac rhythm and the circulation is restored.[118] Although the use of lipid emulsions can be successful in reversing cardiac arrest, their immediate availability does not excuse the anesthesiologist from taking all precautions to prevent systemic injection or absorption when performing the procedure.

Peripheral Nerve Blocks in Children

The introduction of small stimulating needles and ultrasound imaging along with long-acting local anesthetics and continuous catheter techniques in selected cases has resulted in an increase in the use of peripheral nerve blocks in children undergoing orthopedic extremity procedures.[119] The use of stimulating needles permits the anesthesiologist to place the injection after the child is anesthetized.[120] As the child is unresponsive, it is important that the initial injection meets no resistance in order to avoid intraneural injection. Combined ilioinguinal and iliohypogastric nerve blocks performed under ultrasound guidance to reduce the volume of the injection have gained increasing interest for effective pain management in children undergoing inguinal herniorrhaphy.[121]

CONCLUSION

In October 2000, the U.S. Congress designated the decade beginning January 1, 2001, as the Decade of Pain Control and Research. The onus is on dedicated healthcare professionals to provide our patients with the best care possible when it comes to pain and suffering, which applies directly to the perioperative state. Accomplishing this requires integration of information and systems from disparate disciplines within medicine. It challenges physicians to acquire a patient-focused perspective that spans the mind–body spectrum of the perioperative experience. In doing so, clinicians will be challenged to construct systems within hospitals to support such endeavors but will be able to show objective and meaningful outcomes with positive benefits to patients and to healthcare organizations. The cost of ignoring pain and suffering has been widely cited to be in the billions of dollars each, but the cost in suffering is immeasurable. Anesthesiology has led the way in improving the overall pain care of the surgical patient and is positioned to lead medicine into a new era in which perioperative pain management is better, safer, more assured, and consistently available at the highest levels to all.

References

1. United States Agency for Health Care Policy and Research. Acute pain management operative or medical procedures and trauma. Rockville, MD, US Dept of Health and Human Services Public Health Service Agency for Health Care Policy and Research, 1992.
2. American Society of Anesthesiologists Task Force on Acute Pain Management. Practice guidelines for acute pain management in the perioperative setting: An updated report by the American Society of Anesthesiologists Task Force on Acute Pain Management. *Anesthesiology.* 2012;116:248.
3. Wu CL, Naqibuddin M, Rowlingson AJ, et al. The effect of pain on health-related quality of life in the immediate postoperative period. *Anesth Analg.* 2003;97:1078.
4. Joshi GP, Ogunnaike BO. Consequences of inadequate postoperative pain relief and chronic persistent postoperative pain. *Anesthesiol Clin North America.* 2005; 23:21.
5. Carr DB, Goudas LC. Acute pain. *Lancet.* 1999;353:2051.
6. Raja SN, Dougherty PM. Anatomy and physiology of somatosensory and pain processing. In: Benzon HT, Raja SN, Molloy RE, Liu S, Fishman SM, eds. *Essentials of Pain Medicine and Regional Anesthesia,* 2nd ed. Philadelphia, PA: Elsevier, Churchill Livingstone; 2005:1.
7. Wilder-Smith OH, Arendt-Nielsen L. Postoperative hyperalgesia: Its clinical importance and relevance. *Anesthesiology.* 2006;104(3):601.
8. Rowlingson JC. Update on Acute Pain Management. International Anesthesia Research Society Review Course Lectures 2006:95.
9. Lavand'homme P. From preemptive to preventive analgesia: time to reconsider the role of perioperative peripheral nerve blocks? *Reg Anesth Pain Med.* 2011; 36(1):4–6.
10. Taylor DR. Improving outcomes in acute pain management: Optimizing patient selection. *Medscape Neurol Neurosurg.* 2004;6(2).
11. Cepeda MS, Carr DB. Women experience more pain and require more morphine than men to achieve a similar degree of analgesia. *Anesth Analg.* 2003;97(5):1464.
12. Caraceni A, Cherny N, Fainsinger R, et al. Pain measurement tools and methods in clinical research in palliative care: Recommendations of an Expert Working Group of the European Association of Palliative Care. *J Pain Symptom Manage.* 2002; 23(3):239.
13. Portenoy RK, Bennett DS, Rauck R, et al. Prevalence and characteristics of breakthrough pain in opioid-treated patients with chronic noncancer pain. *J Pain.* 2006;7(8):583.
14. Bennett M. The LANSS Pain Scale: the Leeds assessment of neuropathic symptoms and signs. *Pain.* 2001;92(1–2):147.
15. Viscusi ER, Goldstein S, Witkowski T, et al. Alvimopan, a peripherally acting mu-opioid receptor antagonist, compared with placebo in postoperative ileus after major abdominal surgery: Results of a randomized, double-blind, controlled study. *Surg Endosc.* 2006;20(1):64.
16. Angst MS, Clark JD. Opioid-induced hyperalgesia: A qualitative systematic review. *Anesthesiology.* 2006;104(3):570.
17. Budd K. Pain management: Is opioid immunosuppression a clinical problem? *Biomed Pharmacother.* 2006;60:310–7.
18. Gupta K, Kshirsagar S, Chang L, et al. Morphine stimulates angiogenesis by activating proangiogenic and survival promoting signaling and promotes breast tumor growth. *Cancer Res.* 2002;62:4491.
19. Sarhill N, Walsh D, Nelson KA. Hydromorphone: Pharmacology and clinical applications in cancer patients. *Support Care Cancer.* 2001;9(2):84.
20. Mahajan G, Fishman SM. Major opioids in pain management. In: Benzon H, Raja SN, Molloy RE, Liu S, Fishman SM, eds. *Essentials of Pain Medicine and Regional Anesthesia.* Philadelphia, PA: Elsevier, Churchill Livingstone; 2005:94.
21. Mitra S, Sinatra RS. Perioperative management of acute pain in the opioid-dependent patient. *Anesthesiology.* 2004;101(1):212.
22. APS. *Principles of Analgesic Use in the Treatment of Acute Pain and Cancer Pain.* 5th ed. American Pain Society; 2003.
23. Candido KD, Winnie AP, Ghaleb AH, et al. Buprenorphine added to the local anesthetic for axillary brachial plexus block prolongs postoperative analgesia. *Reg Anesth Pain Med.* 2002;27(2):162.
24. Katz JA. NSAIDs and COX-2 Selective Inhibitors. In: Benzon R, Molloy, Liu, Fishman S, eds. *Essentials of Pain Medicine and Regional Anesthesia,* 2nd ed. Elsevier, Churchill Livingston; 2005:141.
25. Marret E, Kurdi O, Zufferey P, et al. Effects of nonsteroidal antiinflammatory drugs on patient-controlled analgesia morphine side effects: Meta-analysis of randomized controlled trials. *Anesthesiology.* 2005;102(6):1249.
26. Nussmeier NA, Whelton AA, Brown MT, et al. Complications of the COX-2 inhibitors parecoxib and valdecoxib after cardiac surgery. *N Engl J Med.* 2005; 352(11):1081.
27. Acute Pain Management: Scientific Evidence, Australian and New Zealand College of Anaesthetists and Faculty of Pain Medicine, 3rd ed., 2010:73.
28. Weinbroum AA. A single small dose of postoperative ketamine provides rapid and sustained improvement in morphine analgesia in the presence of morphine-resistant pain. *Anesth Analg.* 2003;96(3):789.
29. Sveticic G, Gentilini A, Eichenberger U, et al. Combinations of morphine with ketamine for patient-controlled analgesia: A new optimization method. *Anesthesiology.* 2003;98(5):1195.
30. Reeves M, Lindholm DE, Myles PS, et al. Adding ketamine to morphine for patient-controlled analgesia after major abdominal surgery: A double-blinded, randomized controlled trial. *Anesth Analg.* 2001;93(1):116.
31. Wadhwa A, Clarke D, Goodchild CS, et al. Large-dose oral dextromethorphan as an adjunct to patient-controlled analgesia with morphine after knee surgery. *Anesth Analg.* 2001;92(2):448.
32. Sites BD, Beach M, Biggs R, et al. Intrathecal clonidine added to a bupivacaine-morphine spinal anesthetic improves postoperative analgesia for total knee arthroplasty. *Anesth Analg.* 2003;96(4):1083.
33. Gerlach AT, Dasta JF. Dexmedetomidine: an updated review. *Ann Pharmacother.* 2007;41(2):245.
34. Ebert T, Maze M. Dexmedetomidine: another arrow for the clinician's quiver. *Anesthesiology.* 2004;101(3):568.
35. Acute Pain Management: Scientific Evidence, Australian and New Zealand College of Anaesthetists and Faculty of Pain Medicine, 3rd ed., 2010:91.
36. Zhang J, Ho Kok-Yuen, Wang Y. Efficacy of pregabalin in acute postoperative pain: a meta-analysis. *Br J Anaesth.* 2011;106:454–462.
37. Taylor CP. Mechanism of analgesia by gabapentin and pregablain-Calcium channel $\alpha_2\delta$ (Ca_v $\alpha_2\delta$), ligands. *Pain.* 2009;142:13–16.
38. Hurley RW, Cohen SP, Williams KA, et al. The analgesic effects of perioperative gabapentin on postoperative pain: A meta-analysis. *Reg Anesth Pain Med.* 2006; 31(3):237.
39. Menigaux C, Adam F, Guignard B, et al. Preoperative gabapentin decreases anxiety and improves early functional recovery from knee surgery. *Anesth Analg.* 2005;100(5):1394.
40. Turan A, White PF, Karamanlioglu B, et al. Gabapentin: An alternative to the cyclooxygenase-2 inhibitors for perioperative pain management. *Anesth Analg.* 2006;102(1):175.
41. Gilron I. Gabapentin and pregablin for chronic neuropathic and early postsurgical pain: Current evidence and future directions. *Curr Opin Anaesthesiol.* 2007; 20:456–472.
42. Buvanendran A, Kroin JS, Della Valle CJ, et al. Perioperative oral pregabalin reduces chronic pain after total knee arthroplasty: A prospective randomized, controlled trial. *Anesth Analg.* 2010;110:199–207.
43. Kaba A, Laurent SR, Detroz BJ, et al. Intravenous lidocaine infusion facilitates acute rehabilitation after laparoscopic colectomy. *Anesthesiology.* 2007;106(1):11; discussion 15.
44. Koc S, Memis D, Sut N. The preoperative use of gabapentin, dexamethasone, and their combination in varicocele surgery: A randomized controlled trial. *Anesth Analg.* 2007;105:1137.
45. Macintyre PE. Safety and efficacy of patient-controlled analgesia. *Br J Anaesth.* 2001;87(1):36.
46. Gan TJ, Meyer T, Apfel CC, et al. Consensus guidelines for managing postoperative nausea and vomiting. *Anesth Analg.* 2003;97(1):62.
47. Block BM, Liu SS, Rowlingson AJ, et al. Efficacy of postoperative epidural analgesia: A meta-analysis. *JAMA.* 2003;290(18):2455.
48. Bernards CM, Shen DD, Sterling ES, et al. Epidural, cerebrospinal fluid, and plasma pharmacokinetics of epidural opioids (part 1): Differences among opioids. *Anesthesiology.* 2003;99(2):455.
49. Forster JG, Rosenberg PH. Small dose of clonidine mixed with low-dose ropivacaine and fentanyl for epidural analgesia after total knee arthroplasty. *Br J Anaesth.* 2004;93(5):670.
50. Rathmell JP, Lair TR, Nauman B. The role of intrathecal drugs in the treatment of acute pain. *Anesth Analg.* 2005;101(5 suppl):S30.
51. Sites BD, Beach M, Gallagher JD, et al. A single injection ultrasound-assisted femoral nerve block provides side effect-sparing analgesia when compared with intrathecal morphine in patients undergoing total knee arthroplasty. *Anesth Analg.* 2004;99(5):1539.
52. Richman JM, Liu S, Courpas G, et al. Does continuous peripheral nerve block provide superior pain control to opioids? A meta-analysis. *Anesth Analg.* 2006; 102:248.
53. Capdevila X, Pirat P, Bringuier S, et al. Continuous peripheral nerve blocks in hospital wards after orthopedic surgery: A multicenter prospective analysis of the quality of postoperative analgesia and complications in 1,416 patients. *Anesthesiology.* 2005;103(5):1035.
54. Swenson JD, Bay N, Loose E, et al. Outpatient management of continuous peripheral nerve catheters placed using ultrasound guidance: An experience in 620 patients. *Anesth Analg.* 2006;103(6):1436.
55. Winnie AP. Interscalene brachial plexus block. *Anesth Analg.* 1970;49:455.
56. Sinha SK, Abrams JH, Weller RS. Ultrasound-guided interscalene needle placement produces successful anesthesia regardless of motor stimulation above or below 0.5 mA. *Anesth Analg.* 2007;105(3):848.
57. Hadzic A, Williams BA, Karaca PE, et al. For outpatient rotator cuff surgery, nerve block anesthesia provides superior same-day recovery over general anesthesia. *Anesthesiology.* 2005;102(5):1001.
58. Ilfeld BM, Vandenborne K, Duncan PW, et al. Ambulatory continuous interscalene nerve blocks decrease the time to discharge readiness after total shoulder arthroplasty: A randomized, triple-masked, placebo-controlled study. *Anesthesiology.* 2006;105(5):999.
59. Kulenkampf D. Anesthesia of the brachial plexus (German). *Zentralbl Chir.* 1911; 38:1337.

60. Perlas A, Chan VW, Simons M. Brachial plexus examination and localization using ultrasound and electrical stimulation: A volunteer study. *Anesthesiology.* 2003;99(2):429.
61. Soares LG, Brull R, Lai J, et al. Eight ball, corner pocket: the optimal needle position for ultrasound-guided supraclavicular block. *Reg Anesth Pain Med.* 2007;32(1):94.
62. Bigeleisen P, Wilson M. A comparison of two techniques for ultrasound guided infraclavicular block. *Br J Anaesth.* 2006;96(4):502.
63. Dingemans E, Williams SR, Arcand G, et al. Neurostimulation in ultrasound-guided infraclavicular block: a prospective randomized trial. *Anesth Analg.* 2007;104(5):1275.
64. Sandhu NS, Capan LM. Ultrasound-guided infraclavicular brachial plexus block. *Br J Anaesth.* 2002;89(2):254.
65. Sauter AR, Smith HJ, Stubhaug A, et al. Use of magnetic resonance imaging to define the anatomical location closest to all three cords of the infraclavicular brachial plexus. *Anesth Analg.* 2006;103(6):1574.
66. Sandhu NS, Manne JS, Medabalmi PK, et al. Sonographically guided infraclavicular brachial plexus block in adults: A retrospective analysis of 1146 cases. *J Ultrasound Med.* 2006;25(12):1555.
67. Ilfeld BM, Morey TE, Enneking FK. Infraclavicular perineural local anesthetic infusion: A comparison of three dosing regimens for postoperative analgesia. *Anesthesiology.* 2004;100(2):395.
68. Awad IT, Duggan EM. Posterior lumbar plexus block: Anatomy, approaches, and techniques. *Reg Anesth Pain Med.* 2005;30(2):143.
69. Kaloul I, Guay J, Cote C, et al. The posterior lumbar plexus (psoas compartment) block and the three-in-one femoral nerve block provide similar postoperative analgesia after total knee replacement. *Can J Anaesth.* 2004;51(1):45.
70. Kirchmair L, Enna B, Mitterschiffthaler G, et al. Lumbar plexus in children. A sonographic study and its relevance to pediatric regional anesthesia. *Anesthesiology.* 2004;101(2):445.
71. Becchi C, Al Malyan M, Coppini R, et al. Opioid-free analgesia by continuous psoas compartment block after total hip arthroplasty. A randomized study. *Eur J Anaesthesiol.* 2008;25(5):418–423.
72. Horlocker TT, Cabanela ME, Wedel DJ. Does postoperative epidural analgesia increase the risk of peroneal nerve palsy after total knee arthroplasty? *Anesth Analg.* 1994;79(3):495.
73. Capdevila X, Coimbra C, Choquet O. Approaches to the lumbar plexus: Success, risks, and outcome. *Reg Anesth Pain Med.* 2005;30(2):150.
74. Gray AT, Collins AB, Schafhalter-Zoppoth I. An introduction to femoral nerve and associated lumbar plexus nerve blocks under ultrasound guidance. *Tech Reg Anesth Pain Mgmt.* 2004;8(4):155.
75. Nader A, Malik K, Kendall MC, et al. Relationship between ultrasound imaging and eliciting motor response during femoral nerve stimulation. *J Ultrasound Medicine.* 2009;28:345–350.
76. Winnie AP, Ramamurthy S, Durrani Z. The inguinal paravascular technic of lumbar plexus anesthesia: The "3 in-1 block. *Anesth Analg.* 1973;52:989.
77. Anns JP, Chen EW, Nirkava N, et al. A comparison of sartorius versus quadriceps stimulation for femoral nerve block: a prospective randomized double-blind controlled trial. *Anesth Analg.* 2011;112:725–731.
78. Fowler SJ, Symons J, Sabato S, et al. Epidural analgesia compared with peripheral nerve blockade after major knee surgery: A systematic review and meta-analysis of randomized trials. *Br J Anaesth.* 2008;100(2):154.
79. Carli F, Kehlet H, Baldini G, et al. Evidence basis for regional anesthesia in multidisciplinary fast-track surgical care pathways. *Reg Anesth Pain Med.* 2011;36:63–72.
80. Wang AZ, Gu L, Zhou QH, et al. Ultrasound-guided continuous femoral nerve block for analgesia after total knee arthroplasty. *Reg Anesth Pain Med.* 2010;35: 127–131.
81. Krombach J, Gray AT. Sonography for saphenous nerve block near the adductor canal. *Reg Anesth Pain Med.* 2007;32(4):369.
82. Chan VW, Nova H, Abbas S, et al. Ultrasound examination and localization of the sciatic nerve: A volunteer study. *Anesthesiology.* 2006;104(2):309, discussion 305A.
83. Karmakar MK, Kwok WH, Ho AM, et al. Ultrasound-guided sciatic nerve block: Description of a new approach at the subgluteal space. *Br J Anaesth.* 2007;98(3):390.
84. van Geffen GJ, Gielen M. Ultrasound-guided subgluteal sciatic nerve blocks with stimulating catheters in children: A descriptive study. *Anesth Analg.* 2006;103(2):328.
85. Marhofer P, Chan VW. Ultrasound-guided regional anesthesia: Current concepts and future trends. *Anesth Analg.* 2007;104(5):1265.
86. Hunt K, Higgins TF, Carlston CV, et al. Continuous peripheral nerve blockade as postoperative analgesia for open treatment of calcaneal fractures. *J Orthop Trauma.* 2010;24(3):148–155.
87. Zaric D, Boysen K, Christiansen J, et al. Continuous politeal sciatic nerve block for outpatient foot surgery—a randomized, controlled trial. *Acta Anaesthesiol Scand.* 2004;48(3):337.
88. Richardson J. Paravertebral anesthesia and analgesia. *Can J Anaesth.* 2004; 51(6):R1.
89. Naja ZM, El-Rajab M, Al-Tannir MA, et al. Thoracic paravertebral block: Influence of the number of injections. *Reg Anesth Pain Med.* 2006;31(3):196.
90. Karmakar MK, Chui PT, Joynt GM, et al. Thoracic paravertebral block for management of pain associated with multiple fractured ribs in patients with concomitant lumbar spinal trauma. *Reg Anesth Pain Med.* 2001;26(2):169.
91. Evans H, Steele SM, Nielsen KC, et al. Peripheral nerve blocks and continuous catheter techniques. *Anesthesiol Clin North America.* 2005;23(1):141.
92. Hebbard P, Fujiwara Y, Shibata Y, et al. Ultrasound-guided transversus abdominis plane (TAP) block. *Anaesth Intensive Care.* 2007;35(4):616.
93. Brower MC, Johnson ME. Adverse effects of local anesthetic infiltration on wound healing. *Reg Anesth Pain Med.* 2003;28:233.
94. Vendittoli PA, Makinen P, Drolet P, et al. A multimodal analgesia protocol for total knee arthroplasty. *J Bone Joint Surg Am.* 2006;88-A(2):282.
95. McCartney CJL, McLeod GA. Local infiltration analgesia for total knee arthroplasty. *Br J Anaesth.* 2011;107(4):487–489.
96. Horlocker TT, Wedel DJ. Neuraxial block and low-molecular-weight heparin: Balancing perioperative analgesia and thromboprophylaxis. *Reg Anesth Pain Med.* 1998;23(6 suppl 2):164.
97. Horlocker TT, Wedel DJ, Benzon H, et al. Regional anesthesia in the anticoagulated patient: Defining the risks (the second ASRA Consensus Conference on Neuraxial Anesthesia and Anticoagulation). *Reg Anesth Pain Med.* 2003; 28(3):172.
98. Rodgers A, Walker N, Schug S, et al. Reduction of postoperative mortality and morbidity with epidural or spinal anaesthesia: Results from overview of randomised trials. *BMJ.* 2000;321(7275):1493.
99. Tuman KJ, McCarthy RJ, March RJ, et al. Effects of epidural anesthesia and analgesia on coagulation and outcome after major vascular surgery. *Anesth Analg.* 1991;73(6):696.
100. Cheney FW. High-severity injuries associated with regional anesthesia in the 1990's. *ASA Newsletter.* 2001;65(6):6.
101. Hebl JR, Horlocker TT, Sorenson EJ, et al. Regional anesthesia does not increase the risk of postoperative neuropathy in patients undergoing ulnar nerve transposition. *Anesth Analg.* 2001;93(6):1606.
102. Pasternak GW. Incomplete cross tolerance and multiple mu opioid peptide receptors. *Trends Pharmacol Sci.* 2001;22(2):67.
103. Carroll IR, Angst MS, Clark JD. Management of perioperative pain in patients chronically consuming opioids. *Reg Anesth Pain Med.* 2004;29(6):576.
104. Dolin SJ, Cashman JN, Bland JM. Effectiveness of acute postoperative pain management: I. Evidence from published data. *Br J Anaesth.* 2002;89(3):409.
105. Stadler M, Schlander M, Braeckman M, et al. A cost-utility and cost-effectiveness analysis of an acute pain service. *J Clin Anesth.* 2004;16(3):159.
106. Berry PH, Dahl JL. The new JCAHO pain standards: Implications for pain management nurses. *Pain Manag Nurs.* 2000;1(1):3.
107. Kain ZN, Mayes LC, Caldwell-Andrews AA, et al. Preoperative anxiety, postoperative pain, and behavioral recovery in young children undergoing surgery. *Pediatrics.* 2006;118(2):651.
108. Wright KD, Stewart SH, Finley GA, et al. Prevention and intervention strategies to alleviate preoperative anxiety in children: A critical review. *Behav Modif.* 2007;31(1):52.
109. Voepel-Lewis T, Malviya S, Tait AR, et al. A comparison of the clinical utility of pain assessment tools for children with cognitive impairment. *Anesth Analg.* 2008;106(1):72.
110. Taylor EM, Boyer K, Campbell FA. Pain in hospitalized children: A prospective cross-sectional survey of pain prevalence, intensity, assessment and management in a Canadian pediatric teaching hospital. *Pain Res Manag.* 2008;13(1):25.
111. Franck LS, Allen A, Oulton K. Making pain assessment more accessible to children and parents: Can greater involvement improve the quality of care? *Clin J Pain.* 2007;23(4):331.
112. Moir MS, Bair E, Shinnick P, et al. Acetaminophen versus acetaminophen with codeine after pediatric tonsillectomy. *Laryngoscope.* 2000;110(11):1824.
113. Bayrak F, Gunday I, Memis D, et al. A comparison of oral midazolam, oral tramadol, and intranasal sufentanil premedication in pediatric patients. *J Opioid Manag.* 2007;3(2):74.
114. Butkovic D, Kralik S, Matolic M, et al. Postoperative analgesia with intravenous fentanyl PCA vs epidural block after thoracoscopic pectus excavatum repair in children. *Br J Anaesth.* 2007;98(5):677.
115. Saudan S, Habre W, Ceroni D, et al. Safety and efficacy of patient controlled epidural analgesia following pediatric spinal surgery. *Paediatr Anaesth.* 2008; 18(2):132.
116. Wuhrman E, Cooney MF, Dunwoody CJ, et al. Authorized and Unauthorized ("PCA by Proxy") Dosing of Analgesic Infusion Pumps: Position statement with clinical practice recommendations. *Pain Manag Nurs.* 2007;8(1):4.
117. Ecoffey C. Pediatric regional anesthesia—update. *Curr Opin Anaesthesiol.* 2007;20 (3):232.
118. Corman SL, Skledar SJ. Use of lipid emulsion to reverse local anesthetic-induced toxicity. *Ann Pharmacother.* 2007;41(11):1873.
119. Ganesh A, Rose JB, Wells L, et al. Continuous peripheral nerve blockade for inpatient and outpatient postoperative analgesia in children. *Anesth Analg.* 2007;105(5):1234.
120. DeVera HV, Furukawa KT, Matson MD, et al. Regional techniques as an adjunct to general anesthesia for pediatric extremity and spine surgery. *J Pediatr Orthop.* 2006;26(6):801.
121. Weintraud M, Marhofer P, Bosenberg A, et al. Ilioinguinal/iliohypogastric blocks in children: where do we administer the local anesthetic without direct visualization? *Anesth Analg.* 2008;106(1):89.

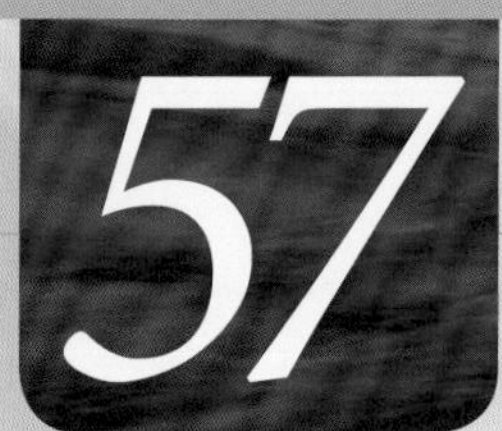

CHAPTER 57

Chronic Pain Management

HONORIO T. BENZON • ROBERT W. HURLEY • TIMOTHY DEER • ASOKUMAR BUVANENDRAN

Key Points

1. A delta and C fibers, under normal conditions, transmit nociceptive (pain) information to the spinal cord from their free nerve endings in the periphery. In chronic pain conditions, the A beta fibers, which normally transmit nonnoxious information, also participate in nociceptive transmission.
2. Most randomized studies on the efficacy of epidural steroid injections show temporary relief of radicular pain. Studies on thermal rhizotomy of the medial branches, for relief of facet syndrome, show benefit that lasts 3 to 12 months. This relief avoids the usage of addicting opioids.
3. Injection of neuraxial local anesthetics and methylprednisolone, when performed 3 to 4 times during the acute stage of herpes zoster, may prevent the development of postherpetic neuralgia. Postherpetic neuralgia is mostly managed pharmacologically, although interventional techniques may be used in resistant cases.
4. Antidepressants are effective in neuropathic pain syndromes but their use is limited because of their side effects. The newer serotonin–norepinephrine reuptake inhibitors have properties that result in less drug interactions and improved efficacy.
5. Anticonvulsants are effective in most neuropathic pain syndromes. Their favorable side effect profile and speed of therapeutic effect makes them the first line of treatment for these syndromes. Their efficacy is improved when combined with an opioid or an antidepressant.
6. Complex regional pain syndrome that does not respond to nerve blocks and physical therapy may respond to spinal cord stimulation.
7. Opioids are the mainstay for cancer pain management and are effective in neuropathic pain although at higher doses.
8. The majority of pain secondary to cancer is effectively managed pharmacologically with opioids, anticonvulsants, and antidepressants. Neurolysis of the visceral sympathetic system for pain secondary to abdominal or pelvic cancer relieves pain, decreases opioid consumption, and improves the patients' quality of life.
9. Vertebroplasty and kyphoplasty are indicated for vertebral compression fractures, although some newer studies question their efficacy.
10. Spinal cord stimulation is effective in patients with failed back syndrome, complex regional pain syndrome, angina, and critical limb ischemia.
11. Intrathecal drug delivery systems are valuable options in patients in whom opioids are ineffective at high doses or cause unacceptable side effects.

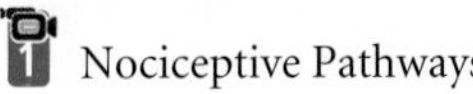

1 Nociceptive Pathways

2 Pain Sensitization

ANATOMY, PHYSIOLOGY, AND NEUROCHEMISTRY OF SOMATOSENSORY PAIN PROCESSING

Primary Afferents and Peripheral Stimulation

A variety of mechanical, thermal, electrical, or chemical stimuli can result in the sensation and perception of pain. Information about these painful or noxious stimuli is transmitted to higher brain centers by receptors and neurons that are often distinct from those that carry innocuous somatic sensory information. The mammalian somatosensory system is subserved by four groups of afferent fibers differentiated by their anatomy, rate of transmission, and sensory modality transduced (Table 57-1).

The first group, the heavily myelinated large-diameter A alpha (Aα) fibers, have specialized terminals incorporated within muscle spindles, Golgi tendon organs, and joints. These fibers and their respective end organs transduce proprioceptive information. The second group, the heavily myelinated large-diameter A beta (Aβ) fibers, have specialized encapsulated nerve endings including the Meissner, Pacinian, and Ruffini corpuscles and the Merkel disc, which transduce innocuous or low-threshold mechanical stimulation. Aα fibers do not ordinarily participate in signaling pain sensations to the central nervous system. However, the activation of Aβ and, possibly, Aα fibers has been invoked as a part of the mechanism for the production of pain relief by transcutaneous electrical nerve stimulators, which may implicate both fibers in a role in pain signal processing.[1] As well, it is becoming increasingly apparent that in chronic pain states, these fibers may indeed participate in pain signaling by adopting a "phenotype" similar to that of a C fiber (vide infra).[2]

The next groups of fibers represent the specialized sensory neurons that respond to actual or potential tissue damage, the *nociceptors.* The lightly myelinated medium-diameter A delta (Aδ) fibers and the unmyelinated small-diameter C fibers have free nerve endings that transduce noxious or high-threshold thermal, mechanical, and chemical stimulation. Patients with a mutation of the tyrosine kinase protein A, which is a component of the nerve growth factor receptor, fail to develop Aβ, Aδ, or C fibers and have no ability to sense pain.[3] Unlike receptors in the first two groups (Aα and Aβ), the Aδ and C fibers respond to stimulation of their receptive fields in a characteristic manner with slow adaptation and residual firing following the withdrawal of the stimulus. Although these two fiber groups respond similarly to stimulation, they mediate different aspects of pain sensation. The rapidly conducting Aδ fibers mediate the "first" pain or *epicritic pain,* which is well localized and is characterized as sharp or prickling. The slowly conducting C fibers mediate the "second" pain or *protopathic pain,* which temporally follows the epicritic pain and is poorly localized or diffuse and is characterized as burning or dull.[4]

The majority of Aδ and C nociceptors are polymodal and therefore are responsible for the transduction of noxious stimuli of different modalities. Nociceptive nerve endings are also located in muscle, the fascia, and adventitia of blood vessels, the knee joint, the dura, and the viscera. Recent evidence suggests that sensory transduction in the skin can include mediation by non-neural skin cells including keratinocytes and epithelial cells. These cells are thought to directly participate in touch and thermal sensation and are believed to communicate with the nerve ending through paracrine transmission.[5] The keratinocytes and epithelial cells may also play a role in neuropathic and inflammatory pain conditions though the release of neuronal activating chemical mediator, or neurotransmitter, including calcitonin gene–related

TABLE 57-1. PRIMARY AFFERENT FIBERS AND THEIR FUNCTION

Modality	Receptor	Fiber Type	Conduction Velocity and Diameter	Rate of Adaptation	Function
Proprioceptive	Golgi and Ruffini endings, muscle spindle afferents	Aα	70–120 m/s 15–20 μm	Slow and rapid	Muscle tension, length, and velocity
Mechanosensitive	Meissner, Ruffini, Pacinian corpuscles, and Merkel disc	Aβ	40–70 m/s 5–15 μm	Rapid (slow—Merkel)	Touch, flutter, motion, pressure, vibration
Thermoreceptive	Free nerve endings	Aδ	10–35 m/s 1–5 μm	Slow	Innocuous cold
	Free nerve endings	C	0.5–1 m/s <1 μm	Slow	Innocuous warmth
Nociceptive	Free nerve endings	Aδ	10–35 m/s 1–5 μm	Slow	Sharp pain
	Free nerve endings	C	0.5–1 m/s <1 μm	Slow	Burning pain

peptide (CGRP).[6] Chemical mediators of pain are numerous. These mediators come from sources intrinsic to the neuron, including various neurotransmitters such as serotonin and substance P, and extrinsic to the nervous system, including substances from inflammatory/immune cells and red blood cells such as prostaglandins, kinins, cytokines, chemokines, and adenosine triphosphate that are released following injury to the tissue.

The primary afferent peripheral (distal) terminals express a variety of specific transducer channels that are sensitive over a range of stimulus intensities. When they are activated by the appropriate stimulus (thermal, chemical, or mechanical) these channels activate voltage-sensitive cation channels (NaV and CaV) and initiate an action potential. The sodium channel is of special interest following the discovery of its involvement in patients that are insensitive to pain. An epidemiologic study identified three Pakistani families with congential insensitivity to pain. All were found to possess nonsense mutations of the SCN9A gene resulting in truncation of the Nav1.7 isoform of the sodium channel.[7] Other mutations of this gene result in the impaired inactivation of this channel resulting in paroxysmal extreme pain disorder or hyperexcitability resulting in erythromelalgia.[8,9]

The understanding of the molecular underpinning of the sensory processing of pain has primarily come from studying two families of proteins, the TRP and the DEG/ENaC channels. The cloning and characterization of the "capsaicin" receptor of the transient receptor potential (TRP) family of nonselective cation channels expanded the field immensely[10] (Table 57-2). Members of this molecular family transduce thermal, mechanical, and chemical information in the periphery. The capsaicin receptor named *TRP vanilloid 1* (TRPV1), which responds not only to capsaicin and other vanilloid compounds, but which is also activated by acid and heat, provides an excellent example of the integration of multiple sensory modalities within a single neuron and is localized to nociceptors.[10] Furthermore, acidic environments can lower the activation threshold of the channel to heat stimuli. Therefore, the TRPV1 receptor may represent an important therapeutic target in inflammatory (acidic) pain conditions. Mice lacking the TRPV1 receptor are deficient in their response to thermal, but not mechanical or other noxious stimuli.[11] These data suggest that this member of the family of TRP channels may play a role in the integration of noxious chemical and thermal stimuli while having relatively less to do with mechanical transduction. Although mechanical transduction has been less well characterized than either thermal or chemical nociceptive transduction, there is evidence of mechanically activated channels in the *degenerins* family of the nematode *Caenorhabditis elegans*. In mammals, studies have provided evidence that the transduction channel is a complex of degenerin and the epithelial Na+ channel (DEG/ENaC)[12] and may have a role in the transduction of mechanical stimuli in humans. The subunit composition of the DEG/ENaC channel may play a role in determining whether a mechanical stimuli is sensed as noxious or innocuous.[13]

Neurochemistry of Peripheral Nerve and the Dorsal Root Ganglion

The nociceptive primary afferents, the Aδ and C fibers, represent the principal target of pharmacologic manipulation by the physician treating pain. Glutamate receptors, as well as opioid, substance P, somatostatin, and vanilloid receptors, have been identified on the peripheral endings of these nerve fibers. Although the transmission of acute nociceptive information is primarily by the Aδ and C fibers, a subset of the Aδ and C fibers are "thermoreceptors" that transduce innocuous cold and warm information, respectively. The cell bodies of primary afferents, regardless of the structure they innervate, make up the *dorsal root ganglia* (DRG) located just outside the spinal cord within the bony foramen.

Primary afferent activation results in a postsynaptic excitatory event in the spinal cord. Glutamate is the primary

TABLE 57-2. MECHANOSENSORY AND THERMOSENSORY TRANSDUCTION CHANNELS FOUND IN MAMMALS

Name	Family	Physical Modality	Additional Activators	Temperature Range (°C)	Neuronal Expression
TRPA1	TRPA	Thermal, mechanical	Icillin, calcium, isothiocyanates	<18	C fibers
TRPC1	TRPC	Mechanical	Receptor-operated	NA	Aβ, Aδ
TRPM8	TRPM	Thermal	Menthol, Icillin	<28	C fibers
TRPV1	TRPV	Thermal, osmotic	Capsaicin, protons, endocannabinoids, diphenyl compounds	>42	C, Aδ, and keratinocytes
TRPV2	TRPV	Thermal, osmotic, mechanical	Diphenyl compounds	>52	Aβ, Aδ, keratinocytes
TRPV3	TRPV	Thermal diphenyl	Camphor, carvacrol,	>34–39	C fibers, keratinocytes
TRPV4	TRPV	Thermal, osmotic acids, epoxyeicosatrienoic acid	Polyunsaturated fatty	>27–34	Aδ, C, keratinocytes, Merkel cells
ASIC1	DEG/ENaC	Mechanical	Protons	NA	Aβ, Aδ, C
ASIC2	DEG/ENaC	Mechanical	Protons	NA	Aβ, Aδ
ASIC3	DEG/ENaC	Mechanical	Protons	NA	Aβ, Aδ
TREK-1	Potassium channel	Thermal, mechanical	Lipids, protons	NA	Aβ, Aδ, C

Adapted from: Lumpkin EA, Caterina MJ. Mechanisms of sensory transduction in the skin. *Nature.* 2007;445:858.

neurotransmitter serving this function. Acute activation events are mediated by the AMPA-type (α-amino-3-hydroxy-5-methyl-4-isoxazole propionic acid) glutamate receptor present on the dorsal horn neurons. This receptor produces a robust, but short-lasting depolarization of the postsynaptic membrane by increasing sodium conductance and augmenting the activation of the NMDA-type (*N*-methyl-D-aspartate) glutamate receptor. In addition to glutamate, populations of primary afferents contain and release a variety of neuropeptides including substance P, calcitonin gene–related peptide, adenosine triphosphate, adenosine, galanin, and somatostatin and growth factors including brain-derived nerve growth factor.[14]

Neurobiology of the Spinal Cord and Spinal Trigeminal Nucleus

Primary afferent fibers enter the gray matter of the spinal cord through the *dorsal root entry zone* and innervate the spinal cord. The majority of heavily myelinated primary afferent fibers (Aα, Aβ) carrying sensory information, including tactile, pressure, and vibratory sense, enter in dorsal roots, traverse across the top of the dorsal horn of the spinal cord (Lissauer's tract), and ascend ipsilaterally within the dorsal column and provide collateral branches into the gray matter of the dorsal horn. The small-diameter lightly myelinated and the small-diameter unmyelinated fibers transmitting temperature and nociceptive information enter Lissauer's tract and innervate the gray matter of the spinal cord. Unlike the heavily myelinated fibers, these fibers may also ascend rostrally or descend caudally through Lissauer's tract before they innervate adjacent spinal levels.

The gray matter of the spinal cord is made up of synaptic terminations of primary afferents and the second-order neurons that form the first stage of processing and integration of sensory information. The gray matter of the spinal cord is divided into 10 laminae on the basis of histologic appearance. The dorsal horn includes laminae I to VI and represents the primary sensory complement of the spinal cord (Fig. 57-1). The ventral horn, including laminae VII to IX and lamina X, is involved in somatic motor and autonomic functions, respectively. *Somatic* C-fiber nociceptive afferent endings primarily terminate in the laminae I and II of the same and/or one to two adjacent spinal segments from which they entered from the periphery, whereas *visceral* C-fiber nociceptive afferents can terminate in the dorsal horn more than five segments rostrally or caudally. They not only terminate in laminae I, II, V, X ipsilaterally but also in laminae V and X contralaterally. Therefore, visceral afferents have a wider branching pattern and the nociceptive information they transmit is less localizable to a particular area of the body.

In addition to the primary afferent endings, neurons of the descending pathways and local interneurons also innervate the superficial dorsal horn (laminae I and II). The outer marginal layer or lamina I contain interneurons and cells that send axonal projections to the brainstem and midbrain structures. The substantia gelatinosa, or lamina II, also contains excitatory and inhibitory interneurons but fewer projection neurons. Laminae III and IV contain interneurons and the second-order neurons that make up the dorsal column pathways relaying nonnociceptive sensory and proprioceptive information. Laminae IV to VI contain interneurons and a modest portion of nociceptive projection neurons that distribute input to the brainstem and thalamus.

Nociceptive somatic input is primarily transmitted by second-order lamina I, IV, and V projection neurons as the contralateral spinothalamic tract (STT) pathway traveling to numerous brainstem regions and the thalamus.[15] There is a nociceptive visceral processing area in laminae III, IV, V, VII, and X. The visceral nociceptive input is relayed by second-order neurons whose axons travel within the dorsal column. Like the fibers transmitting nonnoxious sensory information, these fibers remain uncrossed until relayed with the crossed medial lemniscal fibers to the thalamus. The visceral pain information transmitted by the ventral STT is likely originating from cells also receiving somatic nociceptive input. Nociceptive and nonnociceptive sensory information from the head, neck, and dura transmitted via the trigeminal nerve innervates the dorsal horn of the spinal trigeminal nucleus in the caudal medulla. The organization and neurotransmitter complement of the spinal trigeminal nucleus is similar to that of the spinal dorsal horn.

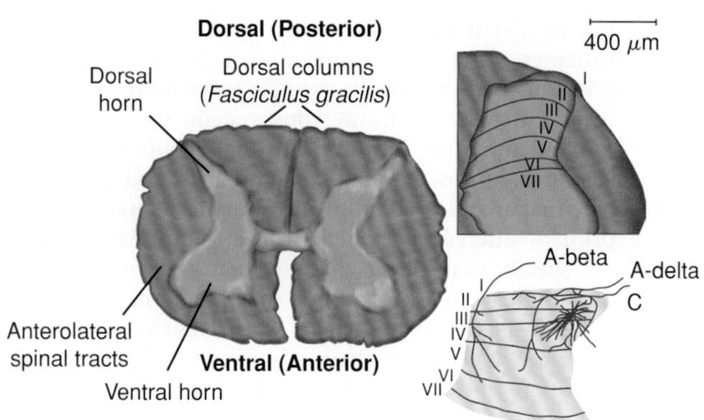

FIGURE 57-1. Anatomy: Histologic sections and schematic diagrams of the spinal dorsal horn. The histologic section at left is from the lumbar segment of the spinal cord. It is labeled to show the relationship between the major spinal somatosensory structures. The histologic section at right is from the rat lumbar spinal cord. The *outer heavy lines* show the boundary of the spinal gray matter while the *inner heavy lines* show the boundaries of Rexed's laminae. These boundaries are established by the histologic characteristics of each zone, and the layers are identified by the Roman numerals. The drawing at the bottom illustrates the pattern of primary afferent innervation to the nonhuman primate spinal dorsal horn. The large myelinated (A-beta) fibers segregate to the dorsal aspect of an entering root and then track medially in the dorsal horn and terminate in layers III to V. The small myelinated (A-delta) fibers and C fibers that carry nociceptive information segregate ventrally in the entering roots, course laterally in the dorsal horn, and then largely terminate in the superficial layers (I and II) of the dorsal horn. (Adapted from: Raja SN, Dougherty PM. Anatomy and physiology of somatosensory and pain processing. In: Benzon HT, Raja SN, Molloy RE, Liu SS, Fishman SM, eds. *Essentials of Pain Medicine and Regional Anesthesia*. 2nd ed. Philadelphia, PA: Elsevier-Churchill Livingstone; 2005;3, with permission.)

Neurobiology of Ascending Pathways

Dorsal Column Tracts

The dorsal column contains the axons of second-order spinal cord projection neurons in addition to the ascending axons of primary afferent neurons relaying touch, pressure, and vibratory sensation. Second-order dorsal column cells in the central visceral processing region of the spinal cord around lamina X also respond to noxious visceral stimulation and converge on some of the thalamic cells receiving nociceptive information from the skin and other somatic structures.

Spinothalamic Tract (STT)

STT neurons are the primary relay cells providing nociceptive input from the spinal cord to supraspinal levels. The axons of

STT cells cross the midline of the spinal cord through the anterior white commissure and ascend primarily in the contralateral and anterolateral tracts. The axons of STT cells terminate primarily in the posterior complex of the thalamus including the ventral posterior lateral and ventral posterior medial nuclei. Nonnoxious sensory input from the same body region converges on the same target thalamic neurons providing somatotopic encoding for localization of the input onto the cortical representation of the specific body region, allowing the ability to locate the source of the nociceptive input. The STT cells receiving noxious somatic input are predominantly situated in lamina I and the lateral aspect of the dorsal horn in laminae IV to V.[15] However, other STT neurons are scattered throughout the deep dorsal horn, intermediate region including lamina X, and even in lamina VII of the ventral horn. These STT cells receive both somatic and visceral nociceptive information.

Spinobulbar Pathways

Major ascending lateral axonal projections relaying information about noxious stimuli terminate in the reticular formation of the ventrolateral medulla. This spinal projection pathway traverses brainstem regions containing catecholaminergic neurons, including the locus coeruleus and A7 nuclei of the dorsolateral pontine tegmentum (DLPT). These catecholaminergic neurons are involved in multiple functions, including modulation of nociceptive transmission through the spinal cord via descending inhibitory input. Connections between the rostral ventromedial medulla (RVM) and the catecholamine cells of the pons and brainstem serotonergic cells also play a role in descending modulation of noxious transmission in the spinal cord.[16] Spinobulbar pathways relaying information about pain also terminate in the parabrachial nucleus, periaqueductal gray (PAG), the RVM, and midline midbrain reticular formation.[17]

Spinohypothalamic, Limbic, and Cortical Connections

Pain is a sensory experience but also has an affective component to the perception of noxious stimuli. Pain can provoke fear, anxiety, and depression, resulting in autonomic responses including increased heart rate and blood pressure as well as the endocrine stress response. These responses to noxious stimuli are thought to be mediated by the spinohypothalamic and spinoamygdalar pathways. In addition to their affective function, these regions are also thought to be involved in antinociception. Ascending axonal projections of these pathways arise predominantly from the spinal cord laminae I and X.

Neurobiology of Descending Pathways

The primary components of this descending pain inhibition system, but certainly not all-inclusive, is the "triad" of the PAG, the RVM, and the DLPT.[17] The PAG is an important site for the production of antinociception following electrical or chemical activation, or the injection of opioid receptor agonists. The endogenous opioid enkephalin is present within this nucleus, and opioid receptors of each subtype are present in this region. The PAG provides dense projections to the RVM, the locus coeruleus, and A7 nuclei.[18] Although each of these regions has direct projections to the spinal cord, it has been proposed that their projections to the RVM are important components in the modulation of nociception. Chemical or electrical inactivation of the RVM results in the attenuation of the antinociceptive effects produced by the activation of these midbrain structures.[19] Although the RVM can function as a relay nucleus in the production of antinociception by more cephalad midbrain structures including the PAG, it also has a primary role in the suppression of nociceptive transmission at the level of the spinal cord. The suppression of nociceptive reflex behavior is mediated by the axons of RVM neurons that descend within the dorsolateral funiculus and terminate bilaterally in laminae I, II, V, VI, and VII of the spinal cord. Anatomic studies have shown that these axons terminate coincident with interneurons of the dorsal horn that are related to nociceptive transmission.[20] Consistent with the anatomic terminations of the RVM axons, physiologic studies have shown that stimulation of the RVM results in the inhibition of a population of nociceptive-specific neurons within the dorsal horn as well as selective inhibition of the nociceptive responses of wide-dynamic range neurons.[21] The neurotransmitters found in the RVM neurons include enkephalin, γ-aminobutyric acid (GABA), glutamate, and substance P.[22] The DLPT is also an important component of spinal cord nociceptive modulation. It contains all of the noradrenergic neurons that project to the RVM and the spinal cord, and electrical stimulation of the DLPT sites produces spinal cord α_2-adrenergic receptor–mediated analgesia.[23]

Neurobiology of Supraspinal Structures Involved in Higher Cortical Processing

Higher cortical centers play a role in the perception of painful stimuli as well as the integration of the sensory-discriminative and affective components of the noxious stimulation. The localization of the neural structures involved in this perception and integration is still in its adolescence. The development of positron emission tomography and functional magnetic resonance imaging technologies has moved this research forward. These imaging technologies produce indirect evidence of neural activity related to pain stimulation. They look for areas of increased blood flow as an indicator of regions of increased activity resulting from the stimulation. The primary and secondary somatosensory cortexes, the anterior cingulate gyrus, the insula, and the prefrontal cortex appear to be involved in the higher processing of somatic and visceral pain.[24] As the primary and secondary cortexes are known to be somatosensory processing regions, the imaging studies are consistent with a sensory-discriminative role of these structures. The insula and frontal cortex may contribute to memory and learning of events related to painful stimuli. The anterior cingulate cortex is thought to be involved in the analysis of the emotional significance of the painful input. Finally, the lentiform nucleus and cerebellum may be involved in the learning of self-protective reflexive motor responsiveness to painful input.

Transition from Acute to Persistent or Chronic Nociception

Pain sensation is unique among the somatosensory modalities in that it does not rapidly adapt to prolonged stimulation as do the other sensory modalities, such as fine touch. In fact, continued stimulation may produce greater noxious sensation or reduce the stimulus threshold or intensity that is necessary for the appreciation of the sensation as noxious. For instance, previously innocuous thermal or mechanical stimulation may be perceived as painful following a prior noxious stimulus. For example, warm water of the shower or the light touch of the towel across sunburned skin produces a painful sensation that may persist for a few minutes following the stimulation. This is termed *allodynia.* Another example of an altered pain state that may follow an acute injury is that of *hyperalgesia,* in which a previously noxious stimulus is perceived as more painful. The sensation of increased intensity of noxious stimulation at the site of the injury is the result of the sensitization of the peripheral nociceptors.

Persistent C fiber, but not Aβ fiber, primary afferent activation of lamina I and lamina V, as occurs with tissue injury and inflammation, has been shown to enhance the response to subsequent stimulation and augment the size of the receptive field of the respective dorsal horn neuron. Therefore, afferent input from adjacent dermatomal areas now produces neuronal excitation. Furthermore, nonnoxious stimulation becomes increasingly able to activate these neurons. This general phenomenon has come to be termed *wind-up* or *central sensitization.*[25] It is these physiologic effects that are believed to underlie the allodynia and hyperalgesia produced by persistent noxious stimulation or tissue injury. This persistent input will lead to cellular damage and migration of inflammatory cells including macrophages and neutrophils into the peripheral tissue. This leads to the release of histamine, bradykinin, prostaglandins, cytokines, growth factors, protons, and peptides that activate or sensitize receptors on the peripheral nociceptor. Activation of these receptors results in depolarization and, under these conditions, spontaneous afferent activity. This activation is thought to explain the allodynia and hyperalgesia observed surrounding the site of injury.

In addition to the alteration of the chemical milieu surrounding the primary afferent distal terminal that results from injury or persistent high-intensity stimulation, axonal sprouting and the formation of neuroma may occur. The neuroma may have an altered complement of ion channels including an up-regulation of sodium channels or a down-regulation of potassium channels that has the net result of increasing neuronal excitability and increasing nociceptive transmission. It has been shown that, following nerve damage, an increase in the expression of sodium channels occurs in the neuroma and the DRG. Numerous sodium channels exist on primary afferents; Nav1.8 and 1.9 subtypes are primarily found on C-fiber DRG cells. Genetic "knock-down" or removal of the Nav1.8 channel had no effect on baseline pain thresholds; however, it reversed nerve injury evoked nociception.[26] Also following nerve damage, potassium currents have been shown to be reduced, suggesting a reduction in these channels contributing to spontaneous nociceptive activity. Consistent with this notion, it has been observed that potassium channel antagonists increase and potassium channel agonists decrease ectopic firing after peripheral nerve injury.[27] The HCN2 ion channel which carries an inward current I_h that is activated by neuronal hyperpolarization may have a significant role in the sensation of chronic pain from neuropathy or inflammation.[28] When this gene product was knocked out of nociceptive primary sensory neurons in mice, the mice failed to express pain behaviors after inflammatory injuries. The mice did not show hyperalgesia or allodynia to mechanical or thermal stimuli in a model of neuropathic injury. The pharmacologic blockade of this channel, or disruption of this gene, could be a potential therapy for those suffering from some conditions of chronic pain.

Neuromas of injured primary afferents have altered sensitivity to a number of humoral factors, including cytokines, prostaglandins, and catecholamines. These factors are released from a variety of cell types including inflammatory cells and neuronal support cells. Cytokines directly activate the nerve and neuroma through receptors that become expressed in the membrane after the nerve injury. A molecule that has been shown to have a prominent role following nerve damage is tumor necrosis factor subunit *alpha* (TNF-α).[29] Shortly after injury, TNF-α decreases potassium conductance, increasing neuronal excitability, while the long-term changes may be produced through the activation of second messenger systems, resulting in altered protein production. Application of TNF-α to the peripheral nerve results in hyperalgesia, while systemic delivery of antibodies to TNF-α or TNF-α–binding protein reduces neuropathic pain.

Prostaglandins are also released from inflammatory cells following nerve and tissue damage. They can enhance the opening of Nav1.8 channels by acting though receptors on the afferent terminal. Nerve growth factor is also released from glial and inflammatory cells after nerve damage, resulting in sprouting of postganglionic sympathetic efferents into the site of injury. Protease-activated receptors isoforms 1, 2, and 4 appear to sensitize TRPV1 channels in nociceptive neurons and are involved in mechanisms of pain and inflammation.[30] These receptors are responsive to thrombin activation and could account for pain resulting from a hematoma. The up-regulation of α_1-adrenergic receptors has been demonstrated in animals with nerve injuries.[31] Stimulation of the postganglionic axons results in the release of catecholamines and excites the injured axon and DRG of the injured axon via α-adrenergic receptors.

Although acute noxious stimuli are transmitted to the spinal cord via Aδ and C fibers, the presence of allodynia is thought to be mediated by the activation of large-diameter Aβ fibers through what has been termed a *phenotypic* switch.[2] Prior to this peripheral injury, the Aβ fibers, unlike the C fibers, do not express substance P. However, following injury these fibers were able to express this neuropeptide.[32] These data therefore implicate Aβ fibers in the transmission of noxious peripheral stimulation and provide further support for the involvement of somatic Aβ fibers in at least some form of the allodynic pain states. Furthermore, the blockade of Aβ fibers results in a reduction in light-touch evoked allodynia.[33] This phenotypic switch of Aβ fibers may represent another avenue for therapeutic intervention; however, the difficulty will be in differentiating between those Aβ fibers involved in noxious versus nonnoxious sensory information.

MANAGEMENT OF COMMON PAIN SYNDROMES

Low Back Pain: Radicular Pain Syndromes

The common causes of low back pain include radicular pain/radiculopathy from herniated disc or spinal/foraminal stenosis, facet syndrome, and internal disc disruption. Myofascial pain syndrome also causes back pain, whereas sacroiliac joint syndrome and piriformis syndrome cause mostly buttock pain but can present as low back pain or radicular pain. Radicular symptoms of pain, paresthesias, and numbness in a typical dermatomal distribution in the presence of objective signs of weakness, diminished reflexes, and positive straight-leg raise are secondary to pathology or dysfunction of the sensory spinal nerve roots. Low back pain, with or without radicular pain, is mostly due to lesions of the intervertebral discs and degenerative spinal disorders. Other causes include spinal metastasis, vertebral body fractures, infections, abdominal aortic aneurysm, and chronic pancreatic lesions.

Low back and radicular pain secondary to a herniated disc is due to mechanical nerve root compression and the subsequent inflammatory process. The presence of a herniated disc does not necessarily result in pain. Up to 36% of the general population[34] and up to 53% of pregnant women[35] can have an asymptomatic herniated disc. Follow-up studies on patients with a herniated disc show spontaneous regression without treatment, absence of symptoms in the presence of more abnormalities, and partial or complete resolution with treatment that includes medications, bed rest, physical therapy, traction, or epidural steroids.[36] If symptomatic, the patient usually presents with low back pain and radicular symptoms that include paresthesias as well as numbness and weakness in the distribution of the involved nerve root. Radicular pain typically travels along a narrow band and has a sharp, shooting, and lancinating quality. Gait disturbances, loss of sensation, reduced muscle strength, and diminished reflexes involve the appropriate affected dermatomal distribution.

Inflammation in the spinal canal secondary to a herniated disc plays an important role in the causation of back and radicular pain. Herniated nucleus pulposus results in local release of cytokines and other inflammatory mediators that cause a chemical radiculitis. High levels of phospholipase A_2 activity were noted in human disc fragments removed at surgery from patients with symptomatic radiculopathy. Increased levels of the inflammatory cytokines interleukin-6 and interleukin-8 were noted from disc material taken from patients with known disc disease.[37] The application of disc material onto spinal nerve roots can induce functional and morphologic changes in the nerves. Disc cells express TNF-α, which, when applied to spinal nerve roots, causes similar changes to those seen after application of disc material; selective inhibition of TNF-α may reduce the intraneural edema.[38] A double-blind, placebo-controlled study showed that an intradiscal injection of 1.5 mg of etanercept, a TNF-α inhibitor, in a pain-generating disc did not reduce the pain scores or disability scores of patients with chronic discogenic pain or lumbosacral radiculopathy.[39]

For patients with radicular symptoms who do not respond to conservative management, including anti-inflammatory medications, epidural steroid injections (ESIs) may be useful. Epidural steroids have an anti-inflammatory effect related to inhibition of phospholipase A_2 activity. In addition, steroids have a local anesthetic and antinociceptive effect. The local application of methylprednisolone blocks transmission of C fibers but not the Aβ fibers. Several prospective, randomized, and controlled studies have demonstrated short-term efficacy of ESIs for treatment of lumbar spine radiculopathy[40–42] while others have not.[43,44] Another study demonstrated less leg pain and sensory deficit with ESI, but the incidence of surgery was the same between the steroid and
2 the control groups.[45] For cervical ESIs, the few studies that have been done are mostly descriptive and their results were the same as in lumbar ESIs, that is, transient relief from the injections. The transient efficacy of the ESIs lasted no more than 3 months. These transient effects were noted by the Therapeutics and Technology Assessment Subcommittee of the American Academy of Neurology,[46] which recommended against the routine use of ESIs. This recommendation has to be viewed against the natural history of patients with herniated disc and spinal stenosis as these patients seem to do well over time with conservative management. The transient relief provided by ESIs may minimize the need for opioids and potent anti-inflammatory medications and their related side effects. ESIs should be a component, and not the sole modality, of the conservative management of radicular pain.

A transforaminal approach can be employed to deposit steroid in the anterolateral epidural space where the herniated disc is located, through the intervertebral foramina, and distally along the nerve root (Fig. 57-2). This approach is especially indicated in radicular pain specific to a single nerve root. Prospective, randomized studies on transforaminal ESIs show the same results as with the interlaminar approach, that is, short-term efficacy of the injection.[47–49] The transforaminal approach has a better rationale than the midline interlaminar approach, and studies that compared the two approaches show better efficacy with the transforaminal approach.[50,51] A study comparing the parasagittal (paramedian approach) and transforaminal approach showed a more ideal spread of the contrast dye in the parasagittal approach although the efficacy was similar between the two techniques.[52]

It is advisable that fluoroscopy be used in ESI, especially with the transforaminal approach, to assure insertion of the needle at the affected vertebral level and document the flow of the contrast

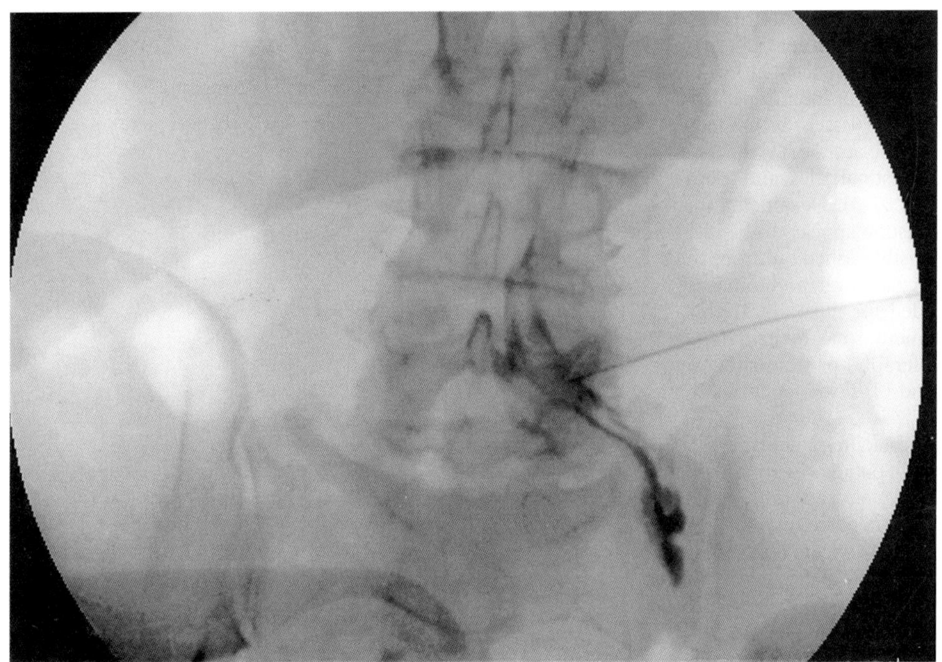

FIGURE 57-2. Right L5 transforaminal epidural injection. Note the spread of the contrast medium proximally into the lateral epidural space and distally along the nerve root.

medium (and the drug). Reassessment should be carried out 2 to 3 weeks after the initial injection. The use of multiple ESIs in a patient, with a short interval between injections, is not advised. If there is no response to an initial injection, it can be repeated once as some patients require a second injection before they respond. If there is partial response, up to three injections can be performed.

The complications of ESI may be due to the technique or from the injected drug, as well as the vehicle and additives. Complications related to the technique include needle trauma, vasospasm, and infection. Glucocorticoids reduce the hypoglycemic effect of insulin and interfere with blood glucose control in patients with diabetes mellitus. Insulin sensitivity may be impaired, there may be no change in the HbA1C levels, or the blood glucose can be increased for 1 week after ESIs. A single dose of 80 mg of methylprednisolone can suppress plasma cortisol levels and the ability to secrete cortisol in response to synthetic corticotropin for up to 3 weeks. Epidural triamcinolone, 80 mg, can suppress serum cortisol and corticotropin levels for up to 7 days after injection. The median recovery to normal levels occurs within 1 month after the last injection, and full recovery is at 3 months.

Injury to the brain or spinal cord can occur with transforaminal ESIs.[53] The cerebral/cerebellar events can be ascribed to trauma to the vertebral artery, vasospasm from the injected steroid or dye, or embolism of the particulate steroid via the vertebral artery.[54,55] The spinal cord injuries can be ascribed to injury to the radicular artery accompanying the nerve root, spasm of the radicular artery from the injected dye or steroid, embolism of the particulate steroid, or from proximal intraneural spread of the injectate. The injection of contrast medium through a radicular artery that passed to the spinal cord or the anterior spinal artery has been demonstrated. The occurrence of adverse events at the lumbar level has been ascribed to intra-arterial injection into an abnormally low-lying artery of the Adamkiewicz. These adverse events have also been described after injection of local anesthetic or dye, without steroid.[55] The use of computed tomography (CT), instead of fluoroscopy, does not assure avoidance of the adverse events.

Huntoon[56] noted that the vertebral, ascending cervical, and deep cervical arteries supply segmental medullary vessels and that the ascending and deep cervical arteries are within 2 mm of the site of insertion of the needle for cervical transforaminal ESIs. The proximity of these arteries to the site of needle placement makes these blood vessels vulnerable to trauma or unintentional sites of injection of the steroid. Occlusion of the vessels occurs from the particulate steroids. Methylprednisolone acetate has the largest particle size, betamethasone the smallest particles, and triamcinolone acetonide is in between[55] (Fig. 57-3). Dexamethasone has no identifiable particles. Dexamethasone appears to be ideal for transforaminal ESIs; however, it is easily washed out from the epidural space, and studies on its efficacy are only preliminary.[57] The following steroids are recommended for ESIs: (1) Methylprednisolone, triamcinolone, or betamethasone for *interlaminar* injections; (2) betamethasone (preferably) or triamcinolone for *lumbar transforaminal* injections; and (3) dexamethasone for *cervical transforaminal* injections.

ESIs are more effective in patients with acute radicular symptoms; however, they are not effective in patients with chronic lumbar radiculopathy.[58] There have been several prospective, randomized controlled studies on the efficacy of surgery in relieving back pain secondary to herniated disc. It appears that surgery for herniated disc produces only short-term relief, whereas the long-term results are comparable with those with conservative management.[59] For spinal stenosis, surgery is associated with greater improvements in most outcome measures.

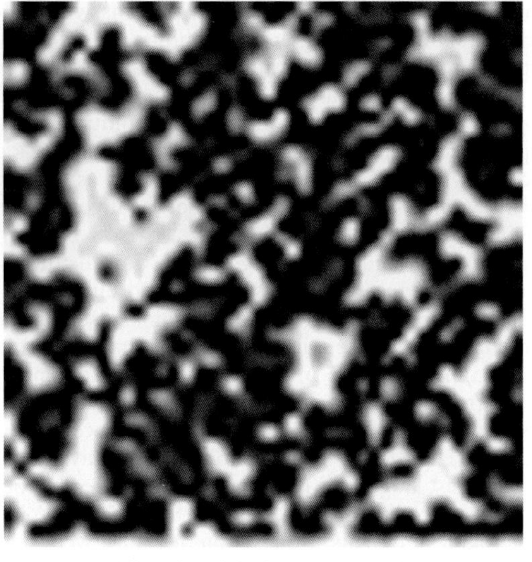

Methylprednisolone 80 mg/mL

Methylprednisolone 40 mg/mL

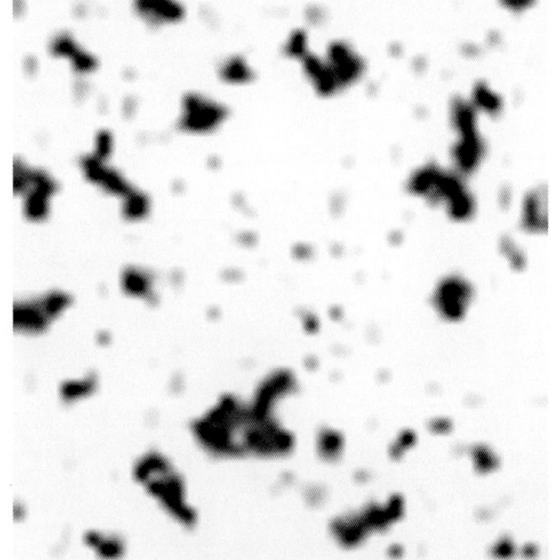

A Triamcinolone 40 mg/mL

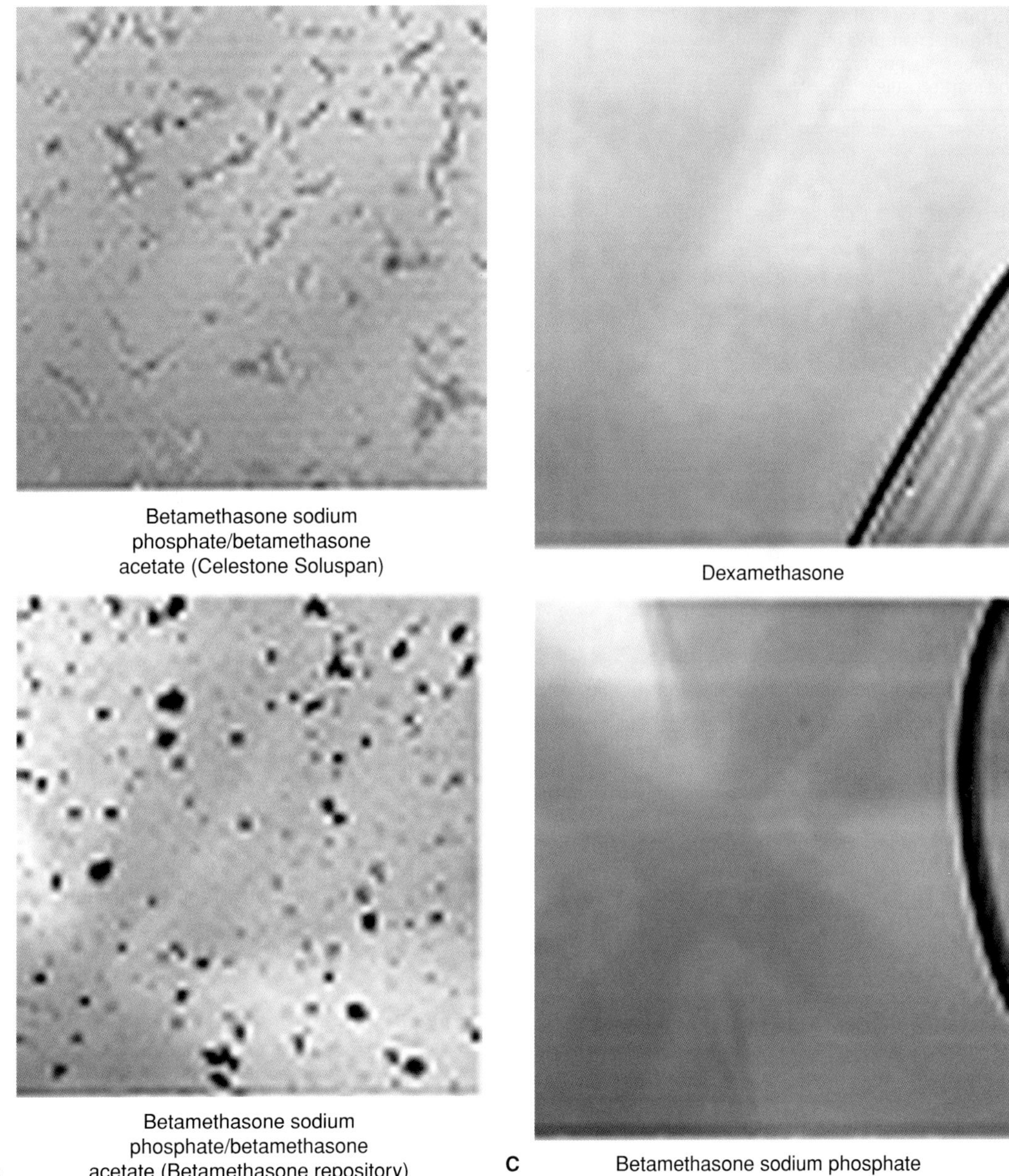

FIGURE 57-3. A: Typical microscopic appearances of methylprednisolone, 80 mg/mL and 40 mg/mL, and triamcinolone 40 mg/mL. The particles are amorphous in appearance. **B:** The particles of commercial betamethasone (Celestone Soluspan) are rodlike and lucent, while those of the compounded betamethasone (betamethasone repository) are amorphous. **C:** Note that dexamethasone is pure liquid. (From: Benzon HT, Chew TL, McCarthy R, et al. Comparison of the particle sizes of the different steroids and the effect of dilution: A review of the relative neurotoxicities of the steroids. *Anesthesiology.* 2007;106:331, with permission.)

Low Back Pain: Facet Syndrome

Patients with low back pain secondary to facet pathology have pain in the low back that radiates to the ipsilateral posterior thigh and usually ends at the knee. On physical examination there is paraspinal tenderness and reproduction of pain with extension–rotation maneuvers of the back. The diagnosis of facet syndrome is arrived at by a combination of the patient's history, physical examination findings, and a positive response to diagnostic medial branch blocks or facet joint injections (Fig. 57-4). For medial branch blocks, some investigators recommend the use of local anesthetics with different durations of effect (e.g., lidocaine and bupivacaine) and to correlate the duration of relief with the known duration of effect of the drug.

Some patients may have a prolonged response to facet joint injections, that is, up to 3 to 6 months. If the patient has a prolonged response, it is best to wait for recurrence of the pain. If the relief is short-lived, especially after medial branch blocks, then thermal

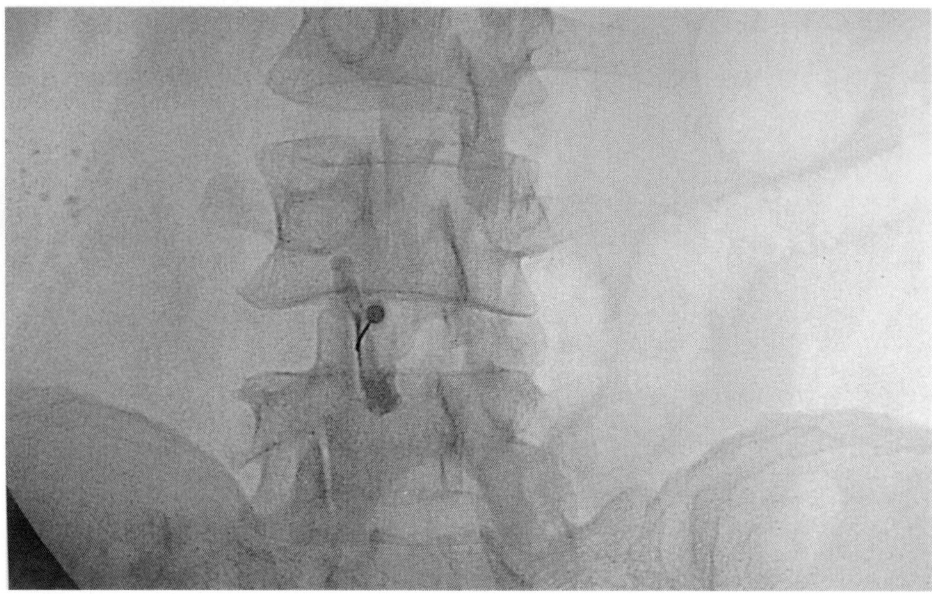

FIGURE 57-4. Left L4 to L5 facet joint injection. The injection of 5 mL of contrast medium demonstrates the extent of the joint capsule.

radiofrequency (RF) rhizotomy of the medial branches should be performed. It appears that there is no relationship between the mean sensory stimulation threshold (which denotes proximity of the electrode to the nerve) during lumbar facet rhizotomy denervation and treatment outcome.[60] Randomized controlled studies have shown improvements after thermal RF of the lumbar medial branches that lasted 3 to 12 months[61–67] (Table 57-3). With regard to cervical facet syndrome, controlled studies on thermal RF of the cervical medial branches have shown different results. Lord et al.[68] showed better results after RF (return to work and relief of pain) while Stovner et al.[69] showed no difference between the RF and sham procedures.

Buttock Pain: Sacroiliac Joint Syndrome and Piriformis Syndrome

The pain of sacroiliac joint syndrome is located in the region of the affected sacroiliac joint and the medial buttock. The pain may

TABLE 57-3. RANDOMIZED, CONTROLLED STUDIES ON RADIOFREQUENCY DENERVATION OF THE MEDIAL BRANCHES (FACET NERVES)

Study (Ref. No.)	Study Population	Results
Gallagher et al.[61]	Patients previously had good or equivocal response to facet joint injections randomized to RF or sham	Significantly better results noted in RF group at 1 and 6 mos
Sanders and Zuurmund[62]	Patients had ≥50% relief after intra-articular lidocaine, randomized to RF of medial branch versus intra-articular RF	At 3 mos: Improvements in both groups
van Kleef et al.[63]	Patients had favorable response to MBB, randomized to RF or sham	Better results noted in the RF group at 3 mos (60% vs. 25%) and at 1 yr (47% vs. 12.5%)
Leclaire et al.[64]	Patients had relief after intra-articular injection, randomized to RF or sham	At 1 mo: Improvements in Roland–Morris scores in the RF group
van Wijk et al.[65]	Patients responded to intra-articular injection, randomized to RF or sham	At 3 mos: ≥50% relief in 62% (RF group) versus 39% (sham)
Tekin et al.[66]	Local anesthetic injection versus conventional RF versus pulsed RF	At 6 mos and 1 year: Decreased in VAS maintained in CRF, patients not using analgesics and patient satisfaction highest in CRF group
Nath et al.[67]	Patients had relief after diagnostic block	At 6 mos: Better results in the RF group compared to sham procedure

RF, radiofrequency; MBB, medial branch block.

Modified from: Benzon HT. Outcomes, efficacy, and complications of the treatment of back pain. In: Benzon HT, Rathmell JP, Wu CL, Turk DC, Argoff CE, eds. *Raj's Practical Management of Pain.* 4th ed. Philadelphia, PA: Mosby Elsevier; 2008;1242, with permission.

radiate to the groin, posterior thigh, and occasionally below the knee. Physical examination usually reveals tenderness over the sacroiliac sulcus, reduction in the joint mobility, and reproduction of the pain when the affected sacroiliac joint is stressed. The most commonly used tests for sacroiliac joint dysfunction include the FABER Patrick, Gaenslen, Yeoman, sacroiliac shear, and Gillet tests. The FABER Patrick and the Yeoman test do not rule out hip pathology while the Yeoman and the shear tests are more specific for sacroiliac joint syndrome. The presence of symptoms and physical examination findings suggestive of SI joint syndrome, pain on three of the tests, and a positive response to sacroiliac joint injection are adequate to make the diagnosis of sacroiliac joint syndrome.

The treatments for sacroiliac joint syndrome include physical therapy, manipulation, intra-articular steroid injections (Fig. 57-5), radiofrequency denervation, and surgical fusion of the joint. Physical therapy and chiropractic manipulations are used extensively for the treatment of sacroiliac joint disease; however, there is no large outcome study validating their use. Intra-articular injections of steroid (40 to 80 mg of methylprednisolone or other depot steroid) and local anesthetic into the sacroiliac joint results in a few months of pain relief, but again, no prospective controlled studies support their use.

Denervation of the lower portion of the sacroiliac joint may be achieved by the creation of bipolar RF strip lesions along the dorsal border of the sacroiliac joint in a leapfrog manner. Local anesthetic blockade of the sensory innervation of the dorsal portion of the sacroiliac joint—the medial branch of the dorsal rami of L5 and the lateral branches of the dorsal rami of S1 to S3—can be performed initially or when the relief from the sacroiliac joint injection is temporary. Relief from the local anesthetic block may last weeks to months when combined with physical therapy. Monopolar and bipolar thermal radiofrequency lesioning of the lateral branches is performed for a more lasting relief. The bigger lesions created by the water-cooled radiofrequency technique (Fig. 57-6)[70] are inherently more effective since it accommodates for the variations in the location of the lateral branches along the lateral border of the sacral foraminas.[71]

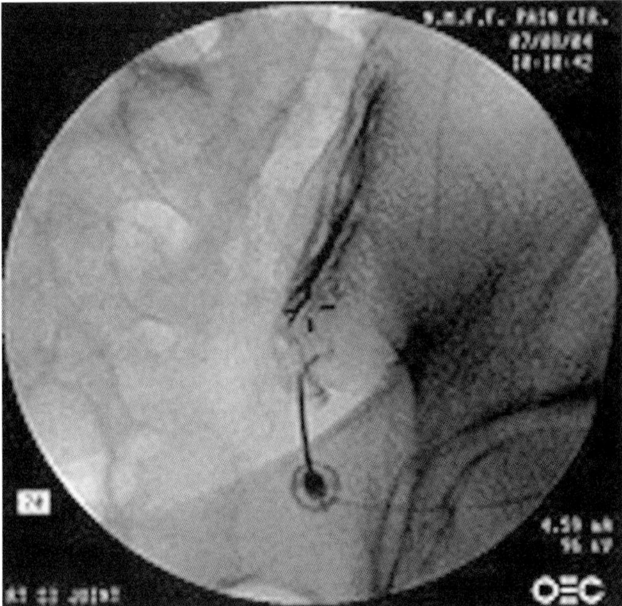

FIGURE 57-5. Sacroiliac joint injection. Note the spread of the contrast medium along the joint. (From: Benzon HT, Nader A. Hip, sacroiliac joint, and piriformis injections. In: Benzon HT, Rathmell J, Wu C, Turk DC, Argoff C, eds. *Raj's Practical Management of Pain*. 4th ed. Philadelphia, PA: Mosby Elsevier; 2008;1070, with permission.)

Piriformis Syndrome

Piriformis syndrome, another pain syndrome that originates in the buttock, comprises 5% to 6% of patients referred for the treatment of back and leg pain. It occurs after trauma, surgery, and infection, or from compression of one of the components of the sciatic nerve as it runs between two divisions of the piriformis muscle.[72] Patients with piriformis syndrome complain of buttock pain with or without radiation to the ipsilateral leg. The buttock pain usually extends from the sacrum to the greater trochanter of the femur whereas irritation of the sciatic nerve results in a buttock pain that radiates to the ipsilateral leg. Prolonged sitting, as in driving or biking, or getting up from a sitting position aggravates the pain. The pain is aggravated by hip flexion, adduction, and internal rotation. Neurologic examination is usually negative. There may be leg numbness when the sciatic nerve is irritated; the straight-leg test may be normal or limited. Three signs confirm the presence of piriformis syndrome[72]: (1) The *Pace sign* wherein there is pain and weakness on resisted abduction of the hip in a patient who is seated with the hip flexed; (2) the *Lasègue sign* wherein there is pain on flexion, adduction, and internal rotation of the hip in a patient who is supine (note that some clinicians call pain on straight-leg raise the Lasègue sign also); and (3) the *Freiberg sign* wherein there is pain on forced internal rotation of the extended thigh. Note that the piriformis is an internal rotator of the flexed hip and an external rotator of the extended hip. The diagnosis of piriformis syndrome is made on clinical grounds. Electromyography may detect myopathic and neuropathic changes including a delay in the H-reflex with the affected leg in a flexed, adducted, and internally rotated (FAIR) position as compared with the same H-reflex in the normal anatomic position.[73] The CT scan of the soft tissues of the pelvis may show an enlarged piriformis muscle, or abnormal uptake by the muscle, and the MRI confirms an enlarged piriformis muscle.

The treatments of piriformis syndrome include physical therapy combined with medications including muscle relaxants, anti-inflammatory drugs, and analgesics to reduce the spasm, inflammation, and pain. Local anesthetic and steroid injections into the piriformis muscle may break the pain/muscle spasm cycle. Although blind injections can be done, more specific techniques involve identification of the piriformis muscle with muscle electromyography, CT guidance, use of a nerve stimulator, or combined fluoroscopy–nerve stimulator guidance.[72] If relief from the local anesthetic does not last, then the piriformis muscle is injected with 100 units of botulinum toxin A in 2 to 3 mL of local anesthetic. The reported complications of botulinum toxin injection include brachial plexopathy, polyradiculoneuritis, and local psoriasiform dermatitis, so precautions should be followed to assure injection of the botulinum toxin into the belly of the piriformis muscle.

Myofascial Pain Syndrome and Fibromyalgia

Myofascial pain syndrome is a painful regional syndrome characterized by the presence of an active trigger point in a skeletal

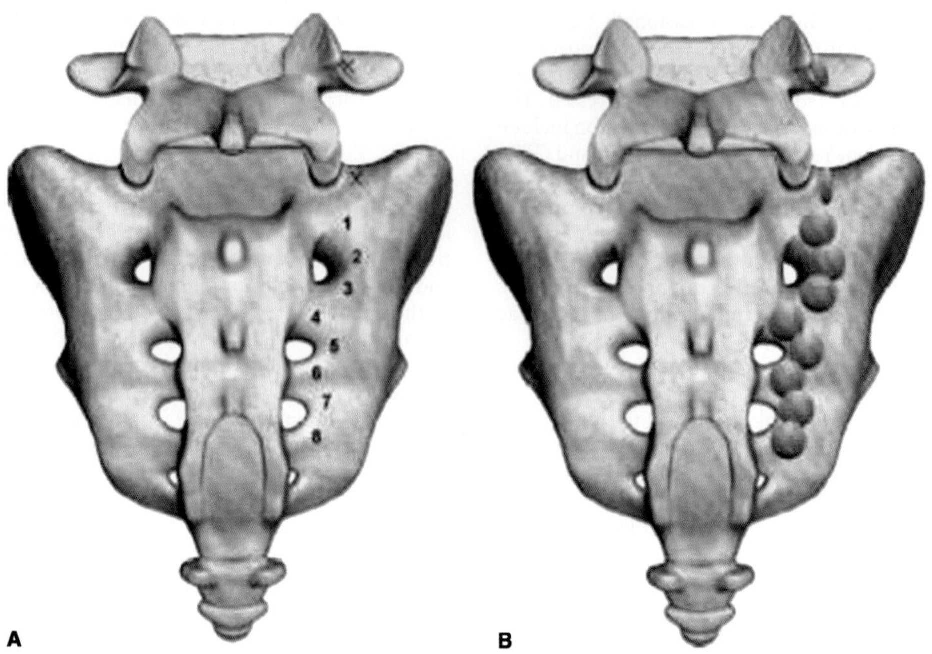

FIGURE 57-6. Target points **(A)** and expected lesions **(B)** from water-cooled radiofrequency denervation at the right L5 medial branch and the S1, S2, and S3 lateral branches (From: Cohen SP, Hurley RW, Buckenmaier CC 3rd, et al. Randomized placebo-controlled study evaluating lateral branch radiofrequency denervation for sacroiliac joint pain. *Anesthesiology.* 2008;109:279–288, with permission.)

muscle. The trigger point can be felt as a palpable taut band and manipulation of the trigger point by digital pressure or by penetration by a needle may induce a twitch response. There is spot tenderness in the taut band, pressure on the tender nodule induces pain that the patient recognizes as an experienced pain pattern, and there may be painful limitation to full passive range of motion of the affected muscle. There is usually an electromyographic demonstration of spontaneous electrical activity characteristic of active loci in the tender nodule of a taut band.

The management of myofascial pain syndrome includes repeated applications of a cold spray over the trigger point in line with the involved muscle fibers, followed by gentle massage of the trigger point and stretching of the affected muscle. Another treatment is local anesthetic injection or dry needling of the trigger point. Trigger point injections may be done under ultrasound but the benefits of this technique have not been proven. Recent studies show that dry needling may be as effective as local anesthetic injection; however, the local anesthetic makes the procedure less painful. Several injections at 1- to 3-week intervals, followed by physical therapy, may result in a long-term benefit. Botulinum toxin injections have been recommended but the results of clinical studies have not been uniform.[74,75] Physical therapy includes improving posture, body mechanics, relaxation techniques, trigger point massage, post-isometric relaxation, and reciprocal inhibition.

Fibromyalgia

The American College of Rheumatology criteria for classification of fibromyalgia,[76] established in 1990, requires two components: A history of widespread pain for at least 3 months and allodynia to digital pressure at 11 or more of 18 anatomically defined tender points. The tender points are located in the occiput, the intertransverse spaces between C5 and C7, trapezii, supraspinatus, the second rib, just lateral to the costochondral junctions, lateral epicondyles, glutei, greater trochanters, and knees. Others employ a whole body pain diagram to indicate areas of pain and obviate the need for tender points.[77] Finally, some clinicians do not require tender points and expand the definition of fibromyalgia to include symptoms of fatigue, sleep disturbance, and cognitive dysfunction.[78]

There is a strong genetic and familial component to the development of fibromyalgia. Also, family members of fibromyalgia patients are also more likely to have irritable bowel syndrome, temporomandibular disorders, headaches, and a host of other regional pain syndromes. They have higher concentrations of substance P and glutamate in CSF compared with normal controls.[79,80]

The opioidergic activity is normal or increased in fibromyalgia, and levels of cerebrospinal fluid enkephalins are roughly twice as high in these patients compared to healthy controls.[81] The increased activity of endogenous opioidergic systems explains the anecdotal experience of clinicians that opioids are ineffective in this syndrome. On the other hand, the principal metabolite of norepinephrine, 3-methoxy-4-hydroxyphenethylene glycol (MPHG), is lower in the CSF of patients with fibromyalgia.[82] This may explain the efficacy of drugs that raises both serotonin and norepinephrine (tricyclic antidepressants, duloxetine, milnacipran, tramadol).

The optimal treatment of fibromyalgia supports a multifaceted program comprising pharmacologic therapy and nonpharmacologic therapy (education, exercise, and cognitive behavioral therapy). Efficacious medications for treatment of fibromyalgia include the two SNRIs, duloxetine and milnacipran.[83,84] Pregabalin, amitriptyline, gabapentin, and gamma-hydroxybutyrate (sodium oxybate) are also effective.[85,86] Exercise programs, specifically low-intensity low-impact programs, appear to be beneficial. Cognitive-behavioral therapy and operant-behavioral therapy also appear to be helpful in these patients.

NEUROPATHIC PAIN SYNDROMES

Herpes Zoster and Postherpetic Neuralgia

Some patients with acute herpes zoster have a prodrome of dermatomal pain before the skin eruptions. The pain of acute herpes zoster is usually moderate in severity and can be managed with analgesics, and the pain usually subsides with healing of the rash. Ten percent to 15% of the patients develop postherpetic neuralgia (PHN), or pain that persists >3 months after resolution of the rash; the incidence rises to 30% to 50% in the elderly. The risk factors for the development of PHN include increased pain during the acute stage, greater severity of the skin lesion, older age, and the presence of a prodrome. The use of antiviral drugs acyclovir, famciclovir, or valacyclovir has been shown to hasten the healing of the rash, reduce the duration of viral shedding, and decrease the increase of PHN.

Most of the studies on the efficacy of neuraxial and peripheral nerve blocks, performed during the acute stage of herpes zoster were either retrospective or case series. Prospective, randomized, and controlled studies provide conflicting results. A study in which epidural methylprednisolone and bupivacaine was compared with acyclovir and prednisolone showed the epidural steroid group to have less pain (1.6% vs. 22%) and less allodynia (4% vs. 12%) at 1 year.[87] Another study in which standard therapy with oral antiviral medications and analgesics was compared with standard therapy and epidural methylprednisolone and bupivacaine noted less pain in the epidural group (48% vs. 58%) at 1 month but not at 3 months (21% vs. 28%).[88] The difference between the two studies is that only one epidural injection was performed in the study that showed no long-term beneficial effect of epidural steroid compared with two to four injections in the study that showed benefit with ESIs. To be effective in preventing PHN, the blocks are preferably done within 2 to 4 weeks of the onset of rash.

3 The mainstay of treatment for PHN is pharmacologic management that includes anticonvulsants, opioids, and antidepressants. Although the antidepressants have been found to be effective, their use is precluded by the frequent occurrence of side effects. The side effects include anticholinergic effects such as tachycardia,
4 dry mouth, constipation, and prostatism in the elderly. Nortriptyline is preferred over amitriptyline because it is equally effective and better tolerated. Studies showed opioids and tramadol to be efficacious.[89–91]

The anticonvulsants gabapentin and pregabalin are usually effective in the management of PHN.[92–94] The side effects of the drugs include somnolence, dizziness, and peripheral edema. Two studies showed that the combination of gabapentin and controlled-release morphine, and gabapentin and nortriptyline, were more effective and at lower daily dosages than either drug given alone.[95,96] Based on efficacy, antidepressants are the first choice for neuropathic pain syndromes, followed by opioids, tramadol, and gabapentin/pregabalin.[97] If quality of life, side effects, pre-
5 vention of addiction, and regulatory issues are important considerations in addition to pain relief, then gabapentin/pregabalin are the first drugs of choice. These are followed by tramadol, opioids, and the tricyclic antidepressants.[97] For the allodynia that accompanies the PHN, lidocaine patch is recommended.

Interventional techniques may be performed if medications do not control the pain of PHN. Intrathecal methylprednisolone, 60 mg in lidocaine, given once a week for 4 times, was noted to be more effective in relieving PHN compared with intrathecal lidocaine or no treatment.[98] The cerebrospinal fluid levels of interleukin-8, a marker of inflammation, decreased by >50% in the intrathecal methylprednisolone group and this correlated with the duration of global pain relief. It should be noted that epidural methylprednisolone is not as beneficial as intrathecal administration.[99] Other interventional techniques for PHN are spinal cord stimulation (SCS) and intrathecal alcohol. When a spinal cord stimulator was placed in 28 patients with intractable PHN for 2 years, long-term pain relief was achieved in 23 patients and the median pain score decreased from 9 to 1.[100] The improvements were confirmed by inactivation, followed by activation of the spinal cord stimulator at quarterly intervals. In resistant cases or when the patient cannot tolerate the medications, pain may be relieved by alcohol neurolysis of the spinal thoracic dermatomes affected by the herpes zoster.[101]

Diabetic Painful Neuropathy

Peripheral neuropathy may be present in approximately 65% of patients with insulin-dependent diabetes, most commonly distal symmetric polyneuropathy, followed by median nerve mononeuropathy at the wrist, and visceral autonomic neuropathy. The incidence of diabetic neuropathy increases with duration of diabetes, age, and degree of hyperglycemia; neuropathies generally develop after persistence of hyperglycemia for several years. The pathophysiology of diabetic neuropathy includes the polyol pathway, microvascular, and glycosylation end-product theories.[102] All pathways result in chronic ischemia of the nerve.

The management of diabetic painful neuropathy (DPN) includes tight control of the patient's blood glucose and pharmacologic therapy. The anticonvulsants gabapentin and pregabalin appear to be effective in the management of DPN, with the efficacy of gabapentin enhanced by the addition of controlled-release morphine or nortriptyline.[95,96] The tricyclic antidepressants are also effective in DPN whereas the selective serotonin reuptake inhibitors are not as effective. The antidepressant duloxetine appears to be effective[103] and, together with its favorable side effect profile compared with the tricyclics, is now widely used in treatment of DPN. The European Federation of Neurological Sciences Task Force and the International Association for the Study of Pain Neuropathic Pain Special Interest group (NeuP-SIG) now recommend the serotonin–norepinephrine reuptake inhibitors (duloxetine, milnacipran) as the first-choice drugs for the treatment of DPN.[104,105] Finally, the opioids and tramadol are also effective in the treatment of DPN.

Complex Regional Pain Syndrome

Complex regional pain syndrome (CRPS) consists of two types. *CRPS type I* was originally termed *reflex sympathetic dystrophy*, whereas *CRPS type II* represents causalgia. The risk factors for the development of CRPS include previous trauma, nerve injury (for causalgia), previous surgery, work-related injuries, and female sex. The signs and symptoms of CRPS include spontaneous pain, hyperalgesia, allodynia, plus trophic, sudomotor, vasomotor abnormalities, and finally, active and passive movement disorders. There may be a discrepancy between the severity of the symptoms and intensity of the inciting injury. The clinical features of CRPS type II are the same as in CRPS type I except there is a preceding nerve injury in CRPS II. The International Association for the Study of Pain (IASP) has proposed standardized diagnostic consensus-based criteria for CRPS. Studies on the validity of the IASP criteria suggest that patients should have (1) at least one symptom in each of the following general categories: Sensory (hyperesthesia-increased sensitivity to a sensory stimulation), vasomotor (temperature abnormalities or skin color changes), sudomotor–fluid balance (sweating abnormalities or edema), or motor (decreased range of movement, weakness, tremor, or neglect); and (2) at least one sign within two or more of the following categories: Sensory (allodynia or hyperalgesia), vasomotor (objective temperature abnormalities or skin color changes), sudomotor–fluid balance (sweating abnormalities or objective edema), or motor (objective decreased range of motion, weakness, tremor or neglect).

The treatments for CRPS include sympathetic blocks, physical therapy, and oral medications. Pharmacologic therapy for CRPS includes gabapentin,[106] memantine (an NMDA blocker), and ketamine infusion. Ketamine can either be given as a 4- to 5-day infusion at 1 to 7 μg/kg/min (5 to 30 mg/hr in a 70-kg patient)[107] or for 4 hours daily for 10 days at an infusion rate of 0.35 mg/kg/hr
6 (24 mg/hr in a 70-kg person).[108] SCS can be entertained if the patient does not respond to these treatments.[109]

Human Immunodeficiency Virus Neuropathy

Symptomatic neuropathy occurs in 10% to 35% of patients who are seropositive for human immunodeficiency virus (HIV), and pathologic abnormalities exist in almost all patients with end-stage AIDS. The sensory neuropathies associated with HIV include distal sensory polyneuropathy, the more common neuropathy related to the viral infection, and antiretroviral toxic neuropathy (ATN) secondary to the treatment. The clinical features of HIV sensory neuropathy typically include painful allodynia and hyperalgesia. The onset is gradual and most commonly involves the lower extremities. The neuropathy and dysesthesia progress from the distal to the more proximal structures. There is minimal subjective or objective motor involvement and this is generally limited to the intrinsic muscles of the foot.

The treatment of HIV sensory neuropathy is symptomatic and includes optimization of the patient's metabolic and nutritional status. Cessation or dose reduction of treatment with nucleoside reverse transcriptase inhibitors may improve the symptoms of ATN. The anticonvulsants, particularly lamotrigine (300 mg/day), can be effective therapy for HIV sensory neuropathy as well as ATN.[110,111] Gabapentin is also effective at doses of 1,200 to 3,600 mg/day.[112]

Phantom Pain

Nearly all patients with amputated extremities experience nonpainful sensations in the absent, phantom limb. As many as 80% of them experience pain. The onset of pain may be immediate but commonly occurs within the first few days following amputation. Approximately 50% of patients experience a decrease of their pain with time, whereas the other 50% report no change or an increase in pain over time. Phantom pain is not felt all the time, only a few days in a month. Phantom pain is caused by both peripheral and central factors. Peripheral mechanisms include neuromas, an increase in C-fiber activity, and sodium channel activation. Central mechanisms include abnormal firing of spinal internuncial neurons and supraspinal involvement secondary to the development of new synaptic connections in the cerebral cortex.

Numerous prophylactic measures have been undertaken in an attempt to reduce the incidence of phantom limb pain, including perioperative epidural infusions of opioids and local anesthetics or clonidine, and continuous brachial plexus blockade with memantine. The treatment of phantom limb pain includes pharmacologic and nonpharmacologic measures. Pharmacologic treatments include the use of opioids; gabapentin, an NMDA antagonist; and the empirical use of antidepressants. The nonpharmacologic measures include transcutaneous electrical nerve stimulation, spinal cord stimulators, and biofeedback. A combination of pharmacologic treatment with physical, psychological, or behavioral intervention is probably most effective approach.[113]

CANCER PAIN

Significant pain is present in up to 25% of patients with cancer who are in active treatment and in up to 90% of patients with advanced cancer. The pain of cancer can be somatic, visceral, or neuropathic. The etiology and characteristics of these pain syndromes are different and they require different treatments. Somatic pain tends to be responsive to opioids, nonsteroidal anti-inflammatory drugs (NSAIDs), or cyclooxygenase 2 inhibitors, and is amenable to treatment with neural blockade. Visceral pain responds to sympathetic blocks, and neuropathic pain is responsive to anticonvulsants, opioids, tricyclic antidepressants, serotonin–norepinephrine reuptake inhibitors, or combinations of these drugs.

Management of cancer pain should be multifaceted and include the following: (1) Antineoplastic treatment, (2) pharmacologic management, (3) interventional management, (4) behavioral and psychological management, and ultimately (5) hospice care. Pharmacologic therapies include opioids, antidepressants, anticonvulsants, NSAIDs, corticosteroids, oral local anesthetics, and topical analgesics. Continuous intravenous opioid infusions can be infused during the later stages of life. Interventional treatments include neurolytic sympathetic blocks and intrathecal opioids; vertebroplasty or kyphoplasty is performed for vertebral compression syndromes.

Opioids are the mainstay of treatment for cancer pain as approximately 70% to 95% of patients are responsive positively when appropriate guidelines are followed. Neurolytic blocks and
7 intrathecal opioids should be considered when pharmacologic agents are not completely effective at maximum tolerated dosages.

Neurolytic Blocks for Visceral Pain from Cancer

Celiac Plexus Block

The celiac plexus innervates all of the abdominal viscera except the left side of the colon and the pelvic viscera. The plexus contains two large ganglia that receive sympathetic fibers from the greater, lesser, and least splanchnic nerves. It also receives parasympathetic fibers from the vagus nerve. The splanchnic nerves are located retroperitoneally at the level of the T12 and L1 vertebrae, and the celiac plexus are anterior to the crura of the diaphragm and surrounds the abdominal aorta and the celiac and superior mesenteric arteries.

Blockade of the celiac plexus can be achieved by the classic retrocrural approach, anterocrural approach, or by neurolysis of the splanchnic nerves.[114] For the procedure, the tip of the needle is directed toward the body of L1 (Fig. 57-7). In the retrocrural approach, the tip of the needle is advanced approximately 1 cm anterior to the anterior and upper border of L1. In anterocrural or transaortic approach, the tip of the needle is advanced through the lower portion of L1 and the aorta on the left side until blood can no longer be aspirated through the needle. For splanchnic nerve block, the tip of the needle is placed at the anterior portion of the

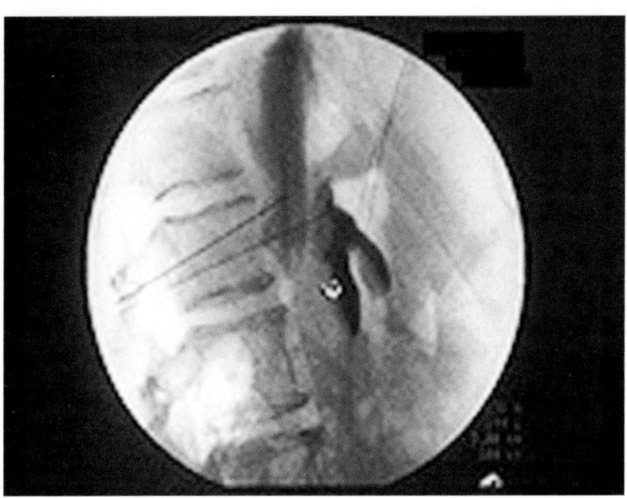

FIGURE 57-7. Retrocrural versus anterocrural approaches to neurolysis of the celiac plexus. Note that the tip of the needle is in the upper third of L1 and about 1 cm beyond the border of the vertebral body for the retrocrural technique; the spread of the contrast medium is cephalad. In contrast, the tip of the needle is the lower third of L1 and about 3 cm beyond the border of the vertebral body for the anterocrural technique; the spread of the contrast medium is caudad and in front of the aorta (*arrow*). (From: de Leon-Casasola OA. Neurolysis of the sympathetic axis for cancer pain management. In: Benzon HT, Rathmell J, Wu C, Turk DC, Argoff C, eds. *Raj's Practical management of Pain.* 4th ed. Philadelphia, PA: Mosby Elsevier; 2008; 918, with permission.)

T12 vertebral body. There appears to be no differences in efficacy between the three approaches.[114] Fluoroscopy is required in the performance of the procedure. CT allows visualization of the diaphragm and aorta, and is used in the transabdominal approach when patients cannot tolerate the prone position. Some clinicians perform an initial diagnostic block with a local anesthetic while others proceed immediately to a neurolytic block since the results of the diagnostic and neurolytic blocks may not be the same. Better results are usually seen with local anesthetics because of better spread (phenol is viscous) and its vascular absorption may relieve pain. Fifty percent alcohol or 6% to 10% phenol is employed for the neurolytic block. The dosages of the neurolytic agents are 30 to 40 mL for the retrocrural and anterocrural approach, and 10 to 15 mL on each side for splanchnic nerve blockade. Complications from the celiac plexus block include orthostatic hypotension, back pain, retroperitoneal hematoma, reactive pleurisy, hiccups, hematuria, transient diarrhea, abdominal aortic dissection, transient motor paralysis, and paraplegia. The paraplegia and transient motor paralysis may be due to spasm of the lumbar segmental arteries that perfuse the spinal cord, direct vascular or neurologic injury, or retrograde spread to the nerve roots or spinal cord.

The efficacy of celiac plexus neurolysis in relieving pain from cancer of the upper abdomen has been noted in randomized,
8 controlled trials.[114–116] The end points of the studies were lower pain scores, less opioid consumption with a lower incidence of side effects, and equal or better quality of life. Better results are achieved when there is better spread of the injectate. A meta-analysis of 21 retrospective studies in 1,145 patients concluded that adequate-to-excellent pain relief was achieved in 89% of the patients during the first 2 weeks following the block and partial-to-complete pain relief continued in 90% of the patients at the 3-month interval.[117]

Superior Hypogastric Plexus Block

Superior hypogastric plexus is indicated for pelvic pain secondary to cancer and chronic nonmalignant conditions. The plexus is located in the retroperitoneum, bilaterally extending from the lower third of the fifth lumbar vertebra to the upper third of the first sacral vertebra. For blockade of the plexus, the patient is placed in the prone position and two 7-cm needles are inserted, under fluoroscopy, in medial and caudal directions until the tips lay anterolateral to the L5 to S1 intervertebral disc space. Alternatively, a single needle can be used through a transdiscal approach. After injection of contrast medium, 6 to 8 mL of local anesthetic is used for a diagnostic block while phenol or alcohol is employed for neurolysis. The complications are minimal and include nerve root blockade secondary to retrograde spread of the injectate. Case reports support the efficacy of neurolytic superior hypogastric plexus block in reducing pelvic pain secondary to cancer and in decreasing opioid consumption.

Ganglion Impar Block

Pain in the perineal area associated with malignancies can be treated with neurolysis of the ganglion impar (Walther's ganglion). The ganglion impar is a solitary retroperitoneal structure located anteriorly to the sacrococcygeal junction. Visceral afferents innervating the perineum, distal rectum, anus, distal urethra, vulva, and distal third of vagina converge at the ganglion. For the procedure, the patient is usually prone and a 22-gauge spinal needle, bent 1 inch from its hub to form a 30-degree angle, is inserted under local anesthesia through the anococcygeal ligament and directed along the midline to reach the sacrococcygeal junction. In the transsacrococcygeal approach, a 20-gauge, 1.5-inch needle is inserted through the sacrococcygeal ligament until the tip of the needle is just anterior to the anterior portion of the sacrum. Four to 8 mL of local anesthetic is used for diagnostic block and 8% to 10% phenol or 50% alcohol is used for neurolysis. Similar to superior hypogastric plexus blocks, there are no controlled studies on its efficacy although case reports confirm its effectiveness in relieving perineal pain secondary to cancer.

PHARMACOLOGIC MANAGEMENT OF PAIN

Opioids

Morphine is the standard for opioid therapy for cancer pain (see Chapter 19). It has a variable oral bioavailability between 10% and 45%. The metabolites of morphine include morphine-6-glucuronide, which causes additional analgesia, and morphine-3-glucuronide, which can cause adverse effects (Table 57-4). Controlled-release preparations are available, reducing the need to take the drug frequently. The *numbers needed to treat* or NNT for 10 mg of morphine for postoperative pain is 2.9 and its *numbers needed to harm* or NNH is 9.1. Hydromorphone, a μ-receptor agonist, is 3 to 5 times more potent than morphine when given orally and 5 to 7 times more potent when given parenterally. Its 3- to 4-hour duration of analgesic effect is similar to that of morphine. Pruritus, sedation, nausea, and vomiting occur less frequently compared with morphine. Its metabolite, hydromorphone-3-glucoronide, lacks analgesic property but possesses properties similar to that of morphine-3-glucuronide.

Methadone has a 60% to 95% bioavailability, high potency, and a long duration of action. It has ideal characteristics that

TABLE 57-4. SELECTED OPIOIDS: ORAL BIOAVAILABILITY, HALF-LIVES, DURATION OF ACTION, AND METABOLITES

Opioid	Availability (%)	Half-Life (h)	Duration (h)	Metabolites
Morphine	10–45	2–3	4–5	M6G, M3G
Oxycodone SR (OxyContin, Purdue Pharma)	60–80	4.5	12	Oxymorphone Noroxycodone
Oxymorphone (Opana ER, Endo Pharmaceuticals)	10	9 ± 3	12	O3G 6-OH-oxymorphone
Hydromorphone	24	2.3	3–4	H3G
Methadone	60–95	8–80 (27)	6–8	

M6G, morphine-6-glucuronide; M3G, morphine-3-glucuronide; O3G, oxymorphone-3-glucuronide; H3G, hydromorphone-3-glucuronide.
From: Cortazzo MH, Fishman SM. Major opioids and chronic opioid therapy. In: Benzon HT, Rathmell JP, Wu CL, Turk DC, Argoff CE, eds. *Raj's Practical Management of Pain.* 4th ed. Philadelphia, PA: Mosby Elsevier; 2008;606, with permission.

include the lack of an active metabolite, additional salutary effects such as acting as an NMDA receptor antagonist and serotonin reuptake inhibitor, and it is inexpensive. Its potency compared with morphine ranges from 1:1 to 1:4 on acute dosing but can be as low as 1:10 with chronic dosing. It has a long and unpredictable half-life of 8 to 80 hours that makes it difficult to achieve steady-state plasma concentrations, increasing the risk of accumulation and the need for careful and individualized dosing. In the United States, there has been an "epidemic" of deaths due to unintentional overdose from methadone when used to treat chronic pain.[118] Many physicians, and most patients, do not appreciate the consequences of the drug's long and unpredictable half-life. Methadone also causes cardiac rhythm abnormalities including QT prolongation and Torsade de pointes. Most reports are based on high-dose maintenance (>120 mg) for the treatment of addiction; however, such occurrences have also been reported with lower dosages. Experts recommend disclosure of the dysrythmogenic property of the drug (especially for patients with cardiac disease), a screening ECG before initiation of therapy, follow-up ECGs in patients who are taking over 100 mg daily, and risk stratification.[119] The risk should be discussed when the QTc interval is 450 to 500 ms and the methadone dose reduced or discontinued when the interval is greater than 500 ms.[119]

Oxycodone is mainly a prodrug, being active after conversion by the enzyme cytochrome P450 2D6 to oxymorphone (a μ-opioid agonist). Noroxycodone is its inactive metabolite. It has a high bioavailability (60%) and is associated with a low incidence of itching and hallucinations. It has an NNT of 2.5 in neuropathic pain; the oxycodone-to-morphine ratio is 1:1.5. The controlled-release preparation (OxyContin) has good analgesic characteristics but has become a popular drug for abuse. Addicts crush the preparation and inhale the powder or inject a solution of the drug into their veins. Oxymorphone has greater affinity to the μ-receptor than morphine and has little or no affinity to the κ-opioid receptor. It is 10 times more potent than morphine when given intravenously. It has low histamine release, similar to fentanyl. Due to extensive first-pass hepatic metabolism, the bioavailability of oxymorphone is only 10%. However, its greater lipid solubility explains its rapid onset of analgesia. It should not be taken with alcohol since this increases its plasma concentration by as much as 300%. The efficacy of oxymorphone in chronic and cancer pain is similar to other opioids.[120] Buprenorphine is a partial agonist at the μ-receptor, a κ-antagonist, and a weak δ-agonist. It has a rapid onset (30 minutes) when given orally and a long duration of action of 6 to 9 hours. There have been increased reports of abuse of the drug.

The weak opioids include codeine, hydrocodone, propoxyphene, and tramadol. Codeine is transformed to morphine via the enzyme cytochrome P450 2D6, and has an NNT of 16.7. Genetic factors can affect the behavior of these drugs. Approximately 9% of white people do not have the enzyme and do not experience analgesia from codeine.[121] Asians have a lower rate of codeine O- demethylation resulting in less morphine formation. Children <12 years of age lack maturity of the enzyme and cannot convert the drug to morphine, experiencing the drug's side effects with minimal analgesia.[122] Hydrocodone reaches peak serum concentrations within 1 to 2 hours and has a half-life of 2.5 to 4 hours. An additive effect is noted when ibuprofen is combined with hydrocodone. The d-isomer of propoxyphene, dextropropoxyphene, a noncompetitive NMDA antagonist, has been withdrawn from the market because of serious side effects.

Tramadol is an opioid agonist and a monoaminergic drug. It has a bioavailability of 80% to 90%, has a low abuse potential, low incidence of constipation, and a minimal risk of fatal respiratory depression that is possibly limited to patients with severe renal failure. It has a dose-dependent efficacy with NNTs of 8.5 for 50 mg, 5.3 for 75 mg, 4.8 for 100 mg, and 2.9 for 150 mg. The maximum dose of tramadol is 400 to 500 mg/day.

The oral equianalgesic doses of morphine 10 mg intravenously or 30 mg orally are (1) 200 mg of codeine, (2) 30 mg of hydrocodone, (3) 20 to 30 mg of oxycodone, (4) 130 mg of propoxyphene, and (5) 120 mg of tramadol. Opioid rotation or substitution, wherein one opioid is changed with another to improve analgesia and decrease side effects, implies knowledge of the equianalgesic dosages of the different opioids.

There is public concern regarding the effect of opioids on driving performance. It appears that cancer patients receiving chronic, stable doses of morphine, up to 290 mg, have minimal or no impairment of their driving abilities.[123] Patients receiving stable doses of transdermal fentanyl over 2 weeks show no significant psychomotor impairment when compared with volunteers.[124] Patients who have their opioid dose increased by >30% over a period of 2 days show worsening of their cognitive performance.[125] Patients receiving stable dose of opioids can probably drive, whereas those who are starting to take opioids and those who had a recent increase in their dose should be warned about the hazards of driving.

Opioids are used mostly for cancer pain, with long-acting opioids supplemented by short-acting ones for breakthrough pain.[126] Opioid monotherapy in cancer pain is rarely successful and adjuvants are usually added for increased efficacy. The use of opioids for treatment of neuropathic pain has been controversial but recent studies show them to be effective, although at higher doses.[89–91] Because of the undesirable issues associated with the use of opioids such as addiction, aberrant behaviors, and regulatory issues,[118] opioids are often a second-line drug for neuropathic pain. The combination of a gabapentin and an opioid has been shown to result in better analgesia, fewer side effects, and lower doses of each drug.[95] For low back pain, it should be noted that while individual studies show the efficacy of opioids in low back pain, a meta-analysis did not show reduced pain when compared with a placebo or a nonopioid control group.[127] Opioids may be efficacious for the short-term relief of acute low back pain, in addition to NSAIDs and muscle relaxants, but the long-term efficacy of opioids (≥16 weeks) is unclear.[127,128] When treating fibromyalgia, only tramadol or a tramadol/acetaminophen combination has been shown to be more effective than placebo. Opioids are usually not effective in pain secondary to spinal cord injury, although intravenous alfentanil has been shown to be better than placebo.

Antidepressants

Tricyclic antidepressants (TCAs) have several mechanisms for their analgesic effects. These include a serotonergic effect (interference with serotonin reuptake and alteration of serotonin binding to receptors in neural tissue), a noradrenergic effect (interaction with α-receptors), an opioidergic effect, blockade of the NMDA receptor complex, inhibition of the uptake of adenosine, and blockade of sodium and calcium channels. TCAs also have an anti-inflammatory effect in animal models of pain. The NNTs of antidepressants are comparable with those of opioids and anticonvulsants. Antidepressants also inhibit the histaminic, cholinergic, muscarinic, and nicotinic receptors resulting in sedation, dry mouth, and urinary retention. TCAs, specifically amitriptyline and nortriptyline, have been shown to be effective in PHN.[102] As stated in "Neuropathic Pain Syndromes," nortriptyline and amitriptyline are both effective in PHN, with nortriptyline having fewer side effects. For DPN, amitriptyline and desipramine appear to be equally effective.[129]

Serotonin and norepinephrine receptor inhibitors (SNRIs) block the reuptake of serotonin and norepinephrine, with duloxetine having increased selectivity for serotonin. Venlafaxine has more serotonergic effects at lower doses but with greater noradrenergic activity at higher dosages. Duloxetine and milnacipran have preferential noradrenergic effect, have longer half-lives (12 and 8 hours respectively), and have no active metabolites. In addition to their antidepressant action, the SNRIs have an antinociceptive effect.[130,131] Duloxetine is effective in DPN and fibromyalgia and has a good safety profile for long-term use.[132,133] Patients with fibromyalgia have been shown improvements in fatigue, physical conditioning, and discomfort after milnacipran[134,135] The efficacy of the SNRIs in DPN and fibromyalgia, coupled with the better side effect profile (free of cholinergic, histaminic, and α-adrenergic receptor effects, and less potential for drug interactions) in comparison to the TCAs are probably the reasons for their increased preferential usage.[130] As stated, the European Federation of Neurological Sciences Task Force and the International Association for the Study of Pain Neuropathic Pain Special Interest group (NeuP-SIG) now recommend the SNRIs as the first-choice drugs for the treatment of DPN.[104,105]

TABLE 57-5. DOSAGES (mg/day) OF THE COMMONLY USED ANTIDEPRESSANTS AND ANTICONVULSANTS[a]

Antidepressants	Anticonvulsants
Amitriptyline: 10–300	Gabapentin: 900–3,600, tid
Doxepin: 30–300	Lamotrigine: 50–150
Nortriptyline: 50–150	Mexiletine: 300–1,350, tid
Desipramine: 25–300	Oxcarbazepine: 300–900, bid
Fluoxetine: 5–40	Pregabalin: 150–600, bid
Paroxetine: 20–40	Topiramate; 50–200, bid
Venlaflaxine: 37.5– 300	
Duloxetine: 60–120	
od or bid	
Milnacipran: 100–200 mg, 50–100 mg bid	

tid, three times a day; bid, twice a day; od, once daily.
[a]Unless indicated, dosing is once a day. Start with smallest possible dose and titrate to efficacy or side effects.

TCAs have an NNT of 2.1 to 2.8 for treatment of PHN, 1.3 to 3.4 for DPN, and 1.7 for central pain. The overall NNT for SNRIs is 15.3, and 5 for paroxetine. The side effects of antidepressants include cholinergic effects such as dry mouth, sedation, and urinary retention. Accidental or intentional overdose can lead to fatal dysrhythmias. Venlafaxine may cause hypertension, mania, and may exacerbate seizures. A gradual withdrawal recommended for duloxetine to prevent agitation, anxiety, confusion, and hypomania. TCAs are more likely to cause weight gain compared with SNRIs. TCAs impair driving ability during the first week of treatment or during dose escalation, but shortly thereafter driving performance returns to baseline.[136] No impairment of driving ability apparently occurs with SNRIs. Other sedating medications should not be prescribed when TCAs are used. The NNHs are 5 to 11 for TCAs and 21 to 24 for SNRIs, showing the better tolerability of the serotonin reuptake inhibitors. Recommended doses for the commonly used antidepressants are shown in Table 57-5.

Anticonvulsants

Neuropathic pain is associated with changes in sodium and calcium channel subunit expression resulting in functional changes. In chronic nerve injury, there is redistribution and alteration of subunit compositions of sodium and calcium channels resulting in spontaneous firing at ectopic sites along the sensory pathway. Sodium channel blockers inhibit spontaneous activities at neuromas, DRG, and at the dorsal horn of the spinal cord. Anticonvulsants block sodium channels, explaining their efficacy in neuropathic pain syndromes. Other anticonvulsants act on ion channel systems, including $GABA_A$ receptor agonists (topiramate and felbamate), $GABA_A$ transaminase blockers (vigabatrin), $GABA_A$

transport blockers (tiagabine), and glutamate receptor antagonists (felbamate and topiramate). The other drugs directly block calcium channels (lamotrigine), T-type calcium channels (topiramate and zonisamide) and α_2-delta subunits (gabapentin and pregabalin).

As noted in the section on "Neuropathic Pain Syndromes," randomized controlled studies demonstrate the efficacy of the anticonvulsants in several neuropathic pain syndromes including trigeminal neuralgia, PHN, DPN, HIV polyneuropathy, phantom limb pain, spinal cord injury pain, and central poststroke pain.

Gabapentin is an effective drug in neuropathic pain (PHN, DPN, and spinal cord injury [SCI]), has few side effects, and lacks drug–drug interactions. Its median effective dose is 900 to 1,800 mg/day. Pregabalin shares the same mode of action as gabapentin but with an improved linear pharmacokinetic profile. It has been shown to be effective in PHN, DPN, and spinal cord injury pain. The maximum dose of pregabalin is 600 mg/day in patients with creatinine clearance >60 mL/min or 300 mg in patients with clearance of 30 to 60 mL/min. The popularity of gabapentin and pregabalin relates to the lack of drug interactions and their perceived speed of onset.[137]

Lamotrigine has been shown to be effective in HIV polyneuropathy, pain from spinal cord injury, and central poststroke pain.[110,111] The most common side effect is rash and its use is limited by the risk of Stevens–Johnson syndrome. Topiramate is effective in migraine prophylaxis, similar to divalproex. Oxcarbazepine is similar in chemical structure to carbamazepine and noted to be effective in trigeminal neuralgia with few side effects[138]; its analgesic effect is fast and pain relief may be noted within 24 to 48 hours. The recommended doses of the commonly used anticonvulsants are in Table 57-5.

The side effects of anticonvulsants include dizziness, fatigue, somnolence, weight gain, peripheral edema (gabapentin and pregabalin); rash (lamotrigine); paresthesia, cognitive effects, weight loss (topiramate); hyponatremia; and low thyroid concentrations (oxcarbazepine).

Lidocaine Patch, Capsaicin Patch, Mexiletine, and Intravenous Lidocaine

The lidocaine patch 5% (Lidoderm, Endo Pharmaceuticals, Inc., Chadds Ford, PA) delivers lidocaine locally at the site of neuropathic pain generation, limiting its systemic effects and reducing its interactions with other concomitantly administered medications; analgesia is by local sodium channel blockade and not by its systemic effects. The patch contains 700 mg of lidocaine inside an adhesive. It is recommended that a maximum of three patches be applied for a maximum of 12 hr/day. Most patients experience pain relief within a few days of application. The occurrence of a delayed response in some patients led to the recommendation that there be a 2-week trial period.[139] Some patients continue to experience relief between patch applications while others have pain when the patch is removed; clinicians recommend using the patch for 16 to 18 hours in these patients. The absorption of lidocaine is limited; only about 3% of the total dose applied is absorbed systemically.[140] The maximum plasma lidocaine concentration is usually achieved on the second day of 12 hr/day of patch application and is significantly lower than concentrations that are cardiotoxic. Clinical experience with the lidocaine patch has shown that it can be used effectively for patients with PHN[139,141] as well as patients with myofascial pain, low back pain, osteoarthritis, and diabetic and nondiabetic polyneuropathy. However, few good research studies exist to verify the efficacy of the patch in these pain syndromes.

Capsaicin has been shown to defunctionalize TRPV1 nerve endings and reduce epidermal nerve fiber density.[142,143] Capsaicin cream (0.25%, 0.075%) requires multiple daily applications for several weeks. It causes burning sensation and results only in modest relief. The newer, higher-concentration capsaicin 8% patch (Qutenza) has been shown to be better than placebo and better than low-concentration (0.04%) capsaicin. It appears to be effective in PHN, DPN, and HIV neuropathy.[144–146] Its NNT, 30% relief, is 12 (6.4 to 70). Because of burning sensation during its placement, local anesthetic cream applied 60 minutes before the patch is applied for 60 to 90 minutes. The 60-minute application is better tolerated and is similar in efficacy. There is an increase in pain 20 to 30 minutes after application which disappears 2 to 3 hours after removal of the patch. Relief can be up to 12 weeks after one application. A maximum of 4 doses can be given at intervals of 12 weeks.[147]

Mexiletine is oral lidocaine. Its efficacy is similar to that of intravenous lidocaine, although a favorable response to intravenous lidocaine does not necessarily mean a similar response to mexiletine. The median recommended dose of mexiletine is 600 mg/per day. Intravenous lidocaine infusions are sometimes used for resistant neuropathic pain syndromes. The median recommended dose of intravenous lidocaine infusions is 5 mg/kg given over 30 minutes. A meta-analysis has shown intravenous lidocaine to be superior to placebo and equal to morphine, gabapentin, and amitriptyline for neuropathic pain.[148] The beneficial effect was noted to be more consistent in patients with peripheral pain secondary to trauma and diabetes and central pain.

Based on original studies, review articles, and meta-analysis publications, the recommended drugs for several different chronic pain syndromes are listed in Table 57-6.

TABLE 57-6. RECOMMENDED DRUGS FOR CHRONIC PAIN SYNDROMES

Postherpetic Neuralgia	Diabetic Painful Neuropathy	Spinal Cord Injury	Fibromyalgia	Human Immunodeficiency Virus
Pregabalin	Duloxetine	Pregabalin	Duloxetine	Lamotrigine
Gabapentin	Pregabalin	Gabapentin	Pregabalin	Gabapentin
Opioid	Gabapentin	Lamotrigine	Milnacipran	
Antidepressants	Antidepressants	IV lidocaine	Tramadol	
Tramadol		Mexilitine (±)		
Lidoderm patch (allodynia)				

INTERVENTIONAL TECHNIQUES

Discography

The symptoms of discogenic pain are nonspecific and include nonradicular back pain that is worse in the standing and sitting positions. The neurologic examination is usually normal including the straight-leg raise. The MRI may show a high-intensity zone on the T2 sagittal images, indicating an annular tear. Treatments include stabilization, exercise training, back education, activity modification, and ESIs.

The American Society of Interventional Pain Physicians has recommended guidelines on when to perform discography.[149] Some of the indications include (1) evaluation of abnormal discs to assess the extent of abnormality or correlation of the abnormality with clinical symptoms, (2) assessment of patients with persistent severe symptoms in whom diagnostic tests have failed to reveal which suspected disc is the source of pain, (3) assessment of discs before fusion to determine which discs within the proposed fusion segment are symptomatic, and (4) confirmation of a contained disc herniation or investigation of contrast distribution pattern before intradiscal procedures. The procedure can be performed on an outpatient basis with fluoroscopic guidance, under light sedation. Antibiotic prophylaxis is recommended and may be administered either intradiscally or intravenously. The specifics of the technique are discussed in textbooks or atlases of pain medicine. Nonionic contrast is injected into the disc, preferably with a controlled injection system with pressure readout. The patient is asked to rate his or her pain on a 0 to 10 scale before and during injection, and whether the pain is *concordant,* that is, similar to the pain for which the patient is being seen.[150] The suggested end points for injection include (1) pain severity of 5/10 or greater that lasts at least 30 seconds, (2) intradiscal pressure of 80 to 100 psi, or (3) a total of 3.5 mL of contrast medium has been injected. Anteroposterior and lateral images are taken to record the distribution of contrast medium and whether the contrast leaked outside the disc through a fissure in the annulus fibrosis. After recovery, the patient is sent for postdiscography CT scan, preferably within 4 hours of the discography.

Discitis is the most feared complication of discography. The incidence of discitis without prophylactic antibiotics is approximately 0.25% and is considerably decreased with prophylactic antibiotic use.[151] The diagnosis of discitis includes worsening back pain the week after discography, and elevated erythrocyte sedimentation rate and C-reactive protein that usually peaks 53 weeks after the procedure. The most common causative organism in discitis is *Staphylococcus aureus.* The possibility of disc injury after discography, resulting in disc degeneration and/or herniation from such procedures[152] may have decreased the frequency with which the procedure is performed.

Intradiscal Electrothermal Therapy

Intradiscal electrothermal therapy (IDET) is a procedure wherein a thermal resistance catheter is placed percutaneously in the posterolateral portion of the disc. Heat causes the collagen of the annulus fibrosis to contract. The intervertebral disc is avascular so that the heat does not travel as easily or dissipate quickly. IDET is performed with a technique similar to discography. The flexible electrode is advanced, contralateral to the lesion, through the introducer until it assumes a circumferential position either between the nucleus pulposus and the annulus fibrosis, or within the annulus fibrosis. The electrode is gradually heated to 90°C, if tolerated, and maintained for 4 minutes. If the patient cannot tolerate 90°C, heating is performed at 85° or 80°C for 5 minutes. The patient rests for 1 to 3 days after the procedure, limits sitting or walking, and wears a corset for 6 to 8 weeks. A gradual increase in activity is encouraged, after which the patient is involved in a physical therapy program. The complications of IDET include catheter kinking or breakage, nerve root injury, nondermatomal leg pain, dural puncture, infection, bleeding, cauda equina syndrome, and spinal cord damage.

The efficacy of IDET has been shown in a meta-analysis[153] and in a randomized study that showed improvements in outcome measures such as pain, physical function, and disability.[154] A review comparing IDET and surgical fusion in patients with intractable discogenic low back pain showed similar improvements in both groups.[155] IDET is now rarely performed since the insurance companies limit payment to patients who fulfill the criteria set in the study by Pauza et al.[154]

Percutaneous Disc Decompression (Nucleoplasty)

Percutaneous disc decompression, a procedure utilized for contained herniated disc, involves removal or coagulation of a portion of the nucleus pulposus.[156] It has been postulated that reducing the intradiscal volume results in a disproportionately higher drop in pressure. Discography may be performed prior to nucleoplasty to help decide which disc is involved. In contrast to IDET, the temperature created by nucleoplasty is in the 40° to 70°C range.

The patient preparation, antibiotic prophylaxis, monitoring, and positioning are similar to discography and IDET. An electrode is passed through the introducer needle and advanced to the interface between the annulus and the nucleus pulposus. Tissue ablation and coagulation are performed with each pass. Six channels ("passes") are usually made through the nucleus, vaporizing a total of 1 cm^3 of intradiscal volume and causing a significant drop in intradiscal pressure. Postoperatively, the patient's activity is restricted. The complications are similar to those with discography and IDET. Complications that are specific to nucleoplasty include probe tip fracture when it is forced against an endplate. The efficacy of nucleoplasty is not well documented.

Minimally Invasive Lumbar Decompression (MILD) Procedure

Spinal stenosis is narrowing of the spinal canal with compression of the nerve roots as demonstrated with an MRI or CT scan. Such canal narrowing can be secondary to hypertrophy of the ligamentum flavum or the facet joint. Low back pain from spinal stenosis is located in the low back area, buttocks, thighs, and/or legs in combination with neurogenic claudication especially with erect posture (due to smaller spinal canal diameter in this position) or walking.[157,158] The MILD procedure is a minimally invasive method of spinal decompression. It is indicated in patients with low back pain and neurogenic claudication associated with MRI or CT evidence of central canal stenosis secondary to facet hypertrophy in the lumbar segments.[159] The procedure involves limited percutaneous laminotomy and thinning of the ligamentum flavum to increase the critical diameter of the stenosed spinal canal. It can be performed under local anesthesia. A one, or more usually, a two-level decompression is performed. In contrast to surgical decompression surgery with fusion wherein there is complete resection of the ligamentum flavum and bony posterior elements compressing the thecal sac and exiting nerve roots, the MILD procedure only partially debulks the ligamentum flavum. In spite of this, initial reports are promising.[160,161]

Vertebroplasty and Kyphoplasty

Vertebroplasty and kyphoplasty are percutaneous interventional modalities to treat vertebral compression fractures (VCFs), a condition usually secondary to osteoporosis in elderly patients. Patients with symptomatic VCFs have decreased vertebral body height, kyphosis, and decreased mobility that may result in atelectasis, pneumonia, and deep venous thrombosis. Most VCFs are asymptomatic although pain may be experienced with bending, lifting, prolonged sitting or standing, or when the patient attempts to stand from a seated position. The pain is usually a deep back pain and there may be intercostal neuralgic symptoms or radiculitis and paravertebral muscle spasm. Pain is relieved by bed rest and the recumbent position. Radiography shows osteopenia or decreased bone mass; MRI is the imaging modality of choice.

Vertebroplasty involves the injection of polymethylmethacrylate (PMMA) into the affected vertebral body; kyphoplasty involves the insertion of a balloon prior to the injection of the cement. These procedures lead to restoration of some of the decreased vertebral height, improved strength of the vertebral body, and decreased stress placed on the adjacent vertebrae. Vertebroplasty is usually performed under fluoroscopic guidance. After administration of prophylactic antibiotic, vertebral body access is obtained through a uni- or bipedicular approach. Some physicians perform venography prior to injection of PMMA to show venous drainage and confirm needle placement into the bony trabeculae. The entire vertebral body does not have to be filled with cement to achieve pain relief as there is no correlation between volumes of cement injected and pain reduction. Usually, 2 to 6 mL of cement is enough for the procedure (Fig. 57-8). The patient remains supine for 3 to 5 hours after the procedure for assessment of neurologic status and observation for the occurrence of bleeding and hematomas. The procedure can be done on an outpatient basis. A CT scan is usually performed afterward for assessment of cement distribution and the occurrence of complications such as bleeding and leakage of the cement. Kyphoplasty involves the percutaneous introduction of a balloon into the vertebral body, inflation of the balloon, then filling the balloon with PMMA that is more viscous than that used for vertebroplasty.

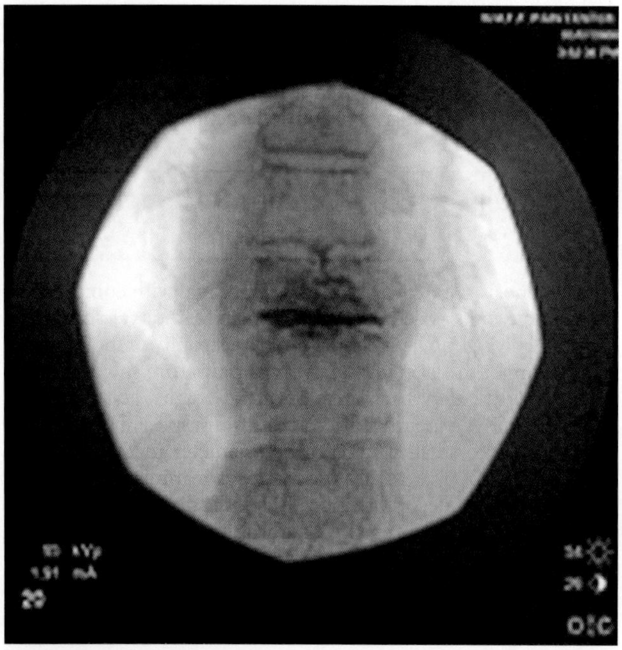

FIGURE 57-8. Vertebroplasty at T10 vertebral level. A total of 5 mL of cement was injected.

The complications of percutaneous vertebral augmentation include leakage of the cement and complications related to the procedure. The factors that contribute to cement leakage include the level of injection, severity of fracture, and the amount of cement injected. Although some leakage of cement is common, severe clinical sequelae occur in a small percentage of patients. Pulmonary embolism may result from leakage of cement into the paravertebral veins and bone marrow, or embolism of fat particles. Neurologic complications include radiculopathy, spinal claudication, and paraplegia. Kyphoplasty is associated with a lower rate of cement extravasation because of the higher viscosity of the PMMA that is used, the lower injection pressure employed, and the inflatable bone trap that seals pathways for cement leakage.[162] Complications related to the procedure include infection, bleeding, and allergic reactions from the PMMA or contrast medium.

Initial results after vertebroplasty and kyphoplasty were good and complications were minimal.[163–167] More recent random-
9 ized, controlled studies have not confirmed the beneficial effects of vertebroplasty in that improvements in pain and pain-related disability were similar to the improvements in the control sham group.[168,169] While the conduct of the studies was criticized appropriately, questions about the mechanism and the effectiveness of this procedure remain unanswered.[170] Two randomized controlled studies showed the superiority of balloon kyphoplasty for VCFs, in patients with osteoporosis or cancer, when compared with a control nonsurgical care group.[171,172] These two randomized studies were partly criticized in that funding of the study came from the maker of the device and that one of the authors was affiliated with the company. Final conclusions on the efficacy of these procedures await additional randomized, controlled studies.

Spinal Cord Stimulation

The analgesic effect of SCS involves the *gate control theory.* Therapeutic effects of neuromodulation are based on the concept that selective excitation of large afferent fiber activity mechanisms control pain.[173] It is hypothesized that SCS increases the input of the large nerve fibers, thus closing the "gate" at the substantia gelatinosa of the dorsal horn of the spinal cord. SCS may alter the local neurochemistry at the dorsal horn, and there may be a decrease of the hyperexcitability of the wide dynamic neurons. It is correlated with increased levels of the inhibitory neurotransmitter GABA and a decrease of the excitatory neurotransmitters glutamate and aspartate.[174] In ischemic pain, the analgesia may be secondary to alteration of the sympathetic tone with restoration of a favorable oxygen supply-and-demand balance.

Indications for SCS implantation include patients with a diagnosis of failed back surgery syndrome, CRPS, neuropathic pain syndromes; angina[175]; chronic critical limb ischemia and pain[176]; patients who failed conservative therapy; patients who had a trial that has demonstrated pain relief; and patients who passed a psychological evaluation.[177] Many patients with chronic pain may have some depressive symptoms and implantation should be avoided in patients with major psychological disorders. There appears to be a high correlation between several items on some psychological tests and a favorable response to trial stimulation. The recommended selection criteria for SCS placement in patients with neuropathic pain are failed trials of pharmacologic management including anticonvulsants, antidepressants, and/or opioids. The general contraindications include systemic or local site of infection and abnormal coagulopathy. Complications include nerve and spinal cord injury, infection, hematoma, and lead breakage or migration.

Studies that examined the efficacy of SCS for chronic pain often lack a randomized control group, have ambiguous entry criteria, few outcome measures, and inadequate follow-up. Although the main use of SCS in the United States is failed back surgery syndrome, it is a treatment for pain secondary to peripheral ischemia in Europe. Meta-analyses concluded that there was sufficient evidence to draw conclusions that prospective randomized studies support the efficacy of SCS[178,179] for persistent back pain. In a randomized study, patients who were candidates for repeat laminectomy were randomized to either SCS or surgery.[180] At 6-month follow-up 67% of patients who had reoperation crossed over to SCS, compared while only 17% in the SCS group crossed over to reoperation. At the 3-year follow-up, the SCS continued to have better outcomes compared with repeat spine surgery. Overall, 47% of patients in the SCS group achieved ≥50% pain relief compared with 12% in the reoperation group ($P < 0.01$). The patients randomized to reoperation used significantly more opioids than those randomized to SCS.
10 Thus, there is sufficient evidence to support the efficacy of SCS for treating failed back syndrome in terms of sustained long-term pain relief with medication reduction, improvement in quality of life, increased patient satisfaction, increased ability to return to work, minimal side effects, cost-effectiveness compared with alternative therapies, and reversibility of the technique.

Studies that examined the efficacy of SCS in CRPS consisted of retrospective case series[181,182] and a prospective randomized controlled study.[183] In the randomized controlled study,[183] patients with a 6-month history of CRPS of the upper extremity had either SCS or physiotherapy. At the 6-month follow-up, patients who were treated with SCS had a significantly greater reduction in pain, and a significantly higher percentage of patients graded their relief as much improved in terms of global perceived effect. A meta-analysis[179] concluded that SCS is an effective tool in the management of CRPS and concluded that a grade A level of evidence supports the efficacy of SCS in CRPS. For pain from peripheral ischemia and angina, most of the published literature consists of a series of case reports.

Commonly SCS trial is carried out on an outpatient basis. The SCS trial and implantation need to be carried out under full aseptic techniques in the operating room to minimize infection. Depending on the pain site (leg or arm) the SCS electrodes are placed via a Touhy needle (Fig. 57-9A and B). It is critical that a shallow angle of entry of the epidural needle be maintained so that the SCS electrode can be placed in the dorsal aspect of the epidural space. The SCS electrodes are advanced under fluoroscopic guidance and the paresthesia obtained should correspond to the topography of the patient's chronic pain. Once this has been achieved, the epidural needle is removed and the electrode position maintained at the same level. The electrodes are secured in place and the patient sent home to determine the efficacy of the SCS trial.

If the SCS trial is successful, permanent implantation should be done in the operating room. Surgical hemostasis is achieved after a midline incision and the Touhy needle placed in the epidural space. Fluoroscopy is critical to determine correct placement of the permanent SCS electrodes. Once appropriate position of the electrodes is confirmed, anchoring is critical to prevent lead migration. The electrodes are then connected to a battery location that is pre-determined by the patient and the implanting surgeon.

Peripheral Nerve Stimulation

Electrical stimulation of a peripheral nerve can be used to treat neuropathic pain, ideally arising from a single nerve. The conditions most amenable to peripheral nerve stimulation (PNS) include occipital neuralgia, supraorbital neuralgia, and peripheral neuropathic pain. Candidates for PNS should have undergone failed or only partially effective multimodal therapy including medical management, anesthetic regional blockade, and physical therapy[184] before consideration for PNS. As with patients who are being evaluated for SCS, neuropsychological testing is valuable. In addition, before permanent implantation of the internal pulse generator, patients should have undergone a successful trial of stimulation with a predetermined therapeutic benefit. There is a surge of PNS or subcutaneous placement of neuromodulation electrodes for chronic axial pain with variable results.

With a more regional subcutaneous stimulation, PNS can affect lower back pain and migraine headache.[185] Similar to SCS, our understanding of the mechanism behind PNS is rooted in Melzack and Wall's gate control theory of pain. Other hypotheses suggest that PNS may result in peripheral nerve blockade or other peripheral changes in action potential kinetics to suppress pain. PNS was traditionally delivered with a cuff electrode wrapped around the target nerve, but this can lead to perineural fibrosis. Trial of PNS placement is ideally done under ultrasound. With surgical implantation, a piece of fascia may be implanted between the electrode and the nerve itself, analogous to the dura mater in the implantation of a spinal cord stimulator.

Occipital Nerve Stimulation

Occipital neurostimulation (ONS) provides reversible and effective therapy for intractable headache. The technique is thought to work via inhibition of central nociceptive impulses by stimulation of the extensions of the trigeminocervical complex, the nerve branches of C2 and C3. Successful electrode implantation for occipital neurostimulation requires knowledge of nerve anatomy and details of the various available devices. Implantation should ideally avoid unpleasant dysesthesias, which can result from superficial placement, and occipital muscle stimulation that causes spasm when electrodes are implanted too deep. As in all forms of neurostimulation, lead migration represents a potential technical failure that can require surgical replacement; this incidence is particularly high with ONS.[186]

Intrathecal Pumps

Intrathecal drug delivery systems (IDDSs) are valuable options in patients in whom oral or transdermal opioids are ineffective at reasonable doses, or cause unacceptable side effects. The main indications for IDDS are cancer pain and pain of spinal origin, with the majority of pumps placed in the United States for failed back surgery syndrome. Baclofen has been administered in patients who have had a significant spinal cord injury or significant spasm with very good successes. In fact the initial drugs for IDDS included baclofen and morphine. Intrathecal drug infusion allows the drug to be directly deposited near the spinal cord receptors, bypassing the blood–brain barrier. By enabling direct access to opioid receptors, an equianalgesic dose is markedly diminished compared with alternative routes. These lower doses result in a
11 marked decrease in side effects and adverse events. The spinal opioid not only interacts with the opioid receptors, the spinal delivery also results in adenosine release in the cerebrospinal fluid.[187]

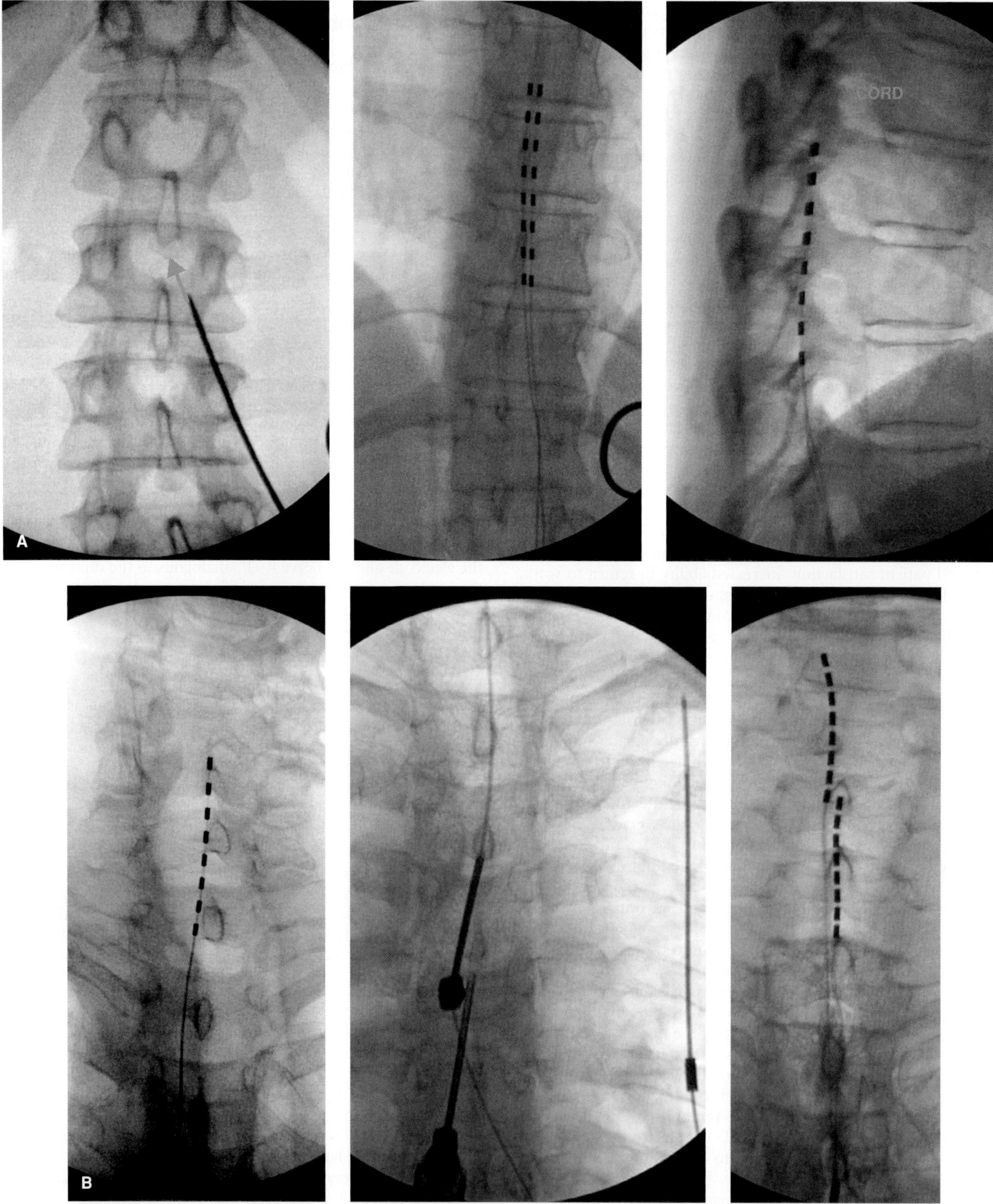

FIGURE 57-9. **A** and **B:** Placement of the epidural needle and the spinal cord electrodes at the thoracic and cervical levels.

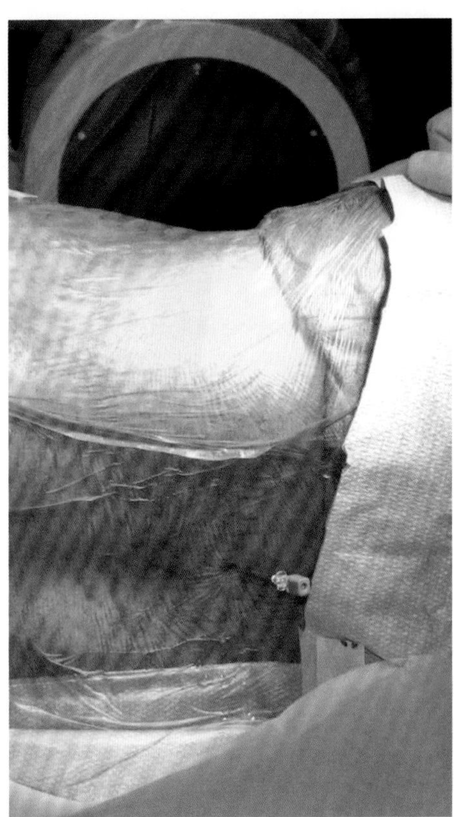
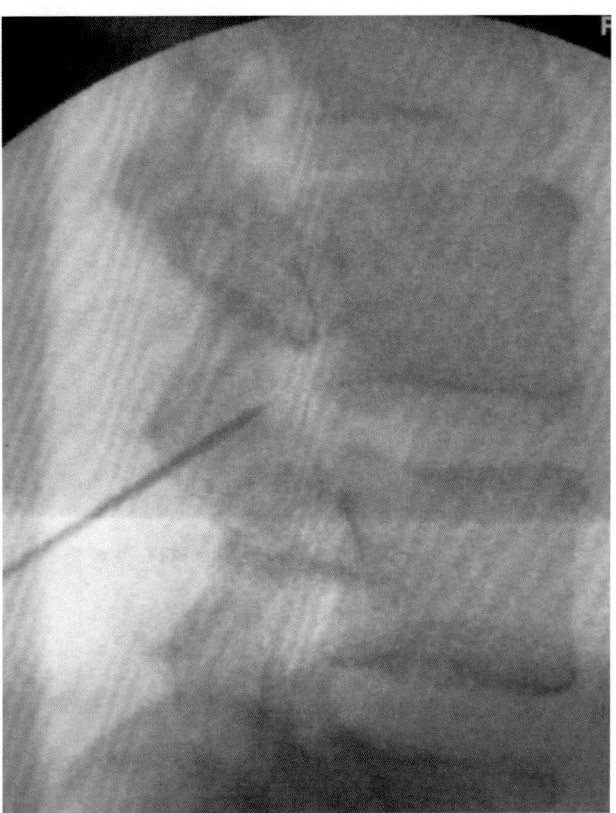

FIGURE 57-10. Placement of the intrathecal needle under fluoroscopy.

For patients with metastatic cancer and severe pain, the use of IDDS becomes invaluable. Several factors should be considered before instituting IDDS for nonmalignant pain including the life span of these patients. A trial period is recommended before an intrathecal pump is permanently placed. A trial can be performed intrathecally or through the epidural space, by a single shot, intermittent bolus, or a continuous infusion. The trial is usually with an opioid and can be performed on an inpatient or outpatient basis. Opioids alone may not be adequate to treat neuropathic or mixed pain syndromes.

Considerations regarding intrathecal (IT) drug pump implantation technique include patient positioning (e.g., lateral decubitus vs. prone; type of anesthetic; IT needle entry point (Fig. 57-10); eventual catheter tip location; site of pump placement; and, a knowledge of the patient's lumbar spine anatomy including prior spine surgery or pathology. The technique to place a permanent pump and catheter should be performed in an operating room under sterile conditions. Intravenous antibiotics should be administered and should cover skin flora. In the majority of patients, the only anatomical location that can reasonably accommodate the size of the pump is the lower quadrant of either side of the abdomen. The anatomic constraints are the bony borders of the iliac crest, the symphysis pubis, and the costal margin. None of these should come in contact with the pump when the patient is seated because of discomfort and risk of damage to the pump or catheter. Therefore, marking the patient in the seated or standing position should be carried out preoperatively. Nonanatomic constraints include the patient's waistline and beltline. With the rise in popularity of patient-activated medication bolusing by remote control, patients may have a preference for abdominal placement on their own left- or right-handedness. It is important not to place the pump too deep because it may lead to problems in interrogation and refilling of the pump. The pump pocket incision should be made to approximate the size of the pump. The incision can be carried down to the rectus fascia in thin patients. This is followed by tunneling through the subcutaneous tissues from the pump pocket to the posterior incision (Fig. 57-11). This must be done carefully to prevent accidental puncture of the peritoneum or even the pleura.

A consensus conference in 2007 resulted in an algorithm that is often used as a guide for patients with intrathecal pumps.[188] The experts recommended morphine and hydromorphone or ziconotide as acceptable first-line agents. If either morphine or hydromorphone does not produce relief or cause side effects, then either one drug is switched to the other first-line drug if the patient has primary nociceptive pain, or clonidine or bupivacaine is added for patients with primary neuropathic or mixed pain syndromes. Fentanyl is a second-line agent because the more hydrophilic agents cause intractable side effects, and because of its apparent granuloma-sparing property, its widespread use and safety.

The complications of IDDS include infection, bleeding, respiratory depression, pump malfunction, catheter failure, hormonal dysfunction including decreased testosterone levels and small gonads, peripheral edema, and formation of an inflammatory mass. Low testosterone levels are managed with transdermal or injectable testosterone. Peripheral edema should be treated with diuretics, compression stockings, extremity elevation, and rotation of the infused drug. An inflammatory mass is a noninfectious eaction that is usually located at the catheter tip.

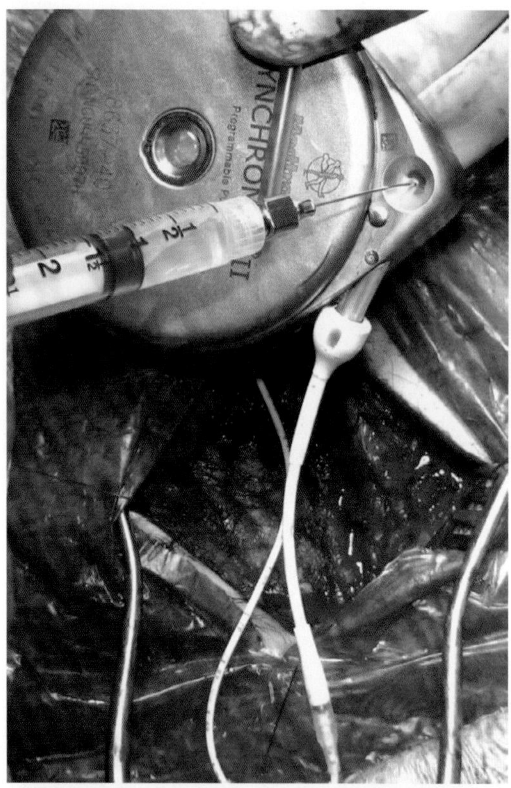
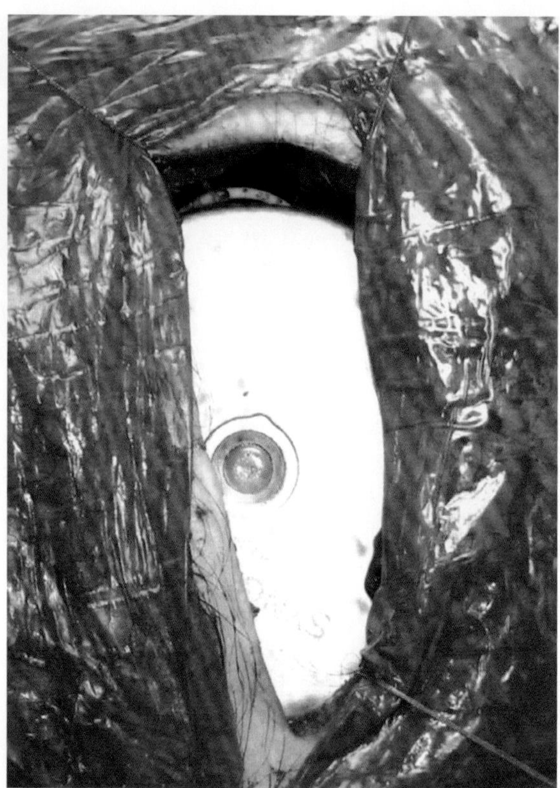

FIGURE 57-11. Connection of the intrathecal catheter to the programmable pump and confirmation of cerebrospinal fluid prior to placement in the pocket.

References

1. Melzack R. Prolonged relief of pain by brief, intense transcutaneous somatic stimulation. *Pain.* 1975;1:357–373.
2. Neumann S, Doubell TP, Leslie T, et al. Inflammatory pain hypersensitivity mediated by phenotypic switch in myelinated primary sensory neurons. *Nature.* 1996;384:360–364.
3. Indo Y, Tsuruta M, Hayashida Y, et al. Mutations in the TRKA/NGF receptor gene in patients with congenital insensitivity to pain with anhidrosis. *Nat Genet.* 1996;13:485–488.
4. Fields HL. *Pain Syndromes in Neurology.* Boston: Butterworths, London; 1990.
5. Lumpkin EA, Caterina MJ. Mechanisms of sensory transduction in the skin. *Nature.* 2007;445:858–865.
6. Hou Q, Barr T, Gee L, et al. Keratinocyte expression of calcitonin gene-related peptide beta: implications for neuropathic and inflammatory pain mechanisms. *Pain.* 2011;152:2036–2051.
7. Cox JJ, Reimann F, Nicholas AK, et al. An SCN9A channelopathy causes congenital inability to experience pain. *Nature.* 2006;444:894–898.
8. Fertleman CR, Baker MD, Parker KA, et al. SCN9A mutations in paroxysmal extreme pain disorder: allelic variants underlie distinct channel defects and phenotypes. *Neuron.* 2006;52:767–774.
9. Rush A, Dib-Hajj SD, Liu S, et al. A single sodium channel mutation produces hyper- or hypoexcitability in different types of neurons. *Proc Natl Acad Sci U S A.* 2006;103:8245–8250.
10. Caterina MJ, Schumacher MA, Tominaga M, et al. The capsaicin receptor: a heat-activated ion channel in the pain pathway. *Nature.* 1997;389:816–824.
11. Caterina MJ, Leffler A, Malmberg AB, et al. Impaired nociception and pain sensation in mice lacking the capsaicin receptor. *Science.* 2000;288:306–313.
12. Suzuki H, Kerr R, Bianchi L, et al. In vivo imaging of C. elegans mechanosensory neurons demonstrates a specific role for the MEC-4 channel in the process of gentle touch sensation. *Neuron.* 2003;39:1005–1017.
13. Chatzigeorgiou M, Yoo S, Watson JD, et al. Specific roles for DEG/ENaC and TRP channels in touch and thermosensation in C. elegans nociceptors. *Nat Neurosci.* 2010;13:861–868.
14. Honda CN, Lee CL. Immunohistochemistry of synaptic input and functional characterizations of neurons near the spinal central canal. *Brain Res.* 1985;343: 120–128.
15. Willis WD, Kenshalo DR, Leonard RB. The cells of origin of the primate spinothalamic tract. *J Comp Neurol.* 1979;188:543–573.
16. Clark FM, Proudfit HK. The projections of noradrenergic neurons in the A5 catecholamine cell group to the spinal cord in the rat: anatomical evidence that A5 neurons modulate nociception. *Brain Res.* 1993;616:200–210.
17. Basbaum AI, Fields HL. Endogenous pain control systems: brainstem spinal pathways and endorphin circuitry. *Annu Rev Neurosci.* 1984;7:309–338.
18. Bajic D, Proudfit HK. Projections of neurons in the periaqueductal gray to pontine and medullary catecholamine cell groups involved in the modulation of nociception. *J Comp Neurol.* 1999;405:359–379.
19. Gebhart GF. Recent developments in the neurochemical bases of pain and analgesia. *NIDA Res Monogr.* 1983;45:19–35.
20. Basbaum AI, Clanton C, Fields HL. Three bulbospinal pathways from the rostral medulla of the cat: An autoradiographic study of pain modulating systems. *J Comp Neurol.* 1978;178:209–224.
21. Duggan AW, Griersmith BT. Inhibition of the spinal transmission of nociceptive information by supraspinal stimulation in the cat. *Pain.* 1979;6:149–161.
22. Antal M, Petko M, Polgar E, et al. Direct evidence of an extensive GABAergic innervation of the spinal dorsal horn by fibres descending from the rostral ventromedial medulla. *Neuroscience.* 1996;73:509–518.
23. Clark FM, Proudfit HK. The projection of noradrenergic neurons in the A7 catecholamine cell group to the spinal cord in the rat demonstrated by anterograde tracing combined with immunocytochemistry. *Brain Res.* 1991;547:279–288.
24. Peyron R, Laurent B, Garcia-Larrea L. Functional imaging of brain responses to pain. A review and meta-analysis. *Neurophysiol Clin.* 2000;30:263–288.
25. Woolf CJ. Evidence for a central component of post-injury pain hypersensitivity. *Nature.* 1983;306:686–688.
26. Lai J, Gold M, Kim CS, et al. Inhibition of neuropathic pain by decreased expression of the tetrodotoxin-resistant sodium channel, NaV1.8. *Pain.* 2002;95: 143–152.
27. Munro G, Dalby-Brown W. Kv7 (KCNQ) channel modulators and neuropathic pain. *J Med Chem.* 2007;50:2576–2582.
28. Emery EC, Young GT, Berrocoso EM, et al. HCN2 ion channels play a central role in inflammatory and neuropathic pain. *Science.* 2011;333:1462–1466.
29. Mulleman D, Mammou S, Griffoul I, et al. Pathophysiology of disk-related sciatica. I.–Evidence supporting a chemical component. *Joint Bone Spine.* 2006;73: 151–158.

30. Vellani V, Kinsey AM, Prandini M, et al. Protease activated receptors 1 and 4 sensitize TRPV1 in nociceptive neurones. *Mol Pain.* 2010;6:61.
31. Novakovic SD, Levinson SR, Schachner M, et al. Disruption and reorganization of sodium channels in experimental allergic neuritis. *Muscle Nerve.* 1998;21: 1019–1032.
32. Basbaum AI. Spinal mechanisms of acute and persistent pain. *Reg Anesth Pain Med.* 1999;24:59–67.
33. Torebjork HE, Lundberg LE, LaMotte RH. Central changes in processing of mechanoreceptive input in capsaicin-induced secondary hyperalgesia in humans. *J Physiol.* 1992;448:765–780.
34. Jensen MC, Brant-Zawadzki MN, Obuchowski N, et al. Magnetic resonance imaging of the lumbar spine in people without back pain. *N Eng J Med.* 1994;331:69.
35. Weinreb JC, Wolbarsht LB, Cohen JM, et al. Prevalence of lumbosacral intervertebral disc abnormalities in MR images of pregnant and asymptomatic nonpregnant women. *Radiology.* 1989;170:125.
36. Borenstein DG, O'Mara JW, Boden SD, et al. The value of magnetic resonance imaging of the lumbar spine to predict low back pain in asymptomatic subjects: A seven-year follow-up study. *J Bone Joint Surg Am.* 2001;83:1306.
37. Burke JG, Watson RWG, McCormack D, et al. Intervertebral discs which cause low back pain secrete high levels of proinflammatory mediators. *J Bone Joint Surg Br.* 2002;84:196.
38. Olmarker K, Rydevik B. Selective inhibition of tumor necrosis factor-alpha prevents nucleus induced thrombus formation, intraneural edema, and reduction of nerve conduction velocity: Possible implications for future pharmacologic treatment strategy of sciatica. *Spine.* 2001;26:863.
39. Cohen SP, Wenzell D, Hurley RW, et al. A double-blind placebo-controlled, dose-response pilot study evaluating intradiscal ethanercept in patients with chronic discogenic low back pain or lumbosacral radiculopathy. *Anesthesiology.* 2007;107:99.
40. Dilke TFW, Burry HC, Grahame R. Extradural corticosteroid injection in management of lumbar nerve root compression. *Br Med J.* 1973;2:635.
41. Arden NK, Price C, Reading I, et al. WEST Study Group: A multicentre randomized controlled trial of epidural corticosteroid injections for sciatica: The WEST study. *Rheumatology.* 2005;44:1399.
42. Wilson-MacDonald J, Burt G, Griffen D, et al. Epidural steroid injection for nerve root compression. A randomized, controlled trial. *J Bone Joint Surg Br.* 2005; 87:352.
43. Snoek W, Weber H, Jorgensen B. Double blind evaluation of extradural methylprednisolone for herniated lumbar discs. *Acta Orthop Scand.* 1977;48:635.
44. Cuckler JM, Bernini PA, Wiesel SW, et al. The use of epidural steroids in the treatment of lumbar radicular pain. *J Bone Joint Surg Am.* 1985;67:63.
45. Carette S, Leclaire R, Marcoux S, et al. Epidural corticosteroid injections for sciatica due to herniated nucleus pulposus. *N Engl J Med.* 1997;336:1634.
46. Armon C, Argoff CA, Samuels J, et al. Assessment: Use of epidural steroid injections to treat radicular lumbosacral pain. *Neurology.* 2007;68:723.
47. Riew KD, Yin Y, Gilula L, et al. The effect of nerve-root injections on the need for operative treatment of lumbar radicular pain. A prospective, randomized, controlled, double-blind study. *J Bone Joint Surg Am.* 2000;82:1589.
48. Karppinen J, Malmivaara A, Kurunlahti M, et al. Periradicular infiltration for sciatica: A randomized controlled trial. *Spine.* 2001;26:1059.
49. Ng L, Chaudhary N, Sell P. The efficacy of corticosteroids in periradicular infiltration for chronic radicular pain: A randomized, double-blind, controlled trial. *Spine.* 2005;30:857.
50. Kraemer J, Ludwig J, Bickert U, et al. Lumbar epidural perineural injection: A new technique. *Eur Spine J.* 1997;6:357.
51. Thomas E, Cyteval C, Abiad L, et al. Effect of transforaminal versus interspinous corticosteroid injection in discal radiculalgia—a prospective, randomized, double-blind study. *Clin Rheumatol.* 2003;22:299.
52. Candido KD, Raghavendra MS, Chintagadda M, et al. A prospective evaluation of iodinated contrast flow patterns with fluoroscopically guided lumbar epidural steroid injections: The lateral parasagittal interlaminar epidural approach versus the transforaminal epidural approach. *Anesth Analg.* 2008;106:638–644.
53. Rathmell JP, April C, Bogduk N. Cervical transforaminal injection of steroids. *Anesthesiology.* 2004;100:1959.
54. Tiso RL, Cutler T, Catania JA, et al. Adverse central nervous system sequelae after selective transforaminal block: the role of corticosteroids. *Spine J.* 2004;4:468.
55. Benzon HT, Chew TL, McCarthy R, et al. Comparison of the particle sizes of the different steroids and the effect of dilution: A review of the relative neurotoxicities of the steroids. *Anesthesiology.* 2007;106:331.
56. Huntoon MA. Anatomy of the cervical intervertebral foramina: Vulnerable arteries and ischemic neurologic injuries after transforaminal epidural injections. *Pain.* 2005;117:104.
57. Dreyfuss P, Baker R, Bogduk N. Comparative effectiveness of cervical epidural steroid injections with particulate and non-particulate corticosteroid preparations for cervical radicular pain. *Pain Med.* 2006;7:237.
58. Iversen T, Solberg TK, Romner B, et al. Effect of caudal epidural steroid or saline injection in chronic lumbar radiculopathy: Muticentre, blinded, randomized controlled trial. *BMJ.* 2011;343:d5278.
59. Weinstein JN, Tosteson TD, Lurie JD, et al. Surgical vs nonoperative treatment for lumbar disk herniation: The Spine Patient Outcomes Research Trial (SPORT): A randomized trial. *JAMA.* 2006;296:2441–2450.
60. Cohen SP, Strassels SA, Kurihara C, et al. Does sensory stimulation threshold affect lumbar facet radiofrequency denervation outcomes: A prospective clinical correlation study. *Anesth Analg.* 2011;113:1233–1341.
61. Gallagher G, Petriccione di Vadi PL, Vedley JR. Radiofrequency facet joint denervation in the treatment of low back pain: A prospective, controlled double-blind study to assess its efficacy. *Pain Clin.* 1994;7:193.
62. Sanders M, Zuurmund WW. Percutaneous intra-articular lumbar facet joint denervation in the treatment of low back pain: A comparison with percutaneous extra-articular lumbar facet denervation. *Pain Clin.* 1999;11:329.
63. van Kleef M, Barendse GA, Kessels A, et al. Randomized trial of radiofrequency lumbar facet denervation for chronic low back pain. *Spine.* 1999;24:1937.
64. Leclaire R, Fortin L, Lambert R, et al. Radiofrequency facet joint denervation in the treatment of low back pain: A placebo-controlled clinical trial to assess efficacy. *Spine.* 2001;26:1411.
65. van Wijk RM, Geurtz JW, Wynne HJ, et al. Radiofrequency denervation of lumbar facet joints in the treatment of chronic low back pain: A randomized, double-blind, sham lesion-controlled trial. *Clin J Pain.* 2005;21:335.
66. Tekin I, Mirzai H, Ok G, et al. A comparison of conventional and pulsed radiofrequency denervation in the treatment of chronic facet joint pain. *Clin J Pain.* 2007;23:524–529.
67. Nath S, Nath CA, Pettersson K. Percutaneous lumbar zygapophyseal (facet) joint neurotomy using radiofrequency current, in the management of chronic low back pain: a randomized double-blind trial. *Spine.* 2008;33:1291–1297.
68. Lord SM, Barnsley L, Wallis BJ, et al. Percutaneous radio-frequency neurotomy for chronic cervical zygapophyseal-joint pain. *N Engl J Med.* 1996;335:1721.
69. Stovner LJ, Kolstad F, Helde G. Radiofrequency denervation of facet joints C2-C6 in cervicogenic headache: a randomized, double-blind-sham-controlled study. *Cephalalgia.* 2004;24:821.
70. Cohen SP, Hurley RW, Buckenmaier CC 3rd, et al. Randomized placebo-controlled study evaluating lateral branch radiofrequency denervation for sacroiliac joint pain. *Anesthesiology.* 2008;109:279–288.
71. Yin W, Willard F, Carreiro J, et al. Sensory stimulation guided sacroiliac joint radiofrequency neurotomy: Technique based on neuroanatomy of the dorsal sacral plexus. *Spine.* 2003;28:2419.
72. Benzon HT, Katz JA, Benzon HA, et al. Piriformis syndrome: Anatomic considerations, a new injection technique, and a review of the literature. *Anesthesiology.* 2003;98:1442.
73. Fishman LM, Zybert PA. Electrophysiologic evidence of piriformis syndrome. *Arch Phys Med Rehabil.* 1992;73:359.
74. Wheeler AH, Goolkasian P, Gretz SS. A randomized, double-blind, prospective pilot study of botulinum toxin injection for refractory, unilateral, cervicothoracic, paraspinal, myofascial pain syndrome. *Spine.* 1998;23:1662.
75. Ferrante FM, Bearn L, Rothrock R, et al. Evidence against trigger point injection technique for the treatment of cervicothoracic myofascial pain with botulinum toxin type A. *Anesthesiology.* 2005;103:377.
76. Wolfe F, Smythe HA, Yunus MB, et al. The American College of Rheumatology 1990 Criteria for the Classification of Fibromyalgia. *Arthritis Rheum.* 1990;33: 160.
77. Macfarlane GJ, Croft PR, Schollum J, et al. Widespread pain: Is an improved classification possible? *J Rheumatol.* 1996;23:1628–1632.
78. Wilke WS. New developments in the diagnosis of fibromyalgia syndrome: Say goodbye to tender points? *Cleve Clin J Med.* 2009;76:345–352.
79. Bradley LA, Alberts KR, Alarcon GS, et al. Abnormal brain regional cerebral blood flow and cerebrospinal fluid levels of Substance P in patients and non-patients with fibromyalgia. *Arthritis Rheum.* 1996;39:1109.
80. Sarchielli P, Di Filippo M, Nardi K, et al. Sensitization, glutamate, and the link between migraine and fibromyalgia. *Curr Pain Headache Rep.* 2007;11:343–351.
81. Baraniuk JN, Whalen G, Cunningham J, et al. Cerebrospinal fluid levels of opioid peptides in fibromyalgia and chronic low back pain. *BMC Musculoskelet Disord.* 2004;5:48.
82. Russell IJ, Vaeroy H, Javors M, et al. Cerebrospinal fluid biogenic amine metabolites in fibromyalgia/fibrositis syndrome and rheumatoid arthritis. *Arthritis Rheum.* 1992;35:550–556.
83. Arnold LM, Lu Y, Crofford LJ, et al. A double-blind, multicenter trial comparing duloxetine with placebo in the treatment of fibromyalgia patients with or without major depressive disorder. *Arthritis Rheum.* 2004;50:2974–2984.
84. Gendreau RM, Thorn MD, Gendreau JF, et al. The efficacy of milnacipran in fibromyalgia. *J Rheumatol.* 2005;32:1975–1985.
85. Crofford LJ, Mease PJ, Simpson SL, et al. Fibromyalgia relapse evaluation and efficacy for durability of meaningful relief (FREEDOM): A 6-month, double-blind, placebo-controlled trial with pregabalin. *Pain.* 2008;136:419–431.
86. Russell IJ, Perkins AT, Michalek JE. Oxybate SXB-26 Fibromyalgia Syndrome Study Group. Sodium oxybate relieves pain and improves function in fibromyalgia syndrome: A randomized, double-blind, placebo-controlled, multicenter clinical trial. *Arthritis Rheum.* 2009;60:299–309.
87. Pasqualucci A, Pasqualucci V, Galla F, et al. Prevention of postherpetic neuralgia: Acyclovir and prednisolone versus epidural local anesthetic and methylprednisolone. *Acta Anaesthesiol Scand.* 2000;44:910.
88. van Wijck AJM, Opstelten W, Moons KGM, et al. The PINE study of epidural steroids and local anaesthetics to prevent postherpetic neuralgia randomized controlled trial. *Lancet.* 2006;367:219.

89. Watson CPN, Babul N. Efficacy of oxycodone in neuropathic pain: A randomized trial in postherpetic neuralgia. *Neurology*. 1998;50:1837.
90. Raja SN, Haythornthwaite JA, Papagallo M, et al. Opioids versus antidepressants in postherpetic neuralgia: A randomized placebo-controlled trial. *Neurology*. 2002; 59:1015.
91. Boureau F, Legallicier P, Kabir-Ahmadi M. Tramadol in postherpetic neuralgia: A randomized, double-blind, placebo-controlled trial. *Pain*. 2003;323.
92. Rice ASC, Maton S. Postherpetic Neuralgia Study group: Gabapentin in postherpetic neuralgia: A randomized, double-blind, placebo-controlled study. *Pain*. 2001; 94:215.
93. Dworkin RH, Corbin AE, Young JP, et al. Pregabalin for the treatment of postherpetic neuralgia: A randomized, placebo-controlled trial. *Neurology*. 2003;60:1274.
94. Freynhagen R, Strojek K, Griesing T, et al. Efficacy of pregabalin in neuropathic pain evaluated in a 12-week, randomised, double-blind, multicentre, placebo-controlled trial of flexible- and fixed-dose regimens. *Pain*. 2005;115:254.
95. Gilron I, Bailey JM, Tu D, et al. Morphine, gabapentin, or their combination for neuropathic pain. *New Engl J Med*. 2005;352:1324.
96. Gilron I, Bailey JM, Tu D, et al. Nortriptyline and gabapentin, alone and in combination for neuropathic pain: A double-blind, randomised controlled crossover trial. *Lancet*. 2009;374:1252–1261.
97. Finnerup NB, Otto M, McQuay HJ, et al. Algorithm for neuropathic pain treatment: An evidence based proposal. *Pain*. 2005;118:289.
98. Kotani N, Kushikata T, Hashimoto H, et al. Intrathecal methylprednisolone for intractable postherpetic neuralgia. *N Engl J Med*. 2000;343:1514.
99. Kikuchi A, Kotani N, Sato T, et al. Comparative therapeutic evaluation of intrathecal versus epidural methylprednisolone for long-term analgesia in patients with intractable postherpetic neuralgia. *Reg Anesth Pain Med*. 1999;24:287.
100. Harke H, Gretenkort P, Ladleif HU, et al. Spinal cord stimulation in postherpetic neuralgia and in acute herpes zoster. *Anesth Analg*. 2002;9:694.
101. Benzon HT, Chekka K, Darnule A, et al. Evidence-based case report: Intrathecal alcohol for postherpetic neuralgia. *Reg Anesth Pain Med*. 2009;34:514–521.
102. Williams KA, Hurley RW, Lin EE, et al. Neuropathic pain syndromes. In: Benzon HT, Rathmell JP, Wu CL, Turk DC, Argoff CE, eds. *Raj's Practical Management of Pain*. 4th ed. Phildelphia, PA: Mosby Elsevier; 2008:427.
103. Goldstein DJ, Lu Y, Detke MJ, et al. Duloxetine vs. placebo in patients with painful diabetic neuropathy. *Pain*. 2005;116:109.
104. Attal N, Cruccu G, Baron R, et al. European Federation of Neurological Sciences. EFNS guidelines on the pharmacological treatment of neuropathic pain: 2010 revision. *Eur J Neurol*. 2010;17:1113–1123.
105. Dworkin RH, O'Connor AB, Audette J, et al. Recommendations for the pharmacologic management of neuropathic pain: An overview and literature update. *Mayo Clin Proc*. 2010;85:S3–S14.
106. van de Vusse AC, Stomp-van den Berg SG, Kessels AH, et al. Randomised controlled trial of gabapentin in complex regional pain syndrome type 1. *BMC Neurol*. 2004;29:4.
107. Sigtermans MJ, van Hilten JJ, Bauer MC, et al. Ketamine produces effective and long-term pain relief in patients with Complex Regional Pain Syndrome Type 1. *Pain*. 2009;145:304–311.
108. Schwartzman RJ, Alexander GM, Grothusen JR, et al. Outpatient intravenous ketamine for the treatment of complex regional pain syndrome: A double-blind placebo controlled study. *Pain*. 2009;147:107–115.
109. Kemler MA, De Vet HC, Barendse GA, et al. The effect of spinal cord stimulation in patients with chronic reflex sympathetic dystrophy: Two years' follow-up of the randomized controlled trial. *Ann Neurol*. 2004;55(1):13–18.
110. Simpson DM, Olney R, McArthur JC, et al. A placebo-controlled trial of lamotrigine for painful HIV-associated neuropathy. *Neurology*. 2000;5411:2115.
111. Simpson DM, McArthur JC, Olney R, et al. Lamotrigine Neuropathy Study HIV Team: Lamotrigine for HIV-associated painful sensory neuropathies: A placebo-controlled trial. *Neurology*. 2003;609:1508.
112. Hahn K, Arendt G, Braun JS, et al. German Neuro-AIDS Working Group: A placebo-controlled trial of gabapentin for painful HIV-associated sensory neuropathies. *J Neurol*. 2004;251:1260.
113. Giummarra MJ, Moseley GL. Phantom limb pain and bodily awareness: Current concepts and future directions. *Curr Opin Anaesthesiol*. 2011;24:524–531.
114. Ischia S, Ischia A, Polati E, et al. Three posterior percutaneous celiac plexus block techniques: A prospective randomized study in 61 patients with pancreatic cancer pain. *Anesthesiology*. 1992;76:534.
115. Mercadante S. Celiac plexus block versus analgesics in pancreatic cancer pain. *Pain*. 1993;52:187.
116. Wong G, Schoeder DR, Carns PE, et al. Effect of neurolytic celiac plexus block on pain relief, quality of life, and survival in patients with unresectable pancreatic cancer. *JAMA*. 2004;291:1092.
117. Eisenberg E, Carr DB, Chalmers TC. Neurolytic celiac plexus block for treatment of cancer pain: A meta-analysis. *Anesth Analg*. 1995;80:290.
118. Okie S. A flood of opioids: A rising tide of deaths. *New Engl J Med*. 2010;383: 1981–1985.
119. Krantz MJ, Martin J, Stimmel B, et al. QTc interval screening in methadone treatment. *Ann Intern Med*. 2009;150:387–395.
120. Mahajan G, Holtsman M. Major opioids in pain management. In: Benzon HT, Raja S, Liu SS, Fishman SN, Cohen SP, eds. *Essentials of Pain Medicine*. 3rd ed. Philadelphia, PA: Elsevier Saunders; 2011:85–96.
121. Somogyi AA, Barratt DT, Coller JK. Pharmacogenetics of opioids. *Clin Pharmacol Ther*. 2007;81:429–444.
122. Williams DG, Patel A, Howard RF. Pharmacogenetics of codeine metabolism in an urban population of children and its implications for analgesic reliability. *Br J Anaesth*. 2002;89:839.
123. Vainio A, Ollila J, Matikainen E, et al. Driving ability in cancer patients receiving long-term morphine analgesia. *Lancet*. 1995;346:667.
124. Sabatowski R, Schwalen S, Rettig K, et al. Driving ability under long-term treatment with transdermal fentanyl. *J Pain Symptom Manage*. 2003;25:38.
125. Bruera E, Macmillan K, Hanson J, et al. The cognitive effects of the administration of narcotic analgesics in patients with cancer pain. *Pain*. 1989;39:13.
126. Ballantyne JC, Mao J. Opioid therapy for chronic pain. *N Engl J Med*. 2003; 349:1943.
127. Martell BA, O'Connor PG, Kerns RD, et al. Systematic review: Opioid treatment for chronic back pain: prevalence, efficacy, and association with addiction. *Ann Int Med*. 2007;146:116.
128. Schnitzer TJ, Ferraro A, Hunsche E, et al. A comprehensive review of clinical trials on the efficacy and safety of drugs for the treatment of low back pain. *J Pain Symptom Manage*. 2004;28:72.
129. Max MB, Lynch SA, Muir J, et al. Effects of desipramine, amitriptyline, and fluoxetine on pain in diabetic neuropathy. *N Engl J Med*. 1992;326:1250.
130. Watson CP, Gilron I, Sawynok J, et al. Nontricyclic analgesics and pain: Are serotonin norpeinephrine reuptake inhibitors (SNRIs) any better? *Pain*. 2011;152: 2206–2210.
131. Bombolt SF, Mikkelsen JD, Blackburn-Munro G. Antinoceptive effects of the antidepressants amitriptyline, duloxetine, mirtazapine and citalopram in animal models of acute, persistent and neuropathic pain. *Neuropharmacology*. 2005;48:252.
132. Rashkin J, Pritchett YL, Wang F, et al. A double-blind, randomized multicenter trial comparing duloxetine with placebo in the management of diabetic peripheral neuropathic pain. *Pain Med*. 2005;6:346.
133. Arnold LM, Rosen A, Pritchett YL, et al. A randomized, double-blind, placebo-controlled trial of duloxetine in the treatment of women with fibromyalgia with or without major depressive disorder. *Pain*. 2005;119:5.
134. Clauw DJ, Mease P, Palmer RH, et al. Milnacipran for the treatment of fibromyalgia in adults: A 15-week, multicenter, randomized, double-blind, placebo-controlled, multiple-dose clinical trial. *Clin Ther*. 2008;30:1988–2004.
135. Mease PJ, Clauw DJ, Gendreau RM, et al. The efficacy and safety of milnacipran for treatment of fibromyalgia. A randomized, double-blind, placebo-controlled trial. *J Rheumatol*. 2009;36:398–409.
136. Ramaekers JG. Antidepressants and driver impairment: Empirical evidence from a standard on-the-road test. *J Clin Psychiatr*. 2003;64:20.
137. Sharma U, Griesing T, Emir B, et al. Time to onset of neuropathic pain reduction: A retrospective analysis of data from nine controlled trials of pregabalin for painful diabetic neuropathy and postherpetic neuralgia. *Am J Ther*. 2010;17:577–585.
138. Zakrewska JM, Patsalos PN. Oxcarbazepine: A new drug in the management of intractable trigeminal neuralgia. *J Neurol Neurosurg Psychiatry*. 1989;52:472.
139. Katz NP, Gammaitoni AR, Davis MW, et al. Lidocaine patch 5% reduces pain intensity and interference with quality of life in patients with postherpetic neuralgia: An effectiveness trial. *Pain Med*. 2002;3:324.
140. Campbell BJ, Rowbotham M, Davies PS, et al. Systemic absorption of topical lidocaine in normal volunteers, patients with post-herpetic neuralgia, and patients with acute herpes zoster. *J Pharm Sci*. 2002;91:1343.
141. Rowbotham MC, Davies PS, Verkempinck C, et al. Lidocaine patch: Double-blind controlled study of new treatment method for postherpetic neuralgia. *Pain*. 1996;65:39.
142. Malmberg AB, Mizisin AP, Calcutt NA, et al. Reduced heat sensitivity and epidermal nerve fiber immunostaining following single applications of a high-concentration capsaicin. *Pain*. 2004;11:360–367.
143. Kennedy WR, Vanhove GF, Lu SP, et al. A randomized, controlled, open-label study of the long-term effects of NGX-4010, a high-concentration capsaicin patch, on epidermal nerve fiber density and sensory function in healthy volunteers. *J Pain*. 2010;11:579–587.
144. Backonja M, Wallace MS, Blonsky ER, et al. NGX-4010C116 Study Group. NGX-4010, a high-concentration capsaicin patch, for the treatment of postherpetic neuralgia: a randomised, double-blind study. *Lancet Neurol*. 2008;7:1106–1112.
145. Backonja MM, Malan TP, Vanhove GF, et al. C102/106 Study Group:NGX-4010, a high-concentration capsaicin patch, for the treatment of postherpetic neuralgia: A randomized, double-blind, controlled study with an open-label extension. *Pain Med*. 2010;11:600–608.
146. Simpson DM, Brown S, Tobias J. NGX-4010 C107 Study Group. Controlled trial of high-concentration capsaicin patch for treatment of painful HIV neuropathy. *Neurology*. 2008;70:2305–2313.
147. Simpson DM, Gazda S, Brown S, et al. NGX-4010 C118 Study Group. Long-term safety of NGX-4010, a high-concentration capsaicin patch, in patients with peripheral neuropathic pain. *J Pain Symptom Manage*. 2010;39:1053–1064.
148. Tremont-Lukats IW, Challapalli V, McNicol ED, et al. Systemic administration of local anesthetics to relieve neuropathic pain: A systematic review and meta-analysis. *Anesth Analg*. 2005;101:1738.
149. Boswell MV, Shah RV, Everett CR, et al. Interventional techniques in the management of chronic spinal pain: Evidence-based practice guidelines. *Pain Physician*. 2005;8:1.

150. Derby R, Lee SH, Kim BJ, et al. Pressure-controlled lumbar discography in volunteers without low back symptoms. *Pain Med.* 2005;6:213.
151. Cohen SP, Larkin TM, Barna SA, et al. Lumbar discography: A comprehensive review of outcome studies, diagnostic accuracy, and principles. *Reg Anesth Pain Med.* 2005;30:163.
152. Carragee EJ, Don AS, Hurwitz EL, et al. 2009 ISSLS Prize Winner: Does discography cause accelerated progression of degeneration changes in the lumbar disc: A ten-year matched cohort study. *Spine.* 2009;34:2338–2345.
153. Appleby D, Andersson G, Totta M. Meta-analysis of the efficacy and safety of intradiscal electrothermal therapy (IDET). *Pain Med.* 2006;7:308.
154. Pauza KJ, Howell S, Dreyfuss P, et al. A randomized, placebo-controlled trial of intradiscal electrothermal therapy for the treatment of discogenic low back pain. *Spine J.* 2004;4:27.
155. Andersson GB, Mekhail NA, Block JE. Treatment of intractable discogenic low back pain. A systematic review of spinal fusion and intradiscal electrothermal therapy (IDET). *Pain Physician.* 2006;9:237.
156. Singh V, Derby R. Percutaneous lumbar disc decompression. *Pain Physician.* 2006;9:139.
157. Markman JD, Gaud KG. Lumbar spinal stenosis in older adults: Current understanding and future directions. *Clin Geriatr Med.* 2008;24:369–388.
158. Kalichman L, Cole R, Kim DH, et al. Spinal stenosis prevalence and association with symptoms: The Framingham Study. *Spine J.* 2009;9:545–550.
159. Deer TR, Kapural L. New image-guided ultra-minimally invasive lumbar decompression method: The mild procedure. *Pain Physician.* 2010;13:35–41.
160. Lingreen R, Grider JS. Retrospective review of patient self-reported improvement and post-procedure findings for mild(R) (minimally invasive lumbar decompression). *Pain Physician.* 2010;13:555–560.
161. Chopko BW. A novel method for treatment of lumbar spinal stenosis in high-risk surgical candidates: Pilot study experience with percutaneous remodeling of ligamentum flavum and lamina. *J Neurosurg Spine.* 2011;14:46–50.
162. Philips FM, Wetzel FT, Leiberman I, et al. An *in vivo* comparison of the potential for extravertebral cement leak after vertebroplasty and kyphoplasty. *Spine.* 2002;27:2173.
163. Diamond TH, Champion B, Clark WA. Management of acute osteoporotic vertebral fractures: A nonrandomized trial comparing percutaneous vertebroplasty with conservative therapy. *Am J Med.* 2003;114:257.
164. Perez-Higueras A, Alvarez L, Rossi RE, et al. Percutaneous vertebroplasty: Long term clinical and radiological outcome. *Neuroradiology.* 2002;44:950.
165. Ledlie JT, Renfro MJ. Balloon kyphoplasty: One year outcomes in vertebral body height restoration, chronic pain, and activity levels. *J Neurosurg.* 2003;98:21.
166. Fourney DR, Schomer DF, Nader R, et al. Percutaneous vertebroplasty and kyphoplasty for painful vertebral body fractures in cancer patients. *J Neurosurg.* 2003;98:21.
167. Coumans JV, Reinhardt MK, Lieberman IH. Kyphoplasty for vertebral compression fractures: 1 year clinical outcomes from a prospective study. *J Neurosurg.* 2003;99:44.
168. Buchbinder R, Osborne RH, Ebeling PR, et al. A randomized trial of vertebroplasty for painful osteoporotic vertebral fractures. *N Engl J Med.* 2009;361:557–568.
169. Kallmes DF, Comstock BA, Heagerty PJ, et al. A randomized trial of vertebroplasty for osteoporotic spinal fractures. *N Engl J Med.* 2009;361:569–579.
170. Muijs SP, van Erkel AR, Dijkstra PD. Treatment of painful osteoporotic vertebral compression fractures: A brief review of the evidence for percutaneous vertebroplasty. *J Bone Joint Surg Br.* 2011;93:1149–1153.
171. Wardlaw D, Cummings SR, Van Meirhaeghe J, et al. Efficacy and safety of balloon kyphoplasty compared with non-surgical care for vertebral compression fracture (FREE): A randomised controlled trial. *Lancet.* 2009;373:1016–1024.
172. Berenson J, Pflugmacher R, Jarzem P, et al. Cancer Patient Fracture Evaluation (CAFE) Investigators. Balloon kyphoplasty versus non-surgical fracture management for treatment of painful vertebral body compression fractures in patients with cancer: A multicentre, randomised controlled trial. *Lancet Oncol.* 2011; 12:225–235.
173. Mazars GJ. Intermittent stimulation of nucleus ventralis posterolateralis for intractable pain. *Surg Neurol.* 1975;4:93–95.
174. Linderoth B, Foreman R. Physiology of spinal cord stimulation: Review and update. *Neuromodulation.* 1999;3:150.
175. Hautvast RW. Spinal cord stimulation in chronic intractable angina pectoris: A randomized, controlled efficacy study. *Am Heart J.* 1998;136:1114–1120.
176. Klomp HM. Spinal cord stimulation in critical limb ischemia: A randomized trial: ESES study group. *Lancet.* 1999;353:1040–1044.
177. Burchiel KJ, Anderson VC, Wilson BJ, et al. Prognostic factors of spinal cord stimulation for chronic back and leg pain. *Neurosurgery.* 1995;36:1101.
178. North R, Wetzel T. Spinal cord stimulation for chronic pain of spinal origin. *Spine.* 2002;22:2584.
179. Taylor RS. Spinal cord stimulation in complex regional pain syndrome and refractory neuropathic back and leg pain/failed back surgery syndrome: Results of a systematic review and meta-analysis. *J Pain Sympt Manage.* 2006;31:S13.
180. North RB, Kidd DH, Farrokhi F, et al. Spinal cord stimulation versus repeated lumbosacral spine surgery for chronic pain: A randomized controlled trial. *Neurosurgery.* 2005;51:106.
181. Calvillo O, Racz G, Didie J, et al. Neuroaugmentation in the treatment of complex regional pain syndrome of the upper extremity. *Acta Orthop Belg.* 1998;1:57.
182. Oakley J, Weiner R. Spinal cord stimulation for complex regional pain syndrome: A prospective study of 19 patients at two centers. *Neuromodulation.* 1999;1:47.
183. Kemler MA, Barendse GA, van Kleef M, et al. Spinal cord stimulation in patients with chronic reflex sympathetic dystrophy. *N Engl J Med.* 2000;343:618.
184. Falco FJ, Berger J, Vrable A, et al. Cross talk: A new method for peripheral nerve stimulation: an observational report with cadaveric verification. *Pain Physician.* 2009;12:965–983.
185. Goroszeniuk T, Kothari S, Hamann W. Subcutaneous neuromodulating implant targeted at the site of pain. *Reg Anesth Pain Med.* 2006;31:168–171.
186. Burns B, Watkins L, Goadsby PJ. Treatment of medically intractable cluster headache by occipital nerve stimulation: Long-term follow-up of eight patients. *Lancet.* 2007;369:1099–1106.
187. Eisenach JC, Hood DD, Curry R, et al. Intrathecal but not intravenous opioids release adenosine from the spinal cord. *Pain.* 2004;5:64.
188. Deer T, Krames ES, Hassenbusch SJ, et al. Polyanalgesic consensus conference 2007: Recommendations for the management of pain by intrathecal (intraspinal) drug delivery: Report of an interdisciplinary expert panel. *Neuromodulation.* 2007; 10:300.

CHAPTER

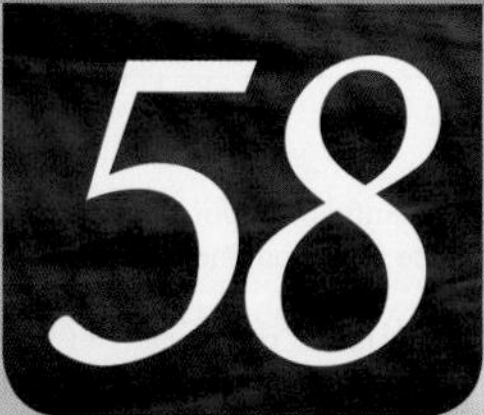

Cardiopulmonary Resuscitation

CHARLES W. OTTO

Key Points

1. Brain adenosine triphosphate is depleted after 4 to 6 minutes of no blood flow. It returns nearly to normal within 6 minutes of starting effective cardiopulmonary resuscitation (CPR).
2. Through living wills and other instruments, patients have begun placing limitations on medical treatment to include do not resuscitate orders.
3. The major components of resuscitation from cardiac arrest are airway, breathing, circulation, drugs, and electrical therapy (ABCDE).
4. Two theories for the mechanism of blood flow during closed-chest compression have been suggested: cardiac pump and thoracic pump.
5. During CPR, myocardial perfusion is 20% to 50% of normal, whereas cerebral perfusion is maintained at 50% to 90% of normal.
6. CPR has limited success, with only approximately 40% of victims being admitted to the hospital and 10% surviving to discharge.
7. End-tidal carbon dioxide has been found to be an excellent noninvasive guide to the adequacy of closed-chest compressions.
8. Effective uninterrupted chest compressions and defibrillation, if appropriate, should take precedence over medications.
9. Although there is some evidence of improved early resuscitation in humans, there is no strong evidence that vasopressors improve long-term survival in human cardiac arrest.
10. After vasopressors, the drugs most likely to be of benefit during CPR are those that help suppress ectopic ventricular rhythms.
11. Ventricular fibrillation is the most common electrocardiogram pattern found during witnessed sudden cardiac arrest in adults.
12. Untreated ventricular fibrillation is a time-sensitive model with three phases: electrical, circulatory, and metabolic.
13. Arrest is less likely to be a sudden event and more likely related to progressive deterioration of respiratory and circulatory function in the pediatric age group.
14. For optimal outcome, successful restoration of spontaneous circulation must be followed by correction of reversible causes of arrest, including immediate coronary reperfusion and aggressive supportive care.

Multimedia

1 Adult Bradycardia Algorithm

2 Tachycardia Algorithm

Treatment of cardiac and respiratory arrest is an integral part of anesthesia practice. The American Board of Anesthesiology indicates in its *Booklet of Information* that the "clinical management and teaching of cardiac, pulmonary and neurologic resuscitation" are some of the activities that define the specialty of anesthesiology. The cardiopulmonary physiology and pharmacology that form the basis of anesthesia practice are applicable to treating the victim of cardiac arrest. However, there is specialized knowledge relating to blood flow, ventilation, and pharmacology under the conditions of a cardiac arrest that must be understood to maintain leadership of the modern cardiopulmonary resuscitation (CPR) team. This chapter concentrates on those aspects of CPR that are different from the more common circumstances requiring cardiovascular support (e.g., shock, dysrhythmias).

HISTORY

Anesthesiologists have contributed many of the elements of modern CPR and continue to be active investigators and teachers in the field. Discoveries leading to current CPR practice have a long history recorded in many famous works.[1,2] The earliest reference may be the Bible story of Elisha breathing life back into the son of a Shunammite woman (2 Kings 4:34). In 1543, Andreas Vesalius[3] described tracheotomy and artificial ventilation. William Harvey's manual manipulation of the heart is well known. Early teaching of resuscitation was organized by the Society for the Recovery of Persons Apparently Drowned, founded in London in 1774. The combined techniques of modern CPR developed primarily from the fortuitous assemblage of innovative clinicians and researchers in Baltimore in the 1950s and early 1960s. Building on the long history of contributions from around the world, these investigators laid the framework for current CPR practice. In the late 1950s, mouth-to-mouth ventilation was established as the only effective means of artificial ventilation.[4–7] The internal defibrillator was developed in 1933,[8] but it was not applied successfully until 1947.[9] It was another decade before general use was made possible by the development of external cross-chest defibrillation.[10,11] Despite these advances, widespread resuscitation from cardiac arrest was not possible until Kouwenhoven et al.[12] described success with closed-chest cardiac massage in a series of patients. The final major component of modern CPR was added in 1963, when Redding and Pearson[13] described the improved success obtained by administering vasopressor drugs.

SCOPE OF THE PROBLEM

Cardiovascular disease remains the most common cause of death in the industrialized world. Although cardiovascular mortality has been declining in the United States since the mid-1960s, >35% of all deaths are due to cardiovascular causes.[14] Of the 860,000 annual cardiovascular deaths, approximately half are related to coronary artery disease, the majority are sudden deaths and 70% occur out of the hospital or in hospital emergency departments. Thus, CPR teaching and research tend to focus on myocardial ischemia as the primary cause of cardiac arrest. However, anesthesiologists are more likely than other practitioners to deal with causes other than myocardial infarction. CPR is symptomatic therapy, aimed at sustaining vital organ function until natural cardiac function is restored. The details of effective resuscitation technique are important. However, search for a remediable cause of the arrest must not be lost in excessive attention to mechanics.

1 Brain adenosine triphosphate (ATP) is depleted after 4 to 6 minutes of no blood flow. It returns nearly to normal within 6 minutes of starting effective CPR. Studies in animals suggest that good neurologic outcome may be possible from 10- to 15-minute periods of normothermic cardiac arrest if good circulation is promptly restored.[15,16] In clinical practice, the severity of the underlying cardiac disease is the major determining factor in the success or failure of resuscitation attempts. Of those factors under control of the rescuers, poor outcomes are associated with long arrest times before CPR is begun, prolonged ventricular fibrillation (VF) without definitive therapy, and inadequate coronary and cerebral perfusion during cardiac massage. CPR begun by bystanders can more than double survival.[17] However, bystanders provide CPR only 25% to 30% of the time in sudden cardiac arrest. Optimum outcome from VF is obtained only if basic life support is begun within 4 minutes of arrest and defibrillation applied within 8 minutes.[18] The importance of early defibrillation has been known for decades and is emphasized in CPR practice.[19,20] What is not as well recognized is the tendency to interrupt chest compressions frequently during a resuscitation attempt. Studies of emergency medical systems suggest that chest compressions are performed <50% of the time during a typical out-of-hospital resuscitation, being interrupted for pulse checks, intubations, starting intravenous catheters, defibrillation attempts, and moving the victim.[21] Because blood flow falls rapidly with cessation of compressions and resumes slowly with reinstitution of compressions, these interruptions are a major contributor to poor survival rates.

With an effective rapid-response emergency medical system, initial resuscitation rates of 40% and survival to hospital discharge of 10% to 15% are possible after out-of-hospital arrests,[18,20] although the median reported survival to discharge with any first recorded rhythm is 6.4%.[22] Rates for survival to discharge from in-hospital arrest are about 18% in adults and 27% in children.[23] Within the hospital, the operating room is the location where CPR has the highest rate of success. Cardiac arrest occurs approximately 7 times for every 10,000 anesthetics.[24] The cause for the arrest is anesthesia related, approximately 4.5 times for every 10,000 anesthetics, but mortality from these arrests is only 0.4 per 10,000 anesthetics. Thus, resuscitation is successful approximately 90% of the time in anesthesia-related cardiac arrests.

ETHICAL ISSUES: DO NOT RESUSCITATE ORDERS IN THE OPERATING ROOM

Although institution of CPR is standard medical care when an individual is found pulseless, terminally ill patients have become increasingly concerned about inappropriate application of life-
2 sustaining procedures, including CPR. Through living wills and other instruments, patients have begun placing limitations on medical treatment to include do not resuscitate (DNR) orders. Such requests are generally accepted, even welcomed, by health care workers. However, the operating room is one area of the hospital where DNR orders continue to cause ethical conflicts between medical personnel and patients.[25,26] There are ethically sound arguments on both sides of the issue as to whether DNR orders should be upheld in the operating room.

The patient's right to limit medical treatment, including refusing CPR, is firmly established in modern medical practice based on the ethical principle of respect for patient autonomy. A terminally ill patient can reject heroic measures such as resuscitation and still choose palliative therapy. If a surgical intervention will ameliorate symptoms or improve quality of life, there is no reason to withhold this treatment. Operative intervention increases the risk of cardiac arrest, and the patient may not want the burden of surviving in a worse condition than preoperatively. The possibility of death under anesthesia may be viewed as especially peaceful. Thus, the time that the DNR order provides the greatest protection against unwanted intervention is during surgery.

Despite these rather strong arguments for treating a DNR status in the operating room the same way it is treated elsewhere in the hospital, many operating room personnel are at least a little uneasy caring for these patients. Many surgeons require that DNR orders be suspended during the perioperative period or assume consent to surgery includes such suspension. There are multiple reasons for the reluctance to accept DNR status during surgery and anesthesia. Approximately 75% of cardiac arrests in the operating room are related to a surgical or anesthetic complication, and resuscitative attempts are highly successful.[24] Ethically, surgeons and anesthesiologists feel responsible for what happens to patients in the operating room: *primum non nocere* (first, do no harm). Although the physicians are highly diligent in monitoring and managing changes in the patient's status, complications and arrests do occur. Honoring a DNR order under these circumstances is frequently viewed as failure to treat a reversible process, and hence, tantamount to killing. This is an ethically sound view if the cause of arrest is readily identifiable and easily reversible and if treatment is likely to allow the patient to fulfill the objectives of coming to surgery.[25]

Institutionally, these ethical conflicts should be addressed by adoption of clear policies by hospitals.[27] For the individual patient, conflicts can be resolved by communication among the patient, family, and caregivers. A mutual decision can often be reached to suspend or severely limit a DNR order in the perioperative period if the patient understands the special circumstances of perioperative arrest, that interventions are brief and usually successful, and that the physicians support the patient's goals in coming to surgery and values in desiring not to prolong death. Many interventions commonly used in the operating room (mechanical ventilation, vasopressors, antidysrhythmics, blood products) may be considered forms of resuscitation in other situations. The only modalities that are not routine anesthetic care are cardiac massage and defibrillation. Therefore, the specific interventions included in a DNR status must be clarified with specific allowance made for methods necessary to perform anesthesia and surgery.

COMPONENTS OF RESUSCITATION

3 The major components of resuscitation from cardiac arrest are airway, breathing, circulation, drugs, and electrical therapy (ABCDE). Traditionally, these have been divided into basic life support (BLS) for those elements that can be performed without additional equipment—basic airway management, rescue breathing, and manual chest compressions (Fig. 58-1)—and advanced cardiac life support (ACLS), encompassing all the cognitive and technical skills necessary for resuscitation (Fig. 58-2). The lines between BLS and ACLS have tended to blur recently with the

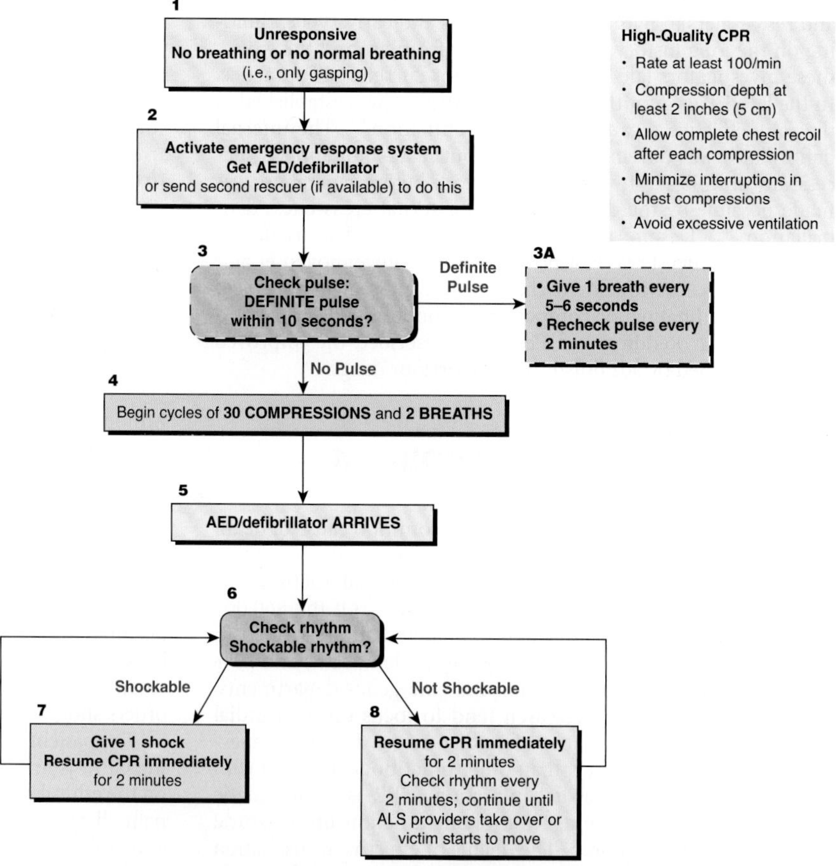

FIGURE 58-1. Adult basic life support (BLS) health care provider algorithm. AED, automatic external defibrillator; CPR, cardiopulmonary resuscitation; ALS, advanced life support. (From 2010 American Heart Association Guidelines for cardiopulmonary resuscitation and emergency cardiovascular care. *Circulation*. 2010;122(Suppl3): S689, with permission.)

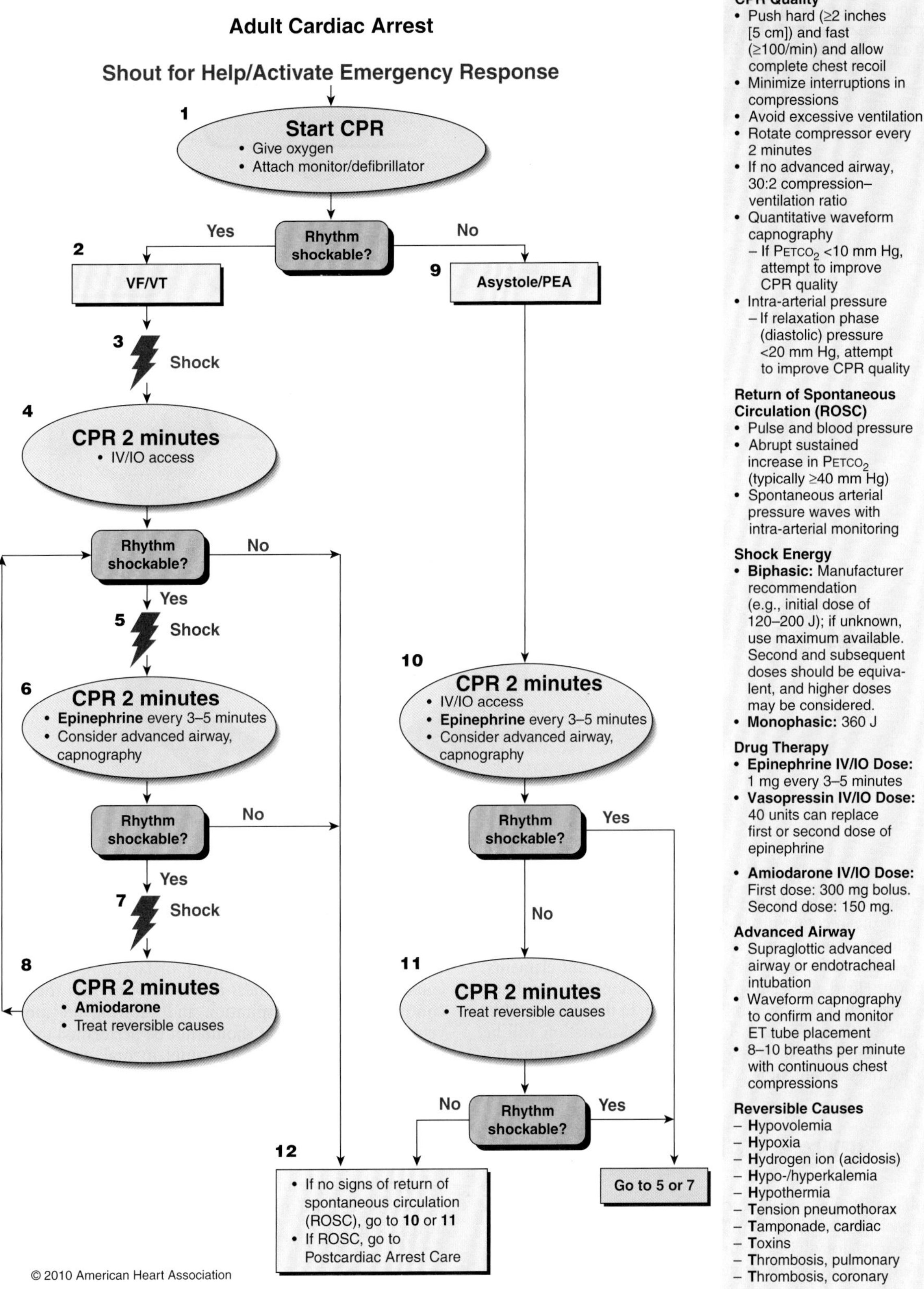

FIGURE 58-2. Adult advanced cardiac life support (ACLS) cardiac arrest algorithm. CPR, cardiopulmonary resuscitation; VF, ventricular fibrillation; VT, ventricular tachycardia; PEA, pulseless electrical activity; IV, intravenous(ly); IO, intraosseous(ly); ROSC, return of spontaneous circulation; $PetCO_2$, partial pressure of end tidal carbon dioxide; J, joules. (From 2010 American Heart Association Guidelines for cardiopulmonary resuscitation and emergency cardiovascular care. *Circulation.* 2010;122(Suppl 3):S736, with permission.)

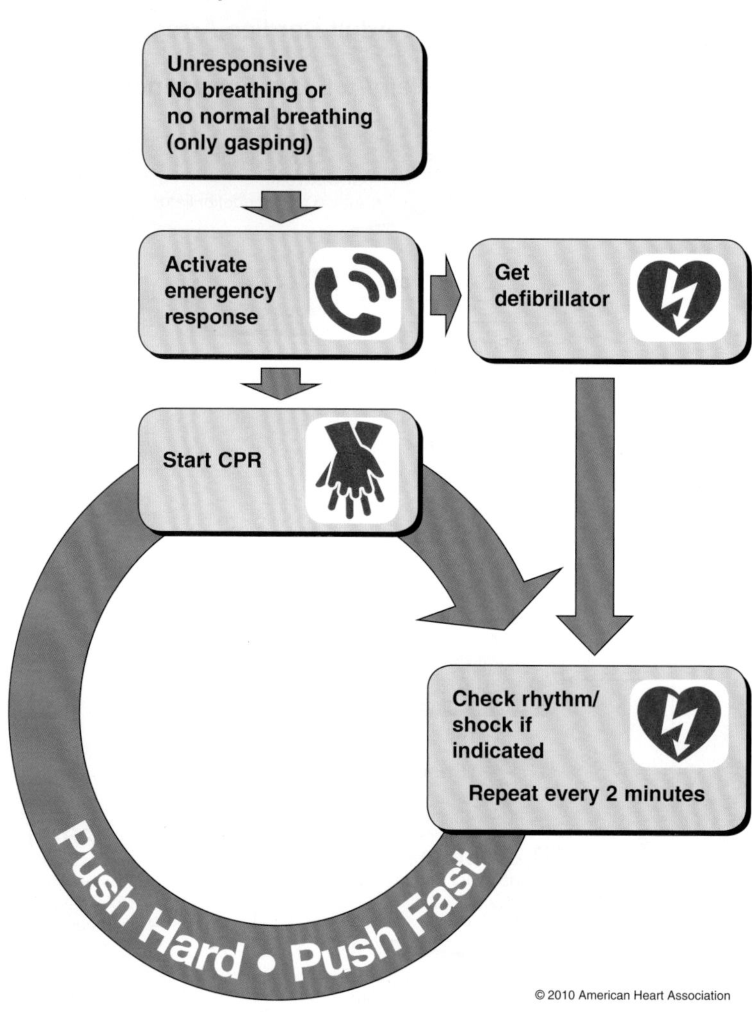

FIGURE 58-3. Simplified adult basic life support algorithm. (From 2010 American Heart Association Guidelines for cardiopulmonary resuscitation and emergency cardiovascular care. *Circulation.* 2010;122(Suppl 3):S687, with permission.)

introduction of public-access automatic external defibrillators (AEDs) and the recognition that careful attention to uninterrupted, effective chest compressions improves outcome more than any advanced therapy. To stress these important elements, the American Heart Association (AHA) has adopted a simplified adult BLS algorithm as shown in Figure 58-3. In the following sections, each of the components involved in resuscitation will be reviewed separately, followed by a discussion of combining the elements for the best outcome.

AIRWAY MANAGEMENT

The problem of airway obstruction caused by the tongue in the unconscious patient is familiar to the anesthesiologist. The techniques used for airway maintenance during anesthesia are applicable to the cardiac arrest victim. The primary method recommended to the public is the same head tilt–chin lift method commonly employed in the operating room.[28] The head is extended by pressure applied to the brow while the mandible is pulled forward by pressure on the front of the jaw, lifting the tongue away from the posterior pharynx. The jaw thrust maneuver (applying pressure behind the rami of the mandible) is an effective alternative. Properly inserted oropharyngeal or nasopharyngeal airways can be useful before intubation, recognizing the danger of inducing vomiting or laryngospasm in the semiconscious victim. Tracheal intubation provides the best airway control, preventing aspiration and allowing the most effective ventilation. However, it should not be performed until adequate ventilation (preferably with supplemental oxygen) and chest compressions have been established. A number of alternative airways designed for blind placement have been described and the laryngeal mask airway and the esophageal-tracheal Combitube (see Chapter 27) have been recommended for use during cardiac arrest by individuals who are not skilled laryngoscopists.[29] When other methods of establishing an airway are unsuccessful, translaryngeal ventilation or tracheotomy by cricothyroid puncture may be necessary.

Foreign Body Airway Obstruction

In 2004, unintentional choking or suffocation accounted for 5,891 deaths in the United States (approximately 0.2% of all deaths) and 725 of the victims were <1 year old.[14] Airway occlusion by a foreign object must be considered in any victim who suddenly stops breathing and becomes cyanotic and unconscious. It occurs most commonly during eating and is usually due to food, especially meat, impacting the laryngeal inlet, at the epiglottis or in the vallecula. Sudden death in restaurants from this cause is frequently mistaken for myocardial infarction, leading to the label cafe coronary. Poorly chewed pieces of food, poor dentition or dentures, and elevated blood alcohol levels are the most common factors contributing to choking. The signs of total airway obstruction are the lack of air movement despite respiratory efforts and the inability of the victim to speak or cough. Cyanosis, unconsciousness, and cardiac arrest follow quickly. Partial airway obstruction will result in rasping or wheezing respirations accompanied by coughing. If the victim has good air movement and is able to cough forcefully, no intervention is indicated. However, if the cough weakens or cyanosis develops, the patient must be treated as if there were complete obstruction.

Mothers and friends have been pounding on the backs of choking victims for centuries. In 1974, Heimlich[30] proposed abdominal thrusts as a better method of relieving airway obstruction and, in 1976, Guildner et al.[31] reported that sternal thrusts were just as effective. Subsequently, there were multiple studies of these maneuvers. In clinical practice, Redding[32] observed that no maneuver was always successful and that each occasionally was successful when another had failed. To minimize confusion from teaching multiple techniques, the AHA has elected to emphasize the abdominal thrust maneuver (with chest thrusts as an alternative for the pregnant and massively obese).[29] This recommendation is made on the twofold premise that the abdominal thrust is at least as effective as other techniques and that teaching one method simplifies education.

For the awake victim, abdominal thrusts are applied in the erect position (sitting or standing). The rescuer reaches around the victim from behind, placing the fist of one hand in the epigastrium between the xiphoid and umbilicus. The fist is grasped with the other hand and pressed into the epigastrium with a quick upward thrust. In the unconscious, thrusts are applied by kneeling astride the victim, placing the heel of one hand in the epigastrium and the other on top of the first hand. Care must be taken to ensure the xiphoid is not pushed into the abdominal contents and that the thrust is in the midline. Sternal thrusts are valuable in the massively obese or in women in advanced pregnancy. In the erect victim, the chest is encircled from behind as in the abdominal maneuver but the fist is placed in the midsternum. For the unconscious, thrusts are applied from the side of the supine victim with a hand position the same as for external cardiac compression. Back blows are applied directly over the thoracic spine between the scapulae. They must be delivered with force. Placing the victim in a head-down position (e.g., leaning over a chair) may help move the obstruction into the pharynx.

Whatever technique is used, each individual maneuver must be delivered as if it will relieve the obstruction. If the first attempt is unsuccessful, repeated attempts should be made because hypoxia-related muscular relaxation may eventually allow success. Complications of thrust maneuvers include laceration of the liver and spleen, gastric rupture, fractured ribs, and regurgitation.

In the unconscious victim, manual dislodgement of the obstruction should be tried only if solid material can be seen obstructing the airway. Grasping the object under direct visualization with a Magill forceps or ordinary instrument (e.g., ice tongs) may be used. Care must be taken not to push the foreign body deeper into the larynx. Blind finger sweeps and blind grasping with instruments are rarely successful and may cause damage to tonsils or other tissue. Finally, if the object cannot be dislodged, a cricothyroidotomy can be lifesaving.

VENTILATION

The standard approach to the unresponsive victim is to follow opening the airway with ventilation. When ventilation is provided in the rescue setting, mouth-to-mouth or mouth-to-nose ventilation is the most expeditious and effective method immediately available. Although inspired gas with this method will contain approximately 4% carbon dioxide and only approximately 17% oxygen (composition of exhaled air), it is sufficient to maintain viability.

Physiology of Ventilation During Cardiopulmonary Resuscitation

In the absence of an endotracheal tube, the distribution of gas between the lungs and stomach during positive pressure ventilation will be determined by the relative impedance to flow into each (i.e., the opening pressure of the esophagus and the lung–thorax compliance). It is likely that esophageal opening pressure during cardiac arrest is no more than that found in anesthetized individuals (approximately 20 cm water [H_2O]), and lung–thorax compliance is likely reduced. To avoid gastric insufflation, inspiratory airway pressures must be kept low.

Insufflation of air into the stomach during CPR leads to gastric distention, impeding ventilation and increasing the risk of regurgitation and gastric rupture. Avoiding gastric insufflation requires that peak inspiratory airway pressures stay below esophageal opening pressure. Partial airway obstruction by the tongue and pharyngeal tissues is a major cause of increased airway pressure contributing to gastric insufflation during CPR. Meticulous attention to airway management is necessary during rescue breathing. Recommended tidal volumes to cause a noticeable rise in the chest wall in most adults is 0.5 to 0.6 L. Each rescue breath should be given over 1 second during a pause in chest compressions.

Techniques of Rescue Breathing

While maintaining an open airway with the head tilt–jaw lift technique, the hand on the forehead pinches the nose, the rescuer takes a normal breath and seals the victim's mouth with the lips and exhales, watching for the chest to rise, indicating effective ventilation. For exhalation, the rescuer's mouth is removed from the victim, and the rescuer listens for escaping air while taking a breath. When both hands are being used in the jaw thrust maneuver of opening the airway, the cheek is used to seal the nose. For mouth-to-nose ventilation, the rescuer's lips surround the nose and the victim's lips are held closed. In some patients, the mouth must be allowed to open for exhalation with this technique. Give one breath over 1 second, take a normal breath, and give a second breath over 1 second. During CPR in adults and one-rescuer CPR in children, a pause for two breaths should be made after each 30 chest compressions. When there are two rescuers with a child victim, a pause for two breaths should be made after each 15 compressions.[29]

Several adjuncts to ventilation are available. Perhaps the most useful adjunct is a common mask, such as that used for anesthesia. The mask can be applied to the face and held in place with the thumbs and index fingers while the other fingers are used to apply jaw thrust. Breathing into the connector port of the mask provides ventilation. Mouth-to-mask ventilation may be more aesthetic than mouth-to-mouth ventilation and can be just as effective in trained hands. Masks are also available with one-way valves that direct the victim's exhaled gas away from the rescuer. Masks with integral nipple adapters are useful for providing supplemental oxygen. An oxygen flow of 10 L/min can raise the inspired concentration to 50%.

The self-inflating resuscitation bag and mask are the most common adjuncts used in rescue vehicles and hospitals. Although these devices have the advantages of noncontact and an ability to use supplemental oxygen, they have been shown to be difficult for a single rescuer to apply properly, preventing substantial gas leak while maintaining a patent airway.[33] Tidal volumes with mouth-to-mouth and mouth-to-mask ventilation are often greater than those with the resuscitation bag. It is now recommended that if this device is to be used, two individuals manage the airway: one to hold the mask and maintain head position and one to squeeze the bag, using both hands.[34] The self-inflating resuscitation bag can also be used with the laryngeal mask airway and the esophageal-tracheal Combitube.

Finally, tracheal intubation provides the best control of ventilation. With an endotracheal tube in place, breathing can proceed without concern for gastric distention or synchronizing ventilation with chest compressions. Blood flow during CPR slows rapidly when chest compressions are stopped and recovers slowly when they are resumed. Consequently, intubation should be accomplished without stopping chest compressions, if possible. Following intubation, no pause should be made for ventilation, and ventilation should be delivered without regard for the compression cycle.

CIRCULATION

Physiology of Circulation During Closed-chest Compression

4 Two theories of the mechanism of blood flow during closed-chest compression have been suggested.[12,35] They are not mutually exclusive, and which mechanism predominates in humans continues to be debated.

Cardiac Pump Mechanism

The cardiac pump mechanism was originally proposed by Kouwenhoven et al.[12] and Jude et al.[36] According to this theory, pressure on the chest compresses the heart between the sternum and the spine. Compression raises the pressure in the ventricular chambers, closing the atrioventricular valves and ejecting blood into the lungs and aorta. During the relaxation phase of closed-chest compression, expansion of the thoracic cage causes a subatmospheric intrathoracic pressure, facilitating blood return. The mitral and tricuspid valves open, allowing blood to fill the ventricles. Pressure in the aorta causes aortic valve closure and coronary artery perfusion.

Thoracic Pump Mechanism

In 1976, Criley et al.[37] reported a patient undergoing cardiac catheterization who simultaneously developed VF and an episode of cough-hiccups. With every cough-hiccup, a significant arterial pressure was noted. This observation of self-administered "cough CPR" prompted further investigations on the mechanism of blood flow, and these studies produced the theory of a thoracic pump mechanism for blood flow during closed-chest compressions.[35] According to this theory, blood flows into the thorax during the relaxation phase of chest compressions in the same manner as that described for the cardiac pump mechanism. During the compression phase, all intrathoracic structures are compressed equally by the rise in intrathoracic pressure caused by sternal depression, forcing blood out of the chest. Backward flow through the venous system is prevented by valves in the subclavian and internal jugular veins and by dynamic compression of the veins at the thoracic outlet by the increased intrathoracic pressure. Thicker, less compressible vessel walls prevent collapse on the arterial side, although arterial collapse will occur if intrathoracic pressure is raised enough.[38] The heart is a passive conduit with the atrioventricular valves remaining open during chest compression. Because there is a significant pressure difference between the carotid artery and jugular vein, blood flow to the head is favored. The lack of valves in the inferior vena cava results in less resistance to backward flow, and pressures in the arteries and veins below the diaphragm are nearly equal. This is consistent with the fact that there is little blood flow to organs below the diaphragm.[39,40]

It seems clear that fluctuations in intrathoracic pressure play a significant role in blood flow during CPR. It is also likely that compression of the heart occurs under some circumstances. Factors that influence the mechanism probably include the compliance and configuration of the chest wall, size of the heart, force of the sternal compressions, duration of cardiac arrest, and other undiscovered factors. Which mechanism predominates varies from victim to victim and even during the resuscitation of the same victim.

Distribution of Blood Flow During Cardiopulmonary Resuscitation

Whatever the predominant mechanism, total body blood flow (cardiac output) is reduced to 10% to 33% of normal during experimental closed-chest cardiac massage. Similar severe reductions in flow are likely during clinical CPR in humans. Nearly all the blood flow is directed to organs above the diaphragm.[39,40]
5 Myocardial perfusion is 20% to 50% of normal, whereas cerebral perfusion is maintained at 50% to 90% of normal. Abdominal visceral and lower extremity flow is reduced to 5% of normal. Total flow tends to decrease with time during CPR, but the relative distribution is not altered. Changes in CPR technique and the use of epinephrine may help sustain cardiac output over time.[40] Epinephrine improves flow to the brain and heart, whereas flow to organs below the diaphragm is unchanged or further reduced.

Gas Transport During Cardiopulmonary Resuscitation

During the low flow state of CPR, excretion of carbon dioxide (CO_2) (milliliters of CO_2 per minute in exhaled gas) is decreased from prearrest levels to approximately the same extent that cardiac output is reduced. This reduced CO_2 excretion is due primarily to shunting of blood flow away from the lower half of the body. The exhaled CO_2 reflects only the metabolism of the part of the body that is being perfused. In the nonperfused areas, CO_2 accumulates during CPR. When normal circulation is restored, the accumulated CO_2 is washed out, and a temporary increase in CO_2 excretion is seen.

Although CO_2 excretion is reduced during CPR, measurement of blood gases reveals an arterial respiratory alkalosis and a venous respiratory acidosis with a markedly elevated arteriovenous CO_2 difference.[41] The primary cause of these changes is the severely reduced cardiac output. Two factors account for the elevation of the venous partial pressure of CO_2 ($PvCO_2$). Buffering acid causes a reduction in serum bicarbonate, so the same blood CO_2 content results in a higher $PvCO_2$. In addition, the mixed venous CO_2 content is elevated. When flow to a tissue is reduced, all the CO_2 produced fails to be removed and CO_2 accumulates, raising the tissue partial pressure of CO_2. This allows more CO_2 to be carried in each aliquot of blood, and mixed venous CO_2 content increases. If flow remains constant, a new equilibrium is established in which all CO_2 produced in the tissue is removed but at a higher venous CO_2 content and partial pressure. In contrast to the venous blood, arterial CO_2 content and partial pressure ($PaCO_2$) are usually reduced during CPR. This reduction accounts for most of the observed increase in arteriovenous CO_2 content difference. Although venous blood may have an increased CO_2, the marked reduction in cardiac output with maintained ventilation results in efficient CO_2 removal.

Decreased pulmonary blood flow during CPR causes a lack of perfusion to many nondependent alveoli. The alveolar gas of these lung units has no CO_2. Consequently, mixed alveolar CO_2 (i.e., end-tidal CO_2) will be low and correlate poorly with arterial CO_2. However, end-tidal CO_2 does correlate well with cardiac output during CPR. As flow increases, more alveoli become perfused, there is less alveolar dead space, and end-tidal CO_2 measurements rise.

Technique of Closed-chest Compression

Cardiac arrest should be assumed in an unresponsive individual with abnormal or absent breathing. The community or institution emergency response system should immediately be activated and chest compressions begun. In emergency circumstances, it is difficult to detect a pulse, even in a major artery (carotid, femoral, axillary). No more than 10 seconds should be taken to check for a pulse and, if a pulse is not definitely felt, chest compressions should be started. Witnessed sudden collapse with unresponsiveness in an adult in the absence of seizure activity is nearly always dysrhythmic cardiac arrest, and chest compressions should be started immediately.

Important considerations in performing closed-chest compressions are the position of the rescuer relative to the victim, the position of the rescuer's hands, and the rate and force of compression. The victim must be supine, the head level with the heart, for adequate brain perfusion. The victim must be on a firm surface. The rescuer should stand or kneel next to the victim's side. Compressions are performed most effectively if the rescuer's hips are on the same level, or slightly above the level of, the victim's chest.

Standard technique consists of the rhythmic application of pressure over the lower half of the sternum. The heel of one hand is placed on the lower sternum, and the other hand is placed on top of the first one. Great care must be taken to avoid pressing the xiphoid into the abdomen, which can lacerate the liver. Even with properly performed CPR, costochondral separation and rib fractures are common. Applying pressure on the ribs by improper hand placement increases these complications and risks puncturing the lung. Pressure on the sternum should be applied through the heel of the hand only, keeping the fingers free of the chest wall. The direction of force must be straight down on the sternum, with the arms straight and the elbows locked into position so the entire weight of the upper body is used to apply force. Inadequate chest recoil due to leaning on the chest during the relaxation phase has been demonstrated to be both common and deleterious to effective chest compressions. During relaxation, care must be taken to remove all pressure from the chest wall, but the hands should not lose contact with the chest wall.

The sternum must be depressed at least 2 inches (5 cm) in the average adult. Occasionally, deeper compressions are necessary to generate a palpable pulse. The duration of compression should be equal to that of relaxation, and the compression rate should be at least 100 times per minute. Push hard and push fast, minimizing interruptions in chest compressions. Allow a brief pause for two 1-second breaths after every 30 compressions. With an advanced airway in place, ventilations at a rate of 8 to 10 breaths per minute should be interposed between compressions without a pause.

Alternative Methods of Circulatory Support

6 As currently practiced, CPR has limited success, with only approximately 40% of victims being admitted to the hospital and 10% surviving to discharge. Despite the occasional success of prolonged resuscitation, standard CPR will sustain most patients for only 15 to 30 minutes. If return of spontaneous circulation has not been achieved in that time, the outcome is dismal. Recognition of these limits and improved understanding of circulatory physiology during CPR have led to several proposals for alternatives to the standard techniques of closed-chest compression. Most, but not all, are based on the thoracic pump mechanism of blood flow. The goals of the new methods are to provide better hemodynamics during CPR and thus improve survival and/or to extend the duration during which CPR can successfully support viability. Unfortunately, none of the alternatives has proved reliably superior to the standard technique.

Simultaneous Ventilation–Compression Cardiopulmonary Resuscitation and Abdominal Binding

According to the thoracic pump theory, elevation of intrathoracic pressure during chest compression should improve blood flow and pressure.[38] Studies with techniques that raise intrathoracic pressure (abdominal binding, simultaneous ventilation–compression) demonstrate that the elevated aortic pressure is offset by similar elevations in right atrial and intracranial pressures, so no improvement in myocardial or cerebral blood flow is found. Most important, survival from cardiac arrest is not improved when these techniques are compared with standard CPR in experimental animals or limited human trials.[42–44]

Interposed Abdominal Compression Cardiopulmonary Resuscitation

Interposed abdominal compression (IAC) is fundamentally different from abdominal binding. With this technique, an additional rescuer applies abdominal compressions manually during the relaxation phase of chest compression.[45] Abdominal pressure is released when chest compression begins. One large randomized trial of out-of-hospital cardiac arrest with IAC CPR found no improvement in survival compared with standard CPR,[46] but a subsequent in-hospital study demonstrated improved outcome.[47] The safety of IAC CPR has been established and is recommended as an alternative to standard CPR for in-hospital resuscitation. Further studies will be needed to establish out-of-hospital efficacy.

Load-distributing Band Cardiopulmonary Resuscitation or Pneumatic Vest Cardiopulmonary Resuscitation

Following the description of "cough CPR" and the development of the thoracic pump theory, a pneumatic vest device was developed that would simulate the events of vigorous coughing.[48]

The technique continues to be investigated with a number of modifications from the original method. Most active investigations use a circumferential chest-compression device composed of a pneumatically or electronically actuated constricting band and backboard. In a preliminary clinical study, aortic and coronary perfusion pressure was better with load-distributing band CPR than with standard CPR.[49] Additional studies are ongoing.

Active Compression–Decompression Cardiopulmonary Resuscitation

The newest proposed alternative technique developed from the anecdotal report of CPR is performed with a plumber's helper applied to the anterior chest wall.[50] This suggested that active decompression of the chest wall might reduce intrathoracic pressure during the relaxation phase of chest compressions, leading to improved venous return, increased stroke volume with compression, and better blood flow. A suction device that can be applied to the chest wall to enable active compression and decompression was developed.[51] Hemodynamic studies in animals and humans with this technique have shown that coronary and cerebral perfusion may be somewhat improved with this method compared with standard CPR, although when epinephrine is used there is no difference between techniques.[51,52] Clinical trials of this technique have had mixed results, with four studies showing improved outcome and five showing no positive or negative effects. No survival benefit of active compression–decompression CPR over standard CPR was found in a meta-analysis of 10 trials involving 4,162 patients in the out-of-hospital setting and in a meta-analysis of two trials involving 826 patients in the in-hospital setting.[53]

Impedance Threshold Device

The impedance threshold device (ITD) is a valve that impedes air entry into the lungs during chest recoil of the relaxation phase of chest compressions, thus reducing intrathoracic pressure and increasing venous return to the thorax. Originally designed to be used with a cuffed endotracheal tube and active compression–decompression CPR (during which it would act to further increase the venous return of active decompression),[54] it has recently been used with conventional CPR and a tight-fitting face mask.[55] Two randomized trials of out-of-hospital cardiac arrest comparing conventional CPR and the ITD with active compression–decompression CPR have shown improvement in short-term resuscitation.[54,56] One randomized trial of 8,718 out-of-hospital cardiac arrest victims undergoing standard CPR with an active versus sham ITD found no difference in short-term or long-term outcomes.[57] Although improved long-term survival has not been demonstrated, the ITD may be a useful adjunct for professionals trained in its use.

Invasive Techniques

In contrast to the closed-chest techniques, two invasive methods have been able to maintain cardiac and cerebral viability during long periods of cardiac arrest. In animal models, open-chest cardiac massage and cardiopulmonary bypass (through the femoral artery and vein using a membrane oxygenator) can provide better hemodynamics, as well as better myocardial and cerebral perfusion, than closed-chest techniques.[58] Prompt restoration of blood flow and perfusion pressure with cardiopulmonary bypass can provide resuscitation with minimal neurologic deficit after 20 minutes of fibrillatory cardiac arrest in canines.[15] However, these techniques must be instituted relatively early (probably within 20 to 30 minutes of arrest) to be effective.[16,59] If open-chest massage is begun after 30 minutes of ineffective closed-chest compressions, survival is no better, although hemodynamics are improved.[60] The need to apply these maneuvers early in an arrest obviously limits the application. Before invasive procedures play a greater role in modern CPR, a method must be developed to predict, early in resuscitation, which patients will and will not respond to closed-chest compressions.

Assessing the Adequacy of Circulation During Cardiopulmonary Resuscitation

The adequacy of closed-chest compression is frequently judged by palpation of a pulse in the carotid or femoral vessels. The palpable pulse primarily reflects systolic pressure. Cardiac output correlates better with mean pressure and coronary perfusion with diastolic pressure. In the femoral area, the palpable pulse is as likely to be venous as arterial. Whenever possible, more accurate means of monitoring the efficacy of chest compressions should be used. The importance of monitoring CPR quality is stressed in the new AHA ACLS circular algorithm (Fig. 58-4).

Return of spontaneous circulation with an arrested heart greatly depends on restoring oxygenated blood flow to the myocardium. In experimental models, a minimum blood flow of 15 to 20 mL/min/100 g of myocardium has been shown to be necessary for successful resuscitation.[61] Obtaining such flow depends on closed-chest compressions developing adequate cardiac output and coronary perfusion pressure. Similar to the beating heart, coronary perfusion during CPR occurs primarily in the relaxation phase (diastole) of chest compressions. In 1906, Crile and Dolley[62] suggested that a critical coronary perfusion pressure was necessary for successful resuscitation. This concept has been confirmed in numerous other reports.[40,61–71] During standard CPR, critical myocardial blood flow is associated with aortic diastolic pressure exceeding 40 mm Hg. Because right atrial pressure can be elevated with some techniques, the aortic diastolic pressure minus the right atrial diastolic pressure is a more accurate reflection of coronary perfusion pressure. The critical coronary perfusion pressure is 15 to 25 mm Hg. When invasive monitoring is available during CPR, adjustments in chest compression technique and epinephrine should be used to ensure critical perfusion pressures are exceeded. Damage to the myocardium from underlying disease may preclude survival no matter how effective the CPR efforts. However, vascular pressures below critical levels are associated with poor results even in patients who may be salvageable (Table 58-1).

Although invasive pressure monitoring may be ideal, it is
7 rarely available during CPR. End-tidal CO_2 also has been found to be an excellent noninvasive guide to the adequacy of closed-chest compressions.[72] CO_2 excretion during CPR with an endotracheal tube in place is flow dependent rather than ventilation dependent. Because alveolar dead space is large in low-flow states, end-tidal CO_2 is very low (frequently <10 mm Hg). If blood flow improves with better CPR technique, more alveoli are perfused and end-tidal CO_2 rises (usually to >20 mm Hg with successful CPR). The earliest sign of return of spontaneous circulation is frequently a sudden increase in end-tidal CO_2 to >40 mm Hg. Within a wide range of cardiac outputs during CPR, end-tidal CO_2 correlates well with cardiac output,[73] coronary perfusion pressure,[74] and initial resuscitation.[75] End-tidal CO_2 correlates with survival in human CPR and can predict a poor outcome.[76,77] Patients with end-tidal CO_2 <10 mm Hg will not be resuscitated successfully. In the absence of invasive monitoring, end-tidal

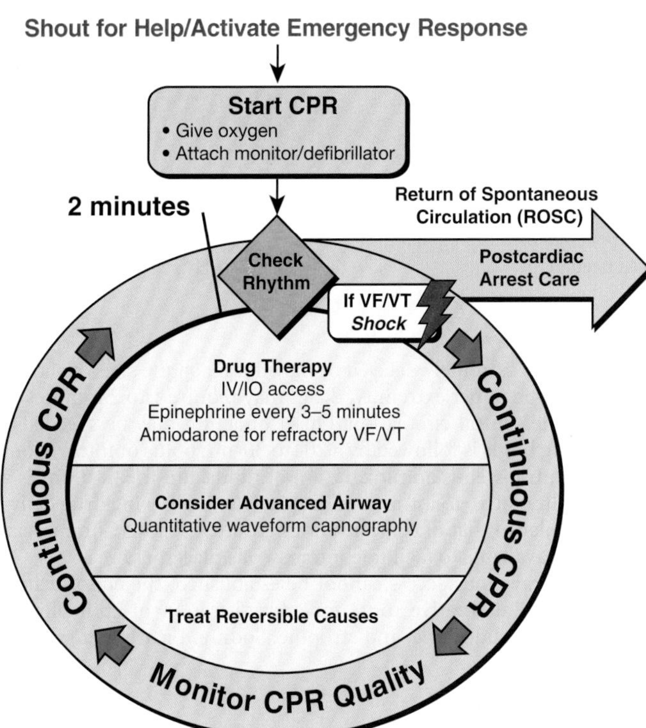

CPR Quality
- Push hard (≥2 inches [5 cm]) and fast (≥100/min) and allow complete chest recoil
- Minimize interruptions in compressions
- Avoid excessive ventilation
- Rotate compressor every 2 minutes
- If no advanced airway, 30:2 compression–ventilation ratio
- Quantitative waveform capnography
  - If P_{ETCO_2} <10 mm Hg, attempt to improve CPR quality
- Intra-arterial pressure
  - If relaxation phase (diastolic) pressure <20 mm Hg, attempt to improve CPR quality

Return of Spontaneous Circulation (ROSC)
- Pulse and blood pressure
- Abrupt sustained increase in P_{ETCO_2} (typically ≥40 mm Hg)
- Spontaneous arterial pressure waves with intra-arterial monitoring

Shock Energy
- **Biphasic:** Manufacturer recommendation (e.g., initial dose of 120–200 J); if unknown, use maximum available. Second and subsequent doses should be equivalent, and higher doses may be considered.
- **Monophasic:** 360 J

Drug Therapy
- **Epinephrine IV/IO Dose:** 1 mg every 3–5 minutes
- **Vasopressin IV/IO Dose:** 40 units can replace first or second dose of epinephrine
- **Amiodarone IV/IO Dose:** First dose: 300 mg bolus. Second dose: 150 mg

Advanced Airway
- Supraglottic advanced airway or endotracheal intubation
- Waveform capnography to confirm and monitor ET tube placement
- 8–10 breaths per minute with continuous chest compressions

Reversible Causes

– **H**ypovolemia	– **T**ension pneumothorax
– **H**ypoxia	– **T**amponade, cardiac
– **H**ydrogen ion (acidosis)	– **T**oxins
– **H**ypo-/hyperkalemia	– **T**hrombosis, pulmonary
– **H**ypothermia	– **T**hrombosis, coronary

FIGURE 58-4. Advanced cardiac life support cardiac arrest circular algorithm. CPR, cardiopulmonary resuscitation; VF, ventricular fibrillation; VT, ventricular tachycardia; IV, intravenous(ly); IO, intraosseous(ly); $PetCO_2$, partial pressure of end tidal carbon dioxide; J, joules. (From 2010 American Heart Association Guidelines for cardiopulmonary resuscitation and emergency cardiovascular care. *Circulation.* 2010;122(Suppl 3):S737, with permission.)

CO_2 using quantitative waveform capnography should be used to judge the effectiveness of chest compressions, whenever possible.[78] Attempts should be made to maximize the measured end-tidal CO_2 by alterations in technique or drug therapy. It should be remembered that sodium bicarbonate administration liberates CO_2 into the blood and causes a temporary increase in end-tidal CO_2. The elevation returns to baseline within 3 to 5 minutes of drug administration and end-tidal CO_2 monitoring can again be used for monitoring effectiveness of closed-chest compressions.

TABLE 58-1. CRITICAL VARIABLES ASSOCIATED WITH SUCCESSFUL RESUSCITATION

Variable	Amount
Myocardial blood flow (mL/min/100 g)	>15–20
Aortic diastolic pressure (mm Hg)	>40
Coronary perfusion pressure (mm Hg)	>15–25
End-tidal carbon dioxide (mm Hg)	>10

PHARMACOLOGIC THERAPY

This discussion of drug therapy is confined to the use of drugs during CPR attempts to restore spontaneous circulation. The use of drugs to support the circulation when there is mechanical cardiac
8 function is discussed elsewhere (see Chapters 15 and 39). During cardiac arrest, drug therapy is secondary to other interventions. Effective uninterrupted chest compressions and defibrillation, if appropriate, should take precedence over medications. Establishing intravenous access and pharmacologic therapy should come as soon as possible but after these critical interventions are estab-
9 lished. Although vasopressors are firmly established as improving survival in animal models and there is some evidence of improved early resuscitation in humans, there is no strong evidence that they improve long-term survival in human cardiac arrest.[79,80] The most common drugs and the appropriate adult doses are shown  in Table 58-2. In addition, pharmacologic and other therapeutic  approaches for the treatment of bradycardia and tachycardia are in Figures 58-5 and 58-6.

TABLE 58-2. ADULT ADVANCED CARDIAC LIFE SUPPORT DRUGS AND DOSES (INTRAVENOUS)

	Dose	Interval	Maximum
Epinephrine	1 mg	Every 3–5 min	None
If dose fails, consider	3–7 mg	Every 3–5 min	None
Vasopressin	40 U	May replace 1st or 2nd dose of epinephrine	—
Amiodarone	300 mg	Repeat 150 mg in 5 min	2 g
Lidocaine	1–1.5 mg/kg	Repeat 0.5–0.75 mg/kg in 5 min	3.0 mg/kg
Sodium bicarbonate	1 mEq/kg	As needed	Check pH

Routes of Administration

The preferred route of administration of all drugs during CPR is intravenous. The most rapid and highest drug levels occur with administration into a central vein. However, peripheral intravenous administration is also effective. The antecubital and external jugular veins are the sites of first choice for starting an infusion during resuscitation because inserting a central catheter usually necessitates stopping CPR. Because of poor blood flow below the diaphragm during CPR, drugs administered in the lower extremity may be extremely delayed or may not reach the sites of action. Even in the upper extremity, drugs may require 1 to 2 minutes to reach the central circulation. Onset of action may be speeded if the drug bolus is followed by a 20- to 30-mL bolus of intravenous fluid. Intraosseous administration of fluids and medications is a good alternative to intravenous cannulation, allowing drug delivery similar to that of central venous administration. Commercial kits are available to facilitate intraosseous placement.

If intravenous access cannot be established, the endotracheal tube is an alternative route for administration of epinephrine, vasopressin, lidocaine, and atropine. Sodium bicarbonate should

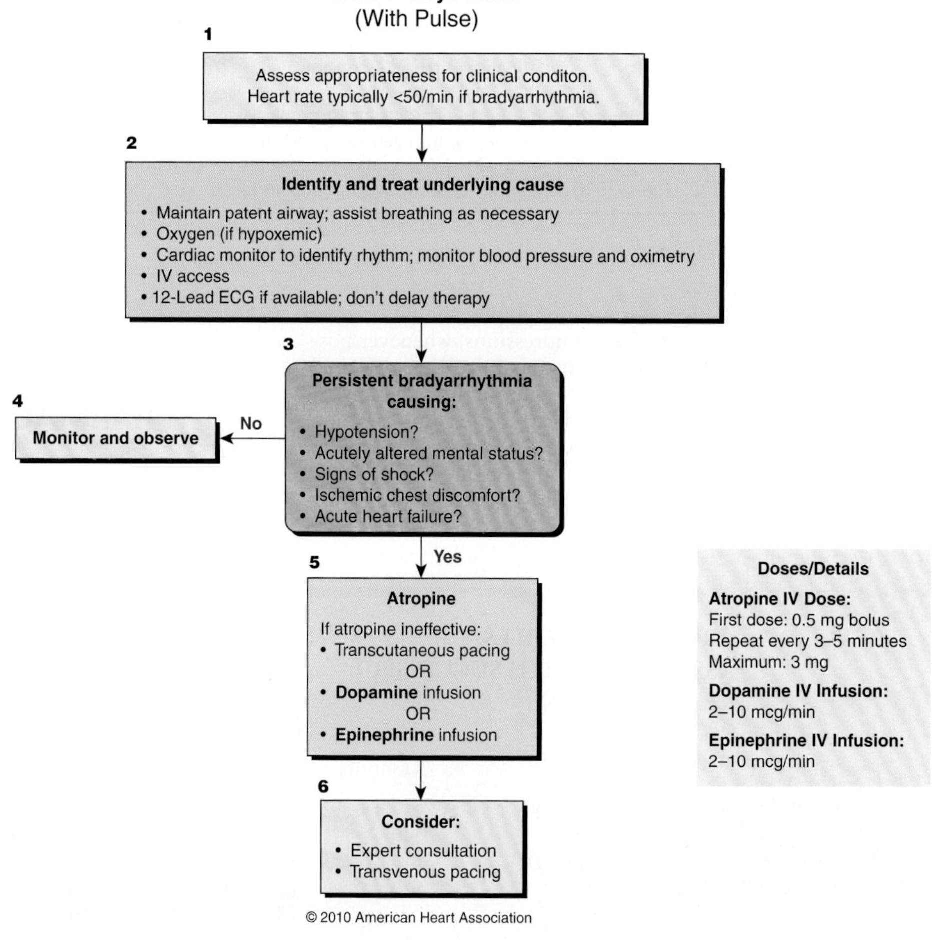

FIGURE 58-5. Adult bradycardia (with pulse) algorithm. ECG, electrocardiogram; IV, intravenous(ly). (From 2010 American Heart Association Guidelines for cardiopulmonary resuscitation and emergency cardiovascular care. *Circulation.* 2010; 122(Suppl 3):S749, with permission.)

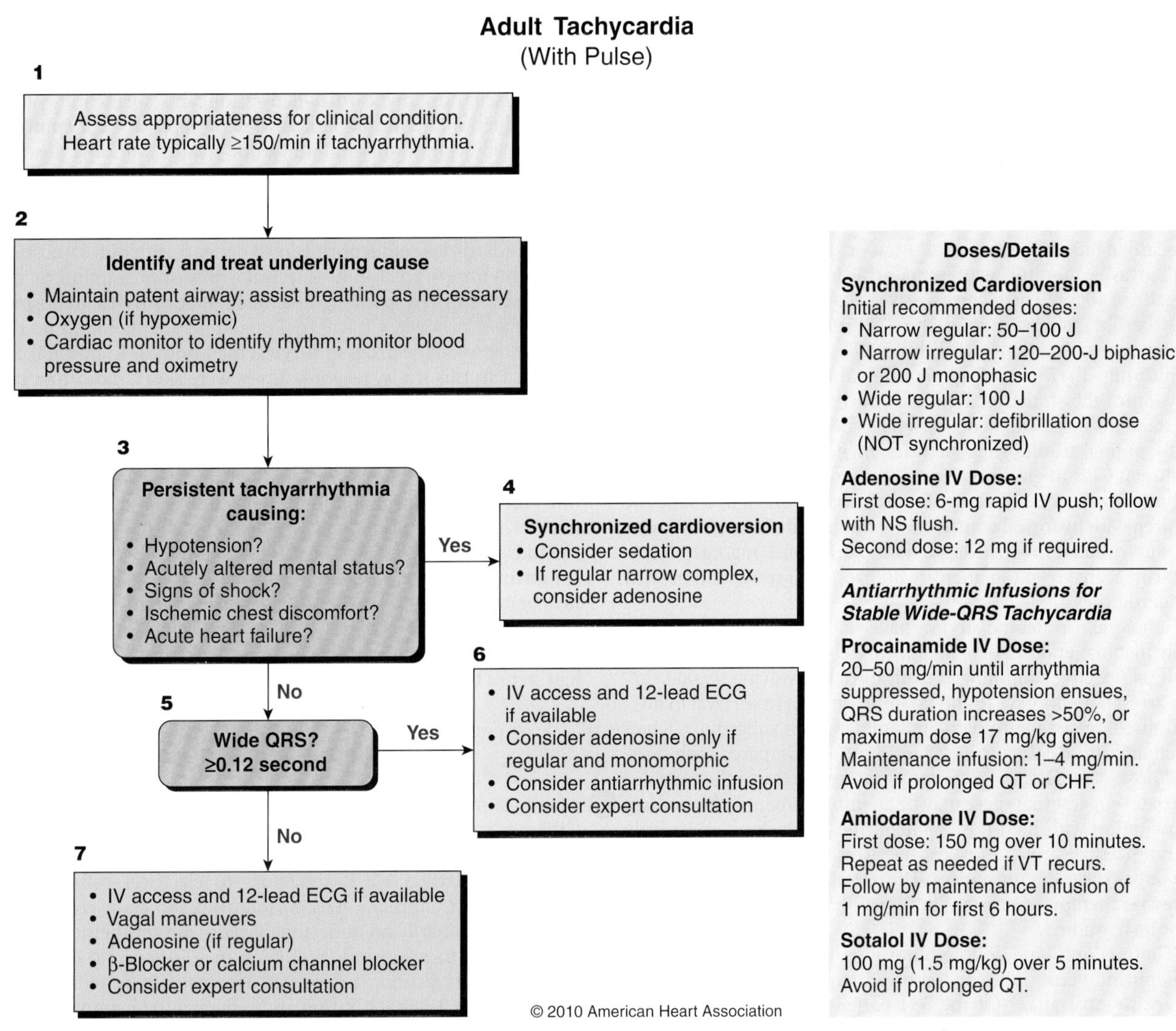

FIGURE 58-6. Adult tachycardia (with pulse) algorithm. ECG, electrocardiogram; IV, intravenous(ly); CHF, congestive heart failure; J, joules. (From 2010 American Heart Association Guidelines for cardiopulmonary resuscitation and emergency cardiovascular care. *Circulation.* 2010;122(Suppl 3):S751, with permission.)

not be given endotracheally. There are no data on endotracheal administration of amiodarone. The time to effect and drug levels achieved are inconsistent with endotracheal drug administration during CPR, so the optimal dose of drug is unknown using this route. In general, doses 2 to 2.5 times higher than the intravenous dose is recommended when this route is used. Better results may be obtained by administering 5- to 10-mL volumes. It is unclear whether deep injection is better than simple instillation into the endotracheal tube.

Catecholamines and Vasopressors

Mechanism of Action

Epinephrine has been used in resuscitation since the 1890s and has been the vasopressor of choice in modern CPR since the studies of Redding and Pearson[13,81] in the 1960s. The efficacy of epinephrine lies entirely in its α-adrenergic properties[68] (see Chapter 15). Peripheral vasoconstriction leads to an increase in aortic diastolic pressure, causing an increase in coronary perfusion pressure and myocardial blood flow.[40,82,83] All strong α-adrenergic drugs (epinephrine, phenylephrine, methoxamine, dopamine, norepinephrine), regardless of β-adrenergic potency, are equally successful in aiding resuscitation, as are strong nonadrenergic vasopressors (vasopressin, endothelin-1).[13,81,84,85] β-Adrenergic agonists without α activity (isoproterenol, dobutamine) are no better than placebo. α-Adrenergic blockade precludes resuscitation, whereas β-adrenergic blockade has no effect on the ability to restore spontaneous circulation.[65,66]

The β-adrenergic effects of epinephrine are potentially deleterious during cardiac arrest. In the fibrillating heart, epinephrine increases oxygen consumption and decreases the endocardial to epicardial blood flow ratio. Myocardial lactate production in the fibrillating heart is unchanged after epinephrine administration during CPR, suggesting that the increased coronary blood flow does not improve the oxygen supply to demand ratio. Large doses of epinephrine increase deaths in swine early after resuscitation because of tachyarrhythmias and hypertension, an effect partially offset by metoprolol treatment. Despite these theoretical considerations, survival and neurologic outcome studies have shown no difference when epinephrine is compared with a pure α-agonist (methoxamine or phenylephrine) during CPR in animals[81,86] or humans.[80,87]

Epinephrine

When added to chest compressions, epinephrine helps develop the critical coronary perfusion pressure necessary to provide enough myocardial blood flow for restoration of spontaneous circulation. With invasive monitoring present during CPR, an arterial diastolic pressure of 40 mm Hg or coronary perfusion pressure of 20 mm Hg must be obtained with good chest-compression technique and/or epinephrine therapy (see Table 58-1). In the absence of such monitoring, the dose of epinephrine must be chosen empirically. Since the studies of Redding and Pearson[13,81] in the 1960s, the standard intravenous dose used has been 0.5 to 1.0 mg. In the 1980s, animal studies suggested that higher doses of epinephrine in human CPR might improve myocardial and cerebral perfusion and improve success of resuscitation. Case reports and a series of children with historical controls were published of return of spontaneous circulation when large doses (0.1 to 0.2 mg/kg) of epinephrine were given to patients who had failed resuscitation with standard doses.

Subsequent outcome studies have not demonstrated conclusively that higher doses of epinephrine will improve survival. Eight adult prospective randomized clinical trials involving >9,000 cardiac arrest patients have found no improvement in survival to hospital discharge or neurologic outcome, even in subgroups, when initial high-dose epinephrine (5 to 18 mg) is compared with standard doses (1 to 2 mg).[88–95] Some of the studies (and the cumulative data) suggest that there may be an improvement in immediate resuscitation with high-dose epinephrine. High doses apparently are not needed early in most cardiac arrests and could be deleterious under some circumstances. The use of high-dose epinephrine as rescue therapy when standard doses have failed has not been rigorously studied.

There is only one double-blind, randomized control trial of epinephrine versus placebo reported from a single ambulance service in Australia.[96] Of the 534 patients, those receiving epinephrine had a 3.4 times greater chance of return of spontaneous circulation than those receiving placebo and a 2.3 times greater chance of hospital admission. Although more than twice as many patients receiving epinephrine survived to hospital discharge, this was not statistically significant because of the low numbers of survivors.

Current recommendations are to give 1 mg intravenously every 3 to 5 minutes in the adult. If this dose seems ineffective or to treat β-blocker or calcium channel blocker overdose, higher doses (3 to 8 mg) may be considered.

Vasopressin

Arginine vasopressin is currently recommended as an alternative to either the first or second dose of epinephrine in a dose of 40 U intravenous/intraosseous (see Chapter 15). Vasopressin is a naturally occurring hormone (antidiuretic hormone) that, when administered in high doses, is a potent nonadrenergic vasoconstrictor, acting by stimulation of smooth muscle V_1 receptors. It is usually not recommended for conscious patients with coronary artery disease because the increased peripheral vascular resistance may provoke angina. The half-life in the intact circulation is 10 to 20 minutes and longer than epinephrine during CPR. Animal studies have demonstrated that vasopressin is as effective as or more effective than epinephrine in maintaining vital organ blood flow during CPR. Repeated doses during prolonged CPR in swine were associated with significantly improved rates of neurologically intact survival compared with epinephrine and placebo. Postresuscitation myocardial depression and splanchnic blood flow reduction are more marked with vasopressin than epinephrine, but they are transient and can be treated with low doses of dopamine.[97] Clinical studies indicate that vasopressin is as effective as epinephrine but have not definitively shown it to be superior. A small randomized, blinded study comparing vasopressin and standard-dose epinephrine in 40 patients with out-of-hospital VF found improved 24-hour survival with vasopressin but no difference in return of spontaneous circulation or survival to hospital discharge.[98] A larger, clinical trial of 200 inpatients found no difference between the drugs in survival for 1 hour or to hospital discharge.[99] In this study, response times were short, indicating that CPR outcome achieved with both vasopressin and epinephrine in short-term cardiac arrest may be comparable. The hemodynamic effects of vasopressin, compared with epinephrine, are especially impressive during long cardiac arrests. Thus, vasopressin may find most use in CPR during prolonged duration resuscitation. A multicenter, randomized study of 1,186 patients comparing vasopressin 40 U and epinephrine 1 mg for the first two doses of vasopressor during resuscitation from out-of-hospital cardiac arrest found no overall difference in survival to hospital admission (36% vs. 31%) or discharge (10% vs. 10%).[100] Overall, evidence currently suggests that, like other potent vasopressors, vasopressin is equivalent to but not better than epinephrine for use during CPR.

Amiodarone and Lidocaine

10 After vasopressors, the drugs most likely to be of benefit during CPR are those that help suppress ectopic ventricular rhythms. Amiodarone and lidocaine are used during cardiac arrest to aid defibrillation when VF is refractory to electrical countershock therapy or when fibrillation recurs following successful conversion. Lidocaine, primarily an antiectopic agent with few hemodynamic effects, tends to reverse the reduction in VF threshold caused by ischemia or infarction. It depresses automaticity by reducing the slope of phase 4 depolarization and reducing the heterogeneity of ventricular refractoriness.

Amiodarone is a pharmacologically complex drug with sodium, potassium, calcium, and α-adrenergic and β-adrenergic blocking properties that is useful for treatment of atrial and ventricular dysrhythmias. Amiodarone can cause hypotension and bradycardia when infused too rapidly in patients with an intact circulation.[101] This can usually be prevented by slowing the rate of drug infusion, or it can be treated with fluids, vasopressors, chronotropic agents, or temporary pacing. There are two randomized, blinded, placebo-controlled clinical trials in shock-resistant cardiac arrest victims demonstrating improved admission alive to hospital with amiodarone treatment, although there was no difference in survival to discharge.[102,103] Although weak, this is more evidence of efficacy than exists for lidocaine.

When VF or pulseless ventricular tachycardia is recognized, defibrillation should be attempted (see Figs. 58-2 and 58-4). No antiarrhythmic agent has been shown to be superior to electrical defibrillation or more effective than placebo in the treatment of VF. Consequently, defibrillation should not be withheld or delayed to establish intravenous access or to administer drugs. When ventricular tachycardia or VF has not responded to or recurred following BLS, epinephrine, and defibrillation, amiodarone should be administered. In cardiac arrest, amiodarone is initially administered as a 300-mg rapid infusion. Supplemental infusions of 150 mg can be repeated as necessary for recurrent or resistant dysrhythmias to a maximum total daily dose of 2 g. (For dysrhythmias with an intact circulation, amiodarone is usually administered as 150 mg intravenously over 10 minutes, followed by 1 mg/min infusion for 6 hours and 0.5 mg/min thereafter.) Although lidocaine has no proven efficacy in cardiac arrest, it has few side effects. It is an alternative therapy in refractory fibrillation if amiodarone is not available. An initial bolus of 1 to 1.5 mg/kg should be given, and additional boluses of 0.5 to 0.75 mg/kg can be given every 5 to 10 minutes during CPR up to a total dose of 3 mg/kg.

Atropine

Atropine sulfate enhances sinus node automaticity and atrioventricular conduction by its vagolytic effects. Although atropine is frequently given during cardiac arrest associated with an electrocardiogram (ECG) pattern of asystole or slow pulseless electrical activity (PEA), neither animal nor human studies provide evidence that it actually improves outcome from asystolic or bradysystolic arrest.[104,105] The predominant cause of asystole and PEA is severe myocardial ischemia. Excessive parasympathetic tone probably contributes little to these rhythms during cardiac arrest in adults. Even in children, it is doubtful that parasympathetic tone plays a significant role during most arrests. Therefore, the most important treatment for asystole and PEA is effective chest compressions, ventilation, and epinephrine to improve coronary perfusion and myocardial oxygenation. There is no evidence that atropine is detrimental during cardiac arrest. However, *routine* use of atropine during cardiac arrest with these rhythms is unlikely to have benefit and is no longer recommended.

Sodium Bicarbonate

Although sodium bicarbonate was used commonly during CPR in the past, little evidence supports its efficacy. Use of sodium bicarbonate during resuscitation has been based on the theoretical considerations that acidosis lowers fibrillation threshold and impairs the physiologic response to catecholamines. But most studies have failed to demonstrate improved success of defibrillation or resuscitation with the use of bicarbonate.[106,107] The lack of effect of buffer therapy may be partially explained by the slow onset of metabolic acidosis during cardiac arrest. As measured by blood lactate or base deficit, acidosis does not become severe for 15 or 20 minutes of the cardiac arrest.[41,108]

In contrast to the lack of evidence that buffer therapy during CPR improves survival, the adverse effects of excessive sodium bicarbonate administration are well documented. In the past, metabolic alkalosis, hypernatremia, and hyperosmolarity were common after administration of bicarbonate during resuscitation attempts.[108,109] These abnormalities are associated with low resuscitation rates and poor outcomes.

Intravenous sodium bicarbonate combines with a hydrogen ion to produce carbonic acid that dissociates into CO_2 and water. The partial pressure of CO_2 in blood is temporarily elevated until the excess CO_2 is eliminated through the lungs. Tissue acidosis during CPR is caused primarily by the low blood flow and accumulation of CO_2 in the tissues.[41] Therefore, concern has been expressed that the liberation of CO_2 by bicarbonate administration would only worsen the existing problem. This is of particular concern within myocardial cells and the brain. CO_2 readily diffuses across cell membranes and the blood–brain barrier, whereas bicarbonate diffuses much more slowly. Thus, it is possible that sodium bicarbonate administration could result in a paradoxical worsening of intracellular and cerebral acidosis by further raising intracellular and cerebral CO_2 without a balancing increase in bicarbonate. Direct evidence for this effect has not been found. Use of clinically relevant doses causes no change in spinal fluid acid–base status or myocardial intracellular pH during bicarbonate administration.[110,111] Therefore, paradoxical acidosis from sodium bicarbonate therapy remains a concern primarily on theoretical grounds.

Routine use of sodium bicarbonate is not recommended for patients in cardiac arrest. Current practice restricts its use to arrests associated with hyperkalemia, severe pre-existing metabolic acidosis, and tricyclic or phenobarbital overdose. It may be considered for use in protracted resuscitation attempts after other modalities have been instituted and failed. When bicarbonate is used in these circumstances, the usual dose is 1 mEq/kg. However, dosing of sodium bicarbonate should be guided by blood–gas determination of acid–base status, whenever possible.

Calcium

With normal cardiovascular physiology, calcium increases myocardial contractility and enhances ventricular automaticity (see Chapter 10). Consequently, it has been advocated as a treatment for asystole and PEA. Early animal studies showed moderate success with calcium chloride in asphyxial arrest, although vasopressors were better.[13] In 1981, Dembo[112] reported dangerously high serum calcium levels (up to 18.2 mg/dL) during CPR and questioned the efficacy of calcium in cardiac arrest. Subsequently, several retrospective studies and prospective clinical trials during out-of-hospital cardiac arrest showed that calcium was no better than placebo in promoting resuscitation and survival from asystole or PEA.[113–116] Consequently, because of potentially deleterious effects, *routine* use of calcium is not recommended during CPR unless specific indications exist. Calcium may prove useful if hyperkalemia, hypocalcemia, or calcium channel blocker toxicity is present. There are no other indications for its use during CPR. When calcium is administered, the chloride salt is recommended because it produces higher and more consistent levels of ionized calcium than other salts. The usual dose is 2 to 4 mg/kg of the 10% solution administered slowly intravenously. Calcium gluconate contains one-third as much molecular calcium as does calcium chloride and requires metabolism of gluconate in the liver.

ELECTRICAL THERAPY

Electrical Pattern and Duration of Ventricular Fibrillation

11 Ventricular fibrillation is the most common ECG pattern found during witnessed sudden cardiac arrest in adults. The only consistently effective treatment is electrical defibrillation. The most important controllable determinant of failure to resuscitate a patient with VF is the duration of fibrillation.[117] Other important factors, such as underlying disease and metabolic status, are largely beyond the control of rescuers. The fibrillating heart has high oxygen consumption, increasing myocardial ischemia and decreasing the time to irreversible cell damage. The longer VF continues, the more difficult it is to defibrillate and the less likely is successful resuscitation.[59,118] If defibrillation occurs within 1 minute of fibrillation, CPR is unnecessary for resuscitation. Initial resuscitation success following out-of-hospital fibrillation and survival to hospital discharge are improved the earlier defibrillation is accomplished.[19,119]

The coarseness of the fibrillatory waves on the ECG may reflect the severity and duration of the myocardial insult and thus have prognostic significance.[120] However, the fibrillation amplitude seen on any one ECG lead varies with the orientation of that lead to the vector of the fibrillatory wave.[121] If the lead is oriented at right angles to the fibrillatory wave, a flat line can be seen. For this reason, the trace from a second lead or from a different position of paddle electrodes should always be inspected before a decision is made not to defibrillate. Low-*amplitude* fibrillatory waveforms are less likely to be associated with successful resuscitation and more likely to convert to asystole following defibrillation.[120] Similarly, low-*frequency* fibrillatory waveforms are associated with poor outcome, and the median frequency of the waveform correlates with myocardial perfusion during CPR and with success of defibrillation.[122,123] Multiple studies in animals and humans have shown that analysis of the VF waveform can predict, with varying reliability, the success of defibrillation attempts.[120,123–126] It is not yet clear whether such waveform analysis can predict success of resuscitation or direct modification of therapy prospectively. Catecholamines with β-adrenergic activity increase the vigor of fibrillation and the amplitude of the electrical activity, leading to the practice of administering epinephrine to make it "easier" to defibrillate. However, experimental work has shown that manipulation of the electrical pattern with epinephrine does not influence the success of defibrillation or reduce the energy needed for defibrillation.[118,127] Consequently, defibrillation should not be delayed for drug administration.

Defibrillators: Energy, Current, and Voltage

Defibrillators derive power from a line source of alternating current or an integral battery. The typical defibrillator consists of a variable transformer that allows selection of a variable voltage potential, an alternating/direct current converter to provide a direct current that is stored in a capacitor, a switch to charge the capacitor, and discharge switches to complete the circuit from capacitor to electrodes. Defibrillators are classified by the current waveform delivered: monophasic (current flows in one direction between electrodes) or biphasic (current reverses direction between electrodes during the shock). Until the past decade, the current waveform of most defibrillators was a monophasic damped half-sinusoid, although some delivered a monophasic truncated exponential waveform. Many of these monophasic defibrillators are still in use, although nearly all new defibrillators, including most AEDs, deliver either a biphasic truncated exponential waveform or a rectilinear biphasic waveform.

The AED is a device that monitors the ECG, recognizes VF, charges automatically, and gives a defibrillatory shock.[128] It has allowed the introduction of defibrillation into first-responder emergency medical system (EMS) networks and public access defibrillation because minimally trained individuals can incorporate defibrillation into BLS skills, improving survival in out-of-hospital arrest by reducing time to delivery of the first shock.[18–20,129] The algorithms these devices use to detect VF are accurate with nearly perfect specificity. They will not defibrillate a nonfibrillatory rhythm. Sensitivity rates are somewhat lower. They sometimes have trouble recognizing low-amplitude VF and can misinterpret pacemaker spikes as QRS complexes. Unfortunately, rhythm analysis can require up to 90 seconds during which chest compressions are not being given. This may adversely influence the outcome in some circumstances.

Defibrillators have been developed that measure transthoracic impedance prior to the shock by passing a low-voltage current through the chest during the charge cycle.[130,131] Although not in clinical use, this technology allows current-based defibrillation by adjusting the delivered energy for the measured resistance, permitting the use of low-energy shocks in appropriate patients and identification of victims needing higher energy.[132]

Defibrillation is accomplished by current passing through a critical mass of myocardium, causing simultaneous depolarization of the myofibrils. However, the output of defibrillators is indicated in energy units (joules or watt-seconds), not current (amperes). The relationships among energy, current, and impedance (resistance) are given by the following equations (standard units are indicated):

$$\text{Energy (joules)} = \text{Power (watts)} \times \text{Duration (seconds)} \quad (58\text{-}1)$$

$$\text{Power (watts)} = \text{Potential (volts)} \times \text{Current (amperes)} \quad (58\text{-}2)$$

$$\text{Current (amperes)} = \text{Potential (volts)/Resistance (ohms)} \quad (58\text{-}3)$$

$$\text{Current (amperes)} = \{\text{Energy (joules)/[Resistance (ohms)} \times \text{Duration (seconds)]}\}^{1/2} \quad (58\text{-}4)$$

From these equations, it can be determined that as the impedance between the paddle electrodes increases, the delivered energy will be reduced. Because internal resistance is low, the primary determinant of delivered energy will be transthoracic impedance. For consistency, the energy level indicated on most commercially available defibrillators is the output when discharged into a 50-ohm load. When transthoracic impedance is higher than that standard, actual delivered energy will be lower. Even at a constant delivered energy, equation 58-4 indicates that delivered current (the critical determinant of defibrillation) will be reduced as impedance increases. At high impedance and relatively low energy levels, current could be too low for defibrillation. Optimal success of defibrillation is obtained by keeping impedance as low as possible.

Transthoracic Impedance

Transthoracic impedance has been measured between 15 and 143 ohms in human defibrillation.[133] (see Chapter 10). The average transthoracic impedance in human defibrillation is 70 to 80 ohms. Many of the important factors in minimizing transthoracic impedance are under the control of the rescuers. Resistance decreases with increasing electrode size, and studies suggest that optimal paddle size may be 13 cm in diameter.[134,135] For adults, handheld paddle electrodes and self-adhesive pad electrodes are most commonly 8 to 12 cm in diameter and work well in practice. Gel pads, electrode paste, or self-adhesive defibrillation or monitor pads specifically designed to conduct electricity in the defibrillation setting must be used.[134,135] When paste is used, it should be applied liberally to the paddle surface, especially the edges, to prevent burns and to obtain the maximum reduction in impedance. Transthoracic impedance is slightly, but significantly, higher during inspiration than during exhalation.[136] Air is a poor electrical conductor. Firm paddle pressure of at least 11 kg reduces resistance by improving paddle-to-skin contact and by expelling air from the lungs.[133] Resistance is probably of little clinical significance when reasonably proper technique and high-energy shocks are used. For lower energy shocks, great care should be taken to minimize resistance.

Adverse Effects and Energy Requirements

Repeated defibrillation with high energy in animals can be associated with dysrhythmias, ECG changes suggesting myocardial damage, and morphologic evidence of myocardial necrosis.[137,138]

Whether similar injuries occur in humans is less certain. Slight elevations in creatine kinase–MB fractions have been measured in patients following cardioversion with high energies.[139] A higher incidence of atrioventricular block has been observed in patients receiving high-energy shocks than in patients receiving low-energy shock.[140] It seems likely that high-energy shocks, especially if repeated at close intervals, may result in myocardial damage. However, if energy is too low, the delivered current may be insufficient for defibrillation, especially when transthoracic impedance is high. There appears to be little risk of significant myocardial injury with currently recommended energy levels.

Older studies using monophasic waveform defibrillators found a general relationship between body size and energy requirements for defibrillation. Geddes et al.[141] observed that the current that is necessary for defibrillation in animals increased with increasing body mass. Children need less energy than adults, perhaps as low as 0.5 J/kg,[142] although the recommended dose is 2.0 to 4.0 J/kg, similar to that for adults.[29] Clinically, over the size range of adults, weight variability is not clinically significant and other factors are more important.[117] Studies of out-of-hospital and in-hospital arrests have demonstrated equal success when using ≤200 J initial energy compared with administering all shocks at energies ≥300 J.[140,143] Both monophasic and biphasic waveforms are successful in terminating VF. Neither waveform has been associated with better return of spontaneous circulation or survival.

Prior to 2005, the AHA recommendation for defibrillation with monophasic waveform devices was to use a stacked shock approach with an initial shock or 200 J followed immediately by a second shock at 200 to 300 J if the first was unsuccessful, followed, if both failed, by a third shock at 300 to 360 J.[144] However, the second and third shocks add limited incremental benefit and caused significant interruptions in chest compressions with reduced survival. With monophasic defibrillators, a single shock of 360 J should be given with immediate resumption of chest compressions (see Figs. 58-2 and 58-4).

Termination of VF with biphasic shocks has occurred at lower energies than any of the monophasic waveforms.[145] Selected energies of 150 to 200 J are generally effective with biphasic truncated exponential waveforms, and a selected energy of 120 J is effective with a rectilinear biphasic waveform. If the specific biphasic device being used has an indicated effective dose, the user should select that dose. If the effective dose for a biphasic device is unknown, a dose of 200 J may be selected. This dose may not be optimal but falls within the effective dose range of nearly all biphasic devices. As with the monophasic devices, a single shock should be delivered with immediate resumption of chest compressions. If additional shocks are necessary, they may be given at the same or higher dose.

PUTTING IT ALL TOGETHER

Since the mid-1970s, CPR has become widely practiced, facilitated by the efforts of the AHA, the International Red Cross, the European Resuscitation Council, and many other organizations around the world. The International Liaison Committee on Resuscitation, in conjunction with the AHA, periodically conducts an international review of the published science regarding CPR and emergency cardiac care. The resulting Consensus on Science and Treatment Recommendations[146] comprises the most complete evidence-based compilation of scientific data related to CPR practice. Individual organizations, including the AHA, use these data to develop guidelines for CPR practice. However, no common infrastructure exists that allows adoption of true international guidelines for CPR.

Following each consensus conference, the AHA refines and publishes specific guidelines for the teaching and practice of CPR in the United States.[29,144] These guidelines are developed because numerous individuals with varying levels of expertise (laypersons, emergency personnel, nurses, and physicians) need to be trained if CPR is to be effective in saving lives. For training to be effective, a standardized approach is needed (see Figs. 58-1 through 58-4). The AHA and other organizations also develop and sponsor courses at different levels of complexity for teaching CPR. The two levels of CPR care are referred to as *basic life support* for ventilation and chest compressions without additional equipment, and *advanced cardiac life support* for using all modalities available for resuscitation. Medical personnel need to be well versed in both levels of care. BLS is also appropriate for laypersons. The algorithms for approaching the patient with cardiac arrest published in the guidelines are familiar to all physicians and are reproduced in this chapter.

CARDIOCEREBRAL RESUSCITATION

The AHA guidelines and algorithms are carefully researched using the best evidence and experts available. Nevertheless, in spite of multiple updates to guidelines for CPR practice and many courses for lay public and health care providers, survival rates are dismal and have remained stagnant for decades.[147] These poor outcomes may be attributable, at least in part, to the fact that standard CPR is being applied to two pathophysiologically distinct entities (respiratory arrest and cardiac arrest) and is not optimal care for either. In the former, arrest occurs because of hypoxemia, and reoxygenating the blood by effective ventilation is mandatory for successful resuscitation. In the latter, arrest occurs because of cardiac dysrhythmia, usually with normal oxygenation, and attempts at ventilation during resuscitation, in fact, are harmful.

What has become clear in the past decade is that improvements in the standard clinical process of CPR may be more important to increase survival than any new intervention.[148] Standardized quality control of CPR practice is mandatory during any clinical trial if meaningful results are to be achieved. A continuous quality-improvement model may be more relevant to improved outcomes than the randomized control trial. Recognizing that the vast majority of cardiac arrests are dysrhythmic in origin, this approach has been taken in Arizona.[149,150] After establishing a statewide database, significant changes to the 2000 AHA standard guidelines were implemented in 2003. This approach to the victim of sudden cardiac death has been called *cardiocerebral resuscitation* (CCR) or *minimally interrupted cardiac resuscitation.* Although the nuances of the technique continue to evolve, the basic outline of CCR as practiced in Tucson is shown in the Figure 58-7. Refinement of the AHA guidelines has aligned the two approaches, but there remain differences from the 2010 AHA cardiac arrest algorithm (see Figs. 58-2 and 58-4).

Time-sensitive Model of Ventricular Fibrillation

12 Weisfeldt and Becker[151] have described untreated VF as a time-sensitive model with three phases: electrical, circulatory, and metabolic. The *electrical phase* occurs during the first 4 to 5 minutes of the arrest, and early defibrillation is critical for success during this time. The *hemodynamic phase* follows for the next 10 to 15 minutes, when perfusing the myocardium and brain with oxygenated blood is critical. This is followed by what has been called

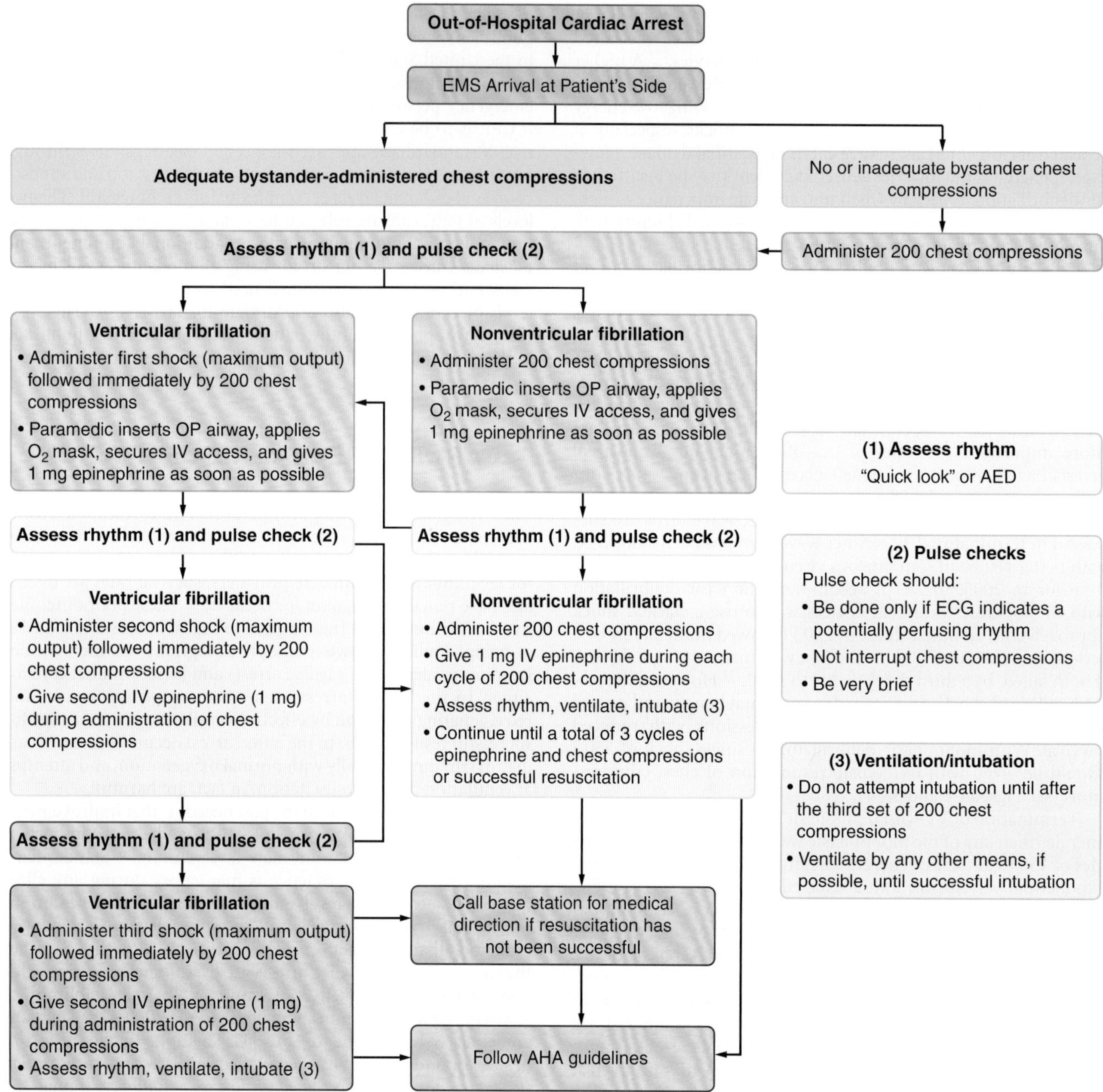

FIGURE 58-7. Cardiocerebral resuscitation algorithm. EMS, emergency medical system; OP, oropharyngeal; O_2, oxygen; IV, intravenous(ly); AHA, American Heart Association.

the *metabolic phase,* when the ischemic injury to the heart is so great that it is not clear what interventions will be successful.

Prompt defibrillation during the electrical phase is when CPR has had the most dramatic effect and why public-access AED has proven beneficial. The longer VF continues, the more difficult it is to defibrillate and the less likely is successful resuscitation. AEDs have been employed successfully in many settings, including airplanes, airports, casinos, and in the community. The success of public access defibrillation was dramatically demonstrated by the results of installing AEDs in Chicago airports where, over the first 2 years, there was a 55% 1-year neurologically intact survival rate.[152] Similarly, when AEDs were installed in Las Vegas casinos and security personnel were instructed in their use, there was a 53% survival to discharge (74% in patients who received the shock within 3 minutes of collapse).[153] If an arrest is witnessed and a defibrillator or AED is immediately available, then defibrillation should be the first priority in resuscitation. However, in the usual out-of-hospital rescue with emergency medical technicians or paramedics doing the defibrillation, a rapid response is to apply the first shock in 6 to 7 minutes, and the time to first shock frequently is more than 10 minutes.

With the onset of VF and cessation of coronary perfusion, the high oxygen consumption of the fibrillating heart causes the rapid depletion of myocardial high-energy phosphates, reducing the time to irreversible cell damage. Myocardial ATP levels during VF correlate with the success of defibrillation and postdefibrillation contractile function.[154] By about 4 minutes, the ATP levels in the heart have fallen to levels that make restoration of normal contractile function problematic. Effective chest compressions help replete or delay reductions in ATP by generating an adequate coronary perfusion pressure to restore myocardial blood flow. Therefore, the most important intervention during the hemodynamic phase of cardiac arrest is producing coronary perfusion with chest compressions before any attempt to defibrillate. In the absence of prompt defibrillation, the most important intervention for neurologically normal survival from cardiac arrest is restoration and maintenance of cerebral and myocardial blood flow. This is the main principle behind the concept of CCR. Because perfusion pressures generated by chest compressions are quite low compared with the intact circulation, any interruption of chest compressions markedly reduces the chances for neurologically normal survival. Therefore, any intervention that interrupts chest compressions is strongly discouraged.

Bystander Cardiopulmonary Resuscitation

Restoration of cerebral and myocardial blood flow must begin at the scene of the cardiac arrest. There are many studies documenting improved survival if bystanders provide CPR to the victim while awaiting arrival of EMS. Unfortunately, the incidence of bystander CPR has been falling for 3 decades. Therefore, a focus of the CCR initiative is to increase bystander participation by making the intervention easier to learn and to perform. The reasons for bystander's reluctance to intervene are multiple but seem to be primarily (a) lack of training, (b) the complexity of the task, and (c) fear of harm. Many of these concerns focus on the mouth-to-mouth ventilation part of the CPR intervention.[155–157] One survey indicated that only 15% of laypersons would perform CPR with mouth-to-mouth ventilation on a stranger. When given the option of doing chest compressions only, 68% indicated they would perform CPR on a stranger.[157]

If the airway remains patent during CPR, chest compressions cause substantial air exchange. Early studies in anesthetized, paralyzed humans suggested that the airway would not remain open in the unconscious,[6,7] leading to the teaching that airway control and artificial ventilation must accompany chest compressions. However, there are considerable data to suggest that eliminating mouth-to-mouth ventilation early in the resuscitation of witnessed fibrillatory cardiac arrest is not detrimental to outcome and may improve survival. Data from the Belgian CPCR Registry has demonstrated that 14-day survival and neurologic outcome are the same if bystanders initiate full BLS or perform chest compressions only. Both are significantly better than if the bystanders only do mouth-to-mouth ventilation or attempt no CPR.[158,159] A recent Japanese study found better survival in victims who received bystander chest compression–only CPR than in those who received both chest compressions and mouth-to-mouth ventilation from bystanders.[160]

The necessity for ventilation during BLS has been studied in animal models. Since 1993, there have been six studies containing data from 169 swine demonstrating that in prolonged fibrillatory cardiac arrest, neurologically intact survival is the same with chest compression–only resuscitation as with idealized standard CPR (as recommended by the 2000 AHA guidelines[144]) with a 15:2 compression-to-ventilation ratio and when compressions are only interrupted for 4 seconds to provide ventilation.[161–164] However, it has been demonstrated that a single lay rescuer interrupts chest compressions for an average of 16 seconds to deliver the two recommended mouth-to-mouth ventilations.[165] When the 15:2 compression-to-ventilation ratio with 16-second pauses for ventilation was tested in the swine model of prolonged fibrillatory arrest, standard CPR resulted in just 13% 24-hour survival compared with 73% in animals receiving chest compressions only.[166]

Recognizing the deleterious effects of prolonged pauses in chest compressions for ventilation, the 2005 AHA guidelines changed the compression-to-ventilation ratio from 15:2 to 30:2, recommending that ventilation be done in 2 to 4 seconds. When the 30:2 ratio with a more realistic 16-second pause for ventilations is compared with continuous chest compressions without ventilation in the animal model, the 24-hour neurologically normal survival is only 42% in the 30:2 group compared with 70% in the continuous compressions group.[167]

Based on these studies, one component of the CCR initiative has been a public education program stressing immediate call to 911 and continuous chest compressions without ventilation in the case of witnessed unexpected sudden collapse in adults. The major advantage of this program is that lay individuals can be taught CCR in a very short period with excellent retention. In Arizona between 2005 and 2009, the rate of bystander CPR increased from 28% to 40%, the rate of chest compression only CPR among bystanders increased from 20% to 76%, and rate of survival to hospital discharge during those years was 7.8% for those receiving standard CPR and 13.3% for those receiving chest compression–only CPR.[168] The importance of minimizing interruptions in chest compressions was emphasized in a science advisory by the AHA recommending "Hands-Only CPR" for the lay public.[169]

Cardiocerebral Resuscitation During Advanced Life Support

Recognizing that dysrhythmic arrest is most common in adults and the importance of establishing blood flow, the most recent AHA guidelines have recommended that CPR be initiated in the unresponsive individual with chest compressions before any attempt at ventilation when a single rescuer is present.[29] The principle of not interrupting chest compressions in order to maintain cerebral and myocardial perfusion applies to resuscitation attempts by health care providers as well as lay bystanders. The adverse hemodynamic consequences of interrupting chest compressions have been well documented.[170] Blood flow stops almost immediately with cessation of chest compressions and returns slowly when they are resumed. Several compressions are necessary before perfusion pressures return to the levels obtained before compressions were stopped. This is particularly true for prolonged, repeated pauses for ventilation. But it is also relevant for the many other interruptions that occur during resuscitation: pulse checks, rhythm analysis, charging the defibrillator, stacked shocks, intubation, patient assessment, and intravenous line placement. Recent reports have documented that paramedics spend only about half the time during a resuscitation doing chest compressions, mostly because they are following the standard guidelines.[21,171]

Consequently CCR emphasizes that chest compressions are to be paused only when absolutely necessary, and then for the shortest time possible. Initial airway management consists of insertion of an oropharyngeal airway and providing oxygen by mask. Intravenous line placement should not require cessation of chest compressions. Pulse checks occur only during pauses for rhythm analysis. Rescue breaths or assisted ventilation or intubation are delayed until return of spontaneous circulation or until at least three cycles of compressions–rhythm analysis–shock are complete. The second rescuer's priorities are obtaining intravenous access, delivering drugs, and relieving the individual giving chest compressions. If there is time and resources for airway management, ventilation and intubation are encouraged to take place while chest compressions continue.

Once ventilation begins, rescuers must be aware of the potentially deleterious effects of positive-pressure ventilation.[172,173] Positive-pressure ventilation increases intrathoracic pressure, reducing venous return, cardiac output, and coronary perfusion pressure and adversely affecting survival. These effects are amplified by the fact that physicians and paramedics often ventilate at rates that are many times the recommended 10 breaths per minute, even after extensive retraining.[171–174]

Rhythm Analysis and Defibrillation

As mentioned previously, after 4 to 5 minutes of VF, the myocardium is so depleted of high-energy phosphates that development of a normal contractile state is difficult, if not impossible. Therefore, immediate defibrillation during the circulatory phase is counterproductive, usually producing either asystole or pulseless electrical activity. In Seattle, it has been noted that patients who had CPR prior to defibrillation had a better survival, and the improvement was accounted for by better results in the group of patients in whom the response time was >4 minutes.[175] In a randomized trial of 200 out-of-hospital cardiac arrests in Oslo, there was a highly significant improvement in outcome if CPR was provided before defibrillation when the response time was >5 minutes.[176] Consequently, during CCR, resuscitation is initiated with 200 continuous chest compressions at a rate of 100 per minute unless bystanders are already providing good chest compressions. Rhythm analysis and defibrillation, if indicated, follow. Pulse checks are done only during the period of rhythm analysis.

The interruption caused by stacked defibrillatory shocks was discussed previously. When combined with time for rhythm analysis and postshock pulse checks, this interruption may be unacceptably long or even fatal when an AED is in use instead of an experienced clinician interpreting the rhythm with a manual defibrillator.[177,178] The postshock pulse check detects a pulse in only 2.5% of the victims. The success rate of a single shock is between 70% and 85% with most monophasic waveform defibrillators and >90% with the newer biphasic waveform units. Recognizing these concerns, both CCR as well as the current AHA guidelines for CPR recommend a single shock at 360 J for monophasic defibrillators and at the manufacturer's recommended power for biphasic units, with immediate resumption of chest compressions.

In prolonged VF arrest, successful defibrillation almost always results in asystole or pulseless electrical activity, as indicated by the extremely small number of victims with a pulse following shocks. In fact, the standard laboratory model for pulseless electrical activity is prolonged VF followed by defibrillation, all without chest compressions. Immediately restarting chest compressions after defibrillation to provide coronary perfusion nearly always results in reversion to a perfusing rhythm.[149] This certainly suggests that the best chance for restoration of spontaneous circulation following defibrillation will be by immediately resuming chest compressions without waiting to check a pulse or reanalyze the ECG rhythm.

Cardiocerebral Resuscitation in Practice

In summary, CCR is an approach to the victim of cardiac arrest that maximizes the chances for restoring and maintaining cerebral and myocardial perfusion at levels that promote neurologically intact survival. For bystanders, it emphasizes activating the EMS as soon as possible and providing continuous chest compressions until help arrives. Immediate defibrillation is encouraged if the collapse is witnessed and a defibrillator or AED is promptly available. If the collapse is not witnessed, 200 continuous chest compressions (100 per minute) are performed before rhythm analysis and defibrillation. If a shockable rhythm exists, a single shock of 360 J monophasic (or the manufacturer's recommended dose biphasic) is administered and continuous chest compressions are immediately resumed. Pulse checks are done only during rhythm analysis. Intravenous administration of drugs is encouraged as soon as possible but without interruption of continuous chest compressions. Most of these principles are also incorporated in the 2010 AHA guidelines for CPR and ECC, although there remain some differences in practice.[29]

Initial results of applying the CCR principles to EMS for out-of-hospital cardiac arrest are beginning to be reported. In rural Rock and Walworth counties in Wisconsin, in the 3 years preceding a change to CCR, there were 92 witnessed out-of-hospital adult cardiac arrests with an initially shockable rhythm, of whom 18 survived and 14 (15%) were neurologically intact. In the first 3 years of using CCR in these counties, there were 89 witnessed out-of-hospital cardiac arrests of whom 42 (47%) survived and 35 (39%) were neurologically intact.[179] In two large metropolitan Arizona cities after institution of minimally interrupted cardiac resuscitation by the EMS, the rate of survival nearly tripled.[180] Among the 886 patients, survival to hospital discharge increased from 1.8% to 5.4% after CCR training, and in the subgroup of 174 patients with witnessed cardiac arrest with VF, survival increased from 4.7% to 17.6%. These highly statistically significant results are encouraging that a significant improvement in outcome from sudden cardiac death is possible.

PEDIATRIC CARDIOPULMONARY RESUSCITATION

The principles of CPR discussed previously also apply to the child
13 in cardiac arrest. Arrest is less likely to be a sudden event and more likely related to progressive deterioration of respiratory and circulatory function in the pediatric age group. Airway and ventilation problems lead to asystole and PEA as the most common presenting rhythms. However, the consequences of myocardial and cerebral ischemia are the same as for the adult, and the basic approach to the unresponsive victim is similar (Fig. 58-8). The specific anatomic and physiologic considerations necessary for the child will be familiar to anesthesiologists. The special circumstance of neonatal resuscitation has been discussed in other chapters.

The problem of airway management in the infant is well known to the anesthesiologist. Effective ventilation is especially critical because respiratory problems are frequently the cause for arrest. Mouth-to-mouth or mouth-to-nose and mouth (for infants) can be used as well as bag-valve–mask devices until intubation is possible. Cardiac compression in the infant is provided with two fingers on the midsternum or by encircling the chest with the hands and using the thumbs to provide compression. For the small child, compression can be provided with one hand on the midsternum.

The algorithm for pulseless arrest in the child is shown in Figure 58-9. Although defibrillation is less frequently necessary in children, the same principles apply as in the adult. However, the recommended starting energy is 2 J/kg (monophasic or biphasic),

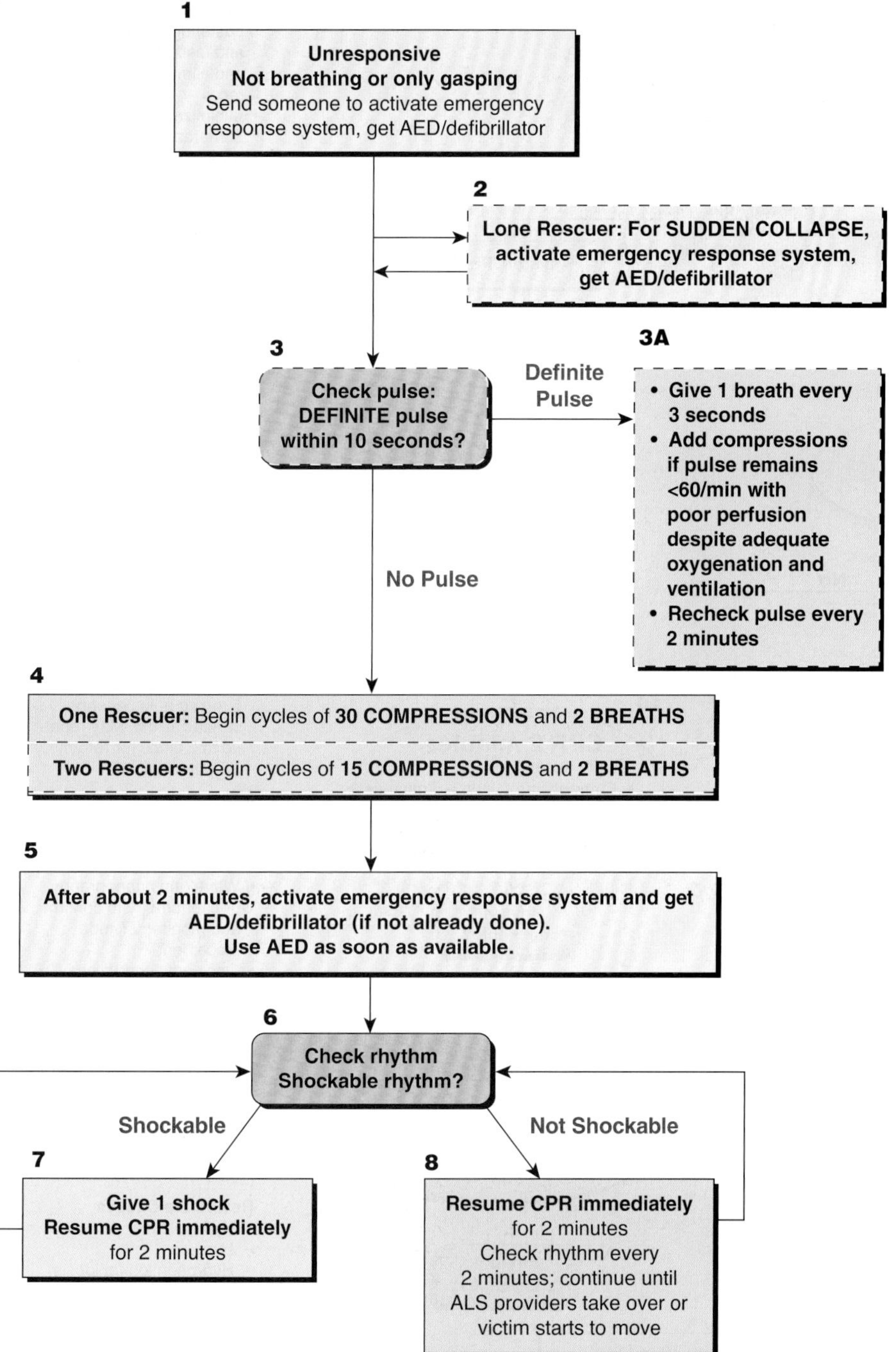

FIGURE 58-8. Pediatric health care provider basic life support algorithm. AED, automatic external defibrillator; CPR, cardiopulmonary resuscitation; ALS, advanced life support. (From 2010 American Heart Association Guidelines for cardiopulmonary resuscitation and emergency cardiovascular care. *Circulation.* 2010;122(Suppl 3):S866, with permission.)

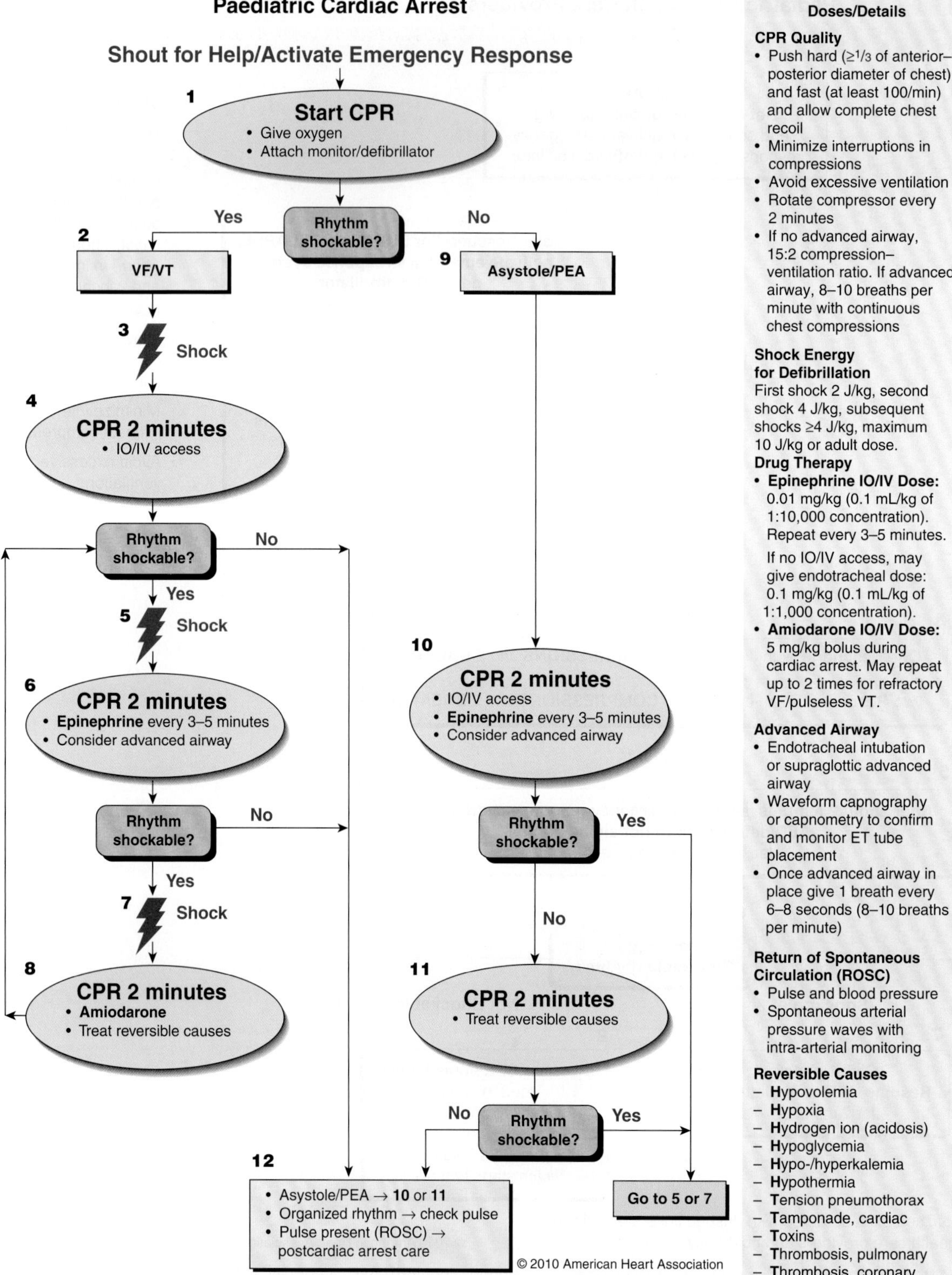

FIGURE 58-9. Pediatric advanced life support pulseless arrest algorithm. CPR, cardiopulmonary resuscitation; VF, ventricular fibrillation; VT, ventricular tachycardia; PEA, pulseless electrical activity; IV, intravenous(ly); IO, intraosseous(ly); J, joules. (From 2010 American Heart Association Guidelines for cardiopulmonary resuscitation and emergency cardiovascular care. *Circulation*. 2010;122(Suppl 3):S885, with permission.)

TABLE 58-3. PEDIATRIC ADVANCED LIFE SUPPORT MEDICATION FOR CARDIAC ARREST AND SYMPTOMATIC ARRHYTHMIAS

Drug	Dosage (Pediatric)	Remarks
Adenosine	0.1 mg/kg (maximum, 6 mg) Repeat: 0.2 mg/kg (maximum, 12 mg)	Monitor ECG during dose Rapid IV/IO bolus
Amiodarone	5 mg/kg IV/IO Repeat up to 15 mg/kg Maximum: 300 mg Use caution when administering with other drugs that prolong QT	Monitor ECG and blood pressure Adjust administration rate to urgency
Atropine	0.02 mg/kg IV/IO 0.04–0.06 mg/kg ET[a] Repeat once if needed Minimum dose: 0.1 mg Maximum single dose: 0.5 mg	Higher doses may be given with organophosphate poisoning
Calcium chloride (10%)	20 mg/kg IV/IO (0.2 mL/kg)	Give slow IV push for hypocalcemia, hypermagnesemia, calcium channel blocker toxicity
Epinephrine	0.01 mg/kg (0.1 mL/kg 1: 10,000) IV/IO 0.1 mg/kg (0.1 mL/kg 1:1,000) ET[a] Maximum dose: 1 mg IV/IO; 2.5 mg ET	May repeat every 3–5 min
Glucose	0.5–1.0 g/kg IV/IO	Newborn: 5–10 mL/kg $D_{10}W$ Children: 2–4 mL/kg $D_{25}W$ Adolescents: 1–2 mL/kg $D_{50}W$
Lidocaine	Bolus: 1 mg/kg IV/IO Maximum dose: 100 mg Infusion: 20–50 μg/kg per minute	—
Magnesium sulfate	25–50 mg/kg IV/IO over 10–20 min; faster in torsades Maximum dose: 2 g	—
Naloxone	≤5 years or ≤20 kg: 0.1 mg/kg IV/IO/ET[a] ≥5 y or >20 kg: 2 mg IV/IO/ET[a]	Use lower doses to reverse respiratory depression associated with therapeutic opioid use (1–5 μg/kg)
Procainamide	15 mg/kg IV/IO over 30 to 60 min Adult dose: 20 mg/min IV infusion up to total maximum dose of 17 mg/kg	Monitor ECG and blood pressure Use caution when administering with other drugs that prolong QT
Sodium bicarbonate	1 mEq/kg IV/IO slowly	After adequate ventilation

ECG, electrocardiogram; IV, intravenous; IO, intraosseous; ET, endotracheal.
[a]Flush with 5 mL of normal saline and follow with five ventilations.
Adapted from 2010 American Heart Association Guidelines for cardiopulmonary resuscitation and emergency cardiovascular care. *Circulation.* 2010;122:S882.

which is doubled if defibrillation is unsuccessful. Considerations for drug administration are the same as for the adult, except that the interosseous route in the anterior tibia is a particularly attractive option in small children. Drug therapy is similar to that of the adult but plays a larger role because electrical therapy is less often needed (Table 58-3). The pediatric algorithms for bradycardia and tachycardia are shown in Figures 58-10 and 58-11.

POSTRESUSCITATION CARE

The major factors contributing to mortality following successful resuscitation are progression of the primary disease and cerebral damage suffered as a result of the arrest. There is growing awareness that many potentially useful interventions during active CPR may not result in improved survival because of the lack of uniform supportive postresuscitation care, allowing progression to multisystem organ dysfunction and death. For optimal outcome, successful restoration of spontaneous circulation must be followed by correction of reversible causes of arrest, including immediate coronary reperfusion and aggressive supportive care (Fig. 58-12). Patients with successful restoration of spontaneous circulation should be transported to a facility with the capability of aggressive postarrest care, including percutaneous coronary intervention, hypothermia, and critical care.

14

Any cardiac arrest, even of brief duration, causes a generalized decrease in myocardial function similar to the regional hypokinesis seen following periods of regional ischemia. This is usually referred to as *global myocardial stunning* and can be mitigated with inotropic agents, if necessary. Active management following resuscitation appears to mitigate postischemic brain damage and improve neurologic outcomes.[181] Although a significant number of patients have severe neurologic deficits following resuscitation, aggressive brain-oriented support does not seem to increase the proportion surviving in vegetative states.

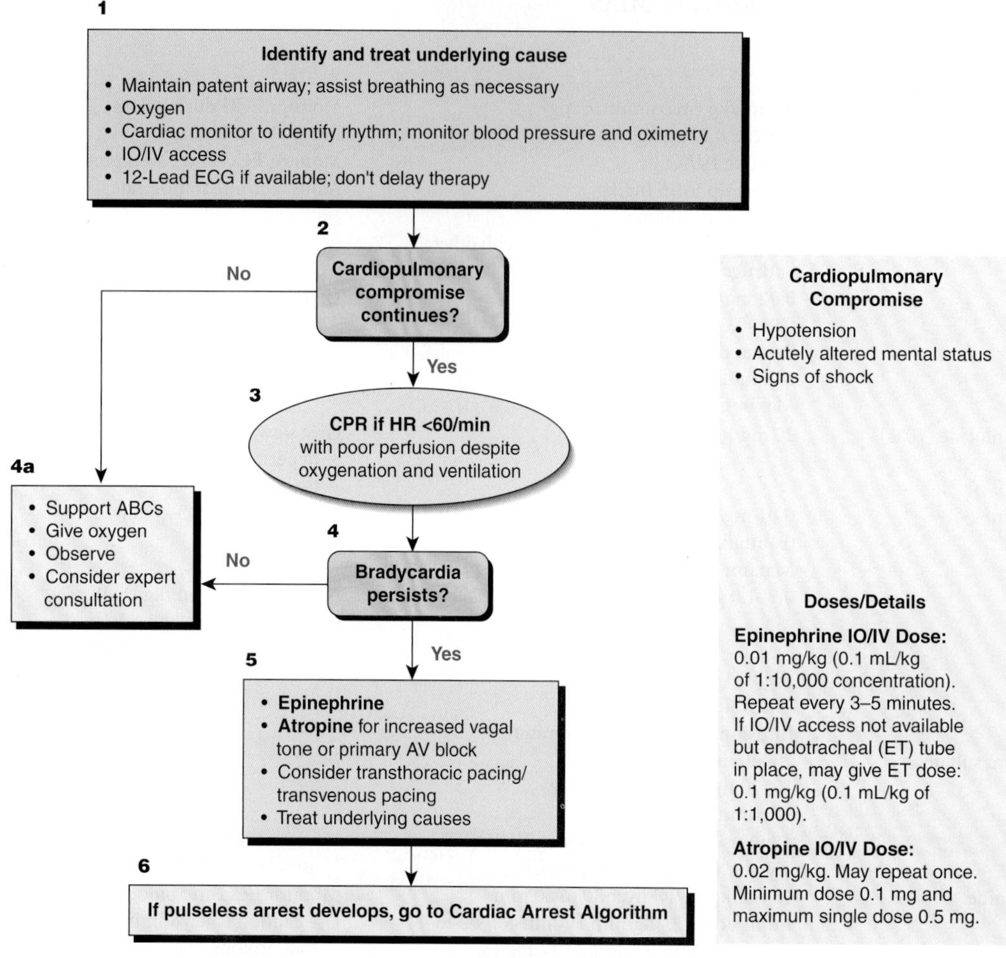

FIGURE 58-10. Pediatric advanced life support bradycardia (with pulse and poor perfusion) algorithm. ABCs, airway, breathing, and circulation; ECG, electrocardiogram; CPR, cardiopulmonary resuscitation; HR, heart rate; IV, intravenous(ly); IO, intraosseous(ly); AV, atrioventricular. (From 2010 American Heart Association Guidelines for cardiopulmonary resuscitation and emergency cardiovascular care. *Circulation.* 2010;122(Suppl 3):S887, with permission.)

Most severely damaged victims die of multisystem failure within 1 to 2 weeks.

When flow is restored following a period of global brain ischemia, three stages of cerebral reperfusion are seen in the ensuing 12 hours. Immediately following resuscitation, there are multifocal areas of the brain with no reflow. Within 1 hour, there is global hyperemia followed quickly by prolonged global hypoperfusion. Elevation of intracranial pressure is unusual following resuscitation from cardiac arrest. However, severe ischemic injury can lead to cerebral edema and increased intracranial pressure in the ensuing days. Seizures are common postresuscitation with or without therapeutic hypothermia.[181] An electroencephalogram for diagnosis of seizure should be done in comatose patients and treatment instituted if indicated.

Postresuscitation support is focused on providing stable oxygenation and hemodynamics to minimize any further cerebral insult. A comatose patient should be maintained on mechanical ventilation for several hours to ensure adequate oxygenation and ventilation. Restlessness, coughing, or seizure activity should be aggressively treated with appropriate medications, including neuromuscular blockers, if necessary. To avoid oxygen toxicity, fraction of inspired oxygen should be titrated to maintain oxygen saturation by pulse oximetry ≥94% or an arterial PaO_2 above 100 mm Hg, and hypocapnia ($PaCO_2$ <30 mm Hg) should be avoided. Because cerebral autoregulation of blood flow is severely attenuated after cardiac arrest, both prolonged hypertension and hypotension are associated with a worsened outcome. Therefore, mean arterial pressure should be maintained at 90 to 110 mm Hg. Hyperglycemia during cerebral ischemia is known to result in increased neurologic damage. Although it is unknown if high serum glucose in the postresuscitation period influences outcome, it seems prudent to control glucose in the 100 to 150 mg/dL range. Specific pharmacologic therapy directed at brain preservation has not been shown to have further benefit. Some animal trials of

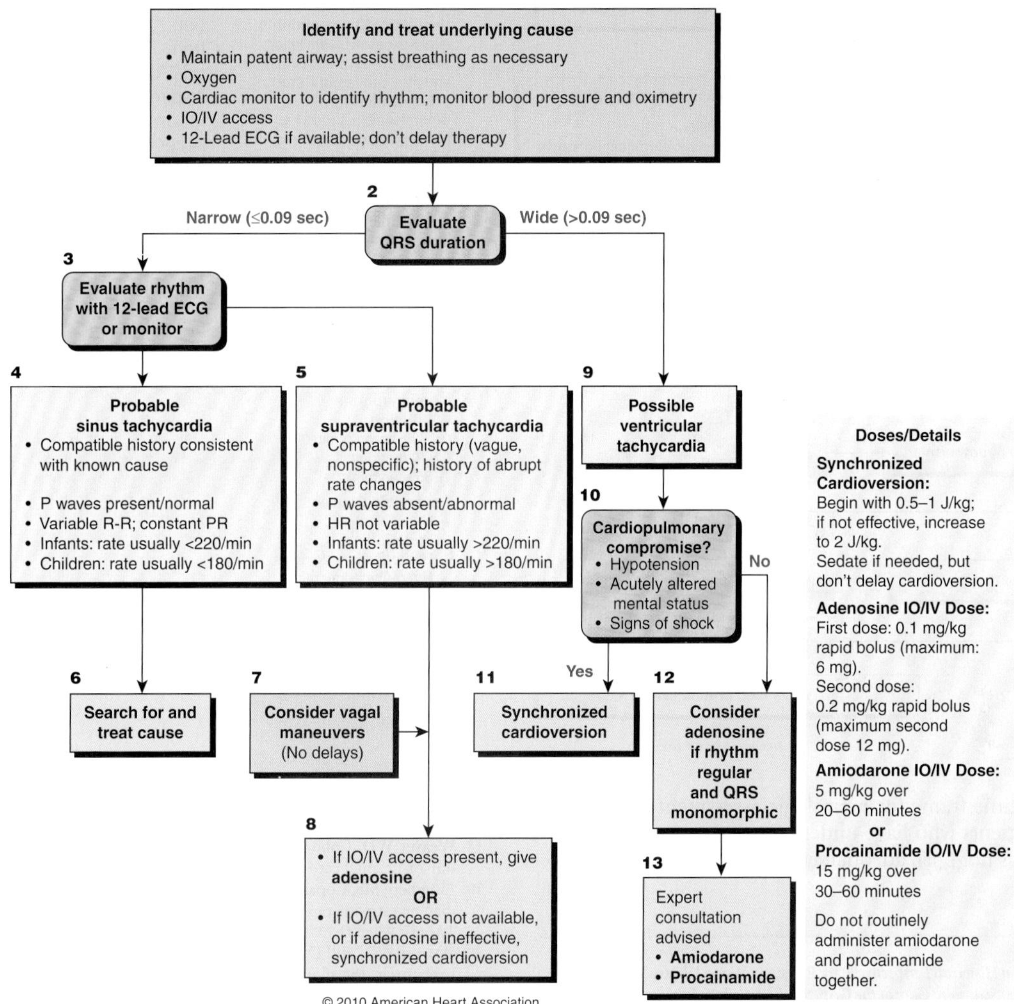

FIGURE 58-11. Pediatric advanced life support tachycardia (with pulse and poor perfusion) algorithm. ECG, electrocardiogram; HR, heart rate; IV, intravenous(ly); IO, intraosseous(ly); J, joules. (From 2010 American Heart Association Guidelines for cardiopulmonary resuscitation and emergency cardiovascular care. *Circulation.* 2010;122(Suppl 3): S888, with permission.)

barbiturates were promising, but a large multicenter trial of thiopental found no improvement in neurologic status when this drug was given following cardiac arrest.[181] Similar results were found with calcium channel blockers. Animal studies were encouraging, but a clinical trial found no improvement in outcome.[182]

In contrast to pharmacologic therapy, two more recent studies have demonstrated improved neurologic outcome when mild therapeutic hypothermia (32°C to 34°C) was induced for 12 to 24 hours in cardiac arrest survivors who remained comatose after admission to the hospital.[183,184] Both investigations studied only patients whose initial rhythm was VF, and the larger of the trials included only witnessed arrests. Nevertheless, these are the first studies to document improved neurologic outcome with a specific postarrest intervention. The International Liaison Committee on Resuscitation now recommends "unconscious adult patients with spontaneous circulation after out-of-hospital cardiac arrest should be cooled to 32 to 34°C for 12 to 24 hours when the initial rhythm was ventricular fibrillation. Such cooling may also be beneficial for other rhythms or in-hospital cardiac arrest."

Prognosis

For the comatose survivor of CPR, the question of ultimate prognosis is important. One older study demonstrated that the chance of ever awakening fell rapidly in the days following arrest.[185] If the patient was not awake by 4 days following arrest, the chance of ever awakening was 20%, and all those awakening had marked neurologic deficits. Most patients who completely recover show rapid improvement in the first 48 hours. Poor outcome cannot be reliably predicted from clinical neurological signs in the first 24 hours. In comatose adults not treated with hypothermia, the absence of both corneal reflexes and pupillary light response at ≥72 hours postarrest reliably predicted poor outcomes.[186] It is

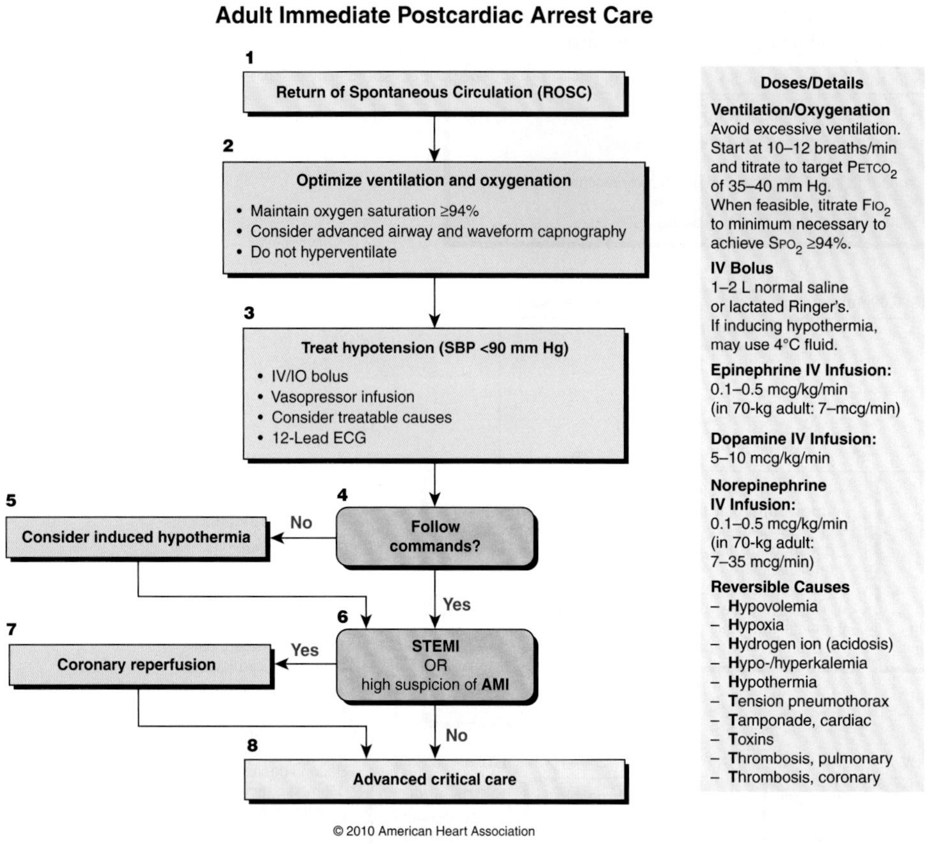

Adult Immediate Postcardiac Arrest Care

1 **Return of Spontaneous Circulation (ROSC)**

2 **Optimize ventilation and oxygenation**

- Maintain oxygen saturation ≥94%
- Consider advanced airway and waveform capnography
- Do not hyperventilate

3 **Treat hypotension (SBP <90 mm Hg)**

- IV/IO bolus
- Vasopressor infusion
- Consider treatable causes
- 12-Lead ECG

4 **Follow commands?**

No → 5 **Consider induced hypothermia**

Yes →

6 **STEMI** OR high suspicion of **AMI**

Yes → 7 **Coronary reperfusion**

No →

8 **Advanced critical care**

Doses/Details

Ventilation/Oxygenation
Avoid excessive ventilation. Start at 10–12 breaths/min and titrate to target P_{ETCO_2} of 35–40 mm Hg.
When feasible, titrate F_{IO_2} to minimum necessary to achieve S_{PO_2} ≥94%.

IV Bolus
1–2 L normal saline or lactated Ringer's.
If inducing hypothermia, may use 4°C fluid.

Epinephrine IV Infusion:
0.1–0.5 mcg/kg/min
(in 70-kg adult: 7–mcg/min)

Dopamine IV Infusion:
5–10 mcg/kg/min

Norepinephrine IV Infusion:
0.1–0.5 mcg/kg/min
(in 70-kg adult: 7–35 mcg/min)

Reversible Causes
- **H**ypovolemia
- **H**ypoxia
- **H**ydrogen ion (acidosis)
- **H**ypo-/hyperkalemia
- **H**ypothermia
- **T**ension pneumothorax
- **T**amponade, cardiac
- **T**oxins
- **T**hrombosis, pulmonary
- **T**hrombosis, coronary

FIGURE 58-12. Postcardiac arrest care algorithm. SBP, systolic blood pressure; ECG, electrocardiogram; STEMI, ST elevation myocardial infarction; AMI, acute myocardial infarction; $PetCO_2$, partial pressure of end tidal carbon dioxide; FiO_2, fraction of inspired oxygen; SpO_2, oxygen saturation by pulse oximetry. (From 2010 American Heart Association Guidelines for cardiopulmonary resuscitation and emergency cardiovascular care. *Circulation.* 2010;122(Suppl 3):S769, with permission.)

likely that the time frame for neurologic assessment needs to be extended in patients who have undergone therapeutic hypothermia, but this has not been adequately studied.

References

1. *Resuscitation: An Historical Perspective.* Park Ridge, IL: Wood Library Museum; 1976.
2. Brooks DK. *Resuscitation: Care of the Critically Ill.* London: Edward Arnold; 1986.
3. Vesalius A. *De Humani Corporis.* Basel: Fabrica, 1543.
4. Elam JO, Brown ES, Elder JD Jr. Artificial respiration by mouth to mask method: A study of the respiratory gas exchange of paralyzed patients ventilated by operator's expired air. *N Engl J Med.* 1954;250:749.
5. Gordon AS, Frye CS, Gittelson L, et al. Mouth-to-mouth versus manual artificial respiration for children and adults. *JAMA.* 1958;167:320.
6. Safar P, Escarraga LA, Elam JO. A comparison of the mouth-to-mouth and mouth-to-airway methods of artificial respiration with the chest-pressure arm-lift methods. *N Engl J Med.* 1958;258:671.
7. Safar P. Failure of manual respiration. *J Appl Physiol.* 1959;14:84.
8. Hooker DR, Kouwenhoven WB, Langworthy OR. The effects of alternating current on the heart. *Am J Physiol.* 1933;103:444.
9. Beck CS, Pritchard WH, Feil HS. Ventricular fibrillation of long duration abolished by electric shock. *JAMA.* 1947;135:985.
10. Zoll PM, Linenthal AJ, Gibson W, et al. Termination of ventricular fibrillation in man by an externally applied electric shock. *N Engl J Med.* 1956;254:727.
11. Kouwenhoven WB, Milnor WR, Knickerbocker GG, et al. Closed-chest defibrillation of the heart. *Surgery.* 1957;42:550.
12. Kouwenhoven WB, Jude JR, Knickerbocker GG. Closed-chest cardiac massage. *JAMA.* 1960;173:1064.
13. Redding JS, Pearson JW. Evaluation of drugs for cardiac resuscitation. *Anesthesiology.* 1963;24:203.
14. Rosamond W, Flegal K, Furie K, et al. Heart disease and stroke statistics 2008 update. A report from the American Heart Association Statistics Committee and Stroke Statistics Subcommittee. *Circulation.* 2008;117:e25.
15. Angelos M, Safar P, Reich H. A comparison of cardiopulmonary resuscitation with cardiopulmonary bypass after prolonged cardiac arrest in dogs: Reperfusion pressures and neurologic recovery. *Resuscitation.* 1991;21:121.
16. Kern KB, Sanders AB, Janas W, et al. Limitations of open-chest cardiac massage after prolonged, untreated cardiac arrest in dogs. *Ann Emerg Med.* 1991;20:761.
17. Wik L, Steen PA, Bircher HB. Quality of bystander cardiopulmonary resuscitation influences outcome after prehospital cardiac arrest. *Resuscitation.* 1994;28:195.
18. Weaver WD, Cobb LA, Hallstrom AP, et al. Factors influencing survival after out-of-hospital cardiac arrest. *J Am Coll Cardiol.* 1986;7:752.
19. Eisenberg MS, Copass MK, Halstrom AP, et al. Treatment of out-of-hospital cardiac arrest with rapid defibrillation by emergency medical technicians. *N Engl J Med.* 1980;302:1379.
20. Weaver WD, Hill D, Fahrenbruch CE, et al. Use of the automatic external defibrillator in the management of out-of-hospital cardiac arrest. *N Engl J Med.* 1988;319:661.
21. Valenzuela TD, Kern KB, Clark LL, et al. Interruptions of chest compressions during emergency medical systems resuscitation. *Circulation.* 2005;112:1259.
22. Nichol G, Stiell IG, Laupacis A, et al. A cumulative meta-analysis of the effectiveness of defibrillator-capable emergency medical services for victims of out-of-hospital cardiac arrest. *Ann Emerg Med.* 2005;46:512.
23. Nadkarni VM, Larkin GL, Peberdy MA, et al. First documented rhythm and clinical outcomes from in-hospital cardiac arrest among children and adults. *JAMA.* 2006;295:50.
24. Olsson GI, Hallen B. Cardiac arrest during anaesthesia: A computer-aided study of 250,543 anaesthetics. *Acta Anaesthesiol Scand.* 1988;32:653.
25. Cohen CB, Cohen PJ. Do-not-resuscitate orders in the operating room. *N Engl J Med.* 1991;325:1879.
26. Walker RM. DNR in the OR: Resuscitation as an operative risk. *JAMA.* 1991;266:2407.
27. Margolis JO, McGrath BJ, Kussin PS, et al. Do no resuscitate (DNR) orders during surgery: Ethical foundations for institutional policies in the United States. *Anesth Analg.* 1995;80:806.
28. Guildner CW. Resuscitation. Opening the airway: A comparative study of techniques for opening an airway obstructed by the tongue. *JACEP.* 1976;5:588.
29. Emergency Cardiac Care Committee, Subcommittees and Task Forces, American Heart Association. 2010 American Heart Association guidelines for cardiopulmonary resuscitation and emergency cardiovascular care. *Circulation.* 2010;122: S640–S946.
30. Heimlich HJ. Pop goes the cafe coronary. *Emerg Med.* 1974;6:154.
31. Guildner CW, Williams D, Subtich T. Airway obstructed by foreign material: The Heimlich maneuver. *JACEP.* 1976;5:675.
32. Redding JS. The choking controversy: Critique of evidence on the Heimlich maneuver. *Crit Care Med.* 1979;7:475.
33. Harrison RR, Maull KI, Keenan RL, et al. Mouth-to-mask ventilation: A superior method of rescue breathing. *Ann Emerg Med.* 1982;11:74.

34. Jesudian MCS, Harrison RR, Keenan RL, et al. Bag-valve-mask ventilation: Two rescuers are better than one: Preliminary report. *Crit Care Med.* 1985;13:122.
35. Babbs CF. New versus old theories of blood flow during CPR. *Crit Care Med.* 1980;8: 191.
36. Jude JR, Kouwenhoven WB, Knickerbocker GG. Cardiac arrest: Report of application of external cardiac massage on 118 patients. *JAMA.* 1961;178:1063.
37. Criley JM, Blaufuss AH, Kissel GL. Cough-induced cardiac compression: Self-administered form of cardiopulmonary resuscitation. *JAMA.* 1976;236:1246.
38. Rudikoff MJ, Maughan WL, Effrom M, et al. Mechanisms of blood flow during cardiopulmonary resuscitation. *Circulation.* 1980;61:345.
39. Holmes HR, Babbs CF, Voorhees WD, et al. Influence of adrenergic drugs upon vital organ perfusion during CPR. *Crit Care Med.* 1980;8:137.
40. Michael JR, Guerci AD, Koehler RC, et al. Mechanisms by which epinephrine augments cerebral and myocardial perfusion during cardiopulmonary resuscitation in dogs. *Circulation.* 1984;69:822.
41. Weil MH, Rackow EC, Trevino R, et al. Difference in acid–base state between venous and arterial blood during cardiopulmonary resuscitation. *N Engl J Med.* 1986;315:153.
42. Kern KB, Carter AB, Showen RL, et al. Twenty-four-hour survival in a canine model of cardiac arrest comparing three methods of manual cardiopulmonary resuscitation. *J Am Coll Cardiol.* 1986;7:859.
43. Kern KB, Carter AB, Showen RL, et al. Comparison of mechanical techniques of cardiopulmonary resuscitation: Survival and neurologic outcome in dogs. *Am J Emerg Med.* 1987;5:190.
44. Kirscher JP, Fine EG, Weisfeld ML, et al. Comparison of prehospital conventional and simultaneous compression–ventilation cardiopulmonary resuscitation. *Crit Care Med.* 1989;17:1263.
45. Babbs CF, Tacker WA. Cardiopulmonary resuscitation with interposed abdominal compression. *Circulation.* 1986;74(Suppl 4):37.
46. Mateer JF, Stueven HA, Thompson BM, et al. Pre-hospital IAC-CPR versus standard CPR: Paramedic resuscitation of cardiac arrests. *Am J Emerg Med.* 1985;3:143.
47. Sack JB, Kesselbrenner MB, Bregman D. Survival from in-hospital cardiac arrest with interposed abdominal counterpulsation during cardiopulmonary resuscitation. *JAMA.* 1992;267:379.
48. Niemann JT, Rosborough JP, Criley JM, et al. Circulatory support during cardiac arrest using a pneumatic vest and abdominal binder with simultaneous high pressure airway inflation. *Ann Emerg Med.* 1984;13:767.
49. Timerman S, Cardoso LF, Ramires JA, et al. Improved hemodynamic performance with a novel chest compression device during treatment of in-hospital cardiac arrest. *Resuscitation.* 2004;61:273.
50. Lurie KG, Lindo C, Chin J. CPR: The P stands for plumber's helper [letter]. *JAMA.* 1990;264:1661.
51. Cohen TJ, Tucker KJ, Lurie KG, et al. Active compression–decompression. A new method of cardiopulmonary resuscitation. *JAMA.* 1992;267:2916.
52. Linder KH, Pfenniger EG, Lurie KG, et al. Effects of active compression–decompression resuscitation on myocardial and cerebral blood flow in pigs. *Circulation.* 1993;88:1254.
53. Lafuente-Lafuente C, Melero-Bascones M. Active chest compression–decompression for cardiopulmonary resuscitation. *Cochrane Database Syst Rev.* 2004;(3): CD002751.
54. Plaisance P, Lurie KG, Payen D. Inspiratory impedance during active compression–decompression cardiopulmonary resuscitation: A randomized evaluation in patients in cardiac arrest. *Circulation.* 2000;101:989.
55. Aufderheide TP, Pirrallo RG, Provo TA, et al. Clinical evaluation of an inspiratory impedance threshold device during standard cardiopulmonary resuscitation in patients with out of hospital cardiac arrest. *Crit Care Med.* 2005;33:734.
56. Plaisance P, Lurie KG, Vicaut E, et al. Evaluation of an impedance threshold device in patients receiving active compression–decompression cardiopulmonary resuscitation for out of hospital cardic arrest. *Resuscitation.* 2004;61:265.
57. Aufderheide TP, Nichol G, Rea TD, et al. A trial of an impedance threshold device in out-of-hospital cardiac arrest. *N Engl J Med.* 2011;365:798.
58. DeBehnke DJ, Angelos MG, Leasure JE. Comparison of standard external CPR, open-chest CPR, and cardiopulmonary bypass in a canine myocardial infarct model. *Ann Emerg Med.* 1991;20:754.
59. Sanders AB, Kern KB, Atlas M, et al. Importance of the duration of inadequate coronary perfusion pressure on resuscitation from cardiac arrest. *J Am Coll Cardiol.* 1985;6:113.
60. Kern KB, Sanders AB, Badylak SF, et al. Long term survival with open-chest cardiac massage after ineffective closed-chest compression in a canine preparation. *Circulation.* 1987;75:498.
61. Ralston SH, Voorhees WD, Babbs CF. Intrapulmonary epinephrine during prolonged CPR: Improved regional blood flow and resuscitation in dogs. *Ann Emerg Med.* 1984;13:79.
62. Crile G, Dolley DH. Experimental research into resuscitation of dogs killed by anesthetics and asphyxia. *J Exp Med.* 1906;8:713.
63. Redding JS. Abdominal compression in cardiopulmonary resuscitation. *Anesth Analg.* 1971;50:668.
64. Pearson JW, Redding JS. Influence of peripheral vascular tone on cardiac resuscitation. *Anesth Analg.* 1965;44:746.
65. Yakaitis RW, Otto CW, Blitt CD. Relative importance of alpha and beta adrenergic receptors during resuscitation. *Crit Care Med.* 1979;7:293.
66. Otto CW, Yakaitis RW, Blitt CD. Mechanism of action of epinephrine in resuscitation from asphyxial arrest. *Crit Care Med.* 1981;9:321.
67. Ditchey RV, Winkler JV, Rhodes CA. Relative lack of coronary blood flow during closed-chest resuscitation in dogs. *Circulation.* 1982;66:297.
68. Otto CW, Yakaitis RW. The role of epinephrine in CPR: A reappraisal. *Ann Emerg Med.* 1984;13:840.
69. Sanders AB, Ewy GA, Taft TV. Prognostic and therapeutic importance of the aortic diastolic pressure in resuscitation from cardiac arrest. *Crit Care Med.* 1984;12:871.
70. Niemann JT, Criley JM, Rosborough JP, et al. Predictive indices of successful cardiac resuscitation after prolonged arrest and experimental cardiopulmonary resuscitation. *Ann Emerg Med.* 1985;14:521.
71. Paradis NA, Martin GB, Rivers EP, et al. Coronary perfusion pressure and the return of spontaneous circulation in human cardiopulmonary resuscitation. *JAMA.* 1990;263:1106.
72. Kalenda Z. The capnogram as a guide to the efficacy of cardiac massage. *Resuscitation.* 1978;6:259.
73. Weil MH, Bisera J, Trevino RP. Cardiac output and end tidal carbon dioxide. *Crit Care Med.* 1985;13:907.
74. Sanders AB, Atlas M, Ewy GA, et al. Expired Pco_2 as an index of coronary perfusion pressure. *Am J Emerg Med.* 1985;3:147.
75. Sanders AB, Ewy GA, Bragg S, et al. Expired PCO_2 as a prognostic indicator of successful resuscitation from cardiac arrest. *Ann Emerg Med.* 1985;14:948.
76. Sanders AB, Kern KB, Otto CW, et al. End-tidal carbon dioxide monitoring during cardiopulmonary resuscitation: A prognostic indicator for survival. *JAMA.* 1989;262:1347.
77. Levine RL, Wayne MA, Miller CC. End-tidal carbon dioxide and outcome of out-of-hospital cardiac arrest. *N Engl J Med.* 1997;337:301.
78. Kern KB, Sanders AB, Raife J, et al. A study of chest compression rates during cardiopulmonary resuscitation in humans: The importance of rate-directed compressions. *Arch Intern Med.* 1992;152:145.
79. Otto CW. Cardiovascular pharmacology II: The use of catecholamines, pressor agents, digitalis, and corticosteroids in CPR and emergency cardiac care. *Circulation.* 1986;74(Suppl 4):80.
80. Larabee TM. Vasopressors in cardiac arrest: A systematic review. *Resuscitation.* 2012;83:932.
81. Redding JS, Pearson JW. Resuscitation from ventricular fibrillation (drug therapy). *JAMA.* 1968;203:255.
82. Schleien CL, Dean JM, Koehler RC, et al. Effect of epinephrine on cerebral and myocardial perfusion in an infant animal preparation of cardiopulmonary resuscitation. *Circulation.* 1986;73:809.
83. Schleien CL, Koehler RC, Gervais H, et al. Organ blood flow and somatosensory-evoked potentials during and after cardiopulmonary resuscitation with epinephrine or phenylephrine. *Circulation.* 1989;79:1332.
84. Otto CW, Yakaitis RW, Redding JS, et al. Comparison of dopamine, dobutamine, and epinephrine in CPR. *Crit Care Med.* 1981;9:640.
85. Lindner KH, Prengel AW, Pfenniger EG, et al. Vasopressin improves vital organ blood flow during closed-chest cardiopulmonary resuscitation in pigs. *Circulation.* 1995;91:215.
86. Brillman JC, Sanders AB, Otto CW, et al. A comparison of epinephrine and phenylephrine for resuscitation and neurologic outcome of cardiac arrest in dogs. *Ann Emerg Med.* 1987;16:11.
87. Silvast T, Saarnivaara L, Kinnunen A, et al. Comparison of adrenaline and phenylephrine in out-of-hospital CPR: A double-blind study. *Acta Anaesthesiol Scand.* 1985;29:610.
88. Linder KH, Ahnefeld FW, Prengel AW. Comparison of standard and high-dose adrenaline in the resuscitation of asystole and electromechanical dissociation. *Acta Anaesthesiol Scand.* 1991;35:253.
89. Stiell IB, Hebert PC, Weitzman BN, et al. High-dose epinephrine in adult cardiac arrest. *N Engl J Med.* 1992;327:1045.
90. Brown CG, Martin DP, Pepe PE, et al. A comparison of standard-dose and high-dose epinephrine in cardiac arrest outside the hospital. *N Engl J Med.* 1992;327:1051.
91. Callaham M, Madsen CD, Barton CW, et al. A randomized clinical trial of high-dose epinephrine and norepinephrine vs standard-dose epinephrine in prehospital cardiac arrest. *JAMA.* 1992;268:2667.
92. Choux C, Gueugniaud P-Y, Barbieux A, et al. Standard doses versus repeated high doses of epinephrine in cardiac arrest outside the hospital. *Resuscitation.* 1995;29:3.
93. Gueugniaud P-Y, Mols P, Goldstein P, et al. A comparison of repeated high doses and repeated standard doses of epinephrine for cardiac arrest outside the hospital. *N Engl J Med.* 1998;339:1595.
94. Lipman J, Wilson W, Kobilski S, et al. High-dose adrenaline in adult in-hospital asystolic cardiopulmonary resuscitation: A double-blind randomized trial. *Anaesth Intensive Care.* 1993;21:192.
95. Sherman BW, Munger MA, Foulke GE, et al. High-dose versus standard-dose epinephrine treatment of cardiac arrest after failure of standard therapy. *Pharmacotherapy.* 1997;17:242.
96. Jacobs IG, Finn JC, Jelinek GA, et al. Effect of adrenaline on survival in out-of-hospital cardiac arrest: a randomised double-blind placebo controlled trial. *Resuscitation.* 2011;82:1138.

97. Prengel AW, Lindner KH, Keller A, et al. Cardiovascular function during the postresuscitation phase after cardiac arrest in pigs: A comparison of epinephrine versus vasopressin. *Crit Care Med.* 1996;24:2014.
98. Lindner KH, Dirks B, Strohmenger HU, et al. Randomized comparison of epinephrine and vasopressin in patients with out-of hospital ventricular fibrillation. *Lancet.* 1997;349:535.
99. Stiell IG, Hebert PC, Wells GA, et al. Vasopressin versus epinephrine for in hospital cardiac arrest: A randomized controlled trial. *Lancet.* 2001;358:105.
100. Wenzel V, Krismer AC, Arntz HR, et al. A comparison of vasopressin and epinephrine for out-of-hospital cardiopulmonary resuscitation. *N Engl J Med.* 2004;350:105.
101. Kowey PR, Levine JH, Herre JM, et al. Randomized, double-blind comparison of intravenous amiodarone and bretylium in the treatment of patients with recurrent hemodynamically destabilizing ventricular tachycardia or fibrillation. *Circulation.* 1995;92:3255.
102. Kudenchuk PJ, Cobb LA, Copass MK, et al. Amiodarone for resuscitation after out of hospital cardiac arrest due to ventricular fibrillation. *N Engl J Med.* 1999;341:871.
103. Dorian P, Cass D, Schwartz B, et al. Amiodarone as compared with lidocaine for shock-resistant ventricular fibrillation. *N Engl J Med.* 2002;346:884.
104. Stueven HA, Tonsfeldt DJ, Thompson BM, et al. Atropine in asystole: Human studies. *Ann Emerg Med.* 1984;13:815.
105. Coon GA, Clinton JE, Ruiz E. Use of atropine for brady-asystolic prehospital cardiac arrest. *Ann Emerg Med.* 1981;10:462.
106. Guerci AD, Chandra N, Johnson E, et al. Failure of sodium bicarbonate to improve resuscitation from ventricular fibrillation in dogs. *Circulation.* 1986;74(Suppl 4):75.
107. Federiuk CS, Sanders AB, Kern KB, et al. The effect of bicarbonate on resuscitation from cardiac arrest. *Ann Emerg Med.* 1991;20:1173.
108. Bishop RL, Weisfeldt ML. Sodium bicarbonate administration during cardiac arrest: Effect on arterial pH, PCO_2, and osmolality. *JAMA.* 1976;235:506.
109. Mattar JA, Weil MH, Shubin H, et al. Cardiac arrest in the critically ill: II. Hyperosmolal states following cardiac arrest. *Am J Med.* 1974;56:162.
110. Sanders AB, Otto CW, Kern KB, et al. Acid–base balance in a canine model of cardiac arrest. *Ann Emerg Med.* 1988;17:667.
111. Kette F, Weil MH, von Planta MS, et al. Buffer agents do not reverse intra-myocardial acidosis during cardiac resuscitation. *Circulation.* 1990;81:1660.
112. Dembo DH. Calcium in advanced life support. *Crit Care Med.* 1981;9:358.
113. Harrison EE, Amey BD. The use of calcium in cardiac resuscitation. *Am J Emerg Med.* 1983;1:267.
114. Stueven HA, Thompson BM, Aprahamian C, et al. Use of calcium in prehospital cardiac arrest. *Ann Emerg Med.* 1983;12:136.
115. Stueven HA, Thompson BM, Aprahamian C, et al. Calcium chloride: Reassessment of use in asystole. *Ann Emerg Med.* 1984;13:820.
116. Stueven HA, Thompson BM, Aprahamian C, et al. Lack of effectiveness of calcium chloride in refractory asystole. *Ann Emerg Med.* 1985;14:630.
117. Kerber RE, Sarnat W. Factors influencing the success of ventricular defibrillation in man. *Circulation.* 1979;60:226.
118. Yakaitis RW, Ewy GA, Otto CW, et al. Influence of time and therapy on ventricular defibrillation in dogs. *Crit Care Med.* 1980;8:157.
119. Weaver WD, Copass MD, Bufi D, et al. Improved neurologic recovery and survival after early defibrillation. *Circulation.* 1984;69:943.
120. Weaver WD, Cobb LA, Dennis D, et al. Amplitude of ventricular fibrillation waveform and outcome after cardiac arrest. *Ann Intern Med.* 1985;102:53.
121. Ewy GA, Dahl CF, Zimmermann M, et al. Ventricular fibrillation masquerading as ventricular standstill. *Crit Care Med.* 1981;9:841.
122. Stewart AJ, Allen JD, Adgey AAJ. Frequency analysis of ventricular fibrillation and resuscitation success. *Q J Med.* 1992;306:761.
123. Brown CG, Griffith RF, Ligten PV, et al. Median frequency—a new parameter for predicting defibrillation success rate. *Ann Emerg Med.* 1991;20:787.
124. Strohmenger HU, Lindner KH, Brown CG. Analysis of the ventricular fibrillation ECG signal amplitude and frequency parameters as predictors of coutershock success in human. *Chest.* 1997;111:584.
125. Povoas HP, Weil MH, Tang W, et al. Predicting the success of defibrillation by electrocardiographic analysis. *Resuscitation.* 2002;53:77.
126. Stromenger HU, Eftestol T, Sunde K, et al. The predictive value of ventricular fibrillation electrocardiogram signal frequency and amplitude variables in patients with out-of-hospital cardiac arrest. *Anesth Analg.* 2001;93:1428.
127. Otto CW, Yakaitis RW, Ewy GA. Effects of epinephrine on defibrillation in ischemic ventricular fibrillation. *Am J Emerg Med.* 1985;3:285.
128. Cummins RO, Eisenberg MS, Bergner L, et al. Sensitivity, accuracy and safety of an automatic external defibrillator: Report of a field evaluation. *Lancet.* 1984;1:318.
129. Cummins RO, Eisenberg MS, Graves JR, et al. Automatic external defibrillators used by emergency medical technicians: A controlled clinical trial. *Circulation.* 1985;72(Suppl 3):8.
130. Kerber RE, Kouba C, Marines J, et al. Advance prediction of transthoracic impedance in human defibrillation and cardioversion: Importance of impedance in determining the success of low energy shocks. *Circulation.* 1984;70:303.
131. Kerber RE, McPherson D, Charbonnier R, et al. Automatic impedance-based energy adjustment for defibrillation: Experimental studies. *Circulation.* 1985;71:136.
132. Lerman BB, DeMarco JP, Haines DE. Current-based versus energy-based ventricular defibrillation: A prospective study. *J Am Coll Cardiol.* 1988;12:1259.
133. Kerber RE, Grayzel J, Hoyt R, et al. Transthoracic resistance in human defibrillation: Influence of body weight, chest size, serial shocks, paddle size and paddle contact pressure. *Circulation.* 1981;63:676.
134. Connel PN, Ewy GA, Dahl CF, et al. Transthoracic impedance to defibrillation discharge: Effect of electrode size and electrode-chest wall interface. *J Electrocardiol.* 1973;6:313.
135. Ewy GA, Taren D. Comparison of paddle electrode pastes used for defibrillation. *Heart Lung.* 1977;6:847.
136. Ewy GA, Hellman DA, McClung S, et al. Influence of ventilation phase on transthoracic impedance and defibrillation effectiveness. *Crit Care Med.* 1980;8:164.
137. Dahl CF, Ewy GA, Warner ED, et al. Myocardial necrosis from direct current countershock. *Circulation.* 1974;50:956.
138. Warner ED, Dahl CF, Ewy GA. Myocardial injury from transthoracic defibrillator countershock. *Arch Pathol.* 1975;99:55.
139. Ehsani A, Ewy GA, Sobel BE. Effects of electrical countershock on serum creatine phosphokinase (CPK) isoenzyme activity. *Am J Cardiol.* 1976;37:12.
140. Weaver WD, Cobb LA, Copass MK, et al. Ventricular defibrillation: A comparative trial using 175-J and 320-J shocks. *N Engl J Med.* 1982;307:1101.
141. Geddes LA, Tacker WA, Rosborough JP, et al. Electrical dose for ventricular defibrillation of large and small animals using precordial electrodes. *J Clin Invest.* 1974;53:310.
142. Gutgesell HP, Tacker WA, Geddes LA, et al. Energy dose for defibrillation in children. *Pediatrics.* 1976;58:898.
143. Kerber RE, Jensen SR, Gascho JA, et al. Determinants of defibrillation: Prospective analysis of 183 patients. *Am J Cardiol.* 1983;52:739.
144. American Heart Association. Guidelines 2000 for cardiopulmonary resuscitation and emergency cardiovascular care: International Consensus on Science. *Circulation.* 2000;102(8):I-1.
145. Bardy GH, Marchlinski FE, Sharma AD, et al. Multicenter comparison of truncated biphasic shocks and standard damped sine wave monophasic shocks for transthoracic ventricular defibrillation. *Circulation.* 1996;94:2507.
146. Hazinski MF, Nolan JP, Billi JE, et al. 2010 international consensus on cardiopulmonary resuscitation and emergency cardiovascular care science with treatment recommendations. *Circulation.* 2010;122(Suppl 2):S250149.
147. Rea TD, Eisenberg MS, Becker LJ, et al. Temporal trends in sudden cardiac arrest: A 25-year emergency medical services perspective. *Circulation.* 2003;107:2780.
148. Sanders AB. Cardiac arrest and the limitations of clinical trials. *N Engl J Med.* 2011;365:850.
149. Ewy GA. Cardiocerebral resuscitation: the new cardiopulmonary resuscitation. *Circulation.* 2005;111:2134.
150. Ewy GA, Kern KB, Sanders AB, et al. Cardiocerebral resuscitation for cardiac arrest. *Am J Med.* 2006;119:6.
151. Weisfeldt ML, Becker LB. Resuscitation after cardiac arrest: a 3-phase time-sensitive model. *JAMA.* 2002;288:3035.
152. Caffrey SL, Willoughby PJ, Pepe PE, et al. Public use of automated external defibrillators. *N Engl J Med.* 2002;347:1242.
153. Valenzulea TD, Roe DJ, Nichol G, et al. Outcomes of rapid defibrillation by security officers after cardiac arrest in casinos. *N Engl J Med.* 2000;343:1206.
154. Kern, KB, Garewal HS, Sanders AB, et al. Depletion of myocardial adenosine triphosphate during prolonged untreated ventricular fibrillation: effect on defibrillation success. *Resuscitation.* 1990;20:221.
155. Ornato JP, Hallagan LF, McMahan SB, et al. Attitudes of BCLS instructors about mouth-to-mouth resuscitation during the AIDS epidemic. *Ann Emerg Med.* 1990;19:151.
156. Brenner BE, Kauffman J. Reluctance of internists and medical nurses to perform mouth-to-mouth resuscitation. *Arch Intern Med.* 1993;153:1763.
157. Locke CJ, Berg RA, Sanders AB, et al. Bystander cardiopulmonary resuscitation: Concerns about mouth-to-mouth contact. *Arch Intern Med.* 1995;155:938.
158. Bossaert L, Van Hoeyweghen R. The cerebral resuscitation study group: Bystander cardiopulmonary resuscitation (CPR) in out-of-hospital cardiac arrest. *Resuscitation.* 1989;17(Suppl):S55.
159. Van Hoeyweghen RJ, Bossaert LL, Mullie A, et al. Quality and efficiency of bystander CPR. *Resuscitation.* 1993;26:47.
160. SOS-KANTO study group. Cardiopulmonary resuscitation by bystanders with chest compression only (SOS-KANTO): An observational study. *Lancet.* 2007;369:920.
161. Berg RA, Kern KB, Sanders AB, et al. Bystander cardiopulmonary resuscitation: Is ventilation necessary? *Circulation.* 1993;88:1907.
162. Berg RA, Wilcoxson D, Hilwig RW, et al. The need for ventilatory support during bystander cardiopulmonary resuscitation. *Ann Emerg Med.* 1995;26:342.
163. Berg RA, Kern KB, Hilwig RW, et al. Assisted ventilation does not improve outcome in a porcine model of single-rescuer bystander cardiopulmonary resuscitation. *Circulation.* 1997;95:1635.
164. Berg RA, Kern KB, Hilwig RW, et al. Assisted ventilation during 'bystander' CPR in a swine acute myocardial infarction model does not improve outcome. *Circulation.* 1997;96:4364.

165. Assar D, Chamberlain D, Colquhoun M, et al. Randomized controlled trials of staged teaching for basic life support: 1. skill acquisition at bronze stage. *Resuscitation.* 2000;45:7.
166. Kern KB, Hilwig R, Berg RA, et al. Importance of continuous chest compressions during cardiopulmonary resuscitation: improved outcome during a simulated single lay-rescuer scenario. *Circulation.* 2002;105:645.
167. Ewy GA, Zuercher M, Hilwig RW, et al. Improved neurological outcome with continuous chest compressions compared with 30: 2 compressions-to-ventilations cardiopulmonary resuscitation in a realistic swine model of out-of-hospital cardiac arrest. *Circulation.* 2007;116:2525.
168. Bobrow BJ, Spaite DW, Berg RA, et al. Chest compression-only CPR by lay rescuers and survival from out-of-hospital cardiac arrest. *JAMA.* 2010;304:1447.
169. Sayre MR, Berg RA, Cave DM, et al. Hands-only (compression-only) cardiopulmonary resuscitation: A call to action for bystander response to adults who experience out-of-hospital sudden cardiac arrest. A science advisory for the public from the American Heart Association Emergency Cardiovascular Care Committee. *Circulation.* 2008;117(16):2162.
170. Berg RA, Sanders AB, Kern KB, et al. Adverse hemodynamic effects of interrupting chest compressions for rescue breathing during cardiopulmonary resuscitation for ventricular fibrillation cardiac arrest. *Circulation.* 2001;104:2465.
171. Wik L, Kramer-Johansen J, Myklebust H, et al. Quality of cardiopulmonary resuscitation during out-of-hospital cardiac arrest. *JAMA.* 2005;293:299.
172. Aufderheide TP, Sigudsson G, Pirrallo RG, et al. Hyperventilation-induced hypotension during cardiopulmonary resuscitation. *Circulation.* 2004;109:1960.
173. Aufderheide TP, Lurie K. Death by hyperventilation: a common and life-threatening problem during cardiopulmonary resuscitation. *Crit Care Med.* 2004; 32(Suppl):S345.
174. Milander MM, Hiscok PS, Sanders AB, et al. Chest compression and ventilation during cardiopulmonary resuscitation: the effects of audible tone guidance. *Acad Emerg Med.* 1995;2:708.
175. Cobb LA, Fahrenbruch CE, Walsh TR, et al. Influence of CPR prior to defibrillation in out-of-hospital ventricular fibrillation. *JAMA.* 1999;281:1182.
176. Wik L, Hansen TB, Fylling F, et al. Delaying defibrillation to give basic cardiopulmonary resuscitation to patients with out-of-hospital ventricular fibrillation. *JAMA.* 2003;289:1389.
177. Berg RA, Hilwig RE, Kern KB, et al. Automated external defibrillation versus manual defibrillation for prolonged ventricular fibrillation: Lethal delays of chest compressions before and after countershocks. *Ann Emerg Med.* 2003; 41:458.
178. Rea Td, Shah S, Kudenchuck PJ, et al. Automated external defibrillators: To what extent does the algorithm delay CPR? *Ann Emerg Med.* 2005;46:132.
179. Kellum MJ, Kennedy KW, Barney R, et al. Cardiocerebral resuscitation improves neurologically intact survival of patients with out-of-hospital cardiac arrest. *Ann Emerg Med.* 2008;52:253.
180. Bobrow BJ, Clark LL, Ewy GA, et al. Minimally interrupted cardiac resuscitation by emergency medical services for out-of-hospital cardiac arrest. *JAMA.* 2008; 299:1158.
181. Abramson NS, Safar P, Detre KM, et al. Randomized clinical study of cardiopulmonary-cerebral resuscitation: Thiopental loading in comatose cardiac arrest survivors. *N Engl J Med.* 1986;314:397.
182. Brain Resuscitation Clinical Trial II study group. A randomized clinical study of a calcium-entry blocker (lidoflazine) in the treatment of comatose survivors of cardiac arrest. *N Engl J Med.* 1991;324:1225.
183. Holzer M. The Hypothermia After Cardiac Arrest Study Group: Mild therapeutic hypothermia to improve the neurologic outcome after cardiac arrest. *N Engl J Med.* 2002;346:549.
184. Bernard SA, Gray TW, Buist MD, et al. Treatment of comatose survivors of out-of-hospital cardiac arrest with induced hypothermia. *N Engl J Med.* 2002; 346:557.
185. Longstreth WT, Inui TS, Cobb LA, et al. Neurologic recovery after out-of-hospital cardiac arrest. *Ann Intern Med.* 1983;98:588.
186. Zandbergen EG, Hijdra A, Koelman JH, et al. Prediction of poor outcome within the first 3 days of postanoxic come. *Neurology.* 2006;66:62.

APPENDIX

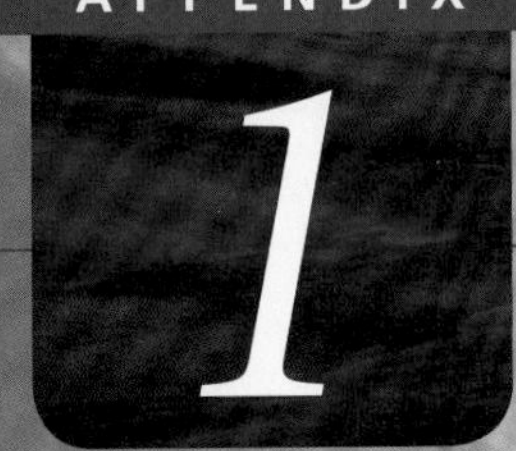

Atlas of Electrocardiography

GINA C. BADESCU • BENJAMIN SHERMAN • JAMES R. ZAIDAN • PAUL G. BARASH

LEAD PLACEMENT

	Electrode	
	Positive	Negative
Bipolar Leads		
I	LA	RA
II	LL	RA
III	LL	LA
Augmented Unipolar		
aVR	RA	LA, LL
aVL	LA	RA, LL
aVF	LL	RA, LA
Precordial		
V_1	4 ICS–RSB	
V_2	4 ICS–LSB	
V_3	Midway between V_2 and V_4	
V_4	5 ICS–MCL	
V_5	5 ICS–AAL	
V_6	5 ICS–MAL	

Abbrev.	Meaning
ICS	Intercostal Space
RSB	Right Sternal Border
LSB	Left Sternal Border
MCL	Midclavicular Line
AAL	Interaxillary Line
MAL	Midaxillary Line

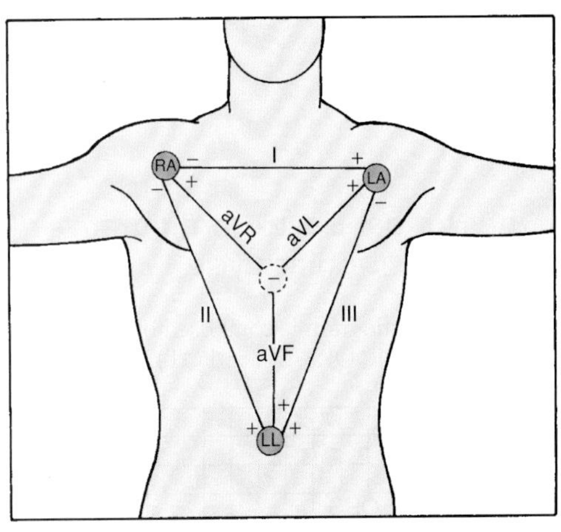

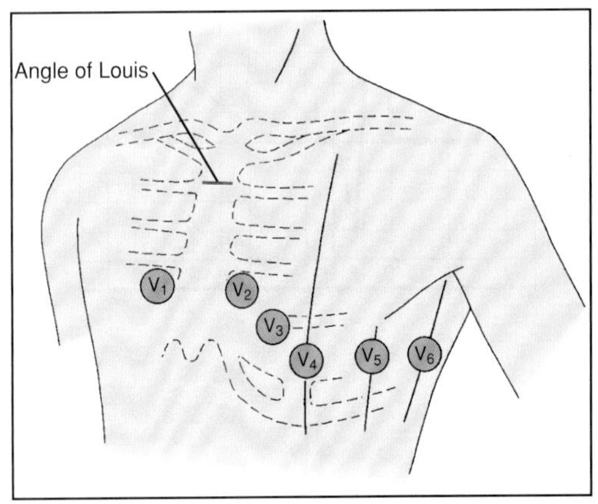

Multimedia

1. Atrial Fibrillation
2. Atrial Flutter
3. Atrioventrcular Block (First Degree)
4. Atrioventricular Block (Second Degree), Mobitz Type I/Wenckebach Block
5. Atrioventricular Block (Second Degree), Mobitz Type II
6. Atrioventricular Block (Third-Degree), Complete Heart Block
7. Bundle Branch Block - Left (LBBB)
8. Bundle Branch Block - Right (RBBB)
9. Transmural Myocardial Infarction
10. Subendocardial Myocardial Infarction (SEMI)
11. Myocardial Ischemia
12. Myocardial Ischemia

Sections and images of this Appendix were developed, in part, for both Barash PG, Cullen BF, Stoelting RK, et al., eds. *Clinical Anesthesia, 7th ed.* Philadelphia: Wolters Kluwer Health/Lippincott Williams & Wilkins; 2013, and Kaplan JA, Reich DL, Savino JS, eds. *Kaplan's Cardiac Anesthesia: The Echo Era.* Philadelphia: Elsevier; 2011 with permission of the editors and publishers.

- 13 Digitalis Effect
- 14 Potassium
- 15 Paroxysmal Atrial Tachycardia (PAT)
- 16 Pericarditis
- 17 Premature Atrial Contraction (PAC)
- 18 Premature Ventricular Contraction (PVC)
- 19 Premature Ventricular Contraction (PVC) - Multifocal
- 20 Premature Ventricular Contraction (PVC) - Triplet
- 21 Premature Ventricular Contraction (PVC) - Bigeminy
- 22 Premature Ventricular Contraction (PVC) - Couplets
- 23 Sinus Bradycardia
- 24 Sinus Bradycardia
- 25 Sinus Bradycardia
- 26 Sinus Arrhythmia
- 27 Sinus Tachycardia
- 28 Torsades De Pointes
- 29 Ventricular Fibrillation
- 30 Ventricular Tachycardia
- 31 Wolff-Parkinson-White Syndrome (WPW)
- 32 Atrial Pacing: Pacemaker Tracings
- 33 Ventricular Pacing
- 34 DDD Pacing

The Normal Electrocardiogram—Cardiac Cycle

The normal electrocardiogram is composed of waves (P, QRS, T, and U) and intervals (PR, QRS, ST, and QT).

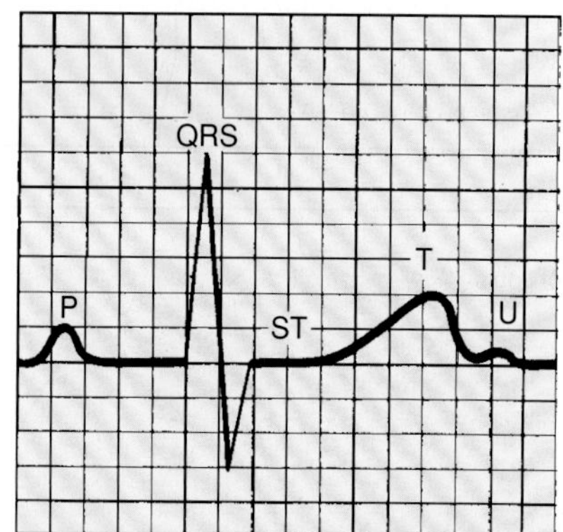

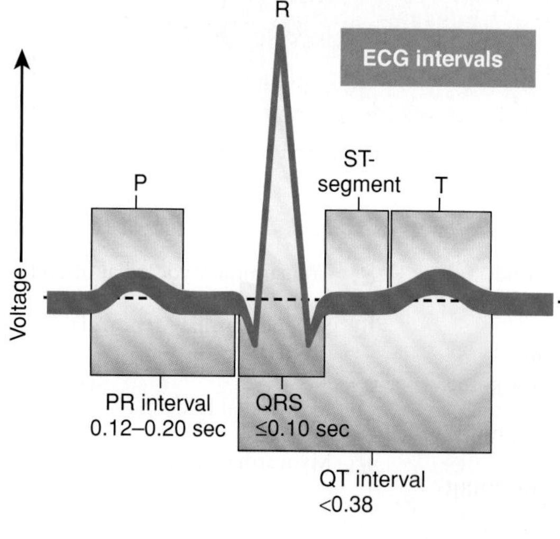

1 Atrial Fibrillation

Rate: Variable (~150–200 beats/min)
Rhythm: Irregular
PR interval: No P wave; PR interval not discernible
QT interval: QRS normal

Note: Must be differentiated from atrial flutter: (1) absence of flutter waves and presence of fibrillatory line; (2) flutter usually associated with higher ventricular rates (>150 beats/min). Loss of atrial contraction reduces cardiac output (10–20%). Mural atrial thrombi may develop. Considered controlled if ventricular rate is <100 beats/min.

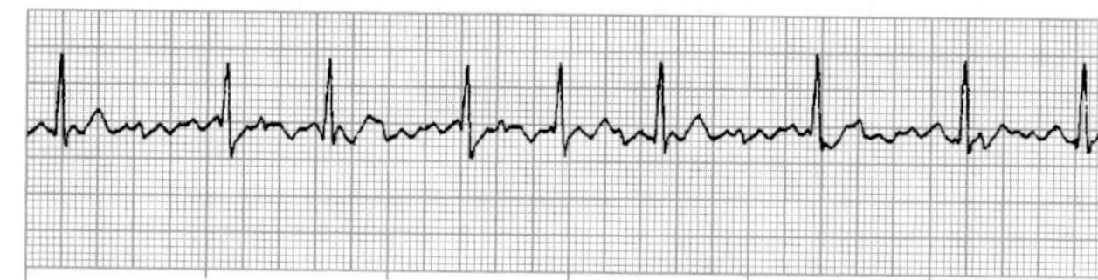

2 Atrial Flutter

Rate: Rapid, atrial usually regular (250–350 beats/min); ventricular usually regular (<100 beats/min)
Rhythm: Atrial and ventricular regular
PR interval: Flutter (F) waves are saw-toothed. PR interval cannot be measured.
QT interval: QRS usually normal; ST segment and T waves are not identifiable.

Note: Vagal maneuvers will slow ventricular response, simplifying recognition of the F waves.

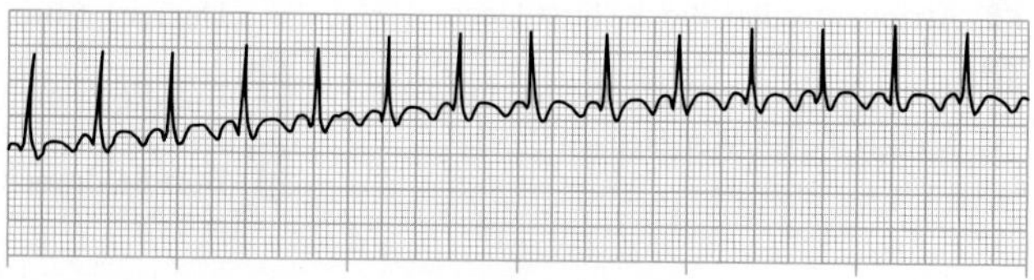

Bundle-Branch Block—Left (LBBB)

Rate: <100 beats/min
Rhythm: Regular
PR interval: Normal
QT interval: Complete LBBB (QRS >0.12 sec); incomplete LBBB (QRS = 0.10–0.12 sec); lead V_1 negative RS complex; I, aVL, V_6 wide R wave without Q or S component. ST segment and T-wave direction opposite direction of the R wave.

Note: LBBB does not occur in healthy patients and usually indicates serious heart disease with a poor prognosis. In patients with LBBB, insertion of a pulmonary artery catheter may lead to complete heart block.

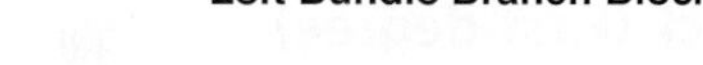

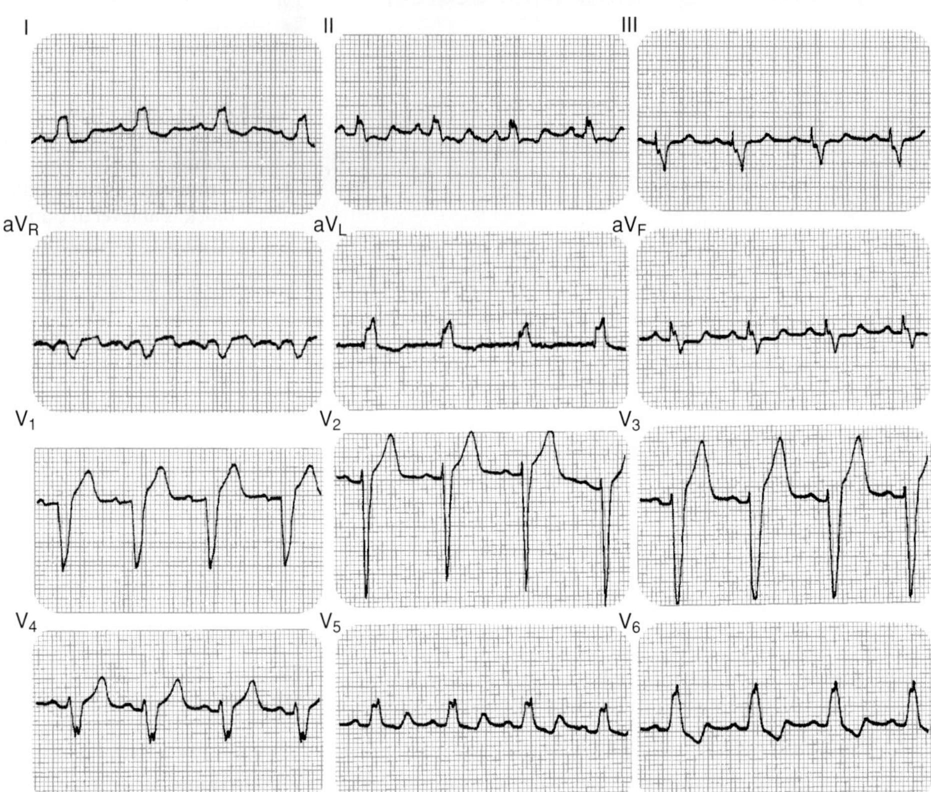

Bundle Branch Block—Right (RBBB)

Rate: <100 beats/min
Rhythm: Regular
PR interval: Normal
QT interval: Complete RBBB (QRS >0.12 sec); incomplete RBBB (QRS = 0.10–0.12 sec). Varying patterns of QRS complex; rSR (V_1); RS, wide R with M pattern. ST segment and T wave opposite direction of the R wave.

Note: In the presence of RBBB, Q waves may be seen with a myocardial infarction.

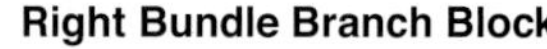

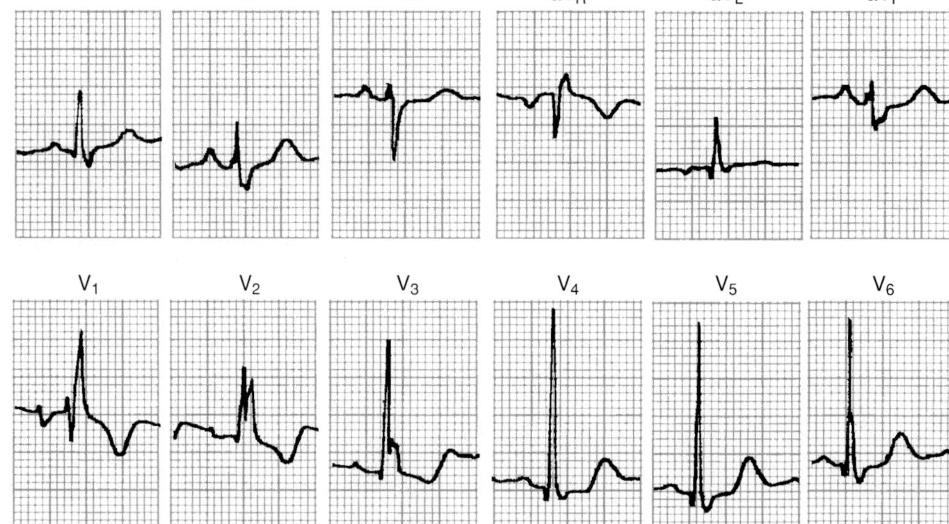

CORONARY ARTERY DISEASE

Transmural Myocardial Infarction (TMI)

Q waves seen on ECG, useful in confirming diagnosis, are associated with poorer prognosis and more significant hemodynamic impairment. Arrhythmias frequently complicate course. Small Q waves may be normal variant. For myocardial infarction (MI), Q waves >0.04 seconds or depth exceeds one third of R wave. For inferior wall MI, differentiate from RVH by axis deviation.

MYOCARDIAL INFARCTION

Anatomic Site	Leads	ECG Changes	Coronary Artery
Inferior	II, III, AVF	Q, ↑ST, ↑T	Right

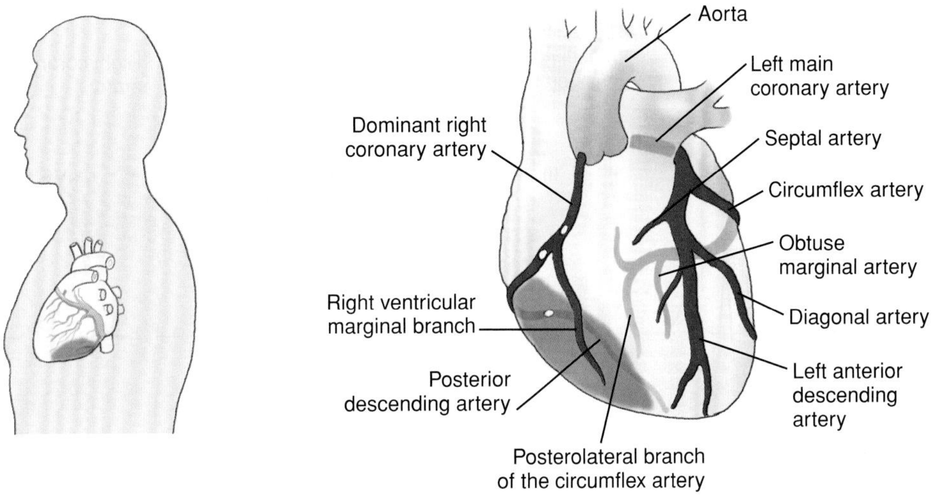

Aorta
Left main coronary artery
Dominant right coronary artery
Septal artery
Circumflex artery
Obtuse marginal artery
Right ventricular marginal branch
Diagonal artery
Posterior descending artery
Left anterior descending artery
Posterolateral branch of the circumflex artery

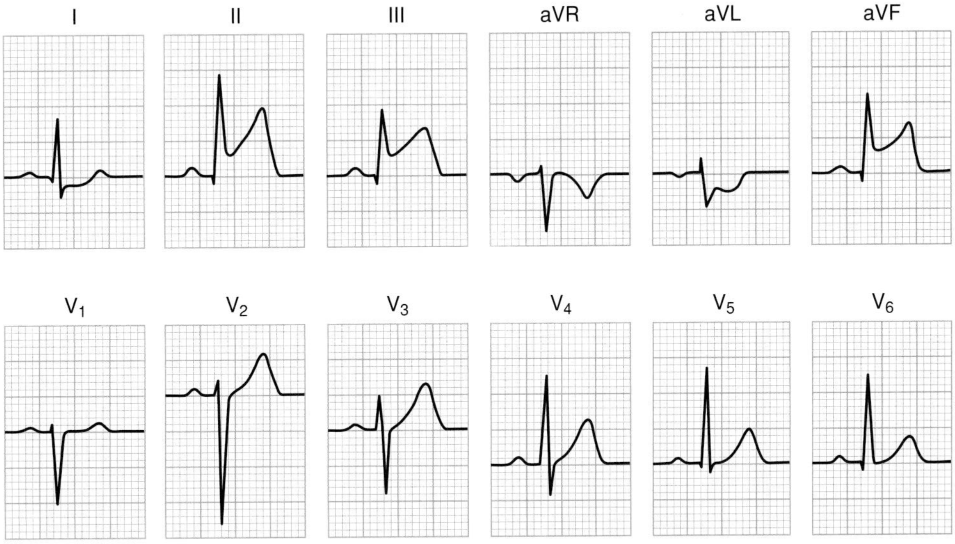

I II III aVR aVL aVF

V_1 V_2 V_3 V_4 V_5 V_6

MYOCARDIAL INFARCTION

Anatomic Site	Leads	ECG Changes	Coronary Artery
Posterior	V_1–V_2	↑R, ↓ST, ↓T	Left circumflex

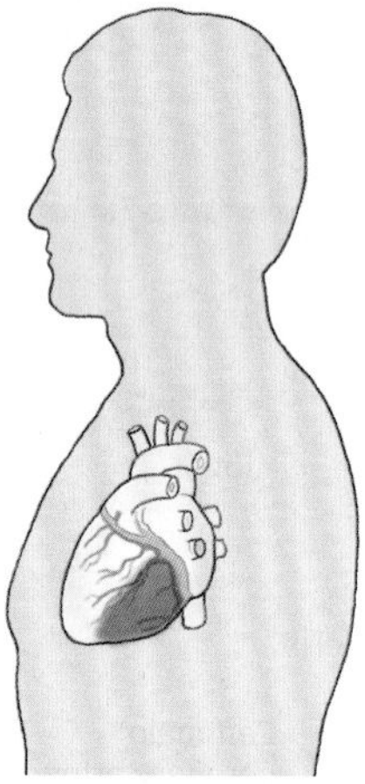

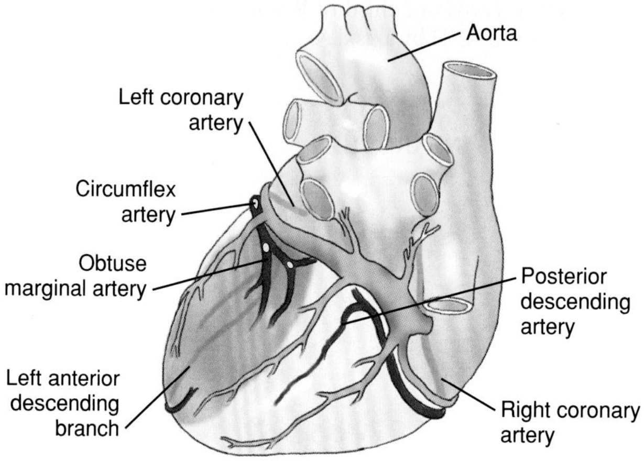

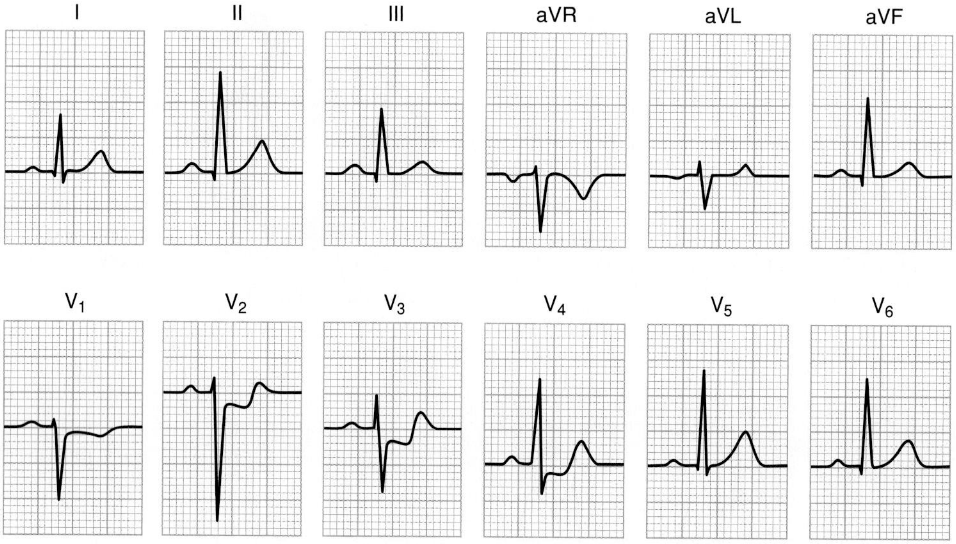

MYOCARDIAL INFARCTION

Anatomic Site	Leads	ECG Changes	Coronary Artery
Lateral	I, aVL, V_5–V_6	Q, ↑ST, ↑T	Left circumflex

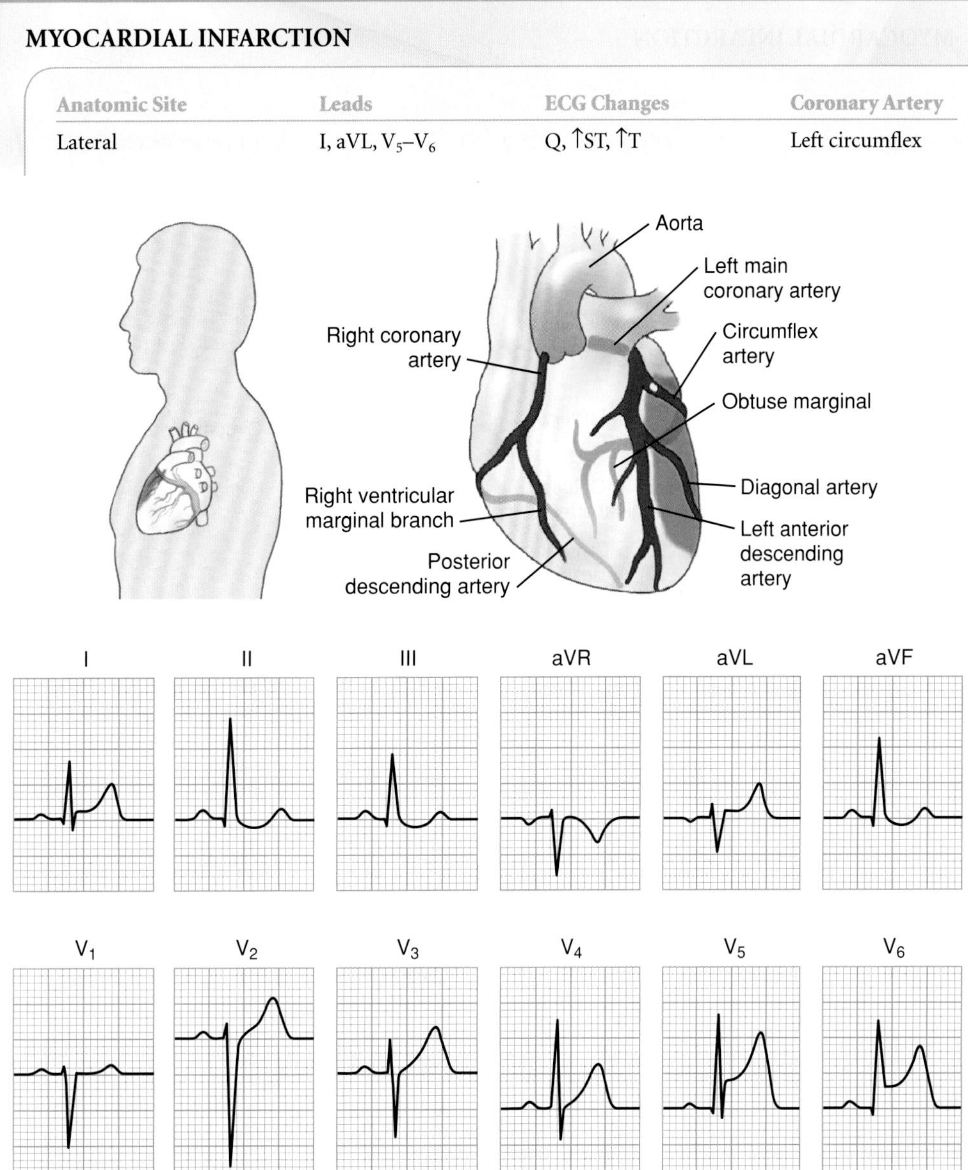

MYOCARDIAL INFARCTION

Anatomic Site	Leads	ECG Changes	Coronary Artery
Anterior	I, aVL, V_1–V_4	Q, ↑ST, ↑T	Left anterior descending

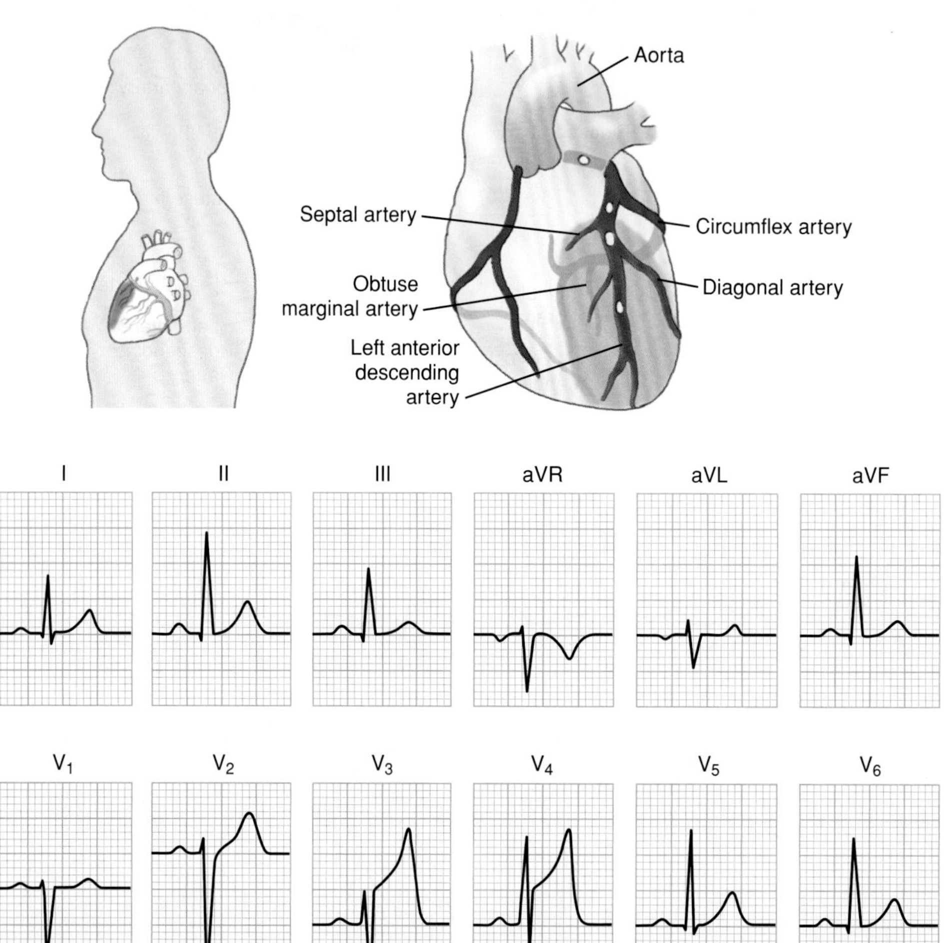

MYOCARDIAL INFARCTION

Anatomic Site	Leads	ECG Changes	Coronary Artery
Anteroseptal	V_1–V_4	Q, ↑ST, ↑T	Left anterior descending

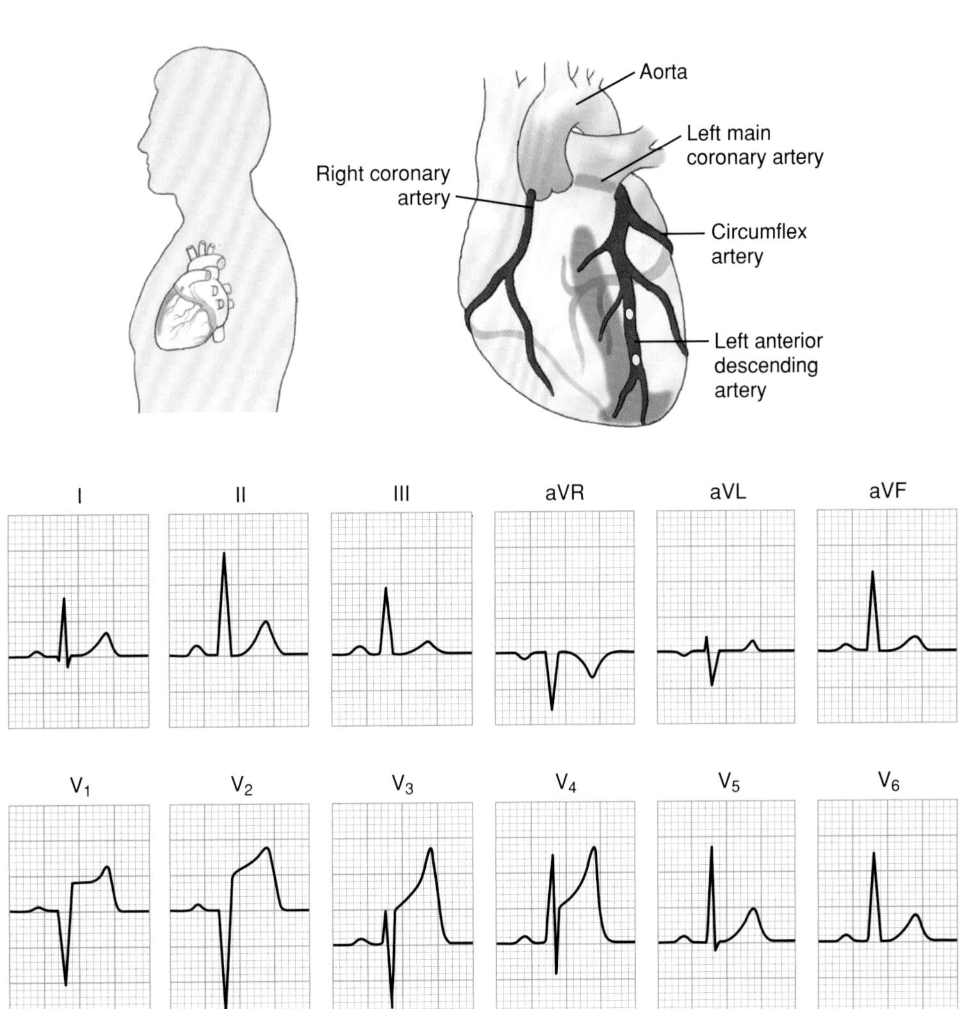

10 Subendocardial Myocardial Infarction (SEMI)

Persistent ST-segment depression and/or T-wave inversion in the absence of Q wave. Usually requires additional laboratory data (e.g., isoenzymes) to confirm diagnosis. Anatomic site of coronary lesion is similar to that of TMI electrocardiographically.

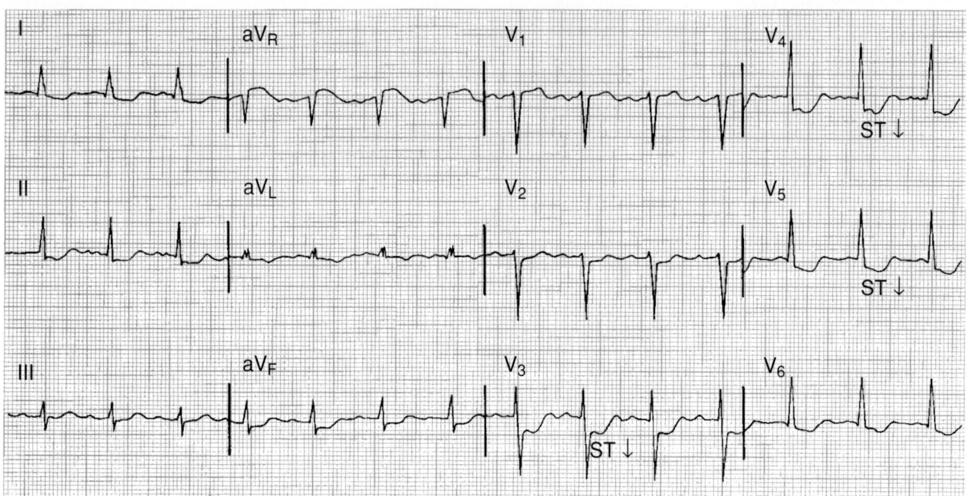

11 Myocardial Ischemia

Rate: Variable
12 **Rhythm:** Usually regular but may show atrial and/or ventricular arrhythmias.
PR interval: Normal
QT interval: ST segment depressed; J-point depression; T-wave inversion; conduction disturbances. (**A**) TP and PR intervals are baseline for ST-segment deviation. (**B**) ST-segment elevation. (**C**) ST-segment depression.

Note: Intraoperative ischemia usually is seen in the presence of "normal" vital signs (e.g., ±20% of preinduction values).

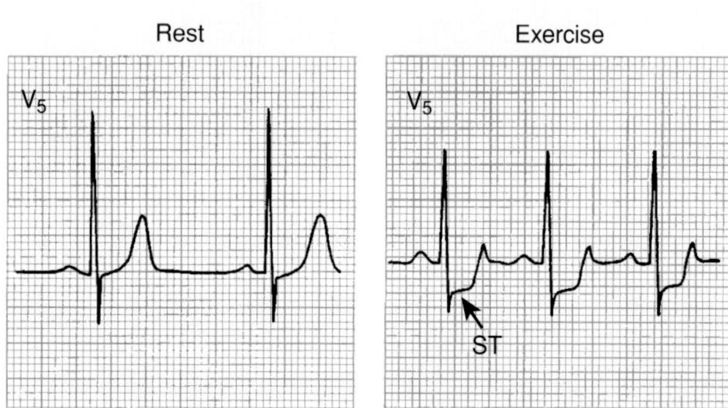

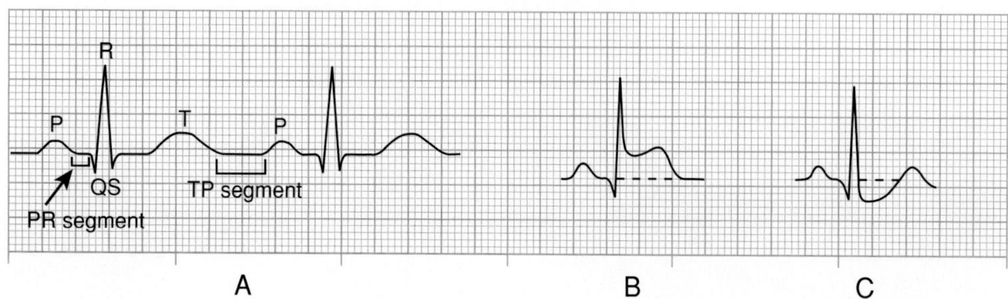

Digitalis Effect

Rate: <100 beats/min
Rhythm: Regular
PR interval: Normal or prolonged
QT interval: ST-segment sloping ("digitalis effect")

Note: Digitalis toxicity can be the cause of many common arrhythmias (e.g., premature ventricular contractions, second-degree heart block). Verapamil, quinidine, and amiodarone cause an increase in serum digitalis concentration.

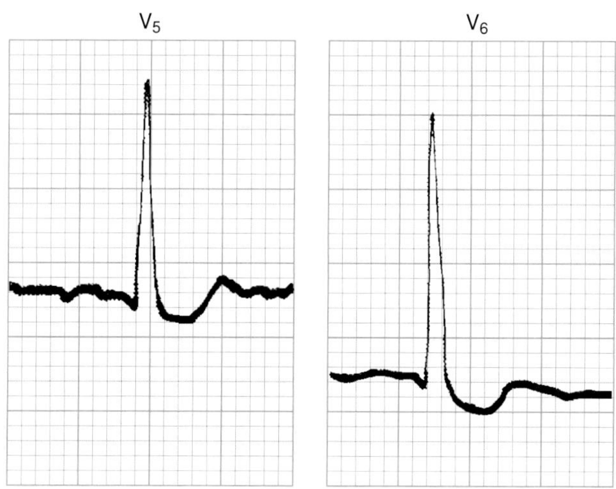

ELECTROLYTE DISTURBANCES

	↓Ca^{22+}	↑Ca^{2+}	↓K^{+}	↑K^{+}
Rate	<100 beats/min	<100 beats/min	<100 beats/min	<100 beats/min
Rhythm	Regular	Regular	Regular	Regular
PR interval	Normal	Normal/-increased	Normal	Normal
QT interval	Increased	Decreased	Normal	Increased
Other			T wave flat U wave	T wave peaked

Note: ECG changes usually do not correlate with serum calcium. Hypocalcemia rarely causes arrhythmias in the absence of hypokalemia. In contrast, abnormalities in serum potassium concentration can be diagnosed by ECG. Similarly, in the clinical range, magnesium concentrations are rarely associated with unique ECG patterns. The presence of a "U" wave (>1.5 mm in height) can also be seen in left main coronary artery disease, with certain medications and long QT syndrome.

Calcium

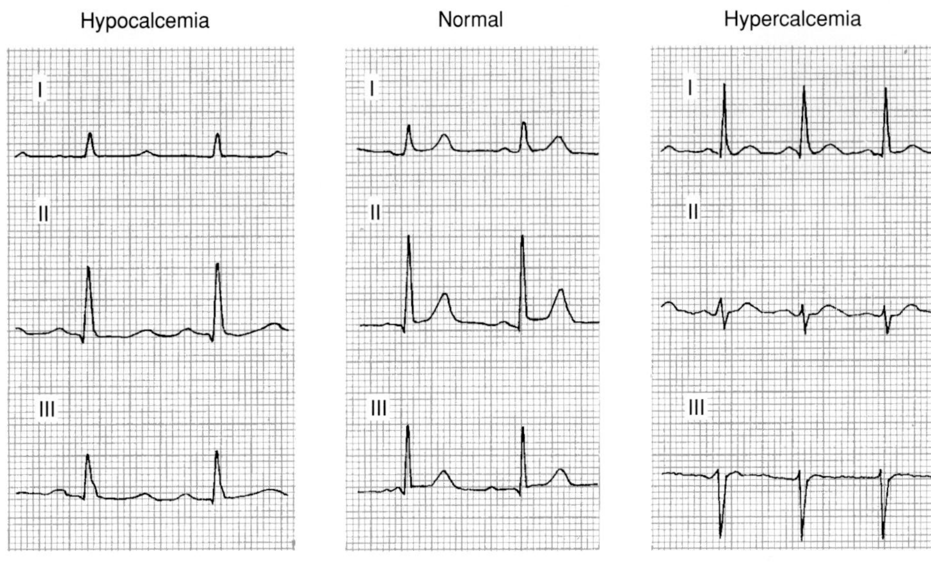

Potassium

Hypokalemia (K+ = 1.9 mEq/L)

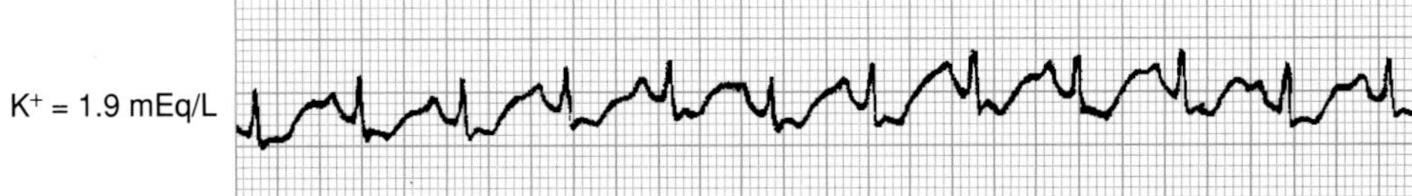

Hyperkalemia (K+ = 7.9 mEq/L)

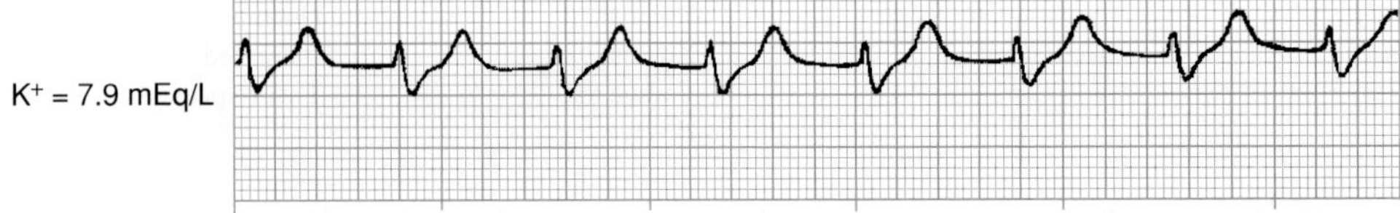

Hypothermia

Rate: <60 beats/min
Rhythm: Sinus
PR interval: Prolonged
QT interval: Prolonged

Note: Seen at temperatures below 33°C with ST-segment elevation (J point or Osborn wave). Tremor due to shivering or Parkinson's disease may interfere with ECG interpretation and may be confused with atrial flutter. May represent normal variant of early ventricular repolarization. (*Arrow* indicates J point or Osborn waves.)

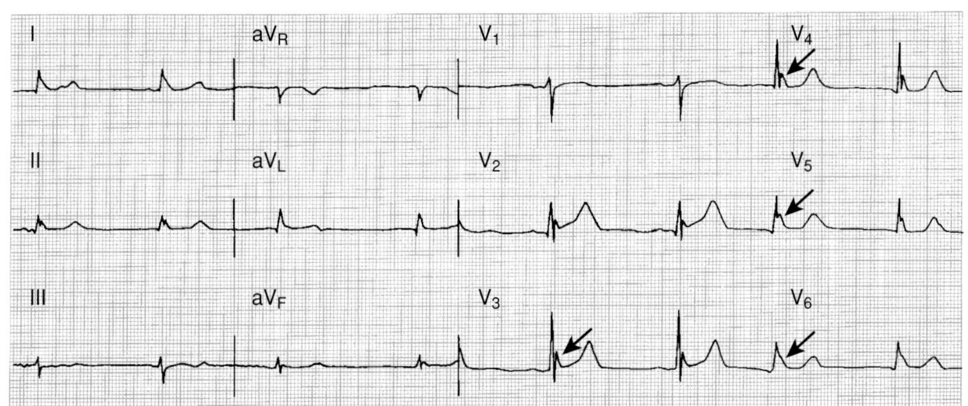

Multifocal Atrial Tachycardia

Rate: 100–200 beats/min
Rhythm: Irregular
PR interval: Consecutive P waves are of varying shape.
QT interval: Normal

Note: Seen in patients with severe lung disease. Vagal maneuvers have no effect. At heart rates <100 beats/min, it may appear as wandering atrial pacemaker. May be mistaken for atrial fibrillation. Treatment is of the causative disease process.

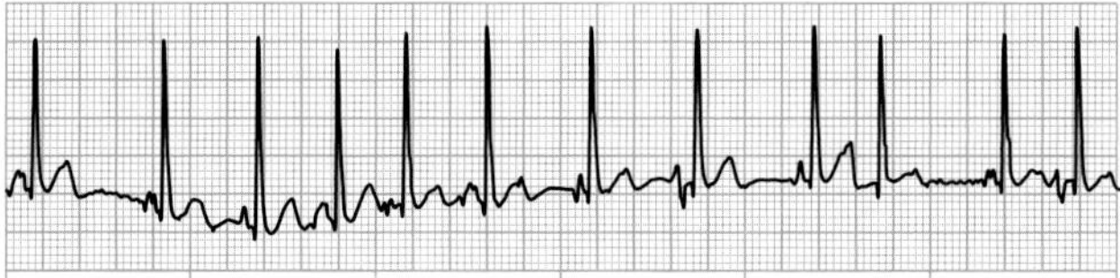

Paroxysmal Atrial Tachycardia (PAT)

Rate: 150–250 beats/min
Rhythm: Regular
PR interval: Difficult to distinguish because of tachycardia obscuring P wave. P wave may precede, be included in, or follow QRS complex.
QT interval: Normal, but ST segment and T wave may be diffcult to distinguish.

Note: Therapy depends on degree of hemodynamic compromise. Carotid sinus massage, or other vagal maneuvers, may terminate rhythm or decrease heart rate. In contrast to management of PAT in awake patients, synchronized cardioversion, rather than pharmacologic treatment, is preferred in hemodynamically unstable anesthetized patients.

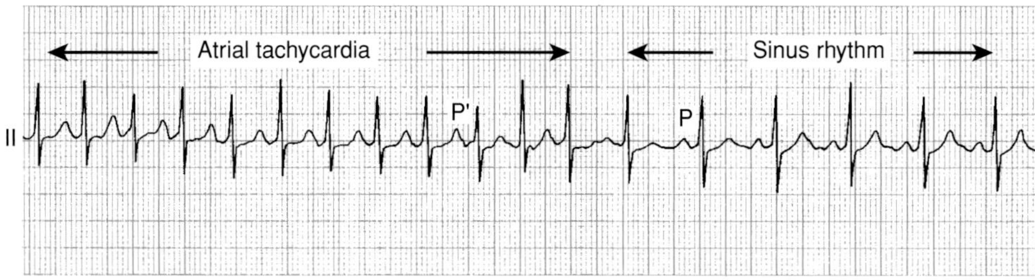

Pericarditis

Rate: Variable
Rhythm: Variable
PR interval: Normal
QT interval: Diffuse ST and T-wave changes with no Q wave and seen in more leads than a myocardial infarction.

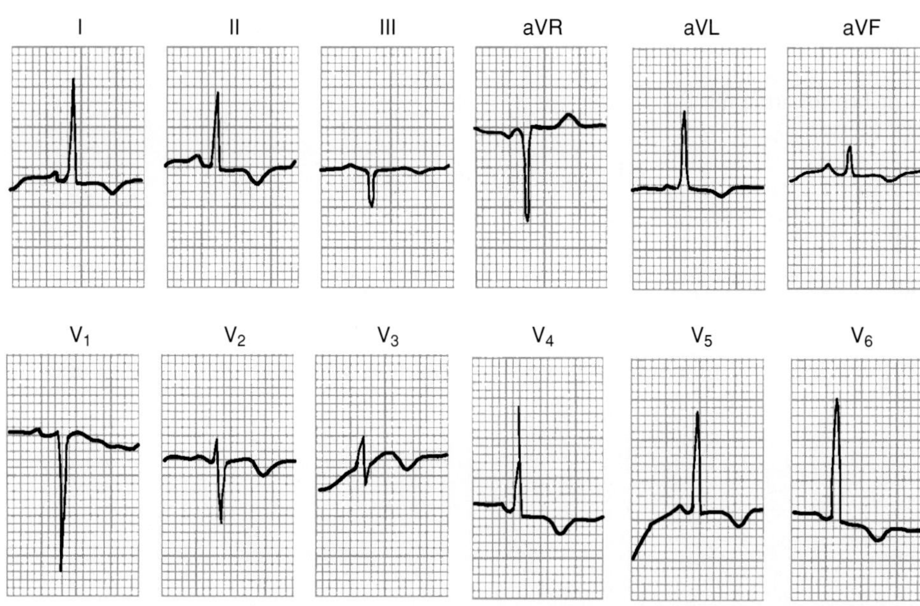

Pericardial Tamponade

Rate: Variable
Rhythm: Variable
PR interval: Low-voltage P wave
QT interval: Seen as electrical alternans with low-voltage complexes and varying amplitude of P, QRS, and T waves with each heart beat.

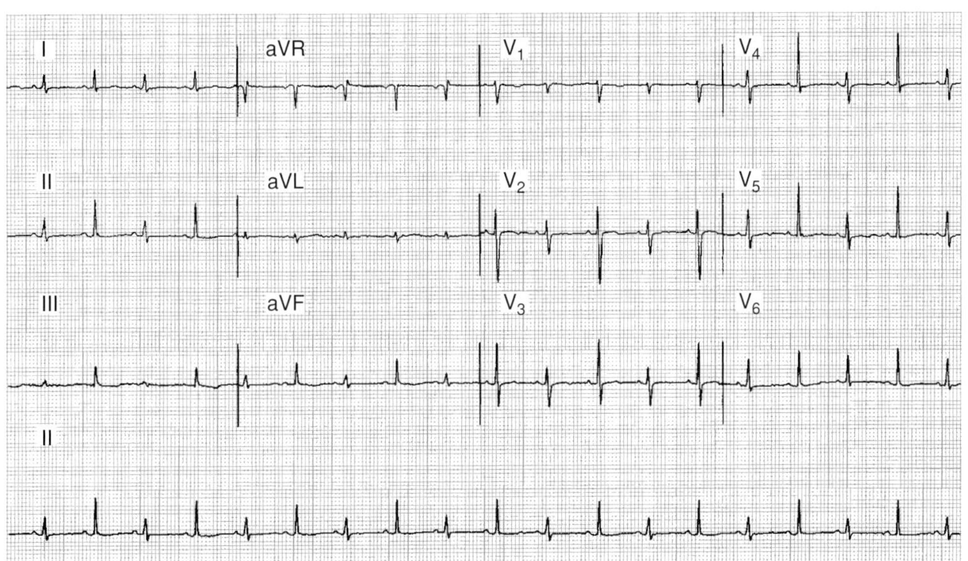

Pneumothorax

Rate: Variable
Rhythm: Variable
PR interval: Normal
QT interval: Normal

Note: Common ECG abnormalities include right-axis deviation, decreased QRS amplitude, and inverted T waves V_1–V_6. Differentiate from pulmonary embolus. May present as electrical alternans; thus, pericardial effusion should be ruled out.

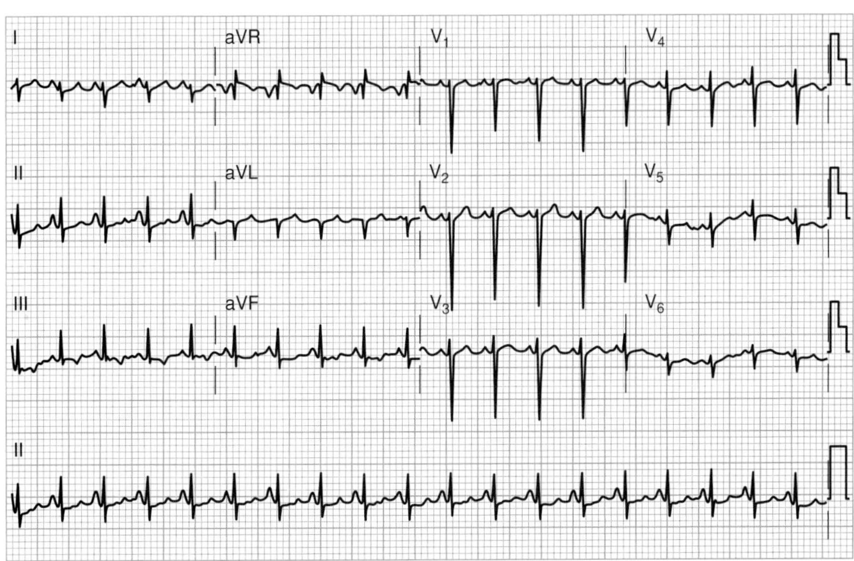

17 Premature Atrial Contraction (PAC)

Rate: <100 beats/min
Rhythm: Irregular
PR interval: P waves may be lost in preceding T waves. PR interval is variable.
QT interval: QRS normal confguration; ST segment and T wave normal.

Note: Nonconducted PAC appearance similar to that of sinus arrest; T waves with PAC may be distorted by inclusion of P wave in the T wave.

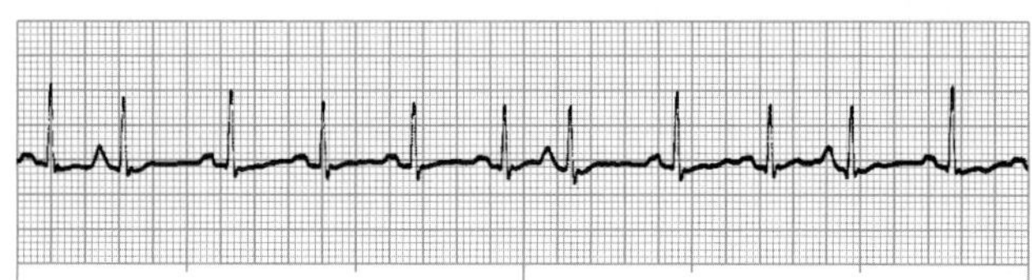

18 Premature Ventricular Contraction (PVC)

19 **Rate:** Usually <100 beats/min
20 **Rhythm:** Irregular
PR interval: P wave and PR interval absent; retrograde conduction of P wave can be seen.
21 22 **QT interval:** Wide QRS (>0.12 sec); ST segment cannot be evaluated (e.g., ischemia); T wave opposite direction of QRS with compensatory pause. Fourth and eighth beats are PVCs.

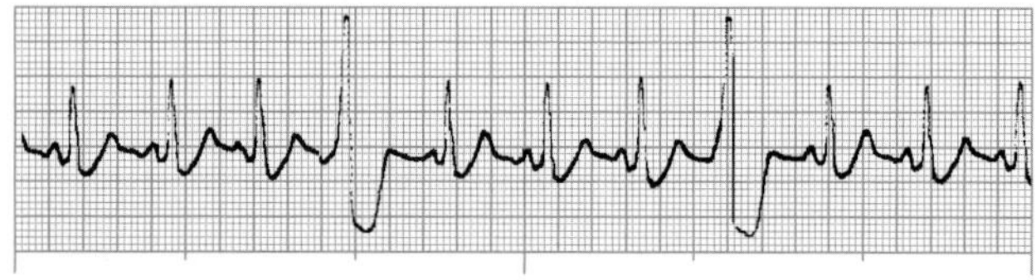

Pulmonary Embolus

Rate: >100 beats/min
Rhythm: Sinus
PR interval: P-pulmonale waveform
QT interval: Q waves in leads III and AVF

Note: Classic ECG signs S1Q3T3 with T-wave inversion also seen in V_1–V_4 and RV strain (ST depression V_1–V_4). May present with atrial fibrillation or flutter.

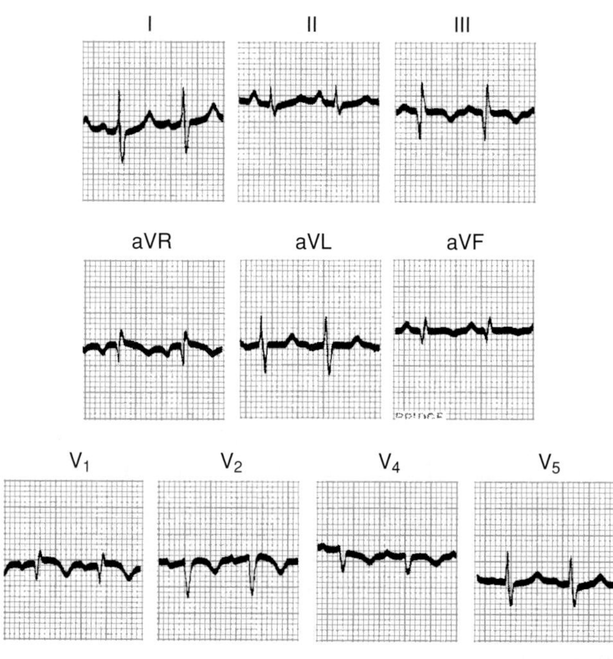

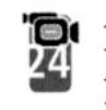

Sinus Bradycardia

Rate: <60 beats/min
Rhythm: Sinus
PR interval: Normal
QT interval: Normal

Note: Seen in trained athletes as normal variant.

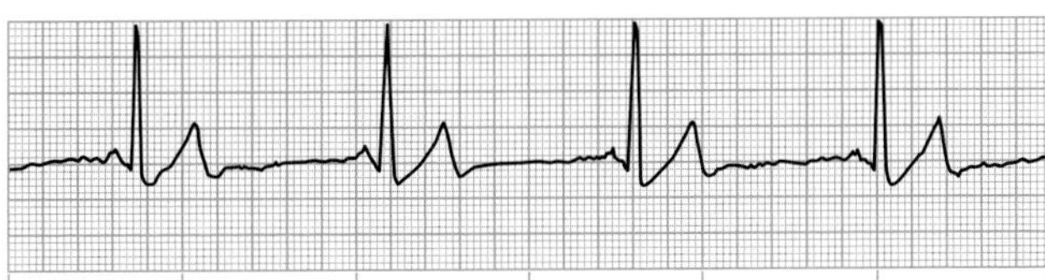

Sinus Arrhythmia

Rate: 60–100 beats/min
Rhythm: Sinus
PR interval: Normal
QT interval: R-R interval variable

Note: Heart rate increases with inhalation and decreases with exhalation + 10–20% (respiratory). Nonrespiratory sinus arrhythmia seen in elderly with heart disease. Also seen with increased intracranial pressure.

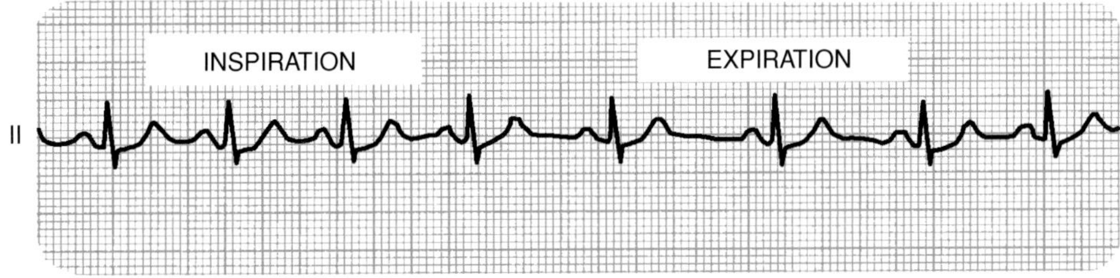

Sinus Arrest

Rate: <60 beats/min
Rhythm: Varies
PR interval: Variable
QT interval: Variable

Note: Rhythm depends on the cardiac pacemaker firing in the absence of sinoatrial stimulus (atrial pacemaker 60–75 beats/min; junctional 40–60 beats/min; ventricular 30–45 beats/min). Junctional rhythm most common. Occasional P waves may be seen (retrograde P wave).

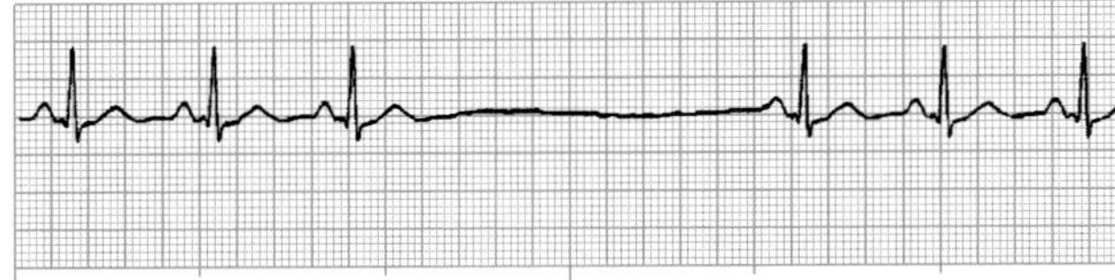

Sinus Tachycardia

Rate: 100–160 beats/min
Rhythm: Regular
PR interval: Normal; P wave may be diffcult to see.
QT interval: Normal

Note: Should be differentiated from paroxysmal atrial tachycardia (PAT). With PAT, carotid massage terminates arrhythmia. Sinus tachycardia may respond to vagal maneuvers but reappears as soon as vagal stimulus is removed.

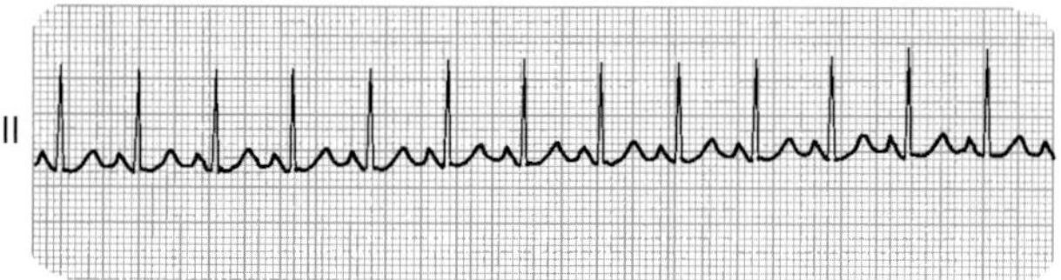

Subarachnoid Hemorrhage

Rate: <60 beats/min
Rhythm: Sinus
PR interval: Normal
QT interval: T-wave inversion is deep and wide. Prominent U waves are seen. Sinus arrythmias are observed. Q waves may be seen and may mimick acute coronary syndrome.

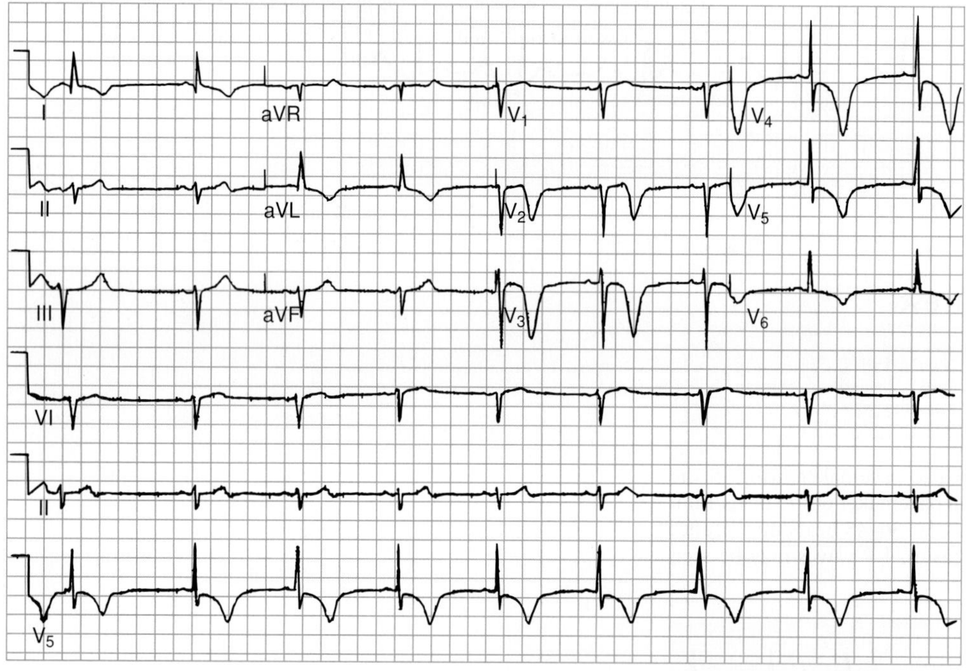

Torsades De Pointes

Rate: 150–250 beats/min
Rhythm: No atrial component seen; ventricular rhythm regular or irregular.
PR interval: P wave buried in QRS complex
QT interval: QRS complexes usually wide and with phasic variation twisting around a central axis (a few complexes point upward, then a few point downward). ST segments and T waves diffcult to discern.

Note: Type of ventricular tachycardia associated with prolonged QT interval. Seen with electrolyte disturbances (e.g., hypokalemia, hypocalcemia, and hypomagnesemia) and bradycardia. Administering standard antiarrhythmics (lidocaine, procainamide, etc.) may worsen torsades de pointes. Prevention includes treatment of the electrolyte disturbance. Treatment includes shortening of the QT interval, pharmacologically or by pacing; unstable polymorphic VT is treated with immediate defibrillation.

Torsades de Pointes: Sustained

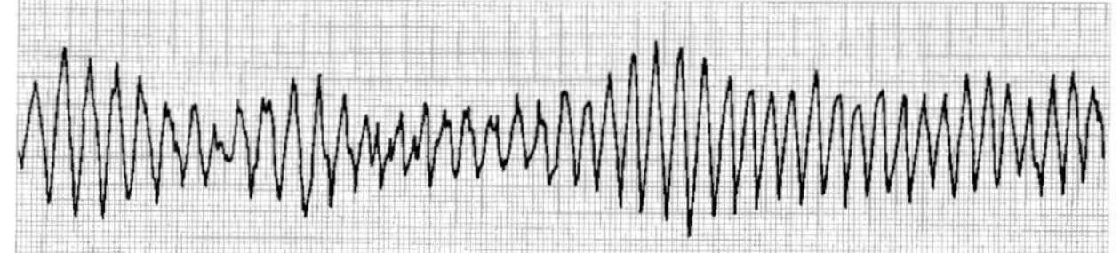

Ventricular Fibrillation

Rate: Absent
Rhythm: None
PR interval: Absent
QT interval: Absent

Note: "Pseudoventricular fibrillation" may be the result of a monitor malfunction (e.g., ECG lead disconnect). Always check for carotid pulse before instituting therapy.

Coarse Ventricular Fibrillation

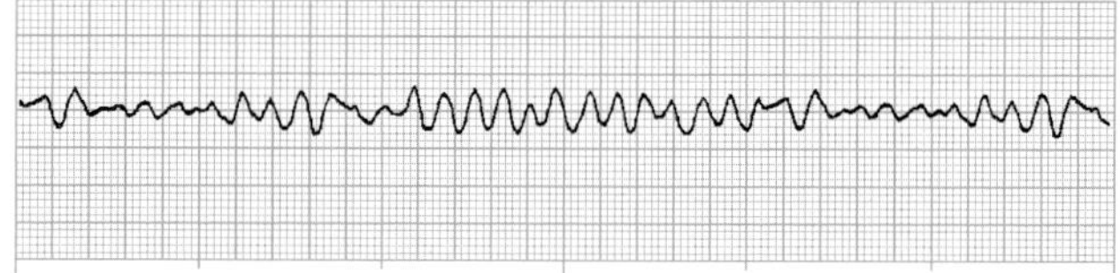

Fine Ventricular Fibrillation

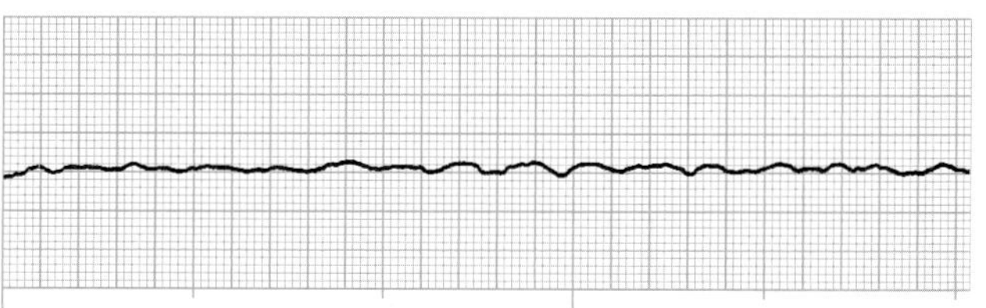

Ventricular Tachycardia

Rate: 100–250 beats/min
Rhythm: No atrial component seen; ventricular rhythm irregular or regular
PR interval: Absent; retrograde P wave may be seen in QRS complex
QT interval: Wide, bizarre QRS complex. ST segment and T wave difficult to determine.

Note: In the presence of hemodynamic compromise, VT with a pulse is treated with immediate synchronized cardioversion, whereas VT without a pulse is treated with immediate defibrillation. If the patient is stable, with short bursts of ventricular tachycardia, pharmacologic management is preferred. Should be differentiated from supraventricular tachycardia with aberrancy (SVT-A). Compensatory pause and atrioventricular dissociation suggest a PVC. P waves and SR' (V_1) and slowing to vagal stimulus also suggest SVT-A.

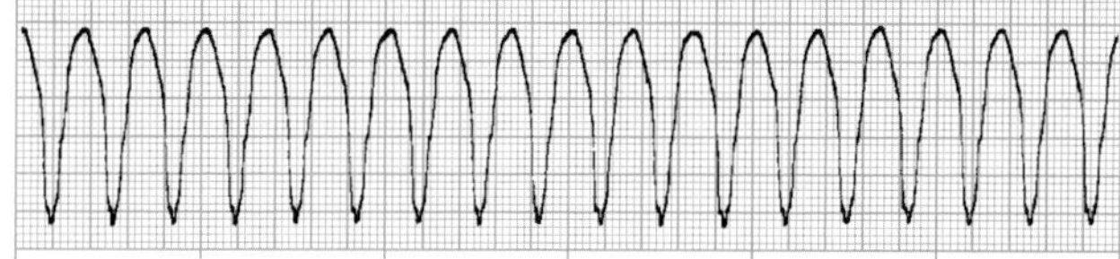

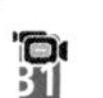

Wolff-Parkinson-White Syndrome (WPW)

Rate: <100 beats/min
Rhythm: Regular
PR interval: P wave normal; PR interval short (<0.12 sec)
QT interval: Duration (>0.10 sec) with slurred QRS complex (delta wave). Type A has delta wave, RBBB, with upright QRS complex V_1. Type B has delta wave and downward QRS-V1. ST segment and T wave usually normal.

Note: Digoxin should be avoided in the presence of WPW because it increases conduction through the accessory bypass tract (bundle of Kent) and decreases AV node conduction; consequently, ventricular fibrillation can occur.

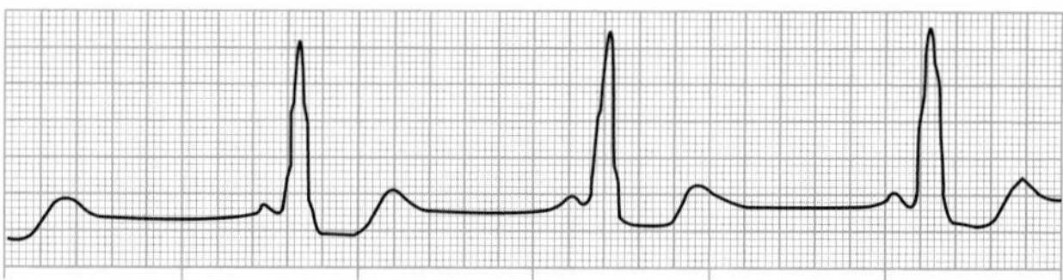

Atrial Pacing

Pacemaker Tracings

Atrial pacing as demonstrated in this figure is used when the atrial impulse can proceed through the AV node. Examples are sinus bradycardia and junctional rhythms associated with clinically significant decreases in blood pressure. (*Arrows* are pacemaker spike.)

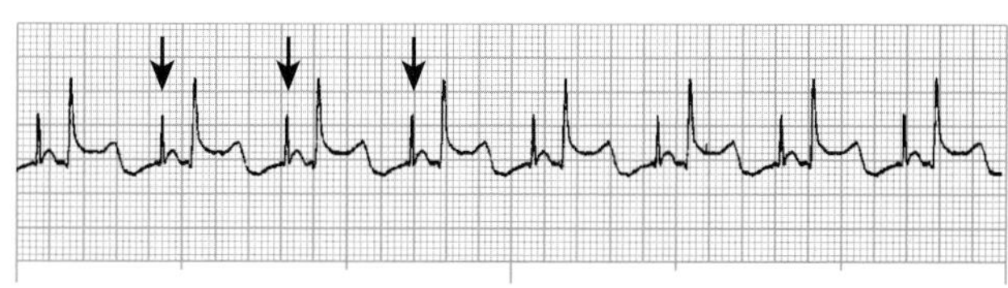

Ventricular Pacing

In this tracing, ventricular pacing is evident by absence of atrial wave (P wave) and pacemaker spike preceding QRS complex. Ventricular pacing is employed in the presence of bradycardia secondary to AV block or atrial fbrillation. (*Arrows* are pacemaker spike.)

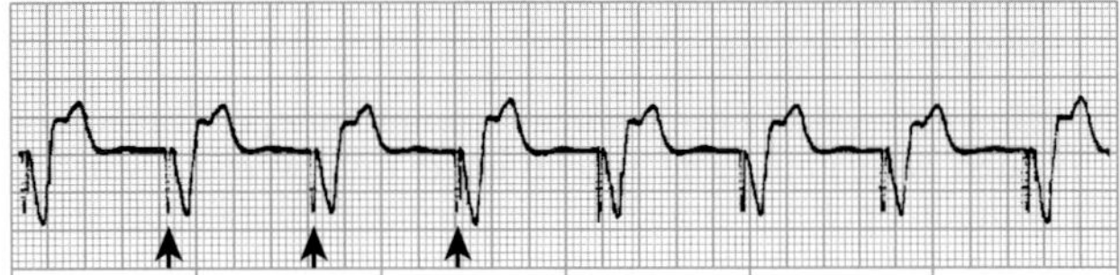

DDD Pacing

DDD pacing, one of the most commonly used pacing modes, paces and senses both the right atrium and right ventricle (A-V Sequential Pacing). Each atrial and the right ventricular complex are preceded by a pacemaker spike.

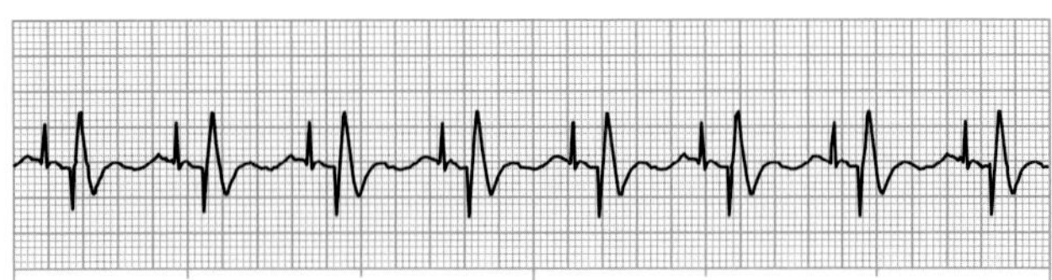

Acknowledgments

Illustrations in the atlas are reprinted from Aehlert B. *ECGs made easy,* 4th ed. St. Louis: Mosby/Elsevier; 2011; Goldberger AL. *Clinical electrocardiography: a simplified approach,* 7th ed. Philadelphia: Mosby/Elsevier; 2006; Groh WJ, Zipes DP. Neurological disorders and cardiovascular disease. In Bonow RO, Mann DL, Zipes DP, et al., eds. *Braunwald's heart disease: a textbook of cardiovascular medicine,* 9th ed. Philadelphia: Saunders/Elsevier; 2012; Huszar RJ. *Basic dysrhythmias: interpretation and management,* 2nd ed. St. Louis: Mosby Lifeline; 1994; and Soltani P, Malozzi CM, Saleh BA, et al. Electrocardiogram manifestation of spontaneous pneumothorax. *Am J Emerg Med* 2009;27:750.e1–5.

Bibliography

1. Thaler MS. *The Only EKG Book You'll Ever Need,* 6th ed. Philadelphia: Wolters Kluwer/Lippincott Williams & Wilkins; 2010:326.
2. Mirvis DM, Goldberger AL. Electrocardiography. In Libby P, Bonow RO, Mann DL, et al., eds. *Braunwald's Heart Disease: A Textbook of Cardiovascular Medicine,* 8th ed. Philadelphia: Saunders Elsevier; 2008:149–194.
3. Drew BJ, Ackerman MJ, Funk M, et al. Prevention of torsade de pointes in hospital settings: A scientific statement from the American Heart Association and the American College of Cardiology Foundation. *Circulation* 2010;121:1047–1060.
4. Huszar RJ. *Basic Dysrhythmias: Interpretation and Management,* 2nd ed. St. Louis: Mosby Lifeline; 1994:453.
5. Aehlert B. *ECGs Made Easy,* 4th ed. Phoenix: Mosby Elsevier; 2011:337.
6. Goldberger AL. *Clinical Electrocardiography: A Simplified Approach,* 7th ed. Philadelphia: Mosby Elsevier; 2006:337.
7. Salonti J, Malozzi CM, Saleh BA, et al. Electrocardiogram manifestation of spontaneous pneumothorax. *Am J Emerg Med* 2009;27:750.e1–e5.
8. Groh WJ, Zipes DP. Neurological disorders and cardiovascular disease. In Libby P, Bonow RO, Mann DL, et al., eds. *Braunwald's Heart Disease: A Textbook of Cardiovascular Medicine,* 8th ed. Philadelphia: Saunders Elsevier; 2008:2135–2154.

APPENDIX

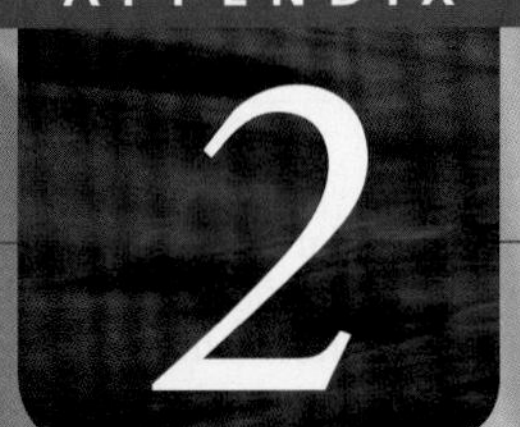

Pacemaker and Implantable Cardiac Defibrillator Protocols

GINA C. BADESCU • BENJAMIN SHERMAN • JAMES R. ZAIDAN • PAUL G. BARASH

TABLE 1. ABBREVIATION TABLE

Abbrev.	Meaning
3D	Three dimensional
ASA	American Society of Anesthesiologists
ATP	Antitachycardia pacing
AV	Atrioventricular
AVB	Atrioventricular block
BPEG	British Pacing and Electrophysiology Group
bpm	Beats per minute
CAD	Coronary Artery Disease
CIED	Cardiac Implantable Electronic Devices
CPB	Cardiopulmonary Bypass
CRP	Current Return Pad
CRT-D	Cardiac Resynchronization Therapy-Defibrillation
CT	Cautery Tool
DCM	Dilated Cardiomyopathy
ECG	Electrocardiogram
ECT	Electroconvulsive Therapy
EF	Ejection Fraction
EMI	Electromagnetic Interference
HCM	Hypertrophic Cardiomyopathy
HR	Heart Rate
HRS	Heart Rhythm Society
HV	HV Interval
ICD	Implantable Cardiac Defibrillators
LV	Left Ventricle
LVOT	Left Ventricular Outflow Tract
MRI	Magnetic Resonance Imaging
NASPE	North American Society of Pacing and Electrophysiology
NBG	N (NASPE), B (BPEG), G (GENERIC)
PG	Pulse Generator
PP	External Cardioversion-Defibrillation Pads or Paddles
RA	Right Atrium
R&R	Rate and Rhythm
RF	Radio frequency
RT	Radiation Therapy
RV	Right Ventricle
SCD	Sudden Cardiac Death
SND	Sinus Node Dysfunction
STEMI	ST-segment elevation myocardial infarction
TUNA	Transurethral Needle Ablation
TURP	Transurethral resection of prostate
VT	Ventricular Tachycardia
VF	Ventricular Fibrillation

Cardiac Implantable Electronic Devices (CIED)—Pacemakers

Pacemakers are devices that deliver electrical energy and control the patient's conduction system when necessary.

Common indications for permanent pacemaker implantation: (For a complete list of indications, please refer to the ACC/ AHA/ HRS 2008 guidelines for Device-Based Therapy of Cardiac Rhythm Abnormalities.)[1]

1. Sinus node dysfunction:
   - Documented symptomatic bradycardia
   - Documented symptomatic chronotropic incompetence
   - Documented symptomatic bradycardia induced by essential medical therapy
   - Syncope of unexplained origin with inducible sinus bradycardia or pauses on electrophysiologic studies.
   - Symptomatic patients with assumed sinus bradycardia and no other possible etiologies
2. Atrioventricular (AV) node dysfunction:
   - Third-degree AV block
   - Type II second-degree AV block
   - Symptomatic type I second-degree AV block
   - Symptomatic first-degree AV block
   - Asymptomatic first-degree AV block with coexisting disease that can impair the conduction system (i.e., sarcoidosis, amyloidosis, neuromuscular diseases)
   - Drug- or medication-induced AV block that is thought to recur despite discontinuation of the drug or medication.
3. Bifascicular block and:
   - Alternating bundle branch block
   - Electrophysiological evidence of a markedly prolonged HV interval ≥100 ms. (His bundle [H] potential and the onset of ventricular activity, also known as the HV, interval, is normally 35–45 ms)
   - Concomitant neuromuscular disease (i.e., myotonic muscular dystrophy, Erb dystrophy)
4. ST-segment elevation myocardial infarction (STEMI) with second- or third-degree AV block
5. Hypersensitive Carotid Sinus Syndrome and Neurocardiogenic Syncope
6. Cardiac transplantation patients who develop persistent inappropriate bradycardia.

3

Atrioventricular Block (First-degree)

Rate: 60–100 beats/min
Rhythm: Regular
PR interval: Prolonged (>0.20 sec) and constant
QT interval: Normal

Note: Usually clinically insignificant; may be early harbinger of drug toxicity.

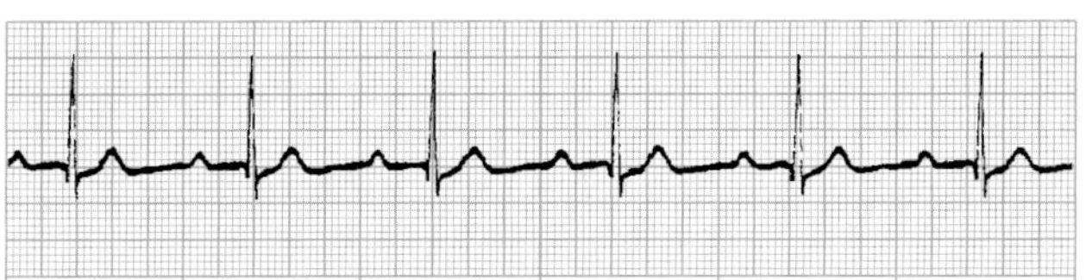

4

Atrioventricular Block (Second-degree), Mobitz Type I/Wenckebach Block

Rate: 60–100 beats/min
Rhythm: Atrial regular; ventricular irregular
PR interval: P wave normal; PR interval progressively lengthens with each cycle until QRS complex is dropped (dropped beat). PR interval following dropped beat is shorter than normal.
QT interval: QRS complex normal but dropped periodically.

Note: Commonly seen in trained athletes and with drug toxicity.

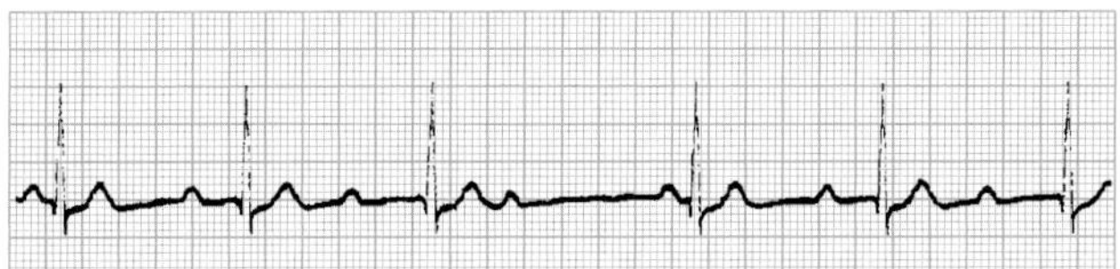

5

Atrioventricular Block (Second-degree), Mobitz Type II

Rate: <100 beats/min
Rhythm: Atrial regular; ventricular regular or irregular
PR interval: P waves normal, but some are not followed by QRS complex.
QT interval: Normal but may have widened QRS complex if block is at level of bundle branch. ST segment and T wave may be abnormal, depending on location of block.

Note: In contrast to Mobitz type I block, the PR and RR intervals are constant and the dropped QRS occurs without warning. The wider the QRS complex (block lower in the conduction system), the greater the amount of myocardial damage.

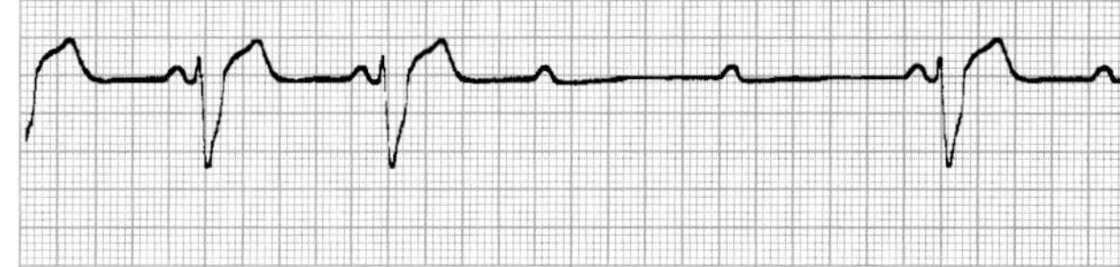

6

Atrioventricular Block (Third-degree), Complete Heart Block

Rate: <45 beats/min
Rhythm: Atrial regular; ventricular regular; no relationship between P wave and QRS complex
PR interval: Variable because atria and ventricles beat independently
QT interval: QRS morphology variable, depending on the origin of the ventricular beat in the intrinsic pacemaker system (atrioventricular junctional vs. ventricular pacemaker). ST segment and T wave normal.

Note: AV block represents complete failure of conduction from atria to ventricles (no P wave is conducted to the ventricle). The atrial rate is faster than ventricular rate. P waves have no relationship to QRS complexes (e.g., they are electrically disconnected). In contrast, with AV dissociation, the P wave is conducted through the AV node and the atrial and ventricular rate are similar. Immediate treatment with atropine or isoproterenol is required if cardiac output is reduced. Consideration should be given to insertion of a pacemaker. Seen as a complication of mitral valve replacement.

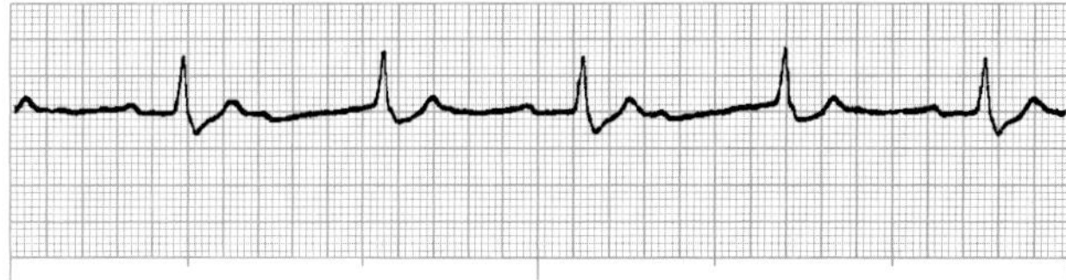

7. Prevention and termination of certain arrhythmias such as:
   - Sustained pause-dependant VT
   - High-risk patients with congenital long-QT syndrome
   - Recurrent refractory symptomatic atrial fibrillation and SND
   - Symptomatic recurrent SVT that is reliably terminated by pacing and catheter ablation and medication management has failed
8. Hemodynamic indications:
   - Cardiac resynchronization therapy (CRT) in patients with NYHA class III or ambulatory class IV heart failure with optimal medical management and an ejection fraction (EF) ≤35% and QRS ≥120 ms
   - Hypertrophic cardiomyopathy with sinus node dysfunction (SND) or AV node dysfunction
9. Congenital heart diseases with associated bradyarrhythmias or AV block.

Cardiac Implantable Electronic Devices (CIEDs)—Implantable Cardiac Defibrillators (ICDs)

Implantable cardiac defibrillators (ICDs) are rhythm management devices that consist of a generator and a lead system.[2] One lead is usually placed in the right atrium and the second lead in the right ventricular apex. A specific type of ICD is the biventricular pacemaker, used for cardiac resynchronization therapy (CRT). This device will have a third lead placed in the coronary sinus to pace the left ventricular (LV) lateral wall in synchrony with the right ventricle (RV), in the patient with EF ≤35% and a QRS duration ≥120 msec.[1,2]

Common indications for ICD implantation: (For a complete list of indications, please refer to the ACC/AHA/HRS 2008 Guidelines for Device-Based Therapy of Cardiac Rhythm Abnormalities.)[1]

1. Prevention of sudden cardiac death (SCD) in survivors of prior cardiac arrest due to VF or unstable VT without a reversible cause.
2. Structural heart disease with spontaneous sustained VT or syncope not otherwise specified.
3. Sustained VT with normal or near normal LV function.
4. Syncope of undetermined origin with clinically relevant, hemodynamically significant, sustained VT or VF induced by an electrophysiological study.
5. Unexplained syncope with significant LV dysfunction and nonischemic DCM.
6. Prior myocardial infarction (not within 40 days) and an EF ≤35%.
7. Nonischemic dialated cardiomyopathy (DCM) and an EF ≤35%.
8. Nonsustained VT due to prior MI with an EF ≤–40% and inducible VF or sustained VT on electrophysiological study.
9. HCM with one or more risk factors for SCD.
10. Arrhythmogenic right ventricular dysplasia/cardiomyopathy with one or more risk factors for SCD.
11. Long QT syndrome with syncope and/or VT due to beta-blocker therapy or other risk factors for SCD.
12. Brugada syndrome with syncope or VT.
13. Catecholaminergic polymorphic VT with syncope while receiving beta-blocker therapy.
14. Diseases associated with cardiac involvement (i.e., Chagas disease, giant cell myocarditis, sarcoidosis)
15. Familial cardiomyopathy associated with SCD.
16. LV noncompaction.

TABLE 2. GENERIC PACEMAKER CODE: NASPE/BPEG REVISED (2002)

Position I, Pacing Chamber(s)	Position II, Sensing Chamber(s)	Position III, Response(s) to Sensing	Position IV, Programmability	Position V, Multisite Pacing
O = none	O = none	O = none	O = none	O = none
A = atrium	A = atrium	I = inhibited	R = rate modulation	A = atrium
V = ventricle	V = ventricle	T = triggered		V = ventricle
D = dual (A + V)	D = dual (A + V)	D = dual (T + I)		D = dual (A + V)

NBG: N refers to North American Society of Pacing and Electrophysiology (NASPE), now called the Heart Rhythm Society (HRS); B refers to British Pacing and Electrophysiology Group (BPEG); and G refers to generic.

Reproduced with permission from Practice advisory for perioperative management of patients with cardiac rhythm management devices: Pacemakers and implantable cardioverter-defibrillators. A report by the American Society of Anesthesiologists Task Force on Perioperative Management of Patients with Cardiac Rhythm Management Devices. *Anesthesiology* 2011;114:247–261.

TABLE 3. GENERIC DEFIBRILLATOR CODE (NBG): NASPE/BPEG

Position I, Shock Chamber(s)	Position II, Antitachycardia Pacing Chamber(s)	Position III, Tachycardia Detection	Position IV,[a] Antibradycardia Pacing Chamber(s)
O = none	O = none	E = electrogram	O = none
A = atrium	A = atrium	H = hemodynamic	A = atrium
V = ventricle	V = ventricle		V = ventricle
D = dual (A + V)	D = dual (A + V)		D = dual (A + V)

[a]For robust identification, position IV is expanded into its complete NBG code. For example, a biventricular pacing-defibrillator with ventricular shock and antitachycardia pacing functionality would be identified as VVE-DDDRV, assuming that the pacing section was programmed DDDRV. Currently, no hemodynamic sensors have been approved for tachycardia detection (position III).

Reproduced with permission from Practice advisory for perioperative management of patients with cardiac rhythm management devices: Pacemakers and implantable cardioverter-defibrillators. A report by the American Society of Anesthesiologists Task Force on Perioperative Management of Patients with Cardiac Rhythm Management Devices. *Anesthesiology* 2011;114:247–261.

Potential Intraoperative Problems with Cardiac Electronic Implantable Devices[3]

Electromagnetic interference (EMI) with a CIED is more likely when electrocautery is used above the umbilicus in a patient with the CIED implanted in the subclavicular region. Current expert opinion further states that the region 15 cm around the generator is the area with the highest risk of EMI interference. For generators placed elsewhere (e.g., abdominal site), the 15-cm rule still applies.

EMI interference leads to:

1. Inhibition of pacemaker by EMI
2. Inappropriate delivery of antitachycardia therapy by ICD
3. Changes in lead parameters:
   a. Atrial mode switching
   b. Inappropriate ventricular sensing
   c. Electrical reset
   d. Increase in ventricular thresholds
4. "Runaway" pacemaker[4]
5. Conversion from VOO back to backup mode (reprogramming).
6. Transient or permanent loss of capture
7. Noise reversal mode
8. Pacemaker failure after direct contact with electrocautery and cardioversion
9. Myocardial burns with increased pacing thresholds if electrocautery travels through leads into the myocardium
10. Rate-adaptive pacing (interaction of minute ventilation sensor with ECG/plethysmography)
11. Oversensing and inhibition with use of lithotripsy
12. Radiofrequency ablation has a high risk of interference due to long episodes of exposure to current.
13. Therapeutic ionizing radiation is especially damaging to CIED's by damaging internal components.

General Principles of Perioperative Management of Patients with CIED[3]

- The perioperative management of the patient with a CIED is via an individualized recommendation, made by the CIED team (electrophysiologist cardiologist), in collaboration with members of the surgical/anesthesia team (perioperative team). The recommendations should not be made by the industry representative without supervision by a physician who is qualified to manage these devices.
- The perioperative team should provide information to the CIED team regarding the upcoming procedure (see Table 4).

TABLE 4. ESSENTIAL ELEMENTS OF THE INFORMATION GIVEN TO THE CIED PHYSICIAN

- Type of procedure
- Anatomic location of surgical procedure
- Patient position during the procedure
- Will monopolar electrosurgery be used? (If so, anatomic location of EMI delivery.)
- Will other sources of EMI likely be present?
- Will cardioversion or defibrillation be used?
- Surgical venue (operating room, procedure suite, etc.)
- Anticipated postprocedural arrangements (anticipated discharge to home <23 hours, inpatient admission to critical care bed, telemetry bed)
- Unusual circumstances: Cardiothoracic or chest wall surgical procedure that could impair/damage or encroach upon the CIED leads, anticipated large blood loss, operation in close proximity to CIED

Reproduced with permission from Crossley GH, Poole JE, Rozner MA, et al. The Heart Rhythm Society (HRS)/American Society of Anesthesiologists (ASA) Expert Consensus Statement on the Perioperative Management of Patients with Implantable Defbrillators, Pacemakers, and Arrhythmia Monitors: Facilities and Patient Management: This document was developed as a joint project with the American Society of Anesthesiologists (ASA), and in collaboration with the American Heart Association (AHA), and the Society of Thoracic Surgeons (STS). *Heart Rhythm* 2011;8(7):1114–1154.

- The CIED team should in turn provide information about the device and a recommendation for perioperative management of the device (see Table 5).

TABLE 5. ESSENTIAL ELEMENTS OF THE PREOPERATIVE CIED EVALUATION TO BE PROVIDED TO THE OPERATIVE TEAM

- Date of last device interrogation
- Type of device: Pacemaker ICD, CRT-D, CRT-P, ILR, implantable hemodynamic monitor
- Manufacturer and model
- Indication for device
  - –Pacemaker: Sick sinus syndrome, AV block, syncope
  - –ICD: Primary or secondary prevention
  - –Cardiac resynchronization therapy
- Battery longevity documented as >3 months
- Are any of the leads <3 months old?
- Programming
  - –Pacing mode and programmed lower rate
  - –ICD therapy
    - –Lowest heart rate for shock delivery
    - –Lowest heart rate for ATP delivery
  - –Rate-responsive sensor type, if programmed on
- Is the patient pacemaker dependent, and what is the underlying rhythm and heart rate if it can be determined?
- What is the response of this device to magnet placement?
  - –Magnet pacing rate for a pacemaker
  - –Pacing amplitude response to magnet function
  - –Will ICD detections resume automatically with removal of the magnet? Does this device allow for magnet application function to be disabled? If so, document programming of patient's device for this feature.
- Any alert status on CIED generator or lead
- Last pacing threshold: Document adequate safety margin with the date of that threshold

Reproduced with permission from Crossley GH, Poole JE, Rozner MA, et al. The Heart Rhythm Society (HRS)/American Society of Anesthesiologists (ASA) Expert Consensus Statement on the Perioperative Management of Patients with Implantable Defibrillators, Pacemakers, and Arrhythmia Monitors: Facilities and Patient Management: This document was developed as a joint project with the American Society of Anesthesiologists (ASA), and in collaboration with the American Heart Association (AHA), and the Society of Thoracic Surgeons (STS). *Heart Rhythm* 2011;8(7):1114–1154.

- The patient with a pacemaker should have had an interrogation of the device in the 12 months prior to the surgical procedure, whereas the patient with an ICD should have had the device interrogated within 6 months prior to the scheduled procedure.
- The inactivation of the ICD or programming of a pacemaker to asynchronous mode is recommended when electromagnetic interference (EMI) is likely to occur.
- In patients in whom the ICD anti-arrhythmia detection is turned off, an external defibrillator should be immediately available and ready to deliver therapy.
- In cases where EMI is likely, the function of the CIED can be altered either by a ferrous magnet or by reprogramming. (See below for magnet response for ICD.)
- Magnet response: Placing a magnet over a pacemaker generator will turn the pacemaker to asynchronous mode in most models. Placing a magnet over an ICD will suspend the arrhythmia detection. It will not switch the pacemaker function to asynchronous mode; therefore, in patients who are pacemaker dependent, the team must be aware of the risk of inhibition of the pacemaker by EMI. If EMI is likely to occur, the recommendation is to reprogram the CIED prior to the operation, by turning off the arrhythmia detection function and programming the pacemaker to asynchronous mode. Due to the fact that a minority of models do not respond to magnet application in the fashion described above, it is always recommended to contact the manufacturer and confirm the response to a magnet for the specific model one is dealing with.

Risk Mitigation Strategies[3]

- Have a magnet available.
- Use bipolar cautery where possible
- Use short bursts of monopolar cautery (5 seconds or less).
- Place the return current pad in such a way to avoid crossing the generator.
- Have rescue equipment, including external pacemaker/defibrillator, immediately available for all patients with a CIED.
- Be aware of other potential sources of EMI in addition to electrocautery.
- Be aware of dislodgement of leads during atrial fibrillation ablations, central intravenous catheter insertions, or other catheter-based procedures.[5]

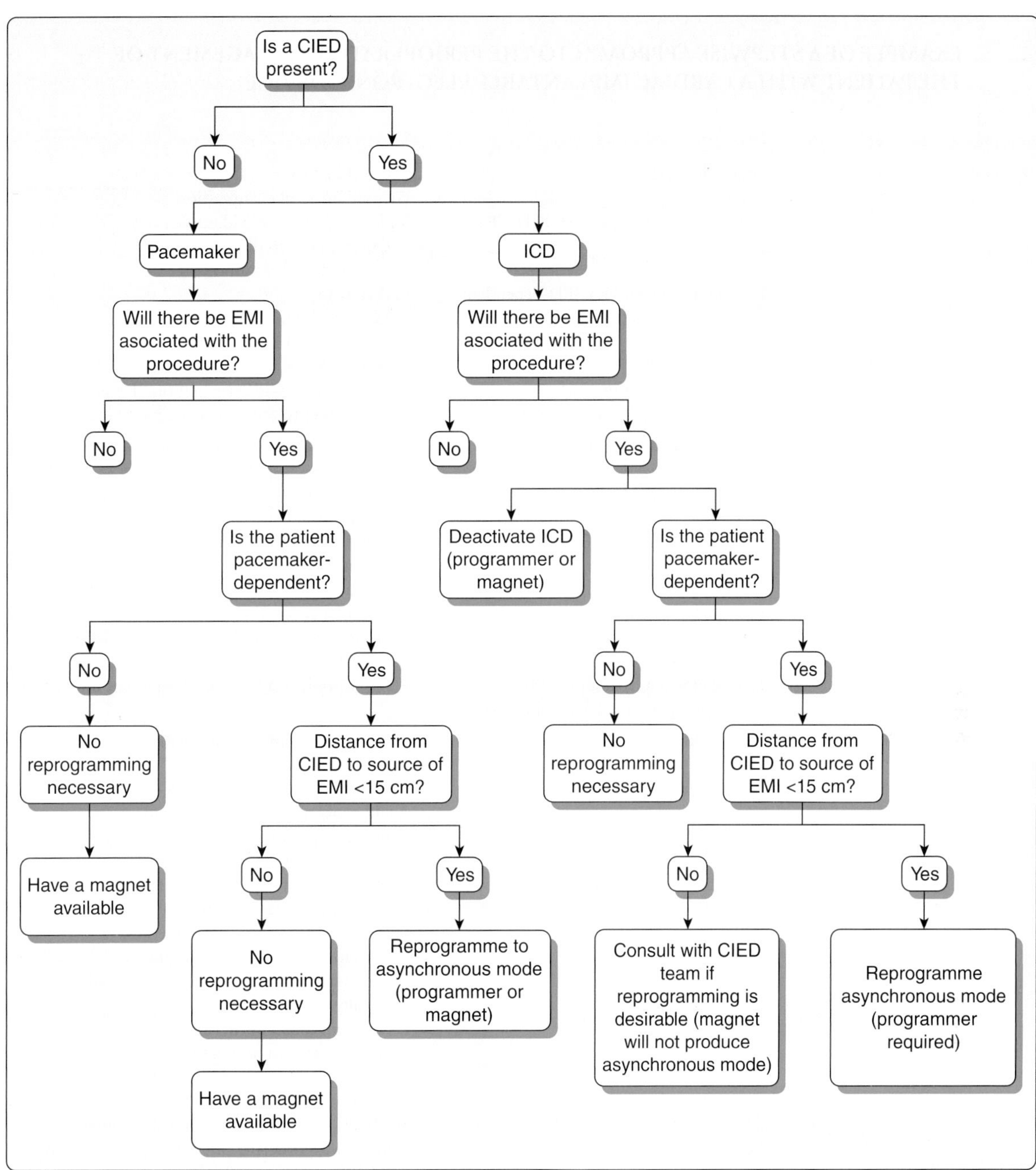

FIGURE 1. Example of an algorithm for perioperative management of patients with CIED. From Stone ME, Salter B, Fischer A. Perioperative management of patients with cardiac implantable electronic devices. *Br J Anaesth* 2011;107(Suppl 1):i16–26, with permission.

TABLE 6. EXAMPLE OF A STEPWISE APPROACH TO THE PERIOPERATIVE MANAGEMENT OF THE PATIENT WITH A CARDIAC IMPLANTABLE ELECTRONIC DEVICE

Perioperative Period	Patient/CIED Condition	Intervention
Preoperative evaluation	Patient has CIED	Focused history Focused physical examination
	Determine CIED type (PM, ICD, CRT)	Manufacturer's CIED identification card Chest x-ray (no data available) Supplemental resources[a]
	Determine if patient is CIED-dependent for pacing function	Verbal history Bradyarrhythmia symptoms Atrioventricular node ablation No spontaneous ventricular activity[b]
	Determine CIED function	Comprehensive CIED evaluation.[c] Determine if pacing pulses are present and create paced beats
Preoperative preparation	EMI unlikely during procedure	If EMI is unlikely, then special precautions are not needed
	EMI likely; CIED is PM	Reprogram to asychronous mode when indicated Suspend rate adaptive functions[d]
	EMI likely; CIED is ICD	Suspend antitachyarrhythmia functions. If patient is dependent on pacing function, then alter pacing function as above
	EMI likely; All CIED	Use bipolar cautery; ultrasonic scalpel Temporary pacing and cardioversion-defibrillation available
	Intraoperative physiologic changes likely (e.g. bradycardia, ischemia)	Plan for possible adverse CIED-patient interaction
Intraoperative management	Monitoring	Electrocardiographic monitoring per ASA standard Peripheral pulse monitoring
	Electrocautery interference	CT/CRP no current through PG/leads Avoid proximity of CT to PG/leads Short bursts at lowest possible energy Use bipolar cautery; ultrasonic scalpel
	RF catheter ablation	Avoid contact of RF catheter with PG/leads RF current path far away from PG/leads Discuss these concerns with operator
	Lithotripsy	Do not focus lithotripsy beam near PG R-wave triggers lithotripsy? Disable atrial pacing
	MRI	Generally contraindicated If required, consult ordering physician, cardiologist, radiologist, and manufacturer
	Radiation therapy	PG/leads must be outside of RT field Possible surgical relocation of PG Verify PG function during/after RT course
	ECT	Consult with ordering physician, patient's cardiologist, a CIED service, or CIED manufacturer
Emergency defibrillation-cardioversion	ICD: magnet-disabled	Terminate all EMI sources Remove magnet to re-enable therapies Observe for appropriate therapies
	ICD: programming disabled	Programming to re-enable therapies or proceed directly with external cardioversion/defibrillation
	ICD: either of above	Minimize current flow through PG/leads PP as far as possible from PG PP perpendicular to major axis PG/leads To extent possible, PP in anterior–posterior location
	Regardless of CIED type	Use clinically appropriate cardioversion/defibrillation energy

TABLE 6. EXAMPLE OF A STEPWISE APPROACH TO THE PERIOPERATIVE MANAGEMENT OF THE PATIENT WITH A CARDIAC IMPLANTABLE ELECTRONIC DEVICE (*continued*)

Perioperative Period	Patient/CIED Condition	Intervention
Postoperative management	Immediate postoperative period Postoperative interrogation and restoration of CIED function	Monitor cardiac R&R continuously Back-up pacing and cardioversion/defibrillation capability Interrogation to assess function Settings appropriate?[e] Is CIED an ICD?[f] Use cardiology/PM-ICD service if needed

Reproduced with permission from Practice advisory for perioperative management of patients with cardiac rhythm management devices: Pacemakers and implantable cardioverter-defibrillators. A report by the American Society of Anesthesiologists Task Force on Perioperative Management of Patients with Cardiac Rhythm Management Devices. *Anesthesiology* 2011;114:247–261.
[a]Manufacturer's databases, pacemaker clinic records, cardiology consultation
[b]With cardiac rhythm management device (CRMD) programmed VVI at lowest programmable rate.
[c]Ideally, CIED function assessed by interrogation, with function altered by reprogramming if required.
[d]Most times this will be necessary; when in doubt, assume so.
[e]If necessary, reprogram appropriate setting.
[f]Restore all antitachycardia therapies.

Recommendations for Postoperative Follow-up of the Patient with CIED (see Tables 7 and 8)

- Note the *Practice Advisory for the Perioperative Management of Patients with Cardiac Implantable Electronic Devices: Pacemakers and Implantable Cardioverter-Defibrillators* states that "postoperative patient management should include interrogating and restoring CIED function in the post anesthesia care unit or intensive care unit."[7]

TABLE 7. SPECIFIC PROCEDURES AND WRITING COMMITTEE RECOMMENDATIONS ON POSTOPERATIVE CIED EVALUATION

Procedure	Recommendation
Monopolar electrosurgery	CIED evaluated[a] within 1 month from procedure unless Table 8 criteria are fulfilled
External cardioversion	CIED evaluated[a] prior to discharge or transfer from cardiac telemetry
Radiofrequency ablation	CIED evaluated[a] prior to discharge or transfer from cardiac telemetry
Electroconvulsive therapy	CIED evaluated[a] within 1 month from procedure unless fulfilling Table 8 criteria
Nerve conduction studies (ENG)	No additional CIED evaluation beyond routine
Ocular procedures	No additional CIED evaluation beyond routine
Therapeutic radiation	CIED evaluated prior to discharge or transfer from cardiac telemetry; remote monitoring optimal; some instances may indicate interrogation after each treatment (see text)
TUNA/TURP	No additional CIED evaluation beyond routine
Hysteroscopic ablation	No additional CIED evaluation beyond routine
Lithotripsy	CIED evaluated[a] within 1 month from procedure unless fulfilling Table 8 criteria
Endoscopy	No additional CIED evaluation beyond routine
Iontophoresis	No additional CIED evaluation beyond routine
Photodynamic therapy	No additional CIED evaluation beyond routine
X-ray/CT scans/ mammography	No additional CIED evaluation beyond routine

CIED, cardiac implantable electronic device; CT, computed tomography; TUNA, Transurethral Needle Ablation; TURP, Transurethral resection of prostate.
[a]This evaluation is intended to reveal electrical reset. Therefore, an interrogation alone is needed. This can be accomplished in person or by remote telemetry.
Reproduced with permission from Crossley GH, Poole JE, Rozner MA, et al: The Heart Rhythm Society (HRS)/American Society of Anesthesiologists (ASA) Expert Consensus Statement on the Perioperative Management of Patients with Implantable Defibrillators, Pacemakers, and Arrhythmia Monitors: Facilities and Patient Management: This document was developed as a joint project with the American Society of Anesthesiologists (ASA), and in collaboration with the American Heart Association (AHA), and the Society of Thoracic Surgeons (STS). *Heart Rhythm* 2011;8(7): 1114–1154.

TABLE 8. INDICATIONS FOR THE INTERROGATION OF CIEDS PRIOR TO PATIENT DISCHARGE OR TRANSFER FROM A CARDIAC TELEMETRY ENVIRONMENT

- Patients with CIEDs reprogrammed prior to the procedure that left the device nonfunctional such as disabling tachycardia detection in an ICD.
- Patients with CIEDs who underwent hemodynamically challenging surgeries such as cardiac surgery or significant vascular surgery (e.g., abdominal aortic aneurysmal repair).[a]
- Patients with CIEDs who experienced significant intraoperative events including cardiac arrest requiring temporary pacing or cardiopulmonary resuscitation and those who required external electrical cardioversion.
- Emergent surgery where the site of EMI exposure was above the umbilicus
- Cardio-thoracic surgery
- Patients with CIEDs who underwent certain types of procedures (Table 7) that emit EMI with a greater probability of affecting device function.
- Patients with CIEDs who have logistical limitations that would prevent reliable device evaluation within one month from their procedure

CIED, cardiac implantable electrical device; EMI, electromagnetic interference; ICD, implantable cardiac defibrillator.
[a]The general purpose of this interrogation is to assure that reset did not occur. In these cases, a full evaluation including threshold evaluations is suggested.
Reproduced with permission from Crossley GH, Poole JE, Rozner MA, et al. The Heart Rhythm Society (HRS)/American Society of Anesthesiologists (ASA) Expert Consensus Statement on the Perioperative Management of Patients with Implantable Defibrillators, Pacemakers, and Arrhythmia Monitors: Facilities and Patient Management: This document was developed as a joint project with the American Society of Anesthesiologists (ASA), and in collaboration with the American Heart Association (AHA), and the Society of Thoracic Surgeons (STS). *Heart Rhythm* 2011;8(7):1114–1154.

Optimization of Pacing after Cardiopulmonary Bypass (CPB)[8]

During separation from CPB, it is not uncommon for a patient to develop a conduction abnormality, ranging from the more benign first-degree AV block or sinus bradycardia to the more severe interventricular delays or third-degree AV block.

Optimizing pacing:

1. **Lead placement:** Right atrial (RA) lead—place at the cephalic atrial wall, between the atrial appendages. Right ventricular lead—place at the level of the right ventricle outflow tract (RVOT). For the patient with obstructive cardiomyopathy, the RV lead is better placed in the RV apex, for less dynamic obstruction of the LVOT. Biventricular pacing can be initiated for patients with intraventricular conduction lesions and dyssynchrony of contraction. The LV lead should be placed at the basal posterolateral wall and the two ventricular leads can be connected through a Y piece to the ventricular output of the temporary pacemaker box.
2. **Rate:** Program to obtain the best improvement in cardiac output and improvement in mixed venous saturation and arterial blood pressure.
3. **AV delay:** In patients with LV dysfunction, we can maximize the contribution of the atria to the preload. Use pulse wave Doppler through the mitral valve infow, and modify the AV delay to obtain a clear E and A waveforms and to ensure that the A wave ends before the onset of the QRS. The closure of the mitral valve should happen at the end of the A wave but before any diastolic mitral regurgitation. If echocardiography is not available, adjust the AV interval to achieve highest cardiac output.
4. **Pacing mode:** Three modes are explained here. In the patient with normal AV conduction, AAI mode allows for increase in HR and a physiological depolarization of the ventricles. If inhibition by electrocautery is a concern, use asynchronous pacing in AOO mode. For the patient with AV conduction delay,

TABLE 9. TREATMENT OF PACEMAKER FAILURE

Rate	Possible Response
Adequate to maintain blood pressure	1. Oxygen, airway control 2. Place magnet over pacemaker 3. Atropine if sinus bradycardia
Severe bradycardia and hypotension	1. Oxygen, airway control 2. Place magnet over pacemaker 3. Other types of pacing if magnet does not activate the pacemaker (transcutaneous, esophageal, or transvenous) 4. Atropine if sinus bradycardia 5. Isoproterenol to increase ventricular rate
No escape rhythm	1. Cardiopulmonary resuscitation 2. Place magnet over pacemaker 3. Other types of pacing if magnet does not activate the pacemaker (transcutaneous, esophageal, or transvenous) 4. Isoproterenol to increase ventricular rate

From Zaidan JR, Youngberg JA, Lake CL, et al., eds. *Pacemakers, Cardiac, Vascular and Thoracic Anesthesia.* New York: Churchill Livingstone; 2000, with permission.

DOO or DDI should be used. DDI mode also avoids tracking of rapid atrial rates in case of post bypass atrial fibrillation.

5. **Biventricular pacing:**[8,9] In patients with EF ≤35% and QRS ≥120 ms, acute biventricular pacing improves torsion and mechanics of contraction, particularly in patients with mitral regurgitation due to papillary muscle dyssynchrony. Speckle-tracking, 3D echocardiography, M-mode definition of septal to wall motion delay, color Doppler tissue imaging and analysis of segmental velocity, are used to characterize ventricular dyssynchrony. Currently available temporary pacemakers only allow biventricular pacing through a Y connection of the two ventricular epicardial wires to the ventricular output of the box. Acute CRT leads to an increase in myocardial performance with a slight decrease in myocardial oxygen consumption.

References

1. Epstein AE, Dimarco JP, Ellenbogen KA, et al. ACC/AHA/HRS 2008 guidelines for Device-Based Therapy of Cardiac Rhythm Abnormalities: Executive summary. *Heart Rhythm* 2008;5:934–955.
2. Stone KR, McPherson CA. Assessment and management of patients with pacemakers and implantable cardioverter defibrillators. *Crit Care Med* 2004;32:S155–S165.
3. Crossley GH, Poole JE, Rozner MA, et al. The Heart Rhythm Society (HRS)/American Society of Anesthesiologists (ASA) Expert Consensus Statement on the perioperative management of patients with implantable defibrillators, pacemakers and arrhythmia monitors: Facilities and patient management this document was developed as a joint project with the American Society of Anesthesiologists (ASA), and in collaboration with the American Heart Association (AHA), and the Society of Thoracic Surgeons (STS). *Heart Rhythm* 2011;8:1114–1154.
4. Heller LI. Surgical electrocautery and the runaway pacemaker syndrome. *Pacing Clin Electrophysiol* 1990;13:1084–1085.
5. Lakkireddy D, Patel D, Ryschon K, et al. Safety and effcacy of radiofrequency energy catheter ablation of atrial fibrillation in patients with pacemakers and implantable cardiac defibrillators. *Heart Rhythm* 2005;2:1309–1316.
6. Stone ME, Salter B, Fischer A. Perioperative management of patients with cardiac implantable electronic devices. *Br J Anaesth* 2011;107(Suppl 1):i16–i26.
7. Practice Advisory for the perioperative management of patients with cardiac implantable electronic devices: Pacemakers and implantable cardioverter-defibrillators. An updated reprot by the American Society of Anesthesiologists Task Force on Perioperative Management of Patients with Cardiac Implantable Electronic Devices. *Anesthesiology* 2011;114(2):247–261.
8. Chua J, Schwarzenberger J, Mahajan A. Optimization of pacing after cardiopulmonary bypass. *J Cardiothorac Vasc Anesth* 2012;26:291–301.
9. Wang DY, Richmond ME, Quinn TA, et al. Optimized temporary biventricular pacing acutely improves intraoperative cardiac output after weaning from cardiopulmonary bypass: A substudy of a randomized clinical trial. *J Thorac Cardiovasc Surg* 2011;141:1002–1008, 8e1.

INDEX

Note: Page number followed by f and t indicates figure and table respectively.

B

D

H

J

K

O

P

W

X

Y

Z